# Encyclopedia of Medical Organizations and Agencies

program for screening persons designated as Hearing Instrument Specialists; administration of a consumer information program; publication of information and research concerning hearing health care; establishment of standards of education, equipment, and techniques in the fitting of hearing aids; cooperation with other professional organizations engaged in hearing health care; cooperation and consultation with government officials and agencies in the development of policies and legislation. Accredits seminars and workshops for the education of hearing aid specialists. Maintains the National Institute for Hearing Instruments Studies as the educational arm of the society. **Pub:** *The Hearing Professional*, bimonthly. Journal. Contains technical articles, business information, and news for hearing health professionals. Includes annual index, chapter news, and book reviews. *Price:* Free to members; $45/year for others; $35 foreign. • *International Hearing Society–Directory of Members*, annual. Membership Directory. Arranged geographically and alphabetically. Includes supplemental directory of manufacturers, suppliers, hearing aid designers, and others. • *International Hearing Society-Professional Association of Hearing Instrument Specialists.* Brochures. • *World of Sound.* Pamphlets. • Books. • Brochures. • Also publishes bylaws and code of ethics. **Frmly:** (1966) Society of Hearing Aid Audiologists; (1990) National Hearing Aid Society.

### ★ 6063 ★ International Rhinologic Society

c/o Prof. P.A.R. Clement
ENT Department
AZ-VUB
Laarbecklaan 101
B-1090 Brussels, Belgium

**Lang(s):** Dutch, English, French. **Desc:** Rhinologists and other medical professionals and researchers with an interest in rhinology. Seeks to advance the study, teaching, research, and practice of rhinology and related disciplines. Serves as a clearinghouse on rhinology. Sponsors research and continuing professional development programs.

### ★ 6064 ★ International Society for Otological Surgery

c/o Dr. O. Nuri Ozgirgin
Department of Otolaryngology
Byindir Medical Centre
TR-06520 Sogutozu, Turkey
**Phone:** 90 312 2879000     **Fax:** 90 312 2850733
**Email:** ozgirgin@politzersociety.org

**Fnded:** 1971. **Mem:** 300. **Desc:** Medical professionals involved in the science and practice of surgery and rehabilitation of diseases and disorders of the ear. Disseminates information. Conducts training programs.

### ★ 6065 ★ Irish Deaf Society (IDS)

30 Blessington St.
Dublin 7, Ireland
**Phone:** 353 1 8601878   •   **Fax:** 353 1 8601960
**Email:** ids@indigo.ie
**Website:** http://www.irishdeafsociety.org

**Lang(s):** English, Irish. **Desc:** A representative organization of the Deaf seeks recognition of Irish sign language and conducts various educational and advocacy campaigns.

### ★ 6066 ★ John Tracy Clinic

704 E Wardlow Rd.
Long Beach, CA 90807
**Phone:** (562)426-2257
**Email:** ewilson@johntracyclinic.org
**Website:** http://www.johntracyclinic.org
Eska Wilson, VP Finance & Admin.

**Fnded:** 1942. **Desc:** Offers parent-centered services to young children with hearing loss advanced courses and practice to professionals in understanding how to work with deaf children. **Pub:** *The John Tracy Clinic Bulletin*, semiannual. Newsletter. Contains news of services, campaigns, and events. *Price:* Free.

### ★ 6067 ★ Judaica Captioned Film Center (JCFC)

PO Box 21439
Baltimore, MD 21208-0439
**Phone:** (410)655-6767     **Free:** 800-735-2258
Lois Lilienfeld-Weiner, Pres.

**Fnded:** 1983. **Desc:** Deaf, hearing impaired individuals, students of English as a second language and other users of captioned films. Locates, produces, and distributes captioned versions of films on Jewish subjects such as the Bible, archaeology, the Holocaust, and Israel. **Pub:** Newsletter, 1-4/year. *Price:* Free.

### ★ 6068 ★ League for the Hard of Hearing

71 W 23rd St.
New York, NY 10010-4162
**Phone:** (917)305-7700     **Fax:** (917)305-7888
**Email:** postmaster@lhh.org
**Website:** http://www.lhh.org

**Fnded:** 1910. **Desc:** Dedicated to improve the life for infants, children and adults with all degrees of hearing loss.

### ★ 6069 ★ Meniere's Network (MN)

1817 Patterson St.
Nashville, TN 37203
**Phone:** (615)284-7807     **Free:** 800-545-HEAR
**Fax:** (615)329-7935
**Email:** ear@earfoundation.org
Bridget Lippard, Exec. Dir.

**Fnded:** 1987. **Mem:** 1,500. **Desc:** Persons suffering from Meniere's disease, an inner ear disorder of unknown cause that results in vertigo, tinnitus, and hearing fluctuation or loss. Seeks to develop a network of peer support groups to help integrate hearing- and balance-impaired people into mainstream society. Operates speakers' bureau and pen pals and "phone buddies" services; offers educational programs and materials. **Pub:** *A Dietary Guidebook for Meniere's Disease; An Introduction to Meniere's Disease; Meniere's Disease-Coping Skills.* Booklets. *Price:* $6.50 pack of 3. • *Steady*, quarterly. Newsletter. Provides medical information and lists selfhelp support groups, pen pals, "phone buddies" and "email buddies". *Price:* $25.

### ★ 6070 ★ Model Secondary School for the Deaf (MSSD)

Gallaudet University
800 Florida Ave. NE
Washington, DC 20002
**Phone:** (202)651-5340     **Fax:** (202)651-5109
**Email:** kajankowski@gallaudet.gallua.edu
**Website:** http://clerccenter.gallaudet.edu/mssd/
Dr. Katherine Jankowski, Dir.

**Fnded:** 1969. **Desc:** Authorized under Model Secondary School for the Deaf Act of 1966. An agreement between the Secretary of Health, Education, and Welfare and Gallaudet College provided for the establishment of the school. Operation was initiated in September 1969, with the intent to provide an exemplary program of instruction and construction of a facility which would exhibit excellence in both architecture and design and would include all innovative auditory and visual devices necessary for education of the deaf. The school's primary service area includes deaf residents of the District of Columbia, Maryland, Virginia, West Virginia, Delaware, and Pennsylvania. Students from all other states may also be accepted as space is available. Additional criteria for admission, such as age level, degree of hearing loss, and previous educational attainment are included in the agreement. U **Pub:** *Family Newsletter.* Newsletter. • *LRC Update*, monthly. Newsletter. Library newsletter. *Price:* Free. • *Perspectives.* Magazine. • *Preview.* Magazine. • *SAERIE.* Magazine. Features literary works by students. • Brochures.

### ★ 6071 ★ National Aphasia Association (NAA)

29 John St., Rm. 1103
New York, NY 10038
**Phone:** (212)267-2814     **Free:** 800-922-4622
**Fax:** (212)267-2812
**Email:** naa@aphasia.org
**Website:** http://www.aphasia.org
Penny Montgomery-West, Response Dir.

**Fnded:** 1987. **Desc:** Works to promote the care, rehabilitation and quality of life of individuals with aphasia, a speech and language disorder caused by stroke, head trauma or other neurological conditions. Conducts public and professional education programs, facilitates the development of community programs to meet the needs of people with aphasia and their families; provides referrals to professionals. **Pub:** *Aphasia Community Group Manual.* Manual. Contains information to aid in the establishment of new support groups. *Price:* $30. • *Listing of Aphasia Community Groups.* Directory. *Price:* $2.75/copy. • *Newsletter of the National Aphasia Association*, semiannual. Newsletter. *Price:* $1. • *Videotape of 3 Community Groups.* Video. *Price:* $10.

### ★ 6072 ★ National Association of the Deaf (NAD)

814 Thayer Ave., Ste. 250
Silver Spring, MD 20910-4500
**Phone:** (301)587-1788     **Fax:** (301)587-1791
**Email:** nadinfo@nad.org
**Website:** http://www.nad.org
Nancy J. Bloch, Exec. Dir.

**Fnded:** 1880. **Mem:** 22,000. **State Groups:** 51. **Desc:** Safeguards accessibility and civil rights of America's deaf population in areas of education, employment, healthcare, and telecommunications. **Pub:** *Deaf American*, annual. Journal. Contains articles on deafness-related topics. *Price:* Included in membership dues; $30/year for nonmembers. • *NAD Broadcaster*, 11/year. Tabloid for and about deaf and hearing impaired persons and their families. Covers political issues, sports, and activities of interest to the deaf. *Price:* Included in membership dues; $30/year for nonmembers. • Also publishes catalog and textbooks on American Sign Language and other systems of manual communication.

### ★ 6073 ★ National Association of the Deaf in Iceland (Felag Heyrnarlausra)

Laugavegur 103
IS-105 Reykjavik, Iceland
**Phone:** 354 5613560     **Fax:** 354 5513567
**Email:** feheyrn@ismennt.is
**Website:** http://www.deaf.is

**Fnded:** 1960. **Mem:** 200. **State Groups:** 1. **Lang(s):** English, Icelandic, Norwegian, Spanish, Swedish. **Desc:** People with hearing impairments, their families, and health care and speech and hearing professionals. Works to improve the quality of life of people with impaired hearing. Works to insure that the legal and economic rights of people with hearing impairments are respected. Conducts research and educational programs on sign language and other means of nonverbal communication. Serves as a liaison with other national and international associations with similar aims. Assists members in obtaining assistive technologies including text telephones, alarm services, and TTD messages. **Pub:** *Doff-laoio*, 3/year. Magazine. • *Doff-postur*, monthly. Newsletter. News regarding the deaf community in Iceland and abroad. • *TDD*, monthly. Magazine. News regarding the deaf community in Iceland and abroad. • *TTP*, 3/year. Newsletter.

### ★ 6074 ★ National Association for Deaf People (NADP)

35 N Frederick St.
Dublin 1, Ireland
**Phone:** 353 1 8723800     **Fax:** 353 1 8723816
**Email:** nad@iol.ie
**Website:** http://www.nadp.ie

**Fnded:** 1963. **Lang(s):** English, Irish. **Desc:** Individuals and organizations. Seeks to improve the quality of life of people with hearing impairments; promotes full recognition of the rights of people with hearing loss. Makes available support and services; conducts educational and advocacy campaigns. Offers a job coaching service; operates Family Resource Centre; conducts sign language classes. **Pub:** *Link*, quarterly. Magazine. Contains information on deaf culture issues plus editorial.

### ★ 6075 ★ National Association of Deafened People

PO Box 50
Amersham HP6 6XB, United Kingdom
**Phone:** 44 1494 724830    **Fax:** 44 1494 431932
**Email:** enquiries@nadp.org.uk
**Website:** http://www.nadp.org.uk

**Fnded:** 1984. **Mem:** 500. **Desc:** People with acquired profound hearing loss and professionals associated with them. Aims to work for improvements in the quality of life of deafened people, by providing a support service of information and advice and promoting an improvement in education, training and rehabilitation opportunities available. It also aims to increase public awareness of the needs and problems of deafened people, and to support research. **Pub:** *An Introduction to Cochlear Implants.* • *Information Booklet.* • *Network*, quarterly. Newsletter.

### ★ 6076 ★ National Association of Future Doctors of Audiology (NAFDA)

c/o Jina Scherer
University of Louisville
School of Medicine
Myers Hall
129 E Broadway
Louisville, KY 40202
**Phone:** (502)852-2620    **Fax:** (502)852-0865
**Email:** nafda@nafda.org
**Website:** http://www.nafda.org/
Jina Scherer, Pres.

**Fnded:** 1998. **Desc:** Audiology students. Provides forum on national, state and regional issues of concern to the AuD student, including opportunity to travel internationally to offer audiologic healthcare to underprivileged nations.

### ★ 6077 ★ National Association of Laryngectomy Clubs

6 Rickett St., Ground Fl.
Fulham
London SW6 1RU, United Kingdom
**Phone:** 44 207 3819993    **Fax:** 44 207 3810025
**Email:** nalc@laryngectomees.inuk.com
**Website:** http://www.laryngectomees.inuk.com

**Fnded:** 1976. **Mem:** 4,000. **Nat'l Groups:** 95. **Desc:** Promotes the welfare of laryngectomees by providing literature to them, their friends and their families and also the relevant professionals. Membership is via a club only. **Pub:** Annual Report, annual. • Newsletter, quarterly. Also publishes emergency resuscitation video and audiotape.

### ★ 6078 ★ National Black Association for Speech-Language and Hearing (NBASLH)

PO Box 50605
Washington, DC 20091
**Phone:** (202)274-6162    **Fax:** (202)274-6350
**Email:** nbaslh@aol.com
**Website:** http://www.nbaslh.org
M. Eugene Wiggins, Exec. Dir.

**Fnded:** 1978. **Mem:** 500. **Desc:** Professionals and other individuals concerned with communicatively handicapped blacks. Strongly encourages the recruitment and training of black professionals to work with individuals suffering from speech, language, and hearing problems; maintains that conditions such as race, socioeconomic class, and cultural differences must be taken into account in order to understand and sensitively study the communicative process, and to treat

communicative disorders. Supports related research; solicits, and provides, financial support for the training of black students in speech-language pathology and audiology. Disseminates information. **Pub:** *Echo*, quarterly. Newsletter. *Price:* $7.

### ★ 6079 ★ National Black Deaf Advocates (NBDA)

PO Box 305288
Charlotte Amalie, VI 00803
**Phone:** (340)774-5899    **Fax:** (340)774-8350
**Email:** rubytim@viaccess.net
**Website:** http://www.nbda.org/
Gwendolyn T. Powell, Pres.

**Fnded:** 1982. **Local Groups:** 20. **Desc:** Advocates for the rights of African-American deaf and hearing impared people. Seeks to promote the well-being, culture and empowerment of African-Americans who are deaf or hard of hearing. Conducts educational outreach programs; offers leadership training and training for interpreters and transliterators of color. Sponsors the Miss NBDA Pageant. **Pub:** *NBDA Network*, quarterly. Newsletter.

### ★ 6080 ★ National Captioning Institute (NCI)

1900 Gallows Rd., Ste. 3000
Vienna, VA 22182
**Phone:** (703)917-7600    **Fax:** (703)917-9853
**Email:** koconnor@ncicap.org
**Website:** http://www.ncicap.org
Gene Chao, Pres. /COO

**Fnded:** 1979. **Desc:** Purpose is to caption television programs for the deaf and hard-of-hearing on behalf of public and commercial television broadcasters, cablecasters, and the home video industry. Makes available captioning services, making use of a "closed captioning" system that allows coded captions not visible on a normal television set to be decoded and made visible by the use of a special adapter which may be attached to a television set.

### ★ 6081 ★ National Center for Stuttering (NCS)

200 E 33rd St.
New York, NY 10016
**Phone:** (212)532-1460    **Free:** 800-221-2483
**Fax:** (212)683-1372
**Email:** martin.schwartz@nyu.edu
**Website:** http://www.stuttering.com
Martin F. Schwartz, Exec. Dir.

**Fnded:** 1974. **Desc:** Furnishes information to parents of children who stutter. Provides treatment for children and adults who stutter and training on the latest practices and theories for speech pathologists. **Pub:** *Annual Review of Published Literature.* • *Stutter No More.* Book. • Newsletter, quarterly. **Frmly:** Center for Speech Pathology.

### ★ 6082 ★ National Cued Speech Association (NCSA)

23970 Hermitage Rd.
Cleveland, OH 44143-4008
**Phone:** (216)292-6213    **Free:** 800-459-3529
**Fax:** (216)292-6213
**Email:** cuedspdisc@aol.com
**Website:** http://www.cuedspeech.org
Pamela Beck, Mgr., NCSA Information Service

**Fnded:** 1982. **Mem:** 1,000. **Reg. Groups:** 2. **State Groups:** 8. **Desc:** Promotes and supports the effective use of Cued Speech for communication, language acquisition, and literacy. Provides information, referral and support for persons with language, hearing, speech, and learning needs. Sponsors instructional programs, exhibits, and family learning vacations. **Pub:** *Cued Speech Journal*, annual. Journal. Covers various aspects of Cued Speech. *Price:* Included in membership dues; $10/year for nonmembers. • *On Cue*, quarterly. Newsletter. Contains calendar of events and regional reports. *Price:* Included in membership dues; $25/year for nonmembers.

### ★ 6083 ★ National Deaf Children's Society

15 Dufferin St.
London EC1Y 8UR, United Kingdom
**Phone:** 44 20 74908656    **Fax:** 44 20 72515020
**Email:** fundraising@ndcs.org.uk
**Website:** http://www.ndcs.org.uk

**Fnded:** 1944. **Mem:** 9,000. **Reg. Groups:** 12. **Local Groups:** 120. **Lang(s):** English. **Desc:** Supports families and young deaf people, chiefly through providing information and advice on education, state benefits, audiology and equipment. **Pub:** *Communication Tips and Terms.* Pamphlet. • *TALK*, quarterly. Magazine. • Annual Report, annual.

### ★ 6084 ★ National Deaf Education Network and Clearinghouse

800 Florida Ave., NE
Washington, DC 20002
**Phone:** (202)651-5051    **Fax:** (202)651-5054
**Email:** clearinghouse.infotogo@gallaudet.edu
**Website:** http://clerccenter.gallaudet.edu
Anita Glibert, Information Specialist

**Desc:** Information dissemination at the Gallaudet University Laurent Clerc National Deaf Education Center on diverse topics related to deaf and hard of hearing children, ages birth to 21 years old. **Pub:** *Odyssey Magazine.* Magazine. Reports on Clerc Center projects and contains peer-reviewed articles from contributors. *Price:* for members. • *World Around You.* Magazine. Provides motivation for independent and assisted reading, creative writing, and drawing for deaf and hard of hearing teens. *Price:* for members.

### ★ 6085 ★ National Education for Assistance Dog Services (NEADS)

PO Box 213
West Boylston, MA 01583
**Phone:** (978)422-9064    **Fax:** (978)422-3255
**Email:** info@neads.org
**Website:** http://www.neads.org
Sheila O'Brien, Exec. Dir.

**Fnded:** 1976. **Mem:** 6,000. **Reg. Groups:** 21. **State Groups:** 5. **Desc:** Interested individuals, clubs, and organizations. Trains dogs to alert deaf or hearing impaired individuals to specific sounds of the environment; also trains dogs to help disabled individuals. After extensive screening, dogs are trained by a professional staff for three to five months, learning: basic obedience; how to respond to household and other sounds including alarm clocks, door bells, smoke alarms, telephone, babies' crying, kettle whistles, oven timer, car horns, and sirens; how to perform assistance tasks such as pulling wheelchairs, using light switches, and retrieving articles from the floor or high shelves. Maintains speakers' bureau. **Pub:** *Hearing Ear Dogs: A Sound Relationship.* Brochure. • *Help Make a Miracle–Participate in Our Puppy Program.* Brochure. • *NEADS Newsletter*, quarterly. Newsletter. • *Service Dogs - Trained to Help the Physically Disabled.* Brochure. • *Sound Friendships - The Story of Willa and Her Hearing Ear Dog.* Book. • *Special Dogs for Special People.* Brochure. **Frmly:** New England Assistance Dog Service; (1989) Hearing Ear Dog Program; (1992) New England Assistance Dog Program.

### ★ 6086 ★ National Hearing Conservation Association (NHCA)

9101 Kenyon Ave., Ste. 3000
Denver, CO 80237
**Phone:** (303)224-9022    **Fax:** (303)770-1812
**Email:** nhca@gwami.com
**Website:** http://www.hearingconservation.org
Karen Wojdyla, Exec. Dir.

**Fnded:** 1977. **Mem:** 500. **Desc:** Individuals holding advanced academic degrees in a discipline involving hearing and hearing loss; professional service organizations engaged in industrial hearing conservation programs; companies that manufacture or sell occupational noise or hearing loss products. Promotes hearing conservation in all sectors of society. Encourages education and standards development among members and industrial groups; monitors legislation and regulatory activities related to hearing conservation. **Pub:** *NHCA Membership Directory*, annual. Membership Directory. Arranged alphabetically, geographically, and by member category. Includes consumer guide. *Price:* Included in membership dues; $25 per issue. • *Resources in Hearing Conservation*, annual. Compilation of references and films listed in previous "Spectrum" issues. *Price:* Included in membership dues; $20/issue. • *Spectrum*, quarterly. Newsletter. Provides information on technology, research, practice, and federal and state legal and regulatory activities. Includes book reviews. *Price:* Included in membership dues; $10/issue; $20 for supplements.

**★ 6087 ★ National Institute on Deafness and Other Communication Disorders Information Clearinghouse**
1 Communication Ave.
Bethesda, MD 20892-3456
**Free:** 800-241-1044 **Fax:** (301)907-8830
**Email:** nidcdinfo@nidcd.nih.gov
**Website:** http://www.nidcd.nih.gov
Dr. Marin Allen, Project Officer
**Fnded:** 1988. **Desc:** Disseminates information on biomedical and behavioral research in human communication. **Pub:** *Information Resources for Human Communication Disorders*, annual. Directory. Encourages networking among those with an interest in deafness and communication disorders. *Price:* Single copies free. • *NIDCD Information Clearinghouse.* Newsletter. • *NIDCD Publications List*, annual. Pamphlet. **Frmly:** (1998) National Committee in Deafness and Other Communication Disorders.

**★ 6088 ★ National Service Dog Center (NSDC)**
c/o Delta Society
289 Perimeter Rd. E
Renton, WA 98055
**Phone:** (425)226-7357 **Fax:** (425)235-1076
**Email:** info@deltasociety.org
**Website:** http://www.deltasociety.org
Tamara Whitehall, Contact
**Fnded:** 1977. **Desc:** A joint program of the American Humane Association and the Delta Society. Provides a national service dog education, advocacy and referral service. Promotes the health benefits of service animals for people with disabilities. **Pub:** *Alert*, bimonthly. Newsletter. Reports on service animals and issues of concern to those who want information about service animals. • *Service Animal Resource Directory*, annual. Directory. Lists service dog training programs and information about selecting a supplier that best meets consumer's needs. • *Service Dogs Welcome!*. Video. **Frmly:** (1983) Hearing Dog Program; (1987) Hearing Dog Project; (1989) National Center for Hearing Dog Information; (1993) Hearing Dog Resource Center.

**★ 6089 ★ National Student Speech Language Hearing Association (NSSLHA)**
10801 Rockville Pike
Rockville, MD 20852
**Phone:** (301)897-5700 **Free:** 800-498-2071
**Fax:** (301)571-0481
**Email:** nsslha@asha.org
**Website:** http://www.nsslha.org
Dawn D. Dickerson, Dir. Of Operations
**Fnded:** 1972. **Mem:** 16,000. **Local Groups:** 285. **Desc:** Preprofessional organization for undergraduate and graduate students in speech-language pathology, speech and hearing sciences, and audiology. **Pub:** *Contemporary Issues in Communication Science and Disorders*, semiannual. Journal. *Price:* Included in membership dues; $20. **Frmly:** National Student Speech and Hearing Association.

**★ 6090 ★ National Stuttering Association (NSP)**
5100 E La Palma Ave., No. 208
Anaheim Hills, CA 92807
**Phone:** (714)693-7480 **Free:** 800-364-1677
**Fax:** (714)693-7554
**Email:** nsastutter@aol.com
**Website:** http://www.nsastutter.org
Annie Bradberry, Exec. Dir.
**Fnded:** 1977. **Mem:** 4,000. **Local Groups:** 79. **Desc:** Selfhelp organization of people who stutter, parents of children who stutter, and speech pathologists. Seeks to provide a safe, supportive environment for stutterers and their families through chapter meetings, special programs, workshops, tape series, and selfhelp groups. Concentrates on issues such as improving self-image and assuming personal responsibility rather than focusing on speech fluency. Educates the public about stuttering and functions as a referral service for those seeking professional help. (Does not provide speech therapy or trained therapists.) Offers consulting in program development and technical assistance to school districts, speech clinics, hospitals, rehabilitation centers, and other agencies involved in speech services. Advises members on how to be wise consumers of speech and related therapies. Maintains speakers' bureau. **Pub:** *Letting Go, Care*, monthly. Publication for parents. • *Letting Go, Stutter Buddies.* Audiotapes. Publication for children. • Audiotapes. • Brochures. • Pamphlets.

**★ 6091 ★ National Temporal Bone, Hearing and Balance Pathology Resource Registry (NIDCD)**
Massachusetts Eye and Ear Infirmary
243 Charles St.
Boston, MA 02114-3096
**Phone:** (617)573-3711 **Free:** 800-822-1327
**Fax:** (617)573-3838
**Email:** tbregistry@meei.harvard.edu
**Website:** http://www.tbregistry.org
Dr. Joseph B. Nadol, Jr., Contact
**Fnded:** 1960. **Reg. Groups:** 25. **Desc:** Promotes research of hearing and balance disorders through the study of the temporal bone and related brain structures. Encourages individuals with hearing or balance disorders to bequeath their temporal bones to scientific research. Serves as a clearinghouse for information on temporal bone research. Develops strategies to conserve human temporal bone collections. Maintains a nationwide network to retrieve donated temporal bone and brain tissue. **Pub:** *The Gift of Hearing, That Others May Hear.* Brochures. • *The Registry*, semiannual. Newsletter. Includes information about temporal bone research and donations. *Price:* Free. **Frmly:** (1992) National Temporal Bone Banks Program of The DRF; (1997) National Temporal Bone Registry; (1999) National Temporal Bone, Hearing and Balance Pathology Registry.

**★ 6092 ★ Nederlandse Federatie van Ouders van Dove Kinderen**
c/o Els van der Zee
PO Box 754
NL-3500 AT Utrecht, Netherlands
**Phone:** 30 2900360
**Email:** fodok@wxs.nl
**Website:** http://www.fodok.nl
**Mem:** 9. **Lang(s):** Dutch. **Desc:** Organizations of parents of deaf children. Addresses the concerns of parents with deaf children; disseminates information.

**★ 6093 ★ Nordic Council for the Deaf (NCD)**
**(Dovas Nordiske Raad — DNR)**
c/o Norwegian Association of the Deaf
B 6850 St. Olausplass
N-0130 Oslo, Norway
**Phone:** 47 22 111775 **Fax:** 47 22 111633
**Fnded:** 1907. **Lang(s):** English. **Desc:** Individuals representing 5 National associations for the deaf from Denmark, Finland, Iceland, Norway, and Sweden. Works for cooperation in cultural, educational, and social matters. Works to establish sign language as the first language of the deaf. Seeks the establishment of special schools for the deaf, an improvement in the interpretation services, and the installment of public

address systems which deaf will understand. Disseminates information about change and development for the deaf.

**★ 6094 ★ Norwegian Association of the Deaf (NAD)**
**(Norges Doveforbund — NDF)**
Postboks 6850
St. Olavs Plass
N-0130 Oslo, Norway
**Phone:** 47 22 111775 **Fax:** 47 22 111633
**Fnded:** 1918. **Mem:** 2,500. **Local Groups:** 35. **Lang(s):** English, Norwegian. **Desc:** Deaf and hearing impaired, family, and friends in Norway. Offers support for the hearing disabled. Addresses concerns of members. **Pub:** *Doves Tidsskrift*, every second week. Magazine.

**★ 6095 ★ Oral Hearing-Impaired Section (OHIS)**
3417 Volta Pl. NW
Washington, DC 20007
**Phone:** (202)337-5220 **Fax:** (202)337-8314
**Email:** webmaster@agbell.org
**Website:** http://www.agbell.org/sections/dhhs/
K. Todd Houston, PhD, Exec. Dir.
**Fnded:** 1964. **Mem:** 345. **Local Groups:** 3. **Desc:** Section of the Alexander Graham Bell Association for the Deaf. Persons who are deaf or hard of hearing predominantly use speech and lipreading work. Encourages deaf young people and their families to use speech, lipreading, and residual hearing. Participates in regional, national, and international conferences on deafness. Appears on television and radio programs to demonstrate communications skills. Seeks to dispel outmoded conceptions about deafness. Supports: richer educational opportunities for the hearing impaired; workshops and outings for deaf or hard of hearing children and their families and teachers; scholarship funds for qualified students with hearing impairments; improved methods for developing better speech, voice, lipreading, and auditory training techniques. **Pub:** *Valta Voices OHIS Section*, bimonthly. Magazine. **Frmly:** (1988) Oral Deaf Adults Section.

**★ 6096 ★ Parents' Section of the Alexander Graham Bell Association for the Deaf (PS)**
c/o Alexander Graham Bell Association for the Deaf
3417 Volta Pl. NW
Washington, DC 20007
**Phone:** (202)337-5220 **Fax:** (202)337-8314
**Email:** lquigley@agbell.org
**Website:** http://www.agbell.org/sections.cfm
Donna Sorkin, Exec. Dir.
**Fnded:** 1958. **Mem:** 2,400. **Local Groups:** 28. **Desc:** Parents of hearing impaired children and individuals concerned with educational, social, pyschological, and vocational needs of hearing impaired children. Encourages and supports parent group action and programs on behalf of hearing impaired children; works for auditory/oral teaching of children who are hearing impaired. Also publishes material concerning the problems of deaf children. **Frmly:** (1989) International Parents' Organization.

**★ 6097 ★ Pax Natura Society for Rehabilitation of the Deaf (PNSRD)**
11460 60th Ave. NW
Edmonton, AB, Canada T6H 1J5
**Phone:** (780)435-7788
**Fnded:** 1975. **Mem:** 100. **Lang(s):** English, French. **Desc:** Individuals working to rehabilitate people with hearing impairment. Seeks to insure availability of social and health care services to people with hearing impairment throughout Canada. Sponsors supported living, educational, and rehabilitative services to people with impaired hearing. Conducts training programs for health care and social workers treating people with hearing impairments. Maintains summer camp and

family retreat programs; undertakes fundraising activities. **Pub:** Annual Report, annual.

★ 6098 ★ **Phone-TTY**
1246 Rte. 46 West
Parsippany, NJ 07054-2121
**Phone:** (973)299-6627          **Free:** 888-332-3889
**Fax:** (973)299-7768
**Email:** phonetty@aol.com
**Website:** http://www.phone-tty.com/
Anna M. Terrazzino, Exec. Dir.

**Fnded:** 1976. **Mem:** 20. **Desc:** Seeks to develop and promote better communication for the deaf using an ordinary telephone and current technology. Installs computerized phone-teletype equipment in the homes of individuals who are deaf, enabling these individuals to communicate with local police, hospitals, answering services, and news services, as well as members of the deaf community who have a PHONE-TTY in their homes. Researches, designs, manufactures, and distributes other communication devices for the deaf. Solicits grants and donations.

★ 6099 ★ **Registry of Interpreters for the Deaf (RID)**
333 Commerce St.
Alexandria, VA 22314
**Phone:** (703)838-0030          **Fax:** (703)838-0454
**Email:** admin@rid.org
**Website:** http://www.rid.org
Clay Nettles, Exec. Dir.

**Fnded:** 1964. **Mem:** 9,300. **Reg. Groups:** 5. **State Groups:** 58. **Desc:** Advocates sign language and oral interpreters. programs. Maintains 34 committees. Compiles statistics. **Pub:** *Registry of Interpreters for the Deaf–Proceedings of National Conventions*, biennial. Proceedings. *Price:* $11.95/copy. • *Views*, monthly. • Also publishes texts and other materials on interpretation, transliteration, and translation. **Frmly:** National Registry of Professional Interpreters and Translators for the Deaf.

★ 6100 ★ **Royal Association for Deaf People (RAD)**
Walsingham Rd.
Colchester CO2 7BP, United Kingdom
**Phone:** 44 1206 509509     **Fax:** 44 1206 769755
**Email:** tom.fenton@royaldeaf.org.uk
**Website:** http://www.yfv16.dial.pipex.com/contact.htm
**Fnded:** 1841. **Desc:** Meets the needs of profoundly deaf people. **Frmly:** (2001) Royal Association in Aid of Deaf People.

★ 6101 ★ **Royal College of Speech and Language Therapists**
2 White Hart Yard
London SE1 1NX, United Kingdom
**Phone:** 44 207 3781200     **Fax:** 44 207 4037254
**Email:** postmaster@rcslt.org
**Website:** http://www.rcslt.org
**Fnded:** 1945. **Mem:** 8,500. **Lang(s):** English. **Desc:** Speech and language therapists, including practising members, non-practising and retired members. All members have a certificate to practise (or its equivalent) issued by the college. Supports qualified speech and language therapists working for the relief of disorders of communication among both adults and children and the accreditation of courses leading to qualification as a speech and language therapist. Careers information available on request. **Pub:** *Bulletin*, monthly. Magazine. Contains clinical articles, news, book reviews, and letters. • *Bulletin Supplement*. • *International Journal of Language and Communication Disorders*, quarterly. Journal. **Frmly:** (1995) College of Speech Therapists; (1997) College of Speech and Language Therapists.

★ 6102 ★ **Royal Institute for Deaf and Blind Children (RIDBC)**
361-365 North Rocks Rd.
North Rocks, NSW 2151, Australia

**Phone:** 61 2 98711233          **Fax:** 61 2 98712196
**Email:** online@ridbc.org.au
**Website:** http://www.ridbc.org.au

**Fnded:** 1860. **Lang(s):** English. **Desc:** Strives to provide the best education possible for children with vision and/or hearing disabilities so that they may achieve their full potential in life. Advances and disseminates knowledge in this field.

★ 6103 ★ **Royal National Institute for Deaf People**
19-23 Featherstone St.
London EC1Y 8SL, United Kingdom
**Phone:** 44 20 72968000     **Fax:** 44 207 2968199
**Email:** helpline@rnid.org.uk
**Website:** http://www.rnid.org.uk

**Fnded:** 1911. **Mem:** 25,455. **Reg. Groups:** 5. **Lang(s):** English. **Desc:** Individual registered members. Provides the following quality services for the deaf, deaf blind and hard of hearing people: information, residential care, training (deaf awareness), specialist telephone services (Typetalk), assistive devices for sale from Sound Advantage, and Communication Support Units. All services are accessed through Regional offices, except Typetalk and Sound Advantage. **Pub:** *One In Seven*, bimonthly. Magazine. News and news relating to deaf & hard of hearing people. Various leaflets and factsheets.

★ 6104 ★ **Selective Mutism Foundation**
c/o Sue Newman
PO Box 450632
Sunrise, FL 33345
**Email:** consultsn@aol.com
**Website:** http://www.orgsites.com/fl/selectivemutismfoundation
Sue Newman, Co-Founder & Dir.

**Fnded:** 1991. **Mem:** 3,000. **Desc:** Individuals and families affected by selective mutism, an inherited anxiety disorder in which children with normal language skills or deficient language skills are unable to speak in school or other social situations. SM is often mistaken for normal shyness, and may go undetected for as long as two years. Promotes awareness and understanding of this condition. Encourages research and treatment. Maintains speakers' bureau. **Pub:** *Selective Mutism, A Silent Cry for Help*. Brochure. *Price:* Free. **Frmly:** (1993) Foundation for Elective Mutism, Inc.

★ 6105 ★ **Self Help for Hard of Hearing People (SHHH)**
7910 Woodmont Ave., Ste. 1200
Bethesda, MD 20814
**Phone:** (301)657-2248          **Fax:** (301)913-9413
**Email:** national@shhh.org
**Website:** http://www.shhh.org
Beth Wilson, Exec. Dir.

**Fnded:** 1979. **Mem:** 12,000. **Reg. Groups:** 10. **State Groups:** 250. **Desc:** Devoted to the welfare and interests of those who cannot hear well, their relatives and friends. Strives to improve quality of hard of hearing people's lives through education, advocacy and self help. **Pub:** *Hearing Loss: The Journal of Self Help for Hard at Hearing People*, bimonthly. Magazine. Contains articles by hearing health professionals and personal narratives by people with hearing loss. Contains information on resources. • *Hospitality for Guests with Hearing Loss: A Guide for Hotel/Motel Compliance with the Americans with Disabilities Act*. • *Operation SHHH: Noise Abuse Prevention Posters*. • *Our Forgotten Children: Hard-of-Hearing Pupils in the Schools*. • *SHHH News*, quarterly. Newsletter. • *Telephone Strategies: A Technical and Practical Guide for Hard of Hearing People*. • Brochures. • Offers various publications on hearing loss, products, and related subjects. **AKA:** SHHH.

★ 6106 ★ **SENSE**
11-13 Clifton Terrace
Finsbury Park
London N4 3SR, United Kingdom

**Phone:** 44 20 72727774     **Fax:** 44 20 72726012
**Email:** enquiries@sense.org.uk
**Website:** http://www.sense.org.uk

**Fnded:** 1955. **Mem:** 650. **Reg. Groups:** 14. **Lang(s):** Welsh. **Desc:** Families, professionals and interested individuals. To provide services for deafblind people, their families, carers and the professionals with whom they work. Campaigns for legislative support for deafblind people. **Pub:** *Publications list*. • *Talking Sense*, quarterly. Magazine. For parents and professionals in the deafblind field. • Books. **Frmly:** (2001) National Deafblind and Rubella Association.

★ 6107 ★ **Signing Exact English Center for the Advancement of Deaf Children (SEE)**
PO Box 1181
Los Alamitos, CA 90720
**Phone:** (562)430-1467          **Fax:** (562)795-6614
**Email:** seectr@aol.com
**Website:** http://www.seecenter.org
Esther Zawolkow, Contact

**Fnded:** 1984. **Desc:** Working to promote early identification and intervention, to develop understanding of principles of Signing, to provide information to parents on deafness and related topics and to foster the positive development of self concept in the deaf child. Conducts workshops, sign skills, evaluations. Provides introductory information.

★ 6108 ★ **Singapore Association for the Deaf**
227 Mountbatten Rd.
Singapore 397998, Singapore
**Phone:** 65 3448274          **Fax:** 65 345706
**Email:** aa@sad.org.sg
**Website:** http://www.sad.org.sg

**Desc:** Works to improve the quality of life for people with impaired hearing. Conducts educational programs.

★ 6109 ★ **Society for Ear, Nose, and Throat Advances in Children (SENTAC)**
Richard D. Wood Center, 1st Fl.
34th St. & Civic Center Blvd.
Division of Otolaryngology
Philadelphia, PA 19104-4399
**Phone:** (215)590-3450          **Fax:** (215)590-3986
**Email:** calandra@email.chop.edu
**Website:** http://www.sentac.org
Linda Miller Calandra, MSN, CPNP, COLRN, Sec.

**Fnded:** 1973. **Mem:** 350. **Desc:** Otolaryngologists, pediatricians, audiologists, speech pathologists, and related professionals. Works to evaluate the science and practice of medicine, surgery, and rehabilitation as related to diseases and disorders of the ear, nose, and throat in infants and children; to improve quality of care; to promote and coordinate research; to foster scientific exchange and coordination among professionals from related disciplines. Sponsors lectures and symposia. Provides forum for interchange of information on practice and research. **Pub:** *Directory and Meeting Abstracts*, annual. Directory. • Brochure.

**Society of Military Otolaryngologists - Head and Neck Surgeons (SMO-HNS)**
*See:* Entry 13467

**Society of Otorhinolaryngology and Head/ Neck Nurses (SOHN)**
*See:* Entry 15774

★ 6110 ★ **Society of Teachers of Speech and Drama**
73 Berry Hill Rd.
Mansfield NG18 4RU, United Kingdom
**Phone:** 44 1623 627636
**Email:** ann.p.jones@btinternet.com
**Website:** http://www.stsd.org.uk

ISSN 0743-4510

# Encyclopedia of Medical Organizations and Agencies

## THIRTEENTH EDITION

A Subject Guide to Organizations, Foundations,
Federal and State Governmental Agencies, Research Centers,
and Medical and Allied Health Schools

**Amanda C. Quick, Project Editor**

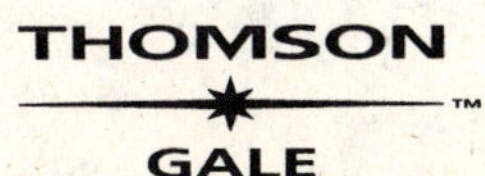



Detroit • New York • San Diego • San Francisco • Cleveland • New Haven, Conn. • Waterville, Maine • London • Munich

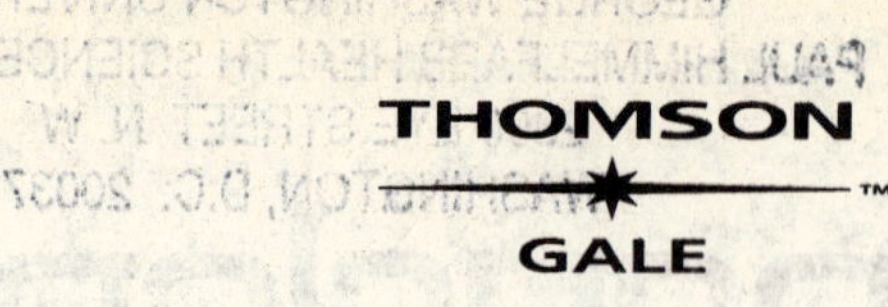


Encyclopedia of Medical Organizations and Agencies, 13th Edition

**Project Editor**
Amanda C. Quick

**Editorial**
Jason Baldwin, Chris Lopez, Rebecca Marlow-Ferguson, Jaime E. Noce, Lynn Pearce

**Editorial Support Services**
Emmanuel T. Barrido, Scott Flaugher

**Product Design**
Michael Logusz

**Composition and Electronic Capture**
Evi Seoud

**Manufacturing**
NeKita McKee



ISBN 0-7876-6321-2
ISSN 0743-4510

# Contents



*Encyclopedia of Medical Organizations and Agencies*

# Highlights

The twelfth edition of the *Encyclopedia of Medical Organizations and Agencies* (EMOA) is a comprehensive guide to medical and health-related organizations, agencies, and institutions, including:

- National, International, and State & Regional Organizations
- Foundations & Other Funding Organizations
- U.S. Federal & State Government Agencies
- Research Centers
- Medical & Allied Health Schools

Entries in EMOA are carefully selected from a wide array of resources to provide a convenient, one-stop source of information on a broad range of topics relating to clinical medicine, basic biomedical sciences, and the technological and socioeconomic aspects of health care. Subjects covered in EMOA include:

- Aging
- Biomedical Engineering
- Child Abuse & Family Violence
- Death & Dying
- Environmental Health
- Family Planning
- Genetics & Genetic Disorders
- Health Care Administration & Financing
- Infectious Diseases
- Mental Health
- Neurology
- Nursing
- Nutrition
- Occupational Health
- Radiology
- Respiratory Diseases
- Sports Medicine
- Substance Abuse
- Transplantation
- and more...

**Features of EMOA**

- More than 21,000 entries arranged within 69 subject-specific chapters, ranging from Aging to Vision.

- Entry cross-references direct users to key entries appearing in other chapters.

- Easy-to-read page design. Catchwords at the top of each page and headings throughout the text help the user quickly locate desired information.

- The **Subject Cross-Index** provides a quick overview of all topics covered in EMOA.

- The **Alphabetical Name and Keyword Index** contains citations to all organizations listed in EMOA, as well as to subject keywords appearing in organization names.

# Introduction

The *Encyclopedia of Medical Organizations and Agencies* (EMOA), now in its thirteenth edition, is a convenient single-volume resource to subject-classified information on medical and health-related organizations, agencies, and institutions. EMOA directs health care professionals and the public alike to a wide variety of organizations, including:

- National & International Organizations
- State & Regional Organizations
- Foundations & Other Funding Organizations
- U.S. Federal Government Agencies
- U.S. State Government Agencies
- Research Centers
- Medical & Allied Health Schools

EMOA provides contact and descriptive information on more than 21,000 such organizations active in clinical medicine, the basic biomedical sciences, or the technological and socioeconomic aspects of health care. The book covers 69 subject areas representing a wide range of contemporary medical interests, including:

- diseases and disorders (birth defects, communicative disorders, infectious diseases, respiratory diseases, etc.);
- medical disciplines (dermatology, neurology, orthopedics, radiology, etc.);
- social health concerns (aging, child abuse, family planning, substance abuse, etc.);
- special aspects of medicine (health care administration, health care financing, the health care industry, and information and communications).

## Content and Arrangement

EMOA consists of descriptive listings and indexes.

- The **Descriptive Listings** are organized within 69 chapters that are arranged alphabetically by subject name. (Consult the "Contents" pages for a complete list of subjects.)  Key entries appearing in other chapters are identified through cross-references appearing throughout the descriptive listings.

- The **Subject Cross-Index**, immediately preceding the descriptive listings, provides thorough access to the subject content of EMOA via chapter names and numbers, synonyms, related terms, and more specific subjects included but not reflected in chapter  titles.

- The **Alphabetical Name and Keyword Index** speeds access to EMOA entries in the book, as well as to significant keywords appearing in organization titles.

For additional information on the content, arrangement, and indexing of EMOA, consult the "User's Guide" following this introduction.

## Method of Compilation

Many sources were used in compiling the twelfth edition of EMOA. Entries relevant to the medical and allied health fields were carefully selected from Gale Group directories, federal government documents, state government publications, and lists and directories supplied by numerous national organizations. Telephone inquiries were also employed to gather data and/or verify information.

# User's Guide

EMOA is organized into 3 parts: **Descriptive Listings** and entry cross-references, which are arranged within subject chapters; a **Subject Cross-Index**, which provides further subject access to the content of EMOA; and an **Alphabetical Name and Keyword Index**, which provides a convenient alphabetical listing of all organizations, agencies, and institutions included in EMOA. Each part is described below.

## Descriptive Listings

Listings are numbered sequentially within 69 subject chapters, as outlined on the "Contents" pages. With the exception of the General Medical section, which is presented first, chapters are arranged alphabetically by subject names.

Entries within subject chapters are grouped according to functional categories. An individual chapter may contain all or only some of the categories, as appropriate to the subject. Consult the "Contents" pages for a listing of the entry categories included in each chapter. Specific information on the content, arrangement, and indexing of each functional category is provided in the following descriptions.

### Federal Government Agencies

**Scope:** Some 105 units of the federal government concerned with medicine and health.
**Entries include:** Agency name, address, telephone number, fax number (when available), and, in many cases, a brief description of the agency's programs and purposes.
**Arrangement:** Alphabetical by agency names.
**Indexed by:** Parent agency and specific unit names, as well as significant intermediate agency names and keywords within names.
**Source:** *United States Government Manual* (published by the U.S. National Archives and Records Administration and available from the U.S. Government Printing Office) and original research by the EMOA editorial staff.

### Foundations and Other Funding Organizations

**Scope:** More than 2,300 U.S. funding organizations, including major private and corporate foundations that provide charitable support to nonprofit organizations, as well as professional associations and special interest groups that administer scholarship, fellowship, and grant programs, and provide other financial assistance for a variety of medical and health-related interests.
**Entries include:** Organization name, address, email and internet addresses (when available), telephone number, toll-free and fax numbers (when available), contact name, and descriptive information on the funding program, including foundation philosophy, giving priorities, typical health-related recipients, and geographic distribution of funds.
**Arrangement:** Alphabetical by organization names within three sections: 1) Private Foundations, 2) Corporate Foundations, and 3) Other Funding Organizations.
**Indexed by:** Organization names and significant keywords within names.
**Source:** *Foundation Reporter* and *Corporate Giving Directory* (both published by the Taft Group), and *Encyclopedia of Associations, Volume 1: National Organizations of the U.S.* (published by Gale).

### Medical and Allied Health Schools

**Scope:** More than 3,800 educational institutions and training programs in 29 occupational categories. Coverage is limited primarily to baccalaureate and advanced degree programs. To obtain information on related educational programs at other levels, consult the section description referred to under the "Arrangement" heading below. Information on schools and programs is also available from the Commission on Accreditation of Allied Health Education Programs (35 E Wacker Dr., Ste. 1970, Chicago, IL 60601-2208, (312)553-9355, http://www.caahep.org), which accredits educational programs in some 18 allied health professions.
**Entries include:** Institution name, address, email and internet addresses (when available), telephone number, and fax number (when available).
**Arrangement:** Geographical by states, then alphabetical by institution names within states. Each section of

schools is accompanied by a brief description of the programs listed there, along with references to professional organizations that may be contacted for general information concerning accreditation or careers in that field.
**Indexed by:** Sponsoring institution names.
**Source:** Lists provided by national organizations and original research by the EMOA editorial staff.

### National and International Organizations

**Scope:** Some 4,400 primarily nonprofit membership groups, including national organizations of the United States, as well as organizations that are international in scope, membership, or interest and are headquartered outside the United States.
**Entries include:** Organization name, address, email and internet addresses (when available), telephone number, toll-free and fax numbers (when available), name and title of the chief official, and a brief description, including founding date, number of members, purpose, publications, and former/alternate organization names (if applicable). In non-U.S. entries, the principal foreign-language name is listed in parentheses following the English-language version of the organization name.
**Arrangement:** Alphabetical by organization names.
**Indexed by:** Organization names, both English- and foreign-language, as well as significant keywords within names.
**Source:** *Encyclopedia of Associations, Volume 1: National Organizations of the U.S.* and *Encyclopedia of Associations: International Organizations* (both published by Gale).

### Research Centers

**Scope:** More than 3,300 research organizations, including: 1) university-related and other nonprofit research centers in the U.S. and Canada that are engaged in medical and health-related research on a continuing basis, and 2) U.S. government research centers and programs, including federal agencies and bureaus that are themselves research organizations, research facilities owned and operated by the federal government, government-owned/contractor-operated facilities, test centers and facilities, cooperative research programs, data collection and analysis activities, and offices that support research by awarding grants and/or contracts.
**Entries include:** Organization or agency name, address, email and internet addresses (when available), telephone number, toll-free and fax numbers (when available), director name, a brief description of principal activities and fields of research, and a listing of publications issued by the research unit.
**Arrangement:** Alphabetical by organization or agency names.
**Indexed by:** Parent organization names, research unit names, significant intermediate organization names, and significant keywords within names.
**Source:** *Research Centers Directory* and *Government Research Directory* (both published by Gale).

### State Government Agencies

**Scope:** More than 1,400 agencies that function in 27 areas relating to medicine and health.
**Entries include:** Agency name, address, telephone number, and fax number (when available).
**Arrangement:** Geographical by states.
**Indexed by:** State designations (Michigan Department of Public Health, Alabama State Board of Pharmacy, etc.) and other keywords within agency names.
**Source:** Lists provided by organizations, as well as original research by the EMOA editorial staff.

### State and Regional Organizations

**Scope:** More than 3,100 entries representing state and regional affiliates of 46 national organizations.
**Entries include:** Organization name, address, email and internet addresses (when available), telephone number, and fax number (when available).
**Arrangement:** Geographical by states, then alphabetical by organization names within states.
**Indexed by:** Organization names, as well as geographic designations and other keywords within names.
**Source:** Lists provided by national organizations and original research by the EMOA editorial staff.

## Entry Cross-References

In a subject-classified compilation such as EMOA, there are many entries that are appropriate for listing in more than one subject chapter. For example, the International Society for Pediatric Neurosurgery applies to three EMOA chapters: Child Health, Neurology, and Surgery. The use of text cross-references in these cases allows the user to locate the names of all organizations concerned with a subject area, while eliminating the need to duplicate complete entries in multiple chapters. In the example cited above, the full entry appears in the Child Health Chapter and cross-references, with the organization name only, are listed in the Neurology and Surgery chapters, referring the user to the full entry in the Child Health Chapter.

## Subject Cross-Index

The **Subject Cross-Index** provides access to the subject content of EMOA by listing chapter names as well as *See* and *See Also* references for synonyms, related terms, and more specific subjects included but not reflected in chapter titles. References are to chapter names and their corresponding chapter numbers.

## Alphabetical Name and Keyword Index

The **Alphabetical Name and Keyword Index** provides access to all entries included in EMOA, as well as to former or alternate names that appear within the text of entries. Each organization, agency, and institution is indexed by the name listed and, when appropriate, by significant keywords that are a part of that name. Index references are to book entry numbers rather than page numbers. Entry numbers appear in the index in boldface type if the reference is to a main entry, and in light-face type if the reference is to a former or alternate name included within the text of the cited entry.

Many of the entries in EMOA use a hierarchical organization name structure, with a parent organization and intermediate sub-units preceding the specific unit name. The Alphabetical Name and Keyword Index offers access to all multiple-part organization names via the parent organization name. Many entries are also referenced under the specific unit name and some under a significant intermediate unit name. Multiple parts of names are separated in index citations by a bullet (•). If several entries have the same parent organization, as is the case with many of the government and university groups listed in EMOA, the related units appear as a group under the name of the parent organization. The parent agencies of most federal government organizations are indexed under "U.S." (e.g., U.S. House of Representatives, U.S. Department of Health and Human Services, etc.).

## Alphabetizing Rules

In both the descriptive listings chapters and the index, organization names are sorted on a word-by-word basis, so that "New York Easter Seal Society" comes before "Newbury College". Initial articles ("A," "An," or "The") are ignored for sorting purposes. Conjunctions, articles, and most prepositions elsewhere in the names are also not considered in alphabetizing. In addition:

- Numbers are sorted as if spelled-out and interfiled alphabetically with other non-number words.

- Abbreviations such as "U.S.," "St.," "Mt.," "Ft.," and "Dr.," are sorted as if spelled-out and interfiled with names in which the full version of those words are used.

- Personal names are sorted under the first name, or initial, within the descriptive listings chapters. In the index, they can be accessed under both the first and last names.

# Key to Abbreviations

| | | | | |
|---|---|---|---|---|
| & | And | | Hwy. | Highway |
| Act. | Acting | | IA | Iowa |
| Adj. | Adjutant | | ID | Idaho |
| Admin. | Administrator | | IL | Illinois |
| AFB | Air Force Base | | IN | Indiana |
| AK | Alaska | | Inc. | Incorporated |
| AL | Alabama | | Info. | Information |
| Apt. | Apartment | | KS | Kansas |
| AR | Arkansas | | KY | Kentucky |
| Asst. | Assistant | | LA | Louisiana |
| Assoc. | Associate | | Lib. | Library |
| Ave. | Avenue | | Libn. | Librarian |
| AZ | Arizona | | Ln. | Lane |
| Bldg. | Building | | MA | Massachusetts |
| Blvd. | Boulevard | | MD | Maryland |
| Br. | Branch | | ME | Maine |
| CA | California | | Med. | Medical |
| CEO | Chief Executive Officer | | Mgr. | Manager |
| Chf. | Chief | | MI | Michigan |
| Chm. | Chairman | | MN | Minnesota |
| Cir. | Circle | | MO | Missouri |
| Clghse. | Clearinghouse | | MS | Mississippi |
| c/o | Care of | | MT | Montana |
| CO | Colorado | | Mt. | Mount |
| Co. | Company | | N. | North |
| Coll. | Collection | | Natl. | National |
| Comdr. | Commander | | NC | North Carolina |
| Commun. | Communication | | ND | North Dakota |
| Coord. | Coordinator | | NE | Nebraska, Northeast |
| Corp. | Corporation | | NH | New Hampshire |
| Couns. | Counselor | | NJ | New Jersey |
| CT | Connecticut | | No. | Number |
| Ct. | Court | | NV | Nevada |
| Ctr. | Center | | NW | Northwest |
| DC | District of Columbia | | NY | New York |
| DE | Delaware | | Off. | Officer |
| Dept. | Department | | OH | Ohio |
| Dir. | Director | | OK | Oklahoma |
| Dr. | Drive | | OR | Oregon |
| E. | East | | PA | Pennsylvania |
| Educ. | Education | | Pkwy. | Parkway |
| Exec. | Executive | | Pl. | Place |
| Expy. | Expressway | | Plz. | Plaza |
| Ext. | Extension | | PO Box | Post Office Box |
| Fl. | Floor | | PR | Puerto Rico |
| FL | Florida | | Pres. | President |
| Ft. | Fort | | Prog. | Program |
| Fwy. | Freeway | | Rd. | Road |
| GA | Georgia | | RD | Rural Delivery |
| Gen. | General | | Ref. | Reference |
| GU | Guam | | Reg. | Regional |
| Hd. | Head | | Res. | Research |
| HI | Hawaii | | RFD | Rural Free Delivery |

| RI | Rhode Island | Supv. | Supervisor |
| Rm. | Room | SW | Southwest |
| RR | Rural Route | Ter. | Terrace |
| Rte. | Route | TN | Tennessee |
| S. | South | Tpke. | Turnpike |
| SC | South Carolina | Trl. | Trail |
| Sci. | Science | TX | Texas |
| SD | South Dakota | Univ. | University |
| SE | Southeast | U.S. | United States |
| Sec. | Secretary | UT | Utah |
| Sect. | Section | VA | Virginia |
| Serv. | Service | VI | Virgin Islands |
| Soc. | Social | VP | Vice President |
| Spec. | Specialist | VT | Vermont |
| Sq. | Square | W. | West |
| Sr. | Senior | WA | Washington |
| St. | Saint, Street | WV | West Virginia |
| Sta. | Station | WY | Wyoming |
| Ste. | Suite, Sainte | | |

# Subject Cross Index

This index provides alphabetical subject access to EMOA by listing chapter names as well as *See* and *See Also* references for synonyms, related terms, and more specific subjects included but not reflected in chapter titles. References are to chapter names and their corresponding chapter numbers.

# Chapter 1
# General Medical

## Federal Government Agencies

**★ 1 ★ Smithsonian Institution**
**National Museum of American History**
**Department of the History of Science and Technology**
**Science, Medicine, and Society Division**
14th St. & Constitution Ave. NW
Washington, DC 20560
**Phone:** (202)357-2700

**Desc:** Division is concerned with the history of public health and pharmacy, 17th-20th century history of medical and dental technology, and 20th century health sciences.

**★ 2 ★ Tennessee Valley Authority**
**Health Services**
20 E 11th St., EB 8A
Chattanooga, TN 37402-2801
**Phone:** (423)751-2091
**Website:** http://www.tva.gov

**★ 3 ★ U.S. Department of Health and Human Services**
200 Independence Ave. SW
Washington, DC 20201
**Phone:** (202)619-0257
**Website:** http://www.dhhs.gov/
Tommy G. Thompson, Secretary

**Desc:** The Department of Health and Human Services is the cabinet-level department of the federal executive branch most concerned with people and most involved with the nation's human concerns. The Secretary of HHS advises the President on health, welfare, and income security plans, policies, and programs of the federal government. Principal operating components of the Department include the Administration for Children and Families, the Health Care Financing Administration, the Administration on Aging, the Centers for Disease Control and Prevention, the Food and Drug Administration, and the National Institutes of Health.

**★ 4 ★ U.S. Department of Health and Human Services**
**Administration for Children and Families (ACF)**
370 L'Enfant Promenade SW
Washington, DC 20447
**Phone:** (202)401-9200
**Website:** http://www.acf.dhhs.gov

**Desc:** The Administration for Children and Families provides national leadership and direction to plan, manage, and coordinate comprehensive support services for vulnerable children and families, Native Americans, people with disabilities, refugees and legalized aliens. The mission of ACF is to promote stability, economic security, responsibility and self-sufficiency. There are seven major program offices: Administration for Children, Youth and Families (ACYF), Administration on Developmental Disabilities, Administration for Native Americans, Office of Family Assistance, Office of Child Support Enforcement, Office of Community Service, and Office of Refugee Resettlement.

**★ 5 ★ U.S. Department of Health and Human Services**
**Administration for Children and Families (ACF)**
**Administration on Children, Youth and Families (ACYF)**
370 L'Enfant Promenade SW
Washington, DC 20447
**Phone:** (202)205-8347
**Website:** http://www.acf.dhhs.gov/programs/acyf/acyf.htm

**Desc:** The Administration for Children, Youth, and Families manages State grant and child care programs including programs to increase child abuse prevention and treatment activities and to develop family preservation and family support services; the Head Start program; programs which provide services for runaway and homeless youth and their families; child welfare training programs; and child abuse and neglect research and demonstration programs.

**★ 6 ★ U.S. Department of Health and Human Services**
**Administration for Children and Families (ACF)**
**Administration for Native Americans (ANA)**
370 L'Enfant Promenade SW
Washington, DC 20447
**Phone:** (202)690-7776
**Website:** http://www.acf.hhs.gov/programs/ana/

**Desc:** The Administration for Native Americans represents and promotes the goal of developmental, social, economic, and lasting self-sufficiency of American Indians, Alaskan Natives; and Pacific Natives.

**★ 7 ★ U.S. Department of Health and Human Services (HRSA)**
**Health Resources and Services Administration (BHPR)**
**Bureau of Health Professions**
Parklawn Bldg.
5600 Fishers Ln.
Rockville, MD 20857
**Phone:** (301)443-1590
**Website:** http://bhpr.hrsa.gov/
Kerry P. Nesseler, Assoc. Administrator

**Desc:** The Bureau provides national leadership in coordinating, evaluating, and supporting the development and utilization of the nation's health personnel. To accomplish this goal, the Bureau provides financial aid to health professions students and support for health professions data analysis and research. It provides leadership for promoting equity in access to health services and health careers for the disadvantaged, and provides technical assistance activities for international projects relevant to domestic health personnel problems.

**★ 8 ★ U.S. Department of Health and Human Services (HRSA)**
**Health Resources and Services Administration (BPHC)**
**Bureau of Primary Health Care**
4350 East West Highway
Bethesda, MD 20814
**Phone:** (301)594-4100   **Fax:** (301)594-5008
**Website:** http://bphc.hrsa.gov/
Sam Shekar, MD, Assoc. Administrator

**Desc:** The Bureau provides national leadership for efforts to increase access to comprehensive preventative and primary health care for underserved and vulnerable populations; provides grants to community, migrant, and school-based health centers, health care for the homeless programs, and public housing primary care programs; and administers the Federal occupational health program of the PHS drug pricing program.

**★ 9 ★ U.S. Department of Health and Human Services**
**Health Resources and Services Administration**
**Maternal and Child Health Bureau**
5600 Fishers Ln.
Rockville, MD 20857
**Phone:** (301)443-2170
**Website:** http://mchb.hrsa.gov/
Peter C. Van Dyck, MD, Assoc. Administrator

**Desc:** The Bureau provides national leadership in supporting, identifying, and interpreting national trends and issues relating to the health needs of mothers, infants, children and adolescents, including those with special health care needs.

**★ 10 ★ U.S. Department of Health and Human Services**
**Indian Health Service (IHS)**
5600 Fishers Ln.
Rockville, MD 20857
**Phone:** (301)443-1083
**Website:** http://www.ihs.gov/
Michael H. Trujillo, MD, Director

**Desc:** The Indian Health Service assures a comprehensive health services delivery system for American Indians and Alaska Natives, with sufficient options to provide for maximum tribal involvement in meeting their health needs. The goal of the Service is to raise the health level of the Indian and Alaska Native people to the highest possible level.

### ★ 11 ★ U.S. Department of Health and Human Services
**National Institutes of Health**
**Clinical Center**
9000 Rockville Pike
Bethesda, MD 20892
**Phone:** (301)496-3227
**Website:** http://www.cc.nih.gov/
John I. Gallin, Director

**Desc:** The Center is designed to bring scientists working in the Center's laboratories into proximity with clinicians caring for patients, so that they may collaborate on problems of mutual concern.

### ★ 12 ★ U.S. Department of Justice
**Bureau of Prisons**
**Health Services Division**
320 1st St. NW
Washington, DC 20534
**Phone:** (202)307-3198     **Free:** 888-317-8455
**Website:** http://www.bop.gov
Kathleen M. Hawk Sawyer, Director

**Desc:** The Health Services Division has oversight responsibility for all medical and psychiatric programs; environmental and occupational health services; food and nutrition services; and farm operations.

### ★ 13 ★ U.S. Department of State
**Office of Medical Services**
2201 C St. NW
Washington, DC 20520
**Phone:** (202)663-1748
**Website:** http://www.state.gov/

**Desc:** The Office develops, manages, and staffs a worldwide primary health care system for U.S. citizen employees and their eligible dependents residing abroad. The Office approves and monitors the medical evacuation of patients, conducts pre-employment and in-service physical examinations, and provides clinical referral and advisory services. The Office also provides for emergency medical response in the event of a crisis at an overseas post.

# Foundations & Other Funding Organizations

## Private Foundations

### ★ 14 ★ A. E. Finley Foundation
PO Box 98266
Raleigh, NC 27624-8266
**Phone:** (919)782-0529     **Fax:** (919)782-6978
**Email:** aeffinc@bellsouth.net
**Website:** http://www.geocities.com/aeffinc
Robert Brown, President

**Fnded:** 1957. **Philosophy:** The A. E. Finley foundation "contributes to and supports charitable, scientific, literary, religious, and educational organizations. It endeavors to contribute to soundly managed and operated qualifying organizations which fundamentally give service with a broad scope and impact, aid all kinds of people, and contribute materially to the general welfare." **Priorities:** *Arts & Humanities:* 4%. Supports art museums, theater, public broadcasting, and historic preservation. *Civic & Public Affairs:* 3%. Supports community foundations and clubs. *Education:* 60%. Funds colleges, universities, leadership training, schools and fellowships. *Environment:* 6%. Supports food distribution programs, senior services, Special Olympics, Young Men's Christian Association's, Young Women's Christian Association and United Way. *International:* 22%. Supports cancer, diabetes, respiratory, Alzheimers disease and hospitals. *Note:* Total contributions made in fiscal 1999. **Typ. Recipients:** Cancer, Children's Health/Hospitals, Hospices, Hospitals, Hospitals (University Affiliated), Medical Education, People with Disabilities, Respiratory, Single-Disease Health Associations, Substance Abuse. **Geo. Dist:** NC; NC, Triangle area; VA.

### ★ 15 ★ A. J. Fletcher Foundation
PO Box 12800
Raleigh, NC 27605
**Phone:** (919)890-6081     **Fax:** (919)890-6279
**Website:** http://www.ajf.org
Thomas McGuire, Jr., Vice President & Executive Director

**Fnded:** 1961. **Philosophy:** Although the primary focus of the foundation has traditionally been on education, communications, and the arts, the foundation will also consider requests from agencies and organizations addressing a wide variety of social issues and charitable endeavors. The foundation has broadened its focus to include health and human services, illiteracy, public education, poverty programs, and statewide service organizations, and has provided seed money for new and emerging nonprofit organizations. In an effort to maintain long-term relationships with grantees, the foundation provides grants for technical assistance, management training, and other developmental programs that benefit an agency long after allocated funds are gone. It also encourages partnerships through seminars and conferences that offer information aimed at fostering financial stability. The foundation will share resources and knowledge in a statewide interactive network that includes other nonprofits and donor groups. **Priorities:** *Arts & Humanities:* 52%. Public television, historic preservation, music, and theater. *Civic & Public Affairs:* 5%. *Education:* About 19%. Primarily to colleges and universities in North Carolina. *Environment:* 22%. Emphasis on child welfare. *International:* 1%. *Note:* Total contributions made in fiscal 1999. **Typ. Recipients:** Children's Health/Hospitals, Eyes/Blindness, Family Planning, People with Disabilities, Public Health, Single-Disease Health Associations. **Geo. Dist:** NC.

### ★ 16 ★ A. L. Mailman Family Foundation
707 Westchester Ave.
White Plains, NY 10604
**Phone:** (914)683-8089     **Fax:** (914)686-5519
**Email:** almf@mailman.org
**Website:** http://www.mailman.org
Luba Lynch, Executive Director & Secretary

**Fnded:** 1980. **Philosophy:** "Recognizing the importance of the early years and the power of prevention, the foundation pays special attention to the needs and potentials of young children and their families. The foundation promotes universal access to high quality, culturally responsive, family-supportive early care and education experiences. The foundation is committed to strengthening families and enhancing their ability to support the healthy development of their children. The foundation is committed to the ideal of social justice and to the development of moral responsibility in children and youth." 1996 Annual Report **Priorities:** *Civic & Public Affairs:* 14%. Public policy groups, legal aid, and minority affairs. *Education:* 44%. Funds colleges, universities and preschool education. Grants focus on early child care. *Environment:* 33%. Child welfare and family services. *International:* 5%. Children's health and hospitals. *Note:* Total contributions made in 1999. **Typ. Recipients:** Alzheimers Disease, Cancer, Children's Health/Hospitals, Clinics/Medical Centers, Domestic Violence, Family Planning, Health Organizations, Medical Education, Mental Health, Nutrition, People with Disabilities, Prenatal Health Issues, Public Health, Research/Studies Institutes. **Geo. Dist:** nationally.

### ★ 17 ★ A. Lindsay and Olive B. O'Connor Foundation
PO Box D
Hobart, NY 13788
**Phone:** (607)538-9248     **Fax:** (607)538-1650
Donald Bishop, II, President & Executive Director

**Fnded:** 1965. **Philosophy:** The foundation gives to a variety of causes that all serve to enhance the quality of life in rural, upstate New York. A majority of donations support organizations concerned with issues affecting civic and public affairs. Educational institutions and the arts also typically receive funding. **Priorities:** *Arts & Humanities:* 29%. Major support for the Hanford Mills Museum. *Civic & Public Affairs:* 31%. Focus on community revitalization projects. *Education:* 3%. Funds education associations and colleges and universities. *Environment:* 1%. Supports family services. *International:* 13%. Primarily supports hospitals. *Note:* Total contributions made in 1998. **Typ. Recipients:** Emergency/Ambulance Services, Heart, Hospices, Hospitals, Medical Education, People with Disabilities, Single-Disease Health Associations. **Geo. Dist:** NY, Delaware County and contiguous rural counties in upstate New York.

### ★ 18 ★ A. V. Hunter Trust, Inc.
650 S Cherry, Ste. 535
Denver, CO 80246-1897
**Phone:** (303)399-5450     **Fax:** (303)399-5499
**Website:** http://www.avhuntertrust.org
Sharon Siddons, Executive Director & Secretary

**Fnded:** 1937. **Philosophy:** In distributing contributions, the trustees adhere to A. V. Hunter's will which states, "the trustees shall from time to time... use the net income from said trust and property included therein, in the aid, support, maintenance and assistance, by gift, donation, or otherwise as to them may seem advisable, of then existing, established nonsectarian, charitable institutions or projects or endeavors located in the State of Colorado...whose objects or purposes are to give aid, comfort, support or assistance to children, or aged persons or indigent adults." **Priorities:** *Civic & Public Affairs:* About 6%. Job resource centers, employment programs for women, and Native American affairs. *Education:* 10%. Outward Bound programs and adult learning. *Environment:* About 61%. Planned Parenthood, youth organizations, and volunteer programs. *International:* 16%. Hospice, health centers, and dentistry programs for the disadvantaged. *Note:* Total contributions made in 1998. **Typ. Recipients:** Adolescent Health Issues, Children's Health/Hospitals, Clinics/Medical Centers, Domestic Violence, Emergency/Ambulance Services, Family Planning, Health Organizations, Hospices, Hospitals, Hospitals (University Affiliated), Medical Rehabilitation, Multiple Sclerosis, Nursing Services, People with Disabilities, Prenatal Health Issues, Public Health, Research/Studies Institutes, Sexual Abuse, Single-Disease Health Associations, Substance Abuse. **Geo. Dist:** Denver, CO.

### ★ 19 ★ Abbot and Dorothy H. Stevens Foundation
PO Box 111
North Andover, MA 01845
**Phone:** (978)688-7211     **Fax:** (978)686-1620
**Email:** 74722.2637@compuserve.com
Elizabeth Beland, Administrator

**Fnded:** 1953. **Philosophy:** The purpose of the Abbot and Dorothy H. Stevens Foundation is to assist local charitable organizations. Grants are made across the major categories of support. Specific interests include the arts, law and justice, colleges, hospitals, churches, conservation/preservation, education, and social services. **Priorities:** *Arts & Humanities:* 30%. Supports museums, art centers, libraries, and performing arts. *Civic & Public Affairs:* 9%. Funds other philanthropic organizations. *Education:* 14%. Funds colleges, universities, and precollege education. *Environment:* 31%. Supports human services and summer youth programs. *International:* 7%. Gives to hospitals and health associations. *Note:* Total contributions made in 1999. **Typ. Recipients:** Cancer, Children's Health/Hospitals, Clinics/Medical Centers, Emergency/Ambulance Services, Home-Care Services, Hospitals, Mental Health, Nursing Services, People with Disabilities, Substance Abuse. **Geo. Dist:** MA, emphasis on Greater Lawrence area.

### ★ 20 ★ Abell Foundation
111 South Calvert St., Ste. 2300
Baltimore, MD 21202
**Phone:** (410)547-1300     **Fax:** (410)539-6579
**Email:** abell@abell.org
**Website:** http://www.abell.org
Robert Embry, Jr., President

**Fnded:** 1953. **Philosophy:** The foundation recognizes the "complex interdependent issues affecting the quality of life in Maryland." From this perspective, the foundation looks to "join others in seeking solutions to pervasive and stubborn social and economic problems, promote the development of fuller human potential and achievement of self-sufficiency through educational opportunities, and strengthen organizations to provide greater access and more effective services." Emphases include educational reform, job creation, tourism, strengthening families, reducing drug addiction, and alleviating hunger and homelessness. **Priorities:** *Arts & Humanities:* 1%. Museums, theater, music, dance, opera, and arts associations. *Civic & Public Affairs:* 12%. Primarily for economic development. *Education:* 40%. Includes the highest grant ($1,684,050) for the Baltimore Curriculum Project supporting six Baltimore City elementary schools. *Environment:* 20%. Child welfare, pregnancy prevention programs, food banks, shelters, youth organizations, job training, and community services. *International:* 21%. Public health concerns. *Note:* Total contributions made in 1999. **Typ. Recipients:** Clinics/Medical Centers, Domestic Violence, Family Planning, Health Organizations, Medical Education, Mental Health, Nutrition, People with Disabilities, Substance Abuse. **Geo. Dist:** Baltimore, MD.

**★ 21 ★ Abell-Hanger Foundation**
PO Box 430
Midland, TX 79702
**Phone:** (915)684-6655 **Fax:** (915)684-4474
**Email:** ahf@abell-hanger.org
**Website:** http://www.abell-hanger.org
David Smith, Executive Director

**Fnded:** 1954. **Philosophy:** The foundation was created to carry on the philanthropic endeavors that Mr. Abell pursued during his professional and civic career. He once commented that "one likes to be successful, not just for the money, but because of what one can do for one's community, one's country, and for mankind. Business success provides the opportunity to do some of the things most of us dream about doing for our community and its various institutions, organizations, and agencies." Since its inception, the foundation has focused its funding on the arts, community and social services (especially for youth and the handicapped), health, social sciences, and higher education. **Priorities:** *Arts & Humanities:* 17%. Supports museums, libraries, and the Midland Odessa Symphony and Chorale. *Civic & Public Affairs:* 10%. Supports community development. *Education:* 38%. Supports schools, colleges and universities. *Environment:* 23%. Supports children's services, senior services, drug abuse centers, food banks and people with disabilities. *International:* 11%. Supports health sciences, hospitals, and disease and disorder centers and ambulance purchases. *Note:* Total contributions made in fiscal 2001. **Typ. Recipients:** AIDS/HIV, Alzheimers Disease, Cancer, Child Abuse, Children's Health/Hospitals, Domestic Violence, Emergency/Ambulance Services, Eyes/Blindness, Family Planning, Health Funds, Health Organizations, Hospices, Hospitals, Medical Education, Medical Education, Medical Rehabilitation, Medical Research, Medical Training, Multiple Sclerosis, Nursing Services, People with Disabilities, Public Health, Single-Disease Health Associations, Substance Abuse. **Geo. Dist:** TX.

**★ 22 ★ Abercrombie Foundation**
PO Box 68
Versailles, KY 40383
**Phone:** (502)873-4477
John Backer, Manager

**Fnded:** 1950. **Philosophy:** "The Board of Trustees of the Foundation has decided to give preference to grant requests from: institutions involved in the education of young people at the secondary and university levels, particularly private universities; organizations working to preserve our natural resources and beautify our environment in rural as well as urban areas; institutions and organizations that provide medical services, information and assistance to the community at large; institutions conducting medical research aimed at alleviating significant current health problems; institutions and organizations that aid children in physical or emotional distress; and institutions and organizations devoted to the education and prevention of substance abuse." **Priorities:** *Arts & Humanities:* 16%. Supports music conservancies. *Education:* 21%. Colleges, universities, and family literacy programs received funding. *Environment:* 17%. Animal welfare, family services, and elder care received grants. *International:* 46%. Supports geriatric health and cancer research. *Note:* Total contributions made in 1999. **Typ. Recipients:** Cancer, Children's Health/Hospitals, Clinics/Medical Centers, Diabetes, Domestic Violence, Family Planning, Geriatric Health, Medical Education, Medical Research, Mental Health, People with Disabilities, Prenatal Health Issues, Research/Studies Institutes, Speech & Hearing, Substance Abuse. **Geo. Dist:** KY.

**★ 23 ★ Abraham and Sonia Rochlin Foundation**
275 Hill St., Ste. 250
Reno, NV 89501
**Phone:** (775)329-1611 **Fax:** (775)329-1983
Heide Marie, President

**Fnded:** 1969. **Philosophy:** The foundation primarily supports civic affairs with Jewish interests. Israeli endowment funds account for most of the giving. Other interests include Jewish religious organizations and universities. **Priorities:** *Arts & Humanities:* 1%. Public broadcasting and an arts foundation. *Civic & Public Affairs:* 9%. Supports the Hebrew Immigrant Aid Society and other civic organizations. *Education:* 9%. Higher education. *International:* 16%. Medical research, cancer centers, geriatric health, and hospices. *Note:* Total contributions made in 1998. **Typ. Recipients:** Alzheimers Disease, Cancer, Clinics/Medical Centers, Hospices, Long-Term Care, Medical Research, Preventive Medicine/Wellness Organizations, Respiratory, Single-Disease Health Associations. **Geo. Dist:** internationally; CA; NV; NY.

**★ 24 ★ Achelis Foundation**
767 3rd Ave., 4th Floor
New York, NY 10017-2023
**Phone:** (212)644-0322 **Fax:** (212)759-6510
**Email:** main@achelis-bodman-fnds.org
**Website:** http://www.fdcenter.org/grantmaker/achelis-bodman
Joseph Dolan, Secretary & Executive Director

**Fnded:** 1940. **Philosophy:** The foundation was created to distribute funds for "charitable, benevolent, educational, and religious uses and purposes." It largely supports youth, social-service agencies, educational institutions (especially school-reform and school-choice programs), major cultural programs, health (including medical research and rehabilitation programs.) Other interests include volunteerism, entrepreneurship, strengthening the two-parent family, fatherhood (and father absence), job training and placement into private-sector jobs, and economic development. Special consideratin is given to leadership development, parental involvement, consumer choice, economic empowerment, independent quality research, prevention and early intervention, advancing the state of art, self-help and self-reliance, innovations and new cost-saving approaches and improving the quality of urban life. The foundation also focuses on returning fathers to their families. Obtaining measurable outcomes of clients and program results in health and social-service agencies is also a goal of the foundation. **Priorities:** *Arts & Humanities:* 9%. Supports museums, dance, and music. *Civic & Public Affairs:* 8%. Including entrepreneurship and job placement. *Education:* 24%. Primary support for education and school reform. *Environment:* 29%. Emphasis on fatherhood, families, restoring marriage, youth, volunteerism, community, and society. *International:* 18%. Supports biomedical research, hospitals, and medical rehabilitation. *Religion:* 5%. Funds Biomedical Research. *Note:* Total contributions made in 1999. **Typ. Recipients:** AIDS/HIV, Alzheimers Disease, Cancer, Children's Health/Hospitals, Clinics/Medical Centers, Domestic Violence, Emergency/Ambulance Services, Eyes/Blindness, Health Funds, Health Organizations, Health-General, Hospitals, Hospitals (University Affiliated), Medical Education, Medical Rehabilitation, Medical Research, Medical Training, Mental Health, Nursing Services, Outpatient Health Care, People with Disabilities, Public Health, Speech & Hearing, Substance Abuse, Transplant Networks/Donor Banks. **Geo. Dist:** New York, NY.

**★ 25 ★ Addison H. Gibson Foundation**
One PPG Place, Ste. 2230
Pittsburgh, PA 15222
**Phone:** (412)261-1611 **Fax:** (412)261-5733
**Email:** ldunbar@gibson-fnd.org
**Website:** http://www.gibson-fnd.org
Lynn Dunbar, Assistant Director

**Fnded:** 1936. **Philosophy:** The foundation's primary interests are health care and higher education. It continues the tradition established by its founder of providing direct assistance on behalf of self-supporting individuals in need of medical care for which they, and their families, cannot afford. The foundation also operates an education loan fund, providing funds at low interest to college and graduate students who have successfully completed one or more full years of their studies. **Priorities:** *Education:* 59%. Supports educational loans. *International:* 41%. Makes grants to medical providers on behalf of individuals who have correctable medical conditions. **Typ. Recipients:** Children's Health/Hospitals, Clinics/Medical Centers, Eyes/Blindness, Health Funds, Health Organizations, Hospitals, Medical Education, Medical Rehabilitation, Medical Research, People with Disabilities, Public Health. **Geo. Dist:** only western Pennsylvania.

**★ 26 ★ Adolph Coors Foundation**
4100 East Mississippi Ave., Ste. 1850
Denver, CO 80246
**Phone:** (303)388-1636 **Fax:** (303)388-1684
**Email:** generalinfo@adolphcoorsfdn.org
Salley Rippey, Executive Director

**Fnded:** 1975. **Philosophy:** The foundation traditionally has funded a variety of organizations. In the area of health, emphasis has been on programs that are preventive in nature and that can demonstrate a reduction in health-care costs. Educational grants usually are directed to private independent four-year colleges and universities that do not receive a significant amount of tax-derived funding. Preservation of historic sites and buildings is funded when there is evidence that a facility will be used by a variety of organizations. Limited grants are made to cultural organizations for capital or special projects. Human service funding targets organizations that help people become self-sufficient and realize their potential. Distribution of the funds from Adolph Coors, Jr.'s, bequest are confined to Colorado. Limited foundation grants for activities outside Colorado were made possible in 1977 with a bequest from the estate of Gertrude Steele Coors. Most of the foundation's activities outside Colorado are directed to institutions and programs that endeavor to preserve and promote traditional values and the principles of a free-market economy. The foundation does not act on behalf of the Adolph Coors Company; nor does it engage in activities for the benefit of the company, its employees, or its distributors. **Priorities:** *Arts & Humanities:* 9%. Funds orchestra and music associations. *Civic & Public Affairs:* 10%. Includes grants to cultural institutions. *Education:* About 30%. Primarily precollege and higher education. *Environment:* 37%. Supports youth activities, community and human services. *International:* 12%. *Note:* Total contributions made in fiscal 1999. **Typ. Recipients:** AIDS/HIV, Children's Health/Hospitals, Clinics/Medical Centers, Domestic Violence, Emergency/Ambulance Services, Health Organizations, Hospitals, Medical Rehabilitation, Medical Research, Mental Health, Mental Health, Nursing Services, People with Disabilities, Preventive Medicine/Wellness Organizations, Public Health, Sexual Abuse, Single-Disease Health Associations, Substance Abuse. **Geo. Dist:** CO.

### ★ 27 ★ Adrian and Jessie Archbold Charitable Trust

401 East 60th St., Ste. 36B
New York, NY 10022
**Phone:** (212)371-1152 **Fax:** (212)753-9327
Myra Mahon, Director

**Fnded:** 1976. **Philosophy:** The trust makes most of its grants in the areas of education, health, and civic affairs. Educational funding favors religious education, colleges and universities, private academies, and law. Health support includes single disease associations, medical centers, health foundations, and hospitals. In civic affairs, interests include foundations and fellowship centers. Other recipient areas also are supported. **Priorities:** *Arts & Humanities:* 8%. Gives to museums and performing arts. *Civic & Public Affairs:* 14%. Suppports public policy and botanical gardens. *Education:* 31%. Gives to higher and precollege education. *Environment:* 4%. Primarily drug abuse programs and united funds. *International:* 23%. Funds hospitals, medical centers, and single-disease health associations. *Note:* Total contributions made in 1998. **Typ. Recipients:** AIDS/HIV, Cancer, Children's Health/Hospitals, Clinics/Medical Centers, Emergency/Ambulance Services, Family Planning, Health Funds, Health Organizations, Health-General, Hospitals, Hospitals (University Affiliated), Medical Education, Medical Rehabilitation, Medical Research, Mental Health, People with Disabilities, Prenatal Health Issues, Public Health, Single-Disease Health Associations, Substance Abuse. **Geo. Dist:** NY, eastern United States.

### ★ 28 ★ Agnes M. Lindsay Trust

660 Chestnut St.
Manchester, NH 03104
**Phone:** (603)669-1366 **Fax:** (603)665-8114
**Email:** admin@lindsaytrust.org
**Website:** http://www.lindsaytrust.org
Susan Bouchard, Administrative Director

**Fnded:** 1939. **Philosophy:** The Agnes M. Lindsay Trust supports colleges, universities, and private secondary schools through scholarship funds. It makes grants for capital needs to certain elementary and secondary schools, especially those schools that serve a special need (for example, to blind, deaf, or learning disabled children). In addition, the foundation supports a number of social welfare organizations, many of which work with special needs populations, health projects, children's hospitals, homes, and youth organizations. **Priorities:** *Arts & Humanities:* 7%. Supports cultural art. *Civic & Public Affairs:* 1%. Supports community affairs. *Education:* 33%. Supports colleges, universities, other educational insitutions, and programs. *Environment:* 44%. Supports YMCA, youth services, and family services. *International:* 15%. Supports hospitals and visiting nurses. *Note:* Contributions were made in 1999. **Typ. Recipients:** AIDS/HIV, Cancer, Children's Health/Hospitals, Clinics/Medical Centers, Domestic Violence, Eyes/Blindness, Geriatric Health, Health Organizations, Heart, Hospices, Hospitals, Long-Term Care, Medical Education, Medical Rehabilitation, Mental Health, Nursing Services, Outpatient Health Care, People with Disabilities, Prenatal Health Issues, Substance Abuse. **Geo. Dist:** ME; MA; NH; VT.

### ★ 29 ★ Ahmanson Foundation

9215 Wilshire Boulevard
Beverly Hills, CA 90210
**Phone:** (310)278-0770
**Website:** http://www.cerritos.edu/cerritos/development/funders_ahmanson.html
Lee Walcott, Jr., Vice President & Managing Director

**Fnded:** 1952. **Philosophy:** "The Foundation concentrates its funding on cultural projects supporting the arts, education at the collegiate and precollegiate levels, medicine and delivery of health care services, specialized library collections, programs related to homelessness and low-income populations, preservation of the environment, and a wide range of human service projects. The vast majority of the Foundation's philanthropy is directed toward organizations and institutions based in and serving the greater Los Angeles community. "Simultaneously, the Foundation is particularly committed to the support of non-profit organizations and institutions which continually demonstrate sound fiscal management, responsibility to efficient operation, and program integrity. "Through such focused interests and a shared vision with the non-profit sector the Foundation endeavors to increase the quality of life in Southern California and to enhance its cultural legacy." **Priorities:** *Arts & Humanities:* 29%. Museums, media, and libraries. *Civic & Public Affairs:* 1%. Supports universities and secondary schools; also religious and humanities education. *Environment:* 3%. Youth and community projects. *International:* 23%. Medical research and hospital equipment, hospitals and clinics. *Religion:* 1%. *Note:* Total contributions made in fiscal 1998. **Typ. Recipients:** Adolescent Health Issues, AIDS/HIV, Alzheimers Disease, Cancer, Children's Health/Hospitals, Clinics/Medical Centers, Domestic Violence, Emergency/Ambulance Services, Eyes/Blindness, Family Planning, Health Organizations, Heart, Hospitals, Long-Term Care, Medical Education, Medical Research, Mental Health, Multiple Sclerosis, Nursing Services, Outpatient Health Care, People with Disabilities, Prenatal Health Issues, Public Health, Research/Studies Institutes, Single-Disease Health Associations, Speech & Hearing, Substance Abuse, Trauma Treatment.

### ★ 30 ★ Alavi Foundation

500 Fifth Ave., 39th Floor
New York, NY 10110
**Phone:** (212)944-8333 **Fax:** (212)921-0325
Dr. Mohammad Geramian, President

**Fnded:** 1973. **Philosophy:** The foundation makes most of its grants in the areas of education, religion, and international organizations. Educational funding favors Muslim and Islamic education, universities, and private schools. Other support goes to major American universities. Religious interests include mosques, temples, and religious centers. **Priorities:** *Arts & Humanities:* Less than 1%. *Civic & Public Affairs:* 2%. Supports ethnic organizations. *Education:* 49%. Supports Islamic education, language schools, and colleges and universities. *Environment:* Less than 1%. *International:* Less than 1%. *Note:* Total contributions were made in fiscal 2000. **Typ. Recipients:** Arthritis, Cancer, Children's Health/Hospitals, Eyes/Blindness, Health Organizations, Heart, Hospitals, Medical Education, Multiple Sclerosis, People with Disabilities, Single-Disease Health Associations, Transplant Networks/Donor Banks. **Geo. Dist:** internationally; nationally.

### ★ 31 ★ Albert and Ethel Herzstein Charitable Foundation

6131 Westview
Houston, TX 77055
**Phone:** (713)681-7868 **Fax:** (713)681-3652
**Email:** albertandethel@herzsteinfoundation.org
**Website:** http://www.herzsteinfoundation.org
L. Hajtman, President

**Fnded:** 1965. **Philosophy:** The foundation gives to a variety of organizations in several fields, but the majority of its donations support education, civic and community, human services and health. **Priorities:** *Arts & Humanities:* 9%. Supports theater, ballet, public broadcasting, and historic preservation. *Civic & Public Affairs:* 1%. Gives to community foundations. *Education:* 9%. Supports colleges and universities, junior achievement, and academies. *Environment:* 28%. Supports family and youth services. *International:* 3%. Supports medical centers. *Religion:* 17%. Funds the Houston Museum of Natural Science. *Note:* Total contributions made in 2000. **Typ. Recipients:** Adolescent Health Issues, AIDS/HIV, Alzheimers Disease, Cancer, Children's Health/Hospitals, Clinics/Medical Centers, Diabetes, Emergency/Ambulance Services, Eyes/Blindness, Health Organizations, Health-General, Heart, Hospitals, Medical Education, Medical Research, Mental Health, Multiple Sclerosis, People with Disabilities, Prenatal Health Issues, Respiratory, Single-Disease Health Associations, Substance Abuse. **Geo. Dist:** Houston, TX.

### ★ 32 ★ Albert Pick, Jr. Fund

30 North Michigan Ave.
Chicago, IL 60602
**Phone:** (312)236-1192
**Email:** info@albertpickjrfund.org
**Website:** http://www.albertpickjrfund.org
Cleopatra Alexander, Executive Director

**Fnded:** 1947. **Philosophy:** The Albert Pick, Jr. Fund makes grants across the major categories of support. In health and human services interests include programs in wellness, community-based health-care delivery, youth, family planning, or geriatric services. Also included are mental health, physical rehabilitation, and crisis care services. Funding for the arts goes to a wide spectrum of organizations, including public broadcasting, festivals, museums, and the performing arts. Educational support includes early childhood education and at-risk intervention, universities, and post-secondary institutions. Civic and community funding supports neighborhood development, environmental affairs, human relations, and minority rights. **Priorities:** *Arts & Humanities:* 5%. Museums, arts festivals, opera, theatre, and performing arts. *Civic & Public Affairs:* 32%. Public interest, housing, zoos, and foundations. *Education:* 28%. Educational programs, learning centers, literacy, career training, and schools. *Environment:* 17%. Youth and family concerns, YMCA/YWCA, shelters and senior services. *International:* 8%. Health centers, hospitals and hospice. *Note:* Total contributions made in 1998. **Typ. Recipients:** AIDS/HIV, Children's Health/Hospitals, Clinics/Medical Centers, Domestic Violence, Emergency/Ambulance Services, Family Planning, Health Organizations, Hospices, Hospitals, Long-Term Care, Medical Training, People with Disabilities, Prenatal Health Issues, Preventive Medicine/Wellness Organizations, Public Health, Sexual Abuse, Single-Disease Health Associations, Substance Abuse. **Geo. Dist:** Chicago, IL.

### ★ 33 ★ Alex Hillman Family Foundation

630 Fifth Ave.
New York, NY 10111
**Phone:** (212)265-3115 **Fax:** (212)765-3134
Rita Hillman, President

**Fnded:** 1966. **Philosophy:** The Alex Hillman Family Foundation makes most of its grants in the areas of arts and education. The foundation's major priority is funding the arts. Interests include museums, music acadamies, film, and public broadcasting. Educational funding supports nursing schools. **Priorities:** *Arts & Humanities:* 18%. Supports music, museum of art, public broadcasting and film and video. *Civic & Public Affairs:* Less than 1%. *Education:* 67%. Supports medical education, and universities. *International:* 12%. Supports hospital, health organizations, and cancer research. *Note:* Total contributions made in 1998. **Typ. Recipients:** Emergency/Ambulance Services, Heart, Hospices, Hospitals, Medical Education, Nursing Services, People with Disabilities. **Geo. Dist:** New York, NY, metropolitan area.

### ★ 34 ★ Alex and Marie Manoogian Foundation

21001 Van Born Rd.
Taylor, MI 48180
**Phone:** (248)649-3400
Gene Gargaro, Vice President & Secretary

**Fnded:** 1942. **Philosophy:** The foundation is very active in the affairs of the Armenian community in the United States. Grants generally are made to Armenian social service organizations and Armenian religious and educational institutions. Funding also is directed to other institutions and organizations in higher and private secondary education, as well as arts organizations. **Priorities:** *Arts & Humanities:* Less then 1%. Supports cultural association. *Civic & Public Affairs:* 5%. Funds ethnic groups. *Education:* Less than 1%. Funds colleges and universities. *International:* 21%. Funds a health center. *Note:* Total contributions made in 1999. **Typ. Recipients:** Cancer, Hospitals, Medical Education, People with Disabilities, Public Health, Substance Abuse. **Geo. Dist:** nationally.

## ★ 35 ★ Alfred I. duPont Foundation

1650 Prudential Dr., Ste. 302
Jacksonville, FL 32207
**Phone:** (904)858-3123
Rosemary Wills, Assistant Secretary & Assistant
    Treasure

**Fnded:** 1936. **Philosophy:** The Alfred I. duPont
Foundation makes most of its grants in the areas of
education, social services, and the arts. Educational
funding favors medical and religious education and
college funds. Social service funding favors homes,
while the support for the arts focuses on galleries and
preservation societies. The foundation will also support health services, civic affairs, and churches. **Priorities:** *Arts & Humanities:* 3%. Supports museums,
historical preservation, and music. *Civic & Public
Affairs:* 14%. Supports law and justice, gardens, and
parks. *Education:* 35%. Supports education funds and
associations, and colleges and universities. *Environment:* 4%. Supports homes, services for the elderly,
and scouting. *International:* 10%. Supports medical
research. *Religion:* 1%. Supports science institute.
*Note:* Total contributions made in 1998. **Typ. Recipients:** Alzheimers Disease, Arthritis, Children's Health/
Hospitals, Clinics/Medical Centers, Emergency/Ambu-
lance Services, Health Organizations, Hospices, Hospices, Long-Term Care, Medical Education, Multiple
Sclerosis, Nursing Services, People with Disabilities,
Public Health, Single-Disease Health Associations.
**Geo. Dist:** southeastern United States; FL.

## ★ 36 ★ Alfred Jurzykowski Foundation

21 East 40th St.
New York, NY 10016
**Phone:** (212)689-2460
Bluma Cohen, Executive Director & Vice President

**Fnded:** 1960. **Philosophy:** The foundation supports
projects and programs in Poland and Brazil. Many
types of U.S. tax-exempt organizations receive support. Interests include the disabled, child welfare,
community service organizations, and family planning.
**Priorities:** *Arts & Humanities:* 8%. Supports public
libraries, theater, art museum, and orchestra society.
*Civic & Public Affairs:* 9%. Support given to civic and
public policy organizations. *Education:* 17%. Funds
educational programs with an international focus.
*Environment:* 10%. Funds youth programs, the homeless, Big Brothers and Big Sisters, and food for the
poor. *Note:* Total contributions made in 1999. **Typ.
Recipients:** AIDS/HIV, Cancer, Children's Health/
Hospitals, Clinics/Medical Centers, Family Planning,
Health Organizations, Home-Care Services, Hospices,
Hospitals, Medical Education, People with Disabilities.
**Geo. Dist:** New York, NY, metropolitan area.

## ★ 37 ★ Alfred P. Sloan Foundation

630 Fifth Ave., Ste. 2550
New York, NY 10111
**Phone:** (212)649-1649          **Fax:** (212)757-5117
**Email:** gassman@sloan.org
**Website:** http://www.sloan.org
Ralph Gomory, President

**Fnded:** 1934. **Philosophy:** The foundation's main
interests and programs are concentrated primarily in
five categories: science and technology, including the
areas of fellowships, direct support of research, and
the history of science and technology; standard of
living and economic performance, including the areas
of industries, nonprofit sectors, the university as a
system and the system of universities, assessment of
government performance, and the family and the
workplace; education and careers in science and
technology, including the areas of careers, the scientific and technical work force, immigration of scientists
and engineers, learning outside the classroom, public
understanding of science and technology, underrepresented minorities, women, and retention; selected
national issues; and civic projects. Recipients are
principally universities, public policy organizations, and
economic associations. Science and Technology are
major interests of the foundation. Programs include
fellowships, direct support of research, and the history
of science and technology. Sloan Research Fellowships are granted in the areas of economics, chemistry, mathematics, neuroscience, computer science,
and physics. The fellowships are made to stimulate
fundamental research by young scholars of outstanding promise at a time in their careers when other
support may be difficult to secure. Candidates are
nominated by department chairmen or other senior
scientists familiar with their work. Another program
area is Education and Careers in Science and Technology. Programs in this area strengthen science and
engineering education and increase interest in these
fields. Issues of main concern include career choice,
developing student interests, learning outside the
classroom, and increasing public understanding. The
foundation also funds programs that involve selected
national issues. It attempts to contribute to other major
national issues including drug abuse, energy and the
environment, and traditional civic programs that benefit the city of New York. **Priorities:** *Arts & Humanities:*
11%. Funding awarded to film institutes and communications projects. *Civic & Public Affairs:* 14%. Supports
standard of living and economic performance, selected national issues, and civic projects. *Education:* 47%.
Supports grants focused on careers in science and
technology. *Environment:* 5%. Supports research on
the effects of women working in families. *International:*
2%. Supports AIDS awareness and research. *Religion:*
20%. Primarily fellowships for research and doctoral
dissertations. *Note:* Total contributions made in 1998.
**Typ. Recipients:** AIDS/HIV, Domestic Violence,
Health Policy/Cost Containment, Medical Education,
Medical Research, Public Health, Research/Studies
Institutes, Substance Abuse. **Geo. Dist:** nationally.

## ★ 38 ★ Alsam Foundation

PO Box 1760
Eagle, ID 83616
**Phone:** (208)854-0414
George Moosman, President

**Fnded:** 1984. **Philosophy:** The foundation typically
funds scholarship programs, religious concerns, arts
organizations, health causes, and civic and community
affairs projects. **Priorities:** *Arts & Humanities:* 2%.
Libraries, performing arts, and public broadcasting.
*Education:* 93%. Scholarships, colleges and universities, and medical education. *Environment:* 3%. Youth
organizations, animal protection, and child welfare.
*Note:* Total contributions made in fiscal 1999. **Typ.
Recipients:** Arthritis, Cancer, Medical Education,
Medical Research, Research/Studies Institutes, Single-Disease Health Associations. **Geo. Dist:** CO; UT.

## ★ 39 ★ Altman Foundation

521 Fifth Ave., 35th Fl.
New York, NY 10175-3599
**Phone:** (212)682-0970
Karen Rosa, Vice President & Executive Director

**Fnded:** 1913. **Philosophy:** "In carrying out its mission, the Altman Foundation seeks to strengthen
communities and enhance the well-being of all New
Yorkers. The Foundation's grants support programs
and institutions that enrich the quality of life within the
five boroughs of New York City, with a particular
interest in initiatives that help individuals, families and
communities benefit from the services and opportunities that will enable them to achieve their full potential." 1997 Guidelines Brochure **Priorities:** *Arts &
Humanities:* 14%. Programs that extend the benefit of
the arts through established and meaningful organizations and institutions, including programs identifying
and providing pre-professional-level training to youngsters in specific art disciplines. *Civic & Public Affairs:*
6%. Funds botanical gardens and community foundations. *Education:* 23%. Independent and non-public
primary and secondary schools, colleges and universities with interest in scholarships and access programs
for promising disadvantaged students. *Environment:*
20%. Social Welfare programs developing long-term
solutions that strengthen communities. *International:*
21%. Voluntary hospitals, health centers and programs in the health field that focus on improving
access to services and providing assistance to those
in need of special care. *Religion:* 3%. Supports
computer and math programs. *Note:* Total contributions were made in 1998. **Typ. Recipients:** AIDS/HIV,
Cancer, Child Abuse, Children's Health/Hospitals,
Clinics/Medical Centers, Domestic Violence, Eyes/
Blindness, Geriatric Health, Health Funds, Health
Organizations, Health Policy/Cost Containment,
Home-Care Services, Hospitals, Medical Education,
Outpatient Health Care, People with Disabilities, Pre-
natal Health Issues, Preventive Medicine/Wellness
Organizations, Public Health. **Geo. Dist:** NY, focusing
on the five boroughs of New York City.

## Amateur Athletic Foundation of Los Angeles

*See:* Entry 5544

## ★ 40 ★ Ambrose Monell Foundation

1 Rockefeller Plaza, Ste. 301
New York, NY 10020
**Phone:** (212)586-0700          **Fax:** (212)245-1863
**Email:** info@aafla.org
**Website:** http://www.monellzetlesen.org
George Rowe, Jr., President

**Fnded:** 1952. **Philosophy:** The foundation was set up
to help improve "the physical, mental, and moral
condition of humanity throughout the world." It pursues
this goal by supporting health, the arts, education,
social services, science, and civic causes. **Priorities:**
*Arts & Humanities:* 21%. Supports public broadcasting, opera, ballet, libraries, symphonies, and museums. *Civic & Public Affairs:* 5%. Public policy groups, a
botanical garden, and legal aid causes. *Education:*
12%. Focus on higher education. *Environment:* 4%.
*International:* About 18%. Includes the highest grant to
the Monell Ohem Senior Center in Philadelphia, PA.
Also supports hospitals, medical research, and single-
disease health associations. *Religion:* 38%. Supports
an earth observatory and research. *Note:* Total contri-
butions made in 1998. **Typ. Recipients:** AIDS/HIV,
Alzheimers Disease, Arthritis, Cancer, Clinics/Medical
Centers, Emergency/Ambulance Services, Eyes/
Blindness, Geriatric Health, Health-General, Hospitals,
Hospitals (University Affiliated), Medical Education,
Medical Rehabilitation, Medical Research, Mental
Health, Public Health, Research/Studies Institutes,
Respiratory, Speech & Hearing. **Geo. Dist:** nationally;
New York, NY, metropolitan area.

## ★ 41 ★ Amelia Peabody Foundation

One Hollis St.
Wellesley, MA 02482
**Phone:** (781)237-6468          **Fax:** (781)237-5014
**Website:** http://www.ameliapeabody.org
Margaret St. Clair, Co-Managing Trustee

**Fnded:** 1985. **Philosophy:** The foundation funds only
charitable organizations in Massachusetts. The foundation's focus is on inner-city disadvantaged youth.
One of the foundation's priorities is urban youth
services with strong leadership, which lives and works
in the community they serve. **Priorities:** *Arts &
Humanities:* 1%. Supports a museum and a theater.
*Civic & Public Affairs:* 4%. Supports public policy,
community foundations, towns and municipalities, and
housing. *Education:* 42%. Supports arts/humanities
education, legal education, schools, and universities.
*Environment:* 31%. Supports Young Men's Christian
AssociationA, youth programs, recreation/athletics,
and emergency relief. *International:* 21%. Funds public
health and medical centers. *Note:* Total contributions
made in 1999. **Typ. Recipients:** Clinics/Medical Centers, Diabetes, Emergency/Ambulance Services,
Health Organizations, Hospitals, Medical Education,
Medical Research, People with Disabilities, Public
Health, Single-Disease Health Associations, Substance Abuse. **Geo. Dist:** MA.

## ★ 42 ★ Amon G. Carter Foundation

201 Main St., Ste. 1945
Fort Worth, TX 76102
**Phone:** (817)332-2783          **Fax:** (817)332-2787
**Email:** jrobinson@agcf.org
**Website:** http://www.agcs.org
John Robinson, Grant Administrator-Executive Vice
Presi

**Fnded:** 1945. **Philosophy:** The foundation supports
visual and performing arts, education, health, and

social services in Fort Worth and Tarrant County, Texas. Current board policy allocates half of annual grant funds to the Amon Carter Museum for general support and acquisitions. Remaining funds are used for the general grant program. Support for education includes primary and secondary education, both public and private. Grants are also made to colleges and universities located in Texas. Contributions in the health field are made to hospitals and to local and national single-disease health organizations. Social service grants emphasize programs that benefit youth, the aged, and the disabled. Recipients include a variety of youth organizations, recreation facilities, homes, and shelters. The foundation provides limited support to civic groups, including police and fire fighter associations, several Fort Worth parks and gardens, and the city zoo. **Priorities:** *Arts & Humanities:* 61%. Supports museum, dance and art gallery. *Civic & Public Affairs:* 5%. Supports public libraries, crime prevention. *Education:* 22%. Supports pubic schools, private schools, religious education, colleges and universities. *Environment:* 10%. Supports Boys & Girls clubs, homeless, family services and the hungry. *International:* 2%. Supports medical research centers and health associations. *Note:* Total contributions made in 1998. **Typ. Recipients:** AIDS/HIV, Alzheimers Disease, Cancer, Children's Health/Hospitals, Clinics/Medical Centers, Diabetes, Emergency/Ambulance Services, Family Planning, Health Organizations, Health Policy/Cost Containment, Hospices, Hospitals, Hospitals (University Affiliated), Medical Education, Medical Rehabilitation, Medical Research, Mental Health, Nursing Services, People with Disabilities, Prenatal Health Issues, Public Health, Research/Studies Institutes, Respiratory, Single-Disease Health Associations, Substance Abuse, Transplant Networks/Donor Banks. **Geo. Dist:** Fort Worth, TX, including Tarrant County.

## ★ 43 ★ Andersen Foundation

100 4th Ave., North
Bayport, MN 55003-1096
**Phone:** (651)642-0127          **Fax:** (651)430-5537
Mary Gillstrom, Assistant Secretary

**Fnded:** 1959. **Philosophy:** The foundation traditionally contributes a significant portion of its funding to education, with emphasis on assisting private colleges who do not accept state and federal funds and local medical projects. **Priorities:** *Arts & Humanities:* 2%. Supports historical preservation and museums. *Education:* 65%. Supports private colleges and universities. *Environment:* 12%. Supports scouts and youth and family services. *International:* 13%. Supports hospitals and medical centers. *Religion:* 3%. Supports a science museum. *Note:* Total contributions made in 1998. **Typ. Recipients:** Cancer, Children's Health/Hospitals, Clinics/Medical Centers, Domestic Violence, Emergency/Ambulance Services, Eyes/Blindness, Health Funds, Health Organizations, Heart, Hospices, Hospitals, Kidney, Medical Research, Mental Health, People with Disabilities, Research/Studies Institutes, Single-Disease Health Associations, Substance Abuse. **Geo. Dist:** nationally; MN.

## ★ 44 ★ Andrew W. Mellon Foundation

140 East 62nd St.
New York, NY 10021
**Phone:** (212)838-8400          **Fax:** (212)223-2778
**Website:** http://www.mellon.org.
Michele Warman, General Counsel, Secretary

**Fnded:** 1969. **Philosophy:** The purpose of the foundation is to "aid and promote such religious, charitable, scientific, literary, and educational purposes as may be in the furtherance of the public welfare or tend to promote the well-doing or well-being of mankind." The foundation currently makes grants on a selective basis in the areas of higher education; culture and the performing arts; population; conservation and the environment; and certain areas of public affairs. It has eliminated its support of public health care. The foundation's overriding interest continues to be in education and is strongly focused on higher education. It includes support for libraries, research institutes, and publishing endeavors that are a part of higher education. Grants to universities stress faculty development

in several ways. The foundation makes grants to encourage outstanding minority students to pursue doctoral degrees in humanities. In addition, the foundation funds other new approaches to graduate education in the arts and sciences. Another aspect of the foundation's interest in higher education is its support for comparative studies of foreign cultures and foreign languages programs. The foundation also supports a variety of programs related directly or indirectly to educational opportunities for minority students and faculty members. These include grants to private black colleges to encourage faculty and curriculum development and to build library collections. The foundation makes a very limited number of educational grants to foreign institutions. In the field of conservation and the environment, the foundation supports research on issues relating to energy, natural resources including ground water and the oceans, global systems, and toxic waste. The foundation "looks for ways to fill gaps in the understanding of basic processes, to encourage good ideas, to provide bridging funds for good programs with temporary financial problems, and to encourage new lines of research." Institution-building and the training of young scientists are priorities. The foundation has a continuing interest in the field of population. It supports organizations that conduct research or provide technical assistance to family-planning programs. It also funds research on contraceptives. however, envision some changes. It would like to see more emphasis placed on the value of research as a guide to grant making. The foundation expects to continue funding for library automation projects, especially through consortia of libraries, publishers, and others concerned with scholarly communication. **Priorities:** *Arts & Humanities:* 22%. Museums, art conservation, the performing arts, libraries, dance, and arts festivals. *Civic & Public Affairs:* 8%. Population issues, public affairs, and botanical garden. *Education:* 49%. Primarily supports higher education programs and scholarships. *International:* 1%. *Religion:* 1%. Supports scientific organizations and general science. *Note:* Total contributions made in 1998. **Typ. Recipients:** Family Planning, Medical Education, Medical Research, Public Health. **Geo. Dist:** nationally.

## ★ 45 ★ Annenberg Foundation

St. Davids Center, Ste. A-200
150 Radnor-Chester Rd.
Saint Davids, PA 19087
**Phone:** (610)341-9066          **Fax:** (610)964-8688
**Website:** http://www.whannenberg.org/
Dr. Gail Levin, Executive Director

**Fnded:** 1989. **Philosophy:** The Annenberg Foundation believes that there is nothing more important than the quality of K-12 education in determining how productive and fulfilling the future will be for America's young people and for society as a whole. Through the Annenberg Challenge grant–its $500 million program in support of systemic public school reform–the foundation and its partner organizations and school districts work to promote school reform nationwide. The Challenge provides 18 matching grants for urban, rural, and arts-centered school reform programs, which are tailored to the needs of individual schools. Serving more than 1.3 million students in largely disadvantaged schools, the Challenge is the largest public/private partnership for school reform in the history of American public education. The Annenberg Foundation's investment in the Challenge program, which was first announced in December 1993, will conclude in 2002. (Additional details about the Challenge sites may be found on the Foundation's web page.) In addition to the Challenge, The Annenberg Foundation still focuses on primary and secondary education, but also has interests in the areas of arts and culture, health care, civic causes, and international institutions. **Priorities:** *Arts & Humanities:* 11%. Museums, historical preservation, and public broadcasting. *Education:* 84%. K-12 education, including curriculum improvement, professional development, and art education. Counseling and mentoring and parent education and involvement are also priorities. *Environment:* 1%. *International:* 2%. *Note:* Total contributions made in fiscal 2000. **Typ. Recipients:** Cancer, Children's Health/Hospitals, Clinics/Medical Centers,

Emergency/Ambulance Services, Family Planning, Health Funds, Health Organizations, Hospitals, Medical Education, Medical Research, Mental Health, Nursing Services, People with Disabilities, Preventive Medicine/Wellness Organizations, Research/Studies Institutes, Substance Abuse. **Geo. Dist:** primarily to national organizations.

## ★ 46 ★ Anschutz Family Foundation

555 17th St., Ste. 2400
Denver, CO 80202
**Phone:** (303)293-2338          **Fax:** (303)299-1235
**Website:** http://www.anschutzfamilyfoundation.org
Sue Anschutz-Rodgers, President & Executive Director

**Fnded:** 1982. **Philosophy:** "The mission of the Anschutz Family Foundation is to support efforts to assist the elderly, the young and the economically disadvantaged with special interest in self-sufficiency and community development in Colorado. The Foundation encourages endeavors which strengthen families and advances individuals to become productive and responsible citizens of society. The goal of the Anschutz Family Foundation is to assist people to help themselves while preserving their self respect." **Priorities:** *Arts & Humanities:* 7%. *Civic & Public Affairs:* 25%. (Civic & Cultural). Supports cultural centers and theaters. *Education:* 2%. Supports educational foundations, literacy, public and charter schools, and colleges. *Environment:* 63%. (Community/Human Services). Funds youth organizations, senior services, homeless shelters, community foundations, nonprofit management, family services, crime prevention, volunteer services, women's issues, and emergency services. *International:* 2%. Funds health associations, clinics and health centers, hospice, services for the disabled, and rehabilitation. *Note:* Total contributions made in fiscal 2000. **Typ. Recipients:** AIDS/HIV, Alzheimers Disease, Cancer, Children's Health/Hospitals, Clinics/Medical Centers, Domestic Violence, Emergency/Ambulance Services, Family Planning, Geriatric Health, Health Organizations, Heart, Home-Care Services, Hospices, Hospitals, Medical Rehabilitation, Medical Research, Mental Health, Multiple Sclerosis, Nursing Services, People with Disabilities, Preventive Medicine/Wellness Organizations, Public Health, Research/Studies Institutes, Single-Disease Health Associations, Substance Abuse, Trauma Treatment. **Geo. Dist:** CO.

## ★ 47 ★ Applebaum Foundation

441 West End Ave.
New York, NY 10024
**Phone:** (212)595-3839          **Fax:** (212)595-3814
Warren Weiss, Vice President

**Fnded:** 1949. **Philosophy:** The Applebaum Foundation makes most of its grants in the areas of education and religion. Educational funding favors specific departments at the University of Miami and educational institutions with Jewish curriculums. Religious funding favors Jewish organizations for Israeli relief and synagogues. The foundation also supports health services and some civic affairs. **Priorities:** *Arts & Humanities:* 1%. *Civic & Public Affairs:* 1%. *Education:* 56%. Primary support for the University of Miami and Jewish education. *Environment:* 8%. Gives to the United Way and to organizations dealing with the disabled. *International:* 12%. Emphasis on a university hospital; also supports research. *Note:* Total contributions made in fiscal 1999. **Typ. Recipients:** Cancer, Children's Health/Hospitals, Geriatric Health, Health Funds, Health Organizations, Health-General, Heart, Hospitals, Kidney, Medical Education, Medical Research, People with Disabilities, Public Health, Respiratory, Single-Disease Health Associations, Transplant Networks/Donor Banks. **Geo. Dist:** nationally; FL; NY.

## ★ 48 ★ Arcadia Foundation

105 East Logan St.
Norristown, PA 19401-3060
**Phone:** (610)275-8460          **Fax:** (610)275-8460
Marilyn Steinbright, President

**Fnded:** 1964. **Philosophy:** The foundation generally supports art, civic, human service, health, and educational organizations working to improve the quality of life in Pennsylvania. **Priorities:** *Arts & Humanities:* 67%. Supports theater, public broadcasting, and music. *Civic & Public Affairs:* 14%. Urban affairs, organizations, and housing. *Environment:* 6%. Focus on community service organizations in eastern Pennsylvania. *International:* 5%. Supports hospitals, health associations, and pediatric health. *Note:* Total contributions made in fiscal 2000. **Typ. Recipients:** Arthritis, Children's Health/Hospitals, Clinics/Medical Centers, Diabetes, Emergency/Ambulance Services, Health Organizations, Hospices, Hospitals, Hospitals (University Affiliated), Long-Term Care, Medical Education, Mental Health, Nursing Services, People with Disabilities, Single-Disease Health Associations. **Geo. Dist:** PA, zip codes 18000 to 19800.

## ★ 49 ★ Arcana Foundation

1401 I St. Northwest, Ste. 530
Washington, DC 20005
**Phone:** (202)789-7280  **Fax:** (202)842-2297
Joan Kennan, Executive Director

**Fnded:** 1986. **Philosophy:** The foundation supports programs in Washington, DC, that work to alleviate poverty and enhance cultural activities. It also makes grants to organizations that Mr. and Mrs. von Hoffman have been actively involved with in the past. **Priorities:** *Arts & Humanities:* 31%. Supports libraries, art museums, music, and public broadcasting. *Civic & Public Affairs:* 9%. Support for community services and housing and employment programs. *Education:* 12%. Supports secondary education. *Environment:* 32%. Funding for the aged, child welfare, substance abuse rehabilitation, and the homeless. *Note:* Total contributions made in fiscal 1999. **Typ. Recipients:** Children's Health/Hospitals, Clinics/Medical Centers, Diabetes, Domestic Violence, Family Planning, Geriatric Health, Health Organizations, Hospices, Long-Term Care, Medical Research, Mental Health, People with Disabilities, Prenatal Health Issues, Public Health, Substance Abuse. **Geo. Dist:** DC.

## ★ 50 ★ Arie and Ida Crown Memorial

222 North LaSalle St., Ste. 2000
Chicago, IL 60601
**Phone:** (312)236-6300  **Fax:** (312)984-1499
**Email:** aicm@crown-chicago.com
Susan Crown, President

**Fnded:** 1947. **Philosophy:** "The Arie and Ida Crown Memorial (AICM) supports projects that offer opportunities to the disadvantaged, strengthen the bond of families and improve the quality of people's lives. As a general rule, the Foundation funds programs that serve members of the Jewish community and residents of Chicago (Cook County)." "In the tradition of its founders, a core purpose of AICM is to bolster the Jewish community. Special emphasis is placed on programs offering assistance to the disenfranchised, promoting Jewish education, fortifying the family unit, strengthening Jewish culture and tradition, assisting in the resettlement efforts and promoting Jewish identity." 1996 Guidelines. **Priorities:** *Arts & Humanities:* 8%. Funds music, opera, arts institutes, museums, and public broadcasting. *Civic & Public Affairs:* 6%. Funds public and foreign policy. *Education:* 34%. Supports education funds and higher education. *Environment:* 7%. Family services, child welfare, and youth organizations, including Jewish welfare organizations. *International:* 9%. Medical centers and single-disease health associations. *Religion:* 4%. *Note:* Total contributions made in 1998. **Typ. Recipients:** Alzheimers Disease, Children's Health/Hospitals, Clinics/Medical Centers, Diabetes, Domestic Violence, Eyes/Blindness, Family Planning, Health Organizations, Hospitals, Hospitals (University Affiliated), Medical Rehabilitation, Medical Research, Mental Health, People with Disabilities, Public Health, Single-Disease Health Associations, Substance Abuse. **Geo. Dist:** Chicago, IL, including Cook County.

## ★ 51 ★ Arkell Hall Foundation

68 Front St.
PO Box 240
Canajoharie, NY 13317-0240
**Phone:** (518)673-5417  **Fax:** (518)673-5493
**Email:** jsantangelo@arkell.org
Joseph Santangelo, Vice President, Treasurer, Administrator

**Fnded:** 1948. **Philosophy:** "The primary mission of the Arkell Hall Foundation is the operation and maintenance of a home for elderly persons. Funds which may become available above the needs of the Home may be distributed annually to organizations providing services within the Target Community." "The most important requirement is significant direct impact in the Western Montgomery County New York community. Projects or organizations not primarily serving the Target Community or with large service areas (such as national or regional) will not qualify for funding." 1997 Grant Program Guidelines **Priorities:** *Arts & Humanities:* 2%. Supports a library, art gallery, and the performing arts. *Civic & Public Affairs:* 10%. Supports community affairs. *Education:* 16%. Supports secondary and training schools, and colleges and universities. *Environment:* 52%. Supports youth services, animal affairs, and social services. *International:* 18%. Supports hospices, hospitals, and disease and disorder awareness programs. *Note:* Total contributions made in fiscal 1997. **Typ. Recipients:** Alzheimers Disease, Cancer, Children's Health/Hospitals, Clinics/Medical Centers, Clinics/Medical Centers, Diabetes, Domestic Violence, Emergency/Ambulance Services, Health Funds, Health Organizations, Health-General, Heart, Hospices, Hospitals, Long-Term Care, Medical Education, Medical Research, Nursing Services, Outpatient Health Care, People with Disabilities, Prenatal Health Issues, Single-Disease Health Associations, Substance Abuse. **Geo. Dist:** NY, Western Montgomery County.

## ★ 52 ★ Arnold and Mabel Beckman Foundation

100 Academy Dr.
Irvine, CA 92612
**Phone:** (949)721-2222  **Fax:** (949)721-2225
**Email:** jdorrance@beckman-foundation.com
**Website:** http://www.beckman-foundation.com
Jacqueline Dorrance, Executive Director

**Fnded:** 1977. **Philosophy:** "The Arnold and Mabel Beckman Foundation makes grants to nonprofit research institutions to promote research in chemistry and the life sciences, broadly interpreted, and particularly to foster the investigation of methods, instruments and materials that will open up new avenues of research in science. The Beckman Young Investigators Program is intended to provide research support to the most promising young faculty members in the early stages of academic careers in the chemical and life sciences." **Priorities:** *Education:* 18%. Supports educational scholarship. *Environment:* 9%. In support of Boy Scouts. *Religion:* 73%. Supports science centers, and organizations with science related interests. *Note:* Contributions made in fiscal 1999. **Typ. Recipients:** Clinics/Medical Centers, Eyes/Blindness, Medical Research, Research/Studies Institutes, Speech & Hearing. **Geo. Dist:** nationally.

## ★ 53 ★ Arthur J. Schmitt Foundation

629 Green Bay Rd., Ste. 1
Wilmette, IL 60091
**Phone:** (847)853-0231
John Donahue, Executive Director

**Fnded:** 1941. **Philosophy:** "Reflecting the strong sense of responsible stewardship to God evidenced in the life of Arthur J. Schmitt, the Arthur J. Schmitt Foundation commits itself to placing its resources toward fashioning a better and more humane world. To this end, and drawing from its founder's quest for leadership, the foundation pledges to support endeavors that will enable the development of human potential, especially in persons in whom notable promise of achievement is discerned. "In its activities, deliberations and decisions, the Arthur J. Schmitt Foundation is rooted in a spirit of Christian concern, with a special, but not exclusive, commitment to the Roman Catholic Tradition, in devotion to country, and in an informed awareness of present day world realities. The foundation realizes that in so doing, it exemplifies the central commitments of Arthur J. Schmitt. "Through this mission the foundation preserves the memory of its founder, Arthur J. Schimitt, and shares his story and his values with those who benefit from the foundation's resources." 1996 Brochure **Priorities:** *Education:* 85%. Supports Catholic educational institutions (49%); scholarships (12%). *Environment:* 3%. Community services, people with disabilities, youth organizations, and shelters. *International:* 1%. Supports home-care services. *Note:* Total contributions made in fiscal 1999. **Typ. Recipients:** AIDS/HIV, Health Funds, Home-Care Services, Hospitals, Long-Term Care, Medical Education, Mental Health, People with Disabilities, Research/Studies Institutes, Substance Abuse. **Geo. Dist:** Chicago, IL, metropolitan area.

## ★ 54 ★ Arthur Vining Davis Foundations

225 Water St., Ste. 1510
Jacksonville, FL 32202-5185
**Phone:** (904)359-0670  **Fax:** (904)359-0675
**Email:** arthurvining@bellsouth.net
**Website:** http://www.jvm.com/davis/
Dr. Jonathan Howe, Executive Director

**Fnded:** 1952. **Philosophy:** Mr. Davis' philanthropic philosophy emphasized higher education and religious activities, with some attention to medicine. The foundations will continue their commitment to Mr. Davis' ideals, again concentrating their funding in the area of private higher education, and, to a lesser extent, to medicine, religion, public television, and secondary education. Grants in private higher education concentrate on institutions with outstanding records of teaching and learning in the liberal arts and sciences, and those with broadly acknowledged academic excellence, adequate financial resources, and a record of good trustee and alumni support. Grants generally range from $100,000 to $200,000 for projects proposed by the applicant college president with the goal of reinforcing institutional excellence. The trustees prefer to give grants in the medical field for programs that encourage caring attitudes in the delivery of health care. Projects should have the potential for widespread practical application and should be of interest to other groups. New ideas are encouraged, especially if they facilitate communications with patients by doctors, nurses, and other caregivers; ameliorate patient anxieties; and foster caring attitudes. Grants range from $50,000 to $200,000. The majority of grants in the field of religion are made to fully accredited by the Association of Theological Schools seminaries that prepare persons for ordained ministry. As with the higher education program, support generally goes to schools known for academic excellence and financial stability. Grants generally range from $75,000-$150,000 for projects proposed by the institutions president or Dean. Support for public television seeks to emphasize the Foundation's interest in education, including television for children. Grants ordinarily are made to provide partial support for a major series of educational programs. A series should be assured of national distribution through the public broadcasting system. Grants in secondary education will be made to professional development programs which strengthen teachers and teaching in high schools. Collaborative partnerships between faculties of colleges and high schools, or combined efforts involving reform organizations, colleges/universities, and high schools are encouraged. **Priorities:** *Arts & Humanities:* 17%. Supports public television specials and series. *Education:* 58%. Supports colleges and higher education. *International:* 10%. *Note:* Total contributions made in 1999. **Typ. Recipients:** Cancer, Children's Health/Hospitals, Clinics/Medical Centers, Health Organizations, Health Policy/Cost Containment, Health-General, Hospices, Hospitals, Hospitals (University Affiliated), Medical Education, Medical Research, Mental Health, Research/Studies Institutes. **Geo. Dist:** nationally.

## ★ 55 ★ Atherton Family Foundation

c/o Hawaii Community Foundation
900 Fort St. Mall, Ste. 1300
Honolulu, HI 96813
**Phone:** (808)556-5508          **Fax:** (808)521-6286
**Email:** lschiff@hcf-hawaii.org
Lissa Schiff, Private Foundation Services Officer
**Fnded:** 1976. **Philosophy:** The foundation supports programs within a broad spectrum of activities, although funding is limited to organizations based in the state of Hawaii. Support of "educational programs, projects, and institutions... continue to have the highest priority, as do those with a religious nature." Organizations concerned with health and social services also are given careful attention. In reviewing proposals, the foundation's directors look for programs that seek to fulfill a "critical need in the community or provide a direct benefit to a group or class of people for the alleviation of a problem, or for the provision of an amenity that enhances life for the people in Hawaii." In addition, the directors have established a scholarship program as a memorial to Juliette M. Atherton. **Priorities:** *Arts & Humanities:* 19%. Supports visual arts, performing arts, folk arts, arts academies, and history and historic preservation. *Civic & Public Affairs:* 8%. *Education:* 42%. Supports Christian K-12 education, educational programs, universities, education councils, literacy, and scholarships. *Environment:* 22%. Supports youth and family services and United Way. *International:* 4%. Gives to hospice, cancer centers, disease and disorders programs, and hospitals. *Note:* Contributions were made in 2000. **Typ. Recipients:** Cancer, Children's Health/Hospitals, Clinics/Medical Centers, Domestic Violence, Emergency/Ambulance Services, Family Planning, Geriatric Health, Health Funds, Health Organizations, Hospices, Hospitals, Long-Term Care, Medical Education, Medical Rehabilitation, Medical Research, Medical Training, Mental Health, Nursing Services, People with Disabilities, Prenatal Health Issues, Substance Abuse. **Geo. Dist:** HI.

## ★ 56 ★ Atkinson Foundation

1100 Grundy Lane, Ste. 140
San Bruno, CA 94066-3030
**Phone:** (650)876-0222          **Fax:** (650)876-0222
**Email:** atkinfdn@aol.com
Elizabeth Curtis, Administrator & Director
**Fnded:** 1939. **Philosophy:** "The Foundation hopes to provide opportunities for people to attain their highest potential in areas of spiritual, educational, social and economic life, to assist their efforts to become independent and self-sufficient and generally to improve the quality of their lives." The foundation gives primary consideration to "nonprofit organizations serving the residents of San Mateo County, CA, through programs that benefit children, youth, families, immigrants, the elderly and the ill, the disadvantaged, needy and homeless, the mentally and physically disabled, and those suffering from drug, alcohol, or physical abuse"; schools and institutions of higher education serving the needs of students in San Mateo County. Selected support for other denominations, religious education and mission programs; U.S. nonprofits providing assistance, support and training abroad for the sustainable development of local food, water and economic resources; for health education and family planning activities; and for emergency relief followed by long range recovery programs. 1999 Annual Report **Priorities:** *Arts & Humanities:* 2%. Funds local library. *Civic & Public Affairs:* 15% Supports community affairs, provides assistance for youths and families, and funds health ministries. *Education:* 15% Supports improving educational opportunities for all students, primarily in the local area. *Environment:* 19%. Supports programs which provide basic human social, physical, and economic services. *International:* 23%. Funds Rehab AssociationS, several disease-specific OrganizationS, and health education. *Note:* Total contributions made in 1999. **Typ. Recipients:** AIDS/HIV, Alzheimers Disease, Children's Health/Hospitals, Domestic Violence, Eyes/Blindness, Family Planning, Health-General, Heart, Hospitals, Medical Rehabilitation, Medical Research, Mental Health, People with Disabilities, Public Health, Substance Abuse. **Geo. Dist:** United

States-based international organizations serving Latin America; CA, San Mateo County.

## ★ 57 ★ Atran Foundation, Inc.

25 East 21st St., 3rd Floor
New York, NY 10010
**Phone:** (718)505-9677
Diane Fischer, President
**Fnded:** 1945. **Philosophy:** The Atran Foundation makes most of its grants in support of Jewish religious organizations, education, and civic affairs. Educational support goes to Jewish universities, medical education, and social science education. In civic affairs, interests include women's affairs, business interests, and community affairs. The foundation supports other recipient areas on a limited basis. **Priorities:** *Arts & Humanities:* 16%. *Education:* 31%. *International:* 2%. *Note:* Total contributions made in fiscal 1999. **Typ. Recipients:** Clinics/Medical Centers, Emergency/Ambulance Services, Geriatric Health, Hospitals, Hospitals (University Affiliated), Long-Term Care, Medical Education, Medical Research, People with Disabilities, Research/Studies Institutes. **Geo. Dist:** NY.

## ★ 58 ★ Audrey and Sydney Irmas Charitable Foundation

16027 Ventura Blvd., Ste. 601
Encino, CA 91436
**Phone:** (818)382-3313          **Fax:** (818)382-3315
Robert Irmas, Administrator & Manager
**Fnded:** 1986. **Philosophy:** The foundation distributes its giving evenly between Jewish religious organizations, civic affairs, the arts, and social services. The foundation also supports health services. **Priorities:** *Arts & Humanities:* 13%. Museums, opera, and photography. *Civic & Public Affairs:* 22%. Law and justice, affordable housing, and feminism studies. *Education:* 6%. *Environment:* 4%. *International:* 3%. *Note:* Total contributions made in 1997. **Typ. Recipients:** Adolescent Health Issues, AIDS/HIV, Cancer, Child Abuse, Children's Health/Hospitals, Clinics/Medical Centers, Diabetes, Eyes/Blindness, Health Organizations, Hospitals, Medical Research, Mental Health, Research/Studies Institutes, Single-Disease Health Associations, Substance Abuse, Transplant Networks/Donor Banks. **Geo. Dist:** Los Angeles, CA.

## ★ 59 ★ Autry Foundation

4383 Colfax Ave.
Studio City, CA 91604
**Phone:** (818)752-7770          **Fax:** (818)752-7779
Jacqueline Autry, President
**Fnded:** 1974. **Philosophy:** The foundation's primary purpose is to support the Autry Museum of Western Heritage. The foundation also supports other arts organizations, health concerns, and educational organizations. **Priorities:** *Arts & Humanities:* 80%. Major support for the Autry Museum of Western Heritage. *Environment:* 20%. Youth organizations, family services, community programs, and recreation and athletics. *Note:* Total contributions made in 1998. **Typ. Recipients:** Alzheimers Disease, Cancer, Child Abuse, Children's Health/Hospitals, Clinics/Medical Centers, Diabetes, Domestic Violence, Eyes/Blindness, Health Organizations, Health-General, Heart, Hospices, Hospitals, Medical Research, People with Disabilities, Prenatal Health Issues, Public Health, Research/Studies Institutes, Respiratory, Single-Disease Health Associations, Speech & Hearing, Substance Abuse. **Geo. Dist:** CA, including southern California.

## ★ 60 ★ B. C. McCabe Foundation

8152 Painter Ave., Ste. 201
Whittier, CA 90602
**Phone:** (562)696-1433          **Fax:** (562)698-5508
James Shepard, Trustee
**Fnded:** 1976. **Philosophy:** The foundation typically supports social service organizations, educational institutions, health concerns, and religious welfare causes within California. **Priorities:** *Arts & Humanities:* 9%. Art center. *Civic & Public Affairs:* 6%.

Women's services. *Education:* 6%. Colleges. *Environment:* 60%. Youth guidance, clubs, and homes. *International:* 19%. Hospitals and health projects. *Note:* Total contributions made in 1998. **Typ. Recipients:** AIDS/HIV, Children's Health/Hospitals, Clinics/Medical Centers, Diabetes, Emergency/Ambulance Services, Health Organizations, Hospitals, Medical Education, Nursing Services, Nutrition, People with Disabilities, Substance Abuse, Trauma Treatment. **Geo. Dist:** CA.

## ★ 61 ★ Ball Brothers Foundation

222 South Mulberry
PO Box 1408
Muncie, IN 47308
**Phone:** (765)741-5500          **Fax:** (765)741-5518
**Email:** ballfoundation@yahoo.com
Douglas Bakken, Executive Director
**Fnded:** 1926. **Philosophy:** "The Foundation was established 'to promote religious, educational or charitable purposes, or all of these, within the State of Indiana." "While Foundation grants support a wide range of Indiana institutions and organizations, the majority of funds have been distributed to Muncie and East Central Indiana." "The Foundation's goal has been to facilitate the building of community. Current areas of funding interest include higher education, K-12 public education, arts, humanities and cultural organizations and outdoor recreation programs, and youth services." "The Foundation, in partnership with other philanthropic entities across Indiana... (facilitates) programs dedicated to stimulating giving and volunteering and seeking ways to enrich and broaden the quality of life in the state." "The Foundation, since 1983, has been the primary funder of the Minnetrista Cultural Foundation, and operator of the Minnetrista Cultural Center, a 70,000 square foot community facility, opened in 1988." "During the past several years, the Foundation has been involved with area public schools in seeking ways to facilitate the introduction of computers and seeking ways to capitalize on the global network, namely (the) Internet." 1997 General Information. **Priorities:** *Arts & Humanities:* 72%. Supports musical performance, museums, libraries, and historical preservation; major grants to the Minnetrista Cultural Foundation and the Ball State University Art Museum. *Civic & Public Affairs:* 9%. Funds community development. *Education:* 10%. Substantial gifts went to Ball State University and local schools. *Environment:* 7%. Supports United Way, Young Men's Christian Association, scouting, and Special Olympics. *International:* 1%. Funds hospitals and preventive medical organizations. *Note:* Total contributions made in 2000. **Typ. Recipients:** AIDS/HIV, Children's Health/Hospitals, Diabetes, Health Organizations, Heart, Hospitals, Medical Rehabilitation, People with Disabilities, Preventive Medicine/Wellness Organizations, Public Health. **Geo. Dist:** IN, East Central Indiana; Muncie, IN.

## ★ 62 ★ Banbury Fund

29 East Gate Rd.
Huntington, NY 11743
**Phone:** (631)367-3121
William Robertson, President
**Fnded:** 1946. **Philosophy:** The fund places an emphasis on educational institutions, environmental causes, civic affairs, and scientific and health care organizations. **Priorities:** *Civic & Public Affairs:* 7%. Supports civic and community development. *Education:* 46%. Supports educational programs, schools, and colleges and universities. *Environment:* 8%. Supports humane studies, United Way, and family and youth services. *International:* 12%. Supports hospices and disease and disorder awareness affairs. *Religion:* 14%. Supports Cold Spring Harbor Laboratory. *Note:* Total contributions made in 1998. **Typ. Recipients:** AIDS/HIV, Cancer, Clinics/Medical Centers, Emergency/Ambulance Services, Eyes/Blindness, Family Planning, Health Organizations, Hospices, Hospitals, Hospitals (University Affiliated), Medical Education, Public Health. **Geo. Dist:** NY.

## ★ 63 ★ Barker Welfare Foundation

PO Box 2
Glen Head, NY 11545
**Phone:** (516)759-5592 **Fax:** (516)759-5497
**Email:** barkersmd@aol.com
Sarane Ross, President & Director

**Fnded:** 1934. **Philosophy:** "The mission of the Barker Welfare Foundation is to make grants to qualified charitable organizations whose initiatives improve the quality of life, with an emphasis on strengthening youth and families and which reflect the philosophy of Catherine B. Hickox, the Founder." The Barker Welfare Foundation gives the majority of its support in the areas of social service and the arts. In the social service category, the foundation emphasizes youth, family services, community centers, and homes. In the arts, a majority of support goes to dance, historic preservation, libraries, museums, music, and theater. The foundation also gives some support to civic causes, health organizations, and educational institutions. In May 1994, the foundation changed its funding policy for the metropolitan Chicago, IL, area. The foundation will no longer accept unsolicited applications for grants; all grants made in that area will be foundation-initiated. **Priorities:** *Arts & Humanities:* 32%. Primary support for music, libraries, museums, opera, ballet, and public broadcasting. *Civic & Public Affairs:* 7%. Emphasis on neighborhood associations and foundations. *Environment:* 52%. Targets youth organizations, family services, child welfare, and people with disabilities. *Note:* Total contributions made in fiscal 1999. **Typ. Recipients:** Adolescent Health Issues, AIDS/HIV, Cancer, Child Abuse, Children's Health/Hospitals, Clinics/Medical Centers, Emergency/Ambulance Services, Family Planning, Heart, Home-Care Services, Hospitals, Long-Term Care, Medical Rehabilitation, Medical Training, Mental Health, Nursing Services, Outpatient Health Care, People with Disabilities, Prenatal Health Issues, Public Health, Substance Abuse. **Geo. Dist:** Chicago, IL; Michigan City, IN; New York, NY.

## ★ 64 ★ Barra Foundation

8200 Flourtown Ave., Ste. 12
Wyndmoor, DE 19038-7976
**Phone:** (302)233-5115 **Fax:** (302)836-1033
William Harral, III, President

**Fnded:** 1963. **Philosophy:** The Barra Foundation seeks to advance knowledge and education, particularly "in the fields of American art history and material culture from the colonial period to 1900." To this end, the foundation supports innovative pilot studies and projects not supported by other agencies or individuals. **Priorities:** *Arts & Humanities:* 66%. Funds museums, historical societies, libraries, public broadcasting, and arts associations. *Civic & Public Affairs:* 12%. Supports career and economic development organizations, zoos and community organizations. *Education:* 9%. Gives to higher education and summer youth education projects. *Environment:* 4%. Funds community services, youth organizations, and united funds. *International:* 6%. Supports medical centers and health associations. *Religion:* 2%. Supports the Academy of Natural Sciences of Philadelphia. *Note:* Total contributions made in 2000. **Typ. Recipients:** Alzheimers Disease, Cancer, Children's Health/Hospitals, Clinics/Medical Centers, Emergency/Ambulance Services, Family Planning, Health Organizations, Health-General, Home-Care Services, Hospices, Hospitals, Hospitals (University Affiliated), Long-Term Care, Medical Education, Medical Rehabilitation, Medical Research, People with Disabilities, Preventive Medicine/Wellness Organizations, Public Health, Single-Disease Health Associations. **Geo. Dist:** Philadelphia, PA.

## ★ 65 ★ Bass Foundation

309 Main St.
Fort Worth, TX 76102
**Phone:** (817)336-0494 **Fax:** (817)332-2176
**Email:** fcabal@sidrichardson.org
Valleau Wilkie, Jr., Executive Director

**Fnded:** 1945. **Philosophy:** The Bass Foundation makes most of its grants in the areas of civic affairs,

the arts, and education. Funding for civic affairs favors zoos and conservation efforts. The arts receive support in the areas of museums, the performing arts, and art councils. Educational funding favors universities, and private education. The foundation also supports medical centers, churches, and social services. **Priorities:** *Arts & Humanities:* 15%. Supports fine arts, arts groups, and an orchestra. *Civic & Public Affairs:* 4%. Supports municipalities. *Education:* 26%. Supports private schools, higher education. *Environment:* 2%. Funds Young Men's Christian Association. *Note:* Total contributions made in 1999. **Typ. Recipients:** Children's Health/Hospitals, Emergency/Ambulance Services, Family Planning, Geriatric Health, Hospitals, Substance Abuse. **Geo. Dist:** Fort Worth, TX.

## ★ 66 ★ Baughman Foundation

PO Box 1356
Liberal, KS 67905-1356
**Phone:** (316)624-1371 **Fax:** (316)624-1371
**Email:** baughman@swko.net
Eugene Slaymaker, President

**Fnded:** 1958. **Philosophy:** The foundation gives to local municipalities and local organizations, primarily providing scholarships and capital or special project support. **Priorities:** *Arts & Humanities:* 7%. Supports libraries, arts and culture. *Civic & Public Affairs:* 36%. Supports community affairs employment, towns, and parks. *Education:* 30%. Supports educational institutions and programs; scholarships. *Environment:* 16%. Supports youth services and social services. *International:* 6%. Supports hospitals and health concerns. *Religion:* 2%. Supports the MidAmerica Air Museum. *Note:* Total contributions made in 1998. **Typ. Recipients:** Alzheimers Disease, Clinics/Medical Centers, Diabetes, Domestic Violence, Emergency/Ambulance Services, Health Organizations, Hospitals, People with Disabilities, Sexual Abuse, Single-Disease Health Associations, Substance Abuse. **Geo. Dist:** Liberal, KS.

## ★ 67 ★ Beatrice P. Delany Charitable Trust

1211 Ave. of the Americas
New York, NY 10036
**Phone:** (212)789-5374
Mr. John Enteman, Administrator

**Fnded:** 1977. **Philosophy:** The trust traditionally supports programs and organizations in the areas of education, religion, civic groups, health, social services, and the arts. **Priorities:** *Arts & Humanities:* 24%. Supports music, with major support given to the Chicago Symphony Orchestra also funds opera, theater, and public broadcasting. *Civic & Public Affairs:* 7%. Major support given to the Devereux Foundation. Also supports botanical gardens & zoos. *Education:* 42%. Supports colleges and universities, religious education, medical education. *Environment:* 4%. Supports young men's christian association, United Way, child welfare, homes, and youth programs. *International:* 10%. Funds hospitals, medical centers, and disease and disorder concerns, hospice and cancer. *Note:* Total contributions made in fiscal 1998. **Typ. Recipients:** Cancer, Children's Health/Hospitals, Clinics/Medical Centers, Health-General, Hospitals, Medical Education, Medical Research, Mental Health, Multiple Sclerosis. **Geo. Dist:** nationally; Chicago, IL.

## ★ 68 ★ Beazley Foundation

3720 Brighton St.
Portsmouth, VA 23707
**Phone:** (757)393-1605 **Fax:** (757)393-4708
**Email:** beazley@norfolk.infi.net
**Website:** http://www.beazleyfoundation.org
Lawrence I'Anson, Jr., President

**Fnded:** 1948. **Philosophy:** "In keeping with the informal policy established by Mr. Beazely, the Trustees of the Beazely Foundation will award grants to organizations that are tax exempt under Section 501(c)(3) of the Internal Revenue Code and which are engaged in educational, charitable and religious activities." "Although there are no set distribution percentages for the three areas of giving, it is expected that the foundation will continue to emphasize grants to

education with a smaller percentage going to charitable projects and a still smaller percentage to religious activities. The Foundation prefers, when making grants to religious activities, to gift ecumenical projects as opposed to grants to individual churches or denominations." "Geographically, the Foundation's goal is to grant the largest percentage of the funds during any one year to projects supporting the citizens of Portsmouth with a majority of the remaining funds to projects within the Tidewater Area preferably, but in the Commonwealth of Virginia at a minimum, with a very small percentage going to organizations outside the Commonwealth." **Priorities:** *Arts & Humanities:* 5%. Museums and cultural centers receive funding. *Civic & Public Affairs:* 7%. Supports anti-crime initiatives, employment, affordable housing, and leadership development. *Education:* 36%. Emphasis on public and private schools, colleges, and academic support. *Environment:* 26%. Primarily supports youth programs. *International:* 21%. Grants are made for operating support for healthcare programs and medical centers. *Note:* Total contributions made in 2000. **Typ. Recipients:** AIDS/HIV, Cancer, Child Abuse, Children's Health/Hospitals, Clinics/Medical Centers, Domestic Violence, Emergency/Ambulance Services, Geriatric Health, Health Organizations, Health-General, Hospitals, Hospitals (University Affiliated), Medical Education, Medical Rehabilitation, People with Disabilities, Public Health, Single-Disease Health Associations, Substance Abuse. **Geo. Dist:** Hampton Roads, VA area; Portsmouth, VA.

## ★ 69 ★ Beinecke Foundation Inc.

8 Sound Shore Dr.
Ste. 120
Greenwich, CT 06830
**Phone:** (203)861-7314 **Fax:** (203)861-7316
John Robinson, President

**Fnded:** 1966. **Philosophy:** "The Beinecke Foundation, Inc. funds two types of programs: 1.Unsolicited projects reflecting an applicant's particular interests. 2.Projects reflecting an applicant's interest which are developed in response to a Foundation call for proposals." The foundation's interests include environmental affairs, higher education, New York City cultural institutions, and Protestant giving. **Priorities:** *Arts & Humanities:* 9%. Supports museums, historical societies, and art centers. *Civic & Public Affairs:* 9%. Supports botanical gardens. *Education:* 47%. Funds higher education. *Environment:* 6%. Funds youth clubs. *International:* 2%. Funds single-disease health associations. *Religion:* 1%. Supports a natural history museum. *Note:* Total contributions made in 1998. **Typ. Recipients:** Cancer, Children's Health/Hospitals, Emergency/Ambulance Services, Family Planning, Health Organizations, Hospitals, Medical Research, Research/Studies Institutes, Single-Disease Health Associations. **Geo. Dist:** CT; NY.

## ★ 70 ★ Beirne Carter Foundation

PO Box 26903
Richmond, VA 23261
**Phone:** (804)521-0272 **Fax:** (804)788-2700
**Email:** bcarterfn@aol.com
**Website:** http://www.bcarterfdn.org
Frederick Willis, Jr., Advisor

**Fnded:** 1986. **Philosophy:** The foundation supports a variety of organizations that have direct impact on Virginia, from Richmond to southern Virginia. Other types of organizations supported include environmental affairs, family services, the disadvantaged, rural arts, and historical programs. **Priorities:** *Arts & Humanities:* 5%. Supports historic preservation, ballet, theater, libraries, museums, arts centers, and public broadcasting. *Civic & Public Affairs:* 12%. Urban renewal, botanical gardens and parks, housing, and legal aid. *Education:* 50%. Funds primary schools and colleges and universities. *Environment:* 16%. Focus on shelters, youth organizations, and family services. *International:* 2%. Single-disease health associations. *Religion:* 1%. Funds science museums and archeological studies. *Note:* Total contributions made in 1999. **Typ. Recipients:** AIDS/HIV, Arthritis, Cancer, Child Abuse, Children's Health/Hospitals, Clinics/Medical Centers, Domestic Violence, Emergency/Ambulance

Services, Family Planning, Hospices, Hospitals, Hospitals (University Affiliated), Medical Education, Medical Research, Mental Health, People with Disabilities, Preventive Medicine/Wellness Organizations, Public Health, Research/Studies Institutes, Respiratory, Single-Disease Health Associations, Transplant Networks/Donor Banks. **Geo. Dist:** VA.

### ★ 71 ★ Ben B. Cheney Foundation

1201 Pacific Ave. South, Ste. 1600
Tacoma, WA 98402
**Phone:** (253)572-2442          **Fax:** (253)572-2902
Dr. William Rieke, Executive Director

**Fnded:** 1955. **Philosophy:** The Ben B. Cheney Foundation "prefers to fund projects that develop new and innovative approaches to community problems, facilitate the improvement of services or programs, or invest in equipment and facilities that will have a lasting impact on community needs." Under its program guidelines, the foundation states that it seeks to disburse funds to civic projects, culture, charity, education, health, social services, youth, and the elderly. **Priorities:** *Arts & Humanities:* 29%. Focus on museums, libraries, historical societies, and the performing arts. *Civic & Public Affairs:* 12%. Funds community development, housing, parks, and an aquarium. *Education:* 21%. Support for colleges, universities, and a scholarship program. *Environment:* 21%. Supports Young Men's Christian Association, food banks, and youth organizations. *International:* 8%. Supports hospitals and mental health. *Religion:* 5%. Funds science centers and science museums. *Note:* Total contributions made in 1999. **Typ. Recipients:** AIDS/HIV, Cancer, Children's Health/Hospitals, Clinics/Medical Centers, Domestic Violence, Emergency/Ambulance Services, Health Funds, Health Organizations, Heart, Hospitals, Medical Training, Mental Health, People with Disabilities, Single-Disease Health Associations, Speech & Hearing, Substance Abuse. **Geo. Dist:** CA, Del Norte, Humboldt, Lassen, Shasta, Siskiyou, and Trinity Counties in northern CA; CA, especially northern CA; OR, especially southwestern OR; WA, especially southwestern WA, Tacoma-Pierce County.

### ★ 72 ★ Ben and Esther Rosenbloom Foundation

106 Old Court Rd., Ste. 302
Baltimore, MD 21208
**Phone:** (410)653-0239
Howard Rosenbloom, Executive Director

**Fnded:** 1982. **Philosophy:** The foundation primarily gives to Jewish human service organizations. **Priorities:** *Arts & Humanities:* 1%. Supports music, art institutes, and museums. *Civic & Public Affairs:* 1%. Funds public policy organizations. *Environment:* 3%. Primarily united funds and community service organizations. *International:* 5%. Funds hospitals and single-disease health associations. *Note:* Total contributions made in 1998. **Typ. Recipients:** AIDS/HIV, Cancer, Domestic Violence, Emergency/Ambulance Services, Eyes/Blindness, Health Organizations, Heart, Hospitals, Hospitals, Kidney, Medical Rehabilitation, People with Disabilities, Single-Disease Health Associations. **Geo. Dist:** Baltimore, MD.

### ★ 73 ★ Beneficia Foundation

1 Pitcairn Place, Ste. 3000
Jenkintown, PA 19046-3593
**Phone:** (215)887-6700          **Fax:** (215)881-6092
**Email:** hm6085@pitcairn.com
Hope Miller, Contact

**Fnded:** 1953. **Philosophy:** "Beneficia's mission is to enhance the quality of life through conservation of the environment and promotion of the arts. Beneficia favors programs which are innovative, catalytic, addressing unmet needs, and striving towards self-sustainability. Priorities for giving in the area of the environment include: inventory, protection and stewardship of high priority ecosystems (especially tropical and marine); creation of economic incentives for the conservation of biodiversity; and policy and legislation. Priorities for the giving in the area of the arts include: performing arts, especially classical music, theater

and opera; and the visual arts with an emphasis on museums and art centers." **Priorities:** *Arts & Humanities:* 13%. Focus on performing arts, museums, and music. *Civic & Public Affairs:* 12%. Supports botanical gardens and zoological societies, and legal concerns. *Education:* 2%. *Note:* Total contributions made in 1998. **Typ. Recipients:** Cancer, Children's Health/Hospitals, Medical Education, Nursing Services, Nutrition, People with Disabilities. **Geo. Dist:** no restrictions.

### ★ 74 ★ Benjamin and Mary Siddons Measey Foundation

PO Box 258
Media, PA 19063
**Phone:** (610)566-5800          **Fax:** (610)566-8197
James Brennan, Member, Board of Managers

**Fnded:** 1958. **Philosophy:** The Benjamin and Mary Siddons Measey Foundation supports two areas of giving: education and health. Educational support favors universities and their medical schools. In health care, interests include university hospitals and health consortiums. **Priorities:** *Education:* 71%. Mainly supports medical education. *International:* 29%. Primarily university hospitals, health consortiums and geriatrics. *Note:* Total contributions made in 1999. **Typ. Recipients:** Cancer, Children's Health/Hospitals, Clinics/Medical Centers, Geriatric Health, Health Funds, Health Organizations, Hospitals, Hospitals (University Affiliated), Medical Education, Medical Research, Public Health. **Geo. Dist:** Philadelphia, PA.

### ★ 75 ★ Benwood Foundation

Suntrust Bank Bldg.
736 Market St., Ste. 1600
Chattanooga, TN 37402
**Phone:** (423)267-4311          **Fax:** (615)267-9049
**Email:** benwoodfnd@benwood.org
Corinne Allen, Executive Director

**Fnded:** 1950. **Philosophy:** The purpose and activities of the foundation, as defined in its charter, cover a wide spectrum of philanthropy. Within this framework, the trustees have discretion to interpret the donor's philanthropic goals in accordance with today's needs. A broad range of organizations receive funding. The foundation contributes in six general areas: social services; health; the environment; education; the arts and humanities; and economic development. **Priorities:** *Arts & Humanities:* 13%. Gives to museums, historical societies, performing arts, public broadcasting, and art associations. *Civic & Public Affairs:* 17%. Funds urban and community affairs, zoos, public safety, and community foundations. *Education:* 28%. Primarily supports colleges and universities, public and private schools, and educational foundations. *Environment:* 13%. United funds, children's organizations, and athletics. *International:* 13%. Funds medical centers and health organizations. *Note:* Total contributions made in 2000. **Typ. Recipients:** Alzheimers Disease, Clinics/Medical Centers, Emergency/Ambulance Services, Health Organizations, Hospitals, Medical Education, Medical Research, Mental Health, People with Disabilities, Public Health, Research/Studies Institutes, Substance Abuse. **Geo. Dist:** Chattanooga, TN.

### ★ 76 ★ Bernard McDonough Foundation

311 Fourth St.
Parkersburg, WV 26101
**Phone:** (304)424-6280          **Fax:** (304)424-6281
James Wakley, President & Director

**Fnded:** 1961. **Priorities:** *Arts & Humanities:* 7%. Supports libraries, museums, and performing arts. *Civic & Public Affairs:* 4%. Funds civic organizations, community foundations, and housing. *Education:* 42%. Colleges, universities, and public schools. *Environment:* 29%. Supports United Way, family causes, aging concerns, people with special needs and social services. *International:* 6%. Supports health, disease and disorder concerns. *Note:* Contributions were made in 1997. **Typ. Recipients:** Alzheimers Disease, Cancer, Children's Health/Hospitals, Clinics/Medical Centers, Emergency/Ambulance Services, Health Or-

ganizations, Health-General, Heart, Hospices, Hospitals, Hospitals (University Affiliated), Mental Health, People with Disabilities, Research/Studies Institutes. **Geo. Dist:** WV.

### ★ 77 ★ Bernard Osher Foundation

909 Montgomery, No. 300
San Francisco, CA 94133
**Phone:** (415)861-5587          **Fax:** (415)677-5868
**Email:** nagle@osherfoundation.com
Patricia Tracy-Nagle, Executive Administrator & Secretary

**Fnded:** 1977. **Philosophy:** "The foundation's objective is to improve the quality of life for Bay Area residents through support of cultural and educational organizations and institutions...The foundation supports programs in these fields of interest: Arts and Humanities (programs which encourage artistic creativity in the visual and performing arts and promote scholarship in the literary arts); and Education (fellowships for colleges, universities, and conservatories for students of exceptional promise, with emphasis on graduate studies, and enrichment programs for schools, grades K-12)." **Priorities:** *Arts & Humanities:* 11%. Emphasis on music, museums, and performing arts. *Civic & Public Affairs:* 2%. Support festivals, zoos, and community foundations. *Education:* 86%. Primary support for the University of California, Berkeley. *Environment:* 1%. Youth organizations, family services, and united funds. *Note:* Total contributions made in 1998. **Typ. Recipients:** AIDS/HIV, Cancer, Diabetes, Family Planning, Health Organizations, Hospitals, Medical Education, Medical Research, Mental Health, People with Disabilities, Substance Abuse. **Geo. Dist:** CA, Alameda County; CA, San Francisco County.

### ★ 78 ★ Bernice Barbour Foundation, Inc.

14434 Laurel Trail
West Palm Beach, FL 33414-7648
**Phone:** (561)791-0861          **Fax:** (561)753-9153
**Email:** bernbar@iesc.net
**Website:** http://www.bernicebarbour.org
Eve Thompson, Secretary & Treasurer

**Fnded:** 1987. **Philosophy:** "The Bernice Barbour Foundation is a private charity established by the late Bernice Wall Barbour. It is a trust to be used for the preservation and care of animals, and prevention of cruelty to animals in the United States." Eve Lloyd Thompson, Treasurer and Secretary **Priorities:** *Civic & Public Affairs:* 16%. Supports zoos and aquariums. *Education:* 33%. Funds colleges and universities for veterinary science. *Environment:* 36%. Supports animal welfare organizations. *Note:* Total contributions made in 1998. **Typ. Recipients:** Clinics/Medical Centers, Emergency/Ambulance Services, Medical Education, Medical Rehabilitation, Medical Research, People with Disabilities. **Geo. Dist:** nationally.

### ★ 79 ★ Billy Rose Foundation

805 3rd Ave., 22nd Floor
New York, NY 10022
**Phone:** (212)407-7745          **Fax:** (212)407-7799
Ms. Terri Mangino, Executive Director

**Fnded:** 1958. **Philosophy:** Of primary interest to the foundation is "making available to the American people works of genius in music, drama, painting, sculpture, all art forms." **Priorities:** *Arts & Humanities:* 41%. Supports arts organizations, music, theater, museums, film & video, ballet, opera, and libraries. *Civic & Public Affairs:* 2%. Funds botanical gardens, civic affairs, and public affairs. *Education:* 9%. Supports arts education, colleges, and universities. *International:* 4%. Supports corrective procedures and nursing services. *Note:* Total contributions made in 1998. **Typ. Recipients:** Cancer, Clinics/Medical Centers, Family Planning, Health Organizations, Hospitals, Medical Rehabilitation, Medical Research, Nursing Services, People with Disabilities, Single-Disease Health Associations, Transplant Networks/Donor Banks. **Geo. Dist:** New York, NY.

## ★ 80 ★ Blandin Foundation
100 North Pokegama Ave.
Grand Rapids, MN 55744
**Phone:** (218)326-0523          **Fax:** (218)327-1949
**Email:** bldnfdtn@uslink.net
**Website:** http://www.blandinfoundation.org
Linda Gibeau, Grants Manager
**Fnded:** 1941. **Philosophy:** "The mission of the Blandin Foundation is to strengthen rural Minnesota communities." The foundation gives in the following areas: Education: "The Foundation's goal is to comprehensively link public schools (K-12) with communities in 24 rural sites. Schools, community members, and educators are being encouraged to work together to increase student achievement and problem solving skills; community involvement in the education process in supportive and responsible ways; and community awareness and utilization of schools, faculty and students as a key community resource." Environmental Stewardship: "Most Minnesota citizens value and protect the state's natural environment. To continue to foster a better understanding of environmental issues, particularly by our young people, the Foundation has a focus on creating a broad base of stewardship for our natural resources. The outcome for this focus is that stewardship, as a key value, will guide public and private decision making and action in 100 communities in rural Minnesota." Safe Communities: "The Foundation provides major funding to address the issue of violence in rural Minnesota in partnership with the Citizen's Council on Crime and Justice... The expected outcome of this work is the reduction of specific violent activity in 25 rural communities in Minnesota over the next five years." Economic Opportunity: " The Foundation supports the development of new technologies with the potential to expand rural employment. (The SOTA TEC Fund) will join with rural Minnesota inventors, entrepreneurs and operating companies to create and fund demand-driven research programs that tap the (University of Minnesota) technical skills and resources. The Foundation also supports access to affordable housing in rural Minnesota." Convening: "The Foundation identifies major areas of interest affecting rural communities and then sponsors various conferences to address these issues. The conferences are designed to develop new ways of approaching problems and taking action on opportunities that strengthen rural communities in Minnesota." 1997 **Priorities:** *Arts & Humanities:* 2%. Supports theater and public broadcasting. *Civic & Public Affairs:* 26%. Supports projects that promote economic opportunity, community safety, and community leadership training. Also supports chambers of commerce, legal aid, and towns/municipalities. *Education:* 39%. Support for public schools, colleges, universities and scholarships. *Environment:* 26%. Funds social and youth services, sexual assault prevention, special Olympics, persons with disabilities, Young Men's Christian Association, and United Way. *International:* 5%. Supports general health care. *Note:* Total contributions made in 1999. **Typ. Recipients:** Clinics/Medical Centers, Domestic Violence, Emergency/Ambulance Services, Health Organizations, Health Policy/Cost Containment, Hospices, Medical Education, Medical Research, Mental Health, Nursing Services, Outpatient Health Care, People with Disabilities, Public Health, Substance Abuse. **Geo. Dist:** Grand Rapids, MN.

## ★ 81 ★ Blum-Kovler Foundation
919 North Michigan Ave., Ste. 2800
Chicago, IL 60611
**Phone:** (312)664-5050          **Fax:** (312)664-8983
**Fnded:** 1957. **Philosophy:** The foundation gives to a wide variety of agencies in the arts, civic affairs, education, health, welfare, and religion categories. **Priorities:** *Arts & Humanities:* 11%. Funds museums, arts centers, arts associations, historical societies, and public broadcasting. *Civic & Public Affairs:* 20%. Funds community development and public policy. *Education:* 18%. Private secondary education and colleges and universities. *Environment:* 14%. Supports child welfare, community services, crime prevention, and people with disabilities. *International:* 18%. Focus on hospitals, medical research, diabetes, and children's health. *Note:* Total contributions made in 1998. **Typ. Recipients:** Cancer, Children's Health/Hospitals, Clinics/Medical Centers, Diabetes, Health Funds, Health Organizations, Hospices, Hospitals, Hospitals (University Affiliated), Medical Education, Medical Rehabilitation, Medical Research, Mental Health, People with Disabilities, Public Health, Research/Studies Institutes, Single-Disease Health Associations, Substance Abuse, Transplant Networks/Donor Banks. **Geo. Dist:** Washington, DC; Chicago, IL, metropolitan area; New York, NY.

## ★ 82 ★ Blumenthal Foundation
PO Box 34689
Charlotte, NC 28234-6080
**Phone:** (704)377-6555          **Fax:** (704)377-9237
**Email:** philipb@vnet.net
**Website:** http://www.blumenthalfoundation.org
Philip Blumenthal, Director
**Fnded:** 1953. **Philosophy:** According to the foundation's literature, it considers grant requests, primarily in the Charlotte/Mecklenburg Co. area of North Carolina, in several fields including the following: religious and interfaith groups, social services, education, the arts and humanities, health care, the environment, and Jewish institutions and philanthropies. The foundation provides grants for seed money, annual operating budgets, capital campaigns, conferences and seminars, special projects, and endowments. **Priorities:** *Arts & Humanities:* 30%. Supports a number of organizations dedicated to fine arts. *Civic & Public Affairs:* 4%. Supports zoological services, community concerns, and leadership organizations. *Education:* 12%. Local and statewide initiatives. *Environment:* 12%. Supports youth. *International:* 1%. *Religion:* 2%. *Note:* Total contributions made in fiscal 1999. **Typ. Recipients:** Adolescent Health Issues, AIDS/HIV, Clinics/Medical Centers, Family Planning, Health Organizations, Hospitals, Mental Health, Single-Disease Health Associations, Substance Abuse. **Geo. Dist:** headquarters; Charlotte, NC. **Frmly:** Blumenthal Foundation for Charity, Religion and Education.

## ★ 83 ★ Bodman Foundation
767 Third Ave., 4th Floor
New York, NY 10017
**Phone:** (212)644-0322          **Fax:** (212)759-6510
**Email:** main@achelis-bodman-funds.org
**Website:** http://www.fducenter.org/grantmaker/achelis-bodman
Joseph Dolan, Secretary & Executive Director
**Fnded:** 1945. **Philosophy:** The foundation was set up to reflect the philanthropic interests of both Mr. and Mrs. Bodman, including religious, educational, and charitable organizations "for the moral, ethical, and physical well-being and progress of mankind." The foundation maintains a strong local orientation. The foundation has adopted a focus on putting responsible, full-time fathers back into two-parent intact families, as well as an emphasis on measurable outcomes of clients and program results in health and social-service agencies. Areas of interest include youth rehabilitation, biomedical research, child welfare, cultural institutions, health and hospitals, social services, education and job training, and job placement into private sector, prevention and early intervention, entrepreneurship, school reform and charter schools. **Priorities:** *Arts & Humanities:* 9%. Community programs and major cultural institutions. *Civic & Public Affairs:* 12%. Supports job training, public policy, and family issues. *Education:* 29%. Primarily precollege education, also supports literacy nad higher education. *Environment:* 17%. Boys and girls clubs, volunteerism, substance abuse programs, family services, and youth programs. *International:* 24%. Biomedical research, hospitals, and single-disease research. *Note:* Total contributions made in 1998. **Typ. Recipients:** Cancer, Child Abuse, Children's Health/Hospitals, Clinics/Medical Centers, Domestic Violence, Emergency/Ambulance Services, Eyes/Blindness, Health Funds, Health Organizations, Hospices, Hospitals, Medical Education, Medical Rehabilitation, Medical Research, Outpatient Health Care, People with Disabilities, Single-Disease Health Associations, Speech & Hearing, Substance Abuse, Transplant Networks/Donor Banks, Trauma Treatment. **Geo. Dist:** NJ, Northern New Jersey; New York, NY, metropolitan area.

## ★ 84 ★ Boettcher Foundation
600 Seventeenth St., Ste. 2210 South
Denver, CO 80202
**Phone:** (303)534-1937
**Email:** grants@boettcherfoundation.org
**Website:** http://www.boettcherfoundation.org
Timothy Schultz, President & Executive Director
**Fnded:** 1937. **Philosophy:** The foundation typically supports education, civic, health, cultural, and community groups. As education is a strong interest of the foundation, educational organizations consistently receive a large percentage of grants. In the area of civic and cultural programs, it emphasizes the economic development of Colorado communities through support of cultural and tourist attractions. In recent years, the foundation's health priorities have focused on programs enhancing cost containment efforts and preventative services, especially in rural areas of Colorado. In 1998, the largest dollar amounts awarded were for capital projects, such as building or equipment needs. The grants most frequently, were in the form of challenges. **Priorities:** *Arts & Humanities:* 9%. Performing arts, museums, historical centers, and archeology. *Civic & Public Affairs:* 5%. Supports gardens and aquariums, with minor support for community development. *Education:* 44%. Universities and educational programs; scholarships. *Environment:* 29%. Youth and child services, food banks, rehabilitation, and the disabled. *International:* 13%. Hospitals and health institutes. *Note:* Total contributions were made in 2000. **Typ. Recipients:** AIDS/HIV, Alzheimers Disease, Children's Health/Hospitals, Clinics/Medical Centers, Domestic Violence, Emergency/Ambulance Services, Eyes/Blindness, Family Planning, Health-General, Hospices, Hospitals, Long-Term Care, Medical Education, Medical Rehabilitation, Mental Health, Multiple Sclerosis, People with Disabilities, Preventive Medicine/Wellness Organizations, Public Health, Sexual Abuse, Single-Disease Health Associations, Substance Abuse. **Geo. Dist:** Denver, CO.

## ★ 85 ★ Booth-Bricker Fund
826 Union St., Ste. 300
New Orleans, LA 70112
**Phone:** (504)581-2430          **Fax:** (504)566-4785
Gray Parker, Chairman
**Fnded:** 1976. **Philosophy:** The Booth-Bricker Fund supports a variety of local organizations, "and makes contributions for the purposes of promoting, developing, and fostering religious, charitable, scientific, literary, or educational programs." Educational support is provided to universities, day schools, and private schools. Health care favors both general care and specialty hospitals in New Orleans. Museums, theater, and public broadcasting are favored areas of support for the arts. The fund also gives to local church organizations and provides general support for social service organizations. **Priorities:** *Arts & Humanities:* 13%. Supports music and museums, historic preservation, and public broadcasting. *Civic & Public Affairs:* 5%. Funds civic groups and public policy organizations. *Education:* 48%. Funds colleges, universities, and pre-college religious education. *Environment:* 14%. Contributes to children's groups, united funds, and community service organizations. *International:* 7%. Gives to medical centers, hospitals, and health associations. *Note:* Total contributions made in 1999. **Typ. Recipients:** Children's Health/Hospitals, Clinics/Medical Centers, Eyes/Blindness, Health Organizations, Hospitals, Hospitals (University Affiliated), Long-Term Care, People with Disabilities, Public Health, Single-Disease Health Associations. **Geo. Dist:** LA, priority given to New Orleans.

## ★ 86 ★ Booth Ferris Foundation
c/o Morgan Guaranty Trust Company of New York
60 Wall St., 46th Floor
New York, NY 10260
**Phone:** (212)809-1630          **Fax:** (212)648-5082
Hildy Simmons, Contact

**Fnded:** 1957. **Philosophy:** The foundation's primary funding area is education, "especially theological, smaller colleges, and independent secondary schools." Social service and cultural activities in New York City receive a limited number of contributions. Civic, social service, education, and religious projects are funded, but to a lesser degree. Support usually goes to established organizations, particularly those in which the donors were interested during their lifetimes. **Priorities:** *Arts & Humanities:* 21%. Funds museums, theaters, and the performing arts. *Civic & Public Affairs:* 12%. Funds community development and public policy. *Education:* 42%. Funds colleges and universities. *Environment:* 8%. Funds youth groups, children's charities, and social services. *Religion:* 5%. Supports a laboratory. *Note:* Total contributions made in fiscal 1998. **Typ. Recipients:** Children's Health/Hospitals, Emergency/Ambulance Services, Eyes/Blindness, Family Planning, Health Organizations, Hospitals, Nutrition, People with Disabilities, Research/Studies Institutes, Substance Abuse. **Geo. Dist:** nationally; New York, NY, metropolitan area.

### ★ 87 ★ Bothin Foundation
PO Box 29906
San Francisco, CA 94129-0906
**Phone:** (415)561-6540          **Fax:** (415)561-6477
**Website:** http://www.pacificfoundationservices.com
Lyman Casey, Executive Director & Treasurer
**Fnded:** 1926. **Philosophy:** With limited funds available, "the foundation traditionally has supported charitable organizations promoting youth, the elderly, the environment, the disabled, health care, minorities, community social services and the arts. Grants for the arts are made only to those groups predominantly serving youth or with heavy emphasis on youth participation. As a rule, the foundation prefers to make grants for capital or building and equipment needs." Annual Report **Priorities:** *Arts & Humanities:* 11%. Funds music, festivals, and art museums. *Civic & Public Affairs:* 15%. Supports civic and public policy. *Education:* 3%. Funds precollege education and educational programs. *Environment:* 50%. Supports food banks, shelters, disabled-citizen concerns, and youth groups. *International:* 4%. Funds health services for disadvantaged youth and children, hospice, and AIDS awareness. *Note:* Total contributions made in 1998. **Typ. Recipients:** AIDS/HIV, Cancer, Clinics/Medical Centers, Domestic Violence, Emergency/Ambulance Services, Eyes/Blindness, Family Planning, Health Organizations, Home-Care Services, Hospices, Hospitals, Kidney, Medical Rehabilitation, Mental Health, People with Disabilities, Prenatal Health Issues, Sexual Abuse, Speech & Hearing, Substance Abuse. **Geo. Dist:** San Francisco, CA, metropolitan area.

### ★ 88 ★ Bradley-Turner Foundation
PO Box 140
Columbus, GA 31902
**Phone:** (706)571-6040          **Fax:** (706)571-3408
Tom Black, Administrator
**Fnded:** 1943. **Philosophy:** The foundation generally funds higher educational institutions, arts and cultural organizations, religious associations, and social services. **Priorities:** *Arts & Humanities:* 4%. Supports museums, music, and historic preservation. *Civic & Public Affairs:* 20%. Supports housing, a cot foundation and towns/municipalities. *Education:* 46%. Supports colleges and universities, public and private schools. literacy and education foundations *Environment:* 14%. Funds youth programs, 4-H, scouting, recreation/athletics United Way, and YMCA. *International:* 6%. Supports hospitals, hospice, children's health, and single disease health associations. *Note:* Total contributions made in 1999. **Typ. Recipients:** Cancer, Child Abuse, Children's Health/Hospitals, Clinics/Medical Centers, Emergency/Ambulance Services, Health Organizations, Hospices, Hospitals, Hospitals (University Affiliated), Long-Term Care, Medical Education, Medical Rehabilitation, Medical Research, Outpatient Health Care, People with Disabilities, Single-Disease Health Associations. **Geo. Dist:** GA.

### ★ 89 ★ Britton Fund
1422 Euclid Ave., Ste. 1010
Cleveland, OH 44115-2078
**Phone:** (216)363-6489
Nick Valentino, Treasurer
**Fnded:** 1952. **Philosophy:** The fund generally supports medical organizations, community services, and educational institutions in the Cleveland, Ohio, area. **Priorities:** *Arts & Humanities:* 6%. Arts centers, music, and museums. *Civic & Public Affairs:* 1%. *Education:* 4%. Primarily for student aid. *Environment:* 18%. Food banks, shelters, family planning, community services, and YMCAs. *International:* 70%. Major grant to University Hospitals in Cleveland, Ohio. Also supports Alzheimer's research, medical rehabilitation, medical centers, and geriatric care. *Note:* Total contributions made in 1998. **Typ. Recipients:** Alzheimers Disease, Cancer, Children's Health/Hospitals, Clinics/Medical Centers, Domestic Violence, Emergency/Ambulance Services, Eyes/Blindness, Family Planning, Geriatric Health, Health Organizations, Hospitals, Hospitals (University Affiliated), Long-Term Care, Medical Education, Medical Rehabilitation, Medical Research, Mental Health, Multiple Sclerosis, Nursing Services, People with Disabilities, Sexual Abuse, Single-Disease Health Associations, Speech & Hearing. **Geo. Dist:** OH, Greater Cleveland including Cayahoga, Geauga, and lake counties.

### ★ 90 ★ Brown Foundation
PO Box 130646
Houston, TX 77219-0646
**Phone:** (713)523-6867          **Fax:** (713)523-2917
**Email:** bfi@brownfoundation.org
**Website:** http://www.brownfoundation.org
Nancy Pittman, Executive Director
**Fnded:** 1951. **Philosophy:** Since its establishment, the foundation has supported a variety of organizations, mostly in the state of Texas. Major areas of giving include education, the arts and humanities, health and medicine, civic & public affairs and human services. In the field of education, the foundation focuses on searching out and supporting non-traditional and innovative approaches designed to improve public education. **Priorities:** *Arts & Humanities:* 17%. Art galleries, arts centers, museums, music, and opera. Major support for the Smithsonian Institute. *Civic & Public Affairs:* 8%. Funds community and neighborhood affairs, housing, and public policy. *Education:* 34%. Engineering education, colleges and universities, faculty endowments, public and private schools, and scholarships. *Environment:* 16%. Funds human services, YMCA, services for the disabled, and youth organizations. *International:* 18%. Supports children's health care, organ donation centers, cancer research, hospitals, health clinics, and drug abuse programs. *Religion:* 2%. Supports science museums. *Note:* Total contributions made in fiscal 2000. **Typ. Recipients:** Adolescent Health Issues, Alzheimers Disease, Cancer, Child Abuse, Children's Health/Hospitals, Clinics/Medical Centers, Domestic Violence, Family Planning, Health Organizations, Heart, Hospices, Hospitals, Medical Education, Medical Research, Mental Health, People with Disabilities, Research/Studies Institutes, Single-Disease Health Associations. **Geo. Dist:** TX.

### ★ 91 ★ Broyhill Family Foundation
PO Box 500
Golfview Park
Lenoir, NC 28645
**Phone:** (828)758-6100
Paul Broyhill, Chairman & Manager
**Fnded:** 1945. **Philosophy:** The Broyhill Family Foundation, formerly the Broyhill Foundation, originally was established to help needy individuals obtain a college education through loans. The foundation also funds civic organizations, community and human services, hospitals and health organizations, and the arts. Although the foundation no longer offers loans directly to students, it is funding a Special Investment Loan Program available through the College Foundation, which provides student aid. **Priorities:** *Arts & Humanities:* 2%. Support given to art and culture. *Civic &*

*Public Affairs:* 27%. Funds community and public affairs. *Education:* 45%. Emphasis on educational institutions and programs, including colleges and universities. *Environment:* 14%. Grants were made to social, family, and youth services. *International:* 6%. Hospices, disease and disorder concerns, single-disease organizations, hospitals, and AIDS causes receive support. *Note:* Total contributions made in 1999. **Typ. Recipients:** Children's Health/Hospitals, Emergency/Ambulance Services, Eyes/Blindness, Health Organizations, Hospices, Hospitals, Medical Education, Medical Research, Mental Health, People with Disabilities, Preventive Medicine/Wellness Organizations, Public Health, Research/Studies Institutes, Substance Abuse. **Geo. Dist:** NC, preference to Cardwell County and surrounding areas.

### ★ 92 ★ The Bryant Foundation
PO Box 1239
Stephens City, VA 22655-1239
**Phone:** (540)662-3800          **Fax:** (540)662-3816
Arthur Bryant, II, President & Treasurer
**Fnded:** 1949. **Philosophy:** The foundation primarily is interested in supporting education in Virginia. Most of the giving focuses, but is not limited to, higher education. Smaller grants are made to other major categories of support. Other interests include libraries, community endowments, health services, religion, and community centers. Many of the foundation's secondary interests support athletic or recreational projects. **Priorities:** *Arts & Humanities:* 7%. Supports historical preservation and museums. *Education:* 88%. Supports colleges and universities and private pre-college schools. *Environment:* 1%. *International:* 3%. Supports hospitals and single-diseae health associations. *Note:* Total contributions made in 1998. **Typ. Recipients:** Cancer, Clinics/Medical Centers, Emergency/Ambulance Services, Health Organizations, Health-General, Hospitals, Long-Term Care, Medical Rehabilitation, Medical Research, Prenatal Health Issues, Public Health, Respiratory, Single-Disease Health Associations. **Geo. Dist:** VA.

### ★ 93 ★ Buchanan Family Foundation
222 East Wisconsin Ave.
Lake Forest, IL 60045
**Phone:** (847)234-0235
Huntington Eldridge, Jr., Treasurer
**Fnded:** 1967. **Philosophy:** The foundation generally supports hospitals and health organizations, cultural and environmental causes, and colleges and universities, all within the metropolitan Chicago, IL, area. **Priorities:** *Arts & Humanities:* 16%. Supports public broadcasting, festivals, libraries, historical society, music, and opera, symphony and theatres. *Civic & Public Affairs:* 15%. Supports aquarium, zoo, parks, and community foundations. *Education:* 19%. Supports colleges and universities, endowments and secondary schools. *Environment:* 8%. Supports community service organizations, scouts, YMCA and United Way. *International:* 25%. Supports hospitals and medical centers; research foundation. *Religion:* 7%. Funds planetarium, science museum. *Note:* Total contributions made in 1999. **Typ. Recipients:** Children's Health/Hospitals, Clinics/Medical Centers, Emergency/Ambulance Services, Family Planning, Health Organizations, Hospitals, Medical Rehabilitation, Medical Research, Nursing Services, Prenatal Health Issues, Single-Disease Health Associations. **Geo. Dist:** Chicago, IL.

### ★ 94 ★ Buhl Foundation (PA)
650 Smithfield St., Ste. 2300
Pittsburgh, PA 15222
**Phone:** (412)566-2711          **Fax:** (412)566-2714
**Email:** buhl@buhlfoundation.com
Doreen Boyce, President
**Fnded:** 1927. **Philosophy:** The foundation's focus is on innovation, with emphasis on funding "opportunities with potential impact beyond the institution which has been funded." The foundation's concerns include "the developing and harnessing of new technologies to address the administration and purposes of organizations or processes of learning and teaching;...the

investigation of problems with a view to generating creative solutions and cooperation among diverse disciplines or organizations;...(and) the generation and dissemination of new knowledge where that knowledge has the possibility of direct practical application." The foundation's board of managers designated that proposals with the following characteristics are of particular interest: educational programs; programs for young people; studies to produce practical applications which make a contribution to basic theory; attempts which relate specialists in a common approach to problems or which call for cooperative efforts among separate agencies; institutional, experimental, or demonstrational approaches to resolving problems when they are innovative; and previously supported and promising programs where time extension or new developments afford opportunity for enhancement of values. **Priorities:** *Arts & Humanities:* 18%. Funds the arts, theater, music, and libraries. *Civic & Public Affairs:* 10%. Funds community education and job training programs, community foundations, and leadership programs. *Education:* 42%. Funds colleges and universities, boards of education, and elementary education programs. *Environment:* 15%. Funds social services, rehabilitation centers, and the United Way. *Note:* Total contributions made in fiscal 2001. **Typ. Recipients:** Cancer, Child Abuse, Children's Health/Hospitals, Emergency/Ambulance Services, Health Organizations, Heart, Hospitals, Mental Health, Nursing Services, People with Disabilities, Sexual Abuse, Substance Abuse. **Geo. Dist:** Pittsburgh, PA, metropolitan area.

### ★ 95 ★ Bunbury Co., Inc.
2 Railroad Place
Hopewell, NJ 08525
**Phone:** (609)333-8800          **Fax:** (609)333-8900
**Email:** BunburyCo@aol.com
**Website:** http://www.bunburycompany.org
Garth Allen, Grants Manager

**Fnded:** 1952. **Philosophy:** "Through its grant making, Bunbury seeks to assist organizations working within a broad spectrum of philanthropic activities. Those organizations include, but are not limited to, those dealing with disadvantaged youth and families; ecology and the natural world, education in the broadest sense; and promotion of the arts." The Bunbury Company Application Guidelines **Priorities:** *Arts & Humanities:* 17%. Supports the performing arts, historical societies, and arts councils. *Civic & Public Affairs:* 17%. Supports community funds, fire departments, and trade organizations. *Education:* 37%. Supports colleges and universities, literacy, and education foundations. *Environment:* 9%. Supports family planning, family and youth services, and housing. *International:* 6%. Supports a medical center. *Note:* Total contributions made in 1999. **Typ. Recipients:** AIDS/HIV, Cancer, Clinics/Medical Centers, Domestic Violence, Emergency/Ambulance Services, Family Planning, Hospitals, Medical Research, Mental Health, Nursing Services, People with Disabilities, Public Health, Substance Abuse. **Geo. Dist:** NJ, Burlington County; NJ, Camden County; NJ, Hunterdon County; NJ, Middlesex County; NJ, Monmouth County; NJ, Ocean County; NJ, Somerset County; NJ, Mercer County.

### ★ 96 ★ Burnett Foundation
801 Cherry St., Ste. 1585
Unit 16
Fort Worth, TX 76102-6881
**Phone:** (817)877-3344          **Fax:** (817)338-0448
Thomas Beech, Executive Vice President

**Fnded:** 1978. **Philosophy:** The Burnett Foundation was founded in 1978 by Anne Burnett Tandy. Since its earliest days the Foundation's grants have reflected the philosophy and special genius of its founder. "Organization-Building grants that help nonprofit organizations become more effective, more responsive and more creative in carrying out their missions. In several instances, the Foundation's support has helped create new organizations. "Community-Building grants that help the citizens of a community capitalize and build on their community's strengths and develop strategies to deal with challenges and opportunities facing them. Most of the Foundation's

Community-Building grants have targeted inner-city neighborhoods. "Grants have been made in the fields of arts and humanities, health, human services, community development and education. Historically, the Foundation has focused its energy and resources in Fort Worth, Texas and in the last few years also in Sante Fe, New Mexico." 1996 Annual Report **Priorities:** *Arts & Humanities:* 75%. Major support is given to museums, also supports music, opera, art festivals, ballet, and the performing arts. *Civic & Public Affairs:* 16%. Supports parks, housing, and community foundation. *Education:* 6%. Supports scholarship and universities. *Environment:* 2%. Supports United Way, food distribution, Young Women's Christian Association, youth programs, and counseling. *International:* 1%. Substance abuse and AIDS prevention. *Note:* Total contributions made in 2000. **Typ. Recipients:** AIDS/HIV, Alzheimers Disease, Cancer, Child Abuse, Children's Health/Hospitals, Clinics/Medical Centers, Domestic Violence, Emergency/Ambulance Services, Family Planning, Health Policy/Cost Containment, Hospitals, Medical Education, Medical Research, Mental Health, People with Disabilities, Prenatal Health Issues, Research/Studies Institutes, Sexual Abuse, Single-Disease Health Associations, Substance Abuse. **Geo. Dist:** occasionally grants are provided nationally, at the trustee's discretion; Santa Fe, NM; Ft. Worth, TX.

### ★ 97 ★ Burton D. Morgan Foundation
PO Box 1500
Akron, OH 44309-1500
**Phone:** (330)258-6512          **Fax:** (330)258-6559
John Frank, President

**Fnded:** 1967. **Philosophy:** The Burton D. Morgan Foundation primarily supports education, including private Episcopal schools and universities. Other interests include churches, arts centers, art associations, and civic affairs in northeastern Ohio. The foundation's present areas of focus include programs to support the free/private enterprise system, economics, education, and mental health. **Priorities:** *Arts & Humanities:* 5%. Supports public broadcasting, music, and history. *Civic & Public Affairs:* 46%. Supports the EAA Aviation Foundation, community foundations, urban and economic development, philanthropic causes, and employment. *Education:* 28%. Focus on colleges and universities and education associations. *Environment:* 3%. Supports Young Men's Christian Association and general social services. *International:* 2%. Supports children's health and hospitals. *Note:* Total contributions made in 2000. **Typ. Recipients:** Children's Health/Hospitals, Domestic Violence, Emergency/Ambulance Services, Family Planning, Health Organizations, Heart, Hospices, Hospitals, Medical Education, Mental Health, Nursing Services, People with Disabilities, Public Health, Research/Studies Institutes, Substance Abuse. **Geo. Dist:** OH, Summit County.

### ★ 98 ★ Burton G. Bettingen Corp.
9777 Wilshire Boulevard, Ste. 615
Beverly Hills, CA 90212
**Phone:** (310)276-4115          **Fax:** (310)276-4693
Patricia Brown, Executive Director

**Fnded:** 1984. **Philosophy:** The current focus of the corporation is child welfare including assistance to child prostitutes, runaways, and abandoned children. The corporation has two separate giving funds: the Haven Fund is committed to supporting child welfare; the General Fund includes support for youth but also supports organizations in several fields including education, health, environment, and welfare. The corporation provides broad types of support including program, capital funds, research, and endowments. **Priorities:** *Arts & Humanities:* 3%. Supports museums and public television. *Civic & Public Affairs:* 10%. Supports community development and philanthropy concerns. *Education:* 14%. Supports educational programs, schools, colleges and universities. *Environment:* 33%. Supports youth services and social services. *International:* 30%. Supports health and medical centers, hospitals, disease and disorder concerns. *Note:* Contributions made in fiscal 1999. **Typ. Recipients:** AIDS/HIV, Alzheimers Disease, Cancer, Child

Abuse, Children's Health/Hospitals, Emergency/Ambulance Services, Family Planning, Health Organizations, Health Policy/Cost Containment, Home-Care Services, Hospitals, Hospitals (University Affiliated), Long-Term Care, Medical Education, Medical Research, Mental Health, People with Disabilities, Preventive Medicine/Wellness Organizations, Research/Studies Institutes, Respiratory, Sexual Abuse, Single-Disease Health Associations, Substance Abuse. **Geo. Dist:** Los Angeles, CA.

### ★ 99 ★ Bush Foundation
E-900 First National Bank Bldg.
332 Minnesota St.
Saint Paul, MN 55101
**Phone:** (651)227-0891          **Fax:** (651)297-6485
**Email:** info@bushfoundation.org
**Website:** http://www.bushfoundation.org
Anita Pampusch, President

**Fnded:** 1953. **Philosophy:** The foundation was incorporated with the broadest possible statement of purpose. It concentrates its grants in the areas of education, humanities and the arts, community and social welfare, health, and leadership development. The foundation is predominantly a regional giver, making grants primarily in Minnesota, North Dakota, and South Dakota. However, it operates two non-regional grant programs, offering grants to historically black private colleges and grants to accredited tribally controlled Indian colleges. The foundation's matching capital grants program and faculty development program for black private colleges is run in cooperation with the William and Flora Hewlett Foundation of Menlo Park, CA. Grants to education programs take the form of faculty development and matching capital grants for undergraduate colleges in Minnesota and the Dakotas; faculty development and matching capital grants to historically black private colleges; grants to encourage elementary and secondary school age girls and all minority students to pursue math and science education; faculty development grants to Indian colleges. In the area of health, the foundation supports programs to improve the quality, accessibility, and efficiency of health care services within its geographic region. Grants are concentrated on training programs for health professionals, efforts to improve access to health care in rural and under-served areas, and the promotion of minority career development in the health field. Human services funding supports programs for troubled and disadvantaged youth; emergency housing and employment counseling services for homeless women with children; programs to assist victims of domestic violence; and programs that provide rehabilitation services for developmentally disabled adults. Other interests include rural economic development, rural family assistance programs, and law and corrections. The Bush Leadership Fellows Program provides full-time mid-career study and development support to emerging leaders in a variety of fields. The Bush Medical Fellows Program seeks to develop physicians' potential for increased competence and leadership in clinical medicine, health care delivery, administration, and education. The Bush Artist Fellowships Program offers stipends to talented artists in literature, visual arts, and the performing arts. Miscellaneous grants are made to community foundations and such areas as public broadcasting and the environment. **Priorities:** *Arts & Humanities:* 16%. Focus on public broadcasting, museums, theaters, music, arts centers, and arts funds. *Civic & Public Affairs:* 20%. Funds community foundations, employment, and housing. *Education:* 34%. Emphasis on colleges and universities primarily in Minnesota, North Dakota, and South Dakota. Fellowships are also supported. *Environment:* 22%. Support for youth organizations, child welfare, immigrant programs, and family services. *International:* 6%. Funds hospitals and direct health care organizations. *Note:* Total contributions made in fiscal 2000. **Typ. Recipients:** AIDS/HIV, Children's Health/Hospitals, Clinics/Medical Centers, Domestic Violence, Family Planning, Health Organizations, Health-General, Medical Education, Medical Rehabilitation, Medical Training, Mental Health, Nursing Services, People with Disabilities, Public Health, Sexual Abuse, Substance Abuse. **Geo. Dist:** nationally; MN; ND; SD.

## ★ 100 ★ Byrne Foundation
35 Rope Ferry Rd.
Hanover, NH 03755
**Phone:** (603)643-4555
Dorothy Byrne, President

**Fnded:** 1993. **Philosophy:** The foundation's primary interests include cancer research, Dartmouth College, and general philanthropy. **Priorities:** *Arts & Humanities:* 2%. Supports public broadcasting. *Civic & Public Affairs:* 4%. Supports community foundations, economic development. *Education:* 27%. Supports secondary schools, Dartmouth College. *Environment:* 6%. Funds community centers, youth programs, services for the elderly. *International:* 57%. Supports cancer research centers. *Note:* Total contributions made in 1998. **Typ. Recipients:** Cancer, Child Abuse, Children's Health/Hospitals, Clinics/Medical Centers, Emergency/Ambulance Services, Health Organizations, Hospices, Hospitals, Medical Rehabilitation, Medical Research, Multiple Sclerosis, People with Disabilities, Public Health, Respiratory, Substance Abuse. **Geo. Dist:** NH, Upper Valley Region; VT, Upper Valley Region.

## ★ 101 ★ Cabot Family Charitable Trust
One Post Office Square
Boston, MA 02109
**Phone:** (617)622-3600
Ruth Scheer, Executive Director

**Fnded:** 1942. **Philosophy:** The trust supports colleges and universities, the arts, scientific organizations, and civic causes. Giving is generally limited to the greater Boston, Massachusetts, area. **Priorities:** *Arts & Humanities:* 16%. Supports orchestra, museums. *Civic & Public Affairs:* 13%. Supports libraries, community foundations. *Education:* 18%. Supports colleges and universities. *Environment:* 28%. Supports family services, YMCA, family planning. *International:* 5%. Supports community health center. *Religion:* 2%. Supports scientific organization. *Note:* Total contributions made in 1998. **Typ. Recipients:** Children's Health/Hospitals, Clinics/Medical Centers, Family Planning, Health Organizations, Hospitals, Medical Education, Mental Health, People with Disabilities, Public Health. **Geo. Dist:** CA; MA.

## ★ 102 ★ The California Endowment
21650 Oxnard St.
Ste. 1200
Woodland Hills, CA 91367
**Phone:** (818)703-3311  **Fax:** (818)703-8640
**Email:** phinz@calendow.org
**Website:** http://www.calendow.org
Peggy Hinz, Vice President

**Fnded:** 1996. **Philosophy:** "The foundation's mission is to improve access to affordable, quality health care for underserved individuals and communities and to promote fundamental improvements in the health status of all Californians." **Priorities:** *Civic & Public Affairs:* 37%. Supports community foundations, legal aid, economic development organizations. *Education:* 3%. Supports medical education. *Environment:* 7% Supports substance abuse coalition, homes, community centers, senior services and the homeless. *International:* 50%. Supports health services, public health institutes and foundations, clinics, hospitals, the uninsured and medically underserved. *Note:* Total contributions made in fiscal 1999. **Typ. Recipients:** Adolescent Health Issues, AIDS/HIV, Cancer, Child Abuse, Children's Health/Hospitals, Clinics/Medical Centers, Domestic Violence, Eyes/Blindness, Family Planning, Geriatric Health, Health Funds, Health Organizations, Health Policy/Cost Containment, Health-General, Hospitals, Medical Rehabilitation, Mental Health, Nutrition, People with Disabilities, Prenatal Health Issues, Public Health, Public Health, Research/Studies Institutes, Respiratory. **Geo. Dist:** CA.

## ★ 103 ★ Callaway Foundation, Inc.
209 Broome St.
PO Box 790
LaGrange, GA 30240
**Phone:** (706)884-7348  **Fax:** (706)884-0201

**Email:** jtgresham@calloway-foundation.org
J. Gresham, President

**Fnded:** 1943. **Philosophy:** The philosophy of the Callaway Foundation was initiated by Fuller E. Callaway, Sr., who had a profound interest in the "health, education, and welfare of the people in the community in which he lived and did business." The foundation is primarily intended for religious, charitable, and educational benefits to the people in Troup County and LaGrange, GA. The foundation prefers to provide capital funds for established and active community organizations, especially those that offer lasting benefit to the community. The foundation also supports organizations and projects considered worthy by others as evidenced by various sources of support. The board of trustees will consider matching funds for such groups and to qualifying churches within the city limits of LaGrange. **Priorities:** *Arts & Humanities:* 10%. Supports arts centers, museums, music, and the performing arts. *Civic & Public Affairs:* 33%. Funds municipalities and housing. *Education:* 38%. Focus on LaGrange College and Georgia Tech. *International:* 6%. Major support for West Georgia Health System. *Note:* Total contributions made in fiscal 2000. **Typ. Recipients:** AIDS/HIV, Alzheimers Disease, Cancer, Clinics/Medical Centers, Emergency/Ambulance Services, Eyes/Blindness, Family Planning, Health Organizations, Health Policy/Cost Containment, Heart, Hospitals, Long-Term Care, Medical Education, Medical Rehabilitation, People with Disabilities, Public Health, Single-Disease Health Associations, Substance Abuse, Transplant Networks/Donor Banks. **Geo. Dist:** LaGrange, GA, including Troup County.

## ★ 104 ★ Camp Airy and Camp Louise Foundation
5750 Park Heights Ave.
Baltimore, MD 21215
**Phone:** (410)466-9010  **Fax:** (410)466-0560
**Email:** airlou@airylouise.org
**Website:** http://www.airylouise.org
Ms. Jan Rivitz, Executive Director

**Fnded:** 1926. **Philosophy:** The foundation owns and operates two summer camps. Revenue is raised by charging those campers able to pay, a tuition. This helps to offset the costs of operating the camps, which is the primary service of the foundation. **Typ. Recipients:** AIDS/HIV, Cancer, Children's Health/Hospitals, Clinics/Medical Centers, Diabetes, Emergency/Ambulance Services, Family Planning, Geriatric Health, Heart, Hospitals, Kidney, Long-Term Care, Medical Research, Multiple Sclerosis, People with Disabilities, Public Health, Single-Disease Health Associations, Substance Abuse. **Geo. Dist:** Washington, DC; Baltimore, MD. **Frmly:** Aaron and Lillie Straus Foundation.

## ★ 105 ★ Carl J. Herzog Foundation
321 Railroad Ave.
Greenwich, CT 06830
**Phone:** (203)629-2424  **Fax:** (203)629-2545
David Babson, Jr., Treasurer & Director

**Fnded:** 1952. **Philosophy:** The Carl J. Herzog Foundation is primarily interested in supporting medical research and dermatology. **Priorities:** *Civic & Public Affairs:* Less than 1%. Supports community foundations. *Education:* About 64%. Primarily supports medical education, primarily in the field of dermatology. *International:* About 35%. Supports international and domestic health care. *Note:* Contributions made in 1998. **Typ. Recipients:** Cancer, Clinics/Medical Centers, Health Funds, Health Organizations, Health-General, Hospitals, Hospitals (University Affiliated), Medical Education, Medical Research, Research/Studies Institutes, Single-Disease Health Associations, Substance Abuse. **Geo. Dist:** nationally.

## ★ 106 ★ Carl and Lily Pforzheimer Foundation
650 Madison Ave., 23rd Floor
New York, NY 10022
**Phone:** (212)223-6500  **Fax:** (212)223-2693
Mary Kitabjian, III, Executive Assistant

**Fnded:** 1942. **Philosophy:** Some of the major responsibilities of the foundation include the continuing publication of scholarly material directly related to the Carl H. Pforzheimer Collection of Shelley and His Circle, previously owned by the foundation and now located at the New York Public Library. It also supports scholarly works by leading university presses of books dealing with fields in which the foundation has a major interest, such as English and American literature. In general, the foundation provides limited support to ongoing programs in education, health care, the arts, and organizations with which the foundation is familiar. While the foundation does not make grants to individuals, it does donate to institutions that may sponsor individuals working in fields or on projects closely identified with the previously mentioned interests. **Priorities:** *Arts & Humanities:* 18%. Funds dance, theater, libraries, music, and cultural concerns. *Civic & Public Affairs:* 3%. Gives to community development, and civic groups. *Education:* 70%. Supports colleges and universities, literacy programs, and precollege education. *Environment:* 3%. Funds children's groups and community centers. *International:* 6%. Supports medical centers. *Note:* Total contributions made in 1998. **Typ. Recipients:** AIDS/HIV, Clinics/Medical Centers, Emergency/Ambulance Services, Eyes/Blindness, Hospitals, Nursing Services, People with Disabilities, Substance Abuse. **Geo. Dist:** nationally; New York, NY.

## ★ 107 ★ Carolyn Foundation
901 Marquette Ave., Ste. 2630
Minneapolis, MN 55402
**Phone:** (612)596-3266  **Fax:** (612)338-2084
**Email:** carolyn@winternet.com
**Website:** http://www.carolynfoundation.org
Carol Fetzer, Foundation Administrator

**Fnded:** 1964. **Philosophy:** The Carolyn Foundation is interested principally in health and welfare, education, the arts, programs addressing social problems, and the environment. It is a regional foundation and limits funding to Minneapolis and St. Paul, MN, and New Haven, CT, and to some national environmental organizations with programs affecting these areas. **Priorities:** *Arts & Humanities:* 20%. Funds ballet, public broadcasting, music, and theater. *Civic & Public Affairs:* 15%. Supports community projects, housing, community development and women's affairs. *Education:* 15%. Gives to universities, prepatory schools, literacy and arts/ humanities education. *Environment:* 29%. Funds family welfare, family planning services, youth programs, and United Way. *International:* 5%. Supports cancer and general health. *Note:* Total contributions made in 2000. **Typ. Recipients:** Child Abuse, Children's Health/Hospitals, Clinics/Medical Centers, Domestic Violence, Emergency/Ambulance Services, Family Planning, Health Organizations, Hospitals, Medical Rehabilitation, Mental Health, Nursing Services, People with Disabilities, Research/Studies Institutes, Substance Abuse. **Geo. Dist:** New Haven, CT; Minneapolis-St. Paul, MN.

## ★ 108 ★ Carrie Estelle Doheny Foundation
707 Wilshire Boulevard, Ste. 4960
Los Angeles, CA 90017
**Phone:** (213)488-1122  **Fax:** (213)488-1544
**Email:** doheny@dohenyfoundation.org
**Website:** http://www.dohenyfoundation.org
Shirley Bernard, Senior Grants Administrator

**Fnded:** 1948. **Philosophy:** The foundation was established "for the advancement of education, medicine, religion, science, the improvement of the health and welfare of infants, children, adults, families, the help and care of the sick, the aged and the incapacitated, and aid to the needy." The foundation supports a variety of local organizations, with emphasis on Roman Catholic groups, medical research, hospital care, education, child health and welfare, and assistance to the sick and needy. **Priorities:** *Education:* 24%. Supports higher and secondary educational institutions and programs. *Environment:* 13%. Supports family services. *International:* 21%. Funds hospitals, medical centers, and disease and disorder concerns. *Note:* Total contributions made in 1998. **Typ. Recipi-**

ents: Cancer, Children's Health/Hospitals, Clinics/ Medical Centers, Domestic Violence, Emergency/Ambulance Services, Eyes/Blindness, Family Planning, Health Organizations, Heart, Hospitals, Long-Term Care, Medical Research, Medical Training, Nutrition, People with Disabilities, Prenatal Health Issues, Public Health, Research/Studies Institutes, Single-Disease Health Associations, Speech & Hearing. **Geo. Dist:** nationally.

## ★ 109 ★ Cele H. and William B. Rubin Family Fund

32 Monadnock Rd.
Wellesley Hills, MA 02481-1338
**Phone:** (781)235-4751          **Fax:** (781)235-4692
Ellen Gordon, President

**Fnded:** 1943. **Philosophy:** The Cele H. and William B. Rubin Family Fund gives across the major categories of support, but primarily focuses on civic affairs and higher education. Civic interests include economic development, housing programs, and zoos and parks. The foundation also supports women's affairs within these categories of support. **Priorities:** *Arts & Humanities:* 67%. Primary support goes to the Old Colony Charitable Fund. Also funds performing arts and libraries. *Civic & Public Affairs:* Less than 1%. Supports women's affairs, ethnic organizations, and other charitable organizations. *Education:* 25%. Colleges, universities, business schools, educational foundations, and private schools. *Environment:* 1%. Funds YMCAs, United Way, youth programs, and food banks. *International:* 4%. Supports single-disease societies and institutes. *Note:* Total contributions made in 2000. **Typ. Recipients:** Alzheimers Disease, Arthritis, Cancer, Clinics/Medical Centers, Diabetes, Health Organizations, Heart, Hospices, Hospitals, Kidney, Medical Education, Medical Rehabilitation, Medical Research, Multiple Sclerosis, People with Disabilities, Prenatal Health Issues, Public Health, Research/Studies Institutes, Single-Disease Health Associations. **Geo. Dist:** nationally.

## ★ 110 ★ Champlin Foundation

300 Centerville Rd., Ste. 300S
Warwick, RI 02886-0226
**Phone:** (401)736-0370          **Fax:** (401)736-7248
**Email:** champlinfdns@worldnet.att.net
**Website:**          http://www.fndcenter.org/grantmaker/ champlin

**Fnded:** 1932. **Philosophy:** The aim of the foundations is to provide funds to Rhode Island organizations helping the broadest possible segment of the population. The foundations are interested in preserving land for recreation and open space. The foundations support land protection efforts in conjunction with the Nature Conservancy, the Rhode Island Department of Environmental Management, and the Audubon Society of Rhode Island. Although cultural projects involving libraries and library services receive considerable support, the foundations generally do not support the arts. Funding is offered instead to organizations with constituencies that are unable to provide monetary support. Some interest is shown for historic preservation efforts. The foundations have developed a scholarship program enabling Rhode Island public high school students to attend Brown University, and have recently instituted a program to fund equipment for Rhode Island public schools. They also have an interest in social service agencies, facilities for youth, hospitals, and health care agencies. **Priorities:** *Arts & Humanities:* 28%. Supports historic preservation, public libraries, museums, and public broadcasting. *Civic & Public Affairs:* 1%. Supports volunteer fire companies. *Education:* 13%. Majority of support to public elementary schools for educational equipment. *Environment:* 28%. Supports housing, family planning, substance abuse prevention, youth and fitness, and animal humane societies. *International:* 8%. Funds construction and mortgage costs for medical facilities. *Note:* Giving analysis provided by foundation. Total contributions made in 2000. **Typ. Recipients:** Clinics/Medical Centers, Emergency/Ambulance Services, Family Planning, Geriatric Health, Health Funds, Health Organizations, Health-General, Heart, Hospices, Hospitals, Long-Term Care, Medical Rehabilita-

tion, Nursing Services, People with Disabilities, Prenatal Health Issues, Public Health, Transplant Networks/ Donor Banks. **Geo. Dist:** Providence, RI.

## ★ 111 ★ Charles A. Dana Foundation

745 Fifth Ave., Ste. 700
New York, NY 10151
**Phone:** (212)223-4040          **Fax:** (212)317-8721
**Email:** danainfo@dana.org
**Website:** http://www.dana.org
William Safire, Chairman & Chief Executive Officer

**Fnded:** 1950. **Philosophy:** In health, the foundation will concentrate on neuroscience, and identify programs and investigators that can apply recent discoveries in neuroscience research to the treatment of the problems of memory loss, genetic basis of manic-depression, and language-based learning disorders. In addition, the foundation will support centers with advanced neuro-imaging capability to train the neuroscience leadership needed to promote the application of such technologies to neuroscience research. Most of the foundation's resources in health will support these efforts. Applicants should be aware that funds for other initiatives will be quite limited. The foundation's education program will seek projects that have an impact on key developments in pre-college education, including the evolution of fundamentally new American schools, the redefinition of public policy to reduce obstacles to school restructuring, the involvement of parents in successful education, and the integration of technology into schools in ways that advance school restructuring. As specific goals in these areas are defined, the foundation anticipates approaching institutions with the demonstrated capacity to mount programs to achieve these goals. The Dana Alliance for Brain Initiatives was created in 1993 to help educate the public and policy makers through the media about brain research and advancements in neuroscience. **Priorities:** *Arts & Humanities:* 3%. Funds libraries and music. *Education:* 23%. Mainly funds college and university projects to support education of the public about the importance of brain research. *International:* 73%. Focus on brain diseases and disorders–long term, multifaceted support, and short-term, flexible support. *Note:* Total contributions made in 1998. **Typ. Recipients:** AIDS/HIV, Cancer, Children's Health/Hospitals, Clinics/Medical Centers, Emergency/Ambulance Services, Geriatric Health, Health Organizations, Health Policy/Cost Containment, Health-General, Heart, Hospitals, Medical Education, Medical Research, Medical Training, Mental Health, Multiple Sclerosis, People with Disabilities, Public Health, Single-Disease Health Associations, Speech & Hearing, Substance Abuse. **Geo. Dist:** nationally.

## ★ 112 ★ Charles A. Frueauff Foundation

Three Financial Center
900 South Shackleford, Ste. 300
Little Rock, AR 72211
**Phone:** (501)219-1410          **Fax:** (501)219-1416
**Website:** http://www.frueaufffoundation.com
Sue Frueauff, Program Officer

**Fnded:** 1950. **Philosophy:** The Charles A. Frueauff Foundation's main areas of support are higher education, social services, health agencies and hospitals. The foundation reports that it is currently focusing on welfare reform and daycare. **Priorities:** *Arts & Humanities:* 11%. Funds libraries and music. *Education:* 42%. Primary support for colleges and universities. *Environment:* 25%. Supports child welfare, family services, people with disabilities, shelters, and youth organizations. *International:* 18%. Supports hospitals, hospices, and single-disease health associations. *Note:* Total contributions made in 1998. **Typ. Recipients:** Children's Health/Hospitals, Clinics/Medical Centers, Emergency/Ambulance Services, Health Organizations, Hospices, Hospitals, Medical Education, Nursing Services, People with Disabilities, Public Health, Substance Abuse, Transplant Networks/Donor Banks. **Geo. Dist:** east of the Rocky Mountains.

## ★ 113 ★ Charles Edison Fund

One Riverfront Plaza, 4th Floor
Newark, NJ 07102
**Phone:** (973)648-0500          **Fax:** (973)675-3345
**Email:** info@charlesedisonfund.org
**Website:** http://www.charlesedisonfund.org
John Keegan, President & Chairman

**Fnded:** 1948. **Philosophy:** "The Charles Edison Fund is an endowed philanthropic institution dedicated to the support of worthwhile endeavors generally within the areas of medical research, science education and historic preservation. The fund is an extension of the benefactions and aspirations of its Founder, a man of discerning foresight, rare achievement and background." "In more recent years a pattern of giving has emerged within the Fund. Its contributions tend to be almost equally divided among medical research projects, science education and historic preservation. Additionally, but with some exceptions, institutions and organizations assisted are based principally in the New York-New Jersey Metropolitan area. This concentration of interest facilitates the efforts of the Trustees to evaluate the work of recipient groups, frequently accomplished by personal visitations." **Priorities:** *Arts & Humanities:* 22%. Supports the Thomas Edison Preservation Society. *Civic & Public Affairs:* 23%. Supports Edison Ford Winter Estates; community foundations. *Education:* 45%. Supports colleges, education institutes, universities and foundations. *Environment:* 2%. Supports a Police Athletic League. *International:* 8%. Supports medical research. *Note:* Total contributions made in 1998. **Typ. Recipients:** Arthritis, Cancer, Children's Health/Hospitals, Clinics/Medical Centers, Diabetes, Eyes/Blindness, Hospitals, Hospitals (University Affiliated), Medical Education, Medical Rehabilitation, Medical Research, Medical Training, Mental Health, People with Disabilities, Prenatal Health Issues, Single-Disease Health Associations, Speech & Hearing, Trauma Treatment. **Geo. Dist:** NJ, primarily metropolitan area; NY, primarily metropolitan area.

## ★ 114 ★ Charles Engelhard Foundation

645 5th Ave.
New York, NY 10022
**Phone:** (212)935-2430          **Fax:** (212)935-2434
Mary Ogorzaly, Contact

**Fnded:** 1949. **Philosophy:** The foundation gives to a variety of cultural, civic, and educational organizations. Less emphasis is placed on religion and social services. **Priorities:** *Arts & Humanities:* 28%. Museums, libraries, and art centers. *Civic & Public Affairs:* 6%. Primary support for foundations. *Education:* 23%. Primarily supports secondary schools. *Environment:* 3%. Supports family programs. *International:* 20%. Hospitals and medical institutes. *Note:* Total contributions made in 1998. **Typ. Recipients:** AIDS/HIV, Cancer, Children's Health/Hospitals, Clinics/Medical Centers, Family Planning, Health Organizations, Health-General, Home-Care Services, Hospices, Hospitals, Medical Education, Medical Research, People with Disabilities, Preventive Medicine/Wellness Organizations, Public Health, Single-Disease Health Associations, Substance Abuse. **Geo. Dist:** nationally; Washington, DC; Missoula, MT; New York, NY; Houston, TX.

## ★ 115 ★ Charles G. Koch Charitable Foundation

655 15th St., Ste. 445
Washington, DC 20005-2001
**Phone:** (202)393-2354          **Fax:** (202)393-2355
Kelly Young, Vice President

**Fnded:** 1981. **Philosophy:** "The Foundation's mission is to advance the well-being of humanity through the development of a free and civil society. To achieve this mission, we essentially fund research and education programs that examine the benefits of using market-process analysis to develop solutions to critical social problems. The Foundation elects to focus specifically on the following issues: environment, labor, legal, and fiscal." **Priorities:** *Arts & Humanities:* 3%. Supports the Kansas Cultural Trust. *Civic & Public Affairs:* 20%. Supports philanthropic causes, civic and community services. *Education:* 71%. Supports education programs, schools and universities. *International:* 3%. Supports the Steadman Sports Medicine Foundation. *Note:* Contributions were made in 1998. **Typ. Recipients:** Clinics/Medical Centers, Medical Research. **Geo. Dist:** nationally; KS; LA; MN; OK; TX.

## ★ 116 ★ Charles Hayden Foundation

130 Liberty St., Ste. 2707
New York, NY 10006-1196
**Phone:** (212)938-0790
Kenneth Merin, President, Chief Executive Officer

**Fnded:** 1937. **Philosophy:** "The Charles Hayden Foundation seeks to promote the mental, moral, and physical development of school-aged youth in the New York and Boston metropolitan areas. Our focus is on those institutions and programs primarily serving youth most a risk of not reaching their full potential, especially youth in low-income communities. Priority is given to programs that intervene early in young people's lives and continuously provide opportunities and support over an extended period. The Foundation looks for the same attributes whether program or capital support is being sought." "Program support grants are focused on efforts to help youth develop the skills and knowledge needed to succeed in school and lay the foundations for satisfying and productive lives. Programs must have well-defined goals that are expected to be met in a specified time frame. Priority is given to: expanding community-based programs offering youth educational, social, recreational and career services (e.g. after school programs); and improving student achievement by strengthening K-12 education, especially elementary and middle school education, for youth in Boston and New York City and in nearby cities of Cambridge, Chelsea, Newark and Jersey City. Most public school support gets to charter schools for capital or for program purposes. K-12 support goes to efforts using independent school resources to expand opportunities for needy inner-city youth. The foundation also supports efforts to strengthen informal education enrichment programs offered outside of schools in institutions such as museums and zoos." "Capital support grants go for renovation, expansion, construction and acquisition of physical facilities and purchase and repair of non-expendable equipment. Emphasis is on assisting those organizations in need of physical facilities to improve the availability and quality of programs for young people. While we acknowledge the problem of deferred maintenance in youth-serving facilities, we will look carefully at the record of past attention to maintenance and an organization's long-term strategy for repair and renovation. Organizations eligible for capital grants include: youth-serving agencies and other community-based organizations whose facilities are largely used by and for youth development; non-public educational institutions serving needy students; charter schools that lack access to significant capital support from local public sources; children's museums, theaters and performing groups; and science and environmental centers with facilities used specifically for youth-oriented activities." 1996 Annual Report **Priorities:** *Arts & Humanities:* 7%. Funds libraries and children's museums. *Civic & Public Affairs:* 25%. Supports nonprofit management organizations, and civic ventures. *Education:* 17%. Supports after school and enrichment programs. *Environment:* 35%. Supports community service organizations, camps, community centers, scouts and at-risk youth programs. *Religion:* 10%. Funds the American Museum of Natural History. *Note:* Total contributions made in fiscal 2000. **Typ. Recipients:** AIDS/HIV, Family Planning, Hospitals, People with Disabilities, Research/Studies Institutes, Substance Abuse. **Geo. Dist:** Boston, MA, metropolitan area; New York, NY, metropolitan area.

## ★ 117 ★ Charles J. Strosacker Foundation

PO Box 471
Midland, MI 48640-0471
**Phone:** (517)839-0300
Karen Willard, Administrative Assistant

**Fnded:** 1957. **Philosophy:** The foundation was established "to assist and benefit political subdivisions of the State of Michigan, and religious, charitable, benevolent, scientific, or educational organizations." **Priorities:** *Arts & Humanities:* 2%. Supports arts centers, museums, visual arts, and historic preservation. *Civic & Public Affairs:* 23%. General civic interests, largely in the Midland, MI, area, including community foundations, parks, and county fairs. *Education:* 37%. Universities, colleges, secondary schools, arts education, legal and medical education, and minority education. *Environment:* 16%. Donates to American Red Cross, domestic violence council, united funds, family services, Young Men's Christian Association, and youth programs. *International:* 18%. Funds medical centers, AIDS organizations, and general health concerns. *Religion:* 3%. Supports the Michigan Molecular Institute. *Note:* Total contributions made in 2000. **Typ. Recipients:** AIDS/HIV, Clinics/Medical Centers, Domestic Violence, Emergency/Ambulance Services, Family Planning, Geriatric Health, Health Organizations, Health Policy/Cost Containment, Hospices, Hospitals, Medical Education, Mental Health, Nursing Services, Public Health, Substance Abuse, Transplant Networks/Donor Banks. **Geo. Dist:** Midland, MI, some statewide funding.

## ★ 118 ★ Charles and M. R. Shapiro Foundation

200 North LaSalle St., Ste. 2100
Chicago, IL 60601
**Phone:** (312)346-3100     **Fax:** (312)621-1750
**Email:** nshubert@muchlaw.com
Norman Shubert, President

**Fnded:** 1958. **Philosophy:** The Charles and M. R. Shapiro Foundation makes most of its grants to Jewish religious organizations. A secondary interest is Jewish education. Minor grants go to civic affairs, health, social services, and the arts. **Priorities:** *Arts & Humanities:* About 4%. *Civic & Public Affairs:* 3%. *Education:* 27%. Religious education, colleges and universities, and special education. *Environment:* 11%. Youth organizations, the elderly, and community services. *International:* 14%. Alzheimer's research, emergency health care, and cancer research. *Note:* Total contributions made in fiscal 1999. **Typ. Recipients:** Alzheimers Disease, Cancer, Emergency/Ambulance Services, Geriatric Health, Hospices, Hospitals, Medical Research, Multiple Sclerosis, People with Disabilities, Single-Disease Health Associations. **Geo. Dist:** nationally; Chicago, IL.

## ★ 119 ★ Charles Stewart Mott Foundation

Office of Proposal Entry
Mott Foundation Bldg.
503 S Saginaw St., Suite 1200
Flint, MI 48502-1851
**Phone:** (810)238-5651     **Fax:** (810)766-1753
**Email:** infocenter@mott.org
**Website:** http://www.mott.org

**Fnded:** 1926. **Philosophy:** Founder Charles Stewart Mott believed that "every person, always, is in a kind of informal partnership with his community. His own success is dependent to a large degree on that community, and the community, after all, is the sum total of the individuals who make it up." Grant making is now organized in four programs: Civil Society, Environment, Flint Area, and Poverty. In addition, the foundation maintains the flexibility to investigate new opportunities through an Exploratory and Special Projects program. Fundamental to all grant making are certain values: learning how people can live together to create a sense of community, whether at the neighborhood level or as a global society; building strong communities through collaboration to provide a basis for positive change; nurturing strong, self-reliant individuals to ensure a well-functioning society; promoting the social, economic, and political empowerment of all individuals to preserve fundamental democratic principles and rights; encouraging responsible citizen participation to help foster social cohesion; developing leadership to build upon the needs and values of people and to inspire the aspirations and potential of others; and respecting the diversity of life to maintain a sustainable human and physical environ-

ment. In the Environment giving area, the goal is "to support efforts of an engaged citizenry working to create accountable and responsive institutions, sound public policies, and appropriate models of development that protect the diversity and integrity of selected ecosystems in North America and around the world". In the Flint Area, the goal is "to foster a well-functioning, connected community that is capable of meeting the economic, social, and racial challenges ahead". Grantmaking is focused in four areas: Developing Public Capital, Creating National Models, Building Upon Legacy, and Effecting Public Policy. Poverty giving focuses on improving life outcomes for children, youth, and families in low-income communities. At its core, this program centers upon the importance of families and communities working together on behalf of children. Its areas of interest are the following: building communities to provide strong, safe environments that nurture and ensure growth opportunities for children, youth, and families; strengthening families so they can nurture children and youth and create strong communities; improving education to enable children, youth, and families to have access to paths out of poverty, and to serve as a resource to strengthen communities; and expanding economic opportunity to provide economic empowerment, job creation, and increased income to enable families to move out of poverty. The Exploratory and Special Projects program is home to a number of grants that the foundation views as special opportunities but that do not easily fit into its program structure. These activities encompass a broad range of fields. **Priorities:** *Civic & Public Affairs:* 44%. *Education:* 21%. *Environment:* Less than 1%. Supports scouting and United Way. **Typ. Recipients:** AIDS/HIV, Family Planning, Health Policy/Cost Containment, Home-Care Services, People with Disabilities, Public Health, Research/Studies Institutes, Substance Abuse. **Geo. Dist:** internationally; nationally; Flint, MI.

## ★ 120 ★ Chatlos Foundation

PO Box 915048
Longwood, FL 32791-5048
**Phone:** (407)862-5077
**Email:** grant-manager@chatlos.org
**Website:** http://www.chatlos.org
William Chatlos, President

**Fnded:** 1953. **Philosophy:** The Chatlos Foundation gives funding priority to Bible colleges, religious causes, medical issues, liberal arts colleges, and social concerns. The foundation prefers to provide program support. As a result, the foundation makes fewer grants to capital funds, conference expenses, administrative costs, multiyear grants or computer projects. **Priorities:** *Education:* 41%. Supports school, colleges, universities, scholarship, and religious education. *Environment:* 2%. Supports scouts, homeless/shelters, young men's christian association, substance abuse, the disabled and the aged, food distribution, and prison alternatives. *International:* 30%. Supports children's health, AIDS, and medical centers. *Note:* Total contributions made in 2000. **Typ. Recipients:** AIDS/HIV, Arthritis, Cancer, Children's Health/Hospitals, Clinics/Medical Centers, Emergency/Ambulance Services, Eyes/Blindness, Health Organizations, Heart, Hospitals, Hospitals (University Affiliated), Long-Term Care, Medical Education, Medical Research, Nursing Services, People with Disabilities, Public Health, Trauma Treatment. **Geo. Dist:** nationally.

## ★ 121 ★ Chauncey and Marion Deering McCormick Foundation

410 North Michigan Ave., Room 590
Chicago, IL 60611
**Phone:** (312)644-6720     **Fax:** (312)644-7555
Lawson Whitesides, Jr., President

**Fnded:** 1957. **Philosophy:** The foundation primarily concentrates on local giving to organizations such as arts institutions, hospitals, universities, museums, wildlife conservation groups, private secondary schools, churches, and social services agencies. The foundation supports capital campaigns, art purchases, library funds, and building funds. **Priorities:** *Arts & Humanities:* 18%. Supports art institutes, libraries, museums, the theater, and the performing arts. *Civic & Public Affairs:* 14%. Supports animal services zoos. *Education:* 23%. Supports schools, colleges and universities. *Environment:* 14%. Supports child welfare, planned parenthood, and the United Way. *International:* 19%. Supports hospices, hospitals, and medical centers. *Religion:* 1%. Supports science research and institutions. *Note:* Total contributions made in fiscal 1999. **Typ. Recipients:** Cancer, Clinics/Medical Centers, Emergency/Ambulance Services, Family Planning, Health Organizations, Hospices, Hospitals, Hospitals (University Affiliated), Medical Education, Medical Rehabilitation, Medical Research, Mental Health, Single-Disease Health Associations. **Geo. Dist:** Chicago, IL, metropolitan area.

★ 122 ★ **Chichester duPont Foundation**
3120 Kennett Pike
Wilmington, DE 19807
**Phone:** (302)658-5244          **Fax:** (302)658-5091
Gregory Fields, Secretary

**Fnded:** 1946. **Philosophy:** The foundation is primarily interested in supporting today's youth. Giving goes to social service organizations for the direct benefit of children. Most of the support is for operating budgets and capital campaigns. Another interest is education at the primary and secondary levels. Giving has been for endowment funds and youth recreation facilities in schools. The foundation also gives to civic affairs and organizations' building funds and operating budgets. The arts and health are minimally supported. **Priorities:** *Arts & Humanities:* 7%. Primarily the performing arts. *Civic & Public Affairs:* 1%. *Education:* 11%. Funds precollege education. *Environment:* 42%. Primarily youth recreation facilities. *International:* 13%. Gives to pediatric health. *Note:* Total contributions made in 1997. **Typ. Recipients:** Arthritis, Cancer, Child Abuse, Children's Health/Hospitals, Clinics/Medical Centers, Emergency/Ambulance Services, Family Planning, Health Organizations, Heart, Hospices, Hospitals, Long-Term Care, Medical Education, Medical Rehabilitation, Medical Research, Nursing Services, People with Disabilities, Preventive Medicine/Wellness Organizations, Public Health, Single-Disease Health Associations, Substance Abuse. **Geo. Dist:** mid-Atlantic United States; northeastern United States.

★ 123 ★ **Chiles Foundation**
111 Southwest Fifth Ave., Ste. 4050
Portland, OR 97204
**Phone:** (503)222-2143          **Fax:** (503)228-7079
**Email:** cf@usnet.net
Earle Chiles, President & Trustee

**Fnded:** 1941. **Philosophy:** "The foundation's principal purposes are to assist and support higher education, medical advancement, and arts and culture." **Priorities:** *Arts & Humanities:* 16%. Supports music, performing arts, museum, dance, and history, and public broadcasting. *Civic & Public Affairs:* 1%. Funds ethnic organizations. *Education:* 64%. Supports school, colleges, universities, and religious education. *Environment:* 4%. Supports recreation. *International:* 8%. Supports hospital, geriatrics, and medical research. *Note:* Total contributions made in 1999. **Typ. Recipients:** Cancer, Clinics/Medical Centers, Emergency/Ambulance Services, Health Funds, Heart, Hospitals, Medical Research, Multiple Sclerosis, Nursing Services, Prenatal Health Issues, Public Health, Single-Disease Health Associations. **Geo. Dist:** primarily Pacific Northwest.

★ 124 ★ **China Medical Board of New York**
750 3rd Ave., 23rd Floor
New York, NY 10017-2701
**Phone:** (212)682-8000          **Fax:** (212)949-8726
**Email:** mschwarz@chinamedicalboard.org
Dr. M. Schwarz, President

**Fnded:** 1928. **Philosophy:** The board's primary interest is supporting medical, nursing, and public health education and research. Contributions are made to eleven different countries and territories in East and Southeast Asia, as directed by its charter. "The Board

is especially interested in grants to advance the recipient institution's pursuit of excellence and for the enhancement of the academic and professional content of medical, nursing, and public health education and training." The board also reports that it has a program for higher education in nursing. Categories of support programs include national fellowship grants, regional fellowship grants, research grants, education grants, and endowment grants. In addition, the Medical Education for Students in Rural Areas project enables students to receive basic medical science education at Chulalongkorn Faculty of Medicine in Bangkok and their clinical education in one of two provincial hospitals. **Priorities:** *Note:* Total contributions made in fiscal 1999. **Typ. Recipients:** Health Organizations, Medical Education, Medical Research. **Geo. Dist:** East and Southeast Asia.

★ 125 ★ **Chisholm Foundation**
114 W 47th St.
New York, NY 10036-1532
**Phone:** (212)852-3834
Vincent Scalice, Contact

**Fnded:** 1960. **Philosophy:** The foundation typically supports secondary and higher education, public policy groups, the arts, and social services. **Priorities:** *Arts & Humanities:* 10%. Museums, arts institutes, theater, and opera received funding. *Civic & Public Affairs:* 19%. Supports public policy organizations, community affairs groups, and arboretums and gardens, and women's affairs. *Education:* 35%. Emphasis on Millsaps College; funds private schools and colleges and universities. *Environment:* 8%. Contributions go to family services, animal rescue, scouts, sexual violence centers, shelters, and United Way. *International:* 24%. Funds hospital and cancer centers. *Note:* Total contributions made in 1999 **Typ. Recipients:** AIDS/HIV, Cancer, Children's Health/Hospitals, Clinics/Medical Centers, Domestic Violence, Emergency/Ambulance Services, Geriatric Health, Health-General, Hospitals, Sexual Abuse, Single-Disease Health Associations, Transplant Networks/Donor Banks. **Geo. Dist:** DC; MS; New York, NY.

★ 126 ★ **Christy-Houston Foundation**
1296 Dow St.
Murfreesboro, TN 37130
**Phone:** (615)898-1140          **Fax:** (615)895-9524
**Email:** christy-houston@mindspring.com
Robert Mifflin, Executive Director

**Fnded:** 1987. **Philosophy:** The foundation is dedicated to the "improvement of the quality of life for the citizens and residents of Rutherford County, TN, with an emphasis on the promotion and enhancement of health care." The foundation has reported that it is placing a greater focus on social services in Rutherford County, TN, and that it plans in the future to fund a Boys and Girls Club, a YMCA, and a senior citizen's center. **Priorities:** *Arts & Humanities:* 7%. Supports museum. *Civic & Public Affairs:* 36%. Supports towns/municipalities and parks. *Education:* 2%. Supports school, universities, and scholarship. *Environment:* 4%. Supports daycare, people with disabilities, and community service organizations. *International:* 51%. Funds nursing homes. *Note:* Total contributions made in fiscal 1999. **Typ. Recipients:** Clinics/Medical Centers, Emergency/Ambulance Services, Health Organizations, Heart, Hospices, Hospitals, Medical Education, Public Health. **Geo. Dist:** Rutherford County, TN.

★ 127 ★ **Claneil Foundation**
630 West Germantown Pike, Ste. 400
Plymouth Meeting, PA 19462-1059
**Phone:** (610)828-6331          **Fax:** (610)828-6405
Dr. Henry Jordan, President & Executive Director

**Fnded:** 1968. **Philosophy:** The foundation typically supports human service organizations, health-related organizations, and civic concerns. **Priorities:** *Arts & Humanities:* 4%. Primarily for historic preservation. *Civic & Public Affairs:* 18%. Community foundations, women's affairs, and economic development. *Education:* 8%. Colleges and universities, faculty development, special education, and minority education. *Environment:* 29%. Community services, family services,

and shelters. *International:* 21%. Trauma treatment, hospitals, prenatal care, geriatrics, and long-term care. *Note:* Total contributions made in 1999. **Typ. Recipients:** AIDS/HIV, Alzheimers Disease, Cancer, Children's Health/Hospitals, Clinics/Medical Centers, Domestic Violence, Family Planning, Geriatric Health, Health Organizations, Home-Care Services, Hospitals, Long-Term Care, Medical Education, Medical Research, Mental Health, Prenatal Health Issues, Preventive Medicine/Wellness Organizations, Single-Disease Health Associations, Substance Abuse, Trauma Treatment. **Geo. Dist:** MA; PA; PA, southeastern.

★ 128 ★ **Clara Blackford Smith and W. Aubrey Smith Charitable Foundation**
330 W Main St.
Denison, TX 75020
**Phone:** (903)415-2300
Linda Hunt, Board Member

**Fnded:** 1985. **Philosophy:** "The Clara Blackford Smith and W. Aubrey Smith Charitable Foundation was established under the will of Mrs. Smith and the funds are to be used exclusively for religious, charitable, educational, scientific and literary purposes. The Foundation is administered by NationsBank of Texas, N.A. The by-laws state the Foundation generally will limit support to non-profit organizations within the State of Texas, primarily in Grayson County." 1997 Grant Application Information Sheet **Priorities:** *Arts & Humanities:* 1%. Supports performing arts and museums. *Civic & Public Affairs:* 34%. Primarily for community organizations in the city of Denison. *Education:* 12%. Public education, colleges, universities, literacy, scholarship, student aid and minority education. *Environment:* 19%. Supports programs for athletics/recreation, camps, shelters, and United Way. *International:* 34%. Funds medical center, public health, and rehabilitation centers. *Note:* Total contributions made in fiscal 2000. **Typ. Recipients:** Cancer, Clinics/Medical Centers, Diabetes, Domestic Violence, Emergency/Ambulance Services, Geriatric Health, Health Funds, Health Organizations, Hospices, Hospitals, Medical Education, Medical Rehabilitation, Medical Research, Nursing Services, People with Disabilities, Public Health, Substance Abuse. **Geo. Dist:** TX, primarily Grayson County.

★ 129 ★ **Clark-Winchcole Foundation**
3 Bethesda Metro Center, Ste. 550
Bethesda, MD 20814
**Phone:** (301)654-3607
Vincent Burke, President & Trustee

**Fnded:** 1964. **Philosophy:** The foundation gives to broad purposes in the Washington, DC, area, with emphasis on social services and the arts. **Priorities:** *Arts & Humanities:* 30%. Supports museums, performing arts, and historical preservation. *Education:* 27%. Student aid, secondary education, and literacy programs. *Environment:* About 13%. Funds social welfare and youth groups. *International:* About 13%. American Red Cross, hospitals, and health foundations. *Note:* Total contributions made in 1998. **Typ. Recipients:** Cancer, Children's Health/Hospitals, Clinics/Medical Centers, Emergency/Ambulance Services, Health Organizations, Hospices, Hospitals, Long-Term Care, Medical Rehabilitation, Mental Health, Nursing Services, People with Disabilities, Public Health, Research/Studies Institutes, Single-Disease Health Associations, Speech & Hearing, Substance Abuse. **Geo. Dist:** Washington, DC, including metropolitan area.

★ 130 ★ **Claude Worthington Benedum Foundation**
1400 Benedum-Trees Bldg.
223 Fourth Ave.
Pittsburgh, PA 15222
**Phone:** (412)288-0360          **Fax:** (412)288-0366
**Website:** http://www.fdncenter.org/grantmaker/benedum
William Getty, President & Trustee

**Fnded:** 1944. **Philosophy:** The foundation operates two grantmaking programs, one in West Virginia and one in the Pittsburgh Region. West Virginia Program: In education, the foundation wants to encourage public education reform with teachers and administrators; support a fundamental reform of teacher education; use the strengths of higher education to serve the needs of the state; and support measures that strengthen the state's independent colleges. In health, the foundation wants to reshape the rural health care delivery by fostering new and more effective systems of service; encourage community-based initiatives in disease prevention and health promotion; foster research and analysis of rural health policy; and support health education to restructure rural health care. In community improvement, the foundation wants to support programs that encourage, enable and empower local residents; understands that local action must include housing, recreation, leisure activities, libraries, small businesses and the arts; recognizes that adequate shelter is the first prerequisite for decent living and development of affordable housing must be a priority. In economic development, the foundation will work with intermediaries to develop alternate economic opportunities; encourages economic development strategies that build upon West Virginia's human, natural, physical, technological and other resources; and encourages the wise use of land and water resources for environmental responsibility and economic gain. In the arts, the foundation seeks to strengthen arts organizations that provide educational, social and economical renewal; believes the major art organizations benefit themselves, their regions and the state by improving their quality and their capacity to reach new audiences; and will work with intermediaries to provide technical assistance to large and small arts organizations. Pittsburgh Region Grants Program: In regional economic development the foundation wants to encourage development focusing on job creation; promote public-private sector collaborations; support initiatives of the Cultural District and its resident art organizations to strengthen their financial viability, improve programs and build new audiences; and provide on-going support to the United Way. **Priorities:** *Arts & Humanities:* 28%. Supports symphony, opera, and ballet. *Civic & Public Affairs:* 19%. Supports economic development and employment/job training. *Education:* 21%. Supports educational foundations, initiatives, programs, and institutions. *Environment:* 19%. Supports homes, family services, domestic violence prevention, and United Way. *International:* 5%. Supports health funds and organizations. *Note:* Total contributions made in 1998. **Typ. Recipients:** Children's Health/Hospitals, Clinics/Medical Centers, Diabetes, Domestic Violence, Emergency/Ambulance Services, Health Organizations, Health Policy/Cost Containment, Hospitals, Medical Education, Nursing Services, Nutrition, People with Disabilities, Prenatal Health Issues, Preventive Medicine/Wellness Organizations, Public Health, Research/Studies Institutes. **Geo. Dist:** Pittsburgh, PA; WV.

### ★ 131 ★ Clay Foundation
1426 Kanawha Boulevard, East
Charleston, WV 25301
**Phone:** (304)344-8656          **Fax:** (304)344-3805
Charles Avampato, President
**Fnded:** 1987. **Philosophy:** The Clay Foundation was established "to promote and enhance the quality of life of the citizens of West Virginia." The foundation's goal is to fund innovative projects or support services which best serve the residents of the state. Although the foundation considers requests from a broad range of organizations, it currently has a special interest in programs in the field of aging; health care research and education; vocational education programs; and services to disadvantaged youth and their families. **Priorities:** *Arts & Humanities:* 53%. Funds art center construction, opera, symphony and museum. *Civic & Public Affairs:* 7%. Supports economic development, community foundations and libraries. *Education:* 32%. Fund higher and precollege education, after school programs and literacy. *Environment:* 8%. Provides funding for housing, United Way and indigent families. *Note:* Total contributions made in 1998. **Typ. Recipients:** Children's Health/Hospitals, Clinics/Medical Centers, Health Organizations, Health Policy/Cost Containment, Hospices, Hospitals, Medical Education,

Mental Health, People with Disabilities, Preventive Medicine/Wellness Organizations, Speech & Hearing. **Geo. Dist:** WV.

### ★ 132 ★ Clayton Fund
PO Box 2558
Houston, TX 77252-8037
**Phone:** (713)216-4513
Charlene Slack, Grants Management
**Fnded:** 1989. **Philosophy:** The trust was created for charitable or educational purposes. These purposes include aid to the needy, especially children; the environment; family planning; education; agriculture; and arts and culture. **Priorities:** *Arts & Humanities:* 4%. Supports opera, theater, and music. *Civic & Public Affairs:* 3%. Urban/community affairs and clubs. *Education:* About 43%. Medical education, colleges and universities, and minority education. *Environment:* About 27%. Planned Parenthood, food banks, and youth organizations. *International:* 3%. Public health issues and children's health. *Note:* Total contributions made in 1998. **Typ. Recipients:** Cancer, Children's Health/Hospitals, Clinics/Medical Centers, Domestic Violence, Emergency/Ambulance Services, Family Planning, Health Organizations, Heart, Hospitals, Hospitals (University Affiliated), Medical Education, Mental Health, People with Disabilities, Prenatal Health Issues, Public Health, Single-Disease Health Associations, Transplant Networks/Donor Banks. **Geo. Dist:** nationally.

### ★ 133 ★ Cleveland H. Dodge Foundation
670 West 247th St.
Bronx, NY 10471
**Phone:** (718)543-1220          **Fax:** (718)543-0737
Phyllis Criscuoli, Executive Director & Treasurer
**Fnded:** 1917. **Philosophy:** The foundation gives priority to organizations supported by the donor and members of his family that continue to perform effective services. In keeping with Cleveland Dodge's philanthropic beliefs, the foundation also funds "institutions aiming to build good moral character in youth without being narrowly sectarian or seeking to proselytize, including social agencies serving needy youth." **Priorities:** *Arts & Humanities:* 20%. Supports libraries and museums. *Civic & Public Affairs:* 20%. Funds parks and gardens. *Education:* 39%. Gives to higher education. *Environment:* 12%. Funds youth groups and community services. *Note:* Total contributions made in 1998. **Typ. Recipients:** Emergency/Ambulance Services, Family Planning, Health Organizations, Nursing Services, People with Disabilities, Public Health. **Geo. Dist:** Northeastern United States; AZ; NM; New York, NY, including metropolitan area.

### ★ 134 ★ Clipper Ship Foundation
Grants Management Associates
77 Summer St., 8th Floor
Boston, MA 02110
**Phone:** (617)426-7172          **Fax:** (617)426-5441
**Email:** philanthropy@grantsmanagement.com
**Website:** http://www.grantsmanagement.com
Anna Karlsson, Foundation Assistant
**Fnded:** 1979. **Philosophy:** The foundation's principal objective is to assist nonprofit, operating organizations serving the Boston community and help them broaden the scope of their activities and fulfill their goals. Special attention will be given to those organizations involved with "the homeless, the destitute, the handicapped, children and the aged, or supplying the special needs of minority, low-income individuals and families." Worldwide disaster relief is also an occasional concern of the foundation. **Priorities:** *Civic & Public Affairs:* 37%. Supports community affairs and economic development. *Environment:* 63%. Funds health and human services. Supports child welfare, people with disabilities, and emergency services. *Note:* Total contributions made in fiscal 1999. **Typ. Recipients:** AIDS/HIV, Clinics/Medical Centers, Domestic Violence, Emergency/Ambulance Services, Eyes/Blindness, Family Planning, Hospices, Hospitals, Long-Term Care, Medical Rehabilitation, Mental Health, Nursing Services, People with Disabilities, Prenatal Health Issues, Preventive Medicine/Wellness

Organizations, Public Health, Speech & Hearing, Substance Abuse. **Geo. Dist:** Boston, MA, within Route 128 area and cities of Brockton, MA.

### ★ 135 ★ Clowes Fund
320 N Meridian, Ste. 316
Indianapolis, IN 46204-1722
**Phone:** (317)833-0144          **Fax:** (317)833-0145
**Email:** staff@dowesfund.org
Elizabeth Casselman, Exec. Dir.
**Fnded:** 1952. **Philosophy:** The fund typically supports higher educational institutions, the performing arts, and social services, primarily in Indiana and Massachusetts. **Priorities:** *Arts & Humanities:* 32%. Supports museums, the performing arts, cultural centers and theaters. *Civic & Public Affairs:* 6%. Funds housing, zoos and parks, and urban affairs. *Education:* 35%. Literacy, scholarships, and endowments. *Environment:* 11%. Supports youth organizations, child welfare, and substance abuse prevention. *International:* 2%. Health associations and funds, and hospitals. *Note:* Total contributions made in 1998. The fund typically does not support environmental causes, health, or religion. **Typ. Recipients:** Child Abuse, Children's Health/Hospitals, Clinics/Medical Centers, Diabetes, Domestic Violence, Family Planning, Health Funds, Health Organizations, Hospices, Hospitals, Hospitals (University Affiliated), Medical Education, Medical Research, Nursing Services, Outpatient Health Care, People with Disabilities, Respiratory, Substance Abuse. **Geo. Dist:** Indianapolis, IN; MA.

### ★ 136 ★ Cockrell Foundation
1600 Smith, Ste. 3900
Houston, TX 77002-7348
**Phone:** (713)209-7500          **Fax:** (713)209-7599
**Email:** mnw@cockrell.com
M. Williams, Executive Vice President
**Fnded:** 1966. **Philosophy:** The Cockrell Foundation is a family organization serving primarily the Houston area. The foundation is required by the last will and testament of Ernest Cockrell, Jr., to give one-half of annual funding to the University of Texas at Austin School of Engineering. It outlines no giving priorities for remaining funds and gives to a variety of areas. **Priorities:** *Arts & Humanities:* About 3%. Natural science and fine arts museums. *Civic & Public Affairs:* About 39%. Community Support. *Education:* 14%. Higher education and continuing education programs. *Environment:* About 26%. Youth and human services. *International:* 18%. Supports hospitals, medical centers, and specified disease organizations. *Note:* Total contributions made in 1999. **Typ. Recipients:** Adolescent Health Issues, Alzheimers Disease, Cancer, Child Abuse, Children's Health/Hospitals, Clinics/Medical Centers, Diabetes, Emergency/Ambulance Services, Eyes/Blindness, Family Planning, Health Organizations, Heart, Hospices, Hospitals, Medical Research, Mental Health, People with Disabilities, Prenatal Health Issues, Single-Disease Health Associations, Speech & Hearing. **Geo. Dist:** Houston, TX.

### ★ 137 ★ Coleman Foundation (IL)
575 West Madison St., Ste. 4605-II
Chicago, IL 60661-2549
**Phone:** (312)902-7120          **Fax:** (312)902-7124
**Email:** Coleman@colemanfoundation.org
**Website:** http://www.colemanfoundation.org
Michael Hennessy, President
**Fnded:** 1953. **Philosophy:** The foundation traditionally supports secondary and higher educational institutions, hospitals, medical training, and health organizations concerned with a single disease. Community and youth-oriented human service organizations are also supported. Limited funding goes to civic and cultural organizations. Program areas funded by the foundation include entrepreneurship awareness education, cancer research in the Midwest, housing and education of the handicapped, and education. **Priorities:** *Arts & Humanities:* 3%. Supports historical museums. *Civic & Public Affairs:* 7%. Supports community development and entrepreneurship. *Education:* 55%. Funds scholarship, universities and colleges, entrepreneurship, society, religious education, arts/humanities edu-

cation, business education, medical education and agricultural education. *Environment:* 2%. Supports community services, Big Brothers/Big Sisters, homes, food distribution, Young Men's Christian Association, and athletics/recreation. *International:* 31%. Supports medical centers, cancer, eyes/blindness, health care organizations, hospice, and hospital. *Note:* Total contributions made in 1999. **Typ. Recipients:** AIDS/HIV, Cancer, Clinics/Medical Centers, Eyes/Blindness, Health Organizations, Hospices, Hospitals, Hospitals (University Affiliated), Medical Education, Medical Rehabilitation, Medical Research, People with Disabilities, Preventive Medicine/Wellness Organizations, Public Health, Research/Studies Institutes, Sexual Abuse, Single-Disease Health Associations. **Geo. Dist:** nationally; especially the midwest; Chicago, IL.

### ★ 138 ★  Collins Foundation
1618 Southwest 1st Ave., Ste. 305
Portland, OR 97201-5708
**Phone:** (503)227-7171          **Fax:** (503)295-3794
**Website:** http://www.collinsfoundation.org
Dr. Jerry Hudson, Executive Vice President

**Fnded:** 1947. **Philosophy:** The foundation was established to use its funds for religious, charitable, and educational purposes within the state of Oregon. It is always open to new ideas and causes which it can support. It looks favorably on small, creative programs that can serve the community. **Priorities:** *Arts & Humanities:* 33%. Supports museums, performing arts, libraries, and public broadcasting. *Civic & Public Affairs:* 4%. Supports community affairs, an aquarium, and housing. *Education:* 18%. Supports higher education and educational programs. *Environment:* 23%. Supports YMCA, youth organizations, and human services. *International:* 8%. Supports hospitals, medical centers, community health, and single disease associations. *Religion:* 2%. Supports a science museum. *Note:* Contributions were made in 1999. **Typ. Recipients:** Alzheimers Disease, Cancer, Children's Health/Hospitals, Clinics/Medical Centers, Emergency/Ambulance Services, Family Planning, Health Funds, Health Organizations, Health Policy/Cost Containment, Heart, Hospices, Hospitals, Hospitals (University Affiliated), Medical Research, Mental Health, People with Disabilities, Prenatal Health Issues, Preventive Medicine/Wellness Organizations, Public Health, Research/Studies Institutes, Substance Abuse, Trauma Treatment. **Geo. Dist:** OR.

### ★ 139 ★  Colorado Trust
1600 Sherman St.
Denver, CO 80203-1604
**Phone:** (303)837-1200          **Fax:** (303)839-9034
**Email:** christie@coloradotrust.org
**Website:** http://www.coloradotrust.org
Christie McElhinney, Senior Communications Officer

**Fnded:** 1985. **Philosophy:** The mission of The Colorado Trust is to involve citizens in community change, develop human potential, and promote the health and well-being of the people of Colorado. To fulfill its mission, the foundation supports innovative projects, conducts studies, develops services and provides education to produce long-lasting benefits. The Trust has developed these initiatives: *Community Action for Health Promotion Initiative (1995-2002)* Designed to increase local health-promotion activities in Colorado and to build the capacity of Colorado communities to identify and address preventable health problems, the initiative is a seven-year $5.2 million program. More than 50 communities in Colorado will receive funding, primarily for these subject areas: adolescent mental health, adolescent pregnancy, child abuse and neglect, chronic disease, congenital abnormalities and infant mortality, dental health, elderly mental health, injuries, low birth-weight, the effects of poverty on child health, reproductive health, substance abuse, tobacco use, and violence. *Colorado Violence Prevention Initiative (1995-2002)* This seven-year, $8.8 million initiative is designed to prevent violence in Colorado communities. The program includes three areas of emphasis: a four-year public education campaign conducted by public television station KRMA-Channel Six; a program of statewide planning and implementation grants for up to 23 communities managed by the

Center for Public-Private Center Cooperation of the University of Colorado at Denver; a collaborative effort with other foundations in the Alliance for Violence Prevention which "seeks to educate grantmakers about the causes of violence and prevention activities that have proven effective; and study gun violence among youth in Colorado." *Coalition for the Medically Underserved (1997-2000)* In 1997, a 35-member coalition, representing health-care providers and agencies, health insurance companies, businesses, and state and county governments began meeting to identify solutions for improving access to quality health care for the medically underserved in Colorado. The Colorado Trust has allocated grants to the coalition to continue its work to remove any substantial differences in access to quality health care by the year 2007. *Community Voices: Healthcare for the Underserved Initiative (1999-2003)* In partnership with the W.K. Kellogg Foundation, The Colorado Trust has awarded Denver Health Medical Center a $2.4 million grant over five years to improve access to health-care services for Denver's medically underserved population. *Assets for Colorado Youth Initiative (1996-2002)* This five-and-one-half year, $10 million initiative is designed to help families, communities, and organizations build "developmental assets" that all young people need to grow up healthy, caring, and responsible. **Priorities:** *Arts & Humanities:* 1%. *Education:* 12%. Focus on health education. *Environment:* 41%. Youth initiatives, child care, family/child development, and violence prevention. *International:* 35%. Supported medically underserved, children's immunization programs, nursing, healthy communities, and local health promotion initiatives. **Typ. Recipients:** Adolescent Health Issues, AIDS/HIV, Children's Health/Hospitals, Clinics/Medical Centers, Domestic Violence, Emergency/Ambulance Services, Family Planning, Geriatric Health, Health Funds, Health Organizations, Health Policy/Cost Care, Medical Education, Medical Research, Mental Health, Nursing Services, Nutrition, People with Disabilities, Prenatal Health Issues, Preventive Medicine/Wellness Organizations, Public Health, Sexual Abuse, Single-Disease Health Associations, Substance Abuse, Transplant Networks/Donor Banks. **Geo. Dist:** CO.

### ★ 140 ★  The Commonwealth Fund
1 East 75th St.
New York, NY 10021-2692
**Phone:** (212)535-0400          **Fax:** (212)606-3500
**Email:** cmwf@cmwf.org
**Website:** http://www.cmwf.org
Andrea Landes, Director, Grants Management

**Fnded:** 1918. **Philosophy:** The fund's current giving is focused on seven areas: improving health care services, advancing the well-being of elderly people, developing the capacities of children and young people, bettering the health of minority Americans, promoting international exchange on health policy, improving the quality of life in New York City, and communicating results to stimulate change. Internationally, since 1925, the fund has also awarded Harkness Fellowships to enable citizens of the United Kingdom, Australia, and New Zealand to study and travel in the United States. In 1998, the fund announced two new programs: The Pediatric Developmental Service Program and the Health Care in New York City Program. **Priorities:** *Civic & Public Affairs:* 13%. Supports economic policy and public policy. *Education:* 42%. Supports medical education. *International:* 45%. Supports medical research, geriatric health, health policy public health and research institutes. *Note:* Total contributions made in 1998. **Typ. Recipients:** Adolescent Health Issues, Cancer, Children's Health/Hospitals, Clinics/Medical Centers, Diabetes, Domestic Violence, Family Planning, Geriatric Health, Health Funds, Health Organizations, Health Policy/Cost Containment, Health-General, Heart, Home-Care Services, Hospitals, Long-Term Care, Medical Education, Medical Research, Medical Training, Mental Health, Nursing Services, Prenatal Health Issues, Preventive Medicine/Wellness Organizations, Public Health, Research/Studies Institutes, Substance Abuse. **Geo. Dist:** national; some emphasis on New York City.

### ★ 141 ★  Compton Foundation
535 Middlefield Rd., Ste. 160
Menlo Park, CA 94025
**Phone:** (650)328-0101          **Fax:** (650)328-0171
**Email:** info@comptonfnd.org
**Website:** http://www.comptonfoundation.org
Edith Eddy, Executive Director

**Fnded:** 1973. **Philosophy:** "In a world in which most problems have become increasingly interrelated and universal in dimension, and where survival of human life under conditions worth living is in jeopardy, the Compton Foundation is concerned first and foremost with the prevention of war, and the amelioration of world conditions that tend to cause conflict. Primary among these conditions are the increasing pressures and destabilizing effects of excessive population growth, the alarming depletion and unequal distribution of the world's natural resources, the tenuous status of human rights, and the steady deterioration of the world's environment." The foundation categorizes these global human survival problems into the areas of Peace and World Order, Population, and the Environment. Other, more limited concerns of the foundation include Equal Educational Opportunity, Community Welfare and Social Justice, and Culture and the Arts. 1997 Policies and Guidelines **Priorities:** *Arts & Humanities:* 10%. Supports arts associations, museums, music, dance, and opera. *Civic & Public Affairs:* 1%. Supports public policy organizations. *Education:* 8%. Supports colleges and universities. *Environment:* 32%. Funds planned parenthood groups, child welfare, and youth organizations. *International:* 1%. Gives to health organizations. *Note:* Total contributions made in 1998. **Typ. Recipients:** AIDS/HIV, Family Planning, Health Organizations, Health Policy/Cost Containment, Medical Education, Public Health. **Geo. Dist:** internationally; nationally; San Francisco, CA, including Marin an Snata Clara Counties.

### ★ 142 ★  Comstock Foundation
PO Box 2127
9th Fl.
Spokane, WA 99210-2127
**Phone:** (509)353-4156

**Fnded:** 1950. **Philosophy:** The foundation carries out Josie Shadle's charitable interests in its current grants program. Almost all grants are made to organizations in Spokane, WA, for specific projects which serve the people of Spokane. Within those limits, the foundation is best characterized by the number and diversity of projects and organizations that it supports. The foundation prefers to make grants for capital projects rather than contribute to operating expenses. Capital grants vary from building and remodeling to providing needed office equipment, such as computers. In special circumstances, the trustees may choose to help a worthy organization with rent, mortgage payments, or other operating costs for short intervals. Whenever possible, the foundation prefers to join with other donors in funding a project, rather than assuming a major portion of the amount needed. **Priorities:** *Arts & Humanities:* 4%. *Civic & Public Affairs:* 1%. *Education:* About 45%. Mainly supports Gonzaga University. *Environment:* 42%. *International:* 8%. *Note:* Contributions made in 1997. **Typ. Recipients:** AIDS/HIV, Cancer, Children's Health/Hospitals, Clinics/Medical Centers, Eyes/Blindness, Health Organizations, Hospitals, Medical Education, Medical Rehabilitation, Multiple Sclerosis, Nursing Services, People with Disabilities, Prenatal Health Issues, Single-Disease Health Associations, Substance Abuse. **Geo. Dist:** Spokane, WA, including metropolitan area and Spokane County.

### ★ 143 ★  Connelly Foundation
One Tower Bridge, Ste. 1450
West Conshohocken, PA 19428
**Phone:** (610)834-3222          **Fax:** (610)834-0866
**Email:** eawilcox@connellyfdn.org
**Website:** http://www.connellyfdn.org
E. Wilcox, Grants Administrator

**Fnded:** 1955. **Philosophy:** The Connelly Foundation is a private grantmaking organization whose mission is to enhance the quality of life in the Delaware Valley.

**Priorities:** *Arts & Humanities:* 8%. Theaters, libraries, museums. *Civic & Public Affairs:* 7%. Rehabilitation for houses. *Education:* 57%. Largely Catholic universities and secondary schools. *Environment:* 11%. Homelessness, addiction, childcare. *International:* 11%. Children's Hospital, cancer therapy, equipment upgrades. *Religion:* 1%. Supports scientific centers and scientific research. *Note:* Total contributions made in 1998. **Typ. Recipients:** AIDS/HIV, Alzheimers Disease, Cancer, Child Abuse, Children's Health/Hospitals, Clinics/Medical Centers, Domestic Violence, Emergency/Ambulance Services, Family Planning, Geriatric Health, Health Funds, Health Organizations, Heart, Home-Care Services, Hospices, Hospitals, Hospitals (University Affiliated), Long-Term Care, Medical Education, Medical Rehabilitation, Medical Research, Nursing Services, Outpatient Health Care, People with Disabilities, Prenatal Health Issues, Preventive Medicine/Wellness Organizations, Public Health, Research/Studies Institutes, Substance Abuse, Transplant Networks/Donor Banks. **Geo. Dist:** Greater Delaware Valley Region; Philadelphia, PA.


### ★ 144 ★ Conrad N. Hilton Foundation

100 West Liberty St., Ste. 840
Reno, NV 89501
**Phone:** (775)323-4221          **Fax:** (775)323-4150
**Email:** cnhf@hiltonfoundation.org
**Website:** http://www.hiltonfoundation.org
Steven Hilton, President

**Fnded:** 1944. **Philosophy:** Conrad Hilton believed, "the practice of charity will bind us...in one great brotherhood. As the funds you will expend here come from many places in the world, so let there be no territorial, religious, or color restrictions on your benefactions, but beware of organized, professional charities with high-salaried executives and a heavy ratio of expenses. Be ever watchful for the opportunity to shelter little children with the umbrella of your charity; be generous to their schools, their hospitals and their places of worship. For, as they must bear the burdens of our mistakes, so are they in their innocence the repositories of our hopes for the upward progress of humanity. Give aid to their protectors and defenders, the Sisters, who devote their love and life's work for the good of mankind, for they appeal especially to me as being deserving of help from the foundation." 2000 Annual Report. The Foundation's mission is to alleviate human suffering. Directors select priority areas including blindness, early childhood development, domestic violence, homelessness, and substance abuse prevention and research. The Foundation focuses upon long-range initiatives. Programs include an international education program for multi-handicapped blind children, their parents, and professionals who work with them (Perkins School for the Blind); nationwide delivery of the Project ALERT curriculum to help middle school students resist drugs (BEST Foundation for a Drug Free Tomorrow); and a comprehensive disease prevention program in Ghana, West Africa, centered around sources of clean water (World Vision). The foundation reports that it has undertaken a global collaborative to control and eliminate trachoma in 10 to 12 countries in Africa and Asia through the Carter Center, World Vision, and Helen Keller International. The foundation is also seeking to improve care and services for infants and toddlers with disabilities through its Early Head Start and Migrant Head Start programs. **Priorities:** *Arts & Humanities:* Less than 1%. *Civic & Public Affairs:* 2%. Funds chambers of commerce, civil rights, ethnic organizations, employment/job training gay/lesbian issues, Hispanic affairs, law and justice, municipalities/towns, philanthropic organizations, women's affairs. *Education:* 41%. Gives to colleges/universities, private education (pre-college). *Environment:* 22%. Supports animal protection, at-risk youth, big brother/big sister, child welfare, domestic violence/child abuse, family services, recreation/athletic organizations, United Way, volunteer services. *International:* 14%. Supports AIDS/HIV organizations, cancer centers, children's health/hospitals, health organizations, hospitals (university affiliated), preventative medicine/wellness organizations, single-disease health associations. *Religion:* Less than 1%. *Note:* Total contributions made in 2000. **Typ. Recipients:** Arthritis, Children's Health/Hospitals, Clinics/

Medical Centers, Diabetes, Domestic Violence, Emergency/Ambulance Services, Eyes/Blindness, Family Planning, Geriatric Health, Health Organizations, Heart, Hospices, Hospitals, Medical Research, Multiple Sclerosis, People with Disabilities, Public Health, Research/Studies Institutes, Single-Disease Health Associations, Substance Abuse, Transplant Networks/ Donor Banks. **Geo. Dist:** internationally; nationally.


### ★ 145 ★ Cooke Foundation

900 Fort St. Mall, Ste. 1300
Honolulu, HI 96813
**Phone:** (808)537-6333          **Fax:** (808)521-6286
**Website:** http://www.hcf-hawaii.org
Lisa Schiff, Grants Administrator

**Fnded:** 1920. **Philosophy:** The foundation is dedicated primarily to culture and the arts; education; social services, including programs for youth; health; and the environment. The foundation is interested in directing financial support to organizations responding to new needs or changing conditions. **Priorities:** *Arts & Humanities:* 63%. Supports art and culture. *Civic & Public Affairs:* 13%. Supports community and public affairs. *Education:* 8%. Supports educational institutions. *Environment:* 10%. Supports family services, youth causes, food banks and social services. *International:* 2%. Supports hospice and health concerns. *Note:* Contributions were made in fiscal 1999. **Typ. Recipients:** AIDS/HIV, Alzheimers Disease, Cancer, Children's Health/Hospitals, Clinics/Medical Centers, Domestic Violence, Emergency/Ambulance Services, Family Planning, Health Organizations, Health Policy/ Cost Containment, Health-General, Heart, Hospices, Hospitals, Medical Research, Mental Health, People with Disabilities, Prenatal Health Issues, Public Health, Single-Disease Health Associations, Substance Abuse. **Geo. Dist:** HI, especially Oahu.


### ★ 146 ★ Corella and Bertram Bonner Foundation

10 Mercer St.
Princeton, NJ 08540
**Phone:** (609)924-6663          **Fax:** (609)683-4626
**Website:** http://www.bonner.org
Wayne Meisel, President

**Fnded:** 1981. **Philosophy:** According to the foundation's literature, its purpose is to "help the person who is hurting." The foundation is primarily interested in directing financial assistance to the basic needs of food, education, and health care. Its goal is "to displace despair with opportunity. ... and it is the intent to develop partners in these programs to ensure the success of all resources invested in each grant." To meet this plan, the foundation focuses on several major areas: crisis ministry, education, medical services, aid to the handicapped, and general relief. The Crisis Ministry Program financially supports initiatives from food-banks and community-based religious organizations and coalitions that are directly involved in the feeding of the hungry. The focus of these initiatives is on religious community leadership against hunger and its underlying causes. In addition to its contributions to numerous food banks throughout the United States, the foundation also supports education. The Bonner Scholars Program supports academically qualified individuals that otherwise would not be able to attend college because of financial need. The foundation works closely with selected colleges to identify and support deserving students. In return, Bonner Scholars are expected to contribute to society by tutoring and mentoring others. The foundation will also consider requests from organizations serving those communities who are in need of emergency or continuing assistance. **Priorities:** *Civic & Public Affairs:* 5%. Supports People in Action. *Education:* 29%. Funds Learn and Serve America. *International:* 57%. Major support for the Lahey Hitchcock Clinic and the Mayo Foundation. *Note:* Total contributions made in fiscal 1999. **Typ. Recipients:** Clinics/Medical Centers, Health Funds, Hospitals, Medical Research, Research/Studies Institutes. **Geo. Dist:** nationally; East Coast region.


### ★ 147 ★ Courtney S. Turner Charitable Trust

PO Box 4119119
Kansas City, MO 64141-6119
**Phone:** (816)979-7481          **Fax:** (816)691-7916
David Ross, Sr., Trust Officer

**Fnded:** 1986. **Philosophy:** The Courtney S. Turner Charitable Trust has two primary interests: education and the arts. Educational funding favors new programs in higher education. Funding for the arts emphasizes music, museums, and theater. Social services are a secondary interest, with minor support to youth organizations. **Priorities:** *Arts & Humanities:* 14%. Supports music, theatre, and public broadcasting. *Civic & Public Affairs:* 12%. Supports gardens. *Education:* 32%. Supports colleges and education funds. *Environment:* 30%. Supports YWCA, scouts, and a community center. *International:* 4%. Supports hospital foundation and a health center. *Religion:* 5%. Supports a science museum. *Note:* Total contributions made in 1998. **Typ. Recipients:** Clinics/Medical Centers, Domestic Violence, Health-General, Heart, Hospitals, Hospitals (University Affiliated), Multiple Sclerosis, People with Disabilities, Public Health, Substance Abuse. **Geo. Dist:** Atchison, MO; Kansas City, MO, metropolitan area.


### ★ 148 ★ Cowles Charitable Trust

PO Box 219
Rumson, NJ 07760
**Phone:** (732)936-9826
Mary Croft, Secretary & Treasurer

**Fnded:** 1948. **Philosophy:** The Cowles Charitable Trust makes most of its grants in the areas of education, arts, health, and environment. Educational funding favors colleges and universities. Funding in the arts emphasizes museums, arts associations, arts centers, music, and theater groups. The trust also will fund civic groups, social services, and health organizations. **Priorities:** *Arts & Humanities:* 34%. Funds arts centers, museums, libraries, opera, and ballet. *Civic & Public Affairs:* 9%. Funds municipalities, parks, and housing. *Education:* 20%. Supports precollege and higher education. *Environment:* 19%. Supports family and children's services. *International:* 14%. Gives to medical centers and health associations. *Note:* Total contributions made in 1999. **Typ. Recipients:** AIDS/HIV, Cancer, Children's Health/Hospitals, Clinics/Medical Centers, Domestic Violence, Emergency/Ambulance Services, Family Planning, Health Organizations, Hospitals, Hospitals (University Affiliated), Medical Research, Mental Health, People with Disabilities, Single-Disease Health Associations, Substance Abuse. **Geo. Dist:** nationally; FL; New York City, NY.


### ★ 149 ★ Crescent Porter Hale Foundation

655 Redwood Highway, Ste. 301
Mill Valley, CA 94941
**Phone:** (415)388-2333          **Fax:** (415)381-4799
Ulla Davis, Executive Director

**Fnded:** 1961. **Philosophy:** The foundation supports organizations devoted to education in the fields of art, music, elementary, secondary, and university education. "The foundation will consider other worthwhile programs which can be demonstrated as serving broad community purposes, leading toward the improvement of the quality of life. Agencies serving disadvantaged youth, the disabled, or the elderly are of particular interest to the foundation." "Emphasis is placed on organizations engaged in Catholic endeavors." **Priorities:** *Arts & Humanities:* 4%. Public libraries and music. *Civic & Public Affairs:* 10% Community organizations and urban parks. *Education:* 37%. Colleges, secondary schools, and educational organizations for religious concerns. *Environment:* 23%. Youth and family services. *International:* 1%. *Note:* Total contributions 1998. **Typ. Recipients:** AIDS/HIV, Arthritis, Cancer, Family Planning, Health Organizations, Hospices, Hospitals, Long-Term Care, Medical Education, Medical Research, Nursing Services, People with Disabilities, Research/Studies Institutes, Sexual Abuse, Single-Disease Health Associations, Substance Abuse. **Geo. Dist:** San Francisco, CA, Bay area.

★ **150 ★ Crestlea Foundation**
100 W 10th St., Ste. 1109
Wilmington, DE 19801
**Phone:** (302)654-2477        **Fax:** (302)654-2323
Stephen Martinenza, Treasurer

**Fnded:** 1955. **Philosophy:** The foundation has three main areas of interest, but does not limit giving to these areas specifically. Secondary and higher education are major interests, followed by support for libraries and museums in Pennsylvania and Delaware. The third main interest is youth activities and family planning. In addition, the foundation distributes the remainder of its support to community affairs, nature conservation, and churches. **Priorities:** *Arts & Humanities:* 8%. Arts funds, libraries, museums, music, and historic preservation. *Civic & Public Affairs:* 43%. Funds civic affairs, free enterprise, community foundations, and housing. *Education:* 30%. Mainly precollege private education and computer equipment. Also supports religious education and literacy. *Environment:* About 11%. United Way, day care programs, people with disabilities, scouts, senior services, and family planning services. *International:* 37%. Supports hospitals, hospice, and health organizations. *Note:* Total contributions made in 1998. **Typ. Recipients:** Alzheimers Disease, Cancer, Children's Health/Hospitals, Clinics/Medical Centers, Family Planning, Geriatric Health, Health Organizations, Hospices, Hospitals, Long-Term Care, Medical Education, People with Disabilities, Public Health, Single-Disease Health Associations. **Geo. Dist:** Wilmington, DE, including surrounding area.

★ **151 ★ Crystal Trust**
1088 Du Pont Bldg.
Wilmington, DE 19898
**Phone:** (302)774-8421
Stephen Doberstein, Director

**Fnded:** 1947. **Philosophy:** The trust has no specific mandate other than that of serving the Wilmington community. It supports a wide variety of causes. Emphasis is on gifts for capital and other one-time special purposes, and against gifts for continuing expenses of operations or deficits. **Priorities:** *Arts & Humanities:* 7%. Museums and historic preservation. *Civic & Public Affairs:* 6%. Primary support for the Delaware Department of State. *Education:* 58%. Includes a major grant to Wilmington College. *Environment:* 16%. Supports people with disabilities, family services, child welfare, youth organizations, and the aged. *International:* 4%. Health centers and single-disease health associations. *Note:* Total contributions made in 1998. **Typ. Recipients:** Cancer, Child Abuse, Clinics/Medical Centers, Domestic Violence, Family Planning, Geriatric Health, Health Funds, Health Organizations, Health-General, Hospices, Hospitals, Long-Term Care, Medical Education, Medical Research, Mental Health, People with Disabilities, Preventive Medicine/Wellness Organizations, Public Health, Single-Disease Health Associations. **Geo. Dist:** nationally.

★ **152 ★ The Cullen Foundation**
PO Box 1600
Houston, TX 77251
**Phone:** (713)651-8600        **Fax:** (713)651-2374
**Website:** http://www.cullenfdn.org
Alan Stewart, Executive Director

**Fnded:** 1947. **Philosophy:** The foundation supports a variety of educational and health institutions, social service programs, and arts groups. **Priorities:** *Arts & Humanities:* 26%. Funds music, museums, the fine arts, and the performing arts. *Civic & Public Affairs:* 5%. Funds nature centers, civic groups and housing. *Education:* 46%. Supports colleges and universities, private religious education and medical education. *Environment:* 6%. Contributes to the United Way, food banks, child welfare, and scouting. *International:* 9%. Funds hospitals and medical centers. *Religion:* 5%. Supports the Houston Museum of Natural Science and science centers. *Note:* Total contributions made in

1998. **Typ. Recipients:** AIDS/HIV, Alzheimers Disease, Cancer, Child Abuse, Children's Health/Hospitals, Clinics/Medical Centers, Emergency/Ambulance Services, Family Planning, Heart, Hospices, Hospitals, Medical Education, Medical Rehabilitation, Medical Research, Speech & Hearing, Substance Abuse. **Geo. Dist:** Houston, TX, including surrounding area.

★ **153 ★ Cuneo Foundation**
9101 Greenwood Ave., Ste. 210
Niles, IL 60714
**Phone:** (847)296-3351        **Fax:** (847)296-3310
John Cuneo, Jr., President

**Fnded:** 1945. **Philosophy:** The two major priorities of the Cuneo Foundation are Catholic churches and social services. Catholic church funding favors churches in Chicago. Support for social services favors children's homes, youth organizations, and support for the needy. Nominal support goes to a number of educational institutions, including private schools, universities, and religious education. Health services, the arts, and civic affairs are lower priorities. **Priorities:** *Arts & Humanities:* 1%. *Civic & Public Affairs:* 3%. *Education:* 18%. Supports parochial schools. *Environment:* 19%. Youth agencies, shelters and food banks are funded. *International:* 12%. Funds single-disease health associations. *Religion:* 1%. *Note:* Total contributions made in 1998. **Typ. Recipients:** Alzheimers Disease, Cancer, Children's Health/Hospitals, Geriatric Health, Health Funds, Heart, Hospices, Hospitals, Long-Term Care, Medical Education, Medical Research, People with Disabilities, Public Health, Single-Disease Health Associations. **Geo. Dist:** Chicago, IL, including metropolitan area.

**D and DF Foundation**
*See:* Entry 10042

★ **154 ★ Daisy Marquis Jones Foundation**
1600 South Ave., Ste. 250
Rochester, NY 14620
**Phone:** (716)461-4950        **Fax:** (716)955-4940
Roger Gardner, President & Trustee

**Fnded:** 1968. **Philosophy:** The foundation considers itself "a citizen of the community and responds to special opportunities to improve local conditions and to help people solve their own problems." The foundation also encourages preventive programs and focuses on projects involving the disadvantaged. The foundation makes grants primarily to improve the quality of health care in Monroe and Yates counties. Other areas of support include community development, senior citizens, youth, men, women, and improving the administration of justice. The foundation "seeks to make the best use of its limited resources and, in keeping with the foundation's 'new directions,' will focus on primary prevention and advocacy issues. The foundation will continue to emphasize projects involving the disadvantaged." **Priorities:** *Arts & Humanities:* 3%. Supports arts councils, public broadcasting, historic preservation, performing arts, and theater. *Civic & Public Affairs:* 14%. Supports housing, community development, employment/job training, philanthropic organizations, women's affairs, law and justice, and botanical gardens/parks. *Education:* 16%. Supports preschools, minority education, and scholarship funds. *Environment:* 29%. Supports Young Men's Christian Association, Big Brothers/Big Sister, senior services, shelters for the homeless, food banks, United Way, and at-risk youth. *International:* 37%. Supports medical centers, children's health, hospice, health organizations, speech and training, AIDS, mental health, and cancer treatment. *Note:* Total contributions made in 2000. **Typ. Recipients:** Adolescent Health Issues, AIDS/HIV, Alzheimers Disease, Cancer, Children's Health/Hospitals, Clinics/Medical Centers, Domestic Violence, Emergency/Ambulance Services, Family Planning, Geriatric Health, Health Organizations, Hospices, Hospitals (University Affiliated), Long-Term Care, Medical Education, Medical Rehabilitation, Mental Health, Nursing Services, Nutrition, Outpatient Health Care, People with Disabilities, Prenatal Health Issues, Preventive Medicine/Wellness

Organizations, Public Health, Research/Studies Institutes, Speech & Hearing, Substance Abuse. **Geo. Dist:** NY, Monroe County; NY, Yates County.

★ **155 ★ Dale J. Bellamah Foundation**
PO Box 36600, Station D
Albuquerque, NM 87176
**Phone:** (505)293-1098        **Fax:** (505)296-7329
Frank Potenziani, Vice President & Director

**Fnded:** 1972. **Philosophy:** The foundation's interests include higher education scholarships, business school programs in international business and law in Eastern Europe, research in diabetes, hospitals, the U.S. Olympic Committee, youth programs, and care of the mentally retarded. **Priorities:** *Civic & Public Affairs:* 1%. Funds ethnic organization. *Education:* 66%. Primarily for scholarships and fellowships. *Environment:* 19%. Funds the U.S. Olympic Committee and training center and a youth organization. *International:* 13%. Supports the American Diabetes Association. *Note:* Total contributions made in 2000. **Typ. Recipients:** Arthritis, Cancer, Diabetes, Hospitals, Medical Education, People with Disabilities, Single-Disease Health Associations. **Geo. Dist:** NM.

★ **156 ★ Dan Murphy Foundation**
PO Box 711267
Los Angeles, CA 90071
**Phone:** (213)623-3120
Daniel Donohue, President

**Fnded:** 1957. **Philosophy:** The Dan Murphy Foundation's primary concerns are the charities and activities of the Roman Catholic church, in the Archdiocese of Los Angeles. Organizations of interest include religious orders, higher education, high schools and elementary schools, social services (especially religious welfare), and medical institutions. **Priorities:** *Education:* 14%. Colleges and schools; religious education. *Environment:* 2%. Charitable youth organizations. *International:* 1%. Healthcare facilities. *Note:* Total contributions made in 1998. **Typ. Recipients:** Cancer, Children's Health/Hospitals, Clinics/Medical Centers, Emergency/Ambulance Services, Eyes/Blindness, Family Planning, Health Organizations, Hospices, Hospitals, Long-Term Care, Medical Education, Medical Research, Mental Health, Nursing Services, People with Disabilities, Prenatal Health Issues, Substance Abuse. **Geo. Dist:** CA; Los Angeles, CA, metropolitan area.

★ **157 ★ Dane G. Hansen Foundation**
110 West Main St.
PO Box 187
Logan, KS 67646
**Phone:** (785)689-4832        **Fax:** (785)689-4833
**Email:** hansentr@ruraltel.net
Russ Beach, Trustee

**Fnded:** 1965. **Philosophy:** The foundation's mission is to "improve the quality of life for citizens of Kansas." Support is provided to a variety of organizations and programs in the arts, civic and public affairs, education, health, and social services. The foundation maintains an education scholarship program to aid students attending Kansas colleges and universities. The foundation also provides scholarships for vocational education and for theological and graduate studies. **Priorities:** *Arts & Humanities:* 2% Supports arts councils and libraries. *Civic & Public Affairs:* 32%. Funds improvements to city and public services. *Education:* 48%. Educational institutions and programs are funded. *Environment:* 11%. Funding went to youth causes, special needs children, and animal training concerns. *International:* 6%. Supports hospice, disease and disorder concerns, hospitals and medical centers. *Note:* Contributions were made in fiscal 1999. **Typ. Recipients:** Cancer, Children's Health/Hospitals, Clinics/Medical Centers, Emergency/Ambulance Services, Eyes/Blindness, Health Organizations, Heart, Hospices, Hospitals, Long-Term Care, Medical Education, Medical Rehabilitation, Medical Research, People with Disabilities, Single-Disease Health Associations. **Geo. Dist:** KS, Northwestern part of state.

## ★ 158 ★ Danforth Foundation

One Metropolitan Square
211 North Broadway, Ste. 2390
Saint Louis, MO 63102
**Phone:** (314)588-1900          **Fax:** (314)588-0035
Dr. Bruce Anderson, President
**Fnded:** 1927. **Philosophy:** "The Danforth Foundation is a private, independent foundation whose mission is to help St. Louis become the leading region in America. Its goals are to do the follow: help established institutions become world class; help organizations which show great promise of making significant contributions to St. Louis; support creation, renovation, and enhancement of selected facilities; and support other projects which promise long-term contributions to the quality of life in the region." The Danforth Foundation also supports four programs with specific purposes. The Danforth Program for Policymakers is a joint project of the Danforth Foundation and three partners: the National Governors Association, the National Conference of State Legislatures, and the Education Commission of the States. Its mission is to help stat and local government officials improve the well-being of high-risk children and their families. A ten-year initiative launched in 1992, the Policymakers Program has helped more than 300 government executives and legislators from 40 states revise ways in which social services are delivered to their residents. The Danforth Program for Successful Schools supported the work of 20 school teams in the states of Missouri, California, Ohio, and Florida in developing action plans to improve student learning. Since the Foundation's change in focus in May 1997, the Ewing Marion Kauffman Foundation in Kansas City has administered the program. Funding from the Danforth Foundation concluded in the 1999 fiscal year. A ten-year initiative which began in 1992, the Danforth Program for Superintendents is designed to develop leadership skills of 60 urban, rural, and suburban superintendents whose school districts have substantial percentages of high-risk students. It also targets women and minority superintendents, who make up about 60 percent of the membership. The Danforth Program for Teachers supported two initiatives designed to improve teaching and learning in the St. Louis metropolitan area: the Action Research Collaborative and the Professional Development Schools Collaborative. Funds for these initiatives were transferred to the St. Louis Regional Professional Development Center as of June 1, 1997. **Priorities:** *Civic & Public Affairs:* 8%. Supports towns/municipalities, policy making, and community foundations. *Education:* 48%. Supports universities, funds early childhood development research and facilities, supports public school systems, teachers training, superintendents, education funds and principals development. *Environment:* 22%. Funds Jackie Joyner-Kersee Youth Center Foundation. *Religion:* 22%. Supports the Donald Danforth Plant Science Center. *Note:* Total contributions made in fiscal 2000. **Typ. Recipients:** Clinics/Medical Centers, Domestic Violence, Family Planning, Health Organizations, Hospitals, Mental Health, Research/ Studies Institutes. **Geo. Dist:** Saint Louis, MO.

## ★ 159 ★ Daniel Foundation of Alabama

820 Shades Creek Parkway, Ste. 1200
Birmingham, AL 35209
**Phone:** (205)879-0902          **Fax:** (205)879-0906
S. Smith, Executive Director
**Fnded:** 1977. **Philosophy:** The concerns of the Daniel Foundation encompass a wide variety of educational, social service, cultural, and community interests in the state of Alabama, particularly in Birmingham. **Priorities:** *Arts & Humanities:* 22%. Gives to Birmingham performing arts groups, museums, and historical societies. *Civic & Public Affairs:* 4%. Funds housing, community foundations, and a botanical garden. *Education:* About 57%. Primarily supports colleges, universities, and secondary schools. *Environment:* 12%. Supports youth groups, anti-substance abuse programs, the aged, and community services. *International:* Less than 1%. Funds medical centers and single-disease health associations. *Note:* Total contributions made in 1998. **Typ. Recipients:** AIDS/ HIV, Cancer, Child Abuse, Clinics/Medical Centers, Eyes/Blindness, Health Organizations, Hospices, Hospitals, Long-Term Care, Medical Education, Medical Rehabilitation, Medical Research, Mental Health, Multiple Sclerosis, People with Disabilities, Research/ Studies Institutes, Single-Disease Health Associations, Substance Abuse. **Geo. Dist:** southeastern states; AL.

## ★ 160 ★ Davenport-Hatch Foundation

PO Box 124
Penfield, NY 14526
**Phone:** (716)546-9289
David Taylor, Contact
**Fnded:** 1952. **Philosophy:** The foundation makes grants across the major categories of support. In the area of health care, interests include hospitals and single-disease health associations. Social services support goes to community service organizations, children and families, and youth organizations. Educational support includes scholarships and capital support, mostly to private schools. Art interests include history and music, and the remainder goes to civic affairs and religion. **Priorities:** *Arts & Humanities:* 10%. Supports philharmonic orchestras, museums, and performing arts. *Civic & Public Affairs:* 9%. Supports the Susan B. Anthony House. *Education:* 21%. Supports colleges, universities, and educational programs. *Environment:* 25%. Supports United Way, child welfare, and youth services. *International:* 22%. Supports hospitals, health services, the elderly, hearing and speech impaired, and disease and disorder concerns. *Religion:* 4%. Supports the Rochester Museum and Science Center. *Note:* Contributions were made in fiscal 1999. **Typ. Recipients:** AIDS/HIV, Alzheimers Disease, Cancer, Clinics/Medical Centers, Domestic Violence, Emergency/Ambulance Services, Family Planning, Geriatric Health, Health Organizations, Health-General, Heart, Home-Care Services, Hospices, Hospitals, Kidney, Long-Term Care, Medical Education, Medical Rehabilitation, Medical Research, Medical Training, Mental Health, Multiple Sclerosis, Nursing Services, People with Disabilities, Prenatal Health Issues, Public Health, Single-Disease Health Associations, Speech & Hearing, Substance Abuse, Trauma Treatment. **Geo. Dist:** Rochester, NY, including surrounding metropolitan area.

## ★ 161 ★ David Geffen Foundation

100 Universal City Plaza
Bldg. 5125
Universal City, CA 91608
**Phone:** (818)733-6333          **Fax:** (818)733-6129
David Geffen, Trustee
**Fnded:** 1986. **Priorities:** *Arts & Humanities:* 33%. Supports libraries fine arts and history. *Civic & Public Affairs:* 1%. Funds civil liberties, gay and lesbian causes and law and justice. *Education:* 25%. Primarily supports colleges and universities. *International:* 28%. Gives to AIDs causes and research, hospitals, children's health concerns, cancer, and respiratory. *Note:* Total contributions made in 1998. **Typ. Recipients:** AIDS/HIV, Cancer, Children's Health/Hospitals, Clinics/Medical Centers, Diabetes, Family Planning, Health Organizations, Health Policy/Cost Containment, Hospices, Hospitals, Medical Education, Medical Research, Public Health, Single-Disease Health Associations, Substance Abuse.

## ★ 162 ★ David Schwartz Foundation

720 Fifth Ave., Ste. 1305
New York, NY 10019
**Phone:** (212)586-4225          **Fax:** (212)586-0649
Richard Schwartz, President
**Fnded:** 1945. **Philosophy:** The David Schwartz Foundation makes most of its grants to education and the arts. Funding supports universities, medical education, and private and day schools. Arts funding goes to the performing arts, historic preservation, and museums. Other areas of support include Jewish religious organizations, civic affairs, health, and social services. **Priorities:** *Arts & Humanities:* 25%. Supports arts funds, theater, museums, and historical societies. *Civic & Public Affairs:* 1%. Philanthropic organizations. *Education:* 59%. Focus on colleges and universities. *Environment:* Less than 1%. *International:* 2%. Funds hospitals. *Note:* Total contributions made in fiscal 1999. **Typ. Recipients:** AIDS/HIV, Cancer, Children's Health/Hospitals, Clinics/Medical Centers, Family Planning, Hospitals, Medical Education, Medical Research, Public Health, Single-Disease Health Associations. **Geo. Dist:** New York, NY.

## ★ 163 ★ Dekko Foundation

PO Box 548
1208 Lakeside Dr.
Kendallville, IN 46755-0548
**Phone:** (219)347-1278          **Fax:** (219)347-7103
**Email:** dekko@dekkofoundation.org
**Website:** http://www.dekkofoundation.org
**Fnded:** 1981. **Philosophy:** The foundation provides grants to charitable organizations primarily in communities where Group Dekko had plants prior to 1992. Education receives the majority of the foundation's giving. The foundation's mission is "to foster economic freedom through education." Approximately 40-60% of all grants will be proactive. **Priorities:** *Arts & Humanities:* 1%. Funds support public libraries and historical organizations. *Civic & Public Affairs:* 10%. Supports community development. *Education:* About 84%. Focus on primary education. *Environment:* 3%. Primarily for the foundation's Youth Initiative, empowering young people to serve their community, and Early Childhood Programs. *Note:* Total contributions made in fiscal 1999. **Typ. Recipients:** Domestic Violence, Emergency/Ambulance Services, People with Disabilities, Public Health. **Geo. Dist:** AL, Limestone County; IN, DeKalb County; IN, Kosciuszko County; IN, LaGrange County; IN, Noble County; IN, Steuben County; IN, Whitley County; IA, Clarke County; IA, Decatur County; IA, Lucas County; IA, Ringgold County; IA, Union County.

## ★ 164 ★ Del E. Webb Foundation

PO Box 3350
Wickenburg, AZ 85358
**Phone:** (520)684-7223          **Fax:** (520)684-5665
Robert Johnson, President & Director
**Fnded:** 1960. **Philosophy:** The foundation primarily applies its resources to preserve and enrich the benefits to be derived by residents of Arizona, Nevada, and California from improved and expanded medical services and medical research. *Del E. Webb Foundation Principles.* Traditional areas of support include health care, health facilities, medical education, and medical research. **Priorities:** *Education:* 10%. Science and math education, medical education, and private precollege education. *Environment:* 6%. Youth organizations, community service organizations, and programs for people with disabilities. *International:* 71%. Medical centers, cancer research, and public health issues. *Note:* Contributions made in 1999. **Typ. Recipients:** Cancer, Children's Health/Hospitals, Clinics/Medical Centers, Diabetes, Emergency/Ambulance Services, Eyes/Blindness, Geriatric Health, Health Funds, Health Organizations, Home-Care Services, Hospitals, Kidney, Long-Term Care, Medical Education, Medical Research, Medical Training, People with Disabilities, Prenatal Health Issues, Preventive Medicine/Wellness Organizations, Public Health, Public Health, Research/Studies Institutes, Single-Disease Health Associations, Speech & Hearing, Trauma Treatment. **Geo. Dist:** AZ; CA; NV.

## ★ 165 ★ Dellora A. and Lester J. Norris Foundation

303 E Main St.
PO Box 4325
Saint Charles, IL 60174
**Phone:** (630)584-2500          **Fax:** (630)584-1020
Eugene Butler, Treasurer
**Fnded:** 1979. **Philosophy:** The foundation gives primarily to health institutions, especially hospitals; social service organizations, where the emphasis is on child welfare, family services, and youth organizations; and higher and secoondary education. The foundation also provides funding to the arts, civic organizations, and churches. Funding is generally limited to organiza-

tions started by or supported by Mr. and Mrs. Norris during their lifetimes. **Priorities:** *Arts & Humanities:* 8%. Museums, libraries, opera, music, arts festivals, and historical societies. *Civic & Public Affairs:* 12. Community foundations. *Education:* 40%. Supports pivate secondary education and colleges and universities. *Environment:* 9%. Youth organizations, family services, and child welfare. *International:* 23%. Focus on health funds, hospitals, and single-disease health associations. *Note:* Total contributions made in 1998. **Typ. Recipients:** AIDS/HIV, Cancer, Children's Health/Hospitals, Clinics/Medical Centers, Diabetes, Health Funds, Health Organizations, Heart, Hospices, Hospitals, Medical Rehabilitation, Medical Research, Mental Health, People with Disabilities, Public Health, Respiratory, Single-Disease Health Associations, Substance Abuse. **Geo. Dist:** nationally; CO; FL; IL.

## ★ 166 ★ DeWitt Wallace-Reader's Digest Fund
2 Park Ave., 23rd Floor
New York, NY 10016
**Phone:** (212)251-9800          **Fax:** (212)679-6990
**Email:** dwrd@wallacefunds.org
**Website:** http://www.wallacefunds.org
M. DeVita, President

**Fnded:** 1965. **Philosophy:** "To foster fundamental improvement in the quality of educational and career development opportunities for all school-age youth and to increase access to these improved services for young people in low-income communities." "These principles guide the translation of the mission of Dewitt Wallace-Readers Digest Fund into specific grantmaking across its program areas: education and career development are lifelong processes that are most effective when they involve active engagement in meaningful pursuits and build on the learner's strengths and current knowledge; education and career development occur in a wide range of settings, including schools, families, community institutions, and the work place; career development is a component of the education process that connects school to work and prepares young people for the productive adulthood; youth are best served when programs to educate and guide them are coordinated and complimentary; increasing young people's access to high quality services requires community institutions to be more inclusive in their outreach and more responsive to the diverse needs of today's youth; improving the quality of services for young people requires investments in the adults who work with and on behalf of youth in schools and community organizations; fundamental improvement in services for youth requires work on several levels of a problem at the same time, combining investments in direct service with complementary efforts to educate leaders in both the public and private sectors." **Priorities:** *Arts & Humanities:* 41%. *Education:* 37%. *Environment:* 22%. Contributions through community based organizations. *Note:* Total contributions made in 2000. Percentages provided by foundation. **Typ. Recipients:** Clinics/Medical Centers, Hospitals, Medical Research, People with Disabilities, Research/Studies Institutes. **Geo. Dist:** nationally; primarily to national organizations.

## ★ 167 ★ Dibner Fund
PO Box 7575
Wilton, CT 06897
**Phone:** (203)761-9904          **Fax:** (203)761-9989
**Email:** Dibnerfund@worldnet.att.net
Marci Sternheim, Executive Director

**Fnded:** 1957. **Philosophy:** The mission of the Dibner Fund is to sustain, in select instances through long term support, institutions or organizations to which the donor was particularly committed, as well as others primarily involved with achieving better understanding of the history of science and technology with primary support of the Dibner Institute and Burndy Library in this field, located in Cambridge, MA. The Fund is uniquely characterized by its highly focused support of unsolicited and internally selected institutions and programs, mostly science driven. Examples of this are those that emphasize education and scholarship in the pure and applied sciences as well as others of special interest to the trustees; institutions, agencies and programs encouraging youth to pursue and sustain careers in science and technology; programs to encourage and assist foreign-born scientists and engineers who emigrate to the US; and other community, educational, health care, environmental and cultural agencies or institutions chosen by the board. In 1998, the Dibner Fund added one new category–peaceful coexistence–and expanded its humanitarian and environmental grantmaking areas. Humanitarian aid focuses on disaster relief and medical aid. Environmental grants focus on fresh water and rivers. The Dibner Fund **Priorities:** *Arts & Humanities:* 29%. Supports public broadcasting, libraries, museums, and history organizations. *Civic & Public Affairs:* 2%. Gives to parks, aquariums, and nonprofit management. *Education:* 18%. Supports colleges and universities and scholarship funds. *Environment:* 3%. Supports aid for people with disabilities and the United Way. *International:* 1%. Supports hospitals. *Religion:* 36%. Major funding goes to the Dibner Institute for the History of Science and Technology. Also funds science centers and scientific history. *Note:* Total contributions made in 1999. **Typ. Recipients:** Cancer, Children's Health/Hospitals, Emergency/Ambulance Services, Emergency/Ambulance Services, Hospices, Hospitals, People with Disabilities, Single-Disease Health Associations. **Geo. Dist:** nationally and internationally.

## ★ 168 ★ Dillon Foundation
PO Box 537
Sterling, IL 61081
**Phone:** (815)626-9000          **Fax:** (815)626-4000
Peter Dillon, President & Director

**Fnded:** 1953. **Philosophy:** The Dillon Foundation makes most of its grants in the area of civic affairs, especially in Sterling Township, IL. Educational institutions, including public schools and universities, are secondary interests. Minor support goes to other charitable recipient areas. **Priorities:** *Civic & Public Affairs:* 48%. Supports City of Sterling. *Education:* 26%. Supports elementary schools, universities, and college associations. *Environment:* 23%. Supports YMCA, senior services and United Way. *International:* 1%. Supports Cancer Center and hospice. *Note:* Total contributions made in 1998. **Typ. Recipients:** Cancer, Children's Health/Hospitals, Clinics/Medical Centers, Emergency/Ambulance Services, Family Planning, Health Organizations, Hospices, Hospitals, Medical Rehabilitation, Medical Research, People with Disabilities, Public Health, Research/Studies Institutes, Single-Disease Health Associations. **Geo. Dist:** Sterling, IL, including metropolitan area.

## ★ 169 ★ Dr. P. Phillips Foundation
PO Box 3753
Orlando, FL 32802
**Phone:** (407)422-6105          **Fax:** (407)422-4952
J. Hinson, President

**Fnded:** 1953. **Philosophy:** The foundation supports a wide variety of charitable organizations in Orange County, FL. Education, social services, the arts, and civic affairs are its main priorities. Social service funding favors child and youth development programs. The foundation supports all categories of the arts, including funds, museums, festivals, symphonies, theaters, and historical societies. Civic affairs in Orlando and Orange County, FL., are also a major interest. Other interests include educational funding for public schools, continuing education programs for youth in Central Florida, and science centers. **Priorities:** *Arts & Humanities:* 13%. *Education:* 17%. Focus on primary and secondary education. *Environment:* 49%. Primarily for youth organizations and recreational activities. *International:* 18%. Emphasis on access to care, mental health services, and rehabilitation services. *Note:* Total contributions made in fiscal 2000. **Typ. Recipients:** AIDS/HIV, Alzheimers Disease, Cancer, Clinics/Medical Centers, Diabetes, Domestic Violence, Emergency/Ambulance Services, Eyes/Blindness, Health Organizations, Hospices, Mental Health, Multiple Sclerosis, People with Disabilities, Prenatal Health Issues, Public Health, Single-Disease Health Associations. **Geo. Dist:** FL, Orange County.

## ★ 170 ★ Dr. Ralph and Marian Falk Medical Research Trust
231 South LaSalle St., Ste. 0260
Chicago, IL 60697-0001
**Phone:** (312)828-4973          **Fax:** (312)987-0806
M. Ryan, Senior Vice President

**Fnded:** 1992. **Philosophy:** "The purpose of the research trust is to provide support for medical research in the areas of diseases for which no definite cure is known." Dr. Ralph and Marian #Falk Medical Research Trust 1998 IRS Form 990 **Priorities:** *Education:* 67%. Supports universities and medical education. *International:* 33%. Supports medical centers and medical research. *Note:* Total contributions made in 1998. **Typ. Recipients:** Arthritis, Cancer, Children's Health/Hospitals, Clinics/Medical Centers, Hospitals, Hospitals (University Affiliated), Medical Education, Medical Rehabilitation, Medical Research, Prenatal Health Issues, Public Health, Research/Studies Institutes. **Geo. Dist:** nationally.

## ★ 171 ★ Dr. Scholl Foundation
11 South La Salle St., Ste. 2100
Chicago, IL 60603-1302
**Phone:** (312)782-5210
Pamela Scholl, President

**Fnded:** 1947. **Philosophy:** The foundation was established, as described in its charter, "for religious, charitable, scientific, literary, and educational purposes, and to do all things necessary or expedient to carry out the foregoing purposes. No part of the activities of the corporation shall be used for propaganda or otherwise to influence legislation." The foundation supports private education at all levels including elementary, secondary, and post-secondary schools; colleges and universities; and medical education. Support is also available for general charitable programs including grants to hospitals, programs for senior citizens, children, and the developmentally disabled. The foundation also shows an interest in civic, cultural, religious, and social welfare projects. **Priorities:** *Arts & Humanities:* 9%. Opera, public broadcasting, libraries, and historical preservation. *Civic & Public Affairs:* 4%. Funds horticultural societies, an aquarium, and employment initiatives. *Education:* 32%. Arts education, colleges and universities, schools, and science education. *Environment:* 12%. Supports youth programs, the disabled, and family services. *International:* 12%. Children's health, blindness, single-disease associations, and infant welfare. *Religion:* 9%. Science museums. *Note:* Total contributions made in 2000. **Typ. Recipients:** Cancer, Children's Health/Hospitals, Clinics/Medical Centers, Eyes/Blindness, Health Funds, Health Organizations, Heart, Hospices, Hospitals, Medical Education, Medical Research, People with Disabilities, Prenatal Health Issues, Research/Studies Institutes, Single-Disease Health Associations, Substance Abuse. **Geo. Dist:** nationally; IL.

## ★ 172 ★ Dr. W. C. Swanson Family Foundation, Inc.
2955 Harrison Boulevard, Ste. 201
Ogden, UT 84403
**Phone:** (801)392-0360          **Fax:** (801)392-0429
**Email:** SwansonFoundation@worldnet.att.net
Cindy Purcell, President

**Fnded:** 1978. **Philosophy:** The stated purpose of the foundation is "for religious, charitable, literary, scientific, or educational purposes, or for the prevention of cruelty to children or animals." Although the foundation's purpose remains the same, the scope of the mission has broadened to include medical research and public information through the use of film and mass media. The foundation developed and sponsored a documentary entitled "A Story of Healing" which won the Academy Award for Documentary-Short Subject, March 1998. **Priorities:** *Arts & Humanities:* 12%. Support for museums, performing arts, arts centers, music, and dance. *Civic & Public Affairs:* 3%. Housing and local government. *Education:* 33%. Primary support for universities in Utah and primary and secondary education. *Environment:* 21%. Emphasis on child welfare, family services, and prevention of domestic violence. *International:* 10%. Focus on pediatric helath and health associations. *Religion:* 1%. Giving to dinosaur park and museum. *Note:* Total contributions made in 1998. **Typ. Recipients:** Cancer, Child Abuse, Children's Health/Hospitals, Domestic Violence, Emergency/Ambulance Services, Health Organizations, Health-General, Heart, Hospices, Hospitals, Medical Education, Medical Rehabilitation, People with Disabilities, Public Health, Sexual Abuse, Substance Abuse, Trauma Treatment. **Geo. Dist:** UT, primarily Northern Utah and Weber County; grants from the rest of Utah are next in priority, then regional requests, and lastly national and international.

### ★ 173 ★ Dodge Jones Foundation
PO Box 176
Abilene, TX 79604
**Phone:** (915)673-6429          **Fax:** (915)673-2028
Lawrence Gill, Grants Administrator
**Fnded:** 1954. **Philosophy:** The foundation focuses its activity in the areas of education, community services, health, civic affairs, historic preservation, and youth organizations. **Priorities:** *Arts & Humanities:* 17%. Supports libraries, public broadcasting, fine arts and museums. *Civic & Public Affairs:* 4%. Supports municipalities and community organizations. *Education:* 46%. Supports colleges, universities and private academies. *Environment:* 17%. Supports children's services, camps, YWCA, scouting and day care. *International:* 11%. Supports hospital and medical centers. *Note:* Total contributions made in 1998. **Typ. Recipients:** AIDS/HIV, Alzheimers Disease, Cancer, Children's Health/Hospitals, Clinics/Medical Centers, Emergency/Ambulance Services, Family Planning, Health Organizations, Health Policy/Cost Containment, Heart, Hospices, Hospitals, Medical Education, Medical Rehabilitation, Medical Rehabilitation, Medical Research, Mental Health, People with Disabilities, Public Health, Speech & Hearing, Substance Abuse. **Geo. Dist:** TX.

### ★ 174 ★ Dolan Family Foundation
340 Crossways Park Dr.
Woodbury, NY 11797
**Phone:** (516)803-9210          **Fax:** (516)393-0158
Marianne Weber, Chairman
**Fnded:** 1987. **Philosophy:** The foundation generally supports educational institutions and health and medical research organizations. **Priorities:** *Education:* About 55%. *Environment:* 8%. Community services. *International:* 27%. **Typ. Recipients:** Hospitals, Medical Research, People with Disabilities. **Geo. Dist:** nationally and internationally; NY.

### ★ 175 ★ Don and Sybil Harrington Foundation
801 South Fillmore, Ste. 700
Amarillo, TX 79101
**Phone:** (806)373-8353          **Fax:** (806)373-3656
**Email:** haf@aaf-hf.org
**Website:** http://www.aaf-hr.org
Jim Allison, President & Executive Director
**Fnded:** 1957. **Philosophy:** The foundation has a wide range of funding interests including health, human services, and education in the Panhandle area of Texas. **Priorities:** *Arts & Humanities:* 21%. Supports performing arts and historical societies. *Civic & Public Affairs:* 7%. Funds community organizations. *Education:* 5%. *Environment:* 10%. Supports United Way and youth organizations. *International:* 24%. Funds medical centers and cancer research. *Religion:* 19%. Supports a discovery center. *Note:* Total contributions made in 1999. **Typ. Recipients:** Arthritis, Cancer, Children's Health/Hospitals, Clinics/Medical Centers, Domestic Violence, Emergency/Ambulance Services, Eyes/Blindness, Geriatric Health, Health Organizations, Hospices, Hospitals, Medical Education, Medical Rehabilitation, Medical Research, People with Disabilities. **Geo. Dist:** TX, 26 Northern Counties in Texas.

### ★ 176 ★ Donald W. Reynolds Foundation
1701 Village Center Circle
Las Vegas, NV 89123-6303

**Phone:** (702)804-6000          **Fax:** (702)804-6099
**Email:** HYSC41A@Prodigy.com
**Website:** http://www.dwreynolds.org
Karine Mayer, Administrative Officer
**Fnded:** 1954. **Philosophy:** "The Donald W. Reynolds Foundation makes grants in Arkansas, Nevada and Oklahoma to qualified charitable organizations that demonstrate a sustainable program, exhibit an entrepreneurial spirit, and assists those served to be health, self-sufficient and productive members of the community." The foundation operates several giving programs. The Capital Grants program is the only one that invites applications. Others are driven by trustee initiative. The foundation decided to devote a substantial portion of resources to capital improvement projects. These projects may include construction of new buildings, renovation of existing structures, capital equipment and furnishings associated with these building projects, and capital equipment and installation projects not associated with new construction or renovation. The foundation may consider being the exclusive funding agency for such capital projects, providing funds for the total cost of the facility. The foundation may, however, issue a challenge grant requiring the applicant to match an appropriate and significant portion of foundation funds to complete a project. While grants focus on capital needs, review includes a comprehensive evaluation of the programmatic, administrative, and organizational aspects of the applicant. A grant should enable the applicant to meet well-documented needs and increase the capacity of the applicant organization to achieve its mission. **Priorities:** *Arts & Humanities:* 11%. Supports public broadcasting, ballet, historic preservation, museums, theater, and arts festivals. *Civic & Public Affairs:* 2%. Supports community foundations, nonprofit management, municipalities/towns, botanical gardens, and womens affairs. *Education:* 72%. Supports universities and colleges, medical education, literacy, legal education, and arts/humanities education. *Environment:* 8%. Supports United Way, youth programs, food distribution, senior services, special Olympics, Big Brothers/Big Sisters, and scouting. *International:* 4%. Supports cancer and heart research, medical centers, and children's health. *Note:* Total contributions made in fiscal 1999. **Typ. Recipients:** AIDS/HIV, Cancer, Clinics/Medical Centers, Emergency/Ambulance Services, Geriatric Health, Health Funds, Health Organizations, Heart, Hospices, Hospitals, People with Disabilities, Single-Disease Health Associations, Substance Abuse. **Geo. Dist:** AR; NV; OK.

### ★ 177 ★ Dora Roberts Foundation
PO Box 2050
Fort Worth, TX 76113
**Phone:** (817)884-4448          **Fax:** (817)884-4294
Rick Piersall, Senior Vice President, Bank One
**Fnded:** 1948. **Philosophy:** The Dora Roberts Foundation makes grants primarily to social services programs, including those for community centers, food and clothing, and the aged. Health support favors rehabilitation, hospitals, and medical centers. Educational interests include junior colleges, high schools, and foundations for education. The foundation also supports religious programs and civic affairs. **Priorities:** *Arts & Humanities:* 7%. Supports history and music. *Civic & Public Affairs:* 14%. Supports safety, clubs, festivals, towns/municipalities, and civic affairs. *Education:* 18%. Supports schools, universities, and colleges. *Environment:* 37%. Supports recreation/athletics, food distribution, animal protection, scouts, community centers, and United Way. *International:* 3%. Supports medical rehabilitation. *Note:* Total contributions made in fiscal 1999. **Typ. Recipients:** Cancer, Heart, Hospices, Hospitals, Medical Education, Medical Rehabilitation, Sexual Abuse. **Geo. Dist:** TX, Big Spring.

### ★ 178 ★ Dorot Foundation
439 Benefit St.
Providence, RI 02903-2934
**Phone:** (401)351-8866          **Fax:** (401)351-4975
**Email:** info@dorot.org
**Website:** http://www.dorot.org
Prof. Ernest Frerichs, Executive Director

**Fnded:** 1958. **Philosophy:** The foundation is a major funder of colleges and universities in New England, Israel, and Canada. Other interests include funding for museums of interest to Israel or the Jewish faith, and other Jewish causes. **Priorities:** *Arts & Humanities:* 33%. Supports the Archives for Historical Documentation with primary support given to the New York Public Library. *Civic & Public Affairs:* 8%. Supports public and civic affairs. *Education:* 43%. Supports primary and secondary educational institutions, colleges, universities, and educational programs. *Environment:* 4%. Supports the 92nd St. YM-YWHA. *International:* 9%. Supports family health, hospice, and alternative medicine. *Note:* Contributions were made in fiscal 1999. **Typ. Recipients:** AIDS/HIV, Clinics/Medical Centers, Hospices, Medical Education, Medical Research, Medical Training, Mental Health, People with Disabilities, Public Health, Substance Abuse. **Geo. Dist:** U.S.-based affiliates of Israeli organizations; northeast United States.

### ★ 179 ★ Dorothy U. Dalton Foundation
Greenleaf Trust Bldg.
490 W South St.
Kalamazoo, MI 49007
**Phone:** (616)388-9800          **Fax:** (616)388-9868
Ronald Kilgore, Secretary & Treasurer
**Fnded:** 1978. **Philosophy:** The Dorothy U. Dalton Foundation primarily supports social service organizations. The foundation supports the YMCA and YWCA, youth organizations, relief for the needy, and united funds. Secondary interests include museums, civic centers, and health clinics in Kalamazoo, MI. **Priorities:** *Arts & Humanities:* 47%. Generally in support of capital campaigns involving theater, the arts, festival, and symphonies. *Civic & Public Affairs:* 14%. Primary support for The Kalamazoo Foundation Center and housing resources. *Education:* 6%. Supports the American Red Cross Building Stronger campaign. *Environment:* 19%. Interests include the United Way, children's organizations, vacation camps, and junior achievement. *International:* 9%. Emphasis mainly on Hospice care of Southwest Michigan. *Note:* Total contributions made in fiscal 1999. **Typ. Recipients:** AIDS/HIV, Alzheimers Disease, Children's Health/Hospitals, Clinics/Medical Centers, Domestic Violence, Emergency/Ambulance Services, Family Planning, Geriatric Health, Health Organizations, Hospices, Hospitals, Long-Term Care, Mental Health, Nursing Services, Nutrition, Outpatient Health Care, People with Disabilities, Sexual Abuse, Substance Abuse. **Geo. Dist:** MI, Kalamazoo County.

### ★ 180 ★ Dorrance Family Foundation
7600 East Doubletree Ranch Rd. Ste. 300
Scottsdale, AZ 85258-2137
**Phone:** (480)367-7233
Carolyn O'Malley, Executive Director
**Fnded:** 1991. **Philosophy:** The foundation provides major support to the Arizona Science Center. Funding also goes to health organizations, arts associations, and community services primarily within Phoenix, AZ. **Priorities:** *Arts & Humanities:* 23%. Primarily for museums and symphonies. *Civic & Public Affairs:* 34%. Supports the Phoenix Zoo and botanical gardens. *Education:* 22%. Private, precollege education, and student aid. *Environment:* 5%. Community centers, united funds, family services, and youth organizations. *International:* 8%. Hospices, medical research, and public health. *Religion:* 8%. Supports the Arizona Science Center. *Note:* Total contributions made in 1998. **Typ. Recipients:** AIDS/HIV, Arthritis, Cancer, Children's Health/Hospitals, Domestic Violence, Family Planning, Health Organizations, Heart, Hospices, Hospitals, Kidney, Medical Research, People with Disabilities, Public Health, Sexual Abuse, Substance Abuse. **Geo. Dist:** AZ.

### ★ 181 ★ Dover Foundation
PO Box 208
Shelby, NC 28151
**Phone:** (704)487-8890          **Fax:** (704)482-6818
**Email:** doverfnd@shelby.net
Hoyt Bailey, President

**Fnded:** 1944. **Philosophy:** The Dover Foundation is primarily interested in supporting higher education in North Carolina, including scholarships. Secondary interests include religious organizations, medical foundations and hospitals, human services, arts and humanities, and youth organizations. **Priorities:** *Arts & Humanities:* 8%. Supports arts councils. *Civic & Public Affairs:* 2%. Funds parks, gardens, and general civic concerns. *Education:* 31%. Supports higher education in North Carolina. *Environment:* 31%. Gives to homes and youth groups. *International:* 13%. Funds hospitals, hospices, and health associations. *Note:* Total contributions made in fiscal 1999. **Typ. Recipients:** Cancer, Child Abuse, Clinics/Medical Centers, Domestic Violence, Emergency/Ambulance Services, Family Planning, Health Funds, Health Organizations, Heart, Hospices, Hospitals, Kidney, Medical Education, Medical Research, Mental Health, Preventive Medicine/Wellness Organizations, Public Health, Research/Studies Institutes, Respiratory. **Geo. Dist:** NC.

## ★ 182 ★ Drue Heinz Trust

PO Box 68
New York, NY 10150
**Phone:** (212)371-5757          **Fax:** (212)759-0479
Julia Shea, Manager

**Fnded:** 1954. **Philosophy:** The Drue Heinz Foundation is primarily interested in supporting the arts, including major support to the Carnegie Museum of Art. The foundation also supports arts associations, museums, libraries, and the performing arts. Other recipient areas are funded on a limited basis. **Priorities:** *Arts & Humanities:* 18%. Supports literary arts, museums, and art education. *Civic & Public Affairs:* 14%. *Education:* 27%. medical education. *Environment:* 3%. *International:* 1%. Medical Centers, and childrens hospitals. *Note:* Total contributions made in 1998. **Typ. Recipients:** AIDS/HIV, Cancer, Children's Health/Hospitals, Clinics/Medical Centers, Emergency/Ambulance Services, Eyes/Blindness, Family Planning, Geriatric Health, Hospitals, Medical Education, Medical Rehabilitation, Medical Research, People with Disabilities, Single-Disease Health Associations. **Geo. Dist:** New York, NY; London.

## ★ 183 ★ Duke Endowment

100 North Tryon St., Ste. 3500
Charlotte, NC 28202-4012
**Phone:** (704)376-0291          **Fax:** (704)376-9336
**Email:** droberson@tde.org
**Website:** http://www.dukeendowment.org
David Roberson, Director, Communications

**Fnded:** 1924. **Philosophy:** Mr. Duke limited his benefaction to North Carolina and South Carolina. Pursuant to the terms of the trust indenture, funds are directed only to four educational institutions (Duke University, Davidson College, Furman University, and Johnson C. Smith University); nonprofit hospitals in North Carolina and South Carolina for operations, programs, and for improving and expanding facilities; nonprofit child care institutions in North Carolina and South Carolina; and the rural United Methodist Church and its pastors in North Carolina; and retired ministers who have served at least five years in an annual conference of the United Methodist Church in North Carolina, and their surviving dependents. The endowment currently addresses health issues that include health care financing, small and rural hospitals, access to primary care, community affiliations, children's health, and care of the indigent. In education, key issues include the problems of private colleges and universities such as endowments, faculty recruitment and retention, student financial aid, and physical plants. In the area of child care, a primary focus involves programs to reunite and strengthen families. Finally, grants to rural churches are centered around community needs, pastoral education, and the construction of churches. **Priorities:** *Education:* 43%. Specifically to four eligible religiously affiliated colleges and universities. *Environment:* 7%. Child care and child welfare programs. *International:* 34%. Hospitals in North and South Carolina. *Note:* Total contributions made in 1999. Analysis provided by foundation. **Typ. Recipients:** Adolescent Health Issues, AIDS/HIV, Alzheimers Disease, Cancer, Children's Health/

Hospitals, Clinics/Medical Centers, Diabetes, Emergency/Ambulance Services, Family Planning, Geriatric Health, Health Organizations, Health Policy/Cost Containment, Heart, Home-Care Services, Hospices, Hospitals, Hospitals (University Affiliated), Long-Term Care, Medical Education, Medical Rehabilitation, Medical Research, Medical Training, Nursing Services, Nutrition, Outpatient Health Care, People with Disabilities, Prenatal Health Issues, Preventive Medicine/Wellness Organizations, Public Health, Respiratory, Substance Abuse. **Geo. Dist:** NC; SC.

## ★ 184 ★ Dumont Foundation

11500 Olympic Blvd., Ste. 340
Los Angeles, CA 90064-1527
**Phone:** (310)478-2888          **Fax:** (310)312-1544
Frances Clarke, President

**Fnded:** 1967. **Priorities:** *Arts & Humanities:* 26%. Museums and art institutes received funding. *Civic & Public Affairs:* 6%. Emphasis on memorial funds and general civic issues. *Education:* 29%. Gives to Colleges and universities mainly for medical research. *International:* 39%. Focus on children's health issues, medical centers, and City of Hope. *Note:* Total contributions in 1999. **Typ. Recipients:** Alzheimers Disease, Arthritis, Children's Health/Hospitals, Clinics/Medical Centers, Eyes/Blindness, Heart, Hospitals, Medical Education, Medical Research. **Geo. Dist:** Los Angeles, CA.

## ★ 185 ★ Dunspaugh-Dalton Foundation

1533 Sunset Dr., Ste. 150
Coral Gables, FL 33143
**Phone:** (305)668-4192          **Fax:** (305)668-4247
William Lane, Jr., President & Trustee

**Fnded:** 1963. **Philosophy:** The primary focus of the foundation's grantmaking is education. Other areas of interest include social services, health, and the arts. **Priorities:** *Arts & Humanities:* 5%. Focus on music, public broadcasting, and museums. *Civic & Public Affairs:* 19%. Funds botanical gardens, aquariums, and community associations. *Education:* About 34%. Primarily for higher education. *Environment:* About 21%. Funds youth concerns and United Way. *International:* 15%. Gives to hospitals, medical centers, hospices, and health associations. *Note:* Total contributions made in 1998. **Typ. Recipients:** Alzheimers Disease, Cancer, Children's Health/Hospitals, Clinics/Medical Centers, Emergency/Ambulance Services, Family Planning, Geriatric Health, Health Organizations, Hospices, Hospitals, Hospitals (University Affiliated), Long-Term Care, Medical Education, Medical Rehabilitation, Medical Research, Mental Health, Nursing Services, People with Disabilities, Research/Studies Institutes, Single-Disease Health Associations, Speech & Hearing, Substance Abuse. **Geo. Dist:** nationally; CA; FL, Dade County; NC.

## ★ 186 ★ Dyson Foundation

25 Halcyon Rd.
Millbrook, NY 12545-9611
**Phone:** (845)677-0644          **Fax:** (845)677-0650
**Email:** info@dyson.org
**Website:** http://www.dyson.org
Dean Stein, Deputy Executive Director

**Fnded:** 1957. **Philosophy:** While the Foundation has continued to support a number of organizations that reflect the special interests of family members, it has increasingly begun to marshal its resources to target specific problems in a more focused manner. Recently the Dyson Foundation has focused special attention on funding organizations in Dutchess County, New York (which is located in the Mid-Hudson Valley). The members of the Foundation's Board of Directors have strong family ties to Dutchess County, and an enduring interest in that community's future and well-being. Through grants to the Mid-Hudson Valley, the foundation seeks to improve and enhance the quality of life by supporting social services, education, health, and arts-related organizations. Through the national and invited grants program, the Foundation supports organizations that make significant differences in the lives of poor and disadvantaged children. Medical services, healthcare, education, social welfare, public policy,

pediatrics and child health are supported. Guidelines for the program were not available at the time of publication. **Priorities:** *Arts & Humanities:* 24%. Libraries, music programs, and dance theater. *Education:* 36%. Funds colleges, universities, and medical school. *Environment:* 10%. Youth organizations, Planned Parenthood organizations, and resource development for youth. *International:* 16%. Hospitals, health education, and medical centers. *Note:* Total contributions made in 1999. **Typ. Recipients:** AIDS/HIV, Cancer, Children's Health/Hospitals, Eyes/Blindness, Family Planning, Health Funds, Health Organizations, Hospitals, Medical Rehabilitation, Medical Research, People with Disabilities, Prenatal Health Issues, Public Health, Substance Abuse, Trauma Treatment. **Geo. Dist:** nationally; NY, Mid-Hudson Valley.

## ★ 187 ★ E. L. Cord Foundation

1 East 1st St., Ste. 901
Reno, NV 89501-1915
**Phone:** (775)323-0373          **Fax:** (775)325-8523
William Bradley, Trustee

**Fnded:** 1962. **Philosophy:** "The E. L. Cord Foundation plans to focus its attention on its interests in the following general fields and activities connected or included therein, as recipients of grants. 1. Charitable 2. Scientific 3. Religious 4. Literacy and 5. Educational" 1997 Grant Policies and Procedures **Priorities:** *Arts & Humanities:* 27%. Supports museums, orchestras, and theaters. *Civic & Public Affairs:* 23%. Funds community and support projects. *Education:* About 25%. SchoolS, universities, and academies receive support. *Environment:* 16%. Supports self help programs, the Humane Society, and recreational activities. *International:* 3%. *Religion:* 3%. *Note:* Total contributions made in 1998. **Typ. Recipients:** Cancer, Children's Health/Hospitals, Clinics/Medical Centers, Diabetes, Domestic Violence, Emergency/Ambulance Services, Health-General, Hospices, Hospitals, Medical Education, Medical Research, People with Disabilities, Single-Disease Health Associations, Substance Abuse. **Geo. Dist:** NV, northern and rural counties.

## ★ 188 ★ E. L. Wiegand Foundation

Wiegand Center
165 West Liberty St.
Reno, NV 89501
**Phone:** (775)333-0310          **Fax:** (775)333-0314
Kristen Avansino, President & Executive Director

**Fnded:** 1982. **Philosophy:** The foundation funds "programs and projects...at educational institutions in the academic areas of science, business, fine arts, law and medicine; and...at health and medical research institutions in the areas of heart, eye, and cancer surgery, treatment, and research, with priority given to programs and projects that benefit children." To a lesser degree, the foundation considers applications from civic and community affairs organizations, public affairs institutions, and cultural institutions. The foundation shows a strong preference for organizations affiliated with the Roman Catholic Church. **Priorities:** *Arts & Humanities:* 12%. Supports libraries, arts foundations, museum, and ballet. *Civic & Public Affairs:* 12%. Supports employment/job training, community foundation, public policy, and law and justice. *Education:* 40%. Funds colleges, universities, science education, religious education, scholarship, and medical education. *Environment:* 8%. Supports athletics/recreation, scouts, and youth programs. *International:* 23%. Supports medical centers, hospital, heart, and home care services. *Religion:* 3%. Supports science museums. *Note:* Total contributions made in fiscal 1998. **Typ. Recipients:** Alzheimers Disease, Cancer, Children's Health/Hospitals, Clinics/Medical Centers, Diabetes, Health Organizations, Health-General, Heart, Hospitals, Long-Term Care, Medical Education, Medical Research, Nursing Services, People with Disabilities, Prenatal Health Issues, Public Health, Respiratory, Single-Disease Health Associations, Substance Abuse. **Geo. Dist:** AZ; CA, Northern California; Washington, DC; ID; NV; New York, NY; OR; UT; WA.

## ★ 189 ★ E and M Charities

PO Box 209
Muscatine, IA 52761
**Phone:** (319)264-8342 **Fax:** (319)264-3363
David Stanley, President

**Fnded:** 1979. **Philosophy:** E and M Charities makes most of its grants in the areas of education and social services. Educational funding favors tax service education, religious education, community colleges, and public school systems. Funding for social services goes to family services and marriage counseling, community centers, and youth organizations. Methodist religious organizations also receive support. Grants to other recipient areas are limited. **Priorities:** *Civic & Public Affairs:* 36%. Legislative exchange programs, nonprofits, economy policy, and community foundations. *Education:* 3%. Supports public schools and colleges. *Environment:* 1%. *Note:* Contributions made in 1998. **Typ. Recipients:** Health Organizations, Respiratory. **Geo. Dist:** nationally.

## ★ 190 ★ E. M. Lynn Foundation

2501 N Military Trl.
Boca Raton, FL 33431
**Phone:** (561)994-1910 **Fax:** (561)994-1910
Christine Lynn, Trustee

**Fnded:** 1977. **Philosophy:** The foundation generally supports a variety of charitable organizations; however, recent giving has been devoted to the Lynn University. **Priorities:** *Arts & Humanities:* 4%. Supports museums and music. *Civic & Public Affairs:* 7%. Supports philanthropic organizations and festivals. *Education:* 45%. Multiple grants to Lynn University. *Environment:* 4%. Funds youth groups and social services. *International:* 40%. Gives to hospitals and single-disease health associations. *Note:* Total contributions made in fiscal 1999. **Typ. Recipients:** AIDS/HIV, Arthritis, Cancer, Clinics/Medical Centers, Diabetes, Emergency/Ambulance Services, Family Planning, Health Funds, Health-General, Heart, Hospices, Hospitals, Hospitals (University Affiliated), Kidney, Medical Education, Medical Research, People with Disabilities, Research/Studies Institutes, Respiratory, Single-Disease Health Associations, Substance Abuse, Transplant Networks/Donor Banks. **Geo. Dist:** FL, Southern Florida.

## ★ 191 ★ E. Rhodes and Leona B. Carpenter Foundation

PO Box 58880
Philadelphia, PA 19102-8880
**Phone:** (215)963-5212
Joseph O'Connor, Jr., Contact

**Fnded:** 1975. **Philosophy:** While education traditionally receives the majority of funding and consideration from the foundation, the foundation maintains a giving pattern to a wide variety of organizations, generally located in the eastern part of the country but stretching to California. It considers requests from museums for the purchase, restoration, and conservation of Asian art and also considers proposals from organizations relating to education in the field of Asian art. The foundation also supports hospices and hospitals. The foundation has outlined a few proposal guidelines for organizations that include the following: public institutions which had direct relationships with Leona or Rhodes Carpenter during their lifetimes, public charities in support of graduate theological education, public charities where E. R. Carpenter Company has had a long-time manufacturing or business facilities including the Richmond, VA, area where requests are limited to the performing arts, museums for the purchase and restoration of Asian art, and organizations involved in providing hospice care. **Priorities:** *Arts & Humanities:* 28%. Supports Arts centers, museums, libraries, ballet and the Virginia Opera. *Civic & Public Affairs:* 1%. Housing and historical preservation projects. *Education:* 43%. Religious schools, secondary schools, and colleges. *Environment:* 8%. Family centers, youth programs and prevention of domestic/sexual abuse. *International:* 15%. Medical centers, hospices, and programs. *Religion:* 1%. *Note:* Total contributions made in 1999. **Typ. Recipients:** AIDS/HIV, Cancer, Children's Health/Hospitals, Clinics/Med-

ical Centers, Domestic Violence, Emergency/Ambulance Services, Health Organizations, Health Policy/Cost Containment, Hospices, Hospitals, Medical Education, Medical Rehabilitation, Nursing Services, People with Disabilities, Public Health, Research/Studies Institutes, Sexual Abuse, Single-Disease Health Associations, Substance Abuse. **Geo. Dist:** east of the Mississippi River; VA.

## ★ 192 ★ Earl C. Sams Foundation

101 North Shoreline Boulevard, Ste. 602
Corpus Christi, TX 78401
**Phone:** (361)884-6485 **Fax:** (361)888-4241
Bruce Hawn, President

**Fnded:** 1946. **Philosophy:** The Earl C. Sams Foundation, Inc., is a charitable foundation focusing primarily on south Texas area needs. The foundation's primary interests are education, medical, social, youth, zoological, and environmental. **Priorities:** *Arts & Humanities:* 9%. Supports museums and dance, and music. *Civic & Public Affairs:* 37%. Funds zoological concerns, aquariums, and parks. *Education:* 7%. Gives to educational foundations, colleges, and elementary education. *Environment:* 23%. Funds youth organizations, united funds, and family and drug counseling. *International:* 7%. Supports hospitals, single-disease health associations, and medical rehabilitation. *Note:* Total contributions made in 1999. **Typ. Recipients:** AIDS/HIV, Alzheimers Disease, Arthritis, Cancer, Child Abuse, Children's Health/Hospitals, Emergency/Ambulance Services, Family Planning, Heart, Kidney, Medical Rehabilitation, Medical Research, Mental Health, People with Disabilities, Substance Abuse, Substance Abuse. **Geo. Dist:** TX, Southern Texas.

## ★ 193 ★ Eden Hall Foundation

600 Grant, Ste. 3232
Pittsburgh, PA 15219
**Phone:** (412)642-6697 **Fax:** (412)642-6698
George. Greer, Grants Manager

**Fnded:** 1984. **Philosophy:** The foundation has four primary areas of interest: "social welfare and the improvement of conditions of the poor and needy; educational programs dedicated to the advancement and dissemination of useful knowledge, and support and maintenance of private colleges, universities, and other educational institutions; the advancement of better health through support and maintenance of hospitals or organizations whose primary purpose is the prevention and alleviation of sickness and disease; and the advancement of good morals." **Priorities:** *Arts & Humanities:* 1%. Supports libraries, museums and theatre. *Civic & Public Affairs:* 5%. Supports economic development, a zoological society and women's affairs. *Education:* 43%. Supports colleges, universities, schools, minority education and scholarships. *Environment:* 36%. Support family services, Big Brother/Big Sister, homes Young Men's Christian Association, and United Way. *International:* 9%. Supports children's health programs, hospital, and health care centers. *Note:* Total contributions made in 2000. **Typ. Recipients:** AIDS/HIV, Arthritis, Cancer, Children's Health/Hospitals, Clinics/Medical Centers, Diabetes, Domestic Violence, Emergency/Ambulance Services, Family Planning, Health Funds, Health Organizations, Hospices, Hospitals, Kidney, Medical Education, Medical Rehabilitation, Mental Health, Multiple Sclerosis, Nursing Services, People with Disabilities, Prenatal Health Issues, Research/Studies Institutes, Single-Disease Health Associations, Substance Abuse. **Geo. Dist:** PA, primarily western area.

## ★ 194 ★ Edgar and Elsa Prince Foundation

190 South River Ave.
Ste. 300
Holland, MI 49423
**Phone:** (616)494-8100 **Fax:** (616)494-8110
Elsa Prince, Director & Trustee

**Fnded:** 1977. **Philosophy:** The foundation typically supports churches, ministries, religious social welfare organizations, and religiously affiliated schools. **Priori-**

ties: *Arts & Humanities:* Less than 1%. *Civic & Public Affairs:* 14%. Supports community foundations, housing, and public policy. *Education:* 12%. Funds Christian schools and educational initiatives. *Environment:* 48%. Supports family services, youth organizations, and community services. *International:* 3%. Supports health services and single-disease associations. Note: Total contributions made in fiscal 2000. **Typ. Recipients:** Children's Health/Hospitals, Emergency/Ambulance Services, Family Planning, Heart, Hospices, Hospitals, Long-Term Care, Medical Rehabilitation, Medical Research, People with Disabilities, Prenatal Health Issues, Public Health, Single-Disease Health Associations, Trauma Treatment. **Geo. Dist:** MI.

## ★ 195 ★ Edmond de Rothschild Foundation

1585 Broadway
New York, NY 10036
**Phone:** (212)969-3000 **Fax:** (212)969-2900
Paul Epstein, President

**Fnded:** 1963. **Philosophy:** The Edmond de Rothschild Foundation is primarily interested in funding organizations located in France and Israel. Major categories of contributions include educational institutions, health care, and the sciences. The foundation also will fund charitable organizations in the United States on a limited basis. **Priorities:** *Education:* 4% Contributes to colleges and universities. *International:* 2% Funds medical centers and hospitals. *Note:* Total contributions made in fiscal 1997. **Typ. Recipients:** Cancer, Clinics/Medical Centers, Emergency/Ambulance Services, Geriatric Health, Hospitals, Medical Education, Multiple Sclerosis, Single-Disease Health Associations. **Geo. Dist:** New York, NY.

## ★ 196 ★ Edna McConnell Clark Foundation

250 Park Ave., Room 900
New York, NY 10177-0026
**Phone:** (212)551-9100 **Fax:** (212)986-4558
**Website:** http://www.emcf.org
Nancy Roob, Vice President & Chief Operating Officer

**Fnded:** 1950. **Philosophy:** Mr. and Mrs. Clark's primary goal in setting up the foundation was "to improve conditions for those people who are least well served by the established institutions of society." They sought to identify specific programs which could make a difference in the lives of the poor and disadvantaged. The trustees concentrate on four areas of funding: children, student achievement, tropical disease research, and New York neighborhoods. The foundation also maintains a small special projects category to respond to important initiatives that fall outside the four program areas. The Program for Children seeks to assure that all children have permanent families. The Community Partnerships for Protecting Children provides support to states and communities to reform their child protection systems. This effort partners public child protective services (CPS) agencies with a broad range of public and private community members to develop a neighborhood-based approach to protecting children. The new approach would reach families earlier, provide preventive and protective services that more closely match the individual needs of families that come to CPS attention, and improve the community's capacity to assure child safety and well-being. Foundation also supports intensive family preservation services (IFPS) as a means of preventing unnecessary placement of children by helping families stay together safely. The Program for New York Neighborhoods (formerly the Program for Homeless Families) seeks to foster neighborhood-based efforts to prevent homelessness among families in New York City. The program focuses primarily on areas of the South Bronx and Central Harlem, where the risk of housing abandonment and homelessness is great. Grantmaking areas include tenant organizing and resident-driven planning projects, family support, and educational programs that increase economic opportunity, community-building activities, and policy-oriented research and advocacy efforts that help to strengthen families and improve the buildings and blocks they live in. The Program for Tropical Disease Research seeks to improve health in the developing world by supporting research to inform health policy and practice. Program emphases include developing a vaccine against onchocerciasis and strengthening national programs for controlling trachoma–the two major infectious causes of blindness. Program staff has also begun to explore formulating a strategy aimed at improving the public health infrastructure in Ghana and Tanzania. The foundation also maintains a venture fund to explore new areas for potential grantmaking and to support projects that are consistent with its mission but that fall outside or cut across its established program areas. **Priorities:** *Civic & Public Affairs:* 33%. Principally for the New York Neighborhoods Program. Also funds institutional field building, justice, the Venture Fund, and communications. *Education:* 16%. Supports the Student Achievement Program. *Environment:* 44%. Primarily for child welfare and youth development. *International:* 7%. Supports Tropical Disease Research. *Note:* Total contributions made in fiscal 2000. **Typ. Recipients:** Child Abuse, Domestic Violence, Eyes/Blindness, Hospitals, Medical Research, Nursing Services, Substance Abuse.

### ★ 197 ★ Educational Foundation of America
35 Church Lane
Westport, CT 06880-3515
**Phone:** (203)226-6498          **Fax:** (203)227-0424
**Email:** efa@efaw.org
Diane Allison, Executive Director

**Fnded:** 1959. **Philosophy:** In general, the foundation makes grants for specific projects in the areas of population issues, the arts, education, the environment, energy, Native American issues, and other interests including medicine and peace. The foundation has recently intensified its activity in population issues, with support for programs enhancing public awareness and parent education, increasing demographic studies, reproductive rights, and strengthening public policy interests. Other civic concerns focus on problems of energy use, conservation, and nonprofit management. Education funding has emphasized nursing programs, science and mathematical programs, special education studies, minority educational projects, international studies, and population and environmental programs. Arts funding has helped institutions and programs in visual arts, dance, music, and theater. **Priorities:** *Arts & Humanities:* 1%. Supports theatre and museum. *Civic & Public Affairs:* 7%. Supports public policy, population, law foundations and organizations. *Education:* 25%. Supports preschool, elementary and secondary education; colleges and universities. *Environment:* 2%. Supports family planning. *Note:* Total contributions made in 1998. **Typ. Recipients:** Cancer, Children's Health/Hospitals, Clinics/Medical Centers, Family Planning, Geriatric Health, Medical Education, Medical Research, Prenatal Health Issues, Public Health, Substance Abuse. **Geo. Dist:** nationally.

### ★ 198 ★ Edward C. Johnson Fund
82 Devonshire St., S3
Boston, MA 02109
**Phone:** (617)563-6806
**Website:** http://www.fidelityfoundation.org
Anne-Marie Soulliere, Foundation Director

**Fnded:** 1964. **Philosophy:** The Edward C. Johnson Fund has made grants to educational institutions, museums, historic preservation and other cultural organizations, for the protection and improvement of the environment, and to community organizations. Purposes include capital campaigns, program support, and special projects. **Priorities:** *Arts & Humanities:* 32%. Museums, historical societies, arts associations, music, and libraries, with major grants to Peabody Essex Museum and Museum of Fine Arts Boston. *Civic & Public Affairs:* 1%. Community projects, foundations, and clubs. *Education:* 49%. Secondary schools and universities, with major grants to Boston College and Garrison Forest School, and economic education. *Environment:* 5%. Supports athletics, Young Men's Christian Association, and homes. *International:* 8%. Hospitals and medical associations. *Note:* Total contributions made in 1999. **Typ. Recipi-**

**ents:** Alzheimers Disease, Cancer, Clinics/Medical Centers, Emergency/Ambulance Services, Eyes/Blindness, Health Organizations, Home-Care Services, Hospitals, Medical Education, Medical Research, Mental Health, Nursing Services, Preventive Medicine/Wellness Organizations, Single-Disease Health Associations. **Geo. Dist:** New England.

### ★ 199 ★ Edward D. and Anna Mitchell Family Foundation
6310 San Vicente Boulevard, Ste. 500
Los Angeles, CA 90048
**Phone:** (213)935-6222          **Fax:** (213)930-1361
Jonathan Mitchell, President

**Fnded:** 1953. **Philosophy:** The foundation's primary interest is Israel-related organizations and education. Other interests include medical research and education. **Priorities:** *Arts & Humanities:* 5%. Supports music, museums, and art centers. *Civic & Public Affairs:* 11%. Emphasis on a charitable trust and a community foundation. *Education:* 9%. Supports educational funds and programs. *Environment:* 5%. Supports united funds, shelters, family planning, and children's welfare programs. *International:* 14%. Focus on AIDS, Parkinsons disease research, hospitals, and health associations. *Note:* Total contributions made in 1998. **Typ. Recipients:** AIDS/HIV, Children's Health/Hospitals, Clinics/Medical Centers, Diabetes, Emergency/Ambulance Services, Family Planning, Health Organizations, Heart, Hospitals, Long-Term Care, Medical Education, Medical Research, Medical Training, People with Disabilities, Single-Disease Health Associations. **Geo. Dist:** Los Angeles, CA; New York, NY.

### ★ 200 ★ Edward G. Schlieder Educational Foundation
313 Carondelet St., 1st Fl.
New Orleans, LA 70130
**Phone:** (504)581-6179          **Fax:** (504)533-3669
Donald Nalty, Chairman

**Fnded:** 1945. **Philosophy:** The foundation primarily supports higher education in Louisiana. **Priorities:** *Arts & Humanities:* 9%. Supports art programs. *Education:* 66%. Supports schools, and colleges. *Environment:* 3%. Supports recreation and athletic programs. *International:* 22%. Supports health programs. *Note:* The foundation reports that 100% of grants are restricted exclusively to educational institutions within the State of Louisiana. While grants may from time to time be specifically designated for special programs or areas of the grantee institution, the foundation indicates that all contributions benefit educational concerns. Total contributions made in 1998. **Typ. Recipients:** Cancer, Children's Health/Hospitals, Health Organizations, Health Policy/Cost Containment, Hospitals (University Affiliated), Medical Education, Medical Research, Nutrition. **Geo. Dist:** LA, limited to educational institutions in Louisiana.

### ★ 201 ★ Edward John Noble Foundation
PO Box 2180
Ardmore, OK 73402
**Phone:** (580)223-5810          **Fax:** (580)221-7362

**Fnded:** 1940. **Philosophy:** The foundation's donor believed that grant making must be a working process and not merely a passive distribution of money; not simply to help others, but to enable others to help themselves. The foundation continues to devote its attention to the arts, education, and health, as Mr. Noble wanted, but is also interested in supporting conservation and preservation of the environment. In the arts, the foundation assists major cultural organizations in New York City and their educational programs. In higher education, the foundation encourages effective interdisciplinary programs of environmental studies. In secondary education, support is given to programs likely to improve educational opportunities for disadvantaged gifted and talented youth in New York City. The foundation supports several conservation projects on St. Catherine's Island and selected other programs which help preserve the natural environment. In the health field, the foundation

primarily supports projects which show the greatest promise of stabilizing the population and providing effective population education. The foundation also considers proposals from established arts organizations interested in management training programs for interns. The foundation sees a developing role in intern programs for efficient administration of institutions and for training the arts managers of the future. **Priorities:** *Arts & Humanities:* 41%. Primary support for museums, performing arts, music, and opera. *Education:* 6%. Colleges, universities, and secondary schools. *Environment:* 1%. Focus on family planning. *International:* 3%. Supports hospitals and medical centers. *Religion:* 15%. Support for a natural history museum. *Note:* Total contributions made in 1998. **Typ. Recipients:** Cancer, Clinics/Medical Centers, Family Planning, Health Organizations, Health-General, Hospitals, Medical Education, Medical Research, Medical Training, Trauma Treatment. **Geo. Dist:** GA, Georgia coast; New York, NY, metropolitan area.

### ★ 202 ★ Edward Mallinckrodt, Jr. Foundation
One North Jefferson
Saint Louis, MO 63103
**Phone:** (314)955-3136          **Fax:** (314)955-2226
Oliver Langenberg, President & Treasurer

**Fnded:** 1953. **Philosophy:** "The basic aim of the Foundation is to dispense that amount required by law for the purpose of advancing knowledge in the various fields of clinical and laboratory research. It is further the general aim to confine contributions to those worthy projects that are in need of initial start-up funding to move the projects foward to the point of other independent support or to support highly promising young investigators at the time when start-up funds are limited and initial progress is dependent on additional funding." **Priorities:** *International:* 100%. Health care and research in major medical universities. *Note:* Total contributions made in 1999. **Typ. Recipients:** Cancer, Children's Health/Hospitals, Clinics/Medical Centers, Emergency/Ambulance Services, Kidney, Medical Research, Speech & Hearing. **Geo. Dist:** nationally.

### ★ 203 ★ Edward S. Moore Foundation
47 Arch St.
Greenwich, CT 06830
**Phone:** (203)629-4591          **Fax:** (203)629-4594
John Cross, III, President

**Fnded:** 1957. **Philosophy:** The foundation distributes donations to a variety of organizations primarily in New York and Connecticut. The foundation typically supports educational institutions, the arts, hospitals and health organizations, and social services, particularly those organizations concerned with the welfare of young people. **Priorities:** *Arts & Humanities:* 20%. Museums, music programs, and historical societies. *Civic & Public Affairs:* 2%. Zoos and aquariums receive funding. *Education:* 21%. Colleges and universities, and mentoring programs. *Environment:* 30%. Primarily supports child welfare and family services organizations. *International:* 9%. Hospitals - mostly children's health concerns. *Religion:* 2%. Funds natural history museums. *Note:* Total contributions made in 1998. **Typ. Recipients:** Children's Health/Hospitals, Clinics/Medical Centers, Health Organizations, Hospitals, Hospitals (University Affiliated), Medical Education, Medical Rehabilitation, Medical Research, Mental Health, People with Disabilities. **Geo. Dist:** CT; NY.

### ★ 204 ★ Edward W. Hazen Foundation
309 Fifth Ave., Second Floor, Room 200-3
New York, NY 10016
**Phone:** (212)889-3034          **Fax:** (212)889-3039
**Website:** http://www.hazenfoundation.org
Barbara Taveras, President

**Fnded:** 1925. **Philosophy:** The Foundation seeks to "assist young people, particularly minorities and those disadvantaged by poverty, to achieve their full potential as individuals and as active participants in a democratic society. This goal remains faithful to Mr. Hazen's original intentions and values – values that honored individual achievement and civic participation." "The Edward W. Haze Foundation has two major grantmaking programs: Public Education and Youth Development. Recognizing that children are best considered within the context of family and community, and reflecting the Foundation's belief in the pivotal role that a strong public education system can play in helping youth fulfill their potential, the Foundation has designed its grantmaking strategy with the following goals in mind: effective schools for all students; and full partnership for parents and communities working to reform and restructure their school systems." To achieve these goals, the Foundation supports new or emerging Community and Parent Organizing initiatives which seek educational equity and improved student achievement; Educational Advocacy efforts which address issues of equity and accountability, including issue analysis, policy recommendations and community education; and Community-based programs which seek to strengthen the connections between schools, families and communities. The Foundation also focuses on youth organizing around concrete social issues. "By fostering new and increased roles for youth in communities and schools the Foundation seeks to contribute to the development of a new generation of grassroots leaders committed to improving conditions in their schools and communities. Toward this end, the Foundation supports new or emerging Leadership Development initiatives which provide advocacy and community organizing skills to middle and high school-age youth; Innovative programs of community based and youth-based organizations which wish to broaden their approach to youth development to include youth organizing around concrete social issues, public education in particular; and school-based programs of community-based and grassroots organizations which help middle and high school age youth develop the interest and skills necessary to become involved in meaningful social change efforts." 1996 Guidelines **Priorities:** *Civic & Public Affairs:* 20%. Supports philanthropic organizations, employment/job training, community affairs, womens issues, civil rights and social justice. *Education:* 45%. Supports education reform, education funds, and leadership training. *Environment:* 26%. Supports family services, homes, and at-risk youth. *Note:* total contributions made in 1999. **Typ. Recipients:** AIDS/HIV, Family Planning, Medical Research, Mental Health, Public Health, Single-Disease Health Associations. **Geo. Dist:** nationally.

## ★ 205 ★ Edwin Gould Foundation for Children

23 Gramercy Park South
New York, NY 10003
**Phone:** (212)982-5200          **Fax:** (212)982-6886
**Email:** bbelfer@ega-ny.org

**Fnded:** 1923. **Philosophy:** "The Foundation is dedicated to improving the educational, personal and professional opportunities of young people. Believing that organizations can achieve more together than they can alone, we collaborate with many other foundations, corporations, nonprofits and a variety of public entities. Through grants and in-kind support as well as leveraging financial and human resources, we nurture programs that we believe can be models of reform." "In Edward Gould's day children typically needed temporary homes, protection against TB, or summer camp opportunities. Today's children face different challenges, including family breakdown, overcrowded schools, a changing job market, a woeful lack of community programs and support systems, and powerful negative peer pressures. Perhaps the most alarming is the growth of what might be called a 'street culture' of drugs, violence, and gangs that confronts young people daily and forces them to make important choices too early and too often in their lives." "As a small foundation in what might be the most challenging urban settings, we have chosen to address these issues in two ways. First we concentrate on a small number of programs and support them over a sustained period. Secondly we have expanded the roles we play in addition to grantmaking. By housing several organizations in our building, we are building a partnership network that encourages the sharing of ideas and resources." Annual Report **Priorities:** *Civic &*

*Public Affairs:* About 20%. Supports aquariums, safety, and business/free enterprise. *Education:* About 78%. Emphasis on the Edwin Gould Academy and a number of other educational associations. Supports scholarship funds. *Environment:* 2%. *Note:* Total contributions made in 1998. **Typ. Recipients:** Health Organizations, Medical Education. **Geo. Dist:** New York, NY.

## ★ 206 ★ Edwin S. Webster Foundation

77 Summer St., Ste. 800
Boston, MA 02110
**Phone:** (617)426-7172          **Fax:** (617)426-5441
**Email:** mjenney@grantsmanagement.com
Michelle Jenney, Foundation Assistant

**Fnded:** 1948. **Philosophy:** The Edwin S. Webster Foundation primarily supports "charitable organizations that are well known to the trustees, with emphasis on hospitals, medical research, education, youth agencies, cultural activities, and programs addressing the needs of minorities." **Priorities:** *Arts & Humanities:* 15%. Supports museums, theater and orchestras. *Civic & Public Affairs:* 10%. Supports gardens and a zoo. *Education:* 24%. Supports education associations, education funds, and public and private schools. *Environment:* 11%. Supports emergency relief, community services, youth services, and family services. *International:* 29%. Supports hospital and medical cneters. *Religion:* 10%. Supports a science laboratory and a museum. *Note:* Total contributions made in 1998. **Typ. Recipients:** Cancer, Children's Health/Hospitals, Clinics/Medical Centers, Diabetes, Emergency/Ambulance Services, Eyes/Blindness, Family Planning, Health Organizations, Heart, Hospitals, Hospitals (University Affiliated), Medical Education, Medical Rehabilitation, Medical Research, Mental Health, People with Disabilities, People with Disabilities, Public Health, Single-Disease Health Associations, Substance Abuse, Trauma Treatment. **Geo. Dist:** New England.

## ★ 207 ★ Edyth Bush Charitable Foundation

199 East Welbourne Ave.
PO Box 1967
Winter Park, FL 32790-1967
**Phone:** (407)647-4322          **Fax:** (407)647-7716
**Email:** dhessler@edythbush.org
David Odahowski, President

**Fnded:** 1966. **Philosophy:** The foundation's original goal was to support charitable, religious, educational, and literary purposes; with special consideration to organizations that help underprivileged or needy people improve themselves or that relieve human suffering. The foundation adheres to the intent of Edyth Bush in its giving patterns, supporting organizations in the areas of education, human services, health, and the arts. Supported art organizations demonstrate nationally recognized quality; strong emphasis is placed on K-12 educational programs. nationally recognized quality; strong emphasis is placed on K-12 educational programs. **Priorities:** *Arts & Humanities:* 4%. Libraries and music. *Civic & Public Affairs:* About 5%. Community foundations and housing. *Education:* 23%. Colleges and universities and secondary schools. *Environment:* 53%. Primarily supports community services, child welfare, family services, counseling centers, and people with disabilities. *International:* 10%. Hospitals and health care centers. *Note:* The foundation also helped to established the Center for Nonprofit Management, a central Florida affiliate of Support Centers of America. Total contributions made in fiscal 1999. **Typ. Recipients:** Alzheimers Disease, Clinics/Medical Centers, Eyes/Blindness, Health Organizations, Hospitals, Mental Health, Nursing Services, People with Disabilities, Single-Disease Health Associations. **Geo. Dist:** FL, Lake County; FL, Orange County; FL, Osceola County; FL, Seminole County.

## ★ 208 ★ Effie and Wofford Cain Foundation

4131 Spicewood Springs Rd., Ste. A-1
Austin, TX 78759
**Phone:** (512)346-7490          **Fax:** (512)346-7491

**Email:** mbratz@cainfoundation.org
Mrs. Lynn Fowler, Executive Director, Secretary & Treasure

**Fnded:** 1952. **Philosophy:** The foundation traditionally focuses its support on educational institutions and programs, social service organizations, medical institutions, and medical research programs. **Priorities:** *Arts & Humanities:* 3%. Cultural institutions. *Civic & Public Affairs:* 3%. Public and community benefit. *Education:* 31%. Educational institutions. *Environment:* 4%. Human needs and services. *Religion:* Scientific and medical institutions. **Typ. Recipients:** Alzheimers Disease, Arthritis, Cancer, Child Abuse, Children's Health/Hospitals, Clinics/Medical Centers, Diabetes, Domestic Violence, Emergency/Ambulance Services, Health Organizations, Heart, Hospitals, Hospitals (University Affiliated), Medical Education, Medical Research, Medical Training, Mental Health, People with Disabilities, Public Health, Respiratory, Single-Disease Health Associations, Substance Abuse. **Geo. Dist:** TX.

## ★ 209 ★ Eisenberg Foundation for Charities

2340 South Arlington Heights Rd., Ste. 615
Arlington Heights, IL 60005
**Phone:** (847)981-0545          **Fax:** (847)981-0548
James Marousis, Secretary, Treasurer & Director

**Fnded:** 1989. **Philosophy:** Foundation makes grants for "medicine and health, education, and physical, emotional and social assistance, primarily for the benefit of underprivileged youth and elderly." **Priorities:** *Civic & Public Affairs:* Less than 1%. *Education:* 8%. Supports universities, medical education, and education foundations. *Environment:* 10%. Supports senior services, youth programs, people with disabilities, homes and children's services. *International:* 69%. Supports medical centers, health care counsels, nursing homes health foundations and medical research. *Note:* Total contributions made in 2000. **Typ. Recipients:** AIDS/HIV, Alzheimers Disease, Cancer, Children's Health/Hospitals, Clinics/Medical Centers, Geriatric Health, Health Organizations, Health Policy/Cost Containment, Hospitals, Hospitals (University Affiliated), Long-Term Care, Medical Education, Medical Rehabilitation, Medical Research, Multiple Sclerosis, People with Disabilities, Prenatal Health Issues, Public Health, Research/Studies Institutes. **Geo. Dist:** IL, DuPage County; Chicago, IL, metropolitan area; Rochester, MN.

## ★ 210 ★ El Pomar Foundation

10 Lake Cir.
Colorado Springs, CO 80906
**Phone:** (719)633-7733          **Fax:** (719)471-6185
**Website:** http://www.elpomar.org
William Hybl, Chairman & Chief Executive Officer

**Fnded:** 1937. **Philosophy:** In general, the foundation supports educational and health institutions; civic, community, and social services; and the arts in Colorado. The foundation places greater emphasis on civic, community, and emergency needs of the poor. The foundation also concentrates on programs designed to promote excellence in nonprofit organizations. **Priorities:** *Arts & Humanities:* 5%. Supports arts centers, opera, museums, and public broadcasting. *Civic & Public Affairs:* 4%. Funds zoos, public foundations, and the Olympics. *Education:* 22%. Supports leadership training, literacy programs, and Colorado colleges. *Environment:* 29%. Gives to safe houses, disaster relief, youth programs, and senior services. *International:* 23%. Funds blood centers, hospitals, and dentistry programs for children. *Religion:* 15%. *Note:* Contributions made in 2000. **Typ. Recipients:** Alzheimers Disease, Arthritis, Cancer, Children's Health/Hospitals, Clinics/Medical Centers, Diabetes, Domestic Violence, Emergency/Ambulance Services, Eyes/Blindness, Health Organizations, Health-General, Hospices, Hospitals, Long-Term Care, Medical Rehabilitation, Medical Research, Mental Health, Nursing Services, People with Disabilities, Preventive Medicine/Wellness Organizations, Public Health, Substance Abuse, Transplant Networks/Donor Banks. **Geo. Dist:** CO.

**★ 211 ★ Elis Olsson Memorial Foundation**
PO Box 311
West Point, VA 23181
**Phone:** (804)843-3300 **Fax:** (804)843-4487
Thelma Downey, Executive Director

**Fnded:** 1966. **Philosophy:** The foundation makes most of its grants to educational institutions. Interests include private high schools, seminaries, universities, medical colleges, and literacy institutes. Secondary interests include family services, historical preservation, and various other charitable organizations. **Priorities:** *Arts & Humanities:* 9%. Supports museums and historic preservation. *Civic & Public Affairs:* 10%. Supports a foundation. *Education:* About 48%. Primarily supports schools in Virginia. *Environment:* 10%. Family services, youth organizations, and the disabled. *International:* About 8%. Focus on medical education and health associations. *Religion:* 6%. For a science museum. *Note:* Total contributions made in 1998. **Typ. Recipients:** Alzheimers Disease, Cancer, Children's Health/Hospitals, Clinics/Medical Centers, Emergency/Ambulance Services, Health Funds, Health Organizations, Health-General, Heart, Hospices, Hospitals, Hospitals (University Affiliated), Long-Term Care, Medical Education, Medical Rehabilitation, Medical Research, People with Disabilities, Public Health, Research/Studies Institutes, Respiratory, Single-Disease Health Associations. **Geo. Dist:** VA.

**★ 212 ★ Elisabeth Severance Prentiss Foundation**
PO Box 5756 Locator 2066
Cleveland, OH 44101-0756
**Phone:** (216)575-2736 **Fax:** (216)575-2695
Michael Galland, Contact

**Fnded:** 1944. **Philosophy:** "The Elisabeth Severance Prentiss Foundation is a charitable trust dedicated to the support and advancement of health care services in the greater Cleveland community. The foundation awards monetary grants to qualifying institutions and agencies for medical research and programs designed to improve the method of health care services." The trust agreement's five objectives are to promote medical and surgical research; to promote public health; to aid hospitals and health institutions in Cuyahoga County, OH, with support for capital and operating expenses; to improve methods of hospital administration; and to promote equitable health care delivery and cost-containment programs. The foundation lacks the resources to provide continuous aid to organizations for operating expenses while at the same time funding new areas of need. Therefore, its primary objective at this time is to support new, essential services that are likely to become self-sustaining. **Priorities:** *Civic & Public Affairs:* Less than 1%. *Education:* 8%. Supports nursing programs and university hospital programs. *Environment:* 6%. Funds neighborhood family practice, Planned Parenthood, and family services. *International:* 86%. Supports health centers, clinics, and foundations, hospices, hospitals, American Red Cross, mental health, children's health, and cancer *Note:* Total contributions made in 1999. **Typ. Recipients:** Adolescent Health Issues, AIDS/HIV, Alzheimers Disease, Cancer, Children's Health/Hospitals, Clinics/Medical Centers, Emergency/Ambulance Services, Eyes/Blindness, Family Planning, Geriatric Health, Health Organizations, Health Policy/Cost Containment, Heart, Hospices, Hospitals (University Affiliated), Long-Term Care, Medical Education, Medical Rehabilitation, Medical Research, Medical Training, Mental Health, Multiple Sclerosis, Nursing Services, Outpatient Health Care, People with Disabilities, Public Health, Research/Studies Institutes, Sexual Abuse, Single-Disease Health Associations, Substance Abuse, Transplant Networks/Donor Banks. **Geo. Dist:** Cleveland, OH, metropolitan area.

**★ 213 ★ Elizabeth Morse Genius Foundation**
PO Box 40
Winter Park, FL 32790

**Phone:** (407)644-0555 **Fax:** (407)644-9504
Harold Ward, III, President & Trustee

**Fnded:** 1959. **Philosophy:** The foundation primarily supports education funds, education associations, and the arts. **Priorities:** *Arts & Humanities:* 5%. Supports arts funds, music, public broadcasting, historic preservation, and libraries. *Education:* 94%. Major support for an education fund and a college. *Note:* Total contributions made in 1998. **Typ. Recipients:** Clinics/Medical Centers, Family Planning, Health Organizations, Hospitals. **Geo. Dist:** Winter Park, FL.

**★ 214 ★ Elizabeth and Stephen Bechtel Jr. Foundation**
PO Box 193809
San Francisco, CA 94119-3809
**Phone:** (415)284-8572 **Fax:** (415)284-8571
Lauren Dachs, Jr., Executive Dir.

**Fnded:** 1957. **Philosophy:** The foundation has traditionally supported higher education organizations, environmental affairs, and cultural activities. Major support from the foundation has been pledged to the California Institute of Technology Campaign for Caltech, the University of California, and Stanford University. **Priorities:** *Civic & Public Affairs:* 7%. *Education:* 30%. *Environment:* 11%. *International:* 5%. *Religion:* 15%. *Note:* Total contributions made in 2000. **Typ. Recipients:** Adolescent Health Issues, Cancer, Children's Health/Hospitals, Clinics/Medical Centers, Emergency/Ambulance Services, Eyes/Blindness, Health Organizations, Hospitals, Hospitals (University Affiliated), Long-Term Care, Medical Education, Medical Research, Multiple Sclerosis, Nutrition, People with Disabilities, Prenatal Health Issues, Research/Studies Institutes, Single-Disease Health Associations, Substance Abuse. **Geo. Dist:** San Francisco, CA, Bay area.

**★ 215 ★ Ella West Freeman Foundation**
PO Box 13218
New Orleans, LA 70185
**Phone:** (504)895-1984 **Fax:** (504)895-1988
**Email:** firstline@compuserve.com
Louis Freeman, Jr., Chairman

**Fnded:** 1940. **Philosophy:** The Ella West Freeman Foundation favors education, primarily Tulane University. Other interests include the arts, civic affairs, and social services. The foundation focuses on programs which produce responses from other donors, especially civic agencies in the New Orleans area. **Priorities:** *Arts & Humanities:* 17%. Funds arts associations and arts preservation. *Civic & Public Affairs:* 3%. Funds community foundations and public policy groups. *Education:* 12%. Gives to math and science education and to colleges and universities. *International:* 68%. Primarily supports medical foundations. *Note:* Total contributions made in 2000. **Typ. Recipients:** Emergency/Ambulance Services, Family Planning, Hospitals, Medical Research, People with Disabilities, Research/Studies Institutes, Substance Abuse. **Geo. Dist:** LA.

**★ 216 ★ Ellen Browning Scripps Foundation**
6121 Terryhill Dr.
La Jolla, CA 92037
**Phone:** 800-326-3776
**Website:** http://www.scrippsfoundation.org
E. Dawson, Sr. Vice President & Manager

**Fnded:** 1935. **Philosophy:** The Ellen Browning Scripps Foundation makes most of its grants in the areas of education, the arts, health, and civic affairs. Educational funding favors Scripps College and private schools. Funding for the arts goes to museums, libraries, and historic preservation. Health interests include research, medical centers, and hospitals. In civic affairs, interests include zoos, women's affairs, and the environment. The foundation also supports a variety of social service interests. **Priorities:** *Arts & Humanities:* About 18%. Museums, libraries, and opera. *Civic & Public Affairs:* About 15%. Primary support given to the San Diego Zoological Society. *Education:* About 23%. Colleges and private educa-

tion. *Environment:* About 14%. Scouting and youth programs, Meals on Wheels, and services for the elderly. *International:* 20%. Hospices and hospitals. *Religion:* 5%. Natural history and maritime museums, aerospace, and oceanography studies. *Note:* Total contributions made in fiscal 1999. **Typ. Recipients:** Children's Health/Hospitals, Eyes/Blindness, Hospices, Hospitals, Medical Research, People with Disabilities, Research/Studies Institutes, Single-Disease Health Associations, Transplant Networks/Donor Banks. **Geo. Dist:** CA, San Diego County.

**★ 217 ★ Ellison Foundation**
1 Memorial Dr.
Cambridge, MA 02142-1300
**Phone:** (617)225-3800 **Fax:** (617)255-3801
Elton Drew, Trustee

**Fnded:** 1952. **Philosophy:** The foundation was formed for the purposes of disbursing funds solely and exclusively for religious, charitable, scientific, literary, or educational purposes, and for the prevention of cruelty to children or animals. Health care receives major support. **Priorities:** *Arts & Humanities:* 14%. Supports historical preservation and museums. *Civic & Public Affairs:* 7%. Supports community foundations. *Education:* 21%. Supports colleges and universities. *Environment:* 4%. Supports youth, and family services. *International:* 48%. Supports hospitals and medical centers. *Note:* Total contributions made in 1998. **Typ. Recipients:** Cancer, Children's Health/ Hospitals, Clinics/Medical Centers, Health Organizations, Hospitals, Hospitals (University Affiliated), Medical Education, Medical Rehabilitation, Nursing Services, People with Disabilities, Public Health, Speech & Hearing. **Geo. Dist:** nationally; MA, primarily.

**★ 218 ★ Ellwood Foundation**
PO Box 550049
Houston, TX 77255
**Phone:** (713)780-7722 **Fax:** (713)780-8833
H. Hightower, Trustee

**Fnded:** 1958. **Philosophy:** The Ellwood Foundation primarily makes grants in the areas of health services and social services. Health support goes to medical research, mental health, hospitals, health foundations, single-disease associations, and health organizations. In social services, funding favors homes, child welfare, the disabled, and youth centers. Grants are made to other recipient areas on a limited basis. **Priorities:** *Arts & Humanities:* 5%. Supports the Institute of Texas Cultures. *Civic & Public Affairs:* 5%. Supports educational programs and institutions. *Environment:* 15%. Supports children and youth services, drug and alcohol abuse assistance, and the disabled. *International:* 53%. Supports hospice, medical centers, hospitals, disease and disorder concerns. *Religion:* 4%. Supports the Institute of Molecular Studies. *Note:* Contributions were made in fiscal 1999. **Typ. Recipients:** Alzheimers Disease, Cancer, Child Abuse, Children's Health/Hospitals, Clinics/Medical Centers, Eyes/Blindness, Health Organizations, Heart, Hospices, Hospitals, Hospitals (University Affiliated), Long-Term Care, Medical Education, Medical Rehabilitation, Medical Research, Mental Health, People with Disabilities, People with Disabilities, Prenatal Health Issues, Public Health, Single-Disease Health Associations, Speech & Hearing, Substance Abuse. **Geo. Dist:** Houston, TX.

**★ 219 ★ Elmer and Mamdouha Bobst Foundation**
c/o Elmer Holmes Bobst Library, New York University
70 Washington Square South, Room 1209
New York, NY 10012-1091
**Phone:** (212)998-2440 **Fax:** (212)995-3679
Ms. Mamdouha Bobst, President

**Fnded:** 1968. **Philosophy:** The foundation's interests include support for the E. and M. Bobst Institute at the Richard Nixon Library, the promotion of health and cancer research, Islamic organizations in the United States and abroad, and youth and community service organizations. **Priorities:** *Civic & Public Affairs:* 1%.

*Education:* 38%. Supports precollege education, colleges and universities. *Environment:* 38%. Supports animal welfare and youth services. *International:* 8%. Hospitals, health funds, and single-disease health associations. *Note:* Total contributions made in 1998. **Typ. Recipients:** AIDS/HIV, Cancer, Children's Health/Hospitals, Clinics/Medical Centers, Emergency/Ambulance Services, Health Funds, Health Organizations, Heart, Hospices, Hospitals, Hospitals (University Affiliated), Medical Research, Public Health, Single-Disease Health Associations, Transplant Networks/Donor Banks. **Geo. Dist:** New York, NY.

### ★ 220 ★ Engelberg Foundation
1050 N Lake Way
Palm Beach, FL 33480
**Phone:** (561)848-7089
Alfred Engelberg, Trustee

**Fnded:** 1991. **Priorities:** *Arts & Humanities:* 11%. Gives to art endowments and performing arts. *Education:* 36%. Focus on art and law education. *Environment:* 7%. Supports programs for the homeless and community service. *International:* 18%. Genetics, hospitals, Medicaid studies, and teen pregnancy prevention programs. *Religion:* 3%. Grants made to research. *Note:* Total contributions in fiscal 1999. **Typ. Recipients:** AIDS/HIV, Cancer, Children's Health/Hospitals, Clinics/Medical Centers, Family Planning, Health Organizations, Hospitals, Long-Term Care, Outpatient Health Care, Public Health. **Geo. Dist:** NY.

### ★ 221 ★ Enid and Crosby Kemper Foundation
PO Box 419692
Kansas City, MO 64141-6692
**Phone:** (816)860-7711          **Fax:** (816)860-5690
**Email:** steven.campbell@umb.com
**Website:** http://www.umb.com
Steve Campbell, Trust Administrator

**Fnded:** 1972. **Philosophy:** The foundation traditionally has placed emphasis on higher and private secondary education and cultural programs, particularly museums and music. Significant support has also been extended to health and youth-related causes. **Priorities:** *Arts & Humanities:* 97%. Primarily to museums, historical societies, and music. *Civic & Public Affairs:* Less than 1%. *Education:* Less than 1%. *Environment:* 2%. Supports the Exploration Place. *International:* Less than 1%. *Note:* Total contributions made in 1999. **Typ. Recipients:** Children's Health/Hospitals, Clinics/Medical Centers, Health Organizations, Hospitals, Kidney, Medical Research, People with Disabilities, Public Health, Single-Disease Health Associations, Speech & Hearing, Substance Abuse. **Geo. Dist:** Kansas City, MO, metropolitan area.

### ★ 222 ★ Ethel Wilson Bowles and Robert Bowles Memorial Fund
301 East Colorado Boulevard, Ste. 900
Pasadena, CA 91101
**Phone:** (626)796-9123
Emrys Ross, Trustee

**Fnded:** 1974. **Philosophy:** The foundation funds medical research, medical schools, and hospitals in California. **Priorities:** *Education:* 46%. Supports medical schools and an institute of technology. *International:* 54%. Funds hospitals and medical centers. *Note:* Total contributions made in 1998. **Typ. Recipients:** Children's Health/Hospitals, Hospitals, Hospitals (University Affiliated), Medical Education, Medical Research, Single-Disease Health Associations. **Geo. Dist:** CA.

### ★ 223 ★ Eugene and Agnes E. Meyer Foundation
1400 16th St. Northwest, Ste. 360
Washington, DC 20036-2217
**Phone:** (202)483-8294          **Fax:** (202)328-6850
**Website:** http://www.meyerfoundation.org
Julie Rogers, President

**Fnded:** 1944. **Philosophy:** The foundation hopes to improve the quality of life in Washington D.C., by supporting community efforts and promoting community responsibility. The foundation takes an innovative and comprehensive approach to the problems and changing needs of the Washington metropolitan area. "We recognize that human needs in a large metropolitan area are always changing and our grant-making process was designed with flexibility in mind." Grants are awarded in six broad program areas: neighborhood development and housing; community service; arts and humanities; education; health and mental health; and law and justice. **Priorities:** *Arts & Humanities:* 16%. Theater, museums, dance, and music. *Civic & Public Affairs:* 56%. Community service grants, neighborhood development/housing, and law and justice programs. *Education:* 23%. Recording for blind and dyslexic, high schools, and multicultural career programs. *International:* 5%. Mental health services, AIDS, and drug/alcohol treatment programs. *Note:* Total contributions made in 1998. **Typ. Recipients:** AIDS/HIV, Children's Health/Hospitals, Clinics/Medical Centers, Domestic Violence, Family Planning, Health Organizations, Health-General, Hospices, Long-Term Care, Mental Health, People with Disabilities, Prenatal Health Issues, Public Health, Substance Abuse. **Geo. Dist:** Washington, DC, metropolitan area; MD, suburban Maryland; VA, Northern Virginia.

### ★ 224 ★ Eugene B. Casey Foundation
800 South Frederick Ave.
Ste. 100
Gaithersburg, MD 20877
**Phone:** (301)948-4595          **Fax:** (301)948-9159
Betty Casey, Chairman, President & Treasurer

**Fnded:** 1981. **Philosophy:** "Grants are primarily restricted to the Maryland and Washington, D.C., area in amounts sufficient to have an impact, and generally limited to the same charitable activities as in the foundation's past years." Major support goes to organizations directly affiliated with the foundation, including the Casey Family Foundation at Washington College and the Eugene B. Casey Center for Diagnostic Cardiolology. Other foundation interests include hospices, mental health, family services, shelters, arts for the disabled and youth, and Washington, D.C., area colleges and universities. **Priorities:** *Arts & Humanities:* 33%. Supports the performing arts and public broadcasting services. *Civic & Public Affairs:* 21%. Supports affordable housing, public policy, Native American affairs, and human rights. *Education:* 13%. Supports educational programs, preparatory schools, colleges and universities, arts & humanities education, literacy, and architects education. *Environment:* 2%. Supports youth services, the homeless, the elderly, battered women, and substance abuse. *International:* 31%. Supports hospices, hospitals, medical centers, medical research, and eyes/blindness. *Note:* Total contributions made in fiscal 2000. **Typ. Recipients:** Cancer, Child Abuse, Children's Health/Hospitals, Clinics/Medical Centers, Domestic Violence, Emergency/Ambulance Services, Eyes/Blindness, Family Planning, Health Funds, Health Organizations, Heart, Hospices, Hospitals, Hospitals (University Affiliated), Medical Education, Medical Research, Mental Health, Nutrition, People with Disabilities, Substance Abuse. **Geo. Dist:** Washington, DC, including metropolitan area.

### ★ 225 ★ Eugene M. Lang Foundation
535 5th Ave., Ste. 906
New York, NY 10017
**Phone:** (212)949-4100          **Fax:** (212)286-8964
Eugene Lang, Contact

**Fnded:** 1963. **Philosophy:** The foundation typically supports education, the arts, health, and civic causes. **Priorities:** *Arts & Humanities:* 2%. Supports opera, theater, music, libraries, museums, and arts festivals. *Civic & Public Affairs:* Less than 1%. *Education:* 50%. Emphasis on colleges and universities. *International:* 41%. Focus on New York Hospital Medical Center and pediatric cancer research. *Religion:* 6%. *Note:* Total contributions made in 1998. **Typ. Recipients:** AIDS/HIV, Cancer, Children's Health/Hospitals, Clinics/Medical Centers, Health Organizations, Hospitals, Medical Rehabilitation, Mental Health. **Geo. Dist:** internationally; nationally; New York, NY.

### ★ 226 ★ The Eugene McDermott Foundation
3808 Euclid
Dallas, TX 75205
**Phone:** (214)521-2924
Mary McDermott Cook, President

**Fnded:** 1972. **Philosophy:** The foundation traditionally has supported medical facilities, science, schools, the arts, educational programs, and cultural organizations. **Priorities:** *Arts & Humanities:* 29%. Supports libraries, music, museums, theater, opera, and dance. *Civic & Public Affairs:* 3%. Urban affairs, zoos, and botanical gardens. *Education:* 53%. Funds colleges and universities, private schools, education funds, and arts education. *Environment:* 9%. Supports youth and senior organizations. *International:* 1%. Hospitals, single-disease health associations, and the American Red Cross. *Note:* Total contributions made in fiscal 1999. **Typ. Recipients:** AIDS/HIV, Cancer, Child Abuse, Children's Health/Hospitals, Clinics/Medical Centers, Domestic Violence, Emergency/Ambulance Services, Family Planning, Hospitals, Hospitals (University Affiliated), Medical Education, People with Disabilities, Prenatal Health Issues, Preventive Medicine/Wellness Organizations, Public Health, Single-Disease Health Associations, Substance Abuse, Transplant Networks/Donor Banks. **Geo. Dist:** Dallas, TX.

### ★ 227 ★ Eva L. and Joseph M. Bruening Foundation
1422 Euclid Ave., Ste. 627
Cleveland, OH 44115-1901
**Phone:** (216)621-2632          **Fax:** (216)621-8198
Janet Narten, Executive Director

**Fnded:** 1988. **Philosophy:** The mission of the foundation is to enhance the quality of life in Cuyahoga County, OH. Priority is given to initiatives designed to educate youth, comfort the aged, and provide encouragement and support to the disabled and disadvantaged. The foundation supports practical programs that meet clearly defined community needs in a creative and efficient manner. The foundation welcomes grant requests for capital, start-up operations, and program support from tax-exempt, non-profit organizations whose goals and objectives match those of the foundation. **Priorities:** *Arts & Humanities:* (Arts/Culture) 5%. Supports opera, ballet, theater, and cultural arts programs. *Civic & Public Affairs:* (Public/Society Benefit) 5%. Funds community programs. *Education:* 12%. Funds secondary schools and education programs. *Environment:* 56%. Supports community services, homes, senior and children's services, and crisis centers. *International:* 20%. Primarily funds clinics. *Note:* Total contributions made in 2000. **Typ. Recipients:** Adolescent Health Issues, AIDS/HIV, Alzheimers Disease, Cancer, Children's Health/Hospitals, Clinics/Medical Centers, Domestic Violence, Emergency/Ambulance Services, Eyes/Blindness, Family Planning, Geriatric Health, Health Organizations, Hospices, Hospitals, Long-Term Care, Nursing Services, People with Disabilities, Prenatal Health Issues, Preventive Medicine/Wellness Organizations, Public Health, Research/Studies Institutes, Sexual Abuse, Single-Disease Health Associations, Speech & Hearing, Substance Abuse. **Geo. Dist:** OH, Cuyahoga County.

### ★ 228 ★ Evelyn and Walter Haas, Jr. Fund
One Market Landmark, Ste. 400
San Francisco, CA 94105
**Phone:** (415)856-1400          **Fax:** (415)856-1500
**Email:** info@haasjr.org
**Website:** http://www.haasjr.org
Clayton Juan, Administrator

**Fnded:** 1953. **Philosophy:** The Evelyn and Walter Haas, Jr. Fund was established to support cultural, educational, and human welfare programs that enrich the lives of residents of the San Francisco area. The 2000 program guidelines reflect the direction of the fund's future grantmaking. Currently, the fund's four program areas are "Strengthening Children, Youth, Families, and the Elderly; Strengthening Neighborhoods; Promoting Diversity and Inclusiveness; and Enhancing Nonprofit Leadership and Governance." "Strengthening Neighborhoods" focuses on efforts to stabilize and improve urban neighborhoods, with a particular emphasis on community development through programs that involve residents and promote leaders who can energize local improvements. In order to reweave community and home safety nets, especially in low-income neighborhoods, "Strengthening Children, Youth, Families, and the Elderly" supports programs that nurture the young to become healthy, productive, caring adults, and enhance elders' well-being and encourage their self-sufficiency. The fund helps ensure that youth have opportunities to enhance their personal development during nonschool hours through activities that include recreation, sports, education, and community service; develops and enhances community-based prevention programs that enable parents to play active roles in their children's development, and foster cooperation between home and school; supports school-linked and community-based approaches that coordinate and leverage resources to effect enduring, systemic improvements in services for healthy child and youth development; and enhances the quality of life for the elderly by strengthening a continuum of independent living services. "Promoting Diversity and Inclusiveness" focuses on promoting a sense of community that respects and embraces diversity with particular interest in strategies designed to overcome barriers caused by racism, seism, and homophobia. Work is done in three arenas: building community; affirming pluralism; and fair and equitable treatment. "Enhancing Nonprofit Leadership and Governance" looks to enhance the effectiveness of local nonprofit groups working in the Fund's interest areas through leadership development, management and technical assistance, and public policy. **Priorities:** *Arts & Humanities:* 6%. Museums, theater, art. *Civic & Public Affairs:* 46%. Neighborhoods and housing. *Education:* 21%. Universities and secondary schools. Includes major grant to UC Berkeley. *Environment:* 21%. Mainly hunger and homelessness. *International:* 2%. *Note:* Total contributions made in 1999. **Typ. Recipients:** Alzheimers Disease, Clinics/Medical Centers, Domestic Violence, Geriatric Health, Health Organizations, Home-Care Services, Hospices, Hospitals, Long-Term Care, Mental Health, Nursing Services, Nutrition, People with Disabilities, Research/Studies Institutes. **Geo. Dist:** CA, Alameda County; CA, San Francisco County.

★ **229 ★ Ewing Halsell Foundation**
711 Navarro, Ste. 537
San Antonio, TX 78205
**Phone:** (210)223-2640      **Fax:** (210)271-9089
Gilbert Denman, Jr., Trustee, Chairman of the Board
**Fnded:** 1957. **Philosophy:** The foundation requires that all contributions be made to help improve the quality of life for Texas citizens. "The foundation makes most of its grants in the San Antonio area and in those Southwestern parts of Texas where a large part of the income producing assets of the foundation are located, and where it can best evaluate needs for assistance." The foundation believes strongly in public involvement and fostering a wide range of philanthropic support. Therefore, matching funds are encouraged but not always required. The foundation may make a challenge grant to stimulate other financial participation. challenge grant to stimulate other financial participation. **Priorities:** *Arts & Humanities:* 51%. Supports public broadcasting, symphony and museum. *Civic & Public Affairs:* 5%. Supports community foundations, housing, zoos and parks. *Education:* 15%. Support public and private schools. *Environment:* 15%. Supports United Way, youth and family services. *International:* 8%. Supports medical research. *Note:* Total contributions made in fiscal 1999. **Typ. Recipients:** AIDS/HIV, Cancer, Children's Health/Hospitals, Clinics/Medical Centers, Domestic Violence, Emergency/Ambulance Services, Family Planning, Geriatric Health, Health Organizations, Heart, Hospitals, Medical Research, Nursing Services, People with Disabilities, Public Health, Single-Disease Health Associations, Substance Abuse. **Geo. Dist:** San Antonio, TX.

★ **230 ★ Ewing Marion Kauffman Foundation**
4801 Rockhill Rd.
Kansas City, MO 64110-2046
**Phone:** (816)932-1000      **Fax:** (816)932-1440
**Email:** acanfiel@emkf.org
**Website:** http://www.emkf.org
Anne Canfield, Communications Director
**Fnded:** 1966. **Philosophy:** "The Ewing Marion Kauffman Foundation is a private foundation that works toward the vision of self-sufficient people in healthy communities. Our mission is to research and identify unfulfilled needs of society and to develop, implement and/or fund breakthrough solutions that have a lasting impact and offer people a choice and hope for the future. The Kauffman Foundation's work is focused on two areas: Youth Development and Entrepreneurial Leadership." "Through partnerships, the Foundation believes it can most effectively support social and economic solutions that support children, their families and communities, and accelerate the development of entrepreneurship in America." **Priorities:** *Arts & Humanities:* 4%. Supports the city museum. *Civic & Public Affairs:* 60%. Funds public policy and entrepreneurial training institutes and education. *Education:* 27%. Funds higher education and educational development programs. *Environment:* 5%. Supports youth development group, including community and economic development centered around youth concerns. *International:* 4%. Supports a health center. *Note:* Total contributions made in 2000. **Typ. Recipients:** Clinics/Medical Centers, Health Policy/Cost Containment, Mental Health, Prenatal Health Issues, Substance Abuse. **Geo. Dist:** Kansas City, MO.

★ **231 ★ F. J. O'Neill Charitable Corp.**
3550 Lander Rd.
Cleveland, OH 44124
**Phone:** (216)464-2121      **Fax:** (216)464-1517
Hugh O'Neill, President
**Fnded:** 1979. **Philosophy:** The corporation's main concerns are higher education and religion. Colleges and universities are funded primarily, as well as churches and religious organizations in Ohio. Of particular interest to the corporation are local concerns and self-help projects. "Applications to the Corporation are considered on their merits. Need and the good to be accomplished are prime considerations." **Priorities:** *Arts & Humanities:* 9%. Museums, historical societies, and theaters. *Civic & Public Affairs:* 3%. Foundations and housing. *Education:* 31%. Supports private precollege education. *Environment:* 21%. Gives to youth concerns, drug abuse programs, and united funds. *International:* 7%. Health care facilities. *Note:* Total contributions made in 1998. **Typ. Recipients:** Cancer, Children's Health/Hospitals, Clinics/Medical Centers, Emergency/Ambulance Services, Eyes/Blindness, Geriatric Health, Health Organizations, Home-Care Services, Hospices, Hospitals, Long-Term Care, Medical Rehabilitation, Medical Research, Nursing Services, People with Disabilities, Public Health, Single-Disease Health Associations, Substance Abuse. **Geo. Dist:** OH, Eastern Ohio.

★ **232 ★ F. M. Kirby Foundation**
17 DeHart St.
PO Box 151
Morristown, NJ 07963-0151
**Phone:** (973)538-4800
**Website:** http://fdncenter.org/grantmaker/kirby/
Mr. F. Kirby, President
**Fnded:** 1931. **Philosophy:** The foundation provides funds to organizations in areas where family members live and work, and to organizations in which Fred M. Kirby, the original donor, had an interest. The foundation states its philosophy as follows: "A distinctive feature of American life, dating back to colonial times, is the remarkable richness and diversity of its voluntary, non-profit sector. Although government has become alarmingly involved in people's lives over the last few decades, we believe people should be encouraged to solve their own problems exclusive of government aid, and on the local level. Private philanthropy is there to help them." **Priorities:** *Arts &*

*Humanities:* 10%. Provides funding to museums, performing arts, and theater. *Civic & Public Affairs:* 1%. Supports individual rights organizations. *Education:* 27%. Funds colleges and universities. *Environment:* 16%. Funds the United Way, family planning and family services, youth organizations, and the prevention of domestic violence. *International:* 43%. Supports medical research, hospitals, single-disease health associations, and health funds. *Note:* Total contributions made in 1999. **Typ. Recipients:** AIDS/HIV, Alzheimers Disease, Arthritis, Cancer, Children's Health/Hospitals, Domestic Violence, Emergency/Ambulance Services, Eyes/Blindness, Family Planning, Geriatric Health, Health Funds, Health-General, Heart, Hospices, Hospitals, Medical Education, Medical Rehabilitation, Medical Research, Nursing Services, People with Disabilities, Public Health, Respiratory, Single-Disease Health Associations, Substance Abuse, Transplant Networks/Donor Banks. **Geo. Dist:** some national organizations; Morristown, NJ; Hillsborough, NC; Wilkes-Barre, PA.

★ **233 ★ F. R. Bigelow Foundation**
600 Norwest Center
55 East Fifth St.
Saint Paul, MN 55101-1797
**Phone:** (651)224-5463      **Fax:** (651)224-8123
Paul Verret, President
**Fnded:** 1934. **Philosophy:** "The F.R. Bigelow Foundation is willing to consider grant applications from all properly qualified nonprofit corporations. Historically, the primary areas of interest have been education, social service, humanities and the arts. The Children, Families, and Community Initiative (CFCI) was established by the trustees in 1990 with a five-year grant of $2.5 million. The purpose of CFCI is to address the needs of children living in the Frogtown and Summit-University neighborhoods in the context of family and community. This program is overseen by an active, multi-cultural Steering Committee of persons who live and/or work in the two neighborhoods. In 1995, the Trustees authorized a second five-year grant of $2.5 million to continue the work of CFCI through the year 2000. In 1998 a majority of CFCI's efforts were devoted to improving the grantmaking process, strengthening internal operations and developing a long-range plan for beyond the year 2000. Over half of grant dollars were directed toward youth leadership, and academic development, collaboration between community-based organizations serving youth, after school and summer enrichment, community building, and neighborhood entrepreneurs." 1998 Annual Report **Priorities:** *Arts & Humanities:* 6%. Performing arts, museums, and historical societies. *Civic & Public Affairs:* 24% Crime prevention efforts, community foundations, and urban affairs. *Education:* 10%. Public education, universities, and lifelong learning support. *Environment:* 42%. Primarily supports youth and family programs. *International:* 6%. Support and expansion of health programs. *Religion:* 10%. Funds a science museum. *Note:* Total contributions made in 1998. **Typ. Recipients:** Alzheimers Disease, Cancer, Children's Health/Hospitals, Emergency/Ambulance Services, Family Planning, Health Organizations, Health-General, Hospices, Hospitals, Medical Rehabilitation, Mental Health, People with Disabilities, Preventive Medicine/Wellness Organizations, Public Health, Research/Studies Institutes, Single-Disease Health Associations, Substance Abuse. **Geo. Dist:** St. Paul, MN.

★ **234 ★ Fan Fox and Leslie R. Samuels Foundation**
350 Fifth Ave., Ste. 4301
New York, NY 10118
**Phone:** (212)239-3030
**Email:** info@samuels.org
**Website:** http://www.samuels.org/
Joseph Mitchell, Director, President, and Treasurer
**Fnded:** 1981. **Philosophy:** The foundation is generally interested in funding organizations in the metropolitan New York area dealing with the performing arts and health. In the performing arts, particular interests are music, especially opera, ballet, dance, theater and programs for young artists. Health-related grants are directed toward improving the delivery of health ser-

vices to the people of New York City, particularly children and the elderly. **Priorities:** *Arts & Humanities:* 57%. Primarily supports performing arts, including theater, ballet, dance, and music. *Education:* 8%. Supports medical and arts education. *Environment:* 5%. Supports human service organizations. *International:* 30%. Funds hospitals and medical centers for the delivery of health services, home-care services, and geriatric health. *Note:* Total contributions made in fiscal 2000. **Typ. Recipients:** Adolescent Health Issues, AIDS/HIV, Alzheimers Disease, Cancer, Children's Health/Hospitals, Clinics/Medical Centers, Diabetes, Geriatric Health, Health Organizations, Health Policy/Cost Containment, Heart, Home-Care Services, Hospices, Hospitals, Long-Term Care, Medical Education, Medical Rehabilitation, Medical Research, Mental Health, Nursing Services, People with Disabilities, Prenatal Health Issues, Public Health, Public Health, Research/Studies Institutes, Respiratory, Substance Abuse. **Geo. Dist:** New York, NY, metropolitan area.

### ★ 235 ★ Faye McBeath Foundation

1020 North Broadway
Milwaukee, WI 53202
**Phone:** (414)272-5805          **Fax:** (414)272-6235
**Email:** mcbeath@execpc.com
**Website:** http://www.fayemcbeath.org
Sarah Dean, Executive Director

**Fnded:** 1964. **Philosophy:** Miss McBeath stipulated specific guidelines when she established the foundation. Under the terms of the trust, grants are made to organizations within the state of Wisconsin for the following purposes: to promote research and education in the fields of medical science and public health; to provide medical, nursing, and hospital care for the sick and disabled; to promote child welfare; to promote research in civic and government affairs directed toward improved efficiency of local government; and to disseminate the results of the research. Currently, the foundation directs special attention to projects consistent with the following priorities: *Welfare of Children:* Grants in this area help to strengthen the family, as the key factor in education, motivation, and development of children, including programs which improve parenting skills and reduce the incidence of child abuse and family violence; to enhance the development and school readiness of preschool children; to stress the development and well-being of children's creativity, imagination, and self-esteem, with emphasis on learning skills and development; to promote experiences which bring excitement and challenge to the learning process and to dramatize the rewards of educational success; to develop quality educational initiatives that prepare youth for employment; to enhance the quality of precollegiate education; and to address special youth problems, such as adolescent pregnancy, unemployment, and teen suicide. *Health Care and Education:* Funding is made to promote improvement in the health of high-risk populations, especially infants, the elderly, and the poor through projects designed to improve prenatal care, encourage healthy lifestyles, and prevent disease; to provide and expand alternatives to institutional and inpatient care; to facilitate access to comprehensive medical care for elderly, youth, minorities, and the indigent; to enhance the development of the Milwaukee Regional Center as a viable resource for the community and state; and to improve the capability of local universities and colleges to educate health-care providers. *Care of Elderly Persons:* Support is given to sustain older persons in their homes and neighborhoods by strengthening alternatives to institutional care, such as support services, special housing, and home care; and to increase access to existing community services for isolated older adults. **Priorities:** *Arts & Humanities:* 6%. Supports museums. *Civic & Public Affairs:* 55%. Supports public policy and community concerns. *Education:* 8%. Supports schools, music education, and colleges and universities. *Environment:* 18%. Supports child care, youth services, planned parenthood, Young Women's Christian Association, and the elderly. *International:* 7%. Funds hospitals, specialty clinics, and disease and disorder concerns. **Typ. Recipients:** AIDS/HIV, Alzheimers Disease, Child Abuse, Children's Health/Hospitals, Clinics/Medical Centers, Domestic Violence, Eyes/Blindness, Family Planning,

Geriatric Health, Health Organizations, Health Policy/Cost Containment, Hospices, Hospitals, Long-Term Care, Medical Education, Medical Rehabilitation, Mental Health, Nursing Services, People with Disabilities, Public Health, Single-Disease Health Associations, Speech & Hearing, Substance Abuse, Transplant Networks/Donor Banks. **Geo. Dist:** WI, particularly the Milwaukee metropolitan area.

### ★ 236 ★ Feldman Foundation

PO Box 1046
Dallas, TX 75221
**Phone:** (214)689-4337
Robert Feldman, Trustee

**Fnded:** 1964. **Philosophy:** Since its inception, the foundation has supported Jewish welfare agencies and organizations that show an interest in Israel. **Priorities:** *Education:* 14%. Includes colleges and universities. *Environment:* 2%. Supports united funds, food banks, and senior concerns. *Note:* Total contributions made in 1998. **Typ. Recipients:** Family Planning, Hospitals, Hospitals (University Affiliated), Long-Term Care, Medical Education, Medical Research, Preventive Medicine/Wellness Organizations, Single-Disease Health Associations. **Geo. Dist:** national organizations for support of Israel; TX.

### ★ 237 ★ Field Foundation of Illinois

200 South Wacker, Ste. 3860
Chicago, IL 60606
**Phone:** (312)831-0910
Handy Lindsey, Jr., President

**Fnded:** 1960. **Philosophy:** "The Field Foundation seeks to provide support for community, civic, and cultural organizations in the Chicago area, enabling both new and established programs to test innovations, to expand proven strengths, or to address specific, time-limited operational needs." **Priorities:** *Arts & Humanities:* 20%. Supports art institutes, galleries, and the opera. *Civic & Public Affairs:* 27%. Supports park development, housing, and community projects. *Education:* 13%. Supports literacy, public schools, and universities. *Environment:* 18%. Supports YMCA, youth services, Hull House, and homeless services. *International:* 16%. Supports HIV facility and health care programs. *Note:* Total contributions made in fiscal 1999. **Typ. Recipients:** AIDS/HIV, Children's Health/Hospitals, Clinics/Medical Centers, Domestic Violence, Emergency/Ambulance Services, Health Organizations, Heart, Hospitals, Hospitals (University Affiliated), Medical Rehabilitation, People with Disabilities, Prenatal Health Issues, Public Health, Sexual Abuse, Substance Abuse. **Geo. Dist:** Chicago, IL, including metropolitan area.

### ★ 238 ★ Figtree Foundation

PO Box 130843
Birmingham, AL 35213
**Phone:** (205)879-0712          **Fax:** (205)879-6382
Jo Morrison, President

**Fnded:** 1986. **Philosophy:** The Figtree Foundation primarily supports religion, targeting a variety of Jewish causes. The foundation also focuses donations on education. Minor interests include civic affairs, health associations, social services, and the arts. **Priorities:** *Arts & Humanities:* 6%. Funds public broadcasting, libraries, and music. *Civic & Public Affairs:* 4%. Supports public policy and advocacy. *Education:* 14%. Primarily Jewish colleges and schools. *International:* 22%. Community support. *International:* 9%. Funds single-disease associations. *Note:* Total contributions made in 1998. **Typ. Recipients:** Cancer, Health-General, Hospices, Medical Rehabilitation, Medical Research, People with Disabilities, Single-Disease Health Associations, Substance Abuse. **Geo. Dist:** Birmingham, AL.

### ★ 239 ★ Fleming Foundation

500 W 7th St., Ste. 1007
Fort Worth, TX 76102-4732
**Phone:** (817)335-3741          **Fax:** (817)338-4844
G. Malcolm Louden, CPA

**Fnded:** 1936. **Philosophy:** The goal of the foundation is to perpetuate Mr. Fleming's community and charitable interests, primarily focusing on educational institutions, the arts, and health services. The foundation also reports that it will no longer provide grants to religious organizations. **Priorities:** *Arts & Humanities:* 94%. Supports performing arts and music. *Education:* 1%. Supports private schools. *Environment:* 2%. Supports boys and girls clubs. *International:* 2%. Supports mental centers. *Note:* Total contributions made in 1999. **Typ. Recipients:** AIDS/HIV, Alzheimers Disease, Cancer, Children's Health/Hospitals, Clinics/Medical Centers, Eyes/Blindness, Family Planning, Health Organizations, Heart, Hospitals, Medical Rehabilitation, Mental Health, People with Disabilities, Research/Studies Institutes, Single-Disease Health Associations, Substance Abuse. **Geo. Dist:** Fort Worth, TX, including Tarrant County.

### ★ 240 ★ Fletcher Jones Foundation

One Wilshire Bldg., Ste. 2900
624 South Grand Ave.
Los Angeles, CA 90017-3335
**Phone:** (213)426-6565          **Fax:** (213)426-6555
**Email:** fletcherjones2@1wilshire.com
Christine Sisley, Executive Director

**Fnded:** 1969. **Philosophy:** According to the foundation, "the trustees of the foundation give consideration to charitable, scientific, literary, and educational areas, plus a minor portion to general-purpose grants. However, from time to time, the trustees may give special emphasis to any one of the above-listed areas. At present, grants are given primarily to private colleges and universities, particularly those in California." The foundation's 1996 annual report stated: "Since the Foundation began making grants about 25 years ago, we have given special emphasis to the private colleges and universities in California. Earlier this year, the Trustees approved a change in that policy. You might call it a slight change. A majority of the Trustees, after considerable thought and discussion, became persuaded that some of our support for education at the college level should go to the public institutions and, in particular, to the University of California." **Priorities:** *Arts & Humanities:* 38%. Supports the performing arts, public broadcasting, museums and libraries. *Civic & Public Affairs:* less than 1%. *Education:* 58%. Largely funds private colleges and universities in California only. *Environment:* 1%. Funds scouting, children's welfare and people with disabilities. *International:* 1%. Supports health associations, hospitals, and speech & hearing. *Religion:* less than 1%. *Note:* Total contributions made in 1999. **Typ. Recipients:** Children's Health/Hospitals, Clinics/Medical Centers, Domestic Violence, Eyes/Blindness, Health Organizations, Health-General, Hospices, Hospitals, Medical Research, Nursing Services, People with Disabilities, Public Health, Research/Studies Institutes, Single-Disease Health Associations. **Geo. Dist:** CA.

### ★ 241 ★ Flinn Foundation

1802 North Central Ave.
Phoenix, AZ 85004
**Phone:** (602)744-6800          **Fax:** (602)274-3194
**Email:** info@flinn.org
**Website:** http://www.flinn.org

**Fnded:** 1965. **Philosophy:** Since the early 1980s, the Flinn Foundation has grown from a modest philanthropic organization whose funds were principally used to support research in cardiovascular disease in Arizona to a sizable statewide foundation supporting a diverse array of projects in health, education, and the cultural arts. The foundation seeks to improve the quality of life in Arizona by enhancing community-based services to local health care needs, especially those for children and youth; strengthening the state's medical education and biomedical research programs; strengthening Arizona's universities through an undergraduate scholarship program for outstanding high school students; and enhancing the visibility and long-term artistic mission of Arizona's principal producing visual and performing arts institutions. Funding goes toward examining specific problems and identifying and testing ways to meet these problems. Most grants support the planning and start-up costs of new initiatives with specific durations and defined operating budgets. **Priorities:** *Arts & Humanities:* 15%. Supports symphony, theatre and ballet. *Education:* 61%. Supports universities and scholarships. *Environment:* 5%. Supports community centers and family planning. *International:* 9%. Supports research. *Religion:* 9%. Supports science center. *Note:* Total contributions made in 1998. **Typ. Recipients:** Adolescent Health Issues, AIDS/HIV, Alzheimers Disease, Child Abuse, Children's Health/Hospitals, Clinics/Medical Centers, Family Planning, Geriatric Health, Health Organizations, Health Policy/Cost Containment, Heart, Hospices, Hospitals, Medical Education, Medical Research, Medical Training, Nursing Services, People with Disabilities, Prenatal Health Issues, Public Health, Research/Studies Institutes, Sexual Abuse, Substance Abuse. **Geo. Dist:** AZ.

**★ 242 ★ The Florence Gould Foundation**
80 Pine St., Ste. 1701
New York, NY 10005-1702
**Phone:** (212)701-3400      **Fax:** (212)269-5420
John Young, President
**Fnded:** 1957. **Philosophy:** The Florence J. Gould Foundation is primarily interested in promoting Franco-American friendship and understanding. **Priorities:** *Arts & Humanities:* 38%. Supports museums, libraries, opera, orchestra, and theater. *Civic & Public Affairs:* 2%. Supports gardens and parks. *Education:* 25%. Supports arts and humanities education, colleges, and universities. *Environment:* 2%. Funds human services. *Religion:* 3%. Supports marine biology. *Note:* Total contributions made in 1999. **Typ. Recipients:** AIDS/HIV, Alzheimers Disease, Children's Health/Hospitals, Clinics/Medical Centers, Geriatric Health, Medical Education, People with Disabilities. **Geo. Dist:** nationally.

**★ 243 ★ Florence V. Burden Foundation**
10 East 53rd St., 32nd Floor
New York, NY 10022
**Phone:** (212)872-1150      **Fax:** (212)872-1149
Marjorie Lipkin, Executive Director
**Fnded:** 1967. **Philosophy:** The Burden Foundation's approach is not just to make grants, but to make productive grants. Initial grants are often applied research projects designed to advance knowledge and practice in the foundation's fields or to demonstrate that a significant advance is feasible. The foundation is interested in issues of broad national importance, looking for projects on the cutting edge of social innovation that will demonstrate new ways to solve basic or enduring problems. The foundation's overall theme is to strengthen families and communities. It has changed priorities replacing crime and justice with a focus on children while continuing its focus on the elderly with its aging program area. For aging, the foundation addresses the following: to support family caregivers, both those caring for frail elders as well as elders caring for grandchildren; and to benefit elders and children, families and communities through intergenerational programs. For children, the foundation addresses the following: to intervene early in children's lives, to build their self-esteem and socialization skills, and to prevent abuse and violence. The foundation will focus on children and youth up to 18 years of age. **Priorities:** *Arts & Humanities:* 9%. Supports the New York Public Library and contemporary art. *Civic & Public Affairs:* 4%. Funds public and community affairs. *Education:* 48%. Primary and secondary education, and colleges and universities. *Environment:* 30%. Senior citizen services, child welfare, youth organizations, crime prevention, and animal welfare. *International:* 6%. Focus on hospitals, centers on aging, gay men's health, and diabetes. *Note:* Total contributions made in 1998. **Typ. Recipients:** AIDS/HIV, Alzheimers Disease, Child Abuse, Children's Health/Hospitals, Clinics/Medical Centers, Diabetes, Domestic Violence, Emergency/Ambulance Services, Eyes/Blindness, Family Planning, Geriatric Health, Health Organizations, Health-General, Hospices, Hospitals, Long-Term Care, People with Disabilities, Single-Disease Health Associations, Substance Abuse,

Transplant Networks/Donor Banks. **Geo. Dist:** Northeast; NY.

**★ 244 ★ Foellinger Foundation**
520 East Berry St.
Fort Wayne, IN 46802
**Phone:** (219)422-2900      **Fax:** (219)422-9436
Cheryl Taylor, President
**Fnded:** 1958. **Philosophy:** The Foundation has a broad range of interests that include Youth and Families, Education and the Arts, Community Development, and Human Services. "The Foundation's Board of Directors emphasizes grant making to support programs and projects that focus on young people and their families, especially the economically disadvantaged. The Foundation encourages applicant organizations to develop linkages with nonprofit agencies and governmental entities in order to more effectively deliver services. Because the Foundation's resources are limited, the Board seeks funding partnerships to provide the maximum leverage for grant effectiveness." The foundation prefers seeking worthy causes rather than merely responding to solicitations. **Priorities:** *Arts & Humanities:* 13%. Supports museums, theaters, and symphonies. *Civic & Public Affairs:* 11%. Funds parks, recreation projects, and community partnerships. *Education:* 40%. Supports universities and public schools. *Environment:* 20%. Supports the United Way, summer park programs, and youth organizations. *International:* 2%. Primary funding goes toward cancer care, health clinics, AIDs prevention and education. *Note:* Contributions made in fiscal 1999. **Typ. Recipients:** AIDS/HIV, Clinics/Medical Centers, Domestic Violence, Health Organizations, Medical Rehabilitation, People with Disabilities, Preventive Medicine/Wellness Organizations, Public Health, Substance Abuse. **Geo. Dist:** Fort Wayne, IN, including Allen County.

**★ 245 ★ Fondren Foundation**
PO Box 2558
Houston, TX 77252-8037
**Phone:** (713)216-4513
Ms. Martie Herrick, Assistant Secretary-Treasurer
**Fnded:** 1948. **Philosophy:** Traditionally, the foundation has focused on education, including higher education and private schools, and health. Major past health recipients have been the Ella F. Fondren Building, a part of Methodist Hospital, as well as university and community hospitals. The foundation also has given generously to the social services, the arts and humanities, and civic and public affairs. **Priorities:** *Arts & Humanities:* 10%. Museums, libraries, historic preservation, performing arts, and music. *Civic & Public Affairs:* 6%. Primarily for a zoo and a park. *Education:* 40%. Supports private primary and secondary schools and colleges and universities. *Environment:* 29%. Provides funding primarily for child welfare and youth organizations. *International:* 12%. Supports children's health and cardiac research. *Religion:* 2%. Supports a health science center and a nature center. *Note:* Total contributions made in fiscal 2000. **Typ. Recipients:** AIDS/HIV, Alzheimers Disease, Cancer, Children's Health/Hospitals, Clinics/Medical Centers, Emergency/Ambulance Services, Family Planning, Geriatric Health, Heart, Hospices, Hospitals, Medical Education, Medical Rehabilitation, Medical Research, Mental Health, People with Disabilities, Prenatal Health Issues, Public Health, Research/Studies Institutes, Single-Disease Health Associations, Speech & Hearing, Substance Abuse, Transplant Networks/Donor Banks. **Geo. Dist:** nationally; Houston, TX.

**★ 246 ★ Ford Family Foundation**
1600 Northwest Stewart Parkway
Roseburg, OR 97470
**Phone:** (541)957-5574      **Fax:** (541)957-5720
**Website:** http://www.tfff.org
Norman Smith, President
**Fnded:** 1957. **Philosophy:** Through grantmaking and internal initiative development, the Ford Family Foundation endeavors to help individuals, through organized learning opportunities, to be contributing and successful citizens; and, to support nonprofit activities,

agencies and projects, with particular emphasis on mid-size and small communities in the state of Oregon and Siskiyou County, California. (Form 990 1998 Grant guidelines) **Priorities:** *Arts & Humanities:* 12%. *Civic & Public Affairs:* 5%. Supports huosing, safety, municipalities/towns, and community foundations. *Education:* 61%. Supports scholarships through the Ford Scholars Program (three scholarship programs in the state of Oregon and Siskiyou County, California.) Foundation also funds grants for technology, colleges, and local school districts. Interests include purchasing computer equipment, literacy projects, athletic programs, and counseling work. *Environment:* 16%. Supports United Way, youth programs, homes, young men's christian association, and food distribution programs. *International:* 5%. Major emphasis on a children's hospital. *Note:* Total contributions made in fiscal 1999. **Typ. Recipients:** Adolescent Health Issues, Cancer, Child Abuse, Children's Health/Hospitals, Clinics/Medical Centers, Domestic Violence, Emergency/Ambulance Services, Health Organizations, Health-General, Hospices, Hospitals, Mental Health, People with Disabilities, People with Disabilities, Prenatal Health Issues, Substance Abuse. **Geo. Dist:** CA, Siskiyou County; OR, rural communities only with population of 30,000 or fewer people.

**★ 247 ★ Ford Foundation**
320 East 43rd St.
New York, NY 10017
**Phone:** (212)573-5000      **Fax:** (212)351-3677
**Email:** office-secretary@fordfound.org
**Website:** http://www.fordfound.org
Barron Tenny, Executive Vice President and Secretary
**Fnded:** 1936. **Philosophy:** "The Ford Foundation is a resource for innovative people and institutions worldwide. Our goals are to: strengthen democratic values; reduce poverty and injustice; promote international cooperation; and advance human achievement." Ford Foundation Annual Report 1999 Program activities are supported primarily within the following broad categories: Asset Building and Community Development; Education, Media, Arts, and Culture; and Peace and Social Justice. Within these three broad categories, the Foundation also funds projects using film, television, and radio to explore public policy issues and uses a limited portion of its capital funds to make program-related investments in enterprises that will advance philanthropic purposes. **Priorities:** *Arts & Humanities:* 8%. Media, Arts and Culture–public broadcasting; promoting a free and responsible news media; independent production of film, video, and radio programming; and strengthening art institutions. *Civic & Public Affairs:* 32%. Community Development, Resource Development and Economic Development–with a focus on development finance and economic security; workforce development; environment and development; and community development. *Education:* 13%. Education, Knowledge and Religion–supports education reform; higher education and scholarship; and religion, society and culture educational initiatives. Major emphasis on education research and reform K-12. *International:* 13%. Human Development and Reproductive Health–funds efforts in the areas of children, youth and families; and sexuality and reproductive health. *Note:* Total contributions made in fiscal 1999. **Typ. Recipients:** AIDS/HIV, Family Planning, Health Organizations, Medical Research, Nutrition, Public Health, Substance Abuse. **Geo. Dist:** internationally, especially Asia, Latin America, and Africa; nationally.

**★ 248 ★ Forest Foundation**
820 A St., Ste. 345
Tacoma, WA 98402
**Phone:** (253)627-1634      **Fax:** (253)627-6249
Frank Underwood, Executive Director
**Fnded:** 1962. **Philosophy:** The Forest Foundation is concerned primarily "with the growth and development of the individual because the individual is primary to solving societal problems and creatively enhancing the human condition. Its focus is on stimulating, encouraging, and supporting activities and programs of established, voluntary non-profit organizations that emphasize individual growth and responsibility." The founda-

tion focuses on these specific program areas: community improvement; culture and the arts; education; the environment; and human services, which includes child welfare, day care, the disabled, drug rehabilitation, hunger/emergency shelter, senior adults, and youth. youth. **Priorities:** *Arts & Humanities:* 29%. Supports museums, theater, historical societies, music, and opera. *Civic & Public Affairs:* 34%. Housing, economic development, and community foundations. *Education:* 29%. Emphasis on secondary schools and education funds. *Environment:* 3%. Focus on child welfare, youth organizaions, and family services. *International:* 1%. Mental health and a blood services center. *Note:* Total contributions made in fiscal 1998. **Typ. Recipients:** AIDS/HIV, Cancer, Child Abuse, Clinics/Medical Centers, Domestic Violence, Emergency/Ambulance Services, Family Planning, Health Funds, Health Organizations, Hospitals, Medical Research, Mental Health, People with Disabilities, Public Health, Single-Disease Health Associations, Transplant Networks/Donor Banks. **Geo. Dist:** WA, southwestern Washington; especially Pierce County.

**★ 249 ★ Forest Lawn Foundation**
1712 South Glendale Ave.
Glendale, CA 91205
**Phone:** (323)340-4703          **Fax:** (213)254-8152
**Website:** http://www.forestlawnfoundation.org
Linda Llewellyn, President & Chief Operating Officer
**Fnded:** 1951. **Philosophy:** The foundation's interests are chiefly focused on social services around Los Angeles. Youth organizations, the Braille Institute, and services for the needy are generally funded. Recently, the foundation has focused more attention on education and youth prevention programs. Although the foundation has other interests, most of the giving goes to community interests and health, including hospitals and hospices. **Priorities:** *Education:* 33%. Supports Junior Achievement, Braille Institute, colleges and universities and scholarships. *Environment:* 49%. Supports scouting, Boy and Girls Clubs, senior citizen programs, emergency relief, and Food distribution programs. *International:* 14%. Supports American Red Cross, medical centers, and hospitals. *Note:* Contributions were made in 1998. **Typ. Recipients:** Child Abuse, Children's Health/Hospitals, Clinics/Medical Centers, Emergency/Ambulance Services, Health Organizations, Heart, Home-Care Services, Hospices, Hospitals, Nursing Services, People with Disabilities, Prenatal Health Issues, Public Health, Single-Disease Health Associations, Substance Abuse. **Geo. Dist:** Los Angeles, CA, including Los Angeles County and Orange County.

**★ 250 ★ Forrest C. Lattner Foundation**
777 East Atlantic Ave., Ste. 317
Delray Beach, FL 33483
**Phone:** (561)278-3781
Susan Lloyd, President & Secretary
**Fnded:** 1982. **Philosophy:** The Forrest C. Lattner Foundation makes most of its grants in the areas of health care, civic affairs, and the arts. Health service funding favors hospitals, mental health, pediatrics, and single-disease associations. Civic affairs funding favors other philanthropic organizations, housing, and botanical gardens. Support for the arts focuses on art centers, museums, and public broadcasting. Minor support is given to education and social services. **Priorities:** *Arts & Humanities:* 17%. Public television, theaters, and library associations. *Civic & Public Affairs:* 19%. Housing and social services. *Education:* 18%. Secondary schools and colleges. *Environment:* 17%. Supports youth organizations, the aged, guidance centers, and the prevention of domestic violence. *International:* 24%. Health clinics, health associations, and medical research. *Note:* Total contributions made in 1996. **Typ. Recipients:** AIDS/HIV, Alzheimers Disease, Cancer, Children's Health/Hospitals, Clinics/Medical Centers, Domestic Violence, Emergency/Ambulance Services, Eyes/Blindness, Family Planning, Health Funds, Health-General, Heart, Home-Care Services, Hospices, Hospitals, Medical Education, Medical Research, Mental Health, People with Disabilities, Public Health, Research/Studies Institutes, Sin-

gle-Disease Health Associations, Substance Abuse, Trauma Treatment. **Geo. Dist:** midwest; FL.

**★ 251 ★ Foster Foundation**
1929 43rd St. East, Ste. 300
Seattle, WA 98112
**Phone:** (206)726-5900
Jill Goodsell, Administrator
**Fnded:** 1984. **Philosophy:** The foundation states that its purpose is to "enhance the quality of life in the Pacific Northwest and Alaska through the support of qualified needs in areas of cultural activities, education, social and community services, health and the environment." The Foster Foundation makes most of its grants in the areas of education, social services, and health. Education support favors the University of Washington and literacy institutes. Support for social services includes children's homes, united funds, youth organizations, and food banks. Health interests include hospitals, AIDS and cancer research, and nursing. The foundation makes grants in other areas of support as well. **Priorities:** *Arts & Humanities:* 20%. Funds Seattle arts organizations. *Civic & Public Affairs:* 12%. Supports homeless shelters. *Education:* 26%. Primarily for private precollege education, literacy, and higher education. *Environment:* 23%. Supports community centers, youth groups, and united funds. *International:* 19%. Gives to hospitals, medical centers, and cancer and AIDS research. *Note:* Total contributions made in 1998. **Typ. Recipients:** AIDS/HIV, Cancer, Children's Health/Hospitals, Clinics/Medical Centers, Emergency/Ambulance Services, Family Planning, Geriatric Health, Health Organizations, Hospitals, Medical Research, Nursing Services, People with Disabilities, Public Health, Research/Studies Institutes, Respiratory, Single-Disease Health Associations. **Geo. Dist:** Seattle, WA.

**★ 252 ★ France-Merrick Foundation**
The Exchange, Ste. 118
1122 Kenilworth Dr.
Towson, MD 21204
**Phone:** (410)832-5700          **Fax:** (410)832-5704
**Email:** fm@france-merrickfdn.org
Robert Schaefer, Executive Director
**Fnded:** 1962. **Philosophy:** The foundation provides most of its support to civic and cultural activities, public education, private and higher education, historic preservation and conservation, and health and social services. **Priorities:** *Arts & Humanities:* 11%. Emphasis on historic preservation. *Civic & Public Affairs:* 20%. Supports foundations and community projects. *Education:* 33%. Primarily supports parochial/private elementary and secondary schools and colleges and universities. *Environment:* 6%. Support for the homeless, child welfare, family services, and united funds. *International:* 16%. *Note:* Total contributions made in fiscal 1999. **Typ. Recipients:** Cancer, Children's Health/Hospitals, Clinics/Medical Centers, Domestic Violence, Health Organizations, Health-General, Hospices, Hospitals, Hospitals (University Affiliated), Medical Education, People with Disabilities, Public Health. **Geo. Dist:** Baltimore, MD, within the metropolitan area.

**★ 253 ★ Frances and Benjamin Benenson Foundation**
708 3rd Ave., 28th Floor
New York, NY 10017
**Phone:** (212)867-0990          **Fax:** (212)983-1952
Charles Benenson, President
**Fnded:** 1983. **Philosophy:** The foundation has two primary interests: the arts and education. Scholarships for minority students is the foundation's chief focus, and other funding for education emphasizes educational foundations and universities. Funding for the arts favors museums, the performing arts, and libraries. Secondary interests include religious organizations and social services. **Priorities:** *Arts & Humanities:* 51%. Supports museums, public libraries, modern art, and the performing arts. *Civic & Public Affairs:* 4%. Assists community development and urban affairs. *Education:* 21%. Supports educational programs,

schools, colleges, and universities. *Environment:* 11%. Supports youth services, the United Way, and social services. *International:* 3%. Supports single-disease associations. *Note:* Contributions made in fiscal 1998. **Typ. Recipients:** AIDS/HIV, Cancer, Children's Health/Hospitals, Clinics/Medical Centers, Diabetes, Emergency/Ambulance Services, Family Planning, Health Organizations, Hospitals, People with Disabilities, Single-Disease Health Associations, Substance Abuse. **Geo. Dist:** New York, NY.

**★ 254 ★ The Frances L. and Edwin L. Cummings Memorial Fund**
501 Fifth Ave., Ste. 708
New York, NY 10017-6103
**Phone:** (212)286-1778          **Fax:** (212)682-9458
Elizabeth Costas, Administrative Director
**Fnded:** 1982. **Philosophy:** The Cummings Fund's philosophy is to assist organizations seeking to "benefit the health and well-being of mankind." The sole giving restriction is that the "cultural arts" may never be the recipient of foundation funds. The primary interest is in the piloting or expansion of new, innovative programs of organizations operating in, or within close proximity to, New York City. The Cummings Fund encourages smaller and lesser-known community-based organizations to submit grant requests which address the sometimes unique needs of that specific community. The fund has a particular interest in programs serving young people. The major fields of interest are as follows: social welfare, especially programs addressing child abuse homelessness, teenage pregnancy, parenting education, and youth employment and job training; education, with a focus on students from disadvantaged backgrounds, especially efforts to reform the public education system or programs that serve public school children; and health care, especially institutions and programs serving economically and socially disadvantaged populations. A minor area of interest is medical research, especially involving AIDS and cancer. **Priorities:** *Education:* 24%. Public education, especially programs serving minorities, the disadvantaged, and the physically and/or mentally disabled. *Environment:* 55%. Child abuse, parent education, juvenile delinquency, teenage pregnancy, youth employment and job training. *International:* 21%. Institutions serving economically and socially disadvantaged populations; cancer and AIDS research. *Note:* Total contributions made in fiscal 2001. **Typ. Recipients:** AIDS/HIV, Cancer, Child Abuse, Children's Health/Hospitals, Clinics/Medical Centers, Family Planning, Health Organizations, Home-Care Services, Hospitals, Medical Rehabilitation, Medical Research, Mental Health, Outpatient Health Care, People with Disabilities, Public Health, Substance Abuse. **Geo. Dist:** New York, NY, including surrounding area.

**★ 255 ★ Frances Wood Wilson Foundation, Inc.**
250 East Ponce de Leon Ste. 702
Decatur, GA 30033
**Phone:** (404)370-0035          **Fax:** (404)370-1624
**Email:** fwilsonfdn@mindspring.com
W. Wingfield, President
**Fnded:** 1954. **Philosophy:** The foundation generally awards its grants to programs and institutions involved in child welfare, religious, civic, health, or educational activities in Georgia, except for programs carried on by Chestnut Hill Benevolent Association in Boston, MA. All grants are made to tax-exempt organizations. Scholarship awards are made to the respective educational institution, rather than to individual students. **Priorities:** *Arts & Humanities:* 8%. Supports historical societies, ballet, and arts centers. *Civic & Public Affairs:* 6%. Supports zoos and parks. *Education:* 36%. Emphasis on colleges and universities. *Environment:* 9%. Recreation and athletics, youth organizations, and child welfare. *International:* 8%. Children's health, hospitals, and cancer causes. *Religion:* 3%. Supports natural history museums. *Note:* Total contributions made in fiscal 2000. **Typ. Recipients:** Cancer, Child Abuse, Children's Health/Hospitals, Clinics/Medical Centers, Health Organizations, Health-General,

Hospices, Hospitals, Medical Education, Medical Rehabilitation, Nursing Services, People with Disabilities, Single-Disease Health Associations. **Geo. Dist:** GA.

**★ 256 ★ Francis Families Foundation**
800 West 47th St., Ste. 717
Kansas City, MO 64112
**Phone:** (816)531-0077          **Fax:** (816)531-8810
**Email:** lyn@francisfoundation.org
**Website:** http://www.francisfoundation.org
Lyn Knox, Program Officer

**Fnded:** 1989. **Philosophy:** The foundation supports post doctoral medical fellowships in pulmonary research and anesthesiology, and educational and cultural institutions in the greater Kansas City metropolitan area. The foundation's fellowship program administrative office, located at the School of Public Health, Department of Environmental Health, Harvard University, is under the direction of Joseph D. Brain, Sc.D. Fellowship awards are made to institutions located throughout the United States and Canada. Grants are awarded to provide a stipend, including fringe benefits and travel expenses. Support for research project cost is not allowed. A fellow must have 75% of his or her time available for research. The foundation also supports educational, art, and cultural institutions in the greater Kansas City, MO, metropolitan area. Areas of interest include theater, art, music, dance, cultural endeavors, and education. Support may be ongoing or a one-time contributions and may include capital campaigns pledges or special projects. However, funding to capital campaigns is limited. The foundation has narrowed the focus in Kansas City to give primary consideration to early childhood development. **Priorities:** *Arts & Humanities:* 19%. Focus on art institutes, museums, and theater. *Civic & Public Affairs:* 46%. Primarily supports child and youth development and community foundations. *Education:* 4%. Supports schools and education centers, and provides fellowships. *Environment:* 11%. Supports youth programs, family services, and United Way. *International:* 19%. Supports hospitals and children's health. *Note:* Total contributions made in 2000. **Typ. Recipients:** Children's Health/Hospitals, Clinics/Medical Centers, Health Organizations, Hospitals, Hospitals (University Affiliated), Medical Education, Medical Research, Prenatal Health Issues, Public Health, Research/Studies Institutes, Respiratory, Single-Disease Health Associations. **Geo. Dist:** nationally; Kansas City, MO.

**★ 257 ★ Frank E. and Seba B. Payne Foundation**
231 South LaSalle St.
Chicago, IL 60697
**Phone:** (312)828-8026          **Fax:** (312)828-1786
M. Ryan, Vice President, Bank of America

**Fnded:** 1962. **Philosophy:** Grants are made solely at the discretion of the trustees for any "religious, charitable, scientific, literary, or educational purposes, and in addition, for the prevention of cruelty to children or animals." **Priorities:** *Arts & Humanities:* 40% Supports music, libraries, theatres and media. *Civic & Public Affairs:* 2% Community projects. *Education:* 35% Scholarships, secondary schools and colleges. *Environment:* 2% Youth and community support. *International:* 17% Hospitals and health centers. *Note:* Total contributions made in fiscal 1999. **Typ. Recipients:** AIDS/HIV, Children's Health/Hospitals, Clinics/Medical Centers, Domestic Violence, Emergency/Ambulance Services, Eyes/Blindness, Family Planning, Hospitals, Nursing Services, People with Disabilities, Public Health, Single-Disease Health Associations, Speech & Hearing, Substance Abuse, Transplant Networks/Donor Banks. **Geo. Dist:** Chicago, IL; Bethlehem, PA.

**★ 258 ★ Frank Loomis Palmer Fund**
777 Main St., CTEH 40222B
Hartford, CT 06115
**Phone:** (860)952-7405          **Fax:** (860)952-7395
Marjorie Davis, Vice President

**Fnded:** 1936. **Philosophy:** The Frank Loomis Palmer Fund distributes its income "to corporations, societies, institutions, and trusts located or operating in the city of New London, CT, which are devoted exclusively to religious, charitable, scientific, literary, historical, or educational purposes, including the encouragement of art. The Fund's purpose is to encourage new projects and to provide seed money rather than to supplement operating expenses; to disseminate the dollars to reach, aid, and assist the largest volume of people." **Priorities:** *Arts & Humanities:* 12%. Funds art centers, museums, and historical preservation. *Civic & Public Affairs:* 22%. Funds community development organizations. *Education:* 21%. Gives to primary and secondary education, and colleges and universities. *Environment:* 28%. Supports drug prevention programs and youth organizations. *International:* 8%. Funds hospitals, hospices, and health groups. *Religion:* 2%. Contributes to science centers and maritime societies. *Note:* Total contributions made in fiscal 1999. **Typ. Recipients:** AIDS/HIV, Children's Health/Hospitals, Domestic Violence, Emergency/Ambulance Services, Family Planning, Health Organizations, Hospices, Hospitals, Medical Rehabilitation, Mental Health, Nursing Services, People with Disabilities, Public Health, Single-Disease Health Associations, Substance Abuse. **Geo. Dist:** New London, CT.

**★ 259 ★ Frank Stanley Beveridge Foundation**
301 Northeast 51st St., Ste. 1130
Boca Raton, FL 33431-4929
**Phone:** (561)241-8388          **Fax:** (561)241-8332
**Email:** administrator@beveridge.org
**Website:** http://www.beveridge.org
Philip Caswell, President

**Fnded:** 1947. **Philosophy:** The foundation was organized "to aid and provide for the benefit of such poor and needy persons...and to aid and provide for the advancement or promotion of science, learning, medicine, surgery, literature, music, art or human welfare." The foundation annually sets aside approximately one-third of funds for the general maintenance of Stanley Park in Westfield, MA, one-third for organizations in Hampden and Hampshire Counties, and one-third for nonprofits located in regions where Beveridge family members reside, namely the Tampa and Palm Beach, FL, areas. The foundation will consider grant proposals from the following institutional/program activity areas: animal welfare, arts and culture, civil rights, community improvement, conservation/environment, crime, disasters/safety, diseases/medical disciplines, medical research, education, employment, food and agriculture, general and rehabilitative health, housing, human services, mental health, crisis intervention, philanthropy/volunteerism, public affairs and society benefit, recreation, religion, science, social sciences, and youth development. **Priorities:** *Arts & Humanities:* 10%. Museums, public broadcasting, music, and libraries. *Civic & Public Affairs:* 54%. Primarily supporting the Stanley Park of Westfield; also funds community foundations. *Education:* 11%. Supports primary and secondary schools, colleges, and special education. *Environment:* 19%. Focus on youth organizations, people with disabilities, and animal welfare. *International:* 2%. Single-disease health associations and hospitals. *Note:* Total contributions made in 1998. **Typ. Recipients:** Cancer, Diabetes, Emergency/Ambulance Services, Eyes/Blindness, Geriatric Health, Health Organizations, Hospices, Hospitals, Medical Education, Mental Health, Nursing Services, People with Disabilities, Public Health, Research/Studies Institutes, Single-Disease Health Associations. **Geo. Dist:** CA, Orange County; FL, Boca Raton; HI, Kauai County; MA, Hampden County; MA, Hampshire County; NH; RI.

**★ 260 ★ Fred L. Emerson Foundation, Inc.**
PO Box 276
Auburn, NY 13021
**Phone:** (315)253-9621          **Fax:** (315)253-5235
Ronald West, Executive Director & Secretary

**Fnded:** 1943. **Philosophy:** "Among the foundation's interests are education (primarily private higher education), hospitals and health programs, community agencies, churches, cultural institutions, youth and community service programs, and social welfare agencies." Support to private colleges and universities is in the form of scholarship endowment and building funds. The foundation generally makes grants for annual campaigns, capital and building funds, equipment and materials, renovation projects, special endowments, research, scholarships, matching and challenge grants, and special local community projects. **Priorities:** *Arts & Humanities:* 6%. Libraries, museums, and the performing arts. *Civic & Public Affairs:* 3%. Supports local commercial and public policy associations. *Education:* 69%. Funds colleges aqnd universities. *Environment:* 22%. Supports local children's programs. *Note:* Total contributions made in 1998. **Typ. Recipients:** Cancer, Emergency/Ambulance Services, Eyes/Blindness, Family Planning, Health Organizations, Health-General, Heart, Hospices, Hospitals, Long-Term Care, Medical Rehabilitation, Medical Research, People with Disabilities, Single-Disease Health Associations, Substance Abuse. **Geo. Dist:** NY, Cayuga County; NY, Upstate; Auburn, NY.

**★ 261 ★ Fred Maytag Family Foundation**
PO Box 366
Newton, IA 50208
**Phone:** (641)791-0395
Ellen Bergeron, Foundation Administrator

**Fnded:** 1945. **Philosophy:** The foundation focuses its funding primarily on higher educational institutions, the arts, health and human service organizations, and civic groups. **Priorities:** *Arts & Humanities:* 8%. Primarily to arts organizations in Des Moines. *Civic & Public Affairs:* 15%. Emphasis on parks and clubs in Iowa. *Education:* 15%. Supports colleges and university foundations. *Environment:* 10%. Funds youth programs in Iowa. *International:* 4%. Mainly to health centers. *Note:* Total contributions made in 1998. **Typ. Recipients:** Cancer, Child Abuse, Children's Health/Hospitals, Clinics/Medical Centers, Emergency/Ambulance Services, Family Planning, Health Organizations, Heart, Hospices, Hospitals, Medical Education, Medical Rehabilitation, Medical Research, Mental Health, People with Disabilities, Single-Disease Health Associations, Substance Abuse. **Geo. Dist:** Des Moines, IA; Newton, IA.

**★ 262 ★ Frederick S. Upton Foundation**
100 Ridgeway
Saint Joseph, MI 49085
**Phone:** (616)982-1905          **Fax:** (616)982-0323
**Email:** supton@qtm.net
Stephen Upton, Chairman, Board of Trustees

**Fnded:** 1954. **Philosophy:** The foundation's primary purpose is local giving, with emphasis on higher education, religion, cultural programs, community funds, and youth organizations. **Priorities:** *Arts & Humanities:* 32%. Supports artists guilds, libraries, and symphonies. *Civic & Public Affairs:* 5%. Supports councils, community centers, and public safety. *Education:* 15%. Funds colleges. *Environment:* 22%. Supports United Funds, women's organizations, and family programs. *International:* 19%. Supports hospitals. *Note:* Total contributions made in 1999. **Typ. Recipients:** AIDS/HIV, Children's Health/Hospitals, Domestic Violence, Family Planning, Geriatric Health, Health Organizations, Hospitals, People with Disabilities, Public Health. **Geo. Dist:** IL; IN; MA; MI, Southwest Michigan; OH; PA; SC; WI.

**★ 263 ★ Freedom Forum International Inc.**
1101 Wilson Boulevard, 21st Flr.
Arlington, VA 22209-2248
**Phone:** (703)528-0800          **Fax:** (703)284-2836
**Email:** news@freedomforum.org
**Website:** http://www.freedomforum.org
Charles Overby, Chairman & Chief Executive Officer

**Fnded:** 1994. **Philosophy:** The Freedom Forum... is dedicated to free press, free speech and free spirit for all people. It is a nonpartisan, international, programmatic foundation. It is a major supporter of journalism education, a leader in assisting the professional development of journalists, a champion of minority and female advancement in media professions and a force in international press freedom programs. The Freedom Forum's major activities include the following: *Freedom Forum Media Studies Center:* Founded in 1985 at Columbia University, New York, NY, the center serves as the nation's preeminent institute for the advanced study of mass communications and media technology. *The Freedom Forum First Amendment Center:* The center was established on December 15, 1991, and is located at Vanderbilt University, Nashville, TN. Its mission is to promote understanding and appreciation of the values of the First Amendment to the U.S. Constitution. *The Pacific Coast Center:* The Pacific Coast Center was established in 1993 in Oakland, CA. Its main activity is to coordinate the foundation's outreach throughout the western United States. *International Operations:* Activities in this area support and encourage an independent free press worldwide. *Journalism Education and Professional Programs:* Activities in this area are dedicated to improving journalism by enhancing the skills of professional journalists, strengthening journalism education, encouraging journalism diversity, and promoting youth journalism, workshops, and minority journalism education. *Other Programs:* Other foundation programs include the *Free Spirit Award* and the *Freedom Forum Journalism Administrator of the Year Award.* **Typ. Recipients:** Domestic Violence, Medical Rehabilitation, People with Disabilities, Substance Abuse. **Geo. Dist:** internationally; nationally.

## ★ 264 ★ Friedman Family Foundation
PMB 719, 204 E 2nd Ave.
San Mateo, CA 94401
**Phone:** (650)342-8750          **Fax:** (650)342-8750
**Email:** fffdn@aol.com
Lisa Kawahara, Program Director

**Fnded:** 1964. **Priorities:** *Civic & Public Affairs:* 51%. Supports public policy organizations and community foundations. *Education:* 6%. Supports after school/enrichment programs and private schools. *Environment:* 20%. Supports youth programs, community service organizations, shelters/homeless and family services. *International:* 1%. Supports single-disease health associations, medical centers and health services. *Note:* Total contributions made in fiscal 1999. **Typ. Recipients:** AIDS/HIV, Child Abuse, Children's Health/Hospitals, Clinics/Medical Centers, Domestic Violence, Emergency/Ambulance Services, Health Organizations, Health Policy/Cost Containment, Heart, Hospitals, Medical Research, Mental Health, People with Disabilities, Public Health, Single-Disease Health Associations. **Geo. Dist:** San Francisco, CA, focus on Bay area.

## ★ 265 ★ Frist Foundation
3319 West End Ave., Ste. 900
Nashville, TN 37203-1076
**Phone:** (615)292-3868          **Fax:** (615)292-5843
**Email:** info@fristfoundation.org
**Website:** http://www.fristfoundation.org
Peter Bird, Jr., Senior Program Officer

**Fnded:** 1982. **Philosophy:** The Frist Foundation makes most of its grants in the areas of education, social services, and the arts. Most of its resources are funneled through its "initiatives", the best-known of which include: The Center for Nonprofit Management: Jointly funded by the United Way of Middle Tennessee, the center offers management training and consulting to nonprofit agencies throughout Middle Tennessee. In providing services, the center utilizes paid professionals along with volunteer business executives from the Nashville community. Youth Leadership and Service: supports a comprehensive effort to promote volunteerism among Nashville's youth and to identify and train young people for roles as community leaders. The Frist Fund for Collaboration: The Frist Foundation awards grants under this program to encourage cooperation and collaboration among Nashville's nonprofit agencies. The Frist Awards of Achievement: This competition, offered annually since 1985, provides unrestricted grants to Nashville organizations best exemplifying improvement and achievement in nonprofit management including innovation,

productivity, and volunteer involvement. Unrestricted grants of $15,000 are awarded to the top agency in each of three categories. The program is a partnership with the Center for Nonprofit Management, and is administered by the CNM. Internship Grants Program: This program is designed to help organizations stretch their capabilities. The foundation offers grants to organizations to enable them to hire student interns to accomplish specific projects. The program is also aimed at introducing college students (graduate and undergraduate) to the nonprofit field while linking nonprofit organizations more closely to college campuses. Technology Grants Program: This program is designed to help nonprofit organizations pursue their missions more efficiently through the acquisition and effective use of new technology. The program, established in 1995, is one of several initiatives to build and recognize excellence in nonprofit management. Teacher and Principal Awards: Administered by the PENCIL Foundation, enables Nashville area teachers to pursue self-designed programs of professional self-improvement. The program is also open to principals seeking to hone their management skills and knowledge. **Priorities:** *Arts & Humanities:* 10%. Major funding for the Frist Center for the Visual Arts; also funds art centers, music, theates, musuems, and ballet. *Civic & Public Affairs:* 10%. Primary support for community affairs organizations. *Education:* 57%. Focus on the Center for Nonprofit Management and education associations and foundations. *Environment:* 7%. Supports health and human services organizations. *Note:* Total contributions made in 1999. **Typ. Recipients:** Child Abuse, Children's Health/Hospitals, Clinics/Medical Centers, Domestic Violence, Emergency/Ambulance Services, Family Planning, Health Funds, Health Organizations, Health Policy/Cost Containment, Medical Education, Medical Training, Mental Health, Nursing Services, People with Disabilities, Public Health, Sexual Abuse, Speech & Hearing, Substance Abuse. **Geo. Dist:** TN; Nashville, TN.

## ★ 266 ★ Frost Foundation
511 Armijo, No. A
Santa Fe, NM 87501
**Phone:** (505)986-0208          **Fax:** (505)986-0430
**Website:** http://www.frostfound.org
Mary Whited-Howell, President

**Fnded:** 1959. **Philosophy:** The focus of the Frost Foundation has expanded over the years to include health groups, social services, humanitarian needs, and the environment. The foundation focuses its charitable giving on three major program areas, namely social service and humanitarian needs, the environment, and education. Social service projects will include, but not be limited to, street and domestic violence, child abuse, specific public health issues such as alcohol and drug abuse, homelessness, and problems of the elderly. Regarding the environment, the foundation will consider programs in research, education, and action to conserve and protect the environment for the well-being and safety of plants, animals, and human beings. Education projects will stress new, innovative, creative, practical programs to address students' and society's needs today, and which will recognize the changing sociological structure and concerns. The foundation favors causes which address urgent and timely needs, utilize funds and personnel creatively and efficiently, promise new ideas for the benefit of humanity, and have far-reaching impact. **Priorities:** *Arts & Humanities:* About 6%. Supports museums, music, and Opera. *Civic & Public Affairs:* 10%. Supports programs that benefit the homeless, and also gives grants towards community projects and nonprofit management. *Education:* 15%. Supports programs that address students' and society's needs today, also those that address the changing sociological structure and concerns and also supports literacy. *Environment:* 35%. Animal protection, prevention of domestic violence and child abuse, early childhood and family support, United Way, Big Brothers/Big Sister, and family planning services. *International:* 18%. Public health issues, hospices, and emergency health organizations. *Note:* Total contributions made in 1998. **Typ. Recipients:** AIDS/HIV, Cancer, Children's Health/Hospitals, Clinics/Medical

Centers, Domestic Violence, Emergency/Ambulance Services, Family Planning, Geriatric Health, Health-General, Hospices, Hospitals, Hospitals (University Affiliated), Medical Rehabilitation, Medical Research, Outpatient Health Care, People with Disabilities, Prenatal Health Issues, Public Health, Research/Studies Institutes, Sexual Abuse, Single-Disease Health Associations, Substance Abuse. **Geo. Dist:** LA; NM.

## ★ 267 ★ Fuller E. Callaway Foundation
209 Broome St.
LaGrange, GA 30241
**Phone:** (706)884-7348          **Fax:** (706)884-0201
**Email:** jtgresham@callaway-foundation.org
J. Gresham, General Manager, President & Treasurer

**Fnded:** 1917. **Philosophy:** The foundation traditionally devotes significant resources to nursing scholarships: the George E. Sims, Jr. Nursing Scholarship Program administered by West Georgia Health System and two foundation-sponsored scholarship programs. The remainder goes to LaGrange area schools and LaGrange College, local community service organizations, and churches. **Priorities:** *Civic & Public Affairs:* 38%. Supports urban and community affairs organizations in La Grange, Georgia. *Education:* 54%. Major support for scholarship programs and education associations. *Environment:* 5%. Focus on child welfare and community service organizations. *Note:* Total contributions made in 2000. **Typ. Recipients:** Arthritis, Cancer, Children's Health/Hospitals, Domestic Violence, Health Organizations, Heart, Hospitals, Medical Education, Multiple Sclerosis, Nursing Services, Respiratory, Single-Disease Health Associations. **Geo. Dist:** LaGrange, GA, including Troup County, GA.

## ★ 268 ★ Fullerton Foundation
PO Box 2208
Gaffney, SC 29342-2208
**Phone:** (864)489-6678          **Fax:** (864)487-9946
**Email:** cjbonner@fullertonfoundation.org
Walter Cavell, Executive Director

**Fnded:** 1954. **Philosophy:** The Fullerton Foundation makes grants in the areas of education, health, and social services. All of the educational funding supports university-level medical training. Health care support goes to medical centers, hospitals, and health associations. Social service funding favors children's homes and community centers. **Priorities:** *Civic & Public Affairs:* 2%. Supports community foundation. *Education:* 52%. Supports medical education and scholarships. *Environment:* 4%. Supports children's organizations and services for the developmentally disabled. *International:* 32%. Funding goes primarily to university-affiliated hospitals. *Note:* Total contributions made in fiscal 2000. **Typ. Recipients:** Cancer, Children's Health/Hospitals, Clinics/Medical Centers, Emergency/Ambulance Services, Family Planning, Geriatric Health, Health Funds, Health Organizations, Health Policy/Cost Containment, Health-General, Hospitals, Hospitals (University Affiliated), Long-Term Care, Medical Education, Medical Research, Nursing Services, Nutrition, Outpatient Health Care, People with Disabilities, Prenatal Health Issues, Preventive Medicine/Wellness Organizations, Public Health, Research/Studies Institutes, Transplant Networks/Donor Banks, Trauma Treatment. **Geo. Dist:** NC; SC.

## ★ 269 ★ Fund for New Jersey
94 Church St., Ste. 303
New Brunswick, NJ 08901
**Phone:** (732)220-8656          **Fax:** (732)220-8654
**Email:** fundnj@worldnet.att.net
**Website:** http://www.fundfornj.org
Mark Murphy, Executive Director & Secretary

**Fnded:** 1969. **Philosophy:** The fund supports "organizations whose efforts have implications for future public policies in New Jersey, organizations that promote public discussion and awareness of New Jersey's neglected problems and that act to rectify them." Social and Economic Opportunity, Environment and Land Use, and Public Affairs in New Jersey are the three fund-designated giving categories. Grants are awarded to inform, demonstrate, publicize, educate, and organize, thus providing essential links for individuals to shape New Jersey's future. "The fund will favor approaches and projects that build consensus by bridging diverse communities and interests; promote prevention and early intervention to address problems, nurture and advance emerging leaders from diverse backgrounds who will bring new perspectives to our public policy debates; pursue the adoption of the 'best' practices and programs; increase the accountability of public institutions and purposes; impact the lives of inner-city residents, particularly youth; help build a sense of community and counteract fragmenting social polarization; prepare individuals, organizations, and communities to exercise authority over important aspects of their lives; demonstrate effective approaches to resolving problems and meeting community needs; and educate the public and governmental leaders on critical issues." "The Fund for New Jersey was a founding member of the Camden Development Collaborative which was created in 1995 to assist the residents of Camden in developing a sustainable economic and social environment for the growth of their children and families." 1996 Annual Report. **Priorities:** *Arts & Humanities:* 1%. *Civic & Public Affairs:* 24%. Support for organizations furthering public policy in New Jersey. *Education:* 45%. Support for college/university programs in public policy. *Environment:* 8%. Emphasis on social and economic opportunity. *International:* 2%. *Note:* Contributions analysis provided by foundation. Total contributions made in 1999. **Typ. Recipients:** AIDS/HIV, Child Abuse, Domestic Violence, Health Organizations, Hospitals, Medical Education, Prenatal Health Issues, Public Health, Substance Abuse. **Geo. Dist:** NJ.

**★ 270 ★ G. Harold and Leila Y. Mathers Charitable Foundation**
103 S Bedford Rd.
Ste. 101
Mount Kisco, NY 10549-3440
**Phone:** (914)242-0465　　　**Fax:** (914)242-0665
James Handelman, Executive Director
**Fnded:** 1975. **Philosophy:** The foundation typically focuses its giving in the field of medical research performed at various hospitals, medical research institutes, and universities throughout the country. **Priorities:** *Civic & Public Affairs:* 6%. Supports *Education:* 30%. Supports colleges and universities and medical education. *Environment:* 1%. Supports family services. *International:* 63%. Supports hospital, single-disese health associations and biomedical research. *Note:* Total contributions made in 1999. **Typ. Recipients:** Cancer, Children's Health/Hospitals, Clinics/Medical Centers, Emergency/Ambulance Services, Health-General, Heart, Hospitals, Hospitals (University Affiliated), Medical Education, Medical Research, Public Health, Research/Studies Institutes, Single-Disease Health Associations. **Geo. Dist:** nationally.

**★ 271 ★ G. Unger Vetlesen Foundation**
One Rockefeller Plaza
Ste. 301
New York, NY 10020
**Phone:** (212)586-0700　　　**Fax:** (212)245-1863
**Website:** http://www.monellvetlesen.org
George Rowe, Jr., President
**Fnded:** 1955. **Philosophy:** The foundation typically supports oceanographic and geological research at scientific institutes. **Priorities:** *Arts & Humanities:* 1%. *Civic & Public Affairs:* 1%. *Education:* 13%. Mainly oceanography and veterinary medicine. *Religion:* 80%. Science museums, oceanography, and observatories. *Note:* Total contributions made in 1998. **Typ. Recipients:** Medical Education, Medical Research. **Geo. Dist:** nationally; MA; NY.

**★ 272 ★ GAR Foundation**
50 South Main St.
PO Box 1500
Akron, OH 44309-1500
**Phone:** (330)643-0201　　　**Fax:** (330)258-6559
**Email:** gar@bdblaw.com
**Website:** http://www.garfdn.org
Robert Briggs, Executive Director

**Fnded:** 1967. **Philosophy:** The foundation supports higher and secondary educational institutions. It also contributes to a variety of programs in the arts, including public broadcasting, music, performing arts, museums, and libraries. Religious organizations, civic groups, and social service agencies are funded on a lesser scale. **Priorities:** *Arts & Humanities:* About 16%. Museums, theaters, public broadcasting, music, historical societies, and art centers. *Civic & Public Affairs:* 59%. Zoos, public policy concerns, and community causes. *Education:* About 16%. Colleges and universities, education funds, and secondary education. *Environment:* 5%. Youth organizations, united funds, homes, people with disabilities, and prevention of domestic violence. *International:* 1%. Health fund. *Note:* Total contributions made in 1998. **Typ. Recipients:** Alzheimers Disease, Cancer, Children's Health/Hospitals, Clinics/Medical Centers, Emergency/Ambulance Services, Eyes/Blindness, Family Planning, Health Funds, Health Organizations, Hospices, Hospitals, Medical Education, Mental Health, Multiple Sclerosis, Nursing Services, People with Disabilities, Prenatal Health Issues, Public Health, Substance Abuse. **Geo. Dist:** OH, Summit County and 5 surrounding counties.

**★ 273 ★ Gates Family Foundation**
3200 Cherry Creek South Dr., Ste. 630
Denver, CO 80209-3247
**Phone:** (303)722-1881　　　**Fax:** (303)698-9031
**Email:** info@gatesfamilyfdn.org
**Website:** http://www.gatesfamilyfdn.org
Tom Kaesemeyer, Executive Director
**Fnded:** 1946. **Philosophy:** The Gates Foundation's purpose is to encourage or initiate "activities which will promote the health and welfare and broaden the education of mankind" through research, grants, publications, its own agencies and activities, and through cooperation with agencies and institutions already involved in such activities. Among the foundation's interests are improvement of the quality of life for Denver residents, including support of cultural activities, provision of better low-cost health care, preservation of parks and historic areas, support of conservation and outdoor recreation programs, and the growth and development of independent schools and colleges. In addition, the foundation supports greater cooperation between the public and private sectors; the development of leadership and managerial skills of elected officials and public sector managers; assessment of and means to address the problems faced by public education; and the development of nonacademic programs for young people, particularly those that encourage the development of character and leadership skills. The foundation continues its interest in organizations that promote free enterprise and constructive public policy dialogue. Programs of special interest to the trustees are occasionally initiated by the foundation. **Priorities:** *Arts & Humanities:* 20%. Theaters, museums, historic preservation, public broadcasting. *Civic & Public Affairs:* 6%. Supports community organizations, foundations, urban issues, and parks. *Education:* 23%. Universities, charter schools. *Environment:* 28%. Funds youth services, including youth organizations; United Way; recreation. *Religion:* 10%. Funds museum and archaeology. *Note:* Total contributions made in 2000. **Typ. Recipients:** Child Abuse, Domestic Violence, Family Planning, Health Policy/Cost Containment, Health-General, People with Disabilities, Substance Abuse. **Geo. Dist:** CO.

**★ 274 ★ Gebbie Foundation**
110 W 3rd St., Ste. 308
Jamestown, NY 14701-5179
**Phone:** (716)487-1062　　　**Fax:** (716)484-6401
Thomas Cardman, Executive Director
**Fnded:** 1964. **Philosophy:** The foundation's mission is "to support appropriate charitable and humanitarian programs to improve the quality of life, primarily in Chautauqua County." Traditionally, the foundation has supported the founder's specific interests and giving patterns. Major initiatives focus on children, youth, and education, "to provide opportunities to young children and families for growth and learning; to encourage them to become productive citizens; assist those

interested in extending their education; and provide funding to enhance educational programs." The foundation also supports arts appreciation and participation, historical societies, and libraries. Human services programs that assist those who suffer from social, economic, or cultural deprivation are of particular interest to the foundation. The foundation provides assistance for community development issues, including the maintenance, preservation, and enhancement of economic, health, and environmental assets. 1997 Annual Report **Priorities:** *Arts & Humanities:* 12%. Theater, libraries, historical societies, ballet, and arts organizations. *Civic & Public Affairs:* 23%. Community development, assistance in bringing new business to the area, legal aid, civic centers, and neighborhood projects. *Education:* 7%. Scholarship funding, preschool education, colleges, environment education, and education reform. *Environment:* 45%. Local YWCA organizations, United Way, youth programs, daycare, family services, food banks, animal protection. *International:* 9%. Supports local hospitals, Chautauqua Health Network, hospice and cancer. *Note:* Total contributions made in fiscal 1999. **Typ. Recipients:** Alzheimers Disease, Cancer, Children's Health/Hospitals, Domestic Violence, Emergency/Ambulance Services, Health-General, Heart, Hospices, Hospitals, Medical Education, Medical Rehabilitation, Medical Research, Mental Health, Nursing Services, People with Disabilities, Prenatal Health Issues, Public Health, Research/Studies Institutes, Speech & Hearing, Substance Abuse. **Geo. Dist:** NY.

**★ 275 ★ George D. Smith Fund**
805 Third Ave.
New York, NY 10022
**Phone:** (212)702-5801
Lawrence Milas, President
**Fnded:** 1956. **Philosophy:** The George D. Smith Fund primarily supports health care services and medical research. Other interests include universities, civil rights, family planning, and public broadcasting. **Priorities:** *Arts & Humanities:* 11%. Public radio. *Civic & Public Affairs:* 6%. Professional/trade associations. *Education:* 36%. Funds universities and secondary public schools. *Environment:* 3%. Planned Parenthood of America. *International:* 31%. Primarily supports medical centers. *Note:* Contributions made in 1998. **Typ. Recipients:** Clinics/Medical Centers, Family Planning, Health Funds, Health Organizations, Hospitals (University Affiliated), Medical Education. **Geo. Dist:** CA; NE; NY; UT.

**★ 276 ★ George F. Baker Trust**
477 Madison Ave., Ste. 1650
New York, NY 10022
**Phone:** (212)755-1890　　　**Fax:** (212)319-6316
Ms. Rocio Suarez, Executive Director
**Fnded:** 1937. **Philosophy:** Grants from the trust are for general charitable giving, largely to institutions in the New York area that have received continuous support over the years from the donor and his family. Special consideration is given to education, hospitals, social services, youth agencies, conservation, and historic preservation. **Priorities:** *Arts & Humanities:* 6%. Supports museums, school libraries, and cultural concerns. *Education:* 75%. Supports secondary and preparatory schools, academies, colleges and universities. *Environment:* 4%. Supports youth services and neighborhood affairs. *International:* 5%. Supports medical centers, rehabilitation centers, and hospitals. *Note:* Contributions were made in 1998. **Typ. Recipients:** AIDS/HIV, Cancer, Children's Health/Hospitals, Clinics/Medical Centers, Diabetes, Emergency/Ambulance Services, Family Planning, Heart, Hospitals, Hospitals (University Affiliated), Medical Education, Medical Rehabilitation, Medical Research, People with Disabilities, Public Health, Substance Abuse. **Geo. Dist:** nationally; New York, NY.

**★ 277 ★ George F. and Sybil H. Fuller Foundation**
1B Central St.
Boylston, MA 01505

**Phone:** (508)869-6723          **Fax:** (508)869-2601
Russell Fuller, Chairman, Treasurer & Trustee
**Fnded:** 1955. **Philosophy:** The foundation generally supports higher educational organizations, cultural institutions, hospitals, historic preservation efforts, and social services. Within the past year, the foundation has placed more emphasis on community service organizations working to improve the quality of life in Massachusetts. **Priorities:** *Arts & Humanities:* 21%. Includes museums, historic preservation, music, and theater. *Civic & Public Affairs:* 25%. Supports Chambers of Commerce, community foundations, safety, and housing. *Education:* 26%. Funds primarily colleges and universities. *Environment:* 18%. Supports the Young Men's Christian Association, Young Women's Christian Association, homes, community centers, and United Way. *International:* 5%. Supports community health associations. *Note:* Total contributions made in 2000. **Typ. Recipients:** Children's Health/Hospitals, Clinics/Medical Centers, Diabetes, Emergency/Ambulance Services, Health Organizations, Health-General, Hospices, Hospitals, Medical Education, Medical Research, Nursing Services, People with Disabilities, Public Health, Single-Disease Health Associations, Substance Abuse. **Geo. Dist:** MA, Worcester County.

★ **278** ★ **George Foundation**
310 Morton St., Ste. C
Richmond, TX 77469-0076
**Phone:** (281)342-6109          **Fax:** (281)341-7635
**Email:** radamson@thegeorgefoundation.org
**Website:** http://www.thegeorgefoundation.org
Roland Adamson, Executive Director
**Fnded:** 1945. **Philosophy:** The George Foundation is "trust for religious, charitable, scientific, literary and/or educational purposes." The founders directed the trustees of their foundation to administer its funds "for the use and benefit of the people of Fort Bend County, primarily, yet the (Trustees) may extend the benefits thereof to the people of other counties in the State of Texas." **Priorities:** *Arts & Humanities:* 6%. supports the Ft. Bend County Museum Association and museums. *Civic & Public Affairs:* 4%. Supports civic and community affairs, philanthropic organizations, and housing. *Education:* 19%. Supports educational programs and institutions, scholarships, and enrichment programs. *Environment:* 32%. Supports youth services planned parenthood, social services, the disabled, and scouts. *International:* 35%. Supports hospitals, family health centers, and disorder and disease concerns. *Note:* Contributions were made in 1998. **Typ. Recipients:** Adolescent Health Issues, AIDS/HIV, Alzheimers Disease, Cancer, Child Abuse, Children's Health/Hospitals, Clinics/Medical Centers, Diabetes, Domestic Violence, Emergency/Ambulance Services, Eyes/Blindness, Family Planning, Geriatric Health, Health Organizations, Hospices, Hospitals, Long-Term Care, Medical Education, Medical Research, Mental Health, Multiple Sclerosis, People with Disabilities, Prenatal Health Issues, Research/Studies Institutes, Single-Disease Health Associations, Speech & Hearing, Substance Abuse, Transplant Networks/Donor Banks. **Geo. Dist:** TX, Fort Bend County and surrounding area.

★ **279** ★ **George and Frances Ball Foundation**
PO Box 1408
Muncie, IN 47308
**Phone:** (765)741-5500          **Fax:** (317)741-5518
Joyce Beck, Administrative Assistant
**Fnded:** 1937. **Philosophy:** The foundation supports higher education and the arts primarily in east central Indiana and the immediate surrounding area. Educational funding goes primarily to colleges and universities, with substantial funding to Ball State University in Muncie, IN. The foundation supports a variety of cultural organizations, especially the Minnetrista Cultural Foundation, also in Muncie. In addition, the foundation funds libraries and museums. Civic affairs and social services also are funded. **Priorities:** *Arts & Humanities:* 44%. *Civic & Public Affairs:* 8%. *Education:* 44%. *International:* 8%. *Note:* Historical percent-

ages 1937-2001. **Typ. Recipients:** Children's Health/Hospitals, Emergency/Ambulance Services, Family Planning, Health Organizations, Hospitals, Medical Education, Medical Rehabilitation, Medical Research, People with Disabilities, Substance Abuse. **Geo. Dist:** IN, Delaware County; IN, East Central Indiana; Muncie, IN.

★ **280** ★ **George Frederick Jewett Foundation**
Russ Bldg.
235 Montgomery St., Ste. 612
San Francisco, CA 94104
**Phone:** (415)421-1351          **Fax:** (415)421-0721
Ann Gralnek, Senior Advisor
**Fnded:** 1957. **Philosophy:** "Following the death of Mary Cooper Jewett Gaiser in 1996, the trustees of the foundation determined to divide the foundation into separate philanthropic entities. During the reorganization and beginning with its 1998 grant cycle, there will be two separate funds within the George Frederick Jewett Foundation divided equally between the two entities. These funds will be directed by the two branches of the Jewett Family and will be known as Jewett Fund A and Jewett Fund B of the George Frederick Jewett Foundation." "The primary interests of the Jewett Fund A within the Foundation are: Arts and Culture, Education, and Environment (with particular emphasis on Land Conservation, Oceanographic Studies, and Population). Some consideration will also be given to Health/Social Services and Medical Research. The Jewett Fund A of the Foundation focuses its grants largely, although not exclusively, to San Francisco, California, and Spokane, Washington." "The priority interests of Jewett Fund B of the Foundation are: Education, Libraries, Music, Preservation, Protection of the Environment, including Population Issues, and Scientific Research. Jewett Fund B of the Foundation focuses its grants largely in geographic areas in which Trustees and family members have knowledge of particular needs." George Frederick Jewett Foundation 1997 Annual Report **Priorities:** *Civic & Public Affairs:* 9%. Supports parks. *Education:* 23%. Supports colleges, universities and private schools. *Environment:* 17%. Supports family planning and community service organizations. *International:* 21%. Supports health clinic and research/studies institute. *Religion:* 18%. Supports science institute and laboratory. *Note:* Total contributions made in 1998. **Typ. Recipients:** Cancer, Clinics/Medical Centers, Diabetes, Emergency/Ambulance Services, Family Planning, Hospitals, Medical Education, Medical Rehabilitation, Nursing Services, People with Disabilities, Prenatal Health Issues, Substance Abuse. **Geo. Dist:** San Francisco, CA; WA, Eastern Washington; Spokane, WA.

★ **281** ★ **George Gund Foundation**
45 Prospect Ave. West
1845 Guildhall Bldg.
Cleveland, OH 44115
**Phone:** (216)241-3114          **Fax:** (216)241-6560
**Email:** dbergholz@gundfdn.org
**Website:** http://www.gundfdn.org
David Bergholz, Executive Director
**Fnded:** 1952. **Philosophy:** The foundation's operations reflect George Gund's belief that creative solutions are needed to cure society's ills. This belief demands the seeking and fostering of innovative ideas to enhance people's understanding of their environment and increase their ability to cope with its ever-changing requirements. The foundation attempts this through its giving to education, human services, economic revitalization, arts, environmental quality, and civic affairs. In education, the foundation supports higher education, primary and secondary education, and early childhood. In human services, the foundation supports programs within Cuyahoga County that enhance the welfare and stability of children and families and promote greater self-sufficiency for persons of low-income. Grantmaking in health focuses primarily on Greater Cleveland programs that seek to prevent infant mortality and improve community health. The foundation also funds national and local family planning and reproductive rights organizations, retinal

degenerative disease research, local AIDS services and educational programs, and national AIDS policy formation. In the arts, the foundation strives to foster a lively and diverse arts community in Greater Cleveland by funding projects that emphasize artistic quality, innovative programming and organizational development and stability. In environmental affairs, primary grantmaking in Greater Cleveland focuses on ecosystems, rivers and watersheds, parks, and open space, and efforts to encourage citizen awareness. Grantmaking in Ohio focuses on state-wide issues and organizations promoting improved public policy or providing coordination and support for local environmental groups. Local grantmaking in the Great Lakes basin emphasizes region-wide protection of environmental resources and strengthening the infrastructure of the environmental community, including programs that develop leadership and management capacity in nonprofit organizations. In civic affairs, the foundation focuses on public policy, increasing governmental effectiveness, and encouraging citizen participation in the Greater Cleveland area. Grantmaking also supports economic and community revitalization efforts at the local and state level, including the creation of jobs. **Priorities:** *Arts & Humanities:* 13%. Supports museums, music, ballet, public broadcasting, dance and theater. *Civic & Public Affairs:* 31%. Supports civil rights, law & justice, festivals, botanical gardens/parks, and public policy. *Education:* 27%. Supports universities, journalism/media education, scholarship, and leadership training. *Environment:* 7%. Supports United Way, family planning services, child welfare and camps. *International:* 11%. Supports AID/HIV, eyes/blindness, medical center. *Religion:* 6%. Supports science museums. *Note:* Total contributions made in 1998. **Typ. Recipients:** AIDS/HIV, Children's Health/Hospitals, Clinics/Medical Centers, Emergency/Ambulance Services, Eyes/Blindness, Family Planning, People with Disabilities, Single-Disease Health Associations. **Geo. Dist:** Cleveland, OH, including northeastern Ohio region.

★ **282** ★ **George H. Deuble Foundation**
PO Box 2288
North Canton, OH 44720
**Phone:** (330)455-0610
Andrew H. Deuble, Secretary
**Fnded:** 1947. **Philosophy:** The foundation makes grants across the major categories of support. Social service support goes to family planning, child welfare, community centers, and employment. Support for education includes scholarships, universities, technical education, and funds. Health support includes brain research, nursing, and single-disease associations. Arts funding favors historic preservation and museums. The foundation also funds civic and religious causes. **Priorities:** *Arts & Humanities:* 26%. Restoration funds, museums, and arts institutes. *Civic & Public Affairs:* 2%. *Education:* About 16%. Primary schools, and colleges and universities. *Environment:* 26%. United funds, youth organizations, the disabled, and YM-YWCAs. *International:* 26%. A medical foundation, hospitals, and medical research. *Note:* Total contributions made in 1994. **Typ. Recipients:** Adolescent Health Issues, Children's Health/Hospitals, Emergency/Ambulance Services, Family Planning, Health Funds, Heart, Hospitals, Medical Education, Medical Research, People with Disabilities, Single-Disease Health Associations, Substance Abuse. **Geo. Dist:** OH, Stark County and metropolitan area.

★ **283** ★ **George Hoag Family Foundation**
11340 West Olympic Blvd., Ste. 300
Los Angeles, CA 90064
**Phone:** (310)473-9050          **Fax:** (310)473-9091
Mr. Charles Smith, Secretary/Executive Director
**Fnded:** 1940. **Philosophy:** The foundation "primarily applies its resources to preserve and enrich the benefits to be derived by California residents, and principally those residing in Orange County, from improved and expanded medical services, opportunities for youth and other humanitarian or similar community projects." **Priorities:** *Arts & Humanities:* 4%. Supports a philharmonic society and ballet. *Civic & Public Affairs:* 14%. Funds community foundations

and housing programs. *Education:* 4%. Funds a college foundation, academic decathlon, and other educational programs. *Environment:* 36%. Supports youth organizations and and food banks. *International:* 35%. Supports hospitals, clinics, and healthcare-related programs. *Note:* Total contributions made in 1998. **Typ. Recipients:** Adolescent Health Issues, AIDS/HIV, Alzheimers Disease, Cancer, Child Abuse, Child Abuse, Children's Health/Hospitals, Clinics/Medical Centers, Diabetes, Domestic Violence, Emergency/Ambulance Services, Eyes/Blindness, Health Organizations, Health-General, Heart, Hospitals, Medical Research, People with Disabilities, Prenatal Health Issues, Preventive Medicine/Wellness Organizations, Public Health, Research/Studies Institutes, Single-Disease Health Associations, Substance Abuse. **Geo. Dist:** CA, Orange County.

**★ 284 ★ George I. Alden Trust**
370 Main St., 12th Fl.
Worcester, MA 01608
**Phone:** (508)798-8621     **Fax:** (508)791-6454
**Email:** trustees@aldentrust.org
**Website:** http://www.aldentrust.org
Mr. Francis Dewey, III, Chairman

**Fnded:** 1912. **Philosophy:** The primary interest of the George I. Alden Trust is education. The focus is on higher education, although a few projects in secondary education are also supported. The trust has funded endowments for scholarship support for students, laboratory and other equipment purchases, and building programs. The trust favors educational institutions combining academic excellence with efficient and economically sound administration. **Priorities:** *Arts & Humanities:* 9%. Supports libraries. *Civic & Public Affairs:* 7%. Supports community foundations. *Education:* 69%. Supports college, universities, and literacy. *Environment:* 14%. Supports Young Men's Christian Association in Massachusetts. *Religion:* 1%. Funds science centers. **Typ. Recipients:** Clinics/Medical Centers, Emergency/Ambulance Services, Family Planning, Health Organizations, Medical Education, Medical Research. **Geo. Dist:** New England area; Worcester, MA.

**★ 285 ★ George Link, Jr. Foundation**
1290 Ave. of the Americas
New York, NY 10104
Michael Cantanzaro, Vice President, Secretary & Director

**Fnded:** 1980. **Philosophy:** The foundation typically supports health organizations, educational institutions, religious causes, and social services. **Priorities:** *Arts & Humanities:* 3%. Museums and cultural centers. *Civic & Public Affairs:* 5%. Housing & Ethnic organizations, and safety. *Education:* 31%. Colleges and high schools. *Environment:* 14%. Community services, primarily organized by religious groups. *International:* 19%. Hospitals and medical centers. *Note:* Total contributions made in 1998. **Typ. Recipients:** Cancer, Children's Health/Hospitals, Clinics/Medical Centers, Health Funds, Health Organizations, Heart, Hospitals, Long-Term Care, Long-Term Care, Medical Education, Medical Rehabilitation, Medical Research, Mental Health, People with Disabilities, Public Health, Single-Disease Health Associations. **Geo. Dist:** Northeast; NJ; NY.

**★ 286 ★ George and Mary Josephine Hamman Foundation**
910 Travis St., state. 1990
Houston, TX 77002-5816
**Phone:** (713)658-8345     **Fax:** (713)658-0980
**Email:** hammanfdn@aol.com
**Website:** http://www.hammanfoundation.org
E. Fritsche, Executive Director

**Fnded:** 1954. **Philosophy:** The foundation makes grants across the major categories of support. Health care interests include single-disease associations, hospices, health organizations, and hospitals. The arts are supported through funding to museums, the performing arts, ballet, and art centers. Educational funding favors private schools, education centers, special education schools for the deaf, colleges, and private universities. Social service interests include family planning, the homeless, homes, child welfare, and the disabled. Other interests include churches and religious groups. **Priorities:** *Arts & Humanities:* 20%. Focus on museums, music, and theater. *Civic & Public Affairs:* 11%. Support for a park, nature center, and community health organization. *Education:* 27%. Primarily to colleges and universities, primary and secondary schools, and scholarships. *Environment:* 14%. Family planning, child welfare, youth organizations, and the homeless. *International:* 19%. Supports single-disease health associations and hospitals. *Note:* Total contributions made in fiscal 1999. **Typ. Recipients:** Alzheimers Disease, Cancer, Children's Health/Hospitals, Clinics/Medical Centers, Domestic Violence, Emergency/Ambulance Services, Eyes/Blindness, Family Planning, Health Organizations, Heart, Hospices, Hospitals, Hospitals (University Affiliated), Medical Education, Medical Rehabilitation, Medical Research, Mental Health, People with Disabilities, Single-Disease Health Associations, Speech & Hearing, Substance Abuse. **Geo. Dist:** Houston, TX.

**★ 287 ★ George S. and Dolores Dore Eccles Foundation**
Deseret Bldg.
79 South Main St., 12th Floor
Salt Lake City, UT 84111
**Phone:** (801)246-5336     **Fax:** (801)350-3510
Lisa Eccles, Contact

**Fnded:** 1958. **Philosophy:** "The George S. and Dolores Dore Eccles Foundation is dedicated to improving the welfare of mankind. It is a foundation which serves the Intermountain West with a particular focus on the State of Utah. The Foundation provides assistance to institutions and organizations with a history of achievement, effectiveness and good management. Moreover, the Foundation supports programs and projects which enrich the quality of life and learning and have the potential to make a significant difference in the community. The Foundation's fields of interest include the arts, community organizations, education and medicineical." **Priorities:** *Arts & Humanities:* 16%. Supports performing arts, and college campus libraries. *Civic & Public Affairs:* 4%. Supports community affairs. *Education:* 60%. Supports educational institutions and programs. *Environment:* 10%. Focus on children and youth services, and a domestic violence prevention facility. *International:* 7%. Supports health concerns. *Note:* Contributions were made in 1998. **Typ. Recipients:** Arthritis, Clinics/Medical Centers, Domestic Violence, Eyes/Blindness, Health Organizations, Hospices, Hospitals, Medical Education, Medical Research, Mental Health, Nursing Services, Outpatient Health Care, People with Disabilities, Preventive Medicine/Wellness Organizations, Public Health, Research/Studies Institutes, Single-Disease Health Associations, Speech & Hearing. **Geo. Dist:** preference for Intermountain area of United States; UT.

**★ 288 ★ George W. Brackenridge Foundation**
711 Navarro St., Ste. 535
San Antonio, TX 78205
**Phone:** (210)224-1011     **Fax:** (210)223-3657
Gilbert Denman, Jr., Trustee

**Fnded:** 1920. **Philosophy:** Foundation support goes to accredited Texas educational organizations for individual scholarips, scholarship programs, and educational facilities and programs. The foundation also supports the arts and zoos. **Priorities:** *Arts & Humanities:* 9%. Supports museums, visual arts, and performing arts. *Civic & Public Affairs:* 1%. Supports zoological and civic affairs. *Education:* 88%. Supports educational programs, colleges, and universities. *International:* 2%. Supports health centers. *Note:* Total contributions made in 1999. **Typ. Recipients:** Clinics/Medical Centers, Medical Education, Medical Training. **Geo. Dist:** TX.

**★ 289 ★ Geraldine R. Dodge Foundation**
163 Madison Ave.
PO Box 1239
Morristown, NJ 07962-1239
**Phone:** (973)540-8442     **Fax:** (973)540-1211
**Email:** info@grdodge.org
**Website:** http://www.grdodge.org
David Grant, Executive Director

**Fnded:** 1974. **Philosophy:** "The foundation works in two ways: one, by responding to imaginative proposals that fall within the declared areas and which promise to have impact, to be replicable, and to effect systemic change; and two, by developing initiatives shaped by close listening to practitioners and resource people in areas where the concentration of funds is likely to improve the quality of life." "Expectations for every project go far beyond the transmittal of funds: they grow out of an extensive review process that continues. Further, we seek to collaborate with other funders, individual, foundation, and corporate, as well as select government units in areas of mutual interest. We often provide seed money that allows a project to take root and find other sources of funding, but we will also willingly follow other funders of successful innovations." "The Foundation seeks to be an enabler, backing persons and ideas and institutions who serve a purpose that transcends self-interest and may contribute to sustain human society and the environment that shelters it." The foundation has five major program areas that receive funding: education, the arts, local projects, the welfare of animals, and public issues. Precollegiate education in the northeastern United States is awarded funds to develop teachers and curriculums and to make good education more accessible. The arts in New Jersey are supported, encouraging art education, promoting the role of the individual artist, supporting public access to the arts, and encouraging stability and development of art institutions. Programs in Morris County, NJ are funded by the focus on local projects. The foundation supports animal welfare projects with national implications, and provides direct assistance to a local animal shelter assistance program. Humane treatment and species conservation are major interests of the foundation. National programs for the environment, including conservation, education, and pollution reduction, are the recipients of public issues funding, with the majority of support for efforts in New Jersey and the Northeast. 1996 Annual Report **Priorities:** *Arts & Humanities:* 26%. Focus on literary arts, performing arts, museums, music, theater, and arts festivals. *Education:* 35%. Primarily for education reform, literacy, higher education, and public education. *Environment:* 16%. Supports family planning organizations, animal protection. *Note:* Total contributions made in 2000. **Typ. Recipients:** Domestic Violence, Family Planning, Medical Education, Medical Research. **Geo. Dist:** nationally; NJ.

**★ 290 ★ Gheens Foundation**
One Riverfront Plaza, Ste. 705
Louisville, KY 40202
**Phone:** (502)584-4650     **Fax:** (502)584-4652
**Email:** lindahw@aye.net
James Davis, Executive Director

**Fnded:** 1957. **Philosophy:** "The Gheens Foundation is one of the largest private foundations in Kentucky and the Trustees oversee the distribution of approximately $4 million each year. Most of the grants are made in the Louisville/New Orleans area and are used to support a wide range of endeavors at all levels, including education, economic development, medical, arts, social/health services, handicapped, mental health programs, etc." *The Gheens Foundation, Inc.: A Brief History* **Priorities:** *Arts & Humanities:* 3%. Primarily for historical societies, museums, and memorial landmarks. *Civic & Public Affairs:* 16%. Support for economic development projects in Louisville. *Education:* 42%. Colleges and universities, primary and secondary education, literacy programs, and education associations. *Environment:* 21%. Supports united funds, youth organizations, and family services. *International:* 7%. Supports medical centers. *Religion:* 2%. Gives to the Louisville Science Center. *Note:* Total contributions made in fiscal 2000. **Typ. Recipients:**

Cancer, Children's Health/Hospitals, Clinics/Medical Centers, Diabetes, Eyes/Blindness, Family Planning, Geriatric Health, Health Organizations, Hospices, Hospitals, Hospitals (University Affiliated), Medical Education, Medical Rehabilitation, Medical Research, Mental Health, People with Disabilities, Preventive Medicine/Wellness Organizations, Public Health, Single-Disease Health Associations, Substance Abuse. **Geo. Dist:** Louisville, KY; LaFourche Parish, LA.

### ★ 291 ★ Gladys and Roland Harriman Foundation

63 Wall St., 31st Floor, Ste. 3101
New York, NY 10005
**Phone:** (212)493-8182       **Fax:** (212)493-5570
William Hibberd, Secretary

**Fnded:** 1966. **Philosophy:** The foundation generally gives a majority of funding to educational institutions, primarily to private secondary schools and colleges and universities. Hospitals and medical research organizations, as well as the arts, are also major beneficiaries. **Priorities:** *Arts & Humanities:* 12%. Supports museums, public broadcasting, performing arts, and libraries. *Civic & Public Affairs:* 12%. Funds community affairs and community development. *Education:* 18%. Supports secondary and preparatory schools, colleges, and universities. *Environment:* 24%. Supports child welfare and services for the elderly; major grant to Boys Club of New York. *International:* 19%. Supports the American Red Cross, medical centers, cancer centers, and hospitals. *Religion:* 8%. Supports American Museum of Natural History. *Note:* Total contributions made in 1999. **Typ. Recipients:** Cancer, Child Abuse, Clinics/Medical Centers, Diabetes, Domestic Violence, Emergency/Ambulance Services, Family Planning, Geriatric Health, Health Organizations, Hospitals, Medical Education, Medical Research, Speech & Hearing, Substance Abuse. **Geo. Dist:** nationally; New York, NY.

### ★ 292 ★ Gleason Foundation

1000 University Ave.
PO Box 22970
Rochester, NY 14692-2970
**Phone:** (716)241-4030       **Fax:** (716)241-4099
**Email:** susy.elniski@gleasonfoundation.org
Ralph Harper, Secretary, Treasurer

**Fnded:** 1959. **Philosophy:** The foundation focuses its interests on education, including secondary education and manufacturing/engineering, research, and technology. It also supports community funds, youth groups, social service agencies, public interest and civic affairs groups, and cultural activities. **Priorities:** *Arts & Humanities:* 4%. Supports museums, historical preservation, libraries and orchestra. *Civic & Public Affairs:* 2%. Supports economic and public policy organizations and community foundations. *Education:* 91%. Supports colleges and universities. *Environment:* 3%. Supports volunteer services, emergency relief and community service organizations. *Note:* Total contributions made in 1998. **Typ. Recipients:** Child Abuse, Children's Health/Hospitals, Clinics/Medical Centers, Domestic Violence, Emergency/Ambulance Services, Family Planning, Medical Rehabilitation, Medical Research, Nursing Services, Nutrition, People with Disabilities. **Geo. Dist:** Rochester, NY. **Frmly:** Gleason Memorial Fund.

### ★ 293 ★ Golden Family Foundation

500 Fifth Ave., 50th Floor
New York, NY 10110
**Phone:** (212)391-8960
William Golden, President

**Fnded:** 1952. **Philosophy:** The Golden Family Foundation makes grants across the major categories of support. Most recently, large contributions were made to civic and public affairs. Other support goes to science, environmental affairs, Jewish religious organizations, higher education, health, the arts, and international organizations. **Priorities:** *Arts & Humanities:* 2%. Supports museums, history, libraries, theater, and music. *Civic & Public Affairs:* 52%. Supports museums, botanical gardens, community foundations,

and civil rights. *Education:* 12%. Supports medical education, science/mathematics education, and universities. *Environment:* 1%. Supports animal protection and family planning services. *International:* 3%. Supports cancer, hospitals, and medical research. *Religion:* 23%. Supports science museums and science labs. *Note:* Total contributions made in 1998. **Typ. Recipients:** Clinics/Medical Centers, Family Planning, Hospitals, Medical Education, Medical Rehabilitation, Medical Research, Research/Studies Institutes, Single-Disease Health Associations. **Geo. Dist:** New York, NY, including metropolitan area.

### ★ 294 ★ The Gordon Fund

125 Broad St.
New York, NY 10004-2498
**Phone:** (212)558-3948       **Fax:** (212)558-3064
Mary Roberts, Trustee

**Fnded:** 1985. **Philosophy:** The foundation makes grants across the major categories of support. The foundation's primary interest is education, with an emphasis on Harvard University and other colleges. Support for civic affairs includes environmental concerns and foreign relations. Health support favors public health and cancer research and treatment. Religious giving focuses on Catholic churches and organizations. Other support goes to social services and the arts. **Priorities:** *Arts & Humanities:* 7%. Supports museums, libraries, opera and orchestra. *Civic & Public Affairs:* 3%. Supports community foundations. *Education:* 71%. Supports colleges, universities and private schools. *Environment:* 5%. Supports community service organizations. *International:* Less than 1%. *Note:* Total contributions made in 1998. **Typ. Recipients:** Cancer, Emergency/Ambulance Services, Health-General, Hospitals, Medical Education, Medical Research, Respiratory, Single-Disease Health Associations. **Geo. Dist:** CT; MA; NY.

### ★ 295 ★ Gordon and Mary Cain Foundation

8 Greenway Plaza, Ste. 702
Houston, TX 77046
**Phone:** (713)960-9283       **Fax:** (713)877-8107
James Weaver, Contact

**Fnded:** 1988. **Philosophy:** The foundation makes grants across the major categories of support. Social service support goes to human services, homes, aid to the homeless, youth organizations, and united funds. Educational funding favors colleges and universities. Various programs also are supported in health care, science, the arts, and civic affairs. **Priorities:** *Education:* 20%. Support secondary schools, medical schools, colleges and universities. *Environment:* 7%. Supports youth programs and services, community centers. *International:* 18%. Funds cancer and heart institutes. *Religion:* 4%. Supports science museums and institutes. *Note:* Total contributions made in 1999. **Typ. Recipients:** AIDS/HIV, Cancer, Children's Health/Hospitals, Clinics/Medical Centers, Diabetes, Emergency/Ambulance Services, Eyes/Blindness, Family Planning, Health Policy/Cost Containment, Heart, Hospices, Hospitals, Medical Education, Medical Rehabilitation, Medical Research, Public Health, Single-Disease Health Associations, Substance Abuse. **Geo. Dist:** Houston, TX; Lake Wales, FL; Linville, NC.

### ★ 296 ★ Gottesman Fund

1818 North St., NW, Ste. 700
Washington, DC 20036
**Phone:** (202)785-2727       **Fax:** (202)331-9306
Milton Gottesman, Vice President

**Fnded:** 1965. **Philosophy:** The fund primarily supports the Jewish religion and higher education, including teaching and medicine. Other interests include organizations involved with Israel and civic foundations. **Priorities:** *Arts & Humanities:* 50%. Museums, the performing arts, and libraries receive funding. *Civic & Public Affairs:* 7%. Grants are made to community foundations and philanthropic organizations. *Education:* 15%. Jewish schools, universities, and day schools are funded. *Environment:* 10%. Monetary

awards are made to youth camps; community centers; day care; and family planning clinics. *International:* 8%. Single-disease organizations are supported. *Note:* Total contributions made in fiscal 1999. **Typ. Recipients:** AIDS/HIV, Arthritis, Cancer, Children's Health/Hospitals, Clinics/Medical Centers, Clinics/Medical Centers, Family Planning, Health Organizations, Hospitals, Hospitals (University Affiliated), Medical Education, Medical Rehabilitation, People with Disabilities, Public Health, Single-Disease Health Associations. **Geo. Dist:** east of the Mississippi River; FL; NY.

### ★ 297 ★ Grable Foundation

650 Smithfield St., Ste. 240
Pittsburgh, PA 15222
**Phone:** (412)471-4550       **Fax:** (412)471-2267
**Email:** grable@grablefdn.org
**Website:** http://www.grablefdn.org
Susan Brownlee, Executive Director

**Fnded:** 1977. **Philosophy:** The foundation's mission is "to help children and youth to become independent, caring, contributing members of society by supporting programs critical to a child's successful development. In order of priority, The Grable Foundation will focus on: improving educational opportunities so that children can achieve their potential; supporting community efforts that create an environment in which children can succeed; strengthening families so they can serve as the core support of children and society." **Priorities:** *Arts & Humanities:* 6%. Supports arts museums, music, and theater. *Civic & Public Affairs:* 18%. Supports public policy and women's affairs. *Education:* 33%. Supports literacy, after school/enrichment programs, universities, and schools. *Environment:* 19%. Supports Young Men's Christian Association, youth organizations, United Way, camps, and day care. *International:* 16%. Supports substance rehabilitation, prenatal health issues, and health organizations. *Religion:* 5%. Funds science centers. *Note:* Total contributions made in 1998. **Typ. Recipients:** Children's Health/Hospitals, Family Planning, Health Organizations, Health-General, Hospitals, Mental Health, Prenatal Health Issues, Substance Abuse. **Geo. Dist:** PA, southwest region.

### ★ 298 ★ Grace and Franklin Bernsen Foundation

15 West 6th St., Ste. 1308
Tulsa, OK 74119
**Phone:** (918)584-4711       **Fax:** (918)584-4713
**Email:** info@bernsen.org
**Website:** http://www.bernsen.org

**Fnded:** 1985. **Philosophy:** The foundation Arts funding "provides grants in support of religious, charitable, scientific, literary or educational purposes, or for the prevention of cruelty to children." Arts funding favors ballet, art centers, museums, and performing arts. Educational funding goes to one university and to programs in Tulsa public schools. Health organizations, youth organizations, community centers, food banks, and the United Way are also supported. **Priorities:** *Arts & Humanities:* 9%. Supports opera, music, museums, and historical societies. *Civic & Public Affairs:* 65%. Community affairs organizations. *Education:* 12%. Primarily for special education and literacy. *Environment:* 1%. Gives to United Way. *International:* 12%. Supports medical centers. *Note:* Total contributions made in fiscal 2000. **Typ. Recipients:** Child Abuse, Children's Health/Hospitals, Clinics/Medical Centers, Domestic Violence, Emergency/Ambulance Services, Health Organizations, Heart, Hospices, Hospitals, Medical Education, Medical Rehabilitation, Medical Research, Mental Health, Multiple Sclerosis, Nursing Services, People with Disabilities, Prenatal Health Issues, Respiratory, Sexual Abuse, Single-Disease Health Associations, Speech & Hearing, Substance Abuse. **Geo. Dist:** Tulsa, OK.

### ★ 299 ★ Graham Foundation for Advanced Studies in the Fine Arts

4 West Burton Place
Chicago, IL 60610-1416
**Phone:** (312)787-4071

**Email:** info@grahamfoundation.org
**Website:** http://www.grahamfoundation.org
Richard Solomon, Director
**Fnded:** 1956. **Philosophy:** "The Graham Foundation is broadly interested in educational areas directly concerned with architecture, primarily at an advanced level, and with other arts that are immediately contributive to architecture. In the past, the foundation has supported a variety of endeavors: fellowship grants to individuals for independent study, normally with some end objective such as a book or monograph; grants to architectural schools for special projects, enrichment programs, new curricula, and assistance to selected graduate students; grants to museums, schools, and libraries for exhibitions, catalogues, and in some cases, for acquisitions; support for publications usually to make an important publication better or more affordable to students and teachers." "The foundation has sponsored fellowships at the American Academy in Rome, architectural internships in museums, student competitions and publications, and seminars and conferences. Its headquarters building in Chicago (Madlener House) is a center for lectures, exhibitions, and conferences. scale. Examples of applications that might fall under this heading would include consideration of historical periods of intense urban revision, such as periods of dynamic political or technological change; the investigation of linkages between urban planning and social, cultural, environmental, physical, and economic contexts; the development of curricula that would re-think preservation, restoration, and sustainability programs to include consideration of the urban scale, or conversely, the development of curricula that would incorporate those concerns in existing urban planning programs; and exhibitions, symposia, or competitions that undertake the development or exposition of paradigmatic solutions to questions of urban replanning. Projects should address the interaction between the past, the present, and the future." 1996 Annual Report and Guidelines In 1996, the foundation awarded the first Carter Manny Award, a dissertation grant that continues to be offered on an annual basis. **Priorities:** *Arts & Humanities:* 46%. Supports arts institutes, museums, and libraries. *Civic & Public Affairs:* 7%. Supports clubs and botanical gardens/parks. *Education:* 40%. Supports universities, scholarship, and journalism/media education. *Note:* Total contributions made in 1998. **Typ. Recipients:** Health Organizations. **Geo. Dist:** internationally; nationally.

## ★ 300 ★ The Grainger Foundation
100 Grainger Parkway
Lake Forest, IL 60045-5201
**Phone:** (847)535-1000
**Website:** http://www.grainger.com
Lee Flory, Vice President & Secretary, Director, As
**Fnded:** 1967. **Philosophy:** While the foundation's funding interests are broad, it places "emphasis on capital funds, and special program funds for higher education (colleges and universities), cultural and historical institutions (art, symphonies, and museums), hospitals, and human service organizations." **Priorities:** *Arts & Humanities:* 5%. Cultural and historical institutions and art museums. *Civic & Public Affairs:* Less than 1%. *Education:* 73%. Colleges and universities, and private secondary education; focus on science and technology education. *Environment:* 2%. Recreation/athletics, crime prevention, youth organizations, and human services. *International:* 19%. Supports hospitals. *Note:* Total contributions made in 2000. **Typ. Recipients:** Cancer, Children's Health/Hospitals, Clinics/Medical Centers, Health Organizations, Hospitals, Medical Education, Medical Research, Research/Studies Institutes, Substance Abuse. **Geo. Dist:** Chicago, IL, including metropolitan area.

## ★ 301 ★ Grayce B. Kerr Fund
117 Bay St.
Easton, MD 21601
**Phone:** (410)822-6652　　　　**Fax:** (410)822-4546
**Email:** gbkf@bluecrab.org
Heather Brady Masone, contact

**Fnded:** 1986. **Philosophy:** "The Grayce B. Kerr Fund, Inc., established in 1986, is a dynamic philanthropic foundation committed to enhancing the quality of life. The Fund awards grants that significantly impact and sustain long term change and growth in organizations and institutions. "Currently, the Fund's principal areas of interest include nurturing educational achievement and excellence, fostering life skills critical to self-sufficiency, and encouraging cultural growth. The Fund supports economic and other research activities directed toward improving the information base available for public policy-making. "Leadership effecting positive change in our community is a goal of Grayce B. Kerr Fund, Inc." Annual Report **Priorities:** *Arts & Humanities:* 12%. *Civic & Public Affairs:* 8%. *Education:* 48%. *Environment:* 5%. *International:* 13%. *Religion:* 14%. **Typ. Recipients:** Cancer, Children's Health/Hospitals, Family Planning, Hospices, Hospitals, Medical Research, Mental Health, Public Health.

## ★ 302 ★ Green Fund
14 East 60th St., Ste. 702
New York, NY 10022
**Phone:** (212)755-2445　　　　**Fax:** (212)755-0021
Bruce Rosenblatt, Contact

**Fnded:** 1947. **Philosophy:** Because the fund initiates its grants program, it will not respond to solicitations. The fund concentrates its donations in the New York metropolitan area, providing general support for social service groups, especially to Jewish welfare organizations, health-related institutions, education, and the arts. **Priorities:** *Arts & Humanities:* 9%. Ballet, opera, music, libraries, public broadcasting, and theater. *Civic & Public Affairs:* 6%. Supports women's rights issues, parks/botanical gardens and housing. *Education:* 28%. Focus on colleges and universities, legal education. *Environment:* 2%. Supports homeless/shelters, family planning services, and child abuse. *International:* 22%. Hospitals, geriatric health, and cancer research are supported. *Religion:* 9%. Supports science centers. *Note:* Total contributions made in fiscal 1999. **Typ. Recipients:** Cancer, Children's Health/Hospitals, Clinics/Medical Centers, Family Planning, Geriatric Health, Health Funds, Health Organizations, Hospices, Hospitals, Medical Education, Medical Rehabilitation, Medical Research, Nursing Services, People with Disabilities, Prenatal Health Issues, Single-Disease Health Associations. **Geo. Dist:** New York, NY.

## ★ 303 ★ Greentree Foundation
400 Madison Ave. Ste. 1001
New York, NY 10017
**Phone:** (212)888-7755　　　　**Fax:** (212)397-4232
John Hannan, Controller

**Fnded:** 1982. **Philosophy:** "The Greentree Foundation supports focused projects initiated by local community groups that provide clearly defined participatory roles for schools, parents, children, and community-based organizations. We seek to reduce educational deficiencies and lessen social and cultural tensions." 1997 Guidelines **Priorities:** *Arts & Humanities:* 11%. Supports museums, libraries, art centers and art institutes. *Civic & Public Affairs:* 7%. Supports gardens and public affairs. *Education:* 47%. Supports colleges and universities private schools and education organizations. *Environment:* 33%. Supports youth programs, shelters, homes and community organizations. *Note:* Total contributions made in 1998. **Typ. Recipients:** Child Abuse, Family Planning, Hospitals, Medical Education, Mental Health, Research/Studies Institutes. **Geo. Dist:** New York, NY, including metropolitan area.

## ★ 304 ★ Greenwall Foundation
2 Park Ave., 24th Floor
New York, NY 10016-9301
**Phone:** (212)679-7266　　　　**Fax:** (212)679-7269
**Website:** http://www.greenwall.org
William Stubing, President

**Fnded:** 1949. **Philosophy:** The foundation primarily supports work in medical research, education, and the arts. Medical funding targets areas of special interest to the foundation including bioethics and basic research in insulin-dependent diabetes mellitus. Educational funding focuses on programs to improve the teaching of mathematics and natural sciences. In the arts, the foundation encourages requests from emerging artists and the development of new artistic work. **Priorities:** *Arts & Humanities:* 1%. Supports theater. *Civic & Public Affairs:* 10%. Supports parks/botanical gardens, towns/municipalities, and law & justice. *Education:* 72%. Supports public schools, educational programs, colleges, universities, and medical education. *International:* 10%. Gives to medical centers, hospitals, the Joslin Diabetes Center, and health organizations. *Religion:* 2%. Supports science academies. *Note:* Contributions were made in 2000. **Typ. Recipients:** Alzheimers Disease, Children's Health/Hospitals, Clinics/Medical Centers, Diabetes, Health Organizations, Health Policy/Cost Containment, Heart, Hospitals, Hospitals (University Affiliated), Long-Term Care, Medical Education, Medical Research, Public Health. **Geo. Dist:** NY.

## ★ 305 ★ Gregg-Graniteville Foundation
PO Box 418
Graniteville, SC 29829
**Phone:** (803)663-7552　　　　**Fax:** (803)663-6435
Patricia Knight, Administrator & Secretary-Treasurer
**Fnded:** 1941. **Philosophy:** The purposes of the foundation are to make contributions or to render financial aid to the churches, schools, colleges, public libraries, and other educational and religious organizations located in Aiken County, SC, and Richmond County, GA; to provide scholarships or to finance other educational training; and to construct, own, operate, and maintain parks, gymnasiums, swimming pools, and other facilities for the benefit of the health and welfare of the people who work in the Graniteville, SC, area. **Priorities:** *Arts & Humanities:* 16%. Dance, music, and libraries. *Civic & Public Affairs:* 9%. Major support for the Gregg Park Civic Center. Also supports clubs. *Education:* 22%. Primarily for colleges and universities and religious education. *Environment:* 10%. Community service organizations, Special Olympics, and atheltics/recreation. *International:* 14%. Medical rehabilitation and single disease health associations. *Note:* Total contributions made in 1998. **Typ. Recipients:** Cancer, Diabetes, Domestic Violence, Geriatric Health, Health Organizations, Hospitals, Hospitals (University Affiliated), Medical Rehabilitation, Mental Health, People with Disabilities, Research/Studies Institutes, Single-Disease Health Associations. **Geo. Dist:** GA, Richmond County; SC, Aiken County.

## ★ 306 ★ Grover Hermann Foundation
1000 Hillgrove, Ste. 200
Western Springs, IL 60558
**Phone:** (708)246-8331　　　　**Fax:** (708)246-8319
Paul Rhoads, President & Director

**Fnded:** 1955. **Philosophy:** The Grover Hermann Foundation funds education, health, community, public policy, and religious programs throughout the United States. In the category of education, higher education receives the greatest consideration, with preference for private rather than tax-supported institutions. Scholarships, fellowships, endowments, challenge grants, and capital grants are considered. Private colleges are strongly favored over tax-supported institutions. In the health category, the foundation considers grants for facilities, basic research, disease-specific organizations, and other health programs having demonstrable significance. Community grants are considered for local development, libraries, organizations for youth, the aged or disadvantaged, and other community-related activities. In the area of public policy, the foundation considers organizations dedicated to the strengthening and improvement of our governmental, economic and social systems and that recognize and promote the values of individual liberty, a strong work ethic, free-market competition and limited government. Religious grants favor established organizations and well-defined secular causes. **Priorities:** *Arts & Humanities:* 3%. Supports ballet and theater. *Civic & Public Affairs:* 79%. Supports public policy and community foundations. *Education:* 11%. Supports education associations, universities, and scholarship foundation. *Environment:* 3%. Supports youth organizations. *International:* 4%. Supports medical research. *Note:* Total contributions made in 1998. **Typ. Recipients:** Child Abuse, Children's Health/Hospitals, Domestic Violence, Health Organizations, Health Policy/Cost Containment, Health-General, Hospices, Hospitals, Long-Term Care, Medical Education, Medical Rehabilitation, Medical Research, Mental Health, Nursing Services, People with Disabilities, People with Disabilities, Single-Disease Health Associations, Speech & Hearing. **Geo. Dist:** CA, Monterey County; Chicago, IL.

### ★ 307 ★ Grundy Foundation

680 Radcliffe St.
PO Box 701
Bristol, PA 19007
**Phone:** (215)788-5460 **Fax:** (215)788-0915
Roland Johnson, Executive Director

**Fnded:** 1961. **Philosophy:** According to the broad directive in Mr. Grundy's will, the foundation considers scientific, literary, educational, and charitable projects in the Commonwealth of Pennsylvania. The board of trustees has limited the foundation's work to Bucks County, primarily to the borough of Bristol. The foundation currently is involved in a variety of projects in support of Bristol's ongoing revitalization program. **Priorities:** *Arts & Humanities:* 47%. Supports historic preservation, museums, and the performing arts. *Civic & Public Affairs:* 8%. Supports fire companies, economic development, and community associations. *Education:* 5%. Supports public education. *Environment:* 37%. Supports United Way, family services, senior services, and youth programs. *Note:* Total contributions made in 1999. **Typ. Recipients:** Cancer, Children's Health/Hospitals, Clinics/Medical Centers, Domestic Violence, Emergency/Ambulance Services, Family Planning, Hospitals, Long-Term Care, Mental Health, People with Disabilities, Public Health, Respiratory, Sexual Abuse, Substance Abuse. **Geo. Dist:** Bristol, PA, and Bucks County.

### ★ 308 ★ Gustavus and Louise Pfeiffer Research Foundation

89 Diamond Spring Rd.
Denville, NJ 07834
**Phone:** (973)983-0480 **Fax:** (973)586-3456
**Website:** http://www.fdncenter.org/grantmaker/pfeiffer
Matthew Herold, Jr., Secretary

**Fnded:** 1942. **Philosophy:** Primary support goes to the advancement of medicine and pharmacy. The foundation generally limits biomedical research to breast, ovarian, and prostate cancer, predictive factors in cardiovascular disease, and gerontological immunology. **Priorities:** *Education:* 47%. Supports medical education. *International:* 53%. Supports medical research in the fields of breast, prostate, and ovarian cancer, and cardiovascular disease. *Note:* Total contributions made in 1998. **Typ. Recipients:** AIDS/HIV, Cancer, Children's Health/Hospitals, Clinics/Medical Centers, Diabetes, Geriatric Health, Health Policy/Cost Containment, Heart, Hospitals, Hospitals (University Affiliated), Kidney, Medical Education, Medical Research, Research/Studies Institutes, Single-Disease Health Associations. **Geo. Dist:** nationally.

### ★ 309 ★ H. A. and Mary K. Chapman Charitable Trust

One Warren Place, Ste. 1816
6100 South Yale Ave.
Tulsa, OK 74136
**Phone:** (918)496-7882 **Fax:** (918)496-7887
Donne Pitman, Trustee

**Fnded:** 1976. **Philosophy:** The bulk of funding goes to health and educational organizations. Most grants are to organizations in Oklahoma, primarily in the metropolitan Tulsa area. **Priorities:** *Arts & Humanities:* 3%. Supports ballet, museums, opera and theater. *Education:* 57%. Colleges, religion education, high schools and education funds. *Environment:* 22%. Supports youth and family services, YWCA, United Way, Goodwill Industries, and youth organizations. *International:* 18%. Hospitals and medical research.

*Note:* Total contributions made in 1999. **Typ. Recipients:** Cancer, Child Abuse, Children's Health/Hospitals, Clinics/Medical Centers, Domestic Violence, Geriatric Health, Health Organizations, Health-General, Hospices, Hospitals, Medical Education, Medical Research, Mental Health, Nursing Services, People with Disabilities, Prenatal Health Issues, Public Health, Research/Studies Institutes, Respiratory, Single-Disease Health Associations, Speech & Hearing, Substance Abuse. **Geo. Dist:** Tulsa, OK.

### ★ 310 ★ H. C. S. Foundation

1801 East 9th St., Ste. 1035
Cleveland, OH 44114-3103
**Phone:** (216)781-3502 **Fax:** (216)781-3504
L. Hiltz, Trustee

**Fnded:** 1959. **Philosophy:** The foundation primarily supports education through capital grants. Other interests include the arts, health services, religion, and social services. **Priorities:** *Arts & Humanities:* 7%. Supports children's theater and public broadcasting. *Civic & Public Affairs:* 54%. Funds Renaissance Village, Cincinnati Zoo and Botanical Garden, community development, and legal concerns. *Education:* 7%. Supports universities. *Environment:* 6%. Funds human services and athletics. *International:* 18%. Supports medical centers, infant care, and hearing and speech centers. *Religion:* 2%. Funds a science center. *Note:* Total contributions made in 2000. **Typ. Recipients:** Cancer, Clinics/Medical Centers, Eyes/Blindness, Family Planning, Health Funds, Health Organizations, Heart, Hospitals, Long-Term Care, Medical Rehabilitation, People with Disabilities, Prenatal Health Issues, Speech & Hearing, Substance Abuse, Trauma Treatment. **Geo. Dist:** MD; Cincinnati, OH.

### ★ 311 ★ H. Leslie Hoffman & Elaine S. Hoffman Foundation

225 South Lake Ave., Ste. 1150
Pasadena, CA 91101
**Phone:** (626)793-0043 **Fax:** (626)793-0047
J. Popovich, Trustee

**Fnded:** 1952. **Philosophy:** The H. Leslie Hoffman and Elaine S. Hoffman Foundation's main focus is educational institutions in the Los Angeles, CA, area. The foundation also supports social service organizations, health concerns, and the arts. **Priorities:** *Arts & Humanities:* 3%. Supports museums, libraries, performing arts. *Civic & Public Affairs:* 1%. Supports municipalities, community foundations, legal aid. *Education:* 74%. Supports colleges and universities. *Environment:* 5%. Supports United Way, YMCA, athletics, and a food bank. *International:* 12%. Supports single-disease health associations, medical research, hospitals. *Note:* Total contributions made in 1999. **Typ. Recipients:** Arthritis, Cancer, Children's Health/Hospitals, Children's Health/Hospitals, Clinics/Medical Centers, Diabetes, Emergency/Ambulance Services, Eyes/Blindness, Health Organizations, Health-General, Heart, Hospices, Hospitals, Medical Education, Medical Research, People with Disabilities, Substance Abuse. **Geo. Dist:** Los Angeles, CA.

### ★ 312 ★ Hagedorn Fund

60 Wall St., 36th Fl.
New York, NY 10260
Monica Neal, Vice President

**Fnded:** 1953. **Philosophy:** The Hagedorn Fund makes most of its grants in two areas: social services and health care. In social services, interests include children, religious charities, homes, and domestic violence. Health care support favors single-disease associations and hospitals. Other areas of interest include religious and legal education, community colleges, minority college funds, libraries, and civic affairs. **Priorities:** *Arts & Humanities:* 5%. Focus on public broadcasting and libraries. *Civic & Public Affairs:* 27%. Supports neighborhood associations and botanical gardens. *Education:* 17%. Primarily scholarship and minority college funds. *Environment:* 25%. Supports youth organizations, homes, and community services. *International:* 13%. Gives to hospitals and AIDs research. **Typ. Recipients:** AIDS/HIV, Arthritis,

Cancer, Children's Health/Hospitals, Clinics/Medical Centers, Diabetes, Emergency/Ambulance Services, Emergency/Ambulance Services, Eyes/Blindness, Family Planning, Health Organizations, Health Policy/Cost Containment, Heart, Hospices, Hospitals, Medical Education, Medical Rehabilitation, Mental Health, Nursing Services, People with Disabilities, Respiratory. **Geo. Dist:** New York, NY.

### ★ 313 ★ Hal and Charlie Peterson Foundation

PO Box 293870
Kerrville, TX 78029-3870
**Phone:** (830)896-2262 **Fax:** (830)896-2283
John Mosty, Secretary-Treasurer

**Fnded:** 1990. **Philosophy:** The foundation generally supports educational institutions, the arts, and health-related causes. Funding is limited to Kerr and adjacent counties in Texas. **Priorities:** *Arts & Humanities:* 13%. Funds museums, theater, and historic preservation. *Civic & Public Affairs:* 8%. Supports municipalities, safety organizations, and housing. *Education:* 29%. Private and public education, medical education, and colleges and universities. *Environment:* 32%. Funds United Way, YMCAs, recreation and athletics, scouting, and people with disabilities. *International:* 9%. Support for hospitals, clinics, and single-disease associations. *Note:* Total contributions made in 2000. **Typ. Recipients:** Alzheimers Disease, Cancer, Clinics/Medical Centers, Emergency/Ambulance Services, Health-General, Hospices, Hospitals, Medical Education, Medical Rehabilitation, Nursing Services, People with Disabilities, Preventive Medicine/Wellness Organizations, Substance Abuse. **Geo. Dist:** TX, Kerr and adjacent counties.

### ★ 314 ★ Hall-Perrine Foundation

115 3rd St. Southeast, Ste. 803
Cedar Rapids, IA 52401-1222
**Phone:** (319)362-9079 **Fax:** (319)362-7220
Jack Evans, President, Chief Executive Officer

**Fnded:** 1953. **Philosophy:** "The foundation is interested in assisting local tax-exempt public institutions and organizations dedicated to the solution of problems of people of all ages. The foundation has a particular interest in all areas of health care. It also has a concern for the advancement of education, seeks to support projects to resolve social problems, and is interested in the encouragement and maintenance of community cultural activities." **Priorities:** *Arts & Humanities:* 6%. Funds libraries, theater, a heritage foundation, and cultural museums. *Civic & Public Affairs:* 24%. Supports chambers of commerce and other foundation's. *Education:* 37%. Colleges and universities, and education foundations. *Environment:* 7%. United Way, scouting, and community centers. *International:* 17%. Supports Mercy Medical Center and Alzheimers. *Religion:* 7%. Supports a science station. *Note:* Contributions made in 1999. **Typ. Recipients:** Clinics/Medical Centers, Domestic Violence, Emergency/Ambulance Services, Family Planning, Geriatric Health, Health Organizations, Heart, Hospitals, Hospitals, People with Disabilities, Substance Abuse. **Geo. Dist:** IA, Linn County; Cedar Rapids, IA.

### ★ 315 ★ Harden Foundation

PO Box 779
Salinas, CA 93902-0779
**Phone:** (831)442-3005 **Fax:** (831)443-1429
Joseph Grainger, Executive Director

**Fnded:** 1963. **Philosophy:** "In general, the Foundation seeks to support not-for-profit organizations that will achieve all or some of the following objectives: improve the well-being of young people; strengthen the family; develop individual self-reliance and health; prevent inappropriate institutionalization of individuals; improve the quality of life through cultural activities; encourage more humane treatment of animals; eliminate duplication and improve coordination of social and community services." 1995-1996 Annual Report **Priorities:** *Arts & Humanities:* 9%. Supports libraries, music, and museum. *Civic & Public Affairs:* 6%. Supports legal aid, clubs, and inner-city developmemt.

*Education:* 2%. Supports agriculture education, education funds. *Environment:* 57%. Supports Big Brothers/Big Sisters, scouts, Young Men's Christian Association, shelters/homelesss, at-risk youth, family services, counseling, and food distribution programs. *International:* 12%. Supports eyes/blindness, hospital, medical funds, AIDS/HIV, and home-care services. *Note:* Contributions made in fiscal 1999. **Typ. Recipients:** AIDS/HIV, Alzheimers Disease, Child Abuse, Children's Health/Hospitals, Clinics/Medical Centers, Domestic Violence, Emergency/Ambulance Services, Eyes/Blindness, Family Planning, Health Funds, Heart, Home-Care Services, Hospices, Hospitals, Long-Term Care, Medical Rehabilitation, Mental Health, Nursing Services, Nutrition, Outpatient Health Care, People with Disabilities, Prenatal Health Issues, Respiratory, Single-Disease Health Associations, Substance Abuse. **Geo. Dist:** CA, Monterey County; Salinas Valley, CA.

## ★ 316 ★ Harold K. Hochschild Foundation

477 Madison Ave.
New York, NY 10022-5802
**Phone:** (212)371-2100  **Fax:** (212)759-2946
Adam Hochschild, Trustee

**Fnded:** 1980. **Philosophy:** The foundation primarily supports the arts, with emphasis on historic preservation, and museums. Civic affairs are a secondary interest, with support to human rights, public policy, and international trade affairs. Other support funds environmental affairs, health care, and social services. The foundation has begun to place a greater emphasis on civil liberties, arms control, and ecology. **Priorities:** *Arts & Humanities:* 15%. Major support to the Adirondack Historical Association of New York, and a matching gifts. *Civic & Public Affairs:* 29%. Foundations public policy, civil rights and safety. *Education:* 6%. Higher education. *Environment:* 1%. *International:* 5%. Health centers. *Religion:* 3%. Federation of American Scientist's Fund. *Note:* Total contributions made in 1998. **Typ. Recipients:** Emergency/Ambulance Services, Family Planning, Health Organizations, Health Policy/Cost Containment, Home-Care Services, Nutrition, Public Health. **Geo. Dist:** internationally; nationally; NY.

## ★ 317 ★ Harold K. L. Castle Foundation

146 Hekili St., Ste. 203A
Kailua, HI 96734
**Phone:** (808)262-9413  **Fax:** (808)261-6918
**Email:** bradenkf@aloha.com
**Website:** http://www.castlefoundation.org
Katherine Braden, Vice President & Treasurer

**Fnded:** 1962. **Philosophy:** The foundation favors private education, the community, health and human services (especially youth), youth concerns, and the arts, in Hawaii. The foundation places more emphasis on programs that can effect true systemic change rather than programs which do not address the cause of the problem. The foundation's giving is becoming more proactive. The foundation is assisting the community to determine its goals and is providing program start-ups and seed money to help the community reach its goals. **Priorities:** *Arts & Humanities:* 7%. Supports museums, fine arts, the performing arts, and music. *Civic & Public Affairs:* 6%. Community development. *Education:* 50%. Public school governance reform, private school development. *Environment:* 13%. Emphasis on youth concerns, United Way, and community services. *International:* 10%. Supports medical centers, the Cancer Society, and Easter Seals Society. *Religion:* 7%. Supports the oceanic institute. *Note:* Total contributions made in 1998. **Typ. Recipients:** AIDS/HIV, Cancer, Child Abuse, Children's Health/Hospitals, Clinics/Medical Centers, Domestic Violence, Emergency/Ambulance Services, Health Organizations, Heart, Hospices, Hospitals, Medical Rehabilitation, Mental Health, People with Disabilities, Prenatal Health Issues, Single-Disease Health Associations, Substance Abuse. **Geo. Dist:** HI, focusing on Windward Oahu.

## ★ 318 ★ Harold McAlister Charitable Foundation

4801 Wilshire Boulevard, Ste. 232
Los Angeles, CA 90010
**Phone:** (323)937-0927  **Fax:** (323)937-4727
Katrina Browne, Secretary

**Fnded:** 1959. **Philosophy:** Health services are a major interest of the foundation, although no specific health field is supported uniformly. Social services organizations also receive regular support, with primary interests in child welfare, animal protection, services for the disabled, and other community-support organizations. Higher education in California also is a major priority. **Priorities:** *Arts & Humanities:* 3%. *Civic & Public Affairs:* Less than 1%. *Education:* 29%. Mainly supports colleges and universities. *Environment:* 16%. Focus on child welfare, youth organizations, family services, and animal protection. *International:* 31%. Supports hospitals, single-disease health associations, and children's health services. *Note:* Total contributions made in fiscal 1999. **Typ. Recipients:** Arthritis, Cancer, Children's Health/Hospitals, Clinics/Medical Centers, Emergency/Ambulance Services, Geriatric Health, Health Organizations, Heart, Hospitals, Kidney, Long-Term Care, Medical Research, Nutrition, People with Disabilities, Public Health, Research/Studies Institutes, Research/Studies Institutes, Respiratory, Sexual Abuse, Single-Disease Health Associations, Speech & Hearing, Substance Abuse. **Geo. Dist:** Los Angeles, CA.

## ★ 319 ★ Harriett Ames Charitable Trust

1600 Market St., 29th Floor
Philadelphia, PA 19103
**Phone:** (215)585-3958  **Fax:** (215)585-5448
**Email:** lynn.brickman@hawthorn-pnc.net
Lynn Brickman, Administrator Officer

**Fnded:** 1952. **Philosophy:** The trust's primary funding interests include hospitals and organizations engaged in medical research, educational institutions, and Jewish welfare organizations. The trust also supports cultural and youth programs. **Priorities:** *Arts & Humanities:* 66%. Supports museums, film, visual arts, music, and arts funds. *Civic & Public Affairs:* 1%. *Education:* 19%. Funds precollege and higher education. *International:* 9%. Supports hospitals and medical centers. *Note:* Total contributions made in 1998. **Typ. Recipients:** Alzheimers Disease, Cancer, Clinics/Medical Centers, Diabetes, Eyes/Blindness, Geriatric Health, Health Funds, Health Organizations, Hospitals, Medical Education, Medical Research, Multiple Sclerosis, People with Disabilities, Research/Studies Institutes, Single-Disease Health Associations, Trauma Treatment. **Geo. Dist:** nationally; NY.

## ★ 320 ★ Harris and Eliza Kempner Fund

2201 Market St., Ste. 601
Galveston, TX 77550-1529
**Phone:** (409)762-1603  **Fax:** (409)762-5435
Elaine Perachio, Executive Director

**Fnded:** 1946. **Philosophy:** The Harris and Eliza Kempner Fund has established three priorities in the Galveston, TX, area which has traditionally received more than 80% of the fund's annual contributions. The fund intends to focus on the needs of children and youth including education, health care, and human services, as well as access to social and cultural enrichment. A second priority is addressing the need for affordable housing for low- to moderate-income families. Finally, economic development will receive particular attention in the coming years. Preference is given to seed money grants, operating funds, and small capital needs. In addition to its general grant program, the fund operates a matching gift program for family members and it began Program Related Investments in 1992. The fund made its first three Program-Related Investments in Galveston. Currently, there are nine volunteer members comprising the board of trustees. Seven are family members and two are non-family. The fund also has established three advisory committees, which review grant requests in education, the environment, or population control and third world development. For the student loans, the fund has narrowed its general application process to a program in which selected colleges recommend a specified number of needy upperclassmen. Historically, the fund provides support to a broad range of activities in the Galveston community. The arts and humanities, human services, and health care have all received substantial contributions. The Galveston County Jewish Welfare Association and the University of Texas Medical Branch (UTMB), which is also located in Galveston, have both received continuing support. UTMB has received more than $2.5 million from the fund over the years. Annually, the fund also provides support to the United Way of Galveston. **Priorities:** *Arts & Humanities:* 14%. Emphasis on opera, historical foundations, and arts centers. *Civic & Public Affairs:* 11%. Supports urban and community affairs projects. *Education:* 16%. Supports medical education, primary and secondary education, and scholarships. *Environment:* 27%. Focus on youth organizations, united funds, and family planning. *International:* 17%. Primary support for a university medical center. *Note:* Total contributions made in 1998 and 1999. Analysis provided by foundation. **Typ. Recipients:** Adolescent Health Issues, AIDS/HIV, Alzheimers Disease, Cancer, Child Abuse, Children's Health/Hospitals, Clinics/Medical Centers, Domestic Violence, Emergency/Ambulance Services, Family Planning, Health Organizations, Heart, Hospices, Medical Education, Mental Health, Nursing Services, People with Disabilities, Prenatal Health Issues, Research/Studies Institutes, Single-Disease Health Associations, Substance Abuse. **Geo. Dist:** TX, Galveston county.

## ★ 321 ★ Harry A. and Margaret D. Towsley Foundation

140 Ashman St., PO Box 349
Midland, MI 48640
**Phone:** (517)837-1100  **Fax:** (517)837-3240
Lynn White, President

**Fnded:** 1959. **Philosophy:** The foundation generally focuses its philanthropic work on the problems and needs of private higher education and health education and services. In this area, the University of Michigan is a primary beneficiary of support. Cultural arts, religion, community services, and innovative projects also receive considerable funding. **Priorities:** *Arts & Humanities:* 13%. Museums, opera, summer festival, and theater. *Civic & Public Affairs:* 11%. Supports community organizations. *Education:* 30%. Mostly colleges and universities, schools, education foundations, and arts/humanities education. *Environment:* 20%. Supports children services, family services, food programs, emergency services, family planning services, and senior services. *International:* 10%. Hospices, health centers, AIDS funds, and hospitals. *Note:* Total contributions made in 2000. **Typ. Recipients:** AIDS/HIV, Alzheimers Disease, Cancer, Child Abuse, Children's Health/Hospitals, Clinics/Medical Centers, Emergency/Ambulance Services, Family Planning, Geriatric Health, Health Organizations, Health-General, Hospices, Hospitals, Medical Education, Medical Rehabilitation, Medical Research, Nursing Services, Public Health, Respiratory, Single-Disease Health Associations, Substance Abuse, Transplant Networks/Donor Banks. **Geo. Dist:** MI, especially Ann Arbor and Washtenaw County.

## ★ 322 ★ Harry C. Moores Foundation

100 South 3rd St.
Columbus, OH 43215
**Phone:** (614)227-8884  **Fax:** (614)227-2390
Mary Cummins, Contact

**Fnded:** 1961. **Philosophy:** The Harry C. Moores Foundation is primarily interested in supporting social services, education, and health. Funding for social services favors food and clothing distribution, homes, and youth organizations. Education interests include universities, colleges, religious education, and minority education. Health funding goes to hospitals, health organizations, and single-disease associations. The foundation also supports the arts, civic affairs, and religion. **Priorities:** *Arts & Humanities:* 5%. Supports art and culture. *Civic & Public Affairs:* 15%. Supports community affairs. *Education:* 11%. Supports educational institutions and programs. *Environment:* 41%.

Supports youth and family services, food banks, abuse and addiction programs. *International:* 16%. Supports health, disease and disorder concerns. *Religion:* 5%. Supports the Center for Science and Industry. *Note:* Contributions made in fiscal 1999. **Typ. Recipients:** Alzheimers Disease, Arthritis, Cancer, Children's Health/Hospitals, Clinics/Medical Centers, Diabetes, Emergency/Ambulance Services, Eyes/Blindness, Health Funds, Health Organizations, Heart, Hospitals, Mental Health, Multiple Sclerosis, People with Disabilities, Respiratory, Single-Disease Health Associations, Speech & Hearing, Substance Abuse. **Geo. Dist:** Columbus, OH, metropolitan area.

### ★ 323 ★ Harry C. Trexler Trust

33 South 7th St., Ste. 205
Allentown, PA 18101
**Phone:** (610)434-9645          **Fax:** (610)437-5721
Thomas Christman, Executive Director

**Fnded:** 1934. **Philosophy:** Following the wishes of the donors, the trustees look to fund organizations which are "of the most benefit to humanity" in Allentown or Lehigh County. Areas of funding are not rigid, but will continually change in response to the needs of the area. Present areas of concern are culture and parks, education, youth, the elderly, and the disadvantaged. **Priorities:** *Arts & Humanities:* About 19%. Contributes to music groups, art associations, public libraries, museums, theater, and historic preservation. *Civic & Public Affairs:* 31%. Principally supports the City of Allentown, PA. Supports economic development, parks, safety, and housing. *Education:* 12%. Primarily funds colleges and art and religious education. Also supports literacy, scholarship, and arts/humanities education. *Environment:* About 16%. Funds youth groups YMCAs, food distribution programs, people with disabilities, daycare, and homes. *International:* 8%. Supports indigent care and blood drives. *Religion:* 4%. Supports science centers. *Note:* Total contributions made in fiscal analysis for 2000 is approximate. **Typ. Recipients:** Children's Health/Hospitals, Clinics/Medical Centers, Emergency/Ambulance Services, Eyes/Blindness, Home-Care Services, Long-Term Care, Medical Rehabilitation, Nursing Services, People with Disabilities, Transplant Networks/Donor Banks. **Geo. Dist:** PA, Lehigh County.

### ★ 324 ★ Harry Frank Guggenheim Foundation

527 Madison Ave., 15th Floor
New York, NY 10022-4304
**Phone:** (212)644-4907          **Fax:** (212)644-5110
**Website:** http://www.hfg.org
Mary-Alice Yates, Secretary

**Fnded:** 1929. **Philosophy:** "The Foundation welcomes proposals from any of the natural and social sciences and the humanities that promise to increase understanding of the causes, manifestations, and control of violence, aggression, and dominance. Highest priority is given to research that can increase understanding and amelioration of urgent problems of violence, aggression, and dominance in the modern world." "Particular questions that interest the Foundation concern violence, aggression, and dominance in relation to social change, the socialization of children, inter-group conflict, drug trafficking and use, family relationships, and investigations of the control of aggression and violence...Priority will also be given to areas and methodologies not receiving adequate attention and support from other funding sources." **Priorities:** *Arts & Humanities:* 3%. Supports general arts organizations and historical societies. *Civic & Public Affairs:* 6%. Funds nonprofit management organizations and foundations. *Education:* 53%. Supports natural and social science research at universities. *Environment:* 9%. Supports community organizations and United Way. *Religion:* 2%. Gives to the National Academy of Sciences. *Note:* Total contributions made in 1999. **Typ. Recipients:** Alzheimers Disease, Child Abuse, Eyes/Blindness, Health Funds, Hospitals, Kidney, Medical Education, Medical Research, People with Disabilities, Substance Abuse. **Geo. Dist:** nationally and internationally.

### ★ 325 ★ Harry and Jeanette Weinberg Foundation

7 Park Center Court
Owings Mills, MD 21117
**Phone:** (410)654-8500          **Fax:** (410)654-3943

**Fnded:** 1959. **Philosophy:** The foundation's current fields of interests are the aged, the homeless, and other disadvantaged groups. It supports building funds, capital campaigns, endowment funds, and special projects. **Priorities:** *Arts & Humanities:* 3%. Supports museums. *Civic & Public Affairs:* 5%. Funds parks. *Education:* 5%. Primarily pre-college education. *Environment:* 14%. Funds organizations serving youth, the elderly, and families. *International:* 18%. Supports hospitals and medical centers. *Religion:* 5%. *Note:* Total contributions made in fiscal 1999. **Typ. Recipients:** Clinics/Medical Centers, Diabetes, Geriatric Health, Health Organizations, Heart, Hospitals, Long-Term Care, Medical Rehabilitation, Mental Health, Public Health. **Geo. Dist:** no restrictions.

### ★ 326 ★ Harry and Maribel G. Blum Foundation

919 North Michigan Ave., Ste. 2800
Chicago, IL 60611
**Phone:** (312)664-5050          **Fax:** (312)664-8983
H. Kovler, Vice President

**Fnded:** 1967. **Philosophy:** The foundation's primary interest is Jewish organizations, including religious and social service organizations. It also supports health care, child welfare, and educational institutions. **Priorities:** *Education:* 12%. Funds Francis W. Parker School. *Environment:* 47%. Supports the Family Institute, jobs for youth, and housing. *International:* 41%. Supports a transplantation center and hospital. *Note:* Total contributions made in 1998. **Typ. Recipients:** Clinics/Medical Centers, Diabetes, Health Organizations, Hospitals, Medical Research, People with Disabilities, Prenatal Health Issues, Single-Disease Health Associations, Transplant Networks/Donor Banks. **Geo. Dist:** nationally; IL.

### ★ 327 ★ Harry S. and Isabel C. Cameron Foundation

Bank of America
PO Box 2518
Houston, TX 77252-2518
**Phone:** (713)247-7865
Diane Guiberteau, Administrator

**Fnded:** 1966. **Philosophy:** The foundation, following the interests of its donors, supports educational institutions in Texas. It also shows an interest in religious organizations and social service agencies. **Priorities:** *Arts & Humanities:* 9%. Major support for the Museum of Fine Arts in Houston. *Civic & Public Affairs:* 11%. Funds urban affairs projects. *Education:* 23%. Focus on Catholic secondary education and colleges and universities. *Environment:* 11%. Provides support for youth organizations, child welfare, United Way, and community services. *International:* 10%. Funds hospitals and single-disease health associations. *Note:* Total contributions made in fiscal 2000. **Typ. Recipients:** AIDS/HIV, Alzheimers Disease, Cancer, Children's Health/Hospitals, Clinics/Medical Centers, Emergency/Ambulance Services, Eyes/Blindness, Health Organizations, Hospices, Hospitals, Medical Education, Medical Rehabilitation, Mental Health, Nursing Services, People with Disabilities, Public Health, Single-Disease Health Associations, Substance Abuse. **Geo. Dist:** Houston, TX, including metropolitan area.

### ★ 328 ★ Harvey Randall Wickes Foundation

4800 Fashion Square Boulevard
Plaza North, Room 472
Saginaw, MI 48604
**Phone:** (517)799-1850          **Fax:** (517)799-3327
**Email:** HRWICKES@concentric.net
James Finkbeiner, President

**Fnded:** 1945. **Philosophy:** In accordance with the donor's wishes, the main purpose of the foundation is to provide buildings and equipment to educational,

health, and social service organizations in the Saginaw, MI, area. Support for the area's three hospitals is also given. The foundation also supports the United Way, and parks and recreation facilities in Saginaw Township. **Priorities:** *Arts & Humanities:* 18%. Supports theater, museums, and orchestra. *Civic & Public Affairs:* 37%. Supports zoos and community foundations. *Education:* 11%. Supports universities and private schools. *Environment:* 11%. Supports youth services, housing, crime prevention, and homes. *International:* 13%. Supports health organizations. *Note:* Total contributions made in 1998. **Typ. Recipients:** Cancer, Child Abuse, Clinics/Medical Centers, Emergency/Ambulance Services, Emergency/Ambulance Services, Eyes/Blindness, Health Funds, Health Organizations, Hospitals, Medical Rehabilitation, People with Disabilities, Public Health, Substance Abuse. **Geo. Dist:** MI, Saginaw County.

### ★ 329 ★ Hattie M. Strong Foundation

1620 Eye St. NW, Ste. 700
Washington, DC 20006
**Phone:** (202)331-1619          **Fax:** (202)466-2894
Judith Cyphers, Secretary & Director of Grants

**Fnded:** 1928. **Philosophy:** The Hattie M. Strong Foundation primarily supports a loan program for American students in their last year of undergraduate or graduate school. The foundation also administers a grant program in support of education projects focusing on the Washington, DC, area. "The foundation considers innovative and effective programs that promote literacy, provide training and basic lifeskills development, and educational enrichment and remedial programs." **Priorities:** *Education:* In fiscal 1999, the foundation gave 100% of its funding to education. About 68% went to loans to college students, and 32% went to organizations in the Washington, DC area that provide educational opportunities for at-risk youth and adults, tutoring, and afterschool programs. **Typ. Recipients:** Medical Rehabilitation, Research/Studies Institutes. **Geo. Dist:** nationally for student loan program; Washington, DC, metropolitan area for community education grant program.

### ★ 330 ★ Hatton W. Sumners Foundation

325 North Saint Paul St., Ste. 3920
Dallas, TX 75201-3814
**Phone:** (214)220-2128          **Fax:** (214)953-0737
Hugh Akin, Executive Director

**Fnded:** 1949. **Philosophy:** The Hatton W. Sumners Foundation "encourages the study, teaching and research into the science and art of self-government, to the end that the American People may understand the fundamental principals of democracy and be guided thereby in shaping governmental policies." The board accomplishes these goals in two ways. First, the foundation supports a scholars program for the study of government, political science, law, history, and public administration. In addition to scholarships, the foundation makes grants "to support programs, projects, or activities that provide personal involvement, or hands-on experience, in the political process and functions of government." The foundation also supports the Hatton W. Sumners Distinguished Lecture Series, sponsored in conjunction with the National Center for Policy Analysis, which focuses on issues of current interest. The foundation has implemented several projects supporting elementary and secondary education teachers, including the Education for Freedom teacher training program on the First Amendment to the U.S. Constitution, and another project focusing on the structure and operations of the Free Enterprise System. Additionally, the foundation has begun the publication of a newsletter, has instituted a new graduate scholarship program at the National Journalism Center, Washington, DC, and sponsors the Texas Citizen Bee Competition Finals. The foundation also supports youth programs, focusing on increasing young people's understanding of, appreciation for, and participation in the American system of government. **Priorities:** *Arts & Humanities:* 1%. Supports public broadcasting. *Civic & Public Affairs:* 4%. For civil liberties and civic values. *Education:* 64%. Primarily supports institutions of higher learning through the Sumners Scholarship Endowment. *Environment:* 16%.

Emphasis on youth organizations and YMCA. *International:* 15%. Health organizations. *Note:* Total contributions made in 1998. **Typ. Recipients:** Health Policy/Cost Containment, Medical Research, Medical Training, Mental Health, People with Disabilities, Substance Abuse. **Geo. Dist:** Southwest USA.

### ★ 331 ★ Hawn Foundation
4809 Cole Ave., Ste. 225
Dallas, TX 75205-3553
**Phone:** (214)219-4809 **Fax:** (214)219-2809
W. Hawn, Jr., President

**Fnded:** 1962. **Philosophy:** The Hawn Foundation primarily makes grants in the areas of education and health care. Educational funding favors universities, religious education, and minority education. In health care, interests include health and research foundations, nursing, single-disease associations, and hospitals. Other recipient areas include social services and the arts. **Priorities:** *Arts & Humanities:* 3%. Funds the Dallas Museum of Art and music. *Civic & Public Affairs:* 9%. Supports Salesmanship Club, housing. *Education:* 5%. Supports schools and universities. *Environment:* 5%. Youth and family services. *International:* 70%. Funds single-disease associations, hospitals, and medical centers. *Religion:* 1%. Funds museum. *Note:* Total contributions made in fiscal 2000. **Typ. Recipients:** Alzheimers Disease, Arthritis, Cancer, Child Abuse, Children's Health/Hospitals, Clinics/Medical Centers, Diabetes, Emergency/Ambulance Services, Eyes/Blindness, Health Funds, Health Organizations, Health-General, Heart, Hospitals, Hospitals (University Affiliated), Long-Term Care, Medical Rehabilitation, Medical Research, Mental Health, Multiple Sclerosis, Nursing Services, People with Disabilities, Public Health, Research/Studies Institutes, Respiratory, Single-Disease Health Associations, Substance Abuse. **Geo. Dist:** Dallas, TX.

### ★ 332 ★ The Hearst Foundation, Inc.
888 7th Ave., 45th Floor
New York, NY 10106-0057
**Phone:** (212)586-5404
Robert Frehse, Jr., Executive Director & Vice President

**Fnded:** 1945. **Philosophy:** Within a general policy of assisting institutions to provide access and opportunity to underrepresented, low-income and minority populations, the Directors of the Hearst Foundations have established the following priorities: "Education: The foundation's primary focus is support of undergraduate education through the establishment of endowed scholarships at private liberal arts colleges and universities. In addition, endowed scholarship support is provided for professional study in teaching, medicine, nursing, engineering, math, science, and the health care professions at the undergraduate and graduate levels. A limited number of proposals are also accepted from K-12 independent schools with outstanding academic programs, and demonstrated track records of outreach to economically disadvantaged students. In general, grants are not made to public schools. However, private organizations or coalitions seeking improvement of public education and broadening access to education will be considered." "Health: The foundation's interests in the health field seek to improve and increase health care, while facilitating wellness, prevention, and rehabilitation. Working largely through leading regional hospitals and medical centers, the Foundation support programs which increase access for underserved urban and rural populations. Areas of interest include perinatology and pediatrics, cancer, stroke, aging, women's health issues, and medical research." "Social Services: Preference is given to well-established, larger agencies, providing comprehensive services. Requests for technical assistance, management training, and leadership development, designed to help nonprofit agencies deliver services more efficiently and effectively are also considered." "Culture: The Foundation's priority in the arts is to increase access and educational opportunities for diverse populations and underserved communities. The major portion of funds endow arts education and/or community outreach programs through major cultural institutions. Special

attention is given to programs which enrich the lives of young people through exposure to the arts." 1997 Guidelines for Grant Applications. **Priorities:** *Arts & Humanities:* 25%. Supports theater, music, the performing arts, opera, libraries, and history. *Education:* 39%. Supports colleges and universities, science/mathematics education, religious education, scholarship, literacy, and schools. *Environment:* 18%. Supports Big Brothers/Big sister, family services, child care services, youth organizations, and community centers. *International:* 16%. Supports emergency/ambulance services, hospital, transplant networks/donor banks, cancor, medical research, and medical center. *Note:* Total contributions made in 1999. **Typ. Recipients:** AIDS/HIV, Cancer, Children's Health/Hospitals, Clinics/Medical Centers, Emergency/Ambulance Services, Heart, Home-Care Services, Hospitals, Hospitals (University Affiliated), Medical Education, Medical Rehabilitation, Medical Research, Mental Health, Nursing Services, People with Disabilities, Prenatal Health Issues, Public Health, Research/Studies Institutes, Single-Disease Health Associations, Substance Abuse. **Geo. Dist:** nationally.

### ★ 333 ★ Helen Brach Foundation
55 W Wacker Dr., Ste. 701
Chicago, IL 60601
**Phone:** (312)372-4417 **Fax:** (312)372-0290
Toni Peville, Associate Director

**Fnded:** 1974. **Philosophy:** Helen Brach established her foundation to be used as the primary vehicle for her annual gifts to charity. The foundation's grants have not been limited to any single area, but "areas of interest, among others, have included efforts to save wildlife, curtail the abuse of children and animals, provide funding for education at the secondary and college level, funding for scientific and literary purposes, and help for those serving the physically and mentally disabled, the poor, the blind, the homeless, the teenaged unwed mother, and the elderly." **Priorities:** *Civic & Public Affairs:* 13%. Supports urban affairs and community foundations. *Education:* 21%. Supports secondary and preparatory schools, colleges, and universities. *Environment:* 31%. Supports child welfare, and social and adult services and churches. *International:* 8%. Supports health care and medical centers. *Note:* Total contributions made in fiscal 1999. **Typ. Recipients:** AIDS/HIV, Children's Health/Hospitals, Clinics/Medical Centers, Geriatric Health, Health Funds, Health Organizations, Hospices, Hospitals, Long-Term Care, Medical Rehabilitation, Medical Research, Mental Health, Nursing Services, Nutrition, People with Disabilities, Preventive Medicine/Wellness Organizations, Public Health, Trauma Treatment. **Geo. Dist:** nationally; IL.

### ★ 334 ★ Helen K. and Arthur E. Johnson Foundation
1700 Broadway, Ste. 2302
Denver, CO 80290-1039
**Phone:** (303)861-4127 **Fax:** (303)861-0607
Stan Kamprath, President & Executive Director

**Fnded:** 1948. **Philosophy:** The foundation supports a wide variety of creative efforts to solve human problems and to enrich the quality of life. It concentrates its efforts on health, education, youth, civic and cultural affairs, community and social services, and senior citizens. **Priorities:** *Arts & Humanities:* 9%. Supports opera, museum, music. *Civic & Public Affairs:* 11%. Supports clubs, community foundations, housing and botanical gardens/parks. *Education:* 22%. Funds student aid, scholarship, school, college, and universities. *Environment:* 22%. Supports senior services, Big Brothers/Big Sisters, shelters/homeless, United Way, scouts, emergency relief and people with disabilities. *International:* 28%. Supports eyes/blindness, respiratory, Alzheimers, hospice and children's hospital, and AIDS. *Religion:* 4%. Supports science museums. **Typ. Recipients:** AIDS/HIV, Alzheimers Disease, Cancer, Children's Health/Hospitals, Clinics/Medical Centers, Eyes/Blindness, Family Planning, Health Organizations, Health-General, Hospices, Hospitals, Long-Term Care, Medical Rehabilitation, Medical Research, Medical Training, Multiple Sclerosis, Nursing Services, People with Disabilities, Public Health, Research/

Studies Institutes, Sexual Abuse, Single-Disease Health Associations, Speech & Hearing, Substance Abuse, Transplant Networks/Donor Banks. **Geo. Dist:** CO.

### ★ 335 ★ Helena Rubinstein Foundation
477 Madison Ave., 7th Floor
New York, NY 10022-5802
**Phone:** (212)750-7310 **Fax:** (212)750-9798
Diane Moss, President & Chief Executive Officer

**Fnded:** 1953. **Philosophy:** When she created the foundation, Ms. Rubinstein wanted to affirm a principle she often expressed, "My fortune comes from women and should benefit them and their children, to better their quality of life." The foundation has developed and broadened its original philanthropic concepts to meet the changing needs of society and continues to support an increasing number of innovative programs in education, the arts, arts-in-education, women's issues, and community services. In 1996, the foundation reported a plan to reduce annual grantmaking and long-term commitments in order to insure future economic stability. Along with this reduction in grantmaking was a commitment to a greater emphasis on school-to-work and welfare-to-work initiatives to prepare young people and poor people for productive futures. The foundation continues to stress the importance of higher education by funding scholarships and remains committed to art education. **Priorities:** *Arts & Humanities:* (Arts/Arts Education) 26%. Funds art museums, the opera, theater, ballet, children's museum, music, dance theater, public broadcasting. *Civic & Public Affairs:* (Community Services) 29%. Supports community affairs, economic development, housing, job training programs, public and women's affairs. *Education:* 38%. Gives to colleges, universities, and educational programs. *International:* 7%. Supports children's health, research, women's health care and aid to the homeless. *Note:* Total contribution made in fiscal 2000. **Typ. Recipients:** AIDS/HIV, Alzheimers Disease, Cancer, Children's Health/Hospitals, Clinics/Medical Centers, Eyes/Blindness, Family Planning, Geriatric Health, Health Organizations, Hospitals, Medical Education, Medical Rehabilitation, Medical Research, Medical Training, Nursing Services, Prenatal Health Issues, Preventive Medicine/Wellness Organizations, Public Health, Single-Disease Health Associations, Substance Abuse. **Geo. Dist:** New York, NY.

### ★ 336 ★ Helmerich Foundation
1579 East 21st St.
Tulsa, OK 74114
**Phone:** (918)742-5531
Walter Helmerich, III, Trustee

**Fnded:** 1965. **Philosophy:** The Helmerich Foundation makes grants to the arts, particularly to the performing arts in Tulsa, Oklahoma, religious organizations, and educational institutions and funds. Other areas of interest include civic concerns, social services, and health foundations and centers. The foundation prefers to make large grants that have an impact on projects. Therefore, other recipient areas are funded on a limited basis. **Priorities:** *Arts & Humanities:* 39%. Primarily for libraries, museums, music, and the performing arts. *Civic & Public Affairs:* 10%. Funds zoological park, community development. *Education:* 15%. Supports schools, education funds, universities. *Environment:* 30%. Funds community and family services and child welfare. *International:* 4%. Funds health centers and health foundations. *Note:* Total contributions made in fiscal 2000. **Typ. Recipients:** AIDS/HIV, Cancer, Children's Health/Hospitals, Clinics/Medical Centers, Diabetes, Domestic Violence, Emergency/Ambulance Services, Eyes/Blindness, Health Organizations, Hospices, Mental Health, Nursing Services, People with Disabilities, Public Health, Respiratory. **Geo. Dist:** Tulsa, OK.

### ★ 337 ★ Henry Ford II Fund
100 Renaissance Center, 34th Floor
Detroit, MI 48243
**Phone:** (313)259-7777 **Fax:** (313)393-7579
David Hempstead, Secretary & Trustee

**Fnded:** 1953. **Philosophy:** The fund reports that "the purpose of each grant or contribution is to provide financial support to corporations, trusts, community chests, funds or foundations, organized and operated solely for religious, charitable, scientific, literary or educational purposes, or for the prevention of cruelty to children or animals." The awards "are generally limited to charitable organizations already favorably known to, and of interest to, the substantial contributors of the foundation." **Priorities:** *Arts & Humanities:* Less than 1%. Supports public broadcasting. *Civic & Public Affairs:* 21%. Supports community organisation and foundations. *Education:* 44%. Supports universities, colleges, education associations, and minority education. *Environment:* 9%. Supports the United Way, food banks, and child welfare. *International:* 14%. Supports children's hospitals. *Religion:* 6%. Funds the Edison Institute. *Note:* Total contributions made in 2000. **Typ. Recipients:** Children's Health/ Hospitals, Emergency/Ambulance Services, Eyes/ Blindness, Health Organizations, Hospitals, Medical Rehabilitation, Medical Research, People with Disabilities. **Geo. Dist:** Detroit, MI.

★ **338** ★ **Henry J. Kaiser Family Foundation**
2400 Sand Hill Rd.
Menlo Park, CA 94025
**Phone:** (650)854-9400          **Fax:** (650)854-4800
**Email:** RWells@kff.org
**Website:** http://www.kff.org
Renee Wells, Grants Manager

**Fnded:** 1948. **Philosophy:** The Kaiser Family Foundation makes approximately $40 million in philanthropic expenditures each year, concentrating its work in three primary areas in the U.S.–Health policy, reproductive health, and HIV. For over a decade, the Foundation has also operated a major program to improve health and health care in South Africa, its only international commitment. **Priorities:** *International:* 100%. Grants support a range of activities, including policy analysis, applied research to define and measure public health problems, demonstration and pilot projects, and communications activities that help sharpen health care debates and improve quality of health information. *Note:* Contributions made in 1998. **Typ. Recipients:** Adolescent Health Issues, AIDS/HIV, Cancer, Clinics/Medical Centers, Emergency/Ambulance Services, Family Planning, Geriatric Health, Health Organizations, Health Policy/Cost Containment, Health-General, Heart, Hospitals, Long-Term Care, Medical Education, Medical Research, Nursing Services, Nutrition, Prenatal Health Issues, Preventive Medicine/Wellness Organizations, Public Health, Research/Studies Institutes, Substance Abuse. **Geo. Dist:** nationally; CA.

★ **339** ★ **Henry Luce Foundation**
111 West 50th St., Ste. 4601
New York, NY 10020-1202
**Phone:** (212)489-7700          **Fax:** (212)581-9541
**Website:** http://www.hluce.org
John Cook, President & Director

**Fnded:** 1936. **Philosophy:** "During the past two years, Public Policy projects have dealt with a range of topics, including citizenship, immigration policy, taxation, youth violence, the environment and the roll of the United Nations." "Grants made through the Higher Education category support special scholarly or educational initiatives that fall outside the guidelines for the foundation's other programs." "The Luce Scholars Program was created to enable young Americans to immerse themselves in Asian culture for a year. The Asia Foundation, the organization that administers the Asian aspects of the program, arranges professional placements for each scholar." "Every year, 67 American colleges and universities nominate candidates who have no formal study of Asia." "The Luce Fund for Asian Studies is a new $12 million initiative designed to strengthen the study of Asia at leading American liberal arts colleges." "The fund provides seed money for junior faculty positions and program development over a four-year period. Project grants support a range of concerns in the humanities and social sciences. Typically, these grants fund research and faculty

development, cultural and scholarly exchange, language and library programs, and policy studies." "The foundation continues to bring attention to the cultural wealth of Asia through art exhibitions that highlight pioneering scholarship." "The Luce Foundation's program in Theology supports activities of faith and learning that strengthen the role of religion in daily life. For more than six decades, the Theology Program has emphasized theological education and scholarship, while also embracing projects that support churches and religious leadership. These activities reflect Henry R. Luce's intent to honor the work of his parents, who were Presbyterian missionary educators in China." "The Luce Fund in American Art funds scholarly exhibitions and publications and is open to all periods and genres of American art history." "Twenty-six dissertation awards for doctoral research in American art continue to assist the next generation of art historians specializing in this field. The primary program provides 10 full fellowships annually through an open national competition administered by the American Council of Learned Societies." "The foundation also makes grants for dissertation research to 30 invited schools that show a strong commitment to American art." "The Women in Science Program offers three categories of funding: undergraduate scholarships, graduate fellowships, and term support for tenure-track junior faculty appointments. The program seeks... to encourage women to enter, study, graduate and teach... in fields where there have been barriers to their advancement. These include physics, chemistry, biology, computer science, meteorology, engineering, and mathematics." "The American Collections Enhancement (ACE) initiative supported small and midsize museums with significant American art holdings. It highlighted collections that were not widely known, but deserved wider attention. This special five-year initiative concluded the end of the year 2000." 1998-1999 Biennial Report. **Priorities:** *Arts & Humanities:* 10%. Focus on museums. *Education:* 29%. Supports higher education. *Note:* Total contributions made in 1999. **Typ. Recipients:** Geriatric Health, Medical Education, Public Health. **Geo. Dist:** nationally; East and Southeast Asia.

★ **340** ★ **Henry and Lucy Moses Fund**
1301 Ave. of the Americas, 40th Fl.
New York, NY 10019-6076
**Phone:** (212)554-7800          **Fax:** (212)554-7700
Irving Sitnick, President & Director

**Fnded:** 1942. **Philosophy:** The foundation reflects the interests of Mr. and Mrs. Moses, now both deceased. Its major concerns are welfare activities, hospitals and health-related causes. Other areas which receive support are education, youth programs, social services, and music. **Priorities:** *Arts & Humanities:* 18%. *Civic & Public Affairs:* 27%. *Education:* 13%. Supports Columbia University and its trustees. *Environment:* 4%. *International:* 17%. *Note:* Contributions made in 1998. **Typ. Recipients:** Cancer, Clinics/ Medical Centers, Family Planning, Health Organizations, Hospitals, Long-Term Care, Medical Education, Medical Research, Nursing Services, People with Disabilities, Single-Disease Health Associations. **Geo. Dist:** some funding nationally; New York, NY, metropolitan area.

★ **341** ★ **Henry and Marilyn Taub Foundation**
300 Frank W Burr Boulevard, 7th Floor
Teaneck, NJ 07666
**Phone:** (201)287-2500          **Fax:** (201)287-2580
**Email:** htaub@aviarycapital.com
Fred Lafer, President & Treasurer

**Fnded:** 1967. **Philosophy:** The Henry and Marilyn Taub Foundation provides funds for Jewish religious organizations. The arts, civic affairs, health services and social services also are supported by the foundation, particularly when they are affiliated with the Jewish faith. **Priorities:** *Arts & Humanities:* 2%. Funds the performing arts. *Education:* 8%. Supports colleges and universities. *International:* 3%. Funds single-disease centers. *Note:* Total contributions made in 1998. **Typ. Recipients:** Cancer, Clinics/Medical Centers, Domestic Violence, Emergency/Ambulance Services,

Eyes/Blindness, Hospitals, Hospitals, Medical Education, Medical Rehabilitation, Medical Research, People with Disabilities, Single-Disease Health Associations, Substance Abuse. **Geo. Dist:** Eastern United States; NJ; NY.

★ **342** ★ **Henry P. and Susan C. Crowell Trust**
620 Southpointe Ct. Ste. 205
Colorado Springs, CO 80906-3861
**Phone:** (719)540-0203          **Fax:** (719)540-0196
**Email:** crowellhp@aol.com
**Website:** http://www.crowellfoundation.org
John Bass, Executive Director & President

**Fnded:** 1927. **Philosophy:** The mission of the trust "is limited to the teaching and active extension of the doctrines of evangelical Christianity through approved grants to qualified organizations." **Priorities:** *Arts & Humanities:* 1%. *Civic & Public Affairs:* 1%. *Education:* 8%. Mainly religious education. *Note:* Contributions made in 1998. **Typ. Recipients:** Clinics/Medical Centers, Hospitals. **Geo. Dist:** national organizations.

★ **343** ★ **Herbert H. and Grace A. Dow Foundation**
1018 West Main St.
Midland, MI 48640-4292
**Phone:** (517)631-3699          **Fax:** (517)631-0675
**Email:** info@hhdowfdn.org
**Website:** http://www.hhdowfdn.org
Margaret Riecker, President

**Fnded:** 1936. **Philosophy:** "The Herbert H. and Grace A. Dow Foundation, while limited in its grant-making to organizations within Michigan, has charter goals to improve educational, religious, economic, and cultural lives of Michigan's people as those needs can be defined in a world which constantly presents new or different challenges and opportunities. The Foundation TrusteeS carefully consider proposals submitted, and look for programs where their contributions can be leveraged. Organizations requesting funding should be sure that they have planned for that programs future self sufficiency." The foundation tends "to support organizations that have clearly stated objectives, strong and purposeful management, and are publicly accountable; have needs which are not normally funded by government or public financing; are not hesitant to explore, initiate, volunteer, or execute, original ideas or concepts; are willing to collaborate with other persons or organizations to give synergy to a common objective or goal; and have purposes which tend to advance private enterprise and the preservation of a free, open, and self-resourceful society." 1999 Herbert H. and Grace A. Dow Foundation, Annual Report. **Priorities:** *Arts & Humanities:* 3%. Funds arts centers and libraries. *Civic & Public Affairs:* 20%. Contributes to municipalities and community foundations. *Education:* 55%. Supports public precollege and higher education. *Environment:* 3%. Gives to united funds and community centers. *International:* 17%. Funds medical centers and health care associations. *Note:* Total contributions made in 1999. **Typ. Recipients:** Children's Health/Hospitals, Clinics/Medical Centers, Emergency/Ambulance Services, Health Policy/Cost Containment, Hospitals, Medical Rehabilitation, People with Disabilities, Public Health, Substance Abuse. **Geo. Dist:** MI, statewide; Midland, MI.

★ **344** ★ **Herbst Foundation**
30 Van Ness Ave., Ste. 3600
San Francisco, CA 94102
**Phone:** (415)252-1220          **Fax:** (415)252-1205
Dwight Merriman, Jr., President

**Fnded:** 1961. **Philosophy:** The foundation's primary purpose is to provide capital support (bricks-and-mortar) to organizations in the city and county of San Francisco. Primary concerns include education and social services. **Priorities:** *Arts & Humanities:* 2%. Funds a museum and the graphic arts. *Civic & Public Affairs:* 6%. *Education:* About 67%. Supports private precollege education and colleges and universities. *Environment:* 10%. Gives to youth organizations. *Note:* Total contributions made in fiscal 1999. **Typ.**

**Recipients:** AIDS/HIV, Alzheimers Disease, Clinics/Medical Centers, Diabetes, Eyes/Blindness, Family Planning, Geriatric Health, Health Organizations, Hospitals, Medical Education, Medical Rehabilitation, Medical Research, People with Disabilities, Speech & Hearing. **Geo. Dist:** nationally; CA, San Francisco County; San Francisco, CA.

### ★ 345 ★ Herman Goldman Foundation
61 Broadway, 18th Floor
New York, NY 10006
**Phone:** (212)797-9090　　　　**Fax:** (212)797-9162
Richard Baron, Executive Director

**Fnded:** 1943. **Philosophy:** From its founding in 1943 until Mr. Goldman's death in 1968, the foundation was modest in size. Through funds from Mr. Goldman's estate, the foundation's assets increased significantly and it established firm guidelines for the distribution of its resources. Those program guidelines emphasize education, social development and justice, health, and the arts. **Priorities:** *Arts & Humanities:* 9%. Supports museums, and performing and visual arts. *Civic & Public Affairs:* 16%. Philanthropic organizations are funded. *Education:* 13%. Funds universities, and educational institutions and programs. *Environment:* 25%. Emphasis is placed on family services. *International:* 18%. Priorities focus on hospitals, geriatric care, medical centers, and disease and disorder concerns. *Note:* Total contributions made in fiscal 1999. **Typ. Recipients:** AIDS/HIV, Cancer, Clinics/Medical Centers, Geriatric Health, Health Funds, Health Organizations, Hospitals, Hospitals (University Affiliated), Long-Term Care, Medical Education, Medical Research, Mental Health, Multiple Sclerosis, People with Disabilities, Prenatal Health Issues, Single-Disease Health Associations. **Geo. Dist:** New York, NY, including metropolitan area.

### ★ 346 ★ Herman T. and Phenie R. Pott Foundation
PO Box 387
Saint Louis, MO 63166
**Phone:** (314)418-2643　　　　**Fax:** (636)537-9267
James Collins, Executive Director

**Fnded:** 1963. **Philosophy:** The foundation makes most of its grants in the areas of social services and education. Social service funding favors shelters, family resource centers, children's services, and united funds. Funding in education emphasizes universities and college funds in St. Louis. The trust also will fund civic affairs, the St. Louis Mercantile Library, and health services. **Priorities:** *Arts & Humanities:* 10%. Supports a library, opera theater, and an arts council. *Civic & Public Affairs:* 4%. Botanical gardens, philanthropic organizations, and employment. *Education:* 13%. Gives to schools, colleges, and universities. *Environment:* 31%. Supports shelters, family resource centers, children's services, youth organizations, the United Way, shelters, Special Olympics and Big Brothers/Big Sisters. *International:* 18%. Pediatric health, mental health, and single-disease health associations. *Note:* Total contributions made in 2000. **Typ. Recipients:** Alzheimers Disease, Child Abuse, Children's Health/Hospitals, Diabetes, Domestic Violence, Emergency/Ambulance Services, Eyes/Blindness, Family Planning, Health Organizations, Heart, Hospitals, Medical Rehabilitation, Medical Research, Mental Health, Multiple Sclerosis, People with Disabilities, Preventive Medicine/Wellness Organizations, Respiratory, Single-Disease Health Associations. **Geo. Dist:** St. Louis, MO.

### ★ 347 ★ Herrick Foundation
840 W Long Lake Rd., Ste. 200
Troy, MI 48098
**Phone:** (248)267-3321　　　　**Fax:** (248)879-2001

**Fnded:** 1949. **Philosophy:** The foundation traditionally supports colleges, universities, educational projects, churches, hospitals, health organizations, civic groups, social service agencies, cultural organizations, and scientific organizations primarily in Michigan. **Priorities:** *Arts & Humanities:* 7%. Supports libraries, public broadcasting, and museums. *Civic &*

*Public Affairs:* 14%. Supports community foundations and fire departments. *Education:* 37%. Supports secondary education and colleges and universities. *Environment:* 16%. Primarily for youth organizations. *International:* 11%. Funds hospitals and health organizations. *Note:* Total contributions made in fiscal 1999. **Typ. Recipients:** Alzheimers Disease, Cancer, Children's Health/Hospitals, Clinics/Medical Centers, Emergency/Ambulance Services, Health Funds, Health Organizations, Health-General, Heart, Hospices, Hospitals, Hospitals (University Affiliated), Kidney, Long-Term Care, Medical Education, Medical Research, Nursing Services, People with Disabilities, Preventive Medicine/Wellness Organizations, Single-Disease Health Associations, Substance Abuse. **Geo. Dist:** MI, Primarily Michigan, occasionally Washington, D.C., Indiana, Mississippi, Ohio, Tennesse, Oklahoma and Wisconsin.

### ★ 348 ★ Hess Foundation
1185 Ave. of the Americas
New York, NY 10036
**Phone:** (212)536-8421
Norma Hess, President

**Fnded:** 1954. **Philosophy:** The foundation concentrates its giving in the areas of higher and secondary education, hospitals, medical research, temples, and social services. **Priorities:** *Arts & Humanities:* 15%. Supports the Lincoln Center Theater, performing arts, museums, the opera, and libraries. *Civic & Public Affairs:* 3%. Supports legal assistance, parks, safety, philanthropic organizations, and womens affairs. *Education:* 22%. Colleges, universitites, educational programs, medical education, art/humanities education, and scholarship. *Environment:* 8%. United Way, YMCA, services for the handicapped, meals on wheels, and recreation/athletics. *International:* 37%. Hospitals, medical centers, gay men's health, hospice, disease and disorder concerns, and childrens health. *Religion:* 19%. *Note:* Contributions were made in fiscal 1999. **Typ. Recipients:** AIDS/HIV, Alzheimers Disease, Children's Health/Hospitals, Clinics/Medical Centers, Clinics/Medical Centers, Emergency/Ambulance Services, Health Organizations, Health-General, Hospices, Hospitals, Medical Education, People with Disabilities, Prenatal Health Issues, Single-Disease Health Associations. **Geo. Dist:** nationally; New York, NY; Paris.

### ★ 349 ★ Hill Crest Foundation
PO Box 530507
Birmingham, AL 35253
**Phone:** (205)870-0400　　　　**Fax:** (205)870-0484
Charles Terry, Sr., Chairman

**Fnded:** 1988. **Philosophy:** The Hill Crest Foundation is primarily engaged in making grants to programs in the field of mental health. In addition to the primary area of support, the officers have decided to support a wide variety of organizations in several fields including the arts, civic and public affairs, education, health care, religion, and social services. The foundation also supports charitable organizations with several grant types including capital, operating support, project, research, and a donation to a scholarship fund. The foundation's grant-making activity is concentrated in Jefferson County, AL, and the surrounding areas. Applications from out of state are given low priority. **Priorities:** *Arts & Humanities:* 8%. Supports museums and music. *Civic & Public Affairs:* 6%. *Education:* About 37%. Primarily to colleges and universities, medical education, religious education, and Social science. *Environment:* 36%. Supports people with disabilities. *International:* 10%. Funds research and specialized services. *Note:* Total contributions made in fiscal 1999. **Typ. Recipients:** AIDS/HIV, Alzheimers Disease, Cancer, Children's Health/Hospitals, Diabetes, Domestic Violence, Eyes/Blindness, Family Planning, Health Funds, Health Organizations, Hospitals, Hospitals (University Affiliated), Medical Education, Medical Rehabilitation, Mental Health, Nutrition, People with Disabilities, Prenatal Health Issues, Public Health, Respiratory, Single-Disease Health Associations, Substance Abuse, Trauma Treatment. **Geo. Dist:** Birmingham, AL, metropolitan area.

### ★ 350 ★ Hillcrest Foundation
PO Box 830241
Dallas, TX 75283-0241
**Phone:** (214)209-1965

**Fnded:** 1959. **Philosophy:** The Hillcrest Foundation was created to help alleviate poverty problems, to aid the advancement of education, and to promote health care in Texas. The grant applicant must be a charitable organization located in Texas, with a purpose compatible with the principles of the foundation. **Priorities:** *Arts & Humanities:* 10%. Supports libraries museum, historical preservation, and film/video *Civic & Public Affairs:* 12%. Supports non-profit management arboretums/botanical gardens, transitional living, philanthropic organizations, and law and justice. *Education:* 36%. Supports religious education, education funds, afterschool programs, technical education, and science education, and student aid. *Environment:* 17%. Supports emergency relief, youth programs, homeless, food distribution, crime prevention, camps, homes, and substance abuse. *International:* 15%. Supports Alzheimers, gereatric health, hospital, hospice, medical centers,, childrens health, hearing, and oral health. *Religion:* 5%. Supports scientific research, observatories, and scientific labs. *Note:* Total contributions made in 1998. **Typ. Recipients:** Alzheimers Disease, Arthritis, Cancer, Child Abuse, Children's Health/Hospitals, Clinics/Medical Centers, Diabetes, Domestic Violence, Emergency/Ambulance Services, Health Organizations, Heart, Hospitals, Long-Term Care, Medical Education, Medical Research, Mental Health, Nursing Services, Outpatient Health Care, People with Disabilities, Prenatal Health Issues, Public Health, Research/Studies Institutes, Respiratory, Single-Disease Health Associations, Substance Abuse. **Geo. Dist:** Dallas, TX.

### ★ 351 ★ Hillman Foundation
2000 Grant Bldg.
Pittsburgh, PA 15219
**Phone:** (412)338-3466　　　　**Fax:** (412)338-3463
**Email:** foundation@hillmanfo.com
Ronald Wertz, President

**Fnded:** 1951. **Philosophy:** The foundation allocates its resources primarily to programs designed to improve the quality of life in Pittsburgh and the southwestern Pennsylvania region. Funding is given to organizations in six program areas, including all levels of education, community and civic affairs, social services, cultural advancement and the arts, health and medicine, and youth and youth services. Over the next several years, the foundation intends to "maintain a contributions program of multiple interests based on the single principal of helping people and organizations to improve themselves and the surrounding region. The current policy of giving priority to requests submitted by qualified organizations located in the Pittsburgh and Southwestern Pennsylvania area will continue." **Priorities:** *Arts & Humanities:* 14%. Supports various arts organizations in Pittsburgh. *Civic & Public Affairs:* 19%. Primarily for community and urban development projects. *Education:* 20%. Colleges and universities, secondary education, and education associations. *Environment:* About 37%. Emphasis is on youth organizations. *International:* 7%. Supports hospitals and health associations. *Note:* Total contributions made in 1998. **Typ. Recipients:** AIDS/HIV, Cancer, Children's Health/Hospitals, Domestic Violence, Eyes/Blindness, Family Planning, Health Organizations, Long-Term Care, Medical Rehabilitation, Medical Research, Mental Health, Nursing Services, Outpatient Health Care, People with Disabilities, Research/Studies Institutes, Sexual Abuse, Single-Disease Health Associations, Speech & Hearing, Substance Abuse. **Geo. Dist:** PA, Southwestern part of state; Pittsburgh, PA.

### ★ 352 ★ Hillsdale Fund
PO Box 20124
Greensboro, NC 27420
**Phone:** (336)274-5471
Eloy Doolan, Vice President

**Fnded:** 1963. **Philosophy:** The Hillsdale Fund makes most of its grants in the areas of civic affairs, education, and social services. Funding for civic affairs favors environmental affairs and community development programs. Educational funding emphasizes public education. Social services favor food and clothing distribution and other relief agencies. The arts are a secondary interest with support to public broadcasting and historical preservation. Health, religion, and other recipient areas are also supported. **Priorities:** *Arts & Humanities:* 29%. Historic preservation, theater, museums, and arts funds. *Civic & Public Affairs:* 16%. Emphasis on parks, public policy organizations, and economic development. *Education:* 17%. Supports secondary schools, colleges, and universities. *Environment:* 7%. Supports child welfare, youth organizations, food banks, and services for the aged. *International:* 6%. Rural health, pediatric health, and single-disease health associations. *Note:* Total contributions made in 1998. **Typ. Recipients:** AIDS/HIV, Alzheimers Disease, Cancer, Children's Health/Hospitals, Emergency/Ambulance Services, Family Planning, Health Organizations, Health-General, Hospices, Hospitals, Multiple Sclerosis, People with Disabilities, Preventive Medicine/Wellness Organizations, Public Health, Single-Disease Health Associations, Substance Abuse. **Geo. Dist:** U.S. Eastern Region; NC.

### ★ 353 ★ Hobby Family Foundation

2131 San Felipe
Houston, TX 77019-5620
**Phone:** (713)521-1163          **Fax:** (713)521-3950
Pamela George, Secretary
**Fnded:** 1945. **Philosophy:** The foundation has shifted its funding toward local cultural and educational organizations in the Houston area. **Priorities:** *Arts & Humanities:* 51%. Supports museums and performing arts; includes major grant to the Houston Music Hall. *Civic & Public Affairs:* 34%. Major support for the Southwest Texas development Foundation. *Education:* 11%. *Environment:* 2%. *Note:* Contributions made in 1998. **Typ. Recipients:** AIDS/HIV, Alzheimers Disease, Cancer, Children's Health/Hospitals, Domestic Violence, Emergency/Ambulance Services, Eyes/Blindness, Family Planning, Health Funds, Health Organizations, Heart, Hospices, Hospitals, Mental Health, People with Disabilities, Single-Disease Health Associations. **Geo. Dist:** Houston, TX.

### ★ 354 ★ Hoblitzelle Foundation

5956 Sherry Lane, Ste. 901
Dallas, TX 75225-6522
**Phone:** (214)373-0462          **Fax:** (214)750-7412
**Website:** http://home.att.net/~hoblitzelle
Paul Harris, Executive Vice President
**Fnded:** 1942. **Philosophy:** The foundation supports educational, scientific, literary, and charitable organizations which "carry out the charitable and philanthropic purposes of the founders." The foundation seeks "to provide the basic tools for people to improve the quality of life in Texas." **Priorities:** *Arts & Humanities:* 15%. Supports arts museum, music, libraries, ballet, and theater. *Civic & Public Affairs:* 14%. Funds botanical gardens/parks, safety clubs, zoos, and women's affairs, and chambers of commerce. *Education:* 29%. Supports religious welfare organizations. *Environment:* 28%. Supports community centers, United Way, emergency relief, shelter/homeless, scouts, family services, food distribution and family planning services. *International:* 8%. Supports eye/blindness, heart associations, arthritis, oral health, and medical centers. *Religion:* 2%. Supports science centers and institutes. *Note:* Total contributions made in 2000. **Typ. Recipients:** AIDS/HIV, Alzheimers Disease, Cancer, Children's Health/Hospitals, Clinics/Medical Centers, Diabetes, Emergency/Ambulance Services, Eyes/Blindness, Family Planning, Health Funds, Health Organizations, Health-General, Hospices, Hospitals (University Affiliated), Long-Term Care, Medical Education, Medical Research, Medical Training, Multiple Sclerosis, Nursing Services, People with Disabilities, Prenatal Health Issues, Public Health, Single-Disease Health Associations, Substance Abuse, Transplant Networks/Donor Banks, Trauma Treatment. **Geo. Dist:** TX; Dallas, TX.

### ★ 355 ★ Homeland Foundation (NY)

230 Park Ave.
PMB 359
New York, NY 10017
**Fax:** (212)949-0543
E. Wyckoff, Jr., President
**Fnded:** 1938. **Philosophy:** "The Homeland Foundation has a threefold purpose: . To maintain Wethersfield House, Wethersfield Gardens, and Wethersfield Stables in Amenia, NY, for the general public, and Wethersfield Farm for open space, scenic enjoyment, and for conservation purposes. . To conduct and fund the cultural and intellectual activities of the Wethersfield Institute and of Homeland Foundation. . To provide financial support to institutions and projects that foster the Roman Catholic Faith, and especially those that strengthen the unity of the Catholic community in the United States with the Holy See; educational initiatives geared to promote Christian culture as it is seen in the history of Western Europe; and projects that address questions touching Christian life, especially major questions of philosophy, theology, political science, and sociology." **Priorities:** *Arts & Humanities:* 10%. Funds libraries, museums, and orchestras. *Civic & Public Affairs:* 10%. Supports public policy, economic development, and job training. *Education:* 35%. Funds higher education. *Environment:* 15%. Contributes to shelters, volunteer services, and youth organizations. *Note:* Total contributions made in fiscal 1999. **Typ. Recipients:** Cancer, Emergency/Ambulance Services, Family Planning, Heart, Hospitals, Long-Term Care, Prenatal Health Issues. **Geo. Dist:** internationally; nationally; NY, metropolitan area.

### ★ 356 ★ Homer and Martha Gudelsky Family Foundation

11900 Tech Rd.
Silver Spring, MD 20904
**Phone:** (301)622-0100          **Fax:** (301)622-3507
Medda Gudelsky, Director
**Fnded:** 1968. **Philosophy:** The foundation's major interests are education and health care. Educational funding favors secondary and higher education in suburban Maryland. The foundation also has interests in the arts, religious groups, and civic projects. **Priorities:** *Arts & Humanities:* 43%. Supports theatre, art centers and public broadcasting. *Civic & Public Affairs:* 1%. Supports municipality. *Education:* 16%. Provides scholarships and supports early childhood development. *Environment:* 3%. Supports community service organization. *International:* 24%. Supports single-disease health associations and medical center. *Note:* Total contributions made in 1998. **Typ. Recipients:** Cancer, Clinics/Medical Centers, Emergency/Ambulance Services, Hospitals, Long-Term Care, Medical Education, Research/Studies Institutes, Substance Abuse. **Geo. Dist:** MD.

### ★ 357 ★ Horace W. Goldsmith Foundation

375 Park Ave., Ste. 1602
New York, NY 10152
**Phone:** (212)319-8700          **Fax:** (212)319-2881
Mr. James Slaughter, Chief Executive Officer & Director
**Fnded:** 1955. **Philosophy:** The foundation is interested in the support of higher education, the performing arts and cultural groups, and social welfare programs. Funding by the foundation is self-initiated. **Priorities:** *Arts & Humanities:* 27%. Museums, libraries, opera, and performing arts centers. *Civic & Public Affairs:* 3%. Supports housing, botanical gardens, and community development. *Education:* 36%. Supports business education, legal education, colleges, and universities. *International:* 14%. Medical centers and hospitals. *Religion:* 3%. Supports science centers and science museums. *Note:* Total contributions made in 1999. **Typ. Recipients:** AIDS/HIV, Cancer, Children's Health/Hospitals, Clinics/Medical Centers, Family Planning, Geriatric Health, Health Organizations, Heart, Hospitals, Hospitals (University Affiliated), Long-Term Care, Medical Education, Medical Rehabilitation, Medical Research, Nursing Services, People with Disabilities, Public Health, Research/Studies Institutes, Single-Disease Health Associations, Substance Abuse. **Geo. Dist:** New York, NY, including metropolitan area.

### ★ 358 ★ Horizons Foundation

4020 East Madison St., Ste. 322
Seattle, WA 98112
**Phone:** (206)323-8061
Ralph Hadac, Executive Director & Treasurer
**Fnded:** 1990. **Philosophy:** The foundation focuses on health organizations, environmental causes, and the arts in the Puget Sound area. **Priorities:** *Arts & Humanities:* 10%. Funds performing arts and outreach programs. *Environment:* 55%. Focus on teen pregnancy prevention, parenting skills, and domestic violence direct services and education. **Typ. Recipients:** Child Abuse, Children's Health/Hospitals, Clinics/Medical Centers, Domestic Violence, Family Planning, Prenatal Health Issues, Sexual Abuse. **Geo. Dist:** WA, Puget Sound region.

### ★ 359 ★ Houston Endowment

600 Travis, Ste. 6400
Houston, TX 77002-3007
**Phone:** (713)238-8100          **Fax:** (713)238-8101
**Website:** http://www.hou-endow.org
H. Nelson, III, President
**Fnded:** 1937. **Philosophy:** The purpose of the endowment "is the support of any charitable, educational or religious undertaking." The directors place priority on organizations and programs serving the greater Houston area and the State of Texas. Support is given to a wide variety of charitable activities, including those in the areas of education, the arts, culture, civic, and human services. "While the Houston Endowment Inc. provides the funds for many scholarships, it does not provide scholarships to individuals on the basis of individual application to the foundation. The foundation's scholarships programs are administered in one of two ways. First, Houston Endowment Inc. funds the Jesse H. Jones and Mary Gibbs Jones High School Scholarship Program." Second, the Endowment provides funding for scholarships in various fields of study by making grants to selected colleges and universities. For a list of colleges and universities and their contact information, refer to the Endowment's website. **Priorities:** *Arts & Humanities:* 17%. Funds visual and performing arts. *Civic & Public Affairs:* 11%. Supports Community enhancement initiatives, including community development, community education, housing, and parks and natural spaces. *Education:* 33%. Supports K-12 and higher education. *Environment:* 23%. Supports health and human services organizations, including services for the elderly and disabled. *International:* 11%. Funds medical facilities and research, and access to healthcare. *Note:* Total contributions made in 2000. **Typ. Recipients:** AIDS/HIV, Cancer, Child Abuse, Children's Health/Hospitals, Clinics/Medical Centers, Diabetes, Domestic Violence, Emergency/Ambulance Services, Family Planning, Geriatric Health, Health Organizations, Health Policy/Cost Containment, Heart, Hospices, Hospitals, Medical Education, Medical Research, Medical Training, Mental Health, Nursing Services, Outpatient Health Care, People with Disabilities, Research/Studies Institutes, Single-Disease Health Associations, Substance Abuse, Transplant Networks/Donor Banks. **Geo. Dist:** Houston, TX.

### ★ 360 ★ Howard Gilman Foundation

111 West 50th St.
New York, NY 10020
**Phone:** (212)408-0486          **Fax:** (212)582-7610
Harry Brown, Program Associate
**Fnded:** 1981. **Philosophy:** The mission of the Howard Gilman Foundation is "to nurture and preserve a vibrant cultural and natural environment." Its grant-making program focuses on conservation, especially wildlife conservation; medicine and health, especially cardiovascular, HIV/AIDS, and sports medicine research; and the preservation and advancement of artistic and cultural endeavors. **Priorities:** *Arts & Humanities:* 24%. Dance, opera, museums, theater (approximately 6% supports the Howard Gilman/Israel

Culture Foundation). *Civic & Public Affairs:* 1%. *Education:* 2%. Universities. *Environment:* 1%. *International:* 54%. Medical Centers, AIDS. *Religion:* 2%. *Note:* Total contributions made in fiscal 1997. **Typ. Recipients:** AIDS/HIV, Children's Health/Hospitals, Clinics/Medical Centers, Health Organizations, Health-General, HRK, Hospitals, Hospitals (University Affiliated), Medical Education, Medical Research, Public Health, Single-Disease Health Associations. **Geo. Dist:** internationally; nationally; New York, NY.

## ★ 361 ★ Howard Heinz Endowment
30 Dominion Tower
625 Liberty Ave.
Pittsburgh, PA 15222-3199
**Phone:** (412)281-5777        **Fax:** (412)281-5788
**Email:** info@heinz.org
**Website:** http://www.heinz.org
Maxwell King, Executive Director
**Fnded:** 1941. **Philosophy:** "Throughout their histories, the Howard and Vira I. Heinz Endowments have been privileged to enjoy a remarkable intimate relationship with the communities and organizations they serve. From this relationship continually emerges two of the Endowments' primary strengths: their sensitivity to the needs of their region, and their willingness to shoulder risks on its behalf. It has been characteristic of the Endowments to want to listen and respond personally to requests for help. We are neighbors, after all, not disinterested observers. For that reason, there has been a reluctance over the years to print formalized program guidelines, suggesting as they might an unfeeling institutionalization of process. We do not intend for that to happen. But we also appreciate how dramatically the philanthropic landscape has changed in recent years. With the demand for philanthropic resources increasing rapidly and with ever greater urgency, we must respond to the call from prospective grantseekers for guidance specificity and direction....The Endowments' present grantmaking reflects over half a century of applied values and experiential learning. Three signature themes emerge from this rich history: leadership, cooperation and enterprise. These themes will continue to guide us in the future." *A Message From the Executive Director* **Priorities:** *Arts & Humanities:* 41%. Supports history, museum, dance, arts festivals, public broadcasting, libraries, theater, music, ballet, and the performing arts. *Civic & Public Affairs:* 21%. Supports public policy, public affairs, and botanical gardens. *Education:* 18%. Supports scholarship, universities, leadership training, continuing education, and literacy. *Environment:* 7%. Supports family services, domestic violence/child abuse, United Way, and food distribution programs. *International:* 3%. Supports hospital, childrens health, and nutrition. *Note:* Total contributions made in 1998. **Typ. Recipients:** Child Abuse, Children's Health/Hospitals, Clinics/Medical Centers, Domestic Violence, Family Planning, Health Organizations, Health Policy/Cost Containment, Hospitals, Medical Education, Medical Rehabilitation, Medical Research, Mental Health, Nursing Services, Nutrition, Prenatal Health Issues, Public Health, Research/Studies Institutes, Substance Abuse. **Geo. Dist:** PA, Southwest Pennsylvania; Pittsburgh, PA.

## ★ 362 ★ Howard Hughes Medical Institute
Office of Grants and Special Programs
4000 Jones Bridge Rd.
Chevy Chase, MD 20815-6789
**Phone:** (301)215-8890        **Fax:** (301)215-8888
**Email:** grantvpr@hhmi.org
**Website:** http://www.hhmi.org
**Fnded:** 1954. **Philosophy:** The largest private initiative in U.S. history to enhance science education at all levels, the Institute disburses grants for preschool through postgraduate training. Through its grants program, the Institute also supports the research of outstanding biomedical scientists outside the United States and provides funding to help medical schools sustain their commitment to research. **Priorities:** *Education:* 100%. Supports science education and research in cell biology, genetics, immunology, neurology, and structural biology. *Note:* Total contributions

made in fiscal 2000. **Typ. Recipients:** Arthritis, Cancer, Hospitals (University Affiliated), Medical Education, Medical Research. **Geo. Dist:** internationally; nationally.

## ★ 363 ★ HRK Foundation
345 Saint Peter St., Ste. 1200
Saint Paul, MN 55102
**Phone:** (651)293-9001        **Fax:** (651)298-0551
**Email:** hrkfoundation@hrkgroup.com
Kathleen Fluegel, Foundation Director
**Fnded:** 1962. **Philosophy:** "HRK Foundation is a family foundation defined and sustained by a sense of spirituality, creativity, and stewardship. Through quiet leadership and philanthropy, the Board seeks to promote healthy families and communities, to enhance the quality of and access to education, and to improve the fabric of our society." "The work of HRK Foundation will be carried out through a commitment to and support for: "The Arts: People and organizations that nourish the human spirit and encourage our connectedness. "Health: Programs that strengthen families and promote healthy lives for children and/or provide services for people affected by HIV/AIDS. "Community Building: Efforts which increase adequate and affordable housing; encourage responsible land use; promote conservation and preservation of community resources; advance the work of neighbors who reach across their differences for the common good. "Education: Educational approaches that promote holistic personal development–intellectual, social, emotional, and spiritual." HRK Foundation Grant Guidelines **Priorities:** *Arts & Humanities:* 47%. Supports libraries, public radio, arts, the opera, and humanities council. *Civic & Public Affairs:* 23%. Civic and public affairs, housing, and community services. *Education:* 21%. Funds Independent School Districts, and Colleges. *International:* 9%. Funds AIDS awareness and health services. *Note:* Contributions were made in 2000. **Typ. Recipients:** AIDS/HIV, Children's Health/Hospitals, Clinics/Medical Centers, Emergency/Ambulance Services, Family Planning, Health Funds, Health Organizations, Hospitals, Medical Education, Medical Rehabilitation, Mental Health, People with Disabilities, Public Health, Single-Disease Health Associations, Substance Abuse, Transplant Networks/Donor Banks. **Geo. Dist:** MN, Twin Cities metropolitan area; WI, St. Croix Valley and Ashland and Bayfield Counties. **Frmly:** Mary Anderson Foundation MAHADH Foundation MAHADH Foundation to HRK Foundation.

## ★ 364 ★ Hugh I. Shott, Jr. Foundation
PO Box 1559
Bluefield, WV 24701
**Phone:** (304)325-8181        **Fax:** (304)325-3727
Richard Wilkinson, President
**Fnded:** 1985. **Philosophy:** The Hugh I. Shott, Jr. Foundation's mission is to "improve social and economic quality of life in the trade area of the Bluefield Daily Telegraph." 1996 application form. Educational funding supports college foundations and public school districts. Civic affairs interests include municipalities, community development, and business. **Priorities:** *Arts & Humanities:* 13%. Performing arts and historic preservation. *Civic & Public Affairs:* 41%. Community programs and foundations, parks and towns/municipalties. *Education:* 20%. College and university foundations mainly in Bluefield, VA. *Environment:* 24%. Supports health organizations and medical centers, sports, youth programs, volunteer projects, and United Way. *International:* About 2%. *Note:* Total contributions made in 1998. **Typ. Recipients:** Clinics/Medical Centers, Emergency/Ambulance Services, Family Planning, Hospices, Hospitals, People with Disabilities, Public Health. **Geo. Dist:** VA, Southwest Virginia; WV, Southern West Virginia.

## ★ 365 ★ Hugh J. Andersen Foundation
PO Box 204
Bayport, MN 55003-0204
**Phone:** (651)439-1557        **Fax:** (651)439-9480
**Email:** kathiwood@scenicriver.org
**Website:** http://www.scenicriver.org
Kathi Wood, Grants Consultant

**Fnded:** 1962. **Philosophy:** "The mission of the Hugh J. Andersen Foundation is to give back to our community through focused efforts that foster inclusivity, promote equality, and lead to increased human independence, self-sufficiency and dignity. To fulfill this mission, the Foundation acts as a grantmaker, innovator, and convenor." 2000 Hugh J. Andersen Foundation Annual Report The foundation places a high priority on organizations that benefit people in St. Croix Valley, which the board has defined as Washington County in Minnesota, and Pierce, Polk, and St. Croix counties in Wisconsin. Projects designed to benefit the people of St. Paul, MN, receive secondary consideration, as will projects serving other parts of Minnesota. Limited consideration will be given to organizations with a national or international scope. The foundation is particularly interested in direct services provided by programs that serve children and youth, especially those that provide personal development activities; that provide various social support services to the community at large; that are engaged in health-related services, other than hospitals and research facilities; and that provide educational opportunities and enrichment to the general community. Consideration will be given to battered women's shelters, special projects or programming in public schools, programs for the developmentally or physically disabled, programs for seniors, and public or civic projects and activities within the St. Croix Valley. **Priorities:** *Arts & Humanities:* 7%. Supports performing arts, theater and arts councils. *Civic & Public Affairs:* 2%. Funds nonprofit management. *Education:* 7%. Supports programs serving children and youth, including children's museums, minority education, and literacy initiatives. *Environment:* 57%. Supports housing, community development, youth groups and camps, women's and family services, support for victims of violence, and United Way. *International:* 20%. Funds health-related services that educate and improve community well-being. *Note:* Total contributions made in fiscal 2000. **Typ. Recipients:** AIDS/HIV, Cancer, Children's Health/Hospitals, Clinics/Medical Centers, Diabetes, Domestic Violence, Emergency/Ambulance Services, Family Planning, Health Organizations, Hospitals, Medical Rehabilitation, Medical Research, People with Disabilities, Sexual Abuse, Single-Disease Health Associations, Substance Abuse. **Geo. Dist:** MN, St. Paul (secondary focus); St. Croix Valley, MN, St. Croix Valley also covers WI; WI, Pierce County; WI, Polk County; WI, St. Croix County.

## ★ 366 ★ Hugh Kaul Foundation Trust
PO Box 11426
Birmingham, AL 35202
**Phone:** (205)326-4696        **Fax:** (205)581-7433
Leah Scalise, Vice President & Trust Officer
**Fnded:** 1990. **Philosophy:** The trust is a private foundation which makes grants to charitable organizations in the Greater Birmingham metropolitan area, in Clay County, and in Coosa County of the state of Alabama. **Priorities:** *Arts & Humanities:* 18%. Funds museums, art councils, and performing arts. *Civic & Public Affairs:* 2%. Community foundations and civic groups. *Education:* 52%. Colleges, universities, precollege education, and education funds. *Environment:* 14%. Gives to YMCAs, YWCAs, children groups, and elder concerns. *International:* 6%. Supports speech and hearing concerns. *Note:* Total contributions were made in 1998. **Typ. Recipients:** Cancer, Children's Health/Hospitals, Eyes/Blindness, Family Planning, Hospitals, Medical Education, Medical Research, Mental Health, Public Health, Single-Disease Health Associations, Speech & Hearing, Substance Abuse. **Geo. Dist:** AL, Coosa County; AL, Jefferson County; Birmingham, AL, Clay County.

## ★ 367 ★ Hunt Alternatives Fund
500 E Eighth Ave.
Denver, CO 80203
**Phone:** (303)722-7606        **Fax:** (303)839-1013
Elsa Holguin, Executive Director
**Fnded:** 1981. **Philosophy:** Among other objectives, The Hunt Alternatives Fund aims to strengthen the role of women in society, accelerate systemic change, nurture coalitions in blighted neighborhoods, and

cultivate the arts (when used as a catalyst for social progress). The Fund concentrates on grassroots efforts in prevention, advocacy and leadership development–particularly those that target the causes, rather than the symptoms. The Fund is especially interested in fostering the long-term viability of non-profit organizations by helping them identify new or increased sources of asistance and develop strategies for self-sufficiency. programs, the individual Leadership and Youth Leadership awards to recognize leadership by individuals in the community. **Priorities:** *Civic & Public Affairs:* 97%. Support a variety of civic causes through the Swanee Hunt Operating Fund. Also funds neighborhood development and women's affairs. *Environment:* 2%. With emphasis on children and families. *International:* 1%. *Note:* Total contributions made in fiscal 1998. **Typ. Recipients:** AIDS/HIV, Cancer, Child Abuse, Children's Health/Hospitals, Clinics/Medical Centers, Domestic Violence, Emergency/Ambulance Services, Family Planning, Health Organizations, Health-General, Medical Education, Mental Health, People with Disabilities, Prenatal Health Issues, Public Health, Respiratory, Sexual Abuse, Single-Disease Health Associations, Substance Abuse. **Geo. Dist:** Denver, CO, metropolitan area.


### ★ 368 ★ Huston Foundation

1 Fayette St., Ste. 190
2 Tower Bridge
Conshohocken, PA 19428-2064
**Phone:** (610)832-4949          **Fax:** (610)832-4960
**Email:** hustonfndn@aol.com
Susan Heilman, Executive Assistant

**Fnded:** 1957. **Philosophy:** "The main purpose of the Huston Foundation's contributions program is to lend financial assistance to help improve social, cultural, intellectual, and economic environments primarily within the continental United States and to Protestant Evangelical Christian organizations worldwide." Grants are divided between religious and secular segments and are primarily made in the categories of health, human services, education, civic affairs, the arts, and community development. The foundation reports that at least 51% of the funding each year supports Protestant Evangelical Christian organizations. **Priorities:** *Arts & Humanities:* 7%. Support visual arts, museum, ballet, and theater. *Civic & Public Affairs:* 12%. Supports nonprofit associations, welfare-to-work, community foundation, botanical gardens, and law and justice. *Education:* 13%. Supports school, colleges, scholarship, arts/humanities, and universities. *Environment:* 13%. Supports YMCA, Big Brothers and Big Sisters organizations, family services, people with disabilities, and camps. *Note:* Total contributions made in 1999. **Typ. Recipients:** Child Abuse, Children's Health/Hospitals, Clinics/Medical Centers, Emergency/Ambulance Services, Eyes/Blindness, Family Planning, Health Organizations, Hospices, Hospitals, Medical Education, Medical Rehabilitation, Nursing Services, People with Disabilities, Public Health, Sexual Abuse, Single-Disease Health Associations. **Geo. Dist:** nationally; PA, Eastern Pennsylvania.


### ★ 369 ★ Hyams Foundation

175 Federal St., 14th Fl.
Boston, MA 02110
**Phone:** (617)426-5600          **Fax:** (617)720-2434
**Email:** info@hyamsfoundation.org
**Website:** http://www.hyamsfoundation.org
Elizabeth Smith, Executive Director

**Fnded:** 1921. **Philosophy:** The mission of the Hyams Foundation is to increase ecomonic and social justice and power within low-income communities. The Hyams Foundation believes that investing in strategies that enable low-income people to increase their economic security, build wealth and become active participants in their communities will have the greatest social return in these times. The Foundation will carry out its mission by these: supporting civic participation by low-income communities; promoting economic development that benefits low-income neighborhoods and their residents; and developing the talents and skills of low-income youth. The Foundation has chosen to focus on civic participation, economic development and young

people, believing that they present three key opportunities for change. Within each priority area, the Foundation will support strategies that reflect several key principles. They are: building capacity within low-income communities and neighborhoods, particularly in communities of color which are disproportionately low-income; connecting low-income communities and neighborhoods to one another and to the broader community at large; identifying and building on those assets and "anchor" institutions that are unique to individual low-income communities; emphasizing the leadership and direct participation of low-income individuals; promoting meaningful diversity and cross-cultural understanding in all communities and institutions; and encouraging comprehensive solutions to achieving economic and social justice while promoting collaboration and cooperation among individuals and organizations. **Priorities:** *Civic & Public Affairs:* 30%. Community development. (Public Policy) 7%. Public policy issues. *Environment:* About 70%. Organizations serving individual or multiple low-income neighborhoods. *Note:* Total contributions made in 1998. **Typ. Recipients:** Adolescent Health Issues, AIDS/HIV, Children's Health/Hospitals, Clinics/Medical Centers, Domestic Violence, Family Planning, Health Funds, Health Organizations, Hospitals, Medical Research, Mental Health, Substance Abuse. **Geo. Dist:** Boston, MA; Chelsea, MA.


### ★ 370 ★ Hyde and Watson Foundation

437 Southern Blvd.
Chatham, NJ 07928
**Phone:** (973)966-6024          **Fax:** (973)966-6404
**Website:** http://www.fdncenter.org/grantmaker/hydeanwatson
Hunter Corbin, President

**Fnded:** 1983. **Philosophy:** The foundation is primarily interested in the support of capital projects that are of lasting value and that will increase the quality, capacity, or efficiency of a grantee's program or services. Typical projects of interest include the purchase, relocation, renovation, or improvement of facilities; purchase of capital equipment; construction; development of materials; and certain areas of medical research. The foundation supports projects in the broad fields of education, health, social services, the arts and humanities, and religion. A substantial portion of the foundation's grant funds each year are allocated to projects for which the foundation's support makes a major contribution. foundation's support makes a major contribution. **Priorities:** *Arts & Humanities:* 13%. Supports public broadcasting, historic preservation, museums and art foundations. *Civic & Public Affairs:* 4%. Supports community foundations and parks. *Education:* 49%. Supports private schools, universities, and educational programs. *Environment:* 16%. Supports family services, scouting, YMCA and animal protection. *International:* 11%. Supports groups with disabilities, single-disease health associations and hospital foundations. *Note:* Total contributions made in 1999. **Typ. Recipients:** Adolescent Health Issues, Alzheimers Disease, Cancer, Children's Health/Hospitals, Clinics/Medical Centers, Domestic Violence, Emergency/Ambulance Services, Eyes/Blindness, Geriatric Health, Health Organizations, Health-General, Heart, Hospices, Hospitals, Hospitals (University Affiliated), Medical Education, Medical Rehabilitation, Medical Research, Nursing Services, People with Disabilities, Prenatal Health Issues, Public Health, Research/Studies Institutes, Respiratory, Single-Disease Health Associations, Speech & Hearing, Substance Abuse, Transplant Networks/Donor Banks, Trauma Treatment. **Geo. Dist:** NJ, Essex County; NJ, Morris County; NJ, Union County; New York, NY, metropolitan area.


### ★ 371 ★ I. A. O'Shaughnessy Foundation

W-1271 First Bank Bldg.
332 Minnesota St.
Saint Paul, MN 55101
**Phone:** (612)222-2323          **Fax:** (612)222-2323
**Email:** iaoshaughnessyfd@qwest.net

**Fnded:** 1941. **Philosophy:** The foundation funds higher education, hospitals, youth organizations, community services, churches, the arts, and sciences.

**Priorities:** *Arts & Humanities:* 8%. Supports art and music. *Civic & Public Affairs:* 2%. Funds community foundations. *Education:* 57%. Largely supports Catholic universities and secondary schools. *Environment:* 15%. Funds centers for families and children. *International:* 10%. Supports psychiatric treatment facilities, a therapeutic riding center, and other medical organizations. *Note:* Total contributions made 2000. **Typ. Recipients:** Alzheimers Disease, Cancer, Children's Health/Hospitals, Clinics/Medical Centers, Domestic Violence, Heart, Hospices, Hospitals, Medical Education, Medical Rehabilitation, People with Disabilities, Prenatal Health Issues. **Geo. Dist:** IL; KS; MN; TX.


### ★ 372 ★ Independence Foundation

Offices at the Bellevue
200 South Broad St., Ste. 1101
Philadelphia, PA 19102
**Phone:** (215)985-4009          **Fax:** (215)985-3989
**Email:** ssherman@independencefoundation.org
Susan Sherman, President

**Fnded:** 1932. **Philosophy:** "True to our charter, the current Directors continue to use and apply the property and the income therefrom, 'exclusively in such charitable, benevolent, scientific, and educational activities as will promote the well-being of mankind and the alleviation of human suffering.' (Charter)." "The interests of the Foundation concentrate on initiatives that demonstrate innovation and make a difference to residents of Philadelphia and the surrounding Pennsylvania counties. These include Nurse Managed Health Care, Culture and the Arts, Legal Aid, and Contemporary Social Problems." "The foundation supports initiatives in community-based and community focused nurse managed primary health care where services to people are not always available. The foundation is particularly interested in promoting wellness through comprehensive primary health care. This may include health promotion, disease prevention, family planning, early intervention and related supportive services that focus particularly on basic human needs of food and shelter. The foundation is also interested in efforts that address the challenge of balancing quality, access and cost in health care." 1996 Annual Report **Priorities:** *Arts & Humanities:* 26%. Funds museums, music associations, and art centers. *Civic & Public Affairs:* 15%. Supports ethnic associations, community councils, zoos, and legal concerns. *Education:* 30%. Supports colleges, particularly nursing and law programs. *Environment:* 14%. Funds health and human service programs, family planning, and associations for people with disabilities. *International:* 15%. Funds single-disease associations, hospitals, and nurse managed primary health care initiatives. *Note:* Total contributions made in 1999. **Typ. Recipients:** AIDS/HIV, Children's Health/Hospitals, Clinics/Medical Centers, Domestic Violence, Emergency/Ambulance Services, Eyes/Blindness, Family Planning, Family Planning, Health Organizations, Health Policy/Cost Containment, Hospitals, Hospitals (University Affiliated), Medical Education, Medical Rehabilitation, Medical Research, Mental Health, Nursing Services, People with Disabilities, Prenatal Health Issues, Preventive Medicine/Wellness Organizations, Public Health. **Geo. Dist:** PA, Bucks County; PA, Chester County; PA, Delaware County; PA, Montgomery County; Philadelphia, PA, metropolitan area.


### ★ 373 ★ International Foundation

170 Changebridge Rd.
Unit C5-4, Second Floor
Montville, NJ 07045
**Phone:** (973)227-6107          **Fax:** (973)227-6821
Dr. Edward Holmes, Grants Chairman

**Fnded:** 1948. **Philosophy:** "The International Foundation exists to help people of the developing world in their endeavors to solve some of their problems, to attain a better standard of living and to obtain a reasonable degree of self-sufficiency." "The Trustees of The International Foundation believe in granting support to those projects which have promise of successfully accomplishing stated objectives to meet defined specific needs." "The Trustees encourage proposals for the developing world which advance a stable social order, provide necessary services for its people, and encourage cultural and artistic endeavors that favor a rising quality of life. "Grants are made in five general areas: agriculture, health, education, social development, and environment. "Some aid to refugees and grants for population planning are also given." The International Foundation Brochure, 1998 **Priorities:** *Note:* Contributions made in 1998. **Typ. Recipients:** Children's Health/Hospitals, Clinics/Medical Centers, Emergency/Ambulance Services, Eyes/Blindness, Family Planning, Health Funds, Health Organizations, Health-General, Hospitals, Medical Rehabilitation, Medical Training, Nutrition, People with Disabilities, Public Health, Public Health, Single-Disease Health Associations. **Geo. Dist:** internationally.

### ★ 374 ★ Ira W. DeCamp Foundation

60 Wall St., 36th Floor
New York, NY 10260
**Phone:** (212)648-9673          **Fax:** (212)648-5082
Lisa Philp, Vice President

**Fnded:** 1975. **Philosophy:** The chief purpose of the foundation is to support health care organizations, medical research, and medical education; social services, and workforce development. **Priorities:** *Arts & Humanities:* 2%. Primarily supports libraries. *Civic & Public Affairs:* 2%. Supports women's affairs and community development. *Education:* 44%. Emphasis on medical education. *Environment:* 8%. Supports child welfare, people with disabilities, youth organizations, and the homeless. *International:* 34%. Primary support for hospitals in New York City. *Religion:* 1%. Funds a laboratory. *Note:* Total contributions made in fiscal 2000. **Typ. Recipients:** AIDS/HIV, Alzheimers Disease, Cancer, Children's Health/Hospitals, Clinics/Medical Centers, Emergency/Ambulance Services, Eyes/Blindness, Geriatric Health, Health Funds, Health Organizations, Heart, Hospices, Hospitals, Hospitals (University Affiliated), Kidney, Long-Term Care, Medical Education, Medical Rehabilitation, Medical Research, Medical Training, Mental Health, Nursing Services, Outpatient Health Care, People with Disabilities, Public Health, Research/Studies Institutes, Single-Disease Health Associations, Speech & Hearing, Substance Abuse, Transplant Networks/Donor Banks. **Geo. Dist:** CT; NJ; NY; New York, NY, including the metropolitan area.

### ★ 375 ★ Ireland Foundation

1422 Euclid Ave.
1030 Hanna Bldg.
Cleveland, OH 44115-2004
**Phone:** (216)363-1033          **Fax:** (216)363-1038
Louise Humphrey, President & Trustee

**Fnded:** 1951. **Philosophy:** The fund generally supports private, secondary schools; the arts; and other philanthropic causes. A majority of funding is distributed within the state of Ohio, but some giving is national. **Priorities:** *Arts & Humanities:* 28%. Historic preservation, museums, and opera. *Civic & Public Affairs:* 5%. Primarily supporting the Archbold Foundation. *Education:* 54%. Supports private precollege education and colleges and universities. *Environment:* 2%. People with disabilities and united funds. *International:* 2%. Cancer research and nursing services. *Religion:* 9%. Fimds Tall Timers Research. *Note:* Total contributions made in 1998. **Typ. Recipients:** Cancer, Children's Health/Hospitals, Clinics/Medical Centers, Family Planning, Health Organizations, Hospitals, Hospitals (University Affiliated), Medical Education, Medical Rehabilitation, Medical Research, Nursing Services, People with Disabilities, Prenatal Health Issues. **Geo. Dist:** Cleveland, OH.

### ★ 376 ★ Irene E. and George A. Davis Foundation

One Monarch Place, Ste. 1450
Springfield, MA 01144
**Phone:** (413)734-8336          **Fax:** (413)734-7845
**Website:** http://www.davisfdn.org
Mary Walachy, Executive Director

**Fnded:** 1970. **Philosophy:** The foundation focuses its grantmaking activities on the local Western Massachu-

setts community with an emphasis on higher education, religious organizations, and the fine arts. The foundation's literature states, "While the Foundation will entertain proposals form all interest areas, the Foundation seeks to support programs which will offer creative responses to the communities' most pressing needs and concerns, which are preeventative and farsighted, and which reach a broad segiment of the community." **Priorities:** *Arts & Humanities:* 3%. Supports museums and public broadcasting. *Civic & Public Affairs:* 20%. Supports community foundations and a zoo. *Education:* 38%. Supports colleges and universities, music education, and public schools. *Environment:* 22%. Supports youth programs, Young Men's Christian AssociationA, services for the elderly, and animal protection. *International:* 8%. Supports disaster relief and hospitals. *Note:* Total contributions made in 1998. **Typ. Recipients:** AIDS/HIV, Children's Health/Hospitals, Clinics/Medical Centers, Domestic Violence, Emergency/Ambulance Services, Geriatric Health, Health Organizations, Hospitals, Mental Health, Nursing Services, People with Disabilities, Prenatal Health Issues, Public Health, Research/Studies Institutes, Single-Disease Health Associations. **Geo. Dist:** MA.

### ★ 377 ★ Irene W. and C. B. Pennington Foundation

8550 United Plaza Blvd., Ste. 1001
Baton Rouge, LA 70809
**Email:** pennogi@bellsouth.net
William Hodgkins, Contact

**Fnded:** 1982. **Philosophy:** The foundation primarily favors social service organizations, with emphasis on youth organizations and community centers. In the past, large grants were given to universities in Louisiana. Minor grants are given to other recipient areas. **Priorities:** *Arts & Humanities:* 4%. Arts centers. *Civic & Public Affairs:* 15%. Foundations and community groups. *Education:* 10%. Gives to private precollege education. *Environment:* 58%. Funds youth groups and YMCAs. *International:* 10%. Support includes the Pennington Medical Foundation. *Note:* Total contributions made in 1998. **Typ. Recipients:** Cancer, Children's Health/Hospitals, Domestic Violence, Emergency/Ambulance Services, Family Planning, Health-General, Hospices, Hospitals, Kidney, Medical Research, Mental Health, Nutrition, Public Health, Sexual Abuse, Substance Abuse. **Geo. Dist:** Baton Rouge, LA.

### ★ 378 ★ Irvine Health Foundation

18301 Von Karman Ave.
Ste. 440
Irvine, CA 92612
**Phone:** (949)253-2959          **Fax:** (949)253-2962
**Email:** ebk@ihf.org
**Website:** http://www.ihf.org
Edward Kacic, President

**Fnded:** 1985. **Philosophy:** "The Irvine Health Foundation is a nonprofit grant-making foundation whose goal is to improve the health, consisting of physical, mental and emotional wellbeing, of the residents of Orange County, California. The foundation is focused on promoting health and wellness, ensuring the availability of accessible, quality, health-related services, working in the area of health policy and supporting research designed to develop new knowledge in areas related to health." **Priorities:** *Civic & Public Affairs:* 10%. Supports law and justice, housing, and community foundation. *Education:* 40%. Supports higher education. *Environment:* 15%. Supports United Way, services for the homeless, and child welfare. *International:* 31%. Supports women's health, medical research, and public health. *Note:* Total contributions made in fiscal 2000. **Typ. Recipients:** AIDS/HIV, Alzheimers Disease, Child Abuse, Children's Health/Hospitals, Clinics/Medical Centers, Domestic Violence, Emergency/Ambulance Services, Family Planning, Geriatric Health, Health Organizations, Health Policy/Cost Containment, Hospices, Hospitals, Medical Education, Medical Research, Mental Health, Multiple Sclerosis, Nursing Services, People with Disabilities, Prenatal Health Issues, Preventive Medicine/Wellness Organizations, Public Health, Respiratory, Sexual Abuse, Single-Disease Health Associa-

tions, Speech & Hearing, Substance Abuse. **Geo. Dist:** CA, Orange County.

### ★ 379 ★ Irving I. Moskowitz Foundation

4201 Long Beach Boulevard, Ste. 304
Long Beach, CA 90807
**Phone:** (562)809-0186          **Fax:** (310)595-4384
Dr. Irving Moskowitz, President

**Fnded:** 1968. **Philosophy:** The foundation primarily supports organizations affiliated with the Jewish faith. **Priorities:** *Civic & Public Affairs:* 56%. Public policy concerns. *Education:* 4%. Colleges, universities, and special education. *Environment:* 12%. Youth organizations, food distribution, and community services. *International:* 6%. *Note:* Total contributions made in 1998. **Typ. Recipients:** Clinics/Medical Centers, Medical Rehabilitation, Mental Health, Single-Disease Health Associations. **Geo. Dist:** nationally.

### ★ 380 ★ Irving S. Gilmore Foundation

136 East Michigan Ave., Ste. 615
Kalamazoo, MI 49007
**Phone:** (616)342-6411          **Fax:** (616)349-3831
**Email:** fritz@isgilmorefoundation.org
**Website:** http://www.isgilmorefoundation.org
Frederick Freund, Executive Director

**Fnded:** 1972. **Philosophy:** "The mission of the Foundation is to support and enrich the cultural, social, and economic life of greater Kalamazoo." **Priorities:** *Arts & Humanities:* 71%. Suuports arts centers, symphonies, arts funds, theater, libraries, and historic preservation. *Civic & Public Affairs:* 9%. Funds community development initiatives, towns/municipalities, and housing. *Education:* 9%. Emphasis on arts education for youth, scholarships and universities. *Environment:* 10%. Focus on community services, youth organizations, the aged, family services, and United Way. *International:* 1%. Hospitals and substance abuse rehabilitation centers, AIDS, and eyes. *Note:* Total contributions made in 1998. **Typ. Recipients:** AIDS/HIV, Clinics/Medical Centers, Emergency/Ambulance Services, Eyes/Blindness, Family Planning, Medical Education, Nursing Services, People with Disabilities, Public Health, Single-Disease Health Associations, Speech & Hearing, Substance Abuse. **Geo. Dist:** Kalamazoo, MI, including greater metropolitan area.

### ★ 381 ★ Island Foundation (MA)

589 Mill St.
Marion, MA 02738-1553
**Phone:** (508)748-2809          **Fax:** (508)748-0991
**Email:** islandfdn@earthlink.net
Julie Early, Executive Director

**Fnded:** 1979. **Philosophy:** "The Island Foundation welcomes proposals in three general categories: the environment, alternative education, and building the capacity of organizations in New Bedford, Massachusetts. Priorities within these areas are described below. Environment: The Island Foundation funds environmental projects within New England (primarily Maine, Massachusetts and Rhode Island) that are (1) regional or statewide collaborative initiatives that improve and/or protect coastal and freshwater resources; or (2) research projects to investigate the environmental impacts of toxic chemicals. In addition, the foundation supports right whale research, university-based ecological economics, and land conservation efforts in southeastern Massachusetts, although the Foundation is not requesting proposals on these topics at this time." "Building Capacity in New Bedford: With a focus on the city of New Bedford, Massachusetts, the Island Foundation seeks local nonprofits that enhance the quality of life of residents, encourage community involvement, and promote sustainable economic development within this city and the surrounding region." "Alternative Education: Through the Year 2001, the Island Foundation has committed its education resources to the *Personal Leadership Development for Making the Right Choices* program at Thompson Island Outward Bound Education Center, located on one of the Boston (Massachusetts) harbor islands...Given the multi-year contribution to the *Choices* program, the Island Foundation is not seeking alternative education proposals at this time." Island

Foundation Guidelines **Priorities:** *Arts & Humanities:* 10%. Funds New Bedford museums. *Civic & Public Affairs:* 9%. Supports community foundations, zoos, and other civic organizations. *Education:* 33%. Supports one multiyear urban Outward Bound education program. *Environment:* 9%. Supports community centers and YMCA. *International:* 3%. Supports therapeutic center. *Note:* Total contributions made in 1999. **Typ. Recipients:** Adolescent Health Issues, AIDS/HIV, Domestic Violence, Family Planning, Kidney, Medical Rehabilitation, People with Disabilities, Substance Abuse. **Geo. Dist:** ME; New Bedford, MA; RI.

### ★ 382 ★ J. Bulow Campbell Foundation
1530 Sun Trust Tower
25 Park Place, Northeast
Atlanta, GA 30303
**Phone:** (404)658-9066          **Fax:** (404)659-4802
John Stephenson, Executive Director

**Fnded:** 1940. **Philosophy:** The J. Bulow Campbell Foundation prefers to give grants to non-governmental organizations "having a program of acknowledged or potential excellence and giving evidence or promise of regional leadership." In considering grants for Presbyterian causes, the foundation follows Mr. Campbell's example "by identifying grant opportunities that are consistent with the purposes of the Southern Presbyterian Church." In considering grants to educational institutions, emphasis is placed on privately supported institutions noted for academic excellence, with priority given to "projects designed to improve the quality of intellectual performance, and the level of spiritual life." The foundation prefers to contribute to projects of a permanent nature or to capital funding rather than to underwrite current operating expenses or recurring programs. In some cases, an exception will be made for an important project which requires startup funds to ensure initial success. It would be expected that the program become self-sustaining after the initial period. In general, the foundation is very selective in its giving decisions. It prefers to give a smaller number of grants to important, well-planned projects rather than to provide assistance to a larger number of less significant projects. The foundation makes all grants anonymously. Although recipients may reveal that a grant has been received, the source must remain confidential. The foundation does not publish an annual report; it does issue a pamphlet with general information and application guidelines. **Priorities:** *Arts & Humanities:* 4%. Supports Robert W. Woodruff Arts Center. *Civic & Public Affairs:* 12%. Funds gardens, zoos. *Education:* 54%. Supports religious education, private schools, colleges and universities. *Environment:* 18%. Supports Scouting, homes, and community centers, United Way. *International:* 9%. Supports Visiting Nurse Associations, Red Cross and medical center. *Note:* Total contributions made in 1999. **Typ. Recipients:** Cancer, Children's Health/Hospitals, Clinics/Medical Centers, Emergency/Ambulance Services, Health Organizations, Hospices, Hospitals, Long-Term Care, Medical Education, Medical Research, Mental Health, Nursing Services, People with Disabilities, Single-Disease Health Associations. **Geo. Dist:** AL; FL; Atlanta, GA, including surrounding area; NC; SC; TN.

### ★ 383 ★ J. E. and Z. B. Butler Foundation
825 3rd Ave.
New York, NY 10082
**Phone:** (212)687-8440
Leon Glaser, Section, Treasurer

**Fnded:** 1958. **Philosophy:** The foundation is committed to supporting social service, health, education, civic, religious, and environmental organizations. The foundation takes a special interest in Jewish causes. **Priorities:** *Civic & Public Affairs:* 44%. Supports community foundations and legal aid. *Education:* 6%. Supports universities and education organizations. *Environment:* 22%. Funds domestic violence, child abuse, battered women and family advocacy programs. *International:* 10%. Supports hospitals and medical centers. *Note:* Total contributions made in 1999. **Typ. Recipients:** AIDS/HIV, Alzheimers Disease, Cancer, Children's Health/Hospitals, Clinics/Medical Centers, Domestic Violence, Family Planning,

Health Organizations, Home-Care Services, Hospitals, Long-Term Care, Nursing Services, People with Disabilities, Prenatal Health Issues, Single-Disease Health Associations, Substance Abuse. **Geo. Dist:** New York, NY.

### ★ 384 ★ J. F Maddox Foundation
PO Box 2588
Hobbs, NM 88241-2588
**Phone:** (505)393-6338          **Fax:** (505)397-7266
**Email:** bobreid@leaco.net
Robert Reid, Executive Director, Secretary

**Fnded:** 1963. **Philosophy:** The foundation seeks to improve the quality of life in southeastern New Mexico and west Texas. The foundation provides support for education, community development, and other social programs. An area of emphasis is to provide support for innovative leadership in the systemic reform of public education. **Priorities:** *Arts & Humanities:* 4%. Supports music, public broadcasting, and museums. *Civic & Public Affairs:* 6%. Supports law/justice, towns/municipalities, and foundations. *Education:* 55%. Supports schools, colleges, universities, religious education, and public schools. *Environment:* 33%. *Note:* Total contributions made in 1999. **Typ. Recipients:** Alzheimers Disease, Cancer, Child Abuse, Diabetes, Domestic Violence, Emergency/Ambulance Services, Hospices, Hospitals, Hospitals (University Affiliated), Nutrition, People with Disabilities, Substance Abuse. **Geo. Dist:** NM, Southeast New Mexico; TX, West Texas.

### ★ 385 ★ J. L. Bedsole Foundation
PO Box 1137
Mobile, AL 36633
**Phone:** (334)432-3369          **Fax:** (334)432-1134
**Email:** bedsole2@bellsouth.net
Mabel Ward, Executive Director

**Fnded:** 1949. **Philosophy:** The J.L. Bedsole Foundation's primary interest is the support of educational institutions in Alabama. The arts, social services, health, and civic groups also receive grants from the foundation. While the foundation has a wide variety of interests, it strictly limits awards on a geographical basis. "Beyond the educational field we give nothing outside of southwest Alabama," explained Mrs. Mabel B. Ward, the foundation's executive director. She emphasized that organizations or projects outside of Alabama are not considered for funding or assistance by the foundation. educational excellence and economic development together are necessary to improve the quality of life in southwest Alabama, the foundation recently established the J.L. Bedsole Scholars Program, which offers scholarships to future leaders from six counties in southwest Alabama. The Scholarship Program recognizes and offers financial assistance to deserving students with recognized leadership ability who desire to pursue a post-secondary education, and will disperse $500,000 in awards annually beginning in academic year 1996-1997. Academic merit is not the most important factor in the selection of the Bedsole Scholars. The Scholars Program was created to meet the needs of average to above average students, with leadership potential, who can demonstrate financial need. The amount of the scholarship varies from a minimum of $2,000 to a maximum of $5,000. **Priorities:** *Arts & Humanities:* 4%. Major funding to arts education. *Civic & Public Affairs:* 37%. Focus on community redevelopment projects in the Mobile, AL, area. *Education:* 17%. Primarily in large gifts to private schools and state universities. *Environment:* 5%. Supports children's charities and volunteer programs. *International:* 1%. Supports hospitals and health organizations. *Religion:* 27%. Gives to Explore Center. *Note:* Total contributions made in 1998. **Typ. Recipients:** Children's Health/Hospitals, Clinics/Medical Centers, Eyes/Blindness, Health Organizations, Health-General, Hospitals, Medical Education, Mental Health, Outpatient Health Care, People with Disabilities, Public Health, Single-Disease Health Associations, Substance Abuse. **Geo. Dist:** AL, Southwest part of the state; Mobile, AL.

### ★ 386 ★ J. M. Kaplan Fund
261 Madison Ave., 19th Fl.
New York, NY 10016
**Phone:** (212)767-0630          **Fax:** (212)767-0639
Peter Davidson, Chairman

**Fnded:** 1945. **Philosophy:** "We maintain our belief that private foundations best serve the general interest when they act with a clear point of view and are willing to take chances so that fresh ideas in both the private and public realms can be safely tested. We believe that only by supporting the positive capacities and assets of individuals and organizations can needs be successfully identified and addressed. To these ends we are loyal to proven efforts and grantees with a track record, and at the same time take pleasure in helping new undertakings get off the ground. We seek to reinforce the honorable tradition of progressive social policy and enable talented people to make wonderful things happen - in city streets and neighborhoods, at the exhibition, in parks, on the printed page, in the classroom and field, and at the official hearing." 1996 Annual Report **Priorities:** *Arts & Humanities:* 14%. Supports libraries, museums, music, architecture and design. *Civic & Public Affairs:* 14%. Supports human rights, and urban and rural restoration organizations. (Public Policy) 7%. *Education:* 12%. Supports colleges, public schools, and literacy campaigns. *Environment:* 8%. Supports human needs, youth services, food banks, AIDS related programs and the homeless. *International:* 36%. *Note:* Total contributions made in 1998. **Typ. Recipients:** AIDS/HIV, Cancer, Children's Health/Hospitals, Family Planning, Health Organizations, Respiratory. **Geo. Dist:** New York, NY.

### ★ 387 ★ J. M. McDonald Foundation
PO Box 3219
Evergreen, CO 80437-3219
**Phone:** (303)674-9300          **Fax:** (303)674-9216
Donald McJunkin, President

**Fnded:** 1952. **Philosophy:** The foundation reflects Mr. McDonald's concerns in greater educational opportunity and educational institutions, the problems of the physically and mentally handicapped and the aged, and the potential for research to improve human conditions. The foundation supports established organizations. Colleges generally receive grants for facilities. The foundation makes grants to social service organizations and has a particular interest in child welfare and care of the aged and needy. The foundation also makes grants to hospitals for facilities. **Priorities:** *Arts & Humanities:* 11%. Supports public broadcasting and museums. *Civic & Public Affairs:* 3%. *Education:* 30%. Funds colleges and education associations. *Environment:* 27%. Supports youth groups and children's services. *International:* 21%. Supports outpatient health care. *Religion:* 6%. Gives to scientific research. *Note:* Total contributions made in 1999. **Typ. Recipients:** Cancer, Child Abuse, Children's Health/Hospitals, Clinics/Medical Centers, Domestic Violence, Emergency/Ambulance Services, Family Planning, Geriatric Health, Health Organizations, Heart, Hospices, Hospitals, Medical Education, Medical Rehabilitation, Medical Research, Mental Health, Outpatient Health Care, People with Disabilities, Public Health, Research/Studies Institutes, Single-Disease Health Associations, Speech & Hearing, Substance Abuse, Substance Abuse. **Geo. Dist:** Northeast USA; primarily upstate NY.

### ★ 388 ★ J. Paul Getty Trust
1200 Getty Center Dr., Ste. 800
Los Angeles, CA 90049-1685
**Phone:** (310)440-7320          **Fax:** (310)440-7703
**Email:** enovotny@getty.edu
**Website:** http://www.getty.edu/grants

**Fnded:** 1953. **Typ. Recipients:** Adolescent Health Issues, Health-General, Health-General. **Geo. Dist:** internationally; nationally.

### ★ 389 ★ J. S. Bridwell Foundation
807 8th St., Ste. 500
Wichita Falls, TX 76301-3365

**Phone:** (940)322-4436     **Fax:** (940)761-3365
Mac Cannedy, President

**Fnded:** 1949. **Philosophy:** The foundation has a broad range of interests that is limited only by its geographic priority of organizations or projects in Texas. Grants primarily are addressed to social services, but the foundation contributes to Southern Methodist University in Dallas, TX, for the Bridwell Library. The foundation has demonstrated a giving pattern of ongoing support to certain established charities, such as the Salvation Army, United Way, and Easter Seals. While the foundation gives to many organizations, it has shown a particular interest in organizations that address the concerns of disadvantaged youth, such as the Methodist Home in Waco, TX. address the concerns of disadvantaged youth, such as the Methodist Home in Waco, TX. **Priorities:** *Arts & Humanities:* 20%. Supports performing arts and museums. *Civic & Public Affairs:* 3%. Gives to volunteer fire departments, and community and public affairs groups. *Education:* 2%. Funds educational programs, with major support given to Midwestern State University. *Environment:* 13%. Emphasis on child and youth services, united funds, food banks, and senior citizen services. *International:* 60%. Rehabilitation centers, hospitals, hospices, and disease and disorder concerns received support. *Note:* Total contributions made in 1999. **Typ. Recipients:** Cancer, Children's Health/Hospitals, Clinics/Medical Centers, Emergency/Ambulance Services, Health Organizations, Heart, Hospices, Long-Term Care, Medical Rehabilitation, Medical Research, Medical Training, People with Disabilities, Single-Disease Health Associations, Substance Abuse. **Geo. Dist:** TX.

**★ 390 ★  J. W. Kieckhefer Foundation**
PO Box 1151
Prescott, AZ 86302
**Phone:** (520)445-4010     **Fax:** (928)445-4012
Eugene Polk, Administrative Officer, Trustee

**Fnded:** 1953. **Philosophy:** The foundation is a general purpose charity which emphasizes social services. The foundation gives grants for annual campaigns, seed money, emergency funds, capital funds (including building funds, equipment, materials, and renovation), special endowments for chairs and lecture series, research-related programs, conferences and seminars, and general purposes. The foundation provides continuous support and gives both one-time and multiple-year grants. **Priorities:** *Arts & Humanities:* 7%. Supports museums, arts centers, and music. *Civic & Public Affairs:* 22%. Emphasis on housing, legal aid, and community development. *Education:* 5%. Universities, education associations, and secondary education. *Environment:* 27%. Primarily supports child welfare, the aged, and people with disabilities. *International:* 27%. Focus on hospitals and medical centers, medical research, and single-disease health associations. *Religion:* 8%. Funds science centers. *Note:* Total contributions made in 1999. **Typ. Recipients:** Alzheimers Disease, Cancer, Child Abuse, Children's Health/Hospitals, Clinics/Medical Centers, Domestic Violence, Eyes/Blindness, Family Planning, Geriatric Health, Health Funds, Health Organizations, Heart, Hospices, Hospitals, Kidney, Medical Education, Medical Rehabilitation, Medical Research, People with Disabilities, Prenatal Health Issues, Public Health, Research/Studies Institutes, Respiratory, Single-Disease Health Associations, Substance Abuse. **Geo. Dist:** nationally; AZ.

**★ 391 ★  J. Willard and Alice S. Marriott**
**Foundation**
PO Box 150
Washington, DC 20058
**Phone:** (301)380-2246     **Fax:** (301)380-8957
**Email:** bonnie.white@marriott.com
Bonnie White, Grant Manager

**Fnded:** 1966. **Philosophy:** The foundation primarily awards grants to local organizations. It also gives to a few general scholarship funds. The majority of funding, however, goes to previously supported organizations. **Priorities:** *Arts & Humanities:* 1%. Gives to arts centers, music, public broadcasting, and performing arts. *Civic & Public Affairs:* 1%. Funds trade associations, municipalities, and civic concerns. *Education:* 62% (Education/Professional Associations). Funds higher education. *Environment:* 28% (Human Services/Civic). Supports youth groups, united funds, and the disabled. *International:* 8% (Health/Medical Research). Focus on health funds, hospitals, and single-disease health associations. *Note:* Total contributions made in 2000. **Typ. Recipients:** AIDS/HIV, Arthritis, Cancer, Children's Health/Hospitals, Clinics/Medical Centers, Emergency/Ambulance Services, Eyes/Blindness, Health Organizations, Heart, Hospitals, Hospitals (University Affiliated), Medical Research, Multiple Sclerosis, Nutrition, People with Disabilities, Prenatal Health Issues, Public Health, Research/Studies Institutes, Speech & Hearing, Substance Abuse, Trauma Treatment. **Geo. Dist:** nationally; Washington, DC, metropolitan area; MD; VA.

**★ 392 ★  Jackson Hole Preserve**
30 Rockefeller Plaza, Room 5600
New York, NY 10112
**Phone:** (212)649-5819
Carmen Reyes, Jr., Contact

**Fnded:** 1940. **Philosophy:** The Jackson Hole Preserve supports organizations involved in the conservation and preservation of wildlife, nature, and land. Recently, the preserve made grants to historic preservation societies in New York. However, most of the funding usually goes to environmental affairs. "Our grant-making activities are directed toward information and action programs that increase public understanding of conservation issues and citizen participation in their resolution." **Priorities:** *Arts & Humanities:* 7%. Supports museum and historic preservation. *Civic & Public Affairs:* 3%. Supports civic planning. *Civic:* 3%. Educational materials development. *Note:* Total contributions made in 1998. **Typ. Recipients:** Hospitals, Single-Disease Health Associations. **Geo. Dist:** NY, Hudson River Valley region; VT; WY.

**★ 393 ★  Jacob and Francis Hiatt**
**Foundation**
PO Box 70562
Worcester, MA 01607
**Phone:** (508)791-2301     **Fax:** (508)792-1578

**Priorities:** *Education:* 100%. Supports higher education, with a focus on the Northeast. *Note:* Contributions were made in fiscal 1998. **Typ. Recipients:** Cancer, Hospitals, Medical Research. **Geo. Dist:** MA.

**★ 394 ★  Jacob G. Schmidlapp Trust No.**
**1**
Charitable Foundations Screening Committee
c/o Fifth Third Bank, MD 109007
Cincinnati, OH 45263
**Phone:** (513)579-6034     **Fax:** (513)744-6997
Lawra Baumann, Foundation Officer

**Fnded:** 1927. **Philosophy:** The Jacob G. Schmidlapp Trust No. 1 believes that funds should be used "for relief in sickness, suffering and distress, the care of young children, or the helpless and afflicted." To this purpose, the trust concentrates on social services, health facilities, and educational institutions that directly or indirectly benefit children, the sick, and the disadvantaged in the Cincinnati area. In the future, the trust expects to elicit proposals for programs which are especially effective in achieving the goals set by Mr. Schmidlapp while at the same time meeting the community needs of today. **Priorities:** *Arts & Humanities:* About 16%. Museums and libraries. *Civic & Public Affairs:* 35%. Supports zoos, botanical gardens, job programs, and housing. *Education:* 19%. Funds colleges and universities and primary and secondary education. *Environment:* 20%. Supports youth organizations, child welfare, and the United Way. *International:* About 3%. Hospitals, hospices, geriatric care, cancer care, and health funds. *Note:* Total contributions made in fiscal 1998. **Typ. Recipients:** Adolescent Health Issues, Arthritis, Cancer, Children's Health/Hospitals, Clinics/Medical Centers, Diabetes, Domestic Violence, Emergency/Ambulance Services, Family Planning, Geriatric Health, Health Funds, Health Organizations, Heart, Hospices, Hospitals, Long-Term Care, Medical Education, Medical Rehabilitation, Mental Health, Nursing Services, People with Disabilities, Prenatal Health Issues, Preventive Medicine/Wellness Organizations, Public Health, Single-Disease Health Associations, Speech & Hearing, Substance Abuse, Trauma Treatment. **Geo. Dist:** Cincinnati, OH, metropolitan area.

**★ 395 ★  Jacob and Hilda Blaustein**
**Foundation**
Blaustein Bldg.
PO Box 238
Baltimore, MD 21203
**Phone:** (410)347-7222     **Fax:** (410)659-0552
**Email:** info@blaufund.org
Betsy Ringel, Contact

**Fnded:** 1957. **Philosophy:** Jewish identity and continuity, health, intergroup relations, and the arts are the foundation's four program areas. **Priorities:** *Arts & Humanities:* 4%. Supports public art organizations, historical organizations, educational broadcasting and libraries. *Civic & Public Affairs:* 10%. Supports the Ellis Island Foundation, rescue services, and civic foundations. *Education:* 20%. Supports education centers, universities, and religious education. *International:* 33%. Supports hospitals, medical centers, and single-disease health organizations. *Note:* Total contributions made in 1998. **Typ. Recipients:** Cancer, Children's Health/Hospitals, Clinics/Medical Centers, Emergency/Ambulance Services, Eyes/Blindness, Health Organizations, Hospitals, Medical Education, Mental Health, People with Disabilities, Preventive Medicine/Wellness Organizations, Public Health, Single-Disease Health Associations, Transplant Networks/Donor Banks. **Geo. Dist:** Baltimore, MD.

**★ 396 ★  James G. Boswell Foundation**
101 West Walnut St.
Pasadena, CA 91103-3642
**Phone:** (626)583-3000     **Fax:** (626)583-3090
Jim Henry, Executive Director

**Fnded:** 1947. **Philosophy:** The foundation generally supports agricultural education and general higher education. Health concerns, precollege private schools, public broadcasting, rural affairs groups, and youth organizations also receive minor support. **Priorities:** *Civic & Public Affairs:* 23%. Supports community and public affairs. *Education:* 53%. Supports educational programs and institutions, with major emphasis given to the Agricultural Education Foundation. *Environment:* 1%. *International:* 23%. Supports health concerns, medical centers and research. *Note:* Contributions were made in 1998. **Typ. Recipients:** Cancer, Clinics/Medical Centers, Health Organizations, Heart, Hospitals, Medical Education, Medical Research, People with Disabilities, Prenatal Health Issues, Public Health. **Geo. Dist:** CA.

**★ 397 ★  James Graham Brown**
**Foundation, Inc.**
4350 Brownsboro Rd.
Ste. 200
Louisville, KY 40207
**Phone:** (502)896-2440     **Fax:** (502)896-1774
**Email:** mason@brownfoundation.com
**Website:** http://www.brownfoundation.com
Mrs. Mason Rummel, Executive Director

**Fnded:** 1943. **Philosophy:** The mission of the foundation is to "foster the well-being, quality of life and image of Louisville and Kentucky." The primary categories of funding of the James Graham Brown Foundation, Inc. are education, civic and economic development, youth, and health and general welfare. Historically, the foundation has supported projects with an emphasis in bricks and mortar and equipment purchases as well as endowment programs for scholarship funds. The foundation also prefers to support organizations located in Kentucky. "Special projects for civic or economic development which have an explicit objective to improve the quality of life of Kentuckians and the image of Kentucky are of particular interest to the Foundation as well." 1996 Guidelines **Priorities:** *Arts & Humanities:* 16%. Supports historical preservation and museums. *Civic & Public Affairs:* 54%. Supports industrial development, employment/job training, municipalities, zoos, economic development and community foundations. *Education:* 22%. Funds colleges, universities and literacy organizations. *Environment:* 5%. Supports United Way, volunteer services, youth services, people with disabilities, scouting, and community centers. *International:* Less than 1%. *Religion:* 2%. Funds a science center. **Typ. Recipients:** Arthritis, Cancer, Children's Health/Hospitals, Clinics/Medical Centers, Emergency/Ambulance Services, Eyes/Blindness, Family Planning, Geriatric Health, Health Organizations, Medical Rehabilitation, Mental Health, Multiple Sclerosis, People with Disabilities, Prenatal Health Issues, Respiratory, Single-Disease Health Associations, Substance Abuse. **Geo. Dist:** KY.

### ★ 398 ★ James H. Cummings Foundation

1807 Elmwood Ave., Rm. 112
Buffalo, NY 14207
**Phone:** (716)874-0040　　　　**Fax:** (716)874-0040
**Email:** INFO@cummings.ncf.org
William McFarland, Executive Director & Secretary

**Fnded:** 1962. **Philosophy:** The foundation was created "to further medical science, medical research, and medical education... to provide services for underprivileged boys and girls" and "to assist aged and infirm persons." Grants are generally for capital expenditures, in particular for the purchase of medical research equipment. The foundation prefers to support organizations that do not receive government funding. Priority is given to medical proposals. **Priorities:** *Arts & Humanities:* 2%. Supports library. *Civic & Public Affairs:* 5%. *Education:* 21%. Supports higher education. *Environment:* 24% Supports underprivileged children aged and infirm persons. *International:* About 40%. Supports medical science, medical research, and medical education. *Note:* Total contributions made in fiscal 1999. **Typ. Recipients:** Cancer, Children's Health/Hospitals, Clinics/Medical Centers, Family Planning, Geriatric Health, Health Organizations, Health-General, Heart, Hospices, Hospitals, Medical Rehabilitation, Medical Rehabilitation, Medical Research, Medical Training, Nursing Services, People with Disabilities, Prenatal Health Issues, Public Health, Respiratory, Speech & Hearing, Substance Abuse. **Geo. Dist:** Buffalo, NY; Hendersonville, NC; Toronto, ON.

### ★ 399 ★ The James Irvine Foundation

One Market, Steuart Tower, Ste. 2500
San Francisco, CA 94105
**Phone:** (415)777-2244　　　　**Fax:** (415)777-0869
**Website:** http://www.irvine.org
Ann Clarke, Director of Grants Administration

**Fnded:** 1937. **Philosophy:** "The James Irvine Foundation is a general purpose private foundation granting funds to support projects and programs for the benefit of California residents. The Foundation is dedicated to enhancing the social, economic, and physical quality of life throughout California and to enriching the state's intellectual and cultural environment." "The James Irvine Foundation: 2000 Summary Information for the Public" The Foundation's funding priorities are Arts; Children, Youth and Families; Civic Culture; Higher Education; Sustainable Communities; and Special Projects. improve the economic and social well-being of the disadvantaged and their communities, foster self-sufficiency, and assist the ethnic minorities to function more effectively as full participants in society To encourage communication, understanding, and cooperation among diverse cultural, ethnic, and socioeconomic groups To promote civic participation, social responsibility, public understanding of issues, and the development of sound public policy To enrich the quality and diversity of educational, cultural, health, and human service programs throughout the State. The Foundation makes grants in seven categorical areas: Arts; Children, Youth and Families; Civic **Priorities:** *Arts & Humanities:* 15%. Museums, dance, and cultural centers. *Civic & Public Affairs:* 39%. Funds community-building, naturalization and civic participa-

tion in California's Central Valley, human and race relations, collaborative regional development, sustainable use of land, and state and local governance reform. *Education:* 11%. Focus on higher education, theological education, and research studies. *Environment:* 9%. Programs for children, youth, and families. *Note:* Total contributions made in 1999. **Typ. Recipients:** AIDS/HIV, Children's Health/Hospitals, Clinics/Medical Centers, Domestic Violence, Family Planning, Health Organizations, Health Policy/Cost Containment, Health-General, Hospitals, Hospitals (University Affiliated), Medical Research, Nursing Services, People with Disabilities, Prenatal Health Issues, Preventive Medicine/Wellness Organizations, Public Health, Research/Studies Institutes. **Geo. Dist:** CA.

### ★ 400 ★ James M. Johnston Trust for Charitable and Educational Purposes

2 Wisconsin Circle, Ste. 600
Chevy Chase, MD 20815
**Phone:** (301)907-0135
Julia Sanders, Office Manager

**Fnded:** 1968. **Philosophy:** The trust, following the interests of its donor, concentrates its grant-making program on education, particularly at the University of North Carolina at Chapel Hill. Support is directed toward scholarship programs, nursing education, and faculty development. **Priorities:** *Civic & Public Affairs:* 2%. Supports a fire department. *Education:* 88%. Funds scholarships, colleges, universities, art education, secondary schools, and academies. *Environment:* 4%. Supports youth organizations, services for the disabled, and the scouts. *International:* 6%. Primary support for hospitals and children's health. *Note:* Total contributions made in 1998. **Typ. Recipients:** Cancer, Children's Health/Hospitals, Diabetes, Emergency/Ambulance Services, Heart, Hospices, Hospitals, Long-Term Care, Medical Education, Medical Rehabilitation, Medical Research, Medical Training, Mental Health, Nursing Services, People with Disabilities, Single-Disease Health Associations. **Geo. Dist:** Washington, DC; NC.

### ★ 401 ★ Janirve Foundation

One North Pack Square, Ste. 416
Asheville, NC 28801
**Phone:** (828)258-1877　　　　**Fax:** (828)258-1837
Met Poston, Chairman, Advisory Committee

**Fnded:** 1964. **Philosophy:** The foundation supports a wide range of charities with emphasis on social services, health, and education. Support also goes to the arts and humanities and environmental causes. The foundation "encourages the submission of proposals which set forth new or different and innovative approaches toward dealing with a problem affecting a significant sector of society." **Priorities:** *Arts & Humanities:* 12%. Supports symphonies, libraries, arts councils, and history. *Civic & Public Affairs:* 21%. Public policy, vocational services, community foundations, and housing. *Education:* 16% Christian colleges and schools, and literacy. *Environment:* 23%. Youth services, child abuse centers, Goodwill Industries, and Special Olympics. *International:* 11%. Hospitals single-disease health organizations, and drug rehabilitation. *Note:* Total contributions made in 1998. **Typ. Recipients:** Adolescent Health Issues, Alzheimers Disease, Cancer, Child Abuse, Children's Health/Hospitals, Clinics/Medical Centers, Domestic Violence, Emergency/Ambulance Services, Family Planning, Geriatric Health, Health Organizations, Health-General, Hospices, Hospitals, Long-Term Care, Medical Education, Medical Rehabilitation, People with Disabilities, Preventive Medicine/Wellness Organizations, Public Health, Single-Disease Health Associations, Transplant Networks/Donor Banks. **Geo. Dist:** Palm Beach, FL; West Palm Beach, FL; NC, Western North Carolina.

### ★ 402 ★ Jay and Betty Van Andel Foundation

333 Bostwick Northeast
Grand Rapids, MI 49503
**Phone:** (616)234-5294　　　　**Fax:** (616)234-5295
Anne Shane, Contact

**Fnded:** 1963. **Philosophy:** The foundation has directed its philanthropy into four main categories–the arts, religious organizations, educational institutions, and civic groups. The foundation's contributions to the arts focus on museums, music, and opera in Grand Rapids, MI. The foundation's religious interests include Christian organizations and missions, churches, and religious welfare organizations. The foundation's educational funding supports religious educational organizations, scholarship funds, and colleges and universities. Its funding to civic groups includes conservative public policy think tanks and a zoological society. **Priorities:** *Arts & Humanities:* About 5%. *Civic & Public Affairs:* About 27%. Zoos, foundations, and free enterprise. *Education:* About 4%. *Environment:* 47%. Community centers, scouting, and family services. *International:* About 5%. *Note:* Contributions made in 1996. **Typ. Recipients:** Alzheimers Disease, Clinics/Medical Centers, Health Organizations, Health-General, Hospices, Hospitals, Long-Term Care, Medical Research, People with Disabilities, Public Health, Research/Studies Institutes. **Geo. Dist:** MI.

### ★ 403 ★ Jay and Rose Phillips Family Foundation

10 Second St., Northeast, Ste. 200
Minneapolis, MN 55413
**Phone:** (612)623-1654　　　　**Fax:** (612)623-1653
**Email:** phillipsfnd@phillipsfnd.org
Patricia Cummings, Executive Director & Secretary

**Fnded:** 1944. **Philosophy:** Jay Phillips, founder of the foundation, died in February 1992, and the foundation reported dramatic changes at that time. Mr. Phillips anticipated the available funds for contributions by establishing long-term gifts for his favorite charities. Thirty-six percent of the allocated funds for giving continue to be distributed in communities where Phillips family members reside. Of particular interest to the foundation are health, higher education, programs for people with disabilities, and programs that address issues of discrimination. Also, during times of severe economic hardship and financial distress, the foundation reports that its primary concern is providing support for projects addressing unmet human and social needs. The foundation awards many grants to local organizations not previously supported. A move from the focus on emergency funding is also taking place. There is more emphasis on providing funding to organizations that find long-term solutions in the area of human services. "The foundations mission is to honor the legacy of its founders, Jay & Rose Phillips, by continuing the the family tradition of sharing resources for the public good, while exercising leadership and flexibility in responding to emerging community needs." **Priorities:** *Arts & Humanities:* 1%. Supports opera, music, theater, history, and public broadcasting. *Civic & Public Affairs:* (Public Policy) 20%. Supports womens affairs, housing, law & justice, native american affairs, civil rights and zoos. *Education:* 21%. Supports school, scholarship, religious education, universities minority education. *Environment:* 13%. Supports senior services, food distribution programs, United Way, young men's christian association, homes, family services, Young Women's Christian Association, scouts, and special olympics. *International:* 5%. Supports medical research hospital, and single-disease health associations. *Note:* Total contributions made in 1999. **Typ. Recipients:** AIDS/HIV, Cancer, Children's Health/Hospitals, Clinics/Medical Centers, Family Planning, Health Organizations, Health-General, Heart, Hospices, Hospitals, Long-Term Care, Medical Education, Medical Rehabilitation, Medical Research, Multiple Sclerosis, People with Disabilities, Prenatal Health Issues, Public Health, Research/Studies Institutes, Sexual Abuse, Single-Disease Health Associations. **Geo. Dist:** MN, seven-county metropolitan area of Minneapolis/St. Paul, MN.

### ★ 404 ★ Jean and Louis Dreyfus Foundation

30 Rockefeller Plaza, Ste. 4340
New York, NY 10112
**Phone:** (212)218-7575　　　　**Fax:** (212)649-5998
Edmee Firth, Executive Director

**Fnded:** 1978. **Philosophy:** The foundation makes grants across the major categories of support. In social services, interests include community and neighborhood centers, crime prevention, and family and children's services. Educational support goes to medical and private education, educational funds, and art education. Museums and other art organizations, civic affairs, and health services are also supported. The foundation no longer gives medical research grants. **Priorities:** *Arts & Humanities:* 25% supports museums, music, theaters, and art centers. *Education:* 25% colleges and research. *Environment:* 25% supports senior services and community centers. *Note:* Total contributions made in 1997. **Typ. Recipients:** Adolescent Health Issues, AIDS/HIV, Alzheimers Disease, Cancer, Children's Health/Hospitals, Clinics/Medical Centers, Family Planning, Geriatric Health, Health Funds, Health Organizations, Health Policy/Cost Containment, Home-Care Services, Hospitals, Long-Term Care, Medical Education, Medical Training, Mental Health, Nursing Services, Nutrition, Prenatal Health Issues, Public Health, Substance Abuse. **Geo. Dist:** New York, NY.

## ★ 405 ★ Jesse Philips Foundation

3870 Honey Hill Lane
Dayton, OH 45405
**Phone:** (937)496-1300
Caryl Philips, President

**Fnded:** 1960. **Philosophy:** The Jesse Philips Foundation makes grants across all major categories of support. The foundation's primary giving interests include social services, health, education, religion, the arts, science, and civic affairs. Religious funding favors Jewish organizations. **Priorities:** *Arts & Humanities:* 9%. Supports theater, ballet, arts centers, and historic preservation. *Civic & Public Affairs:* 1%. *Education:* 73%. Supports universities, scholarships, and general education. *Environment:* 1%. Supports scouting, animal protection, and family planning services. *International:* 3%. Funds medical centers. *Religion:* 4%. Supports science research and science institution. *Note:* Total contributions made in fiscal 1999. **Typ. Recipients:** AIDS/HIV, Cancer, Children's Health/Hospitals, Clinics/Medical Centers, Family Planning, Health Funds, Health Organizations, Hospitals, Medical Research, Mental Health, Respiratory, Single-Disease Health Associations, Transplant Networks/Donor Banks. **Geo. Dist:** OH, Montgomery County.

## ★ 406 ★ Jesselson Foundation

450 Park Ave., Ste. 2603
New York, NY 10022
**Phone:** (212)751-3666 **Fax:** (212)459-9797
Michael Jesselson, Vice President

**Fnded:** 1955. **Philosophy:** The foundation primarily supports Jewish causes, with interest shown for civic, social welfare, and educational organizations. **Priorities:** *Civic & Public Affairs:* 1%. *Education:* 23%. Primarily for Jewish education. *Environment:* 2%. Emphasis on youth organizations. *International:* 1%. *Note:* Total contributions made in fiscal 2000. **Typ. Recipients:** Cancer, Children's Health/Hospitals, Clinics/Medical Centers, Diabetes, Heart, Hospitals, Long-Term Care, Medical Education, Medical Research, Single-Disease Health Associations. **Geo. Dist:** Nationwide.

## ★ 407 ★ Jessie B. Cox Charitable Trust

Donor Services Office
Hemenway & Barnes
60 State St.
Boston, MA 02109-1899
**Phone:** (617)557-9775
**Email:** dso@hembar.com
**Website:** http://www.agmconnect.org/cox.html
Susan Fish, Grants Administrator

**Fnded:** 1982. **Philosophy:** "The purpose of the trust is to increase significantly the ability of New England non-profit organizations to carry out their stated missions in the fields of health, education, the environment, and the development of philanthropy in the community. "In the health field, the trust is particularly interested in supporting primary healthcare, and advocacy projects, and research that will have a positive effect on the prevention and treatment of illness and disability, particularly among children and youth; increased access to appropriate levels of care for New England's underserved populations; and delivery of health services to the poor. In the education area, the trust is particularly interested in supporting projects which will have a significant effect on the availability of academic resources, both traditional and innovative; increased access, incentives and opportunities for educational participation by underserved populations in New England; the availability of instruction and training in the visual and performing arts; and improved academic performance and achievement. "The trust is interested in supporting environmental projects which will have a positive impact on protection of critical natural resources; energy conservation; public awareness of the critical environmental issues facing the region; and protection of the public's health, especially in low-income and minority communities." In philanthropy, the trust seeks to "encourage the development and expansion of emerging community foundations, increase philanthropic resources in underserved areas, and provide modest support for certain special efforts of philanthropic donors." Jessie B. Cox Charitable Trust *Guidelines and Policies* **Priorities:** *Education:* 31%. Supports education associations and colleges and universities. *International:* 30%. Focus on health centers, public health, pediatric health, and single-disease health associations. *Note:* Total contributions made in 1998. **Typ. Recipients:** Adolescent Health Issues, AIDS/HIV, Children's Health/Hospitals, Diabetes, Family Planning, Health Organizations, Health Policy/Cost Containment, Home-Care Services, Hospitals, Hospitals (University Affiliated), Medical Education, Medical Research, Mental Health, Nursing Services, Nutrition, People with Disabilities, Prenatal Health Issues, Preventive Medicine/Wellness Organizations, Public Health, Respiratory, Substance Abuse. **Geo. Dist:** New England.

## ★ 408 ★ Jessie Ball duPont Fund

One Independent Dr., Ste. 1400
Jacksonville, FL 32202-5011
**Phone:** (904)353-0890 **Fax:** (904)353-3870
**Email:** smagill@dupontfund.com
**Website:** http://www.dupontfund.org
Sherry Magill, President

**Fnded:** 1976. **Philosophy:** In 1994, the foundation established the Jessie Ball duPont Fund Making a Difference Award, formerly the Turnaround Award. This award recognizes an individual who can make a difference or literally turn around an organization that meets a critical societal need. In 1991, the foundation launched several new programs. The trustees established the Jessie Ball duPont Fund Award to honor selected individuals at the Fund's eligible institutions. The honorees are chosen for their courage, integrity, creativity, perseverance, and compassion. Their life work focuses on promoting just relations and equality in their communities. The fund also began the Clergy Enrichment Fund, which is designed to respond to the needs of ordained clergy at the fund's eligible religious institutions and includes a sabbatical program and a professional development fund. A strong preference is given to clergy who serve at small, financially-assisted churches. Another program, the Nonprofit Initiative, is a program that addresses the needs of eligible nonprofits with discretionary funds, technical assistance, and a leadership developmental institute. Both programs have their own set of application guidelines. In 1990, the fund launched the Jessie Ball duPont Fund Small Liberal Arts College Initiative. As part of the initiative, the fund has awarded over $3,000,000 to 37 eligible colleges, with an enrollment of fewer than 2,900 students each. In addition to the Small Liberal Arts College Initiative, the fund has application guidelines for a People-In-Need program and a Feasibility Grant program. Through grants to eligible institutions, the fund seeks to help solve the needs of today's society, especially in the South, and to anticipate emerging issues that may become major concerns in the future. The fund's objectives are to enable individuals to reach their full potential in today's society and to enable society to fulfill its obligation to its members; to support projects that are not adequately funded by other sources; and to assist and encourage eligible institutions to work with other organizations to address common problems and achieve common goals. In addition, the fund attempts to enable the eligible institutions to generate additional resources by attracting a broad constituency of donors and volunteer participation; and to preserve and use our historical heritage. **Priorities:** *Civic & Public Affairs:* 39% (Nonprofits). Funds nonprofit management, and broad-based community issues including community economic development and human services organizations. *Education:* 36%. Primarily supports colleges and universities. *Note:* Total contributions made in fiscal 2000. **Typ. Recipients:** AIDS/HIV, Alzheimers Disease, Cancer, Children's Health/Hospitals, Clinics/Medical Centers, Domestic Violence, Emergency/Ambulance Services, Eyes/Blindness, Health Organizations, Heart, Hospitals, Hospitals (University Affiliated), Long-Term Care, Medical Education, Mental Health, Nursing Services, People with Disabilities, Respiratory, Sexual Abuse, Single-Disease Health Associations, Speech & Hearing. **Geo. Dist:** southern states; DE, nationally; FL; VA.

## ★ 409 ★ Jewish Foundation for Education of Women

135 East 64th St.
New York, NY 10021
**Phone:** (212)288-3931 **Fax:** (212)288-5798
**Website:** http://www.jfew.org
Marge Goldwater, Executive Director

**Fnded:** 1984. **Philosophy:** The foundation was established to assist women in achieving their goals through higher education. The foundation is offering the following programs for the School Year 1999/2000: Scholarships for Emigres Training for Careers in Jewish Education. This program is open to emigres from the former Soviet Union who are pursuing careers in Jewish education. Candidates in Jewish education. Candidates in Jewish education, rabbinical and cantorial studies, and Jewish studies are invited to write the foundation for an application. Awards range from $10,000 to $20,000. Approximately seven scholarships will be awarded. Scholarships in the Health Professions. This program will provide scholarships to emigres from the former Soviet Union who are studying medicine, dentistry, nursing, pharmacy, occupational and physical therapy, and physician assistance. Typical awards are $5,000. Approximately 72 scholarships will be awarded. The foundation is offering additional scholarships through the colleges and universities designated below. These scholarships will be awarded through faculty recommendations; students cannot apply directly. CUNY Teacher Incentive Program: This program will provide stipends to CUNY graduates who are studying for a master's degree in education at CUNY and interested in pursuing a teaching career in the New York City public school system. Qualified students should contact the office of the Vice Chancellor for Academic Affairs at CUNY for further information ARTS Scholarships at The Juilliard School, Tisch School of the Arts at New York University, and the Manhattan School of Music: These scholarships are being offered to qualified students enrolled in their programs. Faculty members will select recipients. CUNY Dissertation Fellowships in the Humanities: A small number of fellowships will be awarded through the CUNY Graduate Center to qualified applicants. Barnard College Summer Internships: This program will support summer internships for qualified Barnard College students. Summer stipends are also available for qualified students in Barnard's Double Degree Program with the Jewish Theological Seminary. The foundation also offers scholarships for students of five New York City schools of social work. Faculty members make the decisions. Scholarships are also provided to disadvantaged teens through various social service groups. **Priorities:** *Education:* 100%. Supports higher education. *Note:* Total contributions made in fiscal 1999. **Typ. Recipients:** Medical Education. **Geo. Dist:** NY, five boroughs of New York.

## ★ 410 ★ Jewish Healthcare Foundation

Centre City Tower, Ste. 2330
650 Smithfield St.
Pittsburgh, PA 15222
**Phone:** (412)594-2550     **Fax:** (412)232-6240
**Email:** info@jhf.org
**Website:** http://www.jhf.org
Karen Feinstein, President

**Fnded:** 1991. **Philosophy:** "The Jewish Healthcare Foundation uses its resources to identify and support creative ideas and partnerships with the potential to make our region's health care system one of the best in the country. Our operating principles require that grants build upon proven techniques and the best information available. Funded programs should contribute to reshaping the system and lead to long-term solutions. While addressing ongoing concerns, the foundation will also address emerging health care concerns. The foundation views grants as investments that should strive to have a maximum impact on health status and systems by (1) changing health behaviors, (2) improving networks of care, or (3) generating good public programs. At the Jewish Healthcare Foundation we believe that connecting people with other skilled, informed and inventive people, provides the most direct route to the highest standards in health care. Jewish values compel us to connect system improvements to the Jewish and general communities and their institutions. By working to improve the physical and emotional health of individuals and communities, the JHF honors Jewish heritage and values. Our current agenda focuses on the following funding priorities: Financing Health: Insuring Quality–issues of insurance enrollment, entitlement, coverage and benefits affect access, quality, disease management and early detection. Advancing Health: Information Technology and Medical Research–quality in health care depends increasingly on the speed with which the health sector is transformed into an information driven industry. Integrating Health: Physician, Behavioral, Environmental and Public Health–integrating these elements will improve the health status of all Americans; integrating services for the frail and vulnerable across the continuum of acute rehabilitation, end-of-life, home based and residential services, will produce better outcomes." **Priorities:** *Arts & Humanities:* 3%. Supports public broadcasting. *Civic & Public Affairs:* 34%. Supports general civic affairs, law & justice, philanthropic organizations. *Education:* 5%. Supports universities and medical colleges, and religious education. *Environment:* 6%. Supports scouts and Young Women's Christian AssociationAs. *International:* 19%. Supports hospitals, cancer, respiratory, and medical rehabilitation. *Note:* Total contributions made in 1998. **Typ. Recipients:** Adolescent Health Issues, AIDS/HIV, Alzheimers Disease, Cancer, Children's Health/Hospitals, Clinics/Medical Centers, Domestic Violence, Geriatric Health, Geriatric Health, Health Funds, Health Organizations, Health Policy/Cost Containment, Health-General, Heart, Home-Care Services, Hospitals, Hospitals (University Affiliated), Kidney, Long-Term Care, Medical Education, Medical Research, Medical Training, Mental Health, Nursing Services, Nutrition, People with Disabilities, Prenatal Health Issues, Preventive Medicine/Wellness Organizations, Public Health, Single-Disease Health Associations, Substance Abuse, Transplant Networks/Donor Banks. **Geo. Dist:** PA, Western Pennsylvania.

## ★ 411 ★ JM Foundation

60 East 42nd St., Room 1651
New York, NY 10165
**Phone:** (212)687-7735     **Fax:** (212)697-5495
Carl Helstrom, Senior Program Officer

**Fnded:** 1936. **Philosophy:** The JM Foundation grants program encompasses several related fields, including rehabilitation of people with disabilities, prevention and wellness with an emphasis on individual responsibility for health, and health-related policy research. The foundation also has a strong interest in educational activities which strengthen America's pluralistic system of free markets, entrepreneurship, voluntarism, individual empowerment, and private enterprise. In addition, the foundation directors recognize the importance of the American family and support organiza-tions that reinforce the role of parents; enhance the quality of family life; and provide youth with jobs, healthy lifestyles, and positive character development. The JM Foundation is closely involved with the Philanthropy Roundtable, the State Policy Network, and the National Results Council. **Priorities:** *Civic & Public Affairs:* 35%. Supports public policy, clubs, philanthropic organizations, and urban affairs. *Education:* 11%. Funds education reform, and universities. *Environment:* 23%. Supports people with disabilities, family services, and youth organizations. *International:* 24%. Supports medical research, medical centers, substance abuse rehabilitation, mental health, and medical rehabilitation. *Note:* Total contributions made in 2000. **Typ. Recipients:** Cancer, Children's Health/Hospitals, Clinics/Medical Centers, Eyes/Blindness, Family Planning, Geriatric Health, Health Organizations, Health Policy/Cost Containment, Heart, Hospitals, Medical Education, Medical Rehabilitation, Medical Research, People with Disabilities, Prenatal Health Issues, Preventive Medicine/Wellness Organizations, Public Health, Research/Studies Institutes, Single-Disease Health Associations, Speech & Hearing, Substance Abuse, Trauma Treatment.

## ★ 412 ★ Joe C. Davis Foundation

908 Audubon Dr.
Nashville, TN 37204
**Phone:** (615)297-1030
Anne Fergerson, Contact

**Fnded:** 1976. **Philosophy:** The Joe C. Davis Foundation supports health and education in the Nashville, TN, area. **Priorities:** *Arts & Humanities:* 12%. Funds a local public library. *Civic & Public Affairs:* 6%. *Education:* 33%. Supports secondary education and colleges and universities. *Environment:* 25%. Supports the YMCA in Nashville and other family and children's services. *International:* 24%. Funds a medical school. *Note:* Total contributions made in fiscal 2000. **Typ. Recipients:** Alzheimers Disease, Cancer, Children's Health/Hospitals, Clinics/Medical Centers, Diabetes, Health Organizations, Health Policy/Cost Containment, Hospices, Hospitals, Hospitals (University Affiliated), Medical Education, Medical Research, Public Health, Speech & Hearing, Substance Abuse. **Geo. Dist:** Nashville, TN, including metropolitan area.

## ★ 413 ★ Joe and Emily Lowe Foundation

249 Royal Palm Way, Ste. 502
Palm Beach, FL 33480
**Fax:** (561)655-7130
Ellen Liman, President

**Fnded:** 1949. **Philosophy:** The foundation funds a wide variety of causes in the arts, civic and public affairs, education, health, social services, and religion (emphasizing Jewish causes). **Priorities:** *Arts & Humanities:* 25%. Performing arts, public broadcasting, opera, theater, and ballet. *Civic & Public Affairs:* 6%. Supports legal centers. *Education:* 8%. Colleges and specialty schools. *Environment:* 12%. Youth and family projects. *International:* 20%. Hospitals and health centers. *Note:* Total contributions made in 1999. **Typ. Recipients:** Cancer, Children's Health/Hospitals, Clinics/Medical Centers, Emergency/Ambulance Services, Eyes/Blindness, Family Planning, Heart, Hospices, Hospitals, Kidney, Medical Education, Medical Rehabilitation, Mental Health, People with Disabilities, Single-Disease Health Associations, Substance Abuse. **Geo. Dist:** Palm Beach, FL; New York, NY, metropolitan area.

## ★ 414 ★ John A. and Delia T. Robert Charitable Trust 2

PO Box 10566
Birmingham, AL 35296
**Phone:** (205)558-6717
Arlene Henry, Trust Officer

**Fnded:** 1995. **Priorities:** *Arts & Humanities:* 25%. Funds historic preservation and libraries. *Civic & Public Affairs:* 7%. Supports safety. *Education:* 43%. Supports school and scholarship. *Environment:* 21%. *Note:* Total contributions made in 1999. **Typ. Recipients:** Child Abuse, Health Organizations, Hospitals, People with Disabilities, Public Health. **Geo. Dist:** Birmingham, AL.

## ★ 415 ★ John Ben Snow Memorial Trust

Jefferson Tower
50 Presidential Plaza, Ste. 106
Syracuse, NY 13202
**Phone:** (315)471-5256     **Fax:** (315)471-5256
Jonathan Snow, Trustee

**Fnded:** 1974. **Philosophy:** The John Ben Snow Memorial Trust makes most of its grants in the areas of education, civic affairs, and the arts. Educational funding favors universities and community colleges. Journalism is an area of focus. The arts are supported by grants to historic preservation, museums, and art centers. Grants also are made to other recipient areas, including disabled assistance organizations. **Priorities:** *Arts & Humanities:* 37%. Supports public broadcasting, art centers, and museums. *Civic & Public Affairs:* 14%. Funds community groups and municipalities. *Education:* 29%. Contributes to colleges, universities, law schools, and education associations. *Environment:* 12%. Funds youth groups. *International:* 4%. *Note:* Total contributions made in 1998. **Typ. Recipients:** Cancer, Clinics/Medical Centers, Family Planning, Geriatric Health, Health Funds, Hospitals, Medical Education, Medical Research, People with Disabilities. **Geo. Dist:** Eastern USA; NY.

## ★ 416 ★ John Edward Fowler Memorial Foundation

1725 K St. NW, Ste. 1201
Washington, DC 20006
**Phone:** (202)728-9080     **Fax:** (202)728-9082
**Website:** http://fdncenter.org/grantmaker/fowler
Richard Lee, President

**Fnded:** 1964. **Philosophy:** The Fowler Foundation is interested in supporting "smaller, well managed, non-profit organizations that have innovative ideas about how to help people help themselves." Most grants are limited to grassroots programs in the Washington, DC, area. *John Edward Fowler Memorial Foundation 1999 Grants Report* **Priorities:** *Arts & Humanities:* 7% (Arts in Education). Supports intensive arts outreach programs. *Civic & Public Affairs:* 12%. Primarily for employment and job training programs. *Education:* 22%. Funds after school programs for at-risk youth, and literacy programs. *Environment:* 31%. Primarily supports at-risk youth, shelters, and transitional housing. *International:* 14%. Funds pediatric and low-income health and clinics. *Note:* Total contributions made in 1999. **Typ. Recipients:** AIDS/HIV, Alzheimers Disease, Cancer, Children's Health/Hospitals, Clinics/Medical Centers, Domestic Violence, Emergency/Ambulance Services, Geriatric Health, Hospices, Hospitals (University Affiliated), Long-Term Care, Mental Health, Multiple Sclerosis, Outpatient Health Care, People with Disabilities, Prenatal Health Issues, Public Health. **Geo. Dist:** Washington, DC, including immediate metropolitan area.

## ★ 417 ★ John Ernest Bamberger and Ruth Eleanor Bamberger Memorial Foundation

136 South Main St., Ste. 418
Salt Lake City, UT 84101-1690
**Phone:** (801)364-2045
William Olwell, Secretary & Treasurer

**Fnded:** 1947. **Philosophy:** The foundation provides support primarily for social services, education, including scholarships for undergraduate student nurses, health organizations, and civic causes. **Priorities:** *Arts & Humanities:* 1%. *Civic & Public Affairs:* 10%. Legal aid and Native American affairs. *Education:* 37%. Secondary education, scholarships, literacy, private education, and colleges and universities. *Environment:* 30%. Youth organizations, child welfare, and YMCAs. *International:* 8%. Public health. *Note:* Total contributions made in 1998. **Typ. Recipients:** Alzheimers Disease, Cancer, Clinics/Medical Centers, Domestic Violence, Emergency/Ambulance Services, Family Planning, Health Organizations, Health-General, Hospices, Hospitals, Medical Education, Mental

Health, Multiple Sclerosis, Nursing Services, People with Disabilities, Public Health, Respiratory, Single-Disease Health Associations, Substance Abuse. **Geo. Dist:** Salt Lake City, UT.

**★ 418 ★ John G. and Marie Stella Kenedy Memorial Foundation**
1700 Tower II
Corpus Christi, TX 78478
**Phone:** (361)887-6565   **Fax:** (361)887-6582
**Email:** kmf@kenedy.org
Judy Gilbreath, Office Manager & Grants Officer
**Fnded:** 1960. **Philosophy:** A majority of the foundation's funding supports dioceses and religious organizations in Texas. Educational institutions and social services also receive funding. **Priorities:** *Civic & Public Affairs:* About 4%. Housing. *Education:* 31%. Academic scholarships. *Environment:* 12%. Focus on people with disabilities, child welfare, youth organizations, and substance abuse prevention. *International:* 2%. *Note:* Total contributions made in fiscal 1999. **Typ. Recipients:** AIDS/HIV, Hospitals, People with Disabilities, Substance Abuse. **Geo. Dist:** TX.

**★ 419 ★ John H. and Wilhelmina D. Harland Charitable Foundation**
2 Piedmont Center, Ste. 106
Atlanta, GA 30305
**Phone:** (404)264-9912   **Fax:** (404)266-8834
**Email:** harland@randomc.com
John Conant, Secretary
**Fnded:** 1972. **Philosophy:** The foundation was established to provide ongoing support to organizations personally supported by the donors, as well as to fund other institutions of a similar nature. The Harlands had a particular interest "in causes that serve children and higher education." These remain primary concerns of the foundation, but consideration is given to grant requests that fall within the following categories: education, health, community services, children and youth services, cultural and religious organizations. **Priorities:** *Arts & Humanities:* 17%. Funds arts centers, theatres, museums. *Civic & Public Affairs:* 5%. *Education:* 19%. Supports pre-college education and higher learning. *Environment:* 44%. Gives to youth programs, boys and girls clubs, and family services. *International:* 3%. Children's health. *Religion:* 2%. *Note:* Total contributions made in 1999. **Typ. Recipients:** Child Abuse, Children's Health/Hospitals, Clinics/Medical Centers, Domestic Violence, Emergency/Ambulance Services, Geriatric Health, Health Organizations, Hospitals, Long-Term Care, Medical Education, Mental Health, People with Disabilities, Public Health, Research/Studies Institutes, Single-Disease Health Associations, Speech & Hearing, Substance Abuse. **Geo. Dist:** Atlanta, GA, metropolitan area.

**★ 420 ★ John Huntington Fund for Education**
20620 North Park Boulevard, Ste. 215
Cleveland, OH 44118
**Phone:** (216)321-7185   **Fax:** (216)932-0331
Ann Pinkerton, Treasurer
**Fnded:** 1954. **Philosophy:** The foundation was established to fund student scholarships in the areas of science, nursing, and technology. The foundation makes grants to universities, nursing schools, art institutes, and other scholarship programs in Ohio. **Priorities:** *Education:* 100%. Academic scholarships. *Note:* Contributions made in 1999. **Typ. Recipients:** Hospitals (University Affiliated), Medical Education. **Geo. Dist:** OH, Cuyahoga County.

**★ 421 ★ John M. Olin Foundation**
330 Madison Ave., 22nd Floor
New York, NY 10017
**Phone:** (212)661-2670
**Website:** http://www.jmof.org
James Piereson, Executive Director
**Fnded:** 1953. **Philosophy:** The general purpose of the foundation "is to provide support for projects that reflect or are intended to strengthen the economic, political, and cultural institutions upon which the American heritage of constitutional government and enterprise is based. The foundation also seeks to promote a general understanding of these institutions by encouraging the thoughtful study of the connections between economic and political freedoms, and the cultural heritage that sustains them." The foundation encourages research on the formulation, implementation, and evaluation of public policy in the social and economic fields. Foundation-sponsored projects in this area have included tax policy, monetary policy, welfare policy, and fiscal policy. The foundation supports projects that address the relationship between American institutions and the international context in which they operate. Foundation-sponsored projects in this area have included studies of national security affairs, strategic issues, American foreign policy, and the international economy. The foundation also seeks to promote understanding of the moral, cultural, and institutional foundations of free government. The foundation, therefore, has supported studies of the American Constitution, the operation of the American political institutions, and the moral and cultural principles underlying these institutions. The foundation seeks to deepen understanding of the American judicial system and to preserve the rule of law as the foundation of American constitutional government. Support has gone to public interest law and to studies related to the judicial system, jurisprudence, and the relationship between law and economics. In each of these four areas, the foundation attempts to advance its objectives through research, institutional support, fellowships, professorships, lectures, books, scholarly journals, conferences and seminars, and occasional radio and television programs. **Priorities:** *Arts & Humanities:* 1%. Supports film, libraries, and art associations. *Civic & Public Affairs:* 40%. Supports civil rights and legal aid. *Education:* 44%. Supports education funds and programs. *Environment:* 1%. Primarily supports crime prevention. *International:* 2%. Supports single-disease health associations. *Note:* Total contributions made in 1998. **Typ. Recipients:** Health Organizations, Health Policy/Cost Containment, Single-Disease Health Associations. **Geo. Dist:** internationally; nationally.

**★ 422 ★ John and Mary Franklin Foundation**
3350 Riverwood Parkway, Ste. 2140
Atlanta, GA 30339
**Phone:** (770)933-2144   **Fax:** (770)993-2148
Dr. Marilu McCarty, Executive Secretary
**Fnded:** 1955. **Philosophy:** In 1955, John Franklin wrote that the foundation was to be organized solely for charitable, religious, scientific, and educational purposes. He listed fifteen charities which he and his wife had supported in the preceding year as an indication of their personal preferences. These consisted of health care institutions and social service organizations, primarily for young people. Mr. Franklin also described his and his wife's charitable interests in the fields of science, religion, and education. In the field of science, they were particularly interested in medical research, and listed the Heart Fund, Cancer Fund, and March of Dimes as typical recipients. In education, their primary interest was in educating the disabled so that they might lead fuller lives, listing the Atlanta Speech School and the Muscular Dystrophy Fund as examples. While not specifying any religious charity by name, Mr. Franklin did state that appropriations should be made without respect to denomination, creed, or color and should be governed by the demands of the particular time. The foundation is managed by a nine-member board of trustees which has followed and expanded on the pattern of grants described by John Franklin. Grants generally are limited to the metropolitan Atlanta area, although special grants occasionally are made to institutions in other areas of Georgia and in adjoining states. **Priorities:** *Arts & Humanities:* 4%. Supports ballet, historical preservation, and art centers. *Civic & Public Affairs:* 4%. Funds parks and botanical gardens. *Education:* 76%. Supports schools, colleges and universities, and scholarship funds. *Environment:* 10%. Supports youth organizations and United Way. *International:* 3%. Supports American Red Cross and children's health.

*Note:* Total contributions made in 1999. **Typ. Recipients:** Cancer, Children's Health/Hospitals, Clinics/Medical Centers, Emergency/Ambulance Services, Family Planning, Geriatric Health, Health Policy/Cost Containment, Hospices, Hospitals, Long-Term Care, Medical Education, Medical Research, Medical Training, Mental Health, People with Disabilities, Single-Disease Health Associations. **Geo. Dist:** Atlanta, GA, including metropolitan area.

**★ 423 ★ John P. McGovern Foundation**
2211 Norfolk, Ste. 900
Houston, TX 77098-4044
**Phone:** (713)661-4808   **Fax:** (713)661-3031
Dr. John McGovern, President
**Fnded:** 1961. **Philosophy:** The foundation primarily supports medical research organizations and medical funds, primarily in the area of the prevention of alcohol and substance abuse, with some focus on prevention of allergies. **Priorities:** *Arts & Humanities:* 1%. Supports libraries and museums. *Civic & Public Affairs:* 7%. Funds a foundation and community associations. *Education:* 3%. Supports universities and student exchange programs. *Environment:* 76%. Major gift to McGovern Fund. *International:* 12%. Supports a medical institute and museum of health and medical science. *Note:* Total contributions made in 1999. **Typ. Recipients:** Cancer, Child Abuse, Children's Health/Hospitals, Clinics/Medical Centers, Eyes/Blindness, Health Funds, Health Organizations, Health-General, Heart, Hospitals, Medical Education, Medical Rehabilitation, Medical Research, Mental Health, Public Health, Substance Abuse. **Geo. Dist:** some giving nationally; Houston, TX.

**★ 424 ★ John P. Murphy Foundation**
Terminal Twr.
50 Pulbic Sq., Ste. 924
Cleveland, OH 44113-2203
**Phone:** (216)623-4770   **Fax:** (216)623-4773
Mr. Allan Zambie, Executive Vice President
**Fnded:** 1960. **Philosophy:** The foundation's articles of incorporation state that the foundation will distribute its grants for "charitable, educational, scientific, literary, and religious purposes." Educational grants are usually made to colleges and universities. Artistic and cultural grants generally range from $1,000 to $50,000. Grants to social service organizations typically are below $5,000, and are given to a wide variety of needs. Community service grants also are given to numerous types of organizations. Most of the foundation's health grants are given to hospital building programs. **Priorities:** *Arts & Humanities:* 30%. Includes the highest grant of $5,000,000 to the University of Notre Dame law school. *Civic & Public Affairs:* 6%. Supports community affairs organizations. *Education:* 49%. Primarily supports colleges and universities and educational associations. *Environment:* 4%. United funds, food banks, child welfare, and YMCAs. *International:* 7%. Hospitals, nursing services, clinics, and medical rehabilitation. *Religion:* Less than 1%. *Note:* Total contributions made in 1999. **Typ. Recipients:** Cancer, Children's Health/Hospitals, Clinics/Medical Centers, Family Planning, Health Funds, Health Organizations, Heart, Hospices, Hospitals, Hospitals (University Affiliated), Long-Term Care, Medical Education, Medical Rehabilitation, Medical Research, Mental Health, Nursing Services, People with Disabilities, Preventive Medicine/Wellness Organizations, Public Health, Sexual Abuse, Single-Disease Health Associations, Substance Abuse. **Geo. Dist:** Cleveland, OH, metropolitan area and adjacent counties in Northeastern Ohio.

**★ 425 ★ The John R. Oishei Foundation**
One HSBC Center, Ste. 3650
Buffalo, NY 14203-2805
**Phone:** (716)856-9490   **Fax:** (716)856-9493
**Website:** http://www.oisheifdt.org
Thomas Baker, Executive Director
**Fnded:** 1941. **Philosophy:** "The Foundation's mission is to act as a catalyst for change in the greater Buffalo community by supporting creative programs which attempt to advance the status quo, are strategi-

cally sound and are strongly focused on excellence. Its principal grant-making areas include medical research and care, education, cultural and social needs. The fundamental goal of the Foundation is to enhance the quality of life for members of the Buffalo community as well as to enhance the reputation of the city and the region." **Priorities:** *Arts & Humanities:* 10%. Supports theaters, libraries, music, and arts institutes. *Civic & Public Affairs:* 3%. Major support for the Erie County Bar Association. *Education:* 47%. Supports colleges and universities in Buffalo, NY. *Environment:* 6%. Supports charities, orphanages, youth activities, aid to children, aid to the underprivileged, counseling and Junior Achievement, and the elderly. *International:* 28%. Emphasis on medical research and hospitals. *Note:* Total contributions made in 1999. **Typ. Recipients:** AIDS/HIV, Alzheimers Disease, Children's Health/Hospitals, Emergency/Ambulance Services, Geriatric Health, Health Organizations, Hospices, Hospitals, Long-Term Care, Medical Education, Medical Research, People with Disabilities, Substance Abuse. **Geo. Dist:** NY, Greater Western New York area; Buffalo, NY. **Frmly:** Julia R. and Estelle L. Foundation.

### ★ 426 ★ John Randolph and Dora Haynes Foundation

888 West 6th St., Ste. 1150
Los Angeles, CA 90017-2737
**Phone:** (213)623-9151          **Fax:** (213)623-3951
**Email:** info@haynesfoundation.org
**Website:** http://www.haynesfoundation.org
Diane Cornwell, Administrative Director
**Fnded:** 1926. **Philosophy:** "The Foundation attempts to reflect directly the interests of Dr. and Mrs. Haynes by focusing its resources on the fields which particularly concerned them. Accordingly, the Trustees of the Foundation support study and research in political science, economics, public policy, history, social psychology, and sociology, favoring projects with specific application to the Los Angeles area. By dissemination of the results of the research, and by other means, the Foundation seeks to improve public awareness and understanding of current issues." "Foundation also provides in the social sciences, undergraduate scholarships, graduate fellowships, and faculty research fellowships to selected colleges and universities in the greater Los Angeles area." 2000 Annual Report **Priorities:** *Arts & Humanities:* 17%. Supports historical societies, libraries, and museums. *Civic & Public Affairs:* 4%. *Education:* About 76%. Funds fellowships, internships, and scholarships to colleges and other educational institutions. *Note:* Total contributions made in fiscal 2000. **Typ. Recipients:** Children's Health/Hospitals, Geriatric Health, Health Policy/Cost Containment, Medical Education, Medical Research, Substance Abuse. **Geo. Dist:** Los Angeles, CA, metropolitan area.

### ★ 427 ★ John S. Dunn Research Foundation

3355 West Alabama, Ste. 720
Houston, TX 77098-1718
**Phone:** (713)626-0369          **Fax:** (713)626-0368
Milby Dunn, President
**Fnded:** 1985. **Philosophy:** The foundation typically funds organizations "whose primary efforts are medically related to educational and research activities." **Priorities:** *Civic & Public Affairs:* 1%. *Education:* 4%. Funds medical education and private schools. *Environment:* 12%. Medically-related social service concerns. *International:* 83%. Supports medical research, hospitals, clinics, and single-disease associations. *Note:* Contributions made in 1998. **Typ. Recipients:** Alzheimers Disease, Cancer, Children's Health/Hospitals, Clinics/Medical Centers, Diabetes, Eyes/Blindness, Health Funds, Health Organizations, Heart, Hospices, Hospitals (University Affiliated), Medical Education, Medical Rehabilitation, Medical Research, People with Disabilities, Public Health, Respiratory, Single-Disease Health Associations, Speech & Hearing. **Geo. Dist:** TX.

### ★ 428 ★ John S. and James L. Knight Foundation

One Biscayne Tower, Ste. 3800
2 South Biscayne Boulevard
Miami, FL 33131-1803
**Phone:** (305)908-2600          **Fax:** (305)908-2698
**Email:** publications@knightfdu.org
**Website:** http://www.knightfdn.org
Hodding Carter, III, President & Chief Executive Officer
**Fnded:** 1950. **Philosophy:** "The John S. and James Knight Foundation was established in 1950 as a private foundation independent of the Knight brothers' newspaper enterprises. It is dedicated to furthering their ideals of service to community, to the highest standards of journalistic excellence and to the defense of a free press." "In both their publishing and philanthropic undertakings, the Knight brothers shared a broad vision and uncommon devotion to the common welfare. It is those ideals, as well as their philanthropic interests, to which the Foundation remains faithful. "To heighten the impact of their grantmaking, Knight Foundation's trustees have elected to focus on four programs, each with its own eligibility requirements: Community Initiatives, Journalism, Education and Arts and Culture. "In a rapidly changing world, the Foundation also remains flexible enough to respond to unique challenges, ideas and projects that lie beyond its identified program areas, yet would fulfill the broad vision of its founders. "None of the grantmaking would be possible without a sound financial base. Thus, preserving and enhancing the Foundation's assets through prudent investment management continues to be of paramount importance." Annual Report **Priorities:** *Arts & Humanities:* Supports the symphony orchestra initiative, museums, arts festivals, theater, libraries, dance, opera, ballet, and historic preservation. *Education:* 57%. Primarily for journalism, supporting the education of current and future journalists and defending free press worldwide. Also funds colleges and universities and education reform programs. *Environment:* 20%. Emphasis on child and social welfare literacy, community development, citizenship, homelessness, and disaster relief. *Note:* Total contributions made in 1999. **Typ. Recipients:** Cancer, Children's Health/Hospitals, Emergency/Ambulance Services, Health Organizations, Hospices, Hospitals, Medical Research, Mental Health, Prenatal Health Issues, Substance Abuse. **Geo. Dist:** nationally.  .

### ★ 429 ★ John Simon Guggenheim Memorial Foundation

90 Park Ave.
New York, NY 10016
**Phone:** (212)687-4470          **Fax:** (212)697-3248
**Email:** fellowships@gf.org
**Website:** http://www.gf.org
**Fnded:** 1925. **Philosophy:** The foundation "offers fellowships to further the development of scholars and artists by assisting them to engage in research in any field of knowledge and creation in any of the arts, under the freest possible conditions and irrespective of race, color, or creed." The foundation offers fellowships through two annual competitions: one open to citizens and permanent residents of the United States and Canada, and the other open to citizens and permanent residents of Latin America and the Caribbean. **Priorities:** *Arts & Humanities:* 17%. Supports film/video, dance, history, libraries. *Civic & Public Affairs:* 2%. Supports general civic affairs. *Education:* 79%. Supports religion education, universities, faculty development, arts/humanities education, medical education, and technical education. *Note:* Contributions analysis represents total contributions in 1998. The foundation reports that percentages vary from year to year. **Typ. Recipients:** Medical Education, Medical Research. **Geo. Dist:** nationally; Latin America and the Caribbean.

### ★ 430 ★ John Smith Charities

PO Box 608
Greenville, SC 29608
**Phone:** (864)271-5929          **Fax:** (864)271-5991
Vicki McGartiy, Contact
**Fnded:** 1985. **Philosophy:** John Smith Charities primarily supports education and social services. Educational funding favors colleges, religious education, universities, and private education. Social service support goes to public housing, food distribution, family counseling, and youth camps. Other recipient areas are supported by the foundation are the arts, and health care. **Priorities:** *Arts & Humanities:* 7%. Funds performing arts, symphonies, public broadcasting, theaters, museums, and historical societies. *Civic & Public Affairs:* 40%. Supports community foundations, and women's affairs. *Education:* 39%. Includes a major grant to the South Carolina Governor's School for the Arts. *Environment:* 3%. Supports scouts and YMCA. *Note:* Total contributions made in fiscal 1999. **Typ. Recipients:** Cancer, Clinics/Medical Centers, Emergency/Ambulance Services, Health Organizations, Hospitals, Hospitals (University Affiliated), Long-Term Care, Medical Education, Mental Health, People with Disabilities, Single-Disease Health Associations. **Geo. Dist:** SC, Upstate South Carolina.

### ★ 431 ★ John Steele Zink Foundation

1259 East 26th St.
Tulsa, OK 74114
**Phone:** (918)743-9468
Jacqueline Zink, Trustee
**Fnded:** 1972. **Philosophy:** The John Steele Zink Foundation provides funding to various cultural programs, including museums, theater companies, dance, and music in the Tulsa area. It supports philanthropic organizations, educational funds, and local colleges. The foundation is committed to social service in its contributions to community and youth organizations, as well as to united funds. It also supports local churches. **Priorities:** *Arts & Humanities:* 22%. Mostly funding music programs and theater. *Civic & Public Affairs:* About 37%. Foundation continuing support and operating funds. *Education:* About 11% Colleges and universities in Tulsa OK. *Environment:* 10%. Scouting and youth programs, support groups and humane society. *International:* 17%. Single-disease health associations and emergency health projects. *Note:* Total contributions made in fiscal 1997. **Typ. Recipients:** AIDS/HIV, Child Abuse, Children's Health/Hospitals, Clinics/Medical Centers, Emergency/Ambulance Services, Family Planning, Heart, Hospitals, Mental Health, Multiple Sclerosis, People with Disabilities, Prenatal Health Issues, Sexual Abuse, Speech & Hearing. **Geo. Dist:** Tulsa, OK.

### John Templeton Foundation

*See:* Entry 10046

### ★ 432 ★ John W. Anderson Foundation

402 Wall St.
Valparaiso, IN 46383
**Phone:** (219)462-4611
**Email:** info@templeton.org
**Website:** http://www.templeton.org
William Vinovich, Vice Chairman
**Fnded:** 1967. **Philosophy:** "The John W. Anderson Foundation was created in 1967 for the purpose of supporting such charitable, religious, scientific, literary or educational purposes within the United States as the Trustees, in their discretion, shall determine will best promote the mental, moral, intellectual and physical improvement, assistance and relief of inhabitants of the United States, of all races and creeds and particularly youth who reside in and near Lake and Porter Counties in Northwest Indiana." John W. Anderson Foundation 1999 Annual Report, Grant Application and Guidelines Brochure. **Priorities:** *Arts & Humanities:* 3%. Gives to music and public broadcasting. *Civic & Public Affairs:* 2%. Supports economic development. *Education:* 27%. Funds colleges and universities and education funds. *Environment:* 53%. Supports youth groups, united funds, and social services. *International:* 12%. Contributions go to medical research and health associations. *Note:* Total contributions were made in 2000. **Typ. Recipients:** Cancer, Children's Health/Hospitals, Clinics/Medical Centers, Emergency/Ambulance Services, Family Planning, Health Organizations, Heart, Hospices,

Medical Education, Medical Rehabilitation, Mental Health, Nursing Services, People with Disabilities, Public Health, Research/Studies Institutes, Single-Disease Health Associations. **Geo. Dist:** IL, funds some organizations in Northeastern Illinois; IN.

**★ 433 ★ John W. and Effie E. Speas Memorial Trust**
PO Box 419119
Kansas City, MO 64141-6119
**Phone:** (816)979-7481          **Fax:** (816)979-7916
David Ross, Senior Vice President

**Fnded:** 1947. **Philosophy:** The Speas Memorial Trust supports a variety of health and social service organizations, with some focus on mental health and substance abuse programs. Recently, it has initiated services for the elderly in the Kansas City metropolitan area, with emphasis on helping the elderly to continue to reside in their own homes, and on providing respite care. The trust also contributes to university medical schools. **Priorities:** *Civic & Public Affairs:* 3%. Supports community foundations. *Education:* 30%. Supports healthcare programs at colleges and universities. *Environment:* 18%. Supports family services, United Way, and youth organizations. *International:* 41%. Funds hospitals, medical centers, and cancer research. *Note:* Total contributions made in 1998. **Typ. Recipients:** Cancer, Child Abuse, Children's Health/Hospitals, Clinics/Medical Centers, Emergency/Ambulance Services, Eyes/Blindness, Geriatric Health, Health Organizations, Health Policy/Cost Containment, Heart, Home-Care Services, Hospices, Hospitals, Hospitals (University Affiliated), Kidney, Long-Term Care, Medical Education, Medical Rehabilitation, Medical Research, Medical Training, Mental Health, Multiple Sclerosis, Nursing Services, Nutrition, People with Disabilities, Prenatal Health Issues, Preventive Medicine/Wellness Organizations, Public Health, Single-Disease Health Associations, Speech & Hearing, Substance Abuse, Transplant Networks/Donor Banks. **Geo. Dist:** KS, Johnson County; KS, Wyandotte County; MO, Cass County; MO, Clay County; MO, Jackson County; MO, Platte County.

**★ 434 ★ John Wesley and Anna Hodgin Hanes Foundation**
100 North Main
PO Box 3099
Winston-Salem, NC 27150-7131
**Phone:** (336)770-5000          **Fax:** (336)732-6537
Linda Tilley, Relationship Manager

**Fnded:** 1947. **Philosophy:** The Trust Agreement for the foundation stated that "the income and principal of the Trust shall be used exclusively for such charitable, scientific, literary, or educational purposes...as a majority of the individual trustees...shall determine." The foundation has a primary interest in Winston-Salem and Forsyth county in North Carolina where it is located. "It has always been interested in improving the life of the citizens of North Carolina and will continue to support this interest with funding. However, it is a prime requirement of the foundation that organizations seeking funding show that the community in which the organization is located and the organization's trustees have given substantial financial support prior to consideration by the foundation." **Priorities:** *Arts & Humanities:* 54%. Supports libraries, music, theater, museum, and historic preservation. *Education:* 4%. Supports general education. *Environment:* 15%. Supports Special Olympics, community centers, Young Men's Christian Association, and athletics/recreation. *International:* 17%. Supports medical equipment, Alzheimers research, and children's hospitals. *Religion:* 3%. Funds science centers. *Note:* Total contributions made in 1998. **Typ. Recipients:** AIDS/HIV, Alzheimers Disease, Clinics/Medical Centers, Domestic Violence, Emergency/Ambulance Services, Eyes/Blindness, Family Planning, Health Funds, Hospices, Hospitals, Medical Rehabilitation, People with Disabilities, Public Health, Single-Disease Health Associations, Substance Abuse, Transplant Networks/Donor Banks. **Geo. Dist:** NC, Forsyth County; Winston-Salem, NC.

**★ 435 ★ Joseph Alexander Foundation**
400 Madison Ave., Ste. 906
New York, NY 10017
**Phone:** (212)355-3688
Robert Weintraub, Vice President & Director

**Fnded:** 1960. **Philosophy:** The Joseph Alexander Foundation makes most of its grants in the areas of health, education, and social services. Health funding favors cancer and AIDS research and treatment, hospitals, and geriatric care. Educational support primarily goes to Jewish universities, medical education, and legal education. In social services, interests include the aged, the disabled, homes for children, family services, and community centers. The foundation also makes grants to other recipient areas. **Priorities:** *Arts & Humanities:* 7%. Support for a heritage center. *Civic & Public Affairs:* 5%. Supports community foundations *Education:* 26%. Funds colleges and universities, Jewish studies, and education associations. *Environment:* 5%. Youth programs supported. *International:* 15%. Supports medical research, hospitals, single-disease health associations, and geriatric health. *Religion:* 1%. *Note:* Total contributions made in fiscal 1998. **Typ. Recipients:** AIDS/HIV, Alzheimers Disease, Cancer, Children's Health/Hospitals, Children's Health/Hospitals, Clinics/Medical Centers, Diabetes, Emergency/Ambulance Services, Eyes/Blindness, Family Planning, Geriatric Health, Health Funds, Health Organizations, Hospitals, Kidney, Long-Term Care, Medical Education, Medical Rehabilitation, Medical Research, Mental Health, Multiple Sclerosis, Nursing Services, People with Disabilities, Single-Disease Health Associations, Substance Abuse, Transplant Networks/Donor Banks, Trauma Treatment. **Geo. Dist:** nationally; New York, NY.

**★ 436 ★ Joseph B. Whitehead Foundation**
50 Hurt Plaza, Ste. 1200
Atlanta, GA 30303
**Phone:** (404)522-6755          **Fax:** (404)522-7026
**Email:** fdns@woodruff.org
**Website:** http://www.jbwhitehead.org
Charles McTier, President

**Fnded:** 1937. **Philosophy:** The foundation was established with a particular interest in benefiting children. Its primary areas of giving include human services, particularly for children and youth; elementary and secondary education; health care; economic development and civic affairs; literacy and vocational training; art and cultural activities; and environmental education. **Priorities:** *Civic & Public Affairs:* 8%. General public affairs and philanthropy, and volunteerism. *Education:* 23%. General education programs, primary and secondary, higher education, and special education. *Environment:* 58%. Mostly child/youth welfare, housing and shelter, care of elderly, and the disabled. *International:* Less than 1%. Focus on hospitals and medical care, public and preventive health, and general health. *Note:* Total contributions made in 1998 in the greater Atlanta area. **Typ. Recipients:** Alzheimers Disease, Arthritis, Cancer, Child Abuse, Children's Health/Hospitals, Clinics/Medical Centers, Domestic Violence, Family Planning, Health Organizations, Health Policy/Cost Containment, Health-General, Home-Care Services, Hospitals, Kidney, Medical Rehabilitation, Mental Health, Nursing Services, People with Disabilities, Prenatal Health Issues, Preventive Medicine/Wellness Organizations, Public Health, Respiratory, Single-Disease Health Associations, Substance Abuse, Trauma Treatment. **Geo. Dist:** Atlanta, GA, including metropolitan area.

**★ 437 ★ Joseph and Bessie Feinberg Foundation**
5245 West Lawrence Ave.
Chicago, IL 60630
**Phone:** (773)777-8600
Ruben Feinberg, President

**Fnded:** 1969. **Philosophy:** A majority of the foundation's funding goes to higher education in support of universities and Jewish theological seminaries. Jewish religious organizations are also a major interest. The foundation supports other charitable recipient organizations with minor grants. **Priorities:** *Arts & Humanities:* 4%. Supports public broadcasting, Lyric Opera, and the Ravinia Festival Association. *Civic & Public Affairs:* 1%. Legal affairs. *Education:* 2%. Funds colleges, universities, and educational programs. *Environment:* 1%. *International:* 76%. Supports hospitals, the Gastro Intestinal Research Foundation, and other disease and disorder concerns. *Note:* Total contributions made in fiscal 1998. **Typ. Recipients:** Children's Health/Hospitals, Clinics/Medical Centers, Health Organizations, Heart, Hospitals, Kidney, Medical Education, Medical Research, Multiple Sclerosis, People with Disabilities, Single-Disease Health Associations. **Geo. Dist:** Chicago, IL; NY.

**★ 438 ★ Joseph Drown Foundation**
1999 Ave. of the Stars, Ste. 1930
Los Angeles, CA 90067
**Phone:** (310)277-4488          **Fax:** (310)277-4573
**Email:** staff@jdrown.org
**Website:** http://www.jdrown.org
Wendy Wachtell Schine, Vice President, Program Director

**Fnded:** 1953. **Philosophy:** The foundation's focus remains education and medical research. In education, it funds loan programs in higher education and reform programs in K-12. Some funding is also available for scholarships. The focus on medical and scientific research remains broad, but no unsolicited grant requests in this area are accepted. The grantmaking in community health and social services is geared towards improving life in the local community. The focus is on programs that deal with issues such as high drop-out rates, teen pregnancy, lack of sufficient health care, substance abuse, and violence. The funding in the arts and humanities is limited to outreach and education. **Priorities:** *Arts & Humanities:* 2%. Primarily supports outreach and art education programs. *Civic & Public Affairs:* 3%. Supports legal defense and feminist efforts. *Education:* 30%. Supports public and private education. *Environment:* 11%. Gives to child welfare, youth organizations, and senior services. *International:* 51%. Primary support for single-disease health associations, medical research, and hospitals. *Note:* Total contributions made in fiscal 2000. **Typ. Recipients:** Adolescent Health Issues, Alzheimers Disease, Arthritis, Cancer, Children's Health/Hospitals, Clinics/Medical Centers, Diabetes, Emergency/Ambulance Services, Eyes/Blindness, Family Planning, Health Organizations, Health-General, Heart, Hospitals (University Affiliated), Long-Term Care, Medical Education, Medical Research, Mental Health, Outpatient Health Care, People with Disabilities, Preventive Medicine/Wellness Organizations, Research/Studies Institutes, Single-Disease Health Associations, Speech & Hearing, Substance Abuse. **Geo. Dist:** CA.

**★ 439 ★ Josiah Macy, Jr. Foundation**
44 East 64th St.
New York, NY 10021
**Phone:** (212)486-2424          **Fax:** (212)644-0765
**Website:** http://www.josiahmacyjrfoundation.org
Martha Wolfgang, Vice President

**Fnded:** 1930. **Philosophy:** Traditionally, the Macy Foundation has focused on medicine and health. This stems from Mrs. Ladd's personal interest in these areas. Her instructions, intended to guide the foundation's giving, were concerned with "fundamental aspects of health, of sickness, and of methods for the relief of suffering." "Today the Foundation focuses support on issues that challenge the education of health professionals, such as the increasing need for teamwork, the provision of primary care in the changing environment of health-care management and delivery, and the increasing need for diversity of health-care professionals. In addition, some programs address the fundamental shifts in medical and other health professional education necessitated by the rapid rate of advance in such areas as human genetics." Two recent conferences sponsored by the Foundation focused on ways to improve working relationships between medicine and public health, and the growing challenge of health education posed by rapid advances in genetics. 1997 annual report **Priori-**

**ties:** *Arts & Humanities:* Less than 1%. *Civic & Public Affairs:* 5%. Includes support for other foundations or community programs. *Education:* 56%. Includes support for colleges and universities. *International:* 28%. Includes support for medical training, nursing, health policy organizations, and health professionals training. *Religion:* 9%. Includes support for laboratories. *Note:* Total contributions made in fiscal 2000. **Typ. Recipients:** AIDS/HIV, Cancer, Children's Health/Hospitals, Clinics/Medical Centers, Family Planning, Health Funds, Health Organizations, Health Policy/Cost Containment, Hospitals, Hospitals (University Affiliated), Medical Education, Medical Research, Medical Training, Nursing Services, Public Health, Single-Disease Health Associations, Substance Abuse. **Geo. Dist:** nationally.

### ★ 440 ★ Josiah W. and Bessie H. Kline Foundation

515 S 29th St.
Harrisburg, PA 17104
**Phone:** (717)561-4373     **Fax:** (717)561-0826
John Obrock, CPA

**Fnded:** 1952. **Philosophy:** The foundation makes most of its grants in the areas of education, health, and social services in south-central Pennsylvania. Educational funding supports various small colleges and universities in Pennsylvania. Health interests include medical centers, health foundations, and hospitals. Social service support goes to community centers, family services, and youth organizations. The foundation also makes grants to the arts and civic affairs in south-central Pennsylvania. **Priorities:** *Arts & Humanities:* 20%. Funds public broadcasting, theater, opera, and libraries. *Civic & Public Affairs:* 2%. Supports housing and clubs. *Education:* 22%. Emphasis on Pennsylvania Colleges and Universities, minority education and public education. *Environment:* 21%. Primary support given to organizations such as United Way, the Pennsylvania Special Olympics, organizations that support crippled children. food banks and scouting. *International:* 26%. Supports hospitals, medical centers, hospice and single disease health associations. *Note:* Total contributions made in 1999. **Typ. Recipients:** Alzheimers Disease, Cancer, Children's Health/Hospitals, Clinics/Medical Centers, Diabetes, Emergency/Ambulance Services, Family Planning, Health Organizations, Health-General, Heart, Hospices, Hospitals, Kidney, Medical Rehabilitation, Medical Research, Mental Health, Multiple Sclerosis, Nursing Services, Outpatient Health Care, People with Disabilities, Public Health, Single-Disease Health Associations, Substance Abuse. **Geo. Dist:** PA.

### ★ 441 ★ Joukowsky Family Foundation

410 Park Ave., Ste. 1610
New York, NY 10022
**Email:** info@joukowsky.org
**Website:** http://www.joukowsky.org
Nina Koprulu, Director and President

**Fnded:** 1981. **Philosophy:** The Joukowsky Family Foundation makes most of its grants in the area of education. Additional funding is available for civic affairs, the arts, health care, international affairs, religion, and social services. **Priorities:** *Arts & Humanities:* 5%. Historical associations and music. *Education:* 80%. Primary support for colleges and universities and preparatory schools. *Environment:* 7%. Supports united funds, family planning, child welfare, and the homeless. *Note:* Contributions made in fiscal 2000. **Typ. Recipients:** Diabetes, Domestic Violence, Family Planning, Hospices, Hospitals, Medical Education, Medical Rehabilitation, Medical Research, People with Disabilities, Single-Disease Health Associations. **Geo. Dist:** U.S. Northeast Region; internationally; natioanlly. **Frmly:** The Joukowsky Foundation.

### ★ 442 ★ Judd S. Alexander Foundation

PO Box 2137
Wausau, WI 54402-2137
**Phone:** (715)845-4556     **Fax:** (715)848-9336
Gary Freels, President

**Fnded:** 1973. **Philosophy:** The Judd S. Alexander Foundation makes most of its grants in the areas of social services and civic affairs. Social service interests include youth organizations, recreation, and human development. In civic affairs, funding favors community philanthropic organizations, economic development, and municipalities. Other areas of interest include health care, the arts, and education. **Priorities:** *Arts & Humanities:* 14%. Performing arts, museums, and music. *Civic & Public Affairs:* 31%. Chambers of commerce, county services. *Education:* 29%. Precollege and college education. *Environment:* 14%. Big Brothers, children and youth services. *International:* 4%. *Note:* Total contributions made in fiscal 1998. **Typ. Recipients:** Cancer, Clinics/Medical Centers, Health Funds, Heart, Hospices, Hospitals, Medical Training, People with Disabilities, Public Health, Respiratory, Single-Disease Health Associations. **Geo. Dist:** programs that directly affect and benefit the residents of Marathon County.

### ★ 443 ★ Julius Frankel Foundation

111 West Monroe St., 7 West
Chicago, IL 60603-4003
**Phone:** (312)461-5564     **Fax:** (312)765-1279
**Email:** rebecca.mcdade@harrisbank.com
Rebecca McDade, Vice President

**Fnded:** 1959. **Philosophy:** The foundation principally supports the arts, concentrating on music and dance; higher education; hospitals and health organizations; and social welfare groups. **Priorities:** *Arts & Humanities:* 30%. Supports museums, opera, symphonies, and ballet. *Civic & Public Affairs:* 5%. Funds youth job programs, housing programs, and community foundations. *Education:* 20%. Emphasis on schools and institutes. *Environment:* 20%. Grants are made to youth centers and programs, and family services. *International:* 25% Supports hospitals, medical centers, and rehabilitation centers. *Note:* Total contributions made in fiscal 1999. **Typ. Recipients:** Children's Health/Hospitals, Clinics/Medical Centers, Hospices, Hospitals, Hospitals (University Affiliated), Long-Term Care, Medical Education, Medical Rehabilitation, Medical Research, People with Disabilities, Public Health, Public Health, Speech & Hearing. **Geo. Dist:** IL.

### ★ 444 ★ June Rockwell Levy Foundation

175 Federal St.
Boston, MA 02110
**Phone:** (617)574-3426
Jonathan Loring, Contact

**Fnded:** 1947. **Philosophy:** The June Rockwell Levy Foundation supports a variety of charitable organizations. Health care support favors general hospitals and medical foundations. Private education and colleges are favored for educational support. All areas of social services and civic affairs are supported by the foundation. The arts and international organizations receive minor support. **Priorities:** *Arts & Humanities:* 32%. Supports public libraries, repertory theater, museums, the philharmonic, and symphony orchestras. *Civic & Public Affairs:* 9%. Supports community and civic affairs. *Education:* 14%. Supports educational institutions, services, and programs. *Environment:* 18%. Supports family services, Planned Parenthood, United Way, animal shelters, and social services. *International:* 17%. Supports hospitals, rehabilitation centers, and disease and disorder concerns. *Note:* Contributions were made in 1998. **Typ. Recipients:** AIDS/HIV, Cancer, Children's Health/Hospitals, Clinics/Medical Centers, Diabetes, Domestic Violence, Emergency/Ambulance Services, Family Planning, Geriatric Health, Health Funds, Health Organizations, Home-Care Services, Hospices, Hospitals, Long-Term Care, Medical Education, Medical Rehabilitation, Medical Research, Mental Health, Nursing Services, People with Disabilities, Public Health, Sexual Abuse, Single-Disease Health Associations, Substance Abuse. **Geo. Dist:** MA; RI.

### ★ 445 ★ Jurodin Fund

450 Lexington Ave.
New York, NY 10017
**Phone:** (212)531-1790     **Fax:** (212)531-1982

**Email:** ISJ19BIX@aol.com
Irene Steiner, Secretary

**Fnded:** 1960. **Philosophy:** The Jurodin Fund primarily supports education and religious organizations. Education funding favors colleges and legal education. Jewish religious organizations are also a major priority. Secondary interests include medical centers, civic affairs, and the arts. **Priorities:** *Arts & Humanities:* 1%. Museums, music, libraries, and public broadcasting. *Education:* 88%. Major grant to New York University. *Environment:* 1%. Supports the United Way. *International:* 5%. Funds hospitals. *Note:* Total contributions made in 1998. **Typ. Recipients:** Cancer, Clinics/Medical Centers, Emergency/Ambulance Services, Family Planning, Health Organizations, Hospitals, Medical Education, Medical Rehabilitation, Medical Research, Nursing Services, People with Disabilities, Single-Disease Health Associations. **Geo. Dist:** U.S. Northeast Region; New York, NY.

### ★ 446 ★ Kansas Health Foundation

309 East Douglas
Wichita, KS 67202-3405
**Phone:** (316)262-7676     **Fax:** (316)262-2044
**Email:** nclaassen@khf.org
**Website:** http://www.kansashealth.org
Nancy Claassen, Grants Manager

**Fnded:** 1978. **Philosophy:** The Foundation has three program finding categories: Public Health, Leadership, and Children's Health. The Public Health mission is "to develop and support population-based health in Kansas so preventative measures are utilized to improve the health of Kansans." The Leadership mission is "to build the capacity of individuals to improve the health of all Kansans." The Children's Health mission is "to improve the health of Kansans by creating an environment that puts children first so they become caring, thinking and contributing adults." 2000 Annual Report. **Priorities:** *Education:* 4%. *Leadership. International:* 75%. Funds public health, and childrens health. *Note:* Total contributions made in 1998. **Typ. Recipients:** Adolescent Health Issues, AIDS/HIV, Alzheimers Disease, Cancer, Child Abuse, Children's Health/Hospitals, Clinics/Medical Centers, Domestic Violence, Emergency/Ambulance Services, Geriatric Health, Health Organizations, Health Policy/Cost Containment, Health Policy/Cost Containment, Heart, Home-Care Services, Hospices, Hospitals, Hospitals (University Affiliated), Medical Education, Medical Rehabilitation, Medical Research, Medical Training, Nursing Services, Nutrition, People with Disabilities, Prenatal Health Issues, Preventive Medicine/Wellness Organizations, Public Health, Research/Studies Institutes, Respiratory, Sexual Abuse, Substance Abuse. **Geo. Dist:** KS.

### ★ 447 ★ Kate B. Reynolds Charitable Trust

128 Reynolda Village
Winston-Salem, NC 27106-5123
**Phone:** (336)723-1456     **Fax:** (336)723-7765
**Email:** kbarray@kbr.org
**Website:** http://www.kbr.org
E. Cope, President

**Fnded:** 1947. **Philosophy:** Three-quarters of the total income from the trust is expended through the Health Care Division, which supports innovative health care programs throughout North Carolina, with the remaining 25% of contributions being disbursed through the Poor and Needy Division. Each division has its own advisory board to provide guidance on plans and priorities for the use of funds and to review and recommend approval of specific grant requests. The Health Care Division funds are used to encourage and support innovative programs that increase the availability of health services to under-served groups. This division also provides support for other types of health programs which have merit and which are related to the goal of the division. The Poor and Needy Division funds are used to support organizations which provide for basic needs, such as food, clothing, shelter, and health care. The division also funds efforts that seek to reduce reliance upon support services or that promote maximum levels of functioning for those with chronic problems, and supports other types of programs that have merit and are related to the goal of the division. **Priorities:** *Civic & Public Affairs:* 7%. Funds community foundations. *Education:* 10%. Supports higher education, nursing schools, and boards of education. *Environment:* 34%. Supports United Way, children's organizations, and organizations that assist the poor and needy in Winston-Salem and Forsyth county. *International:* 44%. Funds health care projects, medical centers, community health organizations, and single-disease health associations. *Note:* Total contributions made in fiscal 2000. **Typ. Recipients:** Adolescent Health Issues, AIDS/HIV, Alzheimers Disease, Cancer, Children's Health/Hospitals, Clinics/Medical Centers, Diabetes, Domestic Violence, Emergency/Ambulance Services, Family Planning, Geriatric Health, Health Organizations, Health Policy/Cost Containment, Health-General, Heart, Home-Care Services, Hospices, Hospitals, Long-Term Care, Medical Education, Medical Rehabilitation, Mental Health, Nursing Services, Outpatient Health Care, People with Disabilities, Prenatal Health Issues, Preventive Medicine/Wellness Organizations, Public Health, Single-Disease Health Associations, Speech & Hearing, Substance Abuse. **Geo. Dist:** NC, Forsyth County; grants for the poor and needy; NC, health care grants.

## ★ 448 ★ Katherine Mabis McKenna Foundation

PO Box 186
Latrobe, PA 15650
**Phone:** (724)537-6901          **Fax:** (724)537-6906
Linda Boxx, Chairman

**Fnded:** 1969. **Philosophy:** The Katherine Mabis McKenna Foundation makes grants across the major categories of support. Grants are made primarily to the environment and youth services in western Pennsylvania. **Priorities:** *Arts & Humanities:* 19%. Supports museums, libraries and historical preservation. *Civic & Public Affairs:* 31%. Funds gardens, parks and community foundations. *Education:* 28%. Supports education foundation, local school districts, colleges and universities. *Environment:* 9%. Supports Big Brothers, Big Sisters, scouting and United Way. *Note:* Contributions were made in 1998. **Typ. Recipients:** Arthritis, Cancer, Emergency/Ambulance Services, Hospitals, Medical Rehabilitation, People with Disabilities, Research/Studies Institutes, Single-Disease Health Associations. **Geo. Dist:** PA, Eastern Westmoreland County.

## ★ 449 ★ Kelly Gene Cook, Sr. Charitable Foundation

278 Waterford Way
Montgomery, TX 77356
**Phone:** (936)449-6272
**Email:** pegpool@aol.com
Peggy Pool, President

**Fnded:** 1986. **Philosophy:** The foundation supports higher education, primarily through scholarship programs. Designated programs are coordinated through the financial aid offices at Millsaps College, the University of Mississippi, and Mississippi State University. Other contributions are made on a limited basis to other institutions. **Priorities:** *Education:* 87%. Supports educational institutions and programs including scholarships to colleges and universities. *Environment:* 13%. Supports youth and family services. *Note:* Total contributions made in 1998. **Typ. Recipients:** Domestic Violence, Medical Education, Medical Training. **Geo. Dist:** internationally; nationally; MS.

## ★ 450 ★ Kelvin and Eleanor Smith Foundation

26380 Curtiss Wright Parkway, Ste. 105
Cleveland, OH 44143
**Phone:** (216)289-5789          **Fax:** (216)289-5948
Carol Zett, Grants Manager

**Fnded:** 1955. **Philosophy:** "The Foundation's principal interests are in the fields of non-sectarian education, the free enterprise system, the performing and visual arts, health care, and other activities of the type supported by the United Way Services of Cleveland.

Grants may be made in support of current operations or for special projects; grants for endowment are not made." **Priorities:** *Arts & Humanities:* 47%. Major grant to Case Western Reserve University Kelvin Smith Library. Also museums, public radio, theater, opera, and arts associations. *Civic & Public Affairs:* 19%. An arboretum and zoos. *Education:* 7%. Colleges and universities. *Environment:* 4%. People with disabilities, family services, and child welfare. *International:* 7%. Hospitals and public health. *Note:* Total contributions made in fiscal 1998. **Typ. Recipients:** Cancer, Children's Health/Hospitals, Clinics/Medical Centers, Eyes/Blindness, Family Planning, Health Organizations, Hospices, Hospitals (University Affiliated), Medical Education, Medical Rehabilitation, Mental Health, Nursing Services, People with Disabilities, Prenatal Health Issues, Speech & Hearing, Substance Abuse. **Geo. Dist:** Cleveland, OH, metropolitan area.

## ★ 451 ★ Kenneth T. and Eileen L. Norris Foundation

11 Golden Shore, Ste. 450
Long Beach, CA 90802
**Phone:** (562)435-8444          **Fax:** (562)436-0584
**Email:** savannah@ktn.org
**Website:** http://norrisfoundation.org
Ronald Barnes, Executive Director & Trustee

**Fnded:** 1963. **Philosophy:** When the foundation was established in 1963, grants were focused in two areas: medicine and private education in Southern California. However, "Today's Norris Foundation continues to allocate large portions of its resources to medicine and education but encompasses a broader agenda–one that also includes community and youth programs, science and the arts. In each program area, the sure hand of Ken Norris has shaped the results, producing a pattern of giving designed to encourage, extend, reconfigure or transform projects originating from a diverse assortment of nonprofit recipients." Norris Foundation 1995-1996 Annual Report **Priorities:** *Arts & Humanities:* 13%. Funds theaters, libraries, and museums. *Civic & Public Affairs:* 3%. Supports Las Floristas. *Education:* 39%. Supports colleges and universities; emphasis on medical education. *Environment:* 4%. Emphasis on youth organizations. *International:* 39%. Primary support for the Norris Cancer Center, hospitals and medical centers, single-disease health associations, and pediatric health. *Religion:* 1%. Funds a natural history museum and college scientist achievement rewards. *Note:* Total contributions made in fiscal 1999. **Typ. Recipients:** AIDS/HIV, Alzheimers Disease, Cancer, Children's Health/Hospitals, Clinics/Medical Centers, Diabetes, Emergency/Ambulance Services, Eyes/Blindness, Family Planning, Health Organizations, Heart, Hospices, Hospitals, Kidney, Medical Education, Medical Rehabilitation, Medical Research, People with Disabilities, Research/Studies Institutes, Respiratory, Single-Disease Health Associations, Speech & Hearing, Substance Abuse, Trauma Treatment. **Geo. Dist:** CA, Los Angeles County area.

## ★ 452 ★ Kentland Foundation

PO Box 879
Berryville, VA 22611-1082
**Phone:** (540)955-1268          **Fax:** (540)955-4942
Helene Walker, President

**Fnded:** 1966. **Philosophy:** The Kentland Foundation makes most of its grants to education and religion. Funding favors literacy, religious education, universities, and parochial education. Other significant interests include youth organizations, housing, churches, and health services. **Priorities:** *Civic & Public Affairs:* 1%. *Education:* 29%. Funds pre-college parochial education. *Environment:* 5%. Funds scouting. *International:* 5%. Gives to hospitals and hospice. *Note:* Contributions made in 2000. **Typ. Recipients:** Cancer, Children's Health/Hospitals, Clinics/Medical Centers, Domestic Violence, Emergency/Ambulance Services, Family Planning, Health Funds, Hospices, Hospitals, Long-Term Care, Medical Education, Medical Research, Nutrition, People with Disabilities, Prenatal Health Issues, Preventive Medicine/Wellness Organizations, Preventive Medicine/Wellness Organizations,

Public Health, Research/Studies Institutes, Sexual Abuse. **Geo. Dist:** mid-Atlantic states.

## ★ 453 ★ Kerr Foundation, Inc.

12501 North May Ave.
Oklahoma City, OK 73120
**Phone:** (405)749-7991          **Fax:** (405)749-2877
**Email:** lkerr@ionet.net
**Website:** http://www.thekerrfoundation.org
Robert Kerr, Jr., Trustee

**Fnded:** 1963. **Philosophy:** The foundation's main concern is to support organizations and institutions that provide new or enhanced opportunities to Oklahomans and the Southwest region, particularly the young. The stated areas of interest are "education, health, cultural development, and community service." **Priorities:** *Arts & Humanities:* 21%. Funds museums, art funds, and cultural and historic preservation. *Civic & Public Affairs:* 6%. Gives to public policy organizations and community groups. *Education:* 62%. Supports colleges, universities, education funds, and scholarships. *Environment:* 3%. Funds shelters, youth groups, and senior concerns. *International:* 1%. Contributes to health centers and associations. *Note:* Total contributions made in 1998. **Typ. Recipients:** Cancer, Clinics/Medical Centers, Domestic Violence, Emergency/Ambulance Services, Family Planning, Geriatric Health, Health Organizations, Health-General, Hospitals (University Affiliated), Medical Education, People with Disabilities, Prenatal Health Issues, Public Health, Single-Disease Health Associations, Substance Abuse. **Geo. Dist:** OK.

## ★ 454 ★ Kettering Fund

1560 Kettering Tower
Dayton, OH 45423
**Phone:** (937)228-1021          **Fax:** (937)449-7239
**Email:** ketteringfund@aol.com
Terri Hurd, Director

**Fnded:** 1958. **Philosophy:** The fund supports groups furthering "general philanthropy with an emphasis in higher education and cultural development." **Priorities:** *Arts & Humanities:* 27%. Supports art museums and foundations and Carillon Historical Park. *Civic & Public Affairs:* 10%. Zoos and parks, urban affairs, and civic institutions. *Education:* 30%. Supports higher education. *Environment:* 9%. Focus is on youth activities. *International:* 16%. Supports single-disease health associations, and medical centers. *Religion:* 2%. Funds Dayton Society of Natural History. *Note:* Total contributions made in fiscal 1999. **Typ. Recipients:** Arthritis, Children's Health/Hospitals, Clinics/Medical Centers, Emergency/Ambulance Services, Family Planning, Health Organizations, Hospices, Hospitals, Long-Term Care, Medical Education, Nursing Services, People with Disabilities, Public Health, Transplant Networks/Donor Banks. **Geo. Dist:** OH, especially Dayton.

## ★ 455 ★ Kiplinger Foundation

1729 H St., Northwest
Washington, DC 20006
**Phone:** (202)887-6559          **Fax:** (202)496-1817
Andrea Wilkes, Secretary

**Fnded:** 1948. **Philosophy:** The Kiplinger Foundation makes most of its grants in the areas of education, civic affairs, and the arts. Funding for education is primarily limited to matching gifts made by employees to educational institutions. There is no scholarship funding available. In civic affairs, interests include journalism centers and press associations. Funding for the arts goes to music schools, performing arts, museums, galleries, historic preservation, and theater. Grants also are made to other recipient areas such as welfare and social services, youth agencies, and health organizations on a more limited basis. **Priorities:** *Arts & Humanities:* 30%. Funds symphonies, historical societies, museums, opera, ballet, and arts centers. *Civic & Public Affairs:* 13%. Includes funding for the National Press Foundation. *Education:* 51%. Support mostly given in the form of matching gifts to universities, public and private secondary schools, and education committees. *Environment:* 4%. Supports the United Way, shelters, food banks, and community services. *International:* 1%. Supports health programs. *Religion:* 1%. Supports museums and fairs. *Note:* Total contributions made in 1998. **Typ. Recipients:** Cancer, Children's Health/Hospitals, Emergency/Ambulance Services, Family Planning, Health Organizations, Hospices, Hospitals, Medical Rehabilitation, Mental Health, Nursing Services, People with Disabilities, Public Health, Research/Studies Institutes, Sexual Abuse, Substance Abuse. **Geo. Dist:** Washington, DC, including metropolitan area.

### ★ 456 ★ Kirkpatrick Foundation, Inc.

1200 NW 63rd, Ste. 500
PO Box 268822
Oklahoma City, OK 73126-8822
**Phone:** (405)840-2882          **Fax:** (405)840-2946
**Email:** kfi@compuserve.com
Susan McCalmont, Executive Director

**Fnded:** 1955. **Philosophy:** The Kirkpatrick Foundation makes most of its grants in the areas of civic affairs, the arts and cultural programs, education, and social services. Educational support mainly goes to precollegiate programs. In social services, interests include youth organizations, and child welfare. An emphasis is placed on sharing information between educational and social service organizations. **Priorities:** *Arts & Humanities:* 81%. Supports a variety of art organizations in Oklahoma City. *Education:* 22%. Primary support for arts education. *Religion:* Less than 1%. *Note:* Total contributions made in 2000 **Typ. Recipients:** Children's Health/Hospitals, Clinics/Medical Centers, Domestic Violence, Emergency/Ambulance Services, Family Planning, Heart, Hospitals, Medical Education, Medical Research, People with Disabilities, Public Health, Single-Disease Health Associations. **Geo. Dist:** Oklahoma City, OK, including metropolitan area. **Frmly:** Kirkpatrick Foundation.

### ★ 457 ★ Knapp Foundation, Inc. (MD)

PO Box O
Saint Michaels, MD 21663
**Phone:** (410)745-5660
Ruth Capranica, Vice President

**Fnded:** 1929. **Philosophy:** The Knapp Foundation makes most of its grants in the areas of "wildlife conservation projects and college and university library projects. Several small contributions are disbursed each year that represent a predetermined group of organizations that the foundation has supported for fifty years or more." **Priorities:** *Arts & Humanities:* About 2%. Museums. *Civic & Public Affairs:* 8%. Primarily to aquariums and botanical gardens. *Education:* 17%. Supports colleges and universities. *Environment:* 3%. Primarily for youth organizations and the disabled. *International:* 1%. Supports the American Foundation for the Blind. *Religion:* 7%. Funds natural science museums. *Note:* Total contributions made in 1999. **Typ. Recipients:** Cancer, Children's Health/Hospitals, Emergency/Ambulance Services, Hospitals, Medical Education, People with Disabilities, Research/Studies Institutes, Single-Disease Health Associations. **Geo. Dist:** Eastcoast states.

### ★ 458 ★ Koret Foundation

33 New Montgomery St., Ste. 1090
San Francisco, CA 94105-4509
**Phone:** (415)882-7740          **Fax:** (415)882-7775
**Website:** http://www.koretfoundation.org

**Fnded:** 1966. **Philosophy:** "The Koret Foundation is a Jewish-sponsored charitable trust that seeks to enhance the human spirit by furthering education, economic opportunity and community life in the San Francisco Bay Area and Israel. The Foundation's grant-making objectives are based on ethical values derived from Jewish traditions. The Koret Foundation was created by Joseph and Stephanie Koret, Jewish immigrants from Eastern Europe whose entrepreneurial vision and success provided the resources that have endowed the Koret Foundation's grant-making capabilities. "By enabling the organizations and institutions we support to advance economic opportunity, security and quality of life, the Koret Foundation strives to fulfill its missions to the communities we serve and to the citizens of those communities. "While the majority of funds granted annually by the Koret Foundation go to organizations with established records of successful service, an increasing portion of the Foundation's funding is dedicated to seeding and supporting new and innovative programs that hold the promise of being catalysts for positive change." The foundation's areas of interest include the Local and National Jewish Community with grants to Jewish communal organizations, care for elderly citizens, Jewish cultural identity, Jewish education, and emigre resettlement; the Israel/International Jewish Community with grants to economic reform and development, higher education, and emigre resettlement and career development; and the General Community with grants to cultural and community development, independent living for the elderly, public policy and economic development, youth employment, and higher education. **Priorities:** *Arts & Humanities:* 4%. Emphasis on museums, theater, and opera. *Civic & Public Affairs:* 12%. Primary support for the San Francisco Zoological Society and the Korean Center. *Education:* 10%. Focus on universities in California. *Environment:* 16%. United funds and food banks. *Note:* Total contributions made in 1998. **Typ. Recipients:** Emergency/Ambulance Services, Geriatric Health, Hospitals (University Affiliated), Long-Term Care. **Geo. Dist:** San Francisco, CA, including Bay area.

### ★ 459 ★ Kresge Foundation

3215 West Big Beaver Rd.
PO Box 3151
Troy, MI 48007-3151
**Phone:** (248)643-9630          **Fax:** (248)643-0588
**Website:** http://www.kresge.org
John Marshall, III, President & Chief Executive Officer

**Fnded:** 1924. **Philosophy:** "The Kresge Foundation, an independent private foundation, was created in 1924 by Sebastian S. Kresge 'to promote the well-being of mankind.' Through our grantmaking programs, we seek to strengthen the capacity of charitable organizations to provide effective programs of quality. Our geographic scope is national, and on occasion, international." "The Foundation's grants support a range of organizations reflecting almost the entire breadth of the nonprofit sector. This diverse group is responding to new challenges presented by their communities or sustaining activities that have demonstrated their effectiveness. We believe that a challenge grant toward an organization's capital project does more than just build a building or reward good programs. It presents an opportunity to build institutional capacity by helping an organization broaden and deepen its base of support from the private sector and by encouraging volunteer involvement in the fund-raising effort and beyond." "In December, 1998, The Kresge Foundation Trustees approved the Kresge HBCU Initiative, a five-year, $18 million program to support advancement efforts at historically Black colleges and universities...The ultimate goal of the Initiative is to strengthen HBCUs by increasing ongoing and additional funding sources available to them." 1998 Annual Report **Priorities:** *Arts & Humanities:* 28%. Theater, museums, and cultural activities. *Civic & Public Affairs:* 14%. Includes public affairs programs, and community foundations. *Education:* 25%. Higher education institutions. *Environment:* 15%. Scouting, American Red Cross programs, United Way, and youth organizations. *International:* 9%. Supports hospitals, hospice program, and health-care programs. *Religion:* 4%. Science museums and centers, marine science and The Kresge Foundation Science Initiative. *Note:* Total contributions made in 1999. **Typ. Recipients:** AIDS/HIV, Alzheimers Disease, Cancer, Child Abuse, Children's Health/Hospitals, Clinics/Medical Centers, Diabetes, Domestic Violence, Emergency/Ambulance Services, Eyes/Blindness, Family Planning, Health Organizations, Hospices, Hospitals, Long-Term Care, Medical Education, Medical Rehabilitation, Medical Research, Mental Health, Nursing Services, Outpatient Health Care, People with Disabilities, Preventive Medicine/Wellness Organizations, Research/Studies Institutes, Sexual Abuse, Single-Disease Health Associations, Substance Abuse, Trauma Treatment. **Geo. Dist:** nationally.

### ★ 460 ★ Kulas Foundation

50 Public Square, Ste. 924
Terminal Tower
Cleveland, OH 44113-2203
**Phone:** (216)623-4770          **Fax:** (216)623-4773
Allan Zambie, Vice President, Secretary

**Fnded:** 1938. **Philosophy:** Funding is provided to music programs at colleges and universities, art centers, and community organizations. The foundation identified three categories of grant recipients: musical, educational, and civic and charitable activities. The foundation has made several major grants to support research in the field of music therapy. **Priorities:** *Arts & Humanities:* 45%. Museums, performing arts, visual arts, and public broadcasting. *Civic & Public Affairs:* 2%. Community development projects. *Education:* 18%. Supports colleges and universities. *Environment:* 3%. Supports child welfare, counseling, and community service organizations. *International:* 9%. Medical centers. **Typ. Recipients:** Cancer, Children's Health/Hospitals, Clinics/Medical Centers, Eyes/Blindness, Hospices, Hospitals, Hospitals (University Affiliated), Long-Term Care, Nursing Services. **Geo. Dist:** Cleveland, OH, including metropolitan area.

### ★ 461 ★ L. E. Phillips Family Foundation

3925 N Hastings Way
Eau Claire, WI 54703
**Phone:** (715)839-2139          **Fax:** (715)839-2148
Melvin Cohen, President and Director

**Fnded:** 1943. **Philosophy:** The foundation supports organizations in Wisconsin. Funding has gone primarily to the Melvin S. Cohen Trust for the Minneapolis Federation for Jewish Service. The remainder of funding is disbursed among cultural organizations, educational institutions, health agencies, social service groups, and religious organizations. **Priorities:** *Arts & Humanities:* 3%. *Civic & Public Affairs:* 13%. Focus on the L.E. Phillips Career Development Center. *Education:* 4%. Supports colleges and universities. *Environment:* 23%. Youth organizations and religious welfare. *Note:* Total contributions made in fiscal 1999. **Typ. Recipients:** AIDS/HIV, Children's Health/Hospitals, Geriatric Health, Health Organizations, Health Policy/Cost Containment, Health-General, Heart, Hospitals, Hospitals (University Affiliated), Medical Education, Medical Rehabilitation, Medical Research, People with Disabilities, Public Health, Single-Disease Health Associations, Substance Abuse. **Geo. Dist:** WI, Chippewa County; WI, Eau Claire County; WI, Northwestern Wisconsin;

### ★ 462 ★ L. K. Whittier Foundation

625 South Fair Oaks Ave., Ste. 360
South Pasadena, CA 91030
**Phone:** (626)441-5188          **Fax:** (626)441-3672
Linda Blinkenberg, Secretary & Chief Financial Officer

**Fnded:** 1955. **Philosophy:** The foundation makes grants primarily in Southern California, specifically Los Angeles. The foundation assists in the establishment and development of innovative endeavors in the areas of health and medicine, the sciences, and education. **Priorities:** *Arts & Humanities:* 26%. Supports public broadcasting. *Education:* 20%. Supports technical education and general education. *Environment:* 16%. Supports camps and scouting. *International:* 38%. Funds children's health care. *Note:* Total contributions made in fiscal 1999. **Typ. Recipients:** Cancer, Children's Health/Hospitals, Clinics/Medical Centers, Eyes/Blindness, Family Planning, Geriatric Health, Health Organizations, Hospitals, Medical Education, Medical Research, People with Disabilities, Research/Studies Institutes, Single-Disease Health Associations. **Geo. Dist:** CA, Southern California, particularly Los Angeles.

### ★ 463 ★ Laffey-McHugh Foundation

PO Box 2207
Wilmington, DE 19899-2207
**Phone:** (302)658-9141          **Fax:** (302)658-5614
Arthur Connolly, Jr., President

**Fnded:** 1949. **Philosophy:** The foundation continues to reflect the interests of the original donors by supporting Roman Catholic churches and church-related institutions, including schools, child-welfare agencies, and religious-welfare groups. The foundation also makes grants to institutions of higher education, both sectarian and nonsectarian, and to local hospitals, cultural organizations, and nonsectarian-welfare agencies. **Priorities:** *Arts & Humanities:* 7% Supports public broadcasting, libraries, museums, and the performing arts. *Civic & Public Affairs:* 11%. Community affairs and housing are funded. *Education:* 23%. Supports colleges, universities, religious schools, and educational programs. *Environment:* 31%. Family and childrens services and united funds. *International:* 4%. Supports children's health, hospice, disease and disorder concerns. *Note:* Contributions were made in 1998. **Typ. Recipients:** Alzheimers Disease, Cancer, Child Abuse, Children's Health/Hospitals, Clinics/Medical Centers, Family Planning, Geriatric Health, Heart, Hospices, Hospitals, Long-Term Care, Nursing Services, Outpatient Health Care, People with Disabilities, Preventive Medicine/Wellness Organizations, Public Health, Single-Disease Health Associations, Substance Abuse. **Geo. Dist:** DE.

## ★ 464 ★ Laurel Foundation
Two Gateway Center, Ste. 1800
Pittsburgh, PA 15222
**Phone:** (412)765-2400          **Fax:** (412)765-2407
Donna Panazzi, Vice President

**Fnded:** 1951. **Philosophy:** The Laurel Foundation makes grants to organizations serving southwestern Pennsylvania. In civic affairs, interests include community development, libraries, museums, conservation, and natural resource management. Educational support favors literacy, traditional education centers, vocational training, and apprenticeship programs. Funding for social services goes to health and human services, population control, and youth organizations. The arts are supported by funding to theaters, the performing arts, and festivals. "In response to a considerable increase in grant requests, the Trustees have reviewed the Foundation's priorities and have identified specific goals and objectives with which to guide their deliberations. With an emphasis on outcomes and accountability, grants will focus on programs which offer long-term benefits for participants and the community. The Foundation favors programs that foster individual responsibility and self-sufficiency, exhibit a commitment to sound fiscal and program management, implement collaborative efforts to leverage resources and increase efficiency, and that demonstrate measurable outcomes through the application of conclusive evaluation procedures." 1997 Annual Report **Priorities:** *Arts & Humanities:* 28%. Theater, music, museums, and historic preservation. *Civic & Public Affairs:* 13%. Supports programs dealing with legal issues, community leadership, and the nonprofit sector. Some support given to community development and beautification projects as well. *Education:* 13%. Secondary and higher education. *Environment:* 11%. Animal welfare programs and youth and family services. *International:* 8%. Preventive medicine, and women's and children's health issues. *Note:* Total contributions made in 2000. **Typ. Recipients:** Alzheimers Disease, Children's Health/Hospitals, Clinics/Medical Centers, Emergency/Ambulance Services, Family Planning, Health Funds, Hospitals, Medical Education, Medical Research, Nursing Services, People with Disabilities, Public Health, Substance Abuse. **Geo. Dist:** Pittsburgh, PA, including southwestern PA.

## ★ 465 ★ Leighton-Oare Foundation
211 West Washington Ave., Ste. 2400
South Bend, IN 46601
**Phone:** (219)232-5977          **Fax:** (219)234-5967
Judd Leighton, Secretary & Treasurer

**Fnded:** 1955. **Philosophy:** The Leighton-Oare Foundation is primarily interested in health services, education, and the arts. Health service funding heavily favors health foundations. Educational funding favors colleges and universities. The arts are supported mainly through grants to music and a historical society. Minor interests include civic affairs, religion, and social services. **Priorities:** *Arts & Humanities:* 24%. Funds music, performing arts, historic societies, museums and public broadcasting. *Civic & Public Affairs:* 10%. Gives to community foundations for Endowment for the Advancement of Philanthropy, a botanical garden and clubs. *Education:* 41%. Supports precollege and higher education, and legal education. *Environment:* less than 1%. *International:* 25%. Supports the Memorial Health Foundation, arthritis, and medicine research. *Note:* Total contributions made in 1999. **Typ. Recipients:** Arthritis, Children's Health/Hospitals, Clinics/Medical Centers, Geriatric Health, Health Funds, Hospices, Hospitals, Medical Research, Multiple Sclerosis, Public Health, Research/Studies Institutes. **Geo. Dist:** IN.

## ★ 466 ★ Leland Fikes Foundation
3050 Lincoln Plaza
500 North Akard, Ste. 3050
Dallas, TX 75201-6696
**Phone:** (214)754-0144
Nancy Solana, Vice President & Secretary

**Fnded:** 1952. **Philosophy:** The Fikes Foundation offers support to a wide variety of cultural, civic, educational, health, scientific, and social service organizations. A preference is shown toward local projects and organizations. **Priorities:** *Arts & Humanities:* 18%. Cultural development, symphonies, and museums, libraries, theater, and arts festivals. *Civic & Public Affairs:* 15%. Funds public policy, nonprofit management, housing concerns, zoos, and botanical gardens. *Education:* 12%. Focus on private schools, colleges and universities, and literacy. *Environment:* 21%. Supports youth organizations, family planning, community services, camps, food banks, and family services. *International:* 34%. Primary support for a university hospital. Also supports AIDS, medical research, and mental health. *Note:* Total contributions made in 1998. **Typ. Recipients:** AIDS/HIV, Cancer, Children's Health/Hospitals, Clinics/Medical Centers, Diabetes, Domestic Violence, Eyes/Blindness, Family Planning, Health Organizations, Heart, Hospitals, Hospitals (University Affiliated), Medical Education, Medical Research, Mental Health, Nursing Services, People with Disabilities, Prenatal Health Issues, Public Health, Single-Disease Health Associations, Substance Abuse, Transplant Networks/Donor Banks, Trauma Treatment. **Geo. Dist:** Dallas, TX.

## ★ 467 ★ Leon Lowenstein Foundation
126 East 56th St., 28th Floor
New York, NY 10022
**Phone:** (212)319-0670          **Fax:** (212)319-0670
Robert Bendheim, President

**Fnded:** 1941. **Philosophy:** The foundation provides funding "to higher education and health for the benefit of New York City." **Priorities:** *Arts & Humanities:* 4% supports performing arts, museums, visual arts, art and culture. *Civic & Public Affairs:* 3%. Supports community and public affairs. *Education:* 76%. Supports educational institutions and programs. *Environment:* 2%. Supports meals on wheels, social, children and family services. *International:* 12%. Supports rehabilitation centers, hospitals, disease and disorder concerns. *Note:* Contributions were made in 1998. **Typ. Recipients:** Arthritis, Cancer, Children's Health/Hospitals, Clinics/Medical Centers, Emergency/Ambulance Services, Eyes/Blindness, Health Organizations, Hospitals, Medical Education, Medical Rehabilitation, Medical Research, Mental Health, Nursing Services, People with Disabilities, Single-Disease Health Associations, Substance Abuse. **Geo. Dist:** New York, NY, metropolitan area.

## ★ 468 ★ Lettie Pate Whitehead Foundation
50 Hurt Plaza, Ste. 1200
Atlanta, GA 30303
**Phone:** (404)522-6755          **Fax:** (404)522-7026
**Email:** FDNS@woodruff.org
**Website:** http://www.lpwhitehead.org
Charles McTier, President

**Fnded:** 1946. **Philosophy:** As specified under the will of Conkey Pate Whitehead, the foundation is limited to providing funds for needy female Christian students in Alabama, Florida, Georgia, Louisiana, Mississippi, North Carolina, South Carolina, Tennessee, and Virginia. Grants are made directly to institutions of higher education which, in turn, allocate scholarship funds to individual students. Scholarships are based on financial need. This educational program accounts for about 90% of giving. The remainder of support is given to homes for needy elderly Christian women. **Priorities:** *Civic & Public Affairs:* (Housing & Neighborhood Revitalization) About 12%. For the benefit of needy, elderly Christian women. *Education:* About 88%. Scholarships for needy female Christian students in southern states. *International:* About 12% nursing homes. For the benefit of needy, elderly Christian women. *Note:* Total contributions made in 1997. **Typ. Recipients:** Alzheimers Disease, Cancer, Clinics/Medical Centers, Geriatric Health, Long-Term Care, Medical Education. **Geo. Dist:** AL; FL; GA; LA; MS; NC; SC; TN; VA.

## ★ 469 ★ Lied Foundation Trust
3907 West Charleston Boulevard
Las Vegas, NV 89102
**Phone:** (702)878-1559          **Fax:** (702)878-6469
Christina Hixson, Trustee

**Fnded:** 1972. **Philosophy:** The Lied Foundation Trust traditionally funds three main areas: higher education, religious organizations, and youth organizations in Las Vegas. Major contributions are made to higher education, particularly to Kansas University, the Lied Institute for Real Estate Studies, and the University of Nevada. The Boys and Girls Club of Las Vegas is also a main interest. The foundation also funds other organizations primarily in the areas of social services and education. **Priorities:** *Arts & Humanities:* 16%. Funds performing arts, the Council Bluffs Public Library Foundation and dance theaters. *Civic & Public Affairs:* 10%. Supports Quality Living, Inc. *Education:* 33%. Provides scholarships; supports colleges and universities. *International:* 25%. Supports National Transplant Cener, and House Ear Institute. *Religion:* 1%. Funds museum. *Note:* Total contributions made in 1998. **Typ. Recipients:** Health Organizations, Hospitals (University Affiliated), People with Disabilities, Research/Studies Institutes, Speech & Hearing, Speech & Hearing, Transplant Networks/Donor Banks. **Geo. Dist:** CA; IA; KS; NE; NV; UT; WA.

## ★ 470 ★ Lincy Foundation
150 S Rodeo Dr., Ste. 250
Beverly Hills, CA 90212
**Phone:** (310)271-3490
James Aljian, Chairman

**Fnded:** 1989. **Philosophy:** The Lincy Foundation is primarily interested in aiding Armenian interests through its support of the United Armenian Fund and other organizations. The foundation has also supported care for the elderly with two large grants going to homes for the aged in southern California. **Priorities:** *Arts & Humanities:* 7%. Westwood Playhouse. *Education:* 6%. Supports schools and universities. *Environment:* 10%. Youth, homes for the aged. *International:* 61%. Single-disease research and hospitals. Major donation to American Red Cross. *Note:* Total contributions made in 1999. **Typ. Recipients:** AIDS/HIV, Arthritis, Cancer, Children's Health/Hospitals, Clinics/Medical Centers, Diabetes, Emergency/Ambulance Services, Eyes/Blindness, Geriatric Health, Health Funds, Health Organizations, Heart, Hospices, Hospitals, Hospitals (University Affiliated), Kidney, Long-Term Care, Medical Education, Medical Research, Mental Health, People with Disabilities, Prenatal Health Issues, Public Health, Sexual Abuse, Single-Disease Health Associations, Transplant Networks/Donor Banks. **Geo. Dist:** CA; NV.

## ★ 471 ★ Little Family Foundation
1 Boston Place, AIM 024 0073
Boston, MA 02108
**Phone:** (617)722-6990

**Fnded:** 1946. **Philosophy:** The Little Family Foundation's main emphasis is to promote quality education as a stepping stone to success in the business world. The foundation has established the Little Family Foundation Fellowship Awards in conjunction with the national office of Junior Achievement in Colorado Springs, CO. The foundation also supports arts organizations and conservation minded organizations. **Priorities:** *Arts & Humanities:* 28%. Supports public broadcasting, museums, and music. *Civic & Public Affairs:* 17%. Contributes to zoos and aquariums. *Education:* 24%. Funds business and higher education. *Environment:* About 15%. Funds youth groups and united funds. *International:* 1%. Medical research. *Note:* Total contributions made in 1998. **Typ. Recipients:** AIDS/HIV, Cancer, Domestic Violence, Family Planning, Hospitals, Long-Term Care, Medical Rehabilitation, Medical Research, Nursing Services, People with Disabilities, Single-Disease Health Associations, Substance Abuse. **Geo. Dist:** nationally.

★ **472** ★ **Liz Claiborne and Art Ortenberg Foundation**

650 5th Ave., 15th Floor
New York, NY 10019
**Phone:** (212)333-2536          **Fax:** (212)956-3531
**Email:** lcaof@compuserve.com
James Murtaugh, Program Director

**Fnded:** 1984. **Philosophy:** Environmental concerns top the priority list of the Liz Claiborne and Art Ortenberg Foundation. Typically, the foundation chooses well-established programs with firm reputations, such as the Nature Conservancy, the World Wildlife Fund, and the New York Zoological Society-Wildlife Conservation International. The foundation's board of directors has identified two primary program interests for the future: mitigation of conflict between the land and resource use practices of rural communities and conservation of biological diversity; and, implementation of field-based scientific, technical, and practical training programs in conservation biology for local people. Typically, the foundation funds modest, carefully designed field projects, in which local communities have a substantial proprietary interest. The foundation also provides very limited funding for organizations concerned with health care, social services, education, and the arts. **Priorities:** *Arts & Humanities:* 19%. Supports historic preservation, theater, art museums, public radio and Library of Congress. *Civic & Public Affairs:* 33%. Emphasis on a botanical garden and public policy groups concerned with the protection of native lands. *Education:* 16%. Colleges and universities, and elementary schools. *Environment:* 8%. Youth and family services, community centers, United Way, and YWCA. *International:* 1%.Funds hospital, medical centers, single-disease health associations. *Note:* Total contributions made in fiscal 1999. **Typ. Recipients:** AIDS/HIV, Emergency/Ambulance Services, Family Planning, Health Organizations, Hospitals, People with Disabilities, Single-Disease Health Associations. **Geo. Dist:** internationally especially undeveloped countries; Northern Rockies area and nationally.

★ **473** ★ **Lloyd A. Fry Foundation**

120 S LaSalle St., Ste. 1950
Chicago, IL 60603
**Phone:** (312)580-0310          **Fax:** (312)580-0980
**Email:** info@fryfoundation.org
**Website:** http://www.fryfoundation.org
Jill Darrow, Executive Director

**Fnded:** 1983. **Philosophy:** The foundation focuses its philanthropic efforts in the areas of education, health, civic affairs, social services, and the arts. In education, the foundation is receptive to efforts to improve Chicago inner-city education at the elementary and secondary levels. It works toward this goal through support of programs aimed at Chicago school reform, faculty development programs, and scholarship programs for minority students. The foundation also funds universities, cultural organizations, private agencies, and community groups that improve Chicago public education. Foundation giving in the arts also reflects a commitment to education through the support of arts outreach projects for inner-city students. Chicago's

major cultural institutions and mid-sized arts organizations also receive support. In the area of health, the foundation continues to focus on health education and disease prevention among low-income and minority populations, as well as on efforts to improve health care for the medically indigent in Chicago. Improving health services for low-income children is a special emphasis in this area. Grants to civic and social service organizations reflect foundation interests in monitoring local government, studying the legal system, and providing legal services to needy individuals and organizations. Other concerns include job training and placement for minority youth and neighborhood economic development. **Priorities:** *Arts & Humanities:* 7%. Supports performing arts and public broadcasting. *Civic & Public Affairs:* 13%. Supports urban and community affairs, employment, legal issues, and zoos. *Education:* 31%. Supports private schools, educational foundations and initiatives, public and private colleges and universities. *Environment:* 24%. Supports youth programs, the homeless, community organizations, and family services. *International:* 5%. Supports medical centers and research. *Note:* Total contributions made in fiscal 2000. **Typ. Recipients:** AIDS/HIV, Child Abuse, Children's Health/Hospitals, Clinics/Medical Centers, Domestic Violence, Geriatric Health, Health Organizations, Health Policy/Cost Containment, Heart, Hospitals, Medical Rehabilitation, Mental Health, Nursing Services, People with Disabilities, Prenatal Health Issues, Public Health, Single-Disease Health Associations, Substance Abuse. **Geo. Dist:** Chicago, IL.

★ **474** ★ **Lois U. Horvitz Foundation**

c/o Parkland Management Company
1001 Lakeside Ave., Ste. 900
Cleveland, OH 44114
**Phone:** (216)479-2200          **Fax:** (216)479-2222
Thomas Oden, Contact

**Fnded:** 1988. **Philosophy:** As of August 31, 1998 the Foundation entered into a legal agreement to distribute one-fourth of its assets to each of the H.R.H. Family Foundations: the MJH Foundation, an Ohio charitable trusts; the PTS Family Foundation, a charitable corporation, and the PAH Foundation, a charitable trust. The Foundation retained one-fourth of the Foundations assets. The Foundations new name is the Lois U. Horvitz Foundation, a nonprofit charitable corporation of which Lois U. Horvitz is the sole member. The H.R.H. Family Foundation is obligated to "fund its proportionate share of scholarship payment for any student already in the Scholarship Program as of the date of such notice, until that student has complete college in accordance with the Scholarship Program". "The H.R.H. Family Foundations each agree to participate in Charitable Funds Program until the end of the calendar year in which occurs the fifth anniversary for the Distribution Date." The Distribution Date was September 30, 1998. 1998 Form 990 Addresses for the foundations follow: MJH Foundation, care of Parkland Management Co., 1001 Lakeside Avenue, Suite 900, Cleveland, Ohio 44114 PTS Family Foundation, care of 580, West Germantown Pike #202 Plymouth Metting, Pennsylvania 19462 PAH Foundation, 1705 132nd Avenue N.E., Bellevue, Washington 98005 **Priorities:** *Civic & Public Affairs:* 36%. Supports the Horvitz Newspapers and family business programs. *Education:* 29%. Funds an educational campaign. *Environment:* 34%. Supports family and children's services, philanthropy, and violence prevention. *International:* 1%. Supports a rheumatic disease organization. *Note:* Total contributions made in fiscal 1999. **Typ. Recipients:** Clinics/Medical Centers, Domestic Violence, Hospices, Substance Abuse. **Geo. Dist:** preference is given where Horvitz family members reside. **Frmly:** H.R.H. Family Foundation.

★ **475** ★ **Lon V. Smith Foundation**

9440 Santa Monica Boulevard, Ste. 300
Beverly Hills, CA 90210-4201
**Phone:** (310)276-9306          **Fax:** (310)276-3824
Marguerite Murphy, Secretary & Treasurer

**Fnded:** 1952. **Philosophy:** The primary focus of the foundation is on social services in the Los Angeles area. A variety of organizations are supported, includ-

ing services for the disabled, child welfare programs, youth organizations, family services, shelters, and homes. The foundation also is interested in supporting health services. A variety of health organizations are supported by the foundation, including hospitals, single-disease associations, family clinics, counseling, and pediatrics. **Priorities:** *Civic & Public Affairs:* 13%. Family services, legal associations, and Habitat for Humanity. *Education:* 5%. Educational programs and schools. *Environment:* 38%. Family and youth services including Boy Scouts of America and shelters for abused women. *International:* 33%. Alzheimer's Association, children's health issues and medical centers are funded. *Note:* Total contributions made in 1998. **Typ. Recipients:** Alzheimers Disease, Cancer, Children's Health/Hospitals, Clinics/Medical Centers, Diabetes, Domestic Violence, Emergency/Ambulance Services, Geriatric Health, Health Organizations, Hospitals, Hospitals (University Affiliated), Hospitals (University Affiliated), Long-Term Care, Medical Education, Medical Research, Nursing Services, Nutrition, Outpatient Health Care, People with Disabilities, Prenatal Health Issues, Preventive Medicine/Wellness Organizations, Public Health, Research/Studies Institutes, Single-Disease Health Associations, Speech & Hearing, Substance Abuse. **Geo. Dist:** Los Angeles, CA.

★ **476** ★ **Longwood Foundation**

100 West 10th St., Ste. 1109
Wilmington, DE 19801
**Phone:** (302)654-2477          **Fax:** (302)654-2323
Peter Morrow, Executive Director

**Fnded:** 1937. **Philosophy:** One of the foundation's primary interests has been to support and develop Longwood Gardens, once the home of Pierre du Pont. It is among the finest horticultural gardens open to the public in America. The gardens cover 1,000 acres, and include a conservatory, an arboretum, flower gardens, an open air theater, illuminated fountains, greenhouses, and several other attractions. To a lesser extent, funds traditionally have been given to the Eleutherian Mills Historical Library, a research library which assembles and houses historical documents and records relating to the Brandywine Valley and its development. The foundation also has supported educational institutions for the construction of scientific, engineering training, and library facilities. Local conservation and horticultural groups, hospitals, and a variety of social service agencies have received substantial funding from the foundation. **Priorities:** *Arts & Humanities:* 9%. Supports art funds, art centers, museums, and libraries. *Civic & Public Affairs:* 35%. Includes the foundation's largest grant to Longwood Gardens. *Education:* 5%. Focus on primary and secondary education. *Environment:* 40%. Emphasis on community services, youth organizations, child welfare, united funds, the aged, and family planning. *International:* 4%. Health associations and medical centers. *Note:* Total contributions made in fiscal 1997. **Typ. Recipients:** AIDS/HIV, Cancer, Children's Health/Hospitals, Clinics/Medical Centers, Emergency/Ambulance Services, Family Planning, Geriatric Health, Health Organizations, Hospices, Hospitals, Long-Term Care, Medical Research, People with Disabilities, Preventive Medicine/Wellness Organizations, Public Health, Substance Abuse. **Geo. Dist:** DE; PA, Southern Chester County.

★ **477** ★ **Loren M. Berry Foundation**

3055 Kettering Boulevard, Ste. 418
Dayton, OH 45439
**Phone:** (937)293-0398
William Lincoln, Treasurer & Trustee

**Fnded:** 1960. **Philosophy:** The foundation supports a variety of youth organizations, social and family service organizations, and united funds. The foundation prioritizes higher education and educational foundations. Community affairs, the arts, and health concerns are also important. **Priorities:** *Arts & Humanities:* 14%. Funds art institutes, theater, historical preservation, and public broadcasting. *Civic & Public Affairs:* 12%. Supports public policy and economic development. *Education:* 34%. Supports higher education, education funds, schools, and scholarship programs.

*Environment:* 26%. Grants awarded to Young Men's Christian Association, Planned Parenthood, and services for children and youth. *International:* 1%. Contributes to hospitals, disease and disorder concerns, the American Red Cross, and medical centers. *Religion:* 3%. Supports aviation museum. *Note:* Total contributions made in 2000. **Typ. Recipients:** Alzheimers Disease, Cancer, Children's Health/Hospitals, Clinics/Medical Centers, Domestic Violence, Emergency/Ambulance Services, Eyes/Blindness, Family Planning, Geriatric Health, Health Organizations, Heart, Hospices, Hospitals, People with Disabilities, Single-Disease Health Associations, Transplant Networks/Donor Banks. **Geo. Dist:** Dayton, OH.

## ★ 478 ★ Louis and Anne Abrons Foundation
437 Madison Ave.
New York, NY 10022
**Phone:** (212)756-3376       **Fax:** (212)832-6698
Richard Abrons, President

**Fnded:** 1950. **Philosophy:** The foundation focuses giving on social welfare organizations; civic and public affairs, including environmental causes; educational institutions; and Jewish organizations. **Priorities:** *Arts & Humanities:* 8%. Supports performing arts, museums, and public libraries. *Civic & Public Affairs:* 11%. Supports conservation and community and public affairs. *Education:* 19%. Supports educational programs and universities. *Environment:* 24%. Supports family services and neighborhood concerns, with major support given to the Henry Street Settlement. *International:* 8%. Supports health concerns and single-disease health associations. *Religion:* 1%. Supports the American Museum of Natural History. *Note:* Total contributions made in 1998. **Typ. Recipients:** Cancer, Children's Health/Hospitals, Family Planning, Health Organizations, Hospitals, Medical Education, Medical Research, Mental Health, Nursing Services, Substance Abuse. **Geo. Dist:** New York, NY.

## ★ 479 ★ Louis Calder Foundation
230 Park Ave., Room 1525
New York, NY 10169
**Phone:** (212)687-1680
**Website:** http://www.lcfnyc.org
Allison Sargent, Grant Program Manager

**Fnded:** 1951. **Philosophy:** Foundation grants reflect a high level of social awareness, with particular attention to the problems and needs of those in New York City. The current policy of the foundation is to concentrate "its grantmaking to organizations whose programs and projects are directed to improving the condition of the people of the City of New York. Current funding priorities are grants which support the efforts of community based organizations whose programs are designed to enhance the potential and increase the self sufficiency of New York City's disadvantaged children and youth and their families." **Priorities:** *Arts & Humanities:* 22%. Libraries, public broadcasting, museums, ballet, and music. *Civic & Public Affairs:* 5%. Support law & justice, botanical gardens, and housing. *Education:* 27%. Colleges and universities, private and public pre-college education, literacy, after school enrichment programs, leadership training, education reform, medical education, scholarships, and legal education. *Environment:* 33%. Youth organizations, programs for at-risk youth, family services and child welfare. *International:* 7%. Mainly hospitals. *Note:* Total contributions made in fiscal 2000. **Typ. Recipients:** Adolescent Health Issues, AIDS/HIV, Cancer, Children's Health/Hospitals, Health Organizations, Heart, Hospitals, People with Disabilities, Research/Studies Institutes. **Geo. Dist:** New York City.

## ★ 480 ★ Louis R. Lurie Foundation
555 California St., Ste. 5100
San Francisco, CA 94104
**Phone:** (415)392-2470       **Fax:** (415)421-8669
Robert Lurie, President

**Fnded:** 1948. **Philosophy:** The foundation gives to a wide range of local interests in the San Francisco and Chicago areas. While there is no specific area of focus, the foundation does give substantially to organizations concerned with civic and community issues, the social sciences, education, the arts and humanities, and a variety of health issues. **Priorities:** *Arts & Humanities:* 13%. Supports museums, theater, performing arts, and cultural associations. *Civic & Public Affairs:* 4%. Funds housing and community affairs. *Education:* 9%. Preparatory schools, colleges, and educational programs receive grants. *Environment:* 20%. Family services, child welfare, and food banks receive support. *International:* 13%. Gives to hospitals, medical centers, rehabilitation institutes, elder care, and disease and disorder concerns. *Religion:* 2%. Funds a research center. *Note:* Total contributions made in 1998. **Typ. Recipients:** AIDS/HIV, Alzheimers Disease, Cancer, Child Abuse, Children's Health/Hospitals, Clinics/Medical Centers, Domestic Violence, Emergency/Ambulance Services, Family Planning, Geriatric Health, Health Funds, Health Organizations, Hospitals, Medical Education, Medical Rehabilitation, Medical Research, Mental Health, People with Disabilities, Prenatal Health Issues, Public Health, Single-Disease Health Associations, Substance Abuse. **Geo. Dist:** San Francisco, CA, metropolitan area; Chicago, IL.

## ★ 481 ★ The Louis and Rachel Rudin Foundation, Inc.
345 Park Ave., 33rd Floor
New York, NY 10154
**Phone:** (212)407-2400       **Fax:** (212)407-2540
Robin Avram, Administrator

**Fnded:** 1968. **Philosophy:** The purpose of the foundation is to aid medical and nursing schools in the education and training of doctors and nurses. **Priorities:** *Education:* 100%. Supports medical education through scholarships. *Note:* Contribution made in fiscal 1998. **Typ. Recipients:** Alzheimers Disease, Cancer, Children's Health/Hospitals, Eyes/Blindness, Geriatric Health, Home-Care Services, Medical Education, Medical Training, Mental Health. **Geo. Dist:** NY.

## ★ 482 ★ Louise H. and David S. Ingalls Foundation
301 Tower E
20600 Chagrin Boulevard
Shaker Heights, OH 44122
**Phone:** (216)921-6000       **Fax:** (216)921-7709
Jane Watson, Contact

**Fnded:** 1953. **Philosophy:** The foundation makes most of its grants in the areas of education, health, and the arts. Educational funding favors colleges and private secondary schools. Health care interests include hospital building campaigns, research, and pediatrics. Support for the arts goes to museums, art associations, and the performing arts. Secondary interests include youth organizations and civic affairs. **Priorities:** *Arts & Humanities:* 17%. Funds museums, music, arts festivals, historical societies, and performing arts. *Civic & Public Affairs:* 12%. Supports community foundations, botanical gardens, and clubs. *Education:* 27%. Supports pre-college and higher education. *Environment:* 4% Contributes to youth programs, family services, and community services. *Religion:* 28%. Supports museums. *Note:* Total contributions made in 2000. **Typ. Recipients:** Clinics/Medical Centers, Emergency/Ambulance Services, Eyes/Blindness, Family Planning, Health Organizations, Hospitals, Long-Term Care, Medical Education, Medical Rehabilitation, Nursing Services, People with Disabilities, Single-Disease Health Associations, Transplant Networks/Donor Banks. **Geo. Dist:** CT; NY; OH, Ohio, Connecticut, Virginia, and New York; VT.

## ★ 483 ★ Louise Manoogian Simone Foundation
21001 Van Born Rd.
Taylor, MI 48180
**Phone:** (313)274-8799
Louise Simone, President

**Fnded:** 1962. **Philosophy:** The Simone foundation's principal areas of interest are organizations supporting Armenian culture, religion, and education. The foundation also contributes to the arts, with emphasis on museums. **Priorities:** *Arts & Humanities:* Less than 1%. *Civic & Public Affairs:* 3%. Funds the Fourth Millennium Society and other civic concerns. *Education:* Less than 1%. *Environment:* Less than 1%. *Note:* Total contributions made in fiscal 1998. **Typ. Recipients:** Children's Health/Hospitals, Family Planning, Public Health, Research/Studies Institutes. **Geo. Dist:** nationally, with an emphasis on the eastern states.

## ★ 484 ★ Lowell Berry Foundation
4 Orinda Way, Ste. 140-B
Orinda, CA 94563-2513
**Phone:** (925)254-1944       **Fax:** (925)254-5041
Debbie Coombe, Office Manager

**Fnded:** 1950. **Philosophy:** The primary objective of the foundation is to assist in strengthening Christian ministry at the local church level. Its second purpose is to assist local social service programs in California. The foundation has a large number of ongoing grant programs, and the number of new grants is restricted to programs in California's Contra Costa and northern Alameda counties. The foundation's recipients include evangelical Christian religious programs, higher education, religious welfare organizations, and family services. **Priorities:** *Civic & Public Affairs:* 1%. Funds community affairs and public policy. *Education:* 4%. Supports colleges and universities and education funds. *Environment:* 10%. Gives to youth organizations, animal protection groups, food banks, shelters, and athletic organizations. *International:* 1%. Supports health services and medical centers. *Religion:* 2%. Supports a science center. *Note:* Total contributions made in 2000. **Typ. Recipients:** Cancer, Child Abuse, Children's Health/Hospitals, Clinics/Medical Centers, Domestic Violence, Family Planning, Medical Rehabilitation, Medical Research, People with Disabilities, Public Health, Substance Abuse. **Geo. Dist:** CA, Contra Costa County; CA, Northern Alameda County.

## ★ 485 ★ Lucius N. Littauer Foundation
60 East 42nd St., Ste. 2910
New York, NY 10165
**Phone:** (212)697-2677
William Frost, President

**Fnded:** 1929. **Philosophy:** The primary focus of the foundation is to provide funds for scholars engaged in research in Jewish studies. The foundation established the position of Littauer Hebraica Technical and Research Services Librarian in the Judaica Department of the Harvard College Library. In 1994, the foundation awarded a multi-year grant to Columbia University to establish the Lucius N. Littauer Foundation Professorship of Classical Jewish Civilization. Also, the foundation has founded and contributed to Judaic book funds at colleges and universities throughout the United States. Other current areas of interest are medical ethics and the environment. The foundation also supports some social welfare projects, including federated fund drives, Jewish welfare funds, and selected public interest groups. Some funding is available for health and environmental concerns. **Priorities:** *Arts & Humanities:* 4%. Support includes film, television, museums, libraries and archives, and the performing arts. *Civic & Public Affairs:* 8%. Supports public television specials and series. *Education:* 44%. Supports conferences, programs and workshops held at colleges and universities, scholarships and fellowships. *Environment:* 3%. Supports social welfare. *Note:* Total contributions made in 1998. **Typ. Recipients:** Clinics/Medical Centers, Geriatric Health, Health Organizations, Health Policy/Cost Containment, Hospitals, Hospitals (University Affiliated), Medical Education, People with Disabilities. **Geo. Dist:** internationally; nationally; New York, NY.

## ★ 486 ★ Lund Foundation
535 North Brand Boulevard, Ste. 504
Glendale, CA 91203
**Phone:** (818)291-4000       **Fax:** (818)291-4004
Robert Wilson, Vice President & Secretary

**Fnded:** 1973. **Philosophy:** The foundation typically supports the arts, educational institutions, health oranizations, and social services in the greater Los Angeles area. **Priorities:** *Arts & Humanities:* 50%. Focus on the California Institute of Arts. *Civic & Public Affairs:* 1%. Community foundations. *Education:* 6%. Primarily to colleges and educational foundations. *Environment:* 21%. Funds youth groups, community centers, and family services. *International:* 21%. Hospitals, pediatric health, and single-disease health associations. *Note:* Total contributions made in 1998. **Typ. Recipients:** Arthritis, Cancer, Children's Health/Hospitals, Clinics/Medical Centers, Emergency/Ambulance Services, Hospitals, Medical Research, Mental Health, Multiple Sclerosis, People with Disabilities, Single-Disease Health Associations, Substance Abuse, Trauma Treatment. **Geo. Dist:** CA.

### ★ 487 ★ Lutheran Brotherhood Foundation

625 Fourth Ave. South
Minneapolis, MN 55415
**Phone:** (612)340-8060      **Fax:** (612)340-8447
**Website:** http://www.lutheranbrotherhood.com
Ruth Soby, Grants Specialist
**Fnded:** 1982. **Philosophy:** The Lutheran Brotherhood Foundation provides competitively awarded grants to Lutheran 501(c)(3) organizations and institutions for innovative projects that meet the eligibility requirements and address one of the following funding priorities: Multicultural Ministry: To strengthen Lutheran outreach to minorities, with particular emphasis on the Hispanic population; Church Growth & Evangelism: For innovative projects designed to increase membership growth in the Lutheran Church; Wellness: For projects that address spiritual, mental, and physical health; Leadership Development: To build Lutheran leaders through support for youth, clergy, lay leaders, and leaders within Lutheran institutions and judicatories. Lutheran Brotherhood offers scholarships to Luthern students based on high academic achievement, religious leadership, and financial need. **Priorities:** *Civic & Public Affairs:* 2%. Supports women's affairs. *Education:* 10%. Funds colleges, schools, learning centers and religious education. *Environment:* 1%.Supports camps. *Note:* Contributions made in 2000. **Typ. Recipients:** Health Organizations, Hospitals, Public Health. **Geo. Dist:** nationally.

### ★ 488 ★ Lynde and Harry Bradley Foundation

PO Box 510860
Milwaukee, WI 53203-0153
**Phone:** (414)291-9915      **Fax:** (414)291-9991
**Website:** http://www.bradleyfdn.org
**Fnded:** 1942. **Philosophy:** The programs of the Lynde and Harry Bradley Foundation "support limited, competent government; a dynamic marketplace for economic, intellectual, and cultural activity; and a vigorous defense at home and abroad of American ideas and institutions." Funding is concentrated locally in cultural programs, education, social services, medical programs, health agencies, and public policy. National support goes toward research and education in domestic and international public policy. Grants are also given to higher education, particularly activities that investigate and nurture the moral, cultural, intellectual, and economic institutions which form a free society. The foundation reports that projects that are likely to be supported will "generally share the following assumptions: That free men and women should be treated as self-governing, responsible citizens, not as victims or clients. That the organization's goal should be to restore the intellectual and cultural common sense, wisdom, morality, and personal character, i.e. restoring their roles as reliable guideposts of everyday life. That traditional, local institutions–families, schools, neighborhoods, etc.–need to be reinvigorated, for they provide training of genuine citizenship and that cultivate personal character. That power should be returned to the states and localities, instead of centralized, bureaucratic, national institutions, where citizenship is not fully realized." That any arena of public life may be addressed where citizenship is

understood as an important issue. That the problem of citizenship at home or abroad where the fall of totalitarian regimes has made this issue particularly urgent. That the "projects will aim to improve the life of the community by increasing cultural and educational opportunities, basic economic development, and effective and humane social and health services." *Report of the Lynde and Harry Bradley Foundation* **Priorities:** *Arts & Humanities:* 3%. Supports theaters, symphonies, and art museums. *Civic & Public Affairs:* 29%. Funds neighborhoods and domestic policy programs. *Education:* 50%. Supports scholarship programs, school choice efforts, universities. *Environment:* 1%. Supports family services. *Note:* Total contributions made in 2000. **Typ. Recipients:** Children's Health/Hospitals, Clinics/Medical Centers, Health Policy/Cost Containment, Hospitals, Transplant Networks/Donor Banks. **Geo. Dist:** nationally; WI.

### ★ 489 ★ Lynn R. and Karl E. Prickett Fund

PO Box 20124
Greensboro, NC 27420
Diana Davis, Account Administrator
**Fnded:** 1964. **Philosophy:** The foundation generally supports civic affairs, social service groups, and education. Civic affairs funding favors civil rights, the environment, and municipalities. Funding for social services emphasizes community relations and planned parenthood. Educational funding favors funds, higher education, and political education. The arts and health care are also supported. **Priorities:** *Arts & Humanities:* 5%. Supports art institutes, and music. *Civic & Public Affairs:* 24%. Supports festivals, aquariums, community foundations, civil rights, and legal aid. *Education:* 16%. Mainly supports colleges and universities, education funds, and private secondary schools. *Environment:* 31%. Supports food distribution, youth organizations, and animal protection. *International:* 11%. Primarily supports single-disease health associations. *Religion:* 1%. Supports scientific organizations and research. *Note:* Total contributions made in 1999. **Typ. Recipients:** AIDS/HIV, Cancer, Children's Health/Hospitals, Emergency/Ambulance Services, Eyes/Blindness, Family Planning, Geriatric Health, Health Organizations, Multiple Sclerosis, Single-Disease Health Associations, Substance Abuse. **Geo. Dist:** nationally.

### ★ 490 ★ Lyon Foundation

PO Box 546
Bartlesville, OK 74005
**Phone:** (918)336-0066
James Connor, President
**Fnded:** 1975. **Philosophy:** Recent grants have been made primarily to social service organizations. The foundation favors community centers, youth organizations, and support for services for the disabled. Other recipient areas include health foundations, nutrition programs, and housing. In the past, contributions have been made across all major categories of support. **Priorities:** *Arts & Humanities:* 13%. Funds historical preservation. *Civic & Public Affairs:* 33%. Supports the City of Bartlesville, fire departments, and legal concerns. *Education:* 27%. Supports colleges, nursing scholarships, and community education. *Environment:* 23%. Supports Young Men's Christian Association, a community center, senior citizens organizations, alcohol and drug abuse prevention, and a local Pony League. *International:* 4%. Funds a hospital and family care. *Note:* Total contributions made in 2000. **Typ. Recipients:** Alzheimers Disease, Clinics/Medical Centers, Emergency/Ambulance Services, Geriatric Health, Health Organizations, Hospitals, Medical Education, Medical Rehabilitation, Mental Health, Nutrition, People with Disabilities, Public Health, Substance Abuse. **Geo. Dist:** Bartlesville, OK.

### ★ 491 ★ M. B. and Edna Zale Foundation

3102 Maple Ave., Ste. 225
Dallas, TX 75201-1233
**Phone:** (214)855-0627      **Fax:** (214)220-0633
Leonard Krasnow, President

**Fnded:** 1951. **Philosophy:** The foundation "honors the tradition of its founders through grants that stimulate change. To accomplish this mission, the Foundation acts as a catalyst for collaboration and makes grants in communities where the trustees live or have an interest." M. B. and Edna Zale Foundation 1996 Annual Report. **Priorities:** *Arts & Humanities:* 1%. subpanelports museums, history, theater, and opera. *Civic & Public Affairs:* 5%. Supports civil rights womens affairs, and clubs. *Education:* 10%. Supports colleges and universities, secondary schools, and literacy. *Environment:* 14%. Supports shelters, community services, child welfare, United Way, food distribution programs, family planning services, and people with disabilities. *International:* 15%. Hospital, geriatric health, and clinics. *Religion:* 1%. Supports a science center. *Note:* Total contributions made in 1999. **Typ. Recipients:** Cancer, Children's Health/Hospitals, Clinics/Medical Centers, Diabetes, Emergency/Ambulance Services, Geriatric Health, Health Organizations, Health-General, Heart, Hospitals, Hospitals (University Affiliated), Kidney, Long-Term Care, Medical Education, Mental Health, Nutrition, People with Disabilities, Speech & Hearing. **Geo. Dist:** preference is given to funding organizations in Florida, Georgia, New York, and Texas.

### ★ 492 ★ M. D. Anderson Foundation

PO Box 2558
Houston, TX 77252-8037
**Phone:** (713)216-1457      **Fax:** (713)216-2119
Ms. Ann Trotter, Secretary & Treasurer
**Fnded:** 1936. **Philosophy:** The foundation provides funding for the "improvement of working conditions among workers generally, as well as among particular classes of unskilled, skilled, and agricultural workers; to the establishment, support and maintenance of hospitals, homes and institutions for the care of the sick, the young, the aged, the incompetent and the helpless among the people; to the improvement of living conditions among people generally as well as in particular sections or localities; and to the promotion of health, science, education, and advancement and diffusion of knowledge and understanding among people." **Priorities:** *Arts & Humanities:* 12%. *Civic & Public Affairs:* 19%. *Education:* 46%. *Environment:* 6%. *International:* About 17%. **Typ. Recipients:** Adolescent Health Issues, Cancer, Child Abuse, Children's Health/Hospitals, Clinics/Medical Centers, Emergency/Ambulance Services, Eyes/Blindness, Family Planning, Geriatric Health, Health Organizations, Health Policy/Cost Containment, Heart, Hospices, Hospitals, Medical Education, Medical Rehabilitation, Medical Research, Mental Health, Nursing Services, People with Disabilities, Prenatal Health Issues, Public Health, Research/Studies Institutes, Single-Disease Health Associations, Substance Abuse, Transplant Networks/Donor Banks. **Geo. Dist:** TX, Harris County; Houston, TX; and metropolitan area.

### ★ 493 ★ M. G. and Lillie A. Johnson Foundation

PO Box 2269
Victoria, TX 77902
**Phone:** (512)575-7970      **Fax:** (512)575-2264
**Email:** mgj@cox-internet.com
Robert Halepeska, Executive Vice President
**Fnded:** 1958. **Philosophy:** The foundation's stated priority is support for health and higher education institutions in the Gulf Coast area of Texas. Historically, all grants are made to qualifying entities located in the 13 county area lying between Wharton and San Patricio counties. **Priorities:** *Arts & Humanities:* 10%. Supports the performing arts and libraries. *Civic & Public Affairs:* 18%. Supports municipalities, towns, safety, and parks/gardens. *Education:* 17%. Supports colleges and educational funds. *Environment:* 12%. Includes youth groups, drug abuse programs, food banks, and homes. *International:* 40%. Funds community health care organizations and city/county emergency services. *Note:* Total contributions made in fiscal 1999. **Typ. Recipients:** Clinics/Medical Centers, Domestic Violence, Emergency/Ambulance Services, Eyes/Blindness, Health Funds, Heart, Hospices, Hos-

pitals, Long-Term Care, Medical Education, Medical Rehabilitation, Mental Health, Nursing Services, Nutrition, People with Disabilities, Public Health, Research/Studies Institutes, Substance Abuse, Transplant Networks/Donor Banks, Trauma Treatment. **Geo. Dist:** Gulf Coast between San Patricio and Wharton; TX.


**★ 494 ★ M. J. Murdock Charitable Trust**
PO Box 1618
Vancouver, WA 98668
**Phone:** (360)694-8415          **Fax:** (360)694-1819
**Website:** http://www.murdock-trust.org
John Van Zytveld, Senior Program Director

**Fnded:** 1975. **Philosophy:** "The trust's mission is to enrich the quality of life in the Pacific Northwest by providing grants to organizations that seek to strengthen the region's educational and cultural base in creative and sustainable ways. Although the major funding interests are education and scientific research, grants are also given to a wide variety of organizations, including those that serve the arts, public affairs, health and medicine, human services, and people with disabilities." 1997 Guidelines The trust favors programs aimed at solutions for and the prevention of social problems, either through research or the application of existing knowledge and capabilities. Of major interest are projects which "expand man's knowledge of himself and his world; and which promote those values and activities of society leading to a happier, healthier, freer, and more productive life." The trust's primary function is to "provide 'up-front' or venture capital, along with that of other donors and the applicant's own resources. Funds are provided for the testing and validation of promising concepts, and in the launching of well thought-out programs which have the potential to thrive beyond the stage of initial funding." Science continues to be a major interest of the trust, reflecting Mr. Murdock's own scientific bent. The trust is taking an increasingly informed, active role in improving science and science education in the Pacific Northwest. It will explore additional pre-collegiate science possibilities that address the issue of the diminished supply of science educators and researchers, and will "seek to reinvigorate undergraduate science, and to support research and specialized science-education opportunities that address critical needs" of the region. **Priorities:** *Arts & Humanities:* 10%. Focus on historical societies, theater, and music. *Civic & Public Affairs:* 3%. *Education:* 37%. Interests include higher education, informal education at museums, research at major universities, and natural science research. *Environment:* 33%. Funds human service organizations. *International:* 11%. *Religion:* 18%. Supports scientific research. *Note:* Total contributions made in 1998. **Typ. Recipients:** Alzheimers Disease, Cancer, Children's Health/Hospitals, Clinics/Medical Centers, Emergency/Ambulance Services, Eyes/Blindness, Health Policy/Cost Containment, Hospitals, Hospitals (University Affiliated), Medical Education, Medical Rehabilitation, Medical Research, Mental Health, People with Disabilities, Preventive Medicine/Wellness Organizations, Public Health. **Geo. Dist:** Pacific Northwest USA; AK; ID; MT; OR; WA.


**★ 495 ★ M. R. Bauer Foundation**
208 South LaSalle St., Ste. 1750
Chicago, IL 60604
**Phone:** (312)372-1947          **Fax:** (312)372-2389
**Email:** klawrence@lksu.com
Kent Lawrence, President & Executive Director

**Fnded:** 1994. **Philosophy:** The foundation typically supports judicial system reform projects and programs reducing unwanted pregnancy. Colleges and universities, hospitals and health organizations, civic and public affairs causes, cultural concerns, and social welfare organizations also are supported. **Priorities:** *Arts & Humanities:* 2%. Museums, theater, music, arts associations, and arts festivals. *Civic & Public Affairs:* 22%. Primarily for judicial reform projects. *Education:* 5%. Colleges and universities, and medical education. *Environment:* 20%. Family planning, food and clothing distribution, youth organizations, and community services. *International:* 44%. Hospitals, medical centers, and single-disease health associations. *Note:* Total contributions made in 2000. **Typ. Recipients:** Adoles-

cent Health Issues, Cancer, Children's Health/Hospitals, Clinics/Medical Centers, Emergency/Ambulance Services, Family Planning, Health Organizations, Hospitals, Long-Term Care, Medical Education, Medical Rehabilitation, Medical Research, Mental Health, Multiple Sclerosis, Prenatal Health Issues, Research/Studies Institutes, Single-Disease Health Associations. **Geo. Dist:** Chicago, IL.


**★ 496 ★ M. S. Doss Foundation, Inc.**
PO Box 1677
Seminole, TX 79360-1677
**Phone:** (915)758-2770          **Fax:** (915)758-9591
Joe McGill, President

**Fnded:** 1984. **Philosophy:** The M. S. Doss Foundation primarily supports social service organizations. Recipients include children's homes and youth organizations. The foundation makes grants to other recipient areas, with an emphasis on building funds. **Priorities:** *Arts & Humanities:* 5%. Supports libraries. *Civic & Public Affairs:* 12%. Supports community affairs. *Education:* 4%. Supports educational institutions in Texas. *Environment:* 63%. Supports youth services, food banks, senior services, and women's shelters. *International:* 5%. Supports the Cerebral Palsy Treatment Center and hospitals. *Note:* Contributions were made in 1999. **Typ. Recipients:** Child Abuse, Children's Health/Hospitals, Diabetes, Domestic Violence, Hospices, Hospitals, Medical Education, Medical Rehabilitation, People with Disabilities, Single-Disease Health Associations, Substance Abuse. **Geo. Dist:** NM, eastern New Mexico; TX, western Texas.


**★ 497 ★ Mabel Louise Riley Foundation**
75 State St., 6th Fl.
Boston, MA 02109
**Phone:** (617)951-9100          **Fax:** (617)951-9151
**Website:** http://www.agmconnect.org/riley1.html
Nancy Saunders, Administrative Assistant

**Fnded:** 1972. **Philosophy:** The Mabel Louise Riley Foundation is a general purpose fund with the wide mission of "improving the quality of life for the people of Massachusetts, particularly in Boston." Miss Riley's wish that the trustees give "particular consideration to the needs of children and youth" is a factor in grant decisions. The foundation places an emphasis on education, and also supports youth and young adults through summer activity programs, arts for youth, and various human service programs. Comprehensive community development in low-income and minority neighborhoods is a priority that includes employment and job training, housing, historic preservation, urban affairs, and access to the arts for underserved populations. General city-wide attempts to enhance the quality of life in Boston, activities which have potential for lasting impact upon the Boston population, services to needy constituencies, and cultivation of potentially self-sufficient programs that may serve as models are also supported. **Priorities:** *Arts & Humanities:* 7%. Supports museums, libraries, cultural centers, and arts centers. *Civic & Public Affairs:* 8%. Community affairs, economic development, and housing. *Education:* 9%. Education associations, training organizations, and higher education. *Environment:* 58%. Youth organizations, child welfare, and shelters. *International:* 10%. Community health centers and single-disease health associations. *Note:* Total contributions made in 1999. **Typ. Recipients:** Clinics/Medical Centers, Diabetes, Emergency/Ambulance Services, Family Planning, Health Policy/Cost Containment, Long-Term Care, Medical Education, Mental Health, People with Disabilities, Prenatal Health Issues, Substance Abuse. **Geo. Dist:** Boston, MA.


**★ 498 ★ Malcolm Hewitt Wiener Foundation**
66 Vista Dr.
Greenwich, CT 06830
**Phone:** (203)222-4740
Adelaide Lewis, Contact

**Fnded:** 1984. **Philosophy:** The Malcolm Hewitt Wiener Foundation makes grants across the major categories of support. In civic affairs, interests include

world peace intitiatives, foreign relations, and economics. Arts funding favors art institutes, museums, historical preservation, and libraries. Social service primarily supports family services and family planning. Funding for education supports colleges and universities. Health care contributions include hospitals and health organizations. **Priorities:** *Arts & Humanities:* 30%. Supports ballet, orchestra, performing arts. *Civic & Public Affairs:* 5%. Supports parks, libraries, law and justice organizations. *Education:* 56%. Supports colleges and universities, arts and humanities education. *Environment:* 1%. Supports family planning, United Way. *International:* 6%. Supports New York Hospital-Cornell Medical Center. *Note:* Total contributions made in 1998. **Typ. Recipients:** AIDS/HIV, Children's Health/Hospitals, Children's Health/Hospitals, Clinics/Medical Centers, Emergency/Ambulance Services, Family Planning, Health Organizations, Health-General, Hospitals, Hospitals (University Affiliated), Medical Education, Medical Research, Nursing Services, People with Disabilities, Single-Disease Health Associations, Transplant Networks/Donor Banks. **Geo. Dist:** nationally; New York, NY.


**★ 499 ★ Mamie McFaddin Ward Heritage Foundation**
PO Box 3928
Beaumont, TX 77704-3928
**Phone:** (409)880-1415          **Fax:** (409)880-1437
**Email:** jmoncla@hibernia.com
Jean Moncla, Vice President & Trust Officer

**Fnded:** 1976. **Philosophy:** "The Foundation's primary purpose is to support the McFaddin-Ward House Museum, located in Beaumont, TX. The Foundation may also make grants to non-profit organizations in the local community for educational, cultural and charitable purposes." **Priorities:** *Arts & Humanities:* 2%. Supports historic preservation. *Education:* 4%. Supports legal education and universities. *Environment:* 91%. Supports youth services and food distribution. *International:* 2%. Suports geriatric health. *Note:* Total contributions made in 1999. **Typ. Recipients:** Children's Health/Hospitals, Emergency/Ambulance Services, Geriatric Health, Long-Term Care, Medical Rehabilitation, Medical Research, Nutrition. **Geo. Dist:** TX, Jefferson County.


**★ 500 ★ Mardag Foundation**
600 Norwest Center
55 East 5th St.
Saint Paul, MN 55101-1797
**Phone:** (651)224-5463          **Fax:** (651)224-8123
**Email:** inbox@mardagfoundation.org
Paul Verret, President

**Fnded:** 1969. **Philosophy:** "The Mardag Foundation is committed to making grants to qualified nonprofit organizations within the State of Minnesota that help to enhance and improve the quality of life. Our focus is on children, the elderly and other at-risk populations, education, and the arts. Where appropriate, the Foundation will be an active participant with others in grantmaking programs, and will be proactive in addressing issues as well as responsive to applications for grants." The foundation normally will: make grants for capital, program, or expansion projects of a time-limited nature; help meet start-up costs for promising new programs that demonstrate sound management and clear goals relevant to community needs; support established agencies seeking to expand their services or experiencing temporary financial difficulty; make some grants payable over a number years; provide funds to match resources or offer challenge grants; expect an indication of the general process that will be used to monitor or evaluate the impact or effect of the grants. In recent years, the foundation arranged a partnership with other private and public funders to address the critical needs in education and the problems of illiterate adults in Minnesota, and to achieve a better understanding of the needs of minority students. Included in the foundation's assistance is a three-year statewide program intended to help independent secondary schools improve their economic stability, and develop competitive curricula in an increasingly technological society. Funding for social service projects in Minnesota remains a priority as values, public funding, and local economics continue to change. In 1996, the foundation adopted a provisional policy outlining how it intends to address devolution and changes in public funding. 1996 Annual Report **Priorities:** *Arts & Humanities:* 11%. Arts centers, historical societies, music, and theaters. *Civic & Public Affairs:* 10%. Inner-city development. *Education:* 10%. Colleges and universities, minority education, and education associations. *Environment:* 66%. Child welfare, domestic violence, and family services. *International:* 3%. Public health. *Note:* Total contributions made in 1998. **Typ. Recipients:** Alzheimers Disease, Child Abuse, Domestic Violence, Emergency/Ambulance Services, Family Planning, Geriatric Health, Health Organizations, Hospices, Hospitals, Long-Term Care, Mental Health, People with Disabilities, Public Health, Sexual Abuse, Single-Disease Health Associations, Substance Abuse. **Geo. Dist:** MN.

### ★ 501 ★ Margaret L. Wendt Foundation

40 Fountain Plaza, Ste. 277
Buffalo, NY 14202-2220
**Phone:** (716)855-2146　　　　**Fax:** (716)855-2149
Robert Kresse, Secretary & Trustee

**Fnded:** 1955. **Philosophy:** The foundation makes grants in the following designated areas: schools, religious organizations, hospitals and health organizations, youth programs, the arts, and social and community welfare organizations. **Priorities:** *Arts & Humanities:* 16%. Theater, opera, and public broadcasting. *Civic & Public Affairs:* 22%. Urban programs, community services, and zoos. *Education:* 8%. Colleges and universities. *Environment:* About 19%. Boys and girls clubs, camps, and family support programs. *International:* 17%. Nursing homes, medical centers, and children's hospitals. *Religion:* 1%. *Note:* Total contributions made in fiscal 1998. **Typ. Recipients:** AIDS/HIV, Alzheimers Disease, Children's Health/Hospitals, Clinics/Medical Centers, Emergency/Ambulance Services, Family Planning, Health Funds, Health Organizations, Heart, Home-Care Services, Hospices, Hospitals, Long-Term Care, Medical Education, Medical Research, Mental Health, Nursing Services, Outpatient Health Care, People with Disabilities, Research/Studies Institutes, Single-Disease Health Associations, Speech & Hearing, Substance Abuse. **Geo. Dist:** NY, Western New York state; Buffalo, NY.

### ★ 502 ★ Margaret T. Morris Foundation

PO Box 592
Prescott, AZ 86302
**Phone:** (520)445-4010
Eugene Polk, Trustee

**Fnded:** 1967. **Philosophy:** The foundation supports all areas of philanthropy equally. Acceptable proposals have included arts associations, libraries, community development, support for educational programs at the primary and secondary levels, single-disease health organizations, hospitals, churches and religious community living, youth clubs, shelters, homes, and food and clothing distributors. **Priorities:** *Arts & Humanities:* 8%. Libraries, museums, performing arts and public broadcasting receive funding. *Civic & Public Affairs:* 13%. Supports community development and housing. *Education:* 20%. Emphasis on higher education. *Environment:* 15%. Supports services for youth, seniors, and programs for differently abled groups. *International:* 33%. Hospitals and health services are supported. *Note:* Total contributions made in 1998. **Typ. Recipients:** AIDS/HIV, Alzheimers Disease, Cancer, Children's Health/Hospitals, Clinics/Medical Centers, Emergency/Ambulance Services, Family Planning, Geriatric Health, Health Organizations, Health Policy/Cost Containment, Health-General, Home-Care Services, Hospices, Hospitals, Long-Term Care, Medical Education, Medical Research, Mental Health, People with Disabilities, Prenatal Health Issues, Public Health, Research/Studies Institutes, Single-Disease Health Associations. **Geo. Dist:** nationally.

### ★ 503 ★ Marie H. Bechtel Charitable Remainder Uni-Trust

201 West 2nd St., Ste. 1000
Davenport, IA 52801
**Phone:** (319)328-3333　　　　**Fax:** (319)328-3352
R. Bittner, Trustee

**Fnded:** 1978. **Philosophy:** The Marie H. Bechtel Charitable Remainder Uni-Trust was established with the purpose of serving the needs of the Scott County, IA, community. The trust has a broad range of interests that includes youth, education, public affairs, civic affairs, the arts, health, and social services. Both Harold and Marie Bechtel were lifetime residents of Scott County. Their primary purpose in establishing the trust was "to support all interests which serve to enhance the community, to restore its vitality, and to create meaningful education and employment today and in the future." Since Harold Bechtel's death in 1987, nearly all distributions have been to local organizations or Iowa educational institutions, but there have been several outside of Iowa. **Priorities:** *Arts & Humanities:* 10%. Supports libraries, arts museums, and a music festival. *Civic & Public Affairs:* 8%. Supports urban affairs and development, beautification foundation, and community support. *Education:* 43%. Supports universities, schools, colleges and business school. *Environment:* 23%. Supports Young Men's Christian Association, youth programs, and homes. *International:* 4%. Supports medical centers. *Religion:* 7%. Supports a Natural Science museum. *Note:* Total contributions made in 1999. **Typ. Recipients:** Cancer, Medical Education, Public Health. **Geo. Dist:** IA, Scott County.

### ★ 504 ★ Marion I. and Henry J. Knott Foundation

3904 Hickory Ave.
Baltimore, MD 21211-1834
**Phone:** (410)235-7068　　　　**Fax:** (410)889-2577
**Email:** knott@knottfoundation.org
**Website:** http://www.knottfoundation.org
M. Contori, Jr., Exec. Dir.

**Fnded:** 1986. **Philosophy:** The Marion I. and Henry J. Knott Foundation makes grants to "further Roman Catholic activities and other charitable, cultural, educational, health care, and human service activities." Program areas funded include arts and humanities, Catholic activities, education (limited to Catholic and non-sectarian private schools), health care, and social and human services. The foundation supports the following types of projects: capital/building campaigns, endowment funds (except for arts and humanities), new and/or ongoing programs, and operating expenses. **Priorities:** *Arts & Humanities:* 10%. Museums and arts centers, opera, and historical societies. *Civic & Public Affairs:* 7%. Focus on urban affairs. *Education:* 20%. Primarily supports private primary and secondary education. *Environment:* 14%. Supports shelters, food banks, counseling, and family services. *International:* 1%. Supports health associations. *Note:* Total contributions made in 1998. **Typ. Recipients:** AIDS/HIV, Alzheimers Disease, Cancer, Children's Health/Hospitals, Clinics/Medical Centers, Eyes/Blindness, Health Funds, Health Organizations, Hospices, Medical Education, Medical Rehabilitation, Mental Health, Multiple Sclerosis, Nutrition, People with Disabilities, Prenatal Health Issues, Preventive Medicine/Wellness Organizations, Public Health, Single-Disease Health Associations, Substance Abuse, Trauma Treatment. **Geo. Dist:** MD.

### ★ 505 ★ Marion O. and Maximilian E. Hoffman Foundation

168 Forest Ave.
Locust Valley, NY 11560
Ursula Niarakis, President

**Fnded:** 1984. **Philosophy:** The foundation makes most of its grants in the areas of environmental affairs, education, and the arts. Conservation causes receive major emphasis. Educational funding favors higher education, scholarships, and private schools. Funding for the arts emphasizes film, museums, and theater. Other support also goes to social services. **Priorities:** *Arts & Humanities:* 1%. *Environment:* 2%. *Note:* Total

contributions made in fiscal 1999. **Typ. Recipients:** AIDS/HIV, Cancer, Clinics/Medical Centers, Health Organizations, Hospitals, Medical Research, People with Disabilities, Single-Disease Health Associations. **Geo. Dist:** New York, NY.

### ★ 506 ★ Marriner S. Eccles Foundation

701 Deseret Bldg.
79 South Main St.
Salt Lake City, UT 84111
**Phone:** (801)246-5157
Shannon Toronto, Executive Director

**Fnded:** 1973. **Philosophy:** The foundation's giving is restricted to private, nongovernmental charitable, scientific, and educational organizations located in Utah for the benefit of the citizens of that state. **Priorities:** *Arts & Humanities:* 23%. Supports performing arts, museums, and art centers. *Civic & Public Affairs:* 9%. *Education:* 32%. Funds colleges and unversities. *Environment:* 17%. Includes issues related to teen pregnancy and substance abuse. *International:* 16%. Primarily to hospitals and single-disease health associations. *Note:* Total contributions made in fiscal 1999. **Typ. Recipients:** AIDS/HIV, Arthritis, Cancer, Children's Health/Hospitals, Clinics/Medical Centers, Diabetes, Eyes/Blindness, Family Planning, Geriatric Health, Health Organizations, Hospices, Hospitals, Medical Education, Mental Health, Nursing Services, People with Disabilities, Public Health, Respiratory, Single-Disease Health Associations, Substance Abuse. **Geo. Dist:** UT.

### ★ 507 ★ Mars Foundation

6885 Elm St.
McLean, VA 22101
**Phone:** (703)821-4900　　　　**Fax:** (703)448-9678
Susan Martin, Assistant Secretary

**Fnded:** 1956. **Philosophy:** Grants are generally awarded in the form of unrestricted general support. Though priority is given to programs for children and the environment, other grantees include: educational organizations; fine art associations; and public health organizations, including groups concerned with population problems and medical care and assistance. **Priorities:** *Arts & Humanities:* 12%. Supports the fine arts and historic preservation. *Civic & Public Affairs:* 6%. Urban and economic affairs. *Education:* About 36%. Supports elementary and secondary education and colleges and universities. *Environment:* 20%. Supports family planning organizations, child welfare, animal protection, and youth organizations. *International:* 7%. Primarily for single-disease health associations, hospitals, hospices, and medical training. *Note:* Total contributions made in 1998. **Typ. Recipients:** Cancer, Children's Health/Hospitals, Clinics/Medical Centers, Domestic Violence, Family Planning, Health Funds, Hospices, Medical Education, Medical Research, Nursing Services, People with Disabilities, Single-Disease Health Associations, Substance Abuse. **Geo. Dist:** nationally; Washington, DC, including metropolitan area.

### ★ 508 ★ Martha Holden Jennings Foundation

The Halle Bldg.
1228 Euclid Ave., Ste. 701
Cleveland, OH 44115
**Phone:** (216)589-5700　　　　**Fax:** (216)589-5730
**Website:** http://www.mhjf.org
William Hiller, Executive Director

**Fnded:** 1958. **Philosophy:** The foundation continues its mission to fund projects to "explore new frontiers in elementary and secondary public school education in Ohio and to promote more effective teaching in those schools." In seeking to improve the quality of primary and secondary education, the foundation has "invested heavily in major outreach areas. These include: early childhood education; urban schools; family involvement; improvements in math and science; ... assisting schools with technology; and partnerships involving universities and urban schools in Ohio." Grants also are aimed at programs to build a bridge of understanding and cooperation among colleges, universities, and public schools in order to achieve a higher quality of teaching and improved curricula and materials. The foundation itself administers several programs. These include a grants program for individual teachers and administrators to implement proposals or test new approaches to education designed by the recipients. The foundation also operates an educators' retreat to bring together public school educators, deans of colleges of education, and representatives of the Ohio Department of Education. Other programs offer workshops, lectures, and awards to develop needed skills, provide intellectual stimulation, and recognize outstanding teachers. **Priorities:** *Education:* 100% The Foundation reports its priorities are state initiatives, focusing on technology, and the master teachers program. The state initiatives program encompases three separate initiatives: parent involvement to improve student achievement by strengthening partnerships between families and schools; early childhood with a commitment to operate four Reggio Emilia preschools; and urban schools, with a focus on solving the problems of Large urban schools including early childhood education, prevention of disruptive and dangerous behavior, career planning and placement, assistance for "at-risk" students, intervention and accountability alliance, partnerships with parents and development for educators. The foundation's area of interest focusing on Technology includes programs such as training teachers in technology, software training, preparing high school students for high-tech careers and establishing a distance learning network. Each year the foundation also recognizes three Master Teachers from Ohio that are currently hosting the Jennings Scholar Lecture Series for the master teachers program. *Note:* Total contributions made in 1999. **Typ. Recipients:** Adolescent Health Issues, Heart, Mental Health, People with Disabilities, Preventive Medicine/Wellness Organizations, Substance Abuse. **Geo. Dist:** OH, Cuyahoga County.

### ★ 509 ★ Martin Foundation
500 Simpson Ave.
PO Box 1167
Elkhart, IN 46516
**Phone:** (219)295-3343          **Fax:** (219)523-3636
Elizabeth Martin, Co-President

**Fnded:** 1954. **Philosophy:** "Since its inception, the Martin Foundation has supported many worthy local civic projects and organizations, such as: the Public Library; YM-YWCA; Public Television; Park Development; Civic Plaza; Environmental Center; Midwest Museum of American Art; and the Elkhart County Community Foundation to mention a few." "In addition the Foundation has supported national and international organizations and projects including: University of California, Berkeley, graduate scholarship program; Field Museum of Natural History; Indiana University, South Bend for the endowed professorship in piano; Interlochen Center for the Arts; Massachusetts Institute of Technology for the Lee and Geraldine Martin Professorship in Environmental Studies and the Martin Fund; Nature Conservancy; Samaritan Institute, an international counseling network; and World Wildlife Fund." "The Foundation will continue to fund worthwhile local civic and community projects and has an interest in creative projects at the national level which attempt to address some of the world's challenging problems." 1996/1997 Guidelines and Annual Report **Priorities:** *Arts & Humanities:* 9%. Gives to arts centers, museums, and public broadcasting. *Civic & Public Affairs:* 6%. Funds women's issues, civil rights, and community foundations. *Education:* 63%. Contributes to higher education. Major grant to MIT. *Environment:* 7%. Primarily supports youth concerns, Young Men's Christian Association, and family planning services. *International:* 4%. Supports caregivers, health policy/cost containment, hospitals, and the Red Cross. *Note:* Total contributions made in fiscal 2000. **Typ. Recipients:** AIDS/HIV, Alzheimers Disease, Cancer, Child Abuse, Clinics/Medical Centers, Domestic Violence, Emergency/Ambulance Services, Family Planning, Health-General, Hospices, Hospitals, Medical Education, Medical Research, Medical Training, Mental Health, Nursing Services, People with Disabilities, Public Health, Single-Disease Health Associations, Substance Abuse. **Geo. Dist:** nationally.

### ★ 510 ★ Mary and Daniel Loughran Foundation
601 13th St., Ste. 1000 N
Washington, DC 20005
**Phone:** (202)434-7005          **Fax:** (202)347-4866
F. Burke, Contact

**Fnded:** 1967. **Philosophy:** The foundation primarily supports higher education in Washington, DC, and Virginia. The trustees also support agricultural education and schools for handicapped children. Youth organizations also are a primary focus, with emphasis on infant homes and maternity care. The foundation supports other charitable organizations in addition to its main interests. **Priorities:** *Arts & Humanities:* 15%. Museums and historic building preservation. *Civic & Public Affairs:* 2%. Legal aid. *Education:* 38%. Scholarship, educational instituitions. *Environment:* 24%. Youth organizations and community centers. *International:* 12%. Hospital support. *Note:* Total contributions made in fiscal 1999. **Typ. Recipients:** Adolescent Health Issues, Cancer, Children's Health/Hospitals, Clinics/Medical Centers, Emergency/Ambulance Services, Eyes/Blindness, Family Planning, Heart, Hospitals, Long-Term Care, Medical Education, Medical Rehabilitation, Medical Research, People with Disabilities, Prenatal Health Issues, Sexual Abuse, Single-Disease Health Associations. **Geo. Dist:** DC; MD; VA.

### ★ 511 ★ Mary Duke Biddle Foundation
1044 West Forest Hills Boulevard
Durham, NC 27707
**Phone:** (919)493-5591          **Fax:** (919)489-0118
Dr. James Semans, Chairman

**Fnded:** 1956. **Philosophy:** Mrs. Biddle's interests are still reflected in the foundation's giving pattern. Major recipients include cultural organizations, educational institutions, and community groups. In addition, the foundation shows an interest in aiding the handicapped. The trust agreement establishing the foundation specified that at least one-half of the annual income must go to Duke University for religious, scientific, literary, medical research, or educational purposes. Traditionally, support is given to Duke Memorial United Methodist Church, Durham, NC; Christ Church United Methodist, New York, NY; and Irvington Presbyterian Church, Irvington-on-Hudson, NY. The foundation provides grants for new programs, commissioning new works of art, for feasibility studies, and to organizations that provide assistance to individuals. In addition, challenge grants, planning grants, and start-up grants are made. The trustees are involved in the investigation of proposals and are willing to consider innovative projects and new ventures, even if success cannot be certain. Funding usually takes the form of general, program, and fellowship funds. In the area of music and the cultural arts, the foundation gives grants to organizations that support individual artists. Grants to individuals, however, are not made. Education grants are given to a wide variety of educational efforts in North Carolina and New York. Grants for aid to communities also are made. **Priorities:** *Arts & Humanities:* 32%. Emphasis on the Duke University Institute of Art. Also supports opera, theater, music, libraries, artists guilds, and the performing arts. *Civic & Public Affairs:* 2%. Gives to parks, community foundations and organizations, civil rights and botanical gardens. *Education:* 53%. Primary support for Duke University programs. Also funds scholarship and literacy. *Environment:* 8%. Funds community outreach, family and youth services, Special Olympics and counseling. *International:* 3%. Duke University Medical Center, blindness/eyes, AIDs, and physical therapy. *Note:* Total contributions made in 1999. **Typ. Recipients:** AIDS/HIV, Cancer, Clinics/Medical Centers, Geriatric Health, Health-General, Hospices, Hospitals (University Affiliated), Medical Education, Medical Rehabilitation, Mental Health, People with Disabilities. **Geo. Dist:** NY; NC.

### ★ 512 ★ Mary Hillman Jennings Foundation
625 Stanwix St., Ste. 2203
Pittsburgh, PA 15222
**Phone:** (412)434-5606          **Fax:** (412)434-5907
Paul Euwer, Jr., Executive Director

**Fnded:** 1968. **Philosophy:** The foundation's principal areas of interest are education, social services, and health. In addition, the foundation funds civic, arts, and religious organizations. **Priorities:** *Arts & Humanities:* 9%. Supports museums, ballet, theater, and libraries. *Civic & Public Affairs:* 3%. Supports community foundations and leadership initiatives. *Education:* 25%. Supports colleges and universities. *Environment:* 7%. Supports community service organizations, youth services, and food distribution. *International:* 49%. Supports medical centers and medical research. *Note:* Total contributions made in 1999. **Typ. Recipients:** Alzheimers Disease, Cancer, Children's Health/Hospitals, Clinics/Medical Centers, Diabetes, Domestic Violence, Emergency/Ambulance Services, Family Planning, Health Organizations, Hospices, Hospitals, Long-Term Care, Medical Rehabilitation, Medical Research, Nursing Services, Outpatient Health Care, People with Disabilities, Public Health, Sexual Abuse, Single-Disease Health Associations, Substance Abuse, Trauma Treatment. **Geo. Dist:** Pittsburgh, PA.

### ★ 513 ★ Mary Livingston Griggs and Mary Griggs Burke Foundation
55 East Fifth St.
1400 Norwest Center
Saint Paul, MN 55101-1792
**Phone:** (651)227-7683          **Fax:** (651)602-2670
Marvin Pertzik, Secretary & Treasurer

**Fnded:** 1966. **Philosophy:** The foundation supports the arts, and institutions or programs with a cultural, historical, or educational focus. The foundation has additional interests in social services and conservation, environmental, and beautification efforts. **Priorities:** *Arts & Humanities:* 55%. Supports museum, opera, ballet, libraries, dance, public broadcasting and ethnic/folk art. *Civic & Public Affairs:* 5%. Supports zoological societies botanical gardens and parks. *Education:* 3%. Supports arts/humanities education, minority education, and colleges. *Environment:* 7%. Supports homeless, family planning services, daycare, and United Way. *Religion:* 5%. Supports science museums. *Note:* Total contributions made in fiscal 1999. **Typ. Recipients:** AIDS/HIV, Clinics/Medical Centers, Family Planning, Heart, Hospitals, Medical Research. **Geo. Dist:** Minneapolis, MN; St. Paul, MN; New York, NY.

### ★ 514 ★ Mary Ranken Jordan and Ettie A. Jordan Charitable Foundation
1 US BankPlaza, Ste. 3500
Saint Louis, MO 63101
**Phone:** (314)552-6000          **Fax:** (314)552-7000
Fred Arnold, Chairman, Advisory Committee

**Fnded:** 1958. **Philosophy:** The foundation makes most of its grants in the areas of education, the arts, and children's health and welfare. Educational support favors colleges, universities, special education for the disabled, private secondary education, and art education. Arts interests include the performing arts, museums, historical preservation, and libraries. In social services, support goes to homes, youth organizations, food and clothing distribution, united funds, and community centers. Other recipient areas are funded on a limited basis. **Priorities:** *Arts & Humanities:* 27%. Supports public television, the performing arts, art museums, opera, and theater. *Civic & Public Affairs:* 16%. Supports zoos, parks, botanical gardens, and employment/job training. *Education:* 24%. Mainly supports colleges and universities. *Environment:* 10%. Supports family programs, scouting, people with disabilities, and Young Men's Christian Association. *International:* 19%. Supports health centers, hospitals, and single-disease health organizations. *Religion:* 3%. Supports science academies. *Note:* Contributions were made in 2000. **Typ. Recipients:** Children's Health/Hospitals, Clinics/Medical Centers, Clinics/Medical Centers, Diabetes, Emergency/Ambulance Services, Hospitals, Medical Education, Mental Health, People with Disabilities, Respiratory. **Geo. Dist:** MO, emphasis on St. Louis area.

### ★ 515 ★ Mary S. and David C. Corbin Foundation

910 Key Bldg.
Akron, OH 44308
**Phone:** (330)762-6427          **Fax:** (330)762-6428
**Email:** corbin@nls.net
James Hartenstein, Treasurer

**Fnded:** 1970. **Philosophy:** The foundation primarily supports higher education, health organizations, and civic affairs in the Akron, Ohio, area. **Priorities:** *Arts & Humanities:* 20%. Supports museums and historic preservation. *Civic & Public Affairs:* 29%. Supports botanical gardens, urban affairs, and economic development. *Education:* 4%. Major grant to the University of Akron. *Environment:* 32%. Youth organizations, family services, scouting, and YMCAs receive support. *International:* 6%. Funds hospitals, cardiac care, the American Red Cross, and Multiple Sclerosis. *Note:* Total contributions made in 1999. **Typ. Recipients:** Alzheimers Disease, Arthritis, Cancer, Children's Health/Hospitals, Clinics/Medical Centers, Domestic Violence, Emergency/Ambulance Services, Emergency/Ambulance Services, Health Organizations, Heart, Hospices, Hospitals, Long-Term Care, Mental Health, Multiple Sclerosis, Nursing Services, People with Disabilities, Prenatal Health Issues, Trauma Treatment. **Geo. Dist:** Akron, OH.

### ★ 516 ★ Mary W. Harriman Foundation

63 Wall St., 31st Floor, Ste. 3101
New York, NY 10005
**Phone:** (212)493-8182          **Fax:** (212)493-5570
William Hibberd, Secretary

**Fnded:** 1925. **Philosophy:** Board and family members directly involved with the distribution of funds give to groups that provide "a solid philanthropic benefit to the New York area." **Priorities:** *Arts & Humanities:* 25%. Supports libraries, museums, public broadcasting, the performing arts, and ballet. *Civic & Public Affairs:* 13%. Supports urban development, parks, and botanical gardens. *Education:* 37%. Supports secondary and preparatory schools, colleges and universities, and minority education. *Environment:* 7%. Supports children services, disabled services, social services, and family planning services. *International:* 2%. Supports cancer centers, visiting nurse organizations. *Religion:* 1%. Supports the American Museum of Natural History. *Note:* Total contributions made in 1999. **Typ. Recipients:** AIDS/HIV, Cancer, Child Abuse, Children's Health/Hospitals, Emergency/Ambulance Services, Family Planning, Hospices, Hospitals, Medical Education, Medical Rehabilitation, Mental Health, Nursing Services, People with Disabilities. **Geo. Dist:** New York, NY, metropolitan area.

### ★ 517 ★ Massey Charitable Trust

PO Box 1178
Coraopolis, PA 15108
**Phone:** (412)262-5992
Walter Carroll, Executive Director & Trustee

**Fnded:** 1968. **Philosophy:** The trust makes grants across the major categories of support. In education, funding favors colleges, minority education, and special education for the handicapped. Social service support goes to living services, family services, counseling, youth organizations, and food and clothing distribution. Health support favors single-disease associations, rehabilitation services, and specialty hospitals. In the arts, interests include opera, art centers, historic preservation, and public broadcasting. **Priorities:** *Arts & Humanities:* 22%. Supports symphonies, opera, museums, and arts centers. *Civic & Public Affairs:* 5%. Focus on the Pittsburgh Leadership Foundation, and community and public affairs. *Education:* 24%. Funds colleges, universities, and educational programs. *Environment:* 17%. Supports child and youth services, women's shelters, the disabled, elderly services, and planned parenthood. *International:* 19%. Supports hospitals, visiting nurse foundation, and disease and disorder concerns. *Note:* Total contributions made in 1998. **Typ. Recipients:** Alzheimers Disease, Arthritis, Cancer, Children's Health/Hospitals, Clinics/Medical Centers, Diabetes, Emergency/Ambulance Services, Eyes/Blindness, Family Planning, Health Funds, Health Organizations, Hospices, Hospitals, Hospitals (University Affiliated), Kidney, Long-Term Care, Medical Education, Medical Rehabilitation, Medical Research, Nursing Services, People with Disabilities, Public Health, Sexual Abuse, Single-Disease Health Associations, Substance Abuse. **Geo. Dist:** PA, emphasis on Southwest Pennsylvania; Pittsburgh, PA.

### ★ 518 ★ Massey Foundation

Four N Fourth St. Ste. 100
PO Box 26765
Richmond, VA 23219
**Phone:** (804)288-9500
William Massey, Jr., Contact

**Fnded:** 1957. **Philosophy:** The foundation has traditionally directed its philanthropy to medical, civic, and education activities in the southeastern United States. The foundation's current interests include private and state colleges and universities, as well as selected secondary schools for capital and special needs. The foundation has traditionally given to educational projects in the Appalachian coal fields where the family originated. In addition to educational institutions, the foundation supports religious and charitable organizations. The foundation supports hospitals and selected health care facilities with both capital and program grants. Symphonies, museums, and special arts organizations receive consideration, particularly regional facilities open to the general public. **Priorities:** *Arts & Humanities:* 4%. Richmond Ballet, museums, music, theater and the Virginia Historical Society. *Civic & Public Affairs:* 16%. Renaissance, philanthropy, and a botanical garden. *Education:* 72%. Mostly colleges and universities. Also supports engineering education, educational funds and technical institutes. *Environment:* 1%. Supports a boys home and scouting. *International:* 3%. Hospitals and cancer research. *Religion:* 4%. Virginia Institute of Marine Science and a science museum. *Note:* Total contributions made in fiscal 2000. **Typ. Recipients:** Cancer, Emergency/Ambulance Services, Health Organizations, Hospitals, Hospitals (University Affiliated), Medical Education, Mental Health, Preventive Medicine/Wellness Organizations, Single-Disease Health Associations. **Geo. Dist:** KY; VA; WV.

### ★ 519 ★ Matilda R. Wilson Fund

100 Renaissance Center, 34th Floor
Detroit, MI 48243
**Phone:** (313)259-7777          **Fax:** (313)393-7579
George Miller, Jr., President

**Fnded:** 1954. **Philosophy:** The foundation generally contributes to Southeast Michigan organizations offering services in the following areas: the arts, youth services, education, health, and human services. **Priorities:** *Arts & Humanities:* 16%. Funds a historical society, opera, theatre, and symphony orchestra, a library, and public broadcasting. *Civic & Public Affairs:* 14%. Major support for a zoological society. *Education:* 42%. Supports MI colleges and universities and minority education. *Environment:* 12%. Funds United Way, family services, food distribution, youth programs and shelters. *International:* 5%. Supports hospices, hospitals, and oral health. *Religion:* 5%. Supports the Detroit Science Center. *Note:* Total contributions made in 2000. **Typ. Recipients:** Children's Health/Hospitals, Clinics/Medical Centers, Emergency/Ambulance Services, Eyes/Blindness, Health Organizations, Hospices, Hospitals, Medical Education, People with Disabilities, Public Health, Research/Studies Institutes, Substance Abuse. **Geo. Dist:** nationally; MI.

### ★ 520 ★ Maurice Amado Foundation

3940 Laurel Canyon Boulevard, Ste. 809
Studio City, CA 91604
**Phone:** (818)980-9190          **Fax:** (818)980-9190
**Website:** http://www.mauriceamadofdn.org
Pam Kaizer, Executive Director

**Fnded:** 1961. **Philosophy:** The foundation supports activities that emphasize the Sephardic Jewish heritage, with special interest in cultural and educational projects. **Priorities:** *Arts & Humanities:* 12%. Museums, symphonies, opera, a film festival, history, and a library. *Education:* 17%. Funds a variety of educational institutions; also supports sephardic Jewish studies. **Typ. Recipients:** Cancer, Children's Health/Hospitals, Clinics/Medical Centers, Domestic Violence, Emergency/Ambulance Services, Geriatric Health, Health Organizations, Hospitals, Hospitals (University Affiliated), Long-Term Care, Medical Education. **Geo. Dist:** Los Angeles, CA; New York, NY.

### ★ 521 ★ Max H. Gluck Foundation

10375 Wilshire Boulevard, No. 2
Los Angeles, CA 90024
**Phone:** (310)519-7011
Mrs. Camilla Kocol, Program Director

**Fnded:** 1955. **Philosophy:** The foundation is devoted to supporting the arts through direct support of specific museums and opera companies or by supporting art education. While most of the interests lie in the arts, the foundation also supports children's services, especially day care, health, and public education in California's largest cities. **Priorities:** *Arts & Humanities:* 36%. Supports opera, museums, and libraries. *Civic & Public Affairs:* 3%. *Education:* 56%. Funds music and arts education,literacy, and equipment used in science education. *Environment:* 5%. Supports community centers. *Note:* Total contributions made in fiscal 1999. **Typ. Recipients:** AIDS/HIV, Arthritis, Children's Health/Hospitals, Clinics/Medical Centers, Diabetes, Emergency/Ambulance Services, Family Planning, Hospitals, Medical Education, People with Disabilities, Prenatal Health Issues, Research/Studies Institutes, Single-Disease Health Associations. **Geo. Dist:** Los Angeles, CA, including metropolitan area; NY.

### ★ 522 ★ Max Kade Foundation

450 Park Ave.
New York, NY 10022
**Phone:** (212)752-4693          **Fax:** (212)964-1549
Mr. Hans Hachmann, Contact

**Fnded:** 1944. **Philosophy:** The foundation's primary interest lies in higher education, particularly at the graduate and postdoctoral level. Grants are generally made to universities, colleges, and other educational and research institutions. The foundation seeks to promote international understanding and sharing of knowledge, through the exchange of young postdoctoral research scholars and visiting faculty members between U.S. and European universities. Research scholars are nominated by their home institutions. The foundation's major fields of interest are research and training in medicine or the natural and physical sciences (math, physics, chemistry, and biochemistry), and the study of foreign languages, literature, and culture. **Priorities:** *Arts & Humanities:* 4%. Supports historic preservation. *Education:* 53%. Funds colleges, universities, and educational programs. *International:* 18%. Funds postactoral research exchange programs in hospitals, medical centers, and universities. *Note:* Contributions were made in 1999. **Typ. Recipients:** Cancer, Children's Health/Hospitals, Clinics/Medical Centers, Diabetes, Eyes/Blindness, Geriatric Health, Heart, Hospitals, Medical Education, Medical Research, Medical Training, Nutrition, Research/Studies Institutes. **Geo. Dist:** nationally.

### ★ 523 ★ Max and Victoria Dreyfus Foundation

50 Main St., Ste. 1000
White Plains, NY 10606
**Phone:** (914)682-2008
Lucy Gioia, Office Administrator

**Fnded:** 1965. **Philosophy:** The foundation supports a variety of organizations in the arts, education, social services, health, and civic areas. **Priorities:** *Arts & Humanities:* 24%. Supports arts societies and the performing arts. *Civic & Public Affairs:* 10%. Housing and community programs. *Education:* 17%. Educational programs and funds. *Environment:* 17%. Primarily youth programs. *International:* 24%. Medical research and health care programs. *Religion:* 1%. *Note:* Total contributions made in 1998. **Typ. Recipients:** AIDS/HIV, Cancer, Children's Health/Hospitals, Clinics/Medical Centers, Emergency/Ambulance Services, Eyes/Blindness, Family Planning, Health Organizations, Health Organizations, Health-General, Heart, Home-Care Services, Hospices, Hospitals, Hospitals (University Affiliated), Medical Education, Medical Rehabilitation, Medical Research, Mental Health, People with Disabilities, Sexual Abuse, Single-Disease Health Associations, Substance Abuse. **Geo. Dist:** nationally.

**★ 524 ★ Maximilian E. and Marion O. Hoffman Foundation**
970 Farmington Ave., Ste. 203
West Hartford, CT 06107
**Phone:** (860)521-2949          **Fax:** (860)561-5082
Doris Chaho, President

**Fnded:** 1986. **Philosophy:** The foundation primarily supports health care, public policy, and environmental concerns; however, education, social services, and the arts also receive support from the foundation. **Priorities:** *Arts & Humanities:* 13%. Supports orchestra, theatre and public broadcasting. *Education:* 28%. Supports private education. *Environment:* 5%. Supports people with disabilities and shelters/homes. *International:* 15%. Supports hospital and medical centers. *Religion:* 1%. Supports science center. *Note:* Total contributions made in fiscal 1999. **Typ. Recipients:** Adolescent Health Issues, AIDS/HIV, Alzheimers Disease, Cancer, Child Abuse, Children's Health/Hospitals, Clinics/Medical Centers, Diabetes, Emergency/Ambulance Services, Geriatric Health, Health Organizations, Health-General, Heart, Hospitals, Hospitals (University Affiliated), Kidney, Medical Education, Medical Rehabilitation, Mental Health, Nursing Services, Nutrition, People with Disabilities, Prenatal Health Issues, Research/Studies Institutes, Respiratory, Single-Disease Health Associations, Substance Abuse. **Geo. Dist:** U.S. Northeastern Region.

**★ 525 ★ McBean Family Foundation**
400 S El Camino Real, Ste. 777
San Mateo, CA 94402
**Phone:** (650)558-8480          **Fax:** (650)558-8481
**Email:** mcbeanfamilyfoundation@att.net
Charlene Kleiner, Secretary

**Fnded:** 1955. **Philosophy:** The foundation provides support for health organizations, educational institutions, civic affairs, human services, and the arts. Funding is generally limited to the San Francisco area and Northern California. **Priorities:** *Arts & Humanities:* About 2%. *Civic & Public Affairs:* 16%. *Education:* 25%. *International:* 27%. *Note:* Total contributions made in 2000. Analysis provided by the foundation. **Typ. Recipients:** AIDS/HIV, Alzheimers Disease, Cancer, Child Abuse, Clinics/Medical Centers, Eyes/Blindness, Health Organizations, Hospices, Hospices, Hospitals, Long-Term Care, Medical Education, Medical Research, Sexual Abuse. **Geo. Dist:** CA, San Francisco Bay area.

**★ 526 ★ McCamish Foundation**
3060 Peachtree Rd. Northwest, 19th Floor
Atlanta, GA 30305
**Phone:** (404)261-4418          **Fax:** (404)262-2681
Roy Jones, Chief Operating Officer

**Fnded:** 1989. **Philosophy:** The McCamish Foundation's main concern is social services with multiple grants funding Noah's Ark, an animal protection agency. Other social service concerns include athletics, senior services, and disabled adults. Education also receives large support, including funding for Reinhart College, leadership training, and educational foundations. The foundation also supports religious organizations, public policy groups, and environmental concerns. **Priorities:** *Civic & Public Affairs:* 14%. Supports public policy research, business and legal concerns, and aquariums and botanical gardens. *Education:* 30%. Funds higher education and enrichment programs. *Environment:* 14%. Funds youth groups, services for the elderly, and religious welfare. *International:* 9%. Supports medical centers, rehabilitation, and single-disease associations. *Note:* Total contributions made in 1998. **Typ. Recipients:** Alzheimers Disease, Arthritis, Cancer, Child Abuse, Children's

Health/Hospitals, Clinics/Medical Centers, Domestic Violence, Emergency/Ambulance Services, Health-General, Heart, Hospitals, Medical Education, Medical Rehabilitation, People with Disabilities, Prenatal Health Issues, Preventive Medicine/Wellness Organizations, Public Health, Single-Disease Health Associations. **Geo. Dist:** Atlanta, GA.

**★ 527 ★ McCann Foundation**
35 Market St.
Poughkeepsie, NY 12601
**Phone:** (914)452-3085          **Fax:** (914)452-3093
John Gartland, Jr., President

**Fnded:** 1969. **Philosophy:** The McCann Foundation focuses on the needs of the Dutchess County, NY, community. The foundations awards grants to a number of educational, cultural, religious, social, and recreational organizations "to help them achieve their goals and better serve their communities." As a foundation, their role "is to seek and fund opportunities and projects that benefit the community and everyone who lives, works, studies and visits in Dutchess County." McCann Foundation Annual Report, 1996 During 1996, the foundation directly supported two major community projects. These included the conversion of a former IBM building into a new home for Our Lady of Lourdes High School, as well as a major multipurpose, sports facility expansion of The McCann Recreation Center at Marist College. **Priorities:** *Arts & Humanities:* 1%. Funds public broadcasting. *Civic & Public Affairs:* 3%. Supports public defense, botanical gardens, and community groups. *Education:* 61%. Includes a major grant to Marist College. *Environment:* 25%. Funds recreational activities and community services. *Note:* Total contributions made in 1999. **Typ. Recipients:** Children's Health/Hospitals, Hospices, Hospitals, People with Disabilities, Trauma Treatment. **Geo. Dist:** NY, Dutchess County; Poughkeepsie, NY.

**★ 528 ★ McCasland Foundation**
PO Box 1702
Duncan, OK 73534
**Phone:** (580)252-6559          **Fax:** (580)255-9336
Barbara Braught, Executive Director

**Fnded:** 1952. **Philosophy:** The foundation funds colleges and universities, mostly within Oklahoma, as well as a variety of other organizations. **Priorities:** *Arts & Humanities:* 66%. Funds music, libraries, construction of a museum and statue, and historical societies. *Civic & Public Affairs:* 6%. Urban affairs. *Education:* About 19%. Primarily funds colleges and universities. *Environment:* 5%. Supports united funds and youth groups. *International:* 1%. Pediatric health and health centers. *Religion:* 2%. Gives to science museums. *Note:* Total contributions made in 1998. **Typ. Recipients:** Alzheimers Disease, Cancer, Children's Health/Hospitals, Clinics/Medical Centers, Emergency/Ambulance Services, Health Organizations, Heart, Hospices, Hospitals, Long-Term Care, Medical Education, Medical Rehabilitation, Medical Research, People with Disabilities, Single-Disease Health Associations, Substance Abuse. **Geo. Dist:** OK, primarily Oklahoma.

**★ 529 ★ McConnell Foundation**
PO Box 492050
Redding, CA 96049-2050
**Phone:** (530)226-6200          **Fax:** (530)226-6210
**Email:** info@mcconnellfoundation.org
**Website:** http://www.mcconnellfoundation.org
Lee Salter, President & Executive Director

**Fnded:** 1964. **Philosophy:** Currently, the foundation promotes innovative projects in Shasta and Siskiyou counties in California in the areas of arts and culture, community enrichment, designated special projects, education, environment, health care, recreation, and social services. Within these general giving areas, the foundation has four specific areas of interest including the following: environment, environmental education, and recreation; projects that benefit the working poor; projects for the larger good; and promotion of volunteerism. Support is limited to nonprofit, tax-exempt organizations, public education (high school and above), and governmental entities. **Priorities:** *Arts &*

*Humanities:* 76%. Supports museums, public broadcasting, and libraries. *Civic & Public Affairs:* 6%. Funds community services and redevelopment, parks, women's affairs, and towns/municipalities. *Education:* 3%. Supports public education, scholarships, pre schools, and education foundations,. *Environment:* 10%. Supports family planning services, family services, Young Men's Christian Association, United Way, and senior services. *International:* 5%. Funds hospitals and community health projects. *Note:* Total contributions in 1999. **Typ. Recipients:** Clinics/Medical Centers, Domestic Violence, Emergency/Ambulance Services, Family Planning, Hospices, Hospitals, Medical Rehabilitation, Medical Research, Medical Training, Nutrition, People with Disabilities, Public Health, Substance Abuse. **Geo. Dist:** CA, Shasta County; CA, Siskiyou County.

**★ 530 ★ McCune Foundation**
750 Six PPG Place
Pittsburgh, PA 15222
**Phone:** (412)644-8779          **Fax:** (412)644-8059
**Website:** http://www.mccune.org
Henry Beukema, Executive Director

**Fnded:** 1979. **Philosophy:** The McCune Foundation has a broad mission to support efforts which improve communities. The Distribution Committee emphasizes the following program areas: education, the humanities, human services, and civic affairs. The foundation recognizes the importance of community-based organizations that are working to remedy the effects of economic dislocation, while addressing future issues. With an awareness of limited resources in comparison to growing needs, the Foundation is particularly interested in innovative/collaborative approaches to address regional problems and priorities, primarily in Southwestern Pennsylvania. **Priorities:** *Arts & Humanities:* 9%. Primary support for historic organizations, museums, and theater. *Civic & Public Affairs:* 31%. Funds economic and community development concerns. *Education:* 20%. Focus on colleges. *Environment:* 21%. Focus on services for families and children. *International:* 12%. Funds hospitals. *Religion:* 2%. *Note:* Total contributions made in fiscal 1998. **Typ. Recipients:** AIDS/HIV, Cancer, Children's Health/Hospitals, Clinics/Medical Centers, Domestic Violence, Geriatric Health, Health Funds, Health Organizations, Health Policy/Cost Containment, Hospices, Hospitals, Hospitals (University Affiliated), Medical Education, Medical Rehabilitation, Medical Research, Medical Training, Mental Health, Nursing Services, Nutrition, People with Disabilities, Prenatal Health Issues, Public Health, Single-Disease Health Associations, Substance Abuse. **Geo. Dist:** PA, Southwestern Pennsylvania; Pittsburgh, PA.

**★ 531 ★ McGregor Fund**
333 West Fort St., Ste. 2090
Detroit, MI 48226-3134
**Phone:** (313)963-3495          **Fax:** (313)963-3512
**Email:** dave@mcgregorfund.org
**Website:** http://www.mcgregorfund.org
C. Campbell, President

**Fnded:** 1925. **Philosophy:** "Concern for the needs of the homeless and hungry remains a priority of the fund." In addition, "partnerships and cooperative endeavors which address the critical issues facing greater Detroit continue to be a key element." To these ends, the fund supports a broad range of civic, health, and human service programs in the Detroit area. It also has expanded its interest in the environment and in the arts and humanities. In keeping with Mr. McGregor's belief that education was an essential prerequisite to solving society's ills, the fund supports specific projects at independent elementary and secondary schools serving metropolitan Detroit, colleges and universities in the Detroit area, and Michigan's public research universities. Grants are also awarded under two special programs, one for elementary and secondary schools serving students from low-income families in Detroit and the other for private liberal arts colleges and universities in Michigan and Ohio. In addition to the general and special programs, six discretionary grants are awarded to educational institutions selected each year by the trustees. The

McGregor Fund is a member of several national and statewide service organizations that promote the advancement of the nonprofit sector. The fund is no longer supporting national or local chapters of disease-specific organizations. **Priorities:** *Arts & Humanities:* 21%. Supports symphony orchestra hall, and the Museum of African American History. *Civic & Public Affairs:* 21%. Community affairs. *Education:* 21%. Supports public schools, colleges, universities, and educational programs. *Environment:* 30%. United Way, children's services, food for the needy, and shelters. *International:* 5%. Funds hospitals, AIDS awareness, and American Red Cross. *Religion:* 1%. *Note:* Contributions made in fiscal 1999. **Typ. Recipients:** AIDS/HIV, Children's Health/Hospitals, Emergency/Ambulance Services, Health Organizations, Hospitals, Long-Term Care, Mental Health, People with Disabilities, Prenatal Health Issues, Substance Abuse. **Geo. Dist:** Detroit, MI, metropolitan area.

### ★ 532 ★ McInerny Foundation
PO Box 3170
Honolulu, HI 96802
**Phone:** (808)538-4540          **Fax:** (808)538-4647
**Fnded:** 1937. **Philosophy:** The McInernys established the foundation "in order to promote the welfare of the people of the Hawaiian Islands." Under the terms of the deed of trust creating the foundation, the income is to be used for "charitable, scientific or educational purposes, or for the prevention of cruelty to children or animals." Use of this income is flexible, in order to meet changing conditions, and to "best serve the charitable requirements of the people of the Hawaiian Islands." Grants currently are made in five fields: education, social services, environment, culture and arts, and health and rehabilitation. **Priorities:** *Arts & Humanities:* 3%. Supports museums, arts education, literature, public broadcasting, and the performing arts. *Civic & Public Affairs:* 6%. Supports economic development, housing, legal aid, and community foundations. *Education:* 52%. Supports pre-school through higher education. *Environment:* 28%. Funds United Way, social service organizations, youth groups, and humane societies. *International:* 9%. Supports clinics, medical centers, and single-disease associations. *Note:* Total contributions made in fiscal 1999. **Typ. Recipients:** AIDS/HIV, Cancer, Children's Health/Hospitals, Clinics/Medical Centers, Domestic Violence, Emergency/Ambulance Services, Family Planning, Health Organizations, Home-Care Services, Hospices, Hospitals, Long-Term Care, Medical Education, Medical Rehabilitation, Mental Health, People with Disabilities, Prenatal Health Issues, Public Health, Single-Disease Health Associations, Substance Abuse. **Geo. Dist:** HI.

### ★ 533 ★ McIntosh Foundation
1730 M St. Northwest, Ste. 204
Washington, DC 20036
**Phone:** (202)338-8055          **Fax:** (202)234-0745
Michael McIntosh, President & Director
**Fnded:** 1953. **Philosophy:** With the advent in the past few years of a large number of foundations with hundreds of millions of dollars in assets (and many with billions) almost all of whom are addressing a broad range of social issues, it seemed to make sense that a relatively small foundation like the McIntosh Foundation should think of narrowing its focus. "Accordingly, because of its long-term interest in Southeast Alaska dating back to the early 1970's, several years ago it decided to focus its modest resources on the environment and economic issues (timber, commercial fishing, tourism, etc.) affecting the Tongass National Forest. The Tongass, aside from being by far the U.S.'s largest National Forest, comprises 95% of the land area of the 50,000 square miles that is Southeast Alaska. It is also the last great remaining temperate rainforest on earth." 1999 Philosophy Statement. **Priorities:** *Arts & Humanities:* 3%. Supports historic preservation, libraries, and public broadcasting. *Civic & Public Affairs:* 19%. Supports legal concerns and community foundations. *Education:* 56% Funds higher education. *Environment:* 5%. Funds social welfare. *International:* 4%. Single-disease associations and clinics. *Note:* Total contributions made in

1998. **Typ. Recipients:** Cancer, Clinics/Medical Centers, Clinics/Medical Centers, Geriatric Health, Health Organizations, Hospitals, Nursing Services, People with Disabilities, Single-Disease Health Associations. **Geo. Dist:** AK; AK, Tongass National Forest, Southeast Alaska.

### ★ 534 ★ MCJ Foundation
310 South St.
Morristown, NJ 07960
**Phone:** (973)540-1946          **Fax:** (973)538-8175
**Fnded:** 1983. **Philosophy:** "The MCJ Foundation was founded in the belief that the revitalization of our nation's inner-city neighborhoods through education, social services, economic opportunity and various collaborative efforts that involve the men and women from these communities is essential to ensure the uplifting of our nation's minorities and underprivileged children." "The Foundation currently focuses on programs that encourage and enable the development of mentoring relations, quality education, activities and job training for 'youth at risk,' entrepreneurial opportunities, affordable housing, community service activities, arts and cultural diversity, and health." **Priorities:** *Arts & Humanities:* 14% major support for the New Jersey Performing Arts Center. *Civic & Public Affairs:* 7%. Supports job training and urban affairs organizations. *Education:* 31%. Colleges, universities, and primary and secondary schools. *Environment:* 25%. Focus on youth organizations and child welfare. *International:* 15%. University medical centers and hospitals. *Note:* Total contributions made in fiscal 1998. **Typ. Recipients:** Cancer, Children's Health/Hospitals, Clinics/Medical Centers, Family Planning, Health Funds, Hospitals, Medical Research, People with Disabilities, Public Health, Substance Abuse. **Geo. Dist:** Newark, NJ; New York, NY.

### ★ 535 ★ McKnight Foundation
600 TCF Tower
121 South Eighth St.
Minneapolis, MN 55402
**Phone:** (612)333-4220          **Fax:** (612)332-3833
**Email:** info@mcknight.org
**Website:** http://www.mcknight.org
Richard Scott, Vice President Finance and Administratio
**Fnded:** 1953. **Philosophy:** "Our mission is to improve the quality of life for present and future generations and to seek paths to a more humane and secure world. We support efforts to strengthen communities, families, and individuals, particularly those in need. We contribute to the arts, encourage preservation of our natural environment, and promote research in selected fields. We continually explore innovative ideas to advance our goals in partnership with those we serve." "Making grants in the human services in seven-county Twin Cities metro area is the core of the foundation's work. It seeks to meet the needs of and empower people who are poor or disadvantaged; to identify effective long-term strategies to meet those needs; and to address the underlying problems of the community and the institutional causes of those problems. Within the human services area, the foundation is primarily supporting programs in the following areas: the development of children and young people; the linkage between housing and social services; family stability at a time of change in family structure; employment for people who are hard to employ; community development with an emphasis on enhancing the safety, livability and economic stability of neighborhoods; and greater public understanding of the needs of people confronting these challenges." The foundation has also shown recent interest in community improvement and economic development, affordable housing in the Twin Cities, public affairs, and international development issues (such as women's rights and health and human services). International grant making focuses on relieving the suffering of disadvantaged people in Africa and refugees in Southeast Asia, enhancing international stability with an emphasis on peacekeeping efforts, and improving the understanding of global issues in Minnesota and the upper Midwest. **Priorities:** *Arts & Humanities:* 8%. Supports arts councils, arts education and criticism,

community arts, and dance/film/video. *Civic & Public Affairs:* 15%. Program support to community improvement, housing, public affairs, and family loan programs. *Environment:* 54%. Supports programs providing services to those whose opportunities have been limited by poverty. *International:* 6%. Funds eating disorder research and prevention. *Religion:* 5%. Research and applied science–includes plant and crop research. *Note:* Total contributions made in 2000. **Typ. Recipients:** Adolescent Health Issues, Child Abuse, Domestic Violence, Family Planning, Hospitals, Medical Rehabilitation, Medical Research, Medical Training, Mental Health, People with Disabilities, Sexual Abuse. **Geo. Dist:** environment grants are made within the ten states along the Mississippi River; some funding internationally; MN, emphasis on the Minneapolis-St. Paul metropolitan area.

### ★ 536 ★ McLean Contributionship
945 Haverford Rd., Ste. A
Bryn Mawr, PA 19010-3814
**Phone:** (610)527-6330          **Fax:** (610)527-9733
**Website:** http://fdncenter.org/grantmaker/mclean
Sandra McLean, Executive Director
**Fnded:** 1951. **Philosophy:** The trustees believe the resources of the Contributionship can be used most effectively by making a relatively limited number of grants for projects of long-term benefit rather than by underwriting continuing operating expenses. The trustees focus on capital projects, brick and mortar, and endowments, or will provide seed money for the understanding and preservation of the environment, education, medical purposes, scientific developments, and compassionate care of the elderly. **Priorities:** *Arts & Humanities:* 16%. Supports arts, cultural organizations, historical societies, museums, media, and performing arts. *Education:* 29%. Supports higher education, elementary and secondary education, continuing education, and libraries. *Environment:* 15%. Job training, food/nutrition, recreation, youth development, and United Way. *International:* 13%. Diseases (ALS), Health-general and rehabilitative: hospitals, nursing homes and Programs, rehab, and medical research. *Note:* Total contributions made in 2000. **Typ. Recipients:** AIDS/HIV, Cancer, Children's Health/Hospitals, Diabetes, Domestic Violence, Emergency/Ambulance Services, Eyes/Blindness, Family Planning, Geriatric Health, Health-General, Hospitals, Long-Term Care, Medical Education, Medical Education, Medical Rehabilitation, Medical Research, Mental Health, Nursing Services, People with Disabilities, Prenatal Health Issues, Public Health, Single-Disease Health Associations, Transplant Networks/Donor Banks. **Geo. Dist:** PA, primarily metropolitan Philadelphia.

### ★ 537 ★ McMillen Foundation
6610 Mutual Dr.
Fort Wayne, IN 46825
**Phone:** (260)484-8631          **Fax:** (260)483-0474
John McMillen, President
**Fnded:** 1947. **Philosophy:** The McMillen Foundation makes most of its grants in the areas of social services and education. Social service funding favors recreational support for the benefit of youth. Educational support is directed at health education and outreach programs. Minor grants are given to other recipient areas. **Priorities:** *Arts & Humanities:* 5%. Supports historic preservation and music. *Civic & Public Affairs:* 5%. Major support for the Headwater Park Commission. *Education:* 35%. Emphasis on an education fund and medical education. *Environment:* 52%. Primary support for a recreation association and a YWCA. *Religion:* 2%. Supports science centers. *Note:* Total contributions made in 1998. **Typ. Recipients:** AIDS/HIV, Clinics/Medical Centers, Domestic Violence, Family Planning, Geriatric Health, Health Organizations, Health Organizations, Health-General, People with Disabilities, Public Health, Sexual Abuse, Substance Abuse. **Geo. Dist:** IN, Allen County; Ft. Wayne, IN.

## ★ 538 ★ The Meadows Foundation

3003 Swiss Ave.
Wilson Historic District
Dallas, TX 75204-6090
**Phone:** (214)826-9431  **Fax:** (214)827-7042
**Email:** djones@mfi.org
**Website:** http://www.mfi.org
Bruce Esterline, Vice President, Grants

**Fnded:** 1948. **Philosophy:** The Meadows Foundation looks for "imaginative, innovative ways to solve community problems; for projects leading to organizational self-sufficiency; for capital plans which will enable programs to flourish; and for ways to alleviate pain, to ameliorate social ills, and to promote better human relationships." The foundation continues its tradition of balanced giving in basic areas of human activity and need: the arts, social services, health, education, and civic programs. In 1978, the foundation funded the Algur H. Meadows Award for Excellence in the Arts, established by the Meadows School of the Arts at Southern Methodist University. The annual award of $50,000 is for exceptional achievement or distinguished service in the creative or performing arts. Other grants in arts and culture support various community and educational institutions, including gifts to museums and historic preservation projects. Human services grants support disaster relief, child care, dependency rehabilitation, handicapped, youth, and counseling programs. Educational grants include preschool through postgraduate levels, at both public and private institutions, and numerous community-based organizations. Grants for health services are especially targeted towards disadvantaged or rural citizens. Civic and public affairs grants improve the built or natural environment. The foundation sponsors a program housing nonprofit agencies for creative resource sharing on several unique blocks of turn-of-the-century houses in Dallas. There is an emerging interest in public education, mental health/illness, and the environment. **Priorities:** *Arts & Humanities:* 14%. Focus on museums and fine arts. *Civic & Public Affairs:* 15%. Supports urban affairs, community and public development. *Education:* 12%. Supports institutions that implement programs in literacy, tutoring, drop-out recovery, teacher education, and reading readiness. *Environment:* 34%. Supports child development centers, homeless shelters, food banks, and community centers. *International:* 25%. Emphasis on hospitals, medical centers, and other special cause centers that deal with abuse and rehabilitation. *Note:* Total contributions made in 1999. **Typ. Recipients:** AIDS/HIV, AIDS/HIV, Alzheimers Disease, Cancer, Child Abuse, Children's Health/Hospitals, Clinics/Medical Centers, Domestic Violence, Emergency/Ambulance Services, Eyes/Blindness, Family Planning, Geriatric Health, Health Funds, Health Organizations, Health Policy/Cost Containment, Health-General, Heart, Home-Care Services, Hospices, Hospitals, Hospitals (University Affiliated), Kidney, Long-Term Care, Medical Education, Medical Training, Mental Health, Outpatient Health Care, People with Disabilities, Preventive Medicine/Wellness Organizations, Public Health, Single-Disease Health Associations, Speech & Hearing, Substance Abuse, Transplant Networks/Donor Banks. **Geo. Dist:** TX, emphasis on Dallas.

## ★ 539 ★ Medina Foundation

801 2nd Ave., Ste. 1300
Seattle, WA 98104
**Phone:** (206)652-8783  **Fax:** (206)652-8791
**Email:** info@medinafoundation.org
**Website:** http://www.medinafoundation.org
Gregory Barlow, Executive Director

**Fnded:** 1948. **Philosophy:** The purpose of the foundation is "to aid in improving the human condition in the greater Puget Sound community by fostering positive change and the growth and improvement of people." The foundation specifies four areas of interest: emergency food and shelter; the physically and mentally handicapped and their development; promotion of efficiency and effectiveness of charity-supported and governmental organizations within the foundation's interests; and private education (preschool through grade 12) programs to improve teachers' abilities, programs to improve leadership and develop-

ment, projects fostering communications among various segments of the education community, and support of vocational schools and programs. **Priorities:** *Civic & Public Affairs:* 21%. Housing, community development, resource centers, clubs, and employment/job training. *Education:* 8%. Teacher development, alternative schools, vocational schools, and development of physically and mentally handicapped. *Environment:* 54%. Senior services, youth shelters, alcohol and drug abuse programs, parenting programs, and community services. *International:* 7%. Clinics and services for education and mental health. *Note:* Total contributions made in 1999. **Typ. Recipients:** Children's Health/Hospitals, Clinics/Medical Centers, Domestic Violence, Emergency/Ambulance Services, Geriatric Health, Health Organizations, Hospitals, Medical Education, Medical Rehabilitation, Mental Health, People with Disabilities, Preventive Medicine/Wellness Organizations, Single-Disease Health Associations, Substance Abuse. **Geo. Dist:** WA, greater Puget Sound region.

## ★ 540 ★ Merck Family Fund

303 Adams St.
Milton, MA 02186
**Phone:** (617)696-3580  **Fax:** (617)696-7262
**Email:** merck@merckff.org
**Website:** http://www.merckff.org
Jenny Russell, Executive Director

**Fnded:** 1954. **Philosophy:** The Merck Family Fund is dedicated to protecting the natural environment and addressing the root causes of problems faced by socially and economically disadvantaged people by working to build a sense of community in impoverished neighborhoods. The fund's environmental program focuses on protecting and restoring vital eastern United States ecosystems and promoting economic practices that will assure a sustainable environment for future generations. The fund's community-building program focuses on creating green and open space and meeting the needs of disadvantaged youth. **Priorities:** *Civic & Public Affairs:* 37%. Supports aquariums, gardens, parks, housing, economic development, and minority affairs. *Environment:* 5%. Supports youth and family centers and food banks. *Note:* Total contributions made in 2000. **Typ. Recipients:** Family Planning, Home-Care Services, Hospitals, Long-Term Care, People with Disabilities, Preventive Medicine/Wellness Organizations. **Geo. Dist:** nationally for the Sustainable Economics program; Northern forests, Southern Appalachians, and Southern Coastal Plain for the Eastern Ecosystems program; Boston, MA, community-building program; New York, NY, community-building program; Providence, RI, community-building program.

## ★ 541 ★ Mericos Foundation

625 South Fair Oaks Ave., Ste. 360
South Pasadena, CA 91030
**Phone:** (626)441-5188  **Fax:** (626)441-3672
**Email:** linda@sowest.net
Linda Blinkenberg, Director & Secretary

**Fnded:** 1980. **Philosophy:** Mericos Foundation makes grants across the major categories of support. Educational funding favors universities and public school systems. Education funding also supports science, math, and technology programs. Social services support includes family planning; child welfare; and youth development, citizenship, and responsibility. Arts interests include historic preservation, museums, and arts organizations. Health care support goes to critical health programs, nursing services, and hospices. In civic affairs, interests include the environment as well as zoos and botanical gardens. The foundation reports that it has initiated programs in 1997 to promote youth interest in science, math, and technology. **Priorities:** *Arts & Humanities:* 16%. Historical Society and libraries. *Civic & Public Affairs:* 3%. Community affairs. *Education:* About 49%. High schools and scholarship endowments. *Environment:* 32%. Youth, senior and family program support. *Note:* Total contributions made in 1998. **Typ. Recipients:** Children's Health/Hospitals, Children's Health/Hospitals, Clinics/Medical Centers, Domestic Violence, Family Planning, Health-General, Heart, Hospices,

Medical Research, Nursing Services. **Geo. Dist:** Santa Barbara, CA, including surrounding area.

## ★ 542 ★ Mervin Bovaird Foundation

100 W 5th St., Ste. 800
Tulsa, OK 74103-4291
**Phone:** (918)583-1777
Mr. R. Cooper, President & Trustee

**Fnded:** 1955. **Philosophy:** The purpose of the foundation, as stated in its articles of incorporation, is "to receive and administer funds for scientific, educational and charitable purposes, all for the public welfare." The foundation primarily supports scholarship programs at the University of Tulsa. Funding also is provided for social services, civic causes, and health organizations in the Tulsa, OK, area. **Priorities:** *Arts & Humanities:* 14%. Museums, music, ballet, and opera. *Civic & Public Affairs:* 2%. Primary support for a municipal park. *Education:* 47%. Supports educational concerns mostly in the form of scholarships to students from Tulsa attending the University of Tulsa. *Environment:* 21%. Primary support for family services, child welfare, and youth organizations. *International:* 8%. Hospitals, medical research, and single-disease health associations. *Note:* Total contributions made in 1998. **Typ. Recipients:** Arthritis, Cancer, Children's Health/Hospitals, Clinics/Medical Centers, Domestic Violence, Emergency/Ambulance Services, Family Planning, Health Organizations, Health Policy/Cost Containment, Heart, Hospices, Hospitals, Long-Term Care, Medical Rehabilitation, Medical Research, Mental Health, Multiple Sclerosis, People with Disabilities, Prenatal Health Issues, Sexual Abuse, Single-Disease Health Associations, Speech & Hearing, Substance Abuse. **Geo. Dist:** Tulsa, OK, metropolitan area.

## ★ 543 ★ Meyer Memorial Trust

1515 Southwest Fifth Ave., Ste. 500
Portland, OR 97201
**Phone:** (503)228-5512
**Email:** mmt@mmt.org
**Website:** http://www.mmt.org
Doug Stamm, Executive Director

**Fnded:** 1982. **Philosophy:** Upon creation of the charitable trust, Mr. Meyer stated, "Realizing as I do the uncertainties of the future, I want my trustees to be able to exercise broad discretion in shaping and carrying out charitable programs which can be tailored to fit changing conditions and problems." The trust conducts three types of grant-making activities. General purpose grants are made within Oregon and Clark County, Washington to a broad range of causes, including culture and the arts, education, health, and social services. The trust operates a Small Grants Program, initiated in 1988, under which grants of $500 to $12,000 are awarded for small projects. These grants are limited to Oregon and Clark County, Washington. The trust also makes grants in Support for Teacher Initiatives, a special program initiated in 1994 which provides grants up to $2,000 to individual teachers and $7,000 to teams of teachers for projects that promise to stimulate and facilitate more effective learning by students in the classroom, and is also limited to Oregon and Clark County, Washington. **Priorities:** *Arts & Humanities:* 15%. Museums, symphonies, historic preservation, and cultural centers. *Education:* 16%. Science and math education, private pre-college education, and after school enrichment programs. *Environment:* 28%. Supports programs for workers with disabilities, at-risk family programs, child development services, and youth organizations. *International:* 9%. Mental health services, children's health, and medical centers. *Note:* Total contributions made in fiscal 2001. Contributions analysis was reported by foundation, and includes General Purpose and Small Grants programs. **Typ. Recipients:** AIDS/HIV, Alzheimers Disease, Cancer, Child Abuse, Children's Health/Hospitals, Clinics/Medical Centers, Domestic Violence, Emergency/Ambulance Services, Family Planning, Geriatric Health, Health Organizations, Health Policy/Cost Containment, Heart, Hospices, Hospitals, Long-Term Care, Medical Education, Medical Rehabilitation, Medical Research, Medical Training, Mental Health, Nursing Services, People with

Disabilities, Prenatal Health Issues, Public Health, Sexual Abuse, Single-Disease Health Associations, Substance Abuse. **Geo. Dist:** OR; WA, Clark County.


★ **544** ★ **Middendorf Foundation**

2 East Read St.
Baltimore, MD 21202
**Phone:** (410)752-7088      **Fax:** (410)625-5728
E. Hathaway, President & Trustee

**Fnded:** 1953. **Philosophy:** The foundation's primary interest is supporting health care, specifically the establishment of health clinics. Arts funding favors historical preservation in Maryland. Civic affairs, the Boys Latin School in Baltimore, and family services also are supported. **Priorities:** *Arts & Humanities:* 14%. Restoration and endowments. *Civic & Public Affairs:* 4%. Supports parks, economic development, and community foundations. *Education:* 11%. Universities and secondary schools. *Environment:* 7%. Youth clubs, Special Olympics, and meals on wheels programs. *International:* 35%. Medical centers and health foundations. *Note:* Total contributions made in fiscal 1999. **Typ. Recipients:** Cancer, Child Abuse, Clinics/Medical Centers, Emergency/Ambulance Services, Eyes/Blindness, Family Planning, Geriatric Health, Health Organizations, Health-General, Hospices, Hospitals, Medical Education, Mental Health, People with Disabilities, Prenatal Health Issues, Preventive Medicine/Wellness Organizations, Public Health, Respiratory, Single-Disease Health Associations, Substance Abuse, Trauma Treatment. **Geo. Dist:** MD.


★ **545** ★ **Mildred H. McEvoy Foundation**

370 Main St., Ste. 1200
Worcester, MA 01608
**Phone:** (508)798-8621      **Fax:** (508)791-1201
Sumner Tilton, Jr., Trustee

**Fnded:** 1963. **Philosophy:** "The McEvoy Foundation provides grants to health, educational, cultural and human service organizations that are exempt under Section 501(c)(3) of the Internal Revenue Code and that are based in the Boothbay, Maine area. It supports requests to organizations which are providing solutions to or prevention of problems within the immediate community and which are receiving additional support from other funding sources." 1997 Foundation Guidelines **Priorities:** *Arts & Humanities:* 63%. Multiple grants went to Grand Banks Schooner Museum Trust and the Boothbay Railway Village Museum; other museums and historical societies received support. *Civic & Public Affairs:* 10%. Supports community services and the horticultural society, and botanical gardens. *Education:* 19%. Supports secondary and preparatory schools, colleges, and universities. *Environment:* 4%. Supports Boothbay Region YMCA and child welfare. *International:* 3%. Supports health centers, hospitals, and biomedical research organizations. *Religion:* 1%. Supports the New England Science Center. *Note:* Total contributions made in 1997. **Typ. Recipients:** Cancer, Children's Health/Hospitals, Clinics/Medical Centers, Emergency/Ambulance Services, Family Planning, Hospitals, Hospitals (University Affiliated), Long-Term Care, Medical Research, Nursing Services, Public Health, Single-Disease Health Associations, Substance Abuse. **Geo. Dist:** Boothbay Harbor, ME.


★ **546** ★ **Milken Family Foundation**

1250 4th St., 6th Floor
Santa Monica, CA 90401-1353
**Phone:** (310)998-2800      **Fax:** (310)998-2828
**Email:** admin@mff.org
**Website:** http://www.mff.org
Dr. Julius Lesner, Executive Vice President

**Fnded:** 1982. **Philosophy:** "The purpose of the Milken Family foundaton is to discover and advance inventive and effective ways of helping people help themselves and those around them to lead productive and satisfying lives. The Foundation advances this mission primarily through its work in education and medicine." "In education, the Foundation is committed to: Strengthening the profession by recognizing and rewarding outstanding educators; by expanding their professional leadership and policy influence; and by encouraging talented young people to become educators. Stimulating creativity and productivity among educators and students of all ages–especially by using technology to improve learning and teaching. Fostering the involvement of both the family and the community in schools. Helping build vibrant communities–especially by involving young people who have special needs, or who live in neighborhoods considered disadvantaged, in school-based programs that contribute to the revitalization of their community and to the well-being of its residents." "In medicine, the Foundation is committed to: Advancing and supporting basic and applied medical research–especially in the areas of prostate cancer and epilepsy–and recognizing and rewarding outstanding scientists in these areas. Supporting basic health care programs to assure the well-being of community members of all ages." "A wealth of human potential is represented by individual people of all ages whose vision and purpose make them dynamic forces for change. The Foundation's mission is to help realize this potential by giving support that enables people to create and carry out effective, lasting solutions to the challenges facing our communities." 1997 Funding Guidelines **Priorities:** *Civic & Public Affairs:* 21%. Supports community affairs, urban league, and public policy, safety, and housing. *Education:* 62%. Supports educational programs and institutions, leadership training. *International:* 25%. Supports medical centers and disease and disorder concerns, hospice and childrens health. *Note:* Contributions were made in fiscal 1998. **Typ. Recipients:** AIDS/HIV, Cancer, Children's Health/Hospitals, Clinics/Medical Centers, Eyes/Blindness, Hospitals, People with Disabilities, Single-Disease Health Associations, Substance Abuse. **Geo. Dist:** CA.


★ **547** ★ **Minnie Stevens Piper Foundation**

800 NW Loop 410, Ste. 200 S
San Antonio, TX 78216-5699
**Phone:** (210)525-8494      **Fax:** (210)341-6627
**Email:** cotero@mspf.org
**Website:** http://www.mspf.org
Carlos Otero, Executive Director

**Fnded:** 1950. **Philosophy:** "The foundation was formed to support charitable, scientific or educational undertakings by providing for or contributing toward the education of financially limited but worthy students; by assisting young men and women residents of Texas, attending or wishing to attend colleges and universities in the State of Texas, to complete their education and obtain degrees; by contributing to community chests, and supporting any other nonprofit organization or activity dedicated to the furtherance of the general welfare within the State of Texas." The following continuing programs are presently operated by the foundation: STUDENT LOAN PROGRAM: A revolving fund totaling $2,500,000 with loans limited to amounts repaid to the fund by former borrowers. A total of approximately $350,000 is available yearly. PIPER PROFESSORS PROGRAM: Ten awards of $2,500 each are made annually to professors for superior teaching at the college level. Selection is made on the basis of nominations submitted by each college or university in the State of Texas. STUDENT AID CENTER AND BEXAR COUNTY SCHOLARSHIP CLEARINGHOUSE: The Student Aid Center provides information through the Student Aid Library regarding college admissions, financial assistance, career planning, and international study to students, parents and counselors. The Bexar County Scholarship Clearing House serves as a liaison between applicants and scholarship donors. The purpose of the clearing house is to eliminate unnecessary duplication of work on the part of the counselors, students, donors, and parents; to broaden the scope of scholarship opportunities in this area; to expedite processing of scholarships to an earlier period of the senior year; and to standardize scholarship application forms. PIPER SCHOLARS PROGRAM: Four-year scholarships are awarded to academically promising and superior high school seniors in amounts sufficient for their needs to attend the college or university of their choice in the State of Texas. Applicants must be U.S. Citizens/Permanent Residents and Texas residents. Students selected and named Piper Scholars must maintain a "B" average throughout their undergraduate college career to remain in the program. **Priorities:** *Arts & Humanities:* 2%. Supports libraries, performing arts, public broadcasting and music. *Civic & Public Affairs:* Less than 1%. *Education:* 97%. Provides academic scholarships and awards. *Environment:* Less than 1%. *International:* 1%. Supports medical research and single-disease health associations. *Note:* Total contributions made in 1999. **Typ. Recipients:** Cancer, Eyes/Blindness, Health Organizations, Medical Education, Medical Research, Mental Health, People with Disabilities, Public Health, Substance Abuse. **Geo. Dist:** TX.


★ **548** ★ **Miriam and Peter Haas Fund**

201 Filbert St., 5th Floor
San Francisco, CA 94133
**Phone:** (415)296-9249      **Fax:** (415)296-8842
**Email:** mphf@mphf.org
Cheryl Polk, Executive Director & Secretary

**Fnded:** 1982. **Philosophy:** "The Miriam and Peter Haas Fund, a private foundation located in San Francisco, was incorporated in 1982 and for the first ten years was administered by the trustees. In 1992, the Fund received a large bequest. With new resources, the trustees hired staff, established a more formalized structure and chose early childhood as their primary focus. Based upon research conducted in 1993 and 1994, foundation staff and trustees developed a grantmaking framework to be implemented in stages over several years. It is designed to support activities that provide San Francisco's young (ages 2-5), low-income children and their families with access to high-quality early childhood programs that are a part of a comprehensive, coordinated system. The Fund recognizes the importance of connecting the work of its direct service grants to the ongoing discussions of public policy and will seek specific opportunities to share and collaborate with organizations to improve early childhood settings. The Fund will also continue trustee-initiated grantmaking to arts, education, public affairs and health and human services organizations." "We believe that young children and their families must be able to access high quality early childhood programs which are affordable and part of a comprehensive, coordinated system. Working with others, in long term sustained effort, we believe this vision is attainable." "With this in mind, the Fund's Early Childhood program reflects a multi-level approach. Our strategic support of the field–in areas such as planning, policy, finance, leadership development and comprehensive services–will be complemented by efforts to meet the immediate needs of young children. By weaving these pieces together, we hope to provide thoughtful, responsive and comprehensive grantmaking." "It is our belief that high quality early childhood programs improve children's chances for success in school and life. The Model Centers Initiative is designed to improve the quality of early childhood programs by strengthening and enhancing organizational capacity, service delivery, family involvement, comprehensive services, curriculum, professional and leadership development, and other key components of selected centers over a multi-year period." *Miriam and Peter Haas Fund Statement About the Fund* **Priorities:** *Arts & Humanities:* 13%. Supports arts centers. theater, museums, ballet, and music. *Civic & Public Affairs:* 8%. Supports clubs, law and justice, and housing. *Education:* 28%. Supports universities, religious education. *Environment:* 18%. Supports day care, shelters, athletics/recreation, and United Way. *International:* 8%. Supports multiple sclerosis, childrens health, and cancer. *Note:* Total contributions made in fiscal 1998. **Typ. Recipients:** AIDS/HIV, Cancer, Children's Health/Hospitals, Clinics/Medical Centers, Domestic Violence, Family Planning, Hospitals, Long-Term Care, Medical Rehabilitation, Medical Research, Mental Health, People with Disabilities, Public Health, Research/Studies Institutes, Substance Abuse. **Geo. Dist:** CA, San Francisco County.


★ **549** ★ **Monfort Family Foundation**

PO Box 890
Greeley, CO 80632
**Phone:** (970)454-1357      **Fax:** (970)454-2535
Dave Evans, Administrator

**Fnded:** 1970. **Philosophy:** The foundation primarily supports student programs at the university level. Other educational interests include technical training and support. "Funds are earmarked primarily for projects and/or groups promoting access to education, development of the arts and humanities, conducting scientific research into the causes and/or prevention of life-threatening diseases and the treatment thereof, and providing various forms of aid to the disadvantaged." **Priorities:** *Arts & Humanities:* 1%. *Civic & Public Affairs:* 18%. *Education:* 28%. Mainly scholarships for university students. *Environment:* 50%. Contributes mainly to boys and girls organizations. *International:* 3%. Single-disease health organizations, children's hospitals, and medical centers. *Note:* Total contributions made in 1999. **Typ. Recipients:** AIDS/HIV, Arthritis, Cancer, Children's Health/Hospitals, Clinics/Medical Centers, Hospitals, Medical Rehabilitation, Multiple Sclerosis, People with Disabilities, Prenatal Health Issues, Public Health, Respiratory, Single-Disease Health Associations, Speech & Hearing, Substance Abuse, Trauma Treatment. **Geo. Dist:** CO, Northern Colorado.

### ★ 550 ★ Montgomery Street Foundation
930 Montgomery St., Ste. 1107
San Francisco, CA 94104
**Phone:** (415)398-0600　　　**Fax:** (415)398-0612
Carol Elliott, Secretary & Treasurer
**Fnded:** 1952. **Philosophy:** The foundation primarily supports colleges and universities with moderate grants. Grants to higher education focus on economic education and business schools. Civic interests include law and justice and better business. The foundation also supports a number of social service and health interests. **Priorities:** *Arts & Humanities:* 4% supports historic art, the opera and museum. *Civic & Public Affairs:* 11% supports public and civic affairs. *Education:* 16% supports colleges and universities. *Environment:* 9% supports planned parenthood, handicapped, child sexual abuse treatment, and treatment center for the blind. *International:* 50% supports children's health, and medical research. *Religion:* 7% supports scientific learning center and museum, and science institute. *Note:* Contributions were made in 1998. **Typ. Recipients:** Cancer, Child Abuse, Children's Health/Hospitals, Clinics/Medical Centers, Domestic Violence, Emergency/Ambulance Services, Family Planning, Geriatric Health, Health Funds, Health Organizations, Heart, Hospices, Hospitals, Long-Term Care, Medical Education, Medical Research, People with Disabilities, Public Health, Research/Studies Institutes, Single-Disease Health Associations, Substance Abuse. **Geo. Dist:** San Francisco, CA, metropolitan area.

### ★ 551 ★ Moody Foundation
2302 Postoffice St., Ste. 704
Galveston, TX 77550
**Phone:** (409)763-5333　　　**Fax:** (409)763-5564
**Website:** http://www.moodyf.org
Peter Moore, Grants Director
**Fnded:** 1942. **Philosophy:** In recent years, much of the foundation's funding has supported foundation-initiated projects, primarily through the Transitional Learning Community, a comprehensive head-injury rehabilitation facility, and through Moody Gardens. The Gardens complex, located on Galveston Island, now includes a convention center, a swimming beach, 3-D I-MAX theater, visitors' center, equestrian arena for therapeutic horseback riding, a nine-story glass pyramid biome housing a tropical rainforest the Moody Hospitality Institute and a world class aquarium. The rainforest pyramid provides environmental education while complementing the Gardens' horticultural therapy program. The entire complex has been designed with special attention to the needs of persons with disabilities, both for recreation and employment. The foundation's remaining grants support a wide variety of programs benefiting the people of Texas (mainly in Galveston) in the areas of education, health, social service, law enforcement, civic and public affairs, performing arts and medical research. **Priorities:** *Arts & Humanities:* 1%. Supports performing arts associations and museums. *Education:* 3%. Supports University of Texas Medical Branch, Galveston and scholarships. *Environment:* Less than 1%. *International:* 23%. Supports The Transitional Learning Community, a residential rehabilitation and research facility for the treatment of traumatic brain injuries, mental illness, cancer, and Make-A-Wish Foundation. *Religion:* 73%. *Note:* Total contributions made in 1999. **Typ. Recipients:** AIDS/HIV, Cancer, Children's Health/Hospitals, Domestic Violence, Emergency/Ambulance Services, Eyes/Blindness, Family Planning, Geriatric Health, Health Organizations, Health Policy/Cost Containment, Heart, Hospices, Hospitals, Hospitals (University Affiliated), Kidney, Long-Term Care, Medical Education, Medical Rehabilitation, Medical Research, Mental Health, Nursing Services, People with Disabilities, Prenatal Health Issues, Respiratory, Single-Disease Health Associations, Speech & Hearing, Substance Abuse, Transplant Networks/Donor Banks. **Geo. Dist:** TX; Dallas, TX; Galveston, TX.

### ★ 552 ★ Moriah Fund, Inc.
1 Farragut Square South
1634 I St. Northwest, Ste. 1000
Washington, DC 20006
**Phone:** (202)783-8488　　　**Fax:** (202)783-8499
**Email:** jedwards@moriahfund.org
Janice Edwards, Grants Manager
**Fnded:** 1985. **Philosophy:** "The Moriah Fund was established in 1985; its philosophy of giving is rooted in fundamental Jewish values: a concern for the disadvantaged and an emphasis on self-help; a commitment to equity and justice; and a desire to improve the quality of life for Jews and non-Jews alike. In accordance with these values, the mission and operations of the Moriah Fund incorporate concern for the basic needs of all people-especially the most disadvantaged-and for the well-being and continuation of the Jewish people." "Moriah's grant making program seeks to promote pluralism and democracy, help disadvantaged people gain self-sufficiency and control over their lives, promote sustainable development, women's rights and reproductive health and protect and preserve the environment. Moriah supports programs that strengthen local involvement, leadership and institutional development. The Fund focuses on areas where private funding can make a difference, that is, areas that receive inadequate government funds, or that leverage public and private support through advocacy and the modeling of innovative programs." 1998 Annual Report **Priorities:** *Environment:* 40%. Women's rights and empowering low-income families. *Note:* Analysis excludes a major grant of $90 million which was given to the Central Indiana Community Foundation to Indiana charities. The foundation no longer provides funding in Indianapolis. Total contributions made in 1998. **Typ. Recipients:** Adolescent Health Issues, Children's Health/Hospitals, Clinics/Medical Centers, Family Planning, Health Organizations, Health Policy/Cost Containment, Long-Term Care, Medical Training, Mental Health, People with Disabilities, Prenatal Health Issues, Public Health. **Geo. Dist:** internationally; emphasis on Latin America, particularly Guatemala; Washington, DC; MD; NY.

### ★ 553 ★ Morris Goldseker Foundation of Maryland
Latrobe Bldg.
2 E Read St., 9th Fl.
Baltimore, MD 21202
**Phone:** (410)837-5100　　　**Fax:** (410)837-4701
**Email:** sscott@goldsekerfoundation.org
**Website:** http://www.goldsekerfoundation.org
Sally Scott, Program Officer
**Fnded:** 1974. **Philosophy:** The foundation has established four program areas of interest: community affairs, education, human services, and neighborhood development. In all of these areas, highest priority is given to programs of direct service to disadvantaged people and programs that improve the quality of life, increase access and opportunity, promote self-reliance, encourage creativity, and represent the tradition of private voluntary action beyond peoples' own particular spheres of activity. Also of special interest are programs that strengthen institutions and systems of delivery; address long-term solutions to community

problems; strengthen neighborhoods; strengthen the private nonprofit sector; attract other resources; and improve efficiency of operations. In 1996, the Foundation announced that funding to health interests would be discontinued, and that greater emphasis would be placed on public education. In 2000, the Foundation's Board of Trustees and its Selection Committee adopted a two-track approach to grantmaking. The approach designates priority areas that build on existing experience and investments, but also retains the ability to respond to new ideas and opportunities with established program areas. Between 2001-2003, and possibly beyond, most of the grantmaking funds will focus on the first-track priority areas. In these areas - community development, regionalism, and non-profit sector - the Foundation will be more directly engaged and active partner. The existing grantmaking policies apply to the priority areas. The second track focuses on the Foundation's established program areas - neighborhood development, community affairs, human services, and education. **Priorities:** *Arts & Humanities:* 6%. Supports historic preservation and libraries. *Civic & Public Affairs:* 58%. Supports planning and housing associations, neighborhood development, and community revitalization. *Education:* 23%. Funds colleges and universities, private schools, and scholarship funds. *Environment:* 4%. Funds human services programs, including youth and work programs and food banks. *International:* 1%. Supports a regional health network. *Note:* Total contributions made in 2000. **Typ. Recipients:** Child Abuse, Clinics/Medical Centers, Domestic Violence, Family Planning, Health Organizations, Medical Education, Mental Health, People with Disabilities, Research/Studies Institutes, Substance Abuse. **Geo. Dist:** Baltimore, MD.

### ★ 554 ★ Morris and Gwendolyn Cafritz Foundation
1825 K St. Northwest, Ste. 1400
Washington, DC 20006
**Phone:** (202)223-3100　　　**Fax:** (202)296-7567
**Email:** grantscoord@cafritzfoundation.org
**Website:** http://www.cafritzfoundation.org
Anne Allen, Executive Director
**Fnded:** 1948. **Philosophy:** The foundation has reflected the interests of its founders. The foundation's areas of concern have been the arts and humanities, education, community services, and health in Washington, DC. "The general policy is to concentrate grants to organizations, operating within the Washington metropolitan area, with projects of direct assistance to the District of Columbia." The foundation supports the arts and humanities, gives money for scholarships to local students, and supports education, local health, and community services. This emphasis on the Washington, DC, community is expected to continue. **Priorities:** *Arts & Humanities:* 43%. Supports music, theater, dance, libraries, ethnic and folk art, public broadcasting, and ballet. *Civic & Public Affairs:* 8%. Supports botanical gardens/parks, civil rights, municipalities/towns, community foundation, housing, employment/job training, legal aid, and ethnic organizations. *Education:* 19%. Funds public school, arts/humanities education, education reform, literacy science education, environmental education, and leadership training. *Environment:* 10%. Supports domestic violence, Big Brothers/Big Sisters, daycare, scouts, emergency relif, family services, youth organizations volunteer services, and shelters/homeless. *International:* 6%. Supports children's health, public health, and medical training. *Religion:* 7%. *Note:* Total contributions made in 1999. **Typ. Recipients:** Adolescent Health Issues, AIDS/HIV, Children's Health/Hospitals, Diabetes, Domestic Violence, Emergency/Ambulance Services, Family Planning, Geriatric Health, Health Organizations, Hospices, Hospitals, Long-Term Care, Medical Education, Medical Rehabilitation, Mental Health, Nursing Services, People with Disabilities, Prenatal Health Issues, Single-Disease Health Associations, Substance Abuse. **Geo. Dist:** Washington, DC, including metropolitan area.

### ★ 555 ★ Morris Stulsaft Foundation
100 Bush St., Ste. 825
San Francisco, CA 94104-3911

**Phone:** (415)986-7117       **Fax:** (415)986-2521
**Email:** stulsaft@aol.com
Joseph Valentine, Executive Director

**Fnded:** 1953. **Philosophy:** The foundation, in accordance with its stated goal, is organized to aid and assist needy and deserving children. It has traditionally funded organizations in the broad categories of social services and recreation, education, health, and the arts. Social service funding includes support for child welfare (including adoption services and child abuse prevention); recreational activities (particularly for handicapped youth); traditional youth groups; religious welfare organizations; day care and children's centers; programs for disadvantaged and mentally and physically disabled youth; prevention of substance abuse; family planning and parental services; homes and shelters; job training; volunteer assistance; and immigrant services. In the area of education, interests include minority education, remedial education, tutoring, and drop-out prevention; vocational education; literacy; special education; and preschool, arts, and bilingual education. Health funding includes mental health and child development; pediatric nursing services and in-house care for sick children; respite care; hospitals; and single-disease health associations. Grants in the arts went to public broadcasting, museums, and the performing arts for programs which promote arts appreciation and involve youth (especially minority and low-income youth) in arts activities. **Priorities:** *Arts & Humanities:* 6%. Funds music, museums, and arts. *Education:* 40%. Emphasis on primary and secondary education. *Environment:* 36%. Supports a wide variety of community and social welfare causes in the San Francisco Bay Area. *International:* 17%. Supports hospitals, medical clinics, pediatric health organizations. *Religion:* 2%. *Note:* Total contributions made in fiscal 2000. Percentages provided by foundation and include capital grant contributions. **Typ. Recipients:** Adolescent Health Issues, AIDS/HIV, Cancer, Child Abuse, Children's Health/Hospitals, Diabetes, Domestic Violence, Emergency/Ambulance Services, Eyes/Blindness, Family Planning, Heart, Hospitals, Medical Education, Medical Rehabilitation, Medical Research, Mental Health, Nursing Services, People with Disabilities, Prenatal Health Issues, Preventive Medicine/Wellness Organizations, Public Health, Research/Studies Institutes, Sexual Abuse, Single-Disease Health Associations, Speech & Hearing, Substance Abuse, Trauma Treatment. **Geo. Dist:** CA, Alameda County; CA, Contra Costa County; CA, Marin County; CA, San Francisco County; CA, San Mateo County; CA, Santa Clara County.

### ★ 556 ★ Mr. and Mrs. Lyndon C. Whitaker Charitable Foundation

1034 South Brentwood Boulevard, Ste. 402
Saint Louis, MO 63117
**Phone:** (314)241-4352       **Fax:** (314)726-5735
Betul Ozmat, Executive Director

**Fnded:** 1975. **Philosophy:** "The Foundation funds organizations that promote, contribute, and further develop the cultural heritage and vitality of the St. Louis, MO community. It supports programs and organizations that preserve the natural and cultural heritage of parks and encourage the use of parks. The Foundation supports preventive and primary health care for those in need, and supports medical research that can improve the quality of life for all." **Priorities:** *Arts & Humanities:* 32%. Supports historical preservation, museums, theater, music, and art. *Civic & Public Affairs:* 16%. Supports parks, zoos, and gardens. *Education:* 24%. Supports public schools, and universities. *Environment:* 13%. Supports food distribution and youth programs. *International:* 8%. Supports single-disease health associations. *Note:* Total contributions made in fiscal 1999. **Typ. Recipients:** Alzheimers Disease, Cancer, Clinics/Medical Centers, Family Planning, Health-General, Hospices, Hospitals, Hospitals (University Affiliated), Medical Education, Medical Research, People with Disabilities, Public Health, Respiratory, Single-Disease Health Associations. **Geo. Dist:** St. Louis, MO, metropolitan area.

### ★ 557 ★ Naomi and Nehemiah Cohen Foundation

PO Box 73708
Washington, DC 20056
**Phone:** (202)363-5195       **Fax:** (202)363-5209
**Email:** nncf@starpower.net
Allison McWilliams, Associate Director

**Fnded:** 1959. **Philosophy:** The foundation's primary focus is human services, civic affairs, and Jewish causes. Human service interests include housing, homelessness, and youth programs. Civic affairs include peace initiatives and other international affairs dealing with Israel. Other charitable organizations are also supported with minor grants. **Priorities:** *Arts & Humanities:* 4%. Theater, art galleries/museums, and public television. *Civic & Public Affairs:* 33%. Public policy, human rights, social justice, and economic development. *Education:* 4%. Scholarship funds, foundations, and policy studies. *International:* 6%. Medical centers, planned parenthood programs, and clinics. *Note:* Total contributions made in 1999. Analysis provided by foundation. **Typ. Recipients:** Arthritis, Cancer, Children's Health/Hospitals, Clinics/Medical Centers, Diabetes, Emergency/Ambulance Services, Eyes/Blindness, Family Planning, Health Organizations, Health-General, Heart, Hospices, Hospitals, Hospitals (University Affiliated), Long-Term Care, Medical Education, Mental Health, Prenatal Health Issues, Single-Disease Health Associations, Substance Abuse. **Geo. Dist:** Washington, DC.

### ★ 558 ★ Nelda C. and H. J. Lutcher Stark Foundation

PO Box 909
Orange, TX 77631-0909
**Phone:** (409)883-3513       **Fax:** (409)883-3530
**Email:** starkart@exp.net
**Website:** http://www.starkmuseumofart.org

**Fnded:** 1961. **Philosophy:** The foundation's primary purpose is the operation of the Stark Museum of Art, the Frances Ann Lutcher Theater for Performing Arts, and the W. H. Stark House, the historic home of the Stark family. In addition, the foundation finances scholarships through the Texas Interscholastic League Foundation. Other grants made by the foundation comprise a small percentage of its total operational expenditures. **Priorities:** *Arts & Humanities:* 7%. Supports historical society, opera, libraries, and art. *Education:* 52%. Junior Achievement, educational institutions and programs. *Environment:* 25%. Rehabilitation, youth services and veterans. *International:* 15%. Supports hospices and retina research. *Note:* Contributions were made in fiscal 2000. **Typ. Recipients:** Cancer, Children's Health/Hospitals, Eyes/Blindness, Hospices, People with Disabilities, Single-Disease Health Associations, Transplant Networks/Donor Banks. **Geo. Dist:** LA, Southwest Louisiana; TX, Southeast Texas.

### ★ 559 ★ Neva and Wesley West Foundation

PO Box 7
Houston, TX 77001-0007
**Phone:** (713)520-0400       **Fax:** (713)520-1131
Stuart Stedman, Contact

**Fnded:** 1956. **Philosophy:** The Neva & Wesley West Foundation predominantly supports the arts. Other areas of interest include health and medical organizations, environmental issues, and educational concerns. Traditionally, donations are not granted outside Texas. **Priorities:** *Arts & Humanities:* 56%. Supports museums, opera, threatre, symphony, ballet. *Civic & Public Affairs:* 2%. Supports gardens. *Education:* 5%. Supports schools, colleges. *Environment:* 5%. Supports homes, womens shelters, scouts.' *International:* 6%. Supports medical research. *Religion:* 3%. Supports science museum. *Note:* Total contributions made in 1998. **Typ. Recipients:** Children's Health/Hospitals, Emergency/Ambulance Services, Eyes/Blindness, Eyes/Blindness, Family Planning, Health Organizations, Hospitals, Medical Education, Medical Research, Mental Health, Prenatal Health Issues, Public Health, Speech & Hearing. **Geo. Dist:** Houston, TX.

### ★ 560 ★ New-Land Foundation

1114 Ave. of the Americas, 46th Floor
New York, NY 10036-7798
**Phone:** (212)479-6162       **Fax:** (212)841-6275
**Email:** rschwartz@klwhllp.org
Renee Schwartz, Secretary

**Fnded:** 1941. **Philosophy:** The foundation is currently interested in funding programs in the following areas: civil rights/justice, the environment (other than hazardous waste), population control, and peace and arms control. The foundation does not typically fund programs in medicine, religion, educational institutions, or general social programs, including conferences and symposiums. **Priorities:** *Arts & Humanities:* 16%. Supports music, museums, and art programs. *Civic & Public Affairs:* 22%. Supports public policy, community foundations, and law & justice. *Education:* 5%. Supports educational programs. *Environment:* 1%. Supports Planned Parenthood of New York. *International:* 2%. Funds mental health. *Note:* Total contributions made in 1998. **Typ. Recipients:** Clinics/Medical Centers, Family Planning, Hospitals, Medical Education, Medical Research, Mental Health, Research/Studies Institutes. **Geo. Dist:** primarily to national organizations.

### ★ 561 ★ New York Foundation

350 Fifth Ave., Ste. 2901
New York, NY 10118-2996
**Phone:** (212)594-8009
**Website:** http://www.nyf.org
Madeline Lee, Executive Director

**Fnded:** 1909. **Philosophy:** The foundation supports groups in New York City that are working on problems of urgent concern to disadvantaged communities and neighborhoods. The foundation is particularly interested in start-up grants to new, untested programs that have few other sources of support. The overarching goal of the foundation's grants program is empowerment of the people whose work the foundation supports. The foundation emphasizes activities that enable individuals and groups to become more effective participants in the political and policy-making process. It also emphasizes self-help programs that enable groups to help themselves. In a series of planning meetings, the board reaffirmed the foundation's strong interest in community organizing and advocacy by and on behalf of the populations of concern to the foundation. They also narrowed somewhat the conditions under which the foundation will consider support for direct service programs. Among applicants whose primary aim is direct service, preference will be given to organizations that look likely to move toward advocacy and organizing, and to programs created by newly emerging communities, where service provision is often only the first step to the development of a voice for the community. **Priorities:** *Civic & Public Affairs:* 62%. Focus on poor disadvantaged minorities of the New York City area. *Environment:* 38%. Funds services for disadvantaged groups; including human service organizations serving youth, families, and the elderly. *Note:* Total contributions made in 2000. **Typ. Recipients:** Adolescent Health Issues, AIDS/HIV, Cancer, Domestic Violence, Geriatric Health, Health Organizations, Health Policy/Cost Containment, Heart, Hospitals, Hospitals (University Affiliated), Mental Health, Nutrition, Outpatient Health Care, People with Disabilities, Prenatal Health Issues, Preventive Medicine/Wellness Organizations, Public Health, Single-Disease Health Associations, Substance Abuse. **Geo. Dist:** New York, NY, metropolitan area.

### ★ 562 ★ Norcross Wildlife Foundation

PO Box 0414
Planetarium Station
New York, NY 10024-0414
**Phone:** (212)362-4831       **Fax:** (212)362-4783
**Website:** http://www.norcrossws.org
Richard Reagan, President

**Fnded:** 1964. **Philosophy:** The foundation supports a variety of organizations, but environmental affairs remain the primary focus for its giving program. **Priorities:** *Arts & Humanities:* 1%. Primarily supports libraries. *Civic & Public Affairs:* 20%. Supports community affairs and municipalities. *Education:* 1%. Supports educational institutions. *Environment:* 6%. Supports people with disabilities, and social and youth services. *Religion:* 1%. Funds a natural history society. *Note:* Total contributions made in 1999. **Typ. Recipients:** AIDS/HIV, Children's Health/Hospitals, Clinics/Medical Centers, Emergency/Ambulance Services, Hospitals, Medical Education, People with Disabilities. **Geo. Dist:** nationally.

### ★ 563 ★ Nord Family Foundation
347 Midway Boulevard, Ste. 312
Elyria, OH 44035
**Phone:** (440)324-2822          **Fax:** (440)324-6427
**Email:** exedir@nordff.org
**Website:** http://www.nordff.org
Sharon White, Controller
**Fnded:** 1988. **Philosophy:** The trustees have clarified the foundation's grant-making priorities into the two themes of strengthening the family and strengthening the public service in all of its grant making, and also serve as a general purpose foundation in Lorain County, OH. The foundation has also established three specific priorities for action: improving the county's leadership, education, and physical appearance. An agenda entitled "Lorain County 2020" was recently published with input from the foundation and community leaders. The foundation reports that it is initiating a Grassroots Leadership Program and a Family Investment Fund. **Priorities:** *Arts & Humanities:* 14%. Historical associations, dance, theater, music and public broadcasting. *Civic & Public Affairs:* 8%. Focus on urban affairs, housing, economic development, and job training. *Education:* 30%. Emphasis on primary and secondary education, education associations, minority education and scholarships. *Environment:* 32%. Interests include community service organizations, child welfare, family planning, and food distribution programs, emergency relief. *International:* 2%. Primary support for hospitals and medical centers, single-disease associations, and medical rehabilitation. *Religion:* 4%. Supports science centers. *Note:* Total contributions made in 1999. **Typ. Recipients:** Alzheimers Disease, Cancer, Child Abuse, Children's Health/Hospitals, Clinics/Medical Centers, Domestic Violence, Emergency/Ambulance Services, Eyes/Blindness, Family Planning, Health Organizations, Mental Health, Nursing Services, People with Disabilities, Public Health, Sexual Abuse. **Geo. Dist:** Denver, CO; OH, Cuyahoga County area; OH, Lorain County area; Columbia, SC.

### ★ 564 ★ Norman Foundation
147 East 48th St.
New York, NY 10017
**Phone:** (212)230-9830          **Fax:** (212)230-9849
**Email:** info@normanfdn.org
**Website:** http://www.normanfdn.org
Michelle Lord, Program Director
**Fnded:** 1938. **Philosophy:** The foundation has identified three main areas of interest: economic justice, civil rights/individual liberties and environmental justice. "Economic justice grants are awarded to projects that seek to redress economic inequities or facilitate wider access to employment, education, housing and the like. Grants in the area of civil rights/individual liberties typically fund projects designed to combat systemic discrimination and violence directed against disenfranchised groups, such as racial minorities, women, gays and lesbians, and the disabled. Other grants have gone to projects addressing government and corporate abuses of power, particularly those that create threats to the environment, human health and safety." The foundation encourages cooperation between local groups at the grassroots level and national advocacy groups; a successful proposal would most likely combine a grassroots approach with a strong advocacy component. The foundation provides general support and project-oriented support and places great importance on diversity within organizations. The foundation has an interest in dealing directly in economic, "since the creation of decent, healthy jobs with fair incomes and benefits is not only a good in itself, it empowers people to achieve more" in the foundation's areas of interest. Also of particular interest are strate-

gies on how to engage more Americans in their civic lives and to increase faith and involvement in community institutions. **Priorities:** *Civic & Public Affairs:* 56%. Supports general civil funding and the Welfare Rights Organizing Coalition in Seattle. *Environment:* 19%. Supports youth programs. *International:* 29%. *Note:* Total contributions made in 1998. **Typ. Recipients:** AIDS/HIV, Domestic Violence, Family Planning, Health Policy/Cost Containment, Mental Health, People with Disabilities, Public Health. **Geo. Dist:** nationally.

### ★ 565 ★ Norman and Rosita Winston Foundation
1285 Ave. of the Americas
New York, NY 10019-6064
**Phone:** (212)373-3000          **Fax:** (212)373-2187
John O'Neil, Attorney
**Fnded:** 1954. **Philosophy:** The foundation focuses its funding on higher education, the arts, health and medical research, civic organizations, and social services. **Priorities:** *Arts & Humanities:* About 42%. Supports museums, performing arts, music, ballet, libraries, opera, and public broadcasting. *Civic & Public Affairs:* 3%. Urban affairs projects. *Education:* About 28%. Primary support for colleges, universities, and medical education. *Environment:* 2%. *International:* 9%. Focus on cancer research. *Religion:* 3%. *Note:* Total contributions made in 1996. **Typ. Recipients:** Cancer, Geriatric Health, Hospitals, Long-Term Care, Medical Education, Medical Research, Research/Studies Institutes, Sexual Abuse. **Geo. Dist:** NY.

### ★ 566 ★ Northwest Area Foundation
60 Plato Boulevard E
Saint Paul, MN 55107
**Phone:** (651)224-9635          **Fax:** (651)225-3881
**Email:** kns@nwaf.org
**Website:** http://www.nwaf.org
Karl Stauber, President
**Fnded:** 1934. **Philosophy:** The Northwest Area Foundation seeks to help communities most in need create positive futures - economically, ecologically, and socially. To implement the mission, the Foundation will help communities work toward a balanced system that will reduce poverty; stimulate economic growth; sustain the natural environment; and develop effective institutions, relationships, and individuals. One hundred percent of the Foundation's resources will be devoted to supporting its mission through three programs: Community Ventures: The Foundation will identify approximately 16 communities in which to work intensively. Its commitment to each community will be long-term, as much as 10 years or longer. Investments in these community partnerships will total approximately $150 million over the next decade. Community Connections: The Foundation also will make available an array of shorter-term services, programs, and small grants to an additional number of communities. These will be consistent with the Foundation's new mission. Investments in these activities will total approximately $25 million over the next decade. Community Horizons: Recognizing the dilemma of rural communities where both population and opportunity have been declining for decades, the Foundation will help selected communities develop and retain teams of leaders who can help chart the future. This program, which will be fully operating in three to five years, will total approximately $25 million over the next decade. **Typ. Recipients:** AIDS/HIV, Clinics/Medical Centers, Family Planning, Health Organizations, Health Policy/Cost Containment, Mental Health, Nursing Services, Outpatient Health Care. **Geo. Dist:** ID; IA; MN; MT; ND; OR; SD; WA.

### ★ 567 ★ Ohrstrom Foundation
717 Fifth Ave.
New York, NY 10022
**Phone:** (212)759-5380          **Fax:** (212)486-0935
Ms. Dorothy Barry, Jr., Treasurer
**Fnded:** 1953. **Philosophy:** The Ohrstrom Foundation makes most of its grants in the areas of environmental affairs, education, arts/humanities, health/medical,

community service, civil rights, and religion. In education, interests include technical training, universities, and private schools. **Priorities:** *Arts & Humanities:* 7%. focus on libraries and museums. *Civic & Public Affairs:* 41%. Supports ethnic and community organizations. *Education:* 20%. Funds secondary schools and colleges and universities. *Environment:* 8%. Supports substance abuse programs, animal protection, youth organizations, and community service organizations. *International:* 2%. Supports hospitals and single-disease health associations. *Note:* Total contributions made in fiscal 1997. **Typ. Recipients:** Arthritis, Cancer, Emergency/Ambulance Services, Health Organizations, Heart, Hospices, Hospitals, Medical Research, People with Disabilities, Research/Studies Institutes, Single-Disease Health Associations, Substance Abuse. **Geo. Dist:** nationally; VA.

### ★ 568 ★ Olive B. Cole Foundation
6207 Constitution Dr.
Fort Wayne, IN 46804
**Phone:** (219)436-2182          **Fax:** (219)432-3146
John Hogan, Executive Vice President & Treasurer
**Fnded:** 1954. **Philosophy:** The goal of the Cole Foundation is local giving, chiefly in the areas of education, community projects, and recreation. It strives to fund new organizations and maintain old recipients. **Priorities:** *Arts & Humanities:* 13%. Libraries, historical preservation, museums, music, and public broadcasting. *Civic & Public Affairs:* 34%. Parades/festivals, job training programs, community foundations, a zoo, and parks. *Education:* 10%. Education funds, precollege public education, and colleges and universities. *Environment:* 27%. People with disabilities, community centers, youth organizations, the elderly, and athletics. *Note:* Total contributions made in fiscal 1999. **Typ. Recipients:** AIDS/HIV, Alzheimers Disease, Cancer, Children's Health/Hospitals, Clinics/Medical Centers, Emergency/Ambulance Services, Health Organizations, Home-Care Services, Hospices, People with Disabilities, People with Disabilities, Trauma Treatment. **Geo. Dist:** Kendallville, IN, including surrounding area.

### ★ 569 ★ Oppenstein Brothers Foundation
PO Box 13095
Kansas City, MO 64199-3095
**Phone:** (816)234-8671          **Fax:** (816)234-8690
Sheila Rice, Program Officer
**Fnded:** 1975. **Philosophy:** The Oppenstein Brothers Foundation was created by a bequest of Mr. Michael Oppenstein in order that the accumulated wealth of his brothers and himself might be used "for religious, charitable, scientific and educational purposes serving the public welfare..." The foundation's giving areas include social welfare, education (excluding scholarship assistance), arts (primarily educational programming for children), health (programs that promote wellness), and social services. **Priorities:** *Arts & Humanities:* 37%. Arts outreach, music, and ballet. *Civic & Public Affairs:* 7%. Housing and urban and community affairs. *Education:* 6%. Primary education and colleges and universities *Environment:* 26%. Primary support for child welfare, food banks, shelter, united funds, and youth organizations. *International:* 9%. Health centers and clinics and single-disease health associations. *Note:* Total contributions made in fiscal 1999. **Typ. Recipients:** AIDS/HIV, Alzheimers Disease, Cancer, Child Abuse, Children's Health/Hospitals, Clinics/Medical Centers, Domestic Violence, Emergency/Ambulance Services, Eyes/Blindness, Family Planning, Health Organizations, Heart, Hospices, Hospitals, Medical Rehabilitation, Mental Health, People with Disabilities, Prenatal Health Issues, Public Health, Sexual Abuse, Single-Disease Health Associations, Substance Abuse. **Geo. Dist:** Kansas City, MO, metropolitan area.

### ★ 570 ★ Ordean Foundation
501 Ordean Bldg.
Duluth, MN 55802
**Phone:** (218)726-4785          **Fax:** (218)726-4848
**Email:** ordean@cpinternet.com
Stephen Mangan, Executive Director

**Fnded:** 1933. **Philosophy:** Through his will in 1926, Mr. Ordean directed the founding of "a corporation for the purpose of administering and furnishing relief and charity for the worthy poor...without discrimination as to age, sex, color, or religious inclination. Mr. Ordean also made sizeable bequests to the service of disabled and orphaned children, youth, disadvantaged women, the elderly and infirm." The foundation's mission concentrates on the funding of services and facilities for the needy, treatment of the chronically or temporarily mentally ill, the care and rehabilitation of the physically impaired, and the support of youth guidance programs. **Priorities:** *Arts & Humanities:* 2%. Funds children's museum. *Civic & Public Affairs:* 13%. Supports housing and economic development. *Education:* 8%. Funds colleges. *Environment:* 52%. Emphasis on youth organizations, food and clothing distributions, prevention of domestic violence, child welfare, community centers, and Young Men's Christian Association and Young Women's Christian Association. *International:* 15%. Funding for health centers and single disease health associations. *Note:* Total contributions made in 1999. **Typ. Recipients:** AIDS/HIV, Alzheimers Disease, Children's Health/Hospitals, Clinics/Medical Centers, Domestic Violence, Emergency/Ambulance Services, Family Planning, Health Organizations, Home-Care Services, Medical Education, Medical Rehabilitation, Mental Health, People with Disabilities, Prenatal Health Issues, Public Health, Single-Disease Health Associations, Substance Abuse. **Geo. Dist:** Duluth, MN, Hermantown, and Proctor areas.

### ★ 571 ★ Orville D. and Ruth A. Merillat Foundation

1800 West U.S. 223
PO Box 1946
Adrian, MI 49221
**Phone:** (517)263-6232      **Fax:** (517)265-3041
Mr. John Thurman, Treasurer
**Fnded:** 1983. **Philosophy:** The foundation provides substantial support for a variety of preselected Christian causes. Educational interests include higher education, theological education, and religious schools. Among human services receiving support are Christian service groups, youth organizations, and child welfare and family service agencies. The foundation also supports conferences of churches, crusades, ministries, evangelical associations, and Bible distribution efforts. **Priorities:** *Arts & Humanities:* 3%. Opera and fine arts. *Civic & Public Affairs:* 5%. Public policy and community organizations. *Education:* 27%. Supports colleges and Christian schools. *Environment:* 15%. Family and youth councils and centers. *International:* 3%. Health centers. *Note:* Total contributions made in fiscal 1999. **Typ. Recipients:** Health Funds, Hospices. **Geo. Dist:** MI, particularly Adrian.

### ★ 572 ★ Otto Bremer Foundation

445 Minnesota St., Ste. 2000
Saint Paul, MN 55101-2107
**Phone:** (651)227-8036      **Fax:** (651)312-3550
**Email:** obf@bremer.com
**Website:** http://www.ottobremer.org
John Kostishack, Executive Director
**Fnded:** 1944. **Philosophy:** The Foundation is committed to playing a contributing role in strengthening nonprofits throughout its Service area. Foundation grants favor organizations located in communities serviced by Bremer Banks, which are located in Minnesota, North Dakota, Montana, and Wisconsin. Principal grant recipients within these rural communities are "agencies which address the needs of individuals affected by poverty; activities which address general community needs and encourage citizen participation; educational internships; promotion of individual and community health; and activities of religious organizations which address community needs." The foundation annually reevaluates priorities within these categories in order to remain responsive to the communities' needs. "The current focus areas are...working with nonprofit organizations to bring to communities...providing resources to assist beneficiaries in becoming self supporting organizations that have an impact on the future." Otto Bremer Foundation 1999 Annual Report. **Priorities:** *Note:* Total

contributions made in 1999. **Typ. Recipients:** AIDS/HIV, Clinics/Medical Centers, Diabetes, Domestic Violence, Emergency/Ambulance Services, Geriatric Health, Health Organizations, Hospices, Hospitals, Medical Education, Mental Health, Nursing Services, Outpatient Health Care, People with Disabilities, Public Health, Substance Abuse. **Geo. Dist:** MN; MT; ND; WI.

### ★ 573 ★ Overbrook Foundation

122 East 42nd St., Ste. 2500
New York, NY 10168-2500
**Phone:** (212)661-8710      **Fax:** (212)661-8664
**Email:** Sheila@overbrook.com
M. McGoldrick, Grants Manager
**Fnded:** 1948. **Philosophy:** The foundation reflects the interests of the descendants of Frank and Helen Altschul. Foundation support is often given on a continuing basis. Although the foundation makes some large grants, it prefers to make smaller grants to a variety of institutions. Many of the recipient organizations have a national or international orientation. Major interests of the foundation include Jewish welfare funds, higher and secondary education, hospitals, international relations, cultural programs, and community funds. funding focus. **Priorities:** *Arts & Humanities:* 10% Supports libraries, museums, performing and visual art. *Civic & Public Affairs:* 22%. Supports community and public affairs. *Education:* 28%. Supports educational programs and institutions. *Environment:* 15%. Supports planned parenthood, handgun violence prevention, children's services, and recording services for the blind and dyslexic. *International:* 7%. Supports hospitals, mental health centers, medical centers, gay men's health, and medical research institutes. *Note:* Contributions were made in 1998. **Typ. Recipients:** AIDS/HIV, Emergency/Ambulance Services, Family Planning, Health Organizations, Hospices, Hospitals, Hospitals (University Affiliated), Medical Research, Mental Health, Nursing Services, People with Disabilities, Single-Disease Health Associations, Substance Abuse. **Geo. Dist:** nationally; CT; New York, NY, metropolitan area.

### ★ 574 ★ Oxford Foundation

125D Lancaster Ave.
Strasburg, PA 17579
**Phone:** (717)687-9335      **Fax:** (717)687-9336
**Email:** pcalhoun@oxfordfoundation.org
**Website:** http://www.oxfordfoundation.org
Philip Calhoun, Executive Director
**Fnded:** 1947. **Philosophy:** The Oxford Foundation makes grants across the major categories of support. In education, interests include colleges, universities, public school districts, private education, medical training, and day schools. Health support goes to medical centers, health organizations, and Alzheimer's research. Social service support includes community centers, family services, shelters, and youth organizations. Funding for civic affairs favors foundations, agricultural support, and zoos. **Priorities:** *Arts & Humanities:* 6%. Supports historic preservation, music, museums, and the performing arts. *Civic & Public Affairs:* 14%. Supports fire fighters, gardens, economic policy, and community foundations. *Education:* 17%. Supports schools, educational foundations, and colleges. *Environment:* 25%. Supports child welfare, youth organizations, people with disabilities, senior services, and community partnerships. *International:* 27%. Funds medical centers, community health programs, children's health care, and single-disease health associations. *Note:* Total contributions made in 2000. **Typ. Recipients:** Alzheimers Disease, Arthritis, Cancer, Children's Health/Hospitals, Clinics/Medical Centers, Diabetes, Domestic Violence, Emergency/Ambulance Services, Family Planning, Hospices, Hospitals, Hospitals (University Affiliated), Medical Education, Medical Research, Mental Health, Nursing Services, People with Disabilities, Prenatal Health Issues, Public Health, Sexual Abuse, Single-Disease Health Associations, Substance Abuse. **Geo. Dist:** PA.

### ★ 575 ★ Patrick and Anna M. Cudahy Fund

PO Box 11978
Milwaukee, WI 53211
**Phone:** (414)866-0760      **Fax:** (414)475-0679
**Email:** secretary@cudahyfund.org
**Website:** http://www.cudahyfund.org
Judith Borchers, Executive Director
**Fnded:** 1934. **Philosophy:** The fund supports a broad range of civic, educational, and social service programs, and organizations which are primarily located in the Milwaukee, Madison, and Chicago areas. Current interests include national programs dealing with the environment and other public interest issues, secondary and higher education, religious welfare, and civic and cultural affairs. The fund also supports international social welfare projects. **Priorities:** *Arts & Humanities:* 4%. Supports museums, and art projects. *Civic & Public Affairs:* 14%. Supports housing and public policy. *Education:* 10%. Largely Catholic institutions. *Environment:* 26%. Children's welfare, hunger, and housing. *International:* 10%. Funds clinics and services for the elderly. *Note:* Total contributions made in 1998. **Typ. Recipients:** Clinics/Medical Centers, Domestic Violence, Family Planning, Geriatric Health, Health Organizations, Long-Term Care, People with Disabilities, Preventive Medicine/Wellness Organizations, Public Health, Substance Abuse. **Geo. Dist:** internationally; nationally; Chicago, IL; WI.

### ★ 576 ★ Patrick and Catherine Weldon Donaghue Medical Research Foundation

18 North Main
West Hartford, CT 06107-1919
**Phone:** (860)521-9011      **Fax:** (860)521-9018
**Email:** director@donaghue.org
**Website:** http://www.donaghue.org
**Fnded:** 1989. **Philosophy:** "The Donaghue Medical Research Foundation funds innovative basic biomedical, pre-clinical research, as well as epidemiological, community health and health services research in the areas of cancer, cardiovascular disease, mental health and neurodegenerative diseases." "The Donaghue Foundation, in seeking to promote knowledge of practical benefit to human life through research, conducts several initiatives in support of Connecticut-based health research and related work." "Research in Clinical and Community Health Issues is a funding initiative for biomedical, behavioral and other health-related research projects that address the major medical conditions and social problems influencing the health of individuals, groups, and communities. The Foundation is especially interested in clinical, epidemiological and health service research studies that focus on the development and evaluation of more effective methods for preventing, diagnosing and treating illnesses and conditions that have a major impact on the people of Connecticut." "The Donaghue Investigator Program is an initiative aimed at supporting particularly promising medical researchers holding faculty appointments at Connecticut institutions. The funding emphasis is on the investigator and his or her program of research rather than upon a specific study." "Practical Benefit Initiatives. In these areas the Foundation initiates research projects showing particular promise for producing practical benefit to human life. In areas the Foundation wishes to pursue, an interactive process between the Foundation and prospective investigators is used to develop projects for funding." The Patrick and Catherine Weldon Donaghue Medical Research Foundation 1998 Annual Report **Priorities:** *International:* 100%. The foundation funds individuals at health-research institutions; the giving is distributed as follows: 33% for Research in Clinical and Community Health Issues; 56% for Practical Benefit Initiatives; and 26% for The Donaghue Investigator Program. **Typ. Recipients:** Cancer, Children's Health/Hospitals, Heart, Medical Education, Medical Research, People with Disabilities, Public Health. **Geo. Dist:** CT.

## ★ 577 ★ Paul and Phyllis Fireman Charitable Foundation

1601 Forum Place, Ste. 905
West Palm Beach, FL 33401
**Phone:** (561)684-1900 **Fax:** (561)684-2168
Phyllis Fireman, Trustee

**Fnded:** 1985. **Philosophy:** The foundation's major priority is funding civic affairs organizations, specifically anti-defamation leagues. The foundation is also interested in education and favors Jewish educational institutions, both at the university and secondary levels. Minor support also goes to social services, the arts, and religion. **Priorities:** *Arts & Humanities:* 3%. Supports museums and fine arts. *Civic & Public Affairs:* 62%. Supports Hispanic affairs, philanthropic organizations, human rights, clubs, and ethnic organizations. *Education:* 7%. Funds public schools, colleges and universities. *Environment:* 12%. Supports youth clubs and family services. *International:* 5%. Supports hospitals, single-disease health associations, and medical research. *Note:* Total contributions made in 1998. **Typ. Recipients:** AIDS/HIV, Alzheimers Disease, Arthritis, Cancer, Children's Health/Hospitals, Clinics/Medical Centers, Domestic Violence, Emergency/Ambulance Services, Geriatric Health, Health Organizations, Health-General, Heart, Home-Care Services, Hospices, Hospitals, Medical Education, Medical Rehabilitation, Medical Research, Multiple Sclerosis, Nutrition, People with Disabilities, Preventive Medicine/Wellness Organizations, Public Health, Single-Disease Health Associations, Transplant Networks/Donor Banks. **Geo. Dist:** New York, NY.

## ★ 578 ★ Paul Stock Foundation

PO Box 2020
Cody, WY 82414
**Phone:** (307)587-5275 **Fax:** (307)527-7897
Charles Kepler, President

**Fnded:** 1958. **Philosophy:** The foundation's primary mission is to provide student aid for Wyoming residents to pursue higher education. The foundation also focuses on youth agencies, arts groups, and community activities. **Priorities:** *Arts & Humanities:* 1%. Funds the Buffalo Bill Memorial Association. *Civic & Public Affairs:* 86%. Supports activities in the city of Cody, Wyoming. *Education:* 13%. Student aid, vocational/technical education, and a major endowment to the University of Wyoming. *Note:* Total contributions made in 1999. **Typ. Recipients:** Long-Term Care, Medical Rehabilitation, Research/Studies Institutes. **Geo. Dist:** WY.

## ★ 579 ★ Pauline Allen Gill Foundation

1901 N Akard St.
Dallas, TX 75201
**Phone:** (214)696-3336
Nancy Seay, Vice President

**Fnded:** 1975. **Philosophy:** The foundation gives primarily to health care, educational institutions, and the arts. The foundation also supports social services, religion, civic affairs, and environmental concerns. **Priorities:** *Arts & Humanities:* 1%. Supports music and art museums. *Civic & Public Affairs:* 25%. Supports nonprofit management, housing and gardens and parks. *Education:* 19%. Supports private schools and literacy. *Environment:* 5%. Supports community centers, counseling, family services, and United Way. *International:* 27%. Supports medical centers, hospitals, and visiting nurses. *Note:* Total contributions made in 2000. **Typ. Recipients:** AIDS/HIV, Arthritis, Children's Health/Hospitals, Clinics/Medical Centers, Domestic Violence, Emergency/Ambulance Services, Eyes/Blindness, Family Planning, Health Organizations, Heart, Hospitals, Hospitals (University Affiliated), Kidney, Medical Education, Medical Research, Nursing Services, Nutrition, People with Disabilities, Public Health, Research/Studies Institutes, Single-Disease Health Associations, Substance Abuse, Trauma Treatment. **Geo. Dist:** Dallas, TX.

## ★ 580 ★ Pearl M. and Julia J. Harmon Foundation

PO Box 52568
Tulsa, OK 74152-0568
**Phone:** (918)743-6191
**Website:** http://www.HarmonFoundation.com
George Hangs, Jr., Secretary & Treasurer

**Fnded:** 1962. **Philosophy:** The foundation supports a wide variety of causes, primarily in the Tulsa, OK, area. Major funding is directed to supporting the Harmon Science Center, an interactive science museum in Tulsa, OK. The foundation does not accept applications for outright grants, but rather directs the distribution of funds through interest-free or reduced-rate loans to charitable organizations. It does not restrict funding to set organizations and attempts to respond to the changing needs of the community. **Priorities:** *Arts & Humanities:* 18%. Funds opera, music, and libraries. *Civic & Public Affairs:* 1%. Supports towns/municipalities, safety. *Education:* 18%. Supports universities, education-general, and schools. *Environment:* 22%. Supports food distribution, senior services, and family planning services. *International:* 5%. Supports medical rehabilitation, home-care services, and emergency/ambulance services. *Note:* Total contributions made in 1999. **Typ. Recipients:** Clinics/Medical Centers, Domestic Violence, Emergency/Ambulance Services, Family Planning, Health Organizations, Medical Rehabilitation, Medical Research, Mental Health, Nursing Services, People with Disabilities, Prenatal Health Issues, Sexual Abuse, Substance Abuse. **Geo. Dist:** AR; KS; NM; Tulsa, OK; TX.

## ★ 581 ★ Peery Foundation

2560 Mission College Boulevard, Ste. 101
Santa Clara, CA 95054
**Phone:** (408)980-0130 **Fax:** (408)988-4893
**Website:** http://www.peery.arrillaga.com
Richard Peery, President

**Fnded:** 1977. **Philosophy:** Much of the foundation's support goes to the Church of Latter-day Saints. Other interests focus on youth organizations in a variety of areas, including the arts, scholarships, and social activities. **Priorities:** *Arts & Humanities:* 6%. Supports theater, symphony, historical societies, and arts associations. *Civic & Public Affairs:* 5%. Focus on community affairs. *Education:* 5%. Supports secondary education, colleges, and educational programs. *Environment:* 5%. Supports children and youth services, family services, and food banks. *International:* 4%. Primarily for children's health and single-disease health associations. *Religion:* Less than 1%. *Note:* Total contributions made in fiscal 1997. **Typ. Recipients:** Arthritis, Cancer, Children's Health/Hospitals, Emergency/Ambulance Services, Hospices, Medical Research, People with Disabilities, Prenatal Health Issues, Respiratory, Sexual Abuse, Single-Disease Health Associations, Speech & Hearing. **Geo. Dist:** CA. **Frmly:** Richard T. Peery Foundation.

## ★ 582 ★ Penzance Foundation

237 Park Ave., 21st Floor
New York, NY 10017-3412
John Emery, Vice President

**Fnded:** 1981. **Philosophy:** The foundation's giving program generally supports the preferences of Mrs. Clark, with the majority of funding going to educational institutions and social service organizations, principally to youth groups. Medical facilities are also beneficiaries of the foundation's grant-making program. **Priorities:** *Arts & Humanities:* 22%. Funds museums. *Education:* 48%. Funds colleges, universities, private precollege education, and educational associations. *Environment:* 6%. Funds family services and Boys and Girls clubs. *Note:* Total contributions made in fiscal 2001. **Typ. Recipients:** Family Planning, Health Organizations, Hospitals, Kidney, Medical Rehabilitation, Medical Research. **Geo. Dist:** MA; NY.

## ★ 583 ★ Perkins-Prothro Foundation

2304 Midwestern Parkway, Ste. 200
Wichita Falls, TX 76308

**Phone:** (940)691-7770 **Fax:** (940)691-6304
Joe Prothro, Contact

**Fnded:** 1967. **Philosophy:** The Perkins-Prothro Foundation makes endowments to several universities in Texas in support of higher education. Health services and religion are also of interest to the foundation. Other recipient areas include the arts and community services. **Priorities:** *Arts & Humanities:* 9%. *Civic & Public Affairs:* 1%. *Education:* 37%. Supports a humanities research center and colleges and universities. *Environment:* 20%. Support includes Girls and Boys clubs. *International:* 25%. Hospitals and hospice programs. *Note:* Total contributions made in 1998. **Typ. Recipients:** Cancer, Children's Health/Hospitals, Clinics/Medical Centers, Emergency/Ambulance Services, Health Organizations, Health Policy/Cost Containment, Health-General, Heart, Hospices, Hospitals, Medical Rehabilitation, People with Disabilities, Prenatal Health Issues, Public Health, Single-Disease Health Associations, Substance Abuse. **Geo. Dist:** TX, especially the Wichita Falls area.

## ★ 584 ★ Perot Foundation

12377 Merit Dr., Ste. 1700
Dallas, TX 75251
**Phone:** (972)788-3000 **Fax:** (972)788-3091
Carolyn Rathjen, Director

**Fnded:** 1969. **Philosophy:** The majority of contributions made by the Perot Foundation support higher education, especially medical education at Texas universities. The foundation also supports medical research, religious welfare organizations, and social services. Grants to other recipient areas are made on a limited basis. **Priorities:** *Arts & Humanities:* 8%. Funds music, museums, and opera. *Civic & Public Affairs:* 2%. *Education:* 20%. Emphasis on medical education and scholarship funding. *Environment:* 9%. Funds United Way, scouting, community services, and child welfare. *International:* 55%. Primary support for medical centers, research, nursing services, children's health, and single-disease health associations. *Religion:* Less than 1%. *Note:* Total contributions made in 2000. **Typ. Recipients:** AIDS/HIV, Alzheimers Disease, Cancer, Child Abuse, Children's Health/Hospitals, Emergency/Ambulance Services, Emergency/Ambulance Services, Family Planning, Health Organizations, Heart, Hospitals, Medical Education, Medical Research, Mental Health, Nursing Services, Nutrition, People with Disabilities, Prenatal Health Issues, Public Health, Single-Disease Health Associations, Substance Abuse. **Geo. Dist:** TX, emphasis on Dallas.

## ★ 585 ★ Peter Kiewit Foundation

8805 Indian Hills Dr., Ste. 225
Omaha, NE 68114
**Phone:** (402)344-7890
Lyn Ziegenbein, Executive Director

**Fnded:** 1980. **Philosophy:** The foundation makes charitable contributions in the designated areas of education, community development and service, culture, social welfare, health, and character building and physical improvement. The foundation also maintains a scholarship program for graduating high school seniors in the Omaha area. **Priorities:** *Arts & Humanities:* 9%. Supports public libraries, children's museums, historical societies, and fine art museums. *Civic & Public Affairs:* 43%. Funds Omaha Botanical Center, civic affairs with emphasis on Omaha, and housing. *Education:* 26%. Funds colleges, universities, and educational foundations. *Environment:* 16%. Funds Young Men's Christian Association, United Way, children and youth services, and family services. *International:* Less than 1%. Supports minority health concerns. *Note:* Total contributions made in fiscal 2000. **Typ. Recipients:** AIDS/HIV, Cancer, Clinics/Medical Centers, Emergency/Ambulance Services, Family Planning, Health Organizations, Hospitals, Medical Rehabilitation, Nutrition, People with Disabilities, Trauma Treatment. **Geo. Dist:** Omaha, IA, the portion of Iowa which is within a 100-mile radius of Omaha, NE; NE; Sheridan, WY.

## ★ 586 ★ Pew Charitable Trusts

One Commerce Sq.
2005 Market St., Ste. 1700
Philadelphia, PA 19103
**Phone:** (215)575-9050 **Fax:** (215)575-4776
**Email:** INFO@pewtrusts.com
**Website:** http://www.pewtrusts.com
Rebecca Rimel, President & CEO

**Fnded:** 1948. **Philosophy:** "The Pew Charitable Trusts support the work of nonprofit organizations in the fields of culture, education, the environment, health and human services, public policy, and religion. Through their grantmaking, the Trusts seek to encourage individual development and personal achievement, cross-disciplinary problem solving, and innovative, practical approaches to meeting the changing needs of a global community. The Trusts are based in Philadelphia and maintain a special commitment to the city. The Education program seeks to raise the performance of students at all levels of education, especially their capabilities to learn for understanding and to acquire the literacies they need for productive employment and effective citizenship in an increasingly complex society." "The mission of the Environment program is to promote policies and practices that protect the global atmosphere and preserve healthy forest and marine ecosystems. Much of the Environment program's grantmaking focuses on the development of special initiatives, the mobilization of strategic coalitions to pursue specific policy objectives, and the funding of clusters of projects whose goals reinforce or compliment each other. Because of the program's highly focused nature, the great majority of projects supported are initiated by program staff and/or developed in close collaboration with other foundations and environmental organizations." "The Health and Human Services program is designed to promote the health and well-being of the American people and to strengthen disadvantaged communities." Nationally, the trusts give to biomedical research and training; and a public health initiative is being developed. In the Philadelphia area, the trusts support the Pew Fund for Health and Human Services in Philadelphia and the Fund for Urban Neighborhood Development. "The mission of the Public Policy program is to create sustainable improvements to America's democratic life through promoting improvements in the conduct and financing of elections, research on the causes and consequences of declines in social trust, efforts to call Americans to re-engage in the civic life of their nation and communities, and increases in overall government performance." "The Venture Fund is a unique tool for the Trusts, enabling us to explore opportunities that fall outside the clearly defined goals and objectives of the six program areas." **Priorities:** *Arts & Humanities:* 9%. Supports arts appreciation, artists, and cultural organizations. *Civic & Public Affairs:* (Public Policy) 11%. Seeks to advance and sustain the democratic process. *Education:* 11%. Supports K-12 and higher education. *International:* 18%. Supports biomedical research, scientists, and science policies; also funds human services. *Note:* Total contributions made in 2000. **Typ. Recipients:** Adolescent Health Issues, AIDS/HIV, Cancer, Children's Health/Hospitals, Domestic Violence, Emergency/Ambulance Services, Family Planning, Family Planning, Geriatric Health, Health Organizations, Health Policy/Cost Containment, Home-Care Services, Medical Education, Nutrition, Prenatal Health Issues, Public Health, Substance Abuse. **Geo. Dist:** internationally; nationally; Philadelphia, PA.

## ★ 587 ★ Pfaffinger Foundation

Times Mirror Square
Los Angeles, CA 90053
**Fax:** (213)237-6560
Mary Tower, President

**Fnded:** 1936. **Philosophy:** The foundation primarily assists employees, former employees, and surviving spouses of former employees of the Times Mirror Company, a publishing firm in Los Angeles. Limited support for charitable institutions in the greater Los Angeles area is given when funds are available. **Priorities:** *Environment:* 68%. Food banks, YMCAs, the United Way, youth, family, and senior citizen services. *International:* 30%. Focus on women's, children's, and geriatric health. *Note:* Total contributions made in 1998. **Typ. Recipients:** Child Abuse, Children's Health/Hospitals, Clinics/Medical Centers, Domestic Violence, Emergency/Ambulance Services, Family Planning, Geriatric Health, Health Organizations, Health Policy/Cost Containment, Hospitals, Mental Health, Public Health, Substance Abuse. **Geo. Dist:** CA, Southern California.

## ★ 588 ★ Phil Hardin Foundation

PO Drawer 5533
Meridian, MS 39302-5533
**Phone:** (601)483-4282 **Fax:** (601)483-5665
**Email:** info@philhardin.org
**Website:** http://www.philhardin.org
C. Wacaster, Vice President

**Fnded:** 1964. **Philosophy:** "Our vision is to renew and rebuild communities and their economics by means of education. Our goals to guide efforts to accomplish this vision are: Goal 1: Strengthen the capacity of communities to nurture and educate young children. Goal 2: Strengthen the capacity of higher education institutions to renew communities and their economies. Goal 3: Strengthen the capacity of communities for locally initiated educational improvement and economic development. Goal 4: Strengthen policy and leadership at the local levels that support action and success in regard to the foundation's goals." **Priorities:** *Arts & Humanities:* 7%. Supports historic preservation, history, and museum. *Civic & Public Affairs:* 21%. Supports recently audited financial statement development. *Education:* 63%. Supports colleges, universities, faculty development, tutoring programs, and literacy. *Environment:* 4%. Supports family services. *International:* 1%. Supports speech/hearing. *Note:* Total contributions made in 1998. **Typ. Recipients:** Health Policy/Cost Containment, Hospitals (University Affiliated), Medical Rehabilitation, Medical Research, Outpatient Health Care, People with Disabilities, Speech & Hearing. **Geo. Dist:** nationally; MS.

## ★ 589 ★ Philip L. Graham Fund

1150 15th St., Northwest
Washington, DC 20071
**Phone:** (202)334-6640 **Fax:** (202)334-4498
**Email:** plgfund@washpost.com
Candice Bryant, President

**Fnded:** 1963. **Philosophy:** "From its earliest days, the fund's dual mission has been first, to use its resources for the betterment of the Washington, DC, metropolitan area and second, to provide assistance to activities in the field of journalism and communications." Areas of funding priority reflect the interests of the late Mr. Graham and include: programs enriching the lives of children; projects aiding needy citizens in the community; cultural organizations, especially those promoting the visual or dramatic arts; programs improving pre-college public education; and journalism and communications organizations promoting minority interests and freedom of the press worldwide. **Priorities:** *Arts & Humanities:* 15%. Supports theater, multicultural performing arts, museums, libraries, and arts in education. *Civic & Public Affairs:* (Community Endeavors) 8%. Funds minority and women's affairs, affordable housing, volunteerism, and environment. *Education:* 29%. Supports elementary, secondary, and higher education, early childhood, at-risk youth, and services for the learning disabled. *Environment:* (Health and Human Services) 43%. Funds organizations that address mental health, abused women and children, hunger, shelters, hospitals, vocational training, family services, prenatal care, child care, youth, AIDS, literacy, blindness, and seniors. *Note:* Total contributions made in 2000. Also provides discretionary grants for shelter, food, and other assistance to the poor and homeless. **Typ. Recipients:** AIDS/HIV, Cancer, Children's Health/Hospitals, Clinics/Medical Centers, Diabetes, Domestic Violence, Family Planning, Geriatric Health, Health Organizations, Heart, Home-Care Services, Hospices, Hospitals, Long-Term Care, Mental Health, Outpatient Health Care, People with Disabilities, Prenatal Health Issues, Public Health, Substance Abuse, Transplant Networks/Donor Banks.

**Geo. Dist:** Washington, DC, including metropolitan area.

## ★ 590 ★ Philip L. Van Every Foundation

PO Box 32368
Charlotte, NC 28232
**Phone:** (704)554-1421 **Fax:** (704)556-5636
Sean Jamison, Jr., Executive Director

**Fnded:** 1961. **Philosophy:** The foundation's primary interests are health-related organizations, social welfare causes, and civic concerns in North Carolina. **Priorities:** *Arts & Humanities:* 16%. Supports theatre, public broadcasting, and music. *Civic & Public Affairs:* 10%. Supports community affairs. *Education:* 16%. Supports colleges and universities. *Environment:* 20%. Supports housing, homes, substance abuse services, and YWCA. *International:* 11%. Supports single-disease health associations. *Religion:* 4%. Supports scientific organizations. *Note:* Total contributions made in 1998. **Typ. Recipients:** AIDS/HIV, Arthritis, Cancer, Emergency/Ambulance Services, Emergency/Ambulance Services, Health Organizations, Hospices, Hospitals, Medical Research, Multiple Sclerosis, Single-Disease Health Associations, Speech & Hearing, Substance Abuse, Trauma Treatment. **Geo. Dist:** NC.

## ★ 591 ★ Philip M. McKenna Foundation

PO Box 186
Latrobe, PA 15650
**Phone:** (724)537-6901 **Fax:** (724)537-6906
T. Boxx, Chairman

**Fnded:** 1967. **Philosophy:** The Philip M. McKenna Foundation's "is to support the advancement of a free, prosperous, and well-ordered society based on traditional American civic principles, private enterprise, and the cultural heritage of western civilization. This purpose and public philosophy entails a core commitment to limited constitutional government, free market economics, and moral virture. In conducting this mission, support is directed toward research and educational programs with a long-term focus, as well as public policy programs focused on more immediate concerns. The interests of the foundation also includes support the benefit of the community and scientific, educational, and charitable causes compatible with the foundations heritage and priorities." Mission statement. **Priorities:** *Civic & Public Affairs:* 61%. Supports public policy, legal concerns, and economics. *Education:* 31% Contributes to economic education at colleges and universities. *Environment:* 1%. Supports United Way and youth initiatives. *Religion:* 3%. Funds science museums. *Note:* Total contributions made in 1999. **Typ. Recipients:** Health Policy/Cost Containment, Hospitals, Research/Studies Institutes. **Geo. Dist:** grants to national organizations for public policy; PA, Southwestern Pennsylvania for community and civic programs.

## ★ 592 ★ Pinewood Foundation

30 Rockefeller Plaza, Room 5600
New York, NY 10112
**Fax:** (212)649-5859
Celeste Bartos, President

**Fnded:** 1956. **Philosophy:** The foundation typically funds arts organizations, museums, and cultural programs, and also supports education organizations. **Priorities:** *Arts & Humanities:* 15%. Museums, film and public broadcasting. *Civic & Public Affairs:* 11%. Women's issues, human rights. *Education:* 34%. Colleges and universities. *Note:* Contributions made in fiscal 2000. **Typ. Recipients:** AIDS/HIV, Clinics/Medical Centers, Eyes/Blindness, Family Planning, Health Organizations, Hospices, Hospitals, Hospitals (University Affiliated), Medical Education, Medical Research, Multiple Sclerosis, Prenatal Health Issues, Public Health, Research/Studies Institutes, Single-Disease Health Associations. **Geo. Dist:** New York, NY.

## ★ 593 ★ Pinkerton Foundation

630 Fifth Ave., Ste. 1755
New York, NY 10111
**Phone:** (212)332-3385 **Fax:** (212)332-3399



Encyclopedia of Medical Organizations and Agencies, 13th Edition

**Website:** http://www.fdncenter.org/grantmaker/pinkerton

Joan Colello, Executive Director & Secretary

**Fnded:** 1966. **Philosophy:** The foundation's original mandate was to work to prevent and reduce the incidence of crime and juvenile delinquency and, in the early years, the foundation made grants to a wide range of programs supporting human services and education for the disadvantaged. "Building on the original mandate and concerns of its founder, the foundation concentrates its current grant-making program on two segments of the population: first, economically disadvantaged children and youth and families at risk; and second, severely learning-disabled children and adults of borderline intelligence. Within these groups, the foundation seeks to support programs that develop individual competencies, instill values, and increase opportunities to participate in society. Of particular interest are projects that demonstrate promising new ideas for greater program effectiveness or that replicate projects that have proven effective elsewhere. The foundation supports community-based programs in New York City, with preference given to projects for children, youth, and families that intervene before a pattern of failure has been established. The foundation also occasionally supports research and demonstration projects in its principal program areas. While grants for direct service projects are usually limited to New York City, those with potential for national impact or replication may go beyond this geographic limitation." **Priorities:** *Arts & Humanities:* 3%. *Civic & Public Affairs:* 30%. Funds vocational initiatives and community development. *Education:* 15%. Supports programs for middle and schools. *Environment:* 45% Funds youth services and community centers. *Note:* Contributions made in 2000. **Typ. Recipients:** AIDS/HIV, Clinics/Medical Centers, Domestic Violence, Family Planning, Hospitals, Hospitals (University Affiliated), Nursing Services, Outpatient Health Care, People with Disabilities, Public Health, Research/Studies Institutes. **Geo. Dist:** New York City, NY.


**★ 594 ★ Plough Foundation**
6410 Poplar Ave., Ste. 710
Memphis, TN 38119
**Phone:** (901)761-9180      **Fax:** (901)761-6186
**Email:** mail@plough.org
Noris Haynes, Jr., Executive Director & Trustee

**Fnded:** 1960. **Philosophy:** The foundation supports reform of the public school system and homeless programs in Shelby County, TN. The foundation also plans to place more emphasis on crime prevention and law enforcement. In the area of social services, it has emphasized education reform, Jewish Federation, united funds, homeless projects, youth organizations, and issues related to crime prevention. The foundation's current special interests include: public education, specifically early intervention programs for children; families in crisis, preferably programs and ideas that take a realistic approach to the problems and offer avenues for the participants to become self-sufficient; youth programs, mainly programs that specifically address the needs of and opportunities for young people; stretching the nonprofit dollar, particularly programs and activities that demonstrate unique, innovative ways to maximize resources; homeless programs that are part of a comprehensive system; and crime, specifically programs addressing prevention and law enforcement. The foundation will no longer be making grants to schools of pharmacy. The foundation will, however, continue to make deferred payments to certain institutions. **Priorities:** *Arts & Humanities:* 19%. Ballet, music, arts associations. *Civic & Public Affairs:* 18%. Community affairs and public policy. *Education:* 9%. Public education and education reform. *Environment:* 12%. Family services, united funds, and youth organizations. *International:* 23%. Health centers and hospitals. *Note:* Total contributions made in 1998. **Typ. Recipients:** Cancer, Clinics/Medical Centers, Emergency/Ambulance Services, Hospitals, Medical Education, Mental Health, Outpatient Health Care, People with Disabilities, Single-Disease Health Associations, Substance Abuse. **Geo. Dist:** TN, primarily in Shelby County and Memphis.


**★ 595 ★ Polk Bros. Foundation**
420 North Wabash Ave.
Ste. 204
Chicago, IL 60611
**Phone:** (312)527-4684      **Fax:** (312)527-4681
**Email:** info@polkbrosfdn.org
**Website:** http://www.polkbrosfdn.org
Nikki Stein, Executive Director

**Fnded:** 1957. **Philosophy:** "Founded in 1955, the Foundation remains a Chicago concern. Reflecting the underlying philosophy of the Polk Family, the Foundation supports programs that work directly with populations of need–particularly children. Grants are made for both new and ongoing initiatives in four program areas: social service, education, culture and health." "The goal of the Foundation's grantmaking is to improve the quality of life... (especially in the Chicago area)...with a particular focus on economically-disadvantaged children and youth." "When we look at a grant and the way the money is utilized, we really study three factors. First we consider the quality of the program. We ask ourselves if the idea makes sense and has a reasonable chance of making the impact desired. Equally important is the group's ability to attack the identified problem. Does it have a board and staff committed to the program, competent management and adequate fundraising capability?" "Finally, we analyze an agency's past performance, recognizing that circumstances may dictate the need for flexibility and adjustment and that progress, rather than instant results, may be a more reasonable measure of success during a given time frame. Our own objective then is to blend rigor and realism in developing and utilizing evaluation methods that are useful to grantees as well as to us." Polk Bros. 1995 Annual Report, *Evaluating for Impact* The foundation responds to requests from social service, cultural, educational, and health organizations that provide direct services in Chicago. The foundation has implemented the Full Service Schools Initiative. "The Initiative seeks to meet students' and families' needs for a wide range of educational, health, and social service programs through partnerships between schools and community organizations. By locating programs at schools, we can take advantage of excellent facilities that normally shut down at the end of the school day, while providing families much better access to a wide range of resources." 1996 Annual Report **Priorities:** *Arts & Humanities:* 18%. Supports art and culture. *Civic & Public Affairs:* 9%. Supports community and public affairs. *Education:* 14%. Supports educational institutions and programs. *Environment:* 40%. Supports youth, family, and social services. *International:* 9%. Supports health care centers and services. *Religion:* 1%. Supports museums of natural history, with the majority of support given to the Museum of Science and Industry. *Note:* Contributions were made in fiscal 1999. **Typ. Recipients:** AIDS/HIV, Child Abuse, Clinics/Medical Centers, Health Organizations, Hospitals, Medical Rehabilitation, Mental Health, Nursing Services, People with Disabilities, Prenatal Health Issues, Public Health, Substance Abuse. **Geo. Dist:** Chicago, IL.


**★ 596 ★ Priddy Foundation**
807 8th St.
City National Bldg., Ste. 750
Wichita Falls, TX 76301
**Phone:** (940)723-8720      **Fax:** (940)723-8656
**Email:** info@priddyfdn.org
**Website:** http://www.priddyfdn.org
David Wolverton, President

**Fnded:** 1963. **Philosophy:** The foundation focuses giving on human services, education, the arts, and civic concerns in northern Texas. **Priorities:** *Arts & Humanities:* 1%. Supports theater and arts education. *Civic & Public Affairs:* 80%. Supports community foundations, housing, nonprofit management, womens affairs, and neighborhood groups. *Education:* 4%. Supports higher education. *Environment:* 10%. Supports relief agencies, child welfare, scouting, counseling, senior services, and meals on wheels program. *International:* 2%. Supports a health care center. *Note:* Total contributions made in 1999. **Typ. Recipients:** Alzheimers Disease, Clinics/Medical Centers, Emergency/Ambulance Services, Health Organizations, Hospices, Hospitals, Medical Education, Medical Rehabilitation, Mental Health, People with Disabilities, Prenatal Health Issues. **Geo. Dist:** OK, Southern OK; TX, Northern Texas; Wichita Falls, TX.


**★ 597 ★ Pritzker Foundation**
200 West Madison St., Ste. 3800
Chicago, IL 60606
**Phone:** (312)750-8400      **Fax:** (312)750-8545
Thomas Pritzker, Contact

**Fnded:** 1944. **Philosophy:** The Pritzker Foundation supports Jewish organizations, the arts, health, education, and social services in the Chicago metropolitan area, by providing small grants, ranging from $25 to $1,000, to a large number of organizations. Significant grants are made to a limited number of recipients that include the Jewish United Fund, Crusade of Mercy, several Jewish organizations and synagogues, and programs in support of Israel. In addition, the foundation awards the annual Pritzker Architecture Prize of more than $100,000, administered through the Hyatt Foundation. **Priorities:** *Arts & Humanities:* 7%. Funds public libraries, children's museums, modern & contemporary art museums, the opera, the theater, visual and performing arts. *Civic & Public Affairs:* 1%. Funds community affairs, zoology, aquariums, and primary support given to the Pritzker Family Philanthropic Fund. *Education:* 73%. Supports secondary schools, colleges, universities, and educational programs. *Environment:* Less than 2%. *International:* 9%. Supports medical centers, health centers, and research. *Note:* Total contributions made in 1998. **Typ. Recipients:** Cancer, Children's Health/Hospitals, Clinics/Medical Centers, Domestic Violence, Eyes/Blindness, Family Planning, Health Organizations, Hospitals, Medical Education, Medical Rehabilitation, Medical Research, Mental Health, People with Disabilities, Public Health, Research/Studies Institutes, Single-Disease Health Associations, Substance Abuse. **Geo. Dist:** Chicago, IL, metropolitan area.


**★ 598 ★ Prospect Hill Foundation**
99 Park Ave., Ste. 2220
New York, NY 10016-1601
**Phone:** (212)370-1165
**Website:** http://www.fdncenter.org/grantmaker/prospecthill
Constance Eiseman, Executive Director

**Fnded:** 1960. **Philosophy:** The areas for which the foundation is interested in receiving proposals are nuclear weapons control, environmental conservation, and family planning services in Latin America. The nuclear weapons control grants program seeks to improve communications, understanding, and a sense of mutual risk among leaders in the U.S. and the former Soviet Union; lead to commitments among world leaders to limit and reduce nuclear weapons arsenals; and implement strategies for limiting the proliferation of nuclear weapons, weapons development, and the capacity to manufacture nuclear weapons. The environmental conservation program is concerned with strategies for the preservation of public and private lands and strengthening public policies for environmental protection, water quality, and ecosystem protection in the northeastern U.S. The population program is concerned with programs in Latin America which encourage access to family planning services. Proposals from social services, arts, cultural, and educational institutions are accepted upon invitation only. **Priorities:** *Arts & Humanities:* 11%. Supports historic preservation, museums, music, dance, libraries, and theater. *Civic & Public Affairs:* 4%. Supports zoological societies, botanical gardens, conservancy, and population issues. *Education:* 54%. Supports colleges and preparatory schools. *Environment:* 4%. Focus on community service organizations. *International:* 1%. Supports hospitals. *Note:* Total contributions made in fiscal 1998. **Typ. Recipients:** Emergency/Ambulance Services, Family Planning, Heart, Hospitals, Prenatal Health Issues. **Geo. Dist:** nationally; NY.

## ★ 599 ★ R. C. Baker Foundation

PO Box 6150
Orange, CA 92863-6150
**Phone:** (714)750-8987
Frank Scott, Chairman

**Fnded:** 1952. **Philosophy:** The foundation supports organizations and projects concerned with the arts, education, community services, health, and social services. **Priorities:** *Arts & Humanities:* 8%. Emphasis on museums, the performing arts, and public broadcasting. *Civic & Public Affairs:* 11%. Focus on legal aid, community services, and police officers associations. *Education:* 26%. Supports colleges and universities, education associations, and scholarship funds. *Environment:* 19%. Primary funding for youth organizations and child welfare. *International:* 33%. Primary support for hospitals and single-disease health associations. *Note:* Total contributions made in 2000. **Typ. Recipients:** Cancer, Children's Health/Hospitals, Clinics/Medical Centers, Domestic Violence, Emergency/Ambulance Services, Eyes/Blindness, Health Organizations, Hospitals, Medical Rehabilitation, Medical Research, Mental Health, Multiple Sclerosis, Nursing Services, People with Disabilities, Preventive Medicine/Wellness Organizations, Research/Studies Institutes, Single-Disease Health Associations, Speech & Hearing, Substance Abuse. **Geo. Dist:** western US.

## ★ 600 ★ R. D. and Joan Dale Hubbard Foundation

PO Box 2498
Ruidoso, NM 88355-2498
**Phone:** (505)258-5919          **Fax:** (505)258-3749
James Stoddard, Executive Director

**Fnded:** 1986. **Philosophy:** "From its beginning, the Foundation adopted an entrepreneurial approach to philanthropy that reflects the spirit of (its founders). Both R.D. and Joan Dale Hubbard are Kansas natives and both were teachers in Kansas. They maintain strong ties to education and to the people in the West. ... Together the Hubbards established the Foundation's philanthropic trust, which centers around cultural, education and general benefit to mankind. The foundation's two major categories of support are the arts and humanities, and education." **Priorities:** *Arts & Humanities:* 27%. Supports museum, music, theater, and ballet. *Civic & Public Affairs:* 3%. Funds community foundations. *Education:* 62%. Funds scholarship, universities, colleges, and schools. *Environment:* 3%. Supports Big brothers/Big Sisters and special olympics. *International:* 5%. Supports medical centers, home-care services, hospital. *Note:* Total contributions made in 1998. **Typ. Recipients:** AIDS/HIV, Alzheimers Disease, Cancer, Children's Health/Hospitals, Domestic Violence, Heart, Home-Care Services, Medical Education, Medical Research, Medical Training, People with Disabilities, Single-Disease Health Associations. **Geo. Dist:** CA; KS; NM.

## ★ 601 ★ R. J. McElroy Trust

500 East 4th St., Ste. 318
Waterloo, IA 50703
**Phone:** (319)287-9102          **Fax:** (319)291-1260
**Email:** mcelroy@cedarnet.org
**Website:** http://www.cedarnet.org/mcelroy
Linda Klinger, Executive Director

**Fnded:** 1965. **Philosophy:** The R.J. McElroy Trust assists non-profit organizations which provide educational services to deserving youth, giving high priority to grants which provide seed money to programs rather than capital projects. **Priorities:** *Arts & Humanities:* 13%. Supports libraries, arts forums, theater, the symphony, and public broadcasting. *Civic & Public Affairs:* 22%. Supports community services, urban development, parks and botanical gardens. *Education:* 38%. Supports community schools, colleges, and universities, including scholarships and fellowships. Supports medicine education and science education. *Environment:* 23%. Supports youth and family services, Young Women's Christian Association's, Big Brothers/Big Sisters, community centers and camps. *International:* 2%. *Note:* Total contributions made in 1999. **Typ. Recipients:** AIDS/HIV, Children's Health/

Hospitals, Clinics/Medical Centers, Domestic Violence, Family Planning, Hospices, Hospitals, Medical Education, Medical Training, People with Disabilities, People with Disabilities, Prenatal Health Issues, Research/Studies Institutes, Substance Abuse. **Geo. Dist:** IA, Black Hawk County and rural counties in the Waterloo area; Waterloo, IA.

## ★ 602 ★ R. K. Mellon Family Foundation

One Mellon Bank Center
500 Grant St., Ste. 4106
Pittsburgh, PA 15219-2502
**Phone:** (412)392-2800          **Fax:** (412)392-2849
Michael Watson, Vice President & Director

**Fnded:** 1978. **Philosophy:** According to the foundation's literature, its grant programs support institutions that are focused on the "improvement of the quality of life in Pittsburgh and Western Pennsylvania. The foundation is interested in a broad range of activities with primary emphasis on the fields of education, health care, social and human services, and conservation." **Priorities:** *Arts & Humanities:* 14%. Focus on museums, historic preservation, and music. *Civic & Public Affairs:* 15%. Supports zoos and community services. *Education:* 26%. Primary support for colleges, universities, and private secondary schools. *Environment:* 5%. Community services and youth organizations. *International:* 7%. Hospitals and medical research. *Note:* Total contributions made in 1998. **Typ. Recipients:** AIDS/HIV, Cancer, Clinics/Medical Centers, Domestic Violence, Emergency/Ambulance Services, Health Funds, Hospitals, Hospitals (University Affiliated), Long-Term Care, Medical Education, Medical Rehabilitation, Medical Research, Medical Training, Mental Health, Nursing Services, People with Disabilities, Preventive Medicine/Wellness Organizations, Sexual Abuse, Substance Abuse, Transplant Networks/Donor Banks. **Geo. Dist:** PA, Western Pennsylvania; Pittsburgh, PA.

## ★ 603 ★ Ralph E. Ogden Foundation

Pleasant Hill Rd.
PO Box 290
Mountainville, NY 10953
**Phone:** (845)534-3423          **Fax:** (845)534-5854
Georgene Zlock, Contact

**Fnded:** 1947. **Philosophy:** The foundation's major priority is the arts, with large contributions to the Storm King Art Center, Mountainville, NY. All categories of the arts are supported. Other interests are minor, but include international organizations, education, health, and social services. **Priorities:** *Arts & Humanities:* 90% supports art galleries, museums, opera, and music. *Civic & Public Affairs:* 1% Supports community and civic affairs and public gardens and trails. *Education:* 2% Funds colleges, universities, and educational programs. *Environment:* 1%. Supports health-care and senior welfare. *International:* 1%. Donates to a hospital. *Note:* Contributions were made in 1999. **Typ. Recipients:** Clinics/Medical Centers, Health Organizations, Health Policy/Cost Containment, Hospices, Hospitals, Medical Education, Public Health, Substance Abuse. **Geo. Dist:** nationally; NY.

## ★ 604 ★ Ralph M. Parsons Foundation

1055 Wilshire Boulevard, Ste. 1701
Los Angeles, CA 90017
**Phone:** (213)482-3185          **Fax:** (213)482-8878
**Email:** hoppe@rmpf.org
**Website:** http://www.rmpf.org
Wendy Hoppe, Executive Director & Secretary

**Fnded:** 1961. **Philosophy:** "The Foundation is concerned with the encouragement and support of projects and programs deemed beneficial to humankind in several major areas of interest...The emphasis upon individual categories may vary from year to year, and exceptions to these guidelines may occur solely at the discretion of the Foundation." The foundation's primary areas of interest include the following: higher education, with emphasis on the fields of engineering, technology, and the sciences; social impact, focusing on assistance to socially or economically disadvantaged groups in society; civic and cultural affairs, with a preference for programs that enhance the cultural

life of all people by providing opportunities for access to cultural experiences; civic grants are awarded to address significant concerns which arise in the community; health, with emphasis on services to disadvantaged elderly, families, and youth, through support of programs and medical equipment associated with these services; and special projects, providing giving flexibility through foundation-initiated grants for projects of interest to the Board that are related to the broad purposes of the foundation but fall outside its established areas of interest. **Priorities:** *Arts & Humanities:* About 27%. *Civic & Public Affairs:* 3%. *Education:* 23%. Primarily to colleges and universities for technical education. *Environment:* 37%. Senior services, youth organizations, and day care. *International:* 10%. Supports hospitals, medical research, cancer treatment, and children's health. *Note:* Total contributions made in 1998. **Typ. Recipients:** Adolescent Health Issues, AIDS/HIV, Alzheimers Disease, Cancer, Child Abuse, Children's Health/Hospitals, Clinics/Medical Centers, Domestic Violence, Eyes/Blindness, Family Planning, Geriatric Health, Health Organizations, Heart, Hospitals, Hospitals (University Affiliated), Long-Term Care, Medical Research, Mental Health, People with Disabilities, Prenatal Health Issues, Preventive Medicine/Wellness Organizations, Speech & Hearing, Substance Abuse, Trauma Treatment. **Geo. Dist:** CA, Los Angeles County.

## ★ 605 ★ Ramapo Trust

126 East 56th St., 10th Floor
New York, NY 10022
**Phone:** (212)308-7355          **Fax:** (212)750-0132
**Email:** BkdlFdn@aol.com
**Website:** http://www.ewol.com/brookdale
Stephen Schwartz, Trustee

**Fnded:** 1973. **Philosophy:** The trust "is a charitable institution whose resources have centered on gerontology and geriatrics. The trust will consider innovative projects which serve the aging, or increase knowledge in the field of aging." The trust places emphasis on services for families of Alzheimer's disease patients and for grandparents and other kin raising grandchildren or other relatives children. **Priorities:** *Arts & Humanities:* 13%. Funds performing arts. *Civic & Public Affairs:* 2%. Supports community groups and legal aid. *Education:* 50%. Funds universities, schools, and research. *Environment:* 10%. Supports elder care, services for the disabled, and family services. *International:* 15%. Focus on geriatric medicine; supports medical centers, mental health, and cancer treatment. *Note:* Total contributions made in fiscal 2000. **Typ. Recipients:** Alzheimers Disease, Cancer, Clinics/Medical Centers, Domestic Violence, Geriatric Health, Health Funds, Health Organizations, Health-General, Heart, Hospitals, Hospitals (University Affiliated), Long-Term Care, Medical Education, Medical Research, Mental Health, Nursing Services, Public Health, Substance Abuse. **Geo. Dist:** nationally.

## ★ 606 ★ Raskob Foundation for Catholic Activities

Kennett Pike and Montchanin Rd.
PO Box 4019
Wilmington, DE 19807
**Phone:** (302)655-4440          **Fax:** (302)655-3223
**Website:** http://www.rfca.org
Frederick Perella, Jr., Executive Vice President

**Fnded:** 1945. **Philosophy:** The foundation's purpose is to "engage in such exclusively religious, charitable, literary, and educational activities as will aid the Roman Catholic Church and institutions and organizations identified with it." In determining its own priorities, the foundation takes into account the priorities of the National Conference of Catholic Bishops. It also strives to help the church meet some of the major needs of priests and nuns, and the problems of immigrants and refugees. Toward this end, the foundation supports projects both within the United States and abroad. **Priorities:** *Civic & Public Affairs:* 9%. Funds community leadership. *Education:* 28%. Supports Catholic schools and universities. *Environment:* 24%. Funds family services and youth ministry. *International:* 1%. *Religion:* 1%. *Note:* Total contributions made in 2000. **Typ. Recipients:** Adolescent Health

Issues, AIDS/HIV, Children's Health/Hospitals, Clinics/ Medical Centers, Domestic Violence, Family Planning, Health Organizations, Hospices, Hospitals, Medical Education, Medical Rehabilitation, Mental Health, Nursing Services, People with Disabilities, Preventive Medicine/Wellness Organizations, Public Health, Substance Abuse. **Geo. Dist:** internationally; nationally.

**★ 607 ★ Rauch Foundation**
229 Seventh St., Ste. 306
Garden City, NY 11530-5766
**Phone:** (516)873-9808　　**Fax:** (516)873-0708
**Email:** info@rauchfoundation.org
Nancy Douzinas, President

**Fnded:** 1961. **Philosophy:** "Today, the Foundation concentrates the majority of our grant making to benefit vulnerable young children and their families. The Foundation's mission in this area is to foster the development of programs and policies that promote, strengthen, and maintain the health and well-being of families and their children from conception through age six. Our program interests include family planning, prenatal care, parenting education, income security, family support, and early childhood education. The Foundation encourages proposals for projects that seek to: help families become more self-reliant and build family strengths; change program focus from the child alone to the family as a whole; assist families to remain intact and encourage more fathers to be strong partners in parenting and supporting their children; expand the availability of preventive services and shift existing services from remediation to prevention; extend the reach and effectiveness of current policies or programs; improve policies that impact programs; and streamline the delivery of services." "Environment: The foundation also has initiated two small grant programs in Nassau County and Maryland. The programs will evolve over the next few years, but are expected to focus on community-based efforts to preserve, protect, and clean up the environment. Performing Arts: A modest program is planned for support of music programs in Nassau County next year. The Foundation reported that it is not currently accepting unsolicited proposals in this areas." "Leadership: The Foundation Board will develop a small program focused on leadership over the next year. At this time, the Foundation is not accepting unsolicited proposals in this area." 1997 Guidelines Guidelines **Priorities:** *Civic & Public Affairs:* 14%. Funds community affairs. *Education:* 23%. Supports schools, universities, and literacy programs. *Environment:* 51%. Supports planned parenthood, volunteerism, youth, and family services. *Note:* Total contributions made in fiscal 1999. **Typ. Recipients:** Child Abuse, Family Planning, Hospices, People with Disabilities, Prenatal Health Issues, Public Health. **Geo. Dist:** MD, small environmental program in Maryland; NY, Nassau County.

**★ 608 ★ Ray C. Fish Foundation**
2001 Kirby Dr., Ste. 1005
Houston, TX 77019
**Phone:** (713)522-0741　　**Fax:** (713)529-4033
Barbara Daniel, President

**Fnded:** 1957. **Philosophy:** "Under the charter of the Ray C. Fish Foundation, grants are made for the support, establishment, operation, or advancement of qualified educational, scientific, or other charitable organizations in the state of Texas." The foundation's first large grant, $5 million, was made in 1966 as seed money for the Texas Heart Institute. Other health interests include the American Heart Association, the Living Bank, and various Houston hospitals. Educational interests include colleges, universities, and schools located in Texas, especially those at which there are professorships, chairs, and endowed scholarship funds in the name of Mr. and Mrs. Fish. The foundation supports a broad range of community service programs and organizations. The foundation also supports various Houston museums and performing arts groups. **Priorities:** *Arts & Humanities:* 15%. Supports history, ballet, museum, music, libraries, and historic preservation. *Civic & Public Affairs:* 26%. Supports arboretums, urban affairs, public policy, parks, and nature centers. *Education:* 24%. Primarily

funds colleges and universities, medical education, religious, education, and field specific education. *Environment:* 11%. Emphasis on youth organizations, community affairs, child welfare, food/clothing distribution, sexual abuse, and young men's christian association. *International:* 16%. Supports hospitals, single-disease health associations, and a medical rehabilitation center. *Note:* Total contributions made in fiscal 1999. **Typ. Recipients:** Alzheimers Disease, Cancer, Child Abuse, Clinics/Medical Centers, Emergency/ Ambulance Services, Family Planning, Health Organizations, Heart, Hospices, Hospitals, Hospitals (University Affiliated), Kidney, Medical Education, Medical Rehabilitation, Medical Research, People with Disabilities, Research/Studies Institutes, Single-Disease Health Associations, Single-Disease Health Associations. **Geo. Dist:** Galveston, TX; Houston, TX, including metropolitan area; Kerrville, TX.

**★ 609 ★ Raymond John Wean Foundation**
PO Box 760
Warren, OH 44482-0760
**Phone:** (330)394-5600　　**Fax:** (330)394-5601
**Email:** RJWeanFdn@aol.com
Raymond Wean, Jr., Chairman

**Fnded:** 1949. **Philosophy:** Grants from the foundation primarily support people and communities within the geographic area served. The foundation rewards excellence in those communities and supports groups and projects that empower citizens to meet their full potential. Its main areas of interest include: education, community development, health, the arts, youth and family services, and personal development leading to employment. **Priorities:** *Arts & Humanities:* 17%. Supports art institutes, museums. *Civic & Public Affairs:* 10%. Supports gardens, libraries. *Education:* 60%. Supports public and private schools; colleges and universities, preschool. *Environment:* 3%. Supports camps, youth programs, family services. *International:* 4%. Supports hospitals, medical centers. *Religion:* 1%. Supports science museum. *Note:* Total contributions made in 1998. **Typ. Recipients:** Cancer, Children's Health/Hospitals, Clinics/Medical Centers, Family Planning, Health Organizations, Health Policy/ Cost Containment, Hospices, Hospitals, Long-Term Care, Medical Education, Medical Rehabilitation, Medical Research, Mental Health, Nursing Services, People with Disabilities, Public Health, Single-Disease Health Associations, Substance Abuse. **Geo. Dist:** FL, Southeast Florida; OH, Northeast Ohio; PA, Southeast Pennsylvania.

**★ 610 ★ Regenstein Foundation**
8600 West Bryn Mawr Ave., Ste. 705N
Chicago, IL 60631
**Phone:** (773)693-6464　　**Fax:** (773)693-2480
Robert Mecca, Vice President

**Fnded:** 1950. **Philosophy:** The foundation's primary interests are in arts, music, education, and social services in the Chicago metropolitan area. **Priorities:** *Arts & Humanities:* 15%. Funds public broadcasting, art institutes, music, libraries, history, and opera. *Civic & Public Affairs:* 62%. Supports the Lincoln Park Zoo. *Environment:* 10%. Gives to youth groups, united funds, animal concerns, people with disabilities, food distribution, scouts, and child welfare. *International:* 13%. Funds hospitals. *Note:* Total contributions made in 2000. **Typ. Recipients:** Clinics/Medical Centers, Family Planning, Health Organizations, Heart, Hospitals, Medical Education, Medical Rehabilitation, Mental Health, Nursing Services, People with Disabilities, Prenatal Health Issues, Sexual Abuse, Transplant Networks/Donor Banks. **Geo. Dist:** Chicago, IL, metropolitan area.

**★ 611 ★ Reinberger Foundation**
27600 Chagrin Boulevard
Cleveland, OH 44122
**Phone:** (216)292-2790
Robert Reinberger, Co-Director

**Fnded:** 1968. **Philosophy:** The foundation does not place any restrictions on the types of organizations

which may request a grant; nor does it have a fixed pattern of giving. Priorities are apt to change from year to year. All giving, however, is limited strictly to the greater Cleveland and Columbus areas. The foundation prefers to provide funds for operating purposes and capital improvements. It usually does not provide seed money or fund new projects, preferring to help well-established, traditional organizations. **Priorities:** *Arts & Humanities:* 40%. Supports museums, performing arts, public broadcasting, and cultural affairs. *Civic & Public Affairs:* 12%. Supports zoos, botanical gardens, and community development. *Education:* 16%. Primary support for colleges and universities. *Environment:* 12%. Supports children's services and senior citizen community affairs. *International:* 16%. Supports hospitals, clinics, children's health, and medical rehabilitation. *Religion:* 2%. Supports science museums and science centers. *Note:* Contributions were made in 1998. **Typ. Recipients:** Alzheimers Disease, Cancer, Children's Health/Hospitals, Clinics/Medical Centers, Family Planning, Health Organizations, Health-General, Hospitals, Hospitals (University Affiliated), Long-Term Care, Medical Education, Medical Rehabilitation, Medical Research, People with Disabilities, Public Health, Speech & Hearing. **Geo. Dist:** Cleveland, OH; Columbus, OH.

**★ 612 ★ Research Corp.**
Science Advancement Program
101 North Wilmot Rd., Ste. 250
Tucson, AZ 85711-3332
**Phone:** (520)571-1111　　**Fax:** (520)571-1119
**Email:** awards@rescorp.org
**Website:** http://www.rescorp.org
Carmen Vitello, Editor

**Fnded:** 1912. **Philosophy:** The support of scientific research and experimentation at scholarly institutions is the main activity of Research Corporation. All awards are made within academic settings and within the core physical sciences, chemistry, physics, and astronomy. The emphasis of the foundation has been on support of people and their programs rather than bricks and mortar or broad institutional initiatives. Another goal of Research Corporation is to encourage and support programs that include and motivate students. For instance, the Cottrell College Science Awards encourage research with undergraduates; equipment, summer stipends, and supplies are provided. The Cottrell Scholars Awards reward beginning faculty who wish to excel at both teaching and research; all awards are for $50,000, which can be used largely at the discretion of the scholar. A small group of undergraduate colleges, which have been conspicuously successful at producing science graduates, participate in the Department Development Program; the foundation invites proposals from promising candidates in undergraduate chemistry and physics departments that have the potential to join this group. Research Opportunity Awards are mid-career awards for tenured science faculty aimed at reestablishing vigorous research programs. "Research Corporation is open to opportunities within our fields of activity that fall outside the regular programs. Proposals for support of projects that will enhance science research or that bear on the infrastructure of science can be considered. Occasionally, proposals may also be encouraged for research projects that are exceedingly novel, that run counter to scientific paradigms and are unlikely to achieve support from more traditional sources. Because our resources are limited, only the most challenging and innovative proposals are likely to succeed." 1995 Award Programs Summary **Priorities:** *Religion:* 100%. Supports academic science in two ways: by providing funding for original research in chemistry, physics, and astronomy; and by stressing undergraduate teaching and involvement of students in research: Cottrell College Science program to support projects at predominantly undergraduate institutions (44%); new Research Innovation Awards program (29%); Cottrell Scholars Awards for graduate faculty (12%); Partners in Science program (9%); general grants to research and science education(3%); remaining funds supported the Research Opportunity Awards (3%), given to midcareer scientists to further their research. *Note:* Total contributions made in 1998. **Typ. Recipients:** Health-General,

Medical Education, Substance Abuse. **Geo. Dist:** nationally.

**★ 613 ★ RGK Foundation**
1301 West 25th St.
Ste. 300
Austin, TX 78705—4236
**Phone:** (512)474-9298  **Fax:** (512)474-6389
**Email:** jhampton@rgkfoundation.org
**Website:** http://www.rgkfoundation.org
Gregory Kozmetsky, President, Chairman

**Fnded:** 1966. **Philosophy:** "The RGK Foundation provides support for research in the areas of medicine and education. The foundation additionally supports programs that promote academic excellence in institutions of higher learning; programs that raise literacy levels in our society; programs that promote the health and well-being of children; and programs that attract minority and women students into the fields of math, science, and technology. The foundation has sponsored studies in several areas of national and international concern including health, corporate governance, energy, economic analysis, and technology transfer." 1996 Annual Brochure **Priorities:** *Arts & Humanities:* 5%. Supports film and a children's museum. *Civic & Public Affairs:* 19%. Supports community organizations. *Education:* 45%. Funds schools and higher education. *Environment:* 15%. Funds community centers, youth programs, shelters. *International:* 15%. Funds medical research. *Note:* Total contributions made in 1999. **Typ. Recipients:** Arthritis, Cancer, Child Abuse, Children's Health/Hospitals, Clinics/Medical Centers, Diabetes, Domestic Violence, Eyes/Blindness, Geriatric Health, Health Organizations, Health Policy/Cost Containment, Heart, Hospices, Hospitals (University Affiliated), Kidney, Medical Education, Medical Research, Mental Health, Nursing Services, People with Disabilities, Prenatal Health Issues, Public Health, Research/Studies Institutes, Respiratory, Single-Disease Health Associations, Speech & Hearing, Substance Abuse, Transplant Networks/Donor Banks. **Geo. Dist:** nationally.

**★ 614 ★ Rhodebeck Charitable Trust**
260 Madison Ave., 18th Floor
New York, NY 10167
**Fax:** (212)488-6260
Huyler Held, Trustee

**Fnded:** 1987. **Philosophy:** The Rhodebeck Charitable Trust makes most of its grants in the area of social services. Interests include homes, the homeless, food distribution, and children's services. **Priorities:** *Arts & Humanities:* 10%. *Civic & Public Affairs:* 72%. Legal defense funds, housing programs, jobs for youth, and community service organizations. *Environment:* 8%. Child welfare. *Note:* Total contributions made in fiscal 1999. **Typ. Recipients:** Alzheimers Disease, Child Abuse, Children's Health/Hospitals, Geriatric Health, Health Organizations, Home-Care Services, Mental Health, Nursing Services, Substance Abuse. **Geo. Dist:** New York, NY.

**★ 615 ★ Rice Foundation**
8600 Gross Point Rd.
Skokie, IL 60077-2151
**Phone:** (847)581-9999
Peter Nolan, President

**Fnded:** 1947. **Philosophy:** The foundation generally supports civic organizations and social services in the Chicago metropolitan area. The arts have also been a funding focus. **Priorities:** *Arts & Humanities:* 3%. Supports performing arts and festivals. *Civic & Public Affairs:* 4%. Funds community foundations, zoos, botanical gardens, and arboretums. *Education:* 14%. Funds secondary educational institutions and education foundations. *Environment:* 30%. Supports child and youth services, a crime commission, developmental services, homes, and camps. *International:* 43%. Hospitals, wellness centers, and disease and disorder concerns. *Note:* Total contributions made in 2000. **Typ. Recipients:** Arthritis, Cancer, Children's Health/Hospitals, Clinics/Medical Centers, Geriatric Health, Health Organizations, Health-General, Home-Care Services, Hospitals, Hospitals (University Affiliated),

Long-Term Care, Medical Education, Medical Rehabilitation, Mental Health, People with Disabilities, Prenatal Health Issues, Single-Disease Health Associations. **Geo. Dist:** Chicago, IL.

**★ 616 ★ Rich Foundation**
11 Piedmont Center, Ste. 204
Atlanta, GA 30305
**Phone:** (404)262-2266  **Fax:** (404)266-2123
Anne Berg, Grant Consultant

**Fnded:** 1942. **Philosophy:** The foundation typically supports human service organizations, health organizations, educational institutions, and the arts and humanities. Funding is limited to the metropolitan Atlanta area. **Priorities:** *Arts & Humanities:* 25%. Music, arts centers, theater, opera, and ballet. *Civic & Public Affairs:* 1%. Parks, botanical gardens, and urban affairs. *Education:* 12%. Colleges and universities, primary and secondary education, and education associations. *Environment:* 28%. Emphasis on united funds, family services, child welfare, youth organizations, religious welfare organizations, and the aged. *International:* 20%. Hospitals and medical centers, single-disease health associations, and pediatric health. *Note:* Total contributions made in fiscal 1999. **Typ. Recipients:** Cancer, Child Abuse, Children's Health/Hospitals, Emergency/Ambulance Services, Eyes/Blindness, Health Organizations, Heart, Hospitals, Medical Education, Medical Research, Mental Health, Nursing Services, People with Disabilities, Prenatal Health Issues, Single-Disease Health Associations. **Geo. Dist:** Atlanta, GA, metropolitan area.

**★ 617 ★ Richard and Helen DeVos Foundation**
126 Ottowa Northwest, Ste. 500
Grand Rapids, MI 49503
**Phone:** (616)454-4114  **Fax:** (616)454-0970
**Email:** virginiav@rdvcorp.com
Ginny Vander Hart, Foundation Director

**Fnded:** 1969. **Philosophy:** The foundation primarily funds religious programs and associations, as well as some churches. Education (largely religious) is also a major focus. **Priorities:** *Arts & Humanities:* 4%. Supports art museums, the library of Michigan, symphonies, and performing arts. *Civic & Public Affairs:* 14%. Supports City Vision, city gardens, and community action. *Education:* 34%. Supports colleges, universities, and educational services and programs. *Environment:* 13%. Supports youth services, family services, soup kitchens, and social services. *International:* 2%. Supports health services. *Note:* Contributions were made in 1998. **Typ. Recipients:** Clinics/Medical Centers, Emergency/Ambulance Services, Family Planning, Health Funds, Health Organizations, Health Organizations, Health-General, Hospitals, Long-Term Care, Medical Research, People with Disabilities, Prenatal Health Issues, Public Health, Single-Disease Health Associations, Transplant Networks/Donor Banks. **Geo. Dist:** nationally; FL, including central Florida; Grand Rapids, MI.

**★ 618 ★ Richard King Mellon Foundation**
One Mellon Bank Center
500 Grant St., Ste. 4106
Pittsburgh, PA 15219-2502
**Phone:** (412)392-2800  **Fax:** (412)392-2837
**Website:** http://fdncenter.org/grantmaker/rkmellon/
Michael Watson, Vice President and Director

**Fnded:** 1947. **Philosophy:** The Foundation has two distinct areas of interest: programs that relate to education, human services, medicine and health care, civic affairs, and cultural activities in Pittsburgh and Southwestern Pennsylvania; and the American Land Conservation Program, and conservation of natural areas on a national level. *Education:* Priority is given to for early childhood and preschool education as well as programs designed to change and improve the quality of primary and secondary public school education. After-school programming is also targeted. *Human Services:* Within this area, the sponsor will highlight families and children. Its goal will be the aggressive pursuit of creative approaches to overcoming the

many obstacles now facing disadvantaged families and children, especially through the expansion of successful model programs. The sponsor supports programs that work toward reducing the risks children face, which include substance abuse, violence, poverty, unemployment, illiteracy, poor medical care, lack of family values, and neighborhood deterioration. *Civic Affairs:* Support is available for community development, economic development, and employment development programs. The sponsor welcomes and will continually explore new initiatives. *Medicine:* Support is available for health medicine research. Emphasis is placed on health needs of the disadvantaged. Support of medical facilities will continue with an increased emphasis on the issues of public health. *Cultural Activities:* Operating and capital funds are available to performing arts organizations and major cultural activities located in the Pittsburgh area. *Conservation:* Continues to be the major focus. Of specific significance is a program that focuses on funding acquisitions of significant wilderness areas, both to protect land from development and to assist in wildlife preservation. This program is being pursued on a national basis. *Conservation:* Continues to be the major focus. Of specific significance is a program that focuses on funding acquisitions of significant wilderness areas, both to protect land from development and to assist in wildlife preservation. This program is being pursued on a national basis. **Priorities:** *Arts & Humanities:* 4%. Supports various arts organizations in the Pittsburgh area. *Civic & Public Affairs:* 4%. Economic development. *Education:* 23%. Colleges and universities and public schools. *Environment:* 8%. *International:* 13%. Major support for medical research. *Note:* Total contributions made in 1998. **Typ. Recipients:** AIDS/HIV, Cancer, Children's Health/Hospitals, Clinics/Medical Centers, Domestic Violence, Emergency/Ambulance Services, Family Planning, Geriatric Health, Health Organizations, Health Policy/Cost Containment, Hospices, Hospitals, Long-Term Care, Medical Education, Medical Rehabilitation, Medical Research, Medical Training, Mental Health, Nursing Services, People with Disabilities, Prenatal Health Issues, Preventive Medicine/Wellness Organizations, Public Health, Research/Studies Institutes, Sexual Abuse, Single-Disease Health Associations, Substance Abuse. **Geo. Dist:** nationally for conservation programs; PA, Southwestern Pennsylvania; Pittsburgh, PA.

**★ 619 ★ Richard Lounsbery Foundation**
51 East 63rd St. Ste. 1
New York, NY 10021
**Phone:** (212)319-7033  **Fax:** (212)753-9286
Ms. Marta Norman, Executive Director

**Fnded:** 1959. **Philosophy:** The Richard Lounsbery Foundation makes most of its grants in the area of education. Educational funding favors higher education, with emphasis on scientific research at universities. Other interests include medical and scientific research, international concerns, civic and environmental causes, and the arts. **Priorities:** *Arts & Humanities:* 13%. Supprts museums and music. *Civic & Public Affairs:* 2%. Botanical Gardens and Parks. *Education:* 28%. Colleges/Universities. *Environment:* 5%. *International:* 3%. Single-Disease organizations and healthcare. *Religion:* 26%. Scientific institutions. *Note:* Total contributions made in 1998. **Typ. Recipients:** AIDS/HIV, Cancer, Hospitals, Hospitals (University Affiliated), Medical Education, Medical Rehabilitation, Medical Research, Nutrition, People with Disabilities, Research/Studies Institutes, Respiratory, Single-Disease Health Associations. **Geo. Dist:** internationally; nationally; NY.

**★ 620 ★ Richard and Rhoda Goldman Fund**
One Lombard St., Ste. 303
San Francisco, CA 94111
**Phone:** (415)788-1090  **Fax:** (415)788-7890
**Website:** http://www.goldmanfund.org
Robert Gamble, Executive Director

**Fnded:** 1951. **Philosophy:** "The Richard & Rhoda Goldman Fund is a private foundation reflecting the founders' long-term commitment to support charitable organizations that enhance the quality of life, primarily



Encyclopedia of Medical Organizations and Agencies, 13th Edition

in the Bay Area. The fund is interested in supporting programs that will have a positive impact in an array of fields including: the Environment, Population, Jewish Affairs, Children and Youth, Elderly, Social and Human Services, Health, Education, and the Arts." Richard and Rhoda Goldman Fund Program Priorities **Priorities:** *Arts & Humanities:* 8%. Supports fine arts, museums, opera and ballet. *Civic & Public Affairs:* 10%. Support public policy organizations. *Education:* 9%. Supports colleges and universities. *Environment:* 14%. Supports youth programs, family planning. *International:* 8%. Supports hospital and medical centers. *Note:* Total contributions made in 1998. **Typ. Recipients:** AIDS/HIV, Alzheimers Disease, Cancer, Child Abuse, Children's Health/Hospitals, Clinics/Medical Centers, Domestic Violence, Family Planning, Health Organizations, Health Policy/Cost Containment, Health-General, Heart, Hospices, Long-Term Care, Medical Research, Medical Training, Nursing Services, Public Health. **Geo. Dist:** San Francisco, CA, including metropolitan area.

**★ 621 ★ Richard S. Reynolds Foundation**
1403 Pemberton Rd., Ste. 102
Richmond, VA 23233
**Phone:** (804)740-7350 **Fax:** (804)740-7807
Victoria Pitrelli, Executive Director
**Fnded:** 1965. **Philosophy:** The foundation gives to a variety of groups mainly in the Richmond, VA, area. Education, arts and sciences, religion, and community service groups generally receive a majority of the foundation's giving. **Priorities:** *Arts & Humanities:* 20%. Giving to the performing arts and museums. *Civic & Public Affairs:* 9%. Primarily for housing and community programs. *Education:* 60%. Colleges, universities, and primary and secondary education. *Environment:* 5%. Emphasis on youth organizations and emergency shelters. *International:* 2%. Hospitals, medical research, and single-disease health asssociations. *Religion:* Less than 1%. Supports a science museum. *Note:* Total contributions made in fiscal 1999. **Typ. Recipients:** Cancer, Children's Health/Hospitals, Clinics/Medical Centers, Emergency/Ambulance Services, Health Funds, Heart, Hospitals, Medical Education, Medical Rehabilitation, Medical Research, Mental Health, Multiple Sclerosis, People with Disabilities, Respiratory. **Geo. Dist:** VA, Central Virginia, particularly Richmond.

**★ 622 ★ Rigler-Deutsch Foundation**
PO Box 828
Burbank, CA 91503
**Phone:** (213)878-0283 **Fax:** (213)878-0329
James Rigler, Vice President
**Fnded:** 1966. **Philosophy:** The foundation primarily gives to arts and cultural orgainznations in New York, NY, and Los Angeles, CA. Since 1994 the foundation has contributed a majority of its funding towards the Classic Arts Showcase, which is a twenty-four hour a day classic arts network with an MTV style format. **Priorities:** *Arts & Humanities:* 67%. Primary support for opera, ballet, theaters, and music. *Civic & Public Affairs:* About 3%. Civil rights and public policy. *Education:* 2%. Arts education. *Environment:* 5%. Primary support for Spectrum. *International:* 2%. AIDS and mental health organizations. *Note:* Total contributions made in 1997. **Typ. Recipients:** AIDS/HIV, Cancer, Children's Health/Hospitals, Family Planning, Hospitals, Medical Research, Mental Health, Prenatal Health Issues, Speech & Hearing, Substance Abuse. **Geo. Dist:** Los Angeles, CA; New York, NY.

**★ 623 ★ Rita J. and Stanley H. Kaplan Foundation**
866 United Nations Plaza, No. 306
New York, NY 10017
**Phone:** (212)688-1047 **Fax:** (212)688-6907
**Email:** rskfnd@aol.com
Harriet Botwinick, Associate Director
**Fnded:** 1984. **Philosophy:** The foundation primarily supports the performing arts and Jewish museums. Other recipient areas include medical centers, Jewish religious organizations, and a variety of social services

and civic affairs interests. **Priorities:** *Arts & Humanities:* 15%. Public broadcasting, opera, theater, and museums of fine art. *Civic & Public Affairs:* 13%. Community and urban affairs and clubs. *Education:* 33%. Funds primary and secondary schools with an emphasis on Jewish education. *Environment:* 1%. Supports youth programs. *International:* 20%. Primarily for medicine centers and medical research. *Note:* Total contributions made in 2000. **Typ. Recipients:** Adolescent Health Issues, AIDS/HIV, Cancer, Clinics/Medical Centers, Emergency/Ambulance Services, Family Planning, Health Funds, Health Organizations, Hospitals, Hospitals (University Affiliated), Medical Education, Medical Research, People with Disabilities, Preventive Medicine/Wellness Organizations, Public Health, Single-Disease Health Associations, Transplant Networks/Donor Banks. **Geo. Dist:** New York, NY.

**★ 624 ★ Robert G. Cabell III and Maude Morgan Cabell Foundation**
PO Box 85678
Richmond, VA 23285-5678
**Phone:** (804)780-2000 **Fax:** (804)697-2994
John Werner, Executive Director
**Fnded:** 1957. **Philosophy:** The foundation makes grants across the major categories of support. In education, interests include colleges and universities. Social service support goes to shelters, food banks, senior centers, and youth organizations. Funding for the arts favors historic preservation. Grants also are made to other recipient areas. **Priorities:** *Arts & Humanities:* 29%. Supports museums, libraries, and historical societies. *Civic & Public Affairs:* 38%. Funds neighborhood revitalization, housing, women's affairs, and clubs. *Education:* 8%. Funds colleges and higher education. *Environment:* 12%. Supports the Young Men's Christian Association, family planning services, youth programs, food banks, and family services. *International:* 2%. Supports preventative healthcare. *Religion:* 5%. Suppports a science museum. *Note:* Total contributions made in 2000. **Typ. Recipients:** Alzheimers Disease, Arthritis, Child Abuse, Children's Health/Hospitals, Clinics/Medical Centers, Diabetes, Domestic Violence, Emergency/Ambulance Services, Family Planning, Geriatric Health, Health Organizations, Heart, Hospitals, People with Disabilities, Public Health, Research/Studies Institutes, Single-Disease Health Associations, Transplant Networks/Donor Banks. **Geo. Dist:** Richmond, VA.

**★ 625 ★ Robert J. Kleberg, Jr. and Helen C. Kleberg Foundation**
700 North Saint Mary's St., Ste. 1200
San Antonio, TX 78205
**Phone:** (210)271-3691 **Fax:** (210)299-1541
Robert Washington, Grants Coordinator
**Fnded:** 1950. **Philosophy:** The foundation's goal is to support organizations reflecting the interests of the late donors. The greatest emphasis has been on medical research. Other areas supported by the foundation include veterinary science, wildlife research and preservation, health services, higher education, community organizations, and the arts and humanities. **Priorities:** *Arts & Humanities:* 10%. Funds museums, libraries, performing arts, and music. *Civic & Public Affairs:* 1%. Botanical gardens; park development. *Education:* 53%. Colleges, universities, and secondary education. *Environment:* 4%. *International:* 40%. Primary support for medical research. *Note:* Total contributions made in 1998. **Typ. Recipients:** Alzheimers Disease, Cancer, Children's Health/Hospitals, Clinics/Medical Centers, Domestic Violence, Emergency/Ambulance Services, Eyes/Blindness, Family Planning, Health Organizations, Health-General, Heart, Hospitals, Kidney, Medical Education, Medical Rehabilitation, Medical Research, Nursing Services, People with Disabilities, Research/Studies Institutes, Respiratory, Speech & Hearing, Transplant Networks/Donor Banks, Trauma Treatment. **Geo. Dist:** nationally; TX.

**★ 626 ★ Robert Lehman Foundation**
101 Park Ave.
New York, NY 10178
**Phone:** (212)808-7946 **Fax:** (212)808-7897
**Email:** pguth@kelleydrye.com
Paul Guth, Secretary
**Fnded:** 1943. **Philosophy:** The primary purpose of the foundation is to maintain the Robert Lehman collection at the Metropolitan Museum of Art. The foundation also supports cultural programs and higher educational institutions, with emphasis on arts education. **Priorities:** *Arts & Humanities:* 64%. Supports museums, arts centers and galleries, and historical societies. Major grant to Metropolitan Museum of Art. *Education:* 34%. Primarily supports art education. *Note:* Total contributions made in fiscal 1998. **Typ. Recipients:** AIDS/HIV, Cancer, Children's Health/Hospitals, Clinics/Medical Centers, Emergency/Ambulance Services, Home-Care Services, Hospitals, People with Disabilities. **Geo. Dist:** nationally, particularly the Northeast; New York, NY.

**★ 627 ★ Robert R. McCormick Tribune Foundation**
435 North Michigan Ave., Ste. 770
Chicago, IL 60611
**Phone:** (312)222-3512 **Fax:** (312)222-3523
**Email:** rrmtf@tribune.com
**Website:** http://www.rrmtf.org
**Fnded:** 1990. **Philosophy:** "The Robert R. McCormick Tribune Foundation is dedicated to a democratic society and its quality of life. Its mission is to improve the social and economic environment; to encourage a free and responsible discussion of issues affecting the nation; to enhance the effectiveness of American education; and to stimulate responsible citizenship." The foundation seeks to fulfill its mission through four programs. The Communities program is designed to combine the efforts of the McCormick Tribune Foundation, Tribune Company units, and other organizations to directly impact local communities throughout the country. A complete listing of communities participating in this unique grantmaking program is available at the foundation's website. The Education program is designed focus on the quality of early childhood education; increase the number of accredited preschool programs; enhance the skills and recognition of preschool program directors and teachers; improve the early childhood education system; heighten public understanding of the importance of early childhood education. This program is in the Chicago area. The Journalism program is designed to ensure a viable future for journalism, through research, development and education; promote diversity of news staffing and content; encourage informed coverage of national security issues; and support freedom of expression. This program is nationwide. The Citizenship program is designed to promote patriotism and voluntarism. This program is in the Chicago area. The foundation continues to provide operating support to Cantigny, the former estate of Robert R. McCormick, which is operated as a park in Wheaton, IL. Also, in 1992, the foundation opened, operates, and supports the Cantigny First Division Museum to house and exhibit World War I antiques and memorabilia. **Priorities:** *Civic & Public Affairs:* 75%. Supports the Communities program, which functions through regional partners and which is engaged in stimulating charitable giving from the general public. *Note:* Total contributions made in 2000. **Typ. Recipients:** AIDS/HIV, Cancer, Children's Health/Hospitals, Clinics/Medical Centers, Domestic Violence, Emergency/Ambulance Services, Eyes/Blindness, Health Organizations, Hospitals, Medical Education, Medical Rehabilitation, Medical Research, Mental Health, Multiple Sclerosis, Nursing Services, People with Disabilities, Prenatal Health Issues, Public Health, Respiratory, Single-Disease Health Associations, Substance Abuse. **Geo. Dist:** varies by program area; Chicago, IL, metropolitan area. **Frmly:** Robert R. McCormick Charitable Trust.

**★ 628 ★ Robert R. Meyer Foundation**
PO Box 11426
Birmingham, AL 35202

**Phone:** (205)326-4696        **Fax:** (205)581-7433
Leah Scalise, Vice President & Trustee

**Fnded:** 1923. **Philosophy:** The foundation provides a broad base of support to all types of charitable organizations in the Birmingham area. **Priorities:** *Arts & Humanities:* 19%. Gives to libraries and art festivals. *Civic & Public Affairs:* 6%. Funding includes community development. *Education:* 37%. Funds Alabama universities and colleges. *Environment:* 28%. Supports YMCAs, YWCAs, and youth groups. *International:* 8%. Supports single-health groups and community organizations. *Note:* Total contributions were made in 1998. **Typ. Recipients:** AIDS/HIV, Cancer, Clinics/Medical Centers, Domestic Violence, Eyes/Blindness, Family Planning, Health Organizations, Hospitals, Long-Term Care, Medical Education, Mental Health, Nursing Services, People with Disabilities, Public Health, Research/Studies Institutes, Speech & Hearing, Substance Abuse. **Geo. Dist:** Birmingham, AL, metropolitan area.

### ★ 629 ★ Robert R. Young Foundation
PO Box 1423
Greenwich, CT 06830
**Phone:** (203)359-3336        **Fax:** (203)359-3336
David Wallace, President

**Fnded:** 1959. **Philosophy:** The foundation generally supports colleges and universities, hospitals, and social services in New York and New England. **Priorities:** *Education:* 89%. Supports universities and local schools. *Environment:* 7%. Supports youth programs, youth services, and united way. *International:* 2%. Supports hospitals. *Note:* Total contributions made in 1998. **Typ. Recipients:** Arthritis, Cancer, Children's Health/Hospitals, Clinics/Medical Centers, Diabetes, Emergency/Ambulance Services, Family Planning, Heart, Hospices, Hospitals, Medical Research, Mental Health, Multiple Sclerosis, People with Disabilities, Single-Disease Health Associations, Substance Abuse. **Geo. Dist:** New England; NY.

### ★ 630 ★ Robert Russell Memorial Foundation
1221 Brickell Ave., 21st Fl.
Miami, FL 33131
**Phone:** (305)579-0500        **Fax:** (305)579-0717
Norman Lipoff, Chairman & Trustee

**Fnded:** 1984. **Philosophy:** The foundation primarily supports Jewish organizations in Miami. It also supports educational institutions with Jewish or Middle Eastern studies and programs in Israel. **Priorities:** *Arts & Humanities:* 3%. Supports music and museums. *Education:* 5%. Secondary higher education. *Environment:* 7%. United Way, scouting, and youth programs. *Note:* Contributions made in fiscal 1999. **Typ. Recipients:** Clinics/Medical Centers, Hospitals, Medical Education, Medical Training. **Geo. Dist:** to national and international organizations; FL, emphasis on Dade County.

### ★ 631 ★ Robert S. and Grayce B. Kerr Foundation
PMB 25106
PO Box 2000
Jackson, WY 83001
**Phone:** (307)733-8829        **Fax:** (307)733-9702
Sarah Lacy, Administrative Assistant

**Fnded:** 1986. **Philosophy:** The foundation seeks to identify those people, programs, and policies which best address needs in the arts, education, and the environment (habitat preservation) within Oklahoma and Wyoming. Funding is limited to organizations that benefit these specified fields of interest and geographic affiliations. **Priorities:** *Arts & Humanities:* 51%. Emphasis on museums, public broadcasting, and historical societies. *Civic & Public Affairs:* 11%. Supports a community foundation. *Education:* 18%. Primarily for universities in Oklahoma. *Environment:* 5%. Supports child welfare, family services, and community services organizations. *International:* 8%. Supports medical centers and hospitals. *Religion:* 1%. Supports science museums and centers. *Note:* Total contributions made in 1998. **Typ. Recipients:** AIDS/HIV, Child Abuse, Clinics/Medical Centers, Domestic Violence, Emergency/Ambulance Services, Eyes/Blindness, Health Organizations, Hospices, Hospitals, Long-Term Care, Medical Rehabilitation, Medical Research, Nursing Services, People with Disabilities, Prenatal Health Issues, Substance Abuse. **Geo. Dist:** OH; OK; WY.

### ★ 632 ★ Robert Stewart and Helen Pfeiffer Odell Fund
420 Montgomery St., 5th Fl.
San Francisco, CA 94104
**Phone:** (415)396-3215        **Fax:** (415)834-0604
Gene Ranghiasci, Contact

**Fnded:** 1967. **Philosophy:** The foundation makes most of its grants to benefit youth in California. The primary interest is social services, specifically child welfare programs and youth organizations. Other interests include funding for schools, health care, and the arts. **Priorities:** *Arts & Humanities:* 3%. Contributes to music and historical societies. *Civic & Public Affairs:* 5%. Funds housing, zoos, legal issues, and a festival. *Education:* 51%. Supports private precollege education and scholarship funds. *Environment:* 14%. Funds youth groups and child welfare. *International:* 5%. Supports medical foundations. *Religion:* 1%. Funds exploratorium. *Note:* Total contributions made in 1999. **Typ. Recipients:** Children's Health/Hospitals, Clinics/Medical Centers, Eyes/Blindness, Health Organizations, Hospitals, Medical Rehabilitation, Medical Research, Mental Health, People with Disabilities, Public Health. **Geo. Dist:** CA, Northern California, with emphasis on San Francisco.

### ★ 633 ★ Robert W. Woodruff Foundation
50 Hurt Plz., Ste. 1200
Atlanta, GA 30303
**Phone:** (404)522-6755        **Fax:** (404)522-7026
**Email:** fdns@woodruff.org
**Website:** http://www.woodruff.org/
Charles McTier, President

**Fnded:** 1937. **Philosophy:** The foundation's principal giving interests include education, health care, human services, cultural and civic affairs, and the environment. Preference is given to one-time capital projects. Awards for basic operating expenses usually are avoided. **Priorities:** *Arts & Humanities:* 10%. Supports museums, public broadcasting, orchestra, historical preservation and the Robert W. Woodruff Arts Center. *Civic & Public Affairs:* 4%. Supports legal services programs, community foundations, State of GA, Office of the Governor. *Education:* 18%. Supports colleges and universities, education foundations. *Environment:* 2%. Supports Boys and Girls Clubs, housing. *International:* 51%. Supports the Robert W. Woodruff Health Sciences Center Fund; single-disease health associations. *Religion:* 4%. *Note:* Total contributions made in 2000. **Typ. Recipients:** Alzheimers Disease, Cancer, Children's Health/Hospitals, Emergency/Ambulance Services, Geriatric Health, Health Organizations, Health Policy/Cost Containment, Long-Term Care, Medical Education, Medical Rehabilitation, Medical Research, Mental Health, Nursing Services, Public Health, Trauma Treatment. **Geo. Dist:** Atlanta, GA, some statewide giving.

### ★ 634 ★ Robert Wood Johnson Foundation
College Rd. East
PO Box 2316
Princeton, NJ 08543-2316
**Phone:** (609)243-5986        **Fax:** (609)987-8845
**Email:** rjt@rwjf.org
**Website:** http://www.rwjf.org
Richard Toth, Director, Office of Proposal Management

**Fnded:** 1936. **Philosophy:** The foundation's three objectives are the following: to assure that Americans of all ages have access to basic health care at reasonable cost; to improve the way services are organized and provided to people with chronic health conditions; and to reduce the personal, social and economic harm caused by substance abuse of tobacco, alcohol and illicit drugs. The Substance Abuse Policy Research program helps identify, analyze, and evaluate public- and private-sector policies aimed at reducing the harm caused by abuse of tobacco, alcohol, illegal drugs, and combinations of the three. The foundation assists efforts to fund projects to improve access to care for people with the most serious geographic, cultural, financial, and other barriers to care; to make arrangements for health care more effective and affordable; and to help people maintain or more quickly regain their functional abilities for everyday life. The foundation directs its purpose to focusing upon improving health services; helping those groups most susceptible to disease; addressing individual health problems on a large scale; and promoting bold, creative approaches and solutions to health concerns. The foundation, therefore, explores and funds new areas of medical care concerned with infant, child, and adolescent welfare; chronic illness and disability, particularly among the elderly; AIDS concerns; substance abuse; mental illness; the organization and quality of health services; medical ethical issues; quality and availability of health professionals; and the problems arising from technological advances in medicine. Programs span the areas of education, social services, and civic affairs, yet all related to health interests. The foundation also makes funding available to support research, evaluation, and demonstration projects that will assess the impact of major changes in the financing and organization of health services on health-care costs, quality, and access to care. Additional funds are made available in an effort to strengthen the nation's nursing services, supporting projects that address nursing manpower and educational development. The Health Policy Fellowships Program develops the capacity of outstanding mid-career health professionals in academic and community-based settings to assume leadership roles in health policy and management. Health Tracking is a major initiative that examines and reports on our nation's changing health-care system and how these changes are affecting the American people; and pulls together insights from many foundation programs, as well as from other important groups concerned with health, synthesizing information, and generating new analyses. **Priorities:** *Environment:* 21%. Programs that promote health and reduce the personal, social, and economic harm caused by substance abuse–tobacco, alcohol, and illicit drugs. *International:* 75%. Supports programs that assure that all American have access to basic health care at reasonable cost, and those programs that improve the way services are organized and provided to people with chronic health conditions. *Note:* Contributions made in 2000. **Typ. Recipients:** Adolescent Health Issues, AIDS/HIV, Alzheimers Disease, Cancer, Children's Health/Hospitals, Clinics/Medical Centers, Family Planning, Geriatric Health, Health Organizations, Health Policy/Cost Containment, Heart, Home-Care Services, Hospitals, Long-Term Care, Medical Education, Medical Training, Mental Health, Nursing Services, People with Disabilities, Prenatal Health Issues, Public Health, Research/Studies Institutes, Respiratory, Single-Disease Health Associations, Substance Abuse. **Geo. Dist:** national.

### ★ 635 ★ Robert Z. Hawkins Foundation
One East Liberty St., Ste. 509
Reno, NV 89501
**Phone:** (775)786-1105        **Fax:** (775)786-4886
**Email:** rzhawkins@aol.com
William Wallace, Chairman

**Fnded:** 1980. **Philosophy:** "Grants may be made to organizations operated exclusively for charitable, religious, educational, scientific or literary purposes, or for the prevention of cruelty to children or animals, which hold a letter from the Internal Revenue Service determining that the organization is a qualified Section 501 (c)(3) organization." "Grants may also be made to religious organizations, and to political subdivisions, if made exclusively for public purposes." **Priorities:** *Arts & Humanities:* 8%. Focus on public broadcasting, museums, music and opera. *Civic & Public Affairs:* 32%. Supports The City of Reno and county parks. *Education:* 20%. Supports colleges, universities, medical education, parochial education scholarships and engineering education. *Environment:* 29%. Supports youth organizations, animal welfare, substance abuse, United Way, emergency services and camps. *International:* 4%. Health funds, hospitals, mental illness. *Religion:* 1%. Funds scientific research. *Note:* Total contributions made in 2000. **Typ. Recipients:** Children's Health/Hospitals, Domestic Violence, Emergency/Ambulance Services, Hospitals, Long-Term Care, Medical Education, Mental Health, People with Disabilities, Public Health, Single-Disease Health Associations, Substance Abuse, Substance Abuse, Transplant Networks/Donor Banks. **Geo. Dist:** CA; NV, Northern Nevada; Reno, NV.

## ★ 636 ★ Rockefeller Foundation

420 Fifth Ave.
New York, NY 10018-2702
**Phone:** (212)869-8500      **Fax:** (212)764-3468
**Website:** http://www.rockfound.org
Lynda Mullen, Secretary

**Fnded:** 1913. **Philosophy:** The foundation's stated mission when it was founded in 1913 was, "to promote the well-being of mankind throughout the world." It is dedicated to identifying and attacking the underlying causes of human suffering and need at their source. The foundation carries out its mission through grants and fellowships to individuals and institutions in the following areas: arts and humanities; equal opportunity; agricultural sciences; health sciences; population sciences; global environment; and special African initiatives, including female education. The balance of the foundation's programs support work in building democracy, international security, international philanthropy, and other special interests and initiatives. The foundation operates the Bellagio Study and Conference Center in northern Italy for international conferences and for residencies for artists, scholars and policymakers, and other professionals from around the world. **Priorities:** *Arts & Humanities:* 3%. Supports arts and humanities programs that help to understand and engage difference across changing societies. *Civic & Public Affairs:* About 21%. Equal opportunity to support diverse urban communities, including employment, good schools, freedom from discrimination, and full participation in the democratic process. *Education:* 18%. Supports educational programs, higher education, and school districts for reform policies. *Environment:* 2%. Population sciences, including family planning and reproductive health services. *International:* 19%. Focus on building human capacity for population-based health care in developing nations. *Religion:* 1%. Supports agricultural sciences to increase crop yields of smallholder farmers in developing countries profitably and without degrading natural resources. *Note:* Total contributions made in 2000. **Typ. Recipients:** AIDS/HIV, Family Planning, Health Organizations, Medical Education, Medical Research, Medical Training, Public Health, Research/Studies Institutes. **Geo. Dist:** internationally; nationally.

## ★ 637 ★ Rockwell Fund, Inc.

1330 Post Oak Boulevard, Ste. 1825
Houston, TX 77056
**Phone:** (713)629-9022      **Fax:** (713)629-7702
**Email:** mvogt@rockfund.org
**Website:** http://www.rockfund.org
Martha Vogt, Program Officer

**Fnded:** 1931. **Philosophy:** The fund supports a broad range of activities, with preference for causes in the Houston area. **Priorities:** *Arts & Humanities:* 11%. Supports museums and the theater. *Civic & Public Affairs:* 3%. Supports community services and environmental organizations. *Education:* 35%. Supports independent schools, colleges, and universities. *Environment:* 31%. Supports human services, youth services, and social services. *International:* 20%. Supports hospices, mental health centers, hospitals and emergency care centers. *Note:* Total contributions made in 1999. **Typ. Recipients:** Adolescent Health Issues, AIDS/HIV, Cancer, Child Abuse, Children's Health/Hospitals, Clinics/Medical Centers, Emergency/Ambulance Services, Eyes/Blindness, Family Planning, Health Organizations, Heart, Hospices, Hospitals, Medical Rehabilitation, Medical Research, Mental Health, Nursing Services, People with Disabilities, Prenatal Health Issues, Public Health, Single-Disease

Health Associations, Single-Disease Health Associations, Speech & Hearing, Substance Abuse, Transplant Networks/Donor Banks. **Geo. Dist:** Houston, TX, limited giving outside of the Houston area.

## ★ 638 ★ Rollin M. Gerstacker Foundation

PO Box 1945
Midland, MI 48641-1945
**Phone:** (517)631-6097

**Fnded:** 1957. **Philosophy:** The foundation adheres to Mrs. Gerstacker's belief "that it was the responsibility of private citizens to enrich their communities to the best of their abilities." In accordance with this philosophy, the foundation traditionally has given to homes for the elderly, colleges and universities, the Mid-Michigan Medical Center, research institutions, youth, and community services, particularly in Midland, MI. These areas of interest remain the focus of foundation giving. **Priorities:** *Arts & Humanities:* 5%. Music, museums, theater and historical associations. *Civic & Public Affairs:* 17%. Primarily for public policy institutes, housing. *Education:* 49%. Colleges, universities, and research institutes. *Environment:* 27%. Domestic violence prevention, youth organizations, United Way, and child welfare. *Note:* Total contributions made in 2000. **Typ. Recipients:** AIDS/HIV, Alzheimers Disease, Arthritis, Clinics/Medical Centers, Domestic Violence, Emergency/Ambulance Services, Eyes/Blindness, Hospitals, Medical Rehabilitation, Medical Research, Mental Health, Multiple Sclerosis, Nursing Services, People with Disabilities, Public Health, Research/Studies Institutes, Single-Disease Health Associations, Substance Abuse, Transplant Networks/Donor Banks. **Geo. Dist:** Midland, MI; Cleveland, OH.

## ★ 639 ★ RosaMary Foundation

PO Box 13218
New Orleans, LA 70185
**Phone:** (504)895-1984      **Fax:** (504)895-1988
Richard Freeman, Jr., Chairman

**Fnded:** 1939. **Philosophy:** The foundation supports organizations working toward the betterment of the New Orleans community. Educational institutions and the United Way for the Greater New Orleans area are the major recipients of foundation giving. The foundation also has an interest in the arts and supports various cultural organizations in New Orleans. **Priorities:** *Arts & Humanities:* 11%. Includes museums, music, and arts associations. *Civic & Public Affairs:* 12%. Supports community improvement/development, public affairs concerns, and public protection. *Education:* About 11%. Primarily for colleges and universities. *Environment:* 14%. Focus on youth development, housing/shelter, and other human service organizations. *International:* 52%. Emphasis on mental health and crisis intervention. *Note:* Total contributions made in 1998. **Typ. Recipients:** AIDS/HIV, Clinics/Medical Centers, Eyes/Blindness, Family Planning, Health Organizations, Hospitals, People with Disabilities, Research/Studies Institutes, Transplant Networks/Donor Banks. **Geo. Dist:** New Orleans, LA.

## ★ 640 ★ Rosamond Gifford Charitable Corp.

518 James St., Ste. 280
Syracuse, NY 13203
**Phone:** (315)474-2489      **Fax:** (315)475-4983
**Email:** kgoldfarb@giffordfd.org
**Website:** http://www.giffordfd.org
Kathryn Goldfarb, Executive Director

**Fnded:** 1954. **Philosophy:** "The Rosamund Gifford Charitable Corporation is a philanthropic foundation dedicated to the continuing stewardship of the funds entrusted to our care and committed to using our financial and human resources to build the capacity of individuals, institutions, and associations to enhance the economic vitality and the quality of life of the people of our community." *The Rosamund Gifford Charitable Corporation 1998 Annual Report* "In 1998, The Rosamund Gifford Charitable Corporation adopted a new strategic plan to guide us toward fulfillment of our mission. The continuing vision of the Gifford Foundation, which is reflected in that plan, is to be a

proactive force to bring about a transformation in the philosophy and structures that serve the people, the associations and the institutions of our community. As a focus for changing structures, the Foundation will be convening leaders, building strategic partnerships with other funders, proactively seeking gift recipients and creating a public image as a respected facilitator and agent of community improvement." *The Rosamund Gifford Corporation 1998 Annual Report* **Priorities:** *Arts & Humanities:* 3%. Supports a museum. *Civic & Public Affairs:* 11%. Primarily for municipal services and housing. *Education:* 35%. Supports community schools, higher education, and literacy. *Environment:* 18%. Supports community services and the United Way. *International:* 14%. Major support for the Health Science Center. *Note:* Total contributions made in 1998. **Typ. Recipients:** Alzheimers Disease, Clinics/Medical Centers, Emergency/Ambulance Services, Family Planning, Health Organizations, Health-General, Heart, Hospices, Hospitals, Kidney, Long-Term Care, Medical Research, Mental Health, People with Disabilities, Prenatal Health Issues, Public Health, Sexual Abuse, Single-Disease Health Associations, Substance Abuse. **Geo. Dist:** NY, Syracuse and Onondaga County.

## ★ 641 ★ Rose E. Tucker Charitable Trust

900 Southwest Fifth Ave., 26th Floor
Portland, OR 97204
**Phone:** (503)224-3380      **Fax:** (503)220-2480
**Email:** tuckertrust@stoel.com
Thomas Stoel, Trustee

**Fnded:** 1976. **Philosophy:** The trust makes most of its grants in the areas of social services, education, civic, and the environment. Social service support includes adult care, youth organizations, family planning, and food distribution. Educational funding favors grants, including capital projects and scholarships, to universities and colleges in Oregon. Funding for the arts supports museums, libraries, and the performing arts. **Priorities:** *Arts & Humanities:* 16%. Supports performing arts, museums, theaters, festivals, and historical societies. *Civic & Public Affairs:* 19%. Funds community organizations, policy institutes, and parks and zoos. *Education:* 23%. Funds colleges, universities, and schools. *Environment:* 19%. Funds Young Men's Christian Association, food banks, and youth programs. *International:* 7%. Supports medical aid. *Religion:* 2%. Funds a science museum. *Note:* Total contributions made in fiscal 2000. **Typ. Recipients:** Alzheimers Disease, Clinics/Medical Centers, Emergency/Ambulance Services, Family Planning, Health Funds, Health Organizations, Health-General, Hospitals, Medical Rehabilitation, Mental Health, People with Disabilities, Prenatal Health Issues, Public Health, Single-Disease Health Associations, Substance Abuse. **Geo. Dist:** Portland, OR, metropolitan area; some statewide giving.

## ★ 642 ★ Rose M. Badgeley Residuary Charitable Trust

c/o HSBC Bank, USA
140 Broadway, 11th Fl.
New York, NY 10005
**Phone:** (212)658-7967      **Fax:** (212)658-7790
Roberta Grossman, Vice President

**Fnded:** 1977. **Philosophy:** The trust supports nonprofit organizations with religious, charitable, scientific, literary or educational purposes. **Priorities:** *Arts & Humanities:* 14%. Primarily funds music concerns. Also supports theater. *Civic & Public Affairs:* 4%. Focus on philanthropic organizations. *Education:* 19%. Funds private precollege education. *Environment:* 12%. Supports youth groups and services for the homeless. *International:* 34%. Supports hospitals, medical centers, and cancer research. *Note:* Total contributions made in fiscal 1999. **Typ. Recipients:** AIDS/HIV, Alzheimers Disease, Cancer, Children's Health/Hospitals, Clinics/Medical Centers, Emergency/Ambulance Services, Eyes/Blindness, Geriatric Health, Health Organizations, Heart, Hospitals, Hospitals (University Affiliated), Medical Rehabilitation, Medical Research, Mental Health, Nursing Services, People with Disabilities, Prenatal Health Issues, Single-Disease Health Associations, Substance Abuse,

Transplant Networks/Donor Banks. **Geo. Dist:** NY. **Frmly:** Rose M. Badgeley Charitable Trust.

### ★ 643 ★ Rosenstiel Foundation

575 Madison Ave., 11th Fl.
New York, NY 10022
**Phone:** (212)940-8837          **Fax:** (212)940-6776
Maurice Greenbaum, Secretary & Treasurer

**Fnded:** 1950. **Philosophy:** The Rosenstiel Foundation primarily supports the arts, civic affairs, and health care. Arts funding favors museums, theater, and dance. Support for civic affairs goes to centers for Polish culture and other international affairs. Secondary interests include education with gifts to universities and science education. The foundation also will fund social service organizations. **Priorities:** *Arts & Humanities:* 28%. Funds museums, theaters, symphonies, opera, and arts associations. *Civic & Public Affairs:* 28%. Supports ethnic organizations and public policy associations. *Education:* 29%. Focus on private secondary education, universities, and education funds. *Environment:* 1%. *International:* 7%. Health associations, hospitals, hospices, medical research, and medical rehabilitation. *Note:* Total contributions made in 1999. **Typ. Recipients:** AIDS/HIV, Cancer, Children's Health/Hospitals, Clinics/Medical Centers, Eyes/Blindness, Health Organizations, Health-General, Heart, Hospices, Hospitals, Kidney, Medical Education, Medical Rehabilitation, Medical Research, Nursing Services, People with Disabilities, Public Health, Research/Studies Institutes, Single-Disease Health Associations, Substance Abuse. **Geo. Dist:** Eastern USA; New York, NY.

### ★ 644 ★ Ross Foundation

PO Box 335
Arkadelphia, AR 71923
**Phone:** (870)246-9881          **Fax:** (870)246-9674
**Email:** joe@hsu.edu
Ross Whipple, President

**Fnded:** 1966. **Philosophy:** The Ross Foundation has two primary interests: promoting the economic, cultural, and educational interests of Arkadelphia and Clark County through various projects and programs, as well as promoting conservation and the management of natural resources. The foundation's funding is generated through the timber industry. Therefore, grants are made to support the environment and conservation. **Priorities:** *Arts & Humanities:* About 1%. Supports children's concerts and plays. *Civic & Public Affairs:* 18%. Community foundations, grants to towns, non-profit management and safety. *Education:* 62%. Colleges and universities, science/mathematical education, agricultural education, and environmental education. *Environment:* 7%. United Way, youth activities, and community service organizations. *International:* Less than 1%. *Religion:* 3%. Funds the Arkansas Museum of Science and History. *Note:* Total contributions made in 1998. **Typ. Recipients:** AIDS/HIV, Child Abuse, Clinics/Medical Centers, Domestic Violence, Emergency/Ambulance Services, Hospitals, Public Health, Respiratory, Substance Abuse. **Geo. Dist:** AR, Arkadelphia County; AR, Clark County.

### ★ 645 ★ Roy A. Hunt Foundation

One Bigelow Square, Ste. 630
Pittsburgh, PA 15219-3030
**Phone:** (412)281-8734          **Fax:** (412)281-9463
**Email:** rahfound@aol.com
**Website:** http://www.rahuntfdn.org
Torrence Hunt, Jr., President & Trustee

**Fnded:** 1966. **Philosophy:** The foundation primarily supports the institutions in which the current trustees are interested. **Priorities:** *Arts & Humanities:* 14%. Contributes to arts centers, public broadcasting, historical societies, and the performing arts. *Civic & Public Affairs:* 3%. Funds cultural groups. *Education:* 17%. Supports pre-college education, colleges, and universities. *Environment:* 17%. Funds united funds, community centers, services for the disadvantaged, and YMCAs. *International:* 2%. Funds hospitals and single-disease associations. *Religion:* 2%. Primarily gives to the Boston Museum of Science. *Note:* Total contributions made in fiscal 2000. **Typ. Recipients:**

AIDS/HIV, Alzheimers Disease, Cancer, Children's Health/Hospitals, Clinics/Medical Centers, Family Planning, Health Organizations, Hospitals, Medical Rehabilitation, Mental Health, Single-Disease Health Associations, Substance Abuse. **Geo. Dist:** limited national giving; Boston, MA; Pittsburgh, PA.

### ★ 646 ★ Roy and Christine Sturgis Charitable and Educational Trust (TX)

PO Box 830241
Dallas, TX 75283-0241
**Phone:** (214)209-1965          **Fax:** (214)209-1997
Daniel Kelly, Trust Officer

**Fnded:** 1981. **Philosophy:** The trust's main priorities include education, the arts, health, science, and "the relief of human suffering." Youth and social services and science are also areas of interest. The trust is primarily interested in supplementing needs for capital requirements or special projects, research, and programs that have a measurable beginning and end. Endowments, start-up funds, and limited general operating expenses also are considered. Grants subject to matching requirements receive special consideration. **Priorities:** *Arts & Humanities:* 8%. Supports performing arts, museums, libraries, and historical commissions. *Civic & Public Affairs:* 6%. Funding for parks, zoos, clubs, and restoration. *Education:* 44%. Supports colleges, universities, and literacy. *Environment:* 28%. Funds social services, scouting, youth activities, Young Men's Christian Association camps, and senior citizens. *International:* 6%. Funds hospitals, health centers, nursing and blindness. *Religion:* 3%. Supports a science museum. *Note:* Total contributions made in fiscal 1999. **Typ. Recipients:** Adolescent Health Issues, Alzheimers Disease, Cancer, Children's Health/Hospitals, Clinics/Medical Centers, Diabetes, Domestic Violence, Eyes/Blindness, Health Organizations, Health-General, Heart, Hospices, Hospitals, Hospitals (University Affiliated), Kidney, Medical Education, Nursing Services, People with Disabilities, Single-Disease Health Associations, Substance Abuse. **Geo. Dist:** AR; TX, Dallas County.

### ★ 647 ★ Roy J. Carver Charitable Trust

202 Iowa Ave.
Muscatine, IA 52761-3733
**Phone:** (319)263-4010          **Fax:** (319)263-1547
**Email:** info@carvertrust.org
**Website:** http://www.carvertrust.org
Troy Ross, Executive Administrator

**Fnded:** 1982. **Philosophy:** Roy J. Carver's "commitment to helping young people through educational opportunities and to building a better world through medical and scientific research are cornerstones of the charitable trust. As a matter of policy, the trust favors grants that make its participation a vital factor in the success of the project. Such projects should promote the ethical, intellectual, and physical development of young men and women; establish, equip, or provide for the maintenance of institutions of learning; or contribute to the advancement of knowledge and its practical applications through medical and scientific research." Roy J. Carver Charitable Trust, *Grant Policies and Proposal Guidelines* **Priorities:** *Arts & Humanities:* 11%. Supports historical preservation, public broadcasting, museum. *Civic & Public Affairs:* 7%. Supports public libraries. *Environment:* 5%. Provides resources for handicapped children and YMCA. *International:* 75%. Funds medical research. *Note:* Total contributions made in fiscal 1999. **Typ. Recipients:** AIDS/HIV, Alzheimers Disease, Cancer, Child Abuse, Children's Health/Hospitals, Domestic Violence, Emergency/Ambulance Services, Eyes/Blindness, Hospitals (University Affiliated), Medical Education, Medical Research, Nursing Services, People with Disabilities. **Geo. Dist:** organizations with which the founder had significant involvement; IA.

### ★ 648 ★ Russell Sage Foundation

112 E 64th St.
New York, NY 10021
**Phone:** (212)750-6000          **Fax:** (212)371-4761
**Email:** info@rsage.org

**Website:** http://www.russellsage.org
Eric Wanner, President

**Fnded:** 1907. **Philosophy:** The Russell Sage Foundation functions as a research center, a funding source for various studies, a member of the nation's social science community, and a publisher. Over the years, the foundation has regularly sponsored innovative research in the social sciences, with emphasis on contemporary questions of social policy and scientific development. It also has directed a portion of its funds toward the needs of New York City and the surrounding vicinity. The foundation now dedicates itself exclusively to strengthening the methods, data, and theoretical core of the social sciences as a means of improving social policies. **Priorities:** *Civic & Public Affairs:* 30%. Supports economic policy, census studies, U.S. social policy, and immigration studies. *Education:* 61%. Funds programs in colleges and universities that focus on one or all of the following four areas: (1) research on the future of work, including the causes and consequences of the decline in demand for low-skill workers in advanced economies; (2) research on current U.S. immigration that focuses on the adaptation of the second generation to American society; (3) a joint program with the Andrew W. Mellon Foundation that supports research on curricula designed to foster active literacy among disadvantaged students; and (4) a program on the social psychology of cultural contact that focuses on improving relations between racial and ethnic groups in schools, workplaces, and neighborhood settings. *Environment:* 8%. *Note:* Total contributions made in fiscal 2000. **Typ. Recipients:** Health Policy/Cost Containment, Medical Education, Medical Research, Mental Health. **Geo. Dist:** nationally.

### ★ 649 ★ Ruth and Vernon Taylor Foundation

1670 Denver Club Bldg.
518 17th St., Ste. 1670
Denver, CO 80202
**Phone:** (303)893-5284          **Fax:** (303)893-8263
Friday Green, Trustee

**Fnded:** 1953. **Philosophy:** The foundation's charter decrees the areas of giving to be educational, religious, charitable, and scientific causes. Over the years, the foundation has expanded its interests to include the arts and humanities. **Priorities:** *Arts & Humanities:* 14%. Gives to museums, arts centers, and historic preservation. *Civic & Public Affairs:* 9%. Supports parks, zoos, and aquariums. *Education:* 14%. Primarily colleges and universities. *Environment:* 9%. Supports boys and girls clubs, respite care, and community associations. *International:* 8%. Funds biomedical and single-disease research. *Religion:* 4%. Funds aquariums. *Note:* Total contributions made in fiscal 1999. **Typ. Recipients:** Cancer, Child Abuse, Children's Health/Hospitals, Emergency/Ambulance Services, Family Planning, Health Funds, Health Organizations, Heart, Hospices, Hospitals, Medical Rehabilitation, Medical Research, People with Disabilities, Public Health, Research/Studies Institutes, Single-Disease Health Associations, Substance Abuse. **Geo. Dist:** nationally; Mid-Atlantic states; CO; IL; MT; TX; WY.

### ★ 650 ★ S. H. Cowell Foundation

120 Montgomery St., Ste. 2570
San Francisco, CA 94104
**Phone:** (415)397-0285          **Fax:** (415)986-6786
**Website:** http://www.shcowell.org
Susan Vandiver, Vice President Grants Programs

**Fnded:** 1955. **Philosophy:** The foundation supports a broad array of programs, and "is most interested in awarding grants to agencies which have clearly demonstrated community participation and support as well as evidence of private, non-governmental funding." The foundation's interests include aiding organizations concerned with the welfare of children and minorities; promoting the relative self-sufficiency of physically or mentally handicapped persons; providing general improvement in basic social programs in needy areas; assisting family planning organizations; supporting programs for the prevention of alcoholism; promoting job training programs; and providing for low-income housing. The foundation has recently begun placing greater emphasis on programs that offer affordable housing to the poor and programs that support public primary schools in high-density, low-income areas. It also focuses on the needs of Hispanics in California. Greater emphasis is being placed on serving the needs of children and families at risk in a comprehensive, coordinated way. The foundation's program in support of small arts organizations has been terminated. **Priorities:** *Arts & Humanities:* 1%. Supports the performing arts. *Civic & Public Affairs:* 41%. Funds housing and housing development, population concerns, and arms control. *Education:* 3%. Supports secondary schools and universities. *Environment:* 42%. Community programs, alcoholism, emergency relief, family planning, the United Way, and youth services. *International:* 6%. Funds health-care programs. *Note:* Total contributions made in 1998. **Typ. Recipients:** AIDS/HIV, Cancer, Child Abuse, Children's Health/Hospitals, Clinics/Medical Centers, Domestic Violence, Family Planning, Health Organizations, Medical Research, Nutrition, People with Disabilities, Public Health, Substance Abuse, Trauma Treatment. **Geo. Dist:** CA.

### ★ 651 ★ S. H. and Helen R. Scheuer Family Foundation Inc.

350 Fifth Ave., Ste. 1413
New York, NY 10118
**Phone:** (212)947-9009 **Fax:** (212)947-9770
Linda Ehrlich, Administrative Director

**Fnded:** 1943. **Philosophy:** The foundation gives most of its grants to local Jewish philanthropic, health, welfare, and higher education organizations; other support goes to arts and humanities, education, and social services. **Priorities:** *Arts & Humanities:* 12%. Funds archaeological research, opera, museums and theatre. *Civic & Public Affairs:* 1%. *Education:* 42%. Funds colleges, universities, schools, and education funds. *Environment:* 1%. Includes YMHA/YWHAs. *International:* 2%. Supports medical centers, hospital funds and breast cancer research. *Religion:* 1%. *Note:* Total contributions made in fiscal 1998. **Typ. Recipients:** Clinics/Medical Centers, Family Planning, Geriatric Health, Hospitals, Medical Education, Mental Health, Nursing Services, People with Disabilities. **Geo. Dist:** New York, NY, metropolitan area.

### ★ 652 ★ Sage Foundation

PO Box 1919
Brighton, MI 48116
Melissa Fadim, Chairman, President & Treasurer

**Fnded:** 1954. **Philosophy:** The objective of the Sage Foundation is to make contributions and grants that further charitable, religious, scientific, literary, and educational purposes. The foundation hopes to accomplish these objectives through assisting people and their actions. **Priorities:** *Arts & Humanities:* 51%. Supports music, arts institutes, music, and arts festivals. *Civic & Public Affairs:* 2%. *Education:* 3%. Emphasis on colleges and universities and secondary education. *Environment:* 2%. *International:* 34%. Focus on health funds and medical centers. *Note:* Total contributions made in 1998. **Typ. Recipients:** AIDS/HIV, Alzheimers Disease, Arthritis, Cancer, Children's Health/Hospitals, Clinics/Medical Centers, Domestic Violence, Emergency/Ambulance Services, Geriatric Health, Health Funds, Health Organizations, Heart, Hospices, Hospitals, Hospitals (University Affiliated), Long-Term Care, Medical Research, Mental Health, People with Disabilities, Public Health, Single-Disease Health Associations, Substance Abuse. **Geo. Dist:** nationally.

### ★ 653 ★ Samuel Goldwyn Foundation

9570 W Pico
Los Angeles, CA 90035
**Phone:** (310)860-3100 **Fax:** (310)860-3195
Meyer Gottlieb, Treasurer

**Fnded:** 1947. **Philosophy:** The foundation's trustees generally support all areas of philanthropy. In the past, large grants have been given to the arts. Libraries,

theaters, museums, and public broadcasting have all received funding. Other interests include support for police academies, public education, the aged, child care, and a variety of health concerns. **Priorities:** *Arts & Humanities:* 41%. Supports museums, music, theater, film and video, dance, libraries, and public broadcasting. *Civic & Public Affairs:* 15%. Funds festivals and safety. *Education:* 27%. Supports schools, universities, and literacy. *Environment:* 7%. Supports family planning services and youth organizations. *International:* 3%. Supports diabetes, respiratory, cancer, and clinics. *Note:* Total contributions made in 1999. **Typ. Recipients:** AIDS/HIV, Cancer, Children's Health/Hospitals, Clinics/Medical Centers, Domestic Violence, Emergency/Ambulance Services, Eyes/Blindness, Family Planning, Health Funds, Health Organizations, Heart, Hospitals, Long-Term Care, Mental Health, People with Disabilities, Research/Studies Institutes, Single-Disease Health Associations, Speech & Hearing. **Geo. Dist:** nationally; Los Angeles, CA, including metropolitan area.

### ★ 654 ★ Samuel I. Newhouse Foundation

c/o Paul Scherer & Co.
335 Madison Ave.
New York, NY 10017
**Phone:** (212)588-2200 **Fax:** (212)588-2222

**Fnded:** 1945. **Philosophy:** The foundation principally supports the arts, higher education, Jewish causes, and social services. **Priorities:** *Arts & Humanities:* 42%. Funds art centers, museums, libraries, and performing arts. *Civic & Public Affairs:* 1%. Supports towns and municipalities. *Education:* 21%. Supports higher education and scholarships. *Environment:* 11%. Primarily United Way. Also supports substance abuse and people with disabilities. *International:* 12%. Funds single-disease health associations, hospital, and medical research. *Note:* Total contributions made in fiscal 2000. **Typ. Recipients:** Cancer, Clinics/Medical Centers, Health Organizations, Heart, Hospitals, Medical Education, Medical Research, Mental Health, People with Disabilities, Single-Disease Health Associations, Substance Abuse. **Geo. Dist:** nationally; New York, NY.

### ★ 655 ★ Samuel N. and Mary Castle Foundation

The Pacific Garden Center, Makai Tower
733 Bishop St., Ste. 1275
Honolulu, HI 96813
**Phone:** (808)522-1101 **Fax:** (808)522-1103
**Email:** acastle@aloha.net
**Website:** http://fdncenter.org/grantmaker/castle/
Alfred Castle, Executive Director

**Fnded:** 1925. **Philosophy:** The charter of the Samuel N. and Mary Castle Foundation reflects Mary Tenney Castle's desire "to support such charitable benevolence, religious and education purposes as the Trustees may from time to time decide." The foundation's purpose is "to make grants to appropriate charitable organizations primarily within the state of Hawaii." Through the years the foundation's interests have been primarily in the support of early education and care, private education, Protestant churches and arts and cultural organizations with ties to the Castle family. Mary Castle established the Henry and Dorothy Castle Memorial Fund in 1895, setting aside funds for the training and education of children. In 1953, the memorial became a funding source for organizations providing care and learning opportunities to young children. The foundation reports that projects targeting children (prenatal to age five) and their families are of priority interest. **Priorities:** *Arts & Humanities:* 15%. Music and theater focused on children. *Education:* 61%. Primary and preschool education. *Environment:* 11%. Child welfare. *International:* 6%. National health organizations. *Religion:* 6%. *Note:* Total contributions made in 1999. **Typ. Recipients:** AIDS/HIV, Cancer, Children's Health/Hospitals, Emergency/Ambulance Services, Health Organizations, Hospices, Hospitals, Mental Health, People with Disabilities, Prenatal Health Issues, Respiratory, Speech & Hearing, Substance Abuse. **Geo. Dist:** HI.

### ★ 656 ★ Samuel Roberts Noble Foundation

PO Box 2180
2510 Sam Noble Parkway
Ardmore, OK 73402
**Phone:** (580)223-5810 **Fax:** (580)221-7362
**Email:** macawley@noble.org
**Website:** http://www.noble.org
Michael Cawley, President & Trustee

**Fnded:** 1945. **Philosophy:** Because the trustees were given wide latitude in the activities that could be carried out, the foundation has been successful in adapting to the changing needs of society. By combining in-house research and traditional grant making, the foundation seeks to improve the quality of life in rural and urban communities. The foundation conducts research in the areas of plant biology research and agricultural research, consultation and demonstration. The plant biology division focuses on genetic engineering in plants. The agricultural division continues its interests in conservation, farming techniques, and agricultural economics. In addition to research, the division offers demonstration and consultation programs to regional farmers and ranchers. Although the foundation's main focus includes basic plant biology research and agricultural research, consultation, and demonstration, the foundation also awards grants in other areas when additional funds are available. Other areas of giving focus on capital funding for higher education, health research and delivery systems, and public affairs. Generally, these areas of giving remain geographically limited, with primary emphasis in Oklahoma. The foundation reports that in 1997 a new operating program in forage biotechnology was added to its in-house operations. 1997 Guidelines **Priorities:** *Arts & Humanities:* 3%. Supports historic preservation, music, museums, and art institutes. *Civic & Public Affairs:* 6%. Community affairs and public policy. *Education:* 55%. For research at colleges and universities, school building construction major grant to University of Oklahoma. *Environment:* 3%. Funds day care, Young Men's Christian Association. *International:* 31%. Health research and delivery systems. *Note:* About 70% of total giving supports organizations in Oklahoma. Total contributions made in fiscal 2000. **Typ. Recipients:** Cancer, Child Abuse, Children's Health/Hospitals, Clinics/Medical Centers, Diabetes, Domestic Violence, Emergency/Ambulance Services, Eyes/Blindness, Family Planning, Health Organizations, Health Policy/Cost Containment, Heart, Hospices, Hospitals, Medical Education, Medical Rehabilitation, Medical Research, Mental Health, Nursing Services, People with Disabilities, Preventive Medicine/Wellness Organizations, Public Health, Research/Studies Institutes, Single-Disease Health Associations, Substance Abuse, Transplant Networks/Donor Banks. **Geo. Dist:** Southwestern USA; OK.

### ★ 657 ★ Samuel Rubin Foundation

777 United Nations Plaza
New York, NY 10017
**Phone:** (212)697-8945 **Fax:** (212)682-0886
**Website:** http://www.samuelrubinfoundation.org
Cora Weiss, President

**Fnded:** 1949. **Philosophy:** The foundation's general purpose is to carry on the vision of its founder, Samuel Rubin, whose life was dedicated to the pursuit of peace and justice and the search for an equitable reallocation of the world's resources. The foundation believes that these objectives can be achieved only through the fullest implementation of social, economic, political, civil, and cultural rights for all people. **Priorities:** *Arts & Humanities:* 6%. Supports public broadcasting, cultural projects, and the performing arts. *Civic & Public Affairs:* 55%. Supports community affairs, economic projects, and peace and justice issues. *Education:* 8%. Supports schools, educational programs, and colleges. *International:* 1%. *Note:* Total contributions made in fiscal 2000. **Typ. Recipients:** Domestic Violence, Health-General, Hospitals, Medical Research. **Geo. Dist:** internationally; nationally.

## ★ 658 ★ Samuel S. Fels Fund

1616 Walnut St., Ste. 800
Philadelphia, PA 19103
**Phone:** (215)731-9455 **Fax:** (215)731-9457
**Website:** http://www.samfels.org
Helen Cunningham, Executive Director

**Fnded:** 1935. **Philosophy:** The fund seeks "to initiate and/or to assist any activities or projects of a scientific, educational, or charitable nature which tend to improve human daily life and to bring to the average person greater health, happiness, and a fuller understanding of the meaning and purposes of life." Funding priorities include projects which "prevent, lessen or resolve contemporary social problems," or which are involved in "the provision of service for the improvement of daily life." Grants are given only to organizations located in Philadelphia and that are dedicated to local issues. **Priorities:** *Arts & Humanities:* 20%. Supports theater, ballet, fine arts, music, dance. *Civic & Public Affairs:* 29%. Supports botanical gardens/parks, ethnic organization, law and justice, women's affairs, and urban/community affairs. *Education:* 21%. Supports literacy, religious education, science/mathematics education, and legal education. *Environment:* 20%. Supports homes, community centers, family planning services, Big Sisters, crime prevention, and United Way. *International:* 8%. Supports medical research, AIDS, prenatal health, issues, and clinics/medical centers. *Note:* Total contributions made in 1999. **Typ. Recipients:** Adolescent Health Issues, AIDS/HIV, Cancer, Child Abuse, Children's Health/Hospitals, Clinics/Medical Centers, Diabetes, Domestic Violence, Emergency/Ambulance Services, Family Planning, Health Organizations, Home-Care Services, Hospitals, Long-Term Care, Nutrition, People with Disabilities, Prenatal Health Issues, Public Health. **Geo. Dist:** Philadelphia, PA.

## ★ 659 ★ Sandra Atlas Bass and Edythe and Sol G. Atlas Fund

185 Great Neck Rd.
Great Neck, NY 11021
**Phone:** (516)487-9030 **Fax:** (516)466-6847
Sandra Bass, President

**Fnded:** 1962. **Philosophy:** The fund makes most of its grants in the areas of social services, health, and religion. Social service funding favors programs for the blind and disabled. Health support primarily funds single disease associations, while major support for religion goes to the United Jewish Federation Appeal. Other areas of interest include education, the arts, and international organizations. **Priorities:** *Civic & Public Affairs:* 1%. *Education:* 3%.Supports Veterinary Medical College and scholarships. *Environment:* 22%. Major support goes to animal rights, protection, and animal services. Also supports volunteer services. *International:* 59%. Supports single-disease associations, hospitals, and services for the blind. *Note:* Total contributions made in 1999. **Typ. Recipients:** Cancer, Children's Health/Hospitals, Diabetes, Emergency/Ambulance Services, Hospitals, Hospitals (University Affiliated), Kidney, Medical Education, Medical Research, Multiple Sclerosis, People with Disabilities, Respiratory, Single-Disease Health Associations, Trauma Treatment. **Geo. Dist:** Long Island, NY; New York, NY.

## ★ 660 ★ Sapirstein-Stone-Weiss Foundation

One American Rd.
Cleveland, OH 44144
**Phone:** (216)252-7300 **Fax:** (216)252-6777
Mary Incandela, Financial Administrator

**Fnded:** 1952. **Philosophy:** The foundation is interested in supporting all major support categories for the Jewish faith. Social services, education, and religion are major priorities. Social service funding goes to Jewish community centers. Funding for education supports Jewish religious education and universities. **Priorities:** *Note:* Total contributions made in fiscal 1998. **Typ. Recipients:** Clinics/Medical Centers, Hospitals, Long-Term Care, People with Disabilities. **Geo. Dist:** Eastern USA.

## ★ 661 ★ Sarah and Pauline Maier Foundation

PO Box 6190
Charleston, WV 25362
**Phone:** (304)343-2201 **Fax:** (304)343-2243
**Email:** edhmaier@genrlcorp.com
Edward Maier, President

**Fnded:** 1958. **Philosophy:** The foundation primarily supports higher education in West Virginia, including universities, colleges, legal education, and education funds. Other education related pursuits in Kanawha County, including the arts, a medical center, and civic affairs, are supported. The foundation awarded a 5 year grant of $3,000,000 to the Center for Arts and Sciences of West Virginia, Inc in 1996. **Priorities:** *Arts & Humanities:* 64%. Supports arts associations, theaters, and museums. *Education:* About 36%. Supports West Virginia colleges. *Note:* Total contributions made in fiscal 1999. **Typ. Recipients:** Clinics/Medical Centers, Medical Education. **Geo. Dist:** WV.

## ★ 662 ★ Sarah Scaife Foundation

One Oxford Centre
301 Grant St., Ste. 3900
Pittsburgh, PA 15219-6401
**Phone:** (412)392-2900
**Website:** http://www.scaife.com
Michael Gleba, Vice President, Programs

**Fnded:** 1941. **Philosophy:** The Sarah Scaife Foundation directs its resources primarily to the support of organizations involved in research, publications, and education concerning major domestic and international-public policy issues. The foundation assists a variety of groups that provide decision makers and the general public with informed source material in a timely manner. **Priorities:** *Arts & Humanities:* 1%. Funds a historical society. *Civic & Public Affairs:* 62%. Supports public policy research and legal foundations. *Education:* 22%. Supports programs at colleges and universities, with a focus on domestic public policy and international studies. *Environment:* 1%. Funds Goodwill Industries. *International:* 2%. Funds a health policy institute. *Note:* Total contributions made in 1999. **Typ. Recipients:** Health Policy/Cost Containment, Medical Rehabilitation, People with Disabilities, Substance Abuse. **Geo. Dist:** nationally.

## ★ 663 ★ Sarita Kenedy East Foundation

PO Box 604138
Bay Terrace, NY 11360-4138
**Phone:** (212)701-3292
Margaret Devine, Contact

**Fnded:** 1962. **Philosophy:** The Sarita Kenedy East Foundation's major interest is supporting Roman Catholic churches, monasteries and religious organizations. Few grants are made outside the foundation's primary interest. **Priorities:** *Arts & Humanities:* 3%. Funds cultural and media initiatives. *Education:* 12%. Supports Catholic schools. *Environment:* 18%. Funds human service organizations. *International:* 3%. Supports medical services. *Note:* Total contributions made in 1998. **Typ. Recipients:** Cancer, Nursing Services, Outpatient Health Care. **Geo. Dist:** nationally.

## ★ 664 ★ Sarkeys Foundation

530 East Main St.
Norman, OK 73071
**Phone:** (405)364-3703 **Fax:** (405)364-8191
**Email:** sarkeys@telepath.com
**Website:** http://www.sarkeys.org

**Fnded:** 1962. **Philosophy:** The foundation's mission is "to improve the quality of life in Oklahoma and the Southwest." Major areas of support include higher education, health care and medical research, and cultural and humanitarian programs of regional significance. **Priorities:** *Arts & Humanities:* 22%. Cultural and humanitarian programs of regional significance. Supports arts councils, ballet libraries, theater, opera, and arts institutes. *Civic & Public Affairs:* 10%. Supports housing, community foundations, and zoological societies. *Education:* 34%. Supports scholarship, universities, leadership training, and colleges. *Environment:* 31%. Human services community support, at-

risk youth, daycare, young women's christian association, counseling, domestic violence, camps, and family services. *International:* 3%. Health care medical research, and Alzheimer's. *Note:* Total contributions made in 2000. **Typ. Recipients:** AIDS/HIV, Alzheimers Disease, Cancer, Child Abuse, Children's Health/Hospitals, Clinics/Medical Centers, Diabetes, Domestic Violence, Emergency/Ambulance Services, Eyes/Blindness, Family Planning, Health Organizations, Hospices, Hospitals, Medical Education, Medical Rehabilitation, Medical Research, Mental Health, People with Disabilities, Prenatal Health Issues, Public Health, Sexual Abuse, Single-Disease Health Associations, Speech & Hearing, Substance Abuse. **Geo. Dist:** OK.

## ★ 665 ★ Scaife Family Foundation

One Oxford Centre
301 Grant St., Ste. 3900
Pittsburgh, PA 15219-6401
**Phone:** (412)392-2900 **Fax:** (412)392-2922
**Website:** http://www.scaife.com/scaife.html
Joanne Beyer, Vice President, Secretary & Treasurer

**Fnded:** 1983. **Philosophy:** "The Scaife Family Foundation grant awards will support and develop programs that address the well-being of the family and traditional values. The Foundation will remain flexible in order to offer support in areas of importance as determined by the Trustees. Grant awards are not limited to a particular geographic area, but organizations and projects in the Pittsburgh and Western Pennsylvania area will be given special consideration." **Priorities:** *Arts & Humanities:* 12%. Major support for libraries and opera. *Civic & Public Affairs:* 27%. Supports employment, entrepreneurship, legal affairs issues, housing, economic development, and public policy groups. *Education:* 28%. Supports education funds, medical education, and universities. *Environment:* 21%. Supports family services, child welfare, United Way, youth organizations, and services for the disabled. *International:* 6%. Funds research, health foundations, hospitals, and single-disease associations. *Note:* Total contributions made in 1999. **Typ. Recipients:** Child Abuse, Children's Health/Hospitals, Clinics/Medical Centers, Eyes/Blindness, Family Planning, Health Funds, Health Organizations, Hospices, Hospitals, Kidney, Medical Education, Medical Rehabilitation, Medical Research, Mental Health, Nursing Services, People with Disabilities, Prenatal Health Issues, Public Health, Single-Disease Health Associations, Speech & Hearing, Substance Abuse. **Geo. Dist:** nationally; PA, Western Pennsylvania; Pittsburgh, PA.

## ★ 666 ★ Schumann Fund for New Jersey

21 Van Vleck St.
Montclair, NJ 07042
**Phone:** (973)509-9883 **Fax:** (973)509-1149
**Email:** breisman@worldnet.att.net
Barbara Reisman, Executive Director

**Fnded:** 1988. **Philosophy:** The Schumann Fund for New Jersey has established program priorities that fall into four broad categories to assist nonprofit organizations in New Jersey. The fund supports efforts to encourage academic and social success for young children, especially the urban poor, which enhance the potential for lifelong accomplishment through Early Childhood Development. The fund also supports the protection of natural resources and wildlife through sound land-use planning and balanced economic growth through its Environmental Protection grant program. Essex County, NJ, remains a priority as the fund supports local activities directed at solving community problems, with particular concern for families with young children, education, and social services. The fund also supports efforts to enhance the study, review, and public discussion of important policy issues facing New Jersey through its Public Policy program., particularly in the areas of school reforma nad edicational innovation. Grant proposals that address the fund's priorities receive special consideration if they aim to permanently and positively change the way society deals with a problem, if the proposed project promises to become largely self-sufficient, and if the proposal indicates the recipient has invested a high level of time and/or money to the program.

**Priorities:** *Civic & Public Affairs:* 36%. Supports philanthropic organizations, community foundations, urban/community affairs, law & justice, and public policy. *Environment:* 18%. Supports daycare, at-risk youth, family services, emergency services, and child welfare. *Note:* Total contributions made in 2000. **Typ. Recipients:** AIDS/HIV, Child Abuse, Diabetes, Family Planning, Health Organizations, Mental Health, Prenatal Health Issues, Single-Disease Health Associations. **Geo. Dist:** NJ, Essex County.

**★ 667 ★ Schwartz Foundation**
1650 Arch St., 22nd Floor
Philadelphia, PA 19103-2097
**Phone:** (215)977-2104
Bernard Schwartz, President

**Fnded:** 1983. **Philosophy:** The Schwartz Foundation is primarily interested in supporting Jewish religious organizations. **Priorities:** *Civic & Public Affairs:* 87%. Includes the highest grant to Foundations, Inc., in New Jersey ($1,961,000) and other community concerns. *Education:* 4%. Schools and a Hebrew academy. *Environment:* 3%. Crime prevention, youth services, and United Way. *Note:* Total contributions made in fiscal 1999. **Typ. Recipients:** Alzheimers Disease, Geriatric Health, Multiple Sclerosis, People with Disabilities, Single-Disease Health Associations. **Geo. Dist:** PA, emphasis on Philadelphia.

**★ 668 ★ Scurlock Foundation**
700 Louisiana, Ste. 3920
Houston, TX 77002
**Phone:** (713)236-0550          **Fax:** (713)222-2419
Elizabeth Blanton Wareing, President

**Fnded:** 1954. **Priorities:** *Arts & Humanities:* 16%. Supports museums, opera, dance, fine arts, libraries, and theaters. *Civic & Public Affairs:* 23%. Funds zoos, parks, fire departments, and community organizations. *Education:* 47%. Supports colleges and universities, private secondary education, and special education. *International:* 7%. Supports hospitals, geriatric health, single-disease health associations, and cancer centers. *Note:* Total contributions made in 2000. **Typ. Recipients:** Cancer, Children's Health/Hospitals, Clinics/Medical Centers, Diabetes, Eyes/Blindness, Geriatric Health, Hospices, Hospitals, Hospitals (University Affiliated), Medical Education, Medical Research, Mental Health, Multiple Sclerosis, People with Disabilities, Public Health, Single-Disease Health Associations, Speech & Hearing. **Geo. Dist:** TX.

**★ 669 ★ Seabury Foundation**
208 S LaSalle, Ste., M-14
Chicago, IL 60675
**Phone:** (312)630-6000
Tom Iskalis, Contact

**Fnded:** 1947. **Philosophy:** "The Seabury Foundation is a family foundation that funds projects in the areas of education, social services, health, conservation, and the arts in the city of Chicago. Particular emphasis is placed on programs that nurture strong family relationships, promote individual self-sufficiency, and encourage civic participation. The foundation seeks to improve access of all persons to the education, services, and resources that will support them in living secure, productive, and creative lives." **Priorities:** *Arts & Humanities:* 19%. Supports museums, historical society, theater, music, art, and Shakespeare Repertory. *Civic & Public Affairs:* 13%. Supports neighborhoods, community affairs, and the Chicago Zoological Society. *Education:* 20%. Funds colleges, universities, educational services and programs. *Environment:* 27%. Girls Scouts of America, YMCA, youth and family services. *International:* 10%. Planned Parenthood, community health services, hospitals, hospice, and Down Syndrome National Association. *Note:* Total contributions made in 1998. **Typ. Recipients:** Adolescent Health Issues, Cancer, Children's Health/Hospitals, Clinics/Medical Centers, Domestic Violence, Emergency/Ambulance Services, Family Planning, Hospices, Hospitals, Medical Rehabilitation, Medical Research, Mental Health, Nursing Services, People with Disabilities, Prenatal Health Issues, Public Health,

Single-Disease Health Associations. **Geo. Dist:** Chicago, IL, metropolitan area.

**★ 670 ★ The Seaver Institute**
555 S Flower St. Ste. 4580
Los Angeles, CA 90071
**Phone:** (213)673-2090          **Fax:** (213)673-2089
**Email:** seaverinstitute@aol.com
Victoria Dean, President

**Fnded:** 1955. **Philosophy:** The Seaver Institute provides seed money to highly regarded organizations for particular projects which offer the potential for significant advancement in their fields. Although Science and Education have been the primary recipients of the Institute's benefactions, innovative projects in the Arts and Humanities are equally important. **Priorities:** *Arts & Humanities:* 6%. Funds museums and libraries. *Civic & Public Affairs:* 14%. Supports philanthropy. *Education:* 62%. Primary support for colleges and universities. *Environment:* 1%. *International:* Less than 1% *Religion:* 6%. Emphasis on the California Institute of Technology and the Woods Hole Oceanographic Institute. *Note:* Total contributions made in fiscal 2000. **Typ. Recipients:** Children's Health/Hospitals, Eyes/Blindness, Hospices, Hospitals, Medical Education, Medical Research, Research/Studies Institutes, Single-Disease Health Associations, Substance Abuse, Transplant Networks/Donor Banks. **Geo. Dist:** nationally.

**★ 671 ★ Second Foundation**
1111 Superior Ave. Ste. 1000
Cleveland, OH 44114-2507
**Phone:** (216)696-4200          **Fax:** (216)696-7303
**Email:** pranney@ssrl.com
Phillip Ranney, Secretary

**Fnded:** 1984. **Philosophy:** The Second Foundation makes most of its grants in the areas of higher education, projects related to the environment such as museums and libraries, and organizations located in Cuyahoga County previously supported by the foundation's founder. "Organizations promoting self-help by the recipients are looked upon favorably by the trustees." **Priorities:** *Arts & Humanities:* 46%. Supports libraries and museums with major support for the Case Western Reserve University Library. *Civic & Public Affairs:* 7%. Supports community development and a botanical garden. *Education:* 17%. Supports colleges and universities and scholarships. *Environment:* 5%. Supports Western Reserve Residences, senior citizen services, United Way. *International:* 4%. Funds elder care. *Religion:* 21%. Supports science centers. *Note:* Total contributions made in 1999. **Typ. Recipients:** Child Abuse, Clinics/Medical Centers, Domestic Violence, Health Funds, Hospitals, Hospitals (University Affiliated), Research/Studies Institutes. **Geo. Dist:** OH, Cuyahoga County.

**★ 672 ★ Self Family Foundation**
PO Box 1017
Greenwood, SC 29648-1017
**Phone:** (864)941-4028          **Fax:** (864)941-4091
**Email:** mamienic@greenwood.net
**Website:** http://www.selffoundation.greenwood.net
Mamie Nicholson, Program Officer

**Fnded:** 1942. **Philosophy:** James Self, the founder, and the foundation have "endeavored to incorporate his philosophy in its grant making program – a philosophy that the offering of challenges and tests is the prime ingredient in a successful philanthropic program. Mr. Self viewed grants not as handouts but as catalysts which unearth the latent capabilities of those in need. Consequently, the general philosophy of the foundation is °helping people to help themselves.'" The foundation's core values are "to give back to the communities that have helped make the Foundation possible, to attack root causes rather than symptoms, to view communities as 'systems' with interdependent parts that are only as healthy as their weakest part, and to build self-sufficiency in people and the communities in which they live." The foundation supports projects that mobilize local resources, work collaboratively, and produce measurable results. Education and health care are the primary areas of

focus. In education, the foundation will "concentrate on enhancing children's readiness for school" and will assist schools, families, youth-serving organizations, and other community organizations to work together more effectively to support the intellectual and social development of youth. In health care, the foundation will focus on community wellness and prevention and will provide assistance to community organizations, businesses, public institutions, and local residents who collaborate to revitalize their neighborhood. Secondary interests are activities that support access to the arts or increase the awareness of the culture and history of Greenwood, SC, and the surrounding counties followed by the Upper Piedmont region. 1996 Annual Report **Priorities:** *Arts & Humanities:* 3%. Supports arts councils, libraries, and opera. *Civic & Public Affairs:* 13%. Supports parks, inner-city development, community foundations, and Habitat for Humanity. *Education:* 45%. Supports local schools, literacy, colleges, universities, and enrichment programs. *Environment:* 33%. Supports United Way, domestic abuse, family services, animal protection, scouting, and camps. *International:* 6%. Supports children's health and hospice. *Note:* Total contributions made in 1999. **Typ. Recipients:** Adolescent Health Issues, Alzheimers Disease, Cancer, Child Abuse, Children's Health/Hospitals, Clinics/Medical Centers, Domestic Violence, Family Planning, Heart, Home-Care Services, Hospices, Hospitals, Medical Education, Medical Research, People with Disabilities, Sexual Abuse. **Geo. Dist:** SC, emphasis on Greenwood area.

**★ 673 ★ Sequoia Foundation**
820 A St., Ste. 345
Tacoma, WA 98402
**Phone:** (253)627-1634          **Fax:** (253)627-6249
Frank Underwood, Executive Director

**Fnded:** 1982. **Philosophy:** The current areas of geographic interest for conservation, environment, and social service grants are Mexico, Central America, the Himalayan Mountain region, and the Northwest United States. Grants are given in the foundation's program areas of conservation/environment and social services, where a component of the program is to generate or stabilize economic development. These program areas will tend to remain constant, but the geographic areas on which the foundation will focus its conservation and social service grants will change over time. Because the foundation intends to keep its programs flexible at all times, its focus will vary as conditions change and new needs arise. The Sequoia Foundation focuses its support on established organizations seeking to meet national and international needs rather than on local issues. **Priorities:** *Arts & Humanities:* 3%. *Civic & Public Affairs:* 60%. *Education:* 27%. Primary support for universities and preparatory schools. *Environment:* 7%. Focus on the New Horizon Foundation. *Note:* Total contributions made in fiscal 1999. **Typ. Recipients:** Family Planning, Health Organizations, Hospitals, Medical Education, Medical Rehabilitation, Mental Health, Public Health, Public Health. **Geo. Dist:** nationally, with emphasis on the Western and Northwestern USA; Seattle, WA; Tacoma, WA.

**★ 674 ★ Seth Sprague Educational and Charitable Foundation**
114 W 47th St.
New York, NY 10036
**Phone:** (212)852-1000          **Fax:** (212)852-3377
Elizabeth Irmiter, Financial Officer

**Fnded:** 1939. **Philosophy:** The foundation gives to a broad range of interests, with a focus on education, social services, community affairs, and health. **Priorities:** *Arts & Humanities:* About 17%. Historic preservation, performing arts, and museums. *Civic & Public Affairs:* 16%. Employment and job training, botanical gardens, and community foundations. *Education:* 21%. Private precollege education, legal assistance, and colleges/universities. *Environment:* 15%. Substance abuse programs, youth organizations, and child welfare. *International:* About 20%. Hospitals, AIDS/HIV, and medical centers. *Religion:* 5%. *Note:* Total contributions made in 1996. **Typ. Recipients:** AIDS/HIV, Arthritis, Cancer, Children's Health/Hospitals, Clinics/Medical Centers, Domestic Violence, Emergency/Ambulance Services, Family Planning, Geriatric Health, Health Funds, Health Organizations, Hospices, Hospitals, Medical Education, Medical Rehabilitation, Medical Research, Medical Training, Mental Health, Nursing Services, People with Disabilities, Single-Disease Health Associations, Substance Abuse. **Geo. Dist:** nationally; MA; NY.

### ★ 675 ★ Seymour H. Knox Foundation
1 HSBC Center Ste. 2840
Buffalo, NY 14203
**Phone:** (716)854-6811          **Fax:** (716)856-0517
**Email:** kbojw@aol.com
James Wendel, Assistant Secretary & Assistant Treasure

**Fnded:** 1945. **Philosophy:** The foundation lists the following giving areas: arts and music, universities and schools, hospitals and health organizations, civic organizations, United Way and Red Cross, and religious activities. **Priorities:** *Arts & Humanities:* 15%. Supports historical societies, arts groups, and museums. *Civic & Public Affairs:* 4%. Supports civic groups. *Education:* 51%. Funds colleges, universities, and precollege educational institutions. *Environment:* 12%. Gives to united funds and youth groups. *International:* 6%. Gives to hospitals, hospices, and medical research. *Note:* Total contributions made in 1999. **Typ. Recipients:** Alzheimers Disease, Cancer, Children's Health/Hospitals, Family Planning, Health Funds, Hospices, Hospitals, Medical Education, Medical Rehabilitation, Medical Research, People with Disabilities, Speech & Hearing, Substance Abuse, Trauma Treatment. **Geo. Dist:** nationally; Buffalo, NY.

### ★ 676 ★ Sherman Fairchild Foundation
5454 Wisconsin Ave. Ste. 1205
Chevy Chase, MD 20815
**Phone:** (301)913-5990
Bonnie Himmelman, President

**Fnded:** 1955. **Philosophy:** The foundation generally emphasizes the following areas: education, particularly colleges and universities; health and medical research; and, to a lesser extent, the arts and social services. **Priorities:** *Arts & Humanities:* 29%. Supports libraries, the performing arts, fine arts. *Education:* 49%. Supports colleges, universities, school, and scholarship. *Environment:* 5%. Supports athletics and youth programs. *International:* 15%. Supports hospital and medical research. *Note:* Total contributions made in 1998. **Typ. Recipients:** Cancer, Children's Health/Hospitals, Clinics/Medical Centers, Health Funds, Hospitals, Medical Education, Medical Research. **Geo. Dist:** nationally; New York, NY, including metropolitan area.

### ★ 677 ★ Shoreland Foundation
1 Comac Loop, Unit 9
Ronkonkoma, NY 11779-6816
**Phone:** (516)737-1974          **Fax:** (631)737-1974
Carol-Ann Mealy, Contact

**Fnded:** 1994. **Philosophy:** The foundation focuses on the arts, health care, and education. **Priorities:** *Arts & Humanities:* 24%. Large grant to the Metropolitan Museum of Art in New York, NY. *Civic & Public Affairs:* 2%. Funds women's issues and public safety. *Education:* 70%. Major grant to Wellesley College. *Environment:* 1%. Funds youth programs. *International:* Less than 1%. Funds single-disease health associations. *Religion:* Less than 1%. Supports natural history museum. *Note:* Total contributions made in 1999. **Typ. Recipients:** AIDS/HIV, Alzheimers Disease, Cancer, Children's Health/Hospitals, Eyes/Blindness, Health Organizations, People with Disabilities, Substance Abuse. **Geo. Dist:** nationally.

### ★ 678 ★ Shubert Foundation
234 W 44th St.
New York, NY 10036
**Phone:** (212)944-3777          **Fax:** (212)944-3767
Vicki Reiss, Executive Director

**Fnded:** 1945. **Philosophy:** The goal of the foundation's grants program "is to build and perpetuate the live performing arts, particularly the professional theatre, in the United States. Accomplishment of this goal involves support both of the theatrical institutions and of those other elements of the performing arts and related institutions that are necessary to maintain and support the theatre." Schubert Foundation fiscal 1999 IRS Form 990. Professional resident theater organizations in the United States are the major recipients of Shubert financial support. The foundation also supports "dance because it is a critical performing art form related to and supportive of the theater." The foundation also recognizes the importance of private graduate theater education. **Priorities:** *Arts & Humanities:* 89%. Primarily supports theater organizations. *Education:* 8%. Supports arts education. *Note:* Contributions made in fiscal 2000. **Typ. Recipients:** Clinics/Medical Centers, Hospitals (University Affiliated). **Geo. Dist:** national organizations only.

### ★ 679 ★ Sid W. Richardson Foundation
309 Main St.
Fort Worth, TX 76102
**Phone:** (817)336-0494          **Fax:** (817)332-2176
**Website:** http://www.sidrichardson.org
Mr. Valleau Wilkie, Jr., Executive Vice President & Executive Dir

**Fnded:** 1947. **Philosophy:** The foundation believes it can best serve the state of Texas through its support of both tax-supported groups and nonprofit organizations. In education, it emphasizes support to public elementary and secondary schools, and faculty development programs. Health interests include preventive medicine and efforts to improve the delivery of efficient health care and research. In the areas of the arts, human services, and community projects, the foundation focuses on the needs of the Ft. Worth area. **Priorities:** *Arts & Humanities:* 11%. Art councils and symphony support. *Civic & Public Affairs:* 4%. Housing services, community initiatives and women's centers. *Education:* 30%. Primarily universities. *Environment:* 10%. Supports family services, elderly and youth programs. *International:* 36%. Medical research, universities, and healthcare programs. *Religion:* 1%. *Note:* Total contributions made in 1998. **Typ. Recipients:** Cancer, Children's Health/Hospitals, Clinics/Medical Centers, Diabetes, Emergency/Ambulance Services, Eyes/Blindness, Family Planning, Health Policy/Cost Containment, Health-General, Heart, Hospitals, Hospitals (University Affiliated), Medical Education, Medical Research, Nursing Services, Outpatient Health Care, People with Disabilities, Prenatal Health Issues, Public Health, Research/Studies Institutes, Substance Abuse. **Geo. Dist:** Ft. Worth, TX, some giving in other areas of Texas.

### ★ 680 ★ Sidney Stern Memorial Trust
PO Box 893
Pacific Palisades, CA 90272
**Phone:** (310)459-2117
Peter Hoffenberg, Member, Board of Advisors

**Fnded:** 1974. **Philosophy:** The board of directors of the Sidney Stern Memorial Trust reviews all requests for grants. "The Board endeavors to support soundly managed charitable organizations which give service with broad scope, affect favorably their target populations, and contribute materially to the general welfare. The Board gives priority to the following areas: education, health and science, community service projects, youth, services to the physically and mentally disabled, the arts, and organizations and activities serving California." **Priorities:** *Arts & Humanities:* 1%. Primarily supports public broadcasting. *Civic & Public Affairs:* 12%. Funding for legal aid, public policy organizations, womens affairs, civil rights, zoos, Native American affairs. *Education:* 24%. Supports colleges and universities, special education, literacy, medical schools, religious education, and minority education. *Environment:* 20%. Emphasis on people with disabilities, family services, youth organizations, community services, food distribution programs, child welfare homes, family planning services, young men's christian association, and senior services. *International:* 18%. Supports hospitals, medical clinics, pediatric

health, and medical research. *Note:* Total contributions made in fiscal 2000. **Typ. Recipients:** AIDS/HIV, Arthritis, Children's Health/Hospitals, Clinics/Medical Centers, Domestic Violence, Emergency/Ambulance Services, Eyes/Blindness, Family Planning, Health Organizations, Health-General, Hospitals, Kidney, Long-Term Care, Medical Education, Medical Research, Mental Health, Multiple Sclerosis, People with Disabilities, Prenatal Health Issues, Preventive Medicine/Wellness Organizations, Public Health, Research/Studies Institutes, Single-Disease Health Associations, Substance Abuse. **Geo. Dist:** nationally; CA.

### ★ 681 ★ Siebert Lutheran Foundation
2600 North Mayfair Rd., Ste. 390
Wauwatosa, WI 53226-1392
**Phone:** (414)257-2656          **Fax:** (414)257-1387
**Email:** siebertf@execpc.com
**Website:** http://www.SiebertFoundation.org
Ronald Jones, President

**Fnded:** 1952. **Philosophy:** The foundation concentrates its grant-making activities on the Lutheran community, primarily Lutheran churches and institutions in the state of Wisconsin. Currently, the foundation supports education, and training, community development and outreach, health care, child care, care for the aging, social services with a focus on inner-city service projects, and evangelism and youth. The foundation also sponsors a program which provides financial aid to congregations in Wisconsin on behalf of seminary students. **Priorities:** *Civic & Public Affairs:* 19%. Primarily for community services. *Education:* About 52%. Primarily for religious education, private schools, and education associations. *Environment:* About 3%. Emphasis on child welfare. *Note:* Total contributions made in 1996. **Typ. Recipients:** AIDS/HIV, Cancer, Clinics/Medical Centers, Geriatric Health, Hospitals, Long-Term Care, Nursing Services, People with Disabilities, Public Health. **Geo. Dist:** WI.

### ★ 682 ★ Sierra Health Foundation
1321 Garden Highway
Sacramento, CA 95833
**Phone:** (916)922-4755          **Fax:** (916)922-4024
**Email:** info@sierrahealth.org
**Website:** http://www.sierrahealth.org/
Len McCandliss, President & Chief Executive Officer

**Fnded:** 1984. **Philosophy:** "The foundation engages in an array of activities that support improved health for Northern Californians. Grantmaking, both in well-defined focus areas and for more general purposes, is a major function of the foundation. But equally important is the foundation's drive to stimulate collaboration, promote dialogue and share successful strategies throughout the region. By partnering with other foundations, grant recipients and community leaders, the foundation works to leverage resources and ensure effective outcomes." Currently, the foundation supports three key program areas: health grants, the Community Partnerships for Healthy Children (CPHC) Initiative, and the Conference Program. **Priorities:** *International:* 100%. Supports health and health-related activites in 26 northern California counties. The foundation focuses its giving on local and regional health-related programs and services, influencing public health policy and choices, and stimulating major improvements in California's health care system. *Note:* Total contributions made in 1999. **Typ. Recipients:** Adolescent Health Issues, AIDS/HIV, Cancer, Child Abuse, Children's Health/Hospitals, Clinics/Medical Centers, Domestic Violence, Emergency/Ambulance Services, Eyes/Blindness, Family Planning, Geriatric Health, Health Organizations, Health Policy/Cost Containment, Heart, Hospices, Hospitals, Long-Term Care, Medical Education, Medical Research, Mental Health, Nursing Services, Outpatient Health Care, People with Disabilities, Prenatal Health Issues, Public Health, Research/Studies Institutes, Respiratory, Single-Disease Health Associations, Trauma Treatment. **Geo. Dist:** CA, 26 counties in Northern California.

**★ 683 ★ Skillman Foundation**
600 Renaissance Center, Ste. 1700
Detroit, MI 48243
**Phone:** (313)393-1185　　　　**Fax:** (313)393-1187
**Email:** kschlachtenhaufen@skillman.org
**Website:** http://www.skillman.org
Kari Schlachtenhaufen, President

**Fnded:** 1960. **Philosophy:** "The Skillman Foundation is a resource for improving the lives of children in Metropolitan Detroit. The Foundation applies it resources to foster positive relationships between children and adults, support high quality learning opportunities, and strengthen healthy, safe, and supportive homes and communities. The Foundation's goals are grouped under four broad Program Areas of Interest: Children's Relationships, Learning Opportunities, Home and Community, and Grantmaking Opportunities." 1998 Grantmaking Policies and Procedures **Priorities:** *Arts & Humanities:* 11%. Supports public broadcasting, music, museums, libraries, and theaters. *Civic & Public Affairs:* 19%. Juvenile justice concerns, youth development, and strengthening civic institutions. *Education:* 15%. Primary and secondary education. Also colleges, universities, and minority education. *Environment:* 41%. Children, youth, and family program areas. Also supports basic human needs causes and community services. *International:* 14%. Primarily for child and family health. *Note:* Total contributions made in fiscal 1998. **Typ. Recipients:** Adolescent Health Issues, AIDS/HIV, Child Abuse, Children's Health/Hospitals, Domestic Violence, Family Planning, Health Organizations, Health Policy/Cost Containment, Medical Education, Medical Research, Mental Health, Nursing Services, People with Disabilities, Prenatal Health Issues, Preventive Medicine/Wellness Organizations, Public Health, Research/Studies Institutes, Respiratory, Substance Abuse, Trauma Treatment. **Geo. Dist:** MI, Wayne, Oakland, and Macomb Counties; Detroit, MI.

**★ 684 ★ Slemp Foundation**
PO Box 1118 M.L. 5145
Cincinnati, OH 45201
**Phone:** (513)762-8878

**Fnded:** 1943. **Priorities:** *Arts & Humanities:* 12%. Supports art centers and libraries. *Civic & Public Affairs:* 2%. *Education:* 84%. Supports colleges, universities, and public schools. *Environment:* 2%. Primarily supports scouts. *Note:* Total contributions made in fiscal 1999. **Typ. Recipients:** Cancer, Child Abuse, Children's Health/Hospitals, Clinics/Medical Centers, Emergency/Ambulance Services, Hospices, People with Disabilities. **Geo. Dist:** VA, Lee County; VA, Wise County.

**★ 685 ★ Smart Family Foundation**
74 Pin Oak Lane
Wilton, CT 06897-1329
**Phone:** (203)834-0400　　　　**Fax:** (203)834-0412
Raymond Smart, President

**Fnded:** 1951. **Philosophy:** The foundation funds a wide variety of projects across all major categories. **Priorities:** *Arts & Humanities:* 28%. Supports museums, performing arts centers, libraries, music, and theater. *Civic & Public Affairs:* 13%. Supports civic and public affairs, municipalities. *Education:* 30%. Funds colleges, universities, primary and secondary schools, and educational programs. *Environment:* 5%. Funds YMHA, YWHA, youth councils. *International:* 1%. Supports health research, senior citizen's health. *Religion:* 2%. Supports the Aspen Center for Physics. *Note:* Total contributions made in 1999. **Typ. Recipients:** Eyes/Blindness, Family Planning, Geriatric Health, Health Organizations, Hospitals, Hospitals (University Affiliated), Medical Education, Medical Research, Mental Health, People with Disabilities, Research/Studies Institutes, Substance Abuse. **Geo. Dist:** nationally.

**★ 686 ★ Smith Richardson Foundation**
60 Jesup Rd.
Westport, CT 06880
**Phone:** (203)222-6222　　　　**Fax:** (203)222-6282

**Website:** http://www.srf.org
Peter Richardson, President

**Fnded:** 1935. **Philosophy:** "The Smith Richardson Foundation supports programs that are consistent with the vision of its founder. H. Smith Richardson wrote that 'the need for the time and thought of able men is that they be applied to the increasingly weighty problems of government and the serious social questions which now confront us and will continue to press for solution in the future.' The Foundation's main objective, therefore, is the funding of pragmatic research and programs which seek to inform important public and foreign policy debates. In order to achieve this goal most effectively, the Foundation divides its grant making into two general program areas: international and domestic." "The Foundation's International Affairs program supports programs and research projects on security issues central to the interests of the United States. Such projects seek to define the important challenges facing the United States in the post-cold war security environment, to illuminate key issues affecting U.S. interests in Europe, the former Soviet Union, East Asia and the Middle East, and to underwrite historical research with clear implications or lessons for current policy." "The Foundation's Domestic program supports research on the public policy issues that affect children and families at risk. Accordingly, it supports projects that investigate 'what works' in social programs and that propose and evaluate models for more effective responses to the problems facing children and families in poverty. The Foundation also supports domestic public policy projects in such areas as education and government reform when such projects share similar qualities of pragmatism and applied scholarship." "Generally, the Foundation makes grants only to support research projects. However, a small portion of its funding is reserved for worthy direct service grants within the states of Connecticut and North Carolina, where the Foundation has its offices." **Priorities:** *Civic & Public Affairs:* 29%. Primarily supports foreign public policy programs and international security. *Education:* 40%. Supports educational research at universities. *International:* 10%. Health and education research, hospitals. *Note:* Total contributions made in 1998. **Typ. Recipients:** Cancer, Child Abuse, Children's Health/Hospitals, Domestic Violence, Family Planning, Health Policy/Cost Containment, Long-Term Care, Medical Education, Public Health, Single-Disease Health Associations. **Geo. Dist:** limited giving internationally; primarily to national organizations.

**★ 687 ★ Sol Goldman Charitable Trust**
640 5th Ave., 3rd Floor
New York, NY 10019
**Phone:** (212)265-2280　　　　**Fax:** (212)265-2592
Amy Goldman, Trustee

**Fnded:** 1988. **Priorities:** *Education:* 54%. Supports educational initiatives. *Environment:* 5%. Community groups, children's services, and Special Olympics received funding. *International:* 29%. Supports hospitals, medical research, single-disease causes, and AIDS research. *Note:* Total contributions made in fiscal 1999. **Typ. Recipients:** AIDS/HIV, Cancer, Children's Health/Hospitals, Clinics/Medical Centers, Family Planning, Hospitals, Kidney, Medical Research, Mental Health, Multiple Sclerosis, People with Disabilities, Prenatal Health Issues, Research/Studies Institutes, Single-Disease Health Associations, Speech & Hearing. **Geo. Dist:** NY.

**★ 688 ★ Solon E. Summerfield Foundation, Inc.**
270 Madison Ave., Room 1201
New York, NY 10016
**Phone:** (212)685-5529　　　　**Fax:** (212)685-5526
Clarence Treeger, President

**Fnded:** 1939. **Philosophy:** Education receives the majority of support from the Solon E. Summerfield Foundation. Jewish organizations and groups concerned with blindness and visual impairment also receive large grants from the foundation. Almost 80% of the foundation's funds are set aside for these and other pre-selected organizations. Generally, for new proposals, the foundation makes smaller contributions to many organizations with a wide variety of interests. **Priorities:** *Education:* 56%. Colleges and universities. *Environment:* 25%. Children's welfare organizations are primary recipients. *International:* 5%. Nurse services, hospitals, and foundation for the blind. *Note:* Total contributions made in 1998. **Typ. Recipients:** Child Abuse, Clinics/Medical Centers, Domestic Violence, Emergency/Ambulance Services, Eyes/Blindness, Health Organizations, Hospitals, Long-Term Care, Medical Education, Medical Research, Mental Health, Nursing Services, People with Disabilities, Research/Studies Institutes. **Geo. Dist:** nationally; Northeast USA; New York, NY.

**★ 689 ★ Sosland Foundation**
4800 Main St., Ste. 100
Kansas City, MO 64112-2504
**Phone:** (816)756-1000　　　　**Fax:** (816)756-0494
Debbie Sosland-Edelman, Executive Director

**Fnded:** 1955. **Philosophy:** The foundation supports a wide range of institutions, with at least half of the total awards going to Jewish philanthropies. The purpose of each grant "is to further the causes, whether they be civic, cultural, or religious, of each organization." Grants by the foundation are generally given for unrestricted general support. **Priorities:** *Arts & Humanities:* 15%. *Civic & Public Affairs:* 2%. *Education:* 11%. Focus on education funds, promary and secondary education, Jewish studies, and colleges and universities. *Environment:* 25%. United funds, child welfare, family services, and youth organizations. *International:* 16%. *Religion:* 8%. *Note:* Total contributions made in fiscal 1998. **Typ. Recipients:** AIDS/HIV, Children's Health/Hospitals, Clinics/Medical Centers, Emergency/Ambulance Services, Family Planning, Health Organizations, Hospitals, Medical Rehabilitation, Mental Health. **Geo. Dist:** Kansas City, KS, metropolitan area; Kansas City, MO, metropolitan area.

**★ 690 ★ South Texas Charitable Foundation**
PO Box 2549
Victoria, TX 77902
**Fax:** (512)573-1168
Rayford Keller, Secretary-Treasurer

**Fnded:** 1981. **Philosophy:** The South Texas Charitable Foundation makes most of its grants to Christian religious organizations and social service organizations. Other interests include hospitals, religious education, community emergency services, and counseling. **Priorities:** *Civic & Public Affairs:* 4%. Supports fire departments. *Environment:* 34%. Supports food banks, elderly services, and social service groups. *International:* 11%. Contributes to hospitals and hospices. *Note:* Total contributions made in 1999. **Typ. Recipients:** Cancer, Children's Health/Hospitals, Domestic Violence, Emergency/Ambulance Services, Heart, Hospices, Hospitals, Long-Term Care, Medical Rehabilitation, People with Disabilities, Sexual Abuse, Single-Disease Health Associations. **Geo. Dist:** TX.

**★ 691 ★ Spencer T. and Ann W. Olin Foundation**
7701 Forsyth Boulevard, Ste. 1040
Saint Louis, MO 63105
**Phone:** (314)727-6202　　　　**Fax:** (314)727-6157
Warren Shapleigh, President

**Fnded:** 1957. **Philosophy:** "The principal interests of the foundation are in the fields of higher education, medical education and research, health services and facilities, and environmental conservation...Support is also given to community needs in the metropolitan St. Louis area, including cultural, civic and welfare programs." **Priorities:** *Arts & Humanities:* 1% Supports performing and contemporary art primarily in St. Louis, MO, the symphony and theater. *Civic & Public Affairs:* 14% Supports community and public affairs, philanthropy, and botanical gardens. *Education:* 51% Supports educational programs and institutions, medical education, and arts/humanities education. *Environment:* 24% supports the United Way, youth and family services, the elderly, and disabled, animal protection, Young Men's Christian Association/Young Women's Christian Association and people with disabilities. *International:* 1% Supports hospice, research and treatment fund, Alzheimer's Association and other disease and disorder concerns. *Religion:* Less than 1%. *Note:* Contributions were made in 2000. **Typ. Recipients:** Alzheimers Disease, Arthritis, Cancer, Clinics/Medical Centers, Emergency/Ambulance Services, Family Planning, Geriatric Health, Hospices, Hospitals, Medical Education, Nursing Services, People with Disabilities, Preventive Medicine/Wellness Organizations. **Geo. Dist:** nationally.

### ★ 692 ★ Spring/Close Foundation

308 Springcrest Dr.
Fort Mill, SC 29715
**Phone:** (803)548-2002          **Fax:** (803)548-1797
H.W. Close, Jr., President

**Fnded:** 1968. **Priorities:** *Arts & Humanities:* 7%. Supports art councils and programs. *Civic & Public Affairs:* 16%. Focus on community affairs. *Education:* 42%. Including a large grant to the University of South Carolina - Lancaster. *Environment:* 33%. Primarily supports athletics and recreation, animal protection, people with disabilities, and shelters. *International:* 1%. *Religion:* 1%. Supports science councils. *Note:* Total contributions made in 1998. **Typ. Recipients:** AIDS/HIV, Alzheimers Disease, Clinics/Medical Centers, Diabetes, Emergency/Ambulance Services, Hospices, Hospitals, Mental Health, People with Disabilities, Prenatal Health Issues, Substance Abuse. **Geo. Dist:** NC; Chester Township, SC; Fort Mill Township, SC; Lancaster County, SC.

### ★ 693 ★ Springs Foundation, Inc.

1826 Second Baxter Crossing
Fort Mill, SC 29708
**Phone:** (803)548-2002          **Fax:** (803)548-1797
Mr. H. Close, Jr., President

**Fnded:** 1942. **Philosophy:** The foundation was established to improve the lives of people in areas where Springs Industries plants were located. Colonel Springs was particularly interested in young people and helping them develop their greatest potential. The categories the founder determined to be the most basic to the well-being of individuals were recreation, health care, education, community service, and religion. The foundation continues to give in these five areas. In 1992, the foundation celebrated its 50th anniversary. **Priorities:** *Arts & Humanities:* 4%. Supports arts councils, libraries, and theater. *Civic & Public Affairs:* 1%. Supports clubs, towns, and housing. *Education:* 11%. Supports primary and secondary education and colleges and universities. *Environment:* 51%. Focus on recreation, community services, United Way, Young Men's Christian Association and camps. *International:* 32%. Supports Hospice and emergency services. *Note:* Total contributions made in 2000. **Typ. Recipients:** AIDS/HIV, Cancer, Clinics/Medical Centers, Emergency/Ambulance Services, Health Organizations, Hospices, Hospitals, Medical Education, Mental Health, Nutrition, Prenatal Health Issues, Substance Abuse. **Geo. Dist:** Chester Township, SC; Fort Mill Township, SC; Lancaster County, SC.

### ★ 694 ★ Spunk Fund Inc.

780 3rd Ave., 24th Floor
New York, NY 10017
**Phone:** (212)980-8880          **Fax:** (212)980-8976
**Email:** sfi@spunkfund.com
Marianne Gerschel, President

**Fnded:** 1981. **Philosophy:** "The Spunk Foundation, Inc. is a private foundation created to support initiatives that contribute to the enrichment and well-being of children. Its goal is to fund programs, persons, institutions and ideas of outstanding quality and promise. "The Spunk Fund, Inc. focuses mainly on children's needs in the New York City metropolitan area. It also seeks well-conceived proposals of exceptional merit to benefit children in other nations and in other parts of the United States. Priority is given to programs which are well-integrated into the fabric of their communities and which draw upon existing public and private resources. The Spunk Fund, Inc. welcomes opportunities in which its own involvement will encourage or facilitate the participation of other grantmaking organizations. "While interested in initiatives which impact the overall world of the child, the Spunk Fund, Inc currently concentrates grants in four areas: programs directed toward medical and psychological problems of children; programs which contribute to the general education and cultural expression of children; programs aimed at the prevention and treatment of child abuse and neglect; and programs designed to enhance the quality of life and opportunities for less advantaged children overseas." Spunk Fund, Inc. Philosophy & Guidelines brochure **Priorities:** *Arts & Humanities:* 3% (Culture). Supports public broadcasting, photography, and performing arts. *Education:* 17%. Funds education initiatives focusing on teaching. *Environment:* 11% (Social Services & Policy). Supports services for children and under-served communities. *International:* 69% (Health/Medicine). Supports medical centers and schools of medicine. *Note:* Total contributions for fiscal 2001. Twenty-nine percent of total contributions went to internationally organizations. **Typ. Recipients:** Clinics/Medical Centers, Health Organizations, Heart, Hospitals (University Affiliated), Medical Education, Medical Research, Mental Health, Nutrition, People with Disabilities, Research/Studies Institutes, Substance Abuse. **Geo. Dist:** NY.

### ★ 695 ★ Stackpole-Hall Foundation

44 South Saint Marys St.
Saint Marys, PA 15857
**Phone:** (814)834-1845          **Fax:** (814)834-1869
**Email:** s-hf@ncentral.com
William Conrad, Executive Secretary

**Fnded:** 1951. **Philosophy:** The foundation emphasizes local giving, with major priorities in the fields of education, social services, youth programs, and religious organizations. Educational support includes in-state universities, private education, and minority education funds. Some funding is given to civic causes, medical facilities, and the arts. **Priorities:** *Arts & Humanities:* 1%. Supports historic societies and arts councils. *Civic & Public Affairs:* 35%. Parks and community and municipal services, with major support to St. Mary's and Ridgway, Pennsylvania. *Education:* 19%. Supports schools, universities and religious education. *Environment:* 11%. Supports youth programs, Young Men's Christian Association, and scouting. *International:* 12%. Supports medical services in Pennsylvania. *Note:* Total contributions made in 1999. **Typ. Recipients:** Children's Health/Hospitals, Clinics/Medical Centers, Emergency/Ambulance Services, Family Planning, Health-General, Hospices, Hospitals, Medical Education, Mental Health, Nursing Services, People with Disabilities, Public Health, Speech & Hearing, Substance Abuse. **Geo. Dist:** PA, Elk County.

### ★ 696 ★ Stardust Foundation

6730 North Scottsdale Rd., Ste. 230
Scottsdale, AZ 85253
**Phone:** (480)607-5800          **Fax:** (480)607-5801
Gerald Bisgrove, President

**Fnded:** 1993. **Philosophy:** The foundation provides support for a local Habitat for Humanity, other civic concerns, community services, and education. The foundation promotes individuals responsibility and spiritual values in partnership with God and the community. **Priorities:** *Civic & Public Affairs:* 43%. Primarily for housing, municipalities, and safety organizations. *Education:* 17%. Leadership training and private, secondary education. *Environment:* 25%. Youth organizations, YMCAs, animal protection, and community services. *International:* 3%. Medical rehabilitation. *Note:* Total contributions made in 1997. **Typ. Recipients:** AIDS/HIV, Cancer, Domestic Violence, Family Planning, Health Organizations, Heart, Medical Rehabilitation, Public Health, Substance Abuse. **Geo. Dist:** AZ.

### ★ 697 ★ Starr Foundation

70 Pine St.
New York, NY 10270
**Phone:** (212)770-5202          **Fax:** (212)425-6261
**Email:** grants@starrfoundation.org
**Website:** http://fdncenter.org/grantmaker/starr/
Florence Davis, President & Director

**Fnded:** 1955. **Philosophy:** The foundation's initial activities are "focused on education, particularly the provision of scholarships in the United States and Asia, and local assistance for international studies, community funds, and other civic organizations." This focus continued and grew through the 1970s. In 1980, the foundation added another area of funding: hospitals and health groups. The foundation's current interests are educational institutions and student aid. The foundation also funds health concerns, civic organizations, and cultural activities. **Priorities:** *Arts & Humanities:* 19%. Museums, libraries, and performing arts. *Education:* 37%. Primarily to schools and universities. *Environment:* 15%. *International:* 18%. Funding for medical schools and medical centers. *Religion:* 2%. Supports educational science programs. *Note:* Total contributions made in 1998. **Typ. Recipients:** AIDS/HIV, Cancer, Children's Health/Hospitals, Emergency/Ambulance Services, Eyes/Blindness, Family Planning, Geriatric Health, Health Organizations, Health Policy/Cost Containment, Health-General, Heart, Hospices, Hospitals, Kidney, Long-Term Care, Medical Education, Medical Research, Medical Training, Nursing Services, People with Disabilities, Public Health, Single-Disease Health Associations, Substance Abuse, Transplant Networks/Donor Banks. **Geo. Dist:** internationally; nationally; nationally; internationally; New York, NY; New York, NY, metropolitan area.

### ★ 698 ★ Steele Foundation, Inc.

PO Box 1112
Phoenix, AZ 85001-1112
**Phone:** (602)230-2038
Daniel Cracchiolo, President

**Fnded:** 1980. **Philosophy:** Giving priorities are education and medical research. **Priorities:** *Arts & Humanities:* 23%. Phoenix Symphony, public libraries, and art museums. *Civic & Public Affairs:* 23%. *Education:* 28%. Mainly high schools and prep schools. *Environment:* 4%. Scouting and youth sports programs. *International:* 9%. Cancer treatment programs, heart research, and children's hospitals. *Religion:* 9%. Science centers and observatories. *Note:* Total contributions made in 1998. **Typ. Recipients:** AIDS/HIV, Arthritis, Cancer, Children's Health/Hospitals, Emergency/Ambulance Services, Eyes/Blindness, Health Organizations, Heart, Hospitals, Kidney, Medical Research, People with Disabilities, Prenatal Health Issues, Research/Studies Institutes, Sexual Abuse, Single-Disease Health Associations, Trauma Treatment. **Geo. Dist:** Phoenix, AZ.

### ★ 699 ★ Steele-Reese Foundation

32 Washington Square West
New York, NY 10011
**Phone:** (212)557-7700
William Buice, III, Co-Trustee

**Fnded:** 1955. **Philosophy:** Eleanor Steele Reese established the foundation to honor her and her husband's families. "The attitude behind their giving was as firm and unsentimental as every aspect of their lives on the ranch: they wanted to help people and organizations to help themselves, and they knew that mere handouts often weakened the recipients more than helping them. In developing the foundation's grant policies, the trustees have tried to reflect the personal philosophies of the Reeses." The foundation has a strong preference for projects benefiting rural areas and those directly affecting the people served. "The foundation tends to favor modest, essential, local projects rather than large-scale, glamorous ones." Annual Report **Priorities:** *Arts & Humanities:* 15%. Funds opera, libraries, historical associations, and arts councils. *Civic & Public Affairs:* 20%. Gives to community foundations and rural affairs. *Education:* 23%. Focus on colleges, universities, and primary education. *Environment:* 17%. Supports child welfare, community service organizations, food banks, and an animal foundation. *International:* 19%. Hospitals, hospice, single-disease health associations, and health clinics. *Note:* Total contributions made in fiscal 2000. **Typ. Recipients:** AIDS/HIV, Child Abuse, Clinics/Medical Centers, Emergency/Ambulance Services, Family Planning, Health-General, Heart, Hospices, Hospitals, Medical Rehabilitation, People with Disabilities, Public Health, Single-Disease Health Associations, Substance Abuse, Transplant Networks/Donor Banks. **Geo. Dist:** GA, Northern Georgia; ID; KY, Appalachian region of the state; MT; NC, Appalachian region of the state; TN, Appalachian region of the state; WA.

### ★ 700 ★ Stella and Charles Guttman Foundation
445 Park Ave., 19th Floor
New York, NY 10022
**Phone:** (212)371-7082　　**Fax:** (212)371-8936
**Email:** info@guttmanfdn.org
Elizabeth Olofson, Executive Director

**Fnded:** 1959. **Philosophy:** "The Foundation grant-making is focused on the following program areas: The Foundation funds efforts to improve the educational services available to New York City children and youth, from pre-school to high school. The Foundation also funds collaborative projects among public schools, non-profit education and community based agencies, and institutions of higher education that offer children, youth and their families additional academic and social support, in-school and after-school. The Foundation supports a wide range of traditional education, health and social service programs in Israel. In addition, the Foundation has in recent years supported social and educational programs for Arab Israelis and efforts to promote coexistence among Arabs and Jews in Israel. Through its special grants program, the Foundation is able to respond to project requests and address significant needs outside of its principal program areas. The Foundation also supports a number of cultural institutions that contribute to the quality of life in New York City." Funding Guidelines **Priorities:** *Arts & Humanities:* 3%. Supports public broadcasting, libraries, history, and journalism. *Civic & Public Affairs:* 1%. Supports safety, parks and botanical gardens. *Education:* 18%. Public education, education reform, minority education, faculty development, education, arts education and after school programs. *Environment:* 37%. Recreation and athletics, child welfare, youth organizations, Young Men's Christian Association, food distribution programs, emergency relief services, family planning services, and homes. *International:* 9%. Supports hospitals, AIDS, and emergency services. *Religion:* 2%. Supports science research. *Note:* Contributions made in 1998. **Typ. Recipients:** Adolescent Health Issues, AIDS/HIV, Alzheimers Disease, Cancer, Diabetes, Emergency/Ambulance Services, Family Planning, Geriatric Health, Heart, Hospitals, Medical Education, Medical Research, Mental Health, Nutrition, People with Disabilities, Prenatal Health Issues, Public Health, Single-Disease Health Associations, Substance Abuse. **Geo. Dist:** New York, NY, including metropolitan area.

### ★ 701 ★ Sterling-Turner Foundation
811 Rusk, Ste. 205
Houston, TX 77002-2807
**Phone:** (713)237-1117　　**Fax:** (713)223-4638
**Email:** eyvonne@wt.net
Eyvonne Moser, executive director

**Fnded:** 1956. **Philosophy:** The Sterling-Turner Foundation makes grants primarily in the areas of social services, the arts, and civic affairs. Social service funding favors recreation, youth organizations, the disabled, and child welfare. Funding for the arts includes opera, ballet, theater, and music; large grants are awarded to the Museum of Fine Arts in Houston, TX. Civic affairs interests include housing, zoos, and emergency services. The foundation funds other recipient areas on a limited basis. **Priorities:** *Arts & Humanities:* 15%. Supports arts and culture through museum of Fine Arts in Houston. *Education:* 22%. Supports schools, preschools, religious schools, edu-

cation center and other education organizations. *Environment:* 28%. Provides funding for children and youth services, emergency services, family violence shelters and services. *International:* 10%. Funds local hospice, University of Texas Medical Center and health foundations. *Note:* Total contributions made in 1999. **Typ. Recipients:** AIDS/HIV, Cancer, Children's Health/Hospitals, Clinics/Medical Centers, Emergency/Ambulance Services, Eyes/Blindness, Family Planning, Health Organizations, Hospices, Hospitals, Medical Education, Medical Research, Mental Health, People with Disabilities, Research/Studies Institutes, Single-Disease Health Associations, Speech & Hearing, Substance Abuse. **Geo. Dist:** TX. **Frmly:** Turner Charitable Foundation.

### ★ 702 ★ Stewardship Foundation
PO Box 1278
Tacoma, WA 98401-1278
**Phone:** (253)620-1340　　**Fax:** (253)572-2721
**Email:** info@stewardshipfdn.org
**Website:** http://www.stewardshipfdn.org
Dr. Cary Paine, Executive Director

**Fnded:** 1962. **Philosophy:** The foundation's main objective is to support evangelical Christian institutions whose primary goal is "to bring people into a relationship with God through faith in Jesus Christ." **Priorities:** *Civic & Public Affairs:* 11%. Funds public policy organizations and the National Center for Law and Religious Freedom. *Education:* 13%. Supports colleges, religious education, and leadership development. *Environment:* 13%. Grants funds to Christian youth and family organizations and food distribution agencies. *International:* 1%. Provides funding for the Mercy Medical Airlift. *Note:* Total contributions made in 1999. **Typ. Recipients:** Domestic Violence, Emergency/Ambulance Services, Family Planning, Medical Research, Mental Health, People with Disabilities, Public Health, Substance Abuse. **Geo. Dist:** nationally.

### ★ 703 ★ Stewart Huston Charitable Trust
Lukens Executive office Bldg.
50 S 1st Ave.
Coatesville, PA 19320
**Phone:** (610)384-2666　　**Fax:** (610)384-3396
**Website:** http://www.stewarthuston.org
Scott Huston, Executive Director

**Fnded:** 1989. **Philosophy:** "The purpose of the Trust is to supply funds, technical assistance and collaboration to corporations, of nonprofit associations, trusts, foundations and qualified organizations engaged exclusively in religious, charitable, or educational work; to extend opportunities to deserving, needy persons, and, in general, to promote the establishment of new and innovative religious, charitable, or educational projects." Sixty percent of the annual distributions from the trust are made, as stipulated by Mr. Stewart Huston's will, for the benefit of Trinitarian Evangelical activities. This includes activities carried on by Protestant churches and affiliated or related organizations that follow the Christian Gospel and exemplification of Christian principles through social welfare and other charitable endeavors. Forty percent of the annual distributions from the Trust are to be used for secular charitable activities within one 100 miles of Coatesville, PA. 1997 Annual Report **Priorities:** *Arts & Humanities:* 14%. Supports historical societies, arts outreach, music and libraries. *Civic & Public Affairs:* 27%. Emphasis on community foundations and municipal services. *Education:* 6%. Day schools, public and private education, and colleges. *Environment:* 22%. Community services, youth organizations, family planning, adoption services, and YMCAs. *International:* 3%. *Note:* Total contributions made in 1998. **Typ. Recipients:** AIDS/HIV, Child Abuse, Children's Health/Hospitals, Clinics/Medical Centers, Family Planning, Geriatric Health, Health-General, Medical Rehabilitation, Mental Health, Nursing Services, People with Disabilities, Substance Abuse, Trauma Treatment. **Geo. Dist:** Savannah, GA; PA, Chester County.

### ★ 704 ★ Stoddard Charitable Trust
370 Main St., 12th Floor
Worcester, MA 01608
**Phone:** (508)798-8621　　**Fax:** (508)791-6454
**Email:** wfletcher@ftwlaw.com
Warner Fletcher, Chairman

**Fnded:** 1939. **Philosophy:** The trust does not have a fixed policy regarding the distribution of its funds. It makes grants to organizations in the areas of education, medicine, religion, science, social services, the arts, and civic affairs. Priorities among these areas are apt to vary significantly from year to year. **Priorities:** *Arts & Humanities:* 25%. Museums, theater, and public broadcasting. *Civic & Public Affairs:* 7%. Housing programs, community development, and horticulture. *Education:* 20%. Private schools, colleges and universities, and Junior Achievement. *Environment:* 20%. United funds, renovation projects, community centers, and youth programs. *International:* 14%. Biomedical research and health services and centers. *Religion:* 8%. Biotechnology research. *Note:* Total contributions made in 1999. **Typ. Recipients:** Cancer, Children's Health/Hospitals, Clinics/Medical Centers, Family Planning, Health Funds, Health Organizations, Health-General, Home-Care Services, Hospices, Medical Education, Medical Research, People with Disabilities, Public Health, Sexual Abuse, Substance Abuse. **Geo. Dist:** Worcester, MA.

### ★ 705 ★ Strake Foundation
712 Main St., Ste. 3300
Houston, TX 77002-3291
**Phone:** (713)216-2400　　**Fax:** (713)216-2401
**Email:** foundation@strake.org
George Strake, Jr., President

**Fnded:** 1952. **Philosophy:** The foundation makes grants "primarily to Roman Catholic-affiliated associations, including hospitals and higher and secondary educational institutions; support also for the arts and social services, including programs for youth," primarily in Texas. Grants are made annually and are usually not long-term pledges. They are frequently made to projects whose funding is shared with other contributors. **Priorities:** *Arts & Humanities:* 13%. Cultural organizations. *Education:* 37%. Funds private secondary schools, colleges, and universities. *Environment:* 36%. Supports social services, youth programs, and the United Way. *International:* 10%. Supports hospitals, clinics, and single-disease associations. *Note:* Total contributions made in 2000. **Typ. Recipients:** Cancer, Children's Health/Hospitals, Clinics/Medical Centers, Health Organizations, Health Policy/Cost Containment, Heart, Hospices, Hospitals, Medical Education, Medical Rehabilitation, Medical Research, Mental Health, People with Disabilities, Prenatal Health Issues, Public Health, Single-Disease Health Associations, Speech & Hearing, Substance Abuse, Transplant Networks/Donor Banks. **Geo. Dist:** nationally; TX.

### ★ 706 ★ Stranahan Foundation
4159 Holland-Sylvania Rd., Ste. 206
Toledo, OH 43623
**Phone:** (419)882-5575　　**Fax:** (419)882-2072
**Email:** mail@stranahanfoundation.org
Pamela Roberts, Program Officer

**Fnded:** 1944. **Philosophy:** The foundation primarily supports education, health care, cultural organizations, and community initiatives in northwest Ohio. Preservation of the environment and public policy are secondary concerns. In addition, the foundation supports groups and institutions that give people the tools to become educated, healthy, self-reliant and contributing members of our society. **Priorities:** *Arts & Humanities:* 17%. Supports public broadcasting, music, museum, history, theater, and arts councils. *Civic & Public Affairs:* 5%. Supports clubs, safety, philanthropic organizations and community foundations. *Education:* 26%. Supports scholarship, technical education, after school/enrichment programs, medical education, tutoring, pre-school education, education funds, and minority education. *Environment:* 33%. Supports family planning services, united way, emergency relief, people with disabilities, child welfare, youth programs, and family services. *International:* 14%. Supports mental health, Alzheimers, hospital, hospice, preventative medicine, and medical research. *Religion:* 2%. Supports science labs. *Note:* Total contributions made in 1999. **Typ. Recipients:** AIDS/ HIV, Alzheimers Disease, Children's Health/Hospitals, Clinics/Medical Centers, Emergency/Ambulance Services, Eyes/Blindness, Family Planning, Geriatric Health, Health-General, Hospices, Hospitals, Medical Education, Mental Health, People with Disabilities, Preventive Medicine/Wellness Organizations, Respiratory. **Geo. Dist:** OH, Northwest Ohio.

### ★ 707 ★ Stratford Foundation

125 High St.
Boston, MA 02110
**Phone:** (617)248-7300 **Fax:** (617)248-7100
**Email:** wilsonpa@tht.com
Peter Wilson, Executive Director

**Fnded:** 1983. **Philosophy:** The foundation makes grants "primarily to institutions closely associated with the donor and the donor's family. However, non-donor grants are also actively considered." **Priorities:** *Arts & Humanities:* 17%. Support for museums and major support for the Heartland Film Festival. *Civic & Public Affairs:* 7%. Supports towns/municipalities. *Education:* 29%. Support for coleges and universities, including Christian institutions. *Environment:* 17%. Supports the United Way and other social service organizations. *International:* 7%. Support hospitals and single disease organizations. *Note:* Total contributions made in 1998. **Typ. Recipients:** Cancer, Cancer, Children's Health/Hospitals, Diabetes, Emergency/Ambulance Services, Health Funds, Health Organizations, Heart, Hospitals, Medical Research, People with Disabilities, Single-Disease Health Associations, Substance Abuse. **Geo. Dist:** Boston, MA.

### ★ 708 ★ Strauss Foundation

123 S Broad St., PA 1279
Philadelphia, PA 19109-1199
**Phone:** (215)670-4226 **Fax:** (215)670-4236
**Email:** reginald.middleton@firstunion.com
Reginald Middleton, Assistant Vice President

**Fnded:** 1951. **Philosophy:** The Strauss Foundation makes grants across the major categories of support. In social services, interests include youth camps and youth organizations. Art support favors museums and art institutes. Health-care funding supports medical centers, pediatrics, and research. Religious giving supports Jewish organizations and temples. The foundation also supports civic affairs. **Priorities:** *Arts & Humanities:* 20%. Supports performing arts, museums and public libraries. *Civic & Public Affairs:* 7%. Supports civic groups, including a zoological society. *Education:* 12%. Supports universities and educational opportunities for young people. *Environment:* 13%. Funds services impacting young people. *International:* 12%. Funds single-disease organizations. *Note:* Total contributions made in 1998. **Typ. Recipients:** AIDS/ HIV, Alzheimers Disease, Cancer, Clinics/Medical Centers, Diabetes, Health Organizations, Health Policy/Cost Containment, Health-General, Heart, Hospitals, Medical Education, Medical Research, People with Disabilities, Public Health, Single-Disease Health Associations, Substance Abuse, Transplant Networks/ Donor Banks, Trauma Treatment. **Geo. Dist:** PA.

### ★ 709 ★ Streisand Foundation

1460 Fourth St., Ste. 212
Santa Monica, CA 90401
**Phone:** (310)535-3767 **Fax:** (310)395-9676
**Email:** stfnd@aol.com
Christina Legg, Program Associate

**Fnded:** 1986. **Philosophy:** "Since its inception in 1986, the Streisand Foundation has made grants totaling nearly 10 million dollars. In the early years we have provided assistance to organizations working on the issues of nuclear disarmament, the preservation of the environment, voter education, and the protection of civil liberties and civil rights." "In 1993, the Foundation added additional priorities. We began focusing on women's, children's, and youth-related issues. Under these priorities, we provided assistance to an array of

organizations, including those working to protect the rights of women, and to provide social services to economically disadvantaged children." "Most recently, the Streisand Foundation has made grants to national organizations that promote and support: civil liberties and democratic values; women's issues including choice, pay equity and health-related issues; civil rights and race relations; AIDS research, advocacy, service and litigation; and children's and youth-related issues with a focus on the economically disadvantaged." 1997 Application Guidelines **Priorities:** *Arts & Humanities:* 10%. Funds museums, cinema, music, and literature. *Civic & Public Affairs:* 15%. Supports civil liberties, gay rights, women's advocacy, and democratic values. *Education:* 2%. Funds Teach for America and schools. *Environment:* 11%. Includes support for shelters, anti-violence projects, and human rights groups. *International:* 26%. Focus on women's health and single-disease organizations. *Note:* Total contributions made in 1999. **Typ. Recipients:** AIDS/ HIV, Alzheimers Disease, Cancer, Children's Health/ Hospitals, Domestic Violence, Emergency/Ambulance Services, Eyes/Blindness, Family Planning, Health Organizations, Health-General, Medical Research, Mental Health, Nutrition, Prenatal Health Issues, Research/Studies Institutes, Sexual Abuse, Transplant Networks/Donor Banks. **Geo. Dist:** nationally; Los Angeles, CA; New York, NY.

### ★ 710 ★ Stuart Foundations

50 California St., Ste. 3350
San Francisco, CA 94111
**Phone:** (415)393-1551 **Fax:** (415)393-1552
**Email:** info@stuartfoundation.org
**Website:** http://www.stuartfoundation.org
Theodore Lobman, President

**Fnded:** 1937. **Philosophy:** The Stuart Foundation supports efforts in California and Washington state to help children and youth become capable, responsible citizens. Grants are intended to improve policy and practice in the fields of public education, foster care, and family services. Activities supported include evaluated demonstrations, technical assistance to implement reforms, policy analysis, and advocacy. The foundations generally do not provide capital or general operating support for individual agencies. Most grants are made within three programs. Under Strengthening Public Schools, grants emphasize improving and institutionalizing on-going professional development and better methods for assessing student learning. Grants for Strengthening Systems that Serve Children, Youth, and Families focus on family support programs, including school-linked services and family preservation. Grants for Strengthening the Foster Care System are directed toward removing barriers to permanent placement and assuring that children receive the services they need. **Priorities:** *Civic & Public Affairs:* 20%. *Education:* 45%. *Environment:* 35%. Focus on family services, child welfare, and youth organizations. *International:* 2%. *Note:* Total contributions made in 2001. **Typ. Recipients:** Child Abuse, Children's Health/Hospitals, Children's Health/Hospitals, Clinics/ Medical Centers, Family Planning, Health Policy/Cost Containment, Medical Education, Medical Research, Public Health, Research/Studies Institutes, Sexual Abuse, Substance Abuse. **Geo. Dist:** CA; WA.

### ★ 711 ★ Sulzberger Foundation

229 West 43rd St.
Rm. 1031
New York, NY 10036
**Phone:** (212)556-1755 **Fax:** (212)556-3847
Marian Heiskell, President

**Fnded:** 1956. **Philosophy:** The Sulzberger Foundation makes most of its grants to environmental organizations, zoos and botanical gardens, the arts, and education. Funding categorized as environmental supports think tanks, wilderness councils, and trusts. Contributions to the arts favor museums, the performing arts, libraries, public broadcasting, and arts funds. Educational support goes to medical training, private schools, and education funds. The foundation makes grants to other recipient areas on a limited basis. **Priorities:** *Arts & Humanities:* 24%. Supports museums, public broadcasting, libraries, and theater. *Civic*

*& Public Affairs:* 15%. For foundations and community programs and botanical gardens parks *Education:* 19%. Universities, primary and secondary education, after school programs and study centers. *Environment:* 5%. Supports United Way, family planning services, food distribution programs, and day care. *International:* 4%. Supports cancer, medical centers, AIDS, and hospitals. *Religion:* 2%. Funds natural history museums. *Note:* Total contributions made in 1999. **Typ. Recipients:** AIDS/HIV, Cancer, Clinics/ Medical Centers, Family Planning, Health Organizations, Hospitals, Kidney, Medical Education, Medical Research, Mental Health, People with Disabilities, Sexual Abuse, Single-Disease Health Associations, Substance Abuse. **Geo. Dist:** nationally; internationally.

### ★ 712 ★ Surdna Foundation

330 Madison Ave., 30th Floor
New York, NY 10017-5001
**Phone:** (212)557-0010 **Fax:** (212)557-0003
**Email:** request@surdna.org
**Website:** http://www.surdna.org
Edward Skloot, Executive Director

**Fnded:** 1917. **Philosophy:** For many years, the principal beneficiary of the foundation was the Julia Dyckman Andrus Memorial, a children's home in Yonkers, NY, founded in 1928 in memory of Mrs. Andrus. Today, the foundation continues to provide support for the operations of the home, as well as for the John E. Andrus Memorial, a retirement home established in Hastings-on-Hudson, NY, in honor of Mr. Andrus. The foundation makes grants in four areas with the following objectives: *Environment:* to prevent irreversible damage to the environment; support government, private, and voluntary actions to sustain the environment; and foster a population of environmentally informed citizens. *Community Revitalization:* to increase the availability of affordable housing for low-income individuals; help the disadvantaged move from welfare dependence to economic independence; and strengthen families by enhancing and expanding early childhood initiatives for the zero-to-three population in both child care and parenting education. *Effective Citizenry:* to promote respect, empathy, fairness, and inclusivity in the way individuals and groups interact; motivate individuals to take active roles in their communities; help individuals work together effectively to create joint solutions to serious social and civic problems; and advance participatory decision making and governance in community institutions. *Arts:* to contribute to the ability of young people to explore both their identity and relationship to the world, through high-impact, long-term experiences with artists and the arts; and to deepen the ability of artists and arts organizations to contribute nationally to the needs of young people and educators. deepen the ability of artists and arts organizations to contribute nationally to the needs of young people and educators. **Priorities:** *Arts & Humanities:* 13%. Supports the performing arts, arts centers, and ats institutes. *Civic & Public Affairs:* 24%. Supports employment/job training, public policy, economic policy, business, community development, housing and ethnic organizations. *Education:* 24%. Supports arts/humaintes education, education funds, leadership training, faculty development, public education. *Environment:* 7%. Supports youth programs, daycare, child welfare, at-risk youth. *Note:* Total contributions made in 1999. **Typ. Recipients:** Health Organizations, Long-Term Care, Research/Studies Institutes. **Geo. Dist:** nationally.

### ★ 713 ★ Swalm Foundation

11511 Katy Freeway, Ste. 430
Houston, TX 77079
**Phone:** (281)497-5280 **Fax:** (281)497-7340
**Website:** http://www.swalm.org
Dr. Billy Ward, President

**Fnded:** 1980. **Philosophy:** The Swalm Foundation makes most of its grants in the areas of social services and health care. Social service interests include youth organizations, retirement centers, family services, and drug counseling and rehabilitation. Funding for health care favors rehabilitation centers, mental health, and hospices. The foundation also provides scholarships for dyslexic students. **Priorities:** *Arts & Humanities:* 5%. Funds arts museums. *Civic & Public Affairs:* 5%. Supports job training programs, affordable housing, and Hispanic affairs. *Education:* 12%. Educational programs for at-risk youth, public precollege education, and literacy programs. *Environment:* 66%. Supports programs to prevent child abuse, camps, women's centers, and shelters for the homeless. *International:* 9%. Focus on cancer and AIDS research, children's health programs, and medical clinics for the underserved. *Note:* Contributions made in fiscal 1999. **Typ. Recipients:** AIDS/HIV, Alzheimers Disease, Cancer, Child Abuse, Children's Health/Hospitals, Clinics/Medical Centers, Domestic Violence, Emergency/Ambulance Services, Eyes/Blindness, Family Planning, Health-General, Hospices, Hospitals, Medical Rehabilitation, Mental Health, People with Disabilities, Public Health, Research/Studies Institutes, Speech & Hearing, Substance Abuse. **Geo. Dist:** TX.

### ★ 714 ★ The Swig Foundation
220 Montgomery St., 20th Floor
San Francisco, CA 94104
**Phone:** (415)291-1100          **Fax:** (415)291-8373
Jackie Gianinnow, Foundation Assistant

**Fnded:** 1957. **Philosophy:** The foundation's main interest is promoting education, the arts, and schools for the arts. Other interests include zoological societies, recreational facilites and athletic foundations, and higher education. **Priorities:** *Arts & Humanities:* 16%. Major support to fine arts organization; also supports museums, opera, and art education. *Civic & Public Affairs:* 16%. Funds foundations, public policy. *Education:* 16%. Universities, theology, and precollege private education. *Environment:* 5%. Funds the United Way and other social service organizations. *International:* 19%. Medical centers and cancer research. *Note:* Contributions made in 1998. **Typ. Recipients:** Cancer, Child Abuse, Children's Health/Hospitals, Clinics/Medical Centers, Geriatric Health, Health Funds, Health Organizations, Hospitals, Hospitals (University Affiliated), Medical Research. **Geo. Dist:** CA; NY.

### ★ 715 ★ T. L. L. Temple Foundation
109 Temple Boulevard, Ste. 300
Lufkin, TX 75901
**Phone:** (936)639-5197          **Fax:** (936)634-3333
Wayne Corley, Executive Director

**Fnded:** 1962. **Philosophy:** The T. L. L. Temple Foundation looks favorably upon educational institutions located in the East Texas Pine Timber Belt area. The foundation also supports health care and human services, civic and public affairs, and provides limited funding for the arts. **Priorities:** *Arts & Humanities:* 2%. Supports museums and libraries. *Civic & Public Affairs:* 15%. Supports foundations and fire departments. *Education:* 48%. Supports adult education, colleges, and universities. *Environment:* 8%. Focus on substance abuse services, Special Olympics, women's services, and youth organizations. *International:* 25%. Supports hospitals, medical centers, and single-disease health associations. *Note:* Total contributions made in fiscal 1999. **Typ. Recipients:** Alzheimers Disease, Cancer, Children's Health/Hospitals, Clinics/Medical Centers, Domestic Violence, Emergency/Ambulance Services, Eyes/Blindness, Family Planning, Health Organizations, Heart, Hospices, Hospitals, Hospitals (University Affiliated), Kidney, Medical Education, Medical Rehabilitation, Medical Research, Mental Health, People with Disabilities, Prenatal Health Issues, Research/Studies Institutes, Single-Disease Health Associations, Substance Abuse, Transplant Networks/Donor Banks. **Geo. Dist:** TX, East Texas Pine Timber Belt area.

### ★ 716 ★ Teagle Foundation
10 Rockefeller Plaza, Room 920
New York, NY 10020-1903
**Phone:** (212)373-1970          **Fax:** (212)373-1984
Richard Kimball, Chief Executive Officer & President

**Fnded:** 1944. **Philosophy:** The foundation's major interest is private higher education, including nursing education and theological education, which it supports with project and program grants aimed at strengthening institutions and enhancing the total educational experience of their students. Most grant recipients have relatively small enrollments and modest financial resources. The foundation sponsors a competitive program of college and graduate school scholarships for children of employees of Exxon Corporation and its affiliates. It also makes a few grants to New York City agencies serving youth and matches the gifts of directors and employees to various organizations. In December 1995, the foundation announced its $4 million, invitational Collaborative Ventures Program to encourage institutions of higher learning to work together to make more effective use of academic, administrative, finacial, and physical resources. The first grants, totaling almost $1.5 million, were made in November 1996. **Priorities:** *Education:* 92%. Supports colleges and universities. *Note:* Total contributions made in fiscal 2000. **Typ. Recipients:** Emergency/Ambulance Services, Hospitals, Hospitals (University Affiliated), Medical Education. **Geo. Dist:** nationally.

### ★ 717 ★ Ted Mann Foundation
1801 Century Park East Ste. 1920
Los Angeles, CA 90067
**Phone:** (310)284-8528          **Fax:** (310)551-0604
**Email:** rkipper@usa.net
Rich Kipper, Financial Advisor

**Fnded:** 1985. **Philosophy:** The foundation gives to broad purposes, with emphasis on educational organizations, health care, and youth welfare. **Priorities:** *Arts & Humanities:* 1%. Funds public broadcasting. *Civic & Public Affairs:* 65%. Supports community foundations, housing, and private foundations. *Education:* 21%. Support for higher education, the Mann Center for Education, and education funds. *Environment:* 4%. Supports animal protection, child welfare, family services, and food banks. *International:* 4%. Emphasis on hospitals and medical research at universities. *Note:* Total contributions made in fiscal 2000. **Typ. Recipients:** AIDS/HIV, Alzheimers Disease, Cancer, Clinics/Medical Centers, Diabetes, Eyes/Blindness, Heart, Hospitals, Long-Term Care, Medical Education, Medical Research, Multiple Sclerosis, Preventive Medicine/Wellness Organizations, Public Health, Research/Studies Institutes, Single-Disease Health Associations, Speech & Hearing, Substance Abuse. **Geo. Dist:** nationally; Los Angeles, CA.

### ★ 718 ★ Temple Hoyne Buell Foundation
1666 South University Boulevard, Ste. B
Denver, CO 80210
**Phone:** (303)744-1688          **Fax:** (303)744-1601
**Email:** ssteele@buellfoundation.org
**Website:** http://www.buellfoundation.org
Susan Steele, Executive Director

**Fnded:** 1962. **Philosophy:** "The Temple Hoyne Buell Foundation is an active professional philanthropic organization supporting the healthy development of children, youth and families through grants and partnerships with other sectors of our community. In that regard, the foundation will focus primarily on the State of Colorado." "More emphasis will be placed on long-term programs or system changes that have demonstrated success in helping children thrive." Foundation Annual Report fiscal 1999. **Priorities:** *Arts & Humanities:* 3%. Includes a major grant to the Sangre de Cristo Arts and Conference Center and funding for children's arts & music education. *Civic & Public Affairs:* 8%. Primary support for the Cherokee Ranch and Castle Foundation. *Education:* 46%. Supports Head Start programs, 4-H, home schooling programs, Junior Achievement, and literacy. *Environment:* 32%. Funds programs promoting the social and emotional development of youth, and family stability. *International:* 6%. Emphasis on hospitals and medical centers that treat children and childhood diseases. *Note:* Total contributions made in fiscal 2000. **Typ. Recipients:** Cancer, Children's Health/Hospitals, Diabetes, Domestic Violence, Family Planning, Health Organizations, Heart, Hospitals, Kidney, Mental Health, People with Disabilities, Prenatal Health Issues, Preventive Medicine/Wellness Organizations, Public Health, Research/Studies Institutes, Single-Disease Health Associations, Speech & Hearing. **Geo. Dist:** CO.

### ★ 719 ★ Thelma Doelger Charitable Trust
950 John Daly Boulevard, Ste. 300
Daly City, CA 94015
**Phone:** (650)755-2333
Edward King, Trustee

**Fnded:** 1980. **Philosophy:** The trust traditionally supports California zoos and humane societies with large grants. **Priorities:** *Arts & Humanities:* 4%. Supports museum. *Civic & Public Affairs:* 35%. Supports San Francisco Zoological Society. *Education:* 5%. Supports Stanford University endowment. *Environment:* 35%. Supports animal protection organizations. *International:* 7%. Supports medical centers. *Note:* Total contributions made in 1999. **Typ. Recipients:** Clinics/Medical Centers, Hospitals, Speech & Hearing. **Geo. Dist:** CA, including Bay area.

### ★ 720 ★ Theodore H. Barth Foundation
45 Rockefeller Plaza, 20th Floor, Ste. 2037
New York, NY 10111
**Phone:** (212)332-3466
Ellen Berelson, President

**Fnded:** 1953. **Philosophy:** The foundation's interests focus on higher education, including scholarships; health and hospitals; conservation; Lutheran churches; youth organizations; and the arts. **Priorities:** *Arts & Humanities:* 30%. Funds public library, music, museums, and performing arts in New York City. *Civic & Public Affairs:* 8%. Funds the botanical garden. *Education:* 12%. Supports higher education. *Environment:* 11%. Primarily youth groups. *International:* 34%. Supports hospitals and single-disease health associations. *Note:* Total contributions made in 1998. **Typ. Recipients:** Children's Health/Hospitals, Clinics/Medical Centers, Family Planning, Health Funds, Health Organizations, Hospices, Hospitals, Kidney, Medical Research, Mental Health, Nursing Services, People with Disabilities, Public Health, Research/Studies Institutes, Single-Disease Health Associations, Speech & Hearing, Transplant Networks/Donor Banks. **Geo. Dist:** MA; NY.

### ★ 721 ★ Theresa A. Thomas Memorial Foundation
PO Box 1122
Richmond, VA 23218
**Phone:** (804)697-1200          **Fax:** (804)697-1399
**Email:** rgrier@maysval.com
Richard Grier, Assistant Secretary

**Fnded:** 1975. **Philosophy:** The mission of the foundation is to support organizations providing medical care or assistance with emphasis on primary care provided to medically underserved and uninsured populations within 100 miles of the Richmond Metropolitan area. **Priorities:** *Education:* 35%. Supports medical training. *Environment:* 9%. Camps, senior services, and rescue squads. *International:* 56%. Primarily for clinics and hospitals. *Note:* Total contributions made in fiscal 1999. **Typ. Recipients:** Children's Health/Hospitals, Clinics/Medical Centers, Emergency/Ambulance Services, Family Planning, Health-General, Heart, Home-Care Services, Hospitals, Medical Education, Public Health, Single-Disease Health Associations. **Geo. Dist:** VA.

### ★ 722 ★ Thomas and Agnes Carvel Foundation
35 East Grassy Sprain Rd.
Yonkers, NY 10710
**Phone:** (914)793-7300          **Fax:** (914)793-7381
Ann McHugh, Vice President

**Fnded:** 1976. **Philosophy:** The Thomas and Agnes Carvel Foundation makes most of its grants in the areas of health care and education. Health care funding favors cancer research, hospitals, and pediatric care. Funding for education emphasizes private secondary schools and religious education. **Priorities:** *Arts & Humanities:* 4%. Supports museums, theater, and music. *International:* 72%. Supports medical research, nursing, single-disease health associations, and hospitals. *Note:* Total contributions made in fiscal 2000. **Typ. Recipients:** Cancer, Children's Health/Hospitals, Clinics/Medical Centers, Domestic Violence, Emergency/Ambulance Services, Health-General, Hospices, Hospitals, Medical Rehabilitation, Medical Research, Nursing Services, Nutrition, Outpatient Health Care, Prenatal Health Issues, Prenatal Health Issues, Single-Disease Health Associations, Substance Abuse, Transplant Networks/Donor Banks. **Geo. Dist:** NY, Westchester County.


### ★ 723 ★ Thomas Anthony Pappas Charitable Foundation

PO Box 463
Belmont, MA 02478-0463
**Phone:** (781)862-2802
John Pappas, Director

**Fnded:** 1975. **Philosophy:** The foundation makes most of its grants in the areas of health, education, and the arts. Health interests include hospitals and single-disease associations. Educational funding favors dental schools, universities, technology, and law. Arts support goes primarily to performing arts centers. **Priorities:** *Arts & Humanities:* 2%. Focus on music, museums, and arts centers. *Education:* 64%. Supports colleges and specialized schools. *Environment:* 5%. Youth organizations and child welfare. *International:* 23%. Funds hospitals, single-disease health associations, and pediatric health. *Note:* Total contributions made in 1999. **Typ. Recipients:** Alzheimers Disease, Arthritis, Cancer, Children's Health/Hospitals, Clinics/Medical Centers, Eyes/Blindness, Health Organizations, Health-General, Heart, Hospices, Hospitals, Kidney, Long-Term Care, Medical Education, Medical Rehabilitation, Medical Research, Nursing Services, People with Disabilities, Research/Studies Institutes, Respiratory, Single-Disease Health Associations, Substance Abuse. **Geo. Dist:** MA.


### ★ 724 ★ Thomas and Dorothy Leavey Foundation

10100 Santa Monica Boulevard, Ste. 610
Los Angeles, CA 90067
**Phone:** (310)551-9936          **Fax:** (310)551-9938
Kathleen McCarthy, President

**Fnded:** 1952. **Philosophy:** The foundation originally was established to provide college scholarships. They have broadened their grant-making program to include medical research, churches, and civic groups. **Priorities:** *Civic & Public Affairs:* 2%. Civic and public affairs. *Education:* 60%. Supports higher education and scholarships, with major support going to Loyola Marymount University, and religious pre-college education. *Environment:* 5%. Family services, including those for youth and the elderly. *International:* 3%. Medical centers and hospitals. *Note:* Total contributions made in 1998. **Typ. Recipients:** AIDS/HIV, Cancer, Child Abuse, Children's Health/Hospitals, Clinics/Medical Centers, Domestic Violence, Emergency/Ambulance Services, Family Planning, Health Funds, Health Organizations, Hospitals, Long-Term Care, Medical Education, Medical Research, Nursing Services, People with Disabilities, Prenatal Health Issues, Public Health, Respiratory, Single-Disease Health Associations, Substance Abuse. **Geo. Dist:** Southern California, CA.


### ★ 725 ★ Thomas F. and Kate Miller Jeffress Memorial Trust

PO Box 26688
Richmond, VA 23261-6688
**Phone:** (804)788-3698          **Fax:** (804)788-2700
Dr. Richard Brandt, Advisor

**Fnded:** 1981. **Priorities:** *Religion:* 100%. Funding went to Virginia colleges and universities. The foundation focused its funding toward younger scientists (assistant professors) and change in research directions. *Note:* Contribution made in fiscal 1999. **Typ. Recipients:** Medical Education, Medical Research, Research/Studies Institutes. **Geo. Dist:** VA.


### ★ 726 ★ Thomas J. Emery Memorial

2120 Star Bank Ctr.
425 Walnut St.
Cincinnati, OH 45202
**Phone:** (513)241-5158          **Fax:** (513)651-8403
Lee Carter, Contact

**Fnded:** 1925. **Philosophy:** The memorial makes grants across the major categories of support. In social services, interests include united funds, homes, youth organizations, the disabled, child welfare, and community centers. Educational funding favors universities, high schools, day schools, and nursery schools in Cincinnati. Arts support goes to art institutes, museums, and public broadcasting. Health funding includes children's hospitals and hospices. The memorial also makes grants to other recipient areas. **Priorities:** *Arts & Humanities:* 34%. Supports art associations, theater, and performing arts. *Civic & Public Affairs:* 13%. Grants made to housing and economic development. *Education:* 23%. Funds public and private elementary schools, education funds, colleges, and day school. *Environment:* 13%. Gives to youth groups, shelters, united funds, and family services. *International:* 12%. Emphasis on hospitals, treatment centers, and children's health. *Note:* Total contributions made in 1998. **Typ. Recipients:** Cancer, Children's Health/Hospitals, Clinics/Medical Centers, Diabetes, Domestic Violence, Emergency/Ambulance Services, Family Planning, Health Organizations, Health-General, Hospices, Hospitals, Long-Term Care, Medical Rehabilitation, Mental Health, People with Disabilities, Prenatal Health Issues, Public Health, Research/Studies Institutes, Single-Disease Health Associations, Speech & Hearing, Substance Abuse, Transplant Networks/Donor Banks. **Geo. Dist:** Cincinnati, OH.


### ★ 727 ★ Thompson Charitable Foundation

4823 Old Kingston Pike
PO Box 10516
Knoxville, TN 37939-0516
**Phone:** (865)588-0491
Monica Luke, Foundation Manager

**Fnded:** 1987. **Philosophy:** The foundation's primary focus is health services and sciences, including hospitals and clinics, education, religion, culture, and human services. Major funding also supports capital campaigns and renovation projects for educational institutions. "Reflecting the concerns of the founder, the charitable trust supports programs that seek to improve the quality of life for individuals and communities." **Priorities:** *Arts & Humanities:* 1%. Supports theater groups. *Civic & Public Affairs:* 37%. Focus on Habitat for Humanity. *Education:* 28%. Community colleges, special education, and private precollege education. *Environment:* 16%. Family services, community services, and youth organizations. *International:* 18%. Clinics, hospice programs, and public health. *Note:* Total contributions made in fiscal 1999. **Typ. Recipients:** AIDS/HIV, Cancer, Child Abuse, Children's Health/Hospitals, Clinics/Medical Centers, Family Planning, Geriatric Health, Health-General, Hospices, Hospitals, Medical Rehabilitation, Nursing Services, People with Disabilities, Prenatal Health Issues, Preventive Medicine/Wellness Organizations, Preventive Medicine/Wellness Organizations, Public Health. **Geo. Dist:** KY, Bell County; KY, Clay County; KY, Laurel County; KY, Leslie County; TN, Anderson County; TN, Blount County; TN, Knox County; TN, Scott County; VA, Buchanan County; VA, Tazewell County.


### ★ 728 ★ Thoresen Foundation

2300 West Bay Dr.
Largo, FL 33770-1945
**Phone:** (813)585-1238          **Fax:** (813)581-3625
**Email:** pvoconn@aol.com
Paul O'Connell, Trustee

**Fnded:** 1952. **Priorities:** *Arts & Humanities:* 3% Supports local art festival. *Civic & Public Affairs:* 5%. Supports community foundation. *Education:* 51%. Supports education foundations, colleges and universities, and schools. *Environment:* 15%. Supports ser-

vices for the disabled, youth programs, and athletics. *International:* 8%. Supports emergency care and physician's groups. *Note:* Contributions were made in 2000. **Typ. Recipients:** Cancer, Clinics/Medical Centers, Emergency/Ambulance Services, Health Organizations, Health-General, Home-Care Services, People with Disabilities, Research/Studies Institutes, Respiratory. **Geo. Dist:** FL; IL; NC; VA.


### ★ 729 ★ Tisch Foundation

655 Madison Ave.
New York, NY 10021
**Phone:** (212)521-2930          **Fax:** (212)521-2983
Barry Bloom, Chief Financial Officer

**Fnded:** 1957. **Philosophy:** The foundation was established in 1957 and emphasizes higher education and research programs. It supports Jewish organizations and welfare funds, museums, and secondary schools. It also supports institutions in Israel. **Priorities:** *Arts & Humanities:* 14%. Supports art museums, symphony, theater, and historical preservation. *Civic & Public Affairs:* 5%. Supports community foundations, zoo and gardens. *Education:* 25%. Supports colleges and universities. *Environment:* 7%. Funds family and childrens services organizations, provides aid to the homeless, hungry, and indigent. *International:* 30%. Supports hospitals, medical centers, and medical research organizations. *Note:* Total contributions made in 1998. **Typ. Recipients:** AIDS/HIV, Cancer, Children's Health/Hospitals, Clinics/Medical Centers, Diabetes, Emergency/Ambulance Services, Family Planning, Health Funds, Hospitals, Hospitals (University Affiliated), Long-Term Care, Medical Education, Medical Research, People with Disabilities, Research/Studies Institutes, Single-Disease Health Associations. **Geo. Dist:** nationally; New York, NY.


### ★ 730 ★ Tozer Foundation

First National Bank Bldg.
332 Minnesota St.
Saint Paul, MN 55101
**Phone:** (651)244-0924
Kim Phillips, Contact

**Fnded:** 1946. **Philosophy:** The foundation's primary focus is to provide scholarships for college students. Applications are made usually by seniors at their high school, and recipients are selected on the basis of ability and need by a scholarship committee appointed by the foundation. The scholarships may be renewed annually. Grants are made for educational and other charitable purposes, such as social service organizations and the arts. Most of the funding for social services is awarded to the United Way and youth organizations. Arts funding favors the performing arts in music and theater. The foundation also supports public school districts, civic affairs, health, and religion with smaller grants. **Priorities:** *Education:* About 76%. Supports scholarship programs at colleges and universities. *Note:* Total contributions made in fiscal 1999. **Typ. Recipients:** Clinics/Medical Centers, Hospitals, Medical Rehabilitation. **Geo. Dist:** MN, Kanabec County for scholarship program; MN, Pine County for scholarship program; MN, Washington County for scholarship program.


### ★ 731 ★ The Trull Foundation

404 Fourth St.
Palacios, TX 77465
**Phone:** (512)972-5241          **Fax:** (512)972-1109
**Email:** trullfdn@wcnet.net
**Website:** http://www.trullfoundation.org
Gail Purvis, Executive Director

**Fnded:** 1948. **Philosophy:** "For over forty years (the foundation has) been actively interested in various educational, religious, cultural and social programs, the majority of which have been in the State of Texas. (The foundation has) supported Presbyterian interests, without, however, being limited to those interests. (The foundation has) been concerned with people, with improving the quality of life, especially for those living in poor or oppressed conditions. Currently, the following priorities are set by the Trustees: °A concern for the needs of the Palacios area, where the Foundation has its roots. The senior citizens center, the city paving needs, the Marine Education Center, and other local projects were considered and supported.' °A concern for the pre-adolescent and their families, with special emphasis of family values. Grants were given to help direct and channel lives away from child abuse, from neglect, from hunger, and into an adolescence of good mental and physical growth.' °A concern for Hispanic issues, especially in South Texas. Grants have been made to help hurdle the language barrier, the poverty barrier, and a system which has consistently kept them poor, uneducated and unrepresented.' °A concern for those persons and families devastated by the results of substance abuse.'" 1995-1996 Annual Report **Priorities:** *Arts & Humanities:* 9%. Primary support for historical associations, public broadcasting, and libraries. *Civic & Public Affairs:* 19%. Supports municipalities, population control, and women's issues. *Education:* 45%. Focus on elementary and secondary education, colleges and universities, scholarships, and seminaries. *Environment:* 8%. Supports family services, child welfare, and youth organizations. *International:* 2%. Supports hospitals. *Note:* Total contributions made in 1999. **Typ. Recipients:** AIDS/HIV, Cancer, Children's Health/Hospitals, Domestic Violence, Family Planning, Health Organizations, Health-General, Medical Education, Medical Rehabilitation, Medical Research, Mental Health, Nutrition, Preventive Medicine/Wellness Organizations, Public Health, Substance Abuse. **Geo. Dist:** nationally, although Texas is given preference; TX.

## ★ 732 ★ Tull Charitable Foundation

Hurt Bldg.
50 Hurt Plaza, Ste. 1245
Atlanta, GA 30303
**Phone:** (404)659-7079          **Fax:** (404)659-1223
Ms. Barbara Cleveland, Executive Director

**Fnded:** 1952. **Philosophy:** The foundation trustees prefer to make grants that will "have a significant and lasting impact on an organization as well as its community." The primary focus of the foundation is to respond to needs in Georgia, particularly in the Atlanta metropolitan area, that are strategically important to an organization's growth and capacity, enable the organization to more effectively address important community needs, and are cost-effective. The foundation's areas of primary interest are education, health and human services, civic and community affairs, youth development, and the arts. **Priorities:** *Arts & Humanities:* 3%. Funds arts and culture through history center and symphony orchestra. *Civic & Public Affairs:* 33%. Supports civic and community affairs through housing organizations, junior league and parks. *Education:* 34%. Supports education and youth development through schools, academies, colleges and universities. *Environment:* 19%. Supports boys and girls clubs, homes, youth services and United Way. *International:* 3%. Funds mental health and spinal health. *Religion:* 4%. Supports natural science centers. *Note:* Total contributions made in 2000. **Typ. Recipients:** Alzheimers Disease, Cancer, Children's Health/Hospitals, Clinics/Medical Centers, Domestic Violence, Emergency/Ambulance Services, Eyes/Blindness, Family Planning, Health Organizations, Hospitals, Long-Term Care, Medical Education, Medical Research, Mental Health, Nursing Services, People with Disabilities, Prenatal Health Issues, Public Health, Research/Studies Institutes, Single-Disease Health Associations, Substance Abuse. **Geo. Dist:** GA.

## ★ 733 ★ Turner Foundation

1 CNN Center, Ste. 1090, South Tower
Atlanta, GA 30303
**Phone:** (404)681-9900          **Fax:** (404)681-0172
**Website:** http://www.turnerfoundation.org
Mike Finley, President

**Fnded:** 1990. **Philosophy:** "The Turner Foundation is committed to preventing damage to the natural systems–water, air, and land–on which all life depends." "The foundation makes grants primarily in the areas of the environment and population. The main components of our program are: protection of water and reduction of toxics; improved air quality through promotion of energy efficiency and renewables, and improved transportation policies and practices; protec-

tion of habitats; development and implementation of sound, equitable practices and policies designed to reduce population growth rates." 1996 Annual Grants List Brochure **Priorities:** *Arts & Humanities:* 5%. *Civic & Public Affairs:* 24%. Community development, housing, and women's organizations *Education:* 4%. Universities and research associates. *Environment:* 8%. Pregnancy prevention and family services. *International:* 1%. Centers for disease control and prevention. *Note:* Total contributions made in 1998. **Typ. Recipients:** Adolescent Health Issues, Family Planning, Hospitals, Medical Research, Mental Health, Preventive Medicine/Wellness Organizations. **Geo. Dist:** nationally.

## ★ 734 ★ Valley Foundation

16450 Los Gatos Boulevard, Ste. 210
Los Gatos, CA 95032-5594
**Phone:** (408)358-4545          **Fax:** (408)358-4548
**Email:** applications@valley.org
**Website:** http://www.valley.org
Ervie Smith, Executive Director

**Fnded:** 1984. **Philosophy:** "...the Highest priority...is to provide targeted funding for qualified charitable organizations serving the health care needs of lower income households in Santa Clara County...in the areas of medical research, higher education, social service, programs for youth, aid to senior citiziens, and the arts." The Valley Foundation 2000 Annual Report. **Priorities:** *Arts & Humanities:* 19%. *Education:* 20%. Supports health-related education. *Environment:* 35%. *International:* 26%. *Note:* Contributions analysis from Annual Report for fiscal 2000. **Typ. Recipients:** Adolescent Health Issues, AIDS/HIV, Alzheimers Disease, Cancer, Child Abuse, Children's Health/Hospitals, Clinics/Medical Centers, Diabetes, Domestic Violence, Emergency/Ambulance Services, Geriatric Health, Health Funds, Health Organizations, Health-General, Heart, Hospices, Medical Education, Medical Rehabilitation, Medical Research, Mental Health, Nutrition, People with Disabilities, Prenatal Health Issues, Preventive Medicine/Wellness Organizations, Public Health, Single-Disease Health Associations, Substance Abuse. **Geo. Dist:** CA, Santa Clara County.

## ★ 735 ★ Van Houten Memorial Fund (Edward W. and Stella C.)

190 River Rd., NJ3132
Summit, NJ 07901
**Phone:** (908)598-3577          **Fax:** (908)598-3583
**Email:** talisaifezue@firstunion.com
Ta'Lisa Ifezue, Trust Associate

**Fnded:** 1979. **Philosophy:** The Edward W. and Stella C. Van Houten Memorial Fund provides grants in the areas of human service activities, health care, and higher education. Health care funding favors hospitals and health foundations. Funding for education supports scholarships for medicine and dentistry training. In social services, interests include children's homes, child welfare, and youth organizations. Health and human services are funded in Bergen and Passaic counties only. Children's service organizations and medical and dental scholarships are funded statewide. **Priorities:** *Civic & Public Affairs:* About 3%. *Education:* About 25%. Primary consideration given to accredited medical schools and nursing institutions for assistance in medical, nursing, and child care programs. *Environment:* 10%. Limited to services in Bergen and Passaic counties in New Jersey. Priorities include orphaned/abandoned children, the disabled, and the elderly. *International:* 60% Limited to agencies, hospitals, and healthcare facilities with services located in Bergen and Passaic counties in New Jersey. **Typ. Recipients:** Cancer, Children's Health/Hospitals, Clinics/Medical Centers, Family Planning, Geriatric Health, Hospitals, Hospitals (University Affiliated), Medical Education, Medical Rehabilitation, Medical Research, Mental Health, Multiple Sclerosis, Prenatal Health Issues, Respiratory, Single-Disease Health Associations. **Geo. Dist:** NJ, Bergen County; NJ, Passaic County; NY; PA, children's programs are funded statewide.

## ★ 736 ★ Victor E. Speas Foundation

Bank of America
14 W Tenth St.
Kansas City, MO 64105
**Phone:** (816)979-7481          **Fax:** (816)979-7916
David Ross, Senior Vice President

**Fnded:** 1947. **Philosophy:** The foundation focuses on health and social service programs. It emphasizes the improvement of health-related services in the greater Kansas City metropolitan area. **Priorities:** *Civic & Public Affairs:* 20%. Neighborhood programs and programs that support business/free enterprise. *Education:* 9%. Support for colleges in Kansas City. *Environment:* 54%. Volunteer programs, Goodwill, and family projects, mainly in the Kansas City, MO, area. *International:* 5%. Health education, hospitals, and single-disease health organizations, with an emphasis on children. *Note:* Contributions made in 1998. **Typ. Recipients:** AIDS/HIV, Cancer, Children's Health/Hospitals, Clinics/Medical Centers, Emergency/Ambulance Services, Geriatric Health, Health Funds, Health Organizations, Health Policy/Cost Containment, Heart, Home-Care Services, Hospitals, Medical Education, Medical Rehabilitation, Mental Health, Nursing Services, Nutrition, People with Disabilities, Public Health, Research/Studies Institutes, Sexual Abuse, Single-Disease Health Associations, Speech & Hearing, Substance Abuse, Trauma Treatment. **Geo. Dist:** Kansas City, MO, metropolitan area.

## ★ 737 ★ Vira I. Heinz Endowment

30 Dominion Tower
625 Liberty Ave.
Pittsburgh, PA 15222-3199
**Phone:** (412)281-5777          **Fax:** (412)281-5788
**Email:** info@heinz.org
**Website:** http://www.heinz.org
Maxwell King, Executive Director

**Fnded:** 1986. **Philosophy:** "Throughout their histories, the Howard and Vira I. Heinz Endowments have been privileged to enjoy a remarkable intimate relationship with the communities and organizations they serve. From this relationship continually emerge two of the Endowments' primary strengths: their sensitivity to the needs of their region, and their willingness to shoulder risks on its behalf. It has been characteristic of the Endowments to want to listen and respond personally to requests for help. We are neighbors, after all, not disinterested observers. For that reason, there has been a reluctance over the years to print formalized program guidelines, suggesting as they might an unfeeling institutionalization of process." "We do not intend for that to happen. But we also appreciate how dramatically the philanthropic landscape has changed in recent years. With the demand for philanthropic resources increasing rapidly and with ever greater urgency, we must respond to the call from prospective grantseekers for guidance, specificity and direction....The Endowments' present grantmaking reflects over half a century of applied values and experiential learning. Three signature themes emerge from this rich history: leadership, cooperation and enterprise." *A Message from the Executive Director* **Priorities:** *Arts & Humanities:* 21%. Supports theater, history, museum of art,dance, ballet, the performing arts, libraries, opera, and arts councils. *Civic & Public Affairs:* 30%. Supports employment/job training, rural affairs, urban/community affairs, economic development, municipalities/towns, and philanthropic organizations. *Education:* 15%. Supports school, science education, colleges, universities, after school programs, and economic education. *Environment:* 7%. Supports Big Brothers/Big Sisters, scouts, child services, recreatio/athletics, at-risk youth, and United Way. *International:* 1%. Supports cancer and medical research. *Note:* Total contributions made in 1998. **Typ. Recipients:** Cancer, Children's Health/Hospitals, Domestic Violence, Family Planning, Geriatric Health, Health Organizations, Health Policy/Cost Containment, Hospitals, Medical Education, Medical Research, Mental Health, Sexual Abuse, Single-Disease Health Associations, Substance Abuse. **Geo. Dist:** PA, Southwest Pennsylvania.

## ★ 738 ★ W. Alton Jones Foundation

232 East High St.
Charlottesville, VA 22902-5178
**Phone:** (804)295-2134 **Fax:** (804)295-1648
**Email:** earth@wajones.org
**Website:** http://www.wajones.org
Dr. J. Myers, Director

**Fnded:** 1944. **Philosophy:** The foundation supports efforts to identify and implement solutions to challenges facing humankind which fall into their two program areas: the Secure World Program and the Sustainable Society Program. The first program area emphasizes the need to maintain security while inhibiting the spread of nuclear weapons. The second area focuses on widespread patterns of toxic contamination, sustainment of biological diversity, and climate stabilization through forest protection and appropriate energy policies. In both areas the foundation provides support for programs that identify specific steps to improve the quality and implementation of public policy. The foundation is particularly interested in programs which educate and organize citizens at the grassroots level. Projects which heighten and improve media coverage of the above issues are also encouraged. Other types of activities supported include results-oriented scholarship and research, litigation, and education for policy makers. **Priorities:** *Civic & Public Affairs:* 7%. Funds public policy institutes and associations. *Note:* Total contributions made in 1998. **Typ. Recipients:** Cancer, Children's Health/Hospitals, Medical Education, Mental Health, Respiratory, Substance Abuse.

## ★ 739 ★ W. K. Kellogg Foundation

One Michigan Ave. East
Battle Creek, MI 49017-4058
**Phone:** (616)968-1611 **Fax:** (616)968-0413
**Website:** http://www.wkkf.org

**Fnded:** 1930. **Philosophy:** The W.K. Kellogg Foundation was established in 1930 "to help people help themselves through the practical application of knowledge and resources to improve their quality of life and that of future generations." Its programming activities center around the common visions of a world in which each person has a sense of worth; accepts responsibility for self, family, community, and societal wellbeing; and has the capacity to be productive, and to help create nurturing families, responsive institutions, and healthy communities. To achieve the greatest impact, the foundation targets its grants toward specific focal points or areas. These include health; food systems and rural development; youth development and education, and higher education; and philanthropy and volunteerism. When woven throughout these areas, funding also is provided for leadership; information systems/technology; efforts to capitalize on diversity; and family, neighborhood, and community development programming. Grants are concentrated in the United States, Latin America, the Caribbean, and southern Africa. **Priorities:** *Civic & Public Affairs:* 6%. Social & economic development in the greater Battle Creek MI area. *Education:* 34%. Funds colleges and universities also supports public school systems, education foundations, leadership development, other schools and academics. *Environment:* 6%. Support youth services. *International:* 30%. Healthcare systems organized around public health, prevention, and primary care. *Note:* Total contributions made in fiscal 2000. **Typ. Recipients:** Children's Health/Hospitals, Clinics/Medical Centers, Geriatric Health, Health Organizations, Health Policy/Cost Containment, Hospices, Hospitals, Medical Education, Medical Research, Medical Training, Mental Health, Nursing Services, Nutrition, People with Disabilities, Prenatal Health Issues, Public Health, Research/Studies Institutes, Substance Abuse. **Geo. Dist:** nationally; Caribbean; Latin America.

## ★ 740 ★ W. M. Keck Foundation

555 South Hope St., Ste. 2500
Los Angeles, CA 90071
**Phone:** (213)680-3833 **Fax:** (213)614-0934
**Email:** info@wmkeck.org
**Website:** http://www.wmkeck.org
Maria Pellegrini, Program Director

**Fnded:** 1954. **Philosophy:** The Foundation's grantmaking is focused primarily on the areas of medical research, science, and engineering at colleges and universities nationwide. The Foundation also maintains a program for liberal arts colleges and a Southern California Grant Program that provides support in the areas of civic and community services, health care and hospitals, precollegiate education, and the arts. **Priorities:** *Arts & Humanities:* 3%. Funds public broadcasting. *Civic & Public Affairs:* 2%. Supports community foundation. *Education:* 81%. Supports colleges and universities. *Environment:* 5%. Supports scouting, children's welfare, and United Way. *International:* 7%. Funds clinics and hospitals. *Religion:* 2%. Supports Discovery museum. *Note:* Total contributions made in 1998. **Typ. Recipients:** Clinics/Medical Centers, Geriatric Health, Hospitals, Medical Education, Medical Rehabilitation, Medical Research, People with Disabilities, Speech & Hearing, Substance Abuse. **Geo. Dist:** nationally; CA, southern CA.

## ★ 741 ★ W. O'Neil Foundation

730 Barlow Bldg.
5454 Wisconsin Ave.
Chevy Chase, MD 20815
**Phone:** (301)656-5848
Helene O'Neil Cobb, Vice Chairman, Vice
    President, Assistant

**Fnded:** 1948. **Philosophy:** Grants are given primarily to Catholic organizations for international emergency relief and for programs that bring food, clothing, shelter, basic medical care, and basic education to the poor of the world, preferably though projects that help the poor to help themselves toward these goals. **Priorities:** *Civic & Public Affairs:* 3%. *Education:* 8%. Primarily for private schools. *International:* 5%. Medical clinics and mental health. *Note:* Total contributions made in 1999. **Typ. Recipients:** AIDS/HIV, Emergency/Ambulance Services, Geriatric Health, Health Funds, Hospitals, Long-Term Care, Mental Health, People with Disabilities. **Geo. Dist:** nationally.

## ★ 742 ★ W. W. Smith Charitable Trust

3515 West Chester Pike, Ste. E
Newtown Square, PA 19073
**Phone:** (610)359-1811 **Fax:** (610)359-9717
Frances Tyler, Administrator

**Fnded:** 1977. **Philosophy:** The trust supports four specific programs areas: medical research for heart disease, cancer, and AIDS; hospital indigent medical care; food, clothing, and shelter for children and the aged; and college financial aid. The trust funds research projects for heart disease, cancer, and AIDS that are new or are conducted by investigators before they have qualified for larger National Institutes of Health grants. In its program to provide medical care for the poor and needy, the trust supports hospitals in the cities of Chester and Philadelphia, with an explicit policy of accepting patients with no ability to pay. In its program to provide food, clothing, and shelter for children and the aged, the trust attempts to assist under-supported groups, including ethnic minorities, the elderly, orphans, and abused women and children. It is particularly interested in programs offering respite care to the elderly and in those benefiting older single women who live alone. The trust also supports financial aid programs for college students, prizes for college seniors, and scholarships through the Sea Education Association in Woods Hole, MA. **Priorities:** *Education:* 60%. Scholarships and student aid. *Environment:* 9%. Community services organizations, homeless shelters, and domestic violence. *International:* 26%. AIDS/HIV research, geriatric health, and emergency health care. *Note:* Total contributions made in fiscal 1999. **Typ. Recipients:** AIDS/HIV, Cancer, Diabetes, Domestic Violence, Emergency/Ambulance Services, Geriatric Health, Health Organizations, Heart, Home-Care Services, Hospitals, Long-Term Care, Medical Education, Medical Research, Nursing Services, People with Disabilities, Prenatal Health Issues, Single-Disease Health Associations. **Geo. Dist:** Philadelphia, PA, six-county Philadelphia regional area.

## ★ 743 ★ W. W. W. Foundation

625 Fair Oaks Ave., Ste. 360
South Pasadena, CA 91030
**Phone:** (626)441-5188 **Fax:** (626)441-3672
Linda Blinkenberg, Secretary & Director

**Fnded:** 1981. **Priorities:** *Arts & Humanities:* 5%. Supports a theater. *Education:* 12%. Colleges and universities. *Environment:* 83%. Majority to Helen Woodward Animal Care Center, and the I Have a Dream Foundation. *Note:* Total contributions made in fiscal 1999. **Typ. Recipients:** Child Abuse, Eyes/Blindness, Hospitals, Medical Research, Substance Abuse. **Geo. Dist:** CA, Southern California.

## ★ 744 ★ The Wagnalls Memorial Foundation

150 East Columbus St.
Lithopolis, OH 43136
**Phone:** (614)833-4767 **Fax:** (614)833-4767
**Email:** jneff@clc.lib.oh.us
**Website:** http://www.wagnalls.org
Jerry Neff, Executive Director

**Fnded:** 1924. **Philosophy:** The Wagnalls Scholarship Fund, where most of the funding is given, was established "to encourage and assist student residents of Bloom Township and otherwise eligible to obtain a degree in higher education." The foundation makes grants for undergraduate and post-graduate study. **Priorities:** *Civic & Public Affairs:* 6%. Community projects. *Education:* 94%. Student aid for Lithopolis and Bloom Township, OH, residents. *Note:* Contributions made in fiscal 1998. **Typ. Recipients:** Medical Education. **Geo. Dist:** Bloom Township, OH; Lithopolis, OH.

## ★ 745 ★ Wallace Alexander Gerbode Foundation

470 Columbus Ave., Ste. 209
San Francisco, CA 94133-3930
**Phone:** (415)391-0911 **Fax:** (415)391-4587
**Email:** maildesk@gerbode.org
**Website:** http://fdncenter.org/grantmaker/gerbode
Thomas Layton, President

**Fnded:** 1953. **Philosophy:** The foundation is interested in programs and projects offering potential for significant impact. The primary focus is on the San Francisco Bay area and Hawaii. Interests generally fall under the following categories: arts and culture, environment, population, reproductive rights, citizen participation/building communities/inclusiveness, strength of the philanthropic process and the nonprofit sector, and special projects. **Priorities:** *Arts & Humanities:* 16%. Grants are made to dance, theater, and public broadcasting. *Civic & Public Affairs:* 38%. Issues related to reproductive rights, aid in dying, educational forums, ethnic organizations, and community foundations are funded. *Education:* 4%. Supports universities. *Environment:* 27%. Funding is provided to pro-choice organizations. *Note:* Total contributions made in 1998. **Typ. Recipients:** Children's Health/Hospitals, Domestic Violence, Family Planning, Health Organizations, Health Policy/Cost Containment, Health-General, Hospices, Long-Term Care, People with Disabilities, Public Health. **Geo. Dist:** San Francisco, CA, including Bay area; HI.

## ★ 746 ★ Wallace Genetic Foundation

4900 Massachusetts Ave., Northwest, Ste. 220
Washington, DC 20016
**Phone:** (202)966-2932 **Fax:** (202)966-3370
**Email:** wgfdn@aol.com
**Website:** http://www.wallacegenetic.org
Pat Lee, Co-Executive Director

**Fnded:** 1959. **Philosophy:** Grants are almost entirely limited to organizations associated with the personal interests of present or former trustees which include sustainable agriculture preservation of farmland nearcities, ecology, plant genetic research, biodiversity protection and environmental education. **Priorities:** *Civic & Public Affairs:* 21%. Supports botanical gardens, league of conservation voters, public policy organizations. *Environment:* 5%. Supports animal welfare organizations. *International:* 5%. Supports medical center, childen's hospitals. *Note:* Total contributions made in 1999. **Typ. Recipients:** Cancer, Children's Health/Hospitals, Clinics/Medical Centers, Family Planning, Health Organizations, Health-General, Heart, Hospitals, Hospitals (University Affiliated), Medical Education, Medical Research, Nursing Services, Nutrition, Public Health, Respiratory, Single-Disease Health Associations. **Geo. Dist:** internationally; nationally.

**★ 747 ★ Wallis Foundation**
1880 Century Park East, Ste. 700
Los Angeles, CA 90067
**Phone:** (310)286-9777     **Fax:** (310)826-4476
**Email:** mark@mggcpa.com
Mark Augenstin, Chief Financial Officer & Director
**Fnded:** 1959. **Philosophy:** "The foundation's purpose of all grants and contributions is to aid and promote charitable, educational, scientific, literary and religious projects as well as the arts." 1996 **Priorities:** *Arts & Humanities:* 19%. Supports museums, music, orchestras, and ballet. *Civic & Public Affairs:* 5%. Supports zoos, police foundations, and gardens. *Education:* 13%. Supports private schools, universities, and education foundations. *Environment:* 3%. Funds Boys/Girls clubs, a food bank, and family planning. *International:* 3%. Supports hospitals. *Religion:* 11%. Supports a science museum. *Note:* Total contributions made in 1999. **Typ. Recipients:** AIDS/HIV, Cancer, Cancer, Children's Health/Hospitals, Clinics/Medical Centers, Emergency/Ambulance Services, Health Organizations, Health-General, Hospices, Hospitals, Medical Education, Medical Rehabilitation, Medical Research, Mental Health, Single-Disease Health Associations, Substance Abuse. **Geo. Dist:** CA.

**★ 748 ★ Walter and Elise Haas Fund**
1 Lombard St., Ste. 305
San Francisco, CA 94111-1130
**Phone:** (415)398-4474     **Fax:** (415)986-4779
**Website:** http://www.haassr.org
Bruce Sievers, Executive Director, Secretary & Treasure
**Fnded:** 1953. **Philosophy:** The fund supports a wide variety of programs and activities, primarily in the San Francisco Bay area. According to the late Rhoda H. Goldman, daughter of Walter and Elise Haas and former president of the fund, "we are interested in local programs which promise expansion of access to human services and public affairs, to the arts, humanities, and education." Other priorities include health care and the environment. Grants to the arts include almost every form of performing, literary, and fine arts. Emphasis is placed on extending artistic and cultural programs to children and to the Bay Area community at large. Involvement in civic affairs includes a commitment to projects which are distinguished by imagination and leadership, to the strengthening of important nonprofit institutions, and to citizenship and community service. The fund has shown particular interest in community and service organizations which demonstrate creativity and effectiveness in their approach to meeting human needs, and which encourage individual initiative. The fund also administers the Creative Work Fund for the support of new work in the arts, and a Citizenship and Civic Education program. **Priorities:** *Arts & Humanities:* 13%. Supports museum, visual arts, music, theater, performing arts, dance, opera, and arts festivals. *Civic & Public Affairs:* 23%. Supports women's affairs, philanthropic organizations, civil rights, community foundations. *Education:* 8%. Supports faculty development, school, after school programs, religious education, and minority education. *Environment:* 19%. Funds Big Brothers/Big Sisters, community service organizations, youth organizations, community centers, and family planning services, and United Way. *International:* 1%. Funds mental health. *Note:* Total contributions made in 1998. **Typ. Recipients:** AIDS/HIV, Children's Health/Hospitals, Clinics/Medical Centers, Diabetes, Domestic Violence, Family Planning, Health Organizations, Health-General, Hospitals, Long-Term Care, Mental Health, People with Disabilities, Prenatal Health Issues, Public Health, Substance Abuse. **Geo. Dist:** some national giving;

CA, Alameda County; CA, Marin County; CA, San Mateo County; San Francisco, CA, the Bay area.

**★ 749 ★ Walter and Josephine Ford Fund**
100 Renaissance Center, 34th Floor
Detroit, MI 48243
**Phone:** (313)259-7777     **Fax:** (313)393-7579
David Hempstead, Secretary & Trustee
**Fnded:** 1951. **Philosophy:** The fund reports that "grants are generally limited to charitable organizations already favorably known to, and of interest to, the donors." The fund's designated categories of support are the arts, churches and religious organizations, community chests and other related organizations, hospitals and medical research, education, and miscellaneous organizations. **Priorities:** *Arts & Humanities:* 8%. Supports fine arts, performing arts, historical societies, public broadcasting, and libraries. *Civic & Public Affairs:* 19%. Supports neighborhood societies, community foundations, parks, and philanthropic organizations. *Education:* 37%. Funds support pre-college and higher education, both public and private, and minority education. *Environment:* 10%. Gives to boys and girls clubs, community services, animal causes, United Way, YMCA, and family services. *International:* 7%. Supports hospitals, single-disease associations, and medical centers. *Religion:* 2%. Funds scientific research. *Note:* Total contributions made in 2000. **Typ. Recipients:** Alzheimers Disease, Cancer, Clinics/Medical Centers, Family Planning, Health Organizations, Hospitals, Medical Research, Mental Health, Nursing Services, People with Disabilities, Public Health, Substance Abuse. **Geo. Dist:** ME; Detroit, MI, including metropolitan area; NY.

**★ 750 ★ Walter S. Johnson Foundation**
525 Middlefield Rd., Ste. 110
Menlo Park, CA 94025
**Phone:** (650)326-0485     **Fax:** (650)326-4320
**Email:** info@wsjf.org
**Website:** http://www.wsjf.org
Pancho Chang, Executive Director
**Fnded:** 1968. **Philosophy:** The foundation reflects the interests of Walter S. Johnson by focusing on strengthening public education, assisting young people in the transition from school to career, and enhancing the well-being of children, youth, and families. One of the foundation's highest priorities is enhancing the academic learning of children in the public elementary and secondary schools. The foundation feels that programs promoting the professional development of educators, especially in the context of whole school reform, will best help achieve this goal. The foundation is particularly interested in school reform efforts that feature school-to-career programs aiming to integrate challenging curricula with a real-world context. Working with social-service agencies toward solving problems facing children, adolescents, and families is another of the foundation's primary interests. The foundation gives high priority to projects seeking to promote positive youth development through programs promoting healthy social and emotional development, the prevention of teenage pregnancy, the strengthening of families, and the prevention of drug and alcohol abuse. **Priorities:** *Education:* 50%. Supports professional development of teachers and K-12 school reform. *Environment:* 25%. Supports youth development, family services, and social services. **Typ. Recipients:** Family Planning, Medical Research, Mental Health, Public Health, Research/Studies Institutes, Substance Abuse. **Geo. Dist:** CA, Northern California, including San Francisco Bay Area; Reno, NV, including Washoe County.

**★ 751 ★ Washington Square Health Foundation**
875 North Michigan Ave., Ste. 3516
Chicago, IL 60611-1901
**Phone:** (312)664-6488     **Fax:** (312)664-7787
**Email:** wshf@aol.com
**Website:** http://www.wshf.org
Howard Nochumson, Executive Director

**Fnded:** 1985. **Philosophy:** The Washington Square Health Foundation makes grants and program related investments (PRIs) "in order to promote and maintain access to adequate healthcare for all people in the Chicagoland area regardless of race, sex, creed, or financial need. The foundation meets this goal through its grants for medical and nursing scholarships, medical research, and direct healthcare services." **Priorities:** *International:* 100%. Supports health services, purchases of medical equipment, medical and nursing education, and medical research. *Note:* Total contributions made in fiscal 1998. **Typ. Recipients:** AIDS/HIV, Children's Health/Hospitals, Clinics/Medical Centers, Domestic Violence, Health Organizations, Health Policy/Cost Containment, Hospices, Hospitals, Hospitals (University Affiliated), Medical Education, Medical Rehabilitation, Medical Research, People with Disabilities, Prenatal Health Issues, Preventive Medicine/Wellness Organizations, Public Health, Respiratory, Sexual Abuse, Single-Disease Health Associations. **Geo. Dist:** Chicago, IL.

**★ 752 ★ Wasserman Foundation**
1 Wilshire Blvd., Ste. 2000
Los Angeles, CA 90017
**Phone:** (213)629-7600     **Fax:** (213)624-1376
Edward Landry, Contact
**Fnded:** 1956. **Philosophy:** The foundation generally supports arts groups, educational institutions, religious groups, and medical research. **Priorities:** *Arts & Humanities:* 8%. Supports performing arts centers, libraries, museums, and public broadcasting. *Civic & Public Affairs:* 9%. Supports foundations and legal aid groups. *Education:* 43%. Mostly supports colleges and universities. *Environment:* About 5%. Focus on the disabled, child welfare, and food banks. *International:* 19%. Supports medical centers, AIDS research, diseases that affect women, and diabetes. *Note:* Total contributions made in 1998. **Typ. Recipients:** AIDS/HIV, Cancer, Children's Health/Hospitals, Clinics/Medical Centers, Domestic Violence, Emergency/Ambulance Services, Eyes/Blindness, Family Planning, Health Organizations, Hospitals, Medical Education, Medical Research, Multiple Sclerosis, People with Disabilities, Single-Disease Health Associations, Speech & Hearing, Substance Abuse. **Geo. Dist:** Los Angeles, CA; New York, NY.

**★ 753 ★ Wayne and Gladys Valley Foundation**
1939 Harrison St., Ste. 510
Oakland, CA 94612-3532
**Phone:** (510)466-6060     **Fax:** (510)466-6067
Stephen Chandler, President & Executive Director
**Fnded:** 1977. **Philosophy:** The foundation has established four areas of interest. The areas include the following: Education, including public and private universities' research programs in oceanography; eye diseases; vascular defects, learning disabilities, and physical or mental afflictions affecting children and young adults; medical research concerning the above mentioned health-related programs; community and social services (generally limited to smaller grants to East Bay area projects serving youth or provided by Catholic hospitals, social services, or health care groups); and special projects, which provides the foundation with flexibility in its grant program for worthy projects. The foundation seeks to support organizations that have committed, enthusiastic, and diligent leadership; specifically defined goals and purposes; and reasonable expectations of demonstrating measurable progress and results. The foundation also favors grant requests contingent on receiving matching funding from other sources. Grants generally are payable only in one year. **Priorities:** *Arts & Humanities:* About 13%. Libraries, museums, and public television. *Education:* 18%. Supports science, legal, and mathematical education. *Environment:* 47%. Food banks, childrens services, care centers. *International:* 20%. Cancer research, blindness, and heart disease. *Note:* Total contributions made in fiscal 1999. **Typ. Recipients:** Alzheimers Disease, Cancer, Children's Health/Hospitals, Domestic Violence, Eyes/Blindness, Health Organizations, Heart, Hospitals, Medical Research, Mental Health, People with Disabil-

ities, Prenatal Health Issues, Research/Studies Institutes, Single-Disease Health Associations, Speech & Hearing. **Geo. Dist:** CA, Alameda County; CA, Contra Costa County; CA, East Bay area; CA, Santa Clara County.

### ★ 754 ★ Weingart Foundation

1055 West 7th St., Ste. 3050
Los Angeles, CA 90017-2305
**Phone:** (213)688-7799          **Fax:** (213)688-1515
**Email:** info@weingartfnd.org
**Website:** http://www.weingartfnd.org
Fred Ali, President & Chief Executive Officer

**Fnded:** 1951. **Philosophy:** "The Weingart Foundation's primary area of interest in grant making, is to assist credible agencies and institutions serving children and youth in the Southern California area. A secondary area of interest lies in supporting those agencies and institutions providing services that benefit the entire community regardless of age or other factors. Preferential attention will be given to the support of well-conceived experimental or demonstration projects that promise significant positive results and are likely to produce long-term multiplier effects." 1999 Annual Report **Priorities:** *Arts & Humanities:* 6%. Funds music centers, museums, and the donor adivsed, dance companies. *Civic & Public Affairs:* 13%. Provided major grant to the San Diego Foundation to create Weingart-price fund; supports libraries and zoos. *Education:* 30%. Provides funding for private colleges and universities, and K-12 schools. *Environment:* 20%. Supports youth organizations, domestic violence, substance abuse prevention/ treatment programs, the homeless and community centers. *International:* 25%. Supports hospital, health and hospital foundations. *Religion:* 3%. Supports San Diego Space and Science foundation. *Note:* Total contributions made in fiscal 2000. **Typ. Recipients:** AIDS/HIV, Cancer, Child Abuse, Children's Health/ Hospitals, Clinics/Medical Centers, Diabetes, Domestic Violence, Emergency/Ambulance Services, Eyes/ Blindness, Health Organizations, Hospices, Hospitals, Long-Term Care, Medical Education, Medical Research, Mental Health, Nursing Services, Outpatient Health Care, People with Disabilities, Prenatal Health Issues, Preventive Medicine/Wellness Organizations, Public Health, Speech & Hearing, Substance Abuse. **Geo. Dist:** CA, seven counties in Southern California.

### ★ 755 ★ Welfare Foundation

100 West 10th St.
Wilmington, DE 19801
**Phone:** (302)654-2477          **Fax:** (302)654-2323
Peter Morrow, Executive Director

**Fnded:** 1930. **Philosophy:** The foundation supports social welfare organizations, civic associations, the arts, and educational institutions. **Priorities:** *Arts & Humanities:* 22%. Suppots contemporary arts, museums, opera. *Civic & Public Affairs:* 11%. Supports zoo, libraries, riverfront development organization. *Education:* 25%. Supports colleges and universities, elementary and preschools, after-school programs. *Environment:* 35%. Supports scouting, youth services, food bank, housing, senior services, family planning. *International:* 2%. Supports single-disease health associationss. *Note:* Total contributions made in 1998. **Typ. Recipients:** AIDS/HIV, Cancer, Children's Health/ Hospitals, Clinics/Medical Centers, Emergency/Ambulance Services, Family Planning, Health Organizations, Hospices, Hospitals, Long-Term Care, Medical Education, People with Disabilities, Prenatal Health Issues, Public Health, Single-Disease Health Associations, Substance Abuse. **Geo. Dist:** Wilmington, DE, including surrounding communities; PA, Southern Chester County.

### ★ 756 ★ Whitehall Foundation

PO Box 3423
Palm Beach, FL 33480
**Phone:** (561)655-4474          **Fax:** (561)659-4978
**Email:** Email@Whitehall.org
**Website:** http://www.whitehall.org
Catherine Thomas, Corporate Secretary

**Fnded:** 1937. **Philosophy:** The foundation's policy is to assist areas of basic biological research that are not heavily supported by federal agencies or other specialized foundations. The foundation's current areas of interest are scholarly research in invertebrate and vertebrate neurobiology, specifically investigations of neural mechanisms involved in sensory, motor, and other complex functions of the whole organism as they relate to behavior. Research grants are available to established scientists working in accredited institutions in the United States. The foundation's grants-in-aid program is designed for researchers at the assistant professor level or higher who experience difficulty in competing for research funds, but grants are also available to senior scientists. Funds may be used for personnel, scientific equipment, scientific materials and supplies, publication costs, travel for research purposes, or overhead (limited indirect expenses). The foundation regularly reassesses its areas of interest. However, major changes in programs only occur after several years of consideration and evaluation. **Priorities:** *Education:* 74%. Provides scholarships. *International:* 26%. Supports medical research, primarily at American universities and hospitals. *Note:* Contributions made in 2000. **Typ. Recipients:** Cancer, Children's Health/Hospitals, Clinics/Medical Centers, Hospitals, Medical Education, Medical Research, Substance Abuse. **Geo. Dist:** nationally.

### ★ 757 ★ Whitehead Foundation

67 Wall St.
New York, NY 10005
**Phone:** (212)440-0800          **Fax:** (212)751-5924
Denise Emmett, Grants Administrator

**Fnded:** 1982. **Philosophy:** The Whitehead Foundation makes grants across the major categories of support. In civic affairs, interests include environmental affairs, economic development, national security, international affairs, housing, and public policy. Educational support goes to colleges and universities, and economic and business education. Social service support favors child welfare, youth organizations, the disabled, and employment and job training. Arts funding goes to historic preservation, theaters, galleries, and museums. **Priorities:** *Arts & Humanities:* 14%. Supports libraries, museums, and theater. *Civic & Public Affairs:* 36%. Primary support for philanthropy. *Education:* 22%. Supports colleges, universities, and educational initiatives. *Environment:* 4%. Funds volunteer groups and services for the disabled. *International:* 3%. Focus on medical research. *Note:* Total contributions made in fiscal 2000. **Typ. Recipients:** Hospitals, Medical Research, People with Disabilities, Single-Disease Health Associations, Substance Abuse. **Geo. Dist:** nationally; New York, NY.

### ★ 758 ★ Wilf Family Foundation

820 Morris Turnpike
Short Hills, NJ 07078
**Phone:** (973)467-5000          **Fax:** (973)467-0550
Joseph Wilf, Trustee

**Fnded:** 1964. **Philosophy:** The Wilf Family Foundation primarily supports Jewish organizations in education and religion. Most of the religious organizations are located in New York. Jewish education is supported both at the university and secondary levels. The foundation also supports a number of other recipient areas with Jewish interests. **Priorities:** *Arts & Humanities:* 2%. Funds Jewish museums. *Education:* 10%. Focus on Jewish education. *International:* 4%. Hospitals and single-disease health associations. *Note:* Total contributions made in fiscal 1998. **Typ. Recipients:** Cancer, Children's Health/Hospitals, Clinics/ Medical Centers, Eyes/Blindness, Heart, Hospitals, Long-Term Care, Medical Education, Medical Research, Respiratory, Trauma Treatment. **Geo. Dist:** nationally; New York, NY.

### ★ 759 ★ Willard L. Eccles Charitable Foundation

PO Box 628
Salt Lake City, UT 84110
**Phone:** (801)246-5363
Clark Giles, Contact

**Fnded:** 1981. **Philosophy:** "The specific charitable purposes of the Foundation are to promote, encourage and make available to the public health care services, to aid charitable non-profit hospitals in acquiring appropriate medical equipment for research and for rendering health care services, and to further medical education and research. The Foundation is directed to provide this health care-medical assistance primarily in Utah and particularly in the Ogden area." "In addition to making grants for the above described health care-medical purposes, the Foundation provides funding to charitable organizations for other community charitable purposes and distributes limited grants to qualified charitable organizations as directed by members of the Advisory Committee. These grants are not based on requests submitted to the Foundation without the prior approval of a member of the Advisory Committee." **Priorities:** *Arts & Humanities:* 14%. Focus on theater, libraries, public broadcasting. *Civic & Public Affairs:* 3%. Funds community development. *Education:* 30%. Colleges and universities, and primary and secondary education. *Environment:* 7%. Emphasis on youth organizations and community services. *International:* 4%. Public health care, hospitals, pediatric health, and single-disease health associations. *Note:* Total contributions made in fiscal 2000. **Typ. Recipients:** AIDS/HIV, Alzheimers Disease, Cancer, Children's Health/Hospitals, Clinics/Medical Centers, Domestic Violence, Emergency/Ambulance Services, Eyes/Blindness, Eyes/Blindness, Family Planning, Health Organizations, Health-General, Hospices, Hospitals, Medical Education, Medical Research, Medical Training, Mental Health, Multiple Sclerosis, Nursing Services, People with Disabilities, Prenatal Health Issues, Preventive Medicine/Wellness Organizations, Public Health, Respiratory, Single-Disease Health Associations. **Geo. Dist:** UT, primarily Salt Lake City and Ogden.

### ★ 760 ★ Willard and Pat Walker Charitable Foundation

PO Box 7299
Springdale, AR 72766-7299
**Phone:** (501)751-9083
Willard Walker, Trustee

**Fnded:** 1990. **Philosophy:** The foundation places emphasis on the arts, health, and human services within Arkansas. **Priorities:** *Education:* 47%. Colleges and universities. *Environment:* 15%. Primarily for family services. *International:* 9%. Medical centers and single-disease health associations. *Note:* Total contributions made in 1998. **Typ. Recipients:** Cancer, Clinics/Medical Centers, Single-Disease Health Associations. **Geo. Dist:** AR.

### ★ 761 ★ Willard T. C. Johnson Foundation

630 5th Ave., Ste. 1510
New York, NY 10111
**Phone:** (212)332-7500          **Fax:** (212)332-7510
**Email:** tjici1@tjinc.com
Neil Burmeister, President

**Fnded:** 1979. **Philosophy:** The foundation primarily supports the Arthritits Foundation, Juvenile Diabetes Foundation International, other health organizations, and educational institutions. Other recipients include Opera Festival New Jersey, religious organizations, and social services. **Priorities:** *Arts & Humanities:* 3%. Supports the June Opera Festival of New Jersey. *Civic & Public Affairs:* 18%. Supports the Robin Hood Foundation. *Education:* 18%. Funds a private school. *Environment:* 2%. Funds the Best Friends Foundation. *International:* 60%. Supports the Alliance for Lupus Research. *Note:* Total contributions made in 1999. **Typ. Recipients:** AIDS/HIV, Arthritis, Diabetes, Emergency/Ambulance Services, Family Planning, Health Organizations, Hospitals, Long-Term Care, Single-Disease Health Associations. **Geo. Dist:** Washington, DC; NJ; New York, NY.

### ★ 762 ★ William Bingham Foundation

20325 Center Ridge Rd., Ste. 629
Rocky River, OH 44116-3554
**Phone:** (440)331-6350

**Email:** lauragilbertson@msn.com
**Website:** http://www.fdncenter.org/grantmaker/bing-ham/
Laura Gilbertson, Director

**Fnded:** 1955. **Philosophy:** Since 1977, the foundation has extended its objectives "to include less traditional programs and grantees outside the Cleveland area." Since 1986, the foundation has begun to pay increasing attention to environmental issues. For example, the foundation has supported projects to encourage resolution of environmental problems through negotiation, as well as projects to stop the depletion of the ozone layer of the earth's atmosphere and the "greenhouse effect" which creates global warming. In addition to environmental programs, the foundation continues to contribute to a wide variety of organizations in the areas of education, the arts, health, and welfare, reflecting the diverse interests of the trustees and the needs of the communities in which they live. **Priorities:** *Arts & Humanities:* 12%. Supports public broadcasting, theater and film & radio. *Civic & Public Affairs:* 6%. Supports housing and community affairs. *Education:* 48%. Supports colleges and universities. *Environment:* 23%. Supports YMCA, youth and senior services and community centers. *International:* 2%. Funds hospitals. *Note:* Total contributions approved in 2000. **Typ. Recipients:** Cancer, Clinics/Medical Centers, Diabetes, Domestic Violence, Hospices, Hospitals, Medical Rehabilitation, Multiple Sclerosis, Nursing Services, People with Disabilities, Public Health, Sexual Abuse, Substance Abuse. **Geo. Dist:** United States only; CA; DC; NY; OH; RI.

---

**★ 763 ★  William Bingham Second
    Betterment Fund**
330 Madison Ave. Rm. 3500
New York, NY 10017
**Phone:** (212)557-7700          **Fax:** (212)286-8513
Anna Mosquera, Administrator

**Fnded:** 1955. **Philosophy:** "Although the traditional recipients of Mr. Bingham's benefactions continue to be of special interest and scholarship support continues to be a major activity, the Betterment Fund views the areas of health and education broadly. The Fund will consider requests from qualified institutions and organizations whose activities promote health improvement and education which have the potential for a significant impact on the life of Maine residents in these areas. In recent years the Fund has expanded its areas of concern to include programs which support local communities in their own efforts to increase their capacity to improve the quality of life for residents and programs for the preservation and responsible use of Maine's natural resources." 1997 Statement of Grant Policies and Procedures **Priorities:** *Arts & Humanities:* 14%. Supports libraries, public broadcasting, and historic preservation. *Civic & Public Affairs:* 17%. Funds economic policy, community development, law & justice, and job training. *Education:* 35%. Funds primary and secondary schools, colleges and universities, education associations, literacy, technical colleges, scholarships. *Environment:* 6%. Supports homes, food banks, and community service programs. *International:* 13%. Supports hospitals, medical centers, oral health, public health, medical research, and visiting nurses. *Note:* Total contributions made in 2000. **Typ. Recipients:** Cancer, Children's Health/Hospitals, Clinics/Medical Centers, Diabetes, Family Planning, Health Funds, Health Organizations, Home-Care Services, Hospitals, Long-Term Care, Medical Education, Medical Research, Nursing Services, Preventive Medicine/Wellness Organizations, Public Health, Respiratory, Substance Abuse. **Geo. Dist:** Western Mountain region; ME.

---

**★ 764 ★  William E. Schrafft and Bertha
    E. Schrafft Charitable Trust**
One Financial Center, 26th Floor
Boston, MA 02111-2662
**Phone:** (617)350-6100          **Fax:** (617)350-0038
**Website:** http://www.schraffttrust.org
Karen Faulkner, Executive Director

**Fnded:** 1946. **Philosophy:** "The aim of the Schrafft Charitable Trust continues to be on making a differ-ence in the educational and cultural opportunities for young people in Greater Boston's inner city." The FND's primary focus is on organizations that are involved with the education of indigent or disadvantaged youth in Boston. *Shcrafft Charitable Trust 2000 Annual Report* **Priorities:** *Arts & Humanities:* 15%. Supports dance, theater, music, museums, and fine art. *Civic & Public Affairs:* 17%. Gives to nonprofit management, job training, and an aquarium. *Education:* 25%. Funds scholarships, colleges and universities, charter and alternative schools, and art education. *Environment:* 43%. Supports United Way, youth clubs, camps and organizations, and homeless shelters. *Note:* Total contributions made in 2000. **Typ. Recipients:** Clinics/Medical Centers, Family Planning, Hospitals, Nursing Services, People with Disabilities, Single-Disease Health Associations, Substance Abuse. **Geo. Dist:** Boston, MA.

---

**★ 765 ★  William E. Simon Foundation**
310 South St., PO Box 1913
Morristown, NJ 07962-1913
**Phone:** (973)898-0290          **Fax:** (973)898-4733
**Website:** http://www.wesimonfoundation.org
Sheila Johnston, Contact

**Fnded:** 1967. **Philosophy:** Named after its principal benefactor, the William E. Simon Foundation supports programs that are intended to strengthen the free enterprise system and the moral and spiritual values on which it rests: individual freedom, initiative, thrift, self-discipline, and faith in God. The mission of the Foundation reflects the unique accomplishments of the individual for whom it is named, and the principles of a free society that have made these accomplishments possible. The main charitable purpose of the Foundation is to assist those in need by providing the means through which they may help themselves. The charitable philosophy guiding the Foundation draws heavily on the thoughts expressed a century ago by Andrew Carnegie in *The Gospel of Wealth,* where he wrote: "In bestowing charity, the main consideration should be to help those who will help themselves; to provide part of the means by which those who desire to improve may do so; to give those who desire to rise the aids by which they may rise; to assist, but rarely or never to do all." In implementing this philosophy, and the Foundation seeks to fund programs which are effective in promoting independence and personal responsibility among those in need. **Priorities:** *Education:* 26%. *Environment:* 40%. *Note:* Total contributions made in 1998. **Typ. Recipients:** Cancer, Clinics/Medical Centers, Family Planning, Health Funds, Health Organizations, Hospices, Hospitals, Medical Rehabilitation, Medical Research, Multiple Sclerosis, Nursing Services, People with Disabilities, Public Health, Research/Studies Institutes, Single-Disease Health Associations, Substance Abuse, Transplant Networks/Donor Banks. **Geo. Dist:** nationally, with emphasis in New York Metro, Los Angeles, and the San Francio Bar metropolitan areas. **Frmly:** William E. and Carol G. Simon Foundation.

---

**★ 766 ★  William and Flora Hewlett
    Foundation**
525 Middlefield Rd., Ste. 200
Menlo Park, CA 94025-3495
**Phone:** (650)329-1070          **Fax:** (650)329-9342
**Website:** http://www.hewlett.org
Paul Brest, President

**Fnded:** 1966. **Philosophy:** "In defining programs and establishing "objectives that show promise of realizing the aspirations of the founders," the foundation has restricted its attention to the fields of education, population, conflict resolution, environment, performing arts, family and community development, and U.S.-Latin American relations. A special projects category also was established to provide the foundation with flexibility to respond to proposals of special interest to the board. A large portion of funding has been for the general support of institutions, rather than for project support. Funding has been provided to increase the stability of performing arts organizations, and to strengthen international scholarship and training on university campuses. Institutional recipients have included research universities, liberal arts col-leges, and organizations involved in conflict resolution, the environment, and population. In pursuing the development of public policy options, the foundation has supported institutions and organizations with a record of objective policy research. Some of these grants have gone to public policy organizations working in areas of program interest such as the environment, population, and the urban community. The foundation also has supported community development organizations, youth employment projects, historically black colleges, and a program to increase minority representation in science and engineering. The issues of homelessness and affordable housing are also of interest to the foundation. The foundation has a strong commitment to the voluntary, nonprofit sector. It will therefore assist efforts to improve the financial base and efficiency of organizations and institutions in this category. Proposals that show promise of stimulating private philanthropy are particularly welcome. The foundation's interest in international affairs is reflected primarily in its population program, which supports organizations providing family planning services in less-developed countries and in American population centers. The Hewlett Foundation also supports international and area studies at major research universities." **Priorities:** *Arts & Humanities:* 10%. Supports music, theater, opera, dance, film, and video. *Civic & Public Affairs:* 22%. Focus on the foundation's conflict resolution program; community development, transition to work programs, and employment initiatives. *Education:* About 15%. Supports higher education, elementary education, and secondary education. *Note:* Total contributions made in 1998. **Typ. Recipients:** Adolescent Health Issues, AIDS/HIV, Family Planning, Health Organizations, Health Policy/Cost Containment, Public Health, Research/Studies Institutes. **Geo. Dist:** internationally; nationally; San Francisco, CA, Bay area.

---

**★ 767 ★  William G. Baker, Jr. Memorial
    Fund**
Latrobe Bldg., 9th Floor
2 East Read St.
Baltimore, MD 21202
**Phone:** (410)332-4171          **Fax:** (410)837-4701
Melissa Warlon, Contact

**Fnded:** 1964. **Philosophy:** The William G. Baker, Jr., Memorial Fund donates funds for "charitable purposes such as and limited to religious, charitable, scientific, literary, or educational purposes." **Priorities:** *Arts & Humanities:* 26%. Supports performing arts, museums, and historical societies. *Civic & Public Affairs:* 12%. Gives to neighborhood concerns, economic development, and community foundations. *Education:* 22%. Supports schools, accen programs, and universities. *Environment:* 23%. Supports children, family, and human needs. *International:* 7%. Supports health, and mental health projects. *Note:* Total contributions made in 2000. **Typ. Recipients:** Child Abuse, Children's Health/Hospitals, Clinics/Medical Centers, Emergency/Ambulance Services, Eyes/Blindness, Health Funds, Health Organizations, Heart, Hospices, Hospitals, Mental Health, People with Disabilities, Public Health, Speech & Hearing, Substance Abuse. **Geo. Dist:** Baltimore, MD.

---

**★ 768 ★  William G. Irwin Charity
    Foundation**
711 Russ Bldg.
235 Montgomery St.
San Francisco, CA 94104
**Phone:** (415)362-6954
Michael Gorman, Executive Director

**Fnded:** 1919. **Philosophy:** "The foundation is particularly interested in medical facilities, secondary schools, and cultural and community projects." **Priorities:** *Arts & Humanities:* 13%. Supports museums, history, opera, and music, ballet and theater. *Civic & Public Affairs:* less than 1%. *Education:* 57%. Supports school, religious education, and colleges and medicine education. *Environment:* 5%. Funds United Way, Young Men's Christian Association and youth centers. *International:* 14%. Supports medical research, medical centers, multiple sclerosis, and hospitals. *Note:*

---

Contributions were made in 2000. **Typ. Recipients:** Alzheimers Disease, Arthritis, Cancer, Children's Health/Hospitals, Clinics/Medical Centers, Emergency/Ambulance Services, Eyes/Blindness, Geriatric Health, Health Organizations, Health Organizations, Heart, Hospitals, Long-Term Care, Medical Education, Medical Rehabilitation, Medical Research, Multiple Sclerosis, People with Disabilities, Research/Studies Institutes, Single-Disease Health Associations, Speech & Hearing, Transplant Networks/Donor Banks. **Geo. Dist:** CA; HI.

★ 769 ★ **William G. McGowan Charitable Fund**
PO Box 40515
Washington, DC 20016-0515
**Phone:** (202)364-5030          **Fax:** (202)364-3382
**Email:** goodric@aol.com
**Website:** http://www.mcgowanfund.com
Bernard Goodrich, Executive Director
**Fnded:** 1992. **Philosophy:** The foundation primarily supports organizations engaging in healthcare research, promoting or providing educational opportunities, especially in the business field, or developing the critical skills of undereducated and underdeveloped youth. **Priorities:** *Civic & Public Affairs:* 3%. Supports employment/job training, housing and womens affairs. *Education:* 74%. Colleges and universities, international studies, public education, private secondary education, special education, religious education, student aid and scholarship. *Environment:* 2%. Youth organizations, people with disabilities, homes, united way, at risk youth. *International:* 17%. Supports heart and cancer research, artificial organ development, and transplant networks. *Note:* Total contributions made in fiscal 1997. **Typ. Recipients:** Cancer, Diabetes, Domestic Violence, Health-General, Heart, Medical Education, People with Disabilities, Public Health, Speech & Hearing, Transplant Networks/Donor Banks. **Geo. Dist:** CA, Central, North of San Luis; Washington, DC; Chicago, IL; Kansas City, KS; Baltimore, MD; NY, Western; PA, Northern; Dallas, TX; Houston, TX; San Antonio, TX.

★ 770 ★ **William G. Selby and Marie Selby Foundation**
1800 Second St., Ste. 750
Sarasota, FL 34236
**Phone:** (941)957-0442          **Fax:** (941)957-3135
**Website:** http://www.selbyfdn.org
Debra Jacobs, President
**Fnded:** 1955. **Philosophy:** The purpose of the foundation is to "make grants which will result in the improvement of life in the Sarasota community." Emphasis is placed on social services and education. Organizations and programs serving youth, and programs for the handicapped and the elderly are stressed. The foundation also maintains an extensive scholarship program. Funds are provided to Florida colleges and universities which, in turn, grant scholarships to individuals on the basis of academic excellence and financial need. **Typ. Recipients:** AIDS/HIV, Cancer, Children's Health/Hospitals, Domestic Violence, Emergency/Ambulance Services, Family Planning, Hospices, Medical Research, Mental Health, People with Disabilities, Prenatal Health Issues, Research/Studies Institutes, Single-Disease Health Associations, Substance Abuse. **Geo. Dist:** Sarasota, FL, Manatee, Charlotte, DeSoto Florida counties.

★ 771 ★ **William H. Donner Foundation**
500 Fifth Ave., Ste. 1230
New York, NY 10110-0180
**Phone:** (212)719-9290          **Fax:** (212)302-8734
**Email:** rhgregg@donner.org
**Website:** http://www.donner.org
Rachel Gregg, Program Officer
**Fnded:** 1961. **Philosophy:** In 1998, the foundation reported that its giving philosophy has changed. **Priorities:** *Arts & Humanities:* 3%. Supports art institution. *Civic & Public Affairs:* 63%. Supports public policy and community affairs organizations. *Education:* 23%. Supports universities and education organizations.

*Environment:* 2%. Supports youth services. *Note:* Total contributions made in 1998. **Typ. Recipients:** Adolescent Health Issues, Cancer, Child Abuse, Clinics/Medical Centers, Domestic Violence, Geriatric Health, Health Organizations, Health Policy/Cost Containment, Hospices, Hospitals, Medical Research, Mental Health, People with Disabilities, Prenatal Health Issues. **Geo. Dist:** nationally.

★ 772 ★ **William K. Warren Foundation**
PO Box 470372
Tulsa, OK 74147-0372
**Phone:** (918)492-8100          **Fax:** (918)481-7935
W. Lissau, President & Director
**Fnded:** 1945. **Philosophy:** The foundation reports that it gives preference to "local Catholic health care facilities." Its designated areas of interest are hospitals and medical research centers; churches and related organizations; educational institutions; and other (including youth-related causes, substance abuse prevention, human services, and single-disease health associations). **Priorities:** *Education:* 20%. Supports universities, parochial schools, and educational programs. *Environment:* 1%. Community assistance and youth programs. *International:* 67%. Funds health associations, hospitals, and health societies. *Note:* Total contributions made in 1998. **Typ. Recipients:** Alzheimers Disease, Arthritis, Cancer, Child Abuse, Children's Health/Hospitals, Clinics/Medical Centers, Diabetes, Diabetes, Emergency/Ambulance Services, Eyes/Blindness, Health Organizations, Heart, Hospitals, Medical Rehabilitation, Medical Research, Mental Health, Multiple Sclerosis, People with Disabilities, Prenatal Health Issues, Respiratory, Single-Disease Health Associations, Substance Abuse, Trauma Treatment. **Geo. Dist:** Tulsa, OK.

★ 773 ★ **William Penn Foundation**
2 Logan Sq., 11th Fl.
100 N 18th St.
Philadelphia, PA 19103-2757
**Phone:** (215)988-1830          **Fax:** (215)988-1823
**Email:** info@wpennfdn.org
**Website:** http://www.wpennfdn.org
Kathrine Engebretson, President
**Fnded:** 1945. **Philosophy:** "The Foundation strives to improve the quality of life in the greater Philadelphia area, with particular emphasis upon empowering the neediest residents of the region. It supports programs that nurture families, promote social justice, strengthen communities, help persons participate actively in American democratic life, build a climate of cultural vitality, and foster responsibility for our environment. The Foundation awards grants primarily to non-profit organizations but also makes grants to governments and to churches for community and non-sectarian activities." 1995 Annual Report. In 1998, the foundation reinforced its mission by giving in three responsive grantmaking categories: Children, Youth and Families; Natural and Physical Environment; and Arts and Culture. The foundation also has an initiative grantmaking program to address issues of broad community concerns. Through this program the foundation works in partnership with nonprofits exploring ideas and collaborating on long-term solutions to persistent problems of Philadelphia and the region. **Priorities:** *Arts & Humanities:* 19%. Supports historic preservation, museums and the performing arts. *Civic & Public Affairs:* 20%. Funds community revitalization. *Education:* 18%. Focus is on precollege education. *Environment:* 25%. Supports youth services, housing and urban affairs. *International:* 2%. *Note:* Total contributions made in 1998. **Typ. Recipients:** Child Abuse, Clinics/Medical Centers, Domestic Violence, Family Planning, Geriatric Health, Health Organizations, Nursing Services, Prenatal Health Issues, Public Health. **Geo. Dist:** Philadelphia, PA, including the five suburban counties.

★ 774 ★ **William Randolph Hearst Foundation**
888 7th Ave., 45th Floor
New York, NY 10106-0057
**Phone:** (212)586-5404          **Fax:** (212)586-1917

**Website:** http://hearstfdn.org
Robert Frehse, Jr., Executive Director & Vice President
**Fnded:** 1948. **Philosophy:** Within a general policy of assisting institutions to provide access and opportunity to underrepresented, low-income and minority populations, the Directors of the Hearst Foundations have established the following priorities: "The Foundations' primary focus is support of undergraduate education through the establishment of endowed scholarships at private liberal arts colleges and universities. In addition, endowed scholarship support is provided for professional study in teaching, medicine, nursing, engineering, math, science and the health care professions, at the undergraduate and graduate levels. A limited number of proposals are also accepted from K-12 independent schools with outstanding academic programs, and demonstrated track records of outreach to economically disadvantaged students. In general grants are not made to public schools. However, private organizations or coalitions seeking improvement of public education and broadening access to education may be considered." "The Foundations' interests in the health field seek to improve and increase health care, while facilitating wellness, prevention, and rehabilitation. Working largely through leading regional hospitals and medical centers, the Foundations support programs which increase access for underserved urban and rural populations. Areas of interest include perinatology, pediatrics, cancer, stroke, aging, women's health issues, and research." "In social services, preference is given to well-established, larger agencies, providing comprehensive services. Requests for technical assistance, management training, and leadership development, designed to help non-profit agencies deliver services more efficiently and effectively are also considered." "The Foundations' priority in the arts is to increase access and educational opportunities for diverse populations and underserved communities. The major portion of funds endows arts education and/or community outreach programs through major cultural institutions. Special attention is given to programs which enrich the lives of young people through exposure to the arts." *Guidelines for Grant Applications.* **Priorities:** *Arts & Humanities:* 29%. Supports music, arts centers, ballet, museum, opera, theater, arts festivals and public broadcasting. *Education:* 37%. Funds scholarship, colleges and universities, schools, religious education, minority education, journalism/media education, and medical education. *Environment:* 16%. Supports scouts, child welfare, Big Brothers/Big Sisters, Young Men's Christian Association/Young Women's Christian Association, domestic violence, and family services. *International:* 17%. Supports medical research, hospitals, AIDS, medical centers, heart, and eyes/blindness. *Note:* Contributions analysis provided by foundation. Analysis represents five years of contributions ending with 2000. **Typ. Recipients:** Cancer, Children's Health/Hospitals, Clinics/Medical Centers, Emergency/Ambulance Services, Eyes/Blindness, Geriatric Health, Health Funds, Health Organizations, Home-Care Services, Hospitals, Hospitals (University Affiliated), Medical Education, Medical Rehabilitation, Medical Research, Medical Training, People with Disabilities, Prenatal Health Issues, Public Health, Research/Studies Institutes, Single-Disease Health Associations, Substance Abuse, Transplant Networks/Donor Banks. **Geo. Dist:** nationally.

★ 775 ★ **William Rosenwald Family Fund**
666 3rd Ave.
New York, NY 10017
**Phone:** (212)476-8088          **Fax:** (212)476-8000
David Steinmann, Secretary
**Fnded:** 1938. **Philosophy:** The William Rosenwald Family Fund primarily supports Jewish religious organizations. The fund also supports Jewish education and various other interests on a limited basis. **Priorities:** *Arts & Humanities:* 9%. Historical societies, film, and music. *Civic & Public Affairs:* 3%. Crime prevention, urban parks, and foundations. *Education:* 13%. Secondary schools and colleges. *Environment:* 5%. Youth and family programs. *International:* 9%. Medical schools and health centers. *Note:* Total contributions made in 1998. **Typ. Recipients:** AIDS/HIV, Alzheim-

ers Disease, Cancer, Children's Health/Hospitals, Clinics/Medical Centers, Eyes/Blindness, Family Planning, Geriatric Health, Health-General, Hospitals (University Affiliated), Medical Education, Medical Research, Mental Health, People with Disabilities, Research/Studies Institutes, Substance Abuse, Transplant Networks/Donor Banks. **Geo. Dist:** NY.


## ★ 776 ★ William S. Paley Foundation

1 East 53rd St., Ste. 1400
New York, NY 10022
**Phone:** (212)888-2520          **Fax:** (212)308-7845
Patrick Gallagher, Executive Director
**Fnded:** 1936. **Philosophy:** The founder, William S. Paley, enjoyed strong relationships with a number of charitable organizations during his lifetime. He founded the Museum of Broadcasting in New York, and the foundation continues its support to the organization. Also, the foundation supports the Museum of Modern Art in New York, where Mr. Paley had once served as president. Other art museums and art programs are also of interest to the foundation. **Priorities:** *Arts & Humanities:* 86%. Major support for the Museum of Television and Radio. *Civic & Public Affairs:* 9%. Funds parks and municipalities. *Education:* 2%. Gives to colleges and universities and to primary and secondary education. *Environment:* 2%. *International:* 1%. *Note:* Total contributions made in 1998. **Typ. Recipients:** Alzheimers Disease, Cancer, Children's Health/Hospitals, Clinics/Medical Centers, Family Planning, Health Organizations, Hospices, Hospitals, Hospitals (University Affiliated), Medical Education, Single-Disease Health Associations, Substance Abuse. **Geo. Dist:** New York, NY.


## ★ 777 ★ William Stamps Farish Fund

10000 Memorial Dr., Ste. 920
Houston, TX 77024
**Phone:** (713)686-7373
**Email:** jcc@virginia.edu
Caroline Rotan, Secretary
**Fnded:** 1951. **Philosophy:** The fund primarily gives to local primary education, arts and humanities, social services, and medical research. **Priorities:** *Arts & Humanities:* 6%. Libraries, historical preservation, and art galleries. *Civic & Public Affairs:* 2%. *Education:* 50%. Private secondary education, medical education, and public universities. *Environment:* 24%. Youth organizations, child abuse, and reading programs for the blind. *International:* 15%. Medical centers, cancer research, and hospitals. *Religion:* 1%. Scientific labs and science museums. *Note:* Total contributions made in 1998. **Typ. Recipients:** Cancer, Child Abuse, Clinics/Medical Centers, Emergency/Ambulance Services, Eyes/Blindness, Family Planning, Health Funds, Health Organizations, Health-General, Hospices, Hospitals, Hospitals (University Affiliated), Medical Education, Medical Research, Mental Health, People with Disabilities, Prenatal Health Issues, Public Health, Sexual Abuse, Single-Disease Health Associations, Speech & Hearing, Substance Abuse. **Geo. Dist:** Houston, TX.


## ★ 778 ★ William T. Kemper Charitable Trust

PO Box 419692
Kansas City, MO 64141
**Phone:** (816)860-7711          **Fax:** (816)860-5690
Stephen Campbell, Trust Administrative
**Fnded:** 1989. **Philosophy:** The William T. Kemper Charitable Trust primarily supports the arts, with an emphasis on museums and the performing arts. Civic and community affairs and education are also of interest to the trust. **Priorities:** *Arts & Humanities:* 56%. Supports the Kemper Museum. *Civic & Public Affairs:* 20%. Supports parks and zoos. *Education:* 14%. Supports higher education. *Environment:* 8%. Supports children's centers. *International:* 3%. Supports hospitals. *Note:* Total contributions made in 1999. **Typ. Recipients:** Children's Health/Hospitals, Clinics/Medical Centers, Hospitals, Research/Studies Institutes. **Geo. Dist:** Kansas City, MO.


## ★ 779 ★ William T. Kemper Foundation

PO Box 13095
Kansas City, MO 64199-3095
**Phone:** (816)234-2985          **Fax:** (816)234-8690
Michael Fields, Executive Director
**Fnded:** 1989. **Philosophy:** "The Foundation is dedicated to continuing Mr. Kemper's lifelong interest in improving the human condition and quality of life. Preference is given to projects located in the Midwest, with particular emphasis on his home state of Missouri and the surrounding area." "The philanthropic efforts of the William T. Kemper Foundation concentrate on four broad areas–education, health and human services, civic improvements and the arts." 1997 Brochure **Priorities:** *Arts & Humanities:* 43%. Principal support for museums. *Civic & Public Affairs:* 4%. Major support for a botanical garden, urban and community affairs organizations. *Education:* 35%. Primarily support for colleges and universities, primary and secondary education, and arts education. *Environment:* 7%. Youth organizations, child welfare, and community service organizations. *International:* 7%. Hospitals, single-disease health associations, medical research, and pediatric health. *Note:* Total contributions made in fiscal 2000. **Typ. Recipients:** Cancer, Children's Health/Hospitals, Clinics/Medical Centers, Domestic Violence, Eyes/Blindness, Family Planning, Health Organizations, Hospitals, Hospitals (University Affiliated), Medical Research, Nursing Services, Research/Studies Institutes, Sexual Abuse. **Geo. Dist:** MO.


## ★ 780 ★ William T. Morris Foundation

230 Park Ave., Ste. 622
New York, NY 10169-0622
**Phone:** (212)986-8036          **Fax:** (212)370-1962
Edward Antonelli, President, Chief Executive
    Officer & Dir
**Fnded:** 1937. **Philosophy:** The foundation supports general philanthropy, particularly in the areas of education, health, culture, and youth. **Priorities:** *Arts & Humanities:* 19%. Contributes to music and performing arts. *Civic & Public Affairs:* 5%. Supports other foundations and professional associations. *Education:* 40%. Supports higher education. *Environment:* 1%. Gives to youth groups. *International:* 26%. Funds hospitals, ear and eye research, and medical centers. *Religion:* 1%. Science museums. *Note:* Total contributions made in fiscal 1999. **Typ. Recipients:** Alzheimers Disease, Arthritis, Arthritis, Cancer, Clinics/Medical Centers, Emergency/Ambulance Services, Eyes/Blindness, Health Funds, Heart, Hospitals, Medical Education, Medical Rehabilitation, Medical Research, Multiple Sclerosis, People with Disabilities, Respiratory, Single-Disease Health Associations, Speech & Hearing. **Geo. Dist:** CT; NY; PA.


## ★ 781 ★ Windham Foundation

PO Box 70
Grafton, VT 05146
**Phone:** (802)843-2211          **Fax:** (802)843-2205
**Email:** winfound@sover.net
**Website:** http://www.windham-foundation.org
Stephan Morse, President & Chief Executive Officer
**Fnded:** 1963. **Philosophy:** "The Foundation has a particular interest in innovative programs and furthering proven academic programs that could be replicated in other Vermont locations." "As of January 1, 1998, the Windham Foundation will institute a new grant policy. The Foundation will limit its grant interests to Vermont elementary and secondary education." **Priorities:** *Arts & Humanities:* About 34%. Symphonies, historical preservation, and museums. *Civic & Public Affairs:* 12%. *Education:* 38%. Colleges and universities, high schools, and environmental education. *Environment:* About 13%. Youth organizations, food programs, and family services. *International:* 4%. Hospice programs, hospitals, and cancer research and treatment. *Religion:* 1%. *Note:* Total contributions made in fiscal 1998. **Typ. Recipients:** Arthritis, Cancer, Diabetes, Domestic Violence, Emergency/Ambulance Services, Family Planning, Health Organizations, Health-General, Home-Care Services, Hospices, Hospitals, Kidney, Prenatal Health Issues,

Trauma Treatment. **Geo. Dist:** VT, emphasis on Windham County.


## ★ 782 ★ Wollenberg Foundation

235 MOntgomery St., Ste. 2700
San Francisco, CA 94104
**Phone:** (510)625-9049
Marc Monheimer, Trustee
**Fnded:** 1952. **Philosophy:** The foundation is primarily interested in education and educational funds. Science, medical, and business schools at the university level are supported in addition to public school systems. The foundation also supports a variety of social service programs and civic interests. **Priorities:** *Arts & Humanities:* 1%. Supports the symphony. *Civic & Public Affairs:* 2%. Supports civil rights. *Education:* 92%. Supports education fund, education organizations, colleges and public elementary school programs. *Environment:* 3%. Supports emergency relief and youth services. *Religion:* 1%. Supports a science museum. *Note:* Total contributions made in 1998. **Typ. Recipients:** Domestic Violence, Emergency/Ambulance Services, Family Planning, Hospices, Medical Education, People with Disabilities, Single-Disease Health Associations. **Geo. Dist:** nationally.


## ★ 783 ★ Woods Charitable Fund

PO Box 81309
Lincoln, NE 68501
**Phone:** (402)436-5971          **Fax:** (402)436-4128
**Email:** pbaker@woodscharitable.org
**Website:** http://www.woodscharitable.org
Pam Baker, Executive Director & Secretary
**Fnded:** 1941. **Philosophy:** The fund provides support to nonprofit organizations working to improve living conditions and opportunities for disadvantaged urban residents. A principal goal is to encourage citizen involvement in building a sense of community and in seeking long-term solutions for problems facing Lincoln, NE. The fund is interested in programs that explore policy options in the public interest, and it continues to support cultural and educational programs. Lincoln funding emphasizes education; community development and housing; children, youth, and families; and the arts and humanities. The fund's program for children, youth, and families includes direct-service and policy programs focused on child care, single parenthood, the elderly, family planning, shelter, troubled families, and others. The fund gives special consideration to programs addressing the areas of youth and family violence. The education program looks forward to reviewing proposals from existing educational institutions and from creative new programs to meet the challenge of preparing individuals of all ages for a rapidly changing society. The community development and housing program supports projects that empower less advantaged Lincoln residents to participate in the economic system and that foster community participation and responsibility, thus joining people to solve problems and improve opportunities for all. The program recognizes the growing need in Lincoln for affordable housing and supports projects that expand its availability. Advocacy groups and neighborhood, citizen, and community organizations are avenues to promote citizen involvement and strengthen neighborhoods. The need for individuals to achieve self-sufficiency, including helping people earn an adequate income, has also been identified as a primary community concern. The fund encourages submission of proposals that suggest creative approaches to address this concern. The fund also supports programs in the arts and humanities that enhance or develop the common aesthetic spirit through education, creation, or performance. **Priorities:** *Arts & Humanities:* 27%. Supports performing arts centers, arts councils and associations, orchestras, and public broadcasting. *Civic & Public Affairs:* 8%. Supports leadership organizations and housing. *Education:* 11%. Supports literacy, humanities education, and after-school programs. *Environment:* 52%. Supports youth and family services, food banks, and planned parenthood. *Note:* Total contributions made in 2000. **Typ. Recipients:** AIDS/HIV, Alzheimers Disease, Child Abuse, Clinics/Medical Centers, Domestic Violence, Family Planning, Medical Rehabilitation,

Mental Health, People with Disabilities, Public Health, Single-Disease Health Associations, Substance Abuse. **Geo. Dist:** Lincoln, NE.

## ★ 784 ★ Woods Fund of Chicago
360 N Michigan, Ste. 1600
Chicago, IL 60601
**Phone:** (312)782-2698          **Fax:** (312)782-4155
**Email:** info@woodsfund.org
Todd Dietterle, vice president

**Fnded:** 1993. **Philosophy:** "Woods Fund of Chicago is a grantmaking foundation whose goal is to increase opportunities for less advantaged people and communities in the metropolitan area, including the opportunity to contribute to decisions affecting them. The foundation works primarily as a funding partner with nonprofit organizations. Woods supports nonprofits in their important roles of engaging people in civic life, addressing the causes of poverty and other challenges facing the region, promoting more effective public policies, reducing barriers to equal opportunity, and building a sense of community and common ground." 1998 Annual Report. **Priorities:** *Arts & Humanities:* 6%. Funds dance company, theatre, music. *Civic & Public Affairs:* 68%. Supports organizations for community leadership, economic development, public housing, job training. *Education:* 10%. Funds and after-school programs, pre-schools, and colleges and universities. *Environment:* 7%. Supports family and youth programs, the elderly, programs for the hungry and the homeless. *International:* 4%. Supports adolescent health organizations and medical centers. *Note:* Total contributions made in 1998. **Typ. Recipients:** Adolescent Health Issues, Clinics/Medical Centers, Medical Rehabilitation, Prenatal Health Issues. **Geo. Dist:** Chicago, IL.

## ★ 785 ★ Wortham Foundation
2727 Allen Parkway, Ste. 1570
Wortham Tower
Houston, TX 77019
**Phone:** (713)526-8849          **Fax:** (713)526-7222
Barbara Snyder, Grants Administrator

**Fnded:** 1958. **Philosophy:** Prior to the 1969 Tax Reform Act, the foundation was involved primarily with a research project in cattle fertility. The foundation now carries out its founders' interests in "cultural arts and civic beautification projects and to those projects which benefit the citizens of Houston, Harris County, Texas." Wortham Foundation fiscal 1998 Form 990. **Priorities:** *Arts & Humanities:* 55%. Focus on the performing arts and museums. Also supports public broadcasting and historic preservation. *Civic & Public Affairs:* 19%. Supports parks/recreation organizations, with a focus on civic beautification projects. *Environment:* 11%. Supports youth organizations, YMCA, and United Way. *Religion:* 9%. *Note:* Total contributions made in fiscal 2000. **Typ. Recipients:** Cancer, Children's Health/Hospitals, Clinics/Medical Centers, Emergency/Ambulance Services, Hospitals, Medical Education, Public Health. **Geo. Dist:** Houston, TX.

## ★ 786 ★ Wyomissing Foundation
12 Commerce Dr.
Wyomissing, PA 19610
**Phone:** (610)376-7494          **Fax:** (610)372-7626
**Email:** wfbbec@nni.com
Mrs. C. Walters, Administrator

**Fnded:** 1929. **Philosophy:** The Wyomissing Foundation makes most of its grants in the areas of education, the arts, civic affairs, and social services. Educational funding favors colleges and universities, special education, and literacy. Support for the arts goes to museums, festivals, ballet, libraries, and public broadcasting. Civic affairs support includes environmental affairs and zoos. The majority of the social service funding goes to united funds. Other recipient areas are also supported. **Priorities:** *Arts & Humanities:* 5%. Music, museums, public television, libraries, opera. and historic preservation. *Civic & Public Affairs:* 11%. Community foundations, housing, clubs and safety. *Education:* 4%. Reading/literacy programs, and colleges and universities. *Environment:* 6%. Food banks, scouting, United Way, and youth programs. *Interna-*

*tional:* Less than 1%. *Note:* Total contributions made in 1998. **Typ. Recipients:** AIDS/HIV, Emergency/Ambulance Services, Family Planning, Health Funds, Home-Care Services, Hospitals, Medical Rehabilitation, Nursing Services, People with Disabilities, Prenatal Health Issues. **Geo. Dist:** PA, Berks County and contiguous counties.

## ★ 787 ★ Y. and H. Soda Foundation
2 Theatre Square, Ste. 211
Orinda, CA 94563-3346
**Phone:** (925)253-2630          **Fax:** (925)253-1814
**Email:** Judyed@PacBell.net
Mrs. Judith Murphy, President & Chief Executive Officer

**Fnded:** 1964. **Philosophy:** The foundation focuses on organizations providing the following services in Alameda and Contra Costa Counties, CA: religious welfare (primarily Catholic), health care, human services, youth development, and education. The foundation "seeks to enhance the quality of life for the disadvantaged, to promote their health and welfare, to provide opportunities for education and to support those organizations whose religious philosophy strengthens the spiritual and temporal well-being of those whom they serve." **Priorities:** *Arts & Humanities:* 1%. Supports a museum. *Civic & Public Affairs:* 6%. Funds housing associations, minority affairs, and community organizations. *Education:* 81%. Funds preschool and childcare programs, primary and secondary public and private schools, higher education, and job training programs. *Environment:* 5%. Supports youth development, including services for abused and disadvantaged youth, athletic and mentoring programs, vocational training, camps, and clubs. *International:* 5%. Funds medical centers and hospice. *Note:* Total contributions made in 2000. **Typ. Recipients:** AIDS/HIV, Cancer, Children's Health/Hospitals, Clinics/Medical Centers, Domestic Violence, Geriatric Health, Health Organizations, Hospices, Hospitals, Long-Term Care, People with Disabilities, Prenatal Health Issues, Public Health, Research/Studies Institutes, Sexual Abuse, Single-Disease Health Associations, Speech & Hearing, Substance Abuse. **Geo. Dist:** CA, Alameda and Contra Costa Counties.

## ★ 788 ★ Yawkey Foundation II
990 Washington St.
Dedham, MA 02026
**Phone:** (781)329-7470          **Fax:** (781)329-8195
John Harrington, Trustee

**Fnded:** 1983. **Philosophy:** The foundation primarily supports social services, educational institutions, civic affairs, the arts, and health concerns. **Priorities:** *Arts & Humanities:* 11%. Museums, music, libraries, public broadcasting, and historic preservation. *Civic & Public Affairs:* 14%. Foundations, sports programs, community services, and aquariums. *Education:* 30%. Colleges, secondary schools, and universities. *Environment:* 29%. Youth and family services, athletics/recreation, homes, and people with disabilities. *International:* 7%. Research, medical centers, multiple sclerosis, and hospitals. *Religion:* Less than 1%. Science museums. *Note:* Total contributions made in fiscal 1998. **Typ. Recipients:** Cancer, Children's Health/Hospitals, Clinics/Medical Centers, Eyes/Blindness, Health Organizations, Hospitals, Medical Research, People with Disabilities, Single-Disease Health Associations. **Geo. Dist:** MA; Boston, MA, metropolitan area.

## ★ 789 ★ Z. Smith Reynolds Foundation
101 Reynolda Village
Winston-Salem, NC 27106-5199
**Phone:** (336)725-7541          **Fax:** (336)725-6069
**Email:** tomr@zsr.org
**Website:** http://www.zsr.org
Thomas Ross, Executive Director

**Fnded:** 1936. **Philosophy:** The foundation's original donors intentionally left the terms of its charter broad so that trustees might make grants for a wide array of projects. The foundation is limited, however, to making grants exclusively within the state of North Carolina. The purpose of the foundation, in its own words, is "to enhance the quality of life in North Carolina." It fulfills

this broad-based role by seeking out needy aspects of North Carolina life, and "places higher value on developing new, quality programs, rather than in sustaining well-established, well-funded ones." Areas of interest include economic and community development, pre-collegiate education, minority issues, women's issues, and protection of the environment. Concerns about the persistence of poverty, and the need to develop strategies to ensure greater equity in the accessibility and use of resources are the basis of programs in the area of community and economic development. The foundation's concern in minority affairs focuses on the need to bolster black family life; improve the academic performance of, and opportunities for, black youth; increase political participation; and foster new leadership in the black community. The foundation's concern for women's issues includes eliminating barriers to women's career progress, and raising women's income level. The foundation also is concerned with women in crisis and in the provision of shelters, counseling, and support groups for them. The overall goals of the foundation in the environmental area are to protect North Carolina's land, waters, and air, and to give special attention to the needs of the state's ecologically sensitive areas. The foundation has sponsored conferences in criminal justice, childhood education, housing, black issues, environmental concerns, and the future of rural North Carolina, in order to bring together people with needs and others with knowledge or solutions. In addition, through its sabbatical program, the foundation provides an opportunity for people who have dedicated their careers to public service to enjoy time away from their job responsibilities; they return to their work renewed and often with new ideas for the achievement of their missions. **Priorities:** *Arts & Humanities:* 4%. Supports historic preservation. *Civic & Public Affairs:* 33%. Funds community development initiatives, public policy, housing, self-help programs, and legal aid. *Education:* 43%. Supports literacy programs, alternative learning centers, and colleges and universities. *Environment:* 8%. Funds youth programs, volunteerism, child advocacy programs, domestic violence prevention, and United Way. *Note:* Total contributions made in 1999. **Typ. Recipients:** Adolescent Health Issues, Alzheimers Disease, Child Abuse, Domestic Violence, Family Planning, Health Policy/Cost Containment, People with Disabilities, Prenatal Health Issues, Public Health, Substance Abuse. **Geo. Dist:** NC.

## ★ 790 ★ Zarrow Family Foundation
401 S Boston, Ste. 900
Tulsa, OK 74103
**Phone:** (918)295-8004          **Fax:** (918)295-8049
**Email:** jgillert@zarrow.com
**Website:** http://www.zarrow.com
Jeanne Gillert, Manager

**Fnded:** 1988. **Priorities:** *Arts & Humanities:* 3%. Supports music, museums and the local community ballet theater. *Civic & Public Affairs:* 2%. Supports philanthropy, clubs, community organizations, and zoos. *Education:* 13%. Supports private schools (pre-college), colleges, and universities, education reform and funds, business education, and medical education. *Environment:* 34%. Major support is awarded to Goodwill Industries. Other recipients include community service organizations, youth organizations, senior services, people with disabilities, and food distribution centers. *International:* 16%. Interests include single-disease health associations, mental health foundations, emergency services, clinics and medical centers, and hospitals. *Note:* Total contributions made in 2000. **Typ. Recipients:** Alzheimers Disease, Cancer, Children's Health/Hospitals, Clinics/Medical Centers, Diabetes, Emergency/Ambulance Services, Eyes/Blindness, Geriatric Health, Health Funds, Health Organizations, Heart, Hospices, Hospitals, Medical Education, Medical Research, Mental Health, Multiple Sclerosis, People with Disabilities, Prenatal Health Issues, Respiratory, Single-Disease Health Associations, Substance Abuse. **Geo. Dist:** nationally; Tulsa, OK, supports preselected organizations only.

## ★ 791 ★ Zellerbach Family Fund

120 Montgomery St., Ste. 1550
San Francisco, CA 94104
**Phone:** (415)421-2629    **Fax:** (415)421-6713
Cindy Rambo, Executive Director
**Fnded:** 1956. **Philosophy:** "In 1997, the Fund focused its efforts on programs that: enhance the ability of public systems and institutions to better serve families and children; increase and build upon the strengths and capacities within neighborhoods as residents work together to reduce shared problems; foster the ability of immigrants and refugees to successfully participate in American society; promote culture in its many varieties and traditions; and promote the healthy development of youth." 1997 Annual Report. Grants from the fund are directed largely to needs within the San Francisco Bay Area. The fund is affiliated with the Northern California Grantmakers, and it joins with other foundations, corporations, and nonprofit organizations to be more aware of and responsive to community needs. **Priorities:** *Arts & Humanities:* 28%. Supports ballet, opera, the symphony, and community art organizations. *Civic & Public Affairs:* 26%. Funds botanical gardens, small business development, and urban affairs. *Education:* 19%. Supports education reform and universities. *Environment:* 18%. Supports family services and youth development organizations. *International:* 8%. Supports education reform and universities. *Note:* Total contributions made in 1997. **Typ. Recipients:** AIDS/HIV, Child Abuse, Children's Health/Hospitals, Domestic Violence, Health Organizations, Mental Health, People with Disabilities, Public Health, Research/Studies Institutes, Trauma Treatment. **Geo. Dist:** San Francisco, CA, Bay Area.

## ★ 792 ★ Zemurray Foundation

228 Saint Charles, Ste. 1024
New Orleans, LA 70130
**Phone:** (504)523-4901    **Fax:** (504)571-1024
**Fnded:** 1951. **Philosophy:** The Zemurray Foundation makes most of its grants in the areas of education, civic affairs, and the arts in New Orleans. Educational giving favors colleges and universities. Civic affairs support is given primarily to environmental and regional foundations. The New Orleans Museum of Art is a major recipient along with other art organizations. Minor grants are given to other recipient areas. **Priorities:** *Arts & Humanities:* 21%. Supports art councils, art centers, and museums. *Civic & Public Affairs:* 2%. Supports community foundations, a crime commision, and a civil service league. *Education:* 38%. Supports academics, schools, colleges, and universities. *Environment:* 1%. Supports United Way, YMCA. *Note:* Total contributions made in 1998. **Typ. Recipients:** Cancer, Clinics/Medical Centers, Family Planning, Hospitals, Medical Research, People with Disabilities. **Geo. Dist:** nationally, with some New Orleans, LA.

## Corporate Foundations

## ★ 793 ★ A.O. Smith Foundation, Inc.

PO Box 245007
Milwaukee, WI 53224-9507
**Phone:** (414)359-4042    **Fax:** (414)359-4064
Edward O'Connor, Secretary
**Fnded:** 1955. **Priorities:** *Arts & Humanities:* 16%. Supports museums, libraries, and theater. *Civic & Public Affairs:* 3%. Funds public safety, zoos, and memorials. *Education:* 27%. Emphasis on colleges and universities and independent college funds. *Environment:* 41%. Major emphasis on the United Way. Also supports human services and youth organizations. *International:* 10%. Supports hospitals and single-disease associations. *Note:* Total contributions made in 2000. **Typ. Recipients:** Emergency/Ambulance Services, Hospitals, Medical Education, Medical Rehabilitation, Mental Health, People with Disabilities, Public Health, Substance Abuse. **Geo. Dist:** communities where company has manufacturing facilities.

## ★ 794 ★ Abbott Laboratories Fund

Department 379, Bldg. AP6D-2
100 Abbott Park Rd.
Abbott Park, IL 60064-6048
**Phone:** (847)937-7075    **Fax:** (847)935-5051
**Website:** http://abbott.com/community/lab_fund.html
Cindy Schwab, Vice President
**Fnded:** 1951. **Priorities:** *Arts & Humanities:* (Culture & Arts) 9%. Supports organizations providing cultural enrichment in operating communities. Interests include art, music, and museums. *Civic & Public Affairs:* (Civic, Environment, and Misc.) 15%. Interests include community improvement projects and groups involved in the fields of administration of justice, public policy, safety, and business. *Education:* 22%. Concentrates on colleges and universities possessing the potential to benefit the health care industry, including basic research programs in physical and biological sciences, medicine, pharmacology, nutrition, and diagnostics. Also supports institutions that are potential sources of personnel for the health care industry. *International:* (Health & Welfare) 41%. Supports united funds and community drives funding local institutions, or other specific, well-defined programs in communities where company has a significant number of employees. Supports agencies working with families, disadvantaged youth, and senior citizens, as well as agencies seeking to improve the socioeconomic position of women, minorities, and immigrant populations. Also supports individual hospitals and health-care institutions used frequently by company employees. *Note:* Total contributions in 2000. **Typ. Recipients:** Children's Health/Hospitals, Clinics/Medical Centers, Emergency/Ambulance Services, Geriatric Health, Health Organizations, Health-General, Heart, Hospices, Hospitals, Hospitals (University Affiliated), Kidney, Medical Education, Medical Rehabilitation, Medical Research, Medical Training, Nursing Services, Nutrition, People with Disabilities, Public Health, Research/Studies Institutes, Sexual Abuse, Single-Disease Health Associations, Substance Abuse. **Geo. Dist:** headquarters and operating communities.

## ★ 795 ★ ABC Foundation

1201 Maple St.
Greensboro, NC 27405
**Phone:** (336)379-6220
Mr. Terry Weatherford, Secretary
**Priorities:** *Arts & Humanities:* 8%. Supports the United Arts Council of North Carolina and the Battleship NC monument. *Civic & Public Affairs:* 4%. Favors textile foundations, business foundations, and community organizations. *Education:* 29%. Provides scholarships to college students. Supports colleges, public education, vocational technical schools, and literacy. *Environment:* 55%. Primarily supports various United Ways located in North Carolina, South Carolina and Mississippi. Other support goes to Goodwill Industries, YMCA, and youth organizations. *International:* Less than 1%. Supports public health and hospice programs. *Religion:* 3%. Funds the Institute of Textile Technology. *Note:* Total foundation contributions made in fiscal 2000. **Typ. Recipients:** Emergency/Ambulance Services, Health Organizations, Health-General, Hospices, Multiple Sclerosis, People with Disabilities, Substance Abuse. **Geo. Dist:** operating locations; Greensboro, NC.

## ★ 796 ★ ABC Foundation

77 West 66th St., 20th Floor
New York, NY 10023
**Phone:** (212)456-7011    **Fax:** (212)456-7909
Bernadette Longford, Manager of Corporate Giving
**Fnded:** 1975. **Priorities:** *Arts & Humanities:* 48%. Emphasis is on programs which encourage culturally diverse forms of expression which work to broaden their audiences, with an emphasis on theater and playwrights. Other interests include museums, public broadcasting, film institutes, dance, music, arts associations, and performing arts centers. *Civic & Public Affairs:* 10%. Funding supports professional and trade associations, particularly those related to the news media. Other interests include business, civil rights, women's issues, and public policy. *Education:* 20%.

Supports efforts to bolster private education with emphasis on access and equity. Majority of funding supports colleges and universities, especially in the New York area. Interests include business, medical, journalism, and legal education. Other areas of interest include public education, literacy, minority education, and student aid. *Environment:* 8%. Emphasizes youth organizations. Child welfare, family services, community service organizations, employment, the aged, and religious welfare are also supported. *International:* 12%. Funds single-disease health associations, health centers, and hospitals. *Religion:* 1%. *Note:* Total contributions made in 1999. **Typ. Recipients:** AIDS/HIV, Cancer, Children's Health/Hospitals, Clinics/Medical Centers, Health Organizations, Heart, Hospitals, Hospitals (University Affiliated), Medical Education, Medical Research, Medical Training, People with Disabilities, Single-Disease Health Associations, Substance Abuse, Transplant Networks/Donor Banks. **Geo. Dist:** headquarters and operating communities. **Frmly:** Capital Cities/ABC Foundation.

## ★ 797 ★ Abel Foundation

PO Box 80268
Lincoln, NE 68501
**Phone:** (402)434-1212    **Fax:** (402)434-1799
**Website:** http://www.abelfoundation.org
J. McCown, Vice President
**Fnded:** 1951. **Priorities:** *Arts & Humanities:* 15%. Supports local arts organizations, the performing arts, and historical societies. *Civic & Public Affairs:* 45%. Supports parks, housing, and community foundations. *Education:* 9%. More than half of education grants support Lincoln, NE, area colleges and universities. Also supports public education. *Environment:* 31%. Supports the United Way and community and family services organizations. *Note:* Total contributions made in 1999. **Typ. Recipients:** Children's Health/Hospitals, Domestic Violence, Family Planning, Health Organizations, Health-General, Heart, Hospitals, Mental Health, People with Disabilities, Research/Studies Institutes, Transplant Networks/Donor Banks. **Geo. Dist:** Lincoln, NE.

## Ace Hardware Foundation

*See:* Entry 5568

## ★ 798 ★ Adolph Coors Co.

PO Box 4030, NH 420
Golden, CO 80401-0030
**Phone:** (303)277-6204    **Fax:** (303)277-6132
**Email:** pthom@memo.acehardware.com
**Website:** http://www.coors.com
Buck Boze, Corporate Contributions Manager
**Priorities:** *Voluntarism:* Company supports Volunteers in Community Enrichment (VICE) program. Contact Crystal Adams at (303) 277-3736 for more information. **Typ. Recipients:** AIDS/HIV, Domestic Violence, Emergency/Ambulance Services, Health Funds, Health Organizations, Hospices, Hospitals, Medical Rehabilitation, Mental Health, People with Disabilities, Respiratory, Single-Disease Health Associations, Substance Abuse. **Geo. Dist:** Denver, CO; Memphis, TN; Elkton, VA.

## ★ 799 ★ Advanced Micro Devices, Inc.

5204 E Ben White Blvd.
MailStop 529
Austin, TX 78741
**Phone:** (512)602-5501    **Fax:** (512)602-6985
**Email:** allyson.peerman@AMD.com
**Website:** http://www.amd.com
Allyson Peerman, Manager, Corporate Community Affairs
**Priorities:** *Civic & Public Affairs:* 3%. *Education:* 55%. *Environment:* 34%. Includes health and human services funding. *Voluntarism:* AMD organizes group volunteer activities that provide hundreds of AMD employees with the opportunity to participate in local community events. The company's Grant Incentives for Volunteer Efforts (GIVE) program provides mini-grants to eligible organizations for which AMD employees volunteer. *Note:* Total contributions made in 2000.

**Typ. Recipients:** Clinics/Medical Centers, Hospitals, People with Disabilities. **Geo. Dist:** headquarters and operating communities; CA; TX. **Frmly:** Advanced Micro Devices Charitable Foundation.

### ★ 800 ★ AEGON U.S.A. Charitable Foundation
1111 N Charles St.
Baltimore, MD 21201
**Phone:** (410)576-4576          **Fax:** (410)347-8685
Rosmary Kostmayer, Director, Public Relations and Colorados

**Fnded:** 1988. **Priorities:** *Arts & Humanities:* 15%. Supports orchestras, art museums, historical societies, and public broadcasting. *Civic & Public Affairs:* 7%. Supports chambers of commerce and community/economic development. *Education:* 14%. Gives to Junior Achievement, colleges and universities, public schools, and other education concerns. *Environment:* 41%. Supports United Way, family services, prevention of domestic violence, services for the disabled, YMCAs/YWCAs, and youth groups. *International:* 19%. Supports health foundations and medical centers, and clinics. *Religion:* 3%. Gives to the Science Station. *Note:* Total foundation contributions made in 2000. **Typ. Recipients:** Alzheimers Disease, Arthritis, Children's Health/Hospitals, Diabetes, Domestic Violence, Heart, Hospitals, Prenatal Health Issues, Public Health, Single-Disease Health Associations. **Geo. Dist:** headquarters and operating communities; IA, eastern; KY; MD, central.

### ★ 801 ★ Aetna Foundation
151 Farmington Ave., RE2R
Hartford, CT 06156-3180
**Phone:** (860)273-7580
**Website:** http://www.aetna.com/foundation/
Christopher Montross, Director

**Priorities:** *Arts & Humanities:* 26%. Funds nationally-recognized art museums and performing arts centers. *Civic & Public Affairs:* 5%. Supports public affairs, community/economic development, and workforce development programs. *Education:* 16%. Supports college preparation, school-to-career initiatives, and Junior Achievement. *Environment:* 17%. Supports the United Way, youth organizations, homeless shelters, and other social services. *International:* 35%. Supports cardiovascular disease and cancer prevention, detection, and research initiatives; health funds; public health; maternity health care; and the National Medical Association. *Voluntarism:* The company sponsors the Aetna Volunteers! Program, which makes grants up to $500 to nonprofits where company employees volunteer; grants are initiated by the employee. Also supports the Aetna Volunteer Council, which matches employees with volunteer opportunities. *Note:* Total foundation contributions made in 2000. **Typ. Recipients:** AIDS/HIV, Cancer, Child Abuse, Children's Health/Hospitals, Clinics/Medical Centers, Diabetes, Domestic Violence, Emergency/Ambulance Services, Health Organizations, Heart, Hospitals, Medical Education, Nursing Services, Nutrition, People with Disabilities, Prenatal Health Issues, Public Health, Respiratory. **Geo. Dist:** principally near operating locations and to national organizations; Hartford, CT.

### ★ 802 ★ AFLAC Inc.
1932 Wynnton Rd.
Columbus, GA 31999
**Phone:** (706)323-3431          **Fax:** (706)320-2288
**Website:** http://www.aflac.com
Wendy Hogan, Administrator, Corp. Contributions

**Priorities:** *Arts & Humanities:* About 10%. Supports community arts, historic preservation, and museums. *Civic & Public Affairs:* About 20%. Interests include better government, economic development, public policy, ethnic and minority organizations, and professional associations. *Education:* About 5%. Favors colleges and universities, community and junior colleges, business education, elementary education, and special education. *International:* About 65% of total contributions. Recipients include health organizations, medical research, hospices, single-disease health

organizations, shelters, child welfare, and united funds. Also supports cancer research and treatment, including recent grants to fund chairs in cancer research at various hospitals and to support children's hospitals. **Typ. Recipients:** Health Organizations, Hospices, Medical Research, Single-Disease Health Associations, Substance Abuse. **Geo. Dist:** GA.

### ★ 803 ★ AGL Resources Inc.
817 West Peachtree St. NW, 10th Floor
Atlanta, GA 30308
**Phone:** (404)584-9470          **Fax:** (404)584-3479
**Email:** sbush@aglresources.com
Peter Banks, Vice President, External Affairs

**Priorities:** *Arts & Humanities:* 5% to 10%. Includes arts festivals, music, museums, arts organizations, historic preservation, public broadcasting, and theater arts. *Civic & Public Affairs:* 45% to 50%. Supports better government campaigns, civil rights, consumer affairs, housing, law and justice, professional and trade associations, miscellaneous organizations, community development, economics, and environmental organizations. *Education:* 25% to 30%. Funding favors higher education, agricultural education, secondary, minority, engineering, and journalism education. *International:* About 15%. Recipients include mental health, health organizations, community service organizations, child welfare, youth organizations, and senior services. *Note:* Company also supports United Way. **Typ. Recipients:** Health Organizations, Hospices, Medical Research, Mental Health, Nutrition, People with Disabilities, Public Health, Substance Abuse. **Geo. Dist:** GA.

### ★ 804 ★ Agrilink Foods/Pro-Fac Foundation
PO Box 20670
Rochester, NY 14602-0670
**Phone:** (716)264-3155          **Fax:** (716)383-1606
**Website:**     http://www.agrilinkfoods.com/corp/about/community/index.html
Susan Riker, Secretary

**Priorities:** *Arts & Humanities:* 11%. Supports museums, galleries, history, libraries and theater. *Civic & Public Affairs:* 4%. *Education:* 18%. Supports arts/humanities education, scholarships, colleges, universities and literacy. *Environment:* 54%. Supports people with disabilities, substance abuse programs, youth programs, Special Olympics, scouting, young men's christian association, and camps. *International:* 10%. Supports hospitals, medical, centers, children's health, and nursing services. *Religion:* 2%. *Note:* Total contributions made in 1999. **Typ. Recipients:** Cancer, Children's Health/Hospitals, Clinics/Medical Centers, Domestic Violence, Emergency/Ambulance Services, Family Planning, Geriatric Health, Health Organizations, Heart, Hospices, Hospitals, Medical Rehabilitation, Mental Health, Nursing Services, People with Disabilities, Public Health, Single-Disease Health Associations, Substance Abuse. **Geo. Dist:** headquarters and operating communities.

### ★ 805 ★ Air Products Foundation
7201 Hamilton Boulevard
Allentown, PA 18195-1501
**Phone:** (610)481-6349          **Fax:** (610)481-6642
**Website:** http://www.airproducts.com/social_responsibilities/
Timothy Holt, Contact

**Priorities:** *Arts & Humanities:* (Art and Culture) 11%. Supports museums, music, and the performing arts. Other areas of interest include theaters, festivals, and public broadcasting. *Civic & Public Affairs:* (Community and Economic Development) 10%. Economic development is a major concern, as are environmental affairs, business and free enterprise organizations, and housing rehabilitation. Also supports safety organizations. *Education:* (Pre-college and Higher Education) 45%. Supports engineering and business departments of colleges and universities. Also interested in independent college funds and minority, economic, and arts education. Majority of education funds are in the form of matching gifts. *Environment:* (United Way)

28%. *International:* (Fitness, Health, and Welfare) 6%. Health interests include single-disease health associations and emergency services. *Voluntarism:* VOL Seventy percent of employees volunteer in community activities. Volunteerism is encouraged and recognized by the company, but it does not have a formal volunteer program. *Note:* Above percentages represent fiscal 2000 foundation contributions only. Direct giving program priorities are similar. Matching gifts are included in the analysis. **Typ. Recipients:** Cancer, Children's Health/Hospitals, Domestic Violence, Emergency/Ambulance Services, Health Organizations, Heart, Multiple Sclerosis, Nutrition, People with Disabilities, Single-Disease Health Associations, Substance Abuse. **Geo. Dist:** headquarters and select operating communities.

### ★ 806 ★ Airborne Inc.
PO Box 662
Seattle, WA 98111-0662
**Phone:** (206)285-4600          **Fax:** (206)830-4438
**Website:** http://www.airborne.com
Dave Scheevel, Vice President, Revenue Control

**Priorities:** *Arts & Humanities:* 10%. *Civic & Public Affairs:* 10%. *Education:* 20%. *Environment:* 55%. **Typ. Recipients:** Health-General. **Geo. Dist:** WA, western Washington.

### ★ 807 ★ AK Steel Foundation
703 Curtis St.
Middletown, OH 45043
**Phone:** (513)425-2826          **Fax:** (513)425-2676
Brian Coughlin, Government Affairs Manager;
     Executive Di

**Fnded:** 1990. **Priorities:** *Arts & Humanities:* 1%. Funds community arts, symphonies, and music. *Civic & Public Affairs:* 11%. Support is directed to community foundations and Junior Achievement chapters. *Education:* 16%. Primary interests include colleges and universities, secondary education, and education associations. Also sponsors a scholarship program for children of employees. *Environment:* 54%. Primary support includes funding for the United Way in Ohio and Pennsylvania. *International:* 18%. Supports a medical center. *Note:* Total contributions made in 1999. **Typ. Recipients:** Cancer, Child Abuse, Clinics/Medical Centers, Emergency/Ambulance Services, Heart, Hospices, Hospitals, People with Disabilities, Public Health, Single-Disease Health Associations. **Geo. Dist:** operating locations.

### ★ 808 ★ Alabama Power Foundation
600 N 18th St.
Birmingham, AL 35291
**Phone:** (205)257-2508          **Fax:** (205)257-1860
William Hutchins, III, President

**Fnded:** 1990. **Priorities:** *Arts & Humanities:* 14%. Supports art associations, libraries, symphonies, ballets, and public broadcasting. *Civic & Public Affairs:* 22%. Supports urban and community affairs, service organizations, and business and free enterprise. *Education:* 20%. Primarily supports colleges and universities, scholarships, and K-12 education. Continuing education, economic education, education funds, Junior Achievement, and literacy also receive gifts. *Environment:* 37%. Supports United Way and children and youth organizations. *International:* 5%. Pediatric health, mental health associations, health funds, and single-disease health associations receive support. *Note:* Total foundation contributions made in 2000. **Typ. Recipients:** Cancer, Diabetes, Eyes/Blindness, Health Organizations, Heart, Mental Health, People with Disabilities, Single-Disease Health Associations, Substance Abuse. **Geo. Dist:** headquarters and operating communities.

### ★ 809 ★ Alaska Airlines, Inc.
PO Box 68900
Seattle, WA 98168
**Phone:** (206)433-3383
**Email:** donna.hartman@alaskaair.com
Donna Hartman, Corporate Contribution Administrator

**Priorities:** *Arts & Humanities:* 5%. Gives to theater, art and history museums, music and arts festivals, symphonies and jazz groups, opera, and arts councils. *Civic & Public Affairs:* (Civic/Political) 6%. Supports chambers of commerce and an airport authority. *Education:* 22%. Supports colleges and universities and K-12 education. *Environment:* (Social/Community Services) 30%. Supports youth groups, Make-A-Wish Foundation, career training and placement, a zoo, World Vision, and Mission Aviation Fellowship. *International:* (Medical/Emergency-Research) 29%. Funds single-disease health organizations, Lions Eyebank, medical rescue teams, and Alaska Shriners. *Voluntarism:* Promotes volunteerism through the United Way and its sponsored projects. *Note:* Total corporate contributions made in 2000. **Typ. Recipients:** Health-General, Heart. **Geo. Dist:** headquarters and operating communities.

### ★ 810 ★ Albany International Corp.
PO Box 1907
Albany, NY 12201-1907
**Phone:** (518)445-2200 **Fax:** (518)447-6343
**Email:** ken_pauler@albint.com
**Website:** http://www.albint.com
Ken Pulver, Vice President, Corporate Communications

**Priorities:** *Arts & Humanities:* Funds cultural organizations that further the fine and performing arts. *Education:* Supports capital campaigns for colleges and universities, and paper schools from which company draws employees; also provides scholarships. *Environment:* Funds United Way and human service organizations. *International:* Supports hospital capital campaigns. **Typ. Recipients:** Hospices. **Geo. Dist:** headquarters and operating communities.

### ★ 811 ★ Albertson's Inc.
250 Parkcenter Blvd.
PO Box 20
Boise, ID 83726
**Phone:** (208)395-4382 **Fax:** (208)395-6631
**Website:** http://www1.albertsonss.com/corporate/pr/pr_main.asp?cat=3&subcat=0
Judy McLaughlin, Community Relations Coordinator

**Priorities:** *Education:* Seeks to assure the availability of a pool of trained and educated men and women from which to draw employees; to encourage continuing research and development in academic specialties relevantto the business corporation; and to promote standards of educational excellence. Support includes assistance to public and private higher education institutions, employee matching grants, scholarship programs and related organizations, including those which seek to increase public knowledge of economics and other subjects of special importance to the company. *International:* Goals are to assure the availability of adequate health care and human service support for employees and other corporate constituents; and to promote the development of new, workable responses to human health and welfare needs. Support includes assistance to federated drives, hospitals, youth agencies, and other local health and welfare groups. Customers and employees raise money to support the Muscular Dystrophy Association. **Typ. Recipients:** Emergency/Ambulance Services, Geriatric Health, Hospitals, Medical Rehabilitation, Mental Health, Public Health, Substance Abuse. **Geo. Dist:** headquarters and operating communities.

### ★ 812 ★ Alcoa Foundation
201 Isabella St.
Pittsburgh, PA 15212-5858
**Phone:** (412)553-2348 **Fax:** (412)553-4532
**Website:** http://www.alcoa.com/site/community/homepage/community.asp
Kathleen Buechel, President

**Fnded:** 1952. **Priorities:** *Arts & Humanities:* 4%. Supports arts institutes, libraries, arts associations, museums, music, performing arts and filmmaking and broadcasting. *Education:* 43%. Supports matching gifts, higher education organizations, higher education scholarships and fellowships, and scholarships for children of Alcoa employees. Limited program of

unrestricted funding. Support of quality education and research in public and private educational institutions. Historical interests in engineering and economics; supports newer specialized areas such as ceramics, polymers, and fiber optics. Grants are awarded to help improve both facilities and the quality of teaching at the secondary education level, particularly in the areas of economics, math, and science. *Environment:* 15%. Supports aid to indigent and handicapped persons; community service and welfare organizations; and prevention of cruelty to children and animals. A significant amount of funding goes to youth programs, community organizations, YMCA, the United Way. *International:* (Medical) 2%. Supports, hospitals, and medical organizations. In addition, the foundation supports single-disease health associations, medical research, and aid to patients. *Note:* Total contributions made in 1999. About 15% of the foundation's annual giving is to international organizations that fall within the above categories of giving. **Typ. Recipients:** AIDS/HIV, Cancer, Children's Health/Hospitals, Clinics/Medical Centers, Domestic Violence, Emergency/Ambulance Services, Family Planning, Geriatric Health, Health Funds, Health Organizations, Health Policy/Cost Containment, Hospices, Hospitals, Medical Education, Medical Rehabilitation, Medical Research, Medical Training, Mental Health, People with Disabilities, Prenatal Health Issues, Public Health, Single-Disease Health Associations, Speech & Hearing, Substance Abuse. **Geo. Dist:** principally near operating locations and to national organizations.

### ★ 813 ★ Alexander & Baldwin Foundation
PO Box 3440
Honolulu, HI 96801-3440
**Phone:** (808)525-6642 **Fax:** (808)525-6677
Ms. Meredith Ching, Senior Vice President

**Fnded:** 1992. **Priorities:** *Arts & Humanities:* 17%. Recipients include the performing arts, theater, historical societies, and museums. *Civic & Public Affairs:* 6%. Supports local civic affairs, including economic development, housing, safety programs, minorities, and cultural festivals. *Education:* 12%. Contributes to colleges and universities and private and public education. *Environment:* 53%. Emphasis on United Way. Also supports youth organizations, child welfare, and the disabled. *International:* 11%. Support for hospitals, health services, and single-disease organizations. *Note:* Total contributions made in 2000. **Typ. Recipients:** AIDS/HIV, Children's Health/Hospitals, Clinics/Medical Centers, Emergency/Ambulance Services, Health Organizations, Heart, Hospitals, Medical Rehabilitation, Nutrition, Single-Disease Health Associations, Substance Abuse. **Geo. Dist:** west coast; San Francisco, CA, including bay area; HI.

### ★ 814 ★ Allegheny Technologies Inc. Charitable Trust
1000 Six PPG Place
Pittsburgh, PA 15222
**Phone:** (412)394-2836 **Fax:** (412)394-3010
Jon Walton, Senior Vice President, Secretary & Gener

**Priorities:** *Arts & Humanities:* About 20%. Grants are made to musical organizations, libraries, theaters and arts centers. *Civic & Public Affairs:* 10% to 15%. Primarily supports community and economic development and philanthropic organizations. Interest also shown in professional and trade associations. *Education:* About 15%. Supports colleges and universities, schooladministrations, and high schools in the Pittsburgh area. Also provides employee matching gifts. *Environment:* 50% to 55%. Major support to the United Way in the Northeast and to traditional youth organizations such as the YMCA, Big Brothers and Big Sisters, Boys and Girls Clubs, and the Boy Scouts of America. Limited support also to child welfare organizations, food and clothing distribution, and children's homes. *International:* About 3%. Supports medical rehabilitation, hospitals, and single-disease health associations. **Typ. Recipients:** Children's Health/Hospitals, Emergency/Ambulance Services, Hospitals, Medical Rehabilitation, Mental Health, Nursing Services, People

with Disabilities, Sexual Abuse, Single-Disease Health Associations. **Geo. Dist:** headquarters and operating communities; Pittsburgh, PA, including greater metropolitan area. **Frmly:** Allegheny Teledyne Inc.

### ★ 815 ★ Allfirst Foundation, Inc.
25 South Charles St.
Ste. 1902
Baltimore, MD 21201
**Phone:** (410)244-3949 **Fax:** (410)545-2205
J. Riley, Secretary

**Fnded:** 1967. **Priorities:** *Arts & Humanities:* 20%. Supports art museums and galleries, orchestras, opera, historical societies, and theater. *Civic & Public Affairs:* 18%. Interests include community and urban development, public parks, minority affairs, nonprofit management, and job training and preparation. *Education:* 33%. The majority of education funding is awarded in general support to colleges and universities. The foundation also supports college funds, and matches employee gifts to higher education. *Environment:* 8%. Supports youth, community, and family services, principally in the Baltimore area. *International:* 4%. Supports medical centers. *Religion:* 4%. Gives to a science center. *Note:* Total contributions made in 1999. **Typ. Recipients:** Child Abuse, Clinics/Medical Centers, Hospices, Hospitals, Medical Education, People with Disabilities. **Geo. Dist:** headquarters and operating communities; DE; Washington, DC; Baltimore, MD, including metropolitan area.

### ★ 816 ★ Alliant Techsystems Community Investment Foundation
5050 Lincoln Dr.
Edina, MN 55436-1097
**Phone:** (952)931-6000 **Fax:** (952)931-5423
**Website:** http://www.atk.com
Nancy Darbut, Foundation Section

**Fnded:** 1992. **Priorities:** *Civic & Public Affairs:* (Community Relationships) 4%. Recipients include minority associations, public affairs, civic leagues, management improvement, economic development, and recreation. *Education:* (Increase Pool/Equip Teachers) 30%. Supports business, economic, math, and science education. Public education, colleges and universities, and scholarship funds are other recipients. Focus is on programs that overcome education barriers and equip math and science teachers to improve student performance. Also supports Junior Achievement. *Environment:* (Eliminate Barriers) 43%. Supports organizations and programs that resolve human services issues are barriers to learning. *Note:* Total contributions made in fiscal 2000. **Typ. Recipients:** Cancer, Children's Health/Hospitals, Emergency/Ambulance Services, Medical Education, Medical Research, People with Disabilities, Single-Disease Health Associations. **Geo. Dist:** headquarters and operating communities; Minneapolis, MN; Magna, UT; Seattle, WA.

### ★ 817 ★ Allianz Life Insurance Co. of North America
5701 Golden Hills Dr.
Minneapolis, MN 55416
**Phone:** (763)765-6500 **Fax:** (763)765-6299
**Website:** http://www.allianzlife.com
Julie Letner, Vice President, Human Resources

**Typ. Recipients:** Health Organizations, Heart, Hospitals, People with Disabilities. **Geo. Dist:** near headquarters only.

### ★ 818 ★ Allmerica Financial Charitable Foundation, Inc.
440 Lincoln St.
Worcester, MA 01653
**Phone:** (508)855-1000 **Fax:** (508)855-6332
David Portney, President

**Fnded:** 1991. **Priorities:** *Arts & Humanities:* 4%. Supports performing arts, libraries, and historic preservation. *Civic & Public Affairs:* 15%. Supports urban and community programs, community development, minority and women's affairs, housing, and a fire fighters fund. *Education:* 21%. Funds scholarship funds, music education, colleges and universities, Junior Achievement, and educational programs for public school students. *Environment:* 48%. Includes giving to United Way. Also supports community centers, child advocacy, food and clothing distribution, family services, rape crisis centers, scouting, and sports/recreation programs. *International:* 11%. Funding supports clinics and hospitals, single-disease health associations, and women's health. *Note:* Total contributions made in 1999. **Typ. Recipients:** AIDS/HIV, Cancer, Children's Health/Hospitals, Clinics/Medical Centers, Domestic Violence, Emergency/Ambulance Services, Eyes/Blindness, Health Organizations, Health-General, Heart, Hospitals, Hospitals (University Affiliated), Medical Education, Medical Research, Nursing Services, Public Health, Sexual Abuse, Sexual Abuse, Single-Disease Health Associations, Substance Abuse. **Geo. Dist:** Worcester, MA.

### ★ 819 ★ Allstate Foundation

2775 Sanders Rd., Ste. F-4
Northbrook, IL 60062-6127
**Phone:** (847)402-5502 **Fax:** (847)326-7517
**Email:** allfound@allstate.com
**Website:** http://www.allstate.com/foundation
Jan Epstein, Executive Director

**Priorities:** *Arts & Humanities:* 3%. Supports museums and monuments. *Civic & Public Affairs:* 43%. (Housing & Neighborhood Revitalization) Supported programs that include home fire prevention tips, encourage usage of smoke detectors, security information against burglary, accident prevention within and around the home, and small business safety awareness. Supports affordable housing, building rehabilitation, economic growth, home ownership, and neighborhood improvement. Foundation supports the All-America City Awards program. Company participates in a Neighborhood Partnership Program, partnering with organizations to build stronger and safer neighborhoods. *Education:* 14%. Primarily supports a scholarship foundation. Also provides funding for insurance education programs and other miscellaneous educational programs. *Environment:* 37%. Supports substance abuse prevention programs, youth groups, the United Way, and various social service agencies. *International:* 3%. Gives to hospitals and health programs. *Voluntarism:* Allstate's formal volunteer program, Helping Hands, provides opportunities for employees and agents to volunteer in the community. More than 200 committees nationally and 54 percent of employees and agents partake in volunteer activities. Nonprofit organizations at which Allstate employees volunteer may be eligible for Helping Hands grants from the Allstate Foundation. *Note:* Total contributions made in 2000. **Typ. Recipients:** Children's Health/Hospitals, Children's Health/Hospitals, Clinics/Medical Centers, Domestic Violence, Emergency/Ambulance Services, Health Funds, Health Organizations, Health Policy/Cost Containment, Hospitals, Hospitals (University Affiliated), Medical Education, Medical Research, Prenatal Health Issues, Public Health, Substance Abuse, Trauma Treatment. **Geo. Dist:** nationally.

### ★ 820 ★ AMCORE Foundation

501 7th St., PO Box 1537
Rockford, IL 61110
**Phone:** (815)968-2241 **Fax:** (815)961-7530
**Website:** http://www.amcore.com
James Waddell, Chairman

**Priorities:** *Arts & Humanities:* 18%. Provides major support to the Coronado Theatre. Also funds museums and a dance company. *Civic & Public Affairs:* 24%. Provides a major donation to the Zion Development Corp. for neighborhood building and development of low-income housing. Also funds a community Fourth of July festival. *Education:* 4%. Gives to Junior Achievement, literacy initiatives, public schools, and educational enrichment programs. *Environment:* 51%. Primarily funds a local United Way agency. Also supports youth organizations, a substance abuse treatment facility, food distribution, senior living, and other social service organizations. *International:* 3%. Funds hospice and the Muscular Dystrophy Association. *Note:* Total contributions made in 1999. **Typ.**

**Recipients:** AIDS/HIV, Alzheimers Disease, Cancer, Clinics/Medical Centers, Domestic Violence, Emergency/Ambulance Services, Health Organizations, Health-General, Hospices, Hospitals, Long-Term Care, Medical Education, Mental Health, Nursing Services, Nutrition, People with Disabilities, Public Health, Single-Disease Health Associations, Substance Abuse. **Geo. Dist:** Rockford, IL, including surrounding communities.

### ★ 821 ★ Ameren Corp. Charitable Trust

PO Box 66149, Mail Code 100
Saint Louis, MO 63166-6149
**Phone:** (314)554-4740 **Fax:** (314)554-2888
**Email:** ocowan@ameren.com
**Website:** http://www.ameren.com
Otis Cowan, Manager, Community Relations

**Priorities:** *Arts & Humanities:* 12%. Supports theater, opera, and the Arts and Education fund. *Civic & Public Affairs:* 4%. Supports botanical gardens, parks, and economic development. *Education:* 35%. The majority supports the "Ameren Scholarship" program. *Environment:* 40%. Principal support goes to the United Way of Greater St. Louis. Also supports youth organizations and social/cot services for children and families. *International:* 3%. Funds hospitals, a health foundation, and single-disease health organizations. *Religion:* 2%. Gives to a science center. *Voluntarism:* Ameren Helping Hands where employees and their families volunteer. VIP/TEAMS Program in which small grants ($50-$500) are given to nonprofits for which Ameren employees volunteer. The company also supports the "Ameren Helping Hands" program which involves group volunteer projects at local nonprofit organizations. *Note:* Total contributions made in 2000. **Typ. Recipients:** AIDS/HIV, Children's Health/Hospitals, Domestic Violence, Emergency/Ambulance Services, Health Funds, Health Organizations, Multiple Sclerosis, People with Disabilities. **Geo. Dist:** AmerenUE and AmerenCIPS local district offices; Springfield, IL; St. Louis, MO, near headquarters and service areas in MO and IL.

### ★ 822 ★ America West Airlines Foundation

Corporate Headquarters, 4000 East Sky Harbor Boulevard
Phoenix, AZ 85034
**Phone:** (480)693-3652 **Fax:** (480)693-3715
**Email:** ann.vry@americawest.com
Ann Vry, Coordinator, Community Relations

**Fnded:** 1991. **Priorities:** *Civic & Public Affairs:* 11%. Supports urban and minority affairs and job training organizations. *Education:* 66%. Primarily supports scholarships for higher education. Also funds elementary schools and educational programs. *Environment:* 18%. Gives to family and youth services, parenting programs, and Boys & Girls Clubs. *International:* 5%. Supports the Phoenix Birthing Project. *Voluntarism:* In 1999, over 2,100 volunteers supported communities where America West services. Co. sponsors the "DOCREW" volunteer corps. *Note:* Total foundation contributions made in 1999. **Typ. Recipients:** Health Organizations, Hospitals, Single-Disease Health Associations. **Geo. Dist:** headquarters and operating communities.

### ★ 823 ★ American Express Foundation

World Financial Center
200 Vesey St.
New York, NY 10285-4803
**Phone:** (212)640-5660 **Fax:** (212)693-1033
**Website:** http://home3.americanexpress.com/corp/philanthropy/
Anne Wickham, Director, Cultural Heritage Program

**Priorities:** *Arts & Humanities:* (Cultural Heritage) 29%. *Civic & Public Affairs:* (Economic Independence) 26%. Support is given to economic education, college funds, the Urban League, and global initiatives. *Environment:* (Community Service) 45%. Supports foundations, hospitals and health causes, the Red Cross, YWCAs and YMCAs, United Way, children's concerns, homeless shelters, and domestic peace. *Note:*

Total contributions made in 1999. **Typ. Recipients:** AIDS/HIV, Children's Health/Hospitals, Domestic Violence, Emergency/Ambulance Services, Health Organizations, Hospitals, Hospitals (University Affiliated), People with Disabilities, Single-Disease Health Associations, Substance Abuse. **Geo. Dist:** headquarters and operating communities; international committees South Pacific, South Asia, East Asia, Europe, Middle East, Africa and Latin America/Caribbean; AZ; CA; DC; FL; GA; IL; MA; MN; NY; NC; TX; UT.

### ★ 824 ★ American Fidelity Corp. Founders Fund

2000 Classen Center
Oklahoma City, OK 73106-6092
**Phone:** (405)523-5372 **Fax:** (405)523-5421
Jo Ramsey, Secretary

**Priorities:** *Arts & Humanities:* (Arts/Culture) 18%. Supports museums, art foundations, and the performing arts. *Civic & Public Affairs:* (Urban/Civic) 9%. Supports business and professional organizations, leadership initiatives, youth groups, legal aid, economic development, and community groups. *Education:* 24%. Supports pre-college schools, specialized educational programs, educational funds and universities. *Environment:* (Health/Welfare) 36%. Supports single-disease health organizations, medical centers, shelters for the homeless, food distribution, emergency relief, child welfare, family services, and United Way. *Note:* Total contributions made in 2000. **Typ. Recipients:** AIDS/HIV, Arthritis, Cancer, Child Abuse, Children's Health/Hospitals, Clinics/Medical Centers, Emergency/Ambulance Services, Health Organizations, Heart, Hospitals, Hospitals (University Affiliated), People with Disabilities, Prenatal Health Issues, Single-Disease Health Associations, Substance Abuse. **Geo. Dist:** OK.

### ★ 825 ★ American General Corp.

2929 Allen Parkway
Houston, TX 77019
**Phone:** (713)522-1111 **Fax:** (713)831-3889
**Email:** virginia_tomlinson@agfg.com
**Website:** http://www.americangeneral.com
Virginia Tomlinson, Director, Community Relations

**Priorities:** *Arts & Humanities:* 15% to 20%. *Civic & Public Affairs:* 10% to 15%. *Education:* 25% to 30%. *Environment:* 45% to 50%. United Way and health care. *Voluntarism:* StepUp is American General's employee volunteer program centered on a company-wide commitment to America's Promise. Employees are given time off to volunteer during the work week, allowing them to tutor, mentor, and carry out the goals of America's Promise. **Typ. Recipients:** Health-General.

### ★ 826 ★ American General Finance Foundation

601 NW Second St.
Evansville, IN 47708
**Phone:** (812)468-5854 **Fax:** (812)468-5682
**Website:** http://www.agc.com/agfg2000/agfgweb.nsf
Michelle Dixon, Community Relations Coordinator

**Fnded:** 1958. **Priorities:** *Arts & Humanities:* 7%. Supports Evansville area performing arts organizations, including dance, theater, and the philharmonic. *Civic & Public Affairs:* 16%. Supports community organizations that promote civic pride, as well as improved housing. *Education:* 30%. Primarily supports Indiana colleges and universities. Secondary support is allocated to scholarships for children of employees and a matching gifts program. Also supports secondary education. *Environment:* 43%. More than half supports the United Way and related agencies. Also provides support to a company-sponsored employee volunteer program. The remainder goes to youth organizations and organizations helping the disabled and elderly. *International:* 4%. Supports emergency services and local chapters of national single-disease health organizations in contributions generally less than $1,000. *Voluntarism:* The company's Community Spirit Awards program recognizes employees who demonstrate outstanding volunteer service. Award recipients designate $2,500 grants to the organizations they serve. *Note:* Total contributions made in 1999. **Typ. Recipients:** AIDS/HIV, Alzheimers Disease, Arthritis, Cancer, Children's Health/Hospitals, Children's Health/Hospitals, Diabetes, Domestic Violence, Emergency/Ambulance Services, Heart, Hospices, Hospitals, Medical Rehabilitation, Medical Research, Mental Health, People with Disabilities, Prenatal Health Issues, Single-Disease Health Associations, Substance Abuse. **Geo. Dist:** Evansville, IN, including statewide.

★ 827 ★ **American Snuff Co. Charitable Trust**
701 Main St.
Memphis, TN 38101
**Phone:** (901)523-6200
David Simpson, III, General Counsel

**Fnded:** 1952. **Priorities:** *Arts & Humanities:* 9%. Funds museums and arts councils, public broadcasting, and ballet. *Civic & Public Affairs:* 10%. Supports housing, leadership, and gardens. *Education:* 15%. Colleges, universities, public grade schools, and Junior Achievement are funded. *Environment:* 25%. Youth organizations, food banks, and the United Way receive support. *International:* 16%. Supports hospitals and single-disease associations with a pediatric health focus. *Note:* Total contributions made in 2000. **Typ. Recipients:** Children's Health/Hospitals, Clinics/Medical Centers, Diabetes, Health-General, Kidney, Medical Research, People with Disabilities, Single-Disease Health Associations. **Geo. Dist:** headquarters area only.

★ 828 ★ **American Stock Exchange, Inc.**
86 Trinity Place
10th Fl.
New York, NY 10006-1881
**Phone:** (212)306-1000  **Fax:** (212)306-1152
**Website:** http://www.amex.com
Mike D'Emic, Controller

**Priorities:** *Arts & Humanities:* Museums and the performing arts. *International:* Health care, child welfare, and youth organizations. **Typ. Recipients:** Health-General. **Geo. Dist:** New York, NY, including the metropolitan area.

★ 829 ★ **Ameritas Charitable Foundation**
PO Box 81889
Lincoln, NE 68501
**Phone:** (402)467-1122  **Fax:** (402)467-7939
Scott Stuckey, Assistant Vice President of Corporate Co

**Fnded:** 1985. **Priorities:** *Arts & Humanities:* 2%. Supports performing arts, arts councils, and history/heritage groups. *Civic & Public Affairs:* 42%. Under the foundation's Civic program area, economic development, youth organizations, neighborhood organizations, and community foundations are funded. *Education:* 28%. Supports colleges and universities, secondary education, Junior Achievement, and education associations in Nebraska. *Environment:* 7%. Supports food banks, child advocacy, shelters, and the United Way. *International:* 21%. Medical research, hospitals, and single-disease health associations. **Typ. Recipients:** AIDS/HIV, Children's Health/Hospitals, Clinics/Medical Centers, Emergency/Ambulance Services, Health Organizations, Hospitals, Medical Education, Medical Research, Multiple Sclerosis, People with Disabilities, Public Health, Research/Studies Institutes, Single-Disease Health Associations, Substance Abuse, Transplant Networks/Donor Banks. **Geo. Dist:** Lincoln, NE.

★ 830 ★ **Ameritech Illinois**
225 West Randolph, 30-A
Chicago, IL 60606
**Phone:** (312)727-2080  **Fax:** (312)727-3722
**Email:** ron.c.mori@ameritech.com
Ron Mori, Director of Corporate Contributions

**Typ. Recipients:** Health Organizations, Health Policy/Cost Containment, People with Disabilities, Substance Abuse. **Geo. Dist:** IL.

★ 831 ★ **Amerus Group Co.**
699 Walnut St.
Des Moines, IA 50309
**Phone:** (515)557-3910  **Fax:** (515)283-3269
**Website:** http://www.amerus.com

**Priorities:** *Arts & Humanities:* 5% to 10%. Arts centers, music, the performing arts, art associations, and community arts. *Civic & Public Affairs:* 5% to 10%. Economic development, housing, business interests, and other foundation-related issues. *Education:* 15% to 20%. Public education, community colleges, and general educational programs. *Environment:* 10% to 15%. Community services, family services, the homeless, substance abuse programs, volunteer services, and counseling. *International:* 50% to 55%. Health organizations and hospices. **Typ. Recipients:** Health-General, Hospices, Substance Abuse. **Geo. Dist:** IA.

★ 832 ★ **AMETEK Foundation**
37 North Valley Rd., Bldg. 4
PO Box 1764
Paoli, PA 19301-0801
**Phone:** (610)647-2121
Kathryn Londra, Secretary, Treasurer

**Fnded:** 1960. **Priorities:** *Arts & Humanities:* 18%. Supports libraries and visual and performing arts. *Civic & Public Affairs:* 7%. Supports parks and community foundations. *Education:* 32%. Primarily colleges and universities and technical and engineering institutions and organizations. Other interests include student aid, private secondary education, education funds, and literacy. *Environment:* 20%. Funds the United Way, YMCA, and services for the disabled. *International:* 15%. Health services, cancer centers, single-disease health associations, and hospitals. *Religion:* 1%. Supports science museums. *Note:* Total contributions made in 2000. **Typ. Recipients:** Cancer, Clinics/Medical Centers, Diabetes, Emergency/Ambulance Services, Health Funds, Health Organizations, Hospitals, Medical Education, Medical Rehabilitation, Medical Research, Mental Health, People with Disabilities, Preventive Medicine/Wellness Organizations, Public Health, Single-Disease Health Associations. **Geo. Dist:** headquarters and operating communities; nationally.

★ 833 ★ **Amgen Foundation**
Mailstop 27-4-A
One Amgen Center Dr.
Thousand Oaks, CA 91320-1799
**Phone:** (805)447-4056
**Website:** http://www.amgen.com/community/contributionPrograms.html

**Priorities:** *Arts & Humanities:* 8%. Gives to museums, visual and performing arts, history museums, and arts councils. *Civic & Public Affairs:* 9%. Funds zoos and festivals. *Education:* 43%. Supports precollege and higher education, especially those with a focus on biological science. *Environment:* 4%. Funds senior concerns, the United Way, and youth programs. *International:* 32%. Supports free clinics, the Red Cross, hospice, single-disease health organizations. *Religion:* 2%. Supports science centers. *Voluntarism:* The Amgen Staff Community Involvement Program (SCIP) makes the services of Amgen staff available to nonprofit organizations or needy individuals for community improvement. *Note:* Total contributions made in 1999. **Typ. Recipients:** AIDS/HIV, Alzheimers Disease, Alzheimers Disease, Cancer, Child Abuse, Children's Health/Hospitals, Clinics/Medical Centers, Emergency/Ambulance Services, Health Organizations, Heart, Hospices, Hospitals, Medical Education, Medical Research, People with Disabilities, Preventive Medicine/Wellness Organizations, Single-Disease Health Associations. **Geo. Dist:** headquarters; nationally.

★ 834 ★ **Amon G. Carter Star Telegram Employees Fund**
PO Box 17480
Fort Worth, TX 76102
**Phone:** (817)332-3535
Nenetta Carter Tatum, President

**Fnded:** 1945. **Priorities:** *Arts & Humanities:* 28%. Contributes to museums, arts councils, music, and community theater. *Education:* 17%. Primarily supports universities in Texas. Also operates large scholarship program for the children of employees. *Environment:* 35%. Includes community centers, community service organizations, counseling, and youth organizations. *International:* 19%. Interests include children's hospitals and single-disease health associations. *Religion:* 1%. *Note:* Total contributions made in 1997. **Typ. Recipients:** AIDS/HIV, Cancer, Children's Health/Hospitals, Children's Health/Hospitals, Domestic Violence, Eyes/Blindness, Family Planning, Health Organizations, Hospitals, Hospitals (University Affiliated), Medical Research, Mental Health, Nursing Services, People with Disabilities, Public Health, Research/Studies Institutes, Single-Disease Health Associations, Substance Abuse, Transplant Networks/Donor Banks. **Geo. Dist:** TX, Tarrant County.

★ 835 ★ **AMP Foundation**
MS 140-10
PO Box 3608
Harrisburg, PA 17105-3608
**Phone:** (717)592-4869  **Fax:** (717)592-3043
**Email:** mjrakocz@tycoelectronics.com
**Website:** http://www.amp.com/about/foundation
Mary Rakoczy, Manager, Community Relations & Contribut

**Priorities:** *Arts & Humanities:* (Arts & Culture) 16%. Provides funding for art societies, music, museums, and arts festivals and associations. *Education:* 54%. Support goes to accredited educational institutions, public and private, particularly when grant addresses business or community concerns of Tyco Electronics. Also supports an employee matching gift fund that donates to accredited high schools, colleges, and universities. *Environment:* (Community Impact) 28%. Supports United Way and human service organizations. *Voluntarism:* After employees complete 100 hours of volunteer services in a calendar year with a nonprofit organization, the Dollars for Doers program will authorize a $250 contribution from the Foundation to that organization. This is a yearly maximum of $2,000 to one eligible organization. *Note:* Total contributions made in 2000. **Typ. Recipients:** Cancer, Child Abuse, Children's Health/Hospitals, Clinics/Medical Centers, Emergency/Ambulance Services, Health Organizations, Health-General, Hospices, Hospitals, Mental Health, People with Disabilities, Single-Disease Health Associations, Substance Abuse. **Geo. Dist:** headquarters and operating communities; Triad, NC; PA, central Pennsylvania; VA.

★ 836 ★ **AMR/American Airlines Foundation**
PO Box 619616
Mail Drop 5656
Dallas, TX 75261-9616
**Phone:** (817)967-3540
**Website:** http://www.amrcorp.com/corpinfo.htm
Timothy Doke, Secretary

**Priorities:** *Arts & Humanities:* (Cultural) 3%. Funds activities that exemplify excellence in the visual and/or performing arts, including performances or programs that promote a higher level of understanding of the arts from countries where AMR/American Airlines has a presence. Also aids specific programs designed to highlight the world's diversity of cultures, ethnic background, and national origins. Also gives to art funds that make a significant contribution to the creation of high quality art programs in local communities. *Civic & Public Affairs:* (Civic) 36%. Funds educational programs aimed at increasing awareness and involvement in recycling and other environmental protection activities and projects designed to preserve environmentally sensitive property throughout the world. Partners with environmental organizations, such as the Nature Conservancy. Also sponsors initiatives that promote economic development in company's communities. *Education:* 11%. Supports programs aimed at providing higher education and business career training opportunities to minorities, in particular those that support American's existing national partnership with the United Negro College Fund. Supports efforts to create greater understanding and cooperation between various ethnic groups and activities aimed at educating young adults about world geography. *Environment:* (Health/Welfare) 46%. Funds social services, youth services, meals on wheels, volunteerism, and the United Way. Funding also supports the American Cancer Society, American Red Cross, and Give the Kids the World Foundation. *Voluntarism:* Company reports that no formal volunteer program exists, other than a volunteer recycling program aboard flights and in offices. *Note:* Total contributions made in 1999. **Typ. Recipients:** AIDS/HIV, Cancer, Children's Health/Hospitals, Clinics/Medical Centers, Diabetes, Emergency/Ambulance Services, Eyes/Blindness, Family Planning, Health Funds, Health Organizations, Hospitals, Hospitals (University Affiliated), Kidney, Multiple Sclerosis, Public Health, Single-Disease Health Associations, Substance Abuse. **Geo. Dist:** nationally and internationally.

### ★ 837 ★ Amsted Industries Foundation

205 North Michigan Ave., 44th Floor
Chicago, IL 60601
**Phone:** (312)645-1700
Jerry Gura, Director, Public Affairs

**Fnded:** 1953. **Priorities:** *Arts & Humanities:* 16%. Under the foundation's Cultural program area, support if provided to arts associations (particularly music), opera, orchestras, historical societies, art museums, botanical gardens, zoos, and public broadcasting. *Civic & Public Affairs:* 7%. The foundation's Civic giving encompasses youth activities, animal welfare, environmental causes, anti-defamation groups, legal services, professional organizations, Urban Leagues, city planning and development, and public safety. *Education:* 47%. Major support is given to education, including science and technology at the university level, math and science academies, private precollege schools, education foundations, and colleges and universities. Also supports scholarships and matching gifts. *Environment:* 30%. Funds United Way chapters, food distribution, family planning, family services, research and teaching hospitals, community hospitals serving employees, single-disease health associations, women's health, and special care facilities. *Note:* Total contributions made in fiscal 2000. **Typ. Recipients:** Alzheimers Disease, Clinics/Medical Centers, Family Planning, Health Organizations, Hospitals, Medical Rehabilitation. **Geo. Dist:** headquarters and operating communities; Chicago, IL.

### ★ 838 ★ Anderson Foundation

608 Madison Ave., Ste. 1540
Toledo, OH 43604
**Phone:** (419)243-1706
Ms. Fredi Heywood, Foundation Services
  Administrator

**Priorities:** *Arts & Humanities:* 12%. Primarily supports orchestras and operas. Also funds libraries, museums, public broadcasting, and arts associations. *Civic & Public Affairs:* 12%. Supports economic development, zoos, botanical gardens, and local and community organizations. *Education:* 15%. Supports colleges and universities. Also funds public and private precollege education and agricultural education. *Environment:* 49%. Almost half of the foundation's funding goes to the United Way under Community Chest funding. *International:* 2%. Funds single-disease health organizations, hospitals, and medical centers. *Note:* Total contributions in 1999. **Typ. Recipients:** Clinics/Medical Centers, Emergency/Ambulance Services, Eyes/Blindness, Hospices, Hospitals, Medical Research, Mental Health, Nursing Services, People with Disabilities, Preventive Medicine/Wellness Organizations, Single-Disease Health Associations. **Geo. Dist:** headquarters and operating communities, including plant locations.

### ★ 839 ★ Anheuser-Busch Foundation/ Anheuser-Busch Charitable Trust

1 Busch Place
Saint Louis, MO 63118-1852
**Phone:** (314)577-2453          **Fax:** (314)577-3251
Jayne Nicholson, Specialist, Charitable
  Contributions

**Fnded:** 1975. **Priorities:** *Arts & Humanities:* 16%. Supports libraries, historic preservation, history organizations, and the performing arts. *Civic & Public Affairs:* 8%. Funds urban and community affairs. *Education:* 45%. Primarily supports colleges and universities near company's major facilities. *Environment:* 25%. Primarily supports the United Way, programs for the disabled, and organizations serving youth. *International:* 1%. Gives to hospitals and single-disease health organizations. *Voluntarism:* Through the Anheuser-Busch Employee Volunteer Grant Program, the company supports and recognizes its employees who actively volunteer their time and talents to nonprofit organizations by making grants to these organizations for unusual or special projects. An Employee Matching Gifts Program for educational institutions is also offered through the company's charitable foundation. *Note:* Total contributions made in 2000. **Typ. Recipients:** AIDS/HIV, Alzheimers Disease, Cancer, Children's Health/Hospitals, Emergency/Ambulance Services, Health Organizations, Health Policy/Cost Containment, Heart, Hospitals, Medical Education, Medical Research, People with Disabilities, Public Health, Single-Disease Health Associations, Substance Abuse. **Geo. Dist:** principally near operating locations and to national organizations.

### ★ 840 ★ Anthem Foundation, Inc.

120 Monument Circle
Indianapolis, IN 46204
**Phone:** 800-563-5465
Connie Molland, Secretary

**Fnded:** 1990. **Priorities:** *Arts & Humanities:* 7%. Supports arts funds. *Civic & Public Affairs:* 9%. Funds leadership development and women's affairs organizations. *Education:* 13%. Supports higher education and matching gifts. *Environment:* 29%. Funds the United Way and youth and human services. *International:* 42%. Supports health education, community health initiatives, and single-disease associations. *Note:* Total contributions in 2000. **Typ. Recipients:** AIDS/HIV, Cancer, Child Abuse, Children's Health/Hospitals, Clinics/Medical Centers, Diabetes, Emergency/Ambulance Services, Health Organizations, Health-General, Heart, Hospitals, Medical Education, Medical Rehabilitation, Multiple Sclerosis, Nursing Services, Prenatal Health Issues, Preventive Medicine/Wellness Organizations, Public Health, Respiratory, Single-Disease Health Associations, Substance Abuse, Trauma Treatment. **Geo. Dist:** KY.

### AOL Time Warner Foundation

*See:* Entry 5569

### ★ 841 ★ Aon Foundation

123 North Wacker Dr.
Chicago, IL 60606
**Phone:** (312)701-3000          **Fax:** (312)701-4533
**Email:** aoltwfoundation@aol.com
**Website:** http://aoltwfoundation.org
Carolyn Labutka, Executive Director, AON Foundation

**Priorities:** *Arts & Humanities:* 24%. Supports art museums, historical societies, and performing arts groups. Interests include symphonies, theater, and dance. *Civic & Public Affairs:* 11%. Funds economic and community development, urban affairs, business/professional organizations, and a zoo. *Education:* 26%. Colleges and universities, science, economic and insurance education, private precollege schools, and scholarship funds. *Environment:* 26%. Supports the United Way, child welfare organizations, volunteer groups, youth groups, services for the disabled, and various community service programs. *International:* 5%. Gives to hospitals, single-disease health organizations, pediatric health initiatives, medical research, and health funds. *Note:* Total contributions made in

2000. **Typ. Recipients:** AIDS/HIV, Alzheimers Disease, Cancer, Children's Health/Hospitals, Clinics/Medical Centers, Diabetes, Emergency/Ambulance Services, Health Funds, Hospitals, Hospitals (University Affiliated), Medical Rehabilitation, Medical Research, Multiple Sclerosis, People with Disabilities, Single-Disease Health Associations. **Geo. Dist:** internationally; operating locations.

### ★ 842 ★ APL Ltd.

1111 Broadway
Oakland, CA 94607
**Phone:** (510)272-7208          **Fax:** (510)272-8930
John Pachtner, Director of Corporate
  Communications

**Priorities:** *Arts & Humanities:* 5% to 10%. Funds ballet, theater and the performing arts. *Civic & Public Affairs:* Less than 5%. *Education:* 20% to 25%. Supports colleges, universities and education associations. *Environment:* 50% to 55%. Funds united funds, and youth groups. *International:* 5% to 10%. *Voluntarism:* Employees in the Bay Area are eligible for the pilot volunteer program. They are allowed four hours per month of co. time to volunteer. Co. gives funds through its employee matching gifts volunteer services grant program. Grants of $500 per employee are given to organizations at which employees volunteer their time, limited to four grants per year. **Typ. Recipients:** AIDS/HIV, Cancer, Child Abuse, Children's Health/Hospitals, Clinics/Medical Centers, Domestic Violence, Heart, Hospitals, Medical Research, Multiple Sclerosis, People with Disabilities, Prenatal Health Issues, Public Health, Single-Disease Health Associations. **Geo. Dist:** locations where APL subsidiaries have regional or district offices; Oakland, CA; San Francisco, CA, including Bay area.

### ★ 843 ★ Appleton Papers Inc.

825 East Wisconsin Ave.
PO Box 359
Appleton, WI 54912
**Phone:** (920)991-7448          **Fax:** (920)991-8407
**Email:** dkolb@appletonpapers.com
**Website:** http://www.appletonpapers.com
Donna Kolb, Contribution Committee

**Typ. Recipients:** Domestic Violence, People with Disabilities, Single-Disease Health Associations, Substance Abuse. **Geo. Dist:** headquarters and operating communities; Newton Falls, NY; Dayton, OH; Harrisburg, PA; Roaring Spring, PA; Appleton, WI.

### ★ 844 ★ APS Foundation, Inc.

PO Box 53999
M/S 8010
Phoenix, AZ 85072-3999
**Phone:** (602)250-2888          **Fax:** (602)250-2113
Ms. Charlie Thompson, Manager, Community
  Relations

**Priorities:** *Arts & Humanities:* 18%. Recipients include local theaters, dance companies, museums, historical societies, and arts councils. *Civic & Public Affairs:* 24%. Supports community initiatives, leadership organizations, neighborhood organizations, and a botanical garden. *Education:* 15%. Gives to Junior Achievement, Arizona universities and colleges, and a learning center. *Environment:* 15%. Supports food banks, youth groups, scouts, and animal welfare organizations. *International:* 16%. Supports hospitals, health foundations, and medical centers. *Religion:* 4%. Funds an observatory and a science center. *Voluntarism:* The company matches employee volunteer hours given to nonprofit organizations that provide a service in one of their giving areas. Each hour an APS employee or retiree volunteers is matched at $5, if at least 25 hours in single calendar year have been spent volunteering. *Note:* Total contributions made in 2000. **Typ. Recipients:** Cancer, Children's Health/Hospitals, Clinics/Medical Centers, Domestic Violence, Emergency/Ambulance Services, Eyes/Blindness, Health Funds, Heart, Hospices, Hospitals, Medical Education, Medical Research, People with Disabilities, Prenatal Health Issues, Public Health, Research/Studies Institutes. **Geo. Dist:** near Four Corners Power Plant; AZ, primarily Arizona and New Mexico, near the Four Corners Power Plant; NM.

## ★ 845 ★ Archer-Daniels-Midland Foundation

4666 Faries Parkway
PO Box 1470
Decatur, IL 62526
**Phone:** (217)424-5957　　　　**Fax:** (217)424-5581
**Email:** cmadding@admworld.com
**Website:** http://www.admworld.com
Denise Barry, Contact

**Fnded:** 1953. **Priorities:** *Arts & Humanities:* 2%. Supports arts councils, libraries, orchestras, and cultural exchange between countries. *Civic & Public Affairs:* 24%. Primary interests include public policy organizations, urban affairs groups, and international affairs. Also supports economic development, government improvement, safety, civil rights, housing initiatives, and business organizations. *Education:* 18%. Majority supports colleges and universities. Also supports religious, agricultural, business, and legal education, as well as education funds and associations. *Environment:* 28%. Major support goes to united funds and youth organizations. Other interests include child and family welfare, emergency relief, senior services, and community athletic and recreation programs. *International:* 3%. Funds hospitals, single-disease organizations, and children's health services. *Note:* Total contributions in fiscal 2000. **Typ. Recipients:** Cancer, Children's Health/Hospitals, Emergency/Ambulance Services, Family Planning, Health Organizations, Hospitals, Medical Education, People with Disabilities, Prenatal Health Issues, Substance Abuse. **Geo. Dist:** nationally, principally near operating locations and to national organizations.

## ★ 846 ★ ARCO Foundation

333 South Hope St.
Los Angeles, CA 90071
**Phone:** (213)486-3342　　　　**Fax:** (213)486-0113
Russell Sakaguchi, President

**Priorities:** *Arts & Humanities:* 33%. Supports programs which offer cultural experiences to diverse ethnic groups, or which assist emerging arts organizations in underserved neighborhoods. *Civic & Public Affairs:* 6%. Supports economic development, sustainable development initiatives, and an aquarium. *Education:* 31%. Precollege organizations supported are aimed at promoting: readiness-for-school services, including parent training and early childhood curricula for at-risk children; academic achievement through improvements in school attendance, grades and school-completion levels; increased interest and achievement in mathematics and science resulting in higher enrollment and success rates in college preparatory course-work and in plans to pursue math/science careers; parent effectiveness through increased involvement in public school education, especially among low-income families; professional staff preparation and development through programs that incorporate school restructuring issues as part of the curriculum for teachers, counselors and administrators; programs that improve the qualifications and effectiveness of math and science teachers; and teacher-training curricula on language development and English-language acquisition. Supported higher education programs include special projects at selected research universities and programs that increase the number of minority students entering and completing degree programs in fields related to the energy industry. Also supports policy analysis and scholarship programs. *Environment:* 29%. Supports United Way and social services. *Voluntarism:* Through company's Employee Volunteer Grants Program, employees may request grants of up to $500 for nonprofit organizations to which they give at least 12 hours per month of their own time. *Note:* Total contributions made in 1999. **Typ. Recipients:** Children's Health/Hospitals, Domestic Violence, Research/Studies Institutes. **Geo. Dist:** Southwestern United States; Western United States; AK.

## ★ 847 ★ Arison Foundation

3655 NW 87th Ave.
Miami, FL 33178-2428
**Phone:** (305)599-2600
Maddy Rosenberg, Assistant to the President

**Fnded:** 1981. **Priorities:** *Education:* Less than 1%. *Environment:* 14%. Majority of funding supports United Way International. Also supports senior services and recreational facilities for the disabled. *International:* 10%. Funds Jewish hospitals, medical centers, and medical research organizations in America and Israel. *Note:* Total contributions made in 1999. **Typ. Recipients:** Cancer, Children's Health/Hospitals, Children's Health/Hospitals, Clinics/Medical Centers, Eyes/Blindness, Geriatric Health, Health Organizations, Health-General, Hospices, Hospitals, Medical Education, Medical Research, People with Disabilities, Public Health, Single-Disease Health Associations. **Geo. Dist:** Miami, FL, including surrounding area.

## ★ 848 ★ Aristech Foundation

210 6th Ave.
Pittsburgh, PA 15222
**Phone:** (412)316-1340
Kimberly Weprich, Foundation Administrator

**Fnded:** 1988. **Priorities:** *Arts & Humanities:* 8%. Art institutes; performing arts; public broadcasting in Pittsburgh; libraries; and historical societies. *Civic & Public Affairs:* 5%. Funds economic development, women's concerns, and zoological societies. *Education:* 12%. Higher education, especially universities located in Pittsburgh, PA; education foundations and funds; and small colleges nationwide. *Environment:* 67%. Supports United Way chapters; youth organizations, including boys and girls clubs and the Boy Scouts; and community service organizations. *International:* 3%. Public health. *Religion:* 3%. Gives to the Carnegie Science Center. *Note:* Total contributions in 2000. **Typ. Recipients:** Clinics/Medical Centers, Domestic Violence, Emergency/Ambulance Services, Eyes/Blindness, Hospices, People with Disabilities, Single-Disease Health Associations. **Geo. Dist:** headquarters and operating communities.

## ★ 849 ★ Armstrong Foundation

2500 Columbia Ave.
Lancaster, PA 17603
**Phone:** (717)396-2446
Cathy Witmer, Contributions Administrator

**Priorities:** *Arts & Humanities:* 1%. Support emphasizes libraries and historic preservation. *Civic & Public Affairs:* 36%. Funding supports chambers of commerce, civic associations, and public policy institutions. *Education:* 23%. Funding supports the National Merit Scholarship Corporation, universities, colleges and educational foundations. *Environment:* 26%. Funding supports various United Way chapters, local youth organizations, and local family support services. *Note:* Total contributions made in 2000. **Typ. Recipients:** Cancer, Clinics/Medical Centers, Emergency/Ambulance Services, Eyes/Blindness, Family Planning, Health Organizations, Hospices, Hospitals, Medical Education, Medical Research, Nursing Services, People with Disabilities, Public Health, Single-Disease Health Associations, Substance Abuse. **Geo. Dist:** Lancaster, PA.

## ★ 850 ★ Arthur D. Little Foundation

25 Acorn Park
Cambridge, MA 02140
**Phone:** (617)498-6035　　　　**Fax:** (617)498-7119
Judith Harris, Vice President

**Fnded:** 1953. **Priorities:** *Arts & Humanities:* 9%. Funds libraries and orchestras. *Civic & Public Affairs:* 26%. Supports minority and civic affairs. *Education:* 33%. Foundation makes contributions to nonprofit organizations primarily aimed at improving education, at all levels and across a range of institutional settings. A particular emphasis is placed on improving learning and teaching in the areas of mathematics, science, and technology. In some cases, educational programs in human services, arts and environmental organizations which affect the quality of life in communities

where Arthur D. Little employees live and work will be considered for funding. *Environment:* 21%. Major support for the United Way. *Religion:* 9%. Funds research and science museums. *Note:* Total contributions made in 1997. **Typ. Recipients:** Adolescent Health Issues, AIDS/HIV, Child Abuse, Children's Health/Hospitals, Emergency/Ambulance Services, Hospices, Hospitals, Medical Research, Mental Health, People with Disabilities, Public Health, Sexual Abuse. **Geo. Dist:** operating locations; Cambridge, MA.

## ★ 851 ★ Arvin Foundation

One Noblitt Plaza
PO Box 3000
Columbus, IN 47202-3000
**Fax:** (812)379-3000
John Brown, President

**Priorities:** *Arts & Humanities:* 5%. Supports orchestras, museums, libraries, and several other arts and music groups. *Civic & Public Affairs:* (Civic & Health) 33%. Grants are made to hospitals, health organizations, and single-disease organizations, as well as hospice and home care. Civic concerns include fire departments, environmental projects, historical museums, booster clubs, and public broadcasting. *Education:* 17%. Major support for colleges and universities. Also supports educational foundations, K-12 education, scholarship funds, economic education, and vocational training. *Environment:* (Youth) 28%. Supports scouts, recreational activities and sports, youth foundations, Special Olympics, Junior Achievement, and school-based extracurricular activities. *Note:* Total contributions made in 1999. **Typ. Recipients:** Cancer, Children's Health/Hospitals, Clinics/Medical Centers, Emergency/Ambulance Services, Eyes/Blindness, Health Organizations, Hospices, Hospitals, People with Disabilities, Public Health, Research/Studies Institutes, Respiratory, Single-Disease Health Associations. **Geo. Dist:** headquarters and operating communities; AL; IN; MI; MO; OK; SC; TN.

## ★ 852 ★ Ashland Inc. Foundation

50 East RiverCenter Boulevard
PO Box 391
Covington, KY 41012-0391
**Phone:** (859)815-3630　　　　**Fax:** (859)815-4496
**Email:** sgrice@ashland.com
**Website:** http://www.ashland.com
Charles Whitehead, President

**Priorities:** *Arts & Humanities:* 6%. Funding supports art centers, funds, associations, museums, public broadcasting, and music. *Civic & Public Affairs:* 7%. Funding supports economic development; community affairs; and law and justice. *Education:* 62%. Funding supports colleges, universities, and secondary schools, primarily in operating areas, with a focus on schools preparing students for a career in the industry. Literacy, educational foundations, and community and junior colleges are also of interest. Foundation sponsors scholarships for children of employees, employee matching gifts program to educational institutions, and runs print and broadcast ads promoting education. *International:* 22%. Funds United Way; other recipients include youth organizations, groups concerned with the aged and child welfare, community centers and service agencies, and hospitals and health groups. *Voluntarism:* The company encourages employee volunteerism through activities such as the annual River Sweep, a clean-up of the Ohio River. *Note:* Total contributions made in 1999. **Typ. Recipients:** Cancer, Clinics/Medical Centers, Health Organizations, Hospitals, People with Disabilities, Single-Disease Health Associations, Speech & Hearing. **Geo. Dist:** headquarters and operating communities; KY; MN; OH; WV.

## ★ 853 ★ Associated Food Stores Charitable Foundation

122-20 Merrick Blvd.
Jamaica, NY 11434
**Phone:** (718)978-0764
Harry Laufer, President & Chief Executive Officer

**Fnded:** 1987. **Priorities:** *Arts & Humanities:* 6%. Funds an art museum. *Civic & Public Affairs:* 4%. Supports community funds, a parade, and the Workmens Circle. *Education:* 25%. Supports secondary schools, universities, and communication education. *International:* 2%. Gives to health care centers, geriatric nursing care, and leukemia and cerebral palsy research. *Note:* Total contributions made in 1999. **Typ. Recipients:** Cancer, Children's Health/Hospitals, Clinics/Medical Centers, Diabetes, Eyes/Blindness, Geriatric Health, Hospitals, Long-Term Care, Medical Research, Nursing Services, People with Disabilities, Single-Disease Health Associations. **Geo. Dist:** NY, including metropolitan area.

## ★ 854 ★ AT&T Foundation
32 Ave. of the Americas, 24th Floor
New York, NY 10013
**Phone:** (212)387-4801          **Fax:** (212)387-5098
**Email:** rdabney@attmail.com
**Website:** http://www.att.com/foundation
Ronald Dabney, Communications Manager

**Priorities:** *Arts & Humanities:* 11%. Supports nationally and internationally recognized arts and cultural institutions that foster communication and promote cross-cultural understanding. Organizations must have been professionally managed for at least five years and compensate both artistic and managerial personnel. National arts service organizations are also funded, particularly those that offer technical assistance or professional services to foundation-eligible institutions. Particular interest in the creation, production, and presentation of new work and initiatives that provide access to the arts to all segments of society by bringing the work of women and artists of diverse cultures to wider audiences. The foundation supports two invitation-only initiatives: AT&T: OnStage, for theatrical works; and AT&T: NEAT (New Experiments in Art and Technology), supporting children's and science museums. *Civic & Public Affairs:* 10%. Supports organizations and projects that enhance the effectiveness of the nonprofit sector and promote public policy formulation in matters of children and families, accessibility of health and social services to those in need, the advancement of diversity, and the protection of the environment. Projects should serve as models for other organizations and lend themselves to measurable evaluation, with results that can be disseminated to a wide audience. *Education:* 54%. Supports projects that assist and facilitate lifelong learning, teacher training, and parent participation in education. Emphasis is on initiatives that use technology to connect students, teachers, and institutions of learning; and which stimulate student interests and involvement in mathematics, science and engineering. Through the AT&T Learning Network, funding is provided to organizations that help teachers, students, parents and communities capitalize on technology to enhance education. As part of this effort, funding is provided for the innovative use of technology to foster family involvement in education and provide professional development opportunities for preparation of new teachers. Collaboration among institutions and across communities to promote lifelong learning is encouraged. Invitational grants go to projects that address issues of technology in public policy; education reform; academic standards, assessment and accountability; and access to educational opportunities by all segments of society. *Environment:* 21%. Supports the United Way, youth organizations, scouting, family services, child welfare, the disabled, and community services. *Voluntarism:* Supports the AT&T CARES program, which makes grants to organizations where employees volunteer, and the Telephone Pioneers of America, a volunteer service organization. *Note:* Total foundation contributions made in 1998. **Typ. Recipients:** Children's Health/Hospitals, Emergency/Ambulance Services, Health Policy/Cost Containment, Hospitals, Medical Education, People with Disabilities, Speech & Hearing, Substance Abuse. **Geo. Dist:** headquarters and operating communities; nationally and internationally.

## ★ 855 ★ Atofina Chemicals Foundation
2000 Market St.
Philadelphia, PA 19103-3222
**Phone:** (215)419-7000          **Fax:** (215)419-5494
George Hagar, Executive Secretary

**Fnded:** 1957. **Priorities:** *Arts & Humanities:* 17%. Supports public broadcasting, art museums, historic sites, and performing arts. *Civic & Public Affairs:* 18%. Under the foundation's Civic program area, funding is provided to aquariums, zoos, police/public safety, community art organizations, and science institutes in Philadelphia. *Education:* 31%. Funds the School District of Philadelphia *Environment:* 10%. Funds local United Way agencies. *Religion:* 24%. Supports the Chemical Heritage Foundation and Atofina Chemical initiatives. *Note:* Total foundation contributions in 2000, excluding matching gifts. **Typ. Recipients:** Clinics/Medical Centers, Emergency/Ambulance Services, Hospitals, Medical Rehabilitation, Medical Research, People with Disabilities. **Geo. Dist:** nationally; operating location communities.

## ★ 856 ★ AUL Foundation Inc.
One American Square
PO Box 368
Indianapolis, IN 46206-0368
**Phone:** (317)285-1609          **Fax:** (317)285-1979
James Freeman, Chairman, Committee

**Priorities:** *Arts & Humanities:* 5% to 10%. Provides grants for arts associations, libraries, music, and theater, among other interests. *Civic & Public Affairs:* 5% to 10%. Contributions go to organizations involved with public policy, especially those concerned with minority groups and labor organizations. Interests also include urban and local affairs, and zoos and botanical gardens. *Education:* 35% to 40%. Includes donations to college associations, colleges, universities, and at least one seminary. Economics, law, and physical education are of particular interest. *International:* 35% to 40%. Majority of funding supports the United Way. Also supports hospitals, medical research, health organizations, and social services for the homeless and aged. **Typ. Recipients:** AIDS/HIV, Cancer, Domestic Violence, Health Organizations, Hospitals, Medical Education, Medical Rehabilitation, Medical Research, Medical Training, Mental Health, Nursing Services, People with Disabilities, Public Health, Single-Disease Health Associations, Substance Abuse. **Geo. Dist:** headquarters and operating communities; IN.

## Avery Dennison Foundation
*See:* Entry 5570

## ★ 857 ★ Avon Products Foundation, Inc.
1345 Ave. of the Americas
New York, NY 10105
**Phone:** (212)282-5516          **Fax:** (212)282-6049
**Website:** http://www.avon.com/about/women/foundation/foundation.html
Judy Barker, President

**Fnded:** 1955. **Priorities:** *Arts & Humanities:* 3%. Supports a variety of art interests, including arts associations and centers, theater, music, opera, and museums. *Civic & Public Affairs:* 33%. Funds programs concerned with civil rights, minority business, and women's affairs. Also supports united fund drives, social services programs for women and general community, family, and social service organizations. *Education:* 27%. Primarily supports scholarships to students attending high schools in certain corporate operating locations and scholarship programs targeting women and minorities. Interests also include general support to colleges and universities; education funds; organizations concerned with youth leadership development; minority, business, and economic education; and literacy. *International:* 32%. Funds women's health organizations, programs that deal with early detection of breast cancer, single-disease health organizations, hospice, and hospitals. *Note:* Total contributions made in 1999. **Typ. Recipients:** Cancer, Child Abuse, Children's Health/Hospitals, Domestic Violence, Emergency/Ambulance Services, Health

Funds, Health Organizations, Health-General, Hospices, Hospitals, Medical Education, Medical Rehabilitation, Medical Research, Mental Health, Outpatient Health Care, People with Disabilities, Prenatal Health Issues, Single-Disease Health Associations, Substance Abuse. **Geo. Dist:** headquarters and operating communities.

## ★ 858 ★ B.F. Goodrich Foundation, Inc.
2730 W Tyvola Rd.
Charlotte, NC 28217
**Phone:** (704)423-7080          **Fax:** (704)423-7069
**Email:** marty.visor@goodrich.com
**Website:** http://www.goodrich.com/giving.asp
Ms. Marty Viser, Manager, Community Affairs

**Priorities:** *Arts & Humanities:* (Arts & Culture) 15% to 25%. Supports a variety of interests in major plant communities, including the performing arts, public radio and television, museums, preservation organizations, and historicalsocieties. Sponsors matching gifts programs for cultural organizations located in communities where employees live or work. *Civic & Public Affairs:* (Civic & Community) 15% to 25%. Supports municipalities, trade associations, civic and nonacademic public policy research organizations in plant communities. *Education:* 30% to 40%. Emphasizes support to educational institutions located in major plant locations that provide technical research in areas of company interests or that serve as a major source of personnel. Sponsors matching gifts program and scholarships for children of employees. Also supports education-related public policy research organizations. *Environment:* (Health and Human Services/United Way) 20% to 30%. Emphasis on United Ways in communities where company has operating facilities. Also supports health organizations and privately financed agencies directed to basic human needs, such as youth development and family care. *Voluntarism:* Foundation sponsors a Bonus Volunteer Match program in addition to its Donors Match program. The foundation will make an extra 1 to 1 match of employee gifts to eligible organizations for which the employee volunteers, to a maximum of $1,000. The company also sponsors a school partnership in Charlotte, NC. **Typ. Recipients:** Cancer, Children's Health/Hospitals, Emergency/Ambulance Services, Geriatric Health, Health Organizations, Hospices, Hospitals, Nursing Services, People with Disabilities, Substance Abuse. **Geo. Dist:** nationally; operating locations.

## ★ 859 ★ Badger Meter Foundation
4545 West Brown Deer Rd.
Milwaukee, WI 53223
**Phone:** (414)371-5704          **Fax:** (414)371-5956
Beth McCallister, Secretary

**Priorities:** *Arts & Humanities:* 15%. Interests include festivals, opera, music, the performing arts, and theater. *Civic & Public Affairs:* 5%. Supports a diverse group of community services, including youth organizations, homes, children's centers, museums, and youth recreational activities. *Education:* 24%. Foundation supports colleges, universities, day schools, education funds, engineering education, continuing education, and scholarship funds. *Environment:* 44%. Recipients include rescue missions, aid for the mentally retarded, and food and clothing distribution. Majority of support funds Goodwill Industries. *International:* 4%. Support favors single-disease health associations and hospitals. Also supports pediatric health care, emergency services, community hospitals, and health organizations. *Religion:* Less than 1%. Supports a science museum. *Note:* Total contributions made in 2000. **Typ. Recipients:** Arthritis, Cancer, Domestic Violence, Health Organizations, Heart, Hospitals, Medical Education, Medical Research, Mental Health, People with Disabilities, Preventive Medicine/Wellness Organizations, Single-Disease Health Associations, Speech & Hearing, Substance Abuse, Transplant Networks/Donor Banks. **Geo. Dist:** Milwaukee, WI.

## ★ 860 ★ Baker Hughes Foundation
3900 Essex Lane, Ste. 210
Houston, TX 77027-5133

Phone: (713)439-8600
Isaac Kerridge, Executive Director

**Priorities:** *Arts & Humanities:* 7%. Supports art museums, music, art associations, and dance. *Civic & Public Affairs:* 3%. Provides funding for urban, minority, and women's affairs. *Education:* 28%. Supports colleges and universities, private colleges and schools, technical education, international education, high schools, and Junior Achievement. *Environment:* 46%. Supports United Way, family services, Boys & Girls Clubs, child welfare organizations, substance abuse treatment and prevention, youth organizations, and animal welfare. *International:* 12%. Gives to single-disease health associations, hospitals, and pediatric health. *Religion:* 3%. Funds science museums. *Note:* Total contributions made in 2000. **Typ. Recipients:** Medical Research. **Geo. Dist:** TX.

**★ 861 ★ Ball Corp.**
10 Longs Peak Dr.
Broomfield, CO 80021-2510
Phone: (303)469-5511          Fax: (303)460-2127
Website: http://www.ball.com
Harold Sohn, Vice President, Corporate Relations
**Typ. Recipients:** Health-General. **Geo. Dist:** CO.

**★ 862 ★ Baltimore Gas & Electric
    Foundation**
PO Box 1475
1003 G&E Bldg.
Baltimore, MD 21203-1475
Phone: (410)234-7481          Fax: (410)234-7471
Email: Malinda.B.Small@constellation.com
Website: http://constellationenergy.com
Malinda Small, Director, Corporate Contributions and Co

**Fnded:** 1986. **Priorities:** *Voluntarism:* The company sponsors an employee volunteer program aimed at increasing pride, motivation, and participation by allowing volunteers to direct their own program. **Typ. Recipients:** Child Abuse, Clinics/Medical Centers, Health Organizations, Hospices, Hospitals, Medical Education, People with Disabilities, Public Health. **Geo. Dist:** MD, Central Maryland and other areas where co. has significant business interests.

**★ 863 ★ Bandag, Inc.**
2905 N Hwy. 61
Muscatine, IA 52761-5886
Phone: (563)262-1400          Fax: (319)262-1069
Website: http://www.bandag.com
Jesus Escobebo, Employee Relations Specialist

**Priorities:** *Arts & Humanities:* Less than 5%. Supports arts associations, the performing arts, and community art programs. *Civic & Public Affairs:* About 30%. Contributes to environmental efforts, AfricanAmerican and Hispanic affairs, women's issues, and safety and urban concerns. *Education:* About 40%. Funding is awarded to colleges and universities, business and engineering educational programs, and public education and student aid programs. *International:* About 30%. Supports single-disease health organizations and issues, public health, health care cost containment, and hospitals. Additional support is for community activities and services, child welfare, counseling, and the United Way. **Typ. Recipients:** Adolescent Health Issues, Children's Health/Hospitals, Clinics/ Medical Centers, Domestic Violence, Eyes/Blindness, Health Funds, Health Organizations, Health Policy/ Cost Containment, Health-General, Hospices, Hospitals, Hospitals (University Affiliated), Prenatal Health Issues, Preventive Medicine/Wellness Organizations, Public Health, Speech & Hearing, Substance Abuse. **Geo. Dist:** headquarters and operating communities.

**★ 864 ★ Banfi Vintners Foundation**
1111 Cedar Swamp Rd.
Old Brookville, NY 11545
Frank Savino, Foundation Contact

**Fnded:** 1982. **Priorities:** *Arts & Humanities:* 15%. Supports ballet, art museums, public broadcasting, and a symphony orchestra. *Civic & Public Affairs:* 11%

Funds professional associations and Italian American organizations. *Education:* 62%. Supports colleges, universities, and specialty schools nationwide, with a focus on wine and food education. *Environment:* Less than 1%. Gives to the United Way, people with disabilities, and family services. *International:* 8%. Gives to hospitals and disease research and prevention. *Note:* Total contributions made in 1999. **Typ. Recipients:** Cancer, Diabetes, Eyes/Blindness, Health Organizations, Heart, Hospitals, Medical Research, Multiple Sclerosis, People with Disabilities, Sexual Abuse, Single-Disease Health Associations, Substance Abuse, Trauma Treatment. **Geo. Dist:** New York, NY, Metropolitan Area.

**★ 865 ★ Bank of America Foundation**
NC-007-18-02
100 North Tryon St.
Charlotte, NC 28255
Phone: 888-488-9802
Website: http://www.bankofamerica.com/foundation
Lynn Drury, President

**Priorities:** *Arts & Humanities:* (Arts & Culture) 16%. Interests include music, arts centers, museums, public broadcasting, libraries, and theater. *Civic & Public Affairs:* (Community Development) 13%. Supports community development and economic initiatives, and housing corporations. *Education:* 31%. Gives at the college and university level, as well as the elementary level. Major support goes to scholarship programs and public education. Other interests include economic, medical, and minority education, as well as business/ education partnerships. *Environment:* (Health and Human Services) 25%. Supports youth and family services, women's affairs, and welfare to work programs. Also supports hospitals and various other health organizations. *Voluntarism:* The company sponsors the Volunteer Time for Schools program, which allows each full-time associate to volunteer at a public or private school for up to two hours of paid time per week. The company also sponsors a Volunteer Grants Program. If an associate volunteers 50 or more hours at a nonprofit organization in a calendar year, Bank of America donates $250 to that organization in the associates name; the donation is increased to $500 for those who volunteer 100 or more hours. In addition, the company maintains the Team Bank of America Volunteer Network, which provides volunteer opportunities for Bank of America associates wishing to get involved in any of the approximately 3,000 volunteer events the company sponsors each year. *Note:* Total contributions made in 2000. **Typ. Recipients:** Child Abuse, Children's Health/Hospitals, Clinics/Medical Centers, Emergency/Ambulance Services, Health Organizations, Hospitals, Medical Education, Medical Research, People with Disabilities, Prenatal Health Issues, Substance Abuse. **Geo. Dist:** headquarters and operating communities, except in Washington State.

**★ 866 ★ Bank of Hawaii Charitable
    Foundation**
PO Box 3170
Honolulu, HI 96802-3170
Phone: (808)538-4540          Fax: (808)538-4647
Cheryl Ritchie, Contact

**Fnded:** 1981. **Priorities:** *Arts & Humanities:* 10%. Supports community and cultural arts centers on two islands. The remainder goes to museums and theater. *Civic & Public Affairs:* 22%. Funds community loan funds, economic development, and small business services. *Education:* 25%. Equally supports colleges, private academies, and public education. Additional support goes to a literacy fund. *Environment:* 20%. Supports girl and boy scouts and other youth organizations, family services, and crime prevention initiatives. *International:* 17%. Recipients include hospitals and medical centers. *Note:* Total contributions made in 1999. **Typ. Recipients:** Cancer, Children's Health/ Hospitals, Clinics/Medical Centers, Domestic Violence, Emergency/Ambulance Services, Health Organizations, Hospices, Hospitals, Medical Rehabilitation, Mental Health, Multiple Sclerosis, People with Disabilities. **Geo. Dist:** Honolulu, HI.

**★ 867 ★ Bank of Louisville Charities**
500 W Broadway
PO Box 1101
Louisville, KY 40201
Phone: (502)589-3351          Fax: (502)562-5403
Beth Klein, Senior Vice President, Community Relatio

**Fnded:** 1973. **Priorities:** *Arts & Humanities:* 41%. Supports art funds, ballet, visual and performing arts, and public broadcasting. *Civic & Public Affairs:* 11%. Supports organizations working toward economic development and community improvement projects. *Education:* 11%. Primarily supports public education. *Environment:* 31%. Supports the United Way, family services, youth organizations, senior services, and organizations assisting the disabled. *International:* 1%. Funds hospitals and single-disease health associations. *Religion:* 1%. Funds science centers. *Voluntarism:* Company encourages employee volunteerism; Laura Hillerich is the Employee Activities Coordinator. *Note:* Total contributions made in 2000. **Typ. Recipients:** Cancer, Children's Health/Hospitals, Domestic Violence, Emergency/Ambulance Services, Health-General, Heart, Hospitals, Medical Rehabilitation, Multiple Sclerosis, Nursing Services, People with Disabilities, Prenatal Health Issues, Sexual Abuse. **Geo. Dist:** KY, Jefferson County; Oldham, KY.

**★ 868 ★ Bank of New York Co., Inc.**
1 Wall St.
31st Floor
New York, NY 10286
Phone: (212)635-1802          Fax: (212)635-1799
Pat Bicket, Vice President and Assistant Secretary

**Priorities:** *Arts & Humanities:* About 20%. Support goes to museums, culturalgroups, historic preservation and restoration, public broadcasting, libraries, and the performing arts. *Civic & Public Affairs:* About 60%. Emphasis is on grants supporting housing, youth organizations, drug and alcohol abuse programs, and family and community services. Less than 5%. Emphasis on economic development, civil rights, business and free enterprise, international affairs, and national security. *Education:* About 20%. Private educational institutions receive considerable funding through the company's matching gift program. Support also goes to educational associations, elementary, minority, and liberal arts education. *International:* Less than 5%. Especially supports hospitals, health organizations and nursing services. **Typ. Recipients:** Health Organizations, Hospitals, Nursing Services, Single-Disease Health Associations, Substance Abuse. **Geo. Dist:** DE; NJ; NY.

**★ 869 ★ Bank One, Texas-Houston
    Office**
910 Travis TX2-4240
Houston, TX 77002
Phone: (713)751-3526          Fax: (713)751-3870
Website: http://www.bankone.com
Barbara Harris, Charitable Contributions Coordinator

**Priorities:** *Arts & Humanities:* About 15%. Contributes to performing arts programs, museums, public radio and television, and cultural programs. *Civic & Public Affairs:* About 10%. Interests include business, voter registration and education, civil rights, justice and law, and non-academic research. About 10%. Supports programs and projects in the areas of community and neighborhood improvement, community development, housing and urban revitalization, community-based education, and economic development in low- to moderate-income neighborhoods. *Education:* About 20%. Interests include primary and secondary schools, public and private higher education institutions, adult education programs, scholarship programs, public library systems, and other related organizations. Also operates employee matching gift program to educational institutions. *International:* About 40% of total contributions. Includes assistance to federated drives such as United Way; hospitals; local health and welfare groups; health research organizations; and youth agencies. Also supports nonprofit drug abuse and rehabilitation programs in Houston, and a matching gift program for employee contributions to health and welfare organizations. **Typ. Recipients:** Health Organizations, Health-General, Hospitals, Medical Research, Substance Abuse. **Geo. Dist:** Houston, TX.

### ★ 870 ★ Banta Corp. Foundation
PO Box 8003
Menasha, WI 54952-8003
**Phone:** (920)751-7777　　　　**Fax:** (920)751-7790
Gerald Henseler, President

**Fnded:** 1953. **Priorities:** *Arts & Humanities:* 7%. Supports performing arts, theater, libraries, public radio, a children's museum, and the arts. *Civic & Public Affairs:* 13%. Supports chambers of commerce, free enterprise, and community development. *Education:* 41%. Funds educational programs, scholarship programs, colleges, and universities. *Environment:* 33%. Supports youth organizations and services, family social services, community centers, the Make-A-Wish program, and food distribution. *International:* 4%. Funds community clinics, medical centers, and children's hospitals. *Note:* Total contributions in 2000. **Typ. Recipients:** AIDS/HIV, Cancer, Children's Health/Hospitals, Clinics/Medical Centers, Domestic Violence, Emergency/Ambulance Services, Heart, Hospitals, Medical Education, Mental Health, Nursing Services, People with Disabilities, Substance Abuse. **Geo. Dist:** operating locations; WI.

### ★ 871 ★ Barclays Capital
222 Broadway, 10th Floor
New York, NY 10038
**Phone:** (212)412-3825　　　　**Fax:** (212)412-7300
**Email:** LindaWynns@barcap.com
**Website:** http://www.barcap.com
Linda Wynns, Associate Director, Corporate Communicat

**Priorities:** *Arts & Humanities:* 33%. Donates to performing arts. *Civic & Public Affairs:* 7%. Focuses on improving the community through local community organizations, and neighborhood sports teams. *Education:* 42%. Primarily supports through matching gifts. Also donates to universities, specialized art schools and Junior Achievement. *Environment:* 5%. Majority of support goes to family services and youth organizations. *International:* 11%. Funds the Amyotropic Lateral Sclerosis Association, other disease-specific groups, and hospitals. *Note:* Total contributions in 1997. **Typ. Recipients:** AIDS/HIV, Cancer, Children's Health/Hospitals, Diabetes, Hospices, Hospitals, Medical Research, Single-Disease Health Associations. **Geo. Dist:** New York, NY. **Frmly:** Barclays Bank Foundation.

### ★ 872 ★ Barden Foundation, Inc.
1146 Barnum Ave.
Bridgeport, CT 06610
**Phone:** (203)336-7531　　　　**Fax:** (203)336-6440
Thomas Loughman, Treasurer & Trustee

**Fnded:** 1959. **Priorities:** *Education:* 13%. Funding goes to science education, public education in the headquarters area, and scholarships. *Environment:* 70%. Funds the United Way, youth agencies, local social welfare organizations, national health agencies, hospitals and nursing homes, and local health organizations. *Note:* Total contributions in fiscal 2000. **Typ. Recipients:** Cancer, Children's Health/Hospitals, Clinics/Medical Centers, Emergency/Ambulance Services, Health Organizations, Hospices, Hospitals, Medical Rehabilitation, Nursing Services, People with Disabilities, Single-Disease Health Associations. **Geo. Dist:** Bridgeport, CT; Danbury, CT; Winsted, CT.

### ★ 873 ★ Barnes Group Foundation Inc.
123 Main St.
PO Box 489
Bristol, CT 06011-0489
**Phone:** (860)583-7070　　　　**Fax:** (860)589-7466
Thomas Barnes, Secretary

**Priorities:** *Arts & Humanities:* 11%. Contributes to arts centers, museums, theaters, music, and public broadcasting. *Civic & Public Affairs:* 8%. Recipients include urban affairs, municipalities, leadership councils, and community foundations. *Education:* 40%. About three-fifths of funds supports Citizens Scholarship Foundation for college tuition for children of employees. Also supports colleges and universities, private education, business education, religious high schools, and college funds. *Environment:* 12%. Supports youth organizations, homes for children, guide dogs for the blind, Focus Hope, and family services. Also supports United Way. *International:* 26%. Funds hospitals, cancer centers, and health organizations. *Note:* Total contributions made in 2000. **Typ. Recipients:** Cancer, Children's Health/Hospitals, Emergency/Ambulance Services, Hospitals, Medical Research, People with Disabilities, Single-Disease Health Associations, Substance Abuse, Trauma Treatment. **Geo. Dist:** operating communities.

### ★ 874 ★ Barry Foundation
PO Box 129
Columbus, OH 43216-0129
Marilyn Thomas, Corporate Finance Administrator

**Fnded:** 1963. **Priorities:** *Arts & Humanities:* Less than 1%. Supports museums and cultural programs. *Civic & Public Affairs:* 2%. Gives to community foundations. *Education:* 32%. Supports higher education and educational programs. *Environment:* 11%. Funds youth and social services. *International:* 3%. Funds health care organizations and concerns. *Note:* Total contributions made in 2000. **Typ. Recipients:** AIDS/HIV, Cancer, Children's Health/Hospitals, Diabetes, Emergency/Ambulance Services, Family Planning, Health Funds, Health Organizations, Health-General, Medical Research, People with Disabilities, Single-Disease Health Associations, Speech & Hearing, Substance Abuse. **Geo. Dist:** nationally.

### ★ 875 ★ Bassett Furniture Industries Foundation
PO Box 626
Bassett, VA 24055-0626
**Phone:** (540)629-6200
James Philpott, Vice President & Personnel Director

**Fnded:** 1993. **Priorities:** *Arts & Humanities:* 2%. Supports an arts association. *Civic & Public Affairs:* 18%. Funds a volunteer fire and the Crosby Foundation. *Education:* 44%. Supports college funds and universities. *Environment:* 23%. Supports the United Way and Boy Scouts of America. *International:* 1%. Multiple sclerosis and cancer organizations receive support. *Note:* Total contributions made in fiscal 1999. **Typ. Recipients:** Cancer, Emergency/Ambulance Services, Single-Disease Health Associations. **Geo. Dist:** GA; NC; VA.

### ★ 876 ★ Baxter Allegiance Foundation
One Baxter Parkway
Deerfield, IL 60015-4633
**Phone:** (847)948-4604　　　　**Fax:** (847)948-4026
**Email:** pat_a_morgan@baxter.com
**Website:** http://www.baxter.com
Ms. Patricia Morgan, Executive Director & Secretary

**Priorities:** *Arts & Humanities:* 1%. *Civic & Public Affairs:* 1%. *Education:* 10%. Supports higher education. *Environment:* 11%. Support goes to United Way, community service organizations, and Young Men's Christian Association. *International:* 61%. Supports healthcare access, improving the quality of the healthcare delivery system, and increasing the availability of resources to healthcare providers. Also supports improved cost effectiveness of the delivery system, immunization, and sponsors employees matching gifts to hospitals. *Voluntarism:* Supports Dollars for Doers program, which provides grants to organizations where employees volunteer. *Note:* Total contributions made in 2000. **Typ. Recipients:** AIDS/HIV, Child Abuse, Children's Health/Hospitals, Clinics/Medical Centers, Domestic Violence, Emergency/Ambulance Services, Eyes/Blindness, Health Organizations, Health Policy/Cost Containment, Heart, Home-Care Services, Hospices, Hospitals, Hospitals (University Affiliated), Long-Term Care, Medical Education, Medical Rehabilitation, Medical Research, Mental Health, Nursing Services, People with Disabilities, Prenatal Health Issues, Preventive Medicine/Wellness Organizations, Public Health, Research/Studies Institutes, Respiratory, Sexual Abuse, Substance Abuse. **Geo. Dist:** nationally; Europe; Latin America; Puerto Rico; Chicago, IL.

### ★ 877 ★ Bayer Foundation
100 Bayer Rd., Bldg. 4
Pittsburgh, PA 15205-9741
**Phone:** (412)777-5791　　　　**Fax:** (412)778-4432
**Website:** http://www.bayerus.com
Rebecca Lucore, Executive Director

**Priorities:** *Arts & Humanities:* 15%. Supports visual arts organizations, museums, and performing arts. *Civic & Public Affairs:* 3%. Supports zoos, civic coalitions, and community development organizations. *Education:* 42%. Funds colleges and universities, with a particular emphasis on science, engineering, and chemistry education. *International:* 3%. Gives to AIDs, other single-disease health associations, pediatric health, and medical centers. *Religion:* 1%. Funds chemistry and engineering research organizations and science centers. *Note:* Total contributions made in 1999. **Typ. Recipients:** Clinics/Medical Centers, Diabetes, Health Funds, Health Organizations, Health-General, Hospitals, Medical Education, People with Disabilities, Single-Disease Health Associations. **Geo. Dist:** headquarters and operating communities.

### ★ 878 ★ Bayport Foundation
PO Box 204
Bayport, MN 55003-0204
**Phone:** (651)439-1557　　　　**Fax:** (651)439-9480
**Email:** chloettehaley@scenicriver.org
**Website:** http://www.scenicriver.org
Chloette Haley, Grants Consultant

**Priorities:** *Arts & Humanities:* 7%. Supports orchestras, choirs, and arts centers/councils. *Civic & Public Affairs:* 19%. Funds municipalities, community foundations, and housing initiatives. *Education:* 12%. Focus is on precollege education, with major support typically given to school districts, public and private elementary schools, and arts education for children. Educational television, colleges and universities, and education associations also receive support. *Environment:* 38%. Emphasis on youth organizations. Awards major grants to the United Way and the Salvation Army. Other interests include the aged, community service organizations, recreation and athletics, and volunteer services. *International:* 18%. Supports local hospitals, medical research, and single-disease health organizations. **Typ. Recipients:** Cancer, Children's Health/Hospitals, Clinics/Medical Centers, Emergency/Ambulance Services, Eyes/Blindness, Family Planning, Health Funds, Health Organizations, Hospitals, Kidney, Medical Rehabilitation, Medical Research, People with Disabilities, Public Health, Single-Disease Health Associations, Speech & Hearing, Substance Abuse. **Geo. Dist:** MN, East Metro area; MN, Washington County; WI, Barron County; WI, Burnett County; WI, Dunn County; WI, Pierce County; WI, Polk County; WI, St. Croix County.

### ★ 879 ★ BD
1 Becton Dr.
Franklin Lakes, NJ 07417
**Phone:** (201)847-7065　　　　**Fax:** (201)847-5305
**Website:** http://www.bd.com/responsibility/
Jennifer Farrington, Manager, Community Partnerships

**Priorities:** *Voluntarism:* BD employees and retirees who volunteer their time to charitable organizations are honored through the company's Community Service Awards Program. The program provides financial contributions to the non-profit organization to which BD associates have donated their time. **Typ. Recipients:** Hospitals, Medical Education, Medical Research, Medical Training, Nursing Services. **Geo. Dist:** principally near operating locations and to national organizations.

## ★ 880 ★ Beckman Coulter, Inc.

4300 N Harbor Boulevard
PO Box 3100
C-30-B
Fullerton, CA 92835-3100
**Phone:** (714)871-4848 **Fax:** (714)773-7743
**Website:** http://www.beckman.com
Tracy Hatt, Manager, Community Affairs

**Priorities:** *Education:* Scientific education, science, and research-related healthcare. **Typ. Recipients:** AIDS/HIV, Alzheimers Disease, Arthritis, Cancer, Diabetes, Heart, Kidney, Medical Research, Multiple Sclerosis, Respiratory. **Geo. Dist:** headquarters and operating communities.

## ★ 881 ★ BellSouth Foundation

1155 Peachtree St., NE, Room 7H08
Atlanta, GA 30309-3610
**Phone:** (404)249-2396 **Fax:** (404)249-5696
**Email:** grants.manager@bellsouth.com
**Website:** http://www.bellsouth.com/foundation
Greg Norton, Grants Administrator

**Fnded:** 1986. **Priorities:** *Education:* 100%. The foundation has the sole priority of improving the quality of education in its Southeastern service area and in Latin America. The foundation conducts a target requests for proposals process accepted for two special initiatives; limited funds are available for Opportunity Grants, or unsolicited requests that address the two initiatives. The first initiative is Closing the Divides: an equity agenda for student learning and achievement and for community well-being. Supported projects are for disadvantaged high school students, college-bound minorities, and technology-disadvantaged communities. The second initiative is Forging New Paths: a capacity-building agenda for innovation and opportunity. Supported projects benefit Latin America's children, teachers and leaders, and technology and learning. *Note:* Company also maintains a substantial direct giving program, which makes contributions within the company's service area in the categories of education, 51%; health and human services, 29%; arts and culture, 13%; civic and community, 6%; and miscellaneous interests, 1%. **Typ. Recipients:** Health-General, Medical Education. **Geo. Dist:** principally near operating locations and to national organizations.

## ★ 882 ★ Belo Foundation

PO Box 655237
Dallas, TX 75265-5237
**Phone:** (214)977-6661 **Fax:** (214)977-6620
**Website:** http://www.belo.com/phil.html
Judith Garrett Sequra, President, Executive Director

**Fnded:** 1952. **Priorities:** *Arts & Humanities:* 46%. Supports broadcasting associations and museums, history/heritage organizations, cultural centers, art museums, and performing arts. *Civic & Public Affairs:* 31%. Primarily funds freedom of speech/press initiatives and professional journalism organizations. Also gives to community development, urban planning, public policy organizations, and police associations. *Education:* 9%. Funds colleges and universities, with a focus on media law and journalism education. *Environment:* 13%. Supports United Way agencies in metropolitan Dallas, youth organizations, and a veteran's memorial. *Note:* Total foundation contributions made in 1999. **Typ. Recipients:** Family Planning, Health Organizations, Hospitals. **Geo. Dist:** headquarters area only; principally near operating locations and to national organizations; Sacramento, CA; Owensboro, KY; New Orleans, LA; Tulsa, OK; Bryan, TX; College Station, TX; Dallas, TX; Ft. Worth, TX; Houston, TX; Hampton, VA; Norfolk, VA; Seattle, WA; Tacoma, WA. **Frmly:** Dallas Morning News-WFAA Foundation A. H. Belo Corp. FND.

## ★ 883 ★ Bemis Co. Foundation

222 South 9th St., Ste. 2300
Minneapolis, MN 55402
**Phone:** (612)376-3093 **Fax:** (612)376-3150
**Email:** ajkirchner@bemis.com
Gene Seashore, Trustee

**Priorities:** *Civic & Public Affairs:* (Cultural & Civic) 16%. Funds civic concerns include economic development, environmental affairs, safety, and business and free enterprise groups. Also supports cultural interests including public broadcasting, theater, arts centers, music, and museums. *Education:* 27%. Supports employee educational matching gifts, scholarship programs for children of employees, and independent college associations in states where company facilities are located. *Environment:* (Social Welfare & Health) 57%. Major support goes to united fund drives in operating locations. Another priority is food shelves and food banks (the company also sponsors an employee matching gifts program to food banks). Other social welfare interests include child welfare and youth organizations, the aged, employment, and community service organizations. Health interests include hospitals and single-disease health organizations. *Note:* Total foundation contributions in 2000. **Typ. Recipients:** Clinics/Medical Centers, Diabetes, Domestic Violence, Emergency/Ambulance Services, Family Planning, Health Funds, Health Organizations, Health Policy/Cost Containment, Hospitals, Medical Education, Nursing Services, People with Disabilities, Prenatal Health Issues, Public Health, Single-Disease Health Associations, Speech & Hearing, Substance Abuse. **Geo. Dist:** principally near operating locations and to national organizations; Minneapolis, MN.

## ★ 884 ★ Benjamin Jacobson & Sons Foundation

40 Wall St., 45th Floor
New York, NY 10005
**Phone:** (212)952-1012 **Fax:** (212)952-0920
Robert Jacobson, Sr., President

**Priorities:** *Arts & Humanities:* 16%. Funds museums, performing arts centers, music, and public broadcasting. *Civic & Public Affairs:* 3%. Supports philanthropic organizations, researchfunds, and community affairs. *Education:* 4%. Funds colleges and universities, student aid, and private education. *Environment:* 19%. Favors youth organizations, the needy, child welfare, family services, and community services organizations. *International:* 36%. Supports cancer research, hospitals, single-disease health associations, and health organizations. *Note:* Contributions made in fiscal 1999. **Typ. Recipients:** Arthritis, Cancer, Children's Health/Hospitals, Clinics/Medical Centers, Diabetes, Emergency/Ambulance Services, Health Organizations, Hospitals, Medical Education, Medical Research, People with Disabilities, Public Health, Single-Disease Health Associations, Substance Abuse. **Geo. Dist:** nationally; New York, NY.

## ★ 885 ★ Berwind Group

3000 Centre Square West
1500 Market St.
Philadelphia, PA 19102
**Phone:** (215)563-2800 **Fax:** (215)563-1493
**Email:** mlarue@berwind.com
**Website:** http://www.berwind.com
Mary LaRue, Chairperson, Contributions Committee

**Typ. Recipients:** Family Planning, Health-General, Hospitals. **Geo. Dist:** headquarters area only.

## ★ 886 ★ Bethlehem Steel Foundation

1170 Eighth Ave.
Rm. 1711, Martin Tower
Bethlehem, PA 18016-7699
**Phone:** (610)694-6940 **Fax:** (610)694-1509
**Email:** kostecky@bethsteel.com
**Website:** http://www.bethsteel.com/about/foundation.shtml
James Kostecky, Executive Director

**Priorities:** *Arts & Humanities:* 10%. Focus is on the cultural resources that provide contribute to the vitality and quality of life in operating communities. Funds the performing arts and public broadcasting. *Civic & Public Affairs:* 9%. Supports organizations that study important issues impacting the company and the steel industry, and provide government, industry, and the public with the results of investigations. Funds organizations and programs devoted to government improvement, community revitalization, public safety, economic development, and community planning. *Education:* 17%. Goal of giving is to maintain and improve the quality of pre-K through higher educational programs and institutions; to support research facilities important to the company's business interests; to ensure appropriate numbers of high-quality graduates, and to improve the level of understanding of the free enterprise system, particularly among young people during their formative years. Foundation also provides scholarships to the children of employees and matches gifts to higher education. *Environment:* 59%. Supports United Way, urban renewal groups, boys and girls clubs, substance abuse clinics, disease-specific organizations and community organizations. *International:* 1%. Supports hospitals, medical centers, and health clinics. *Note:* Total foundation contributions made in 2000. **Typ. Recipients:** Domestic Violence, Emergency/Ambulance Services, Geriatric Health, Health Organizations, Health Policy/Cost Containment, Hospitals, Medical Research, Nursing Services, Nutrition, People with Disabilities, Public Health, Substance Abuse. **Geo. Dist:** headquarters and operating communities.

## ★ 887 ★ Binney & Smith Inc.

PO Box 431
1100 Church Ln.
Easton, PA 18042-0431
**Phone:** (610)559-6607 **Fax:** (610)559-6691
**Email:** mvoden@binney-smith.com
**Website:** http://www.binney-smith.com
Mary Ellyn Volden, Director, Global Philanthropy

**Priorities:** *Arts & Humanities:* Supports art organizations that help ensure a higher quality of life for all citizens. Considers requests to organizations that stress excellence and community participation, especially with children. Also considers support for performing arts and public broadcasting. *Civic & Public Affairs:* Funds organizations that encourage a better working relationship between business and the community. Also funds local environmental and ecological issues. *Education:* Focus on early childhood development and quality arts in education initiatives. Grants may be made for start-up programs. Limited support for special programs. Assistance is given to programs for the physically and mentally disabled. *International:* Majority of contributions go to the United Way. Limited support towards preventive health measures. Funding also given to human service programs, services for children, the elderly and the disabled, and programs that assist disadvantaged children. *Voluntarism:* The company provides volunteers for special events. **Typ. Recipients:** Children's Health/Hospitals, Domestic Violence, Emergency/Ambulance Services, Health-General, Sexual Abuse, Speech & Hearing. **Geo. Dist:** Easton, PA.

## ★ 888 ★ Binswanger Foundation

2 Logan Square, 4th Floor
Philadelphia, PA 19103
**Phone:** (215)448-6000 **Fax:** (215)448-6238
**Email:** info@cbbi.com
John Binswanger, President

**Priorities:** *Arts & Humanities:* 17%. Supports public broadcasting, music, literature, libraries, history organizations, historic preservation, and the performing arts. *Civic & Public Affairs:* 7%. Funds public parks, community funds, voting right, economic development, and legal assistance organizations. *Education:* 10%. Supports universities, schools, and arts/humanities education. *Environment:* 1%. Supports the American Red Cross, food distribution, Planned Parenthood, and orphan services. *International:* 16%. Supports hospital, cancer research, children's health and medical centers. *Religion:* 1%. Funds natural science research. *Note:* Total contributions made in 1999. **Typ. Recipients:** Cancer, Cancer, Children's Health/Hospitals, Emergency/Ambulance Services, Family Planning, Health Organizations, Hospitals, Hospitals (University Affiliated), Medical Research, Mental Health, People with Disabilities, Public Health, Single-Disease Health Associations, Substance Abuse. **Geo. Dist:** PA.

### ★ 889 ★ Blade Foundation
541 N Superior St.
Toledo, OH 43660
**Phone:** (419)724-6210
William Block, Jr., President & Trustee

**Priorities:** *Arts & Humanities:* 33%. Supports ballet, museum, opera, theater, history, arts centers. *Civic & Public Affairs:* 10%. Funds urban affairs, parks, local initiatives, and entrepreneurism. *Education:* 15%. Supports literacy, scholarships, minority education. *Environment:* 31%. Supports family planning services, United Way, scouts, volunteer services, special olympics, and animal protection. *International:* 5%. Funds Red Cross and single-disease health associations. *Voluntarism:* Company actively promotes employee volunteerism through participation in the United Way, Read for Literacy, and in activities with the Sherman School, its adopted school. *Note:* Total contributions made in 1999. **Typ. Recipients:** Alzheimers Disease, Arthritis, Children's Health/Hospitals, Clinics/Medical Centers, Emergency/Ambulance Services, Family Planning, Medical Education, Medical Education, Multiple Sclerosis, Preventive Medicine/Wellness Organizations, Respiratory, Single-Disease Health Associations. **Geo. Dist:** Toledo, OH.

### ★ 890 ★ Blount International, Inc.
PO Box 949
Montgomery, AL 36101-0949
**Phone:** (334)244-4000          **Fax:** (334)271-8175
**Email:** jdm@blount.com
Rodney Blanenship, CFO

**Priorities:** *Arts & Humanities:* 15%. Interests include historic preservation, opera, ballet, museums, and arts associations. Grants typically range from $100 to $5,000. A small percentage of funds is disbursed through a matching grants program. *Civic & Public Affairs:* 4%. Interests include economic development, municipalities, and safety organizations. Sponsors small matching grants program. *Education:* 60%. General goals of education grants are to prepare students for careers in business, government, and education; to advance knowledge in science and technology; and to enhance educational opportunities for minorities and the disadvantaged. One-half of contributions support colleges and universities. Also shows interest in economic education, private and public education, and education associations. Matching grants comprise about one third of education funding. *Environment:* 11%. Funds YMCA and children's organizations. *International:* 2%. Interests include hospitals and health associations. *Religion:* 5%. *Note:* Total contributions made in 1998. **Typ. Recipients:** Arthritis, Cancer, Domestic Violence, Emergency/Ambulance Services, Eyes/Blindness, Health Organizations, Hospices, Hospitals, Medical Education, Mental Health, Single-Disease Health Associations, Substance Abuse. **Geo. Dist:** principally near operating locations and to national organizations; Montgomery, AL.

### ★ 891 ★ Blue Bell Foundation
PO Box 21488
Greensboro, NC 27420
**Phone:** (910)373-3412
Charles Conkin, Vice President, Human Resources

**Priorities:** *Arts & Humanities:* 16%. Supports museums and libraries. *Civic & Public Affairs:* 6%. Recipients include municipalities, environmental efforts, and community affairs organizations. *Education:* 41%. Emphasis is on the National Merit Scholarship Corporation, colleges and universities. Also supports preschools, high schools (public and private), education funds, and community education programs. The foundation operates a large matching gift program for company employees who wish to contribute to educational institutions. *Environment:* 34%. Supports United Way chapters and community service organizations. Housing, food distribution, and youth activities are also major priorities. *International:* 2%. Funds single-disease health associations, Ronald McDonald House, dental health, and health centers. *Note:* total contributions made in 2000. **Typ. Recipients:** Cancer, Child Abuse, Children's Health/Hospitals, Clinics/Medical

Centers, Diabetes, Domestic Violence, Emergency/Ambulance Services, Heart, Hospices, Hospitals, Medical Rehabilitation, Medical Research, People with Disabilities, Prenatal Health Issues, Public Health, Respiratory, Single-Disease Health Associations, Substance Abuse. **Geo. Dist:** principally near operating locations and to national organizations.

### ★ 892 ★ Blue Cross & Blue Shield of Michigan Foundation
600 Lafayette E, X520
Detroit, MI 48226-2927
**Phone:** (313)225-8706          **Fax:** (313)225-7730
**Email:** nmaloy@bcbsm.com
**Website:** http://www.bcbsm.com/foundation.shtml
Nancy Szydlowski, Executive Assistant

**Priorities:** *Civic & Public Affairs:* 1%. *Education:* 3%. Supports student awards program in public health, medicine, and health policy. *Environment:* 26%. Funds went to projects that addressed domestic violence, through the Request for Proposals Program. *International:* 76%. Goals for giving are to enhance the quality and appropriate use of healthcare services, improve access to appropriate health services, and control healthcare costs. Supports the following programs: the Investigator Initiated Research Program, which supports healthcare researchers interested in finding ways to improve healthcare in Michigan by funding projects which address healthcare costs, quality, and access to services; the Matching Initiative Program, which supports a variety of innovative health service projects and attempts to foster collaboration among foundations and other funding organizations, and which matches grants for conferences and seminars; the Request for Proposals Program; the Physician Investigator Research Award, for projects that include physician-led pilot studies, feasibility studies, or small research studies in clinical or health services research; the Student Award Program, which offers one-year grants for health-care research to doctoral and medical students in Michigan universities; the Proposal Development Award, which helps community nonprofit organizations develop proposals for improving healthcare delivery; and the Excellence in Research Awards, which honors researchers who make significant contributions toward improving health care delivery in Michigan. *Note:* Total foundation contributions made in 2000. **Typ. Recipients:** AIDS/HIV, Cancer, Children's Health/Hospitals, Diabetes, Domestic Violence, Geriatric Health, Health Organizations, Health Policy/Cost Containment, Health-General, Heart, Hospitals, Medical Education, Medical Research, Mental Health, People with Disabilities, Prenatal Health Issues, Preventive Medicine/Wellness Organizations, Single-Disease Health Associations. **Geo. Dist:** MI.

### ★ 893 ★ Blue Cross & Blue Shield of Minnesota Foundation Inc.
PO Box 64560
Saint Paul, MN 55164-0560
**Phone:** (612)662-1580          **Fax:** (612)662-1570
**Email:** community@bluecrossmn.com
**Website:** http://www.bluecrossmn.com
Daniel Johnson, Director, Community Affairs

**Fnded:** 1986. **Priorities:** *Environment:* 25%. Funds the United Way. *International:* 75%. Supports programs and organizations that reduce tobacco use, particularly use by youths; help individuals with chronic illness to navigate the health care system; promote fitness, nutrition, and safety; increase childhood immunization; and other miscellaneous health objectives. *Voluntarism:* Volunteer Council manages employee volunteer efforts. *Note:* Total foundation contributions made in 2000. **Typ. Recipients:** AIDS/HIV, Cancer, Children's Health/Hospitals, Clinics/Medical Centers, Diabetes, Domestic Violence, Emergency/Ambulance Services, Health Funds, Health Organizations, Health Organizations, Health Policy/Cost Containment, Health-General, Heart, Hospitals, Kidney, Medical Education, Medical Rehabilitation, Medical Research, Medical Training, Mental Health, Multiple Sclerosis, Nutrition, People with Disabilities, Prenatal Health Issues, Preventive Medicine/Wellness Organizations,

Public Health, Respiratory, Single-Disease Health Associations, Trauma Treatment. **Geo. Dist:** MN.

### ★ 894 ★ Borden Foundation, Inc.
180 East Broad St.
Columbus, OH 43215-3799
**Phone:** (614)225-4580          **Fax:** (614)225-4066
Ms. Frankie Nowland, President, Director of Social Responsibi

**Fnded:** 1944. **Priorities:** *Arts & Humanities:* 12%. Contributions are considered for arts organizations and activities within budgetary limitations. *Civic & Public Affairs:* 15%. Grants for selected community activities are considered within budgetary limitations. *Education:* 9%. Supports post-secondary educational institutions through grants to select national umbrella agencies. *Environment:* 28%. Majority of support funds large grants to united funds and youth organizations, and considerable support to religious welfare organizations. Special consideration given to nutrition education and food programs for children and projects that improve living conditions for children or provide them with adequate shelter and/or health care. Foundation also supports parenting and early childhood education programs; sports, recreation, and camping programs sponsored by youth-serving agencies; and programs that enable disadvantaged children to participate in the arts through programming by community arts institutions. Interests also include community services, shelters, and aid to the homeless. *International:* 20%. Supports research for heart disease, diabetes, respiratory illness, and AIDS. *Religion:* 15%. Gives to science centers and museums. *Note:* The foundation focuses on funding direct services and programs for disadvantaged youth across all program areas. Total contributions made in 1998. **Typ. Recipients:** AIDS/HIV, Arthritis, Cancer, Children's Health/Hospitals, Diabetes, Domestic Violence, Emergency/Ambulance Services, Eyes/Blindness, Hospitals, Medical Research, Mental Health, People with Disabilities, Prenatal Health Issues, Public Health, Single-Disease Health Associations, Speech & Hearing. **Geo. Dist:** principally near operating locations and to national organizations.

### ★ 895 ★ Borman's Inc. Fund
20500 Civic Center Dr., Ste. 2750
Southfield, MI 48076
**Phone:** (248)350-0300          **Fax:** (248)350-2920
Gilbert Borman, Secretary & Treasurer

**Priorities:** *Arts & Humanities:* 1%. Supports the Detroit Symphony Orchestra. *Civic & Public Affairs:* 8%. Supports public policy institutes. *Education:* 16%. Colleges and universities, religious education, and private precollege education are funded. *Environment:* 2%. Funds United Way. *International:* 1%. Primarily funds single-disease health organizations and national health societies. *Note:* Total foundation contributions made in 1998. **Typ. Recipients:** AIDS/HIV, Alzheimers Disease, Alzheimers Disease, Cancer, Children's Health/Hospitals, Domestic Violence, Emergency/Ambulance Services, Eyes/Blindness, Family Planning, Geriatric Health, Health Organizations, Hospices, Hospitals, Long-Term Care, Mental Health, Multiple Sclerosis, People with Disabilities, Single-Disease Health Associations, Substance Abuse. **Geo. Dist:** MI, Southeastern Michigan.

### ★ 896 ★ Boston Globe Foundation
135 Morrissey Boulevard, 2nd Floor
Boston, MA 02107
**Phone:** (617)929-2895          **Fax:** (617)929-2041
**Email:** foundation@globe.com
Suzanne Maas, Executive Director

**Priorities:** *Education:* 6%. Supports scholarship funds, internships, student aid, colleges and universities. *Environment:* 41%. Supports the Globe Santa Fund, for the purchase and distribution of holiday gifts for needy children. Also supports the United Way and human service agencies. *Note:* Total foundation contributions made from July 31, 1999 through December 31, 2000. **Typ. Recipients:** AIDS/HIV, Children's Health/Hospitals, Clinics/Medical Centers, Domestic Violence, Health Organizations, Hospitals, Medical

Education, Medical Research, Mental Health, Nutrition, People with Disabilities, Substance Abuse. **Geo. Dist:** Boston, MA; Cambridge, MA; Chelsea, MA; Somerville, MA.

**★ 897 ★ Boswell Foundation, Inc.**
PO Box 104
Lebanon, MO 65536
**Phone:** (417)588-4151 **Fax:** (417)588-3344
Paul Walker, Secretary

**Fnded:** 1985. **Priorities:** *Civic & Public Affairs:* 14%. Subpanel Zoos. *Education:* 25%. Subpanel Colleges/universities, private education. *Environment:* 19%. Contributes to animal protection, social services for women and children. *International:* 14%. Subpanel single-disease health associations. *Note:* Total contributions made in fiscal 1998. **Typ. Recipients:** Arthritis, Cancer, Family Planning, Health-General, Medical Education, Prenatal Health Issues, Public Health, Single-Disease Health Associations. **Geo. Dist:** nationally; Palm Beach, FL; Lebanon, MO.

**★ 898 ★ Bourns Foundation**
1200 Columbia Ave.
Riverside, CA 92507
**Phone:** (909)781-5606 **Fax:** (909)781-5273
Gordon Bourns, President

**Priorities:** *Arts & Humanities:* 1%. *Civic & Public Affairs:* 2%. *Education:* 97%. Funds public and private pre-college and private colleges and universities focusing on engineering. *Environment:* Less than 1%. *International:* Less than 1%. *Note:* Total foundation contributions made in fiscal 2000. **Typ. Recipients:** Cancer, Children's Health/Hospitals, Diabetes, Health-General, Hospices, Hospitals, Mental Health. **Geo. Dist:** CA, focusing on Inland Empire area of Southern California; UT.

**★ 899 ★ Bowater Inc.**
55 East Camperdown Way
Greenville, SC 29601-3597
**Phone:** (864)271-7733 **Fax:** (864)282-9482
**Website:** http://www.bowater.com
Gordon Manuel, Director, Government Affairs

**Priorities:** *Arts & Humanities:* 10% to 15%. Museums, libraries, community arts, theater, and the performing arts. *Civic & Public Affairs:* About 5%. Supports economic development, environmental affairs, urban and community affairs, and zoos and botanical gardens. *Education:* About 25%. Colleges, universities, community colleges, continuing education programs, economic education, business education, and education for minorities. *International:* 45% to 50%. Hospitals, hospices, health organizations, aid for the disabled, community centers, drug abuse programs, shelters, and community service organizations. A large portion of funds in this category support the United Way. **Typ. Recipients:** Health Organizations, Hospitals. **Geo. Dist:** headquarters and operating communities.

**★ 900 ★ BP Amoco Foundation**
200 East Randolph Dr.
Chicago, IL 60601
**Phone:** (312)856-6306 **Fax:** (312)616-0826
Sonya Jackson, President

**Priorities:** *Arts & Humanities:* 15% to 20%. Supports museums, music, art, theaters, and artscenters. Also funds visual and performing arts when these organizations enhance the quality of life, strengthen neighborhoods by bringing art to disadvantaged individuals and communities, and present performances and instructions in schools, community centers, and neighborhoods. *Civic & Public Affairs:* About 10%. Interests include employment, economic growth, public policy groups, government and tax issues, public safety, housing, youth leadership, and urban redevelopment issues. Supports programs that strengthen communities by promoting and investing in economic growth, and a healthy environment. Programs that promote minorities, emergency relief efforts, and the United Way receive funding under this category. Also sup-

ports major health facilities, programs that help the disadvantaged receive health-care, and hospices when these programs reflect the educational and community objectives of the foundation. *Education:* 30% to 35%. To foster an effective educational system and adequate workforce pool that reflects the diversity of the people in Amoco communities. Supports university programs that target disciplines required in Amoco's business; precollege programs that focus on math, science, and economic education; programs that promote minority participation in technical fields; and national and local school reform efforts. Also supports precollege and higher education through matching gifts and volunteer efforts. *Environment:* 30% to 35%. Includes United Way and family and community service organizations. *International:* Less than 5%. *Religion:* About 1%. **Typ. Recipients:** Children's Health/Hospitals, Clinics/Medical Centers, Emergency/Ambulance Services, Health-General, Hospitals, People with Disabilities, Public Health, Research/Studies Institutes, Single-Disease Health Associations. **Geo. Dist:** headquarters and operating communities, nationally and internationally. **Frmly:** Amoco Foundation.

**★ 901 ★ Brayton Wilbur Foundation**
345 California St., 27th Floor
San Francisco, CA 94104-2644
**Phone:** (415)772-4006 **Fax:** (415)772-4005
Brayton Wilbur, Jr., President

**Fnded:** 1947. **Priorities:** *Arts & Humanities:* 85%. Primary support for museums, opera, symphonies, arts associations, and art institutes. *Environment:* 5%. Funds the United Way and community services. *Note:* Total contributions made in 1999. **Typ. Recipients:** Clinics/Medical Centers, Emergency/Ambulance Services, Family Planning, Health Organizations, Health-General, Hospices, Hospitals, People with Disabilities, Single-Disease Health Associations, Substance Abuse. **Geo. Dist:** headquarters and operating communities.

**★ 902 ★ The Bridgestone/Firestone Trust Fund**
50 Century Boulevard
Nashville, TN 37214
**Phone:** (615)872-1415 **Fax:** (615)872-1414
**Email:** bfstrustfund@bfsusa.com
Bernice Csaszar, Administrator

**Fnded:** 1952. **Priorities:** *Arts & Humanities:* 13%. Primarily gives to arts councils and institutions. *Civic & Public Affairs:* 27%. Supports community and neighborhood improvement, environment and energy conservation, law and justice, housing and urban revitalization, civil rights and equal opportunity, voter registration and education, and job training. *Education:* 23%. Priorities include colleges, universities, and youth development programs. Contributions support programs that assure availability of trained persons, encourage research in areas relevant to the corporation, and promote excellence. Other interests include education-related organizations that expand public knowledge of the free enterprise system; public and private higher education; adult education programs; fellowships; and scholarships. Also sponsors employee matching gifts program. *Environment:* 29%. Supports the United Way, youth organizations, human welfare programs, and community groups. *International:* 5%. Contributes to organizations that provide adequate healthcare for employees and their communities, and that promote the development of new approaches to health needs. *Note:* Total foundation contributions made in 2000. **Typ. Recipients:** Children's Health/Hospitals, Emergency/Ambulance Services, Family Planning, Health Organizations, Hospices, Hospitals, Medical Education, Medical Research, Nursing Services, People with Disabilities, Single-Disease Health Associations, Substance Abuse. **Geo. Dist:** headquarters and operating communities.

**★ 903 ★ Briggs & Stratton Corp. Foundation**
12301 West Wirth St.
Wauwatosa, WI 53222
**Phone:** (414)259-5333 **Fax:** (414)259-5773
Kasandra Preston, Secretary & Treasurer

**Priorities:** *Arts & Humanities:* 17%. Supports the United Performing Arts Fund, museums, theater, and music. *Civic & Public Affairs:* 18%. Supports community and economic development projects in Milwaukee, festivals and parks, public policy, business and free enterprise, and industry concerns. *Education:* 17%. Support includes funding for scholarships to employees' children. Other interests include colleges and universities, schools in communities where the company has plants, precollege programs, and agricultural education. *Environment:* 38%. Majority of support goes to the United Way; also funds human services for families and youth. *International:* 6%. Supports children's health organizations. *Religion:* 1%. *Note:* Total foundation contributions made in fiscal 2000. **Typ. Recipients:** Children's Health/Hospitals, Health Funds, Health Organizations, Health-General, Heart, Long-Term Care, Medical Education, Nursing Services, Speech & Hearing, Substance Abuse, Trauma Treatment. **Geo. Dist:** principally near operating locations and to national organizations; Milwaukee, WI.

**★ 904 ★ Bristol-Myers Squibb Foundation Inc.**
345 Park Ave.
New York, NY 10154
**Website:** http://www.bms.com/aboutbms/founda/data/founda.html
John Damonti, Contact

**Fnded:** 1990. **Priorities:** *Arts & Humanities:* 3%. Provides support on very selective basis to prominent cultural institutions. Emphasis is on nationally recognized performing arts centers and major natural history, science, and art museums. Also considers organizations with broad appeal in operating communities. *Civic & Public Affairs:* 5%. Seeks to support organizations that help strengthen economic and community development and provide equal opportunity and job training for socially disadvantaged groups, as well as to improve operation of our system of law and justice. Also supports united funds and public policy research that advances understanding of the free enterprise system. Other interests include youth, the aged, and the disabled. *Education:* 35%. Directs support toward: advancement of higher education; math and science education; independent state and regional associations; graduate schools of business with which company coordinates recruitment programs; programs widening opportunities for minorities and women; schools with programs of special interest to company and divisions; and selected national programs to advance and improve quality of education and broaden educational opportunities. Also emphasizes support for secondary education, particularly programs that focus on math, science, and health education, and the shortage of qualified teachers in these subjects. *Environment:* 19%. Funds United Way and youth organizations. *International:* 22%. Select grants to support unrestricted medical research at leading national and international institutions. Since 1977, company has committed funding through its unrestricted grant programs to support research in cancer, nutrition, orthopedics, cardiovascular medicine and related metabolic diseases, infectious diseases, and neuroscience. Has established a Women's Health Education Initiative. Funding also goes to research into alternatives to the use of animals in testing. Other health interests include hospitals, and organizations working to solve administrative, economic, and public policy problems in health care in areas of company operations. No grants are made available for individual research projects. *Religion:* 1%. *Note:* Total foundation giving in 1999. **Typ. Recipients:** AIDS/HIV, Cancer, Children's Health/Hospitals, Clinics/Medical Centers, Diabetes, Emergency/Ambulance Services, Geriatric Health, Health Organizations, Health-General, Heart, Hospitals, Medical Education, Medical Rehabilitation, Medical Research, Medical Training, Mental Health, Nutrition, People with Disabilities, Public

Health, Research/Studies Institutes, Substance Abuse, Transplant Networks/Donor Banks. **Geo. Dist:** headquarters and operating communities; internationally; nationally.

### ★ 905 ★ Browning-Ferris Industries Inc.
757 N Eldridge
Houston, TX 77079
**Phone:** (713)671-1507          **Fax:** (281)870-7182
**Email:** argentina.james@bfi.com
Maryann McGuire, Director Corporate Affairs
**Typ. Recipients:** Health Funds, Health Organizations, Hospices, Single-Disease Health Associations. **Geo. Dist:** headquarters and operating communities.

### ★ 906 ★ Brunswick Foundation
One North Field Court
Lake Forest, IL 60045
**Phone:** (847)735-4667
Carol Stame, President
**Priorities:** *Arts & Humanities:* 1%. Support given to cultural arts and music. *Civic & Public Affairs:* Less than 1%. *Education:* 92%. Majority of funding supports scholarships to children of company employees. Also provides grants to colleges and universities. *Environment:* 4%. Supports youth and child services, volunteer programs, and recreation and scouting. *International:* 3%. Supports American Red Cross Disaster Relief Fund, hospitals, and health care organizations. *Note:* Total foundation contributions made in 2000. **Typ. Recipients:** Cancer, Children's Health/Hospitals, Clinics/Medical Centers, Diabetes, Emergency/Ambulance Services, Family Planning, Health Organizations, Heart, Hospices, Hospitals, Mental Health, Nursing Services, People with Disabilities, Prenatal Health Issues, Single-Disease Health Associations, Substance Abuse. **Geo. Dist:** principally near operating locations and to national organizations.

### ★ 907 ★ Bucyrus-Erie Foundation
1020 Broadway
Milwaukee, WI 53202
**Phone:** (414)272-5805          **Fax:** (414)272-6235
**Email:** milwfdn@execpc.com
Mr. Sigfredo Gutieriez, Administrator, Program Officer
**Priorities:** *Arts & Humanities:* 29%. Funds museums, performing arts, public broadcasting, and libraries. *Civic & Public Affairs:* 9%. Supports public policy, environmental affairs, business/free enterprise, and urban and community affairs. *Education:* 11%. Emphasis on higher education institutions. Interests include technical and engineering education at the university level. Also supports scholarships, education funds, arts education, student aid, literacy programs, and public and private precollege education. *Environment:* 48%. Majority of funding supports united funds, youth programs, and community service organizations in Milwaukee County. Other interests include the handicapped, the prevention of domestic violence, homes, employment programs, and family service organizations. *International:* 2%. Focus on hospitals, pediatric health, and single-disease associations. *Note:* Total foundation contributions made in 2000. **Typ. Recipients:** Children's Health/Hospitals, Clinics/Medical Centers, Domestic Violence, Health Organizations, Hospitals, Medical Education, Medical Rehabilitation, Medical Research, People with Disabilities, Single-Disease Health Associations, Substance Abuse. **Geo. Dist:** WI, Milwaukee County; Milwaukee, WI, South Milwaukee.

### Burlington Resources Foundation
*See:* Entry 11424

### ★ 908 ★ Business Men's Assurance Co. of America
BMA Tower, PO Box 419458
Kansas City, MO 64141
**Phone:** (816)751-5742          **Fax:** (816)751-5710
**Website:** http://www.bma.com
Simonetta Balzer, Chair for Community Giving

**Typ. Recipients:** Health-General. **Geo. Dist:** headquarters; Kansas City, MO, metropolitan area.

### ★ 909 ★ Butler Manufacturing Co. Foundation
PO Box 419917, BMA Tower
Kansas City, MO 64141-0917
**Phone:** (816)968-3208          **Fax:** (816)968-3211
**Email:** blfay@butlermfg.org
Barbara Fay, Foundation Administrator
**Priorities:** *Arts & Humanities:* About 15%. Primarily supports major art groups that broaden the cultural experience where Butler has a presence. Recipients include museums, theater, arts associations, symphonies, and ballet. Some interest in minority groups and cultural opportunities for the economically disadvantaged. Foundation also operates an employee matching gift program for arts interests. *Civic & Public Affairs:* 55% to 60%. Foundation makes contributions to communities where company has employees and significant capital investment. Supports the United Way. Also supports minority assistance, youth programs, special-interest hospitals and health care programs, and neighborhoods and non-residential building. *Education:* 20% to 25%. Majority of funding supports scholarship programs operated by the foundation. Awards are given to children of Butler employees attending four-year accredited colleges. Also provides matching gifts to colleges and universities. Institutions receiving grants must provide opportunities for continuing education to Butler employees, or have programs that provide education to residents of the city where a Butler plant operates. Foundation also gives assistance to minority education and marketable career skills for youth. **Typ. Recipients:** Cancer, Children's Health/Hospitals, Clinics/Medical Centers, Emergency/Ambulance Services, Health Organizations, Health Policy/Cost Containment, Hospitals, Medical Education, Medical Rehabilitation. **Geo. Dist:** Kansas City, MO.

### ★ 910 ★ C.R. Bard Foundation
730 Central Ave.
Murray Hill, NJ 07974
**Phone:** (908)277-8182          **Fax:** (908)277-8098
**Email:** linda.hrevnack@crbard.com
**Website:** http://www.crbard.com/about/foundation.html
Ms. Linda Hrevnack, Manager, Community Affairs & Contributio
**Fnded:** 1988. **Priorities:** *Arts & Humanities:* (Culture & Art) 4%. Funds theater and children's arts groups. *Civic & Public Affairs:* Less than 1%. Supports the Washington Legal Foundation. *Education:* 19%. Supports colleges, universities, and independent college funds. Focus on medical education and research, and programs which benefit the health-care industry. *International:* (Health & Welfare) 58%. Majority of health funding supports health-related united funds. Supports programs specializing in cardiology, urology, and oncology. Other interests include health-care associations, hospitals, and emergency services. Welfare organizations receiving support include children's groups, camps, and clubs; food banks; and other community and social services. *Note:* Total contributions made in 1999. **Typ. Recipients:** AIDS/HIV, Cancer, Children's Health/Hospitals, Clinics/Medical Centers, Clinics/Medical Centers, Diabetes, Domestic Violence, Emergency/Ambulance Services, Geriatric Health, Health Funds, Health Organizations, Health-General, Heart, Hospices, Hospitals, Hospitals (University Affiliated), Kidney, Medical Education, Medical Rehabilitation, Medical Research, People with Disabilities, Preventive Medicine/Wellness Organizations, Public Health, Single-Disease Health Associations, Speech & Hearing, Substance Abuse. **Geo. Dist:** headquarters and operating communities.

### ★ 911 ★ Cabot Corp. Foundation
Two Seaport Ln., Ste. 1300
Boston, MA 02210
**Phone:** (617)342-6004          **Fax:** (617)342-6312
**Email:** dorothy_forbes@cabot-corp.com
Dorothy Forbes, Executive Director, Vice President

**Priorities:** *Arts & Humanities:* 4%. Supports museums that promote science education and community arts organizations, including visual and performing arts groups in company operating communities. *Civic & Public Affairs:* 10%. Includes civic, health and welfare concerns. Priority is given to community projects involving company employees and retirees. Typical recipients include youth organizations, urban and community affairs groups, safety organizations, the handicapped, and hospitals. *Education:* 28%. Supports higher educational science and technology programs, placing priority on mathematics, physics, chemistry, and special disciplines, including ceramics, materials and polymer sciences, and chemical and metallurgical engineering. Special interest is in schools that encourage research by students and junior faculty. Also supports secondary school science and mathematics education, particularly programs focused on gifted students. Other interests include colleges and universities in company operating communities; skills development and occupational retraining, especially for minorities, women, and the handicapped; and, to a lesser degree, applied economics programs at all levels of education. Also supports educational public broadcasting and Junior Achievement. *Environment:* 23%. Supports child and youth services, and the United Way. *International:* 2%. Supports hospitals, medical centers and single-disease concerns. *Religion:* 11%. Supports American Association for the Advancement of Science; Massachusetts State Science Fair. *Note:* Total contributions in 1999. **Typ. Recipients:** Cancer, Clinics/Medical Centers, Diabetes, Domestic Violence, Health Organizations, Health-General, Heart, Hospitals, People with Disabilities, Prenatal Health Issues, Substance Abuse. **Geo. Dist:** principally near operating locations and to national organizations.

### ★ 912 ★ California Bank & Trust
Community Development Department
11622 El Camino Real, Ste. 200
San Diego, CA 92130
**Phone:** (858)793-7470          **Fax:** (858)793-7438
Lynda Buckner, Vice President and Manager
**Priorities:** *Voluntarism:* Employees are encouraged to become involved in their communities through participation in local civic and government groups and whose primary focus is to improve economic development in the community. **Typ. Recipients:** Health Organizations, People with Disabilities. **Geo. Dist:** headquarters area only; CA, Southern and Northern regions.

### ★ 913 ★ Callaway Golf Co. Foundation
2180 Rutherford Rd.
Carlsbad, CA 92008
**Phone:** (760)930-8686          **Fax:** (760)929-9780
**Website:** http://www.callawaygolf.com
Karen Smelkinson, Executive Director
**Fnded:** 1994. **Priorities:** *Arts & Humanities:* 3%. Supports a museum. *Civic & Public Affairs:* 7%. Supports entrepreneurship and technical training. *Education:* 16%. Funds literacy, scholarships, technical schools, and mentoring programs. *Environment:* 44%. Major support for at-risk youth. Also funds family violence prevention and services, counseling, shelters, and programs for the disabled. *International:* 27%. Supports dental care, clinics, hospitals, and hospice, with a focus on children's health. *Voluntarism:* Committee supports the Callaway Golf Community Program, which organizes one community services project per month for employee volunteers. *Note:* Total foundation contributions made in 2000. **Typ. Recipients:** Alzheimers Disease, Cancer, Child Abuse, Children's Health/Hospitals, Domestic Violence, Eyes/Blindness, Health-General, Hospices, Medical Rehabilitation, Medical Research, People with Disabilities, Prenatal Health Issues. **Geo. Dist:** CA, San Diego County.

### ★ 914 ★ Calvin Klein Foundation
205 West 39th St.
New York, NY 10018

**Phone:** (212)719-2600 **Fax:** (212)292-9787
Joel Semel, Foundation Manager

**Priorities:** *Arts & Humanities:* 15%. Supports art museums, performing arts, photography, and art associations. *Civic & Public Affairs:* 15%. Funds women's and minority affairs, fashion trade organizations and awards, and legal defense funds. *Education:* 7%. Gives to colleges and universities, and institutions providing fashion design education. *Environment:* 23%. Funds youth organizations, food/clothing distribution, substance abuse treatment, and recreational and athletic associations. *International:* 36%. Supports medical centers, children's health, and single-disease health associations with a focus on cancer and AIDS research and treatment. *Note:* Total contributions made in fiscal 1999. **Typ. Recipients:** AIDS/HIV, Alzheimers Disease, Cancer, Children's Health/Hospitals, Clinics/Medical Centers, Diabetes, Health Organizations, Hospitals, Medical Research, Mental Health, Multiple Sclerosis, People with Disabilities, People with Disabilities, Prenatal Health Issues, Single-Disease Health Associations, Substance Abuse.

**★ 915 ★ Campbell Soup Foundation**
Campbell Place
Camden, NJ 08103-1799
**Phone:** (856)342-4800
J. Buckley, Chairman

**Priorities:** *Arts & Humanities:* 5%. Supports arts centers and performing arts in Camden and plant communities. *Civic & Public Affairs:* 34%. Supports family centers, trade associations, housing, economic development, and minority affairs. *Education:* 5%. Emphasis on Camden area public education. Also supports colleges and universities that specialize in medical, engineering, and business education. *Environment:* 50%. Grants support Camden youth organizations and the United Way. Also funds family services, recreation, and people and disabilities. *International:* 2%. Funds medical research, pediatric health care, and eye care center *Voluntarism:* Foundation operates a Dollars for Doers fund to support and reward company employees who volunteer in their communities; also supports a program in which employees tutor disadvantaged youth. Giving to the United Way is determined by employee involvement. *Note:* Total contributions made in fiscal 1999. **Typ. Recipients:** Cancer, Children's Health/Hospitals, Clinics/Medical Centers, Diabetes, Emergency/Ambulance Services, Eyes/Blindness, Health-General, Heart, Hospitals, Kidney, Medical Education, Medical Research, Nutrition, Single-Disease Health Associations. **Geo. Dist:** headquarters and operating communities.

**★ 916 ★ Cargill Foundation**
PO Box 5626
Minneapolis, MN 55440-5650
**Phone:** (952)742-6213
**Website:** http://www.cargill.com/commun/found.htm
James Hield, Executive Director

**Priorities:** *Arts & Humanities:* 9%. *Civic & Public Affairs:* 11%. *Education:* 42%. Funds higher education and Junior Achievement. *Environment:* 32%. Supports United Way and family and youth services. *International:* 4%. *Note:* Total foundation contributions in 1999. **Typ. Recipients:** AIDS/HIV, Cancer, Children's Health/Hospitals, Clinics/Medical Centers, Domestic Violence, Emergency/Ambulance Services, Eyes/Blindness, Family Planning, Health Organizations, Hospitals, Medical Education, People with Disabilities, Substance Abuse. **Geo. Dist:** headquarters and operating locations; internationally; nationally; Minneapolis, MN, including western and northern suburbs.

**★ 917 ★ Caring Foundation**
c/o Blue Cross and Blue Shield of Alabama
450 Riverchase Pkwy. East
Birmingham, AL 35244
**Phone:** (205)220-2100
**Email:** tkellogg@bcbsal.org
Mr. Terry Kellogg, Vice President

**Priorities:** *Arts & Humanities:* 9%. Emphasis on the symphony, ballet, and opera. *Civic & Public Affairs:* 11%. Supports community foundations, Rotary Clubs, and a poison control center. *Education:* 14%. Provides major support to the University of Alabama. Also funds other institutions of higher education, Junior Achievement, education foundations, and public pre-college schools. *Environment:* 45%. Supports youth agencies, child welfare, and the United Way. *International:* 21%. Primarily supports single-disease health organizations. *Note:* Total contributions in 2000. **Typ. Recipients:** AIDS/HIV, Alzheimers Disease, Arthritis, Cancer, Children's Health/Hospitals, Domestic Violence, Emergency/Ambulance Services, Eyes/Blindness, Health Organizations, Health-General, Heart, Hospitals, Kidney, Medical Research, Multiple Sclerosis, People with Disabilities, Prenatal Health Issues, Public Health, Respiratory, Single-Disease Health Associations, Speech & Hearing, Substance Abuse, Trauma Treatment. **Geo. Dist:** AL.

**★ 918 ★ Carrier Corp.**
PO Box 4808
Syracuse, NY 13221
**Phone:** (315)432-6000 **Fax:** (315)432-7898
**Website:** http://www.utc.com/commun
Dan Fessenden, Director, Community Relations

**Priorities:** *Arts & Humanities:* 13%. Interests include performing arts groups, museums, arts education, dance, opera, historical societies, arts centers, orchestras, libraries, theater, and public broadcasting. *Civic & Public Affairs:* 13%. Support goes to community and public policy groups. *Education:* 33%. Supports various colleges and universities, professional and technical schools, and non-public secondary schools that include at least grades 9-12. *Environment:* 24%. Supports united funds, health organizations, rehabilitation, and programs for the mentally retarded. Emphasis is also on geriatric care and programs for the disabled. Some support is provided for youth groups and community service organizations. *Note:* Total contributions made in 2000. **Typ. Recipients:** Health Organizations, Hospitals, Medical Rehabilitation, Mental Health, People with Disabilities. **Geo. Dist:** principally near operating locations and to national organizations.

**★ 919 ★ Carris Corp. Foundation**
PO Box 696
Rutland, VT 05702-0696
**Phone:** (802)773-9111
Karen O'Brien, Foundation Bookkeeper

**Fnded:** 1990. **Priorities:** *Arts & Humanities:* 32%. Supports performing arts centers, fine arts studios and museums, historical societies, libraries, and arts councils. *Civic & Public Affairs:* 13%. Funds housing initiatives, community festivals, civil rights organizations, and the Civil Air Patrol. *Education:* 31%. Supports academies, colleges, and youth education programs for specific areas of study, including environmental, business, and civics education. *Environment:* 14%. Supports Meals on Wheels, United Way agencies, criminal rehabilitation, family social services, youth groups, recreational and sporting events for the mentally and physically disabled, and violence prevention. *International:* 5%. Funds mental health services, pediatric hospitals, diabetes organizations, and research and services for the blind. *Religion:* 1%. Funds the Salk Institute for Biological Studies and the Vermont Institute of Natural Science. *Note:* Total contributions made in 2000. **Typ. Recipients:** AIDS/HIV, Cancer, Child Abuse, Children's Health/Hospitals, Diabetes, Emergency/Ambulance Services, Health Organizations, Health-General, Hospitals, Nursing Services, People with Disabilities, Prenatal Health Issues, Public Health, Single-Disease Health Associations, Substance Abuse. **Geo. Dist:** headquarters and operating communities.

**★ 920 ★ Carter-Wallace Foundation**
1345 Ave. of the Americas
New York, NY 10105-0302
**Phone:** (212)339-5010 **Fax:** (212)339-5100

**Priorities:** *Arts & Humanities:* 14%. Grants benefit a wide variety of recipient types. Interests include opera and other music-oriented organizations, performing arts centers, libraries, and museums. *Civic & Public Affairs:* 2%. Funds zoos, botanical gardens, and professional associations. *Education:* 24%. Supports colleges and universities in northeastern United States. Medical and dental education are among the highest priorities. Grants are also made to education funds, scholarship funds, and Junior Achievement. *Environment:* 11%. Funds anti-substance abuse organizations, United Way, and youth organizations. *International:* 44%. Priority is given to hospitals, medical centers, and single-disease health associations. *Religion:* 1%. Supports science museums. *Note:* Total contributions made in fiscal 1999. **Typ. Recipients:** Arthritis, Cancer, Clinics/Medical Centers, Eyes/Blindness, Family Planning, Health Organizations, Hospitals, Hospitals (University Affiliated), Medical Education, Medical Research, Medical Research, Mental Health, People with Disabilities, Public Health, Single-Disease Health Associations, Speech & Hearing, Substance Abuse. **Geo. Dist:** CT; Decatur, IL; NJ; NY.

**★ 921 ★ Caterpillar Foundation**
100 NE Adams St.
Peoria, IL 61629-1480
**Phone:** (309)675-4418 **Fax:** (309)675-5815
**Website:** http://www.cat.com/about_cat/social_responsibility/05_ca ring_for_our_communities/images/foundationar.pdf
Henry Holling, Vice President

**Fnded:** 1952. **Priorities:** *Arts & Humanities:* 7%. Provides capital and operating grants. Recipients include music groups, public broadcasting, arts centers, and theaters. Also sponsors matching gifts program, which accounts for the largest share of cultural giving. *Civic & Public Affairs:* 7%. Supports community and economic development programs, environmental organizations, criminal justice, and race relations. The majority of funding in this area is awarded directly by the company and primarily goes to public policy issues and urban affairs. *Education:* 59%. Supports colleges and universities, business, economic, and engineering education; student aid; universities and colleges; and education funds. *International:* 18%. United Ways in plant communities receive the majority of funding. Also makes capital grants to local health institutions and human service agencies, including youth organizations, homes, and programs for drug and alcohol abuse prevention. *Note:* Total contributions made in 2000. **Typ. Recipients:** Cancer, Emergency/Ambulance Services, Health Organizations, Hospices, Hospitals, Medical Education, Medical Rehabilitation, Mental Health, People with Disabilities, Sexual Abuse, Single-Disease Health Associations, Substance Abuse. **Geo. Dist:** operating locations; educational matching gifts program is international.

**★ 922 ★ CBS Foundation**
51 West 52nd St.
New York, NY 10019
**Phone:** (212)975-3773
Helene Blieberg, Vice President

**Priorities:** *Arts & Humanities:* 40%. Supports public broadcasting, theaters and performing arts centers, film, art museums, film/broadcasting museums, and libraries. *Civic & Public Affairs:* 11%. Funds broadcasting and entertainment industry professional organizations, community organizations, minority affairs, and public policy groups. *Education:* 45%. Provides major support for the United Negro College Fund. Also funds colleges and universities, foundations promoting higher education, and broadcasting education. *Environment:* 2%. Primarily supports United Way agencies in operating locations. Some funding also supports other social service organizations. *Religion:* 1%. The California Science Center receives support. *Note:* Total contributions made in 1999. **Typ. Recipients:** People with Disabilities. **Geo. Dist:** markets where CBS has major ownership presence.

## ★ 923 ★ CCB Foundation

PO Box 931
Durham, NC 27702-0931
**Phone:** (919)683-7251　　　**Fax:** (919)682-3870
John Ramsey, President

**Fnded:** 1985. **Typ. Recipients:** Cancer, Emergency/Ambulance Services, Health Organizations, Health-General, Hospitals. **Geo. Dist:** headquarters area only.

## ★ 924 ★ Centex Corp.

PO Box 199000
Dallas, TX 75219
**Phone:** (214)981-5000　　　**Fax:** (214)981-6859
**Website:** http://www.centex.com
Amy Nation, Secretary to the Chairman & Chief Execut

**Priorities:** *Arts & Humanities:* 15%. *Civic & Public Affairs:* 59%. The Company supports Habitat for Humanity and Hearts and Hammers. *Education:* 12%. *International:* 14%. **Typ. Recipients:** Health-General. **Geo. Dist:** Dallas, TX, including metropolitan area.

## ★ 925 ★ Central Maine Power Co.

83 Edison Dr.
Augusta, ME 04336
**Phone:** (207)623-3521　　　**Fax:** (207)623-5908
**Website:** http://www.cmpco.com
John H. Carroll, Community Relations Specialist

**Priorities:** *Civic & Public Affairs:* (United Funds & United Way) About 30%. Company favors contributions to organizations such as United Ways which channel assistance to agencies active in service area. Employee involvement, number of customers served, population density, plus the number of organizations, communities, and services provided by each United Way will determine amount of support. 5% to 10%. General support to groups improving the quality of life in areas where employees work and live. *Education:* About 15%. Supports colleges, universities, and technical schools in Maine on a case-by-case basis. Also supports educational programs outside Maine offering programs of interest to company, such as: energy seminars; secondary schools, including public and private institutions for special programs; economic education; and a limited scholarship program. *Environment:* Less than 5%. Supports youth organizations and activities that guide, counsel, and enrich the lives of young people. Recipients include 4-H, community centers, scouting, Junior Achievement, summer camps, camps for disabled children, child welfare, and children's homes. *International:* About 20%. Supports capital campaigns conducted by hospitals and health care centers in service area for new facilities, expansion or renovation, or specialized equipment. Also supports annual operating gifts, single-disease health associations, and health organizations active in service area. *Note:* Company reports that 15% of its contributions budget is given at the discretion of its local divisions. **Typ. Recipients:** Domestic Violence, Emergency/Ambulance Services, Family Planning, Geriatric Health, Health Organizations, Health-General, Hospices, Hospitals, Medical Rehabilitation, Mental Health, Nutrition, People with Disabilities, Public Health, Single-Disease Health Associations, Substance Abuse. **Geo. Dist:** ME, primarily central and southern Maine.

## ★ 926 ★ Central National-Gottesman Foundation

3 Manhattanville Rd.
Purchase, NY 10577
**Phone:** (914)696-9153　　　**Fax:** (914)696-1066
Joshua Eisentein, Treasurer

**Fnded:** 1981. **Priorities:** *Arts & Humanities:* 10%. Supports museums, libraries, and arts societies. *Civic & Public Affairs:* 4%. Funds housing, clubs, and safety. *Education:* 31%. Majority of funding supports scholarships for employees' children; also funds special programs at universities. *Environment:* 30%. Funds child welfare organizations and services for the disadvantaged. *International:* 3%. *Note:* Total foundation contributions made in 2000. **Typ. Recipients:** Cancer, Children's Health/Hospitals, Diabetes, Health Funds, Heart, Hospices, Hospitals, Medical Education, Mental Health, Multiple Sclerosis, People with Disabilities, Research/Studies Institutes, Single-Disease Health Associations, Substance Abuse. **Geo. Dist:** NY.

## ★ 927 ★ Central & South West Foundation

PO Box 660164
Dallas, TX 75266-0164
**Phone:** (214)777-1115　　　**Fax:** (214)777-3067
Kenneth Raney, Vice President, Associate General Counse

**Priorities:** *Arts & Humanities:* 38%. Primarily supports museums. *Civic & Public Affairs:* 1%. Support includes community foundations, public policy and youth organizations. *Education:* 42%. Funds numerous colleges and universities. Majority of support is donated through matching gifts. *Environment:* 17%. Supports youth groups and child welfare organizations. *International:* 2%. Funds medical research. *Note:* Total contributions made in fiscal 1999. **Typ. Recipients:** Clinics/Medical Centers, Emergency/Ambulance Services, Health Organizations, Health-General, Medical Education, Medical Research, Nursing Services, Public Health, Substance Abuse. **Geo. Dist:** nationally.

## ★ 928 ★ CertainTeed Corp. Foundation

PO Box 860
Valley Forge, PA 19482-0101
**Phone:** (610)341-7000　　　**Fax:** (610)341-7777
Dorothy Wackerman, Vice President

**Fnded:** 1955. **Priorities:** *Arts & Humanities:* 40%. Funds museums, historical societies, public broadcasting, and the performing arts. *Civic & Public Affairs:* 8%. Supports community centers, economic development, clubs, urban affairs and community services. *Education:* 21%. Supports schools, colleges and universities. *Environment:* 11%. Funds United Way, youth organizations, and social services. *International:* 9%. Funding supports health organizations, hospitals, pediatric healthcare, and single-disease associations. *Note:* Approximately 42% of total contributions are for matching gifts. Total foundation contributions made in 2000. **Typ. Recipients:** Alzheimers Disease, Cancer, Child Abuse, Children's Health/Hospitals, Clinics/Medical Centers, Domestic Violence, Emergency/Ambulance Services, Health Organizations, Heart, Hospices, Hospitals, Medical Education, Medical Research, Multiple Sclerosis, People with Disabilities, Prenatal Health Issues, Public Health, Single-Disease Health Associations, Substance Abuse. **Geo. Dist:** principally near operating locations and to national organizations.

## ★ 929 ★ Cessna Foundation, Inc.

PO Box 7706
Wichita, KS 67277-7706
**Phone:** (316)517-7810　　　**Fax:** (316)517-7812
Marilyn Richwine, Secretary & Treasurer

**Fnded:** 1952. **Priorities:** *Arts & Humanities:* 9%. Supports arts associations, museums, history, music, and theater. *Education:* 49%. Funding supports colleges and universities, primarily in Kansas. Other interests include vocational, economic, and medical education. Administers employee matching gifts program to education, and administers Del Roskam Scholarship program for children or grandchildren of Cessna employees. *Environment:* 39%. Funding supports united funds and youth organizations. Other interests include athletic programs, people with disabilities, emergency relief, and food and clothing distribution. *International:* 3%. Funding supports health, including mental health and single disease health associations. *Note:* Total foundation contributions made in 2000. **Typ. Recipients:** AIDS/HIV, Cancer, Children's Health/Hospitals, Clinics/Medical Centers, Emergency/Ambulance Services, Emergency/Ambulance Services, Health Funds, Health Organizations, Heart, Hospices, Hospitals, Medical Education, Multiple Sclerosis, People with Disabilities, Preventive Medicine/Wellness Organizations, Single-Disease Health Associations, Substance Abuse. **Geo. Dist:** principally near operating locations and to national organizations; Wichita, KS, including surrounding area.

## ★ 930 ★ The Charitable Foundation of Frost National Bank

PO Box 1600
San Antonio, TX 78296
**Phone:** (210)220-4353　　　**Fax:** (210)220-5144
Melissa Adams, Assistant Vice President, Corporate Dona

**Fnded:** 1981. **Typ. Recipients:** Domestic Violence, Hospices, Hospitals, Medical Education, Medical Rehabilitation, Medical Research, Mental Health, People with Disabilities, Public Health, Single-Disease Health Associations, Substance Abuse. **Geo. Dist:** TX.

## ★ 931 ★ Charles Schwab Corp. Foundation

101 Montgomery St., 28th Floor
San Francisco, CA 94104
**Phone:** 877-408-5438
**Email:** corporation.foundation@schwab.com
**Website:** http://www.schwabfoundation.org
Amanda Flores-White, Manager, Community Investor Services

**Priorities:** *Arts & Humanities:* 14%. Emphasis on educational and community-based programs. *Civic & Public Affairs:* 2%. Supports nonprofit organizations and public concerns. *Education:* 14%. Contributions support K-12 education especially school-to-career programs and literacy. *Environment:* 68%.Supports Health and Human Services. Recipients include HIV/AIDS programs, children and youth programs, women and minority programs, and community service organizations such as Meals on Wheels, Big Brothers and Big Sisters, retarded children association, and food banks. *Note:* Total foundation contributions made in fiscal 1999. **Typ. Recipients:** AIDS/HIV, Cancer, Children's Health/Hospitals, Clinics/Medical Centers, Diabetes, Domestic Violence, Emergency/Ambulance Services, Family Planning, Health Organizations, Home-Care Services, Hospices, Kidney, Medical Research, Multiple Sclerosis, Nursing Services, People with Disabilities, Prenatal Health Issues, Single-Disease Health Associations, Transplant Networks/Donor Banks. **Geo. Dist:** communities where there are Schwab branch offices; San Francisco, CA.

## ★ 932 ★ Charter Manufacturing Co. Foundation

411 East Wisconsin Ave., Ste. 2040
Milwaukee, WI 53202-4497
**Phone:** (414)277-5000
Linda Mellowes, President

**Priorities:** *Arts & Humanities:* 3%. Funds performing arts, art museums, and public broadcasting. *Civic & Public Affairs:* 10%. Funds community and neighborhood development, community foundations, and botanical gardens. *Education:* 27%. Supports higher education, Junior Achievement, and medical and engineering education. *Environment:* 55%. Support for United Way, YMCA/YWCA, animal welfare, and family planning. *International:* 5%. Funds hospitals and health foundations. *Note:* Total contributions in 2000. **Typ. Recipients:** Cancer, Children's Health/Hospitals, Domestic Violence, Family Planning, Health Organizations, Hospitals, Medical Education, Medical Research, People with Disabilities, Single-Disease Health Associations, Transplant Networks/Donor Banks. **Geo. Dist:** WI, WI.

## ★ 933 ★ Chemed Foundation

255 East 5th St., 2600 Chemed Center
Cincinnati, OH 45202
**Phone:** (513)762-6912
Sandra Laney, President & Director

**Fnded:** 1993. **Priorities:** *Arts & Humanities:* 8%. Supports arts funds, museums, music, and theater. *Civic & Public Affairs:* 15%. Funds housing, land use, and justice issues. *Education:* 41%. Supports colleges, universities, schools, and Junior Achievement. *Environment:* 15%. Funds scouting and youth organizations, services for the disabled, and the United Way. *International:* 21%. Supports hospitals and cancer research. *Voluntarism:* Company employees help rehabilitate homes for community housing projects. *Note:* Total foundation contributions made in 2000. **Typ. Recipients:** Cancer, Children's Health/Hospitals, Emergency/Ambulance Services, Eyes/Blindness, Health-General, Medical Education, People with Disabilities, Single-Disease Health Associations, Speech & Hearing. **Geo. Dist:** headquarters and operating communities.

## ★ 934 ★ Chesapeake Corp. Foundation

PO Box 2350
Richmond, VA 23218
**Phone:** (804)697-1132        **Fax:** (804)697-1199
Louis Matherne, Secretary & Treasurer

**Priorities:** *Arts & Humanities:* 3%. Funding emphasizes libraries and museums; also supports arts councils and performing arts. *Civic & Public Affairs:* 9%. Supports municipal initiatives, housing coalitions, fire departments and emergency squads, and other community services. *Education:* 68%. Funds elementary and secondary schools; educational associations; and higher education through scholarships for children of employees, an employee matching gifts program for education; and direct grants to colleges and universities. *Environment:* 5%. Supports Boy Scouts, domestic abuse services, and youth organizations. *International:* 7%. Supports hospitals and medical centers, therapeutic riding, and single-disease associations. *Religion:* 6%. Funds a planetarium and a science museum. *Note:* Total contributions in 1999. **Typ. Recipients:** Cancer, Children's Health/Hospitals, Clinics/Medical Centers, Diabetes, Domestic Violence, Emergency/Ambulance Services, Health Organizations, Hospitals, Medical Rehabilitation, Mental Health, People with Disabilities, Research/Studies Institutes. **Geo. Dist:** operating locations.

## ★ 935 ★ ChevronTexaco Corp.

575 Market St.
San Francisco, CA 94105
**Phone:** (415)894-7700        **Fax:** (415)894-3583
**Website:** http://www.chevronTEXACO.com/social_responsibility/grant_guidelines
Skip Rhodes, Jr., Manager, Corporate Contributions

**Fnded:** 2001. **Priorities:** *Arts & Humanities:* 8%. Supports visual, literary, performing arts and cultural institutions in communities where company has significant operations, principally in California. Also supports local arts funds and councils, community concerts, historic preservation, libraries, national and regional art associations, cultural centers, and theaters. *Civic & Public Affairs:* 12%. Contributes to policy research and planning organizations and business/free enterprise groups; organizations that deal with individual initiatives, volunteerism, and philanthropy; and groups that promote community involvement and civic pride, law and justice, better government, and public safety. Other interests include urban planning and development programs and agricultural expositions and fairs. *Education:* 34%. Colleges and universities in fields of science, engineering, computer science, business, economics, communications, human resource development, equal access and quality in schools, and other disciplines of interest to the company. Funds are for scholarships, fellowships, department support, and research. Also supports a variety of educational organizations and funds. While most contributions continue to go to higher education, support for targeted programs that improve the quality of public education at the primary and secondary levels is increasing. Provides support for disadvantaged and under-represented minority students requiring accelerated instruction in grades K-12. Also matches gifts to education. *International:* 23%. Health funding emphasizes hospitals and various local health organizations. Human services includes youth organizations; united funds; social welfare organizations that meet the needs of the homeless and abused and neglected children; groups that promote equal opportunity, equity,and access to the mainstream of society; job-readiness and employ-

ment programs; and programs targeted to the elderly. *Note:* Total giving in 1998. **Typ. Recipients:** AIDS/HIV, Clinics/Medical Centers, Domestic Violence, Emergency/Ambulance Services, Health Funds, Health Organizations, Health Policy/Cost Containment, Hospices, Hospitals, Medical Rehabilitation, Mental Health, People with Disabilities, Public Health, Single-Disease Health Associations, Substance Abuse. **Geo. Dist:** corporate operating locations nationally and internationally.

## ★ 936 ★ Chicago Sun-Times Charity Trust

401 N Wabash Ave.
Chicago, IL 60611
**Phone:** (312)321-2213        **Fax:** (312)321-0629
**Email:** pdudek@hollingerintl.com
**Website:** http://www.suntimes.com
Patricia Dudek, Vice President and Manager, Community &

**Fnded:** 1936. **Priorities:** *Education:* 10%. Funds precollege education and literacy. *Environment:* 83%. Primary support for youth groups, food banks, and social services. *International:* 7%. Supports cancer organizations and a pediatric health foundation. *Note:* Total contributions in fiscal 2000. **Typ. Recipients:** Child Abuse, Children's Health/Hospitals, Domestic Violence, Health-General, People with Disabilities. **Geo. Dist:** Chicago, IL, including metropolitan area.

## ★ 937 ★ Chicago Title and Trust Co. Foundation

171 N Clark St., 9TF
Chicago, IL 60601-3294
**Phone:** (312)335-9442
Eileen Hughes, Treasurer

**Fnded:** 1951. **Priorities:** *Arts & Humanities:* 27%. Supports major cultural institutions such as theaters, art institutes, festivals, and libraries. Also operates an Employee Matching Gift for PBS Programs with grants to Chicago stations and others throughout the United States. *Civic & Public Affairs:* 24%. Focus on strengthening the social and economic position of the community. Funds housing projects, services for the disadvantaged through job training, mentoring, and help programs. Supports parks, cultural diversity, and economic development. *Education:* 10%. Supports higher education, primarily through an employee matching gift program. Other education support includes Junior Achievement, grants for improvement of existing facilities, and for specific objectives with established needs evidenced by stable or growing enrollment. *Environment:* 37%. Emphasis on supporting youth by developing mentoring programs and youth groups. Recipients include United Way, youth programs, and Planned Parenthood. *International:* 2%. Limited funding supports American Red Cross, disease-specific organizations, and hospitals. *Religion:* Less than 1%. *Note:* Total foundation contributions made in 2000. **Typ. Recipients:** Cancer, Child Abuse, Children's Health/Hospitals, Clinics/Medical Centers, Diabetes, Emergency/Ambulance Services, Eyes/Blindness, Family Planning, Health Organizations, Hospitals, Medical Education, Multiple Sclerosis, Respiratory, Single-Disease Health Associations, Trauma Treatment. **Geo. Dist:** Chicago, IL.

## ★ 938 ★ Chicago Tribune Foundation

435 N Michigan Ave., Ste. 200
Chicago, IL 60611-4041
**Phone:** (312)222-4300        **Fax:** (312)222-3751
**Email:** ctcommunityrelations@tribune.com
**Website:** http://www.chicagotribune.com/communityrelations
Frank Gihan, President

**Priorities:** *Arts & Humanities:* 17%. Support is directed to programs for disadvantaged children who would not otherwise have access to the arts, and to organizations that foster diversity. Some general support is given to select cultural institutions in Chicago. Grants support programs that lead to journalistic excellence, promote diversity in the newspaper industry, and protect press freedoms. Support goes to professional

associations, including minority associations; student groups and universities; and public policy institutes. *Civic & Public Affairs:* 17%. Grants support civic efforts in the Chicago area led by the business community. *Education:* 23%. Supports programs that provide basic literacy and employment skills and GED preparation. Funds scholarship. *Environment:* 41%. Major support goes to the United Way/Crusade of Mercy. Grants in this area are by invitation only. *International:* 1%. *Note:* The company also helps raise money for Chicago area causes through the Chicago Tribune Charities Program by sponsoring local fundraising events. The program works in partnership with the Robert R. McCormick Tribune Foundation; focuses are employment and literacy. The Chicago Tribune Holiday Fund generates contributions from the public to address basic human needs for children, people with developmental disabilities, the homeless, and the hungry. Total contributions made in 1998. **Typ. Recipients:** AIDS/HIV, Child Abuse, Children's Health/Hospitals, Domestic Violence, Emergency/Ambulance Services, Health Organizations, People with Disabilities, Prenatal Health Issues, Substance Abuse, Transplant Networks/Donor Banks. **Geo. Dist:** Chicago, IL, including metropolitan area.

## ★ 939 ★ CHS Cooperatives Foundation

5500 Cenex Dr.
Inver Grove Heights, MN 55077
**Phone:** (651)451-5481        **Fax:** (651)451-5073
**Email:** wnels@chsco-ops.com
William Nelson, President

**Fnded:** 1947. **Priorities:** *Civic & Public Affairs:* 3%. Funds economic development in rural areas. *Education:* 90%. Supports agricultural education, with a focus on cooperative education, 4-H, and scholarships. *Note:* Total contributions made in 2000. **Typ. Recipients:** Emergency/Ambulance Services, Health-General, Medical Research, People with Disabilities. **Geo. Dist:** CO; ID; IA; KS; MN; MT; NE; ND; OR; SD; UT; WA; WA; WI.

## ★ 940 ★ CIGNA Foundation

2 Liberty Place
1601 Chestnut St., TL06B
Philadelphia, PA 19192-2066
**Phone:** (215)761-4881        **Fax:** (215)761-5632
**Email:** deborah.veney-robinson@cigna.com
**Website:** http://www.cigna.com/general/about/community/index.html
Deborah Robinson, Director, Civic Affairs

**Priorities:** *Arts & Humanities:* 11%. Grants go to arts councils, ballet, museums, orchestras, science academies, and theaters in Philadelphia and Hartford. Significant portion of funding supports the foundation's matching gifts program. *Civic & Public Affairs:* 16%. Emphasis on public policy research, urban and minority affairs groups, safety, and the environment. *Education:* 24%. Support is provided to colleges and universities, with a special interest in minority education and insurance-related curricula. Limited support given to literacy and arts education projects. Substantial support is given to the foundation's matching gifts program. *International:* 49%. CIGNA's primary focus is on women's health and infant maternal care, with an emphasis on programs that reduce infant mortality and low-birthweight. **Typ. Recipients:** Adolescent Health Issues, Cancer, Children's Health/Hospitals, Clinics/Medical Centers, Health Organizations, Health-General, Medical Education, People with Disabilities, People with Disabilities, Prenatal Health Issues, Public Health. **Geo. Dist:** Hartford, CT, including metropolitan area; Philadelphia, PA, including metropolitan area.

## ★ 941 ★ Cincinnati Bell Foundation, Inc.

ML 102-560, 201 East Fourth St.
Cincinnati, OH 45202
**Phone:** (513)397-7545        **Fax:** (513)723-9815
Robert Horine, Contact

**Priorities:** *Arts & Humanities:* 41%. Supports performing arts, museums, historical preservation, libraries, music, and arts funds. *Civic & Public Affairs:* 27%. Funds zoos and nature centers. *Education:* 20%. Majority to colleges and universities in communities where Cincinnati Bell operates. Other recipients include educational funds which help disadvantaged youth. Many grants are part of the matching gifts program. *Environment:* 9%. Supports youth organizations, Habitat for Humanity, work and rehabilitation centers. *International:* 3%. Supports hospitals, hospice, medical centers, and American Red Cross Disaster Relief Fund. *Note:* Total foundation contributions made in 2000. **Typ. Recipients:** Cancer, Children's Health/Hospitals, Clinics/Medical Centers, Emergency/Ambulance Services, Hospices, Hospitals, Medical Education, People with Disabilities, Public Health, Single-Disease Health Associations, Speech & Hearing. **Geo. Dist:** areas where employees live and work.

### ★ 942 ★ Cinergy Foundation

139 E 4th St.
Cincinnati, OH 45202
**Phone:** (513)287-1251     **Fax:** (513)651-9196
**Email:** kking@cinergy.com
**Website:** http://www.cinergy.com/Community/default.asp
Karol King, Foundation Manager

**Fnded:** 1992. **Priorities:** *Arts & Humanities:* Supports visual and performing arts, cultural programs, and arts education in company's service area. *Civic & Public Affairs:* Supports projects that help communities help themselves. Supports the environment through environmental education, park development and enhancement, resource preservation, reforestation, and recycling; and youth development. *Education:* Supports two primary areas: workforce development and staff development. Workforce development projects create a fundamental, seamless, results-based system that enhances the way youth are prepared to meet the demands of a highly skilled workforce, including school-to-work and career development initiatives; increase academic standards; and encourage lifelong learning. Staff development projects encourage continuous improvement in teaching and expanded leadership roles for all teachers, including providing peer assistance and review; training for teachers to take on new roles within the school as mentors, facilitators, community liaisons,curriculum development and assessment experts; enhance educators' ability to observe exemplary teaching practices, conduct and review research, plan for school improvement, and integrate technlogy; individualize instruction; and facilitate schools' efforts to reach out effectively to parents and the community. *International:* Supports health and social service programs which promotehealthy lifestyles and preventative medical care. Major support to the United Way. **Typ. Recipients:** Children's Health/Hospitals, Emergency/Ambulance Services, Health-General, Hospitals, Mental Health, People with Disabilities, Prenatal Health Issues, Single-Disease Health Associations, Substance Abuse. **Geo. Dist:** IN, company service area); KY, Northern Kentucky (company service area); OH, company service area. **Frmly:** PSI Energy Foundation.

### ★ 943 ★ Circuit City Foundation

9950 Mayland Dr.
Richmond, VA 23233
**Phone:** (804)527-4000     **Fax:** (804)527-4173
Cassandra Stoddart, Co-EXE Director

**Priorities:** *Arts & Humanities:* 19%. Major emphasis is on public broadcasting, which typically accounts for nearly three-quarters of total arts giving. Considerable support also goes to symphonies and museums. *Civic & Public Affairs:* 28%. Funding is provided to community affairs organizations, police agencies and volunteer fire departments, environmental organizations, African-American affairs, and women's groups. *Education:* 20%. Foundation focused its education giving to concentrate on public education reform; support also goes to higher education. *Environment:* 16%. United Ways throughout the Eastern states and California receive the majority of this support. Other interests include youth organizations and aid to persons with disabilities. *International:* 1%. Grants generally benefit hospitals, single-disease health organizations, and the American Red Cross. *Religion:* 8%. Funds science museums. *Note:* Total contributions made in 1999.

**Typ. Recipients:** Emergency/Ambulance Services, Heart, Multiple Sclerosis, People with Disabilities, Sexual Abuse, Single-Disease Health Associations, Transplant Networks/Donor Banks. **Geo. Dist:** communities where employees live and work.

### ★ 944 ★ CIT Group Foundation

1211 Ave. of the Americas
New York, NY 10036
**Phone:** (973)740-5000     **Fax:** (973)740-5264
Corinne Taylor, Assistant Secretary

**Priorities:** *Arts & Humanities:* 15%. Supports music, performing arts, libraries, historical preservation, and museums. *Civic & Public Affairs:* 3%. Emphasis is on economic development, minority affairs, and industry concerns. *Education:* 33%. Supports scholarships, schools, business education, student aid, private education, and education reform. Other interests include minority education, enrichment programs, and education funds. Also supports matching gifts to colleges and universities. *Environment:* 28%. Majority of funding supports United Way and youth organizations. Also supports community centers, people with disabilities, and substance abuse organizations. *International:* 20%. Supports clinics, hospitals, hospice, single-disease associations, emergency care, and children's healthcare. *Note:* Total foundation contributions made in 2000. **Typ. Recipients:** AIDS/HIV, Arthritis, Cancer, Children's Health/Hospitals, Clinics/Medical Centers, Emergency/Ambulance Services, Health Organizations, Heart, Hospitals, Medical Research, Mental Health, People with Disabilities, Single-Disease Health Associations, Substance Abuse, Transplant Networks/Donor Banks, Trauma Treatment. **Geo. Dist:** nationally, with an emphasis on headquarters area only.

### Citigroup Foundation
*See:* Entry 11426

### ★ 945 ★ Citizens Bank-Flint

328 South Saginaw St.
Flint, MI 48502
**Phone:** (810)766-7500     **Fax:** (810)766-7634
**Website:** http://www.cbclientsfirst.com
David Albert, Assistant Vice President

**Typ. Recipients:** Adolescent Health Issues, Children's Health/Hospitals, Clinics/Medical Centers, Family Planning, Health-General, Medical Education, People with Disabilities. **Geo. Dist:** headquarters and operating communities.

### ★ 946 ★ Citizens Charitable Foundation

1 Citizens Plaza
Providence, RI 02903-1339
**Phone:** (401)456-7285     **Fax:** (401)456-7644
D. Sanders, Senior Vice President

**Priorities:** *Arts & Humanities:* 8%. Supports museums, music, and the performing arts. *Civic & Public Affairs:* 28%. Supports economic development organizations, a tax clinic, low-income housing, minority affairs, and business groups. *Education:* 19%. Funds colleges and universities, medical schools, economic education, and programs for community education. Also provides scholarships. *Environment:* 38%. Supports United Way, child welfare, youth organizations, community centers, day care, and community service organizations. *International:* 1%. Supports medical information dissemination and general medical organizations. *Note:* Total contributions made in 2000. **Typ. Recipients:** AIDS/HIV, Children's Health/Hospitals, Clinics/Medical Centers, Emergency/Ambulance Services, Geriatric Health, Health Organizations, Hospices, Hospitals, Medical Education, Medical Rehabilitation, Medical Research, Mental Health, Nursing Services, People with Disabilities, Public Health, Sexual Abuse, Single-Disease Health Associations, Substance Abuse. **Geo. Dist:** RI.

### ★ 947 ★ CLARCOR Foundation

2323 6th St.
Rockford, IL 61125
**Phone:** (815)962-8867     **Fax:** (815)962-0417
David Lindsay, Chairman

**Priorities:** *Arts & Humanities:* 15%. Includes support for music, theater, historic preservation projects, and dance groups. *Civic & Public Affairs:* 7%. Gives to economic development and neighborhood/community enhancement projects. *Education:* 25%. Supports business education and colleges and universities. *Environment:* 39%. Supports the United Way, child welfare and youth organizations, veterans groups, and family services. *International:* 1%. Recipients include health organizations, hospitals, and mental health centers. *Note:* Total contributions made in 2000. **Typ. Recipients:** Cancer, Clinics/Medical Centers, Emergency/Ambulance Services, Health Funds, Health Organizations, Hospices, Hospitals, Long-Term Care, Mental Health, Nursing Services, People with Disabilities, Public Health, Respiratory. **Geo. Dist:** operating locations only.

### ★ 948 ★ The Cleveland-Cliffs Foundation

1100 Superior Ave.
Cleveland, OH 44114
**Phone:** (216)694-5407     **Fax:** (216)694-6741
David Gardner, Vice President, Assistant Treasurer

**Priorities:** *Arts & Humanities:* 17%. Supports natural history museums, music, theater, public libraries, and art funds. *Civic & Public Affairs:* 11%. Interests include municipalities, urban leagues, legal foundations, better business, and economic development. *Education:* 53%. Education foundations and college funds, including business, economic, minority, private, and public education. Supports matching gifts to education institutions. *Environment:* 18%. Supports YMCA, family services, child welfare, Boys/Girls Scouts, homes, people with disabilities, athletics, and United Way. *International:* 1%. Largest contribution supports United Way. Other recipients include health foundations, community child care services, cancer society, hospitals, the aged, youth organizations, athletics, and community service organizations. *Note:* Total contributions in 1999. **Typ. Recipients:** Cancer, Children's Health/Hospitals, Clinics/Medical Centers, Emergency/Ambulance Services, Health Organizations, Heart, Hospitals, People with Disabilities, Preventive Medicine/Wellness Organizations, Public Health. **Geo. Dist:** nationally; MI; MN; OH; nationally.

### ★ 949 ★ Clorox Co. Foundation

1221 Broadway, 13th Floor
Oakland, CA 94612-1888
**Phone:** (510)271-2199     **Fax:** (510)271-7757
**Email:** community.relations@clorox.com
**Website:** http://www.clorox.com/company/foundation
Carmella Johnson, Contributions Manager

**Fnded:** 1980. **Priorities:** *Arts & Humanities:* 7%. Funding is awarded to music, theater, community arts, and dance organizations in California. Other interests include museums, opera, painting/sculpture, ethnic arts, and arts festivals and centers. *Civic & Public Affairs:* 5%. Civic interests include civil rights, low-income housing, law and justice, economic development, parks and the environment, technical assistance, volunteer development, and conflict resolution programs. *Education:* 25%. Emphasis is on quality of education for all young people from kindergarten through college, particularly public school reform with attention to minority and low-income youth. Education grants will increasingly focus on K-12, as well as preschool and early childhood development programs that emphasize prevention and intervention through mentoring, tutoring, and parent involvement. Of special interest are drop-out prevention, programs designed to help students develop tools for learning, programs that actively involve parents and the community in the educational process, job readiness and career development, and programs that provide for and nurture students from infancy through high school and beyond. Matches employee contributions to higher education. Supports programs such as the East Oakland Youth Development Center, which provide a place for youth to go for recreation and personal and intellectual enrichment. Funds the Clorox Partners Scholarships for college education. Also supports arts outreach activities, reading camps, and leadership development programs. *Environment:* 62%. Primarily funds United Way and youth organizations. Supports family counseling, and programs which promote positive relationships among youth from diverse cultural and ethnic groups. Includes support for employee matching gifts. *International:* 1%. Supports disaster relief. *Voluntarism:* The company reports that more than one-third of employees in its General Offices and its Technical Center volunteer time at more than 375 agencies. The Clorox Employee Volunteer Program identifies volunteer opportunities, disseminates information about community agencies and programs to employees, and helps match volunteers with organizations. Company awards $200 grants to organizations where employees volunteer. *Note:* Total foundation contributions made in fiscal 2000. **Typ. Recipients:** Children's Health/Hospitals, Clinics/Medical Centers, Domestic Violence, Emergency/Ambulance Services, Family Planning, Geriatric Health, Health Funds, Health Organizations, Hospices, Mental Health, People with Disabilities, Prenatal Health Issues, Public Health, Research/Studies Institutes, Single-Disease Health Associations, Substance Abuse. **Geo. Dist:** operating locations; Oakland, CA; San Francisco, CA, including metropolitan area.

## ★ 950 ★ CNA Foundation

CNA Plaza
Chicago, IL 60685
Andrea Sinisi, Executive Director

**Fnded:** 1995. **Priorities:** *Arts & Humanities:* 10%. Provides funding to a variety of causes, including music, theater, and art institutes. *Civic & Public Affairs:* 31%. Grants support professional organizations (especially those related to the insurance industry) and encourage community economic development and the advancement of sound civic policy. Funds programs that address affordable housing, leadership development, job creation and overall economic development in depressed neighborhoods. *Education:* 31%. The company encourages pre-collegiate education programs that strengthen public schools and school reform through the advancement of basic curriculum, enhanced learning opportunities and faculty development. Another area of interest is pre-collegiate mathematics and science. Emphasis is placed on programs that encourage innovations in the teaching and learning of mathematics and science. Provides matching gifts to higher education institutions. *Environment:* 22%. Primary support for the United Way. Also funds child welfare and youth organizations, food distribution, and other social services. *International:* 1%. Supports health organizations located in communities where the company has a presence. *Note:* Total contributions in 2000. **Typ. Recipients:** AIDS/HIV, Child Abuse, Children's Health/Hospitals, Health Organizations, Health-General, Heart, Hospitals, Medical Research, Mental Health, People with Disabilities. **Geo. Dist:** in communities where co. has a presence.

## ★ 951 ★ Coca-Cola Foundation

PO Drawer 1734
Atlanta, GA 30301
**Phone:** (404)676-2568      **Fax:** (404)676-8804
**Website:** http://www2.coca-cola.com/citizenship/foundation.html
Donald Greene, President

**Fnded:** 1984. **Priorities:** *Arts & Humanities:* 5%. Supports historical preservation and the performing arts. *Civic & Public Affairs:* 9%. Funds national parks. *Education:* 73%. Supports public and private colleges and universities, elementary and secondary schools, teacher training programs, educational programs for minority students, arts and environmental education programs and educational programs that serve a global constituency. Grants span the traditional areas of giving–arts, civic, health, and social service–but projects must have some basis in education. Special interests include pipeline programs that encourage students to stay in school and proceed on to college and graduate school, scholarship programs that support graduate and undergraduate students, minority advancement through scholarships, urban and cultural diversity programs and global exchange programs

which encourage international studies, global understanding, or student exchange. The foundation is also interested in programs that introduce art education curricula into public schools and programs which collaborate between higher education, cultural institutions, and K-12 public schools. *Environment:* 4%. Funds youth and family organizations. *Religion:* 4%. Supports science centers and museums. *Voluntarism:* Company sponsors an employee volunteer reaching-out program. *Note:* Total foundation contributions made in 1999. **Typ. Recipients:** Medical Education. **Geo. Dist:** internationally; nationally.

## ★ 952 ★ Colgate-Palmolive Co.

300 Park Ave.
New York, NY 10022
**Phone:** (212)310-2175      **Fax:** (212)310-2873
Sally Phipps, Contributions Manager
**Typ. Recipients:** Health-General.

## ★ 953 ★ Collins & Aikman Foundation

701 McCullough Dr.
Charlotte, NC 28232
**Phone:** (704)548-2389      **Fax:** (704)548-2391
Arlene Bookman, Administrator

**Priorities:** *Arts & Humanities:* 3%. Major interests are music, arts outreach programs, and performing arts. *Civic & Public Affairs:* 6%. Supports civic foundations and urban affairs. *Education:* 34%. Majority of grants benefit colleges and universities, with limited support to Junior Achievement. Also funds educational matching gifts and scholarships. *Environment:* 50%. Majority of funding supports United Ways in various communities. Remaining funds generally support youth organizations, family services, and crime prevention. *International:* 7%. Funding supports hospitals and single-disease health organizations. *Note:* Total contributions in 2000. **Typ. Recipients:** AIDS/HIV, Cancer, Clinics/Medical Centers, Eyes/Blindness, Health Organizations, Hospices, Hospitals, Medical Research, Nursing Services, People with Disabilities, Public Health, Single-Disease Health Associations, Substance Abuse, Trauma Treatment. **Geo. Dist:** operating locations.

## ★ 954 ★ Colonial Foundation

PO Box 576
Savannah, GA 31402
**Phone:** (912)236-1331
Francis Brown, Vice President, Finance & Chief Financia

**Fnded:** 1986. **Priorities:** *Arts & Humanities:* 39%. Supports historic preservation, museums, and performing arts. *Civic & Public Affairs:* 5%. Funds citizen advocacy groups, low-income housing, and chambers of commerce. *Education:* 11%. Funds higher education, scholarship programs, Junior Achievement, family literacy, and private pre-college education. *Environment:* 37%. Primarily funds United Way and youth groups. *International:* 6%. Gives to cancer organizations and hospice. *Religion:* Less than 1%. Funds a science museum. *Note:* Total contributions in 2000. **Typ. Recipients:** Arthritis, Cancer, Children's Health/Hospitals, Diabetes, Emergency/Ambulance Services, Health Organizations, Health-General, Hospices, Long-Term Care, People with Disabilities, Prenatal Health Issues, Respiratory, Sexual Abuse, Single-Disease Health Associations. **Geo. Dist:** GA.

## ★ 955 ★ Colonial Life & Accident Insurance Co.

1200 Colonial Life Blvd.
PO Box 1365
Columbia, SC 29202
**Phone:** (803)213-7424      **Fax:** (803)213-7427
Melanie Marmo, Community Relations Specialist

**Priorities:** *Arts & Humanities:* About 20%. Favors local ballet, symphony, and museums. *Civic & Public Affairs:* 20%%. Supports government, economic development, housing, community affairs, and national security. *Education:* 20%. Interests include teacher training and development programs, college scholarships, K-12 mentoring programs, and colleges, univer-

sities, and community colleges. *International:* 30%. Interests include homeless shelters, AIDS and drug abuse education projects, child abuse prevention, and elder-care. **Typ. Recipients:** Domestic Violence, Emergency/Ambulance Services, Family Planning, Geriatric Health, Health Policy/Cost Containment, Hospices, Hospitals, Medical Research, Medical Training, Mental Health, Nursing Services, People with Disabilities, Public Health, Single-Disease Health Associations, Substance Abuse. **Geo. Dist:** SC.

## ★ 956 ★ Comdisco Foundation

6111 North River Rd.
Rosemont, IL 60018
**Phone:** (847)698-3000
Barbara Herman, Executive Assistant

**Fnded:** 1994. **Priorities:** *Arts & Humanities:* 2%. Funds children's museums and libraries. *Civic & Public Affairs:* 2%. Supports community foundations and municipalities. *Education:* 31%. Funds private schools, Junior Achievement, and education foundations. *Environment:* 36%. Supports Special Olympics, family services, and child and youth organizations. *International:* 27%. Hospitals, children's health, hospice, and single-disease associations receive funding. *Note:* Total foundation contributions made in fiscal 2000. **Typ. Recipients:** Cancer, Child Abuse, Children's Health/Hospitals, Clinics/Medical Centers, Emergency/Ambulance Services, Hospices, Hospitals, Hospitals (University Affiliated), Long-Term Care, Medical Rehabilitation, Mental Health, People with Disabilities, Single-Disease Health Associations. **Geo. Dist:** headquarters area only.

## ★ 957 ★ Comerica Charitable Foundation

500 Woodward Ave., MC 3352
Detroit, MI 48275-3352
**Phone:** (313)222-3571      **Fax:** (313)222-8720
**Email:** caroline_chambers@comerica.com
Caroline Chambers, Corporate Contributions Vice President

**Fnded:** 1997. **Priorities:** *Arts & Humanities:* 20%. Recipients include museums, opera, arts centers and institutes, and libraries. *Civic & Public Affairs:* (Housing & Neighborhood Revitalization) 33%. Contributes to revitalize the cities near operating locations, including projects to rehabilitate or construct housing in low-to moderate-income neighborhoods, and efforts to stimulate business growth. *Education:* 9%. Supports minority and independent college funds, colleges and universities, United Negro College Fund, public broadcasting, science centers, and business and free enterprise education programs for youth. Matches employee gifts to higher education. *Environment:* 28%. Supports United Way and federated campaigns, youth organizations, and food banks. *International:* 7%. Recipients include hospitals and single-disease health associations. *Religion:* 2%. *Voluntarism:* Company offers Comerica Cares program in which employees participate in volunteer activities of community organizations. *Note:* Total foundation contributions made in 2000. **Typ. Recipients:** Cancer, Children's Health/Hospitals, Health Organizations, Hospices, Hospitals, Medical Rehabilitation, Mental Health, Single-Disease Health Associations. **Geo. Dist:** CA; FL; MI, especially southeastern MI; TX. **Frmly:** Comerica Foundation.

## ★ 958 ★ Commerce Bancshares Foundation

PO Box 13095
Kansas City, MO 64199-3095
**Phone:** (816)234-2985

**Fnded:** 1952. **Priorities:** *Arts & Humanities:* 10% to 15%. Supports Kansas City arts organizations, including music, public television, and a museum. *Civic & Public Affairs:* 10% to 15%. Supports housing and economic development, civil rights, public protection, employment, and local civic organizations. *Education:* 10% to 15%. Supports institutions of higher education in Missouri, including colleges, universities, military schools, and education funds. Provides some support for public education. Also supports science and social science programs. *Environment:* 60% to 65%. Primarily supports the United Way, recreation, youth development, food distribution, and other human service organizations. *Voluntarism:* The company actively encourages employee volunteerism. Employees and executives also are active in United Way, Habitat for Humanity, and numerous community organizations. **Typ. Recipients:** Cancer, Children's Health/Hospitals, Clinics/Medical Centers, Domestic Violence, Emergency/Ambulance Services, Family Planning, Health Organizations, Hospitals, Public Health, Single-Disease Health Associations, Substance Abuse. **Geo. Dist:** West Central, IL; KS; MO.

### ★ 959 ★ Commercial Intertech Foundation

PO Box 239
Youngstown, OH 44501
**Phone:** (330)746-8011　　　**Fax:** (330)746-0422
Mary Tanner, Executive Assistant to Chief
　Executive O

**Priorities:** *Arts & Humanities:* 8%. Supports symphonies, art associations, public radio, and public television. *Civic & Public Affairs:* 6%. *Education:* 28%. Gives to colleges and universities, primarily in Ohio. *Environment:* 50%. Primarily gives to United Way; also supports drug abuse prevention. *International:* 7%. Supports hospices and medical centers. *Note:* Total foundation contributions in fiscal 1998. **Typ. Recipients:** Cancer, Children's Health/Hospitals, Clinics/Medical Centers, Diabetes, Domestic Violence, Emergency/Ambulance Services, Family Planning, Health Organizations, Health-General, Heart, Home-Care Services, Hospices, Hospitals, Long-Term Care, Multiple Sclerosis, People with Disabilities, Public Health, Single-Disease Health Associations, Speech & Hearing, Substance Abuse. **Geo. Dist:** OH.

### ★ 960 ★ Commonwealth Edison Co.

PO Box 767
Chicago, IL 60690
**Phone:** (312)394-3060　　　**Fax:** (312)394-3552
**Email:** leslie.jackson@exeloncorp.com
Mr. Leslie Jackson, Corporate Affairs Associate

**Priorities:** *Arts & Humanities:* 12%. Supports a wide variety of activities; largest contributions are awarded to major institutions within service area. Offers modest contributions to broad range of smaller organizations. *Civic & Public Affairs:* 35%. Primarily United Funds & United Way with emphasis on Metropolitan Crusade of Mercy. Other interest include urban development, particularly in low-income areas of northern Illinois. *Education:* 32%. Priority is higher education, particularly private institutions within company's service area. *Environment:* 18%. Supports various welfare and community organizations. *International:* 3%. Emphasis is on hospitals, which generally receive only capital support; also limited support for other health activities. *Note:* Total contributions made in 1997. **Typ. Recipients:** Health Organizations, Hospitals, Single-Disease Health Associations, Substance Abuse. **Geo. Dist:** Chicago, IL, including surrounding area.

### ★ 961 ★ Compaq Computer Corp.

20555 SW 249. MS05 0204
Houston, TX 77070-2698
**Phone:** (281)370-0670　　　**Fax:** (281)514-9953
**Email:** cpg.contributions@compaq.com
**Website:** http://www.compaq.com/corporate/community
Brenda Ellis, Director, Corporate Community Relations

**Fnded:** 1989. **Priorities:** *Civic & Public Affairs:* Community programs focus on healthcare and community services, environment, and arts and culture. *Education:* Contributed resources to support education. Continues support to technology in the classroom. Also supports K-12 education for math and science programs, porfession development for teachers, and programs for education enrichment (i.e., mentoring and homework centers). *Voluntarism:* The company provides technology assistance through employee volunteers. *Note:* Call (281) 514-0527 for recent priorities. **Typ. Recipients:** AIDS/HIV, Cancer, Children's Health/Hospitals, Diabetes, Eyes/Blindness, Heart, Medical Rehabilitation, Medical Research, Mental Health, Multiple Sclerosis, People with Disabilities, Single-Disease Health Associations, Substance Abuse. **Frmly:** Compaq Computer Foundation.

### ★ 962 ★ Compass Bank Foundation

PO Box 10566
15 S 20th St.
Birmingham, AL 35296
**Phone:** (205)933-3960　　　**Fax:** (205)933-3336
Jerry Powell, Jr., Contact

**Fnded:** 1981. **Priorities:** *Arts & Humanities:* 1%. Supports humanities, children's theater, festivals, and arts councils. *Civic & Public Affairs:* 3%. Funds botanical gardens, public affairs, urban revitalization programs, and community foundations. *Education:* 60%. Funds higher education, scholarships, and Junior Achievement. *Environment:* 20%. Primarily supports United Way, youth and social services. *International:* 9%. Funds community health, hospice, American Red Cross, and single-disease associations. *Religion:* 4%. Supports science museums. *Note:* Total foundation contributions made in 1999. **Typ. Recipients:** Cancer, Children's Health/Hospitals, Clinics/Medical Centers, Diabetes, Emergency/Ambulance Services, Health Funds, Health Organizations, Heart, Hospices, Hospitals, Mental Health, Multiple Sclerosis, People with Disabilities, Transplant Networks/Donor Banks. **Geo. Dist:** AL; TX.

### ★ 963 ★ Computer Associates International, Inc.

1 Computer Associates Plaza
Islandia, NY 11749
**Phone:** (631)342-3562　　　**Fax:** (631)342-5013
**Email:** bonnie.burk@ca.com
**Website:** http://www.ca.com/charity
Bonnie Burk, Administrative Assistant

**Typ. Recipients:** Health-General. **Geo. Dist:** internationally; nationally.

### ★ 964 ★ ConAgra Foundation

1 ConAgra Dr.
Omaha, NE 68102-5001
**Phone:** (402)595-4000　　　**Fax:** (402)595-4595
**Website:** http://www.conagra.com/conagra_foundation.jsp
Lynn Phares, Vice President, Corporate Relations

**Priorities:** *Arts & Humanities:* 27%. Supports theater, museums, arts festivals, opera. *Civic & Public Affairs:* 13%. Supports housing, safety, municipalities/towns, botanical centers. *Education:* 29%. Supports scholarships, colleges, universities, literacy, schools, and minority education. *Environment:* 27%. Supports United Way, scouting, shelters, food banks, child welfare, Special Olympics, young men's christian association. *International:* 3%. *Note:* Total contributions made in 1999. **Typ. Recipients:** Clinics/Medical Centers, Emergency/Ambulance Services, Health Organizations, Hospices, Nursing Services, Nutrition, People with Disabilities, Substance Abuse. **Geo. Dist:** primarily in locations where there are major ConAgra facilities.

### ★ 965 ★ Consolidated Natural Gas System Foundation

CNG Tower
Dominion Tower, 625 Liberty Ave.
Pittsburgh, PA 15222-3199
**Phone:** (412)690-1231　　　**Fax:** (412)690-7608
James Mesloh, Executive Directory

**Priorities:** *Arts & Humanities:* 10%. Funds music, public broadcasting, historic groups, and museums and galleries. *Civic & Public Affairs:* 25%. Supports municipalities and towns, community foundations, urban and community affairs, and economic development. *Education:* 15%. Supports colleges and universities, education funds, and secondary education. *Environment:* 41%. Primarily supports the United Way in operating areas; also funds youth and family services. *International:* Less than 1%. Supports emergency health organizations and health policy foundations. *Religion:* 2%. Supports science centers. *Note:* Total foundation contributions made in 2000. **Typ. Recipients:** Cancer, Children's Health/Hospitals, Clinics/Medical Centers, Domestic Violence, Emergency/Ambulance Services, Health Organizations, Health Policy/Cost Containment, Hospitals, People with Disabilities, Substance Abuse. **Geo. Dist:** national organizations; Washington, DC; LA; OH; OK; PA; VA; WV.

### ★ 966 ★ Consolidated Papers Foundation, Inc.

PO Box 3
Wisconsin Rapids, WI 54495-0003
**Phone:** (715)424-3004　　　**Fax:** (715)424-1314
Susan Feith, President

**Fnded:** 1951. **Priorities:** *Arts & Humanities:* 12%. Supports public broadcasting, public libraries, arts councils, and historic preservation and renovation, primarily in Wisconsin. *Education:* 65%. Primarily independent, accredited four-year colleges and universities in Wisconsin. Support includes unrestricted and capital grants. Special interests include science, technology, and engineering education relating to the pulp and paper industry. Also supports minority and independent college funds and merit scholarship programs. *Environment:* 22%. Funds Planned Parenthood, youth services, women's shelters, and the United Way. *Note:* Total contributions made in 1999. **Typ. Recipients:** AIDS/HIV, Emergency/Ambulance Services, Eyes/Blindness, Family Planning, Health Organizations, Hospices, Hospitals, Medical Education, Medical Rehabilitation, People with Disabilities, Preventive Medicine/Wellness Organizations, Trauma Treatment. **Geo. Dist:** WI, headquarters and operating communities.

### ★ 967 ★ Consumers Energy Foundation

212 W Michigan Ave.
Jackson, MI 49201
**Phone:** (517)788-0432　　　**Fax:** (517)788-2281
**Email:** foundation@consumersenergy.com
**Website:** http://www.consumersenergy.com/community/foundation/index.htm
Carolyn Bloodworth, Secretary/Treasurer

**Priorities:** *Arts & Humanities:* 23%. Interests include museums, opera, public broadcasting, symphonies, and theater. *Civic & Public Affairs:* 28%. Supports economic development and job training, housing, and public affairs. *Education:* 22%. Supports Michigan colleges and universities, K-12 education, specialized educational foundations, and programs that improve the curricula for business, economics, engineering, math, and the natural and physical sciences. *Environment:* 17%. The majority of support goes to the Unifed Way. Other interests include family and children services, YMCAs, volunteer programs, senior services, and food distribution programs. *International:* 2%. Supports American Red Cross. *Note:* Total contributions made in 1998. **Typ. Recipients:** Alzheimers Disease, Cancer, Children's Health/Hospitals, Emergency/Ambulance Services, Hospitals, People with Disabilities, Substance Abuse. **Geo. Dist:** nationally; MI.

### ★ 968 ★ ContiGroup Companies Foundation

277 Park Ave.
New York, NY 10172-0003
**Phone:** (212)207-5470　　　**Fax:** (212)207-5163
Susan McIntyre, Assistant Secretary

**Priorities:** *Arts & Humanities:* 21%. Supports performing arts, museums, and The Library of Congress. *Civic & Public Affairs:* 7%. Funds leadership development and community development. *Education:* 35%. Supports colleges and universities, business education, scholarship funds, and education foundations. *Environment:* 20%. Supports youth organizations, including YMCAs and Girl Scouts councils. *International:* 2%. Gives to single-disease health organizations. *Note:* Total contributions made in fiscal 2001. **Typ. Recipients:** Cancer, Children's Health/Hospitals, Clinics/Medical Centers, Emergency/Ambulance Services, Hospitals, Multiple Sclerosis, Nursing Services, People with Disabilities, Single-Disease Health Associations, Substance Abuse. **Geo. Dist:** Midwest; NY.

**★ 969 ★ Cooper Industries Foundation**
PO Box 4446
Houston, TX 77210-4446
**Phone:** (713)209-8800          **Fax:** (713)209-8982
**Email:** evans@cooperindustries.com
Jennifer Evans, Manager, Corporate Giving Programs

**Priorities:** *Arts & Humanities:* 34%. Majority of support funds museums, music, opera, and theaters. Other beneficiaries include cultural centers, arts associations, arts funds, and libraries. *Civic & Public Affairs:* 3%. Primarily supports civic improvement, environmental affairs organizations, and public policy research organizations. Other interests include business, international, and women's affairs organizations; zoos; and botanical gardens. *Education:* 37%. Primarily supports colleges and universities; also scholarships, education funds and associations, and economic education. *Environment:* 24%. Funds United Way and social services. *International:* 2%. Primarily supports single-disease health associations. *Note:* Total contributions mmade by the foundation in 1999. **Typ. Recipients:** Cancer, Children's Health/Hospitals, Emergency/Ambulance Services, Health Funds, Health Organizations, Heart, Hospices, Hospitals, Medical Education, Medical Education, Mental Health, People with Disabilities, Single-Disease Health Associations. **Geo. Dist:** operating locations.

**★ 970 ★ Cooper Tire & Rubber Foundation**
Lima & Western Ave.
Findlay, OH 45840
**Phone:** (419)423-1321          **Fax:** (419)424-4212
**Website:** http://www.cooperindustries.com/about/index.htm
Philip Weaver, Trustee

**Priorities:** *Arts & Humanities:* 5%. Supports arts associations, public broadcasting, and museums. *Civic & Public Affairs:* 10%. Supports job training and trade associations. *Education:* 44%. Funding supports universities, technical colleges, secondary education, and business education. *Environment:* 39%. Emphasis is on united funds, youth organizations, and senior services. *International:* 1%. Funds single-disease health organizations and hospitals. *Note:* Total contributions made in 2000. **Typ. Recipients:** Health-General, Hospitals, Medical Rehabilitation, People with Disabilities, Public Health. **Geo. Dist:** operating locations; OH.

**★ 971 ★ Courts Foundation**
1530 SunTrust Tower
25 Park Pl., NE
Atlanta, GA 30303-2917
**Phone:** (404)658-9066          **Fax:** (404)659-4802
John Stephenson, Executive Director

**Fnded:** 1950. **Priorities:** *Arts & Humanities:* 9%. Funds arts centers and festivals, museums, and dance. *Civic & Public Affairs:* 29%. Supports community foundations, a botanical garden, economic development, and legal affairs. *Education:* 43%. Funds precollege and higher education. *Environment:* 6%. Supports United Way, scouting, and family services. *International:* 2%. Supports hospitals, hospice, and single-disease health associations. *Note:* Total foundation contributions made in 2000. **Typ. Recipients:** Cancer, Children's Health/Hospitals, Clinics/Medical Centers, Diabetes, Emergency/Ambulance Services, Eyes/Blindness, Health Organizations, Heart, Hospices, Hospitals, Medical Education, Mental Health, People with Disabilities. **Geo. Dist:** headquarters and operating communities.

**★ 972 ★ Cowen Foundation**
1221 Ave. of the Americas
New York, NY 10020
Robert Greenberger, Director, Taxes

**Fnded:** 1990. **Priorities:** *Arts & Humanities:* 2%. Supports museums and music. *Civic & Public Affairs:* 2%. *Education:* 42%. Supports colleges, universities, schools, and educational funds. *Environment:* 18%. Supports United Way, scouting, youth programs, and human services. *International:* 21%. Supports medical centers, hospitals, and medical research. *Note:* Total foundation contributions made in 2000. **Typ. Recipients:** AIDS/HIV, Cancer, Children's Health/Hospitals, Clinics/Medical Centers, Diabetes, Emergency/Ambulance Services, Eyes/Blindness, Health Organizations, Heart, Hospitals, Hospitals (University Affiliated), Long-Term Care, People with Disabilities, Single-Disease Health Associations, Transplant Networks/Donor Banks. **Geo. Dist:** NY; PA.

**★ 973 ★ CPI Corp. Philanthropic Trust**
1706 Washington Ave.
Saint Louis, MO 63103
**Phone:** (314)231-1575          **Fax:** (314)231-2398
Fran Scheper, Executive Vice President, Human Resource

**Priorities:** *Civic & Public Affairs:* 100%. Supports organizations that provide job training, preparation, and placement for youth and minorities. *Note:* Total contributions made in fiscal 2000. **Typ. Recipients:** Children's Health/Hospitals, Domestic Violence, Eyes/Blindness, Geriatric Health, Hospitals, Multiple Sclerosis, People with Disabilities, Respiratory. **Geo. Dist:** near headquarters.

**★ 974 ★ Crane & Co. Fund**
30 South St.
Dalton, MA 01226
**Phone:** (413)684-2600          **Fax:** (413)684-1820
Liz Pomeroy, Executive Secretary

**Fnded:** 1953. **Priorities:** *Arts & Humanities:* 36%. Supports museums, theater, historic preservation, music, and the performing arts. *Civic & Public Affairs:* 3%. Supports business organizations, Native American affairs, community affairs, and local trade associations. *Education:* 20%. Funds the Zenas Crane Fund for Student Aid. Colleges and universities and educational programs also receive funding. *Environment:* 22%. Majority supports youth organizations. Additional recipients include organizations for people with disabilities, religious welfare, and community centers. *International:* 12%. A local medical center, health organizations, and emergency services receive funding. *Note:* Total contributions made in 2000. **Typ. Recipients:** Cancer, Child Abuse, Children's Health/Hospitals, Clinics/Medical Centers, Diabetes, Emergency/Ambulance Services, Eyes/Blindness, Health Funds, Health Organizations, Health-General, Heart, Hospices, Hospitals, Hospitals (University Affiliated), Kidney, People with Disabilities, Public Health, Respiratory, Single-Disease Health Associations, Substance Abuse. **Geo. Dist:** MA, Berkshire County and near headquarters.

**★ 975 ★ Crane Foundation**
100 First Stamford Pl.
Stamford, CT 06902
**Phone:** (203)363-7300          **Fax:** (203)363-7295
Gil Dickoff, Treasurer

**Fnded:** 1951. **Priorities:** *Arts & Humanities:* 11%. Supports arts councils, libraries, museums, historical preservation, and the performing arts. *Civic & Public Affairs:* 16%. Legal affairs, municipalities, zoos and parks receive support. *Education:* 45%. Funds colleges, universities, and private pre-college education. *Environment:* 9%. Funds family services and athletic organizations. *International:* 12%. Supports hospitals, medical services, and healthcare. *Note:* Total foundation contributions made in 2000. **Typ. Recipients:** Cancer, Child Abuse, Diabetes, Domestic Violence, Emergency/Ambulance Services, Eyes/Blindness, Health Organizations, Hospitals, Medical Research, Mental Health, Multiple Sclerosis, People with Disabilities, Public Health, Single-Disease Health Associations, Substance Abuse, Transplant Networks/Donor Banks. **Geo. Dist:** NY; PA.

**★ 976 ★ Cranston Foundation**
1381 Cranston St.
Cranston, RI 02920
**Phone:** (401)943-4800          **Fax:** (401)943-3971
**Email:** cpw@cpw.com
Carolyn Lake, Administrator

**Priorities:** *Arts & Humanities:* 4%. Interests include museums, libraries, music, historic preservation, and arts councils. *Civic & Public Affairs:* 8%. Favors housing projects, youth organizations, and ambulance and fire safety services. *Education:* 63%. Majority of funding supports scholarships to colleges and universities, primarily for children of company employees. Also, a few direct grants are given to education. Foundation also operates matching grants program. *International:* 25%. Focus on community service organizations, homes for the elderly, and health foundations and associations. One-third supports the United Jewish Appeal. Other interests include community centers, municipal funds for community needs and health. *Note:* Total contributions made in 1998. **Typ. Recipients:** Emergency/Ambulance Services, Hospitals, Kidney, Medical Education, Prenatal Health Issues. **Geo. Dist:** LA; MA; NY; RI.

**★ 977 ★ Credit Suisse First Boston Foundation Trust**
11 Madison Ave.
New York, NY 10010
**Phone:** (212)325-2389          **Fax:** (212)325-6665
**Email:** casey.karel@csfb.com
Casey Karel, Vice President

**Fnded:** 1959. **Priorities:** *Arts & Humanities:* 10% to 15%. Support is for major nationally oriented groups and community-based organizations. Supports museums and performing arts centers. *Education:* About 50%. Grants support educational initiatives and inner-city youth programs. *Environment:* 10% to 15%. Supports organizations in the New York area or in cities where company has branch offices. Other areas of interest include shelters for the homeless, child welfare, volunteer services, and youth organizations, including those serving at-risk youth. *International:* 10% to 15%. *Note:* Total contributions made in 1996. **Typ. Recipients:** Cancer, Children's Health/Hospitals, Clinics/Medical Centers, Emergency/Ambulance Services, Hospitals, Medical Research, Mental Health, People with Disabilities, Prenatal Health Issues, Single-Disease Health Associations, Transplant Networks/Donor Banks. **Geo. Dist:** headquarters and operating communities; nationally; New York, NY.

**★ 978 ★ Crestar Foundation**
919 East Main St.
Richmond, VA 23219
**Phone:** (804)782-5000          **Fax:** (804)782-5191
Brenda Skidmore, President

**Priorities:** *Arts & Humanities:* 15%. Supports museums, performing arts and literary groups, historic preservation, and arts funds and centers. Public broadcasting and libraries are also of interest. Includes matching gifts. *Civic & Public Affairs:* 35%. Economic development in operating communities is primary focus. Also supports national organizations that promote public understanding of economics and free enterprise. *Education:* 24%. Primarily supports private colleges and universities through independent college funds. Supports private secondary and elementary schools that are important to communities served by Crestar. Support is also provided in the form of employee matching gifts. *International:* 25%. Major emphasis is on United Way organizations serving Crestar communities. Awards capital and other grants to hospitals, religious welfare organizations such as the Salvation Army, youth homes, and scouting. *Note:* Total contributions in 1998. **Typ. Recipients:** AIDS/HIV, Cancer, Children's Health/Hospitals, Clinics/Medical Centers, Domestic Violence, Emergency/Ambulance Services, Eyes/Blindness, Health Funds, Health Organizations, Health Policy/Cost Containment, Heart, Hospices, Hospitals, Medical Education, Mental Health, Multiple Sclerosis, People with Disabilities, Speech & Hearing. **Geo. Dist:** headquarters and operating communities.

## ★ 979 ★ Croft-Leominster Foundation

Canton House, 300 Water St.
Baltimore, MD 21202
**Phone:** (410)576-0100          **Fax:** (410)576-8232
**Email:** jyoo@croft-leominster.com
L. Croft, Chairman

**Fnded:** 1990. **Priorities:** *Arts & Humanities:* Less than 1%. *Civic & Public Affairs:* 4%. Supports foundations, volunteer programs, and housing. *Education:* 81%. Supports colleges, universities, and education organizations. *Environment:* 1%. Supports community programs for the hungry, for senior citizens, and for families. *International:* Less than 1%. *Note:* Total foundation contributions made in 2000. **Typ. Recipients:** Alzheimers Disease, Emergency/Ambulance Services, Health-General, Heart, Hospitals, Single-Disease Health Associations, Substance Abuse. **Geo. Dist:** Baltimore, MD.

## ★ 980 ★ CSX Corp.

1 James Ctr.
901 E Cary St.
Richmond, VA 23219-5629
**Phone:** (804)782-1490          **Fax:** (804)783-1356
**Email:** Steven_larson@csx.com
**Website:** http://www.csx.com
Steve Larson, Vice President, General Counsel, Corpora

**Typ. Recipients:** Health-General. **Geo. Dist:** nationally.

## ★ 981 ★ Cummings Properties Foundation

200 West Cummings Park
Woburn, MA 01801
**Phone:** (617)935-8000
**Email:** leasing@cummings.com
**Website:** http://www.cummings.com/mck_info.html
Rob Nigro, Managing Trustee

**Fnded:** 1986. **Priorities:** *Arts & Humanities:* 4%. Funds museums, societies, and collections. *Civic & Public Affairs:* 6%. Funds civic associations. *Education:* 19%. Funds colleges and universities. *Environment:* 30%. Supports youth organizations, human services, and United Way. *International:* 7%. Supports hospitals and single-disease health organizations. *Religion:* 2%. *Note:* Total contributions in 1999. **Typ. Recipients:** Cancer, Children's Health/Hospitals, Clinics/Medical Centers, Diabetes, Health Organizations, Heart, Hospices, Hospitals, Medical Education, Medical Research, Nursing Services, People with Disabilities, Respiratory, Single-Disease Health Associations, Substance Abuse. **Geo. Dist:** Woburn, MA.

## ★ 982 ★ Cummins Foundation

Box 3005, Mail Code 60909
Columbus, IN 47202-3005
**Phone:** (812)377-3746          **Fax:** (812)377-3265
Tracy Souza, President

**Priorities:** *Civic & Public Affairs:* (United Funds & United Way) About 25%. (Public Policy) Less than 5%. *Education:* About 40%. Supports private, public, and religious elementary and secondary education, colleges, and universities. Also supports youth groups, Big Brothers/Big Sisters, YMCA's, and community foundations. Provides scholarships and matches employee gifts. *Note:* Above priorities reflect foundation giving. **Typ. Recipients:** Children's Health/Hospitals, Domestic Violence, Eyes/Blindness, Family Planning, Heart, Hospices, Hospitals, Mental Health, Preventive Medicine/Wellness Organizations, Public Health, Research/Studies Institutes, Substance Abuse. **Geo. Dist:** operating locations.

## ★ 983 ★ CUNA Mutual Foundation, Inc.

5910 Mineral Point Rd.
PO Box 391
Madison, WI 53701-0391
**Phone:** (608)231-7908          **Fax:** (608)238-2449
Terri Fiez, Executive Director

**Priorities:** *Arts & Humanities:* 7%. Supports theater, orchestras, pubic broadcasting, and history organizations. *Civic & Public Affairs:* 17%. Funds housing, legal and economic concerns, and civic institutions and events. *Education:* 11%. Emphasis on minority vocational training, fields related to CUNA Mutual business, employee recruitment, quality projects that do not receive tax support, and projects that link business need with educational development. *Environment:* 58%. Majority of funding supports United Way. Emphasis is on basic resources (food/shelter/clothing); employment and training; minority and underprivileged youth; transportation; and community assistance. *International:* 6%. Emphasis is on cost containment, wellness and prevention, family support and services access, and local-level services. *Note:* Total contributions in 1997. **Typ. Recipients:** AIDS/HIV, Cancer, Children's Health/Hospitals, Clinics/Medical Centers, Diabetes, Emergency/Ambulance Services, Health Organizations, Health Policy/Cost Containment, Hospitals, Medical Rehabilitation, Medical Research, Mental Health, Nursing Services, People with Disabilities, Prenatal Health Issues, Public Health, Single-Disease Health Associations, Single-Disease Health Associations. **Geo. Dist:** generally in communities where CUNA Mutual is located; Pomona, CA; Duluth, GA; Waverly, IA; Southfield, MI; Bloomington, MN; Albany, NY; Dallas, TX; Madison, WI.

## ★ 984 ★ Curtis L. Carlson Family Foundation

301 Carlson Parkway, Ste. 102
Minnetonka, MN 55305
**Phone:** (952)404-5604          **Fax:** (952)404-5601
Donna Snyder, Secretary

**Fnded:** 1959. **Priorities:** *Arts & Humanities:* 4%. Supports museums, libraries, music, theater, and public broadcasting. *Civic & Public Affairs:* 3%. Funds women's issues and neighborhood development. *Education:* 71%. Funds universities and private and public pre-college education. *Environment:* 19%. Supports United Way, YMCA, and Boys/Girls Clubs. *International:* 3%. Supports hospitals and cardiac care. *Note:* Total foundation contributions made in 2000. **Typ. Recipients:** AIDS/HIV, Cancer, Children's Health/Hospitals, Clinics/Medical Centers, Diabetes, Emergency/Ambulance Services, Eyes/Blindness, Health Organizations, Heart, Hospitals, Medical Research, Multiple Sclerosis, People with Disabilities, Public Health, Research/Studies Institutes, Single-Disease Health Associations, Substance Abuse. **Geo. Dist:** MN.

## ★ 985 ★ D.B. Reinhart Family Foundation

PO Box 2228
La Crosse, WI 54602-2228
**Phone:** (608)782-4999          **Fax:** (608)782-5084
Nancy Hengel, Manager

**Priorities:** *Arts & Humanities:* 10%. Supports arts funds, music, and children's museums. *Civic & Public Affairs:* 7%. Funds community and economic development and clubs. *Education:* 50%. Supports colleges and high schools. *Environment:* 9%. Supports United Way, community services, traditional youth organizations, and children's services. *International:* 12%. Primarily supports hospitals and medical institutes. *Note:* Total foundation contributions made in fiscal 2000. **Typ. Recipients:** Cancer, Children's Health/Hospitals, Clinics/Medical Centers, Diabetes, Emergency/Ambulance Services, Eyes/Blindness, Heart, Hospitals, Medical Education, Medical Research, People with Disabilities, Prenatal Health Issues, Public Health, Single-Disease Health Associations, Substance Abuse. **Geo. Dist:** WI.

## ★ 986 ★ DaimlerChrysler Corp. Fund

CIMS: 485-02-46
1000 Chrysler Dr.
Auburn Hills, MI 48326-2766
**Phone:** (248)512-2502          **Fax:** (248)512-2503
**Website:** http://www.fund.daimlerchrysler.com/data/fund/main.nsf
Lynn Feldhouse, Vice President & Secretary

**Fnded:** 1953. **Priorities:** *Arts & Humanities:* 17%. Supports local and national cultural organizations, with emphasis on the performing arts. Recipients include performing arts centers, historical societies, music groups, libraries, museums, and public broadcasting. *Civic & Public Affairs:* 9%. Supports organizations that work for improvement of the economy and quality of life in operating communities. Other interests include economic research and development, traffic safety, trade-related issues, minority and women's affairs, and groups that fight racism and bigotry. *Education:* 35%. About one-half of education support reaches precollege education programs and institutions, K-12 education, and community colleges. The other half supports colleges and universities, with special emphasis on business, automotive design, and engineering programs; state associations of colleges and universities; tax and economic education, minority education programs; and national educational organizations. Also provides scholarships for employees' children and matching gifts. The goal of the fund's educational spending is to prepare the future workforce. *Environment:* 21%. Supports organizations serving youth and the disadvantaged, community centers, and United Way. *International:* 4%. Supports the American Red Cross, single-disease health organizations and medical research. *Religion:* 6%. Supports science centers. *Note:* Total contributions made by DaimlerChrysler Corp. Fund in 1999. **Typ. Recipients:** Cancer, Diabetes, Emergency/Ambulance Services, Eyes/Blindness, Health Organizations, Hospices, Hospitals, People with Disabilities, Speech & Hearing, Substance Abuse. **Geo. Dist:** headquarters and operating communities and nationally.

## ★ 987 ★ Dain Rauscher Foundation

Dain Rauscher Plz.
PO Box 1160
Minneapolis, MN 55440-1160
**Phone:** (612)371-2765          **Fax:** (612)371-7933
**Website:** http://www.dain.com
Sherry Koster, Charitable Giving Specialist Senior

**Fnded:** 1961. **Priorities:** *Arts & Humanities:* About 25%. Interests include art institutes, associations, and centers; public broadcasting; theater; music; and programs that generate an appreciation of diverse cultures. *Civic & Public Affairs:* 13%. Supports community youth organizations and foundations. *Education:* About 21%. Emphasizes helping young people understand our country's economic system and helping disadvantaged youth. Supports K-12 programs that impact students of color or the economically disadvantaged. *Environment:* 32%. Supports the United Way. Special Olympics, family services, family planning, domestic violence concerns, and food distribution. Focuses on fostering economic independence, self-sufficiency, breaking the cycle of poverty, and strengthening the family. *International:* 9%. Supports the Courage Center and children's hospital. **Typ. Recipients:** AIDS/HIV, Cancer, Children's Health/Hospitals, Clinics/Medical Centers, Diabetes, Domestic Violence, Emergency/Ambulance Services, Family Planning, Health Organizations, Health-General, Heart, Hospices, Hospitals, Kidney, Medical Rehabilitation, Medical Research, People with Disabilities, Prenatal Health Issues, Public Health, Research/Studies Institutes, Sexual Abuse, Single-Disease Health Associations, Substance Abuse. **Geo. Dist:** headquarters and operating communities; Minneapolis, MN; Saint Paul, MN.

## ★ 988 ★ Dana Corp. Foundation

PO Box 1000
Toledo, OH 43697
**Phone:** (419)535-4601          **Fax:** (419)535-4896
Mr. Don Decker, Administrator

**Priorities:** *Arts & Humanities:* 20%. Emphasis on public broadcasting, arts associations, museums, and music. *Civic & Public Affairs:* 5%. Interests include business and free enterprise, public policy, and zoos and botanical gardens. Other areas of concern include civil rights, environmental affairs, and urban and community affairs. *Education:* 8%. Funding primarily supports colleges and universities. Also supports private, public, and precollege education, and medical and technical education. *Environment:* 63%. Majority of funding supports united funds. Other interests include youth organizations, child welfare, community centers, community service organizations, drug and alcohol programs, and emergency relief. *International:* 2%. Supports hospitals, hospices, health organizations, pediatric health, and medical research. *Note:* Total contributions in fiscal 1999. **Typ. Recipients:** AIDS/HIV, Alzheimers Disease, Cancer, Emergency/Ambulance Services, Eyes/Blindness, Family Planning, Health Organizations, Hospices, Hospitals, Medical Education, People with Disabilities, Preventive Medicine/Wellness Organizations, Single-Disease Health Associations, Substance Abuse. **Geo. Dist:** principally near operating locations and to national organizations.

**★ 989 ★ Danis Foundation**
Two River Place
PO Box 725
Dayton, OH 45401
**Phone:** (937)228-1225
John Danis, President

**Fnded:** 1957. **Priorities:** *Arts & Humanities:* 28%. Supports museums, music, and the performing arts. *Civic & Public Affairs:* 23%. Funds urban affairs, clubs, and festivals. *Education:* 19%. Supports high schools, colleges, and universities. *Environment:* 10%. Supports community centers and shelters. *International:* 6%. Funds children's health care. *Note:* Total foundation contributions made in 1999. **Typ. Recipients:** Alzheimers Disease, Arthritis, Cancer, Children's Health/Hospitals, Clinics/Medical Centers, Health Funds, Health Organizations, Heart, Hospices, Hospitals, Medical Education, Medical Research, People with Disabilities, Public Health, Single-Disease Health Associations. **Geo. Dist:** OH.

**★ 990 ★ Dayton Power and Light Co. Foundation**
Courthouse Plaza Southwest
PO Box 1247
Dayton, OH 45401
**Phone:** (937)259-7131      **Fax:** (937)259-7245
**Website:** http://www.waytogo.com/support_community.html
Vicki Shortal, Foundation Administrator

**Priorities:** *Arts & Humanities:* 46%. Supports arts centers, opera, dance, theater, and orchestras. *Civic & Public Affairs:* 24%. Supports ecomonic development efforts, community improvement, historical societies, and crime prevention. *Education:* 7%. Support includes colleges and universities, public schools, and scholarships. *Environment:* 23%. Supports united funds and other health related organizations and youth organizations, including a large amount of support to YMCA's. *Note:* Total foundation contributions in 1999. **Typ. Recipients:** Alzheimers Disease, Cancer, Children's Health/Hospitals, Domestic Violence, People with Disabilities, Substance Abuse, Transplant Networks/Donor Banks. **Geo. Dist:** headquarters and operating communities.

**★ 991 ★ DeKalb Genetics Foundation**
3100 Sycamore Rd.
DeKalb, IL 60115
**Phone:** (815)758-9116
Bob Pritchard, Contact

**Fnded:** 1964. **Priorities:** *Civic & Public Affairs:* 4%. Supports civic improvements and agricultural issues. *Education:* 5%. Funds colleges and universities and agricultural education programs. *Environment:* 89%. Major grant to YMCA; also funds the United Way. *International:* 1%. Supports hospitals and medical centers. *Note:* Total contributions made in fiscal 1999. **Typ. Recipients:** Cancer, Clinics/Medical Centers, Emergency/Ambulance Services, Health Policy/Cost Containment, Health-General, Heart, Hospices, Hospitals, Mental Health, Preventive Medicine/Wellness Organizations, Substance Abuse. **Geo. Dist:** headquarters and operating communities.

**★ 992 ★ Delta Air Lines Foundation**
Hartsfield Atlanta International Airport
Department 979
Atlanta, GA 30320
**Phone:** (404)715-7922      **Fax:** (404)715-5876
**Email:** mike.young-air@deltaair.com
**Website:** http://www.delta-air.com/inside/community/index.jsp
Michael Young, Vice President, Community Affairs

**Priorities:** *Arts & Humanities:* 13%. Supports theater, performing arts, music, and art. *Civic & Public Affairs:* 13%. Supports community affairs and neighborhood development. *Education:* 26%. Funds educational programs, colleges and universities, and a matching gift program. *Environment:* 38%. Supports homeless, youth and social services, and the United Way. *International:* 10%. *Note:* Total contributions in fiscal 1999. **Typ. Recipients:** AIDS/HIV, Children's Health/Hospitals, Clinics/Medical Centers, Diabetes, Emergency/Ambulance Services, Health Organizations, Heart, Hospitals, Medical Education, Medical Education, People with Disabilities. **Geo. Dist:** headquarters and operating communities.

**★ 993 ★ Deluxe Corp. Foundation**
PO Box 64235
Saint Paul, MN 55164-0235
**Phone:** (651)483-7842      **Fax:** (651)481-4371
**Email:** jenny.anderson@deluxe.com
**Website:** http://www.dlx.com/foundation.cfm
Jennifer Anderson, Director of Foundations

**Fnded:** 1952. **Priorities:** *Arts & Humanities:* 23%. Supports public broadcasting, museums, theater, arts associations and centers, music, dance, and arts appreciation. *Civic & Public Affairs:* 7%. Funds economic development and industrialization, minority affairs/services, and a zoo. *Education:* 28%. Funding supports colleges and universities, education in the arts, student aid, education funds, and scholarships that are administered through the National Merit Scholarship Corporation, National Hispanic Scholarship Fund, and the United Negro College Fund. Also supports literacy initiatives, primary and secondary education, and Junior Achievement. *Environment:* 27%. Major support goes to the United Way. Also supports youth programs, with emphasis on at-risk youth; programs that serve the mentally challenged, with a special focus on employment programs; programs that serve people who are physically challenged; programs for senior citizens e.g., home delivered meals, companionship, chore services and other programs that enable seniors to remain in their homes; programs for victims of domestic abuse; transitional housing programs; programs that provide emergency needs, e.g., clothing, food, housing; programs that assist financially disadvantaged people; and programs that serve people of color. *International:* 2%. Funds women's cancer research, pediatric health and diseases, health centers, and suicide prevention. *Religion:* 7%. Majority of support is given to science museums. *Note:* Total contributions in 1999. **Typ. Recipients:** AIDS/HIV, Cancer, Children's Health/Hospitals, Clinics/Medical Centers, Domestic Violence, Emergency/Ambulance Services, Eyes/Blindness, Health Organizations, Medical Education, Medical Rehabilitation, People with Disabilities, Single-Disease Health Associations, Substance Abuse. **Geo. Dist:** headquarters and operating communities.

**★ 994 ★ Demoulas Foundation**
286 Chelmsford St.
Chelmsford, MA 01824
**Phone:** (978)224-1024      **Fax:** (978)640-8392
T. Demoulas, Contact

**Fnded:** 1964. **Priorities:** *Arts & Humanities:* 4%. Supports a variety of arts organizations, including ballet and operas, music, arts centers, and museums. *Civic & Public Affairs:* 1%. A majority of funding supports urban affairs and revitalization projects. Also supports philanthropic organizations. *Education:* 13%. Majority of funding supports colleges and universities in the New England area. Also supports religious education and private secondary education. *Environment:* 12%. Funds community centers, recreation, and

youth organizations. Community service organizations, the disabled, food and clothing distribution, and housing also receive funds. *International:* 20%. The majority of support funds hospitals. Also supports medical rehabilitation for burn victims, pediatric health, and single-disease health associations. *Note:* Total contributions in 1999. **Typ. Recipients:** Cancer, Children's Health/Hospitals, Diabetes, Health Organizations, Hospices, Hospitals, Long-Term Care, Medical Education, Medical Rehabilitation, Medical Research, People with Disabilities, Respiratory, Single-Disease Health Associations, Substance Abuse, Trauma Treatment. **Geo. Dist:** primarily New England.

**★ 995 ★ Deposit Guaranty Foundation**
1 Deposit Guaranty Plz.
Jackson, MS 39215
**Phone:** (601)354-8571      **Fax:** (601)354-8192
James Moore, Senior Vice President, Public Affairs

**Priorities:** *Arts & Humanities:* 5% to 10%. Supports arts associations, dance, museums, music, theater, opera, community and performing arts, and symphonies. *Civic & Public Affairs:* Less than 5%. Funding supports housing, community development, and youth organizations. *Education:* 50% to 55%. Majority supports Mississippi colleges and universities. Other interests include public education, education funds, international studies, and private education. *Environment:* 25% to 30%. Supports family services, food banks, youth services, and the United Way. *International:* Less than 5%. Supports medical centers and single-disease associations. *Note:* Total contributions in fiscal 1999. **Typ. Recipients:** Children's Health/Hospitals, Diabetes, Health Organizations, Hospitals, People with Disabilities, Single-Disease Health Associations, Substance Abuse, Transplant Networks/Donor Banks. **Geo. Dist:** MS.

**★ 996 ★ Deutsch Foundation**
2444 Wilshire Blvd., Ste. 600
Santa Monica, CA 90403
**Phone:** (310)453-0055      **Fax:** (310)453-6467
Lester Deutsch, Executive Vice President

**Priorities:** *Arts & Humanities:* 7%. Interests include music centers, museums, dance societies, and public broadcasting. *Civic & Public Affairs:* 5%. Supports women's affairs, gardens, community foundations, and environmental concerns. *Education:* 13%. Supports colleges and universities, public and private precollege education, art schools, and education associations. *Environment:* 10%. Youth organizations are major recipients. Other interests include sexual abuse issues, substance abuse prevention programs, aid for the homeless, athletics, and animal welfare. *International:* 16%. Interests include single-disease health organizations, pediatric and geriatric medicine, and health centers. *Note:* Total contributions in fiscal 1999. **Typ. Recipients:** Arthritis, Cancer, Children's Health/Hospitals, Clinics/Medical Centers, Eyes/Blindness, Family Planning, Geriatric Health, Health Organizations, Health-General, Hospitals, Hospitals (University Affiliated), Medical Rehabilitation, Medical Research, Mental Health, People with Disabilities, Public Health, Research/Studies Institutes, Sexual Abuse, Single-Disease Health Associations, Speech & Hearing, Substance Abuse, Trauma Treatment. **Geo. Dist:** CA, including southern California.

**★ 997 ★ Dexter Corp. Foundation**
1 Elm St.
Windsor Locks, CT 06096
**Phone:** (860)627-9051      **Fax:** (860)292-7669
Lani Kretschmar, Coordinator

**Priorities:** *Arts & Humanities:* 16%. Areas of interest include arts associations, historic preservation, museums, music, opera, public broadcasting, theater, dance, history, and libraries. *Civic & Public Affairs:* 7%. Interests include economic development, public policy, safety, and urban and women's affairs organizations. *Education:* 23%. Foundation primarily gives funds in the form of matching gifts. Direct support goes to education funds, colleges and universities, minority education organizations, public secondary schools, religious education, and community and junior colleges. *Environment:* 37%. Most support goes to the United Way in the form of employee matching gifts; other interests include shelters for the homeless, organizations that help the abused, youth organizations, food and clothing distribution, and volunteer services. *International:* 13%. Interests include hospitals, single-disease health associations, health funds, mental health organizations, pediatric health, and nursing services. *Note:* Total contributions made in 1999. **Typ. Recipients:** Children's Health/Hospitals, Clinics/Medical Centers, Domestic Violence, Emergency/Ambulance Services, Health Funds, Health Organizations, Hospitals, Mental Health, Nursing Services, People with Disabilities, Public Health, Single-Disease Health Associations, Substance Abuse. **Geo. Dist:** CT, headquarters and operating communities, including Dexter; Hartford, CT.

### ★ 998 ★ Dickson Foundation
301 South Tryon St., Ste. 1800
Charlotte, NC 28202
**Phone:** (704)372-5404          **Fax:** (704)372-6409
Susan Patterson, Secretary & Treasurer

**Priorities:** *Arts & Humanities:* 8%. Funds visual arts centers, museums, and the Arts and Sciences Council. *Civic & Public Affairs:* 11%. Funds business and free enterprise, minority affairs, municipalities, and community affairs. *Education:* 42%. Primarily supports colleges and universities in North Carolina, specifically the University of North Carolina, Wake Forest University, and North Carolina University. Also supports education funds, faculty development, medical education, and secondary schools. *Environment:* 12%. Supports United Way and family and youth services. *International:* 10%. Supports medical centers, hospitals, and hospices; single-disease health associations also receive support. *Religion:* 1%. *Note:* Contributions made in 2000. **Typ. Recipients:** Clinics/Medical Centers, Health Organizations, Health-General, Heart, Hospices, Hospitals, Medical Education, Medical Research, Preventive Medicine/Wellness Organizations, Single-Disease Health Associations, Substance Abuse. **Geo. Dist:** FL; GA; NC; SC; TN.

### ★ 999 ★ Diebold, Inc.
PO Box 3077
5995 Mayfair Rd.
North Canton, OH 44720-8077
**Phone:** (330)490-4000          **Fax:** (330)490-4549
**Email:** scheurc@diebold.com
**Website:** http://www.diebold.com
Charles Scheurer, Vice President, Human Resources

**Typ. Recipients:** Health-General. **Geo. Dist:** headquarters and operating communities.

### ★ 1000 ★ Dixie Yarns Foundation, Inc.
PO Box 751
Chattanooga, TN 37401
**Phone:** (423)698-2501          **Fax:** (423)493-7450
Ms. Starr Klein, Secretary, Treasurer & Trustee

**Priorities:** *Arts & Humanities:* 18%. Gives to art councils, museums, and public broadcasting. *Civic & Public Affairs:* 3%. Supports housing for the disadvantaged, community foundations, urban development, and a conference center. *Education:* 34%. Gives to variety of educational organizations, including colleges and universities, minority education, private precollege education, and Junior Achievement. *Environment:* 35%. Majority of contributions support United Way chapters near company's headquarters and operating locations. Also gives to youth organizations, YMCAs, community service organizations, and religious welfare. *International:* 1%. Provides funding to a mental health initiative for the homeless. *Note:* Total contributions made in 1999. **Typ. Recipients:** Children's Health/Hospitals, Clinics/Medical Centers, Health Organizations, Hospitals, Medical Research, Mental Health, Substance Abuse. **Geo. Dist:** Chattanooga, TN.

### ★ 1001 ★ Dominion Resources, Inc.
PO Box 26532
Richmond, VA 23261

**Phone:** (804)819-2580          **Fax:** (804)819-2217
**Email:** reneejohnson@dom.com
**Website:** http://www.dom.com/about/foundation/index.html
Renee Johnson, Contributions Coordinator

**Priorities:** *Arts & Humanities:* 10% to 15%. Supports theater, ballet, symphonic and choral music, opera, art councils, museums, multicultural arts associations, and public broadcasting. *Education:* 15% to 20%. Supports early childhood and precollege basics programs, accredited private colleges and universities, independent college funds, job creation and training programs. *International:* 40% to 50%. Supports United Way, health care groups, volunteer fire and rescue squads, Red Cross, civic groups, neighborhood improvement, cultural diversity groups, shelters, programs for older Americans, literacy programs, and programs for the homeless. **Typ. Recipients:** Emergency/Ambulance Services, Health Organizations, Hospices, Hospitals, Mental Health, People with Disabilities, Substance Abuse. **Geo. Dist:** operating locations.

### ★ 1002 ★ Donaldson Foundation
PO Box 1299 MS 100
Minneapolis, MN 55440
**Phone:** (612)703-4999          **Fax:** (612)887-3005
**Email:** donaldsonfoundation@mail.donaldson.com
Norman Linnell, President & Trustee

**Priorities:** *Arts & Humanities:* 3%. Supports public broadcasting, arts centers, arts institutes, museums, theater, and historical preservation. *Civic & Public Affairs:* 8%. *Education:* 35%. Support goes to the foundation's scholarship program. Other interests include minority education funds, colleges and universities, engineering, law economics, and public education. *Environment:* About 39%. Supports general charities, including United Way, health relief organizations, and community centers. Counseling and rehabilitation receive limited support; interests include opportunity workshops, homes, family planning, welfare transition, religious charity groups, and resources for women. *International:* 5%. **Typ. Recipients:** Children's Health/Hospitals, Clinics/Medical Centers, Domestic Violence, Emergency/Ambulance Services, Family Planning, Health Funds, Health Organizations, Hospices, Hospitals, Medical Rehabilitation, Mental Health, People with Disabilities, Preventive Medicine/Wellness Organizations, Public Health, Substance Abuse. **Geo. Dist:** headquarters and operating communities.

### ★ 1003 ★ Dow Chemical Co. Foundation
47 Bldg.
Midland, MI 48667
**Phone:** (517)636-6891          **Fax:** (517)638-7238
**Website:** http://www.dow.com/about/corp.corp.htm
Mr. Jerold Ring, Director of Global Contributions & Commu

**Priorities:** *Arts & Humanities:* 7%. Funds children's museums, the performing arts, museums, and arts centers. *Civic & Public Affairs:* 10%. Supports community development, economic concerns, and engineering organizations. *Education:* 38%. Highest priority of foundation. Chemical science education is main focus. Supports basic research and education in the physical and natural sciences at U.S. colleges and universities. Funding includes chemical engineering faculty support. A limited number of universities receive grants for undergraduate scholarships in the physical and natural sciences. Also supports science-based institutions and organizations such as the National Science Resource Center, American Chemical Society, Council for Chemical Research, and the Mathematical Association. K-12 education grants support math and science, teacher training, and parental involvement; educational initiatives include the Hands-On Science Program, Keystone Summer Initiatives Workshop, MATHCOUNTS, and Presidential Classroom. *Environment:* 20%. Supports domestic violence and sexual abuse centers, community centers, youth and child services, and the United Way. *Religion:* 7%. Funds science centers and associations. *Note:* Percentages reflect foundation grants made in 2000. Through direct giving programs, company and divisions disburse

approximately 60% of support to Education, 30% to Health and Community Betterment, about 5% to Arts and Culture, and the remaining 5% to miscellaneous recipients. Company operating divisions administer independent contributions programs. Divisions support community projects (United Way and groups concerned with child welfare, health care, drug abuse prevention, etc.) and cultural activities in areas in which they are located. **Typ. Recipients:** Domestic Violence. **Geo. Dist:** nationally.

### ★ 1004 ★ Dow Corning Foundation
Midland, MI 48686-0994
**Phone:** (517)496-6290          **Fax:** (517)496-4393
**Email:** a.m.deboer@dowcorning.com
Anne DeBoer, Executive Director

**Priorities:** *Arts & Humanities:* 4%. Supports arts centers. *Civic & Public Affairs:* 32%. Supports job training, parks, zoos, community foundations, and fire departments. *Education:* 21%. Supports both privately endowed and tax-supported colleges and universities. The majority of aid to education is directed toward institutions that have been sources of new employees, have strong, effective minority programs, or provide science and math improvements in K-12 education. *Environment:* 43%. Funds family and community centers. *Note:* Percentages reflect foundation contributions made in 1999. **Typ. Recipients:** Child Abuse, Medical Research. **Geo. Dist:** headquarters and operating communities.

### ★ 1005 ★ DTE Energy Foundation
2000 Second Ave., 1046 WCB
Detroit, MI 48226
**Phone:** (313)235-9271          **Fax:** (313)235-0285
**Email:** hallk@dteenergy.com
**Website:** http://www.dteenergy.com/community/dte-foundation.html
Karla Hall, Secretary & Manager

**Priorities:** *Arts & Humanities:* (Culture) 18%. Primarily supports region's major cultural institutions. Interests include music, theater, arts centers and funds, libraries, museums, historical societies, and public broadcasting. Youth educational programs and event or project sponsorship are preferable to general operating support. *Civic & Public Affairs:* 21%. Interests include economic development, crime prevention, race relations, public policy research, zoos, environmental programs, and neighborhood revitalization. Urban and community development coalitions are a high priority. Particular interest in local citizen and community self-help initiatives and projects where funds can complement support from the public sector. *Education:* 23%. Funds school readiness (pre-school), K-12 education improvement, vocational education, school-to-work and career awareness programs, citizenship education, environmental education, and higher education. In higher education, emphasis is placed on business and engineering and programs that increase student participation and retention, including pre-college math and science enrichment programs, and student tutoring and mentoring programs. *Environment:* (Health and Human Services) 38%. Funds the United Way, emergency food and shelter, teen pregnancy prevention and parenting skills. *Note:* Total cash contributions made in 1998. Percentages provided by foundation. **Typ. Recipients:** Children's Health/Hospitals, Emergency/Ambulance Services, Eyes/Blindness, Health Funds, Health Organizations, Hospices, Hospitals, Medical Education, Mental Health, Public Health, Single-Disease Health Associations, Substance Abuse. **Geo. Dist:** MI, headquarters and operating communities; Detroit, MI.

### ★ 1006 ★ Duchossois Foundation
845 Larch Ave.
Elmhurst, IL 60126-1196
**Phone:** (847)381-6278          **Fax:** (847)381-4102
Kimberly Duchossois, President

**Priorities:** *Arts & Humanities:* 11%. Supports the development and enrichment fine arts, cultural and educational museums, theater, music, and dance. *Civic & Public Affairs:* 13%. Supports public policy, Habitat for Humanity, zoos, and community services.

*Education:* 32%. Funds colleges and universities. *Environment:* 19%. Supports programs that seek to enhance the emotional growth and development of children and youth. *International:* 21%. Supports research, education, and advocacy in three primary areas: AIDS, cancer, and mental health. Major support is for cancer research at the University of Chicago. *Note:* Total contribution in 1998. **Typ. Recipients:** AIDS/HIV, Cancer, Children's Health/Hospitals, Clinics/Medical Centers, Geriatric Health, Health Funds, Health Organizations, Hospices, Hospitals, Hospitals (University Affiliated), Medical Rehabilitation, Medical Research, Mental Health, People with Disabilities, Prenatal Health Issues, Research/Studies Institutes, Single-Disease Health Associations, Speech & Hearing, Substance Abuse. **Geo. Dist:** Chicago, IL.


**★ 1007 ★ Duke Energy Foundation**
422 S Church St.
Charlotte, NC 28202-1904
**Phone:** (704)382-7200          **Fax:** (704)382-7600
**Email:** cecarter@duke-energy.com
**Website:** http://www.duke-energy.com/decorp/content/community/deip22.asp?RBU=1
Christopher Carter, Jr., Director

**Priorities:** *Arts & Humanities:* 15% to 20%. Primarily focuses on museums, art associations, galleries, and art funds. *Civic & Public Affairs:* 5%. Focus is on building strategic capacities of non-profit organizations in operating communities and leadership development. Interests include economic development, zoos and botanical gardens. *Education:* About 40%. Supports colleges and universities, public schools, and educational funds and foundations. Focus is on K-12 science and math instruction. *Environment:* 20% to 25%. Primarily supports United Way chapters. Other interests include youth organizations, food and clothing distribution, and community service organizations. *Voluntarism:* Community Volunteer Grants provide $1,000 for materials for employees and retirees who volunteer time to one-time, hands-on projects, and $1,000 grants to organizations where employees help achieve significant strategic objectives. *Note:* Total contributions made in 1999. **Typ. Recipients:** Adolescent Health Issues, Child Abuse, Domestic Violence, Emergency/Ambulance Services, Family Planning, Health Organizations, Health Policy/Cost Containment, Hospices, Hospitals, Medical Education, Mental Health, Nutrition, People with Disabilities, Single-Disease Health Associations, Substance Abuse. **Geo. Dist:** headquarters and operating communities; NC; SC. **Frmly:** Duke Power Co. Foundation.


**★ 1008 ★ Dun & Bradstreet Corp. Foundation, Inc.**
1 Diamond Hill Rd.
Murray Hill, NJ 07974
**Phone:** (908)665-8052          **Fax:** (908)665-5022
Rosa Guzman, Executive Administrator

**Priorities:** *Arts & Humanities:* Areas of interest include music, art centers, libraries, museums, and the performing arts. *Civic & Public Affairs:* Areas of interest include business, economics, civil rights, law and justice, and public policy. *Education:* Interests include independent and minority college funds, higher education associations, and business education. *Environment:* Majority of funding supports United Way campaigns. Other areas of interest include child welfare, youth groups, and community service organizations. *International:* Supports the American Red Cross, AIDS research, and single-disease health associations. **Typ. Recipients:** AIDS/HIV, Cancer, Emergency/Ambulance Services, Health Organizations, Hospitals, Mental Health, People with Disabilities, Single-Disease Health Associations, Speech & Hearing, Substance Abuse. **Geo. Dist:** nationally.


**★ 1009 ★ Duracell International**
Research Dr.
Berkshire Corporate Park
Bethel, CT 06801
**Phone:** (203)796-4000          **Fax:** (203)796-4483
**Website:** http://www.duracell.com
Jane Steiner, Corporate Contributions Administration

**Typ. Recipients:** Health-General. **Geo. Dist:** principally near operating locations and to national organizations.


**★ 1010 ★ Dynamet, Inc.**
195 Museum Rd.
Washington, PA 15301
**Phone:** (724)228-1000          **Fax:** (724)229-4195
**Website:** http://www.dynamet.com
Sharon Blackford, Exec. Sec. to Pres.

**Priorities:** *Arts & Humanities:* 3%. Supports museums, cultural resources, performing arts, music, and theater. *Education:* 52%. Funds educational programs, and colleges and universities. *Environment:* 3%. Supports handicapped services, volunteer services, senior care, people with mental disabilities, YM/YWCA, and youth services. *International:* 5%. Supports hospitals, rehabilitation centers, and single-disease concerns. *Religion:* 1%. Funds the Carnegie Institute, for scientific research. *Note:* Total contributions in 1998. **Typ. Recipients:** Cancer, Children's Health/Hospitals, Clinics/Medical Centers, Diabetes, Emergency/Ambulance Services, Eyes/Blindness, Health Organizations, Hospices, Hospitals, Kidney, Medical Rehabilitation, Medical Research, Mental Health, People with Disabilities, Single-Disease Health Associations, Substance Abuse. **Geo. Dist:** Pittsburgh, PA.


**★ 1011 ★ E.I. du Pont de Nemours & Co.**
1007 Market St., Room 11046
Wilmington, DE 19898
**Phone:** (302)774-2036          **Fax:** (302)773-2919
**Website:** http://www.dupont.com/corp/community.html
Pat Eggert, Contributions Coordinator

**Priorities:** *Arts & Humanities:* 5% to 10%. Supports local museums, libraries, and other cultural organizations. A limited number of high visibility national organizations also receive funding. *Civic & Public Affairs:* Focus on neighborhood revitalization, economic development, and minority businesses. *Education:* About 45%. Almost all grants are made at the initiative of the Committee on Educational Aid, not in response to proposals or requests. Most support falls within six main categories: University Science and Engineering Grants, supporting undergraduate business, science, and engineering departments and interdisciplinary programs in such areas as occupational and environmental health; Minority Education Grants, to colleges and universities for scholarships and programs to advance the science and engineering education of minorities and to K-12 programs to help prepare minority students for engineering and technical careers; Young Faculty Grants, for research assistants; College Science Grants, to liberal arts colleges producing significant numbers of graduates who go on to advanced studies in science; Business and Economic Grants, supporting training and research at business schools; and Secondary School Grants, emphasizing improvement of teaching in science and economics. The bulk of funding is awarded in the first two categories listed above. The educational program emphasizes physical and life sciences, with grants awarded on the basis of scope, quality of institution's teaching and research, and company's research and recruitment needs. The goals of the program include the following: stimulating applied and basic research; improving higher, secondary, and special educational support programs for minorities in science, engineering, and business management; increasing the number of top graduates, minority scholars, and prospective employees in the fields of company enterprise; and promoting programs to improve the national science policy. Additional areas funded in recent years include energy policy, materials science, and computer-based science applications. Other educational support activities include sponsorship of visiting and adjunct professorships and postdoctoral appointments in DuPont research labs. Does not award direct grants to individuals; endowment and capital grants do not fall within preferred areas of giving. *International:* 15% to 20%. Primarily supports United Way programs. Strong support is also given to hospital capital campaigns and health projects in operating locations. Other contributions go toward occupational medicine, the elderly, and the disabled. **Typ. Recipients:** Domestic Violence, Emergency/Ambulance Services, Geriatric Health, Health Organizations, Health Policy/Cost Containment, Hospices, Hospitals, Medical Rehabilitation, Medical Research, Medical Training, Mental Health, People with Disabilities, Single-Disease Health Associations, Substance Abuse. **Geo. Dist:** headquarters and operating communities.


**★ 1012 ★ E.L. Craig Foundation**
PO Box 1404
Joplin, MO 64802
**Phone:** (417)624-6644
Ethel Humphreys, President

**Fnded:** 1960. **Priorities:** *Civic & Public Affairs:* 81%. Supports business institutions, as well as policy groups and think-tanks. *Education:* 19%. Funds the Institute for Humane Studies and universities. *Note:* Total contributions made in fiscal 2000. **Typ. Recipients:** Cancer, Hospitals, People with Disabilities, Public Health, Single-Disease Health Associations. **Geo. Dist:** nationally; Joplin, MO.


**★ 1013 ★ Eastern Bank Charitable Foundation**
217 Essex St.
Salem, MA 01970
**Phone:** (978)740-6319          **Fax:** (978)740-6329
Sumner Jones, Executive Vice President

**Fnded:** 1985. **Priorities:** *Arts & Humanities:* 12%. Funds public broadcasting, libraries, museums, theaters, and community centers. *Civic & Public Affairs:* 9%. Supports housing and community and economic development. *Education:* 10%. Supports scholarship funds, colleges and universities, public and private elementary and secondary schools, and public libraries. *Environment:* 54%. Supports YMCAs, United Way, children and family services, food banks, and services and activities for the mentally and physically challenged. *International:* 12%. Funds hospitals and medical centers, single-disease organizations, and mental health centers. *Note:* Total contributions in 1999. **Typ. Recipients:** AIDS/HIV, Cancer, Children's Health/Hospitals, Clinics/Medical Centers, Domestic Violence, Health Organizations, Health-General, Heart, Hospices, Hospitals, Medical Education, Mental Health, People with Disabilities, Preventive Medicine/Wellness Organizations, Single-Disease Health Associations. **Geo. Dist:** MA, market area.


**★ 1014 ★ Eastman Chemical Co.**
PO Box 431
Kingsport, TN 37662
**Phone:** (423)229-1413          **Fax:** (423)229-8280
**Email:** p.montgomery@eastman.com
**Website:** http://www.eastman.com
Paul Montgomery, Manager, Community Relations

**Typ. Recipients:** Health-General. **Geo. Dist:** headquarters and operating communities.


**★ 1015 ★ Eastman Kodak Charitable Trust**
343 State St.
Rochester, NY 14650-0517
**Phone:** (716)724-2434          **Fax:** (716)724-1376
**Website:** http://www.kodak.com/US/en/corp/community.shtml
Essie Calhoun, President

**Priorities:** *Arts & Humanities:* 13%. Funds museums, film and photography institutes, and the performing arts. *Civic & Public Affairs:* Less than 1%. Civic interests include youth programs, community centers, zoos, environmental conservation, economic development, home and neighborhood rehabilitation, employment programs, promotion of equal opportunities, and examination of key social issues. Also supports culture and the arts. *Education:* 1%. Supports colleges, universities, preschool, and K-12 educational programs nationwide, with emphasis on science and engineering education. University funding includes seed money or start-up grants for research in the areas of U.S. manufacturing competitiveness, optics, imaging science, biotechnology, electronics, and material processing. Also provides scholarships. Kodak Fellows program provides grants to graduate students and specific departments of science and engineering. Educational organizations supported include minority and independent college funds, economics, and minority engineering associations. On the precollege level, focuses on academic opportunities in scientific, mathematics, and technical disciplines. Sponsors partnerships between the company and precollege educational institutions in local Kodak communities to improve science and mathematics achievement for all students. Also funds school-based initiatives that aim at acquainting students with opportunities in manufacturing. *Environment:* 53%. Principally supports the United Way. Youth groups, local and national health organizations, job training, homes and shelters, child welfare, and services for the aged and the handicapped are also supported. *International:* 1%. *Voluntarism:* Company offers "Dollars for Doers" program through which it makes small donations to nonprofit organizations where company employees serve as volunteers; supports Global Service Day; when all employees are encouraged to volunteer in their communities. *Note:* Total contributions made by the foundation in 1999. **Typ. Recipients:** Clinics/Medical Centers, Emergency/Ambulance Services, Health Organizations, Health-General, Hospitals, Medical Rehabilitation, Mental Health, Nursing Services, People with Disabilities, Single-Disease Health Associations. **Geo. Dist:** nationally, especially in operating locations.

### ★ 1016 ★ Eaton Charitable Fund
1111 Superior Ave.
Cleveland, OH 44114-2584
**Phone:** (216)523-4452          **Fax:** (216)479-7013
**Website:** http://www.eaton.com/about/report.html
James Mason, Vice President, Public & Community Affai

**Fnded:** 1953. **Priorities:** *Civic & Public Affairs:* 30%. Within Eaton's Community Improvement giving area, the foundation contributes to organizations that help people become self-sufficient, strengthen families, encourage neighborhood and economic development, and enhance the qualify of life through civic, cultural and arts programs. Contributes to housing, shelters and social services, youth activities, health care facilities, and visual and performing arts institutions, public radio and television, civic improvements, and humanitarian efforts. *Education:* 24%. Gifts go to educational institutions for programs that help students prepare for careers in business and industry, particularly in engineering. Supports programs that attract students at all grade levels to the study of math, science, and technology. Contributes to programs that help students overcome barriers to academic achievement and complete their education. Awards scholarships for minority engineering students. *Environment:* 35%. Supports the United Way, primarily in Eaton operating communities. *Voluntarism:* Volunteer services of all types are encouraged. Volunteers support many causes including teaching reading to the illiterate, coaching little league softball, organizing school aid programs, serving food at hunger centers, building houses for the needy, and chairing United Way campaigns. Company sponsors the James R. Stover Awards to recognize employee volunteers, and makes cash grants to organizations where employees contribute their time and talents. *Note:* Contributions made in 2000. **Typ. Recipients:** Cancer, Clinics/Medical Centers, Emergency/Ambulance Services, Health Funds, Health Organizations, Health Policy/Cost Containment, Hospices, Hospitals, Hospitals (University Affiliated), Nursing Services, People with Disabilities, Public Health, Single-Disease Health Associations. **Geo. Dist:** corporate operating locations.

### ★ 1017 ★ Echoing Green Foundation
24 East 21st St.
New York, NY 10016
**Phone:** (212)689-1165          **Fax:** (212)689-9010
**Website:** http://www.echoinggreen.org
Sandra Jones, Director of Search & Selection

**Fnded:** 1987. **Typ. Recipients:** AIDS/HIV, Domestic Violence, Emergency/Ambulance Services, Health Organizations, Medical Education, Mental Health, Public Health, Substance Abuse. **Geo. Dist:** NY, emphasis on New York.

### ★ 1018 ★ Eckerd Corp. Foundation
PO Box 4689
Clearwater, FL 33758
**Phone:** (727)395-6289          **Fax:** (727)395-7934
**Email:** webmaster@eckerd.com
Tami Alderman, Community and Public Relations Project M

**Priorities:** *Arts & Humanities:* 1%. *Civic & Public Affairs:* 6%. *Education:* 25%. Supports United Negro College Fund and Colleges of Pharmacy. *Environment:* 56%. Supports United Way and children's organizations. *International:* 8%. Funds national health organizations. *Note:* Total contributions made in fiscal 1999. **Typ. Recipients:** Cancer, Clinics/Medical Centers, Diabetes, Emergency/Ambulance Services, Family Planning, Health Funds, Health Organizations, Heart, Hospices, Hospitals, Medical Education, Multiple Sclerosis, People with Disabilities, Prenatal Health Issues, Public Health. **Geo. Dist:** CT; DE; FL; GA; KS; LA; MD; MS; MO; NJ; NY; NC; OH; OK; PA; SC; TN; TX; VA; WV.

### ★ 1019 ★ Edison International
Edison International
2244 Walnut Grove Ave.
PO Box 800
Rosemead, CA 91770
**Phone:** (626)302-9853          **Fax:** (626)302-8114
**Email:** Lucia.Galindo@.sce.com
**Website:** http://www.edison.com
Lucia Galindo, Manager, Corporate Contributions

**Typ. Recipients:** Geriatric Health, Health Organizations, Hospices, Hospitals, Nursing Services, People with Disabilities, Substance Abuse. **Geo. Dist:** CA, primarily in company's Southern CA service area; strategic giving outside traditional service territory.

### ★ 1020 ★ EDS Corp.
5400 Legacy Dr., H3-6F-47
Plano, TX 75024
**Phone:** (972)605-0329          **Fax:** (972)605-8625
**Website:** http://www.eds.com/about_eds/about_eds_community.shtml
Dale McKay, Manager, Community Contributions

**Priorities:** *Voluntarism:* Each year, the company sponsors a "Global Volunteer Day," an annual day of celebration for ongoing volunteerism and giving back. As the volunteerism movement has grown worldwide, EDS' program has grown in interest and participation. **Typ. Recipients:** People with Disabilities, Substance Abuse. **Geo. Dist:** headquarters and operating communities.

### ★ 1021 ★ El Paso Energy Foundation
1001 Louisiana St.
Houston, TX 77002
**Phone:** (713)420-2878          **Fax:** (713)420-4993
Karen King, Manager

**Fnded:** 1992. **Priorities:** *Arts & Humanities:* 20%. Cultural support includes the performing arts, visual arts, historical centers, public and educational broadcasting, and other related activities. *Civic & Public Affairs:* 3%. Supports economic and community development and ethnic affairs organizations. Other interests include organizations that are government-related, community-based organizations concerned with crime prevention, and parks and recreation facilities. *Education:* 34%. Supports public and private colleges and universities throughout its service region. Also provides major support for a summer school for the arts. Generally, contributions are directed toward the improvement of the quality of education. Funds a scholarship program. *Environment:* 40%. Major support for the United Way and community chests. Also supports youth organizations, programs assisting runaway youth, scouting, clubs, YMCA/YWCA, chemical

dependency prevention, senior citizens, spouse and child abuse prevention, offender programs, and women's programs. *International:* 1%. Supports hospitals and medical facilities and programs such as hospital building, equipment, and improvement campaigns. Also funds the American Red Cross. *Note:* Total foundation contributions made in 1999. **Typ. Recipients:** Alzheimers Disease, Cancer, Child Abuse, Domestic Violence, Hospices, Hospitals (University Affiliated), Medical Rehabilitation, Medical Research, Nursing Services, People with Disabilities, Public Health, Substance Abuse. **Geo. Dist:** nationally, AZ; CA; CO; NM; TX, western area.

### ★ 1022 ★ Eli Lilly Foundation
Lilly Corporate Center
Indianapolis, IN 46285
**Phone:** (317)276-3177          **Fax:** (317)277-6719
**Email:** tom@lilly.com
**Website:** http://www.lilly.com/about/community/foundation/
Thomas King, President

**Priorities:** *Arts & Humanities:* 11%. Priorities include Indianapolis music and theater groups. Also supports arts funds and associations, historic preservation, museums, children's museums and concerts, and dance. Focus is on plant-site communities. *Civic & Public Affairs:* 5%. Supports zoos and other interests such as public policy, local economic development, diversity, and urban and community affairs. *Education:* 45%. Major support goes to pharmaceutical and medical education, colleges and universities, and higher education associations. Also funds minority education and precollege education. Focus is on science and technical education. *Environment:* 20%. Primarily to the United Way. *International:* 10%. Primary support goes to united funds in corporate communities. Supports medical research, medical centers, and local health organizations, primarily in Indiana. Also funds national health organizations concerned with health and human services related to Lilly's major theraputic interests. Foundation provides matching gifts to the United Way. *Note:* Percentages are based on cash grants only. **Typ. Recipients:** AIDS/HIV, Cancer, Children's Health/Hospitals, Diabetes, Emergency/Ambulance Services, Health Organizations, Health Policy/Cost Containment, Heart, Medical Education, Medical Research, Mental Health, People with Disabilities, Prenatal Health Issues, Public Health, Public Health, Single-Disease Health Associations, Trauma Treatment. **Geo. Dist:** headquarters and operating communities; international organizations; national organizations.

### ★ 1023 ★ Emerson Charitable Trust
8000 West Florissant Ave.
PO Box 63136
Saint Louis, MO 63136
**Phone:** (314)553-2000
Ms. Joann Harmon, Senior Vice President

**Priorities:** *Arts & Humanities:* 14%. Almost all awards support organizations in the St. Louis area. Areas of interest are symphonies, arts centers, dance, historical societies, museums, and opera. Administers small matching gifts program in the arts. *Civic & Public Affairs:* 19%. Areas of interest include minority representation in professional organizations, zoos and botanical gardens, business and free enterprise, public policy, and urban affairs. *Education:* 37%. The majority is awarded to colleges and universities. Emphasis is on business, engineering, and technical education, with some interest in legal and medical education and public school systems. The majority of grants in this category are awarded in communities near company operating locations. Company administers employee matching grants program in education, and sponsors an educational scholarship program for children of employees. *Environment:* 24%. Supports youth development through mentoring, scouting, and related organizations. *International:* About 4%. Emphasis on united funds and youth organizations near company operating locations. Other areas of interest include community centers, homes, animal welfare, recreation and athletics, and substance abuse prevention and treatment. *Note:* Foundation giving accounts for 80% of contributions; direct giving, 20%. Above priorities reflect foundation giving in fiscal 1999. **Typ. Recipients:** AIDS/HIV, Alzheimers Disease, Children's Health/Hospitals, Eyes/Blindness, Health Organizations, Hospitals, Long-Term Care, Medical Education, Medical Research, People with Disabilities, Single-Disease Health Associations, Substance Abuse. **Geo. Dist:** nationally, emphasizing operating locations.

★ 1024 ★ **Employers Insurance of Wausau, A Mutual Co.**
2000 Westwood Dr.
PO Box 8017
Wausau, WI 54402-8017
**Phone:** (715)845-5211          **Fax:** (715)843-3690
**Website:** http://www.wausau.com
Brad Zweck, Senior Public Relations Coordinator

**Typ. Recipients:** Health-General. **Geo. Dist:** primarily at headquarters and operating communities.

★ 1025 ★ **Employers Mutual Charitable Foundation**
PO Box 712
Des Moines, IA 50303
**Phone:** (515)280-2788
Joe Smith, Manager, Executive Director

**Priorities:** *Arts & Humanities:* 26%. Funds art centers, music, and historic preservation. *Civic & Public Affairs:* 12%. Supports community foundations and a zoo. *Education:* 22%. Focus on higher education. *Environment:* 38%. Funds United Ways, YMCAs, and youth organzations. *International:* 1%. *Religion:* 1%. *Note:* Total contributions made in 1999. **Typ. Recipients:** Children's Health/Hospitals, Diabetes, Emergency/Ambulance Services, Eyes/Blindness, Health Policy/Cost Containment, Health-General, Hospices, Hospitals, Multiple Sclerosis, People with Disabilities. **Geo. Dist:** IA.

★ 1026 ★ **Ensign-Bickford Foundation**
10 Mill Pond Rd.
Simsbury, CT 06070
**Phone:** (860)658-4411          **Fax:** (860)843-2805
**Website:** http://www.e-bind.com/community.html
Linda Angelastro, Executive Director, Corporate Communicat

**Fnded:** 1952. **Priorities:** *Arts & Humanities:* 10%. Supports libraries, arts associations and councils, theater, dance and museums. *Civic & Public Affairs:* 8%. Supports municipalities and towns, public parks, fire companies and police forces, civic clubs, chambers of commerce, and community developments, including an ice rink. *Education:* 46%. Supports public and private schools, especially high school activities. Also provides a small number of community scholarships. *Environment:* 4%. Supports united funds, YMCA, scouting, Boy Scouts, Big Brothers/Big Sisters, and sports and recreation for youth. *International:* 6%. Funds hospitals. *Religion:* 11%. Supports a science center and the Mineral Information Institute. *Note:* Total foundation contributions made in 1999. **Typ. Recipients:** Cancer, Children's Health/Hospitals, Health Organizations, Hospitals, Medical Education, Multiple Sclerosis, People with Disabilities, Single-Disease Health Associations. **Geo. Dist:** primarily in areas of company operations; Avon, CT; Simsbury, CT.

★ 1027 ★ **Entergy Corp.**
PO Box 61000
New Orleans, LA 70161
**Phone:** (504)576-5785          **Fax:** (504)576-2190
**Email:** drodri2@energy.com
**Website:** http://www.entergy.com/contributions
Deanna Rodriguez, V. P. Corp. Contributions

**Priorities:** *Voluntarism:* Entergy sponsors Community Connectors, an employee volunteer program. Employees and retirees who volunteer as Connectors can earn grants through their volunteer hours (up to $250 on an individual basis and $500 per team) and designate those grants to a qualified organization of

their choice. *Note:* Dollar for dollar matching funds must be secured for the requested grant amount. **Typ. Recipients:** Health-General. **Geo. Dist:** company's service area; AR; LA; MS; TX.

★ 1028 ★ **Enterprise Rent-A-Car Foundation**
600 Corporate Park Dr.
Saint Louis, MO 63105
**Phone:** (314)512-2754          **Fax:** (314)512-4754
**Email:** cconrad@erac.com
JoAnn Kindle, President

**Priorities:** *Arts & Humanities:* 7%. Gives to symphonies, orchestras, and operas. Also supports art museums, art fairs, historical societies, and public broadcasting. Generally, giving for the arts has been limited to the St. Louis, MO, area. *Civic & Public Affairs:* 5%. Areas of interest include urban renewal, housing, community festivals, and zoos. *Education:* 24%. Primarily supports colleges and universities within Missouri. Also supports technology education and college preparation. *Environment:* 62%. Supports United Ways, projects designed to aid children, parent and family services, and Special Olympics. *International:* 1%. Supports single-disease health associations, medical centers, and children's hospitals and health organizations. *Voluntarism:* All employees are encouraged to participate in community and national programs. *Note:* Total contributions in fiscal 2000. **Typ. Recipients:** Alzheimers Disease, Cancer, Children's Health/Hospitals, Clinics/Medical Centers, Diabetes, Domestic Violence, Emergency/Ambulance Services, Family Planning, Health Organizations, Hospitals, Mental Health, Preventive Medicine/Wellness Organizations, Single-Disease Health Associations.

★ 1029 ★ **Equifax Foundation**
1550 Peachtree St. NW
Atlanta, GA 30309
**Phone:** (404)885-8012          **Fax:** (404)885-8215
**Email:** karen.gaston@equifax.com
Kirby Thompson, Contact

**Priorities:** *Arts & Humanities:* 12%. Funding goes to museums, art centers, art funds, and choirs. *Civic & Public Affairs:* 15%. Supports economic development programs, chamber of commerce, Habitat for Humanity, zoos and botanical gardens, and business associations. *Education:* 10%. Supports universities, Junior Achievement, United Negro College Fund, literacy programs and K-12 education. *Environment:* 60%. Funds United Way. *International:* 37%. Youth groups, YMCA, and the Boys and Girls Club. *Note:* Total contributions made in 1999. **Typ. Recipients:** Cancer, Children's Health/Hospitals, Emergency/Ambulance Services, Health Organizations, Health-General, Heart, Hospices, Hospitals, Kidney, Medical Education, Medical Rehabilitation, Nursing Services, People with Disabilities, Prenatal Health Issues, Public Health, Research/Studies Institutes, Single-Disease Health Associations, Substance Abuse. **Geo. Dist:** GA.

★ 1030 ★ **Equitable Resources, Inc.**
One Oxford Center Ste. 3300
301 Grant St.
Pittsburgh, PA 15219
**Phone:** (412)553-7739          **Fax:** (412)553-5757
**Website:** http://www.eqt.com/about_EQT/Community.asp
Estelle Christian, Executive Assistant to CEO

**Priorities:** *Education:* Focuses support on education. *Environment:* Primary support to United Way. **Typ. Recipients:** Arthritis, Children's Health/Hospitals, Domestic Violence, Health-General, Hospitals, Hospitals (University Affiliated), Medical Education, People with Disabilities. **Geo. Dist:** headquarters area only.

★ 1031 ★ **Erb Foundation**
PO Box 3013
Birmingham, MI 48012-3013
**Phone:** (248)644-5300
Gary Robinette, President

**Priorities:** *Arts & Humanities:* 8%. Supports art museums, the performing arts, and public broadcasting. *Civic & Public Affairs:* 1%. Supports community foundations, zoos, and parks. *Education:* 1%. Supports colleges, universities and private educational institutions. *Environment:* 4%. Funds youth organizations, violence prevention, and United Way. *International:* 83%. Supports hospitals, single-disease health orgs, and hospice programs. *Religion:* 1%. Funds the Cranbrook Institute of Science. *Note:* Total contributions made in 2000. **Typ. Recipients:** Alzheimers Disease, Cancer, Children's Health/Hospitals, Eyes/Blindness, Family Planning, Hospices, Hospitals, Medical Research, Mental Health, People with Disabilities, Substance Abuse. **Geo. Dist:** MI.

★ 1032 ★ **Ethyl Corp.**
330 S 4th St.
Richmond, VA 23219
**Phone:** (804)788-5720          **Fax:** (804)788-5636
Henry Page, Jr., Vice President, Human Resources & Extern

**Priorities:** *Arts & Humanities:* About 25%. Supports programs to improve the quality of life, particularly those designed to make a community more attractive to prospective employees. *Civic & Public Affairs:* 5% to 10%. Emphasis is on economic education and better government organizations. *Education:* 40% to 45%. Supports public and private institutions, with emphasis on those that serve as a potential source of employees or those which are of significance to employee family members. Administers matching gifts program and scholarship program for employee family members. Supports secondary, undergraduate, and graduate level study. *International:* About 25%. Emphasizes programs of direct benefit to employees in the areas of health, social services, recreation, and physical fitness. Includes support for United Way. **Typ. Recipients:** Emergency/Ambulance Services, Health Organizations, Hospitals. **Geo. Dist:** headquarters and operating communities.

★ 1033 ★ **Excel Corp.**
151 North Main St.
Wichita, KS 67202
**Phone:** (316)291-2500          **Fax:** (316)291-3499
**Email:** contactexcel@cargill.com
Ron Minihan, Excel Cares Chairperson

**Typ. Recipients:** Health-General, Medical Rehabilitation. **Geo. Dist:** headquarters and operating communities.

★ 1034 ★ **Extendicare Foundation**
111 W Michigan St.
Milwaukee, WI 53203
**Phone:** (414)908-8230
Dr. Ronald Retzke, Vice President, Community Relations

**Fnded:** 1985. **Priorities:** *International:* 100%. Funds education and research on Alzheimer's disease, caregiver education and quality of life initiatives. **Typ. Recipients:** Alzheimers Disease, Geriatric Health, Health Organizations, Health Policy/Cost Containment, Long-Term Care, Mental Health, Nursing Services, Public Health. **Geo. Dist:** headquarters and operating communities.

★ 1035 ★ **Exxon Mobil Foundation**
5959 Las Colinas Boulevard
Irving, TX 75039-2298
**Phone:** (972)444-1104          **Fax:** (972)444-1405
**Website:** http://www.exxon.mobil.com
Edward Ahnert, Manager, Contributions

**Priorities:** *Arts & Humanities:* 14%. Supports programs that strengthen the community-building power of the arts. Special emphasis is placed on supporting organizations and programs that reach out to nontraditional audiences, provide greater access to arts and cultural institutions and programs, and incorporate the arts and culture into local schools. *Civic & Public Affairs:* 4%. Supports organizations dealing with public policy alternatives with direct bearing on the company's business operations and interests, as well as legal policy research and education, environmental policy, and regulation. Also supports community foundations and local civic organizations. *Education:* 44%. Supports pre-college and higher education through grants to colleges and universities, junior achievement, local schools, and minority education. *Environment:* 3%. Supports community service organizations, community centers, and minority and women-oriented service organizations. *International:* 4%. Supports research projects on topics related to the company's business operations; occupational health education, especially for traditionally underrepresented populations; outreach to local institutions in ExxonMobil communities; and health matters affecting the workforce. *Note:* Total contributions made in 1999. **Typ. Recipients:** Cancer, Clinics/Medical Centers, Emergency/Ambulance Services, Health Organizations, Hospitals, Medical Education, Medical Rehabilitation, Medical Research, Medical Training, Nursing Services, Public Health, Substance Abuse. **Geo. Dist:** internationally; nationally. **Frmly:** Exxon Education Foundation.

## ★ 1036 ★ F.K. Bemis Family Foundation
PO Box 901
Sheboygan Falls, WI 53085-0901
**Phone:** (920)467-4621　　　**Fax:** (920)467-8573
**Email:** corp@BemisMfg.com
Richard Bemis, President

**Fnded:** 1953. **Priorities:** *Arts & Humanities:* 23%. Funds arts centers, museums, libraries, and public broadcasting. *Civic & Public Affairs:* 2%. Gives to municipalities, job training initiatives, and civic groups such as Jaycees. *Education:* 44%. Supports colleges and universities. *Environment:* 30%. Supports United Way, activities for youth, and the American Red Cross. *International:* 1%. Funds medical centers and single-disease associations. *Note:* Total contributions in 2000. **Typ. Recipients:** Cancer, Children's Health/Hospitals, Clinics/Medical Centers, Emergency/Ambulance Services, Hospitals, Medical Research. **Geo. Dist:** WI, Sheboygan County.

## ★ 1037 ★ Fabri-Kal Foundation
Plastics Place
Kalamazoo, MI 49001-4880
**Phone:** (616)385-5050　　　**Fax:** (616)385-0197
Robert Kittredge, Chairman & Chief Executive Officer

**Priorities:** *Arts & Humanities:* 2%. Supports arts councils. *Civic & Public Affairs:* 11%. Funds parks, community organizations and municipalities. *Education:* 19%. Funds educational grants for the children of company employees and educational initiatives. *Environment:* 50%. Funds the United Way, children's organizations, and human services. *International:* 16%. Supports hospice. *Note:* Total contributions made in 2000. **Typ. Recipients:** Emergency/Ambulance Services, Health-General, Hospices, Medical Education, Nursing Services, People with Disabilities, Substance Abuse. **Geo. Dist:** Kalamazoo, MI; Hazleton, PA; Greenville, SC.

## ★ 1038 ★ Fannie Mae Foundation
North Tower, Ste. One
4000 Wisconsin Ave., NW
Washington, DC 20016-2804
**Phone:** (202)274-8000　　　**Fax:** (202)274-8111
**Website:** http://www.fanniemaefoundation.org

**Fnded:** 1979. **Priorities:** *Arts & Humanities:* 7%. *Civic & Public Affairs:* (Housing & Neighborhood Revitalization) 58%. Reflecting the corporation's role as a national provider of mortgages, the foundation's grantmaking is focused on identifying and properly preparing the next generation of homeowners; reaching out to lower-income families, individuals, and communities to revitalize the neighborhoods and create affordable housing opportunities; and preparing the next generation of leaders in the affordable housing industry in communities across America. The foundation sponsors the Maxwell Awards of Excellence Program, a national grants program to acknowledge and reward

outstanding examples of the work of nonprofit organizations in providing quality housing for low-income families and individuals. Sponsors the New Americans Initiative, designed to help immigrants break down the information barrier to become homeowners, the Native American Financial Education Initiative, and the Adult Homeownership Education Initiative. Also participates in a partnership with the National Basketball Association to support community development, and funds a fellowship program at the John F. Kennedy School of Government. The foundation's Research Grant Program funds policy analysis and empirical or theoretical research that contributes to the state of knowledge on housing policy, housing finance, and community development issues related to the Foundation's focus areas. *Education:* 19%. Supports urban planning and economics programs at colleges and universities. *Environment:* 4%. Supports United Way, community outreach, and services for families. **Typ. Recipients:** Single-Disease Health Associations. **Geo. Dist:** national organizations; operating locations; Washington, DC.

## ★ 1039 ★ Farber Foundation
1845 Walnut St., Ste. 800
Philadelphia, PA 19103
**Phone:** (215)569-9900　　　**Fax:** (215)569-9979
Jack Farber, Chairman & President

**Priorities:** *Arts & Humanities:* 19%. Supports museums, music organizations, and the performing arts. *Civic & Public Affairs:* 19%. Funds philanthropic and community based organizations. *Education:* 6%. Funds colleges and universitites. *International:* 8%. Primarily supports single-disease causes. *Note:* Total contributions in 1999. **Typ. Recipients:** Alzheimers Disease, Arthritis, Cancer, Children's Health/Hospitals, Diabetes, Emergency/Ambulance Services, Health Policy/Cost Containment, Hospitals, Kidney, Long-Term Care, Medical Rehabilitation, Medical Research, Multiple Sclerosis, People with Disabilities, Single-Disease Health Associations, Substance Abuse. **Geo. Dist:** PA.

## ★ 1040 ★ Federal-Mogul Corp.
Corporate Communications
26555 Northwestern Highway
Southfield, MI 48034
**Phone:** (248)354-1916　　　**Fax:** (248)354-8450
Kim Welch, Vice President Corporate Communications

**Priorities:** *Arts & Humanities:* About 15%. Supports bands and orchestras in Detroit, public broadcasting, arts centers and institutes, libraries, and dramatic arts groups. *Civic & Public Affairs:* 20% to 25%. Recipients include business/free enterprise, zoological parks, community development, public policy, civil rights, safety, and urban affairs organizations. *Education:* About 15%. A large portion goes to colleges and universities. Other interests include education funds; business, technical, and minority education; and education associations. Also administers employee matching gifts program. *Environment:* 30% to 35%. Majority of funding supports united funds. Organizations concerned with the disabled and youth also are supported. *International:* 10% to 15%. Recipients include medical research, single-disease health organizations, hospitals, and pediatric health. *Note:* Above priorities are for the foundation only. The company now gives directly, and solely supports three charities: Big Brothers and Big Sisters, the Karmanos Institute, and the United Way. **Typ. Recipients:** Cancer, Children's Health/Hospitals, Clinics/Medical Centers, Diabetes, Health Funds, Health Organizations, Hospices, Hospitals, Medical Research, People with Disabilities, Prenatal Health Issues, Single-Disease Health Associations, Substance Abuse. **Geo. Dist:** headquarters and operating communities; nationally. **Frmly:** Federal-Mogul Corp. Charitable Trust Fund.

## ★ 1041 ★ Federated Department Stores Foundation
7 West Seventh St.
Cincinnati, OH 45202
**Phone:** (513)579-7569　　　**Fax:** (513)579-7185

**Email:** dbarker@fds.com
**Website:** http://www.federated-fds.com
Dixie Barker, Manager, Corporate Contributions & Execu

**Priorities:** *Arts & Humanities:* 17%. Supports orchestras, dance, and art museums. *Civic & Public Affairs:* 10%. Funds minority affairs, zoos, and community and economic development. *Education:* 7%. Supports elementary, secondary, and higher education. *Environment:* 60%. Priorities are the United Way, people with disabilities, and youth. *International:* 6%. Supports the Pediatric Aids Foundation. *Voluntarism:* Partners in Time program established in 1989 as a vehicle to organize and stimulate volunteerism activities. Multi divisional projects involve employees from divisions in the same city working together on a unified project. *Note:* Total contributions made in fiscal 2000. **Typ. Recipients:** AIDS/HIV, Cancer, Children's Health/Hospitals, Domestic Violence, Eyes/Blindness, Family Planning, Health Funds, Hospices, Medical Education, People with Disabilities, Single-Disease Health Associations, Substance Abuse. **Geo. Dist:** headquarters and operating communities. **Frmly:** Robert Campeau Family Foundation (U.S.) Ilse and Robert Campeau Family Foundation.

## ★ 1042 ★ Federated Mutual Insurance Foundation
121 E Park Sq.
Owatonna, MN 55060
**Phone:** (507)455-5200
Richard Kraus, Director, Human Resources

**Priorities:** *Arts & Humanities:* 4%. Funds community arts, performing arts, arts centers and institutes. *Civic & Public Affairs:* 43%. Supports community foundations and professional trade organizations. *Education:* 18%. Supports colleges and universities and after-school enrichment programs. *Environment:* 33%. Supports causes under the foundation's Human Services (28%) and Youth (5%) programs. *International:* 1%. Funds health and wellness organizations. *Note:* Contributions Analysis provided by foundation. Total contributions made in 1999. **Typ. Recipients:** Cancer, Children's Health/Hospitals, Emergency/Ambulance Services, Geriatric Health, Health Organizations, Health Policy/Cost Containment, Health-General, Heart, Home-Care Services, Medical Research, People with Disabilities, Public Health, Substance Abuse. **Geo. Dist:** operating locations.

## ★ 1043 ★ Ferro Foundation
1000 Lakeside Ave.
Cleveland, OH 44114-1183
**Phone:** (216)641-8580　　　**Fax:** (216)696-5803
James Hill, Secretary & Treasurer

**Fnded:** 1959. **Priorities:** *Arts & Humanities:* 17%. Supports performing arts, museums, music, public broadcasting, and historical preservation. Recipients include Musical Arts Association, Playhouse Square Foundation and Western Reserve Historical Association. *Civic & Public Affairs:* 15%. Supports employment and job training, towns and municipalities, and economic development. Recipients include Urban League of Northern Cleveland and Cleveland Technical Services Council. *Education:* 17%. Supports private pre-college education and college and universities. *Environment:* 48%. Supports united funds, youth programs, and family services. *International:* 2%. *Note:* Total foundation contributions made in fiscal 2000. **Typ. Recipients:** Alzheimers Disease, Cancer, Children's Health/Hospitals, Clinics/Medical Centers, Diabetes, Emergency/Ambulance Services, Health-General, Hospitals, Hospitals (University Affiliated), Medical Rehabilitation, Mental Health, Multiple Sclerosis, Nursing Services, People with Disabilities, Prenatal Health Issues, Substance Abuse. **Geo. Dist:** Cleveland, OH.

## ★ 1044 ★ Fidelity Investments Charitable Gift Fund Foundation, Inc.
82 Devonshire St., R22C
Boston, MA 02109
**Phone:** (617)563-6806　　　**Fax:** (617)476-4234

**Website:** http://www.fidelityfoundation.org
Margaret Morton, Program Director

**Priorities:** *Arts & Humanities:* 41%. Supports museums, music, theaters, dance, art institutes, and historic preservation. *Civic & Public Affairs:* 6%. Community development interests include neighborhood housing services, economic development, environmental, nonprofit management, shelters family services, child welfare, the elderly, and the handicapped. *Education:* 45%. Majority of support goes to matching gifts. Also supports universities, colleges and educational funds. *Environment:* 7%. Funds youth organizations, shelters, and volunteerism. *International:* 1%. Supports medical research in health organizations and hospitals. *Note:* Total foundation contributions made in 1999. **Typ. Recipients:** Cancer, Child Abuse, Children's Health/Hospitals, Clinics/Medical Centers, Health Organizations, Hospices, Hospitals, Medical Research, Mental Health, People with Disabilities. **Geo. Dist:** Covington, KY; Marlborough, MA; Merrimack, NH; New York, NY; New York, NY; Cincinnati, OH; Cincinnati, OH; Smithfield, RI; Smithfield, RI; Dallas, TX; Salt Lake City, UT; Toronto, ON; Toronto, ON.


## ★ 1045 ★ Fifth Third Foundation
38 Fountain Square Plaza
Maildrop 1090D7
Cincinnati, OH 45263
**Phone:** (513)579-6034          **Fax:** (513)579-5461
Lawra Baumann, Foundation Officer

**Priorities:** *Arts & Humanities:* 19%. Major support for music, arts funds, museums, and arts centers. Historic preservation, the performing arts, theater, and public broadcasting are also supported. *Civic & Public Affairs:* 24%. Contributes to a variety of causes, including housing, law and justice, business, minority interests, and zoos. *Education:* 9%. Majority of funding goes to colleges and universities, generally in grants of $5,000 or less. Other areas of interest include arts education, education funds, and youth, medical, precollege, and religious education. *Environment:* 35%. Majority of funding supports United Way chapters. Major grants are also made to various youth organizations, especially those supporting scouting. Other interests include religious welfare, the aged, the disabled, and family services. *International:* 5%. *Religion:* 2%. *Note:* Total contributions in fiscal 1998. **Typ. Recipients:** Children's Health/Hospitals, Emergency/Ambulance Services, Health Funds, Health Organizations, Hospices, Hospitals, Medical Education, Medical Rehabilitation, People with Disabilities, Single-Disease Health Associations, Speech & Hearing. **Geo. Dist:** Cincinnati, OH, including metropolitan area.


## ★ 1046 ★ FINA Foundation
15710 JFK Boulevard
Houston, TX 77032
**Fax:** (281)227-5000
Ms. Carolyn Sanders, Vice President

**Fnded:** 1974. **Priorities:** *Arts & Humanities:* 13%. Recipients include opera, public broadcasting, and museums. Also supports dance and theater. *Civic & Public Affairs:* 15%. Emphasis on philanthropic organizations, community development, and nonprofit management. *Education:* 20%. Favors universities and minority education. Foundation operates matching gift program to accredited institutions of higher learning. *Environment:* 39%. Supports United Way in Texas. Also supports youth organizations, community service organizations, and community centers. *International:* 4%. Supports medical centers and cancer treatment and research. *Religion:* 7%. Supports science museums. *Note:* Total foundation contributions made in 1999. **Typ. Recipients:** Cancer, Clinics/Medical Centers, Health Organizations, Hospitals, Hospitals (University Affiliated), Public Health. **Geo. Dist:** operating communities.


## ★ 1047 ★ Fireman's Fund Foundation
777 San Marin Dr.
Novato, CA 94998-1406
**Phone:** (415)899-2757          **Fax:** (415)899-2126
Barbara Friede, Secretary & Director

**Fnded:** 1953. **Priorities:** *Arts & Humanities:* 23%. Supports the performing arts, projects, concerts, and exhibitions that make the arts accessible to youth, the low-income, the disabled, and senior citizens. Matches employee contributions to cultural groups. *Civic & Public Affairs:* 24%. Interests include projects that improve the quality of community life. *Education:* 15%. Funds match employee contributions to institutions of higher, secondary, and elementary learning. *Environment:* 31%. Priorities include programs concerned with youth, the disabled, drugs and alcohol, the homeless, family services, mental health, United Way and the aged. *International:* 4%. Mental health, preventive medicine, and single-disease health associations. *Religion:* 2%. Recipients include science museums and scientific institutes. *Note:* Total contributions in 1999. **Typ. Recipients:** AIDS/HIV, Alzheimers Disease, Domestic Violence, Health Organizations, Home-Care Services, Hospitals, Medical Rehabilitation, Mental Health, People with Disabilities, Preventive Medicine/Wellness Organizations, Substance Abuse. **Geo. Dist:** CA, Marin and Sonoma Counties.


## ★ 1048 ★ First Evergreen Foundation
14329 Blue Spruce Court
Orland Park, IL 60462
**Phone:** (708)460-7357
Kenneth Ozinga, Manager

**Fnded:** 1985. **Priorities:** *Civic & Public Affairs:* 6%. Supports leadership initiatives, legal affairs, and clubs. *Education:* 42%. Supports Christian schools and universities. *International:* 51%. Funds medical centers and hospitals. *Note:* Total foundation contributions made in 2000. **Typ. Recipients:** Clinics/Medical Centers, Hospitals, Medical Rehabilitation, Mental Health, Prenatal Health Issues. **Geo. Dist:** Chicago, IL, southwest area.


## ★ 1049 ★ First Financial Foundation
1305 Main St.
Stevens Point, WI 54481
**Phone:** (715)341-0400
Wanda Lay, Assistant Secretary

**Fnded:** 1977. **Priorities:** *Arts & Humanities:* 6%. Supports libraries, the performing arts, and arts councils. *Civic & Public Affairs:* 8%. Funds housing and neighborhood development. *Education:* 15%. Recipients include higher education and enrichment programs. *Environment:* 65%. Major support for United Ways; youth activities, including YMCA's are also funded. *International:* 5%. Funds hospitals and health clinics. *Note:* Total contributions in 1998. **Typ. Recipients:** AIDS/HIV, Cancer, Children's Health/Hospitals, Clinics/Medical Centers, Domestic Violence, Family Planning, Geriatric Health, Health Funds, Hospitals, Medical Research, Nursing Services, People with Disabilities, Public Health, Single-Disease Health Associations. **Geo. Dist:** IL, areas of business; WI, areas of business.


## ★ 1050 ★ First Hawaiian Foundation
999 Bishop St., 29th Floor
Honolulu, HI 96813
**Phone:** (808)525-7766          **Fax:** (808)525-7750
Lily Yao, President

**Priorities:** *Arts & Humanities:* 12%. Supports museums, arts centers, film, and music. *Civic & Public Affairs:* 2%. Supports housing and memorials. *Education:* 34%. Funds colleges and universities. Private and public precollege education receives most support through capital campaigns and grants used to renovate or refurbish facilities. *Environment:* 30%. Majority of giving supports united funds. Funds also provided for services for youth, shelters and food banks, and drug prevention. *International:* 8%. Supports health clinics, hospitals, single-disease health associations, and health organizations. *Voluntarism:* Company supports employee volunteerism through the YesTeam. *Note:* Total foundation contributions made in 1999. **Typ. Recipients:** Cancer, Children's Health/Hospitals, Clinics/Medical Centers, Domestic Violence, Emergency/Ambulance Services, Health Organizations, Hospices, Hospitals, Medical Rehabilitation, People with Disabilities, Research/Studies Institutes, Single-

Disease Health Associations, Substance Abuse. **Geo. Dist:** HI.


## ★ 1051 ★ First National Bank in Wichita Charitable Trust
PO Box One
Wichita, KS 67201
**Phone:** (316)383-1236          **Fax:** (316)383-5879
**Email:** dmiseman@intrustbank.com
**Website:** http://www.intrustbank.com
Diane Iseman, marketing officer

**Priorities:** *Arts & Humanities:* 1%. Supports arts centers, museums and galleries, and music and operas. *Civic & Public Affairs:* 1%. Supports community foundations. *Education:* 6%. Supports public education and colleges and universities. *Environment:* 52%. Supports child welfare, youth organizations, family services, community services, neighborhood revitalization, and the United Way. *International:* 2%. Supports health and wellness concerns and Cerebal Palsy research. *Voluntarism:* INTRUST recruits employees to volunteer in school classrooms during regular work hours. *Note:* Total contributions in 1999. **Typ. Recipients:** Cancer, Children's Health/Hospitals, Health Organizations, Health-General, Hospices, Hospitals, Mental Health, People with Disabilities, Preventive Medicine/Wellness Organizations, Preventive Medicine/Wellness Organizations, Single-Disease Health Associations. **Geo. Dist:** operating locations.


## ★ 1052 ★ First Source Foundation
Care of First Source Bank
PO Box 1602
South Bend, IN 46601
**Phone:** (219)235-2790          **Fax:** (219)235-2771
Mary Sonneborn, Trust Officer

**Fnded:** 1952. **Priorities:** *Arts & Humanities:* 34%. Supports art museums, performing arts, and fine arts foundations and councils. *Civic & Public Affairs:* 17%. Funds community foundations, local community activities, and fire departments. *Education:* 12%. Gives to high schools, Junior Achievement, scholarship funds, colleges and universities. *Environment:* 33%. Supports local United Ways, Boys and Girls Clubs, animal welfare organizations, and rescue missions. *International:* 4%. Funds hospice programs, hospitals, and a health foundation. *Note:* Total contributions in 1999. **Typ. Recipients:** Child Abuse, Children's Health/Hospitals, Health Funds, Health Organizations, Hospices, Hospitals, Medical Education, Mental Health, People with Disabilities, Preventive Medicine/Wellness Organizations, Public Health, Substance Abuse. **Geo. Dist:** IN.


## ★ 1053 ★ First Tennessee Foundation
PO Box 84
Memphis, TN 38101
**Phone:** (901)523-4352          **Fax:** (901)523-4354
**Email:** jtlee@ftb.com
J. Lee, Senior Vice President, Corporate Communi

**Priorities:** *Note:* Focus of priorities is shifting toward emphasis on education and parental involvement in education. **Typ. Recipients:** Hospitals. **Geo. Dist:** TN, headquarters and operating communities.


## ★ 1054 ★ First Union Foundation
PO Box 1357
Richmond, VA 23218-1357
**Phone:** (804)649-2311          **Fax:** (804)782-6698
**Website:** http://www.firstunionsec.com

**Priorities:** *Arts & Humanities:* 12%. Funds symphony, performing arts, educational television, theater, and historic preservation. *Civic & Public Affairs:* 23%. Supports municipalities, environmental concerns, and a business council. *Education:* 40%. Funds are distributed to colleges and universities, primarily in Virginia, Pennsylvania, Maryland, and North Carolina. Also supports scholarship funds and higher education organizations. *Environment:* 15%. Supports the United Way and youth organizations. *Note:* Total foundation contributions in 1998. **Typ. Recipients:** Cancer, Children's Health/Hospitals, Clinics/Medical Centers,

Emergency/Ambulance Services, Eyes/Blindness, Health Organizations, Heart, Hospitals, Long-Term Care, Medical Education, Medical Research, People with Disabilities, Prenatal Health Issues, Single-Disease Health Associations. **Geo. Dist:** headquarters and operating communities; Richmond, VA, change in giving area due to merger. **Frmly:** Wheat Foundation Wheat, First Securities/Butcher & Singer Foundation.

★ 1055 ★ **Firstar Milwaukee Foundation**
777 E Wisconsin Ave.
Milwaukee, WI 53202
**Phone:** (414)765-4579          **Fax:** (414)765-6667
Dennis Fredrickson, Secretary & Treasurer
**Priorities:** *Arts & Humanities:* 30%. Primarily supports a performing arts fund. Also gives to museums, ballet, historic preservation, opera, symphonies, and libraries. *Civic & Public Affairs:* 5%. About one-half supports economic and community development in Milwaukee. The remainder supports a variety of interests, including civil rights, professional organizations, public policy, nonprofit management, and zoos. *Education:* 14%. Supports colleges and universities, exclusively in the state of Wisconsin. *Environment:* 47%. Recipients include youth organizations, religious welfare groups, community centers, child welfare, and programs for the aged. *International:* 3%. Supports single-disease health associations, medical research, nursing services, and health funds. *Voluntarism:* The Company has an active employee volunteer program. *Note:* Total contributions made in 1998. **Typ. Recipients:** Children's Health/Hospitals, Clinics/Medical Centers, Emergency/Ambulance Services, Family Planning, Health Organizations, Health-General, Heart, Hospices, Hospitals, Medical Education, Nursing Services, People with Disabilities, Single-Disease Health Associations, Substance Abuse, Transplant Networks/Donor Banks. **Geo. Dist:** Milwaukee, WI.

★ 1056 ★ **FirstEnergy Corp.**
76 South Main St.
Akron, OH 44308-1890
**Phone:** (330)761-4246          **Fax:** (330)761-4203
**Email:** valentined@firstenergycorp.com
**Website:** http://www.firstenergycorp.com/community
Donna Valentine, Director of Contributions
**Priorities:** *Arts & Humanities:* (Arts & Culture) 21%. Supports museums, orchestras, art centers, libraries, historical societies. *Civic & Public Affairs:* 14%. Funds community groups, zoos, botanical gardens, community festivals, business development and international affairs. *Education:* 14%. Gives to colleges and universities, secondary schools, Junior Achievement programs, and specialized education, including business and performing arts education programs. *Environment:* (Health and Human Services) 51%. Supports scouts, hospitals and clinics, youth services, United Way, YMCA, and volunteer programs. *Note:* Total contributionss made in 1999. **Typ. Recipients:** Health-General. **Geo. Dist:** headquarters and operating communities.

★ 1057 ★ **Fisher Brothers Foundation, Inc.**
299 Park Ave.
New York, NY 10017
**Phone:** (212)752-5000          **Fax:** (212)940-6207
Mr. Richard Fisher, Director
**Fnded:** 1981. **Priorities:** *Arts & Humanities:* 36%. Supports performing arts, museums, art associations, and public broadcasting. *Civic & Public Affairs:* 4%. Funds the Anti-defamation League, public safety/law enforcement, and other civic organizations. *Education:* 1%. Provides grants for colleges and universities, and private secondary education. *Environment:* 1%. Supports local United Way agencies, YMCA/YWCA, and Boy Scouts of America. *International:* 52%. Major funding for New York Presbyterian Hospital. *Note:* Total contributions made in 1999. **Typ. Recipients:** AIDS/HIV, Cancer, Children's Health/Hospitals, Diabetes, Geriatric Health, Health-General, Hospitals, Medical Education, People with Disabilities, Single-Disease Health Associations, Transplant Networks/

Donor Banks. **Geo. Dist:** New York, NY, metropolitan area.

★ 1058 ★ **FleetBoston Financial Foundation**
100 Hundred Federal St.
Boston, MA 02110
**Phone:** (617)434-2629          **Fax:** (617)434-6072
**Website:** http://www.fleet.com
Michele Courton-Brown, President
**Priorities:** *Arts & Humanities:* Funding in this area includes sponsorship of initiatives from major exhibits to community and grassroots performances; educational outreach to low- and moderate-income youth; and projects that promote increased access to the arts. *Civic & Public Affairs:* Funding in civic and public affairs focuses on economic opportunity, with a particular focus on community development programs; microenterprise, entrepreneurial, and small business development; job creation and employment training; affordable housing initiatives and homebuyer seminars; and selected programs that serve low- and moderate-income individuals. *Education:* Funds public education programs, emphasizing programs that support literacy programs, business and finance education, transition from school to career, and long-term education reform efforts. *Environment:* Supports youth development, including programs that promote healthy development, adult mentoring support, job readiness and skill building, and leadership skills through community service. *Note:* Contribution priorities were derived from the foundation's Grantmaking Guidelines. **Typ. Recipients:** AIDS/HIV, Children's Health/Hospitals, Clinics/Medical Centers, Domestic Violence, Emergency/Ambulance Services, Family Planning, Heart, Hospices, Hospitals, Hospitals (University Affiliated), Medical Research, Nutrition, People with Disabilities, Prenatal Health Issues, Substance Abuse. **Geo. Dist:** CT; FL, in limited areas; ME; MA; NH; NJ; NY; RI.

★ 1059 ★ **Florida Rock Industries Foundation**
PO Box 4667
Jacksonville, FL 32201
**Phone:** (904)355-1781          **Fax:** (904)366-1866
**Email:** frih.b.horner@aol.com
H. Horner, Secretary
**Priorities:** *Arts & Humanities:* 10%. Supports historical societies and performing arts. *Civic & Public Affairs:* 22%. Supports urban leagues, public policy associations and the Police Athletic League. *Education:* 17%. Funds scholarships and universities. *Environment:* 31%. Supports the United Way, youth organizations, and homeless centers. *International:* 13%. Supports single-disease health organizations and local children's hospital. *Note:* Total contributions made in fiscal 1999. **Typ. Recipients:** Alzheimers Disease, Cancer, Children's Health/Hospitals, Clinics/Medical Centers, Geriatric Health, Health Organizations, Medical Research, Multiple Sclerosis, People with Disabilities, Single-Disease Health Associations. **Geo. Dist:** FL; GA.

★ 1060 ★ **Fluor Foundation**
One Enterprise Dr., F2C
Aliso Viejo, CA 92656-2606
**Phone:** (949)349-6797
**Email:** community.relations@fluordaniel.com
Ms. Suzanne Esber, Manager Community Relations
**Priorities:** *Arts & Humanities:* 2%. Funds performing arts and arts associations. *Civic & Public Affairs:* 2%. Supports urban and community affairs, professional associations for engineers, zoos and botanical gardens, business and free enterprise groups, and public policy organizations. *Education:* 58%. Majority of funding supports colleges and universities, with emphasis on science and technology education. Other interests include engineering education and minority education. Also sponsors employee matching gifts program. *Environment:* 34%. Major priority is United Way. The remainder is disbursed among youth organizations, child welfare, and community service organi-

zations. *International:* 3%. Supports emergency services, hospitals, and some single-disease health organizations. *Religion:* 1%. Funds science centers. *Voluntarism:* "The Fluor Community Involvement Team," is a corporate volunteer program in which employees, retirees, and their family and friends carry out service projects in local communities. Employees also volunteer for many education programs: Junior Achievement, school partnerships, mentoring, and classroom presentations. *Note:* Total foundation contributions made in fiscal 1999. **Typ. Recipients:** Cancer, Children's Health/Hospitals, Clinics/Medical Centers, Diabetes, Emergency/Ambulance Services, Hospitals, Medical Education, Substance Abuse. **Geo. Dist:** operating locations.

★ 1061 ★ **Forbes Foundation**
60 5th Ave.
New York, NY 10011
**Phone:** (212)620-2248          **Fax:** (212)633-1958
Mr. Leonard Yablon, Secretary & Treasurer
**Fnded:** 1979. **Priorities:** *Arts & Humanities:* 6%. Funds arts associations, museums, libraries, and historical preservation. *Civic & Public Affairs:* 11%. Business, public policy, and professional organizations receive support. *Education:* 74%. Colleges, universities, and private precollege education are funded. *Environment:* 1%. Supports athletics and youth organizations. *International:* 5%. Supports hospitals, medical education, and pediatric health. *Note:* Total contributions made in 1999. **Typ. Recipients:** AIDS/HIV, Arthritis, Cancer, Clinics/Medical Centers, Diabetes, Emergency/Ambulance Services, Family Planning, Health Funds, Health Organizations, Hospices, Hospitals, Medical Education, Medical Research, Mental Health, Nursing Services, Single-Disease Health Associations, Substance Abuse. **Geo. Dist:** New York, NY, including metropolitan area.

★ 1062 ★ **Ford Meter Box Foundation**
PO Box 443
775 Manchester Ave.
Wabash, IN 46992
Marta Gidley, Secretary
**Fnded:** 1988. **Priorities:** *Arts & Humanities:* 1%. Museums, opera, music, and arts associations receive funding. *Civic & Public Affairs:* 56%. Supports community-oriented philanthropic organizations and business and free enterprise. *Education:* 1%. Focus on higher education, education funds, and public education. *Environment:* 40%. Funds youth organizations, homes, child welfare, and community service organizations. *International:* About 1%. Heart associations and cancer agencies are funded. *Note:* Total contributions in 1999. **Typ. Recipients:** Cancer, Child Abuse, Children's Health/Hospitals, Domestic Violence, Emergency/Ambulance Services, Eyes/Blindness, Geriatric Health, Health Organizations, Heart, Hospices, Hospitals, Medical Research, Mental Health, Outpatient Health Care, Prenatal Health Issues, Single-Disease Health Associations, Substance Abuse. **Geo. Dist:** IN, Wabash County and surrounding area.

★ 1063 ★ **Ford Motor Co. Fund**
One American Rd.
PO Box 1899
Dearborn, MI 48126
**Phone:** 888-313-0102
**Website:** http://www.ford.com/en/ourCompany/corporateCitizenship/fordMotorCompanyFund/default.htm
Sandy Ulsh, Vice President and Executive Director
**Priorities:** *Arts & Humanities:* 11%. Large part of this support goes to performing arts groups in areas such as music, opera, dance, and theater, mostly in the Detroit area. The remainder primarily supports museums, libraries, public broadcasting, and arts councils and centers. *Civic & Public Affairs:* 11%. Emphasis on community improvement, which includes economic development, urban groups, and business associations. Other priorities are public policy research and youth groups. Employment training, traffic safety, housing, and education related to the free enterprise and economics also are of interest. *Education:* 47%. Major support goes to engineering, scientific, and

technical education. Other priorities include business education, state and national education associations and funds, minority education, and general education (including, colleges and universities, public schools, and other organizations). Company also sponsors employee matching gifts program in this area, makes student loans to children of employees, and sponsors a program to promote scientific research. *Environment:* 10%. Majority of support goes to United Way. The remainder supports social service groups such as food banks, shelters, recreation programs, and organizations serving children, the elderly, and the disabled. *International:* 4%. Interests include hospitals, substance abuse programs, and other health organizations. *Voluntarism:* Ford Motor Company offers every Ford salaried employee 16 hours of paid time off per year to volunteer in teams of co-workers at various agencies. *Note:* Total contributions made in 2000. Above priorities are those of the Ford Motor Company Fund. Company also sponsors a direct giving program. Company reports that direct giving goes to a variety of organizations, but priorities are similar to those of the fund. **Typ. Recipients:** Cancer, Emergency/Ambulance Services, Health Organizations, Health Policy/Cost Containment, Hospices, Hospitals, Kidney, People with Disabilities, Prenatal Health Issues, Public Health, Substance Abuse. **Geo. Dist:** headquarters and operating communities; national organizations.

### ★ 1064 ★ Fortis Foundation
1 Chase Manhattan Plaza, 41st Floor
New York, NY 10005
**Phone:** (212)859-7000      **Fax:** (212)859-7010
**Website:** http://www.fortisfoundation.com
Jackie Gentile, Directory

**Fnded:** 1982. **Priorities:** *Education:* 98%. Matches employee gifts to education and provides scholarships for employees' children. *Note:* Total contributions made in fiscal 1999. **Typ. Recipients:** AIDS/HIV, Cancer, Children's Health/Hospitals, Emergency/Ambulance Services, Family Planning, Multiple Sclerosis, Single-Disease Health Associations. **Geo. Dist:** nationally health-related organizations; NY.

### ★ 1065 ★ Fortis Insurance Foundation
501 West Michigan Ave.
Milwaukee, WI 53203-3050
**Phone:** (414)299-7702      **Fax:** (414)299-6900
Jack Gochenaur, President

**Fnded:** 1973. **Priorities:** *Arts & Humanities:* 10%. Funds museums, libraries, and art programs. *Civic & Public Affairs:* 10%. Gives to economic and community development organizations and a zoo. *Education:* 12%. Supports higher education, literacy services, and secondary schools in Wisconsin. *Environment:* 38%. Supports United Way, caregivers' associations, food banks, and community centers. *International:* 15%. Supports single-disease associations. *Voluntarism:* The foundation supports employee volunteer activities, with special consideration given to organizations where employees volunteer that fall within the foundation's focus areas. The foundation does consider grants to organizations where employees volunteer but are not within the foundation focus. However, grants of this nature are limited to $100 per organization, with priority given to programs providing education, training, and direct services. *Note:* Total contributions in 2000. **Typ. Recipients:** AIDS/HIV, Alzheimers Disease, Children's Health/Hospitals, Children's Health/Hospitals, Clinics/Medical Centers, Domestic Violence, Family Planning, Geriatric Health, Health Organizations, Health Policy/Cost Containment, Hospitals, Medical Rehabilitation, Medical Research, Mental Health, Nutrition, People with Disabilities, Public Health, Respiratory, Single-Disease Health Associations, Substance Abuse. **Geo. Dist:** WI, Southeastern Wisconsin. **Frmly:** Fortis Insurance Foundation.

### ★ 1066 ★ Fortune Brands International, Inc.
1700 East Putnam Ave.
Old Greenwich, CT 06870
**Phone:** (203)698-5211      **Fax:** (203)698-5577

**Email:** jm@fortunebrands.com
Joan McGrath, Contributions Administrator
**Typ. Recipients:** Emergency/Ambulance Services, Health Organizations, Hospitals, Medical Research, People with Disabilities, Public Health, Single-Disease Health Associations, Substance Abuse. **Geo. Dist:** headquarters and operating communities.

### ★ 1067 ★ FPL Group Foundation, Inc.
9250 West Flagler St.
Miami, FL 33174
**Phone:** (305)552-4806      **Fax:** (305)552-4722
**Email:** John_Kitchens@fpl.com
**Website:** http://www.fpl.com
John Kitchens, Contributions Administrator

**Fnded:** 1989. **Priorities:** *Arts & Humanities:* 1%. Supports performing arts centers, museums, and music. *Civic & Public Affairs:* 9%. Funds economic development, community affairs, and municipalities. *Education:* 27%. Sponsors a matching gifts program to schools and universities; funding also goes to community colleges, and technology institutes. *Environment:* 57%. Supports United Way organizations and emergency relief, low-income family services and youth services. *International:* 2%. Funds diabetes and cancer research. *Note:* Total contributions in 2000. **Typ. Recipients:** Cancer, Cancer, Emergency/Ambulance Services, Geriatric Health, Health Organizations, Medical Rehabilitation, People with Disabilities. **Geo. Dist:** company service areas.

### ★ 1068 ★ Fred C. and Mary R. Koch Foundation, Inc.
PO Box 2256
Wichita, KS 67201
**Phone:** (316)828-7483      **Fax:** (316)828-5739
**Email:** ramseyer@kochind.com
**Website:** http://www.kochind.com/community.asp
Roger Ramseyer, Directory

**Priorities:** *Arts & Humanities:* 20%. Supports arts centers and the arts and humanities council. *Education:* 27%. Supports universities, colleges and scholarship funds in Kansas. Particularly funds programs involving economic and scientific problem solving. *Environment:* 53%. Funds youth organizations. Supports programs that promote self-sufficiency, responsibility, and tolerance for others. *Note:* Total contributions made in 1999. **Typ. Recipients:** Cancer, Children's Health/Hospitals, Hospices, People with Disabilities, Single-Disease Health Associations. **Geo. Dist:** KS; Baton Rouge, LA; St. Paul, MN; Oklahoma City, OK; Corpus Christi, TX; Houston, TX; Calgary, AB.

### ★ 1069 ★ Freddie Mac Foundation
Mailstop A-40
8250 Jones Branch Dr.
Mc Lean, VA 22102
**Phone:** (703)918-5788      **Fax:** (703)903-3585
**Website:** http://www.freddiemacfoundation.org
Shane Falter, Director of Foundation Giving

**Fnded:** 1990. **Priorities:** *Arts & Humanities:* 1%. Arts council supported. *Civic & Public Affairs:* 15%. Supports numerous child welfare and advocacy groups/programs. *Education:* 22%. Focus on early childhood education programs that address the developmental needs of children ages 0-6 and prepare them for learning. Includes early intervention services, strengthening day care and home day care systems; efforts to stimulate parental involvement in their child's educational development; school-based services for families, particularly pregnant or parenting teens; programs that enhance academic performance; initiatives to reform public education systems and advocate for stronger schools, including professional development opportunities and training for teachers; and programs that help children envision a successful future by providing teachers; and programs that help children envision a successful future by providing training and/or exposure to career opportunities. *Environment:* 50%. Focus on prevention of abuse (physical, sexual, emotional) and neglect. Targets factors leading to child abuse, including poor parenting skills,

young inexperienced parents, stressful living situations and financial hardship, domestic violence, and substance abuse. Encourages grant requests in the following areas: parent training, eduation and support groups, home visitor programs, public awareness campaigns, comprehensive family support services, mental health services, teenage pregnancy prevention, services to parentsand children who are victims of domestic violence, father involvement programs, support services to parents who are substance abusers, treatment programs that enable families to stay together during the treatment period, and advocacy and system reform initiatives related to preventing child abuse through the strengthening of families and communities, as well as professional development opportunities for social workers. *International:* 10%. Funding supports children's hospital and single-disease organizations. *Note:* Total contributions made in 1998. **Typ. Recipients:** AIDS/HIV, Child Abuse, Children's Health/Hospitals, Clinics/Medical Centers, Domestic Violence, Family Planning, Health Organizations, Heart, Hospices, Mental Health, People with Disabilities, Prenatal Health Issues, Public Health, Substance Abuse. **Geo. Dist:** nationally organizations; Washington, DC, including metropolitan area; MD, Frederick County; MD, Howard County; MD, Montgomery County; MD, Prince Georges County; VA, Loudoun and Prince William Counties; Alexandria, VA; Arlington, VA; Fairfax, VA.

### ★ 1070 ★ Freeport-McMoRan Foundation
1615 Poydras St.
New Orleans, LA 70112
**Phone:** (504)582-4000      **Fax:** (504)582-4028
Ursula Joseph, Administrative Assistant

**Priorities:** *Arts & Humanities:* 10% to 15%. Supports historical societies, museums, community arts funds, and music. Recipients include the New Orleans Museum of Art, the Acadiana Symphony, and Young Aspirations/Young Artists, Inc. *Civic & Public Affairs:* 15% to 20%. Supports community revitaization, housing, and anti-crime activities. Supports Louisiana Executive Corp and the Greater New Orleans Foundation. *Education:* 40% to 45%. Focus on science, math, and economic education in elementary, secondary and higher education. *International:* About 30%. Major support to the United Way. Recipients include organizations providing health care, shelter, food, and clothing. Also supports innovative environmental programs and recreation. *Note:* Above priorities are for the foundation's 1999 contributions. Company also gives directly, through subsidiaries, and through the newly-created Research, Environmental, and Corporate Fund. **Typ. Recipients:** AIDS/HIV, Cancer, Children's Health/Hospitals, Clinics/Medical Centers, Domestic Violence, Emergency/Ambulance Services, Eyes/Blindness, Health Organizations, Heart, Hospitals, Medical Research, Mental Health, Nutrition, People with Disabilities, Prenatal Health Issues, Single-Disease Health Associations, Substance Abuse. **Geo. Dist:** principally near operating locations and to national organizations.

### ★ 1071 ★ G.D. Searle and Co. Charitable Trust
PO Box 1045
Skokie, IL 60076
**Phone:** (847)581-6769      **Fax:** (847)581-4032
Dr. William Greener, Jr., Trust Administrator

**Priorities:** *Arts & Humanities:* 19%. Supports museums, historical societies, and the performing arts and fine arts. *Civic & Public Affairs:* 31%. Supports zoos, botanical gardens, parks, legal and urban issues, and community foundations. *Education:* 9%. Provides funding for medical education, primary and secondary education, and junior achievement. *Environment:* 9%. Supports family services, homeless shelters, and youth foundations. *International:* 15%. Funds single-disease health organizations, patient rights, and medical research. *Religion:* 1%. *Note:* Total foundation contributions made in 1999. **Typ. Recipients:** AIDS/HIV, Cancer, Children's Health/Hospitals, Clinics/Medical Centers, Health Organizations, Heart, Hospitals (University Affiliated), Long-Term Care, Medical Education, Medical Research, Nursing Services, People with Disabilities, Public Health, Single-Disease Health Associations. **Geo. Dist:** nationally, with emphasis on operating communities.

---

★ **1072** ★ **Gallo Foundation**
PO Box 1130
Modesto, CA 95353
**Phone:** (209)341-3111          **Fax:** (209)341-3324
Ouida McCullough, Secretary

**Priorities:** *Civic & Public Affairs:* 2%. *Education:* 36%. Majority of funds support universities and public secondary education. *Environment:* 6%. Interests include youth organizations, child welfare, food banks and farming associations. *International:* 37%. Primarily supports single-disease health associations. *Note:* Total contributions in 1999. **Typ. Recipients:** AIDS/HIV, Alzheimers Disease, Cancer, Child Abuse, Children's Health/Hospitals, Clinics/Medical Centers, Diabetes, Domestic Violence, Emergency/Ambulance Services, Geriatric Health, Health Organizations, Heart, Hospices, Hospitals, Medical Research, Multiple Sclerosis, People with Disabilities, Prenatal Health Issues, Public Health, Single-Disease Health Associations, Substance Abuse, Transplant Networks/Donor Banks. **Geo. Dist:** nationally; CA.

---

★ **1073** ★ **Galter Foundation**
215 E Chicago Ave.
Chicago, IL 60611
**Phone:** (312)664-5370
Dollie Galter, Director

**Fnded:** 1943. **Priorities:** *Arts & Humanities:* 76%. Primarily supports libraries. *International:* 19%. Funding for rehabilitation. *Note:* Contributions made in 1998. **Typ. Recipients:** AIDS/HIV, Arthritis, Cancer, Children's Health/Hospitals, Clinics/Medical Centers, Diabetes, Health Organizations, Heart, Home-Care Services, Hospitals, Hospitals (University Affiliated), Kidney, Medical Education, Medical Rehabilitation, Medical Research, Multiple Sclerosis, People with Disabilities, Prenatal Health Issues, Public Health, Respiratory, Single-Disease Health Associations. **Geo. Dist:** Chicago, IL.

---

★ **1074** ★ **GATX Corp.**
500 West Monroe St.
Chicago, IL 60661-3676
**Phone:** (312)621-6222          **Fax:** (312)621-6698
**Email:** communityaffairs@gatx.com
**Website:** http://www.gatx.com
Jesse Kane, Supervisor, Community Affairs

**Priorities:** *Education:* Supports a variety of educational programs for economically disadvantaged children and youth. Programs focus on intellectual and emotional development, academic and social preparation for high school and college, academic support to youth in higher education, arts education, and adult literacy education. *Environment:* Supports programs that provide adults with skills training and placement services, prevent domestic and community violence, provide families with access to quality health care, enhance family communications and improve parenting capabilities, and work to provide affordable housing to families. *Voluntarism:* GATX employees nationwide are recognized for volunteer efforts from tutoring students to building playgrounds. GATX presents its Spirit of Volunteerism Award twice a year to honor those whose best exemplify principles of community service, teamwork, and good corporate citizenship. **Typ. Recipients:** AIDS/HIV, Cancer, Child Abuse, Clinics/Medical Centers, Domestic Violence, Geriatric Health, Health Organizations, Hospices, Hospitals, Medical Rehabilitation, Mental Health, Nutrition, People with Disabilities, Public Health, Single-Disease Health Associations, Substance Abuse. **Geo. Dist:** operating locations; Chicago, IL.

---

★ **1075** ★ **GE Fund**
3135 Easton Turnpike
Fairfield, CT 06431
**Phone:** (203)373-3216          **Fax:** (203)373-3029
**Email:** gefund@corporate.ge.com

**Website:**          http://www.ge.com/community/fund/index.html
Joyce Hergenhan, President

**Priorities:** *Arts & Humanities:* 7%. Fund's objective is to further arts education, particularly through partnerships of arts organizations with public schools. *Civic & Public Affairs:* 6%. Funding in this category is focused on public policy organizations promoting international business, economic development, and employment opportunities. Regional planning associations in operating locations are also supported. Minority groups are supported through job training and business education. *Education:* 55%. Supports colleges and universities, and education associations and organizations. The fund's graduate fellowship program awards grants to colleges and universities for support of first-year doctoral students which include stipends and departmental grants. The forgivable loan program supports doctoral candidates. Under this program, 25% of the loan is forgiven for each year the recipient serves as a faculty member at a college or university. Provides scholarships to children of employees through the fund's STAR/ACE programs. Also makes direct grants to colleges, universities, and education associations for science and engineering program development and business curriculum development. Other initiatives include increased educational opportunities for women and minorities, with emphasis on engineering, management, and finance. Support includes sponsorship of a minority engineering scholarship program, funding for Hispanic scholarship programs, scholarships for first-year female engineering students, and aid for minority educational associations and institutions (including schools of engineering and faculty development). Grants on the precollege level emphasize improving math and science teaching and curricula and raising students' abilities in these subject areas. Also, the foundation supports school projects involving GE volunteers. Much support is in the form of matching gifts to colleges and universities. The GE Fund also supports international education. *Environment:* 18%. Primarily supports United Way. *Voluntarism:* GE supports the United Way and United Way-sponsored agencies where GE volunteers perform a variety of services, including agency clean-ups, refurbishing day care centers, and building houses through Habitat for Humanity. GE also supports Elfun, a global organization of GE employees and retirees who work to improve the company and communities through volunteerism, leadership, and camaraderie. GE volunteer hours approach $500,000 in billable hours. *Note:* Total contributions made in 2000. Contributions analysis excludes matching gifts through the Corporate Alumni Program and More Gifts...More Givers Program. **Typ. Recipients:** Clinics/Medical Centers, Emergency/Ambulance Services, Health Organizations, Health Policy/Cost Containment, Hospitals, Hospitals (University Affiliated), Medical Education, Medical Research, People with Disabilities, Substance Abuse. **Geo. Dist:** headquarters and operating communities; international organizations; national organizations. **Frmly:** GE Foundations.

---

★ **1076** ★ **GEICO Philanthropic Foundation**
One Geico Plz.
Washington, DC 20076
**Phone:** (301)986-2387          **Fax:** (301)718-5239
**Website:**          http://www.geico.com/infocenter/goodworks.htm
Karen Watson, Administrator

**Priorities:** *Arts & Humanities:* 1%. Supports performing arts, public television, museums, and historical societies. *Civic & Public Affairs:* 54%. Majority of funding supports the National Safety Association and other safety programs. Other grants support environmental projects, professional organizations, and groups promoting better government. *Education:* 31%. Supports colleges and universities, with emphasis on business education. Also matches employee gifts to higher education. Other recipients include educational fundraising organizations and scholarship foundations. *Environment:* 6%. Primarily supports united funds. Other major recipients include child welfare and recreation groups, programs for the mentally retarded

and disabled, and family services. *International:* 8%. Funds go primarily to hospitals and single-disease research organizations. Some support goes to hospices and other facilities. *Note:* Total foundation contributions made in 2000. **Typ. Recipients:** Cancer, Children's Health/Hospitals, Emergency/Ambulance Services, Heart, Hospices, Hospitals, Medical Rehabilitation, Medical Research, Mental Health, People with Disabilities, Public Health, Single-Disease Health Associations, Substance Abuse. **Geo. Dist:** organizations serving operating locations.

---

★ **1077** ★ **GenAmerican Foundation**
700 Market St.
Saint Louis, MO 63101
**Phone:** (314)444-0520          **Fax:** (314)444-0681
**Email:** cendicott@genam.com
**Website:** http://www.genamerica.com
Cheryl Endicot, Contributions Specialist

**Priorities:** *Arts & Humanities:* Interests include arts education, museums, dance and the St. Louis Symphony. *Civic & Public Affairs:* A variety of causes are supported, including philanthropic organizations, urban affairs organizations, and botanical gardens. *Education:* Emphasis on colleges and universities. Interests include minority scholarships, medical education, and Junior Achievement programs. *Environment:* Primarily supports United Way. *Voluntarism:* Company executives and associates have assumed leadership roles in a variety of civic and charitable causes. **Typ. Recipients:** AIDS/HIV, Alzheimers Disease, Cancer, Children's Health/Hospitals, Clinics/Medical Centers, Diabetes, Domestic Violence, Emergency/Ambulance Services, Family Planning, Heart, Hospitals, Hospitals (University Affiliated), Medical Education, Medical Rehabilitation, Medical Research, People with Disabilities, Preventive Medicine/Wellness Organizations, Public Health, Single-Disease Health Associations, Substance Abuse. **Geo. Dist:** St. Louis, MO. **Frmly:** General American Foundation.

---

★ **1078** ★ **GenCorp Foundation**
175 Ghent Rd.
Fairlawn, OH 44333-3300
**Phone:** (330)869-4289          **Fax:** (330)869-4227
**Email:** tcarter@gencorp.com
Theresa Carter, Director

**Priorities:** *Arts & Humanities:* 3%. Supports organizations and programs rich in diversity that provide educational experiences, and performances and events that broaden awareness and appreciation for the arts. *Civic & Public Affairs:* 17%. Supports projects that address important issues and are designed to improve the quality of life in operating communities, including select urban renewal projects, working collaboratively with community leaders and organizations; drug and crime prevention, and safety issues; and projects that promote community awareness of key issues and community educational opportunities. *Education:* About 40%. Supports K-12 schools that address specific improvements and opportunities for academic excellence in areas such as: reading and economic literacy programs as basic educational needs, math and science, school-to-work readiness, initiatives that encourage professional development for teachers, parental involvement, and programs that advance state-of-the-art technologies. Also supports a select number of colleges and universities, elementary and secondary school programs, and state and local educational organizations whose activities support and encourage educational excellence in polymer science and engineering, and other endeavors related to GenCorp's core technology competencies. Supports adult literacy programs in communities where GenCorp employees take an active role as tutors and volunteers. Funds technology partnership grants, student achievement awards, scholarships, and internships. *Environment:* 20%. Funds United Way, disaster relief, and community needs. *International:* 15%. Funds hospitals, in limited, targeted, and pro-active ways. *Religion:* 5%. *Voluntarism:* Company gives the Community Leadership Award to recognize employee volunteer efforts; award includes a cash grant to the organization where employee volunteers. *Note:* Total contributions in fiscal 1997. **Typ. Recipients:** Cancer,

Children's Health/Hospitals, Diabetes, Emergency/Ambulance Services, Hospitals, Hospitals (University Affiliated), Mental Health, Nursing Services, Research/Studies Institutes. **Geo. Dist:** nationally, with emphasis on corporate operating locations.

**★ 1079 ★ Genentech Foundation for Biomedical Sciences**
1 DNA Way
South San Francisco, CA 94080
**Phone:** (650)225-2487    **Fax:** (650)225-2414
**Website:** http://www.gene.com/about_genentech/responsibility/
Bunnie Jack, Foundation Coordinator
**Fnded:** 1988. **Priorities:** *Education:* 79% of total contributions. Funds and matches education programs in the San Francisco Bay area. Typical recipients include the University of California and Mills College. Also supports scholarship programs for math and science education. *Environment:* Less than 1%. *International:* 3%. *Religion:* 17%. Support in this category includes grants to Stanford University School of Medicine for scientific scholarships; Science 2000 City School Service Fund in Redwood City, CA, for scientific educational kits; and to the University of California, San Francisco, Science and Health Educational Partnership for scientific educationalkits. *Note:* Contributions made in fiscal 1999. **Typ. Recipients:** Kidney, Medical Education. **Geo. Dist:** CA, northern California.

**★ 1080 ★ General Accident Charitable Trust**
One Beacon St.
Boston, MA 02108
**Phone:** (617)725-6000
Tom Ford, Vice President of Association Relations
**Fnded:** 1987. **Priorities:** *Arts & Humanities:* Less than 1%. Support goes to historical preservation. *Civic & Public Affairs:* Less than 1%. *Education:* 8%. Gives to private schools and seminaries. Also supports colleges, universities, education funds, and high schools. *Environment:* 34%. Funds scouting, youth organizations, and United Way. *International:* 20%. Funds medical centers, single-disease associations, and the American Red Cross. *Religion:* Less than 1%. *Note:* Total foundation contributions made in 1999. **Typ. Recipients:** Cancer, Children's Health/Hospitals, Clinics/Medical Centers, Diabetes, Emergency/Ambulance Services, Hospitals, Long-Term Care, Medical Research, Multiple Sclerosis, People with Disabilities, Prenatal Health Issues, Single-Disease Health Associations, Substance Abuse. **Geo. Dist:** nationally.

**★ 1081 ★ General Mills Foundation**
PO Box 1113
Minneapolis, MN 55440
**Phone:** (612)540-2579    **Fax:** (612)540-4114
**Website:** http://www.generalmills.com/explore/community/
Reatha Clark King, President and Executive Director
**Fnded:** 1954. **Priorities:** *Arts & Humanities:* 21%. Foundation supports the performing and visual arts, public broadcasting, and cultural centers. *Civic & Public Affairs:* 2%. Supports economic development, community foundations, nonprofit management, and housing. *Education:* 29%. Supports Junior Achievement, literacy projects, pre-college programs, scholarship funds, colleges and universities. The foundation makes grants to programs which emphasize student academic achievement, particularly at the K-12 level, and on efforts to improve the quality and efficiency of educational services. *Environment:* 42%. Foundation supports programs which strengthen families, nurture children, support youth development, address the needs of individuals with disabilities, and improve communities. Violence prevention initiatives will be favored. The foundation allocates grants to the United Way. Also supports the development and maintenance of domestic and international food distribution systems serving low-income families. *International:* 6%. The foundation supports programs that promote healthy lifestyles in underserved communities and

educate individuals on self-care techniques. *Voluntarism:* General Mills' Volunteer Connection and Retirement PLUS programs promote employee volunteerism by matching volunteers with projects, and the Volunteer Advisory Board Steers Company involvement in volunteer endeavors. *Note:* Total contributions made in 2001. **Typ. Recipients:** Cancer, Cancer, Children's Health/Hospitals, Clinics/Medical Centers, Domestic Violence, Emergency/Ambulance Services, Family Planning, Geriatric Health, Health Organizations, Health Policy/Cost Containment, Hospitals, Medical Education, Medical Rehabilitation, Medical Research, Mental Health, Nutrition, People with Disabilities, Substance Abuse. **Geo. Dist:** nationally; operating locations.

**★ 1082 ★ General Motors Foundation**
600 Renaissance Center
Detroit, MI 48265-3000
**Phone:** (313)665-2992    **Fax:** (313)665-0746
**Website:** http://www.generalmotors.com/company/community_involvement
Lorna Utley, Vice-Chairperson
**Priorities:** *Arts & Humanities:* 3%. Supports museums and the performing arts. *Civic & Public Affairs:* 25%. Major support for the National Safety Council. Gives to disaster relief, and supports urban development and community action programs designed to improve communities in which the company operates. Responds to a variety of community needs. Interests include urban and community affairs, youth groups, and economic development. Public Policy giving specifically targets economic policies. *Education:* 17%. More than half of annual educational cash contributions are given to colleges and universities on GM's Key Institutions list, schools from which GM recruits, and institutions with which GM has research and development contracts. Supports graduate, undergraduate, and precollege engineering, science, and business education. Precollege education supported through such organizations as MathCounts, Detroit Area Precollege Engineering Program, Summer Training and Education Programs, and The LEAD Program in business. At the higher education level, supports colleges and universities and provides scholarships in engineering, including major support to women and minorities. Promotes the participation of minorities in handling their legal affairs through special grants at six university law schools; and develops Hispanic student involvement in high-technology and business careers. Also matches employee contributions to higher education. *Environment:* 17%. Major funding for the United Way. Supports special programs and projects, anti-drug activities, mentoring, and community service organizations. *International:* 33%. Supports cancer research, including the Karmanos Cancer Institute and the GM Cancer Research Foundation. Also supports the Children's National Medical Center and the American Red Cross. *Religion:* 3%. *Voluntarism:* GM loans employees for such projects as Habitat for Humanity building projects and answering telephones for public television telethons. *Note:* A high percentage of grants are awarded through domestic and international subsidiaries and divisions, which have decision-making autonomy for gifts of less than $5,000. Total contributions made 1999. **Typ. Recipients:** Alzheimers Disease, Cancer, Children's Health/Hospitals, Clinics/Medical Centers, Emergency/Ambulance Services, Health Organizations, Hospices, Hospitals, Medical Rehabilitation, Medical Training, Mental Health, People with Disabilities, Public Health, Single-Disease Health Associations, Substance Abuse. **Geo. Dist:** nationally; operating locations.

**★ 1083 ★ George Kress Foundation**
1700 N Webster Ave.
Green Bay, WI 54301
**Phone:** (920)433-5113
John Kress, Secretary & Treasurer
**Fnded:** 1953. **Priorities:** *Arts & Humanities:* 13%. Funds symphonic and performing arts, creativity programs, and art and historical museums. *Civic & Public Affairs:* 10%. Supports botanical gardens/parks, community foundations, economic development, and professional and trade associations. *Education:* 40%.

Funds colleges and universities, minority education funds, literacy initiatives, and scholarship funds. *Environment:* 17%. Supports the United Way, animal protection, children's programs, volunteer services, and family services. *International:* 13%. Supports hospitals, single-disease health associations, and public health. *Note:* Total contributions made in 2000. **Typ. Recipients:** Children's Health/Hospitals, Emergency/Ambulance Services, Health Organizations, Hospitals, Hospitals (University Affiliated), Medical Education, People with Disabilities, Public Health, Single-Disease Health Associations. **Geo. Dist:** occasionally to state aside from Wisconsin; WI, primarily Green Bay.

**★ 1084 ★ Georgia-Pacific Foundation**
133 Peachtree St. Northeast
Atlanta, GA 30303
**Phone:** (404)652-4000    **Fax:** (404)584-1470
**Website:** http://www.gp.com/center/community/index.html
Curley Dossman, Jr., President
**Priorities:** *Arts & Humanities:* 18%. Special interest in art museums and music. Also supports arts associations, and historic preservation and history groups. *Civic & Public Affairs:* 18%. Provided a major grant to Habitat for Humanity. Also supports minority affairs, job training and placement, botanical gardens, community parks, and zoos. *Education:* 32%. Sponsors Georgia-Pacific Foundation Merit Scholarships. Other areas of interest include colleges and universities, literacy programs, school-to-work programs, higher education funds and associations, public schools, Junior Achievement, and technology education. *Environment:* 21%. Foundation generally emphasizes United Way chapters. Other recipients include programs for the disabled and recreational activities for youth. *International:* Less than 1%. *Voluntarism:* Employee volunteers serve such organizations as United Way, American Red Cross, Boy Scouts of America, Girl Scouts, Better Business Bureaus and councils, and Keep America Beautiful. *Note:* Total foundation contributions made in 2000. **Typ. Recipients:** Children's Health/Hospitals, Emergency/Ambulance Services, Eyes/Blindness, Health Funds, Health Organizations, Health-General, Hospitals, Hospitals (University Affiliated), Medical Rehabilitation, Medical Research, People with Disabilities, Single-Disease Health Associations, Substance Abuse. **Geo. Dist:** operating locations.

**★ 1085 ★ Georgia Power Foundation**
241 Ralph McGill Boulevard
Bin No. 10130
Atlanta, GA 30308-3374
**Phone:** (404)506-6784    **Fax:** (404)506-1485
Judy Anderson, Foundation President
**Fnded:** 1930. **Priorities:** *Arts & Humanities:* 9%. Primarily supports arts organizations, historic preservation, and museums. *Civic & Public Affairs:* 17%. Emphasis on chambers of commerce. Also funds a variety of activities including community affairs and development groups, trade associations, and civil rights organizations. *Education:* 25%. Primarily supports colleges and universities, education funds, and secondary education. Interests include business, medical, engineering, technical, and legal education. *International:* 40%. Focus on health and human services. Majority of funding supports the United Way. Interests also include traditional youth organizations, the YMCA and YWCA, hospitals and clinics, national health organizations, medical research, and the American Red Cross. *Religion:* 1%. *Voluntarism:* Company sponsors the Citizens of Georgia Power, a group of employees and retirees that volunteers with nonprofit groups throughout the state. OrganizationS supported include Habitat for Humanity, the March of Dimes, and the American Red Cross. *Note:* Total contributions in 2000. **Typ. Recipients:** Cancer, Child Abuse, Children's Health/Hospitals, Clinics/Medical Centers, Emergency/Ambulance Services, Family Planning, Geriatric Health, Health Organizations, Hospices, Hospitals, Medical Education, Medical Rehabilitation, Medical Research, Mental Health, People with Disabilities, Public Health, Single-Disease Health Associa-

tions, Substance Abuse. **Geo. Dist:** GA, operating locations and service area.

### ★ 1086 ★ Giant Eagle Foundation
101 Kappa Dr.
Pittsburgh, PA 15238
**Phone:** (412)963-6200          **Fax:** (412)963-2540
Jody Clark, Administrator

**Priorities:** *Arts & Humanities:* 8%. Funding supports performing arts organizations, museums, symphony, opera, ballet, theater, and dance. *Civic & Public Affairs:* 6%. Supports community development, municipalities, and zoos. *Education:* 17%. Favors educational foundations and the University of Pittsburgh. Other recipients include private precollege education, Junior Achievement, and minority education funds. Provides scholarships to children of employees. *Environment:* 7%. Contributes to youth organizations including Big Brothers and Big Sisters and scouting; supports family services, food banks, and the United Way. *International:* 5%. Supports AIDS concerns, pediatric health-care facilities, medical rehabilitation, cancer organizations, and medical research. *Note:* Total contributions in fiscal 2000. **Typ. Recipients:** AIDS/HIV, Cancer, Children's Health/Hospitals, Diabetes, Domestic Violence, Emergency/Ambulance Services, Geriatric Health, Health Organizations, Heart, Hospitals, Kidney, Medical Rehabilitation, Medical Research, Mental Health, People with Disabilities, Prenatal Health Issues, Public Health, Sexual Abuse, Single-Disease Health Associations, Substance Abuse. **Geo. Dist:** Pittsburgh, PA.

### ★ 1087 ★ Giant Food Foundation
PO Box 1804, D-599
Washington, DC 20013
**Phone:** (301)341-4561          **Fax:** (301)618-4972
**Website:** http://www.giantfood.com/community.htm
Caron Sisson, Foundation Coordinator

**Fnded:** 1950. **Priorities:** *Arts & Humanities:* 3%. Supports music and ballet, theater, museums, public broadcasting, arts festivals, and arts education. *Civic & Public Affairs:* Less than 1%. Majority of funding supports united funds and religious welfare projects. Other interests include urban affairs organizations and organizations aiding minorities, youth, the elderly, and the handicapped. *Education:* 9%. Interests include colleges and universities, private schools, medical and minority education, and education funds. *Environment:* 52%. Funds the United Way. *International:* 4%. Primarily supports medical research for single diseases, hospitals, health and mental health organizations, andorganizations concerned with the handicapped. *Note:* Contributions made in fiscal 1999. **Typ. Recipients:** Alzheimers Disease, Cancer, Children's Health/Hospitals, Clinics/Medical Centers, Geriatric Health, Health Organizations, Heart, Hospices, Hospitals, Medical Education, Mental Health, People with Disabilities, Prenatal Health Issues, Single-Disease Health Associations, Substance Abuse. **Geo. Dist:** DE; DC; MD; NJ; VA.

### ★ 1088 ★ Giddings & Lewis Foundation
PO Box 590
Fond du Lac, WI 54936-0590
**Phone:** (920)921-9400
Heike Franke, Treasurer

**Fnded:** 1952. **Priorities:** *Arts & Humanities:* 10%. Funds art centers, symphonies, historical societies, and an arts council. *Civic & Public Affairs:* 8%. Funds community development, an aviation center, and fire departments. *Education:* 35%. Supports scholarships, schools, universities. *Environment:* 36%. Supports youth athletics, children's homes, and United Way. *International:* 5%. Supports hospitals, hospice, the American Red Cross, and single-disease health associations. *Religion:* 1%. *Note:* Total foundation contributions made in 1999. **Typ. Recipients:** AIDS/HIV, Cancer, Emergency/Ambulance Services, Heart, Hospices, Hospitals, Multiple Sclerosis, Nursing Services, People with Disabilities, Prenatal Health Issues, Single-Disease Health Associations, Substance Abuse, Transplant Networks/Donor Banks. **Geo. Dist:** CA; MI; OH; WI.

### ★ 1089 ★ Gilbert and Ildiko Butler Foundation, Inc.
767 5th Ave.
New York, NY 10153
**Phone:** (212)980-0606          **Fax:** (212)759-0876
Gilbert Butler, President

**Fnded:** 1988. **Priorities:** *Arts & Humanities:* 9%. Funds museums, libraries, historic preservation, and performing arts. *Civic & Public Affairs:* 11%. Supports parks, gardens, and housing. *Education:* 56%. Supports colleges and universities. *Environment:* 1%. Supports United Way. *International:* 8%. Supports hospitals and medical research. *Religion:* 1%. *Note:* Total foundation contributions made in 1999. **Typ. Recipients:** Cancer, Eyes/Blindness, Hospitals, Mental Health. **Geo. Dist:** headquarters area only.

### ★ 1090 ★ Gillette Co.
Prudential Tower Bldg., 49th Floor
Boston, MA 02199-8004
**Phone:** (617)463-8608          **Fax:** (617)421-8484
**Email:** cathy_chizauskas@gillette.com
**Website:** http://www.gillette.com/community/corpcontributions.asp
Cathleen Chizauskas, Director, Civic Affairs

**Priorities:** *Voluntarism:* Company employees volunteer with Making Strides for Breast Cancer, Walk for Hunger, and the AIDS Walk. **Typ. Recipients:** Clinics/Medical Centers, Emergency/Ambulance Services, Hospitals. **Geo. Dist:** operating locations; Boston, MA.

### ★ 1091 ★ Glaxo Wellcome Foundation
5 Moore Dr.
Research Triangle Park, NC 27709
**Phone:** (919)483-2140          **Fax:** (919)315-3015
**Website:** http://www.glaxowellcome.com/gwfound
Marilyn Foote-Hudson, Executive Director

**Fnded:** 1986. **Priorities:** *Arts & Humanities:* 25%. Supports the National Humanities Center and the North Carolina Museum of Art. *Education:* 70%. Supports North Carolina colleges and universities, with an emphasis on medical, health, and pharmacy programs at the University of North Carolina. *International:* 5%. Gives to the Leukemia Society of Leukemia. *Voluntarism:* Glaxo's Investment in Volunteer Excellence (GIVE) matches employees' volunteer hours with monetary donations. GIVE grants are $500 for fifty or more hours volunteered during a 12 month period. The Glaxo Wellcome Foundation's primary interests are organizations and programs that fall within the fields of education, science, and health. Primary focus is seed funds for new and worthwhile educational programs. Supports Glaxo Wellcome Women in Science Scholars Program, which awards grants of $1,000 to women pursuing careers in science. Normally awards 3 or 4 grants annually. *Note:* Total foundation contributions made in 1999. **Typ. Recipients:** Cancer, Clinics/Medical Centers, Eyes/Blindness, Eyes/Blindness, Health Organizations, Health Policy/Cost Containment, Hospitals, Medical Education, Medical Research, People with Disabilities, Preventive Medicine/Wellness Organizations, Research/Studies Institutes, Single-Disease Health Associations, Substance Abuse. **Geo. Dist:** NC, Triangle Park area.

### ★ 1092 ★ Glickenhaus Foundation
100 Dorchester Rd.
Scarsdale, NY 10583
**Phone:** (212)953-7800          **Fax:** (212)983-8436
Nancy Pier, President

**Fnded:** 1960. **Priorities:** *Arts & Humanities:* 16%. Supports craft museums and councils, theater, orchestras, opera, and museums of fine art. *Civic & Public Affairs:* 1%. Funds legal awareness and services, and community affairs. *Education:* 37%. Primarily funds colleges and universities, as well as educational foundations and funds. *Environment:* 9%. Supports youth services, Planned Parenthood, United Way and senior funds. *International:* 10%. Supports single-disease health associations, psychotherapy organizations, medical research, and medical centers throughout New York. *Religion:* 6%. Funds scientific research

and a museum of natural history. *Note:* Total contributions made in 1999. **Typ. Recipients:** AIDS/HIV, Cancer, Children's Health/Hospitals, Clinics/Medical Centers, Emergency/Ambulance Services, Family Planning, Geriatric Health, Health Organizations, Hospitals, Kidney, Medical Education, Medical Research, Mental Health, People with Disabilities, Single-Disease Health Associations. **Geo. Dist:** nationally; NY.

### ★ 1093 ★ Global Community Partnerships
One Franklin Plaza
PO Box 7929
Philadelphia, PA 19101-7929
**Phone:** (215)751-4668          **Fax:** (215)751-7655
**Email:** community.partnership@gsk.com
**Website:** http://corp.gsk.com/community/working-with.htm
Doug Bauer, Director, Global Community Partnerships

**Fnded:** 2001. **Priorities:** *Arts & Humanities:* 7%. Supports libraries, theater; museum; public broadcasting, and history. *Education:* 85%. Supports colleges, schools, secondary education, universities, and religious education. *Environment:* 2%. Supports community services. *International:* 3%. Supports hospitals, medical centers, and childrens health. *Note:* Total contributions made in 1998. **Typ. Recipients:** AIDS/HIV, Cancer, Children's Health/Hospitals, Diabetes, Emergency/Ambulance Services, Health Funds, Health Organizations, Hospitals, Long-Term Care, Medical Education, Medical Research, People with Disabilities, Single-Disease Health Associations, Substance Abuse. **Geo. Dist:** internationally; nationally.

### ★ 1094 ★ GlobalSantaFe Corp.
Two Lincoln Centre
5420 LBJ Freeway, Ste. 1100
Dallas, TX 75240-2648
**Phone:** (972)701-7820          **Fax:** (972)701-7600
**Website:** http://www.sfdreill.com
Joe Boyd, Vice President, Corporate Affairs

**Typ. Recipients:** Health-General.

### ★ 1095 ★ Globe Foundation
6730 North Scottsdale Rd., Ste. 250
Scottsdale, AZ 85253-4424
**Phone:** (480)991-0500          **Fax:** (480)991-1912
James Johnson, Treasurer & Assistant Secretary

**Fnded:** 1958. **Priorities:** *Arts & Humanities:* 19%. Support goes to historical preservation, art museums, ballet, and other performing arts. *Civic & Public Affairs:* 10%. Gives to community and historical foundations, zoos, and botanical gardens. *Education:* 40%. Supports schools, Junior Achievement, colleges and universities, religious education, and medical education. *Environment:* 5%. Supports United Way, YMCA, youth organizations, and humane societies. *International:* 24%. Funding goes to a variety of causes including health foundations, hospitals, medical research, and education. *Note:* Total foundation contributions made in 2000. **Typ. Recipients:** AIDS/HIV, Arthritis, Cancer, Children's Health/Hospitals, Clinics/Medical Centers, Diabetes, Domestic Violence, Family Planning, Health Funds, Health Organizations, Heart, Hospices, Hospitals, Medical Education, Medical Rehabilitation, Medical Research, Nursing Services, People with Disabilities, Public Health, Research/Studies Institutes, Single-Disease Health Associations. **Geo. Dist:** AZ; IL.

### ★ 1096 ★ Golub Foundation
PO Box 1074
Schenectady, NY 12301
**Phone:** (518)356-9450
Melissa Pabis, Foundation Administrator

**Fnded:** 1981. **Priorities:** *Arts & Humanities:* 10%. Supports theaters, performing arts centers, and music. *Civic & Public Affairs:* About 16%. Contributes to safety, community affairs, and public policy groups. *Education:* 13%. Major interest in public education. Also supports colleges, literacy, and technology programs. Operates scholarship program for students attending colleges in New York, Massachusetts, Pennsylvania, Connecticut, and Vermont. *Environment:* 8%. Favors community centers, united funds, community recreation and athletics, the disabled, and family services. *International:* 7%. Contributes to hospitals, medical centers, children's health, and single-disease health associations. *Note:* Contributions made in fiscal 1999. **Typ. Recipients:** Arthritis, Cancer, Children's Health/Hospitals, Clinics/Medical Centers, Eyes/Blindness, Health Organizations, Hospices, Hospices, Hospitals, Medical Education, Medical Rehabilitation, People with Disabilities, Prenatal Health Issues, Single-Disease Health Associations. **Geo. Dist:** headquarters and operating communities.

**★ 1097 ★ Gosiger Foundation**
108 McDonough St.
Dayton, OH 45402
**Phone:** (937)228-5174          **Fax:** (937)463-7718
Mrs. J. Haley, President

**Fnded:** 1992. **Priorities:** *Arts & Humanities:* 14%. Supports cultural programs, museums, and art institute. *Civic & Public Affairs:* 67%. Funds economic development, foundations, and an aboretum. *Education:* 16%. Focus is on universities and schools. *Environment:* 2%. *International:* Less than 1%. *Note:* Contributions made in 1998. **Typ. Recipients:** Cancer, Children's Health/Hospitals, Heart. **Geo. Dist:** headquarters area only.

**★ 1098 ★ Grace Foundation Inc.**
7500 Grace Dr.
Columbia, MD 21044
**Phone:** (410)531-4000
Mary Helen Johnson, Contact

**Priorities:** *Arts & Humanities:* Less than 5%. Interest in major museums and similar institutions that perform a specialized function in the fields of art, history, or science. *Civic & Public Affairs:* 20% to 25%. Interest in major national programs designed to improve the quality of life in cities and the general welfare of minorities, with emphasis on youth organizations. Also supports conservation programs and local zoos and parks. Company supportsunited funds nationwide with emphasis on employee communities. *Education:* 55% to 60%. Supports colleges and universities with undergraduate and graduate schools of business and major departments of chemistry. Other priorities include special education, with emphasis on math and science. Sponsors employee matching gifts program for higher and secondary education institutions, which accounts for about 15% of contributions in this category. Scholarship program is available for children of company employees. *Environment:* 15% to 20%. Foundation interests include primary health-care facilities that serve the communities in which the company operates,hospitals whose activities are national in scope or unique in type of care delivered, major national medical research programs deemed vital to social welfare, major national organizations whose objective is the betterment of societal welfare, and a variety of community service organizations. *Note:* Above priorities are for foundation giving. Company facilities also make grants in local communities; priorities may vary. **Typ. Recipients:** Health Funds, Health Organizations, Hospices, Hospitals, Medical Education, Medical Rehabilitation, Medical Research, People with Disabilities, Substance Abuse. **Geo. Dist:** corporate operating locations; nationally.

**★ 1099 ★ Graco Foundation**
PO Box 1441
Minneapolis, MN 55440-1441
**Phone:** (612)623-6000          **Fax:** (612)623-6944
Robert Mattison, Vice President & Secretary

**Priorities:** *Civic & Public Affairs:* 12%. Supports affordable housing, neighborhood organizations, economic development, employment services, and refugee support. *Education:* 25%. Gives to scholarship funds, colleges and universities, economic education, private schools, and alternative schooling. *Environment:* 58%. Supports youth organizations, day care, and United Way. Achievement and the Business Economics Education Foundation. Graco's program also included year-round volunteer assignments (on

boards, etc.) with Junior Achievement, the United Way, Metro Paint-a-Thon, and other events of interest to employees. The company has a Volunteer Coordinator. *Voluntarism:* In the past, employees have volunteered time for education associations such as Junior Achievement and the Business Economics Education Foundation. Graco's program also included year-round volunteer assignments (on boards, etc.) with Junior Achievement, the United Way, Metro Paint-a-Thon, and other events of interest to employees. The company has a Volunteer Coordinator. *Note:* Total contributions in 1999. **Typ. Recipients:** Cancer, Children's Health/Hospitals, Clinics/Medical Centers, Diabetes, Domestic Violence, Health Organizations, Hospitals, Medical Education, Medical Rehabilitation, People with Disabilities, Research/Studies Institutes. **Geo. Dist:** operating locations; MN; Sioux Falls, SD.

**★ 1100 ★ Grand Marnier Foundation**
1 Whitman Ct.
Teaneck, NJ 07666
**Phone:** (201)342-4663
Jerry Ciraulo, Treasurer

**Priorities:** *Arts & Humanities:* 55%. Funds performing arts, repertory theater, public television, fine arts museums, and film festivals. *Civic & Public Affairs:* 4%. Supports clubs and women's organizations. *Education:* 12%. Funds educational programs, colleges, and universities. *Environment:* 10%. Supports youth and child services, Meals on Wheels, social services, and youth and family counseling services. *International:* 3%. Support goes to single-disease organizations, medical centers, and hospitals. *Note:* Total foundation contributions made in 1999. **Typ. Recipients:** AIDS/HIV, Cancer, Child Abuse, Children's Health/Hospitals, Clinics/Medical Centers, Emergency/Ambulance Services, Health Organizations, Hospitals, Medical Education, Medical Research, Nutrition, Single-Disease Health Associations. **Geo. Dist:** nationally; CA; MD; NY.

**★ 1101 ★ Grede Foundation**
9898 West Bluemound Rd.
Milwaukee, WI 53226-0499
**Phone:** (414)257-3600
Burleigh Jacobs, President

**Priorities:** *Civic & Public Affairs:* 20%. Funds public policy, legal issues, taxpayers' and workers rights, and economic research. *Education:* 35%. Supports colleges and universities; medical, technology, and engineering education; and private pre-college education. *Environment:* 44%. Primary support is for the United Way; also funds activities benefiting youth, including YMCAs, cultural programs, community centers, and family services. *International:* Less than 1%. Supports single-disease health associations and the Visiting Nurse Foundation. *Note:* Total contributions in 2000. **Typ. Recipients:** Cancer, Children's Health/Hospitals, Clinics/Medical Centers, Hospitals, Medical Education, Medical Research, People with Disabilities, Single-Disease Health Associations, Speech & Hearing, Transplant Networks/Donor Banks. **Geo. Dist:** WI.

**Griffith Laboratories Foundation**
*See:* Entry 5574

**★ 1102 ★ Group Health Foundation**
36 Four Seasons Center, Ste. 274
Chesterfield, MO 63017
**Phone:** (314)205-0115
Dr. Robert Swanson, Secretary & Vice President

**Fnded:** 1986. **Priorities:** *Education:* 34%. Supports medical education programs and provides nursing scholarships. *Environment:* 13%. Funds family services and services for the mentally disabled. *International:* 53%. Supports health centers, infant health, childhood immunization, and promotion of healthy lifestyles. *Note:* Total contributions made in fiscal 2000. **Typ. Recipients:** Adolescent Health Issues, AIDS/HIV, Alzheimers Disease, Arthritis, Cancer, Children's Health/Hospitals, Clinics/Medical Centers, Diabetes, Emergency/Ambulance Services, Eyes/Blindness, Geriatric Health, Health Organizations,

Health Policy/Cost Containment, Health-General, Heart, Hospices, Hospitals, Hospitals (University Affiliated), Kidney, Long-Term Care, Medical Education, Medical Rehabilitation, Medical Research, Medical Training, Mental Health, Multiple Sclerosis, Nursing Services, Nutrition, People with Disabilities, Prenatal Health Issues, Preventive Medicine/Wellness Organizations, Public Health, Respiratory, Single-Disease Health Associations, Speech & Hearing, Substance Abuse, Transplant Networks/Donor Banks, Trauma Treatment. **Geo. Dist:** headquarters and operating communities.

**★ 1103 ★ Guardian Life Insurance Co. of America**
7 Hanover Square
New York, NY 10004-2616
**Phone:** (212)598-7499          **Fax:** (212)919-2944
**Email:** karen_olvany@glic.com
**Website:** http://www.glic.com
Karen Olvany, Assistant Corporate Secretary

**Priorities:** *Arts & Humanities:* About 8%. Funding supports historic preservation, libraries, museums, music, theater, and community arts. *Civic & Public Affairs:* 8%. Supports economic development through free enterprise organizations, zoos and aquariums, and urban and community affairs. *Education:* 29%. Primarily supports colleges, universities, education funds and literacy organizations. *Environment:* 29%. Recipients include united funds, youth organizations, and substance abuse prevention centers. *International:* About 12%. Recipients include hospices, medical research, and single-disease health associations. *Note:* Total contributions made in 1999. **Typ. Recipients:** Health Policy/Cost Containment, Hospices, Medical Research, Single-Disease Health Associations, Substance Abuse. **Geo. Dist:** headquarters and operating communities.

**★ 1104 ★ Guess? Foundation**
1444 South Alameda St.
Los Angeles, CA 90021
**Phone:** (213)765-3100          **Fax:** (213)765-5927
Lena Chin, Accounting Manager

**Fnded:** 1995. **Priorities:** *Arts & Humanities:* 3%. Supports museums. *Civic & Public Affairs:* 7%. Funds women's affairs and law and justice concerns. *Education:* 12% Funds schools, vocational training, and scholarship programs. *Environment:* 33%. Funds child welfare, scouting, and community services. *International:* 6%. Supports single-disease organizations, hospitals, and AIDS/HIV. *Note:* Total contributionss made in 1999. **Typ. Recipients:** AIDS/HIV, Cancer, Clinics/Medical Centers, Diabetes, Diabetes, Geriatric Health, Health Organizations, Heart, Medical Education, Medical Research, Multiple Sclerosis, People with Disabilities, Prenatal Health Issues, Substance Abuse. **Geo. Dist:** limited to headquarters area only.

**★ 1105 ★ Guinness/UDV**
6 Landmark Square
Stamford, CT 06901-0778
**Phone:** (203)682-7700
Brian Gordon, Contact

**Fnded:** 1960. **Priorities:** *Arts & Humanities:* About 22%. A local arts council, museums, music, and historical preservation associations. *Civic & Public Affairs:* 4%. Environmental, urban, andwomen's affairs organizations. *Education:* 13%. Scholarship program for company employees' children, colleges and universities, economic and minority education, and education funds. *Environment:* 54%. Major support goes to the United Way and other federated campaigns. Also funds youth organizations, shelters, food distribution programs, and other community service organizations. *International:* 3%. Community health care centers, hospitals, and health organizations. *Note:* Contributions made in 1998. **Typ. Recipients:** AIDS/HIV, Child Abuse, Children's Health/Hospitals, Health Funds, Health Organizations, Hospitals, People with Disabilities, Prenatal Health Issues, Substance Abuse. **Geo. Dist:** principally near operating locations and to national organizations. **Frmly:** Heublein Foundation Inc.

## ★ 1106 ★ Gulf Power Foundation

1 Energy Place
Pensacola, FL 32520-0786
**Phone:** (850)444-6806
John Hodges, Jr., Chairman

**Fnded:** 1987. **Priorities:** *Arts & Humanities:* 9%. Supports libraries, historical societies and arts councils. *Civic & Public Affairs:* 7%. Gives to chambers of commerce and community organizations. *Education:* 27%. Funds scholarships, colleges and universities, and education associations. *Environment:* 38%. Primarily funds United Way and youth concerns. *International:* 17%. Supports single-disease health associations; hospice programs; blood banks; and speech, hearing, and blindness centers. *Voluntarism:* Company reports that it supports, "Junior Achievement, (charity) runs and holiday shopping." *Note:* Total contributions made in 2000. **Typ. Recipients:** Cancer, Children's Health/Hospitals, Emergency/Ambulance Services, Health Organizations, Hospices, Hospitals, People with Disabilities, Prenatal Health Issues, Public Health, Single-Disease Health Associations, Substance Abuse. **Geo. Dist:** Northwest Florida.

## ★ 1107 ★ H.B. Fuller Co. Foundation

PO Box 64683
1200 Willow Lake Blvd.
Saint Paul, MN 55164-0683
**Phone:** (612)236-5217
**Website:** http://www.hbfuller.com
Karen Muller, Director of Community Affairs

**Priorities:** *Arts & Humanities:* 14%. Focus on youth and creativity. Also supports arts institutions in headquarters area. *Civic & Public Affairs:* (Public Benefit; Employee Community Leadership Fund) 2%. Supports nonprofit resources, urban affairs and leadership development. *Education:* 14%. Supports programs for economically disadvantaged youth which provide the basics in literacy and vocational training. *International:* (Health and Human Services) 70%. Funds programs which provide activities and health care for disadvantaged youth, with the dual purpose of involving community adults and the development of local youth. *Note:* Company gives through facilities, which respond to community needs. Above priorities reflect year 2000 foundation giving only. **Typ. Recipients:** Child Abuse, Clinics/Medical Centers, Domestic Violence, Emergency/Ambulance Services, Health Organizations, Mental Health, People with Disabilities, Research/ Studies Institutes, Substance Abuse. **Geo. Dist:** internationally; headquarters and operating communities; nationally.

## ★ 1108 ★ H.J. Heinz Co. Foundation

PO Box 57
Pittsburgh, PA 15230-0057
**Phone:** (412)456-5772　　　　**Fax:** (412)456-7868
**Website:** http://www.heinz.com/jsp/foundation.jsp
Loretta Oken, Program Director

**Fnded:** 1951. **Priorities:** *Arts & Humanities:* 15%. Funds ballet, opera, theater, symphonies, and history groups, primarily in the Pittsburgh area. *Civic & Public Affairs:* 4%. Funds community and economic development organizations and professional organizations, especially those associated with the food industry. *Education:* 18%. Includes support to pre-college and college education, educational foundations. An educational focus is on food science and restaurant education. *Environment:* 11%. Supports the United Way, youth and family services, substance abuse treatment and awareness, and food banks. *International:* 13%. Supports hospital foundations, children's health concerns, medical centers, hospice, and community health centers. *Religion:* 9%. Primarily funds food science research. *Note:* Total contributions made in 1999. **Typ. Recipients:** AIDS/HIV, Cancer, Children's Health/Hospitals, Clinics/Medical Centers, Family Planning, Health Organizations, Heart, Home-Care Services, Hospices, Hospitals, Medical Education, Medical Rehabilitation, Medical Research, Nutrition, People with Disabilities, Public Health, Single-Disease Health Associations, Substance Abuse. **Geo. Dist:** principally near operating locations and to national organizations.

## ★ 1109 ★ Halliburton Foundation, Inc.

3600 Lincoln Plaza
500 N Akard St.
Dallas, TX 75201
**Phone:** (214)978-2600　　　　**Fax:** (214)978-2611
**Email:** pat.george@halliburton.com
**Website:** http://www.halliburton.com/corp/about.asp
Celeste Colgan, Vice President & Secretary

**Priorities:** *Arts & Humanities:* 1%. Gives to the Oklahoma City Memorial Foundation. *Education:* 89%. Primarily supports faculty, equipment acquisition, and content development initiatives within engineering, technical or business departments of major colleges and universities. Limited unrestricted support. *Environment:* 5%. A small number of grants support youth organizations and the United Way. *Religion:* 2%. Supports a natural science museum. *Note:* Contributions made in 1999. **Typ. Recipients:** Cancer, Hospitals, Medical Education, Substance Abuse. **Geo. Dist:** Southwest; TX.

## ★ 1110 ★ Hallmark Corporate Foundation

PO Box 419580
Department 323
Kansas City, MO 64141-6580
**Phone:** (816)274-8508　　　　**Fax:** (816)274-8547
Karen Bartz, Community Development Manager

**Priorities:** *Arts & Humanities:* 23%. The company expresses strong interest in the arts through the support of local professional arts organizations which have an impact on a broad segment of the community. Emphasis is on culturally diverse audiences and involving youth. *Civic & Public Affairs:* 14%. Support for organizations which represent business interests or which promote community development, such as neighborhood preservation and redevelopment, especially neighborhoods adjacent to Hallmark facilities or in the urban core; business support groups/economic development; and social investments in support of housing or other redevelopment activities. *Education:* 22%. Assistance is given to local schools, adult education, support of public television, and projects designed to improve teaching and learning. Systemic educational reform efforts are of special interest. In addition, the company has a strong interest in the area of design education, initiating grants to art and design schools which are a source of talent for Hallmark Cards Inc. *International:* 37%. Support includes contributions to human service programs and/or agencies which serve minorities, low income, the homeless, disadvantaged youth, infant care, the disabled, AIDS patients, and others; primary support of such programs is through company contributions to local United Way campaigns. While the company does not make grants to governmental agencies, partnerships with the public sector in support of human service programs can be considered. *Voluntarism:* Supports the Volunteer Involvement Pays Program, through which a $200 grant is contributed to a 501(c)3 organization that has benefited from employee volunteers. Grant applications are employee initiated, and employees must volunteer at least 25 hours of service within a six-month period. *Note:* Company prefers to respond to requests on a case-by-case basis and has not established target levels for contribution categories. **Typ. Recipients:** AIDS/HIV, Cancer, Children's Health/Hospitals, Domestic Violence, Emergency/Ambulance Services, Health Organizations, Hospices, Hospitals, Long-Term Care, Mental Health, People with Disabilities, Public Health, Sexual Abuse, Substance Abuse. **Geo. Dist:** headquarters; principally near operating locations and to national organizations; Metamora, IL; Leavenworth, KS; Topeka, KS; Kansas City, MO; Liberty, MO.

## ★ 1111 ★ H&R Block Foundation

4435 Main St., Ste. 500
Kansas City, MO 64111
**Phone:** (816)932-8324　　　　**Fax:** (816)753-1585
Barbara Lebedun, President

**Fnded:** 1974. **Priorities:** *Arts & Humanities:* (Arts & Culture) 18%. Supports theaters, symphonies, operas, dance, art museums, and art concerts and festivals. *Civic & Public Affairs:* (Neighborhood Development) 22%. Funds efforts to support neighborhood development with a focus on grassroots needs, community activities, environmental improvements, and safety in core city neighborhoods of Greater Kansas City, MO. *Education:* 24%. Major interest in supporting education through Kansas and Missouri college funds. Considers requests for specific projects and capital improvements from higher education institutions and independent primary and secondary schools. Also funds adult literacy initiatives, special education programs for at-risk youths, and job training. *Environment:* (Corporate Social Responsibility and High-Rish Youth) 13%. Corporate Social Responsibility grants focus on parks and recreation, community services, minority/religious affairs, and nonprofit management. High-Risk Youth program funds organizations that provide services to high-risk, vulnerable, or emotionally disturbed youth. *International:* (Health & Mental Health) 17%. Considers requests for special projects from hospitals and neighborhood health centers. Also interested in mental health centers and educational programs to prevent mental illness. Places a focus on access to health care, substance abuse treatment, counseling services, and shelter for abused women and children. *Voluntarism:* Individual H&R Block associates actively participate in community programs such as Habitat for Humanity and United Way. The foundation provides strategic support, rewards, and recognition for volunteer efforts. *Note:* Total contributions made in 2000. **Typ. Recipients:** AIDS/HIV, Cancer, Children's Health/Hospitals, Clinics/Medical Centers, Domestic Violence, Family Planning, Geriatric Health, Health Funds, Health Organizations, Heart, Hospices, Hospitals, Medical Rehabilitation, Mental Health, Multiple Sclerosis, People with Disabilities, Prenatal Health Issues, Public Health, Research/Studies Institutes, Single-Disease Health Associations, Substance Abuse. **Geo. Dist:** Kansas City, MO.

## ★ 1112 ★ Hannaford Charitable Foundation

PO Box 1000
Portland, ME 04104
**Phone:** (207)885-3834　　　　**Fax:** (207)885-2859
**Website:** http://www.hannaford.com/community/index.htm
Donna Boyce, Secretary

**Fnded:** 1994. **Priorities:** *Arts & Humanities:* 8%. Funds support museums, libraries, art associations, and performing arts. *Education:* 21%. Provides scholarships through the Hannaford Scholarship Program. Supports college education that focuses on food marketing, pharmacy, or other programs that meet Hannaford's needs for associates. *Environment:* 44%. Primarily funds United Way or United Way supported agencies. Provides support to family services and youth organizations. *International:* 2%. Supports medical centers, hospitals, and hospice programs. *Note:* Total contributions made in 2000. **Typ. Recipients:** AIDS/HIV, Alzheimers Disease, Cancer, Children's Health/Hospitals, Clinics/Medical Centers, Emergency/Ambulance Services, Health Organizations, Heart, Hospices, Hospitals, Hospitals (University Affiliated), Medical Research, Research/Studies Institutes. **Geo. Dist:** headquarters and operating communities.

## ★ 1113 ★ Harcourt General Charitable Foundation

27 Boylston St.
Chestnut Hill, MA 02467
**Phone:** (617)278-5220　　　　**Fax:** (617)731-2354
Kay Kilpatrick, Director of Corporate Giving

**Fnded:** 1990. **Typ. Recipients:** Cancer, Children's Health/Hospitals, Clinics/Medical Centers, Diabetes, Domestic Violence, Eyes/Blindness, Health Funds, Hospices, Hospitals, Hospitals (University Affiliated), Medical Education, Medical Research, People with Disabilities, Prenatal Health Issues, Research/Studies Institutes, Substance Abuse. **Geo. Dist:** Boston, MA, including metropolitan area.

**★ 1114 ★ Harnischfeger Industries Foundation**
PO Box 554
Milwaukee, WI 53201-0554
**Phone:** (414)319-8506      **Fax:** (414)319-8520
Sandy McKenzie, Executive Assistant
**Fnded:** 1989. **Priorities:** *Arts & Humanities:* 19%. Supports museums, performing arts, libraries, the orchestra, and the theater. *Civic & Public Affairs:* 10%. Funds programs for ethnic and racial minorities, women's groups, foundations, and city offices. *Education:* 7%. Supports education programs, colleges, and secondary schools. *Environment:* 49%. Major grant to the United Way. Also gives to programs for the blind, youth clubs, Special Olympics, and community athletic and social clubs. *International:* 11%. Funds single-disease health organizations and organizations focusing on pediatric health/pediatric disease. *Religion:* 1%. Funds Discovery World - The James Lovell Museum of Science, Economic, and Technology. *Note:* Total contributions made in fiscal 2000. **Typ. Recipients:** AIDS/HIV, Cancer, Children's Health/Hospitals, Clinics/Medical Centers, Diabetes, Domestic Violence, Emergency/Ambulance Services, Health Organizations, Heart, Long-Term Care, Medical Education, Medical Research, Mental Health, People with Disabilities, Prenatal Health Issues, Single-Disease Health Associations. **Geo. Dist:** AZ; DC; IL; MD; MI; MN; NY; PA; TX; VA; WI.

**★ 1115 ★ Harold Simmons Foundation, Inc.**
5430 LBJ Freeway, Ste. 1700
Dallas, TX 75240-2697
**Phone:** (972)991-2400      **Fax:** (972)448-1456
Lisa Simmons Epstein, President
**Fnded:** 1988. **Priorities:** *Arts & Humanities:* 3%. Recipients include symphonies, opera, public broadcasting, theater, and museums. *Civic & Public Affairs:* 6%. Funding supports economic development, community philanthropic organizations, women's affairs, housing, and nonprofit management. *Education:* 5%. Funding supports colleges and universities, public and private secondary schools, and education reform. *Environment:* 72%. Funding supports the disabled, youth organizations, family services, child welfare, drug rehabilitation, and violence prevention. *International:* 10%. Recipients include community clinics, single-disease health organizations, nursing associations, and medical research. *Note:* Total contributions made in 1999. **Typ. Recipients:** AIDS/HIV, Cancer, Children's Health/Hospitals, Clinics/Medical Centers, Domestic Violence, Family Planning, Health Organizations, Hospitals, Hospitals (University Affiliated), Kidney, Medical Education, Medical Research, Mental Health, Multiple Sclerosis, Nursing Services, People with Disabilities, Prenatal Health Issues, Public Health, Single-Disease Health Associations, Substance Abuse, Transplant Networks/Donor Banks. **Geo. Dist:** Dallas, TX, including metropolitan area.

**★ 1116 ★ Harris Bank Foundation**
111 W Monroe St.
PO Box 755
Chicago, IL 60690-0755
**Phone:** (312)461-5834      **Fax:** (312)987-4702
Donna Streibich Curtis, Secretary & Treasurer
**Fnded:** 1953. **Priorities:** *Arts & Humanities:* 26%. Focus on promoting cultural diversity while providing access to the arts for underserved communities. Supports both the major cultural institutions and smaller art groups in Chicago, including museums, dance, theater, music, and zoos and parks. *Civic & Public Affairs:* 27%. Civic focus is on race relations, business and economic issues, infrastructure and environmental concerns, and strategic planning efforts. Community revitalization grants support programs which increase or improve housing for low/moderate income people in Chicago, and which promote commercial and industrial activity in low income neighborhoods. *Education:* 16%. Supports higher education, particularly in Chicago. Also supports organizations advocating for training and/or public school reform; technical and science education;

urban education; and opportunities for inner-city youth. Provides scholarships for children of employees. *Environment:* 28%. Grants go to new projects or programs which provide direct services to underserved, financially disadvantaged populations. Includes grants to community revitalization organizations. *International:* 3%. Grants are designed to improve hospitals and health care delivery systems. *Note:* Above priorities are for foundation giving in 2000. The company and its subsidiaries also make cash and nonmonetary donations; priorities vary according to community needs. **Typ. Recipients:** Clinics/Medical Centers, Domestic Violence, Health Organizations, Hospices, Medical Rehabilitation, Mental Health, People with Disabilities. **Geo. Dist:** Chicago, IL.

**★ 1117 ★ Harris Foundation**
1025 West NASA Boulevard
Melbourne, FL 32919
**Phone:** (407)727-9163      **Fax:** (407)727-9222
Richard Ballantyne, Secretary
**Priorities:** *Arts & Humanities:* Less than 1%. Museums, music, and arts associations. *Civic & Public Affairs:* 1%. Housing, safety, and urban affairs. *Education:* 93%. Matching gift program to secondary and higher education. *Environment:* 5%. Child welfare, scouts, and food and clothing distribution. *International:* 1%. Single-disease health associations, children's hospitals, and ambulance services. *Religion:* Less than 1%. *Note:* Above percentages reflect foundation giving in 1999 only. Company administers a direct giving program and a foundation. Both programs direct funds to eligible nonprofit organizations in Brevard County, FL, primarily through united funds, civic organizations, and various community serviceorganizations. **Typ. Recipients:** Cancer, Children's Health/Hospitals, Clinics/Medical Centers, Diabetes, Domestic Violence, Emergency/Ambulance Services, Health Organizations, Hospitals, Prenatal Health Issues, Substance Abuse. **Geo. Dist:** principally near operating locations and to national organizations; FL.

**★ 1118 ★ Harsco Corp. Fund**
PO Box 8888
Camp Hill, PA 17001-8888
**Phone:** (717)763-7064
**Website:** http://www.harsco.com/about1/community.html
Robert Yocum, Chairman & Trustee
**Priorities:** *Arts & Humanities:* 12%. Supports public broadcasting, the Harrisburg Symphony, libraries, arts centers and associations, and the performing arts. *Civic & Public Affairs:* 3%. Funds local civic organizations. *Education:* 58%. Includes colleges, universities, other higher education organizations, and educational programs such as 4-H. Supports the National Merit Scholarship Corporation with a large grant for scholarships for employees' children. *Environment:* 15%. Supports the United Way, Goodwill Industries, and YMCA/YWCA. *International:* 11%. Supports hospitals, cancer organizations, mental health, and health foundations. *Note:* Total contributions in 1999. **Typ. Recipients:** Cancer, Children's Health/Hospitals, Clinics/Medical Centers, Diabetes, Emergency/Ambulance Services, Family Planning, Health Organizations, Hospices, Hospitals, Medical Education, Medical Research, Mental Health, People with Disabilities, Public Health, Sexual Abuse, Single-Disease Health Associations, Substance Abuse. **Geo. Dist:** headquarters and operating communities.

**★ 1119 ★ Hartford Financial Services Group, Inc.**
Hartford Place
690 Asylum Ave.
Hartford, CT 06115
**Phone:** (860)547-5000      **Fax:** (860)547-3799
**Email:** Lynn.Jurgenson@thehartford.com
**Website:** http://www.thehartford.com
Lynn Jurgenson, Director, Community Affairs
**Priorities:** *Arts & Humanities:* 22%. Supports museums, public television, arts and the symphony orchestra. *Civic & Public Affairs:* 10%. Funds organizations

that provide programs to develop self-sufficiency to individualss with disabilities and to mature Americans. Also supports programs that provide employment training, job creation, housing, business development, transportation, neighborhood development, and law enforcement. *Education:* 31%. Supports mostly colleges and universities, primarily for scholarships, development of academic programs, business education, and insurance education. Also supports job training and career advancement for minorities and the disadvantaged. Employee matching gifts to colleges and universities amount to nearly one third of all educational grants. **Typ. Recipients:** AIDS/HIV, Children's Health/Hospitals, Clinics/Medical Centers, Domestic Violence, Eyes/Blindness, Geriatric Health, Health Organizations, Health Policy/Cost Containment, Hospices, Hospitals, Medical Education, Medical Rehabilitation, Medical Research, People with Disabilities, Prenatal Health Issues, Preventive Medicine/Wellness Organizations, Public Health, Substance Abuse. **Geo. Dist:** principally near operating locations and to national organizations, grant monies are allocated based on the size of the operation; Hartford, CT, Greater Hartford area.

**★ 1120 ★ Hartmarx Charitable Foundation**
101 North Wacker Dr.
Chicago, IL 60606
**Phone:** (312)357-5331
**Website:** http://www.hartmarx.com
Kay Nalbach, President
**Priorities:** *Arts & Humanities:* 21%. Supports music, museums, arts festivals, dance, public broadcasting, libraries, history organizations, and theater. *Civic & Public Affairs:* 5%. Funds business organizations, community development, housing, professional associations, public policy, women's and minority affairs, zoos, and aquariums. *Education:* 7%. Gives to colleges and universities, education associations, minority education, and education funds. Also sponsors an educational matching gifts program. *Environment:* 54%. Primary support is awarded to local United Ways in or near company operating locations. Other areas of support are youth organizations, legal aid, recreation and athletics, child welfare, and services for seniors. *International:* 2%. Funds national single-disease health organizations, hospitals, and pediatric health. *Note:* About 60% of contributions are made from corporate headquarters; 40% is allocated and disbursed through operating companies. Total foundation contributions made in fiscal 2000. **Typ. Recipients:** AIDS/HIV, Cancer, Child Abuse, Children's Health/Hospitals, Clinics/Medical Centers, Diabetes, Domestic Violence, Emergency/Ambulance Services, Family Planning, Health Organizations, Hospitals, Nursing Services, People with Disabilities, Prenatal Health Issues, Public Health, Respiratory, Sexual Abuse, Single-Disease Health Associations. **Geo. Dist:** headquarters and operating communities.

**★ 1121 ★ Harvest Charities**
Wachovia Bank, NA
C. Gerald Lane
Holman St.
Columbia, SC 29226
**Phone:** (803)765-3671
**Fnded:** 1944. **Priorities:** *Arts & Humanities:* 7%. Funds museums, performing arts, and historical society. *Civic & Public Affairs:* 1%. *Education:* 20%. Supports private pre-college and higher education. *Environment:* 19%. Funds United Way, youth groups, and social services. *International:* 7%. Supports hospitals, clinics, and cancer research. *Note:* Total contributions in 1999. **Typ. Recipients:** Cancer, Clinics/Medical Centers, Emergency/Ambulance Services, Health Organizations, Hospitals, Medical Education, Medical Research, Sexual Abuse, Single-Disease Health Associations. **Geo. Dist:** headquarters and operating communities. **Frmly:** Belk Simpson Foundation.

## ★ 1122 ★ Harvey Hubbell Foundation

PO Box 549
584 Derby-Milford Rd.
Orange, CT 06477-4024
**Phone:** (203)799-4100　　　**Fax:** (203)799-4333
Harry Rowell, Trustee

**Fnded:** 1959. **Priorities:** *Arts & Humanities:* 1%. Funds youth symphony assocation and the arts. *Civic & Public Affairs:* 8%. Supports parks and recreational facilities, festivals. *Education:* 35%. Contributes to several universities, and also supports medical education and scholarship programs. *Environment:* 35%. Majority supports various United Way agencies in Connecticut. Other recipients include boys clubs and homes, scouting programs, community centers, and food and clothing distribution. *International:* 20%. Interests include hospitals, emergency services, medical rehabilitation, and single disease organizations. *Note:* Total contributions made in 1999. **Typ. Recipients:** Cancer, Children's Health/Hospitals, Domestic Violence, Emergency/Ambulance Services, Health Organizations, Hospices, Hospitals, Hospitals (University Affiliated), Medical Education, Medical Rehabilitation, Mental Health, Nursing Services, People with Disabilities, Public Health, Respiratory, Single-Disease Health Associations. **Geo. Dist:** principally near operating locations and to national organizations.

## ★ 1123 ★ Hasbro Charitable Trust Inc.

1027 Newport Ave.
Pawtucket, RI 02862
**Phone:** (401)727-5429　　　**Fax:** (401)721-7275
**Website:** http://www.hasbro.org
Karen Davis, Director

**Priorities:** *Arts & Humanities:* 11%. Funds museums, museums, public art, and history organizations/monuments. *Civic & Public Affairs:* 22%. Supports community and neighborhood associations, economic development, public parks/playgrounds, and urban, minority, and legal affairs. *Education:* 10%. Funds higher education, public education, and Junior Achievement in Rhode Island. *Environment:* 45%. Funds United Way, scouting, children's services, food banks, community centers, recreation programs, and services for the disabled. *International:* 5%. Funds children's health, the Red Cross, hospitals and rehabilitation centers, and single-disease health associations. *Note:* Total foundation giving in 2000. **Typ. Recipients:** AIDS/HIV, Alzheimers Disease, Cancer, Child Abuse, Children's Health/Hospitals, Clinics/Medical Centers, Diabetes, Emergency/Ambulance Services, Eyes/Blindness, Family Planning, Geriatric Health, Health Organizations, Heart, Hospices, Hospitals, Hospitals (University Affiliated), Kidney, Medical Education, Medical Rehabilitation, Medical Research, Multiple Sclerosis, Nursing Services, People with Disabilities, Prenatal Health Issues, Public Health, Research/Studies Institutes, Sexual Abuse, Single-Disease Health Associations, Single-Disease Health Associations, Substance Abuse, Transplant Networks/Donor Banks. **Geo. Dist:** headquarters and operating communities.

## ★ 1124 ★ Hawaiian Electric Industries Charitable Foundation

900 Richards St.
Honolulu, HI 96813
**Phone:** (808)543-7350
**Website:** http://www.heicf/heicf.html
Curtis Harada, Treasurer

**Priorities:** *Arts & Humanities:* 17%. Supports public broadcasting, museums, and historical societies. *Civic & Public Affairs:* 21%. Supports economic development, housing, and the Better Business Bureau. *Education:* 23%. Education funds are directed to programs at Hawaiian colleges, universities, and secondary schools. *Environment:* 19%. Supports youth organizations, food banks, Special Olympics, and volunteer services. *International:* 12%. Contributes to the American Heart Association, American Cancer Society, and hospitals and medical centers. *Voluntarism:* Company sponsors an employee volunteerism program, including the Great Aloha Run, and the Special Olympics; small grants are awarded to non-profits where employees volunteer through the Volun-

teer Recognition Program. *Note:* Total giving in 1999. **Typ. Recipients:** AIDS/HIV, Cancer, Children's Health/Hospitals, Clinics/Medical Centers, Emergency/Ambulance Services, Health Organizations, Heart, Hospices, Hospitals, Medical Rehabilitation, Mental Health, People with Disabilities, Public Health, Single-Disease Health Associations, Speech & Hearing, Substance Abuse. **Geo. Dist:** HI.

## ★ 1125 ★ HCR Manor Care Foundation

PO Box 10086
Toledo, OH 43699-0086
**Phone:** (419)252-5578　　　**Fax:** (419)252-5521
**Email:** jsteiner@hcr-manorcare.com
**Website:** http://www.hcr-manorcare.org
Jennifer Steiner, Executive Director

**Priorities:** *Education:* 4%. *Environment:* 24%. Priorities include family services, and senior services. *International:* 48%. Supports the Alzheimer's Association, the Arthritis Foundation, the American Heart Association, Red Cross, hospice, and the Mayo Foundation. *Note:* Contributions made in fiscal 1999. **Typ. Recipients:** Alzheimers Disease, Arthritis, Emergency/Ambulance Services, Geriatric Health, Heart, Home-Care Services, Hospices, Long-Term Care, Medical Education, Medical Rehabilitation, Nursing Services, Public Health, Research/Studies Institutes. **Geo. Dist:** the 32 states in which the company operates. **Frmly:** Manor Care Health SVS, Inc.

## ★ 1126 ★ Hercules Inc.

1313 N Market St.
Wilmington, DE 19894-0001
**Phone:** (302)594-5137　　　**Fax:** (302)594-6909
**Email:** kchiomento@herc.com
Kim Chiomento, Community Relations Representative

**Typ. Recipients:** Health-General. **Geo. Dist:** principally near operating locations and to national organizations; DE.

## ★ 1127 ★ Hewlett-Packard Co. Foundation

PO Box 10301
Palo Alto, CA 94304-1185
**Phone:** (650)857-3053
**Email:** bess_stephens@hp.com
**Website:** http://www.hp.com/go/grants
Mr. Bess Stephens, Director, Corporate Philanthropy

**Priorities:** *Arts & Humanities:* 2%. Supports the arts. *Civic & Public Affairs:* 2%. Funds community foundations and civic institutions. *Education:* 70%. The majority of this support takes the form of equipment grants to more than 100 colleges and universities, supporting science, engineering, business, and medical education. Focus is on science and mathematics in primary and secondary schools; and science, engineering, medicine, and business in colleges and universities. *Environment:* 4%. Supports the United Way, the Red Cross and substance abuse prevention. *International:* 20%. Support goes to health organizations. *Note:* Overall priorities for both cash and equipment grants are programs that advance understanding of science and enhance the human environment through health, human services, and the arts. Total contributions made in 1999. **Typ. Recipients:** Emergency/Ambulance Services, Eyes/Blindness, Health-General, Hospitals, Medical Education, Public Health, Single-Disease Health Associations, Substance Abuse. **Geo. Dist:** international principally near operating locations and to national organizations; nationally; U.S. principally near operating locations and to national organizations.

## ★ 1128 ★ High Meadow Foundation

PO Box 955
Stockbridge, MA 01262
**Phone:** (413)243-1474　　　**Fax:** (413)243-1067
Tamara Stevens, Administrator

**Priorities:** *Arts & Humanities:* 70%. Over one-half of contributions for the arts support theater and performing arts. Other interests include chamber music, operas, symphonies, museums, art associations,

dance, and public broadcasting. *Civic & Public Affairs:* 1%. Support community service organizations. *Education:* 19%. The majority of giving supports private and public precollege education. Also donates to colleges and universities, including scholarships, agricultural education, arts education, educational associations and funds, international studies, legal education, and minority education. *Environment:* 5%. Funds child welfare, the diasble, family planning and services, shelters, and united funds. *Note:* Total contributions made in fiscal 1999. **Typ. Recipients:** AIDS/HIV, Children's Health/Hospitals, Clinics/Medical Centers, Emergency/Ambulance Services, Family Planning, Hospices, Hospitals, Nursing Services, People with Disabilities, Public Health. **Geo. Dist:** MA, Berkshire County, MA.

## ★ 1129 ★ Hitachi Foundation

1509 22nd St., NW
Washington, DC 20037
**Phone:** (202)457-0588　　　**Fax:** (202)296-1098
**Website:** http://www.hitachi.org

**Fnded:** 1985. **Priorities:** *Civic & Public Affairs:* 35% to 40%. Foundation is interested in helping to develop a wider definition of and vision for communities and community development. Supports projects that enable people and organizations to identify their collective needs and then develop strategies for addressing those needs. Also seeks to support projects that develop and engage community leadership; bring a variety of community actors to the table; facilitate the building of strong and accountable community institutions; actively seek to explore innovative strategies, creative use of resources, and new organizational roles or institutional mechanisms to build community capacity, particularly at the local level in an integrative way; and make more effective use of existing resources while mobilizing new financial, material, and human resources for community development. The company sponsors the Yoshiyama Award to individuals for exemplary service to community. and private institutions, communities, and individuals. *Education:* 35% to 40%. Foundation encourages projects that support children, youth, adults, and educators as they learn to participate in an increasingly pluralistic and complex society. Projects that further these goals include those that foster an understanding of diversity and global issues across disciplines, explore the role of museums and the arts in effective education, connect learning objectives with community service, and work force development. The majority of the foundation's education dollars are targeted toward the precollegiate level, with support at the post-secondary level directed mainly toward assisting institutions to build collaborative and cooperative programs with communities or the K-12 schools. Education projects that receive support reflect the necessity to prepare individuals to participate more fully as citizens and productive members of society; recognize that schools can play a significant role in building and stabilizing communities; improve and develop the connections between schools, parents, and communities; recognize the diversity of learning styles and pedagogical approaches needed to educate all of America's students; incorporate the arts or museums as an educator and provider of increased opportunities for creativity and problem solving; link education to economic opportunity; and utilize community resources, such as arts organizations, corporations, churches and synagogues, and community service organizations. In the area of education, the foundation does not support math and science programs that are not interdisciplinary and do not build upon emerging and existing research on teaching and learning; projects that focus on schools, teachers, and students in a vacuum, seeing them as separate from the community; or efforts to "internationalize" curricula, programs, or institutions at the post-secondary level. *Religion:* 5% to 10%. Foundation makes grants to organizations for support programs that address technology-related issues in education and community development. Grants are not solely for acquisition or use of technology, nor for equipment purchase. **Typ. Recipients:** Domestic Violence, Medical Education, Substance Abuse. **Geo. Dist:** continental United States; parent company gives internationally.

★ 1130 ★ **Hoffmann-La Roche Foundation**
340 Kingsland St.
Nutley, NJ 07110-1199
**Phone:** (973)562-2055      **Fax:** (973)562-2999
**Website:** http://www.rocheusa.com
Vivian Beetle, Director Corporate Relations, Contributi
**Fnded:** 1945. **Priorities:** *Arts & Humanities:* 1%. Funds a science library. *Civic & Public Affairs:* 18%. Supports community foundations, industry organizations, drug use prevention, and minority affairs. *Education:* 31%. Primarily gives to universities, with priority placed on scientific research in medicine and biology. Supports education funds, including the Independent College Fund of New Jersey. Also funds educational programs that encourage math and science literacy. *Environment:* 7%. Supports general social programs. *International:* 36%. Grants emphasize medical research and training. Supports hospitals, health organizations, and similar groups. Does not support medical delivery of services. *Religion:* 7%. Supports research foundations. *Note:* Above priorities are based on foundation giving only. Company also sponsors a direct giving program, which is considerably larger than the foundation program. Financial data for the direct giving program is not available; interests include health promotion and education, and math and science literacy. **Typ. Recipients:** AIDS/HIV, Cancer, Children's Health/Hospitals, Emergency/Ambulance Services, Health Organizations, Health Policy/Cost Containment, Hospices, Hospitals, Medical Education, Medical Research, Medical Training, Mental Health, People with Disabilities, Public Health, Single-Disease Health Associations, Substance Abuse, Transplant Networks/Donor Banks. **Geo. Dist:** NJ.

★ 1131 ★ **Honeywell Foundation**
PO Box 524
Minneapolis, MN 55440-0524
**Phone:** (612)951-2368      **Fax:** (612)951-0433
**Website:** http://www.honeywell.com/merger/page_3_2.html
Andre Lewis, Executive Director
**Priorities:** *Arts & Humanities:* 10% to 15%. Provides capital grants, general support, and employee matching gifts to public radio and television. Other interests include theaters, arts centers and associations, and music and dance groups. Focuses on major arts organizations and aselect group of new and emerging arts programs. *Civic & Public Affairs:* About 5%. The foundation's contributions support affordable housing, crime prevention in theneighborhood, and training and employment preparedness. Disbursements outside of Minneapolis are determined by the individual community needs. (United Funds & United Way) 15% to 20%. Foundation supports United Ways in operating areas. *Education:* About 25%. Emphasis on early childhood development and elementary and secondary education programs in major Honeywell locations. Other interests include business, engineering, and increased educational opportunities for women and minorities in technical disciplines. Grant types include scholarship funds (to institutions, not individuals), general support, endowment, and employee matching gifts. Also supports independent college and minority education funds, education associations, and precollegiate programs in technological sciences. *International:* Less than 5%. **Typ. Recipients:** Adolescent Health Issues, Cancer, Children's Health/Hospitals, Domestic Violence, Family Planning, Health Organizations, Hospitals, Hospitals (University Affiliated), Mental Health, People with Disabilities, Prenatal Health Issues, Public Health, Research/Studies Institutes, Substance Abuse. **Geo. Dist:** major principally near operating locations and to national organizations; MN, organizations in Minnesota receive about 50% of total contributions.

★ 1132 ★ **Household International Inc.**
2700 Sanders Rd.
Prospect Heights, IL 60070
**Phone:** (847)564-6010      **Fax:** (847)564-7094
**Email:** dmfunk@household.com
**Website:** http://www.household.com
Donna Funk, Director, Employee & Philanthropic Servi
**Priorities:** *Arts & Humanities:* 11%. Focus is on headquarters community. Nonprofit groups in this category must demonstrate how their organization and its programming efforts enhance the quality of life, educational readiness, or economic vitality of the community. *Civic & Public Affairs:* 24%. Company takes particular interest in the economic vitality and physical rehabilitation of key communities around the nation where customers and employees live and work. Funded programs focus on helping those who need assistance in basic skills and job training; stabilizing or improving housing; and revitalizing neighborhoods. Also supports diversity initiatives for women, minorities, and young people, as well as work and family programs. *Education:* 24%. Supports economic education, strengthening consumer education, and preparing students and adults to be financially responsible. Funds efforts of local school systems to improve education in operating communities. It does not provide direct operating grants to secondary or elementary schools. Scholarship awards and financial aid is available for the children of company employees. The company also allocates a portion of its company-wide education budget for grants to select colleges and universities from which it recruits its employees, and for institutions that maintain outstanding research departments in topics of relevance to its industry. Unsolicited proposals from post-secondary institutions are not accepted. *Environment:* 20%. Company may support the needs of senior citizens, the physically disabled, and providers of crisis and shelter care services. Company makes analysis contributions to the United Ways in its operating locations communities. *International:* 41%. Company takes interest in the direct delivery of health care and human services and may make grants to community-based agencies which address the diverse needs of children and their families, the physically disabled, and senior citizens. Funds United Ways in operating communities. *Voluntarism:* Co. supports a Volunteer Incentive Plan that provides $100 grants to organizations where employees volunteer; also supports United for Hope Campaign and Junior Achievement Program. *Note:* Total domestic contributions made in 2000. **Typ. Recipients:** Health Organizations, Medical Rehabilitation, Mental Health, People with Disabilities, Substance Abuse. **Geo. Dist:** headquarters area only.

★ 1133 ★ **Housen Foundation**
120 E Main St.
Erving, MA 01344
**Phone:** (978)544-3335      **Fax:** (978)544-2865
Denis Emmett, Treasurer
**Fnded:** 1968. **Priorities:** *Arts & Humanities:* 1%. Gives to a community arts fund. *Civic & Public Affairs:* 17%. Supports community foundations, parks, and a fire department. *Education:* 65%. Primary interest in Brandeis University. Also funds a community college, elementary schools, and scholarships. *Environment:* 3%. Gives to the United Way and YMCAs. *International:* Less than 1%. Funds the Franklin Medical Center. *Note:* Total contributions made in 2000. **Typ. Recipients:** Cancer, Child Abuse, Clinics/Medical Centers, Domestic Violence, Emergency/Ambulance Services, Health-General, Heart, Home-Care Services, Hospices, Hospitals, Hospitals (University Affiliated), Medical Education, Preventive Medicine/Wellness Organizations. **Geo. Dist:** MA.

★ 1134 ★ **HSB Group Inc.**
1 State St.
PO Box 5024
Hartford, CT 06102-5024
**Phone:** (860)722-5040      **Fax:** (860)493-1038
**Email:** justine_long@hsb.com
**Website:** http://www.hsb.com
Justine Long, Contact
**Priorities:** *Education:* 100%. The company matches employee gifts to accredited colleges and independent secondary and elementary shools. Interests also include business education, literacy programs, and education funds. **Typ. Recipients:** AIDS/HIV, Emergency/Ambulance Services, Health Organizations, Hospitals, Medical Rehabilitation, People with Disabilities, Substance Abuse. **Geo. Dist:** headquarters area only.

★ 1135 ★ **HSBC in the Community (USA) Inc. Foundation**
425 5th Ave.
New York, NY 10018
**Phone:** (212)525-8239      **Fax:** (212)525-6875
**Website:** http://www.us.hsbc.com
Kristen Alvanson, Assistant VP Group Public Affairs
**Priorities:** *Civic & Public Affairs:* Provides some support for Community and Economic Development, with a focus on the needs of low-to-moderate income people in HSBC communities. Funding interests include community-based organizations that develop affordable housing, create business opportunities, and address other important community needs, and local and national organizations that help such community-based organizations succeed; organizations that provide small business loans or technical assistance to small business/entrepreneurs; cityand county-wide nonprofit organizations that provide technical assistance to community-based groups that serve low and moderate income people, and community-based groups that provide homeownership counseling to this target population. *Education:* Supports underprivileged young people and schools in economically deprived areas; K-12 public schools and post secondary institutions; and adult education. K-12 education funding may target students, teachers, or parents. Higher education grants give priority to scholarship programs, especially those that support disadvantaged students. Schools, colleges, universities, and other educational institutions also receive support. **Typ. Recipients:** Health-General. **Geo. Dist:** headquarters and operating communities.

★ 1136 ★ **Hubbard Foundation**
3415 University Ave.
Saint Paul, MN 55114
**Phone:** (612)642-4300      **Fax:** (612)642-4103
Gerald Deeney, Secretary
**Priorities:** *Arts & Humanities:* 14%. Supports symphonic music, arts centers, theaters, historic preservation and arts associations. *Civic & Public Affairs:* 1%. Funds neighborhood housing services, community services, and zoology. *Education:* 63%. Colleges and universities receive primary support. Other priorities include Junior Achievement and education funds. *Environment:* 9%. Youth organizations are primary concern. United funds and child welfare organizations also received significant support. *International:* 5%. Primarily supports hospitals. Grants are also made to single-disease health associations, health organizations, and medical education and research. *Note:* Total contributions made in fiscal 1999. **Typ. Recipients:** Arthritis, Cancer, Children's Health/Hospitals, Family Planning, Health Funds, Health Organizations, Hospitals, Kidney, Medical Education, Medical Rehabilitation, Medical Research, Mental Health, People with Disabilities, Preventive Medicine/Wellness Organizations, Research/Studies Institutes, Single-Disease Health Associations, Speech & Hearing, Substance Abuse. **Geo. Dist:** nationally; principally near operating locations and to national organizations.

★ 1137 ★ **Huffy Foundation, Inc.**
225 Byers Rd.
Miamisburg, OH 45342
**Phone:** (937)865-2820      **Fax:** (937)865-5484
Pamela Booher, Secretary
**Priorities:** *Arts & Humanities:* 2%. Supports art institutes, dance, classical music, and theater. *Civic & Public Affairs:* (Civic & Community) 53%. Supports local community affairs, historical societies, parks, housing, and women's and minority affairs. Also supports public policy, the Red Cross, and public broadcasting. *Education:* 17%. Supports colleges and universities. Minor support for secondary education. Provides scholarships to children of employees. *Environment:* 27%. Supports the United Way, combined

charities, and United Cerebral Palsy. Less than 5%. Supports sports, Boys and Girls Clubs, scouting, and Junior Achievement. *International:* 1%. Supports hospitals, research, hospices, community health, and single-disease health associations. *Note:* Total contributions made in 2000. **Typ. Recipients:** Alzheimers Disease, Cancer, Children's Health/Hospitals, Emergency/Ambulance Services, Family Planning, Health Funds, Health Organizations, Health-General, Hospices, Hospitals, Medical Research, People with Disabilities, Single-Disease Health Associations, Substance Abuse. **Geo. Dist:** headquarters; principally near operating locations and to national organizations; Dayton, OH.

### ★ 1138 ★ Humana Foundation
500 West Main St.
Louisville, KY 40202
**Phone:** (502)580-3613            **Fax:** (502)580-1256
**Email:** BWright@Humana.com
**Website:** http://www.humanafoundation.org

**Priorities:** *Arts & Humanities:* 11%. Almost exclusively gives major grants to arts groups in Louisville, KY, such as Actors Theatre of Louisville, Louisville Orchestra, and the Greater Louisville Fund for the Arts. Also funds public broadcasting, historic preservation, and historical societies. *Civic & Public Affairs:* 4%. Supports economic development, business and free enterprise, philanthropic organizations, and urban and community affairs. *Education:* 61%. Major support goes to colleges and universities, including medical education programs. Other interests include public and private precollege education, education funds and associations, and business and economic education. *Environment:* 10%. Major support goes to the Metro United Way of Louisville, KY. Other recipients include youth organizations, recreation and athletics, child welfare, the aged, and community services. *International:* 9%. Recipients include hospitals, single-ease health associations, and mental health organizations. *Religion:* 4%. Supports a science center. *Note:* Total contributions in 2000. **Typ. Recipients:** AIDS/HIV, Cancer, Children's Health/Hospitals, Clinics/Medical Centers, Emergency/Ambulance Services, Eyes/Blindness, Family Planning, Health Organizations, Heart, Hospitals, Medical Education, Medical Research, Mental Health, Nursing Services, People with Disabilities, Prenatal Health Issues, Public Health, Respiratory, Single-Disease Health Associations. **Geo. Dist:** principally near operating locations and to national organizations; Phoenix, AZ; Tucson, AZ; Clearwater, FL; Daytona, FL; Ft. Lauderdale, FL; Ft. Myers, FL; Jacksonville, FL; Miami, FL; Orlando, FL; St. Petersburg, FL; Tampa, FL; West Palm Beach, FL; Atlanta, GA; Chicago, IL; Louisville, KY; Louisville, KY; Kansas City, MO; Cincinnati, OH; Austin, TX; Corpus Christi, TX; Dallas, TX; Houston, TX; San Antonio, TX; Green Bay, WI; Milwaukee, WI.

### ★ 1139 ★ Humanitas Foundation
1114 Ave. of the Americas, 28th Floor
New York, NY 10036
**Phone:** (212)704-2304            **Fax:** (212)704-2301
Peter Robinson, Executive Director, Vice President

**Fnded:** 1979. **Priorities:** *Arts & Humanities:* Less than 1%. Gives to a community youth music group. *Civic & Public Affairs:* 6%. Supports organizations that promote social justice and peace. *Education:* 14%. Gives to Catholic founded colleges, universities, and precollege educational institutions. *Environment:* 6%. Funds family services, temporary shelters, and other social services. *International:* 10%. Funds Catholic health organizations with a focus on services for AIDS victims. *Note:* Total contributions made in 1999. **Typ. Recipients:** AIDS/HIV, Children's Health/Hospitals, Domestic Violence, Family Planning, Geriatric Health, Health Organizations, Health-General, Long-Term Care, Medical Education, Outpatient Health Care, Prenatal Health Issues, Public Health. **Geo. Dist:** nationally.

### ★ 1140 ★ Huntington Bancshares Inc.
41 S High St.
Columbus, OH 43215
**Phone:** (614)480-8300
**Website:** http://www.huntington.com
Elfi DiBella, Executive Vice President, Director of CO

**Typ. Recipients:** Alzheimers Disease, Arthritis, Cancer, Children's Health/Hospitals, Eyes/Blindness, Geriatric Health, Health-General, Heart, Hospices, Hospitals, Hospitals (University Affiliated), Long-Term Care, Medical Research, Multiple Sclerosis, Respiratory, Speech & Hearing. **Geo. Dist:** headquarters area only; States where company has business locations.

### ★ 1141 ★ IBJ Foundation
1251 Ave. of the Americas
New York, NY 10020-1104
**Phone:** (212)282-4190            **Fax:** (212)354-7355
Ms. Lesley Harris Palmer, Executive Director

**Priorities:** *Arts & Humanities:* 26%. Supports children's museums. *Civic & Public Affairs:* 39%. Funds programs designed to improve and enhance the quality of life in urban neighborhoods, focusing on housing, childcare, and economic development. *Education:* 13%. Supports educational programs that foster among Americans a deeper understanding of the profound changes now occurring in an evolving global society. Funds teacher recruitment, community in school programs, and the National Geographic Society Education Foundation. *Environment:* 17%. *Religion:* 2%. *Note:* Total contributions made in 1999. **Typ. Recipients:** Children's Health/Hospitals, Home-Care Services. **Geo. Dist:** principally near operating locations and to national organizations; Los Angeles, CA; San Francisco, CA; Atlanta, GA; Chicago, IL; New York, NY; Houston, TX.

### ★ 1142 ★ IBM International Foundation
New Orchard Rd.
Armonk, NY 10504
**Phone:** (914)499-6420            **Fax:** (914)499-7624
**Website:** http://www.ibm.com/ibm/ibmgives
Paula Baker, Director, Corporate Community Relations

**Fnded:** 1985. **Priorities:** *Arts & Humanities:* 10%. *Civic & Public Affairs:* 3%. *Education:* 70%. Through the Reinventing Education Program, the company's K-12 focus, IBM promotes fundamental school restructuring and broad-based systemic change to improve student performance. The program motivates and enables districts to use technology to teach as well as restructure. Also promotes adult education, job training, literacy, and helping disadvantaged youth acquire education and skill technology. Contributions take place within the context of large-scale, district-wide reform efforts initiated locally. The program offers equipment, technical and consultant services and volunteer support. Also funds the KidSmart Early Learning Program and Project FIRST initiatives. and Project FIRST initiatives. *Environment:* 10%. Corporate and employee contributions of cash and equipment aid local United Way and other community-based organizations. Areas of support include child care, substance abuse, hunger and homelessness, illiteracy and education, physical and developmental disabilities, children and youth at risk, the elderly, as well as disaster relief. *International:* 6%. *Voluntarism:* The IBM Fund for Community Service recognizes and encourages the involvement of IBM employees and their spouses as volunteers in their local communities. Through the Fund, IBM makes financial and IBM product grants to specific projects of eligible community organizations and schools, provided an employee, retiree or spouse is actively involved on a continuing basis. *Note:* Total contributions made in 2000. **Typ. Recipients:** Health Organizations, Health Policy/Cost Containment, Hospitals, Mental Health, People with Disabilities, Single-Disease Health Associations, Substance Abuse. **Geo. Dist:** principally near operating locations and to national organizations. **Frmly:** IBM South Africa Project Fund.

### ★ 1143 ★ Idaho Power Co.
Idaho Power Corporate Contributions Committee
1221 Idaho St.
PO Box 70
Boise, ID 83707
**Phone:** (208)388-2530            **Fax:** (208)388-6903
**Website:** http://www.idahopower.com
Fran Martin, Executive Assistant

**Priorities:** *Arts & Humanities:* Funds historic preservation and cultural centers. *Civic & Public Affairs:* Supports housing, animal welfare, and community recreation. *Environment:* Social services organizations receive funding. *Voluntarism:* Co. supports employee volunteerism and notifies employees of community events and projects. **Typ. Recipients:** Health-General. **Geo. Dist:** headquarters and operating communities; ID, Southern Idaho; OR, Eastern Oregon.

### ★ 1144 ★ IFF Foundation Inc.
521 West 57th St.
New York, NY 10019
**Phone:** (212)765-5500            **Fax:** (212)708-7144
Douglas Wetmore, Treasurer

**Priorities:** *Arts & Humanities:* 36%. Supports fine art institutions, with major support benefiting the Whitney Museum of American Art. Also supports opera, ballet, art festivals, and historic preservation. *Civic & Public Affairs:* 25%. Within its Civic program area, the foundation funds women's affairs; fire departments, rescue squads, and police departments; senior, youth, and family services; and citizen groups. *Education:* 16%. Supports colleges and universities, private precollege education, and education in the fields of agriculture, food chemistry, and sciences studying sensory perception (particularly the senses of taste and smell). The company also supports an employee matching gifts program for educational institutions. *International:* 23%. Primarily supports cancer research; also funds hospitals, medical centers, single-disease health associations, and fundraising events for health organizations. *Note:* Total contributions made in 2000. **Typ. Recipients:** AIDS/HIV, Cancer, Child Abuse, Clinics/Medical Centers, Diabetes, Domestic Violence, Emergency/Ambulance Services, Eyes/Blindness, Family Planning, Health Policy/Cost Containment, Heart, Hospitals, Medical Research, Mental Health, People with Disabilities, Single-Disease Health Associations, Substance Abuse, Trauma Treatment. **Geo. Dist:** New York, NY.

### ★ 1145 ★ IKON Office Solutions Foundation, Inc.
70 Valley Stream Parkway
Malvern, PA 19355
**Phone:** (610)408-7285            **Fax:** (610)408-7022
**Website:** http://www.ikon.com
Kathy Fortebono, Manager, Strategic Services

**Priorities:** *Civic & Public Affairs:* About 4%. Support goes to zoological societies, other philanthropic organizations, women's issues, and civil rights. *Education:* 71%. Majority of support goes to matching gifts to universities and colleges. The remainder goes directly to private schools and education funds. *Environment:* About 19% of total contributions. Primarily supports United Way chapters across the country. The remainder supports youth organizations and community service groups. *International:* 6%. Support includes single-disease organizations, nurses associations, Easter Seals, and hospitals. *Note:* Total contributionss ade in 1999. **Typ. Recipients:** AIDS/HIV, Alzheimers Disease, Cancer, Children's Health/Hospitals, Emergency/Ambulance Services, Health Funds, Health Organizations, Heart, Multiple Sclerosis, Nursing Services, Prenatal Health Issues, Sexual Abuse, Single-Disease Health Associations, Substance Abuse. **Geo. Dist:** nationally; Philadelphia, PA, including greater metropolitan area.

### ★ 1146 ★ Illinois Tool Works Foundation
3600 West Lake Ave.
Glenview, IL 60025
**Phone:** (847)657-4092            **Fax:** (847)657-4505
**Email:** mmallahan@itw.com
Mary Mallahan, Manager, Community Relations

**Priorities:** *Arts & Humanities:* 11%. Primarily supports the Chicago Symphony Orchestra, Newberry Library, and the Shedd Aquarium. Museums, theater, music, dance, and public broadcasting also receive funding.

*Civic & Public Affairs:* 11%. Supports the Commerical Club of Chicago Civic Committee. Also makes matching grants to various civic organizations. Other interests include economic development, government improvement, professional and business organizations, and zoos. *Education:* 20%. Colleges and universities receive the majority of funds, largely in the form of matching grants. Other interests include education associations and funds and student aid. *Environment:* 35%. Primarily supports united funds; youth organizations also receive substantial support. Other interests include child welfare, volunteer services, and employment services. *International:* 1%. Supports hospitals and medical centers. *Religion:* 20%. Supports museums. *Note:* Total contributions made in fiscal 1999. **Typ. Recipients:** Cancer, Children's Health/Hospitals, Clinics/Medical Centers, Family Planning, Heart, Hospitals, Medical Rehabilitation, Medical Research, Mental Health, Nursing Services, People with Disabilities, Substance Abuse. **Geo. Dist:** principally near operating locations and to national organizations; IL.

## ★ 1147 ★ Inland Foundation, Inc.

4030 Vincennes Rd.
Indianapolis, IN 46268-0937
**Phone:** (317)879-4220 **Fax:** (317)337-8865
**Email:** vperkin@iccnet.com
Vicki Perkins, Director

**Priorities:** *Arts & Humanities:* About 4%. Particular interest in projects with strong educational components, which promote access to cultural opportunities for young people or the economically disadvantaged, and which advocate community involvement. *Civic & Public Affairs:* About 5%. Of particular interest are programs that address environmental issues, leadership development, job creation, community safety, and economic development in depressed neighborhoods. *Education:* 47%. Emphasis is placed on improving educational opportunities at public schools, especially those public schools that have established a partnership with Inland and with which company employees actively volunteer. Grants are designed to strengthen basic educational programs in reading, math, and science, as well as for the professional development of teachers, with primary emphasis on elementary schools. Colleges that provide specialized education in the fields of pulp, paper, packaging, and graphics are supported. Other targeted activities are those aligned to company's interests and the specialized educational needs of local plant communities, including literacy programs and programs designed to benefit minorities and at-risk young people. Scholarships are provided for the children of company employees. *Environment:* 39%. Major support goes to the United Way. Supports initiatives that emphasize quality health care, particularly for the benefit of the disadvantaged, disabled, minority populations, children, and families. Supports youth organizations which improve the quality of life for young people, particularly those most at risk. **Typ. Recipients:** Children's Health/Hospitals, Health Organizations, Hospices, Hospitals, Mental Health, People with Disabilities, Single-Disease Health Associations, Substance Abuse. **Geo. Dist:** headquarters and operating communities; Indianapolis, IN.

## ★ 1148 ★ Inman-Riverdale Foundation

PO Box 207
Inman, SC 29349
**Phone:** (803)472-2121
Patricia Robbins, Secretary

**Priorities:** *Arts & Humanities:* 6%. Supports community arts organizations and music. *Civic & Public Affairs:* 5%. Gives to county foundations, affordable housing, community parks, and civic organizations. *Education:* 34%. Funds colleges and universities, private precollege schools, adult education, and scholarship funds. *Environment:* 23%. Favors United Way, food banks, youth organizations, scouting programs, and the disabled. *International:* 7%. Supports hospitals and medical centers, a free clinic, and single-disease associations. *Religion:* 1%. Supports a children's science museum. *Note:* Total contributions made in 2000. **Typ. Recipients:** AIDS/HIV, Clinics/Medical Centers, Emergency/Ambulance Services, Health Organiza-

tions, Heart, Hospices, Medical Research, People with Disabilities, Research/Studies Institutes, Single-Disease Health Associations. **Geo. Dist:** SC.

## ★ 1149 ★ Intel Foundation

5200 NE Elam Young Parkway, AG6-601
Hillsboro, OR 97124-6497
**Phone:** (503)696-8080
**Email:** intel.foundation@intel.com
**Website:** http://www.intel.com/education/grants/index.htm
Lisa Siewert, Program Administrator

**Fnded:** 1988. **Priorities:** *Civic & Public Affairs:* (Community) 11%. Community programs, the Intel Computer Clubhouse Network, disaster relief efforts, arts organizations, and environmental causes are supported under the Community Organizations program area. *Education:* 89%. Of all education grants, 60% went to higher education and 29% went to K-12 education. Supports colleges and universities through equipment donations, research grants, a visiting faculty program, Distinguished Lectures in Technology Series, and employee matching gifts. Goals are to enhance education in math and science, increase the use of technology in community schools, and develop a future work force that represents the diversity of operating communities. Grants support curriculum development that involves math, science, and technology. *Voluntarism:* Intel sponsors a Volunteer Matching Grant Program; for every 20 hours of volunteer time donated to local schools by Intel employees, Intel gives the school $200. *Note:* Total contributions made in 2000. **Typ. Recipients:** Emergency/Ambulance Services. **Geo. Dist:** headquarters and operating communities; nationally; operating locations; AZ; CA; CO; MA; NM; OR; TX; UT; WA.

## ★ 1150 ★ International Paper Co. Foundation

2 Manhattanville Rd.
Purchase, NY 10577
**Phone:** (914)397-1500 **Fax:** (914)397-1684
**Website:** http://www.internationalpaper.com
Sandra Wilson, Vice President, Corporate Communications

**Priorities:** *Arts & Humanities:* 13%. Supports a variety of local arts groups, museums, historical societies, and libraries, with a special interest in the visual arts. *Civic & Public Affairs:* 27%. Supports municipalities and counties, as well as local groups concerned with community and economic development and volunteerism. Donations of $100 to $500 are available to organizations that have a significant number of International Paper Company volunteers. Also supports professional/trade associations associated with paper production and forestry. *Education:* 43%. For precollege education, focus is on improving the quality of teaching and learning in operating communities. Most contributions support the foundation's Education and Community Resources Program (EDCORE), which assists selected public school districts in areas where company employees are concentrated. Also gives to other precollege programs and institutions. The bulk of funding for higher education is disbursed through an employee matching gifts program. Also sponsors fellowship programs at selected institutions. Minority education receives between 5% and 10% of total annual contributions, including programs, funds, and institutions, with an emphasis on increasing career opportunities for minorities in the fields of science and engineering. Economic education also receives between 5% and 10% of total annual contributions. *Environment:* 4%. Supports youth organizations and other social services. *International:* Less than 1%. *Religion:* 4%. Funds science centers. *Note:* Total foundation contributions made in 2000. Company direct giving is about the same amount as foundation giving. Priorities are educational institutions, professional and trade associations relating to company's business interests, local youth and community organizations, hospitals, civic organizations, and arts groups. **Typ. Recipients:** Children's Health/Hospitals, Clinics/Medical Centers, Emergency/Ambulance Services, Health Organizations, Hospitals, Substance Abuse.

**Geo. Dist:** nationally; principally near operating locations and to national organizations.

## ★ 1151 ★ Invacare Foundation

One Invacare Way
Elyria, OH 44036
**Phone:** (440)329-6201 **Fax:** (440)365-4558
Debra Warden, Assistant Secretary

**Fnded:** 1994. **Priorities:** *Arts & Humanities:* 2%. Funds music and theater. *Civic & Public Affairs:* 2%. Job training, municipalities, and parks. *Education:* 8%. Gives to colleges, private secondary schools, public schools, and school-sponsored activities. *Environment:* 21%. Supports local United Way agencies, senior services, youth organizations, and people with disabilities. *International:* 66%. Primarily for single-disease health associations. *Voluntarism:* Company participates in the United Way Day of Sharing. *Note:* Total contributions made in 2000. **Typ. Recipients:** Alzheimers Disease, Arthritis, Cancer, Children's Health/Hospitals, Children's Health/Hospitals, Clinics/Medical Centers, Diabetes, Health Funds, Health-General, Heart, Hospices, Hospitals, Medical Education, Medical Rehabilitation, Multiple Sclerosis, Nursing Services, People with Disabilities, Prenatal Health Issues, Respiratory, Single-Disease Health Associations. **Geo. Dist:** headquarters and operating communities.

## ★ 1152 ★ J.C. Bradford and Co. Foundation

530 Belle Meade Boulevard
Nashville, TN 37205
**Phone:** (615)748-9302
**Email:** jimmy@jcbradford.com
James Bradford, Jr., President

**Fnded:** 1986. **Priorities:** *Arts & Humanities:* 10%. Supports public broadcasting, historic preservation, museums, opera, symphonies, and theater. *Civic & Public Affairs:* 50%. Supports community foundations, neighborhood development, zoos, parks, botanical gardens, public policy and civic affairs. *Education:* 16%. Supports educational programs and higher education. *Environment:* 14%. Supports child and family services, United Way, humane society, centers for victims of sexual and drug abuse. *International:* 3%. Supports American Red Cross, hospitals, single-disease health associations, and health care concerns. *Note:* Total contributions made in 2000. **Typ. Recipients:** Arthritis, Cancer, Children's Health/Hospitals, Health Funds, Heart, Hospices, Hospitals, Medical Education, Prenatal Health Issues, Sexual Abuse, Single-Disease Health Associations. **Geo. Dist:** Nashville, TN.

## ★ 1153 ★ J.C. Penney Co. Fund

PO Box 10001
Dallas, TX 75301-8101
**Phone:** (972)431-1349 **Fax:** (972)431-1355
**Email:** jsiegel@jcpenney.com
**Website:** http://www.jcpenney.net/company/commrel/index.htm
Jeannette Siegel, Community Relations and Contributions Ma

## ★ 1154 ★ J.D. Edwards Foundation

One Technology Way
Denver, CO 80237
**Phone:** (303)334-4807 **Fax:** (303)799-1705
**Email:** leslie_testa@jdedwards.com
Leslie Testa, Foundation Assistant

**Fnded:** 1991. **Priorities:** *Arts & Humanities:* Less than 1%. *Civic & Public Affairs:* 22%. Supports housing, employment initiatives, and urban affairs. *Education:* 23%. Funds private education, tutoring, and economic education. *Environment:* 25%. Funds youth programs, services for the disabled and disadvantaged, and United Way. *International:* 5%. Supports health centers and foundations. *Voluntarism:* Company provides employee volunteers for the Habitat for Humanity Summer Build Program. *Note:* Total foundation contributions made in 1999. **Typ. Recipients:** Cancer, Children's Health/Hospitals, Clinics/Medical Centers,

Family Planning, People with Disabilities, Prenatal Health Issues, Public Health, Substance Abuse. **Geo. Dist:** Denver, CO.


### ★ 1155 ★ J. F. Shea Co. Foundation
655 Brea Canyon Rd.
Walnut, CA 91789
**Phone:** (909)594-0941          **Fax:** (909)869-0849
Ronald Lakey, Chief Financial Officer

**Fnded:** 1967. **Priorities:** *Arts & Humanities:* 1%. Focus on museums, libraries, public broadcasting, and arts outreach. *Civic & Public Affairs:* 3%. Women's affairs, community affairs, and job training receive support. *Education:* 52%. Majority of funding supports school districts in California and Arizona. *Environment:* 32%. Emphasis on United Way, youth organizations, domestic violence, and family services. *International:* 8%. Supports single-disease health organizations, hospitals, and children's health. *Note:* Total contributions in 1998. **Typ. Recipients:** Arthritis, Cancer, Children's Health/Hospitals, Domestic Violence, Emergency/Ambulance Services, Eyes/Blindness, Health-General, Hospitals, Hospitals (University Affiliated), Kidney, Mental Health, Multiple Sclerosis, Nutrition, People with Disabilities, Single-Disease Health Associations, Speech & Hearing, Transplant Networks/Donor Banks. **Geo. Dist:** AZ; CA.


### ★ 1156 ★ J.P. Morgan Charitable Trust
60 Wall St., 46th Floor
New York, NY 10260
**Phone:** (212)648-9673          **Fax:** (212)648-5082
**Website:**     http://www.jpmorganchase.com/chase/gx.cgi/     Applogic%2bFTContentServer?pagename=Chase/Href&urlname=jpmc/community
Hildy Simmons, Managing Director, Community Relations

**Priorities:** *Arts & Humanities:* 15%. Supports both major cultural institutions and smaller, less established programs. Trust promotes groups which bring the arts to new audiences, particularly underserved populations and neighborhoods that lack cultural enrichment. Also supports those organizations that enrich the quality of life in New York City and encourage cultural diversity. Funds theater, dance, music, film and visual arts groups. Other recipients include libraries, arts in education, and programs which provide assistance to art organizations. Foundation matches gifts to arts organizations. *Civic & Public Affairs:* 26%. Supports organizations that seek to improve the quality of life in New York City. Interests include the preservation and development of affordable housing, assisting the economic development of the community, and projects that strengthen the neighborhoods by creating and preserving jobs, work readiness and employment training programs. Other interests include organizations that build on the strength of New York's racial and ethnic diversity, secure and maintain civil rights, and promote cooperation among diverse people. Also supports programs that provide training, strategic planning, and other technical assistance. *Education:* 30%. Supports colleges and universities from which company recruits its workforce, that provide educational opportunities for disadvantaged students, or that work collaboratively with the New York City public school system. Increasing attention paid to programs designed to improve public education, especially programs that can be replicated throughout the educational system. Promotes programs that develop student skills, teacher training and support, professional development, educational advocacy, and parental involvement. Also funds literacy programs and minority education programs that provide opportunity and access to independent secondary and higher education. Foundation matches gifts to education organizations. Foundation matches gifts to education organizations. *Environment:* (Health and Human Services) 24%. Human services funding supports children and youth services, food centers, Planned Parenthood, YMCA, United Funds & United Way, and basic social services. The major goal of health care giving is to make health care available to everyone, particularly low-income families in New York. Supports community-based primary care programs, health education,

disease prevention, and AIDS programs. Also gives to programs that provide self-sufficiency for low-income families, promote child care, and fight against homelessness, hunger, and violence. *International:* (See social services.) *Voluntarism:* Employee volunteers work with social service agencies, educational institutions, arts organizations, and hospitals. Company administers two volunteer-support programs: "Volunteer Center," which assists employees in finding suitable volunteer work, and "Volunteer Involvement Fund," which enhances employee volunteer efforts with cash grants of $100 to $1,000. *Note:* Total foundation contributions made in 2000. **Typ. Recipients:** Cancer, Clinics/Medical Centers, Domestic Violence, Emergency/Ambulance Services, Family Planning, Geriatric Health, Health Organizations, Health Policy/Cost Containment, Hospitals, Medical Education, Medical Research, People with Disabilities, Public Health, Sexual Abuse, Transplant Networks/Donor Banks. **Geo. Dist:** some funding internationally; some funding nationally; New York, NY.


### ★ 1157 ★ J.P. Morgan Chase Foundation
1 Chase Manhattan Plaza, 5th Floor
New York, NY 10081
**Phone:** (212)552-4892
Steven Gelston, Secretary

**Priorities:** *Arts & Humanities:* 4%. Major recipients include arts centers and programs in the visual arts. Other support goes to dance and music groups, arts councils, museums, and zoos. The company seeks to support effective arts in education programs, strong audience development and community outreach programs, and programs which encourage the emerging artist and the creative process through the creation and presentation of new work or through the support of developing artists. *Civic & Public Affairs:* 19%. A portion of the philanthropic budget goes to stabilize distressed neighborhoods and improve the lives of those communitys residents. Focus is on developing housing and jobs for low- and moderate-income people and addressing the diverse needs of the homeless. Other recipients include hospitals, youth organizations, aid to the aged and handicapped, recreation and athletic programs, community service organizations, and employment programs. Recipients include groups concerned with economic development, urban affairs, economic education, and the homeless and hungry. Funds an assortment of nonprofit organizations in the New York area, Connecticut, the U.S. Virgin Islands, and Hong Kong. The grants support local neighborhood projects and nonprofits. U.S. Virgin Islands, and Hong Kong. The grants support local neighborhood projects and nonprofits. *Education:* 18%. Supports development funds of colleges and universities. Other interests include graduate and undergraduate education, literacy programs, and minority education. Precollege education is a major priority. The company supports preK-12 programs, primarily in the public school arena, which: provide research and advocacy promoting education reform; develop the leadership skills of school administrators; increase effective pedagogy; or collaborate with schools to address the social, emotional and health needs of children so as to remove barriers to learning. Foundation also sponsors scholarships for children of employees. *Environment:* 51%. Supports youth and social services and United Way. *International:* 2%. Supports health care organizations. *Voluntarism:* Several thousand company employees volunteer in programs serving the communities in which they live and work, in a diverse set of activities that range from serving as mentors for at-risk teenagers to working as "huggers" for hospital boarder babies, from delivering meals to the homebound elderly to serving on numerous nonprofit boards. *Note:* Total contributions made in 1999. **Typ. Recipients:** AIDS/HIV, Cancer, Children's Health/Hospitals, Clinics/Medical Centers, Diabetes, Domestic Violence, Emergency/Ambulance Services, Eyes/Blindness, Family Planning, Geriatric Health, Health Organizations, Health Policy/Cost Containment, Hospitals, Medical Education, Medical Rehabilitation, People with Disabilities, Prenatal Health Issues, Public Health, Sexual Abuse, Substance Abuse, Transplant Networks/Donor Banks. **Geo. Dist:** internationally; nationally; primarily headquarters and

operating communities; AZ; CA; CT; DE; FL; MA; NJ; NY; OH.


### ★ 1158 ★ J.R. Simplot Foundation
PO Box 27
Boise, ID 83707
**Phone:** (208)336-2110
Connie Shields, Executive Secretary, Public Relations De

**Priorities:** *Arts & Humanities:* 79%. Supports museum and music, with major gift to Simplot Agriculture museum. *Civic & Public Affairs:* 5%. Supports community foundations and botanical gardens. *Environment:* 8%. Supports youth programs, homes, and scouts United Way. *Note:* Total foundation contributions made in fiscal 2000. **Typ. Recipients:** Cancer, Clinics/Medical Centers, Diabetes, Diabetes, Health Organizations, Prenatal Health Issues. **Geo. Dist:** headquarters and operating communities.


### ★ 1159 ★ J.T. Tai and Co. Foundation, Inc.
18 E 67th St.
New York, NY 10021
**Phone:** (212)288-5242          **Fax:** (212)737-4105
Ping Tai, Co-President & Co-Treasurer

**Priorities:** *Civic & Public Affairs:* 3%. Supports community programs. *Education:* 57%. Primarily supports colleges, universities, and medical schools throughout the country. *Environment:* 3%. Focuses on at-risk youth and community service organizations. *International:* 26%. Supports cancer research, other single-disease health organizations, and hospitals. *Note:* Total foundation contributions made in 2000. **Typ. Recipients:** Cancer, Children's Health/Hospitals, Clinics/Medical Centers, Emergency/Ambulance Services, Health Organizations, Heart, Hospitals, Hospitals (University Affiliated), Medical Education, Medical Research, People with Disabilities, Public Health. **Geo. Dist:** Northeastern United States; NY.


### ★ 1160 ★ J.W. Burress Foundation
380 Knollwood St., Ste. 610
Winston-Salem, NC 27103
**Phone:** (336)767-6900
**Email:** jwburress@jwburress.com
John Burress, III, President & Treasurer

**Fnded:** 1986. **Priorities:** *Arts & Humanities:* 7%. Funds arts councils, music, historic preservation, and a children's museum. *Education:* 73%. Supports colleges and universities, a military institute, and private pre-college education. *Environment:* 10%. Gives to the United Way, a children's home, senior services, and community centers. *Note:* Total contributions made in 2000. **Typ. Recipients:** Cancer, Child Abuse, Children's Health/Hospitals, Eyes/Blindness, Hospices, Single-Disease Health Associations, Transplant Networks/Donor Banks. **Geo. Dist:** NC.


### ★ 1161 ★ J. Walter Thompson Co. Fund
466 Lexington Ave.
New York, NY 10017
**Phone:** (212)210-7000          **Fax:** (212)210-6852
Donald Gammon, Secretary

**Priorities:** *Arts & Humanities:* 22%. Gives to libraries. *Civic & Public Affairs:* 55%. Supports The Advertising Council. *Education:* 12%. Funds scholarship funds. *Environment:* 11%. Supports child welfare organizations. *Note:* Requests in areas other than the arts and education are considered by the relevant offices of the co. Such contributions in most cases are made to organizations that in some way are connected with the co.'s business or because the request is client-related. Total contributions made in 2000. **Typ. Recipients:** Cancer, Clinics/Medical Centers, Diabetes, Health-General, Heart, Hospitals, Medical Education, Medical Rehabilitation, Medical Research, Single-Disease Health Associations, Speech & Hearing, Substance Abuse. **Geo. Dist:** nationally.

**★ 1162 ★ Jack and Bessie Fiterman Foundation**
5600 N Highway 169
Minneapolis, MN 55428
**Phone:** (612)536-6636 **Fax:** (612)536-6694
**Email:** davidlenzen@libertydiversified.com
David Lenzen, Executive Vice President

**Fnded:** 1966. **Priorities:** *Arts & Humanities:* 1%. Supports arts centers and historic preservation. *Civic & Public Affairs:* 3%. Supports recreation, community organizations, and foundations. *Environment:* 32%. Funds children's clubs, United Way, and social service organizations. *International:* 2%. Funds single-disease associations. *Note:* Minor support given to the areas of science and education. Total contributions made in fiscal 1999. **Typ. Recipients:** AIDS/HIV, Alzheimers Disease, Cancer, Children's Health/Hospitals, Diabetes, Health Organizations, Long-Term Care, Medical Research, People with Disabilities, Substance Abuse. **Geo. Dist:** MN.

**★ 1163 ★ Jacobs Engineering Foundation**
1111 South Arroyo Parkway
Pasadena, CA 91105
**Phone:** (626)449-2171 **Fax:** (626)578-6837
John Prosser, Jr., Senior Vice President, Finance & Adminis

**Priorities:** *Arts & Humanities:* 6%. Supports public broadcasting. *Civic & Public Affairs:* 27%. Supports community foundations and public policy. *Education:* 10%. Educational programs, educational funds, and universities. *Environment:* 32%. Funding is awarded to the United Way, senior centers, and youth programs. *International:* 8%. Funding goes primarily to hospitals. *Note:* Total contributions in 1999. **Typ. Recipients:** Alzheimers Disease, Cancer, Children's Health/Hospitals, Clinics/Medical Centers, Health Organizations, Health-General, Heart, Hospices, Hospitals, Medical Research, Multiple Sclerosis, Preventive Medicine/Wellness Organizations, Public Health, Research/Studies Institutes, Single-Disease Health Associations, Substance Abuse. **Geo. Dist:** headquarters area only.

**★ 1164 ★ James S. Copley Foundation**
7776 Ivanhoe Ave.
PO Box 1530
La Jolla, CA 92038-1530
**Phone:** (858)454-0411

**Priorities:** *Arts & Humanities:* 60%. Support goes to San Diego area arts organizations such as the symphony, opera, and museum of art. The remainder, in grants generally less than $5,000, supports arts funds and festivals, historical societies, theaters, and dance. *Civic & Public Affairs:* 4%. Gives to zoos, police organizations, and community foundations. *Education:* 6%. Funds colleges and universities, private precollege education, scholarship programs, and education associations; supports journalism education and literacy. Also gives matching gifts. *Environment:* 24%. Primarily supports united funds and youth organizations. Also funds recreation, senior programs, assistance for the disadvantaged and various community service organizations. Supports religious organizations that help the disadvantaged. *International:* 4%. Funds hospitals and hospices. Occasionally gives to single-disease health associations and blood banks. *Note:* Total contributions made in 2000. **Typ. Recipients:** AIDS/HIV, Alzheimers Disease, Child Abuse, Children's Health/Hospitals, Clinics/Medical Centers, Hospices, Hospitals, Medical Education, Medical Rehabilitation, Mental Health, People with Disabilities, Preventive Medicine/Wellness Organizations, Public Health, Research/Studies Institutes, Single-Disease Health Associations, Substance Abuse. **Geo. Dist:** in immediate circulation areas only.

**★ 1165 ★ James S. Kemper Foundation**
One Kemper Dr.
Long Grove, IL 60049-0001
**Phone:** (847)320-2847 **Fax:** (847)320-7996
**Email:** thellie@kemperinsurance.com
**Website:** http://jskemperfoundation.org
Thomas Hellie, Executive Director

**Priorities:** *Arts & Humanities:* 2%. Arts institutes, museums, and opera. *Education:* 91%. Grants are made to colleges and universities primarily for projects dealing with undergraduate or graduate business education. The Kemper Scholars grant program is offered in partnership with specific colleges and universities. The Foundation's Nursing Student grants are presently administered at Baylor University, Crouse-Irving Memorial Hospital School of Nursing, Massachusetts General Hospital Institute of Health Professions, and the University of Texas Austin. Fellowships are also supported at certain universities. *Note:* Priorities reflect foundation giving in fiscal 1998. Direct giving supports youth, health and cultural activities. **Typ. Recipients:** Emergency/Ambulance Services, Hospitals, Medical Education, Medical Rehabilitation, Medical Research, People with Disabilities, Single-Disease Health Associations, Substance Abuse. **Geo. Dist:** nationally; Chicago, IL, including metropolitan area.

**★ 1166 ★ Jefferson Smurfit Corp. Charitable Trust**
PO Box 66820
Saint Louis, MO 63166
**Phone:** (314)746-1151 **Fax:** (314)746-1259
Lyle Meyer, Contact

**Fnded:** 1951. **Priorities:** *Arts & Humanities:* 2%. Supports various arts organizations located in the St. Louis area. *Civic & Public Affairs:* 11%. Supports economic development, women's affairs, and zoos. *Education:* 9%. Supports colleges, universities, and business education. *Environment:* 32%. Awards major support to Boys Hope; also supports the United Way and youth organizations. *International:* 7%. Interests include single-disease health associations. *Note:* Total foundation contributions made in 2000. **Typ. Recipients:** Alzheimers Disease, Cancer, Children's Health/Hospitals, Diabetes, Hospices, Mental Health, Multiple Sclerosis, Respiratory, Single-Disease Health Associations. **Geo. Dist:** St. Louis, MO.

**★ 1167 ★ Jeld-wen Foundation**
PO Box 1329
Klamath Falls, OR 97601
**Phone:** (541)882-3451 **Fax:** (541)885-7454
Carol Chesnut, Contact

**Priorities:** *Arts & Humanities:* 15%. Recipients include museums, libraries, and arts associations. *Civic & Public Affairs:* 13%. Grants support community organizations, business and economic associations, and housing. *Education:* 7%. Most grants support higher education, including community colleges and universities; provides scholarships. Some funding supports secondary institutions, such as preparatory schools. *Environment:* 44%. United Way contributions account for the majority of grants in this category. Also funds children's organizations, community centers such as YMCAs, and recreational and athletic groups. *International:* 19%. Recipients include family and child medical centers; also supports healthcare policy organizations. *Note:* Total foundation contributions made in 1999. **Typ. Recipients:** Children's Health/Hospitals, Clinics/Medical Centers, Emergency/Ambulance Services, Health Organizations, Health Policy/Cost Containment, Hospices, Hospitals, Medical Rehabilitation, People with Disabilities, Prenatal Health Issues, Public Health, Substance Abuse. **Geo. Dist:** major principally near operating locations and to national organizations.

**★ 1168 ★ The Jochum-Moll Foundation**
PO Box 368022
Cleveland, OH 44136-9722
**Phone:** (330)225-2600 **Fax:** (330)225-0896
Chris Proto, Executive Administrator

**Priorities:** *Arts & Humanities:* 1%. Funds an art museum and music. *Civic & Public Affairs:* 26%. Supports civic instiitutions and women's affairs. *Education:* 34%. Supports colleges, religious education, secondary schools, education funds, minority and private education. *Environment:* 17%. Funds youth activities and the United Way. *International:* 17%. Funding supports hosptials and medical centers. *Note:* Total contributions in fiscal 1999. **Typ. Recipients:** Cancer, Clinics/Medical Centers, Diabetes, Health Organizations, Hospitals, People with Disabilities, Prenatal Health Issues, Research/Studies Institutes, Sexual Abuse. **Geo. Dist:** OH.

**★ 1169 ★ John Deere Foundation**
1515 River Dr.
Moline, IL 61265
**Phone:** (309)765-4137 **Fax:** (309)765-9855
**Email:** DP51104@deere.com
**Website:** http://www.deere.com/en_US/compinfo/johndeere_foundations/contributions_index.html?sidenavstate= 00000000001
Darlene Ellis, Contributions Representative

**Priorities:** *Arts & Humanities:* 6%. Supports historical societies, museums, cultural centers, orchestras, and other cultural activities. *Civic & Public Affairs:* 17%. Supports organizations concerned with public policy, business and free enterprise, civil rights, law and justice, and economic development. *Education:* 42%. Supports higher education, K-12 programs, minority education associations, and economic, science, and technical education. Emphasis is on recruiting, research, and retraining programs. *Environment:* 31%. Majority supports united funds. Other interests include youth organizations, programs for drug and alcohol abuse, child welfare, and the disabled. *International:* Less than 1%. *Religion:* Less than 1%. *Note:* Total foundation contributions made in fiscal 1999. **Typ. Recipients:** Emergency/Ambulance Services, Health Organizations, Health Policy/Cost Containment, Health-General, Hospices, Outpatient Health Care, People with Disabilities, Public Health, Substance Abuse, Transplant Networks/Donor Banks. **Geo. Dist:** principally near operating locations and to national organizations.

**★ 1170 ★ John Hancock Financial Services**
Box 111, T-58
Boston, MA 02117
**Phone:** (617)572-0451 **Fax:** (617)572-6290
**Email:** cfulp@jhancock.com
**Website:** http://www.jhancock.com
Carol Fulp, 2nd Vice President of Community Relation

**Priorities:** *Arts & Humanities:* 12%. In general, supports arts programs that have special initiatives for inner-city residents. Music, dance, community arts, and performing arts are of interest. Boston, MA, area. *Education:* 34%. Supports public schools through partnerships in Boston, MA. Emphasizes career/vocational training, and programs for the advancement of women, minorities, and the handicapped. *Environment:* 40%. Funds youth organizations, hunger/housing/homelessness programs, human services, and violence prevention. *International:* 10%. Supports local hospitals, neighborhood health centers, and emergency services. *Voluntarism:* Supports HERO (Hancock Employees Reaching Out), a program which organizes group volunteer projects. Outreach programs include Community Sports Initiative; educational programs, such as Operation Math Corps, Adopt-a-Class, Summer of Opportunity, and Financial Wizard Program; and community service programs, including the Incredible Sandwich Making Event (for food banks), Habitat for Humanity building projects, and holiday relief efforts. *Note:* Contributions analysis provided by the company. Beginning in 2000, giving will focus on programs that serve Boston's youth, particularly educational, after-school and recreational programs. **Typ. Recipients:** Health Policy/Cost Containment, Hospitals, Medical Education, Medical Research, Nutrition, People with Disabilities, Public Health, Single-Disease Health Associations, Substance Abuse. **Geo. Dist:** Boston, MA.

**★ 1171 ★ John Wiley & Sons, Inc.**
111 River St.
Hoboken, NJ 07030
**Phone:** (201)748-6000 **Fax:** (201)748-6088

**Website:** http://www.wiley.com
Deborah Wiley, Senior Vice President Corp. Comm.
**Priorities:** *Voluntarism:* Voluntarism is promoted through the Corporate ServiceMatch Program, through which the company provides small grants to organizations where employees volunteer. **Typ. Recipients:** AIDS/HIV, Diabetes, Medical Education. **Geo. Dist:** headquarters area only.


### ★ 1172 ★ Johnson Controls Foundation

PO Box 591, M/S x-46
Milwaukee, WI 53201-0591
**Phone:** (414)524-2296          **Fax:** (414)524-3200
**Website:** http://www.johnsoncontrols.com
Valerie Adisek, Foundation Coordinator

**Priorities:** *Arts & Humanities:* 34%. Primarily to Milwaukee-based arts organizations. Priorities include public broadcasting, museums, ballet, and visual, performing, and literary arts organizations and funds. Sponsors matching gifts program. *Civic & Public Affairs:* 4%. Mainly supports community and neighborhood development, parks, justice and law, civil rights and equal opportunity, citizenship, safety, and environmental affairs. *Education:* 8%. Primarily supports public and private colleges and universities. Other interests include adult education, education associations, and programs that seek to increase public knowledge of economics. Supports a matching gifts program. *Environment:* 49%. Major support to the United Way. Youth organizations are also a primary concern. Other interests include child welfare, the disabled, homes, the aged, and family and community centers. Also matches employee gifts to United Ways. *International:* 2%. Primarily supports hospitals and single-disease health associations. Will consider grants to capital fund programs supporting hospitals only if programs have been approved by appropriate health planning agencies. *Religion:* Less than 1%. Science museums. *Note:* Total contributions made in 2000. **Typ. Recipients:** Cancer, Children's Health/Hospitals, Clinics/Medical Centers, Health Organizations, Heart, Hospitals, Medical Education, Medical Research, People with Disabilities, Public Health, Single-Disease Health Associations, Substance Abuse, Transplant Networks/Donor Banks. **Geo. Dist:** in areas where company has a significant presence.


### ★ 1173 ★ Johnson & Johnson Family of Companies Contribution Fund

One Johnson & Johnson Plaza
New Brunswick, NJ 08933
**Phone:** (732)524-3255          **Fax:** (732)524-3300
**Website:** http://www.johnsonandjohnson.com/who_is_jnj/sr_index.html
Michael Bzdak, Director, Corporate Contributions

**Priorities:** *Arts & Humanities:* 6%. Supports the arts worldwide, with an emphasis on operating locations. *Civic & Public Affairs:* 11%. Supports urban, women's, and minority affairs and public policy. Also supports law and justice, public safety, and economic development. *Education:* 21%. Supports higher education, particularly medical and minority education. Also supports early learning programs and math and science education. *International:* About 45%. Supports health and medical research. *Note:* Total contributions made in 1999. **Typ. Recipients:** Cancer, Clinics/Medical Centers, Diabetes, Geriatric Health, Health Organizations, Hospitals, Hospitals (University Affiliated), Medical Research, People with Disabilities, Single-Disease Health Associations, Substance Abuse. **Geo. Dist:** internationally; nationally; principally near operating locations and to national organizations.


### ★ 1174 ★ The Jostens Foundation Inc.

5501 Norman Center Dr.
Minneapolis, MN 55437
**Phone:** (612)830-3235          **Fax:** (612)897-4116
**Email:** ourtown@jostens.com
**Website:** http://www.jostens.com
Lynda Michielutti, Executive Director

**Priorities:** *Arts & Humanities:* 6%. Interests include arts associations and centers, music, and theater. Emphasis is on programs for youth. *Civic & Public*

*Affairs:* 7%. *Education:* 53%. Funds economic and business education. Supports education funds, public education, and minority grants. Also supports the Junior Achievement and Reading Is Fundamental programs. Sponsors the Jostens Scholars and Holt Memorial Programs for dependents of employees and sales agents. *Environment:* 15%. Supports the United Way. *International:* About 10%. Supports youth organizations, disability centers, pediatric health clinics, single-disease health associations, and drug and substance abuse services. *Religion:* 2%. *Note:* Above priorities reflect foundation giving. The company also supports regional giving, directed by employees on Plant Contribution Committees. The company supports Jostens Renaissance Program, designed to recognize academic achievement through a business approach to education. Contributions made in 1998. **Typ. Recipients:** AIDS/HIV, Arthritis, Cancer, Child Abuse, Children's Health/Hospitals, Clinics/Medical Centers, Diabetes, Emergency/Ambulance Services, Eyes/Blindness, Health-General, Hospices, Hospitals, Medical Education, Multiple Sclerosis, People with Disabilities, Prenatal Health Issues, Public Health, Single-Disease Health Associations, Substance Abuse, Trauma Treatment. **Geo. Dist:** principally near operating locations and to national organizations.


### ★ 1175 ★ Journal-Gazette Foundation, Inc.

701 South Clinton St.
Fort Wayne, IN 46802-1806
**Phone:** (219)424-5257          **Fax:** (219)426-0949
Richard Inskeep, President

**Fnded:** 1985. **Priorities:** *Arts & Humanities:* 15%. Supports historic preservation, fine arts, performing arts, libraries, and public broadcasting in Ft. Wayne, IN. *Civic & Public Affairs:* 18%. Supports fairgrounds, community foundations, and minority organizations. *Education:* 23%. Major support goes to the Indiana University Foundation. Also contributes to Junior Achievement, secondary and higher education, and literacy programs. *Environment:* 34%. Support goes to the YMCA, the United Way, food banks, Planned Parenthood, and youth organizations. *International:* 4%. Primarily supports hospitals and the American Red Cross. Also supports health services and an AIDS task force. *Religion:* 2%. Supports a science museum. *Note:* Total contributions made in 2000. **Typ. Recipients:** AIDS/HIV, Cancer, Child Abuse, Children's Health/Hospitals, Clinics/Medical Centers, Emergency/Ambulance Services, Family Planning, Geriatric Health, Health Organizations, Hospitals, Kidney, Medical Education, Mental Health, People with Disabilities, Research/Studies Institutes, Single-Disease Health Associations, Substance Abuse. **Geo. Dist:** IN, Northeast Indiana.


### ★ 1176 ★ JSJ Foundation

700 Robbins Rd.
Grand Haven, MI 49417-2651
**Phone:** (616)842-6350          **Fax:** (616)847-3112
**Email:** sherwoodl@jsjcorp.com
Lynne Sherwood, Secretary & Trustee

**Priorities:** *Arts & Humanities:* 5%. Supports arts, museums, and music. *Civic & Public Affairs:* 20%. Supports civic programs, libraries, and a diversity program. *Education:* 36%. Supports higher education. *Environment:* 33%. Supports humane society, united funds and United Way, and youth services. *International:* 6%. Supports hospice. *Note:* Total contributions made in 2000. **Typ. Recipients:** Cancer, Health Organizations, Health Policy/Cost Containment, Hospices, Substance Abuse, Transplant Networks/Donor Banks. **Geo. Dist:** CA, southern; FL; MI; TX; WI.


### ★ 1177 ★ Julius and Ray Charlestein Foundation

3600 Horizon Dr.
King of Prussia, PA 19406
**Phone:** 888-773-6872          **Fax:** (610)239-6172
Morton Charlestein, President

**Fnded:** 1963. **Priorities:** *Arts & Humanities:* 2%. *Education:* 6%. *Environment:* 8%. *International:* 23%.

Funds oral health, diabetes, eyes/blindness, and geriatrics, and single diseases health associations. *Note:* Total contributions made in fiscal 1999. **Typ. Recipients:** Alzheimers Disease, Children's Health/Hospitals, Diabetes, Eyes/Blindness, Family Planning, Geriatric Health, Health Organizations, Health-General, Hospitals (University Affiliated), Medical Education, Medical Rehabilitation, Medical Research, Nursing Services, People with Disabilities, Public Health, Single-Disease Health Associations. **Geo. Dist:** nationally; PA.


### ★ 1178 ★ Katten, Muchin & Zavis Foundation

525 West Monroe St., Ste. 1600
Chicago, IL 60661-3693
**Phone:** (312)902-5200
Mark Broutman, Contributions

**Fnded:** 1982. **Priorities:** *Arts & Humanities:* 13%. Supports museums, opera, theater, and local arts organizations. *Civic & Public Affairs:* 26%. Primarily funds legal aid organizations for minorities, women, and the disadvantaged. Also supports community groups, and business/professional organizations. *Education:* 4%. Supports business education and colleges and universities. *International:* 7%. Supports youth organizations, the United Way, and numerous community service organizations. *International:* 9%. Primarily supports hospitals, health care, pediatric health organizations, and local chapters of single-disease health associations. *Note:* Total contributions in 1999. **Typ. Recipients:** AIDS/HIV, Alzheimers Disease, Alzheimers Disease, Cancer, Child Abuse, Children's Health/Hospitals, Clinics/Medical Centers, Diabetes, Emergency/Ambulance Services, Health Organizations, Hospitals, Kidney, Medical Research, Mental Health, Multiple Sclerosis, People with Disabilities, Public Health, Single-Disease Health Associations, Substance Abuse. **Geo. Dist:** nationally and internationally; Chicago, IL.


### ★ 1179 ★ Kellogg Co. Twenty-Five Year Employees' Fund Inc.

One Kellogg Square
Battle Creek, MI 49016-3599
**Phone:** (616)961-3125          **Fax:** (616)961-3494
Timothy Knowlton, Director

**Typ. Recipients:** Clinics/Medical Centers, Emergency/Ambulance Services, Health Organizations, Hospices, Hospitals, People with Disabilities, Substance Abuse. **Geo. Dist:** MI.


### ★ 1180 ★ Kellwood Foundation

600 Kellwood Parkway
Chesterfield, MO 63017
**Phone:** (314)576-3431          **Fax:** (314)576-3439
Terri Wise, Secretary, Treasurer & Director

**Fnded:** 1965. **Priorities:** *Arts & Humanities:* 1%. Supports art centers. *Civic & Public Affairs:* 1%. Supports housing and botanical gardens. *Education:* 85%. Supports colleges, universities, and educational funds. *Environment:* 10%. Supports child welfare, homes, food distribution, YMCA, and substance abuse programs. *International:* 1%. Supports single-disease health associations, and medical research. *Note:* Total contributions made in fiscal 1999. **Typ. Recipients:** AIDS/HIV, Cancer, Children's Health/Hospitals, Diabetes, Emergency/Ambulance Services, Eyes/Blindness, Health-General, People with Disabilities, Single-Disease Health Associations, Substance Abuse, Transplant Networks/Donor Banks. **Geo. Dist:** St. Louis, MO, including greater metropolitan area.


### ★ 1181 ★ Kelly Services Foundation

999 W Big Beaver
Troy, MI 48084
**Phone:** (248)244-5419          **Fax:** (248)244-5516
**Email:** kennelb@kellyservices.com
Lori Beirne-Kennedy, Foundation Administrator

**Fnded:** 1994. **Priorities:** *Arts & Humanities:* 2%. Funds festivals, performing arts, and cultural centers. *Civic & Public Affairs:* 19%. Funds foundations, professional associations, and a zoological institute. *Education:* 13%. Supports schools, academies, and the United Negro College Fund. *Environment:* 49%. Supports child abuse prevention, Boys & Girls Clubs, Ronald McDonald House, Make-A-Wish Foundation, and various other organizations. *International:* 17%. Supports hospitals and single-disease associations. *Note:* Total contributions made in 1998. **Typ. Recipients:** Alzheimers Disease, Cancer, Children's Health/Hospitals, Clinics/Medical Centers, Emergency/Ambulance Services, Eyes/Blindness, Health-General, Heart, Home-Care Services, Hospices, Hospitals, Long-Term Care, People with Disabilities. **Geo. Dist:** MI.

**★ 1182 ★ Kennametal Foundation**
PO Box 231
Route 981 South
Latrobe, PA 15650
**Phone:** (724)539-5203      **Fax:** (724)539-5024
Richard Gibson, Secretary & Treasurer

**Priorities:** *Arts & Humanities:* 20%. Supports libraries, music, public broadcasting, and historic preservation. *Civic & Public Affairs:* 5%. Primarily supports community foundations and organizations for economic development. Other interests include free enterprise, minority affairs, taxation, and environmental affairs. *Education:* 51%. Majority of funding supports the National Merit Scholarship Corporation and the Foundation of Independent Colleges of Pennsylvania. The remainder supports Eastern colleges and universities. *Environment:* 13%. Primarily supports the United Way. Family services, youth organizations, and people with disabilities also receive support. *International:* 1%. Major support to emergency services, hospitals, and single-disease health organizations. *Religion:* 1%. Supports science institutes. *Note:* Total contributions made in fiscal 1999. **Typ. Recipients:** Cancer, Cancer, Diabetes, Health Organizations, Heart, Hospitals, Medical Research, Mental Health, People with Disabilities, Single-Disease Health Associations. **Geo. Dist:** East coast.

**★ 1183 ★ Kerr-McGee Foundation**
PO Box 25861
Kerr McGee Center
Oklahoma City, OK 73125
**Phone:** (405)270-1313      **Fax:** (405)270-3940
Martha Brady, Administrator, Contributions

**Priorities:** *Arts & Humanities:* 13%. Supports arts funds, museums, and performing artsorganizations. Major grants are awarded in Oklahoma City. *Civic & Public Affairs:* 38%. Principal concerns include safety, economics, and professional organizations, as well as groups concerned with legal and public policy issues. *Education:* 31%. Interests include state universities in Oklahoma; technical, mining, and engineering education; independent and minority college funds; and economic education associations. *International:* 18%. Interests include hospitals, health organizations, single-disease health associations, and health funds. Also supports united funds, legal aid organizations, youth agencies, and community services. **Typ. Recipients:** Health Funds, Health Organizations, Hospices, Hospitals, Medical Research, Medical Training, People with Disabilities, Single-Disease Health Associations. **Geo. Dist:** operating locations; Oklahoma City, OK. **Frmly.** Kerr-McGee Foundation Corp.

**★ 1184 ★ KeySpan Energy Delivery New England**
201 Rivermoor St.
Boston, MA 02132
**Phone:** (617)723-5512      **Fax:** (617)742-3042
**Email:** scarlson@keyspanenergy.com
**Website:** http://www.keyspanenergy.com/community/index.cfm
Susan Carlson, Manager Corporate & Foundation Giving

**Typ. Recipients:** Health-General. **Geo. Dist:** MA, Central Massachusetts; MA, Eastern Massachusetts.

**KeySpan Foundation**
*See:* Entry 11444

**★ 1185 ★ Kimberly-Clark Foundation**
PO Box 619100
Dallas, TX 75261-9100
**Phone:** (972)281-1200      **Fax:** (972)281-1490
**Email:** foundation@keyspanenergy.com
**Website:** http://www.kimberly-clark.com/aboutus/comm_involvement.a sp
Carolyn Mentesana, Vice President

**Priorities:** *Arts & Humanities:* 1%. Supports symphony associations, museums, the theater, and programs for writers. *Civic & Public Affairs:* 37%. Interests include community foundations, municipalities, legal affairs, women's causes, and philanthropy. *Education:* 37%. Major support to colleges and universities as capital and operating grants, scholarships, and to minority education programs. *Environment:* 8%. Emphasis on United Ways in operating communities. Other recipients include youth and the aged, services for the handicapped, and programs for the treatment and prevention of alcohol and drug abuse. *International:* 4%. Support includes hospitals and health agencies, such as single-disease health associations. *Voluntarism:* Foundation makes grants to organizations where employees and their spouses volunteer through the Community Partners program. *Note:* Total foundation contributions made in 2000. **Typ. Recipients:** Adolescent Health Issues, Cancer, Children's Health/Hospitals, Clinics/Medical Centers, Diabetes, Domestic Violence, Emergency/Ambulance Services, Geriatric Health, Health Funds, Health Organizations, Health-General, Hospitals, Hospitals (University Affiliated), Medical Education, Medical Research, Multiple Sclerosis, Nursing Services, People with Disabilities, Public Health, Single-Disease Health Associations, Substance Abuse. **Geo. Dist:** national organizations; operating locations.

**★ 1186 ★ Kinder Morgan Foundation**
370 Van Gordon St.
Lakewood, CO 80228-8304
**Phone:** (303)763-3471      **Fax:** (303)984-3306
**Email:** maureen_bulkley@kindermorgan.com
**Website:** http://www.kindermorgan.com
Maureen Bulkley, Community Relations Coordinator
**Fnded:** 1990. **Priorities:** *Education:* Higher education, including community colleges, is a priority; also funds preschoo1, K-12, and enrichment programs. *Environment:* Supports youth activities. *Voluntarism:* The Foundation funds the KM for Kids program, through which youth programs throughout Kinder Morgan's retail communities receive funding and volunteer support. **Typ. Recipients:** Children's Health/Hospitals, Emergency/Ambulance Services, Family Planning, Health Organizations, Health-General, Hospitals, People with Disabilities, Public Health. **Geo. Dist:** AR; CO; IA; KS; LA; MO; MT; NE; NM; OK; TX; UT; WY.

**★ 1187 ★ Kingsbury Fund**
80 Laurel St.
Keene, NH 03431-4207
**Phone:** (603)352-5212      **Fax:** (603)357-7419
**Website:** http://www.kingsburycorp.com
James O'Neil, Vice President, Corporate Relations
**Fnded:** 1952. **Priorities:** *Arts & Humanities:* About 37%. Historic preservation, public broadcasting, art centers, and visual and performing arts. *Civic & Public Affairs:* 8%. Urban and community affairs and urban safety programs. *Education:* 30%. Colleges and universities, scholarship funds, and secondary education. *Environment:* 24%. United Ways, YMCAs, youth organizations, and athletic programs. *International:* 1%. Cancer centers and health care facilities. *Note:* Contributions analysis reflects typical annual distribution of funds. **Typ. Recipients:** Cancer, Children's Health/Hospitals, Clinics/Medical Centers, Emergency/Ambulance Services, Health Organizations, Heart, Hospices, Medical Research, Substance Abuse. **Geo. Dist:** NH, Cheshire County.

**★ 1188 ★ Kirkland & Ellis Foundation**
200 E Randolph Dr.
Chicago, IL 60601
**Phone:** (312)861-2038      **Fax:** (312)861-2200
Willard Fraumann, President

**Fnded:** 1981. **Priorities:** *Arts & Humanities:* 7%. Opera, museums, and theater. *Civic & Public Affairs:* 23%. Legal aid, civil rights, public policy, and minority affairs. *Education:* 63%. Majority of funding supports legal education. Also supports minority education and colleges. *International:* 4%. Single-disease health organizations. **Typ. Recipients:** Cancer, Health-General, Substance Abuse. **Geo. Dist:** headquarters and operating communities.

**★ 1189 ★ Koch Foundation**
10 South 11th Ave.
Evansville, IN 47744
**Phone:** (812)465-9800      **Fax:** (812)465-9613
Edward Koch, II, President

**Fnded:** 1945. **Priorities:** *Arts & Humanities:* 1%. Supports Evansville area arts organizations, with interests in theater, music, and public broadcasting. *Civic & Public Affairs:* 8%. Supports housing and economic development, organizations that promote civic pride, Right to Life, and local parks and zoos. *Education:* 39%. Supports public education, independent college funds, and colleges and universities. Provides scholarships at several local higher education institutions. Also sponsors a scholarship program for employees' children, totaling about one-quarter of education contributions. Co. matches gifts to educational and medical research organizations. *Environment:* 13%. Supports youth organizations and the United Way. *International:* 7%. Primarily supports hospitals and medical centers. *Religion:* Less than 1%. Supports science museums. *Note:* Total contributions made in 2000. **Typ. Recipients:** Cancer, Children's Health/Hospitals, Clinics/Medical Centers, Emergency/Ambulance Services, Hospitals, Medical Rehabilitation, Mental Health, People with Disabilities, Public Health, Single-Disease Health Associations, Substance Abuse. **Geo. Dist:** IN; KY, especially western KY. **Frmly:** George Koch Sons Foundation.

**★ 1190 ★ Kraft Foods, Inc.**
Three Lakes Dr.
Northfield, IL 60093-2753
**Phone:** (847)646-2000
**Website:** http://www.kraftfoods.com
Wanda Goin, Manager, Community Affairs

**Typ. Recipients:** Health Organizations, Medical Research. **Geo. Dist:** nationally and in operating communities. **Frmly:** Kraft General Foods Foundation.

**★ 1191 ★ The Kroger Co. Foundation**
1014 Vine St.
Cincinnati, OH 45202-1100
**Phone:** (513)762-4000      **Fax:** (513)762-4370
**Website:** http://www.kroger.com/corpnewsinfo_charitablegiving_art3.htm
Janet Ausdenmoore, Administrator

**Priorities:** *Arts & Humanities:* 4%. Supports a broad spectrum of disciplines in operating locations. *Civic & Public Affairs:* 8%. Funds community revitalization projects, parks, and employment projects. *Education:* 3%. Interests include colleges and universities, with emphasis on nutrition and food-related education. Minority and independent college funds also supported. *Environment:* (United Funds & United Way) 72%. Most of this supports local united funds. Other interests include substance abuse programs, youth organizations, human services, food and clothing distribution, and crime prevention. *International:* 12%. Supports the American Red Cross, hospitals, and single disease organizations. *Note:* Kroger targets its giving program to domestic problems related to food and pharmaceuticals by donating products to emergency community services, food banks, soup kitchens, and shelters for the homeless; drug abuse prevention and education programs; and nutrition consumer education. Contributionsc were made in 1999. **Typ. Recipients:** Arthritis, Cancer, Children's Health/Hospitals,

Diabetes, Emergency/Ambulance Services, Eyes/ Blindness, Health Organizations, Hospices, Hospitals, Medical Education, Medical Rehabilitation, Medical Research, Nutrition, People with Disabilities, Prenatal Health Issues, Single-Disease Health Associations, Substance Abuse. **Geo. Dist:** principally near operating locations and to national organizations. **Frmly:** Kroger Co. Foundation.

## ★ 1192 ★ La-Z-Boy Foundation
1284 N Telegraph Rd.
Monroe, MI 48162
**Phone:** (734)242-1444          **Fax:** (734)457-2005
Donald Blohm, Administrator

**Fnded:** 1953. **Priorities:** *Arts & Humanities:* (Humanities-Art-Cultural) 7%. Supports libraries and public television. *Civic & Public Affairs:* (Public Benefit) 37%. Supports economic development, community foundations, and clubs. *Education:* (Education-Libraries) 27%. Supports schools and colleges. *Environment:* (Human Services) 23%. United funds, YMCA's, and youth groups receive majority of funding. *International:* 4%. Major grants benefit hospitals and the American Red Cross. *Note:* Total contributions made in 2000. **Typ. Recipients:** Children's Health/Hospitals, Clinics/ Medical Centers, Diabetes, Emergency/Ambulance Services, Emergency/Ambulance Services, Health Organizations, Hospices, Hospitals, Single-Disease Health Associations. **Geo. Dist:** operating locations; Siloam Springs, AR; Redlands, CA; Monroe, MI; Leland, MS; Newton, MS; Neosho, MO; Lincolnton, NC; Florence, SC; Dayton, TN; Tremonton, UT.

## ★ 1193 ★ Lancaster Lens Foundation
37 West Broad St.
Columbus, OH 43215
**Phone:** (614)224-7141          **Fax:** (614)469-8219
Clarence Clapham, Secretary

**Fnded:** 1953. **Priorities:** *Civic & Public Affairs:* 100%. Primary support made to economic development. *Note:* Total contributions in fiscal 1999. **Typ. Recipients:** Cancer, Heart, Medical Research, Respiratory, Single-Disease Health Associations, Substance Abuse. **Geo. Dist:** OH.

## ★ 1194 ★ Lance Foundation
PO Box 32368
Charlotte, NC 28232-2368
**Phone:** (704)554-5529          **Fax:** (704)556-5636
Mr. Zean Jamison, Jr., Director

**Priorities:** *Arts & Humanities:* 17%. Arts associations, museums, public broadcasting, and arts centers are supported. *Civic & Public Affairs:* 8%. Emphasis is on community affairs, housing, women's affairs, trade associations, and safety issues. *Education:* 26%. Colleges and universities, education funds, business, minority, agricultural, economic, and public education receive support. *Environment:* 43%. Majority of funding supports the United Way. Senior services, youth organizations, crime prevention, family services, and community service organizations also receive support. *International:* About 2%. Supports medical research, trauma treatment, emergency services, and single-disease health organizations. *Note:* Contributions were made in fiscal 1999. **Typ. Recipients:** Adolescent Health Issues, Cancer, Emergency/Ambulance Services, Family Planning, Health Organizations, Medical Research, Mental Health, Multiple Sclerosis, Nutrition, People with Disabilities, Single-Disease Health Associations, Trauma Treatment. **Geo. Dist:** NC.

## ★ 1195 ★ LandAmerica Foundation
101 Gateway Center Parkway
Richmond, VA 23235
**Phone:** (804)267-8330          **Fax:** (804)267-8827
W. Riker Purcell, Trustee, Vice President and
  Regulatory C

**Priorities:** *Arts & Humanities:* 1%. Supports public broadcasting and museums. *Civic & Public Affairs:* 21%. Funds foundations, women's causes, gay and lesbian support programs, community activities, eco-

nomic development, and housing. *Education:* 45%. Funds private and public colleges, universities, and college educational foundations. *Environment:* 25%. Supports United Way, children's programs, and food banks. *International:* 5%. Supports single-disease associations. *Voluntarism:* Co. encourage its employees to volunteer on a housing project with local colleges. *Note:* Total contributions made in 1998. **Typ. Recipients:** Cancer, Clinics/Medical Centers, Diabetes, Emergency/Ambulance Services, Heart, Hospitals, Single-Disease Health Associations. **Geo. Dist:** operating locations.

## ★ 1196 ★ Landmark Communications Foundation
150 W Brambleton Ave.
Norfolk, VA 23510
**Phone:** (757)446-2011          **Fax:** (757)446-2489
**Email:** Lhyatt@Lcimedia.com
Linda Hyatt, Executive Director

**Priorities:** *Arts & Humanities:* 15%. The highest priorities are museums, arts centers and associations. Also supports performing arts, such as music and theater. *Civic & Public Affairs:* 20%. Supports a wide variety of interests, including professional organizations (primarily journalistic), environmental projects, leadership programs, and other community affairs organizations. *Education:* 28%. Most grants support colleges and universities, often funding journalism programs. Business and minority education, literacy, and education funds also receive support. *Environment:* 34%. Majority of funds support the United Way. Other interests include youth organizations, athletic and recreational programs, and community service organizations. *International:* 1%. Supports hospitals and health organizations. *Note:* Contributions made in 1999. **Typ. Recipients:** Emergency/Ambulance Services, Hospitals, People with Disabilities, Research/ Studies Institutes. **Geo. Dist:** Las Vegas, NV; Greensboro, NC; Nashville, TN; Norfolk, VA; Roanoke, VA.

## ★ 1197 ★ Lee Foundation
215 North Main St.
Davenport, IA 52801
**Phone:** (319)383-2102          **Fax:** (319)326-2972
Russel Kennel, Secretary & Director

**Fnded:** 1962. **Priorities:** *Arts & Humanities:* 16%. Emphasis on museums, art centers, theaters, and historical societies. *Civic & Public Affairs:* 18%. Community foundations, zoos, parks, urban and community affairs, and economic development. *Education:* 48%. Primary support for colleges and universities. *Environment:* 6%. Youth organizations, scouting, YMCAs, and the disabled. *International:* 5%. Supports the Allied Health Consortium and children's health. *Religion:* 1%. Science museums. *Note:* Total contributions made in fiscal 1999. **Typ. Recipients:** Children's Health/Hospitals, Clinics/Medical Centers, Emergency/Ambulance Services, Family Planning, Geriatric Health, Health-General, Hospitals, Medical Education, Public Health, Single-Disease Health Associations. **Geo. Dist:** IL; IA; MT; ND; OR; WI.

## ★ 1198 ★ Lehigh Portland Cement Co.
7660 Imperial Way
Allentown, PA 18195
**Phone:** (610)366-4764          **Fax:** (610)366-4684
**Email:** christ@lehighcement.com
**Website:** http://www.lehighcement.com
Corliss Hirst, communications co-ordinator

**Typ. Recipients:** Cancer, Children's Health/Hospitals, Domestic Violence, Emergency/Ambulance Services, Health Organizations, Health-General, Heart, Hospices, Hospitals, People with Disabilities, Prenatal Health Issues, Sexual Abuse, Substance Abuse, Transplant Networks/Donor Banks. **Geo. Dist:** headquarters and operating communities. **Frmly:** Lehigh Portland Cement Co.

## ★ 1199 ★ Lennox Foundation
PO Box 799900
Dallas, TX 75379

**Phone:** (972)497-5000          **Fax:** (972)497-5268
Dorothy Henson, Contact

**Priorities:** *Civic & Public Affairs:* 5%. *Education:* 28%. Majority goes to Grinnell College in Grinnell, IA. Other support goes to the US Academic Decathlon and the National Merit Scholarship Corporation. *Environment:* 19%. Primarily to community service organizations and family planning. *International:* 18%. Supports women's health, mitochondial disease foundation, and other health concerns. *Religion:* 4%. *Note:* Contributions were made in fiscal 1999. **Typ. Recipients:** Diabetes, Emergency/Ambulance Services, Family Planning, Health Funds, Health Organizations, Hospitals, Public Health, Single-Disease Health Associations. **Geo. Dist:** nationally.

## ★ 1200 ★ Leo Burnett Co. Charitable Foundation
35 West Wacker Dr.
Chicago, IL 60601
**Phone:** (312)220-5959          **Fax:** (312)220-6523
Christian Kimball, Vice President

**Priorities:** *Arts & Humanities:* 3%. Supports art institutes, museums, art funds, and groups such as symphonies and theater players in the Chicago area. *Civic & Public Affairs:* 1%. Contributions go to groups in the field of advertising and organizations that benefit the Chicago area, including anti-defamation groups and projects devoted to urban safety and improvement. *Education:* 14%. Funds support colleges, universities, and business education. Also supports educational funds, high schools and other institutes in the Chicago region, and independent programs such as literacy promotion campaigns. Emphasis is placed on programs that support the field of advertising. *Environment:* 29%. Majority of funds support United Way. Also supports youth recreation and welfare organizations. *International:* 6%. Funds health organizations, hospitals, and single-disease associations. *Voluntarism:* Company sponsors "Give Back Day," a day when about 500 employees volunteer in local schools. *Note:* Total foundation contributions made in 2000. **Typ. Recipients:** AIDS/HIV, Cancer, Children's Health/ Hospitals, Clinics/Medical Centers, Emergency/Ambulance Services, Family Planning, Health Organizations, Hospices, Hospitals, Medical Education, Multiple Sclerosis, Single-Disease Health Associations. **Geo. Dist:** Chicago, IL.

## ★ 1201 ★ Levi Strauss Foundation
1155 Battery St., 7th Fl.
San Francisco, CA 94111
**Phone:** (415)501-6579          **Fax:** (415)501-6575
**Email:** lsf@levi.com
**Website:** http://www.levistrauss.com/responsibility/ foundation/
Theresa Fay-Bustillos, Executive Director

**Fnded:** 1952. **Priorities:** *Arts & Humanities:* 1%. *Civic & Public Affairs:* 44%. Support is provided in four areas: Economic Development, AIDS and Disease Prevention, Social Justice, and Youth Empowerment. In economic development, the foundation seeks to enhance economic opportunities for low-income people, including the working poor. Priorities include job creation and community-based economic development; job training, placement, and access; leadership development; and micro-enterprise. In the category of AIDS and Disease Prevention, priorities include direct assistance to persons with AIDS and their caregivers; risk reduction education for those with high-risk behaviors. The Social Justice program seeks to break down barriers that prevent low-income and disenfranchised people from realizing their basic human rights. The Youth Empowerment initiative supports programs that challenge and involve youth in improving social and economic prospects, and which engage them as decision-makers. The company supports programs that seek to remove racial and other discriminatory barriers; ease tension between groups; promote diversity in community leadership; and prevent violent acts of racial and cultural prejudice. *Education:* 16%. Supports educational programs and university scholarships. *Environment:* 11%. More than half of social service contributions support the United Way in the

Bay Area. Other funds support YWCA, and social services. *International:* 5%. Majority of support given to AIDS education organizations. *Note:* Total contributions in 1997. **Typ. Recipients:** AIDS/HIV, Cancer, Clinics/Medical Centers, Domestic Violence, Emergency/Ambulance Services, Family Planning, Health Organizations, Health-General, Long-Term Care, People with Disabilities, Public Health, Research/Studies Institutes, Respiratory, Sexual Abuse. **Geo. Dist:** operating communities.

**★ 1202 ★ Leviton Foundation New York**
59-25 Little Neck Parkway
Little Neck, NY 11362-2531
**Phone:** (718)229-4040      **Fax:** (718)281-6401
**Email:** hleviton@leviton.com
Stephen Sokolow, Vice President

**Fnded:** 1952. **Priorities:** *Arts & Humanities:* Less than 1%. Funds a children's museum and the World War II Memorial Fund. *Civic & Public Affairs:* 9%. Gives to community foundations, parades, and other civic causes. *Education:* 21%. Supports colleges, universities, college/scholarship funds. *Environment:* 22%. Provides major support to the United Way of Southeastern New England. Also supports youth organizations and family services. *International:* 24%. Supports hospitals, medical centers, and single-disease associations. *Note:* Total contributions made in 2000. **Typ. Recipients:** Arthritis, Cancer, Children's Health/Hospitals, Heart, Hospices, Hospitals, Kidney, Medical Education, Medical Research, Medical Research, Multiple Sclerosis, Respiratory, Single-Disease Health Associations. **Geo. Dist:** NY; RI.

**★ 1203 ★ Liberty Corp. Foundation**
PO Box 789
Greenville, SC 29602
**Phone:** (864)609-8398      **Fax:** (864)609-3176
**Email:** svergas@libertycorp.com
Sophia Vergas, Secretary

**Priorities:** *Arts & Humanities:* 31%. Support goes to performing arts, libraries, and visual arts. *Civic & Public Affairs:* 9%. Primary support to economic development, urban affairs, and business concerns. *Education:* 15%. Supports colleges, universities, and pre-college education. *Environment:* 39%. Primarily supports United Ways, YMCA, and Boy Scouts. *Note:* Total contributions in fiscal 1999. **Typ. Recipients:** Cancer, Children's Health/Hospitals, Clinics/Medical Centers, Emergency/Ambulance Services, Health Organizations, Hospitals, People with Disabilities, Research/Studies Institutes, Single-Disease Health Associations. **Geo. Dist:** nationally; SC.

**★ 1204 ★ Liberty Mutual Insurance Group**
175 Berkeley St.-10B
Boston, MA 02117
**Phone:** (617)357-9500      **Fax:** (617)574-6688
Melissa MacDonnell, Dir. & Asst. Sec., Corp. Public Affairs

**Priorities:** *Arts & Humanities:* 9%. Supports the orchestra, museums, and arts institutes. *Civic & Public Affairs:* 3%. Supports community and neighborhood service. *Education:* 14%. Supports universities and colleges. *Environment:* 46%. Supports child and youth services, and the United Way. *Note:* Contributions analysis provided by the company. **Typ. Recipients:** Health-General. **Geo. Dist:** headquarters and operating communities.

**★ 1205 ★ Lincoln Financial Group Foundation**
1300 South Clinton St.
PO Box 7863
Fort Wayne, IN 46801-7863
**Phone:** (219)455-3879      **Fax:** (219)455-4004
**Email:** mjohnson@lnc.com
**Website:** http://www.lfg.com
Mary Johnson, Assistant Vice President

**Priorities:** *Arts & Humanities:* 30% to 35%. Support covers cultural spectrum: dance, museums, art exhib-

its, orchestras, theater, and historic preservation. *Education:* 30% to 35%. Focus on higher education. Supports colleges and universities, higher education associations, and actuarial scholarships. Also gives to the Local Education Fund, Junior Achievement, and preschool education. Provides matching gifts to higher education. *Environment:* 30% to 35%. Supports united funds, community services, the elderly, domestic violence, and youth programs. Also funds food banks, homeless shelters, drug treatment programs, and AIDS education programs. *International:* Less than 5%. Supports medical research, with focus on AIDS. *Voluntarism:* Volunteer Involvement Program retains a liaison linking employees with community non-profit organizations and activities. **Typ. Recipients:** AIDS/HIV, Domestic Violence, Medical Research, Mental Health, Single-Disease Health Associations, Substance Abuse. **Geo. Dist:** communities where their employees live and work.

**★ 1206 ★ Lipton Foundation**
800 Sylvan Ave.
Englewood Cliffs, NJ 07632
**Phone:** (201)894-7405      **Fax:** (201)871-8198
Suzanne Cuff, Contact

**Fnded:** 1952. **Priorities:** *Arts & Humanities:* 5% to 10%. Arts centers and institutes, historic preservation, museums, libraries, public broadcasting, and the performing arts. Also matches employee contributions to arts organizations. *Civic & Public Affairs:* About 30%. Community groups, environmental affairs, civil rightsorganizations, and others. *Education:* About 30%. National scholarship programs, higher education institutions, food sciences and nutrition, and technology and business education. Also sponsors matching gifts program. *International:* About 30%. Nutrition programs, united funds, youth organizations, legal aid agencies, family planning, recreation and athletics, community service organizations, hospitals, single-disease health organizations, and medical research groups. *Note:* Priorities remain flexible in an effort to respond to community needs. **Typ. Recipients:** Cancer, Children's Health/Hospitals, Clinics/Medical Centers, Diabetes, Family Planning, Health Funds, Health Organizations, Heart, Hospices, Hospitals, Medical Education, Medical Rehabilitation, Medical Research, Medical Training, Mental Health, Multiple Sclerosis, Nutrition, People with Disabilities, Prenatal Health Issues, Single-Disease Health Associations, Substance Abuse. **Geo. Dist:** primarily near corporate headquarters and plant locations.

**★ 1207 ★ Liz Claiborne Foundation**
1441 Broadway Ave.
New York, NY 10018
**Phone:** (212)626-5767      **Fax:** (212)626-8060
**Website:** http://www.lizclaiborne.com/lizinc/foundation
Melanie Lyons, Director

**Fnded:** 1981. **Priorities:** *Arts & Humanities:* 15%. Supports museums, libraries, public braodcasting, and the performing arts. *Civic & Public Affairs:* 29%. To help women and families in need gain their self-sufficiency through long-term, broad-based solutions to poverty; improve opportunities for women through multi-dimensional job readiness, adult education, vocational training, career advancement, and enterprise development programs. *Education:* 16%. Supports schools, educational programs and organizations. *Environment:* 25%. Supports organizations that provide comprehensive services to aid abused women and children in their recovery; address the causes of violence and abuse against women and children, and work toward prevention. To expand opportunities for economically disadvantaged children and teens to meet their full potential through innovative child care and educational approaches, and through exceptional programs providing solid preparation for higher education and the world of work. *International:* 4%. To enhance services to meet the special needs of HIV-positive women and their children; increase access to effective education and prevention programs targeting women and girls. *Note:* Total contributions made in 1999. **Typ. Recipients:** AIDS/HIV, Cancer, Child Abuse, Clinics/Medical Centers, Domestic Violence,

Eyes/Blindness, Health Organizations, Hospitals, Long-Term Care, Medical Education, Prenatal Health Issues, Public Health, Single-Disease Health Associations. **Geo. Dist:** Montgomery, AL; NJ, Hudson County; New York, NY.

**★ 1208 ★ Loctite Corp.**
1001 Troutbrook Crossing
Rocky Hill, CT 06067-3910
**Phone:** (860)571-5100      **Fax:** (860)571-5294
**Email:** don.atencio@loctite.com
**Website:** http://www.loctite.com
Don Atencio, Administrator, Corporate Contributions,

**Priorities:** *Arts & Humanities:* About 10%. *Civic & Public Affairs:* Less than 5%. *Education:* About 65%. About one-third of educational funding supports pre-high school education, including infant and pre-kindergarten programs. *International:* About 20% **Typ. Recipients:** Health-General. **Geo. Dist:** areas where the company has offices.

**★ 1209 ★ Loews Foundation**
667 Madison Ave.
New York, NY 10021
**Phone:** (212)521-2950      **Fax:** (212)521-2329
Peter Keegan, Senior Vice President & Chief Financial

**Fnded:** 1957. **Priorities:** *Arts & Humanities:* 3%. Support goes to museums; libraries; public broadcasting; arts organizations; and music, dance and performing arts groups. *Civic & Public Affairs:* 27%. Interests include professional and trade associations, economic development groups, consumer affairs groups, and zoological societies. *Education:* 15%. Supports higher education; provides scholarships and matching gifts. *Environment:* 7%. Funds the United Way, family planning, and youth concerns. *International:* 5%. Supports hospitals, single-disease associations, and medical research. *Religion:* 2%. Supports American Museum of Natural History. *Note:* Total contributions made in 1998. **Typ. Recipients:** AIDS/HIV, Cancer, Children's Health/Hospitals, Clinics/Medical Centers, Diabetes, Emergency/Ambulance Services, Family Planning, Geriatric Health, Health Organizations, Health-General, Hospitals, Hospitals (University Affiliated), Medical Education, Medical Rehabilitation, Medical Research, Medical Research, Mental Health, Multiple Sclerosis, Nutrition, People with Disabilities, Prenatal Health Issues, Public Health, Research/Studies Institutes, Single-Disease Health Associations, Speech & Hearing. **Geo. Dist:** operating locations; NY.

**★ 1210 ★ Lotus Development Philanthropy Program**
55 Cambridge Parkway
Cambridge, MA 02142
**Phone:** (617)693-1667      **Fax:** (617)693-3728
Patty Olan, Lotus Philanthropy Program

**Priorities:** *Civic & Public Affairs:* Supports projects with an action component which prevent or combat the development of biased and prejudicial attitudes regarding race, primarily, and class, secondarily. Focus on direct civic participation, public policy initiatives, or demonstrated leadership. Focus on efforts to educate and mobilize community residents to advocate, speak out, and takecontrol over a particular challenge; causes receiving support have been welfare rights, lead poisoning initiatives, housing, public safety, job creation, entrepreneurship, and economic development. Supports the rights of families and individuals to live violence-free and with adequate support, particularly in communities of color and inner-city neighborhoods. *International:* Addresses racial and class inequities of the health care environment, and increased access to public health services, such as pre- and post-natal education and treatment; AIDS advocacy, education, and treatment; and preventative health care. *Religion:* Supports the extension of computer-related skills and technologies to people and organizations otherwise not enjoying access to such technologies and training. Both individual skill development programs and technological enhancement and capacity-building projects are supported. **Typ. Recipients:**

AIDS/HIV, Domestic Violence, Family Planning, Health Organizations, Mental Health, Nutrition, People with Disabilities, Prenatal Health Issues, Public Health. **Geo. Dist:** headquarters and operating communities.


### ★ 1211 ★ Louisiana Land & Exploration Co. Foundation

PO Box 4239
Houston, TX 77210-3239
**Phone:** (713)624-9366     **Fax:** (713)624-9645
Dee McBride, Contact

**Priorities:** *Arts & Humanities:* 4%. Majority of funding supports city of New Orleans, arts funds, historic preservation, and housing. *Civic & Public Affairs:* 4%. *Education:* 59%. Highest priority is colleges and universities, both in unrestricted support and through scholarships; also awards major grants through multi-year commitments to universities. Employee matching gifts account for a significant portion of education contributions (about one-third). Other interests include Junior Achievement and various education associations. Also sponsors scholarship programs for children of employees. *Environment:* 21%. Majority of funding supports united funds. Youth organizations also receive significant support. *International:* 1%. Funds American Red Cross. *Religion:* 2%. Supports research and science centers. *Note:* Total foundation contributions in 1997. **Typ. Recipients:** Diabetes, Emergency/Ambulance Services, Health Organizations, Hospices, Medical Research, Single-Disease Health Associations, Substance Abuse. **Geo. Dist:** operating locations.


### ★ 1212 ★ Lowe's Charitable and Educational Foundation

PO Box 1111
North Wilkesboro, NC 28656
**Phone:** (336)658-4000
David Oliver, Director, Community Relations

**Priorities:** *Arts & Humanities:* 4%. Supports libraries. *Civic & Public Affairs:* 12%. Funds foundations, associations, and public offices. *Education:* 13%. Supports colleges, universities, and secondary schools. *Environment:* 70%. Funds youth programs, community programs, and united funds. *International:* 1%. Funds hospitals, hospices, and health services. *Note:* Total contributions made in fiscal 1998. **Typ. Recipients:** Cancer, Children's Health/Hospitals, Health-General, Hospices, Hospitals, Medical Education. **Geo. Dist:** headquarters and operating communities.


### ★ 1213 ★ LTV Foundation

200 Public Square, 38-506
Cleveland, OH 44114-2308
**Phone:** (216)622-5000     **Fax:** (216)622-4578
Laura Stacko, Director

**Priorities:** *Arts & Humanities:* 10%. Funds theater, dance, musical performances and music museums, and art museums. *Civic & Public Affairs:* 12%. Supports employment/job training, minority business, economic development, urban/community affairs, law & justice, and African American affairs. *Education:* 23%. Supports public education (precollege), secondary education (public and private), science/mathematics education, and student aid. *Environment:* 45%. Recipients include the United Way, food/clothing distribution, local YMCAs, scouts, child welfare, and senior groups and services. *International:* 7%. Recipients include clinics/medical centers, children's health/hospitals, health organizations, and single-disease associations with some emphasis on cerebral palsy and cancer research. *Religion:* 2%. Funds the Great Lakes Science Center and a natural history museum. *Note:* Total contributions in 2000. **Typ. Recipients:** Alzheimers Disease, Cancer, Children's Health/Hospitals, Clinics/Medical Centers, Domestic Violence, Eyes/Blindness, Health Funds, Health Organizations, Health Policy/Cost Containment, Heart, Hospitals (University Affiliated), Kidney, Medical Research, Mental Health, People with Disabilities, Prenatal Health Issues, Public Health, Single-Disease Health Associations, Substance Abuse. **Geo. Dist:**

principally near operating locations and to national organizations.


### ★ 1214 ★ The Lubrizol Foundation

29400 Lakeland Boulevard
Drop No. 053A
Wickliffe, OH 44092-2298
**Phone:** (440)347-5080     **Fax:** (440)347-1858
**Email:** kmi@lubrizol.com
**Website:** http://www.lubrizol.com/aboutlubrizol/lz_foundation/index.html
Kenneth Iwashita, President & Chief Operating Officer

**Priorities:** *Arts & Humanities:* 10%. Funds the arts, music, and public broadcasting. *Education:* 58%. Major support for higher education. Through the scholarship program, the foundation selects the colleges and universities and designates the fields of study. Emphasis is on chemistry, chemical engineering, and mechanical engineering. Also makes grants for capital and operating purposes to colleges and universities and private and secondary schools. Grants are also made to educational programs and combined educational funds. *Environment:* 30%. Supports united funds and human services groups providing basic human needs. Supports organizations which grant youth the opportunity to enjoy healthy recreation and experience leadership and responsible citizenship. *International:* 2%. Provides direct capital and operating support for health organizations in its primary communities. Grants go to hospitals and specialized health care providers. *Note:* Contributions made in 1999. **Typ. Recipients:** Alzheimers Disease, Children's Health/Hospitals, Clinics/Medical Centers, Emergency/Ambulance Services, Eyes/Blindness, Geriatric Health, Health Organizations, Hospices, Hospitals, Long-Term Care, Medical Rehabilitation, Mental Health, Nursing Services, People with Disabilities, Public Health, Single-Disease Health Associations. **Geo. Dist:** OH, metropolitan area; Houston, TX, metropolitan area.


### ★ 1215 ★ Madison Gas & Electric Foundation

PO Box 1231
Madison, WI 53701-1231
**Phone:** (608)252-7279
Bonnie Juul, Grants Coordinator

**Fnded:** 1966. **Priorities:** *Arts & Humanities:* 6%. Supports theater, music, and historical preservation. *Civic & Public Affairs:* 33%. Funds political conferences, municipalities, and public safety. *Education:* 14%. Supports schools, educational funds, higher education, and scholarships. *Environment:* 33%. Supports United Way, YMCA and community centers, youth organizations, and human services. *International:* 3%. Funds hospice and single-disease associations. *Religion:* 9%. Funds a science center. *Note:* Total foundation contributions made in 2000. **Typ. Recipients:** AIDS/HIV, Cancer, Children's Health/Hospitals, Domestic Violence, Health Organizations, Heart, Hospices, Hospitals, Medical Research, People with Disabilities, Prenatal Health Issues, Public Health, Single-Disease Health Associations. **Geo. Dist:** WI.


### ★ 1216 ★ Mamiye Foundation

PO Box 320
Keasbey, NJ 08832
**Phone:** (732)417-9400     **Fax:** (732)346-3694
Charles Mamiye, Vice President

**Fnded:** 1982. **Priorities:** *Civic & Public Affairs:* 2%. *International:* 1%. *Note:* Total foundation contributions made in 2000. **Typ. Recipients:** AIDS/HIV, Cancer, Children's Health/Hospitals, Geriatric Health, Health Organizations, Hospitals, Medical Research, Single-Disease Health Associations. **Geo. Dist:** NJ.


### M&T Charitable Foundation

*See:* Entry 5580


### ★ 1217 ★ Manulife Financial

73 Tremont St., Ste. 1300
Boston, MA 02108

**Phone:** (617)854-4345     **Fax:** (617)854-4304
**Email:** aricco@manualifeusa.com
**Website:** http://www.manulife.com/corporate/corporate2.nsf/Public/uscommunity.html
Alison Ricco, Manager, Corporate Giving Programs

**Typ. Recipients:** Arthritis, Cancer, Health Organizations, Health-General, Heart, Hospitals, Medical Research, Public Health, Single-Disease Health Associations. **Geo. Dist:** headquarters and operating communities.


### ★ 1218 ★ Marcus Corp. Foundation

250 East Wisconsin Ave., Ste. 1700
Milwaukee, WI 53202-4220
**Phone:** (414)905-1503
Stephen Marcus, President

**Priorities:** *Arts & Humanities:* 42%. Recipients include performing arts, music, film, and arts associations. Also funds public broadcasting and museums. *Civic & Public Affairs:* 19%. Funding supports parades, festivals, and economic development in operating areas. Other recipients include African American affairs and community programs. *Education:* 8%. Supports colleges, universities, and educational programs. *Environment:* 15%. Supports United Way, child welfare, youth organizations, and people with disabilities. *International:* 15%. Primarily supports hospitals and single-disease health organizations. *Note:* Contributions made in 2000. **Typ. Recipients:** AIDS/HIV, Alzheimers Disease, Arthritis, Cancer, Child Abuse, Children's Health/Hospitals, Clinics/Medical Centers, Diabetes, Domestic Violence, Health Organizations, Heart, Hospitals, Kidney, Medical Education, Medical Research, Multiple Sclerosis, People with Disabilities, Prenatal Health Issues, Public Health, Respiratory, Single-Disease Health Associations, Transplant Networks/Donor Banks, Trauma Treatment. **Geo. Dist:** Milwaukee, WI.


### ★ 1219 ★ Maritz Inc.

1375 North Highway Dr.
Fenton, MO 63099
**Phone:** (636)827-4000     **Fax:** (636)827-5505
**Website:** http://www.maritz.com/maritz/about/asp/community.asp
Norm Schwesig, Senior Vice President, Corporate Communi

**Priorities:** *Arts & Humanities:* About 20%. Supports a broad spectrum of community arts organizations, including libraries, museums, the performing arts, theater, and public broadcasting. *Civic & Public Affairs:* About 15%. Interests include economic development, business and free enterprise, civil rights, environmental affairs, public policy, andmunicipalities. *Education:* 30% to 35%. Interests include colleges and universities, economic education, literacy, minority education, and precollege education at all levels. *Environment:* About 5% of contributions. Focus on the United Way and Toys for Tots. *International:* 25% to 30%. Major support to youth organizations. Also supports child welfare, drug and alcohol prevention, united funds, food and clothing distribution, and employment and job training. **Typ. Recipients:** Domestic Violence, Health-General, Hospitals, Mental Health, People with Disabilities, Substance Abuse. **Geo. Dist:** headquarters and operating communities.


### ★ 1220 ★ Mark IV Industries Foundation

PO Box 810
Amherst, NY 14226-0810
**Phone:** (716)689-4972     **Fax:** (716)689-6098
Joanne Eckert, Executive Assistant

**Fnded:** 1976. **Priorities:** *Arts & Humanities:* 4%. Funds a theater company, ballet, and public broadcasting. *Civic & Public Affairs:* 4%. Supports citizens groups, women's affairs, and parks. *Education:* 49%. Funds higher education. *Environment:* 1%. Supports youth services. *International:* 37%. Gives to hospitals, pediatric health organizations, and single-disease concerns. *Note:* Total contributions made in fiscal 2000. **Typ. Recipients:** Cancer, Children's Health/Hospitals, Diabetes, Emergency/Ambulance Services, Heart, Hospices, Hospitals, Medical Education, Multiple Sclerosis, People with Disabilities, Prenatal Health Issues,

Single-Disease Health Associations, Speech & Hearing, Substance Abuse. **Geo. Dist:** Buffalo, NY.

**★ 1221 ★ Marshall & Ilsley Foundation, Inc.**
770 North Water St.
Milwaukee, WI 53202
**Phone:** (414)765-7805          **Fax:** (414)765-7899
Rebecca Lonergan, Assistant Secretary
**Fnded:** 1958. **Priorities:** *Arts & Humanities:* 23%. Musical and theatrical organizations, arts funds, and history and arts associations. *Civic & Public Affairs:* 8%. Urban and community affairs, zoos and botanical gardens, housing, and professional and trade organizations. *Education:* 20%. Largely funds colleges and universities, and supports scholarships and scholarship funds. Interests also include arts and music education, and business, elementary, and private precollege education. *Environment:* 37%. Primarily funds youth organizations, united funds, and child welfare. Interests also include community services and centers, volunteer services, family services, and organizations concerned with the disabled. *International:* 6%. Funds hospitals and health centers, medical research, single-disease health organizations, and nursing services. *Note:* Total foundation contributions made in 2000. **Typ. Recipients:** Cancer, Children's Health/Hospitals, Clinics/Medical Centers, Family Planning, Health Organizations, Hospitals, Long-Term Care, Medical Education, Medical Research, Medical Training, Mental Health, Nursing Services, People with Disabilities, Research/Studies Institutes, Single-Disease Health Associations, Transplant Networks/Donor Banks, Trauma Treatment. **Geo. Dist:** WI, emphasis on Milwaukee.

**★ 1222 ★ Masco Corp. Foundation**
21001 Van Born Rd.
Taylor, MI 48180
**Phone:** (313)274-7400          **Fax:** (313)792-6262
**Website:** http://www.masco.com
**Priorities:** *Arts & Humanities:* (Culture/Arts) 28%. Supports museums, historical societies, opera, and arts organizations. *Civic & Public Affairs:* (Civic/Community) 30%. Supports accounting aid, economic development, and community groups. *Education:* 12%. Funds private schools, colleges and universities, minority education and education foundations. *Environment:* (Health & Human Services) 10%. Gives to health-care systems, cancer research, youth organizations, food distribution, and the United Way. *Voluntarism:* The company sponsors a Habitat for Humanity/Masco Home Build volunteer program. *Note:* Total of foundation and corporate giving contributions made in 2000. Does not include giving by subsidiaries. **Typ. Recipients:** Cancer, Health Organizations, Hospitals, Hospitals (University Affiliated), Medical Education, Medical Research, Public Health. **Geo. Dist:** some giving nationally; MI, Southeastern Michigan.

**★ 1223 ★ The MassMutual Foundation for Hartford, Inc.**
140 Garden St.
ATTN: H356
Hartford, CT 06154
**Phone:** (860)987-2085          **Fax:** (860)987-2493
**Email:** rcopes@massmutual.com
Ronald Copes, Executive Director
**Priorities:** *Arts & Humanities:* 19%. Supports music, libraries, theater, and fine arts institutions which educate, inspire, and enrich the lives of Springfield and Hartford residents. *Civic & Public Affairs:* 27%. Emphasizes violence prevention, youth leadership development, clean streets, civic pride, ethnic and cultural diversity, youth activities, employment, and downtown events in Springfield and Hartford. Goal is to improve the economic and residential viability of neighborhoods. Promotes small business growth and first-time home ownership. Supports the Urban League, housing, and youth employment. *Education:* 8%. Supports business and school partnerships, teacher and student training, incentives for academic achievement in Springfield and Hartford schools, and

colleges through scholarships. Grants emphasize school improvement, including academic excellence, safety, and scholarship opportunities. *Environment:* 35%. Supports the United Way, Salvation Army, family services, child welfare, and shelters. *Voluntarism:* Company sponsors volunteer activities, such as Junior Achievement, literacy, and tutor/mentor programs. Supports the volunteers in Action Program, which awards cash grants to organizations where employees actively volunteer. *Note:* Total foundation contributions in 2000. **Typ. Recipients:** AIDS/HIV, Children's Health/Hospitals, Clinics/Medical Centers, Hospitals, Medical Research, Multiple Sclerosis, Substance Abuse. **Geo. Dist:** Hartford, CT; Springfield, MA.

**★ 1224 ★ Mattel Foundation**
333 Continental Blvd.
Mail Stop M1-1418
El Segundo, CA 90245-5012
**Phone:** (310)252-3530          **Fax:** (310)252-3802
**Website:** http://www.mattel.com
Paul Millman, Foundation Directory
**Priorities:** *Arts & Humanities:* Less than 5%. Supports orchestra groups, libraries, ballet, and performing arts. *Civic & Public Affairs:* 2%. Primarily supports housing, philanthropic organizations, free enterprise, and community foundations. *Education:* 69%. Interests include literacy, math education, private education, and colleges, universities and scholarships. Supports the Mattel Family Learning Program, which promotes computer literacy, and the Hand in Hand program, which promotes volunteerism in school systems. *Environment:* 17%. Majority supports direct care services for youth and children. Other areas of interest include aid for the handicapped, family services, food banks, substance abuse prevention programs, and volunteer services. *International:* 5%. Major support for the Mattel Children's Hospital at UCLA. Funds single-disease health organizations and clinics. *Voluntarism:* Employees may apply for Employee Volunteer Grants. Grants amounts are linked to the length of service of requesting employee, and by number of other Mattel employees volunteering within the organization. The Foundation coordinates more than 30 volunteer activities annually to encourage employee volunteerism. *Note:* Above priorities are for foundation only. **Typ. Recipients:** AIDS/HIV, Cancer, Children's Health/Hospitals, Clinics/Medical Centers, Diabetes, Geriatric Health, Health Funds, Health Organizations, Heart, Hospitals, Medical Education, Medical Rehabilitation, Multiple Sclerosis, People with Disabilities, Prenatal Health Issues, Public Health, Single-Disease Health Associations, Substance Abuse. **Geo. Dist:** Southern California and Western New York; Los Angeles, CA.

**★ 1225 ★ Mazda Foundation (USA), Inc.**
1025 Connecticut Ave., Ste. 910
Washington, DC 20036
**Phone:** (202)467-5088          **Fax:** (202)233-6490
**Website:** http://www.mazdafoundation.org
Barbara Nocera, Program Director
**Priorities:** *Arts & Humanities:* 3%. Funds educational public broadcasting programs. *Education:* 86%. Supports schools, universities, literacy programs, resource conservation education, and organizations that promote study abroad. *International:* 11%. Supports the Juvenile Diabetes Foundation and an organization that addresses mental/emotional health issues for minority children. *Note:* Total contributions made in fiscal 2000. **Typ. Recipients:** Children's Health/Hospitals, Medical Research, People with Disabilities, Substance Abuse. **Geo. Dist:** headquarters and operating communities.

**★ 1226 ★ MBIA Inc.**
113 King St.
Armonk, NY 10504
**Phone:** (914)273-4545          **Fax:** (914)765-3375
**Email:** sue.voltz@mbia.com
**Website:** http://www.mbia.com
Susan Voltz, Director
**Priorities:** *Arts & Humanities:* About 10%. Funds arts associations, historic preservation, libraries, museums, and the performing arts. *Civic & Public Affairs:* About 20%. Recipients include ethnic and minority

affairs, housing programs, municipalities, and women's affairs. *Education:* About 30%. Supports business, elementary, and legal education. Also funds colleges and universities. Employee matching gift program supports institutions of higher education. *International:* About 40%. Interests include geriatric health, health organizations, medical research, single-disease associations, family services, community service organizations, volunteer services, youth organizations, and other social services. *Note:* Primary focus is on programs for children, which receive half of all contributions. **Typ. Recipients:** Family Planning, Geriatric Health, Health Organizations, Health-General, Medical Research, People with Disabilities, Single-Disease Health Associations, Substance Abuse. **Geo. Dist:** generally in tri-state area where employees live.

**McCormick & Co. Inc.**
*See:* Entry 18222

**★ 1227 ★ McDonald Investments Foundation**
800 Superior Ave.
Cleveland, OH 44114-2603
**Phone:** (216)443-2981          **Fax:** (216)443-3865
Thomas Clevidence, Senior Managing Director
**Priorities:** *Arts & Humanities:* 13%. Supports museums, theater, music, and art. *Civic & Public Affairs:* 27%. Supports community and neighborhood development, clubs, and community foundations. *Education:* 13%. Funds higher education, education foundations, and education programs. *Environment:* 22%. Supports youth services, the disabled, social services, and United Way. *International:* 15%. Supports hospitals, medical centers, single-disease associations, and AIDS prevention. *Note:* Total contributions made in fiscal 1999. **Typ. Recipients:** AIDS/HIV, Alzheimers Disease, Cancer, Children's Health/Hospitals, Diabetes, Domestic Violence, Emergency/Ambulance Services, Eyes/Blindness, Family Planning, Health Organizations, Health-General, Hospices, Hospitals, Medical Research, Mental Health, Multiple Sclerosis, Nursing Services, People with Disabilities, Sexual Abuse, Single-Disease Health Associations, Speech & Hearing, Substance Abuse. **Geo. Dist:** headquarters and operating communities.

**★ 1228 ★ McGraw-Hill Companies, Inc.**
1221 Ave. of the Americas
New York, NY 10020-1095
**Phone:** (212)512-6480          **Fax:** (212)512-3611
**Email:** teresa_white@mcgraw-hill.com
**Website:**    http://www.mcgraw-hill.com/community/community/html
Susan Wallman, Manager, Corporate Contributions
**Typ. Recipients:** AIDS/HIV, Clinics/Medical Centers, Eyes/Blindness, Health Organizations, Hospitals, Hospitals (University Affiliated), People with Disabilities, Substance Abuse, Transplant Networks/Donor Banks. **Geo. Dist:** national organizations; primarily headquarters and operating communities; New York, NY.

**★ 1229 ★ McKesson Foundation**
1 Post St.
San Francisco, CA 94104
**Phone:** (415)983-9325          **Fax:** (415)983-7590
**Website:** http://www.mckesson.com/wt/brochure.php
Ms. Marcia Argyris, President
**Priorities:** *Arts & Humanities:* 5%. Supports museums, symphonies, and the performing arts in the San Francisco Bay Area. *Civic & Public Affairs:* 11%. Employee committees in operating communities evaluate and recommend grants. 5% to 10%. Supports volunteer centers and public broadcasting. Less than 5%. Primarily encourages and supports employee volunteers. The company has created special grant programs: the Community Action Team Fund Grant program, which supports nonprofit organizations in which five or more McKesson employees and retirees are involved on a volunteer basis (grants range from $500 to $5,000); the Community Action Fund Grant program, which funds nonprofits with grants for specific items or special programs (grants range up to

$1,000 and are limited to organizations where employees, retirees, or their spouses volunteer); and the Neil Harlan Award for Community Service program, which awards grants to organizations appointed by chosen employees who are being honored for community service (grants to nonprofits range from $300 to $5,000 and employees must work for company for one year). *Education:* 27%. Contributions support colleges, universities, and other educational institutions, both in the form of grants and through the employee matching gifts program. Supports scholarships with a focus on the children of employees. The foundation also funds youth educational enrichment programs, especially those that deal with the prevention of substance abuse, development of decision-making skills, exploration of career directions, after-school community service projects, and K-12 public school education. *Environment:* 32%. Supports Youth with Special Needs, comprised of Learning Exchange (a tutoring program), Work Experience Program, and Summer Youth Employment Program. Emphasis is on pre-teen and adolescent age groups. Also funds Human Services, including emergency services for families in crisis, including emergency food programs, services for runaway youth, and shelter for mothers and children in temporary crisis situations. The Youth and Families Initiative, a regional program, focuses on youth services and medical care. mothers and children in temporary crisis situations. *International:* 17%. Supports health programs for at-risk children. *Note:* Total contributions made in fiscal 2001. **Typ. Recipients:** AIDS/HIV, Children's Health/Hospitals, Clinics/Medical Centers, Emergency/Ambulance Services, Health Organizations, Health-General, Hospitals, Medical Education, People with Disabilities, Prenatal Health Issues, Preventive Medicine/Wellness Organizations, Public Health, Single-Disease Health Associations, Substance Abuse. **Geo. Dist:** communities where company has a sizable employee representation; CA, San Francisco Bay area.

**★ 1230 ★ McWane Foundation**
2900 Highway 280, Ste. 300
Birmingham, AL 35223
**Phone:** (205)414-3100          **Fax:** (205)414-3180
Jeanette Sommers, Corporate Secretary
**Fnded:** 1961. **Priorities:** *Arts & Humanities:* 5%. Supports museums, dance, historical preservation, libraries, and music. *Civic & Public Affairs:* 59%. Supports the McWane Center, community development, free enterprise, housing, and civil rights organizations. *Education:* 23%. Supports colleges, universities, scholarships, Junior Achievement, and educational foundations. *Environment:* 4%. Supports youth organizations and family services. *International:* 8%. Supports health organizations and medical associations. *Note:* Total foundation contributions made in 2000. **Typ. Recipients:** Arthritis, Cancer, Children's Health/Hospitals, Diabetes, Diabetes, Emergency/Ambulance Services, Health Organizations, Heart, Hospitals, Mental Health, Multiple Sclerosis, Single-Disease Health Associations, Substance Abuse. **Geo. Dist:** AL.

**MDU Resources Foundation**
*See:* Entry 5581

**★ 1231 ★ Mead Corp. Foundation**
Courthouse Plaza, Northeast
Dayton, OH 45463
**Phone:** (937)495-3849          **Fax:** (937)495-4103
**Email:** benzw@mduresources.com
**Website:** http://www.mead.com/am/cc_frset.html
R.F. Budzik, Executive Director
**Fnded:** 1957. **Priorities:** *Arts & Humanities:* 24%. Supports visual, performing, and literary arts, and historical preservation. Funds efforts to reach underserved audiences and arts education. Recipients include dance, historic sites, libraries, museums, opera, performing arts funds, public broadcasting, classical music, and theaters. *Civic & Public Affairs:* 12%. Seeks to encourage growth and development for communities, improve opportunities for citizens, encourage volunteerism, and preservation of natural

resources. Main interests are chambers of commerce, economic development organizations, urban re-development, volunteer fire and rescue squads, voter participation and education projects, parks and recreation, and Nature Conservancy. *Education:* 36%. Seeks to improve elementary and secondary public education, support colleges and universities, and provide opportunities for students to learn about basic business and economic principles. Emphasis is on math, science, forestry, engineering, and computer science education, as well as programs designed to develop critical thinking and problem solving skills. *International:* 24%. Emphasis is placed on meeting critical human needs that arise from emergencies, homelessness, domestic violence and child abuse, substance abuse, dependent day care, and a wide range of youth programs. Funds United Way, American Red Cross, Big Brothers/Big Sisters, Goodwill, anti-domestic violence coalitions, scouting, and Young Men's Christian Association. *Note:* Giving priorities are based on foundation grants in 1999. **Typ. Recipients:** Diabetes, Domestic Violence, Emergency/Ambulance Services, Health-General, Hospices, Public Health. **Geo. Dist:** operating locations; Cottonton, AL; Phenix City, AL; Stevenson, AL; Buena Park, CA; Garden Grove, CA; Atlanta, GA; Bridgeview, IL; Rumford, ME; South Lee, MA; Escanaba, MI; Kalamazoo, MI; St. Joseph, MS; Potsdam, NY; Chillicothe, OH; Dayton, OH; Washington Court House, OH; Alexandria, PA; Spartanburg, SC; Lewisburg, TN; Garland, TX; Menasha, WI; Milwaukee, WI.

**★ 1232 ★ Mellon Financial Corp.**
One Mellon Ctr., Ste. 1830
Pittsburgh, PA 15258
**Phone:** (412)234-2732          **Fax:** (412)234-0831
**Website:** http://www.mellon.com
James McDonald, President
**Priorities:** *Arts & Humanities:* 20%. Supports museums, arts centers and festivals, music groups, and programs concerned with historic preservation. *Civic & Public Affairs:* 19%. Favors community initiatives that attract and develop business and jobs. Also supports efforts to promote affordable housing, homeownership, and economic development in low and moderate income areas. *Education:* 25%. Interests include business education, literacy and minority education funds. Matches employee gifts to colleges and universities. *International:* 15%. Health grants given to hospitals, health centers, special care facilities, and health cost containment programs. Human service grants include organizations concerned with the disabled, drug and alcohol abuse, and food distribution. *Voluntarism:* VOL Mellon Volunteer Professionals - a volunteer program that supports nonprofit initiatives at certain Mellon communities. Mellon also has an active Retiree Volunteer program in its Pittsburgh location. *Note:* Total contributions made in 2000. **Typ. Recipients:** Health Organizations, People with Disabilities. **Geo. Dist:** retail location areas; DE; Boston, MA; Philadelphia, PA; Pittsburgh, PA.

**★ 1233 ★ Memphis Light Gas & Water Division**
PO Box 430
Memphis, TN 38101-0430
**Phone:** (901)528-4151          **Fax:** (901)528-4321
**Website:** http://www.mlgw.com
Doris Douglas, Jr., Admin. Asst.
**Priorities:** *Voluntarism:* Company employees volunteer their time with United Way. *Note:* Most giving is through employee campaigns and fundraising efforts. **Typ. Recipients:** Cancer, Children's Health/Hospitals, Health-General, Mental Health, Prenatal Health Issues, Transplant Networks/Donor Banks. **Geo. Dist:** Memphis, TN.

**★ 1234 ★ Menasha Corp. Foundation**
PO Box 367
Neenah, WI 54957-0367
**Phone:** (920)751-1217          **Fax:** (920)751-1236
**Website:** http://www.menasha.com/about/foundation/
Steven Kromholz, President

**Priorities:** *Arts & Humanities:* 11%. Supports museums, theater, historical societies and history organizations, public broadcasting, and opera. *Civic & Public Affairs:* 18%. Interests include urban and community affairs and local clubs, chambers of commerce, parks, and municipalities, with a focus on community redevelopment. *Education:* 10%. Funds universities and colleges in Wisconsin, economic education, education funds, minority education, literacy programs, public and private precollege schools, and youth educational programs. *Environment:* 49%. Supports local United Way agencies, senior services, and youth organizations including YMCAs, Boys and Girls Clubs, and scouting. *International:* 7%. Gives to medical centers, residency programs, medical foundations, hospice, and single-disease health associations. *Voluntarism:* Foundation gives Employee Volunteer Awards, donating cash grants to select organizations where employees volunteer. *Note:* Total foundation contributions made in 2000. **Typ. Recipients:** Child Abuse, Children's Health/Hospitals, Clinics/Medical Centers, Domestic Violence, Emergency/Ambulance Services, Health Organizations, Health-General, Hospices, Hospitals, Nursing Services, People with Disabilities, Public Health, Sexual Abuse, Substance Abuse. **Geo. Dist:** headquarters and operating communities.

**★ 1235 ★ The Mercantile Foundation**
PO Box 387
Saint Louis, MO 63166
**Phone:** (314)418-2643
Edward Higgins, Chairman

**Priorities:** *Arts & Humanities:* 25%. Main support to symphony, museums, and arts councils. *Civic & Public Affairs:* 24%. Supports botanical gardens, clubs, jobs, and foundations. *Education:* 16%. Colleges and universities mainly. *Environment:* 10%. Supports United Way, YMCA, scouts, and food distribution. *International:* 19%. Funds medical centers, hospitals, and health foundations. *Religion:* 3%. Gives to science centers and museums. *Note:* Total foundation contributions made in fiscal 1999. **Typ. Recipients:** Cancer, Children's Health/Hospitals, Clinics/Medical Centers, Emergency/Ambulance Services, Health-General, Hospitals, Medical Education, Medical Training, People with Disabilities, Public Health. **Geo. Dist:** headquarters and operating communities only; St. Louis, MO, metropolitan area.

**★ 1236 ★ Merck Co. Foundation**
One Merck Dr.
PO Box 100 (WS1AF-35)
Whitehouse Station, NJ 08889-0100
**Phone:** (908)423-2042          **Fax:** (908)423-1987
**Website:** http://www.merck.com
John Taylor, Executive Vice President

**Priorities:** *Civic & Public Affairs:* About 30%. Funds social services through the United Way, and health interests such as hospitals, medical centers, children's health; the arts and the environment receive minor support. Some civic groups also receive funding. (Public Policy) About 10%. Mainly supports groups concerned with health policy issues. Also supports organizations dealing with the pharmaceutical business, economics, and health care cost containment. *Education:* About 50%. Supports programs designed to increase knowledge of medicine and science. Also emphasizes the creation of education opportunities for minorities. Support to secondary and primary science education in selected locations. **Typ. Recipients:** AIDS/HIV, Cancer, Children's Health/Hospitals, Clinics/Medical Centers, Emergency/Ambulance Services, Geriatric Health, Health Organizations, Health Policy/Cost Containment, Heart, Hospitals, Hospitals (University Affiliated), Medical Education, Medical Research, Medical Training, Public Health, Research/Studies Institutes, Respiratory, Single-Disease Health Associations, Substance Abuse. **Geo. Dist:** internationally; nationally; primarily headquarters and operating communities.

**★ 1237 ★ Merit Gasoline Foundation**
551 West Lancaster Ave.
Haverford, PA 19041

**Phone:** (610)527-7900
Robert Harting, Executive Director
**Fnded:** 1956. **Priorities:** *Arts & Humanities:* 3%. Supports museums and art centers, orchestra, and the performing arts. *Civic & Public Affairs:* 4%. Supports public safety, job training, and community development. *Education:* 11%. Primarily funds universities and colleges. *Environment:* 22%. Focus on the United Way and child welfare. *International:* 8%. Supports medical services and single-disease associations. *Note:* Total foundation contributions made in fiscal 2000. **Typ. Recipients:** Arthritis, Children's Health/Hospitals, Clinics/Medical Centers, Diabetes, Domestic Violence, Emergency/Ambulance Services, Health Organizations, Health-General, Hospitals, Medical Education, Multiple Sclerosis, Public Health, Single-Disease Health Associations, Substance Abuse. **Geo. Dist:** cities in the Mid-Atlantic and New England states where company has operating gasoline stations.

**★ 1238 ★ Merrill Lynch & Co.**
    **Foundation Inc.**
Global Philanthropy and Community Relations
2 World Financial Center, 6th Floor
New York, NY 10281
**Phone:** (212)614-5277
**Email:** p22@exchange.ml.com
**Website:** http://philanthropy.ml.com
Eddy Bayardelle, Director, Philanthropic Programs
**Fnded:** 1950. **Priorities:** *Arts & Humanities:* 22%. Major areas of support include music, ethnic and folk museums, arts centers and institutes, dance theaters, libraries, history organizations and memorials, and botanical gardens. *Civic & Public Affairs:* 11%. Interests include business organizations, civil rights, job training, urban and community affairs, housing initiatives, and women's and minority affairs. *Education:* 35%. Supports education reform, minority education, student aid, colleges and universities, and business and technical education. Additionally, awards scholarships to children of employees based both on merit and need. *Environment:* 21%. Gives to a variety of local and national social service organizations, with emphasis on youth and community service organizations. Other interests include substance abuse programs, YMCAs, and people with disabilities. About 3% of total contributions is provided to the United Way. *International:* 11%. Donations fund single-disease health associations, hospitals and health organizations, clinics and medical centers, geriatric health groups, children's health concerns, and emergency services. *Voluntarism:* The company sponsors an Employee Community Involvement Program, which provides grants of $100 to $1,000 to organizations where employees volunteer. *Note:* Total contributions made in 2000. **Typ. Recipients:** AIDS/HIV, Cancer, Children's Health/Hospitals, Clinics/Medical Centers, Emergency/Ambulance Services, Geriatric Health, Health Organizations, Heart, Hospitals, Medical Research, People with Disabilities, Research/Studies Institutes, Single-Disease Health Associations, Substance Abuse, Transplant Networks/Donor Banks. **Geo. Dist:** national organizations; primarily in areas where Merrill Lynch & Co. maintains offices; New York, NY, metropolitan area.

**★ 1239 ★ MetLife Foundation**
1 Madison Ave.
New York, NY 10010
**Phone:** (212)578-6272          **Fax:** (212)685-1435
**Website:** http://www.metlife.com/Companyinfo/Community/index.html
Sibyl Jacobson, President & Chief Executive Officer
**Priorities:** *Arts & Humanities:* 24%. Foundation aims to bring enriching cultural experiences to diverse audiences across the country. Grants are made for arts education, as well as tours, traveling exhibitions, cultural broadcasts, public broadcasting, national arts centers, museums, journalism, and the written, performing and visual arts. Funding is also provided for creation of new work and initiatives that foster greater understanding and appreciation of diversity. *Civic & Public Affairs:* 18%. The foundation awards civic affairs grants to help organizations meet the pressing

economic and social needs of their communities. Targeted to low- and moderate-income areas, these grants are earmarked for affordable housing, economic development, job training, open spaces, family and youth programs, and business, economic, and public policy research organizations. Volunteer activity, especially among young people and MetLife employees, is also supported. *Education:* 17%. Focus is on strengthening the quality of education by supporting activities and programs that improve the education system, include the classroom teacher in the process, involve parents in their children's education, and provide all children–especially those who have been traditionally underserved and disadvantaged–with the resources and opportunities they need to succeed. Grants are made in the areas of teacher preparation, school-to-work transition, and youth violence prevention, with support also given to business, insurance and economic education. *Environment:* 7%. Supports the United Way. *International:* 18%. Foundation funds public information campaigns to provide individuals and communities with the facts they need to preserve and enhance physical health. Grants support national health education and promotion initiatives that reach large audiences, particularly youth, minorities and other at-risk populations. Areas of focus are substance abuse prevention, school health education and promoting healthy lifestyles, and Alzheimer's disease research. *Voluntarism:* Recognizes company volunteers with the MetLife Volunteer ServiceAwards; also sponsors an employee volunteer program that helps employees find volunteer opportunities with nonprofits, schools, and other public agencies. There is a full-time volunteer coordinator at the headquarters location, and several branch offices have structured volunteer programs. Company makes small grants to organizations where employees actively volunteer, through the Volunteer Ventures program. *Note:* Above priorities include 2000 foundation and direct giving. **Typ. Recipients:** AIDS/HIV, Alzheimers Disease, Cancer, Children's Health/Hospitals, Clinics/Medical Centers, Health Funds, Health Organizations, Health Policy/Cost Containment, Heart, Hospitals, Medical Education, Medical Research, Medical Training, Nursing Services, Nutrition, Prenatal Health Issues, Public Health, Research/Studies Institutes, Respiratory, Substance Abuse, Transplant Networks/Donor Banks. **Geo. Dist:** programs that are national in scope; special consideration to communities in which Metropolitan has a major presence.

**★ 1240 ★ MGIC Investment Corp.**
PO Box 488
Milwaukee, WI 53202
**Phone:** (414)347-6577          **Fax:** (414)347-4866
**Email:** john_ludwick@mgic.com
John Ludwick, Vice President Human Resources
**Priorities:** *Arts & Humanities:* 25%. *Civic & Public Affairs:* 20%. *Education:* 15%. *International:* 40%. Funds health and welfare organizations. **Typ. Recipients:** Domestic Violence, Hospitals, Single-Disease Health Associations, Substance Abuse. **Geo. Dist:** Milwaukee, WI.

**★ 1241 ★ Milacron Foundation**
2090 Florence Ave.
Cincinnati, OH 45206
**Phone:** (513)487-5912          **Fax:** (513)487-5586
John Francy, Assistant Treasurer
**Priorities:** *Arts & Humanities:* 16%. Gives to museums, opera, and arts funds. *Civic & Public Affairs:* 9%. Supports urban development, organizations that promote racial equality, employment services, public safety, and zoos. *Education:* 13%. Supports higher education with an emphasis on technology, engineering, and science education. Also funds a school for the deaf. *Environment:* 58%. Majority of funding supports United Way campaigns near operating locations. Other interests include youth organizations and services for senior citizens. *International:* 3%. Funds a children's hospital and wellness initiatives. *Religion:* 1%. Gives to a science fair and a plastics center. *Note:* Total contributions made in 1999. **Typ. Recipients:** Cancer, Children's Health/Hospitals, Children's Health/Hospitals, Emergency/Ambulance Services,

Health Organizations, Hospices, Preventive Medicine/Wellness Organizations. **Geo. Dist:** principally near operating locations and to national organizations. **Frmly:** Cincinnati Milacron Inc.

**★ 1242 ★ Milliken Foundation**
153 E 53rd St.
New York, NY 10043
Sid Nichols, Executive Director
**Fnded:** 1945. **Priorities:** *Arts & Humanities:* 2%. Supports arts associations and councils, libraries, theater, ballet, public broadcasting, and historic preservation. *Civic & Public Affairs:* 15%. Primarily supports public policy and organizations for better government; also supports business and free enterprise organizations and several local fire departments and municipalities. *Education:* 19%. Main interests are colleges and universities, and scientific and technology institutions, particularly schools for textile research. Other interests include private precollege and special education. *Environment:* 55%. The majority of social services giving went to united funds and the Boys' Club of New York. Other interests include recreation, athletics, community service organizations, food and clothing distribution, and programs for the disabled. *International:* 3%. Supports the March of Dimes, Alzheimer's research, and hospitals and clinics. *Religion:* 2%. Major interests include scientific research and science institutes, particularly those involved in textile research. *Note:* Total contributions made in 1999. **Typ. Recipients:** Alzheimers Disease, Children's Health/Hospitals, Clinics/Medical Centers, Emergency/Ambulance Services, Family Planning, Hospitals, Medical Education, Medical Rehabilitation, People with Disabilities, Prenatal Health Issues, Public Health, Single-Disease Health Associations, Substance Abuse. **Geo. Dist:** headquarters and operating communities; nationally.

**★ 1243 ★ The Millipore Foundation**
80 Ashby Rd.
Bedford, MA 01730-2271
**Phone:** (781)533-2210          **Fax:** (781)533-3301
**Email:** Charleen_Johnson@millipore.com
**Website:** http://www.millipore.com/foundation
Charleen Johnson, Executive Director

**Priorities:** *Arts & Humanities:* 22%. Funds public libraries, performing arts, museums, and fine arts. *Civic & Public Affairs:* 8%. Support for the resolution of key industrial policy issues at local, national, and international levels. *Education:* 37%. Supports selected organizations, universities, institutions, and teaching hospitals engaged in research and training, primarily in the fields of chemistry, biochemistry and engineering. Supports programs in minority education (national organizations that extend opportunities for minorities at all educational levels), and awards scholarships each year to employees' children. *Environment:* 22%. Supports and youth development, especially regional programs that provide employment and self-development, particularly for inner-city youth. Center, The Massachusetts Volunteer Network, and local charitable organizations. It acts as a clearinghouse between 500 agencies and the volunteers. Employees and others are matched with nonprofit agencies and organizations that can benefit from their specific skills, talent and knowledge. *International:* 7%. Funds hospitals, medical centers, and biomedical research. *Religion:* 4%. Supports science museums. *Voluntarism:* Under the Voluntary Service Grant Program, employees who are currently doing volunteer work in their communities can petition the foundation for funds to support a special need or program of the organization where they volunteer. The program now provides a grant of up to $5,000 to support specific projects of eligible community organizations in which the Millipore employee is actively involved. The Skills-Bank program is open to current employees, retirees, and family members who want to get involved in volunteer work. SkillsBank is a computerized program linked to the United Way's Voluntary Action Center, The Massachusetts Volunteer Network, and local charitable organizations. It acts as a clearinghouse between 500 agencies and the volunteers. Employees and others are matched with nonprofit agencies and organizations that can benefit from their specific skills, talent and knowledge. *Note:* Total contributions made in fiscal 2000, excluding matching gifts. **Typ. Recipients:** AIDS/HIV, Cancer, Children's Health/Hospitals, Clinics/Medical Centers, Diabetes, Emergency/Ambulance Services, Health Organizations, Home-Care Services, Hospitals, Medical Education, Medical Research, Medical Training, Mental Health, People with Disabilities, Public Health, Single-Disease Health Associations, Substance Abuse. **Geo. Dist:** matching gifts awarded nationally; MA, cash grants made primarily in Massachusetts.

### ★ 1244 ★ Mine Safety Appliances Co. Charitable Foundation

PO Box 426
Pittsburgh, PA 15230
**Phone:** (412)967-3000          **Fax:** (412)967-3452
Dennis Zeitler, Vice President

**Priorities:** *Arts & Humanities:* 10%. Funds music, ballet, opera, theater, museums, and libraries. *Civic & Public Affairs:* 17%. Emphasis on economic development and public policy. Supports business, professional, and safety organizations in addition to those with an emphasis on urban and community affairs. *Education:* 9%. Pittsburgh area colleges and universities receive funding. Also supports economic, engineering, and minority education and independent college funds. *Environment:* 50%. Primarily supports united funds. Also funds shelters, youth organizations, emergency relief, child welfare, and the disabled. *International:* 11%. Supports hospitals, pediatric health, rehabilitation centers, and single-disease health associations. *Religion:* 1%. *Note:* Total foundation contributions made in 2000. **Typ. Recipients:** Children's Health/Hospitals, Diabetes, Emergency/Ambulance Services, Health Funds, Health Organizations, Hospitals, Kidney, Long-Term Care, Medical Rehabilitation, Mental Health, Multiple Sclerosis, People with Disabilities, Single-Disease Health Associations. **Geo. Dist:** operating location communities; Pittsburgh, PA.

### ★ 1245 ★ Minnesota Mutual Foundation

400 Robert St. North
Saint Paul, MN 55101-2098
**Phone:** (651)665-3501          **Fax:** (651)665-3551
**Email:** lori.koutsky@minnesotamutual.com
**Website:** http://www.minnesotamutual.com
Lori Koutsky, Manager

**Priorities:** *Arts & Humanities:* 15%. Supports chamber orchestras and united arts funds. *Civic & Public Affairs:* 10%. Gives to civic groups in operating locations, particularly business-related causes. *Education:* 25%. Interests include colleges and universities, business and economic education, literacy, and science education. Supports college scholarship programs. *Environment:* 45%. Support the United Way, family services, and child welfare. *International:* Less than 5%. Supports health-care services for the disadvantaged, and medical research. *Voluntarism:* Company conducts a special program that recognizes employee volunteerism with $100 donations to organizations where employees volunteer their time. *Note:* Total contributions made in 1999. **Typ. Recipients:** AIDS/HIV, Child Abuse, Domestic Violence, Emergency/Ambulance Services, Health Funds, Hospices, Long-Term Care, Medical Rehabilitation, Medical Research, Nursing Services, People with Disabilities, Prenatal Health Issues, Public Health, Research/Studies Institutes, Substance Abuse. **Geo. Dist:** Minneapolis, MN, metropolitan area; St. Paul, MN, metropolitan area.

### ★ 1246 ★ Mitsubishi Electric America Foundation

1560 Wilson Boulevard, Ste. 1150
Arlington, VA 22209
**Phone:** (703)276-8240          **Fax:** (703)276-8260
**Email:** rayna.aylward@mevs.mea.com
**Website:** http://www.meaf.org
Rayna Aylward, Executive Director

**Fnded:** 1991. **Priorities:** *Environment:* 100%. Funding supports a range of projects addressing the needs

of people with disabilities. Grants have supported internships of visually impaired students, exploration of career opportunities, online meeting places for children with disabilities, and training for teachers to improve their ability to assist disabled students. *Voluntarism:* To recognize growing interest in volunteerism among Mitsubishi Electric America employees, the foundation administers the MEA Foundation Starfish Enterprise Award program. The foundation also donates $10 per volunteer hour contributed to eligible projects by employees, their friends, and family members. *Note:* Total contributions made in 1999. **Typ. Recipients:** AIDS/HIV, Cancer, Children's Health/Hospitals, Diabetes, Eyes/Blindness, Heart, Medical Rehabilitation, People with Disabilities, Prenatal Health Issues, Single-Disease Health Associations. **Geo. Dist:** nationally; operating locations.

### ★ 1247 ★ Monsanto Fund

800 N Lindbergh Blvd.
Saint Louis, MO 63167
**Phone:** (314)694-4596          **Fax:** (314)694-7658
**Website:** http://www.monsantofund.org
Deborah Patterson, President

**Priorities:** *Arts & Humanities:* 3%. Supports music, public broadcasting, libraries, historical societies, and arts education. *Civic & Public Affairs:* 15%. Funds parks, zoos, botanical gardens, employment, economic development, and municipalities. *Education:* 5%. Supports both precollege and higher educational institutions, with strong emphasis on science, agriculture, biotechnology, and sustainable development. Focus is on innovative science education programs, training for teachers, collaborations in science literacy, and development of new curricula. *Environment:* 13%. Supports the United Way, youth services, and health and human services organizations. *International:* 1%. *Religion:* 61%. Major grant to the Plant Science Institute. Focus is supporting "Agricultural Abundance": increasing agricultural productivity, yields, and nutritional value; capital projects which increase infrastructure and farmers' linkages to local markets; reducing the pressures of agriculture on fragile areas; training, information dissemination, and extension services. *Note:* Total fund contributions made in 1999. **Typ. Recipients:** AIDS/HIV, Alzheimers Disease, Cancer, Children's Health/Hospitals, Clinics/Medical Centers, Diabetes, Domestic Violence, Emergency/Ambulance Services, Health Organizations, Health Policy/Cost Containment, Hospitals, Medical Research, Research/Studies Institutes, Substance Abuse. **Geo. Dist:** operating facilities.

### ★ 1248 ★ Montana Power Foundation

40 E Broadway St.
Butte, MT 59701
**Phone:** (406)497-2602          **Fax:** (406)497-2451
**Email:** bcain@mtpower.com
**Website:** http://www.mtpower.com/community/cm_foundation.htm
William Cain, Director Corporate Community Relations

**Fnded:** 1985. **Priorities:** *Arts & Humanities:* 3%. Supports local museums, libraries, cultural centers, and the performing arts. *Civic & Public Affairs:* 7%. Supports business organizations, employment initiatives, community activities, special events, and civic improvement. *Education:* 51%. Supports the University Excellence Program. Funds are applied to higher education at public and private colleges, universities, and vocational and technical programs within the state. Additional grants were made for capital programs, matching gifts, and scholarships to these same schools and additional primary and secondary schools in the state in the fields of math, science, and youth leadership. *Environment:* 35%. Majority of support is given to the United Way. Other funds go toward community services, youth organizations, services for seniors, and YMCA. *International:* 3%. Supports hospitals and single-disease health associations. *Voluntarism:* In 1998, Montana Power announced the launch of an official corporate volunteer program. The Montana Power Company Hearts and Hands Employee Volunteer Program will acknowledge employee volunteer efforts through the new Dollars for Doers program, by which donations of $250 will be made to

non-profit organizations supported by employee volunteers. *Note:* Contributions analysis based on foundation giving only. Total contributions made in 1999. **Typ. Recipients:** Cancer, Children's Health/Hospitals, Clinics/Medical Centers, Diabetes, Domestic Violence, Emergency/Ambulance Services, Family Planning, Health Organizations, Hospitals. **Geo. Dist:** headquarters and operating communities.

### ★ 1249 ★ The MONY Life Insurance of New York

1740 Broadway
New York, NY 10019
**Phone:** (212)708-2136          **Fax:** (212)708-2001
**Website:** http://www.mony.com/AboutMONY/Inside-MONY/Foundation
Lynn Stekas, President

**Priorities:** *Arts & Humanities:* 4%. Supports performing arts. *Civic & Public Affairs:* 10%. Funds economic development. *Education:* 14%. Supports higher education relevant to the insurance industry, magnet and private schools, Junior Achievement, and AIDS education. *Environment:* 53%. Funds the United Way and services for youth and families. *International:* 19%. Interests include AIDS, cancer, and children's health. *Voluntarism:* The company sponsors the Volunteer Incentive at MONY (VIM) program, which encourages employee volunteerism at nonprofit organizations by providing semi-annual grants to those served by MONY Group volunteers. Another program, the Volunteer Incentive Award Program (VIP), makes an annual monetary award to a nonprofit social service agency in the community of each of its two major sites to encourage volunteer programs that effectively maximize their recourses by creatively utilizing employed volunteers. *Note:* Total contributions in 1999. **Typ. Recipients:** AIDS/HIV, Cancer, Clinics/Medical Centers, Emergency/Ambulance Services, Family Planning, Health Organizations, Health-General, Hospices, Medical Research, Mental Health, People with Disabilities, Prenatal Health Issues, Public Health, Research/Studies Institutes, Single-Disease Health Associations, Substance Abuse. **Geo. Dist:** headquarters and operating communities; New York, NY; Syracuse, NY.

### ★ 1250 ★ Motorola Foundation

1303 E Algonquin Rd.
Schaumburg, IL 60196
**Phone:** (847)576-7895          **Fax:** (847)576-3997
**Website:**          http://www.motorola.com/GSS/
SSTG.motinAZ/Giving.html
Judy Adkins, Program Administrator

**Priorities:** *Arts & Humanities:* 7%. Funds public broadcasting and provides major support for the National Underground Railroad Foundation. *Civic & Public Affairs:* 4%. Supports foundations, economic development, minority affairs, public communications, and public affairs. *Education:* 52%. Supports engineering, technology, and science programs at universities; historically minority colleges and universities, based upon emphasis in engineering and science; programs providing technical assistance, research, and statistical information on the state of science and engineering education; strengthening science and mathematics education at the pre-college level; programs reaching traditionally under-represented groups in the areas of math, science, engineering, and business; pre-K programs; parental involvement in education programs; and educational programs that promote and support preserving the environment. *Environment:* 24%. Supports volunteer programs and United Way. *Religion:* 1%. Funds natural history and science museums and efforts to increase funds for scientific awareness. *Voluntarism:* The company sponsors volunteer programs that enable employees to support local organizations and schools in their communities. The foundation sponsors a volunteer grants program. *Note:* Total contributions made in 2000. **Typ. Recipients:** Emergency/Ambulance Services, Hospices, Hospitals, People with Disabilities, Single-Disease Health Associations, Substance Abuse. **Geo. Dist:** headquarters community, plant locations, and to select national organizations.

**★ 1251 ★ Mutual of Omaha Insurance Co.**
Mutual of Omaha Plz.
Omaha, NE 68175
**Phone:** (402)342-5263     **Fax:** (402)351-2407
**Website:** http://www.mutualofomaha.com
Pam Shafer, Comm Affairs & Corp. Contributions Admin

**Priorities:** *Arts & Humanities:* 20%. *Civic & Public Affairs:* 20%. Distributed equally among the arts, health and human services, and civic organizations. *Education:* 40%. *International:* 20%. **Typ. Recipients:** AIDS/HIV, Domestic Violence, Health-General, Heart, Hospices, People with Disabilities. **Geo. Dist:** major business locations.


**★ 1252 ★ Nabisco Foundation Trust**
Nabisco Plaza
Parsippany, NJ 07054
**Phone:** (973)682-7098     **Fax:** (973)682-6265
Henry Sandbach, Director OF Contributions

**Fnded:** 1953. **Priorities:** *Arts & Humanities:* 15%. Funds performing arts and community theater. *Civic & Public Affairs:* 10%. Contributes to a citizen action group. *Education:* 18%. Supports universities and scholarship funds. *Environment:* 38%. Supports youth services and a food bank. *International:* 19%. Funds hospitals and medical centers. *Note:* Total foundation contributions made in 2000. **Typ. Recipients:** Clinics/Medical Centers, Health Organizations, Hospitals, Hospitals, Medical Education, Nutrition, People with Disabilities. **Geo. Dist:** headquarters and operating communities.


**★ 1253 ★ National City Bank Foundation**
PO Box E1919
Minneapolis, MN 55480
**Phone:** (612)904-8503     **Fax:** (612)904-8016
Gloria Noetzelman, Secretary

**Fnded:** 1970. **Priorities:** *Arts & Humanities:* 15%. Supports arts centers, the performing arts, and film. *Civic & Public Affairs:* 24%. Funds housing, women's concerns, and community groups. *Education:* 6%. Supports arts education and ACORN. *Environment:* 44%. Funds United Way and youth concerns. *International:* 2%. Funds children's health initiatives. *Note:* Total contributions in 1998. **Typ. Recipients:** AIDS/HIV, Children's Health/Hospitals, Emergency/Ambulance Services, Family Planning, Health Organizations, Kidney, Medical Rehabilitation, Research/Studies Institutes, Substance Abuse. **Geo. Dist:** Minneapolis, MN.


**★ 1254 ★ National City Bank of Ohio**
1900 E 9th St.
Locator 01-2157
Cleveland, OH 44114
**Phone:** (216)222-2995     **Fax:** (216)222-2670
**Website:** http://www.nationalcity.com
Joanna Clark, Assistant Vice President, Corporate Publ

**Typ. Recipients:** Health Organizations, Health-General, Hospitals. **Geo. Dist:** operating community.


**★ 1255 ★ National City Bank of Pennsylvania**
20 Stanwix, 25-146
Pittsburgh, PA 15222-4802
**Phone:** (412)644-8083     **Fax:** (412)644-8099
**Website:** http://www.national-city.com/natcity/otherdocs/about/community.html
Angie Longa, Vice President, Public Affairs

**Priorities:** *Arts & Humanities:* Supports local museums, theater, and arts festivals. *Civic & Public Affairs:* Emphasis on revitalization of low-to-modrate-income housing and neighborhoods. *Education:* Provides scholarships to children of employees. Matches employee contributions to secondary schools and colleges and universities. *Environment:* Supports the United Way and a variety of community service programs. *International:* Priorities include children's health and health services for the indigent. **Typ.**

**Recipients:** Health-General. **Geo. Dist:** headquarters and operating communities in western PA.


**★ 1256 ★ National City Corp. Charitable Foundation**
c/o Corporate Public Affairs Department
PO Box 5756
Cleveland, OH 44101
**Phone:** (216)575-2994     **Fax:** (216)575-2670
Allen Waddle, Senior Vice President

**Priorities:** *Arts & Humanities:* (Art & Culture) 12%. Supports art institutions, museums, galleries, festivals, music, theater, and dance. *Civic & Public Affairs:* (Civic & Community) 30%. Supports a wide range of civic causes promoting financial cooperation among government, business, and community leaders. Major support goes to economic development concerns, including neighborhood revitalization, inner-city and community development, and public-private partnerships. Also supports public policy organizations, parks, minority affairs, and organizations concerned with violent crime. *Education:* 19%. Supports universities and colleges, providing capital and operating support. Supports business education through Inroads and Junior Achievement. Also supports economic, arts, and minority education, and private precollege education. Bank matches employee contributions to education. *Environment:* (Health and Human Services) 21%. Primarily supports community service and religious welfare organizations, community centers, food and clothing distribution, and a range of organizations that provide services for the elderly, families, youth, and children. Has supported groups devoted to researching diseases including cancer, arthritis, cystic fibrosis, and kidney ailments. *Note:* Total contributions made in 2000. **Typ. Recipients:** Cancer, Children's Health/Hospitals, Clinics/Medical Centers, Emergency/Ambulance Services, Geriatric Health, Hospices, Hospitals, Hospitals (University Affiliated), Medical Rehabilitation, Mental Health, Prenatal Health Issues, Public Health, Substance Abuse. **Geo. Dist:** considers national organizations on an individual basis; IL; IN; KY; MI; OH; PA.


**★ 1257 ★ National Life Group**
One National Life Dr.
Montpelier, VT 05604
**Phone:** (802)229-3333     **Fax:** (802)229-7006
**Website:** http://www.nationallife.com
Brian Vachon, Vice President, Communications

**Priorities:** *Voluntarism:* Company promotes employee volunteerism by providing support to organizations at which employees volunteer, as well as by allowing time off during the work day. **Typ. Recipients:** Domestic Violence, Health-General, Medical Research, Mental Health, Single-Disease Health Associations, Substance Abuse. **Geo. Dist:** VT, Central Vermont.


**★ 1258 ★ National Machinery Foundation, Inc.**
161 Greenfield St.
Tiffin, OH 44883
**Phone:** (419)447-5211     **Fax:** (419)443-2380
Don Bero, Assistant Secretary

**Priorities:** *Arts & Humanities:* 17%. Supports theaters and libraries. *Civic & Public Affairs:* 6%. Gives to career counseling/preparation, community fairs and festivals, public transportation, and a fire department. *Education:* 14%. Supports public high schools, private education, universities, and Junior Achievement. *Environment:* 49%. Primary support is for a stadium project. Other interests include community service organizations, substance abuse treatment and prevention, youth organizations, and the United Way. *International:* 12%. Funds rehabilitation centers, hospitals, nursing homes, hospices, and single-disease health associations. *Note:* Total contributions made in 1999. **Typ. Recipients:** AIDS/HIV, Cancer, Children's Health/Hospitals, Clinics/Medical Centers, Domestic Violence, Emergency/Ambulance Services, Geriatric Health, Health Organizations, Health-General, Heart, Hospices, Hospitals, Medical Rehabilitation, Nursing

Services, Single-Disease Health Associations, Substance Abuse. **Geo. Dist:** OH, Seneca County.


**★ 1259 ★ National Service Foundation**
1420 Peachtree St., NE
Atlanta, GA 30309-3002
**Phone:** (404)853-1000     **Fax:** (404)858-1015
James Balloun, President, Chairman & Chief Executive Of

**Fnded:** 1969. **Priorities:** *Arts & Humanities:* 15%. Supports arts centers, the performing arts, and libraries. *Civic & Public Affairs:* 20%. Funds economic development and civic organizations. *Education:* 8%. Supports colleges and universities, minority education, and Junior Achievement. *Environment:* 25%. Funds United Way and youth concerns. *International:* 6%. Funds hospitals and single-disease health associations. *Note:* Total contributions made in fiscal 2000. **Typ. Recipients:** Arthritis, Cancer, Child Abuse, Diabetes, Domestic Violence, Heart, Hospitals, Medical Education, Medical Rehabilitation, Medical Research, Multiple Sclerosis, People with Disabilities, Prenatal Health Issues. **Geo. Dist:** GA.


**★ 1260 ★ National Starch & Chemical Foundation**
10 Finderne Ave.
Bridgewater, NJ 08807
**Phone:** (908)685-5001     **Fax:** (908)685-5096
Carmen Ortiz, Contact

**Fnded:** 1968. **Priorities:** *Arts & Humanities:* 3%. Supports theater and performing arts, musical groups such as symphonies, museums and historical societies, and arts associations and festivals. *Civic & Public Affairs:* 11%. Funds professional associations, public policy, urban leagues, business groups, and environmental organizations. *Education:* 27%. Elementary and secondary schools, colleges and universities, and junior achievement. Also supports math and science education programs for minorities. Matching gifts constitute a large number of grants to colleges. Foundation provides scholarships to the children of employees. *Environment:* 42%. United Way organizations in various company-operating communities, child welfare and recreational groups, volunteer organizations, food banks, services for the elderly and disabled, and others. *International:* 15%. Hospitals, research, foundations, and single-disease health organizations. *Voluntarism:* In the counties surrounding company headquarters in Bridgewater, NJ, National actively supports the Science Alliance Program. Senior staffers devote their time and expertise to help teach middle school and high school students about science in an interesting and hands-on fashion. In Woodruff, SC, employees help nurture the growth and aspirations of children by serving as positive role models, confidants and supporters. Volunteerism extends to international National Starch and Chemical employees in England, Italy, and South Africa. *Note:* Total contributions made in 1999. **Typ. Recipients:** Cancer, Clinics/Medical Centers, Emergency/Ambulance Services, Health Funds, Health Organizations, Hospitals, Medical Rehabilitation, Medical Training, Nursing Services, Public Health, Substance Abuse. **Geo. Dist:** primarily in headquarters and operating communities.


**★ 1261 ★ Nationwide Foundation**
1 Nationwide Plaza
Mail Drop 1-36-13
Columbus, OH 43215-2220
**Phone:** (614)249-5095     **Fax:** (614)677-0320
**Website:** http://www.nationwide.com/about_us/involve/fndatn.htm
Stephen Rish, President

**Fnded:** 1959. **Priorities:** *Arts & Humanities:* 11%. Supports libraries, musical performance, ballet, theater, art councils, museums, and history. *Civic & Public Affairs:* 12%. Funds urban affairs, public safety, economic development, housing initiatives, and community organizations. *Education:* 23%. Supports colleges, universities, economic education, education funds, scholarships, and literacy. *Environment:* 52%.

Supports child abuse programs, youth programs, shelters, food banks, YMCAs, family planning services and major support to United Way. *Note:* Total contributions made in 2000. **Typ. Recipients:** AIDS/HIV, Alzheimers Disease, Cancer, Child Abuse, Children's Health/Hospitals, Emergency/Ambulance Services, Eyes/Blindness, Family Planning, Health Organizations, Heart, Hospitals, Long-Term Care, Medical Research, Mental Health, Nursing Services, People with Disabilities, Single-Disease Health Associations, Speech & Hearing, Substance Abuse. **Geo. Dist:** OH, Central Ohio and near state operating locations. **Frmly:** Nationwide Insurance Enterprise Foundation.

### ★ 1262 ★ NCR Foundation

1700 S Patterson Boulevard
Dayton, OH 45479
**Phone:** (937)445-2577          **Fax:** (937)445-0636
Mary Karr, Vice President, Director

**Fnded:** 1953. **Priorities:** *Arts & Humanities:* 11%. Supports arts programs for children, a cultural council, and an outdoor history museum. *Civic & Public Affairs:* 35%. Supports economic development. *Education:* 24%. Supports schools and universities, and provides scholarships for minority students. *Environment:* 29%. Supports emergency relief organizations and the United Way. *International:* 1%. Funds the American Red Cross and the Cancer Hope Network. *Note:* Total contributions made in 1999. **Typ. Recipients:** Cancer, Emergency/Ambulance Services, Health Organizations. **Geo. Dist:** headquarters and operating communities; Dayton, OH.

### ★ 1263 ★ NCS Pearson, Inc.

5601 Green Valley Dr.
Bloomington, MN 55437
**Phone:** (952)681-3000          **Fax:** (952)681-3040
**Website:** http://www.ncspearson.com
David Hakensen, Corporate Contributions Program Manager

**Priorities:** *Arts & Humanities:* 15% to 20%.Supports arts and humanities, including art appreciation, art centers, and art institutes. Focus is on larger, established, highly-visible institutions. *Civic & Public Affairs:* About 20%. Contributions fund economic development, professional associations, nonprofit management, public policy, environmental affairs, and urban affairs. *Education:* 25% to 30%. Recipients include arts education, business education, career/vocational education, and colleges and universities. *International:* 35% to 40%. Supports public health, hospitals, health care cost containment, and health maintenance services. Additional funding goes to child welfare agencies, chemical abuse treatment centers, employment programs for the handicapped, community services, youth and family organizations, shelters, united funds, and volunteer action. **Typ. Recipients:** Domestic Violence, Family Planning, Health Policy/Cost Containment, Health-General, Hospices, Hospitals, Nutrition, People with Disabilities, Public Health, Single-Disease Health Associations, Substance Abuse. **Geo. Dist:** headquarters and operating communities.

### ★ 1264 ★ Nestle U.S.A. Inc.

800 North Brand Boulevard
Glendale, CA 91203
**Phone:** (818)549-6000          **Fax:** (818)549-6952
**Fnded:** 1952. **Priorities:** *Arts & Humanities:* 10%. Supports music and museums. *Civic & Public Affairs:* 5%. Supports women's affairs and justice. *Education:* 55%. Supports literacy, universities, and college funds. *Environment:* 24%. Primarily supports United Way. *International:* 2%. Supports health centers and organizations. *Note:* Total contributions made in 1998. **Typ. Recipients:** Clinics/Medical Centers, Emergency/Ambulance Services, Hospitals, Nutrition, People with Disabilities, Preventive Medicine/Wellness Organizations. **Geo. Dist:** manufacturing facility areas.

### ★ 1265 ★ New England Bio Labs Foundation

32 Tozer Rd.
Beverly, MA 01915
**Phone:** (978)927-2404          **Fax:** (978)921-1350
**Email:** cataldo@nebf.org
**Website:** http://www.nebf.org
Martine Kellett, Executive Director

**Fnded:** 1982. **Priorities:** *Arts & Humanities:* 5%. Supports music, dance, and community arts organizations, primarily in Massachusetts. *Education:* 8%. Funds the reuse of textbooks in international locations, and a college of art. *Environment:* 13%. Supports self-sufficiency, youth, and health initiatives internationally, and funds youth and family services domestically. *Religion:* 3%. Gives to the Sustainable Sciences Institute. *Note:* Total contributions made in fiscal 2000. The foundation reports that 75% of its grants were made to international organizations, 24% were made to domestic community organizations, and 1% were made to national organizations. **Typ. Recipients:** Clinics/Medical Centers, Eyes/Blindness, Health Organizations, Health-General, Nutrition, Prenatal Health Issues, Preventive Medicine/Wellness Organizations, Public Health. **Geo. Dist:** internationally; MA.

### ★ 1266 ★ New England Financial

501 Boylston St., 5th Fl.
Boston, MA 02116-3700
**Phone:** (617)578-2119          **Fax:** (617)536-5566
**Email:** bspence@nefn.com
**Website:** http://www.nefn.com
Bryan Spence, Director, Charitable Contributions

**Priorities:** *Arts & Humanities:* 5% to 10%. Supports art institutes that reach a large population and contribute to the community, art programs in the Boston Public schools, and organizations that make cultural events accessible to the community. *Civic & Public Affairs:* (United Funds & United Way) Supports the United Way of Massachusetts Bay. (Housing & Neighborhood Revitalization) 10% to 15%. Provides grants to agencies that develop affordable, permanent, transitional, and shelter housing, and those that support community development initiatives. *Education:* 25% to 30%. Supports Boston public schools, particularly in the area of basic skills that impact company's partnership schools, Jeremiah E. Burke High School and the Mather Elementary School. Also gives direct grants to Greater Boston  area colleges and universities for special projects. *Environment:* 25% to 30%. Supports organizations that focus on social and economic issues involving the community. Emphasis on youth programs, mentoring, jobtraining, women's issues, and other community-based programs. *International:* 15% to 20%. Supports programs that are community-based, increase community access, targets underserved populations, and promote efficient care delivery. **Typ. Recipients:** AIDS/HIV, Cancer, Children's Health/Hospitals, Clinics/Medical Centers, Domestic Violence, Family Planning, Geriatric Health, Health Organizations, Hospitals, Medical Rehabilitation, Medical Research, Mental Health, Nutrition, People with Disabilities, Prenatal Health Issues, Public Health, Substance Abuse. **Geo. Dist:** Boston, MA, metropolitan area.

### ★ 1267 ★ New Jersey Natural Gas Foundation

PO Box 1464
Wall, NJ 07719
**Phone:** (732)938-1134          **Fax:** (732)938-7183
Tom Kononowitz, Senior Vice President

**Priorities:** *Civic & Public Affairs:* 12%. Supports community safety initiatives, Urban Leagues, minority affairs, law enforcement organizations, parks, environmental organizations, and community foundations. *Education:* 15%. Funds colleges, universities, community colleges, and programs that assist minority students. *Environment:* 38%. Supports the United Way, youth organizations, family services, and drug abuse prevention. Company also sponsors a "Gift of Warmth" program. *International:* 26%. Gives to medical centers, hospitals, single-disease health associations (particularly the American Cancer Society), American Red Cross, health care foundations, and pediatric health. *Note:* Total contributions made in fiscal 2000. **Typ. Recipients:** Cancer, Children's Health/Hospitals, Clinics/Medical Centers, Diabetes, Emergency/Ambulance Services, Health Organizations, Health-General, Hospitals, People with Disabilities, Prenatal Health Issues, Public Health, Single-Disease Health Associations, Substance Abuse. **Geo. Dist:** company's service area; NJ, Monmouth County; NJ, Ocean County; NJ, portions of Morris County. **Frmly:** New Jersey Resources Foundation, Inc.

### ★ 1268 ★ New York Life Foundation

51 Madison Ave.
New York, NY 10010
**Phone:** (212)576-6902
**Email:** NYLFoundation@newyorklife.com
**Website:** http://www.newyorklife.com/foundation
Peter Bushyeager, President

**Priorities:** *Arts & Humanities:* (Arts & Culture) 3%. Recipients include performing arts centers, libraries, and public broadcasting. *Civic & Public Affairs:* (Civic & Community Affairs) 12%. Supports community development programs, civil rights, women's groups, philanthropic organizations, and others. *Education:* 61%. Supports higher education, literacy, Junior Achievement, YMCAs, Boys & Girls Clubs, and arts education. Provides matching gifts to educational institutions. *Environment:* (Health & Human Services) 24%. Supports the United Way, child welfare, recreation organizations, single-disease health associations, and volunteer groups. *Voluntarism:* Provides grants to local grassroots organizations where employees volunteer. *Note:* Total contributions made in 2000. **Typ. Recipients:** AIDS/HIV, Clinics/Medical Centers, Domestic Violence, Emergency/Ambulance Services, Eyes/Blindness, Geriatric Health, Health Organizations, Hospitals, Medical Education, Medical Rehabilitation, Medical Research, Medical Training, Mental Health, Nursing Services, People with Disabilities, Single-Disease Health Associations, Substance Abuse. **Geo. Dist:** nationally; New York, NY.

### ★ 1269 ★ New York Mercantile Exchange Charitable Foundation

Executive Committee
1 North End Ave.
World Financial Center
New York, NY 10282-1101
**Phone:** (212)299-2517
Madeline Boyd, Chairman

**Fnded:** 1989. **Priorities:** *Arts & Humanities:* 3%. Supports public broadcasting and a music outreach program. *Civic & Public Affairs:* 6%. Funds public parks and community resource foundations. *Education:* 7%. Gives to education foundations, universities, precollege schools, and a school for autistic children. *Environment:* 43%. Supports disaster relief efforts, summer camps, and family/youth/senior services. *International:* 26%. Supports single-disease health organizations, hospitals and medical centers, and pediatric health initiatives. *Note:* Total contributions made in 2000. **Typ. Recipients:** AIDS/HIV, Cancer, Children's Health/Hospitals, Clinics/Medical Centers, Diabetes, Domestic Violence, Emergency/Ambulance Services, Health-General, Hospitals, Medical Education, Medical Rehabilitation, Multiple Sclerosis, People with Disabilities, Public Health, Research/Studies Institutes, Single-Disease Health Associations, Substance Abuse, Trauma Treatment. **Geo. Dist:** principally near operating locations and to national organizations.

### ★ 1270 ★ Newman's Own Foundation

246 Post Rd. East
Westport, CT 06880-3615
**Phone:** (203)222-0136          **Fax:** (203)227-5630
**Website:**     http://www.newmansown.com/sa_giving.html
Aaron Hotchner, Vice President & Director

**Fnded:** 1989. **Priorities:** *International:* 100%. Supports the Sydney Children's Hospital in Australia. *Note:* Total contributions in fiscal 1999. **Typ. Recipients:** Arthritis, Child Abuse, Children's Health/Hospitals, Domestic Violence, Health Funds, Hospices, Hospitals, Medical Rehabilitation, People with Disabilities, Single-Disease Health Associations. **Geo. Dist:** internationally, where Newman's Own is sold.

**★ 1271 ★ Niagara Mohawk Foundation**
300 Erie Boulevard
Syracuse, NY 13202
**Phone:** (315)428-5691
Carolyn May, Contact

**Priorities:** *Arts & Humanities:* 9%. Support goes to public broadcasting, libraries, art museums, and the performing arts. *Civic & Public Affairs:* 8%. Supports local initiatives and community services. *Education:* 15%. Supports universities and colleges. *Environment:* 40%. Major support for the United Way; also funds youth organizations and human services. *International:* 21%. Funds American Red Cross, hospice, and hospitals. *Religion:* 1%. Supports museums of science and technology. *Voluntarism:* Sponsors a volunteer grant program and a community action team. *Note:* Total foundation contributions made in 2000. **Typ. Recipients:** Cancer, Children's Health/ Hospitals, Emergency/Ambulance Services, Health-General, Heart, Hospices, Hospitals, People with Disabilities, Prenatal Health Issues. **Geo. Dist:** service areas; NY, Upstate New York.


**Nissan Foundation**
*See:* Entry 5584


**★ 1272 ★ Nomura America Foundation**
2 World Financial Center, Bldg. B
New York, NY 10281-1198
**Phone:** (212)667-9433
**Website:** http://www.nissandriven.com/insidenissan/corporateoutreach/
P. Johnson, Director, Advertising & Public Relations

**Fnded:** 1994. **Priorities:** *Civic & Public Affairs:* 59%. Supports public policy institutes and think tanks, enterprise initiatives, parks and community foundations. *Education:* 29%. Supports colleges and universities and private precollege education. *Environment:* 7%. Supports youth organizations. *International:* 4%. Gives to the National Multiple Sclerosis Society. *Note:* Total contributions made in 2000. **Typ. Recipients:** Arthritis, Cancer, Emergency/Ambulance Services, Health Funds, Hospitals, Medical Education, Multiple Sclerosis, Single-Disease Health Associations, Transplant Networks/Donor Banks. **Geo. Dist:** headquarters and operating communities.


**★ 1273 ★ Nordson Corp. Foundation**
28601 Clemens Rd.
Westlake, OH 44145-1148
**Phone:** (440)892-1580          **Fax:** (440)892-9507
**Email:** kladiner@nordson.com
**Website:**          http://www.nordson.com/corporate/grants.html
Constance Haqq, Executive Director

**Priorities:** *Arts & Humanities:* 24%. Funding is given to established arts organizations that actively seek to broaden their audience bases in Nordson communities. Supports museums, musical groups, art programs, public broadcasting, performing arts, and enhanced multicultural awareness. *Civic & Public Affairs:* 21%. Supports minority affairs, housing, economic development, and job training and placement. Efforts to involve citizens in community improvement are also a priority. *Education:* 35%. Supports education reform, colleges, minority education, student aid, and secondary public and private education. *Environment:* 12%. Funding supports organizations that promote prevention, crisis intervention, life transition opportunities, and systemic policy change. Also, supports family services and united funds. Other interests include services for the aged, and youth organizations. Each year, two or three organizations are chosen to receive intense assistance for one year in the form of grant money, emergency funding, equipment donations, and volunteer time. *International:* 5%. Funds clinics, hearing and speech and blindness organizations, and nursing associations. *Religion:* 1%. Supports a hands-on science museum. *Voluntarism:* Company operates the Time'n Talent (T'nT) program, which links employ-

ees with volunteer opportunities in the community and generates new community service projects. *Note:* Total contributions made in fiscal 2000. **Typ. Recipients:** Clinics/Medical Centers, Domestic Violence, Emergency/Ambulance Services, Hospices, Medical Education, Medical Research, Mental Health, Nursing Services, People with Disabilities, Single-Disease Health Associations, Speech & Hearing, Substance Abuse. **Geo. Dist:** headquarters and operating communities; Atlanta, GA; OH.


**★ 1274 ★ Norfolk Southern Foundation**
PO Box 3040
Norfolk, VA 23514-3040
**Phone:** (757)629-2640          **Fax:** (757)629-2361
**Email:** dhwyld@nscorp.com
**Website:** http://www.nscorp.com
Deborah Wyld, Executive Director

**Priorities:** *Arts & Humanities:* 25%. Supports music, theater and performing arts. *Civic & Public Affairs:* 21%. Urban affairs and community foundations. *Education:* 29%. Supports scholarship programs and education funds. *Environment:* 25%. Supports United Way. *Note:* Total contributions made in 1999. **Typ. Recipients:** Cancer, Children's Health/Hospitals, Emergency/Ambulance Services, Health Organizations, Heart, Hospitals, Medical Education, Medical Research, Research/Studies Institutes, Single-Disease Health Associations. **Geo. Dist:** headquarters and operating communities within the company's 22-state territory.


**★ 1275 ★ Northeast Utilities**
PO Box 5563
Hartford, CT 06102-5563
**Phone:** (860)721-4063          **Fax:** (860)721-4331
**Email:** allsoth@nu.com
**Website:** http://www.nu.com
Teresa Allsop, Director Community Relations

**Priorities:** *Arts & Humanities:* Programs are funded which provide services to children and youth, the elderly, or other traditionally underserved groups. *Environment:* Supports education and training programs, including developing technically skilled people, develop basic budgeting skills and skills needed for entry-level jobs. Also funds economic development programs, social services and public safety issues, and services thatenable people to function independently. *International:* Supports income assistance and energy assistance programs and efforts to maintain and improve basic prevention and rehabilitative health service. **Typ. Recipients:** Domestic Violence, Emergency/Ambulance Services, Hospitals, Mental Health, Nutrition, People with Disabilities, Substance Abuse. **Geo. Dist:** company service areas.


**★ 1276 ★ Northern Indiana Public Service Co.**
801 E 86th Ave.
Merrillville, IN 46410
**Phone:** (219)647-6388          **Fax:** (219)647-6380
**Email:** rbiddings@nisource.com
**Website:** http://www.nipsco.com
Regina Biddings, Director, Communications and Community R

**Priorities:** *Arts & Humanities:* Less than 5%. Symphonies, united arts organizations, art centers, science exhibits and fairs, museums, performing arts, and historic preservation. *Civic & Public Affairs:* 10% to 15%. Civic organization membership. Funds also support nature preservation through assistance to wildlife organizations, and humane societies. *Education:* 10% to 15%. Schools, colleges, and universities, including agricultural education, engineering, literacy, vocational education, liberal arts and technology, and student aid. *International:* 55% to 60%. Organizations promoting health and safety, as well as individuals and families confronted with various health issues, including cancer, arthritis, heart disease, and lung disease. Includes social service funding that supports services for the good of the community, including youth organizations, food and clothing distribution, community service organizations, civil rights

advocacy, and community centers. **Typ. Recipients:** Hospices, Hospitals, Nursing Services, People with Disabilities, Single-Disease Health Associations. **Geo. Dist:** headquarters and operating communities; IN, northern third of Indiana.


**★ 1277 ★ Northern Trust Co. Charitable Trust**
50 S LaSalle St., M-14
Chicago, IL 60675
**Phone:** (312)630-6000
Marjorie Lundy, Vice President, Community Affairs

**Priorities:** *Arts & Humanities:* 16%. Priority is given to programs which reach out to the community, making cultural opportunities more accessible for hard-to-reach and disadvantaged populations. Art museums; music, dance, and theater organizations; and libraries receive support. *Civic & Public Affairs:* 12%. Supports projects designed to serve communities which have both limited local resources and the potential for significant development. Priority is given to programs which improve and increase affordable housing for low-income Cook County residents, and promote commercial and industrial development that creates and sustains jobs in low and moderate income neighborhoods. Recipients include community development organizations; zoos, aquariums, and horticultural societies; and minority organizations receive support. *Education:* 20%. Contributes to higher education in the Chicago area, and nationally through the employee matching gifts program. Other priorities are groups which focus on prevention of school failure through early intervention, work to improve the Chicago public school system, and help the economically disadvantaged stay in school and further their education. *Environment:* 20%. Priority is given to programs which help the unemployed and underemployed break out of the cycle of poverty and public dependency; and provide services to victims of domestic abuse. Youth groups, services for families and the disabled, substance abuse treatment facilities, community centers, and shelters receive support. *International:* 20%. Priority is given to programs which make primary health care services more accessible and affordable to low-income Cook County residents. Primarily funds hospitals, medical centers, and health foundations. *Religion:* 12%. Supports science centers and museums, and a planetarium. *Voluntarism:* Company supports a volunteer grants program which makes grants to organizations where employees volunteer. *Note:* Total contributions made in 1999. **Typ. Recipients:** Adolescent Health Issues, AIDS/HIV, Children's Health/Hospitals, Clinics/Medical Centers, Domestic Violence, Family Planning, Health Funds, Health Organizations, Hospices, Hospitals, Medical Rehabilitation, Medical Training, Mental Health, Nutrition, People with Disabilities, People with Disabilities, Public Health, Research/Studies Institutes, Sexual Abuse, Substance Abuse. **Geo. Dist:** Chicago, IL, metropolitan area, with priority given to Cook County.


**★ 1278 ★ Northrop Grumman Corp.**
1840 Century Park E, 131/cc
Los Angeles, CA 90067-2199
**Phone:** (310)553-6262          **Fax:** (310)556-4510
**Website:** http://www.northgrum.com/com_rel/community_main.html
Cheryl Horn, Community Relations Manager

**Typ. Recipients:** Health-General. **Geo. Dist:** emphasis on company plants and employee living areas.


**★ 1279 ★ Northwest Natural Gas Co.**
220 Northwest 2nd Ave.
Portland, OR 97209
**Phone:** (503)226-4211          **Fax:** (503)220-2584
**Email:** george.richardson@nwnatural.com
Marie Krasnow, Administrative Assistant

**Priorities:** *Arts & Humanities:* About 5%. Supports arts centers and funds, museums, music, performing arts, and visual arts. *Civic & Public Affairs:* (United Funds & United Way) About 45% of total funding. Primary means for disbursement of funds. Also funded by employee matching gifts. 5% to 10%. Funding goes to economic development, housing, urban and community affairs, environmental concerns, and women's affairs. 5% to 10%. Supports community needs and concerns. *Education:* 10% to 15%. Primary support goes to business education, colleges and universities, elementary education, and minority education. *International:* 10% to 15%. Supports hospices and hospitals, medical rehabilitation, mental health, the aged, child welfare, community centers, the disabled, food and clothing distribution, and traditional youth groups. **Typ. Recipients:** Health Organizations, Health-General, Hospices, Hospitals, Medical Rehabilitation, Mental Health, People with Disabilities, Single-Disease Health Associations, Substance Abuse. **Geo. Dist:** headquarters and operating communities.

### ★ 1280 ★ Norton Co. Foundation
One New Bond St.
PO Box 15008
Worcester, MA 01615
**Phone:** (508)795-2605          **Fax:** (508)795-2761
Judith Cutts, Contributions Coordinator

**Fnded:** 1953. **Priorities:** *Arts & Humanities:* 3%. Recipients include historical preservation societies, arts centers, museums, public broadcasting stations, libraries, theaters, and community arts groups. *Civic & Public Affairs:* 5%. Interests include safety, nonprofit management, providing housing to the homeless, and urban affairs. Also supports zoos and botanical gardens, job training, and community foundations. *Education:* 23%. The majority of funds go to colleges and universities, and teaching programs for learning basic skills at primary and secondary levels. Other interests include arts, business, economic, public, religious, and secondary education. *International:* 34%. Supports various health and human service interests, including hospices, emergency/ambulance services, single-disease health organizations, United Way and youth organizations. *Note:* Total foundation contributions made in 2000. **Typ. Recipients:** AIDS/HIV, Cancer, Children's Health/Hospitals, Clinics/Medical Centers, Domestic Violence, Emergency/Ambulance Services, Family Planning, Geriatric Health, Health Organizations, Health Policy/Cost Containment, Hospices, Hospitals, Medical Education, Medical Rehabilitation, Medical Research, Mental Health, Nursing Services, Nutrition, People with Disabilities, Prenatal Health Issues, Public Health, Sexual Abuse, Single-Disease Health Associations, Substance Abuse. **Geo. Dist:** headquarters and operating communities.

### ★ 1281 ★ NSTAR Foundation
800 Boylston St. (P-1701)
Boston, MA 02199-2599
**Phone:** (617)424-2235          **Fax:** (617)424-2736
**Email:** Ann_Cardello@bedison.com
**Website:** http://www.bedison.com/community/index.htm
Ann Cardello, Foundation Administrator

**Priorities:** *Arts & Humanities:* 5% to 10%. Supports area museums, art centers, and cultural organizations that enhance the quality of life in the Boston area, that generally attract a broad segment of the public, and that are of interest to the company's employees. *Civic & Public Affairs:* 10% to 15%. Main concern is economic development and business and free enterprise, but also supports environmental efforts, civil rights, and minority organizations. Also, supports science museums and local churches. *Education:* 30% to 35%. Major support awarded to private colleges and universities and higher education associations located within company's service area that supply an appreciable number of employees, or have a significant relationship to the company or the electric utility industry. Other areas of interest include student aid; business, arts, legal, religious, and continuing education; education funds; and faculty development. Educational programs that address significant community needs (particularly those related to the unemployed, handicapped,minorities, and women) are also supported. *International:* 40% to 45%. Supports hospitals, health centers, nursing services, United Way, Youth organizations, and hospices. **Typ. Recipients:** AIDS/HIV, Alzheimers Disease, Cancer, Clinics/Medical Centers, Emergency/Ambulance Services, Health Or-

ganizations, Hospices, Hospitals, Long-Term Care, Nursing Services, People with Disabilities, Single-Disease Health Associations. **Geo. Dist:** MA, Eastern Massachusetts; Boston, MA.

### ★ 1282 ★ NYSEG Foundation
PO Box 5224
Binghamton, NY 13902-5224
**Phone:** (607)762-7333
**Website:** http://www.nyseg.com/nysegweb/main.nsf/Doc/community
Paul Karakantas, Treasurer/Secretary

**Priorities:** *Arts & Humanities:* 6%. Supports arts councils, living history centers, community arts organizations, opera, and libraries. *Civic & Public Affairs:* 5%. Gives to community foundations, The American Ireland Fund, and community initiatives. *Education:* 8%. Funding goes to schools for higher learning. *Environment:* 65%. Primarily supports the American Red Cross and United Ways. Also funds YMCAs and youth organizations. *International:* 8%. Funds medical centers and hospitals, hospice programs, and health foundations. *Religion:* 6%. Supports the Paleontological Research Institute and science centers. *Note:* Total contributions made in fiscal 2000. **Typ. Recipients:** Emergency/Ambulance Services, Health-General. **Geo. Dist:** headquarters and operating communities.

### ★ 1283 ★ Occidental Petroleum Charitable Foundation
10889 Wilshire Boulevard
Los Angeles, CA 90024
**Phone:** (310)443-6506          **Fax:** (310)443-6977
Christel Pauli, Assistant Corporate Secretary

**Priorities:** *Arts & Humanities:* 29%. Emphasis on the performing arts. Other interests include museums, theaters, music, public broadcasting, arts funds, literary groups, and libraries. *Civic & Public Affairs:* 1%. Gives to minority affairs organizations and professional organizations, an urban league, and a legal foundation. *Education:* 40%. Contributions distributed primarily through matching gifts program to colleges and universities. Also supports secondary education and literacy programs. *Environment:* 8%. Supports youth services, children's rights, and the United Way. *International:* 20%. Supports an eye institute, single-disease health associations, and hospitals. *Voluntarism:* Supports employee volunteerism with grants to nonprofit groups of $250 to $2,000 where employees volunteer. *Note:* Total contributions made in 2000. **Typ. Recipients:** Cancer, Children's Health/Hospitals, Clinics/Medical Centers, Diabetes, Domestic Violence, Emergency/Ambulance Services, Eyes/Blindness, Heart, Hospices, Hospitals, Medical Rehabilitation, Mental Health, Multiple Sclerosis, People with Disabilities, Sexual Abuse, Single-Disease Health Associations, Speech & Hearing, Substance Abuse. **Geo. Dist:** headquarters and operating communities.

### ★ 1284 ★ Ohio National Foundation
PO Box 237
Cincinnati, OH 45201
**Phone:** (513)794-6594
Anthony Esposito, Vice President, Human Resources & Corpor

**Fnded:** 1987. **Typ. Recipients:** AIDS/HIV, Alzheimers Disease, Cancer, Children's Health/Hospitals, Clinics/Medical Centers, Diabetes, Eyes/Blindness, Health Policy/Cost Containment, Health-General, Heart, Home-Care Services, Hospices, Hospitals, Medical Rehabilitation, Medical Research, Multiple Sclerosis, People with Disabilities, Public Health, Substance Abuse. **Geo. Dist:** Cincinnati, OH.

### ★ 1285 ★ Oklahoma Gas & Electric Co. Foundation
Box 321
Oklahoma City, OK 73101
**Phone:** (405)553-3196          **Fax:** (405)553-3567
Erma Elliot, Secretary & Treasurer

**Fnded:** 1957. **Priorities:** *Arts & Humanities:* 23%. Supports historic preservation, museums, and arts

funds. *Civic & Public Affairs:* 8%. Economic and community development are typical areas of funding, with support also going to environmental, urban, and community affairs. *Education:* 48%. Supports colleges and universities, public and private secondary schools. Large grants consistently are given to Oklahoma City University, the University of Oklahoma, and Oklahoma State University. *Environment:* 15%. Primary concern is youth organizations. Other interests include community services, family planning, recreation and athletics, and organizations concerned with the elderly and children. *International:* 6%. Funds hospitals, medical research, and pediatric health. *Note:* Total contributions made in 1999. **Typ. Recipients:** Children's Health/Hospitals, Clinics/Medical Centers, Emergency/Ambulance Services, Family Planning, Health Organizations, Heart, Hospitals, Medical Education, Medical Research, People with Disabilities, Public Health. **Geo. Dist:** headquarters and operating communities; OK.

### ★ 1286 ★ The Oklahoman Foundation
PO Box 25125
Oklahoma City, OK 73125
**Phone:** (405)475-3298          **Fax:** (405)475-3128
**Email:** lbrown@oklahoman.com
Linda Brown, Executive Assistant

**Fnded:** 1990. **Priorities:** *Arts & Humanities:* 36%. Major support for the National Cowboy Hall of Fame. Also supports various arts organizations, including an arts fund. *Civic & Public Affairs:* 1%. Supports the US Olympic Committee. *Education:* 31%. Funds Oklahoma universities. *Environment:* 21%. Supports the United Way and American Red Cross. *International:* 7%. Primarily supports medical research. *Religion:* 4%. Supports the Omniplex Science Museum. *Note:* Total contributions made in 2000. **Typ. Recipients:** Child Abuse, Children's Health/Hospitals, Clinics/Medical Centers, Emergency/Ambulance Services, People with Disabilities, Public Health. **Geo. Dist:** Oklahoma City, OK.

### ★ 1287 ★ Old National Bank Charitable Trust
PO Box 207
Evansville, IN 47702
**Phone:** (812)464-1441          **Fax:** (812)464-1505
**Email:** prudence_pekinpaugh@oldnational.com
Prudence Pekinpaugh, Public Relations Representative

**Fnded:** 1957. **Priorities:** *Arts & Humanities:* 6%. Supports Evansville area arts organizations, including museums, theaters, music, and arts councils. *Civic & Public Affairs:* 8%. Supports community affairs organizations, development, zoos, and housing. *Education:* 39%. Major support goes to colleges and universities. Other interests include private and public education at the elementary and secondary school levels. *Environment:* 31%. Primarily supports the United Way and youth organizations. *International:* 15%. Supports medical rehabilitation, health centers, and various health organizations. *Voluntarism:* The company encourages employee volunteerism through an informal volunteer program. *Note:* Total contributions made in 1999. **Typ. Recipients:** Adolescent Health Issues, Cancer, Children's Health/Hospitals, Clinics/Medical Centers, Emergency/Ambulance Services, Family Planning, Health Organizations, Health-General, Home-Care Services, Hospitals, Medical Education, Medical Rehabilitation, People with Disabilities, Respiratory, Single-Disease Health Associations, Substance Abuse. **Geo. Dist:** IL, Gibson County; IL, Perry County; IL, Posey County; IL, Spencer County; IL, Vandeburg County; IL, Wabash County; IL, Warrick County; IL, White County; KY, Henderson County.

### ★ 1288 ★ ONDEO Nalco Foundation
ONDEO Nalco Center
Naperville, IL 60563-1198
**Phone:** (630)305-1566          **Fax:** (630)305-2896
**Email:** foundation@nalco.com
**Website:** http://www.ondeo-nalco.com
Ellen DeLordo, President

**Priorities:** *Arts & Humanities:* 10%. Funds go to art institutes, community theater, performing arts, the symphony, and public broadcasting. *Civic & Public Affairs:* 30%. Supports boys and girls clubs, housing assistance, career training, and youth issues. *Education:* 35%. Supports junior achievement, pre-college and college education, arts education, training for disabled, and scholarship awards. *International:* 25%. Support goes to AIDs programs, single-disease research, equipment needs, substance abuse programs, care for the disabled, hospitals, and medical centers. **Typ. Recipients:** AIDS/HIV, Alzheimers Disease, Cancer, Children's Health/Hospitals, Clinics/Medical Centers, Domestic Violence, Emergency/Ambulance Services, Geriatric Health, Health Organizations, Health Policy/Cost Containment, Heart, Home-Care Services, Hospices, Hospitals, Hospitals (University Affiliated), Medical Education, Medical Rehabilitation, Medical Research, Mental Health, People with Disabilities, Prenatal Health Issues, Preventive Medicine/ Wellness Organizations, Public Health, Single-Disease Health Associations, Substance Abuse, Trauma Treatment. **Geo. Dist:** Carson, CA; IL, DuPage County; Chicago, IL, metropolitan area; Garyville, LA; Freeport, TX; Sugarland, TX.

## ★ 1289 ★ ONEOK, Inc.

PO Box 871
Tulsa, OK 74102-0871
**Phone:** (918)588-7000     **Fax:** (918)588-7490
**Website:** http://www.oneok.com
Ginny Creveling, Administrator, Corporate Responsibility
**Typ. Recipients:** Health-General.

## ★ 1290 ★ Orange & Rockland Utilities, Inc.

1 Blue Hill Plaza
Pearl River, NY 10965
**Phone:** (845)577-2545     **Fax:** (845)577-6913
**Email:** fegerl@oru.com
**Website:** http://www.oru.com
Linda Vessa-Feger, Manager, Corporate Programs
**Typ. Recipients:** Cancer, Health-General, Heart, Hospitals, Medical Research, People with Disabilities, Respiratory. **Geo. Dist:** headquarters and operating communities.

## ★ 1291 ★ Orchard Foundation

PO Box 2587
South Portland, ME 04116
**Phone:** (207)799-0686     **Fax:** (207)799-0686
**Email:** orchard@maine.rr.com
**Website:** http://www.orchardfoundation.org
Brigitte Kingsbury, Executive Director
**Priorities:** *Civic & Public Affairs:* 5%. Interests include Native Americans and community affairs organizations. *Education:* 57%. Major support for the Buckingham Browne and Nichols Schools. Also supports Boston area higher education institutions and private secondary schools. Focus is on enrichment programs for children of all ages, and literacy projects. *Environment:* 8%. Interests include children, youth, and family welfare. Focus is on basic parenting skills and support. *International:* 3%. Supports a children's hospital and various health organizations. *Note:* Total contributions in 1999. **Typ. Recipients:** AIDS/HIV, Alzheimers Disease, Arthritis, Child Abuse, Children's Health/Hospitals, Clinics/Medical Centers, Domestic Violence, Family Planning, Health Funds, Hospices, Hospitals, Medical Education, Medical Research, Multiple Sclerosis, Nursing Services, Outpatient Health Care, People with Disabilities. **Geo. Dist:** New England area; NY.

## ★ 1292 ★ Orscheln Industries Foundation, Inc.

PO Box 698
Moberly, MO 65270
**Phone:** (816)263-4377     **Fax:** (816)269-3520
Gerald Orscheln, Director
**Fnded:** 1968. **Priorities:** *Arts & Humanities:* 1%. *Education:* 26%. Supports local schools and colleges,

as well as religious colleges. Also sponsors scholarship awards program for Randolph County High School seniors, and provides scholarships to children of employees. *Environment:* 10%. Grants are made to the United Way, child welfare organizations, youth groups, community centers, and a variety of other programs. *International:* 2%. Funds support hospitals, single-disease health organizations, and similar health groups. *Note:* Total contributions in fiscal 1999. **Typ. Recipients:** Alzheimers Disease, Arthritis, Health Funds, Health Organizations, Hospitals, Medical Education, Prenatal Health Issues, Public Health, Single-Disease Health Associations. **Geo. Dist:** MO, especially Randolph County.

## ★ 1293 ★ OSG Foundation

1114 Ave. of the Americas
511 5th Ave.
New York, NY 10017
**Phone:** (212)578-1822     **Fax:** (212)578-1832
Luis Alicea, Secretary
**Priorities:** *Arts & Humanities:* 2%. Supports museums, symphonies, and arts centers. *Civic & Public Affairs:* 1%. Funds are divided between philanthropic organizations, housing, and child welfare. *Education:* 2%. Majority of grants benefit colleges and universities. Substantial interest in arts education and medical education. *Environment:* 1%. *International:* 71%. Highest grants were given to Mount Sinai Medical Center, and NuBeth Israel Medical Center. Remaining funds benefit medical research and single-disease health organizations. *Note:* Total contributions made in 1998. **Typ. Recipients:** AIDS/HIV, Cancer, Children's Health/Hospitals, Clinics/Medical Centers, Diabetes, Geriatric Health, Health Policy/Cost Containment, Heart, Hospitals, Medical Education, Medical Research, Mental Health, People with Disabilities, Respiratory, Single-Disease Health Associations, Substance Abuse, Transplant Networks/Donor Banks. **Geo. Dist:** New York, NY, metropolitan area.

## ★ 1294 ★ Oshkosh B'Gosh Foundation Inc.

112 Otter Ave.
Oshkosh, WI 54901
**Phone:** (920)231-8800     **Fax:** (920)231-8621
**Website:** http://www.oshkoshbgosh.com
Michael Wachtel, Executive Vice President
**Priorities:** *Arts & Humanities:* 5%. The Paine Art Center and Arboretum in Oshkosh, WI, receives major support. Music and dance are also funded. *Civic & Public Affairs:* 32%. Supports community affairs and organizations. *Education:* 24%. Supports colleges and universities and educational foundations and programs. A significant amount is devoted to scholarships, awarded to high school graduates from cities with company operating locations. *Environment:* 18%. Major support goes to the United Way. Additional funds support community service organizations and youth activities. *International:* 21%. Supports hospitals, health societies, and single-disease health associations. *Note:* Total contributions in 1999. **Typ. Recipients:** Cancer, Child Abuse, Children's Health/Hospitals, Clinics/Medical Centers, Diabetes, Domestic Violence, Emergency/Ambulance Services, Eyes/Blindness, Health Organizations, Heart, Medical Education, Medical Rehabilitation, Mental Health, People with Disabilities, Respiratory, Sexual Abuse, Single-Disease Health Associations, Speech & Hearing. **Geo. Dist:** operating locations.

## ★ 1295 ★ Owens Corning Foundation, Inc.

One Owens Corning Parkway
Toledo, OH 43659
**Phone:** (419)248-6719
**Email:** em.ross@owenscorning.com
Mr. Emerson Ross, President, Treasurer
**Priorities:** *Arts & Humanities:* (Arts & Culture) 10%. Supports museums and galleries, music, and the performing arts. Also gives to arts associations and community arts groups. *Civic & Public Affairs:* (Civic and Community) 14%. Primary interests are business and

free enterprise organizations and civil rights groups. Also supports organizations concerned with safety, public policy, and environmental, urban, and women's affairs. *Education:* 27%. Emphases include colleges and universities; business, economic, and engineering education; public and private precollege education programs; at-risk children's achievement programs; junior achievement; and minority education. Other interests include faculty development, literacy, community and junior colleges, and science and technology education. *Environment:* (Health & Human Services) 49%. Priority is affordable housing. Supports human service organizations in communities with major employee populations. Also supports united funds, community centers, organizations concerned with domestic violence and substance abuse, youth organizations, family services, the aged, deliquency and crime, health organizations, hospitals, and health-care cost containment. *International:* 6%. Supports *Voluntarism:* VOL The company sponsors the Owens Corning Volunteer of the Year award to recognize employee and retiree volunteer efforts. The Owens Corning Foundation provides grants in honor of the Volunteer of the Year finalists to charities of their choice. *Note:* Total contributions made in 2000. **Typ. Recipients:** Cancer, Medical Research, Mental Health, Preventive Medicine/Wellness Organizations, Respiratory, Substance Abuse. **Geo. Dist:** headquarters and operating communities.

## ★ 1296 ★ Owens-Illinois Inc.

1 Seagate
Toledo, OH 43666
**Phone:** (419)247-1386     **Fax:** (419)247-1436
**Email:** cheryl.johnson@owens-ill.com
Cheryl Johnson, Contributions Administrator
**Priorities:** *Note:* Support for minority education is given only in areas of company operation. **Typ. Recipients:** Health-General. **Geo. Dist:** headquarters and operating communities.

## ★ 1297 ★ PACCAR Foundation

PO Box 1518
Bellevue, WA 98009-1518
**Phone:** (425)468-7400
**Website:** http://www.paccar.com/corp/foundation.asp
Norm Proctor, Vice President & General Manager
**Fnded:** 1951. **Priorities:** *Arts & Humanities:* 10%. Supports arts councils, orchestras, and art museums. *Civic & Public Affairs:* 5%. Supports community foundations, business and free enterprises, and public policy groups. *Education:* 20%. Primarily supports colleges and universities, including major support to independent college foundations. Also awards matching giftsand supports economic education. *Environment:* 57%. Major support for the United Way and Boy Scout troops; also funds youth organizations, child welfare, adult daycare services, and family services. *International:* 3%. Funds cancer organizations and cancer research, medical centers, and single-disease health associations addressing diseases that affect children. *Religion:* 3%. Supports science centers. *Note:* Total contributions made in 2000. **Typ. Recipients:** AIDS/HIV, Cancer, Children's Health/Hospitals, Clinics/Medical Centers, Emergency/Ambulance Services, Health Organizations, Hospitals, Medical Research, Mental Health, People with Disabilities, Research/Studies Institutes, Substance Abuse. **Geo. Dist:** headquarters and operating communities.

## ★ 1298 ★ Pacific Life Foundation

700 Newport Center Dr.
Newport Beach, CA 92660-6397
**Phone:** (949)219-3787
**Website:** http://www.pacificlife.com/about/community/index.asp
Robert Haskell, President
**Priorities:** *Arts & Humanities:* (Arts and Culture) 18%. Supports museums, symphonies, ballets, gardens and musical endeavors. *Civic & Public Affairs:* (Civic, Community, and Environment) 14%. Includes support for cultural diversity programs, urban affairs, community development organizations, and ecological and environmental concerns. *Education:* 20%. Supports

universities, graduate schools and drop-out programs. Also includes matching gifts to institutions of higher learning. *International:* (Health and Human Services) 48%. Supports the United Way, shelters, hospitals and single disease organizations such as the American Cancer Society and the American Heart Association. Funding also goes to children's advocacy groups and AIDS education/home care. *Note:* Total contributions made in 2000. **Typ. Recipients:** AIDS/HIV, Alzheimers Disease, Cancer, Child Abuse, Children's Health/Hospitals, Domestic Violence, Emergency/Ambulance Services, Eyes/Blindness, Family Planning, Geriatric Health, Health Organizations, Health Policy/Cost Containment, Heart, Hospices, Hospitals, Medical Education, Medical Research, Medical Training, Mental Health, Multiple Sclerosis, Nutrition, People with Disabilities, Public Health, Single-Disease Health Associations, Speech & Hearing, Substance Abuse, Trauma Treatment. **Geo. Dist:** primarily to organizations in areas with large concentrations of company employees; some funding nationally; Phoenix, AZ; CA, Orange County, and some statewide organizations.

★ **1299** ★ **PacifiCare Health System Foundation**
3120 Lake Center Dr.
Mail Stop LC01-320
PO Box 25186
Santa Ana, CA 92799
**Phone:** (714)825-5233        **Fax:** (714)825-5028
Riva Gebel, Director

**Fnded:** 1996. **Priorities:** *Arts & Humanities:* 1%. Funds a theater. *Civic & Public Affairs:* 2%. Supports affordable housing and municipalities. *Education:* 15%. Supports universities, public school districts, and educational foundations. *Environment:* 15%. Supports the United Way, youth and family services, prevention of rape and child abuse, community counseling organizations, senior services. *International:* 65%. Provides major support to the American Diabetes Association. Also supports children's health, hospitals and clinics, blood banks, dental health, and health initiatives for seniors. *Note:* Total foundation contributions made in 1999. **Typ. Recipients:** Adolescent Health Issues, AIDS/HIV, Alzheimers Disease, Arthritis, Cancer, Child Abuse, Children's Health/Hospitals, Clinics/Medical Centers, Diabetes, Domestic Violence, Geriatric Health, Health Funds, Health Organizations, Health-General, Heart, Hospices, Hospitals, Long-Term Care, People with Disabilities, Preventive Medicine/Wellness Organizations, Public Health, Sexual Abuse, Single-Disease Health Associations. **Geo. Dist:** CA, within company service area; FL, within company service area; OK, within company service area; OR, within company service area; TX, within company service areas; WA, within company service areas.

★ **1300** ★ **PacifiCorp Foundation**
825 NE Multnomah, Ste. 2000
Portland, OR 97232
**Phone:** (503)813-7257        **Fax:** (503)813-7249
**Email:** ernie.bloch@pacificorp.com
**Website:**        http://www.pacificorp.com/paccomp/commsvc
Ernest Bloch, II, Executive Director

**Fnded:** 1988. **Priorities:** *Arts & Humanities:* 21%. Supports the performing arts, the visual arts, historic preservation, and public broadcasting. *Civic & Public Affairs:* 13%. Funds community chests, parks, recreation facilities, crime prevention, chemical dependency treatment and prevention programs, and senior citizens centers. *Education:* 5%. Provides funds to educational and research institutions, both public and private, from elementary through university level. *Environment:* 57%. Funds youth organizations, United Way, runaway youth services, and domestic violence treatment and prevention. *International:* 4%. Supports medical centers and hospitals. *Note:* Total contributions made in fiscal 2000. **Typ. Recipients:** Children's Health/Hospitals, Emergency/Ambulance Services, Family Planning, Health Organizations, Hospitals, People with Disabilities, Public Health. **Geo. Dist:** CA, Northern California; ID; NV; OR; UT; WA; WY.

★ **1301** ★ **Paine Webber Foundation**
1285 Ave. of the Americas
New York, NY 10019
**Phone:** (212)352-4324
Elaine Conte, Foundation Contact

**Fnded:** 1879. **Priorities:** *Arts & Humanities:* 44%. Major support for the New York Public Library; also supports art museums. *Education:* 7%. Funds mentoring and educational programs. *Environment:* 31%. Emphasis on the homeless and youth organizations. *International:* 18%. Major support for the New York Foundling Hospital. *Voluntarism:* The company sponsors a national volunteer initiative through which employees can access volunteer opportunities at local and national nonprofit organizations via the PaineWebber's intranet system. *Note:* Total contributions in 1999. **Typ. Recipients:** AIDS/HIV, Arthritis, Cancer, Children's Health/Hospitals, Diabetes, Emergency/Ambulance Services, Health Organizations, Hospices, Hospitals, Medical Research, People with Disabilities, Public Health, Single-Disease Health Associations, Substance Abuse, Transplant Networks/Donor Banks. **Geo. Dist:** New York, NY.

★ **1302** ★ **Park National Corp. Foundation**
PO Box 3500
Newark, OH 43058-3500
**Phone:** (614)349-8451
Stuart Parsons, Trust Officer

**Priorities:** *Arts & Humanities:* 5%. Supports historical preservation and the performing arts. *Civic & Public Affairs:* 3%. Supports festivals and community development organizations. *Education:* 20%. Supports local school associations. *Environment:* 59%. Supports Scouting, family services, and assistance for the needy. *International:* 8%. Supports health organizations. *Note:* Total contributions made in 1999. **Typ. Recipients:** Cancer, Domestic Violence, Emergency/Ambulance Services, Hospitals, Mental Health, Prenatal Health Issues, Public Health, Single-Disease Health Associations, Substance Abuse. **Geo. Dist:** OH.

★ **1303** ★ **Parker Hannifin Foundation**
6035 Parkland Boulevard
Cleveland, OH 44124-1290
**Phone:** (216)896-3000        **Fax:** (216)896-4057
Chris Semik, Administrative Assistant

**Priorities:** *Arts & Humanities:* About 15%. Major support goes to theater groups. Other recipients include arts centers, museums, and music and dance groups. *Civic & Public Affairs:* 35% to 40%. Emphasis is on economic development organizations. Other recipients include environmental affairs organizations and police and fire departments in plant communities. *Education:* About 40%. Funds matching gifts to educational institutions. Major support is provided to colleges, universities, and funds for higher education. Focus on economic education. *Environment:* 1% to 5%. Majority of funds go to United Way drives in plant communities. Also provides substantial support to youth organizations, particularly to local Boy Scouts/Girl Scouts, YMCA/YWCA, and Junior Achievement chapters. Other recipients include organizations concerned with child welfare, the handicapped, and recreation and athletics, as well as local chapters of the Salvation Army and the Red Cross. *International:* About 10%. Focus is on hospitals. Other interests include single-disease health organizations, clinics, and medical centers. Remaining funds support ambulance services, pediatric health, mental health, and medical research programs. **Typ. Recipients:** Children's Health/Hospitals, Emergency/Ambulance Services, Health Funds, Health Organizations, Hospitals, Medical Research, Mental Health, Nursing Services, Outpatient Health Care, Single-Disease Health Associations, Substance Abuse. **Geo. Dist:** nationally.

★ **1304** ★ **Pella Rolscreen Foundation**
102 Main St.
Pella, IA 50219
**Phone:** (515)628-1000        **Fax:** (515)628-6487

**Email:** mavzante@pella.com
Mary Van Zante, Director

**Priorities:** *Arts & Humanities:* 9%. Primarily supports historical organizations, museums, and libraries. *Civic & Public Affairs:* 10%. Interests include economic development, municipalities, and environmental affairs. *Education:* About 41%. Majority of education funds support colleges and universities in Iowa in the form of scholarship and capital grants. Also sponsors a scholarship program for children of company employees. *Environment:* 21%. Most contributions are made to recreational and athletic programs and centers, and to nondenominational religious welfare organizations. Also supports child welfare, community service organizations, and united funds. *International:* 15%. Funding supports hospitals, emergency services, and single-disease health associations. *Note:* Contributions analysis reflects Pella's typical grant distribution. **Typ. Recipients:** AIDS/HIV, Cancer, Child Abuse, Clinics/Medical Centers, Emergency/Ambulance Services, Health Policy/Cost Containment, Hospitals, Outpatient Health Care, People with Disabilities, Substance Abuse, Transplant Networks/Donor Banks. **Geo. Dist:** IA, central and western Iowa.

★ **1305** ★ **PEMCO Foundation**
325 Eastlake Ave. E
Seattle, WA 98109
**Phone:** (206)628-7916
Stan McNaughton, Foundation Administrator

**Priorities:** *Arts & Humanities:* 4%. Supports art museums, musical performance, public broadcasting, history museums, and art councils. *Civic & Public Affairs:* 2%. Funds crime prevention and community affairs. *Education:* 30%. Supports public and private secondary education, colleges and universities, education foundations, and a school for the hearing impaired. *Environment:* 42%. Supports the United Way, youth organizations, people with disabilities, senior services, child welfare, and family services. *International:* 11%. Gives to pediatric health, medical centers, medical rehabilitation, and single-disease organizations. *Religion:* 2%. Funds a science center. *Note:* Total contributions made in fiscal 2000. **Typ. Recipients:** Cancer, Children's Health/Hospitals, Clinics/Medical Centers, Domestic Violence, Emergency/Ambulance Services, Emergency/Ambulance Services, Geriatric Health, Health Funds, Health Organizations, Health-General, Heart, Home-Care Services, Hospices, Hospitals, Kidney, Medical Rehabilitation, Multiple Sclerosis, People with Disabilities, Research/Studies Institutes, Respiratory, Single-Disease Health Associations, Trauma Treatment. **Geo. Dist:** WA.

★ **1306** ★ **Penn Mutual Life Insurance Co.**
C3A
600 Dresher Rd.
Horsham, PA 19044
**Phone:** (215)956-8060        **Fax:** (215)956-8347
**Website:** http://www.pennmutual.com
Donna Beath, Contributions Coordinator

**Priorities:** *Voluntarism:* Employee volunteers support United Way related events. **Typ. Recipients:** Health-General. **Geo. Dist:** DE; NJ; NY; PA.

★ **1307** ★ **Pennzoil-Quaker State Co.**
PO Box 2967
Houston, TX 77252-2967
**Phone:** (713)546-8590
Barbara Tambakakis, Coordinator, Contributions & Community R

**Priorities:** *Arts & Humanities:* About 15%. Supports performing and visual arts, museums, zoos, libraries, and other cultural activities that are broadly supported and that benefit a large segment of the population in local communities. *Civic & Public Affairs:* 5% to 10%. Supports selected organizations that work to improve the quality of life in company communities. *Education:* About 50%. Emphasis is on accredited colleges and universities in communities where company has significant operations, where it recruits employees, or where research relevant to company's business is conducted. Related disciplines including accounting, geology, and engineering are priorities. Also administers matching gifts program. *Environment:* About 15%. Local united funds are principal vehicles of support. Well-established, widely supported service organizations (including those for the handicapped) that are not members of united funds are also eligible forconsideration. *International:* About 10%. Supports local hospitals, clinics, rehabilitation centers, and other health-related organizations. Contributions are restricted to building programs, equipment additions, or unusual research programs. Contributions to single-disease health associations also may be considered. **Typ. Recipients:** Emergency/Ambulance Services, Health Organizations, Hospices, Hospitals, Medical Rehabilitation, Medical Research, People with Disabilities, Single-Disease Health Associations, Substance Abuse. **Geo. Dist:** communities in which company has plants, warehouses, or refineries; rarely gives nationally, internationally.

**★ 1308 ★ Pentair Foundation**
1500 County Rd. B2 West
Saint Paul, MN 55113-3105
**Phone:** (651)636-7920    **Fax:** (651)639-5203
**Website:** http://www.pentair.com/ci/ci_pf.htm
Jeanne Kavanaugh, Foundation Manager

**Priorities:** *Arts & Humanities:* 11%. Funds programs that provide a solid cultural base and offer opportunities to experience art in many different forms. Encourages development and preservation of artistic and cultural traditions; broadening and expanding the audience base for the arts so they are accessible for all; and development and expansion of programs that offer educational and developmental opportunities in literature, music, and theater. *Civic & Public Affairs:* 29%. Supports mentoring and tutoring opportunities for youth, together with general guidance and recreation; programs which encourage economic self-reliance among individuals; job training for youth, the disadvantaged, and the disabled; and low-income housing. *Education:* 19%. Supports elementary, secondary, and higher education programs that provide innovative education opportunities for youth; target socially and economically disadvantaged youth; bring business concepts, practices, and principles into the classroom; and provide a trade curriculum to add skilled workers to the work force. *Environment:* 33%. Funds United Ways, disaster relief organizations, youth organizations, services for the disabled, Girl and Boy Scouts, and senior centers. *International:* 5%. Supports programs which ensure access to adequate health care and health care education, including rehabilitation services for the disabled, particularly youth; effective, low-cost health care services for those who are unable to afford adequate health care; and educational information and promotion of sound physical and mental health and development. *Religion:* 1%. Supports a science museum. *Note:* Total contributions made in 2000. **Typ. Recipients:** Emergency/Ambulance Services, Health-General, Medical Rehabilitation. **Geo. Dist:** headquarters and operating communities; Minneapolis, MN, metropolitan area; St. Paul, MN, metropolitan area.

**★ 1309 ★ Peoples Energy Corp.**
130 E Randolph Dr.
Chicago, IL 60601
**Phone:** (312)240-7516    **Fax:** (312)240-4389
Richard Turner, Manager, Corporate Contributions

**Priorities:** *Arts & Humanities:* About 5%. Supports museums, historical societies, libraries, visual and performing arts. *Civic & Public Affairs:* 45%. Support of civic and neighborhood causes includes study and research projects. Support of programs in the areas of social services, housing, employment, education, and economic development is designed to help economically distressed neighborhoods and communities. *Education:* 45%. Invests in higher education – public and private colleges and universities – by making annual contributions to selected institutions. In addition, support goes to outreach efforts, such as educational television and community outreach programs within the public school system. *International:* 5%. Generally, contributions go to programs through the

Metropolitan Crusade of Mercy and various United Way funds. Other donations are earmarked for health and welfare agencies, hospitals, research projects, and medical programs. *Note:* Contributions analysis provided by foundation. **Typ. Recipients:** Health Organizations, Hospitals. **Geo. Dist:** company service area.

**★ 1310 ★ PepsiCo Foundation, Inc.**
700 Anderson Hill Rd.
Purchase, NY 10577
**Phone:** (914)253-3153    **Fax:** (914)253-3553
Jacqueline Millan, Vice President, Contributions

Fnded: 1962. **Priorities:** *Arts & Humanities:* 5%. Supports opera, dance, theater, museums, and historical societies. *Civic & Public Affairs:* 11%. Funds the National Urban League, community and neighborhood affairs. *Education:* 57%. Support is given to major colleges and universities; education programs for minorities, including scholarships and leadership development; and scholarships for children of employees. *Environment:* 24%. Provides major support to the United Way. Also supports youth organizations, senior services and other social service organizations. *Voluntarism:* Contributions are matched dollar for dollar to institutions and organizations that are determined tax-exempt by the I.R.S. When an employee volunteers in addition to a financial contribution, the foundation will double the match. Employee Community Involvement Grants are made to non-profit organizations where employees volunteer. *Note:* Total contributions made in 1999, excluding matching gifts. **Typ. Recipients:** Cancer, Children's Health/Hospitals, Emergency/Ambulance Services, Family Planning, Health Organizations, Hospitals, Medical Research, Multiple Sclerosis, People with Disabilities, Substance Abuse. **Geo. Dist:** headquarters and operating communities.

**★ 1311 ★ Pfizer Foundation**
235 East 42nd St.
New York, NY 10017-5755
**Phone:** 800-733-4717
**Website:** http://www.pfizer.com/pfizerinc/philanthropy
Rick Luftglass, Grants Coordinator

**Priorities:** *Arts & Humanities:* 8%. Priority is given to arts and cultural organizations identified as making a positive contribution to the cultural life of a Pfizer operating community. Primary focus is on New York City. Cultural organizations eligible for funding include, but are not limited to, art education programs, museums, performing arts organizations, and cultural and performing arts centers. Programs that strive to develop working relationships between business and the arts community also are funded. *Civic & Public Affairs:* 12%. Focus is on New York City. Grants support programs such as community organizations and development, botanical gardens, aquariums, and non-profit management assistance providers. Through this fund, the company invests in nonprofit organizations dedicated to breaking the cycle of poverty through innovative, entrepreneurial programs that create wealth in local communities. Funds organizations that address urgent community needs, seek long-term solutions to community issues, and strengthen to cultural vitality of diverse communities. *Education:* 33%. Preference given to schools at which Pfizer recruits; to schools located in Pfizer facility communities; and to educational programs that relate to the company's business operations in math and science-based disciplines. Focus is on science and math K-12 education, especially improving understanding of scientific principles and the importance of scientific innovation. Supports organizations that develop and apply systematic, sustainable strategies to improve teaching and learning, such as implementation of hands-on, inquiry-based science curricula, teacher training, and the upgrading of labs. Supports exhibits and educational outreach programs at various science-rich institutions as well as collaborations between Pfizer sites and local schools. *International:* 44%. Supports patient education programs; programs that help people live healthier, more productive lives; therapeutic programs including those targeting hypertension, diabetes and depression; community health centers; social service providers; technical assistance

providers; health communications technology to provide access to up-to-date health information; projects for changing the health care system; maternal and child health; and women's health issues. Focus is on community-based efforts to improve the health of those at greatest risk for poor health outcomes. *Note:* Total contributions made in 2000. **Typ. Recipients:** Adolescent Health Issues, AIDS/HIV, Alzheimers Disease, Child Abuse, Children's Health/Hospitals, Clinics/Medical Centers, Emergency/Ambulance Services, Eyes/Blindness, Geriatric Health, Health Funds, Health Organizations, Health Policy/Cost Containment, Health-General, Home-Care Services, Hospices, Hospitals, Medical Education, Medical Rehabilitation, Medical Research, Mental Health, People with Disabilities, Preventive Medicine/Wellness Organizations, Public Health, Single-Disease Health Associations, Substance Abuse, Transplant Networks/Donor Banks. **Geo. Dist:** principally near operating locations and to national organizations; New York, NY.

**★ 1312 ★ Pharmacia Foundation**
7000 Portage Rd.
Kalamazoo, MI 49001
**Phone:** (616)833-4929
Phillip Carra, Secretary

**Priorities:** *Arts & Humanities:* 23%. Supports symphonies, arts funds, performing arts, art institutes, and art festivals. *Civic & Public Affairs:* 25%. Funds urban and community affairs, chambers of commerce, and nonprofit management. *Education:* 18%. Primarily to colleges and universities, minority scholarship funds, and arts and pharmaceutical education. *Environment:* 2%. Focus on the United Way and youth organizations. *International:* 31%. Supports health foundations, biomedical research, pediatric health, and American Red Cross chapters. *Religion:* less than 1%. Funds the American Association for Laboratory Animal Science. *Note:* Total contributions in 1999. **Typ. Recipients:** AIDS/HIV, Cancer, Children's Health/Hospitals, Emergency/Ambulance Services, Family Planning, Health Organizations, Hospices, Hospitals, Medical Education, Medical Research, Mental Health, Nursing Services, Nutrition, People with Disabilities, Prenatal Health Issues, Public Health, Research/Studies Institutes, Single-Disease Health Associations, Substance Abuse, Transplant Networks/Donor Banks. **Geo. Dist:** headquarters and operating communities; internationally; product donations go only to Third World countries; Kalamazoo, MI. **Frmly:** Pharmacia & Upjohn Foundation.

**★ 1313 ★ Phelps Dodge Foundation**
2600 N Central Ave.
Phoenix, AZ 85004
**Phone:** (602)234-8100    **Fax:** (602)234-8082
**Email:** phx-communityaffairs@phelpsdodge.com
**Website:** http://www.phelpsdodge.com/index-community.html
Ann Gibson, Community Affairs

**Priorities:** *Arts & Humanities:* 15%. Funding supports symphonies, opera, museums, performing arts, and historic preservation. Limited support to art funds and centers. *Civic & Public Affairs:* 5%. Supports community safety and community development initiatives. *Education:* 49%. Majority of funding supports scholarships to colleges and universities. Funding also emphasizes scientific, technological, mining, and business education. Interests include minority and independent college funds, community colleges, and medical education. *Environment:* 10%. Supports the United Way. *International:* 14%. Supports children's health centers, electrical safety, hospitals, crisis nurseries, prevention of domestic violence, and public health and safety. *Note:* Total contributions made in 2000. **Typ. Recipients:** Cancer, Children's Health/Hospitals, Clinics/Medical Centers, Domestic Violence, Emergency/Ambulance Services, Family Planning, Geriatric Health, Health Funds, Health Organizations, Hospitals, Kidney, Medical Education, Medical Research, Medical Training. **Geo. Dist:** communities where company maintains major operating facilities.

**Pheonix Foundation**
*See:* Entry 17784

**★ 1314 ★ Philips Electronics North America Corp.**
1251 Ave. of the Americas
New York, NY 10020
**Phone:** (212)536-0500
**Fnded:** 1979. **Priorities:** *Education:* 100%. The company's charitable activities go directly to support a scholarship program. *Note:* Total contributions made in 1998. **Typ. Recipients:** Hospitals, Medical Education. **Geo. Dist:** operating areas.

**★ 1315 ★ Physicians Mutual Insurance Co. Foundation**
2600 Dodge St.
Omaha, NE 68131
**Phone:** (402)633-1000        **Fax:** (402)633-1096
Jerome Coon, Secretary/Treasurer
**Priorities:** *Arts & Humanities:* 7%. Supports public broadcasting, theater, museums and historic preservation. *Civic & Public Affairs:* 19%. Supports community foundations and civic policy. *Education:* 33%. Supports colleges, universities and higher education. *Environment:* 36%. Supports food banks, family services, scouting organizations, and United Way. *International:* 4%. Funds single-disease health associations. *Note:* Total contributions made in 2000. **Typ. Recipients:** Alzheimers Disease, Arthritis, Cancer, Children's Health/Hospitals, Diabetes, Emergency/Ambulance Services, Health Organizations, Health Policy/Cost Containment, Health-General, Heart, Hospices, Hospitals, Long-Term Care, Medical Research, Multiple Sclerosis, Nursing Services, People with Disabilities, Public Health, Respiratory, Single-Disease Health Associations, Substance Abuse. **Geo. Dist:** NE.

**★ 1316 ★ Piedmont Charitable Foundation**
7 Piedmont Center, Ste. 100
Atlanta, GA 30305
**Phone:** (404)816-5205        **Fax:** (404)816-3537
J. Robinson, President
**Fnded:** 1957. **Priorities:** *Arts & Humanities:* 8%. Historic preservation and art centers are funded. *Civic & Public Affairs:* 4%. Funds chambers of commerce and business forums. *Education:* 67%. Supports higher education, literacy, and educational enrichment. *Environment:* 11%. Supports services for youth. *Note:* Total contributions in 1999. **Typ. Recipients:** Cancer, Clinics/Medical Centers, Geriatric Health, Hospitals, Single-Disease Health Associations. **Geo. Dist:** GA.

**★ 1317 ★ Pillsbury Co. Foundation**
200 South, 6th St.
Minneapolis, MN 55402-1464
**Phone:** (612)330-5046
Rebecca Erdahl, Executive Director
**Fnded:** 1957. **Priorities:** *Civic & Public Affairs:* 7%. Organizations and programs that offer educational and employment skills young people need to achieve self-sufficiency. Typically funds school and community organization education programs, academic support, career awareness/work readiness, life skills, and employment programs. *Education:* 9%. Funds public and private precollege and higher education. Also provides scholarships to children of employees. *Environment:* 81%. Supports the United Way, youth groups, and organizations that build and sustain ongoing relationships with caring adults and at-risk young people. Typically funds mentoring programs. *International:* Less than 1%. *Voluntarism:* Company offers employee volunteer opportunities, and gives priority to organizations where employees volunteer. *Note:* Total contributions in fiscal 2000. **Typ. Recipients:** Children's Health/Hospitals, Clinics/Medical Centers, Family Planning, Hospitals, Medical Rehabilitation, Nutrition, Prenatal Health Issues. **Geo. Dist:** headquarters and operating communities.

**★ 1318 ★ Pioneer Investments Management USA Inc.**
60 State St., 5th Fl.
Boston, MA 02109
**Phone:** (617)742-7825        **Fax:** (617)422-4293
**Website:** http://www.pioneerfunds.com
Susan Bullock, Sr. Corporate Paralegal
**Typ. Recipients:** Clinics/Medical Centers, Health-General. **Geo. Dist:** headquarters and operating communities.

**★ 1319 ★ Pittway Corp. Charitable Foundation**
200 S Wacker Dr., Ste. 700
Chicago, IL 60606-5802
**Phone:** (312)831-1070        **Fax:** (312)831-0808
Paul Gauvreau, Treasurer
**Priorities:** *Arts & Humanities:* 10%. Emphasis on public broadcasting, museums, history, and arts institutes. *Civic & Public Affairs:* 4%. Funds economic development, business and free enterprise, promotion of democracy, and urban and community programs. *Education:* 34%. Supports colleges and universities, early education, literacy programs, and education funds. *Environment:* 35%. Focuses on programs working to break the intergenerational transmission of poverty. Family planning and family services receive much of this funding, as well as united funds. Child welfare, food and clothing distribution, and youth organizations are also supported. *International:* 10%. Funds support hospitals, various single-disease health organizations, pediatric health, and other facilities. *Religion:* 1%. Funds laboratories and institutes specializing in biological, cancer, neurobiology and plant genetics research. *Note:* Total foundation contributions made in fiscal 2000. **Typ. Recipients:** Alzheimers Disease, Cancer, Children's Health/Hospitals, Clinics/Medical Centers, Family Planning, Health Funds, Hospices, Hospitals, Medical Education, Medical Rehabilitation, Medical Research, Mental Health, Nursing Services, People with Disabilities, Prenatal Health Issues, Single-Disease Health Associations, Substance Abuse. **Geo. Dist:** emphasis on communities near company's manufacturing sites.

**★ 1320 ★ Playboy Foundation**
680 N Lake Shore Dr.
Chicago, IL 60611
**Phone:** (312)751-8000        **Fax:** (312)266-8506
**Email:** giving@playboy.com
**Website:** http://www.playboy.com/corporate/foundation/index.html
Cleo Wilson, Executive Director
**Typ. Recipients:** Domestic Violence, Family Planning, Medical Research, People with Disabilities, Single-Disease Health Associations. **Geo. Dist:** nationally.

**★ 1321 ★ PNC Foundation**
Two PNC Plaza, 34th Floor
620 Liberty Ave.
Pittsburgh, PA 15222-2729
**Phone:** (412)762-7076        **Fax:** (412)705-1062
**Email:** marianna.hallett@pnc.com
**Website:** http://www.pnc.com/aboutus/pncfoundation.html
Mia Hallett, Vice President and Manager
**Fnded:** 1970. **Priorities:** *Arts & Humanities:* 20% to 25%. Supports local symphony organizations and music groups, public broadcasting, libraries, performing arts, museums, opera, and arts associations, festivals, and centers. *Civic & Public Affairs:* 15% to 20%. Primary support to economic development and urban affairs. Other interests include international affairs, public policy, economics, civil rights, women's interests, and business and free enterprise. *Education:* 5% to 10%. Major support goes to local colleges and universities. Also gives to public and private precollege education, minority education, and education funds. *Environment:* 40% to 45%. Most of this supports united funds in southwestern Pennsylvania. Also matches employee gifts to colleges and universities. Also contributes to organizations concerned with youth, the

elderly, the disabled, food distribution, community and family services, religious welfare, and emergency relief. *International:* Less than 5%. Primarily supports local hospitals. Other interests include single-disease health associations, health funds and organizations, medical rehabilitation, and pediatric health. **Typ. Recipients:** Cancer, Children's Health/Hospitals, Domestic Violence, Health Organizations, Home-Care Services, Hospices, Hospitals, Long-Term Care, Medical Rehabilitation, People with Disabilities, Single-Disease Health Associations. **Geo. Dist:** areas served by PNC Bank Corp. and affiliates. **Frmly:** PNC Bank Foundation.

**★ 1322 ★ Polaroid Foundation**
784 Memorial Dr.
Cambridge, MA 02139
**Phone:** (781)386-9400        **Fax:** (781)386-9818
**Email:** Polaroid.Foundation@polaroid.com
**Website:** http://www.polaroid.com/polinfo/foundation
Donna Eidson, Executive Director
**Priorities:** *Arts & Humanities:* 28%. Funding to historical and arts museums and public television. *Civic & Public Affairs:* 4%. Community support Massachusetts. *Education:* 45%. Primarily technical colleges, universities, and program support for educational incentives. *Environment:* 12%. YMCA, women's shelters, United Way and programs for children. *Religion:* 11%. *Voluntarism:* Polaroid employees who volunteer 50+ hours of personal time per calendar year at a nonprofit organization can apply to the Polaroid Foundation for a $1,000 grant for that organization. Information on Polaroid's Volunteer Action Program is available from (800)480-4438. Polaroid employees also have the opportunity to volunteer on grantmaking committees; on company time, employee volunteers review grant proposals, visit agencies, and make funding recommendations under the direction of foundation staff members. **Typ. Recipients:** AIDS/HIV, Clinics/Medical Centers, Diabetes, Domestic Violence, Eyes/Blindness, Heart, Hospices, Hospitals, Medical Education, Medical Research, Mental Health, Nursing Services, People with Disabilities, Public Health, Speech & Hearing. **Geo. Dist:** internationally for product donations; nationally for product donations; nationally: considers funding outside of Massachusetts to historically black educational institutions; Boston, MA, metropolitan area; Cambridge, MA; New Bedford, MA, including surrounding area; Waltham, MA.

**★ 1323 ★ Post and Courier Foundation**
134 Columbus St.
Charleston, SC 29403-4800
**Phone:** (843)937-5789
J. Donehue, Administrator
**Priorities:** *Arts & Humanities:* 14%. Museums, historic foundations, music, ballet, and art associations receive support. *Civic & Public Affairs:* 6%. Primary support goes to ethnic affairs, trade associations, and community affairs. *Education:* 10%. Recipients include South Carolina colleges, secondary schools, and educational organizations. *Environment:* 19%. Majority of funding supports Carolina Youth Development Center and the United Way. *International:* 16%. Supports health care centers, single-disease associations, and hospice. *Note:* Total contributions made in 1999. **Typ. Recipients:** Cancer, Health-General, Hospices, Medical Rehabilitation, People with Disabilities, Preventive Medicine/Wellness Organizations, Speech & Hearing. **Geo. Dist:** headquarters area only.

**★ 1324 ★ PPG Industries Foundation**
One PPG Pl.
Pittsburgh, PA 15272
**Phone:** (412)434-2453
Sue Sloan, Senior Program Officer
**Priorities:** *Arts & Humanities:* (Culture) 11%. Pittsburgh arts organizations, including symphonies, libraries, and museums. Also supports local performing arts organizations and public broadcasting. *Civic & Public Affairs:* (Civic & Community Affairs) 4%. Research, education, and the dissemination of information related to the areas of economic education and develop-

ment, and public policy issues. Large grants are awarded to support economic development and public policy groups. Other recipients include business and free enterprise, and civil rights groups. *Education:* 53%. Most grants support higher education, with emphasis on private colleges and universities, especially those in plant communities and those with engineering and science programs. Of special interest are science-based efforts that attract students to chemistry, business, and engineering; education for minorities; and support of students achieving high academic standards. Other areas receiving major gifts include college funds, minority engineering and other education associations, and precollege education. Awards include capital and operating support. *Environment:* (Human Services) 29%. Primarily United Way campaigns, which receive about two-thirds of human service funds. Other grants are allocated for capital projects and special programs to provide support for new facilities and changing services. *International:* (Health & Safety) 3%. Improved patient care, effective delivery of services, and educational programs. *Voluntarism:* VOL Sponsors the GIVE Program to recognize employee involvement in volunteerism. Employees may apply for one grant of $250 annually to benefit an eligible non-profit organization for whom they volunteer. **Typ. Recipients:** Clinics/Medical Centers, Emergency/Ambulance Services, Eyes/Blindness, Health Organizations, Health Policy/Cost Containment, Hospitals, Long-Term Care, Medical Rehabilitation, Mental Health, Nursing Services, People with Disabilities, Public Health, Single-Disease Health Associations. **Geo. Dist:** headquarters and operating communities; nationally; Pittsburgh, PA.

### ★ 1325 ★ Praxair Foundation
39 Old Ridgebury Rd.
Danbury, CT 06810-5113
**Phone:** (203)837-2000 **Fax:** (203)837-2550
Nigel Muir, President & Director
**Fnded:** 1995. **Priorities:** *Arts & Humanities:* 3%. Funds public libraries. *Civic & Public Affairs:* 28%. Supports minority/women's organizations and professional associations (particularly associations of engineers and scientists), gardens, municipalities, economic development, and public policy. *Education:* 15%. Primarily supports universities and colleges, especially those that focus on science, technology, and engineering education. *Environment:* 4%. Supports scouts, youth sports and recreation programs, YMCAs, and youth welfare organizations. *International:* 41%. Funds hospice programs, single-disease health organizations, and medical centers, with cancer, AIDS, and multiple sclerosis organizations receiving significant funding. *Religion:* 2%. Supports science institutes and museums. *Note:* Total contributions made in fiscal 2000. **Typ. Recipients:** AIDS/HIV, Cancer, Children's Health/Hospitals, Clinics/Medical Centers, Emergency/Ambulance Services, Hospices, Hospitals, Medical Education, Medical Rehabilitation, Multiple Sclerosis, Single-Disease Health Associations, Transplant Networks/Donor Banks.

### ★ 1326 ★ Premcor
8182 Maryland Ave.
Saint Louis, MO 63105
**Phone:** (314)854-9804 **Fax:** (314)854-1580
Suzanne Miller, Charitable Contributions Coordinator
**Typ. Recipients:** AIDS/HIV, Alzheimers Disease, Arthritis, Cancer, Children's Health/Hospitals, Clinics/Medical Centers, Diabetes, Eyes/Blindness, Health-General, Multiple Sclerosis. **Geo. Dist:** headquarters and operating communities.

### ★ 1327 ★ Premier Industrial Foundation
2829 Euclid Ave.
Cleveland, OH 44115
**Phone:** (216)875-6500 **Fax:** (216)875-6580
Morton Mandel, Trustee
**Fnded:** 1953. **Priorities:** *Arts & Humanities:* 9%. Museums performing arts groups including theatre and music. *Civic & Public Affairs:* 84%. Supports nonprofit management and promotion of philanthropic

activity. *Education:* 16%. Provides scholarships to individuals. *Environment:* 40%. Organizations that build homes and supply clothing to the needy, volunteer organizations, children's recreation groups such as Boy Scouts, and United Way organizations. *International:* 2%. *Note:* Total contributions made in 1999. **Typ. Recipients:** AIDS/HIV, Clinics/Medical Centers, Domestic Violence, Emergency/Ambulance Services, Eyes/Blindness, Health Organizations, Hospices, Hospitals, Medical Education, Nursing Services, Public Health, Substance Abuse. **Geo. Dist:** OH, Northeast Ohio with emphasis on Cleveland.

### ★ 1328 ★ Presto Foundation
3925 North Hastings Way
Eau Claire, WI 54703
**Phone:** (715)839-2119 **Fax:** (715)839-2122
Norma Jaenke, Executive Director
**Priorities:** *Arts & Humanities:* 29%. Primarily supports public television stations. Also supports libraries, historical museums, theater, dance, and symphonies. *Civic & Public Affairs:* 16%. Funds community development, job training, and advocacy issues. *Education:* 38%. Supports colleges and universities, scholarships to employee's children, career/vocational education, and public pre-college education. *Environment:* 7%. Primarily supports the United Way. Also funds organizations concerned with personal growth, such as Special Olympics, youth recreation and athletic activities, and Big Brothers/Big Sisters. *International:* 8%. Supports hospitals, pediatric health, and single-disease health associations. *Note:* Total contributions made in fiscal 2001. **Typ. Recipients:** Cancer, Children's Health/Hospitals, Emergency/Ambulance Services, Health Funds, Heart, Hospitals, Medical Research, Multiple Sclerosis, People with Disabilities, Single-Disease Health Associations. **Geo. Dist:** headquarters and operating communities; WI, Northwestern Wisconsin, especially Eau Claire and Chippewa Counties.

### ★ 1329 ★ Principal Financial Group Foundation, Inc.
711 High St.
Des Moines, IA 50392-0001
**Phone:** (515)247-5091 **Fax:** (515)246-5475
**Website:** http://www.principal.com/about/giving/index.htm
Michele Walstrom, Contributions Consultant
**Fnded:** 1987. **Priorities:** *Arts & Humanities:* 25%. Support of the greater Des Moines area and selected visual and performing arts organizations, museums, cultural centers, public television, arts-related organizations, and other cultural groups. *Civic & Public Affairs:* 18%. Supports civic and public policy. *Education:* 18%. Support of local universities and colleges, the Iowa College Foundation, various actuarial scholarships and programs at select universities, economic education programs, and education-related organizations. Supports education matching gifts program for employees and qualified agents/brokers of The Principal Financial Group. *Environment:* 36%. Support of human services organizations, youth organizations, family services, the United Way, and special projects. *International:* Less than 1%. Primarily supports single-disease health associations. *Religion:* Less than 1%. Supports a science museum. *Note:* Total contributions made in 2000. **Typ. Recipients:** AIDS/HIV, Alzheimers Disease, Cancer, Children's Health/Hospitals, Emergency/Ambulance Services, Family Planning, Health Organizations, Health Policy/Cost Containment, Health-General, Hospices, Medical Research, Mental Health, People with Disabilities, Respiratory, Single-Disease Health Associations, Substance Abuse. **Geo. Dist:** occasional nationally and internationally; operating locations; Des Moines, IA.

### ★ 1330 ★ Procter & Gamble Cosmetics Foundation
11050 York Rd.
Hunt Valley, MD 21030
**Phone:** (410)785-7300 **Fax:** (410)316-8025
Marian Lubbert, Administrator

**Fnded:** 1951. **Priorities:** *Arts & Humanities:* (Culture & the Arts; Museums) 19%. Supports art museums, music, theater, and community arts organizations. *Civic & Public Affairs:* 2%. Supports community youth organizations and civic organizations. *Education:* 18%. Funds colleges and universities, Catholic colleges and precollege schools, arts education, and scholarship funds. *International:* 22%. Supports hospitals and single-disease health associations, with a focus on pediatric health. *Note:* Total contributions made in 2000. **Typ. Recipients:** AIDS/HIV, Cancer, Children's Health/Hospitals, Clinics/Medical Centers, Diabetes, Domestic Violence, Emergency/Ambulance Services, Health Organizations, Hospitals, Medical Education, Medical Rehabilitation, Mental Health, Nursing Services, People with Disabilities, Public Health, Respiratory, Single-Disease Health Associations, Substance Abuse. **Geo. Dist:** some support to nationally organizations with local chapters; NY: New York City; Baltimore, MD, metropolitan area.

### ★ 1331 ★ Procter & Gamble Fund
PO Box 599
Cincinnati, OH 45201-0599
**Phone:** (513)945-8454
**Website:** http://www.pg.com/about_pg/corporate/community/community_submain.jhtml
Brenda Ratliss, Contributions & Community Relations
**Priorities:** *Arts & Humanities:* 6%. Promotes cultural enrichment, educational programs, and entertainment. Supports theater, dance, music, and the visual arts. *Civic & Public Affairs:* About 11%. Goals are to promote economic stimulation and enrichment for all parts of the community. Supports youth programs, chambers of commerce, the Urban League, libraries, zoos, and museums. *Education:* 60%. Major support to scholarship programs and grants to public and private colleges and universities. Also supports employee matching gifts; public policy, research, and economic education organizations; scholarships for employees' children, and K-12 initiatives. *International:* About 1%. Supports United Way, the Salvation Army, Red Cross, hospitals, food banks, and social service agencies. *Note:* Contributions made in 1999. **Typ. Recipients:** Cancer, Emergency/Ambulance Services, Health Organizations, Hospitals, Nutrition, People with Disabilities, Substance Abuse. **Geo. Dist:** headquarters and operating communities, nationally and internationally.

### ★ 1332 ★ Providence Journal Charitable Foundation
75 Fountain St.
Providence, RI 02902-9985
**Phone:** (401)277-7597 **Fax:** (401)277-7529
**Email:** mary_ellen_ahern@projo.com
Mary Ahern, Community Services and Gift Committee Di
**Priorities:** *Arts & Humanities:* 10% to 15%. Grants support performing arts groups, libraries, public broadcasting, philharmonic orchestras, and historic preservation. *Civic & Public Affairs:* 5% to 10%. Environment is a major area of concern; trade associations, housing, public parks, and economic developmentgroups also receive funding. *Education:* About 15%. Local colleges and universities, preparatory schools, and Junior Achievement receive support. *Environment:* 40% to 45%. Majority of funding supports the United Way. Other interests include religious welfare, youth organizations, food banks and shelters, and women's and family services. *International:* 15% to 20%. Supports hospitals, single-disease health organizations, and adolescent health associations. **Typ. Recipients:** Adolescent Health Issues, AIDS/HIV, Cancer, Emergency/Ambulance Services, Family Planning, Health Organizations, Hospices, Hospitals, Long-Term Care, Medical Rehabilitation, Mental Health, Nursing Services, People with Disabilities, Research/Studies Institutes, Sexual Abuse, Single-Disease Health Associations, Substance Abuse. **Geo. Dist:** MA; RI.

### ★ 1333 ★ Provident Mutual Life Insurance Co.

1000 Chesterbrook Boulevard
Berwyn, PA 19312
**Phone:** (610)407-1501    **Fax:** (610)407-1718
**Email:** khopson@providentmutual.com
**Website:** http://www.providentmutual.com
Kathy Hopson, Administrative Assistant to Chief Executive

**Typ. Recipients:** Health-General. **Geo. Dist:** Philadelphia, PA, metropolitan area.

### ★ 1334 ★ Prudential Foundation

Prudential Plaza
751 Broad St., 15th Floor
Newark, NJ 07102-3777
**Phone:** (973)802-4791    **Fax:** (973)802-3345
**Email:** community.resources@prudential.com
**Website:** http://www.prudential.com/community
Lata Reddy, Secretary

**Priorities:** *Civic & Public Affairs:* (Ready to Work) 15% to 20%. Promotes job entry skills that are acquired through initiatives that focus on school-to-work transition, workforce development and adherence-to-work; job creation strategies that include access to capital, nonprofit/for-profit ventures, adult and youth entrepreneurship, financial training, business attraction/development/retention; decent, affordable housing that is created through programs that focus on either housing strategies or neighborhood-based activities. Housing strategies include investment/grant partnerships with Prudential's Social Investment Program, community development financial institutions, or technical assistance to Community Housing Development Organizations. Neighborhood-based activities include community organizing, neighborhood strategic planning, leadership development, and community security. *Education:* (Ready to Learn) 15% to 20%. Supports education efforts that strengthen early childhood education initiatives; support professional development for preK-3 teachers; build strong school leadership, with a particular emphasis on parental involvement; provide school-based health and human services that reduce the barriers to learning; or create safe school environments through conflict resolution programs. Within this framework, the foundation emphasizes the creation of model schools, arts education, and literacy. *Environment:* (Ready to Live) 25% to 30%. Supports community health and safety efforts that include community-based culture/arts programs in New Jersey; initiatives that build healthy families; community-based health care and human services for economically disadvantaged populations; high-impact national projects that address major health or human services issues affecting children and families; and youth development programs that foster leadership skills. Also supports the Greater Newark AIDS Initiative. *Voluntarism:* Company supports Prudential CARES (Community, Action Renewal Efforts) which provides individual and team building volunteer programs for Prudential employees and retirees at local nonprofits. Also supports Global Volunteer Day. **Typ. Recipients:** AIDS/HIV, Child Abuse, Children's Health/Hospitals, Clinics/Medical Centers, Emergency/Ambulance Services, Family Planning, Geriatric Health, Health Organizations, Health Policy/Cost Containment, Hospitals, Medical Education, Medical Rehabilitation, Medical Training, Mental Health, People with Disabilities, Public Health, Research/Studies Institutes, Substance Abuse. **Geo. Dist:** headquarters and operating communities; nationally; Los Angeles, CA; Jacksonville, FL; Atlanta, GA; Minneapolis, MN; NJ, particularly Newark; Philadelphia, PA; Houston, TX.

### ★ 1335 ★ Prudential Securities Foundation

One New York Plaza
New York, NY 10292
**Phone:** (212)214-4884    **Fax:** (212)214-5541
Elizabeth Longley, Vice President

**Priorities:** *Arts & Humanities:* 50%. Supports museums, libraries, dance, orchestras, opera, arts associations, and art education. *Civic & Public Affairs:* 14%. Supports community development, housing, employment, and parks. *Education:* 21%. Funds colleges and universities, literacy programs, scholarship funds, schools, and education associations. *Environment:* 10%. Supports youth organizations, athletics, substance abuse education, and food distribution. *International:* 5%. Most contributions go to hospitals and single-disease associations. Foundations involved with mental health, children, cancer, general health, emergency relief, and fitness also receive funding. *Note:* Total foundation contributions made in fiscal 2000. **Typ. Recipients:** Arthritis, Children's Health/Hospitals, Health Organizations, Heart, Hospitals, Medical Research, Mental Health, Outpatient Health Care, People with Disabilities, Single-Disease Health Associations, Substance Abuse, Transplant Networks/Donor Banks. **Geo. Dist:** CT; NJ; NY.

### ★ 1336 ★ Pulitzer Foundation

900 North Tucker Boulevard
Saint Louis, MO 63101
**Phone:** (314)340-8440    **Fax:** (314)340-3133
Ronald Ridgway, Secretary & Treasurer

**Priorities:** *Arts & Humanities:* 20%. Primarily supports St. Louis area cultural institutions. Funds the St. Louis Symphony, historic preservation, music, opera, theater, arts funds and associations, and dance. *Civic & Public Affairs:* 16%. Supports press associations, First Amendment issues, business/free enterprise organizations, and botanical gardens. *Education:* 32%. Supports colleges and universities, principally in St. Louis and elsewhere in Missouri. Remaining funds support journalism studies, education funds, minority education, technical education, and student aid. Scholarships are limited to St. Louis area minority students who are either high school graduates or in junior college. Scholarships are for attending the University of Missouri Journalism School. *Environment:* 30%. Majority of funding supports the United Way of Greater St. Louis. Also supports traditional youth organizations, community services, employment, emergency relief, and the aged. *International:* 1%. Funds hospitals, hospices, and single-disease associations. *Note:* Total foundation contributions made in 2000. **Typ. Recipients:** AIDS/HIV, Cancer, Children's Health/Hospitals, Emergency/Ambulance Services, Family Planning, Home-Care Services, Hospices, Hospitals, Long-Term Care, Medical Education, Mental Health, Multiple Sclerosis, Respiratory, Single-Disease Health Associations. **Geo. Dist:** St. Louis, MO, metropolitan area.

### ★ 1337 ★ Putnam Investors Fund

c/o Public Relations
1 Post Office Square, Mail Stop A-4-E
Boston, MA 02109
**Phone:** (617)292-1000    **Fax:** (617)760-8048
Margaret Leipsitz, Manager, Community Relations Assistant V

**Priorities:** *Arts & Humanities:* 10%. Boston area arts and cultural organizations receive funding. Interests include the fine arts, museums, public broadcasting, music, and dance. *Civic & Public Affairs:* 5%. Supports housing, city improvement projects, charitable gift funds, a taxpayer's foundation, and organizations that provide job skills training. *Education:* 24%. Primarily supports colleges and universities, particularly highly recognized business schools; technology education; scholarship funds; and literacy initiatives. *Environment:* 55%. Supports youth organizations, the United Way, family services, homeless shelters, and organizations assisting the disabled and at-risk. *International:* 1%. Funds hospitals, pediatric health, and cancer research and treatment. *Note:* Total foundation contributions made in 2000. **Typ. Recipients:** AIDS/HIV, Arthritis, Cancer, Child Abuse, Children's Health/Hospitals, Clinics/Medical Centers, Diabetes, Heart, Hospices, Hospitals, Medical Research, Multiple Sclerosis, People with Disabilities, Prenatal Health Issues, Single-Disease Health Associations. **Geo. Dist:** Boston, MA; Quincy, MA.

### ★ 1338 ★ Quaker Chemical Foundation

Elm and Lee St.s
Conshohocken, PA 19428
**Phone:** (610)832-4127    **Fax:** (610)832-4282
Kathleen Lasota, Secretary

**Priorities:** *Arts & Humanities:* 30%. Supports arts outreach, opera, arts funds, library funds, and art centers. *Civic & Public Affairs:* 18%. Emphasis is on women's affairs, job training, and community affairs. *Education:* 29%. Majority of education contributions are in the form of scholarships to employees and individuals in the community. Focus is on chemistry and the physical sciences. Other funding supports colleges and universities. *International:* (Health and Welfare) 23%. Funding supports hospital foundations, nursing services, and health organizations. Also funds family services, counseling, food distribution, and victims of sexual abuse. *Note:* Total foundation contributions made in fiscal 2000. **Typ. Recipients:** Eyes/Blindness, Health Organizations, Heart, Hospices, Hospitals, Medical Research, Nursing Services, Nutrition, People with Disabilities, Sexual Abuse, Single-Disease Health Associations. **Geo. Dist:** headquarters and operating communities.

### ★ 1339 ★ Quanex Foundation

1900 West Loop S, Ste. 1500
Houston, TX 77027
**Phone:** (713)961-4600
Sandy Hatcher, Director Corporate Communications

**Fnded:** 1951. **Priorities:** *Arts & Humanities:* 11%. Supports museums, orchestras, and art centers. *Civic & Public Affairs:* 2%. Supports festivals. *Education:* 26%. Supports scholarships funds, colleges and universities, schools, and Junior Achievement. *Environment:* 50%. Funds United Way, shelters, and scouting. *International:* 9%. Supports American Red Cross, hospice, and single-disease groups. *Note:* Total foundation contributions made in 2000. **Typ. Recipients:** AIDS/HIV, Cancer, Children's Health/Hospitals, Clinics/Medical Centers, Diabetes, Emergency/Ambulance Services, Eyes/Blindness, Health Organizations, Heart, Hospices, Hospitals, Kidney, Medical Research, Nutrition, People with Disabilities, Public Health, Research/Studies Institutes, Single-Disease Health Associations. **Geo. Dist:** TX.

### ★ 1340 ★ Questar Corp.

180 East 1st South St.
PO Box 45433
Salt Lake City, UT 84145-0433
**Phone:** (801)324-5435    **Fax:** (801)324-5483
**Email:** janb@questar.com
**Website:** http://www.questar.com
Janice Bates, Director, Community Affairs

**Priorities:** *Arts & Humanities:* 20% to 25%. Funding goes to dance and music, historic preservation, museums and galleries, and performing arts. *Civic & Public Affairs:* 10% to 15%. Funds programs for better government and economic development. *Education:* About 30%. Business education, colleges and universities, and economic education are all supported. *International:* 25% to 30%. Support goes to hospitals, single-disease health associations, child welfare, community service organizations, traditional youth groups, the United Way, and food and clothing distribution. **Typ. Recipients:** Health Organizations, Hospitals, People with Disabilities. **Geo. Dist:** CO, limited funding; OK, limited funding; TX, limited funding; UT; WY.

### ★ 1341 ★ Ralph's-Food 4 Less Foundation

PO Box 54143
Los Angeles, CA 90054
**Phone:** (310)884-6205    **Fax:** (310)884-2590
Jan Golleher, Executive Director

**Fnded:** 1992. **Priorities:** *Arts & Humanities:* Less than 1%. Supports music, the performing arts, libraries, and arts funds/foundations. *Civic & Public Affairs:* 10%. Funds urban leagues, public safety, minority affairs, and legal aid. *Education:* 14%. Supports colleges and universities, and educational programs for pre-college education. *Environment:* 49%. Supports day care, food distribution, family services, scouting, community sports, and violence and substance abuse prevention. *International:* 18%. Supports children's health organizations, medical centers, and single-disease health organizations. *Note:* Total foundation contributions made in 2000. **Typ. Recipients:** AIDS/HIV, Cancer, Child Abuse, Children's Health/Hospitals, Clinics/Medical Centers, Diabetes, Domestic Violence, Eyes/Blindness, Family Planning, Health Organizations, Medical Education, Mental Health, Multiple Sclerosis, People with Disabilities, Prenatal Health Issues, Single-Disease Health Associations, Substance Abuse. **Geo. Dist:** CA, southern California.

### ★ 1342 ★ Ralston Purina Trust Fund

Checkerboard Square
Saint Louis, MO 63164
**Phone:** (314)982-3234 **Fax:** (314)982-2752
Fred Perabo, Secretary

**Priorities:** *Arts & Humanities:* 6%. Supports museums, music, and public broadcasting. *Civic & Public Affairs:* 7%. Supports urban affairs, community development, parks, and chambers of commerce. *Education:* 20%. Supports colleges and universities, scholarship programs, and Junior Achievement. *Environment:* 54%. Supports the United Way, humane societies, youth concerns, and service groups. *International:* 1%. Funds the Alzheimer's Association and the March of Dimes. *Note:* Total foundation contributions made in fiscal 2000. **Typ. Recipients:** Alzheimers Disease, Children's Health/Hospitals, Domestic Violence, Family Planning, Health Organizations, Health Policy/Cost Containment, Hospices, Hospitals, Medical Education, Medical Research, Nursing Services, People with Disabilities, Single-Disease Health Associations, Substance Abuse. **Geo. Dist:** headquarters and operating communities; St. Louis, MO.

### ★ 1343 ★ Rayonier Foundation

50 North Laura St., Ste. 1900
Jacksonville, FL 32202
**Phone:** (904)357-9100
Jay Fredericksen, Vice President

**Fnded:** 1952. **Priorities:** *Arts & Humanities:* Less than 1%. *Civic & Public Affairs:* 29%. Supports community service organizations, chambers of commerce, fire departments, and free enterprise. *Education:* 44%. Supports individual scholarship programs including the Black Scholar Awards, the Four Year Scholarship Program, the Timber County Scholarship Program, and the Rayonier College Scholarship. Other areas of interests include colleges and universities, elementary and secondary schools, and Head Start programs. *Environment:* 25%. Supports United Way, YMCA, youth organizations, and volunteer programs. *International:* Less than 1%. Contributes to hospitals and health-care organizations. *Note:* Total foundation contributions made in 1999. **Typ. Recipients:** Child Abuse, Domestic Violence, Hospices, Hospitals, Mental Health, People with Disabilities, Substance Abuse. **Geo. Dist:** headquarters area only.

### ★ 1344 ★ Reader's Digest Foundation

1 Reader's Digest Rd.
Pleasantville, NY 10570
**Phone:** (914)244-5370 **Fax:** (914)244-7642
Jan Braun, Program Manager

**Priorities:** *Arts & Humanities:* 31%. Primarily supports libraries. *Civic & Public Affairs:* 21%. Supports community services. *Education:* 23%. The company supports such initiatives as the Putnam Valley School's early intervention reading program, the Links to Literacy program, the Westchester Education Coalition, and the Horizons Student Summer Enrichment program. The company also maintains a national scholarship program and the Tall Tree Initiative for Libraries. *International:* 24%. Supports children's health organizations and a clinic. *Voluntarism:* Reader's Digest employees, employee spouses, and retirees can receive grants for nonprofit groups where they actively volunteer. The company operates a Double-Match Gift Program where employees and retirees may give up to $10,000 per year to charities of their choice. *Note:*

Contributions made in 1998. Percentages exclude matching gifts, scholarship, and volunteer program investments. **Typ. Recipients:** Children's Health/Hospitals, Clinics/Medical Centers. **Geo. Dist:** nationally.

### ★ 1345 ★ Red Wing Shoe Co. Foundation

314 Main St.
Red Wing, MN 55066-2300
**Phone:** (651)385-1203 **Fax:** (651)385-1760
Shirley Perkins, Secretary

**Priorities:** *Arts & Humanities:* 2%. Supports arts associations, historic preservation, orchestral music, theater, and public broadcasting. *Civic & Public Affairs:* 21%. Supports community development, municipalities, an auditorium, and parks. *Education:* 21%. Major support for Red Wing School District #256; colleges, economic education, and education reform receive minor funding. *Environment:* 53%. Primarily supports the YMCA and United Way. Youth organizations, family services, and Special Olympics also receive support. *International:* 1%. Health organizations, single disease associations, and medical centers. *Religion:* 1%. Science Museum of Minnesota. *Note:* Total foundation contributions made in 2000. **Typ. Recipients:** Cancer, Children's Health/Hospitals, Clinics/Medical Centers, Emergency/Ambulance Services, Health Organizations, Hospices, Medical Rehabilitation, People with Disabilities, Preventive Medicine/Wellness Organizations, Single-Disease Health Associations, Substance Abuse. **Geo. Dist:** Danville, KY; Minneapolis, MN; Red Wing, MN; St. Paul, MN; Potosi, MO.

### ★ 1346 ★ The Reebok Human Rights Foundation

1895 J.W Foster Blvd.
Canton, MA 02021
**Phone:** (781)401-7946 **Fax:** (781)401-4806
**Email:** geri.noonan@reebok.com
Geri Noonan, Manager

**Priorities:** *Civic & Public Affairs:* Company supports human rights organizations. The majority of company's international giving is through its Human Rights Award. Foundation supports a short list of major national organizations devoted to furthering the achievement of social and economic equality of communities of color. Grants are made by invitation only. *Environment:* Contributions go to organizations in Boston serving the needs of underserved youth population, especially programs that educate, improve self-esteem, and protect the rights of African-American, Hispanic and Asian people. New proposals are not currently being accepted for this program. **Typ. Recipients:** Children's Health/Hospitals, Clinics/Medical Centers, Diabetes, Domestic Violence, Medical Education, Public Health. **Geo. Dist:** internationally through Human Rights Awards; principally near operating locations and to national organizations; Boston, MA. **Frmly:** The Reebok Foundation.

### ★ 1347 ★ Reilly Foundation

300 North Meridian St., Ste. 1500
Indianapolis, IN 46204-1763
**Phone:** (317)248-6464 **Fax:** (317)248-6472
Rand Brooks, Trustee

**Fnded:** 1962. **Priorities:** *Arts & Humanities:* 9%. Supports museums, galleries, and the performing arts. *Civic & Public Affairs:* 4%. Supports neighborhood organizations and leadership development. *Education:* 40%. Supports colleges and universities, education funds and associations. Foundation offers scholarships and an employee matching gifts program. *Environment:* 25%. Funding primarily supports the United Way. Other interests include youth activities, child welfare, homelessness, and food distribution. *International:* 5%. Supports health education, community clinics, and Ronald McDonald House. *Note:* Total foundation contributions made in 2000. **Typ. Recipients:** Cancer, Children's Health/Hospitals, Clinics/Medical Centers, Family Planning, Health Organizations, Hospitals, Long-Term Care, Long-Term Care, Medical Rehabilitation, Medical Research, People with

Disabilities, Public Health, Transplant Networks/Donor Banks. **Geo. Dist:** company operating locations.

### ★ 1348 ★ Reily Foundation

640 Magazine St.
New Orleans, LA 70130
**Phone:** (504)524-6131 **Fax:** (504)539-5417
Robert Reily, President

**Priorities:** *Arts & Humanities:* 17%. Emphasis on arts funds, museums, orchestras, historic preservation, and public broadcasting. *Civic & Public Affairs:* 27%. Majority of funding supports community foundations, public policy, botanical gardens, and professional trade associations in New Orleans. *Education:* 18%. Supports universities; public and private, secondary and elementary education; education reform; minority education; and Junior Achievement. *Environment:* 25%. Provides funding for United Way, youth groups, family services, crime prevention, and food distribution. Also supports criminal rehabilitation and at-risk youth. *International:* 2%. Single-disease health organizations, hospitals and clinics receive support. **Typ. Recipients:** AIDS/HIV, Clinics/Medical Centers, Family Planning, Health Organizations, Hospitals, Medical Education, People with Disabilities, Single-Disease Health Associations. **Geo. Dist:** LA.

### Reliant Energy Foundation

*See:* Entry 5587

### ★ 1349 ★ ReliaStar Foundation

20 Washington Ave. South, Ste. 0941
Minneapolis, MN 55401
**Phone:** (612)342-7443 **Fax:** (612)342-3578
**Email:** terry.egge@reliastar.com
**Website:** http://www.reliantenergy.com/company/community/
Teresa Egge, Community Relations & Reliastar Foundati

**Priorities:** *Arts & Humanities:* 10% to 15%. Priority given to organizations providing free or subsidized access to low-income people, the elderly, or school children. Supports performing and visual arts, including theaters, museums, and musical organizations; public radio and television; and programs designed to enhance the cultural life of the community. *Civic & Public Affairs:* 15% to 20%. Funds urban and civic affairs. Grants in this category will generally serve the needs of minorities, families, and people of low income and will be directed to organizations that take a proactive approach to alleviating existing social problems or preventing problems by: promoting economic development; promoting self sufficiency; promoting the general well-being and improved status of minorities, women and children of low income; strengthening families; increasing low-cost housing; developing job opportunities for the unemployed, underemployed, or hard-to-employ; or providing development opportunities for young people. *Education:* 35% to 40%. Supports preschool through higher education in the areas of business, economics, and minority education. Priority is given to programs supporting youth, women, people of color, disabled people, and people of low income. Focuses on preparing young people for the workforce. Also offers a matching gift program for post-secondary education and a scholarship program for dependents of employees. *Environment:* 20% to 25%. Supports the United Way in communities with significant numbers of employees. *Voluntarism:* ReliaStar offers employees a variety of opportunities to volunteer their time and talents to help others in the community. These programs include tutoring, food and clothing distribution, and community cleanup. **Typ. Recipients:** Health Funds. **Geo. Dist:** near headquarters and subsidiaries, and to a limited number of national organizations in health fields.

### ★ 1350 ★ Revlon Foundation Inc.

625 Madison Ave.
New York, NY 10022
**Phone:** (212)527-5000 **Fax:** (212)527-6977
Joan Horton, Corporate Events

**Fnded:** 1955. **Priorities:** *Arts & Humanities:* 2%. Supports a performing arts center. *Civic & Public Affairs:* 3%. Gives to African-American affairs groups and to urban affairs. *Education:* 83%. Supports colleges and universities. Matching grants also are made in the area of education. *International:* 12%. Support goes to medical centers. *Note:* Total contributions made in 1997. **Typ. Recipients:** AIDS/HIV, Cancer, Clinics/Medical Centers, Hospitals, Medical Education, People with Disabilities, Single-Disease Health Associations. **Geo. Dist:** headquarters and operating communities; nationally.

★ **1351** ★ **Rexford Fund**
1 Whitehall St., 17th Floor
New York, NY 10004
**Phone:** (212)483-1500          **Fax:** (212)363-7265
Douglas Schloss, Chairman & Chief Executive Officer

**Fnded:** 1967. **Priorities:** *Arts & Humanities:* 28%. Funds art and history museums, theater and other performing arts, and libraries. *Civic & Public Affairs:* 5%. Supports parks and conservatories, community clubs, and community loan funds. *Education:* 20%. Funds colleges and universities, nursery and primary education, and scholarship funds. *Environment:* 32%. Supports family and youth centers. *Note:* Total contributions made in 1999. **Typ. Recipients:** Adolescent Health Issues, Cancer, Clinics/Medical Centers, Emergency/Ambulance Services, Family Planning, Health Organizations, Hospices, Hospitals, Hospitals, Mental Health, Multiple Sclerosis, People with Disabilities, Public Health, Single-Disease Health Associations, Substance Abuse. **Geo. Dist:** NY.

★ **1352** ★ **Reynolds Metals Co. Foundation**
PO Box 27003
Richmond, VA 23261-7003
**Phone:** (804)281-2222          **Fax:** (804)281-4160
Linda Fowler, Administrator

**Priorities:** *Arts & Humanities:* 9%. Supports museums, symphonies, opera, theater, historical societies, and public broadcasting. *Civic & Public Affairs:* 13%. Supports economic and business development, public affairs, and a botanical garden. *Education:* 22%. Major support goes to colleges and universities with strong business, science, and engineering programs, and to middle and secondary schools and organizations which demonstrate initiative in preparing and recruiting quality students for those career tracks. The foundation sponsors a matching gifts program for graduate or professional schools, four-year colleges, two-year junior or community colleges, and independent and public secondary schools. *Environment:* 34%. Provides major support for the United Way; also funds YMCAs. *International:* 10%. Primary interest is the American Red Cross, hospitals, and services for families of hospital patients. *Religion:* 10%. Gives to a science museum. *Note:* Total contributions in 1999. **Typ. Recipients:** Cancer, Children's Health/Hospitals, Domestic Violence, Emergency/Ambulance Services, Health-General, Hospitals, Medical Rehabilitation, Medical Research, People with Disabilities, Public Health, Single-Disease Health Associations, Substance Abuse, Transplant Networks/Donor Banks. **Geo. Dist:** headquarters and operating communities.

★ **1353** ★ **Reynolds & Reynolds Co. Foundation**
PO Box 2608
Dayton, OH 45401
**Phone:** (937)485-4409          **Fax:** (937)485-3831
**Email:** alice_davisson@reyrey.com
**Website:** http://www.reyrey.com/about/commun.html
Alice Davisson, Administrator

**Priorities:** *Arts & Humanities:* 16%. Foundation supports a variety of arts and cultural organizations that enrich the quality of life for area residents. Funds museums, theater, and music. *Civic & Public Affairs:* 17%. Grants encourage strategic community economic development in company's operating areas, including community foundations and urban affairs. *Educa-*

tion: 17%. Funding emphasizes support for programs geared toward at-risk children in grades K-12. Foundation allocates funds to educational institutions and nonprofit organizations that help keep children in school and prepare them for employment, college, technical training, or the military. *Environment:* 50%. Majority of support reaches the United Way; also funds YMCA and youth organizations. *Voluntarism:* Employee "Spirit Award" offered to employees dedicating 50+ hours per calendar year to a non-profit agency. Agency receives $200 grant in employee's name. *Note:* Total foundation contributions made in fiscal 2000. **Typ. Recipients:** Arthritis, Cancer, Children's Health/Hospitals, Emergency/Ambulance Services, Health Organizations, Hospices, Trauma Treatment. **Geo. Dist:** OH.

★ **1354** ★ **Rich Family Foundation**
PO Box 245
Buffalo, NY 14240-0245
**Phone:** (716)878-8363          **Fax:** (716)878-8775
David Rich, Executive Director

**Fnded:** 1961. **Priorities:** *Arts & Humanities:* 8%. Contributes to music and the performing arts. *Civic & Public Affairs:* 4%. Supports business concerns. *Education:* 67%. Supports the University of Buffalo Foundation in New York, NY, and other regional colleges and universities, scholarship funds, and schools. *Environment:* 9%. The United Way receives the majority of grants. Also supports child welfare organizations. *International:* 3%. Funds hopitals and single-disease associations. *Note:* Total foundation contributions made in 2000. **Typ. Recipients:** Alzheimers Disease, Cancer, Children's Health/Hospitals, Clinics/Medical Centers, Diabetes, Emergency/Ambulance Services, Health Organizations, Health-General, Heart, Hospitals, Medical Rehabilitation, Multiple Sclerosis, Prenatal Health Issues, Public Health, Single-Disease Health Associations, Substance Abuse. **Geo. Dist:** Buffalo, NY.

★ **1355** ★ **Riggs Bank NA**
800 17th St., NW, 2nd Floor
Washington, DC 20006
**Phone:** (202)835-4495          **Fax:** (202)835-5184
**Email:** marybeth-jones@riggsbank.com
**Website:** http://www.riggsbank.com
Marybeth Jones, Corporate Events Manager

**Priorities:** *Arts & Humanities:* Supports organizations that provide artistic enrichment to the community or reach underserved audiences, including museums and visual and performing arts groups. *Civic & Public Affairs:* Supports organizations committed to the safety, welfare, and well-being of the community. Physical revitalization of the community; economic development; groups with monitor legal, consumer, and governmental issues; boys and girls clubs; and community associations are supported. Supports organizations dedicated to affordable housing initiatives, neighborhood development, small-business development and enhancement, and job training and development programs. *Education:* Supports formal education and community-based organizations for educational purposes. *International:* Supports mental and physical medical care and basic human services. Supports hospitals, clinics, food banks, shelters for the homeless, and federated campaigns. **Typ. Recipients:** Clinics/Medical Centers, Kidney, Single-Disease Health Associations. **Geo. Dist:** Washington, DC, metropolitan area.

★ **1356** ★ **Robert I. Wishnick Foundation**
1 American Lane
Greenwich, CT 06831
**Phone:** (203)371-1844
William Wishnick, President & Director

**Priorities:** *Arts & Humanities:* 24%. Interests include theaters, museums, ballet, and opera. *Civic & Public Affairs:* 9%. Funds Native American issues and peace initiatives. *Education:* 16%. Primarily supports colleges and universities, private secondary education, and art, science and math education programs. *Environment:* 2%. Supports people with disabilities, family planning, programs protecting the homeless, and shelters. *Inter-*

national: 6%. Primary interests include hospitals, clinics and medical centers, and medical research. *Note:* Total contributions in 1999. **Typ. Recipients:** AIDS/HIV, Cancer, Children's Health/Hospitals, Clinics/Medical Centers, Emergency/Ambulance Services, Family Planning, Family Planning, Geriatric Health, Home-Care Services, Hospitals, Medical Education, Medical Research, Multiple Sclerosis, People with Disabilities, Single-Disease Health Associations. **Geo. Dist:** operating communities.

★ **1357** ★ **Robert W. Baird & Co. Foundation**
777 East Wisconsin Ave., 28th Floor
Milwaukee, WI 53202
**Phone:** (414)765-3500          **Fax:** (414)765-3600

**Fnded:** 1967. **Priorities:** *Arts & Humanities:* 12%. Funding goes to art institutions and museums, the performing arts, theaters, and libraries. Also funds events under the category of "entertainment" including cultural festivals and parades. *Education:* 19%. Supports business education, colleges and universities, education reform, minority education and private education. *Environment:* 15%. Supports child welfare issues, scouting, the United Way, youth organizations, and delinquency and criminal rehabilitation. *International:* 12%. Funding goes to cancer research, children's health issues, health organizations, hospitals, and medical research. *Note:* Total contributions made in 1999. **Typ. Recipients:** Cancer, Children's Health/Hospitals, Diabetes, Domestic Violence, Emergency/Ambulance Services, Health Organizations, Health-General, Heart, Hospitals, Medical Education, Medical Rehabilitation, Medical Research, People with Disabilities, Public Health. **Geo. Dist:** headquarters and operating communities.

★ **1358** ★ **Rockwell International Corp. Trust**
777 E Wisconsin Ave., Ste. 1400
Milwaukee, WI 53202
**Phone:** (414)212-5258
Christine Rodriguez, Contact

**Priorities:** *Arts & Humanities:* 7%. Supports museums, public broadcasting, arts alliances, and the performing arts, including theater, music, and opera. *Civic & Public Affairs:* 12%. Supports chambers of commerce, law and justice, civil rights, public policy, Native American Affairs, and housing. *Education:* 46%. Supports colleges, universities, education reform, educational associations, minority education, scholarships, and education funds. *Environment:* 33%. Supports United Way, Young Men's Christian Association, youth programs, scouting, and volunteer services. *International:* 1%. *Religion:* Less than 1%. *Note:* Total foundation contributions made in fiscal 2000. **Typ. Recipients:** Cancer, Children's Health/Hospitals, Domestic Violence, Emergency/Ambulance Services, Health Organizations, Health Policy/Cost Containment, Hospices, Hospitals, Medical Rehabilitation, Mental Health, People with Disabilities, Public Health, Single-Disease Health Associations, Substance Abuse. **Geo. Dist:** headquarters and operating communities; nationally to education.

★ **1359** ★ **Rohm & Haas Co.**
Corp. Contributions
100 Independence Mall West
Philadelphia, PA 19106-2399
**Phone:** (215)592-3644          **Fax:** (215)592-6808
**Email:** asamuels@rohmhaas.com
**Website:** http://www.rohmhaas.com
Alexandra Samuels, Manager, Civic & Philanthropic Affairs

**Priorities:** *Arts & Humanities:* 17%. Funding primarily supports Philadelphia arts organizations, including public broadcasting stations, music groups, and museums. *Civic & Public Affairs:* 11%. Typically funds organizations concerned with civil rights, urban affairs, business and free enterprise. *Education:* 39%. Support for higher education includes programs that encourage minority youths to enter the fields of chemistry and engineering. Also supports career and vocational training programs, economic education, and matching gifts to precollege and higher education. *International:* About 32% of total annual contributions. Primaily supports united funds in company operating locations, the handicapped and youth. **Typ. Recipients:** Health-General. **Geo. Dist:** principally near operating locations and to national organizations; where employees live.

## ★ 1360 ★ Rouse Co. Foundation

10275 Little Patuxent Pkwy.
Columbia, MD 21044
**Phone:** (410)992-6000        **Fax:** (410)992-6363
**Email:** mpm@therousecompany.com
**Website:**    http://therousecompany.com/whoweare/community/index.html
Margaret Mauro, Executive Director, Secretary & Treasure

**Fnded:** 1967. **Priorities:** *Arts & Humanities:* 28%. Supports the performing arts, orchestra, and museums. *Civic & Public Affairs:* 25%. Funds community services, housing, and foundations. *Education:* 15%. Gives to education foundations, colleges and universities, scholarship funds, with an emphasis on arts education. *Environment:* 18%. Supports United Way, youth services, and domestic violence centers. *International:* 8%. Supports single-disease health organizations, hospitals and medical centers, hospice programs, and health care for the disadvantaged. *Religion:* 3%. Funds science centers. *Voluntarism:* The company encourages its employees to volunteer time to nonprofit groups and organizations through its Volunteer Contributions Program. Through this program, the company provides grants of up to $1,000 to nonprofit organizations at which the Rouse employees volunteer. Volunteer grants are awarded in the fields of health, education, human services, arts and humanities, community affairs, museums, conservation and preservation. *Note:* Total foundation contributions made in 1999. **Typ. Recipients:** Cancer, Clinics/Medical Centers, Domestic Violence, Hospices, Hospitals, Hospitals (University Affiliated), People with Disabilities, People with Disabilities, Prenatal Health Issues, Preventive Medicine/Wellness Organizations, Sexual Abuse, Single-Disease Health Associations, Substance Abuse. **Geo. Dist:** MD, Central Maryland.

## ★ 1361 ★ Royal & SunAlliance Insurance Foundation, Inc.

9300 Arrowpoint Blvd.
PO Box 1000
Charlotte, NC 28201-1000
**Phone:** (704)522-2056        **Fax:** (704)522-2055
Fred Dabney, Executive Director

**Fnded:** 1989. **Priorities:** *Arts & Humanities:* 21%. Funds arts councils, theaters, museums with educational programs, and performing arts. *Civic & Public Affairs:* 1%. Supports scouting organizations and the Charlotte/Mechlenburg Urban League. *Education:* 25%. Supports universities, colleges, and education funds. Focus on business and insurance courses. Also supports early childhood intervention, drop-out prevention, and Junior Achievement. Provides education matching gifts. *International:* 53%. Funds a variety of health and human services organizations. Interests include the homeless, the developmentally and mentally disabled, the elderly, single-disease health organizations, child welfare, medical centers, and the United Way. *Voluntarism:* Company actively encourages employee volunteerism, including an Education Week. Special consideration is given to requests for funding if an employee is involved in the organization in a meaningful voluntary capacity. *Note:* Total contributions in 1999. **Typ. Recipients:** Adolescent Health Issues, Cancer, Child Abuse, Children's Health/Hospitals, Emergency/Ambulance Services, Geriatric Health, Health Funds, Health Organizations, Health-General, Heart, Home-Care Services, Hospices, Hospitals, Mental Health, People with Disabilities, Public Health, Single-Disease Health Associations, Substance Abuse. **Geo. Dist:** areas where producers, employees, and customers reside.

## ★ 1362 ★ Rubbermaid Foundation

1147 Akron Rd.
Wooster, OH 44691-0800
**Phone:** (330)264-6464        **Fax:** (330)287-2864
Richard Gates, Administrator

**Priorities:** *Arts & Humanities:* 45%. Major support for the Wayne Center for the Arts; other interests include historic preservation, art appreciation, and the literary arts. *Civic & Public Affairs:* 3%. Interests include professional and trade associations, business and free enterprise. A majority of this type of giving is in the form of general operating support. *Education:* 9%. Most educational giving is provided in the form of matching gifts to universities and colleges. *Environment:* 43%. Majority of support goes to local United Ways, Boy Scouts, and other social services agencies located in areas where Rubbermaid operates. *International:* Less than 1%. *Note:* Total foundation contributions made in 1999. **Typ. Recipients:** Cancer, Children's Health/Hospitals, Clinics/Medical Centers, Emergency/Ambulance Services, Health Organizations, Hospices, Hospitals, People with Disabilities, Substance Abuse. **Geo. Dist:** headquarters and operating communities.

## ★ 1363 ★ Russer Foods/Zemsky Family Trust

6420 SE Harbor Circle
Stuart, FL 34996-1958
**Phone:** (407)225-1602
Sam Zemsky, Manager

**Fnded:** 1987. **Priorities:** *Arts & Humanities:* 35%. Supports museums, performing arts, libraries, public broadcasting, orchestra, and festivals. *Civic & Public Affairs:* 4%. Supports community activities. *Education:* 9%. Funds schools and universities. *Environment:* 10%. Supports United Way, YMCA, Planned Parenthood, and youth programs. *International:* 8%. Funds hospice, care for the aging, and single-disease associations. *Religion:* 1%. *Note:* Total foundation contributions made in 2000. **Typ. Recipients:** Alzheimers Disease, Arthritis, Cancer, Children's Health/Hospitals, Diabetes, Domestic Violence, Geriatric Health, Health Organizations, Heart, Hospices, Hospitals, Medical Research, Mental Health, Multiple Sclerosis, People with Disabilities, Prenatal Health Issues, Public Health, Research/Studies Institutes, Respiratory, Single-Disease Health Associations, Substance Abuse. **Geo. Dist:** Buffalo, NY.

## ★ 1364 ★ Ryder System Charitable Foundation

3600 NW 82nd Ave.
Miami, FL 33166
**Phone:** (305)500-3031        **Fax:** (305)593-4579
Ross Roadman, Executive Director

**Priorities:** *Arts & Humanities:* 26%. Provides basic support to numerous established organizations, including museums, theater, and music organizations. Priority is broadening access to cultural events to school children, the economically disadvantaged, and others. *Civic & Public Affairs:* 10%. Supports community centers, urban and minority affairs, and zoos. Supports revitalizing communities through economic development programs and improved housing facilities. *Education:* 22%. Supports public and private educational programs from kindergarten through graduate school. Contributes to educational programs and employment opportunities for minorities in America. *Environment:* 33%. Provides funding for United Way, private social service agency programs, and counseling services and other coping mechanisms to those in crisis situations. *International:* 8%. Supports research and cancer care. *Religion:* 1%. *Voluntarism:* Company actively supports employee volunteerism, and encourages management to volunteer in organizations it supports. *Note:* Total foundation contributions made in 1999. **Typ. Recipients:** Cancer, Children's Health/Hospitals, Hospitals, People with Disabilities, Research/Studies Institutes, Single-Disease Health Associations, Substance Abuse. **Geo. Dist:** Los Angeles, CA, through community initiative program; FL, Dade County; Miami, FL, metropolitan area Miami; Atlanta, GA, through community initiative program; St. Louis, MO, through community initiative program; Cincinnati, OH, through community initiative program; Dallas, TX, through community initiative program.

## ★ 1365 ★ S.C. Johnson Fund

1525 Howe St.
Racine, WI 53403
**Phone:** (262)260-2119        **Fax:** (262)260-2652
**Website:** http://www.scjohnsonwax.com/community/
Colleen Cribari, Program Administrator

**Priorities:** *Arts & Humanities:* 10%. Supports music, museums, dance, and theater. *Civic & Public Affairs:* 23%. Funds community development, urban centers, municipalities, housing, gardens, and justice concerns. *Education:* 23%. Majority of funding supports scholarships and fellowships for employee children, and minority students in a variety of fields. Also supports capital campaigns and specific programs at local colleges and universities. Education funds, associations, high schools, and INROADS/Wisconsin's Racine Youth Leadership Academy receive funding as well. *Environment:* 6%. Supports Young Men's Christian Association, food banks, human service agencies, and women's centers. *International:* Less than 1%. *Note:* Total contributions made in fiscal 2000. Priorities based on contributions made by S.C. Johnson Fund only. Corporation also sponsors the Johnson Foundation, a private operating foundation. The Johnson Foundation hosts conferences (known as Wingspread conferences) devoted to the improvement of society in several key areas: international understanding, educational excellence, improvement of the human environment, and intellectual and cultural growth. The foundation carries out program extension activities and publications through which it shares with a wider audience the information generated in these conferences. The corporation also offers limited direct contributions. Direct contributions are made to worthy causes for education, social welfare, culture and the arts, youth activities, health and medical concerns, preservation of the environment, emergency and disaster relief, and the disadvantaged. **Typ. Recipients:** AIDS/HIV, Cancer, Children's Health/Hospitals, Clinics/Medical Centers, Health Organizations, Hospitals, Medical Education, Medical Research, Medical Training, Nutrition, Single-Disease Health Associations, Substance Abuse. **Geo. Dist:** Racine, WI. **Frmly:** S.C. Johnson Wax Fund, Inc.

## ★ 1366 ★ SAFECO Corp.

SAFECO Plaza
Seattle, WA 98185
**Phone:** (206)545-5015        **Fax:** (206)545-5730
**Email:** roslin@afeco.com
**Website:** http://www.safeco.com/safeco/about/giving/giving.asp
Rose Lincoln, Manager Community Relations

**Priorities:** *Arts & Humanities:* 10% to 15%. Interests include theater, music, dance, museums, arts federations, visual arts, and community festivals. *Civic & Public Affairs:* About 30%. Supports economic development, public safety, civic improvement and neighborhood development. *Education:* About 20%. Interests include adult education, job readiness, and consumer education in financial areas. *Environment:* 30% to 35%. Major support goes to United Way in operating communities. Supports traditional social services, youth development, family relationships, and natural disaster preparedness. **Typ. Recipients:** Health Organizations, Health Policy/Cost Containment, Mental Health, Nutrition, People with Disabilities, Public Health, Single-Disease Health Associations, Substance Abuse. **Geo. Dist:** headquarters and operating communities in the United States.

## ★ 1367 ★ Safeguard Scientifics Foundation

800 Safeguard Bldg., 435 Devon Park Dr.
Wayne, PA 19087-1945
**Phone:** (610)293-0600
Gerald Hogan, Director, Corporate Administration

**Priorities:** *Arts & Humanities:* 12%. Supports performing arts, humanities councils, and museums. *Civic &*

*Public Affairs:* 39%. Supports community and economic development, business affairs, public policy, municipal services, women's affairs, housing issues, and gardens/parks. *Education:* 18%. Supports colleges and universities, secondary and special education, and economic and arts education. *Environment:* 14%. Supports United Way, children's issues, community centers, and scouting. *International:* 17%. Supports children's health, hospitals, and single-disease health associations. *Note:* Total foundation contributions made in 2000. **Typ. Recipients:** AIDS/HIV, Cancer, Children's Health/Hospitals, Children's Health/Hospitals, Diabetes, Emergency/Ambulance Services, Health Organizations, Heart, Hospices, Medical Education, Medical Rehabilitation, People with Disabilities, Single-Disease Health Associations.

### ★ 1368 ★ Saint Paul Companies Inc.

385 Washington St., MC514D
Saint Paul, MN 55102
**Phone:** (651)310-7911          **Fax:** (651)310-2327
**Website:** http://www.stpaul.com
Deb Anderson, Community Affairs Administrator

**Priorities:** *Arts & Humanities:* 23%. Supports a variety of art groups to ensure expression of diverse cultures and to enhance efforts in education and neighborhood development. Funding includes annual operating support on a three-year basis, capital support (excluding endowment) and special project funds for activities that advance the company's other community affairs goals. Interests include museums, music and art funds, which combine resources to support small- and medium-sized organizations. *Civic & Public Affairs:* 27%. Focus on low-income housing opportunities, leadership skills, and economic viability of city neighborhoods. Interests include philanthropic organizations, neighborhood development, neighborhood-based health clinics, and housing. Company sponsors the Leadership Initiatives in Neighborhoods (LIN) Program, which provides grants to individuals who do community action work. Goals are to encourage citizen participation in, and improve the effectiveness of, the nonprofit voluntary. sector. Foucs includes improving financial development capabilities, enhancing informaiton management systems, consolidation administrative functions and project activities with other nonprofits, and improving lleadership opportunities. Interests include nonprofit management, volunteer services, ethnic/minority organizations ans youth organizations. *Education:* About 25%. General operating support to private colleges and secondary schools in Minnesota through federated fund drives; support of private college capital and endowment fund drives in Minnesota; support of community-based education, including early childhood development, K-12 initiatives, and employment programs, and support of opportunities for minorities. *Environment:* 25%. Major support for the United Way. *Note:* Total contributions in 1999. **Typ. Recipients:** Adolescent Health Issues, AIDS/HIV, Cancer, Clinics/Medical Centers. **Geo. Dist:** select areas where company has large business presence; MD, Baltimore area; Minneapolis, MN; St. Paul, MN.

### ★ 1369 ★ S&T Bancorp Charitable Foundation

Main Office
PO Box 190
Indiana, PA 15701-0190
**Phone:** (724)465-1443
James Miller, President

**Fnded:** 1993. **Priorities:** *Arts & Humanities:* 6%. Supports historical societies, arts councils, museums, dance, symphonies, and libraries. *Civic & Public Affairs:* 27%. Supports community and economic development, fire departments, public safety, and community fairs and festivals. *Education:* 9%. Supports colleges, Head Start, and economic education. *Environment:* 39%. Funds United Way, senior services, youth organizations, and community centers. *International:* 19%. Supports single-disease health organizations, hospitals and medical centers, and children's health issues. *Note:* Total foundation contributions made in 2000. **Typ. Recipients:** Cancer, Children's Health/Hospitals, Clinics/Medical Centers,

Diabetes, Emergency/Ambulance Services, Heart, Hospitals, Nursing Services, People with Disabilities, Public Health. **Geo. Dist:** headquarters and operating communities.

### ★ 1370 ★ Sanford C. Bernstein & Co. Foundation, Inc.

767 5th Ave., 22nd Fl.
New York, NY 10153
**Phone:** (212)486-5800          **Fax:** (212)486-8430
Zalman Bernstein, Trustee

**Priorities:** *Arts & Humanities:* 19%. Supports historical preservation, opera, arts institutes, and the performing arts. *Education:* 7%. Mostly supports pre-college education, including inner-city scholarship funds, tutoring, minority education, Jewish schools, day schools, and high schools. *Environment:* 66%. Supports youth programs with emphasis on disadvantaged youth, as well as shelters, immigration projects, and family planning services. *International:* 7%. Support favors hospitals, medical research, single-disease associations, nursing homes, camps for the disabled, and pediatric health. *Note:* Total foundation contributions in 2000. **Typ. Recipients:** AIDS/HIV, Arthritis, Cancer, Child Abuse, Children's Health/Hospitals, Clinics/Medical Centers, Diabetes, Eyes/Blindness, Family Planning, Geriatric Health, Health Organizations, Heart, Hospices, Hospitals, Long-Term Care, Medical Research, Nursing Services, People with Disabilities, Prenatal Health Issues, Preventive Medicine/Wellness Organizations, Single-Disease Health Associations, Speech & Hearing. **Geo. Dist:** Los Angeles, CA; San Francisco, CA; CT; FL; NJ; NY; Dallas, TX.

### ★ 1371 ★ Sara Lee Foundation

3 First National Plaza
Chicago, IL 60602-4260
**Phone:** (312)558-8448          **Fax:** (312)419-3192
**Website:** http://www.saraleefoundation.org
Robin Tryloff, President, Executive Director

**Priorities:** *Arts & Humanities:* 64%. Provides cash support for new, emerging arts groups as well as for major, established institutions in Chicago. Funds performing arts, libraries, art institutes and the visual arts, and culture and the humanities. *Civic & Public Affairs:* 8%. Supports housing, women's causes, community services, and employment. *Education:* 8%. Supports educational programs, minority education and scholarship programs, colleges, and universities. *Environment:* 17%. Gives to organizations that aid the homeless, hungry, youth, and victims of family violence. Also provides major support to the United Way. *Religion:* 2%. Funds the Field Museum of Natural History, the Museum of Science and Industry, and food industry related research. *Voluntarism:* Company maintains a 15 to 20 person "Employee Volunteerism Committee," which is responsible for organizing approximately eight programs per year. Also sponsors a "Board Placement Program," through which company executives in the Chicago area are recruited to serve on nonprofit boards. These organizations also may be eligible for a $1,000 grant. *Note:* Total foundation contributions made in fiscal 2000. In addition to foundation's programs, operating companies and divisions administer giving programs based on assessment of needs in the communities where they operate. They contribute cash and product donations to local and national organizations. Divisions and employees also participate in community-based projects. **Typ. Recipients:** Cancer, Domestic Violence, Family Planning, Health Organizations, Hospitals, Nutrition, People with Disabilities, Prenatal Health Issues, Substance Abuse. **Geo. Dist:** principally near operating locations and to national organizations; Chicago, IL, metropolitan area.

### ★ 1372 ★ Sara Lee Hosiery, Inc.

5650 University Parkway
Winston-Salem, NC 27105
**Phone:** (336)519-3427          **Fax:** (336)519-7555
**Email:** contributions@slkp.com
**Website:** http://www.saralee.com
John Cox, Manager Community Relations

**Priorities:** *Civic & Public Affairs:* 67%. Supports minority and women's programs. *Environment:* 33%. Supports children's programs. *Note:* Total contributions made in 1999. **Typ. Recipients:** Domestic Violence, Emergency/Ambulance Services, Health Organizations, Health-General, Hospices, Hospitals, People with Disabilities, Public Health, Substance Abuse. **Geo. Dist:** headquarters and operating communities.

### ★ 1373 ★ SBC Foundation

175 East Houston, Ste. 200
San Antonio, TX 78205
**Phone:** 800-591-9663          **Fax:** (210)351-2259
**Website:** http://www.sbc.com/Community/SBC_Foundation
Gloria Delgado, President

**Priorities:** *Arts & Humanities:* About 16%. Supports initiatives that promote cultural and arts education, broaden access to arts and cultural activities and help promote community pride. Areas of focus include broad-based performing arts and cultural programs that promote cultural diversity and community outreach, and partnerships between arts and cultural institutions and schools that provide educational programs for K-12 students and underserved communities. *Civic & Public Affairs:* About 5%. Supports initiatives designed to promote the sustained economic growth of our communities and build the capacity of community-based organizations to serve their clients. Areas of focus are programs that broaden economic growth opportunities for the whole community; technology-based programs that enhance a community's infrastructure or improve the efficiency and productivity of community-based organizations; community coalitions that stimulate business retention and expansion, especially in economically disadvantaged areas; programs that address adult literacy, job training and leadership skill development. *Education:* 28%. Supports K-12 and higher education initiatives that can improve and strengthen the education process, produce sustained improvement in student learning, broaden educational opportunity and increase the potential for each student to succeed. Areas of focus include programs that support strategic and systemic change in K-12 education and can be linked to improved student achievement; programs that integrate innovative approaches to instruction with a focus on creative technology applications for enhanced learning and improved school effectiveness; programs that support at-risk students and encourage parental involvement in student achievement; public or private colleges and universities with an emphasis on collaborations to improve teacher preparedness, expand the use of technology in the classroom, promote excellence in math, science, and engineering, and support student success and achievement. *Environment:* 41%. Funds the United Way. *Note:* Total contributions in 1998. **Typ. Recipients:** Alzheimers Disease, Cancer, Children's Health/Hospitals, Emergency/Ambulance Services, Health Organizations, Health-General, Hospitals, Medical Education, Medical Research, Mental Health, People with Disabilities. **Geo. Dist:** nationally; AR; CA; CT; DC; IL, central Illinois; Chicago, IL; KS; KS; Baltimore, MD; MA, western Massachusetts; Boston, MA; MO; NV; NY, Upstate; OK; RI; TX. **Frmly:** Southwestern Bell Foundation.

### ★ 1374 ★ Schering-Plough Foundation

One Giralda Farms
Madison, NJ 07940-1010
**Phone:** (973)822-7414          **Fax:** (973)822-7349
Christine Fahey, Assistant Secretary

**Priorities:** *Arts & Humanities:* 8%. Support is awarded to galleries, museums, arts centers, exhibitions, and performing arts organizations. *Civic & Public Affairs:* 10%. Supports affordable housing, women's shelters, public policy, and the environment. *Education:* 48%. Supports higher and secondary education. Interests include medical and pharmaceutical schools, medical research, and public health education. Also awards funding to establish scholarships in the natural sciences and biomedical studies, and to support traditional scholarship programs and education funds. Also supports management education, education associations, and student aid programs. *Environment:* 3%. Supports YMCAs, anti-drug campaigns, and other social service organizations. *International:* 9%. Supports hospitals and healthcare programs most used by employees and their families, American Red Cross, healthcare services to low-income working people, and university schools of pharmacy. *Religion:* Less than 1%. Supports science research and laboratories. *Voluntarism:* Provides small grants through its Dollar for Volunteer program most used by employees and their families, American Red Cross, health-care services to low-income working people, and university schools of pharmacy. *Note:* Total foundation contributions made in 2000. **Typ. Recipients:** Alzheimers Disease, Cancer, Children's Health/Hospitals, Clinics/Medical Centers, Domestic Violence, Emergency/Ambulance Services, Health Policy/Cost Containment, Health-General, Hospices, Hospitals, Hospitals (University Affiliated), Long-Term Care, Medical Education, Medical Rehabilitation, Medical Research, Medical Training, Mental Health, Public Health, Research/Studies Institutes, Single-Disease Health Associations, Substance Abuse, Transplant Networks/Donor Banks. **Geo. Dist:** principally near operating locations and to national organizations.

**★ 1375 ★ Schlumberger Foundation**
277 Park Ave.
New York, NY 10172-0266
**Phone:** (212)350-9400          **Fax:** (212)350-9440
Arthur Alexander, Secretary & Treasurer

**Priorities:** *Arts & Humanities:* 3%. Majority of support funds music and museums. Dance organizations, arts centers, and performing arts organizations also receive support. *Civic & Public Affairs:* 2%. Environmental efforts, women's issues, and law and justice are supported. *Education:* 61%. Funding primarily supports colleges and universities for professorships, research programs, and facilities grants. Interest is also shown in minority education, and scholarships and fellowships. *Environment:* 12%. Supports community service organizations with emphasis on neighborhoods and homelessness. Youth clubs and people with disabilities also receive funding. *International:* 7%. Interests include geriatric health, single-disease health associations, and hospitals. *Religion:* 6%. Funding supports the Houston Museum of Natural Science. *Note:* Total contributions made in 1998. **Typ. Recipients:** Alzheimers Disease, Cancer, Children's Health/Hospitals, Eyes/Blindness, Family Planning, Hospices, Hospitals, Medical Education, Medical Research, People with Disabilities, Single-Disease Health Associations, Substance Abuse. **Geo. Dist:** nationally to education; New York, NY.

**★ 1376 ★ Schoeneckers Foundation**
PO Box 1610
Minneapolis, MN 55440
**Phone:** (612)835-4800          **Fax:** (612)844-4033
L. Schoenecker, President

**Fnded:** 1979. **Priorities:** *Civic & Public Affairs:* 2%. Supports philanthropic organizations and fire and rescue squads. *Education:* 93%. Supports universities and private schools. *Environment:* 3%. Supports youth organizations, food pantries and shelters, and United Way. *International:* Less than 1%. *Note:* Total foundation contributions made in fiscal 2000. **Typ. Recipients:** Alzheimers Disease, Cancer, Children's Health/Hospitals, Diabetes, Emergency/Ambulance Services, Health Organizations, Heart, Hospices, Hospitals, Multiple Sclerosis, Respiratory, Single-Disease Health Associations. **Geo. Dist:** MN.

**★ 1377 ★ Schurz Communications Foundation**
225 West Colfax Ave.
South Bend, IN 46626
**Phone:** (219)236-1773          **Fax:** (219)236-1765
Todd Schurz, President

**Fnded:** 1940. **Priorities:** *Arts & Humanities:* 28%. Historical societies, museums, arts centers, music, and arts festivals. *Civic & Public Affairs:* 16%. Primarily for community foundations and economic develop-

ment. *Education:* 13%. Colleges and universities and business education. *Environment:* Emphasis on the United Way; also supports child welfare and youth organizations. **Typ. Recipients:** Hospices. **Geo. Dist:** South Bend, IN.

**★ 1378 ★ Schwebel Family Foundation**
PO Box 6018
Youngstown, OH 44501
**Phone:** (330)783-2860
Joseph Schwebel, President

**Fnded:** 1989. **Priorities:** *Arts & Humanities:* 5%. Funds arts councils and a theater. *Civic & Public Affairs:* 4%. Supports Junior League and other civic organizations. *Education:* 25%. Supports colleges and universities, public schools, and arts education. *Environment:* 22%. Supports the United Way, youth organizations, YMCAs, substance abuse organizations, planned parenthood, and food distribution services. *International:* 22%. Supports single-disease health organizations, hospitals, hospice, and health funds. *Note:* Total contributions made in 1998. **Typ. Recipients:** Cancer, Children's Health/Hospitals, Diabetes, Family Planning, Health Organizations, Health-General, Heart, Hospices, Hospitals, Multiple Sclerosis, People with Disabilities, Single-Disease Health Associations, Speech & Hearing. **Geo. Dist:** OH.

**★ 1379 ★ Scientific-Atlanta, Inc.**
5030 Sugarloaf Pkwy.
Lawrenceville, GA 30042
**Phone:** (770)236-4607          **Fax:** (770)236-4725
**Email:** bill.mccargo@sciatl.com
**Website:** http://www.sciatl.com
Bill McCargo, Directory, Community Relations

**Priorities:** *Arts & Humanities:* 15%. *Civic & Public Affairs:* 15%. *Education:* 40%. *International:* 30%. **Typ. Recipients:** Health-General. **Geo. Dist:** headquarters and operating communities.

**★ 1380 ★ Security Benefit Life Insurance Co. Charitable Trust**
700 Southwest Harrison St.
Topeka, KS 66636-0001
**Phone:** (785)431-3215
Krysta Congrove, Contact

**Fnded:** 1976. **Priorities:** *Arts & Humanities:* 14%. Supports arts organizations in Topeka. *Civic & Public Affairs:* 41%. Gives to the United Way, the Boy Scouts of America, and Big Brothers and Big Sisters. Also supports women's resources, community affairs, and Friends of the Topeka Zoo. *Education:* 20%. Major support given to colleges and secondary schools, primarily in Topeka, KS. *Environment:* 25%. Supports scout troops, youth and senior organizations, and animal welfare. *Note:* Total contributions made in 1999. **Typ. Recipients:** Cancer, Children's Health/Hospitals, Diabetes, Emergency/Ambulance Services, Family Planning, Health Organizations, Hospices, People with Disabilities, Prenatal Health Issues, Single-Disease Health Associations. **Geo. Dist:** Topeka, KS, some giving in other areas of Kansas.

**★ 1381 ★ Sempra Energy**
101 Ash St.
San Diego, CA 92101-3017
**Phone:** (619)696-4297          **Fax:** (619)696-1868
**Email:** community@sempra.com

**Priorities:** *Arts & Humanities:* About 15%. Supports arts appreciation, artsassociations, art centers, visual arts, opera and music, and historic preservation. Emphasis is on making the arts accessible to underserved or disadvantaged groups. *Civic & Public Affairs:* About 20%. Supports consumer affairs, economic development, environmental affairs, urban and community affairs, and ethnic and minority affairs. Emphais on crime prevention. *Education:* 25% to 30%. Primary support goes to business education, colleges and universities, elementary education, literacy programs, and minority education. *International:* 35% to 40%. Supports the aged and geriatric health, hospices and hospitals, medical research, single-disease health

associations, child welfare, community centers and community service organizations, family services, and traditional youth organizations. Major emphasis is on drug abuse prevention. *Voluntarism:* The company promotes employee volunteerism through Team San Diego Gas & Electric, a group of nearly 1,200 employees and family members who volunteer in hands-on community service projects. **Typ. Recipients:** Geriatric Health, Health Organizations, Hospices, Hospitals, Medical Education, Medical Research, Mental Health, People with Disabilities, Single-Disease Health Associations, Substance Abuse. **Geo. Dist:** CA, Southern California.

**★ 1382 ★ Sentry Insurance Foundation Inc.**
1800 N Point Dr.
Stevens Point, WI 54481
**Phone:** (715)346-6000          **Fax:** (715)346-6405
Margie Coker-Nelson, Executive Director, Vice President

**Priorities:** *Arts & Humanities:* 1%. *Civic & Public Affairs:* 1%. *Education:* 33%. Supports scholarships and higher education. *Environment:* 30%. Supports the United Way and human service organizations. *International:* 2%. *Note:* Total foundation contributions made in 1999. **Typ. Recipients:** Cancer, Health Organizations, Heart, Hospitals, Medical Research, People with Disabilities, Public Health, Substance Abuse. **Geo. Dist:** nationally; areas with large employee populations.

**★ 1383 ★ Servco Foundation**
PO Box 2788
Honolulu, HI 96803
**Phone:** (808)521-6511          **Fax:** (808)523-3937
Sandra Wong, Corporate Secretary

**Fnded:** 1986. **Typ. Recipients:** Cancer, Child Abuse, Clinics/Medical Centers, Diabetes, Emergency/Ambulance Services, Health Organizations, Health-General, Heart, Hospitals, Medical Rehabilitation, Single-Disease Health Associations, Substance Abuse. **Geo. Dist:** nationally; HI.

**★ 1384 ★ ServiceMaster Foundation**
1 ServiceMaster Way
Downers Grove, IL 60515
**Phone:** (708)271-1300
Claire Buchan, Vice President, Corporate Communications

**Fnded:** 1987. **Priorities:** *Education:* 61%. Supports higher education, including religious training, and enrichment programs. *Environment:* 10%. Social services and youth activities receive support. *International:* 3%. *Note:* Total contributions in 1997. **Typ. Recipients:** Family Planning, Health-General, Hospitals. **Geo. Dist:** headquarters area only.

**★ 1385 ★ Shaw Industries Inc.**
PO Box 2128
Dalton, GA 30722
**Phone:** (706)278-3812          **Fax:** (706)275-1129
**Email:** crollins@shawninc.com
**Website:** http://www.shawinc.com
Carl Rollins, Vice President, Administration

**Typ. Recipients:** Health-General. **Geo. Dist:** headquarters and operating communities.

**★ 1386 ★ Shaw's Supermarkets Charitable Foundation**
140 Laurel St.
PO Box 600
East Bridgewater, MA 02333
**Phone:** (508)350-3316          **Fax:** (508)350-3112
**Website:** http://www.shaws.com/about_us/community_commitment.html
Bernard Rogan, Corporate Communications Director

**Fnded:** 1959. **Priorities:** *Arts & Humanities:* 20%. Supports museums, libraries, and performing arts, with an emphasis on children's programs. *Civic & Public Affairs:* 7%. Supports fire fighters, law enforcement, and a zoo. *Environment:* 45%. Supports local United Ways, YMCAs, and Boys and Girls Clubs. Also funds food banks, shelters, youth organizations, and adult day care centers. *International:* 14%. Interests include hospitals, medical centers, and nurse associations. *Religion:* 13%. Funds a science museum. *Note:* Total contributions in fiscal 2000. **Typ. Recipients:** Children's Health/Hospitals, Clinics/Medical Centers, Emergency/Ambulance Services, Geriatric Health, Health Organizations, Hospitals, Nursing Services, Public Health, Single-Disease Health Associations. **Geo. Dist:** headquarters and operating communities; CT; ME; MA; NH; RI.

### ★ 1387 ★ Shell Oil Co. Foundation

One Shell Plaza
Box 2099
Houston, TX 77252
**Phone:** (713)241-1595　　**Fax:** (713)241-3329
**Website:** http://www.countonshell.com/community/involvement/shell_foundation.html
Terry Garland, Administrative Assistant

**Fnded:** 1953. **Priorities:** *Arts & Humanities:* About 10%. Primarily gives in communities where company employees live. Supports a variety of disciplines, with emphasis on cultural centers, music, museums, opera, public TV/radio, dance, art councils, performing arts, theaters, and libraries. *Civic & Public Affairs:* 5% to 10%. Interest in national and local development, community improvement, research organizations, environmental efforts, public policy, justice and law, and minority needs. *Education:* 45% to 50%. Emphasis on support of higher education through established programs (by invitation only). Shell Doctoral Fellowships encourage outstanding students to seek teaching careers in engineering and the sciences. Shell Faculty Career Initiation Funds support untenured faculty in science and engineering research. Shell Departmental Grants are designed to strengthen activities in specified areas related to teaching and/or research. Shell Career Counseling Grants are used to enhance career counseling and placement activities in colleges and universities with well-established programs. Precollege programs focus on math and science programs. Shell Incentive Funds are targeted to undergraduate minority students, with emphasis on technical and business education. National education funds, education organizations, and economic education receive substantial support. Also sponsors matching gifts program, and scholarships for children of employees. *International:* About 35%. Primary support goes to united funds. Support also goes to national health agencies, national welfare agencies, youth organizations and local health and welfare agencies. A priority is hospitals which serve employees, particularly through capital support. *Voluntarism:* Company sponsors "Shell Employees and Retirees Volunteerism Effort" (SERVE), through which company employees and retirees have participated in housing rehabilitation projects, educational television solicitations, school clothing drives, and picnics for mentally handicapped children. Employees also serve on the boards of various organizations and loaned executives work with United Way campaigns. **Typ. Recipients:** Children's Health/Hospitals, Clinics/Medical Centers, Eyes/Blindness, Health Funds, Health Organizations, Heart, Hospices, Hospitals, Hospitals (University Affiliated), Medical Education, Medical Rehabilitation, Medical Research, Mental Health, People with Disabilities, Single-Disease Health Associations, Substance Abuse. **Geo. Dist:** nationally, with emphasis on communities where Shell employees are located.

### ★ 1388 ★ Shelter Insurance Foundation

1817 West Broadway
Columbia, MO 65218
**Phone:** (573)214-4290　　**Fax:** (573)446-5727
Raymond Jones, Secretary & Director

**Fnded:** 1981. **Priorities:** *Arts & Humanities:* 1%. *Civic & Public Affairs:* 3%. *Education:* 91%. Almost all funding went towards scholarships. *Environment:* 2%. Supports scouting, crime prevention, and programs for the elderly. *International:* 2%. *Note:* Total contributions in fiscal 1999. **Typ. Recipients:** Alzheimers Disease, Cancer, Children's Health/Hospitals, Heart, Medical

Education, Medical Research, People with Disabilities, Single-Disease Health Associations. **Geo. Dist:** AK; CO; IL; IN; IA; KS; KY; LA; MS; MO; Columbia, MO; NE; OK; TN.

### ★ 1389 ★ Sherman-Standard Register Foundation

600 Albany St., PO Box 1167
Dayton, OH 45408
**Phone:** (937)443-1540　　**Fax:** (937)221-3431
Kathryn Lamme, Corporate Vice President, Secretary and

**Fnded:** 1955. **Priorities:** *Arts & Humanities:* 3%. Supports arts organizations. *Civic & Public Affairs:* 9%. Supports women's causes, community development, parks, and clubs. *Education:* 6%. Provides funds for high schools and Junior Achievement. *Environment:* 50%. Supports the United Way, scouting, YMCA, and youth organizations. *International:* 7%. Funds cancer organizations, blood banks, neuroscience, and the American Red Cross. *Religion:* 4%. Funds a natural history museum. *Note:* Total foundation contributions made in fiscal 2000. **Typ. Recipients:** Cancer, Children's Health/Hospitals, Clinics/Medical Centers, Emergency/Ambulance Services, Health Funds, Health-General, Hospices, Hospitals, Public Health, Transplant Networks/Donor Banks. **Geo. Dist:** OH.

### ★ 1390 ★ Sherwin-Williams Foundation

101 Prospect Ave. Northwest
Cleveland, OH 44115
**Phone:** (216)566-2511　　**Fax:** (216)566-3266
Barbara Gadosik, Director, Corporate Contributions

**Priorities:** *Arts & Humanities:* 14%. Supports museums, art associations, and performing arts associations in Cleveland, OH, area. *Civic & Public Affairs:* 7%. Funds development programs for Cleveland, OH, professional associations, sports and recreation, and matching gifts for volunteer leaders. *Education:* 34%. More than half of education support is given in the form of matching gifts. Also supports universities, independent college funds, and official scholarship programs. *Environment:* 33%. Funds the United Way in operating locations. Youth, the disabled, and other human services organizations also receive support. *International:* 5%. Supports hospitals and the American Red Cross. *Note:* Total foundation contributions made in 1999. **Typ. Recipients:** Cancer, Emergency/Ambulance Services, Hospices, Hospitals, Hospitals (University Affiliated), Long-Term Care, Medical Education, Medical Rehabilitation, People with Disabilities, Public Health, Single-Disease Health Associations. **Geo. Dist:** headquarters and operating communities, primarily Cleveland.

### ★ 1391 ★ Shoney's Inc.

1727 Elm Hill Pike
Nashville, TN 37210
**Phone:** (615)231-2253　　**Fax:** (615)231-2734
**Email:** sue_downs@shoneys.com
**Website:** http://www.shoneys.com
Richard Schafstall, General Counsel

**Priorities:** *Arts & Humanities:* About 10%. Interests include festivals, art institutes, community arts, ethnic arts, performing arts, music, opera, theater, and public broadcasting. *Civic & Public Affairs:* About 35%. Supports civic and public affairs groups near headquarters and operating locations. *Education:* 40% to 45%. Recipients include public and private education, business education, colleges and universities, community colleges, education funds, and scholarship programs. The company is also an active supporter of United Negro College Fund and is a sponsor of the annual Bootstrap Awards Scholarship Program. *International:* About 10%. Supports health funds, hospitals, health organizations, mental health, and public health. **Typ. Recipients:** Domestic Violence, Health Funds, Health Organizations, Hospitals, Public Health, Substance Abuse. **Geo. Dist:** headquarters and operating communities.

### ★ 1392 ★ Sierra Pacific Foundation

PO Box 496028
Redding, CA 96049-6028
**Phone:** (530)378-8000　　**Fax:** (916)378-8109
Stephanie Donham, Contact

**Fnded:** 1978. **Priorities:** *Arts & Humanities:* 6%. Supports museums. *Civic & Public Affairs:* 19%. Supports fire departments, agriculture, public safety, community foundations, media affairs, and county fairs. *Education:* 55%. Scholarships are awarded to children of employees for higher education. Also supports local high schools, colleges, and universities. *Environment:* 11%. Supports scouting, YMCA, athletics, and community youth organizations. *International:* 5%. Funds hospitals and the American Red Cross. *Religion:* 2%. Supports a planetarium. *Note:* Total foundation contributions made in fiscal 2000. **Typ. Recipients:** Cancer, Emergency/Ambulance Services, Health Organizations, Heart, Hospices, Hospitals, Medical Research, Nutrition, Single-Disease Health Associations, Transplant Networks/Donor Banks. **Geo. Dist:** headquarters and operating communities.

### ★ 1393 ★ Sierra Pacific Resources Charitable Foundation

PO Box 30150
Reno, NV 89520
**Phone:** (702)367-5748
**Email:** kfoster@sppc.com
Karen Foster, Secretary, Treasurer

**Fnded:** 1988. **Priorities:** *Arts & Humanities:* 14%. Supports art museums and foundations, classical music, humanities councils, libraries, and an opera house. *Civic & Public Affairs:* 13%. Gives to municipality, minority and women's affairs, and state sponsored events, including a rodeo. *Education:* 32%. Primarily supports colleges and universities, with an emphasis on technology, mining and geology, and environmental science. Also supports science fairs and pre K-12 education schools and programs. *Environment:* 36%. Mainly supports youth organizations including scouting, Boys & Girls Clubs, YMCAs and athletic/recreational activities. Also funds senior services, food distribution, and the United Way. *International:* 3%. Primarily funds national health organizations and single-disease associations. *Voluntarism:* Company employees are active in the community, participating in the Day of Caring, blood drives, and events such as the Special Olympics and the March of Dimes WalkAmerica. *Note:* Total contributions made in 1999. **Typ. Recipients:** Alzheimers Disease, Cancer, Children's Health/Hospitals, Diabetes, Emergency/Ambulance Services, Family Planning, Heart, Hospitals, Mental Health, People with Disabilities, Respiratory, Single-Disease Health Associations. **Geo. Dist:** headquarters and operating communities; CA, Northeastern California; NV, Northern Nevada.

### ★ 1394 ★ Simpson Fund

1301 5th Ave., No. 2800
Seattle, WA 98101
**Phone:** (206)224-5198　　**Fax:** (206)436-1852
**Email:** cmusgra@smpsn.com
**Website:** http://www.simpson.com
Colleen Musgrave, Administrator

**Priorities:** *Arts & Humanities:* 10%. Funds museums, performing arts, and art councils. *Civic & Public Affairs:* 10%. Support focuses on zoological societies and the community. *Education:* 23%. Colleges and universities are primary recipients. *Environment:* 38%. Most support goes to united funds, shelters, and food banks. *International:* 10%. Interests include hospitals. *Religion:* 1%. Supports the Pacific Science Center in Seattle. *Voluntarism:* The company sponsors a United Way "Day of Caring" program where employees volunteer their time to help a designated United Way organization. *Note:* Total contributions made in 2000. **Typ. Recipients:** Arthritis, Child Abuse, Children's Health/Hospitals, Clinics/Medical Centers, Emergency/Ambulance Services, Geriatric Health, Health Organizations, Hospices, Hospitals, Nursing Services, Sexual Abuse, Substance Abuse, Transplant Networks/Donor Banks, Trauma Treatment. **Geo. Dist:**

CA, Del Norte County; CA, Humboldt County; OR, Lincoln County; OR, Tillamook County; WA, Grays Harbor County; WA, King County; WA, Mason County; WA, Pierce County; WA, Thurston County.

**★ 1395 ★ SIT Investment Associates Foundation**
4600 Norwest Center
90 S 7th St.
Minneapolis, MN 55402
**Phone:** (612)332-3223 **Fax:** (612)342-2018
Paul Rasmussen, Chief Financial Officer

**Typ. Recipients:** Children's Health/Hospitals, Emergency/Ambulance Services, Health Organizations, Heart, Hospices, Medical Rehabilitation, People with Disabilities, Single-Disease Health Associations, Substance Abuse. **Geo. Dist:** MN.

**★ 1396 ★ Slant/Fin Foundation**
100 Forest Dr.
Greenvale, NY 11548
**Phone:** (516)484-2600 **Fax:** (516)484-8906
Ray Blaquiere, Controller

**Fnded:** 1985. **Priorities:** *Arts & Humanities:* 2%. Interests include art associations, museums, music, and performing arts. *Civic & Public Affairs:* 2%. Emphasis on community development and civic affairs. *Education:* 6%. Supports colleges, universities, and foundations. *Environment:* 1%. *International:* 3%. Supports hospitals, medical centers, and single-disease health associations. *Note:* Total contributions made in 1998. **Typ. Recipients:** Alzheimers Disease, Cancer, Children's Health/Hospitals, Clinics/Medical Centers, Geriatric Health, Health-General, Hospices, Hospitals, Medical Education, Medical Rehabilitation, Medical Research, People with Disabilities, Public Health, Single-Disease Health Associations. **Geo. Dist:** nationally; NY.

**★ 1397 ★ Solo Cup Foundation**
1700 Old Deerfield Rd.
Highland Park, IL 60035
**Phone:** (847)831-4800 **Fax:** (847)831-5849
Ronald Whaley, Foundation Administrator

**Fnded:** 1959. **Priorities:** *Civic & Public Affairs:* 2%. Supports volunteer organizations and civic initiatives. *Education:* 13%. Funds private precollege education. *Environment:* 7%. Supports United Way, homes for the disabled, substance abuse recovery programs, religious welfare, and youth groups. *International:* 7%. Supports hospitals and medical research. *Note:* Total foundation contributions made in fiscal 2001. **Typ. Recipients:** Cancer, Children's Health/Hospitals, Hospitals, People with Disabilities, Prenatal Health Issues, Public Health, Single-Disease Health Associations, Substance Abuse. **Geo. Dist:** IL.

**★ 1398 ★ Sonoco Foundation**
One North 2nd St., Mail Stop A09
Hartsville, SC 29550
**Phone:** (843)383-7851 **Fax:** (843)383-7008
**Email:** joyce.beasley@sonoco.com
**Website:** http://www.sonoco.com/sonoco_foundation.htm
Joyce Beasley, Manager, Community Affairs

**Priorities:** *Arts & Humanities:* 3%. Supports historic preservation, museums, arts councils, and arts festivals. *Civic & Public Affairs:* 8%. Majority of giving supports urban and community development projects designed to improve and revitalize communities, and promote the general well-being of all citizens. *Education:* 60%. Primarily supports colleges and universities, college funds, private and public secondary education, business education, and humanities education. Focus is on institutions from which the company recruits. *Environment:* 28%. Emphasis on YMCAs and the United Way. *International:* 1%. Single-disease health associations and emergency services. *Note:* Total contributions in 1998. **Typ. Recipients:** Cancer, Children's Health/Hospitals, Domestic Violence, Emergency/Ambulance Services, Eyes/Blindness, Health Organizations, Health-General, Hospitals, Medical Rehabil-

itation, Medical Research, Mental Health, Multiple Sclerosis, People with Disabilities, Research/Studies Institutes, Single-Disease Health Associations, Substance Abuse. **Geo. Dist:** counties in which employees reside; SC.

**★ 1399 ★ Sony U.S.A. Foundation Inc.**
Sony U.S.A. Foundation
550 Madison Ave., 35th Floor
New York, NY 10022
**Phone:** (212)833-6872 **Fax:** (212)833-6869
Ken Nees, President

**Priorities:** *Arts & Humanities:* 1%. Supports music, opera, museums, and public broadcasting in New York City. *Civic & Public Affairs:* 19%. Supports urban and community affairs including civic organizations, foundations, and employment training. Includes efforts to promote the advancement and recognition of minorities. *Education:* 29%. Funding supports institutions and programs that bring commitment and innovation to the task of strengthening education at the primary and secondary school levels, with consideration also given to selected higher education initiatives. Also supports efforts that promote literacy and basic educational competency, and encouragement of the technical and scientific skills required of tomorrow's work force. Also funds arts education. Scholarships are awarded to the children of employees. *Environment:* 41%. Majority of funds support the United Way. Additional funding supports youth organizations and other human services. *International:* 10%. Supports hospitals and healthcare organizations. *Note:* Above priorities are for Sony USA Foundation in 2000. Sony Corp. of America subsidiaries run independent giving programs. **Typ. Recipients:** Child Abuse, Children's Health/Hospitals, Diabetes, Emergency/Ambulance Services, Eyes/Blindness, Health Organizations, Hospitals, Medical Rehabilitation, Mental Health, Multiple Sclerosis, People with Disabilities, Prenatal Health Issues, Preventive Medicine/Wellness Organizations, Public Health. **Geo. Dist:** headquarters and operating communities; nationally.

**★ 1400 ★ Southwest Gas Corp. Foundation**
PO Box 98510
5241 Spring Mountain Rd.
Las Vegas, NV 89193-8510
**Phone:** (702)876-7247 **Fax:** (702)876-7037
Suzanne Farinas, Assistant to the Chief Executive Officer

**Priorities:** *Arts & Humanities:* 6%. Support includes local orchestras, symphonies, museums, public broadcasting, and performing arts. *Civic & Public Affairs:* 17%. Funding supports a variety of legal and business associations, youth programs, and public safety. *Education:* 30%. Education program emphasizes universities, colleges, scholarship funds, and literacy. *Environment:* 39%. Major support for the United Way. Also supports community service organizations, a volunteer center, seniors, low-income services, shelters and food banks, and emergency relief. Supports youth agencies, scholarships, and scouting. *International:* 6%. Funds single-disease health associations and university medical centers. *Voluntarism:* The company sponsors an employee volunteer team that works on various projects. *Note:* Total foundation contributions made in 2000. **Typ. Recipients:** Arthritis, Cancer, Children's Health/Hospitals, Clinics/Medical Centers, Diabetes, Domestic Violence, Emergency/Ambulance Services, Eyes/Blindness, Heart, Hospices, Hospitals, Medical Research, People with Disabilities, Prenatal Health Issues, Respiratory, Single-Disease Health Associations. **Geo. Dist:** AZ, Southern and Central Arizona; Barstow, CA; Big Bear, CA; Victorville, CA; NV, Northern and Southern Nevada (except Reno).

**★ 1401 ★ Sovereign Bank Foundation**
Two Aldwyn Center
Lancaster Ave. & Route 30
Villanova, PA 19085
**Phone:** (610)526-6226
John Killen, Manager

**Priorities:** *Arts & Humanities:* 1%. Supports libraries, museums, and performing arts. *Civic & Public Affairs:* 72%. Supports housing and community and economic development. *Education:* 7%. Funds colleges, universities, scholarship funds, and schools. *Environment:* 18%. Supports homeless shelters and youth organizations. *International:* 2%. *Note:* Total foundation contributions made in 2000. **Typ. Recipients:** AIDS/HIV, Clinics/Medical Centers, Domestic Violence, Family Planning, Health-General, Hospitals, People with Disabilities, Public Health, Sexual Abuse, Single-Disease Health Associations. **Geo. Dist:** bank or service areas; NJ, Mercer County.

**★ 1402 ★ Springs Industries, Inc.**
PO Box 70
Fort Mill, SC 29716
**Phone:** (803)547-3736 **Fax:** (803)547-3740
**Website:** http://www.springs.com
Ted Matthews, Vice President, Corporate Contributions

**Priorities:** *Arts & Humanities:* About 10%. Priorities include arts associations and historic preservation. Other interests include a museum, galleries, and community arts. *Civic & Public Affairs:* 25%. Primary interest is organizations concerned with business or free enterprise. Interests also include economic development, professional and trade associations, and public policy organizations. *Education:* 55%. Major priorities include improvement in higher education and adult education. Other interests include business education, elementary and secondary education, economic education, and public and private education organizations. *International:* 10%. Major welfare interests include community service, family service, and youth organizations. Major health interests include hospitals and single disease health associations. Smaller contributions go to organizations promoting health care cost containment, child welfare, drug and alcohol abuse prevention, and united funds. **Typ. Recipients:** Hospices, Hospitals, Single-Disease Health Associations, Substance Abuse. **Geo. Dist:** principally near operating locations and to national organizations.

**★ 1403 ★ Sprint/United Telephone**
125 N Main
Sidney, OH 45365
**Phone:** (419)755-8011 **Fax:** (937)498-0066
**Website:** http://www.sprint.com
Dave Brown, Budget Administrator & Public Affairs Ma

**Typ. Recipients:** Children's Health/Hospitals, Emergency/Ambulance Services, Health-General. **Geo. Dist:** limited to areas of service.

**★ 1404 ★ SPX Foundation**
700 Terrace Point Dr.
Muskegon, MI 49443-3301
**Phone:** (231)724-5000 **Fax:** (231)724-5720
Tina Betlejewski, President

**Fnded:** 1984. **Priorities:** *Arts & Humanities:* About 5%. Major support to art museums, theaters, music, public radio, and the performing arts. *Civic & Public Affairs:* Less than 1%. Supports local iniatives and chambers of commerce. *Education:* About 17%. Primarily supports community colleges and public and private higher education. Interests also include business, science, and minority education. Company also matches employee gifts to higher education. *Environment:* 47%. Supports the United Way and youth organizations. *International:* 31%. Supports community hospitals and cancer research. *Note:* Total contributions made in 1998. **Typ. Recipients:** Cancer, Child Abuse, Diabetes, Emergency/Ambulance Services, Family Planning, Health Organizations, Health-General, Hospitals, Multiple Sclerosis, People with Disabilities, Substance Abuse. **Geo. Dist:** primarily in plant communities.

**★ 1405 ★ Square D Foundation**
1415 South Roselle Rd.
Palatine, IL 60067

**Phone:** (847)397-2610 **Fax:** (847)397-2804
James White, Secretary

**Priorities:** *Arts & Humanities:* 1%. Supports museums, arts councils, arts festivals, and arts funds. *Education:* 63%. Primarily supports colleges and universities. Also supports education funds, scholarships, endowments for faculty, acquisition of equipment, and operating support. Interests include engineering, business, economics, and minority education. Matching gifts account for a significant portion of funding. Supports the National Merit Scholarship Corporation for children of employees. *Environment:* 30% to 35%. Supports united funds and child welfare, as well as youth organizations, rural affairs, and community service organizations. About 10% of giving is in the form of matching gifts. *International:* About 6%. Interests include hospitals, single-disease health associations, medical research, and geriatric health. *Note:* Total contributions made in 1998. **Typ. Recipients:** Cancer, Children's Health/Hospitals, Clinics/Medical Centers, Emergency/Ambulance Services, Health Funds, Hospitals, Long-Term Care, Medical Research, Mental Health, People with Disabilities, Single-Disease Health Associations. **Geo. Dist:** manufacturing facility communities.


★ **1406** ★ **Standard Products Co.
Charitable Foundation**
701 Lima Ave.
Findlay, OH 45840
**Phone:** (419)424-4320
Philip Weaver, Trustee

**Fnded:** 1984. **Priorities:** *Arts & Humanities:* 9%. Supports museums and music. *Civic & Public Affairs:* 14%. Supports economic development and urban and community affairs. *Education:* 16%. Supports higher education and literacy programs. *Environment:* 47%. Most grants are given to the United Way. Also supports community and family service organizations. *International:* 10%. Primarily supports hospitals. *Religion:* 4%. Funds a science center. *Note:* Total foundation contributions made in fiscal 2000. **Typ. Recipients:** Cancer, Children's Health/Hospitals, Clinics/Medical Centers, Emergency/Ambulance Services, Health Organizations, Hospitals, Medical Research, People with Disabilities, Prenatal Health Issues, Single-Disease Health Associations, Substance Abuse, Transplant Networks/Donor Banks. **Geo. Dist:** headquarters and operating communities.


★ **1407** ★ **Stanley Works**
1000 Stanley Dr.
New Britain, CT 06053
**Phone:** (860)827-3566 **Fax:** (860)827-3581
**Email:** plevenson@stanley.com
**Website:** http://www.stanleyworks.com

**Typ. Recipients:** Cancer, Children's Health/Hospitals, Emergency/Ambulance Services, Hospitals, Medical Research, People with Disabilities, Substance Abuse. **Geo. Dist:** operating location communities.


★ **1408** ★ **Star Bank NA, Cincinnati
Foundation**
777 E Wisconsin Ave.
Milwaukee, WI 53202
**Phone:** (414)765-5717 **Fax:** (414)765-6111
Jennie Carlson, Contact

**Priorities:** *Arts & Humanities:* 13%. Supports fine and performing arts and museums. *Civic & Public Affairs:* 15%. Supports chambers of commerce, community foundations, and housing. *Education:* 17%. Funds higher education and junior achievement. *Environment:* 46%. Supports youth groups and organizations, including scouts, sports groups, and Boys and Girls Clubs. Also funds organizations dealing with chemical dependency and the United Way. *International:* 6%. Funds hospitals and homecare services. *Note:* Contributions made in 1999. **Typ. Recipients:** Cancer, Children's Health/Hospitals, Clinics/Medical Centers, Eyes/Blindness, Health Organizations, Heart, Home-Care Services, Hospitals, Long-Term Care, Medical Education, Medical Research, People with Disabilities,

Single-Disease Health Associations. **Geo. Dist:** IN, prefabricated; KY; OH.


★ **1409** ★ **Starwood Hotels & Resorts
Worldwide, Inc.**
1111 Westchester Ave.
White Plains, NY 10604
**Phone:** (914)640-8198 **Fax:** (914)640-8134
**Email:** Katherine.Condits@starwoodhotels.com
**Website:** http://www.starwoodhotels.com
Katherine Condits, Senior Vice President Corporate Affairs

**Priorities:** *Arts & Humanities:* Supports a variety of local arts groups, centers, and funds. Also supports museums and public broadcasting. *Civic & Public Affairs:* Sponsors awards and assistance program to recognize and support ideas for local civic improvement. Also supports civil rights and minority affairs groups and urban affairs organizations. *Education:* Highest priority. Areas of interest include independent and minority college funds, business education, and education associations. Also supports programs in creative management and computer technology. Administers matching gifts program. *Environment:* Emphasis on youth programs. Also supports organizations concerned with the disabled, emergency relief, alcohol and drug abuse, the aged, community service, and delinquency and crime. *International:* Supports a variety of medical research programs, as well as hospitals and other health organizations. **Typ. Recipients:** Domestic Violence, Emergency/Ambulance Services, Geriatric Health, Hospices, Medical Research, Nutrition, People with Disabilities, Single-Disease Health Associations, Substance Abuse. **Geo. Dist:** headquarters and operating communities.


★ **1410** ★ **State Street Foundation**
225 Franklin St.
Boston, MA 02110-2804
**Phone:** (617)664-3381 **Fax:** (617)451-6315
**Email:** gabowman@statestreet.com
George Bowman, Jr., Vice President, Community Affairs

**Priorities:** *Arts & Humanities:* 12%. *Civic & Public Affairs:* 31%. Supports initiatives to increase housing availability for low and moderate income persons and make their neighborhoods safer, more prosperous places to live and work. *Education:* 24%. Supports initiatives to improve educational quality and opportunities for students in areas where State Street has operations. Funds programs that help students succeed and prepare for advancement to higher education, and that increase jobs and job opportunities. Funds adult/family literacy and job skills training and development initiatives that help prepare under-employed and displaced workers to participate successfully in the changing workforce. *Environment:* 23%. Supports initiatives addressing high school dropout prevention and teen pregnancy and parenting issues; major support for the United Way. *International:* 9%. *Note:* Total contributions in 1998. **Typ. Recipients:** Adolescent Health Issues, AIDS/HIV, Cancer, Child Abuse, Children's Health/Hospitals, Clinics/Medical Centers, Diabetes, Domestic Violence, Eyes/Blindness, Geriatric Health, Health Funds, Health Organizations, Health Policy/Cost Containment, Hospitals, Medical Education, Medical Rehabilitation, Mental Health, People with Disabilities, Public Health. **Geo. Dist:** Boston, MA, including surrounding communities.


★ **1411** ★ **Stauffer Communications
Foundation**
616 Southeast Jefferson
Topeka, KS 66607
**Phone:** (785)295-1111 **Fax:** (785)295-1144
Stan Stauffer, Chairman

**Priorities:** *Arts & Humanities:* 19%. Primarily for the literary arts. *Civic & Public Affairs:* 38%. Support for a community foundation, philanthropic organizations, public policy groups, and civil rights causes. *Education:* 17%. Colleges and universities, medical education, public and private secondary education, and

vocational education. *Environment:* 15%. Community centers, YM/YWCAs, scouting, child welfare, and youth organizations. *Religion:* 8%. *Note:* Total contributions made in 1998. **Typ. Recipients:** Alzheimers Disease, Cancer, Child Abuse, Children's Health/Hospitals, Clinics/Medical Centers, Emergency/Ambulance Services, Health Organizations, Hospitals, Medical Education, People with Disabilities. **Geo. Dist:** KS; OK.


★ **1412** ★ **Steelcase Foundation**
PO Box 1967
Location CH-4E
Grand Rapids, MI 49501-1967
**Phone:** (616)246-4695 **Fax:** (616)475-2200
**Email:** sbroman@steelcase.com
Susan Broman, Executive Director

**Priorities:** *Arts & Humanities:* 13%. Supports theaters, ballet, museums, and arts centers. The Grand Rapids symphony is a major recipient. *Civic & Public Affairs:* 25%. Supports community and economic development programs. *Education:* 17%. Funds colleges, universities, and higher education foundations. Company also matches employee gifts to education. *Environment:* 40%. Supports child welfare and family services primarily. *International:* 1%. *Note:* Total contributions in 1999. **Typ. Recipients:** AIDS/HIV, Child Abuse, Children's Health/Hospitals, Clinics/Medical Centers, Domestic Violence, Emergency/Ambulance Services, Family Planning, Geriatric Health, Health Organizations, Health Policy/Cost Containment, Hospices, Medical Rehabilitation, Mental Health, Nutrition, People with Disabilities, Prenatal Health Issues, Public Health, Single-Disease Health Associations, Substance Abuse. **Geo. Dist:** communities in which company has manufacturing operations: AL: Athens,CA: Tustin, MI: Grand Rapids, NC: Fletcher, ON: Markham.


★ **1413** ★ **Stonecutter Foundation**
Dallas St.
PO Box 157
Spindale, NC 28160
**Phone:** (828)286-2341
Van Lonon, Staff Assistant

**Priorities:** *Civic & Public Affairs:* 7%. Employee legal affairs, economic development, and housing. *Education:* 83%. Emphasis on colleges and universities and private secondary education. *Environment:* 3%. Focus on scouting, the United Way, and crime prevention. *International:* 2%. Hospices and medical research. *Note:* Total foundation contributions made in fiscal 2001. **Typ. Recipients:** Domestic Violence, Hospices, Hospitals, Medical Research. **Geo. Dist:** NC.


★ **1414** ★ **StorageTek Foundation**
2270 S 88th St., MS-4341
Louisville, CO 80028-4310
**Phone:** (303)673-6833 **Fax:** (303)673-8876
**Website:** http://www.storagetek.com/about_us/foundation/
Arlyce Lewis, Manager, Community Relations

**Priorities:** *Arts & Humanities:* 8%. Supports orchestras, outreach programs, arts education, and children's programs. Supports projects that extend cultural opportunities that benefit a broad population base and enhance the quality of life. *Education:* 29%. Supports Junior Achievement, scholarships, leadership and outreach programs, women and minority engineering programs, computer labs and networking, educational media, matching gifts, and Boulder Valley public schools. Focus is on innovative programs that strengthen the educational process in the areas of science, math, engineering, management, and technology. Supports literacy, including computer literacy and reading skills. *Environment:* 61%. Support includes health and human services. Major support to the YMCA in Boulder, CO. *Voluntarism:* Employees actively volunteer for a variety of corporate-sponsored activities, including Meals on Wheels, Boy Scouts, community hospitals, food banks, high schools and elementary schools, 4-H clubs, and wildlife and rescue groups. The company initiated the Volunteers in Partnership with the Community (VIP.COM) program in 1998. The program not only encourages employees to volunteer commitments, but also generates additional funds from the company for nonprofit organizations to which employees dedicate time. *Note:* Total contributions made in 1998. **Typ. Recipients:** Arthritis, Cancer, Children's Health/Hospitals, Clinics/Medical Centers, Domestic Violence, Emergency/Ambulance Services, Health Funds, Health Organizations, Health-General, Heart, Hospices, Hospitals, Medical Rehabilitation, Mental Health, Multiple Sclerosis, Nutrition, People with Disabilities, Public Health, Single-Disease Health Associations, Substance Abuse, Transplant Networks/Donor Banks. **Geo. Dist:** headquarters area only.

**★ 1415 ★  Strear Family Foundation**
6825 E Tennessee Ave., Ste. 235
Denver, CO 80224
**Phone:** (303)399-4631        **Fax:** (303)388-9125
Leonard Strear, Chairman, President & Chief
  Executive Of
**Fnded:** 1987. **Priorities:** *Arts & Humanities:* 3%. Supports arts leagues, history, libraries, and public broadcasting. *Civic & Public Affairs:* 10%. Supports zoos, cemeteries, and botanical gardens. *Education:* 4%. Supports schools. *Environment:* 5%. Supports food banks, Special Olympics, and family planning services. *International:* 8%. Supports cancer research and treatment, hospice, and hospitals. *Note:* Total foundation contributions made in fiscal 2000. **Typ. Recipients:** Cancer, Children's Health/Hospitals, Diabetes, Hospices, Hospitals, Medical Research, People with Disabilities, Speech & Hearing, Substance Abuse. **Geo. Dist:** CO.

**★ 1416 ★  Stride Rite Foundation**
Review Committee
400 Atlantic Ave.
Boston, MA 02110
**Phone:** (617)574-4169        **Fax:** (617)574-6595
Ellen Sahl, Contact
**Fnded:** 1953. **Priorities:** *Arts & Humanities:* 1%. Grants often support museums, art centers, theater, dance, operas, and symphonies. *Civic & Public Affairs:* 22%. Recipients include civic and public affairs groups and community organizations. Supports other grant-making foundations. *Education:* 27%. Majority of funding supports precollege education. *Environment:* 48%. Supports United Way, Big Brothers/Big Sisters, and children and family social service organizations. Recipients also include child recreational groups, including volunteer groups and community centers. *Note:* Total foundation contributions made in fiscal 2000. **Typ. Recipients:** Cancer, Child Abuse, Children's Health/Hospitals, Clinics/Medical Centers, Diabetes, Hospitals, Nursing Services, People with Disabilities, Prenatal Health Issues, Public Health, Substance Abuse. **Geo. Dist:** operating locations; Boston, MA; Cambridge, MA.

**★ 1417 ★  Stupp Brothers Bridge & Iron Co. Foundation**
120 S Central Ave., Ste. 1650
Saint Louis, MO 63105
**Phone:** (314)638-5000        **Fax:** (314)721-6334
Robert Stupp, Trustee
**Priorities:** *Arts & Humanities:* 2%. Supports and arts fund. *Civic & Public Affairs:* 12%. Primarily supports Operation P.R.I.D.E. Zoos, parks, botanical gardens, and specialized foundations also received support. *Education:* 39%. Colleges, universities, and secondary schools received support, as well as education funds and foundations. *Environment:* 23%. Major support is given to the United Way. Other interests include traditional youth organizations, community service groups, and child welfare. *International:* 19%. Funds children's hospitals, hospice, and health care concerns. *Note:* Total foundation contributions made in fiscal 2000. **Typ. Recipients:** Cancer, Children's Health/Hospitals, Family Planning, Health Organizations, Hospices, Hospitals, Medical Research, People with Disabilities, Public Health, Single-Disease Health Associations, Substance Abuse. **Geo. Dist:** MO.

**★ 1418 ★  Sun Microsystems Foundation, Inc.**
Mail Stop PAL1-462
901 San Antonio Rd.
Palo Alto, CA 94303
**Phone:** (650)336-0545        **Fax:** (650)856-2114
**Email:** corpaffr@corp.sun.com
**Website:** http://www.sun.com/aboutsun/comm_invest/giving/foundation.html
Gary Serda, President, Executive Director
**Fnded:** 1990. **Priorities:** *Arts & Humanities:* Less than 1%. *Civic & Public Affairs:* 11%. Supports the Sun Training and Employment Program (STEP) for Solaris. The goal of the program is to give people in low-income and underrepresented communities the chance to participate in the "Net economy." STEP grants are available on an invitation-only basis. Foundation supports projects that close the gap in the current employment development system; projects which help reverse conditions of high unemployment and low income; provide job placement and counseling; work closely with the industry; and provide training for occupations that are in high demand. *Education:* 18%. Supports 7-12 education which prepares young people for the workforce and for lifelong learning. Supported programs incorporate target population's needs and interests; programs designed to increase education; projects that reverse unsatisfactory academic school performance; engage students in activities that enable them to make experiential connections between learning and real life; foster motivation and improve academic skills; and improve college readiness. Overall goals for education giving include increased enrollment in college preparatory courses; heightened interest in high-tech careers; improved achievement in mathematics, science, engineering, and computer-related courses; and higher enrollment in 4-year colleges or universities. The Open Gateways Program focuses on providing Sun products and teacher professional development through partnerships with K-12 schools. Also supports higher education through equipment donations, collaborative and sponsored research; and university affiliate programs. *International:* Less than 1%. *Voluntarism:* Sun Microsystem's Community Action Volunteer Program provides employees with a wide range of volunteer opportunities. Through the Open Gateways program, employees volunteer to provide technical support and training for schools and teachers to make meaningful use of technology in the classroom. The Community Partnership Program provides financial support for organizations where employees volunteer; the company and organization form a year-long partnership. Employee volunteers also participate in the Sun Foundation's grant review process. Worldwide Volunteer Week allows for more concentrated efforts by company volunteers. *Note:* Total foundation contributions made in fiscal 2000. **Typ. Recipients:** AIDS/HIV, AIDS/HIV, Cancer, Children's Health/Hospitals, Emergency/Ambulance Services, Heart, Hospitals, People with Disabilities. **Geo. Dist:** South San Francisco, CA, Bay Area; Denver, CO, the Front Page Communities (up to and including Longmont); MA, Merrimack Valley; West Lothian District.

**★ 1419 ★  SunTrust Bank Atlanta Foundation**
Mail Code 041
PO Box 4418, Mail Code 041
Atlanta, GA 30302
**Phone:** (404)588-8246        **Fax:** (404)230-5550
William Bowdoin, Jr., First Vice President/Secretary
**Priorities:** *Arts & Humanities:* 19%. Supports major Atlanta arts organizations and centers through direct grants and arts funds. Interests include dance, history, and public broadcasting. *Civic & Public Affairs:* 10%. Interests include urban and community affairs, economic development, municipalities, philanthropic organizations, botanical gardens, and zoos. *Education:* 18%. Primarily supports colleges and universities. Private schools are also major recipients, including religious institutions. The remainder supports business and economic education, minority education, international studies, and secondary education. Also sponsors matching gifts program. *Environment:* 49%. Supports human service organizations primarily through the United Way of Metropolitan Atlanta. Other interests include youth organizations, child welfare, community service organizations, family services, and recreation and athletics. *International:* Less than 1%. *Religion:* 1%. *Note:* Total foundation contributions made in 2000. **Typ. Recipients:** Alzheimers Disease, Children's Health/Hospitals, Clinics/Medical Centers, Domestic Violence, Emergency/Ambulance Services, Geriatric Health, Health Organizations, Hospitals, Medical Education, Medical Rehabilitation, Medical Training, Mental Health, Nursing Services, People with Disabilities, Public Health, Single-Disease Health Associations, Substance Abuse. **Geo. Dist:** Atlanta, GA, metropolitan area.

**★ 1420 ★  SunTrust Banks Foundation**
PO Box 3838
Orlando, FL 32802
David Hanson, Contact
**Priorities:** *Civic & Public Affairs:* 20%. Funds a statewide leadership organization and a zoo. *Education:* 14%. Supports an educational foundation and Florida community colleges. *Environment:* 9%. Funds services for families, youth, and the disabled. *International:* 57%. Supports Florida medical centers and hospitals. *Note:* Total contributions made in 2000. **Typ. Recipients:** Cancer, Clinics/Medical Centers, Hospitals, People with Disabilities, Substance Abuse. **Geo. Dist:** FL.

**★ 1421 ★  Susquehanna-Pfaltzgraff Foundation**
140 East Market St.
York, PA 17401
**Phone:** (717)848-5500        **Fax:** (717)771-1440
John Finlayson, Vice President, Finance &
  Administration
**Fnded:** 1966. **Priorities:** *Arts & Humanities:* 17%. Supports museums, theaters, and historical societies. *Civic & Public Affairs:* 22%. Funds community foundations. *Education:* 16%. Funds colleges, minority education, and private primary and secondary schools. *Environment:* 34%. Supports the United Way, youth organizations, Make a Difference conferences, and YMCAs. *International:* 2%. Supports a hospital. *Note:* Total contributions made in 1998. **Typ. Recipients:** Cancer, Children's Health/Hospitals, Children's Health/Hospitals, Eyes/Blindness, Health-General, Hospitals, People with Disabilities, Public Health, Single-Disease Health Associations. **Geo. Dist:** headquarters and operating communities.

**★ 1422 ★  Sverdrup Corp. Charitable Trust**
13723 Riverport Dr.
Maryland Heights, MO 63043
**Phone:** (314)466-3439
Thomas Wehrle, Treasurer
**Fnded:** 1951. **Priorities:** *Arts & Humanities:* 23%. Supports performing arts and arts councils. *Civic & Public Affairs:* 14%. Funds professional trade organizations, county fairs, and the Better Business Bureau. *Education:* 33%. Supports scholarship funds, colleges and universities, technical and engineering education, and Junior Achievement. *Environment:* 24%. Supports the United Way and Goodwill Industries. *International:* Less than 1%. Supports Race for the Cure. *Note:* Total contributions made in 2000. **Typ. Recipients:** Cancer, Children's Health/Hospitals, People with Disabilities, Single-Disease Health Associations. **Geo. Dist:** nationally; Saint Louis, MO.

**Synetic Foundation**
*See:* Entry 5589

**★ 1423 ★  Synovus Charitable Trust**
PO Box 120
Columbus, GA 31902
**Phone:** (706)649-2679        **Fax:** (706)649-5986
William Slaughter, Contact

**Priorities:** *Arts & Humanities:* 1%. Funds museums and historical preservation. *Civic & Public Affairs:* 9%. Supports community affairs and development, parks and gardens. *Education:* 14%. Supports higher education. *Environment:* 59%. Funding supports United Way, youth organizations, recreation, and family services. *International:* 9%. Contributions favor medical centers and community-focused health organizations. *Note:* Total foundation contributions made in 2000. **Typ. Recipients:** Alzheimers Disease, Cancer, Child Abuse, Children's Health/Hospitals, Clinics/Medical Centers, Domestic Violence, Emergency/Ambulance Services, Eyes/Blindness, Family Planning, Geriatric Health, Health Organizations, Health-General, Heart, Hospices, Hospitals, Long-Term Care, Medical Education, Medical Rehabilitation, Mental Health, Multiple Sclerosis, Outpatient Health Care, Single-Disease Health Associations, Substance Abuse. **Geo. Dist:** Columbus, GA.

### ★ 1424 ★ T. Rowe Price Associates Foundation
100 E Pratt St., 8th Fl.
Baltimore, MD 21202
**Phone:** (410)345-3603          **Fax:** (410)345-2848
Albert Hubbard, Jr., Program Director

**Priorities:** *Arts & Humanities:* 32%. Supports theaters, museums, galleries, music, art associations, and historic preservation. *Civic & Public Affairs:* 18%. Funds public policy, environmental affairs, and urban and community affairs. *Education:* 31%. Supports colleges and universities, public and private schools for precollege education, art education, business education, literacy, after-school and summer education programs, education scholarship funds and minority education. *Environment:* (Health and Human Services) 20%. Supports United Way chapters, community and family service organizations, child welfare, shelters for abused women and children, food distribution, mentoring programs for at-risk children, homeless shelters, single-disease health organizations, blood banks, Make-a-Wish, and health and wellness organizations. *Note:* Total contributions in 2000. **Typ. Recipients:** Child Abuse, Emergency/Ambulance Services, Health Organizations, Heart, Hospitals, Mental Health, People with Disabilities, Single-Disease Health Associations. **Geo. Dist:** headquarters and operating communities.

### ★ 1425 ★ Target Foundation
1000 Nicollet Mall, TPS-3080
Minneapolis, MN 55403
**Phone:** (612)696-6098          **Fax:** (612)696-5088
**Email:** bridget.mcginnis@target.com
**Website:** http://www.targetfoundation.org
Bridget McGinnis, Associate Specialist

**Fnded:** 1918. **Priorities:** *Arts & Humanities:* 15%. Supports professional nonprofit arts organizations in all disciplines. Typically supported are arts centers and museums, public broadcasting, orchestras and opera, theater, and children's arts organizations. support professional nonprofit arts institutions and/or individual artists, and whose services are integral to the continued well-being of the arts fields they serve. *Civic & Public Affairs:* 21%. Supports community volunteer resources, chambers of commerce, economic and neighborhood development, minority affairs, immigrant services, job training, nonprofit management, public parks/playgrounds, and other civic interests. *Education:* 33%. Funds scholarship funds, colleges and universities, primary school programs, and literacy initiatives. *Environment:* 17%. Supports the United Way, youth and family services, prevention of child abuse, disaster relief, and recreation programs. *International:* 13%. Funds hospitals, medical centers, and camps for children with cancer and terminal illnesses and single-disease health organizations. *Voluntarism:* Each division of the company has its own volunteer program. Company-wide, Target Corp. jointly sponsors "Day of Giving" in the spring/summer. *Note:* Total contributions made in fiscal 2000. Target stores (Mervyn's California, Target, Dayton's, Hudson's, and Marshall Field's) also support giving programs. **Typ. Recipients:** AIDS/HIV, Children's Health/Hospitals, Domestic Violence, Family Planning, Health Organiza-

tions, People with Disabilities, Research/Studies Institutes. **Geo. Dist:** Minneapolis, MN; Saint Paul, MN. **Frmly:** Dayton Hudson Corporate.

### ★ 1426 ★ TCF Foundation
200 Lake St. East (EXO-02-T)
Wayzata, MN 55391-1693
**Phone:** (952)745-2755          **Fax:** (952)745-2775
**Email:** ksack@mailbox1.tcfbank.com
Kelly Sack, Contact

**Priorities:** *Civic & Public Affairs:* 11%. Supports employment initiatives. *Environment:* 89%. Supports YMCA. *Voluntarism:* The company encourages employee volunteerism through local divisions, including programs such as March of Dimes, paint-a-thons, and home-repair days. *Note:* Total foundation contributions made in 2000. **Typ. Recipients:** Children's Health/Hospitals, Clinics/Medical Centers, Health Funds, Health Organizations, Health-General, Heart, Hospitals, Medical Rehabilitation, Public Health, Substance Abuse. **Geo. Dist:** headquarters and operating communities.

### ★ 1427 ★ Teleflex Foundation
630 West Germantown Pike, Ste. 461
Plymouth Meeting, PA 19462
**Phone:** (610)831-6301
Thelma Fretz, Executive Director

**Priorities:** *Arts & Humanities:* 4%. Funds a children's museum and a musical concert series. *Civic & Public Affairs:* 32%. Supports zoos, women's affairs, public safety, community foundations, career training, and free enterprise. *Education:* 27%. Funds major universities, private precollege schools, and Junior Achievement. *Environment:* 19%. Supports youth organizations, substance abuse education, child welfare, food banks, senior services, volunteer corps, Special Olympics, and animal welfare. *International:* 11%. Supports hospice, children's health, burn treatment, poison control, hospitals, and single-disease associations. *Note:* Total contributions made in 2000. **Typ. Recipients:** Children's Health/Hospitals, Health-General, Hospices, Nursing Services, People with Disabilities, Public Health, Single-Disease Health Associations, Substance Abuse. **Geo. Dist:** headquarters and operating communities.

### ★ 1428 ★ Temple-Inland Foundation
303 South Temple Dr.
Diboll, TX 75941
**Phone:** (936)829-7950
M. Warner, Vice President

**Priorities:** *Arts & Humanities:* 16%. Under the Arts program area, the foundation supports libraries, historical societies, public broadcasting, performing arts, and art museums/centers. Also funds civic groups, community programs, and environmental and nature programs under the foundation's Cultural program area. *Education:* 58%. Supports institutions of higher learning and private schools, and provides scholarships for children of company employees. *International:* 26%. Funds single-disease health associations, services for the disabled, medical research organizations, child welfare initiatives, and recreational youth programs that contribute to healthy growth. *Note:* Total contributions made in fiscal 2000. Grant awards comprise 55% to 60% of total foundation giving; employee scholarships and other scholastic awards, 20% to 25%; and matching gifts, 15% to 20%. **Typ. Recipients:** Cancer, Children's Health/Hospitals, Clinics/Medical Centers, Health Organizations, Hospices, Hospitals, Medical Research, People with Disabilities, Substance Abuse. **Geo. Dist:** headquarters.

### ★ 1429 ★ Tenet Healthcare Foundation
PO Box 31907
Santa Barbara, CA 93105-1907
**Phone:** (805)563-6845          **Fax:** (805)898-9104
**Email:** foundation@tenethealth.com
Barbara Luton, Executive Director

**Priorities:** *Arts & Humanities:* 2%. Provides some support for arts organizations. *Civic & Public Affairs:*

6%. Funds civic and community organizations. *Education:* 26%. Funding goes to general education programs and to programs leading to careers in medicine, nursing, or health care administration; institutions that train future health care professionals, and provide continuing education of health care professionals; and programs to support advancement and improvement of health care education. *Environment:* 14%. Funds human service programs and United Way. *International:* 51%. Majority of support goes to health care projects and programs, including organizations that improve the efficiency of the healthcare delivery system; organizations that promote individual and community education in health; organizations and institutions the develop medical research programs, publications, conferences and seminars; organizations that seek to develop cures for debilitating diseases and conditions; and human service programs that benefit the aging, the handicapped, and persons unable to obtain adequate medical care. *Note:* Total contributions made in fiscal 2001. **Typ. Recipients:** Health Organizations, Medical Education, Medical Research, Medical Training, Mental Health, Nursing Services, People with Disabilities, Single-Disease Health Associations. **Geo. Dist:** principally near operating locations and to national organizations.

### ★ 1430 ★ TENNANT Co. Foundation
PO Box 1452
Minneapolis, MN 55440
**Phone:** (612)540-1240          **Fax:** (612)540-1616
**Email:** carol.vanlith@tennantco.com
Carol A. Van Lith, Secretary/Administrator

**Fnded:** 1973. **Priorities:** *Arts & Humanities:* 17%. Supports Minneapolis/St. Paul area arts organizations. Interests include the performing arts, opera, music, and public broadcasting. *Civic & Public Affairs:* 8%. Supports youth organizations, housing, shelters, neighborhood improvement projects, citizens groups, and women's issues. *Education:* 4%. Supports public and private higher education and education organizations. Company also sponsors a scholarship program for eligible children of employees. *Environment:* 54%. Supports learning disabilities, children services, YMCA, food for the hungry, and the United Way. *Voluntarism:* The Volunteer Gift-Matching Program was established to recognize the volunteer work of company employees. The program matches 40 hours or more per year of volunteer hours to a single agency with a $200 gift, if that agency would otherwise be eligible for foundation grants. In 1997, the program supported over 850 hours of volunteer work by TENNANT employees. *Note:* Total foundation contributions made in 2000. **Typ. Recipients:** Clinics/Medical Centers, Domestic Violence, Family Planning, Health Organizations, Health Policy/Cost Containment, Medical Rehabilitation, Mental Health, People with Disabilities, Single-Disease Health Associations, Substance Abuse. **Geo. Dist:** headquarters and operating communities.

### ★ 1431 ★ Tenneco Automotive, Inc.
500 North Field Dr.
Lake Forest, IL 60045
**Phone:** (847)482-5000          **Fax:** (847)482-5940
**Website:** http://www.tenneco-automotive.com
Jane Ostrander, Corporate Communications

**Typ. Recipients:** Emergency/Ambulance Services, Health Organizations, Hospices, Hospitals, Medical Research, Mental Health, Nutrition, People with Disabilities, Single-Disease Health Associations, Substance Abuse. **Geo. Dist:** headquarters and operating communities.

### ★ 1432 ★ Tension Envelope Foundation
819 East 19th St., 3rd Floor
Kansas City, MO 64108
**Phone:** (816)471-3800          **Fax:** (816)283-1498
Eliot Berkley, Secretary

**Fnded:** 1954. **Priorities:** *Arts & Humanities:* 4%. Museums, public broadcasting, symphonies and theaters are supported. *Civic & Public Affairs:* 22%. Supports housing, community foundations, crime prevention, industry/professional organizations, botanical gardens, and neighborhood and economic development. *Education:* 15%. Primarily supports child development, colleges, and universities. *Environment:* 23%. Funds the United Way, and family and youth services. *International:* Less than 1%. Funds mental health services, the Alzheimer's Association, and health foundations. *Note:* Total contributions in fiscal 2000. **Typ. Recipients:** Clinics/Medical Centers, Domestic Violence, Family Planning, Health Organizations, Hospices, Hospitals, Mental Health, People with Disabilities, Public Health, Substance Abuse. **Geo. Dist:** MO.

**★ 1433 ★ Texas Instruments Foundation**
PO Box 650311, M/S 3906
Dallas, TX 75265
**Phone:** (972)917-4505　　　**Fax:** (972)917-4583
**Website:** http://www.ti.com/corp/docs/company/citizen/index.shtml
Ann Minnis, Grants Administrator
**Priorities:** *Arts & Humanities:* 2%. Funds performing arts, music and cultural centers. *Civic & Public Affairs:* 1%. Funds minority affairs, job training programs, zoos, and arboretums. *Education:* 76%. Supports educational programs, colleges and universities. *Environment:* 21%. Major support given to United Way; also supports child welfare, youth organizations, and drug abuse treatment. *Religion:* Less than 1%. Supports science museums. *Note:* Total foundation contributions made in 2000. **Typ. Recipients:** Clinics/Medical Centers, Hospitals, Hospitals (University Affiliated), Medical Education, Medical Research, Nursing Services, People with Disabilities, Research/Studies Institutes, Substance Abuse. **Geo. Dist:** nationally; TX, emphasis on Texas-based organizations; Dallas, TX.

**★ 1434 ★ Textron Charitable Trust**
40 Westmintster St.
Providence, RI 02903
**Phone:** (401)457-2430　　　**Fax:** (401)457-3598
Ellie Weston, Contributions Coordinator
**Priorities:** *Arts & Humanities:* 13%. Funds the arts centers and music receive primarysupport. Other interests include arts associations, dance, historical preservation and restoration, and museums and galleries. Also includes matching gifts to arts institutions and organizations. *Civic & Public Affairs:* 8%. Organizations involved in civil rights, women's issues and urban development. *Education:* 46%. Majority of funding consists of matching grants. Substantial amounts also support student aid organizations, such as the National Merit Scholarship program and College Scholarship Service. Limited support goes to colleges, universities, and minority education. *Environment:* 10%. Support typically includes scouting organizations, youth employment services, and YMCA/YWCAs and united funds. *International:* 22%. Hospitals receive the largest amount of health care funds, through both general support and matching grants. Health organizations, single-disease health associations, hospices, and pediatric health also are supported. **Typ. Recipients:** Cancer, Children's Health/Hospitals, Emergency/Ambulance Services, Family Planning, Health Organizations, Health Policy/Cost Containment, Hospices, Hospitals, Medical Education, Medical Rehabilitation, People with Disabilities, Prenatal Health Issues, Single-Disease Health Associations, Substance Abuse. **Geo. Dist:** headquarters and operating communities.

**★ 1435 ★ Thomasville Furniture Industries Foundation**
PO Box 339
Thomasville, NC 27360
**Phone:** (336)472-4000　　　**Fax:** (336)472-4085
**Email:** vholder@thomasville.com
Vickie Holder, General Manager
**Fnded:** 1960. **Priorities:** *Arts & Humanities:* 1%. Supports a memorial monument. *Education:* 9%. Provides scholarships for higher education and gives to elementary schools. *Environment:* 78%. Major support is awarded to United Way and Young Men's Christian Association. *International:* 11%. Gives to hospitals. *Voluntarism:* Thomasville employees volunteer in Communities in Schools and Chamber programs and in local school systems and YMCA's. *Note:* Total contributions made in 2000. **Typ. Recipients:** Emergency/Ambulance Services, Hospitals, Medical Research. **Geo. Dist:** NC.

**★ 1436 ★ 3M Foundation**
3M Community Affairs
591-30-02 3M Ctr.
Saint Paul, MN 55144-1000
**Phone:** (651)733-0144　　　**Fax:** (651)737-3061
**Email:** cfkleven@mmm.com
**Website:** http://www.3M.com/profile/community
Cynthia Kleven, Manager Contributions
**Fnded:** 1953. **Priorities:** *Arts & Humanities:* 7%. Supports arts organizations with emphasis on educational achievement and also community outreach programs. *Civic & Public Affairs:* 7%. Supports local initiatives in 3M communities. *Education:* 54%. Supports elementary through graduate education, where science, technology, and business are targeted educational areas. K-12 programs focus on programs that stimulate student interest and achievement. Teacher training is also an area of support. *International:* (Health and Human Services) 32%. Especially interested in programs that support families and have an emphasis on youth development, including parenting skills and employment training. Health care initiatives are supporting patient safety issues. *Voluntarism:* Through 3M GIVES (Grants Initiated by Volunteer Service), the company donates $200 to each employee or retiree volunteer's qualifying non-profit organization, matching 25 hours of volunteer service. The company also sponsors the 3M Community Volunteer Award, which annually recognizes 25 of the company's outstanding employee and retiree volunteers with a $1,000 donation to a qualified nonprofit organization of each winner's choice. *Note:* Total contributions made in 2000. **Typ. Recipients:** Clinics/Medical Centers, Domestic Violence, Emergency/Ambulance Services, Geriatric Health, Health Organizations, Health Policy/Cost Containment, Hospices, Hospitals, Medical Education, Medical Rehabilitation, Mental Health, People with Disabilities, Public Health, Substance Abuse, Transplant Networks/Donor Banks. **Geo. Dist:** headquarters and operating communities.

**★ 1437 ★ Ticketmaster Foundation**
3701 Wilshire Blvd., 7th Floor
Los Angeles, CA 90010
**Phone:** (310)360-6000　　　**Fax:** (310)383-8714
Claire Rothman, Executive Vice President & General Manag
**Fnded:** 1994. **Priorities:** *Arts & Humanities:* 25%. Funds museums, art institutes, and music centers. *Civic & Public Affairs:* 24%. Funds civic and community foundations. *Education:* 13%. Funds universities, colleges, and learning centers. *Environment:* 5%. Supports Big Brother/Big Sisters, US Olympic Committee, and United Way. *International:* 10%. Funds health centers, hospice, AIDS groups, single-disease health associations. *Note:* Total contributions made in 1998. **Typ. Recipients:** AIDS/HIV, Children's Health/Hospitals, Clinics/Medical Centers, Diabetes, Health Organizations, Medical Research, Multiple Sclerosis, Respiratory.

**★ 1438 ★ The Timken Co. Charitable Trust**
1835 Dueber Ave. Southwest
Canton, OH 44706
**Phone:** (330)471-4062　　　**Fax:** (330)471-4041
Mr. Ward Timken, Office of Vice President
**Priorities:** *Arts & Humanities:* 6%. Supports arts funds and historic preservation. *Civic & Public Affairs:* 13%. Supports chambers of commerce, low-income housing, community funds, and civic groups. *Education:* 33%. Funds education reform, Junior Achievement, business education, and several colleges and universities. *Environment:* 48%. Primarily funds United Way agencies in Ohio communities. *International:* Less than 1%. Supports the Alzheimer's Association. *Note:* Total contributions made in 2000. **Typ. Recipients:** Arthritis, Emergency/Ambulance Services, Health Organizations, Substance Abuse. **Geo. Dist:** communities where company operates plants, with an emphasis on Ohio.

**★ 1439 ★ Tippins Foundation**
1090 Freeport Rd.
Pittsburgh, PA 15238
**Phone:** (412)784-8804　　　**Fax:** (412)782-7210
George Tippins, Trustee
**Priorities:** *Arts & Humanities:* 13%. Funds museums, opera, theater, historical preservation, and public broadcasting. *Civic & Public Affairs:* 15%. Supports economic development, philanthropy, and parks and zoos. *Education:* 16%. Funds schools, colleges, and universities. *Environment:* 15%. Supports shelters, scouting, human service organizations, and humane societies. *International:* 34%. Funds single-disease associations, hospitals, and the American Red Cross. *Note:* Total foundation contributions made in 2000. **Typ. Recipients:** Alzheimers Disease, Arthritis, Cancer, Children's Health/Hospitals, Clinics/Medical Centers, Diabetes, Emergency/Ambulance Services, Health Organizations, Heart, Hospitals, Kidney, Medical Rehabilitation, People with Disabilities, Public Health, Single-Disease Health Associations. **Geo. Dist:** PA.

**★ 1440 ★ Titan Industrial Foundation**
555 Madison Ave., 10th Fl.
New York, NY 10022
**Phone:** (212)421-6700
Jerome Siegel, President & Treasurer
**Fnded:** 1951. **Priorities:** *Arts & Humanities:* 6%. Supports museums, art centers, and performance centers. *Civic & Public Affairs:* 3%. Gives to civil rights organizations and minority affairs. *Education:* 59%. Funds institutions of higher learning, leadership development for educators, and major support to Sarah Lawrence College. *Environment:* 16%. Supports Big Brothers/Big Sisters, volunteer programs, shelters, food banks, and YMCA. *International:* 2%. Supports hospitals and single-disease health associations. *Note:* Total contributions made in fiscal 2000. **Typ. Recipients:** AIDS/HIV, Cancer, Clinics/Medical Centers, Clinics/Medical Centers, Eyes/Blindness, Health Organizations, Hospitals, Mental Health, People with Disabilities, Research/Studies Institutes, Single-Disease Health Associations. **Geo. Dist:** NY.

**★ 1441 ★ TJX Foundation, Inc.**
770 Cochituate Rd., Route 1E
Framingham, MA 01701
**Phone:** (508)390-3199　　　**Fax:** (508)390-2091
**Email:** christy_strickland@tjx.com
**Website:** http://www.tjmaxx.com
Christine Strickland, Foundation Manager
**Priorities:** *Arts & Humanities:* 6%. Proposals that bring art or artists to new audiences; also supports initiatives that encourage people, especially the handicapped, elderly, young, or disadvantaged, to express themselves through art. *Civic & Public Affairs:* 23%. Supports programs which promote improved race relations, community development and housing. *Education:* 21%. Funds programs that benefit children of preschool age through college, which provide scholarship or vocational education for the disadvantaged; strengthen leadership in public schools; teach people to speak, read, and write English; and encourage collaboration between community agencies and schools. *Environment:* 37%. Families and children are main beneficiaries. Priority is given to programs that strengthen the family unit, help single-parent families, encourage families to adopt or accept foster children, and help the physically impaired; also funds programs that provide shelter for victims of domestics violence. *International:* 13%. Supports health care initiatives for underserved populations; seeks programs that provide early and comprehensive prenatal services, immunizations and health screening for children who lack them, and preventative care and alternatives to hospitalization. *Note:* Total contributions made in fiscal 2001. **Typ. Recipients:** AIDS/HIV, Cancer, Children's Health/Hospitals, Clinics/Medical Centers, Diabetes,

Domestic Violence, Emergency/Ambulance Services, Health Organizations, Health-General, Heart, Hospices, Hospitals, Medical Education, Medical Rehabilitation, Medical Research, Mental Health, Nursing Services, People with Disabilities, Prenatal Health Issues, Public Health, Single-Disease Health Associations, Substance Abuse. **Geo. Dist:** principally near operating locations and to national organizations; Boston, MA.

## ★ 1442 ★ Tomkins Corp. Foundation
4801 Springfield St.
Dayton, OH 45431
**Phone:** (937)476-0359          **Fax:** (937)476-0439
Greg Kirchhoff, Vice President

**Fnded:** 1989. **Priorities:** *Arts & Humanities:* 12%. Supports museums and libraries. *Civic & Public Affairs:* 3%. Gives to legal foundations and community foundations. *Education:* 34%. Aids public and private education (precollege), student aid, colleges and universities, and Junior Achievement. *Environment:* 49%. Supports the United Way, united funds, YMCAs, emergency relief services, and scouting organizations. *International:* 2%. Funds health foundations, cancer research, and juvenile diabetes. *Note:* Total contributions made in fiscal 2000, excluding matching gifts. **Typ. Recipients:** Alzheimers Disease, Cancer, Child Abuse, Children's Health/Hospitals, Clinics/Medical Centers, Diabetes, Emergency/Ambulance Services, Health Organizations, Hospices, Hospitals, Medical Research, People with Disabilities, Prenatal Health Issues, Public Health, Single-Disease Health Associations, Substance Abuse. **Geo. Dist:** Dayton, OH. **Frmly:** Philips Industries Foundation.

## ★ 1443 ★ Torchmark Corp.
2001 3rd Ave. South
Birmingham, AL 35233
**Phone:** (205)325-4243          **Fax:** (205)325-4198
**Email:** c.mccoy@torchmarkcorp.com
**Website:** http://www.torchmarkcorp.com
Carol McCoy, Associate Counsel & Secretary

**Priorities:** *Education:* About 30%. Colleges and universities. *Environment:* About 35%. United appeals in communities where home office and district offices are located. *International:* About 20%. Health organizations in the Birmingham area. **Typ. Recipients:** Health Organizations, Hospitals, Medical Rehabilitation, People with Disabilities, Single-Disease Health Associations. **Geo. Dist:** Birmingham, AL.

## ★ 1444 ★ Toyota U.S.A. Foundation
19001 South Western Ave.
Torrance, CA 90509
**Phone:** (310)618-4000          **Fax:** (310)618-7809
**Website:** http://www.toyota.com/html/about/community_care/
Gloria Jahn, Corporate Manager, Corporate Philanthrop

**Fnded:** 1987. **Priorities:** *Civic & Public Affairs:* 7%. Funds educational programs at an aquarium. *Education:* 66%. Supports science and math education at universities; math, science, and environmental precollege educational programs; and teacher development and training in math, science, and environmental curricula. *Religion:* 14%. Supports natural history and science museums. *Note:* Total foundation contributions made in fiscal 2000. **Typ. Recipients:** Health Organizations, Nutrition, People with Disabilities, Substance Abuse. **Geo. Dist:** nationally for foundation contributions; major operating facility areas for corporate contributions.

## ★ 1445 ★ Trace International Holdings, Inc. Foundation
375 Park Ave.
New York, NY 10152
**Phone:** (212)715-8619          **Fax:** (212)593-1363
Judith Hershon, Vice President

**Priorities:** *Arts & Humanities:* 22%. Major recipients include museums, libraries, dance, orchestras, and art centers. *Civic & Public Affairs:* 2%. Supports parks and chambers of commerce. *Education:* 3%. Primarily supports colleges and universities in the Northeast. Educational foundations and Junior Achievement also receive grants. *Environment:* 27%. Majority of grants made to child welfare organizations. Organizations that give aid to the homeless also receive support. *International:* 13%. Support medical research, single-disease health organizations, hospitals, and medical centers. *Note:* Total foundation contributions made in 1998. **Typ. Recipients:** Alzheimers Disease, Cancer, Children's Health/Hospitals, Clinics/Medical Centers, Emergency/Ambulance Services, Eyes/Blindness, Geriatric Health, Health Organizations, Hospitals, Hospitals (University Affiliated), Medical Education, Medical Research, People with Disabilities, Single-Disease Health Associations, Substance Abuse. **Geo. Dist:** New York, NY.

## ★ 1446 ★ Tribune New York Foundation
450 West 33rd St., 3rd Floor
New York, NY 10001
**Phone:** (212)210-2100
John Campi, Vice President, Promotions

**Fnded:** 1958. **Priorities:** *Arts & Humanities:* 63%. Supports the theater, music, dance, museums, film, and arts centers. *Civic & Public Affairs:* 14%. Funds minority and journalism interests. *Education:* 7%. Supports a college. *Environment:* 13%. Supports shelters, meals-on-wheels, and drug use prevention and rehabilitation. *Note:* Total foundation contributions made in 1999. **Typ. Recipients:** Cancer, Family Planning, Hospitals, Long-Term Care, Medical Research, People with Disabilities, Single-Disease Health Associations, Substance Abuse. **Geo. Dist:** New York, NY. **Frmly:** Daily News Foundation.

## ★ 1447 ★ True Foundation
PO Box 2360
Casper, WY 82602
**Phone:** (307)237-9301
Cherie Miller, Secretary

**Priorities:** *Civic & Public Affairs:* 16%. Funds legal aid and research, economic policy, and public policy. *Education:* 7%. Supports colleges, universities, and funds for scholarships. *Environment:* 60%. Under the foundation's Community & Social Services program area, provides support to united funds, hunger relief, children's issues, community centers, alumni associations, community arts organizations, and religious welfare organizations. *International:* 17%. Gives to medical rehabilitation centers, cancer treatment centers, and children's hospitals receive funding. *Note:* Total contributions made in fiscal 2000. **Typ. Recipients:** Alzheimers Disease, Cancer, Cancer, Children's Health/Hospitals, Clinics/Medical Centers, Diabetes, Emergency/Ambulance Services, Health Funds, Hospitals, Medical Rehabilitation, Medical Research, Public Health, Respiratory, Single-Disease Health Associations. **Geo. Dist:** WY.

## Truland Foundation
*See:* Entry 5590

## ★ 1448 ★ Trustmark Foundation
400 Field Dr.
Lake Forest, IL 60045
**Phone:** (847)615-1500          **Fax:** (847)615-5860
Warren Schreier, Trustee

**Priorities:** *Arts & Humanities:* 4%. Supports museums, festivals, and zoos. *Education:* 20%. Supports various colleges and universities, mostly within Illinois, Wisconsin, and Indiana; and programs associated with technology, finance or actuarial studies, and minority scholarships and endowments. *Environment:* 44%. Supports family and youth services, United Way and social services. *Voluntarism:* The company encourages employee volunteerism by loaning executives to the United Way and through Community IMPACT, a program in which volunteers teach seventh graders about healthy lifestyles. *Note:* Total contributions made in 2000. **Typ. Recipients:** Adolescent Health Issues, AIDS/HIV, Clinics/Medical Centers, Diabetes, Domestic Violence, Health-General, Hospices, Hospitals, Medical Research, People with Disabilities, Prenatal Health Issues, Preventive Medicine/Wellness Organizations, Sexual Abuse, Single-Disease Health Associations, Substance Abuse. **Geo. Dist:** headquarters and operating communities.

## ★ 1449 ★ TRW Foundation
1900 Richmond Rd.
Cleveland, OH 44124
**Phone:** (216)291-7160          **Fax:** (216)291-7632
**Website:** http://www.trw.com
Alan Senger, Vice President

**Priorities:** *Arts & Humanities:* 21%. Supports the performing arts, museums, theaters, arts centers, and dance and music groups. *Civic & Public Affairs:* 21%. Supports professional trade associations, economic development, and urban and community affairs. *Education:* 28%. Supports colleges and universities. Special interests include mathematics, engineering, computer science, and business administration. Also funds minority education and scholarship programs. *Environment:* 19%. Supports United Ways in company operating locations and in areas with a significant number of TRW employees. Also funds YMCA and youth organizations. *International:* 5%. Supports research institutes, emergency services, hospitals, youth organizations, and volunteer services. *Religion:* 6%. Funds science centers. *Note:* Total foundation contributions made in 2000. In addition to foundation giving, the company also makes direct grants. Foundation generally represents about 90% of the total TRW contributions program. Direct giving priorities are the same as those of the foundation. **Typ. Recipients:** Alzheimers Disease, Children's Health/Hospitals, Clinics/Medical Centers, Emergency/Ambulance Services, Health Organizations, Health Policy/Cost Containment, Hospices, Hospitals, Hospitals (University Affiliated), Medical Rehabilitation, Mental Health, People with Disabilities, Research/Studies Institutes. **Geo. Dist:** principally near operating locations and to national organizations and internationally organizations.

## ★ 1450 ★ Tyson Foundation, Inc.
2210 Oaklawn Dr.
Springdale, AR 72762-6999
**Phone:** (501)290-4955          **Fax:** (501)290-7984
**Email:** comments@tysonfoundation.org
**Website:** http://www.tysonfoundation.org
Cheryl Tyson, President

**Priorities:** *Arts & Humanities:* 3%. Funds arts centers and music. *Civic & Public Affairs:* 3%. Supports towns and fire departments. *Education:* 72%. Support goes to a large scholarship program, colleges and universities. *Environment:* 22%. Supports family services. *Note:* Total foundation contributions made in 2000. **Typ. Recipients:** Children's Health/Hospitals, Emergency/Ambulance Services, Health Organizations, Heart, Medical Education, Sexual Abuse, Single-Disease Health Associations, Substance Abuse. **Geo. Dist:** AR.

## ★ 1451 ★ Ukrop Foundation
600 Southlake Boulevard
Richmond, VA 23236
**Phone:** (804)327-7521          **Fax:** (804)379-7368
Gail Long, Assistant to the President

**Fnded:** 1983. **Priorities:** *Arts & Humanities:* 15%. Primarily supports historic preservation. *Civic & Public Affairs:* 26%. Major support to business and economic development organizations. Also supports community affairs organizations, professional organizations, cities and counties, and housing. *Education:* 28%. Funds colleges and universities, with emphasis on business education; community-school partnerships; and literacy. *Environment:* 22%. Major support goes to the United Way. Also supports recreation, athletics programs, community service organizations, and the disabled. *International:* 1%. Supports a free clinic and single-disease health associations. *Note:* Total contributions made in fiscal 1999. **Typ. Recipients:** Cancer, Clinics/Medical Centers, Emergency/Ambulance Services, Hospitals, Medical Education, Medical Research, Public Health, Single-Disease Health Associations. **Geo. Dist:** Richmond, VA.

## ★ 1452 ★ Unilever Foundation

390 Park Ave.
New York, NY 10022
**Phone:** (212)888-1260  **Fax:** (212)906-4666
**Website:** http://www.unilever.com/so/co.html
John Gould, Jr., Director, Corporate Affairs

**Fnded:** 1952. **Priorities:** *Arts & Humanities:* 5%. Supports museums, libraries, performing arts organizations, public broadcasting, and historic preservation. *Civic & Public Affairs:* 44%. Interests include community improvement, the environment, legal organizations, economic development, and public policy. *Education:* 12%. Supports school-based programs for K-12 children; scholarships for children of employees and minorities; colleges, universities and graduate schools that have research, recruiting, scholarship programs or special minority-help programs; programs that combat illiteracy; job training or retraining programs; scientific research groups whose activities are directly related to the participating companies' interests; consumer and economic research and education programs; and programs that promote free enterprise. *Environment:* 20%. Supports United Way, homeless and feeding programs; programs that address needs of minorities, the disadvantaged, and victims of domestic violence; programs for the prevention and treatment of substance abuse; youth and senior citizens groups; and organizations that are directly related to participating companies' interest. *International:* 9%. Supports hospitals and healthcare. **Note:** Total foundation contributions made in 1999. **Typ. Recipients:** Cancer, Children's Health/Hospitals, Clinics/Medical Centers, Emergency/Ambulance Services, Health Organizations, Hospitals, Medical Education, Medical Research, People with Disabilities, Single-Disease Health Associations, Substance Abuse, Trauma Treatment. **Geo. Dist:** headquarters and operating communities.

## ★ 1453 ★ Union Carbide Foundation

Corporate Center L4-507
39 Old Ridgebury Rd.
Danbury, CT 06817-0001
**Phone:** (203)794-6945
Deborah Surat, Manager, Corporate Contributions

**Priorities:** *Arts & Humanities:* 11%. Promotes museums, art centers, and libraries. *Civic & Public Affairs:* 12%. Supports public policy research, safety organizations, and diversity initiatives. *Education:* 65%. Support's public education reform and secondary and elementary programs that promote math, science, and engineering. Also funds higher education with a focus on science and engineering. Particular interest in encouraging minority students, women, and at-risk youth in engineering education and careers. *Environment:* 4%. Supports family services and programs for at-risk youth. *International:* 2%. Supports hospitals, hospice programs, and health related issues. *Religion:* 5%. Funds science centers and chemical research. *Voluntarism:* Company sponsors an employee volunteer mentoring program for children. **Note:** Total foundation contributions made in 2000. **Typ. Recipients:** Clinics/Medical Centers, Home-Care Services, Hospices, Hospitals, Medical Education, Medical Rehabilitation, People with Disabilities. **Geo. Dist:** nationally; Danbury, CT; Taft, LA; Central Area, NJ; Seadrift, TX; Texas City, TX; Kanawha Valley, WV.

## ★ 1454 ★ Union Pacific Foundation

1416 Dodge St., Room 802
Omaha, NE 68179
**Phone:** (402)271-5600  **Fax:** (402)271-5477
**Website:** http://www.up.com/found/index.htm
Darlynn Herweg, Director

**Priorities:** *Arts & Humanities:* 8%. Supports a broad range of activities and organizations with emphasis on museums and performing arts groups. Grants most often awarded for specific project support. *Education:* 29%. Support is given largely to private colleges and universities and independent college funds. Also supports a variety of programs through capital projects, annual giving funds, scholarships, and special research projects related to company business. *International:* 43%. Includes health and human services

grants. Funds hospitals for building, equipment, or project support, and supports hospices and rehabilitation facilities. United funds receive the majority of support. Also funds youth organizations and child welfare groups, as well as services for the handicapped and the disadvantaged, and a variety of other community service agencies. **Note:** Total foundation contributions made in 1999. **Typ. Recipients:** Alzheimers Disease, Cancer, Children's Health/Hospitals, Clinics/Medical Centers, Domestic Violence, Emergency/Ambulance Services, Health Organizations, Hospices, Hospitals, Long-Term Care, Medical Rehabilitation, Medical Research, Mental Health, People with Disabilities, Prenatal Health Issues, Public Health, Substance Abuse. **Geo. Dist:** AR; CA; CO; DE; Washington, DC; FL; GA; ID; IL; IN; IA; KS; LA; MD; MI; MN; MS; MT; NE; NV; NJ; NM; NY; NC; OH; OK; OR; PA; TN; TX; UT; VA; WA; WI.

## ★ 1455 ★ United Co. Charitable Foundation

PO Box 1280
Bristol, VA 24203
**Phone:** (540)466-3322  **Fax:** (540)645-1427
William Miller, Vice President, Marketing & Communicatio

**Fnded:** 1986. **Priorities:** *Arts & Humanities:* 5%. Supports arts centers and museums. *Civic & Public Affairs:* 3%. Funds community foundations. *Education:* 63%. Supports colleges and universities. *Environment:* 7%. Supports YMCAs and youth organizations. *International:* 3%. Supports clinics and health foundations. **Note:** Total contributions made in 2000. **Typ. Recipients:** Cancer, Clinics/Medical Centers. **Geo. Dist:** VA.

## ★ 1456 ★ United Dominion Foundation

2300 One First Union Center
Charlotte, NC 28202
**Phone:** (704)347-6800  **Fax:** (704)347-6900
William Holland, President

**Priorities:** *Arts & Humanities:* 38%. Major support for the Arts and Science Council. Also funds music, theater, ballet, and history/cultural museums. *Civic & Public Affairs:* 9%. Supports the Carolinas Partnership. Also funds housing and building initiatives, nonprofit management, and community organizations. *Education:* 17%. Funds universities, college funds, Junior Achievement, precollege education, and preschools. *Environment:* 26%. Supports United Way, Boy Scouts of America, youth organizations, senior services, family services, and community recreational activities. *International:* 5%. Supports single-disease health associations and clinics. *Religion:* 1%. Gives to the North Carolina Museum of Natural Sciences. **Note:** Total foundation contributions made in 1998. **Typ. Recipients:** AIDS/HIV, Alzheimers Disease, Cancer, Children's Health/Hospitals, Clinics/Medical Centers, Domestic Violence, Eyes/Blindness, Family Planning, Heart, Hospices, Hospitals, Medical Research, People with Disabilities, Single-Disease Health Associations, Substance Abuse. **Geo. Dist:** headquarters and operating communities.

## ★ 1457 ★ U.S. Bancorp Piper Jaffray Foundation

222 S Ninth St.
Minneapolis, MN 55402
**Phone:** (612)342-5501  **Fax:** (612)342-6085
**Website:** http://www.piperjaffray.com/about/community_involve.html
Marina Lyon, Director, Public Affairs

**Fnded:** 1993. **Priorities:** *Arts & Humanities:* 2%. Funds art museums, opera, public radio, film institute, and performing art. *Civic & Public Affairs:* 25%. Funds urban leagues, economic development, employment initiatives, and neighborhood services. *Education:* 30%. Funds educational programs, literacy initiatives, parent involvement in education, preparatory schools, and colleges. *Environment:* 32%. Funds youth services, YMCA/YWCAs, and food banks. **Note:** Total foundation contributions made in fiscal 2000. **Typ. Recipients:** Cancer, Children's Health/Hospitals, Do-

mestic Violence, Emergency/Ambulance Services, Family Planning, Hospitals, Long-Term Care, Medical Rehabilitation, Multiple Sclerosis, People with Disabilities, Public Health. **Geo. Dist:** headquarters; MN, Twin Cities area. **Frmly:** Piper Jaffray Companies Inc.

## ★ 1458 ★ United States Sugar Corp. Charitable Trust

PO Box 1207
Clewiston, FL 33440
**Phone:** (863)983-8121  **Fax:** (863)983-9827
**Website:** http://www.ussugar.com/aboutus/aboutus_frame.html
Jane Parrish, Community Affairs Assistant

**Fnded:** 1952. **Priorities:** *Arts & Humanities:* 28%. Supports history organizations and libraries. *Civic & Public Affairs:* 20%. Funds municipalities, community redevelopment projects, business/free enterprise programs, low-income housing, and leadership development. *Education:* 32%. More than one-half of giving supports colleges and universities. Other areas of interest include agricultural education, business education, health and physical education, and public education (elementary and precollege). *Environment:* 17%. Child welfare and youth organizations, community centers, the disabled, family services, and united funds receive contributions. *International:* 3%. Supports the Cystic Fibrosis Foundation and Parkinson's Action Network. **Note:** Total contributions made in 2000. **Typ. Recipients:** Alzheimers Disease, Cancer, Children's Health/Hospitals, Clinics/Medical Centers, Diabetes, Emergency/Ambulance Services, Eyes/Blindness, Health Organizations, Heart, Hospices, Hospitals, Medical Rehabilitation, Mental Health, People with Disabilities, Public Health, Single-Disease Health Associations, Substance Abuse. **Geo. Dist:** headquarters and operating communities.

## ★ 1459 ★ U.S. Trust Corp. Foundation

114 West 47th St.
New York, NY 10036-1532
**Phone:** (212)852-1400  **Fax:** (212)852-1341
**Email:** foundation@ustrust.com
Carol Strickland, Chairman, Corporate Contributions Commit

**Priorities:** *Arts & Humanities:* 36%. Contributions are equally distributed between cultural jewels of New York City and institutions supporting the work of emerging artists. U.S. Trust is interested in institutions which make their art accessible to all New Yorkers. *Civic & Public Affairs:* 8%. Supports economic development and community and neighborhood organizations. *Education:* 40%. Supports private pre-college education, colleges, and universities. Most funding to education is provided through employee participation in the matching gift program. *Environment:* 11%. A substantial portion of the trust's support for human services is allocated through the United Way system. Also funds organizations serving children and the disadvantaged. *International:* 5%. Supports children's health and services for seniors. **Note:** Total foundation contributions made in 2000. **Typ. Recipients:** AIDS/HIV, Cancer, Children's Health/Hospitals, Geriatric Health, Health Funds, Health Organizations, Health Policy/Cost Containment, Hospitals, Long-Term Care, Medical Rehabilitation, Nursing Services, Nutrition, People with Disabilities, People with Disabilities, Substance Abuse. **Geo. Dist:** New York, NY, metropolitan area.

## ★ 1460 ★ United Technologies Corp.

One Financial Plaza
MS 503
Hartford, CT 06101
**Phone:** (860)728-7904  **Fax:** (860)728-7041
**Website:** http://www.utc.com
Jacqueline Strayer, Director, Contribution & Communication S

**Priorities:** *Arts & Humanities:* 10% to 15%. National touring museum exhibitions, art education, dance companies, opera, historical societies, art centers, libraries, museums, public radio and television, and historic architectural restoration projects. *Civic & Pub-*

*lic Affairs:* 10% to 15%. Primarily organizations involved in community development activities in operating locations.Supports civic projects, minority and women's programs, and public policy organizations. Particular interest in agencies willing to form alliances with other groups to improve the community. *Education:* 45%. Colleges and universities, including company's 22 "focus" schools. Emphasis is on institutions from which company recruits employees and quality engineering programs, including those directed at women and minorities. Other interests include basic research related to company's fields of business and continuing education for company employees. Additional support provided through precollegiate math and science programs and teacher enrichment programs. Education is the company's major priority. *International:* 20% to 25%. Major support to United Ways and hospitals. Also supports preventive medical treatment groups and activities for the mentally and physically handicapped,senior citizens, youth groups, and health care cost containment. Some funding seeks to establish links between traditional funding areas; for example, funding for a human service organization might be contingent on help they provide an educational or civic group. Grants favored in states where company has operations. **Typ. Recipients:** Health Organizations, Health Policy/Cost Containment, Hospitals, People with Disabilities, Substance Abuse. **Geo. Dist:** communities with major facilities and substantial employee residence population; East Hartford, CT; Hartford, CT; Middletown, CT; Stratford, CT; Windsor Lock, CT; Washington, DC; Palm Beach, FL; Bloomington, IN; Dearborn, MI; Syracuse, NY.

### ★ 1461 ★ United Wisconsin Services Foundation

401 West Michigan St.
Milwaukee, WI 53203
**Phone:** (414)226-5756          **Fax:** (414)226-2637
Tom Luljak, Executive Director

**Fnded:** 1984. **Priorities:** *Arts & Humanities:* About 20%. Supports cultural education, museums, and theaters. *Civic & Public Affairs:* 13%. Funds public and civic foundations. *Education:* 10%. Supports scholarship funds and other educational programs. *Environment:* 32%. Major support given to the United Way. Also funds Big Brothers/Big Sisters, the Boys and Girls Club, crime prevention programs, and child welfare issues. *International:* 25%. Supports children's health education programs, mental health associations, research studies, and other health organizations. **Typ. Recipients:** Alzheimers Disease, Arthritis, Cancer, Children's Health/Hospitals, Clinics/Medical Centers, Eyes/Blindness, Geriatric Health, Health Organizations, Health Policy/Cost Containment, Heart, Medical Education, Medical Research, Mental Health, Prenatal Health Issues, Public Health, Respiratory, Single-Disease Health Associations, Substance Abuse. **Geo. Dist:** WI.

### ★ 1462 ★ Universal Leaf Foundation

PO Box 25099
Richmond, VA 23260
**Phone:** (804)359-9311          **Fax:** (804)254-3594
Nancy Powell, Manager, Corporate Relations

**Priorities:** *Arts & Humanities:* 9%. Supports theater, art and history museums, symphonies, dance, and events promoting the arts. *Civic & Public Affairs:* 19%. Funds community foundations, professional women's organizations, fire departments, minority affairs, and economic and community development. *Education:* 33%. Supports scholarship funds, universities, middle schools, high schools, literacy programs, and business education. *International:* (Health & Welfare) 38%. Contributes to single-disease health associations, pediatric health and pediatric disease research, hospice programs, youth groups and activities, and United Way agencies. *Note:* Total foundation contributions made in fiscal 2001. **Typ. Recipients:** Children's Health/Hospitals, Clinics/Medical Centers, Emergency/Ambulance Services, Eyes/Blindness, Family Planning, Health Funds, Health Organizations, Hospices, Kidney, Multiple Sclerosis, People with Disabilities, Single-Disease Health Associations, Transplant Networks/Donor Banks. **Geo. Dist:** headquarters and operating communities; NC; VA.

### ★ 1463 ★ Universal Studios Foundation

100 Universal City Plaza
Universal City, CA 91608
**Phone:** (818)777-1208
**Email:** unistudios@isearch.com
**Website:** http://www.universalstudios.com/home-page/html/about_us/
Helene Giambone, Foundation Contact

**Fnded:** 1956. **Priorities:** *Arts & Humanities:* 54%. Supports theater/performing arts, film and filmmaker organizations, and the World War II Memorial. *Civic & Public Affairs:* 8%. Provides funding for ethnic affairs and the Greater Los Angeles Zoo. *Education:* 4%. Funds universities and environmental education. *Environment:* 9%. Supports child welfare, youth organizations, and the American Red Cross. *International:* 25%. Supports single-disease health associations, hospitals, and health foundations. *Voluntarism:* The company holds a company-wide annual Volunteer Day during which employees volunteer to work in food banks, build houses with Habitat for Humanity, beautify schools and parks, and provide books to school libraries. In addition, the company sponsors Education is Universal, through which employee volunteers tutor children in schools, provide students with job shadowing opportunities, and hold career days to introduce students to careers within the entertainment industry. *Note:* Total contributions made in fiscal 2000. **Typ. Recipients:** Cancer, Children's Health/Hospitals, Clinics/Medical Centers, Diabetes, Emergency/Ambulance Services, Eyes/Blindness, Family Planning, Health Organizations, Health-General, Medical Education, Medical Research, Mental Health, Multiple Sclerosis, People with Disabilities, Research/Studies Institutes, Single-Disease Health Associations, Substance Abuse. **Geo. Dist:** major operating locations; Los Angeles, CA; New York, NY.

### ★ 1464 ★ Unocal Foundation

14141 Southwest Freeway
Sugar Land, TX 77478
**Phone:** (281)287-7917
Stephen Hayes, Contact

**Priorities:** *Education:* 53%. Education grants are also disbursed through the company's matching gifts program for employees, retirees, and company directors. Also gives graduate and undergraduate scholarships and fellowships that aim to strengthen student interest in disciplines vital to the petroleum industry. Supports regional associations of independent colleges. Awards scholarships to children of employees. *Environment:* 47%. Primarily supports the United Way. *Note:* Total foundation contributions made in fiscal 2000. **Typ. Recipients:** Arthritis, Children's Health/Hospitals, Clinics/Medical Centers, Emergency/Ambulance Services, Health Organizations, Hospitals, Medical Education, Medical Rehabilitation, Medical Research, Medical Training, Mental Health, People with Disabilities, Single-Disease Health Associations, Substance Abuse. **Geo. Dist:** nationally, with preference given to locations with Unocal corporate facilities.

### ★ 1465 ★ UNUM Foundation

2211 Congress St.
Portland, ME 04122
**Phone:** (207)575-4478
Sheila Coyne, Grant Administrator

**Priorities:** *Arts & Humanities:* (See Civic funding.) *Civic & Public Affairs:* 61%. Support is for initiatives that promote economic development and leadership within the state of Maine and enhance the role of art organizations as economic enterprises. *Education:* 17%. Support is directed to programs focused on long-term, systemic restructuring K-12 public schools that are committed to outcome-based education, accountability, and community involvement. *Environment:* 7%. Funds are primarily given to United Way organizations in company headquarters, and in affiliate and field office communities. Supports programs that help the elderly maintain their independence and quality of life. Initiatives with an emphasis on intergenerational collaborations will be given a high priority. *International:* Less than 1%. Supports single-disease health associations and organizations that provide health services to the disabled. *Voluntarism:* Company provides cash grants to nonprofits where employees volunteer. Also supports Heart-to-Heart, an employee-managed volunteer program that researches, develops, and coordinates activities for employees. *Note:* Total foundation contributions made in 2000, excluding matching gifts. **Typ. Recipients:** AIDS/HIV, Alzheimers Disease, Cancer, Clinics/Medical Centers, Domestic Violence, Emergency/Ambulance Services, Health Policy/Cost Containment, Medical Rehabilitation, Medical Research, People with Disabilities. **Geo. Dist:** Portland, ME.

### ★ 1466 ★ UPS Foundation

55 Glenlake Pkwy., NE
Atlanta, GA 30328
**Phone:** (404)828-6374          **Fax:** (404)828-7435
**Website:** http://www.community.ups.com
Ms. Evern Cooper, Executive Director

**Priorities:** *Arts & Humanities:* 4%. Supports historical societies, art and history museums, and libraries. *Civic & Public Affairs:* 25%. Funds women's groups, ethnic and minority organizations, urban leagues, municipalities, economic development, job training and placement, and affordable housing initiatives. *Education:* 41%. Supports academic research, programs that raise the level of educational effectiveness, enhance the quality of instruction, family learning opportunities, literacy, and school involvement projects. Scholarship programs include The Citizen's Scholarship Foundation of America, Inc. and The National Merit Scholarship Corporate. *Environment:* 19%. Supports programs for families and children in crisis, food shelters, the economically or culturally disadvantaged, the physically or mentally challenged, community development programs, YMCAs, United Way, and organizations dealing with domestic violence. *Voluntarism:* The UPS Neighbor to Neighbor program matches employees and their family members interested in volunteer opportunities with community service projects based upon their interests, skills, and schedules. *Note:* Total foundation contributions made in 1999. **Typ. Recipients:** AIDS/HIV, Child Abuse, Domestic Violence, Family Planning, Medical Education, Medical Rehabilitation, Nursing Services, People with Disabilities, Single-Disease Health Associations. **Geo. Dist:** nationally.

### ★ 1467 ★ US Bank, Washington

1420 5th Ave., Ste. 800
PO Box 720 PD-WA-T8CR
Seattle, WA 98111-0720
**Phone:** (206)344-2360          **Fax:** (206)340-8554
**Email:** mary.moore@usbank.com
**Website:** http://www.usbank.om/comm_relations
Mary Moore, Vice President & Manager, Community Rela

**Priorities:** *Arts & Humanities:* 25%. Funds organizations and programs that build audiences of arts organizations; bring the arts to underserved populations; bring select and limited civic amenities to underserved, rural communities; and promote the arts in education. *Civic & Public Affairs:* 25%. Funds economic opportunity by supporting affordable housing, welfare-to-work transitioning, and employment and skills training. Also supports small business development and expansion, commercial revitalization, and job creation. *Education:* 25%. Funds organizations that work in collaboration with K-12 schools (public or private) that develp and/or deliver innovative programs addressing dropout prevention, economic education, mentoring, and curriculum innovation. *Environment:* 25%. United Way. **Typ. Recipients:** Adolescent Health Issues, AIDS/HIV, Cancer, Children's Health/Hospitals, Domestic Violence, Health-General, Hospices, Mental Health, People with Disabilities, Prenatal Health Issues, Sexual Abuse, Substance Abuse. **Geo. Dist:** WA.

★ 1468 ★ **USAA Foundation, A Charitable Trust**

c/o Community Relations (D-3-E)
Office of the Chairman
9800 Fredericksburg Rd.
San Antonio, TX 78288-0115
**Phone:** (210)498-1225    **Fax:** (210)498-8216
Barbara Gentry, Vice President, Community Affairs

**Priorities:** *Arts & Humanities:* Museums and cultural centers, public radio and television stations, and visual and performing arts organizations. *Civic & Public Affairs:* New businesses and new community services. *Education:* Organizations committed to improving education and supporting the literacy effort, as well scholarship assistance in school programs. *Environment:* United Way, health care facilities, youth organizations, services for the elderly and disadvantaged, and family support agencies. *International:* Research and treatment institutions primarily in the San Antonio area. Areas include research in cancer, heart disease, diabetes, genetics, Alzheimer's disease, and AIDS. **Typ. Recipients:** AIDS/HIV, Cancer, Children's Health/Hospitals, Hospitals, Medical Research. **Geo. Dist:** operating locations; TX.

★ 1469 ★ **USAA Foundation, A Charitable Trust**

9800 Fredericksburg Rd., Tax Department F3E
San Antonio, TX 78288
**Phone:** (210)498-1225    **Fax:** (210)498-8216
**Website:** http://www.usaaedfoundation.org
Barbara Gentry, Community Affairs, D-3-E

**Fnded:** 1994. **Priorities:** *Arts & Humanities:* 5%. Supports music, museums, libraries, and public broadcasting. *Civic & Public Affairs:* 24%. Supports housing, women's issues, aquariums, and law and justice. *Education:* 7%. Funds scholarships, religious education, colleges and universities, and educational programs. *Environment:* 34%. Supports crime prevention, United Way, animal protection, youth programs, community service organizations, and relief agencies. *International:* 11%. Supports preventative medicine, cancer, Alzheimer's, diabetes and hospice. *Religion:* 13%. Supports scientific and medical research facilities. *Note:* Total contributions made in 2000. **Typ. Recipients:** Cancer, Children's Health/Hospitals, Emergency/Ambulance Services, Health Funds, Hospitals, Medical Research, Medical Research. **Geo. Dist:** headquarters and operating communities.

★ 1470 ★ **USG Foundation**

PO Box 6721
Chicago, IL 60680-6721
**Phone:** (312)606-4297    **Fax:** (312)606-5316
Harold Pendexter, Jr., President

**Priorities:** *Arts & Humanities:* 18%. Supports performing arts, museums, and historical preservation. Matches employee contributions to the arts. *Civic & Public Affairs:* 16%. Funds crime prevention, legal and justice issues, urban affairs, housing, parks, and economic development. *Education:* 21%. Funds organizations committed to educational improvement, colleges and universities, and scholarship programs. Matches employee contributions to education. *Environment:* 35%. Funds family services, youth organizations, and services for the disabled. *International:* 8%. Supports hospice, hospitals, health education, and single-disease associations. *Note:* Total foundation contributions made in 2000. **Typ. Recipients:** AIDS/HIV, Cancer, Children's Health/Hospitals, Clinics/Medical Centers, Diabetes, Eyes/Blindness, Health Organizations, Heart, Hospices, Hospitals, Long-Term Care, Medical Research, Medical Training, Mental Health, People with Disabilities, Public Health, Single-Disease Health Associations, Substance Abuse. **Geo. Dist:** IL, nationally, with emphasis on corporate operating locations.

★ 1471 ★ **UST Inc.**

100 W Putnam Ave.
Greenwich, CT 06830
**Phone:** (203)661-1100    **Fax:** (203)863-7259
**Email:** mminton@usthq.com

**Website:** http://www.ustshareholder.com
Mary Minton, Manager, Corporate Contributions & Commu

**Typ. Recipients:** Domestic Violence, Health Organizations, Medical Research, Substance Abuse. **Geo. Dist:** headquarters and operating communities; on rare occasions will consider awards to national organizations.

★ 1472 ★ **USX Foundation, Inc.**

600 Grant St., Rm. 685
Pittsburgh, PA 15218
**Phone:** (412)433-5237    **Fax:** (412)433-6847
James Hamilton, III, General Manager

**Priorities:** *Arts & Humanities:* (Public, Cultural, and Scientific Affairs) 18%. Support is allocated to the performing arts, particularly symphonies and operas; art and science museums; historic preservation; and community groups and initiatives. *Education:* 43%. Supports a higher educational programs focusing on engineering, science, and business. Interests include stimulating voluntary educational support, supporting private institutions, and assisting higher education associations. *Environment:* (Health and Human Services). 39%. A large portion of Human Services is provided to the United Way. Also funds single-disease health associations, pediatric health, substance abuse treatment, community centers, and youth groups. *Note:* Contributions analysis represents fiscal 2000 contributions, excluding scholarships and matching gifts. **Typ. Recipients:** Health Organizations, Medical Rehabilitation, Mental Health, People with Disabilities, Single-Disease Health Associations, Substance Abuse, Trauma Treatment. **Geo. Dist:** nationally, with emphasis on communities where USX Corp. and its subsidiaries operate.

★ 1473 ★ **Valmont Foundation**

One Valmont Plaza
Omaha, NE 68154-5215
**Phone:** (402)963-1000    **Fax:** (402)963-1095
Robert Daugherty, Director

**Fnded:** 1976. **Priorities:** *Arts & Humanities:* 3%. Funds museums, history organizations, and the performing arts. *Civic & Public Affairs:* 15%. Supports community foundations, economic development, zoos, and fairs/festivals. *Education:* 41%. Funds colleges and universities, and public and private secondary educational institutions. *Environment:* 35%. Supports the United Way and youth groups, and family services. *International:* 3%. Gives to single-disease health organizations and hospitals. *Note:* Total contributions made in fiscal 2000. **Typ. Recipients:** AIDS/HIV, Arthritis, Children's Health/Hospitals, Diabetes, Emergency/Ambulance Services, Heart, Hospitals, Kidney, Medical Rehabilitation, Nutrition, People with Disabilities, Single-Disease Health Associations, Substance Abuse. **Geo. Dist:** limited giving nationally; NE.

★ 1474 ★ **Valspar Foundation**

1700 Foshay Tower
821 Marquette Ave.
Minneapolis, MN 55402
**Phone:** (612)337-5903    **Fax:** (612)337-5904
**Email:** gleifeld@valspar.com
Gwen Leifeld, Administrator

**Priorities:** *Arts & Humanities:* 17%. Supports public radio, theater, music and art museum. *Civic & Public Affairs:* 30%. Supports clubs, Native American Affairs, and housing. *Education:* 10%. Supports scholarships to children of Valspar employees. *Environment:* 33%. Supports United Way, Young Men's Christian Association, Big Brothers/Big Sisters and Scouts. *International:* 4%. *Religion:* 5%. *Note:* Total contributions made in 1999. **Typ. Recipients:** Cancer, Hospitals, Medical Research, People with Disabilities, Single-Disease Health Associations. **Geo. Dist:** communities with manufacturing facilities only.

★ 1475 ★ **Van Leer U.S. Foundation**

101 Merritt 7
Norwalk, CT 06856

**Phone:** (203)849-4128    **Fax:** (203)849-4133
Marvin Witham, Treasurer

**Priorities:** *Education:* 26%. Funds colleges and universitites. *Environment:* 74%. Supports community organizations and programs for children and families. *Note:* Total contributions made in 1998. **Typ. Recipients:** Family Planning, Medical Research, Public Health.

★ 1476 ★ **Vanguard Group Foundation**

PO Box 2600
Valley Forge, PA 19482-2600
**Phone:** (610)669-1000
Ralph Packard, Principal & Chief Financial Officer

**Fnded:** 1994. **Priorities:** *Arts & Humanities:* 9%. Funds historical monuments, historical societies, art museums and centers, libraries, and performing arts. *Civic & Public Affairs:* 10%. Supports fire departments and public safety, public policy organizations, economic development, community foundations, constitutional law, community revitalization, and botanical gardens, parks, and zoos. *Education:* 13%. Gives to colleges and universities, pre-college education, Junior Achievement, business and economic education, and private/religious schools. *Environment:* 65%. Supports the United Way, American Red Cross, youth organizations, and general social service organizations. *International:* 2%. Gives to single-disease health organizations, hospitals, rehabilitation services, and community health initiatives. *Religion:* Less than 1%. Funds science centers. *Note:* Total contributions made in 2000. **Typ. Recipients:** Cancer, Heart, Nursing Services, People with Disabilities.

★ 1477 ★ **Varian Medical Systems, Inc.**

3100 Hansen Way
Palo Alto, CA 94304
**Phone:** (650)424-6444    **Fax:** (650)424-6822
Spencer Sias, Commincations Directory

**Priorities:** *Education:* About 50%. Colleges and universities with strong programs in engineering, science, business, and medicine, as well as to those institutions that participate in scientific research important to company. *International:* About 40%. United Way fund drives in operating locations, as well as special projects. Company also matches employee donations to the United Way. Limited support to non-United Way organizations, provided services do not duplicate United Way efforts. **Typ. Recipients:** Health Organizations, Mental Health, People with Disabilities, Public Health. **Geo. Dist:** headquarters and operating communities.

★ 1478 ★ **Verizon Delaware Inc.**

901 Tatnall St., 2nd Floor
Wilmington, DE 19801
**Phone:** (302)576-5322    **Fax:** (302)576-1132
**Email:** lauren.a.petrusky@verizon.com
**Website:** http://www.verizon.com/foundation
Lauren Petrusky, Co-Manager, Corporate Contributions/Even

**Priorities:** *Arts & Humanities:* 32%. *Civic & Public Affairs:* 2%. *Education:* 48%. *Environment:* 15%. **Typ. Recipients:** Health-General. **Geo. Dist:** DE; DC; ME; MD; MA; NH; NJ; NY; PA; RI; VT; VI; WV.

★ 1479 ★ **Viad Corp. Fund**

15501 North Dial Boulevard
Scottsdale, AZ 85260-1619
**Phone:** (480)754-4090    **Fax:** (480)754-8003
Cindy Demers, Vice President, Corp. /Gov. Affairs

**Fnded:** 1987. **Priorities:** *Civic & Public Affairs:* 23%. Supports economic development, urban and community affairs, and public policy. *Education:* 13%. Supports colleges and universities. *Environment:* 45%. Supports youth organizations, family services, and community service organizations. *International:* 4%. Supports the American Lung Association and single-disease associations. *Note:* Total contributions in 1999. **Typ. Recipients:** Alzheimers Disease, Arthritis, Cancer, Child Abuse, Children's Health/Hospitals, Diabetes, Domestic Violence, Emergency/Ambulance

Services, Eyes/Blindness, Family Planning, Health Funds, Health Organizations, Heart, Hospices, Hospitals, Kidney, Medical Rehabilitation, People with Disabilities, Prenatal Health Issues, Preventive Medicine/Wellness Organizations, Respiratory, Sexual Abuse, Single-Disease Health Associations, Substance Abuse. **Geo. Dist:** AZ, statewide; Phoenix, AZ.

### ★ 1480 ★ Vivendi Universal Foundation

375 Park Ave., 5th Floor
New York, NY 10152-0192
**Phone:** (212)572-7240
Richard Marker, Vice President

**Fnded:** 1951. **Priorities:** *Arts & Humanities:* 13%. Funds museums, history, music, opera, and theater. *Civic & Public Affairs:* 5%. Supports housing and urban affairs, zoos, and nature centers. *Education:* 16%. Supports Jewish studies, colleges, public schools, and universities. *Environment:* 4%. Youth organizations and camps receive the majority of funding. Also supports United Way. *International:* 3%. Funds hospitals and AIDS research. *Note:* Total foundation contributions made in fiscal 2001. **Typ. Recipients:** AIDS/HIV, Cancer, Clinics/Medical Centers, Medical Education, Medical Research, Mental Health, Substance Abuse. **Geo. Dist:** New York, NY.

### ★ 1481 ★ Vodafone-US Foundation

1 California St., 17th Fl.
San Francisco, CA 94111-5401
**Phone:** (415)658-2080          **Fax:** (415)658-2332
Sam Ginn, Chairman & President

**Fnded:** 1993. **Priorities:** *Arts & Humanities:* 22%. Funds art museums and associations, ballet, opera, and other performing arts. *Civic & Public Affairs:* (Civic Projects and Community)21%. Funds public safety, community foundations, public policy, zoos, legal aid, and voter education. *Education:* 8%. Supports minority education and art, science, and economics education. *Environment:* (Safe Communities and Transitional Assistance) 22%. Supports youth organizations, safety initiatives, and welfare transition groups. *International:* 3%. Gives to a children's hospital, cancer research, and an organization that provides guide dogs for the blind. *Voluntarism:* Company actively promotes and encourages volunteerism, both through its grantmaking and internal policies. *Note:* Total contributions made in 2000. **Typ. Recipients:** AIDS/HIV, Cancer, Children's Health/Hospitals, Emergency/Ambulance Services, Eyes/Blindness, Family Planning, Public Health, Research/Studies Institutes. **Geo. Dist:** areas where company provides cellular and paging operations; AZ; CA; San Francisco, CA; Walnut Creek, CA; CO; Washington, DC; Atlanta, GA; ID; IA; MI; MN; NE; NM; ND; OH; OR; Dallas, TX; UT; WA; WY.

### ★ 1482 ★ Vulcan Materials Co. Foundation

PO Box 385014
Birmingham, AL 35253-5014
**Phone:** (205)298-3130          **Fax:** (205)298-2960
**Website:** http://www.vulcanmaterials.com
Joy Phillips, Community Relations

**Priorities:** *Arts & Humanities:* 14%. Large grants support theater and neighborhood growth/economic development projects. Also supports museums, arts festivals, and public broadcasting. Civic interests include business, safety, and urban affairs organizations. *Civic & Public Affairs:* 11%. Interests include economic development, public policy, and urban and community affairs. *Education:* 34%. Supports educational interests in operating areas, including education funds, scholarships, public and private precollege education, and minority education. *Environment:* 33%. Primarily gives to united funds. Also interested in programs for unemployed youth, employment, and youth organizations. *International:* 4%. Supports hospitals. *Religion:* 1%. Supports science museums. *Note:* Total contributions made in fiscal 1999. **Typ. Recipients:** Cancer, Children's Health/Hospitals, Clinics/Medical Centers, Emergency/Ambulance Services, Health Organizations, Mental Health, People with

Disabilities, Substance Abuse. **Geo. Dist:** states in which company has operations.

### ★ 1483 ★ The Wachovia Foundation, Inc.

100 North Main St.
Winston-Salem, NC 27102-7203
**Phone:** (336)732-5252

**Priorities:** *Arts & Humanities:* 14%. Recipients include festivals, art museums, living history sites, performing arts, and community arts organizations. *Civic & Public Affairs:* 12%. Supports chambers of commerce, business organizations, economic and community development, and community organizations. *Education:* 27%. Funds colleges and universities, precollege programs and schools, school readiness programs, and community involvement in schools. *Environment:* 36%. Supports traditional youth organizations, senior services, food distribution, and other human welfare agencies. Major support goes to united funds in North Carolina. *International:* 3%. Supports single-disease health organizations, public health, and medical research. **Typ. Recipients:** Emergency/Ambulance Services, Family Planning, Health Funds, Health Organizations, Hospices, Hospitals, Medical Education, People with Disabilities, Respiratory, Substance Abuse. **Geo. Dist:** GA; NC; SC.

### ★ 1484 ★ Waffle House Foundation, Inc.

5986 Financial Dr.
PO Box 6450
Norcross, GA 30071
**Phone:** (770)729-5700          **Fax:** (770)729-5900
Alice Johnson, President

**Priorities:** *Arts & Humanities:* 5%. Funds museums and history programs. *Civic & Public Affairs:* 8%. Women's affairs, African American affairs, foundations, and housing. *Education:* 16%. Funds K-12 education and literacy efforts. *Environment:* 21%. Funds family services and youth organizations, community service organizations, the homeless and domestic violence. *International:* 37%. Single-disease centers and foundations receive support. *Note:* Total contributions made in 1999. **Typ. Recipients:** AIDS/HIV, Alzheimers Disease, Arthritis, Cancer, Child Abuse, Children's Health/Hospitals, Domestic Violence, Emergency/Ambulance Services, Eyes/Blindness, Health Organizations, Heart, Hospices, Hospitals, Medical Rehabilitation, Mental Health, Multiple Sclerosis, Nursing Services, People with Disabilities, Prenatal Health Issues, Preventive Medicine/Wellness Organizations, Sexual Abuse, Single-Disease Health Associations, Trauma Treatment. **Geo. Dist:** Atlanta, GA, including metropolitan area.

### ★ 1485 ★ Wal-Mart Foundation

702 Southwest Eighth St.
Bentonville, AR 72716-8071
**Phone:** (501)277-1905          **Fax:** (501)273-6850
**Email:** fndatn@wal-mart.com
**Website:** http://www.walmartfoundation.org
Betsy Reithemeyer, Foundation Director

**Priorities:** *Arts & Humanities:* 2%. *Civic & Public Affairs:* 41%. *Education:* 18%. *Environment:* 33%. Focus on United Way. *International:* 5%. *Note:* Total contributions made in fiscal 1999. **Typ. Recipients:** Cancer, Children's Health/Hospitals, Domestic Violence, Emergency/Ambulance Services, Eyes/Blindness, Geriatric Health, Health Funds, Health Organizations, Hospices, Hospitals, Medical Education, Medical Rehabilitation, Medical Research, Mental Health, Nutrition, People with Disabilities, Public Health, Single-Disease Health Associations, Substance Abuse. **Geo. Dist:** headquarters and operating communities.

### ★ 1486 ★ Walgreen Benefit Fund

200 Wilmot Rd.
Mail Stop 2255
Deerfield, IL 60015-4681
**Phone:** (847)914-3550          **Fax:** (847)914-3417
**Email:** ed.king@walgreens.com
**Website:** http://www.walgreens.com
Edward King, Vice President

**Priorities:** *Arts & Humanities:* 4%. Funds museums and music. *Civic & Public Affairs:* 1%. *Education:* 1%. *Environment:* 6%. Focus is on youth organizations. *International:* 12%. Supports single-disease associations. *Note:* Total foundation contributions made in fiscal 2000. **Typ. Recipients:** AIDS/HIV, Cancer, Children's Health/Hospitals, Health-General, Mental Health, People with Disabilities, Single-Disease Health Associations, Substance Abuse. **Geo. Dist:** company operating locations; Chicago, IL, including metropolitan area.

### ★ 1487 ★ Walt Disney Co. Foundation

500 South Buena Vista St.
Burbank, CA 91521-0987
**Phone:** (818)560-1006
Tillie Baptie, Executive Director

**Priorities:** *Arts & Humanities:* 6%. Supports music and the performing arts. *Civic & Public Affairs:* 2%. Supports minority affairs and special funds. *Education:* 40%. Supports special pre-college education, colleges and universities, minority education, and college funds. Also supports the Disney scholarship program. *Environment:* 13%. Supports youth and community services, including the United Way. *International:* 10%. Grants support single-disease health funds, hospitals and other facilities in company operating areas. Focus is on children's health *Note:* Total foundation contributions made in fiscal 2000. **Typ. Recipients:** Cancer, Children's Health/Hospitals, Clinics/Medical Centers, Diabetes, Domestic Violence, Emergency/Ambulance Services, Eyes/Blindness, Health Organizations, Health-General, Hospitals, Medical Education, Medical Rehabilitation, Mental Health, People with Disabilities, Public Health, Single-Disease Health Associations, Substance Abuse. **Geo. Dist:** headquarters and operating communities; CA, Los Angeles County; CA, Orange County; FL, Orange County; FL, Osceola County.

### ★ 1488 ★ Walter Foundation

1500 North Dale Mabry
PO Box 31601
Tampa, FL 33631-3601
**Phone:** (813)871-4168          **Fax:** (813)871-4094
W. Baker, Trustee

**Fnded:** 1966. **Priorities:** *Arts & Humanities:* 1%. Music and visual arts. *Civic & Public Affairs:* 8%. Support goes to community foundations and neighborhood improvement. *Education:* 45%. Major interests include Catholic education, colleges and universities, and private secondary education. *Environment:* 30%. Majority of support goes to youth groups, including Boys and Girls Clubs, and the United Way. *International:* 9%. Interests include cancer research, hospitals, clinics, and medical centers. *Note:* Total contributions in fiscal 1999. **Typ. Recipients:** Cancer, Children's Health/Hospitals, Clinics/Medical Centers, Emergency/Ambulance Services, Health Organizations, Heart, Hospices, Hospitals, Medical Research, People with Disabilities, Respiratory, Single-Disease Health Associations, Substance Abuse. **Geo. Dist:** headquarters and operating communities; Tampa, FL.

### ★ 1489 ★ Washington Group Foundation, Inc.

PO Box 73
Boise, ID 83729
**Phone:** (208)386-5201
Marlene Puckett, Administrator, Director, Secretary

**Priorities:** *Arts & Humanities:* 7%. Supports museums, theater, and public television. *Civic & Public Affairs:* 8%. Supports housing, justice, and community foundations. *Education:* 8%. Supports colleges, universities, and scholarships. *Environment:* 12%. Supports child welfare, Boy Scouts, food distribution, shelters, and senior centers. *International:* 5%. Supports hospices, medical centers, and single-disease health associations. *Note:* Total foundation contributions made in 2000. **Typ. Recipients:** Cancer, Children's Health/Hospitals, Clinics/Medical Centers, Diabetes, Domestic Violence, Emergency/Ambulance Services, Health Organizations, Health-General, Hospices, Hospitals, Long-Term Care, Medical Rehabilitation, Medical Research, Multiple Sclerosis, People with Disabilities, Public Health, Respiratory, Single-Disease Health Associations. **Geo. Dist:** nationally; operating locations; ID.


### ★ 1490 ★ Washington Mutual Bank Foundation

1201 Third Ave., WMT1213
Seattle, WA 98101
**Phone:** (206)377-4508          **Fax:** (206)377-5723
Christine Park, Vice President, Community
Relations

**Priorities:** *Arts & Humanities:* 4%. Supports cultural enhancement in operating communities. *Civic & Public Affairs:* 46%. Supports rural and urban housing in areas where the company operates. Focus is on increasing the amount of long-term affordable housing in the community. Also supports community development organizations. *Education:* 21%. Supports systemic change to improve the delivery of educational services to students, and encourages model K-12 programs that improve academic success in core subjects; supports programs which increase parental involvement, or train or diversify teaching corps. *Environment:* 20%. Major support for the United Way. Also funds food banks, child welfare, and YMCA/YWCA. *Note:* Total foundation contributions made in 1999. **Typ. Recipients:** AIDS/HIV, Cancer, Children's Health/Hospitals, Clinics/Medical Centers, Domestic Violence, Emergency/Ambulance Services, Long-Term Care, Mental Health, Public Health. **Geo. Dist:** company operating areas; OR, Western Oregon; WA.


### ★ 1491 ★ Washington Mutual Fund

1000 Wilshire, 22nd Fl., Ste. 695
Los Angeles, CA 90017
**Phone:** (626)814-7924          **Fax:** (626)814-5659
Randy Robinson, Vice President, Corporate Giving
& Commi

**Priorities:** *Arts & Humanities:* About 5%. General support for arts organizations in California. *Civic & Public Affairs:* About 50%. The company's specific focus is on housing. Supports neighborhood improvement, community reinvestment, and diversity. (United Funds & United Way) About 5%. General support to various United Way chapters. *Education:* About 20%. The company's main priority is its "Career Awareness Program," which focuses on the problem of high unemployment among teenagers. *International:* About 20%. Majority of funding supports Alzheimer's research and treatment. Also supports scouting. Includes support to youth programs, homeless centers, soup kitchens, health care, battered women's centers, daycare, and alcohol and drug recovery programs. **Typ. Recipients:** Health-General, Medical Research, Single-Disease Health Associations. **Geo. Dist:** headquarters and operating communities; CA.


### ★ 1492 ★ Washington Trust Bank Foundation

PO Box 2127
Spokane, WA 99210
**Phone:** (509)353-3820
Susan Rowe-Adler, Director Community Affairs

**Priorities:** *Arts & Humanities:* 17%. Primary support is for the Spokane Symphony in Spokane, WA. Other interests include a ballet company, civic theater, and concert and arts associations. *Civic & Public Affairs:* 15%. Funds community foundations and civic and women's affairs. *Education:* 23%. Major support to St. George's School in Spokane, WA. The remainder of funds support other universities, specialty schools, and education funds in Washington state. *Environment:* 38%. Primary support goes to the United Way. Other support goes to traditional youth groups and community services. *Religion:* 1%. Funds the Pacific Science Center. *Note:* Total contribution in 1998. **Typ. Recipients:** AIDS/HIV, Cancer, Children's Health/Hospitals, Clinics/Medical Centers, Heart, Hospitals, Multiple Sclerosis, Nursing Services, People with Disabilities, Research/Studies Institutes. **Geo. Dist:** Spokane, WA, metropolitan area.


### ★ 1493 ★ Waste Management Inc.

1001 Fannin, Ste. 4000
Houston, TX 77002
**Phone:** (713)512-6200          **Fax:** (713)287-2616
**Website:** http://www.wm.com
Marilyn Brown, Director, Community Relations

**Typ. Recipients:** Health Funds, Hospitals, Medical Research, Mental Health, Single-Disease Health Associations. **Geo. Dist:** principally near operating locations and to national organizations.


### ★ 1494 ★ Weil, Gotshal & Manges Foundation

767 5th Ave.
New York, NY 10153
**Phone:** (212)310-8000
Jesse Wolff, Treasurer & Director

**Fnded:** 1983. **Priorities:** *Arts & Humanities:* 3%. Supports performing arts, museums, symphonies, and libraries. *Civic & Public Affairs:* 29%. Primarily for legal aid, parks, and urban affairs. *Education:* 23%. Focus on law schools and private primary and secondary education. *Environment:* 19%. Funds the United Way, family services, and youth organizations. *International:* 5%. Funds healthcare, blood centers, and Make-a-Wish Foundation. *Note:* Total foundation contributions made in 1999. **Typ. Recipients:** AIDS/HIV, Cancer, Children's Health/Hospitals, Emergency/Ambulance Services, Family Planning, Heart, Medical Research, Prenatal Health Issues, Public Health, Single-Disease Health Associations, Transplant Networks/Donor Banks. **Geo. Dist:** NY.


### ★ 1495 ★ Wellmark Foundation

636 Grand Ave., Station 150
Des Moines, IA 50309-2502
**Phone:** (515)245-4572          **Fax:** (515)245-5092
**Email:** wmfoundation@wellmark.com
**Website:** http://www.wellmark.com
Dr. Sheila Riggs, Executive Director

**Fnded:** 1991. **Priorities:** *International:* 100%. Funding is given for the purpose of measurably improving the health of communities in Iowa and South Dakota. **Typ. Recipients:** Alzheimers Disease, Arthritis, Cancer, Child Abuse, Children's Health/Hospitals, Clinics/Medical Centers, Domestic Violence, Emergency/Ambulance Services, Eyes/Blindness, Family Planning, Health Organizations, Health-General, Home-Care Services, Hospices, Hospitals (University Affiliated), Medical Education, Mental Health, Multiple Sclerosis, Nursing Services, People with Disabilities, Prenatal Health Issues, Preventive Medicine/Wellness Organizations, Public Health, Respiratory, Substance Abuse. **Geo. Dist:** IA; SD.


### ★ 1496 ★ Wells Fargo Bank Nebraska, N.A.

1919 Douglas St.
PO Box 3408
Omaha, NE 68103
**Phone:** (402)536-2329          **Fax:** (402)536-2812
**Website:** http://www.wellsfargo.com
Richard Schenck, Vice President & Director of Contributio

**Priorities:** *Arts & Humanities:* 10% to 15%. Contributes to theaters, arts festivals, ballet, symphonies, and arts centers. *Civic & Public Affairs:* About 15%. Supports parades and community arts events. 5% to 10%. Primarily supports philanthropic associations and economic development. *Education:* 20% to 25%. Supports colleges and universities, public high schools, education foundations, religious colleges, and Junior Achievement programs. *Environment:* 40% to 45%. Majority of funds support United Way agencies throughout Nebraska. Also supports religious organizations, community service organizations, scouting and other youth organizations, Planned Parenthood, and community centers. **Typ. Recipients:** Family Planning, Health Organizations, Mental Health, People with Disabilities, Public Health, Single-Disease Health Associations. **Geo. Dist:** operating communities.


### ★ 1497 ★ Wells Fargo Foundation

550 California St., 7th Floor
San Francisco, CA 94163
**Phone:** (415)222-5235          **Fax:** (415)975-6260
**Website:** http://www.wellsfargo.com/about/charitable.jhtml
Tim Hanlon, Contact

**Priorities:** *Civic & Public Affairs:* Programs that help provide affordable housing for low and moderate income individuals; promote economic development by financing small businesses or small farms that meet size eligibility standards for the SBA's Development Company Program or have gross annual revenues of $1,000,000 or less; provide job training programs that assist low and moderate income individuals to find and retain employment; or help revitalize or stabilize low and moderate income communities. *Education:* Prekindergarten through twelfth grade institutions, as well as for nonprofits whose primary focus is to assist them, when the primary purpose of the grant is to promoteacademic achievement to low and moderate income students in the areas of math and science, literacy, and history of the American West. Also considers support of programs that work to encourage school partnerships with parents/guardians, the community in which the school is located, and the business community, as well as to programs that provide staff training for teachers and administrators working with low and moderate income students. *Environment:* Organizations whose work primarily benefits low and moderate income individuals. Issues of interest include child care, health services and education, and basic needs assistance. **Typ. Recipients:** AIDS/HIV, People with Disabilities, Single-Disease Health Associations. **Geo. Dist:** AZ; CA, headquarters and operating communities; CO; ID; NV; NM; OR; TX; UT; WA.


### ★ 1498 ★ Western-Southern Enterprise Fund

400 Broadway
Cincinnati, OH 45202-3341
**Phone:** (513)629-2121
**Website:** http://www.westernsouthern.com/giving-to.htm
Richard Taulbee, Assistant Treasurer

**Fnded:** 1990. **Priorities:** *Arts & Humanities:* 5%. Majority of funding supports museums, arts funds, arts festivals, and historic preservation in Cincinnati, OH. *Civic & Public Affairs:* 6%. Contributes community development, parks, urban affairs, a zoo and botanical garden, and professional and trade associations promoting the insurance business. *Education:* 58%. Primarily supports higher education, with an emphasis on institutions located in Ohio. Major funding goes to Xavier University. Other interests include minority and economic education. *Environment:* 13%. Majority of funding supports various United Way agencies in Ohio. Other recipients include youth organizations and food and clothing distributors, and people with disabilities. *International:* 4%. Emphasis is on single-disease health associations, long-term care, and preventative medicine. *Note:* Total foundation contributions made in 1999. **Typ. Recipients:** Cancer, Children's Health/Hospitals, Diabetes, Emergency/Ambulance Services, Health Organizations, Home-Care Services, Hospices, Hospitals, Long-Term Care, Mental Health, Multiple Sclerosis, People with Disabilities, Prenatal Health Issues, Single-Disease Health Associations. **Geo. Dist:** OH.


### ★ 1499 ★ Westvaco Foundation Trust

299 Park Ave.
New York, NY 10171
Roger Holmes, Contact

**Priorities:** *Arts & Humanities:* 1%. Supports public broadcasting, opera, and arts funds. *Civic & Public Affairs:* 15%. Supports public policy organizations, business and free enterprise, and urban and community affairs groups. *Education:* 24%. Supports universities and colleges, education funds, technology and minority education, and education associations. Some interest in pulp and paper sciences and forestry. Also includes matching grants to educational institutions. *Environment:* 44%. Primarily supports united funds.

Recipients of smaller amounts include youth organizations, drug and alcohol programs, community service organizations, and recreation and athletics. *International:* 4%. Primarily supports hospitals and medical centers. Other interests include single-disease health associations, health organizations, and medical research. *Note:* Total contributions in fiscal 2000. **Typ. Recipients:** Cancer, Health Funds, Health Organizations, Hospitals, Medical Education, Medical Rehabilitation, Medical Research, People with Disabilities, Single-Disease Health Associations, Substance Abuse. **Geo. Dist:** headquarters and operating communities.

### ★ 1500 ★ Whirlpool Foundation

2000 North M-63
Benton Harbor, MI 49022
**Phone:** (616)923-5583 **Fax:** (616)923-3214
**Website:** http://www.whirlpoolcorp.com/whr/foundation/index.html
Jay Van Den Berg, President

**Priorities:** *Arts & Humanities:* 2%. Primarily supports museums, arts centers, symphony orchestras, and arts institutes. *Civic & Public Affairs:* 22%. Supports cultural diversity organizations and civic and community groups. *Education:* 36%. Supports colleges and universities, with interests in science, technological, business, minority education, arts and humanities education and higher education associations. Provides scholarships for children of employees who exhibit exceptional academic achievement. *Environment:* 20%. Provides major support for the United Way. *International:* (Health & Human Services) 4%. Supports traditional youth groups, community services, family planning, single-disease health organizations, hospitals, and programs for the handicapped, the elderly, and children. *Note:* Total contributions made in fiscal 1999. **Typ. Recipients:** Cancer, Clinics/Medical Centers, Domestic Violence, Emergency/Ambulance Services, Family Planning, Health Organizations, Hospitals, Medical Education, People with Disabilities, Public Health, Sexual Abuse, Substance Abuse. **Geo. Dist:** operating locations.

### ★ 1501 ★ Whitman Corp. Foundation

3501 Algonquin Rd.
Rolling Meadows, IL 60008
**Phone:** (847)818-5000 **Fax:** (847)818-5046
Karen Golden, President

**Priorities:** *Arts & Humanities:* 1%. Supports the symphony. *Civic & Public Affairs:* 14%. Urban and community affairs. *Education:* 80%. Includes matching gifts to educational institutions. Majority of funding supports colleges and universities nationwide. *Environment:* 4%. United funds, YMCA's youth organizations, and child welfare. *International:* 1%. Emergency relief, health policy, hospitals, and single-disease health associations. *Note:* Total contributions in 1998. **Typ. Recipients:** Cancer, Child Abuse, Children's Health/Hospitals, Diabetes, Emergency/Ambulance Services, Eyes/Blindness, Health Organizations, Health Policy/Cost Containment, Hospitals, Hospitals (University Affiliated), Kidney, Medical Rehabilitation, People with Disabilities, Prenatal Health Issues, Single-Disease Health Associations. **Geo. Dist:** nationally; Chicago, IL.

### ★ 1502 ★ William Blair & Co. Foundation

222 West Adams St.
Chicago, IL 60606
**Phone:** (312)236-1600
E. Coolidge, III, Chief Executive Officer

**Fnded:** 1980. **Priorities:** *Arts & Humanities:* 23%. Arts institutes, dance, museums, historical societies, opera, and theater. *Civic & Public Affairs:* 18%. Primarily for community affairs programs, zoos, and a horticultural society. *Education:* 17%. Emphasis on colleges and universities, secondary schools, and education associations. *Environment:* 25%. Focus on youth organizations, child welfare, and recreation projects. *International:* 5%. Hospitals, medical centers, and medical rehabilitation. *Religion:* 3%. *Note:* Total contributions for fiscal 1999. **Typ. Recipients:** Children's Health/Hospitals, Clinics/Medical Centers, Health Or-

ganizations, Health-General, Hospitals, Hospitals (University Affiliated), Medical Rehabilitation, Medical Research, People with Disabilities, Single-Disease Health Associations, Substance Abuse. **Geo. Dist:** Chicago, IL.

### ★ 1503 ★ Williams

2800 Post Oak Boulevard
Houston, TX 77056
**Phone:** (713)215-3132 **Fax:** (713)215-2340
**Email:** charlene.c.floyd@williams.com
**Website:** http://www.williams.com
Charlene Floyd, Manager, Community Relations

**Priorities:** *Arts & Humanities:* About 15%. Programs that benefit the greatest number of people in the community. *Civic & Public Affairs:* 10% to 15%. Organizations that address diverse contemporary issues and challenges facing society, including conservation and preservation, crime prevention, community revitalizations, and thedevelopment of public policy. *Education:* About 35%. Direct grants to colleges and universities where the company actively recruits and to those institutions that provide education to their employees; K-12 education with focus on adopt-a-school programs, character education, math, science, and technology education, and literacy; and economic education programs that promote the understanding of economics and the free enterprise systems. Additionally, the company matches employee gifts to eligible educational institutions and sponsors a scholarship program for employee children. *Environment:* About 35%. Majority to United Way. Also supports disaster relief efforts, programs for the disabled, prevention of child abuse, and youth organizations. *International:* Less than 5%. Organizations where employees are directly involved and hospitals near operating locations. **Typ. Recipients:** Domestic Violence, Hospices, Medical Research, Mental Health, People with Disabilities, Substance Abuse. **Geo. Dist:** headquarters and operating communities.

### ★ 1504 ★ The Williams Companies Foundation

PO Box 2400
Tulsa, OK 74102
**Phone:** (918)573-2106
Sylvia Schmidt, Director, Community Relations

**Priorities:** *Arts & Humanities:* 10% to 15%. Performing arts organizations, museums, ethnic arts, and historical preservation. *Civic & Public Affairs:* 15% to 20%. Primarily supports environmental affairs and urban and community affairs. Also supports business, philanthropy, minority affairs, public policy, and women's organizations. *Education:* 20% to 25%. Majority of funds support colleges and universities. Remaining support goes to engineering and economic education, education funds, and business education. *Environment:* 20% to 25%. Funds Meals on Wheels, children and youth services, YMCA, and social services. *International:* 10%. More than three-fourths supports united funds, American Red Cross, and family service organizations. Other interests include youth organizations, drug and alcohol abuse, the disabled, and child welfare organizations. Health interests include medical centers, medical research, and single-disease health associations. *Note:* Above giving reflects corporate donations. In 2000, the foundation donated 95% of funds to a community foundation, and 5% to higher education. **Typ. Recipients:** AIDS/HIV, Children's Health/Hospitals, Clinics/Medical Centers, Domestic Violence, Family Planning, Health Funds, Health Organizations, Hospitals, People with Disabilities, Prenatal Health Issues, Single-Disease Health Associations, Substance Abuse. **Geo. Dist:** areas near company headquarters and operating communities.

### ★ 1505 ★ Winn-Dixie Stores Foundation

PO Box B
Jacksonville, FL 32203-0297
**Phone:** (904)783-5000 **Fax:** (904)783-5235
**Website:** http://www.winn-dixie.com/company/community/main.asp
August Toscano, Foundation President & Director, Matchin

**Priorities:** *Arts & Humanities:* 4%. Funds performing arts, public broadcasting, arts councils, and art museums. *Civic & Public Affairs:* 22%. Supports urban leagues, housing, economic development, zoos, and Lion's Clubs. *Education:* 16%. Support for colleges, college funds, minority education, and elementary and secondary schools. *Environment:* 15%. Supports the United Way, YMCA/YWCA, recreation, Junior Achievement, scouting, and professional sports charities. *International:* 40%. Supports hospitals, hospices, national disease associations, and mental health. *Note:* About half of foundation giving is in the form of employee matching gifts. Total contributions made in 2000. **Typ. Recipients:** Alzheimers Disease, Cancer, Children's Health/Hospitals, Clinics/Medical Centers, Diabetes, Emergency/Ambulance Services, Heart, Hospices, Hospitals, Medical Education, Mental Health, People with Disabilities, Prenatal Health Issues, Public Health, Single-Disease Health Associations, Substance Abuse. **Geo. Dist:** primarily in the company's 14-state trade area; generally within the Southern United States; AL; FL; GA; IN; KY; LA; MS; NC; OH; OK; SC; TN; TX; VA.

### ★ 1506 ★ Winthrop Foundation

1 Liberty Lane
Hampton, NH 03842
**Phone:** (603)926-5911 **Fax:** (603)929-2248
Spencer Stokes, President

**Priorities:** *Arts & Humanities:* 10% to 15%. Supports the performing arts and music. A variety of museums also receive substantial support, including those which focus on automobiles, modern art, and American art. *Civic & Public Affairs:* 10% to 15%. Recipients include philanthropic organizations, civil rights, and law and justice. *Education:* 20% to 25%. Supports colleges, universities and private precollege education. *Environment:* 5% to 10%. Primarily supports united funds and youth organizations. Foundation also funds family counseling, daycare, and hospices. *International:* 20% to 25%. Interests include medical foundations, single-disease health associations, medical centers, and hospitals. Also funds disabled veterans. *Religion:* Less than 5%. Supports the American Museum of Natural History. **Typ. Recipients:** Cancer, Clinics/Medical Centers, Diabetes, Emergency/Ambulance Services, Health Organizations, Hospices, Hospitals, Medical Education, Medical Research, People with Disabilities, Research/Studies Institutes, Single-Disease Health Associations, Speech & Hearing, Transplant Networks/Donor Banks. **Geo. Dist:** headquarters and operating communities.

### ★ 1507 ★ Wiremold Foundation

60 Woodlawn St.
West Hartford, CT 06110
**Phone:** (860)233-6251 **Fax:** (860)523-3699
John Murphy, President

**Fnded:** 1967. **Priorities:** *Arts & Humanities:* 16%. Funds public broadcasting, arts councils, music, and historic preservation. *Civic & Public Affairs:* 4%. Supports housing and community development. *Education:* 17%. Focus is on higher education; also supports 4-H, Junior Achievement, and schools for the deaf and blind. *Environment:* 44%. Supports youth organizations, including scouting and camps; and human services, such as food banks, shelters, and family services. *International:* 6%. Supports hospitals and the American Red Cross. *Religion:* 1%. *Note:* Total foundation contributions made in 1999. **Typ. Recipients:** AIDS/HIV, Children's Health/Hospitals, Clinics/Medical Centers, Emergency/Ambulance Services, Health Organizations, Health-General, Hospitals, People with Disabilities, Public Health. **Geo. Dist:** headquarters area only.

### ★ 1508 ★ Wisconsin Energy Corp. Foundation, Inc.

231 West Michigan St.
Milwaukee, WI 53290-0001
**Phone:** (414)221-2106 **Fax:** (414)221-2412
**Email:** carolyn.simpson@wepco.com
**Website:** http://foundation.wisconsinenergy.com
Carolyn Simpson, Foundation Coordinator

**Priorities:** *Arts & Humanities:* 21%. Supports the performing arts, community arts, and arts centers. Museums also receive significant support. *Civic & Public Affairs:* 4%. Funds community/economic development initiatives, civil rights, and business and free enterprise groups. *Education:* 34%. Majority of education support is given to general programs at colleges and universities in Wisconsin. Other recipients include education reform programs, education funds, engineering programs, minority education, and business education projects. Also sponsors an employee matching gifts program for contributions to higher education institutions. *Environment:* 38%. Provides major support to the United Way in Wisconsin communities. Also supports youth groups and community centers. Other interests include the aged and community service organizations. *Religion:* 2%. Funds a science museum. *Voluntarism:* Company actively promotes volunteerism through the Employee Volunteer Program, including mentoring programs, a speakers bureau, and other volunteer activities. *Note:* Total contributions made in 2000. **Typ. Recipients:** Children's Health/Hospitals, Clinics/Medical Centers, Health Organizations, Hospitals, Medical Education, Medical Rehabilitation, Medical Research, Mental Health, People with Disabilities, Public Health, Respiratory, Single-Disease Health Associations, Trauma Treatment. **Geo. Dist:** headquarters and operating communities.

**★ 1509 ★ Wisconsin Power & Light Foundation, Inc.**
222 West Washington Ave.
PO Box 219
Madison, WI 53701-0192
**Phone:** (608)252-5545          **Fax:** (608)283-6991
Joann Healy, Foundation Administrator

**Priorities:** *Arts & Humanities:* 21%. Cultural interests include history, museums, and libraries. Art interests include performing arts events, music, dance, community ensembles, small theaters, arts and crafts centers, and visual arts. *Civic & Public Affairs:* 4%. Supports neighborhood improvement, community business funds, parks and environmental projects, community affairs, fire safety. *Education:* 43%. Supports colleges and universities in areas where the company operates, and funds agricultural and technical programs. Supports matching gifts, and scholarship funds. *Environment:* 31%. Most support goes to social services, with about one-third awarded to united fund drives in local communities. Also supports youth organizations and family services. *International:* 1%. *Note:* Total foundation contributions made in 1999. **Typ. Recipients:** Cancer, Children's Health/Hospitals, Clinics/Medical Centers, Emergency/Ambulance Services, Health Organizations, Hospitals, Nursing Services, People with Disabilities, Public Health, Single-Disease Health Associations. **Geo. Dist:** WI, near headquarters and service areas (central and south central Wisconsin).

**★ 1510 ★ Wisconsin Public Service Foundation, Inc.**
PO Box 19001
Green Bay, WI 54307-9001
**Phone:** (920)448-7260          **Fax:** (414)433-1693
**Website:** http://www.wpsr.com/foundat/index.html
Larry Weyers, President & Chief Executive Officer

**Priorities:** *Arts & Humanities:* About 5%. Supports historical societies and historical preservation, music, dance, and museums. *Civic & Public Affairs:* 16%. Funds cities, parks, and public affairs organizations. *Education:* About 30%. Major support is for colleges and universities. Also funds health, technical, and religious education, and educational associations. Foundation makes scholarships, as well. *Environment:* 34%. Supports united funds, Salvation Army, youth organizations including clubs, camps, sports, and Christian youth organizations, and family services. *International:* 7%. Supports hospitals and health organizations. *Voluntarism:* The company sponsors employee volunteer programs in association with the United Way at Work Committee, Adopt-a-Classroom, and the Lyle Kingston Environmental Group. *Note:* Total contributions in 1998. **Typ. Recipients:** Children's Health/Hospitals, Clinics/Medical Centers, Domestic Violence, Emergency/Ambulance Services, Health Organizations, Health-General, Hospitals, Medical Education, Medical Rehabilitation, People with Disabilities, Prenatal Health Issues, Single-Disease Health Associations, Substance Abuse. **Geo. Dist:** MI, Northern Michigan; WI, Northeast Wisconsin.

**★ 1511 ★ Wm. Jr. Wrigley Co. Foundation**
410 North Michigan Ave.
Chicago, IL 60611
**Phone:** (312)645-3950          **Fax:** (312)661-1267
William Piet, President

**Priorities:** *Arts & Humanities:* 6%. Funds arts outreach, war memorials. *Civic & Public Affairs:* 7%. Supports NAACP, conservation associations, and neighborhood and community development. *Education:* 10%. Funds groups concerned with minority education, education funds and nursing scholarships. Company provides scholarships for children of employees. Makes no direct grants to colleges or universities. *Environment:* 39%. Supports United Way, youth and family services, child abuse prevention, and social services. *International:* 27%. Supports medical centers, health care, single-disease associations, elder care, and American cancer Society. *Religion:* 2%. Supports Chicago Academy of Science, and Museum of Science & Industry. *Note:* Total contributions made in 1999. **Typ. Recipients:** AIDS/HIV, Alzheimers Disease, Cancer, Child Abuse, Clinics/Medical Centers, Diabetes, Domestic Violence, Eyes/Blindness, Health Funds, Health Organizations, Heart, Hospitals, Medical Education, Nursing Services, People with Disabilities, Prenatal Health Issues, Public Health, Single-Disease Health Associations, Substance Abuse. **Geo. Dist:** nationally; Chicago, IL.

**Wolfe Associates, Inc.**
*See:* Entry 5591

**★ 1512 ★ Wolverine World Wide Foundation**
9341 Courtland Dr.
Rockford, MI 49351
**Phone:** (616)866-5500
**Email:** comrel@dispatch.com
**Website:** http://www.dispatch.com
Robert Sedrowski, Vice President Human Resources

**Typ. Recipients:** Clinics/Medical Centers, Emergency/Ambulance Services, Eyes/Blindness, Health Organizations, Health-General, Heart, Hospitals. **Geo. Dist:** MI.

**★ 1513 ★ WorldCom Education Foundation**
22001 Loudoun County Parkway
G1-3-3288
Ashburn, VA 20147
**Phone:** (703)886-2353          **Fax:** (703)415-7175
Laura Gundert, Director

**Fnded:** 1986. **Priorities:** *Arts & Humanities:* 16%. Supports libraries, museums, and art institutes. *Education:* 59%. Supports the integration of Internet technology into K-12 education to enhance the process of learning. *Religion:* 25%. Supports associations and societies. *Note:* Total foundation contributions made in 2000. **Typ. Recipients:** Arthritis, Cancer, Emergency/Ambulance Services, Family Planning, Health Organizations, Hospitals, Medical Education, Medical Training, People with Disabilities, Single-Disease Health Associations. **Geo. Dist:** headquarters and operating communities.

**WPWR-TV Channel 50 Foundation**
*See:* Entry 11698

**★ 1514 ★ Wyman-Gordon Foundation**
370 Main St., Ste. 1100
Worcester, MA 01608
**Phone:** (508)798-8621          **Fax:** (508)791-6454

**Email:** mail@wpwr50fund.org
Warner Fletcher, Jr., Director

**Priorities:** *Arts & Humanities:* 14%. Contributes to museums, historic preservation, historic sites, and libraries, as well as general art activities. *Civic & Public Affairs:* 2%. Supports community and civic needs in operating locations, including community groups, housing, and legal aid. *Education:* 5%. Supports technical and vocational schools, colleges and universities, primarily in Massachusetts. *Environment:* 71%. The majority of funding supports the United Way. Additional funds support traditional youth organizations, food banks, community recreation, and people with disabilities. *International:* 2%. Funds are awarded to public health associations and centers, and for disease research and prevention. *Religion:* 6%. Supports biology research, science centers and fairs, and an environmental science museum. *Note:* Total contributions made in 2000. **Typ. Recipients:** AIDS/HIV, Cancer, Children's Health/Hospitals, Emergency/Ambulance Services, Health-General, Hospices, Hospitals, Medical Research, Multiple Sclerosis, Nursing Services, People with Disabilities, Public Health. **Geo. Dist:** principally near operating locations and to national organizations.

**★ 1515 ★ Xcel Energy Foundation**
800 Nicollet Mall Ste. 2900
Minneapolis, MN 55402
**Phone:** (612)330-5500          **Fax:** (612)330-6947
**Website:**    http://www.xcelenergy.com/community/Community.asp
John Pacheco, Director

**Priorities:** *Arts & Humanities:* 8%. Contributions provide opportunities for all individuals and families to learn and grow from the arts. Supports a broad spectrum of cultural activities, including theater, dance, music and arts organizations. Historic preservation and museums also supported. Emphasis on programs designed to increase accessibility to community performances for special populations. *Civic & Public Affairs:* 35%. Contributions build stronger neighborhoods by providing opportunities for members of the community to rebuild their neighborhoods. Interests include urban and community affairs. 10% to 15%. Generally smaller grants made at the local level. Priorities will vary according to community needs. *Education:* 14%. Contributes to education-focused programs to provide access to life-long learning, and opportunities for youth and adults to become contributing members of the workforce. Primarily supports postsecondary scholarship and financial assistance programs for low-income groups, minorities, and women. Emphasis onlearning-disabled children and adults. Capital grants awarded to higher education institutions. Also sponsors matching gifts program in education. *Environment:* 31%. Contributions focus on building the capacity of families and individuals of all ages to become stronger, more independent and self sufficient members in the community. Major support for programs that remove barriers for the economically or socially disadvantaged, including social services to special population groups; employment assistance; and short-term and crisis assistance programs such as food shelves, battered women's shelters, and crisis nurseries. Youth organizations, community centers, and organizations concerned with the elderly are also supported, as well as health care for under-served population groups. **Typ. Recipients:** AIDS/HIV, Cancer, Clinics/Medical Centers, Domestic Violence, Health Organizations, Hospitals, Mental Health, Nursing Services, People with Disabilities, Single-Disease Health Associations, Substance Abuse. **Geo. Dist:** near headquarters and service areas only.

**★ 1516 ★ Yellow Corp. Foundation**
10990 Roe Ave.
Overland Park, KS 66211-1213
**Phone:** (913)696-6123          **Fax:** (913)696-6116
Steve Richards, Managing Director

**Priorities:** *Civic & Public Affairs:* 3%. Supports National World War II Memorial. *Education:* 29%. Administers matching gifts program to accredited colleges and universities. Major interests include education concerned with traffic and logistics, business education, and arts education. Substantial funding is also awarded to education associations, economic education, literacy programs, and faculty development. *Environment:* 60%. Major interests include united funds, community centers, and youth organizations. Yellow Corporation matches United Way contributions. *International:* 8%. Funds hospitals, health organizations. *Note:* Total contributions made in 1999. **Typ. Recipients:** Cancer, Children's Health/Hospitals, Domestic Violence, Health Organizations, Heart, Multiple Sclerosis, Public Health. **Geo. Dist:** headquarters and operating communities; Kansas City, MO.

**★ 1517 ★ York Federal Savings & Loan Foundation**
c/o York Federal Savings & Loan Foundation
101 South George St.
York, PA 17401
**Phone:** (717)846-8777    **Fax:** (717)846-5590
Robert Pullo, Chairman & Chief Executive Officer
**Priorities:** *Arts & Humanities:* 27%. Supports theater, performing arts, libraries, community art projects, and art funds. *Civic & Public Affairs:* 7%. Interests include immigrant services and community foundations. *Education:* 24%. Funds Penn State York, public and private preK-12 schools, scholarship funds, and Junior Achievement. *Environment:* 25%. Major funding for the United Way; also supports youth organizations and social service agencies. *International:* 13%. Supports hospitals, a mental health association, and single-disease health associations. *Note:* Total contributions made in fiscal 2000. **Typ. Recipients:** Children's Health/Hospitals, Clinics/Medical Centers, Emergency/Ambulance Services, Health Organizations, Heart, Hospices, Hospitals, Mental Health, Multiple Sclerosis, People with Disabilities, Prenatal Health Issues, Public Health, Sexual Abuse, Single-Disease Health Associations, Substance Abuse. **Geo. Dist:** York, PA.

**★ 1518 ★ Young & Rubicam Foundation**
1114 Ave. of the Americas, 12th Floor
New York, NY 10036
**Phone:** (212)798-1039
**Fnded:** 1955. **Priorities:** *Arts & Humanities:* 25%. Museums, theaters, and libraries. *Civic & Public Affairs:* 14%. The Advertising Council, with other funding directed to community and economic development. *Education:* 38%. Primarily in the form of employee matching gifts. Remaining support goes to education funds in New York, NY. *Environment:* 10%. United Way of New York City, youth and family services, and disaster relief. *International:* 5%. Hospitals, community service programs, and disease-specific foundations. *Religion:* 3%. Donates to science museums and centers. *Note:* Total contributions made in 1999. **Typ. Recipients:** AIDS/HIV, Arthritis, Cancer, Children's Health/Hospitals, Clinics/Medical Centers, Diabetes, Emergency/Ambulance Services, Family Planning, Geriatric Health, Heart, Hospitals, Medical Education, Medical Research, Multiple Sclerosis, Nursing Services, People with Disabilities, Prenatal Health Issues, Public Health, Respiratory, Single-Disease Health Associations, Substance Abuse, Transplant Networks/Donor Banks. **Geo. Dist:** NY.

**★ 1519 ★ The Zachry Foundation**
310 South St. Mary's St., Ste. 2500
San Antonio, TX 78205
**Phone:** (210)554-4663    **Fax:** (210)554-4605
Pamela O'Connor, Executive Director
**Fnded:** 1960. **Priorities:** *Arts & Humanities:* 10% to 15%. Performing arts, libraries, and museums and galleries. *Education:* 30% to 40%. Public education, colleges and universities, and private education. *Environment:* 35% to 40%. United funds, child welfare, and family services. **Typ. Recipients:** Cancer, Children's Health/Hospitals, Clinics/Medical Centers, Diabetes, Domestic Violence, Health Organizations, Health-General, Hospices, Hospitals, Hospitals (University Affiliated), Medical Education, Medical Rehabilitation, Medical Research, People with Disabilities, Speech & Hearing, Substance Abuse. **Geo. Dist:** TX, higher

education grants are given throughout the state; San Antonio, TX.

## Other Funding Organizations

**★ 1520 ★ American Academy of Physician Assistants (AAPA)**
950 N Washington St.
Alexandria, VA 22314-1552
**Phone:** (703)836-2272    **Fax:** (703)684-1924
**Email:** aapa@aapa.org
**Website:** http://www.aapa.org
Kevin D. Bayes, Asst. Dir.
**Desc:** Physician assistants and other interested parties. Seeks to promote quality, cost-effective, and accessible healthcare, and the professional and personal development of PAs. Provide services for members. Organizes annual National PA Day. Develops research and education programs; compiles statistics. **Awards:** Scholarship.

**★ 1521 ★ American Academy on Physician and Patient**
6728 Old McLean Village Dr.
Mc Lean, VA 22101
**Phone:** (703)556-9222    **Fax:** (703)556-8729
**Email:** aappatient@degnon.org
**Website:** http://www.physicianpatient.org
**Desc:** Research and education professionals. Dedicated to research, education and improving professional standards in doctor-patient communication. Sponsors scholarships and grants. **Awards:** Grant; scholarship.

**★ 1522 ★ American Association for Chronic Fatigue Syndrome (AACFS)**
515 Minor Ave., Ste. 18
Seattle, WA 98104
**Phone:** (206)781-3544    **Fax:** (206)749-9052
**Email:** info@aacfs.org
**Website:** http://www.aacfs.org
Benjamin H. Natelson, MD, Pres.
**Desc:** Research scientists, physicians and other health care professionals, and institutions with an interest in chronic fatigue syndrome (CFS). Seeks to advance the diagnosis and treatment of CFS. Facilitates exchange of information among members; sponsors research; serves as a clearinghouse on CFS diagnosis and patient care. Maintains speakers' bureau. **Awards:** Junior Investigator Award (biennial); Rudy Perpich Award (biennial).

**★ 1523 ★ American Association of Small Ruminant Practitioners (AASRP)**
1910 Lyda Ave., No. 200
Bowling Green, KY 42104
**Phone:** (270)793-0781    **Fax:** (270)782-0188
**Email:** aasrp@assrp.org
**Website:** http://www.aasrp.org
Richard W. Stobaeus, Jr., Pres.
**Desc:** Practicing veterinarians and veterinary students; associate members are producers, feeders, hobbyists, and others interested in sheep, goats, llamas, deer, and exotic small ruminants. Aims are to: elevate standards of practice in the field; further research programs that will assist in solving small ruminant health problems; foster communication between veterinarians, owners, and researchers in order to improve small ruminant health management programs. Sponsors specialized education programs. Conducts educational programs. Maintains speakers' bureau. **Awards:** George McConnell Award (biennial) professional service; Sam Guss Memorial Awards for student research and extern purposes.

**★ 1524 ★ American College of Medical Physics**
11250 Roger Bacon Dr., Ste. 8
Reston, VA 20190-5202
**Phone:** (703)481-5001    **Fax:** (703)435-4390
**Email:** acmpwebmaster@radiationphysics.com

**Website:** http://www.acmp.org
Richard A. Guggolz, Exec. Dir.
**Desc:** Covers socioeconomic aspects of practice, management issues, reimbursement, licensure, and practice standards. **Awards:** ACMP Graduate Scholarship Award (annual).

**★ 1525 ★ American Medical Student Association (AMSA)**
1902 Association Dr.
Reston, VA 20191
**Phone:** (703)620-6600    **Free:** 800-767-2266
**Fax:** (703)620-5873
**Email:** amsa@amsa.org
**Website:** http://www.amsa.org
Jaya Agrawal, Pres.
**Desc:** Medical students; local, state, and national organizations; premedical students, interns, and residents. Seeks to improve medical education by making it relevant to today's needs and by making the process by which physicians are trained more humanistic. Contributes to the improvement of health care of all people; involves its members in the social, moral, and ethical obligations of the profession of medicine. Serves as a mechanism through which students may actively participate in the fields of community health through various student health programs. Addresses political issues relating to the nation's health care delivery system and other medical and health issues. Maintains standing committees and interest groups which publish newsletters, organize educational workshops, and initiate special projects. **Awards:** Paul R. Wright Excellence in Medical Education Award (annual).

**★ 1526 ★ American Polarity Therapy Association**
PO Box 19858
Boulder, CO 80308-2858
**Phone:** (303)545-2080    **Fax:** (303)545-2161
**Email:** hq@polaritytherapy.org
**Website:** http://www.polaritytherapy.org
E. Simmons, Exec. Dir.
**Desc:** Polarity therapy education. Dedicated to the advancement of polarity therapy. (Polarity therapy is a non-diagnostic holistic health system supplementing and supporting medical treatment. Polarity techniques include bodywork, diet, exercise and self awareness for health maintenance.) Develops and disseminates educational and support materials; registers practitioners; holds competitions. **Awards:** Dr. Stone Award (annual).

**★ 1527 ★ American School Health Association (ASHA)**
PO Box 708
7263 State Route 43
Kent, OH 44240
**Phone:** (330)678-1601    **Free:** 800-445-2742
**Fax:** (330)678-4526
**Email:** asha@ashaweb.org
**Website:** http://www.ashaweb.org
Cynthia Symons, Pres.
**Desc:** School physicians, school nurses, dentist, nurses, nutritionists, health educators, dental hygenist, school-based professionals and public health workers. Promotes coordinated school health programs that include health education, health services, a healthful school environment, physical education, nutrition services, and psycho-social health services offered in schools collaboratively with families and other members of the community. Offers professional reference materials. Conducts pilot programs that inform materials developement, provides technical assistance to school professionals, advocates for school health, and complies statistics. **Awards:** ASHA Scholarship for college juniors, seniors, and graduate students majoring in health education, nursing, adolescent/pediatric medicine, or dentistry; Distinguished Service Award (annual) for outstanding contributions to the child health field through ASHA; William A. Howe Award (annual) for distinguished service in school health.

## ★ 1528 ★ American Society for Clinical Investigation (ASCI)

35 Research Dr., Ste. 300
Ann Arbor, MI 48103
**Phone:** (734)222-6050 **Fax:** (734)222-6058
**Email:** asci@the-jci.org
**Website:** http://www.asci-jci.org/asci
Dr. Chi Van Dang, Pres.

**Desc:** Physician scientists with meritorious original clinical investigations. Active members are doctors under age 50; senior members are those over age 50. Promotes cultivation of clinical research by methods of natural sciences, correlation of science with the art of medical practice, encouragement of scientific investigation by medical practitioners, and publication of papers on the methods and results of clinical research. **Awards:** ASCI Award (annual).

## ★ 1529 ★ Animal Health Foundation (AHF)

3615 Bassett Rd.
Pacific, MO 63069
**Website:** http://www.animalhealthfoundation.com
Donald M. Walsh, D.V.M., Pres.

**Desc:** Individuals interested in finding the causes, treatments, and cure for the crippling equine disease laminitis/founder syndrome. (Laminitis is an inflammation of the laminae, the semi-rigid internal supporting structures of the horse's foot; founder is the crippling result of laminitis in which the coffin bone in the horse's foot puts pressure on the sole of the foot, and sometimes actually penetrates the sole.) These ailments affect horses of any age or breed, and are counted by the AHF as the second ranking disease leading to the need to euthanize horses. Supports extensive research and collects a range of related data. **Awards:** Grant.

## ★ 1530 ★ Association of Physician Assistant Programs (APAP)

950 N Washington St.
Alexandria, VA 22314-1552
**Phone:** (703)548-5538 **Fax:** (703)684-1924
**Website:** http://www.apap.org
David P. Asprey, Pres.

**Desc:** Represents physician assistant (PA) educational programs in the United States. Assists PA educational programs-institutions with training programs for physician assistants to primary care and surgical physicians. Assists in the development and organization of educational curricula for PA programs to assure the public of competent PAs. Contributes to defining the roles of PAs in the field of medicine to maximize their benefit to the public; serves as a public information center on the profession; coordinates program logistics such as admissions and career placements; and is currently initiating a centralized application service for PA applicants. Sponsors the Annual Survey of Physician Assistant Educational Programs in the United States. Conducts and sponsors research projects; compiles statistics; offers ongoing training for PA leadership and faculty. **Awards:** APAP Partnership Award (annual) for contribution to excellence in PA education by an individual or institution outside of PA program circles; J. Peter Nyquist Student Writing Award Competition (annual) for student submissions dealing with clinical medicine or us issues impacting the PA profession; Master Teacher Award (annual) for excellence in clinical or classroom teaching, scholarship and/or professional service; Outstanding Service Award (annual) for exceptional service or leadership to APAP, or contributions to the profession through scholarly, teaching or advocate activit.

## ★ 1531 ★ Association of Polysomnographic Technologists (APT)

PO Box 14861
Lenexa, KS 66285-1991
**Phone:** (913)541-1991 **Fax:** (913)541-0156
**Email:** soneal@goamp.com
**Website:** http://www.aptweb.org
Sheila O'Neal, Exec. Dir.

**Desc:** Individuals who practice polysomnography in research or clinical settings. (Polysomnographic technology deals with the measurement and recording of multiple physiological activity, such as eye movement and heart rate, during sleep.) Seeks to establish standards for polysomnographic technology and provide education and training for people entering in the field. Acts as a forum for communication among members. **Awards:** Carskadon Research (annual).

## ★ 1532 ★ Association for Research in Otolaryngology (ARO)

c/o Susan Whitehouse
19 Mantua Rd.
Mount Royal, NJ 08061
**Phone:** (856)423-0041 **Fax:** (856)423-3420
**Email:** headquarters@aro.org
**Website:** http://www.aro.org
Susan Whitehouse, Exec. Dir.

**Desc:** Medical professionals, scientists, and researchers with an interest in otolaryngology. Promotes increased understanding of basic science and clinical practice associated with hearing, speech, balance, the senses of taste and smell, and diseases of the head and neck. Conducts educational programs; facilitates exchange of information among members. **Awards:** Midwinter Meeting Travel Award (annual) medical residents and students of otolaryngology.

## ★ 1533 ★ Association for Women Veterinarians (AWV)

PO Box 2039
Starkville, MS 39760-2039
**Phone:** (662)312-0893 **Fax:** (662)323-3280
**Email:** lapancho@ra.msstate.edu
**Website:** http://www.awv-women-veterinarians.org
Dr. Shirley Johnston, Pres.

**Desc:** Works to support veterinary medicine by providing leadership in women's issues. **Awards:** AWV Service Award (annual) to individual contributing to the advancement of women in veterinary medicine; Outstanding Woman Veterinarian (annual) for contributions to veterinary medicine; Student Scholarship (annual) for second or third year veterinary students.

## ★ 1534 ★ Auxiliary to the National Medical Association (ANMA)

1012 10th St. NW
Washington, DC 20001
**Phone:** (202)371-9008 **Fax:** (202)289-2662
**Email:** info@anma-online.org
**Website:** http://www.anma-online.org
Mrs. Maurce W. Ayton, Pres.

**Desc:** Spouses of active members of the National Medical Association (see separate entry); widows and widowers of former members. Purposes are to: create a greater interest in the NMA; assist and encourage the medical profession in its efforts to educate and serve the public in matters of sanitation and health; develop and promote a national program on health and education with subcategories in community needs, legislation, and human relations. Conducts workshops on teenage pregnancy, breast self-examinations, high blood pressure screening, and sickle cell anemia screening. Plans and implements an annual youth forum under the auspices of the March of Dimes Birth Defects Foundation . Provides youth with professional guidance and the opportunity for peer exchange in the areas of mental and physical health; deals with the health of newborns, health services, nutrition, and teenage pregnancy. Also conducts programs for youth on parenting, socially transmitted diseases, nutrition, birth defects, and continued education after pregnancy. **Awards:** Alma Wells Givens Scholarship (annual) to medical students; Omega Mason Memorial Scholarship to outstanding student nurses.

## ★ 1535 ★ Bill and Melinda Gates Foundation

PO Box 23350
Seattle, WA 98102
**Phone:** (206)709-3140

**Email:** libraryinfo@gatesfoundation.org
**Website:** http://www.gatesfoundation.org
Richard Akeroyd, Exec. Dir.

**Desc:** Strives to help improve people's lives through health and learning and looks for strategic opportunities to extend the benefits of modern science and technology to people around the world. **Awards:** Grant.

## ★ 1536 ★ Boston International Foundation for Medical Exchange

c/o Joseph J. Vitale, MD
784 Massachusetts Ave.
Boston, MA 02118-2317
**Phone:** (617)414-4829
**Email:** jjvitale@bu.edu
**Website:** http://www.bifme.org
Joseph J. Vitale, Chm.

**Desc:** Supports senior medical students, medical and surgical residents and junior faculty from Harvard, Tufts and Boston University, who successfully complete a minimum two to six month elective at a foreign medical center acceptable to the respective medical school administration and the foundation. Support is intended to defray travel and living expenses. Believes this experience provides useful and practical insight into cultural, moral and ethnic perceptions of health care in our multi-ethnic and multi-cultural society. **Awards:** Scholarship (3/year) 4th year medical student completing a 2-3 month overseas elective.

## ★ 1537 ★ Clinical Magnetic Resonance Society (CMRS)

4550 Post Oak Pl., Ste. 342
Houston, TX 77027
**Phone:** (713)623-8336 **Free:** 877-841-2522
**Fax:** (713)960-0488
**Email:** cmrs@one.net
**Website:** http://www.cmrs.com
Darcee Brown, Acct. Exec.

**Desc:** Offers experience-based credentialing for physicians who practice MRI. Provides a forum for networking among members. Defines procedure protocols and safety information. **Awards:** Recognition (annual); scholarship (annual) for physicians in training.

## ★ 1538 ★ Entertainment Industries Council (EIC)

1760 Reston Pky., Ste. 415
Reston, VA 20190
**Phone:** (703)481-1414 **Fax:** (703)481-1418
**Email:** eiceast@eiconline.org
**Website:** http://eiconline.org
Brian L. Dyak, Pres.

**Desc:** Corporations and representatives of the entertainment industry including actors, agents, publicists, producers, directors, and writers. Goal is to utilize the power and influence of the entertainment industry in a national campaign to combat and deglamorize substance abuse, especially among young people. Seeks to identify and provide celebrity role models for young people. Hopes to increase youth awareness of drug abuse through television, radio, music, and motion pictures. Develops projects to aid in eliminating substance abuse problems within the entertainment industry. Conducts seminars and training sessions on drug abuse prevention; also conducts radio interview series, television specials, outreach programs, and employee assistance and fundraising programs. Collects and disseminates information on progress made by the entertainment industry in drug abuse prevention. In conjunction with IMMEDIA Foundation, coordinates network of 400 radio stations involved in public affairs projects designed to discourage substance abuse. Provides celebrity speakers' bureau on drug prevention, seat belt awareness, and intravenous drug use/AIDS. Bestows EIC Drug Prevention Award annually to a leader from entertainment industry contributing to drug awareness. **Awards:** Prism Awards (annual); Prism Generation Next (annual).

**★ 1539 ★ Fellowship of Associates of Medical Evangelism (FAME)**
PO Box 34800
Indianapolis, IN 46234
**Phone:** (317)272-5937          **Fax:** (317)272-5940
**Email:** medicalmissions@fameworld.org
**Website:** http://www.fameworld.org
Kevin Dooley, Exec. Dir.

**Desc:** Builds hospitals and clinics and provides mobile medical units for Christian missionaries outside the U.S.; secures and ships medicine and medical supplies. Conducts charitable programs; maintains speakers' bureau. **Awards:** Scholarship for individuals who have been accepted into medical school and are committed to missionary work.


**★ 1540 ★ Healthcare Forum**
180 Montgomery St., Ste. 1520
San Francisco, CA 94104-4230
Kathryn E. Johnson, CEO & Pres.

**Desc:** Healthcare leaders and executives. Promotes visionary leadership and motivation in healthcare. Conducts leadership development education programs; produces computer based educational materials. Sponsors research activities. **Awards:** Healthier Communities (annual).


**★ 1541 ★ Hospitalized Veterans Writing Project (HVWP)**
5920 Nall, Rm. 105
Mission, KS 66202
**Phone:** (913)432-1214
Barbara Sauvan, Pres.

**Desc:** Individuals and organizations united to encourage hospitalized U.S. veterans to write for pleasure and rehabilitation during their hospital stay. Maintains speakers' bureau and slide program with commentary. Conducts writing sessions in hospitals. **Awards:** Monetary (3/year) for prose, poetry, cartoon and drawing, and photographs.


**★ 1542 ★ Howard Hughes Medical Institute (HHMI)**
4000 Jones Bridge Rd.
Chevy Chase, MD 20815-6789
**Phone:** (301)215-8500
**Email:** webmaster@hhmi.org
**Website:** http://www.hhmi.org

**Desc:** Works to help enhance biomedical science education at all levels. Conducts research. **Awards:** Grant.


**★ 1543 ★ International College of Applied Kinesiology - U.S.A. (ICAK-USA)**
6405 Metcalf Ave., Ste. 503
Shawnee Mission, KS 66202-3929
**Phone:** (913)384-5336          **Fax:** (913)384-5112
**Email:** icak@dci-kansascity.com
**Website:** http://www.icakusa.com
Andria Dibbern, Membership Services

**Desc:** Promotes the science of applied kinesiology. Applied Kinesiology is the system of evaluating the structural, chemical, and mental aspect of human heath, involving muscle health, nutrition, manipulation, diet, acupressure, and exercise. Conducts educational programs, research programs, and training seminars. **Awards:** Scholarship (annual).


**★ 1544 ★ International Federation of Societies for Histochemistry and Cytochemistry (IFSHC)**
c/o Dr. Denis G. Baskin
Department of Biological Structure
Univ. of Washington
PO Box 357420
Seattle, WA 98195-9420
**Phone:** (206)616-5894          **Fax:** (206)616-5842
**Email:** baskindg@u.washington.edu

**Website:** http://www.ifshc.org
Prof.Dr. Denis G. Baskin, Sec. Gen.

**Desc:** National societies for histochemistry and cytochemistry. Seeks to promote communication and cooperation among scientists throughout the world and establish histochemistry and cytochemistry institutes. Promotes histochemistry and cytochemistry as basic, independent sciences and advocates their teaching in universities. Appoints committees for the study of scientific matters requiring international collaboration. **Awards:** David Glick Lectureship (quadrennial) for significant contribution to histochemistry; Young Histochemist Awards (quadrennial) for new investigators from societies with paid-up dues to travel to International Congress of Histochemistry & Cytochemistry.


**★ 1545 ★ International Society for Mountain Medicine**
c/o Peter Hackett, MD
610 Sabeta Dr.
Ridgway, CO 81432-9335
**Phone:** (970)626-2477          **Fax:** (970)626-2467
**Email:** hackett@ismmed.org
**Website:** http://www.ismmed.org

**Desc:** Brings together scientists and physicians, and allied trade professionals interested in mountain medicine. Encourages research on all aspects of mountains, mountain peoples and mountaineers. **Awards:** ISMM Research Prize (biennial) for scientific merit.


**★ 1546 ★ Islamic Medical Association of North America (IMANA)**
950 75th St.
Downers Grove, IL 60516
**Phone:** (630)852-2122          **Fax:** (630)435-1429
**Email:** imana@aol.com
**Website:** http://www.imana.org
Khursheed Mallick, MD, Exec. Dir.

**Desc:** Muslim physicians and allied health professionals. Unites Muslim physicians and allied health professionals in the U.S. and Canada for the improvement of professional and social contact; provides assistance to Muslim communities worldwide. Charitable programs include: donation of books, journals, and educational and research materials to medical institutions; donation of medical supplies and equipment to charity medical institutions in Muslim countries. Maintains speakers' bureau to present Islamic viewpoints on medical topics; sponsors placement service; offers assistance in orientation. **Awards:** Scholarship.


**★ 1547 ★ Laboratory Animal Management Association (LAMA)**
7300 Metro Blvd., Ste. 585
Edina, MN 55439
**Phone:** (952)250-6201          **Fax:** (952)835-4774
**Email:** imartinez@rcm.upr.edu
**Website:** http://www.lama-online.org
Ivette Martinez-Palma, Pres.

**Desc:** Laboratory animal facility managers. Seeks to evaluate and update basic and advanced management techniques and to educate laboratory animal facility managers. Makes available resource material; coordinates exchange programs for management personnel. Offers consulting on management techniques. **Awards:** Charles River Medallion for distinguished contributions to the field by an administrator/manager who is a current member of LAMA and engaged in laboratoryanimal management; LAMA Foundation Award to qualified members within laboratory animal management for the futherance of his or her education in the field; U. Kristina Stephens Award awarded to a LAMA Member for outstanding and exceptional service to LAMA.


**★ 1548 ★ Lesbian Health Fund (LHF)**
459 Fulton St., Ste. 107
San Francisco, CA 94102
**Phone:** (415)255-4547          **Fax:** (415)255-4784
**Email:** info@glma.org
**Website:** http://www.glma.org/

**Desc:** Works to recognize the unique healthcare needs of lesbians; seeks to strengthen the health of lesbians and their families through health and medical research grants and education. **Awards:** Lesbian Health Research Grant (semiannual).


**★ 1549 ★ Medical Group Management Association (MGMA)**
104 Inverness Terr. E
Englewood, CO 80112-5306
**Phone:** (303)799-1111          **Free:** 877-275-6462
**Fax:** (303)643-4439
**Email:** infocenter@mgma.com
**Website:** http://www.mgma.com
William F. Jessee, MD, CEO

**Desc:** For professionals involved in the business management of groups in medical practice. Products and services include education, benchmarking, surveys, national advocacy and networking opportunities for members. **Awards:** Recognition (annual); scholarship (annual).


**★ 1550 ★ Narcolepsy Network**
10921 Reed Hartman Highway
Cincinnati, OH 45242
**Phone:** (513)891-3522          **Fax:** (513)891-3836
**Email:** narnet@aol.com
**Website:** http://www.websciences.org/narnet
Robert L. Cloud, Exec. Dir.

**Desc:** Individuals with narcolepsy, their friends and families, sleep professionals, and interested others. Seeks to improve the quality of life of individuals who have narcolepsy. Works to educate members and the general public about narcolepsy. Fosters communication among members. Offers referral service. Supports research; disseminates information. **Awards:** Grant (periodic) for research.


**★ 1551 ★ National Alopecia Areata Foundation (NAAF)**
PO Box 150760
San Rafael, CA 94915-0760
**Phone:** (415)472-3780          **Fax:** (415)472-5343
**Email:** info@naaf.org
**Website:** http://www.naaf.org
Vicki Kalabokes, CEO

**Desc:** Individuals concerned about alopecia areata, a disease causing partial scalp hair loss, total scalp hair loss (alopecia totalis), or total loss of body hair (alopecia universalis); cause and cure are unknown and the course of the disease is unpredictable. Objectives are to: develop public awareness of the disease; provide a support network; raise funds for research; keep patients medically informed with explanations about AA and the latest treatments. Maintains medical advisory board; operates information booth at meetings of the American Academy of Dermatology. **Awards:** National Alopecia Areata Foundation Research Grants (annual) for research on Alopecia Areata.


**★ 1552 ★ National Arab American Medical Association (NAAMA)**
801 S Adams Rd., Ste. 208
Birmingham, MI 48009-7018
**Phone:** (248)646-3661          **Fax:** (248)646-0617
**Email:** naama@naama.com
**Website:** http://www.naama.com
Ellen R. Potter, Exec. Dir.

**Desc:** Medical professionals of Arab descent. Fosters exchange of scientific information. Encourages continuing education for members. Provides financial and technical support for medical students and institutions in the United States and in Arab countries. Offers medical assistance to needy individuals of Arab descent. **Awards:** Monetary (semiannual) for the medical resident submitting the best paper.

**★ 1553 ★ National Board of Medical Examiners (NBME)**
3750 Market St.
Philadelphia, PA 19104-3190
**Phone:** (215)590-9500          **Fax:** (215)590-9555
**Email:** webmail@nbme.org
**Website:** http://www.nbme.org
Donald E. Melnick, MD, Pres.

**Desc:** Purposes are: to prepare and administer qualifying examinations either independently or in conjunction with other organizations, of such high quality that legal agencies governing the practice of medicine within each state may, in their discretion, grant a license without further examination for those who have successfully completed such examinations; to cooperate with and, where appropriate, to make its specialized services available to the examining boards of the states, specialty boards, and other organizations concerned with the education and qualification of personnel in the fields of health; to assist medical schools, hospitals and related organizations and institutions in evaluation of the effectiveness of their educational programs; to initiate, develop, and participate in research designed to evaluate the effectiveness of educational programs and techniques, and to assess ever more precisely the knowledge, competence, and qualification of professionals in public health care; to provide educational opportunities for professional personnel in the methods, techniques, and values of testing methods related to knowledge and competence in the broad field of medicine. **Awards:** Medical Education Research Fund (annual).

**★ 1554 ★ National Center for FarmWorker Health**
1770 FM 967
Buda, TX 78610-2884
**Phone:** (512)312-2700          **Fax:** (512)312-2600
**Email:** mckay@ncfh.org
**Website:** http://www.ncfh.org
Mimi McKay, Library and Information Resources Dir.

**Desc:** Seeks to make quality primary health care accessible to migrant and seasonal farm workers. Supports the establishment of a national network of migrant health centers through the production, processing, and distribution of information, including information on health problems specific to or more prevalent in the migrant community. Works to provide technical assistance for health development and research. Develops collaborative working relationship between agencies serving migrant farmworkers. Maintains job/resume bank, biographical archives, and library. Bestows awards; operates placement service; compiles statistics. biographical archives, library, and speakers' bureau. Bestows awards; operates placement service; compiles statistics. **Awards:** Migrant Health Scholarship (annual) work in migrant health center.

**★ 1555 ★ National CFIDS Foundation**
103 Althea Rd.
Needham, MA 02492
**Phone:** (781)449-3535          **Fax:** (781)449-8606
**Email:** info@ncf-net.com
**Website:** http://www.ncf-net.org
Gail R. Kansky, Pres.

**Desc:** Provides education, advocacy and fundraising for research. **Awards:** Grant.

**★ 1556 ★ National Medical Fellowships (NMF)**
5 Handover Sq., 15th Fl.
New York, NY 10004
**Phone:** (212)483-8880          **Fax:** (212)483-8897
**Email:** info@nmfonline.org
**Website:** http://www.nmfonline.org
Vivian Fox, Pres. /CEO

**Desc:** Promotes education of minority students in medicine. Provides need-based scholarships, special merit awards, and leadership opportunities to medical students of African American, Native American, Mexican American and mainland Puerto Rican heritage.

**Awards:** Recognition (annual) for third- and fourth-year minority medical students; scholarship (annual).

**★ 1557 ★ National Sleep Foundation**
1522 K St., NW, Ste. 500
Washington, DC 20005
**Phone:** (202)347-3471          **Fax:** (202)347-3472
**Email:** nsf@sleepfoundation.org
**Website:** http://www.sleepfoundation.org
Richard L. Gelula, Exec. Dir.

**Desc:** Works to improve the quality of life of people suffering from sleep disorders and to prevent accidents related to sleep disorders. (Sleep disorders include: insomnia, narcolepsy, sleep apnea syndrome, sudden infant death syndrome, stroke, epilepsy, and other disorders of sleep and daytime alertness.) Educates health care professionals and the public about the existance and treatment of sleep disorders. Promotes the development of patient services, community resources, and support groups for individuals affected by sleep disorders. Sponsors educational and research programs. **Awards:** Pickwick Club and Narcolepsy Fellowships (annual); scholarship.

**★ 1558 ★ Pan American Medical Association (PAMA)**
c/o William E. Sorrel, M.D. Pres.
263 W End Ave., Ste. 1A
New York, NY 10023
**Phone:** (212)362-0159
William E. Sorrel, M.D., PhD, Pres.

**Desc:** Fosters the exchange of medical information and research results among physicians in Western Hemisphere countries. **Awards:** P.A.M.A. Medal for distinguished medical service; Postgraduate Medical Fellowship (annual) for postgraduate students with M.D. degree.

**★ 1559 ★ Phi Chi Medical Fraternity (PCMF)**
1201 E Spring St.
New Albany, IN 47150
**Phone:** (812)948-0581          **Free:** 800-800-7442
**Fax:** (812)941-8850
**Email:** phichi@phi-chi.org
**Website:** http://www.phi-chi.org
Daniel H. Cannon, MD, Chm., Exec. Trustees

**Desc:** Professional fraternity - medicine. Maintains Phi Chi Welfare Association, which accepts voluntary contributions to a student loan fund and other services. **Awards:** Recognition (annual); scholarship (annual).

**★ 1560 ★ RGK Foundation**
1301 W 25th St., Ste. 300
Austin, TX 78705-4236
**Phone:** (512)474-9298          **Fax:** (512)474-7281
**Website:** http://www.rgkfoundation.org
Gregory A. Kozmetsky, Pres.

**Desc:** Works to promote medical research. **Awards:** Grant.

**★ 1561 ★ Royal Society of Medicine Foundation (RSMF)**
207 E Westminster Rd. Ste. 201
Lake Forest, IL 60045-1860
**Phone:** (847)234-6782
**Website:** http://www.rsm.ac.uk
Richard S. Wilbur, MD, Exec. Officer

**Desc:** Serves as a forum for the discussion of topics relevant to the medical community in the U.S. and the United Kingdom. Sponsors conference series and exchange programs in conjunction with the Royal Society of Medicine. **Awards:** Hewitt (semiannual) lifetime achievement.

**★ 1562 ★ Seventh-Day Adventist Dietetic Association (SDADA)**
1 Angwin Ave.
Angwin, CA 94508

**Phone:** (916)782-5200          **Fax:** (916)782-5458
**Email:** rubyh@rsvl.ah.com

**Desc:** Seventh-Day Adventist registered dietitians; dietitians working in Seventh-Day Adventist institutions. Strives to motivate members to attain high professional standards and to actively promote Seventh-Day Adventist health principles. Provides resources and guidance concerning vegetarian lifestyles to dietitians. Disseminates nutrition information. **Awards:** Dietetic Studetn Scholarship Awards; scholarship for Seventh-Day adventist dietetic students.

**★ 1563 ★ Society of Critical Care Medicine (SCCM)**
701 Lee St., Ste. 200
Des Plaines, IL 60016
**Phone:** (847)827-6869          **Fax:** (847)827-6886
**Email:** info@sccm.org
**Website:** http://www.sccm.org
David Julian Martin, CEO/Exec. VP

**Desc:** Physicians, nurses, scientists, technicians, respiratory therapists, engineers, pharmacists, and physicians assistants involved in the field of critical care medicine. Purposes are: to improve care for acute life-threatening illnesses and injuries; to promote development of optimal care facilities; to guarantee high educational standards in critical care medicine. SCCM has initiated self-assessment testing program in an effort to establish core curriculum and assist physicians in self-evaluation. SCCM established American College of Critical Care Medicine in 1988. **Awards:** American College of Critical Care Medicine Distinguished Investigator Award (annual) honors the meritorious and pioneering research of an SCCM established clinical investigator with a $10,000 award; Christer Grenvik Memorial Award (annual) honors an SCCM member who has promoted the ethical and humane delivery of critical care medicine with a $1000 cash award; ICU Design Citation (annual) honors a critical care unit that combines functional ICU design with the humanitarian delivery of critical care with a $1500 award; In-Training Fellow Award (annual) honors an author participating in a critical care fellowship training program or who has completed a program not more than a year before the annual Symposium with a $3000 cash award; Norma J. Shoemaker Award (annual) award of $1000 presented to the nurse member who demonstrates excellence in clinical practice, education, and/or administration; Norma J. Shoemaker Grant (annual) $15,000 nursing research award; Young Investigator's Award.

**★ 1564 ★ Society for Medical Decision Making (SMDM)**
c/o George Washington University Medical Center
2300 K St. NW
Office of Continuing Medical Education in the Health
Professions
Washington, DC 20037
**Phone:** (202)994-8929          **Fax:** (202)994-1791
**Email:** smdm-office@smi.stanford.edu
**Website:** http://www.gwu.edu/~smdm
Daniel E. Reichard, Admin. Dir.

**Desc:** Individuals with an interest in "developing rational and systematic approaches" to medical decision making, including educators, clinicians, managers, and policy makers. Promotes improvement in all aspects of medical decision making. Evaluates decision making applications and disseminates conclusions. Facilitates multidisciplinary scholarship and research; conducts continuing professional education programs. **Awards:** Career Achievement Award (annual); Distinguished Service Award (annual); Lee B. Lusted Student Prizes (annual) outstanding research presented at SMDM annual meeting; Outstanding Short Course; Young Investigator Award (annual).

**★ 1565 ★ Surfer's Medical Association**
PO Box 1210
Aptos, CA 95001
**Phone:** (831)684-0916          **Fax:** (831)684-0916
**Email:** smacentral@aol.com

**Website:** http://www.damoon.net/sma/index.html
Paula Smith, Exec. Dir.

**Desc:** Surfer-health professionals and surfers interested in the health and medical aspects of surfing. Works to educate surfers and medical practitioners on the unique health problems of surfers. Represents the sport of surfing in the fields of medicine and science and also works to preserve the environment of beaches and oceans. Established the first international network of surfing health professionals. Sponsors members' research in this field. **Awards:** Scholarship (periodic) to a fijian village student.

★ **1566** ★ **Tissue Banks International (TBI)**
815 Park Ave.
Baltimore, MD 21201-4887
**Phone:** (410)783-0183 **Free:** 800-756-4824
**Fax:** (410)454-4457
**Email:** tbi@tbionline.org
**Website:** http://www.tbionline.org
Gerald Cole, Pres. /CEO

**Desc:** A non-profit network of medical eye and tissue banks. Provides eye tissue for sight-restoring corneal transplant surgery. Also distributes bone, skin, and other soft tissues. Assists members with operational areas. Provides grants for research into the causes and cures of blindness. Distributes information on eye, tissue, and organ donation. Conducts educational and charitable programs. **Awards:** Grant.

★ **1567** ★ **United Mitochondrial Disease Foundation (UMDF)**
8085 Saltsburg Rd., Ste. 201
Pittsburgh, PA 15239
**Phone:** (412)793-8077 **Fax:** (412)793-6477
**Email:** info@umdf.org
**Website:** http://www.umdf.org
Antoinette Renda Beasley, Fin. Svcs. Coord.

**Desc:** Patients, parents or guardians, friends, relatives, medical professionals, hospitals, and other organizations. Promotes research for cures and treatments of mitochondrial disease; provides support to patients and families. Patient registry database includes information from symptoms and treatment to diagnostic methods and specific disorders. **Awards:** Research Award (annual).

★ **1568** ★ **Velo-Cardio-Facial Syndrome (VCFS)**
c/o Dr. Robert J. Shprintzen
Upstate Medical University
University Hospital
708 Jacobsen Hall (CDU)
750 E Adams St.
Syracuse, NY 13210
**Phone:** (315)464-6590 **Fax:** (315)464-6593
**Email:** vcfsef@mail.upstate.edu
**Website:** http://www.vcfsef.org
Dr. Robert J. Shprintzen, Exec. Dir.

**Desc:** Committed to educating the lay and professional public, offers family programs, provides parent-to-parent networking; promotes the diagnosis and treatment of individuals with VCF; distributes educational materials about Velo-Cardio-Facial (also known as Shprintzen Syndrome, DiGeorge Sequence, and Catch 22); and distributes questionnaire regarding the medical diagnosis and management of individuals with this disorder. **Awards:** Caitlin Lynch Memorial Fund Award (annual); Tony Lipson Memorial Fund Award (annual) helps members from Australia attend annual meetings.

★ **1569** ★ **Vietnamese Medical Association of the U.S.A.**
c/o B.S. NguyenleHieu, M.D.
Shelton Medical Clinic
302 C St.
PO Box 476
Shelton, NE 68876
**Phone:** (308)647-6828 **Fax:** (308)647-5219
B.S. Nguyenlehieu, MD, Contact

**Desc:** Vietnamese-American medical professionals. Promotes mutual support and fellowship among its members, while fostering and maintaining medical ethics. Assures the provision of equal educational and professional opportunities for its members and the welfare of the general Vietnamese community. Supports and assists the Vietnamese victims of the Vietnamese communist regime. **Awards:** Pham bieu Tam MD Award (biennial) for contribution to advancing medical knowledge for Vietnamese.

★ **1570** ★ **W.M. Keck Foundation**
550 S Hope St., Ste. 2500
Los Angeles, CA 90071
**Phone:** (213)680-3833
**Website:** http://www.wmkeck.org
Robert A. Day, Pres.

**Desc:** Works to support medical research, science, and engineering. **Awards:** Grant.

★ **1571** ★ **William H. Donner Foundation**
500 Fifth Ave., Ste. 1230
New York, NY 10110-0180
**Phone:** (212)719-9290 **Fax:** (212)302-8734
**Website:** http://www.donner.org

**Desc:** Strives to fund thoughtful and creative medical-related projects. **Awards:** Grant.

# Medical & Allied Health Schools

## Medicine

*The following are accredited U.S. medical schools. Professional associations to contact for further information on medical education include the Association of American Medical Colleges (2450 N St. NW, Washington, DC 20037-1126, (202)828-0400, http://www.aamc.org/) and the American Medical Association (515 N State St., Chicago, IL 60610, (312)464-5000, http://www.ama-assn.org/).*

### Alabama

★ **1572** ★ **University of Alabama, Birmingham School of Medicine**
1813 6th Ave., S
Birmingham, AL 35294-3293
**Phone:** (205)934-4011 **Fax:** (205)934-0333
**Website:** http://www.uab.edu/uasom
William B. Deal, MD, Director
**Fnded:** 1945.

★ **1573** ★ **University of South Alabama College of Medicine**
307 University Blvd.
Mobile, AL 36688
**Phone:** (334)460-7174 **Fax:** (334)460-6073
**Website:** http://www.southalabama.edu
Robert A. Kreisberg, MD, Director
**Fnded:** 1973.

### Alberta

★ **1574** ★ **University of Alberta Faculty of Medicine and Dentistry**
2J2 Walter Mackenzie Health Sciences Center
8440 112th St.
Edmonton, AB, Canada T6G 2R7
**Phone:** (780)492-6350 **Fax:** (780)492-7303
**Website:** http://www.med.ualberta.ca
D. L. J. Tyrrell, MD,PhD, Director
**Fnded:** 1913.

★ **1575** ★ **University of Calgary Faculty of Medicine**
3330 Hospital Dr., NW
Calgary, AB, Canada T2N 4N1
**Phone:** (403)220-6848 **Fax:** (403)283-4740
**Email:** staylors@ucalgary.ca
**Website:** http://www.med.ucalgary.ca/
D. G. Gall, MD, Director
**Fnded:** 1970.

### Arizona

★ **1576** ★ **University of Arizona College of Medicine**
PO Box 245018
Tucson, AZ 85724-5018
**Phone:** (520)626-6214 **Fax:** (520)626-4884
**Website:** http://www.ahsc.arizona.edu/
Raymond L. Woolsey, MD,PhD, Director
**Fnded:** 1967.

### Arkansas

★ **1577** ★ **University of Arkansas College of Medicine**
4301 W Markham St.
Little Rock, AR 72205
**Phone:** (501)686-5000 **Fax:** (501)686-8160
**Website:** http://www.uams.edu/com/
John P. Shock, MD, Director
**Fnded:** 1879.

### British Columbia

★ **1578** ★ **University of British Columbia Faculty of Medicine**
317-2194 Health Sciences Mall
Vancouver, BC, Canada V6T 1Z3
**Phone:** (604)822-2421 **Fax:** (604)822-6061
**Website:** http://www.med.ubc.ca
John A. Cairns, MD, Director
**Fnded:** 1950.

### California

★ **1579** ★ **Loma Linda University School of Medicine**
Loma Linda, CA 92350
**Phone:** (909)558-4462 **Fax:** (909)558-0292
**Email:** cbender@som.llu.edu
**Website:** http://www.llu.edu/llu/medicine/
Brian S. Bull, MD, Director
**Fnded:** 1961. **Frmly:** (1909) College of Medical Evangelists.

★ **1580** ★ **Stanford University School of Medicine**
300 Pasteur Dr.
Stanford, CA 94305-5519
**Phone:** (650)725-3900 **Fax:** (650)725-7368
**Website:** http://www.med.stanford.edu
Philip A. Pizzo, MD, Director
**Fnded:** 1908.

★ **1581** ★ **University of California, Davis School of Medicine**
Davis, CA 95616
**Phone:** (916)752-0331 **Fax:** (916)752-3512
**Website:** http://www.med.ucdavis.edu/
Dr. Joseph Silva, Jr., Director
**Fnded:** 1968.

★ **1582** ★ **University of California, Irvine College of Medicine**
Irvine, CA 92697-3950
**Phone:** (949)824-6119 **Fax:** (949)824-2676
**Website:** http://www.ucihs.uci.edu
Thomas C. Cesario, MD, Director

**Fnded:** 1965. **Frmly:** (1898) California College of Medicine.

★ **1583 ★ University of California, Los Angeles**
**UCLA School of Medicine**
10833 Le Conte Ave.
Los Angeles, CA 90024
**Phone:** (310)825-9111 **Fax:** (310)206-5046
**Website:** http://www.medsch.ucla.edu
Gerald S. Levey, MD, Director
**Fnded:** 1951.

★ **1584 ★ University of California, San Diego**
**School of Medicine**
Office of Admissions, 0621
La Jolla, CA 92093
**Phone:** (858)534-3713 **Fax:** (858)534-6573
**Website:** http://medicine.ucsd.edu
Edward W. Holmes, MD, Director
**Fnded:** 1968.

★ **1585 ★ University of California, San Francisco**
**School of Medicine**
513 Parnassus Ave., Rm. S-224
San Francisco, CA 94143-0410
**Phone:** (415)476-9000 **Fax:** (415)476-0689
**Website:** http://www.som.ucsf.edu
Haile T. Debas, MD, Director
**Fnded:** 1873. **Alt. Contact:** Admissions, c-200, Box 0408, San Francisco, CA 92350; (415)476-4044. **Frmly:** (1864) Toland Medical College.

★ **1586 ★ University of Southern California**
**Keck School of Medicine**
1975 Zonal Ave.
Los Angeles, CA 90033
**Phone:** (323)442-1900 **Fax:** (323)442-2722
**Website:** http://www.usc.edu/schools/medicine
Stephen J. Ryan, MD, Director
**Fnded:** 1885.

## Colorado

★ **1587 ★ University of Colorado, Denver**
**School of Medicine**
4200 E 9th Ave.
Box C290
Denver, CO 80262
**Phone:** (303)372-0000 **Fax:** (303)315-8494
**Email:** som@uchsc.edu
**Website:** http://www.uchsc.edu/sm/sm
Richard D. Krugman, MD, Director
**Fnded:** 1883.

## Connecticut

★ **1588 ★ University of Connecticut**
**School of Medicine**
263 Farmington Ave.
Farmington, CT 06030
**Phone:** (860)679-2000 **Fax:** (860)679-1371
**Website:** http://www.uchc.edu
Peter J. Deckers, MD, Director
**Fnded:** 1968.

★ **1589 ★ Yale University**
**School of Medicine**
PO Box 208055
333 Cedar St.
New Haven, CT 06520-8055
**Phone:** (203)785-4672 **Fax:** (203)785-7437
**Website:** http://info.med.yale.edu/
David A. Kessler, MD, Director
**Fnded:** 1813.

## District of Columbia

★ **1590 ★ George Washington University**
**School of Medicine and Health Sciences**
2300 Eye St. NW
Washington, DC 20037
**Phone:** (202)994-1000 **Fax:** (202)994-0926
**Website:** http://www.gwu.edu/~gwumc
Dr. John F. Williams, Jr., Director
**Fnded:** 1974. **Frmly:** (1821) Medical Department of the Columbian College.

★ **1591 ★ Georgetown University**
**School of Medicine**
3900 Reservoir Rd. NW
Washington, DC 20007
**Phone:** (202)687-1612 **Fax:** (202)687-2792
**Website:** http://www.dml.georgetown.edu/schmed/
S. Ray Mitchell, MD, Director
**Fnded:** 1851.

★ **1592 ★ Howard University**
**College of Medicine**
520 W St. NW
Washington, DC 20059
**Phone:** (202)806-6270 **Fax:** (202)806-7934
**Website:** http://www.med.howard.edu
Floyd J. Malveaux, MD,PhD, Director
**Fnded:** 1867.

## Florida

★ **1593 ★ University of Florida**
**College of Medicine**
Box 100014, JHMHC
Gainesville, FL 32610-0014
**Phone:** (352)392-2761 **Fax:** (352)392-9395
**Website:** http://www.med.ufl.edu
Kenneth I. Burns, MD,PhD, Director
**Fnded:** 1956.

★ **1594 ★ University of Miami**
**School of Medicine**
PO Box 016099 (R699)
1600 NW 10th Ave.
Miami, FL 33101
**Phone:** (305)243-6545 **Fax:** (305)243-4888
**Email:** jclarkson@miami.edu
**Website:** http://www.miami.edu
John G. Clarkson, MD, Director
**Fnded:** 1952.

★ **1595 ★ University of South Florida**
**College of Medicine**
12901 Bruce B. Downs Blvd., MDC 2
Tampa, FL 33612-4742
**Phone:** (813)974-2196 **Fax:** (813)974-3886
**Website:** http://www.med.usf.edu/med.html
Dr. Robert M. Daugherty, Jr., Director
**Fnded:** 1971.

## Georgia

★ **1596 ★ Emory University**
**School of Medicine**
Woodruff Health Sciences Center Administration Bldg.
1440 Clifton Rd., NE
Atlanta, GA 30322-4510
**Phone:** (404)727-5640 **Fax:** (404)727-0473
**Website:** http://www.emory.edu/WHSC/MED/med.html
Thomas J. Lawley, MD, Director
**Fnded:** 1854.

★ **1597 ★ Medical College of Georgia**
**School of Medicine**
1120 15th St.
Augusta, GA 30912
**Phone:** (706)721-0211 **Fax:** (706)721-7035
**Website:** http://www.mcg.edu/SOM/index.html
Betty B. Ray, MD, Director
**Fnded:** 1833. **Frmly:** (1828) Medical Academy of Georgia.

★ **1598 ★ Mercer University**
**School of Medicine**
1550 College St.
Macon, GA 31207
**Phone:** (912)301-2600 **Fax:** (912)301-2547
**Website:** http://www.mercer.edu
Ann C. Jobe, MD, Director
**Fnded:** 1972.

★ **1599 ★ Morehouse School of Medicine**
720 Westview Dr. SW
Atlanta, GA 30310
**Phone:** (404)752-1500 **Fax:** (404)752-1594
**Website:** http://www.msm.edu/
Louis W. Sullivan, MD, Director
**Fnded:** 1978.

## Hawaii

★ **1600 ★ University of Hawaii, Manoa**
**John A. Burns School of Medicine**
1960 East-West Rd.
Honolulu, HI 96822
**Phone:** (808)956-8287 **Fax:** (808)956-5506
**Website:** http://www.hawaiimed.hawaii.edu
Edwin C. Cadman, MD, Director
**Fnded:** 1965.

## Illinois

★ **1601 ★ Finch University of Health Sciences/Chicago Medical School**
3333 Green Bay Rd.
North Chicago, IL 60064
**Phone:** (847)578-3301 **Fax:** (847)578-3343
**Email:** barsanoc@finchcms.edu
**Website:** http://www.finchcms.edu
Charles P. Barsano, MD,PhD, Director
**Fnded:** 1912.

★ **1602 ★ Loyola University, Chicago**
**Stritch School of Medicine**
2160 S First Ave.
Maywood, IL 60153
**Phone:** (708)216-9000 **Fax:** (708)216-4305
**Website:** http://www.meddean.luc.edu/
Stephen Slogoff, MD, Director
**Fnded:** 1915.

★ **1603 ★ Northwestern University**
**Medical School**
303 E Chicago Ave.
Chicago, IL 60611-3008
**Phone:** (312)503-8649 **Fax:** (312)503-7757
**Website:** http://www.nums.nwu.edu
Lewis Landsberg, MD, Director
**Fnded:** 1859.

★ **1604 ★ Rush University**
**Rush Medical College**
1653 W Congress Pkwy
Chicago, IL 60612
**Phone:** (312)942-6913 **Fax:** (312)942-2828
**Email:** medcol@rush.edu
**Website:** http://www.rush.edu
Larry J. Goodman, MD, Director
**Fnded:** 1837.

**★ 1605 ★ Southern Illinois University School of Medicine**
801 N Rutledge
PO Box 19230
Springfield, IL 62794-9230
**Phone:** (217)782-3318          **Fax:** (217)524-0786
**Email:** cgetto@siumed.edu
**Website:** http://www.siumed.edu
Carl J. Getto, MD, Director
**Fnded:** 1969.

**★ 1606 ★ University of Chicago Division of the Biological Sciences Pritzker School of Medicine**
5841 S Maryland Ave.
Chicago, IL 60637
**Phone:** (773)702-9000          **Fax:** (773)702-1897
**Website:** http://www.uchicago.edu
Bruce Weir, MD, Director
**Fnded:** 1968. **Frmly:** (1927) The School of Medicine of the University of Chicago.

**★ 1607 ★ University of Illinois, Chicago College of Medicine**
1853 W Polk St. (M/C 784)
Chicago, IL 60612
**Phone:** (312)996-3500          **Fax:** (312)996-9006
**Website:** http://www.uic.edu/depts/mcam/
Gerald S. Moss, MD, Director
**Fnded:** 1900. **Frmly:** (1881) College of Physicians and Surgeons of Chicago.

### Indiana

**★ 1608 ★ Indiana University School of Medicine**
Indiana University Medical Center
1120 South Dr.
Indianapolis, IN 46202-5114
**Phone:** (317)274-8157          **Fax:** (317)274-8439
**Website:** http://www.medicine.iu.edu
D. Craig Brater, MD, Director
**Fnded:** 1903.

### Iowa

**★ 1609 ★ University of Iowa College of Medicine**
200 Medicine Admin. Bldg.
100 Medicine Admin. Bldg.
Iowa City, IA 52242-1101
**Phone:** (319)335-8050          **Fax:** (319)335-8049
**Website:** http://www.medadmin.uiowa.edu
Robert P. Kelch, MD, Director
**Fnded:** 1850.

### Kansas

**★ 1610 ★ University of Kansas School of Medicine**
3901 Rainbow Blvd.
Kansas City, KS 66160-7300
**Phone:** (913)588-5200          **Fax:** (913)588-5259
**Website:** http://www.kumc.edu/som
Deborah E. Powell, MD, Director
**Fnded:** 1906.

### Kentucky

**★ 1611 ★ University of Kentucky College of Medicine**
A. B. Chandler Medical Center
800 Rose St. (MN-150)
Lexington, KY 40536-0298
**Phone:** (859)323-5000          **Fax:** (859)323-2039
**Website:** http://www.mc.uky.edu/medicine
Emery A. Wilson, MD, Director
**Fnded:** 1960.

**★ 1612 ★ University of Louisville School of Medicine**
Health Sciences Center
Abell Administration Center
323 E Chestnut St.
Louisville, KY 40202
**Phone:** (502)852-5184          **Fax:** (502)852-6849
**Website:** http://www.louisville.edu/medschool/
Joel A. Kaplan, MD, Director
**Fnded:** 1833.

### Louisiana

**★ 1613 ★ Louisiana State University School of Medicine in New Orleans**
1542 Tulane Ave.
New Orleans, LA 70112-2822
**Phone:** (504)568-4007          **Fax:** (504)568-4008
**Website:** http://www.lsumc.edu
Robert L. Marier, MD, Director
**Fnded:** 1931.

**★ 1614 ★ Louisiana State University School of Medicine in Shreveport**
Office of Student Admissions
PO Box 33932
Shreveport, LA 71130-3932
**Phone:** (318)675-5000          **Fax:** (318)675-5244
**Website:** http://lib-sh.lsumc.edu
John C. McDonald, MD, Director
**Fnded:** 1965.

**★ 1615 ★ Tulane University School of Medicine**
1430 Tulane Ave.
New Orleans, LA 70112
**Phone:** (504)588-5462          **Fax:** (504)584-2945
**Email:** medsch@tmcpop.tmc.tulane.edu
**Website:** http://www.mcl.tulane.edu/tumc
Ian L. Taylor, MD, Director
**Fnded:** 1834.

### Manitoba

**★ 1616 ★ University of Manitoba Faculty of Medicine**
753 McDermot Ave.
Winnipeg, MB, Canada R3E 0W3
**Phone:** (204)789-3557          **Fax:** (204)789-3928
B. K. Hennen, MD, Director
**Fnded:** 1883.

### Maryland

**★ 1617 ★ Johns Hopkins University School of Medicine**
720 Rutland Ave.
Baltimore, MD 21205
**Phone:** (410)955-5000          **Fax:** (410)955-0889
**Website:** http://www.hopkins.med.jhu.edu
Dr. Edward D. Miller, Jr., Director
**Fnded:** 1893.

**★ 1618 ★ Uniformed Services University of the Health Sciences F. Edward Hebert School of Medicine**
4301 Jones Bridge Rd.
Bethesda, MD 20814-4799
**Phone:** (301)295-3016          **Fax:** (301)295-3542
**Website:** http://www.usuhs.mil
Val G. Hemming, MD, Director
**Fnded:** 1972.

**★ 1619 ★ University of Maryland School of Medicine**
655 W Baltimore St.
Baltimore, MD 21201
**Phone:** (410)706-3100          **Fax:** (410)706-0235
**Email:** deanmed@som.umaryland.edu
**Website:** http://medschool.umaryland.edu
Donald E. Wilson, MD, Director
**Fnded:** 1807.

### Massachusetts

**★ 1620 ★ Boston University School of Medicine**
715 Albany St.
Boston, MA 02118
**Phone:** (617)638-8000          **Fax:** (617)638-5258
**Website:** http://www.bumc.bu.edu
Aram V. Chobanian, MD, Director
**Fnded:** 1873.

**★ 1621 ★ Harvard Medical School**
25 Shattuck St.
Boston, MA 02115
**Phone:** (617)432-1000          **Fax:** (617)432-3907
**Website:** http://www.med.harvard.edu
Joseph B. Martin, MD, PhD, Director
**Fnded:** 1782.

**★ 1622 ★ Tufts University School of Medicine**
136 Harrison Ave.
Boston, MA 02111
**Phone:** (617)636-7000          **Fax:** (617)636-0375
**Email:** jharrington@infonet.tufts.edu
**Website:** http://www.tufts.edu/med
John T. Harrington, MD, Director
**Fnded:** 1893.

**★ 1623 ★ University of Massachusetts Medical School**
55 Lake Ave. N
Worcester, MA 01655
**Phone:** (508)856-8100          **Fax:** (508)856-8181
**Email:** aaron.lazare@umassmed.edu
**Website:** http://www.umassmed.edu
Aaron Lazare, MD, Director
**Fnded:** 1962.

### Michigan

**★ 1624 ★ Michigan State University College of Human Medicine**
A-110 East Fee Hall
East Lansing, MI 48824
**Phone:** (517)353-1730          **Fax:** (517)355-0342
**Website:** http://www.chm.msu.edu
Glenn C. Davis, MD, Director
**Fnded:** 1964.

**★ 1625 ★ University of Michigan Medical School**
1301 Catherine Rd.
Medical Science Bldg. I
Ann Arbor, MI 48109-0624
**Phone:** (734)763-9600          **Fax:** (734)763-4936
**Website:** http://www.med.umich.edu/medschool
Allen S. Lichter, MD, Director
**Fnded:** 1850.

**★ 1626 ★ Wayne State University School of Medicine**
540 E Canfield
Detroit, MI 48201
**Phone:** (313)577-1460          **Fax:** (313)577-8777
**Website:** http://www.med.wayne.edu
John D. Crissman, MD, Director
**Fnded:** 1956. **Frmly:** (1868) Detroit Medical College.

### Minnesota

**★ 1627 ★ Mayo Medical School**
200 First St. SW
Rochester, MN 55905

**Phone:** (507)284-3671    **Fax:** (507)284-2634
**Website:** http://www.mayo.edu/mms
Anthony J. Windebank, MD, Director
**Fnded:** 1972.

**★ 1628 ★ University of Minnesota,
Duluth
School of Medicine**
10 University Dr.
Duluth, MN 55812
**Phone:** (218)726-7571    **Fax:** (218)726-7383
**Email:** med@d.umn.edu
**Website:** http://www.d.umn.edu/medweb/
Richard J. Ziegler, PhD, Director
**Fnded:** 1972.

**★ 1629 ★ University of Minnesota,
Minneapolis
Medical School**
Mayo Mail Code 293
420 Delaware St. SE
Minneapolis, MN 55455
**Phone:** (612)624-1188
**Website:** http://www.med.umn.edu
Alfred F. Michael, MD, Director
**Fnded:** 1888.

### Mississippi

**★ 1630 ★ University of Mississippi
School of Medicine**
2500 N State St.
Jackson, MS 39216-4505
**Phone:** (601)984-1000    **Fax:** (601)984-1011
**Website:** http://umc.edu
A. Wallace Conerly, MD, Director
**Fnded:** 1903.

### Missouri

**★ 1631 ★ Saint Louis University
School of Medicine**
1402 S Grand Blvd.
Saint Louis, MO 63104
**Phone:** (314)577-8000    **Fax:** (314)577-8645
**Website:** http://www.slu.edu/colleges/med/
Patricia L. Monteleone, MD, Director
**Fnded:** 1903. **Frmly:** Marion Sims-Beaumont College
of Medicine.

**★ 1632 ★ University of Missouri,
Columbia
School of Medicine**
MA202 Medical Sciences Bldg.
1 Hospital Dr.
Columbia, MO 65212
**Phone:** (573)882-2923    **Fax:** (573)884-4808
**Website:** http://www.muhealth.org
Daniel H. Winship, MD, Director
**Fnded:** 1841.

**★ 1633 ★ University of Missouri, Kansas
City
School of Medicine**
2411 Holmes St.
Kansas City, MO 64108-2792
**Phone:** (816)235-1808    **Fax:** (816)235-5277
**Website:** http://www.med.umkc.edu
Betty M. Dress, MD, Director
**Fnded:** 1971.

**★ 1634 ★ Washington University
School of Medicine**
660 S Euclid Ave., Box. 8106
Saint Louis, MO 63110
**Phone:** (314)362-5000    **Fax:** (314)367-6666
**Website:** http://medinfo.wustl.edu
William A. Peck, MD, Director

**Fnded:** 1891.

### Nebraska

**★ 1635 ★ Creighton University
School of Medicine**
2500 California Plaza
Omaha, NE 68178
**Phone:** (402)280-2900    **Fax:** (402)280-4027
**Website:** http://medicine.creighton.edu
M. Roy Wilson, MD, Director
**Fnded:** 1892.

**★ 1636 ★ University of Nebraska
College of Medicine**
986545 Nebraska Medical Ctr
Omaha, NE 68198-6545
**Phone:** (402)559-4000    **Fax:** (402)559-4148
**Website:** http://www.unmc.edu
James O. Armitage, MD, Director
**Fnded:** 1902. **Frmly:** (1881) Omaha Medical College.

### Nevada

**★ 1637 ★ University of Nevada
School of Medicine**
2040 W Charleston Blvd.
Ste. 400
Reno, NV 89557-0046
**Phone:** (775)784-6001    **Fax:** (702)671-2277
**Website:** http://www.unr.edu/med/
Robert H. Miller, MD, Director
**Fnded:** 1969.

### New Hampshire

**★ 1638 ★ Dartmouth Medical School**
7020 Remsen, Rm. 306
Hanover, NH 03755-3833
**Phone:** (603)650-1481    **Fax:** (603)650-1202
**Website:** http://www.dartmouth.edu/dms
John C. Baldwin, MD, Director
**Fnded:** 1797.

### New Jersey

**★ 1639 ★ University of Medicine and
Dentistry of New Jersey
New Jersey Medical School**
185 S Orange Ave.
Newark, NJ 07103-2714
**Phone:** (973)972-4300    **Fax:** (973)972-7104
**Website:** http://njms.umdnj.edu/
Russell T. Joffe, MD, Director
**Fnded:** 1965. **Frmly:** (1954) Seton Hall College of
Medicine and Dentistry.

**★ 1640 ★ University of Medicine and
Dentistry of New Jersey
Robert Wood Johnson Medical School**
125 Paterson St., Ste. 1400
New Brunswick, NJ 08901
**Phone:** (732)235-5600    **Fax:** (732)235-6315
Harold L. Paz, MD, Director
**Fnded:** 1970.

### New Mexico

**★ 1641 ★ University of New Mexico
School of Medicine**
Albuquerque, NM 87131
**Phone:** (505)272-2321    **Fax:** (505)272-6581
**Website:** http://medlab1.unm.edu
Paul B. Roth, MD, Director
**Fnded:** 1961.

### New York

**★ 1642 ★ Albany Medical College**
47 New Scotland Ave.
Albany, NY 12208
**Phone:** (518)262-5582    **Fax:** (518)262-6515
**Website:** http://www.amc.edu
Vincent P. Verdile, MD, Director
**Fnded:** 1839.

**★ 1643 ★ Columbia University
College of Physicians and Surgeons**
630 W 168th St.
New York, NY 10032
**Phone:** (212)305-3592    **Fax:** (212)305-3545
**Website:** http://www.columbia.edu
Gerald D. Fischbach, MD, Director
**Fnded:** 1814.

**★ 1644 ★ Cornell University
Joan and Sanford I. Weill Medical
College
Graduate School of Medical Sciences**
New York, NY 10021
**Phone:** (212)746-5454    **Fax:** (212)746-8424
**Email:** dean@mail.med.cornell.edu
**Website:** http://www.med.cornell.edu
Dr. Antonio M. Gotto, Jr., Director
**Fnded:** 1898.

**★ 1645 ★ New York Medical College**
Administration Bldg.
Valhalla, NY 10595
**Phone:** (914)594-4000    **Fax:** (914)594-4145
**Website:** http://www.nymc.edu
Francis L. Belloni, PhD, Director
**Fnded:** 1860.

**★ 1646 ★ New York University
Mount Sinai School of Medicine**
1 Gustave L. Levy Pl.
New York, NY 10029-6574
**Phone:** (212)241-6500    **Fax:** (212)410-6111
**Website:** http://www.mssm.edu
Nathan Kase, MD, Director
**Fnded:** 1963.

**★ 1647 ★ New York University
School of Medicine**
550 1st Ave.
New York, NY 10016
**Phone:** (212)263-7300    **Fax:** (212)545-8846
**Website:** http://www.med.nyu.edu
Robert M. Glickman, MD, Director
**Fnded:** 1841.

**★ 1648 ★ State University of New York,
Buffalo
School of Medicine and Biomedical
Sciences**
3435 Main St.
Buffalo, NY 14214
**Phone:** (716)829-2771    **Fax:** (716)829-3395
**Website:** http://www.smbs.buffalo.edu
John R. Wright, MD, Director
**Fnded:** 1846.

**★ 1649 ★ State University of New York
Downstate Medical Center
College of Medicine**
450 Clarkson Ave., Box 97
Brooklyn, NY 11203-2098
**Phone:** (718)270-1000    **Fax:** (718)270-4074
**Email:** efeigelson@netmail.hscbklyn.edu
**Website:** http://www.downstate.edu
Eugene B. Feigelson, MD, Director
**Fnded:** 1860.

**★ 1650 ★ State University of New York, Stony Brook**
**Health Sciences Center**
**School of Medicine**
HSC Level 4-170
Level 4, Rm. 170
Stony Brook, NY 11794-8430
**Phone:** (631)444-2080          **Fax:** (631)444-6266
**Website:** http://www.uhmc.sunysb.edu/hsc/
Norman H. Edelman, MD, Director
**Fnded:** 1971.

**★ 1651 ★ State University of New York**
**Upstate Medical Center**
**College of Medicine**
750 E Adams St.
Syracuse, NY 13210-2399
**Phone:** (315)464-9720          **Fax:** (315)464-9721
**Website:** http://www.upstate.edu
Michael F. Roizen, MD, Director
**Fnded:** 1834.

**★ 1652 ★ University of Rochester**
**School of Medicine and Dentistry**
601 Elmwood Ave.
Rochester, NY 14642
**Phone:** (716)275-7181          **Fax:** (716)256-1131
**Website:** http://www.rochester.edu
Edward M. Hundert, MD, Director
**Fnded:** 1920.

**★ 1653 ★ Yeshiva University**
**Albert Einstein College of Medicine**
1300 Morris Park Ave.
Bronx, NY 10461
**Phone:** (718)430-2000          **Fax:** (718)430-8822
**Website:** http://www.aecom.yu.edu
Dominick P. Purpura, MD, Director
**Fnded:** 1955.

### Newfoundland

**★ 1654 ★ Memorial University of**
**Newfoundland**
**Faculty of Medicine**
Health Sciences Centre
Prince Philip Dr.
Saint John's, NF, Canada A1B 3V6
**Phone:** (709)777-6602          **Fax:** (709)777-6746
**Website:** http://www.med.mun.ca/med
M. I. Bowmer, MD, Director
**Fnded:** 1967.

### North Carolina

**★ 1655 ★ Duke University**
**School of Medicine**
PO Box 2927
Durham, NC 27710
**Phone:** (919)684-2455          **Fax:** (919)684-0208
**Website:** http://www.mc.duke.edu/depts/som
R. Sanders Williams, MD, Director
**Fnded:** 1390.

**★ 1656 ★ East Carolina University**
**Brody School of Medicine**
Greenville, NC 27858-4354
**Phone:** (252)816-2201          **Fax:** (252)816-3192
**Website:** http://www.med.ecu.edu
Peter J. Kragel, MD, Director
**Fnded:** 1972.

**★ 1657 ★ University of North Carolina,**
**Chapel Hill**
**School of Medicine**
Chapel Hill, NC 27599
**Phone:** (919)966-4161          **Fax:** (919)966-8623

**Website:** http://www.med.unc.edu
Jeffrey L. Houpt, MD, Director
**Fnded:** 1879.

**★ 1658 ★ Wake Forest University**
**School of Medicine**
Medical Center Blvd.
Winston-Salem, NC 27157
**Phone:** (336)716-2011          **Fax:** (336)716-5139
**Website:** http://isnet.is.wfu.edu
James N. Thompson, MD, Director
**Fnded:** 1902.

### North Dakota

**★ 1659 ★ University of North Dakota**
**School of Medicine and Health Sciences**
501 N Columbia Rd.
Box 9037
Grand Forks, ND 58202-9037
**Phone:** (701)777-2514          **Fax:** (701)777-3527
**Website:** http://www.med.und.nodak.edu
H. David Wilson, MD, Director
**Fnded:** 1905.

### Nova Scotia

**★ 1660 ★ Dalhousie University**
**Faculty of Medicine**
Clinical Research Ctr
5849 University Ave
Halifax, NS, Canada B3H 4H7
**Phone:** (902)494-6592          **Fax:** (902)494-7119
**Website:** http://www.medicine.dal.ca
N. MacDonald, MD, Director
**Fnded:** 1868.

### Ohio

**★ 1661 ★ Case Western Reserve**
**University**
**School of Medicine**
10900 Euclid Ave.
Cleveland, OH 44106-4915
**Phone:** (216)368-2000          **Fax:** (216)368-3013
**Website:** http://mediswww.cwru.edu
Nathan A. Berger, MD, Director
**Fnded:** 1843. **Frmly:** Cleveland Medical College.

**★ 1662 ★ Medical College of Ohio**
PO Box 10008
Toledo, OH 43699-0008
**Phone:** (419)383-4172          **Fax:** (419)383-6100
**Website:** http://www.mco.edu/smed
Amira F. Gohara, MD, Director
**Fnded:** 1967. **Frmly:** (1964) Toledo State College of Medicine.

**★ 1663 ★ Northeastern Ohio Universities**
**College of Medicine**
4209 State Rte. 44
PO Box 95
Rootstown, OH 44272-0095
**Phone:** (330)325-2511          **Fax:** (330)325-5919
**Website:** http://www.neoucom.edu
Robert S. Blacklow, MD, Director
**Fnded:** 1973.

**★ 1664 ★ Ohio State University**
**College of Medicine and Public Health**
200A Meiling Hall
370 W 9th Ave.
Columbus, OH 43210
**Phone:** (614)292-2220          **Fax:** (614)292-1301
**Website:** http://www.med.ohio-state.edu
Fred Sanfilippo, MD, Director
**Fnded:** 1914.

**★ 1665 ★ University of Cincinnati**
**College of Medicine**
PO Box 670555
Cincinnati, OH 45267-0555
**Phone:** (513)558-7391          **Fax:** (513)558-1165
**Website:** http://www.med.uc.edu
John J. Hutton, MD, Director
**Fnded:** 1819.

**★ 1666 ★ Wright State University**
**School of Medicine**
PO Box 927
Dayton, OH 45401-0927
**Phone:** (937)775-3010          **Fax:** (937)775-2211
**Email:** howard.part@wright.edu
**Website:** http://www.med.wright.edu
Howard M. Part, MD, Director
**Fnded:** 1973.

### Oklahoma

**★ 1667 ★ University of Oklahoma**
**College of Medicine**
PO Box 26901
Oklahoma City, OK 73190
**Phone:** (405)271-2265          **Fax:** (405)271-3032
**Website:** http://medicine.ouhsc.edu
Jerry B. Vannatta, MD, Director
**Fnded:** 1900.

### Ontario

**★ 1668 ★ McMaster University**
**Faculty of Health Sciences**
1200 Main St. W
Hamilton, ON, Canada L8S 4J9
**Phone:** (905)525-9140          **Fax:** (905)546-0800
J. G. Kelton, MD, Director
**Fnded:** 1967.

**★ 1669 ★ Queen's University**
**Faculty of Health Sciences**
Kingston, ON, Canada K7L 3N6
**Phone:** (613)533-2542          **Fax:** (613)553-6884
**Website:** http://meds.queensu.ca
David M. C. Walker, MD, Director
**Fnded:** 1854.

**★ 1670 ★ University of Ottawa**
**Faculty of Medicine**
451 Smyth Rd.
Ottawa, ON, Canada K1H 8M5
**Phone:** (613)562-5400          **Fax:** (613)562-5457
Peter Walker, MD, Director
**Fnded:** 1945.

**★ 1671 ★ University of Toronto**
**Faculty of Medicine**
1 King's College Cr.
Toronto, ON, Canada M5S 1A8
**Phone:** (416)978-6585          **Fax:** (416)978-1774
**Email:** medicine.web@utoronto.ca
**Website:** http://utl2.library.utoronto.ca/www/medicine
C. D. Naylor, MD, Contact
**Fnded:** 1843.

**★ 1672 ★ University of Western Ontario**
**Faculty of Medicine and Dentistry**
Richmond St., N
London, ON, Canada N6A 5C1
**Phone:** (519)661-3744          **Fax:** (519)661-3797
C. P. Herbert, MD, Director
**Fnded:** 1882.

## Oregon

**★ 1673 ★ Oregon Health Sciences University**
**School of Medicine**
3181 SW Sam Jackson Park Rd.
Portland, OR 97201-3098
**Phone:** (503)494-8311　　**Fax:** (503)494-3400
**Website:** http://www.ohsu.edu/som
Dr. Joseph E. Robertson, Jr., Director
**Fnded:** 1887.

## Pennsylvania

**★ 1674 ★ MCP Hahnemann School of Medicine**
**Medical Program**
2900 Queen Lane
Philadelphia, PA 19129
**Phone:** (215)991-8560　　**Fax:** (215)843-0214
**Website:** http://www.mcphu.edu
Warren E. Ross, MD, Director
**Fnded:** 1998.

**★ 1675 ★ Pennsylvania State University**
**College of Medicine**
500 University Dr.
PO Box 850
Hershey, PA 17033
**Phone:** (717)531-8521　　**Fax:** (717)531-5351
**Email:** dkirch@psu.edu
**Website:** http://www.hmc.psu.edu
Darrell G. Kirch, MD, Director
**Fnded:** 1963.

**★ 1676 ★ Temple University**
**School of Medicine**
3420 N Broad St.
Philadelphia, PA 19140
**Phone:** (215)707-7000　　**Fax:** (215)707-8431
**Email:** tusmdean@vm.temple.edu
**Website:** http://www.temple.edu/medschool/
Leon S. Malmud, MD, Director
**Fnded:** 1901.

**★ 1677 ★ Thomas Jefferson University**
**Jefferson Medical College**
1025 Walnut St.
Philadelphia, PA 19107-5083
**Phone:** (215)955-6000　　**Fax:** (215)503-2654
**Email:** dean.jmc@mail.tju.edu
**Website:** http://www.tju.edu
Thomas J. Nasca, MD, Director
**Fnded:** 1824.

**★ 1678 ★ University of Pennsylvania**
**School of Medicine**
36th and Hamilton Walk
Philadelphia, PA 19104-6055
**Phone:** (215)898-8034　　**Fax:** (215)573-2030
**Website:** http://www.med.upenn.edu
Arthur H. Rubenstein, MBBCh, Director
**Fnded:** 1765.

**★ 1679 ★ University of Pittsburgh**
**School of Medicine**
Alan Magee Scaife Hall of the Health Professions
Pittsburgh, PA 15261
**Phone:** (412)648-9891　　**Fax:** (412)648-1236
**Website:** http://www.omed.pitt.edu
Arthur S. Levine, MD, Director
**Fnded:** 1908. **Frmly:** (1886) Western Pennsylvania Medical College.

## Puerto Rico

**★ 1680 ★ Ponce School of Medicine**
PO Box 7004
Ponce, PR 00732
**Phone:** (787)840-2575　　**Fax:** (787)840-9756
**Email:** psm004@caribe.net
**Website:** http://www.psm.edu
Manuel Martinez-Maldonado, MD, Director
**Fnded:** 1977. **Alt. Contact:** Fax: (787)841-1040.

**★ 1681 ★ Universidad Central del Caribe**
**School of Medicine**
PO Box 60-327
Bayamon, PR 00960-6032
**Phone:** (787)798-3001　　**Fax:** (787)798-4990
**Website:** http://www.ucaribe.edu
Helen Rosa, MD, Director
**Fnded:** 1976.

**★ 1682 ★ University of Puerto Rico**
**School of Medicine**
Medical Sciences Campus
PO Box 365067
San Juan, PR 00936-5067
**Phone:** (787)758-2525　　**Fax:** (787)756-8475
**Email:** fjoglar@rcm.upr.edu
**Website:** http://www.rcm.upr.edu
Francisco M. Joglar, MD, Director
**Fnded:** 1950.

## Quebec

**★ 1683 ★ Laval University**
**Faculty of Medicine**
Quebec City, QC, Canada G1K 7P4
**Phone:** (418)656-2331　　**Fax:** (418)656-5062
Marc Desmeules, MD, Director
**Fnded:** 1852.

**★ 1684 ★ McGill University**
**Faculty of Medicine**
3655 Promenade Sir-William-Osler
Montreal, QC, Canada H3G 1Y6
**Phone:** (514)398-3515　　**Fax:** (514)398-3595
**Email:** recepmed@med.mcgill.ca
**Website:** http://www.med.mcgill.ca
Abraham Fuks, MD, Director
**Fnded:** 1829.

**★ 1685 ★ University of Montreal**
**Faculty of Medicine**
2900 Blvd. Edouard-Montpetit
PO Box 6128, Succ. Centre-ville
Montreal, QC, Canada H3C 3J7
**Phone:** (514)343-6267　　**Fax:** (514)343-2068
**Email:** vinaypa@alize.ere.umontreal.ca
Patrick Vinay, MD,PhD, Director
**Fnded:** 1843.

**★ 1686 ★ University of Sherbrooke**
**Faculty of Medicine**
3001 12th Ave. N
Sherbrooke, QC, Canada J1H 5N4
**Phone:** (819)564-5200　　**Fax:** (819)564-5420
**Website:** http://www.crc.cuse.usherb.ca/facmed
Michel Baron, MD, Director
**Fnded:** 1961.

## Rhode Island

**★ 1687 ★ Brown University**
**School of Medicine**
97 Waterman St.
Providence, RI 02912
**Phone:** (401)863-3971　　**Fax:** (401)863-3431
**Website:** http://biomedics.biomed.brown.edu
Donald J. Marsh, MD, Director
**Fnded:** 1973.

## South Carolina

**★ 1688 ★ Medical University of South Carolina**
**College of Medicine**
171 Ashley Ave.
Charleston, SC 29425
**Phone:** (843)792-2300　　**Fax:** (843)792-2967
**Website:** http://www2.musc.edu
J. G. Reves, MD, Director
**Fnded:** 1824.

**★ 1689 ★ University of South Carolina**
**School of Medicine**
Columbia, SC 29208
**Phone:** (803)733-3200　　**Fax:** (803)733-3335
**Email:** faulkner@med.sc.edu
**Website:** http://www.med.sc.edu
Larry R. Faulkner, MD, Director
**Fnded:** 1973.

## South Dakota

**★ 1690 ★ University of South Dakota**
**School of Medicine**
1400 W 22nd
Sioux Falls, SD 57105-1570
**Phone:** (605)357-1300　　**Fax:** (605)357-1311
**Website:** http://www.usd.edu/med/som
Robert C. Talley, MD, Director
**Fnded:** 1907.

## Tennessee

**★ 1691 ★ East Tennessee State University**
**James H. Quillen College of Medicine**
PO Box 70694
Johnson City, TN 37614
**Phone:** (423)439-1000　　**Fax:** (423)439-8090
**Email:** medcom@etsu.edu
**Website:** http://www.qcom.etsu.edu
Ronald D. Franks, MD, Director
**Fnded:** 1974.

**★ 1692 ★ Meharry Medical College**
**School of Medicine**
1005 Dr. D.B. Todd Jr. Blvd.
Nashville, TN 37208
**Phone:** (615)327-6204　　**Fax:** (615)327-6568
**Email:** meharrysom@ccvax.mmc.edu
**Website:** http://www.mmc.edu
A. Cherrie Epps, PhD, Director
**Fnded:** 1876.

**★ 1693 ★ University of Tennessee Health Science Center**
**College of Medicine**
62 S Dunlap, Rm. 420
Memphis, TN 38163
**Phone:** (901)448-5529　　**Fax:** (901)448-7683
**Website:** http://www.utmem.edu
Henry G. Herrod, MD, Director
**Fnded:** 1851.

**★ 1694 ★ Vanderbilt University**
**School of Medicine**
21st Ave. S at Garland Ave.
Nashville, TN 37232
**Phone:** (615)322-5000　　**Fax:** (615)343-7286
**Email:** steven.gabbe@mcmail.vanderbilt.edu
**Website:** http://www.mc.vanderbilt.edu/medschool/
Steven G. Gabbe, MD, Director
**Fnded:** 1875.

## Texas

### ★ 1695 ★ Baylor College of Medicine
1 Baylor Plaza
Houston, TX 77030
**Phone:** (713)798-4951 **Fax:** (713)798-8811
**Website:** http://www.bcm.tmc.edu
Bobby R. Alford, MD, Director
**Fnded:** 1969.

### ★ 1696 ★ Texas A&M University Health Science Center College of Medicine
147 Joe H. Reynolds Medical Bldg.
College Station, TX 77843-1114
**Phone:** (979)845-7743 **Fax:** (979)847-8663
**Website:** http://tamushsc.tamu.edu
Nancy W. Dickey, MD, Director
**Fnded:** 1971.

### ★ 1697 ★ Texas Tech University Health Sciences Center School of Medicine
3601 4th St.
Lubbock, TX 79430
**Phone:** (806)743-1000 **Fax:** (806)743-3021
**Website:** http://www.ttuhsc.edu
Joel Kupersmith, MD, Director
**Fnded:** 1969.

### ★ 1698 ★ University of Texas Houston Medical School
6431 Fannin
Houston, TX 77030
**Phone:** (713)500-5160 **Fax:** (713)500-0602
**Website:** http://www.med.uth.tmc.edu/
L. Maximilian Buja, MD, Director
**Fnded:** 1969.

### ★ 1699 ★ University of Texas Medical Branch University of Texas Medical School at Galveston
301 University Blvd.
Galveston, TX 77555-0133
**Phone:** (409)772-1011 **Fax:** (409)772-9598
**Email:** smlemon@utmb.edu
**Website:** http://www.utmb.edu
Stanley M. Lemon, MD, Director
**Fnded:** 1881.

### ★ 1700 ★ University of Texas, San Antonio Medical School
7703 Floyd Curl Dr.
San Antonio, TX 78284-7790
**Phone:** (210)567-4420 **Fax:** (210)567-6962
**Website:** http://www.uthscsa.edu/som/som_main.htm
Steven A. Wartman, MD, Director
**Fnded:** 1959.

### ★ 1701 ★ University of Texas Southwestern Medical Center, Dallas
5323 Harry Hines Blvd.
Dallas, TX 75390
**Phone:** (214)648-3111 **Fax:** (214)648-8955
**Website:** http://www.swmed.edu
Robert J. Alpern, MD, Director
**Fnded:** 1972. **Frmly:** (1943) Southwestern Medical College.

## Utah

### ★ 1702 ★ University of Utah School of Medicine
50 N Medical Dr.
Salt Lake City, UT 84132
**Phone:** (801)581-7201 **Fax:** (801)585-3300
**Website:** http://www.med.utah.edu/som
A. Lorris Betz, MD,PhD, Director
**Fnded:** 1905.

## Vermont

### ★ 1703 ★ University of Vermont College of Medicine
Burlington, VT 05405
**Phone:** (802)656-2150 **Fax:** (802)656-8577
**Website:** http://salus.uvm.edu
Joseph B. Warshaw, MD, Director
**Fnded:** 1803.

## Virginia

### ★ 1704 ★ Medical College of Hampton Roads Eastern Virginia Medical School
PO Box 1980
Norfolk, VA 23501
**Phone:** (757)446-5600 **Fax:** (757)446-8444
**Website:** http://www.evms.edu
Evan R. Farmer, MD, Director
**Fnded:** 1964.

### ★ 1705 ★ University of Virginia School of Medicine
Health System
PO Box 800793, McKim Hall
Charlottesville, VA 22908-0793
**Phone:** (804)924-0211 **Fax:** (804)982-0874
**Website:** http://www.med.virginia.edu
Robert M. Carey, MD, Director
**Fnded:** 1825.

### ★ 1706 ★ Virginia Commonwealth University School of Medicine
PO Box 980565
Richmond, VA 23298
**Phone:** (804)828-9000 **Fax:** (804)371-7628
**Website:** http://www.medschool.vcu.edu
Dr. Heber H. Newsome, Jr., Director
**Fnded:** 1838.

## Washington

### ★ 1707 ★ University of Washington School of Medicine
Box 356340
Seattle, WA 98195
**Phone:** (206)543-1515 **Fax:** (206)543-3639
**Website:** http://www.washington.edu/medical.som
Paul G. Ramsey, MD, Director
**Fnded:** 1945.

## West Virginia

### ★ 1708 ★ Marshall University Joan C. Edwards School of Medicine
1600 Medical Center Dr., Ste. 3400
Huntington, WV 25701-3655
**Phone:** (304)691-1700 **Fax:** (304)691-1726
**Website:** http://musom.marshall.edu/
Dr. Charles H. McKown, Jr., Director
**Fnded:** 1972.

### ★ 1709 ★ West Virginia University School of Medicine
Robert C. Byrd Health Sciences Center
Box 9000
Morgantown, WV 26506-9000
**Phone:** (304)293-0111 **Fax:** (304)293-4973
**Email:** cwhyte@hsc.wvu.edu
**Website:** http://www.hsc.wvu.edu
Robert M. D'Alessandri, MD, Director
**Fnded:** 1902.

## Wisconsin

### ★ 1710 ★ Medical College of Wisconsin
8701 Watertown Plank Rd.
Milwaukee, WI 53226
**Phone:** (414)456-8296 **Fax:** (414)456-6560
**Website:** http://www.mcw.edu
Michael J. Dunn, MD, Director
**Fnded:** 1913.

### ★ 1711 ★ University of Wisconsin Medical School
1300 University Ave.
Madison, WI 53706
**Phone:** (608)263-4900 **Fax:** (608)262-2327
**Website:** http://www.biostat.wisc.edu
Philip M. Farrell, MD,PhD, Director
**Fnded:** 1979.

# Physician Assistant

*The physician assistant educational programs listed in this section are accredited by the Commission on Accreditation of Allied Health Education Programs, 35 E Wacker Dr., Ste. 1970, Chicago, IL 60601-2208, (312)553-9355, http://www.caahep.org/. For information on the profession, contact the Association of Physician Assistant Programs, 950 N Washington St., Alexandria, VA 22314, (703)548-5538, or the American Academy of Physician Assistants, 950 N Washington St., Alexandria, VA 22314 (703)836-2272, http://www.aapa.org/.*

## Alabama

### ★ 1712 ★ University of Alabama, Birmingham School of Health Related Professions Surgical Physician Assistant Program
SHR2 Annex
1530 3rd Ave. S
Birmingham, AL 35294-1270
**Phone:** (205)934-4407
**Email:** wilsonc@shrp.uab.edu

### ★ 1713 ★ University of South Alabama College of Allied Health Professions Department of Physician Assistant Studies
1504 Springhill Ave., Ste. 4410
Mobile, AL 36604-3273
**Phone:** (334)434-3641 **Fax:** (334)434-3646
**Email:** pastudies@usamail.usouthal.edu

## Arizona

### ★ 1714 ★ Arizona School of Health Sciences Physician Assistant Program
3210 W Camelback Rd.
Phoenix, AZ 85017
**Email:** paprogram@ashs.edu

### ★ 1715 ★ Midwestern University Physician Assistant Program
Office of Admissions
19555 N 59th Ave.
Glendale, AZ 85308
**Phone:** (623)572-3215

## California

### ★ 1716 ★ Charles R. Drew University of Medicine and Science College of Health Sciences Physician Assistant Program
1621 E 120th St.
Los Angeles, CA 90059
**Phone:** (323)563-5879

**Email:** belassit@cdrewu.edu
**Website:** http://www.cdrewu.edu

**★ 1717 ★ Loma Linda University**
**School of Allied Health Professions**
**Physician Assistant Program**
Nichol Hall, Rm. 2033
Loma Linda, CA 92350
**Phone:** (909)558-7295

**★ 1718 ★ Riverside County Regional**
**Medical Center/Riverside Community**
**College**
**Primary Care PA Program**
16130 Lasselle St.
Moreno Valley, CA 92551
**Phone:** (909)485-6100

**★ 1719 ★ Samuel Merritt College**
**Physician Assistant Program**
370 Hawthorne Ave.
Oakland, CA 94609
**Phone:** (510)869-6576
**Email:** admission@samuelmerritt.edu

**★ 1720 ★ Stanford University**
**School of Medicine**
**Primary Care Associate Program**
703 Welch Rd., Ste. F-1
Palo Alto, CA 94304-1760
**Phone:** (650)723-7043
**Email:** pcap-information@lists.standford.edu

**★ 1721 ★ University of California, Davis**
**Medical Center**
**Department of Family and Community**
**Medicine**
**Physician Assistant Program/Family**
**Nurse Practitioner Program**
2516 Stockton Blvd., Ste. 254
Sacramento, CA 95817-2297
**Phone:** (916)734-3551
**Email:** patty.frank@ucdmc.ucdavis.edu
**Website:** http://www-med.ucdavis.edu/adm_edu/fnp_pa_program/index.htm

**★ 1722 ★ University of Southern**
**California**
**Keck School of Medicine**
**Primary Care Physician Assistant**
**Program**
1975 Zonal Ave., KAM B-29
Los Angeles, CA 90089-9039
**Phone:** (323)442-1328

**★ 1723 ★ Western University of Health**
**Sciences**
**Primary Care Physician Assistant**
**Program**
College Plaza
Pomona, CA 91766-1854
**Phone:** (909)469-5378
**Email:** admissions@westernu.edu

### Colorado

**★ 1724 ★ Red Rocks Community College**
**Physician Assistant Program**
13300 W 6th Ave.
Campus Box 38
Lakewood, CO 80228-1255
**Phone:** (303)914-6386
**Email:** Arlene.duran@rrr.ccoes.edu
**Website:** http://www.rrcc.cccoes.edu/academic/health/pa.html

**★ 1725 ★ University of Colorado**
**School of Medicine**
**Child Health Associate/Physician**
**Assistant Program**
4200 E 9th Ave.
Box C-219
Denver, CO 80262
**Phone:** (303)315-4614
**Email:** chapa-info@uchsc.edu
**Website:** http://www.uchsc.edu/sm/chapa

### Connecticut

**★ 1726 ★ Quinnipiac University**
**Physician Assistant Program**
Office of Graduate Admission
Hamden, CT 06518
**Phone:** (203)582-8672
**Email:** graduate@quinnipiac.edu
**Website:** http://www.quinnipiac.edu/grad_adm/physicn.html

**★ 1727 ★ Yale University**
**School of Medicine**
**Physician Associate Program**
47 College St., Ste. 220
New Haven, CT 06510
**Phone:** (203)785-4252
**Email:** janet.liscio@yale.edu
**Website:** http://info.med.yale.edu/phyassoc/

### District of Columbia

**★ 1728 ★ George Washington University**
**Physician Assistant Program**
2175 K St. NW, Ste. 820
Washington, DC 20037
**Phone:** (202)530-2390
**Email:** npamag@gwumc.edu
**Website:** http://www.gwu.edu/~gwu_pa

**★ 1729 ★ Howard University**
**College of Pharmacy, Nursing, and Allied**
**Health Sciences**
**Physician Assistant Program**
Sixth and Bryant Sts. NW, Annex I
Washington, DC 20059
**Phone:** (202)806-7536
**Email:** mbarnard@howard.edu
**Website:** http://www.howard.edu/CollegeAlliedHealth/paprog.html

### Florida

**★ 1730 ★ Barry University**
**School of Graduate Medical Sciences**
**Physician Assistant Program**
11300 NE 2nd Ave.
Miami Shores, FL 33161
**Phone:** (305)899-3964
**Email:** mweinter@mail.barry.edu
**Website:** http://www2.barry.edu/vpaa-gms/pa/paprog.htm

**★ 1731 ★ Miami-Dade Community**
**College**
**Physician Assistant Program**
Medical Center Campus
950 NW 20th St.
Miami, FL 33127-4693
**Phone:** (305)237-4051
**Email:** taylow@mdcc.edu
**Website:** http://www.mdcc.edu/medical/

**★ 1732 ★ Nova Southeastern University**
**Physician Assistant Program**
3200 S University Dr.
Fort Lauderdale, FL 33328
**Phone:** (954)262-1250
**Email:** redavis@nova.edu

**Website:** http://www.nova.edu/cwis/centers/hpd/pap

**★ 1733 ★ University of Florida**
**Physician Assistant Program**
PO Box 100176
Gainesville, FL 32610-0176
**Phone:** (352)265-7955
**Email:** ops@pap.ufl.edu
**Website:** http://www.med.ufl.edu/pap

### Georgia

**★ 1734 ★ Emory University**
**School of Medicine**
**Physician Assistant Program**
1462 Clifton Rd. NE, Ste. 280
Atlanta, GA 30322
**Phone:** (404)727-7825
**Email:** ljohn07@learnlink.emory.edu
**Website:** http://www.cc.emory.edu/MED/AH/ah.pa.html

**★ 1735 ★ Medical College of Georgia**
**Physician Assistant Program**
AE 1032
Physician Assistant Department
Augusta, GA 30912
**Phone:** (706)721-2725
**Email:** underadm@mail.mcg.edu
**Website:** http://www.mcg.edu/SAH/PhyAsst/index.html

**★ 1736 ★ South College**
**Physician Assistant Program**
9 Mall Ct.
Savannah, GA 31406
**Phone:** (912)691-6023
**Email:** southcollege@southcollege.edu
**Website:** http://www.southcollege.edu

### Idaho

**★ 1737 ★ Idaho State University**
**Physician Assistant Program**
Campus Box 8253
Pocatello, ID 83209-8253
**Phone:** (208)282-4726
**Email:** ruchanit@isu.edu

### Illinois

**★ 1738 ★ Finch University of Health**
**Sciences/Chicago Medical School**
**Physician Assistant Program**
3333 Green Bay Rd., Bldg. 51
North Chicago, IL 60064-3095
**Phone:** (847)578-3312
**Website:** http://www.finchcms.edu

**★ 1739 ★ Malcolm X College /Cook**
**County Hospital**
**Physician Assistant Program**
1900 W Van Buren St., Ste. 3241
Chicago, IL 60612
**Phone:** (312)850-7255
**Website:** http://www.ccc.edu/malcolmx/malcolmx1/CD_physassist.htm

**★ 1740 ★ Midwestern University**
**Physician Assistant Program**
555 W 31st St.
Downers Grove, IL 60515
**Free:** 800-458-6253
**Email:** admissil@midwestern.edu
**Website:** http://www.midwestern.edu

**★ 1741 ★ Southern Illinois University, Carbondale**
**Physician Assistant Program**
Lindegren Hall, Rm. 129
MC 6516
Carbondale, IL 62901-6516
**Phone:** (618)453-5527
**Website:** http://www.siu.edu/~hcp/pa.html

### Indiana

**★ 1742 ★ Butler University/Clarian Health**
**College of Pharmacy and Health Sciences**
**Physician Assistant Program**
4600 Sunset Ave.
Indianapolis, IN 46208
**Phone:** (317)940-9969
**Email:** tepp@butler.edu
**Website:** http://www.butler.edu/www/cophs

**★ 1743 ★ University of Saint Francis**
**Physician Assistant Program**
2701 Spring St.
Fort Wayne, IN 46808
**Email:** jroth@sf.edu
**Website:** http://www.sf.edu

### Iowa

**★ 1744 ★ Des Moines University**
**Osteopathic Medical Center**
**Physician Assistant Program**
3200 Grand Ave.
Des Moines, IA 50312
**Phone:** (515)271-1603
**Email:** pam.chambers@dmu.edu
**Website:** http://www.dmu.edu/cohs/pa/index.htm

**★ 1745 ★ University of Iowa**
**College of Medicine**
**Physician Assistant Program**
5167 Westlawn
Iowa City, IA 52242
**Phone:** (319)335-8922
**Email:** paprogram@uiowa.edu
**Website:** http://www.medicine.uiowa.edu/pa/pa.htm

### Kansas

**★ 1746 ★ Wichita State University**
**College of Health Professions**
**Physician Assistant Program**
Campus Box 43
Wichita, KS 67260-0043
**Phone:** (316)978-3011
**Email:** biddle@chp.twsu.edu
**Website:** http://twsuvm.uc.twsu.edu/~chpwww/Passt.htm

### Kentucky

**★ 1747 ★ University of Kentucky**
**Physician Assistant Program**
121 Washington Ave., Rm. 105
Lexington, KY 40536-0003
**Phone:** (606)323-1100
**Email:** mspas-dgs@lsc.uky.edu
**Website:** http://www.mc.uky.edu/pa/home.htm

### Louisiana

**★ 1748 ★ Louisiana State University**
**Health Sciences Center**
**School of Allied Health Professions**
**Physician Assistant Program**
1501 Kings Hwy.
PO Box 33932
Shreveport, LA 71130-3932
**Phone:** (318)675-7317

**Email:** kwili6@lsuhsc.edu
**Website:** http://www.lsuhsc.edu/

### Maine

**★ 1749 ★ University of New England**
**Physician Assistant Program**
11 Hills Beach Rd.
Biddeford, ME 04005
**Phone:** (207)283-0171
**Email:** dfarrell@mailbox.une.edu
**Website:** http://www.une.edu

### Maryland

**★ 1750 ★ Anne Arundel Community College**
**School of Health Professions, Wellness, and Physical Education**
**Physician Assistant Program**
101 College Pkwy.
Arnold, MD 21012
**Phone:** (410)315-7310
**Email:** pdfalkenstein@mail.aacc.cc.md.us
**Website:** http://www.aacc.cc.md.us/ahd/physasst.html

**★ 1751 ★ Community College of Baltimore-Essex**
**Physician Assistant Program**
7201 Rossville Blvd.
Baltimore, MD 21237
**Phone:** (410)780-6579
**Email:** sshaw@ccbc.cc.md.us
**Website:** http://www.ccbc.cc.md.us/campuses/essex/academics/career/cert/pa/e_pa_prog. htm

**★ 1752 ★ University of Maryland, Eastern Shore**
**Physician Assistant Program**
Modular 934-5 Backbone Dr.
Princess Anne, MD 21853
**Phone:** (410)651-7584

### Massachusetts

**★ 1753 ★ Massachusetts College of Pharmacy and Health Sciences**
**Physician Assistant Studies Program**
179 Longwood Ave., WB01
Boston, MA 02115
**Phone:** (617)732-2140
**Email:** cfasser@mcp.edu

**★ 1754 ★ Northeastern University**
**Physician Assistant Program**
202 Robinson Hall
Boston, MA 02115
**Phone:** (617)373-3195
**Website:** http://www.dac.neu.edu/pap/physasst.html

**★ 1755 ★ Springfield College/Baystate Health System**
**Physician Assistant Program**
263 Alden St.
Springfield, MA 01109
**Free:** 800-343-1257
**Website:** http://www.springfieldcollege.edu/home-page.nsf

### Michigan

**★ 1756 ★ Central Michigan University**
**Physician Assistant Program**
Foust Hall
Mount Pleasant, MI 48859
**Phone:** (989)774-1237
**Email:** chpadmit@cmich.edu
**Website:** http://www.cmich.edu/pa-pro.html

**★ 1757 ★ Grand Valley State University**
**Mental Education and Research Center**
**Physician Assistant Program**
1000 Monroe NW
Grand Rapids, MI 49503
**Phone:** (616)233-6500
**Email:** pas@gvsu.edu
**Website:** http://www4.gvsu.edu/pas/index.htm

**★ 1758 ★ University of Detroit Mercy**
**Physician Assistant Program**
8200 Outer Dr.
PO Box 19900
Detroit, MI 48219-0900
**Phone:** (313)993-6177
**Email:** vitalel@udmercy.edu
**Website:** http://www.udmercy.edu

**★ 1759 ★ Wayne State University**
**College of Pharmacy and Allied Health Professions**
**Department of Physician Assistant Studies**
Detroit, MI 48202
**Phone:** (313)577-1368
**Email:** ab4754@wayne.edu
**Website:** http://wizard.pharm.wayne.edu/pastudies/pa.htm

**★ 1760 ★ Western Michigan University**
**Physician Assistant Program**
Kalamazoo, MI 49008-5138
**Phone:** (616)387-5314
**Website:** http://www.wmich.edu/paprog/

### Minnesota

**★ 1761 ★ Augsburg College**
**Physician Assistant Program**
2211 Riverside Ave.
Campus Box 149
Minneapolis, MN 55454
**Phone:** (612)330-1039
**Email:** paprog@augsburg.edu
**Website:** http://www.augsburg.edu/pap/index.html

### Missouri

**★ 1762 ★ Saint Louis University**
**School of Allied Health Professions**
**Physician Assistant Program**
3437 Caroline St.
Saint Louis, MO 63104
**Phone:** (314)577-8521
**Email:** mayj@slu.edu
**Website:** http://www.slu.edu/colleges/AH/PA

**★ 1763 ★ Southwest Missouri State University**
**Department of Physician Assistant Studies**
901 S National Ave.
Springfield, MO 65804
**Phone:** (417)836-6151
**Email:** physicianassststudies@smsu.edu

### Montana

**★ 1764 ★ Rocky Mountain College**
**Physician Assistant Program**
1511 Poly Dr.
Billings, MT 59102-1797
**Phone:** (406)657-1190
**Email:** bentss@rocky.edu
**Website:** http://www.rocky.edu

## Nebraska

**★ 1765 ★ Union College**
**Physician Assistant Program**
3800 S 4th St.
Lincoln, NE 68506
**Phone:** (402)486-2527
**Email:** paprog@ucollege.edu
**Website:** http://www.college.edu/pa/home.htm

**★ 1766 ★ University of Nebraska Medical Center**
**Physician Assistant Program**
Box 984300
Omaha, NE 68198-4300
**Phone:** (402)559-5266
**Email:** dklandon@unmc.edu
**Website:** http://www.unmc.edu/AlliedHealth/pa

## New Hampshire

**★ 1767 ★ Notre Dame College**
**Physician Assistant Program**
Office of Graduate Admissions and Continuing
  Education
2321 Elm St.
Manchester, NH 03104-2299
**Phone:** (603)222-7210
**Website:** http://www.notredame.edu

## New Jersey

**★ 1768 ★ Seton Hall University**
**University of Medicine and Dentistry of New Jersey**
**Physician Assistant Program**
400 South Orange Ave.
South Orange, NJ 07079-2689
**Phone:** (973)761-7145
**Website:** http://www.shu.edu/academic/arts_sci/Undergraduate/biology/pa.html

**★ 1769 ★ University of Medicine and Dentistry of New Jersey**
**Physician Assistant Program**
65 Bergen St.
Newark, NJ 07107-3001
**Phone:** (973)972-5954

**★ 1770 ★ University of Medicine and Dentistry of New Jersey / Rutgers, the State University of New Jersey / New Jersey Institute of Technology**
**Robert Wood Johnson Medical School**
**Physician Assistant Program**
675 Hoes Ln.
Piscataway, NJ 08854-5635
**Phone:** (732)235-4444
**Website:** http://www2.umdnj.edu/paweb

## New Mexico

**★ 1771 ★ University of New Mexico**
**School of Medicine**
**Department of Family & Community Medicine**
**Physician Assistant Program**
2400 Tucker NE
Albuquerque, NM 87131-5241
**Phone:** (505)272-9678
**Email:** paprogram@salud.unm.edu
**Website:** http://hsc.unm.edu/fcm/

**★ 1772 ★ University of St. Francis**
**Physician Assistant Program**
4401 Silver Ave. SE, Ste. B
Albuquerque, NM 87108
**Phone:** (505)266-5565
**Email:** pa@stfrancis.edu

## New York

**★ 1773 ★ Albany Medical College/Hudson Valley Community College**
**Physician Assistant Program**
47 New Scotland Ave.
Mail Code 4
Albany, NY 12208
**Phone:** (518)262-5251
**Email:** daisr@mail.amc.edu
**Website:** http://www.hvcc.edu/academ/schools/health/pas/pas.html

**★ 1774 ★ Bronx Lebanon Hospital Center**
**Physician Assistant Program**
1650 Selwyn Ave., Ste. 11D
Bronx, NY 10457
**Phone:** (718)960-1255

**★ 1775 ★ Brooklyn Hospital Center/Long Island University**
**Physician Assistant Program**
121 DeKalb Ave.
Brooklyn, NY 11201
**Phone:** (718)250-8144    **Fax:** (718)260-2780
**Email:** tbhcpap@aol.com
**Website:** http://www.brooklyn.liunet.edu/cwis/bklyn/health/bsphyass.html

**★ 1776 ★ City University of New York, Harlem Hospital Center**
**Sophie Davis School of Biomedical Education**
**Physician Assistant Program**
Women's Pavilion, Rm. 619
506 Malcolm X Blvd.
New York, NY 10037
**Phone:** (212)939-2525
**Email:** shrcc@cunyvm.cuny.edu
**Website:** http://www.ccny.cuny.edu/undergrad_bulletin_97/Sophie_Davis.html

**★ 1777 ★ Daemen College**
**Physician Assistant Department**
4380 Main St.
Amherst, NY 14226-3592
**Free:** 800-462-7652
**Email:** admissions@daemen.edu
**Website:** http://www.daemen.edu/departments/pa

**★ 1778 ★ D'Youville College**
**Physician Assistant Program**
320 Porter Ave.
Buffalo, NY 14201
**Phone:** (716)881-7713
**Website:** http://www.dyc.edu/academics/

**★ 1779 ★ Le Moyne College**
**Physician Assistant Program**
Department of Biology
1419 Salt Springs Rd.
Syracuse, NY 13214-1399
**Phone:** (315)445-4745
**Email:** simonpa@mail.lemoyne.edu
**Website:** http://www.lemoyne.edu/academic_affairs/programs/pa/PApage.htm
Patricia Simone, Contact

**★ 1780 ★ Mercy College**
**Graduate Program in Physician Assistant Studies**
555 Broadway
Dobbs Ferry, NY 10522
**Phone:** (914)674-7635
**Email:** paprogram@mercynet.edu

**★ 1781 ★ New York Institute of Technology**
**Physician Assistant Program**
PO Box 8000
Old Westbury, NY 11568-8000
**Phone:** (516)686-3881
**Email:** sbarese@nyit.edu

**★ 1782 ★ Pace University, Lenox Hill Hospital**
**Physician Assistant Program**
1 Pace Plaza, Rm. Y-31
New York, NY 10038
**Phone:** (212)346-1357
**Email:** paprogram@pace.edu

**★ 1783 ★ Rochester Institute of Technology**
**Physician Assistant Program**
85 Lomb Memorial Dr.
Rochester, NY 14623-5603
**Phone:** (716)475-2978
**Email:** hbmscl@rit.edu
**Website:** http://www.rit.edu/~930www/Proj/UGrad/UGradCat/colleges/cos/phyassist.html

**★ 1784 ★ St. Vincent Catholic Medical Centers of New York**
**Brooklyn and Queens Region**
**Physician Assistant Program**
175-05 Horace Harding Expressway
Fresh Meadows, NY 11365
**Phone:** (718)357-0500
**Email:** tsimone@cmcny.com

**★ 1785 ★ St. Vincent Catholic Medical Centers of New York**
**Physician Assistant Program**
75 Vanderbilt Ave.
Staten Island, NY 10304-3850
**Phone:** (718)354-5570

**★ 1786 ★ State University of New York, Brooklyn**
**Downstate Medical Center**
**Health Science Center**
**Physician Assistant Program**
450 Clarkson Ave.
Box 1222
Brooklyn, NY 11234
**Phone:** (718)270-2324
**Email:** admissions@downstate.edu
**Website:** http://www.hscbklyn.edu/CHRP/pa.html

**★ 1787 ★ State University of New York, Stony Brook**
**School of Health Technology and Management**
**Physician Assistant Program**
Health Sciences Center, L2-052
Stony Brook, NY 11794-8202
**Phone:** (631)444-3190
**Email:** paprogram@sunysb.edu
**Website:** http://www.uhmc.sunysb.edu/shtm/pa/pa_welcome.html

**★ 1788 ★ Touro College**
**School of Health Sciences**
**Physician Assistant Program**
1700 Union Blvd.
Bay Shore, NY 11706
**Phone:** (631)665-1600
**Website:** http://www.touro.edu

★ **1789** ★ **Touro College-Manhattan Campus**
**School of Health Sciences**
**Physician Assistant Program**
27-33 W 23rd St.
New York, NY 10010
**Phone:** (212)463-0400
**Email:** ngraff@touro.edu

★ **1790** ★ **Wagner College / Staten Island University Hospital**
**Physician Assistant Program**
74 Melville St.
Staten Island, NY 10309-4035
**Phone:** (718)226-2928
**Email:** nlowy@siuh.edu
**Website:** http://www.siuh.edu/pa/pa.html

★ **1791** ★ **Weill Cornell Medical College**
**Physician Assistant Program**
1300 York Ave., F-1919
New York, NY 10021
**Phone:** (212)746-5133
**Email:** jdrawls@mail.med.cornell.edu
**Website:** http://www.med.cornell.edu/dept/index.html

### North Carolina

★ **1792** ★ **Duke University Medical Center**
**Physician Assistant Program**
DUMC 3848
Durham, NC 27710
**Phone:** (919)681-3155
**Email:** paadmission@mc.duke.edu
**Website:** http://dmi-www.mc.duke.edu/cfm/pap

★ **1793** ★ **East Carolina University**
**School of Allied Health Sciences**
**Physician Assistant Program**
West Research Campus
1157 VOA Site "C" Rd.
Greenville, NC 27834
**Phone:** (252)744-1100
**Website:** http://www.ecu.edu/pa

★ **1794** ★ **Methodist College**
**Physician Assistant Program**
5107B College Centre Dr.
Fayetteville, NC 28311
**Phone:** (910)630-7495
**Email:** paprog@methodist.edu
**Website:** http://www.apcnet.com/methodist/methodist.html

★ **1795** ★ **Wake Forest University**
**School of Medicine**
**Physician Assistant Program**
Medical Center Blvd.
Winston Salem, NC 27157-1006
**Phone:** (336)716-4356
**Email:** shfoster@wfubmc.edu
**Website:** http://mero.lib.wfubmc.edu/paprogram/

### North Dakota

★ **1796** ★ **University of North Dakota**
**School of Medicine and Health Sciences**
**Department of Community Medicine and Rural Health**
**Physician Assistant Program**
PO Box 9037
Grand Forks, ND 58202-9037
**Phone:** (701)777-2344
**Email:** mcdaniel@medicine.nodak.edu
**Website:** http://www.med.und.nodak.edu/depts/Commed/Home.html
Rhonda McDaniel, Contact

### Ohio

★ **1797** ★ **Cuyahoga Community College**
**Surgical Physician Assistant Program**
11000 Pleasant Valley Rd.
Parma, OH 44130
**Phone:** (216)987-5363
**Email:** joyce.janicek@tri-c.cc.oh.us

★ **1798** ★ **Kettering College of Medical Arts**
**Physician Assistant Program**
3737 Southern Blvd.
Kettering, OH 45429
**Phone:** (937)296-7238
**Email:** neida.rowland@kmcnetwork.org
**Website:** http://www.kcma.edu/

★ **1799** ★ **Medical College of Ohio**
**School of Allied Health**
**Physician Assistant Program**
3015 Arlington Ave.
Toledo, OH 43614-5803
**Phone:** (419)383-5408
**Email:** tlangenderfe@mco.edu
**Website:** http://www.mco.edu

★ **1800** ★ **University of Findlay**
**Physician Assistant Program**
1000 N Main St.
Findlay, OH 45840-3695
**Phone:** (419)424-4529
**Email:** davis@mail.Findlay.edu

### Oklahoma

★ **1801** ★ **University of Oklahoma**
**Health Sciences Center**
**Physician Associate Program**
Health Sciences Center
PO Box 26901
Oklahoma City, OK 73190
**Phone:** (405)271-2058
**Website:** http://www.medicine.ouhsc.edu/education/pafset.html

### Oregon

★ **1802** ★ **Oregon Health Sciences University**
**Physician Assistant Program**
3181 SW Sam Jackson Park Rd.
Mailcode GH219
Portland, OR 97201-3098
**Phone:** (503)494-1484
**Email:** paprgm@ohsu.edu
**Website:** http://www.ohsu.edu/ah-pa

★ **1803** ★ **Pacific University**
**School of Physician Assistant Studies**
**Physician Assistant Program**
2043 College Way
Forest Grove, OR 97116
**Phone:** (503)359-2900
**Email:** pa@pacificu.edu
**Website:** http://www.pacificu.edu/academics/pa.html

### Pennsylvania

★ **1804** ★ **Arcadia University**
**Physician Assistant Program**
Brubaker Hall, Health Science Center
450 S Easton Rd.
Glenside, PA 19038
**Phone:** (215)572-2082
**Email:** paruchg@camelot.beaver.edu
**Website:** http://www.beaver.edu/programs/passist.htm

★ **1805** ★ **Chatham College**
**Physician Assistant Program**
Woodland Rd.
Pittsburgh, PA 15232
**Phone:** (412)365-1412
**Email:** admissions@chatham.edu
**Website:** http://www.chatham.edu/academic/PA/pac1.html

★ **1806** ★ **DeSales University**
**Physician Assistant Program**
2755 Station Ave.
Center Valley, PA 18034-9568
**Phone:** (610)282-1100
**Email:** Pamela.wertman@desales.edu

★ **1807** ★ **Duquesne University**
**John G. Rangos Sr. School of Health Sciences**
**Physician Assistant Program**
323 Health Sciences Bldg.
Pittsburgh, PA 15282
**Free:** 800-456-0590
**Email:** pinevich@duq.edu
**Website:** http://www.duq.edu/healthsciences/pa/pa-home.html

★ **1808** ★ **Gannon University**
**Physician Assistant Program**
109 University Sq.
Erie, PA 16541-0001
**Phone:** (814)871-7420
**Website:** http://WWW.GANNON.EDU/PROGRAMS/UNDER/phyasst.html

★ **1809** ★ **King's College**
**Physician Assistant Program**
133 N River St.
Wilkes Barre, PA 18711
**Phone:** (570)208-5853
**Email:** sesedon@kings.edu
**Website:** http://www.kings.edu/home/majors/pa_program.htm

★ **1810** ★ **Lock Haven University**
**Physician Assistant Program in Rural Primary Care**
Lock Haven, PA 17745
**Phone:** (570)893-2541
**Email:** weisenha@lhup.edu
**Website:** http://www.lhup.edu/academic/acad_affairs/academ_grad_phyas.html

★ **1811** ★ **Marywood University**
**Physician Assistant Program**
2300 Adams Ave.
Scranton, PA 18509
**Phone:** (570)348-6298
**Email:** ugadm@ac.marywood.edu
**Website:** http://www.marywood.edu/ug_cat/departments/phys_asst.stm

★ **1812** ★ **MCP Hahnemann University**
**College of Nursing and Health Professions**
**Physician Assistant Program**
245 N 15th St.
Mail Stop 504
Philadelphia, PA 19102-1192
**Phone:** (215)762-7135
**Email:** enroll@mcphu.edu
**Website:** http://www.auhs.edu/shp/shpprogs/physasst.html
**Frmly:** Allegheny University of Health Profession

**★ 1813 ★ Pennsylvania College of Technology**
**Physician Assistant Program**
1 College Ave., DIF 123
Williamsport, PA 17701-5799
**Phone:** (570)327-4779
**Email:** kmayer@pct.edu
**Website:** http://www.pct.edu

**★ 1814 ★ Philadelphia College of Osteopathic Medicine**
**Department of Physician Assistant Studies**
4170 City Ave., Ste. 005
Evans Hall
Philadelphia, PA 19131
**Phone:** (215)871-6772
**Email:** kennethha@pcom.edu
**Website:** http://www.pcom.edu/academicprograms/pa/index.html

**★ 1815 ★ Philadelphia University**
**Physician Assistant Program**
School House Ln. and Henry Ave.
Philadelphia, PA 19144
**Phone:** (215)951-2908
**Email:** mccombs@philau.edu
**Website:** http://www.philau.edu

**★ 1816 ★ Saint Francis University**
**Department of Physician Assistant Sciences**
PO Box 600
Loretto, PA 15940-0600
**Phone:** (814)472-3020
**Email:** admissions@francis.edu
**Website:** http://www.sfcpa.edu

**★ 1817 ★ Seton Hill College**
**Physician Assistant Program**
College Ave.
Greensburg, PA 15601
**Free:** 800-826-6234
**Email:** admit@setonhill.edu
**Website:** http://maura.setonhill.edu/~msct/fmsc15.htm

## South Carolina

**★ 1818 ★ Medical University of South Carolina**
**College of Health Professions**
**Physician Assistant Program**
PO Box 250856
Charleston, SC 29425
**Phone:** (843)792-0376
**Email:** jonesmo@musc.edu
**Website:** http://www.musc.edu/pa_program

## South Dakota

**★ 1819 ★ University of South Dakota**
**School of Medicine**
**Physician Assistant Studies Program**
414 E Clark St.
Vermillion, SD 57069-2390
**Phone:** (605)677-5128
**Email:** usdpa@usd.edu
**Website:** http://www.usd.edu/med/som/somdept/pa

## Tennessee

**★ 1820 ★ Bethel College**
**Physician Assistant Program**
325 Cherry Ave.
McKenzie, TN 38201
**Phone:** (901)352-4004

**★ 1821 ★ Trevecca Nazarene University**
**Physician Assistant Program**
333 Murfreesboro Rd.
Nashville, TN 37210-2877
**Phone:** (615)248-1225
**Website:** http://www.trevecca.edu/academics/nas/gradphysasst/

## Texas

**★ 1822 ★ Academy of Health Sciences**
**Interservice Physician Assistant Program**
3151 Scott Rd., Ste. 1202
Attn: MCCS HMP
Fort Sam Houston, TX 78234-6138
**Phone:** (210)221-8004

**★ 1823 ★ Baylor College of Medicine**
**Physician Assistant Program**
1 Baylor Plaza, Rm. 633E
Houston, TX 77030
**Phone:** (713)798-4619
**Website:** http://www.bcm.tmc.edu

**★ 1824 ★ Texas Tech University Health Sciences Center**
**School of Allied Health**
**Department of Diagnostic and Primary Care**
**Physician Assistant Program**
3600 N Garfield
Midland, TX 79705
**Phone:** (915)686-4213
**Email:** jrunyan@midland.cc.tx.us

**★ 1825 ★ University of North Texas Health Science Center**
**Physician Assistant Studies**
3500 Camp Bowie Blvd.
Fort Worth, TX 76107-2699
**Phone:** (817)735-2301
**Email:** pa_program@hsc.unt.edu
**Website:** http://www.hsc.unt.edu/departments/fammed/assist.htm

**★ 1826 ★ University of Texas Southwestern Medical Center**
**Physician Assistant Program**
6011 Harry Hines Blvd.
Dallas, TX 75235-9090
**Phone:** (214)648-1701
**Email:** isela.perez@utsouthwestern.edu
**Website:** http://www.swmed.edu/home_pages/allied/hcpa.htm

**★ 1827 ★ University of Texas Health Science Center, San Antonio**
**Department of Physician Assistant Studies**
**Physician Assistant Program**
7703 Floyd Curl Dr.
Mail Code 6249
San Antonio, TX 78229-3900
**Phone:** (210)567-8811
**Email:** blessing@uthscsa.edu

**★ 1828 ★ University of Texas Medical Branch**
**School of Allied Health Sciences**
**Physician Assistant Program**
301 University Blvd.
Galveston, TX 77555-1028
**Phone:** (409)772-3046
**Email:** rrahr@utmb.edu
**Website:** http://www.sahs.utmb.edu/sahs/physician_assistant_studies

**★ 1829 ★ University of Texas-Pan American**
**Physician Assistant Program**
1201 W University Dr.
Edinburg, TX 78539
**Phone:** (956)381-2292

## Utah

**★ 1830 ★ University of Utah**
**Physician Assistant Program**
375 Chipeta Way
Salt Lake City, UT 84108
**Phone:** (801)581-7764
**Email:** drobinson@upap.utah.edu
**Website:** http://www.utah.edu/upap/

## Virginia

**★ 1831 ★ College of Health Sciences**
**Physician Assistant Program**
920 S Jefferson St.
Roanoke, VA 24016
**Phone:** (540)985-4016
**Email:** pa@health.chs.edu
**Website:** http://www.chs.edu

**★ 1832 ★ Eastern Virginia Medical School**
**Physician Assistant Program**
700 W Olney Rd.
PO Box 1980
Norfolk, VA 23501-1980
**Phone:** (757)446-7158
**Email:** paprog@evmsmail.evms.edu
**Website:** http://www.evms.edu/hlthprof/mpa.html

**★ 1833 ★ James Madison University**
**Department of Health Sciences**
**Physician Assistant Program**
MSC-4301
Harrisonburg, VA 22807
**Phone:** (540)568-2395
**Email:** paprogram@jmu.edu

## Washington

**★ 1834 ★ University of Washington**
**MEDEX Northwest**
**Physician Assistant Program**
4245 Roosevelt Way NE
Seattle, WA 98105-6920
**Phone:** (206)598-2600
**Website:** http://www.washington.edu/medical/som/depts/medes

## West Virginia

**★ 1835 ★ Alderson-Broaddus College**
**Physician Assistant Program**
PO Box 2036
Philippi, WV 26416
**Phone:** (304)457-6283
**Email:** holt_m@ab.edu
**Website:** http://blue.ab.edu/

**★ 1836 ★ Mountain State University**
**Physician Assistant Program**
PO Box AG
Beckley, WV 25802
**Phone:** (304)253-7351
**Website:** http://www.cwv.edu/nhs/pa/index.html

## Wisconsin

**★ 1837 ★ Marquette University**
**College of Health Sciences**
**Department of Physician Assistant**
**Studies**
1700 Bldg.
PO Box 1881
Milwaukee, WI 53201-1881
**Phone:** (414)288-5688
**Website:** http://www.marquette.edu/chs/phas/

**★ 1838 ★ University of Wisconsin—**
**LaCrosse**
**Gunderson Lutheran Medical Foundation/**
**Mayo School of Health Related**
**Sciences**
**Physician Assistant Program**
1725 State St.
4031 Health Science Center
La Crosse, WI 54601-3767
**Phone:** (608)785-6620
**Email:** paprogram@uwlax.edu
**Website:** http://www.uwlax.edu/SAH/PhysicianAssistant/

**★ 1839 ★ University of Wisconsin,**
**Madison**
**Physician Assistant Program**
1300 University Ave.
Medical Sciences Center, Rm. 1050
Madison, WI 53706
**Phone:** (608)263-5620
**Website:** http://www.medsch.wisc.edu/pa/

# National & International Organizations

**★ 1840 ★ Academy for Health Services**
**Research and Health Policy**
1801 K St. NW, Ste. 701-L
Washington, DC 20006-1301
**Phone:** (202)292-6700          **Fax:** (202)292-6800
**Email:** info@ahsrhp.org
**Website:** http://www.academyhealth.org
David Helms, Pres.

**Fnded:** 1981. **Mem:** 2,800. **Desc:** Individuals and organizations concerned with health services research. Objectives are to educate the public concerning the need for and contribution of health services research in improving health care in the U.S.; to foster productive cooperation among researchers, public and private funding agencies, health professionals, policymakers, and the public; to represent the views of members in the development and implementation of national legislative and administrative policies concerning health services research. Disseminates research findings to public and private sector officials. **Pub:** *HSR Reports*, quarterly. Newsletter. Covers legislative news and association activities. Includes conference calendar, employment listings, and training opportunities. *Price:* Free with membership. **Frmly:** (2002) Association for Health Services Research.

**★ 1841 ★ Academy for International**
**Health Studies (AIHS)**
621 Georgetown Pl.
Davis, CA 95616
**Phone:** (530)758-8600          **Fax:** (916)313-3410
**Email:** jlewis@aihs.com
**Website:** http://www.aihs.com
Jonathan C. Lewis, Pres.

**Fnded:** 1993. **Desc:** Senior health care executives from multinational health industries including health plans, health care providers, medical device manufacturers, pharmaceutical companies, and information technology vendors. Seeks to improve understanding of the international health care market and the American health system. Brings together members for the discussion of matters of mutual concern; serves as a clearinghouse on the health care industries; organizes trade and study missions. Operates Mexico-U.S.A. CrossBorder Health Insurance Initiative, which assists in the development of commercially viable health insurance for Mexican nationals living in the United States. Maintains speakers' bureau; functions as the North American Office of the International Federation of Health Funds. **Pub:** *Modern Healthcare International*, weekly. Magazine.

**★ 1842 ★ Academy of Managed Care**
**Providers (AMCP)**
1945 Palo Verde Ave. Ste. 202
Long Beach, CA 90815-3445
**Phone:** (562)596-8660          **Free:** 800-297-2627
**Fax:** (562)799-3355
**Email:** members@academymcp.org
**Website:** http://www.academymcp.org
Dr. John Russell, Pres.

**Fnded:** 1993. **Mem:** 2,500. **Desc:** Clinicians and Managed Care Industry executives. Provides a mulititude of services to members. Awards diplomate status to qualified members who meet criteria and pass written exam. **Pub:** *Managed Care Times*, monthly. Newsletter. Contains update on all aspects of the healthcare industry. *Price:* *imd.

**★ 1843 ★ Accessibility Equipment**
**Manufacturers Association (AEMA)**
PO Box 380
Metamora, IL 61548-0380
**Free:** 800-514-1100          **Fax:** (309)923-7964
**Email:** host@aema.com
**Website:** http://www.aema.com/

**Fnded:** 1990. **Desc:** Promotes awareness of accessibility equipment, including the design, installation and servicing of vertical, inclined and horizontal conveying systems that are used to provide access and/or egress for physically challenged people in public and residential areas. Accessibility products are platform lifts, wheelchair lifts, access elevators, residence elevators, stairway chairlifts, and similar products.

**★ 1844 ★ Accreditation Association for**
**Ambulatory Health Care (AAAHC)**
3201 Old Glenview Rd., Ste. 300
Wilmette, IL 60091
**Phone:** (847)853-6060          **Fax:** (847)853-9028
**Email:** info@aaahc.org
**Website:** http://www.aaahc.org
John E. Burke, PhD, Exec. Dir.

**Fnded:** 1979. **Mem:** 15. **Desc:** Operates a voluntary, peer-based accreditation and consulting program for ambulatory health care organizations as a means of assisting them in efficiently providing a high level of care for patients. Distributes free lists of accredited organizations. **Pub:** *Accreditation Handbook for Ambulatory Health Care*, biennial. Standards for accreditation of ambulatory health care centers. Includes subject index. *Price:* $90/copy prepaid. • Also publishes related survey materials.

**★ 1845 ★ Accreditation Council for**
**Continuing Medical Education (ACCME)**
515 N State St., Ste. 2150
Chicago, IL 60610
**Phone:** (312)464-2500          **Fax:** (312)464-2586
**Email:** postmaster@accme.org
**Website:** http://www.accme.org
Murray Kopelow, MD, Exec. Dir.

**Fnded:** 1981. **Desc:** Acts as an accrediting agency for sponsors of continuing medical education for physicians. Sponsoring participants are: American Board of Medical Specialties; American Hospital Association; American Medical Association; Association of American Medical Colleges; Association for Hospital Medical Education; Council of Medical Specialty Societies; Federation of State Medical Boards of the United States. **Frmly:** Liaison Committee on Continuing Medical Education.

**★ 1846 ★ Accreditation Review**
**Commission on Education for**
**Physician Assistants (ARC-PA)**
1000 N Oak Ave.
Marshfield, WI 54449-5788
**Phone:** (715)389-3785          **Fax:** (715)387-5163
**Email:** mccartyj@mfldclin.edu
**Website:** http://www.arc-pa.org
John E. McCarty, Exec. Dir.

**Fnded:** 1971. **Mem:** 16. **Desc:** Serves as an accrediting body for physician assistant education nationwide. **Frmly:** (1972) Joint Review Committee on Educational Programs for Physician's Assistants; (1987) Joint Review on Educational Programs for Physician Assistants; (1989) Accreditation Committee on Education for Physicians Assistants; (2000) Accreditation Review Committee on Education for Physician Assistants.

**★ 1847 ★ Action in International**
**Medicine (AIM)**
125 High Holborn
London WC1V 6QA, United Kingdom
**Phone:** 44 171 4053090          **Fax:** 44 171 4053093
**Email:** actintmed@aol.com

**Fnded:** 1988. **Mem:** 100. **Lang(s):** English. **Desc:** Health care institutions and health services. Promotes adoption of of "CCI," a self-help health improvement program which empowers local communities to address their health and poverty issues. Works to establish health care infrastructure in developing areas; provides support and assistance to grass roots health services. **Pub:** *AIM Bulletin*, quarterly. Newsletter.

**★ 1848 ★ Action for Victims of Medical**
**Accidents**
44 High St.
Croydon CR0 14B, United Kingdom
**Phone:** 44 208 6868333
**Website:** http://www.avma.co.uk

**Desc:** Provides independent advice and support to anyone who has suffered a medical accident.

**★ 1849 ★ Ad Hoc Group for Medical**
**Research Funding (AHGMRF)**
c/o Association of American Medical Colleges
2450 N St. NW
Washington, DC 20037-1126
**Phone:** (202)828-0525          **Fax:** (202)862-6218
**Email:** adhoc@aamc.org
**Website:** http://www.aamc.org/research/adhocgp/start.htm
Richard M. Knapp, PhD, Chmn.

**Fnded:** 1982. **Mem:** 300. **Desc:** Organizations engaged in or supporting biomedical and behavioral research. Goals are to assess federal funding for biomedical and behavioral research and advocate appropriate funding for the National Institutes of Health. **Pub:** *Annual Funding Proposal*, annual. Brochure. • *NIH Resource Guide*, biennial. Directory. • Annual Report. *Price:* Free.

**★ 1850 ★ Adelaide Hospital Society**
c/o Adelaide and Meath Hospital
Tallaght
Dublin 24, Ireland
**Phone:** 353 1 4142072          **Fax:** 353 1 4142070
**Website:** http://www.adelaide.ie

**Fnded:** 1839. **Mem:** 1,000. **Desc:** Promotes the participation of the Protestant community in the Irish health system. Makes available financial support to Adelaide and Meath Hospital. Conducts fundraising activities; sponsors charitable programs.

**★ 1851 ★ Aesculapian Club (AC)**
c/o Dr. Sam Kim
25 Shattuck St., Bldg. A Rm. 206
Boston, MA 02115
**Phone:** (617)726-8858
Dr. Sam Kim, Contact

**Desc:** Social organization of graduates of Harvard Medical School or physicians who have held teaching appointments there for three years.

**★ 1852 ★ African Medical and Research Foundation - Denmark (AMRFD)**
12 H.C. Andersens Blvd.
DK-1553 Copenhagen V, Denmark
**Phone:** 45 33157533          **Fax:** 45 33156802
**Lang(s):** Danish, English. **Desc:** Medical and public health professionals. Seeks to identify and address health needs in rural Africa. Develops, implements, and evaluates public health programs; encourages enhancement of local administrative capacities through training.

**★ 1853 ★ African Medical and Research Foundation - France (AMRFF)**
38 rue des Sablons
F-75116 Paris, France
**Phone:** 33 1 45538684          **Fax:** 33 1 46422321
**Website:** http://www.amref.org
**Lang(s):** English, French. **Desc:** Medical and public health professionals. Seeks to identify and address health needs in rural Africa. Develops, implements, and evaluates public health programs; encourages enhancement of local administrative capacities through training.

**★ 1854 ★ African Medical and Research Foundation - Italy (AMREF - It) (Fondazione Africana per la Medicina e la Ricerca)**
Via Settembrini, 30
I-00195 Rome, Italy
**Phone:** 39 6 3202222          **Fax:** 39 6 3202227
**Email:** info@amref.it
**Website:** http://www.amref.it
**Fnded:** 1988. **Mem:** 30,000. **Lang(s):** French, German, Italian, Spanish. **Desc:** Provides health care services to people in eastern Africa. Identifies health needs and evaluates and implements methods and programs to meet those needs. Maintains projects which emphasize affordable health care for people in underdeveloped, rural areas. Operates mobile health service facilities, airborn support for health centers in remote areas, and radio communication services with over 100 two-way radio stations. Conducts training programs for rural health care workers and research into the control of hydatid disease, malaria, and sleeping sickness. Applies knowledge from the behavioral and social sciences to health care improvement initiatives. Writes articles and information for training manuals, health education materials, and medical journals. Disseminates information. Offers consultancy services. **Pub:** *Amref News*, every four months. Newsletter. Eight pages of information about our projects and general conditions and problems of the Horn of Africa Where AMREF works.

**★ 1855 ★ African Medical and Research Foundation - Kenya (AMREF)**
PO Box 30125
Nairobi, Kenya
**Phone:** 254 2 501301          **Fax:** 254 2 609518
**Email:** amref.info@amref.org
**Website:** http://www.amref.org
**Fnded:** 1957. **Nat'l Groups:** 5. **Lang(s):** English, Kiswahili. **Desc:** Purpose is to improve the health of people living in 5 east and south African countries. Focuses efforts on developing low-cost healthcare for people in rural areas. Program includes: training of community health workers; planning and evaluation of health projects; consulting services; primary health-care education; operation of a medical radio communi-

cation network within the region; ground mobile health services for nomadic and pastoral peoples; the Flying Doctor Service (funded by the Flying Doctors' Society of Africa), which provides airborne support for remote medical, surgical, and public health facilities. Conducts medical research, particularly into the control of malaria, sleeping sickness, and hydatid disease; applies behavioral and social sciences in health improvement. Offers computerized services. **Pub:** *Afya*, quarterly. Journal. Covers developments in medical education. • *AMREF Annual Report*, annual. Annual Report. **Frmly:** Flying Doctors Service.

**★ 1856 ★ African Medical and Research Foundation - Sweden (AMREF - Sw)**
Djurgardsvagen 230
S-115 21 Stockholm, Sweden
**Phone:** 46 8 6620910          **Fax:** 46 8 6674494
**Email:** amref@bok.bonnier.se
**Website:** http://www.amref.org
**Desc:** Aims to improve the health of people in eastern Africa. Seeks to indentify health needs and develop, implement, and evaluate methods and programmes to meet those needs through service, training and research. Programmes include: primary health care; training of community health workers; training of rural health staff through continuing education, teacher training and correspondence courses; development, printing, and distribution of training manuals, medical journals, and health education materials; application of behavioral and social sciences to health improvement; airborne support for remote health facilities, including surgical, medical, and public health services; grounds mobile health services for nomadic pastoralists; medical research into the control of hydatid disease, and malaria.

**★ 1857 ★ Afro-Asia-Oceania Association of Anatomists (AAOAA)**
Room No 1025 PC Block, Ansari Nagar
New Delhi 110 029, India
**Fnded:** 1985.

**★ 1858 ★ Aid for International Medicine (AIM)**
PO Box 119
Rockland, DE 19732
**Phone:** (302)655-8290          **Fax:** (302)655-0487
Dr. John Levinson, Pres.
**Fnded:** 1965. **Mem:** 25. **Reg. Groups:** 2. **Desc:** To extend medical help through areas where one or more members of the board have personally served and documented a need. Funding and/or materials have been provided for hospitals, medical schools, and orphanages in Asia, Africa, and the U.S. Has established medical textbook program which makes available new books to medical schools and hospitals.

**★ 1859 ★ Air Medical Physician Association (AMPA)**
c/o Pat Petersen
383 F St.
Salt Lake City, UT 84103
**Phone:** (801)408-3699          **Fax:** (801)408-1668
**Email:** patp@ampa.org
**Website:** http://www.ampa.org
Pat Petersen, Exec. Dir.
**Mem:** 400. **Desc:** Physicians and professionals involved in medical transport. Promotes safe and effective patient transportation through medical direction, research, education, leadership and collaboration. **Pub:** *Air Medical Journal*, quarterly. Journal. Peer-reviewed journal. • *Air Medical Physician Handbook.* Handbook. *Price:* $65 for nonmembers; $50 additional copies for members.

**★ 1860 ★ Algerian Ostomy Association**
c/o Rachid Rezgui, Pres.
Clinique Mohamed Boudiaf
12, rue Kesri Amar
Tizi-Ouzou, Algeria

**Phone:** 213 26 227521          **Fax:** 213 26 227361
**Email:** aoa@djaznir-connect.com
**Fnded:** 1988. **Mem:** 600. **Nat'l Groups:** 1. **State Groups:** 1. **Local Groups:** 2. **Lang(s):** English, French. **Desc:** Works to put into the disposition of ostomates in Algeria the different medical apparatus they need and to provide information on therapies and medical assistance in our clinics.

**★ 1861 ★ Alliance for Continuing Medical Education (ACME)**
1025 Montgomery Hwy., Ste. 105
Birmingham, AL 35216
**Phone:** (205)824-1355          **Fax:** (205)824-1357
**Email:** acme@acme-assn.org
**Website:** http://www.acme-assn.org
Bruce J. Bellande, PhD, Contact
**Fnded:** 1978. **Mem:** 2,500. **Desc:** Professionals engaged in continuing medical educational programs. Seeks to "educate and support continuing medical education professionals and to promote leadership in the development of continuing medical education to improve health care outcomes and the performance of health care providers." Facilitates exchange of information among members; makes available educational and continuing professional development opportunities; works to "shape and influence policy in the field of continuing medical education." Makes available discounts on product and services to members. **Pub:** *Almanac*, monthly. Newsletter. • *Journal of Continuing Education in the Health Professions*, quarterly. Journal.

**★ 1862 ★ Alliance of Independent Academic Medical Centers (AIAMC)**
c/o Glenn Craig Davis
233 E Erie St., Ste. 306
Chicago, IL 60611
**Phone:** (312)874-2181          **Fax:** (312)874-2180
**Email:** nancie@aiamc.org
**Website:** http://www.aiamc.org
Dr. Glenn Craig Davis, Pres.
**Fnded:** 1989. **Desc:** Independent academic medical center that sponsor four or more accredited residency programs, supports an institutional research program, and serves as a major affiliate for a significant number of medical school student clerkships. Promotes the roles and contributions of independent academic medical centers, fosters professional collegiality among their leaders, and works with other professional organizations to achieve mutual goals.

**★ 1863 ★ Alpha Omega Alpha Honor Medical Society**
525 Middlefield Rd., Ste. 130
Menlo Park, CA 94025
**Phone:** (650)329-0291          **Fax:** (650)329-1618
**Email:** eharris@alphaomegaalpha.org
**Website:** http://www.alphaomegaalpha.org
Edward D. Harris, Jr., Exec. Sec.
**Fnded:** 1902. **Mem:** 72,000. **Reg. Groups:** 124. **Desc:** Honor society for men and women studying medicine at graduate and postgraduate levels. Sponsors "Leaders in American Medicine" videotape series; underwrites visiting professorships. Also sponsors student research, student essay, and medical student service project awards. **Pub:** *The Pharos*, quarterly. Journal. Contains nontechnical articles of medical interest. **Frmly:** Alpha Omega Alpha.

**★ 1864 ★ America Association of Integrative Medicine**
2750 E Sunshine
Springfield, MO 65804
**Phone:** (417)881-9995          **Free:** 877-718-3053
**Fax:** (417)881-6414
**Email:** info@aaimedicine.com
**Website:** http://www.aaimedicine.com
Jennifer Leimkuehler, Ch. Assn. Off.
**Fnded:** 2000. **Mem:** 200. **Desc:** Seeks to bring together health care providers of both traditional and nontraditional medicine, from varied backgrounds

such as acupuncture, massage therapy, herbology, pain management, pastoral counseling. **Pub:** Newsletter, monthly.

★ **1865** ★ **America Society of Internal Medicine**
190 N Independence Mall
Philadelphia, PA 19106-1572
**Phone:** (215)351-2600          **Free:** 800-523-1546
**Email:** interpub@mail.acponline.org
**Website:** http://www.acponline.org
**Fnded:** 1915. **Reg. Groups:** 77. **Desc:** Dedicated to high standards in medical education, practice, and research. **Pub:** *ACP-ASIM Observer*, monthly. Contains news, legistlation, and economics for internists. *Price:* included in membership dues, except for Medical Student Members. • *Annals of Internal Medicine*, semimonthly. Journal. Delivers major review articles, research, editorials, exchange of medical opinion, and commentary. *Price:* included in membership dues, except Medical Student Members.

★ **1866** ★ **American Academy of Ambulatory Care**
2813 S Hiawassee Rd., Ste. 206
Orlando, FL 32835
**Phone:** (407)521-5789          **Fax:** (407)521-5790
**Email:** info@ambulatorymedicine.org
**Website:** http://www.ambulatorymedicine.org
Franz Ritucci, Jr. MD, Dir.
**Fnded:** 1997. **Desc:** Licensed practitioners advancing the profession of Ambulatory Care/Acute Care Medicine by elevating standards through education, basic and advanced training, and board certification. Contributes to the field in the areas of professional growth, scientific and medical research, and medical education, to improve the overall quality of medical care. **Pub:** *AAAC Newsletter*, quarterly. Newsletter. Features current issues and relevant reviews on ambulatory medicine.

★ **1867** ★ **American Academy of Family Physicians (AAFP)**
11400 Tomahawk Creek Pkwy.
Leawood, KS 66211-2672
**Phone:** (913)906-6000          **Free:** 800-274-2237
**Fax:** (913)906-6077
**Email:** fp@aafp.org
**Website:** http://www.aafp.org
Douglas E. Henley, MD, Exec. VP
**Fnded:** 1947. **Mem:** 90,000. **State Groups:** 55. **Local Groups:** 200. **Desc:** Professional society of family physicians who provide continuing comprehensive care to patients. **Pub:** *AAFP Reporter*, monthly. Newsletter. Covers socioeconomic issues and legislative news affecting medicine; includes member news. Available to selected media. • *American Family Physician*, 16/year. Journal. Includes book reviews, newsletter, calendar of events, and therapeutic, product, and subject indexes. *Price:* Free to qualified recipients; $50/year for nonmembers. • *Family Practice Management*, 10/year. Covers practice management and socioeconomic issues. • Annual Report. **Frmly:** (1971) American Academy of General Practice.

★ **1868** ★ **American Academy of Health Physics (AAHP)**
1313 Dolley Madison Blvd., Ste. 402
Mc Lean, VA 22101
**Phone:** (703)790-1745          **Fax:** (703)790-2672
**Email:** aahp@burkinc.com
**Website:** http://www.hps1.org/aahp
**Desc:** Certified Health Physicists. Works to promote the profession. Actively participates in the certification program.

★ **1869** ★ **American Academy of Pain Management**
13947 Mono Way, No. A
Sonora, CA. 95370
**Phone:** (209)533-9744          **Fax:** (209)533-9750

**Email:** aapm@aapainmanage.org
**Website:** http://www.aapainmanage.org
Kathryn A. Weiner, PhD, Exec. Dir.
**Fnded:** 1988. **Mem:** 6,000. **Desc:** To establish the core body of knowledge necessary to become a pain management professional. Provides educational and research programs and a speakers bureau. **Pub:** *American Journal of Pain Management*, quarterly. Journal. • *Pain Management A Practical Guide for Clinicians*. Textbook. • *The Pain Practitioner*, quarterly. Newsletter.

★ **1870** ★ **American Academy of Physician Assistants (AAPA)**
950 N Washington St.
Alexandria, VA 22314-1552
**Phone:** (703)836-2272          **Fax:** (703)684-1924
**Email:** aapa@aapa.org
**Website:** http://www.aapa.org
Kevin D. Bayes, Asst. Dir.
**Fnded:** 1968. **Mem:** 36,000. **Reg. Groups:** 5. **State Groups:** 57. **Local Groups:** 59. **Desc:** Physician assistants and other interested parties. Seeks to promote quality, cost-effective, and accessible healthcare, and the professional and personal development of PAs. Provide services for members. Organizes annual National PA Day. Develops research and education programs; compiles statistics. **Pub:** *AAPA News*, biweekly. Newsletter. News on physician assistant programs, AAPA's activities, and employment information and opportunities. • *Journal of the American Academy of Physician Assistants*, monthly, 12/year. Journal. Covers clinical and scholarly research. Includes book reviews. *Price:* Included in membership dues; $50/year for nonmembers; $75/year for institutions. • *Legislative Watch*, monthly. • Membership Directory, annual.

★ **1871** ★ **American Academy on Physician and Patient**
6728 Old McLean Village Dr.
Mc Lean, VA 22101
**Phone:** (703)556-9222          **Fax:** (703)556-8729
**Email:** aappatient@degnon.org
**Website:** http://www.physicianpatient.org
**Desc:** Research and education professionals. Dedicated to research, education and improving professional standards in doctor-patient communication. Sponsors scholarships and grants.

★ **1872** ★ **American Academy of Wound Management (AAWM)**
1255 23rd St., NW, No. 200
Washington, DC 20037-1174
**Phone:** (202)521-0368          **Fax:** (202)833-3636
**Email:** woundnet@aawm.org
**Website:** http://www.aawm.org
Melissa T. Forburger, Exec. Dir.
**Fnded:** 1995. **Mem:** 2,000. **Nat'l Groups:** 1. **Desc:** Medical practitioners, representing numerous professional specialties, with an interest in wound management. Seeks to advance the study and practice of wound treatment. Formulates standards of wound management practice; sponsors examinations and confers certification. Conducts continuing professional education programs. **Pub:** *AAWM Quarterly News Briefing*, quarterly. Journal. • *National Registry of Board Certified Wound Specialists*, annual. • Brochure.

★ **1873** ★ **American Association of Anatomists (AAA)**
9650 Rockville Pike
Bethesda, MD 20814
**Phone:** (301)571-8314          **Fax:** (301)571-0619
**Email:** exec@anatomy.org
**Website:** http://www.anatomy.org
John Fallon, Pres.
**Fnded:** 1888. **Mem:** 2,500. **Desc:** Professional society of anatomists and scientists in related fields. **Pub:** *Anatomical News*, quarterly. Newsletter. Includes list of employment opportunities. *Price:* Included in mem-

bership dues. • *Anatomical Record*, monthly. • *Developmental Dynamics*, monthly. • *Directory, Departments of Anatomy, U.S. and Canada*, triennial. Directory.

★ **1874** ★ **American Association for Chronic Fatigue Syndrome (AACFS)**
515 Minor Ave., Ste. 18
Seattle, WA 98104
**Phone:** (206)781-3544          **Fax:** (206)749-9052
**Email:** info@aacfs.org
**Website:** http://www.aacfs.org
Benjamin H. Natelson, MD, Pres.
**Fnded:** 1992. **Mem:** 500. **Nat'l Groups:** 1. **Desc:** Research scientists, physicians and other health care professionals, and institutions with and interest in chronic fatigue syndrome (CFS). Seeks to advance the diagnosis and treatment of CFS. Facilitates exchange of information among members; sponsors research; serves as a clearinghouse on CFS diagnosis and patient care. Maintains speakers' bureau. **Pub:** *AACF'S Newsletter*, quarterly. Newsletter. • Position papers and conference proceedings.

★ **1875** ★ **American Association of Clinical Anatomists (AACA)**
c/o R. Benton Adkins, Jr.
Vanderbilt University Medical Center
D5220 Medical Center N
1161 21st Ave. S
Nashville, TN 37232-2577
**Phone:** (731)500-6169          **Fax:** (731)500-0621
**Email:** benton.adkins@mcmail.vanderbilt.edu
**Website:** http://www.clinicalanatomy.org/
Dr. Lawrence M. Ross, Sec.
**Desc:** Dedicated to the advancement of science and art of clinical anatomy; encourages research and publication in the field and maintaining high standards in teaching of anatomy. **Pub:** *Clinical Anatomy*. Journal. Provides a medium for the exchange of current information between anatomists and clinicians.

★ **1876** ★ **American Association of Drugless Practitioners (AADP)**
708 Madalaine Dr.
Gilmer, TX 75644
**Phone:** (903)843-6401          **Free:** 888-764-AADP
**Email:** join@aadp.net
**Website:** http://www.aadp.net
Donald A. Rosenthal, PhD, Dir.
**Fnded:** 1990. **Mem:** 1,000. **Desc:** Health care professionals including physicians, chiropractors, nurses, and herbalists. Promotes drugless health care and the professional advancement of members. Serves as a clearinghouse on drugless health care; sponsors educational and training programs for health care professionals interested in drugless practice. Conducts examinations and bestows certification upon qualified drugless practitioners.

★ **1877** ★ **American Association for Health Education (AAHE)**
1900 Association Dr.
Reston, VA 20191
**Phone:** (703)476-3437          **Free:** 800-213-7193
**Fax:** (703)476-6638
**Email:** aahe@aahperd.org
**Website:** http://www.aahperd.org/aahe
Becky J. Smith, PhD, Exec. Dir.
**Fnded:** 1937. **Mem:** 7,500. **Desc:** Professionals who have responsibility for health education in schools, colleges, communities, hospitals and clinics, and industries. Purposes are advancement of health education through program activities and federal legislation; encouragement of close working relationships between all health education and health service organizations; achievement of good health and well-being for all Americans automatically, without conscious thought and endeavor. Member of the American Alliance for Health, Physical Education, Recreation and Dance. **Pub:** *Directory of Institutions Offering Undergraduate and Graduate Degree Programs in*

*Health Education*, biennial. Directory. Features appearence in the Journal of Health Education. • *HE-XTRA*, 5/year. Reports on health education programs across the nation. Includes association news and research updates. *Price:* Included in membership dues. • *Journal of Health Education*, bimonthly. Journal. • Books. • Handbooks. • Reports. • Videos. • Also publishes guides and educational packets, and produces microcomputer software. **Frmly:** (1974) School Health Division of American Association for Health, Physical Education and Recreation; (1997) Association for the Advancement of Health Education.

★ **1878** ★ **American Association for Klinefelter Syndrome Information and Support (AAKSIS)**
2945 W Farwell Ave.
Chicago, IL 60645-2925
**Phone:** (773)761-5298
**Email:** xxxyinfo@aakis.org
**Website:** http://www.aaksis.org
Roberta Rappaport, Contact
**Fnded:** 1999. **Desc:** Volunteers, those affected by the disease. Provides support, information and resources. Promotes public awareness.

★ **1879** ★ **American Association of Medical Assistants (AAMA)**
20 N Wacker Dr., Ste. 1575
Chicago, IL 60606-2963
**Phone:** (312)899-1500          **Free:** 800-228-2262
**Fax:** (312)899-1259
**Website:** http://www.aama-ntl.org
Donald A. Balasa, Exec. Dir.
**Fnded:** 1956. **Mem:** 20,000. **State Groups:** 46. **Desc:** Medical assistants are allied health professionals who work primarily in anbilatory (out patient) settings and perform clinical and administrative procedures. Activities include a certification program consisting of study and an examination, passage of which entitles the individual to become credentialed as a Certified Medical Assistant. Conducts accreditation of one- and two-year programs in medical assisting in conjunction with the commission on Accreditation of Allied Health Education Programs. Provides assistance and information to institutions of higher learning desirous of initiating courses for medical assistants. Awards continuing education units for selected educational programs. **Pub:** *Accounts Receivable and Collection for the Medical Practice. Price:* $20 for members; $30 for nonmembers. • *AIDS Concepts for Medical Assistnts – Part I. Price:* $15 for member; $25 for nonmember. • *Human Relations for the Medical Office. Price:* $30 for member; $50 for nonmember. • *Law for the Medical Office. Price:* $30 for member; $50 for nonmember. • *Managing Managed Care. Price:* $15 for member; $25 for nonmember. • *Medical Office Management – Part I. Price:* $22 for member; $32 for nonmember. • *PMA*, bimonthly. Journal. Includes association news, index of advertisers, continuing education articles, and calendar of events. *Price:* Included in membership dues; $30/year for nonmembers and students. • *Urinalysis Today. Price:* $30 for member; $50 for nonmember. • Brochures. • Pamphlets.

★ **1880** ★ **American Association of Medical Society Executives (AAMSE)**
515 N State St.
Chicago, IL 60610
**Phone:** (312)464-2555          **Fax:** (312)464-2467
**Email:** aamse@aamse.org
**Website:** http://www.aamse.org
William M. Guertin, Pres.
**Fnded:** 1947. **Mem:** 1,200. **Desc:** Professional society of executives of national, state, regional, or county medical and specialty societies. Conducts continuing education seminars. Makes available management resources and operational evaluations. **Pub:** *Hotline*, monthly. • *Who's Who in Medical Society Management*, annual. **Frmly:** Medical Society Executives Association.

★ **1881** ★ **American Association of Professional Ringside Physicians (AAPRP)**
40 Heights Rd.
Darien, CT 06820-4132
**Phone:** (914)699-2020          **Fax:** (914)699-2025
**Email:** mcs@clnn.com
**Website:** http://www.aaprp.org
Mana Camille Sclafani, Exec. Dir.
**Fnded:** 1997. **Desc:** Physicians who provide ringside services during boxing matches. Seeks to create and develop protocols and guidelines for ringside physicians; works to ensure the safety and protection of professional boxers. Facilitates communication and cooperation among members; develops standards of practice for ringside physicians; serves as a clearinghouse on the medical aspects of boxing.

★ **1882** ★ **American Association for World Health (AAWH)**
1825 K St., NW, Ste. 1208
Washington, DC 20006
**Phone:** (202)466-5883          **Fax:** (202)466-5896
**Email:** staff@aawnworldhealth.org
**Website:** http://www.aawhworldhealth.org
Richard L. Wittenberg, Pres. & CEO
**Fnded:** 1953. **Mem:** 1,200. **Desc:** Individuals and organizations interested in strengthening U.S. commitment to world health. To inform Americans about world health issues and to strengthen public support for activities and programs that improve health conditions worldwide. Supports programs of the World Health Organization, Pan American Health Organization, and other agencies. Sponsors: World Health Day in U.S.; World AIDS Day, and World No-Tobacco Day. **Pub:** *AAWH Quarterly*, quarterly. Newsletter. Covering international health policy issues; includes news of the AAWH and WHO. *Price:* Included in membership dues. • *Tobacco Alert*, annual. Newsletter. *Price:* Free. • *World AIDS Day Action Kit*, annual. Booklet. *Price:* First copy free. • *World Health Day Planning Kit*, annual. Booklet. *Price:* First copy free. **AKA:** U.S. Committee for the World Health Organization. **Frmly:** (1966) National Citizens Committee for the World Health Organization.

★ **1883** ★ **American Board of Family Practice (ABFP)**
2228 Young Dr.
Lexington, KY 40505-4294
**Phone:** (859)269-5626          **Free:** 888-995-5700
**Fax:** (859)335-7501
**Email:** general@abfp.org
**Website:** http://www.abfp.org
Robert F. Avant, MD, Exec. Dir.
**Fnded:** 1969. **Desc:** Certifying board for physicians specializing in family practice. Conducts certification/recertification examinations. **Pub:** *Journal of the American Board of Family Practice*, bimonthly. Journal. *Price:* $60 institution; $35 physician.

★ **1884** ★ **American Board of Health Physics (ABHP)**
1313 Dolley Madison Blvd., Ste. 402
Mc Lean, VA 22101-3926
**Phone:** (703)790-1745          **Fax:** (703)790-2672
**Email:** aahp@burkinc.com
**Website:** http://www.aahp-abhp.org
Richard J. Burk, Jr., Exec. Sec.
**Fnded:** 1960. **Mem:** 8. **Desc:** Certifying body. Promotes the health physics profession by establishing standards and procedures for certification and conducting certification examinations. Issues written proof of certification.

★ **1885** ★ **American Board of Internal Medicine (ABIM)**
501 Walnut St., Ste. 1700
Philadelphia, PA 19106-3699
**Phone:** (215)446-3500          **Free:** 800-441-2246
**Fax:** (215)446-3470
**Email:** request@abim.org
**Website:** http://www.abim.org
Harry R. Kimball, Pres.
**Fnded:** 1936. **Mem:** 25. **Desc:** Certification board established to determine the qualifications of, administer examinations to, and certify as specialists in internal medicine those doctors meeting its standards of clinical competence. Board members are elected from certified leaders in internal medicine. The board has certified approximately 150,000 internists and 65,000 subspecialist diplomates and issued 15,000 recertification certificates. **Pub:** *Policies and Procedures*, annual.

★ **1886** ★ **American Board of Medical Specialties (ABMS)**
1007 Church St., Ste. 404
Evanston, IL 60201-5913
**Phone:** (847)491-9091          **Fax:** (847)328-3596
**Email:** info@abms.org
**Website:** http://www.abms.org
Stephen H. Miller, M.D., M.P.H., Exec. VP
**Fnded:** 1933. **Mem:** 30. **Desc:** Primary medical specialty boards and conjoint boards; organizations with related interests are associate members. Acts as spokesman for approved medical specialty boards as a group; is actively concerned with the establishment, maintenance, and elevation of standards for the education and qualification of physicians recognized as specialists through the certification procedures of its members; cooperates with other groups concerned in establishing standards, policies, and procedures for ensuring the maintenance of continued competence of such physicians. Compiles statistics. **Pub:** *ABMS Directory of Board Certified Medical Specialists*, annual. Directory. Four volumes listing over 500,000 specialists certified by 24 U.S. medical specialty boards. Arranged by specialty, name, and location. *Price:* $485/copy. • *ABMS Record*, quarterly. Newsletter. Reports on legislative-judicial events related to medical education. Includes meeting reports. *Price:* Free. • *American Board of Medical Specialties–Annual Report and Reference Handbook*, annual. Guide to medical specialty boards and specialty certification. *Price:* $10. • Also publishes text publications on evaluating physicians.

★ **1887** ★ **American Board of Quality Assurance and Utilization Review Physicians (ABQAURP)**
2120 Range Rd.
Clearwater, FL 33765-2125
**Phone:** (727)298-8777          **Free:** 800-998-6030
**Fax:** (727)449-0555
**Email:** abqaurp@abqaurp.org
**Website:** http://www.abqaurp.org
Arthur I. Border, MD, Chair
**Fnded:** 1977. **Mem:** 6,351. **Desc:** Seeks to maintain and improve the process of health care and management through development, administration, and supervision of a certification program in the field. Provides evaluation services in connection with certification examinations for physicians and coordinators and makes available study material. **Pub:** *Diplomat Focus*, quarterly. Newsletter. Contains information on ABQAURP and issues important to diplomats. *Price:* Free with diplomat status. • Books.

★ **1888** ★ **American Bureau for Medical Advancement in China (ABMAC)**
45 John St. No.1100
New York, NY 10038
**Phone:** (212)233-0608          **Fax:** (212)233-0614
**Email:** phyllis@abmac.org
**Website:** http://www.abmac.org
Phyllis Scarnozzino, Exec. Dir.
**Fnded:** 1937. **Mem:** 52. **Desc:** Cooperates with medical and health personnel to support a broad program of medical and health services for the Chinese people. Provides, upon request from Republic of China institutions, consultants for development projects and visiting specialists for longer term teaching and clinical assignments in Taiwan. Sponsors Republic of China postgraduate fellowships for study,

research, and observation in the U.S. Organizes research projects for treatment of diseases prevalent in Southeast Asia. Offers placement services for Chinese doctors and nurses interested in postgraduate study in the U.S.

### ★ 1889 ★ American Clinical and Climatological Association (ACCA)

Univ. of Cincinnati Medical Center
231 Albert Sabin Way
PO Box G70557
Cincinnati, OH 45267-0557
**Phone:** (513)558-4231     **Fax:** (513)558-0852
Dr. Robert Luke, Sec/Treas.

**Fnded:** 1884. **Mem:** 375. **Desc:** Internists interested in the clinical study of disease. **Pub:** *Transactions*, annual.

### ★ 1890 ★ American College Health Association (ACHA)

PO Box 28937
Baltimore, MD 21240-8937
**Phone:** (410)859-1500     **Fax:** (410)859-1510
**Email:** pcrone@sacha.org
**Website:** http://www.acha.org
Col. Doyle E. Randol, MS, Exec. Dir.

**Fnded:** 1920. **Mem:** 3,438. **Local Groups:** 11. **Desc:** Institutions (930) and individuals (2500). Provides an organization in which institutions of higher education and interested individuals may work together to promote health in its broadest aspects for students and all other members of the college community. Offers continuing education programs for health professionals. Maintains placement listings for physicians and other personnel seeking positions in college health. Compiles statistics. Conducts seminars and training programs. **Pub:** *ACHA Action*, quarterly. Newsletter. Includes calendar of events, college health resource listings, annual report, and leadership directory. • *Health Information Series*. Pamphlets. • *Journal of American College Health*, bimonthly. Journal. • *Membership Profile Directory*, periodic. Directory. • Catalog.Lists publications. • Monographs. • Reports. • Also publishes guidelines. **Frmly:** American Student Health Association.

### ★ 1891 ★ American College of Home Health Administrators (ACHHA)

c/o Thomas R. O'Donovan
701 Lee St., No. 600
Des Plaines, IL 60016-4516
Renee S. Schleisher, Pres.

**Fnded:** 1957. **Mem:** 3,500. **Reg. Groups:** 7. **Desc:** Home health administrators, executives, and managers at all levels. Promotes professional indentification within the home health care field and seeks to facilitate the career and professional development of members. Represents the interests of the home health care industry within the medical community and before government agencies and the public; makes available to members discounts on educational programs conducted by the ACHHA or the American Academy of Medical Administrators; offers professional referral services; holds examinations and confers professional certification. **Pub:** *Executive*, monthly. Newsletter.

### ★ 1892 ★ American College of International Physicians (ACIP)

c/o Sally Askew, Exec.Dir.
307 S Lowe Ave., Ste. A-309
Cookeville, TN 38501
**Phone:** (931)526-8675     **Fax:** (931)525-6769
**Email:** acip@citlink.net
**Website:** http://www.acip.org
Sally Askew, Exec. Dir.

**Fnded:** 1975. **Mem:** 1,200. **State Groups:** 8. **Desc:** Physicians and surgeons interested in initiatives to promote national efforts in international health, education, research, training, and welfare. Promotes the betterment of the health of all peoples and seeks to advance the art and science of medicine. Emphasizes the international character of medicine and the educa-

tion of international physicians. Seeks parity for foreign medical graduates. Supports relief programs to areas struck by natural calamities or epidemic diseases. **Pub:** *International Medical Journal*, semiannual. Newsletter. • *The International Physician*, quarterly. Newsletter.

### ★ 1893 ★ American College of Medical Quality (ACMQ)

4334 Montgomery Ave.
Bethesda, MD 20814
**Phone:** (301)913-9149     **Free:** 800-924-2149
**Fax:** (301)913-9142
**Email:** ACMQ@acmq.org
**Website:** http://www.acmq.org
Bridget Brodie, Exec. VP

**Fnded:** 1973. **Mem:** 1,000. **Reg. Groups:** 4. **Desc:** Physicians, affiliates, and institutions. Seeks to set standards of competence in the field of quality assurance and utilization review. Conducts educational seminars and workshops in quality assurance and utilization review. Offers placement services. Maintains speakers' bureau. **Pub:** *American College of Medical Quality Newsletter - Focus*, bimonthly. Newsletter. Includes topical articles and college and chapter news. *Price:* Included in membership dues. • *American Journal of Medical Quality*, bimonthly. Journal. Covers topics concerning evaluation of quality in health care, DRGs, Medicare and Medicaid, risk management, and other areas of interest. *Price:* Included in membership dues; $151/year for nonmembers. **Frmly:** (1988) ACURP.

### ★ 1894 ★ American College of Medicine (ACM)

4711 Golf Rd., Ste. 408
Skokie, IL 60076
**Phone:** (847)568-1500     **Free:** 800-621-4002
**Fax:** (847)568-1527
**Email:** iaos@aol.com
Randall T. Bellows, MD, Dir.

**Fnded:** 1981. **Desc:** Promotes and recognizes the specific needs of general practitioners and provides continuing medical education programs to physicians for maintaining competence in the practice of medicine. **Pub:** *Comprehensive Therapy*, monthly. **Frmly:** (1984) American College of General Practice.

### ★ 1895 ★ American College of Physicians (ACP)

190 N Independence Mall West
Philadelphia, PA 19106-1572
**Phone:** (215)351-2600     **Free:** 800-523-1546
**Fax:** (215)351-2448
**Email:** neilk@mail.acponline.org
**Website:** http://www.acponline.org
Sara E. Walker, MD, Pres.

**Fnded:** 1915. **Mem:** 85,000. **Desc:** Professional society of medical doctors specializing in internal medicine and closely related specialties such as dermatology, neurology, psychiatry, cardiology, gastroenterology, and public health. Sponsors annual postgraduate courses for practicing physicians. Sponsors teaching and research scholarship competition. **Pub:** *ACP Journal Club*, bimonthly. • *Annals of Internal Medicine*, biweekly. Journal. *Price:* $131/year. • *Medical Knowledge Self-Assessment*, triennial. • *Observer*, monthly. • Directory, periodic.

### ★ 1896 ★ American Correctional Health Services Association (ACHSA)

6 Royale Dr.
Lake Saint Louis, MO 63367
**Phone:** (636)561-8857     **Free:** 800-918-1842
**Fax:** (636)625-6356
**Email:** achsa@mindspring.com
**Website:** http://www.corrections.com/achsa
Sandy Collier, Exec. Dir.

**Fnded:** 1975. **Mem:** 1,100. **State Groups:** 8. **Desc:** Health care providers, individuals, or organizations interested in improving the quality of correctional health services. Aims are: to promote the provision of

health services to incarcerated persons consistent in quality and quantity with acceptable health care practices; to promote and encourage continuing education and provide technical and professional guidance for correctional health care personnel; to establish a forum for the sharing and discussion of correctional health care issues. Conducts conferences on correctional health care management, nursing, mental health, juvenile corrections, dentistry, and related subjects. Maintains placement service. **Pub:** *CORHEALTH*, bimonthly. Newsletter. Includes book reviews, conference calendar, list of new members, and chapter news. *Price:* Included in membership dues. • Brochures.Provides information on policy matters.

### ★ 1897 ★ American Council for Health Care Reform (ACHCR)

3554 Chain Bridge Rd., Ste. 101
Fairfax, VA 22030-2709
**Phone:** (703)908-9220     **Free:** 800-240-6423
**Fax:** (703)908-9467
William Shaker, Pres.

**Fnded:** 1982. **Mem:** 500,000. **Desc:** Organized to eliminate what the council terms unnecessary and costly federal and state health care regulations and laws, such as certificate of public need restrictions that limit public choice in the selection of health care providers. Supports health care reform, based on Consumer choice. Testifies before congressional and state legislative committees. Coordinates grass roots support for free market approaches to health care delivery and health, safety, and consumer-oriented projects. Works to achieve public access to medical practice information. Supports medical savings accounts.

### ★ 1898 ★ American Electrology Association (AEA)

106 Oakridge Rd.
Trumbull, CT 06611
**Phone:** (203)374-6667     **Free:** 877-746-9723
**Fax:** (203)372-7134
**Email:** info@electrology.com
**Website:** http://www.electrology.com
Teresa E. Petricca, Exec. Dir.

**Fnded:** 1958. **Mem:** 2,000. **Nat'l Groups:** 2. **State Groups:** 27. **Desc:** Electrologists united for education, professional advancement, protection of public welfare. Promotes uniform legislative standards throughout the states. Coordinates efforts of affiliated associations in dealing with problems of national scope. Sponsors the International Board of Electrologist Certification and Council on Accreditation of Electrology Schools/Programs. Maintains referral, reference, advisory, and consulting services. **Pub:** *American Electrology Association–Roster*, annual. Membership Directory. Arranged geographically. Includes modalities used. *Price:* Included in membership dues. • *Direct Line*, periodic. Bulletin. Provides communication between AEA executives and board members. Includes meeting minutes, committee reports, and program status reports. *Price:* Available to board members and committee chairs. • *Electrolysis World*, quarterly. Newsletter. Includes calendar of events. *Price:* available to members only. • *Infection Control Standards for the Practice of Electrology*. • *Journal of the American Electrology Association*, semiannual. Journal. Includes case studies. *Price:* $10/issue. • *Medical/Professional News*, semiannual. • Brochures. **Frmly:** (1986) American Electrolysis Association.

### ★ 1899 ★ American Federation of Home Health Agencies (AFHHA)

1320 Fenwick Ln., Ste. 100
Silver Spring, MD 20910
**Fax:** (301)588-4732
**Email:** afhha@his.com
Betty Leake, Pres.

**Fnded:** 1980. **Mem:** 325. **Desc:** Agencies providing therapeutic services such as nursing, speech therapy, and physical therapy in the home; associate members are corporations and individuals that support the federation. Promotes home health by influencing public policy. Presents the concerns of home health agencies to Congress and the Health Care Financing Administration; helps members work with their fiscal intermediary. Pub: *Insider*, semimonthly. Newsletter. *Price:* Included in membership dues.

★ **1900** ★ **American Foundation for Health (AFH)**
2107 Dwight Way
Berkeley, CA 94704
**Phone:** (510)644-3366
Leonard Stryker, Exec. Dir.

**Fnded:** 1979. **Mem:** 17,,000. **Desc:** Individuals interested in improving the delivery of health care services. Encourages recording of personal medical data. Conducts educational research projects and activities. Pub: *Health Features*, periodic. Newsletter.

★ **1901** ★ **American Foundation of Traditional Chinese Medicine (AFTCM)**
PO Box 330267
San Francisco, CA 94133
**Phone:** (415)392-7002    **Fax:** (415)392-7003
**Email:** aftcm@earthlink.net
Barbara Bernie, CEO

**Fnded:** 1982. **Desc:** Works to promote global human health through creating services and healing enviroments that demonstrate practices and teachings of the world's systems of health and healing. Also provides consultation to hospitals and clinics expending their services to include traditional Chinese herbal medicine, acupuncture, and other health care practices including teaching Qi Gong to Elementary school childern. incorporating traditional Chinese, Western, and other medicines at this center, patients will have available a wide variety of diagnosis and treatment options which will result in reducing the cost of healthcare. **Pub:** *Chinese Medicine*.

★ **1902** ★ **American Health Assistance Foundation (AHAF)**
15825 Shady Grove Rd., Ste. 140
Rockville, MD 20850
**Phone:** (301)948-3244    **Free:** 800-437-2423
**Fax:** (301)258-9454
**Email:** aphillips@ahaf.org
**Website:** http://www.ahaf.org
Angelia Ragsdale, Head Receptionist

**Fnded:** 1973. **Desc:** Established to support medical research. Four programs within the foundation are Alzheimer's Family Relief Program, Coronary Heart Disease Research, National Glaucoma Research, and Alzheimer's Disease Research. **Pub:** *Alzheimer's Research Review*, quarterly. Newsletter. Updates the work of Alzheimer's disease researchers. Provides tips for families with members who have the disease.

★ **1903** ★ **American Health Quality Association (AHQA)**
1140 Conneticut Ave. NW, Ste. 1050
Washington, DC 20036
**Phone:** (202)331-5790    **Fax:** (202)331-9334
**Email:** info@ahqa.org
**Website:** http://www.ahqa.org
Amanda D. Scott, Admin. Asst.

**Fnded:** 1973. **Mem:** 1,400. **State Groups:** 53. **Local Groups:** 11. **Desc:** Institutions and individuals. Purpose is to develop communications programs for physicians, institutions, and others interested in peer review organizations (PROs). Provides a national forum for the interchange of ideas, techniques, and information relating to medical quality assessment. Conducts courses and on-site educational programs to increase physicians' involvement and leadership in PROs, improve practice patterns through review, understand and use PRO data to improve service delivery, pre-admission review, profile analysis, retrospective review, and organizational development. Sponsors placement service; maintains a speakers' bureau and a library. **Pub:** *AHQA Bulletin*, periodic. Bulletin. Covers medical regulatory and legislative developments. *Price:* Included in membership dues. •

*Legislative Monitor*, periodic. *Price:* Free, available to members only. • *Physician Advisor Manual*. • *Quality Advocate*, quarterly. Newsletter. Includes Policy Outlook, Innovation, Washington Update, Legislative Update, Calendar of Events columns and job announcements. *Price:* Included in membership dues; $75/year for nonmembers. • *Resource Document and Private Review Manual*. • *Tapes of Conference Programs*. • Membership Directory, annual. **Frmly:** (1982) American Association of Professional Standards Review Organizations; (1997) American Medical Peer Review Association.

★ **1904** ★ **American Hernia Society (AHS)**
PO Box 536544
Orlando, FL 32853-6544
**Phone:** (407)898-1695    **Fax:** (407)894-2312
**Email:** wilkesmgmt@aol.com
**Website:** http://www.americanherniasociety.org
Shelburn M. Wilkes, Exec. Dir.

**Fnded:** 1997. **Mem:** 400. **Desc:** Surgeons interested in the mangement of hernias. Seeks to advance the diagnosis and treatment of hernias; promotes continuing professional development of members. Serves as a forum for the exchange of information among members; gathers and disseminates information on emerging methods of hernia surgery and management. **Pub:** *Hernia*, quarterly. Journal. *Price:* $35.

★ **1905** ★ **American International Health Alliance (AIHA)**
1212 New York Ave. NW, Ste. 750
Washington, DC 20005
**Phone:** (202)789-1136    **Fax:** (202)789-1277
**Email:** aiha@aiha.com
**Website:** http://www.aiha.com
James Smith, Exec. Dir.

**Fnded:** 1992. **Desc:** Institutional health care providers. Promotes increased availability of health care services in previously underserved areas worldwide. Creates partnerships between hospitals in the United States and their counterparts abroad to facilitate sharing of technology and expertise; sponsors educational programs; serves as a clearinghouse on international health issues and emerging medical technologies and practices. **Pub:** *Commonhealth*, monthly. Newsletter. Focuses on topics of concern to healthcare providers/practitioners in the countries of the former Soviet Union and Central and Eastern Europe. *Price:* Free.

★ **1906** ★ **American Lebanese Medical Association (ALMA)**
3654 E Imperial Hwy.
Lynwood, CA 90262
**Phone:** (619)937-3071    **Fax:** (619)937-3081
**Email:** eayoub@hotmail.com
**Website:**    http://www.ALMAmater.org/ALMA/Default.html
Joe F. Jabre, MD, Contact

**Fnded:** 1994. **Desc:** Health care professionals with Lebanese heritage, or with and interest in providing assistance to the people of Lebanon. Promotes increased access to improved health care for all religious and cultural communities in Lebanon. Fosters development of medical education institutions and health care facilities in Lebanon. Gathers and distributes Lebanese medical and scientific publications; conducts continuing professional education programs for members. Plans to operate library in conjunction with the Lebanese Medical Association.

★ **1907** ★ **American Lyme Disease Foundation (ALDF)**
Mill Pond Offices
293 Rte. 100
Somers, NY 10589
**Phone:** (914)277-6970    **Free:** 800-876-LYME
**Fax:** (914)277-6974
**Email:** inquire@aldf.com
**Website:** http://www.aldf.com
David L. Weld, Contact

**Fnded:** 1990. **Nat'l Groups:** 1. **Desc:** Health care professionals and other individuals with an interest in Lyme Disease, a disorder transmitted to humans by the deer tick. Works to control the spread of Lyme Disease, and to improve treatments for the disorder. Maintains physician referral service; produces educational materials and conducts public and professional education programs; supports Lyme Disease research. **Pub:** Newsletter, periodic. *Price:* Included in membership dues. • Video.Educational videos for use in schools, libraries, and camps.

★ **1908** ★ **American Medical Association (AMA)**
515 N State St.
Chicago, IL 60610
**Phone:** (312)464-5000    **Free:** 800-AMA-3211
**Fax:** (312)464-4184
**Website:** http://www.ama-assn.org/

**Fnded:** 1847. **Mem:** 297,,000. **State Groups:** 54. **Desc:** County medical societies and physicians. Disseminates scientific information to members and the public. Informs members on significant medical and health legislation on state and national levels and represents the profession before Congress and governmental agencies. Cooperates in setting standards for medical schools, hospitals, residency programs, and continuing medical education courses. Offers physician placement service and counseling on practice management problems. Operates library which lends material and provides specific medical information to physicians. Ad-hoc committees are formed for such topics as health care planning and principles of medical ethics. **Pub:** *American Medical News*, weekly. Newspaper. Covers news and opinions on key issues of political, social, and economic significance concerning the practice and delivery of medical care. *Price:* Included in membership dues; $99/year for nonmembers; $49.50/year for medical students, interns, and residents. • *Archives of Dermatology*, monthly. Journal. Oriented to the dermatologic clinician. Includes book reviews, employment opportunity listings, annual index, and index of advertisers. *Price:* $67.50/year for members; $135/year for nonmembers; $67.50/year for residents and medical students. • *Archives of Family Medicine*, monthly. Oriented to physicians in family and general practice. *Price:* $47.50 for members; $95 for nonmembers. • *Archives of General Psychiatry*, monthly. Journal. Oriented toward the psychiatric clinician. Includes employment opportunity listings, book reviews, annual index, and index of advertisers. *Price:* $47.50/year for members; $95/year for nonmembers; $47.50/year for residents and medical students. • *Archives of Internal Medicine*, semimonthly. Journal. Oriented toward physicians in internal medicine. Includes employment opportunity listings, annual index, and index of advertisers. *Price:* $57.50/year for members; $115/year for nonmembers; $57.50/year for residents and medical students. • *Archives of Neurology*, monthly. Journal. Oriented toward the neurologic clinician. Includes employment opportunity listings, annual index, and index of advertisers. *Price:* $72.50/ year for members; $145/year for nonmembers; $72.50/year for residents and medical students. • *Archives of Ophthalmology*, monthly. Journal. Includes employment opportunity listings, case reports, book reviews, annual index, and index of advertisers. *Price:* $55/year for members; $110/year for nonmembers; $55/year for residents and medical students. • *Archives of Otolaryngology–Head and Neck Surgery*, monthly. Journal. Ori.

★ **1909** ★ **American Medical Association Alliance (AMAA)**
515 N State St.
Chicago, IL 60610-0174
**Phone:** (312)464-5000    **Fax:** (312)464-5020
**Website:** http://www.ama-assn.org
Hazel J. Lewis, Exec. Dir.

**Fnded:** 1922. **Mem:** 70,000. **Nat'l Groups:** 100. **State Groups:** 46. **Local Groups:** 815. **Desc:** Physicians' spouses. Serves as the volunteer arm of the American Medical Association. Promotes the goals of the medical profession and works to meet public health needs.

Raises more than $2 million annually for the American Medical Association Education and Research Foundation (see separate entry), which provides assistance to medical schools and students. Sponsors the Shape Up for Life Campaign, a nationwide auxiliary program to promote good health. Maintains Project Bank, an information clearinghouse of community projects initiated by auxiliaries across the country. Implements community health projects on such concerns as child abuse prevention, adolescent health, family violence, AIDS education, seatbelt usage, pre- and postnatal care, drug abuse, suicide prevention, proper nutrition, drunk driving prevention, venereal disease awareness, and services to the aging. Works with the AMA to promote sound health legislation; conducts public education programs, letter-writing campaigns, and personal interviews with legislators involved in health matters. **Pub:** *Facets Magazine*, bimonthly. Magazine. Includes information on community health projects, public health issues, socioeconomic health care issues, and physician family concerns. *Price:* Included in membership dues; $7/year for nonmembers. • *Horizons Newsletter*, bimonthly. Newsletter. Covers topics of concern to the families of resident physicians and medical students. *Price:* Free to resident physicians and medical students. • *Newsline*, bimonthly. Includes information on health periodicals and health projects. *Price:* Included in membership dues. **Frmly:** (1975) Women's Auxilliary to the American Medical Association; (1993) American Medical Association Auxilliary.

★ **1910** ★ **American Medical Association Foundation**
515 N State St.
Chicago, IL 60610
**Phone:** (312)464-4543          **Fax:** (312)464-5973
**Email:** amafoundation@ama-assn.org
**Website:** http://www.ama-assn.org/ama/pub/category/3119.html
Kathleen MacArthur, Exec. Dir.

**Fnded:** 1962. **Desc:** Foundation managed by Directors of the American Medical Association . Receives and distributes funds to benefit medical education in U.S. medical schools and to support education, research and service progams within the community of medicine. Foundation funds consist of contributions from physicians, medical societies and auxiliaries, of other foundations, private industry, and the public. Accepts bequests and other gifts for allocation to various projects in medicine. **Frmly:** (1999) American Medical Association Education and Research Foundation.

★ **1911** ★ **American Medical Electroencephalographic Association (AMEEGA)**
PO Box 757
Pewaukee, WI 53072-0757
**Phone:** (414)797-7800          **Fax:** (414)782-8788
**Email:** medassn@aol.com
Michael J. Herzog, Contact

**Fnded:** 1964. **Mem:** 700. **Desc:** Works to advance clinical electroencephalography and to promote the development of clinical and technical training programs. **Pub:** *Clinical EEG*, quarterly.

★ **1912** ★ **American Medical Group Association (AMGA)**
1422 Duke St.
Alexandria, VA 22314-3430
**Phone:** (703)838-0033          **Fax:** (703)548-1890
**Email:** roconnor@amga.org
**Website:** http://www.amga.org
Dr. Donald W. Fisher, CAE, Pres. /CEO

**Fnded:** 1949. **Mem:** 300. **Desc:** Trade association for group practice integrate a delivery systems and IPAS representing more than 45,000 physicians. Provides public policy advocacy, compiles statistics on group practice, sponsors research, patient education, insurance programs. **Pub:** *Group Practice Journal*, 10/year. Journal. Covers market trends, health care policy and legislation, and management topics affecting the medical profession. Includes advertiser index. *Price:* Includ-

ed in membership dues; $75/year for nonmembers. **Frmly:** American Group Practice Association; (1974) American Association of Medical Clinics.

★ **1913** ★ **American Medical Student Association (AMSA)**
1902 Association Dr.
Reston, VA 20191
**Phone:** (703)620-6600          **Free:** 800-767-2266
**Fax:** (703)620-5873
**Email:** amsa@www.amsa.org
**Website:** http://www.amsa.org
Jaya Agrawal, Pres.

**Fnded:** 1950. **Mem:** 30,000. **Local Groups:** 140. **Desc:** Medical students; local, state, and national organizations; premedical students, interns, and residents. Seeks to improve medical education by making it relevant to today's needs and by making the process by which physicians are trained more humanistic. Contributes to the improvement of health care of all people; involves its members in the social, moral, and ethical obligations of the profession of medicine. Serves as a mechanism through which students may actively participate in the fields of community health through various student health programs. Addresses political issues relating to the nation's health care delivery system and other medical and health issues. Maintains standing committees and interest groups which publish newsletters, organize educational workshops, and initiate special projects. **Pub:** *The New Physician*, 9/year. Magazine. *Price:* $25/year. **Frmly:** (1975) Student American Medical Association.

★ **1914** ★ **American Medical Women's Association (AMWA)**
801 N Fairfax St., Ste. 400
Alexandria, VA 22314
**Phone:** (703)838-0500          **Fax:** (703)549-3864
**Email:** info@amwa-doc.org
**Website:** http://www.amwa-doc.org
Omega C. Logan Silva, MD, Pres.

**Fnded:** 1915. **Mem:** 10,000. **Reg. Groups:** 10. **Local Groups:** 160. **Desc:** Women holding a M.D. or D.O. degree from approved medical colleges; women interns, residents, and medical students. Promotes women's health issues in medical education and public policy. Seeks to find solutions to problems common to women studying or practicing medicine, such as career advancement and the integration of professional and family responsibilities. Provides student members with educational loans and personal counseling. Sponsors continuing medical education programs. **Pub:** *What's Happening in AMWA*, semiannual. Newsletter. *Price:* Included in membership dues. • Journal, bimonthly. • Newsletter, quarterly.

★ **1915** ★ **American Obesity Association (AOA)**
1250 24th St., NW
No. 300
Washington, DC 20037
**Phone:** (202)776-7711          **Free:** 800-986-2373
**Fax:** (202)776-7712
**Email:** executive@obesity.org
**Website:** http://www.obesity.org
Morgan Downey, Exec. Dir.

**Fnded:** 1995. **Mem:** 450. **Desc:** Health professionals. Supports research and education about obesity including the discrimination against the obese. Actively seeks government funding and is an advocate for insurance coverage for the obese. **Pub:** *AOA Report*, quarterly. Newsletter.

★ **1916** ★ **American Osler Society (AOS)**
c/o Charles S. Bryan
University of South Carolina School of Medicine
2 Medical Park, Ste. 502
Columbia, SC 29203
**Phone:** (803)540-1000          **Fax:** (803)540-1075
**Email:** trout@abanet.org
**Website:** http://www.americanosler.org/
Charles S. Bryan, Sec. -Treas.

**Fnded:** 1970. **Mem:** 135. **Desc:** Physicians, librarians, and scientists united to further a humanistic approach to the study and practice of medicine as exemplified in the life work of Sir William Osler (1849-1919). **Pub:** *Osler Biographical Directory*, annual. Directory. • *The Persisting Osler*. Book. • *The Persisting Osler II*. Book. • Also publishes books on Sir William Osler, medical humanism, and the history of medicine.

★ **1917** ★ **American Pain Foundation**
111 S Calvert St., Ste. 2700
Baltimore, MD 21202
**Website:** http://www.painfoundation.org
James N. Campbell, MD, Chm.

**Fnded:** 1998. **Desc:** Foundations, individuals and pharmaceutical companies. Aims to improve the quality of life with pain. Publishes and distributes practical information, sponsors initiatives to reduce regulatory and other barriers to effective pain management.

★ **1918** ★ **American Physicians Association of Computer Medicine (APACM)**
19 Crossover Rd.
Fairport, NY 14450-1209
**Phone:** (716)586-8147          **Fax:** (716)586-8147
Lawrence B. Tilis, MD, Pres.

**Fnded:** 1984. **Mem:** 350. **Desc:** Physicians, interns, and medical students. Encourages the use of computers in medicine. Seeks to inform physicians about the computer and its applications in patient care, education, and research. Conducts lectures.

★ **1919** ★ **American Professional Practice Association (APPA)**
Hillsboro Executive Center N
350 Fairway Dr., Ste. 200
Deerfield Beach, FL 33441-1834
**Phone:** (954)571-1877          **Free:** 800-221-2168
**Fax:** (954)571-8582
**Email:** membership@assnservices.com
**Website:** http://www.appa-assn.com
Joseph P. Santol, Jr., Mgr., Membership Services

**Fnded:** 1963. **Mem:** 70,000. **Desc:** Provides physicians with economic benefits and financial services including the following: unsecured loan plans; group insurance discounts; accounts receivable collections; electronic credit services; continuing medical education. **Pub:** *Association's Digest*, semiannual. Newsletter. Provides business advice on private practice; also covers APPA activities. *Price:* Included in membership dues.

★ **1920** ★ **American Registry of Medical Assistants (ARMA)**
69 Southwick Rd.
Westfield, MA 01085-4729
**Phone:** (413)562-7336          **Free:** 800-527-2762
**Fax:** (413)562-9021
Annette H. Heyman, Dir.

**Fnded:** 1950. **Mem:** 10,000. **Desc:** Medical assistants who have completed an accredited medical assistant training course or who have trained with a physician for a minimum of three years. Objectives are to: establish and maintain high training standards for medical assistants; promote greater efficiency within the profession; raise awareness of medical assistants within the medical community. **Pub:** *The Medical Assistant*, annual. Journal. Information of interest to the medical community. • *Registry Connection*, quarterly. • *200 Ways to Put Your Talent To Work in the Health Field*. Pamphlet. *Price:* Free. • Brochures.*Price:* Included in application fee and annual fee of; Members.

★ **1921** ★ **American Rheumatism Association**
1314 Spring St. NW
Atlanta, GA 30309
**Phone:** (404)872-7100
Lynn Bonifiglio, Exec. Sec.

**Desc:** Health care professionals with an interest in rheumatism and related disorders; people with rheumatic diseases and their families. Seeks to improve the quality of life of people with rheumatism and related disorders; promotes improved diagnosis and treatment of rhuematic diseases. Serves as a clearinghouse on rheumatism and related disorders; provides support and assistance to people with rheumatic diseases and their families.

### ★ 1922 ★ American School Health Association (ASHA)

PO Box 708
7263 State Route 43
Kent, OH 44240
**Phone:** (330)678-1601     **Free:** 800-445-2742
**Fax:** (330)678-4526
**Email:** asha@ashaweb.org
**Website:** http://www.ashaweb.org
Cynthia Symons, Pres.

**Fnded:** 1927. **Mem:** 2,500. **State Groups:** 16. **Desc:** School physicians, school nurses, dentist, nurses, nutritionists, health educators, dental hygienst, school-based professionals and public health workers. Promotes coordinated school health programs that include health education, health services, a healthful school environment, physical education, nutrition services, and psycho-social health services offered in schools collaboratively with families and other members of the community. Offers professional reference materials. Conducts pilot programs that inform materials developement, provides technical assistance to school professionals, advocates for school health, and complies statistics. **Pub:** *Building Effective Coalitions to Prevent the Spread of HIV.* Book. • *Guide to Developing and Evaluating Medicine Education Programs. Price:* $7 for members; $10 for nonmembers. • *Guidelines for Comprehensive School Heath Programs.* Book. • *Guidelines for Protecting Confidential Student Health Information,* periodic. Journal. *Price:* $13 for members; $19 for nonmembers. • *Health Counseling.* Book. • *Healthy Students 2000: An Agenda for Continuous Improvement in America's Schools.* Book. • *Journal of School Health,* 10/year. Journal. Includes articles, research papers, reports, commentaries, teaching techniques, and health service application. *Price:* $85/year; $95/year for institutions; $110/year outside U.S.; $8.50/copy for members. • *The PULSE,* quarterly. *Price:* Included in membership. • *The Role of the Nurse in the School Setting: A Historical Perspective.* Book. • *School-Based HIV Prevention: A Multidisciplinary Approach.* Book. • *School Health in America.* Survey. • *Science and Health Experiments and Demonstrations in Smoking Education.* Book. • *Sexuality Education Within Comprehensive School Health Education.* Book. • *Standards of School Nursing Practice.* Book. • *Teaching Human Sexuality.* Book. • *Thinking Ahead: Preparing for Controversy.* Book. • *Topical Index of Articles From the Journal,* annual. Journal. **Frmly:** (1936) American Association of School Physicians.

### ★ 1923 ★ American Society of Bariatric Physicians (ASBP)

5453 E Evans Pl.
Denver, CO 80222-5234
**Phone:** (303)770-2526     **Fax:** (303)779-4834
**Email:** info@asbp.org
**Website:** http://www.asbp.org
Beth A. Little, CAE, Interim Exec. Dir.

**Fnded:** 1950. **Mem:** 1,000. **State Groups:** 2. **Desc:** Physicians with a special interest in the study and treatment of obesity and associated conditions. Encourages excellence in the practice of bariatric medicine through exchange of information, research, and continuing education. Sponsors regional courses and clinical research programs. Offers a physician referral service. **Pub:** *The Bariatrician,* quarterly. Journal. Includes articles on health, fitness, nutrition, and current treatments for obesity. *Price:* $48/year in U.S.; $72/year outside U.S. • *Membership Directory,* annual. Membership Directory. • *News from ASBP,* bimonthly. Newsletter. *Price:* available to members only.

• Manuals. • Pamphlets. **Frmly:** (1972) The Obesity Foundation.

### ★ 1924 ★ American Society Bioethics and Humanities

4700 W Lake Ave.
Glenview, IL 60025-1485
**Phone:** (847)375-4745     **Free:** 877-734-9385
**Fax:** 877-734-9385
**Email:** info@asbh.org
**Website:** http://www.asbh.org
Richard G. Muir, Exec. Dir.

**Fnded:** 1998. **Mem:** 1,500. **Desc:** Promotes the exchange of ideas and fosters multidisciplinary, interdisciplinary, and interprofessional scholarship, research, teaching, policy development, professional development, and collegiality among people engaged in all of the endeavors related to clinical and academic bioethics and the health-related humanities. **Pub:** *Core Competencies for Health Care Ethics Consultation.* Report. *Price:* $12.00. • Membership Directory, annual.

### ★ 1925 ★ American Society for Clinical Investigation (ASCI)

35 Research Dr., Ste. 300
Ann Arbor, MI 48103
**Phone:** (734)222-6050     **Fax:** (734)222-6058
**Email:** asci@the-jci.org
**Website:** http://www.asci-jci.org/asci
Dr. Chi Van Dang, Pres.

**Fnded:** 1909. **Mem:** 2,600. **Desc:** Physician scientists with meritorious original clinical investigations. Active members are doctors under age 50; senior members are those over age 50. Promotes cultivation of clinical research by methods of natural sciences, correlation of science with the art of medical practice, encouragement of scientific investigation by medical practitioners, and publication of papers on the methods and results of clinical research. **Pub:** *Journal of Clinical Investigation,* biweekly. Journal. • Newsletter, quarterly.

### ★ 1926 ★ American Society of Gene Therapy

611 E Wells St.
Milwaukee, WI 53202
**Phone:** (414)278-1341     **Fax:** (414)276-3349
**Email:** info@asgt.org
**Website:** http://www.asgt.org
Elizabeth Dooley, CAE, Exec. Dir.

**Fnded:** 1996. **Mem:** 3,000. **Desc:** Engages exclusively in scientific and educational activities including specifically, but not limited to, promoting and fostering the exchange and diffusion of information and ideas relating to gene therapy and encouraging the general field of clinical research. **Pub:** *The Journal of Molecular Therapy,* monthly. Journal.

### ★ 1927 ★ American Society for Medicine and Science (ASMS)

875 Providence Hwy.
Dedham, MA 02026-6868
**Phone:** (781)326-7800     **Free:** 800-972-7777
**Fax:** (781)326-2921
**Email:** medical@colpittswt.com
Alan M. Krensky, Contact

**Desc:** Not an association. Organizes medical and scientific conventions worldwide for nonprofit organizations. **Frmly:** (1998) American Academy of Medicine and Science.

### ★ 1928 ★ American Subacute Care Association (ASCA)

1255 23rd St. NW, Ste. 200
Washington, DC 20037-1152
**Phone:** (305)864-0396     **Fax:** (305)868-0905
**Email:** ASCAMail@aol.com
Mike Freedman, Pres.

**Fnded:** 1993. **Mem:** 375. **Desc:** Executives of subacute care companies, vendors, and allied legal and financial professionals; physicians, nurses, physical therapists, occupational therapists, and other healthcare professionals involved in subacute care. Dedicated to advancing the field of subacute care. **Pub:** *ASCA Quarterly,* quarterly. Newsletter. *Price:* Included in membership dues.

### ★ 1929 ★ Americans for Free Choice in Medicine (AFCM)

1525 Superior Ave., Ste. 100
Newport Beach, CA 92663
**Phone:** (949)645-2622     **Fax:** (949)645-4624
**Email:** mail@afcm.org
**Website:** http://www.afcm.org

**Fnded:** 1993. **Desc:** Patients, Medicare recipients, physicians, nurses and health care professionals, insurance industry professionals, pharmacists and pharmaceutical industry professionals, financial services professionals, businessmen, employee benefits professionals, and hospital staff. Promote the philosophy of individual rights, personal responsibility and free market economics in the health care industry. Sponsors educational programs, lectures and town hall meetings, as well as "The Andrew Lewis Show", a weekly radio show.

### ★ 1930 ★ Americans for Medical Progress Educational Foundation (AMPEF)

908 King St., Ste. 201
Alexandria, VA 22314-3067
**Phone:** (703)836-9595     **Free:** 800-426-7872
**Fax:** (703)836-9594
**Email:** info@amprogress.org
**Website:** http://www.amprogress.org
Jacqueline Calnan, Pres.

**Fnded:** 1990. **Mem:** 3,000. **Desc:** Works to ensure the public supports the role of animals in medical research. Supports scientists' ability to search for cures and treatments for injury, illness, and disease. **Pub:** *News and Notes,* quarterly. Newsletter. *Price:* Included in membership dues. • Brochures. • Also, publishes bimedical research fact sheets and other educational materials.

### ★ 1931 ★ Amputee Coalition of America

900 E Hill Ave., Ste. 285
Knoxville, TN 37915-2568
**Phone:** (865)524-5669     **Free:** 888-AMP-KNOW
**Fax:** (865)525-7917
**Email:** acainfo@amputee-coalition.org
**Website:** http://www.amputee-coalition.org
John Miller, CEO and Pres.

**Fnded:** 1989. **Desc:** Information clearinghouse and cooperative program of the Centers for Disease Control & Prevention and the Amputee Coalition of America. Serves people who have limb differences, their families, and friends, healthcare providers, and the general public. Provides information on adapting to limb loss, directs referrals to groups/agencies and programs. Offers informative resources, technical assistance and education for consumer and professional groups. **Pub:** *First Step - A Guide For Adapting To Limb Loss.* • *inMotion,* bimonthly. Magazine. • Books. • Videos.

### ★ 1932 ★ Anatomical Society of West Africa (ASWA)

Department of Anatomy
University of Ibadan
Ibadan, Oyo, Nigeria
**Phone:** 234 22 400550

**Lang(s):** English. **Desc:** Anatomists and anatomy educators and students. Seeks to advance the study and teaching of anatomy. Facilitates exchange of information among members; conducts research and educational programs.

## ★ 1933 ★ Andean Rural Health Care (ARHC)

224 E Martin St.
Raleigh, NC 27601-1818
**Phone:** (828)452-3544　　**Fax:** (828)452-7790
**Email:** sarale@haywood.main.nc.us
David Shanklin, Exec. Dir.

**Desc:** Volunteers united to improve the health care available to people living in rural areas of Bolivia. Collaborates with Bolivian health organizations and government agencies to develop and expand health care services. Trains indigenous people to operate and maintain public health services. Conducts research to determine health care needs in rural Bolivia. Maintains home visitation programs; sponsors volunteer work teams from the U.S. to support Bolivian health care services.

## ★ 1934 ★ Aneurysm Outreach (AOI)

17222 Hwy. 929
Prairieville, LA 70769
**Phone:** (225)673-0682　　**Fax:** (225)622-1577
**Email:** aneurysmoutreach@aneurysm-help.org
**Website:** http://aneurysm-help.org
Sheila G. Arrington, Pres.

**Fnded:** 1999. **Nat'l Groups:** 1. **Local Groups:** 1. **Desc:** Volunteers, family and friends affected or at risk. Provide a support network. Promote public awareness; funds research through advocacy and tax-deductible donations.

## ★ 1935 ★ Applied Research Ethics National Association (ARENA)

132 Boylston St.
Fourth Fl.
Boston, MA 02116
**Phone:** (617)423-4112　　**Fax:** (617)423-1185
**Email:** info@arena.org
**Website:** http://www.arena.org
Sanford Chodosh, Pres.

**Fnded:** 1983. **Mem:** 1,400. **Reg. Groups:** 6. **Desc:** Professionals concerned with ethical issues for humans and animals. Promotes the protection of humans and the humane care and treatment of animals. Sponsors national and regional meetings, disseminates research information and assists with the development of regional networks.

## ★ 1936 ★ Arab Centre for Medical Literature (ACML)

Box 5225
Safat 13053, Kuwait
**Phone:** 965 5338610　　**Fax:** 965 5338618

**Lang(s):** Arabic, English. **Desc:** Physicians and medical writers. Promotes dissemination of medical knowledge. Encourages publication of medical texts; sponsors research and educational programs; facilitates communication among doctors in the Arab World.

## ★ 1937 ★ Arab Forum for Primary Health Care and Community Based Rehabilitation

32 avenue Tour Hassan, Apt. 7
Rabat, Morocco
**Phone:** 212 7 726336　　**Fax:** 212 7 726340

**Lang(s):** Arabic, English. **Desc:** Health care organizations and institutions. Promotes increased availability of quality primary health care and rehabilitation services in the Arab World. Facilitates communication and cooperation among members; conducts public health programs; sponsors research and educational initiatives.

## ★ 1938 ★ Arab Medical Union (AMU)

Union des Medecins Arabes
Mahrajene
PO Box 290
1082 Tunis, Tunisia
**Phone:** 216 1 886800　　**Fax:** 216 1 889293

**Lang(s):** Arabic, English. **Desc:** Physicians and other health care professionals. Seeks to increase availability and quality of health care services in the Arab World; promotes professional advancement of members. Makes available health services; sponsors research; conducts continuing professional development courses.

## ★ 1939 ★ Argentina Association of Medical Advisers (AAMA) (Association Agentes de Propaganda Medica de la Republica Argentina — AAPMRA)

Avenida Avellanda 2144
Capital Federal
Buenos Aires, Argentina
**Phone:** 54 1 6337878　　**Fax:** 54 1 6339336

**Lang(s):** Spanish. **Desc:** Medical advisers. Promotes professional advancement of members. Represents members' interests before industrial organizations, government agencies, and the public.

## ★ 1940 ★ Argentine Association of Biology and Nuclear Medicine (Asociacion Argentina de Biologia y Medicina Nuclear)

Bulnes 1878 6 to.23
1425 Buenos Aires, Argentina
**Fax:** 54 1 48272340
**Email:** correo@aabymn.org.ar
**Website:** http://www.aabymn.org.ar

**Fnded:** 1963.

## ★ 1941 ★ Argentine Association of Mycology (Asociacion Argentina de Micologia)

Paraguay 2155
1121 Buenos Aires, Argentina
**Phone:** 54 1 9627274　　**Fax:** 54 1 9625404
**Fnded:** 1960.

## ★ 1942 ★ ASEAN Institute for Health Development

25/5 Phutthamonthon 4 Rd.
Salaya
Mahidol University
Nakorn Pathom 73170, Thailand
**Phone:** 66 2 8496311　　**Fax:** 66 2 8496237
**Email:** orbsw@mahidol.ac.th
**Website:** http://www.mahidol.ac.th

**Fnded:** 1982. **Lang(s):** English, Thai. **Desc:** International health agencies. Seeks to improve the availability and quality of primary health care services in Southeast Asia. Facilitates establishment of local health services and facilities; serves as a clearinghouse on public health policies and programs. **Pub:** *Journal of Primary Health Care*, quarterly. Journal. Articles/research on primary health care.

## ★ 1943 ★ ASEAN Otorhinolaryngolical - Head and Neck Federation

Sinraj Hospital
Faculty of Medicine
Department of Otorhinolaryngology
Bangkok 10700, Thailand
**Phone:** 66 2 4113254

**Lang(s):** English, Thai. **Desc:** Otorhinolaryngologists and other health care professionals with an interest in diseases of the head and neck. Seeks to advance otorhinolaryngological study, teaching, and practice. Facilitates exchange of information among members; sponsors continuing professional development courses.

## ★ 1944 ★ ASEAN Poulty Disease Research and Training Centre

59 Jalan Sultan Azlan Shah
Perak Darul Ridzuan
31400 Ipoh, Malaysia

**Lang(s):** English, Malay. **Desc:** Veterinarians and poultry growers and processors. Seeks to advance the prevention, diagnosis, and treatment of poultry diseases. Serves as a clearinghouse on poultry and avian medicine; conducts continuing professional development courses for veterinarians.

## Asian Academy of Craniomandibular Disorders (AACD)

*See:* Entry 13554

## ★ 1945 ★ Asian Federation of Catholic Medical Associations (AFCMA)

Catholic University Medical College
505 Banpo-dong
Sochu-ku
Seoul 137 701, Republic of Korea
**Phone:** 82 2 5935141　　**Fax:** 82 2 5323112

**Lang(s):** English, Korean. **Desc:** Catholic medical associations. Seeks to increase the availability of quality health care services in previously underserved areas of Asia; promotes adherence to high standards of ethics and practice among Catholic health care services and institutions. Facilitates communication and cooperation among members; makes available health services; conducts exchange and continuing professional development programs.

## ★ 1946 ★ Asian Federation for Medical Chemistry (AFMC)

c/o Korean Chemical Society
Science and Technology Bldg., Rm. 703
635-4 Yoksam-dong
Kangnam-gu
Seoul 135 703, Republic of Korea
**Phone:** 82 2 34533781　　**Fax:** 82 2 34533785
**Email:** kcschem@neon.kcsnet.or.kr

**Fnded:** 1946. **Mem:** 5,000. **Reg. Groups:** 13. **Lang(s):** English, Korean. **Desc:** Chemists, physicians, and other scientists and health care personnel with an interest in medical chemistry. Promotes medical chemistry research and scholarship. Serves as a clearinghouse on medical chemistry; conducts research and educational programs. **Pub:** *Bulletin of the Korean Chemical Society*, monthly. Journal. • *Chemical Education*, quarterly. Magazine. • *ChemWorld*, monthly. Magazine. • *Journal of the Korean Chemical Society*, bimonthly. Journal. • *Korean Journal of Medicinal Chemistry*, semiannual. Journal.

## ★ 1947 ★ Asian-Pacific Resource and Research Centre for Women (ARROW)

Ground Floor, Block G
Anjung Felda
Jalan Maktab
54000 Kuala Lumpur, Malaysia
**Phone:** 60 3 26929913　　**Fax:** 60 3 26929958
**Email:** arrow@arrow.po.my

**Fnded:** 1993. **Lang(s):** English, Malay. **Desc:** Advocate to reorient health, population and reproductive health policies with women's gender perspectives and to ensure that health services are comprehensive, accessible and affordable for women in Malaysia. **Pub:** *Arrows for Change*, 3/year. Bulletin. Focuses on the gender dimension of women and health. • *Gender and Women's Health: Information Package, No. 2, 1997.* • *Reappraising Population Policies and Family Planning Programmes: An Annotated Bibliography Series 1, 1994.* • *Towards Women-Centered Reproductive Health: Information Package No. 1, 1994.* • *Women-Centered and Gender-Sensitive Experiences: Changing Our Perspectives, Policies, and Programmes on Womens Health in Asia and the Pacific Ref. Kit.*

## ★ 1948 ★ Asociacion Medica Argentina

Santa Fe 1171
1059 Buenos Aires, Argentina
**Phone:** 54 1 411633
**Fnded:** 1891.

## ★ 1949 ★ Associacao Medica Brasileira

CP 8904
01333 Sao Paulo, Brazil
**Phone:** 55 11 2893511
**Fnded:** 1951.


## ★ 1950 ★ Association of Academic Health Centers (AHC)

1400 16th St. NW, Ste. 720
Washington, DC 20036
**Phone:** (202)265-9600          **Fax:** (202)265-7514
**Email:** ahc@acadhlthctrs.org
**Website:** http://www.ahcnet.org
Roger J. Bulger, MD, Pres.

**Fnded:** 1969. **Mem:** 102. **Desc:** Chief executive officers of university-based academic health centers in the U.S. and Canada. Interdisciplinary in focus, with a primary interest in total health manpower education. Sponsors task forces and forums to advance public policy dialogue on health and science issues. Develops research and education programs. Publishes, reports, books, and issues papers. **Pub:** *General Meetings*, periodic. • *Directory*, periodic. • *Reports.* Provides information on special projects. **Frmly:** Organization of University Health Center Administrators.


## ★ 1951 ★ Association for the Advancement of Blacks in Health Sciences (AABHS)

42 Charles St. E
Toronto, ON, Canada M4Y 1T4
**Phone:** (416)928-9201          **Fax:** (416)928-3325
**Fnded:** 1993. **Desc:** Health care professionals, researchers, graduate, undergraduate students, non-health professionals. Promotes the pursuit of higher education in health science fields to black youth; strives to optimize health care services and information to black community. Supports the following initiatives: Health Sciences Summer Mentorship Program, Visions of Science Forums, Camp Jumoke, Black Medical Student Association (BMSA), and community outreach programs.


## ★ 1952 ★ Association for the Advancement of Wound Care (AAWC)

950 West Valley Rd., Ste. 2800
Wayne, PA 19087
**Free:** (866)229-2999          **Fax:** (610)688-8050
**Email:** aawchelp@voicenet.com
**Website:** http://www.aawcone.com
Tina Thomas, Assoc. Liaison

**Fnded:** 1996. **Mem:** 900. **Desc:** Works to advance the cause of wound care through education, research, clinical practice and public policy. Provides a forum for communication and partnership among all people involved in wound care. **Pub:** *AAWC Newsletter*, quarterly. Newsletter. Contains updates on wound care. *Price:* Free for members. • *Ostomy/Wound Management*, monthly. Journal. *Price:* Free for members. • *Wound Care Clinic Directory*, annual. Directory. *Price:* $10 for members; $20 for nonmembers. • *Wounds*, bimonthly. Journal. *Price:* Free for members.


## ★ 1953 ★ Association of American Indian Physicians (AAIP)

1225 Sovereign Row, Ste. 103
Oklahoma City, OK 73108-1854
**Phone:** (405)946-7072          **Fax:** (405)946-7651
**Email:** aaip@aaip.com
**Website:** http://www.aaip.com
Margaret Knight, Exec. Dir.

**Fnded:** 1971. **Mem:** 270. **Desc:** Physicians (M.D. or D.O.) of American Indian descent. Encourages American Indians to enter the health professions. Provides a forum for the interchange of ideas and information of mutual interest to physicians of Indian descent. Establishes contracts with government agencies to provide consultation and other expert opinion regarding health care of American Indians and Alaskan Natives; receives contracts and grant monies and other forms of assistance from these sources. Supports and encourages all other agencies and organizations, Indian and non-Indian, working to improve health conditions of American Indians and Alaskan Natives. Locates scholarship funds for Indian professional students; provides counseling assistance; preserves American Indian culture. Conducts seminars for students interested in health careers and for counselors in government and other schools where American Indian children are taught. **Pub:** Newsletter, quarterly.


## ★ 1954 ★ Association of American Medical Colleges (AAMC)

2450 N St. NW
Washington, DC 20037-1136
**Phone:** (202)828-0400          **Fax:** (202)828-1125
**Email:** amcas@aamc.org
**Website:** http://www.aamc.org
Jordan J. Cohen, MD, Pres.

**Fnded:** 1876. **Mem:** 2,200. **Desc:** Medical schools, graduate affiliate medical colleges, academic societies, teaching hospitals, and individuals interested in the advancement of medical education, biomedical research, and healthcare. Provides centralized application service. Offers management education program for medical school deans, teaching hospital directors, department chairmen, and service chiefs of affiliated hospitals. Develops and administers the Medical College Admissions Test (MCAT). Operates student loan program. Maintains information management system and institutional profile system. Compiles statistics. **Pub:** *Academic Medicine*, monthly. Journal. Provides scholarly articles on physician education and workforce issues. *Price:* $120/year in U.S.; $180 Canada and foreign. • *Directory of American Medical Education*, annual. Directory. • *Medical School Admission Requirements*, annual. • *Reports*, annual. • *Reports*, semiannual.


## ★ 1955 ★ Association of American Medical Colleges-Women in Medicine Program (AAMC-WIM)

c/o Janet Bickel
2450 N St. NW
Washington, DC 20037-1126
**Phone:** (202)828-0521          **Fax:** (202)828-1125
**Email:** jbickel@aamc.org
**Website:**          http://www.aamc.org/about/progemph/wommed
Janet Bickel, MA, Assoc. VP & Dir.

**Desc:** Dedicated to increasing women's leadership in academic medicine. **Pub:** *Membership Directory*. • *Women in Medicine Update*, quarterly.


## ★ 1956 ★ Association of American Physicians and Surgeons (AAPS)

1601 N Tucson Blvd., Ste. 9
Tucson, AZ 85716
**Phone:** (520)327-4885          **Free:** 800-635-1196
**Fax:** (520)326-3529
**Email:** jorient@mindspring.com
**Website:** http://www.aapsonline.org/
Jane M. Orient, MD, Exec. Dir.

**Fnded:** 1943. **Mem:** 4,500. **Desc:** Physicians dedicated to preserving and promoting quality medical care. Represents physicians in the socioeconomic and legal aspects of medical practice such as medical economics, public relations, and legislation. Makes available legal consultation services. **Pub:** *AAPS News*, monthly. Newsletter. Covers developments affecting health care and the profession. Includes legislative news, calendar of events, and health law commentary. *Price:* Included in membership dues; $35/year for nonmembers. • *The Medical Sentinel*, quarterly. Journal. Peer-reviewed journal. • Audiotapes.


## ★ 1957 ★ Association of Asian/Pacific Community Health Organizations (AAPCHO)

429 23rd St.
Oakland, CA 94612-2025
**Phone:** (510)272-9536          **Fax:** (510)272-0817
**Email:** info@aapcho.org
**Website:** http://www.aapcho.org
Jeffrey Caballero, Interim Exec. Dir.

**Fnded:** 1987. **Mem:** 14. **Desc:** Works to improve access to culturally and linguistically appropriate health care in order to improve the health status of Asians and Pacific Islanders with a special focus on the medically underserved. **Pub:** *Hepatitis B.* Brochure. • *Parent's Guide to Common Childhood Illnesses.* Brochure. • *Thalassemia Among Asians.* Brochure.


## ★ 1958 ★ Association of Canadian Medical Colleges (ACMC) (Association des Facultes de Medecine du Canada — AFMC)

774 Echo Dr.
Ottawa, ON, Canada K1S 5P2
**Phone:** (613)730-0687          **Fax:** (613)730-1196
**Email:** dhawkins@acmc.ca
**Website:** http://www.acmc.ca

**Lang(s):** English, French. **Desc:** Colleges of medicine. Promotes excellence in the study and teaching of medicine; seeks to advance the profession of medicine through improved medical education programs. Conducts research and educational programs; facilitates exchange of information among members.


## ★ 1959 ★ Association for Chemoreception Sciences (AChemS)

744 Duparc Cir.
Tallahassee, FL 32312-1409
**Phone:** (850)531-0854
**Email:** sjf24@columbia.edu
**Website:** http://achems.org
Dr. Stuart J. Firestein, Pres.

**Fnded:** 1979. **Mem:** 649. **Desc:** Research scientists, experimental psychologists, and industrial researchers. Purpose is to study chemoreception (the physiological reception of chemical stimuli) by the senses of taste and smell. Conducts research on the differences in human and animal perception of chemical stimuli in taste and smell. Offers seminars, fellowships, and workshops. Maintains placement service. Bestows annual Best Student Presentation at conference. **Pub:** Newsletter, biennial.


## ★ 1960 ★ Association of Community Health Councils for England and Wales (ACHCEW)

Earlsmead House
30 Drayton Park
London N5 1PB, United Kingdom
**Phone:** 44 20 76098405          **Fax:** 44 207 7001152
**Email:** mailbox@achcew.org.uk
**Website:** http://www.achcew.org.uk

**Fnded:** 1977. **Mem:** 204. **Desc:** Community Health Councils set up to monitor the National Health Service. Provides forum for member CHCs, provides information and advisory services to CHCs and represents the user of health services at a national level. **Pub:** *CHC News*, 10/year. • *Factsheets for the Public*, periodic. • *Health News Briefings*, 10/year. • *Perspectives - Brief Topic Papers*, 10/year. Papers.


## ★ 1961 ★ Association for Continence Advice (ACA)

Winchester House
Cramer Rd.
The Oval
London SW9 6EJ, United Kingdom
**Phone:** 44 171 8208113          **Fax:** 44 171 8200442

**Fnded:** 1981. **Mem:** 755. **Desc:** Professionals with an interest in the health and social care of people with continence problems. Aims to provide a means of communication and support between members and other interested groups; to promote educational activities; to produce and distribute a newsletter; to promote research activities and disseminate research findings; to liaise and maintain dialogue with relevant manufacturers; to promote public awareness and positive attitudes within society. **Pub:** Newsletter. • Pamphlets.


★ **1962** ★ **Association of Family Practice Administrators (AFPA)**
11400 Tomahawk Creek Parkway
Leawood, KS 66211
**Phone:** (913)906-6000          **Free:** 800-274-2237
**Fax:** (913)906-6092
**Email:** cweber@aafp.org
**Website:** http://www.uams.edu/afpa/afpa1.htm
Cynthia W. Weber, Exec. Sec.

**Fnded:** 1984. **Mem:** 375. **Nat'l Groups:** 1. **Desc:** Administrators and coordinators of family practice residency training programs. Promotes professionalism in family practice administration. Serves as a network for sharing of information and fellowship among members. Provides technical assistance to members; functions as a liaison to related professional organizations. **Pub:** *Connections*, quarterly. Newsletter.


★ **1963** ★ **Association of French-Speaking Physicians of Canada (AFSPC)**
**(Association des Medicins de Langue Francaise du Canada — AMLFC)**
8355 Boulevard Saint-Laurent
Montreal, QC, Canada H2P 2Z6
**Phone:** (514)388-2228          **Free:** 800-387-2228
**Fax:** (514)388-5335
**Email:** info@amlfc.org
**Website:** http://www.amlfc.org

**Lang(s):** English, French. **Desc:** French-speaking physicians practicing in Canada. Seeks to increase availability and quality of health care in French-speaking areas of Canada; promotes professional advancement of members. Makes available health services in underserved areas; facilitates communication and cooperation among members.


★ **1964** ★ **Association for Health-Care Institutions**
**(Verbond der Verzorgingsinstellingen — VVI)**
Guimardstraat 1
B-1040 Brussels, Belgium
**Phone:** 32 2 5118008          **Fax:** 32 2 5135269
**Email:** post@vvi.be

**Fnded:** 1938. **Mem:** 500. **Lang(s):** Dutch, English, French. **Desc:** Hospitals; psychiatric hospitals; nursing homes; homes for elderly people. Promotes high standards of health service. Fosters exchange and cooperation; offers consultative services; makes recommendations to government authorities. **Pub:** *Hospitalia*, quarterly. Magazine. • *VVI-Information*, 11/year.


★ **1965** ★ **Association of Healthcare Philanthropy (AHP)**
259 Beattie Ave.
Summerside, PE, Canada C1N 2A9
**Phone:** (902)432-2547          **Fax:** (902)436-1501
**Email:** jmhierlihy@ihis.org
**Website:** http://www.ahpcanada.com/

**Mem:** 3,100. **Desc:** Promotes healthcare fundraising professionals; dedicated to supporting members ability to perform philanthropic work for healthcare organizations; develops career opportunities.


★ **1966** ★ **Association of Independent Care Advisors**
6 West Mount Close
Southwick
Brighton BN42 4SR, United Kingdom
**Phone:** 44 1483 203066     **Fax:** 44 1483 202535
**Website:** http://www.aica.org.uk

**Fnded:** 1994. **Mem:** 8. **Nat'l Groups:** 1. **Desc:** Members provide advice to individuals about their care options, either in their own homes or in residential homes.


★ **1967** ★ **Association of International Health Researchers (AIHR)**
2665 Pleasant Valley Rd.
Mobile, AL 36606
**Phone:** (251)473-3946
Dr. Roy E. Kadel, Pres.

**Fnded:** 1982. **Mem:** 123. **Reg. Groups:** 5. **Desc:** Individuals interested in quality health research. Works to: promote a better understanding of scientifically effective research techniques and methodologies; encourage interaction among individuals in international health research. Compiles statistics.


★ **1968** ★ **Association of Massage Therapists Australia (AMTA)**
PO Box 358
Prahran, VIC 3181, Australia
**Phone:** 61 3 95103930          **Fax:** 61 3 95213209
**Email:** amta@amta.asn.au
**Website:** http://www.amta.asn.au

**Fnded:** 1989. **Mem:** 1,750. **Reg. Groups:** 9. **Lang(s):** English. **Desc:** Professional massage therapists and those studying professional massage. Promotes the professional interests of massage therapists in Australia.


★ **1969** ★ **Association of Medical Doctors of Asia (AMDAI)**
310-1 Nazaru
Okayama 701-12, Japan
**Phone:** 81 86 2847730          **Fax:** 81 86 2848959
**Website:** http://www.amda.or.jp

**Fnded:** 1984. **Mem:** 665. **Lang(s):** English, French, Japanese, Spanish. **Desc:** Physicians, medical students, and organizations are members; nurses and other health care personnel and organizations are associate members. Promotes and works to strengthen partnership among Asian doctors. Seeks to insure adequate medical care for people in underserved areas. Conducts emergency relief and rehabilitation operations in areas affected by natural disasters or human conflicts; implements community health development programs in rural areas; facilitates continuing professional education and training of members. **Pub:** *AMDA International*, quarterly. Newsletter. • *Harukanaru Yume*. Book. • *International Collaboration of Medical Care*, monthly. Journal. • *International Medical Cooperation - Proceedings of the Hayabashibara Forum 1993*. Proceedings. • *Proceedings of the 1994 Okayama NGO Summit*. Proceedings. • *Ruwandakarano Shogen*. Book. • *Tobidase! AMDA*. Report.


★ **1970** ★ **Association for Medical Education in the Eastern Mediterranean Region (AMEEMR)**
Jordan University of Science and Technology
PO Box 3030
Irbid, Jordan
**Phone:** 962 2 7095111          **Fax:** 962 2 7095123
**Email:** hijazi@just.edu.jo

**Lang(s):** English. **Desc:** Medical schools, educators, and students. Seeks to advance medical scholarship and practice. Serves as a clearinghouse on medical education; encourages communication and cooperation among members; sponsors research programs and continuing professional development courses.


★ **1971** ★ **Association for Medical Education in Europe (AMEE)**
Centre for Medical Education
University of Dundee
Tay Park House
484 Perth Rd.
Dundee DD2 1LR, United Kingdom
**Phone:** 44 1382 631953     **Fax:** 44 1382 645748
**Email:** amee@dundee.ac.uk
**Website:** http://www.amee.org

**Lang(s):** English. **Desc:** Medical schools, educators, and students. Seeks to advance medical scholarship and practice. Serves as a clearinghouse on medical education; encourages communication and coopera-

tion among members; sponsors research programs and continuing professional development courses. **Pub:** *Medical Teacher*, bimonthly. Journal.


★ **1972** ★ **Association for Medical Education in the Western Pacific Region (AMEWPR)**
Seoul National University
College of Medicine
28 Yong-Dong, Chongno-Gu
Seoul 110-799, Republic of Korea
**Phone:** 82 2 7602552          **Fax:** 82 2 7476779
**Email:** kimyi@plaza.snu.ac.kr

**Lang(s):** English, Japanese. **Desc:** Medical schools, educators, and students. Seeks to advance medical scholarship and practice. Serves as a clearinghouse on medical education; encourages communication and cooperation among members; sponsors research programs and continuing professional development courses.


★ **1973** ★ **Association of Medical Research Charities (AMRC)**
61 Gray's Inn Rd.
London WC7X 8TL, United Kingdom
**Phone:** 44 20 72698820          **Fax:** 44 20 72698821
**Email:** info@amrc.org.uk
**Website:** http://www.amrc.org.uk

**Fnded:** 1987. **Mem:** 111. **Lang(s):** English. **Desc:** Medical research charities. Furthers the advancement of medical research in the United Kingdom. Focuses attention on the collective effectiveness of members. Provides information, advice and guidance to members and others. **Pub:** *Handbook*, annual. Booklet. Lists member charities that award funding for medical research. • Newsletter. Features member information.


★ **1974** ★ **Association of Medical Schools in Africa (AMSA)**
Easterna and Southern Africa Regional Office
  UNICEF
United Nations Office
Gigiri
Nairobi, Kenya

**Lang(s):** English. **Desc:** Medical schools. Seeks to advance medical scholarship and practice. Facilitates communication and exchange among members; sponsors research and educational programs.


★ **1975** ★ **Association of Medical Schools in Europe (AMSE)**
University of Vienna
Wahringerstrabe 13
A-1090 Vienna, Austria
**Phone:** 43 1 4088366          **Fax:** 43 1 40480224

**Fnded:** 1979. **Lang(s):** English. **Desc:** Deans of medical schools; representatives of medical deans in 25 countries. Provides a forum for the exchange of ideas and information. Objectives are: to address important questions concerning medical education, with special emphasis on policies affecting the future of medical education in Europe; to discuss practical issues such as admission criteria and organizational problems; to analyze the relationship between medical schools and health service organizations; to assess the impact of medical science on medical education. **Pub:** *AMSE Newsletter*, quarterly. Newsletter. **Frmly:** (1992) Association of Medical Deans in Europe.


★ **1976** ★ **Association of Minority Health Professions Schools (AMHPS)**
507 Capitol Court, Ste. 200
Washington, DC 20002
**Phone:** (202)544-7499          **Fax:** (202)546-7105
**Website:** http://svmc107.tusk.edu/amphs2.html
Dale P. Dirks, Wash. Rep.

**Fnded:** 1978. **Mem:** 11. **Desc:** Predominantly black health professions schools. Seeks to: increase the number of minorities in health professions; improve the health of blacks in the U.S.; increase the federal resources available to minority schools and students.

Provides information to the U.S. Congress; conducts educational programs. **Pub:** *Study of the Health Status of Minorities in the U.S.*, periodic.

**★ 1977 ★ Association of Morphologists**
BP 184
F-54505 Vanduvre-les-Nancy, France
**Phone:** 33 3 83592833     **Fax:** 33 3 83446065
**Email:** grignon@facmed.u-nancy.fr
**Fnded:** 1899. **Desc:** Encourages discussion and publication of papers on anatomy, histology, embryology, and odontology.

**★ 1978 ★ Association of Native American Medical Students (ANAMS)**
1225 Sovereign Row, Ste. 103
Oklahoma City, OK 73108
**Phone:** (405)946-7072     **Fax:** (405)946-7651
**Email:** aaip@aaip.com
**Website:** http://www.aaip.com/anams
**Desc:** Committed to Native American medical students.

**★ 1979 ★ Association of Nigerian Physicians in the Americas (ANPA)**
6876 Indiana Ave., Ste. F
Riverside, CA 92501-4010
**Phone:** (909)778-0716     **Fax:** (909)778-0717
**Email:** dokita@anpa.org
**Website:** http://www.anpa.org
Alphonsus Obayuwana, Pres.
**Fnded:** 1995. **Desc:** Physicians and surgeons of Nigerian descent practicing in the United States and Canada. Promotes professional advancement of members; seeks to stimulate interest in matters affecting the health of people of Nigerian descent; encourages adherence to high standards of professional ethics and practice by members. Serves as a clearinghouse on professional opportunities available to physicians of Nigerian descent in North America; conducts charitable, social, educational, and scientific activities. **Pub:** *Directory of Nigerian Physicians in the United States and Canada*, annual. Directory. • *Quarterly News Bulletin*, quarterly. Newsletter.

**★ 1980 ★ Association of Otolaryngology Administrators (AOA)**
PO Box 503269
Saint Louis, MO 63150-3269
**Phone:** (636)394-6262     **Fax:** (636)394-3501
**Email:** cgfears@earthlink.net
**Website:** http://www.oto-online.org
Patricia E. Brown-Oliver, Pres.
**Fnded:** 1983. **Mem:** 730. **Reg. Groups:** 8. **Desc:** Persons employed in a managerial capacity for private or academic group medical practices specializing in otolaryngology (the study of the ear, nose, and throat). Seeks to: promote the concept of professional management in otolaryngology; provide a forum for interaction and exchange of information between otolaryngological managers; present educational programs. Maintains data exchange service for members researching specific topics. **Pub:** *Oto's Scope*, 3/year.

**★ 1981 ★ Association of Pakistani Physicians (APPNA)**
6414 S Cass Ave.
Westmont, IL 60559
**Phone:** (630)968-8585     **Fax:** (630)968-8677
**Email:** appna@appna.org
**Website:** http://www.appna.org
Dr. Mohammad Saleman, Pres.
**Fnded:** 1976. **Mem:** 1,200. **Desc:** Physicians and dentists who are native to Pakistan but now live and practice in North America. Purposes are: to support medical education and research and advance the interests of medicine and medical organizations; to foster scientific development and education in order to improve the quality of medicine and health care; to facilitate better relations among Pakistani physicians and between them and the people of North America.

Assists Pakistani physicians newly arrived in North America in orientation and adjustment. Arranges for donation of medical literature and medical supplies to Pakistan, and for lecture tours, medical conferences, and seminars to be held there. Participates in medical relief and charitable activities in Pakistan and North America; cooperates with other medical organizations in North America. Offers scientific programs for which continuing medical education credits are awarded. **Pub:** Bulletin, monthly. • Newsletter, quarterly.

**★ 1982 ★ Association for Palliative Medicine of Great Britain and Ireland**
11 Westwood Rd.
Southampton SO17 1DL, United Kingdom
**Phone:** 44 23 80672888     **Fax:** 44 23 80672888
**Email:** apmsecretariat@claranet.co.uk
**Website:** http://www.palliative-medicine.org
**Fnded:** 1985. **Mem:** 760. **Desc:** Aims to promote the advancement and development of palliative medicine and is recognized as representing physicians at all grades who work in palliative medicine and those with an interest in the specialty.

**★ 1983 ★ Association of Philippine Physicians in America (APPA)**
PO Box 452164
Los Angeles, CA 90045
**Fax:** (310)677-7238
**Email:** masmd@aboutappa.org
**Website:** http://www.aboutappa.org/
Alfonso Nillas, MD, Pres.
**Fnded:** 1972. **Mem:** 3,000. **Nat'l Groups:** 27. **State Groups:** 27. **Desc:** Individuals from the Philippines who are licensed to practice medicine in the U.S. Seeks to: render free medical care to indigent persons; establish a continuing medical education program for physicians; provide aid for education of physicians; support medical research. Sends medical missions to the Philippines. Provides medical residency program placement service. Maintains speakers' bureau; compiles statistics. **Pub:** *Directory of Physicians*, biennial. Directory. • *Leadership Roster of Officers*, annual. • *Philippine Physician*, periodic. Association and professional newsletter. *Price:* Free. • Also publishes CME abstracts; plans to publish journal of medicine. **Frmly:** (1986) Association of Philippine Practicing Physicians in America.

**★ 1984 ★ Association of Physician Assistant Programs (APAP)**
950 N Washington St.
Alexandria, VA 22314-1552
**Phone:** (703)548-5538     **Fax:** (703)684-1924
**Website:** http://www.apap.org
David P. Asprey, Pres.
**Fnded:** 1972. **Mem:** 123. **Reg. Groups:** 6. **Desc:** Represents physician assistant (PA) educational programs in the United States. Assists PA educational programs-institutions with training programs for physician assistants to primary care and surgical physicians. Assists in the development and organization of educational curricula for PA programs to assure the public of competent PAs. Contributes to defining the roles of PAs in the field of medicine to maximize their benefit to the public; serves as a public information center on the profession; coordinates program logistics such as admissions and career placements; and is currently initiating a centralized application service for PA applicants. Sponsors the Annual Survey of Physician Assistant Educational Programs in the United States. Conducts and sponsors research projects; compiles statistics; offers ongoing training for PA leadership and faculty. **Pub:** *Annual Report on Physician Assistant Education in the U.S.*, annual. Report. Provides data on physician assistant education, employment, and trends affecting the profession. Includes statistics. *Price:* $50/copy. • *APAP Update*, monthly. Newsletter. For physician assistant program faculty and others concerned with curricula and government/legislative developments affecting the profession. *Price:* Included in membership dues. • *Physician Assistant Programs Directory*, annual. Directory. De-

scribes curriculum, university and institutional affiliations, entrance requirement's, selection factors, credentials awarded, and financial aid. *Price:* $35/copy.

**★ 1985 ★ Association of Professional Schools of International Affairs (APSIA)**
c/o Marcus Grundahl
420 W 118 St., Rm. 1415A
New York, NY 10027
**Phone:** (212)854-3952     **Free:** 877-409-5510
**Fax:** (212)864-4847
**Email:** apsia@erols.com
**Website:** http://www.apsia.org/main.html
Marcus Grundahl, Dir.
**Desc:** Dedicated to advancing global understanding and cooperation by preparing men and women to assume positions of leadership in world affairs; serves as a source of information on professional international affairs education, represents the interests of professional international affairs education in national and international forums, and coordinates activities among and for its member institutions.

**★ 1986 ★ Association of Professors of Medicine (APM)**
2501 M St. NW, Ste. 550
Washington, DC 20037-1308
**Phone:** (202)861-7700     **Fax:** (202)861-9731
**Email:** apm@im.org
**Website:** http://www.im.org/apm
Tod Ibrahim, Exec. Dir.
**Fnded:** 1954. **Mem:** 152. **Desc:** Heads of departments of internal medicine in medical schools. Conducts educational programs; compiles statistics. **Pub:** *APM Update*, quarterly. Newsletter. • *Federal Health Policy Update*, quarterly. • Directory, annual. **Frmly:** Academic Medicine Club.

**★ 1987 ★ Association of Program Directors in Internal Medicine (APDIM)**
2501 M St. NW Ste. 550
Washington, DC 20037
**Phone:** (202)887-9450     **Free:** 800-622-4558
**Fax:** (202)887-9447
**Email:** wkidd@bmc.org
**Website:** http://apdim.med.edu
Wayne R. Kidd, Dir., Communications/Membership
**Fnded:** 1977. **Mem:** 1,400. **Desc:** Physicians in internal medicine including departmental chairmen and directors of internal medicine, directors of residency training programs, associate program directors, medical education directors, and chiefs of medical service. Advances medical education through assisting accredited hospital internal medicine residency training programs in the United States and Puerto Rico. Conducts annual course for chief residents and program directors. Offers consulting services. **Pub:** *APDIM Directory*, annual. Membership Directory. • *Careers in Internal Medicine*, quarterly. • Membership Directory, annual. • Newsletter, quarterly. Profiles successful residency programs and summarizes developments in the field of internal medicine. *Price:* Included in membership dues.

**★ 1988 ★ Association of Reflexologists**
27 Old Gloucester St.
London WC1N 3XX, United Kingdom
**Phone:** 44 870 5673320     **Fax:** 44 1989 567676
**Email:** aor@assocmanagement.co.uk
**Website:** http://www.aor.org.uk
**Fnded:** 1984. **Mem:** 6,700. **Reg. Groups:** 43. **Desc:** Promotes reflexology to the public. **Pub:** *Reflexions*, quarterly. Journal.

**★ 1989 ★ Association of Schools of Allied Health Professions (ASAHP)**
1730 M St. NW, Ste. 500
Washington, DC 20036
**Phone:** (202)293-4848     **Fax:** (202)293-4852
**Email:** asahp3@asahp.org

**Website:** http://www.asahp.org
Thomas W. Elwood, PhD, Exec. Dir.

**Fnded:** 1967. **Mem:** 750. **Desc:** National allied health professional membership organizations, clinical service programs, academic institutions, and other institutions and organizations whose interests include the advancement of allied health education, research, and service delivery. Aims include: to provide communication among schools and colleges of allied health professions; to promote development of new programs; to encourage research and to provide liaison with other health organizations, professional groups, and educational and governmental institutions. Sponsors short-term institutes for allied health education, administration, and practice. Conducts research programs. programs. **Pub:** *Allied Health Trends*, monthly. Newsletter. *Price:* $55. • *Journal of Allied Health*, quarterly. Journal. *Price:* $75. • Directory, annual. **Frmly:** (1974) Association of Schools of Allied Health Professions; (1992) American Society of Allied Health Professions.

---

### ★ 1990 ★ Association for the Study of Medical Education (ASME)

12 Queen St.
Edinburgh EH2 1JE, United Kingdom
**Phone:** 44 131 2259111     **Fax:** 44 131 2259444
**Email:** info@asme.org.uk

**Fnded:** 1957. **Mem:** 970. **Lang(s):** English. **Desc:** Individuals engaged in medical education at the undergraduate, postgraduate, and continuing professional development levels. Promotes "knowledge and expertise in medical education." Facilitates information exchange and the establishment of formal networks linking schools; serves as a forum for the debate of issues impacting the field of medical education. **Pub:** *ASME Bulletin*, bimonthly. Newsletter. • *Journal of Medical Education*, monthly. Journal.

---

### ★ 1991 ★ Association for the Study of Obesity (ASO)

20 Brook Meadow Close
Woodford Green IG8 9NR, United Kingdom
**Phone:** 44 29 85032042     **Fax:** 44 29 85032042
**Email:** cahawkins@compuserve.com
**Website:** http://www.aso.org.uk

**Fnded:** 1967. **Mem:** 420. **Lang(s):** English. **Desc:** Scientists, researchers, dieticians, health education workers, and students in England. Promotes information exchange between members; promotes research into the causes, prevention and treatment of obesity; seeks to encourage action to reduce the prevalence of obesity and to enhance treatment.

---

### ★ 1992 ★ Association of Telemedicine Service Providers (ATSP)

4702 SW Scholls Ferry Rd., No. 400
Portland, OR 97225-2008
**Phone:** (503)222-2406     **Fax:** (503)223-7581
**Email:** info@atsp.org
**Website:** http://www.atsp.org

**Desc:** Companies providing telemedical services. Seeks to advance the practice of telemedicine and to stimulate the development of more effective telemedical technologies. Provides educational, business leadership, and marketing services to members; facilitates networking among members; makes available discounts on products and services to members; represents members before government agencies, industry organizations, and the public. **Pub:** *ATSP Annual Survey*, annual. Report.

---

### ★ 1993 ★ Attention Deficit Information Network (ADIN)

c/o Moira Munns
475 Hillside Ave.
Needham, MA 02494
**Phone:** (781)455-9895     **Fax:** (781)444-5466
**Email:** adin@gis.net
**Website:** http://www.addinfonetwork.com

**Fnded:** 1988. **Reg. Groups:** 41. **State Groups:** 20. **Desc:** People with Attention Deficit Disorders (ADD), their families, and other individuals with an interest in ADD. Promotes improved quality of life for people with ADD. Works to expand home, school, and work-based strategies for aiding people with ADD; advocates for improved responsiveness to the needs of people with ADD by schools, businesses, and organizations. Provides support and information to families of people with ADD; conducts educational programs; maintains speakers' bureau. **Pub:** *AD-IN*. Brochure.

---

### ★ 1994 ★ Australasian College of Tropical Medicine (ACTM)

PO Box 123
Red Hill, QLD 4059, Australia
**Phone:** 61 7 38722246     **Fax:** 61 38564727
**Email:** actm@tropmed.org

**Fnded:** 1991. **Desc:** Encourages education and exchange of knowledge in tropical medicine; promotes research.

---

### ★ 1995 ★ Australian Council for Health, Physical Education and Recreation (ACHPER)

214 Port Rd.
Hindmarsh, SA 5007, Australia
**Phone:** 61 8 83403388     **Fax:** 61 8 83403399
**Email:** membership@achper.org.au
**Website:** http://www.achper.org.au

**Mem:** 3,300. **State Groups:** 8. **Desc:** Professionals dedicated to healthy lifestyles. Promotes healthy lifestyles in schools and the community; develops public awareness through political process and media; supports research and projects aimed at creating healthy lifestyle awareness. **Pub:** *Active & Healthy*. Magazine. • *Australian Journal of Science and Medicine in Sport*. Journal.

---

### ★ 1996 ★ Australian Medical Association (AMA)

42 Macquarie St.
Barton, ACT 2600, Australia
**Phone:** 61 6 2705400     **Fax:** 61 6 2705499
**Email:** ama@com.au

**Fnded:** 1962.

---

### ★ 1997 ★ Australian Medical Council (AMC)

PO Box 4810
Kingston, ACT 2604, Australia
**Phone:** 61 2 62709777     **Fax:** 61 2 62709799
**Email:** amc@amc.org.au
**Website:** http://www.amc.org.au

**Fnded:** 1984. **Lang(s):** English. **Desc:** Academic and governmental groups associated with Australian medical standards. Functions as a national standards body for primary medical training. Advises and makes recommendations to State and Territory Medical Boards; maintains a national network of medical registers; provides advice to the Australian Health Ministry Advisory Council.

---

### ★ 1998 ★ Australian Medical Students' Association (AMSA)

Level 3, 33 Lincoln Square South
Carlton, VIC 3053, Australia
**Phone:** 61 3 93479566     **Fax:** 61 3 93478577
**Email:** mail@amsa.org.au
**Website:** http://www.amsa.org.au

**Mem:** 8,500. **Lang(s):** English. **Desc:** Medical students in Australia. Provides social activities, supplements members' intellectual development, and offers support for discovering life in the workforce.

---

### ★ 1999 ★ Australian and New Zealand Forensic Medicine Society (ANZFMS)

PO Box 2019
Templestowe Heights 3107, Australia
**Email:** ed.ogden@bigpond.com

---

### ★ 2000 ★ Australian and New Zealand Society of Nuclear Medicine (ANZSNM)

PO Box 7108
Upper Fern Tree Gulley, VIC 3156, Australia
**Phone:** 61 3 97560128     **Fax:** 61 3 97536372
**Email:** anzsnm@21century.com.au
**Website:** http://www.anzsnm.org.au

**Fnded:** 1969.

---

### ★ 2001 ★ Australian Physiotherapy Association

24 Logan Rd.
Woolloongabba, VIC 4102, Australia
**Phone:** 61 7 33917100     **Fax:** 61 7 33917283
**Email:** nationaloffice@physiotherapy.asn.au
**Website:** http://www.physiotherapy.asn.au

**Mem:** 10,200. **Nat'l Groups:** 11. **Lang(s):** English. **Desc:** Physiotherapists. Seeks to improve public health through advancing the science and practice of physiotherapy. Establishes standards of ethics, training, and practice for physiotherapists. Represents members' interests within the national health care system; supports research; conducts continuing professional development courses.

---

### ★ 2002 ★ Australian Society for Medical Research (ASMR)

145 Macquarie St.
Sydney, NSW 2000, Australia
**Phone:** 61 2 92565450     **Fax:** 61 2 92520294
**Email:** asmr@world.net
**Website:** http://www.asmr.org.au

**Fnded:** 1961. **Mem:** 1,200. **Lang(s):** English. **Desc:** Persons who are or have been engaged in the practice of medical research, including postgraduate students. Fosters excellence in Australian health and medical research and promotes community understanding and support. **Pub:** Newsletter, 3/year.

---

### ★ 2003 ★ Australian Women's Health Network (AWHN)

PO Box 400
Dickson, ACT 2609, Australia
**Phone:** 61 3 54447569     **Fax:** 61 3 54447977
**Website:** http://www.awhn.org.au/about.htm

**Fnded:** 1986. **Desc:** Aims to maintain and increase a national focus on women's health issues. Aims to be a national advocacy and information sharing organization.

---

### ★ 2004 ★ Auxiliary to the National Medical Association (ANMA)

1012 10th St. NW
Washington, DC 20001
**Phone:** (202)371-9008     **Fax:** (202)289-2662
**Email:** info@anma-online.org
**Website:** http://www.anma-online.org
Mrs. Maurce W. Ayton, Pres.

**Fnded:** 1935. **Mem:** 1,000. **Reg. Groups:** 6. **State Groups:** 14. **Local Groups:** 40. **Desc:** Spouses of active members of the National Medical Association; widows and widowers of former members. Purposes are to: create a greater interest in the NMA; assist and encourage the medical profession in its efforts to educate and serve the public in matters of sanitation and health; develop and promote a national program on health and education with subcategories in community needs, legislation, and human relations. Conducts workshops on teenage pregnancy, breast self-examinations, high blood pressure screening, and sickle cell anemia screening. Plans and implements an annual youth forum under the auspices of the March of Dimes Birth Defects Foundation . Provides youth with professional guidance and the opportunity for peer exchange in the areas of mental and physical health; deals with the health of newborns, health services, nutrition, and teenage pregnancy. Also conducts programs for youth on parenting, socially transmitted diseases, nutrition, birth defects, and continued education after pregnancy. **Pub:** Book.Covers standard procedures. • Membership Directory, periodic. *Price:* available to members only. • Newsletter, quarterly. **Frmly:** (1975) Women's Auxiliary to the National Medical Association.

**★ 2005 ★ Bangladesh Medical Association of North America (BMA)**
c/o S. Hasan
43700 Woodward, Ste. 210
Bloomfield Hills, MI 48302
**Fax:** (248)338-9520
**Website:** http://www.heartburnnet.com
F. Hasan, MD, Sec.

**Fnded:** 1982. **Mem:** 200. **Desc:** Physicians who are from Bangladesh or have graduated from a medical college in Bangladesh. Seeks to bring together and improve communication between physicians who are of Bangladeshi origin or have trained in Bangladesh, and are currently residents of the United States or Canada, and other physicians. Assists medical students and physicians in obtaining specialized medical training and in post-training job placement in North America.

**★ 2006 ★ Bangladesh Medical Studies and Research Institute (BMSRI)**
35 H Rd., No. 14 A
Dhanmondi Residential Area
Dhaka, Bangladesh
**Phone:** 880 2 9120792      **Fax:** 880 2 9125655
**Email:** bmch@bangla.net
**Website:** http://www.bmcbd.org

**Fnded:** 1984. **Mem:** 15. **Lang(s):** English. **Desc:** Promotes medical studies and research with the object of raising the standard of medical education in Bangladesh. Encourages growth in Bangladesh's pharmaceutical, medical, and surgical instrument industries. Conducts research in disease prevention and treatment and on medical applications of indigenous plants and herbs. Offers refresher courses and monthly academic seminar; organizes conferences, lectures, seminars, and study groups. Operates speakers' bureau. Maintains the Bangladesh Medical College which grants degrees in medicine and surgery and the Dental College which grants degrees in dentistry. **Pub:** *Annual Report and Prospectus*, annual. Directory. • *Bangladesh Medical College*, quarterly. Journal.

**★ 2007 ★ Barbados Association of Medical Practitioners (BAMP)**
c/o Dr. Ermine Belle, Pres.
BAMP Complex
Spring Garden
Saint Michael, Barbados
**Phone:** (246)429-7569      **Fax:** (246)435-2328
**Email:** bamp@sunbeach.net
**Website:** http://www.bamp.org.bb

**Mem:** 375. **Desc:** Promotes the medical and allied sciences and better health education of the community. Aims to maintain the honor and interests of the medical profession.

**★ 2008 ★ Berufsverband der Pharmaberater (BP)**
Europahaus
Postfach 18 30
D-67547 Worms, Germany
**Phone:** 49 6241 24239      **Fax:** 49 6241 24239
**Email:** bdp-wo@t-online.de
**Website:** http://www.pharmaberater-bdp.de

**Fnded:** 1973. **Mem:** 1,500. **Lang(s):** German. **Desc:** Medical advisers. Promotes professional advancement of members. Represents members' interests before industrial organizations, government agencies, and the public.

**★ 2009 ★ Berufsverband der Pharmarefenten Osterreichs (BPO)**
Geidorfgurtel 22/24/111
A-8010 Graz, Austria
**Phone:** 43 316 377800      **Fax:** 43 316 377800

**Lang(s):** German. **Desc:** Medical advisers. Promotes professional advancement of members. Represents members' interests before industrial organizations, government agencies, and the public.

**★ 2010 ★ Bill and Melinda Gates Foundation**
PO Box 23350
Seattle, WA 98102
**Phone:** (206)709-3140
**Email:** libraryinfo@gatesfoundation.org
**Website:** http://www.gatesfoundation.org
Richard Akeroyd, Exec. Dir.

**Desc:** Strives to help improve people's lives through health and learning and looks for strategic opportunities to extend the benefits of modern science and technology to people around the world.

**★ 2011 ★ Boston International Foundation for Medical Exchange**
c/o Joseph J. Vitale, MD
784 Massachusetts Ave.
Boston, MA 02118-2317
**Phone:** (617)414-4829
**Email:** jjvitale@bu.edu
**Website:** http://www.bifme.org
Joseph J. Vitale, Chm.

**Fnded:** 1996. **Mem:** 6. **Desc:** Supports senior medical students, medical and surgical residents and junior faculty from Harvard, Tufts and Boston University, who successfully complete a minimum two to six month elective at a foreign medical center acceptable to the respective medical school administration and the foundation. Support is intended to defray travel and living expenses. Believes this experience provides useful and practical insight into cultural, moral and ethnic perceptions of health care in our multi-ethnic and multi-cultural society.

**★ 2012 ★ Brazilian Society of Aesthetic Medicine (Sociedade Brasileira de Medicina Estetica)**
Av Rio Branco, 257 Ste. 906
20040-009 Rio de Janeiro, Brazil
**Fax:** 55 21 5244401
**Email:** sbme@congregare.com.br

**Fnded:** 1987. **Desc:** Organizes post-graduate courses of aesthetic medicine in association with the School of Medicine "Souza Marques" in Rio de Janeiro and Sao Paulo.

**★ 2013 ★ British In Vitro Diagnostics Association (BIVDA)**
1 Queen Anne's Gate
London SW1H 9BT, United Kingdom
**Phone:** 44 20 79574633      **Fax:** 44 20 79574644
**Email:** bvida@compuserve.com

**Lang(s):** English. **Desc:** Individuals and organizations in the IVD industry in the UK. Promotes the awareness of the value of diagnostics in the wider theatre of healthcare. Represents members' interests to the government, professional bodies, the public, and the European Diagnostic Manufacturers Association.

**★ 2014 ★ British Medical Association (BMA)**
Tavistock Sq.
London WC1H 9JP, United Kingdom
**Phone:** 44 20 73874499      **Fax:** 44 20 73836400
**Website:** http://www.bma.org.uk

**Fnded:** 1832. **Mem:** 124,000. **Local Groups:** 202. **Lang(s):** English. **Desc:** Doctors' trade union. A scientific and educational body and a publishing house. **Pub:** *BMA News Review*, monthly. Magazine. • *BMJ Specialist Journals*. Journal. • *British Medical Journal*, weekly. Journal. • *Student BMJ*. Journal. Reports and recommendations.

**★ 2015 ★ British Performing Arts Medicine Trust**
196 Shaftesbury Ave.
London WC2H 8JF, United Kingdom
**Phone:** 44 20 72403331      **Fax:** 44 20 72403335
**Email:** bpamt@dial.pipex.com

**Fnded:** 1987. **Mem:** 700. **Reg. Groups:** 2. **Desc:** Provides helpline and free assessment and diagnosis for performers with performance-related injuries and illnesses. **Frmly:** (2001) British Association for Performing Arts Medicine.

**★ 2016 ★ British Support Group - Inter-African Committee Against Harmful Traditional Practices**
Russell Lodge
Parkend
Lydney GL15 4HS, United Kingdom
**Phone:** 44 1594 562617
**Email:** johnholman@namloh.fsnet.co.uk

**Fnded:** 1990. **Lang(s):** English. **Desc:** Expresses solidarity with African women who struggle against traditional health practices which are harmful to their lives, health, and personal dignity. Raises funds and conducts research. Arouses public awareness through the media. Offers educational programs related to the population in Africa and African immigrants in Britain. **Pub:** Newsletter, bimonthly.

**★ 2017 ★ Business Alliance for Commerce in Hemp (IASPA) (Associazione Italiana Informatori Scientifici del Farmaco — AIISF)**
Via Turati 19
Casella Post. 4331
I-50136 Florence, Italy
**Phone:** 39 55 691166      **Fax:** 39 55 6503736

**Lang(s):** Italian. **Desc:** Businesses, consumers, and other individuals and organizations with an interest in hemp and hemp products. Promotes "full and unrestricted restoration of hemp as a sustainable farm crop and industrial resource;" seeks to legalize therapeutic use of marijuana and regulate adult consumption. Conducts lobbying, community organization, and outreach activities supporting hemp producers and consumers; consulting services; disseminates information on the commercial and industrial uses of hemp and the therapeutic benefits of marijuana.

**★ 2018 ★ Canadian Association for Anatomy, Neurobiology and Cell Biology (CAANCB)**
Department of Oral Biology, College of Dentistry
Univ. of Saskatchewan
107 Wiggins Rd.
Saskatoon, SK, Canada S7N 5E5
**Phone:** (306)966-5137      **Fax:** (306)966-5126
**Email:** devonr@duke.usask.ca

**Fnded:** 1957. **Mem:** 125. **Desc:** Represents members' interests. **Pub:** *Bulletin of the CAANCB/A-CANBC*, annual. Bulletin.

**★ 2019 ★ Canadian Association for Entrostomal Therapy (CAET)**
PO Box 48069
60 Dundas St., E
Mississauga, ON, Canada L5A 1W4
**Phone:** (905)270-8433      **Fax:** (905)270-8963
**Email:** caet@on.aibn.com
**Website:** http://www.caet.ca

**Fnded:** 1979. **Mem:** 280. **Reg. Groups:** 5. **Lang(s):** English, French. **Desc:** Health care professionals and medical facilities providing enterostomal therapy. Seeks to advance the practice of enterostomal therapy. Serves as a clearinghouse on enterostomal therapy; conducts continuing professional education courses. **Pub:** *Link*. Newsletter. Includes updates of focus groups and regional or membership news. • Journal, quarterly. Contains articles pertaining to wound, ostomy, incontinence and professional issues.

**★ 2020 ★ Canadian Association of Internes and Residents (CAIR)**
151 Slater St., Ste. 412
Ottawa, ON, Canada K1P 5H3
**Phone:** (613)234-6448     **Fax:** (613)234-5292
**Email:** cair@magma.ca
**Website:** http://www.cair.ca
**Fnded:** 1973. **Mem:** 6,000. **Lang(s):** English, French. **Desc:** Medical residents, interns, and other physicians-intraining. Promotes professional advancement of members. Represents members' interests before medical organizations, government agencies, and the public in matters including medical education, licensure, certification, and entry into practice.

**★ 2021 ★ Canadian Association for School Health (CASH)**
2835 Country Woods Dr.
Surrey, BC, Canada V4P 9P9
**Phone:** (604)535-7664     **Fax:** (604)531-6454
**Email:** dmccall@netcom.ca
**Website:** http://www.schoolfile.com/CASH.htm
**Lang(s):** English, French. **Desc:** School health services. Promotes increased availability and quality of school health programs. Serves as a clearinghouse on school health services; facilitates communication and cooperation among members.

**Canadian Council on Multicultural Health (CCMH)**
**(Conseil Canadien de la Sante Multiculturelle — CCSM)**
*See:* Entry 17929

**★ 2022 ★ Canadian Critical Care Society (CCCS)**
**(La Societe Canadienne de Soins Intensifs — SCSI)**
9 Eaton North, Rm. 242
Toronto General Hospital
Toronto, ON, Canada M5G 2C4
**Phone:** (416)340-3573     **Fax:** (416)595-9486
**Email:** deborah.wilson@uhn.on.ca
**Website:** http://www.canadiancriticalcare.org
**Lang(s):** English, French. **Desc:** Health care professionals specializing in the provision of critical care. Seeks to advance the practice of critical and intensive care; promotes ongoing professional development of members. Serves as a forum for the exchange of information among members; conducts continuing professional education courses.

**★ 2023 ★ Canadian Friends of the American-Israel Medical Foundation (CFAIMF)**
600 University Ave., Ste. 474
Toronto, ON, Canada M5G 1X5
**Phone:** (416)586-4473     **Fax:** (416)586-4507
**Lang(s):** English, French, Hebrew. **Desc:** Supporters of the American-Israel Medical Foundation and its programs. Seeks to advance the practice of medicine. Provides support and assistance to the programs of the American-Israel Medical Foundation.

**★ 2024 ★ Canadian Friends of Bikur Cholim Hospital of Jerusalem**
579 Old Orchard Grove
Toronto, ON, Canada M5M 2H2
**Phone:** (416)783-5773     **Fax:** (416)537-0487
**Fnded:** 1976. **Lang(s):** French. **Desc:** Solicits and collects donations to help support the Bikur Cholim Hospital. **Pub:** Newsletter.

**★ 2025 ★ Canadian Health Care Guild (CHCG)**
**(Guilde Canadienne de Soins de la Sante)**
4208 97th St., NO. 203
Edmonton, AB, Canada T6E 5Z9
**Phone:** (780)483-5800     **Fax:** (780)483-7404
**Lang(s):** English, French. **Desc:** Medical technicians, ambulance drivers, and other health care personnel. Seeks to obtain optimal conditions of employment for members. Represents members in negotiations with employers.

**★ 2026 ★ Canadian Home Care Association (CHCA)**
**(Association Canadienne de Soins et Services a Domicile — ACSSD)**
17 York St., Ste. 401
Ottawa, ON, Canada K1N 9J6
**Phone:** (613)569-1585     **Fax:** (613)569-1604
**Email:** chca@cdnhomecare.on.ca
**Website:** http://www.cdnhomecare.on.ca
**Lang(s):** English, French. **Desc:** Providers of home health care services. Promotes excellence in the practice of home care. Represents members' interests before medical organizations, government agencies, and the public. Conducts continuing professional development courses for home care personnel. Sponsors promotional programs. **Pub:** *Cnez Nous, At Home,* quarterly. Newsletter.

**★ 2027 ★ Canadian Institute of Stress (CIS)**
Medcan Clinic Office
Ste. 1500, 150 York St.
Toronto, ON, Canada M5H 3S5
**Phone:** (416)236-4218
**Email:** earle@idirect.com
**Website:** http://www.stresscanada.org
**Fnded:** 1979. **Lang(s):** English. **Desc:** Works to educate workplaces, communities, and individuals in change-abilities and risk management strategies for successful, not stressful transitions. Provides clinical assessment, counseling, and coaching; develops specialized change and risk management services; conducts research; and sponsors professional certification programs.

**★ 2028 ★ Canadian Intramural Recreation Association (CIRA)**
740-B, rue Befast
Ottawa, ON, Canada K1G 0Z5
**Phone:** (613)244-1594     **Fax:** (613)244-4738
**Email:** cira@intramurals.ca
**Website:** http://www.intramurals.ca
**Fnded:** 1977. **Mem:** 800. **Lang(s):** English, French. **Desc:** Seeks to encourage, promote and develop active living, healthy lifestyle and personal growth through intramural and recreational programs within the educational community. **Pub:** Catalog, periodic. Contains more than 160 resources. • Bulletin, 8/year.

**★ 2029 ★ Canadian Medical Association**
1867 Alta Vista Dr.
Ottawa, ON, Canada K1G 5W8
**Free:** 800-457-4205     **Fax:** (613)236-8864
**Email:** cmamsc@cma.ca
**Website:** http://www.cma.ca
**Desc:** Seeks to improve medical care for persons living in Canada. Works to maintain high standards of hospital care and health related services. Encourages constant improvement in the medical profession.

**★ 2030 ★ Canadian Medical Protective Association (CMPA)**
**(Association Canadienne de Protection Medicale — ACPM)**
PO Box 8225, Sta. T
Ottawa, ON, Canada K1G 3H7
**Phone:** (613)725-2000     **Free:** 800-267-6522
**Fax:** (613)725-1300
**Website:** http://www.cmpa.org
**Lang(s):** English, French. **Desc:** Physicians and other health care professionals. Seeks to protect the commercial and professional interests of members. Provides support and assistance to medical professionals; advocates legal reform.

**★ 2031 ★ Canadian Organization for Rare Disorders (CORD)**
PO Box 814
Coaldale, AB, Canada T1M 1M7
**Phone:** (403)345-4544     **Free:** 877-302-7273
**Fax:** (403)345-3948
**Email:** office@cord.ca
**Website:** http://www.cord.ca
**Fnded:** 1987. **Lang(s):** English. **Desc:** People suffering from rare disorders and their families. Works to enhance the lives of all persons affected by rare disorders through an educational and informational support network. Provides information on more than 6,000 rare disorders.

**★ 2032 ★ Canadian Post-MD Education Registry (CAPER)**
774 Echo Dr.
Ottawa, ON, Canada K1S 5P2
**Phone:** (613)730-1204
**Email:** caper@acmc.ca
**Website:** http://www.caper.ca
**Lang(s):** English, French. **Desc:** National data source concerning post-MD (residency) training. Provides information concerning the number and type of residents in Canadian training programs. **Pub:** *CAPER Annual Census of Post-M.D. Trainees,* annual. Directory.

**★ 2033 ★ Canadian Sleep Society (CSS)**
3080 Yonge St., Ste. 5055
Toronto, ON, Canada M4N 3N1
**Phone:** (416)483-6260     **Fax:** (416)483-7081
**Website:** http://www.css.to
**Fnded:** 1986. **Mem:** 226. **Lang(s):** English, French. **Desc:** Scientists, health care professionals, students, and other individuals with an interest in sleep; corporations manufacturing sleep-related products. Promotes increased understanding of sleep and sleep disorders and their treatment. Sponsors research and educational programs. **Pub:** *Vigilance,* 3/year. Newsletter. • Brochure.

**★ 2034 ★ Canadian Society of Internal Medicine (CSIM)**
**(Societe Canadienne de Medicine Interne — SCMI)**
774 Echo Dr.
Ottawa, ON, Canada K1S 5N8
**Phone:** (613)730-6244     **Fax:** (613)730-1116
**Email:** csim@rcpsc.edu
**Website:** http://www.csim.medical.org
**Fnded:** 1984. **Mem:** 700. **Lang(s):** English, French. **Desc:** Physicians with an interest in internal medicine. Seeks to advance the study and practice of internal medicine. Serves as a forum for the exchange of information among members; sponsors research and educational programs. **Pub:** *The General Internist,* quarterly. Newsletters.

**★ 2035 ★ Canadians for Health Research (CHR)**
**(Canadiens pour la Recherche Medicale — CRM)**
PO Box 126
Westmount, QC, Canada H3Z 2T1
**Phone:** (514)398-7478     **Fax:** (514)398-8361
**Email:** info@chrcrm.org
**Website:** http://www.chrcrm.org
**Fnded:** 1976. **Mem:** 400. **Lang(s):** English, French. **Desc:** Health care professionals and scientists with an interest in health research. Seeks to advance medical research; promotes continuing professional development of members. Serves as a forum for the exchange of information among members; sponsors research and educational programs. **Pub:** *The Diary,* quarterly. Newsletter. Contains information devoted to experi-

mental animal issues, including summaries of national and international animal rights activities. • *Future Health/Perspectives Sante*, quarterly. Magazine. Contains Canadian health research news.

---

**★ 2036 ★ Carers Association**
c/o St. Mary's Community Center
Richmond Hill
Rathmines
Dublin 6, Ireland
**Phone:** 353 1 4974498     **Fax:** 353 1 4976108
**Email:** carers@tinet.ie
**Fnded:** 1987. **Mem:** 8,000. **Reg. Groups:** 42. **Desc:** Care-givers who provide high levels of care in their own homes for family members and neighbors. Provides home-based respite services. Disseminates information; conducts educational programs. **Pub:** Journal, quarterly.

---

**★ 2037 ★ Carers National Association**
Ruth Pitter House
20-25 Glass House Yard
London EC1A 4JS, United Kingdom
**Phone:** 44 207 4908818     **Fax:** 44 207 4908824
**Website:** http://www.carersuk.demon.co.uk
**Fnded:** 1988. **Mem:** 12,000. **Reg. Groups:** 120. **Desc:** Provides information and support to carers, persons who provide assistance and support to ill, disabled, or elderly individuals. Encourages carers to recognize and work towards meeting their own needs as caregivers through actively participating in social issues and legislative development that affects care givers and recipients. Offers training programs for professionals. **Pub:** *The Carer*, bimonthly. Newsletter. • Brochures, bimonthly.

---

**★ 2038 ★ Catholic Health Association of Canada**
1247 Kilborn Pl.
Ottawa, ON, Canada K1H 6K9
**Phone:** (613)731-7148     **Fax:** (613)731-7797
**Email:** chac@web.ca
**Website:** http://www.chac.ca
**Fnded:** 1939. **Lang(s):** English, French. **Desc:** Works to administer Christian principles within the Canadian healthcare system. Fosters competent and efficient health care services. Disseminates health information.

---

**★ 2039 ★ Catholic Health Association of the United States (CHA)**
4455 Woodson Rd.
Saint Louis, MO 63134-3797
**Phone:** (314)427-2500     **Fax:** (314)427-0029
**Email:** webmaster@chausa.org
**Website:** http://www.chausa.org
Rev. Michael D. Place, Pres. & CEO
**Fnded:** 1915. **Mem:** 2,000. **Desc:** Catholic hospitals, health care facilities, religious orders, health care systems, and extended care facilities. Aims to participate in the life of the Church by advancing the healthcare ministry and assert leadership within the Church and society through programs of advocacy, facilitation, and education. Conducts surveys; compiles statistics. **Pub:** *Catholic Health Care in the USA*, periodic. Directory. Current online listing of Catholic organizations providing care and sponsoring or operating facilities. • *Catholic Health World*, bimonthly, except Jan. and Aug.Newspaper. Reports on the health care ministry. Includes *Catholic Health Association Assembly. Price:* Included in membership dues; $35/year for nonmembers. • *Catholic Long-Term Care Facilities and Services Online Directory*, periodic. Directory. Online directory that details current list of facilities and services for long term care needs. • *Health Progress*, bimonthly. Journal. Addresses the administrative, ethical, financial, legal, and political problems faced by Catholic health care administrators. *Price:* Included in membership dues; $50/year for nonmembers. **Frmly:** Catholic Hospital Association of U.S. and Canada; (1979) Catholic Hospital Association.

---

**★ 2040 ★ Catholic Medical Association (CMA)**
PO Box 757
N27 W23957 Paul Rd., Ste. 202
Pewaukee, WI 53072
**Phone:** (262)523-6201     **Fax:** (262)523-6211
**Email:** info@cathmed.org
**Website:** http://www.cathmed.org
Michael J. Herzog, Exec. Dir.
**Fnded:** 1932. **Mem:** 3,500. **Local Groups:** 90. **Desc:** Catholic physicians and dentists dedicated to upholding the principles of the Catholic faith in the practice of medicine. **Pub:** *The Linacre Quarterly*, quarterly. Journal. Bioethics journal. **Frmly:** (1998) National Federation of Catholic Physicians Guilds.

---

**★ 2041 ★ Center for Medical Consumers (CMC)**
130 MacDougal St.
New York, NY 10012-5030
**Phone:** (212)674-7105     **Fax:** (212)674-7100
**Email:** medconsumers@earthlink.net
**Website:** http://www.medicalconsumers.org
Arthur Aaron Levin, Dir.
**Fnded:** 1976. **Desc:** Advocacy group on health and medical information at the state and local legislative level. **Pub:** *HealthFacts*, monthly. Newsletter. Helps consumers determine the risks and effectiveness of common medical procedures. Presents all treatment options, including nonmedical. *Price:* $25/year. • Reports. **Frmly:** (1998) Center for Medical Consumers and Health Care Information.

---

**★ 2042 ★ Centra-Cam Vocational Training Association (CCVTA)**
PO Box 1443
Camrose, AB, Canada T4V 1X4
**Phone:** (780)672-9995     **Fax:** (780)672-0534
**Email:** cctva@centracam.ca
**Fnded:** 1979. **Mem:** 25. **Lang(s):** English, French. **Desc:** Individuals with an interest in the vocational training of adults with disabilities. Seeks to improve the quality of life of people with disabilities; encourages employers to hire qualified people with disabilities. Assists in the integration of adults with disabilities into society; sponsors training programs for people providing vocational education to individuals with disabilities.

---

**★ 2043 ★ Central American Health Institute (ICAS)**
Apartado 6-2010
Zapote
San Jose, Costa Rica
**Phone:** 506 221 5278     **Fax:** 506 258 3843
**Email:** costarico@icas.net
**Website:** http://www.icas.net
**Fnded:** 1993. **Mem:** 25. **Reg. Groups:** 3. **Lang(s):** English, Spanish. **Desc:** Promotes improvement to the health of the population of Central America.

---

**★ 2044 ★ Centre for Health Education, Training and Nutrition Awareness (CHETNA)**
Lilavatiben Laibhai's Bungalow
Civil Camp Rd.
Shahibaug
Ahmedabad 380 004, Gujarat, India
**Phone:** 91 79 2866695     **Fax:** 91 79 2866513
**Email:** chetna@iccnet.net.in
**Lang(s):** English, Gujarati, Hindi. **Desc:** Promotes development of regional health programs with a feminist perspective. Works to expand understanding of women's health beyond matters of maternal and child health; examines gender relations as they impact on women's health; develops local health care capabilities through encouragement of appropriate traditional treatments; trains women to manage local and regional health care programs. Main program areas include: early childhood care and development; school health; adolescent health; women's health and development; promotion of traditional health practices; and gender

---

and development. Activities include: training; documentation of innovative efforts; creating educational material, and networking and advocacy. **Pub:** *CHETNA News*, quarterly. Newsletter. Contain current activity profiles. • *List of Material.* Directory. • Manual. Also publishes manuals, posters, and charts.

---

**★ 2045 ★ Centre Muraz**
01 Boite Postale 153
Bobo-Dioulasso 01, Burkina Faso
**Phone:** 226 970102     **Fax:** 226 970457
**Email:** direction.muraz@fasonet.bf
**Website:** http://www.multimania.com/centremuraz
**Lang(s):** English, French. **Desc:** Medical researchers and health care professionals. Promotes improved diagnostic techniques and treatments of common diseases. Conducts research and educational programs; makes available health services.

---

**★ 2046 ★ Centre for Women's Health**
6 Sandyford Pl.
Sauchiehall St.
Glasgow G3 7NB, United Kingdom
**Phone:** 44 141 2116700     **Fax:** 44 141 2116702
**Email:** cfwh@dial.pipex.com
**Website:** http://www.sandyford.com
**Fnded:** 1994. **Desc:** Seeks to promote women's health. Offers counseling services and groups for women. Provides a training center and meeting place. Conducts studies on the quality of existing women's health services. Disseminates information and provides an extensive information an library service and links to health service and local authority prevision.

---

**★ 2047 ★ Chi Delta Mu**
PO Box 1
River Edge, NJ 07661-0001
**Phone:** (201)842-1111     **Free:** 800-484-7593
**Fax:** (201)842-0222
**Email:** mollynj@hotmail.com
**Website:** http://www.geocities.com/westhollywood/heights/7396/
Tracy M. Walton, Jr., Sec.
**Fnded:** 1913. **Mem:** 650. **State Groups:** 7. **Desc:** To improve relationships among physicians, dentists, and pharmacists so that they may better serve their respective communities. Maintains revolving loan funds. **Pub:** *Chi Delta Mu News*, quarterly. Newsletter. • *Dragon*, annual. Magazine. • Proceedings, annual.

---

**★ 2048 ★ China Medical Board of New York (CMBNY)**
750 3rd Ave., 23rd Fl.
New York, NY 10017-2703
**Phone:** (212)682-8000     **Fax:** (212)949-8726
**Email:** administrator@chinamedicalboard.org
**Website:** http://www.chinamedicalboard.org/
M. Roy Schwarz, MD, Pres.
**Fnded:** 1928. **Desc:** Purpose is to support programs of medical, nursing, and public health education and research. Assists institutions in East and Southeast Asia in improving the health levels and services in Asian societies. Seeks to improve the quality and increase the numbers of appropriate health practitioners in these societies. Has programs in Korea, Taiwan, Hong Kong, the Philippines, Thailand, Malaysia, Myanmar, Singapore, Indonesia, Mongolia, Vietnam, Laos, and China. Endowed by the Rockefeller Foundation and controlled by an independent board of trustees who serve without compensation. Formerly devoted entire income to support of Peking Union Medical College, nationalized in 1949 by People's Republic of China. **Pub:** *China Medical Board of New York–Annual Report.* Includes list of grants and endowments made during year of report. *Price:* Free.

---

**★ 2049 ★ Chinese American Medical Society (CAMS)**
c/o Dr. H.H. Wang
281 Edgewood Ave.
Teaneck, NJ 07666

**Phone:** (201)833-1506          **Fax:** (201)833-8252
**Email:** hw5@columbia.edu
**Website:** http://www.camsociety.org
Dr. Daisy Saw, MD, Pres.

**Fnded:** 1962. **Mem:** 850. **Reg. Groups:** 4. **Desc:** Physicians of Chinese origin residing in the U.S. and Canada. Seeks to advance medical knowledge, scientific research, and interchange of information among members and to promote the health status of Chinese Americans. Conducts educational meetings; supports research. Maintains placement service. Sponsors limited charitable program. **Pub:** *Chinese American Medical Society–Newsletter*, 3-4/year. Newsletter. Includes membership news, annoucements, and calendar of events. *Price:* Included in membership dues. • Membership Directory, annual. **Frmly:** (1985) American Chinese Medical Society.

★ **2050** ★ **Chinese Association of Integrated Traditional and Western Medicine**
18 Beixincang, Dongzhimennei
Beijing, People's Republic of China
**Phone:** 852 10 64014411

★ **2051** ★ **Chinese Medical Association**
42 Dongsi Xidajie
Beijing 100710, People's Republic of China
**Phone:** 86 10 65250394    **Fax:** 86 10 65123754
**Email:** infor@chinamed.com.cn
**Website:** http://www.chinamed.com.cn
**Fnded:** 1915. **Mem:** 250,000. **Desc:** Physicians in the People's Republic of China. Promotes the advancement of medical science and technology. Conducts information exchanges among physicians in China and in other countries. Conducts and analyzes medical research programs. Gathers and disseminates medical research data. Develops and approves medical terminology. Offers training programs to members.

★ **2052** ★ **Chinese Society for Anatomical Sciences**
c/o Xu Qunyuan, Pres.
42 Dongsi Xidajie
Beijing 100710, People's Republic of China
**Phone:** 86 10 65257568    **Fax:** 86 10 65257568
**Email:** csas@public.bta.net.cn
**Mem:** 7,000. **Desc:** Seeks to enhance the friendship and cooperation between anatomists not only domestic but also international members and groups, to promote the development of the Anatomical Sciences.

★ **2053** ★ **Christian Health Association of Kenya (CHAK)**
PO Box 30690
Nairobi, Kenya
**Phone:** 254 2 441920    **Fax:** 254 2 440306
**Email:** chak@insightkenya.com
**Fnded:** 1930. **Mem:** 230. **Reg. Groups:** 4. **Lang(s):** English. **Desc:** Fosters improved health in Kenya through programs in health education. Compiles statistics on youth and population. Disseminates information. Organizes training courses in health, AIDS/HIV prevention, essential drugs program and family planning. Provides forum for members to network. Acts as advocate with the government Ministry of Health and donors on behalf of members. **Pub:** *AIDS for Health Workers*. Manuals. • *CHAK Quarterly News*, quarterly. Newsletter.

★ **2054** ★ **Christian Medical and Dental Associations (CMDA)**
PO Box 7500
Bristol, TN 37621
**Phone:** (423)844-1000    **Fax:** (423)844-1005
**Email:** main@cmdahome.org
**Website:** http://www.cmdahome.org
David Stevens, MD, Exec. Dir.
**Fnded:** 1931. **Mem:** 15,000. **Reg. Groups:** 6. **Desc:** Serves as a voice and ministry for Christian doctors. Its mission is to "change the heart of healthcare."

Promotes positions and addresses policies on health care issues; conducts overseas and domestic medical mission projects; coordinates a network of Christian doctors for fellowship and professional growth; sponsors student ministries in medical and dental schools; distributes educational and inspirational resources; holds marriage and family conferences; provides Third World missionary doctors with continuing education resources; and conducts academic exchange programs overseas. **Pub:** *Christian Doctor's Digest*, 8/year. Magazine. • *Today's Christian Doctor*, quarterly. Journal. Contains articles on medical and ethical issues. *Price:* Included in membership dues. • Brochure. • SCAN is distributed free to doctors serving in foreign countries; public service announcements - CMDS Healthwise (quarterly, CD format). **Frmly:** (1988) Christian Medical Society; (1998) Medical Group Missions of the Christian Medical and Dental Society; (2000) Christian Medical and Dental Society; (2000) Global Health Outreach of the Christian Medical and Dental Society.

★ **2055** ★ **Christian Medical and Dental Society of Canada (CMDS)**
23 Old Hastings Rd.
PO Box 160
Warkworth, ON, Canada K0K 3K0
**Phone:** (705)924-3246    **Free:** 888-256-8653
**Fax:** (705)924-3384
**Email:** cmdsemas@oncomdis.on.ca
**Website:** http://www.cmdsemas.ca
**Fnded:** 1970. **Mem:** 1,300. **Reg. Groups:** 14. **Lang(s):** English, French. **Desc:** Christian physicians, dentists, and medical and dental students. Seeks to present "a positive witness of God our Father and our Saviour, Jesus Christ, to the medical and dental professions and to the recipients of health care." Serves as a Christian voice within the medical community and before government agencies, medical and dental associations, policy makers, and patients. Facilitates communication among members; makes available to members opportunities for overseas voluntary service; sponsors social and fellowship activities. **Pub:** *Focus*, 3/year. Magazine. • *NUCLEUS*, quarterly. Journal. • *Spotlight*, periodic. Newsletter.

★ **2056** ★ **Christian Medical Foundation International (CMF)**
4009 N Lynn Ave.
Tampa, FL 33603
**Phone:** (813)932-3688    **Fax:** (813)232-4745
**Email:** cmfintl@aol.com
**Website:** http://www.wwmedical.com/cmf/
William Standish Reed, MD, Pres.
**Fnded:** 1962. **Mem:** 4,854. **State Groups:** 4. **Desc:** Physicians, nurses, clergy, and laity. Seeks to: investigate and promote the Christian spiritual care of those who are ill; educate doctors, nurses, and medical students regarding Christian medical and ethical principles. Maintains speakers' bureau, placement service, biographical archives, and 2500 volume library; sponsors charitable programs. **Pub:** *Progress Notes*, bimonthly. • Also publishes books and monographs.

★ **2057** ★ **Chronic Fatigue Immune Dysfunction Syndrome (CFIDS) Activation Network (CAN)**
PO Box 345
Larchmont, NY 10538
**Phone:** (212)280-4726    **Fax:** (914)636-6515
**Email:** cfidsnet@aol.com
Ms. Jane Perlmutter, Contact
**Fnded:** 1991. **Mem:** 1,000. **Desc:** Works to prompt government into action on research issues concerning Chronic Fatigue Immune Disfunction Syndrome (CFIDS). (CFIDS is a disease that affects women more than men and causes flu-like symptoms such as aches, pains, and muscle weakness.) Promotes public awareness and knowledge of the disease. Provides information on CFIDS on local and national television and radio. Maintains political action committee to obtain government funding for further research. Compiles statistics. **Pub:** *CAN Bulletin*, monthly. Newsletter. Contains advocacy updates. *Price:* Free.

★ **2058** ★ **Chronic Pain Support Group (CPSG)**
PO Box 148
Peninsula, OH 44264
**Phone:** (216)526-1530
**Email:** cps.group@cpsg.22n.com
**Website:** http://www.chronicpainsupport.org/
Karen Moss Hale, Dir.
**Fnded:** 1985. **Desc:** Individuals suffering from chronic pain and their families and friends. Provides a forum for pain sufferers to help themselves through communication with other members. Promotes public awareness of chronic pain and its victims; encourages medical research on causes and treatments. Operates speakers' bureau; conducts educational programs. **Pub:** *Stop Pain*, monthly. Newsletter. Covers coping skills. *Price:* $25/year.

★ **2059** ★ **Churches Medical Council (CMC)**
PO Box 3269
Boroko, Papua New Guinea
**Phone:** 675 3252362    **Fax:** 675 3013898
**Email:** cmcpng@datron.com.pg
**Fnded:** 1960. **Mem:** 24. **Nat'l Groups:** 1. **Reg. Groups:** 4. **State Groups:** 18. **Lang(s):** English. **Desc:** Health care programs and services operated by religious organizations. Promotes effective delivery of health care to previously underserved populations. Facilitates communication and cooperation among members. Sponsors public health and educational programs; makes available health services.

★ **2060** ★ **City of Hope (COH)**
1500 E Duarte Rd.
Duarte, CA 91010
**Phone:** (626)359-8111    **Free:** 800-826-HOPE
**Fax:** (626)301-8115
**Email:** kkoga@coh.org
**Website:** http://www.cityofhope.org
Elaine Goehner, Contact
**Fnded:** 1913. **Desc:** Supports the National Pilot Medical Center and the Beckman Research Institute, which are engaged in treatment, research, and medical education in catastrophic diseases including cancer; leukemia; blood, heart and lung diseases; certain hereditary maladies; and metabolic disorders, such as diabetes. Patient care is available on a national and nonsectarian basis. Provides physician referrals. Offers free consulting service to doctors and hospitals. Seeks to influence medicine and science through 80 pilot research programs. From its staff and 200 laboratories, during the past decade over 3000 original findings have emerged in diseases treated as well as studies in diabetes, Alzheimer's disease, AIDS, Huntington's disease, genetics, and brain and nerve function. Receives nationwide support from nearly 500 chartered auxiliaries in over 230 cities, 32 states and Washington, DC, and from management, labor, fraternal and benevolent organizations, individuals, and special campaigns.

★ **2061** ★ **Clinical Directors Network (CDN)**
54 W 39TH St Fl 11
New York, NY 10018-3808
**Email:** info@cdnetwork.org
**Website:** http://www.cdnetwork.org
Jonathan N. Tobin, Exec. Dir.
**Fnded:** 1985. **Mem:** 15. **Desc:** Provides clinical leaders and staff at community, migrant, HIV and homeless health centers with educational meetings and peer support activities. Also, improves access of minority communities to clinical research. **Pub:** Annual Report, annual. • Brochure, annual.

**★ 2062 ★ Clowns Without Borders**
Payasos Sin Fronteras
Passatge Prunera, 3
08004 Barcelona, Spain
**Phone:** 34 93 4230494 **Fax:** 34 93 4268697
**Email:** psf@clowns.org
**Website:** http://www.clowns.org
**Fnded:** 1993. **Mem:** 700. **Desc:** Seeks to improve the psychological condition of populations living in refugee camps and areas of conflict, by organising volunteer artist preformances and sociocultural workshops; and to raise our society's awareness of the situation of affected populations and to promote a spirit of solidarity.

**★ 2063 ★ Coalition for Healthy Korean Americans (COHKA)**
196 Harvard Ave., Ste. 4
Allston, MA 02134
**Email:** sonnykim@cohka.org
**Desc:** Promotes better health through education. Health care services include cancer screening and dental care. Also offers health insurance, HIV prevention, immunization, and smoking cessation programs.

**★ 2064 ★ Coalition of National Health Education Organizations (CNHEO)**
c/o Ellen M. Capwell, PhD, CHES
Otterbein College
Department of Health & Physical Education
Rike Center
Westerville, OH 43081
**Phone:** (614)823-3535 **Fax:** (614)823-1966
**Email:** ecapwell@otterbein.edu
**Website:** http://hsc.usf.edu/CFH/cnheo/
Ellen M. Capwell, PhD, Coordinator
**Fnded:** 1972. **Desc:** Nine national health education organizations, each represented by a delegate and an alternate. Facilitates coordination, collaboration and communication among the member organizations, to identify and discuss profession wide issues. Formulates recommendations, takes appropriate action, communicates information to the health education field, and serves as a focus for collaborative initiatives.

**★ 2065 ★ Coalition for Nonprofit Health Care Research and Development (CNHCRD)**
c/o T.J. Sullivan
1301 K St. NW, Ste. 900E
Washington, DC 20005-3317
**Phone:** (202)408-7170 **Fax:** (202)289-1504
**Email:** info@cnhc.org
**Website:** http://www.cnhc.org
Boone Powell, Jr., Chr.
**Fnded:** 1997. **Mem:** 27. **Desc:** Nonprofit health care institutions and systems. Seeks to "ensure the continued survival of a primarily nonprofit, tax exempt health care delivery system." Works to improve communication between health care providers, plans, community organizations, and government agencies. Conducts grass roots public education programs; sponsors advocacy campaigns; undertakes research projects. **Pub:** *Coalition for Nonprofit Health Care.* Brochure.

**★ 2066 ★ College of Family Physicians of Canada (CFPC)**
**(College des Medecins de Famille du Canada — CMFC)**
2630 Skymark Ave.
Mississauga, ON, Canada L4W 5A4
**Phone:** (905)629-0900 **Fax:** (905)629-0893
**Email:** info@cfpc.ca
**Website:** http://www.cfpc.ca
**Fnded:** 1954. **Mem:** 15,000. **State Groups:** 10. **Lang(s):** English, French. **Desc:** National medical association of family physicians and general practitioners. Members must maintain a minimum of 50 hours of continuing medical education credits annually. Works to maintain standards of family medicine training in the 16 Canadian medical schools through support of the

Departments of Family Medicine and the accreditation of family practice residency programs. Administers certification examinations in emergency medicine and family medicine. Runs practice assessment program. Offers public education programs on family medicine topics. **Pub:** *Canadian Family Physician,* monthly. Journal. • *CFPC-Liaison Newsletter,* quarterly. Newsletter. • *Self-Evaluation,* bimonthly. Home study program.

**★ 2067 ★ Command Trust Network (CTN)**
PO Box 17082
Covington, KY 41017-0082
**Fax:** (606)331-0055
Kathleen Anneken, Exec. Officer
**Fnded:** 1988. **Desc:** Individuals concerned with the effects of silicone breast implants. Seeks to inform the public and motivate women with implants to consider all possible options. Disseminates information on medical studies, legal referrals, research, choosing a doctor, implant removel procedures, and other related topics. Maintains speakers' bureau for consumer, medical, or legal meetings on breast implants. **Pub:** Newsletter, quarterly.

**★ 2068 ★ Committee of Interns and Residents (CIR)**
386 Park Ave. S, Rm. 1502
New York, NY 10016
**Phone:** (212)725-5500 **Free:** 800-247-8877
**Fax:** (212)779-2413
**Email:** info@cirseiu.org
**Website:** http://www.cirseiu.org
Mark Levy, Exec. Dir.
**Fnded:** 1957. **Mem:** 11,000. **Desc:** Medical and dental interns, residents, chief residents, and fellows (collectively referred to as house staff officers) at 60 member hospitals located in California, Florida, New York, New Jersey, and Washington, DC. Purposes include representing house staff in matters pertaining to compensation, benefits, hours, working conditions, and other issues affecting their employment, education, training, and the quality of health services and patient care. **Pub:** *CIR News,* quarterly. Newsletter. **Frmly:** (1974) Committee of Interns and Residents in New York City.

**★ 2069 ★ The Commonwealth Fund**
1 E 75th St.
New York, NY 10021
**Phone:** (212)606-3800 **Fax:** (212)606-3500
**Email:** cmwf@cmwf.com
**Website:** http://www.cmwf.org/
Karen Davis, Pres.
**Desc:** Social scientists, health care professionals, and other individuals and organizations with an interest in health and social issues. Seeks to improve the quality and availability of health care services in the United States, particularly among elderly, minority, and economically disadvantaged communities. Conducts research on health and social issues; assists government agencies and health care organizations seeking to reform public health policies and delivery systems in the United States.

**★ 2070 ★ Commonwealth Medical Association (CMA)**
BMA House
Tavistock Sq.
London WC1H 9JP, United Kingdom
**Phone:** 44 20 72728492 **Fax:** 44 20 72721663
**Email:** office@commat.org
**Website:** http://www.commat.org
**Fnded:** 1962. **Mem:** 38. **Nat'l Groups:** 38. **Reg. Groups:** 6. **Lang(s):** English. **Desc:** National medical associations in Commonwealth countries. Provides technical assistance and cooperation to the national medical associations of Commonwealth developing countries. Offers educational programs and conducts projects in areas such as reproductive health, women's health, youth health, medical ethics and human rights. Conducts studies; acts as a clearinghouse for

news and information. **Pub:** *Manual on Ethics and Human Rights Standards for Health Professionals.*

**★ 2071 ★ Comprehensive Health Education Foundation (CHEF)**
22419 Pacific Hwy. S
Seattle, WA 98198
**Phone:** (206)824-2907 **Free:** 800-323-2433
**Fax:** (206)824-3072
**Email:** chefstaff@chef.org
**Website:** http://www.chef.org
Larry Clark, Pres. & CEO
**Fnded:** 1974. **Desc:** Encourages and supports improvement of health through education. Seeks to improve health education in the schools and community, enhance the public image of health educators, and stimulate community support of health education. Produces and disseminates health education information and materials. Initiates and supports innovations in health education. Supports the Health Education Fund, which sponsors pilot programs, offers scholarships for health education studies, and bestows leadership/recognition and professional enrichment awards.

**★ 2072 ★ Consortium of Institutes of Higher Education in Health and Rehabilitation in Europe (COHEHRE)**
Elfde Liniestraat 24
B-3500 Hasselt, Belgium
**Fnded:** 1990.

**★ 2073 ★ Council for International Organizations of Medical Sciences (CIOMS)**
**(Conseil des Organisations Internationales des Sciences Medicales)**
World Health Org.
Ave. Appia
CH-1211 Geneva 27, Switzerland
**Phone:** 41 22 7913406 **Fax:** 41 22 7913111
**Email:** cioms@who.ch
**Website:** http://www.cioms.ch
**Fnded:** 1949. **Mem:** 103. **Lang(s):** English, French. **Desc:** International organizations of medical sciences. Promotes and coordinates medical and scientific activities of member associations and national institutions affiliated with the council. Maintains collaborative relations with the World Health Organization and United Nations Educational, Scientific and Cultural Organization. Serves the scientific interests of the international biomedical community. **Pub:** *International Nomenclature of Diseases.* • *Proceedings of Round Table Conferences.* • Directory, periodic.

**★ 2074 ★ Council of Medical Specialty Societies (CMSS)**
51 Sherwood Ter., Ste. M
Lake Bluff, IL 60044-2232
**Phone:** (847)295-3456 **Fax:** (847)295-3759
**Email:** mailbox@cmss.org
**Website:** http://www.cmss.org
Rebecca R. Gschwend, MA,MBA, Exec. VP
**Fnded:** 1965. **Mem:** 17. **Desc:** National medical specialty societies representing 325,000 physicians. Purpose is to improve the quality of medical care in the United States and to foster excellence in the education of physicians. Provides a forum for discussion by specialty societies of national issues affecting the practice and teaching of medicine. Promotes communication among specialty organizations involved in the principal disciplines of medicine. **Frmly:** Tri-College Council.

**★ 2075 ★ Council for Professions Supplementary to Medicine**
Park House
184 Kensington Park Rd.
London SE11 4BU, United Kingdom
**Phone:** 44 171 5820866 **Fax:** 44 171 8209684

**Website:** http://www.cpsm.org.uk

**Fnded:** 1960. **Mem:** 110,000. **Desc:** Those wishing to practise as state registered arts therapists, chiropodists, dietitians, medical laboratory scientific officers, occupational therapists, orthoptists, prosthetists/orthotists, physiotherapists, radiographers, clinical scientists, paramedics, or speech and language pathologists must register at CPSM. State Registration is required for the NHS. and Local Authority Social Services and is a universal kitemark of professional excellence. To implement as effectively as possible the Professions Supplementary to Medicines Act, 1960, and EC Directives 89/48 and 92/51 with particular reference to the duty laid on the Council at Boards by Parliament, of promoting high standards of professional education and professional conduct. **Pub:** Annual Report, annual.

### ★ 2076 ★ Cushing's Support and Research Foundation (CSRF)

c/o Louise Pace
65 E India Row, Ste. 22-B
Boston, MA 02110
**Phone:** (617)723-3674
**Email:** csrf@world.std.com
**Website:** http://world.std.com/~csrf/welcome.html
Louise Pace, Pres.

**Mem:** 300. **Desc:** Provides information and support for Cushing's Disease and Cushing's Syndrome patients and their families; increases awareness, educates the public about Cushing's Disease and Cushing's Syndrome; provides information and support to health care professionals; raises and distribute funds for Cushing's Disease and Cushing's Syndrome research. **Pub:** Newsletter.

### ★ 2077 ★ Cyprus Medical Representatives Association (CMRA)

PO Box 2134
Nicosia, Cyprus

**Lang(s):** English, Greek, Turkish. **Desc:** Medical advisers. Promotes professional advancement of members. Represents members' interests before industrial organizations, government agencies, and the public.

### ★ 2078 ★ Czech Medical Association (CzMA) (Ceska Lekarska Spolecnost)

Sokolskoi 31
PO Box 88, Sokolska 31
CZ-120 26 Prague, Czech Republic
**Phone:** 42 2 24266201          **Fax:** 42 2 24266212
**Email:** cls@cls.cz
**Website:** http://www.cls.cz

**Fnded:** 1868. **Mem:** 32,000. **Reg. Groups:** 102. **Local Groups:** 40. **Lang(s):** English, French, German, Spanish. **Desc:** Physicians, pharmacists, and other medical personnel. **Pub:** *Medical Congresses and Symposia*, annual. • Journals, monthly. Thirty various medical journals.

### ★ 2079 ★ DEBRA European

c/o Debra House
13 Wellington Business Park
Duke's Ride
Crowthorne RG45 6LS, United Kingdom
**Phone:** 44 1344 771961     **Fax:** 44 1344 762661
**Email:** john.dart@btinternet.com
**Website:** http://www.debra-international.org

**Fnded:** 1992. **Mem:** 20. **Desc:** Umbrella organization of patient support groups for people whose lives have been affected by Epidemidysis Bullosa (EB). Activities include peer support, workshops, and dissemination of research findings. **Frmly:** (2001) EUR Network of EB Support Groups.

### ★ 2080 ★ Doctors Ought to Care (DOC)

5615 Kirby Dr., Ste. 440
Houston, TX 77005

**Phone:** (713)528-1487          **Free:** 800-362-9340
**Fax:** (713)528-2146
**Email:** d-o-c@texas.net
**Website:** http://www.bcm.tmc.edu/doc
Eric Solberg, M.A., Pres.

**Fnded:** 1977. **Mem:** 1,374. **Local Groups:** 76. **Desc:** A physician-led organization of medical students, teachers, parents, and other concerned individuals working to counteract the promotion of unhealthy products, primarily tobacco and alcohol. Works through school programs, health professionals' offices, hospitals, media, and Super Health 2000, a health promotion effort which attempts to counter the effects of advertising unhealthy products. Seeks to launch a broad health promotion effort aimed at educating the public, particularly teenagers and children, on the "lethal" lifestyles of tobacco and alcohol use. Campaigns through television commercials, radio, sports events, posters and t-shirts, and its speakers' bureau to promote the image of good health through community-wide reinforcement of the positive role model of the health professional. Serves as a resource center on tobacco and alcohol issues. **Pub:** *The Journal of Medical Activism*, quarterly. Newsletter. Fights advertising and promotion of unhealthy products by the tobacco and alcohol industry. Includes information on the pro-health community.

### ★ 2081 ★ Ecological Physicians Association (Okologischer Arztebund eV Ecological Physicians Association)

Bundesgeschaftsstelle
Fedelhoren 88
D-28203 Bremen, Germany
**Phone:** 49 421 4984251     **Fax:** 49 421 4984252
**Email:** oekologischer.aerztebund@t-online.de
**Website:** http://www.oekologischer-aerztebund.de

**Fnded:** 1987. **Mem:** 500. **Desc:** Promotes the return to a natural life existence as well as the preservation of human health. Provides information and treatment. Seeks to contribute to building ecological awareness. German section of the International Doctors for the Environment (ISDE). **Pub:** *Umwelt Medizin-Gesellschdft*, quarterly. Journal. Environment medicine society.

### ★ 2082 ★ Educational Commission for Foreign Medical Graduates (ECFMG)

3624 Market St., 4th Fl.
Philadelphia, PA 19104-2685
**Phone:** (215)386-5900          **Fax:** (215)387-9963
**Website:** http://www.ecfmg.org
Nancy E. Gary, MD, Pres. & CEO

**Fnded:** 1956. **Mem:** 20. **Desc:** Sponsoring organizations are American Board of Medical Specialties; American Medical Association; Association of American Medical Colleges; Association for Hospital Medical Education; the Federation of State Medical Boards of the U.S.; National Medical Association. Aims to provide information to graduates of foreign medical schools regarding entry into graduate medical education and the U.S. health care system; evaluate the qualifications of graduates of foreign medical schools; identify the cultural and professional needs of graduates of foreign medical schools and assist in the establishment of educational policies and programs; provides international access to testing and evaluation programs to meet theses needs. Sponsors exchange visitor program to enable physicians from other countries to participate in graduate medical education or training. Gathers and disseminates data about graduates of foreign medical schools. **Pub:** *Educational Commission for Foreign Medical Graduates–Annual Report*, annual. Annual Report. Details organizations history and programs. *Price:* Free. • *Educational Commission for Foreign Medical Graduates–Information Booklet*, annual. Booklet. Provides procedures for fulfilling ECFMG examination and certification requirements. *Price:* Free. **Frmly:** (1974) Educational Council for Foreign Medical Graduates.

### ★ 2083 ★ Egg Nutrition Center (ENC)

1050 17th St., NW, Ste. 560
Washington, DC 20036
**Phone:** (202)833-8850          **Fax:** (202)463-0102
**Website:** http://www.enc-online.org
Donald J. McNamara, PhD, Exec. Dir.

**Fnded:** 1984. **Desc:** Commercial egg producers and processors, health promotion agencies, and consumers. Provide scientifically accurate information on egg nutrition and the role of eggs in health and nutrition. Monitor nutrition research reports and nutrition policy development. **Pub:** *Nutrition Close-Up*, quarterly. Newsletter. Reviews and summarizes recent research reports.

### ★ 2084 ★ Estonian Medical Association (Eesti Arstide Liit)

Pepleri 32
EE-51010 Tartu, Estonia
**Phone:** 372 7 430029          **Fax:** 372 7 430029
**Email:** eal@arstideliit.ee
**Website:** http://www.arstideliit.ee

**Fnded:** 1921. **Mem:** 2,550. **Reg. Groups:** 20. **Desc:** Promotes the educational and professional interests of physicians. **Pub:** *Esti Arstide Liidu Teataja*, monthly. Journal. **Frmly:** Estonian Doctor's Association.

### ★ 2085 ★ European Advisory Committee on Health Research (EACHR)

Scherfigsvej 8
DK-2100 Copenhagen, Denmark
**Phone:** 45 1 290111          **Fax:** 45 1 181120

**Fnded:** 1975.

### ★ 2086 ★ European Association of Clinical Anatomy

Faculte de Medecine
F-59045 Lille, France
**Phone:** 33 3 20626940
**Email:** cfontaine@chru-lille.fr

### ★ 2087 ★ European Association for the History of Medicine and Health (EAHMH)

4, rue Kirschleger
F-67085 Strasbourg, France

**Fnded:** 1991. **Desc:** Fosters research and education in the history of medicine and health; encourages scientific cooperation.

### ★ 2088 ★ European Association of Human Ecology (EAHE)

Ave de Laerbeek 103
B-1090 Brussels, Belgium
**Phone:** 32 2 4774964          **Fax:** 32 2 4774925
**Email:** gronsse@meko.vub.ac.be
**Website:** http://vub.vub.ac.be/~gronsse/index.html

**Fnded:** 1987. **Desc:** Supports cooperation in the field.

### ★ 2089 ★ European Association of New Medical Techniques (EANMT) (Association Europeenne de Methodes Medicales Nouvelles — AEMMN)

Route d'Esch 7
L-1470 Luxembourg, Luxembourg
**Phone:** 352 250226
**Email:** grinberg@pt.lu

**Fnded:** 1987. **Mem:** 300. **Lang(s):** English, French, German. **Desc:** Physicians and other health care professionals. Promotes advancement of medical practice through the introduction of new techniques and technologies. Identifies and evaluates new medical methods and equipment; sponsors research; conducts training programs for health care personnel.

**★ 2090 ★ European Association for the Promotion of the Hand Hygiene**
46 Rue Lieutenant Liedel
B-1070 Brussels, Belgium
**Fax:** 32 2 5212099
**Fnded:** 1983.

**★ 2091 ★ European Association of Transactional Analysis (EATO)**
c/o Martine Huon
Les Toits de l'Aune Bat. E
3, rue Hugo Ely
F-13090 Aix-en-Provence, France
**Email:** info@eatanews.org
**Desc:** Promotes knowledge and research of transactional analysis. Seeks to develop standards of practice and certification. Conducts research; disseminates information. **Pub:** Newsletter, periodic.

**★ 2092 ★ European Council of Integrated Medicine (ECIM)**
71 Rue des Echevins
1050 Brussels, Belgium
**Fax:** 32 2 6483480

**★ 2093 ★ European Federation for Primatology (EFP)**
Station biologique
F-35380 Paimpont, France
**Phone:** 33 2 99618188
**Email:** deputte@univ-rennes1.fr
**Fnded:** 1993. **Desc:** Coordinates actions related to primatology between European societies.

**★ 2094 ★ European Forum for Good Clincal Practice**
Schoolberenstraat 47
B-3010 Kessel-LO, Belgium
**Phone:** 32 16 350369       **Fax:** 32 16 350369
**Email:** info@efgcp.org
**Website:** http://www.efgcp.org
**Fnded:** 1995. **Mem:** 145. **Desc:** Individuals with a professional interest or involvement in clinical or biomedical research. Promotion of "good clinical practice" through education and to develop high quality standards in clinical research.

**★ 2095 ★ European Medical Association (EMA)**
Place de Jamblinne de Meux 12
1030 Brussels, Belgium
**Phone:** 32 2 7342135       **Fax:** 32 2 7342980
**Email:** contact@emanet.org
**Website:** http://www.emanet.org
**Fnded:** 1991. **Desc:** Improves information and transparency; encourages collaboration and mobility for doctors; aims to influence actively the development of European health care.

**★ 2096 ★ European Science Foundation (ESF)**
1, quai Lezay Marnesia
F-67080 Strasbourg Cedex, France
**Phone:** 33 3 88767100     **Fax:** 33 3 88370532
**Email:** esf@esf.org
**Website:** http://www.esf.org
**Fnded:** 1971. **Mem:** 24. **Lang(s):** English. **Desc:** Association of 67 member organisations devoted to scientific research in 24 European countries. Core purpose is to promote high quality science at a European level. Committed to facilitating cooperation and collaboration in European science on behalf of its principal stakeholders. Combines both 'top-down' and 'bottom-up' approaches in the long-term development of science. Provides scientific leadership through its networking expertise and by ensuring that there is a European added value to all of its initiatives and projects. pertaining to research grants in those areas. *Human Genome Research: A Review of European and International Contributions, Report on Genome Research,* and *Clinical Research Training in Europe.* **Frmly:** (2001) European Medical Research Councils.

**★ 2097 ★ European Society for Gender Specific Medicine (ESGSM)**
Wahringer Gurtel 18-20
A-1090 Vienna, Austria
**Phone:** 43 1 404002813       **Fax:** 43 1 4060840
**Email:** jhuber@akh-wien.ac.at
**Website:** http://www.esgsm.com
**Lang(s):** English, French, German, Italian. **Desc:** Promotes the study of gender-specific diseases and conditions such as sexually transmitted diseases, hormones, specific neoplasias, and pregnancy, among others.

**★ 2098 ★ European Society of Intensive Care Medicine (ESICM)**
40 Ave. Joseph Wybran
B-1070 Brussels, Belgium
**Phone:** 32 2 5590350       **Fax:** 32 2 5270062
**Email:** public@esicm.org
**Website:** http://www.esicm.org
**Fnded:** 1982. **Mem:** 2,772. **Lang(s):** English, French. **Desc:** Physicians, nurses, physiotherapists, and students with an interest in intensive care medicine. Seeks to advance study, teaching, research, and practice in the field. Facilitates exchange of information among members; serves as a clearinghouse on intensive care medicine; conducts continuing professional development and other educational programs for members. Sponsors intensive care medical research; conducts examinations. **Pub:** *Intensive Care Medicine,* monthly. Journal. Includes original articles, pediatrics, experimental reports, and current topics.

**★ 2099 ★ European Society of Pediatric Otorhinolaryngology (ESPO)**
Via Belpoggio 2
I-34123 Trieste, Italy
**Phone:** 39 40304798       **Fax:** 39 40304798
**Email:** fiorfior@tin.it
**Fnded:** 1979. **Mem:** 250. **Desc:** Aims to foster clinical research work in the field of medicine surgery of diseases and disorders of the ear, nose and throat in children.

**★ 2100 ★ European Union of Medical Specialists (UEMS)**
20, ave. de la Couronne
B-1050 Brussels, Belgium
**Phone:** 32 2 6495164     .**Fax:** 32 2 6403730
**Email:** uems@skynet.be
**Website:** http://www.uems.be
**Fnded:** 1958. **Nat'l Groups:** 25. **Lang(s):** English, French. **Desc:** Representative national associations of medical specialists in all European countries. Works to ensure high quality care for patients. Fosters communication among members; promotes members' interests.

**★ 2101 ★ European Wound Management Association (EWMA)**
PO Box 864
London SE1 8TT, United Kingdom
**Phone:** 44 171 8723496
**Fnded:** 1991. **Lang(s):** English. **Desc:** Health care professionals, scientists, and pharmaceutical manufacturers with an interest in wound healing. Seeks to "address clinical and scientific issues associated with wound healing," in areas including the native epidemiology, pathology, diagnosis, prevention, and management of wounds. Serves as a clearinghouse on wound healing; facilitates exchange of information among members; sponsors research and educational programs.

**★ 2102 ★ Family Health Care Association of America**
c/o James Mark Reynolds
PO Box 1208
Jamestown, NC 27282
**Phone:** (910)887-3484
**Email:** fitaa@juno.com
**Fnded:** 1996. **Desc:** Provides educational, charitable, and research programs. Also offers a speakers bureau.

**★ 2103 ★ Family and Health Section of the National Council on Family Relations (FHS)**
3989 Central Ave. NE, Ste. 550
Minneapolis, MN 55421
**Phone:** (763)781-9331       **Free:** 888-781-9331
**Fax:** (763)781-9348
**Email:** ncfr3989@ncfr.com
**Website:** http://www.ncfr.org
Michael Benjamin, PhD, Exec. Dir.
**Fnded:** 1984. **Mem:** 345. **Desc:** A section of the National Council on Family Relations. Health and education professionals. Serves as a forum for all professionals involved in interdisciplinary work in the family and health fields. Presents clinical research and educational programs at NCFR conferences. **Pub:** *Family Health News,* periodic. Newsletter. **Frmly:** (1991) Family and Health Section.

**★ 2104 ★ Family Research Institute (FRI)**
PO Box 62640
Colorado Springs, CO 80962-2640
**Phone:** (303)681-3113       **Fax:** (303)681-3427
**Website:** http://familyresearchinst.org
Dr. Paul Cameron, Exec. Officer
**Fnded:** 1982. **Mem:** 1,900. **Desc:** Promotes information about sexual, family, and substance abuse issues. Conducts research and educational programs. Maintains speakers' bureau; compiles statistics. **Pub:** *Family Research Report,* bimonthly. Newsletter. *Price:* $25/year.

**★ 2105 ★ Federal Physicians Association (FPA)**
9001 Braddock Rd., No. 380
Springfield, VA 22151
**Phone:** (703)426-8100       **Free:** 800-403-3374
**Fax:** 800-528-3492
**Email:** info@fedphy.org
**Website:** http://www.fedphy.org
Dennis W. Boyd, Exec. Dir.
**Fnded:** 1978. **Mem:** 500. **Nat'l Groups:** 1. **Reg. Groups:** 1. **State Groups:** 1. **Desc:** Physicians employed by or retired from the federal government. Objectives are: to improve the health care of patients served by federal physicians; to advance the practice of medicine within the federal government; to better the working conditions and benefits of federal physicians. Conducts specialized education programs. **Pub:** *The Federal Physician,* bimonthly. Newsletter. *Price:* $37.50/year. **Frmly:** (1982) American Academy of Federal Civil Service Physicians.

**★ 2106 ★ Federation of Asian and Oceanian Physiological Societies**
PO Box 2609
Sydney, NSW 2001, Australia
**Phone:** 61 2 92411478       **Fax:** 61 92513552
**Email:** physiol98@icmsaust.com.au

**★ 2107 ★ Federation of Associations of Regulatory Boards (FARB)**
1603 Orrington Ave., Ste. 2080F
Evanston, IL 60201
**Phone:** (847)328-7909       **Fax:** (847)864-0588
**Email:** farb@farb.org
**Website:** http://www.farb.org
Dale Atkinson, Contact

**Fnded:** 1973. **Mem:** 13. **Desc:** National associations of regulatory boards united to exchange information and engage in programs and joint activities relating to the education and licensing of professionals and to cooperate in solving the mutual problems of members. Conducts attorney certification course. **Pub:** *FARB Facts*, periodic. **Frmly:** (1985) Federation of Associations of Health Regulatory Boards.

★ **2108** ★ **Federation of European Societies for Tropical Medicine and International Health (FESTMIH)**

25, rue du Docteur Roux
F-75724 Paris, France
**Phone:** 33 1 45668869      **Fax:** 33 1 45664485
**Email:** socpatex@club-internet.fr
**Fnded:** 1995. **Desc:** Fosters cooperation between societies dedicated to tropical medicine and international health.

★ **2109** ★ **Federation of Hungarian Medical Societies**

**(Magyar Orvostudomanyi Tarsasagok es Egyesuletek Szovetsege — MOTESZ)**
PO Box 145
H-1443 Budapest, Hungary
**Phone:** 36 1 3123807      **Fax:** 36 1 3837918
**Email:** motesz@elender.hu
**Website:** http://www.motesz.hu
**Fnded:** 1966. **Mem:** 93. **Lang(s):** English, German, Hungarian. **Desc:** Medical and Dental professionals. Works to enhance the medical sciences in Hungary. Encourages the development of Hungarian health care, medical, dental and closely related social sciences. Promotes the development of international relations in the field of health. Conducts educational programs. **Pub:** *MOTESZ Calendar*, annual. Brochure. Information on Medical Congresses. • *MOTESZ Magazine*, monthly. Journal of Medical Scientific and Medical Policy issues.

★ **2110** ★ **Federation of Medical Societies of Hong Kong**

Duke of Windsor Social Service Bldg., 4/F
15 Hennessy Rd.
Hong Kong, People's Republic of China
**Phone:** 852 25278898      **Fax:** 852 28650345
**Email:** info@fmshk.com.hk
**Website:** http://www.fmshk.com.hk
**Fnded:** 1965. **Mem:** 111. **Lang(s):** Chinese, English. **Desc:** Medical and dental associations and related professional organizations. Promotes advancement of the medical, dental, and related sciences. Represents the interests of the medical community. Coordinates activities of members; conducts educational programs. **Pub:** *Hong Kong Medical Diary*, monthly. Bulletin. • *Medical and Dental Directory of Hong Kong*, quadrennial. Directory.

★ **2111** ★ **Federation of State Medical Boards of the United States (FSMB)**

PO Box 619850
Dallas, TX 75261-9850
**Phone:** (817)868-4000      **Fax:** (817)868-4099
**Email:** fsmb@fsmb.org
**Website:** http://www.fsmb.org
**Fnded:** 1912. **Mem:** 69. **State Groups:** 69. **Desc:** State medical examining and licensing boards (including fourteen osteopathic boards). **Pub:** *Exchange*, triennial. Journal. Listing of MD and DO licensing requirements in each state of US. *Price:* $25 each volume; $60 for set of three volumes. • *Federation Journal*, quarterly. Journal. • *FSMB NewsLine*, monthly. • *Handbook*, annual. Directory.

★ **2112** ★ **Federation of Women's Health Councils - New Zealand**

103 Old Porirua Rd.
Ngaio
Wellington, New Zealand
**Phone:** 64 4 4795852      **Fax:** 64 4 4795752

**Email:** teenah@handiside.wn.planet.gen.nz
**Fnded:** 1990. **Reg. Groups:** 15. **Lang(s):** English. **Desc:** Women's health councils united to develop a national health policy for women. Coordinates information sharing and networking among member organizations. Monitors the provision of women's health care services to ensure that doctors and health professionals are accountable to consumers. Defends women's rights to control their bodies; supports access to free abortions. Fosters research activities. **Pub:** *Accident Compensation: A Women's Issue*. Monograph. • *Consumer Consultation, Representation and Participation*. Monograph. • *Ensuring the Cervical Screening Programme Survives the Health Changes*. Monograph. • Newsletter, bimonthly.

★ **2113** ★ **Fellowship of Associates of Medical Evangelism (FAME)**

PO Box 34800
Indianapolis, IN 46234
**Phone:** (317)272-5937      **Fax:** (317)272-5940
**Email:** medicalmissions@fameworld.org
**Website:** http://www.fameworld.org
Kevin Dooley, Exec. Dir.
**Fnded:** 1970. **Desc:** Builds hospitals and clinics and provides mobile medical units for Christian missionaries outside the U.S.; secures and ships medicine and medical supplies. Conducts charitable programs; maintains speakers' bureau. **Pub:** *Spreading the Fame of Christ*, quarterly. Newsletter.

★ **2114** ★ **Fenway Community Health Center**

Lesbian/Gay Family & Parenting Services
7 Haviland St.
Boston, MA 02115-2608
**Phone:** (617)267-0900      **Free:** 888-242-0900
**Email:** drockwell@fenwayhealth.org
**Website:** http://www.fenwayhealth.org
**Desc:** Strives to treat every client as a whole and unique person to receive the best health care available, including HIV prevention, treatment, and research; women's health, particularly understanding the needs of lesbians; and the health care needs of gays and lesbians.

★ **2115** ★ **Finnish Medical Association (Suomen Laakariliitto)**

Makelankatu 2
PO Box 49
SF-00501 Helsinki, Finland
**Phone:** 358 9 393091      **Fax:** 358 9 3930794
**Email:** fma@fimnet.fi
**Website:** http://www.laakariliitto.fl
**Fnded:** 1910. **Mem:** 18,000. **Nat'l Groups:** 26. **State Groups:** 5. **Local Groups:** 60. **Lang(s):** English, Finnish, Swedish. **Desc:** Physicians' organizations to safeguard physicians' economic interests and working conditions. Promotes formation and implementation of effective national health policies. Develops and administers national training programs for physicians and confers professional certification. Conducts research on health systems and services. Facilitates international cooperation in the provision of health care in underserved areas. Aims at maintaining a high standard of professional ethics. **Pub:** *Finnish Medical Journal*, 36/year. Journal. • *Information Newsletter*, 15/year. Newsletter. • *Newsletter for the General Press*, 15/year. Newsletter. • Books. • Manuals. **Frmly:** (2000) Finnish Medical Association.

★ **2116** ★ **Fitness for Life (FFL)**

5060 Cascade Rd. SE, Ste. A
Grand Rapids, MI 49546
Dan Distin, Contact
**Fnded:** 1984. **Desc:** Personal Fitness Training Massages. **Pub:** *On Purpose*, quarterly. Newsletter. • *On Purpose Manual*. Manual.

★ **2117** ★ **Flying Physicians Association (FPA)**

PO Box 677427
Orlando, FL 32867
**Phone:** (407)359-1423      **Fax:** (407)359-1167
**Email:** fpahq@aol.com
**Website:** http://www.fpadrs.org
Lawrence O. Grahagan, MD, Pres.
**Fnded:** 1954. **Mem:** 1,200. **Reg. Groups:** 5. **Desc:** Doctors of medicine who have a current pilot certificate and are members of an ethical medical organization. Promotes the interests of medicine in aviation, safety, and education. **Pub:** *The Flying Physician*, quarterly. Magazine. For physicians with pilot's certificates covering medical and aviation topics; also includes association activities, book reviews, and calendar. *Price:* Included in membership dues; $50/year for nonmembers. • *Flying Physicians Association–Bulletin*, monthly. Newsletter. Membership activities newsletter. *Price:* Included in membership dues. • *Flying Physicians Association–Directory*, annual. Directory. *Price:* Included in membership dues.

★ **2118** ★ **Forum for Medical Affairs (FORUM)**

760 Riverside Ave.
Jacksonville, FL 32204-3335
**Fax:** (904)353-1247
Donald F. Foy, Sr., Exec. VP
**Fnded:** 1944. **Mem:** 800. **Desc:** Presidents, presidents-elect, and past presidents of state medical associations, members of the American Medical Association and the House of Delegates, editors of state medical association journals, executive directors of state medical associations, and representatives of AMA-recognized medical specialty societies. **Frmly:** (1972) Conference of Presidents and Officers of State Medical Associations.

★ **2119** ★ **Foundation for Advances in Medicine and Science (FAMS)**

PO Box 832
Mahwah, NJ 07430-0832
**Phone:** (201)818-1010      **Free:** 800-443-0263
**Fax:** (201)818-0086
**Email:** scanning@fams.org
**Website:** http://www.scanning-fams.org/profile.html
Tony Bourgholtzer, Bd. Chm.
**Fnded:** 1983. **Mem:** 400. **Desc:** Clinical cardiologists, scientists, and scanning electron microscopists. Disseminates resource information in clinical medicine and science. Funds research projects. **Pub:** *Clinical Cardiology*, monthly. Journal. Contains peer-reviewed articles for practicing cardiologists. *Price:* $80/year in U.S.; $126.50/year outside U.S.; $15.50/single copy. • *Scanning*, 6/year. *Price:* $175/year in U.S.; $185/year outside U.S.; $325/year, institutional in the U.S.; $40/single copy. **Frmly:** (1990) Foundation for Advances in Clincal Medicine and Science.

★ **2120** ★ **Foundation for Health (FFH)**

337 East Ave.
Watertown, NY 13601-3829
**Phone:** (315)782-6664      **Free:** 800-724-7460
**Fax:** (315)782-6664
**Email:** gbonadio@imcnet.net
George Bonadio, Exec. Dir.
**Fnded:** 1972. **Desc:** Gathers and disseminates information regarding health; seeks to publicize "natural" laws of health in an effort to make excellent health and long, useful lives common throughout the world. Proclaims the simplicity and inexpensiveness of maintaining one's health in contrast to the complexity and expense of disease. Researches and develops nutrition and health related projects and programs. **Pub:** *Ask the Nutritionist*, weekly. Newspaper. • *Seven Disciplines of Health*. • Also contributes weekly health column to newspapers; plans to publish book.

### ★ 2121 ★ Foundation for Informed Medical Decision Making
PO Box 5457
Hanover, NH 03755-5457
**Phone:** (603)650-1180 **Fax:** (603)650-1125
**Email:** judith.m.fitzpatrick@dartmouth.edu
Judith Fitzpatrick, Admin. Dir.

**Fnded:** 1989. **Desc:** Gathers and contributes scientific research information for use in videotape programs on shared decision making topics. **Pub:** Video.

### ★ 2122 ★ Foundation for Innovation in Medicine (FIM)
411 North Ave. E
Cranford, NJ 07016
**Phone:** (908)272-2967 **Fax:** (908)272-4583
**Email:** fundefelice@aol.com
**Website:** http://www.fimdefelice.org/
Stephen L. DeFelice, MD, Chair

**Fnded:** 1976. **Desc:** Seeks to regenerate interest in medical discovery and innovation, which the foundation believes flourished in the U.S. in the 1940s and 1950s, but has since declined despite "vastly increased public and private expenditures in research and development." Intends to monitor the state of innovation by conducting seminars and conferences. Encourages clinical research on natural substances and substances with little commercial value. **Pub:** *From Oysters to Insulin: Nature and Medicine at Odds.* Book. *Price:* $15.95. • *Nutraceutical White Paper. Price:* $10.

### ★ 2123 ★ Foundation for International Self Help Development (FISH)
19 Gordon Town Rd.
Kingston, Jamaica
**Phone:** (809)927-6715

**Fnded:** 1985. **Lang(s):** English. **Desc:** Seeks to improve the health and nutrition of the needy in Jamaica. Maintains medical, dental, and eye care clinic. Plans to operate programs in areas including community development, reforestation, and energy conservation and alternative fuels.

### ★ 2124 ★ Foundation for the Support of International Medical Training (FSIMT)
417 Center St.
Lewiston, NY 14092
**Phone:** (716)754-4883 **Fax:** (716)836-3412
**Email:** iamat@sentex.net
**Website:** http://www.sentex.net/~iamat
Mrs. M. A. Uffer, Pres.

**Fnded:** 1960. **Mem:** 6000,000. **Desc:** Individuals and corporations organized to provide information regarding the availability of competent medical care overseas and information concerning sanitary conditions, health hazards, and climatic conditions in various parts of the world. Offers detailed guidance on vaccination and immunization requirements and tropical diseases. **Pub:** *Be Aware of Schistosomiasis.* • *How to Protect Yourself Against Malaria*, annual. • *Immunization Chart*, annual. • *Set of 24 World Climate Charts*, annual. • *Traveller Clinical Chart*, annual. • *When Hiking Through Latin America, Be Alert to Chagas' Disease*, annual. • *World Malaria Risk Chart*, annual. • *World Schistosomiasis Risk Chart*, annual. • Brochure, annual. • Directory, annual.

### ★ 2125 ★ Foundation for Women's Health Research and Development (FORWARD)
40 Eastbourne Terrace
London W2 3QR, United Kingdom
**Phone:** 44 171 7252606 **Fax:** 44 171 7252796
**Email:** forward@dircon.co.uk
**Website:** http://www.forward.dircon.co.uk
**Fnded:** 1983. **Mem:** 951. **Nat'l Groups:** 10. **Reg. Groups:** 10. **Lang(s):** English. **Desc:** Promotes the studies of women's health research and development throughout Europe and other western countries. Supports the rights of women and children. Promotes the

prevention of early childhood marriage that contributes to VVF and RVF. Protects women and children from becoming victims of abuse. Opposes and fights for the elimination of the practice of gential mutilation of young girls. Disseminates information. Conducts training programs. **Pub:** *Another Form of Physical Abuse: Prevention of Female Genital Mutilation in the United Kingdom.* Video. • *Child Protection and Female Genital Mutilation: Advice for Health, Education, and Social Work Professionals.* Book. • *Cutting the Rose: Female Genital Mutilation - The Practice and its Prevention.* • *Female Genital Mutilation Proposals for Change.* • *Holistic Care for Women: A Practical Guide for Midwives.* Offers detailed advice for midwives caring for women affected by FGM. • *Out of Sight, Out of Mind?.* Report of a survey into inter-agency policies and procedures relating to female genital mutilation in England and Wales. • *Report on the First Study Conference on Genital Mutilation of Girls in Europe July 1992 in London.* Position papers and reports.

### ★ 2126 ★ Friends of Celiac Disease Research
8832 N Port Washington Rd., No. 204
Milwaukee, WI 53217
**Phone:** (414)540-6679 **Fax:** (414)540-0587
**Email:** friends@aero.net
**Website:** http://www.friendsofceliac.com
Dana Tehako-Esser, Exec. Dir.

**Fnded:** 1999. **Desc:** Devoted to assisting people with celiac disease and dermatitis herpetiformis; supports research and education.

### ★ 2127 ★ Fundacion ALFA-1 de Puerto Rico
PO Box 6729
Bayamon, PR 00960-9007
**Phone:** (787)743-0268 **Fax:** (787)743-0268
**Email:** fundacion.alfa1@alfa1.org
**Website:** http://www.alfa1.org
Elaine Alfonzo, Coord.

**Fnded:** 1996. **Desc:** Offers support and education for the Spanish speaking Alpha 1-Antitrypsin Deficiency patients and their families. Distributes Spanish educational materials. Works to increase awareness about Alpha 1-Antitrypsin Deficiency and the importance of early detection and treatment. **Frmly:** (1999) Puerto Rico Alpha 1 Support Group.

### ★ 2128 ★ General Medical Council
178 Great Portland St.
London W1N 5JE, United Kingdom
**Phone:** 44 207 5807642 **Fax:** 44 207 9153641
**Email:** gmc@gmc.uk.org
**Fnded:** 1858. **Mem:** 102. **Desc:** Doctors elected by UK doctors or appointed by UK universities with medical schools and by Royal Colleges. Lay members nominated by Privy Council. Protects the public by overseeing medical education, keeping a register of qualified doctors and taking action where a doctor's fitness to pratise is in doubt. **Pub:** *Duties of a Doctor - Guidance on Professional Ethics.* • *GMC News Review*, semiannual. Newsletter. • *Medical Register*, annual. • Annual Report, annual.

### ★ 2129 ★ German Women Physicians Association (Deutscher Arztinnenbund)
Herbert-Lewin-Str. 1
D-50931 Cologne, Germany
**Phone:** 49 221 4004540 **Fax:** 49 221 4004541
**Email:** gsdaeb@aol.com
**Website:** http://www.aerztinnen.de
**Fnded:** 1924. **Mem:** 2,100. **Reg. Groups:** 33. **Lang(s):** Dutch, English, Portuguese. **Desc:** Promotes solidarity among women doctors. Represents members' interests in the medical sphere. Cultivates international contacts. **Pub:** *Aerztin*, bimonthly. Magazine.

### ★ 2130 ★ Global Alliance for Women's Health
823 UN Plaza, Ste. 712
New York, NY 10017
**Phone:** (212)286-0424 **Fax:** (212)286-9561
**Email:** webmaster@gawh.org
**Website:** http://www.gawh.org
Elaine M. Wolfson, PhD, Pres.

**Desc:** Individuals and organizations working to improve the quality of women's health worldwide. Gathers and disseminates information on topics including primary health care, education of health care providers, cultural practices affecting the health of women and girls, occupational health and safety, sexually transmitted diseases, domestic violence, and mental health. Develops model health programs addressing women's needs. Conducts research; compiles statistics. **Pub:** *Women's Health Compendium.* Book.

### ★ 2131 ★ Global Health Action (GHA)
2250 N Druid Hills Rd., Ste. 130
Atlanta, GA 30329-3118
**Phone:** (404)634-5748 **Fax:** (404)634-9685
**Email:** gha@globalhealthaction.org
**Website:** http://www.globalhealthaction.org
Robin C. Davis, Exec. Dir.

**Fnded:** 1972. **Desc:** Provides health education and leadership training for participants from over 87 countries worldwide. Programs include: international health management and leadership courses, community health worker training and goat farmer training programs in Haiti, village health worker trainers' programs and AIDS education program in India and neighboring countries, short-term workshops throughout the world. Participants include health and developmental professionals, community health workers, and community leaders. New initiatives include training community-based and faith-based health educators and lay health leaders working in under-served U.S. communities. Consultation services available. Conducts annual health & leadership training programs in Atlanta, Georgia, USA. **Pub:** *A Great and Mighty Tree.* Video. • *Global Health Action Newsletter*, semiannual. Newsletter. Primarily for donor education and publicity. **Frmly:** (1985) International Nursing Services Association; (1993) INSA, The International Service Association for Health.

### ★ 2132 ★ Global Health Council
1701 K St. NW, Ste. 600
Washington, DC 20006-1503
**Phone:** (202)833-5900 **Fax:** (202)833-0075
**Email:** ghc@globalhealth.org
**Website:** http://www.globalhealth.org/
Nils Daulaire, Pres. /CEO

**Fnded:** 1971. **Mem:** 1,600. **Desc:** Membership organization made up of private voluntary organizations, health and medical associations, universities, government agencies, foundations, corporations, consulting firms, and individuals interested in promoting greater and more effective U.S. participation in practical international health and development programs. Seeks to strengthen U.S. public and private sector participation in international health activities. Areas of concern include: HIV/AIDS; women's health; improving primary health care worldwide; environmental health; population and family planning; tropical and preventive medicine; appropriate health technology. Supports improved health and development legislation. Conducts career service in conjunction with annual conference. **Pub:** *AIDS Link*, bimonthly. Newsletter. Contains the latest global information on HIV/AIDS issues. • *Career Network*, monthly. Bulletin. Contains listings of employment opportunities in International Health. • *Directory of U.S.-Based Agencies Involved in International Health Assistance*, periodic. Directory. Lists geographical areas served and types of workers sought by U.S. health agencies. *Price:* $60 non-members; $30 members. • *Global Learning for Health.* Paper. *Price:* $16.95 for members; $26.95 for non-members. • *Healthlink*, 10/year. Contains information on international health policy issues and calendar of events. *Price:* available to members only. • *NCIH Membership Directory*, periodic. Membership

Directory. Contains individual and organizational members with phone numbers and key contacts. **Frmly:** (1999) National Council for International Health.

★ **2133** ★ **Global Health Ministries (GHM)**
7831 Hickory St. NE
Minneapolis, MN 55432-2500
**Phone:** (763)586-9590          **Fax:** (763)586-9591
**Email:** ghm@compuserve.com
**Website:** http://www.ghm.org/
**Desc:** Provides Lutheran health care work overseas; gathers and sends medical supplies around the world, recruits health related personnel; funds training of national health care givers. **Pub:** Newsletter. • Annual Report.

★ **2134** ★ **Global Vaccine Awareness League (GVAL)**
25422 Trabuco Rd., Ste. 105-230
Lake Forest, CA 92630
**Phone:** (949)929-1191
**Email:** michelle@gval.com
**Website:** http://www.gval.com/
Michelle Helms, Founder
**Fnded:** 1995. **Mem:** 160. **Desc:** Dedicated to disseminating information on the serious side effects of government sponsored vaccinations. Conducts educational programs; promotes parents right to choose whether or not to vaccinate their children; supports research; conducts fundraising events. **Pub:** Newsletter.

★ **2135** ★ **Guam Lytico and Bodig Association**
PO Box 1458
Hagatna, GU 96932
**Phone:** (671)477-2293          **Fax:** (671)477-2294
**Email:** lyticobodig@hotmail.com
**Website:** http://lytico.tripod.com/
Madeleine Z. Bordallo, Pres.
**Fnded:** 1983. **Mem:** 18. **Desc:** Provides supportive services and information to individuals stricken with disease.

★ **2136** ★ **Harveian Society of London**
11 Chandos St.
London W1M 0EB, United Kingdom
**Phone:** 44 20 75801043
**Fnded:** 1831. **Mem:** 350. **Lang(s):** English. **Desc:** Promotes discussion of the medical, surgical, and philosophical subjects connected with medical subjects.

★ **2137** ★ **Harvey Society (HS)**
c/o Dr. Savio L.C. Woo
Mt. Sinai School of Medicine
Institute of Gene Therapy
1425 Madison Ave., PO Box 1496
New York, NY 10029
**Phone:** (212)659-8260          **Fax:** (212)849-2572
**Email:** Savio.Woo@mssm.edu
Dr. Savio Woo, Prof. /Dir.
**Fnded:** 1905. **Mem:** 1,600. **Desc:** Persons with a Ph.D. or M.D. degree active or interested in making contributions to the literature of medical and biological science. Seeks to disseminate knowledge and promote the development of the biomedical sciences. Sponsors a series of public lectures delivered by leaders in the field. Society is named after William Harvey (1578-1657), who identified the circulation of blood. **Pub:** Harvey Lectures, annual. Book. Contains lectures given during the year.

★ **2138** ★ **Health and Development International (HDI)**
PO Box 382077
Cambridge, MA 02238-2077
**Phone:** (617)864-2042          **Fax:** (617)864-7757
**Email:** anders@hdi.no

**Website:** http://www.hdi.no/
Dr. Anders R. Seim, Founder
**Desc:** Works to free the world of guinea worm and lymphatic filariasis (elephantiasis).

★ **2139** ★ **Health Economics Association of Ireland (HEAI)**
c/o Mr. Brendan McElroy
Department of Economics and General Practice
University College Cork
Cork, Ireland
**Email:** c.oneill2@ulst.ac.uk
**Lang(s):** English. **Desc:** Promotes health economics in Ireland.

★ **2140** ★ **Health First International (HFI)**
508 N 1st St.
Sartell, MN 56377
Elsie Harper, Exec. Dir.
**Fnded:** 1989. **Mem:** 250. **Reg. Groups:** 1. **State Groups:** 3. **Local Groups:** 1. **Desc:** Disseminates information on low-cost health care. Offers classes in nutrition, diet management, stress and anger control, family life, drug abuse recognition, and how to stop smoking; holds well-baby clinics. Compiles statistics. Plans to conduct cooking, physical therapy, and exercise classes.

★ **2141** ★ **Health Information Resource Center (HIRC)**
c/o Carole Klein-Alexander
621 E Park Ave.
Libertyville, IL 60048
**Phone:** (847)816-8660          **Free:** 800-828-8225
**Fax:** (847)816-8662
**Email:** info@healthawards.com
**Website:** http://www.healthawards.com
Patricia Henze, Exec. Dir.
**Fnded:** 1993. **Desc:** Clearinghouse for consumer health information. Provides information and referral services to many organizations that use or produce consumer health information materials. Conducts market research. **Pub:** Consumer Health Information Online, annual. Price: $29.95. • Consumer Health Information: The Professional Guide to the Nations Best Consumer Health Information Programs and Materials, annual. • Health and Medical Media '99, annual. Sourcebook of health and medical media contacts. Price: $149. • The Health Events Calendar, annual. Planning guide to national health events. Price: $19.95.

★ **2142** ★ **Health Ministries (HM)**
Board for Human Care Ministries
1333 S Kirkwood Rd.
Saint Louis, MO 63122-7295
**Free:** 888-843-5267          **Fax:** (314)965-0277
**Email:** bruce.hartung@lcms.org
**Website:** http://humancare.lcms.org/hm/hm.htm
Bruce M. Hartung, PhD, Dir.
**Desc:** Consultants to all boards and commissions of the Lutheran Church-Missouri Synod having a relationship to the "healing mission" of the church and health issues of professional church workers. **Pub:** AIDS Alert. Newsletter. • Cross and Caduceus, 3/year. Newsletter. Focuses on health and wellness issues. Price: Free. • Gesundheit. Newsletter. • Parish Nurse, quarterly. Newsletter. **Frmly:** (1969) Council for Christian Medical Work; (1981) Commission on Health and Healing; (1986) Health and Healing Ministries.

★ **2143** ★ **Health Occupations Students of America (HOSA)**
6021 Morris Rd., No. 111
Flower Mound, TX 75028
**Free:** 800-321-HOSA          **Fax:** (972)874-0063
**Email:** info@hosa.org
**Website:** http://www.hosa.org
Dr. Jim Koeninger, Contact
**Fnded:** 1975. **Mem:** 52,000. **State Groups:** 36. **Local Groups:** 2100. **Desc:** Secondary and postsecondary students enrolled in health occupations education programs; health professionals and others interested in assisting and supporting the activities of HOSA; alumni of health occupations education programs and individuals who have made significant contributions to the field. Primary aim is to improve the quality of healthcare for all Americans by urging members to develop self-improvement skills. Operates within health occupation education programs in public high schools and postsecondary institutions. Encourages members to develop an understanding of current healthcare issues, environmental concerns, and survival needs worldwide. Conducts programs to help individuals improve their occupational skills and develop leadership qualities. Conducts exhibits, management workshops, and medical facility tours; provides social and recreational activities. Maintains speakers' bureau; compiles statistics. **Pub:** HOSA Leaders Directory, annual. Directory. • HOSA Leaders' Update, quarterly. • HOSA News Magazine, quarterly. Magazine. • Story of HOSA. Video. • Brochure. • Handbook. • Also publishes recruitment package. **AKA:** National HOSA.

★ **2144** ★ **Health Physics Society (HPS)**
1313 Dolley Madison Blvd., Ste. 402
Mc Lean, VA 22101-3926
**Phone:** (703)790-1745          **Fax:** (703)790-2672
**Email:** hps@burkinc.com
**Website:** http://www.hps.org/
Richard J. Burk, Jr., Exec. Sec.
**Fnded:** 1956. **Mem:** 6,890. **Local Groups:** 41. **Desc:** Persons engaged in some form of activity in the field of health physics (the profession devoted to radiation protection). To improve public understanding of the problems and needs in radiation protection; to promote health physics as a profession. Maintains Elda E. Anderson Memorial Fund to be used for teachers, researchers, and others. Provides placement service at annual meeting. Cosponsors American Board of Health Physics for certification of health physicists. **Pub:** Health Physics Journal, monthly. Journal. • Health Physics Society–Membership Handbook, annual. • Health Physics Society–Newsletter, monthly. Newsletter.

★ **2145** ★ **Health Professions Council Zimbabwe**
PO Box A410 Avondale
Harare, Zimbabwe
**Phone:** 263 754930          **Fax:** 263 756731
**Lang(s):** English. **Desc:** Statutory body registering health practitioners. Promotes and coordinates members' activities; facilitates communication among members. Issues certification; formulates and enforces standards of conduct and practice among members.

★ **2146** ★ **Health Research Council of New Zealand (HRC)**
PO Box 5541
Wellesley St.
Auckland, New Zealand
**Phone:** 64 9 3798227          **Fax:** 64 9 3779988
**Email:** jrankine@hrc.govt.nz
**Website:** http://www.hrc.govt.nz
**Fnded:** 1990. **Mem:** 12. **Desc:** Initiates and supports general health-related research, including the biomedical, public health, Maori, and clinical fields in New Zealand. Coordinates health research on a national basis and administers and disburses government research funding. Bestows awards. **Pub:** HRC Annual Report. Annual Report. • HRC Newsletter, quarterly. Newsletter. Contains information on health research in New Zealand. • Maori Health Research Newsletter, semiannual. Newsletter. **Frmly:** (1937) Medical Research Council of New Zealand.

★ **2147** ★ **Health Research and Educational Trust (HRET)**
1 N Franklin
Chicago, IL 60606
**Phone:** (312)422-2600          **Fax:** (312)422-4568

**Email:** mpittman@aha.org
**Website:** http://www.aha.org/hret
Mary A. Pittman, Dr.PH, Pres.

**Fnded:** 1944. **Desc:** Encourages and engages in educational, research, and demonstration activities to improve the management of hospital and health services. **Pub:** *Health Services Research*, bimonthly. • Books. • Manuals. • Monographs. **Frmly:** (1959) Educational Trust of the American Hospital Association; (2002) Hospital Research and Educational Trust.

**★ 2148 ★ Health and Social Policy Corp. (Corporacion de Salud y Politicas Sociale — CORSAPS)**
Roman Diez 228 Of. 401
Providencia
Santiago, Chile
**Phone:** 56 2 2641261          **Fax:** 56 2 2352312
**Email:** corsaps@reuna.cl
**Fnded:** 1990. **Lang(s):** English, Spanish. **Desc:** Promotes health reform and the development of related social policy for the citizens of Chile. Focuses primarily on the health concerns of young people and women. Supports applied research.

**★ 2149 ★ Health Workers Union of the Russian Federation**
Lenin Ave. 42
117119 Moscow, Russia
**Phone:** 7 95 9388443          **Fax:** 7 95 9388134
**Email:** ckprz@online.ru
**Fnded:** 1990. **Mem:** 3100,022. **Reg. Groups:** 78. **Local Groups:** 23094. **Lang(s):** English, Russian. **Desc:** Physicians, nurses, pharmacists, paramedical personnel, and medical students and trainees. Promotes professional advancement of members; works to maintain high standards of practice and ethics in the field of medicine. Represents members' interests before government agencies; promulgates and enforces standards of practice and conduct. **Pub:** *Profsoiuznaya Tema*, quarterly. Information on protection of health workers' rights and interests.

**★ 2150 ★ HealthCare Ministries (HCM)**
521 W Lynn St.
Springfield, MO 65802
**Phone:** (417)866-6311          **Fax:** (417)866-4711
**Email:** ivainio@hcmdfm.org
**Website:** http://www.healthcareministries.org
**Desc:** Medical missions arm of the Assemblies of God Foreign Missions. Strives to demonstrate and teach love and compassion in all aspects of the ministry. Conducts seminars, short-term medical evangelism teams and teaches health education.

**★ 2151 ★ Healthlink Worldwide**
Cityside
40 Adler St.
London E1 1EE, United Kingdom
**Phone:** 44 20 75391570      **Fax:** 44 20 75391580
**Email:** info@healthlink.org.uk
**Website:** http://www.healthlink.org.uk
**Fnded:** 1977. **Mem:** 70. **Lang(s):** English. **Desc:** Works in partnership with organisations in developing countries seeking to improve the health and well-being of poor and vulnerable communities by strengthening the provision, use, and impact of information. Offers expertise in various aspects of health and disability-related communications, including development of print and electronic materials, resource centre, and database development. **Pub:** *AIDS Action*, quarterly. Newsletter. • *Annual Report*. • *Child Health Dialogue*, quarterly. Newsletter. • *Disability Dialogue*, quarterly. Newsletter. **Frmly:** Appropriate Health Resources and Technologies Action Group.

**★ 2152 ★ Hesperian Foundation (HF)**
1919 Addison St., Ste. 304
Berkeley, CA 94704
**Phone:** (510)845-1447      **Fax:** (510)845-9141
**Email:** hesperian@hesperian.org

**Website:** http://www.hesperian.org
Sarah Shannon, Exec. Dir.
**Fnded:** 1973. **Desc:** Promotes good health in the developing world and in poor communities in the U.S. through community-based, informed self-care. Fosters constructive dialogue on health care and social change. Originally established to help launch Project Piaxtla, a health care network, and Project Projimo, a community-based rehabilitation center for spinal cord injuries, in western Mexico. The foundation now focuses on publishing community self-help health care books that are used throughout the world. Analyzes and criticizes existing social, political, and economic systems that prevent the poor from obtaining adequate standards of life and health. Operates gratis book fund, in which third world health care workers in the developing world receive Hesperian publications at no charge. **Pub:** *A Book for Midwives*. Book. *Price:* $22. • *Disabled Village Children*. Book. *Price:* $22. • *Helping Health Workers Learn*. Book. *Price:* $20. • *Where There Is No Dentist*. Book. *Price:* $9. • *Where There Is No Doctor*. Book. *Price:* $17. • *Where Women Have No Doctor*. Book. *Price:* $20. • *The Women's Health Exchange*, quarterly. Newsletter. *Price:* Free.

**★ 2153 ★ Hong Kong Institute of Family Medicine**
18 Fu Kin St.
Tai Wai
Shatin
Hong Kong, People's Republic of China
**Phone:** 852 26083311          **Fax:** 852 26053334
**Fnded:** 1994. **Lang(s):** Chinese, English. **Desc:** Seeks to advance the study, theory, and practice of family medicine; encourages professional advancement of individuals engaged in the provision of family medical services. Conducts research and continuing professional development programs.

**★ 2154 ★ Hong Kong Laboratory Technicians' Association**
PO Box 80401
Cheung Sha Wan Post Office
Hong Kong, People's Republic of China
**Phone:** 852 23611551          **Fax:** 852 27252793
**Email:** hklta@bigfoot.com
**Fnded:** 1972. **Mem:** 400. **Lang(s):** Chinese, English. **Desc:** Medical and laboratory technicians. Promotes professional competence in the practice of medical and laboratory technology. Seeks to secure optimal conditions of employment for members. Formulates and enforces standards of practice and ethics for the field. Represents members in negotiations with employers. Conducts continuing professional development and other educational and training programs for members; sponsors research projects. Provides laboratory equipment, job referral, and discount shopping services to members. **Pub:** *Laboratory and Labtek*, monthly. Newsletter.

**★ 2155 ★ Hong Kong Medical Association**
Duke of Windsor Social Service Bldg., 5/F
15 Hennessy Rd.
Hong Kong, People's Republic of China
**Phone:** 852 25278285          **Fax:** 852 28650943
**Email:** hkma@hkma.com.hk
**Website:** http://www.hkma.org
**Fnded:** 1920. **Mem:** 5,500. **Lang(s):** Chinese, English. **Desc:** Physicians and other health care professionals. Seeks to advance the profession and practice of medicine. Promotes professional advancement of members. Represents members' interests before government agencies and the public. Conducts continuing professional development courses; sponsors research projects; holds social and charitable activities. **Pub:** *HK Medical Journal*, quarterly. Journal. Features official journal of Hong Kong Medical Association and Hong Kong Academy of Medicine. • *HKMA News*, monthly. Newsletter. **Frmly:** (1970) Hong Kong Chinese Medical Association.

**★ 2156 ★ Hospice Foundation of America (HFA)**
2001 S St. NW, Ste. 300
Washington, DC 20009
**Free:** 800-854-3402          **Fax:** (202)638-5312
**Email:** david@hospicefoundation.org
**Website:** http://www.hospicefoundation.org
David Abrams, Pres.
**Fnded:** 1982. **Desc:** Works to promote the philosophy and application of hospice care for terminally ill people and improve the American health system. Advocates the hospice concept of care; offers professional development and educational programs; sponsors research on ethical issues; participates in public policy initiatives; provides technical assistance to hospices **Pub:** *Choosing Hospice*. Booklet. Provides consumer information on Hospices. *Price:* Free. • *Hospice Care and the Military Family*. Brochure. • *Hospice Forum*, bimonthly. Newsletter. Provides information on research, regulatory issues, public policy, legislation, and state hospice programs. *Price:* $105/year for nonmembers; included in membership dues. • *Volunteering in Hospice*. Booklet. *Price:* Free.

**★ 2157 ★ Hospital Consultants and Specialists Association (HCSA)**
1 Kingsclere Rd.
Overton
Basingstoke RG25 3JA, United Kingdom
**Phone:** 44 1256 771777      **Fax:** 44 1256 770999
**Email:** conspec@hcsa.com
**Fnded:** 1948. **Desc:** Membership is open to hospital consultants, associate specialists, senior registrars, and staff grade doctors working in the National Health Service. Concerned with the interests of senior hospital doctors and their patients. Aims to improve the conditions of service of members, informing them on matters affecting their practice and endeavouring to ensure that key health decisions are taken with due regard to their views. **Pub:** *The Consultant*, annual. • *Consultant Newsletter*, 10/year. Newsletter. • Yearbook.

**★ 2158 ★ Hospital Doctors' Association**
Old Court House
London Rd.
Ascot SL5 7EN, United Kingdom
**Phone:** 44 1344 26613
**Fnded:** 1966. **Mem:** 600. **Desc:** All hospital doctors below consultant level. The organisation exclusively representing junior doctors interests. It is concerned with their pay and terms and condition of service. At present it is concerned with the changes in specialist training and the reduction in hours of work **Pub:** *Official Reference Directory*, annual. Directory.

**★ 2159 ★ Imagine World Health (IWH)**
105 E Dolphin Blvd.
Ponte Vedra Beach, FL 32082-1714
**Phone:** (904)285-0240
**Email:** imagineuldhealth@aol.com
**Website:** http://www.imagineworldhealth.org
David Stearns, Contact
**Fnded:** 1998. **Desc:** Strives to educate and promote good health and fitness in mind, body and spirit.

**★ 2160 ★ Incurably Ill for Animal Research (IIFAR)**
PO Box 27454
Lansing, MI 48909
**Phone:** (517)887-1141          **Fax:** (517)887-1550
**Email:** info@iifar.org
**Website:** http://www.iifar.org/
Gregory A. Maas, CEO
**Fnded:** 1985. **Mem:** 2,500. **Local Groups:** 18. **Desc:** Persons who have health problems and interested individuals who are concerned that animal research for medical purposes will be stopped or severely limited due to the efforts of animal rights activists. Supports the use of animals for the purpose of medical research, teaching, and testing. Seeks to educate the public regarding the role animals serve in biomedical

research and improving human and animal health. Maintains speakers' bureau. **Pub:** *Have You Benefited?*. Brochure. • *How Can You Show Your Support?*. Brochure. • *iiFAR Update*, monthly. Includes local chapter news and information on legislation and the activities of animal rights activists. • *iiFARsighted Report*, quarterly. Report. • *Why Should You Care?*. Brochure. • Also distributes educational literature and student information packets.

### ★ 2161 ★ Independent Citizens Research Foundation for the Study of Degenerative Diseases (ICRFSDD)

PO Box 97
Ardsley, NY 10502
**Phone:** (914)591-4374          **Fax:** (914)591-7090
Mark Bereday, Exec. Dir.

**Fnded:** 1957. **Desc:** Individuals united to seek and publish information of aid to those affected by degenerative diseases. Makes available in bulletin form documented information on the multiple and contributing causes of degenerative diseases, testing procedures for their early detection, and possible approaches to therapy and prevention. Seeks out factors in the environment that are detrimental to health. Supports research on calibrated transcutaneous electric nerve stimulation and preventive medicine techniques. Maintains 400 volume library on maintenance of health and prevention of disease. Seeks out factors in the environment that are detrimental to health. **Pub:** Newsletter, bimonthly. • Also publishes authorized transcripts of radio lectures on nutrition.

### ★ 2162 ★ Independent Healthcare Association

Westminster Tower
3 Albert Embankment
London SE1 7SP, United Kingdom
**Phone:** 44 207 794620     **Fax:** 44 207 8203738
**Website:** http://www.iha.org.uk

**Fnded:** 1987. **Mem:** 1,000. **Desc:** Independent hospitals and homes registered under the 1984 Registered Homes Act. The representative body for independently-owned healthcare providers, whether voluntary or private, funded largely by member subscriptions based on a fee per bed. Its charitable status derives from its objectives to promote high standards of care in the independent sector. **Pub:** *Focus*, quarterly. • Bulletin, monthly.

### ★ 2163 ★ Indian Association of General Practitioners (IAGP)

c/o Mohan's Clinic
No. 613, 2nd Main
1 Stage, Indirangar
Bangalore 560 038, Karnataka, India
**Email:** docmohan@vsnl.com

**Fnded:** 1979. **Mem:** 500. **Desc:** Represents the interests of family physicians in India. Works to strengthen partnership between Indian doctors. **Pub:** Journal, bimonthly.

### ★ 2164 ★ Indian Council of Medical Research (ICMR)

PO Box 4911
New Delhi 110 029, India
**Phone:** 91 11 6963980     **Fax:** 91 11 6868662
**Email:** icmrhqd@ren.nic.in

**Fnded:** 1911.

### ★ 2165 ★ Indian Society for Medical Statistics (ISMS)

Ansari Nagar
New Delhi 110 029, India
**Phone:** 91 11 6516003     **Fax:** 91 11 6862663
**Email:** karimassery@netscape.net

**Fnded:** 1983. **Desc:** Facilitates communication among those engaged in medical research and teaching of medical statistics; enhances the development and use of statistics in medicine and public health.

### ★ 2166 ★ Indians Into Medicine (INMED)

University of North Dakota
School of Medicine and Health Services
PO Box 9037
Grand Forks, ND 58202-9037
**Phone:** (701)777-3037     **Fax:** (701)777-3277
**Email:** inmed@medicine.nodak.edu
**Website:**          http://www.med.und.edu/depts/inmed/home.htm
Eugene DeLorme, J.D., Dir.

**Fnded:** 1973. **Desc:** Support program for American Indian students. Seeks to: increase the awareness of and interest in healthcare professions among young American Indians; recruit and enroll American Indians in healthcare education programs; place American health professionals in service to Indian communities. Coordinates financial and personal support for students in healthcare curricula. Provides referral and counseling services. Maintains 2000 volume library. Provides summer enrichment sessions at the junior high, high school and pre-medical levels as well as academic year support for college and professional level students. **Pub:** *Serpent, Staff and Drum*, quarterly. Newsletter. *Price:* Free. • Also publishes program information and motivational materials.

### ★ 2167 ★ Inflammation Research Association (IRA)

c/o Richard J. Griffiths, Secretary
Pfizer Global R&D
Eastein Point Rd.
Groton, CT 06340
**Phone:** (860)441-6124          **Fax:** (860)270-5114
**Email:** Richard_J_Griffiths@groton.pfizer.com
**Website:** http://www.inflammationresearch.org
Richard D. Dyer, PhD, Pres.

**Fnded:** 1970. **Desc:** Brings together scientists with an interest in inflammation research. Encourages the communication and discussion of science. **Pub:** *IRA Newsletter*, quarterly. Newsletter. Exchanges information between the Association and its members. • *Official Journal: Inflammation Research*. Journal.

### ★ 2168 ★ Institut Pierre Richet

01 Boite Postale 1500
Bouake, Cote d'Ivoire
**Phone:** 225 633746          **Fax:** 225 632738
**Email:** ipr@ird.ci
**Website:** http://www.ird.ci/ird/richet.html

**Lang(s):** English, French. **Desc:** Medical researchers and health care professionals. Promotes improved diagnostic techniques and treatments of common diseases. Conducts research and educational programs; makes available health services.

### ★ 2169 ★ Institute of Arctic Medicine

c/o University of Oulu
PO Box 5000
90014 University of Oulu
FIN-90220 Oulu 22, Finland
**Phone:** 358 8 5533568     **Fax:** 358 8 5376203
**Email:** juhani.hassi@oulu.fi
**Website:** http://cc.oulu.fi

**Fnded:** 1969. **Mem:** 6. **Lang(s):** English, Finnish, Swedish. **Desc:** Promotes research into arctic medicine; encourages cooperation among researchers. Disseminates reports and other information to persons engaged in arctic medicine. **Pub:** *International Journal of Circumpolar Health*, quarterly. Journal. • Monographs. • Proceedings. **Frmly:** Nordic Council for Artic Medical Research.

### ★ 2170 ★ Institute of Health Promotion and Education

University Dental Hospital
Department of Oral Health and Development
Higher Cambridge St.
Manchester M15 6FH, United Kingdom
**Phone:** 44 161 2756610     **Fax:** 44 161 2756299
**Email:** anthony.blinkhorn@man.ac.uk
**Website:** http://www.ihpe.org.uk

**Fnded:** 1962. **Mem:** 1,000. **Desc:** Members are individuals concerned with the promotion of health and the prevention of illness in all sections of the community at home, school, work and leisure. **Pub:** *International Journal of Health Promotion and Education*, quarterly. Journal.

### ★ 2171 ★ Institute for Research on Women's Health

c/o Deborah Brower
PMB 4013
1825 I St., Ste. 400
Washington, DC 20006
**Phone:** (202)429-2025     **Fax:** (301)564-0987
**Email:** djbrower2@earthlink.net
**Website:** http://www.irwh.org
Deborah J. Brower, Exec. Dir.

**Fnded:** 1984. **Desc:** Scholarly research, education, and policy work related to the health of women. Promotes work related to the physical and mental health of women.

### ★ 2172 ★ Institute of Sterile Services Management

c/o Frank Waller
Sterile Services Department
Royal Cornwall Hospitals Trust
Treslike Hospital
Treslike
Truro TR1 3LJ, United Kingdom
**Phone:** 44 1872 252816     **Fax:** 44 1872 260470
**Email:** frank.waller@rcht.swest.nhs.uk
**Website:** http://www.issm.org.uk

**Desc:** Different grades of membership - Fellow, Member, Student member, Associate, Corporate, Honorary, Associate Technician. Aims to organise and initiate training programmes for members/students, with the object of achieving high professional standards; provides a forum for members through regional branches to consider and discuss matters relating to sterilization and disinfection and promotes and encourages research and development in the world of sterile service. **Pub:** *The ISSM Journal*, quarterly. Journal. • *Official Reference Book*, annual. • *Training Handbook for Steril Service Personnel*.

### ★ 2173 ★ Intensive Care Society (ICS)

9 Bedford Sq.
London WC1B 3RE, United Kingdom
**Phone:** 44 20 76318890     **Fax:** 44 20 76318897
**Email:** admin@ics.ac.uk
**Website:** http://www.ics.ac.uk

**Fnded:** 1970. **Mem:** 2,000. **Lang(s):** English. **Desc:** Medical and scientific specialists in the field of intensive care. Seeks to provide the scientific and professional basis necessary for the research activities related to intensive care issues, and to make advice and information available to interested parties. Promotes communication among related organizations. **Pub:** *Fire Safety in the Intensive Care Unit*. Book. • *ICS Newsletter*, quarterly. Newsletter. • *Recommendations for Training in Intensive Care*. Book. • *Transport of the Critically Ill*. Book.

### ★ 2174 ★ Interamerican College of Physicians and Surgeons (ICPS)

915 Broadway, Ste. 1105
New York, NY 10010
**Phone:** (212)777-3642     **Fax:** (212)777-5000
**Email:** icps@icps.org
**Website:** http://www.icps.org
Dr. Rene F. Rodriguez, MD, Pres.

**Fnded:** 1979. **Mem:** 4,000. **Desc:** Physicians in countries of the Americas. Encourages understanding and communication among members concerning all aspects of medical practice. Promotes health education in Hispanic communities in the Western Hemisphere. Maintains library of Spanish language medical books. **Pub:** *Interamerican Medical Directory*, biennial. Directory. • *Medico Interamericano*, monthly. Journal.

**★ 2175 ★ Interamerican Medical and Health Association (IMHA)**
3025 St. James Dr.
Boca Raton, FL 33434
**Phone:** (561)483-7682     **Fax:** (561)483-3239
Dr. Maurizio Luca-Moretti, Pres.
**Fnded:** 1989. **Mem:** 4,000. **Desc:** Academicians of national academies of medicine, deans of medical facilities, and professors of medical science. Promotes the work of biomedical and health scientists and the effectiveness of science in the promotion of human welfare. Facilitates networking among members and their institutions. Conducts research programs on medical and public health issues; current research focuses on nutrition and AIDS. **Pub:** *Journal of the Interamerican Medical and Health Association*, 3/year. Journal. *Price:* $60/year for institutions in North America; $60/year for insititutions in Europe and Japan; $30/year for individuals in North America; $30/year for individuals in Europe and Japan.

**★ 2176 ★ Interchurch Medical Assistance (IMA)**
College Ave. at Blue Ridge
Box 429
New Windsor, MD 21776
**Phone:** (410)635-8720     **Fax:** (410)635-8726
**Email:** imainfo@interchurch.org
**Website:** http://www.interchurch.org
Paul Derstine, Pres.
**Fnded:** 1961. **Mem:** 12. **Desc:** Denominational-founded autonomous organization for the solicitation, collection, and distribution of pharmaceutical, medical, dental, and hospital supplies for use in the overseas charity medical programs of American Protestant churches, relief agencies, and other American charitable organizations. **Pub:** *Interchurch Medical Newsletter*, monthly. Newsletter. Electronic newsletter. • Annual Report, annual.

**★ 2177 ★ Intermed International**
420 Lexington Ave., Ste. 2331
New York, NY 10170
**Phone:** (212)687-3620     **Fax:** (212)599-6137
**Email:** dooleyfdn@aol.com
Verne Chaney, MD, Founder & Pres.
**Fnded:** 1961. **Desc:** Assists Third World countries in the development of medical care systems through self-help projects in disease prevention, health education, personnel development, and research and medical aid to refugees. Presently operates programs in Laos, Honduras, Nepal, and Nicaragua. **Pub:** *Intermed Journal*, semiannual. Brochure. • *INTERMED Journal*, semiannual. Journal. **Frmly:** Dooley Foundation/INTERMED; (1962) Dr. Thomas A. Dooley Foundation; (1978) Thomas A. Dooley Foundation; (1980) Thomas A. Dooley Foundation/INTERMED U.S.A.

**★ 2178 ★ International Academy of Cytology (IAC)**
Department of Obstetrics and Gynecology
University of Freiburg
Burgunderstr. 1
D-79104 Freiburg, Germany
**Phone:** 49 761 2923802     **Fax:** 49 761 2703122
**Email:** centraloffice@cytology-iac.org
**Website:** http://www.cytology-iac.org
**Fnded:** 1957. **Mem:** 1,900. **Lang(s):** English, French, German, Japanese, Spanish. **Desc:** Doctors of medicine concerned with research in clinical cytology (the scientific study of the structure, organization, and function of cells, particularly for cancer diagnosis); cytotechnologists actively engaged in the practice of cytodiagnosis and research. Encourages cooperation among persons engaged in the practice of clinical cytology; facilitates international exchange of information on specialized problems in this field; standardizes terminology; stimulates development of all phases of clinical cytology and encourages research. **Pub:** *Acta Cytologica*, bimonthly. • *Analytic and Quantitative Cytology and Histology*, bimonthly. • Newsletter, periodic.

**★ 2179 ★ International Academy of Gnathology-American Section (IAG)**
3868 Riviera Dr.
San Diego, CA 92109-6351
Dr. James M. Benson, Sec. -Treas.
**Fnded:** 1964. **Mem:** 200. **Desc:** Dentists and educators interested in the science of gnathology. (Gnathology is the science that treats the biology of chewing and the jaws and cheeks as related to the rest of the body.) Areas of concern include morphology, anatomy, psychology, physiology, pathology, and therapy of the mouth. **Pub:** *Journal of Gnathology*, annual. Journal.

**★ 2180 ★ International Academy of Health Care Professionals (IAHCP)**
333 Glen Cove Rd., Ste. 180
Old Brookville, NY 11545
**Phone:** (516)759-4630     **Fax:** (516)931-3163
Dr. Henry H. Reiter, Pres.
**Fnded:** 1984. **Mem:** 38. **Desc:** Nurses, psychologists, social workers, and medical and health care professionals. Provides for educational exchange among members. Offers research and educational materials to Third World health care institutions. **Pub:** *Membership Brochure*. Brochure. • Newsletter, periodic.

**★ 2181 ★ International Adhesions Society (IAS)**
c/o David Wiseman
Synechion, Inc.
6757 Arapaho Rd., Ste. 711 No. 238
Dallas, TX 75248
**Phone:** (972)931-5596     **Fax:** (972)931-5476
**Email:** david.wiseman@adhesions.org
**Website:** http://www.adhesions.org
Dr. David Wiseman, Contact
**Desc:** Promotes treatment for adhesions and chronic pelvic pain. Adhesions are scars that form an abnormal connection between two parts of the body, including non-surgical insults such as endometriosis, infection, chemotherapy, radiation and cancer, or from surgical procedures. Assists formation of support groups. **Pub:** Video.Set of lecture tapes from the March 12, 2001 IAS conference held in Detroit, Michigan. *Price:* Included with $50 member donation.

**★ 2182 ★ International Alliance of Healthcare Educators (IAHE)**
11211 Prosperity Farms Rd., Ste. D-325
Palm Beach Gardens, FL 33410
**Phone:** (561)622-4334     **Free:** 800-233-5880
**Fax:** (561)622-4771
**Email:** upledger@upledger.com
**Website:** http://www.upledger.com/know/iahe.htm
**Fnded:** 1996. **Desc:** Health care instructors and curriculum developers; seeks to advance innovative therapies through continuing education.

**★ 2183 ★ International Association for Accident and Traffic Medicine (IAATM)**
IAATM Offuce
Schit Ersan cad 28/6
Cankaya
TR-06680 Ankara, Turkey
**Phone:** 90 312 2850202     **Fax:** 90 312 2872390
**Fnded:** 1960. **Mem:** 370. **Reg. Groups:** 7. **Lang(s):** English. **Desc:** Physicians and other professionals in 56 countries who are interested in motor vehicle and traffic related accidents; national associations for accident and traffic medicine. Fosters communication among governments and other organizations concerned with traffic problems. Conducts research; disseminates information. **Pub:** *Congress Proceedings*. Proceedings. • *Journal of Traffic Medicine*, quarterly. Journal.

**★ 2184 ★ International Association of Healthcare Practitioners (IAHP)**
11211 Prosperity Farms Rd., Ste. D-325
Palm Beach Gardens, FL 33410
**Phone:** (561)622-4334     **Free:** 800-233-5880
**Fax:** (561)622-4771
**Email:** upledger@upledger.com
**Website:** http://www.upledger.com/know/iahp.htm
**Desc:** Osteopathic physicians, medical doctors, doctors of Chiropractic, doctors of Oriental medicine, naturopathic physicians, nurses, psychiatric specialists, psychologists, dentists, speech pathologists, physical acupuncturists, massage therapists and other professional bodyworkers. Dedicated to offering innovative therapies and solutions in healthcare; provides a united voice to legislative bodies, insurance regulators, patients, clients and other healthcare providers. **Pub:** Directories.

**★ 2185 ★ International Association of Holistic Medicine**
BernaDean University
4842 Whitsett Ave.
Valley Village, CA 91607-3544
Adele Kadans, Pres.
**Fnded:** 1954. **Desc:** Works to: establish standards for public retreats for the study of health practices; operate health havens as pilot studies; approve and supervise retreats operated by others. **Pub:** *Holistic Health Quarterly*, quarterly. Journal. **Frmly:** (1998) Holistic Health Havens.

**★ 2186 ★ International Association for Hospice and Palliative Care (IAHPC)**
c/o Josefina B. Magno
1515 Holcombe Blvd., Box 08
Houston, TX 77030
**Phone:** (713)339-2006     **Fax:** (713)339-9041
**Email:** sitemngr@hospicecare.com
**Website:** http://www.hospicecare.com/
Josefina B. Magno, MD, Founder & Pres.
**Desc:** Promotes availability and access to high quality hospice and palliative care for patients and families in order to alleviate physical and psychosocial suffering associated with progressive, incurable illness throughout the world. Provides communication and education for patients, professionals, health care providers and policy makers. **Pub:** Reports.

**★ 2187 ★ International Association for Medical Research and Cultural Exchange (AIRMEC) (Association Internationale pour la Recherche Medicale et les Echanges Culturels — AIRMEC)**
2, blvd. Pershing
F-75017 Paris, France
**Phone:** 33 1 55379015     **Fax:** 33 1 55379040
**Fnded:** 1956. **Mem:** 2,000. **Lang(s):** French. **Desc:** Medical and pharmaceutical professionals. Fosters and participates in the development of medical research. Initiates scientific exchange among members throughout the world. Organizes activities such as conferences, conventions, and workshops to facilitate medico-pharmaceutical comparison. Promotes and contributes to postgraduate medical and pharmaceutical study. **Pub:** *Medecine d'Afrique Noire*, monthly.

**★ 2188 ★ International Association of Medical Science Educators (IAMSE)**
One Crested Butte Dr., Ste. 100
Huntington, WV 25705
**Phone:** (304)733-1270     **Fax:** (304)733-6203
**Email:** julie@iamse.org
**Website:** http://www.iamse.org
Julie Hewett, Bus. Mgr.
**Fnded:** 1997. **Mem:** 390. **Desc:** Dedicated to sharing experiences and strategies for teaching the fundamental sciences of medicine. **Pub:** *Basic Science Educator*, semiannual. Journal. Written specifically for medical science educators.

### ★ 2189 ★ International Association of Neuro-Linguistic Programming (IANLP)

42 Spruce Ridge
Route 9P
Saratoga Springs, NY 12866
**Email:** info@inlpa.org
**Website:** http://www.ia-nlp.org
Laura Shaw, Mgr.

**Fnded:** 1983. **Mem:** 1,300. **Reg. Groups:** 9. **Desc:** Certified neuro-linguistic programming practitioners and programmers (355); certified master programmers (393); certified NLP trainers (152); individuals with some training in NLP (400). (NLP is a discipline that examines the structure of human thought and response and is used in counseling, psychotherapy, and business applications.) Provides an international network for the exchange of ideas, materials, and services. Sets standards for the ethical use of NLP and for NLP training and certification. Encourages and supports research and development; fosters utilization of new technologies in NLP; seeks to integrate the skills and ideas of other disciplines with those of NLP. Promotes greater public understanding of NLP and its objectives. Sponsors NLP workshops. Cooperates with other professional organizations. **Pub:** *IANLP*, annual. Membership Directory. • Newsletter, bimonthly. **Frmly:** (1991) International Association for Neuro-Linguistic Programming; (1993) International Association of Neuro-Linguistic Programming; (1995) North American Association of Neuro-Linguistic Programming.

### ★ 2190 ★ International Association of Physicians and Health Care Professionals

PO Box 13089
Tallahassee, FL 32317
R.S. Rhinehart, Pres. /CEO

**Fnded:** 1996. **Mem:** 85. **Desc:** Organization for physicians and allied health care workers.

### ★ 2191 ★ International Biodegradable Products Manufacturers Association (IBPMA)

Eglantierlaan 5a
B-2020 Antwerp, Belgium
**Phone:** 32 3 8357728          **Fax:** 32 3 8257726
**Email:** bertlemmes@ibpma.be

**Desc:** Promotes members' interests.

### ★ 2192 ★ International Center for the Health Sciences (ICHS)

Barracks Hill
PO Box 4744
Charlottesville, VA 22904-4744
**Phone:** (804)971-7605          **Fax:** (804)971-7605
**Email:** info@ichsciences.org
**Website:** http://www.ichsciences.org
Warren E. Grupe, MD, Medical Dir.

**Fnded:** 1991. **Desc:** Works to improve the health of all people through creative health education programs designed to meet the unique needs and capabilities of communities around the world. Sponsors collaborative research; develops and strengthens current preventative and curative care; manages and implements health science education programs in cooperation with US institutions in Central America, Africa and the former Soviet Union; advocates for the health care needs of all people.

**International Child Care - Canada (ICC)**
*See:* Entry 5693

### ★ 2193 ★ International Christian Federation for the Prevention of Alcoholism and Drug Addiction (Federation Chretienne Internationale pour la Prophylaxie de l'Alcoolisme et des Autres Toxicomanies)

c/o Johnathan N. Gnanadasn
20A Ancienne Route. Apt. 42
Grand Succonex
CH-1218 Geneva, Switzerland
**Phone:** 41 22 7888158
**Email:** canada@intlchildcare.org
**Website:** http://www.gospelcom.net/icc/

**Fnded:** 1980. **Mem:** 34. **Lang(s):** English, French, German, Spanish. **Desc:** Churches and federations of churches in membership with the World Council of Churches; national temperance councils or regional groups working in the field of alcohol and drugs; other supporting churches or federations of churches. Seeks to: promote worldwide educational and remedial work through the churches, "teaching the wisdom of sobriety for the welfare of society"; act as a resource agency focusing on the Christian concern related to alcohol and drug abuse by sharing research, educational work, and experience; provide a means whereby informed Christian thought and experience is related to the World Health Organization and is expressed by member churches. Organizes charitable and training programs. **Pub:** *Newsletter*, periodic. Newsletter.

### ★ 2194 ★ International Congress on Tropical Medicine and Malaria (Congres International de Medicine Tropicale et de Paludisme)

c/o Dr. E.C. Garcia
Institute of Public Health
University of the Philippines
PO Box EA-460
Manila, Philippines

**Lang(s):** English, Tagalog. **Desc:** Health care professionals and medical researchers with an interest in tropical medicine. Seeks to advance research and practice in tropical medicine; promotes development of improved methods of prevention, diagnosis, and treatment of tropical disorders. Serves as a clearinghouse on tropical medicine; sponsors research; conducts educational and continuing professional development courses.

### ★ 2195 ★ International Council on Alcohol and Addictions (ICAA) (Conseil International sur les Problemes de l'Alcoolisme et des Toxicomanies — CIPAT)

Case Postale 189
CH-1001 Lausanne, Switzerland
**Phone:** 41 21 3209865          **Fax:** 41 21 3209817
**Email:** secretariat@icaa.ch
**Website:** http://www.icaa.de/

**Fnded:** 1907. **Mem:** 450. **Lang(s):** English, French, German, Spanish. **Desc:** Persons and organizations interested in or working with problems of alcoholism or drug addiction in 80 countries. Encourages interdisciplinary exchange of information and experience in research, prevention, treatment, and rehabilitation for alcoholism and drug addiction. Organizes international conferences on the prevention and treatment of alcohol and drug dependence. Also focusses on issues related to tobacco dependence and gambling. **Pub:** *Alcoholism*, semiannual. Journal. • *ICAA News*, quarterly. **Frmly:** (1935) International Bureau Against Alcoholism; (1968) International Union Against Alcoholism.

**International Council on Alcohol, Drugs and Traffic Safety (ICADTS)**
*See:* Entry 19295

### ★ 2196 ★ International Council for Control of Iodine Deficiency Disorders (ICCIDD)

72 King William Rd.
North Adelaide, SA 5006, Australia
**Phone:** 61 8 2047021          **Fax:** 61 8 2047221
**Email:** iccidd@ao11.aone.net.au
**Website:** http://www.people.virginia.edu/~jtd/iccidd

**Fnded:** 1986. **Desc:** Promotes development of national iodine deficiency disorders, assists and promotes adaptive research, practical validation and transfer of technology.

### ★ 2197 ★ International Council of Prison Medical Services (ICPMS) (Conseil International des Services Medicaux Penitentiaires)

750 W Broadway, Ste. 1417
Vancouver, BC, Canada V5Z 1J4
**Phone:** (604)872-8719

**Fnded:** 1976. **Mem:** 200. **Nat'l Groups:** 1. **Lang(s):** English, French, Spanish. **Desc:** Medical and health care professionals; associate members are administrators of prison health care agencies. Promotes discussion among prison health professionals. Strives to improve health care worldwide; encourages postgraduate training for doctors working in prison settings. **Pub:** Proceedings.

### ★ 2198 ★ International Electrology Educators (IEE)

c/o SCME
132 Great Rd., No. 200
Stow, MA 01775
**Phone:** (978)461-0313          **Fax:** (617)237-9039
**Email:** scme@scmeweb.org
**Website:** http://www.scmeweb.org/ieeabou.htm
Lauren Hunte, Contact

**Fnded:** 1979. **Mem:** 55. **Desc:** Electrology schools and teachers. Purposes are to instruct teachers and standardize the curriculum and teaching of electrology. Conducts educational programs and regional educational conferences for electrology educators. **Pub:** *IEE Directory of Schools*, periodic. Directory. • *Perspectives*, quarterly. **Frmly:** (1982) National Electrology Educators; (1985) International Electrology Educators; (1993) Institute of Electrology Educators.

### ★ 2199 ★ International Enneagram Association (IEA)

1060 N 4th St.
San Jose, CA 95113
**Phone:** (408)971-5905          **Fax:** (408)999-0344
**Email:** ieastaff@intl-enneagram-assn.org
**Website:** http://www.intl-enneagram-assn.org
Debi Goddard, Adm.

**Desc:** Working to promote the highest human values through the insights of the Enneagram. Sponsors open and constructive interactions among various schools of Enneagram thought; encourages innovative application of the Enneagram and builds community through grass roots regional participation.

### ★ 2200 ★ International Federation of the Blue Cross (IFBC) (Federation Internationale de la Croix-Bleue — FICB)

Lindenrain 5A
PO Box 6813
CH-3001 Bern, Switzerland
**Phone:** 41 31 3005860          **Fax:** 41 31 3005869
**Email:** ifbc.bern@bluewin.ch
**Website:** http://www.eurocare.org/bluecross/

**Fnded:** 1877. **Mem:** 72,946. **Nat'l Groups:** 33. **Reg. Groups:** 2170. **Lang(s):** English, French, German, Portuguese. **Desc:** National societies and local groups representing individuals in 50 countries. Works to help alcoholics and drug addicts. Disseminates information concerning alcoholism. Operates cure homes and clinics. **Pub:** *Editorial*, bimonthly. Newsletter. • *INFO*, semiannual. **Frmly:** (1983) International Federation of the Temperance Blue Cross Societies.

**★ 2201 ★ International Federation of Health Plans (FHP)**
46 Grosvenor Gardens
London SW1W 0EB, United Kingdom
**Phone:** 44 20 78819281  **Fax:** 44 20 77309234
**Email:** administrator@fhf.com
**Website:** http://www.fhf.com
**Fnded:** 1968. **Mem:** 100. **Lang(s):** English. **Desc:** Nongovermental organizations involved in the execution of independent health care finance (100); associations of health funds (11) and individuals (26) in 20 countries. Promotes the study and development of independent health care services. Encourages research and the exchange of information. Operates conferences and meetings; information and research; sharing of infromation in cohesive network of member health funds. Offers study tours and educational programmes. **Pub:** *Conference Proceedings*, biennial. • *Membership Directory*, annual. Directory. • *National Commentaries*, biennial. • *Newsletter*, quarterly. Newsletter. • Booklets, periodic. **Frmly:** (1989) International Federation of Voluntary Health Service Funds; (1999) International Federation of Health Funds.

**★ 2202 ★ International Federation of Societies for Histochemistry and Cytochemistry (IFSHC)**
c/o Dr. Denis G. Baskin
Department of Biological Structure
Univ. of Washington
PO Box 357420
Seattle, WA 98195-9420
**Phone:** (206)616-5894  **Fax:** (206)616-5842
**Email:** baskindg@u.washington.edu
**Website:** http://www.ifshc.org
Prof.Dr. Denis G. Baskin, Sec. Gen.
**Fnded:** 1960. **Mem:** 22. **Nat'l Groups:** 22. **Desc:** National societies for histochemistry and cytochemistry. Seeks to promote communication and cooperation among scientists throughout the world and establish histochemistry and cytochemistry institutes. Promotes histochemistry and cytochemistry as basic, independent sciences and advocates their teaching in universities. Appoints committees for the study of scientific matters requiring international collaboration. **Pub:** *Proceedings*, quadrennial. • Also publishes scientific journals.

**★ 2203 ★ International Foundation for Homeopathy (IFH)**
PO Box 7
Edmonds, WA 98020
**Fax:** (425)776-1499
**Email:** ifh@nwlink.com
Niedra North, Exec. Dir.
**Fnded:** 1978. **Mem:** 2,000. **Desc:** Medical professionals (700) and laypersons (1300) interested in homeopathy. Promotes homeopathy and provides the public with a better understanding of health and diseases through homeopathy. (The word "homeopathy" is taken from the Greek "homeos", meaning "similar", and "pathos", meaning "suffering." Homeopathy therefore means "to treat with something that produces an effect similar to the suffering.") Works to: increase public and professional education; promote acceptance and teaching of homeopathy in medical schools. Sponsors research; conducts annual courses for licensed medical professionals and serious students of homeopathy. Maintains referral service. **Pub:** *International Foundation for Homeopathy–Resonance*, bimonthly. Magazine. Contains information on case histories and clinical advances in research, medicine, and technology. Includes book reviews and calendar of events. *Price:* Included in membership dues. • *Proceedings of Professional Case Conference*, annual. Book. Contains presentation of cured cases. *Price:* $34.50. **Frmly:** (1981) International Foundation for the Promotion of Homeopathy.

**★ 2204 ★ International Guild of Professional Electrologists (IGPE)**
803 N Main St., Ste. A
High Point, NC 27262
**Phone:** (336)841-6631  **Free:** 800-830-3247
**Fax:** (336)841-5187
**Website:** http://www.igpe.org
Trudy Brown, Pres.
**Fnded:** 1978. **Mem:** 2,200. **Reg. Groups:** 5. **Desc:** Electrologists; electrology schools; manufacturers and suppliers of electrolysis equipment. Works to improve the image of electrolysis and promote it as an acceptable allied health profession. Promotes licensing of electrologists. Provides referral service. Conducts seminars. **Pub:** *A Complete Guide to Hair Removal*. Brochure. • *A Doctor Answers Questions About Hair Removal*. Brochure. • *Consumer Health Guidelines*. Brochure. • *Everything You Ever Wanted to Know About Hair Removal But Were Afraid to Ask*. Brochure. • *International Directory*, annual. Directory. • *International Guild of Professional Electrologists*, quarterly. Newsletter. Includes biennial conference reports. *Price:* Free to members. • *Physical Methods for the Management of Hirsutism*. Brochure. • *Selecting an Electrologist: Thermolysis for Permanent Hair Removal*. Brochure.

**★ 2205 ★ International Health Foundation**
6501 Bright Mountain Rd.
Mc Lean, VA 22101
**Fax:** (703)356-4143
**Email:** eyedoc2000@hotmail.com
**Website:** http://www.ihf.nl/
Kenneth D. Hansen, MD, Exec. Dir.
**Fnded:** 1972. **Desc:** Provides governmental organizations and health providers with methods for improving health services. Focuses on medical systems and medical and legal affairs. Offers assistance to developing countries. Sponsors educational programs; conducts research. Maintains speakers' bureau. Distinct from organization of same name listed in index.

**★ 2206 ★ International Health and Safety Association for Radio and Television (IHSART)**
c/o Andre Vincke
VRT-2N20
52, Auguste Reyers
B-1043 Brussels, Belgium
**Phone:** 32 2 7413681  **Fax:** 32 2 7349351
**Email:** aslak.savolainen@yle.fi
**Fnded:** 1980. **Mem:** 14. **Lang(s):** English, French. **Desc:** Broadcasting corporations; organizations and individuals interested in the radio and television fields. Seeks to: improve the physical and mental health of radio and television employees; promote safety, hygiene, and preventive medicine as well as better working facilities for radio and television personnel; advance ergonomics, rehabilitation for the handicapped, and the disciplines of industrial medicine. Encourages the collection of statistical and nosological information on the health of television and radio personnel. Conducts research on ergonomics and occupational therapy and medicine. **Pub:** *Newsletter*, annual. Newsletter. • Papers, periodic. Containing information on science and applied medical and paramedical technology. **Frmly:** International Medical Association for Radio and Television.

**★ 2207 ★ International Maritime Health Association (IMHA)**
Italielei 51
2000 Antwerp, Belgium
**Phone:** 32 3 2252038  **Fax:** 32 3 2290776
**Email:** imha@online.be
**Website:** http://www.imha.net/
**Fnded:** 1997. **Desc:** Fosters scientific research and the quality of maritime medicine worldwide; creates a forum for people, ideas, efforts, research and questions regarding maritime health.

**★ 2208 ★ International Medical Informatics Association for Latin America and the Caribbean (IMIA-LAC)**
PO Box 6005
13081-970 Campinas, Brazil
**Phone:** 55 19 2899800  **Fax:** 55 19 2894959
**Email:** sabbatin@nib.unicamp.br
**Website:** http://www.imia-lac.org
**Fnded:** 1983.

**★ 2209 ★ International Network Towards Smoke-free Hospitals**
c/o John Bickerstaff, Gen.Sec.
45 Brookscroft
Linton Glade
Croydon CR0 9NA, United Kingdom
**Phone:** 44 20 86515436  **Fax:** 44 20 86513428
**Email:** jbickerstaff@cix.co.uk
**Fnded:** 1991. **Lang(s):** English. **Desc:** Physicians, nurses, hospital administrators, healthcare workers, and other interested parties. Seeks to protect, preserve, and improve the health of patients, visitors, and person working in hospitals or in connection with health services, in the U.K. and overseas, by promoting smoke-free environments in hospitals and other healthcare facilities. Provides advice and briefings to hospitals wishing to become smoke-free. **Pub:** *Making Hospitals Smoke Free*. • *Smoke-Free Hospitals International*.

**★ 2210 ★ International Organization for Cooperation in Health Care (IOCHC) (Medicus Mundi Internationalis — MMI)**
64, rue des Deux Eglises
B-1210 Brussels, Belgium
**Phone:** 32 2 2310605  **Fax:** 32 2 2311852
**Email:** medicusmundi@ngonet.be
**Website:** http://medicusmundi.org
**Fnded:** 1963. **Mem:** 11. **Nat'l Groups:** 8. **Lang(s):** English, French. **Desc:** National branches and organizations of physicians and paramedical personnel. Promotes the fields of health care and disease prevention as a necessary part of development of all nations. Encourages primary health care through comprehensive, integrated, long-term health programs. Documents socio-medical information on developing countries to assess the medical needs and demands of those countries. Other aims include: encouraging dialogue with the Third World; strengthening relations between national branches and European governments; profiling experts serving IOHC; providing field workers with practical conclusions, recommendations, and moral support regarding new strategies, methods, or operations. Offers training programs. **Pub:** Newsletter, quarterly. • Proceedings, periodic. Contains meeting reports.

**★ 2211 ★ International Organization for Medical Physics (IOMP)**
c/o Gary D. Fullerton, PhD
Department of Radiology
MSC 7800
7703 Floyd Curl Dr.
San Antonio, TX 78229-3900
**Phone:** (210)567-5551  **Fax:** (210)567-5549
**Email:** fullertson@uthscsa.edu
**Website:** http://www.iomp.org/
Gary D. Fullerton, PhD, Sec. Gen.
**Fnded:** 1963. **Mem:** 56. **Desc:** A member of the International Union of Physical and Engineering Sciences in Medicine. National organizations of medical physics representing 10,000 individuals. Fosters international cooperation in medical physics; promotes communication between various branches of medical physics and allied subjects. Conducts training programs. Has established 43 libraries in developing countries. **Pub:** *Clinical Physics and Physiological Measurement*, bimonthly. • *Medical Physics World*, semiannual. • *Physics in Medicine and Biology*, monthly.

**International Paediatric Pathology Association**
*See:* Entry 5696

**International Regional Organization of Plant Protection and Animal Health (OIRSA)**
**(Organismo Internacional Regional de Sanidad Agropecuaria — OIRSA)**
*See:* Entry 20632

★ **2212** ★ **International Research Group on Biochemistry of Exercise**
Av Paul Heger 28
1000 Brussels, Belgium
**Phone:** 32 2 6504209          **Fax:** 32 2 6502195
**Email:** jrpoortma@ulb.ac.be
**Website:** http://www.oirsa.org.sv

★ **2213** ★ **International Society for Artificial Organs (ISAO)**
8937 Euclid Ave.
Cleveland, OH 44106
**Phone:** (440)358-1102        **Fax:** (440)358-1104
Dr. S. Nitta, MD, Dir.
**Fnded:** 1977. **Mem:** 1,000. **Reg. Groups:** 4. **Desc:** Medical doctors, technicians, bioengineers, and researchers. Publishes materials covering all aspects of artificial organs; conducts research. Maintains museum. **Pub:** *Artificial Organs*, bimonthly. • Also publishes books.

★ **2214** ★ **International Society for the History of Medicine (ISHM)**
20, rue Armagis
F-78105 St.-Germain-en-Laye, France
**Email:** alain.lellouch@wanadoo.fr

★ **2215** ★ **International Society of Internal Medicine (ISIM)**
**(Societe Internationale de Medecine Interne)**
c/o Dr. Rolf A. Streuli
Regional Hospital
CH-4900 Langenthal, Switzerland
**Phone:** 41 62 9163102        **Fax:** 41 62 9164155
**Email:** r.streuli@sro.ch
**Website:** http://www.acponline.org/isim/
**Fnded:** 1948. **Mem:** 3,000. **Nat'l Groups:** 54. **Lang(s):** English. **Desc:** Internal medicine specialists. Promotes scientific knowledge in internal medicine; furthers the education of young internists; encourages friendship among physicians in all countries. Federation of Societies of Internal Medicine from 43 countries.

★ **2216** ★ **International Society for the Investigation of Stress (ISIS)**
Level 1
South Wing
A and RMC, Repat Campus
Heidelberg West, VIC 3081, Australia
**Phone:** 61 3 94964105        **Fax:** 61 3 94964107

★ **2217** ★ **International Society for Medical Education - United States**
c/o S.H.K. Reddy, MD.
200 Medical Center Dr., Ste. 3A
Hazard, KY 41701-9422
**Phone:** (606)439-4767        **Fax:** (606)439-4768
**Email:** shkreddy@lname.com
T.S. Reddy, MD., Pres.
**Fnded:** 1992. **Mem:** 7. **Reg. Groups:** 1. **Desc:** Works to provide medical education and health care in underdeveloped and third-world countries by establishing medical schools and hospitals. Provides free medical education, and charity medical care. Establishes women's welfare centers.

★ **2218** ★ **International Society for Mountain Medicine**
c/o Peter Hackett, MD
610 Sabeta Dr.
Ridgway, CO 81432-9335
**Phone:** (970)626-2477        **Fax:** (970)626-2467
**Email:** hackett@ismmed.org
**Website:** http://www.ismmed.org
**Fnded:** 1985. **Mem:** 450. **Desc:** Brings together scientists and physicians, and allied trade professionals interested in mountain medicine. Encourages research on all aspects of mountains, mountain peoples and mountaineers. **Pub:** *High Altitude Medicine and Biology*, quarterly. Journal. Provides information about high altitude/mountain physiology and clinical medicine.

★ **2219** ★ **International Society for Orthomolecular Medicine**
16 Florence Ave.
Toronto, ON, Canada M2N 1E9
**Phone:** (416)733-2117        **Fax:** (416)733-2352
**Email:** centre@orthomed.org
**Website:** http://www.orthomed.org/isom/isom.htm
**Fnded:** 1994. **Desc:** Aims to further the advancement of Orthomolecular medicine throughout the world, to raise awareness of this rapidly growing and cost effective practice of health care, and to unite the many and various groups already operating in this field.

★ **2220** ★ **International Society for Research in Human Milk and Lactation**
c/o Frank R. Greer
Meriter Hospital
Perinatal Center
202 S Park St.
Madison, WI 53715
**Phone:** (608)262-6561        **Fax:** (608)267-6377
**Email:** frgreer@facstaff.wisc.edu
**Website:** http://www.isrhml.org/
Dr. Frank R. Greer, Sec. Treas.
**Desc:** Promotes research and dissemination of findings in the field of human milk and lactation. Establishes liaisons with government agencies, public health authorities, industry, and other organizations; provides listserver for communication of information among members.

★ **2221** ★ **International Society for the Study of Tension in Performance**
c/o 28 Emperor's Gate
Kingston University
School of Music
London SW7 4HS, United Kingdom
**Phone:** 44 207 3737307        **Fax:** 44 207 3735440
**Email:** carogrindea@yahoo.com
**Fnded:** 1981. **Mem:** 360. **Nat'l Groups:** 3. **Lang(s):** English, Russian, Spanish. **Desc:** Musicians, actors, dancers, medical practitioners, consultants, psychologists, physiotherapists, Alexander Technique, yoga, Feldenkrais disciplines teachers and practitioners and others interested in the subject and in the problems created by muscular and nervous tensions, physical injuries, among instrumentalists. Aims to collect and disseminate information regarding the debilitating effects of excess anxiety and tensions experienced by musicians, actors, dancers, public speakers, sportsmen, etc; to foster research and related activities; to provide advisory service for members and to assist performers with their physical or psychological problems offering free consultations. **Pub:** Journal, annual.

★ **2222** ★ **International Society for Telemedicine (IST)**
c/o Arvid Overgard
PO Box 1233
N-9262 Oslo, Norway
**Phone:** 47 77 638460        **Fax:** 47 77 610866
**Email:** isft.coordinator@trollnet.no
**Website:** http://www.isft.org
nbweb391 020328BA NKSTON.N 020328 X International Society for Telemedicine, Contact

**Desc:** Aims to promote the development of telemedicine, telecare and telehealth around the world. Seeks to work with existing national telemedicine societies, and encourage the formation of new national societies where they do not currently exist. **Frmly:** (2000) International Conference on the Medical Aspects of Telemedicine.

★ **2223** ★ **International Spa Association**
2365 Harrodsburg Rd., Ste. A325
Lexington, KY 40504
**Phone:** (859)226-4326        **Free:** 888-651-4772
**Fax:** (859)226-4445
**Email:** ispa@hostcommunications.com
**Website:** http://www.experienceispa.com
Lynne Walker, Exec. Dir.
**Fnded:** 1991. **Mem:** 1,450. **Reg. Groups:** 2. **Desc:** Professional association and voice of the spa industry. Forms and maintains alliances that educate, set standards, provide resources, influence policy and build coalitions for the industry. Raises awareness of the spa industry and educates the public and industry professionals about the benefits of the spa experience.

★ **2224** ★ **International Union for Health Promotion and Education (IUHPE)**
**(Union Internationale de Promotion de la Sante et d'Education pour la Sante — UIPES)**
2, rue Auguste Comte
F-92170 Vanves, France
**Phone:** 33 1 46450059        **Fax:** 33 1 46450045
**Email:** iuhpemcl@worldnet.fr
**Website:** http://www.iuhpe.org
**Fnded:** 1951. **Mem:** 2,000. **Reg. Groups:** 6. **Lang(s):** English, French, Spanish. **Desc:** Promotes global health and contributes to the achievement of equity in health among all countries of the world. Builds and operates an independent, global professional network of individuals and institutions to encourage free exchange of ideas, knowledge, and development of relevant collaboration at the global and regional levels. **Pub:** *Conference Proceedings*, triennial. • *The Evidence of Health Promotion Effectiveness*, periodic. Report. Report for the European Commission on the health, social, economic, and political impacts of health promotion. • *Promotion & Education*, quarterly. Journal. Contains articles on the theory and practice of health promotion and health education as well as international news about major events. • Brochure, periodic. • Newsletters, periodic.

★ **2225** ★ **International Union of Medical Advisers Associations (IUMAA)**
**(Union Internationale des Associations de Delegues Medicaux — UIADM)**
c/o Angelo De Rita
Via F. Turati, 19
I-50136 Florence, Italy
**Phone:** 39 55 691166        **Fax:** 39 55 650736
**Fnded:** 1974. **Lang(s):** French. **Desc:** Medical advisers and related scientific and medical personnel. Promotes professional advancement of members; seeks to facilitate medical and scientific research. Represents the interests of medical advisers before industrial organizations, government agencies, scientific and medical bodies, and the public. Formulates codes of ethics and practice for members.

★ **2226** ★ **Interstate Postgraduate Medical Association of North America (IPMANA)**
PO Box 5474
Madison, WI 53705
**Phone:** (608)231-9045        **Fax:** (608)231-9045
**Email:** ipma@chorus.net
H. B. Maroney, Exec. Dir.
**Fnded:** 1916. **Desc:** Presents annual four-day teaching program in various branches of medicine and medical research, aimed at the family practitioner who must keep up with new developments in a short time away from his practice.

**★ 2227 ★ Irish Medical Organisation (IMO)**
10 Fitzwilliam Pl.
Dublin 2, Ireland
**Phone:** 353 1 6767273   **Fax:** 353 1 6612758
**Email:** imo@imo.ie
**Mem:** 5,000. **Lang(s):** English, Irish. **Desc:** Physicians and medical students and their families. Seeks to develop a "caring, efficient and effective health service." Serves as a professional body representing physicians in Ireland; facilitates exchange of information among members; encourages medical research. **Pub:** *Irish Medical Journal.* Journal.

**★ 2228 ★ Irish Society of Chartered Physiotherapists**
Royal College of Surgeons
St. Stephen's Green
Dublin 2, Ireland
**Phone:** 353 1 4022148   **Fax:** 353 1 4022160
**Email:** info@iscp.ie
**Website:** http://www.iscp.ie
**Fnded:** 1983. **Mem:** 1,600. **Reg. Groups:** 8. **Desc:** Physiotherapists.

**★ 2229 ★ Islamic Medical Association of North America (IMANA)**
950 75th St.
Downers Grove, IL 60516
**Phone:** (630)852-2122   **Fax:** (630)435-1429
**Email:** imana@aol.com
**Website:** http://www.imana.org
Khursheed Mallick, MD, Exec. Dir.
**Fnded:** 1967. **Mem:** 6,000. **Desc:** Muslim physicians and allied health professionals. Unites Muslim physicians and allied health professionals in the U.S. and Canada for the improvement of professional and social contact; provides assistance to Muslim communities worldwide. Charitable programs include: donation of books, journals, and educational and research materials to medical institutions; donation of medical supplies and equipment to charity medical institutions in Muslim countries. Maintains speakers' bureau to present Islamic viewpoints on medical topics; sponsors placement service; offers assistance in orientation. **Pub:** *Al-Itiknga*, quarterly. Newsletter. • *The Journal of IMA*, quarterly. Journal. *Price:* $50/year. • *The Mediview*, quarterly. Newsletter. **Frmly:** (2001) Islamic Medical Association.

**★ 2230 ★ Islamic Organization for Medical Sciences (IOMS)**
PO Box 31280
Sulaibekhat 90803, Kuwait
**Phone:** 965 4834984   **Fax:** 965 4837854
**Email:** ioms@kuwait.net
**Website:** http://www.islamset.com
**Fnded:** 1984. **Mem:** 432. **Reg. Groups:** 6. **Lang(s):** English. **Desc:** Promotes human health standards through collaborative activities in Islamic countries and Muslim communities throughout the world, focusing on medical ethics, healthy lifestyles, and herbal medicine, as well as the fight against endemic and emerging diseases.

**★ 2231 ★ Israel Society for Microbiology (ISM)**
PO Box 9095
52190 Ramat Efal, Israel
**Phone:** 972 3 6355038   **Fax:** 972 3 5351103
**Email:** mrgzur@ibm.net
**Website:** http://ism.md.huji.ac.il
**Lang(s):** English, Hebrew. **Desc:** Microbiologists in Israel. Seeks to unite its members to ensure the scientific and professional standards are upheld; advances the science of microbiology and its research. Strengthens ties with similar societies.

**★ 2232 ★ Italian Society of Anatomy (ISA) (Societa Italiana di Anatomia — SIA)**
Istituto di Anatomia Umana Normale
Via A. Borelli No. 50
I-00161 Rome, Italy
**Phone:** 39 6 4462623   **Fax:** 39 6 4452349
**Email:** pietro.motta@uniroma1.it
**Fnded:** 1929. **Mem:** 400. **Lang(s):** English, Italian. **Desc:** Fosters the study of anatomy, histology, and embryology in Italy. **Pub:** *Italian Journal of Anatomy and Embriology*, quarterly. Journal. • Papers, periodic.

**★ 2233 ★ Jacobs Institute of Women's Health**
409 12th St. SW
Washington, DC 20024-2188
**Phone:** (202)863-4990   **Fax:** (202)488-4229
**Website:** http://www.jiwh.org/
**Mem:** 2,000. **Desc:** Works to improve health care for women through research, dialogue and education. **Pub:** *In Touch*, quarterly. Newsletter. • *Women's Health Data Book.* Book. Third edition.

**★ 2234 ★ Japan Medical Women's Association (Nihon Joi Kai)**
3rd Floor, Aoyama-Shrinefield Bldg.
Shibuya 2-8-7
Shibuya-ku
Tokyo 150-0002, Japan
**Phone:** 81 3 34980571   **Fax:** 81 3 34988769
**Email:** jmwa@jade.dti.we.jp
**Desc:** Women working in the medical profession. Works to maintain high standards.

**★ 2235 ★ Japan Overseas Christian Medical Cooperative Service (JOCS)**
2-3-18-23 Nishiwaseda
Shinjuku-ku
Tokyo 169-0051, Japan
**Phone:** 81 3 32082416   **Fax:** 81 3 32326922
**Email:** jocs-net@jocs.mxe.mesh.ne.jp
**Fnded:** 1960. **Lang(s):** English, Japanese. **Desc:** Works to coordinate the efforts of Christian sects providing medical services in Bangladesh, Cambodia, India, Indonesia, Nigeria, Pakistan, and Taiwan. Organization believes that Japan is indebted to the rest of Asia due to atrocities committed during World War II. Does not conduct evangelical programs, providing medical services without reference to a patients race, religion, color, or creed.

**★ 2236 ★ Japanese Association for Acute Medicine (JAAM)**
Department of Emergency Medicine
Osaka University School of Medicine
2-2 Yamadaoka
Suita City
Osaka 565, Japan
**Phone:** 81 6 8793331   **Fax:** 81 6 8783540
**Desc:** Medical practitioners involved in acute medicine. Represents members' interests. **Pub:** *Journal of he Japanese Association for Acute Medicine.* Journal.

**★ 2237 ★ Jeffrey Modell Foundation (JMF)**
c/o Vicki Modell
43 W 47th St.
New York, NY 10036
**Phone:** (212)819-0200   **Fax:** (212)764-4180
**Email:** info@jmfworld.org
**Website:** http://www.jmfworld.com/
Vicki Modell, Co-Founder
**Desc:** Devoted to primary immune deficiency, including research, physician and patient education, patient support, and public awareness.

**★ 2238 ★ Joint Commission on Accreditation of Healthcare Organizations (JCAHO)**
1 Renaissance Blvd.
Oakbrook Terrace, IL 60181
**Phone:** (630)792-5000   **Fax:** (630)792-5005
**Email:** doleary@jcaho.org
**Website:** http://www.jcaho.org
Dennis S. O'Leary, MD, Pres.
**Fnded:** 1951. **Desc:** Strives to improve the safety and quality of care provided to the public through the provision of health care accreditation and related services that support performance improvement in health care organizations. Evaluates and accredits nearly 20,000 health care organizations and programs in the United States, including hospitals, networks, home care, long term care, assisted living, behavioral health care, laboratory and ambulatory care services. **Pub:** *Accreditation Manuals for all Programs.* Manuals. • *Ambulatory Care Advisor.* Newsletter. Covers ambulatory care accreditation program, survey processes, standards and programs for ambulatory care. *Price:* Free. • *BHC Accreditation News*, 3/year. Newsletter. Covers the behavioral health care accreditation program. Includes information about survey processes for behavioral health care and substance abuse. *Price:* Free. • *Long Term Care Update*, 3/year. Newsletter. • *Sentinel Event Alert*, bimonthly. Newsletter. • *This Month*, monthly. Newsletter. • Also publishes educational materials, software, and videos. **Frmly:** (1987) Joint Commission on Accreditation of Hospitals.

**★ 2239 ★ Landmine Survivors Network (LSN)**
1420 K St. NW, Ste. 650
Washington, DC 20005-3960
**Phone:** (202)464-0007   **Fax:** (202)464-0011
**Email:** lsn@landminesurvivors.org
**Website:** http://www.landminesurvivors.org
**Fnded:** 1997. **Desc:** Survivors of landmines.

**★ 2240 ★ Latin American and Caribbean Women's Health Network**
Casilla Postal 50610
Santiago 1, Chile
**Phone:** 56 2 2237077   **Fax:** 56 2 2231066
**Email:** rsmlac@mail.bellsouth.cl
**Website:** http://www.reddesalud.web.cl
**Fnded:** 1984. **Mem:** 2,000. **Lang(s):** English, Spanish. **Desc:** Members include groups and organizations working directly or indirectly in fields related to women's health. Seeks to establish contacts among women and organizations active in women's health issues at the local, regional, and national levels. Promotes the sharing of information, experiences, and ideas through the development of communication networks. Coordinates common activities. Encourages informational campaigns on such subjects as reproductive rights, medicine, the environment, and other health topics of interest to women. Participates in conferences, seminars, and meetings. **Pub:** *Cuadernos Mujer Salud*, annual. Magazine. • *Revista Mujer Salud*, quarterly. Magazine. • *Women's Health Collection*, annual. Magazine.

**★ 2241 ★ Latin American Diabetes Association (Asociacion Latinoamericana de Diabetes — ALAD)**
Apartado Postal 25
Curridabat
San Jose 2300, Costa Rica
**Desc:** Promotes the study of diabetes. Works for the cure and prevention of diabetes.

**★ 2242 ★ Lebanese Ostomy Association (LOA)**
c/o Dr. Michel Daher
PO Box 166378
St. George's Hospital
Beirut, Lebanon

**Phone:** 961 1 581714          **Fax:** 961 3 422125
**Email:** mdaher@lb.refer.org
**Fnded:** 1993. **Mem:** 43. **Desc:** Medical professionals representing the interests of ostomy patients. Makes available training to nurses for ostomy care. Fosters communication and exchange.


★ 2243 ★ **Let's Face it U.S.A. (LFASU)**
c/o Betsy Wilson
PO Box 29972
Bellingham, WA 98228-1972
**Phone:** (360)676-7325
**Email:** letsfaceit@faceit.org
**Website:** http://www.faceit.org
Betsy Wilson, Dir.
**Fnded:** 1987. **Desc:** An information and support network for people who have or who care for those with facial disfigurement. Web site and annual publication with over 150 resources for medicfal and educational professionals and families. Links to all related networks for specific conditions ie. Genetic Disorders, Burns, Cancer, etc. Resource can be downloaded in Adobe format from web site or send a self addressed 9" by 12" envelop stamped with a $3.50 stamp with a note telling of information need. **Pub:** *Resources for People with Facial Difference*, annual. Report.


★ 2244 ★ **Life and Liberty for Women**
PMB 213
1015-M S Taft Hill Rd.
Fort Collins, CO 80521
**Phone:** (970)416-6872
**Website:** http://www.lifeandlibertyforwomen.org
**Desc:** Women. Advocates for safe abortion. Provides newsletters, research and information covering abortion issues.


★ 2245 ★ **Long-term Medical Conditions Alliance (LMCA)**
Unit 212
16 Baldwins Gardens
London EC1N 7RJ, United Kingdom
**Phone:** 44 2078133637          **Fax:** 44 2078133640
**Email:** alliance@lmca.demon.co.uk
**Website:** http://www.lmca.org.uk
**Fnded:** 1989. **Mem:** 115. **Desc:** Umbrella body working with member organisations towards better lives for people with long-term health conditions. Aims to gain recognition of people's needs and ensure resources are available to meet them, to campaign to achieve change in areas of common concern, to develop effective partnerships between service providers and service users, and to promote participation by individuals in their own care and treatment.


★ 2246 ★ **Loops for Lupus**
390 Hawk Ln.
Basalt, CO 81621-9788
**Phone:** (970)927-3983          **Fax:** (970)963-0590
**Email:** tommy@loopsforlupus.org
**Website:** http://www.loopsforlupus.org/
**Desc:** Committed to raising funds and heighten awareness about the disease Lupus.


**Make Today Count (MTC)**
*See:* Entry 10215


★ 2247 ★ **Malaysian Medical Association (MMA)**
MMA House, 4th Fl.
124 Jalan Pahang
53000 Kuala Lumpur, Malaysia
**Phone:** 60 3 40411375          **Fax:** 60 3 40418187
**Email:** mma@tm.net.my
**Website:** http://www.mma.org.my
**Fnded:** 1952. **Mem:** 8,000. **Lang(s):** English, Indonesian. **Desc:** Conducts educational programs for medical professionals; sponsors research and charitable activities. **Pub:** *Berita MMA*. Newsletter. • *Medical Journal of Malaysia*, quarterly. Journal.


★ 2248 ★ **MAP International (MAP)**
2200 Glynco Pky.
PO Box 215000
Brunswick, GA 31521-6800
**Phone:** (912)265-6010          **Free:** 800-225-8550
**Fax:** (912)265-6170
**Email:** map@map.org
**Website:** http://www.map.org
Michael J. Nyenhuis, Pres. /CEO
**Fnded:** 1954. **Reg. Groups:** 5. **Desc:** Non-profit Christian relief and development organization that promotes the health of people living in the world's poorest communities. Works with partners in the areas of community health development, disease prevention and eradication, relief and rehabilitation and global health advocacy. Promotes access to health services and essential medicines in more than 100 countries each year. **Pub:** *MAP International Report*, bimonthly. Newsletter. • *Our Health*, semiannual. Magazine. • Annual Report. **Frmly:** (1976) Medical Assistance Programs.


★ 2249 ★ **Medical Association of Jamaica (MAJ)**
19a Windsor Ave.
Kingston 5, Jamaica
**Phone:** (876)946-1105          **Fax:** (876)946-1102
**Email:** medassnjam@kasnet.com
**Website:** http://www.maj.org.jm
**Fnded:** 1967. **Mem:** 660. **Reg. Groups:** 5. **Lang(s):** English. **Desc:** Health care professionals. Works to ensure availability of medical care and to maintain high standards of practice in all medical specialties. Makes available professional and advisory services to members. Gathers and disseminates information.


★ 2250 ★ **Medical Association of Malta**
Federation of Professional Bodies
Alamein Rd.
Pembroke GZR 06, Malta
**Phone:** 356 312888          **Fax:** 356 331713
**Email:** mam@synapse.net.mt
**Website:** http://www.synapse.net.mt/mam/
**Fnded:** 1954. **Mem:** 700. **Lang(s):** English. **Desc:** Represents the interests of doctors and their patients in the differing spheres of professional activity at a national and international level.


★ 2251 ★ **Medical Association of South Africa (MASA)**
**(Mediese Vereniging van Suid Afrika — MVSA)**
PO Box 20272
Alkantrant
Pretoria 0005, Republic of South Africa
**Phone:** 27 12 4812000          **Fax:** 27 12 4812100
**Email:** masaceo1@iafrica.co
**Fnded:** 1927. **Mem:** 12,000. **Reg. Groups:** 20. **Lang(s):** Afrikaans, English. **Desc:** Registered medical doctors and residents. Represents and protects interests of the medical profession in South Africa and promotes the medical and allied sciences. Makes representations on health policy and medico-political and social issues; advises members on matters affecting medical practice. Operates charitable program for dependents of deceased colleagues; awards loans to medical students. Holds symposia and clinical meetings; offers medical refresher courses. Bestows awards. **Pub:** *South African Journal of Continuing Medical Education*, monthly. Journal. • *South African Medical Journal*, biweekly. Journal. Also publishes booklets and brochures.


★ 2252 ★ **Medical Council of India**
Aiwan-e-Galib Marg
Kotla Rd.
New Delhi, India
**Phone:** 91 11 3235178          **Fax:** 91 11 3236604
**Fnded:** 1933.


★ 2253 ★ **Medical Education for South African Blacks (MESAB)**
120 Albany St., Ste. 810
New Brunswick, NJ 08901-2163
**Phone:** (732)745-1292          **Fax:** (732)745-9794
**Email:** mesab@mesab.org
**Website:** http://www.mesab.org/
James W. Scott, Pres.
**Fnded:** 1985. **Desc:** Supports the training of South African black health professionals to bring better health care to all South Africans. Provides scholarships for black students in the health professions at South African universities. Develops health-related training programs, rural outreach programs, and offers scholarship support for nurses enrolled in university-level nursing programs. **Pub:** *Annual Report.* • *MESAB News*, 1-2/year. Newsletter. Includes information about the organization and its programs. *Price:* Free.


★ 2254 ★ **Medical Foundation**
Edward Ford Bldg., A27
University of Sydney
Sydney, NSW 2006, Australia
**Phone:** 61 2 93517315          **Fax:** 61 2 93513299
**Email:** medfdn@med.usud.edu.au
**Website:** http://www.medicalfoundation.usyd.edu.au
**Fnded:** 1958. **Desc:** Aims to improve the health of Australians of all ages.


★ 2255 ★ **Medical Research Modernization Committee (MRMC)**
PO Box 201791
Cleveland, OH 44120
**Phone:** (216)283-6702          **Fax:** (216)283-6702
**Email:** stkaufman@mindspring.com
**Website:** http://www.mrmcmed.org
Stephen R. Kaufman, MD, Co-Chair
**Fnded:** 1987. **Mem:** 1,000. **Desc:** Individuals, primarily scientists and clinicians, who evaluate the medical and/or scientific merit of research modalities in an effort to identify outdated research methods and to promote sensible, reliable, and efficient methods. Represents positions to the public, health care professionals, and government officials. Maintains speakers' bureau; distributes literature to the public. **Pub:** *A Critical Look at Animal Experimentation*, annual. Booklet. *Price:* Free to members; $1/copy for nonmembers. • *MRMC Report*, quarterly. Newsletter. *Price:* Free to members; $2/copy for nonmembers. • *Perspectives on Medical Research*, annual. Monograph. Includes essays and commentary. *Price:* $10/paperback; $16/hardback.


★ 2256 ★ **Medical Sciences Historical Society**
117 Woodland Dr.
Cassiobury
Watford WD17 3DA, United Kingdom
**Fnded:** 1981. **Mem:** 60. **Desc:** Holds four annual meetings. Publishes two newsletters and a journal. **Pub:** Newsletter, semiannual. • Journal, periodic.


★ 2257 ★ **Medical Society of Copenhagen**
**(Det Medicinske Selskab i Copenhagen)**
Trondhjemsgade 9
DK-2100 Copenhagen, Denmark
**Phone:** 45 31380984          **Fax:** 45 35448503
**Fnded:** 1772.


★ 2258 ★ **Medical Women's Federation**
Tavistock Sq.
Tavistock House North
London WC1H 9HX, United Kingdom
**Phone:** 44 171 3877765          **Fax:** 44 171 3877765
**Email:** lyn@m-w-f.demon.co.uk
**Fnded:** 1917. **Mem:** 2,000. **Local Groups:** 20. **Desc:** Women doctors and medical students. The professional association of women doctors in the UK. **Pub:** *Medical Woman*, 3/year. Newsletter.

**★ 2259 ★ Medical Women's International Association (MWIA)**
Wilhelm-Brand-Str. 3
D-44141 Dortmund, Germany
**Phone:** 49 231 9432771　　**Fax:** 49 231 9432773
**Email:** mwia@aol.com
**Website:** http://members.aol.com/mwia

**Fnded:** 1919. **Mem:** 14,000. **Nat'l Groups:** 44. **Reg. Groups:** 8. **Lang(s):** English. **Desc:** Women involved in or interested in medicine in 70 countries. Provides women with an opportunity to exchange information about medical problems with worldwide implications; promotes friendship and understanding between women; secures members' cooperation in matters relating to international health. Seeks to encourage women to enter the field of medicine and allied sciences and to overcome discrimination against female physicians. Aids women in developing countries in obtaining fellowships and grants for research and travel; offers information and advice to members visiting other countries. **Pub:** *Congress Report*, triennial. Report. • *MWIA Update*, quarterly. Newsletter. • *Women Physicians of the World*. Book.

**★ 2260 ★ MedicAlert Foundation (MAFI)**
2323 Colorado Ave.
Turlock, CA 95382
**Phone:** (209)668-3333　　**Free:** 888-633-4298
**Fax:** (209)669-2495
**Email:** customer_service@medicalert.org
**Website:** http://www.medicalert.org
Tanya J. Glazebrook, Pres. /CEO

**Fnded:** 1956. **Mem:** 4700,000. **Desc:** Medical information service open to all. Computerized, confidential medical file, MedicAlert emblem on pendant or bracelet engraved with primary medical condition and can call collect number to access 24-hour Emergency Response Center. Information is uses to speed diagnosis, accurate treatment and save lives. Conducts continuous public and professional education program. **Pub:** *MedicAlert Foundation*, semiannual. Newsletter.

**★ 2261 ★ Melpomene Institute**
1010 University Ave.
Saint Paul, MN 55104
**Phone:** (651)642-1951　　**Fax:** (651)642-1871
**Email:** health@melpomene.org
**Website:** http://www.melpomene.org
Judy Mahle Lutter, Pres.

**Fnded:** 1982. **Mem:** 1,350. **Desc:** Individuals professionally trained in healthcare, physical activity, and sports for girls and women. Conducts research and disseminates information on issues such as body image, osteoporosis, athletic amenorrhea, exercise and pregnancy, and aging. Offers undergraduate and graduate internships, and volunteer programs. Provides consulting services for program evaluations. Operates speakers' bureau. **Pub:** *The Bodywise Woman*. Book. Provides information for women on physical activity and health. *Price:* $16.95. • *Breast Cancer: A Handbook*. Book. • *Heroes: Growing Up Female and Strong*. Video. Concerns self-esteem in adolescent girls. *Price:* $19.95; $29.95 curriculum. • *HRT: Is It For Me?*. Booklet. Helps individuals make a more informed decision about Hormone Replacement Therapy. *Price:* $2.50. • *Let's Get Moving*. Booklet. Contains information about physical activity for women over 50. *Price:* $4.50. • *Melpomene Journal*, 3/year. Journal. Examines the relationship between physical activity and lifestyles. Features research reports, scientific bibliographies, and personal profiles. *Price:* Included in membership dues; $5/issue for nonmembers. • *Of Heroes, Hopes and Level Playing Fields*. Book. *Price:* $10. **Frmly:** (2002) Melpomene Institute for Women's Health Research.

**★ 2262 ★ Mercy Ships International Operations Center**
PO Box 2020
Garden Valley, TX 75771-2020
**Phone:** (903)939-7000　　**Free:** 800-MERCYSHIPS
**Fax:** (903)882-0336

**Email:** info@mercyships.org
**Website:** http://www.mercyships.org
**Desc:** Working to bring physical and spiritual healing to the poor and needy in port cities around the world.

**★ 2263 ★ Microsoft Healthcare Users Group (MS-HUG)**
3300 Washtenaw Ave.
Ann Arbor, MI 48104
**Phone:** (734)973-1995　　**Fax:** (734)973-1996
**Email:** kmalecki@ic.net
**Website:** http://www.mshug.org
**Desc:** Forum for the exchange of ideas. Promotes learning, and sharing solutions for information systems using Microsoft technologies. "Works to provide industry leadership, drive appropriate standards and develop associated requirements in support of healthcare solutions."

**★ 2264 ★ Migraine Association of Ireland**
Coleraine House
Coleraine St.
Dublin 7, Ireland
**Phone:** 353 1 8724137　　**Fax:** 353 1 8724157
**Email:** info@migraine.ie
**Website:** http://www.migraine.ie
**Fnded:** 1994. **Mem:** 1,700. **Nat'l Groups:** 1. **Reg. Groups:** 1. **State Groups:** 1. **Lang(s):** English. **Desc:** Seeks to share information and provide support for those affected by chronic migraine headaches in Ireland. Encourages medical research; lobbies for a national headache/migraine specialist clinic in Ireland; maintains relationships with other related societies and associations. **Pub:** *Migraine Association of Ireland*, 3/year. Newsletter. Features information on migraine.

**★ 2265 ★ Milton Helpern Institute of Forensic Medicine (MHIFM)**
520 1st Ave.
New York, NY 10016
**Phone:** (212)447-2030　　**Fax:** (212)447-2716
Dr. Charles S. Hirsch, Chief Med. Exam.

**Fnded:** 1968. **Mem:** 405. **Desc:** Operated by New York University and the city of New York to strengthen teaching and research in forensic medicine and forensic pathology. Trains postgraduate students; sponsors symposia, seminars, lectures, and courses; conducts research projects and undertakes investigations and related studies of sudden, suspicious, and violent deaths. Maintains Milton Helpern Library of Legal Medicine. **Frmly:** (1978) Institute of Forensic Medicine.

**★ 2266 ★ Mitochondria Research Society (MRS)**
c/o Keshav K. Singh
Johns Hopkins Oncology Center
School of Medicine
Bunting-Blaustein Cancer Research Bldg.
1650 Orleans St., Rm. 1-143
Baltimore, MD 21231-1000
**Phone:** (410)614-5128　　**Fax:** (410)502-7234
**Email:** singhke@jhmi.edu
**Website:** http://www.mitoresearch.org/contribu.htm
Keshav K. Singh, PhD, Contact
**Desc:** Scientists and physicians. Committed to finding a cure for mitochondrial diseases; promotes research on basic science of mitochondria, mitorchonrial pathogenesis, prevention, diagnosis and treatment throughout the world; fosters public education, training and provides a platform for communication and dissemination of knowledge among scientists, physicians and others interested in mitochondria. **Pub:** *Mitochondria Matters*, semiannual. Newsletter. Includes highlights of research, products, new developments in prevention, diagnosis and treatment of diseases associated with mitochondria. *Price:* included in membership dues. • *Mitochondrion*. Journal.

**★ 2267 ★ National Academy of Medicine (Academia Nacional de Medicina)**
Apdo Aereo 23224
Santa Fe de Bogota, Colombia
**Phone:** 57 1 2493122

**Fnded:** 1890.

**★ 2268 ★ National Alliance for Autism Research (NAAR)**
99 Wall St., Research Park
Princeton, NJ 08540
**Phone:** (609)430-9160　　**Free:** 888-777-NAAR
**Fax:** (609)430-9163
**Email:** naar@naar.org
**Website:** http://www.naar.org
Karen Margulis London, Pres.

**Fnded:** 1994. **Desc:** Dedicated to finding the causes, prevention, effective treatment and, ultimately, cure of the autism spectrum disorders. **Pub:** *NAARATIVE*, 3/year. Newsletter. Includes autism research articles.

**★ 2269 ★ National Ankylosing Spondylitis Society (NASS)**
PO Box 179
Mayfield TN20 6ZL, United Kingdom
**Phone:** 44 1435 873527　　**Fax:** 44 1435 873027
**Email:** nass@nass.co.uk
**Website:** http://www.nass.co.uk
**Fnded:** 1976. **Mem:** 8,000. **Reg. Groups:** 115. **Lang(s):** English. **Desc:** Promotes patient education in the medical and social aspects of the condition. Provides support through local UK groups for supervised physiotherapy one evening per week.

**★ 2270 ★ National Arab American Medical Association (NAAMA)**
801 S Adams Rd., Ste. 208
Birmingham, MI 48009-7018
**Phone:** (248)646-3661　　**Fax:** (248)646-0617
**Email:** naama@naama.com
**Website:** http://www.naama.com
Ellen R. Potter, Exec. Dir.

**Fnded:** 1974. **Mem:** 2,000. **State Groups:** 23. **Desc:** Medical professionals of Arab descent. Fosters exchange of scientific information. Encourages continuing education for members. Provides financial and technical support for medical students and institutions in the United States and in Arab countries. Offers medical assistance to needy individuals of Arab descent. **Pub:** *Al Hakeem*, quarterly. Newsletter. *Price:* Included in membership dues; $12/year. **Frmly:** (1997) Arab Americam Medical Association.

**★ 2271 ★ National Asian Women's Health Organization (NAWHO)**
250 Montgomery St., Ste. 900
San Francisco, CA 94104
**Phone:** (415)989-9747　　**Fax:** (415)989-9758
**Email:** nawho@nawho.org
**Fnded:** 1993. **Desc:** Asian American women. Promotes increased awareness of the unique health needs of Asian American women among health care professionals and the public. Serves as a clearinghouse on Asian American women's health issues; conducts advocacy campaigns; compiles statistics.

**★ 2272 ★ National Association of Advisors for the Health Professions (NAAHP)**
PO Box 1518
Champaign, IL 61824-1518
**Phone:** (217)355-0063　　**Fax:** (217)355-1287
**Email:** naaphtrevor@aol.com
**Website:** http://www.naahp.org
Susan Maxwell, Exec. Dir.

**Fnded:** 1974. **Mem:** 1,275. **Reg. Groups:** 4. **Desc:** College and university faculty who advise and counsel students on health careers. Seeks to improve and preserve advisement at all educational levels of the health professions. Fosters and coordinates communication among the health professions and advisers. Marshalls resources; provides services concerning health professions advisement. Goals include: informed counseling for students seeking careers in the health professions; proper preparation of student evaluations for the professional schools; participation of advisers in curriculum development; improved communication between secondary and undergraduate institutions; coordination of record keeping and information exchange among undergraduate schools and local, state, and regional preprofessional programs. Makes available Advisor's Supplementary Student Evaluation Tool software program; conducts surveys. **Pub:** *Directory of the National Association of Advisors for the Health Professions*, annual. Directory. Includes health professional school announcements and order forms. *Price:* $25/issue. • *The Medical School Interview.* • *National Association of Advisors for the Health Professions–The Advisor*, quarterly. Focuses on manpower statistics, financial aid, admission procedures, curriculum, advising, recruitment, counseling practice, and ethics. *Price:* $70/year. • *Strategy for Success: A Handbook for Prehealth Students*. Handbook. • *Write for Success.* • Audiotapes. • Videos.

### ★ 2273 ★ National Association of Community Health Centers (NACHC)

1330 New Hampshire Ave. NW, Ste. 122
Washington, DC 20036
**Phone:** (202)659-8008          **Fax:** (202)659-8519
**Email:** info@nachc.com
**Website:** http://www.nachc.com
Leslyn Phelps, Sec.

**Fnded:** 1970. **Mem:** 950. **Desc:** Advocacy organization of ambulatory healthcare centers, administrators, clinicians, and consumers. Works to assure the continued growth and development of community-based healthcare delivery programs for medically underserved populations by providing technical assistance and education and training opportunities for health center staff and board members. Disseminates information and research data and provides representation in legislative and professional arenas. Sponsors educational institutes, workshops, and seminars throughout the year. **Pub:** *NACHC Link.* Newsletter. *Price:* Included in membership dues. • *The Vanguard*, quarterly. Newsletter. • *Washington Update*, monthly. Newsletter. **Frmly:** National Association of Directors and Administrators; (1977) National Association of Neighborhood Health Centers.

### ★ 2274 ★ National Association of General Practitioner Veterinarians (Bundesverband Praktischer Tierarzte — BPT)

Hahnstr. 70
D-60528 Frankfurt, Germany
**Phone:** 49 69 6698180          **Fax:** 49 69 6668170
**Email:** bptev@tonline.de
**Website:** http://www.tieraerzteverband.de

**Fnded:** 1951. **Mem:** 6,500. **Desc:** Veterinarians in Germany. Represents the professional, economic, and social interests of members. Advocates for animal health and welfare.

### ★ 2275 ★ National Association for Healthcare Quality (NAHQ)

4700 W Lake Ave.
Glenview, IL 60025-1485
**Phone:** (847)375-4720          **Free:** 800-966-9392
**Fax:** 877-218-7939
**Email:** dsimmons@nahq.com
**Website:** http://www.nahq.org
Diane K. Simmons, Exec. Dir.

**Fnded:** 1976. **Mem:** 6,800. **State Groups:** 47. **Desc:** Healthcare professionals in quality assessment and improvement, utilization and risk management, case management, infection control, managed care, nursing, and medical records. Objectives are: to encourage, develop, and provide continuing education for all persons involved in health care quality; to give the patient primary consideration in all actions affecting his or her health and welfare; to promote the sharing of

knowledge and encourage a high degree of professional ethics in health care quality. Offers accredited certification in the field of healthcare quality, utilization, and risk management. Facilitates communication and cooperation among members, medical staff, and health care government agencies. Conducts educational seminars and conferences. **Pub:** *Journal for Healthcare Quality*, bimonthly. Journal. *Price:* $125/year. • *NAHQ Guide to Quality Management.* • *NAHQ News*, quarterly. Newsletter. • Membership Directory, annual. **Frmly:** (1979) National Association of Utilization Review Coordinators; (1991) National Association of Quality Assurance Professionals.

### ★ 2276 ★ National Association of Health Career Schools (NAHCS)

750 1st St. NE, Ste. 940
Washington, DC 20002
**Phone:** (202)842-1595          **Fax:** (202)842-1565
**Email:** nahcs@aol.com
Jeanne Russell, Exec. Dir.

**Fnded:** 1980. **Mem:** 180. **Desc:** Private, vocational, technical, and junior colleges training allied health personnel. Objectives are to: promote the interests and general welfare of health career training schools and their students accredited by the Accrediting Bureau of Health Education Schools; conduct and promote research for the advancement of the educational offerings of such schools; cooperate with local, state, and federal authorities and organizations engaged in the healing arts and the allied health sciences and with business, commerce, and industry in the maintenance of proper standards and sound policies in the field of health career training. Compiles statistics; develops curricula for allied health programs. **Pub:** *News Update.* • Newsletter, monthly.

### ★ 2277 ★ National Association of Hispanic-Serving Health Professions Schools

c/o Elena Rios, MD
1411 K St., NW, Ste. 200
Washington, DC 20005
**Phone:** (202)783-5262          **Fax:** (202)628-5898
**Email:** hishps@aol.com
**Website:** http://www.hshps.com
Elena Rios, MD, Dir.

**Fnded:** 1996. **Mem:** 22. **Desc:** Represents 16 medical schools. Seeks to strengthen the nation's capacity to educate and increase then numbers of high-quality Hispanic health care providers to serve and improve the health status of Hispanics and other populations. Develops educational opportunities in health professions schools in curriculum, research, and clinical experiences that will enable Hispanic and non-Hispanic health professions students to provide excellent health care to Hispanic populations. Promotes collaboration at the regional and national levels between educational institutions, communities, and other partners.

### ★ 2278 ★ National Association of Local Boards of Health (NALBOH)

c/o Ned Baker
1840 E Gypsy Lane Rd.
Bowling Green, OH 43402
**Phone:** (419)353-7714          **Fax:** (419)352-6278
**Email:** nalboh@nalboh.org
**Website:** http://www.nalboh.org
Marie M. Fallon, Exec. Dir.

**Fnded:** 1992. **Mem:** 800. **State Groups:** 11. **Desc:** Represents the interests of local boards of health throughout the United States and relates their concerns to individuals responsible for developing public health policy at the national level. Offers educational programs and speakers' bureau. **Pub:** *NewsBrief*, quarterly. Newsletter.

### ★ 2279 ★ National Association of Medical Advisers of Morocco (NAMAA) (Association Nationale des Delegues Medicaux du Maroc — ANDMM)

Boite Postale 15808
Casablanca 20000, Morocco
**Phone:** 212 2 293576

**Lang(s):** Arabic, French. **Desc:** Medical advisers. Promotes professional advancement of members. Represents members' interests before industrial organizations, government agencies, and the public.

### ★ 2280 ★ National Association of Professionals in Women's Health (NAPWH)

300 W Adams St., Ste.328
Chicago, IL 60606-5107

**Desc:** Health care professionals from a broad range of disciplines with a common interest in improving health outcomes for women. Seeks to "promote excellence and provide leadership, resources, and collegial support to all professionals who influence, develop, and champion quality health care programs for women." Works with community organizations to increase awareness of health care issues among women; sponsors continuing professional development courses for members; designs and implements community education programs.

### ★ 2281 ★ National Association of Residents and Interns (NARI)

350 Fairway Dr., Ste. 200
Deerfield Beach, FL 33441-1834
**Phone:** (954)571-1877          **Free:** 800-221-2168
**Fax:** (954)571-8582
**Email:** membership@assnservices.com
**Website:** http://www.nari-assn.com
Joseph P. Santoli, Jr., Manager, Membership Services

**Fnded:** 1959. **Mem:** 40,000. **Desc:** Medical and dental students, interns, residents, and fellows. Contributes to the economic welfare of members through unsecured loan plans, affordable group insurance, group purchase discounts, and continuing medical education programs. **Pub:** *Association's Digest.* • *NARI Stethoscope*, semiannual. Newsletter. Provides advice on business interests and benefits news. *Price:* Included in membership dues.

### ★ 2282 ★ National Black Women's Health Project (NBWHP)

600 Pennsylvania Ave. SE, Ste. 310
Washington, DC 20003
**Phone:** (202)548-4000          **Fax:** (202)543-9743
**Email:** nbwhp@nbwhp.org
**Website:** http://www.BlackWomensHealth.org
Lorraine Cole, PhD, Pres.

**Fnded:** 1981. **Mem:** 2,000. **Reg. Groups:** 5. **State Groups:** 26. **Local Groups:** 150. **Desc:** Education, advocacy, research, and leadership development organization focusing on health issues affecting Black women across their lifespan. groups. Also notes that black infant mortality is twice that of whites and that black women are often victims of family violence. Offers seminars outlining demographic information, chronic conditions, the need for health information and access to services, and possible methods of improving the health status of black women. Sponsors Center for Black Women's Wellness. Maintains library, database, and speakers' bureau. Conducts gender and race specific health research programs. Plans to: establish black women's wellness centers; develop Empowerment Through Wellness curriculum. **Pub:** *It's Ok to Peek.* Video. • *It's Up to Us.* Video. • *On Becoming a Woman: Mothers and Daughters Talking Together.* Video. • *Vital Signs*, quarterly. Newsletter. *Price:* Included in membership dues. • Annual Report. • Also publishes conference reports, brochures, and health fact sheets. Makes available educational films. **Frmly:** (1984) Black Women's Health Project.

**★ 2283 ★ National Board of Medical Examiners (NBME)**
3750 Market St.
Philadelphia, PA 19104-3190
**Phone:** (215)590-9500 **Fax:** (215)590-9555
**Email:** webmail@nbme.org
**Website:** http://www.nbme.org
Donald E. Melnick, MD, Pres.
**Fnded:** 1915. **Mem:** 75. **Desc:** Purposes are to: prepare and administer qualifying examinations either independently or in conjunction with other organizations, of such high quality that legal agencies governing the practice of medicine within each state may, in their discretion, grant a license without further examination for those who have successfully completed such examinations; to cooperate with and, where appropriate, to make its specialized services available to the examining boards of the states, specialty boards, and other organizations concerned with the education and qualification of personnel in the fields of health; to assist medical schools, hospitals and related organizations and institutions in evaluation of the effectiveness of their educational programs; to initiate, develop, and participate in research designed to evaluate the effectiveness of educational programs and techniques, and to assess ever more precisely the knowledge, competence, and qualification of professionals in public health care; to provide educational opportunities for professional personnel in the methods, techniques, and values of testing methods related to knowledge and competence in the broad field of medicine. **Pub:** *National Board Examiner*, quarterly. Newsletter. Reports on new medical evaluation programs and new directions in the research and development of examinations. *Price:* Free. • Annual Report. • Also publishes information bulletins and policy statements.

**★ 2284 ★ National Business Coalition on Health**
1015 18th St. NW, Ste. 730
Washington, DC 20036-5214
**Phone:** (202)775-9300 **Fax:** (202)775-1569
**Email:** mcornejo@nbch.org
**Website:** http://www.nbch.org
Greg Lehman, Pres. /CEO
**Fnded:** 1992. **Mem:** 100. **Desc:** Employer-led coalitions that group-purchase health care benefits for employees and measure and improve health care quality.

**★ 2285 ★ National Center for FarmWorker Health**
1770 FM 967
Buda, TX 78610-2884
**Phone:** (512)312-2700 **Fax:** (512)312-2600
**Email:** mckay@ncfh.org
**Website:** http://www.ncfh.org
Mimi McKay, Library and Information Resources Dir.
**Fnded:** 1975. **Desc:** Seeks to make quality primary health care accessible to migrant and seasonal farm workers. Supports the establishment of a national network of migrant health centers through the production, processing, and distribution of information, including information on health problems specific to or more prevalent in the migrant community. Works to provide technical assistance for health development and research. Develops collaborative working relationship between agencies serving migrant farmworkers. Maintains job/resume bank, biographical archives, and library. Bestows awards; operates placement service; compiles statistics. biographical archives, library, and speakers' bureau. Bestows awards; operates placement service; compiles statistics. **Pub:** *Migrant Health Newsline*, bimonthly. Newsletter. Includes clinical supplement. • *Migrant Health Referral Directory*, annual. Directory. • *Migrant Health Resource Catalog*. Catalogs. • Books. • Directory. • Videos. **Frmly:** (1989) National Migrant Referral Project.

**★ 2286 ★ National Center for Health Education (NCHE)**
240 W 30th St., 10th Fl.
New York, NY 10001
**Phone:** (212)594-8001 **Free:** 800-551-3488
**Fax:** (212)594-8023
**Email:** nche@nche.org
**Website:** http://www.nche.org
Lynne Whitt, Exec. VP
**Fnded:** 1975. **Desc:** Professionals promoting health education in schools, communities, and family settings. Aims to "extend the reach and power of education for health." Advocates health education and health promotion; builds coalitions of private and public sector groups; documents, develops, and disseminates model programs. Develops and manages Growing Healthy, a comprehensive school health education curriculum for kindergarten through grade six and "Starting Healthy" pre-kindergarten curriculum. **Pub:** *Growing Healthy (K-6)*. Book. Contains school health education. • *Starting Healthy (Pre-K)*. Book. Contains school health education.

**★ 2287 ★ National Certification Council for Activity Professionals (NCCAP)**
PO Box 62589
Virginia Beach, VA 23466
**Phone:** (757)552-0653
**Email:** info@nccap.org
**Website:** http://www.nccap.org
**Desc:** Activity professionals. Serves as a credentialing body setting standards and criteria to ensure that those served have optimal life experiences. Member of the National Registry of Certified Activity Professionals. **Pub:** Newsletter, quarterly.

**★ 2288 ★ National Chronic Care Consortium (NCCC)**
8100 26th Ave. S, Ste. 120
Bloomington, MN 55425
**Phone:** (952)858-8999
**Website:** http://www.nccconline.org
**Desc:** Nonprofit plans and providers. Aims to develop real-world solutions in chronic illness care. Serves as an operational laboratory for members in developing innovative care programs and as a national resource center.

**★ 2289 ★ National Commission on Correctional Health Care (NCCHC)**
1300 W Belmont Ave.
Chicago, IL 60657
**Phone:** (773)880-1460 **Fax:** (773)880-2424
**Email:** ncchc@ncchc.org
**Website:** http://www.ncchc.org
Edward A. Harrison, Pres.
**Fnded:** 1983. **Mem:** 35. **Desc:** Professional organizations in the fields of medical and health care. Works to improve the quality of and set standards for medical care in correctional institutions in the U.S. including prisons, jails, and detention and juvenile facilities. Acts as an accrediting body for such facilities; develops training programs and conducts seminars; provides technical assistance; organizes special task forces on issues such as suicide and AIDS; annually bestows Award of Merit for achievement in the field of correctional health care. Compiles statistics; conducts research; disseminates information. **Pub:** *CorrectCare*, quarterly. Newspaper. • *Journal of Correctional Care*, semiannual. Journal. Contains articles on correctional health care topics including law, medicine, and ethics. *Price:* $30/year for individuals; $65/year for institutions. • *Prison Health Care: Guidelines for the Management of an Adequated Delivery System*. Manuals. • Films. • Monographs. • Proceedings.

**★ 2290 ★ National Federation of Opticianry Schools (NFOS)**
c/o Randall L. Smith
9604 Escada Ct.
Chesterfield, VA 23832
**Phone:** (804)790-0026 **Fax:** (804)790-0026

**Email:** rlsmitl@jsr.cc.va.us
**Website:** http://www.nfos.org/
Randall L. Smith, Pres.
**Desc:** Promotes formal opticianry education offered by accredited educational institutions. Strives to develop formal education programs in identified areas of need; upgrade standards of opticianry education; facilitate exchange of teaching methods; achieve uniformity of formal education in opticianry; and assist national opticianry organizations.

**★ 2291 ★ National Health Care for the Homeless Council (NHCHC)**
HCH Clinicians' Network
PO Box 60427
Nashville, TN 37206-0427
**Phone:** (615)226-2292 **Fax:** (615)226-1656
**Email:** council@nhchc.org
**Website:** http://www.nhchc.org
Mr. John Lozier, Exec. Dir.
**Mem:** 455. **Desc:** Agencies (35) and clinicians (425) with an interest in providing health care services to the homeless. Promotes increased availability of primary health care services to homeless people; seeks to prevent homelessness. Works to reform the U.S. health care system to best serve the needs of the homeless and indigent; cooperates with other organizations and agencies working to eradicate homelessness. Facilitates networking, information sharing, and peer support among members; conducts educational programs. **Pub:** *HCH Mobilizer*. Newspaper. *Price:* $15. • *Healing Hands*. Newsletter. *Price:* $25.

**★ 2292 ★ National Health Council (NHC)**
1730 M St. NW, Ste. 500
Washington, DC 20036
**Phone:** (202)785-3910 **Fax:** (202)785-5923
**Email:** info@nhcouncil.org
**Website:** http://www.nhcouncil.org
Myrl Weinberg, Pres.
**Fnded:** 1920. **Mem:** 115. **Desc:** National membership association of voluntary and professional societies in the health field; national organizations and business groups with strong health interests. Seeks to improve the health of patients, particularly those with chronic diseases, through conferences, publications, policy briefings and special projects. Distributes printed material on health careers and related subjects. Promotes standardization of financial reporting for voluntary health groups. **Pub:** *Council Currents*, bimonthly. Books. *Price:* Free. • *Directory of Health Groups in Washington*. Directory. • *Guide to America's Voluntary Health Agencies*. Directory. • *Standards of Accounting and Reporting for Voluntary Health and Welfare Organizations (The Black Book)*. Book. • *300 Ways to Put Your Talent to Work in the Health Field*. Book.

**★ 2293 ★ National Health Federation (NHF)**
PO Box 688
Monrovia, CA 91017
**Phone:** (626)357-2181 **Fax:** (626)303-0642
**Email:** raivennhf@msn.com
**Website:** http://www.thenhf.com/
Raiven Blanca, Exec. Dir.
**Fnded:** 1955. **Mem:** 6,000. **Local Groups:** 123. **Desc:** Persons interested in individual freedom of choice in matters relating to health. Represents belief "that organized medicine, the pharmaceutical industry, and other special interests have been responsible for many laws, rules, and regulations which very often better serve the interests of these groups than the interests of the American public." Seeks to serve as a "watch dog" and to institute corrective measures through investigation, education, legislation, and coordination of organizations with similar purposes. Supports research in areas such as laetrile testing; supports numerous educational foundation programs. Conducts lobbying activities. **Pub:** *Health Freedom News*, bimonthly. Magazine. *Price:* $3.95.

**★ 2294 ★ National Health and Medical Research Council (NHMRC)**
Office of the NHMRC
GPO Box 9848
Canberra, ACT 2601, Australia
**Phone:** 61 2 62899184　　**Fax:** 61 2 62899197
**Email:** exec.sec@nhmrc.gov.au
**Fnded:** 1936. **Mem:** 30. **Lang(s):** English. **Desc:** Representatives from state and territory health authorities, professional and scientific colleges and associations, unions, universities, industry, business and consumer groups, welfare organizations, and the commonwealth administration. Evaluates reports from committees, expert panels, working parties and disseminates results. **Pub:** *Annual Report of NHMRC*, annual. Report. Contains research results.

**★ 2295 ★ National Health Policy Forum (NHPF)**
2131 K St. NW, Ste. 500
Washington, DC 20037
**Phone:** (202)872-1390　　**Fax:** (202)862-9837
**Email:** nhpf@gwu.edu
**Website:** http://www.nhpf.org
Judith Miller Jones, Dir.
**Fnded:** 1971. **Desc:** Nonpartisan education program serving primarily senior federal legislative and regulatory health staff but also addressing the interests of state officials and their Washington representatives. Seeks to foster more informed government decision making. Helps decision makers forge the personal acquaintances and understanding necessary for cooperation among government agencies and between government and the private sector. Provides technical assistance to staff and grantees of its sponsoring foundations and corporate contributors. **Pub:** *Background Papers*. Papers. • *Issue Briefs*, 25-30/year. • *Site Visit Reports*. Reports.

**★ 2296 ★ National Hispanic Medical Association**
c/o Elena Rios, MD
1411 K St. NW, Ste. 200
Washington, DC 20005
**Phone:** (202)628-5895　　**Fax:** (202)628-5898
**Email:** nhma@nhmamd.net
**Website:** http://home.earthlink.net/~nhma
Elena Rios, MD, Contact
**Fnded:** 1994. **Desc:** Hispanic physicians. Works to improve health care for Hispanics and underserved populations. Promotes Hispanic health policy issues in relevant forums. Conducts continuing education programs.

**★ 2297 ★ National Incontinentia Pigmenti Foundation (NIPF)**
c/o Susanne Bross Emmerich
30 E 72nd St.
New York, NY 10021
**Phone:** (212)452-1231　　**Fax:** (212)452-1406
**Email:** ipif@ipif.org
**Website:** http://imgen.bcm.tmc.edu/NIPF/
Susanne Bross Emmerich, Exec. Dir.
**Fnded:** 1995. **Desc:** Patients, physicians, educators, parents, relatives, volunteers. Strives to support research, education and funding for Incontinentia Pigmenti; provides family support and education; seeks to develop accurate and safe prenatal diagnostic testing; and develop database to assess clinical variation, natural history, and prognostic indicators. **Pub:** Newsletter. • Reports.

**★ 2298 ★ National Institute for Jewish Hospice (NIJH)**
444 San Vincente Blvd.
Los Angeles, CA 90048
**Phone:** (323)467-7423　　**Free:** 800-446-4448
Shirley Lamm, Exec. Dir.
**Fnded:** 1985. **Mem:** 43,320. **Desc:** Individuals, business firms, and organizations concerned about terminally ill Jewish people. Serves as a resource center

that seeks to help terminal patients and their families deal with their grief by providing information on traditional Jewish views on death, dying, and managing the loss of a loved one. Offers guidance and training to patients and interested hospice personnel, health care professionals, clergy, and family members who work with terminally ill Jewish people. Maintains speakers' bureau; conducts research programs. Jewish living will, booklets and tapes are available. **Pub:** *At Bedside.* • *Caring for the Jewish Terminally Ill.* • *For Families of the Jewish Terminally Ill.* • *Hemlock Is Poison for Society.* • *How to Console.* • *Introduction to Jewish Hospice.* • *The Jewish Living Will.* • *The Jewish Orphaned Adult.* • *Realities of the Dying.* • *Self-Healing and Hospice Care.* • *The Spiritual Component Cannot Be Ignored.* • *Strategies for Jewish Care.* • *The Undying Hope.*

**★ 2299 ★ National Latina Health Organization (NLHO)**
PO Box 7567
Oakland, CA 94601
**Phone:** (510)534-1362　　**Fax:** (510)534-1364
**Email:** latinahlth@aol.com
**Website:** http://clnet.ucr.edu/women/nlho
Luz Alvarez Martinez, Exec. Dir.
**Fnded:** 1986. **Desc:** Puerto Rican, Chicana, Mexican, Cuban, Caribbean and South and Central American women. Works to increase awareness of health issues among Latin American women. Works to achieve bilingual access to quality health care and self-empowerment of Latinas through culturally sensitive educational programs, health advocacy, outreach, research, and the development of public policy. Cooperates with other organizations to defend reproductive rights, affordable birth control, sex education, prenatal care, and freedom from sterilization abuse. Offers technical training for community health facilitators. Organizes forums. **Pub:** Newsletter, periodic. Includes Latina health issues, legislation affecting Latinas, and calendar of events and activities on health and reproductive rights.

**★ 2300 ★ National Lupron Victims Network (NLVN)**
PO Box 193
Collingswood, NJ 08108
**Phone:** (856)858-2131　　**Fax:** (856)858-2131
**Email:** nlvn@lupronvictims.com
**Website:** http://www.lupronvictims.com
Linda Abend, Founder
**Fnded:** 1993. **Desc:** Works to provide information and support to men and women who have medical problems from taking the drug Lupron.

**★ 2301 ★ National Medic-Card Systems (NMCS)**
1070 Commerce St., Ste. D
San Marcos, CA 92069
**Phone:** (760)744-1560　　**Fax:** (760)744-1569
**Email:** mikeb@bhprint.com
Michael C. Barksdale, Sales Mgr.
**Fnded:** 1978. **Desc:** Produces wallet-size medical cards that have five sections, fold into the size of a credit card, and describe individuals' medical conditions in detail. **Frmly:** (1986) National Medic-Card Society.

**★ 2302 ★ National Medical Association (NMA)**
1012 10th St. NW
Washington, DC 20001
**Phone:** (202)204-1223　　**Fax:** (202)898-2510
**Email:** brainhardt@nmanet.org
**Website:** http://www.nmanet.org
Patricia Norman, Contact
**Fnded:** 1895. **Mem:** 22,000. **Reg. Groups:** 6. **State Groups:** 42. **Local Groups:** 93. **Desc:** Professional society of black physicians. Maintains 24 scientific sections representing major specialties of medicine. Plans to establish library. Conducts symposia and workshops. **Pub:** *Journal of the National Medical*

*Association*, monthly. Journal. Contains scientific articles. *Price:* $35. • *National Medical Association Newsletter*, quarterly. Newsletter.

**★ 2303 ★ National Medical Fellowships (NMF)**
5 Handover Sq., 15th Fl.
New York, NY 10004
**Phone:** (212)483-8880　　**Fax:** (212)483-8897
**Email:** info@nmfonline.org
**Website:** http://www.nmfonline.org
Vivian Fox, Pres. /CEO
**Fnded:** 1946. **Reg. Groups:** 2. **Desc:** Promotes education of minority students in medicine. Provides need-based scholarships, special merit awards, and leadership opportunities to medical students of African American, Native American, Mexican American and mainland Puerto Rican heritage. **Pub:** *NMF Update*, quarterly. • Newsletter. • Annual Report. **Frmly:** (1952) Provident Medical Associates.

**★ 2304 ★ National Necrotizing Fasciitis Foundation**
c/o Donna Batdorff
2731 Porter SW
Grand Rapids, MI 49509-2140
**Phone:** (616)261-2538　　**Fax:** (616)261-2539
**Email:** dbatdorff@nnff.org
**Website:** http://www.nnff.org
Donna Batdorff, Contact
**Fnded:** 1997. **Desc:** Strives to educate and offer support to those affected by necrotizing fasciitis (flesh eating bacteria).

**★ 2305 ★ National Organization for Competency Assurance (NOCA)**
2025 M St. NW, Ste. 800
Washington, DC 20036
**Phone:** (202)367-1165　　**Fax:** (202)367-2165
**Email:** info@noca.org
**Website:** http://www.noca.org
Wade Delk, Exec. Dir.
**Fnded:** 1977. **Mem:** 300. **Desc:** Organizations conducting certification programs for occupations and professionals and trade associations representing these professionals. Seeks to increase public awareness, understanding, and acceptance of private sector credentialing as an alternative to licensure; promotes nonlicensed but certified practitioners as a means to achieving high quality and cost containment. **Pub:** *NOCA News*, quarterly. Newsletter. *Price:* $95/year. **Frmly:** (1989) National Commission for Health Certifying Agencies.

**★ 2306 ★ National Organization for Rare Disorders (NORD)**
PO Box 8923
New Fairfield, CT 06812-8923
**Phone:** (203)746-6518　　**Free:** 800-999-6673
**Fax:** (203)746-6481
**Email:** orphan@rarediseases.org
**Website:** http://www.rarediseases.org
Susan Olivo, Admin. Assistant
**Fnded:** 1983. **Mem:** 65,000. **Nat'l Groups:** 130. **Desc:** Doctors, professionals, academics, voluntary health organizations, and individuals interested in rare disorders. Serves as a clearinghouse for information concerning rare disorders. Objectives are: to monitor the Orphan Drug Act; to link individuals with rare disorders together for mutual support; to stimulate research on rare diseases; to foster communication among voluntary agencies, health-related industries, and government bodies. (Orphan drugs are used in the treatment of rare disorders. Since their use is not widespread, most drug companies cannot expect to profit from the development and manufacture of these drugs. The Orphan Drug Act gives financial assistance and tax incentives to drug companies that develop these drugs.) Provides information on rare disorders and referrals to organizations. **Pub:** *NORD On-Line Bulletin*, monthly. Newsletter. Updating service for voluntary health agency members on legislation and

other issues related to orphan drugs and diseases. Includes meeting schedule. *Price:* Included in membership dues, for organizations. • *NORD Resource Guide.* An alphabetical listing of national support groups and foundations that service the needs of people with rare disorders and disabilities. • *Orphan Disease Update*, 3/year. Newsletter. For individual members updating information on orphan diseases and orphan drug research; discusses legislative issues related to health. *Price:* Included in membership dues. • *Physician Guide to Rare Diseases.* Book.

**★ 2307 ★ National Physician's Association (NPA)**
PO Box 35189
Chicago, IL 60707-0189
**Phone:** (773)283-3880          **Fax:** (708)453-0083
**Email:** npa@rentamark.com
**Website:** http://www.rentamark.com/npa/
L. Stollen, Contact

**Fnded:** 1975. **Nat'l Groups:** 1. **Desc:** Physicians. Seeks to increase members' public visibility and professional influence. Provides trademark licensing and product and service endorsement services to support members' activities. A platform for doctors to find new patients and receive information about the latest healthcare "breakthroughs", and receive advice on healthcare matters. **Pub:** *National Physicians Journal*, quarterly. Journal. NPA invites authors to submit articles in Word format via email for publication. *Price:* for members.

**★ 2308 ★ National Potter Syndrome Support Group**
c/o Evy Wright
541-B Bitteroot Cir.
Anchorage, AK 99504
**Phone:** (907)333-4475
**Email:** potters_syndrome@mailcity.com
**Website:**                                    http://www.potterssyndromesupport.homestead.com/potters.html
Evy Wright, Contact

**Fnded:** 1995. **Mem:** 105. **Desc:** Supports and disseminates information to families affected with Potter Syndrome. **Pub:** *National Patter Syndrome Support Group Newsletter*, biennial. Newsletter.

**★ 2309 ★ National Resident Matching Program (NRMP)**
2501 N St. NW, Ste. 1
Washington, DC 20037-1127
**Phone:** (202)828-0677          **Fax:** (202)828-1121
**Email:** nrmp@aamc.org
**Website:** http://www.aamc.org/nrmp
Robert L. Beran, PhD, Exec. Dir.

**Fnded:** 1951. **Desc:** National clearinghouse for matching the preferences of medical school graduates for medical residencies in the U.S. with the hospitals' choices of applicants. Runs matches for 17 medical sub-specialty fellowships. **Pub:** *NRMP Data*, annual. Booklet. *Price:* $35. **Frmly:** (1953) National InterAssociation Committee on Internships; (1968) National Intern Matching Program; (1978) National Intern and Resident Matching Program.

**★ 2310 ★ National Rural Health Association (NRHA)**
One W Armour Blvd., Ste. 203
Kansas City, MO 64111
**Phone:** (816)756-3140          **Fax:** (816)756-3144
**Email:** mail@nrharural.org
**Website:** http://www.nrharural.org
Rob McVay, Contact

**Fnded:** 1978. **Mem:** 2,000. **Desc:** Administrators, physicians, nurses, physician assistants, health planners, academicians, and others interested or involved in rural health care. Creates a better understanding of health care problems unique to rural areas; utilizes a collective approach in finding positive solutions; articulates and represents the health care needs of rural America; supplies current information to rural health

care providers; serves as a liaison between rural health care programs throughout the country. Offers continuing education credits for medical, dental, nursing, and management courses. **Pub:** *Journal of Rural Health*, quarterly. Journal. Includes rural health research, book reviews, abstracts of published research, and research reviews. *Price:* Included in membership dues; $45 for nonmembers; $90 for institutions. • Also publishes many other resources.

**★ 2311 ★ National Rural Recruitment and Retention Network (3R Net)**
2536 Kendall Ave.
Madison, WI 53705
**Phone:** (715)343-8244          **Free:** 800-787-2512
**Email:** info@3rnet.org
**Website:** http://www.3rnet.org/
**State Groups:** 45. **Desc:** 45 member state organizations. Strives to assist health professionals locate practice sites in rural areas throughout the United States.

**★ 2312 ★ National Special Needs Network**
c/o Jeffrey H. Minde
8041 W McNab Rd.
Tamarac, FL 33321
**Phone:** (954)721-1020          **Fax:** (954)721-3555
**Email:** nsnn@aol.com
**Website:** http://www.nsnn.com/
Jeffrey H. Minde, Pres.

**Desc:** Special needs professionals. Dedicated to providing the finest and most complete special needs support services in America, including individuals and families with developmental and acquired disabilities, mental illnesses, and chronic medical conditions.

**★ 2313 ★ National Subacute Care Association (NSCA)**
1960 Gallows Rd., Ste. 210
Vienna, VA 22182
**Phone:** (703)790-8989          **Fax:** (703)790-8485
**Email:** info@nsca.net
**Website:** http://www.nsca.net
Sanford. J. Hill, Exec. Dir.

**Fnded:** 1995. **Mem:** 1,500. **Desc:** Hospitals, nursing facilities, professionals and suppliers. Works to serve and represent the subacute and transitional healthcare industry. Provides information on subacute healthcare; promotes high level of ethics; develops standards. **Pub:** *NSCA News*, quarterly. Newsletter. • *Subacute Care*, quarterly. Journal. • Also issues InfoFaxes and Government Affairs Updates.

**★ 2314 ★ National Union of Medical Advisers Associations (NUMAA) (Syndicat National Professionel Autonome des Delegues Visiteurs Medicaux — SNPADVM)**
63, rue Bichat
F-75010 Paris, France
**Phone:** 33 1 4247462          **Fax:** 33 1 60039577
**Lang(s):** French. **Desc:** Medical advisers. Promotes professional advancement of members. Represents members' interests before industrial organizations, government agencies, and the public.

**★ 2315 ★ National Vulvodynia Association**
PO Box 4491
Silver Spring, MD 20914-4491
**Phone:** (301)299-0775          **Fax:** (301)299-3999
**Email:** mate@nva.org
**Website:** http://www.nva.org
Phyllis Mate, Exec. Dir.

**Fnded:** 1994. **Mem:** 2,500. **Nat'l Groups:** 80. **Desc:** Strives to improve the lives of individuals affected by Vulvodynia, a spectrum of chronic vulvar pain disorders. **Pub:** *NVA News*, 3/year. Newsletter. *Price:* $35 included with donation, $5 for back issues.

**★ 2316 ★ National Women's Health Network (NWHN)**
514 10th St. NW, Ste. 400
Washington, DC 20004
**Phone:** (202)347-1140          **Fax:** (202)347-1168
**Website:** http://www.womenshealthnetwork.org
Cynthia Pearson, Exec. Dir.

**Fnded:** 1975. **Mem:** 12,000. **Desc:** An advocacy organization giving women a greater voice in the health care system in the United States. It is the only such membership organization and has a 25-year history of accomplishments on behalf of all women. Provides women with unbiased health information through its clearinghouse. Also monitors federal legislation to ensure that women's needs are not overlooked. **Pub:** *National Women's Health Network–Network News*, bimonthly. Newsletter. Keeps readers informed about the important developments in womens health, provides ways to improve one's health, recommends books. *Price:* Included in membership dues. • Also publishes health information packets, booklets, and brochures.

**★ 2317 ★ Native American Women's Health Education Resource Center**
PO Box 572
Lake Andes, SD 57356-0572
**Phone:** (605)487-7072          **Fax:** (605)487-7964
**Email:** nativewoman@igc.apc.org
**Website:** http://www.nativeshop.org/nawherc.html

**Desc:** Individuals and organizations interested in the health status of Native American women. Promotes improved health and access to health services for Native American women. Works to redress Eurocentrism in American society. Gathers and disseminates information on women's health and related topics. Conducts educational programs. **Pub:** Newsletter, periodic.

**★ 2318 ★ Nature of Wellness**
PO Box 10400
Glendale, CA 91209-3400
**Phone:** (818)790-6384          **Free:** 800-519-9996
**Fax:** (818)790-9660
**Email:** supress@earthlink.net
**Website:** http://home.earthlink.net/~supress/

**Desc:** Seeks to inform the public about medical and scientific invalidity of animal experimentation and testing; investigates the impact of reliance by the medical/pharmaceutical/petrochemical industry on animal experimentation (in biomedical research) and animal testing (to assess the safety of drugs, pesticides and other chemicals) has on the health care system, environment and economy.

**★ 2319 ★ Netherlands Dietetic Association (NVD) (Nederlandse Vereniging van Dietisten)**
Postbus 341
NL-5340 AH Oss, Netherlands
**Phone:** 31 412 624543          **Fax:** 31 412 637736
**Website:** http://www.nvdietist.nl

**Fnded:** 1941. **Mem:** 2,500. **Desc:** Strives to maintain high professional standards for dieticians working in the Netherlands. Represents members interests. Offers postgraduate training courses. **Pub:** *Dutch Journal for Dietitians*, periodic. Journal. • Brochures.

**★ 2320 ★ Netherlands Society of Tropical Medicine (Societe Nederlandaise de Medecine Tropicale)**
c/o Nadamo Bos
PO Box 244
NL-3970 AE Driebergen Rijsenburg, Netherlands
**Phone:** 31 343 517126
**Email:** nadamo@worldaccess.nl

**Fnded:** 1907. **Mem:** 950. **Desc:** Physicians, nurses, midwives, social scientists, biologists, public relations officers, economists, and others working in the field of tropical medicine. Promotes research education and practice of tropical medicine and other related sciences. Areas of interest include: health care in developing countries, tropical surgery, topical pediatrics, maternal health and family planning. Collaborates with national and international organizations concerned with tropical health care. **Pub:** *Medicus Tropicus*, bimonthly. Magazine. • *Tropical Medicine and International Health*, monthly. Journal.

★ 2321 ★ **Network for Continuing
    Medical Education (NCME)**
One Harmon Plaza
Secaucus, NJ 07094
**Phone:** (201)867-3550          **Free:** 800-223-0272
**Fax:** (201)867-2491
**Website:** http://www.ncme.com
Paul Gersh, Pres.

**Fnded:** 1965. **Mem:** 800. **Desc:** Hospitals that subscribe to receive NCME services. Produces and distributes monthly course package including videotape, posters, program brochure, and workbook to members. Course packages cover the full spectrum of medical topics and are designed to provide category 1 continuing medical education credit to physicians. **Pub:** *Video Journal Dermatology*, quarterly. • *Video Journal Oncology*, quarterly.

★ 2322 ★ **New Zealand Medical
    Association (NZMA)**
26 The Terrace
PO Box 156
Wellington, New Zealand
**Phone:** 64 4 4724741          **Fax:** 64 4 4710838
**Email:** nzma@nzma.org.nz
**Website:** http://www.nzma.org.nz

**Desc:** Members come for all disciplines within the medical profession. Aims to provide advocacy on behalf of doctors and their patients. Provides support and services to members and their practices.

★ 2323 ★ **NHS Consultants Association**
Hill House
Banbury
Oxon OX17 1QH, United Kingdom
**Phone:** 44 1295 750407          **Fax:** 44 1295 750407
**Email:** nhsca@pop3.poptel.org.uk
**Website:** http://www.nhsca.org.uk

**Fnded:** 1976. **Mem:** 600. **Desc:** Senior doctors committed to the NHS and the basic principles on which it was founded. Acts as a pressure group lobbying politicians and other, publishing arenas. **Frmly:** (2001) National Health Service Consultants Association.

★ 2324 ★ **Nordic Federation for Medical
    Education**
Tagensvej 18
DK-2200 Copenhagen, Denmark
**Phone:** 45 35375252          **Fax:** 45 31357043
**Email:** nofenfre@inet.uni.c.dk
**Fnded:** 1966.

★ 2325 ★ **Nordic Society for Disaster
    Medicine**
c/o Karl-Axel Wallman
AneQual
Kallgardsv 5
S-230 42 Tygelsjo, Sweden
**Phone:** 46 40 49546
**Email:** kale@wallman.nu
**Desc:** Dedicated to improving medical disaster relief.

★ 2326 ★ **Nordic Telemedicine
    Association (NTA)**
c/o Siri Birgitte Uldal
National Centre for Telemedicine
University Hospital of Tromso
PO Box 35
N-9038 Tromso, Norway
**Phone:** 47 77 75 41 49          **Fax:** 47 77 75 40 99
**Email:** tmasbu@rito.no

**Website:** http://www.telemedicine.dk
**Fnded:** 1999. **Desc:** Telemedicine organizations. Strives to strengthen and expand telemedicine activities; promotes collaboration with telemedicine groups worldwide.

★ 2327 ★ **North American Association
    for Ambulatory Urgent Care (NAFAC)**
18870 Rutledge Rd.
Wayzata, MN 55391
**Phone:** (612)868-8417          **Fax:** (952)476-0646
**Email:** health1@aol.com
**Website:** http://www.nafac.com
William H. Wenmark, Pres.

**Fnded:** 1981. **Mem:** 200. **State Groups:** 6. **Desc:** Governing body for urgent care in North America. Representatives of hospital, corporate, and independently owned ambulatory urgent care centers. Seeks to: establish operational standards for such centers; in order for members to provide lower cost and more convenient outpatient urgent medical care; make the public aware of the concept of ambulatory urgent care centers and their usefulness in problem-based and episodic care. Cooperates with medical organizations; conducts public relations activities and studies on the industry as well as education programs and business support services. **Pub:** *Factor Studies*, triennial. Reports. National Research on Industry. **Frmly:** (1981) National Association of Centers for Urgent Treatment; (1984) National Association of Freestanding Emergency Centers; (2000) National Association for Ambulatory Care Medicine; (2002) North American Association of Urgent Care Medicine.

★ 2328 ★ **North American Primary Care
    Research Group (NAPCRG)**
11400 Tomahawk Creek Pky.
Leawood, KS 66211-2672
**Phone:** (913)906-6000          **Free:** 800-274-2237
**Fax:** (913)906-6096
**Email:** napcrg@stfm.org
**Website:** http://www.napcrg.org
Stacy Brungardt, Exec. Dir.

**Fnded:** 1972. **Mem:** 700. **Desc:** Physicians and other individuals interested in primary care research. (Primary care is the type of medicine practiced by physicians who do not require patient referrals from other physicians.) Promotes research on primary care topics. Maintains 11 special interest groups including: Ambulatory Sentinel Practice; Clinical Decision Making; Health Status Group. Disseminates information and serves as a forum for exchange of ideas on research projects. Maintains speakers' bureau. **Pub:** *Glossary of Primary Care Terms*. • *Process Classification for Family Care*. • Newsletter, quarterly. • Proceedings. • Reports.

★ 2329 ★ **ODPHP National Health
    Information Center (NHIC)**
PO Box 1133
Washington, DC 20013-1133
**Phone:** (301)565-4167          **Free:** 800-729-6686
**Fax:** (301)984-4256
**Email:** info@nhic.org
**Website:** http://www.health.gov/nhic

**Fnded:** 1979. **Desc:** A health information referral service which links consumers and health professionals who have health questions with organizations best able to provide answers. Funded by the Office of Disease Prevention and Health Promotion, Public Health Service, U.S. Department of Health and Human Services. Maintains an online directory of more than 1,100 health-related organizations that can provide health information. These include Federal and State agencies, voluntary associations, self-help and support groups, trade associations and professional societies. Prints directories and resource guides on a variety of health topics. **Pub:** *National Health Observances Planner*, annual. • *Prevention Report*, quarterly. Newsletter. **Frmly:** (1986) National Health Information Clearinghouse; (1987) ODPHP Health Information Center.

★ 2330 ★ **Organic Living Association**
St. Mary's Villa
Hanley Swan
Worcester WR8 0EA, United Kingdom
**Fnded:** 1971. **Mem:** 200. **Nat'l Groups:** 1. **Desc:** Aims to integrate the production and consumption of vegetables, fruit, cereals and dairy produce grown on healthy, naturally fertilized soil. Promotes human health by whatever humane means may be necessary; promotes establishment of ecological, self-reliant, self-sufficient villages. Disseminates knowledge of alternatives to allopathic medicine. **Pub:** Newsletter, bimonthly.

★ 2331 ★ **Organization for Integration of
    Women in Development (WID)**
PO Box 31802
Addis Ababa, Ethiopia
**Phone:** 251 1 118460          **Fax:** 251 1 514682
**Email:** britcoun.dis@telecom.net.et

**Fnded:** 1993. **Mem:** 100. **Lang(s):** English, French, German. **Desc:** Promotes increased availability of nutrition and family planning services. Conducts primary health care and nutrition programs, HIV/AIDS prevention programs and counseling, community based urban/rural poverty alleviation programs, child welfare, education/vocational training for youth/school dropout girls. **Pub:** *Gender & Development*.

★ 2332 ★ **Organization Internationale de
    Cooperation pour la Sante**
153, rue de Charonne
F-75011 Paris, France
**Phone:** 33 1 43732904
**Website:** http://www.cirad.nc

**Desc:** Promotes health care and disease prevention efforts in developing nations. Conducts research.

★ 2333 ★ **Orthodox Christian Association
    of Medicine, Psychology and Religion
    (OCAMPR)**
PO Box 958
Cambridge, MA 02238
**Phone:** (617)868-6557          **Fax:** (617)495-7728
John T. Chirban, PhD, Pres.

**Fnded:** 1986. **Mem:** 2. **Desc:** Professionals in medicine, psychology, and religion. Facilitates interdisciplinary programs and community understanding of Orthodox Christianity concerning interdisciplinary studies. Encourages Christian fellowship among professionals. Sponsors charitable activities. Operates research center. **Pub:** *Conference Proceedings*, annual. Proceedings. Contains formal papers and reports of ethical, medical, and religious issues. • *Membership Directory*, periodic. Directory. Contains listing of Orthodox Health Professionals. *Price:* $2.50. • *Synergia*, quarterly. Newsletter.

★ 2334 ★ **Osterreichischer Verein fur
    Suizidpravention, Krisenintervention, un
    donfliktbewaltigung (OVSKK)**
c/o Prime Dr. Claudius Stein
Kriseninterrentiousfuntrum
A-1090 Vienna, Austria
**Phone:** 43 1 406959523          **Fax:** 43 1 406959514
**Fnded:** 1986. **Mem:** 80. **Lang(s):** English, German. **Desc:** Professionals and interested individuals concerned with the prevention of suicide. Maintains crisis intervention, conflict resolving, and suicide prevention services and programs. **Pub:** *Krise aktuell*, semiannual. Journal. Contains information about the association and about suicide prevention in Austria in general.

★ 2335 ★ **Ostomy Association of China
    (OAC)**
c/o Dr. Yu De-Hong MD, Pres.
174 Chang Hai Rd.
Shanghai 200433, People's Republic of China
**Phone:** 86 21 25070965          **Fax:** 86 21 65492727

Fnded: 1988. Mem: 400. Nat'l Groups: 1. Reg. Groups: 22. Local Groups: 23. Lang(s): English. Desc: Doctors, stoma nurses, and ostomates. Promotes the care of ostomates in China. Offers medical and practical advice and provides a way for ostomates to exchange information about their experiences. Operates the Ostomy Museum of China in Shanghai. Pub: *Friend of Ostomates*, monthly. • *From Anti Cancer*, bimonthly. Newspaper.

**★ 2336 ★ Pan American Sanitary Bureau**
525 23rd St. NW
Washington, DC 20037
Phone: (202)974-3000          Fax: (202)974-3663
Website: http://www.paho.org/

Desc: Dedicated to improving and maintaining a healthy environment for people of the Americas; aims to develop a course to sustainable human development. Works as the Secretariat of the Pan American Health Organization.

**★ 2337 ★ Pan American Health Organization (PAHO)**
525 23rd St. NW
Washington, DC 20037
Phone: (202)974-3000          Fax: (202)974-3663
Email: webmaster@paho.org
Website: http://www.paho.org
Dr. Bryna Brennan, Dir., Public Information

Fnded: 1902. Mem: 41. Desc: Governments of Western Hemisphere nations united to improve physical and mental health in the Americas. Coordinates regional activities combating disease including exchange of statistical and epidemiological information, development of local health services, and organization of disease control and eradication programs. Encourages development in health systems and technology; provides consulting services; conducts educational courses on public health topics including environmental health, food and nutrition, and tropical diseases. Has established Emergency Preparedness and Disaster Relief Coordination Program in order to increase the ability of health institutions to effectively handle emergencies. Operates the Natural Disaster Relief Voluntary Fund to support disaster relief activities. Maintains the Pan American Sanitary Bureau, the regional office for the Americas of the World Health Organization. Develops health documentaries and coordinates teleconferences. Pub: *Disaster Preparedness in the Americas*, quarterly. Newsletter. PAHO Emergency Preparedness and Disaster Relief Coordination Program. Covers disaster preparedness, mitigation, and management. Price: Free. • *EPI Newsletter*, bimonthly. Newsletter. Provides information on immunization programs in the Americas. Covers new technologies available for the execution of programs. Price: Distributed free to health workers. • *Epidemiological Bulletin*, bimonthly. Bulletin. Disseminates epidemiological information regarding communicable and noncommunicable diseases of public health importance. Price: Free. • *Health in the Americas*, quadrennial. • *Revista Panamericana de Salud Publica/Pan American Journal of Public Health*, monthly. Journal. Serves as a reference source regarding health problems in the Americas and progress made toward solutions. Includes book reviews and results. Price: $75/year. • Manuals. • Monographs. • Reports. • Also publishes scientific books and technical paper.

**★ 2338 ★ Pan American Health Organization - Costa Rica (Organizacion Panamericana de la Salud - Costa Rica)**
Apartado 3745
San Jose, Costa Rica
Phone: 503 2338878          Fax: 503 2338061
Desc: Works to improve the health and standard of living for individuals in Costa Rica. Pub: *Bulletin*, quarterly.

**★ 2339 ★ Pan American Health Organization - Mexico**
Apartado Postal 10-880
110000 Mexico City, DF, Mexico
Phone: 52 1 2028200          Fax: 52 1 5208868
Email: cervante@servidor.dgsca.unam.mx
Lang(s): English, French. Desc: Promotes the well-being and health of individuals in Mexico. Sponsors health education programs.

**★ 2340 ★ Pan American Medical Association (PAMA)**
c/o William E. Sorrel, M.D. Pres.
263 W End Ave., Ste. 1A
New York, NY 10023
Phone: (212)362-0159
William E. Sorrel, M.D., PhD, Pres.

Fnded: 1925. Mem: 6,000. Nat'l Groups: 58. Desc: Fosters the exchange of medical information and research results among physicians in Western Hemisphere countries. Pub: *Journal of the Pan American Medical Association*, biennial. Journal. Price: Free. For members only. AKA: Associacion Medica Pan Americana.

**★ 2341 ★ Parenteral Society**
99 Ermin St.
Stratton St. Margaret
Swindon SN3 4NL, United Kingdom
Phone: 44 1793 824254          Fax: 44 1793 832551
Email: secretary@parenteral.demon.org.uk
Website: http://www.parenteral.co.uk
Fnded: 1981. Mem: 1,250. Desc: Fosters the advancement in the interests of public health, the practice and science of parenteral therapy and to preserve and improve the integrity and standards of the parenteral industry.

**★ 2342 ★ Parkinson's Association of Ireland**
Carmichael Centre
N Brunswick St.
Dublin, Ireland
Phone: 353 1 8722234          Fax: 353 1 8735737
Website: http://www.officeobjects.com/PARKINSONS/
Lang(s): English. Desc: Seeks to provide comfort and assistance to those living with Parkinson's Disease in Ireland.

**★ 2343 ★ Parkinson's Disease Foundation (PDF)**
710 West 168th St.
3rd Fl.
New York, NY 10032
Phone: (212)923-4700          Free: 800-457-6676
Fax: (212)923-4778
Email: info@pdf.org
Website: http://www.pdf.org/
Robin Elliott, Exec. Dir.

Fnded: 1957. Mem: 95,000. Local Groups: 500. Desc: Raises funds for support of scientific research into causes, prevention, and cure of Parkinson's disease. Supports its own laboratories for research in Parkinsonism. Prepares and distributes information on patient care and rehabilitation including list of clinics where treatment is available, and a list of patient selfhelp groups. Supports a brain bank to permit anatomical and chemical studies. Sponsors scientific symposia. Offers patient and family counseling and advocacy services. Maintains research advisory board. Sponsors summer fellowship program for medical students and undergraduate. Pub: *Exercises for the Parkinson Patient and Hints for Daily Living*. • *Health Care Manual for the Professional Team*. Price: $10. • *Information Packet*. Booklets. Price: Free. • *PDF Newsletter*, 3-4/year. Newsletter. Covers developments in Parkinson's disease research, hints for daily living, and advice to health care professionals. Includes case studies. Price: Free. • *Progress, Promise, and Hope: The Parkinson Patient at Home*. •

Brochures. Frmly: (1999) United Parkinson Foundation.

**★ 2344 ★ Partnership for Patient Safety (P4PS)**
c/o Martin Hatlie
1 W Superior St., Ste. 2410
Chicago, IL 60610
Phone: (312)274-9695          Fax: (312)274-9696
Email: info@p4ps.com
Website: http://www.p4ps.org
Martin Hatlie, Pres.

Desc: People and organizations involved in health care. Dedicated to reducing the harm caused by healthcare errors.

**★ 2345 ★ Pathological Society of Great Britain and Ireland**
2 Carlton House Terrace
London SW1Y 5AF, United Kingdom
Phone: 44 207 9761260          Fax: 44 207 9761267
Email: administrator@pathsoc.ac.uk
Website: http://www.pathsoc.org.uk

Fnded: 1906. Mem: 1,700. Desc: Those engaged in research or teaching in connection with pathology or allied science. Holds two scientific meetings each year. Pub: *Journal of Medical Microbology*, monthly. Journal. • *Journal of Pathology*, monthly. Journal. • *Reviews in Medical Microbiology*, quarterly.

**★ 2346 ★ People-to-People Health Foundation (HOPE)**
Project HOPE Health Sciences
Educ. Center
225 Carter Hall Ln.
Millwood, VA 22646
Phone: (540)837-2100          Free: 800-544-HOPE
Fax: (540)837-1813
Email: webmaster@projecthope.org
Website: http://www.projecthope.org
Dr. John Howe, Pres. &CEO

Fnded: 1958. Desc: Promotes better world health and understanding through the training of medical, nursing, dental, and allied health personnel in developing areas of the world. Operates the Center for Health Affairs, which provides research and policy analysis to help develop solutions to problems in worldwide health systems. Develops programs which include the use of volunteer doctors, nurses, and allied health professionals to teach modern techniques in health sciences education, health services delivery systems, health facilities management, and health-related humanitarian assistance. Programs are currently operating in 37 countries, located in Africa, Asia, Eastern Europe, and North, Central, and South America. Pub: *Health Affairs*, quarterly. Journal. Covers domestic and international health policies; annual and five-year indexes available. Price: $45/year for individuals; $75/year for institutions. • *HOPE News*, quarterly. Newsletter. Covers Project HOPE's international and domestic programs. Includes calendar of events and news of fundraising activities. Price: Free. • Annual Report. AKA: Project HOPE.

**★ 2347 ★ People's Medical Society (PMS)**
462 Walnut St.
Allentown, PA 18102
Phone: (610)770-1670          Free: 800-624-8773
Fax: (610)770-0607
Email: mad1@peoplesmed.org
Website: http://www.peoplesmed.org
Pamela Maraldo, Chair

Fnded: 1982. Mem: 80,000. Desc: Promotes citizen involvement in the cost, quality, and management of the American health care system. Seeks to: train and encourage individuals to study local health care systems, practitioners, and institutions and promote preventive health care and medical cost control by these groups; address major policy issues and control health costs; encourage more preventive practice and research; promote self-care and alternative health care procedures; launch an information campaign to assist individuals in maintaining personal health and to prepare them for appointments with medical professionals. **Pub:** *Allergies: Questions You Have...Answers You Need.* • *Alzheimer's and Dementia: Questions You Have...Answers You Need.* • *Arthritis: Questions You Have, Answers You Need.* • *Asthma: Questions You Have, Answers You Need.* • *Breathe Better, Feel Better.* • *The Consumer's Medical Desk Reference.* • *Depression: Questions You Have, Answers You Need.* • *Headaches: 47 Ways to Stop the Pain.* • *Hearing Loss: Questions You Have, Answers You Need.* • *Long-Term Care and Alternatives.* • *Medicare Made Easy.* • *Medicine on Trial.* • *Misdiagnosis: Woman as a Disease.* • *Natural Recipes for the Good Life.* • *150 Ways to Be a Savvy Medical Consumer.* • *People's Medical Society Newsletter,* bimonthly. Newsletter. Includes membership activities information. *Price:* Included in membership dues. • *Prostate: Questions You Have...Answers You Need.* • *77 Ways to Beat Colds and Flu.* • *So You're Going to be a Mother.* • *Tai Chi Made Easy.* • *Take This Book to the Gynecologist With You.* • *Take This Book to the Hospital With You.* • *28 Days to a Better Body.* • *Vitamins & Minerals: Questions You Have, Answers You Need.* • *Your Complete Medical Record.* • Bibliographies. • Bulletins.

### ★ 2348 ★ Periodic Paralysis Association (PPA)

1024 Royal Oaks Dr., Ste. 620
Monrovia, CA 91016
**Phone:** (626)303-3244          **Fax:** (626)337-1966
**Email:** info@periodicparalysis.org
**Website:** http://www.periodicparalysis.org
Patrick E. Cochran, Pres.

**Fnded:** 1997. **Desc:** Offers information, support to those inflicted with periodic paralysis and brings awareness to the public of this disorder.

### ★ 2349 ★ Phi Alpha Sigma

313 S 10th St.
Philadelphia, PA 19107
**Phone:** (215)625-2650
**Email:** philip.torina@jefferson.edu
Dr. Thomas Griffin, Pres.

**Fnded:** 1886. **Mem:** 120. **Nat'l Groups:** 1. **Reg. Groups:** 1. **State Groups:** 1. **Local Groups:** 1. **Desc:** Professional fraternity - medicine. **Pub:** *Bubbling Rales,* annual. Newsletter. *Price:* Free to alumni.

### ★ 2350 ★ Phi Chi Medical Fraternity (PCMF)

1201 E Spring St.
New Albany, IN 47150
**Phone:** (812)948-0581          **Free:** 800-800-7442
**Fax:** (812)941-8850
**Email:** phichi@phi-chi.org
**Website:** http://www.phi-chi.org
Daniel H. Cannon, MD, Chm., Exec. Trustees

**Fnded:** 1889. **Mem:** 40,818. **Local Groups:** 12. **Desc:** Professional fraternity - medicine. Maintains Phi Chi Welfare Association, which accepts voluntary contributions to a student loan fund and other services. **Pub:** *Constitution and Statutes.* • *Officers' Manual.* Manual. • *PC Chronicles,* semiannual. Magazine. Provides chapter news and information. *Price:* Included in membership dues. • *Phi Chi Directory.* Directory. • *Phi Chi History, 1889-1989.* • *Phi Chi Songs.* **Frmly:** (1989) Phi Chi.

### ★ 2351 ★ Phi Delta Epsilon Medical Fraternity

2228 E Solano Dr.
Phoenix, AZ 85016
**Free:** 800-347-3713
**Email:** phide@phide.org
**Website:** http://www.phide.org
George Craft, MD, Exec. Dir.

**Fnded:** 1904. **Mem:** 25,000. **Local Groups:** 41. **Desc:** Professional fraternity - medicine. **Pub:** *Phi*

*Delta Epsilon News and Scientific Journal,* quarterly. Journal.

### ★ 2352 ★ Phi Lambda Kappa Medical Fraternity

3060 Bristol Rd., No. 239
Bensalem, PA 19020
**Phone:** (215)949-8700
Eleanor G. Halprin, Exec. Sec.

**Fnded:** 1907. **Mem:** 4,800. **Reg. Groups:** 17. **Local Groups:** 20. **Desc:** Professional fraternity - medicine. **Pub:** *Quarterly.*

### ★ 2353 ★ Phi Rho Sigma Medical Society

PO Box 90264
Indianapolis, IN 46290
**Phone:** (317)334-8720          **Fax:** (317)334-8721
**Email:** hrodenbe@wpo.iupui.edu
Harriet Rodenberg, MD, Central Office Admin.

**Fnded:** 1890. **Mem:** 31,260. **Reg. Groups:** 13. **State Groups:** 12. **Desc:** Professional society - medicine. **Pub:** *Journal of Phi Rho Sigma,* quarterly. Journal. *Price:* Free. For members only.

### ★ 2354 ★ Physicians Committee for Responsible Medicine (PCRM)

5100 Wisconsin Ave., Ste. 400
Washington, DC 20016
**Phone:** (202)686-2210          **Fax:** (202)686-2216
**Email:** pcrm@pcrm.org
**Website:** http://www.pcrm.org
Neal D. Barnard, MD, Pres.

**Fnded:** 1985. **Mem:** 110,000. **Desc:** Physicians, scientists, healthcare professionals, and interested others. Increases public awareness about the importance of preventive medicine and nutrition, and raises scientific and ethical questions pertaining to the use of humans and animals in medical research. Supports research into U.S. agricultural and public health policies. Promotes the New Four Food Groups, a no-cholesterol, low-fat alternative to U.S.D.A. dietary recommendations. Maintains the Gold Plan program which includes information on low-fat, cholesterol-free entrees and nutrition for institutional food services. Offers fact sheets on nutrition, preventive medicine, and non-animal research topics. Maintains speakers' bureau. **Pub:** *Alternatives in Medical Education.* • *Best in the World (Cookbook).* Book. • *Eat Right, Live Longer.* • *Food for Life.* • *Foods That Fight Pain.* • *Good Medicine,* quarterly. Magazine. Provides information about preventive medicine, nutrition, public health policy, medical/nutrition research updates, and AIDS research. *Price:* Included in membership dues. • *The Power of Your Plate.* • Brochures. • Also publishes fact sheets.

### ★ 2355 ★ Physicians Who Care (PWC)

12125 Jones Maltsberger Rd., No. 607
San Antonio, TX 78247
**Phone:** (210)545-5840          **Free:** 800-545-9305
**Fax:** (210)545-4475
**Email:** pwc@pwc.org
**Website:** http://www.pwc.org
Dr. Stephen C. Cohen, Exec. VP

**Fnded:** 1985. **Mem:** 3,500. **Desc:** A patient advocacy group devoted to protecting the traditional doctor-patient relationship and ensuring quality health care. Believes the responsibility for medical care belongs to physicians, as provider of care, and patients, who have the choice of determining the type of treatment received. Promotes communication between members and their patients on health care issues. **AKA:** (1989) National Organization of Physicians Who Care.

### ★ 2356 ★ Physiological Society of New Zealand (PSNZ)

c/o Dr. P. A. Cragg
Department of Physiology
University of Otago

PO Box 913
Dunedin, New Zealand

**Fnded:** 1972. **Mem:** 180. **Lang(s):** English. **Desc:** Physiological scientists in New Zealand. Seeks to enhance the quality of physiological and related research in New Zealand by establishing links with similar societies throughout the world, enhancing the effectiveness of all levels of education in the teaching of physiological, biological and related sciences, and by acting as a national body to provide advice and information to the government and the community. Provides career advice and fosters career opportunities for graduate and postgraduate students.

### ★ 2357 ★ Polish Anatomical Society (PAS) (Polskie Towarzystwo Anatomiczne — PTA)

Department of Anatomy
University School of Medical Sciences
6 Swiecicki St.
PL-60 781 Poznan, Poland
**Phone:** 48 61 8699181          **Fax:** 48 61 8658985
**Email:** wwozniak@usoms.poznan.pl

**Fnded:** 1926. **Mem:** 500. **Local Groups:** 12. **Lang(s):** English, French. **Desc:** Encourages scientific activities dealing with the morphological sciences, including anatomy, cell biology, embryology, histochemistry, histology, and zoology. Promotes modernization of educational methods. Conducts research. **Pub:** *Advances in Cell Biology,* quarterly. • *Folia Morphologica,* quarterly. **Frmly:** Polish Anatomical and Zoological Society.

### ★ 2358 ★ Polish Medical Association (Polski Towarzystwo Lekarskie)

Al. Ujazdowskie St. 24
PL-00-478 Warsaw, Poland
**Phone:** 48 26 288699          **Fax:** 48 26 288699
**Website:** http://www.polmed.org

**Fnded:** 1820. **Mem:** 30,000. **Reg. Groups:** 50. **Local Groups:** 284. **Lang(s):** Polish. **Desc:** Aims to maintain high professional and ethical standards in the medical profession. **Pub:** *Polski Tygodnik Lekavski also cited as: Polish Medical Weekly,* weekly. Magazine. • *Przeyład Lekavski also cited as: Medical Review.* • *Wiadomoici Leharshie also cited as: News for Physicians.*

### ★ 2359 ★ Population and Community Development Association (PDA)

6 Sukhumvit Rd., SOI-12
Bangkok 10110, Thailand
**Phone:** 66 2 2294611          **Fax:** 66 2 2294632
**Email:** pda@mozart.inet.co.th
**Website:** http://www.pda.or.th

**Fnded:** 1974. **Mem:** 483. **Local Groups:** 16. **Lang(s):** English, Thai. **Desc:** Seeks to improve the quality of life and increase economic levels in rural areas of Thailand. Coordinates development projects focusing on family planning, primary health care, and rural development. Offers training courses on the management of community-based development programs; conducts population research; educates communities on AIDS prevention. Maintains the Asian Center for Population and Community Development. Worked to popularize birth control practices through socially entertaining programs such as condom-blowing contests and the Cops and Rubbers Project. Over the past 15 years Thailand's population growth has been cut in half through these types of programs. **Pub:** *From Condoms to Cabbages.* Book. An authorized biography of Mechai Viravaidya. • *PDA,* 3/year. Newsletter. • *Strategies to Strengthen NGO Capacity in Resource Mobilization through Business Activities.* UNAIDS best practice collection. • *TBIRD: News,* 3/year. Newsletter. Features TBIRD project activities. **Frmly:** (1977) Community-Based Family Planning Services.

### ★ 2360 ★ Premenstrual Society

PO Box 429
Addlestone KT15 1DZ, United Kingdom

**Phone:** 44 1932 872560

**Fnded:** 1986. **Mem:** 500. **Reg. Groups:** 10. **Lang(s):** English. **Desc:** Seeks to provide advice and support for sufferers of premenstrual syndrome (PMS). Provides support for local groups and professionals in the field. **Pub:** *Premsul*, semiannual. Newsletter.

★ **2361** ★ **Professional Association of German Internists (Berufsverband Deutscher Internisten)**
Schone Aussicht 5
D-65193 Wiesbaden, Germany
**Phone:** 49 611 181330     **Fax:** 49 611 1813350
**Email:** info@bdi.de
**Website:** http://www.bdi.de
**Fnded:** 1959. **Mem:** 29,000. **Reg. Groups:** 23. **Local Groups:** 77. **Lang(s):** English, French. **Desc:** Protects and represents the interests of internal medicine specialists in Germany. Promotes continuing education. **Pub:** *BDI - Ruudschveiben*, monthly. Newsletter. • *Der Internist*, monthly. Magazine.

★ **2362** ★ **Professional Association of Medical Advisers (PAMA) (Association Professionelle des Delegues Medicaux — APDM)**
Boite Postale 30
1014 El Menzah, Tunisia
**Phone:** 216 1 785000     **Fax:** 216 1 781401
**Lang(s):** Arabic, French. **Desc:** Medical advisers. Promotes professional advancement of members. Represents members' interests before industrial organizations, government agencies, and the public.

★ **2363** ★ **Professional Union of French-Speaking Medical Advisers (PUFSMA) (Union Professionelle des Delegues Medicaux Francophones — UPDMF)**
32, rue de la Foriere
B-4100 Seraing, Belgium
**Phone:** 32 4 3361167     **Fax:** 32 4 3361167
**Lang(s):** French. **Desc:** Medical advisers. Promotes professional advancement of members. Represents members' interests before industrial organizations, government agencies, and the public.

★ **2364** ★ **Professional Women Health Society**
PO Box 2319
Hong Kong, People's Republic of China
**Phone:** 852 28132625     **Fax:** 852 25372218
**Fnded:** 1991. **Mem:** 100. **Desc:** Women working in healthcare fields, including nursing, rehabilitative therapy, alternative medicine, psychology, nutrition, social work, administration/finance, academics/research, and insurance.

★ **2365** ★ **Project Concern Hong Kong**
Shop 105, Lei Cheng Uk Shopping Arcade
Lei Cheng Uk Estate
Hong Kong, People's Republic of China
**Phone:** 852 27769081     **Fax:** 852 27769083
**Email:** medcare@projectconcern.org.hk
**Fnded:** 1961. **Mem:** 12. **Nat'l Groups:** 35. **Local Groups:** 10. **Lang(s):** Chinese, English. **Desc:** National branch of the international organization. Health care practitioners and other interested individuals. Seeks to reduce morbidity and mortality, particularly among women and children. Establishes and operates medical and dental clinics and provides social services in economically disadvantaged areas. Sponsors charitable activities. **Pub:** *Project Concern Hong Kong Annual Report*, annual. Annual Report.

★ **2366** ★ **Project Concern International (PCI)**
3550 Afton Rd.
San Diego, CA 92123

**Phone:** (858)279-9690     **Free:** 877-PCI-HOPE
**Fax:** (858)694-0294
**Email:** postmaster@projectconcern.org
**Website:** http://www.projectconcern.org
Barbara Burgess Soltz, Board Chair
**Fnded:** 1961. **Desc:** Works with communities worldwide to ensure low-cost, basic health care for those most in need, particularly mothers and children. Provides education, training, and medical assistance to safeguard the world's impoverished children. Works with volunteers to prepare local communities to care for their own children with long-term, self-sustaining projects. Maintains programs in Bolivia, Guatemala, El Salvador, Honduras, Nicaragua, India, Indonesia, Romania, Zambia and the United States. **Pub:** *Concern News*, quarterly. Newsletter. Includes news about the organization, special events and donors. *Price:* Free. • *Project Concern International–Annual Report*. Annual Report. Contains financial statements. *Price:* Free. **Frmly:** (1978) Project Concern, Inc.

★ **2367** ★ **Re-Solv, the Society for the Prevention of Solvent and Volatile Substance Abuse (RS)**
30A High St.
Stone STl5 8AW, United Kingdom
**Phone:** 44 1785 817885     **Fax:** 44 1785 813205
**Email:** information@re-solv.org
**Website:** http://www.re-solv.org
**Fnded:** 1984. **Mem:** 300. **Lang(s):** English. **Desc:** Promotes increased awareness on the part of parents, local authorities, retailers, and law enforcement officials of the problem of the "sniffing" of solvents and volatile substances. Acts as an information clearinghouse on solvent abuse. Liaises with other agencies, the Home Office, and other government bodies in the dissemination of information. Supports legislation that seeks to control solvent abuse. Provides videos and other materials for use in primary and secondary schools and by parents, teachers, doctors, social workers, retailers, and law enforcement personnel. doctors, social workers, retailers, and law enforcement personnel. doctors, social workers, retailers, and law enforcement personnel. **Pub:** *The Adolescent Epidemic*. Video. • *Chicken!*. Video. Video for young people; presents the story of how substance abuse affects the lives of young people and their families. • *Guide for the Carer*. Book.

★ **2368** ★ **Recovered Medical Equipment for the Developing World (REMEDY)**
c/o Darryl Rotman Kuperstock
PO Box 208051
New Haven, CT 06520
**Phone:** (203)737-5356     **Fax:** (203)785-6664
**Email:** remedy@yale.edu
**Website:** http://www.remedyinc.org/
Darryl Rotman Kuperstock, Exec. Dir.
**Fnded:** 1991. **Mem:** 250. **Desc:** Dedicated to achieving safe, efficient, and cost effective methods for recovering opened, but unused materials from hospital operating rooms. Provides teaching problem solving, and networking assistance. Sponsors the Agencies for International Relief E-mail (AIRE-mail) program that works to quickly fulfill the needs of urgent situations and special circumstances.

★ **2369** ★ **Research! America**
908 King St. No. 400E
Alexandria, VA 22314-3067
**Phone:** (703)739-2577     **Free:** 800-366-CURE
**Fax:** (703)739-2372
**Email:** info@researchamerica.org
**Website:** http://www.researchamerica.org
Mary Woolley, Pres. & CEO
**Fnded:** 1989. **Mem:** 450. **Desc:** Academia, voluntary health organizations, professional and scientific societies, hospitals and independent research institutes, businesses and industries, and foundations and philanthropists. Works to increase public awareness of the benefits to humankind of medical and health research and to build a strong base of citizen support for research into he cure, treatment, and prevention of

physical and mental disorders. Seeks to stimulate interest in medical research careers. Appeals to institutions and the government to provide essential funding for medical and health research. Engages in multimedia communications programs and serves as a clearinghouse and source of information to members, the media, the general public, and elected officials including public opinion data. **Pub:** *Membership Matters*, monthly. Newsletter. *Price:* Included in membership dues.

★ **2370** ★ **Research-Based Dietary Ingredient Association (RDIA)**
1722 Eye St. NW
Washington, DC 20006
**Email:** info@rdia.org
**Website:** http://www.rdia.org/
**Desc:** Life sciences companies and organizations. Dedicated to advancing the role and safety of functional foods, medical foods, nutraceuticals, dietary supplements, and other dietary ingredients in the public health system of the U.S. and other countries.

★ **2371** ★ **RGK Foundation**
1301 W 25th St., Ste. 300
Austin, TX 78705-4236
**Phone:** (512)474-9298     **Fax:** (512)474-7281
**Website:** http://www.rgkfoundation.org
Gregory A. Kozmetsky, Pres.
**Desc:** Works to promote medical research.

★ **2372** ★ **Royal Academy of Medicine in Ireland (RAMI)**
6 Kildare St.
Dublin 2, Ireland
**Phone:** 353 1 6767650     **Fax:** 353 1 6611684
**Email:** secretary@rami.ie
**Website:** http://www.rami.ie
**Fnded:** 1882. **Mem:** 2,000. **Lang(s):** English, Irish. **Desc:** Physicians, medical researchers, and other scientists with an interest in medicine. Seeks to advance medical study, teaching, and practice. Serves as a forum for the exchange of information among members; sponsors research and educational programs. **Pub:** *Irish Journal of Medical Science*, periodic. Journal.

★ **2373** ★ **Royal Australasian College of Physicians (RACP)**
145 Macquarie St.
Sydney, NSW 2000, Australia
**Phone:** 61 2 92565444     **Fax:** 61 2 92523310
**Fnded:** 1938.

★ **2374** ★ **Royal College of General Practitioners**
14 Princes Gate
Hyde Pk.
London SW7 1PU, United Kingdom
**Phone:** 44 207 5813232     **Fax:** 44 207 2253047
**Email:** info@rcgp.org.uk
**Website:** http://www.rcgp.org.uk
**Fnded:** 1952. **Mem:** 18,400. **Desc:** General practitioners. Responsible for the promotion of high quality general practice through education, research and standard setting. **Pub:** *British Journal of General Practice*, monthly. Journal.

★ **2375** ★ **Royal College of Pathologists**
2 Carlton House Terrace
London SW1Y 5AF, United Kingdom
**Phone:** 44 20 74516700     **Fax:** 44 20 74516701
**Email:** info@rcpath.org
**Website:** http://www.rcpath.org
**Fnded:** 1962. **Mem:** 7,500. **Lang(s):** English. **Desc:** Postgraduate medical and scientific graduates who have successfully completed all or part of the college's examinations following a specified period of approved training, or elected under specified college ordinances. Advances the science and practice of pathology,

furthers public education, promotes study and research work in pathology and related subjects and publishes the results of such study and research. **Pub:** *College Bulletin*, quarterly. Journal. • *Manpower and Management Policy Documents.* • *Training and Examination Guidelines.* • Reports.


**★ 2376 ★ Royal College of Physicians (RCP)**
11 St. Andrew's Pl.
Regent's Park
London NW1 4LE, United Kingdom
**Phone:** 44 20 79351174     **Fax:** 44 20 74867038
**Email:** linda.cuthbertson@rcplondon.ac.uk
**Website:** http://www.rcplondon.ac.uk
**Fnded:** 1518. **Mem:** 8,000. **Lang(s):** English. **Desc:** Individuals in 64 countries. Responsible for the postgraduate education and training of physicians in England, Wales, and Northern Ireland. Committed to maintaining the highest standards of medical practice. Advises the government, public, and members of the profession on health and medical issues. Conducts educational and training programs; organizes examinations; operates clinical effectiveness unit. **Pub:** *Annual Report.* • *College List*, annual. • *Working Party Reports.* • Journal, bimonthly.


**★ 2377 ★ Royal College of Physicians of Ireland**
6 Kildare St.
Dublin 2, Ireland
**Phone:** 353 1 6616677     **Fax:** 353 1 6762920
**Email:** info@rcpi.ie
**Fnded:** 1654. **Mem:** 4,500. **Desc:** Makes available post graduate medical education and training.


**★ 2378 ★ Royal College of Physicians and Surgeons of Canada (RCPSC)**
774 Echo Dr.
Ottawa, ON, Canada K1S 5N8
**Phone:** (613)730-8177     **Free:** 800-668-3740
**Fax:** (613)730-8830
**Email:** pierrette.leonard@rcpsc.edu
**Website:** http://rcpsc.medical.org
**Fnded:** 1929. **Mem:** 33,178. **Lang(s):** English, French. **Desc:** Medical fellows (22,339); surgical fellows (10,839). Founded by the Canadian Medical Association. Prescribes requirements of specialty training in 58 medical, laboratory, and surgical specialties and subspecialties. Accredits specialty residency programs in Canada, judges the acceptability of residency education, and conducts the certifying examinations. Also assists its members (fellows) to maintain their specialty competence through continuing medical education and the maintenance of Certification Program. Intervenes in matters involving health and public policy and biomedical ethics; it is not a licensing or disciplinary body. **Pub:** *Annals RCPSC*, 8/year. Journal. Peer reviewed scientific articles. • *Annual Meeting Scientific Programme*, annual. • *RC Report*, semiannual. Report.


**★ 2379 ★ Royal College of Physicians and Surgeons of Glasgow**
232-242 St. Vincent St.
Glasgow G2 5RJ, United Kingdom
**Phone:** 44 141 2216072     **Fax:** 44 141 2211804
**Website:** http://www.rcpsglasg.ac.uk
**Fnded:** 1599. **Mem:** 7,060. **Desc:** Physicians, surgeons, and dentists. Conducts educational and training programs. **Pub:** Annual Report.


**★ 2380 ★ Royal College of Physicians and Surgeons of the United States of America (RCPS)**
485 Allard Rd.
PO Box 24224
Grosse Pointe, MI 48236
**Phone:** (313)882-0641     **Fax:** (313)882-0979
**Website:** http://www.royalcollegeusa.com
Martin Savitz, Exec. Dir.

**Fnded:** 1984. **Mem:** 2,500. **Nat'l Groups:** 32. **Reg. Groups:** 30. **State Groups:** 4. **Local Groups:** 28. **Desc:** Physicians and allied health professionals interested in tropical medicine. Provides postgraduate continuing medical education; confers certificates and diplomas. Maintains speakers' bureau and hall of fame and provides placement services. Conducts research and educational programs; compiles statistics. **Pub:** *Bare Facts for Practicing Doctors*, semiannual. Magazine. Provides clinical info to doctors in tropical countries. • *Journal of the Royal College of Physicians and Surgeons*, semiannual. Journal. Focuses on continuing medical education and certificate/diploma award. *Price:* $50 for members; $75 for nonmembers; $110 institutions. • *JRCP&S*, periodic. Newsletter. • *Proceedings of the Royal College of Physicians and Surgeons*, semiannual. *Price:* $100.


**★ 2381 ★ Royal Medical Society**
Student Centre
5/5 Bristol Sq.
Edinburgh EH8 9AL, United Kingdom
**Phone:** 44 131 6502672
**Email:** royalmedsoc@btinternet.com
**Website:** http://www.royalmedsoc.btinternet.co.uk
**Fnded:** 1737. **Mem:** 2,500. **Desc:** Mainly medical students. Fellows and Life Members are medical graduates. An educational charity for medical students, run by medical students. **Pub:** *Res Medica*, periodic.


**★ 2382 ★ Royal Society of Medicine**
1 Wimpole St.
London W1G 0AE, United Kingdom
**Phone:** 44 207 2902900     **Fax:** 44 207 2902992
**Email:** webmaster@rsm.ac.uk
**Website:** http://www.roysocmed.ac.uk
**Fnded:** 1805. **Mem:** 18,000. **Desc:** Doctors, dentists, vets and lay members with interest in medicine. **Pub:** *The AIDS Letter*, bimonthly. • *International Journal of STD and AIDS*, bimonthly. Journal. • *Journal of Medical Biography*, quarterly. Journal. • *Journal of Royal Society of Medicine*, monthly. Journal. • *Journal of Telemedicine and Telecare*, quarterly. Journal. • *Tropical Doctor*, quarterly.


**★ 2383 ★ Royal Society of Medicine Foundation (RSMF)**
207 E Westminster Rd. Ste. 201
Lake Forest, IL 60045-1860
**Phone:** (847)234-6782
**Website:** http://www.rsm.ac.uk
Richard S. Wilbur, MD, Exec. Officer
**Fnded:** 1967. **Mem:** 3,500. **Desc:** Serves as a forum for the discussion of topics relevant to the medical community in the U.S. and the United Kingdom. Sponsors conference series and exchange programs in conjunction with the Royal Society of Medicine. **Pub:** *Digest*, quarterly.


**★ 2384 ★ Royal Society for the Promotion of Health**
38A St. George's Dr.
London SW1V 4BH, United Kingdom
**Phone:** 44 207 6300121     **Fax:** 44 207 9766847
**Email:** rshealth@rshealth.org.uk
**Website:** http://www.rsph.org
**Fnded:** 1876. **Mem:** 7,000. **Desc:** Members are drawn from a wide variety of professions and occupations with an interest in improving the health of the population. They range from architects and engineers, the health related profession, to food scientists and caterers. Aims to improve the quality and dignity of human life worldwide and to promote the continuous improvement of health and safety through education communication and the encouragement of scientific research. **Pub:** *JRSH*, quarterly. Journal. **Frmly:** (1999) Royal Society of Health.

**★ 2385 ★ Safety Assessment Federation**
Nutmeg House
60 Gainsford St. Butlers
London SE1 2NY, United Kingdom
**Phone:** 44 20 74030987     **Fax:** 44 20 74030137
**Email:** info@safed.co.uk
**Website:** http://www.safed.co.uk
**Fnded:** 1995. **Mem:** 17. **Desc:** Represents the interests of companies that undertake the independent safety inspection and certification of machinery plant and equipment. **Pub:** *Fact sheets*.


**★ 2386 ★ Salvation Army Medical Fellowship (SAMF)**
c/o Gen. Paul Rader
101 Queen Victoria St.
London EC4P 4EP, United Kingdom
**Phone:** 44 171 3320101
**Fnded:** 1943. **Mem:** 10,648. **Lang(s):** English, French, German, Norwegian, Swedish. **Desc:** Purpose is to support members of the International Headquarters of the Salvation Army involved in the field of medicine, particularly those involved in nursing.


**★ 2387 ★ Samaritans - Western Australia**
60 Bagot Rd.
Subiaco, WA 6008, Australia
**Phone:** 61 8 93815555     **Fax:** 61 9 3882368
**Email:** samarita@starwon.com.au
**Website:** http://www.thesamaritans.org.au
**Fnded:** 1967. **Mem:** 90. **Nat'l Groups:** 3. **Reg. Groups:** 3. **State Groups:** 2. **Local Groups:** 1. **Lang(s):** Chinese, English, German, Indonesian. **Desc:** National branch of Befrienders International Samaritans Worldwide. Offers supportive listening, usually by phone for suicidal and/or despairing people, and education for young persons who have attempted suicide and their families. Provides support and information services to health care professionals. **Pub:** *Directory of Youth Services*, annual. Directory. • *Information Handbook for Youth at Risk.* • *Survivor's Kit.* • *Teen Suicide Guidelines for Parents.* **Frmly:** (1998) Samaritan Befrienders.


**★ 2388 ★ Scientific Society of Microbiology**
Katedra po Microbiologia
V.Levski 16
BG-1000 Sofia, Bulgaria
**Phone:** 359 2 449894
**Fnded:** 1991. **Desc:** Fosters research in microbiology.


**★ 2389 ★ Scottish Association of Health Councils**
24 A Palmerston Place
Edinburgh EH12 5AL, United Kingdom
**Phone:** 44 131 2204101     **Fax:** 44 131 2204108
**Email:** admin1@sahc.sol.co.uk
**Website:** http://www.show.scot.nhs.uk/sahc
**Fnded:** 1977. **Mem:** 16. **Desc:** Membership is open to all 16 health councils in Scotland. Provides information, training resources and development of public participation to all health related matters. The organization is the focal point between Local Health Councils, the Scottish Executive and Health Department and other national organizations, SAHC is voluntary and funded by LHC's subscriptions. **Pub:** Papers.


**★ 2390 ★ Scottish Society of the History of Medicine**
Red Gable
Denhead
Saint Andrews KY16 8PB, United Kingdom
**Email:** jdmac74@aol.com
**Fnded:** 1948. **Mem:** 200. **Desc:** Aims to further the general history of medicine with particular attention to Scottish medicine. **Pub:** *Report of Proceedings*, semiannual. Proceedings.

**★ 2391 ★ SEAMEO Regional Centre for Medical Microbiology, Parasitology and Entomology (SEAMEO TRO)**
c/o Institute of Medical Research
Jalan Pahang
Kuala Lumpur, Malaysia
**Email:** seameo@imr.gov.my
**Fnded:** 1970. **Desc:** A project of the Southeast Asian Ministers of Education Organization. Works to improve medical education and related programs in southeast Asia. Encourages study and research in the field. Conducts training programs and 2 graduate programs in medical microbiology and parasitology/entomology.

**★ 2392 ★ Seventh-Day Adventist Dietetic Association (SDADA)**
1 Angwin Ave.
Angwin, CA 94508
**Phone:** (916)782-5200          **Fax:** (916)782-5458
**Email:** rubyh@rsvl.ah.com
**Fnded:** 1956. **Mem:** 505. **Desc:** Seventh-Day Adventist registered dietitians; dietitians working in Seventh-Day Adventist institutions. Strives to motivate members to attain high professional standards and to actively promote Seventh-Day Adventist health principles. Provides resources and guidance concerning vegetarian lifestyles to dietitians. Disseminates nutrition information. **Pub:** Diet Manual. Includes vegetarian options. Price: $54.95. • SDADA News, quarterly. Price: available to members only. • Seventh-Day Adventist Dietetic Association Diet Manual. • The Vegetarian Advantage. Brochure.

**★ 2393 ★ Shwachman-Diamond Syndrome International**
PMB 162
5195 Hampsted Village Center Way
New Albany, OH 43054-8331
**Free:** 877-737-4685          **Fax:** (614)939-0752
**Email:** 4sskids@shwachman-diamond.org
**Website:** http://www.shwachman-diamond.org/
**Fnded:** 1994. **Desc:** Provides emotional support to patients and their families; educates the medical community and general public about Schwachman-Diamond Syndrome; encourages training of and research by medical professionals; advocates support of research; links families through exchange of experience and ideas; disseminates current medical information; supports an International Patient Registry/Database. **Pub:** Newsletter.

**★ 2394 ★ Sleep/Wake Disorders Canada (SWDC)**
**(Affections du Sommeil/Eveil Canada)**
3080 Yonge St., Ste. 5055
Toronto, ON, Canada M4N 3N1
**Phone:** (416)483-9654          **Fax:** (416)483-7081
**Email:** swdc@globalserve.net
**Website:** http://swdca.org
**Fnded:** 1985. **Mem:** 1,000. **Lang(s):** English, French. **Desc:** People with narcolepsy, insomnia, and other sleeping disorders and their families. Promotes self-help for people with sleep disorders; seeks to increase public awareness of sleep disorders and their causes and treatment. Encourages and facilitates establishment of local self-help and support groups for people with sleep disorders; conducts fundraising activities; sponsors National Sleep Awareness Week. Serves as a clearinghouse on sleep disorders; maintains register of sleep laboratories; functions as liaison between members and the Canadian Sleep Society, the national organization of doctors and sleep researchers. **Pub:** Good Night/Good Day, quarterly. Newsletter. • Sleep Solutions. Booklet. • Books. • Brochures.

**★ 2395 ★ Sociedad de Anestesiologla de Chile**
Casilla 4259
Santiago, Chile
**Fnded:** 1946.

**★ 2396 ★ Sociedade Brasileira de Engenharia Biomedica (SBEB)**
Caixa Postal 68.510, Centro de Tecnologia - COPPE/UFRJ
21945-970 Rio de Janeiro, Brazil
**Email:** sbeb@peb.ufrj.br
**Website:** http://www.peb.ufrj.br/~sbeb

**★ 2397 ★ Society of Apothecaries of London**
Apothecaries Hall
Black Friars Ln.
London EC4V 6EJ, United Kingdom
**Phone:** 44 207 2361189          **Fax:** 44 207 3293177
**Email:** clerk@apothecaries.org
**Website:** http://www.apothecaries.org
**Fnded:** 1617. **Mem:** 1,700. **Desc:** Members of the medical profession. Functions as City of London Livery Company and medical examining body.

**★ 2398 ★ Society for Clinical and Medical Hair Removal (SCME)**
7600 Terrace Ave., Ste. 203
Middleton, WI 53562
**Phone:** (608)831-8009          **Fax:** (608)831-5122
**Email:** scme@reesgroupinc.com
**Website:** http://www.scmhr.org
Lisia Walch, Pres.
**Fnded:** 1985. **Mem:** 1,000. **Reg. Groups:** 10. **Desc:** Professional society of electrologists (persons engaged in the removal of superfluous hair by galvanic blend or short wave methods for cosmetic and medical purposes). Conducts continuing education and leadership development seminars. **Pub:** Perspectives, periodic. • SCME Directory of Membership, annual. Membership Directory. • SCME Newsletter, quarterly. Newsletter. **Frmly:** (2002) Society of Clinical and Medical Electrologists.

**★ 2399 ★ Society for Clinical Trials (SCT)**
600 Wyndhurst Ave.
Baltimore, MD 21210
**Phone:** (410)433-4722          **Fax:** (410)435-8631
**Email:** sctbalt@aol.com
**Website:** http://www.sctweb.org
Mary C. Burke, Contact
**Fnded:** 1978. **Mem:** 1,450. **Desc:** Persons with training and expertise in behavioral science, bioethics, biostatistics, computer science, dentistry, epidemiology, law, management, medicine, nursing, and pharmacology. To promote the development and dissemination of knowledge about the design and conduct of clinical trials and other research employing similar methods. **Pub:** Controlled Clinical Trials, bimonthly. Journal.

**★ 2400 ★ Society of General Internal Medicine (SGIM)**
2501 M St. NW, Ste. 575
Washington, DC 20037-1126
**Phone:** (202)887-5150          **Free:** 800-822-3060
**Fax:** (202)887-5405
**Email:** karlsond@sgim.org
**Website:** http://www.sgim.org
David Karlson, PhD, Exec. Dir.
**Fnded:** 1978. **Mem:** 3,000. **Reg. Groups:** 8. **Desc:** Physicians combining clinical practice with research. Promotes improved patient care, research, and teaching in primary care and general internal medicine. Sponsors research and educational programs. **Pub:** Directory of Primary Care Internal Medicine Residency Programs and Fellowship Training Programs, annual. Directory. Descriptiojns of 146 primary care general internal medicine programs. Lists 60 fellowship programs in general internal medicine. • Journal of General Internal Medicine, monthly. Journal. • SGIM Forum, monthly. Newsletter. **Frmly:** (1987) Society for Research and Education in Primary Care Internal Medicine.

**★ 2401 ★ Society for Health and Human Values (SHHV)**
4700 W Lake Ave.
Glenview, IL 60025
**Email:** shhv@aol.com
George K. Degnon, Exec. Officer
**Fnded:** 1969. **Mem:** 900. **Desc:** Educators in the health professions united to develop new understandings, concepts, and programs in the area of human values and medicine with special emphasis on the education of health professionals. Conducts programs at national association meetings. Acts as resource service for educational institutions. **Pub:** Advance Directives in Medicine. Book. • Literature and Medicine: A Claim for a Discipline. Book. • The Meaning of AIDS: Implications for Medical Science, Clinical Practice and Public Health Policy. Book. • Medicine & Religion: Strategies of Care. Book. • Ministers in Medical Education. Book. • Nurshing the Humanities in Medicine: Interactions with the Social Sciences. Book. • Of Value, quarterly. • The Visual Arts and Medical Education. Book.

**★ 2402 ★ Society for Healthcare Consumer Advocacy of the American Hospital Association**
One North Franklin
Chicago, IL 60606
**Phone:** (312)422-3999          **Fax:** (312)422-4580
**Email:** mhogan@aha.org
**Website:** http://www.shca-aha.org
Michaeleen Hogan, Exec. Dir.
**Fnded:** 1972. **Mem:** 960. **State Groups:** 31. **Desc:** To advance the development of effective patient representative and advocacy programs in health care institutions. Conducts seminars and workshops. **Pub:** In The Name of the Patient: Consumer Advocacy in Healthcare. Book. Price: $35 for members; $45 for nonmembers. • Membership Roster, annual. **Frmly:** (1981) Society of Patient Representatives; (1988) National Society of Patient Representatives of the American Hospital Association; (1998) National Society of Patient Representation and Consumer Affairs of the American Hospital Association.

**★ 2403 ★ Society for Human Ecology (SHE)**
c/o Melville Cote
College of the Atlantic
105 Eden St.
Bar Harbor, ME 04609
**Phone:** (207)288-5015          **Fax:** (207)288-4126
**Email:** inquiry@ecology.coa.edu
**Website:** http://www.coa.edu
Melville P. Cote, Exec. Dir.
**Fnded:** 1981. **Mem:** 150. **Desc:** Educators, health practitioners, scientists, and other professionals in 30 countries studying human ecology and its applications. Focuses attention on the consequences of human action on manufactured, natural, and social environments. Promotes interdisciplinary collaboration; facilitates the exchange of information; identifies problems and recommends solutions from an ecological perspective. Conducts workshops and symposia. Participates in human ecology consortium. Organization is distinct from the International Organization for Human Ecology, formerly known as the Society for Human Ecology. **Pub:** Human Ecology: A Gathering of Perspectives. Proceedings. Proceedings from SHE's First International Conference, held in 1985. • Human Ecology and Decision Making: An International and Interdisciplinary Collaboration. • Human Ecology Bulletin, semiannual. • Human Ecology–Coming of Age: An International Overview. Proceedings. Proceedings of the symposium organized at the International Congress of Ecology in 1990. • Human Ecology: Crossing Boundaries. Selected papers from the 6th conference of SHE. • Human Ecology: Research and Applications. Proceedings. Proceedings from SHE's Second International Conference, held in 1988. • Human Ecology: Steps to the Future. Proceedings. Proceedings from SHE's Third International Conference. • Human Ecology: Strategies for the Future. Selected papers from the 4th conference of the SHE,

held in 1990. • *International Directory of Human Ecologists*, periodic. Directory. Lists over 700 human ecologists worldwide, with descriptions of their work, research, and activities; includes addresses and phone numbers. • Brochure.

### ★ 2404 ★ Society for Medical Decision Making (SMDM)

c/o George Washington University Medical Center
2300 K St. NW
Office of Continuing Medical Education in the Health
Professions
Washington, DC 20037
**Phone:** (202)994-8929　　**Fax:** (202)994-1791
**Email:** smdm-office@smi.stanford.edu
**Website:** http://www.gwu.edu/~smdm
Daniel E. Reichard, Admin. Dir.

**Fnded:** 1979. **Mem:** 1,000. **Desc:** Individuals with an interest in "developing rational and systematic approaches" to medical decision making, including educators, clinicians, managers, and policy makers. Promotes improvement in all aspects of medical decision making. Evaluates decision making applications and disseminates conclusions. Facilitates multidisciplinary scholarship and research; conducts continuing professional education programs. **Pub:** *Medical Decision Making*, bimonthly. Journal. • Newsletter, semiannual.

### ★ 2405 ★ Society for Medicine and Law in Israel

c/o A. Carmi, Pres.
PO Box 6451
Haifa, Israel
**Phone:** 972 4 8375219　　**Fax:** 972 4 8381587
**Email:** acarmi@research.haifa.ac.il

**Fnded:** 1972. **Mem:** 1,600. **Lang(s):** English. **Desc:** Promotes the advancement of medicine and law in Israel. **Pub:** *Refuah Umishpat*, semiannual. Journal.

### ★ 2406 ★ Society of Rural Physicians of Canada (SRPC)

RR 5
Shawville, QC, Canada J0X 2Y0
**Phone:** (819)647-3971　　**Fax:** (819)647-3971
**Email:** admin@srpc.ca
**Website:** http://www.srpc.ca

**Fnded:** 1992. **Mem:** 1,200. **Reg. Groups:** 5. **Lang(s):** English, French. **Desc:** Physicians practicing in rural areas of Canada. Promotes delivery of health care services to individuals in remote areas nationwide. Seeks to ensure suitable working conditions for members. Sponsors annual continuing professional development course. Develops model policies for regulation and delivery of health care in rural areas; encourages medical research; provides support and services to members and to communities seeking to improve their health care resources; plans to establish a library. Offers free membership to students, residents, and honourary members. **Pub:** *Canadian Journal of Rural Medicine*, periodic. Newsletter.

### ★ 2407 ★ Society of Teachers of the Alexander Technique (STAT)

129 Camden Mews
London NW1 9AH, United Kingdom
**Phone:** 44 20 72843338　　**Fax:** 44 20 74825434
**Email:** info@stat.org.uk
**Website:** http://www.stat.org.uk

**Fnded:** 1958. **Mem:** 1,737. **Nat'l Groups:** 1. **Lang(s):** English. **Desc:** Teachers (1150), students (230) and others (360) in 24 countries. Works to maintain professional standards and gain wider recognition of the Alexander Technique (a means of posture re-education). Encourages research and communication among members. **Pub:** *Alexander Journal*, periodic. Journal. • *List of Teachers*, triennial. Directory. • *STATNEWS*, 3/year. Newsletter.

### ★ 2408 ★ Society of Teachers of Family Medicine (STFM)

11400 Tomahawk Creek Pkwy., Ste. 540
Leawood, KS 66211
**Phone:** (913)906-6000　　**Free:** 800-274-2237
**Fax:** (913)906-6096
**Email:** admstaff@stfm.org
**Website:** http://www.stfm.org
Roger A. Sherwood, CAE, Exec. Dir.

**Fnded:** 1967. **Mem:** 5,000. **Desc:** Physicians involved in teaching or promoting family medicine; individuals in related fields. Organized to promote public welfare by maintaining and improving standards and practices of medical service, especially in the field of family medicine. Promotes these objectives by: supporting and expressing the tenets of family medicine as an academic discipline; maintaining and continually improving the quality of instructional and scientific skills and knowledge in the field of family medicine; providing a forum for the interchange of experience and ideas among its members and other interested persons; and encouraging research and teaching in family medicine. medicine. medicine. **Pub:** *Family Medicine*, monthly. Journal. Includes annual index, book reviews, and employment opportunities. *Price:* Included in membership dues; $12.50/copy for nonmembers; $88/year for individual nonmembers; $120/year for institutions. • *STEM Membership Directory*, biennial. Membership Directory. • *STFM Membership Directory*, biennial. Membership Directory. Arranged alphabetically and geographically. *Price:* Included in membership dues; $25 for nonmembers. • *STFM Messenger*, bimonthly. Newsletter. Covers general information related to family medicine issues. Includes research and education columns. *Price:* Included in membership dues. • Monographs.

### ★ 2409 ★ Society for Women's Health Research

1828 L St. NW, Ste. 625
Washington, DC 20036
**Phone:** (202)223-8224　　**Fax:** (202)833-3472
**Email:** info@womenshealth.org
**Website:** http://www.womens-health.org
Phyllis Greenberger, MSW, Exec. Dir.

**Fnded:** 1990. **Desc:** Seeks to improve the health of women by promoting equity in research. Advocates policies which promotes the inclusion of women in clinical trials; informs government agencies and private industry of issues affecting women's health and sex-based biology; educates women consumers on conditions that affect women; promotes funding for women's health research. **Pub:** *Journal of Women's Health*, 10/year. Journal. **Frmly:** (2001) Society for the Advancement of Womens Health Research.

### ★ 2410 ★ South Pacific Underwater Medicine Society (SPUMS)

Australian and New Zealand College of Anaesthetists
630 St. Kilda Rd.
Melbourne, VIC 3004, Australia
**Phone:** 61 3 2485950　　**Fax:** 61 6 2485950
**Website:** http://www.spums.org.au

**Fnded:** 1972. **Mem:** 1,000. **Lang(s):** English. **Desc:** Physicians and interested individuals in 10 countries. Serves to promote diving medicine. Organizes Project Stickybeak. **Pub:** *SPUMS Journal*, quarterly. Journal.

### ★ 2411 ★ Spanish Alpha 1-Antitypsin Deficiency Association

Apartado de Correos 96
Valladolid
E-47320 Tudela de Duero, Spain
**Phone:** 34 983 682043　　**Fax:** 34 626 367468
**Email:** deficit.alfa1@retemail.es
**Website:** http://www.alfa1.org

**Fnded:** 1999. **Desc:** Offers support and education for the Spanish speaking Alpha 1-Antitrypsin Deficiency patients and their families. Distributes Spanish educational materials. Works to increase awareness of Alpha 1-Antitrypsin Deficiency and the importance of early detection and treatment.

### ★ 2412 ★ Spanish Confederation of Medical and Technical Advisers Associations (SCMTAA)

### (Confederacion Espanola de Asociaciones de Informadores Tecnicos Sanitarios — CEATIMEF)

Calle Mauricio Legendre, 2-3-I
E-28046 Madrid, Spain
**Phone:** 34 956 010025　　**Fax:** 34 956 226919
**Email:** presidencia@ceatimef.es

**Fnded:** 1977. **Mem:** 12,000. **Reg. Groups:** 34. **Lang(s):** Spanish. **Desc:** Medical advisers. Promotes professional advancement of members. Represents members' interests before industrial organizations, government agencies, and the public.

### ★ 2413 ★ Stickler Involved People (SIP)

15 Angelina Dr.
Augusta, KS 67010
**Phone:** (316)775-2993
**Email:** sip@stickler.org
**Website:** http://sticklers.org/sip/

**Desc:** Dedicated to early diagnosis and treatment of Stickler Syndrome; provides support, medical information and offers ways in which to cope. **Pub:** Newsletter, quarterly.

### ★ 2414 ★ Student National Medical Association (SNMA)

5113 Georgia Ave. NW
Washington, DC 20011
**Phone:** (202)882-2881　　**Fax:** (202)882-2886
**Email:** snmamain@msn.com
**Website:** http://www.snma.org
Annette McLane, Exec. Dir.

**Fnded:** 1964. **Mem:** 5,000. **Reg. Groups:** 10. **Local Groups:** 155. **Desc:** Medical students, residents, and undergraduates of color. Seeks to help students in recruitment, admission, and retention in medical school and publishes information on problems and achievement in this area. Conducts annual research forum and community service projects. **Pub:** *Journal of the Student National Medical Association*, quarterly. Journal. • *SNMA News*, quarterly.

### ★ 2415 ★ Suicide Information and Education Centre (SIEC)

1615 10th Ave. SW, Ste. 201
Calgary, AB, Canada T3C 0J7
**Phone:** (403)245-3900　　**Fax:** (403)245-0299
**Email:** siec@suicideinfo.ca
**Website:** http://www.suicideinfo.ca

**Fnded:** 1982. **Lang(s):** English. **Desc:** Information center whose users include researchers, educators, students, health care professionals, social service agencies, librarians, and the general public. Obtains and provides access to a comprehensive collection of more than 27,000 English language documents on suicide and suicidal behaviors. Provides information to all professions and public on specific topics such as adolescent suicide and bereavement. **Pub:** *Counselling the Bereaved: Caregiver Handbook*. Booklets. • *Reach Out With Hope*. Videos. • *SIEC Newspaper Clipping Service*, bimonthly. Bulletin. Contains news clippings on suicide. • *Youth Suicide and You*. Booklet.

### ★ 2416 ★ Surfer's Medical Association

PO Box 1210
Aptos, CA 95001
**Phone:** (831)684-0916　　**Fax:** (831)684-0916
**Email:** smacentral@aol.com
**Website:** http://www.damoon.net/sma/index.html
Paula Smith, Exec. Dir.

**Fnded:** 1986. **Mem:** 1,000. **Reg. Groups:** 2. **Desc:** Surfer-health professionals and surfers interested in the health and medical aspects of surfing. Works to educate surfers and medical practitioners on the unique health problems of surfers. Represents the sport of surfing in the fields of medicine and science and also works to preserve the environment of beaches and oceans. Established the first international-al network of surfing health professionals. Sponsors members' research in this field. **Pub:** *Collected Surf Medicine Works*, 1-2/year. Book. *Price:* for members only, included in membership dues. • *Surfing Medicine*. Journal.

### ★ 2417 ★ Swedish Medical Association (Sveriges Laekarfoerbund)

c/o Dr.Anders Milton
Villagatan 5
PO Box 5610
S-114 86 Stockholm, Sweden
**Phone:** 46 8 7903300          **Fax:** 46 8 205718
**Email:** info@slf.se
**Website:** http://www.ronden.se/slf

**Fnded:** 1903. **Mem:** 35,500. **Reg. Groups:** 29. **Desc:** Union of physicians in Sweden. Advocates collective negotiations on physicians' employment conditions, health policy, and medical education issues. Maintains professional and specialist groups. **Pub:** *Laekartidningen*, weekly. Journal.

### ★ 2418 ★ Swiss Association of Medical Advisers (SWMA) (Association Suisse Delegues Medicaux — ASDM)

Case Postale 8149
CH-3001 Bern, Switzerland
**Phone:** 41 32 846554          **Fax:** 41 32 26421

**Lang(s):** French, German, Italian. **Desc:** Medical advisers. Promotes professional advancement of members. Represents members' interests before industrial organizations, government agencies, and the public.

### ★ 2419 ★ Swiss Tropical Institute (STI) (Bureau Appui Sante Environnement — BASE)

Socinstrasse 57 Postfasch
CH-4002 Basel, Switzerland
**Phone:** 41 61 2848111          **Fax:** 41 61 2718654
**Website:** http://www.sti.unibas.ch/index.htm

**Fnded:** 1987. **Lang(s):** French. **Desc:** Swiss organizations and government agencies concerned with international development and relief operations. Promotes improved health and quality of life in Chad. Seeks to develop local administrative capacities to ensure sustained economic and social development. Facilitates cooperation among development agencies; works to increase awareness of development issues among people in developing areas. Makes available health care services; conducts training courses to enable local communities to maintain autonomous primary health care facilities. Monitors environmental impact of development programs.

### ★ 2420 ★ Syllogos Iatrikon Episkepton Elladas (SIEE)

Halkondyli 56
GR-10432 Athens, Greece
**Phone:** 30 1 5224070          **Fax:** 30 1 5235331

**Lang(s):** Greek. **Desc:** Medical advisers. Promotes professional advancement of members. Represents members' interests before industrial organizations, government agencies, and the public.

### ★ 2421 ★ Systematics Association

c/o Dr. Zofia Lawrence
CABI Bioscience UK Centre
Bakeham Lane
Egham TW20 9TY, United Kingdom
**Phone:** 44 1491 829080     **Fax:** 44 1491 829100
**Email:** z.lawrence@.cabi.org
**Website:** http://www.systass.org

**Fnded:** 1937. **Mem:** 600. **Desc:** Aims to provide a forum for discussing systematic problems and integrated new information from genetics, ecology and other specific fields into concepts and activities. **Pub:**

Newsletter, quarterly. Contains association news and events.

### ★ 2422 ★ Tenovus - Scotland (TS)

234 St. Vincent St.
Glasgow G2 5RJ, United Kingdom
**Phone:** 44 141 2216268     **Fax:** 44 1292 311433
**Email:** gen.sec@talk21.com
**Website:** http://www.tenovus-scotland.org.uk

**Fnded:** 1967. **Reg. Groups:** 4. **Local Groups:** 1. **Lang(s):** English. **Desc:** Individuals and organizations. Promotes advancement of medical research projects undertaken by Scottish hospitals and university medical schools. Provides financial support and other assistance to medical research programs. Conducts fundraising activities. **Pub:** Newsletter, semiannual. • Brochure.

### ★ 2423 ★ Thalidomide Society

c/o Ms. Vivien Kerr
19 Central Ave.
Middlesex
Pinner HA5 5BT, United Kingdom
**Phone:** 44 20 88685309     **Fax:** 44 20 88685309
**Email:** info@thalsoc.demon.co.uk

**Fnded:** 1962. **Mem:** 330. **Desc:** Provides support, advice and information to thalidomide and similarly disabled people living in the U.K.

### ★ 2424 ★ Trauma Foundation at San Francisco General Hospital

c/o Andrew McGuire
Bldg. 1, Rm. 300
San Francisco, CA 94110
**Phone:** (415)821-8209
**Email:** tf@tf.org
**Website:** http://www.tf.org/
Andrew McGuire, Exec. Dir.

**Fnded:** 1973. **Desc:** Dedicated to improving the lives of survivors of traumatic injuries and injury prevention issues and policies, including fire safe cigarettes, automobile safety, gun control and alcohol policy. **Pub:** Videos.

### ★ 2425 ★ Tropical Health and Education Trust (THET)

21 Edenhurst Ave.
London SW6 3PD, United Kingdom
**Phone:** 44 20 79272411     **Fax:** 44 20 76374314
**Email:** vpthet1@aol.com

**Fnded:** 1989. **Lang(s):** English. **Desc:** Medical training institutions specializing in tropical medicine. Seeks to advance the study, teaching, and practice of tropical medicine. Serves as a liaison linking medical education institutions in Europe and the developing world; sponsors research and educational programs. **Pub:** *THET Annual Review*. Annual Report.

### ★ 2426 ★ Ukrainian Medical Association of North America (UMANA)

2247 W Chicago Ave., 2nd Fl.
Chicago, IL 60622
**Phone:** (773)278-6262     **Free:** 888-RXUMANA
**Fax:** (773)278-6962
**Email:** info@umana.org
**Website:** http://www.umana.org
George Hrycelak, Exec. Dir.

**Fnded:** 1950. **Mem:** 1,000. **Nat'l Groups:** 1. **Reg. Groups:** 19. **Local Groups:** 1. **Desc:** Physicians, surgeons, dentists, and persons in related professions who are of Ukrainian descent. Provides assistance to members; sponsors lectures. Maintains placement service, museum, biographical and medical archives, and library of 1800 medical books and journals in Ukrainian. **Pub:** *Journal of the Ukrainian Medical Association of North America (JUMANA)*, quarterly. Journal. Contains medical research articles and news. *Price:* Free to members; $10 otherwise. • *Newsletter to Membership*, quarterly. Newsletter. • *Umana News*. **Frmly:** American Ukrainian Medical Society.

### ★ 2427 ★ Undersea and Hyperbaric Medical Society (UHMS)

10531 Metropolitan Ave.
Kensington, MD 20895
**Phone:** (301)942-2980          **Fax:** (301)942-7804
**Email:** uhms@uhms.org
**Website:** http://www.uhms.org
Donald R. Chandler, Exec. Dir.

**Fnded:** 1967. **Mem:** 2,500. **Reg. Groups:** 4. **Desc:** Diving physiologists, physicians, biologists, and bioengineers with subsea or hyperbaric interests. Seeks to: develop and advance undersea and hyperbaric medicine and its supporting sciences; provide channels of scientific communication among researchers dedicated to the safe penetration of the oceans by man; disseminate information on diving problems. Conducts courses on diving medicine for physicians. **Pub:** *Case Histories of Diving and Hyperbaric Accidents*. • *Directory of Hyperbaric Chambers*. • *Diving Accident Management*. • *Diving Physiology in Plain English*. • *Fitness to Dive*. • *Flying After Diving*. • *Handbook and Membership Directory*, biennial. Directory. • *Hyperbaric Oxygen Therapy: A Committee Report*. • *Journal: Undersea & Hyperbaric Medicine*, quarterly. Journal. *Price:* $85. • *Key Documents of the Biomedical Aspects of Deep Diving*. • *Near Drowning*. • *Pressure*, bimonthly. Newsletter. Includes book reviews and obituaries. *Price:* $30/year. • *Treatment of Decompression Illness*. • *Underwater and Hyperbaric Medicine: Abstracts from the Literature*, bimonthly. *Price:* $100. • *Women in Diving*. • Are Astmatics Fit to Dive **Frmly:** (1986) Undersea Medical Society.

### ★ 2428 ★ Uniformed Services Academy of Family Physicians (USAFP)

2301 N Parham Rd., Ste. 4
Richmond, VA 23229
**Phone:** (804)968-4436          **Fax:** (804)968-4418
**Email:** fpnet@msn.com
**Website:** http://www.usafp.org/
Christy Duncan, Asst. Exec. Dir.

**Fnded:** 1973. **Mem:** 2,000. **Desc:** Family physicians, teachers of family medicine, medical students, and residents in the armed services, public health service, or Indian health service. Sponsors continuing education program. Sponsors educational programs.

### ★ 2429 ★ Union of American Physicians and Dentists (UAPD)

1330 Broadway, Ste. 730
Oakland, CA 94612
**Phone:** (510)839-0193          **Free:** 800-622-0909
**Fax:** (510)763-8756
**Email:** uapd@uapd.com
**Website:** http://www.uapd.com
Gary Robinson, Exec. Dir.

**Fnded:** 1972. **Mem:** 10,000. **Nat'l Groups:** 1. **Reg. Groups:** 1. **State Groups:** 1. **Local Groups:** 3. **Desc:** Independent national labor organization made up of self-employed medical doctors and dentists as well as those employed by hospitals, teaching institutions, counties, and municipalities. Seeks to: provide optimum medical care for the people; ensure quality facilities for the provision of medical care; enable physicians to give of themselves, unhindered by extraneous forces, for the welfare of their patients; ensure reasonable compensation for physicians commensurate with their training, skill, and the responsibility they bear for the life and health of their fellow human beings. **Pub:** *UAPD Report*, monthly. Newsletter. *Price:* Free with membership. • Also publishes materials on socioeconomic issues. **Frmly:** Union of American Physicians and Dentists.

### ★ 2430 ★ Union Nationale des Associations de Soins et Service a Domicile (UNASSAD)

108-110 rue St. Maur
F-75011 Paris, France
**Phone:** 33 1 49238252     **Fax:** 33 1 43385533
**Email:** umanaol@wanadoo.fr

**Fnded:** 1970. **Mem:** 1,700. **Lang(s):** English, French. **Desc:** Organizations providing home health care for the elderly or disabled and their families. Promotes high industry standards.

## ★ 2431 ★ United Methodist Association of Health and Welfare Ministries (UMA)

601 W Riverview Ave.
Dayton, OH 45406-5543
**Phone:** (937)227-9494          **Free:** 800-411-9901
**Fax:** (937)222-7364
**Email:** uma@umassociation.org
**Website:** http://www.umassociation.org
Mr. Dean W. Pulliam, CEO

**Fnded:** 1940. **Mem:** 400. **Desc:** Membership association for 400 United Methodist related hospitals, retirement homes, community based ministries, youth and family service organizations, children's homes, churches, and individuals. Offers communications and church relations guidance. Provides leadership development training for health and human service professionals in United Methodist related organizations and agencies. Develops ethical and theological statements on institutional care. Operates Educational Assessment Guidelines Leading Toward Excellence (EAGLE), a self-assessment and peer review accreditation program. Operates a Field Consultation Program; members may access skilled professionals to assist with governance questions. Offers audiovisual services to members. Administers the Order of Good Shepherds program designed to recognize ministry in the workplace by employees at member organizations. Maintains speakers' bureau; compiles statistics. **Pub:** *Articles depicting innovative ministries by member organizations*, quarterly. Magazine. Professional journal related to operation of United Methodist related institutional ministries. *Price:* $40/year member; $60/year nonmember. • *Children, Youth, & Family Services Section Salary & Benefit Study.* • *National Directory of all United Methodist Related Health and Welfare Ministries*, annual. *Price:* $17/year for members; $27/year for nonmembers. • *Older Adult Ministries Section Salary & Benefit Study.* • *The UMA Journal*, quarterly. Magazine. Depicts innovative ministries by member organizations. **Frmly:** (1968) Board of Hospitals and Homes of The Methodist Church; (1972) Division of Health and Welfare Ministries of The United Methodist Church; (1983) National Association of Health and Welfare Ministries of The United Methodist Church.

## ★ 2432 ★ Vietnamese Medical Association of the U.S.A.

c/o B.S. NguyenleHieu, M.D.
Shelton Medical Clinic
302 C St.
PO Box 476
Shelton, NE 68876
**Phone:** (308)647-6828          **Fax:** (308)647-5219
B.S. Nguyenlehieu, MD, Contact

**Fnded:** 1989. **Mem:** 498. **Nat'l Groups:** 1. **State Groups:** 10. **Desc:** Vietnamese-American medical professionals. Promotes mutual support and fellowship among its members, while fostering and maintaining medical ethics. Assures the provision of equal educational and professional opportunities for its members and the welfare of the general Vietnamese community. Supports and assists the Vietnamese victims of the Vietnamese communist regime.

## ★ 2433 ★ Voluntary Euthanasia Society of Scotland

17 Hart St.
Edinburgh EH1 3RN, United Kingdom
**Phone:** 44 131 5564404          **Fax:** 44 131 5574403
**Website:** http://www.euthanasia.org

**Fnded:** 1980. **Desc:** Aims to make dying with dignity an option available to anyone, to protect patients and doctors alike in upholding the humanity of dying well, to seek legal reform, where necessary, and to introduce safeguards regarding voluntary euthanasia.

## W.M. Keck Foundation

*See:* Entry 4612

## ★ 2434 ★ Wellness Councils of America

9802 Nicholas St., Ste. 315
Omaha, NE 68114
**Phone:** (402)827-3590          **Fax:** (402)827-3594
**Email:** wellworkplace@welcoa.org
**Website:** http://www.welcoa.org
David Hunnicutt, Pres.

**Fnded:** 1988. **Mem:** 500. **Reg. Groups:** 10. **Desc:** Conducts health education at the workplace. Offers advisory services; maintains educational programs. **Pub:** *The Well Workplace*, monthly. Newsletter.

## ★ 2435 ★ Wellness International

5800 Democracy Dr.
Plano, TX 75024
**Phone:** (972)312-1100          **Fax:** (972)943-5260
**Email:** webmaster@winltd.com
**Website:** http://web.winltd.com
Susan Shapiro, Contact

**Desc:** Promotes application of the precepts of health maintenance organizations to public health problems in developing areas. Provides technical assistance to health services operating in developing regions.

## ★ 2436 ★ Wilderness Medical Society (WMS)

3595 E Fountain Blvd., Ste. A1
Colorado Springs, CO 80910
**Phone:** (719)572-9255          **Fax:** (719)572-1514
**Email:** wms@wms.org
**Website:** http://www.wms.org
David Just, Exec. Dir.

**Fnded:** 1983. **Mem:** 4,200. **Desc:** Regular membership for persons with advanced degrees in the biomedical or life sciences with an interest in the medical, behavioral, and life sciences aspects of wilderness environments. Objectives are to promote research and educational activities that increase scientific knowledge about human activities in wilderness environments; stimulate interest and research in health consequences of wilderness activities; serve as central information source. Areas of interest include treatment of accident victims and victims of bites and stings, exotic infectious diseases and toxic plants, desert survival, avalanche control, and search and rescue. **Pub:** *Wilderness and Environmental Medicine*, quarterly. Journal. • *Wilderness Medicine Letter*, quarterly. Newsletter. *Price:* Included in membership dues.

## ★ 2437 ★ William H. Donner Foundation

500 Fifth Ave., Ste. 1230
New York, NY 10110-0180
**Phone:** (212)719-9290          **Fax:** (212)302-8734
**Website:** http://www.donner.org

**Fnded:** 1961. **Desc:** Strives to fund thoughtful and creative medical-related projects.

## ★ 2438 ★ Williams Syndrome Association (WSA)

PO Box 297
Clawson, MI 48017-0297
**Phone:** (248)541-3630          **Fax:** (248)541-3631
**Email:** tmonkaba@aol.com
**Website:** http://www.williams-syndrome.org
Terry Monkaba, Exec. Dir.

**Fnded:** 1983. **Mem:** 8,000. **Reg. Groups:** 11. **State Groups:** 50. **Desc:** Individuals with Williams Syndrome and their families; medical and health care professionals; educators. (Williams Syndrome is characterized by similar facial features, low birth weight, heart disorders, hearing sensitivity, talkative personality, mild to severe learning disabilities, and developmental delays.) Provides support and assistance to families with a WS child. Conducts networking in the medical, scientific, educational, and professional communities for referral and study of newly-diagnosed WS individuals. Encourages medical behavior and supports research into all aspects of the syndrome. Compiles statistics. **Pub:** *Ben's Big Decision.* Book. Storybook and tape. *Price:* $19.95. • *Facts Brochure.* Brochures. *Price:* Free. • *Information for Teachers.* Handbook. For parents and professionals. *Price:* $4. •

*The Promenade: A Story about Adolescents with Williams Syndrome.* Provides testing and evaluations for WSA. *Price:* $15; $4 for parents and professors. • *Williams Syndrome Association National Newsletter*, 4/year. Newsletter. Includes research updates and parent and professional forums. *Price:* $15/year.

## ★ 2439 ★ Women's Health

52 Featherstone St.
London EC1Y 8RT, United Kingdom
**Phone:** 44 171 2516580          **Fax:** 44 20 72504152
**Email:** womenshealth@pop3.poptel.org.uk
**Website:** http://www.womenshealthlondon.org.uk

**Fnded:** 1982. **Mem:** 250. **Lang(s):** English. **Desc:** Women's health information organization in the UK. Works to empower women to make informed decisions about health and reproductive issues. Promotes a pro-choice perspective on women's health issues, including abortion. Informs women of their reproductive rights; provides information about women's health issues. Develops and promotes a feminist perspective of women's health and reproductive rights. **Pub:** *Annual Report.* • *Women's Health*, quarterly. Newsletter. Covers information about women's health and reproductive issues.

## ★ 2440 ★ Women's Health and Economic Development Association (WHEDA)

3B Ekpo Obot St.
PO Box 2665
Uyo, Nigeria
**Phone:** 234 85 203944
**Email:** wheda@fordwa.linkserve.com

**Fnded:** 1988. **Mem:** 18,000. **Nat'l Groups:** 4. **State Groups:** 20. **Local Groups:** 180. **Lang(s):** English. **Desc:** Works to prevent health problems of women in rural Nigerian communities. Provides education and counseling on nutritional and family planning issues. Encourages economic independence for women through supportive programs and activities. **Pub:** Articles. In newspapers and magazines. **Frmly:** (1988) Rural Women Health Association.

## ★ 2441 ★ Working Group on Health and Development Issues (DEAG) (Werkgroep Medische Ontwikkelingssamenwerking — WEMOS)

Postbus 1693
NL-1000 BR Amsterdam, Netherlands
**Phone:** 31 20 4688388          **Fax:** 31 20 4686008
**Email:** wemos@antenna.nl
**Website:** http://www.wemos.nl

**Fnded:** 1980. **Lang(s):** Dutch, English. **Desc:** Provides information on health problems in Third World countries: women's issues, pharmaceuticals, availability of basic health care, and nutrition. **Pub:** *Exposed Deadly Exports: The Story of European Community Exports of Banned or Withdrawn Drugs to the Third World.* Book. • *WEMOScoop*, bimonthly. Magazine. • Books.

## ★ 2442 ★ World Apheresis Association (WAA)

1, av Claude Vellefaux
F-75475 Paris, France
**Phone:** 33 1 42499210          **Fax:** 33 1 42409314
**Email:** ets-bussel@chu-stlouis.fr

## ★ 2443 ★ World Federation of Catholic Medical Associations (FIAMC) (Federation Internationale des Associations Medicales Catholiques — FIAMC)

Palazzo San Calisto
V-00120 Vatican City, Vatican City
**Phone:** 39 6 69887372          **Fax:** 39 6 69887372
**Email:** fiamc@pcn.net
**Website:** http://www.fiamc.org

**Fnded:** 1950. **Mem:** 52. **Nat'l Groups:** 64. **Reg. Groups:** 5. **Lang(s):** English, French. **Desc:** National associations and guilds of Catholic physicians. Seeks to: coordinate the efforts of Catholic medical associations worldwide; promote Christian principles throughout the medical profession; discuss and find new ethical approaches to biotechnological problems. Encourages the development of Catholic medical associations globally to assist in the moral, spiritual, and technical advancement of the Catholic physician; participates in the development of the medical profession. Maintains speakers' bureau. **Pub:** *Catholic Medical Quarterly*, quarterly. • *Decisions*, 3/year. Newsletter. • *Linacre Bulletin*, quarterly. • Journal, quarterly.

**★ 2444 ★ World Federation of Doctors Who Respect Human Life (United States Section) (WFDRHL)**
PO Box 101501
Pittsburgh, PA 15237
**Phone:** (724)444-8045 **Fax:** (724)444-8013
Dr. Brain Donnelly, Sec. -Treas.
**Fnded:** 1976. **Mem:** 1,400. **Desc:** Physicians united to restore the "traditional Hippocratic medical position" through firm opposition to abortion, suicide, and direct euthanasia. Sponsors educational programs and seminars. Presently inactive. **Pub:** *Primum Non Nocere*, quarterly. Newsletter.

**★ 2445 ★ World Federation for Medical Education (WFME) (Federation Mondiale pour l'Enseignement Medical — FMEM)**
Univ. of Copenhagen
Faculty of Health Sciences
Blegdamsvej 3
DK-2200 Copenhagen, Denmark
**Phone:** 45 35327103 **Fax:** 45 35327070
**Email:** wfme@adm.ku.dk
**Website:** http://www.sund.ku.dk/wfme/
**Fnded:** 1972. **Reg. Groups:** 6. **Lang(s):** English. **Desc:** Regional medical associations and associations of medical schools. Promotes the integrated study of medical education worldwide. Evaluates the effectiveness of medical education in meeting the needs of contemporary society. Acts as international representative of medical education before the World Health Organization, UNICEF, UNESCO, United Nations Development Programme, and the World Bank. **Pub:** *Report of the World Conference on Medical Education, Edinburgh, 1988/Proceedings of the World Summit on Medical Education, Edinburgh, 1994*. Report. • *Report of the World Summit on Medical Education, Edinburgh, 1994*. Report.

**★ 2446 ★ World Health Organization (WHO) (Organisation Mondiale de la Sante — OMS)**
20, ave. Appia
CH-1211 Geneva 27, Switzerland
**Phone:** 41 22 7912111 **Fax:** 41 22 7910746
**Website:** http://www.who.org
**Fnded:** 1948. **Mem:** 192. **Reg. Groups:** 6. **Lang(s):** Arabic, Chinese, English, French, Russian, Spanish. **Desc:** International health agency of the United Nations consisting of countries working toward the goal of "health for all," seeking to obtain the highest level of health care for all people. Believes health is a fundamental right of every human being without distinction of race, religion, political belief, economic situation, or social conditions and holds that all people deserve equal access to health services to enable them to lead socially and economically productive lives. Objectives are to: act as directing and coordinating authority on international health work; ensure valid and productive technical cooperation; promote research; prevent and combat diseases; generate and transfer information. Strives to eliminate poverty. Emphasizes the health needs of developing countries lacking resources and funds for modern medical technologies; works toward developing new techniques that will fulfill these needs by utilizing available resources, integrating education-

al, agricultural, town planning, and sanitation programs with health programs, combining peripheral health services and existing health systems, and applying appropriate technologies at reasonable costs. Establishes standards for food, biological, and pharmaceutical needs, develops standardized diagnostic procedures, and determines environmental health criteria. Promotes 8 elements of primary health care including: health education on prevention and cures; proper food supply and nutrition; adequate supply of safe water and sanitation; maternal and child health care; immunization; control of endemic diseases; and provisions of essential drugs. Acts as clearinghouse; coordinates activities with the United Nations on health and socioeconomic development; works with international nongovernmental organizations in the health sector. Supports International Agency for Research on Cancer. Maintains expert and scientific committees. **Pub:** *Bulletin of WHO*, bimonthly. Bulletin. • *International Digest of Health Legislation*, quarterly. • *World Health*, 10/year. Magazine. • *World Health Statistics Quarterly*. Includes summaries in Arabic, Chinese, Russian, and Spanish.

**★ 2447 ★ World Health Organization - Regional Office for the Eastern Mediterranean (EMRO)**
Abdul Razzak Al Sanhouri St.
PO Box 7608
Nasr City
Cairo 11371, Egypt
**Phone:** 20 2 6702535 **Fax:** 20 2 6702492
**Email:** postmaster@emro.who.int
**Website:** http://www.emro.who.int
**Fnded:** 1948. **Mem:** 22. **Lang(s):** Arabic, English, Farsi, French, Urdu. **Desc:** Regional office of the World Health Organization. Works to ensure that WHO programs effectively meet the particular public health needs of the Eastern Mediterranean; serves as a liaison between national and local public health agencies and the WHO. **Pub:** *Eastern Mediterranean Health Journal*, bimonthly. Journal. Contains information on public health and health systems research. Additional publications available on request.

**★ 2448 ★ World Health Organization - Regional Office for Europe (EURO)**
8 Scherfigsvej
DK-2100 Copenhagen 0, Denmark
**Phone:** 45 39171717 **Fax:** 45 39171818
**Email:** webmaster@who.dk
**Website:** http://www.who.dk
**Lang(s):** Danish, English. **Desc:** Regional office of the World Health Organization. Works to ensure that WHO programs effectively meet the particular public health needs of Europe; serves as a liaison between national and local public health agencies and the WHO.

**★ 2449 ★ World Health Organization - Regional Office for South-East Asia (SEARO)**
World Health House
Indraprastha Estate
Mahatma Gandhi Rd.
New Delhi 110 002, Delhi, India
**Phone:** 91 11 33870804 **Fax:** 91 11 3379507
**Email:** pandeyh@whosea.org
**Website:** http://www.who.org
**Desc:** Regional branch of the World Health Organization. Works to ensure that WHO programs effectively meet the particular public health needs of southeast Asia; serves as a liaison between national and local public health agencies and the WHO.

**★ 2450 ★ World Medical Association (WMA) (Association Medicale Mondiale — AMM)**
13 Ch. du Levant
BP 63
F-01212 Ferney-Voltaire, France
**Phone:** 33 450 407575 **Fax:** 33 450 405937
**Email:** info@wma.net

**Website:** http://www.wma.net
**Fnded:** 1947. **Mem:** 73. **Reg. Groups:** 6. **Lang(s):** English, French, Spanish. **Desc:** Federation of national medical associations throughout the world. Goal is to achieve the highest international standards in medical education, medical science, medical ethics, and health care for people worldwide. Promotes closer ties and better communication among medical organizations and doctors of the world; studies professional problems in different countries. Represents and protects the rights and interests of physicians and people internationally. Encourages proper nutrition in developing countries; urges the teaching of human values in the practice of medicine. Seeks to improve maternal and child health care. Issues declarations on ethical topics including: abortion; AIDS; abuse of children and the elderly; euthanasia; genetic engineering; organ transplantation; the use and misuse of psychotropic drugs; torture; biomedical research on human subjects; medical care in rural areas; an international code of medical ethics; and rights of the patient. **Pub:** *World Medical Journal*, bimonthly. Journal. Contains medical and medico-political articles.

**★ 2451 ★ World Medical Mission (WMM)**
PO Box 3000
Boone, NC 28607
**Phone:** (828)262-1980 **Fax:** (704)266-1055
**Email:** jcastle@samaritan.org
**Website:** http://www.samaritan.org
W. Franklin Graham, III, Pres.
**Fnded:** 1977. **Desc:** Coordinates medical activities of the evangelical group Samaritan's Purse. Places Christian physicians who serve voluntarily in evangelical mission hospitals overseas and conducts emergency medical relief. Provides assistance in refurbishing and equipping mission hospitals and conducts training sessions. **Pub:** *On Call*, quarterly. • *The PaceMaker*, quarterly. • *World Medical Mission Newsletter*, 6/year. Newsletter. • Brochures.

**★ 2452 ★ World Organization of Family Doctors (WONCA)**
Collins St. East Post Office
Locked Bag 11
Melbourne, VIC 8003, Australia
**Phone:** 61 3 96500235 **Fax:** 61 3 96500236
**Email:** enquiries@wonca.org
**Website:** http://www.globalfamilydoctor.commm
**Fnded:** 1972. **Mem:** 56. **Reg. Groups:** 5. **Lang(s):** English, French, German, Spanish. **Desc:** Colleges, academies, or organizations in 53 countries concerned with the academic aspects of general family practice. Objectives are to: promote and maintain high standards of general family practice through education and research; foster worldwide communication and understanding among general practitioners; represent the academic and research activities of general practitioners to other worldwide bodies concerned with health or medical care. **Pub:** *The Family Doctor*, semiannual. Magazine. • *International Classification of Health Problems in Primary Care*. Book. • *Membership Directory*, annual. Directory. • *WONCA News*, bimonthly. **Frmly:** (1999) World Organization of National Colleges, Academies, and Academic Associations of General Practitioners/Family Physicians.

## Research Centers

**★ 2453 ★ Advanced Medical Research Foundation, Inc.**
333 Longwood Ave.
Boston, MA 02115-5711
**Phone:** (617)278-1800 **Fax:** (617)264-2400
**Email:** amrf333@msn.com
Nile L. Albright, MD, Pres.
**Activities/Fields:** Medical and cancer research and science education.

## ★ 2454 ★ Albert Einstein College of Medicine
**General Clinical Research Center**
Jack and Pearl Resnick Campus
Forchheimer Bldg., Rm. G47
1300 Morris Park Ave.
Bronx, NY 10461
**Phone:** (718)430-8800     **Fax:** (718)430-8998
**Email:** shamoon@aecom.yu.edu
**Website:** http://gcrcweb.aecom.yu.edu/gcrc
Harry Shamoon, MD, Prog. Dir.

**Activities/Fields:** Major areas of investigation include cancer, diabetes, gastrointestinal disorders, hematology, immunology. liver disease and renal disease.

## ★ 2455 ★ Alberta Centre for Active Living
11759 Groat Rd., 3rd Fl.
Edmonton, AB, Canada T5M 3K6
**Phone:** (780)427-6949     **Fax:** (780)455-2092
**Email:** active.living@ualberta.ca
**Website:** http://www.centre4activeliving.ca
Judith Moodie, Dir.

**Activities/Fields:** Physical activity in Alberta, Canada. **Pub:** *Research Update Bulletin*, quarterly. • *Well-Spring*, quarterly. **Frmly:** Alberta Centre for Well-Being.

## ★ 2456 ★ Alton Ochsner Medical Foundation
1516 Jefferson Hwy.
New Orleans, LA 70121
**Phone:** (504)842-3000     **Fax:** (504)842-2152
**Email:** rre@ochsner.org
**Website:** http://www.ochsner.org
Richard N. Re, MD, Dir.

**Activities/Fields:** Hypertension, oncology, cardiovascular research, immunology, orthopedics, renal stones, gastrointestinal physiology (motility and perfusion), depression, and clinical pharmacology.

## ★ 2457 ★ American Council on Science and Health
1995 Broadway, 2nd Fl.
New York, NY 10023-5860
**Phone:** (212)362-7044     **Fax:** (212)362-4919
**Email:** whelan@acsh.org
**Website:** http://www.acsh.org
Elizabeth Whelan, Pres.

**Activities/Fields:** Relationship between human health and chemicals, foods, nutrition, lifestyle factors, including cigarette smoking, the environment and human health. Activities include studies on animal-to-man extrapolation in laboratory testing, smoking cessation, Lyme disease, Reye's syndrome, hay fever, microwave ovens, infant mortality, life expectancy, AIDS, and automobile occupant restraint systems. **Pub:** *Media Update.* • *Priorities Quarterly Magazine.*

## ★ 2458 ★ American Federation for Medical Research
227 Massachusetts Ave. NE, Ste. 303
Washington, DC 20002
**Phone:** (202)543-7032     **Fax:** (202)543-7062
**Email:** admin@afmr.org
**Website:** http://www.afmr.org
Kevin D. O'Brien, Pres.

**Activities/Fields:** Clinical and laboratory medicine, including cardiovascular, dermatology, endocrinology, gastroenterology, genetics, hematology, immunology and connective tissue, infectious disease, metabolism, neoplastic disease, patient care, pulmonary, renal, and electrolytes. **Pub:** *Journal of Investigative Medicine*, bimonthly.

## ★ 2459 ★ American Medical Association Foundation
515 N State St.
Chicago, IL 60610
**Phone:** (312)484-5000     **Free:** 800-262-3211
**Fax:** (312)484-5973
**Email:** amafoundation@ama-assn.org
**Website:** http://www.ama-assn.org/amafoundation
Kathleen MacArthur, Exec. Dir.

**Activities/Fields:** Receives and distributes funds to benefit medical education in the U.S. Also supports medical research and innovative health care programs.

## ★ 2460 ★ Association of International Health Researchers
2665 Pleasant Valley Rd.
Mobile, AL 36606
**Phone:** (334)473-3946
**Email:** roykadel@mobis.com
Dr. Roy E. Kadel, Contact

**Activities/Fields:** International health research, focusing on quality, education, techniques and methodologies.

## ★ 2461 ★ Atlanta Research and Education Foundation, Inc.
1670 Clairmont Rd., 151F
Decatur, GA 30033-4004
**Phone:** (404)728-7772     **Fax:** (404)235-3061
**Email:** aref@mindspring.com
**Website:** http://www.atlaref.org
Antonio Laracuente, Exec. Dir.

**Activities/Fields:** Cardiology, pulmonary medicine, HIV/AIDS, infectious diseases, Alzheimer's disease, rehabilitation, and cancer.

## ★ 2462 ★ Bassett Healthcare Research Institute
1 Atwell Rd.
Cooperstown, NY 13326
**Phone:** (607)547-3048     **Fax:** (607)547-3061
**Email:** research.institute@bassett.org
Allan Green, PhD, Dir.

**Activities/Fields:** Basic, clinical, and population studies in the following areas: obesity; biochemistry of serum albumin; molecular biology of autoimmune diseases; experimental pathology of cancer; immunology and antigen processing; cardiovascular epidemiology; rural health education; neuroendocrine regulation of breast cancer; nutrition; health care delivery systems; and gut hormones.

## ★ 2463 ★ Beth Israel Deaconess Medical Center
**General Clinical Research Center**
330 Brookline Ave., Rm. GZ 800
Boston, MA 02215
**Phone:** (617)667-5576     **Fax:** (617)667-5953
**Email:** sfreedma@caregroup.harvard.edu
**Website:** http://research.caregroup.org/gcrc
Steven Freedman, MD, Prog. Dir.

**Activities/Fields:** Biomedicine, cardiology, endocrinology, gastroenterology, gerontology, hematology, nephrology, neurology, nutrition, obstetrics, pulmonary physiology, psychiatry, and surgery.

## ★ 2464 ★ Boston University
**General Clinical Research Center**
East Newton Campus, Evans 8
Boston Medical Ctr.
715 Albany St., E-860
Boston, MA 02118
**Phone:** (617)414-1960     **Fax:** (617)414-1969
**Email:** jkopp@bu.edu
**Website:** http://www.bumc.bu.edu/Departments/HomeMain.asp?DepartmentID=291
Janice Kopp, Admin.

**Activities/Fields:** Cardiovascular disease, collagen vascular disease, diabetes, gastrointestinal disease, nephrology, pediatrics, dermatology, AIDS, psoriasis, amyloidosis, and drug abuse.

## ★ 2465 ★ Brigham and Women's Hospital
**General Clinical Research Center**
221 Longwood Ave., 2nd Fl.
Boston, MA 02115
**Phone:** (617)732-5661     **Fax:** (617)732-5666
**Email:** gwilliams@partners.org
Dr. Gordon Williams, Prog. Dir.

**Activities/Fields:** Support facility for clinical investigation of diseases in humans.

## ★ 2466 ★ California Institute for Medical Research
2260 Clove Dr.
San Jose, CA 95128
**Phone:** (408)998-4554     **Fax:** (408)998-2723
**Email:** admin@cimr.org
**Website:** http://cimr.org
Pat Barnett, Oper. Dir.

**Activities/Fields:** Medical research, including infectious diseases, stroke, analytical tools for pharmacokinetic study of anticoagulant drugs, neurological disorders, tumor biology, and AIDS. Drugs useful in the treatment of heart diseases.

## ★ 2467 ★ California Pacific Medical Center Research Institute
2340 Clay
San Francisco, CA 94115
**Phone:** (415)600-1601     **Fax:** (415)600-1753
**Email:** dfielder@cooper.cpmc.org
**Website:** http://www.cpmc.org
David R. Fielder, VP

**Activities/Fields:** Medical sciences, including basic clinical research on heart and lung disease, organ transplantation, neurology, laboratory medicine, cancer, arthritis, neonatology, gene therapy (non-viral), complementary medicine, and gastroenterology. **Pub:** *California Pacific Currents.* **Frmly:** Medical Research Institute of San Francisco.

## ★ 2468 ★ Case Western Reserve University
**General Clinical Research Center**
11100 Euclid Ave.
Cleveland, OH 44106
**Phone:** (216)844-4902     **Fax:** (216)844-1522
**Email:** jpd@po.cwru.edu
**Website:** http://gcrc.meds.cwru.edu
Nathan A. Berger, MD, Principal Investigator

**Activities/Fields:** Clinical investigations in humans, including specific, carefully planned studies of illnesses of voluntarily participating adult and pediatric patients. **Frmly:** Metabolic Research Unit.

## ★ 2469 ★ Center for Medical Consumers
130 MacDougall St.
New York, NY 10012-5030
**Phone:** (212)674-7105     **Fax:** (212)674-7100
**Email:** medconsumers@earthlink.net
**Website:** http://www.medicalconsumers.org
Arthur Levin, Dir.

**Activities/Fields:** Mainstream and alternative medical treatments. **Pub:** *HEALTHFACTS*, monthly.

## ★ 2470 ★ Children's Hospital (Boston)
**General Clinical Research Center**
300 Longwood Ave., 7 East
Boston, MA 02115
**Phone:** (617)355-7541     **Fax:** (617)264-9896
**Email:** kristine.jordan@tch.harvard.edu
**Website:** http://web2.tch.harvard.edu/clinresearch
Kristine Jordan, Admin. Mgr.

**Activities/Fields:** Protocols in bone marrow transplantation, immunodeficiencies, pediatric endocrinology, bone and mineral metabolism, pediatric hematology, neuroimmunology, oncology, and pediatric gastroenterology. **Pub:** *Grand Rounds*, occasionally.

**★ 2471 ★ CIIT Centers for Health Research**
6 Davis Dr., Box 12137
Research Triangle Park, NC 27709-2137
**Phone:** (919)558-1200
**Email:** CIITinfo@ciit.org
**Website:** http://www.ciit.org/
Bob Nellis, Contact

**Activities/Fields:** Potential adverse effects of chemicals, pharmaceuticals, and consumer products on human health. Research is structured into four programs: Chemical Carcinogenesis Program; Endocrine, Reproductive and Developmental Toxicology Program; Neurotoxicology Program; and Respiratory Toxicology Program. **Pub:** *Articles.* • *CIIT Activities Newsletter*, monthly. • *CIIT Annual Report.*

**★ 2472 ★ City of Hope**
**National Medical Center and Beckman Research Institute**
1500 E Duarte Rd.
Duarte, CA 91010
**Phone:** (626)301-8164          **Fax:** (626)930-5300
**Website:** http://www.cityofhope.org
Theodore G. Krontiris, MD, Interim Exec. VP

**Activities/Fields:** Biology, including cell biology, molecular biology, developmental biology; molecular genetics; molecular immunology; gene regulation; and theoretical biology; immunology; molecular medicine; virology; information sciences; hematology research; radiation research, including radioimmunotherapy; surgical research; experimental therapeutics diabetes research.

**★ 2473 ★ Cleveland Clinic Foundation**
**Lerner Research Institute**
9500 Euclid Ave.
Cleveland, OH 44195
**Phone:** (216)444-3900          **Fax:** (216)444-3279
**Email:** starkg@ccf.org
**Website:** http://www.lri.ccf.org/
George R. Stark, PhD, Chm.

**Activities/Fields:** Molecular biology; structure and function in regulation of viral and cellular genes and (proto)oncogenes, and interferon signaling mechanisms; cancer biology and genetics, including Wilms' tumor, cellular gene regulation, transgenic models, and use of newly patented 2-5A antisense technology; cell biology, including vessel wall pathophysiology, lipoprotein oxidation, regulation of gene expression and intracellular signaling pathways. Studies also include immunology, biologic response modifiers in tumor growth and regression, chemokines, nitric oxide synthase; neurosciences emphasizing cellular and genetic mechanisms in multiple sclerosis, effects of AIDS; epilepsy; neuronal signaling in cardiovascular neurobiology and diagnostic methods in cerebrovascular disease and hypertrophy, studies of lipoprotein(a), computerized modeling of protein structures, G-proteins, and study of the basis of hypertension; biomedical engineering, including musculoskeletal biology, imaging research, biomaterials and biocompatibility, and total artificial heart and heart assist devices; and biostatistics and epidemiology. **Pub:** *Notations*, bimonthly. Newsletter.

**★ 2474 ★ Clinical Research Institute of Montreal**
110 Pine Ave. W
Montreal, QC, Canada H2W 1R7
**Phone:** (514)987-5500          **Fax:** (514)987-5789
**Email:** GuindoY@ircm.qc.ca
**Website:** http://www.ircm.qc.ca
Dr. Yvan Guindon, CEO/Sci. Dir.

**Activities/Fields:** Causes, mechanisms, and more effective treatments of diseases in many fields of medicine, including research on hypertension, neurobiology and behavior, hyperlipidemias and atherosclerosis, proteins and peptides hormones, lipid metabolism, biomedical engineering, molecular biology, immunology, molecular genetics, bioethics, reproduction, chemical biology and polypeptides, hematopoiesis

and leukemia, cancer, and bio-organic chemistry. **Pub:** *Annual Report.* • *Scientific Brochure*, biennially.

**★ 2475 ★ Colorado State University**
**Hypo-Hyperbaric Chamber Facility**
Department of Physiology
Fort Collins, CO 80523
**Phone:** (970)491-6187          **Fax:** (970)491-7569
**Email:** alan.tucker@colostate.edu
**Website:** http://www.cvmbs.colostate.edu/cvmbs/hypo.html
Dr. Alan Tucker, Contact

**Activities/Fields:** High altitude physiology, altitude illness, pulmonary hypertension, human performance at various altitudes, hyperbaric physiology, and human and animal studies.

**★ 2476 ★ Columbia University**
**Center for Health Promotion**
Box 114
Teachers College
New York, NY 10027
**Phone:** (212)678-3960          **Fax:** (212)678-8259
**Email:** jpa1@columbia.edu
John P. Allegrante, PhD, Dir.

**Activities/Fields:** Health promotion and disease prevention, focusing on the effects on health of personal behavior and lifestyle, including physical activity and fitness, nutrition, alcohol and other drugs; mental health and mental disorders violent and abusive behavior; and how educational and community-based programs can be used to improve health and prevent premature death and disability throughout the human life span through schools, patient care, workplace, and other community settings.

**★ 2477 ★ Columbia University**
**Irving Center for Clinical Research**
Columbia-Presbyterian Medical Center
622 W 168th St., PH-10
New York, NY 10032
**Phone:** (212)305-9562          **Fax:** (212)305-3213
**Email:** hng1@columbia.edu
**Website:** http://cpmcnet.columbia.edu/dept/irving_center
Dr. Henry N. Ginsberg, Prog. Dir.

**Activities/Fields:** Multidisciplinary studies of human disease and clinical pharmacology. Areas include arrhythmia control, heart failure, atherosclerosis, nutrition, metabolism, clinical pharmacology, dermatology, endocrinology, hypertension, immunology, mineral metabolism and skeletal disease, neuromuscular disease, physiology, pulmonary disease, pulmonary physiology, reproductive research studies, neurology (including dementia, stroke, and seizure disorders), oncology, AIDS/infectious disease, geriatrics, epidemiology, and substance abuse.

**★ 2478 ★ Columbia University**
**New York Obesity Research Center**
St. Luke's-Roosevelt Hospital
1090 Amsterdam Ave., 14th Fl.
New York, NY 10025
**Phone:** (212)523-4196          **Fax:** (212)523-3416
**Email:** fxp1@columbia.edu
**Website:** http://cpmcnet.columbia.edu/dept/obesectr/NYORC/
Dr. F. Xavier Pi-Sunyer, Dir.

**Activities/Fields:** Obesity, including molecular genetics, regulation of food intake, nutrient uptake and oxidation, body composition, stable isotope methodology, exercise physiology, diabetes, and insulin resistance.

**Cornell University**
**General Clinical Research Center— Children**
*See:* Entry 5789

**★ 2479 ★ Cornell University**
**Weill Medical College**
**General Clinical Research Center**
1300 York Ave., Rm. Baker 2006
New York, NY 10021
**Phone:** (212)746-4745          **Fax:** (212)746-8922
**Email:** jimperat@mail.med.cornell.edu
**Website:** http://www.tc.faa.gov
Dr. Julianne Imperato-McGinley, MD, Prog. Dir.

**Activities/Fields:** Cancer prevention, cardiovascular diseases, dermatology, diabetes and metabolism, digestive diseases, endocrinology, gene therapy, hematology, immunology and infectious diseases, neurology and neuroscience, oncology, pharmacology, and psychiatry.

**★ 2480 ★ Dalhousie University**
**Atlantic Health Promotion Research Centre (AHPRC)**
6090 University Ave.
Halifax, NS, Canada B3H 3J5
**Phone:** (902)494-2240          **Fax:** (902)494-3594
**Email:** ahprc@dal.ca
**Website:** http://www.medicine.dal.ca/ahprc
Renee F. Lyons, Dir.

**Activities/Fields:** Physical, mental, social, and spiritual health of individuals and communities by increasing control over health issues by combining personal choice and social responsibility, and contributes to the health and well being of Atlantic Canadians. **Pub:** *General Guidelines for Health Promotion Research Proposals.* • *Health Promotion Atlantic Newsletter*, 3/year.

**★ 2481 ★ Dalhousie University**
**Population Health Research Unit (PHRU)**
Department of Community Health & Epidemiology
Faculty of Medicine
5849 University Ave.
Halifax, NS, Canada B3H 4H7
**Phone:** (902)494-3860          **Fax:** (902)494-1597
**Email:** george.kephart@dal.ca
**Website:** http://www.medicine.dal.ca/che/phru/
George Kephart, Dir.

**Activities/Fields:** Health and social sciences, particularly population health, health services utilization and their interrelationships.

**★ 2482 ★ Department of Veterans Affairs**
**Medical Center (Portland, OR)**
**Research & Development Service**
3710 SW Veterans Hospital Rd.
PO Box 1034
Portland, OR 97201
**Phone:** (503)273-5125          **Fax:** (503)273-5351
**Email:** michael.davey@med.va.gov
Dr. Michael P. Davey, Assoc. Ch., Res.

**Activities/Fields:** Genetics of alcoholism and substance abuse, osteoporosis in men, virology (CMV, HIV), immunology, diabetes, multiple sclerosis, hematology-oncology, spinal cord regeneration, tardive dyskinesia, Parkinson Disease, Hepatitis C, neurology health services research, hypertension, dermatology (malignant melanoma), etiology of rheumatoid arthritis, Alzheimer's disease, audiology, stroke, depression, schizophrenia, BI-polor disorders, and colon cancer. **Pub:** *R&D Newsletter*, quarterly. • *Research News*, quarterly. • *VA Regeneration Research Newsletter*, semiannually.

**★ 2483 ★ Donald Guthrie Foundation for Education and Research**
1 Guthrie Sq.
Sayre, PA 18840
**Phone:** (570)882-4620          **Fax:** (570)882-5151
**Email:** raronsta@ghs.guthrie.org
**Website:** http://www.guthrie.org/research
Dr. Robert Aronstam, Sci. Dir.

**Activities/Fields:** Cell communication and signal transduction and clinical research in immunology, virology, cancer biology, lung cancer, and neuroscience. **Pub:** *Guthrie Medical Journal*, quarterly.

★ **2484** ★ **Duke University**
**Center for Hyperbaric Medicine and Environmental Physiology**
Medical Center
PO Box 3823
Durham, NC 27710
**Phone:** (919)684-5514          **Fax:** (919)684-6002
**Email:** pbennett@dan.duke.edu
**Website:** http://hyperbaric.mc.duke.edu
Dr. Peter B. Bennett, Exec. Dir.

**Activities/Fields:** Hypobaric and hyperbaric medicine and physiology, including studies of how increased hydrostatic pressure affects cells, tissues, organs, and intact organisms; studies of morphological and metabolic effects of oxygen pressures; clinical investigations of use of hyperbaric oxygen therapy; study of effects of pressure on respiratory and cardiovascular systems and thermal homeostasis; and investigations of causes, mechanisms, and prevention of effects of decompression sickness.

★ **2485** ★ **Duke University**
**General Clinical Research Center**
Medical Center
PO Box 3068
Durham, NC 27710
**Phone:** (919)684-6263          **Fax:** (919)684-8676
**Email:** marke001@mc.duke.edu
**Website:** http://igg1.mc.duke.edu/Gaveston/
Dr. M. Louise Markert, Prog. Dir.

**Activities/Fields:** Multidisciplinary, clinical research into the cause, progression, prevention, control, and cure of human disease. Sample projects have studied immunodeficiency diseases, Alzheimer's disease, food allergy, X-linked hypophosphatemic rickets, and cardiovascular disease. **Frmly:** Rankin Clinical Research Unit.

★ **2486** ★ **Duke University**
**Institute on Care at the End of Life**
023 New Divinity Bldg.
Divinity School
Durham, NC 27708
**Phone:** (919)660-3553          **Fax:** (919)660-3544
**Email:** iceol@duke.edu
**Website:** http://www.iceol.duke.edu
Keith G. Meador, MD, Dir.

**Activities/Fields:** Care of the dying and their families, with an emphasis on underserved and diverse populations with varied religious and spiritual practices regarding the issue of dying.

★ **2487** ★ **Dwight David Eisenhower Army Medical Center**
**Department of Clinical Investigation**
Bldg. 300
Fort Gordon, GA 30905-5650
**Phone:** (706)787-4273          **Fax:** (706)787-5216
**Email:** kent.plowman@se.amedd.army.mil
**Website:** http://www.ddeamc.amedd.army.mil/clinical/investigation/clin_inv.htm
Col. Kent M. Plowman, Ch.

**Activities/Fields:** Osteomyelitis in rat tibias, fibroblast attachment to teeth, periodontal implants, pharmacotherapy in burns, hormonal influence of bone growth, synthetic bone grafting materials, wound healing, and markers for malignancy. **Pub:** *Annual Progress Report*.

★ **2488** ★ **East Carolina University**
**Center for Health Services Research and Development (CHSR&D)**
Physician Quadrangle, Bldg. N
Greenville, NC 27858-4354
**Phone:** (252)816-2785          **Fax:** (252)816-3259
**Email:** mansfieldc@mail.ecu.edu
**Website:** http://www.chsrd.med.ecu.edu
Christopher J. Mansfield, PhD, Dir.

**Activities/Fields:** Health care needs of rural North Carolina, including understanding epidemiology; the organization, finance, and delivery of health services; patient-provider interaction; professional workforce issues; and the effectiveness of clinical practices. **Pub:** *Eastern Carolina Health Care Atlas.* • *Physicians Directory.*

★ **2489** ★ **Emory University**
**Center for Cell and Molecular Signaling**
School of Medicine
1648 Pierce Dr.
Atlanta, GA 30322
**Phone:** (404)727-7421          **Fax:** (404)727-0329
**Email:** deaton@emory.edu
**Website:** http://www.emory.edu/WHSC/MED/CCMS/
Douglas C. Eaton, PhD, Dir.

**Activities/Fields:** Cellular signaling or cellular signal transduction, which is the process by which cells recognize external events and respond to the events with appropriate changes within the cell.

★ **2490** ★ **Emory University**
**General Clinical Research Center (GCRC)**
Emory University Hospital, Ste. GG-23
1364 Clifton Rd. NE
Atlanta, GA 30322
**Phone:** (404)712-7258          **Fax:** (404)727-5563
**Email:** wmitch@emory.edu
**Website:** http://www.emory.edu/WHSC/MED/RESEARCH/GCRC/index.htm
William E. Mitch, MD, Dir.

**Activities/Fields:** Nutrition, molecular cell biology, gene therapy, calorimetry.

★ **2491** ★ **Emory University**
**General Clinical Research Center**
School of Medicine
1364 Clifton Rd., Ste. GG23
Atlanta, GA 30322
**Phone:** (404)712-7258          **Fax:** (404)727-5563
**Email:** wmitch@emory.edu
**Website:** http://www.emory.edu/WHSC/MED/RESEARCH/GCRC/
William Mitch, Dir.

**Activities/Fields:** Disorders of amino acid, and protein metabolism; branch-chain ketoacid abnormalities; mitochondrial myopathies; clinical nutrition; energy metabolism; metabolic consequences of diabetes and obesity; effects of low protein diets and blood pressure control on the progression of renal disease; and growth disorders. **Frmly:** W. Dean Warren Clinical Research Center.

★ **2492** ★ **Emory University**
**Yerkes Regional Primate Research Center**
**Applied Research for Improving Behavioral Management of Captive Chimpanzees**
954 N Gatewood Rd. NE
Atlanta, GA 30329
**Phone:** (404)624-5990          **Fax:** (404)627-7514
**Email:** mbloomsmith@zooatlanta.org
Mollie A. Bloomsmith, PhD, Prin. Investigator

**Activities/Fields:** Improvement in the care and management of captive chimpanzees. Studies identify factors that influence the production of successful breeders from captive-born animals, identify improvements in the care and behavioral management of chimpanzees, and objectively evaluate forms of environmental enrichment and animal training.

★ **2493** ★ **Florida State University**
**Sensory Research Institute**
B-340, NHMFL
1800 E Paul Dirac Dr.
Tallahassee, FL 32306-2741
**Phone:** (850)644-2637          **Fax:** (850)645-3295
**Email:** fsusri@psy.fsu.edu

**Website:**          http://www.psy.fsu.edu/~fsusri/welcome.html
Dr. James C. Walker, Dir.

**Activities/Fields:** Human and animal sensory response to airborne chemicals.

★ **2494** ★ **Frontier Science and Technology Research Foundation**
1244 Boylston St.
Chestnut Hill, MA 02467
**Phone:** (617)632-2000          **Fax:** (617)632-2001
**Email:** fstrf@fstrf.org
**Website:** http://www.fstrf.org
Dr. Marvin Zelen, Contact

**Activities/Fields:** Conducts joint research projects with cooperative clinical trial groups and other organizations. Provides biostatistical support and collaboration, data management and processing, project management, and administrative support to researchers.

★ **2495** ★ **General Clinical Research Center**
Department of Medicine
Tulane/LSU Medical Center
1430 Tulane Ave.
Medicine SL-12
New Orleans, LA 70112
**Phone:** (504)585-4000          **Fax:** (504)585-4045
**Email:** lerclpha@tulane.edu
**Website:** http://www.som.tulane.edu/gcrc
Juan J. Lertora, MD, Prog. Dir.

**Activities/Fields:** Major areas of investigation include AIDS immunosuppression, cardiac diseases, clinical immunology and allergy, gastroenterology and hepatic diseases, neuroendocrinology, oncology and renal diseases.

★ **2496** ★ **Georgetown University**
**Division of Comparative Medicine**
3950 Reservoir Rd. NW, Rm. G05
Washington, DC 20007
**Phone:** (202)687-2488          **Fax:** (202)687-6256
Stephen P. Schiffer, DVM, Dir.

**Activities/Fields:** Medical sciences, with particular reference to surgical aspects, including basic studies of tissue transplantation, neuroscience, techniques of extracorporeal circulation, magnetic resonance imaging (MRI) techniques, and technique of perfusion of orbital artery and heart/lung transplantation. Also designs and develops valvular devices and other cardiac instrumentation and evaluates vascular prosthetic devices. **Frmly:** Surgical Research Laboratory; Research Resources Facility.

★ **2497** ★ **Georgia State University**
**Center for Brain Sciences and Health (CBH)**
University Plaza
Atlanta, GA 30303
**Phone:** (404)463-9611
**Website:** http://www.gsu.edu/~wwwcbh/
Dr. Elliott Albers, Dir.

**Activities/Fields:** Brain injury; obesity, eating disorders and energy balance; aggression/ violence; sleep and attention disorders.

★ **2498** ★ **Hamot Medical Center**
**Research Center**
Hamot Professional Bldg.
104 E 2nd St.
Erie, PA 16507
**Phone:** (814)877-6026          **Fax:** (814)877-5089
**Email:** phyllis.kuhn@hamot.org
**Website:** http://www.hamot.org
Phyllis Kuhn, PhD, Dir.

**Activities/Fields:** Drug evaluations, medical devices and diagnostic products, orthopedics, infection control, and microbiology.

**★ 2499 ★ Heimlich Institute**
311 Straight St.
Cincinnati, OH 45219
**Phone:** (513)559-2391          **Fax:** (513)559-2403
**Email:** heimlich@lglou.com
**Website:** http://www.heimlichinstitute.org
Henry J. Heimlich, MD, Pres.

**Activities/Fields:** Malaria therapy for cancer and Lyme disease, rehabilitation of swallowing, and transtracheal oxygen therapy for chronic lung diseases, including oxygen-dependent emphysema, black lung, cystic fibrosis, and interstitial fibrosis. Developments include Heimlich Maneuver for choking and drowning, Heimlich chest drainage valve, Heimlich Micro-Trach, and Heimlich operation for esophageal replacement. **Pub:** *Newsletter.* **Frmly:** Dysphagia Foundation.

**★ 2500 ★ Hektoen Institute for Medical Research**
627 S Wood St., Ste. 201
Chicago, IL 60612-3810
**Phone:** (312)738-3100          **Fax:** (312)738-3102
**Email:** LabHektoen@aol.com
**Website:** http://www.themeasurementgroup.com/edcpage/hektoen.html
Peter Friedell, MD, Chm.

**Activities/Fields:** Medicine and surgery, including laboratory and clinical studies in cancer metabolism, kidney disease, virology, hematology, microbiology, bacteriology, endocrinology, pediatric cardiology, neurology, immunology, pathology, gastroenterology, orthopedic surgery, congenital heart diseases, infectious diseases, and hypertension. Specific investigations include treatment of cancer by new modalities, incidence of perinatal mortality and effect of neonatal care, metabolic aspects of renal disease, cell surface alterations in cancer and their effects on metastasis, effects of different hormones in breast carcinoma, influence of hormone receptors on several varieties of soft tissue sarcomas and malignant melanomas, and the immunological aspects of prostatic cancer. **Pub:** *Biennial Report.*

**★ 2501 ★ Howard Hughes Medical Institute**
4000 Jones Bridge Rd.
Chevy Chase, MD 20815-6789
**Phone:** (301)215-8855          **Fax:** (301)215-8863
**Email:** potterr@hhmi.org
**Website:** http://www.hhmi.org
Thomas R. Cech, PhD, Pres.

**Activities/Fields:** Molecular biology, especially genetics, immunology, cell biology, structural biology, neuroscience, and computational biology. Conducts research with scientists and staff at over 70 academic medical centers, universities and other research organizations. **Pub:** *Annual report.* • *H HMImagazine*, quarterly.

**★ 2502 ★ Howard University General Clinical Research Center**
Howard University Hospital, 4th Fl., West
2041 Georgia Ave. NW
Washington, DC 20060
**Phone:** (202)865-7272          **Fax:** (202)865-1933
**Email:** orandall@howard.edu
**Website:** http://www.gcrc.howard.edu
Otelio S. Randall, MD, Prog. Dir.

**Activities/Fields:** Major areas of investigation include cardiovascular diseases, dermatology, endocrinology, genetic disorders, geriatrics and gerontology, infectious diseases, metabolism, hyperlipidemia and obesity, neurology and nutrition. **Pub:** *GCRC Newsletter*, quarterly.

**★ 2503 ★ Indiana University Bowen Research Center**
Long Hospital, 2nd Fl.
1110 W Michigan St.
Indianapolis, IN 46202
**Phone:** (317)278-0300
**Email:** diallen@iupui.edu

**Website:** http://www.bowenresearchcenter.iupui.edu/bowen3.htm
Debbie Allen, MD, Dir.

**Activities/Fields:** Quality-of-life issues, lifestyle changes to prevent disease; health care costs, access to healthcare services for rural and underserved populations.

**★ 2504 ★ Indiana University General Clinical Research Center**
550 N University Blvd.
Indianapolis, IN 46202
**Phone:** (317)274-4356          **Fax:** (317)274-7346
**Email:** mpeacock@iupui.edu
**Website:** http://www.gcrc.iupui.edu
Dr. Munro Peacock, Dir.

**Activities/Fields:** AIDS, alcohol, amyloidosis, bone disease, cancer, cardiology, diabetes, gene therapy, genetics, hypertension, infectious disease, metabolism, neonatalogy, neurology, pharmacology, psychiatry, and transplantation.

**★ 2505 ★ Indiana University—Northwest Northwest Center for Medical Education**
School of Medicine
3400 Broadway
Gary, IN 46408
**Phone:** (219)980-6550          **Fax:** (219)980-6566
**Email:** wbaldwin@meded.iun.indiana.edu
**Website:** http://www.medlib.iupui.edu/nwcme/nwcme.html
William W. Baldwin, PhD, Dir.

**Activities/Fields:** Diabetes, mitochondria enzymes, lymphocyte activation microvessels, corneal innervation, autonomic nervous system, blood coagulation, neuroglialneuron interactions, membrane-bound transport enzymes, erthrocyte membrane skeletal proteins, avian musculoskeletal funtional morphology, bacterial growth, immunoglobulin molecular biology.

**★ 2506 ★ Indiana University-Purdue University at Indianapolis Center for Enhancing Quality of Life in Chronic Illness (CEQL)**
School of Nursing
1111 Middle Dr., NU 337B
Indianapolis, IN 46202-5107
**Phone:** (317)278-0511
**Email:** joausti@iupui.edu
**Website:** http://nursing.iupui.edu/Research/
Joan K. Austin, Contact

**Activities/Fields:** Improvement in the health-related quality of life in persons with chronic conditions across the life span. **Pub:** *Newsletter.*

**★ 2507 ★ Iowa State University of Science and Technology Bessey Microscopy Facility**
Bessey Hall, Rm. 1
Ames, IA 50011-1020
**Phone:** (515)294-8635          **Fax:** (515)294-1337
**Email:** hth@iastate.edu
**Website:** http://www.biotech.iastate.edu/facilities/BMF/
Prof. Harry T. Horner, Dir.

**Activities/Fields:** Applications of microscopy in areas of biology, biomedicine, botany, agronomy, animal science, biotechnology, and engineering.

**★ 2508 ★ Jackson Laboratory Cryopreservation of Murine Germplasm**
600 Main St.
Bar Harbor, ME 04609-1500
**Phone:** (207)288-6373          **Fax:** (207)288-6005
**Email:** lem@jax.org
**Website:** http://www.jax.org
Larry E. Mobraaten, PhD, Prin. Investigator

**Activities/Fields:** Cryopreservation of mouse embryos and spermatozoa.

**★ 2509 ★ Jacobs Institute of Women's Health**
409 12th St. SW
Washington, DC 20024-2188
**Phone:** (202)863-4990          **Fax:** (202)488-4229
**Email:** mromans.@acog.org
**Website:** http://www.jiwh.org
Martha C. Romans, Exec. Dir.

**Activities/Fields:** Women's health care issues, focusing on the interaction of medical and social systems. **Pub:** *InTouch*, quarterly. Newsletter. • *Women's Health Issues*, bimonthly. Journal.

**★ 2510 ★ John P. Robarts Research Institute**
100 Perth Dr.
PO Box 5015
London, ON, Canada N6A 5K8
**Phone:** (519)663-5777          **Fax:** (519)663-3789
**Email:** iposliff@rri.on.ca
**Website:** http://rri.on.ca
Dr. Mark J. Poznansky, Pres. /Sci. Dir.

**Activities/Fields:** Cardiovascular sciences, immunology, neuroscience, imaging, clinical trials, and gene therapy and molecular virology. Research is conducted into major causes of death and disability such as stroke, heart disease, Alzheimer's, organ failure, and diabetes, with the goal to develop new treatments and cures as a result of advances in genetic medicine and diagnostic imaging techniques. **Pub:** *Annual Report.* • *Research Report.*

**★ 2511 ★ John P. Robarts Research Institute Imaging Research Laboratories**
100 Perth Dr.
PO Box 5015
London, ON, Canada N6A 5K8
**Phone:** (519)663-3833          **Fax:** (519)663-3403
**Email:** afenster@irus.rri.uwo.ca
**Website:** http://www.irus.rri.on.ca/
Dr. Aaron Fenster, Dir.

**Activities/Fields:** Medical imaging systems and techniques, including diagnostic X-rays, computed tomography, ultrasound, and magnetic resonance imaging. Develops new diagnostic imaging systems and techniques focusing on vascular imaging research, three dimensional image processing and display, multimodality display, image guided surgery and therapy, prostate and breast cancer.

**★ 2512 ★ Johns Hopkins University Biomedical Instrumentation Laboratory**
Department of Biomedical Engineering
School of Medicine
720 Rutland Ave.
Baltimore, MD 21205
**Phone:** (410)955-0077          **Fax:** (410)955-0549
**Email:** nthakor@bme.jhu.edu
**Website:** http://www.bme.jhu.edu/~nthakor/Lab/
Nitish V. Thakor, PhD, Contact

**Activities/Fields:** Medical instrumentation, signal analysis, and computer modeling and simulation to develop novel diagnostic and therapeutic technologies for cardiovascular diseases and neurological injury.

**★ 2513 ★ Johns Hopkins University Center for American Indian and Alaskan Native Health**
School of Public Health
621 N Washington St.
Baltimore, MD 21205
**Phone:** (410)955-6931          **Fax:** (410)955-2010
**Website:** http://ih.jhsph.edu/cnah/mission.htm
Mathuram Santosham, MD, Dir.

**Activities/Fields:** Health and well being of American Indians and Alaskan Natives.

**★ 2514 ★ Johns Hopkins University Center for Clinical Trials**
615 N Wolfe St., Rm. 5010
Baltimore, MD 21205
**Phone:** (410)955-8175     **Fax:** (410)955-0932
**Email:** cctmail@jhsph.edu
**Website:** http://www.jhsph.edu/Research/Centers/CCT/
Curtis L. Meinert, PhD, Dir.

**Activities/Fields:** Design, conduct, and analysis of clinical medical trials; analysis of longitudinal data and other methods of analyzing results from trials; publication process; and the language and nomenclature of clinical trials.

**★ 2515 ★ Johns Hopkins University Center for Computational Medicine and Biology**
Department of Biomedical Engineering
710 Traylor Research Bldg.
720 Rutland Ave.
Baltimore, MD 21205
**Phone:** (410)614-6685     **Fax:** (410)614-8796
**Email:** ccmb@bme.jhu.edu
**Website:** http://www.bme.jhu.edu/ccmb/
Prof. Raimond L. Winslow, Co-Dir.

**Activities/Fields:** Understanding the integrative function in biological systems, including human, through development and application of computational models, and the application of these models to the design of novel therapeutics.

**★ 2516 ★ Johns Hopkins University Division of Comparative Medicine**
720 Rutland Ave.
Baltimore, MD 21205
**Phone:** (410)955-3273     **Fax:** (410)502-5068
**Website:** http://www.hopkinsmedicine.org/comparativemedicine
Dr. Janice E. Clements, Interim Dir.

**Activities/Fields:** Comparative pathology, laboratory animal medicine, retrovirus biology, transgenic biology, infectious diseases, and oncology. Research activities focus on naturally occurring diseases of animals as models of human disease, molecular biology and pathogenesis of lentiviral infections, aquatic toxicology, and benign prostatic hyperplasia.

**★ 2517 ★ Johns Hopkins University General Clinical Research Center**
Osler
Johns Hopkins Hospital
600 N Wolfe St.
Baltimore, MD 21205
**Phone:** (410)955-2132     **Fax:** (410)955-0801
**Email:** csaudek@jhu.edu
**Website:** http://gcrc.med.jhmi.edu/gcrc
Christopher D. Saudek, MD, Prog. Dir.

**Activities/Fields:** Major areas of investigation include anesthesiology, cardiology, clinical pharmacology, emergency medicine, endocrinology, gene therapy, genetic diseases, geriatrics and gerontology, hematology, hypertension, infectious diseases, liver diseases, musculoskeletal disorders, neonatal medicine, nephrology, neurology, nutrition, oncology, psychiatry and behavioral sciences, pulmonary diseases and sleep studies.

**★ 2518 ★ Johns Hopkins University Institute for Global Tobacco Control**
School of Public Health
615 N Wolfe St.
Baltimore, MD 21205
**Phone:** (410)614-5378     **Fax:** (410)955-0863
**Email:** jsamet@jhsph.edu
**Website:** http://www.jhsph.edu/~o-gtc/
Dr. Jonathan M. Samet, Dir.

**Activities/Fields:** Prevention of death and disease from tobacco use around the world.

**★ 2519 ★ Johns Hopkins University Institute for Vaccine Safety (IVS)**
School of Public Health
615 N Wolfe St., Ste. 5515
Baltimore, MD 21205-2179
**Email:** info@vaccinesafety.edu
**Website:** http://www.vaccinesafety.edu
Neal A. Halsey, MD, Dir.

**Activities/Fields:** Vaccine safety issues. **Pub:** *Newsletter*, quarterly.

**★ 2520 ★ Johns Hopkins University Medical Imaging Laboratory**
Departments of Biomedical Engineering & Radiology
School of Medicine
720 Rutland Ave.
Baltimore, MD 21205
**Phone:** (410)502-6958     **Fax:** (410)955-0549

**Activities/Fields:** Development of new imaging techniques and advanced applications of existing techniques to solve problems in medicine and biology.

**★ 2521 ★ Johns Hopkins University Parkinson's Disease Research Center (PDRC)**
Carnegie 214
600 N Wolfe St.
Baltimore, MD 21287
**Phone:** (410)614-3359     **Fax:** (410)614-9568
**Website:** http://www.med.jhu.edu/pdrc
Dr. Ted M. Dawson, Dir.

**Activities/Fields:** Cause and treatment of Parkinson's Disease.

**★ 2522 ★ Johns Hopkins University Phoebe R. Berman Bioethics Institute**
Hampton House 352
624 N Broadway
Baltimore, MD 21205-1996
**Phone:** (410)955-3018     **Fax:** (410)614-9567
**Email:** bioethic@jhsph.edu
**Website:** http://www.med.jhu.edu/bioethics_institute
Ruth R. Faden, PhD, Exec. Dir.

**Activities/Fields:** Moral and policy issues in biomedical science, health care, and health policy, and the development of thoughtful solutions for the benefit of society.

**★ 2523 ★ Kaiser Permanente Center for Health Research**
3800 N Interstate Ave.
Portland, OR 97227-1098
**Phone:** (503)335-2400     **Fax:** (503)335-2424
**Email:** mary.durham@kpchr.org
**Website:** http://www.kpchr.org/
Mary L. Durham, PhD, Dir.

**Activities/Fields:** Organization, financing, costs and quality of medical care in an HMO; mental health; medical informatics; patient safety; health behavior interventions; epidemiology; effectiveness of alternative therapies and services; nutrition; genetics; dental research; and biometry and research methods. **Pub:** *Annual Report.* ● *The Chronicle*, 3/year. Newsletter. ● *Current Studies*, annually. Brochure.

**★ 2524 ★ Lahey Clinic Foundation**
41 Mall Rd.
Burlington, MA 01805
**Phone:** (781)273-5100     **Fax:** (781)273-8999
**Website:** http://www.lahey.org
Dr. David Barett, Dir.

**Activities/Fields:** Medical, surgical, and radiological techniques, with special emphasis on clinical applications, including studies on high and mega voltage radiation, treatment of cancer with drugs and immunotherapy, cancer cell kinetics, electronic measurement of bacterial growth, pancreatic and renal transplantation, cardiac surgery, diagnostic radiology, amino acid absorption, treatment of pancreatitis, and hospital and prolonged storage by freezing of blood for transfusion. Maintains a clinic for patient care and application of research results and an educational division for postgraduate medical training and residency, both at the clinic and at local hospitals and medical schools. **Pub:** *Lahey Clinic Foundation Bulletin*, quarterly.

**★ 2525 ★ Laval University Medical Research Centre**
2705 Blvd. Laurier
Sainte Foy, QC, Canada G1V 4G2
**Phone:** (418)654-2296     **Fax:** (418)654-2735
**Email:** fernand.labrie@crchul.ulaval.ca
Dr. Fernand Labrie, Hd.

**Activities/Fields:** Family medicine, rheumatology and immunology, infectious diseases, health and environment, genetics and molecular medicine, ontogeny and reproduction, molecular endocrinology, hypertension, diabetes, lipids, ophthalmology, pediatrics, hormonal bioregulation, and public health.

**★ 2526 ★ Laval University Medical Research Centre Family Medicine Research Group**
2705 Blvd. Bay-tree
Sainte Foy, QC, Canada G1V 4G2
**Phone:** (418)654-2701     **Fax:** (418)654-2138
**Email:** lucie.baillargeon@crchul.ulaval.ca
Lucie Baillargeon, Dir.

**Activities/Fields:** Causes of, and therapeutic alternatives to, overuse of hypnotic and anxiolytic drugs; family physicians treatment of patients who are facing domestic violence; evaluation of validity of international prostatic symptoms scale; physicians knowledge of diabetic retinopathy; risk of severe perineal tears in relation to median episiotomy; clinical trials on antibiotherapy for various infectious diseases; and smoking cessation.

**★ 2527 ★ Laval University Saint-Sacrement Hospital Research Centre**
1050 Chemin Ste-Foy
Quebec, QC, Canada G1S 4L8
**Phone:** (418)682-7390     **Fax:** (418)682-7949
**Email:** lucie.huart@gre.ulaval.ca

**Activities/Fields:** Epidemiology and public health, experimental organogenesis, hematology, and clinical research in gynecology, obstetrics, respiratory diseases, and breast cancer.

**★ 2528 ★ Lexington Clinic Foundation for Medical Education and Research Inc.**
1221 S Broadway St.
Lexington, KY 40504
**Phone:** (859)258-4000
James W. Bard, MD, Pres.

**Activities/Fields:** Cancer therapy, muscle physiology and athletic injury, diabetes, and cardiac surgery.

**★ 2529 ★ Los Amigos Research and Education Institute, Inc.**
PO Box 3500, Los Amigos Sta.
Downey, CA 90242
**Phone:** (562)401-8111     **Fax:** (562)803-5569
**Email:** julial@larei.org
Julia F. LaPlount, Admin. Off.

**Activities/Fields:** Clinical medicine, including multidisciplinary study of severe chronic disabilities in pulmonary and respiratory functions, cardiology, spinal cord injury, orthopedic disabilities, environmental health, stroke, pathokinesiology, liver disease, neuromuscular stimulation and control, rehabilitation of severely disabled persons, cerebral palsy, problem amputations, arthritis, and diabetes. Treats effects of atmospheric pollutants on human lung function, investigates possible causes of Alzheimer's disease, and explores new methods and procedures for care and treatment of gerontology patients.

**★ 2530 ★ Louisiana Health and Hospitals Department**
**Research and Development**
250 University Blvd., Ste. 122
Baton Rouge, LA 70821-2870
**Phone:** (225)342-2964 **Fax:** (225)278-0900
**Email:** dgmarrer@iupui.edu
Dr. David G. Marrerro, Actg. Dir.
**Activities/Fields:** Health, hospitals.

**★ 2531 ★ Lovelace Respiratory Research Institute**
2425 Ridgecrest Dr. SE
Albuquerque, NM 87108-5127
**Phone:** (505)348-9400 **Fax:** (505)348-8542
**Email:** rrubin@lrri.org
**Website:** http://www.lrri.org
Dr. Robert W. Rubin, Pres. /CEO
**Activities/Fields:** Respiratory disease (primarily asthma and cancer), respiratory pharmaceuticals, inhalation drug delivery, inhalation toxicology, aerosol science, animal models of human respiratory disease, and health risks from inhaled materials in the workplace, home, and general environment. **Pub:** *Gift of Breath*, quarterly. **Frmly:** Lovelace Medical Foundation; The Lovelace Institutes.

**★ 2532 ★ Maine Medical Center**
**Research Institute (MMCRI)**
81 Research Dr.
Scarborough, ME 04074
**Phone:** (207)885-8100 **Fax:** (207)885-8110
**Email:** lovete@mail.mmc.org
**Website:** http://zappa.mmcri.mmc.org
Edmund J. Lovett, III, Assoc. VP, Res. Dir.
**Activities/Fields:** Laboratory, clinical, and epidemiologic research on molecular genetics, hematology, infectious diseases, endocrinology, cardiology and nephrology. **Pub:** *Inquiry Newsletter*.

**★ 2533 ★ Maisonneuve-Rosemont**
**Hospital Research Centre**
5415 de l'Assomption Blvd.
Montreal, QC, Canada H1T 2M4
**Phone:** (514)252-3557 **Fax:** (514)252-3430
**Email:** yleroux@hmr.qc.ca
**Website:** http://www.guybernier.com
Dr. Alain Bonnardeaux, MD, Dir.
**Activities/Fields:** Reproductive biology, including epididymal maturation, acrosome reaction, fertilization, and implantation; immunology, including bone marrow transplantation, transplantation of encapsulated cells, DNA repair, lymphocyte function and ontogeny, immunogenetics, and cytokines; hypertension, including angiotensinogen gene; calcium metabolism; kidney physiology; cancer, including prostate and leukemias; nuclear medicine; and neurology, including cerebrovascular diseases and aphasia.

**★ 2534 ★ Marshfield Medical Research**
**Foundation**
1000 N Oak Ave.
Marshfield, WI 54449-5790
**Phone:** (715)387-5241 **Fax:** (715)389-3131
**Website:** http://research.marshfieldclinic.org
Richard A. Leer, MD, Ch.
**Activities/Fields:** Diagnosis and treatment of human disease, including basic and/or applied studies on respiratory disease, human angiotensinogen and renin in hypertension, infertility, human genome mapping, epidemiology and biostatistics, clinical drug trials, searching for tumor suppressor genes, infectious disease and vaccine development, zoonotic illness and food safety, genetic epidemiology and pharmacogenomics. Operates the Center for Medical Genetics, which conducts population-based epidemiologic research; the National Farm Medicine Center, which is designed to improve the quality of life; the Center for

Personalized Medicine, which conducts research in genetic epidemiology and pharmacogenetics; and the Epidemiological Research Center which conducts population-based studies using a 90,000-patient study cohort. **Pub:** *Marshfield Medical Journal*.

**Masonic Medical Research Laboratory (MMRL)**
*See:* Entry 5117

**★ 2535 ★ Massachusetts General Hospital**
**Mallinckrodt General Clinical Research Center**
55 Fruit St., WHT 13
Boston, MA 02114-2696
**Phone:** (617)726-4272 **Fax:** (617)724-3299
**Email:** farefield.william@mgh.harvard.edu
**Website:** http://www.mgh.harvard.edu/GCRC
William Z. Farefield, Admin. Dir.
**Activities/Fields:** The Center's major areas of investigation are aging, diabetes, endocrinology, gastroenterology, genetic diseases, infectious diseases, neuroendocrinology, neurology, neuropsychiatry, oncology, pediatrics, psychiatry, reproductive endocrinology and gynecology and rheumatology.

**★ 2536 ★ Massachusetts Institute of Technology**
**Center for Biomedical Engineering (CBE)**
77 Massachusetts Ave., Rm. 56-341
Cambridge, MA 02139
**Phone:** (617)258-8949 **Fax:** (617)258-0204
**Email:** cbe-www@mit.edu
**Website:** http://web.mit.edu/cbe/
Prof. Alan Grodzinsky, Dir.
**Activities/Fields:** Molecular medicine, including molecular engineering, cell and tissue engineering, and physiological systems engineering.

**★ 2537 ★ Massachusetts Institute of Technology**
**General Clinical Research Center**
Bldg. E17-445
77 Massachusetts Ave.
Cambridge, MA 02142
**Phone:** (617)253-3091 **Fax:** (617)253-6882
**Email:** dick@mit.edu
**Website:** http://web.mit.edu/crc/www
Dr. Richard J. Wurtman, Prog. Dir.
**Activities/Fields:** Normal human metabolism, physiology, and behavior, including studies on hormones, fates of deuterated amino acids, behavioral and neuroendocrine effect of foods (carbohydrate, protein, and caffeine), effects of drugs on memory and other behaviors, and endocrine and metabolic effects on aging. Also studies human diseases such as obesity, Alzheimer's disease, brain injury, Parkinson's disease, use of brain imaging techniques to follow metabolic events, and infectious diseases (HIV).

**★ 2538 ★ Mayo Clinic and Foundation**
**General Clinical Research Center**
St. Mary's Hospital
1216 2nd St. SW
Rochester, MN 55902
**Phone:** (507)255-6122 **Fax:** (507)255-7445
**Email:** andresen@mayo.edu
**Activities/Fields:** Allergy, endocrinology, gastrointestinal disease, lipid disorders, osteoporosis, pediatrics, pharmacology, renal disease, surgery, cardiovascular disease, oncology, neurology, hypertension, and nutrition.

**★ 2539 ★ McGill University**
**Centre for Nonlinear Dynamics in Physiology and Medicine**
McIntyre Medical Science Bldg.
3655 Drummond St.
Montreal, QC, Canada H3G 1Y6
**Phone:** (514)398-4336 **Fax:** (514)398-7452
**Email:** mackey@cnd.mcgill.ca
**Website:** http://www.cnd.mcgill.ca
Michael C. Mackey, Dir.
**Activities/Fields:** Understanding the origin of dynamic behavior in health and disease, focusing on cyclical hematopoiesis, neurological tremor, and cardiac arrythmias.

**★ 2540 ★ McGill University**
**Health Centre Research Institute**
**Clinical Research Centre (CRC)**
1650 Cedar Ave., Ste. D13 173
Montreal, QC, Canada H3G 1A4
**Phone:** (514)937-6011 **Fax:** (514)934-8338
**Email:** muhc.crc@mcgill.ca
**Website:** http://crcmgh.com
Dr. Phil Gold, Exec. Dir.
**Activities/Fields:** All therapeutic areas of medicine.

**★ 2541 ★ McGill University**
**Lady Davis Institute for Medical Research**
3755 Chemin de la Cote-Sainte-Catherine
Montreal, QC, Canada H3T 1E2
**Phone:** (514)340-8260 **Fax:** (514)340-7502
**Email:** wainberg@ldi.jgh.mcgill.ca
**Website:** http://www.jgh.ca/research/ldi/index.html
Mark A. Wainberg, MD, Dir.
**Activities/Fields:** AIDS, Aging, Cognitive Neuroscience, Molecular Oncology, Pharmacology of Cancer, Endocrinology and Metabolism, Human Genetics, Iron Metabolism, Cardiovascular Diseases, Clinical Epidemiology, Health Services Research, Psychosocial Aspects of Illness. **Pub:** *Annual Scientific Activity Report*.

**★ 2542 ★ Medical College of Georgia**
**Georgia Prevention Institute (GPI)**
HS-1640
Augusta, GA 30912-3710
**Phone:** (706)721-4534 **Fax:** (706)721-7150
**Email:** ftreiber@mail.mcg.edu
**Website:** http://www.mcg.edu/institutes/gpi
Dr. Frank A. Treiber, Dir.
**Activities/Fields:** Health promotion and disease prevention, mainly in youth, particularly pediatric antecedents of cardiovascular and metabolic disease that are ordinarily manifested in the adult years.

**★ 2543 ★ Medical College of Wisconsin**
**Center for the Study of Bioethics**
8701 Watertown Plank Rd.
Milwaukee, WI 53226
**Phone:** (414)456-8498 **Fax:** (414)456-6511
**Email:** rshapiro@mcw.edu
**Website:** http://www.mcw.edu/bioethics/
Robyn Shapiro, JD, Dir.
**Activities/Fields:** Ethics studies, with special emphasis on AIDS, abortion, drug testing, euthanasia, fetal rights, genetics, technology assessment and allocation of resources, and multicultural approaches to bioethics. **Pub:** *Bioethics Bullentin*, biennially.

**★ 2544 ★ Medical College of Wisconsin**
**General Clinical Research Center**
9200 W Wisconsin Ave.
Milwaukee, WI 53226
**Phone:** (414)805-7325 **Fax:** (414)805-7330
**Email:** gsonnen@mcw.edu
**Website:** http://www.mcw.edu/gcrc/
Gabriele E. Sonnenberg, MD, Prog. Dir.
**Activities/Fields:** Physiology and pathophysiology of disease in areas of metabolism, endocrinology, gastroenterology, kidney, central nervous system, con-

nective tissues, hematopietic system, and bone, respiratory, and cardiovascular disorders.

**★ 2545 ★ Medical and Health Research Association of New York City, Inc. (MHRA)**
40 Worth St., Ste. 720
New York, NY 10013-2988
**Phone:** (212)285-0220      **Fax:** (212)385-0565
**Email:** erautenberg@mhra.org
**Website:** http://www.mhra.org
Ellen Rautenberg, Pres. /CEO

**Activities/Fields:** Obstetrics, gynecology, midwifery, nursing, prenatal care and diagnoses, maternity care, infant care, infant mortality, pediatric care, family planning, childhood immunizations, health and HIV education, and nutrition for persons living in New York City. **Pub:** *MHRA News*, semiannually. Newsletter.

**★ 2546 ★ Medical University of South Carolina**
**General Clinical Research Center**
96 Jonathan Lucas St., Ste. 213
PO Box 250609
Charleston, SC 29425
**Phone:** (843)792-3256      **Fax:** (843)792-2601
**Email:** keyl@musc.edu
**Website:** http://www.gcrc.musc.edu
Dr. L. Lyndon Key, Jr., Prog. Dir.

**Activities/Fields:** Bone and mineral metabolism, cardiology, diabetes, endocrinology, gastroenterology, hypertension, nutrition, obstetrics and gynecology, oncology, hematology, pharmacology, pulmonary medicine, and rheumatology and immunology. Provides medical scientists with the opportunity for clinical research in all aspects of biomedicine. **Pub:** *Annual Report to National Institute of Health*.

**★ 2547 ★ Meharry Medical College**
**Clinical Research Center**
1005 D.B. Todd Blvd.
Nashville, TN 37208
**Phone:** (615)327-6353      **Fax:** (615)327-5835
**Email:** jhinds@mmc.edu
Joseph Hinds, MD, Dir.

**Activities/Fields:** Clinical research, including pulmonary studies, AIDS, sickle cell disease, hypertension, body composition, coronary artery disease, infectious diseases, and oncology.

**★ 2548 ★ Methodist Research Institute**
1701 N Senate Blvd.
PO Box 1367
Indianapolis, IN 46206
**Phone:** (317)962-3554      **Fax:** (317)962-5954
**Email:** gzaloga@clarian.org
**Website:** http://mri.clarian.com
Gary P. Zaloga, MD, Med. Dir.

**Activities/Fields:** Pharmaceutical and device clinical trials, experimental cell research, cell signalling, ion channel physiology, immunology. Other research involves heart, kidney, lung, pancreas, and liver transplants; biliary and renal extracorporeal shock wave lithotripsy; and clot lysis programs. **Pub:** *Journal of Hemato-therapy & Stem Cell Research*, monthly. • *News from the Methodist Research Institute*, quarterly.

**★ 2549 ★ Michigan State University**
**Institute of International Health**
B-301 West Fee Hall
East Lansing, MI 48824-1315
**Phone:** (517)353-8992      **Fax:** (517)355-1894
**Email:** petropou@msu.edu
**Website:** http://www.rnsu.edu/unit/iih
Dr. Evangelos A. Petropoulos, Dir.

**Activities/Fields:** World health problems, including overseas health studies. Specific projects include: the Training and Research on Environmental and Occupational Health in the Balkans project focusing on Bulgaria; Minority International Research Training (MIRT), for undergraduate, graduate, and professional level minority students and faculty in biomedical and behavioral research in 12 research sites in nine countries; the Medical Informatics Training in Malawi project; and the Environmental Sciences Training in Japan project. The IIH has conducted research and training on schistosomiasis with Egyptians scientists and worked on the management and prevention of cardiovascular diseases in Bulgaria and has helped develop country background information on health in Sub-Saharan Africa for the World Bank. **Pub:** *Newsletter*, bimonthly.

**★ 2550 ★ Michigan State University**
**Office of Medical Education Research and Development (OMERAD)**
East Fee Hall, Rm. A-217
College of Human Medicine
East Lansing, MI 48824-1316
**Phone:** (517)353-7791      **Fax:** (517)353-8926
**Email:** ander113@msu.edu
**Website:** http://www.msu.edu/unit/omerad/
William A. Anderson, PhD, Dir.

**Activities/Fields:** Medical education evaluation and research including evaluation of innovative educational programs, measures of physician competence, health policy forums, and faculty development. Utilizes an interdisciplinary faculty representing the fields of psychology, anthropology, statistics, and education. Office capabilities include research design and analysis support, faculty development, and program evaluation. **Pub:** *Vital Signs*, semiannually. Newsletter.

**★ 2551 ★ Middle Tennessee Research Institute**
3400 Lebanon Rd.
Murfreesboro, TN 37130
**Phone:** (615)327-0938      **Fax:** (615)321-6305
Gary Linn, Dir.

**Activities/Fields:** Medical clinical trials. **Frmly:** Nashville Research Institute, Inc.

**★ 2552 ★ Midwest Biomedical Research Foundation**
4801 E Linwood Blvd., Ste. 103
Kansas City, MO 64128-2226
**Phone:** (816)921-8311      **Fax:** (816)861-1110
**Email:** kimberly.collins@med.va.gov
**Website:** http://www.midwestbiomed.org
Kimberly Collins, Exec. Dir.

**Activities/Fields:** Clinical studies, focusing on improving treatments and cures of health problems prevalent among veteran patients and the general population.

**★ 2553 ★ Minneapolis Medical Research Foundation**
600 HFA Bldg.
914 S 8th St.
Minneapolis, MN 55404
**Phone:** (612)347-7680      **Fax:** (612)337-7189
**Email:** info@mmrf.org
**Website:** http://www.mmrf.org
Michael West, MD, Pres.

**Activities/Fields:** Medicine, surgery, pediatrics, neurology, urology, renal transplant, endocrinology, nephrology, dialysis, anesthesia, hyperbaric medicine, program evaluation and outcomes research, addiction, AIDS, Alzheimer's disease, trauma, and health care policy. **Pub:** *Research Connections*.

**★ 2554 ★ Minnesota Center for Health Care Ethics**
601 25th Ave. S
Minneapolis, MN 55454
**Phone:** (612)690-7895      **Fax:** (612)690-7774
**Email:** jarobbins@stkate.edu
**Website:** http://www.stkate.edu/mnethx
Karen G. Gervais, PhD, Dir.

**Activities/Fields:** Diverse faith and cultural perspectives, end-of-life decision making, health care reform, emerging technologies. **Pub:** *Ethical Challenges in Managed Care: A Casebook.* • *A Role Playing Exercise in Managed Care Decision Making.*

**★ 2555 ★ Mount Sinai Hospital**
**Samuel Lunenfeld Research Institute**
600 University Ave.
Toronto, ON, Canada M5G 1X5
**Phone:** (416)586-4800      **Fax:** (416)586-8857
**Email:** pawson/rossant@mshri.on.ca
**Website:** http://www.mshri.on.ca
Dr. Tony Pawson, Interim Co-Dir.

**Activities/Fields:** Cancer biology, cell biology, clinical epidemiology, endocrinology, hemopoiesis, musculoskeletal diseases, bone mineral metabolism, genetics, developmental biology, immunology, perinatology, neurobiology, physiology, molecular biology, bioinformatics, proteomics, biochemistry, gastroenterology, respiratory research, and hearing research. **Pub:** *Annual Report.* • *Scientific Report*. **Frmly:** Mount Sinai Hospital Research Institute.

**★ 2556 ★ Mount Sinai School of Medicine of City University of New York**
**General Clinical Research Center**
1184 5th Ave., Box 1027
New York, NY 10029
**Phone:** (212)241-6045      **Fax:** (212)348-5811
**Website:** http://www.mssm.edu/gcrc/
Dr. Hugh A. Sampson, Prog. Dir.

**Activities/Fields:** Nature and treatment of human diseases through clinical investigation, including studies on Gaucher disease, Parkinson's disease, Fabry's disease, Alzheimer's disease, nutrition, energy expenditure, AIDS, lipid metabolism, peptide and steroid hormones, lead poisoning, and pediatric food allergy.

**★ 2557 ★ National Council for Reliable Health Information**
300 E Pink Hill Rd.
Independence, MO 64057
**Phone:** (816)228-4595      **Fax:** (816)228-4995
**Email:** drrenner@msn.com
Dr. John H. Renner, Pres.

**Activities/Fields:** Clinical medicine, health fraud and quakery, patient education, toxicology, history of medicine, medicine in art, and therapeutics. **Pub:** *Bulletin Board*, bimonthly. • *NCAHF Newsletter*, bimonthly. • *Position Papers.* • *Recommended Antiquackery Publications*. **Frmly:** National Council Against Health Fraud.

**★ 2558 ★ Nemours Foundation**
**Nemours Research Programs**
PO Box 269
Wilmington, DE 19899
**Phone:** (302)651-6819      **Fax:** (302)651-6810

**Activities/Fields:** Programs are composed of two research departments: the Department of Applied Science and Engineering, which applies technology to the development of communication, mobility, robotic, and therapeutic interactive devices to aid in independent living, education, and employment of disabled children; the Department of Clinical Science conducts medical research in the various fields of basic science as well as physician-directed projects with direct clinical applications. **Frmly:** Alfred I. DuPont Institute.

**★ 2559 ★ Neuro Immuno Therapeutic Research Foundation**
1092 Boiling Springs Rd.
Spartanburg, SC 29303
**Phone:** (864)591-0944      **Fax:** (864)591-0622
**Email:** nitrf@aol.com
**Website:** http://members.aol.com/nitrf
Dr. H. Hugh Fudenberg, Dir.

**Activities/Fields:** Immunology, Alzheimer's disease, AIDS, autism, and chronic fatigue syndrome. **Pub:** *Scientific Reference Journal*, occasionally. Journal.

**★ 2560 ★ New England Medical Center Hospitals, Inc.**
**Division of Clinical Care Research**
Box 63
750 Washington St.
Boston, MA 02111
**Phone:** (617)636-5009 **Fax:** (617)636-8023
**Email:** hselker@lifespan.org
**Website:** http://www.nemc.org/dccr
Harry P. Selker, MD, Ch.

**Activities/Fields:** Ongoing research programs in clinical trials in emergency room based cardiovascular health services research, mathematical modeling and statistics, meta-analysis and other evidence-based research methodologies. **Frmly:** Center for Health Services Research and Study Design.

**★ 2561 ★ New England Medical Center Hospitals, Inc.**
**General Clinical Research Center**
Box 831
750 Washington Ave.
Boston, MA 02111
**Phone:** (617)636-6149 **Fax:** (617)636-8397
**Email:** dj.greenblatt@tufts.edu
**Website:** http://www.nemc.org/gcrc/gcrc.htm
Dr. David Greenblatt, Prog. Dir.

**Activities/Fields:** Biomedicine, including endocrinology and metabolism, hematology, neurology, nutrition, oncology, immunology, and infectious disease.

**★ 2562 ★ New Mexico Clinical Research and Osteoporosis Center**
300 Oak NE
Albuquerque, NM 87106
**Phone:** (505)855-5505 **Fax:** (505)855-5506
**Email:** medsitenm@aol.com
**Website:** http://www.nmbonecare.com
Lance Rudolph, MD, Dir.

**Activities/Fields:** Health care quality, health promotion, clinical research, and continuing medical education. **Pub:** *Newsletter*, quarterly. **Frmly:** New Mexico Medical Group; Research and Education Foundation.

**★ 2563 ★ New York University**
**General Clinical Research Center**
New York University Medical Center
550 1st Ave., New Bellevue 8E, Rm. 36
New York, NY 10016
**Phone:** (212)263-6479 **Fax:** (212)263-8501
**Email:** romw01@med.nyu.edu
**Website:** http://gcrc.med.nyu.edu/gcrc/
Dr. William N. Rom, Dir.

**Activities/Fields:** The unit is a hospital within a hospital that allows investigators to observe patients for extended lengths of time. Projects include studies in endocrinology and metabolism, rheumatology, immunology, genetics, hypertension, hematology, neurology, neurosurgery, respiratory medicine, and infectious diseases. Focuses on cancer, AIDS, and tuberculosis research. Maintains a nursing staff and laboratories to facilitate research.

**★ 2564 ★ North Carolina State University**
**North Carolina Ergonomics Resource Center (NCERC)**
703 Tucker St.
Raleigh, NC 27603
**Phone:** (919)515-2052
**Email:** goehring@ncerc.com
**Website:** http://www.ncerc.com/
Anita R. Goehringer, MS, Exec. Dir.

**Activities/Fields:** Ergonomic deficiencies in the workplace.

**★ 2565 ★ Northern California Institute for Research and Education (NCIRE)**
4150 Clement St. (151NC)
San Francisco, CA 94121-1545
**Phone:** (415)750-6954 **Fax:** (415)750-9358

**Email:** askncire@ncire.org
**Website:** http://www.ncire.org/
Jack Nagan, CEO
**Activities/Fields:** New medical treatments and procedures, new drugs, rehabilitation, health services delivery, geriatrics, etc.

**★ 2566 ★ Northwestern University**
**Center for Sleep and Circadian Biology**
Department of Neurobiology & Physiology
2153 N Campus Dr., Hogan 2-160
Evanston, IL 60208
**Phone:** (847)491-2865 **Fax:** (847)467-4065
**Email:** fturek@northwestern.edu
**Website:** http://www.northwestern.edu/cscb/
Fred W. Turek, Dir.

**Activities/Fields:** Circadian rhythms and sleep, including the elucidation of the fundamental mechanisms that underlie circadian dysfunctional for human health, safety and productivity and development of treatments to alleviate symptons of circadian dysfunction. **Frmly:** Center for Circadian Biology and Medicine.

**★ 2567 ★ Northwestern University**
**General Clinical Research Center**
10E Feinberg
Northwestern Memorial Hospital
251 E Huron St.
Chicago, IL 60611
**Phone:** (312)503-2539 **Fax:** (312)926-8450
**Email:** wlowe@northwestern.edu
William L. Lowe, Jr., Prog. Dir.

**Activities/Fields:** Diabetes insipidus, malabsorption in AIDS, cardiac arrhythmias, effects of diabetes on pregnancy, pituitary tumors, tumoral calcinosis, gastrointestinal malabsorption of carbohydrates and other nutrients, monoclonal antibodies in diagnosis and therapy of cancer, and Phase I and II drug trials. **Pub:** *Annual Report*.

**★ 2568 ★ Ohio State University**
**General Clinical Research Center**
200 Meiling Hall
370 W 9th Ave.
Columbus, OH 43210
**Phone:** (614)292-1200
**Email:** sanfilippo.5@osu.edu
Dr. Fred Sanfilippo, Sr. VP

**Activities/Fields:** Diabetes, heart disease, endocrine and metabolic disorders, nutrition, neuroendocrine tumors, osteoporosis, cancer, eating disorders, affective disorders and depression, and renal disease.

**★ 2569 ★ Olive View-UCLA Education and Research Institute, Inc.**
Research Administration Office
14445 Olive View Dr.
Sylmar, CA 91342-1438
**Phone:** (818)364-3434 **Fax:** (818)364-3465
**Email:** denisetritt@ix.netcom.com
Denise Tritt, Bus. Mgr.

**Activities/Fields:** Perinatal issues, dopamine and alcoholics, genetics, AIDS, pneumonia, and diabetics (including foot infection).

**★ 2570 ★ Oregon Health and Science University**
**General Clinical Research Center**
3181 SW Sam Jackson Pk. Rd., CR107
Portland, OR 97201-3098
**Phone:** (503)494-7601 **Fax:** (503)494-0165
**Email:** pillowe@ohsu.edu
**Website:** http://www.ohsu.edu/gcrc/
Eric Orwoll, MD, Prog. Dir.

**Activities/Fields:** Cardiovascular disease, collagen vascular disease and immunology, endocrinology, hematology, hypertension, metabolism, neurology, oncology, pediatric nephrology, pharmacology, psychiatry, renal disease, and rheumatology. Testing services

include steroid receptor analysis, membrane receptor analysis, radioimmunoassay, and spectrophotometric analyses.

**★ 2571 ★ Ottawa Hospital**
**Ottawa Health Research Institute**
725 Parkdale Ave.
Ottawa, ON, Canada K1Y 4E9
**Phone:** (613)761-4395 **Fax:** (613)761-4920
**Email:** rworton@ohri.ca
**Website:** http://www.ohri.ca
Dr. Ronald Worton, CEO/Sci. Dir.

**Activities/Fields:** Neurosciences, clinical epidemiology, growth hormone development, diabetes, cancer, genetics, thyroid disease, molecular medicine, and diseases of ageing. **Frmly:** Loeb Health Research Institute.

**★ 2572 ★ Pacific Health Research Institute**
Thomas Sq. Ctr.
846 S Hotel St., Ste. 303
Honolulu, HI 96813
**Phone:** (808)524-4411 **Fax:** (808)524-5559
**Email:** vshamba@phri.hawaii-health.com
**Website:** http://www.phrihawaii.org
Dr. J. David Curb, CEO/Med. Dir.

**Activities/Fields:** Health services and clinical research, including breast cancer, hypertension, osteoporosis, diabetes, heart attacks, drug studies, effects of chemical exposure, and cost-effectiveness analysis. Specific studies focus on risk factors associated with breast cancer, methods of delaying or preventing postmenopausal osteoporosis, isolated systolic hypertension among the elderly, outcomes research, leprosy, interactive videodiscs, geriatrics, and prostate, lung, colorectal, and ovarian cancer screening. Participates in a statewide consortium of hospitals to address quality and cost of care. Hawaii MEDTEP (Medical Treatment Effectiveness Program) Research Center, outcomes research with a focus on minority populations. **Frmly:** Straub Medical Research Institute.

**★ 2573 ★ Pennsylvania State University**
**Doctors Kienle Center for Humanistic Medicine**
Milton S Hershey Medical Center
500 University Dr.
Hershey, PA 17033-0850
**Phone:** (717)531-8592 **Fax:** (717)566-8593
**Email:** dhufford@psu.edu
David J. Hufford, PhD, Dir.

**Activities/Fields:** Developing programs in humanistic medicine, including medical curriculum concerning the patients experience of care, phenomonology of care, and human diversity and medicine.

**★ 2574 ★ Pennsylvania State University**
**General Clinical Research Center**
Milton S Hershey Medical Center
500 University Dr.
PO Box 850
Hershey, PA 17033
**Phone:** (717)531-5154 **Free:** 800-336-2591
**Fax:** (717)531-1792
**Email:** lsinoway@psu.edu
**Website:** http://www.hmc.psu.edu/gcrc
Lawrence I. Sinoway, MD, Prog. Dir.

**Activities/Fields:** Major areas of investigation include cardiovascular metabolic responses, diabetes and metabolism, gastrointestinal research, pediatric metabolism, pulmonary metabolic responses, sleep-related metabolic responses and women's health.

**★ 2575 ★ Pennsylvania State University**
**Motor Control Laboratory**
Recreational Bldg., 20
State College, PA 16801
**Phone:** (814)863-4424 **Fax:** (814)863-4424
**Email:** mll11@psu.edu

**Website:** http://www.personal.psu.edu/faculty/m/l/mll11/mcl.html
Prof. Mark L. Latash, PhD, Dir.
**Activities/Fields:** Multi-joint limb movements, postural control, multi-limb coordination; changes in movement and posture coordination with age; and neurological disorders. **Pub:** *Refereed publications.*

**★ 2576 ★ Pennsylvania State University**
**Noll Physiological Research Center**
**General Clinical Research Center (GCRC)**
112 Elmore Research Wing
University Park, PA 16802-6501
**Phone:** (814)865-4302          **Fax:** (814)865-0351
**Email:** gcrc@psu.edu
**Website:** http://www.gcrc.psu.edu/
Jan Ulbrecht, MD, Assoc. Prog. Dir.
**Activities/Fields:** Pathogenic mechanisms of disease and strategies for health promotion and disease prevention.

**★ 2577 ★ Polyclinic Associates**
22401 Foster-Winter Dr.
Southfield, MI 48075
**Phone:** (248)423-1481          **Fax:** (248)423-1482
**Email:** polyclinic@neastic.net
Dr. Claude Oster, CEO
**Activities/Fields:** Epidemiology of musculoskeletal pain, especially its neurochemical and metabolic and biochemical causes. Examines stress and other psychiatric components of pain, tests experimental groups for certain metabolic disorders such as porphyria and hypoglycemia, and conducts longitudinal studies for occupational hazards. After recognizing an individual's pain, the Institute seeks treatment of both its mental and physical causes through a team system utilizing specialists in pain management, physical medicine and rehabilitation, orthopedics, nursing, internal medicine, Rheumatology, neurology, neurosurgery, anesthesiology, psychiatry, and psychology, as necessary. **Frmly:** Pain Research and Control Institute; Institute for Pain Management.

**★ 2578 ★ Portland VA Research**
**Foundation, Inc.**
PO Box 69539
Portland, OR 97201-0539
**Phone:** (503)273-5228          **Fax:** (503)402-2866
**Email:** david.hickam@med.va.gov
David Hickam, MD, Pres.
**Activities/Fields:** Medicine and medical research.

**★ 2579 ★ Primate Foundation of Arizona**
PO Box 20027
Mesa, AZ 85277-0027
**Phone:** (480)832-3780          **Fax:** (480)830-7039
**Email:** jopfa@qwest.net
Jo Fritz, Prin. Investigator
**Activities/Fields:** Improvement in the captive management of chimpanzees. **Pub:** *Newsletter*, quarterly.

**★ 2580 ★ Providence Ambulatory Center**
5050 NE Hoyt St., Ste. 540
Portland, OR 97213
**Phone:** (503)215-6258          **Fax:** (503)215-6857
**Email:** dgilbert@providence.org
David N. Gilbert, MD, Dir.
**Activities/Fields:** Clinical and basic investigations in cancer immunology, cardiovascular diseases, infectious diseases, and diabetes and metabolism. **Pub:** *Annual Report.*

**★ 2581 ★ Public Responsibility in**
**Medicine and Research**
132 Boylston St., 4th Fl.
Boston, MA 02116
**Phone:** (617)423-4112          **Fax:** (617)423-1185
**Email:** info@primr.org
**Website:** http://www.primr.org
Joan Rachlin, Exec. Dir.

**Activities/Fields:** Medical research, focusing on education of public responsibility and regulation of research. **Pub:** *Conference proceedings.* • *Educational Materials.* • *IRB/IACUC Mailing Lists.*

**Purdue University**
**Botanical Center for Age-Related**
**Diseases**
*See:* Entry 3065

**★ 2582 ★ Rat Resource and Research**
**Center**
University of Missouri—Columbia
Columbia, MO 65211
**Phone:** (573)884-9469          **Fax:** (573)884-7521
**Email:** critserj@missouri.edu
**Website:** http://www.radil.missouri.edu/rrrc
John K. Critser, PhD, Prin. Investigator
**Activities/Fields:** Rats as animal models, particularly development of efficacious methods for nuclear transfer in the rat; development of efficient methods for genome resource banking and strain/stock reconstitution, including ovarian tissue preservation and transplantation in combination with artificial insemination with cryopreserved spermatozoa; and improved methods for health monitoring of rats using molecular diagnostics and environmental monitoring.

**★ 2583 ★ Research Institute of Palo Alto**
**Medical Foundation**
Ames Bldg.
795 El Camino Real
Palo Alto, CA 94301
**Phone:** (650)326-8120          **Fax:** (650)329-9114
**Email:** ohearnk@pamf.org
**Website:** http://www.pamf.org
Dr. Allen D. Cooper, Dir.
**Activities/Fields:** Clinical and general medical sciences, including immunology, infectious diseases, health services research, cardiac physiology, metabolism, atherosclerosis, and cancer cell biology. **Pub:** *News*, quarterly. **Frmly:** Palo Alto Medical Research Foundation.

**★ 2584 ★ Rockefeller University**
**General Clinical Research Center**
Rockefeller University Hospital
1230 York Ave.
Box 327
New York, NY 10021-6399
**Phone:** (212)327-7730          **Fax:** (212)327-7157
**Email:** kruegej@rockefeller.edu
**Website:** http://clinfo.rockefeller.edu
James G. Krueger, MD, Dir.
**Activities/Fields:** Chronic immune disorders, dermatology, gastrointestinal motility, lipid metabolism, metabolic disorders, medical biochemistry, cystic fibrostic, AIDS, tuberculosis, neurological disorders, and obesity and nutrition.

**★ 2585 ★ Rush Primary Care Institute**
**Center for Health Services Research**
Rush-Presbyterian-St. Luke's Medical Center
1653 W Congress Pky.
Chicago, IL 60612
**Phone:** (312)942-3576          **Fax:** (312)432-1915
**Email:** rpci@rush.edu
Dr. Whitney Addington, Dir.
**Activities/Fields:** Primary care, education, and community outreach.

**★ 2586 ★ Rutgers University**
**Institute for Health, Health Care Policy,**
**and Aging Research**
30 College Ave.
New Brunswick, NJ 08901-1293
**Phone:** (732)932-8413          **Fax:** (732)932-6872
**Email:** caboyer@rci.rutgers.edu
**Website:** http://www-ihhcpar.rutgers.edu/
Dr. David Mechanic, Dir.

**Activities/Fields:** Research divisions include and focus on the following activities: the Division of Health studies the impact of stress on emotional states and health and risk behaviors and how these latter factors influence the immune system and morbidity and mortality, and studies how stress and emotional states affect symptom appraisal and the decision to use health care; the Division of Health Care Policy analyzes the health and cost outcomes of the current allocation of health and resources, with emphasis on preventive care and chronic illnesses; analyses the evolution of managed care and its impact on patient outcomes, medical professions and utilization of services; examines trust relationships among consumers and physicians and managed care organizations; the Division on Aging measures income inequality, investigates the role of instrumental and social support as buffers against stress and chronic illness, and identifies predictors of poor self-assessments of health among the elderly; the AIDS Policy Research Group measures health care utilization and cost among patients with HIV illness; the Center for Research on the Organization and Financing of Care for the Severely Mentally Ill provides a structure for interdisciplinary research and training on mental health services and policy for persons with severe and persistent mental illness and examines the human services and family support systems that shape outcomes for patients and their families. Multi-investigator research teams work in the areas of successful community living, organization and financing incentives in treatment programs, service systems integration, and managed care and rationing; the Center for State Health Policy is a recent initiative established to create a formal capacity within the university for policy analysis, research, training, facilitation, and consultation on state health policy. The center informs, supports, and stimulates sound and creative state health policy in New Jersey and around the nation.

**★ 2587 ★ Sansum Medical Research**
**Institute**
2219 Bath St.
Santa Barbara, CA 93105
**Phone:** (805)682-7638          **Fax:** (805)682-3332
**Email:** ljovanovic@sansum.org
**Website:** http://www.sansum.org
Lois Jovanovic, MD, Dir.
**Activities/Fields:** Diabetes mellitus, immunology, cancer, gastrointestinal disorders and physiology.

**★ 2588 ★ Scripps Research Institute**
10550 N Torrey Pines Rd.
La Jolla, CA 92037
**Phone:** (858)784-1000          **Fax:** (858)784-9899
**Email:** info@scripps.edu
**Website:** http://www.scripps.edu
Richard A. Lerner, MD, Pres.
**Activities/Fields:** Immunology and immunopathology, biochemistry, cell biology, molecular biology, structural biology, oncology, autoimmune diseases, cardiopulmonary diseases, hematology, diabetes and endocrinology, virology, preclinical neuroscience, neuropharmacology, vascular biology, synthetic bioorganic chemistry, biocatalysis and protein design, plant biology, and synthetic and vaccine development. **Pub:** *Scientific Report.* **Frmly:** Research Institute of Scripps Clinic.

**★ 2589 ★ Scripps Research Institute**
**General Clinical Research Center**
10550 N Torrey Pines Rd., 311N
La Jolla, CA 92037
**Phone:** (858)554-2281          **Fax:** (858)554-2252
**Email:** fchisari@scripps.edu
**Website:** http://www.scripps.edu/mem/gcrc
Francis V. Chisari, MD, Prog. Dir.
**Activities/Fields:** Develops and evaluates new and experimental therapeutic procedures, including therapies for cancer, vascular disease, thrombotic disease, sleep disorders, multiple sclerosis, hepatitis, inflammatory bowel disease, asthma, alcoholism and depres-

sion, and autoimmune diseases such as rheumatoid arthritis and systemic lupus erythematosus.

**★ 2590 ★ Shute Medical Clinic**
367 Princess Ave.
London, ON, Canada N6B 2A7
**Phone:** (519)432-1884 **Fax:** (519)432-1886
**Email:** shutemedical@lweb.net
Dr. Julian Oates, Contact
**Activities/Fields:** Total approach to patient care, vitamin dosage response, use of vitamin E for burn treatment, and medicinal use of d-alpha tocopheryl in diabetes, stroke, angina, coronary artery diseases, and intermittent claudication and phlebitis.

**★ 2591 ★ Southern Illinois University at Carbondale**
**Center for Rural Health and Social Service Development (CRHSSD)**
Office of Economic & Regional Development, MC 6892
Carbondale, IL 62901-6892
**Phone:** (618)453-1262 **Fax:** (618)453-5040
**Email:** tessh@siu.edu
**Website:** http://www.siu.edu/~crhssd/
Tess D. Heiple, PhD, Dir.
**Activities/Fields:** Health care and social service issues that impact the lives and productivity of the citizens in the state and nation, including alternative service delivery systems and policy alternatives. Studies include rural primary health care, rural safety and health promotion, and rural environmental health.

**★ 2592 ★ Southwest Foundation for Biomedical Research**
**Southwest Regional Primate Research Center**
PO Box 760549
San Antonio, TX 78245-0549
**Phone:** (210)258-9885 **Fax:** (210)258-9883
**Email:** stardif@sfbr.org
**Website:** http://www.srprc.org
John L. VandeBerg, PhD, Dir.
**Activities/Fields:** Nonhuman primate models of human diseases, including common chronic diseases and infectious diseases; genetic and environmental effects on physiological processes and on susceptibility to specific diseases.

**★ 2593 ★ Stanford University**
**General Clinical Research Center**
300 Pasteur Dr., Unit H1
Stanford, CA 94305-5251
**Phone:** (650)729-6427 **Fax:** (650)725-1420
**Email:** brandy@stanford.edu
**Website:** http://www.stanford.edu/dept/gcrc
Branimir I. Sikic, MD, Prog. Dir.
**Activities/Fields:** Clinical research on nutrition, diabetes, growth hormone deficiencies and growth hormone therapies, oncology, monoclonal antibodies, lupus nephritis, epidermolysis bullosa, pharmokinetics of drugs, interferon, infectious diseases, human immunodeficiency virus (HIV), and sleep disorders; physiological and pathophysiological adaptations of prematurely born infants, critically ill term infants, and normal infants. Also focuses on computer modelling of pressure-limited mechanical ventilation, infant heme catabolism, modulation of circadian rhythmicity in preterm infants, treatment of perinatal infectious diseases such as neonatal herpes simplex infection and AIDS, markers of basement membrane disruption, late pulmonary sequelae of BPD, treatment of newborn skin, cystic fibrosis, and extra corporeal membrane oxygenation (ECMO).

**★ 2594 ★ Stanford University**
**Stanford Center for Narcolepsy Research**
Department of Psychiatry & Behavioral Sciences
Stanford University Medical Center/Sleep Research Center
701 B Welch Rd., Rm. 143
Palo Alto, CA 94304-5742
**Phone:** (650)725-6517 **Fax:** (650)725-4913
**Email:** mignot@stanford.edu
Dr. Emmanuel Mignot, Dir.
**Activities/Fields:** Narcolepsy, from pharmacological treatments for patients to isolating the genes.

**★ 2595 ★ State University of New York at Binghamton**
**Institute for Primary and Preventative Health Care**
Academic Bldg. B, Rm. 116
PO Box 6000
Binghamton, NY 13902-6000
**Phone:** (607)777-6086 **Fax:** (607)777-6162
**Email:** gdjames@binghamton.edu
**Website:** http://www.binghamton.edu/ipph/abou-tipph.html
Gary D. James, Dir.
**Activities/Fields:** Causes and consequences of health and disease; implementation, organization, and effectiveness of primary and preventative health care regimens.

**State University of New York at Binghamton**
**Roger L. Kresge Center for Nursing Research**
*See:* Entry 15783

**State University of New York at Buffalo**
**Infectious and Chronic Disease Center (ICDC)**
*See:* Entry 11877

**★ 2596 ★ State University of New York**
**Health Science Center at Brooklyn**
**Diabetes Diagnostic and Research Center**
Box 123
450 Clarkson Ave.
Brooklyn, NY 11203
**Phone:** (718)270-2813 **Fax:** (718)270-3240
**Email:** rjgenco@acsu.buffalo.edu
**Website:** http://research.sdm.buffalo.edu/
Dr. Marianne Banerji, Actg. Dir.
**Activities/Fields:** Diabetes, endocrinology, immunology and metabolism, nephrology, and carcinoid syndrome. **Frmly:** General Clinical Research Center.

**★ 2597 ★ State University of New York**
**Health Science Center at Stony Brook**
**Center for Photographic Images of Medicine and Health Care**
Media Services, Level 3, Rm. 044
Health Science Center
Stony Brook, NY 11794-8030
**Phone:** (631)444-3228 **Fax:** (631)444-6172
**Email:** kgebhart@uhmc.sunysb.edu
Kathleen Gebhart, Dir.
**Activities/Fields:** Houses 3,000 photographic images of medical practices. Activities include searching historical records and archives for additional photographs. **Pub:** *Illustrated Catalog of the Slide Archive of Historical Medical Photographs at Stony Brook.*

**★ 2598 ★ State University of New York**
**Health Science Center at Stony Brook**
**General Clinical Research Center**
University Hospital, 12 South
Stony Brook, NY 11794
**Phone:** (631)444-6900 **Fax:** (631)444-6930
**Email:** marie.gelato@stonybrook.edu
**Website:** http://webster.gcrc.sanysb.edu
Marie C. Gelato, MD, Prog. Dir.
**Activities/Fields:** Major areas of investigation include aging, diabetes, Dupuytren Disease, Lyme Disease, metabolism, osteoporosis, psychiatry and renal failure.

**★ 2599 ★ State University of New York**
**Upstate Medical University at Syracuse**
**Clinical Research Unit**
University Hospital
750 E Adams St., Rm. 8602
Syracuse, NY 13210-2375
**Phone:** (315)464-9000 **Fax:** (315)464-9002
**Email:** mosesa@upstate.edu
**Website:** http://www.hscsyr.edu
Arnold M. Moses, MD, Dir.
**Activities/Fields:** Endocrinology, gastroenterology, metabolism, nephrology, oncology, nutrition, and neurology.

**★ 2600 ★ Temple University**
**General Clinical Research Center**
3401 N Broad St.
Philadelphia, PA 19140
**Phone:** (215)707-3086 **Fax:** (215)707-1560
**Email:** gcrc@bm.temple.edu
Guenther Boden, MD, Prog. Dir.
**Activities/Fields:** Gastroenterology, cardiology, metabolism, nephrology, neurology, AIDS, pulmonary research, and social phobias.

**★ 2601 ★ Thomas Jefferson University**
**Center for Research in Medical Education and Health Care**
Jefferson Medical College
1025 Walnut St., Rm. 119
Philadelphia, PA 19107-5083
**Phone:** (215)955-8907 **Fax:** (215)923-6939
**Email:** daniel.louis@mail.tju.edu
**Website:** http://www.tju.edu/jmc/crmehc
Joseph S. Gonnella, MD, Dir.
**Activities/Fields:** Medical education process and factors affecting the quality of cost of health care. Medical education research focuses on the following areas: measurement of physician competence; long-term follow-up study of graduates; program evaluation; specialty choice; and refinement of evaluation methods. Health services research focuses on the concept and system of disease staging for classification of severity of illness, cost, and quality of care. **Pub:** *ABSTRACTS: Longitudinal Study of Medical Students and Graduates.* • *Annual Report.*

**★ 2602 ★ Torrey Pines Institute for Molecular Studies (TPIMS)**
3550 General Atomics Ct.
San Diego, CA 92121-1122
**Phone:** (858)455-3803 **Fax:** (858)455-3804
**Email:** houghten@tpims.org
**Website:** http://www.tpims.org/home.html
Richard A. Houghten, Pres.
**Activities/Fields:** Treatments for major medical conditions, including multiple sclerosis, AIDS, Alzheimer's disease, pain, heart disease, many types of cancer, and more.

**★ 2603 ★ Totts Gap Medical Research Laboratories, Inc.**
1430 Totts Gap Rd.
Bangor, PA 18013
**Phone:** (610)588-0572 **Fax:** (610)588-8452
**Email:** tottsgap@epix.net
Stewart Wolf, MD, Dir.
**Activities/Fields:** Neural regulation of visceral function, emphasizing current focus on the cardiovascular system. Specific projects involve the study of the mechanisms of cardiac arrhythmia and sudden death and other aspects of neurocardiology. **Frmly:** Stewart Wolf Medical Research Foundation.

**★ 2604 ★ U.S. Department of the Air Force**
**Wilford Hall USAF Medical Center**
**Clinical Investigation Facility**
ATTN: WHMC/MSR
1255 Wilford Hall Loop
Lackland AFB, TX 78236-5319
**Phone:** (210)292-7141 **Fax:** (210)292-6053
**Email:** willard.mollerstrom@59mdw.whmc.af.mil
Col. Willard Mollerstrom, Comdr.

**Activities/Fields:** Medical research includes biological, behavioral, and psychological studies. Investigative efforts have contributed to improved disease prevention, diagnosis, and treatment modalities, including: advances in the application of hyperbaric oxygen therapy in a variety of conditions; better biochemical characterization of disease leading to enhanced understanding of underlying mechanisms in a spectrum of non-cancer diseases; improved procedures for cancer chemo-, immuno-, radiotherapy, and surgical techniques; pioneer development of extracorporeal membrane oxygenation, high frequency ventilation, and organ transplantation techniques; and selection of improved dental procedures through critical evaluation of safety and effectiveness.

**★ 2605 ★ U.S. Department of Energy**
**Department of Energy Program Offices—**
  **Nuclear Energy, Science and**
  **Technology**
**Office of Science**
**((Office of High Energy and Nuclear**
  **Physics)**
**Division of High Energy Physics)**
19901 Germantown Rd.
Germantown, MD 20874
**Phone:** (301)903-3624 **Fax:** (301)903-2597
**Email:** john.ofallon@science.doe.gov
**Website:** http://doe-hep.hep.net/home.html
John R. O'Fallon, Dir.

**Activities/Fields:** Continuing research and development in the study of elementary particle physics, understanding both the experimental and theoretical consequences of this research.

**★ 2606 ★ U.S. Department of Energy**
**Department of Energy Program Offices—**
  **Nuclear Energy, Science and**
  **Technology**
**Office of Science**
**((Office of High Energy and Nuclear**
  **Physics)**
**Division of Nuclear Physics)**
19901 Germantown Rd., SC-23
Germantown, MD 20874-1290
**Phone:** (301)903-3613 **Fax:** (301)903-3833
**Email:** dennis.kovar@science.doe.gov
**Website:** http://www.sc.doe.gov/production/henp/np/index.html
Dennis Kovar, Dir.

**Activities/Fields:** Understanding the fundamental forces and particles of nature as manifested in nuclear matter.

**★ 2607 ★ U.S. Department of Health and**
  **Human Services**
**Academy for Educational Development**
**Center for Community-Based Health**
  **Strategies**
1825 Connecticut Ave., NW
Washington, DC 20009-5721
**Phone:** (202)884-8862 **Fax:** (202)884-8474
**Email:** fbeadle@aed.org
**Website:** http://www.healthstrategies.org
Frank Beadle de Palomo, Dir.

**Activities/Fields:** Needs assessment, intervention effectiveness, process evaluation.

**★ 2608 ★ U.S. Department of Health and**
  **Human Services**
**Agency for Health Care Policy and**
  **Research**
**Center for Outcomes and Effectiveness**
  **Research**
6010 Executive Blvd., Ste. 300
Rockville, MD 20852
**Phone:** (301)594-1485 **Fax:** (301)594-3211
**Email:** hhubbard@ahrq.gov
Heddy Hubbard, MD, Actg. Dir.

**Activities/Fields:** Awards grants and contracts for patient outcomes research and studies on practice variations, outcomes research methodologies, and other medical effectiveness research topics. Monitors the work of patient outcomes research teams and the MEDTEP research centers on minority populations.

**★ 2609 ★ U.S. Department of Health and**
  **Human Services**
**Food and Drug Administration**
**Office of Orphan Products Development**
5600 Fishers Ln.
HF-35
Rockville, MD 20857
**Phone:** (301)827-3666 **Fax:** (301)443-4915
**Email:** mhaffner@oc.fda.gov
**Website:** http://www.fda.gov/orphan/index.htm
Marlene E. Haffner, Dir.

**Activities/Fields:** Availability of orphan products. Orphan products are defined as drugs, biologics, medical devices, and foods for medical purposes which are indicated for a rare disease or condition (i.e., one affecting fewer than 200,000 people in the U.S.). Grants and contracts support clinical research intended to provide safety and efficacy data acceptable to the FDA which will either result in or substantiaily contribute to the approval of the products. **Pub:** *Request for Applications in the Federal Register*, annually.

**★ 2610 ★ U.S. Department of Health and**
  **Human Services**
**Food and Drug Administration**
**Office of Women's Health**
HF-8
Rm. 16-65
5600 Fishers Ln.
Rockville, MD 20857
**Phone:** (301)827-0350
**Website:** http://www.fda.gov/womens/

**Activities/Fields:** Funds research on women's health issues including breast and ovarian cancer, women and HIV, women and cardiovascular disease, osteoporosis, breast implant safety, the effects of estrogen, and on the safe and effective use of medications, therapeutic products, medical devices, food and cosmetics. Conducts intramural research on gender effects and regulatory science. Encourages industry to include women in their studies and promotes participation of women in clinical trials of FDA-regulated products. Encourages the analysis of clinical trial data for gender differences.

**★ 2611 ★ U.S. Department of Health and**
  **Human Services**
**National Cancer Institute**
**Macromolecular Crystallography**
  **Laboratory**
Bldg. 536, Rm. 5
PO Box B
Frederick, MD 21702-1201
**Phone:** (301)846-5036 **Fax:** (301)846-6128
**Email:** wlodawer@ncifcrf.gov
**Website:** http://mcl1.ncifcrf.gov/
Dr. Alexander Wlodawer, Dir.

**Activities/Fields:** Macromolecular crystallography and its applications.

**★ 2612 ★ U.S. Department of Health and**
  **Human Services**
**National Center for Chronic Disease**
  **Prevention and Health Promotion**
**Chronic Disease Control and Community**
  **Intervention Division**
1600 Clifton Rd. NE
Atlanta, GA 30333
**Phone:** (770)488-5403 **Fax:** (770)488-5971
**Email:** dvm0@cdc.gov
David McQueen, Assoc. Dir.

**Activities/Fields:** Chronic diseases, including maternal and child health, breast and cervical cancer, diabetes, smoking, adolescents and school health, AIDS and women, and reproductive health. **Pub:** *Chronic Disease Notes and Reports.*

**★ 2613 ★ U.S. Department of Health and**
  **Human Services**
**National Center for Health Statistics**
**Office of Vital and Health Statistics**
  **Systems**
**Health Care Statistics Division**
Presidential Bldg., Rm. 952
6525 Belcrest Rd.
Hyattsville, MD 20782
**Phone:** (301)458-4369 **Fax:** (301)458-4031
**Email:** ttm1@cdc.gov
Thomas McLemore, Dep. Dir.

**Activities/Fields:** Division's data collection and analysis program administers provider-based health care surveys, which monitor the nation's use of health care resources (including hospitals, nursing homes, and physicians). Specific areas of interest are health statistics, epidemiology, and health services research. Division comprised of branches for ambulatory care statistics, hospital care statistics, long-term care statistics, and technical services. **Pub:** *Vital and Health Statistics Report Series 13.*

**★ 2614 ★ U.S. Department of Health and**
  **Human Services**
**National Center for Health Statistics**
**Office of Vital and Health Statistics**
  **Systems**
**Health Examination Statistics Division**
6525 Belcrest Rd., Rm. 1000
Hyattsville, MD 20782
**Phone:** (301)436-7068 **Fax:** (301)436-5431
Clifford Johnson, Contact

**Activities/Fields:** Nutritional status for adults and children, growth and development of children, nominative or descriptive physiological data for children and adults, chronic disease in adults, and some environmental exposures. **Pub:** *Vital and Health Statistics Series II.*

**★ 2615 ★ U.S. Department of Health and**
  **Human Services**
**National Center for Health Statistics**
**Office of Vital and Health Statistics**
  **Systems**
**Health Interview Statistics Division**
6525 Belcrest Rd., Rm. 850
Hyattsville, MD 20782
**Phone:** (301)436-7085 **Fax:** (301)436-3484
**Email:** jgentleman@cdc.gov
Jane Gentleman, Dir.

**Activities/Fields:** Conducts the National Health Interview Survey (NHIS), a major data collection program of the National Center for Health Statistics. In accordance with the National Health Survey Act of 1956, NHIS provides continuing survey and special follow-up studies on major current health issues affecting the civilian noninstitutionalized population of the United States. NHIS data are obtained through personal interviews with household members conducted each week throughout the year in a probability sample of households; interviewing is performed by a staff employed by the Bureau of the Census. Specific activities involve collection and analysis of data concerning the incidence of acute illness and injuries, prevalence of chronic conditions and impairments, extent of disability, utilization of health care services, and other health-related topics. Data collected over a one-year period form the basis for the development of annual estimates of the health characteristics of the population and for the analysis of trends in those characteristics. Division comprises branches for Illness and Disability Statistics, Survey Planning and Development, Systems and Programming, and Utilization and Expenditures Statistics. **Pub:** *Advanced Data Reports.* • *Public use data files; peer-reviewed journal articles.* • *Vital and Health Statistics Series Reports.* **Frmly:** (2000) Health Interview Statistics Division.

**★ 2616 ★ U.S. Department of Health and Human Services**
**National Institutes of Health**
1 Center Dr., MSC 0148
Bethesda, MD 20892-0148
**Phone:** (301)496-4000
**Email:** rk25n@nih.gov
**Website:** http://www.nih.gov
Dr. Ruth Kirschstein, Act. Dir.

**Activities/Fields:** Principal medical research arm of the federal government, with a mission to improve the health of the nation by increasing understanding of the processes underlying human health and by acquiring new knowledge to help prevent, detect, diagnose, and treat disease. NIH accomplishes this mission by: supporting research in universities, medical schools, hospitals, and research institutions in this country and abroad; conducting research in its own laboratories and clinics; supporting training for promising young researchers; helping to develop and maintain research resources; identifying research findings that can be applied to the care of patients and helping to transfer such advances to the health care system; promoting effective ways to communicate biomedical information to scientists, health practitioners, and the public; and developing and recommending policies related to the conduct and support of biomedical research. To carry out these functions, NIH is organized into 17 research Institutes (National Cancer Institute; National Eye Institute; National Heart, Lung and Blood Institute; National Institute on Aging; National Institute on Alcohol Abuse and Alcoholism; National Institute of Allergy and Infectious Diseases; National Institute of Arthritis and Musculoskeletal and Skin Diseases; National Institute of Child Health and Human Development; National Institute on Deafness and Other Communication Disorders; National Institute of Dental and Craniofacial Research; National Institute of Diabetes and Digestive and Kidney Diseases; National Institute on Drug Abuse; National Institute of Environmental Health Sciences; National Institute of General Medical Sciences; National Institute of Mental Health; National Institute of Neurological Disorders and Stroke; National Institute of Nursing Research); two divisions (Computer Research and Technology, and Research Grants); National Center for Nursing Research; the Warren Grant Magnuson Clinical Center; the John E. Fogarty International Center for Advanced Study in the Health Sciences; the National Center for Research Resources; and the National Library of Medicine.

**★ 2617 ★ U.S. Department of Health and Human Services**
**National Institutes of Health**
**Fogarty International Center for Advanced Study in the Health Sciences**
NIH Bldg. 31-B2C29
31 Center Dr., MSC 2220
Bethesda, MD 20892-2220
**Phone:** (301)496-2075          **Fax:** (301)594-1211
**Email:** ficinfo@nih.gov
Irene Edwards, Info. Off.

**Activities/Fields:** Promotes international cooperation in biomedical and behavioral research through grants, fellowships, exchange awards, and int ernational agreements. **Pub:** *Directory of International Grants and Fellowships in the Health Sciences.*

**★ 2618 ★ U.S. Department of Health and Human Services**
**National Institutes of Health**
**Fogarty International Center for Advanced Study in the Health Sciences**
**Division of International Training and Research**
Bldg. 31, Rm. B2C39
31 Center Dr., MSC 2220
Bethesda, MD 20892
**Phone:** (301)496-1653          **Fax:** (301)402-0779
**Email:** kb16r@nih.gov
**Website:** http://www.nih.gov/fic/programs.html
Kenneth Bridbord, Dir.

**Activities/Fields:** Funds extramural research in order to enhance collaborative projects between U.S. principal investigators and non-U.S. principal investigators through research grants, fellowships, and training grants. Efforts are also made to foster scientific exchange between countries in all areas of biomedical and behavioral research.

**U.S. Department of Health and Human Services**
**National Institutes of Health**
**National Cancer Institute**
**Analytical Chemistry Laboratory**
*See:* Entry 10509

**U.S. Department of Health and Human Services**
**National Institutes of Health**
**National Cancer Institute**
**Protein Chemistry Laboratory**
*See:* Entry 10564

**★ 2619 ★ U.S. Department of Health and Human Services**
**National Institutes of Health**
**National Heart, Lung, Blood Institute**
**Laboratory of Biochemistry**
Bldg. 3, Rm. 222
3 Center Dr., MSC 0340
Bethesda, MD 20892
**Phone:** (301)496-2073
**Email:** bc50r@nih.gov
**Website:** http://www.nhlbi.nih.gov/labs/biochemistry/index.htm
Dr. Boon Chock, Ch.

**Activities/Fields:** Studies on the role of oxygen free radical mediated oxidation of enzymes in aging and various diseases (especially those involved in pulmonary dysfunction and arteriosclerosis); characterization of several bacterial selenoproteins, mechanism of biosynthesis of selenophosphate and 2-selenouridine including EPR studies; regulation of protein ubiquitinating proteins, formation and utilization of free radicals, and cytosolic calcium oscillation; biochemical studies of the HIV-1 protease.

**★ 2620 ★ U.S. Department of Health and Human Services**
**National Institutes of Health**
**National Heart, Lung, Blood Institute**
**Laboratory of Lymphocyte Biology**
Bldg. 10, Rm. 5D49
10 Center Dr., MSC 1586
Bethesda, MD 20892
**Phone:** (301)402-6786          **Fax:** (301)480-1792
**Email:** biererb@nih.gov
**Website:** http://www.nhlbi.nih.gov/labs/lymphocyte-bio/index.htm
Dr. Barbara Bierer, Dir.

**Activities/Fields:** Understanding of lymphocyte signal transduction and immune function.

**★ 2621 ★ U.S. Department of Health and Human Services**
**National Institutes of Health**
**National Heart, Lung, Blood Institute**
**Laboratory of Molecular Biology**
Bldg. 10, Rm. 7B14
10 Center Dr.
Bethesda, MD 20892
**Phone:** (301)496-5817
**Email:** finkelt@nhlbi.nih.gov
**Website:** http://www.nhlbi.nih.gov/labs/molecularbiology/index.htm
Dr. Toren Finkel, Ch.

**Activities/Fields:** Understanding the role of reactive oxygen species (ROS) as intracellular signaling molecules.

**★ 2622 ★ U.S. Department of Health and Human Services**
**National Institutes of Health**
**National Heart, Lung, Blood Institute**
**Laboratory of Molecular Immunology**
Bldg. 10, Rm. 7N244
10 Center. Dr.
Bethesda, MD 20892
**Phone:** (301)496-0098
**Email:** wl2w@nih.gov
**Website:** http://www.nhlbi.nih.gov/labs/molecularimmunology/index.htm
Dr. Warren Leonard, Ch.

**Activities/Fields:** T-cell activation process in normal and pathological states, including the elucidation of the interleukin-2 including the molecular regulation of the expression of its protein subunits.

**★ 2623 ★ U.S. Department of Health and Human Services**
**National Institutes of Health**
**National Heart, Lung, Blood Institute**
**Vascular Biology Branch**
Bldg. 10, 8C103
10 Center Dr.
Bethesda, MD 20892
**Phone:** (301)496-1518          **Fax:** (301)402-7560
**Email:** enabel@nih.gov
**Website:** http://www.nhlbi.nih.gov/labs/vascularbiology/index.htm
Dr. Elizabeth Nabel, Sci. Dir. of Clin. Res.

**Activities/Fields:** Pathophysiology of vascular diseases and novel therapeutics. Emphasis is on vessel wall biology and cell cycle regulation focusing on endothelial and smooth muscle cell biology.

**★ 2624 ★ U.S. Department of Health and Human Services**
**National Institutes of Health (NIH)**
**National Institute on Aging**
**Intramural Research Programs**
**(Molecular Dynamics Section)**
Gerontology Research Center
5600 Nathan Shock Dr.
Baltimore, MD 21224
**Phone:** (410)558-8168          **Fax:** (410)558-8173
**Email:** rifkindj@grc.nia.nih.gov
**Website:** http://www.grc.nia.nih.gov/branches/lcmb/mds/mds.htm
Joseph M. Rifkind, PhD, Ch.

**Activities/Fields:** Research on the interplay between structure dynamics and how these influence biological function.

**★ 2625 ★ U.S. Department of Health and Human Services**
**National Institutes of Health**
**National Institute of Child Health and Human Development**
**Division of Intramural Research**
**(Research Animal Management Branch)**
Bldg. 6, Rm. 434
Bethesda, MD 20892
**Phone:** (301)496-9733
**Email:** barthoj@mail.nih.gov
**Website:** http://dir2.nichd.nih.gov/labs/lab.php3?19
John Bartholomew, Hd.

**Activities/Fields:** Animal disease control programs, including diagnosis, therapy, and prevention of disease from animals to humans (zoonoses).


**★ 2626 ★ U.S. Department of Health and Human Services**
**National Institutes of Health**
**National Institute of Child Health and Human Development**
**Division of Intramural Research**
**(Laboratory of Physical and Structural Biology)**
12A/2041
Bethesda, MD 20892
**Phone:** (301)496-6561
**Email:** aparsegi@helix.nih.gov
**Website:** http://dir2.nichd.nih.gov/labs/lab.php3?16
V.A. Parsegian, Ch.

**Activities/Fields:** Aims to understand biological structures through the physical forces that animate them, in order to measure force vs. separation between molecules from all classes of bio-matter.


**★ 2627 ★ U.S. Department of Health and Human Services**
**National Institutes of Health**
**National Institute of Child Health and Human Development**
**Division of Intramural Research**
**(Laboratory of Integrative and Medical Biophysics)**
Bldg. 12A, Rm. 2001
Bethesda, MD 20892
**Phone:** (301)435-9233
**Email:** rjn@helix.nih.gov
**Website:** http://dir2.nichd.nih.gov/labs/lab.php3?11
Ralph Nossal, Ch.

**Activities/Fields:** Understanding basic biophysical mechanisms underlying cell and tissue function.


**★ 2628 ★ U.S. Department of Health and Human Services**
**National Institutes of Health**
**National Institute of Dental and Craniofacial Research**
**Division of Extramural Research**
**(Craniofacial Anomalies and Injury Branch)**
Bldg. 45, Rm. 4AN-24
45 Center Dr., MSC 6402
Bethesda, MD 20892-6402
**Phone:** (301)594-9898          **Fax:** (301)480-8318
**Email:** rochelle.small@nih.gov
**Website:** http://www.nidcr.nih.gov/research/extramural/cranio.asp
Rochelle K. Small, PhD, Actg. Ch.

**Activities/Fields:** Understanding the development of head, face, and neck and to identify genetic and environmental contributions to craniofacial anomalies including biology of tooth and bone.


**★ 2629 ★ U.S. Department of Health and Human Services**
**National Institutes of Health**
**National Institute of Diabetes and Digestive and Kidney Diseases**
**Division of Diabetes, Endocrinology, and Metabolic Diseases**
**(Developmental Biology Research Program)**
2 Democracy Plz., Rm. 6105
Bethesda, MD 20892
**Phone:** (301)594-8811
**Email:** satos@extra.niddk.nih.gov
**Website:** http://www.niddk.nih.gov/fund/program/A-Elist.htmdevelop
Sheryl Sato, PhD, Dir.

**Activities/Fields:** Understanding the signaling pathways and transcriptional programs underlying the formation of tissues and organs.


**★ 2630 ★ U.S. Department of Health and Human Services**
**National Institutes of Health**
**National Institute of Diabetes and Digestive and Kidney Diseases**
**Division of Diabetes, Endocrinology, and Metabolic Diseases**
**(Complications of Diabetes Program)**
2 Democracy Plz., Rm. 699
Bethesda, MD 20892
**Phone:** (301)594-0021
**Email:** linderb@extra.niddk.nih.gov
**Website:** http://www.niddk.nih.gov/fund/program/A-Elist.htmcomplications
Barbara Linder, MD, Dir.

**Activities/Fields:** Classical diabetic complications and the effect of diabetes on any organ system.


**★ 2631 ★ U.S. Department of Health and Human Services**
**National Institutes of Health**
**National Institute of Diabetes and Digestive and Kidney Diseases**
**Division of Diabetes, Endocrinology, and Metabolic Diseases**
**(Behavioral Research Program)**
2 Democracy Plz.
Bethesda, MD 20892
**Email:** garfields@extra.niddk.nih.gov
**Website:** http://www.niddk.nih.gov/fund/program/A-Elist.htmbehavioral
Sanford Garfield, Sr. Adv.

**Activities/Fields:** Individual, family, and community-based strategies aimed at prevention of diabetes and its complications through lifestyle modifications, education, and other behavioral interventions, particularly on development of culturally sensitive, lifestyle interventions to prevent or treat diabetes in diverse high-risk populations including African-Americans, Hispanic Americans, and Native Americans.


**★ 2632 ★ U.S. Department of Health and Human Services**
**National Institutes of Health**
**National Institute of Diabetes and Digestive and Kidney Diseases**
**Division of Digestive Diseases and Nutrition**
**(Clinical Nutrition Research Unit)**
MSC 5461
6707 Democracy Blvd.
45 Center Dr.
Bethesda, MD 20892
**Phone:** (301)594-8822          **Fax:** (301)480-3768
**Email:** hubbardv@extra.niddk.nih.gov
**Website:** http://www.niddk.nih.gov/fund/program/A-Elist.htmCNRU
Van S. Hubbard, MD, Dir.

**Activities/Fields:** Research, educational, and service activities focused on human nutrition in health and disease; serves as focal point for an interdisciplinary approach to clinical nutrition research and for the stimulation of research in areas such as improved nutritional support of acutely and chronically ill persons, assessment of nutritional status, effects of disease states on nutrient needs, and effects of changes in nutritional status on disease.


**★ 2633 ★ U.S. Department of Health and Human Services**
**National Institutes of Health**
**National Institute of Environmental Health Sciences**
**Division of Extramural Research and Training**
**(Program Analysis Branch)**
PO Box 12233
Research Triangle Park, NC 27709
**Phone:** (919)541-7752          **Fax:** (919)541-2843
**Email:** vanhout1@niehs.nih.gov
**Website:** http://www.niehs.nih.gov/dert/dertpab/pabmisn.htm
Dr. Bennett VanHouten, Ch.

**Activities/Fields:** Conducts long and short-term scientific analyses of grants portfolio; provides basis for priority setting, decision making, and strategic planning; develops methodologies to conduct impact analyses; identifies emerging emphasis areas for program development.


**★ 2634 ★ U.S. Department of Health and Human Services**
**National Institutes of Health**
**National Institute of Environmental Health Sciences**
**Laboratory of Signal Transduction**
**(Cell Biology Group)**
PO Box 12233
Research Triangle Park, NC 27709
**Phone:** (919)541-3873          **Fax:** (919)541-3385
**Email:** murphy1@niehs.nih.gov
**Website:** http://dir.niehs.nih.gov/dirlst/groups/murphy.htm
Dr. Elizabeth Murphy, Hd.

**Activities/Fields:** Stress induced alterations in signaling pathways and ionic homeostasis that induce protection and/or death.


**★ 2635 ★ U.S. Department of Health and Human Services**
**National Institutes of Health**
**National Institute of Environmental Health Sciences**
**Laboratory of Signal Transduction**
**(Receptor Tyrosine Kinsase Signaling and Regulation Group)**
PO Box 12233
Research Triangle Park, NC 27709
**Phone:** (919)541-3619          **Fax:** (919)541-1898
**Email:** obryan@niehs.nih.gov
**Website:** http://dir.niehs.nih.gov/dirlst/groups/o-bryan.htm
Dr. John P. O'Bryan, Hd.

**Activities/Fields:** Integration of signal transduction cascades by adaptor proteins, particularly those which modulate the function of receptor tyrosine kinases.


**★ 2636 ★ U.S. Department of Health and Human Services**
**National Institutes of Health**
**National Institute of Environmental Health Sciences**
**Laboratory of Signal Transduction**
**(Membrane Biophysics Group)**
PO Box 12233
Research Triangle Park, NC 27709
**Phone:** (919)541-0062          **Fax:** (919)541-1898
**Email:** armstro3@niehs.nih.gov

**Website:** http://dir.niehs.nih.gov/dirlst/groups/armstrong.htm
Dr. David L. Armstrong, Hd.

**Activities/Fields:** Patch clamp techniques; ion channel modulation at the molecular level.

**★ 2637 ★ U.S. Department of Health and Human Services**
**National Institutes of Health**
**National Institute of Environmental Health Sciences**
**Laboratory of Signal Transduction**
**(Studies in Polypeptide Hormone Action Group)**
PO Box 12233
Research Triangle Park, NC 27709
**Phone:** (919)541-4899 **Fax:** (919)541-4571
**Email:** black009@niehs.nih.gov
**Website:** http://dir.niehs.nih.gov/dirlst/groups/blackshear.htm
Dr. Perry J. Blackshear, MD, Hd.

**Activities/Fields:** Signal transduction mechanisms and intracellular responses to surface acting agonists, with particular emphasis on the PKC pathway and on rapid transcriptional responses.

**★ 2638 ★ U.S. Department of Health and Human Services**
**National Institutes of Health**
**National Institute of Environmental Health Sciences**
**Laboratory of Signal Transduction**
PO Box 12233
Research Triangle Park, NC 27709
**Phone:** (919)541-1564 **Fax:** (919)541-1367
**Email:** cidlowski@niehs.nih.gov
**Website:** http://dir.niehs.nih.gov/dirlst/
Dr. John Cidlowski, Ch.

**Activities/Fields:** Mechanisms by which environmental agents can affect physiological processes and cause pathological outcomes by disrupting signal transduction pathways.

**★ 2639 ★ U.S. Department of Health and Human Services**
**National Institutes of Health**
**National Institute of Environmental Health Sciences**
**Laboratory of Structural Biology**
**(Nuclear Magnetic Resonance Group)**
PO Box 12233
Research Triangle Park, NC 27709
**Phone:** (919)541-4879 **Fax:** (919)541-5707
**Email:** london@niehs.nih.gov
**Website:** http://dir.niehs.nih.gov/dirlsb/nmrhome.htm
Robert E. London, PhD, Prin. Investigator

**Activities/Fields:** Structural characterizations of adducts which form between chemicals of environmental or pharmacological interest, and macromolecular targets or model systems; studies of intracellular ions and development of methods to determine ion levels in cells; intracellular magnesium and its measurement.

**★ 2640 ★ U.S. Department of Health and Human Services**
**National Institutes of Health**
**National Institute of General Medical Sciences**
45 Center Dr., MSC 6200
Bethesda, MD 20892-6200
**Phone:** (301)594-2172 **Fax:** (301)402-0156
**Email:** cassmanm@nigms.nih.gov
**Website:** http://www.nigms.nih.gov/
Dr. Marvin Cassman, Dir.

**Activities/Fields:** Non-disease-targeted research and research training in the basic biomedical sciences; maintains no intramural (in-house) research. Program focuses on the areas of cell biology and biophysics; genetics and developmental biology; phamacology,

physiology, and biological chemistry; and minority opportunities in research. The Institute fosters multidisciplinary approaches to research and employs the full range of support mechanisms–research project grants, program-project grants, research center grants, research career development awards, awards to new investigators, and institutional and individual fellowships.

**★ 2641 ★ U.S. Department of Health and Human Services**
**National Institutes of Health**
**National Institute of Mental Health**
**Laboratory of Neurotoxicology**
**(Section on Analytical Biochemistry)**
10 Center Dr., Rm. 3D42
Bethesda, MD 20892-1262
**Phone:** (301)496-4022 **Fax:** (301)480-0198
**Email:** nimhinfo@nih.gov
**Website:** http://intramural.nimh.nih.gov/research/lnt/sab.html
Jeffrey A. Kowalak, PhD, Mgr.

**Activities/Fields:** Analytical methods for the characterization and quantification of bioactive components in physiological fluids and tissues.

**★ 2642 ★ U.S. Department of Health and Human Services**
**National Institutes of Health (NIH)**
**National Library of Medicine**
**National Center for Biotechnology Information**
**(Computational Biology Branch)**
Bldg. 45, Rm. 6AN12J
45 Center Dr., MSC 6510
Bethesda, MD 20892-6510
**Phone:** (301)435-5981 **Fax:** (301)480-2918
**Email:** landsman@ncbi.nlm.nih.gov
**Website:** http://www.ncbi.nlm.nih.gov/CBBresearch/
David Landsman, PhD, Ch.

**Activities/Fields:** Theoretical, analytical and applied approaches to a broad range of fundamental problems in molecular biology. **Pub:** *Papers.* • *Reports.*

**★ 2643 ★ U.S. Department of Health and Human Services**
**National Institutes of Health**
**Office of Dietary Supplements**
Bldg. 31, Rm. 1B29
31 Center Dr., MSC 2086
Bethesda, MD 20892-2086
**Phone:** (301)435-2920 **Fax:** (301)480-1845
**Email:** ods@nih.gov
**Website:** http://dietary-supplements.info.nih.gov/
Paul M. Coates, PhD, Dir.

**Activities/Fields:** Explore the role of dietary supplements to improve health care and promote scientific study of dietary supplements in maintaining health and preventing chronic disease. **Pub:** *Bibliography of Significant Advances in Dietary Supplements*, annually.

**★ 2644 ★ U.S. Department of Health and Human Services**
**National Institutes of Health**
**Office of Extramural Research**
NIH Bldg. 1, Rm. 144
1 Center Dr., Mail Stop 0152
Bethesda, MD 20892
**Phone:** (301)496-1096 **Fax:** (301)402-3469
**Email:** wendy_baldwin@nih.gov
**Website:** http://www.nih.gov/grants/oer.htm
Wendy Baldwin, PhD, Dep. Dir.

**Activities/Fields:** Administers the development and coordination of NIH policies and procedures for awarding funds in support of biomedical research, including policies for the conduct of biomedical and behavioral research involving human subjects or vertebrate animals; and provides policy guidance for the Research Grants Division.

**★ 2645 ★ U.S. Department of Health and Human Services**
**Public Health Service**
**Agency for Health Care Policy and Research**
Executive Office Center, Ste. 600
2101 E Jefferson St., Rm. 600
Rockville, MD 20852
**Phone:** (301)594-6662 **Free:** 800-358-9295
**Fax:** (301)594-2168
**Email:** info@ahrq.gov
**Website:** http://www.ahrq.gov
Dr. Carolyn M. Clancy, Actg. Dir.

**Activities/Fields:** Develops and disseminates research-based information to increase the scientific knowledge needed to enhance consumer and clinical decisionmaking, improve health care quality, and promote efficiency in the organization of public and private systems of health care delivery. Its programs evaluate the effectiveness of medical treatments and other health services and improve access to new scientific and technical information for health care practitioners, policymakers, administrators, insurers, researchers, educators, and consumers. AHRQ supports and conducts research and evaluation projects in eight areas: consumer choice; clinical improvement; health care cost, financing, and access; health information technology; outcomes and effectiveness of health care; health care organization and delivery; quality measurement and improvement; and technology assessment. **Frmly:** (2000) Agency for Health Care Policy and Research.

**★ 2646 ★ U.S. Department of Health and Human Services**
**Public Health Service**
**Agency for Health Care Policy and Research**
**Center for General Health Services Extramural Research**
Executive Office Center, Rm. 502
Rockville, MD 20852-4993
**Phone:** (301)594-1349 **Fax:** (301)594-2155
Linda Demlo, Actg. Dir.

**Activities/Fields:** Delivery of health care service in rural areas and frontier areas; and the health of low-income groups, minority groups, and the elderly. Emphasizes the effectiveness, efficiency, and quality of health care services; the outcomes of health care services and procedures; clinical practice, including primary care and practice-oriented research; health care technologies, facilities, and equipment; health care costs, productivity, and market forces; health promotion and disease prevention; health statistics and epidemiology; and medical liability. **Pub:** *proceedings.* • *Research reports.*

**★ 2647 ★ U.S. Department of Health and Human Services**
**Social Security Administration**
**Office of Research and Statistics**
**Division of RSDI Research Statistics**
Rm. 4-C 16, Operations Bldg.
6401 Security Blvd.
Baltimore, MD 21235
**Phone:** (410)965-0156 **Fax:** (410)966-3308
Barbara Lingg, Dir.

**Activities/Fields:** Preparation of statistical and analytical data pertaining to RSDI benefit provisions of Title II of the Social Security Act. **Frmly:** Division of RSD1 Research Statistics; (2001) Office of Research and Statistics; Division of RSDI Statistics and Evaluation Analysis.

**★ 2648 ★ U.S. Department of Health and Human Services**
**Warren Grant Magnuson Clinical Center**
NIH Bldg. 10
6100 Executive Blvd., Rm. 2C6-146
Bethesda, MD 20892
**Phone:** (301)496-2563 **Fax:** (301)402-2984

**Email:** jg21z@nih.gov
**Website:** http://www.cc.nih.gov
John I. Gallin, MD, Dir.

**Activities/Fields:** Designed to place patient care facilities close to research laboratories to promote the quick transfer of new findings of basic and clinical scientists to the treatment of patients. The Center provides high-quality patient care necessary for intramural clinical research conducted at the National Institutes of Health; performs research on methods and systems involved in patient care and study; disseminates information to professionals and to the public relevant to clinical investigation; develops and maintains training programs in the techniques and ethics of biomedical and clinical research; and interacts with scientists and physicians, nationally and internationally, on such mutual problems of clinical research as policy, education, ethics, and priorities. To be considered for admission to the Clinical Center, patients should be referred by their private physician and they can be admitted only if their medical condition meets the precise requirements of a specific research protocol. **Pub:** *Current Clinical Studies.* • *Medicine for the Public Booklets.* • *Patient Admission Procedures at NIH.*

### ★ 2649 ★ University of Alabama at Birmingham
**Pittman General Clinical Research Center**
619 19th St. S, 907 M
Birmingham, AL 35294-6909
**Phone:** (205)934-4852          **Fax:** (205)975-6616
**Email:** gcrc@uab.edu
**Website:** http://gcrc.hs.uab.edu
Larry W. Moreland, MD, Prog. Dir.

**Activities/Fields:** Patient care and laboratory support of clinical investigations for all departments and divisions of the Medical Center, including the Schools of Medicine and Dentistry. Studies are conducted on metabolism, cardiology, hematology, rheumatology, infectious diseases, virology, immunology, pulmonary medicine, renal medicine, gastroenterology, oncology, neurosurgery, AIDS, and the mechanisms of disease.

### ★ 2650 ★ University of Alaska Anchorage
**Institute for Circumpolar Health Studies (ICHS)**
3211 Providence Dr., Ste. DPL 530
Anchorage, AK 99508
**Phone:** (907)786-6575          **Fax:** (907)786-6576
**Email:** anbls@uaa.alaska.edu
**Website:** http://ichs.uaa.alaska.edu
Brian Saylor, Contact

**Activities/Fields:** Health problems and issues facing Alaskans and other populations in the circumpolar north, including epidemiologic studies of population health problems; studies of health services need, access and utilization; and evaluation of health policy and the effectiveness of new health programs.

### ★ 2651 ★ University of Alberta
**Centre for the Cross-Cultural Study of Health and Healing**
c/o 13-15 Tory Bldg.
Edmonton, AB, Canada T6G 2H4
**Phone:** (780)492-4008          **Fax:** (780)492-5273
Dr. Denise L. Spitzer, Co-Dir.

**Activities/Fields:** Multicultural health issues, including healing practices and efficacy of traditional healers, and developing a cross-cultural model for understanding similarities and differences among traditional healers; documentation and assessment of alternative healing practices; how societies deal with relationships among traditional, alternative and modern biomedicine; and programs which can best meet the needs of all Canadians, including aboriginals, established ethnic groups, and new immigrants.

### ★ 2652 ★ University of Alberta
**Centre for Health Promotion Studies**
5-10 University Extension Centre
8303-112 St.
Edmonton, AB, Canada T6G 2T4
**Phone:** (780)492-4039          **Fax:** (780)492-9579
**Email:** donna.richardson@ualberta.ca
**Website:** http://www.chps.ualberta.ca
Dr. Leah Achout, Dir.

**Activities/Fields:** Health promotion.

### ★ 2653 ★ University of Alberta
**Centre for Studies in Clinical Education (CSCE)**
3-48 Corbett Hall
Faculty of Rehabilitation Medicine
Edmonton, AB, Canada T6G 2G4
**Phone:** (780)492-2903          **Fax:** (780)492-1626
**Email:** vivien.hollis@ualberta.ca
**Website:** http://www.rehabmed.ualberta.ca/csce/
Vivien Hollis, PhD, Dir.

**Activities/Fields:** Clinical education, curriculum development, supervisor effectiveness.

### ★ 2654 ★ University of Arizona
**Native American Research and Training Center**
1642 E Helen
Tucson, AZ 85719
**Phone:** (520)621-5075          **Fax:** (520)621-9802
**Email:** lclore@u.arizona.edu
**Website:** http://www.ahsc.arizona.edu/nartc
Jennie R. Joe, PhD, Dir.

**Activities/Fields:** Health and rehabilitation of disabled and chronically ill Native Americans. Core areas include the following: needs assessment, service delivery, and evaluation as determined by or in cooperation with the tribal community and empowerment that is sensitive to Indian values and needs. Also studies the impact of government policy on the delivery of health care. Promotes self determination and parity among Native Americans in health and rehabilitation. Serves as a national resource for all North American tribes and Alaska natives. **Pub:** *Books.* • *Dual track videotapes.* • *Reports.*

**University of British Columbia**
**Centre for Community Health and Health Evaluation Research**
*See:* Entry 5816

### ★ 2655 ★ University of British Columbia
**G.F. Strong Research Laboratory for Medical Research**
Division of Infectious Diseases
2733 Heather St., Rm. 452, Fl. D
Vancouver, BC, Canada V5Z 3J5
**Phone:** (604)875-4588          **Fax:** (604)875-4013
**Email:** ethan@interchange.ubc.ca
**Website:** http://www.bcricwh.bc.ca/child-health
Dr. Reiner, Dir.

**Activities/Fields:** Infectious diseases, immunology, toxic shock syndrome, HIV/AIDS, host defense, macrophage cell regulation, tuberculosis, and leishmaniasis.

### ★ 2656 ★ University of British Columbia
**Institute of Health Promotion Research**
Library Processing Centre, Rm. 324
2206 East Mall
Vancouver, BC, Canada V6T 1Z3
**Phone:** (604)822-2258          **Fax:** (604)822-9210
**Email:** info@ihpr.ubc.ca
**Website:** http://www.ihpr.ubc.ca/aboutus.htm
C. James Frankish, Actg. Dir.

**Activities/Fields:** Social, behavioral, and environmental determinants of health and the factors that predispose, enable, and reinforce individual and collective actions in relation to these determinants. Research projects include policy analyses, epidemio-

logical study of social and behavioral causes of health and disease or injury, design and evaluation of innovative approaches to bring about change in these factors, and studies of the implementation and diffusion of these innovations by policymakers, institutions, agencies, communities, practitioners, and populations.

### ★ 2657 ★ University of British Columbia
**Jack Bell Research Centre**
Vancouver Hospital & Health Sciences Centre
2660 Oak St.
Vancouver, BC, Canada V6H 3Z6
**Phone:** (604)875-5840          **Fax:** (604)875-5684
**Email:** dmclean@vanhosp.bc.ca
Dr. David McLean, VP, Res.

**Activities/Fields:** Steroid hormone receptors, cancer chemotherapy, immunogenetics, kinases, micro-surgical procedures for repairing the bladder and urethra after an injury, and lung hazards in the work place and their effects on workers. Research also focuses on improving patient care, determining causes and treatments of diseases, detecting cancer at an early stage, and improving facilities for specialized surgery.

### ★ 2658 ★ University of California at Berkeley
**Center for Family and Community Health**
140 Warren Hall
Berkeley, CA 94720-7360
**Phone:** (510)643-7314          **Fax:** (510)643-5136
**Email:** ibt@uclink.berkeley.edu
**Website:** http://socrates.berkeley.edu/~sph/CFCH
Joel Moskowitz, PhD, Dir.

**Activities/Fields:** Health issues such as AIDS; breast, cervical and prostate cancer; cardiovascular disease; alcohol and tobacco use; and the geographic distribution of health problems.

### ★ 2659 ★ University of California, Davis
**Center for Neuroscience**
1544 Newton Ct.
Davis, CA 95616
**Phone:** (530)757-8708          **Fax:** (530)757-8827
**Email:** ejones@ucdavis.edu
**Website:** http://neuroscience.ucdavis.edu/
Edward G. Jones, PhD, Dir.

**Activities/Fields:** Single-cell recordings; neuronal populations in isolation; human perception, attention, memory, language; and the nature of consciousness.

### ★ 2660 ★ University of California, Los Angeles
**Center for Public Health and Disaster Relief (CPHDR)**
School of Public Health
10911 Weyburn Ave., Ste. 206
Los Angeles, CA 90024
**Phone:** (310)794-8064
**Website:** http://www.ph.ucla.edu/cphdr/
Steven J. Rottman, MD, Dir.

**Activities/Fields:** How natural and human generated disasters affect the public's health.

### ★ 2661 ★ University of California, Los Angeles
**Center for Sleep Research**
**Siegel Laboratory**
Neurobiology Research 151A3
Department of Psychiatry
North Hills, CA 91343
**Phone:** (818)891-7711
**Email:** jsiegel@ucla.edu
**Website:** http://www.bol.ucla.edu/~jsiegel/
Jerry Siegel, PhD, Contact

**Activities/Fields:** Evolution, function, and disorders of REM sleep.

**★ 2662 ★ University of California, Los Angeles**
**General Clinical Research Center**
27-066B CHS
Center for Health Sciences
10833 Le Conte Ave.
Los Angeles, CA 90095-1697
**Phone:** (310)794-9224          **Fax:** (310)206-9440
**Email:** isalusky@mednet.ucla.edu
**Website:** http://www.gcrc.medsch.ucla.edu
Isidro B. Salusky, MD, Prog. Dir.

**Activities/Fields:** Cardiovascular system, dermatology, endocrinology and metabolism, gastroenterology, genetic disease, gynecology, hematology, immunology and rheumatology, nephrology, neurology, oncology, and pulmonary physiology.

**★ 2663 ★ University of California, Los Angeles**
**Harbor-UCLA Medical Center**
**General Clinical Research Center**
1000 W Carson St.
Box 16
Torrance, CA 90509
**Phone:** (310)222-2503          **Fax:** (310)533-6297
**Email:** wang@gcrc.rei.edu
Dr. Christina Wang, MD, Prog. Dir.

**Activities/Fields:** Biomedicine, endocrinology, reproductive physiology, gastroenterology, genetics, immunology and infectious disease, nephrology, obstetrics and gynecology, labor and delivery, diabetes, metabolism, oncology, pediatrics, nutrition, psychiatry, neurology, AIDS research and neonatology.

**★ 2664 ★ University of California, San Diego**
**General Clinical Research Center**
UCSD Medical Center, 8203
200 W Arbor Dr.
San Diego, CA 92103-8203
**Phone:** (619)543-6180          **Fax:** (619)543-5536
**Email:** mziegler@ucsd.edu
**Website:** http://medicine.ucsd.edu/GCRC/
Michael G. Ziegler, MD, Dir.

**Activities/Fields:** Cardiovascular disease, endocrinology, gastroenterology, genetic disease, immunology, infectious disease, metabolism, neurological disease, oncology, pulmonary medicine, renal disease, reproductive endocrinology, rheumatology, hypertension, and gene therapy.

**★ 2665 ★ University of California, San Francisco**
**Cardiovascular Research Institute**
513 Parnassus Ave.
San Francisco, CA 94143-0130
**Phone:** (415)476-6174          **Fax:** (415)476-8173
**Email:** couglin@cvrimail.ucsf.edu
**Website:** http://cvri.ucsf.edu/default.html
Dr. Shaun R. Coughlin, Dir.

**Activities/Fields:** Physiology, biochemistry, pharmacology, cell biology, molecular biology, and immunology of the cardiovascular, pulmonary, respiratory, and renal systems; circulation, respiration, lung development, and metabolism of the fetus and newborn; membrane transduction systems; lipoprotein metabolism; growth factors and atherosclerosis; water and electrolyte transport; physical chemistry of contraction/relaxation of muscle; lung injury and repair; myocardial growth and development; macromolecular conformation; and mathematical analysis of biological systems.

**★ 2666 ★ University of California, San Francisco**
**General Clinical Research Center—Adults**
1202 Moffitt Hospital
505 Parnassus Ave.
San Francisco, CA 94143-0126
**Phone:** (415)476-9232          **Fax:** (415)476-0986
**Email:** tierneyc@gcrc.ucsf.edu

**Website:** http://www.gcrc.ucsf.edu
Joel Palefsky, MD, Prog. Dir.

**Activities/Fields:** Cardiovascular disease, hypertension, clinical pharmacology, lipid metabolism, nephrology, nutrition, oncology, acid-base physiology, dermatology, infectious diseases, reproductive endocrinology, AIDS, potassium metabolism, osteoporosis, recombinant human hemoglobin, liver disease, aging, psychopharmacology, hereditary fructose intolerance, gene theraphy, and wound healing.

**University of California, San Francisco**
**General Clinical Research Center—Children**
*See:* Entry 5817

**★ 2667 ★ University of California, San Francisco**
**Osher Center for Integrative Medicine (OCIM)**
1701 Divisadero St., Ste. 150
San Francisco, CA 94115-3010
**Phone:** (415)353-7700          **Fax:** (415)353-7711
**Email:** ocim@ocim.ucsf.edu
**Website:** http://www.ucsf.edu/ocim/
Susan Folkman, PhD, Dir.

**Activities/Fields:** Integrative medicine which seeks the most effective treatments for patients by combining non-traditional and traditional approaches that address all aspects of their health and wellness: biological, psychological, social, and spiritual.

**★ 2668 ★ University of Central Florida**
**Center for Discovery of Drugs and Diagnostics (CD3)**
12722 Research Pky.
Orlando, FL 32826-3227
**Phone:** (407)384-2818          **Fax:** (407)384-2062
**Email:** jgood@mail.ucf.edu
John Goodchild, PhD, Dir.

**Activities/Fields:** Molecular medicine, leading to the identification of new drugs and diagnostic procedures. Greatest emphasis is placed on preventing and treating diseases of most concern to the citizens of Florida.

**★ 2669 ★ University of Chicago**
**General Clinical Research Center**
MC 1027
5841 S Maryland Ave.
Chicago, IL 60637
**Phone:** (773)702-6980          **Fax:** (773)702-6952
**Email:** mfavus@medicine.bsd.uchicago.edu
**Website:** http://gcrc.bsd.uchicago.edu
Murray J. Favus, Dir.

**Activities/Fields:** Endocrinology, including insulin metabolism in health and disease, evaluation and treatment of hormonal disorders of growth and puberty, and polycystic ovary syndrome; psychiatry, including substance abuse; pharmacology; oncological research chemotherapies in the treatment of malignancies; investigations into human circadian rhythms; and genetics of diabetes, osteoporosis, and asthma.

**★ 2670 ★ University of Chicago**
**Institute for Mind and Biology**
940 E 57th St.
Chicago, IL 60637
**Phone:** (773)702-2579
**Email:** MKM1@midway.uchicago.edu
**Website:** http://socialpsy.uchicago.edu/imb.htm
Martha K. McClintock, Dir.

**Activities/Fields:** Relationship between the mind, the brain and the body in health and disease.

**★ 2671 ★ University of Cincinnati**
**Noyes-Giannestres Biomechanics Laboratories**
893 Engineering Research Center
Biomedical Engineering Department

College of Engineering
PO Box 210048
Cincinnati, OH 45221-0048
**Phone:** (513)556-4171          **Fax:** (513)556-4162
**Email:** david.butler@uc.edu
David L. Butler, Contact

**Activities/Fields:** Promotes graduate student involvement in biomechanics research, including functional tissue engineering, human body dynamics, joint mechanics and kinematics, soft tissue mechanics, robotics, ergonomics, mechanical stresses in the work place, and sports medicine. **Frmly:** Center for Biomechanics Studies and Research.

**★ 2672 ★ University of Colorado**
**Center for Human Nutrition**
CB C225
4200 E 9th
Denver, CO 80262
**Phone:** (303)315-4084
**Email:** james.hill@uchsc.edu
**Website:** http://www.uchsc.edu/nutrition/cnru.htm
James O. Hill, PhD, Dir.

**Activities/Fields:** Obesity and diabetes, developmental aspects of nutrient utilization and function, and micronutrient absorption and bioavailability.

**★ 2673 ★ University of Colorado**
**General Clinical Research Center—Adults**
Health Science Center
4200 E 9th Ave., B-141
Denver, CO 80262
**Phone:** (303)372-8799          **Fax:** (303)372-5866
**Email:** robert.eckel@uchsc.edu
**Website:** http://www.uchsc.edu/gcrc
Robert H. Eckel, MD, Prog. Dir.

**Activities/Fields:** Cardiovascular disease, connective tissue disease, dermatology, endocrinology, gastroenterology, hematology, immunology, metabolism and nutrition, nephrology, neurology, oncology, psychiatry, and pulmonary disease.

**★ 2674 ★ University of Connecticut**
**Center for Health Fitness**
359 Mansfield Rd., Rm. 105
Storrs, CT 06269-2034
**Phone:** (860)486-2763          **Fax:** (860)486-2776
**Email:** camaione@uconn.edu
Dr. David N. Camaione, Dir.

**Activities/Fields:** Biophysical and social sciences, including the complex interaction between physiology and behavioral responses related to physical activity and health. **Pub:** *Brochures.* • *Newsletters.*

**★ 2675 ★ University of Connecticut Health Center**
**Center for Biomaterials**
MC 1615
263 Farmington Ave.
Farmington, CT 06030-1615
**Phone:** (860)679-3743          **Fax:** (860)679-1370
**Email:** goldberg@nso1.uchc.edu
**Website:** http://it.uchc.edu/biomaterials/General.html
A. Jon Goldberg, Dir.

**Activities/Fields:** Structure, properties, and function of biomaterials, especially material-tissue interfacial behavior for use in restoration, reconstruction, biosensors, and drug delivery systems in the areas of orthopedics, endocrinology, prosthodontics, restorative dentistry, oral surgery, surgery, orthodontics, endodontics and pharmacology.

**★ 2676 ★ University of Connecticut Health Center**
**General Clinical Research Center**
263 Farmington Ave.
Farmington, CT 06030-3805
**Phone:** (860)679-4145          **Fax:** (860)679-1454
**Email:** raisz@nso.uchc.edu
Dr. Lawrence G. Raisz, Prog. Dir.

**Activities/Fields:** Major areas of investigation include asthma, cardiology, diabetes, endocrinology, genetic diseases, obstetrics and gynecology, oncology, pediatrics, psychiatry and rheumatology.

## ★ 2677 ★ University of Florida
### Center for Research on Women's Health
Box 100171
Gainesville, FL 32610-0171
**Phone:** (352)392-9000     **Fax:** (352)392-9018
**Email:** crwh@vpha.health.ufl.edu
**Website:** http://www.medinfo.ufl.edu/other/crwh/
Leslie Sue Lieberman, PhD, Exec. Dir.

**Activities/Fields:** Women's health and disease processes.

## ★ 2678 ★ University of Florida
### Florida Center for Health Promotion
PO Box 118211, FLG-23
Gainesville, FL 32611-8211
**Phone:** (352)392-0583     **Fax:** (352)392-1909
**Email:** hse@hhp.ufl.edu
**Website:**     http://www.hhp.ufl.edu/hse/main/flcntrhp.htm
W. William Chen, PhD, Dir.

**Activities/Fields:** Health promotion strategies for racial, ethnic and cultural groups of all ages.

## ★ 2679 ★ University of Florida
### General Clinical Research Center
1600 SW Archer Rd.
PO Box 100322
Gainesville, FL 32610-0322
**Phone:** (352)265-8909     **Fax:** (352)265-8910
**Email:** stacpool@gcrc.ufl.edu
**Website:** http://www.gcrc.ufl.edu
Dr. Peter W. Stacpoole, Prog. Dir.

**Activities/Fields:** Allergy, immunology, rheumatology, cardiology, endocrinology, gastroenterology, hematology, metabolism, obstetrics and gynecology, oncology, and surgery.

## ★ 2680 ★ University of Florida
### Health Science Center-Jacksonville
### Office for Research Affairs
653 1 W 8th St.
Jacksonville, FL 32209
**Phone:** (904)244-6693     **Fax:** (904)244-6844
**Email:** paula.fuqua@jax.ufl.edu
Paula S. Fuqua, Dir.

**Activities/Fields:** Clinical medicine, including cardiology, obstetrics and gynecology, pediatrics, gastroenterology, hematology/oncology, nephrology, neurology, and fetal medicine.

## ★ 2681 ★ University of Georgia
### Resource Center for Biomedical Complex Carbohydrates
Complex Carbohydrate Research Center
220 Riverbend Rd.
Athens, GA 30602-4712
**Phone:** (706)542-4404     **Fax:** (706)542-4412
**Email:** palbersh@ccrc.uga.edu
**Website:** http://www.ccrc.uga.edu/
Dr. Peter Albersheim, Prin. Investigator

**Activities/Fields:** Characterization of complex carbohydrates.

## ★ 2682 ★ University of Houston
### Biological Clocks Program
Department of Biology and Biochemistry
Houston, TX 77204-5513
**Phone:** (713)743-2652     **Fax:** (713)743-2636
**Email:** phardin@uh.edu
**Website:** http://www.bchs.uh.edu/research/clocks/
Prof. Paul Hardin, Contact

**Activities/Fields:** Cellular and molecular clock mechanisms in animal nervous systems, including behavioral, physiological, biochemical, genetic, and molecular studies of invertebrates and vertebrates.

## ★ 2683 ★ University of Illinois
### Health Systems Research
College of Medicine
1601 Parkview Ave.
Rockford, IL 61107
**Phone:** (815)395-5639     **Fax:** (815)395-5602
**Email:** joelc@uic.edu
Joel B. Cowen, Asst. Dean

**Activities/Fields:** Community health, including primary care, public health, geriatrics, substance abuse, evaluation of delivery of health services, survey research, focus groups, demographic studies, health care planning, program evaluation, and feasibility studies.

## ★ 2684 ★ University of Illinois at Chicago
### Center for Health Services Research
MC 922
2121 W Taylor St., Rm. 211
Chicago, IL 60612-7260
**Phone:** (312)996-1047     **Fax:** (312)996-0065
Judith A. Cooksey, Dir.

**Activities/Fields:** New health care tehnologies, medical informatics, health manpower, observation unit medicine in the hospital emergency room, and performance of preventive through tertiary healthcare delivery at the systems, program, and specific intervention levels. Studies focus on access, appropriateness, acceptibility, cost, safety, availability, effectiveness, benefits, and overall quality of healthcare. Specific topics include clinical decision-making, health information management, psychological and social sciences, and public health policy analysis. **Frmly:** Center for Study of Patient Care and Community Health.

## ★ 2685 ★ University of Illinois at Chicago
### Center for Narcolepsy Research (CNR)
College of Nursing, M/C 802
845 S Damen Ave., Rm. 215
Chicago, IL 60612-7350
**Phone:** (312)996-5176     **Fax:** (312)996-7008
**Email:** narcolep@listserv.uic.edu
**Website:** http://www.uic.edu/depts/cnr/
Dr. Sharon L. Merritt, Dir.

**Activities/Fields:** Biobehavioral impact of narcolepsy, defined as excessive daytime sleepiness, on persons and their families.

## ★ 2686 ★ University of Illinois at Chicago
### Health Promotion and Disease Prevention Research Center (HPDPRC)
850 W Jackson Blvd., Ste. 400
Chicago, IL 60607
**Phone:** (312)996-1167     **Fax:** (312)996-2703
**Email:** slevy@uic.edu
Susan R. Levy, PhD, Dir.

**Activities/Fields:** Real-world effectiveness and dissemination of health promotion and disease prevention interventions.

## ★ 2687 ★ University of Illinois at Chicago
### Midwest Latino Health, Research, Training, and Policy Center (MLHRC)
Jane Addams College of Social Work
1640 W Roosevelt, Ste. 636
Chicago, IL 60608
**Phone:** (312)413-1952     **Fax:** (312)996-3212
**Email:** aida@uic.edu
**Website:**     http://www.uic.edu/jaddams/mlhrc/mlhrc.html
Aida L. Giachello, PhD, Dir.

**Activities/Fields:** Latino health and health services, in Chicago and throughout the Midwest region.

## ★ 2688 ★ University of Iowa
### General Clinical Research Center
157 Medical Research Facility
University of Iowa Hospitals
Iowa City, IA 52242
**Phone:** (319)384-8305     **Fax:** (319)384-8325
**Email:** william-haynes@uiowa.edu
**Website:** http://www.medicine.uiowa.edu/gcrc
William A. Haynes, MD, Prog. Dir.

**Activities/Fields:** Major areas of investigation include cardiology, clinical pharmacology, endocrinology, gastroenterology, infectious diseases, neonatology, nephrology, neurology, nutrition, oncology and hematology, opthalmology, orthopedics, otolaryngology, pediatrics, psychiatry, pulmonary diseases, rheumatology, urology and women's studies.

## ★ 2689 ★ University of Kentucky
### General Clinical Research Center
University of Kentucky Medical Center, Rm. MN578
800 Rose St.
Lexington, KY 40536-0293
**Phone:** (859)323-6623     **Fax:** (859)257-9560
**Email:** cwcrick@pop.uky.edu
**Website:** http://www.gcrc.uky.edu
Hartmut Malluche, MD, Prog. Dir.

**Activities/Fields:** Major areas of investigation include aging, behavioral science, cardiology and biomedical engineering, gastroenterology, infectious diseases, neurology, nutrition, obstetrics and gynecology, oncology, pharmacy, psychiatry, pulmonary disorders and renal diseases.

## ★ 2690 ★ University of Louisiana at Lafayette
### New Iberia Research Center
4401 W Admiral Dr.
New Iberia, LA 70560
**Phone:** (318)482-0225     **Fax:** (318)373-0057
**Email:** tjr7173@usl.edu
Dr. Thomas J. Rowell, Dir.

**Activities/Fields:** Human disease research, animal models development, and pharmacology/toxicology research.

## ★ 2691 ★ University of Manitoba
### Manitoba Centre for Health Policy and Evaluation (MCHPE)
Department of Community Health Sciences
Faculty of Medicine
S101-750 Bannatyne Ave.
Winnipeg, MB, Canada R3E 0W3
**Phone:** (204)789-3819     **Fax:** (204)789-3910
**Email:** c_black@umanitoba.ca
**Website:** http://www.umanitoba.ca/centres/mchpe/
Charlyn Black, Co-Dir.

**Activities/Fields:** How health care services are used by Manitobans. It examines patterns of illness in the population, and studies how people use health care services. It also researches the factors that affect health, since there is considerable evidence that many factors influence physical well-being, including income, education, employment, and social status, as well as nutrition, early childhood programs and even highway safety. **Pub:** Annual report. • Newsletter.

## ★ 2692 ★ University of Manitoba
### Northern Health Research Unit
Department of Community Health Sciences
750 Bannatyne Ave.
Winnipeg, MB, Canada R3E 0W3
**Phone:** (204)789-3250     **Fax:** (204)975-7783
**Email:** cahr@umanitoba.ca
**Website:** http://www.umanitoba.ca/centres/cahr
John D. O'Neil, Dir.

**Activities/Fields:** Problems relevant to the health of Aboriginal and northern peoples in Canada.

**★ 2693 ★ University of Maryland**
**Center for Fluorescence Spectroscopy**
**(CFS)**
Department of Biochemistry & Molecular Biology
School of Medicine
725 W Lombard St.
Baltimore, MD 21201
**Phone:** (410)706-8409 **Fax:** (410)706-8408
**Email:** lakowicz@cfs.umbi.umd.edu
**Website:** http://cfs.umbi.umd.edu/cfs/index.html
Joseph R. Lakowicz, PhD, Dir.

**Activities/Fields:** Development and application of advanced fluorescence concepts and measurements to biochemical questions, especially the use of fluorescence to quantify structural features of biological molecules.


**★ 2694 ★ University of Maryland**
**Women's Health Research Group (WHRG)**
Howard Hall, Rm. 100E
Department of Epidemiology & Preventive Medicine
660 W Redwood St.
Baltimore, MD 21201
**Phone:** (410)706-3251
**Email:** plangenb@epi.umaryland.edu
**Website:** http://medschool.umaryland.edu/womenshealth/
Patricia Langenberg, PhD, Dir.

**Activities/Fields:** Women's health issues, including menopause, hip fracture, breast cancer, osteoporosis, hormone replacement therapy, uterine fibroids, hysterectomy, caregiving, ovarian functioning, genetics, environmental toxins, health promotions, nutrition, and mental health.


**★ 2695 ★ University of Massachusetts**
**Lowell**
**Center for Chronic Disease Control**
**(CCDC)**
3 Solomont Way, Ste. 4
Lowell, MA 01854-5125
**Phone:** (978)934-4501 **Fax:** (978)934-3025
**Email:** robert.nicolosi@uml.edu
Dr. Robert J. Nicolosi, Dir.

**Activities/Fields:** Chronic diseases with a focus on the diagnosis, treatment and prevention of heart disease, cancer, and neurodegenerative diseases including Alzheimer's disease. Also develops, evaluates, and assesses whole foods and certain micro nutrients with medical benefits and conventional pharmaceuticals, and medical devices and procedures.


**★ 2696 ★ University of Medicine and**
**Dentistry of New Jersey**
**Robert Wood Johnson Medical School**
**Clinical Research Center**
One Robert Wood Johnson Pl.
PO Box 19
New Brunswick, NJ 08903-0019
**Phone:** (732)418-8479 **Fax:** (732)418-8480
**Email:** gottliab@umdnj.edu
**Website:** http://www.crctrials.org
Alice B. Gottlieb, PhD, Dir.

**Activities/Fields:** Immunology, dermatology, adult and pediatric clinical pharmacology, psoriasis.


**★ 2697 ★ University of Michigan**
**General Clinical Research Center**
University Hospital, A7119
PO Box 0108
Ann Arbor, MI 48109-0108
**Phone:** (734)936-8080 **Fax:** (734)936-4024
**Email:** jwiley@umich.edu
**Website:** http://www.med.umich-edu/gcrc/
Dr. John Wiley, Dir.

**Activities/Fields:** Multicategorical research program geared to research on humans in support of clinical studies at department or subspecialty sectional level throughout the Medical School and the Hospital.


**★ 2698 ★ University of Michigan**
**Protein Folding and Stability Research**
**Laboratory**
Institute of Gerontology
300 N Ingalls St., Rm. 947
Ann Arbor, MI 48109-2007
**Phone:** (734)936-2156 **Fax:** (734)936-2116
**Email:** arigafni@umich.edu
**Website:** http://www.umich.edu/~protein/
Dr. Ari Gafni, Prin. Investigator

**Activities/Fields:** Mechanisms of protein folding and stability.


**★ 2699 ★ University of Minnesota**
**General Clinical Research Center**
420 Delaware St. SE, MC 8504
Minneapolis, MN 55455
**Phone:** (612)626-0476 **Fax:** (612)626-2456
**Email:** gcrc@gcrc.umn.edu
**Website:** http://www.gcrc.med.umn.edu
Dr. David M. Brown, Prog. Dir.

**Activities/Fields:** Human disease, including normal and abnormal physiology and biochemistry in the human being, AIDS, cystic fibrosis, organ transplantation, human growth, carbohydrate metabolism, and a broad range of other medical areas.


**★ 2700 ★ University of Montreal**
**Research Centre, Hospital du Sacre-**
**Coeur**
5400 blvd. Gouin W
Montreal, QC, Canada H4J 1C5
**Phone:** (514)338-2172 **Fax:** (514)338-2694
**Email:** abastado@crhsc.umontreal.ca
**Website:** http://www.crhsc.umontreal.ca
Diane Abastado, Dir.

**Activities/Fields:** Biomedical modelling, pharmacology, and clinical studies of cardiac arrhythmias, with the aim of describing the spatial distribution of cardiac arrhythmias, their relationship to the nervous system, and their treatment by pharmacologic and noninvasive surgical methods. Centre also studies occupational respiratory diseases, biology of asthma, sleep disorders and neuropsychobiology, and molecular genetics of kidney diseases.


**★ 2701 ★ University of Montreal Health**
**Centre**
**Research Centre**
3850 Rue Saint-Urbain
Montreal, QC, Canada H2W 1T8
**Phone:** (514)890-8110 **Fax:** (514)412-7204
**Email:** hamet@umontreal.ca
Dr. Pavel Hamet, Dir.

**Activities/Fields:** AIDS, burns and after-effects, cancer and nutrition, cardiovascular diseases and hypertension, diabetes and nutrition, epidemiology, gastroenterology-heptology, hormone signaling and metabolism, imaging, immunology and host defense, medical genetics, respiratory electrophysiology, pulmonary diseases and anesthesia, gene and cellular therapy, including cardiovascular biochemistry, cellular biology of hypertension, experimental surgery, locomotion, microbiology, molecular endocrinology, gene medicine, molecular oncopathology, neurological sciences, nuclear medicine, oncology, pain and health research, clinical pharmacology and pharmacogenetics, pharmacoepidemiology and pharacoeconomics, population health and genetics, rheumatology, toxicology, and transplantation. **Frmly:** Montreal Research Centre, Hotel-Dieu.


**★ 2702 ★ University of New Mexico**
**Artificial Muscle Research Institute**
**(AMRI)**
School of Engineering
School of Medicine
Albuquerque, NM 87131
**Phone:** (505)277-3966 **Fax:** (505)277-1571
**Email:** amri@unm.edu
**Website:** http://www.unm.edu/~amri/
Dr. Mohsen Shahinpoor, Dir.

**Activities/Fields:** Electrically and chemically controlled artificial muscles.


**★ 2703 ★ University of New Mexico**
**General Clinical Research Center**
915 Camino de Salud NE
Albuquerque, NM 87131
**Phone:** (505)272-2366 **Fax:** (505)272-0266
**Email:** klegoza@salud.unm.edu
**Website:** http://www.unm.edu/~gcrc
Katherine M. Legoza, Prog. Mgr.

**Activities/Fields:** Diabetes, renal diseases, arthritis, premature infants, asthma, depression, hypertension. Provides inpatient, outpatient, and neonatal facilities (including laboratory, dietary, and nursing support) in support of clinical research.


**★ 2704 ★ University of North Carolina at**
**Chapel Hill**
**Cecil G. Sheps Center for Health**
**Services Research**
CB 7590
725 Airport Rd.
Chapel Hill, NC 27599-7590
**Phone:** (919)966-5011 **Fax:** (919)966-5764
**Email:** tim_carey@unc.edu
**Website:** http://www.shepscenter.unc.edu
Timothy S. Carey, MD, Dir.

**Activities/Fields:** Aging, disability, and long-term care; child health services; health care economics and finance; health care organization; medical practice; mental health and substance abuse services and systems research; health professions and primary care; preventive health services; rural health research; and women's health research. **Pub:** *Consensus in DHHS Region IV: Women and Infant Health Indicators for Planning and Evaluation.* • *North Carolina Health Professions Data Book.* • *North Carolina Health Professions Fact Sheet.*


**★ 2705 ★ University of North Carolina at**
**Chapel Hill**
**Center for Research on Chronic Illness**
**(CRCI)**
Carrington Hall, CB 7460
School of Nursing
Chapel Hill, NC 27599
**Phone:** (919)966-0453 **Fax:** (919)966-0456
**Email:** crci@unc.edu
**Website:** http://www.unc.edu/depts/crci/
Prof. Joanne S. Harrell, PhD, Dir.

**Activities/Fields:** Prevention and management of chronic illness in vulnerable people.


**★ 2706 ★ University of North Carolina at**
**Chapel Hill**
**Clinical Research Unit**
809 Ruggles Dr.
Raleigh, NC 27603
**Phone:** (919)733-5227 **Fax:** (919)733-5869
**Email:** jlieberman@med.unc.edu
**Website:** http://www.psychiatry.unc.edu/CRU/Cru.htm
Jeffery Lieberman, MD, Dir.

**Activities/Fields:** Schizophrenia, including but not limited to treatments dealing with first episode psychosis and treatment for refractory schizophrenia patients.


**★ 2707 ★ University of North Carolina at**
**Chapel Hill**
**General Clinical Research Center**
CB 7600, APCF
101 Manning Dr.
Chapel Hill, NC 27599-7600
**Phone:** (919)966-1435 **Fax:** (919)966-1576
**Email:** pbwatkins@med.unc.edu
**Website:** http://verne.med.unc.edu/home.html
Paul B. Watkins, MD, Dir.

**Activities/Fields:** Human physiology and pharmacology, including research on growth hormone, hemophilia, AIDS and other sexually transmitted diseases, stress and cardiovascular physiology, cystic fibrosis, drug metabolism and disposition in patients with hepatic and renal dysfunction, glomerular diseases, the neuropsychopharmacologic correlates of depression and other mental illnesses, cancer chemotherapy and immunotherapy, sickle cell anemia and related red blood cell diseases, and cardiac diseases such as congestive failure and arrhythmias.

## ★ 2708 ★ University of North Carolina at Chapel Hill
**Mutant Mouse Regional Resource Center**
221 Fordham Hall, CB 3280
Program in Molecular Biology & Biotechnology
Chapel Hill, NC 27599-3280
**Phone:** (919)962-2145          **Fax:** (919)962-4296
**Email:** tvdlab@med.unc.edu
Terry A. VanDyke, PhD, Prin. Investigator
**Activities/Fields:** Mouse models, especially in the areas of development and genomics, cardiovascular, and cancer; development of the ability to efficiently clone mice from somatic cells; development of reporter mouse strains that facilitate rapid phenotyping within particular cell/tissue types.

## ★ 2709 ★ University of Oklahoma
**Baboon Research Resources**
Division of Animal Resources
Health Sciences Center
940 SL. Young Blvd., BMSB 203
Oklahoma City, OK 73190
**Phone:** (405)271-5185          **Fax:** (405)271-2660
**Email:** gary-white@ouhsc.edu
Gary L. White, DVM, Prin. Investigator
**Activities/Fields:** Captive baboons.

## ★ 2710 ★ University of Oklahoma Health Sciences Center
**Center for American Indian Health Research**
College of Public Health
801 NE 13th St.
PO Box 26901
Oklahoma City, OK 73190
**Phone:** (405)271-3090
**Email:** chris-mcglory@ouhsc.edu
**Website:**                    http://w3.ouhsc.edu/coph/CophSub/CAIHRtxt.htm
Chris McGlory, Contact
**Activities/Fields:** Chronic disease, particularly diabetes and cardiovascular disease, health education and promotions, infectious disease, social/behavioral epidemiology, genetic disorders, molecular epidemiology, and injury epidemiology among Native Americans.

## ★ 2711 ★ University of Ottawa
**Ottawa Health Research Institute (OHRI)**
725 Parkdale Ave.
Ottawa, ON, Canada K1Y 4E9
**Phone:** (613)761-4395          **Fax:** (613)761-4920
**Email:** info@ohri.ca
**Website:** http://www.ohri.ca/
Dr. Ronald G. Worton, CEO/Sci. Dir.
**Activities/Fields:** Health and disease, particularly increasing understanding what is happening at the molecular and cellular level in complex disease states, and best practices in the delivery of health care.

## ★ 2712 ★ University of Pennsylvania
**Center for Bioethics**
3401 Market St., Ste. 320
Philadelphia, PA 19104-3308
**Phone:** (215)898-7136          **Fax:** (215)573-3036
**Email:** caplan@mail.med.upenn.edu
**Website:** http://www.med.upenn.edu/bioethics/center/index.html
Prof. Arthur Caplan, PhD, Dir.

**Activities/Fields:** Improvement in the practices and delivery of medical care. **Pub:** *PennBioethics*, semiannually.

## ★ 2713 ★ University of Pennsylvania
**Center for Human Appearance**
Medical Center
Penn Tower Hotel, 10th Fl.
3400 Spruce St.
Philadelphia, PA 19104
**Phone:** (215)662-7095          **Free:** 800-234-7366
**Fax:** (215)349-5895
**Email:** linton.whitaker@uphs.upenn.edu
Dr. Linton A. Whitaker, Dir.
**Activities/Fields:** Treatment of appearance-related problems, including reconstructive and cosmetic procedures to correct aesthetic and functional problems of the face, body, and extremities resulting from birth defects, traumatic injury, and diseases such as cancer and other tumors. The Center is divided into six patient treatment sections: craniofacial, to correct severe deformities of facial areas above the jaws; dentofacial, to correct dental and bone abnormalities of the lower portion of the face; interface, to improve variations in normal facial form; aging, to correct facial, body, and skin changes caused by the aging process; body contour, to improve the appearance of various areas of the body for both medical and cosmetic reasons; and self-image, to counsel patients with body image problems.

## University of Pennsylvania
**Center for Research on Reproduction and Women's Health**
*See:* Entry 18413

## ★ 2714 ★ University of Pennsylvania
**General Clinical Research Center**
160 Dulles Bldg.
3400 Spruce St.
Philadelphia, PA 19104-4283
**Phone:** (215)662-2641          **Fax:** (215)662-2643
**Email:** garret@spirit.gcrc.upenn.edu
**Website:** http://www.gcrc.upenn.edu/
Garret A. FitzGerald, MD, Dir.
**Activities/Fields:** AIDS, cardiovascular research, chemical senses, chronobiology and sleep, dermatology, endocrinology, gene therapy, metabolism, neonatal medicine, neurology, oncology, psychiatry, and women and minority health issues.

## ★ 2715 ★ University of Pittsburgh
**Center for Injury Research and Control (CIRCL)**
200 Lothrop St., Ste. B400-PUH
Pittsburgh, PA 15213
**Phone:** (412)648-2600          **Fax:** (412)648-8924
**Email:** circl@pitt.edu
**Website:** http://www.circl.pitt.edu
Dr. Donald W. Marion, Dir.
**Activities/Fields:** Understanding of injuries and the reduction of their occurrence, severity, and consequences, including traumatic brain injury and spinal cord injury. **Pub:** *Frontlines Newsletter*, quarterly.

## ★ 2716 ★ University of Pittsburgh
**Center for Nursing Research**
School of Nursing
3500 Victoria St., Rm. 360
Pittsburgh, PA 15261
**Phone:** (412)624-4854          **Fax:** (412)624-1201
**Email:** mek1@pitt.edu
**Website:** http://cnr.nursing.pitt.edu/
Prof. Mary E. Kerr, PhD, Dir.
**Activities/Fields:** Health care of individuals across the life span, including adolescent health, chronic disorders, critical care, and health care outcomes. **Pub:** *Newsletter*, quarterly.

## ★ 2717 ★ University of Pittsburgh
**Center for Research in Chronic Disorders (CRCD)**
460 Victoria Bldg.
School of Nursing
3500 Victoria St.
Pittsburgh, PA 15261
**Phone:** (412)624-7838          **Fax:** (412)624-1508
**Email:** crcd@pitt.edu
**Website:** http://crcd.nursing.pitt.edu/
Jaqueline Dunbar-Jacob, PhD, Dir.
**Activities/Fields:** Chronic disorders, with particular emphasis on quality of life, functional status, cognitive function, and adherence to treatment regimens as they are impacted by and impact management of those disorders. Additionally, the center is interested in the moderating effects of comorbid conditions and sociodemographic characteristics on these four outcomes.

## ★ 2718 ★ University of Pittsburgh
**General Clinical Research Center**
Montefiore University Hospital
200 Lothrop St.
Pittsburgh, PA 15213-2582
**Phone:** (412)648-6691          **Fax:** (412)648-6697
**Email:** branch@msx.dept-med.pitt.edu
Robert A. Branch, MD, Prog. Dir.
**Activities/Fields:** Cardiology, connective tissue disease, diabetes, endocrinology, hematology and oncology, hypertension, infectious disease, pulmonary physiology, nephrology, transplantation, behavioral medicine, psychiatry and women's health.

## ★ 2719 ★ University of Quebec
**National Institute for Scientific Research-Armand-Frappier Institute**
531 Blvd. des Prairies
Laval, QC, Canada H7V 1B7
**Phone:** (450)686-5010          **Fax:** (450)686-5501
**Email:** jean-guy.bisaillon@inrs-iaf.uquebec.ca
Jean-Guy Bisaillon, Contact
**Activities/Fields:** Human and animal health, including prevention of infectious diseases, virology, immunology, and applied microbiology; environmental health, including cancer epidemiology, biodegradation, professional diseases, and electromagnetism and cancer. **Pub:** *Annual report.* • *A Retrospect*, occasionally.

## ★ 2720 ★ University of Rochester
**General Clinical Research Center**
Strong Memorial Hospital, 4th Fl.
601 Elmwood Ave.
Rochester, NY 14642
**Phone:** (716)275-5295          **Fax:** (716)461-4737
**Email:** clinfomgr@cln1.medicine.rochester.edu
**Website:**          http://www.urmc.rochester.edu/smd/crc/crcweb.html
John E. Gerich, MD, Prog. Dir.
**Activities/Fields:** Studies of normal and deranged tissue and organ function in humans, including endocrinology, metabolism, neurology, gastroenterology, immunology, pulmonary disease, cardiology, hematology, psychiatry, dermatology, infectious disease, oncology, and pediatrics. Functions as a resource for Medical Center faculty.

## ★ 2721 ★ University of Saskatchewan
**Saskatchewan Stroke Research Centre**
Royal University Hospital
Saskatoon, SK, Canada S7N 0W8
**Phone:** (306)966-7695          **Fax:** (306)966-7685
**Email:** kalraj@sdh.sk.ca
**Website:** http://www.usask.ca/medicine/ssrc
Dr. J. Kalra, Dir.
**Activities/Fields:** Treatment and prevention of strokes.

**★ 2722 ★ University of South Carolina**
**South Carolina Rural Health Research**
**Center**
800 Sumter St., Ste. 116
Columbia, SC 29208
**Phone:** (803)777-6096          **Fax:** (803)777-1836
**Email:** msamuels@sph.sc.edu
**Website:** http://hadm.sph.sc.edu/rhr/
Dr. Michael E. Samuels, Dir.
**Activities/Fields:** Inequities in health status among
the population of the rural U.S. with an emphasis on
factors related to socioeconomic status, race and
ethnicity, and access to healthcare services.


**★ 2723 ★ University of Southern**
**California**
**John T. Nicoloff General Clinical**
**Research Center**
LACUSC Medical Center
1200 N State St., Ward 6800
Los Angeles, CA 90033
**Phone:** (323)226-4632          **Fax:** (323)226-2796
**Email:** buchanan@hsc.usc.edu
**Website:** http://www.usc.edu/hsc/gcrc/
Dr. Thomas Buchanan, Prog. Dir.
**Activities/Fields:** Clinical endocrinology, infectious
diseases, cancer, cardiology, rheumatology, neurology, obstetrics and gynecology, surgery, pediatrics,
psychiatry, and radiology, including studies on thyroid
hormone metabolism, reproductive endocrinology, role
of aldosterone and renin in system, growth hormone
metabolism, calcium and bone metabolism, water and
electrolyte metabolism, androgen metabolism, obesity,
hypertension, diabetes, fasting, and neuromuscular
disease. Specific research includes a study on the
mechanism by which smoking and contraceptive pills
combine to produce cardiovascular disease in women,
and the thyroid function, association of obesity, diabetics, and hypertension in fasting and nonthyroidal
illnesses. **Pub:** *Annual Report.*


**★ 2724 ★ University of Southern Maine**
**Edmund S. Muskie School of Public**
**Service**
**Maine Rural Health Research Center**
**(MRHRC)**
96 Falmouth St.
PO Box 9300
Portland, ME 04104-9300
**Phone:** (207)780-4435          **Fax:** (207)780-4417
**Email:** andyc@usm.maine.edu
**Website:**        http://www.muskie.usm.maine.edu/re-
search/ruralheal/
Andrew F. Coburn, PhD, Dir.
**Activities/Fields:** Rural health services, with special
focus on rural mental health services, institutional and
community-based services for rural elders, and private
and public health insurance in rural areas. **Pub:**
*Research and policy briefs.* • *Working papers.*


**★ 2725 ★ University of Tennessee**
**General Clinical Research Center**
777 Washington Ave.
Memphis, TN 38105
**Phone:** (901)570-3380          **Fax:** (901)448-7608
**Email:** bsalpert@utmem.edu
**Website:** http://www.utmem.edu/crc
Bruce Alpert, MD, Dir.
**Activities/Fields:** Provides general clinical research
facilities for controlled inpatient and outpatient studies
on human subjects with various disorders, including
sickle cell anemia, diabetes mellitus, hyperandrogen-
ism and other endocrine disorders, kidney disease,
liver disorders, hypertension, brain tumors, muscular
dystrophy, obesity, metabolic bone diseases, psychiatric disorders, osteoporosis, Reye's syndrome, hirsutism, sexual disorders, reproduction problems, thyroid
disorders, breast cancer, and leukemia. Also studies
the physiology of hypertension and the metabolic
effect of exercise. **Pub:** *Annual Report.*


**★ 2726 ★ University of Tennessee,**
**Knoxville**
**Community Health Research Group**
**(CHRG)**
Conference Center Bldg., Ste. 309
Knoxville, TN 37996-4133
**Phone:** (865)974-4511          **Fax:** (865)974-4521
**Email:** chrg@utk.edu
**Website:** http://web.utk.edu/~chrg/hit/chrghome.htm
Sandra L. Putnam, PhD, Dir.
**Activities/Fields:** Social and medical epidemiology
and the planning, organization, delivery, financing, and
quality of health care, at local, regional and national
levels. **Pub:** *Reports.*


**★ 2727 ★ University of Texas at**
**Arlington**
**Human Performance Institute**
PO Box 19180
Arlington, TX 76019-0180
**Phone:** (817)273-2335
**Email:** gvk@hpi.uta.edu
**Website:** http://www-ee.uta.edu/hpi/
Dr. George Kondraske, Dir.
**Activities/Fields:** Methods of measurement of human
performance, including performance theory, human
performance conceptual framework, and specialized
instrumentation; studies have broad applications in the
fields of space, rehabilitation, the military, and industry. Fundamental focus is on the human system-task
interface. Projects include development of a computer-
automated system to measure basic elements of
human performance, testing of both normal and
impaired individuals, and the development of methods
for automated, objective disability determination. Conducts longitudinal studies of patients to characterize
disease history. Also studies human performance in
relation to spasmodic dysphonia, athletes, post-polio
syndrome, and head injuries. Develops software tools
for automated assessment of complex sets of measurements. **Pub:** *Newsletter,* semiannually. • *Progress
Report,* annually.


**★ 2728 ★ University of Texas Health**
**Science Center at Houston**
**University Clinical Research Center**
Robertson Pavilion, Rm. 658
6411 Fannin
Houston, TX 77030
**Phone:** (713)704-4137          **Fax:** (713)704-6417
**Email:** ann.ince@uth.tmc.edu
**Website:** http://oac.hsc.uth.tmc.edu/uth_orgs/crc
Charles Forbes, Mgr.
**Activities/Fields:** Major areas of investigation include
allergy and immunology, endocrinology, genetic dis-
eases, hematology, hypertension, infectious diseases,
metabolic disorders, nephrology, neurology, oncology,
psychiatry and behavioral sciences, pulmonary disor-
ders and critical care and rheumatology.


**★ 2729 ★ University of Texas Medical**
**Branch at Galveston**
**General Clinical Research Center**
301 University Blvd.
Rte. 0331
Galveston, TX 77555
**Phone:** (409)772-1950          **Fax:** (409)772-8097
**Email:** wmeyer@utmb.edu
**Website:** http://www2.utmb.edu/gcrc
Dr. Walter J. Meyer, III, Prog. Dir.
**Activities/Fields:** Aging, AIDS, burn injuries, cardio-
vascular disease, endocrinology, exercise, gastroen-
terology, geriatrics, gynecology, immunology, infec-
tious diseases, metabolism, nutrition, obstetrics, on-
cology, ophthalmology, preventive medicine and occupational health, pulmonary diseases, rare diseases,
rheumatology, sleep and space medicine.


**★ 2730 ★ University of Texas**
**Southwestern Medical Center at Dallas**
**Center for Developmental Biology (CDB)**
5323 Harry Hines Blvd.
Dallas, TX 75390-9133
**Phone:** (214)648-1951          **Fax:** (214)648-1960
**Email:** luis.parada@utsouthwestern.edu
**Website:**        http://www2.utsouthwestern.edu/devbio/
center_frame.htm
Luis F. Parada, PhD, Dir.
**Activities/Fields:** Embryonic development, especially
intracellular signaling pathways.


**★ 2731 ★ University of Texas**
**Southwestern Medical Center at Dallas**
**Center for Immunology**
Department of Microbiology
5323 Harry Hines Blvd.
Dallas, TX 75390-9093
**Phone:** (214)648-7330          **Fax:** (214)648-7331
**Email:** edward.wakeland@utsouthwestern.edu
**Website:** http://www.swmed.edu/home_pages/immu-
nology
Prof. Edward K. Wakeland, PhD, Dir.
**Activities/Fields:** Characterization of animal models
of human diseases, with an emphasis on the delinea-
tion of molecular mechanisms mediating normal and
abnormal immune functions.


**★ 2732 ★ University of Texas**
**Southwestern Medical Center at Dallas**
**General Clinical Research Center**
5323 Harry Hines Blvd.
Dallas, TX 75390-8891
**Phone:** (214)590-7783          **Fax:** (214)590-4091
**Email:** khashayar.sakhaee@email.swmed.edu
**Website:** http://crcdec.swmed.edu
Khashayar Sakhaee, MD, Prog. Dir.
**Activities/Fields:** Calcium metabolism, cardiopulmo-
nary system, endocrinology, liver diseases, lipid disor-
ders, nephrology, neurology, oncology, and pharma-
cology.


**★ 2733 ★ University of Texas**
**Southwestern Medical Center at Dallas**
**Hamon Center for Basic Research in**
**Cancer**
Department of Molecular Biology, MC-9148
5323 Harry Hines Blvd.
Dallas, TX 75390-9148
**Phone:** (214)648-1187          **Fax:** (214)648-1196
**Email:** eolson@hamon.swmed.edu
**Website:** http://hamon.swmed.edu/
Eric Olson, PhD, Ch.
**Activities/Fields:** Understanding mechanisms that
control normal and abnormal cell growth and differenti-
ation during development and disease.


**★ 2734 ★ University of Toronto**
**Centre for Health Promotion**
Banting Institute
100 College St., Rm. 207
Toronto, ON, Canada M5G 1L5
**Phone:** (416)978-1809          **Fax:** (416)971-1365
**Email:** centre.healthpromotion@utoronto.ca
**Website:** http://www.utoronto.ca/chp/
Dr. Suzanne Jackson, Actg. Dir.
**Activities/Fields:** Health promotion, including tobacco
research, quality of life issues, health communication,
evaluation, best practices in health promotion, health
policy, policy development, and workplace health
policy. **Pub:** *Centre for Health Promotion Annual
Report,* annually. • *The Health Communication Update,* quarterly. • *Information Update,* 3/year. • *Series
and Health Promotion.*

★ **2735** ★ **University of Toronto**
**Centre for Health Promotion**
**Quality of Life Research Unit**
256 Mccaul St., Ste. 404
Toronto, ON, Canada M5T 1W5
**Phone:** (416)978-1457          **Fax:** (416)978-4363
**Email:** quality.oflife@utoronto.ca
**Website:** http://www.utoronto.ca/qol
Rebecca Renwick, Dir.

**Activities/Fields:** Quality of life, defined as factors that make living both meaningful and enjoyable, for seniors, adolescents, people with developmental disabilities, persons with physical disabilities, and adults in the general population.

★ **2736** ★ **University of Toronto**
**Institute of Medical Science**
Medical Science Bldg., Rm. 7213
1 King's College Cir.
Toronto, ON, Canada M5S 1A8
**Phone:** (416)978-8886          **Fax:** (416)971-2253
**Email:** dir.medscience@utoronto.ca
Dr. Mel Silverman, Dir.

**Activities/Fields:** Multidisciplinary research in clinical and basic medical science and related fields. Research is focused in three distinct areas: molecular; clinical investigation of whole organ integrative biology, and clinical investigation of quantitative methodological approaches to health outcomes. Studies focus around fields such as cardiovascular sciences, bioethics, membrane biology, respiratory medicine, and psychosomatic medicine. Collaborative programs include: bioethics; cardiovascular sciences; history of medicine; neurosciences; toxicology; and alcohol, tobacco, and other psychoactive substances.

★ **2737** ★ **University of Utah**
**General Clinical Research Center**
50 N Medical Dr., Rm. 4R210
Salt Lake City, UT 84132
**Phone:** (801)581-6736          **Fax:** (801)585-1461
**Email:** jkushner@crc.med.utah.edu
**Website:** http://crc-gw.med.utah.edu
James P. Kushner, MD, Dir.

**Activities/Fields:** Provides facilities for School of Medicine faculty conducting clinical investigations in the areas of renal and cardiac failure, cardiac transplantation, genetic diseases, nutrition and cancer, atherosclerosis, diabetes and obesity, psychiatric and neuromuscular disorders, disorders of intermediary metabolism (porphyrins, carbohydrates, lipids, trace elements), diseases of the endocrine system (adrenal, pituitary, gonad, thyroid, and pancreas), infectious disease, and drug therapy of human diseases.

★ **2738** ★ **University of Vermont**
**General Clinical Research Center**
111 Colchester Ave.
Burlington, VT 05401
**Phone:** (802)847-2777          **Fax:** (802)847-5562
**Email:** rgalbrai@zoo.uvm.edu
**Website:**          http://www.vtmednet.org/~g195040/
gcrcpage.htm
Dr. Richard A. Galbraith, Dir.

**Activities/Fields:** Various medical and surgical problems. Provides research facility for individual research studies.

★ **2739** ★ **University of Virginia**
**Center for the Engineering of Wound**
**   Prevention and Repair**
Health Science Center, Box 377
Department of Biomedical Engineering
School of Engineering & Applied Science
Charlottesville, VA 22908
**Phone:** (434)924-0270          **Fax:** (434)982-3780
**Email:** tskalak@virginia.edu
**Website:**          http://yakko.bme.virginia.edu/wound/index.html
Thomas Skalak, Dir.

**Activities/Fields:** Principles governing mechanical and biological events in chronic skin wounds, to eradicate chronic wounds in hospital settings, to apply these principles to accelerate the repair of acute skin wounds caused by trauma, and to improve therapies for skin flap procedures, intestinal ulcers, and neurological injury.

★ **2740** ★ **University of Virginia**
**Center for Structural Biology (CSB)**
Molecular Physiology & Biological Physics
PO Box 10011
Charlottesville, VA 22906-0011
**Phone:** (434)924-5926
**Email:** aps2n@virginia.edu
**Website:**          http://olenka.med.virginia.edu/newcsb2/
Consort.html
Andrew P. Somlyo, Dir.

**Activities/Fields:** Cellular and macromolecular structure, function and interactions.

★ **2741** ★ **University of Virginia**
**General Clinical Research Center**
School of Medicine
PO Box 800787
Charlottesville, VA 22908
**Phone:** (434)982-3160          **Fax:** (434)924-9960
**Email:** pfs2h@virginia.edu
Dr. Johannes D. Veldhuis, Dir.

**Activities/Fields:** Endocrinology, neurology, surgery, gastroenterology, ophthalmology, cardiology, obstetrics/gynecology, immunology, renal diseases, and ear, nose, and throat studies. Special interests include neuroendocrinology, hypertension, vascular disease, juvenile diabetes mellitus, genetic disorders, fertility disorders, digestive and growth disorders, sleep disorders, asthma and pulmonary disorders, congestive heart failure, arrhythmias, and epilepsy. Personnel are trained in rapid blood sampling and blood processing and a biostatistician is available to assist in research protocol design. Serves as a general clinical center for use by entire faculty of the School for any type of clinical investigation.

★ **2742** ★ **University of Virginia**
**Surgical Therapeutic Advancement Center**
**Tissue Adhesive Center**
MR 4 Bldg., Rm. 3122
PO Box 801373
Charlottesville, VA 22908-1373
**Phone:** (434)243-0315          **Fax:** (434)243-0318
**Email:** uvatac@virginia.edu
**Website:** http://hsc.virginia.edu/tac/
William D. Spotnitz, MD, Dir.

**Activities/Fields:** Tissue adhesives for the clinical care of patients, and especially cellular biology, adhesive strength profiling, and animal modeling.

★ **2743** ★ **University of Washington**
**Center for Health Education and**
**   Research (CHER)**
901 Boren Ave., Ste. 1100
Seattle, WA 98104
**Phone:** (206)221-4944          **Fax:** (206)221-4945
**Email:** marnae@u.washington.edu
**Website:** http://depts.washington.edu/cherweb/
King K. Holmes, MD, Dir.

**Activities/Fields:** Health and quality of life of individuals and communities.

★ **2744** ★ **University of Washington**
**Center for Women's Health Research**
**   (CWHR)**
Box 357261
T624 Health Sciences Bldg.
Seattle, WA 98195-7261
**Phone:** (206)543-1414          **Free:** 877-543-1414
**Fax:** (206)543-4091
**Email:** cwhr@u.washington.edu
**Website:** http://www.uw-cwhr.org
Margaret Heitkemper, Dir.

**Activities/Fields:** Health of women across the life span. **Pub:** *Newsletter*.

★ **2745** ★ **University of Washington**
**General Clinical Research Center**
1959 NEPacific St., Rm. SS732
Seattle, WA 98195-6178
**Phone:** (206)598-4700          **Fax:** (206)598-2890
**Email:** brunzell@u.washington.edu
**Website:** http://www.crc.washington.edu
John D. Brunzell, MD, Prog. Dir.

**Activities/Fields:** Conducts a diversified research program designed to make possible precise, laboratory-type measurements of patients' disease states and their progress under various types of treatment.

★ **2746** ★ **University of Washington**
**Rural Health Research Center (RHRC)**
Box 354696
Department of Family Medicine
Seattle, WA 98195-4696
**Phone:** (206)685-0402          **Fax:** (206)616-4768
**Email:** jhansen@fammed.washington.edu
**Website:** http://www.fammed.washington.edu/wwam-irhrc/
L. Gary Hart, PhD, Dir. /Prin. Investigator

**Activities/Fields:** Rural health care. Research focuses on the training and supply of rural health care providers and content and outcomes of the care they provide; the availability and quality of care for rural women and children, including obstetric and perinatal care; and access to high-quality care for vulnerable and minority rural populations.

★ **2747** ★ **University of Washington**
**Washington Regional Primate Research**
**   Center (WaRPRC)**
I-421 Health Sciences
Box 357330
Seattle, WA 98195-7330
**Phone:** (206)543-1430          **Fax:** (206)685-0305
**Email:** pattir@bart.rprc.washington.edu
**Website:** http://www.rprc.washington.edu/
William R. Morton, DVM, Dir.

**Activities/Fields:** Use of nonhuman primates for biomedical research on AIDS, developmental biology, neurobiological and behavioral sciences, cardiovascular physiology, molecular and cell biology, immunology, virology, transplantation and stem cell biology, genomics and primate disease models.

★ **2748** ★ **University of Wisconsin—**
**   Madison**
**Center for Human Performance and Risk**
**   Analysis (CHPRA)**
456 Mechanical Engineering Bldg.
1513 University Ave.
Madison, WI 53706-1572
**Phone:** (608)263-7456          **Fax:** (608)265-9094
**Email:** chpra@engr.wisc.edu
**Website:** http://www.engr.wisc.edu/centers/chpra/
Prof. Vickie M. Bier, Dir.

**Activities/Fields:** Issues of human performance and the role human performance plays in industrial accidents. **Pub:** *The Human Element Newsletter*, quarterly.

★ **2749** ★ **University of Wisconsin—**
**   Madison**
**General Clinical Research Center**
School of Medicine
600 Highland Ave.
Madison, WI 53792-6736
**Phone:** (608)263-6183          **Fax:** (608)263-3104
**Email:** wwb@medicine.wisc.edu
Dr. William W. Busse, Prog. Dir.

**Activities/Fields:** Major areas of investigation include immunology, oncology, pediatrics, pulmonary medicine, sleep disorders, surgery and whole-body hyperthermia.

★ 2750 ★ **University of Wisconsin—Madison**
**Laboratory of Genetics**
445 Henry Mall
Madison, WI 53706
**Phone:** (608)262-3112     **Fax:** (608)262-2976
**Email:** mrculber@facstaff.wisc.edu
**Website:** http://www.wisc.edu/genetics/
Prof. Michael Culbertson, Chm.

**Activities/Fields:** Genetics, including molecular, human, nematode, population, microbial, behavioral, and plant genetics, cytogenetics, yeast genetics, somatic cells, zebrafish, genomics, and other areas ranging from theoretical genetics to agricultural and medical genetics.

★ 2751 ★ **University of Wisconsin—Madison**
**Office of International Health Affairs**
1760 MSC
1300 University Ave.
Madison, WI 53706
**Phone:** (608)263-4150     **Fax:** (608)262-2327
**Email:** jlladins@facstaff.wisc.edu
Dr. Judith L. Ladinsky, Dir.

**Activities/Fields:** International health issues. **Pub:** *Newsletter*.

★ 2752 ★ **Van Andel Research Institute (VARI)**
333 Bostwick NE
Grand Rapids, MI 49503
**Phone:** (616)234-5000     **Fax:** (616)234-5001
**Email:** george.vandewoude@vai.org
**Website:** http://www.vai.org/vari/home.htm
George F. Vande Woude, PhD, Dir.

**Activities/Fields:** Improvement of human health, especially determination of the causes and treatment of cancer.

★ 2753 ★ **Vanderbilt University**
**Center for Clinical and Research Ethics**
319 Oxford House
Vanderbilt University Medical Center
Nashville, TN 37232-4350
**Phone:** (615)936-2686     **Fax:** (615)936-3800
**Email:** med.ethics@mcmmail.vanderbilt.edu
**Website:** http://www.mc.vanderbilt.edu/ethics/
Stuart G. Finder, Dir.

**Activities/Fields:** Moral and ethical issues.

★ 2754 ★ **Vanderbilt University**
**General Clinical Research Center**
21st Ave. S
Nashville, TN 37232-2195
**Phone:** (615)343-6499     **Fax:** (615)343-8649
**Email:** david.robertson@mcmail.vanderbilt.edu
**Website:** http://www.mc.vanderbilt.edu/gcrc/
Dr. David Robertson, Dir.

**Activities/Fields:** Human physiology and diseases, including studies in medicine, neuroscience, molecular biology, pharmacology, hematology, cardiovascular diseases, genetics, obstetrics and gynecology, pediatrics, psychiatry, surgery, and psychology. Activities focus on hypertension, hypotension, arrhythmias, carcinoid syndrome, and disorders of the autonomic nervous system. **Pub:** *Elliot Newman Handbook*.

★ 2755 ★ **Veterans Affairs Medical Center (Danville, IL)**
**Research and Development Service**
1900 E Main St.
Danville, IL 61832
**Phone:** (217)442-5534     **Fax:** (217)554-4836
**Email:** mukund.prabhudesai@med.va.gov
Mukund Prabhudesai, MD, R&D Coord.

**Activities/Fields:** Alcoholism, rehabilitation, psychology, drugs, and nutrition. Also studies health care management and psychiatry.

★ 2756 ★ **Veterans Affairs Medical Center (Martinez, CA)**
**Research Administration Office**
150 Muir Rd.
Martinez, CA 94553
**Phone:** (925)372-2484     **Fax:** (925)228-5738
**Email:** gakaysen@ucdavis.edu
Dr. George Kaysen, Assoc. Ch

**Activities/Fields:** Basic and clinical biomedical research.

★ 2757 ★ **Veterans Affairs Medical Center (Minneapolis, MN)**
1 Veterans Dr.
Minneapolis, MN 55417-2300
**Phone:** (612)725-2033     **Fax:** (612)725-2093
**Email:** michael.levitt@med.va.gov
Dr. Michael D. Levitt, MD, Ch. of Res.

**Activities/Fields:** Health services, including cooperative clinical trials, psychiatry, prostate cancer, and kidney disease.

★ 2758 ★ **Veterans Affairs Medical Center (Omaha, NE)**
**Research and Development Service**
4101 Woolworth Ave.
Omaha, NE 68105
**Phone:** (402)346-8800     **Fax:** (402)449-0604
**Email:** nowling.stephan_d@omaha.va.gov
Lynell W. Klassen, MD, Assoc. Ch.

**Activities/Fields:** Immunology, infectious disease, oncology, liver disease, diabetes, orthopedics, pulmonary disease, gastroenterology, and endocrinology. Utilizes rats, mice, and rabbits, as animal models.

★ 2759 ★ **Veterans Affairs Medical Center (Reno, NV)**
**Research Service**
1000 Locust St.
Reno, NV 89502-2597
**Phone:** (775)328-1486     **Fax:** (775)328-1816
Dr. Jon Schrage, PhD, Dir. of Res.

**Activities/Fields:** Alzheimer's disease, bone marrow transplantation, cancer, cardiology, clinical trials of investigational drugs, diabetes, in-utero transplantation of blood-forming cells, nephrology, pulmonary medicine, stress in employment, health services, and surgery.

★ 2760 ★ **Veterans Affairs Pittsburgh Health Care System**
**Research Service**
University Dr. C
Pittsburgh, PA 15240
**Phone:** (412)688-6104     **Fax:** (412)688-6945
**Email:** sax.martin@pittsburgh.va.gov
**Website:** http://www.research.vares-pitt.org
Dr. Martin Sax, Assoc. Chf. of Staff, Res. Development

**Activities/Fields:** Oncogene expression in colon cancer, immunochemical targeting of tumors, dermatology, vascular surgery, three-dimensional structure of bacterial toxins, and transplantation. Neurosciences studies focus on epilepsy, hypertension, and schizophrenia and rehabilitation.

★ 2761 ★ **Veterans Affairs Salt Lake City Health Care System**
**Research Service**
500 Foothill Dr.
Salt Lake City, UT 84148
**Phone:** (801)584-1271     **Fax:** (801)583-9624
**Email:** richard.straight@med.va.gov
Richard C. Straight, PhD, Dir.

**Activities/Fields:** Diabetes, cancer, arthritis, aging and alcoholism, stroke and rehabilitation, dermatitis, neuroimmunological diseases, myasthenia gravis, tumors, dementia, laser medicine and surgery, herpes, genetics, cardiology, immunology, basic science, molecular biology, national cooperative drug studies, and rehabilitation research and development of artificial limbs, and clinical outcomes research. **Pub:** *Scientific Journal*, annually. Journal.

★ 2762 ★ **Veterans Health Administration**
**Office of Research and Development**
**Health Services Research and Development Service**
**Center of Excellence**
VA Medical Center, 152
3801 Miranda Ave.
Palo Alto, CA 94304
**Phone:** (650)617-2746     **Fax:** (650)617-2736
**Email:** janice.beyer@med.va.gov
**Website:** http://www.chce.research.med.va.gov
Dr. Rudolf Moos, Dir.

**Activities/Fields:** Organization and delivery of health care services; diagnostic assessment, screening, and clinical decision making; evaluation of treatments for substance abuse and psychiatric disorders; health services research methodology. Current project involve improving HIV screening policies; implementing practice guidelines; evaluating the effectiveness and cost-effectiveness of interventions for alcohol abuse, drug abuse, and depression. **Pub:** *Newsletter*.

★ 2763 ★ **Via Christi Research, Inc.**
1100 N St. Francis, Ste. 200
Wichita, KS 67214-2878
**Phone:** (316)291-4900     **Fax:** (316)291-7704
**Email:** dale_horst@via-christi.org
**Website:** http://www.viamtec.org
Dr. W. Dale Horst, Dir.

**Activities/Fields:** Psychiatry; phase I, II, and III clinical drug studies; orthopedic research; biomedical device and materials research and development; technology transfer and product development; hospital operations research; and pharmacoeconomic research. **Frmly:** St. Francis Research Institute, Inc.

★ 2764 ★ **Virginia Commonwealth University**
**General Clinical Research Center**
PO Box 980155
Richmond, VA 23298
**Phone:** (434)828-9228     **Fax:** (434)828-5002
**Email:** clore@hsc.vcu.edu
John N. Clore, MD, Prog. Dir.

**Activities/Fields:** Endocrinology, gastroenterology, infectious disease, metabolism, neurology, pediatrics, pharmacology, psychiatry, pulmonary physiology, and surgery.

★ 2765 ★ **Virginia Mason Research Center**
1201 9th Ave.
Seattle, WA 98101-2795
**Phone:** (206)583-6525     **Fax:** (206)223-7543
**Email:** info@vmresearch.org
**Website:** http://www.vmresearch.org
Dr. Gerald T. Nepom, Dir.

**Activities/Fields:** Immunology, diabetes and clinical research. **Pub:** *Bulletin of the Virginia Mason Clinic*.

★ 2766 ★ **Wake Forest University**
**Comparative Medicine Clinical Research Center**
School of Medicine
Medical Center Blvd.
Winston Salem, NC 27157-1040
**Phone:** (336)716-2673     **Fax:** (336)716-6279
**Email:** rstclair@wfubmc.edu
**Website:** http://www.wfubmc.edu/research/comp_med.html
Richard W. St. Clair, PhD, Contact

**Activities/Fields:** Animal models of human disease studies, including research in heart disease, osteoporosis, women's health, and arteriosclerosis. Also studies relationship between aggression and low cholesterol levels.

## ★ 2767 ★ Wake Forest University General Clinical Research Center

Medical Center Blvd.
Winston Salem, NC 27157
**Phone:** (336)716-9750 **Fax:** (336)716-5055
**Email:** chmcall@wfubmc.edu
**Website:** http://www.gcrc.wfubmc.edu
Charles E. McCall, MD, Prog. Dir.

**Activities/Fields:** Major areas of investigation include anesthesiology, autoimmune diseases, endocrinology, gastroenterology, genetics, geriatrics and gerontology, hematology and oncology, hypertension, infectious diseases, nephrology, neurology, obstetrics and gynecology, pediatrics, psychiatry, pulmonary diseases, and women's health.

## ★ 2768 ★ Wake Forest University Pain Mechanisms Laboratory

Gray Bldg.
Medical Center Blvd.
Winston Salem, NC 27157
**Phone:** (336)716-2591 **Fax:** (336)716-3220
**Email:** eisenach@wfubmc.edu
**Website:** http://www.wfubmc.edu/painlab/main.html
James C. Eisenach, MD, Dir.

**Activities/Fields:** Pain and analgesia.

## ★ 2769 ★ Wake Forest University Women's Health Center of Excellence

Medical Center Blvd.
PO Box 573050
Winston Salem, NC 27157-3050
**Phone:** (336)713-4220
**Website:** http://www.wfubmc.edu/women/whcoe/mission.html
Sally A. Shumaker, PhD, Dir.

**Activities/Fields:** Diseases that affect women, delivery of health care services to women, and health education for women. **Pub:** *Newsletter*, monthly.

## ★ 2770 ★ Washington University in St. Louis General Clinical Research Center

4th Floor Barnes Hospital
Box 8071
Saint Louis, MO 63110
**Phone:** (314)362-7617 **Fax:** (314)362-7989
**Email:** pcryer@imgate.wustl.edu
**Website:** http://gcrc.wustl.edu
Dr. Philip E. Cryer, Dir.

**Activities/Fields:** Provides clinical research facilities for faculty members of the School.

## ★ 2771 ★ Wayne State University Center for Health Research

317 Cohn
College of Nursing
5557 Cass Ave.
Detroit, MI 48202-3515
**Phone:** (313)577-4135 **Fax:** (313)577-5777
**Email:** nursinginfo@wyne.edu
**Website:** http://www.nursing.wayne.edu/
Mary A. Nies, Assoc. Dean, Res.

**Activities/Fields:** Nursing, urban health, pain reduction in hospitalized children, adolescent health, teen pregnancy, aging, chronicity, health education and promotion (e.g. smoking cessation), community health, psychosocial oncology, health behavior, self care, stress and coping, parent/child health, family health, caregivers of aged individuals, drug use, violence and abuse, sleep patterns, risk-taking with respect to teen pregnancy and sexually transmitted diseases (including HIV), and transcultural nursing. Multidisciplinary studies involve health professionals and faculty members from disciplines such as nursing, psychology, sociology, anthropology, medicine, and epidemiology. **Frmly:** Center for Nursing Research.

## ★ 2772 ★ Wesley Medical Research Institutes

3306 E Central
Wichita, KS 67208
**Phone:** (316)686-7172 **Fax:** (316)687-0033
**Email:** wmriks@aol.com
Dr. Sechin Cho, Pres.

**Activities/Fields:** Maternal and fetal medicine, respiratory distress syndrome in neonates, obstetrical and gynecologic oncology, infant nutrition, genetics, sickle cell anemia, heart disease, cancer, birth defects, and infertility. **Pub:** *The Investigator*, semiannually.

## ★ 2773 ★ The Western Pennsylvania Hospital Foundation

4818 Liberty Ave.
Pittsburgh, PA 15224
**Phone:** (412)578-5153 **Fax:** (412)578-4428
**Email:** bbeisgen@wpahs.org
**Website:** http://trfn.clpgh.org/wphf/
Arlene Apfel Snyder, Pres.

**Activities/Fields:** Oncology, infertility, cardiology, genetics, geriatrics, pharmaceutical studies, and other health research. **Pub:** *Outcomes*, semiannually. Newsletter.

## ★ 2774 ★ Yale University General Clinical Research Center—Adults

Yale New Haven Hospital, East Pavilion
20 York St.
PO Box 208076
New Haven, CT 06520-8076
**Phone:** (203)688-4106 **Fax:** (203)688-3100
**Website:** http://www.info.med.yale.edu/crc/gcrc/
Gerald I. Shulman, PhD, Dir.

**Activities/Fields:** Endocrinology, gastroenterology, mineral metabolism, oncology, psychology and pharmacology, respiratory psychology, and rheumatology.

**Yale University General Clinical Research Center— Children**
*See:* Entry 5841

# State Government Agencies

## <u>Medical Boards</u>

## ★ 2775 ★ Alabama State Board of Medical Examiners

848 Washington Ave.
PO Box 946
Montgomery, AL 36101-0946
**Phone:** (334)242-4116 **Fax:** (334)242-4155
**Email:** bme@albme.org
**Website:** http://www.albme.org/

## ★ 2776 ★ Arizona State Board of Medical Examiners

9545 E Doubletree Ranch Rd.
Scottsdale, AZ 85258-5539
**Phone:** (480)551-2700 **Free:** 877-255-2212
**Website:** http://www.bomex.org/index.htm

## ★ 2777 ★ Arkansas State Medical Board

2100 Riverfront Dr.
Little Rock, AR 72202
**Phone:** (501)296-1802 **Fax:** (501)296-1805
**Email:** office@armedicalboard.org
**Website:** http://www.armedicalboard.org/

## ★ 2778 ★ Bureau of Health Services Michigan Board of Medicine

PO Box 30670
Lansing, MI 48909
**Phone:** (517)335-0918 **Fax:** (517)241-2635
**Email:** bhserinfo@cis.state.mi.us
**Website:** http://www.michigan.gov/cis/

## ★ 2779 ★ California Medical Board

1426 Howe Ave. Ste. 54
Sacramento, CA 95825-3236
**Phone:** (916)263-2382
**Email:** Webmaster@medbd.ca.gov
**Website:** http://www.medbd.ca.gov/

## ★ 2780 ★ Colorado State Board of Medical Examiners

1560 Broadway, Ste. 1300
Denver, CO 80202
**Phone:** (303)894-7690 **Fax:** (303)894-7692
**Email:** medical@dora.state.co.us
**Website:** http://www.dora.state.co.us/Medical/
Susan Miller, Contact

## ★ 2781 ★ Connecticut Department of Public Health Physician Licensure

PO Box 340308
410 Capitol Ave., MS No. 12APP
Hartford, CT 06134-0308
**Phone:** (860)509-7563
**Website:** http://www.ct-clic.com/detail.asp?code=1759

## ★ 2782 ★ Delaware Board of Medical Practice

Cannon Bldg., Ste. 203
861 Silver Lake Blvd.
Dover, DE 19904
**Phone:** (302)744-4520 **Fax:** (302)739-2711
**Email:** gfranzolino@.state.de.us
**Website:** http://www.professionallicensing.state.de.us/boards/
Gayle Franzolino, Contact

## ★ 2783 ★ District of Columbia Board of Medicine

825 North Capital St, NE, 2nd Fl
Washington, DC 20002
**Phone:** (202)442-4777 **Fax:** (202)442-9431
**Website:** http://dchealth.dc.gov/index.asp

## ★ 2784 ★ Florida Board of Medicine

4052 Bald Cypress Way, Bin C03
Tallahassee, FL 32399-3253
**Phone:** (850)245-4131 **Fax:** (850)488-9325
**Email:** MQA_medicine@doh.state.fl.us
**Website:** http://www9.myflorida.com/Mqa/medical/me_home.html

## ★ 2785 ★ Georgia Composite State Board of Medical Examiners

2 Peachtree St.
Atlanta, GA 30303
**Phone:** (404)656-3913
**Website:** http://www.sos.state.ga.us/ebd-medical/default.htm
Karen Mason, Contact

## ★ 2786 ★ Hawaii Board of Medical Examiners Department of Commerce & Consumer Affairs

DCCA-PVL
PO Box 3469
Honolulu, HI 96801
**Phone:** (808)586-2708
**Email:** medical@dcca.state.hi.us
**Website:** http://www.state.hi.us/dcca/pvl/areas_medical.html
Constance Cabral-Makanani, Contact

**★ 2787 ★ Idaho State Board of Medicine**
1755 Westgate Dr.
PO Box 83720
Boise, ID 83720-0058
**Phone:** (208)327-7000 **Fax:** (208)327-7005
**Email:** info@bom.state.id.us
**Website:** http://www.bom.state.id.us/

**★ 2788 ★ Illinois Department of Professional Regulation**
**Board of Medicine (Licensing)**
320 W Washington St.
Springfield, IL 62786
**Phone:** (217)785-0800 **Fax:** (217)782-7645
**Website:** http://www.dpr.state.il.us

**★ 2789 ★ Indiana Health Professions Bureau**
**Medical Licensing Board**
402 W Washington, Rm. W041
Indianapolis, IN 46204
**Phone:** (317)234-2060 **Fax:** (317)233-4236
**Email:** hpb3@hpb.state.in.us
**Website:** http://www.in.gov/hpb/boards/mlbi/
Angela Smith-Jones, Director

**★ 2790 ★ Iowa State Board of Medical Examiners**
400 SW 8th St., Ste. C
Des Moines, IA 50309-4686
**Phone:** (515)242-6039 **Fax:** (515)242-5908
**Email:** ann.mowery@ibme.state.ia.us
**Website:** http://www.docboard.org/ia/ia_home.htm
Ann E. Mowery, PhD, Director

**★ 2791 ★ Kansas Board of Healing Arts**
235 SW Topeka Blvd.
Topeka, KS 66603-3068
**Phone:** (785)296-7413 **Fax:** (785)296-0852
**Email:** Healer3@ink.org
**Website:** http://www.ksbha.org/

**★ 2792 ★ Kentucky Board of Medical Licensure**
310 Whittington Pkwy, Ste 1B
Louisville, KY 40222-4916
**Phone:** (502)429-8046 **Fax:** (502)429-9923
**Email:** kbml@mail.state.ky.us
**Website:** http://www.state.ky.us/agencies/kbml/

**★ 2793 ★ Louisiana State Board of Medical Examiners**
630 Camp St.
PO Box 30250
New Orleans, LA 70190-0250
**Phone:** (504)568-6820 **Fax:** (504)599-0503
**Email:** lsbmever@lsbme.org
**Website:** http://www.lsbme.org/

**★ 2794 ★ Maine Board of Licensure in Medicine**
137 State House Station
1 Bangor St.
Augusta, ME 04333-0137
**Phone:** (207)287-3601
**Website:** http://www.docboard.org/me/me_home.htm
Randal Manning, Director

**★ 2795 ★ Maryland Board of Physician Quality Assurance**
4201 Patterson Ave.
Baltimore, MD 21215-0095
**Phone:** (410)764-4777 **Free:** 800-492-6836
**Fax:** (410)358-2252
**Email:** bpqa@erols.com
**Website:** http://www.bpqa.state.md.us/

**★ 2796 ★ Massachusetts Board of Registration in Medicine**
10 W St., 3rd Fl.
Boston, MA 02111
**Phone:** (617)727-3086 **Fax:** (617)451-9568
**Email:** webmaster@massmedboard.org
**Website:** http://www.massmedboard.org/

**★ 2797 ★ Minnesota Board of Medical Practice**
2829 University Ave. SE, Ste. 400
Minneapolis, MN 55414-3246
**Phone:** (612)617-2130 **Free:** 800-657-3709
**Fax:** (612)617-2166
**Email:** medical.board@state.mn.us
**Website:** http://www.bmp.state.mn.us/

**★ 2798 ★ Mississippi State Board of Medical Licensure**
1867 Crane Ridge Dr., Ste. 200-B
PO Box 9268
Jackson, MS 39286-9268
**Phone:** (601)987-3079 **Fax:** (601)987-4159
**Email:** mboard@msbml.state.ms.us
**Website:** http://www.msbml.state.ms.us/

**★ 2799 ★ Missouri State Board of Registration for the Healing Arts**
3605 Missouri Blvd.
PO Box 4
Jefferson City, MO 65102
**Phone:** (573)751-0098 **Fax:** (573)751-3166
**Email:** healarts@mail.state.mo.us
**Website:** http://www.ecodev.state.mo.us/pr/healarts/
Tina Steinman, Director

**★ 2800 ★ Nebraska Department of Health and Human Services**
PO Box 95044
Lincoln, NE 68509-5044
**Phone:** (402)471-2306 **Fax:** (402)471-3577
**Email:** hhs_system_information@hhs.state.ne.us
**Website:** http://www.hhs.state.ne.us/

**★ 2801 ★ Nevada State Board of Medical Examiners**
1105 Terminal Way, Ste. 301
PO Box 7238
Reno, NV 89510
**Phone:** (775)688-2559 **Fax:** (775)688-2321
**Email:** nsbme@govmail.state.nv.us
**Website:** http://www.state.nv.us/medical/

**★ 2802 ★ New Hampshire Board of Medicine**
2 Industrial Park Dr., Ste. 8
Concord, NH 03301-8520
**Phone:** (603)271-1203
**Website:** http://www.state.nh.us/medicine/index.html
Cynthia Cooper, President

**★ 2803 ★ New Jersey Department of Law and Public Safety**
**New Jersey State Board of Medical Examiners**
PO Box 183
Trenton, NJ 08625-0183
**Phone:** (609)826-7100
**Website:** http://www.state.nj.us/lps/ca/medical.htmbme5
William Roeder, Director

**★ 2804 ★ New Mexico State Board of Medical Examiners**
Lamy Bldg., 2nd Fl.
491 Old Santa Fe Trail
Santa Fe, NM 87501

**Phone:** (505)827-5022 **Free:** 800-945-5845
**Fax:** (505)827-7377
**Website:** http://www.state.nm.us/nmbme/

**★ 2805 ★ New York State Board for Medicine Licensing**
Office of the Professions
State Education Bldg., 2nd Fl.
Albany, NY 12234
**Phone:** (518)474-3817 **Fax:** (518)486-4846
**Email:** medbd@mail.nysed.gov
**Website:** http://www.op.nysed.gov/med.htm
Thomas J. Monahan, Contact

**★ 2806 ★ New York State Department of Health**
**New York State Board for Professional Medical Conduct (Discipline)**
433 River St. ste. 303
Troy, NY 12180
**Phone:** (518)402-0855 **Free:** 800-663-6114
**Fax:** (518)402-0866
**Email:** nyhealth@health.state.ny.us
**Website:** http://www.health.state.ny.us/
Dennis Graziano, Contact

**★ 2807 ★ North Carolina Medical Board**
1201 Front St, ste.100
Raleigh, NC 27609-7533
**Phone:** (919)326-1100 **Free:** 800-253-9653
**Fax:** (919)326-1130
**Email:** public.affairs@ncmedboard.org
**Website:** http://www.ncmedboard.org/
Shannon Kingston, Contact

**★ 2808 ★ North Dakota State Board of Medical Examiners**
418 E Broadway, Ste. 12
City Center Plaza
Bismarck, ND 58501
**Phone:** (701)328-6500 **Fax:** (701)328-6505
**Website:** http://www.ndbomex.com/
Rolf P. Sletten, J.D., Contact

**★ 2809 ★ Ohio State Medical Board**
77 S High St., 17th Fl.
Columbus, OH 43215-6127
**Phone:** (614)466-3934 **Free:** 800-554-7717
**Fax:** (614)728-5946
**Website:** http://www.state.oh.us/med/

**★ 2810 ★ Oklahoma State Board of Medical Licensure and Supervision**
5104 N Francis, Ste. C
PO Box 18256
Oklahoma City, OK 73154-0256
**Phone:** (405)848-6841 **Free:** 800-381-4519
**Fax:** (405)848-8240
**Email:** executive@osbmls.state.ok.us
**Website:** http://www.osbmls.state.ok.us

**★ 2811 ★ Oregon Board of Medical Examiners**
1500 SW 1st Ave., Ste. 620
Portland, OR 97201-5826
**Phone:** (503)229-5770 **Free:** 877-254-6263
**Fax:** (503)229-6543
**Email:** bme.info@state.or.us
**Website:** http://www.bme.state.or.us/

**★ 2812 ★ Pennsylvania State Board of Medicine**
PO Box 2649
Harrisburg, PA 17105-2649
**Phone:** (717)783-1400 **Fax:** (717)787-7769
**Email:** medicine@pados.dos.state.pa.us
**Website:** http://www.dos.state.pa.us/bpoa/cwp/view.asp?a=1104&q=432799

**★ 2813 ★ Puerto Rico Board of Medical Examiners**
Call Box 13969
San Juan, PR 00908
**Phone:** (787)782-8989    **Fax:** (787)782-8733

**★ 2814 ★ Rhode Island Board of Medical Licensure and Discipline**
Department of Health
3 Capitol Hill, Room 205
Providence, RI 02908
**Phone:** (401)222-3855    **Fax:** (401)222-2158
**Website:** http://www.docboard.org/ri/main.htm

**★ 2815 ★ South Carolina Department of Labor, Licensing and Regulation**
Board of Medical Examiners
Synergy Business Park
Kingstree Bldg.
110 Centerview Dr., Ste. 202
PO Box 11289
Columbia, SC 29211-1289
**Phone:** (803)896-4500    **Fax:** (803)896-4515
**Email:** medboard@mail.llr.state.sc.us
**Website:** http://www.llr.state.sc.us/POL/Medical/Default.htm

**★ 2816 ★ South Dakota State Board of Medical and Osteopathic Examiners**
1323 S Minnesota Ave.
Sioux Falls, SD 57105
**Phone:** (605)334-8343    **Fax:** (605)336-0270
**Email:** kachenba@sdsma.org
**Website:** http://www.state.sd.us/dcr/medical/medhorn.htm
Paul Jensen, Contact

**★ 2817 ★ Tennessee State Board of Medical Examiners**
Cordell Hull Bldg., 3rd Fl.
425 Fifth Ave. N
Nashville, TN 37247
**Phone:** (615)532-3202    **Free:** 888-310-4650
**Fax:** (615)532-5369
**Email:** DDenton@mail.state.tn.us
**Website:** http://170.142.76.180/bmf-bin/BMFprofgen.pl

**★ 2818 ★ Texas State Board of Medical Examiners**
333 Guadaloupe, Tower 3, Ste. 610
PO Box 2018
Austin, TX 78701
**Phone:** (512)305-7010    **Free:** 800-248-4062
**Fax:** (512)305-7008
**Website:** http://www.tsbme.state.tx.us/

**★ 2819 ★ Utah Department of Commerce**
Div. of Occupational & Professional Licensure
160 E 300 S, 4th Fl.
PO Box 146741
Salt Lake City, UT 84114-6741
**Phone:** (801)530-6628    **Free:** 888-275-3675
**Fax:** (801)530-6511
**Email:** commerce@br.state.ut.us
**Website:** http://www.commerce.state.ut.us/dopl/dopl1.htm

**★ 2820 ★ Vermont Board of Medical Practice**
109 State St.
Montpelier, VT 05609-1106
**Phone:** (802)828-2673    **Fax:** (802)828-5450
**Email:** gloria.hurd@medbd.state.vt.us
**Website:** http://www.docboard.org/vt/vermont.htm
Gloria Hurd, Contact

**★ 2821 ★ Virgin Islands Board of Medical Examiners**
Virgin Islands Department of Health
48 Sugar Estate
St Thomas, VI 00802
**Phone:** (340)774-0117    **Fax:** (340)777-4001
Lydia Scott, Contact

**★ 2822 ★ Virginia Board of Medicine**
6606 W Broad St., 4th Fl.
Richmond, VA 23230-1717
**Phone:** (804)662-9908    **Free:** 800-533-1560
**Fax:** (804)662-9517
**Email:** medbd@dhp.state.va.us
**Website:** http://www.dhp.state.va.us/medicine/default.htm
William L. Harp, MD, Contact

**★ 2823 ★ Washington State Department of Health**
Health Professions Quality Assurance
1300 SE Quince St.
PO Box 47860
Olympia, WA 98504-7860
**Phone:** (360)236-4700    **Fax:** (360)586-4818
**Email:** glenda.moore@doh.wa.gov
**Website:** http://www.doh.wa.gov/Medical/default.htm

**★ 2824 ★ West Virginia State Board of Medicine**
101 Dee Dr.
Charleston, WV 25311
**Phone:** (304)558-2921    **Fax:** (304)558-2084
**Email:** crystalwvbom@citynet.net
**Website:** http://www.wvdhhr.org/wvbom/
Ronald D. Walton, Contact

**★ 2825 ★ Wisconsin Medical Examining Board**
Department of Regulation & Licensing
1400 E Washington Ave., Rm. 173
PO Box 8935
Madison, WI 53708-8935
**Email:** web@drl.state.wi.us
**Website:** http://www.drl.state.wi.us/

**★ 2826 ★ Wyoming Board of Medicine**
Colony Bldg., 2nd Fl.
211 W 19th St.
Cheyenne, WY 82002
**Phone:** (307)778-7053    **Free:** 800-438-5784
**Fax:** (307)778-2069
**Email:** wyomedical@wyomedicalboard.org
**Website:** http://wyomedboard.state.wy.us/

# State & Regional Organizations

## Lyme Disease

*State chapters of the Lyme Alliance are listed below. The national office is located at PO Box 454, Concord, MI 49237. Additional information can be obtained by calling the national office at (517) 563-3582, or by consulting their web site at http://www.lymealliance.org/.*

### California

**★ 2827 ★ Lyme Disease Resource Center**
PO Box 707
Weaverville, CA 96093
**Email:** info@lymedisease.org
**Website:** http://www.lymedisease.org/index.html
Nancy Brown, President

### Connecticut

**★ 2828 ★ Lyme Disease Foundation**
1 Financial Plaza
Hartford, CT 06103-2601
**Phone:** (860)525-2000    **Free:** 800-886-5963
**Fax:** (860)525-8425
**Email:** Lymefnd@aol.com
**Website:** http://www.lyme.org

### Massachusetts

**★ 2829 ★ Massachusetts Lyme Disease Coalition**
Cape Cod Lyme Disease Awareness Association
PO Box 1916
Mashpee, MA 02649
**Phone:** (508)563-7033
John Coughlan, President

### Michigan

**★ 2830 ★ Lyme Alliance, Inc.**
PO Box 454
Concord, MI 49237
**Phone:** (517)563-3582    **Fax:** (517)524-7250
**Email:** barbfitz@concentric.net
**Website:** http://www.lymealliance.org

### Minnesota

**★ 2831 ★ Lyme Disease Coalition of Minnesota**
902 Grandview Ave.
Duluth, MN 55812-1146
**Phone:** (218)728-3914
**Email:** lymenet_mn@yahoo.com
**Website:** http://www.freeyellow.com/members2/olivierlynn/page3.html
Tom Grier, President

### New Jersey

**★ 2832 ★ Lyme Disease Association**
5019 Megill Rd.
Farmingdale, NJ 07727
**Phone:** (732)938-4834
**Email:** lymeliter@aol.com
**Website:** http://www.lymediseaseassociation.org
Pat Smith, President

# Medicine

*Listed below are state medical associations. The national organization is the American Medical Association, 515 N State St., Chicago, IL 60610, (312)464-5000, http://www.ama-assn.org/.*

### Alabama

**★ 2833 ★ Medical Association of the State of Alabama**
19 S Jackson St.
Montgomery, AL 36104
**Phone:** (334)954-2500    **Fax:** (334)269-5200
**Email:** cary@MASALINK.org
**Website:** http://www.MASALINK.org

### Alaska

**★ 2834 ★ Alaska State Medical Association**
4107 Laurel St.
Anchorage, AK 99508
**Phone:** (907)562-0304    **Fax:** (907)561-2063
**Email:** ASMA@alaska.net
**Website:** http://www.akmed.org

## Arizona

**★ 2835 ★ Arizona Medical Association**
810 W Bethany Home Rd.
Phoenix, AZ 85013
**Phone:** (602)246-8901  **Fax:** (602)242-6283
**Website:** http://www.azmedassn.org

## Arkansas

**★ 2836 ★ Arkansas Medical Society**
PO Box 55088
Little Rock, AR 72215
**Phone:** (501)224-8967  **Fax:** (501)224-6489
**Website:** http://www.arkmed.org

## California

**★ 2837 ★ California Medical Association**
PO Box 7690
San Francisco, CA 94120
**Phone:** (415)541-0900  **Fax:** (415)882-3349
**Website:** http://www.cmanet.org
Steve Thompson, Vice President

## Colorado

**★ 2838 ★ Colorado Medical Society**
PO Box 17550
Denver, CO 80217-0550
**Phone:** (720)859-1001  **Fax:** (720)859-7509
**Website:** http://www.cms.org

## Connecticut

**★ 2839 ★ Connecticut State Medical Society**
160 St. Ronan St.
New Haven, CT 06511
**Phone:** (203)865-0587  **Fax:** (203)865-4997
**Website:** http://www.csms.org

## Delaware

**★ 2840 ★ Medical Society of Delaware**
131 Continental Dr., Ste. 405
Newark, DE 19713
**Phone:** (302)658-7596  **Fax:** (302)658-9669
**Website:** http://www.medsocdel.org

## District of Columbia

**★ 2841 ★ Medical Society of the District of Columbia**
2175 K St. NW, Ste. 200
Washington, DC 20037
**Phone:** (202)466-1800  **Fax:** (202)452-1542
**Website:** http://www.msds.org

## Florida

**★ 2842 ★ Florida Medical Association**
113 E College Ave.
PO Box 10269
Tallahassee, FL 32302
**Phone:** (850)224-6496  **Fax:** (850)222-8030
**Website:** http://www.fmaonline.org

## Georgia

**★ 2843 ★ Medical Association of Georgia**
1330 W Peachtree St. NW, Ste. 500
Atlanta, GA 30309-2904
**Phone:** (404)876-7535  **Fax:** (404)881-5073
**Website:** http://www.mag.org
David A. Cook, Director

## Hawaii

**★ 2844 ★ Hawaii Medical Association**
1360 S Beretania St., 2nd Fl.
Honolulu, HI 96814
**Phone:** (808)536-7702  **Fax:** (808)528-2376
**Website:** http://www.hma-assn.org

## Idaho

**★ 2845 ★ Idaho Medical Association**
305 W Jefferson St.
Boise, ID 83701
**Phone:** (208)344-7888  **Fax:** (208)344-7903
**Email:** ima@micron.net
**Website:** http://www.idmed.org

## Illinois

**★ 2846 ★ Illinois State Medical Society**
20 N Michigan Ave., Ste. 700
Chicago, IL 60602
**Phone:** (312)782-1654  **Fax:** (312)782-2023
**Email:** info@isms.org
**Website:** http://www.isms.org

## Indiana

**★ 2847 ★ Indiana State Medical Association**
322 Canal Walk, Canal Level
Indianapolis, IN 46202
**Phone:** (317)261-2060  **Fax:** (317)261-2076
**Website:** http://www.ismanet.org

## Iowa

**★ 2848 ★ Iowa Medical Society**
1001 Grand Ave.
West Des Moines, IA 50265
**Phone:** (515)223-1401  **Fax:** (515)223-0590
**Website:** http://www.iowamedical.org

## Kansas

**★ 2849 ★ Kansas Medical Society**
623 SW 10th Ave.
Topeka, KS 66612
**Phone:** (785)235-2383  **Fax:** (785)235-5114
**Email:** ksmedsoc@inlandnet.net
**Website:** http://www.kmsonline.org

## Kentucky

**★ 2850 ★ Kentucky Medical Association**
4965 U.S. Hwy. 42, Ste. 2000
Louisville, KY 40222
**Phone:** (502)426-6200  **Fax:** (502)426-6877
**Website:** http://www.kyma.org

## Louisiana

**★ 2851 ★ Louisiana State Medical Society**
6767 Perkins Rd.
Baton Rouge, LA 70808
**Phone:** (225)763-8500  **Fax:** (225)763-6122
**Website:** http://www.lsms.org
Sharon Knight, JD, Director

## Maine

**★ 2852 ★ Maine Medical Association**
PO Box 190
Manchester, ME 04351
**Phone:** (207)622-3374  **Fax:** (207)622-3332
**Website:** http://www.mainemed.com

## Maryland

**★ 2853 ★ Medical and Chirurgical Faculty of Maryland (MedChi)**
Maryland State Medical Society
1211 Cathedral St.
Baltimore, MD 21201
**Phone:** (410)539-0872  **Fax:** (410)547-0915
**Website:** http://www.medchi.org

## Massachusetts

**★ 2854 ★ Massachusetts Medical Society**
860 Winter St.
Waltham Woods Corporate Ctr.
Waltham, MA 02451-1423
**Phone:** (781)893-4610  **Fax:** (781)893-8009
**Website:** http://www.massmed.org

## Michigan

**★ 2855 ★ Michigan State Medical Society**
120 W Saginaw
East Lansing, MI 48823
**Phone:** (517)337-1351  **Fax:** (517)337-2490
**Website:** http://www.msms.org

## Minnesota

**★ 2856 ★ Minnesota Medical Association**
3433 Broadway St. NE, Ste. 300
Minneapolis, MN 55413-1761
**Phone:** (612)378-1875  **Fax:** (612)378-3875
**Website:** http://www.mnmed.org

## Mississippi

**★ 2857 ★ Mississippi State Medical Association**
PO Box 2548
Ridgeland, MS 39158-2548
**Phone:** (601)853-6733  **Fax:** (601)853-6746
**Website:** http://www.msmaonline.com

## Missouri

**★ 2858 ★ Missouri Medical Association**
113 Madison St.
PO Box 1028
Jefferson City, MO 65102
**Phone:** (573)636-5151  **Fax:** (573)636-8552
**Website:** http://www.msma.org

## Montana

**★ 2859 ★ Montana Medical Association**
2021 11th Ave., Ste. 1
Helena, MT 59601
**Phone:** (406)443-4000  **Fax:** (406)443-4042
**Website:** http://www.mmaoffice.com

## Nebraska

**★ 2860 ★ Nebraska Medical Association**
233 S 13th St., Ste. 1512
Lincoln, NE 68508
**Phone:** (402)474-4472  **Fax:** (402)474-2198
**Email:** nma@inetnebr.com
**Website:** http://www.nebmed.org

## Nevada

**★ 2861 ★ Nevada State Medical Association**
3660 Baker Ln., Ste. 101
Reno, NV 89509
**Phone:** (702)825-6788  **Fax:** (702)825-3202
**Email:** nvstmeda@aol.com
**Website:** http://www.nsmadocs.org/index.html

## New Hampshire

**★ 2862 ★ New Hampshire Medical Society**
7 N State St.
Concord, NH 03301
**Phone:** (603)224-1909 **Fax:** (603)226-2432
**Website:** http://www.nhms.org

## New Jersey

**★ 2863 ★ Medical Society of New Jersey**
2 Princess Rd.
Lawrenceville, NJ 08648
**Phone:** (609)896-1766 **Fax:** (609)896-1368
**Email:** info@msnj.org
**Website:** http://www.msnj.org

## New Mexico

**★ 2864 ★ New Mexico Medical Society**
7700 Jefferson NE, Ste. 400
Albuquerque, NM 87109
**Phone:** (505)828-0237 **Fax:** (505)828-0336
**Email:** nmms@nmms.org
**Website:** http://www.nmms.org/nmms/

## New York

**★ 2865 ★ Medical Society of the State of New York**
420 Lakeville Rd.
Lake Success, NY 11042-5404
**Phone:** (516)488-6100 **Fax:** (516)488-1267
**Website:** http://www.mssny.org
Gerard L. Conway, Director

## North Carolina

**★ 2866 ★ North Carolina Medical Society**
222 N Person St.
PO Box 27167
Raleigh, NC 27611
**Phone:** (919)833-3836 **Fax:** (919)833-2023
**Website:** http://www.ncmedsoc.org
Stephen W. Keene, Director

## North Dakota

**★ 2867 ★ North Dakota Medical Association**
1025 3rd St. N
PO Box 1198
Bismarck, ND 58502-1198
**Phone:** (701)223-9475 **Fax:** (701)223-9476
**Website:** http://www.ndmed.com

## Ohio

**★ 2868 ★ Ohio State Medical Association**
3401 Mill Run Dr.
Hilliard, OH 43026
**Phone:** (614)527-6762 **Fax:** (614)527-6763
**Website:** http://www.osma.org
Tim I. Maglione, Director

## Oklahoma

**★ 2869 ★ Oklahoma State Medical Association**
601 NW Grand. Blvd.
Oklahoma City, OK 73118
**Phone:** (405)843-9571 **Fax:** (405)842-1834
**Website:** http://www.okmed.org

## Oregon

**★ 2870 ★ Oregon Medical Association**
5210 SW Corbett St.
Portland, OR 97201
**Phone:** (503)226-1555 **Fax:** (503)241-7148
**Website:** http://www.ormedassoc.org
Scott C. R. Gallant, BA, Director

## Pennsylvania

**★ 2871 ★ Pennsylvania Medical Society**
777 E Park Dr.
PO Box 8820
Harrisburg, PA 17105-8820
**Phone:** (717)558-7750 **Fax:** (717)558-7840
**Website:** http://www.pamedsoc.org

## Puerto Rico

**★ 2872 ★ Asociacion Medica de Puerto Rico**
Ave. Fernandez Juncos No. 1305
Santurce, PR 00908
**Phone:** (787)721-6969 **Fax:** (787)722-1191
**Website:** http://www.asociacionmedicapr.com/in-dice.htm
**Alt. Contact:** PO Box 9387, San Juan, PR 00908.

## Rhode Island

**★ 2873 ★ Rhode Island Medical Society**
106 Francis St.
Providence, RI 02903
**Phone:** (401)331-3207 **Fax:** (401)751-8050
**Email:** RIMS@ids.net
**Website:** http://www.rimed.org

## South Carolina

**★ 2874 ★ South Carolina Medical Association**
PO Box 11188
Columbia, SC 29211
**Free:** 800-327-1021 **Fax:** (803)772-6783
**Website:** http://www.scmanet.org
Jan McKellar, Director

## South Dakota

**★ 2875 ★ South Dakota State Medical Association**
1323 S Minnesota Ave.
Sioux Falls, SD 57105
**Phone:** (605)336-1965 **Fax:** (605)336-0270
**Website:** http://www.usd.edu/med/sdsma

## Tennessee

**★ 2876 ★ Tennessee Medical Association**
PO Box 120909
Nashville, TN 37212
**Phone:** (615)385-2100 **Fax:** (615)383-5918
**Website:** http://www.medwire.org/

## Texas

**★ 2877 ★ Texas Medical Association**
401 W 15th St.
Austin, TX 78701-1680
**Phone:** (512)370-1300 **Fax:** (512)370-1693
**Website:** http://www.texmed.org

## Utah

**★ 2878 ★ Utah Medical Association**
540 E 500 S
Salt Lake City, UT 84102
**Phone:** (801)355-7477 **Fax:** (801)532-1550
**Website:** http://www.utahmed.org
Val Bateman, Exec VP

## Vermont

**★ 2879 ★ Vermont Medical Society**
PO Box 1457
Montpelier, VT 05601-1457
**Phone:** (802)223-7898 **Fax:** (802)223-1201
**Website:** http://www.vtmd.org

## Virginia

**★ 2880 ★ Medical Society of Virginia**
4205 Dover Rd.
Richmond, VA 23221
**Phone:** (804)353-2721 **Fax:** (804)355-6189
**Website:** http://www.msv.org

## Washington

**★ 2881 ★ Washington State Medical Association**
2033 6th Ave., Ste. 1100
Seattle, WA 98121
**Phone:** (206)441-9762 **Fax:** (206)441-5863
**Website:** http://www.wsma.org
Len Eddinger, Director

## West Virginia

**★ 2882 ★ West Virginia State Medical Association**
4307 MacCorkle Ave. SE
PO Box 4106
Charleston, WV 25364
**Phone:** (304)925-0342 **Fax:** (304)925-0345
**Website:** http://www.wvsma.com

## Wisconsin

**★ 2883 ★ State Medical Society of Wisconsin**
PO Box 1109
Madison, WI 53701
**Phone:** (608)257-6781 **Fax:** (608)283-5401
**Website:** http://www.wismed.org

## Wyoming

**★ 2884 ★ Wyoming Medical Society**
1920 Evans Ave.
PO Box 4009
Cheyenne, WY 82003
**Phone:** (307)635-2424 **Fax:** (307)632-1973
**Website:** http://www.wyomed.org

# Chapter 2
# Aging

## Federal Government Agencies

**★ 2885 ★ U.S. Department of Health and Human Services**
**Administration on Aging (AOA)**
330 Independence Ave. SW
Washington, DC 20201
**Phone:** (202)401-4541     **Fax:** (202)619-3759
**Website:** http://www.aoa.dhhs.gov/
**Desc:** The Administration on Aging is the principal agency designated to carry out the provisions of the Older Americans Act of 1965. It is responsible for all issues involving the elderly. The Administration develops policies, plans, and programs designed to promote the welfare of the elderly; promotes their needs by planning programs and developing policy; provides policy, procedural direction, and technical assistance to States and Native American tribal governments.

**★ 2886 ★ U.S. Department of Health and Human Services**
**National Institutes of Health (NIH)**
**National Institute on Aging (NIA)**
9000 Rockville Pike
Bethesda, MD 20892
**Phone:** (301)496-1752
**Website:** http://www.nih.gov/nia/
Richard J. Hodes, MD, Director
**Desc:** The Institute conducts and supports biomedical and behavioral research to increase the knowledge of the aging process and associated physical, psychological, and social factors resulting from advanced age. Alzheimer's Disease, health and retirement, menopause, and fraility are among the areas of special concern.

## Foundations & Other Funding Organizations

### <u>Private Foundations</u>

**California Wellness Foundation**
*See:* Entry 5547

**★ 2887 ★ Charles H. Farnsworth Trust**
PO Box 351, M-3
Boston, MA 02101
**Phone:** (617)664-3261
**Website:** http://www.tcwf.org
Marilyn Wales, Vice President
**Fnded:** 1930. **Philosophy:** The purpose of the Charles H. Farnsworth Trust "is to assist elderly persons to live in dignity and with independence. In describing the purpose of his legacy, Mr. Farnsworth made clear his interest in housing, particularly in affordable housing options providing support services to the elderly. Program interests include services to the elderly in their homes, such as health care, homemaker assistance, and nutritional support; collective and supportive housing and services; and research, planning, and communication to better inform individuals, institutions, and the community at large of ways to improve the quality and quantity of housing and support services for the elderly." 1998 Form 990 Supplement **Priorities:** *Arts & Humanities:* 4%. Supports community music centers. *Civic & Public Affairs:* 10%. Supports housing, legal aid, and community development. *Environment:* 53%. Gives to elderly causes and senior services. *International:* 33%. Funds visiting nurses associations and health services to the elderly. *Note:* Total contributions made in fiscal 2001. **Typ. Recipients:** Alzheimers Disease, Clinics/Medical Centers, Diabetes, Emergency/Ambulance Services, Eyes/Blindness, Geriatric Health, Health Funds, Health Organizations, Home-Care Services, Hospices, Hospitals, Hospitals (University Affiliated), Long-Term Care, Medical Research, Mental Health, Nursing Services, People with Disabilities, Prenatal Health Issues, Public Health, Speech & Hearing. **Geo. Dist:** MA.

**★ 2888 ★ Clara and Spencer Werner Foundation**
711 South Main St.
PO Box 493
Paris, IL 61944
**Phone:** (217)466-1215     **Fax:** (217)466-1017
**Email:** cswernerf@tigerpaw.com
Jerry Klug, President
**Fnded:** 1953. **Philosophy:** The foundation gives only to Lutheran organizations; its primary interest is religious education. **Priorities:** *Education:* 84%. Provides for scholarship fund and religious education. *Note:* Total contributions made in fiscal 1999. **Typ. Recipients:** Alzheimers Disease. **Geo. Dist:** IL, including surrounding states.

**The Commonwealth Fund**
*See:* Entry 140

**★ 2889 ★ Fannie E. Rippel Foundation**
180 Mt. Airy Rd., Ste. 200
Basking Ridge, NJ 07920-2021
**Phone:** (908)766-0404
**Email:** rippel@gti.net
**Website:** http://www.fdncenter.org/grantmaker/rippel
Edward Probert, President & Chief Executive Officer
**Fnded:** 1953. **Philosophy:** The objectives of the Fannie E. Rippel Foundation were specified in the will of Julius S. Rippel and in the foundation's certificate of incorporation. These objectives are "to aid, assist, fund, equip, and provide for maintenance of corporations, institutions or associations, organizations or societies which are maintained for the relief and care of aged women; to provide and furnish funds for the erection of...hospitals; to provide and furnish funds for the equipment of...hospitals either in whole or in part; to aid or provide for the maintenance of hospitals in whole or in part; to provide and furnish funds for corporations, institutions and other organizations organized, maintained and existing for the purpose of treatment of and/or research concerning heart disease; to provide and furnish funds for corporations, institutions and other organizations organized, maintained and existing for the purpose of treatment of and/or research concerning cancer." Fannie E. Rippel Foundation Fiscal 2000 IRS Form 990 The foundation states that it is also interested in strategies to reach under-served rural and urban populations, women's health, prevention and strategies to change the behavior of populations including research and access to preventative care, humanistic medicine and mind-body-spirit connections as relating to the healing process. **Priorities:** *Arts & Humanities:* 3%. *Education:* 36%. *International:* 61%. *Note:* Total contributions made in fiscal 2000. **Typ. Recipients:** Cancer, Children's Health/Hospitals, Clinics/Medical Centers, Diabetes, Emergency/Ambulance Services, Eyes/Blindness, Geriatric Health, Health Organizations, Health-General, Heart, Hospitals, Hospitals (University Affiliated), Medical Education, Medical Rehabilitation, Medical Research, Public Health, Research/Studies Institutes. **Geo. Dist:** nationally; Middle Atlantic Seaboard.

**Florence V. Burden Foundation**
*See:* Entry 243

**Harry C. Trexler Trust**
*See:* Entry 323

**Henry Luce Foundation**
*See:* Entry 339

**Jack N. and Lilyan Mandel Foundation**
*See:* Entry 8539

**John A. Hartford Foundation**
*See:* Entry 9850

**Lucius N. Littauer Foundation**
*See:* Entry 485

**★ 2890 ★ Marty and Dorothy Silverman Foundation**
150 East 58th St., 29th Floor
New York, NY 10155
**Fax:** (212)755-1410
**Email:** mail@jhartfound.org
**Website:** http://www.jhartfound.org
Lorin Silverman, Treasurer
**Fnded:** 1986. **Philosophy:** The foundation provides grants to programs that address the needs of indigent senior citizens including nursing homes and hospitals. Additionally, grants may be made to other educational, scientific, cultural, and health and welfare agencies. **Priorities:** *Arts & Humanities:* About 2%. The performing arts and museums. *Civic & Public Affairs:* About 17%. Legal assistance, urban affairs, and housing.

*Education:* 17%. Emphasis on legal education. *Environment:* 29%. Primarily for services for the aged. *International:* 11%. Supports hospitals, health associations, and geriatric health concerns. *Note:* Total contributions made in fiscal 1998. **Typ. Recipients:** AIDS/HIV, Alzheimers Disease, Cancer, Child Abuse, Clinics/Medical Centers, Domestic Violence, Family Planning, Geriatric Health, Health Organizations, Health Policy/Cost Containment, Heart, Hospitals, Long-Term Care, Medical Education, Medical Research, Mental Health, Nursing Services, People with Disabilities, Public Health, Single-Disease Health Associations. **Geo. Dist:** New York, NY.

**Mary Duke Biddle Foundation**
*See:* Entry 511

**Maurice Amado Foundation**
*See:* Entry 520

★ 2891 ★ **Max Factor Family Foundation**
9777 Wilshire Boulevard, Ste. 1011
Beverly Hills, CA 90212
**Phone:** (310)274-8193　　　**Fax:** (310)274-9058
**Website:** http://www.mauriceamadofdn.org
Barbara Bentley, Trustee
**Fnded:** 1941. **Philosophy:** The foundation's primary concerns lie in geriatric health, research grants for doctors, scholarships for minorities in health-related fields, Jewish welfare organizations, and children's diseases. **Priorities:** *Education:* 7%. Gives to literacy programs and educational development programs. *Environment:* 13%. Funds support anti-violence programs, senior services, and children's concerns, including a $5,000 grant to Children of the Night in California. *International:* 47%. Supports medical centers and clinics. *Note:* Total contributions made in 1999. **Typ. Recipients:** Cancer, Children's Health/Hospitals, Clinics/Medical Centers, Diabetes, Domestic Violence, Emergency/Ambulance Services, Eyes/Blindness, Geriatric Health, Health Funds, Health Organizations, Health-General, Heart, Hospitals, Long-Term Care, Medical Research, Mental Health, People with Disabilities, Public Health, Single-Disease Health Associations, Single-Disease Health Associations, Speech & Hearing, Substance Abuse. **Geo. Dist:** CA.

**Nathan Cummings Foundation**
*See:* Entry 18215

★ 2892 ★ **Retirement Research Foundation**
8765 West Higgins Rd., Ste. 430
Chicago, IL 60631-4170
**Phone:** (773)714-8080　　　**Fax:** (773)714-8089
**Email:** info@rrf.org
**Website:** http://www.rrf.org
Marilyn Hennessy, President
**Fnded:** 1950. **Philosophy:** The foundation is particularly interested in innovative programs in aging that have the potential for national and regional impact. Funding interests fall into four areas: to improve the availability and quality of community-based and institutional long term care; to provide new and expanded opportunities for older adults to engage in meaningful roles in society such as employment and volunteerism that will strengthen community activities including advocacy, community leadership, community services, and intergenerational programs; to seek causes and solutions to significant problems of older adults through support of basic, applied, and policy research for which federal funding is not available; and to increase the number of professionals and para-professionals adequately prepared to serve the elderly population through support of selected education and training initiatives which enhance knowledge and skills of participants. The foundation currently operates the Congregational Connection Program (CCP) and the Organizational Capacity Building Program (OCB). **Priorities:** *Arts & Humanities:* 1%. Supports public broadcasting libraries. *Civic & Public Affairs:* 9%.

Supports Native American issues, Asian American affairs, safety, and legal aid. *Education:* 13%. Supports religious education, universities, fellowships, colleges, faculty development, literary, and medical education. *Environment:* 21%. Supports senior services, community service organizations shelters/homeless, family services. *International:* 46%. Supports Alzheimers, medical research, geriatric health, public health, hospital, health organizations, and hospices. *Note:* Total contributions made in 1998. **Typ. Recipients:** Alzheimers Disease, Alzheimers Disease, Cancer, Children's Health/Hospitals, Clinics/Medical Centers, Diabetes, Emergency/Ambulance Services, Family Planning, Geriatric Health, Health Organizations, Health Policy/Cost Containment, Heart, Home-Care Services, Hospices, Hospitals, Long-Term Care, Medical Education, Medical Research, Mental Health, Nursing Services, People with Disabilities, Preventive Medicine/Wellness Organizations, Public Health, Single-Disease Health Associations, Speech & Hearing, Transplant Networks/Donor Banks. **Geo. Dist:** nationally; Midwest: direct service projects; FL, direct service projects; Chicago, IL, metropolitan area.

**Schwartz Foundation**
*See:* Entry 667

**Vira I. Heinz Endowment**
*See:* Entry 737

## Corporate Foundations

★ 2893 ★ **Ameritech Michigan**
444 Michigan Ave., Room 1700
Detroit, MI 48226
**Phone:** (313)223-5747　　　**Fax:** (313)496-9337
**Email:** info@heinz.org
**Website:** http://www.sbc.com
Lisa Hamway, Director, Corporate Contributions
**Typ. Recipients:** Family Planning, Geriatric Health, Hospitals. **Geo. Dist:** MI, emphasis on the Detroit metropolitan area.

**FPL Group Foundation, Inc.**
*See:* Entry 1067

**Kupferberg Foundation**
*See:* Entry 5577

**Mamiye Foundation**
*See:* Entry 1216

★ 2894 ★ **Wachtell, Lipton, Rosen & Katz Foundation**
51 West 52nd St.
New York, NY 10019
**Phone:** (212)403-1000　　　**Fax:** (212)403-2000
**Email:** John_Kitchens@fpl.com
**Website:** http://www.fpl.com
Hillary Rappaport, Coordinator, Charitable Contributions
**Fnded:** 1981. **Priorities:** *Civic & Public Affairs:* 25%. Legal services, citizen committees, and local public affairs. *Education:* 40% to 45%. Law schools, legal education programs and conferences, and private preparatory schools. *Environment:* Less than 5%. Supports the homeless and social services. *International:* Less than 5%. Supports medical centers. **Typ. Recipients:** Geriatric Health, Hospitals (University Affiliated), Long-Term Care, Medical Education, Speech & Hearing. **Geo. Dist:** New York, NY, metropolitan area.

## Other Funding Organizations

**Alzheimer's Association**
*See:* Entry 13859

★ 2895 ★ **American Federation for Aging Research (AFAR)**
70 W 40th St.
New York, NY 10018
**Phone:** (212)703-9977　　　**Free:** 800-330-4660
**Fax:** (212)997-0330
**Email:** amfedaging@aol.com
**Website:** http://www.afar.org
Hadley C. Ford, Chair
**Desc:** Physicians, scientists, and other individuals involved or interested in research in aging and associated diseases. Purpose is to stimulate and fund research on aging. Facilitates communication among scientists in the field. Fosters public education regarding the need for support of related research. **Awards:** AFAR Research Grant (annual) to individuals conducting research; Irving Wright Distinghished Achievement Award (annual); Merck/AFAR Fellows in Gevatric Clinical Pharmacology (annual) to individual; Paul Beeson Physician Faculty Scholar in Aging Research.

★ 2896 ★ **American Foundation for Aging Research (AFAR)**
North Carolina State University
Biochemistry Department
128 Polk Hall
Raleigh, NC 27695-7622
**Phone:** (919)515-5679　　　**Fax:** (919)515-2047
**Email:** afar@bchserver.bch.ncsu.edu
**Website:** http://www4.ncsu.edu/unity/users/a/agris/afar/afar.htm
Dr. Paul F. Agris, Pres.
**Desc:** Supports basic research and educational opportunities for the study of age-related diseases and the biology of aging. Supports projects emphasizing modern biological, genetic, biochemical, and biophysical techniques and approaches to the problems of age-associated diseases and the understanding of aging. **Awards:** AFAR Fellowship (annual) for graduate students; Cecille Gould Memorial Fund for Cancer Research (annual); Glaxo Wellcome Fellowship; MaWren Wilson Fulton Memorial Scholarship (annual) for undergraduates.

★ 2897 ★ **American Geriatrics Society (AGS)**
350 5th Ave., Ste. 801
New York, NY 10118
**Phone:** (212)308-1414　　　**Free:** 800-247-4779
**Fax:** (212)832-8646
**Email:** info.amger@americangeriatrics.org
**Website:** http://www.americangeriatrics.org
Linda Hiddemen Barondess, Exec. VP
**Desc:** Professional society of physicians and other health care professionals interested in problems of the aged. Encourages and promotes the study of geriatrics; stresses the importance of medical research in the field of aging. Conducts seminars. **Awards:** Edward Henderson Student Award (annual); Milo D. Leavitt Student Award (annual); Nascher/Manning Award (biennial) for excellence in clinical geriatrics; New Investigator Award (annual); Student Travel Stipend (annual).

★ 2898 ★ **Donald W. Reynolds Foundation**
1701 Village Center Cir.
Las Vegas, NV 89134
**Phone:** (702)804-6000　　　**Fax:** (702)804-6099
**Email:** generalquestions@dwrf.org
**Website:** http://www.dwreynolds.org
**Desc:** Works to provide support for cardiovascular clinical research and aging and quality of life programs. **Awards:** Grant.

★ 2899 ★ **Gray Panthers (GP)**
733 15th St. NW, Ste. 437
Washington, DC 20005
**Phone:** (202)737-6637　　　**Free:** 800-280-5362
**Fax:** (202)737-1160
**Email:** info@graypanthers.org

**Website:** http://www.graypanthers.org
Tim Fuller, Exec. Dir.

**Desc:** Consciousness-raising activist group of older adults and young people. Aims to combat ageism - the discrimination against persons on the basis of chronological age. Believes that both the old and the young have much to contribute to make our society more just and humane. Advises, acts as acatalyst for, and organizes local groups of young, middle-aged, and older persons to work on issues of their choosing. Conducts work on eight national interests: national health care, affordable housing, environmental preservtion, peace, ending discrimination, education, economic and tax justice, and social justice. **Awards:** Mahler Grant (semiannual).

### ★ 2900 ★ John A. Hartford Foundation
55 E 59th St., 16th Fl.
New York, NY 10022-1178
**Phone:** (212)832-7788       **Fax:** (212)593-4913
**Email:** mail@jhartford.org
**Website:** http://www.jhartfound.org
Corinne H. Rieder, Exec. Dir.

**Desc:** Works to promote health care, training, research, and service related to older adults. **Awards:** Grant.

### ★ 2901 ★ National Caucus and Center on Black Aged (NCBA)
1200 L St. NW, Ste. 800
Washington, DC 20005
**Phone:** (202)637-8400       **Fax:** (202)347-0895
**Email:** info@ncba-aged.org
**Website:** http://www.ncba-blackaged.org
Samuel J. Simmons, Pres.

**Desc:** Seeks to improve living conditions for low-income elderly Americans, particularly blacks. Advocates changes in federal and state laws in improving the economic, health, and social status of low-income senior citizens. Promotes community awareness of problems and issues effecting low-income aging population. Operates an employment program involving 2000 older persons in 14 states. Sponsors, owns, and manages rental housing for the elderly. Conducts training and intern programs in nursing home administration, long-term care, housing management, and commercial property maintenance. **Awards:** Recognition; scholarship.

**National Gerontological Nursing Association**
*See:* Entry 14932

### ★ 2902 ★ North American Menopause Society (NAMS)
PO Box 94527
Cleveland, OH 44101
**Phone:** (440)442-7550       **Fax:** (440)442-2660
**Email:** info@menopause.org
**Website:** http://www.menopause.org
Wulf H. Utian, MD,PhD, Exec. Dir.

**Desc:** Physicians, scientists, research and clinical personnel, and other health care professionals are active members; student or physicians serving residencies or fellowships are associate members. Promotes understanding of menopause in women. Advances the exchange of research plans and experience between members. Offers educational programs. **Awards:** Grant (annual).

### ★ 2903 ★ Retirement Research Foundation (RRF)
8765 W Higgins Rd., Ste. 430
Chicago, IL 60681-4170
**Phone:** (773)714-8080       **Fax:** (773)714-8089
**Email:** info@rrf.org
**Website:** http://www.rrf.org
Edward J. Kelly, Chm.

**Desc:** Works to promote aging and retirement issues. Supports efforts that improve care for the aging, and enable older adults to live at home or in residential settings that facilitate independent living. **Awards:** Grant.

### ★ 2904 ★ Society of Geriatric Cardiology
Heart House
9111 Old Georgetown Rd.
Bethesda, MD 20814
**Phone:** (301)581-3449       **Fax:** (301)581-3408
**Email:** sgc@sgcard.org
**Website:** http://www.sgcard.org
Jane M. Dunne, Mgr.

**Desc:** Geriatric cardiologists and physicians in related fields are fellows; medical practitioners certified in specialties other than geriatrics or cardiologists are members; other individuals with an interest in geriatric cardiology are nonphysician members. Works to improve the clinical and therapeutic management of older individuals with cardiovascular disease; encourages use of preventive measures to avert the onset of cardiovascular aging and disease. Promotes more effective public policy and education regarding cardiac health. Conducts educational programs for physicians, other health care professionals, and the public. Supports research into cardiovascular aging and diseases relevant to older people. Serves as a clearinghouse on geriatric cardiology. Sponsors competitions. **Awards:** Merck Geriatric Cardiology Award (annual) for applicant reviewed by Research Committee.

# National & International Organizations

### ★ 2905 ★ African Gerontological Society (AGS)
c/o Dr. Nana Apt, PRes.
PO Box 01803
Osa
Accra, Ghana
**Phone:** 233 21 556382       **Fax:** 233 21 228397
**Lang(s):** English. **Desc:** Health care professionals with an interest in gerontology. Seeks to advance the study, teaching, and practice of gerontology. Serves as a forum for the exchange of information among members; sponsors continuing professional development courses.

### ★ 2906 ★ Age Action Ireland
30/31 Lower Camden St.
Dublin 2, Ireland
**Phone:** 353 1 4756989       **Fax:** 353 1 476011
**Email:** ageact@indigo.ie
**Website:** http://indigo.ie/~ageact
**Fnded:** 1992. **Mem:** 950. **Reg. Groups:** 1. **Local Groups:** 54. **Desc:** Works to improve the quality of life of older people, especially those who are most vulnerable and frail, by enabling them to live full, independent and satisfying lives. Membership is open to all organizations and individuals concerned with aging and older people. Main activities include information and library services, education and training, innovative projects, research, policy development and campaigning.

### ★ 2907 ★ Age - Belgium
111 rue Froissart
B-1040 Brussels, Belgium
**Phone:** 32 2 2801470       **Fax:** 32 2 2801522
**Email:** age.information@skynet.be
**Fnded:** 1982. **Mem:** 140. **Lang(s):** Dutch, English, French, German, Italian, Portuguese, Spanish. **Desc:** Works to improve the quality of life of older people. Gathers and disseminates information on issues including social issues, pensions, and employment. **Pub:** *Eurolink Age Bulletin*, 5/year. Bulletin. Conference reports, fact sheets, and policy papers.

### ★ 2908 ★ Age Concern England (ACE)
Astral House
1268 London Rd.
London SW16 4ER, United Kingdom
**Phone:** 44 20 87657200       **Fax:** 44 20 87657211
**Email:** infodep@ageconcern.org.uk
**Website:** http://www.ageconcern.org.uk
**Fnded:** 1940. **Mem:** 98. **Local Groups:** 1100. **Lang(s):** Dutch, English, French, German, Spanish. **Desc:** Involved in campaigning, parliamentary work, policy analysis, research, specialist information and advice provision and publishing. Raises funds. Member of the federation of over 400 Age Concern organizations operating in England. Provides both financial and development support to assist the other members in their provision of vital local services. **Pub:** *Information Bulletin*, monthly. Journal. • Books, periodic. • Pamphlets, periodic. • Papers, periodic.

### ★ 2909 ★ Age Concern Institute of Gerontology
King's College London
Waterloo Bridge Wing, Rm. 4.28
Franklin-Wilkins Bldg.
Waterloo Rd.
London SE1 9NN, United Kingdom
**Phone:** 44 40 78483035       **Fax:** 44 20 78483235
**Email:** aciog@kcl.ac.uk
**Website:** http://www.kcl.ac.uk/kis/schools/life_sciences/health/gerontology/top.html
**Lang(s):** English. **Desc:** Health care professionals treating the elderly; scientists and clinicians with an interest in the aging process and diseases of the aged. Works to insure high standards of research and practice in gerontology, and to maximize availability of gerontological services. Conducts research and educational activities. **Frmly:** (1997) British Society of Gerontology.

### ★ 2910 ★ Age Concern Scotland (ACS)
113 Rose St.
Edinburgh EH2 3DT, United Kingdom
**Phone:** 44 131 2203345       **Fax:** 44 131 2202779
**Email:** enquiries@acsinfo3.freeserve.co.uk
**Website:** http://www.ace.org.uk
**Fnded:** 1943. **Mem:** 593. **Nat'l Groups:** 1. **Local Groups:** 278. **Lang(s):** English. **Desc:** Individuals and organizations concerned with the quality of life and improving services available for senior citizens in Scotland. Supports a network of local Age Concern groups providing practical services and friendships for elderly individuals. Compiles statistics; sponsors research. **Pub:** *Adage*, bimonthly. Newsletter. Incorporates network notes. • Brochures, periodic.

### ★ 2911 ★ Aging in America (AIA)
1500 Pelham Pky. S
Bronx, NY 10461
**Phone:** (718)824-4004       **Fax:** (718)409-8781
William Smith, CEO

**Fnded:** 1979. **Desc:** Research and service organization for professionals in gerontology. Objectives are: to produce, implement, and share effective and affordable programs and services that improve the quality of life for the elderly community; to better prepare professionals and students interested in, or currently involved with, aging and the aged. Conducts research projects, educational and training seminars, and inservice curricula for long-term and acute care facilities. Operates: Education and Training Program to educate professionals and para-professionals; Projects With Industry Program to help both able-bodied and disabled elderly individuals enter into the work force. Conducts local programs in New York City including: In-Home Services, which provides Meals-on-Wheels, transportation, and housekeeping; Alzheimer's Day Care; Respite and Long-Term Residence; Self-Governing Senior Centers. Provides social services, including case management, information, referral, and advocacy; Research. Maintains speakers' bureau; compiles statistics. **Pub:** *Sharing Newsletter*, quarterly. Newsletter. • Brochure.Outlines various programs. **Frmly:** (1952) Morningside House.

## ★ 2912 ★ Albanian Association of Gerontology and Geriatrics

Rruga Mine Peza, Pall 1
Shk1., Ap 1.
Tirana, Albania
**Phone:** 355 42 26423          **Fax:** 355 42 32200
**Fnded:** 1996. **Lang(s):** Albanian, English. **Desc:** Provides services to the aged.

## ★ 2913 ★ Alliance for Aging Research (AAR)

2021 K St. NW, Ste. 305
Washington, DC 20006-1003
**Phone:** (202)293-2856          **Free:** 800-497-0360
**Fax:** (202)785-8574
**Email:** info@agingresearch.org
**Website:** http://www.agingresearch.org
Daniel Perry, Exec. Dir.
**Fnded:** 1986. **Desc:** Gerontologists and other medical professionals, executives, and members of Congress are participants. Works to increase private and public research into aging. Supports policies concerning: productive aging; independence for older Americans; successful aging; human genome initiative. **Pub:** *Age-Related Macular Degeneration.* Report. • *Aging Research on the Threshold of Discovery.* • *Alliance Reports.* Reports. • *Americans' View on Aging.* • *Health Care Options under MEDICARE: The Choice is Yours.* Report. • *Independence for Older Americans: Task Force for Aging Research Funding.* • *Investing in Older Women's Health.* • *Is it Time for a Heart to Heart?.* An educational kit for CHF. • *Issue Reports*, periodic. • *Last Year of Life: Exposing Seven Deadly Myths About the High Costs of Dying in America.* Report. • *Meeting the Medical Needs of the Senior Boom: The National Shortage of Geriatricians.* • *Putting Aging on Hold–Delaying the Diseases of Old Age.* • *Report on Public Opinion.* Report. • *The Research Gap.* • *Will You Still Treat Me When I'm 65?.* Report.

## ★ 2914 ★ Almshouse Association

c/o National Association of Almshouses
Billingbear Lodge
Wokingham RG40 5RU, United Kingdom
**Phone:** 44 1344 452922          **Fax:** 44 1344 862062
**Email:** naa@almshouses.org
**Website:** http://www.almshouses.org
**Fnded:** 1946. **Mem:** 1,850. **Desc:** Members are almshouse foundations which provide accommodation for the elderly. Advises members on any matters, concerning almshouses and the welfare of the elderly; promotes improvements in almshouses; promotes study and research into all matters affecting alms-houses; makes grants or loans to members. **Pub:** *The Almshouses Gazette*, quarterly.

## ★ 2915 ★ Alzheimer Society of Canada (ASC)

20 Eglington Ave. W, Ste. 1200
Toronto, ON, Canada M4R 1K8
**Phone:** (416)488-8772          **Free:** 800-616-8816
**Fax:** (416)488-3778
**Email:** info@alzheimer.ca
**Website:** http://www.alzheimer.ca
**Fnded:** 1978. **Mem:** 10. **Nat'l Groups:** 1. **State Groups:** 10. **Local Groups:** 145. **Lang(s):** English, French. **Desc:** Volunteers with an interest in helping individuals with Alzheimer's disease. Promotes an improved quality of life for people with Alzheimer's disease and their families. Supports research and educational programs; undertakes fundraising; creates awareness of Alzheimer's disease.

**Alzheimer's Association of Australia**
*See:* Entry 13894

**Alzheimer's Association NSW**
*See:* Entry 13895

## ★ 2916 ★ American Academy of Anti-Aging Medicine (A4M)

c/o Dr. Ronald Klatz
2415 North Greenview Ave.
Chicago, IL 60614
**Phone:** (773)528-4333          **Fax:** (773)528-5390
**Email:** media@worldhealth.net
**Website:** http://www.worldhealth.net
Dr. Ronald Klatz, Pres.
**Fnded:** 1993. **Mem:** 10,000. **Desc:** Dedicated to the advancement of technology to detect, prevent, and treat aging related disease and to promote research into methods to retard and optimize the human aging process. Also educates physicians, scientists and members of the public on anti-aging issues. Seeks to disseminate information concerning innovative science and research as well as treatment modalities designed to prolong human lifespan. **Pub:** *Anti-Aging Medical News*, quarterly. Newsletter. • *Report of the Medical Committee on Aging Research & Education*, quarterly. Newsletter.

## ★ 2917 ★ American Aging Association (AGE)

c/o The Sally Balin Medical Center
110 Chesley Dr.
Media, PA 19063
**Phone:** (610)627-2626          **Fax:** (610)565-9747
**Email:** ameraging@aol.com
**Website:** http://www.americanaging.org
Arthur K. Balin, MD, Exec. Dir.
**Fnded:** 1970. **Mem:** 500. **Desc:** Laymen and scientists primarily in the biomedical field. Dedicated to "helping people live better, longer" by promoting biomedical aging studies directed toward slowing down the aging process, informing the public of the progress of aging research and of practical means of achieving a long and healthy life, and increasing knowledge of gerontology among physicians and other health workers. **Pub:** *Age News*, quarterly. Newsletter. • *Journal of the American Aging Association*, quarterly. Journal. Covers biomedical aging research. *Price:* $50/year for individuals; $70/year outside U.S.

## ★ 2918 ★ American Association for Geriatric Psychiatry (AAGP)

7910 Woodmont Ave., Ste. 1050
Bethesda, MD 20814-3004
**Phone:** (301)654-7850          **Fax:** (301)654-4137
**Email:** main@aagpgpa.org
**Website:** http://www.aagpgpa.org
David Greenspan, MD, Sec.
**Fnded:** 1978. **Mem:** 1,468. **Desc:** Psychiatrists interested in promoting better mental health care for the elderly. Maintains placement service and speakers' bureau. **Pub:** *AAGP Membership Directory*, annual. Membership Directory. • *American Journal of Geriatric Psychiatry*, quarterly. Journal. • *Geriatric Psychiatry News*, bimonthly. Newsletter. Provides brief articles on psychiatric topics and case reports pertaining to elderly patients; includes association news, and employment listings. • *Growing Older and Wiser.* Covers consumer and general public information. *Price:* 14.

## ★ 2919 ★ American Association of Homes and Services for the Aging (AAHSA)

2519 Connecticut Ave. NW
Washington, DC 20008-1520
**Phone:** (202)783-2242          **Fax:** (202)783-2255
**Email:** info@aahsa.org
**Website:** http://www.aahsa.org
Michele Lacher, Communications Coor.
**Fnded:** 1961. **Mem:** 5,600. **Reg. Groups:** 3. **State Groups:** 40. **Desc:** Commmitted to advancing the vision of healthy, affordable, ethical long-term care for America. Represents 5,600 mission-driven, not-for-profit nursing homes, continuing care retirement communities, assisted living and senior housing facilities, and community service organizations. Serves its members through interaction with Congress and Federal agencies. Strives to enhance the professionalism of practitioners and facilites through the certification

program for retirement housing professionals, the Continuing Care Accreditation Commission, conferences and programs, and publications representing current thinking in the long-term care and retirement housing fields. Seeks to enhance its members' financial strength through group purchasing and the AAHSA Development Council. **Pub:** *American Association of Homes and Services for the Aging Publications Catalog*, 2/year. Catalog. • *Best Practices*, quarterly. Magazine. • *Directory of Members*, annual. Membership Directory. • *Washington Report*, biweekly. Report. Provides legislative and regulatory highlights. *Price:* Included in membership dues. **Frmly:** American Association of Homes for the Aging.

## ★ 2920 ★ American Association for International Aging (AAIA)

1900 L St., NW, Ste. 510
Washington, DC 20036-5002
**Phone:** (202)833-8893          **Fax:** (202)833-8762
Helen K. Kerschner, PhD, Pres.
**Fnded:** 1983. **Desc:** Advocates for the aged; organizations, corporations, foundations, and individuals concerned about the interests and needs of the aged worldwide, particularly in the Third World. Seeks to improve the socioeconomic conditions of older, low-income persons in developing countries through self-help, mutual support, and economic development activities. Sponsors international developmental education programs for retired Americans. Provides small grants assistance to economic-development projects for Third World aging; sponsors an information exchange program. **Pub:** *Aging and the Global Agenda for Women: Conversations in Nairobi.* • *American Association for International Aging Reports*, quarterly. Newsletter. Highlights activities benefiting aging persons worldwide. • *International Directory of Organizations in Aging.* Directory. • *Retired Americans Look at International Development.*

## ★ 2921 ★ American Disabled for Attendant Program Today (ADAPT)

201 S Cherokee St.
Denver, CO 80223-1836
**Phone:** (303)733-9324          **Fax:** (303)733-6211
**Email:** national@adapt.org
**Website:** http://www.adapt.org/
Mike Auberger, Dir.
**Fnded:** 1983. **Mem:** 5,000. **State Groups:** 34. **Local Groups:** 50. **Desc:** Promotes federal funding of in-home support services for the elderly and disabled in an effort to decrease the number of individuals being placed in nursing homes. **Pub:** *Incitement*, 6/year. Newsletter. **Frmly:** (1991) American Disabled for Accessible Public Transit.

## ★ 2922 ★ American Federation for Aging Research (AFAR)

70 W 40th St.
New York, NY 10018
**Phone:** (212)703-9977          **Free:** 800-330-4660
**Fax:** (212)997-0330
**Email:** amfedaging@aol.com
**Website:** http://www.afar.org
Hadley C. Ford, Chair
**Fnded:** 1981. **Reg. Groups:** 1. **Desc:** Physicians, scientists, and other individuals involved or interested in research in aging and associated diseases. Purpose is to stimulate and fund research on aging. Facilitates communication among scientists in the field. Fosters public education regarding the need for support of related research. **Pub:** *AFAR Newsletter*, biennial. Newsletter. Includes profiles of members. *Price:* Free. • *The Paul Besson Physician Faculty Scholars in Aging Research Report*, annual. Reprint. Contains scientific research projects of physician scientists.

## ★ 2923 ★ American Foundation for Aging Research (AFAR)

North Carolina State University
Biochemistry Department

128 Polk Hall
Raleigh, NC 27695-7622
**Phone:** (919)515-5679 **Fax:** (919)515-2047
**Email:** afar@bchserver.bch.ncsu.edu
**Website:** http://www4.ncsu.edu/unity/users/a/agris/
afar/afar.htm
Dr. Paul F. Agris, Pres.
**Fnded:** 1979. **Mem:** 295. **Desc:** Supports basic
research and educational opportunities for the study of
age-related diseases and the biology of aging. Supports projects emphasizing modern biological, genetic,
biochemical, and biophysical techniques and approaches to the problems of age-associated diseases
and the understanding of aging. **Pub:** *News From
AFAR*, quarterly. Newsletter. *Price:* Included in membership dues.

★ 2924 ★ **American Geriatrics Society
 (AGS)**
350 5th Ave., Ste. 801
New York, NY 10118
**Phone:** (212)308-1414 **Free:** 800-247-4779
**Fax:** (212)832-8646
**Email:** info.amger@americangeriatrics.org
**Website:** http://www.americangeriatrics.org
Linda Hiddemen Barondess, Exec. VP
**Fnded:** 1942. **Mem:** 6,022. **Reg. Groups:** 3. **State
Groups:** 23. **Desc:** Professional society of physicians
and other health care professionals interested in
problems of the aged. Encourages and promotes the
study of geriatrics; stresses the importance of medical
research in the field of aging. Conducts seminars.
**Pub:** *AGS Newsletter*, bimonthly. Newsletter. Includes
information on public policy issues of concern to
members, upcoming courses, events, publications,
and annual meeting. *Price:* Free. • *Annals of Long-
Term Care*, monthly. Journal. Contains articles, abstracts and meeting notices. *Price:* $60 for medical
students; $95 for nonmembers. • *Geriatrics Review
Syllabus: A Core Curriculum in Geriatric Medicine.*
*Price:* Call for information. • *Journal of the American
Geriatrics Society*, monthly. Journal. Includes original
articles, abstracts of geriatric literature, book reviews,
employment listings, and notices of meetings,
courses, and symposia. *Price:* Included in membership dues; $175/year for nonmembers in U.S.; $313/
year for institutions in U.S.; $80/year for nonmember
residents and interns in U.S.

★ 2925 ★ **American Senior Citizens
 Association (ASCA)**
PO Box 41
Fayetteville, NC 28302
**Phone:** (910)323-3641 **Free:** 800-323-6525
**Fax:** (910)323-4343
Ben Sutton, Exec. VP
**Fnded:** 1982. **Mem:** 35,000. **Desc:** Senior citizens.
Purpose is to promote the physical, mental, emotional,
and economic well-being of senior citizens. Believes
that senior citizens have a right to live with compe-
tence, security, and dignity. Promotes activities that
help senior citizens to be active participants in their
communities. Seeks affiliations with state senior citizens associations. **Pub:** *Senior Citizens Voice*, quarterly. Newspaper.

★ 2926 ★ **American Society on Aging
 (ASA)**
833 Market St., Ste. 511
San Francisco, CA 94103-1824
**Phone:** (415)974-9600 **Fax:** (415)974-0300
**Email:** info@asaging.org
**Website:** http://www.asaging.org
Gloria H. Cavanaugh, Exec. Dir.
**Fnded:** 1954. **Mem:** 10,000. **Desc:** Health care and
social service professionals, educators, researchers,
administrators, businesspersons, students, and senior
citizens. Works to enhance the well-being of older
individuals and to foster unity among those working
with and for the elderly. Offers 25 continuing education
programs for professionals in aging-related fields.
**Pub:** *Aging Today*, bimonthly. Newspaper. Tabloid
covering critical events and issues in the field of aging,

including legislative news, new products and designs,
and research. *Price:* Included in membership dues;
$14.95/year for nonmembers. • *Generations*, quarter-
ly. Journal. Provides practical, current information in
the field of aging, with emphasis on medical and social
practice, research, and policy. *Price:* Included in
membership dues; $38/year for nonmember individu-
als; $50 for institutions. **Frmly:** (1985) Western Geron-
tological Society.

★ 2927 ★ **Association of Brethren
 Caregivers (ABC)**
1451 Dundee Ave.
Elgin, IL 60120
**Phone:** (847)742-5100 **Free:** 800-323-8039
**Fax:** (847)742-5160
**Email:** abc@brethren.org
**Website:** http://www.brethren.org/abc/
Steve Mason, Exec. Dir.
**Fnded:** 1968. **Mem:** 24. **Desc:** Develops resources,
leadership, and programs within the caring ministries
of the Church of the Brethren and the wider communi-
ty. **Pub:** *Caregiving*, quarterly. Newsletter. Contains
information for the Church of the Brethren on caregiv-
ing issues. *Price:* $10/year. **Frmly:** (1989) Church of
the Brethren Homes and Hospitals Association; (1990)
Board of Brethren Homes and Older Adult Ministries;
(1993) Brethren Homes and Older Adult Ministries.

★ 2928 ★ **Association of Gerontology
 (India) (AGI)**
Banaras Hindu University
Department of Zoology
Varanasi 221 005, Uttar Pradesh, India
**Phone:** 91 542 307149 **Fax:** 91 542 368174
**Email:** agi@banaras.ernet.in
**Fnded:** 1982. **Mem:** 205. **Reg. Groups:** 6. **Lang(s):**
English. **Desc:** Health care professionals treating the
elderly; scientists and clinicians with an interest in the
aging process and diseases of the aged. Works to
insure high standards of research and practice in
gerontology, and to maximize availability of geronto-
logical services. Conducts research in biological,
clinical and psycho-social aspects of gerontology.

★ 2929 ★ **Association Internationale
 Francophone des Aines (AIFA)**
39 Dalhousie
Quebec, QC, Canada G1K 8R8
**Phone:** (418)646-9117 **Fax:** (418)644-7670
**Email:** cvfa@cvfa.ca
**Website:** http://www.cvfa.ca
**Fnded:** 1981. **Mem:** 125. **Lang(s):** French. **Desc:**
Individuals in 9 countries belonging to associations or
organizations that provide services to senior citizens.
Aims to: unite associations of senior citizens in
French-speaking areas; encourage participation by
senior citizens in social life; foster independent living;
promote the use of French and an understanding of
francophone culture; encourage information exchange
and visits to French-speaking areas. **Pub:** *Maturite*,
quarterly.

★ 2930 ★ **Association of Jewish Aging
 Services (AJAS)**
316 Pennsylvania Ave. SE, Ste. 402
Washington, DC 20003
**Phone:** (202)543-7500 **Fax:** (202)543-4090
**Email:** jodi@ajas.org
**Website:** http://ajas.org
Jodi L. Lyons, Pres.
**Fnded:** 1960. **Mem:** 200. **Desc:** Nonprofit charitable
Jewish homes and nursing homes; retirement and
housing units; independent and assisted living, geriat-
ric hospitals, and special facilities for Jewish aged and
chronically ill. Conducts institutes and conferences;
undertakes legislative activities; compiles statistics.
**Pub:** *Escribe Newsletter*, quarterly. Newsletter. •
Membership Directory, annual. **Frmly:** (1982) National
Association of Jewish Homes for the Aged; (1998)
North American Association of Jewish Homes and
Housing for the Aging.

★ **Australasian Menopause Society (AMS)**
*See:* Entry 16655

★ 2931 ★ **Australian Association of
 Gerontology (AAG-IAG)**
Centre for Ageing Studies
Mark Oliphant Bldg.
Laffer Dr.
Bedford Park, SA 5042, Australia
**Phone:** 61 8 82017552 **Fax:** 61 8 82017551
**Email:** aag.secre@flinders.edu.au
**Website:** http://www.cas.flinders.edu.au/aag
**Fnded:** 1961. **Mem:** 950. **Desc:** Focuses on issues
related to aging and the aging process.

★ 2932 ★ **Beverly Foundation (BF)**
566 El Dorado St., No. 100
Pasadena, CA 91101-2560
**Phone:** (626)792-2292 **Fax:** (626)792-6117
**Email:** bf3@ix.netcom.com
**Website:** http://www.beverlyfoundation.org/
Helen Kerschner, Pres.
**Fnded:** 1978. **Desc:** Develops education and research programs and policy studies to facilitate long-
term health care and supportive services and life
quality of people with chronic-care needs, particularly
older adults, their families, and caregivers. The focus
is on optimal functional independence and an informed
public. Unrestricted income is derived from product
sales, interest, dividends, donations, and grants. Restricted funds are sought to support new program
developments which focus on improving service systems and methods of long-term care. Sells educational
materials to health care industry. Maintains library.
**Pub:** *Pioneering Times*, biennial. Newsletter. *Price:*
Free.

★ 2933 ★ **British Geriatrics Society**
31 St. John's Sq.
London EC1M 4DN, United Kingdom
**Phone:** 44 20 76081369 **Fax:** 44 20 76081041
**Email:** info@bgs.org.uk
**Website:** http://www.bgs.org.uk
**Fnded:** 1947. **Mem:** 2,500. **Reg. Groups:** 17.
**Lang(s):** English. **Desc:** Consultant geriatricians and
other doctors, scientists, and professionals with an
interest in geriatric medicine and care of the elderly.
To promote scientific developments of geriatric medicine, improve medical and social services for elderly
people and promote measures which will improve
health throughout adult life to ensure better fitness on
achieving old age. **Pub:** *Age and Ageing*, bimonthly.

★ 2934 ★ **British Society for Research
 on Ageing (BSRA)**
PO Box 2316
Cardiff CF23 5YY, United Kingdom
**Phone:** 44 29 20744847 **Fax:** 44 29 20744276
**Email:** secretary@bsra.org.uk
**Website:** http://www.bsra.org.uk
**Fnded:** 1945. **Mem:** 150. **Lang(s):** English. **Desc:**
Biological scientists and clinicians involved in the
study of aging. Promotes knowledge of the biology of
aging and effective treatment of age-related diseases.
Works to increase public awareness of the aging
process. Sponsors annual postgraduate award com-
petition. **Pub:** *Lifespan*, semiannual. Newsletter. •
*Newsletter*, periodic. Newsletter.

★ 2935 ★ **Canada's Association for the
 Fifty-Plus (CARP)**
27 Queen St. E, Ste. 300
Toronto, ON, Canada M5C 2M6
**Phone:** (416)363-8748 **Free:** 800-363-9736
**Fax:** (416)363-8747
**Email:** info@50plus.com
**Website:** http://www.fifty-plus.net
**Fnded:** 1976. **Mem:** 380,000. **Reg. Groups:** 8.
**Lang(s):** English. **Desc:** Canadians who are at least
50 years old. Promotes the rights and seeks to
improve the quality of life of older people. Provides

products and services to members; represents members in public forums. **Pub:** *CARPNEWS*, bimonthly. Magazine. **Frmly:** (1999) Canadian Association of Retired Persons.


★ **2936** ★ **Canadian Alliance of British Pensioners (CABP)**
605 Royal York Rd., Ste.202
Toronto, ON, Canada M8Y 4G5
**Phone:** (416)253-6402  **Fax:** (416)253-6402
**Email:** info@britishpensions.com
**Website:** http://www.britishpensions.com
**Fnded:** 1991. **Lang(s):** English. **Desc:** Senior citizens and British expatriates in Canada. Works to safeguard the interests of senior citizens. Campaigns to end pension discrimination such as freezing of British pension for those residents in Canada. **Pub:** *Quarterly View*, quarterly. Newsletter. **Frmly:** British Pensioners Association.


★ **2937** ★ **Canadian Association of Gerontology (CAG)**
824 Meath St., Ste. 100
Ottawa, ON, Canada K1Z 6E8
**Phone:** (613)728-9347  **Fax:** (613)728-8913
**Email:** info@cagacg.ca
**Website:** http://www.cagacg.ca
**Fnded:** 1973. **Mem:** 1,000. **Desc:** Focuses on the problems and process of aging. **Pub:** *CAG Newsletter*, quarterly. Newsletter. • *Canadian Journal on Aging*, quarterly. Journal.


★ **2938** ★ **Canadian Association of Pre-Retirement Planners (CAPP)**
289 Greenwood Dr.
Stratford, ON, Canada N5A 7K6
**Phone:** (519)273-5616  **Fax:** (519)273-6097
**Email:** cappnational@cyg.net
**Website:** http://www.retirementplanners.ca
**Fnded:** 1981. **Reg. Groups:** 6. **Lang(s):** English. **Desc:** Organizations that provides pre- or post-retirement services, seminars or workshops, and individuals who are lifestyle planners, human resource personnel, financial planners, counselors, adult educators, health professionals, leisure and fitness personnel, program planners, gerontologists, and others. Promotes the retirement planning industry. Provides information and networking opportunities; encourages high standards of performance and ethical behavior; seeks to improve public awareness; encourages members to become registered with the Professional Retirement Planners Registry.


★ **2939** ★ **Canadian Geriatrics Society (Societe Canadienne de Geriatrie — SCG)**
100-824 Meath St.
Ottawa, ON, Canada K1Z 6E8
**Phone:** (613)728-9347  **Fax:** (613)728-8913
**Email:** wbdalziel@ottawahospital.on.ca
**Fnded:** 1980. **Mem:** 200. **Lang(s):** English, French. **Desc:** Health care professionals with an interest in geriatric medicine. Seeks to advance the practice of gerontology; promotes ongoing professional development of members. Facilitates exchange of information among members; conducts continuing professional education courses. **Frmly:** (2001) Canadian Society of Geriatric Medicine.


**Canadian Gerontological Nursing Association (CGNA) (Association Canadienne des Infirmiers et Infirmieres en Gerontologie — ACIG)**
*See:* Entry 15688


★ **2940** ★ **Canadian Hispanic Senior Services (CHSS)**
1829 54th St. SE, Ste. 200
Calgary, AB, Canada T2B 1N5
**Phone:** (403)569-0133  **Fax:** (403)569-0133
**Email:** cgna@home.com

**Website:** http://www.cgna.net
**Lang(s):** English, French. **Desc:** Individuals and organizations providing services to senior citizens. Promotes increased availability of senior services among Canadians of Hispanic descent. Provides support and services to Hispanic Canadians.


★ **2941** ★ **The Center for Social Gerontology (TCSG)**
2307 Shelby Ave.
Ann Arbor, MI 48103
**Phone:** (734)665-1126  **Fax:** (734)665-2071
**Email:** tcsg@tcsg.org
**Website:** http://www.tcsg.org
Clifford Douglas, Pres.
**Fnded:** 1971. **Desc:** Purpose is to advance the well-being of older people in the U.S. through research, education, technical assistance, and training. Focuses primarily on legal rights, guardianship and alternative protective services, delivery of legal services, and issues of tobacco and older persons. Provides consulting services. Develops and researches standards for the provision of guardianship services for older people; works to improve the court processes for determining the need for guardianship through development and evaluation of a new model. Conducts periodic training on Legal rights and Legal resources, for legal advocates, nonlawyers who work with the elderly, and older consumers. **Pub:** *Adult Guardianship Mediation.* Manuals. • *Adult Guardianship Mediation: An Introduction.* Videos. • *Best-Practice Notes on Delivery of Legal Services to Older Persons*, quarterly. Bulletin. • *Comprehensive Guide to Delivery of Legal Assistance to Older Persons.* • *Guidelines for Planning and Evaluating Legal Assistance Programs Funded Under the Older Americans Act.* • Audiotapes. • Reports. • Adult Guardianship Mediation Manual, Guardianship & Alternatives: A Guide to Personal, Health Care & Financial Management Options, and National Study of Guardianship Systems: Findings & recommendations. **Frmly:** (1985) International Center for Social Gerontology.


★ **2942** ★ **Center for the Study of Aging of Albany (CSA)**
706 Madison Ave.
Albany, NY 12208
**Phone:** (518)465-6927  **Fax:** (518)462-1339
**Email:** apaas@aol.com
**Website:** http://www.rit.edu/~pjr0120/csa/iapaas/main.html
Norm Thompson, Dir. Office of Mgmt.
**Fnded:** 1957. **Desc:** Participants include behavioral scientists, educators, gerontologists, physicians, and other health professionals. Promotes education, research, and training; provides leadership in the field of health and fitness for older people. Includes: programs for volunteers and professionals in aging, gerontology, geriatrics, wellness, physical fitness, and mental health; consultant services include adult day care, nutrition, physical and mental fitness, nursing home, housing, and retirement; speakers' bureau. Develops national and international conferences on health, fitness, and prevention. Provides expert assistance in research, institutional and community program development, planning, and organization; offers consultation addressing the development of library resource centers and collections of books on aging. Conducts seminars and offers information and referral services. **Pub:** *Classics in Aging.* Book. • *Environment and Aging.* Book. • *Physical Activity, Aging and Sports - Volume I: Scientific and Medical Research.* • *Physical Activity, Aging and Sports - Volume II: Practice, Program, and Policy.* • *Physical Activity Aging and Sports - Volume III: International Perspectives Toward Healthy Aging, Part I Physiological and Biomedical Aspects.* • *Physical Activity, Aging and Sports - Volume IV: Toward Healthy Aging, Part 2 Psychology, Motivation and Programs.* • *Safe Therapeutic Exercise for the Frail Elderly: An Introduction.* Manual. • *Senior Citizen School Volunteer Program: A Manual for Program Implementation.* • *Series: Life Long Health and Fitness-Volume I-Prevention and Human Aguiy*, annual. Bibliographies. Covers health and fitness. •

*Who? Me!? Exercise: Safe Exercise for Over Fifty.* 48 pp. exercises illustrations. • Books. **AKA:** International Association of Physical Activity.


★ **2943** ★ **Centre for Policy on Ageing (CPA)**
19-23 Ironmonger Row
London EC1V 3QP, United Kingdom
**Phone:** 44 207 5536500  **Fax:** 44 207 5536501
**Email:** cpa@cpa.org.uk
**Website:** http://www.cpa.org.uk
**Fnded:** 1947. **Mem:** 90. **Lang(s):** English. **Desc:** Health care professionals; social workers; academics. Promotes policies in England which will result in higher standards of care and a better lifestyle for the elderly. Encourages informed debate about issues affecting older people and stimulates public awarenesss of their needs. Conducts studies and makes recommendations to policy makers. Maintains CPA Information Service which keeps readers abreast of trends in policy, practice, and research development. Areas of interest include residential care policy, educational and recreational activities for the elderly, and elderly people in ethnic minorities. Strives to address the needs of housebound and vulnerable elderly people and integrate all older people into the community. Currently investigating possible methods of providing for homeless elderly people. Has established the Niccol Center in Cirencester. Works closely with the University of the Third Age. **Pub:** *Age Info CD-ROM.* CD-Rom which provides information from 3 different databases, covering all aspects of aging. • *Aging and Society*, quarterly. • *CPA Papers*, periodic. • *CPA Report*, periodic. • *New Literature on Old Age*, bimonthly. • *Old Age: A Register of Social Research*, periodic. • *Policy Studies in Ageing*, periodic.


★ **2944** ★ **Centro Gerontologico Latino/ Latino Gerontological Center (CGL)**
120 Wall St., 23rd Fl.
New York, NY 10005-4001
**Phone:** (212)344-9636  **Fax:** (212)480-9734
**Email:** info@gerolatino.org
**Website:** http://www.gerolatino.org
Mario E. Tapia, Pres. & CEO
**Fnded:** 1991. **Mem:** 300. **Desc:** Works to improve the quality of life of Hispanic seniors. Provides Thanksgiving meals to needy families; operates cable television show in Manhattan, NY. Writes question and answer column in New York paper "El Diario" to provide information to hispanic seniors.


★ **2945** ★ **Children of Aging Parents (CAPS)**
Woodbourne Office Campus, Ste. 302A
1609 Woodbourne Rd.
Levittown, PA 19057-1511
**Phone:** (215)945-6900  **Free:** 800-227-7294
**Fax:** (215)945-8720
**Email:** caps4caregivers@aol.com
**Website:** http://www.caps4caregivers.org/
Lorraine Sailor, Contact
**Fnded:** 1977. **Mem:** 1,300. **Desc:** National information and referral service for caregivers of the elderly. Provides a speakers bureau as part of its educational outreach mission to churches, service clubs, schools, hospitals, TV/radio and colleges. Conducts workshops, seminars, and conferences for lay individuals and professionals in the field of aging. Publishes a bimonthly newsletter and numerous fact sheets on various topics of interest to caregivers. Organizes and promotes caregivers' support groups, and responds to requests for assistance nationally. **Pub:** *The Capsule*, bimonthly. Newsletter. Reports on concerns of elderly persons and their families. Includes publications listing, book reviews, and research news. *Price:* Included in membership dues. • *Guide to Selecting a Nursing Home.* • *How to Start A Self Group for Caregivers.* • *Instant Aging–Sensory Deprivation Manual.* Manual. • Bibliographies. • Publishes fact sheets on caregiving issues.

**★ 2946 ★ Chilean Gerontological Study Group (CGSG)**
Avenida Presidente Riesco 6007
Classifiacdor 1
Correo 27
Santiago, Chile
**Lang(s):** English, Spanish. **Desc:** Health care professionals treating the elderly; scientists and clinicians with an interest in the aging process and diseases of the aged. Promotes gerontological research and increased availability of gerontological care; facilitates training of gerontology specialists. Represents the interests of gerontologists and gerontological organizations.

**★ 2947 ★ Christian Association of Primetimers**
PO Box 777
Saint Charles, IL 60174
**Phone:** (630)443-0050 **Free:** 800-443-0227
**Fax:** (630)444-0087
**Email:** email@christianprimetimers.org
**Website:** http://christianprimetimers.org
Roland Johnson, Pres.
**Fnded:** 1993. **Mem:** 50,000. **Desc:** Seeks to improve, encourage and provide a better quality of life to those ages 50 and older; offers discount travel and volunteer opportunities. **Pub:** *PrimeTimer Newsletter*, bimonthly. Newsletter. Provides updates on new benefits, travel opportunities, and CAP activities.

**Commission for Certification in Geriatric Pharmacy (CCGP)**
*See:* Entry 17533

**★ 2948 ★ Costa Rican Gerontology Association (CRGA)**
**(Asociacion Gerontologica Costarricense — AGECO)**
Apartado Postal 5956
San Jose 1000, Costa Rica
**Phone:** 506 2210310 **Fax:** 506 2220348
**Email:** info@ccgp.org
**Website:** http://www.ticofiesta.com
**Fnded:** 1980. **Mem:** 54. **Nat'l Groups:** 120. **Reg. Groups:** 40. **Local Groups:** 80. **Lang(s):** Spanish. **Desc:** Health care professionals treating the elderly; scientists and clinicians with an interest in the aging process and diseases of the aged. Promotes gerontological research and increased availability of gerontological care; facilitates training of gerontology specialists. Represents the interests of gerontologists and gerontological organizations. **Pub:** *Ejercicios en la Tercera Edad*, biennial. Manual. • *Envejecer Sano Con Una Buena Allimentacion*, biennial. Bulletin. • *La Voz de Ageco*, biennial. Bulletin. • *Manual de Consejos Practicos en la III Edad Y Otros*, biennial. Bulletin.

**★ 2949 ★ Cuban Society of Geriatrics and Gerontology (CSGG)**
**(Sociedad Cubana de Gerontologia y Geriatria — SCGG)**
Calle L, No. 406, entre 23 Y
25 Vedado
PO Box 10400
Havana, Cuba
**Phone:** 53 7 333864 **Fax:** 53 7 333319
**Email:** cited@infomed.sld.cu
**Mem:** 200. **Lang(s):** Spanish. **Desc:** Health care professionals treating the elderly; scientists and clinicians with an interest in the aging process and diseases of the aged. Promotes gerontological research and increased availability of gerontological care; facilitates training of gerontology specialists. Represents the interests of gerontologists and gerontological organizations.

**★ 2950 ★ Danish Gerontological Association (DGA)**
Aurehojvej 24
DK-2900 Hellerup, Denmark
**Phone:** 45 39627627 **Fax:** 45 39626627
**Email:** dgs@geroinst.dk
**Website:** http://www.gerodan.dk
**Lang(s):** Danish, English. **Desc:** Health care professionals treating the elderly; scientists and clinicians with an interest in the aging process and diseases of the aged. Promotes gerontological research and increased availability of gerontological care; facilitates training of gerontology specialists. Represents the interests of gerontologists and gerontological organizations.

**★ 2951 ★ Daughters of the Elderly Bridging the Unknown Together (DEBUT)**
c/o Pat Meier
3616 E Homestead Dr.
Bloomington, IN 47401
**Phone:** (812)339-2092
Pat Meier, Facilitator
**Fnded:** 1981. **Mem:** 10. **Local Groups:** 1. **Desc:** Women involved in caring for elderly parents; individuals preparing for future roles as caregivers. Provides: nonjudgmental support; education in all areas of caring, coping, and in the complex process of aging. Stresses the importance of nursing center advocacy, community outreach, and intergenerational dialogue between adult children and their parents. Delivers presentations at local gerontological functions. **Pub:** *Daughters of the Elderly: Building Partnerships in Caregiving*. Book. *Price:* $9.95.

**★ 2952 ★ Ebenezer Society (ES)**
2722 Park Ave.
Minneapolis, MN 55407-1043
Mark Thomas, Pres.
**Fnded:** 1917. **Mem:** 45. **Desc:** Lutheran congregations and their delegates. Works to provide quality services and facilities for older people with varying needs; to make their lives more healthful, meaningful, and secure. Services are not limited to Lutheran clients. Offers nursing home care for low-income elderly; provides home services, including medical treatment, to help persons remain in their own homes as long as possible. Sponsors Ebenezer Center for Aging and Human Development which provides consultative services, conducts educational events and applied research, and issues publications. Maintains Ebenezer Foundation as the support arm of the society. Compiles research statistics; offers placement service. Ebenezer means "stone of help."

**★ 2953 ★ Elder Craftsmen (EC)**
610 Lexington Ave.
New York, NY 10022
**Phone:** (212)319-8128 **Fax:** (212)319-8141
**Email:** eldercraftsmen@mindspring.com
**Website:** http://www.eldercraftsmen.org/
Janet Langlois, Exec. Dir.
**Fnded:** 1955. **Desc:** Helps men and women 55 and older be creative, productive, and independent. Seeks broader recognition by the general public of the skills and capabilities of older people. Sponsors craft training workshops for representatives of Senior Centers. Sponsors community service projects with older adults making items for people in need. **Pub:** *What's This Got to do With Quilting: Nine Stories of Southern Women Quilters*. Booklet.

**★ 2954 ★ Energy Action (EA)**
IDA Unit 14
Newmarket
Dublln 8, Ireland
**Phone:** 353 1 4545464 **Fax:** 353 1 4549797
**Email:** info@energyaction.ie
**Website:** http://www.energyaction.ie
**Fnded:** 1988. **Mem:** 14. **Reg. Groups:** 8. **Lang(s):** English, Irish. **Desc:** Individuals interested in meeting the energy needs of the elderly. Seeks to improve energy efficiency in the homes of elderly people. Provides home insulation services at no cost to elderly individuals. Trains unemployed people to install insulation in accordance with building codes and safety standards.

**★ 2955 ★ Episcopal Society for Ministry on Aging (ESMA)**
PO Box 3065
Meridian, MS 39303
**Phone:** (601)485-0311
**Email:** info@esmanet.com
**Website:** http://www.episcopalchurch.org/episcopal-life/RetClose.html
**Fnded:** 1964. **Desc:** Develops and supports Episcopal Church by strengthening God's people for ministry throughout the entire life span. Publishes resources and provides education and training for clergy and lay leaders; offers consultations to seminaries on development of curricula in gerontology; develops Age in Action educational materials for parishes. Operates a national network of clergy and lay volunteers for the dissemination of information and for program development at grass-roots level. **Pub:** *Affirmative Aging*. Book. Includes study guide. • *Directory of Episcopal Related Housing for the Aging*. Directory. • *ESMA's Network News*, 3/year. Newsletter. • *Large Print Book of Common Prayer*. • *Older Adult Ministry: A Resource for Program Development*. • Distributes *(In)Dignity of Aging* (videotape).

**★ 2956 ★ ESHEL - The Association for the Planning and Development of Services for the Aged in Israel (ESHEL)**
**(Haagudah Letichnun Vepituach Sherutim Lemaan Hazaken Beyisrael)**
JDC Hill
PO Box 3489
IL-91034 Jerusalem, Israel
**Phone:** 972 2 6557128 **Fax:** 972 2 5662716
**Email:** eshelnet@jointnet.org.il
**Website:** http://www.jointnet.org.il/eshelnet/
**Fnded:** 1969. **Local Groups:** 115. **Lang(s):** Hebrew. **Desc:** Develops and plans services for the aged in Israel, including daycare centers, homes for the aged, sheltered housing projects, supportive neighborhoods, respite care centers, health promotion programs, volunteer-based services, and others. Conducts training programs for managers, professionals, paraprofessionals, and others who work with the aged in Israel and abroad. Develops computer based information services to improve access to information, products and services. Conducts research and develops products to improve the quality of life of the elderly in Israel. Publishes books and pamphlets and produces videos on aging. **Pub:** *Aging as an Academic Field: Aging and SocioAnthropological Studies*. Book. • *The Association for the Elderly: A Guide for Establishing a Public Organization*. Book. • *Between Ourselves and Our Parents: A Reader on the Relationship betwe en Children and their Elderly Parents*. Book. • *Day Center for the Elderly*. Book. • *Guidelines for the Planning of Homes for the Aged in Israel*. Book. • *Suggested Activities for the Teaching of Aging as a High School Subject*. Book. • Audiotapes. • Pamphlets. • Videos.

**★ 2957 ★ Eurolink Age - England**
1268 London Rd.
London SW16 4ER, United Kingdom
**Phone:** 44 208 7657717 **Fax:** 44 208 6796727
**Email:** eurolink@ace.org.uk
**Website:** http://www.eurolinkage.org
**Fnded:** 1981. **Mem:** 100. **Lang(s):** Dutch, English, French, German, Italian, Spanish. **Desc:** Works to improve the quality of life of the elderly. Gathers and disseminates information on issues including social benefits, pensions, and employment. **Pub:** *Eurolink Age Bulletin*, bimonthly. Journal. Frmly: Eurolink Age - England.

## ★ 2958 ★ European Federation of the Elderly
### (Federation Europeenne des Personnes Agees)
Secretariat General
Wielandgasse 9
A-8010 Graz, Austria
**Phone:** 43 316 814608 **Fax:** 43 316 814767
**Email:** eurag.europe@aon.at

**Fnded:** 1962. **Mem:** 350. **Lang(s):** English, French, German, Italian. **Desc:** Self-help groups working with older people; volunteers, physicians, psychologists, sociologists, social workers, researchers, and para-medical personnel helping the elderly in 33 countries. Promotes the well-being of the aged by working to improve their socioeconomic status; encourages the elderly to attain independence and become self-reliant by developing practical skills. Works to heighten public awareness of older people's needs. Cooperates with European organizations on questions regarding aging and the aged. Stimulates contacts and information exchange among members; compiles bibliographic information on aging. Sponsors colloquia. **Pub:** *EURAG Information*, monthly. • *EURAG Newsletter*, quarterly. **Frmly:** (1996) European Federation for the Welfare of the Elderly.


### European Society of Surgical Geriatrics
*See:* Entry 19552


## ★ 2959 ★ Federation of Active Retirement Association (FARA)
Shamrock Chambers
59-61 Dame St.
Dublin 2, Ireland
**Phone:** 353 1 6792142 **Fax:** 353 1 6792142

**Fnded:** 1995. **Mem:** 110,000. **Reg. Groups:** 65. **Local Groups:** 69. **Desc:** Retired individuals over 55 years of age. Encourages member to "lead a full, happy and healthy retirement." Organizes outings, social activities, sports activities, educational pro-grams, and community service activities. **Pub:** Bulle-tin, monthly.


## ★ 2960 ★ French Society of Gerontology (FSG)
### (Societe Francaise de Gerontologie — SFG)
Faculte de Medecine Pite-Salpetriere - 91
Boulevard de l'Hopital
F-75013 Paris, France
**Phone:** 33 1 40779645 **Fax:** 33 1 40779644
**Email:** michel-frossard@umpf.grenoble.fr

**Fnded:** 1961. **Lang(s):** French. **Desc:** Health care professionals treating the elderly; scientists and clini-cians with an interest in the aging process and diseases of the aged. Works to insure high standards of research and practice in gerontology, and to maximize availability of gerontological services. Con-ducts research and educational activities.


## ★ 2961 ★ Gerontological Society of America (GSA)
1030 15th St. NW, Ste. 250
Washington, DC 20005-1503
**Phone:** (202)842-1275 **Fax:** (202)842-1150
**Email:** cschutz@geron.org
**Website:** http://www.geron.org
Carol A. Schutz, Exec. Dir.

**Fnded:** 1945. **Mem:** 5,000. **Desc:** Physicians, physiol-ogists, psychologists, anatomists, biochemists, sociol-ogists, social workers, psychiatrists, pharmacologists, nurses, geneticists, zoologists, endocrinologists, econ-omists, administrators, and other professionals inter-ested in improving the well-being of older people by promoting scientific study of the aging process, pub-lishing information for professionals about aging, and bringing together groups interested in aging research. Encourages research and education on the aging process. **Pub:** *Aging and Sensory Change: An Anno-tated Bibliography*. Bibliography. • *CommonStake.* •

*The Gerontologist*, bimonthly. Journal. Includes book and media reviews and abstracts of papers to be presented at the annual meeting. *Price:* $77/year for nonmembers in U.S.; $145/year for institutions in U.S. • *Gerontology News*, monthly. Newsletter. Includes employment listings, information on fellowship oppor-tunities and new books, and conference calendar. *Price:* Included in membership dues; $50/year for nonmembers. • *Journal of Gerontology - Series B*, bimonthly. Journal. *Price:* $73 $85/year for domestic nonmembers; $175/year for institutions. • *Journals of Gerontology - Series A*, monthly. Journal. Contains two individual journals entitled *Biological Sciences*, *Medical Sciences*. *Price:* Included in mem-bership dues; $161/year for domestic nonmembers; $350/year for domestic institutions. • *Membership Directory*, periodic. **Frmly:** (1980) Gerontological Soci-ety.


## ★ 2962 ★ Gerontological Society of the Russian Academy of Sciences
NN Petrov Research Institute of Oncology, 68
Leningradskaya St., Pesochny-2
189646 Saint Petersburg, Russia
**Phone:** 7 812 5968607 **Fax:** 7 812 5968947
**Email:** aging@mail.ru
**Website:** http://www.gerontology.spb.ru

**Fnded:** 1994. **Mem:** 1,500. **Reg. Groups:** 38. **Desc:** Facilitates research in Russian gerontological science and related fields of physiology and biology. Liaises with other scientific gerontological organizations. **Pub:** *Advances in Gerontology*, 3 volumes/year. Journal. Contains peer-reviewed articles about gerontology. • *Herald of Gerontological Society*, monthly. Newsletter.


## ★ 2963 ★ Grace and Compassion Benedictines
St. Joseph's
Albert Rd.
Bognor Regis PO21 1NJ, United Kingdom
**Phone:** 44 1273 680720 **Fax:** 44 1273 680527
**Email:** generalate@graceandcompassion.co.uk
**Website:** http://www.dabnet.org/gcb.htm

**Fnded:** 1954. **Mem:** 198. **Reg. Groups:** 14. **Lang(s):** English. **Desc:** Individuals, Benedictine congrega-tions, and long-term care facilities for the elderly. Seeks to improve the quality of life of elderly people requiring residential care and other living assistance. Maintains network of nursing homes, group resi-dences, and shelters for the elderly. Provides charita-ble assistance to the elderly, frail and sick. **Pub:** *Our Lady's Newsletter*, quarterly. Newsletter.


## ★ 2964 ★ Gray Panthers (GP)
733 15th St. NW, Ste. 437
Washington, DC 20005
**Phone:** (202)737-6637 **Free:** 800-280-5362
**Fax:** (202)737-1160
**Email:** info@graypanthers.org
**Website:** http://www.graypanthers.org
Tim Fuller, Exec. Dir.

**Fnded:** 1970. **Mem:** 40,000. **Local Groups:** 60. **Desc:** Consciousness-raising activist group of older adults and young people. Aims to combat ageism - the discrimination against persons on the basis of chrono-logical age. Believes that both the old and the young have much to contribute to make our society more just and humane. Advises, acts as acatalyst for, and organizes local groups of young, middle-aged, and older persons to work on issues of their choosing. Conducts work on eight national interests: national health care, affordable housing, environmental pres-ervtion, peace, ending discrimination, education, eco-nomic and tax justice, and social justice. **Pub:** *Gray Panther Network*, bimonthly. Newsletter. Contains articles on ageism, health care, housing, disarma-ment, and other intergenerational issues. *Price:* In-cluded in membership dues; $20/year for nonmem-bers; $35/year for organizations. • *Network Newslet-ter*, bimonthly. Covers national Gray Panther issues like housing, health care, and environmental protec-tion. **AKA:** Gray Panthers Project Fund.

## ★ 2965 ★ Health Promotion Institute (HPI)
c/o National Council on the Aging
409 3rd St. SW, 2nd Fl.
Washington, DC 20024
**Phone:** (202)479-1200 **Fax:** (202)479-0735
**Email:** info@ncoa.org
**Website:** http://www.ncoa.org
Glendale Johnson, Contact

**Fnded:** 1986. **Mem:** 700. **Desc:** A program of the National Council on the Aging. Seeks to aid profes-sionals who are interested in developing and imple-menting health promotion programs for senior citizens and serving older consumers. Promotes optimal quali-ty of life for older adults, including physical, emotional, and mental health as well as social and spiritual well-being. Advocates for and empowers older adults to achieve health and well-being through a multidisciplin-ary approach. Provides information and materials on health promotion programs. **Frmly:** (1991) National Center for Health Promotion and Aging.


## ★ 2966 ★ Hellenic Association of Gerontology and Geriatrics (HAGG)
Kaningos 23
GR-10677 Athens, Greece
**Phone:** 30 1 3811612 **Fax:** 30 1 3840317
**Email:** hagg@compulink.gr
**Website:** http://users.compulink.gr/hagg

**Fnded:** 1977. **Mem:** 168. **Lang(s):** English, French, Greek. **Desc:** Focuses on the problems and the process of aging. **Pub:** *Alzheimer's Disease.* Booklet. • *Depression for the Elderly.* Booklet. Guides to geriatric health and nutrition. **Frmly:** (1994) Hellenic Association for Geronontoolgy and Geriatrics.


## ★ 2967 ★ Help the Aged
1300 Carling Ave., Ste. 205
Ottawa, ON, Canada K1Z 7L2
**Phone:** (613)232-0727 **Free:** 800-648-1111
**Fax:** (613)232-7625
**Email:** helpage@cyberus.ca
**Website:** http://www.cyberus.ca/~helpage/

**Fnded:** 1975. **Mem:** 10,000. **Lang(s):** English, French. **Desc:** Individuals and organizations united to provide assistance to the destitute elderly. Works to increase public awareness of issues facing older people in Canada and in the developing world. **Pub:** *Agecare*, annual. Newspaper.


## ★ 2968 ★ Helpage International
PO Box 32832
London N1 9ZN, United Kingdom
**Phone:** 44 207 2787778 **Fax:** 44 207 8431840
**Email:** hai@helpage.org

**Fnded:** 1983. **Mem:** 65. **Reg. Groups:** 5. **Lang(s):** English, French, Russian, Spanish. **Desc:** Works with and for disadvantaged older people worldwide, to achieve lasting improvement in the quality of their lives. Supports the development of "grass roots" activity and the growth of local organisations working with older people. Projects focus on health, social services, residential, community and home care, in-come generation, advocacy, training and organisation-al development. **Pub:** *Adding Health to Years*. Hand-book. • *Helpage International News*, 3/year. Newslet-ter. • *Opening a Residential Home for Elderly People.* Handbook.


## ★ 2969 ★ Helpage International - Thailand
c/o Asia/Pacific Regional Development Centre
Faculty of Nursing
Chiang Mai University
Chiang Mai 50200, Thailand
**Phone:** 66 53 894805 **Fax:** 66 53 894214
**Email:** helpage@helpageasia.com
**Website:** http://www.helpageasia.com

**Fnded:** 1988. **Mem:** 16. **Lang(s):** English. **Desc:** Works to improve quality of life of older persons. Initiates and supports programs worldwide designed to help older persons meet their financial, material, medical, and social needs. **Pub:** *New Age Asia*, semiannual. Newsletter. A contact point for the network of members and non-member organisations of HelpAge International in order to promote age care in Asia region. • *Withichiwit (Thai Ageways)*, quarterly. Magazine. Magazine with pratical information on ageing issues for those working with older people.

### ★ 2970 ★ Helpage Latin America
c/o Valerie Mealla
Regional Centre for Latin America
Casilla 2217
La Paz, Bolivia
**Email:** helpage.bolivia@unete.com

**Fnded:** 1991. **Desc:** Works to improve quality of life for the aged. Initiates and supports programs worldwide designed to help the aged meet their financial, material, medical, and social needs. **Pub:** *Latin America Quarterly Magazine*, quarterly. Magazine. Features information about the exchange of experiences at the regional level.

### ★ 2971 ★ Hong Kong Association of Gerontology
GPO Box 10020
Hong Kong, People's Republic of China
**Phone:** 852 25581181          **Fax:** 852 25581181
**Email:** info@hkag.org
**Website:** http://www.hkag.org

**Fnded:** 1987. **Mem:** 500. **Lang(s):** Chinese, English. **Desc:** Health care professionals treating the elderly; scientists and clinicians with an interest in the aging process and diseases of the aged. Works to insure high standards of research and practice in gerontology, and to maximize availability of gerontological services. Conducts research and educational activities. **Pub:** *Hong Kong Journal of Gerontology*, biennial. Journal.

### ★ 2972 ★ Hungarian Gerontological Association (HGA)
PO Box 45
H-1428 Budapest, Hungary
**Phone:** 36 1 3294630          **Fax:** 36 1 3291206
**Email:** csaszalb@hiete.hu

**Fnded:** 1966. **Mem:** 215. **Local Groups:** 5. **Lang(s):** English, German, Hungarian. **Desc:** Health care professionals treating the elderly; scientists and clinicians with an interest in the aging process and diseases of the aged. Promotes gerontological research and increased availability of gerontological care; facilitates training of gerontology specialists. Represents the interest of gerontologists and gerontological organizations, and civil organizations of the Pensioners and Elderly.

### ★ 2973 ★ Indonesian Society of Gerontology
Jalan Iskandarsyah Raya 7
12160 Jakarta, Indonesia

**Lang(s):** English, Indonesian. **Desc:** Health care professionals treating the elderly; scientists and clinicians with an interest in the aging process and diseases of the aged. Works to insure high standards of research and practice in gerontology, and to maximize availability of gerontological services. Conducts research and educational activities.

### ★ 2974 ★ International Association of Biomedical Gerontology (IABG)
c/o Denham Harman, MD
Department of Medicine
84635 Nebraska Medical Center
Omaha, NE 68198-4635
**Phone:** (402)559-4416          **Fax:** (402)559-7330

**Fnded:** 1985. **Mem:** 200. **Desc:** Promotes the study of biomedical gerontology.

### ★ 2975 ★ International Association of Gerontology (IAG)
c/o Secretariat: Gerontology Research Centre
Simon Fraser University
2800 - 515 W Hastings St.
Vancouver, BC, Canada V6B 5K3
**Phone:** (604)291-5062          **Fax:** (604)291-5066
**Email:** iag@sfu.ca
**Website:** http://www.sfu.ca/iag

**Fnded:** 1950. **Mem:** 65. **Lang(s):** English. **Desc:** National gerontological societies. Promotes basic and applied research on aging and the aged and members interests on international issues. Fosters training of highly qualified personnel. Organizes a World Congress every four years and auspices other events. Has a consultative status with the UN and collaborates regularly with the UN's Programme on Aging, the WHO's Ageing and Life Course Programme and with other international agencies concerned with the well being of aging persons. **Pub:** *Bulletin*, annual. Bulletin.

### ★ 2976 ★ International Association of Gerontology European Region (IAG)
c/o Permanent Secretariat
PO Box 9191
28080 Madrid, Spain
**Phone:** 34 91 334 51 56   **Fax:** 34 91 334 51 50
**Email:** eriag@eriag.org
**Website:** http://www.eriag.org/

**Desc:** Gerontology research, including biological, medical, behavioral, and social. Provides training in fields of aging.

### ★ 2977 ★ International Federation on Ageing (IFA)
c/o Mr. Ivan Hale
425 Viger Ave. W, Ste. 520
Montreal, QC, Canada H2Z 1X2
**Phone:** (514)396-3358          **Fax:** (514)396-3378
**Email:** ifa@citenet.net
**Website:** http://www.ifa-fiv.org

**Fnded:** 1973. **Mem:** 215. **Nat'l Groups:** 1. **Reg. Groups:** 1. **Lang(s):** English, French, Spanish. **Desc:** Federation of voluntary organizations from close to 50 countries that represents the elderly as their advocate and/or provide services to them. Purposes are: to serve as an international advocate for the aging; to exchange information on a cross-national level of developments in aging of primary interest to the practitioner. **Pub:** *EAGLE*, 3/year. Bulletin. Covers legal issues and related policy questions affecting older people around the world. • *Empowering Older People*. Book. • *IFA Journal on Ageing*, quarterly. Journal. Contains news about older persons around the world. Provides coverage of trends; contains international conference calendar. • *Network News*, semiannual. Newsletter. Contains information about midlife and older women. Includes reviews of publications and calendar.

### ★ 2978 ★ International Federation of the Little Brothers of the Poor (IFLBP) (Federation Internationale des Petits Freres des Pauvres — FIPFP)
c/o Dr. R. Scott Walker
64, ave. Parmentier
F-75011 Paris, France
**Phone:** 33 1 47007968          **Fax:** 33 1 48062867
**Email:** federation@petits-freres.org
**Website:** http://www.PETITS-FRERES.org

**Fnded:** 1979. **Mem:** 8. **Nat'l Groups:** 8. **Lang(s):** English, French, Spanish. **Desc:** National Little Brothers organizations from Canada, France, Germany, Mexico, Morocco, Spain, Republic of Ireland, and the United States. Provides material and emotional support to older people who are handicapped, isolated, or destitute. Believes that old age should not prevent people from leading satisfying and fulfilling lives. Coordinates the efforts of volunteers and professionals to assist the elderly in areas such as housing, travel, and social and cultural activities.

### ★ 2979 ★ International Institute on Ageing
117 St. Paul's St.
Valletta VLT 07, Malta
**Phone:** 356 21 243044          **Fax:** 356 21 230248
**Email:** inia@maltanet.net
**Website:** http://www.inia.org.mt

**Lang(s):** English. **Desc:** Gerontologists and other individuals with an interest in the aging process. Seeks to advance medical understanding of aging; promotes development of new gerontological practices to improve the quality of life of the elderly. Serves as a forum for the exchange of information among members; sponsors research and educational programs.

**International Menopause Society**
*See:* Entry 16695

### ★ 2980 ★ International Psychogeriatric Association (IPA)
550 Frontage Rd., Ste. 2820
Northfield, IL 60093
**Phone:** (847)784-1701          **Fax:** (847)784-1705
**Email:** ipa@ipa-online.org
**Website:** http://www.ipa-online.org
Fern Finkel, Exec. Dir.

**Fnded:** 1981. **Mem:** 1,500. **Reg. Groups:** 2. **Desc:** To improve the mental health of the aging world population through information dissemination, research, professional development, advocacy and service development. Multidisciplinary health care professionals and scientists from 70 countries with an interest in the behavioral and biological aspects of mental in the elderly. Works to keep members abreast of developments in research and clinical practice in the field of geriatric mental health. **Pub:** *International Psychogeriatrics*, quarterly. Journal. *Price:* available to members only. • *IPA Bulletin*, quarterly. Newsletter. • Books. • Pamphlets.

### ★ 2981 ★ International Senior Citizens Association (ISCA)
255 S Hill St., Ste. 409
Los Angeles, CA 90012
Chris Valante, CEO

**Fnded:** 1964. **Mem:** 500. **Reg. Groups:** 20. **Desc:** Individuals over 50 years of age. Provides coordination on the international level to safeguard interests and needs of senior citizens; establishes means of communication among older citizens for educational and cultural developments; acts as a catalyst and presents forums through which older persons may contribute to world betterment. Conducts educational programs. Represents seniors before the United Nations. **Pub:** *Forum*, quarterly. Newsletter. Includes calendar of events. • Brochure.

### ★ 2982 ★ Irish Gerontological Society (IGS)
J. Connolly Memorial Hospital
Blanchardstown 15, Dublin, Ireland

**Desc:** Health care professionals treating the elderly; scientists and clinicians with an interest in the aging process and diseases of the aged. Promotes gerontological research and increased availability of gerontological care; facilitates training of gerontology specialists. Represents the interests of gerontologists and gerontological organizations.

### ★ 2983 ★ Israel Gerontological Society (IGS)
Habonim 8
IL-52462 Ramat Gan, Israel
**Phone:** 972 3 7513620          **Fax:** 972 3 5756748
**Email:** leglober@weizmann.weizmann.ac.il
**Website:** http://jointnet.org.il/eshelnet/igs

**Lang(s):** English, Hebrew. **Desc:** Health care professionals treating the elderly; scientists and clinicians with an interest in the aging process and diseases of the aged. Works to insure high standards of research and practice in gerontology, and to maximize availability of gerontological services. Conducts research and educational activities.

★ **2984** ★ **Japan Gerontological Society (JGS)**
Kyorin Bldg., Ste. 702
4-2-1 Yushima
Bunkyo-ku
Tokyo 113, Japan
**Lang(s):** English, Japanese. **Desc:** Health care professionals treating the elderly; scientists and clinicians with an interest in the aging process and diseases of the aged. Promotes gerontological research and increased availability of gerontological care; facilitates training of gerontology specialists. Represents the interests of gerontologists and gerontological organizations.

★ **2985** ★ **Jewish Association for Services for the Aged (JASA)**
132 W 31st St., 15th Fl.
New York, NY 10001
**Phone:** (212)273-5272      **Fax:** (212)695-4206
David J. Stern, Exec. VP

**Fnded:** 1968. **Local Groups:** 61. **Desc:** Social welfare organization whose objective is to provide the services necessary to enable the older adult to remain in the community. Maintains 18 community service offices and 24 local senior citizens centers in New York City and Nassau and Suffolk Counties, NY. Services include: case management; information and referral to appropriate health, welfare, educational, social, recreational, and vacation services, and on government benefits and entitlements; personal counseling; financial assistance; health and medical service counsel; counsel on housing and long-term care; homemaker service; group educational and recreational activities through senior citizens centers; information and guidance for social action on legislative issues affecting the elderly; hot lunch programs; referral to summer camps; legal services; protective services; reaching out to the isolated; programs for independent senior clubs; volunteer service opportunities. Conducts programs for elderly Soviet Jewish immigrants. Sponsors housing for the elderly: Friendset Apartments, Brookdale Village; Scheuer Houses of Coney Island, Brighton Beach, and Manhattan Beach; Green Residences at Far Rockaway and Cooper Square, NY. Operates home attendant agencies in Brooklyn and Queens, NY. Trains students from the New York University School of Social Work, Hunter College School of Social Work, Yeshiva University School of Social Work, and Adelphi University School of Social Work. **Pub:** *JPAC Action Memo/Senior Citizens Advocate*, 10/year. Addresses the issues of interest to senior citizens, especiall y those with low income. *Price:* Free.

★ **2986** ★ **Jewish Council for the Aging (JCA)**
c/o David Gamse
11820 Parklawn Dr., No. 200
Rockville, MD 20852-2511
**Phone:** (301)255-4200      **Fax:** (301)231-9360
**Email:** jcagw@jcagw.org
**Website:** http://www.jcagw.org
David N. Gamse, Exec. Dir.

**Fnded:** 1973. **Mem:** 17,000. **Desc:** Seeks to assist the elderly of all faiths lead independent lives. Provides transportation, job search assistance, fitness training, computer training and information and referral. Conducts educational programs. Maintains speakers' bureau. **Pub:** *JCA Today Newsletter*, 6/year. Newsletter.

★ **2987** ★ **John A. Hartford Foundation**
55 E 59th St., 16th Fl.
New York, NY 10022-1178
**Phone:** (212)832-7788      **Fax:** (212)593-4913
**Email:** mail@jhartford.org
**Website:** http://www.jhartfound.org
Corinne H. Rieder, Exec. Dir.

**Fnded:** 1929. **Desc:** Works to promote health care, training, research, and service related to older adults.

★ **2988** ★ **Leadership Council of Aging Organizations (LCAO)**
c/o National Council of Senior Citizens
8403 Colesville Rd., Ste. 1200
Silver Spring, MD 20910-3314
**Phone:** (301)578-8800      **Fax:** (301)578-8999
**Website:** http://www.lcao.org
Steve Protulis, Exec. Dir.

**Fnded:** 1978. **Mem:** 37. **Desc:** Professional groups serving older persons. Objective is to further the public's understanding of the potential and needs of older persons. Responds to public or private initiatives concerning the aging. Acts as coordinating body in reviewing and acting on public policy issues. Compiles statistics on aging. **Pub:** Monographs. • Papers.

★ **2989** ★ **Lemko Housing Organization (LHO)**
603 S Ann St.
Baltimore, MD 21231
**Phone:** (410)342-7200      **Fax:** (410)276-1233
Dr. Ivan Dornic, Pres.

**Desc:** Individuals and organizations. Promotes availability of housing and living assistance for elderly people or people with disabilities of Slavic descent. Purchases property and constructs housing and assisted care facilities; provides programs and services to people with disabilities and the elderly.

★ **2990** ★ **Lifespan Resources (LR)**
1212 Roosevelt
Ann Arbor, MI 48104
**Phone:** (734)663-9891      **Fax:** (313)973-7645
Carol Tice, Pres.

**Fnded:** 1979. **Desc:** Designs, implements, and develops innovations for programs involving interaction between youth and senior citizens, emphasizing mentoring. Develops policy initiatives to assist states in determining their intergenerational program needs. Is concerned with multicultural issues and economic development for youth and senior citizens. Conducts surveys; operates speakers' bureau. **Pub:** *Guide for Mentoring At-risk Youths*, daily. Manuals. • *Guide to Intergenerational Programs.* Booklets. • *What We Have.* Film. • Reports. **Frmly:** (1990) New Age.

★ **2991** ★ **Little Brothers - Friends of the Elderly**
954 W Washington Blvd., 5th Fl.
Chicago, IL 60607
**Phone:** (312)829-3055      **Fax:** (312)829-3099
**Email:** national@littlebrothers.org
**Website:** http://www.littlebrothers.org/
Tina Stretch, Exec. Dir.

**Fnded:** 1959. **Mem:** 1,000. **Reg. Groups:** 7. **Desc:** Participants are individuals over 70 years old who live alone, have limited incomes, and do not receive emotional and physical support from relatives. Seeks to combat the isolation and loneliness often experienced by elderly people by providing friendship and special assistance. Sponsors visitation programs, holiday and birthday parties, and summer vacations. Provides transportation for shopping and doctor's visits, food packages, and other "special touches." Also offers information, referrals, and contacts with other public or private agencies. Maintains vacation homes. **Pub:** *Reaching Out*, 3/year. Newsletter. For donors and volunteers. • *Volunteer Newsletter.* Newsletter. • Annual Report. • Brochure. **AKA:** Little Brothers of the Poor.

★ **2992** ★ **Mature Market Resource Center (MMRC)**
c/o Janet Jesse
621 E Park Ave.
Libertyville, IL 60048
**Phone:** (847)816-8660      **Free:** 800-828-8225
**Fax:** (847)816-8662

**Email:** info@healthawards.com
**Website:** http://www.seniorprograms.com
Janet Jesse, Assoc. Dir.

**Fnded:** 1992. **Desc:** Acts as a clearinghouse of resources for the mature market. Provides research and information on new trends and discoveries in senior health and fitness. Produces resource books. National Senior Health and Fitness Day and various Mature Fitness Awards USA. **Pub:** *Mature Market Calendar of Events*, annual. Directory. • *Mature Markets*, annual. Directory. • *Mature Markets Online*, annual. Directory. • *Resources for Senior Programs Catalog*, annual. • *What's New in senior Health and Fitness Action Cards*, annual.

★ **2993** ★ **Mature Outlook (MO)**
PO Box 9390
Des Moines, IA 50306-9519
**Free:** 800-336-6330

**Fnded:** 1984. **Mem:** 600,000. **Desc:** Individuals over 50 years of age. **Pub:** *Mature Outlook Magazine*, bimonthly. Magazine.

★ **2994** ★ **Medicare Rights Center**
1460 Broadway, 11th Fl.
New York, NY 10036-7393
**Phone:** (212)869-3850      **Fax:** (212)869-3532
**Email:** info@medicarerights.org
**Website:** http://www.medicarerights.org
Robert Hayes, Pres.

**Fnded:** 1989. **Mem:** 23. **Desc:** Seeks to ensure the rights of senior citizens and people with disabilities to quality, affordable health care. Provides counseling services to people with Medicare with health insurance problems and questions; compiles information on inquiries to detect issues and systemic problems in Medicare claims administration. Educates consumers, advocates, providers, and social workers about developments in Medicare law and how to handle problems. Monitors trends and changes in Medicare laws, regulations, and guidelines. **Pub:** *"Lets Learn Medicare!" Training and Reference Manual.* A sense of Medicare educational materials for consumers and professionals. *Price:* $125 plus shipping and handling $15.00. • *The Medicare Survival Kit: Medicare Answers.* A sense of Medicare educational materials for consumers and professionals. *Price:* $25 plus shipping and handling $6.00. **Frmly:** (1997) Medicare Beneficiaries Defense Fund.

**Mutual Help Home Association (MHHA) (Association d'Entraide vive Chez Nous — AECN)**
*See:* Entry 15918

★ **2995** ★ **National Academy for Teaching and Learning About Aging**
University of North Texas
PO Box 310919
Denton, TX 76203-0919
**Phone:** (940)565-3450      **Fax:** (940)565-3141
**Email:** natla@scs.unt.edu
**Website:** http://www.unt.edu/natla
Dr. Donna P. Couper, Dir. -NE Office

**Fnded:** 1983. **Mem:** 250. **Desc:** Professionals in gerontology, education, health care, and other fields interested in developing aging education and intergenerational programming. Seeks to dispel myths about aging and old age; encourages communication among generations and works to create a social environment where people of all ages can live together. Serves as a clearinghouse of information on issues of aging and intergenerational programs; provides consultation and presentation services to individuals or groups that wish to develop aging education programs. Maintains resources for aging education and intergenerational programming. **Pub:** *AgeShare.* • *Schools in an Aging Society.* Six interrelated curriculum guides which provide education, for, with, and about older adults. *Price:* $55. • *Teaching about Aging: Enriching Lives across the Lifespan* (published by the National Retired Teachers Association; free & available from NRTA/AARP).

**Frmly:** Center for Understanding Aging; (1996) Center for Understanding Aging.

### ★ 2996 ★ National Adult Day Services Association

c/o National Council on the Aging
409 3rd St. SW
Washington, DC 20024
**Phone:** (202)479-1200 **Fax:** (202)479-0735
**Email:** info@ncoa.org
**Website:** http://www.ncoa.org/nadsa
James P. Firman, Pres.

**Fnded:** 1979. **Mem:** 1,200. **Reg. Groups:** 10. **Desc:** Adult daycare practitioners; health and social service planners; individuals involved in planning and providing services for older persons. (Daycare centers offer services in a group setting ranging from active rehabilitation to social and health care.) Promotes and enhances adult daycare programs; provides services and activities for disabled older persons on a long-term basis; provides training and technical assistance and consultation services for daycare personnel; organizes funding; develops standards and guidelines for adult daycare programs; encourages adult daycare centers to participate in local area health planning activities to heighten the effectiveness of adult daycare. Plans and conducts training events for annual meeting and related conferences; maintains annotated bibliography; lobbies for approved public policy positions; surveys state adult daycare regulations and legislation. **Pub:** *Developing Adult Day Care: An Approach to Maintaining Independence for Impaired Older Persons.* • *NCOA Networks,* bimonthly. Newsletter. Reports on adult day care and other aging issues with a focus on public policy. *Price:* Free, for members only. • *Standards for Adult Day Care.*

### ★ 2997 ★ National Alliance of Senior Citizens (NASC)

2525 Wilson Blvd.
Arlington, VA 22201
**Fax:** (703)528-4380
Peter J. Luciano, CEO

**Fnded:** 1974. **Mem:** 117,000. **Desc:** Persons advocating the advancement of senior Americans through sound fiscal policy and through belief in the American system of individuality and personal freedom. Purpose is to inform the membership and the American public of the needs of senior citizens and of the programs and policies being carried out by the government and other specified groups. Represents the views of senior Americans before Congress and state legislatures. Maintains Golden Age Hall of Fame honoring individuals for outstanding service to the senior community. Conducts educational program; compiles statistics. Project "Life with Dignity: Compassionate Care for the Dying" helps to improve quality of life for people with terminal illness. Advocates living will and patients rights. **Pub:** *Senior Guardian,* bimonthly.

### ★ 2998 ★ National Asian Pacific Center on Aging (NAPCA)

PO Box 21668
Seattle, WA 98101
**Phone:** (206)624-1221 **Fax:** (206)624-1023
**Email:** napca@napca.org
**Website:** http://www.napca.org/
Clayton Fong, Exec. Dir.

**Fnded:** 1979. **Reg. Groups:** 4. **Desc:** Goals are to: ensure and improve the delivery of health and social services to elderly Pacific/Asians; increase the capabilities of community-based services by expanding their information and technical base; include Pacific/Asians in planning and organizational activities, thus maintaining a strong link between the center and the community. Provides technical assistance to the generic service delivery system on program development and organizational capacity building and training. Compiles statistics. **Pub:** *Asian Pacific Affairs,* bimonthly. Newsletter. • *Demographic & Socio-Economic Characteristics of Elderly Asian & Pacific Island Americans.* • *Directory of Pacific/Asian Media Sources.* Directory. • *Pacific/Asian Elderly Bibliography.* Directory. • *Registry of Services for Pacific/Asian Elderly,* biennial. Directory. **Frmly:** (1993) National Pacific/Asian Resource Center on Aging.

### ★ 2999 ★ National Association of Activity Professionals (NAAP)

PO Box 23909
Jackson, MS 39225
**Phone:** (601)853-3722 **Fax:** (601)853-3536
**Email:** naap1@aol.com
Catherine R. Selman, Exec. Dir.

**Fnded:** 1981. **Mem:** 2,800. **Desc:** Those who are or have been therapists, activity directors, and activity consultants in nursing homes, senior centers, retirement housing, or adult day care programs; other interested individuals. Purposes are to promote quality care and services for elderly and/or handicapped persons; to assist in the delivery of activity services; to foster research and the production of relevant literature; to upgrade educational programs. Sets standards and has established a certification process. Compiles statistics; maintains speakers' bureau, placement service, and resource review; sponsors National Activity Professional Day. Offers correspondence courses. **Pub:** *NAAP News: News of the Activity Profession,* monthly. Newsletter. Includes information on new members, upcoming events, and educational opportunities. *Price:* Included in membership dues.

### ★ 3000 ★ National Association of Area Agencies on Aging (NAAAA)

927 15th St., 6th Fl.
Washington, DC 20005
**Phone:** (202)296-8130 **Fax:** (202)296-8134
**Email:** info@n4a.org
**Website:** http://www.n4a.org
Sandy Markwood, CEO

**Fnded:** 1975. **Mem:** 665. **Desc:** Members are Area Agencies on Aging, established under the provisions of the Older Americans Act of 1965; also offers corporate and cooperating memberships. Promotes the achievement of a reasonable and realistic national policy on aging; assists the process of partnership and regular communication within a national network on aging. Acts as advocate for the needs of older persons at the national level. Maintains communication among members to enable an effective response to federal legislation and regulations. Disseminates information to the federal government, the private sector, and the public. Provides general administrative, training, and technical assistance to area agencies. **Pub:** *In Step with N4A,* monthly. Newsletter. • *National Directory for Eldercare Information and Referral,* biennial. Manuals. Contains listings of all area agencies throughout the US. *Price:* $50.

### ★ 3001 ★ National Association of County Aging Programs

440 1st St. NW
Washington, DC 20001
**Phone:** (202)942-4260 **Fax:** (202)942-4281
**Email:** msanz@naco.org
**Website:** http://www.naco.org/affils/affils.cfm?code=A20
Sandra Reinsel-Markwood, Staff Liaison

**Fnded:** 1978. **Desc:** Affiliated with the National Association of Counties. Assists counties in their plans for providing services to the aging of the community.

### ★ 3002 ★ National Association for Mental After-care in Residential Care Homes

Silverwells House
1 Old Mill Rd.
Bothwell
Glasgow G71 8AY, United Kingdom
**Phone:** 44 1698 852771 **Fax:** 44 1698 854712
**Email:** silverwellshouse@btinternet.com
**Lang(s):** English. **Desc:** Promotes services for people with mental health problems. Provides help and advice.

### ★ 3003 ★ National Association of Nutrition and Aging Services Programs (NANASP)

1101 Vermont Ave., Ste. 1001
Washington, DC 20005
**Phone:** (202)682-6899 **Fax:** (202)682-3984
**Website:** http://www.nanasp.org/

**Desc:** Dedicated to supporting a broad, comprehensive range of nutrition and other support services for the aging living in community dwellings; helps shape national policy; provides training for service providers; advocates on behalf of senior citizens.

### ★ 3004 ★ National Association of Professional Geriatric Care Managers (PGCM)

1604 N Country Club Rd.
Tucson, AZ 85716-3102
**Phone:** (520)881-8008 **Fax:** (520)325-7925
**Email:** info@caremanager.org
**Website:** http://www.caremanager.org
Laury Adsit Gelardi, Exec. Dir.

**Fnded:** 1984. **Mem:** 1,700. **Reg. Groups:** 1. **State Groups:** 11. **Desc:** Promotes quality services and care for elderly citizens. Provides referral service and distributes information to individuals interested in geriatric care management. Maintains referral network. **Pub:** *GCM Journal,* quarterly. Journal. *Price:* $75/year. • *Inside GCM,* quarterly. Newsletter. • Membership Directory, annual. **Frmly:** National Association of Private Geriatric Care Managers.

### ★ 3005 ★ National Association of Senior Companion Project Directors (NASCPD)

c/o Lynne Brown-Zounes
Community Teamwork, Inc.
167 Dutton St.
Lowell, MA 01852
**Phone:** (978)459-0551
**Email:** brown@comteam.org
**Website:** http://www.nascpd.org/
Dwight Rasmussen, Contact

**Fnded:** 1978. **Mem:** 187. **Reg. Groups:** 5. **Desc:** Project directors from the Corp. for National Service's Senior Companion Program. Works to address the needs of SCP. Provides opportunities for expression and education for and by SCP project directors. Fosters communication between project directors, organizations, and agencies serving the SCP and the Corp. for National Service offices. Encourages the support and exchange of services among programs benefiting the aging. Seeks to prevent duplication and maximize the quality and level of services. Expands and promotes opportunities for senior companions worldwide. Assists in preserving government funding for SCP projects; works for increased stipends for volunteers. Works with Washington representatives on behalf of legislative changes affecting Corp. for National Service's and the SCP. Offers professional training and development. Conducts surveys. Operates speakers' bureau; compiles statistics. **Pub:** *NASCPD Newsletter,* periodic. Newsletter.

### ★ 3006 ★ National Association of State Units on Aging (NASUA)

1201 15th St. NW, No. 300
Washington, DC 20005
**Phone:** (202)898-2578 **Fax:** (202)898-2583
**Email:** info@nasua.org
**Website:** http://www.nasua.org/
Daniel A. Quirk, PhD, Exec. Dir.

**Fnded:** 1964. **Mem:** 57. **Desc:** Public interest organization that provides information, technical assistance, and professional development support to State Units on Aging. (A state unit is an agency of state government designated by the governor and state legislature to administer the Older Americans Act and to serve as a focal point for all matters relating to older people.) Serves as organized channel for officially designated state leadership in aging to exchange information and mutual experiences, and to join together for appropriate action on behalf of the elderly. Services include:

information on federal policy and program developments in aging; training and technical assistance on a wide range of program and management issues; liaison with organizations representing the public and private sectors. **Pub:** *Directory of State Units on Aging,* periodic. Directory. • Books. • Manuals. • Reports. • Also publishes materials on aging policy and programs, policy briefs, legislative updates, and technical assistance documents.

### ★ 3007 ★ National Caucus and Center on Black Aged (NCBA)

1200 L St. NW, Ste. 800
Washington, DC 20005
**Phone:** (202)637-8400          **Fax:** (202)347-0895
**Email:** info@ncba-aged.org
**Website:** http://www.ncba-blackaged.org
Samuel J. Simmons, Pres.

**Fnded:** 1970. **Mem:** 3,000. **Local Groups:** 45. **Desc:** Seeks to improve living conditions for low-income elderly Americans, particularly blacks. Advocates changes in federal and state laws in improving the economic, health, and social status of low-income senior citizens. Promotes community awareness of problems and issues effecting low-income aging population. Operates an employment program involving 2000 older persons in 14 states. Sponsors, owns, and manages rental housing for the elderly. Conducts training and intern programs in nursing home administration, long-term care, housing management, and commercial property maintenance. **Pub:** *Golden Page,* quarterly. Newsletter. Reports developments concerning elderly blacks; includes association news and legislative update. *Price:* Included in membership dues. • Bulletin.

### ★ 3008 ★ National Coalition on Rural Aging (NCRA)

409 3rd St. SW, No. 200
Washington, DC 20024
**Phone:** (202)479-1200          **Fax:** (202)479-0735
**Email:** info@ncoa.org
**Website:** http://www.ncoa.org
James P. Firman, Pres.

**Fnded:** 1978. **Mem:** 500. **Desc:** Planners and providers of services for the aging, academicians and students, and others interested in issues related to older persons living in rural areas. Purposes are to develop social and public policies related to the needs and interests of rural older adults; to improve and increase services to rural older adults by working with national organizations and government agencies at all levels; to provide guidance to supportive organizations and communities; to encourage action on legislative, public policy, and service delivery issues. Disseminates information and promotes research and demonstration projects on the aging in rural America. Conducts training for individuals working with rural older adults, emphasizing the cultural mores of rural America and the methods of service provision which have proven adaptable to rural areas. Provides technical assistance and consultation significant to rural program planning and implementation. **Frmly:** (1999) National Center on Rural Aging.

### ★ 3009 ★ National Committee for the Prevention of Elder Abuse (NCPEA)

c/o Bob Blancato
1101 Vermont Ave., NW, Ste. 1001
Washington, DC 20002
**Phone:** (202)682-4140          **Fax:** (202)682-3984
**Email:** ncpea@erols.com
**Website:** http://www.preventelderabuse.org
Rosalie S. Wolf, Pres.

**Fnded:** 1987. **Mem:** 450. **State Groups:** 3. **Local Groups:** 10. **Desc:** Established to promote a greater understanding of the problem and the development of services to protect older persons and disabled adults in order to reduce the likelihood of their abuse and neglect. Performs research, advocacy, public awareness, and training services. **Pub:** *Journal of Elder Abuse & Neglect,* quarterly. Journal. • *nexus,* 3/year. • Membership Directory.

### ★ 3010 ★ National Committee for Senior Americans (NCSA)

PO Box 9009
Valley Forge, PA 19485
**Fax:** (215)648-9345
John E. Baumgardner, Dir.

**Fnded:** 1989. **Desc:** Individuals concerned with providing representation for senior citizens to assure a dignified retirement, including adequate health care and pension plans. Areas of interest include social security, medicare, extended health care, crime reduction, and the environment. Provides benefits and free services to increase members' functioning. **Pub:** *Senior Sentinel,* quarterly.

### ★ 3011 ★ National Council on the Aging (NCOA)

409 3rd St. SW, Ste. 200
Washington, DC 20024
**Phone:** (202)479-1200          **Free:** 800-424-9046
**Fax:** (202)479-0735
**Email:** info@ncoa.org
**Website:** http://www.ncoa.org
Dr. James Firman, Pres. and CEO

**Fnded:** 1950. **Mem:** 7,500. **Desc:** Individuals and organizations who work on behalf of older Americans, including individuals in business and industry, organized labor, and the health professions; social workers, librarians, the clergy, and educators; housing, research, and government agencies; state and local agencies on the aging. Cooperates with other organizations to promote concern for older people and develop methods and resources for meeting their needs. Provides a national information and consultation center; holds conferences and workshops. Operates Family Friends Program, which recruits and trains older volunteers to work with families with chronically ill or disabled children. Conducts research and demonstration programs on issues important to older people such as: training and placement of older workers; economic security; services for the frail elderly living in their own homes; access to health and social services; increasing opportunities for socialization and participation in artistic, cultural, and educational programs and services; corporate programs; senior centers. Maintains the National Association of Older Worker Employment Services, Health Promotion Institute, National Center on Rural Aging, National Adult Day Services Association, National Institute on Community-Based Long-Term Care, National Institute of Senior Centers, National Institute of Senior Housing, National Interfaith Coalition on Aging, and National Institute on Financial Issues and Services for Elders. **Pub:** *Abstracts in Social Gerontology: Current Literature on Aging,* quarterly. Journal. Features books, reports, and articles on a variety of aging issues. Includes author and subject index. *Price:* Free to members. • *Innovations in Aging,* quarterly. Magazine. Covers issues and developments in the field of aging. *Price:* available to members only. • Books. • Brochures. • Pamphlets. **Frmly:** (1960) National Committee on Aging of National Social Welfare Assembly.

### National Eye Care Project (NECP)
*See:* Entry 21034

### National Gerontological Nursing Association
*See:* Entry 15752

### ★ 3012 ★ National Hispanic Council on Aging (NHCoA)

2713 Ontario Rd. NW
Washington, DC 20009
**Phone:** (202)265-1288          **Fax:** (202)745-2522
**Email:** nhcoa@worldnet.att.net
**Website:** http://www.nhcoa.org
Marta Sotomayor, PhD, Pres.

**Fnded:** 1980. **Mem:** 50,000. **Nat'l Groups:** 25. **Reg. Groups:** 4. **State Groups:** 38. **Local Groups:** 20. **Desc:** Individuals and groups who work in administrative, planning, direct services, research, or educational areas who have a concern for the Hispanic elderly. Fosters the well-being of the Hispanic elderly through research, policy analysis, demonstration projects, development of educational resources, and training. Compiles research data and provides a network for organizations and community groups interested in the Hispanic elderly. Maintains speakers' bureau. **Pub:** *The Hispanic Elderly: A Cultural Signature, Latino Elderly: Issues and Solutions for 20th Centry Triple Jeopardy: Aged, Hispanic Women,* quarterly. Book. *Price:* $18.45 portage per book. • *Hispanic Elderly: Issues and Solutions for the 21st Century.* Book. • *Noticias on Hispanic Elderly Issues,* quarterly. Newsletter. Publicizes the activities of NHCoA. Includes calendar of events, legislative news, and notices of publications available. *Price:* $25/year. • *Triple Jeopardy: Hispanic Older Women.* Book.

### ★ 3013 ★ National Indian Council on Aging (NICOA)

10501 Montgomery Blvd. NE, Ste. 210
Albuquerque, NM 87111
**Phone:** (505)292-2001          **Fax:** (505)292-1922
**Email:** info@nicoa.org
**Website:** http://www.nicoa.org
Dave Baldridge, Exec. Dir.

**Fnded:** 1976. **Mem:** 1,037. **Desc:** Native American/Alaska Native populations. The National Indian Council on Aging seeks to bring about improved comprehensive services to the American Indian and Alaska Native elderly. Objectives include: interaction with service provider agencies and advocacy organizations in the aging network, disseminate information to Indian communities and provide technical assistance and training opportunities to organizations. Research activities performed, as well as acting as a clearinghouse for current issues affecting the American Indian and Alaska Native elderly. **Pub:** *Elder Voices,* quarterly. Newsletter. *Price:* $5 for nonmembers. • *Mapping Indian Elders.* Reports. *Price:* $25. • Monographs. • Proceedings.

### ★ 3014 ★ National Institute on Community-Based Long-Term Care (NICLC)

c/o National Council on the Aging
409 3rd St. SW
Washington, DC 20024
**Phone:** (202)479-1200          **Fax:** (202)479-0735
**Email:** info@ncoa.org
**Website:** http://www.ncoa.org/niclc/niclc.htm
Carol McClendon, Contact

**Fnded:** 1984. **Mem:** 1,100. **Desc:** A unit of the National Council on the Aging. Seeks to promote a comprehensive long-term care system that will integrate home-and community-based services, enabling older adults to live in their own homes as long as it is medically, socially, and economically feasible. Serves as information clearinghouse for long-term care professionals. Advocates public policies that support home and community-based services. Maintains speakers' bureau; offers educational sessions; compiles statistics. **Pub:** *Care Management Standards.* Book. • *NCOA Networks,* bimonthly. Newsletter. • *Perspective on Aging,* periodic. Journal. Provides information on aging issues.

### ★ 3015 ★ National Institute of Senior Centers (NISC)

c/o National Council on the Aging
409 3rd St. SW
Washington, DC 20024
**Phone:** (202)479-1200          **Free:** 800-424-9046
**Fax:** (202)479-0735
**Email:** info@ncoa.org
**Website:** http://www.ncoa.org/nisc/nisc.htm
Peter Wyckoff, Exec. Dir.

**Fnded:** 1970. **Mem:** 3,000. **Desc:** Individuals or organizations who are affiliated with senior centers at the local, state, or national level. (Senior centers are places where senior citizens can go for services, recreation, and information on topics such as nutrition, employment, and housing.) Assists senior centers, organizations, and communities in developing new centers and upgrading existing operations. Promotes professionalism within the senior center field and develops standards for senior centers nationwide. Maintains advocacy and public policy positions for senior centers; provides management training for persons working with senior centers. **Pub:** *NCOA Network*, bimonthly. Newspaper. Reports on senior citizen centers, including legislative updates, program and funding information, and current issues. *Price:* Free, for members only. • *Senior Center Operation: A Guide to Organization and Management.* • *Senior Center Standards.*

**★ 3016 ★ National Interfaith Coalition on Aging (NICA)**
409 3rd St. SW
Washington, DC 20024
**Phone:** (202)479-1200          **Free:** 800-424-9046
**Fax:** (202)479-0735
**Website:** http://www.ncoa.org/nica/nica.htm
Rita Chow, Dir.

**Fnded:** 1972. **Mem:** 300. **Desc:** Shares administrative capabilities and resources with National Council on the Aging. Religious and secular organizations and individuals concerned with the U.S. religious community's response to the problems of aging, and about the spiritual well-being of the elderly. Promotes communication and cooperative effort among religious organizations and individuals concerned about older people; assists churches and synagogues that attempt to respond to the needs of the elderly; identifies and supports programs and services for the elderly that are best implemented by religious organizations; facilitates continued participation in community affairs by the elderly. Serves as a resource and gerontological training agency for clergy and religious workers. **Pub:** *Journal of Religious Gerontology*, quarterly. Journal. Contains articles about developments in religious gerontology and religious concerns of aging. Includes book reviews and research reports. *Price:* $40/year.

**★ 3017 ★ National Meals on Wheels Foundation**
PO Box 1727
Iowa City, IA 52244
**Phone:** (319)354-0862          **Fax:** (319)354-0845
**Email:** info@nationalmealsonwheels.org
**Website:** http://www.nationalmealsonwheels.org/
Connie Benton Wolfe, Exec. Dir.

**Fnded:** 1977. **Mem:** 1,000. **Desc:** Grants-making organization. **Pub:** *Collection of Innovative Models.* • *Monthly Membership Updates*, monthly. • *NANASP News*, quarterly. Newsletter. Contains legislative and membership updates, and new product information. *Price:* Included in membership dues. • *National Standards for Congregate Meals.* • *National Standards for Home-Delivered Meals.* • *Preparing Nutrition Programs for the Nineties.* • *Special Bulletins*, monthly. Bulletin. • *Special Report to Members*, quarterly. Newsletter. *Price:* Included in membership dues. • Annual Report, annual. **Frmly:** (1978) National Association of Title Seven Directors.

**★ 3018 ★ National PACE Association (NPA)**
801 N Fairfax St., Ste. 309
Alexandria, VA 22314
**Phone:** (703)535-1565          **Fax:** (703)535-1566
**Email:** info@npaonline.org
**Website:** http://www.natlpaceassn.org

**Desc:** Promotes the availability of healthcare services to older adults through the Program of All-inclusive Care for the Elderly (PACE) and similar care models.

**★ 3019 ★ National Pensioners and Senior Citizens Federation (NPSCF)**
PO Box 393
Hanley, SK, Canada S0G 2E0
**Phone:** (306)544-2737          **Fax:** (306)544-2757
**Email:** helen.decoste@ns.sympatico.co

**Fnded:** 1945. **Mem:** 600. **Nat'l Groups:** 750. **Lang(s):** English, French. **Desc:** Senior citizens' and pensioners' clubs. Seeks to stimulate public interest in the welfare of older Canadians. Provides services to improve the quality of life of senior citizens, including counselling and education. **Pub:** *National News*, quarterly. Newsletter. Seniors issues. • Brochure. • Papers.

**★ 3020 ★ National Senior Citizens Law Center (NSCLC)**
1101 14th St. NW, Ste. 400
Washington, DC 20005
**Phone:** (202)289-6976          **Fax:** (202)289-7224
**Email:** nsclc@nsclc.org
**Website:** http://www.nsclc.org
Edward King, Exec. Dir.

**Fnded:** 1972. **Desc:** Legal services support center specializing in the legal problems of the elderly poor. Acts as advocate on behalf of elderly, poor clients in litigation and administrative affairs. Sponsors conferences and workshops on areas of the law affecting the elderly. **Pub:** *Nursing Home Law Letter*, quarterly. • *Washington Weekly*, weekly. Newsletter. • Also publishes handbooks, guides, and testimonies.

**★ 3021 ★ New England Gerontological Association (NEGA)**
1 Cutts Rd.
Durham, NH 03824-3102
**Phone:** (603)868-5757
**Email:** genetsr@attbi.com
**Website:** http://www.negaonline.org
Dr. Eugene E. Tillock, Exec. Dir.

**Fnded:** 1958. **Mem:** 125. **Reg. Groups:** 1. **Desc:** Promotes the study of the aging process. Conducts educational programs in aging, health service administration and long-term care administration. **Pub:** *Gerontology Topics*, quarterly. Newsletter.

**★ 3022 ★ New Zealand Association of Gerontology**
Auckland Hospital
Private Bag 92024
Auckland, New Zealand
**Phone:** 64 9 3074949          **Fax:** 64 9 3754344
**Email:** apoulter@adhb.govt.nz

**Fnded:** 1981. **Mem:** 400. **Nat'l Groups:** 1. **Reg. Groups:** 4. **Local Groups:** 4. **Desc:** Gerontologists in New Zealand. Studies ageing in all aspects. Encourages training for individuals caring for older people. Promotes gerontological research. **Pub:** *NZAG Newsletter*, quarterly. Newsletter. Includes information, feedback, and upcoming events.

**Old Lesbians Organizing for Change (OLOC)**
*See:* Entry 18908

**P.R.I.D.E. Foundation - Promote Real Independence for the Disabled and Elderly (P.R.I.D.E.)**
*See:* Entry 20166

**★ 3023 ★ Philippine Association of Gerontology**
4th St. BBB Marulas
Valenzuela Metro Manila, Metro Manila, Philippines
**Phone:** 63 2 2916801          **Fax:** 63 2 29167113
**Email:** fgc@pacific.net.ph
**Website:** http://www.sfu.ca/iag/

**Fnded:** 1998. **Mem:** 65. **Desc:** Seeks to improve the welfare of senior citizens. Supports and encourages research in gerontology. Fosters communication and exchange among members.

**★ 3024 ★ Pre-Retirement Association (PRA)**
9 Chesham Rd.
Surrey
Guildford GU2 3LS, United Kingdom
**Phone:** 44 1483 301170          **Fax:** 44 1483 300981
**Email:** info@pra.uk.com
**Website:** http://www.pra.uk.com

**Fnded:** 1964. **Mem:** 404. **Local Groups:** 16. **Desc:** People with associated interests in a personal or professional capacity and companies willing to be associated with the development of retirement/redundancy advice/mid life planning. Promoting awareness of the needs of all those preparing for retirement. It provides education, planning and support services that relate to the successful management of transitional changes from an increasing diversity of employment patterns. Runs a course leading to a certificate in pre-retirement education with life planning. **Pub:** *Directory of Midlife/Pre-Retirement Courses, U.K.*, annual. Directory. • *PRA Resources Unit News*, quarterly. Newsletter. • *Preparation for Retirement: The Employer's Guide.* • *Your Retirement*, annual. Features basic information for retirees. **Frmly:** (2001) Pre-Retirement Association of Great Britain and Northern Ireland.

**★ 3025 ★ Relatives and Residents Association**
5 Tavistock Place
London WC1H 9SN, United Kingdom
**Phone:** 44 20 76924302          **Fax:** 44 20 79166093
**Email:** relres@totalise.co.uk

**Fnded:** 1992. **Mem:** 2,500. **Nat'l Groups:** 2. **Local Groups:** 30. **Lang(s):** English. **Desc:** Provides advice and support to relatives and friends of older people in residential care homes, nursing homes and long stay hospitals. Also offers training to homes in order to promote good practice through involvement of relatives. **Pub:** *The Relatives & Residents Association*, 3/year. Newsletter. Contains news and updates nationally and within the organization.

**★ 3026 ★ Retirement Income Association**
PO Box 21957
Santa Barbara, CA 93121-1957
James J. Maher, Pres.

**Fnded:** 1994. **Mem:** 250,000. **Desc:** Acts as a liaison between retired consumers and service and product providers. Offers access to insurance packages and health-related products and services. **Pub:** *Retirement Income Newsletter*, bimonthly. Newsletter. *Price:* $12.95. • *Retirement Today*, bimonthly. Newsletter. *Price:* $12.95/year.

**★ 3027 ★ Retirement Research Foundation (RRF)**
8765 W Higgins Rd., Ste. 430
Chicago, IL 60681-4170
**Phone:** (773)714-8080          **Fax:** (773)714-8089
**Email:** info@rrf.org
**Website:** http://www.rrf.org
Edward J. Kelly, Chm.

**Desc:** Works to promote aging and retirement issues. Supports efforts that improve care for the aging, and enable older adults to live at home or in residential settings that facilitate independent living.

**★ 3028 ★ Royal Surgical Aid Society**
47 Great Russell St.
London WC1B 3PB, United Kingdom
**Phone:** 44 2076374577          **Fax:** 44 2073236878
**Email:** enquiries@agecare.org.uk
**Website:** http://www.agecare.org.uk

**Fnded:** 1862. **Mem:** 17. **Desc:** Seeks to improve the care and well being of older people who are physically frail or suffering from dementia, through a combination of continuous development of good practice in it's own homes, seeking pre-eminence in education and training, supporting research and innovation, providing awards for excellence, and continuing in the exchange of knowledge and ideas.

**★ 3029 ★ Scottish Pensions Association (SPA)**
54A Fountainbridge
Edinburgh EH3 9PT, United Kingdom
**Phone:** 44 131 2291886     **Fax:** 44 131 2291886
**Email:** spa@tinyworld.co.uk
**Fnded:** 1937. **Mem:** 10,000. **Reg. Groups:** 3. **Local Groups:** 90. **Lang(s):** English. **Desc:** Pensioners and those interested in issues affecting older peoples' lives, rights, and welfare. Aims to improve the quality of life for older people and urges that the State Pension should rise annually in line with prices or average earnings. Provides opportunities for members to gain a voice on the key issues affecting older people.

**★ 3030 ★ Seniors Coalition (TSC)**
9001 Braddock Rd., Ste. 200
Springfield, VA 22151
**Phone:** (703)239-1960     **Fax:** (703)239-1985
**Email:** tsc@senior.org
**Website:** http://www.senior.org
Mary Martin, Exec. Dir.
**Fnded:** 1989. **Desc:** Represents the interests and concerns of America's senior citizens at state and federal levels. **Pub:** *The Advocate,* quarterly. Magazine.

**★ 3031 ★ 60 Plus Association**
1655 N Ft. Myers Dr., Ste. 355
Arlington, VA 22209
**Phone:** (703)807-2070     **Fax:** (703)807-2073
**Email:** webmaster@60plus.org
**Website:** http://www.60plus.org
James L. Martin, Pres.
**Fnded:** 1992. **Mem:** 500,000. **Desc:** Individuals aged 60 years or older. Promotes adoption of a "less government, less taxes approach to seniors' issues." Conducts lobbying and advocacy activities. **Pub:** *Scorecard,* periodic. Report. • *Senior Voice,* periodic. Newsletter.

**★ 3032 ★ Slovak Society of Gerontology and Geriatrics (SSGG)**
c/o Zoltan Mikes
Department of Geriatrics
Faculty of Medicine
Dumbierska 3
SK-831 01 Bratislava, Slovakia
**Phone:** 421 7 59545232     **Fax:** 421 7 59546263
**Email:** mikes@fmed.uniba.sk
**Fnded:** 1995. **Lang(s):** English, Slovak. **Desc:** Health care professionals and other individuals with an interest in the well-being of the elderly. Promotes delivery of improved health and social services to older people. Encourages professional advancement of health care practitioners. Makes available preventive and primary health care services; conducts research; maintains Geriatric Center.

**★ 3033 ★ Society of the Destitute Aged**
PO Box DH 53
Egypt Lines
Highfield, Zimbabwe
**Phone:** 263 884525
**Fnded:** 1968. **Mem:** 50. **Desc:** Aims to improve living conditions for elderly destitute people in Zimbabwe. Conducts community sponsorship programs.

**★ 3034 ★ Society of Geriatric Cardiology**
Heart House
9111 Old Georgetown Rd.
Bethesda, MD 20814
**Phone:** (301)581-3449     **Fax:** (301)581-3408
**Email:** sgc@sgcard.org
**Website:** http://www.sgcard.org
Jane M. Dunne, Mgr.
**Fnded:** 1986. **Mem:** 500. **Desc:** Geriatric cardiologists and physicians in related fields are fellows; medical practitioners certified in specialties other than geriatrics or cardiology are members; other individuals with an interest in geriatric cardiology are nonphysician members. Works to improve the clinical and therapeutic management of older individuals with cardiovascular disease; encourages use of preventive measures to avert the onset of cardiovascular aging and disease. Promotes more effective public policy and education regarding cardiac health. Conducts educational programs for physicians, other health care professionals, and the public. Supports research into cardiovascular aging and diseases relevant to older people. Serves as a clearinghouse on geriatric cardiology. Sponsors competitions. **Pub:** *American Journal of Geriatric Cardiology,* bimonthly. Journal. • *News Brief,* 3/year. Newsletter. **Frmly:** (1999) Council on Geriatric Cardiology.

**★ 3035 ★ Society of Gerontology of the Republic Serbia**
Gerontolosko Drustvo Srbije
Krfska 7
YU-11000 Belgrade, Serbia
**Phone:** 381 11 415734     **Fax:** 381 11 415734
**Email:** gerontolog@yahoo.com
**Fnded:** 1973. **Mem:** 210. **Local Groups:** 8. **Lang(s):** English. **Desc:** Individuals who professionally deal with the problems of the aged and aging and their social, medical, legal, sociological, psychological, sociopolitical, economic, and other aspects. Seeks to improve gerontological theory and practice and to contribute to the implementation of the gerontological knowledge in the humanization of living conditions of the aged and aging.

**★ 3036 ★ Society of Prospective Medicine (SPM)**
c/o Dr. Gerald C. Hyner
Purdue University
The Lambert Bldg.
West Lafayette, IN 47907-1362
**Phone:** (765)494-3151     **Fax:** (765)496-1239
**Email:** info@spm.org
**Website:** http://www.spm.org
Dr. Gerald C. Hyner, Pres.
**Fnded:** 1972. **Mem:** 250. **Desc:** Physicians, allied health workers, scientists, and others committed to extending the useful life expectancy of persons by identifying actual and potential health hazards and by developing and implementing risk assessment techniques and risk reduction programs. Conducts research; compiles statistics. Develops education programs and supplies information concerning diseases that frequently cause death and disability. Maintains speakers' bureau. **Pub:** *An Ounce of Prevention–Newsletter,* quarterly. Newsletter. Reports on developments in health hazard appraisal. Includes calendar of events. *Price:* Included in membership dues; $20/year for nonmembers. • *Health Risk Appraisal Book.* Book. • *Proceedings of Annual Meeting.* Proceedings. *Price:* $35. • *SPM Handbook of Health Risk Appraisal.* Directory. *Price:* $35.

**★ 3037 ★ Sozialverband Vdk Deutschland**
WurzerstraBe 4a
D-53175 Bonn, Germany
**Phone:** 49 228 820930     **Fax:** 49 228 8209343
**Email:** kontakt@vdk.de
**Website:** http://www.vdk.de
**Fnded:** 1950. **Mem:** 1100,000. **Reg. Groups:** 14. **Lang(s):** English, French, German. **Desc:** Victims of accidents and violence, elderly citizens, pensioners, mentally disabled individuals, victims of war or military service, and their dependents. Provides legal representation, accident and death insurance, and convalescent care; works to achieve social and vocational integration. Organizes recreational activities for members including: cultural events, parties, and travel excursions. Conducts public sensitization campaigns. Lobbying at national and European level. **Pub:** *Behinderte und Arbeitswelt.* • *Sozialrecht & Praxis,* periodic. Journal. Developments in social legislation and policy. • *Vdk Zeitung,* monthly. Journal. **Frmly:** German Organization of Victime of War and Military Service, Disabled People and Pensioners.

**★ 3038 ★ Swedish Society for Geriatric Medicine and Gerontology**
c/o Dr. Gunnar Akner
Nutrition and Pharmacotherapy Unit A1:05
Department of Geriatric Medicine
Karolinska Hospital
Karolinska Institute
S-17176 Stockholm, Sweden
**Phone:** 46 8 6510129     **Fax:** 46 8 6511441
**Email:** gunnar.akner@chello.se
**Website:** http://www.svls.se/sektioner/age/
**Fnded:** 1999. **Mem:** 625. **Lang(s):** English. **Desc:** Geriatricians, physicians, nurses, and paramedics. Supports the development of Swedish geriatric medicine and gerontology. Formulates the core curriculum for specialist training in geriatric medicine and serves as a center for international cooperation regarding scientific and educational matters.

**★ 3039 ★ Ukrainian Gerontology and Geriatrics Society (UGGS)**
Vyshgorodskaya St. 67
254114 Kiev, Ukraine
**Phone:** 380 44 4304068     **Fax:** 380 44 4329956
**Email:** direct@geront.freenet.kiev.ua
**Fnded:** 1965. **Mem:** 500. **Reg. Groups:** 10. **Lang(s):** English, Russian, Ukrainian. **Desc:** Health care professionals treating the elderly; scientists and clinicians with an interest in the aging process and diseases of the aged. Promotes gerontological research and increased availability of gerontological care; facilitates training of gerontology specialists. Represents the interests of gerontologists and gerontological organizations. **Pub:** *Problems of Aging & Longevity,* quarterly. Journal. Contains biology of aging, clinical gerontology and geriatrics, social gerontology and gerohygiene. **Frmly:** (1963) Gerontological & Geriatric Society of the USSR.

**★ 3040 ★ United Seniors Association (USA)**
3900 Jermantown Rd., Ste. 450
Fairfax, VA 22030-4900
**Phone:** (703)359-6500     **Free:** 800-8US-AUSA
**Fax:** (703)359-6510
**Email:** usa@unitedseniors.org
**Website:** http://www.unitedseniors.org
Charles W. Jarvis, Pres. & CEO
**Fnded:** 1991. **Mem:** 550,000. **Nat'l Groups:** 1. **Desc:** Seeks to educate and mobilize senior citizens about Social Security, Medicare taxes, and other related issues. **Pub:** *The Senior American and On the Issues,* 4/year. Newsletter.

**★ 3041 ★ United Seniors Health Cooperative**
409 Third St. SW, Ste. 200
Washington, DC 20024
**Phone:** (202)479-6973     **Free:** 800-637-2604
**Fax:** (202)479-6660
**Email:** ushc@unitedseniorhealth.org
**Website:** http://WWW.unitedseniorshealth.org
Ann Werner, Pres. & CEO
**Fnded:** 1984. **Mem:** 10,000. **Desc:** The elderly, their families, and interested others. Assists elderly persons in independent living, health and insurance issues. Provides information resources for professionals serving seniors. **Pub:** *United Seniors Health Report,* periodic. Newsletter. Provides information on important topics for seniors. *Price:* $15.

# Research Centers

**Aging Research Institute**
*See:* Entry 15926

**★ 3042 ★ Alzheimer Treatment Research Center**
279 Norman Dr.
Cranberry Twp., PA 16066-4229
**Phone:** (412)683-1181
**Email:** jrgrace@kahsa.org
**Website:** http://www.kahsa.org
Arthur C. Walsh, MD, Pres.

**Activities/Fields:** Senility, Alzheimer's disease, and hypochondriasis in the elderly, particularly brain dysfunction related to impaired circulation, psychiatric aspects of senility, treatment of chronic schizophrenia, and the effect of anticoagulant therapy. **Pub:** *Mental Capacity: Medical and Legal Aspects of Aging*, annually. **Frmly.** Center for Senility Studies: Alzheimer's Disease Treatment Research.

**★ 3043 ★ American Federation for Aging Research**
1414 Ave. of the Americas, 18th Fl.
New York, NY 10019
**Phone:** (212)752-2327          **Fax:** (212)832-2298
**Email:** amfedaging@aol.com
**Website:** http://www.afar.org
Dr. Odette Vanderwillik, Contact

**Activities/Fields:** Aging and associated diseases. **Pub:** *Newsletter*, semiannually.

**★ 3044 ★ American Foundation for Aging Research**
128 Polk Hall, Box 7622
Biochemistry Department
North Carolina State University
Raleigh, NC 27695-7622
**Phone:** (919)515-5679          **Fax:** (919)515-2047
**Email:** afar@bchserver.bch.ncsu.edu
**Website:** http://www4.ncsu.edu/unity/users/a/agris/afar/afar.htm
Paul F. Agris, Contact

**Activities/Fields:** Age-related diseases and the biology of aging, focusing on modern biological, genetic, biochemical, and biophysical techniques and approaches to the problems of age-associated diseases and the understanding of aging. **Pub:** *Newsletter*, quarterly.

**★ 3045 ★ Baylor College of Medicine Roy M. and Phyllis Gough Huffington Center on Aging**
MC M-320
1 Baylor Plz.
Houston, TX 77030-3498
**Phone:** (713)798-5804          **Fax:** (713)798-6688
**Email:** rsmith@bcm.tmc.edu
**Website:** http://www.hcoa.org
Roy G. Smith, PhD, Dir.

**Activities/Fields:** Cell and molecular biology of aging, cardiovascular disease, and ethics in long-term care.

**★ 3046 ★ Buck Institute**
8001 Redwood Blvd.
Novato, CA 94945
**Phone:** (415)209-2000          **Fax:** (415)899-1810
**Website:** http://www.buckinstitute.org/
Dale E. Bredesen, MD, Pres. /CEO

**Activities/Fields:** The aging process and age-associated diseases.

**★ 3047 ★ Case Western Reserve University University Center on Aging and Health**
10900 Euclid Ave.
Cleveland, OH 44106-7131
**Phone:** (216)368-2692          **Fax:** (216)368-6389
**Email:** dxf5@po.cwru.edu
Dr. May L. Wykle, Dir.

**Activities/Fields:** Conducts, supports, and facilitates research at the University Center on Aging and Health, including the effects of stress and strains, and elderly physical health on persons over 65 years of age.

Emphasizes prevention, diagnosis, treatment, management of illness or disability, and service utilization of care giver. **Pub:** *Newsletter*, semiannually.

**★ 3048 ★ Center for the Study of Aging, Inc.**
706 Madison Ave.
Albany, NY 12208-3604
**Phone:** (518)465-6927          **Fax:** (518)462-1339
**Email:** iapaas@aol.com
**Website:** http://members.aol.com/iapaas
Sara Harris, Exec. Dir.

**Activities/Fields:** Social and medical research on aging, including physical activity and aging, housing for the elderly, geriatric cardiology, nutrition, mental health, oral history, public policy, caregiving, prevention and respite care for the frail elderly. **Pub:** *Aging and Sports.* • *Environment Aging.* • *Physical Activity.* • *Safe Therapeutic Exercise for the Frail Elderly.* • *Who? Me?! Exercise? - Safe Exercise for People Over 50.* Book.

**Columbia-Presbyterian Medical Center Gertrude H. Sergievsky Center**
*See:* Entry 14178

**★ 3049 ★ Columbia University Stroud Center for Geriatrics and Gerontology**
100 Haven Ave., Tower 3-30F
New York, NY 10032
**Phone:** (212)781-0600          **Fax:** (212)795-7696
**Email:** bjg1@columbia.edu
**Website:** http://cpmcnet.columbia.edu/dept/sergievsky
Dr. Barry Gurland, Dir.

**Activities/Fields:** Methodological, epidemiological and clinical research in geriatrics/gerontology and long-term care. Specific studies are directed toward mental disorders, psychosocial problems, and funtional impairments of the elderly. The Center has developed model projects using a comprehensive assessment instrument that has been refined for use in various settings. The Center is also active in cross-national research with a collaborating group in London. **Frmly.** Long-Term Care Gerontology Center.

**★ 3050 ★ Cornell University Cornell Gerontology Research Institute (CGRI)**
G58 MVR Hall
Ithaca, NY 14853
**Phone:** (607)255-0838          **Fax:** (607)255-9856
**Email:** pem3@cornell.edu
**Website:** http://www.blcc.cornell.edu/cagri/
Phyllis Moen, Co-Dir.

**Activities/Fields:** Social integration of older Americans. **Pub:** *CAGRI Newsletter*.

**★ 3051 ★ Duke University Center for the Study of Aging and Human Development**
Medical Center
PO Box 3003
Durham, NC 27710
**Phone:** (919)660-7500          **Fax:** (919)684-8569
**Email:** ray00004@mc.duke.edu
**Website:** http://www.geri.duke.edu
Harvey Jay Cohen, MD, Dir.

**Activities/Fields:** Human and animal physiology, immunology, neuroendocrinology, pharmacology, carcinogenesis, enzyme biochemistry, free radical effects, membrane and receptor function, bone metabolism and osteoporosis, central nervous system structure and function, Alzheimer's disease, dementia, cognitive processes, psychometrics, human personality and behavior, family structure and intergenerational relationships, social factors and illness, epidemiology of aging and chronic illness, stress and coping, cell growth and differentiation, signal transduction, and the demographics and economics of aging populations.

The Aging Center coordinates research, training, and clinical services in aging for the University. The Division of Geriatrics focuses research on the basic and clinical aspects of aging, emphasizing neoplasia, bone and musculoskeletal disorders and rehabilitation involved, immunology, cardiovascular diseases, cerebrovascular disease/dementia, enzymatic and cellular basis for aging, and health services delivery for the aged. **Pub:** *Center Report*, quarterly. • *Long Term Care Advances.*

**Hospital for Joint Diseases Orthopaedic Institute Geriatric Hip Fracture Research Group**
*See:* Entry 16948

**★ 3052 ★ Indiana University Center for Aging Research (CAR)**
The Regenstrief Institute
1050 Wilshire Blvd.
Indianapolis, IN 46202
**Phone:** (317)630-7200          **Fax:** (317)287-3798
**Email:** ccallahan@regenstrief.org
**Website:** http://iucar.iu.edu/
Christopher M. Callahan, MD, Dir.

**Activities/Fields:** Aging, improvement of quality of life for older adults, how to disseminate health information to older adults and enhance self-care behaviors.

**Indiana University Center for Alzheimer's Disease and Related Disorders**
*See:* Entry 14205

**★ 3053 ★ Indiana University Bloomington Center on Aging and Aged**
2805 E 10th St.
Bloomington, IN 47408-2698
**Phone:** (812)855-0815          **Fax:** (812)855-6194
**Email:** hawkinsb@indiana.edu
**Website:** http://www.indiana.edu/~caa/
Barbara Hawkins, Dir.

**Activities/Fields:** Gerontology, including developmentally disabled, handicapped, minorities, rural-isolated, and mainstream aging populations.

**Institute of Developmental Neuroscience and Aging**
*See:* Entry 14207

**John P. Robarts Research Institute Stroke and Aging Group Neurobiology Group**
*See:* Entry 14211

**★ 3054 ★ Johns Hopkins Bayview Medical Center General Clinical Research Center**
B3NW, Rm. 310
4940 Eastern Ave.
Baltimore, MD 21224
**Phone:** (410)550-1850          **Fax:** (410)550-1227
**Email:** pouyang@jhmi.edu
**Website:** http://www.jhbmc.jhu.edu/gcrc/gcrc.html
Pamela Ouyang, MD, Prog. Dir.

**Activities/Fields:** Major areas of investigation include aging and cardiovascular diseases.

**★ 3055 ★ Lankenau Institute for Medical Research (LIMR)**
100 Lancaster Ave.
Wynnewood, PA 19096
**Phone:** (610)645-3475          **Fax:** (610)645-8533
**Email:** cristofalov@mlhs.org
**Website:** http://www.mainlinehealth.org/limr/
Vincent J. Cristofalo, PhD, Pres. /CEO

**Activities/Fields:** Biological mechanisms of aging and the diseases associated with it, including but not limited to cancer, cardiovascular disease, osteoporosis and age-related neurodegenerative disorders. The focus of this research is to improve the health and quality of life for all, with particular emphasis on older persons. **Pub:** *Papers.* • *Abstracts.* • *Newsletters.*

### ★ 3056 ★ McGill University
### Centre for Studies in Aging
Douglas Hospital
6825 La Salle Blvd.
Verdun, QC, Canada H4H 1R3
**Phone:** (514)766-2010          **Fax:** (514)888-4050
**Email:** jpoiri@pobxo.mcgill.ca
**Website:** http://www.mcgill.ca/mcsa
Dr. Judes Poirier, Dir.

**Activities/Fields:** Alzheimer's disease, including diagnostic methods, drug trials, brain banking, and genetic studies; Parkinson's disease; autonomous nervous dysfunction in aging; cellular models of aging; community health and epidemiology; bioethics; nutrition in aging; and social gerontology. **Pub:** *Geronto-McGill Newsletter.*

### ★ 3057 ★ McMaster University
### R. Samuel McLaughlin Centre for Research and Education in Aging and Health
1200 Main St. West
Chedoke Campus, Bldg 74
Hamilton, ON, Canada L8N 3Z5
**Phone:** (905)521-2100          **Fax:** (905)318-6556
**Email:** bodden@mcmaster.ca
**Website:** http://www.fhs.mcmaster.ca/mcah
Dr. Larry W. Chambers, Dir.

**Activities/Fields:** Health promotion and disease prevention, focusing on health promotion and disease prevention for seniors in the practices of family physicans; aging brain, focusing on dementia, risk factors for dementia, and the impact on caregiver health; aging, mobility and participation, focusing on ways to keep seniors active so they may order their own lives; and pharmacology and therapeutics, focusing on finding ways to reduce polypharmacy. **Pub:** *Quarterly Newsletter.*

### ★ 3058 ★ National Institute on Aging
### Gerontology Research Center
5600 Nathan Shock Dr.
Baltimore, MD 21224
**Phone:** (410)558-8110          **Fax:** (410)558-8137
**Email:** longod@grc.nia.nih.gov
Dr. Dan L. Longo, MD, Dir.

**Activities/Fields:** Gerontology research, including molecular genetics, human physiology, neurosciences, cardiovascular, personality, behavioral research, and Alzheimer's disease studies.

### ★ 3059 ★ New York University Medical Center
### William and Sylvia Silberstein Aging and Dementia Research Center (ADRC)
550 1st Ave., Rm. THN-314
New York, NY 10016
**Phone:** (212)263-8088
**Email:** steve.ferris@med.nyu.edu
**Website:** http://aging.med.nyu.edu/
Steven Ferris, PhD, Exec. Dir.

**Activities/Fields:** Memory problems attributed to normal aging; the diagnosis, causes, and treatment of Alzheimer's disease.

### ★ 3060 ★ Northwestern University
### Buehler Center on Aging
750 N Lake Shore Dr., Ste. 601
Chicago, IL 60611-2611
**Phone:** (312)503-3087          **Fax:** (312)503-5868
**Email:** miris@nwu.edu

**Website:** http://www.nwu.edu/aging/index.htm
Dr. Madelyn Iris, Interim Dir.

**Activities/Fields:** Gerontology and geriatrics to improve the medical/social/emotional functioning and status of the elderly. **Pub:** *Buehler Center on Aging Quarterly Newsletter.* • *Geriatrics Resource Guide.* • *Monograph series.* • *Videos.*

### ★ 3061 ★ Northwestern University
### Multipurpose Arthritis and Musculoskeletal Diseases Center
303 E Chicago Ave., Ward 3-315
Chicago, IL 60611
**Phone:** (312)503-8003          **Fax:** (312)503-0994
**Email:** rmp158@northwestern.edu
Dr. Richard M. Pope, Dir.

**Activities/Fields:** Biomedical, educational, and health services research in the musculoskeletal diseases.

### ★ 3062 ★ Oklahoma Medical Research Foundation
### Free Radical Biology and Aging Research Program
825 NE 13th St.
Oklahoma City, OK 73104
**Phone:** (405)271-6673          **Fax:** (405)271-3980
**Email:** robert-floyd@omrf.ouhsc.edu
**Website:** http://www.omrf.org/OMRF/Research/13/Program.asp
Robert A. Floyd, PhD, Prog. Hd.

**Activities/Fields:** Mechanistic basis of aging as well as several diseases of aging including neurodegenerative diseases, cardiovascular disease, cancer and diabetes. Much of the research involves the action of reactive oxygen and nitric oxide species and free radical aspects of signal transduction.

### Oregon Health and Science University
### Oregon Aging and Alzheimer's Disease Center (OADC)
*See:* Entry 14258

### ★ 3063 ★ Orentreich Foundation for the Advancement of Science, Inc.
Biomedical Research Station
Rd. 2, Box 375
855 Rte. 301
Cold Spring, NY 10516
**Phone:** (845)265-4200          **Fax:** (845)265-4210
**Email:** ofas1@juno.com
**Website:** http://www.ohsu.edu/som-alzheimers/
Rozlyn Krajcik, Asst. Dir.

**Activities/Fields:** Dermatology, aging, endocrinology, and serum markers for human diseases. **Pub:** *Report of the Director.*

### ★ 3064 ★ Pennsylvania State University
### Gerontology Center
S-105 Henderson Bldg.
University Park, PA 16802
**Phone:** (814)865-1710          **Fax:** (814)863-9423
**Email:** gero@psu.edu
**Website:** http://geron.psu.edu
Dr. K. Warner Schaie, Dir.

**Activities/Fields:** Aging, including cognition in aging, developmental methodology, family and informal supports, human services for the elderly, caregiving, urinary incontinence, and the use of pharmaceutical products. **Pub:** *Annual preprint/reprint catalog*, biennially. • *Newsletter*, biennially.

### ★ 3065 ★ Purdue University
### Botanical Center for Age-Related Diseases
Stone Hall
West Lafayette, IN 47907
**Phone:** (765)494-8237          **Fax:** (765)494-0674
**Email:** weavercm@cfs.purdue.edu

**Website:** http://nccam.nih.gov/nccam/fi/research/desc.htmlbot1
Connie M. Weaver, PhD, Prin. Investigator

**Activities/Fields:** Health effects of polyphenols, a diverse group of chemical components widely distributed in plants, including soy, grapes, green tea, and several herbs. Research is focused on heart disease and cancer, and to two leading causes of diminished quality of life, osteoporosis and cognitive decline.

### ★ 3066 ★ Rehabilitation Research and Training Center on Aging With a Disability
Rancho Los Amigos National Rehabilitation Center
7601 E Imperial Hwy., Bldg. 800-W
Downey, CA 90242
**Phone:** (562)401-7402          **Fax:** (562)401-7011
**Email:** gracefg@agingwithdisability.org
**Website:** http://www.agingwithdisability.org
Bryan Kemp, PhD, Dir.

**Activities/Fields:** Problems people face as they age with disabilities, including those who are post-polio, have rheumatoid arthritis, cerebral palsy, or have suffered a stroke. **Pub:** *Fact Sheet: Aging with a Disability Instrument Development.* • *A Life Course Perspective: Aging with Long-Term Disability.* • *A Research Perspective: Next Steps in Bridging the Gap Between Aging and Disability.* • *Resource List: Wellness, Self-Care, Exercise and Aging with Disability.*

### Rockefeller University
### Fisher Center for Research on Alzheimer's Disease
*See:* Entry 14265

### ★ 3067 ★ Rush University
### Rush Institute for Healthy Aging
1645 W Jackson Blvd., Ste. 675
Chicago, IL 60612
**Phone:** (312)942-3350          **Fax:** (312)942-2861
**Email:** devans2@rush.edu
**Website:** http://www.rockefeller.edu/graduate/cenzach.htm
Dr. Denis A. Evans, Co-Dir.

**Activities/Fields:** Epidemiology of Alzheimer's disease, community-based studies of Alzheimer's disease and other common problems of older persons, physical functions among older persons, and statistical methods in aging research.

### St. Boniface General Hospital Research Centre
*See:* Entry 5137

### ★ 3068 ★ Sherbrooke University
### Gerontology and Geriatrics Research Centre
1036 Belvedere South
Sherbrooke, QC, Canada J1H 4C4
**Phone:** (819)829-7131          **Fax:** (819)829-7141
**Email:** cdrgg@courrier.usherb.ca
**Website:** http://www.usherb.ca/cdrgg
Dr. Rejean Hebert, Dir.

**Activities/Fields:** Biology of aging, rehabilitation, Alzheimer's disease, diabetes, nutrition, epidemiology and prevention of functional decline, physical activity, gait and balance, psycho-sociology of aging, and sleep disorders.

### Southern Illinois University at Carbondale
### Center for Alzheimer Disease and Related Disorders (CADRD)
*See:* Entry 14274

**★ 3069 ★ Temple University**
**Institute on Aging**
1601 N Broad St.
Philadelphia, PA 19130
**Phone:** (215)204-6834          **Fax:** (215)204-6733
**Email:** neuro@siumed.edu
**Website:** http://www.temple.edu/aging
Kathy Segrist, PhD, Exec. Dir.

**Activities/Fields:** Changes in adaptive capabilities during aging, anti-aging effects of dehydroepiandrosterone (DHEA), the influences of characteristics of elderly disabled clients on their experiences in case management, minority/ethnic aging research, and service management and services to the frail elderly. **Frmly:** Aging Research Center.


**★ 3070 ★ U.S. Department of Health and**
**Human Services**
**National Institute on Aging**
Public Information Office
Bldg. 31., Rm. 5C27
31 Center Dr., MSC 2292
Bethesda, MD 20892-2292
**Phone:** (301)496-1752          **Free:** 800-222-2225
**Fax:** (301)496-2525
**Email:** hodesr@31.nia.nih.gov
**Website:** http://www.nia.nih.gov
Dr. Richard J. Hodes, Dir.

**Activities/Fields:** Biomedical, social, and behavioral aspects of aging. The Intramural Research Program is primarily conducted at the Gerontology Research Center in Baltimore, MD. In addition, the Institute's Neurosciences Laboratory operates basic and clinical research programs from the NIH Clinical Center in Bethesda, MD. The principal NIA extramural programs are the Behavioral and Social Research Program, the Biology of Aging Program, the Geriatrics Program, and the Neuroscience and Neuropsychology of Aging Program. Areas included in the program are: diagnostic assessment of the geriatric patient, dementia, incontinence, fall injuries, and musculoskeletal disorders producing functional disability in the geriatric population, among others.


**★ 3071 ★ U.S. Department of Health and**
**Human Services**
**National Institute on Aging**
**Behavioral and Social Research Program**
Gateway Bldg., Rm 533
7201 Wisconsin Ave.
MSC 9205
Bethesda, MD 20892-9205
**Phone:** (301)496-3131          **Fax:** (301)402-0051
**Email:** BSRquery@EXMUR.NIA.NIH.GOV
**Website:** http://www.nia.nih.gov/research/extramural/behavior/
Dr. Richard M. Suzman, Assoc. Dir.

**Activities/Fields:** Social, psychological, cultural, demographic, and economic factors that affect both the process of growing old and the place of older people in society, as well as the ways in which behavioral and social processes interacting with biomedical processes influence particular aspects of health and functioning as people age. Its goals are to prolong the productive, healthy, middle years of life and to prevent or reverse such decrements of old age as memory loss, chronic ill health, sensory deficits, low self-esteem, and withdrawal from active participation in social and economic roles. The program focuses primarily on three broad categories: adult psychological development, with research supported that investigates social and behavioral influences upon cognitive functioning, personality, attitudes, and interpersonal relations over the adult life course, with emphasis on research relevant to maintaining and improving well being and independent functioning; social science research on aging, which is directed at understanding the social and environmental conditions influencing health, well being, and functioning of people in their middle and later years as well as the influence of social structures on aging and the interactions among psychosocial and biological processes on health and functioning; and demography and population epidemiology, involving research on the dynamics and consequences of

population aging and aims to describe and understand the older population in terms of its social, demographic, economic, health, and functional characteristics and the impact of these changes on society as a whole.


**★ 3072 ★ U.S. Department of Health and**
**Human Services**
**National Institute on Aging**
**Biology of Aging Program**
7201 Wisconsin Ave., Ste. 2C-231
Bethesda, MD 20892
**Phone:** (301)496-6402          **Fax:** (301)496-4996
**Email:** bapquery@nia.nih.gov
**Website:** http://www.nih.gov/research/extramural/biology
Dr. Richard L. Sprott, Assoc. Dir.

**Activities/Fields:** Basic mechanisms involved in aging processes and age-related disease. It funds research and training in ten main areas: biochemistry; genetics; endocrinology; immunology; nutrition and metabolism; molecular biology; pathobiology; cell biology, physiology; and biomarkers of aging. The Program also supports facilities that provide investigators with aging animals and cell cultures for use in aging research. **Frmly:** (1990) Biomedical Research and Clinical Medicine Program.


**★ 3073 ★ U.S. Department of Health and**
**Human Services**
**National Institute on Aging**
**Biology of Aging Program**
**Biology Branch**
Gateway Bldg., Ste. 2C231
7201 Wisconsin Ave., MSC 9205
Bethesda, MD 20892-9205
**Phone:** (301)496-6402          **Fax:** (301)402-0010
**Website:** http://www.nih.gov/research/extrmural/biology/programs.htm
Francis L. Bellino, Dep. Assoc. Dir.

**Activities/Fields:** Cellular aging research, which involves research using differentiated human cells in culture and the study of age-associated alterations in differentiated functions that are expressed by cells in vitro; fundamental molecular and genetics research and research training on the biology and mechanisms of aging at the cellular level and on vertebrate and invertebrate organisms, with particular interest in research that emphasizes the use of mammalian and human models; immunological research on the effects of aging on the various functions of the immune system; and research on age-related changes in endocrine function. **Frmly:** Molecular and Cell Biology Branch.


**★ 3074 ★ U.S. Department of Health and**
**Human Services**
**National Institute on Aging**
**Epidemiology, Demography, and Biometry**
**Program**
7201 Wisconsin Ave., Ste. 3C-309
Bethesda, MD 20892
**Phone:** (301)496-1178          **Fax:** (301)496-4006
**Email:** havlikr@gw.nia.nih.gov
**Website:** http://www.nia.nih.gov/research/intramural/edb
Richard J. Havlik, MD, Assoc. Dir.

**Activities/Fields:** Health and illness in older populations, including hip fractures and osteoporosis, dementia and other cognitive impairments, sleep disorders, predictive factors of mortality, bereavement behaviors, and events and conditions common among older persons prior to death. Gathers demographic information on the current and projected health, economic, social, and occupational status of older people.

**★ 3075 ★ U.S. Department of Health and**
**Human Services**
**National Institute on Aging**
**Geriatrics Program**
7201 Wisconson Ave., St. 3E-327
Bethesda, MD 20892-9205
**Phone:** (301)496-1033          **Fax:** (301)402-1784
Dr. Evan Hadley, Chf.

**Activities/Fields:** Epidemiology, etiology, pathophysiology, diagnostic evaluation, and treatment of urinary incontinence in the elderly; studies on obesity, with particular interest in the effects of obesity on health and longevity, treatment of obesity, and contribution of overnutrition to aging of organ systems; research on infectious diseases in the elderly (cosponsored with the National Institute of Allergy and Infectious Diseases); studies on aspects of diabetes mellitus related to aging and the elderly and studies on the epidemiology of diabetes; and nutrition in relation to health of the aged and the aging process. Research also includes investigation of the function of the aging musculoskeletal system (including support for animal models or clinical studies in exercise physiology or orthopedic research); studies on enteral and parenteral nutritional support in elderly patients in acute and long-term care facilities (announced with five other institutes); research on the causes of age-related cardiovascular changes (and changes in risk factors for cardiovascular disease) and on the role of cardiovascular factors in age-related physiologic and pathologic changes; and studies on exercise physiology and aging.


**★ 3076 ★ U.S. Department of Health and**
**Human Services**
**National Institute on Aging**
**Intramural Research Program**
Gerontology Research Center
5600 Nathan Shock Dr.
Baltimore, MD 21224
**Phone:** (410)558-8110          **Fax:** (410)558-8137
Dr. Dan L. Longo, Dir.

**Activities/Fields:** Process of aging in animals and man. Projects include the Baltimore Longitudinal Study of Aging, which involves the biennial observation of the same human subjects to determine changes and elucidate mechanisms underlying these changes. Program components include Behavioral Sciences Laboratory; Biological Chemistry Laboratory; Cardiovascular Science Laboratory; Cellular and Molecular Biology Laboratory; Clinical Physiology Laboratory; Longitudinal Studies Branch; Molecular Genetics Laboratory; Neurosciences Laboratory; and Personality and Cognition Laboratory.


**★ 3077 ★ U.S. Department of Health and**
**Human Services**
**National Institute on Aging**
**Intramural Research Program**
**Longitudinal Studies Section**
**(Laboratory of Clinical Investigation)**
Gerontology Research Center
5600 Nathan Shock Dr.
Baltimore, MD 21224
**Phone:** (410)558-8364          **Fax:** (410)558-8321
**Email:** jf72d@nih.gov
**Website:** http://www.grc.nia.nih.gov
Jerome L. Fleg, MD, Interim Dir.

**Activities/Fields:** Longitudinal research on aging, particularly physiological and psychological aspects. **Pub:** *Proceedings.* • *Research reports.*


**★ 3078 ★ U.S. Department of Health and**
**Human Services**
**National Institute on Aging**
**Laboratory of Cardiovascular Science**
Gerontology Research Center, Rm. 3B03
5600 Nathan Shock Dr.
Baltimore, MD 21224
**Phone:** (410)558-8650          **Fax:** (410)558-8137
Dr. Edward G. Lakatta, Chf., Behavioral
Hypertension

**Activities/Fields:** Basic mechanisms that control myocardial and vascular function. Studies are extended to describe the influence of age and age-related chronic pathologic conditions in studies conducted in human and animal models. In humans, laboratory seeks to identify the adaptive changes in cardiovascular structure and function that occur with normative aging as well as those changes that predict or accompany the development of cardiovascular disease. Studies in animal models involve isolated cardiac and vascular cells and subcellular organelles. The biophysical mechanisms that govern excitation and contraction of myocardial cells are investigated with techniques that allow the simultaneous recording of contra c tility, cytosolic and membrane potential, or current in a single myocyte. Current research includes a program to study molecular mechanisms of vascular cell functions and pathology using molecular and tissue culture techniques. Also studies whether the blood vessels of adults and animals respond differently to injury by altered gene expression of growth factors and extracellular matrix proteins, and whether age alters endothelial cell growth and differentiation of in vivo systems. Also investigates the effects produced by cytokines, second messengers, aging, and cell cycle of in vitro models for angiogenesis.

★ 3079 ★ **U.S. Department of Health and Human Services**
**National Institute on Aging**
**Laboratory of Cardiovascular Science**
**Membrane Biology Section**
Gerontology Research Center, Rm. 1B04
5600 Nathan Shock Dr.
Baltimore, MD 21224
**Phone:** (410)558-8110          **Fax:** (410)558-8137
Dr. Jeffrey Froehlich, Chf.

**Activities/Fields:** Ion and metabolite transport across biological membranes; studies how the translocation mechanisms are regulated by hormones, pharmacological agents, diet, and other pathophysiological effectors; and explores the mechanisms by which these systems are modified during the aging process and in age-associated disease. Also studies angiogenesis and smooth muscle function with special emphasis on intracellular ion metabolism. intracellular and extracellular environment and metabolism (involving identification, characterization, and regulation of membrane transport systems largely, but not exclusively, in the kidney).

★ 3080 ★ **U.S. Department of Health and Human Services**
**National Institute on Aging**
**Laboratory of Cellular and Molecular Biology**
Gerontology Research Center
Rm. 1-B-02, Stop 12
5600 Nathan Shock Dr.
Baltimore, MD 21224
**Phone:** (410)558-8443          **Fax:** (410)558-8335
**Email:** gorospem@grc.nia.nih.gov
**Website:** http://www.grc.nia.nih.gov/branches/lcmb/lcmb.htm
Myriam Gorospe, Actg. Ch.

**Activities/Fields:** Basic biological and biochemical mechanisms of aging. Activities include research into the mechanism of stress responses, hormone/neurotransmitter, signal transduction, neurodegeneration/protection, behavior, erythrocyte oxyradical production and aging, and NMR methodology and applications. Nutritional, pharmacological, exercise and other interventions into the aging process are also employed. Four groups make up the laboratory: Gene Expression and Aging Section; Molecular Dynamics Section; Molecular Physiology and Genetics Section; and NMR Unit. **Pub:** *Proceedings.*

★ 3081 ★ **U.S. Department of Health and Human Services**
**National Institute on Aging**
**Laboratory of Clinical Physiology**
Gerontology Research Center
5600 Nathan Shock Dr.
Baltimore, MD 21224
**Phone:** (410)558-8193          **Fax:** (410)558-8113
Dr. Reubin Andres, Chf.

**Activities/Fields:** Physiologic changes occurring over the entire adult lifespan. The Laboratory comprises sections on Applied Physiology, Clinical Immunology, Endocrinology, and Metabolism. The Applied Physiology Section studies age changes in specific human systems, including renal, bone, and musculoskeletal. Investigations are concerned with interrelationships between age effects in different organ systems and in overall physiological changes in individuals, and efforts are made to differentiate between pathological disease changes and those secondary to pure age effects. In addition, Section develops and adapts computer techniques for kinetic modeling of physiological systems for the analysis of longitudinal data. In the Clinical Immunology Section, studies are conducted on the decline in host immune responsiveness that is seen in aging. These studies involve the development of diagnostic procedures for the detection of relative immunodeficiencies in humans and the investigation of the mechanisms of these deficiencies in humans and experimental animals. The Endocrinology Section conducts studies on the molecular basis of age-related changes of hormone responses, especially those related to the biochemistry of the adenylate cyclase system and hormone receptors, aging and the endocrinology of the reproductive system, and neuroendocrinology. Clinical studies are conducted on subjects from the Baltimore Longitudinal Study of Human Aging; and studies on rodents are done on tissues from a variety of organs. The Metabolism Section emphasizes clinical research on such metabolic variables as: glucose-insulin homeostatic mechanisms and diabetes mellitus; obesity, patterns of fat distribution, and body composition; acute and sustained effects of physical activity; dietary and nutritional evaluation; and the interactive effects of these variables on rates of aging, disease developments, and longevity.

★ 3082 ★ **U.S. Department of Health and Human Services**
**National Institute on Aging**
**Laboratory of Molecular Genetics**
5600 Nathan Shock Dr.
Baltimore, MD 21224-6823
**Phone:** (410)558-8162          **Fax:** (410)558-8157
**Email:** vbohr@nih.gov
Dr. Vilhelm A. Bohr, Chf.

**Activities/Fields:** Fundamental nature of aging at the molecular level, including studies on changes in gene structure and function with aging. Researchers utilize the techniques of molecular genetics to examine age-related alterations in cellular function and the DNA repair processes.

★ 3083 ★ **U.S. Department of Health and Human Services**
**National Institute on Aging (NIA)**
**Laboratory of Neurosciences**
NIH Bldg. 10, Rm. 6N202
10 Center Dr., MSC 1582
Bethesda, MD 20892-1582
**Phone:** (301)496-1765          **Fax:** (301)402-0074
**Email:** sir@helix.nih.gov
Dr. Stanley Rapoport, Chf.

**Activities/Fields:** Function, structure, physiology, biochemistry, and pharmacology of the central and peripheral nervous system. Laboratory also examines changes that take place in these systems during development and aging in animal models and humans. The Laboratory comprises the Brain Aging and Dementia Section, the Cerebral Physiology and Metabolism Section, and the Neurochemistry and Brain Transport Section. The Brain Aging and Dementia

Section operates an eight-bed Patient Care Unit at the Clinical Center as well as an outpatient Dementia and Aging Clinic. Clinical methods involve positron emission tomography. Research activities focus primarily on aging of the central nervous system and on dementia and associated neurological diseases as these relate to the elderly. Subject groups include outpatient healthy men and women between 18 and 90 years of age, with syndrome and chronic hypertension. The Cerebral Physiology and Metabolism Section conducts fundamental research on animal models of human brain aging and disease using molecular biology, clinical in vivo brain imaging, neurochemistry involving phospholipid metabolism, electrophysiology, and cell culture techniques. The Neurochemistry and Brain Transport Section studies transport and regulation at the blood-brain and blood-nerve barriers, focusing on amino acids, toxic metals, and fatty acids. **Pub:** *Proceedings.*

★ 3084 ★ **U.S. Department of Health and Human Services**
**National Institute on Aging**
**Laboratory of Personality and Cognition**
Gerontology Research Center
5600 Nathan Shock Dr.
Baltimore, MD 21224
**Phone:** (410)558-8220          **Fax:** (410)558-8108
**Email:** lpcpsc@helix.nih.gov
**Website:** http://www.grc.nia.nih.gov/branches/lpc/lpc.htm
Dr. Paul T. Costa, Chf.

**Activities/Fields:** Individual differences in cognitive and personality processes and traits. Also investigated are the influence of age on these variables and their reciprocal influence on health, well-being, and adaptation. Studies employ longitudinal, experimental, and epidemiological methods in the analysis of psychological and psychosocial issues of aging, including health and health care needs, predictors of intellectual competence and decline, models of adult personality, and correlates of disease risk factors. Laboratory comprises sections on: Cognition and Personality, Stress, and Coping. The Cognition Section studies the psychological mechanisms underlying age-related changes in memory, learning, problem solving, and information processing. In addition, the roles of psychological and physiological characteristics in age differences and age changes in cognitive performance are analyzed. The Personality, Stress, and Coping Section deals with the dimensions of personality and their influence on processes of adaptation in adult men and women. The objective is to determine methods and strategies for coping with the stresses of adult life and evaluate the effects of different coping mechanisms and personality dispositions on such outcomes as subjective well-being, social functioning, physical and psychiatric health and personality and psychological processes.

★ 3085 ★ **U.S. Department of Health and Human Services**
**National Institute on Aging**
**Neuroscience and Neuropsychology of Aging Program**
NIH Gateway Bldg., Ste. 3C307
7201 Wisconsin Ave. MSC9205
Bethesda, MD 20892-9205
**Phone:** (301)496-9350          **Fax:** (301)496-1494
Marcelle Moorison-Bogorad, Assoc. Dir.

**Activities/Fields:** Normal and pathological aging of the nervous system and its behavioral consequences. Etiology or pathogenesis of Alzheimer's disease, improve diagnosis, and eventually provide a sound basis for effective therapy. Areas of particular interest are: differential diagnosis; clinical and basic studies of cerebral circulation, metabolism, neurochemistry, and neuroendocrinology; genetics; population studies; immunology-virology; and animal and other model systems. Other areas of interest include: research on role of infectious agents and immunolgoical processes that cause degeneration in the aging brain; identification of biological markers in the diagnosis of diseases, such as Alzheimer's; epidemiological investigations of Alzheimer's disease and other dementing disorders of older age; research on diagnostic screening; development and validation of new measures for the diagnosis of Alzheimer's disease; studies designed to examine the nature and extent of age-related sensory and motor changes in older people, such as hearing and understanding of everyday speech, visual perception, taste, and smell as related to the effective functioning of older people in everyday contexts; neurobiological processes as they relate to the aging nervous system and behavior neuropsychological processes in aging animals and humans; sleep and circadian rhythms in aging and the treatment of disturbances; neural plasticity; and mechanisms underlying neural growth, survival, and death in the aging brain. **Frmly:** Physiology of Aging Branch.

### ★ 3086 ★ U.S. Department of Health and Human Services
**National Institute on Aging**
**Office of Extramural Affairs**
Gateway Bldg. 2C218
7201 Wisconsin Ave.
MSC 9205
Bethesda, MD 20892-9205
**Phone:** (301)496-9322      **Fax:** (301)402-2945
**Email:** mk46u@nih.gov
**Website:** http://www.nia.nih.gov
Dr. Miriam F. Kelty, Assoc. Dir.

**Activities/Fields:** Administers the funding programs through which NIA supports research and research training. Specific NIA funding mechanisms include: Research Project Grants; Research Program Project Grants; Research Career Development Awards; Clinical Investigator Awards; Academic Awards; National Research Service Awards; Physician Scientist Awards; Geriatric Leadership Academic Awards; Small Business Innovative Research Program; and Academic Research Enhancement Awards.

**U.S. Department of Health and Human Services**
**National Institute of Mental Health**
**Division of Clinical and Treatment Research**
**Mental Disorders of the Aging Research Branch**
*See:* Entry 12719

**U.S. Department of Health and Human Services**
**National Institutes of Health (NIH)**
**National Cancer Institute (NCI)**
**Division of Basic Sciences**
**((Laboratory of Biosystems and Cancer) Cancer and Aging Section)**
*See:* Entry 10511

**U.S. Department of Health and Human Services**
**National Institutes of Health (NIH)**
**National Eye Institute (NEI)**
**Intramural Research**
**((Laboratory of Mechanisms of Ocular Diseases) Aging and Ocular Disease)**
*See:* Entry 21161

### ★ 3087 ★ U.S. Department of Health and Human Services
**National Institutes of Health**
**National Institute on Aging**
**Extramural Programs**
**(Geriatrics Program)**
Bldg. 31, Rm. 5C27
31 Center Dr., MSC 2292
Bethesda, MD 20892
**Phone:** (301)496-1752
**Email:** gpquery@exmur.nia.nih.gov

**Website:** http://www.nia.nih.gov/research/extramural/geriatrics

**Activities/Fields:** Pathophysiology, diagnosis, treatment, and prevention of age-related diseases, degenerative conditions, and disabilities, especially physical frailty (deficits in strength, mobility, balance, and endurance); new diseases of old age; development of interventions and testing in controlled clinical trials.

### ★ 3088 ★ U.S. Department of Health and Human Services
**National Institutes of Health (NIH)**
**National Institute on Aging**
**Intramural Research Programs**
**(Brain Physiology and Metabolism Section)**
Gateway
7201 Wisconsin Ave., Ste. 3C309
Bethesda, MD 20892-9205
**Phone:** (301)496-1765      **Fax:** (301)402-0074
**Email:** sir@helix.nih.gov
**Website:** http://www.grc.nia.nih.gov/branches/lns/cpms.htm
Stanley I. Rapoport, MD, Ch.

**Activities/Fields:** Brain structure and function with regard to development, aging, drug activation of second messenger systems involving phospholipids, acute and chronic sensory deprivation and lesions, and basic mechanisms of brain function; molecular biology of regional brain vulnerability to Alzheimers' diseases; electrophysiologic assessment of animal models for Down's syndrome, and the effect of Beta-amyloid and other toxic substances on cell membranes.

### ★ 3089 ★ U.S. Department of Health and Human Services
**National Institutes of Health (NIH)**
**National Institute on Aging**
**Intramural Research Programs**
**(Laboratory of Molecular Gerontology)**
Nathan W Shock Laboratories
Rm. 2-D-09, Stop 01
Baltimore, MD 21224
**Phone:** (410)558-8223      **Fax:** (410)558-8157
**Email:** bohrv@grc.nia.nih.gov
**Website:** http://www.grc.nia.nih.gov/branches/lmg/lmg.htm
Vilhelm A. Bohr, MD, Ch.

**Activities/Fields:** Molecular basis for aging and age-dependent diseases, notably cancer.

### ★ 3090 ★ U.S. Department of Health and Human Services
**National Institutes of Health (NIH)**
**National Institute on Aging**
**Intramural Research Programs**
**(Laboratory of Immunology)**
5600 Nathan Shock Dr.
Baltimore, MD 21224
**Phone:** (410)558-8159      **Fax:** (410)558-8284
**Email:** taubd@grc.nia.nih.gov
**Website:** http://www.grc.nia.nih.gov/branches/li/li.htm
Dennis D. Taub, PhD, Actg. Ch.

**Activities/Fields:** Dedicated to understanding the biological, biochemical, and molecular alterations in immune functions that occur within individuals during both normal and disease-associated aging processes.

### ★ 3091 ★ U.S. Department of Health and Human Services
**National Institutes of Health (NIH)**
**National Institute on Aging**
**Intramural Research Programs**
**(Cell Stress and Aging Section Program)**
Gerontology Research Center
5600 Nathan Shock Dr.
Baltimore, MD 21224
**Phone:** (410)558-8446
**Email:** holbroon@intra.nia.nih.gov

**Website:** http://www.grc.nia.nih.gov/branches/lbc/gea/gea.htm
Nikki Holbrook, PhD, Ch.

**Activities/Fields:** Cellular responses to stress and how they become altered with age.

### ★ 3092 ★ U.S. Department of Health and Human Services
**National Institutes of Health (NIH)**
**National Institute on Aging**
**Intramural Research Programs**
**(Behavioral Hypertension Section)**
Gerontology Research Center
5600 Nathan Shock Dr.
Baltimore, MD 21224-6825
**Email:** andersond@grc.nia.nih.gov
**Website:** http://www.grc.nia.nih.gov/branches/lcs/bhs.htm
David E. Anderson, PhD, Ch.

**Activities/Fields:** Strives to clarify role of behavior in the etiology and pathogenesis of selected disorders of aging, to elucidate physiological and biochemical pathways by which behavioral factors influence disorders of aging, and to develop and apply behavioral interventions to prevent, ameliorate, or reverse disorders of aging.

### ★ 3093 ★ U.S. Department of Health and Human Services
**National Institutes of Health (NIH)**
**National Institute on Aging**
**Intramural Research Programs**
**(Cardiac Function Unit)**
Gerontology Research Center
5600 Nathan Shock Dr.
Baltimore, MD 21224
**Phone:** (410)558-8110
**Email:** lakattae@grc.nia.nih.gov
**Website:** http://www.grc.nia.nih.gov/branches/lcs/cardfunc/cardfunc.htm
Edward G. Lakatta, MD, Ch.

**Activities/Fields:** Cardiac dynamics and basic studies on isolated myocardial cells, including the influence of age on the intact cardiovascular system, especially the human myocardium; also studies the vascular structure, function, and mechanics of atherosclerosis, as well as gene therapy for age-related cardiovascular disease.

### ★ 3094 ★ U.S. Department of Health and Human Services
**National Institutes of Health**
**National Institute on Aging**
**Intramural Research Programs**
**(Laboratory of Epidemiology, Demography, and Biometry)**
Gateway
7201 Wisconsin Ave., Ste. 3C309
Bethesda, MD 20892-9205
**Phone:** (301)496-1752
**Website:** http://www.nia.nih.gov/research/intramural/edb
Richard J. Havlik, MD, Assoc. Dir.

**Activities/Fields:** Chronic diseases and functional status and disability in the older population; physiologic risk factors for different dimensions of the dementing process, including cognitive decline and structural brain changes; geriatric epidemiology in areas of metabolism and nutritional risk factors, chronic inflammation, and comorbidity as they relate to functional outcomes, disease endpoints, and mortality in older persons; mathematical, statistical, and numerical aspects of aging and health.

**★ 3095 ★ U.S. Department of Health and Human Services**
**National Institutes of Health**
**National Institute of Mental Health**
**Experimental Therapeutics Branch**
**(Geriatric Psychiatry Branch)**
MSC 1275
Bldg. 10, Rm. 3N226
Bethesda, MD 20892
**Phone:** (301)496-0948      **Fax:** (301)496-2847
**Email:** nimhinfo@nih.gov
**Website:** http://intramural.nimh.nih.gov/research/gpb/
P. Trey Sunderland, MD, Ch.

**Activities/Fields:** Alzheimer's disease (AD); tests for therapeutic synergy among available drugs, such as monoamine oxidase inhibitor selegline, cholinergic agent physostigmine, and serotonin uptake inhibitor fluoxetine.


**U.S. Department of Health and Human Services**
**Office of Family, Community and Long-Term Care Policy**
**Division of Disability, Aging and Long-Term Care Policy**
*See:* Entry 8201


**U.S. Department of Veterans Affairs**
**Rehabilitation Research and Development Service**
**Center of Excellence on Geriatric Rehabilitation**
*See:* Entry 8204


**★ 3096 ★ U.S. Department of Veterans Affairs**
**Rehabilitation Research and Development Service**
**Center of Excellence on Healthy Aging with Disabilities**
Houston VA Medical Center
2002 Holcombe Blvd.
Houston, TX 77030
**Phone:** (713)794-7254      **Fax:** (713)794-7623
**Email:** healthyaging@bcm.tmc.edu
**Website:** http://www.healthyagingva.org/
Trilok N. Monga, MD, Med. Dir.

**Activities/Fields:** Process of aging with disabilities in order to design, implement, and evaluate strategies that enhance the health, functioning, and well-being of veterans aging with disabilities, with an ultimate goal of establishing best rehabilitation practices for the benefit of veterans.


**★ 3097 ★ University of Akron**
**Institute for Life-Span Development and Gerontology**
326 Polsky
Akron, OH 44325-4307
**Phone:** (330)972-7243      **Fax:** (330)972-5174
**Email:** hsterns@uakron.edu
**Website:** http://www.uakron.edu/ilsdg
Dr. Harvey L. Sterns, Dir.

**Activities/Fields:** Improving older adult cognitive functioning, aging and work, career development, training and retraining adult and older adult workers, mental retardation and aging, gender identity, human development, health and aging, and family and aging. Programs concentrate on aging changes in perception, perceptual style, selective attention, and learning and memory. Other studies focus on performance appraisal and selection of older adult workers. **Pub:** *Continuum Newsletter.*


**★ 3098 ★ University of Alabama at Birmingham**
**Center for Aging**
201 Community Health Services Bldg.
933 S 19th St.
Birmingham, AL 35294-2041
**Phone:** (205)934-9261      **Fax:** (205)934-7354
**Email:** rallman@uab.edu
**Website:** http://www.aging.uab.edu
Richard M. Allman, MD, Dir.

**Activities/Fields:** Aging, including immobility and its complications, genito-urinary disorders, health policy and aging, the social-behavioral aspects of Alzheimer's disease, atherosclerosis, muscoskeletal disease, and age-related cancer. **Pub:** *Insight on Aging.*


**★ 3099 ★ University of Alabama at Birmingham**
**Center for Research in Applied Gerontology**
Campbell Hall, Ste. 201
Department of Psychology
1300 University Blvd.
Birmingham, AL 35294-1170
**Phone:** (205)934-3850
**Email:** kball@uab.edu
**Website:** http://main.uab.edu/show.asp?durki=6771
Dr. Karlene Ball, Dir.

**Activities/Fields:** Gerontology, particularly interventions which will allow older individuals to remain independent and to experience a high quality of life. The research of the center is designed to evaluate the ways in which improved visual, attentional and cognitive functions enhance everyday activities, focusing on the area of mobility.


**★ 3100 ★ University of Calgary**
**Vision and Aging Laboratory**
Administration 237
Department of Psychology
2500 University Dr. NW
Calgary, AB, Canada T2N 1N4
**Phone:** (403)220-4969      **Fax:** (403)282-8249
**Email:** donkline@ucalgary.ca
**Website:** http://www.psych.ucalgary.ca/PACE/VA-Lab/
Prof. Donald Kline, PhD, Dir.

**Activities/Fields:** Aging effects on vision, optical and neural aspects of visual aging, visual aging, human factors & everyday tasks; visual health, refractive surgery, vision change and quality-of-life, visual testing.


**University of California, Los Angeles**
**Alzheimer's Disease Center (ADC)**
*See:* Entry 14397


**★ 3101 ★ University of California, San Diego**
**Sam and Rose Stein Institute for Research on Aging**
MC 0664
School of Medicine
9500 Gilman Dr.
La Jolla, CA 92093-0664
**Phone:** (858)534-6299      **Fax:** (858)534-5475
**Email:** steininstitute@ucsd.edu
**Website:** http://medschool.ucsd.edu/sira
Dr. Dennis A. Carson, Dir.

**Activities/Fields:** Aging and Alzheimer's disease, arthritis, osteoporosis, cardiovascular disease, sleep disorders, genetics, and mind, body, and health relationships. Investigates the relationships between the deterioration of the central nervous system and speech, hearing, and sleep problems; studies the effects of aging on production of hormones; evaluates alternatives to nursing home confinement; investigates immune system deteriorations; and studies the genetic and biochemical basis for long and healthy lifespans and the genetic basis of human diseases of accelerated aging. Also conducts studies of the elderly's

susceptibility to infections, loss of bone minerals, changes in the vascular system and the development of glaucoma. **Pub:** *Newsletter,* monthly.


**★ 3102 ★ University of Florida**
**Center for Gerontological Studies**
2326 Turlington Hall
PO Box 117335
Gainesville, FL 32611-7335
**Phone:** (352)392-2116      **Fax:** (352)392-8524
**Email:** pkricos@csd.ufl.edu
**Website:** http://www.geron.ufl.edu/
Dr. Patricia Kricos, Dir.

**Activities/Fields:** Interdisciplinary studies on family economic status, labor force participation and survivorship in life course perspective, alternative living arrangements for older people, political attitudes and policy issues in aging, fall prevention, rehabilitation, nutritional status of elderly, memory fitness and intelligence in adulthood and old age, training needs of counselors and physician assistants, geriatric dentistry, health care for older persons, care giving and demography. **Pub:** *Outlook on Aging: Florida.* • *Pathways to Aging.*


**University of Florida**
**Center for Neurobiology of Aging**
*See:* Entry 14414


**★ 3103 ★ University of Florida**
**Claude D. Pepper Center for Research on Oral Health in Aging**
JHMHSC
PO Box 100416
Gainesville, FL 32610
**Phone:** (352)392-6796      **Fax:** (352)846-0588
**Email:** mheft@dental.ufl.edu
**Website:** http://www.cop.ufl.edu/centers/cna/cna.htm
Dr. Marc Heft, Dir.

**Activities/Fields:** Health services research and basic oral-health functions of the elderly, including the development of periodontal disease, the effects of medications on saliva production, and the effects of aging on the senses.


**★ 3104 ★ University of Illinois at Chicago**
**Center for Research on Health and Aging (CRHA)**
Health Research & Policy Centers, M/C 275
850 W Jackson Blvd., Ste. 400
Chicago, IL 60607-3025
**Phone:** (312)996-1473      **Fax:** (312)996-2703
**Email:** shughes@uic.edu
**Website:** http://www.uic.edu/depts/ovcr/hrpc/centers/rha.html
Prof. Susan L. Hughes, Co-Dir.

**Activities/Fields:** Health issues for older persons, including prevention, health maintenance, and the cost, quality and effectiveness of health care delivery systems such as long-term care and managed care.


**★ 3105 ★ University of Illinois at Chicago**
**Rehabilitation Research and Training Center on Aging with Developmental Disabilities (RRTCADD)**
Department of Disability & Human Development
1640 W Roosevelt Rd.
Chicago, IL 60608-6904
**Phone:** (312)413-1520      **Free:** 800-996-8845
**Fax:** (312)996-6942
**Email:** theller@uic.edu
**Website:** http://www.uic.edu/orgs/rrtcamr/index.html
Tamar Heller, PhD, Dir.

**Activities/Fields:** How age-related changes in physical and psychological well being affect a person's ability to function in the community; the changing support needs of adults with developmental disabilities and their families as they age; and the effectiveness of innovative public policies and services in addressing later life needs. Research priorities include promoting health and wellness; understanding women's health issues; understanding family, including sibling caregiving roles across residential settings; developing effective approaches that support individuals and their families in making future plans; identifying gaps in age-related health resources and employment; and developing universal design and assistive technology capabilities to maintain employability and enhance functioning in the community. **Pub:** *A/DDVANTAGE*, semiannually.

**★ 3106 ★ University of Iowa**
**Gerontological Nursing Interventions**
**    Research Center**
410 Nursing Bldg.
College of Nursing
Iowa City, IA 52242
**Phone:** (319)335-7133          **Fax:** (319)353-5535
**Email:** toni-reimer@uiowa.edu
**Website:** http://www.nursing.uiowa.edu/gnirc
Dr. Toni Tripp-Reimer, Dir.

**Activities/Fields:** Nursing intervention in care of the elderly. **Pub:** *Advances in Gerontological Nursing*, annually. • *Iowa Aging News*, quarterly.

**★ 3107 ★ University of Kansas**
**Center on Aging**
Kansas University Medical Center
5026 Wescoe Pavillion
3901 Rainbow Blvd.
Kansas City, KS 66160-7117
**Phone:** (913)588-1203          **Fax:** (913)588-1201
**Email:** rnudo@kumc.edu
**Website:** http://www2.kumc.edu/coa
Randolph Nudo, PhD, Interim Dir.

**Activities/Fields:** Provides support for interdisciplinary research on issues of age and aging.

**★ 3108 ★ University of Kentucky**
**Sanders-Brown Center on Aging**
101 Sanders-Brown Bldg.
Lexington, KY 40536-0230
**Phone:** (859)257-1412          **Fax:** (859)323-2866
**Email:** wmarkesbery@aging.coa.uky.edu
**Website:** http://www.coa.uky.edu
William R. Markesbery, MD, Dir.

**Activities/Fields:** Biology of aging, including studies on aging nervous systems, Alzheimer's disease, stroke, hypertension in the elderly, immunology, geriatrics, and social-behavioral science. **Pub:** *Kentucky Atlas of the Elderly.* • *Sounding Board*, quarterly. **Frmly:** Multidisciplinary Center on Gerontology.

**University of Maryland**
**Division of Infectious Diseases**
*See:* Entry 11947

**University of Maryland**
**Lamy Center on Drug Therapy and Aging**
*See:* Entry 17394

**University of Miami**
**Center on Aging and Disabilities**
*See:* Entry 6909

**★ 3109 ★ University of Michigan**
**Biomechanics Research Laboratory (BRL)**
3216 G.G. Brown Bldg.
2350 Hayward St.
Ann Arbor, MI 48109-2125
**Phone:** (734)936-0366          **Fax:** (734)763-9332
**Email:** jaam@umich.edu
**Website:** http://www.engin.umich.edu/dept/meam/brl/
Dr. James A. Ashton-Miller, Dir.

**Activities/Fields:** How the brain coordinates and controls a myriad of muscles in human locomotion and how aging affects that control.

**★ 3110 ★ University of Michigan**
**Institute of Gerontology**
300 N Ingalls
Ann Arbor, MI 48109-2007
**Phone:** (734)764-3493          **Fax:** (734)936-2116
**Email:** brcarl@umich.edu
**Website:** http://www.IOG.umich.edu
Bruce M. Carlson, MD, Dir.

**Activities/Fields:** Gerontological research studies in the behavioral, biological, clinical, and social sciences and the humanities. **Pub:** *Annual Report.*

**★ 3111 ★ University of Nevada, Reno**
**Sanford Center for Aging**
Reno, NV 89557
**Phone:** (775)784-4774          **Fax:** (775)784-1814
**Email:** weisslj@unr.edu
**Website:** http://www.unr.edu/hcs/sanford/
Dr. Lawrence J. Weiss, Dir.

**Activities/Fields:** Aging, especially as it relates to health ecology, nutrition psychology, sociology, nursing, and medicine.

**★ 3112 ★ University of North Carolina at**
**    Greensboro**
**Institute for Health, Science, and Society**
**    (IHSS)**
PO Box 26170
Greensboro, NC 27402-6170
**Phone:** (336)334-4775          **Fax:** (336)334-4794
**Email:** health_institute@uncg.edu
**Website:** http://www.uncg.edu/ihs/
Jennifer Kimbrough, Asst. Dir.

**Activities/Fields:** Health and health care needs, especially child/adolescent health, obesity prevention, alcohol/tobacco prevention, genomic medicine. **Pub:** *Guilford County Health Trends 1991-1998.* • *Wellness Council Directory.*

**★ 3113 ★ University of North Texas**
**    Health Science Center at Fort Worth**
**Geriatrics Education and Research**
**    Institute (GERI)**
3500 Camp Bowie Blvd.
Fort Worth, TX 76107-2699
**Phone:** (817)735-0158          **Fax:** (817)735-0167
**Email:** tfairchi@hsc.unt.edu
**Website:** http://www.hsc.unt.edu/research/aging.cfm
Thomas J. Fairchild, PhD, Dir.

**Activities/Fields:** Biology of aging, including fundamental chemical and molecular biological changes that may cause aging; health promotion in older adults including health programs promoting physical, psychological, and social well being; geriatric care and practice including evaluation of new clinical programs, physical/mental functions, long term care system development focusing on case management, and in-home health screen/assessment of home-bound elderly. **Frmly:** Texas Institute for Research and Education on Aging.

**★ 3114 ★ University of Pennsylvania**
**Institute on Aging**
3615 Chestnut St.
Philadelphia, PA 19104-6006
**Phone:** (215)898-3163          **Fax:** (215)573-8684
**Email:** trojanow@mail.med.upenn.edu
**Website:** http://www.uphs.upenn.edu/~aging
John Q. Trojanowski, MD, Dir.

**Activities/Fields:** Biomedical and social science research on aging, including cellular mechanisms of aging, Alzheimer's disease, sleep disturbances, arthritis, osteoporosis, population demographics of aging, nursing home quality, organization and structure of life care communities, social security, and social support systems for the aged. **Pub:** *Newsletter*, quarterly. **Frmly:** Center for the Study of Aging.

**★ 3115 ★ University of Quebec at Trois-**
**    Rivieres**
**Departmental Laboratory of Gerontology**
PO Box 500
Trois-Rivieres, QC, Canada G9A 5H7
**Phone:** (819)376-5090          **Fax:** (819)376-5195
**Email:** micheline_dube@uqtr.uquebec.ca
**Website:** http://www.uqtr.uquebec.ca/psycho/gerontologie/
Micheline Dube, Dir.

**Activities/Fields:** Gerontology and the elderly, including personal goals, suicidal ideas and behavior, self-actualization and well-being, grief and bereavement, and prevention of osteoporosis, grand-parenthood and the AIDS epidemic.

**★ 3116 ★ University of South Florida**
**Institute on Aging**
13201 Bruce B. Downs Blvd., MDC-56
Tampa, FL 33612-3899
**Phone:** (813)974-9808          **Fax:** (813)974-7047
**Email:** nhallfor@hsc.usf.edu
**Website:** http://www.hsc.usf.edu/ioa/
James A. Mortimer, Dir.

**Activities/Fields:** Needs and knowledge of senior citizens, especially regarding Alzheimer's disease where researchers contribute to understanding the biological, epidemiological, clinical and social aspects of this illness.

**★ 3117 ★ University of Western Ontario**
**Dementia Study Group**
University Hospital
London, ON, Canada N6A 5C1
**Phone:** (519)663-3035
Harold Merskey, Dir.

**Activities/Fields:** Clinical, pathological, and neuro-chemical analyses of normal aging in the human nervous system and in organic senile dementias, especially Alzheimer's disease. Clinical trials.

**★ 3118 ★ USDA Human Nutrition**
**    Research Center on Aging**
Tufts University
711 Washington St.
Boston, MA 02111-1524
**Phone:** (617)556-3330          **Fax:** (617)556-3344
**Website:** http://www.hnrc.tufts.edu
Robert M. Russell, MD, Dir.

**Activities/Fields:** Investigates the relationship of nutrition to aging, including research programs in nutrient metabolism, nutrient requirements, nutritional epidemiology, functional systems, and drug-nutrient interactions. **Pub:** *HNRC Newsletter*, monthly.

**Veterans Affairs Medical Center**
**    (Birmingham, AL)**
**Research and Development Service**
*See:* Entry 17407

**Veterans Health Administration**
**Geriatric Research, Education and**
**    Clinical Center-Gainesville**
*See:* Entry 17408

**★ 3119 ★ Virginia Commonwealth**
**    University**
**Virginia Center on Aging**
Medical College of Virginia Campus
520 N 12th St., Rm. B-25
PO Box 980229
Richmond, VA 23298-0229
**Phone:** (434)828-1525          **Fax:** (434)828-7905
**Email:** eansello@nsc.vcu.edu
**Website:** http://views.vcu.edu/vcoa
Edward F. Ansello, PhD, Dir.

**Activities/Fields:** Mental and physical health of the elderly, focusing on community-living and health-related factors of aging. Studies include: eldercare responsibilities of employed family caregivers, inter-system cooperation in delivery of human services, impact of aging of adults with developmental disabilities, minority healthcare utilization, caregiving of demented elders, research and documentation project on rural geropharmacy. **Pub:** *AGE In Action Newsletter*, quarterly.


### ★ 3120 ★ Wake Forest University
### J. Paul Sticht Center on Aging and Rehabilitation
North Carolina Baptist Hospitals, Inc.
Medical Center Blvd.
Winston Salem, NC 27157
**Phone:** (336)713-8570          **Fax:** (336)713-8588
**Email:** mpahor@wfubmc.edu
**Website:** http://www.wfubmc.edu
Marco Pahor, MD, Dir.
**Activities/Fields:** Metabolic and biomedical research in aging and rehabilitation, focusing on physical disabilities and problems in the elderly.


**Washington University in St. Louis**
**Alzheimer's Disease Research Center**
*See:* Entry 14483


### ★ 3121 ★ Yeshiva University
### Resnick Gerontology Center
Bldg. R, Rm. 343
Albert Einstein College of Medicine
1165 Morris Park Ave.
Bronx, NY 10461
**Phone:** (718)430-3888          **Fax:** (718)430-3870
**Email:** adrc@neuro.wustl.edu
**Website:** http://www.adrc.wustl.edu
Richard B. Lipton, Dir.
**Activities/Fields:** Alzheimer's disease and other dementia. Conducts the Bronx Aging Study, a ten-year longitudinal study of the Bronx elderly. Also conducts a teaching nursing project, a biochemical research assessment program, and drug studies.


# State Government Agencies

## Aging

### ★ 3122 ★ Alabama Department of Senior Services
770 Washington Ave. RSA Plaza Ste. 470
Montgomery, AL 36130
**Phone:** (334)242-5743          **Free:** 877-425-2243
**Fax:** (334)242-5594
**Email:** ageline@adss.state.al.us
**Website:** http://www.adss.state.al.us/
Melissa Mauser Galvin, Director
**Frmly:** Alabama Commission on Aging.


### ★ 3123 ★ Alaska Department of Administration
### Division of Senior Services
### Alaska Commission on Aging
PO Box 110209
Juneau, AK 99811-0209
**Phone:** (907)465-3250          **Fax:** (907)465-4716
**Email:** bob_taylor@admin.state.ak.us
**Website:** http://www.alaskaaging.org/
Bob Taylor, PhD, Director


### ★ 3124 ★ American Samoa Territorial Administration on Aging
Government of American Samoa
Pago Pago, American Samoa 96799
**Phone:** (684)633-2207          **Fax:** (684)633-2533
**Website:** http://www.aoa.gov/aoa/pages/state.html
Fa'oalatia Siatu'u, Director


### ★ 3125 ★ Arizona Department of Economic Security
### Aging and Adult Administration
1789 W Jefferson St., Site Code 950A
Phoenix, AZ 85007
**Phone:** (602)542-4446          **Fax:** (602)542-6575
**Email:** askdesaaa@mail.de.state.az.us
**Website:** http://www.de.state.az.us/links/aaa/


### ★ 3126 ★ Arkansas Department of Human Services
### Division of Aging and Adult Services
1417 Donaghey Plaza South, 7th and Main Sts.
PO Box 1437, Slot S-530
Little Rock, AR 72203-1437
**Phone:** (501)682-2441          **Fax:** (501)682-8155
**Email:** herb.sanderson@mail.state.ar.us
**Website:** http://www.state.ar.us/dhs/aging/
Herb Sanderson, Director


### ★ 3127 ★ California Department of Aging
1600 K St.
Sacramento, CA 95814
**Phone:** (916)322-3887          **Fax:** (916)324-4989
**Email:** Webmaster@aging.ca.gov
**Website:** http://www.aging.state.ca.us/


### ★ 3128 ★ D.C. Office on Aging
441 4th St., NW, Ste. 900 South
Washington, DC 20001
**Phone:** (202)724-5622          **Fax:** (202)724-4979
**Website:** http://www.ftc.gov/bcp/conline/states/dc.htm


### ★ 3129 ★ Delaware Department of Health and Social Services
### Delaware Division of Services for Aging and Adults with Physical Disabilities
Admin. Bldg., First Floor Annex, 1901 N Dupont Hwy.
New Castle, DE 19720
**Phone:** (302)255-9390          **Free:** 800-223-9074
**Fax:** (302)255-4445
**Email:** dsaapdinfo@state.de.us
**Website:** http://www.dsaapd.com/index.htm
Carolee Burton Kunz, Director


### ★ 3130 ★ Department of Public Health & Social Services
### Division of Senior Citizens
PO Box 2816
Hagatna, GU 96932
**Phone:** (671)475-0263          **Fax:** (671)477-2930
**Email:** tommyt@mail.gov.gu
**Website:** http://www.dphss.govguam.net/dsc/srd/srdindex.htm
Dennis G. Rodriguez, Director


### ★ 3131 ★ Florida Department of Elder Affairs
4040 Esplanade Way
Tallahassee, FL 32399-7000
**Phone:** (850)414-2000          **Free:** 800-963-5337
**Fax:** (850)414-2002
**Email:** information@elderaffairs.org
**Website:** http://elderaffairs.state.fl.us/doea/ea.html
Terry F. White, Secretary


### ★ 3132 ★ Georgia Department of Human Resources
### Division of Aging Services
2 Peachtree St. NW, Ste. 9-385
Atlanta, GA 30303-3142
**Phone:** (404)657-5258          **Fax:** (404)657-5285
**Website:** http://www.state.ga.us/Departments/dhr/aging.html


### ★ 3133 ★ Hawaii Executive Office on Aging
250 S Hotel St., Rm 406
Honolulu, HI 96813-2831
**Phone:** (808)586-0100          **Fax:** (808)586-0185
**Email:** eoa@mail.health.state.hi.us
**Website:** http://www2.state.hi.us/eoa/
Marilyn R. Seely, Director


### ★ 3134 ★ Idaho Commission on Aging
3380 Americana Terrace, Ste. 120
Boise, ID 83706
**Phone:** (208)334-3833          **Free:** 877-471-2777
**Fax:** (208)334-3033
**Email:** senglesby@icoa.state.id.us
**Website:** http://www2.state.id.us/icoa
Y. Sue Englesby, Contact


### ★ 3135 ★ Illinois Department on Aging
421 E Capitol Ave., Ste. 100
Springfield, IL 62701
**Phone:** (217)785-3356          **Free:** 800-252-8966
**Fax:** (217)785-4477
**Email:** ilsenior@aging.state.il.us
**Website:** http://www.state.il.us/aging/
Margo E. Schreiber, Director
**Alt. Contact:** Chicago Office, 312-814-2630.


### ★ 3136 ★ Indiana Family and Social Services Administration
### Bureau of Aging & In-Home Services
PO Box 7083, MS-21
Indianapolis, IN 46207-7083
**Phone:** (317)232-7000          **Free:** 800-986-3505
**Fax:** (317)232-7867
**Email:** dlewers@fssa.state.in.us
**Website:**      http://www.in.gov/fssa/elderly/aging/index.html
Deborah Lewers, Contact


### ★ 3137 ★ Iowa Department of Elder Affairs
Clemens Bldg., 3rd Fl.
200 10th St.
Des Moines, IA 50309-3609
**Phone:** (515)242-3333          **Fax:** (515)242-3300
**Email:** Sherry.James@dea.state.ia.us
**Website:** http://www.state.ia.us/elderaffairs/
Mark A. Haverland, Director


### ★ 3138 ★ Kansas Department on Aging
New England Bldg.
503 S Kansas Ave.
Topeka, KS 66603-3404
**Phone:** (785)296-4986          **Free:** 800-432-3535
**Fax:** (785)296-0256
**Email:** wwwmail@aging.state.ks.us
**Website:** http://www.k4s.org/kdoa
Connie Hubbell, Director


### ★ 3139 ★ Kentucky Cabinet for Health Services
### Office of Aging Services
275 E Main St., 5-C
Frankfort, KY 40621
**Phone:** (502)564-6930          **Fax:** (502)564-4595
**Website:** http://chs.state.ky.us/aging/
Jerry Whitley, Director


### ★ 3140 ★ Maine Bureau of Elder and Adult Services
### Department of Human Services
11 State House Station
442 Civic Center Dr.
Augusta, ME 04333
**Phone:** (207)287-9200          **Free:** 800-262-2232
**Fax:** (207)287-9229
**Email:** webmaster.beas@state.me.us
**Website:** http://www.state.me.us/dhs/beas

**★ 3141 ★ Maryland Department of Aging**
301 W Preston St., Ste 1007
Baltimore, MD 21201
**Phone:** (410)767-1100      **Free:** 800-243-3425
**Fax:** (410)333-7943
**Email:** ptc@mail.ooa.state.md.us
**Website:** http://www.mdoa.state.md.us/
Sue Fryer Ward, Director

**★ 3142 ★ Michigan Office of Services to the Aging**
7109 West Saginaw, First Floor
PO Box 30676
Lansing, MI 48909-8176
**Phone:** (517)373-8230      **Fax:** (517)373-4092
**Website:** http://www.miseniors.net/
Lynn Alexander, Director

**★ 3143 ★ Minnesota Board on Aging**
444 Lafayette Rd. North
Saint Paul, MN 55155-3843
**Phone:** (651)296-2770      **Free:** 800-882-6262
**Fax:** (651)297-7855
**Email:** mba@state.mn.us
**Website:** http://www.mnaging.org/
Jim Varpness, Director

**★ 3144 ★ Missouri Department of Health and Senior Services**
PO Box 570
Jefferson City, MO 65102
**Phone:** (573)751-6400      **Free:** 800-235-5503
**Fax:** (573)751-6041
**Email:** info@dhss.state.mo.us
**Website:** http://www.dhss.state.mo.us/
Jerry Simon, Director

**★ 3145 ★ Montana Senior and Long Term Care Division**
**Department of Public Health & Human Services**
111 North Sanders, Rm. 210
Helena, MT 59604
**Phone:** (406)444-4077      **Free:** 800-332-2272
**Fax:** (406)444-7743
**Email:** mhanshew@state.mt.us
**Website:** http://www.dphhs.state.mt.us/sltc
Mike Hanshew, Director

**★ 3146 ★ Nebraska Health and Human Services**
**Division of Aging and Disability Services**
**State Unit on Aging**
PO Box 95044
301 Centennial Mall South, 5th Floor
Lincoln, NE 68509-5044
**Phone:** (402)471-4623      **Free:** 800-942-7830
**Fax:** (402)471-4619
**Email:** joann.weis@hhss.state.ne.us
**Website:** http://www.hhs.state.ne.us/ags/agsindex.htm
Joann Weis, Contact

**★ 3147 ★ Nevada Division for Aging Services**
3100 West Sahara Ave., Ste. 103
Las Vegas, NV 89102
**Phone:** (702)486-3545      **Fax:** (702)486-3572
**Email:** dasvegas@aging.state.nv.us
**Website:** http://www.nvaging.net/
Mary Liveratti, Director

**★ 3148 ★ New Hampshire Department of Health and Human Services**
**Division of Elderly and Adult Services**
129 Pleasant St.
Concord, NH 03301-3857
**Phone:** (603)271-4680      **Free:** 800-351-1888
**Fax:** (603)271-4643

**Website:** http://www.dhhs.state.nh.us/DHHS/DEAS/default.htm

**★ 3149 ★ New Jersey Division of Senior Affairs**
PO Box 807
Trenton, NJ 08625-0807
**Phone:** (609)943-3437      **Free:** 800-792-8820
**Fax:** (609)588-3601
**Website:** http://www.state.nj.us/health/senior/srafffair.htm
Nancy Day, Director

**★ 3150 ★ New Mexico State Agency on Aging**
228 E Palace Ave.
Santa Fe, NM 87501
**Phone:** (505)827-7640      **Free:** 800-432-2080
**Fax:** (505)827-7649
**Email:** nmaoa@state.nm.us
**Website:** http://www.nmaging.state.nm.us/
Michelle Lujan Grisham, Director

**★ 3151 ★ New York State Office for the Aging**
112 State St., Room 710
Albany, NY 12207-2069
**Phone:** (518)447-7179      **Free:** 800-342-9871
**Fax:** (518)447-7188
**Website:** http://aging.state.ny.us/index.htm
Patricia P. Pine, Ph.D, Director

**★ 3152 ★ North Carolina Division of Aging**
693 Palmer Dr.
2101 Mail Service Ctr.
Raleigh, NC 27699-2101
**Phone:** (919)733-3983      **Fax:** (919)733-0443
**Email:** karen.gottovi@ncmail.net
**Website:** http://www.dhhs.state.nc.us/aging/home.htm
Karen E. Gottovi, Director

**★ 3153 ★ North Dakota Department of Human Services**
**Aging Services Division**
600 S 2nd St., Ste. 1C
Bismarck, ND 58504-5729
**Phone:** (701)328-8910      **Free:** 800-451-8693
**Fax:** (701)328-8989
**Email:** dhsaging@state.nd.us
**Website:** http://lnotes.state.nd.us/dhs/dhsweb.nsf/ServicePages/AgingServices
Linda Wright, Director

**★ 3154 ★ Office of Adult and Veterans Services**
**Division of Aging and Adult Services**
1575 Sherman St., Ground Floor
Denver, CO 80203
**Phone:** (303)866-2800      **Fax:** (303)866-2696
**Email:** viola.mcneace@state.co.us
**Website:** http://www.cdhs.state.co.us/oss/aas/index1.html
Rita Barreras, Director

**★ 3155 ★ Ohio Department of Aging**
50 W Broad St., 9th Fl.
Columbus, OH 43215-3363
**Phone:** (614)466-5500      **Free:** 800-282-1206
**Fax:** (614)466-5741
**Email:** ODAMAIL@age.state.oh.us
**Website:** http://www.state.oh.us/age/
Joan W. Lawrence, Director

**★ 3156 ★ Oregon Department of Human Resources**
**Seniors & People with Disabilities Division**
500 Summer St. NE, EO2
Salem, OR 97301-1073
**Phone:** (503)945-5811      **Free:** 800-282-8096
**Fax:** (503)373-7823
**Email:** sdsd.info@state.or.us
**Website:** http://www.sdsd.hr.state.or.us/
Lydia Lissman, Director

**★ 3157 ★ Pennsylvania Department of Aging**
555 Walnut St., 5th Fl.
Harrisburg, PA 17101-1919
**Phone:** (717)783-1550      **Free:** 800-225-7223
**Fax:** (717)783-6842
**Email:** aging@state.pa.us
**Website:** http://www.aging.state.pa.us/
Larissa B. Johnson, Contact

**★ 3158 ★ Puerto Rico Governor's Office of Elderly Affairs**
PO Box 50063 Old San Juan Station
Call Box 50063
San Juan, PR 00902
**Phone:** (787)721-5710      **Fax:** (787)721-6510
**Email:** thooker@ban-gate.aoa.dhhs.gov
**Website:** http://www.aoa.dhhs.gov/RegionsI-II/stpr.htm
Ruby Rodriguez Ramirez, MHSA, Director

**★ 3159 ★ Rhode Island Department of Elderly Affairs**
160 Pine St.
Providence, RI 02903
**Phone:** (401)222-2858      **Fax:** (401)222-1490
**Email:** larry@dea.state.ri.us
**Website:** http://www.dea.state.ri.us/
Barbara Rayner, Director

**★ 3160 ★ South Carolina Department of Health and Human Services**
**Office of Senior and Long Term Care Service**
PO Box 8206
Columbia, SC 29202-8206
**Phone:** (803)898-2500      **Fax:** (803)898-4515
**Email:** adams@dhhs.state.sc.us
**Website:** http://www.dhhs.state.sc.us/offices/long_term_care/ltcindex.htm
Elizabeth M. Fuller, Director

**★ 3161 ★ South Dakota Department of Social Services**
**Office of Adult Services and Aging**
Richard F. Kneip Bldg.
700 Governors Dr.
Pierre, SD 57501-2291
**Phone:** (605)773-3656      **Free:** (866)854-5465
**Fax:** (605)773-6834
**Email:** asaging@dss.state.sd.us
**Website:** http://www.state.sd.us/social/ASA/index.htm
Gail Ferris, Dir of Admin

**★ 3162 ★ State of Connecticut**
**Department of Social Services**
**Elderly Services Division**
25 Sigourney St.
Hartford, CT 06106
**Phone:** (860)424-5233      **Free:** 800-443-9946
**Fax:** (860)424-4966
**Website:** http://www.ctelderlyservices.state.ct.us/
Christine M. Lewis, Director

**★ 3163 ★ Tennessee Commission on Aging & Disability**
Andrew Jackson Bldg.
500 Deaderick St., 9th Fl.
Nashville, TN 37243-0860
**Phone:** (615)741-2056          **Fax:** (615)741-3309
**Email:** ldunn5@mail.state.tn.us
**Website:** http://www.state.tn.us/comaging/
James S. Whaley, Director


**★ 3164 ★ Texas Department on Aging**
4900 N Lamar Blvd., 4th Fl.
PO Box 12786
Austin, TX 78711
**Phone:** (512)424-6840          **Fax:** (512)424-6890
**Email:** Mary.Sapp@tdoa.state.tx.us
**Website:** http://www.tdoa.state.tx.us/
Mary Sapp, Director


**★ 3165 ★ US Virgin Islands Department of Human Services**
**Senior Citizens Division**
Knud Hansen Complex, Bldg. A 1303
Hospital Ground
Saint Thomas, VI 00802
**Phone:** (340)774-0930          **Fax:** (340)774-3466
**Email:** humanservices@usvi.org
**Website:**      http://www.usvi.org/humanservices/index.html
Ms. Sedonie Halbert, Director


**★ 3166 ★ Utah Division of Aging and Adult Services**
120 N 200 West, Rm. 325
Salt Lake City, UT 84103
**Phone:** (801)538-3910          **Fax:** (801)538-4395
**Email:** DAAS@utah.gov
**Website:** http://www.hsdaas.state.ut.us/


**★ 3167 ★ Vermont Department of Aging and Disabilities**
Waterbury Complex
103 S Main St.
Waterbury, VT 05671-2301
**Phone:** (802)241-2400          **Fax:** (802)241-2325
**Email:** webmaster@dad.state.vt.us
**Website:** http://www.dad.state.vt.us
Patrick Flood, Director


**★ 3168 ★ Virginia Department for the Aging**
1600 Forest Ave., Ste. 102
Richmond, VA 23229
**Phone:** (804)662-9333          **Free:** 800-552-3402
**Fax:** (804)662-9354
**Email:** aging@vdh.state.va.us
**Website:** http://www.aging.state.va.us/
Jay W. DeBoer, J.D., Director


**★ 3169 ★ Washington Department of Social and Health Services**
**Aging and Adult Services Administration**
PO Box 45040
Olympia, WA 98504-5050
**Phone:** (360)725-2310          **Free:** 800-422-3263
**Fax:** (360)438-8633
**Email:** wongma@dshs.wa.gov
**Website:** http://www.aasa.dshs.wa.gov/
Kathy Leitch, Director


**★ 3170 ★ West Virginia Bureau of Senior Services**
Holly Grove, Bldg. 10
1900 Kanawha Blvd. E
Charleston, WV 25305-0160
**Phone:** (304)558-3317          **Fax:** (304)558-0004
**Email:** astottlemyer@boss.state.wv.us
**Website:** http://www.state.wv.us/seniorservices/
Ann M. Stottlemyer, Director


**★ 3171 ★ Wyoming Department of Health**
**Aging Division**
259B North Bldg.
6101 Yellowstone Rd.
Cheyenne, WY 82002
**Phone:** (307)777-7986          **Free:** 800-442-2766
**Fax:** (307)777-5340
**Email:** cnoon@state.wy.us
**Website:** http://wdhfs.state.wy.us/aging/index.htm
Colleen Noon, Contact

# Chapter 3
# Allergy & Immunology

## Federal Government Agencies

★ **3172** ★ **U.S. Department of Health and Human Services**
**Centers for Disease Control and Prevention**
**National Immunization Program Office**
1600 Clifton Rd. NE
Atlanta, GA 30333
**Phone:** (404)639-3311
**Website:** http://www.cdc.gov/nip/

★ **3173** ★ **U.S. Department of Health and Human Services**
**National Institutes of Health (NIH)**
**National Institute of Allergy and Infectious Diseases (NIAID)**
9000 Rockville Pike
Bethesda, MD 20892
**Phone:** (301)496-5717          **Fax:** (301)496-4409
**Website:** http://www.niaid.nih.gov/
Anthony S. Fauci, MD, Director
**Desc:** NIAID conducts and supports research, research training, and clinical evaluations on the causes, treatment and prevention of a wide variety of infectious, allergic, and immunologic diseases. Areas of special emphasis include AIDS; asthma and allergic diseases; immunologic diseases; transplantation; emerging and reemerging infectious diseases; sexually transmitted diseases; enteric diseases such as hepatitis; food-borne diseases; influenza and other respiratory infections; malaria and other parasitic diseases; and tuberculosis.

## Foundations & Other Funding Organizations

### Other Funding Organizations

★ **3174** ★ **American Academy of Allergy, Asthma and Immunology (AAAAI)**
611 E Wells St.
Milwaukee, WI 53202
**Phone:** (414)272-6071          **Fax:** (414)272-6070
**Email:** membership@aaaai.org
**Website:** http://www.aaaai.org
Audrey Mudek, Membership Service Mgr.
**Desc:** Professional society of physicians specializing in allergy and allergic diseases. Sponsors annual two-day postgraduate course and three-day scientific session. Conducts research and educational programs. Maintains speakers' bureau; operates placement service; compiles statistics. **Awards:** Grant (annual); recognition for research.

★ **3175** ★ **American Autoimmune Related Diseases Association**
22100 Gratiot Ave.
East Detroit, MI 48021-2227
**Phone:** (586)776-3900          **Free:** 800-598-4668
**Fax:** (810)776-3903
**Email:** aarda@aol.com
**Website:** http://www.aarda.org
Virginia Ladd, Exec. Dir.
**Desc:** Promotes national focus and collaborative efforts among state and national volunteer health groups on autoimmunity, the major cause of serious chronic diseases. Offers research and educational programs; maintains speakers' bureau. **Awards:** Grant for nonprofit organizations and foundations doing work on autoimmunity and basic autoimmunity research.

★ **3176** ★ **Asthma and Allergy Foundation of America (AAFA)**
1233 Twentieth St. NW, Ste. 402
Washington, DC 20036
**Phone:** (202)466-7643          **Free:** 800-7-ASTHMA
**Fax:** (202)466-8940
**Email:** info@aafa.org
**Website:** http://www.aafa.org
C. Ben Hadden, Pres.
**Desc:** Dedicated to finding a cure for and controlling asthma and allergic diseases. AAFA serves the estimated 50 million Americans with asthma and allergic diseases through the support of research, patient and public education programs, public and governmental advocacy, and a nationwide network of chapters and education/support groups. **Awards:** Investigator Grants (annual) researchers referred by NIH.

★ **3177** ★ **CFIDS Association of America**
PO Box 220398
Charlotte, NC 28222-0398
**Free:** 800-442-3437          **Fax:** (704)365-9755
**Email:** info@cfids.org
**Website:** http://www.cfids.org
Kim Kenney, Exec. Officer
**Desc:** Individuals with chronic fatigue and immune dysfunction syndrome (chronic viral illness associated with dysfunction of the immune system; formerly called chronic Epstein-Barr virus); doctors, nurses, and government officials. Advocates continued research into the cause and cure of the syndrome. Funds pilot medical research projects. **Awards:** Grant for research.

★ **3178** ★ **Clinical Immunology Society (CIS)**
611 E Wells St.
Milwaukee, WI 53202
**Phone:** (414)224-8095          **Fax:** (414)276-3349
**Email:** cis@execinc.com
**Website:** http://www.clinimmsoc.org
Ken Janowski, Assoc. Exec. Dir.
**Desc:** Investigators and clinicians concerned with immunologic diseases. Promotes research on: the causes and mechanisms of immunologic diseases; improved treatment, evaluation, and prevention of diseases related to immunity. Facilitates exchange of ideas and findings; fosters excellence in research and medical practice. Works to increase public awareness and knowledge of immunologically-mediated diseases. Conducts scientific, educational programs. **Awards:** CIS Science Recognition Award for New Investigators (annual) based on abstract submissions.

★ **3179** ★ **Immune Deficiency Foundation (IDF)**
40 W Chesapeake Ave., Ste. 308
Towson, MD 21204
**Phone:** (410)321-6647          **Free:** 800-296-4433
**Fax:** (410)321-9165
**Email:** idf@primaryimmune.org
**Website:** http://www.primaryimmune.org
Thomas L. Moran, Pres.
**Desc:** Immune deficiency patients, their families, and medical professionals. Promotes education and research in primary immune deficiency diseases. Holds medical symposia; bestows patient scholarship and research awards. **Awards:** Immune Deficiency Foundation Scholarship (annual) primary immune deficiency diagnosis; Novartis Fellowship (annual).

★ **3180** ★ **International Society for Neuroimmunomodulation**
c/o Craig C. Smith
National Institute of Health
36 Convent Dr., Rm. 1A23/MSC 4020
Bethesda, MD 20892-4020
**Phone:** (301)496-4561          **Fax:** (301)496-6095
**Email:** ccs@codon.nih.gov
**Website:** http://www.isnim.org
Craig C. Smith, Exec. Dir.
**Desc:** Professional society for scientists involved in interdisciplinary research in the molecular and cellular aspects of neurobiology, neuroendocrinology, immunology, and the behavioral sciences. Interests focus on discerning the integrative elements underlying communication and modulation between the central nervous, endocrine, and immune systems, and upon related disease states. **Awards:** Novera Herbert Spector Lectureship (annual) for significant contributions in both leadership and research to the field of Neuroimmunomodulation.

★ **3181** ★ **National Chronic Fatigue Syndrome and Fibromyalgia Association (NCFSFA)**
PO Box 18426
Kansas City, MO 64133
**Phone:** (816)313-2000          **Fax:** (816)524-6782
**Email:** information@ncfsfa.org
**Website:** http://www.ncfsfa.org
Orvalene Prewitt, Pres.
**Desc:** Individuals suffering from chronic fatigue syndrome and Fibromyalgia health care professionals. Chronic fatigue syndrome, also known as Chronic Epstein-Barr Virus syndrome, is characterized by persistent, recurring feelings of general weakness; other symptoms include sore throat, unexplained

muscle pain, new headaches, devastating fatigue, impaired memory or concentration, tender lymph nodes, unrefreshing sleep and post-exertion malaise. Fibromyalgia is characterized as pain, generally felt all over, and can be compounded by fatique, sleep disturbances, changes in mood, headaches and gastro-intestinal problems. Sponsors educational programs. Maintains speakers' bureau. **Awards:** Research Grant (annual).

### ★ 3182 ★ National Sjogren's Syndrome Association (NSSA)

PO Box 22066
Beachwood, OH 44122-0066
**Phone:** (216)292-3866　　　**Free:** 800-395-6772
**Fax:** (216)433-9838
**Email:** nickofohio@aol.com
**Website:** http://www.sjogrenssyndrome.org/
Barbara Henry, Exec. Dir.

**Desc:** Promotes public awareness of Sjogren's Syndrome; encourages research into the cause and cure of the disorder. (Sjogren's Syndrome is an autoimmune disorder characterized by dryness of all mucous membranes resulting from deficient secretion of the glands. Approximately 50% of Sjogren's Syndrome patients also have rheumatoid arthritis.) Sponsors chapters and offers information to the medical community. Conducts educational and research programs; maintains speakers' bureau. **Awards:** Fellow in Rheumatology (annual); Student of Ophotolomology (annual).

### ★ 3183 ★ World Allergy Organization (WAO)

611 E Wells St.
Milwaukee, WI 53202
**Phone:** (414)276-1791　　　**Fax:** (414)276-3349
**Email:** info@worldallergy.org
**Website:** http://www.worldallergy.org/
Gail Bast, Exec. Dir.

**Desc:** Umbrella organization for 59 international allergy association representing 27,000 health professionals. **Awards:** Lectureship Grant (annual) to hold a national scientific meeting.

# National & International Organizations

### Academy of Veterinary Allergy and Clinical Immunology (AVA)

*See:* Entry 20527

### ★ 3184 ★ Action Against Allergy (AAA)

PO Box 278
Twickenham
Middlesex
Twickenham TW1 4QQ, United Kingdom
**Phone:** 44 20 8922711　　　**Fax:** 44 20 8924950
**Email:** aaa@freeserve.co.uk
**Website:** http://www.avaci.org

**Fnded:** 1978. **Mem:** 1,200. **Lang(s):** English, French, German, Italian. **Desc:** Campaigns for diagnosis and treatment of allergies through the British national health service institutions and physicians. Provides information to chronic allergy sufferers. Coordinates medical reference center. **Pub:** *Allergy Newsletter*, 3/year. Newsletter. • Brochures, periodic. • Directory, periodic. Information on suppliers of additive-free and non-allergenic foods and materials.

### ★ 3185 ★ Albanian Association in Support of Asthma and Allergy Patients

c/o Aristo Uruci
Rr. Anastas Kullorioti 8/1
Tirana, Albania
**Phone:** 355 42 69200　　　**Fax:** 355 42 69200
**Email:** aasap@icc-al.org

**Desc:** Protects the interests of asthma and allergy patients. Conducts educational programs; offers medical advice to patients. **Pub:** Booklet.

### ★ 3186 ★ Allergy/Asthma Information Association (AAIA)

PO Box 100
Toronto, ON, Canada M9W 5K9
**Phone:** (416)679-9521　　　**Free:** 800-611-7011
**Fax:** (416)679-9524
**Email:** national@aaia.ca
**Website:** http://www.aaia.ca/aaia/index.htm

**Fnded:** 1964. **Mem:** 6,000. **Reg. Groups:** 5. **Local Groups:** 85. **Lang(s):** English, French. **Desc:** Seeks to develop societal awareness of the seriousness of allergic disease, including asthma, and to enable allergic individuals, their families, and caregivers to increase control over allergy symptoms. Provides leadership in information, education, and advocacy through partnership with healthcare professionals, businesses, industry, and government. Maintains speakers' bureau. **Pub:** *Awareness and Info Allergie*, quarterly. Magazine. Provides the latest medical finding and coping tips. Also publishes info-letters on allergies, asthma and oraphylaxis.

### Allergy and Asthma Network/Mothers of Asthmatics (AAN/MA)

*See:* Entry 5601

### ★ 3187 ★ Allergy Society of South Africa (ALLSA)

PO Box 88
Observatory 7935
Cape Town, Republic of South Africa
**Phone:** 27 21 44790919　　　**Fax:** 27 21 4480846
**Email:** aanma@aol.com
**Website:** http://www.aanma.org

**Desc:** Works to advance the practice of allergy and immunology. Fosters education and research.

### ★ 3188 ★ American Academy of Allergy, Asthma and Immunology (AAAAI)

611 E Wells St.
Milwaukee, WI 53202
**Phone:** (414)272-6071　　　**Fax:** (414)272-6070
**Email:** membership@aaaai.org
**Website:** http://www.aaaai.org
Audrey Mudek, Membership Service Mgr.

**Fnded:** 1943. **Mem:** 6,200. **Desc:** Professional society of physicians specializing in allergy and allergic diseases. Sponsors annual two-day postgraduate course and three-day scientific session. Conducts research and educational programs. Maintains speakers' bureau; operates placement service; compiles statistics. **Pub:** *American Academy of Allergy Asthma and Immunology–Abstract Book*, annual. Journal. Contains abstracts of papers presented at annual meeting. *Price:* $30/copy. • *American Academy of Allergy, Asthma and Immunology–Academy News*, bimonthly. Newspaper. *Price:* Included in membership dues. • *American Academy of Allergy, Asthma and Immunology–Membership Directory*, biennial. Membership Directory. *Price:* Included in membership dues; $200/copy for nonmembers. • *Journal of Allergy and Clinical Immunology*, monthly. Journal. *Price:* Included in membership dues. **Frmly:** (1982) American Academy of Allergy.

### ★ 3189 ★ American Academy of Otolaryngic Allergy Foundation (AAOA)

1990 M St. NW, Ste. 680
Washington, DC 20036
**Phone:** (202)955-5010　　　**Fax:** (202)955-5016
**Email:** aaoa@aaoaf.org
Jami Lucas, Exec. Dir.

**Fnded:** 1941. **Mem:** 2,300. **Desc:** Otolaryngologists who are interested in the study, research, and practice of otolaryngic allergy. Offers research fellowship in allergy related to the head and neck. Sponsors scientific meetings and continuing medical education

programs. **Pub:** *AAOA News*, quarterly. Newsletter. *Price:* Free. • Directory, annual. **Frmly:** American Society of Ophthalmologic and Otolaryngologic Allergy.

### ★ 3190 ★ American Allergy Association (AAA)

3104 E Camelback, Ste. 459
Phoenix, AZ 85016
**Fax:** (480)368-1238
**Email:** allergyaid@aol.com
Carol Rudoff, Pres.

**Fnded:** 1978. **Desc:** Allergy and asthma patients and their families, health care professionals, and others interested in problems created by foods, allergies, and asthma. Disseminates information on diet, environmental control, and other facets of allergy and asthma advice. **Pub:** *Allergy Products Directory*. Directory. Features 5 volumes practical information, publications, on-line listings, suppliers, resources, finding help, libraries, hotlines, and support groups. • *Asthma Resources Directory*. Directory. Contains listing of resources, companies, products, services, classes, support groups, mail order, and recipe books for asthma sufferers. • *Food Allergy Resources*. Directory. Lists resources, companies, recipe books, and mail order information for allergy sufferers. • *Guide to Gluten-Free Diets*. Handbook. • *Living With Allergies*, annual. Handbook. Includes articles on maintaining an allergen-free diet and enviroment, allergen-free recipes, book reviews, and pollen data. *Price:* $18. • Pamphlets.

### ★ 3191 ★ American Apitherapy Society (AAS)

5390 Grande Rd.
Hillsboro, OH 45133-9188
**Phone:** (937)364-1108　　　**Fax:** (937)364-9109
**Email:** aasoffice@in-touch.net
**Website:** http://www.apitherapy.org/
Linda Day, Contact

**Fnded:** 1989. **Mem:** 2,500. **Reg. Groups:** 9. **Desc:** Beekeepers, physicians, scientists, and others interested in apitherapy, the therapeutic use of honey bee products. Purpose is to collect and disseminate information in the field and to provide a forum for researchers to present the results of their work. Encourages investigation of hive products in order to provide a scientific foundation for their curative properties and use in human medicine. Seeks to prove the effectiveness of bee venom in treating inflammatory diseases such as arthritis and rheumatism. Gains funding for clinical laboratory studies through contributions. Supports selected research and fundraising projects for the investigation of apitherapeutic agents. Compiles statistics. **Pub:** *BeeWell Newsletter - Bee Informed*, quarterly. Newsletter. *Price:* Free with membership. • Brochures.Contains information on bee venom, honey, pollen, and beeswax. • Journal, annual. • Proceedings, annual. *Price:* Free. **Frmly:** (1989) North American Apio-Therapy Society.

### ★ 3192 ★ American Association of Certified Allergists (AACA)

85 W Algonquin Rd. Ste. 550
Arlington Heights, IL 60005
**Phone:** (847)427-8111　　　**Fax:** (847)427-1294
Richard Slawny, Exec. Dir.

**Fnded:** 1968. **Mem:** 510. **Desc:** Physicians specializing in allergy and clinical immunology. Objectives are to: improve expertise in allergy treatment; disseminate information pertaining to undergraduate and graduate education in allergology; promote improved standards for the practice and teaching of allergy; exchange information between physicians facing similar problems under different circumstances. **Pub:** Newsletter, 3/year. *Price:* Included in membership dues.

### ★ 3193 ★ American Association of Immunologists (AAI)

9650 Rockville Pike
Bethesda, MD 20814-3994

**Phone:** (301)530-7178 **Fax:** (301)571-1816
**Email:** infoaai@aai.faseb.org
**Website:** http://mercury.faseb.org/aai/default.asp
M. Michele Hogan, PhD, Contact
**Fnded:** 1913. **Mem:** 5,500. **Desc:** Scientists engaged in immunological research including aspects of virology, bacteriology, biochemistry, genetics, and related disciplines. Goals are to advance knowledge of immunology and related disciplines and to facilitate the interchange of information among investigators in various fields. Promotes interaction between laboratory investigators and clinicians. Conducts training courses, symposia, workshop, and lectures. Compiles statistics. **Pub:** *AAI Newsletter*, bimonthly. Newsletter. • *Journal of Immunology*, semimonthly. Journal. Reports on original research efforts on cellular immunology; clinical immunology and immunopathology; cytokines, mediators, and regulatory molecules. *Price:* Included in membership dues; $200 for nonmembers in USA.

**American Autoimmune Related Diseases Association**
*See:* Entry 13540

**★ 3194 ★ American Board of Allergy and Immunology (ABAI)**
510 Walnut, Ste. 1701
Philadelphia, PA 19106-3699
**Phone:** (215)592-9466 **Fax:** (215)592-9411
**Email:** abai@abai.org
**Website:** http://www.abai.org
John W. Yunginger, Jr., Exec. Sec.
**Fnded:** 1971. **Mem:** 4,859. **Desc:** Examining and credentialing body whose primary function is to establish qualifications and examine physician candidates who meet the requirements for training and experience and grant certification to those who pass the examination. Does not recommend specialists and cannot offer advice on individual allergic or immunologic problems. Member board of the American Board of Medical Specialties and conjoint board of the American Board of Internal Medicine and the American Board of Pediatrics. **Pub:** *Policies and Procedures*, biennial.

**★ 3195 ★ American College of Allergy, Asthma and Immunology (ACAAI)**
85 W Algonquin Rd., Ste. 550
Arlington Heights, IL 60005-4425
**Phone:** (847)427-1200 **Fax:** (847)427-1294
**Email:** mail@acaai.org
**Website:** http://www.allergy.mcg.edu
James R. Slawny, Exec. Dir.
**Fnded:** 1942. **Mem:** 3,900. **Desc:** Practicing allergists, educators, researchers, and clinical immunologists united to: encourage the study, improve the practice, and advance the cause of clinical immunology and allergy; promote association of and highest possible standards among medical scientists and physicians specializing in clinical immunology and in research, teaching, and treatment of allergy; promote dissemination of information regarding clinical immunology and allergy. Maintains a special program for allergy assistants such as nurses, technologists, and clinic aides of lectures, conferences, seminars, participatory workshops, peer-group discussions, poster programs, and technical and scientific exhibits. **Pub:** *ACAAI News*, bimonthly. Newsletter. • *Annals of Allergy, Asthma and Immunology*, 12/year. Journal. Includes original articles by experts in the field, abstracts, reviews, and editorials. *Price:* $50/year for individuals; $75/year for institutions; $78/year outside the U.S. • Membership Directory, biennial. **Frmly:** (1996) American College of Allergy and Immunology.

**★ 3196 ★ American In-Vitro Allergy/ Immunology Society**
PO Box 341461
Bethesda, MD 20827-1461
**Phone:** (301)263-0703 **Fax:** (301)263-0776
**Email:** aiais@erols.com

**Website:** http://www.invitroallergy.org
Barbara Buchman, Admin.
**Fnded:** 1988. **Mem:** 210. **Desc:** Physicians, scientists, and other health professionals who study or use in-vitro technology in the diagnosis and treatment of allergic and immunologic disorders; individuals engaged in activities related to the treatment of allergies or the advancement of immunological science. Promotes the appropriate use of in-vitro procedures in allergy and immunology; explores and refines allergy and immunology in-vitro techniques; fosters research in and development of in-vitro procedures that enhance the diagnosis and management of allergy or immune dysfunction. Acts as forum on information regarding new scientific information, research, and application of in-vitro techniques in allergy and immunology practice; represents members in professional and public relations; operates physician referral service. Offers services in third party payer negotiation and in-vitro testing standardization. Conducts continuing medical education. **Pub:** Brochure. • Newsletter, quarterly.

**★ 3197 ★ American Society for Histocompatibility and Immunogenetics (ASHI)**
1700 Commerce Pky., Ste. C
Mount Laurel, NJ 08054
**Phone:** (856)638-0428 **Fax:** (856)439-0525
**Email:** lmorrisey@ashi-hla.org
**Website:** http://www.ashi-hla.org
Len Morrissey, Exec. Dir.
**Fnded:** 1968. **Mem:** 1,000. **Desc:** Scientists, physicians, and technologists involved in research and clinical activities related to histocompatibility testing (a state of mutual tolerance that allows some tissues to be grafted effectively to others). Conducts proficiency testing and educational programs. Maintains liaison with regulatory agencies; offers placement services and laboratory accreditation. Has co-sponsored development of histocompatability specialist and laboratory certification program. **Pub:** *ASHI Quarterly*, quarterly. Includes calendar of events, employment listings, certification data, and notices of awards. *Price:* Included in membership dues; $30/year for nonmembers. • *Human Immunology*, monthly. Journal. • *Laboratory Procedures Manual*. Manual. Covers laboratory procedures. • Membership Directory. • Papers. • Proceedings. **Frmly:** American Association for Clinical Histocompatibility Testing.

**★ 3198 ★ Arthritis and Research Campaign**
Copeman House
St. Mary's Court
St. Mary's Gate
Chesterfield S41 7TD, United Kingdom
**Phone:** 44 1246 558033 **Fax:** 44 1246 558007
**Email:** info@arc.org.uk
**Website:** http://www.arc.org.uk
**Fnded:** 1936. **Mem:** 40,000. **Desc:** Voluntary helpers, donators and support staff. Conducts research and education to find the cause of rheumatic disease. In pursuit of these objectives mounts a wide ranging research program involving people, projects and centers - usually at university medical schools. Currently running at over 15 million pounds per year. The income raised to meet this commitment comes entirely from voluntary donations. **Pub:** *Arthritis Today*, 3/year. Booklets. • Booklets. **Frmly:** Arthritis and Rheumatism Council for Research.

**★ 3199 ★ Association of Latin Languages Allergologists and Immunologists (LLSA) (Groupement des Allergologistes et Immunologistes de Langues Latines — GAILL)**
c/o CAIC
Rua Sampaio e Pina 16-4
P-1070 Lisbon, Portugal
**Phone:** 351 1 3874201 **Fax:** 351 1 3858202

**Fnded:** 1969. **Mem:** 300. **Reg. Groups:** 8. **Lang(s):** English, French, Italian, Portuguese, Spanish. **Desc:** Latin-language-speaking medical doctors and holders of doctoral and master's degrees in 14 countries. Promotes and disseminates information on allergic and immunologic diseases. Facilitates personal contacts between scientists. Sponsors charitable program. Provides research and travel grants. Operates speakers' bureau and placement service. **Pub:** *Allergie et Immunologie*, quarterly. Journal. • *Cadernos Luso-Brasileiros de Alergia e Imunologia*, quarterly. Journal. • *GAILL Directory*, annual. Directory.

**★ 3200 ★ Asthma and Allergy Foundation of America (AAFA)**
1233 Twentieth St. NW, Ste. 402
Washington, DC 20036
**Phone:** (202)466-7643 **Free:** 800-7-ASTHMA
**Fax:** (202)466-8940
**Email:** info@aafa.org
**Website:** http://www.aafa.org
C. Ben Hadden, Pres.
**Fnded:** 1953. **Reg. Groups:** 12. **Desc:** Dedicated to finding a cure for and controlling asthma and allergic diseases. AAFA serves the estimated 50 million Americans with asthma and allergic diseases through the support of research, patient and public education programs, public and governmental advocacy, and a nationwide network of chapters and education/support groups. **Pub:** *ADVANCE*, bimonthly. Newsletter. • Also publishes educational pamphlets. **Frmly:** (1957) American Foundation for Allergic Diseases; (1978) Allergy Foundation of America.

**Asthma Society of Ireland (ASI)**
*See:* Entry 18736

**★ 3201 ★ Bath Institute for Rheumatic Diseases**
Trim Bridge
Bath BA1 1HD, United Kingdom
**Phone:** 44 1225 448444 **Fax:** 44 1225 336809
**Email:** asthma@indigo.ie
**Website:** http://www.asthmasociety.ie
**Desc:** Promotes the study of rheumatic diseases.

**Body Positive**
*See:* Entry 11745

**★ 3202 ★ British Society for Immunology**
Triangle House
Broomhill Rd.
London SW18 4HX, United Kingdom
**Phone:** 44 208 8752400 **Fax:** 44 181 8752424
**Email:** bsi@immunology.org
**Website:** http://immunology.org
**Fnded:** 1956. **Mem:** 4,000. **Reg. Groups:** 18. **Lang(s):** English. **Desc:** Immunologists. To advance the science of immunology for the benefit of the public. **Pub:** *Clinical & Experimental Immunology*, monthly. Journal. • *Immunology*, monthly. Journal. • *Immunology News*, bimonthly. Newsletter.

**★ 3203 ★ British Society for Rheumatology**
41 Eagle St.
London WC1R 4TL, United Kingdom
**Phone:** 44 207 2423313 **Fax:** 44 207 2423277
**Email:** bsr@rheumatology.org.uk
**Website:** http://www.rheumatology.org.uk
**Fnded:** 1984. **Mem:** 1,500. **Lang(s):** English. **Desc:** Hospital doctors, non-clinical scientists, general practitioners, other professions allied to medicine. Promotes the treatment and prevention of rheumatic diseases, education and research. **Pub:** *Rheumatology*, monthly. Journal.

### ★ 3204 ★ Bulgarian Society for Immunology of Reproduction (IBIR-BAN)

73, Tzangradsko Shosse
BG-1113 Sofia, Bulgaria
**Phone:** 359 2 722386　　　**Fax:** 359 2 720022
**Fnded:** 1989. **Mem:** 32. **Desc:** Conducts research in reproduction immunology.

### ★ 3205 ★ Canadian Society of Allergy and Clinical Immunology (CSACI)

774 Echo Dr.
Ottawa, ON, Canada K1S 5N8
**Phone:** (613)730-6272　　　**Fax:** (613)730-1116
**Email:** csaci@rcpsc.edu
**Website:** http://csaci.medical.org
**Fnded:** 1945. **Lang(s):** English, French. **Desc:** Allergists, immunologists, and others with an interest in the diagnosis and treatment of allergic and immunological disorders. Seeks to advance the understanding and treatment of allergic and immunological diseases. Conducts continuing professional education courses; sponsors research. **Pub:** *Canadian Journal Allergy and Clinical Immunology*, periodic. Journal. • Newsletter, periodic.

### ★ 3206 ★ Canadian Society for Immunology (CSI)

### (Societe Canadienne d'Immunologie — SCI)

795 McDermot Ave.
Winnipeg, MB, Canada R3E 0W3
**Phone:** (204)789-3316　　　**Fax:** (204)789-3921
**Email:** michael.ratcliffe@utoronto.ca
**Website:** http://www.csi.ucalgary.ca
**Fnded:** 1980. **Mem:** 300. **Lang(s):** English, French. **Desc:** Immunologists and other health care professionals and scientists with an interest in immunology. Seeks to advance immunological study, research, and practice. Promotes ongoing professional development of members. Serves as a network linking members; sponsors research and educational programs.

### Cancer Federation (CFI)
*See:* Entry 10144

### CDC National Prevention Information Network (NPIN)
*See:* Entry 11754

### ★ 3207 ★ Clinical Immunology Society (CIS)

611 E Wells St.
Milwaukee, WI 53202
**Phone:** (414)224-8095　　　**Fax:** (414)276-3349
**Email:** cis@execinc.com
**Website:** http://www.clinimmsoc.org
Ken Janowski, Assoc. Exec. Dir.
**Fnded:** 1986. **Mem:** 840. **Desc:** Investigators and clinicians concerned with immunologic diseases. Promotes research on: the causes and mechanisms of immunologic diseases; improved treatment, evaluation, and prevention of diseases related to immunity. Facilitates exchange of ideas and findings; fosters excellence in research and medical practice. Works to increase public awareness and knowledge of immunologically-mediated diseases. Conducts scientific, educational programs. **Pub:** *Clinical Immunology*, monthly. Journal. *Price:* Included with membership. • *Immunology News*, quarterly. Newsletter. Includes brief highlights of activities within the society, such as, meeting activities, a letter from the president and a listing of new members. *Price:* Free. For members only.

### ★ 3208 ★ EFA

c/o Susana Palkonen
Allergia-ja Astnaliito
Pacuiksenkatu 19
FIN-00270 Helsinki, Finland
**Phone:** 358 9 47335303　　　**Fax:** 358 9 47335390
**Email:** susanna.palkonen@allergia.com
**Fnded:** 1991. **Desc:** Represents the interests of allergy patients in Europe.

### ★ 3209 ★ European Academy of Allergology and Clinical Immunology (EAACI)

### (Academie Europeenne d'Allergologie et d'Immunologie Clinique)

c/o Dr. Frew
Southhampton General Hospital
Tremona Rd.
Southampton SO16 6YD, United Kingdom
**Phone:** 44 23 80794069　　　**Fax:** 44 23 80777996
**Email:** a.j.frew@soton.ac.uk
**Website:** http://www.eaaci.org
**Fnded:** 1950. **Mem:** 3,000. **Nat'l Groups:** 38. **Lang(s):** English, French, German. **Desc:** Medical doctors in 38 countries. Facilitates the exchange of ideas and information in the field of allergy and clinical immunology; assists and promotes international initiatives among European workers in related fields. Conducts training courses. **Pub:** *Allergy - The European Journal of Allergy and Clinical Immunology*, bimonthly. Journal.

### ★ 3210 ★ European Federation for Immunogenetics (EFI)

c/o Department of Immunohematology and Blood Transfusion
Leiden University Medical Centre
Bldg. 1 E3-Q
PO Box 9600
NL-2300 RC Leiden, Netherlands
**Email:** ihbsecr@euronet.nl
**Fnded:** 1985. **Mem:** 630. **Desc:** Individuals working in the field of immunogentics, histocompatibility testing, and transplantation. Seeks to advance the development of immunogenetics in Europe. Fosters the organization and and use of immunogenitic and histocompability databases. Provides a forum for the exchange of scientific information. **Pub:** Newsletter, quarterly.

### ★ 3211 ★ European Federation of Immunological Societies (EFIS)

c/o Anna Erdei, Sec.Gen.
Department of Immunology
Eotvos Lorand University
1/C Pazmany S
H-1117 Budapest, Hungary
**Phone:** 36 1 3812175　　　**Fax:** 36 1 3812176
**Email:** anna.erdei@freemail.hu
**Website:** http://www.efis.org
**Fnded:** 1975. **Mem:** 16,000. **Nat'l Groups:** 25. **Desc:** Immunological societies from around the world focusing on Europe. Promotes the advancement of research and education in immunology.

### ★ 3212 ★ European Society for Immunodeficiencies (ESID)

c/o Dr. Bert Gerritsen
St. Clara Hospital
Olympiaweg 350
NL-3078 HT Rotterdam, Netherlands
**Phone:** 31 10 2911911　　　**Fax:** 31 10 2911026
**Email:** gerritsene@clarazhs.nl
**Fnded:** 1983. **Desc:** Facilitates the exchange of immunological information among doctors, nurses, biomedical investigators, patients, and other individuals interested in immunodeficiency diseases. Fosters excellence in research and medical practice.

### ★ 3213 ★ European Society of Paediatric Allergy and Clinical Immunology

University Children's Hosptial
Augustenburger Platz 1
D-13353 Berlin, Germany
**Phone:** 49 30 45066643　　　**Fax:** 49 30 45066931
**Email:** brigitte.michel@charite.de
**Website:** http://www.espaci.de
**Fnded:** 1988. **Desc:** Aims to promote the development of pediatric allergy and immunology by several means.

### ★ 3214 ★ European Society of Reproductive and Development Immunology (ESRADI)

c/o Dr. M. Kurpisz
General Institute of Human Genetics
Polish Academy of Sciences
Strzeszynska 32
PL-60-479 Poznan, Poland
**Fax:** 48 61 8233235
**Desc:** Promotes fundamental and applied research concerning immunological processes in reproductive and developmental physiology and morphology, pathology and therapeutics. Fosters cooperation between laboratories involved in experimental and clinical research. Facilitates the exchange of research workers and training of students.

### Evans Syndrome Research and Support Group
*See:* Entry 13590

### ★ 3215 ★ Federation of Hungarian Associations for Asthmatic and Allergic Patients (ABOSZ)

Szoboszia u. 2-4
H-1126 Budapest, Hungary
**Phone:** 36 1 3551049　　　**Fax:** 36 1 3551049
**Email:** lnalou@aol.com
**Website:** http://www.legalnurseassociates.com
**Fnded:** 1995. **Mem:** 24. **Desc:** Works to improve early identification and awareness of asthma and allergies. Seeks to improve living conditions and treatment for members and nonmembers. Disseminates information.

### ★ 3216 ★ Federation of Immunological Societies of Asia-Oceania (FIMSA)

Ansari Nagar
New Delhi 110 029, India
**Phone:** 91 11 6967588　　　**Fax:** 91 11 6862663
**Email:** nkmehra@medinst.ernet.in
**Fnded:** 1992. **Desc:** Facilitates exchange of scientific information and personnel, organizes workshops and conferences.

### ★ 3217 ★ Food Allergy and Anaphylaxis Network

10400 Eaton Pl., Ste. 107
Fairfax, VA 22030-2208
**Phone:** (703)691-3179　　　**Free:** 800-929-4040
**Fax:** (703)691-2713
**Email:** faan@foodallergy.org
**Website:** http://www.foodallergy.org
**Fnded:** 1991. **Mem:** 25,000. **Desc:** Individuals with food allergies; health care professionals with an interest in allergology. Seeks to increase public awareness of food allergies and their treatment. "Works with government agencies, health professionals, food manufacturers, restaurant associations, and schools to educate them about the needs of food allergic individuals." **Pub:** *Food Allergy News*, bimonthly. Newsletter. • *Food Allergy News for Kids*, periodic. Newsletter. **Frmly:** (2001) Food Allergy Network.

### Gay Men's Health Crisis (GMHC)
*See:* Entry 11774

### Health Education Resource Organization (HERO)
*See:* Entry 12084

**★ 3218 ★ Hungarian Society of Allergology and Clinical Immunology**
c/o National Institute Rheumatology
PO Box 54
H-1525 Budapest, Hungary
**Phone:** 36 1 3350915 **Fax:** 36 1 3350915
**Email:** nekamker.allergy@mail.datanet.hu
**Website:** http://www.gmhc.org
**Fnded:** 1989. **Mem:** 400. **Lang(s):** English, German. **Desc:** Incorporates all health providers interested and active in diagnosis, therapy, prevention, epidemiology, rehabilitation, under- and post-graduate education, national and international basic and clinical research in the field of allergology and clinical immunology. **Pub:** *Nutrition - Allergy - Diet*, bimonthly. Journal.

**★ 3219 ★ Immune Deficiency Foundation (IDF)**
40 W Chesapeake Ave., Ste. 308
Towson, MD 21204
**Phone:** (410)321-6647 **Free:** 800-296-4433
**Fax:** (410)321-9165
**Email:** idf@primaryimmune.org
**Website:** http://www.primaryimmune.org
Thomas L. Moran, Pres.
**Fnded:** 1980. **Mem:** 11,500. **State Groups:** 19. **Local Groups:** 14. **Desc:** Immune deficiency patients, their families, and medical professionals. Promotes education and research in primary immune deficiency diseases. Holds medical symposia; bestows patient scholarship and research awards. **Pub:** *Guide for Nurses.* • *IDF Newsletter*, quarterly. Newsletter. Contains announcements of patient scholarship and research awards. Includes health insurance information and calendar of events. *Price:* Free. • *Our Immune System.* • *Patient and Family Handbook.* • *Primer for Physicians.*

**International Association of Asthmology (INTERASMA)**
**(Asociacion Internacional de Asmología — INTERASMA)**
*See:* Entry 18745

**International Cytokine Societies (ICS)**
*See:* Entry 10190

**★ 3220 ★ International Society for Immunology of Reproduction (ISIR)**
c/o JNU Campus
Shahid Jeet Sing Marg
New Delhi 110067, India
**Phone:** 91 11 6184446 **Fax:** 91 11 6184447
**Email:** talwar@icgebnd.erner.in
**Website:** http://www.asmanet.com/interasma.html
**Fnded:** 1976. **Mem:** 250. **Reg. Groups:** 12. **Lang(s):** English. **Desc:** Scientists and physicians interested in the immunological processes involved in all aspects of reproduction. Seeks to encourage and develop research on immunological processes through scientific publications, workshops, and colloquia. **Pub:** *American Journal of Reproductive Immunology.* Journal. • *ISIR Newsletter*, semiannual. Newsletter. Provides minutes of meetings, notices of upcoming meetings, and general news updates. • *Journal of Reproductive Immunology.* Journal.

**★ 3221 ★ International Union of Immunological Societies (IUIS)**
c/o Dr. Fritz Melchers
Basel Institute for Immunology
Postfach
Grenzacherstrasse 487
CH-4005 Basel, Switzerland
**Phone:** 41 61 6051237 **Fax:** 41 61 6051300
**Email:** iuispres@bii.ch
**Website:** http://www.qimr.edu.au/iuis/
**Fnded:** 1969. **Mem:** 53. **Reg. Groups:** 4. **Lang(s):** English. **Desc:** National professional societies of basic and applied immunologists. Encourages the orderly development and utilization of the science of immunol-

ogy. Promotes the application of new developments to clinical and veterinary problems and standardizes reagents and nomenclature. Conducts educational symposia and scientific meetings. **Pub:** *The Immunologist*, bimonthly. Journal.

**★ 3222 ★ Joint Council of Allergy, Asthma and Immunology (JCAAI)**
50 N Brockway, Ste. 3-3
Palatine, IL 60067
**Phone:** (847)934-1918 **Fax:** (847)934-1820
**Email:** info@caai.org
**Website:** http://www.jcaai.org
David F. Graft, MD, Pres.
**Fnded:** 1975. **Mem:** 2,350. **Desc:** Physicians specializing in allergy or clinical immunology. Members must belong to the American Academy of Allergy and Immunology or the American College of Allergy and Immunology. Serves as political and socioeconomic arm for these sponsoring organizations. **Pub:** *JCAAI Reports*, periodic. Newsletter. **Frmly:** (1977) Joint Council of Socio-Economics of Allergy.

**Names Project Foundation (NPF)**
*See:* Entry 11804

**★ 3223 ★ National Coalition for Adult Immunization (NCAI)**
4733 Bethesda Ave., Ste. 750
Bethesda, MD 20814-5228
**Phone:** (301)656-0003 **Fax:** (301)907-0878
**Email:** ncai@nfid.org
**Website:** http://www.nfid.org/ncai
David A. Neumann, PhD, Dir.
**Fnded:** 1988. **Mem:** 126. **Desc:** Medical associations, advocacy groups, vaccine manufacturers and government health agencies. Dedicated to promoting adolescent and adult immunization and to raise immunization levels in high-risk and other target groups. Promotes and supports National Adult Immunization Awareness Week and the objectives of the U.S. Healthy People 2010 initiative. Educates physicians and public on vaccines for diptheria, hepatitis A and B, influenza, measles, mumps, pneumococcal pneumonia, rubella (German measles), tetanus, and chickenpox. **Pub:** *National Adult Immunization Awareness Week Campaign Kit*, annual. • *Resource Guide for Adolescent and Adult Immunization*, semiannual.

**★ 3224 ★ National Foundation for the Chemically Hypersensitive (NFCH)**
4407 Swinson Rd.
Rhodes, MI 48652
**Phone:** (517)689-6369 **Fax:** (517)689-6877
**Email:** fred-nelson@mcsrelief.com
**Website:** http://www.mcsrelief.com
Fred Nelson, Dir.
**Fnded:** 1986. **Mem:** 16,000. **Reg. Groups:** 40. **State Groups:** 40. **Desc:** Individuals suffering from chemical hypersensitivity, their families, and friends; health care professionals; interested others. Promotes public awareness of chemical hypersensitivity disorders, such as multiple chemical sensitivities, environmental illness, food intolerance, total allergy syndrome, candida, and chronic fatigue. Disseminates information on symptoms of chemical hypersensitivity and the potential sources of exposure to the toxic substances that can result in hypersensitivity. Facilitates networking among those afflicted with chemical hypersensitivity. Compiles case histories and statistics; conducts research and educational programs; operates health care and legal referral services. Provides assistance in handling Social Security and worker's compensation claims and locating low-cost housing resources. Maintains speakers' bureau.

**National Jewish Medical and Research Center**
*See:* Entry 18753

**★ 3225 ★ National Pemphigus Foundation**
Atrium Plz., Ste. 203
828 San Pablo Ave.
Albany, CA 94706
**Phone:** (510)527-4970
**Email:** pvnews@aol.com
**Website:** http://www.pemphigus.org
Jean B. Barish, Esq., Pres.
**Desc:** People living with pemphigus and their families, friends, and the general public. Information forum for medical community and general public, provides general support and counseling for those in need, raises funds for research. **Pub:** Newsletter, quarterly. *Price:* $50.

**★ 3226 ★ National Sjogren's Syndrome Association (NSSA)**
PO Box 22066
Beachwood, OH 44122-0066
**Phone:** (216)292-3866 **Free:** 800-395-6772
**Fax:** (602)433-9838
**Email:** nickofohio@aol.com
**Website:** http://www.sjogrenssyndrome.org/
Barbara Henry, Exec. Dir.
**Fnded:** 1990. **Mem:** 4,500. **Desc:** Promotes public awareness of Sjogren's Syndrome; encourages research into the cause and cure of the disorder. (Sjogren's Syndrome is an autoimmune disorder characterized by dryness of all mucous membranes resulting from deficient secretion of the glands. Approximately 50% of Sjogren's Syndrome patients also have rheumatoid arthritis.) Sponsors chapters and offers information to the medical community. Conducts educational and research programs; maintains speakers' bureau. **Pub:** *Learning to Live with Sjogren's Syndrome*. Video. *Price:* $25. • *Patient Education Series*, quarterly. • *Sjogren's Digest*, quarterly. Newsletter. *Price:* Included in membership dues.

**★ 3227 ★ National Society for Research into Allergy**
PO Box 45
Hinckley LE10 1JY, United Kingdom
**Phone:** 44 1455 851546 **Fax:** 44 1455 851546
**Email:** nsra.allergy@virgin.net
**Fnded:** 1980. **Mem:** 1,000. **Desc:** Main aim is to educate the populace on the devastating effects of allergy/intolerance and to see effective treatment in all teaching hospitals.

**National Vaccine Information Center**
*See:* Entry 5734

**★ 3228 ★ Nightingale Research Foundation (NRF)**
c/o Dr. Byron Hyde, Chair
121 Iona St.
Ottawa, ON, Canada K1Y 3M1
**Phone:** (613)523-1958
**Email:** nightingale@nightingale.ca
**Website:** http://www.nightingale.ca/index.shtml
**Fnded:** 1988. **Mem:** 8,000. **Lang(s):** English, French. **Desc:** Individuals with Myalgic Encephalomyelitis (Chronic Fatigue Syndrome); health care providers and medical researchers with an interest in non-HIV acquired immune deficiency syndromes. Seeks to advance scientific knowledge of the causes of non-HIV immune deficiency syndromes, and to develop more effective treatments for these diseases. Conducts research and educational programs for the public, health care professionals, and medical researchers; sponsors fundraising activities. **Pub:** *Nightingale*, annual. Newsletter. • Booklets. • Brochure.

**★ 3229 ★ Norwegian Immune Deficiency Foundation (NIDF)**
**(Norsk Immunsviktforening — NI)**
c/o Eva Brox
Borgundveien 478
N-6015 Alesund, Norway

**Phone:** 47 70 146565　　**Fax:** 47 70 146566
**Email:** evabrox@online.no
**Website:** http://immunsvikt.no
**Fnded:** 1983. **Mem:** 120. **Nat'l Groups:** 1. **Lang(s):** Norwegian. **Desc:** Persons with primary immunological disorders and their families; private companies. Acts as support group. Disseminates information. **Pub:** *Immunsvikt hos Voksne og Barn,* periodic. • *Primary Antibody Deficiency and Self-Administration Home Therapy with s.c. immunoglobulin..* Video.

### ★ 3230 ★ Pan-American Allergy Society (PAAS)

PO Box 947
Fredericksburg, TX 78624
**Phone:** (830)997-9853　　**Fax:** (830)997-8625
**Email:** info@paas.org
**Website:** http://www.paas.org
Ann Brey, Exec. Sec.
**Fnded:** 1956. **Mem:** 500. **Desc:** Physicians who include allergy diagnosis and management in their practice. Purpose is to serve as a forum for physicians who actively participate in the diagnosis and treatment of allergic disorders. Seeks to provide a means of social communication among members, thereby promoting interspecialty cooperation and an increase in individual excellence. Sponsors continuing medical education programs annually. **Pub:** *Pan American Allergy Society Report,* semiannual. Newsletter. • Membership Directory, biennial. **Frmly:** (1976) Gulf Coast Allergy Study Group.

### ★ 3231 ★ Polish Society for Immunology (PSI)

### (Polskie Towarzystwo Immunologii Doswiadczalnej i Klinicznej)

Institute of Human Genetics
Polish Academy of Sciences
Strzeszynska 32
60-479 Poznan, Poland
**Phone:** 48 61 8233011　　**Fax:** 48 61 8233235
**Email:** kurpimac@man.poznan.pl
**Website:** http://www.pkidik.medianus.net
**Fnded:** 1969. **Mem:** 547. **Local Groups:** 10. **Lang(s):** English, Polish. **Desc:** Researchers. Encourages, coordinates, and supervises immunological research activities in Poland. Assists instruction at universities and medical centers. Disseminates scientific information. Conducts educational and research programs. **Pub:** *Bulletin,* periodic. Bulletin. • *Central European Journal of Immunology,* quarterly.

### ★ 3232 ★ Practical Allergy Research Foundation (PARF)

1421 Colvin Blvd.
Buffalo, NY 14223
**Phone:** (716)875-0398　　**Free:** 888-895-7277
**Fax:** (716)875-5399
**Website:** http://www.drrapp.com
Dr. Doris J. Rapp, MD, Pres.
**Desc:** Seeks to enhance public awareness of allergies, their symptoms, and remedies; fosters research in allergy. Produces and distributes teaching aids; participates in allergy teaching programs and seminars worldwide. Maintains speakers' bureau. **Pub:** *Allergies and the Hyperactive Child.* Book. • *Allergies and Your Family.* Book. • *Allergies Do Alter Activities and Behavior.* Video. • *The Impossible Child.* Book. • *Impossible Child or Allergic Child?.* Video. • *Recognize and Manage Your Allergies.* Book. • *Why An Environmentally Clean Classroom?.* Video. • *Why Some Children Can't Learn or Behave.* Video. • Audiotapes. • Catalog.

### Sjogren's Syndrome Foundation (SSF)

*See:* Entry 13665

### ★ 3233 ★ Society for Leukocyte Biology (SLB)

9650 Rockville Pike
Bethesda, MD 20814

**Phone:** (301)571-5703　　**Fax:** (301)571-5704
**Email:** slb@faseb.org
**Website:** http://www.biosci.ohio-state.edu/~slb
Debbie Weinstein, PhD, Exec. Mgr.
**Fnded:** 1954. **Mem:** 1,025. **Desc:** Persons holding M.D. and/or Ph.D. degrees who conduct research with universities; private, industrial, and government institutes; hospital clinics; members of the pharmaceutical industry. Facilitates the association of persons studying the reticuloendothelial system; fosters research in the field. (The reticuloendothelial system comprises all the cells of the blood and body tissues, including macrophages, lymphocytes, and granulocytes. It is involved in the immune response and in inflammation and functions in host defense against such problems as malignancies, infection, and environmental pathogens.) Sponsors workshop on macrophage methodology. **Pub:** *Directory and Constitution,* annual. Directory. • *Journal of Leukocyte Biology,* monthly. Journal. • Books. • Newsletter, quarterly. **Frmly:** (1988) Reticuloendothelial Society.

### ★ 3234 ★ Society for Mucosal Immunology

4350 E West Hwy., Ste. 401
Bethesda, MD 20814-4411
**Phone:** (301)718-6516　　**Fax:** (301)656-0989
**Email:** smi@paimgmt.com
**Website:** http://www.socmucimm.org
Peter Ernst, Contact
**Fnded:** 1987. **Mem:** 700. **Nat'l Groups:** 37. **Desc:** Clinician-scientists and basic scientists comprised of immunologists, physicians, dentists, veterinarians, biochemists and others interested in the immunology of the gastrointestinal, respiratory and urogential tracts, as well as the eye. Formed to advance research and education related to the field of mucosal immunology. **Pub:** *Mucosal Immunology Update.*

### ★ 3235 ★ Wegener's Granulomatosis Support Group International

PO Box 28660
Kansas City, MO 64188-8660
**Phone:** (816)436-8211　　**Free:** 800-277-9474
**Fax:** (816)436-8211
**Email:** wgsg@wgassociation.org
**Website:** http://www.wgsg.org
Iva N. Roe, Pres. & Exec. Dir.
**Fnded:** 1986. **Mem:** 5,000. **Local Groups:** 50. **Desc:** Seeks to raise public awareness of Wegener's Granulomatosis. Alleviates the isolation of having the disease. Wegener's Granulomatosis is an uncommon life threatening disease, a form of vasculitis and an autoimmune disease. Disseminates information. **Pub:** *Wegener's Granulomatosis Support Group, Inc. International,* bimonthly. Newsletter. **Frmly:** (1999) Wegener's Granulomatosis Support Group.

### ★ 3236 ★ World Allergy Organization (WAO)

611 E Wells St.
Milwaukee, WI 53202
**Phone:** (414)276-1791　　**Fax:** (414)276-3349
**Email:** info@worldallergy.org
**Website:** http://www.worldallergy.org/
Gail Bast, Exec. Dir.
**Fnded:** 1951. **Mem:** 27,000. **Nat'l Groups:** 49. **Reg. Groups:** 4. **Desc:** Umbrella organization for 59 international allergy association representing 27,000 health professionals. **Pub:** *Allergy and clinical immunology International,* bimonthly. Journal. Includes research updates. *Price:* $44/year for members; $68/year for nonmembers. • *Progress in allergy and Clinical Immunology,* triennial. Proceedings. **Frmly:** (1980) International Association of Allergology; (2002) International Association of Allergology and Clinical Immunology.

### World Association of Veterinary Microbiologists, Immunologists, and Specialists in Infectious Diseases (WAVMI)

### (Association Mondiale des Veterinaires Microbiologistes, Immunologistes et Specialistes des Maladies Infectieuses — AMVMI)

*See:* Entry 20665

## Research Centers

### ★ 3237 ★ Allergy Research Foundation

11620 Wilshire Blvd., No. 200-210
Los Angeles, CA 90025
**Phone:** (310)312-5050　　**Fax:** (310)575-9292
**Email:** joncorren@hotmail.com
Jonathan Corren, MD, Dir.
**Activities/Fields:** Allergies, asthma, urticaria.

### Arthritis and Immune Disorder Research Centre (AIDRC)

*See:* Entry 13680

### Arthritis and Immune Disorder Research Centre

### Arthritis Community Research and Evaluation Unit (ACREU)

*See:* Entry 13681

### ★ 3238 ★ Baylor College of Medicine Center for Allergy and Immunological Disorders

Feigin Center, 4th Fl.
1102 Bates, Ste. 450
Houston, TX 77030
**Phone:** (832)798-4295　　**Fax:** (832)825-1260
**Email:** wshearer@bcm.tmc.edu
**Website:** http://www.bcm.tmc.edu/cfar
William T. Shearer, MD, Ch.
**Activities/Fields:** Allergy and immunological disorders, including basic and clinical projects in cancer immunology, immunoreconstitution of immunodeficient children, immunoregulation of cellular and humoral immune responses, immune complex diseases, immunotherapy of neoplastic diseases, pulmonary immunology, rheumatic diseases, allergic diseases of children, and AIDS. Facilities available for specialty training of pre- and postdoctoral students on either a research or clinical level.

### Blood and Marrow Transplant Laboratory

*See:* Entry 20349

### ★ 3239 ★ Brigham and Women's Hospital

### Asthma and Allergic Diseases Cooperative Research Center

Smith Bldg., 6th Fl.
1 Jimmy Fund Way
Boston, MA 02115
**Phone:** (617)525-1300　　**Fax:** (617)525-1310
**Email:** fausten@rics.bwh.harvard.edu
K. Frank Austen, MD, Contact
**Activities/Fields:** Clinical areas include allergy, clinical immunology, rheumatology, immunodermatology, and pre-clinical areas include mast cell biology, biology of human peripheral blood, leukocytes including eosinophils, neutrophils and monocytes, arachidonic acid metabolism by the 5-lipoxygenase pathway, and complement biology.

### Brigham and Women's Hospital Center for Neurologic Diseases

*See:* Entry 14162

**★ 3240 ★ Bucknell University Immunobiology Research Laboratory**
Department of Biology
Lewisburg, PA 17837
**Phone:** (570)577-1135 **Fax:** (570)577-3537
**Email:** pearson@bucknell.edu
**Website:** http://www.bucknell.edu
Dr. David D. Pearson, Dir.

**Activities/Fields:** Autoimmune diseases, particularly the causes of rheumatoid arthritis and type I diabetes. Studies techniques to detect the disease, including protein blotting on nitro-cellulose, binding of oligosaccharides to lectins, enzyme-linked immunoabsorbent assay tests, and the relationships between fat metabolism and the immune response with possible involvement of leptin. Also studies methods to detect small quantities of antibodies secreted from single cells and a small number of immunoassays in developmental stages for small amounts of proteins.

**★ 3241 ★ Center for Allergy and Immunology Research**
Rush Medical College
1725 W Harrison, Ste. 207
Chicago, IL 60612
**Phone:** (312)942-6296 **Fax:** (312)563-2201
**Email:** jmoy@rush.edu
James N. Moy, MD, Contact

**Activities/Fields:** Allergy, asthma, basic immunology, and product testing, including therapeutic agent evaluation, allergenic extract developments, immunodeficiency, adverse food reaction pathogensis, Samter Syndrome etiology and pathogenesis, urticaria/angiodema etiology, laboratory assay development, and hypogammaglobulinemia treatment. **Frmly:** Allergy/Immunology Service.

**★ 3242 ★ Center for Molecular Medicine and Immunology**
520 Belleville Ave.
Belleville, NJ 07109
**Phone:** (973)844-7000 **Fax:** (973)844-7020
**Email:** gscancer@att.net
Dr. David M. Goldenberg, Pres.

**Activities/Fields:** Molecular immunology, nuclear medicine, immunobiology, and molecular genetics. Seeks to advance cancer detection techniques and translate them into methods of treatment and control.

**★ 3243 ★ Creighton University Center for Allergy, Asthma, and Immunology**
2500 California Plz.
Omaha, NE 68178
**Phone:** (402)280-2940 **Fax:** (402)280-1843
**Email:** rtownley@creighton.edu
**Website:** http://medicine.creighton.edu/allergy/home-page.html
Robert G. Townley, MD, Ch.

**Activities/Fields:** Multidisciplinary research in asthma, allergic rhinitis, allergic diseases, clinical and basic immunology, clinical and basic pharmacology and physiology, airway reactivity in patients with asthma, and allergies. Laboratory research consists of studies of human lung, eosinophils, mast cells, lymphocytes, and platelets to correlate adrenergic and cholinergic receptors and receptor mechanisms; and role of pro-inflamatory cytokines, leukotrienes and platelet activating factor on airway reactivity and in asthma and animal models of asthma. Focuses on mechanisms of immediate hypersensitivity and the late allergic reaction. **Pub:** *Allergy Principles & Practice*, quadrennially.

**Dana-Farber Cancer Institute Department of Cancer Immunology and AIDS**
*See:* Entry 11851

**★ 3244 ★ Duke University Pediatric Asthma and Allergic Disease Center**
Medical Center
PO Box 2898
Durham, NC 27710
**Phone:** (919)684-2922 **Fax:** (919)681-7979
**Email:** buckl003@mc.duke.edu
Rebecca H. Buckley, Div. Ch.

**Activities/Fields:** As a unit of NIAID, the Center seeks to integrate the concepts of immunology, genetics, biochemistry, and pharmacology into clinical investigations of patients with asthma and allergic diseases. Specific projects include studies on immunoregulation in atopic eczema and in vitro studies of human immunoglobulin E (IgE) synthesis, including lymphocyte phenotypes and their function in humans with allergic diseases and excessively high IgE antibody production. Functional studies include proliferative responses, in vitro IgE production and the effects of various cytokines on it, and epidermal T cell interactions in atopic dermatitis.

**★ 3245 ★ Emory University Emory Vaccine Research Center**
954 Gatewood Rd.
Atlanta, GA 30322
**Phone:** (404)727-3774 **Fax:** (404)727-8199
**Email:** jfine03@rmy.emory.edu
**Website:** http://www.emory.edu/WHSC/YERKES/VRC/
Jacqueline Fine, PhD, Prog. Admin.

**Activities/Fields:** Immunology and vaccines, especially new technologies to prevent AIDS, tuberculosis, malaria, influenza, and respiratory illnesses.

**★ 3246 ★ Gamble Program for Clinical Studies**
Children's Hospital Medical Center
3333 Burnet Ave., CH1
Cincinnati, OH 45229-3039
**Phone:** (513)636-4578 **Fax:** (513)636-7682
**Email:** schigo@chmcc.org
Gilbert M. Schiff, MD, Dir.

**Activities/Fields:** Virology and immunology, including studies on rubella and rubella vaccines, anti-influenza agents, basic virology of influenza, herpes virus latency, role of complement in sickle cell disease and burn wounds, and basic and clinical studies on rotaviruses, hepatitis, and human immunodeficiency virus. **Frmly:** Christ Hospital Institute of Medical Research; James N. Gamble Institute of Medical Research at the Children's Hospital.

**General Clinical Research Center**
*See:* Entry 2495

**★ 3247 ★ Georgetown University International Center for Interdisciplinary Studies of Immunology**
318 Kober-Cogan Bldg.
3800 Reservoir Rd. NW
Washington, DC 20007
**Phone:** (202)687-8227 **Fax:** (202)784-3597
**Email:** bellantj@georgetown.edu
**Website:** http://www.som.tulane.edu/gcrc
Dr. Joseph A. Bellanti, MD, Dir.

**Activities/Fields:** Immunobiology, immunochemistry, immunogenetics, immunopharmacology, and immunopathology, including the clinical disciplines of allergy and immunology, infectious diseases, respiratory diseases, and disorders of immune regulation. The center's program emphasizes pediatrics. **Frmly:** Center for Interdisciplinary Research on Immunologic Diseases.

**★ 3248 ★ Gladstone Institute of Virology and Immunology**
San Francisco General Hospital
PO Box 419100
San Francisco, CA 94141-9100
**Phone:** (415)826-7500 **Fax:** (415)826-1514
**Email:** wgreene@gladstone.ucsf.edu
**Website:** http://gladstone.ucsf.edu
Dr. Warner C. Greene, Dir.

**Activities/Fields:** Human virology and immunology with a focus on HIV and AIDS. **Pub:** *Annual Report.* • *Focus*, quarterly.

**★ 3249 ★ Harvard University Laboratory of Immunology**
Harvard Medical Sch.
200 Longwood Ave., 5th Fl., D-530
Boston, MA 02115
**Phone:** (617)432-1978 **Fax:** (617)432-2789
**Email:** martin_dorf@hms.harvard.edu
Dr. Martin Dorf, Dir.

**Activities/Fields:** Indentification of chemokines and their receptors. Applications to autoimmunity.

**HIV Center for Clinical and Behavioral Studies**
*See:* Entry 12691

**★ 3250 ★ John P. Robarts Research Institute London Clinical Trials Research Group**
100 Perth Dr.
PO Box 5015
London, ON, Canada N6A 5K8
**Phone:** (519)663-3400 **Fax:** (519)663-3807
**Email:** lctrg@lctrg.com
**Website:** http://www.lctrg.com
Dr. Feagan, Dir.

**Activities/Fields:** Evaluates new medications and treatments in a variety of medical fields. Provides biostatistics and data coordination for national and international trials.

**★ 3251 ★ John P. Robarts Research Institute Viral Immunology and Pathogenesis**
100 Perth Dr.
PO Box 5015
London, ON, Canada N6A 5K8
**Phone:** (519)663-5777 **Fax:** (519)663-3789
Dr. Calvin Stiller, Dir.

**Activities/Fields:** Molecular biology of immune system, with emphasis on genetic factors of abnormal autoimmune response and control mechanisms of normal immune system. Studies focus on juvenile diabetes, transplant rejection, multiple sclerosis, rheumatoid arthritis, and AIDS.

**★ 3252 ★ Johns Hopkins University Asthma and Allergy Center**
5501 Hopkins Bayview Cir.
Baltimore, MD 21224
**Phone:** (410)550-2101 **Fax:** (410)550-1733
**Website:** http://www.med.jhu.edu/allergy/
Dr. Lawrence M. Lichtenstein, Dir.

**Activities/Fields:** Allergic diseases and individuals with allergic diseases, pulmonary diseases and individuals with pulmonary diseases, and diseases involving inflammation and immunological processes.

**★ 3253 ★ Johns Hopkins University Center for Immunization Research**
Hampton House, Rm. 217A
Johns Hopkins School of Public Health
624 N Broadway
Baltimore, MD 21205-1901
**Phone:** (410)614-5960 **Fax:** (410)502-6898
**Email:** dburke@jhsph.edu
**Website:** http://ih.jhsph.edu/cir/
Dr. Donald Burke, Dir.

**Activities/Fields:** Influenza, parainfluenza, respiratory syncytial virus, AIDS, and rotavirus vaccines, hepatitis B, immunoglobulins, and antiviral drug efficacy studies. Uses volunteers 18 years of age or older for vaccine studies and children from the ages of 1 month to 48 months for pediatric vaccine studies.

### ★ 3254 ★ La Jolla Institute for Allergy and Immunology

10355 Science Center Dr.
San Diego, CA 92121
**Phone:** (858)558-3500 **Fax:** (858)558-3525
**Website:** http://www.liai.org
Dr. Howard Grey, Pres.

**Activities/Fields:** Increased knowledge of the immune system including the study of the regulatory mechanisms involved in the onset and maintenance of immune response, and the development of new, more sophisticated and precise strategies and/or therapies for managing various immunological and allergic disorders.

**La Jolla Institute for Molecular Medicine**
*See:* Entry 10361

**Laboratory of Tumor Antigen Immunochemistry**
*See:* Entry 10363

**Loyola University Chicago**
**Heart Transplant and Heart Failure Program**
*See:* Entry 20350

### ★ 3255 ★ Mayo Clinic and Foundation Allergic Diseases Research Laboratory

200 1st St. SW
Rochester, MN 55905
**Phone:** (507)284-2789 **Fax:** (507)284-5045
**Email:** gleich@mayo.edu
**Website:** http://www.mayo.edu
Gerald J. Gleich, MD, Dir.

**Activities/Fields:** Provides a focus for research into the causes, prevention, and management of allergic diseases such as asthma, allergies, contact hypersensitivity, immune deficiencies and infection, and autoimmune disorders plus related studies of fundamental immune mechanisms involving immune cells, antibodies, genetic factors, and immune regulatory systems. Projects focus on functions of the eosinophilic leukocyte, immunotherapy of patients with pollen allergies, and clinical studies of passive immunotherapy in patients allergic to honeybee stings who fail to respond to venom immunotherapy and who are members of beekeeping families.

**McGill University**
**Centre for the Study of Host Resistance**
*See:* Entry 11864

**McGill University**
**Division of Transplantation**
*See:* Entry 20351

### ★ 3256 ★ National Jewish Medical and Research Center

1400 Jackson St.
Denver, CO 80206
**Phone:** (303)388-4461 **Free:** 800-222-5864
**Fax:** (303)270-2165
**Email:** taussigl@njc.org
**Website:** http://www.nationaljewish.org
Lynn M. Taussig, MD, Pres./CEO

**Activities/Fields:** Etiology, progression, manifestation, treatment, rehabilitation, and prevention of pulmonary, allergic, and immunologic diseases. Studies encompass cellular and molecular biology. Pub: *ARIA (Allergy, Rheumatology, Immunology, Asthma)* Newsletter. • *National Jewish Center Scientific Annual Report.* • *New Directions Newsletter.* **Frmly:** National Jewish Center for Immunology and Respiratory Medicine.

### ★ 3257 ★ Ohio State University Division of Pulmonary and Critical Care Medicine

201 Heart & Lung Research Institute
Department of Internal Medicine
473 W 12th Ave.
Columbus, OH 43210-1228
**Phone:** (614)293-4925 **Fax:** (614)293-4799
**Website:** http://www.intmed.med.ohio-state.edu/pulmo/pulmonary_homepage.htm
Mark D. Wewers, MD, Dir.

**Activities/Fields:** Mechanisms of allergic, immunologic, and inflammatory diseases, including ventilatory control and respiratory failure, inflammatory mechanisms in adult respiratory distress syndrome, cystic fibrosis, emphysema, staging and therapy of pulmonary neoplasms, respiratory distress in HIV, and occupational lung diseases. Collaborates with the departments of physiology and exercise physiology and with the cardiopulmonary unit of the School of Veterinary Medicine at the University.

### ★ 3258 ★ Ohio State University Transplant Sciences Laboratories

355 Means Hall
1654 Upham Dr.
Columbus, OH 43210
**Phone:** (614)293-3212 **Fax:** (614)293-4541
**Email:** orosz-1@medctr.osu.edu
Dr. Charles Orosz, Dir.

**Activities/Fields:** Transplantation related immunobiology, inflammation, clinical histocompatibility testing and post-transplant immunologic monitoring, clinical and experimental immunosuppression, and application of complexity theory to immunology, including agent-based computer simulation of immune behavior. **Frmly:** Therapeutic Immunology Laboratories.

**Oklahoma Medical Research Foundation**
**Arthritis/Immunology Research Program**
*See:* Entry 13701

**Oklahoma Medical Research Foundation**
**Immunobiology and Cancer Research Program**
*See:* Entry 10395

### ★ 3259 ★ Oklahoma Medical Research Foundation Molecular Immunogenetics Research Program

825 NE 13th St.
Oklahoma City, OK 73104
**Phone:** (405)271-6673 **Fax:** (405)271-7510
**Email:** donald-capra@omrf.ouhsc.edu
**Website:** http://www.omrf.org/OMRF/Research/05/CapraJD.asp
J. Donald Capra, MD, Prog. Hd.

**Activities/Fields:** Molecular mechanisms of the immune system.

**Oregon Health and Science University**
**Transplant and Immunogenetics Laboratory**
*See:* Entry 20354

### ★ 3260 ★ Rockefeller University Laboratory of Bacteriology, Pathogenesis and Immunology

1230 York Ave., DWB 800
New York, NY 10021-6399
**Phone:** (212)327-8157 **Fax:** (212)327-8960
**Email:** ecg@rockvax.rockefeller.edu
Emil C. Gotschlich, MD, Dir

**Activities/Fields:** Investigates the parasitic mechanisms used by pathogenic bacteria, especially streptococci and neisseria. Also studies the derangements of the human immune system which lead to chronic

diseases such as rheumatic fever and glomerulonephritis as a result of infection with streptococci.

### ★ 3261 ★ Rockefeller University Laboratory of Cellular Physiology and Immunology

1230 York Ave.
New York, NY 10021-6399
**Phone:** (212)327-7763 **Fax:** (212)327-8875
**Email:** steinm@rockvax.rockefeller.edu
Dr. Ralph Steinman, Contact

**Activities/Fields:** Functional properties of eukaryotic cells and their role in physiologic and pathologic events. Using the tools of immunology, cell biology, and biochemistry, the Lab studies problems of inflammation, the immune response, and host defense against parasites and tumor cells.

### ★ 3262 ★ Rockefeller University Laboratory of Clinical Microbiology and Immunology

1230 York Ave., Box 255
New York, NY 10021
**Phone:** (212)327-8155 **Fax:** (212)327-7579
**Email:** zabrisk@mail.rockefeller.edu
Dr. John B. Zabriskie, Dir.

**Activities/Fields:** Microbe-induced autoimmunity and human genetics, including molecular biology emphasizing eukaryotic systems, protein chemistry, and immunology.

**Rush University**
**Rush Arthritis and Orthopedics Institute**
*See:* Entry 13704

**St. Clare's Hospital and Health Center**
**Spellman Center for HIV-Related Disease**
*See:* Entry 11875

### ★ 3263 ★ Scripps Research Institute W.M. Keck Autoimmune Diseases Center

10666 N Torrey Pines Rd.
La Jolla, CA 92037
**Phone:** (858)784-1000 **Fax:** (858)784-8118
**Email:** emtan@scripps.edu
**Website:** http://www.rush.edu/arthritis/
Eng Tan, MD, Dir.

**Activities/Fields:** Immunologic studies on the development of allergic disorders, especially aspirin and related drug sensitivities, bisulfite-sensitivity in asthma, and hereditary angioedema. Investigates the role of leukotrienes in the development of allergic disorders and conducts studies on drug-induced lupus reactions and the role specific autoantibodies may play in the development of the disease. Emphasizes immunology and molecular biology of autoimmunity related to lupus, scleroderma, Sjogren's syndrome, dermatomyositis, and polymyositis.

**Stanford University**
**Laboratory for Transplantation Immunology**
*See:* Entry 20355

**Temple University**
**Center for Neurovirology and Cancer Biology**
**Laboratory of Neuro-Immunology (LNI)**
*See:* Entry 14285

**Thomas Jefferson University**
**Lupus Center**
*See:* Entry 13708

**Thomas Jefferson University**
**Scleroderma and Arthritis Research**
**  Center**
*See:* Entry 13709


**★ 3264 ★ Trudeau Institute, Inc.**
100 Algonquin Ave.
PO Box 59
Saranac Lake, NY 12983
**Phone:** (518)891-3080        **Fax:** (518)891-5126
**Email:** scooper@trudeauinstitute.org
**Website:** http://www.trudeauinstitute.org
Susan Cooper, Dir., Inst. Advancement
**Activities/Fields:** Cellular immunology and infectious disease, particularly tuberculosis, influenza, cancer, the opportunistic infections in the AIDS patient and the effects of aging on immunity, vaccines, immune memory, and other immunotherapies. **Pub:** *Annual Report.* • *Focus Newsletter.*


**★ 3265 ★ Tufts University**
**Asthma and Allergic Diseases**
**  Cooperative Research Center**
Sch. of Medicine New England Medical Center
750 Washington St.
Boston, MA 02111
**Phone:** (617)636-5333        **Fax:** (617)636-4843
**Email:** johman@lifespan.org
Dr. John Ohman, Ch.
**Activities/Fields:** Studies of the release of histamine (a body chemical best known for its ability to cause itching, nasal symptoms, hives, or asthma during an allergy attack) to determine whether patients with various allergic disorders either are more sensitive to the effects of histamine or release larger quantities than normal; studies of endothelial cells, which line blood vessels in the human body, and possible interaction of this type of cell with immune system cells and the role of this interaction in an inflammatory disease of blood vessels known as vasculitis; and studies of a type of blood cell known as the eosinophil frequently found in and around the site of an allergic reaction and the interaction of this cell with other immune system functional cells known as lymphocytes.


**★ 3266 ★ Tulane University**
**Clinical Immunology Section**
1700 Perdido St., 3rd Fl.
New Orleans, LA 70112
**Phone:** (504)588-5578        **Fax:** (504)584-3686
**Email:** malopez@tulane.edu
Prof. Manuel Lopez, MD, Dir.
**Activities/Fields:** Provides a focus for research into the causes, prevention, and management of diseases such as asthma, allergies, immune deficiencies and infections, and autoimmune disorders, plus related studies of fundamental immune mechanisms involving immune cells, antibodies, genetic factors, and immune regulatory systems, especially as they relate to the lung. Investigates tobacco smoke products as possible allergens, mechanisms of AIDS, and immunologic mechanisms of occupational and environmental lung disease.


**★ 3267 ★ U.S. Department of Defense**
**Army Medical Research and Materiel**
**  Command**
**Walter Reed Army Institute of Research**
**Communicable Diseases and Immunology**
**  Division**
Bldg. 40, Rm. 2129
Washington, DC 20307-5100
**Phone:** (202)782-3561        **Fax:** (202)782-0748
Col. Charles H. Hoke, Jr., Dir.
**Activities/Fields:** Ecology, etiology, pathogenesis, diagnosis, prevention, and therapy of selected diseases of military importance and develop, validate, and apply methods of disease control through the use of immunizing agents (including studies of modification induced in the host by exposure to disease agents);

develop methods of production (including actual emergency manufacture) and methods of assaying the biologicals required by the Armed Forces; and provide reference and consultative services on the diagnosis, epidemiology, control, and chemotherapy of infectious diseases of military importance. Divisional components include departments of Bacterial Diseases, Biologics Research, Enteric Infections, Entomology, Immunology, and Virus Disea ses.


**★ 3268 ★ U.S. Department of Health and**
**  Human Services**
**Centers for Disease Control and**
**  Prevention**
**Antinuclear Antibody Reference**
**  Laboratory**
1600 Clifton Rd. NE, Rm. 17-3040
Mailstop A-25
Atlanta, GA 30333
**Phone:** (404)639-2727        **Fax:** (404)639-2108
**Email:** mgb1@cdc.gov
Dr. J. Steven McDougal, Chf.
**Activities/Fields:** Collaborating scientists from the Arthritis Foundation and CDC have prepared for distribution eleven antisera to nuclear components useful in the diagnosis and classification of certain autoimmune diseases. These reference antisera have been used in approximately 1900 laboratories and can be obtained by writing to the ANA Reference Laboratory at the above address. The eleven antisera currently available are: Homogeneous Pattern Antinuclear Antibody (ANA) and anti-native DNA; Speckled ANA (anti-SSB/La); Speckled ANA; Anti-U-1 RNP; Anti-Sm; Anti-Nucleolar; Anti-SSA/RO; Anti-centromere; Anti-Scl-70; Anti-Jo-1; Anti-PM-Scl.


**★ 3269 ★ U.S. Department of Health and**
**  Human Services**
**Centers for Disease Control and**
**  Prevention**
**National Centers for Prevention Services**
**National Immunization Program**
Mail Stop E-05
CDC NIP 1600 Clifton Rd, NE
Atlanta, GA 30333
**Phone:** (404)639-8200        **Fax:** (404)639-8626
**Email:** wa01@CDC.GOV
Dr. Walter A. Orenstein, Dir.
**Activities/Fields:** Vaccine-preventable disease control.


**U.S. Department of Health and Human**
**  Services**
**Centers for Disease Control and**
**  Prevention**
**National Institute for Occupational Safety**
**  and Health**
**National Occupational Research Agenda**
**(Indoor Environment)**
*See:* Entry 16813


# Chapter 34

**U.S. Department of Health and Human**
**  Services**
**Food and Drug Administration**
**Center for Bilogics Evaluation and**
**  Research**
**Laboratory Cellular Immunology**
**(Division of Cellular and Gene Therapies)**
*See:* Entry 4696


**U.S. Department of Health and Human**
**  Services**
**Food and Drug Administration**
**Center for Biologics Evaluation and**
**  Research**
**Division of Allergenic Products and**
**  Parasitology**
*See:* Entry 4700

**U.S. Department of Health and Human**
**  Services**
**Food and Drug Administration**
**Center for Biologics Evaluation and**
**  Research**
**Laboratory of Immuno-Chemistry**
*See:* Entry 4714


**U.S. Department of Health and Human**
**  Services**
**Food and Drug Administration**
**Center for Biologics Evaluation and**
**  Research**
**Laboratory of Immunobiochemistry**
*See:* Entry 4715


**U.S. Department of Health and Human**
**  Services**
**Food and Drug Administration**
**Center for Biologics Evaluation and**
**  Research**
**Laboratory of Immunoregulation**
*See:* Entry 4716


**U.S. Department of Health and Human**
**  Services**
**Food and Drug Administration**
**Center for Biologics Evaluation and**
**  Research**
**Laboratory of Molecular and**
**  Developemental Immunology**
*See:* Entry 4717


**U.S. Department of Health and Human**
**  Services**
**Food and Drug Administration**
**Center for Biologics Evaluation and**
**  Research**
**Laboratory of Molecular Immunology**
*See:* Entry 4718


**U.S. Department of Health and Human**
**  Services**
**National Cancer Institute**
**Laboratory of Immunobiology**
*See:* Entry 10487


**U.S. Department of Health and Human**
**  Services**
**National Cancer Institute**
**Laboratory of Molecular Biology**
*See:* Entry 10490


**U.S. Department of Health and Human**
**  Services**
**National Cancer Institute**
**Laboratory of Molecular**
**  Immunoregulation**
*See:* Entry 10492


**U.S. Department of Health and Human**
**  Services**
**National Cancer Institute**
**Laboratory of Tumor Immunology and**
**  Biology**
**Laboratory of Tumor Immunology and**
**  Biology**
*See:* Entry 10497

## ★ 3270 ★ U.S. Department of Health and Human Services
### National Center for Prevention Services
### National Immunization Program
### Epidemiology and Surveillance Division
1600 Clifton Rd. NE, No. E-05
Atlanta, GA 30333
**Phone:** (404)639-8549　　　　**Fax:** (404)639-8626
**Email:** js141c@nih.gov
**Website:** http://rex.nci.nih.gov/RESEARCH/basic/ltib/ltibpage.htm
Stephen C. Hadler, Chf.

**Activities/Fields:** Incidence of diseases preventable by vaccination; and conducts studies on the safety and efficacy of new or existing vaccines. **Pub:** *Research Reports.*

## ★ 3271 ★ U.S. Department of Health and Human Services
### National Institute of Allergy and Infectious Diseases
### Asthma and Allergic Diseases Cooperative Research Center (NIAID)
NIH, Bldg. 10, Rm. 11C205
10 Center Dr. MSC1881
Bethesda, MD 20892-1881
**Phone:** (301)496-2165　　　　**Fax:** (301)480-8384
**Email:** dean_metcalfe@nih.gov
Dr. Dean Metcalfe, Chf.

**Activities/Fields:** Studies of the mast cell and its role in causing various allergic diseases, including asthma; and study of mast cell disorders including mastocytosis. **Frmly:** Asthma and Allergic Diseases Cooperative Research Center.

## ★ 3272 ★ U.S. Department of Health and Human Services
### National Institute of Allergy and Infectious Diseases
### Division of Allergy, Immunology, and Transplantation
6700-B, Rm. 5142-MSC7640
Rockledge Dr.
Bethesda, MD 20892-7640
**Phone:** (301)496-1886　　　　**Fax:** (301)402-2571
**Email:** dr17g@nih.gov
**Website:** http://www.nih.niaid.gov/research/diat.htm
Dr. Daniel Rotrosen, Ch.

**Activities/Fields:** Immune system as it functions in the maintenance of health and as it malfunctions in the production of disease. The Division provides leadership in the identification, design, and implementation of basic and clinical research initiatives encompassing a wide range of disorders including: autoimmune diseases such as childhood diabetes, rheumatoid arthritis and multiple sclerosis, allergic diseases such as asthma and occupational and environmental disorders and organ transplant rejection. **Frmly:** Immunology Allergic, and Immunologic Diseases Program, Allergy, Immunology, and Transplantation Program.

## ★ 3273 ★ U.S. Department of Health and Human Services
### National Institute of Allergy and Infectious Diseases
### Division of Allergy, Immunology, and Transplantation
### Asthma, Allergy, and Inflamation Branch
6700-B Rockledge Dr.
Rm. 5142, MSC 7640
Bethesda, MD 20892-7640
**Phone:** (301)496-1886　　　　**Fax:** (301)402-0175
**Email:** DR17G@NIH.GOV
Dr. Daniel Rotrosen, Chf.

**Activities/Fields:** Branch supports (through grants, cooperative agreements, career development awards, fellowships, and other mechanisms) basic and clinical research on the etiology, pathogenesis, diagnosis, prevention and treatment of allergic diseases and asthma; it also supports research on mucosal immunity, phagocyte biology and complement. Basic investigations include a study of the regulation of IgE antibody synthesis and IgE interactions with IgE receptors and other IgE binding molecules; studies of the epitopes of allergens and T cells that mediate allergic reations; assessment of the role of cytokines and adhesion molecules in regulating IgE synthesis and allergic inflammation in vitro and in vivo; and molecular and biochemical characterization of molecules expressed on, and in, mast cells, basophils and eosinophils. The diseases studies include asthma, allergic rhinitis, otitis, atopic dermatitis, and urticaria/angioedema. Also studies diseases induced by immune responses to specific antigens, notably IgE-mediated and T cell-mediated reactions to insect venoms, foods, industrial chemicals, contact sensitizers, airborne allergens, and drug hypersensitivity. The Asthma, Allergy and Inflammation Branch supports eight centers for the National Cooperative Inner City Asthma Study (NCICAS), which focuses on determining the mechanisms for the high morbidity and mortality from asthma of African American and Hispanic children ages 4-9 living in inner cities, and defining effective interventions to reduce that high morbidity and mortality. In addition, the Branch supports 15 (of 21) Asthma, Allergic and Immunologic Diseases Cooperative Research Centers, which integrate investigations of basic and clinical research related to human asthma, allergic diseases, and other immunologic diseases.

## ★ 3274 ★ U.S. Department of Health and Human Services
### National Institute of Allergy and Infectious Diseases
### Division of Allergy, Immunology, and Transplantation
### Basic Immunology Branch
6700 B Rockledge Dr.
MSC 7640
Bethesda, MD 20892
**Phone:** (301)496-7551　　　　**Fax:** (301)402-2571
**Email:** hq1t@nih.gov
Dr. Helen Quill, Chf.

**Activities/Fields:** Biology and chemistry of the immune system and its products. Immunobiologic studies include: the origin, maturation, localization, and interactions of immunocyte (lymphocyte, plasmocyte, macrophage) populations and subpopulations; the cellular and biochemical mechanisms responsible for antigen processing, tolerance, and enhancement; research in the mechanisms responsible for induction and regulation of the immune response; and studies on lymphokines and other substances produced by immunocytes and other cells that regulate the immune system. Immunochemical studies include: the chemical structure and function of the immunoglobulin components of body fluids; the chemical structure, function, and biologic importance of naturally occurring antigens; the mechanisms of antigen-antibody reactions and the chemical basis of immunologic specificity; the regulation of immunoglobulin synthesis; the chemistry and function of immunopharmacologic agents; and chemical characterization of the molecular components and the function of accessory systems that participate in the immune response. **Frmly:** Immunobiology and Immunochemistry Branch.

## ★ 3275 ★ U.S. Department of Health and Human Services
### National Institute of Allergy and Infectious Diseases
### Division of Allergy, Immunology, and Transplantation
### Clinical Immunology Branch
6700 B Rockledge Dr.
Room 5135
Bethesda, MD 20892
**Phone:** (301)496-7104　　　　**Fax:** (301)402-2571
**Email:** ecollier@niaid.nih.gov
Dr. Elaine Collier, Chf.

**Activities/Fields:** Underlying cellular and molecular mechanisms responsible for the pathogenesis of immunologic diseases, as well as the application of basic knowledge to the etiology, prevention, and management of immunologic disorders, including autoimmune, immune complex, and immunodeficiency diseases and immunoregulatory dysfunctions. A special feature of this program is the support of Asthma, Allergic and Immunologic Disease Cooperative Research Centers (AAIDCRCs). An objective of AAIDCRCs is to accelerate the clinical application of new knowledge of the immune system. Programs are designed to integrate and coordinate research projects in clinical immunology that are being pursued in clinical specialties with those in basic research. AAIDCRC grants are awarded to an institution on behalf of a program director for support of a broadly based, multidisciplinary long-term research program that has a specific objective or basic theme. An AAIDCRC generally involves the organized efforts of groups of investigators who conduct research projects related to the overall program objective. The grant can provide support for the projects and for certain basic resources shared by individuals in a program where the sharing facilitates the total research effort. NIAID currently supports five CIRIDs (see following entries).

## ★ 3276 ★ U.S. Department of Health and Human Services
### National Institute of Allergy and Infectious Diseases (NIAID)
### Division of Allergy, Immunology, and Transplantation
### Genetics and Transplantation Branch
6700B Rockledge Dr., Rm. 5142
Bethesda, MD 20892-7640
**Phone:** (301)496-1886　　　　**Fax:** (301)402-2571
**Email:** dr17g@nih.gov
**Website:** http://www.niaid.nih.gov/organization/daitorg.htm
Dr. Daniel Rotrosen, Ch.

**Activities/Fields:** Genetic and immunologic mechanisms that are involved in responses to foreign substances such as infecting microorganisms and engrafted tissues. These mechanisms determine susceptibility or resistance to various diseases and the success or failure of organ or tissue grafts. The program supports investigations in animal species ranging from invertebrates to man, and the development of technologies and reagents. Research in genetics and transplantation is supported through the award of both grants and contracts. The research grant program supports studies on the molecular genetics of the immune system. The contract program in transplantation immunology supports the acquisition and distribution of reagents useful in research in immunogenetics and transplantation, evaluation of methodologies currently in use at the laboratory and the clinical level in those fields, development of new and more effective technologies for histocompatibility testing and immunologic manipulation, and collection and analysis of data to permit assessment of the efficacy of various transplant procedures.

## ★ 3277 ★ U.S. Department of Health and Human Services
### National Institute of Allergy and Infectious Diseases
### Division of Extramural Activities
6700 B Rockledge Dr.
Bethesda, MD 20892
**Phone:** (301)496-7291　　　　**Fax:** (301)402-0369
Dr. John McGowan, Dir.

**Activities/Fields:** Coordinates and provides administrative support for all NIAID program activities in the extramural area. The DEA staff work closely with scientific program staff, grantees, and potential grantees in providing management information, advice, and consultation as needed to fulfill the broad objectives of the NIAID research grants and contracts programs. DEA also directs and carries out the scientific and technical merit review of proposals and applications for research contracts, program projects, special research grants, and research training. Activities are organized in branches for contract management, grants management, program and project review, and research manpower development.

**★ 3278 ★ U.S. Department of Health and Human Services**
**National Institute of Allergy and Infectious Diseases**
**Division of Extramural Activities**
**Contract Management Branch**
6700-B Rockledge Dr., Rm. 2115
Bethesda, MD 20892
**Phone:** (301)496-0612          **Fax:** (301)402-0972
**Email:** bv4y@nih.gov
**Website:** http://www.niaid.nih.gov/contract/default.htm
Brenda J. Velez, Chf.

**Activities/Fields:** Contract management.

**★ 3279 ★ U.S. Department of Health and Human Services**
**National Institute of Allergy and Infectious Diseases**
**Division of Extramural Activities**
**Grants Management Branch**
National Inst. of Health
6700 B Rockledge Dr. Room 2116
Bethesda, MD 20892-7614
**Phone:** (301)402-6400          **Fax:** (301)480-3780
Mary Kirker, Chf.

**Activities/Fields:** Supports research activities through grant management.

**★ 3280 ★ U.S. Department of Health and Human Services**
**National Institute of Allergy and Infectious Diseases**
**Division of Intramural Research**
NIH Bldg. 10, Rm. 4A-31
10 Center Dr., MSC 1356
Bethesda, MD 20892-1356
**Phone:** (301)496-3006          **Fax:** (301)480-9324
**Email:** tk9c@nih.gov
**Website:** http://www.niaid.nih.gov/dir/default.htm
Dr. Thomas Kindt, Dir.

**Activities/Fields:** Causes of allergic, immunologic, and infectious diseases; research that has developed to the point of clinical application is pursued through clinical trials, performed at the Clinical Center of NIH or in collaboration with university centers. The NIAID Intramural Program has diverse components covering medical research relevant to the Institute's mission and includes laboratories for: Cellular and Molecular Immunology; Clinical Investigation; Host Defense; Immunogenetics; Immunology; Immunopathology; Immunoregulation; Infectious Diseases; Molecular Microbiology; Parasitic Diseases; Viral Diseases; Persistant Viral Diseases and Allergic Diseases. and Function Laboratory; and Persistant Viral Diseases. **Pub:** *Opportunities in the division of Intramural Research, NIAID, Annual Report.*

**★ 3281 ★ U.S. Department of Health and Human Services**
**National Institute of Allergy and Infectious Diseases**
**Laboratory of Cellular and Molecular Immunology**
NIH Bldg. 4, Rm. 111
9000 Rockville Pike
Bethesda, MD 20892-0420
**Phone:** (301)496-1257          **Fax:** (301)496-0877
**Email:** rs34r@nih.gov
Ronald H. Schwartz, Chf.

**Activities/Fields:** Cellular and molecular immunology.

**★ 3282 ★ U.S. Department of Health and Human Services**
**National Institute of Allergy and Infectious Diseases**
**Laboratory of Clinical Investigation**
NIH Bldg. 10, Rm. 11N228
10 Center Dr., MSC 1888
Bethesda, MD 20892-1888
**Phone:** (301)496-5807          **Fax:** (301)496-7383
Dr. Stephen E. Straus, Chf.

**Activities/Fields:** Allergic, immunologic, and infectious diseases. Specific areas of research interest are: the molecular biology, pathogenesis, prevention and antiviral treatment of herpes virus infections in humans; the role of host defense mechanisms in prevention of infections; the pathogenesis, treatment, and prevention of cryptococcal and candida infections; the molecular basis of macrophage responses to infection; identification of genes that contribute to virulence in E. coli; mechanisms of regulation of immune reactivity in normal individuals and patients with immunologically mediated diseases; the biochemical response in lymphoid cells following antigenic stimulation in normal and immunologically impaired subjects; the immunologic abnormalities of asthma and other allergic diseases mechanisms of regulation of mucosal immune responses; the pathogenesis of inflammatory bowel diseases; the pathogenesis of immunodeficiency diseases; the biology of the mast cell; and the diagnosis and effective management of systemic mastocytosis.

**★ 3283 ★ U.S. Department of Health and Human Services**
**National Institute of Allergy and Infectious Diseases**
**Laboratory of Immunogenetics**
NIAID Twinbrook Facility
12441 Parklawn Dr., Rm. 200B
Rockville, MD 20852
**Phone:** (301)496-9589          **Fax:** (301)402-0259
**Email:** spierce@niaid.nih.gov
**Website:** http://www.niaid.nih.gov/dir/labs/lig.htm
Susan K. Pierce, PhD, Chf.

**Activities/Fields:** Multigene families that are involved in the control of immune function. Research emphasizes the structure and function of the genes and their products as well as mechanisms for gene regulation. Studies involve structural, serologic, and molecular genetic investigations. Techniques used include quantitative radioimmunoassays, protein structure determinations, recombinant DNA technologies (gene cloning and nucleotide sequencing) assays for DNA regulatory elements, and DNA-mediated gene transfer into mammalian cells; preparation and study of T- and B-cell hybridomas; and a variety of immunologic assays for cellular and humoral components of the immune response.

**★ 3284 ★ U.S. Department of Health and Human Services**
**National Institute of Allergy and Infectious Diseases**
**Laboratory of Immunology**
NIH Bldg. 10, Rm. 11N311
10 Center Dr. MSC 1892
Bethesda, MD 20892-1892
**Phone:** (301)496-5046          **Fax:** (301)496-0222
**Website:** http://www.nih.gov
William Paul, MD, Chf.

**Activities/Fields:** Various aspects of cellular, molecular, and developmental biology of lymphocytes; the regulation of immune responses; immunogenetics; and immunochemistry. Emphasis is on developing an understanding of how the various elements of the immune system function normally and of the role of immune mechanisms in the prevention and pathogenesis of diseases. Studies utilize a variety of techniques, including production and use of monoclonal antibodies, cloning and long-term growth of lymphocyte lines; molecular genetic analysis of cells of the immune system; and cell biological analysis of lymphocyte activation and differentiation. **Pub:** *Proceedings.*

**★ 3285 ★ U.S. Department of Health and Human Services**
**National Institute of Allergy and Infectious Diseases**
**Laboratory of Immunopathology**
NIH Bldg. 7, Rm. 304
7 Center Dr., MSC 0760
Bethesda, MD 20892-0760
**Phone:** (301)496-1150          **Fax:** (301)402-0077
Dr. Herbert C. Morse III, Chf.

**Activities/Fields:** Mechanisms by which retroviruses and adenoviruses induce disease. Activities involve: evaluation of the genetic organization of viruses in relation to their pathogenic properties; definition of the characteristics of normal target cell population and the effects of viruses on these cells; and identification of host characteristics that influence the outcome of virus infections. Methods involve molecular technology as well as in vivo analyses of viral pathogenicity in mice and hamsters, and immunologic studies of cells from normal, mutant, and virus-infected mice.

**★ 3286 ★ U.S. Department of Health and Human Services**
**National Institute of Allergy and Infectious Diseases**
**Laboratory of Immunoregulation**
NIH Bldg. 10, Rm. 11B13
9000 Rockville Pike
Bethesda, MD 20892
**Phone:** (301)496-1124          **Fax:** (301)402-0070
Dr. Anthony S. Fauci, Chf.

**Activities/Fields:** Mechanisms of activation and immunoregulation of human immune responses in normal individuals and in a variety of disease states characterized by abnormalities of immune function. Recent areas of research interest have included: acquired immunodeficiency syndrome (AIDS); immunoregulation of human lymphocyte function in normal and disease states; immunopathogenic features of immune-mediated diseases; clinical, immunopathogenic, and therapeutic studies in the spectrum of vasculitis; molecular biologic approach to the immune system; and immunopathogenesis of *Chlamydia trachomatis* infection. **Pub:** *Proceedings.*

**★ 3287 ★ U.S. Department of Health and Human Services**
**National Institute of Allergy and Infectious Diseases (NIAID)**
**Laboratory of Molecular Structure**
Twinbrook II
12441 Parklawn Dr., Rm. 205
Rockville, MD 20852
**Phone:** (301)496-8247          **Fax:** (301)480-2818
**Email:** jcoligan@niaid.nih.gov
John E. Coligan, PhD, Section Chf.

**Activities/Fields:** Molecular basis of the immune response. Also studies structural biology of immunologically relevant molecules. **Frmly:** Biological Resources Branch.

**★ 3288 ★ U.S. Department of Health and Human Services**
**National Institute of Allergy and Infectious Diseases**
**Office of Administrative Management**
**Extramural Administrative Management Branch**
6700 B. Rockledge Dr.
Bethesda, MD 20892
**Phone:** (301)496-7151          **Fax:** (301)402-0520
Marilyn Kunzweiler, Chf.

**Activities/Fields:** Extramural administrative management.

**★ 3289 ★ U.S. Department of Health and Human Services**
**National Institute of Allergy and Infectious Diseases**
**Office of Communications**
NIH Bldg. 31, Rm. 7A50
31 Center Dr., MSC2520
Bethesda, MD 20892-2520
**Phone:** (301)496-5717          **Fax:** (301)402-0120
**Email:** lf7j@nih.gov
**Website:** http://www.niaid.nih.gov/cgi-shl/contacts/contacts.cfm
Leslie Fink, Dir.
**Activities/Fields:** Supports the communication of research activities in the areas of AIDS, allergy, immunology, and infectious diseases.

**★ 3290 ★ U.S. Department of Health and Human Services**
**National Institute of Allergy and Infectious Diseases**
**Office of Policy Analysis**
NIH Bldg. 31, Rm. 7A52
9000 Rockville Pike
Bethesda, MD 20892
**Phone:** (301)496-6752          **Fax:** (301)402-0492
**Email:** lh28q@nih.gov
**Website:** http://www.niaid.nih.gov/cgi-shl/contacts/contacts.cfm
Lynn C. Hellinger, Actg. Dir.
**Activities/Fields:** Allergies and infectious diseases.
**Pub:** *Profile*, annually.

**★ 3291 ★ U.S. Department of Health and Human Services**
**National Institute of Allergy and Infectious Diseases**
**Rocky Mountain Laboratories**
**Administrative and Facilities Management Section**
903 S 4th St.
RML/8207
Hamilton, MT 59840
**Phone:** (406)363-9324          **Fax:** (406)363-9218
**Email:** ps144e@nih.gov
**Website:** http://www.niaid.nih.gov/dir/labs.htm
Patricia A. Stewart, Chf.
**Activities/Fields:** Components include the Microbial Structure and Function Laboratory; Microscopy Branch; the Persistent Viral Diseases Laboratory; and Intracellular Parasites Laboratory. **Frmly:** Rocky Mountain Operations Branch.

**U.S. Department of Health and Human Services**
**National Institute of Neurological Disorders and Stroke**
**Division of Intramural Research (Clinical Neurosciences Program)**
**Neuroimmunology Branch**
*See:* Entry 14314

**U.S. Department of Health and Human Services**
**National Institutes of Health**
**National Cancer Institute**
**Division of Basic Sciences**
**((Laboratory of Experimental Immunology)**
**Leokocyte Cell Biology Section)**
*See:* Entry 10513

**U.S. Department of Health and Human Services**
**National Institutes of Health**
**National Cancer Institute**
**Division of Basic Sciences**
**((Laboratory of Experimental Immunology)**
**Cellular and Molecular Immunology Section)**
*See:* Entry 10514

**U.S. Department of Health and Human Services**
**National Institutes of Health**
**National Cancer Institute**
**Division of Basic Sciences**
**((Laboratory of Experimental Immunology)**
**Experimental Therapeutics Section)**
*See:* Entry 10515

**U.S. Department of Health and Human Services**
**National Institutes of Health**
**National Cancer Institute**
**Division of Basic Sciences**
**((Experimental Immunology Branch)**
**Dinah Singer Laboratory)**
*See:* Entry 10523

**U.S. Department of Health and Human Services**
**National Institutes of Health**
**National Cancer Institute**
**Division of Basic Sciences**
**((Experimental Immunology Branch)**
**Alfred Singer Laboratory)**
*See:* Entry 10524

**U.S. Department of Health and Human Services**
**National Institutes of Health**
**National Cancer Institute**
**Division of Basic Sciences**
**((Experimental Immunology Branch)**
**Andre Nussenzweig Laboratory)**
*See:* Entry 10525

**U.S. Department of Health and Human Services**
**National Institutes of Health**
**National Cancer Institute**
**Division of Basic Sciences**
**((Experimental Immunology Branch)**
**Richard Hodes Laboratory)**
*See:* Entry 10526

**U.S. Department of Health and Human Services**
**National Institutes of Health**
**National Cancer Institute**
**Division of Basic Sciences**
**((Experimental Immunology Branch)**
**Pierre Henkart Laboratory)**
*See:* Entry 10527

**U.S. Department of Health and Human Services**
**National Institutes of Health**
**National Cancer Institute**
**Division of Basic Sciences**
**((Experimental Immunology Branch)**
**Michael Kuehn Laboratory)**
*See:* Entry 10528

**U.S. Department of Health and Human Services**
**National Institutes of Health**
**National Cancer Institute**
**Division of Basic Sciences**
**((Experimental Immunology Branch)**
**Paul Roche Laboratory)**
*See:* Entry 10529

**U.S. Department of Health and Human Services**
**National Institutes of Health**
**National Cancer Institute**
**Division of Basic Sciences**
**((Experimental Immunology Branch)**
**Gene Shearer Laboratory)**
*See:* Entry 10530

**U.S. Department of Health and Human Services**
**National Institutes of Health**
**National Cancer Institute**
**Division of Basic Sciences**
**((Experimental Immunology Branch)**
**Stephen Shaw Laboratory)**
*See:* Entry 10531

**U.S. Department of Health and Human Services**
**National Institutes of Health**
**National Cancer Institute**
**Division of Basic Sciences**
**((Experimental Immunology Branch)**
**David Segal Laboratory)**
*See:* Entry 10532

**U.S. Department of Health and Human Services**
**National Institutes of Health (NIH)**
**National Institute on Aging**
**Intramural Research Programs**
**(Laboratory of Immunology)**
*See:* Entry 3090

**★ 3292 ★ U.S. Department of Health and Human Services**
**National Institutes of Health**
**National Institute of Allergy and Infectious Diseases (NIAID)**
NIH Bldg. 31, Rm. 7A03
31 Center Dr., MSC2520
Bethesda, MD 20892-2520
**Phone:** (301)496-2263          **Fax:** (301)402-0120
**Email:** afauci@niaid.nih.gov
**Website:** http://www.niaid.nih.gov
Dr. Anthony S. Fauci, MD, Dir.
**Activities/Fields:** Causes of allergic, immunologic, and infectious diseases and to the development of better means of preventing, diagnosing, and treating illnesses. Its mission involves studies on: genetic control, maturation, characteristics, and manipulation of the immune system; disorders of the immune system, including asthma and other allergies, immuno-deficiency states, and autoimmunity; the role of the immune system in the pathogenesis of chronic diseases such as arthritis, the etiology, epidemiology, and pathogenesis of all types of infections (including those caused by viruses, mycoplasma, bacteria, fungi, and parasites) involving a variety of organ systems; the diagnosis, treatment, and prevention of all types of infections (including research on antimicrobial, antifungal, and antiviral therapy, and vaccines); and the role and mechanism of nucleic acid recombination in microbial agents. Fields of research include microbiology, parasitology, virology, bacteriology, genetics and transplantation biology, and mycology. The Institute is also concerned with enteric diseases and tropical diseases research. NIAID's program includes both in-

house (intramural) research and research conducted through grants, contracts, and interagency agreements (extramural). NIAID's extramural divisions are the Division of Acquired Immunodeficiency Syndrome (DAIDS), Division of Allergy, Immunology, and Transplantation (DAIT), and the Division of Microbiology and Infectious Diseases. NIAID's Division of Intramural Research (DIR) comprises 17 laboratories in Bethesda, MD, and the Rocky Mountain Laboratories in Hamilton, MT. Also supports a 52-bed inpatient service and outpatient research facility on the NIH campus.

**★ 3293 ★ U.S. Department of Health and Human Services**
**National Institutes of Health**
**National Institute of Dental and Craniofacial Research**
**Division of Intramural Research (Peptide and Immunochemistry Unit)**
Bldg. 30, Rm. B17B
30 Convent Dr., MSC 4340
Bethesda, MD 20892-4340
**Phone:** (301)496-4779        **Fax:** (301)402-0823
**Email:** frank.robey@nih.gov
**Website:** http://wwwdir.nidcr.nih.gov/dirweb/opcb/piu.asp
Dr. Frank Robey, Ch.

**Activities/Fields:** AIDS and cancer immunology, including immunosuppression in oral cancer.

**★ 3294 ★ University of Alabama at Birmingham**
**Division of Clinical Immunology and Rheumatology**
Tinsley Harrison Tower, 429A
Birmingham, AL 35294-0006
**Phone:** (205)934-5306        **Fax:** (205)934-1564
**Email:** robert.kimberly@ccc.uab.edu
**Website:** http://info.dom.uab.edu/rheum/index.htm
Dr. Robert P. Kimberly, Dir.

**Activities/Fields:** Rheumatic diseases and clinical immunology, including clinical studies on antibody receptor structure and function, glycopeptide chemistry, chemistry and physiology of complement, biochemical and biophysical properties of immunoglobulins, molecular biology of genetic risk factors, and pathophysiology of bone calcification. Conducts laboratory investigations in macromolecular physical chemistry, protein structure, polysaccharide chemistry, and immunology. **Pub:** *Arthritis Today Newsletter*, biennially.

**★ 3295 ★ University of Calgary**
**Health Science Centre**
**Immunology Research Group**
3330 Hospital Dr. NW
Calgary, AB, Canada T2N 4N1
**Phone:** (403)220-8558        **Fax:** (403)283-1267
**Email:** pkubes@acs.ucalgary.ca
**Website:** http://www.csi.ucalgary.ca/irg.nsf
Dr. Paul Kubes, Chm.

**Activities/Fields:** Characteristics and modulation of immune and inflammatory responses in normal and disease states. **Pub:** *Annual Report*.

**★ 3296 ★ University of California, Davis**
**Allergy-Clinical Immunology Program**
Sch. of Medicine, TB 192
1 Shields Ave.
Davis, CA 95616
**Phone:** (530)752-2884        **Fax:** (530)754-6047
**Email:** ssteuber@ucdavis.edu
Dr. Suzanne S. Teuber, Dir.

**Activities/Fields:** Cellular immunology and immunochemistry, especially the immunopathogenesis of systemic rheumatic diseases and autoimmune disorders, and the immunobiology of food allergies.

**★ 3297 ★ University of California, Los Angeles**
**Harbor-UCLA Medical Center**
**UCLA Center for Vaccine Research**
1124 W Carson St., Bldg. E6
Torrance, CA 90502
**Phone:** (310)222-2346        **Fax:** (310)782-8776
**Email:** joelward@ucla.edu
Dr. Joel Ward, Dir.

**Activities/Fields:** Clinical, epidemiologic, laboratory, and pharmacoeconomic studies of vaccines vaccine preventable dieases (all age groups, normal and high risk populations). Evaluation of mechanisms of immune responses to vaccines. Design and conduct multicenter trials nationally and internationally.

**★ 3298 ★ University of California, San Diego**
**Raz Laboratory**
126 Stein Clinical Research Bldg., MC 0663
9500 Gilman Dr.
La Jolla, CA 92093-0663
**Phone:** (858)534-5444        **Fax:** (858)534-5399
**Email:** eraz@ucsd.edu
**Website:** http://www.raz.ucsd.edu/
Eyal Raz, MD, Prin. Investigator

**Activities/Fields:** Immunostimulatory DNA sequences, both the basic science of how and why these sequences function and the applied science of how to prevent and treat human disease using their immunologic properties.

**★ 3299 ★ University of California, San Francisco**
**Immunogenetics and Transplantation Laboratory**
Main Hospital, Level B
Davies Medical Center
45 Castro St.
San Francisco, CA 94114
**Phone:** (415)476-3883        **Fax:** (415)476-0379
**Email:** baxterlowel@surgery.uscf.edu
Lee Ann Baxter-Lowe, PhD, Dir.

**Activities/Fields:** Immunogenetics and transplantation, including immunopharmacology of immunosuppressive agents.

**★ 3300 ★ University of California, San Francisco**
**Multiple Sclerosis Center**
350 Parnassus Ave., Ste. 908
San Francisco, CA 94117
**Phone:** (415)514-1684        **Fax:** (415)514-2443
**Website:** http://mscenter.ucsf.edu
Douglas S. Goodin, MD, Dir.

**Activities/Fields:** Cause and treatment of multiple sclerosis.

**University of Chicago**
**Gwen Knapp Center for Lupus and Immunology Research**
*See:* Entry 13723

**University of Cincinnati**
**Cincinnati Rheumatic Disease Study Group**
*See:* Entry 13724

**★ 3301 ★ University of Colorado**
**Immunology Center**
Division of Allergy & Clinical Immunology
4200 E 9th Ave., B164
Denver, CO 80262
**Phone:** (303)315-7601        **Fax:** (303)315-7642
**Email:** ffinkelman@mem.po.com
Dr. Brian L. Kotzin, Dir.

**Activities/Fields:** Provides a focus for research into the causes, prevention, and management of diseases such as asthma, allergies, systemic lupus erythematosus, rheumatoid arthritis, immune deficiencies and infection, plus related studies of fundamental immune mechanisms involving immune cells, antibodies, genetic factors, and immune regulatory systems. Ongoing studies include investigations of the genetic bais of autoimmunity, T cell activation in immuno-mediated diseases, mast cell activation in allergic and infectious diseases, the effects of benzopyrenes (from tobacco smoke) on T cell function, mechanisms underlying recurrent miscarriages, the role of soluble T cell receptors in contact hypersensitivity, and xenotransplantation of pancreatic islets.

**★ 3302 ★ University Hospital of Quebec**
**Pavilion CHUL Research Center**
**Rheumatology and Immunology Research Center**
2705 Blvd. Laurier, Rm. T 1-49
Sainte Foy, QC, Canada G1V 4G2
**Phone:** (418)654-2772        **Fax:** (418)654-2765
**Email:** sec.crri@crchul.ulaval.ca
**Website:** http://www.crchul.ulaval.ca/crchul/en/acti/Unite/rhum.htm
Pierre Borgeat, Dir.

**Activities/Fields:** Tissue damage in rheumatoid arthritis, regulation of leukotriene synthesis, arachidonic acid metabolism, regulation of antibody production, identification of major surface antigens, molecular mechanisms of neutrophil activation, effects of virus-leukocyte interactions on cell functional responses, regulation of apoptosis, MHC class II-mediated cell signaling, and importance of cellular compatibility.

**★ 3303 ★ University of Illinois at Chicago**
**Institute for Tuberculosis Research**
College of Pharmacy, MC 964
833 S Wood St.
Chicago, IL 60612-7231
**Phone:** (312)355-1715        **Fax:** (312)355-2693
**Email:** sgf@uic.edu
**Website:** http://itr.pharm.uic.edu
Scott G. Franzblau, PhD, Dir.

**Activities/Fields:** New drugs for tuberculosis, leprosy, and othe mycobacterial diseases, including tetracyclines, dications, efflux pump inhibitors, and natural products from plant and microbial sources. Drug delivery systems for established and experimental drugs are also researched. **Pub:** *Annual Reports*. • *Chicago Symposium Proceedings (1973-82)*.

**★ 3304 ★ University of Kansas**
**Allergy and Immunology Clinic**
3901 Rainbow Blvd.
Kansas City, KS 66160-7317
**Phone:** (913)588-3904        **Fax:** (913)588-3994
**Email:** dstechsc@kumc.edu
Dr. Daniel J. Stechschulte, Dir.

**Activities/Fields:** Studies of the normal mechanism that attract and inhibit the accumulation of WBG (type of defense cells) in the lungs and synovial membranes, clinical trials to evaluate the effectiveness of less toxic drugs in the treatment of systemic lupus erythematosus and rheumatoid arthritis, and studies on the role of mediators in the disease course of asthma.

**University of Kansas**
**Center for Neurobiology and Immunology Research (CNIR)**
*See:* Entry 14420

**★ 3305 ★ University of Maryland at Baltimore**
**Center for Celiac Research (CFCR)**
22 S Greene St., Box 140
Baltimore, MD 21201
**Phone:** (410)706-8021
**Email:** afasano@umaryland.edu

**Website:** http://www.celiaccenter.org/
Alessio Fasano, MD, Co-Med. Dir.

**Activities/Fields:** Celiac disease, including the prevalence of the disease worldwide; pathophysiology, autoimmune mechanisms, inflammatory processes, genetics of the disease; association with other autoimmune diseases; complications including infertility, osteoporosis and malignant transformation; and challenges of the treatment of the disease.

**University of Michigan
Immunology Laboratory**
*See:* Entry 6641

★ 3306 ★ **University of Minnesota
Bone Marrow Transplant Program**
420 Delaware St. SE, MMC 366
Minneapolis, MN 55474-0374
**Phone:** (612)626-2961          **Fax:** (612)626-4074
**Email:** ramsa001@umn.edu
**Website:** http://www.peds.umn.edu/divisions/bmt/directory.html
Dr. Norma Ramsay, Pediatric Dir.

**Activities/Fields:** Bone marrow transplantation.

★ 3307 ★ **University of North Carolina at Chapel Hill
Histocompatibility Laboratory**
1011 Anderson Pavilion
Department of Immunology
101 Manning Dr.
Chapel Hill, NC 27514
**Phone:** (919)966-4057          **Fax:** (919)966-4086
**Email:** jschmitz@unch.unc.edu
Dr. John Schmitz, Dir.

**Activities/Fields:** Diseases associated with histocompatibility antigens.

**University of North Carolina at Chapel Hill
Thurston Arthritis Research Center**
*See:* Entry 13733

★ 3308 ★ **University of Quebec
National Institute for Scientific Research-
Armand-Frappier Institute
Human Health Research Centre**
531, Blvd. des Prairies
Laval, QC, Canada H7V 1B7
**Phone:** (450)687-5010          **Fax:** (450)686-5501
**Email:** pierre.talbot@inrs-iaf.uquebec.ca
**Website:** http://www.inrs-iaf.uquebec.ca
Dr. Pierre Talbot, Dir.

**Activities/Fields:** Microbiology and immunity, including host-pathogen interactions, functions of regulators of immunity; environmental health, including toxicology and epidemiology; molecular pharmacochemistry, including peptides, natural products, and control of doping in sports.

★ 3309 ★ **University of Sherbrooke
Immunobiology Research Group
Clinical Research Center**
Faculty of Medicine
3001 N 12 Ave.
Sherbrooke, QC, Canada J1H 5N4
**Phone:** (819)346-1110          **Fax:** (819)564-5215
**Email:** mrolaple@courrier.usherb.ca
Dr. Marek Rola-Pleszczynski, Dir.

**Activities/Fields:** Immunoglobulin gene expression and control, lymphocyte activation pathways and second messangers, stem cell biology, cytokine receptor physiology, structure-function studies of lipid mediator receptors, natural cytotoxicity against tumor cells, ultraviolet-irradiation and immune functions, and immune interactions in atherosclerosis.

★ 3310 ★ **University of Southern California
Division of Rheumatology and Immunology**
2011 Zonal Ave., HMR 711
Los Angeles, CA 90033
**Phone:** (323)442-1946          **Fax:** (323)442-2874
**Email:** dhorwitz@hsc.usc.edu
David A. Horwitz, MD, Dir.

**Activities/Fields:** Pathogensis and treatment of human autoimmune diseases emphasizing systemic lupus erythematosus. The potential of regulatory T cells generated ex-vivo as a therapy for autoimmune diseases, for graft-versus-host disease associated with adoptive immunotherapy, and for the long-term survival or organ grafts.

**University of Tennessee, Knoxville
Human Immunology and Cancer Program
(HICP)**
*See:* Entry 10631

★ 3311 ★ **University of Virginia
Asthma and Allergic Diseases Center**
Division of Asthmas, Allergy & Immunology
University of Virginia Health System
Charlottesville, VA 22908
**Phone:** (434)924-5917          **Fax:** (434)924-5779
**Email:** tap2z@virginia.edu
**Website:** http://www.med.virginia.edu/medicine/clinical/internal/allergy/
Thomas A.E. Platts-Mills, MD, Dir.

**Activities/Fields:** Allergic and immunologic respiratory and skin diseases, especially asthma, hives, immunodeficiency diseases, respiratory fungal diseases, drug allergies, hay fever, and insect venom sensitivity.

★ 3312 ★ **University of Virginia
Beirne Carter Center for Immunology
Research**
Health Science Center
PO Box 801386
Charlottesville, VA 22908-1386
**Phone:** (434)924-9233          **Fax:** (434)924-1221
**Email:** lbm6b@galen.med.virginia.edu
**Website:** http://www.med.virginia.edu/cic
Dr. Thomas J. Braciale, Dir.

**Activities/Fields:** Basic and clinical immunology, infectious diseases, cancer, auto-immune diseases, and cell signaling in the immune system. **Pub:** *Annual report.* • *Research and training brochure.*

★ 3313 ★ **University of Wisconsin—
Madison
Allergy/Asthma Clinical Research Unit**
Medical School, K4/952 CSC
600 Highland Ave.
Madison, WI 53792-9988
**Phone:** (608)262-2804          **Fax:** (608)265-9890
**Email:** mjb@medicine.wisc.edu
**Website:** http://www.medicine.wisc.edu/sections/allergy/
Dr. William W. Busse, Dir.

**Activities/Fields:** Relationship between viruses and asthma using correlative studies derived from animal models and human experiments. In particular, the effect of virus infections on beta-adrenergic receptor structure, airway mechanics, mediator release from pulmonary alveolar cells, and the late phase reaction are studied. Research also involves characterization of B cell isotype repertoire responses to viral antigens. **Frmly:** Asthma and Allergic Diseases Cooperative Research Center.

# State & Regional Organizations

## Asthma & Allergies

*State chapters of the Asthma and Allergy Foundation of America are listed below. The national office is located at 1233 Twentieth St. NW, Ste. 402, Washington, DC 20036. Additional information can be obtained by calling the national office at (800) 7-ASTHMA or by consulting their web site at http://www.aafa.org.*

### Alaska

★ 3314 ★ **Asthma and Allergy
Foundation of America
Alaska Chapter**
PO Box 201927
Anchorage, AK 99520-1927
**Phone:** (907)696-4810
**Email:** aafaalaska@gci.net
Suzi Jackson, Exec Director

### California

★ 3315 ★ **Asthma and Allergy
Foundation of America
Northern California Chapter**
2269 Chestnut St., Ste. 481
San Francisco, CA 94123
**Phone:** (415)339-8880          **Fax:** (415)339-8881
**Email:** aafanorcal@yahoo.com
Ben Loewy, Exec Director

★ 3316 ★ **Asthma and Allergy
Foundation of America
Southern California Chapter**
5900 Wilshire Blvd., Ste. 2330
Los Angeles, CA 90036
**Phone:** (323)937-7859          **Free:** 800-624-0044
**Fax:** (323)937-7815
**Email:** aafasocal@aol.com
**Website:** http://www.aafasocal.com
Francene Lifson, Exec Director

### Florida

★ 3317 ★ **Asthma and Allergy
Foundation of America
Florida Chapter**
11700 N 58th St., Ste. J
Tampa, FL 33617
**Phone:** (813)983-0244          **Fax:** (813)983-9057
**Email:** johnlittle@aafaflorida.org
**Website:** http://www.aafaflorida.org

### Maryland

★ 3318 ★ **Asthma and Allergy
Foundation of America
Maryland-Greater Washington, D.C.,
Chapter**
1777 Reisterstown Rd., Ste. 370
Baltimore, MD 21208
**Phone:** (410)653-2880          **Fax:** (410)653-9611
**Email:** info@aafa-md.org
**Website:** http://www.aafa-md.org
Linda R. Boyer, Exec Director

### Massachusetts

★ 3319 ★ **Asthma and Allergy
Foundation of America
New England Chapter**
220 Boylston St.
Chestnut Hill, MA 02467
**Phone:** (617)965-7771          **Fax:** (617)965-8886

Email: aafane@aol.com
Patricia Goldman, Exec Director

## Michigan

★ 3320 ★ Asthma and Allergy
Foundation of America
**Michigan State Chapter**
17520 W 12 Mile Rd., Ste. 102
Southfield, MI 48076-1943
**Phone:** (248)557-8050      **Free:** 888-444-0333
**Fax:** (248)557-8768
**Email:** aafamich@aol.com
Karen Katz, Exec Director

## Missouri

★ 3321 ★ Asthma and Allergy
Foundation of America
**Greater Kansas City Chapter**
9140 Ward Parkway, Ste. 120
Kansas City, MO 64114
**Phone:** (816)333-6608      **Free:** 888-542-8252
**Fax:** (816)333-6608
**Email:** infor@aafakc.org
**Website:** http://www.aafakc.org
Noel Albert, Exec Director

★ 3322 ★ Asthma and Allergy
Foundation of America
**Saint Louis Chapter**
1500 S Big Bend, Ste. 1
Saint Louis, MO 63117
**Phone:** (314)645-2422      **Fax:** (314)645-2022
**Email:** aafa@mindspring.com
**Website:** http://postwebsites.com/stlouis/aafa
Patricia Williams, Exec Director

## New Jersey

★ 3323 ★ Asthma and Allergy
Foundation of America
**Southeastern Pennsylvania Chapter**
PO Box 115
32 Caspertown St.
Gibbstown, NJ 08027
**Phone:** (856)224-9547      **Fax:** (856)224-5893
**Email:** aafasepa@prodigy.net
Debi Maines, Exec Director

## Oregon

★ 3324 ★ Asthma and Allergy
Foundation of America
**Oregon Chapter**
14530 SW 144th Ave.
Tigard, OR 97224-1445
**Phone:** (503)579-8375

Email: hensches@teleport.com
Sandra L. Henschel, Exec Director

## Texas

★ 3325 ★ Asthma and Allergy
Foundation of America
**North Texas Chapter**
155 Southwood
Burleson, TX 76028
**Phone:** (817)483-8131      **Free:** 888-932-2232
**Email:** aafantx@hotmail.com
**Website:** http://www.aafa-ntx.org
Joan Hart, Exec Director

## Washington

★ 3326 ★ Asthma and Allergy
Foundation of America
**Washington State Chapter**
108 S Jackson St., Ste. 205
Seattle, WA 98104
**Phone:** (206)368-2866      **Free:** 800-778-2232
**Fax:** (206)368-2941
**Email:** aafawa@aafawa.org
**Website:** http://www.aafawa.org
Penny Nelson, Exec Director
**Remarks:** Based in Seattle. Serves the state of Washington.

# Federal Government Agencies

★ **3327** ★ **U.S. Department of Health and Human Services (NIH)**
**National Institutes of Health (NCCAM)**
**National Center for Complimentary and Alternative Medicine**
9000 Rockville Pike
Bethesda, MD 20892
**Phone:** (301)435-5042
**Website:** http://www.nccam.nih.gov

**Desc:** The Center works to prevent and alleviate human suffering by stimulating, developing, conducting, and supporting research on complimentary and alternative medicine. Research training programs develop skilled investigators necessary to conduct rigorous and relevant research to determine which complimentary and alternative medicine practices work, which do not, and why.

# Foundations & Other Funding Organizations

## Other Funding Organizations

★ **3328** ★ **American Holistic Nurses Association (AHNA)**
PO Box 2130
Flagstaff, AZ 86003-2130
**Phone:** (520)526-2196    **Free:** 800-278-2462
**Fax:** (520)526-2752
**Email:** ahna-flag@flaglink.com
**Website:** http://www.ahna.org
Doris Rager, Exec. Dir.

**Desc:** The AHNA is a 501(c) (3) non-profit educational organization whose membership is open to nurses and other individuals interested in holistically-oriented health care practices throughout the United States and the world. ASHNA supports the education of nurses, allied health practitioners, and the general public on health-related issues. The American Holistic Nurses' Association embraces nursing as a lifestyle and a profession and provides a means to create bonds within the nursing community. Because true healing comes from within, the AHNA recognizes that nurses must first heal themselves before they can facilitate the healing of others. **Awards:** Scholarship (annual).

★ **3329** ★ **Association for Applied Psychophysiology and Biofeedback (AAPB)**
10200 W 44th Ave., Ste. 304
Wheat Ridge, CO 80033
**Phone:** (303)422-8436    **Free:** 800-477-8892
**Fax:** (303)422-8894
**Email:** fbutler@resourcecenter.com

**Website:** http://www.aapb.org
Francine Butler, PhD, Pres.

**Desc:** Persons interested in the "interrelationship of external feedback systems, states of consciousness, and the physiological mechanisms involved." Promotes rapid interchange of ideas and information among members. Offers Continuing Education Training Programs. Maintains numerous committees. **Awards:** AAPB Foundation Award; Distinguished Scientist Award; Mary Brazier Scholarship; Student Travel Scholarship.

★ **3330** ★ **Biomagnetic Therapy Association (BTA)**
PO Box 394
Lyons, CO 80540
**Phone:** (303)823-0307
**Email:** info@biomagnetic.org
**Website:** http://www.biomagnetic.org
Suzy Balliett, Contact

**Desc:** Health care professionals and other individuals with an interest in biomagnetic therapy. Biomagnetic therapy is the art and science of applying and removing magnetic fields for health benefits. Seeks to advance the study and practice of biomagnetic therapy; promotes increased use of biomagnetic therapy in the treatment of a wide variety of disorders. Serves as a clearinghouse on biomagnetic and related therapies; conducts continuing professional education programs; sponsors research. **Awards:** William Philpott (annual).

★ **3331** ★ **Complementary Medicine Association (CMA)**
c/o Mary Wolken-Rodriguez
4649 E Malvern
Tucson, AZ 85711-4249
**Phone:** (602)323-6291    **Fax:** (602)323-0264
**Email:** compmeded@aol.com
Mary Wolken-Rodriguez, Exec. Off.

**Desc:** Provides education and supports cooperation between all medical disciplines. Fosters and teaches cost effective and more natural systems of medicine to professionals and the public. Focuses on homeopathic, acupuncture, herbal medicines, kinesiology and learning/memory improvement research and education. **Awards:** AIDS Education (annual).

★ **3332** ★ **Flower Essence Society (FES)**
PO Box 459
Nevada City, CA 95959
**Phone:** (530)265-9163    **Free:** 800-736-9222
**Fax:** (530)265-0584
**Email:** mail@flowersociety.org
**Website:** http://www.flowersociety.org
Patricia A. Kaminski, Pres.

**Desc:** Project of Earth-Spirit Inc. Health centers, holistic health practitioners, and interested individuals. Seeks to increase public awareness of Nature and the evolving spiritual relationship between human beings and the earth. Promotes the use of flower essences as catalysts to health and important tools "for personal and planetary evolution." Seeks to establish a worldwide network among health practitioners and others using flower essences. Encourages intuitive and scientific investigation of the essences and the creation of a center for educational and research programs. Organizes introductory weekends and annual weeklong intensives for professional and lay health practitioners. Sponsors lectures and research, educational, and experimental activities on topics concerning scientific and spiritual approaches to nature, preparation and use of flower essences, practical skills for flower essence practitioners, and recent developments in the field. Maintains library and referral service. Conducts seven-day professional training seminar and wildflower preservation and naturalist program. **Awards:** Scholarship (annual) for our certification program.

★ **3333** ★ **National Association for Holistic Aromatherapy**
4509 Interlake Ave., N, No. 233
Seattle, WA 98103
**Phone:** (206)547-2164    **Free:** 888-ASK-NAHA
**Fax:** (206)547-2680
**Email:** info@naha.org
**Website:** http://www.naha.org/
Jade Shutes, Pres.

**Desc:** Seeks to establish and promote the art and science of aromatherapy as a health care alternative. Works to elevate and maintain high standards of aromatherapy eduction. Works to raise public awareness of the benefits of aromatherapy. Fosters communication and exchange among members. Offers educational programs. Maintains speakers' bureau. **Awards:** Student Education Scholarship (annual).

★ **3334** ★ **National Center for Complementary and Alternative Medicine (NCCAM)**
PO Box 7923
Gaithersburg, MD 20898
**Phone:** (301)519-3153    **Free:** 888-644-6226
**Fax:** (866)464-3616
**Email:** info@nccam.nih.gov
**Website:** http://nccam.nih.gov/
Stephen E. Straus, MD, Dir.

**Desc:** Committed to exploring complementary and alternative healing practices, including but not limited to acupuncture, herbs, homeopathy, therapeutic massage, and traditional oriental medicine; trains CAM researchers; conducts biomedical research; disseminates information. Programs focus on evaluating the safety and efficacy of natural products, supporting pharmacological studies to determine potential interactive effects with standard treatment medications, evaluates CAM practices such as acupuncture and chiropractic. Acts as the NCCAM Clearinghouse. **Awards:** National Research Service Award Institutional Training Grants to eligible institutions to develop or enhance research training in specified areas of biomedical and behavioral research.

★ **3335** ★ **Nurse Healers Professional Associates International (NH-PAI)**
3760 Highland Dr., No. 429
Salt Lake City, UT 84106

**Phone:** (801)273-3399    **Fax:** (801)693-3537
**Email:** nh-pai@therapeutice-touch.org
**Website:** http://www.therapeutic-touch.org
Rebecca M. Good, MA, RN, LPC, Coor.
**Desc:** Official organization for Therapeutic Touch (TT). Healthcare professionals and lay persons united to promote a holistic approach to healing and health maintenance and nontraditional healing methods. Disseminates information on therapeutic touch. Maintains speakers' bureau; conducts research and educational programs for Therapeutic Touch. Sets standards and scope of practice for TT and recognition program for Qualified Therapeutic Touch teachers and practitioners. **Awards:** Healer's Award (annual); scholarship (annual) outstanding accomplishments in working for the advancement of complementary therapics through research, practice, education and/or publications.

★ 3336 ★ **The Radiance Technique International Association**
PO Box 40570
Saint Petersburg, FL 33743
**Phone:** (727)347-2106    **Free:** 888-878-7733
**Fax:** (727)347-2106
**Email:** trtia@aol.com
**Website:** http://www.trtia.org
Shoshanna Shay, Dir. Office Services
**Desc:** Protects and preserves the science known as The Radiance Technique, an Authentic Reiki "science of universal energy which harmonizes and aligns the mind-body-spirit dynamic." Provides a network for those interested in The Radiance Technique. Maintains speakers' bureau. Compiles statistics and conducts research on the effectiveness of The Radiance Technique. Creates and promotes Radiant Peace Projects and sponsors the International Day of Radiant Peace on June 22 every year. **Awards:** Peace Education Awards (annual) for elementary-school children writing on the selected theme about peace; Peace Profiles for people and organizations who have made a definite contribution towards peace locally or globally.

# Medical & Allied Health Schools

## Alternative Health Care

*Listed below are schools of alternative health. Individual specialties and techniques are listed for each school.*

### Alabama

★ 3337 ★ **The PATH Foundation, Birmingham**
1207 18th Ave. S
Birmingham, AL 35205
**Phone:** (205)322-7284
Cheryl W. Martin, Contact
**Program(s):** Hypnotherapy.

★ 3338 ★ **Red Mountain Institute for the Healing Arts Inc.**
1900 20th Ave. S, Ste. 220
Birmingham, AL 35209
**Phone:** (205)836-2024    **Fax:** (205)278-8802
Kitty Flewelling, Director
**Program(s):** Ayurvedic Medicine; Deep Tissue Massage; Massage Therapy; Neuromuscular Therapy; Swedish Massage.

### Alaska

★ 3339 ★ **Acupressure Institute of Alaska**
119 Second St.
Juneau, AK 99801

**Phone:** (907)463-5560
Alexander Majewski, Director
**Program(s):** Acupressure; Aromatherapy; CranioSacroTherapy; Jin Shin Do; Qigong; Shiatsu.

★ 3340 ★ **Gatekey School of Mind-Body Integration Studies**
4041 B St., Flr. 300
Anchorage, AK 99503-5945
**Phone:** (907)561-7327    **Fax:** (907)561-6582
Carol Stiles, Contact
**Program(s):** Body-Mind Integration; Energy Work; Massage Therapy; Reiki.

### Alberta

★ 3341 ★ **Calgary College of Holistic Health and Clinics, Inc.**
412 Silver Valley Rd. NW
Calgary, AB, Canada T3B 4B9
**Phone:** (403)288-4511    **Fax:** (403)288-0114
John Neumann, Contact
**Program(s):** Acupressure; Aromatherapy; Energy Work; Hypnotherapy; Massage Therapy; Reflexology; Shiatsu.

★ 3342 ★ **Foothills College of Massage Therapy**
7330 Fisher St., Ste. 400
Calgary, AB, Canada T2H 2H8
**Phone:** (403)255-4445    **Fax:** (403)255-4074
Beth Checkley, Contact
**Program(s):** Massage Therapy.

★ 3343 ★ **Mount Royal College Centre for Complementary Haelth Education**
2204 2nd St. SW
Calgary, AB, Canada T2S 1F5
**Phone:** (403)503-4886    **Fax:** (403)503-4899
Attiya Ghani, Contact
**Program(s):** Acupressure; Aromatherapy; Herbal Medicine; Massage Therapy; Reflexology; Sports Massage.

★ 3344 ★ **School of Homeopathy-Devon, England**
4 Oakvale Pl. SW
Calgary, AB, Canada T2V 1H4
**Phone:** (403)281-7976    **Fax:** (403)281-7976
Hana Stastny, Contact
**Program(s):** Anatomy and Physiology; Homeopathy; Pathology and Disease.

★ 3345 ★ **Yoga Association of Alberta**
Percy Page Center
11759 Groat Rd.
Edmonton, AB, Canada T5M 3K6
**Phone:** (403)427-8776    **Fax:** (403)427-0524
Margo Balog, Contact
**Program(s):** Yoga Teacher Training.

### Arizona

★ 3346 ★ **Arizona School of Integrative Studies**
753 N Main St.
Cottonwood, AZ 86326
**Phone:** (520)639-3455    **Fax:** (520)639-3694
Jamie Rongo, Director
**Program(s):** Acupressure; Aromatherapy; CranioSacral Therapy; Energy Work; Homeopathy; Hydrotherapy; Massage Therapy; Polarity Therapy; Qigong; Reflexology; Shiatsu; Sports Massage; Structural Integration.

★ 3347 ★ **Bonnie Prudden School of Physical Fitness and Myotherapy, LLC**
4725 E Sunrise Dr., Ste. 346
Tucson, AZ 85718
**Phone:** (520)529-3979    **Free:** 800-221-4634
**Fax:** (520)529-6679
**Email:** info@bonnieprudden.com
Bonnie Prudden, Director
**Program(s):** Exercise Therapy; Myotherapy.

★ 3348 ★ **Desert Institute of the Healing Arts**
639 N 6th Ave.
Tucson, AZ 85705-8330
**Phone:** (520)882-0899    **Free:** 800-733-8098
**Fax:** (520)624-2996
**Website:** http://www.diha.com
Margaret Avery Moon, Director
**Program(s):** Aromatherapy; Hydrotherapy; Massage Therapy; Reflexology; Shiatsu; Sports Massage.

★ 3349 ★ **Foundation for Holistic Health Therapy**
80 Farmer Brothers Dr.
Sedona, AZ 86336
**Phone:** (520)204-1968    **Free:** 800-578-7312
**Fax:** (520)204-1968
**Email:** drbrown@cybertrails.com
**Website:** http://www.sedona-web.com/Lymphatic
William N. Brown, PhD, Director
**Program(s):** Energy Work; Lymphatic Massage.

★ 3350 ★ **Institute for Natural Therapeutics**
217 W University Dr.
Mesa, AZ 85201
**Phone:** (602)844-2255    **Fax:** (602)962-9907
Amy K. Hatch, Contact
**Program(s):** Aromatherapy; CranioSacral Therapy; Deep Tissue Massage; Massage Therapy; Reflexology; Reiki; Shiatsu.

★ 3351 ★ **International Foundation of Bio-Magnetics**
5447 E 5th st., Ste. 111
Tucson, AZ 85711
**Phone:** (520)751-7751    **Fax:** (520)751-7751
John Munno, Contact
**Program(s):** Bio-Magnetic Touch Healing; Energy Work.

★ 3352 ★ **International Yoga Studies**
13833 S 31st Pl.
Phoenix, AZ 85048
**Phone:** (602)759-1972    **Fax:** (602)704-9656
Sandra Summerfield Kozak, Director
**Program(s):** Ayurvedic Medicine; Yoga Teacher Training.

★ 3353 ★ **Jin Shin Jyutsu, Inc.**
8719 E San Alberto Dr.
Scottsdale, AZ 85258
**Phone:** (602)998-9331    **Fax:** (602)998-9335
David Burmeister, Director
**Program(s):** Jin Shin Jyutsu.

★ 3354 ★ **Phoenix Institute of Herbal Medicine and Acupuncture**
7501 E Oak, Ste. 114-115
Scottsdale, AZ 85252
**Phone:** (602)994-3648    **Fax:** (602)439-1511
Mary Beth Madden, Contact
**Program(s):** Acupuncture; Herbal Medicine; Traditional Chinese Medicine.

**★ 3355 ★ Phoenix Therapeutic Massage College**
609 N Scottsdale Rd.
Scottsdale, AZ 85257
**Phone:** (480)945-9461  **Fax:** (480)425-8247
Rose Taylor, Contact
**Program(s):** Massage Therapy; Swedish Massage.

**★ 3356 ★ RainStar College**
4130 N Goldwater Blvd.
Scottsdale, AZ 85251
**Phone:** (602)423-0375  **Fax:** (602)945-9824
Edvard R. Richards, Director
**Program(s):** Acupressure; Aromatherapy; Breathwork; Chinese Herbal Medicine; CranioSacral Therapy; Geriatric Massage; Herbal Medicine; Homeopathy; Hydrotherapy; Hypnotherapy; Iridology; Lymphatic Massage; Massage Therapy; Myofascial Release; On-Site Massage; Oriental Medicine; Pediatric Massage; Pregnancy Massage; Qigong; Reflexology; Reiki; Shiatsu; Spa Therapies; Sports Massage; Traditional Chinese Medicine; Trigger Point Therapy.

**★ 3357 ★ Southwest College of Naturopathic Medicine and Health Sciences**
2140 E Broadway Rd.
Tempe, AZ 85282
**Phone:** (602)858-9100  **Fax:** (602)858-9116
**Website:** http://www.scnm.edu
Melissa Winquist, Contact
**Program(s):** Acupuncture; Naturopathic Medicine.

**★ 3358 ★ Southwest Institute of Healing Arts**
1402 N Miller Rd., Ste. D-2
Scottsdale, AZ 85257
**Phone:** (602)994-9244  **Fax:** (602)994-3228
K.C. Miller, Director
**Program(s):** Acupressure; Acupuncture; Aromatherapy; Ayurvedic Medicine; Body-Mind Psychology; Childbirth Educator; CranioSacral Therapy; Doula; Energy Work; Equine Massage; Holistic Health; Herbal Medicine; Hypnotherapy; Massage Therapy; Oriental Medicine; Polarity Therapy; Qigong; Reflexology; Reiki; Shiatsu; Sports Massage; Traditional Chinese Medicine; Yoga Teacher Training.

**★ 3359 ★ University of Arizona, College of Medicine**
**Program of Integrative Medicine**
1249 N Mountain
Tucson, AZ 85724-5153
**Phone:** (520)626-7222  **Fax:** (520)626-6484
**Website:** http://www.ahsc.arizona.edu/integrative_medicine
Andrew Weil, MD, Contact
**Program(s):** Integrative Medicine.

**★ 3360 ★ Wesland Institute**
3367 N Country Club Rd.
Tucson, AZ 85716-1349
**Phone:** (520)881-1530  **Fax:** (520)881-1530
Richard Corvino, Director
**Program(s):** Hypnotherapy; Neuro-Linguistic Programming.

## Arkansas

**★ 3361 ★ American Academy of Healing Arts**
**School of Massage Therapy**
1501 N University, Ste. 570
Little Rock, AR 72207
**Phone:** (501)666-9100  **Free:** 888-666-9101
**Fax:** (501)666-3133
Eileen Joyce, Contact

**Program(s):** CranioSacral Therapy; Deep Tissue Massage; Energy Work; Hydrotherapy; Massage Therapy; Polarity Therapy; Reflexology; Shiatsu.

**★ 3362 ★ Body Wellness Therapeutic Massage Academy**
11323 Arcade Dr.
Little Rock, AR 72212
**Phone:** (501)219-2639  **Fax:** (501)221-7626
**Email:** bodywellness@aristotle.net
Donna McGriff, Contact
**Program(s):** Acupressure; Aromatherapy; Ayurvedic Medicine; Deep Muscle Massage; Energy Work; Massage Therapy; Myofascial Release; Polarity Therapy; Reflexology; Reiki; Sports Massage; Swedish Massage.

**★ 3363 ★ Center for Wellbeing**
101 W Mountain
GCM Bldg., Ste. 107
Fayetteville, AR 72701
**Phone:** (501)442-2026  **Fax:** (501)442-2897
**Email:** cbeckerphd@aol.com
Chandana Becker, PhD, Director
**Program(s):** Polarity Therapy; Somatic Experiencing (Shock Trauma Renegotiaation Therapy).

**★ 3364 ★ A Healing Touch, Inc.**
**Clinic and School of Massage Therapy**
2201 Rogers Ave., Ste. F
Fort Smith, AR 72901
**Phone:** (501)783-7566
Wendy L. Morgan, Contact
**Program(s):** Acupressure; Aromatherapy; CranioSacral Therapy; Deep Tissue Massage; Energy Work; Herbal Medicine; Hypnotherapy; Massage Therapy; Shiatsu; Traditional Chinese Medicine.

**★ 3365 ★ Hot Springs School of Therapy Technology**
1415 N Moore Rd.
Hot Springs, AR 71913
**Free:** 800-844-0667
Ronald L. Wallace, Contact
**Program(s):** Acupressure; Aromatherapy; Herbal Medicine; Hydrotherapy; Massage Therapy; Reflexology; Shiatsu.

**★ 3366 ★ Jean's School of Therapy Technology, Inc.**
655 Park Ave.
Hot Springs, AR 71901
**Phone:** (501)623-9686  **Fax:** (501)623-0070
Jean R. Miller, Contact
**Program(s):** Acupressure; Deep Tissue Massage; Massage Therapy; Reflexology; Reiki; Shiatsu.

**★ 3367 ★ White River School of Massage**
48 Colt Square Dr.
Fayetteville, AR 72703
**Phone:** (501)521-2550  **Fax:** (501)521-2558
Ellen May, Director
**Program(s):** Aromatherapy; CranioSacral Therapy; Energy Work; Massage Therapy; Myofascial Release; Neuromuscular Therapy; Reflexology; Shiatsu; Sports Massage.

## British Columbia

**★ 3368 ★ Canadian College of Acupuncture and Oriental Medicine**
855 Cormorant St.
Victoria, BC, Canada V8W 1R2
**Phone:** (250)384-2942  **Fax:** (250)360-2871
Diane St. Hilair, Contact
**Program(s):** Acupressure; Acupuncture; Herbal Medicine; Oriental Medicine; Traditional Chinese Medicine.

**★ 3369 ★ Dominion Herbal College**
7527 Kingsway
Burnaby, BC, Canada V3N 3C1
**Phone:** (604)521-5822  **Fax:** (604)526-1561
Bernice Birzneck, Contact
**Program(s):** Aromatherapy; Herbal Medicine.

**★ 3370 ★ Meridian Institute**
225 Canada Ave., Ste. 105
Duncan, BC, Canada V9L 1T6
**Phone:** (250)748-3588  **Fax:** (250)748-3578
Doris Gray, Contact
**Program(s):** Hypnotherapy.

**★ 3371 ★ Vancouver Homeopathic Academy**
PO Box 34095, Stn D
Vancouver, BC, Canada V6J 4M1
**Phone:** (604)708-9387  **Fax:** (604)708-1547
Kim Boutilier, Contact
**Program(s):** Homeopathy.

**★ 3372 ★ West Coast College of Massage Therapy**
555 W Hastings St., 6th Flr.
Vancouver, BC, Canada V6B 4N6
**Phone:** (604)689-3854  **Free:** 888-449-2242
**Fax:** (604)689-9804
Christine Mullie, Contact
**Program(s):** Acupuncture; Herbal Medicine; Humanistic Counseling; Hydrotherapy; Massage Therapy; Reflexology; Shiatsu.Nturopathic Medicine; Traditional Chinese Medicine.

## California

**★ 3373 ★ Academy of Chinese Culture & Health Sciences**
1601 Clay St.
Oakland, CA 94612
**Phone:** (510)763-7787  **Fax:** (510)834-8646
**Email:** acchs@best.com
**Program(s):** Acupuncture; Herbal Medicine; Traditional Chinese Medicine.

**★ 3374 ★ Academy for Guided Imagery**
311 Miller Ave., Ste. G
PO Box 2070
Mill Valley, CA 94942
**Free:** 800-726-2070  **Fax:** (415)389-9342
**Website:** http://www.healthy.net/agi
Martin Rossman, MD, Director
**Program(s):** Guided Imagery.

**★ 3375 ★ Academy of Health Professions**
6784 El Cajon Blvd., Ste. G
San Diego, CA 92105
**Phone:** (619)464-3570  **Fax:** (619)461-5375
Karen Croft, Contact
**Program(s):** Aromatherapy; Deep Tissue Massage; Energy Work; Hawaiian Massage; Herbal Medicine; Holistic Health; Hypnotherapy; Massage Therapy; Nutrition; Passive Joint Movement; Pregnancy Massage; Reflexology; Reiki; Shiatsu; Sports Massage; Structural Alignment; Swedish Massage; Tui Na.

**★ 3376 ★ Academy of Professional Careers**
8376 Hercules St.
La Mesa, CA 91942
**Phone:** (619)461-5100  **Fax:** (619)461-1401
Juanita Cherry, Contact
**Program(s):** Energy Work; Holistic Health; Massage Therapy; Neuromuscular Therapy; Nutrition; Reflexology; Reiki; Shiatsu; Sports Massage.

**★ 3377 ★ Acupressure Institute: Shiatsu, Massage & Asian Bodywork Trainings**
1533 Shattuck Ave.
Berkeley, CA 94709
**Phone:** (510)845-1059    **Fax:** (510)845-1496
**Email:** colburn@acupressure.com
**Website:** http://www.acupressure.com
Pat Colburn, Contact

**Program(s):** Acupressure; Emotional Balancing; Energy Work; Massage Therapy; Oriental Medicine; Shiatsu; Sports Massage; Thai Massage; Traditional Chinese Medicine; Yoga Teacher Training.


**★ 3378 ★ Advanced School of Massage Therapy**
1414 E Thousand Oaks Blvd., Ste. 211, 213
Thousand Oaks, CA 91362
**Phone:** (805)495-1353    **Fax:** (805)379-1408
Jan Suckut, Contact

**Program(s):** CranioSacral Therapy; Energy Work; Facial Massage; Infant Massage; Massage Therapy; Pregnancy Massage; Reflexology; Sports Massage; Trigger Point Therapy.


**★ 3379 ★ Alexander Educational Center**
St. John Presbyterian Church
2727 College Ave., Rm. 207
Berkeley, CA 94705
**Phone:** (925)937-5746
Giora Pinkas, Director

**Program(s):** Alexander Technique.


**★ 3380 ★ Alexander Training Institute of Los Angeles**
1526 14th St., Ste. 110
Santa Monica, CA 90404
**Phone:** (310)395-9170
Lyn Charlsen, Director

**Program(s):** Alexander Technique.


**★ 3381 ★ Alexander Training Institute of San Francisco**
ACT
30 Grant Ave., 8th Fl.
San Francisco, CA 94108
**Phone:** (415)439-2465
Frank Ottiwell, Director

**Program(s):** Alexander Technique.


**★ 3382 ★ Alive & Well! Institute of Conscious BodyWork**
100 Shaw Dr.
San Anselmo, CA 94960
**Phone:** (415)258-0402    **Fax:** (415)258-0635
**Email:** alivewel@aol.com
Jocelyn Olivier, Director

**Program(s):** Acupressure; Aromatherapy; CranioSacral Therapy; Massage Therapy; Neuromuscular Reprogramming; Polarity Therapy; Qigong; Reflexology; Synergetic Studies.


**★ 3383 ★ American Academy of Reflexology**
606 E Magnolia Blvd., Ste. B
Burbank, CA 91501-2618
**Phone:** (818)841-7741    **Fax:** (818)841-2346
Bill Flocco, Contact

**Program(s):** Reflexology.


**★ 3384 ★ American College of Traditional Chinese Medicine**
455 Arkansas St.
San Francisco, CA 94107
**Phone:** (415)282-7600    **Fax:** (415)282-0856
**Email:** lhuang@actcm.org
**Website:** http://www.actcm.org
Lixin Huang, Contact

**Program(s):** Acupuncture; Herbal Medicine; Qigong; Traditional Chinese Medicine.


**★ 3385 ★ American Institute of Hypnotherapy**
16842 Von Karman Ave., Ste. 475
Irvine, CA 92606
**Phone:** (949)261-6400    **Free:** 800-872-9996
**Fax:** (949)251-4632
Guy Robert, Contact

**Program(s):** Hypnotherapy.


**★ 3386 ★ American Institute of Massage Therapy, Inc., Costa Mesa**
2156 Newport Blvd.
Costa Mesa, CA 92627
**Phone:** (949)642-0735    **Fax:** (949)642-1729
M.K. Hungerford, PhD, Contact

**Program(s):** Acupressure; Aromatherapy; CranioSacral Therapy; Massage Therapy; Neuromuscular Therapy; Reflexology; Reiki; Shiatsu; Sports Massage; Swedish Massage; Thai Massage.


**★ 3387 ★ Ayurveda Institute of Massage and Spa Services**
3140 Stone Station
Sebastopol, CA 95472
**Phone:** (707)523-9923    **Fax:** (707)824-4778
Dharmini Zelin, Contact

**Program(s):** Ayurvedic Medicine; Energy Work; Massage Therapy; Polarity Therapy; Reflexology; Spa Therapies.


**★ 3388 ★ Belavi Institute for Facial Massage**
1500 N Coast Hwy.
Laguna Beach, CA 92651
**Phone:** (714)443-1954    **Free:** 800-235-2844
**Fax:** (714)443-2292
Belle Tuckerman, Contact

**Program(s):** Facial Massage; Spa Therapies.


**★ 3389 ★ Biofeedback Institute of Los Angeles**
3710 S Robertson Blvd., Ste. 216
Culver City, CA 90232-2351
**Phone:** (310)841-4970    **Free:** 800-246-3526
**Fax:** (310)840-0923
Marjorie K. Toomin, PhD, Director

**Program(s):** Biofeedback; Neuromuscular Therapy.


**★ 3390 ★ Biofeedback Training Institute - Stens Corp.**
6451 Oakwood Dr.
Oakland, CA 94611
**Free:** 800-257-8367    **Fax:** (510)339-2222
**Email:** stensco@aol.com
Wendy Kesseler, Contact

**Program(s):** Biofeedback.


**★ 3391 ★ Body Therapy Center**
368 California Ave.
Palo Alto, CA 94306
**Phone:** (650)328-9400    **Fax:** (650)328-9478
Laura Skinner, Contact

**Program(s):** CranioSacral Therapy; Deep Tissue Massage; Esalen Massage; Massage Therapy; On-Site Massage; Reflexology; Reiki; Shiatsu; Sports Massage; Swedish Massage.


**★ 3392 ★ Body Therapy Institute of Santa Barbara**
835 N Milpas St.
Santa Barbara, CA 93103
**Phone:** (805)966-5802
Gael Ashwood, Contact

**Program(s):** Accupressure; CranioSacral Therapy; Deep Tissue Massage; Energy Work; Holistic Health; Massage Therapy; Polarity Therapy; Qigong; Reflexology; Reiki; Shiatsu.


**★ 3393 ★ Breema Center**
6076 Claremont Ave.
Oakland, CA 94618
**Phone:** (510)428-0937    **Fax:** (510)428-9235
Mary Cunio, Contact

**Program(s):** Breema Bodywork.


**★ 3394 ★ British Institute of Homeopathy and Complementary Medicine**
520 Washington Blvd., Ste. 423
Marina Del Rey, CA 90292
**Phone:** (310)557-2235    **Fax:** (310)577-0296
**Email:** bihus@thegrid.net
Dr. Trevor Cook, Contact

**Program(s):** Animal Therapy; Flower Essences; Herbal Medicine; Homeopathy.


**★ 3395 ★ Calaveras College of Therapeutic Massage**
96 Court St.
PO Box 274
San Andreas, CA 95249
**Phone:** (209)754-4876
Michelle Olkowski, Contact

**Program(s):** Acupressure; Aromatherapy; CranioSacral Therapy; Massage Therapy; Reflexology; Shiatsu; Swedish Massage.


**★ 3396 ★ California College of Ayurveda**
1117A E Main St.
Grass Valley, CA 95945
**Phone:** (530)274-9100    **Fax:** (530)274-7350
Marc Halpern, Contact

**Program(s):** Aromatherapy; Ayurvedic Medicine; Herbal Medicine.


**★ 3397 ★ California College of Physical Arts, Inc.**
18582 Beach Blvd., Ste. 11
Huntington Beach, CA 92648
**Phone:** (714)964-7744    **Fax:** (714)962-3934
**Email:** calcopa@gte.net
**Website:** http://www.fyi.com
Deborah S. Mulholland, Director

**Program(s):** Acupressure; Alexander Technique; Aromatherapy; Herbal Medicine; Holistic Health; Massage Therapy; Oriental Medicine; Reflexology; Reiki; Shiatsu; Sports Massage.


**★ 3398 ★ California Graduate Institute**
1145 Gayley Ave., Ste. 322
Los Angeles, CA 90024
**Phone:** (310)208-4240    **Fax:** (310)208-0684
Terry Oleson, PhD, Contact

**Program(s):** Biofeedback; Hypnotherapy.


**★ 3399 ★ California Institute of Integral Sciences**
1453 Mission St.
San Francisco, CA 94103
**Phone:** (415)575-6126    **Fax:** (415)575-1264
**Email:** iang@ciis.edu
**Website:** http://www.ciis.edu
Ian Grand, Director

**Program(s):** Somatic Education.


**★ 3400 ★ California Institute of Massage and Spa Services**
139 E Napa St.
730 Broadway
Sonoma, CA 95476
**Phone:** (707)939-9431
Kate Alves, Director

Program(s): Acupressure; Aromatherapy; CranioSacral Therapy; Energy Work; Massage Therapy; Polarity Therapy; Reflexology; Shiatsu; Spa Therapies; Swedish Massage.

**★ 3401 ★ California Naturopathic College**
1228 Camino Del Mar
Del Mar, CA 92014
**Phone:** (619)259-1222        **Fax:** (619)259-0730
Bettina Yelman, Contact

Program(s): Acupressure; Aromatherapy; Ayurvedic Medicine; CranioSacral Therapy; Energy Work; Herbal Medicine; Holistic Health; Homeopathy; Hypnotherapy; Massage Therapy; Naturopathic Medicine; Nutrition; Oriental Medicine; Polarity Therapy; Reflexology; Reiki; Shiatsu; Sports Massage.

**★ 3402 ★ California School of Herbal Studies**
9309 Hwy. 116
Forestville, CA 95436
**Phone:** (707)887-7457
James Green, Director

Program(s): Aromatherapy; Herbal Medicine.

**★ 3403 ★ Calistoga Massage Therapy School**
5959 Commerce Blvd., Ste. 13
Rohnert Park, CA 94928
**Phone:** (707)586-1953
Dr. Steven L. Ticen, Contact

Program(s): Massage Therapy.

**★ 3404 ★ Caring Hands School of Massage**
1484 E Main St.
Ventura, CA 93001
**Phone:** (805)643-3032

Program(s): Acupressure; LomiLomi Massage; Massage Therapy; Shiatsu.

**★ 3405 ★ Center for the Alexander Technique**
714 Nash Ave.
Menlo Park, CA 94025
**Phone:** (650)328-4736
Edward Avak, Director

Program(s): Alexander Technique.

**★ 3406 ★ Center for Conscious Touch - Lupin Massage Institute**
PO Box 1274
Los Gatos, CA 95031
**Phone:** (408)353-4231
Stuart Grace, Contact

Program(s): Acupressure; Anatomy and Phisiology; CranioSacral Therapy; Esalen Massage; Manual Lymph Drainage; Massage Therapy; Swedish Massage; Visceral Massage.

**★ 3407 ★ Center for Hypnotherapy Certification**
455 Newton Ave., Ste. 1
Oakland, CA 94606
**Phone:** (510)839-4800        **Free:** 800-398-0034
**Fax:** (510)836-0477
Marilyn Gordon, Director

Program(s): Hypnotherapy.

**★ 3408 ★ Central California School of Body Therapy**
1330 Southwood Dr., Ste. 7
San Luis Obispo, CA 93401
**Phone:** (805)783-2200        **Fax:** (805)783-2200
**Email:** siouxsun1@aol.com
Susan E. Stocks, Contact

Program(s): Acupressure; CranioSacral Therapy; Herbal Medicine; Homeopathy; Hypnotherapy; Massage Therapy; Shiatsu.

**★ 3409 ★ Charles R. Drew University of Medicine and Sciences**
**College of Allied Health Sciences**
**Nurse-Midwifery Education Program**
1621 E 120th St.
Los Angeles, CA 90059
**Phone:** (213)563-4951
H. Frances Hayes-Cushenberry, Director

Program(s): Midwifery.

**★ 3410 ★ Chico Therapy: Wellness Center**
1215 Mangrove Ave., Ste. B
Chico, CA 95926
**Phone:** (530)891-4301        **Fax:** (530)891-4359
Mike L. Metzger, Contact

Program(s): Acupressure; Aromatherapy; Ayurvedic Medicine; Deep Tissue Massage; Herbal Medicine; Infant Massage; Manual Lymph Drainage; Massage Therapy; Neuromuscular Therapy; Prenatal Massage; Reflexology; Shiatsu; Traditional Chinese Medicine.

**★ 3411 ★ Chopra Center for Well Being**
7630 Fay Ave.
La Jolla, CA 92037
**Phone:** (619)551-7788        **Fax:** (619)551-9570
David Simon, MD, Director

Program(s): Ayurvedic Medicine; Childbirth Education; Herbal Medicine; Meditation; Mind-Body Medicine.

**★ 3412 ★ Circle of Friends**
704 N Hwy. 101
Leucadia, CA 92024
**Free:** 800-434-9642        **Fax:** (619)753-5785
**Email:** rudra@unit.edu
Rudi M. Kadre, Director

Program(s): Yoga Teacher Training; Meditation.

**★ 3413 ★ Cleveland Chiropractic College, Los Angeles**
590 N Vermont Ave.
Los Angeles, CA 90004
**Phone:** (213)660-6166        **Free:** 800-466-2252
**Fax:** (213)660-5387
Carl S. Cleveland, Contact

Program(s): Chiropractic.

**★ 3414 ★ College of Bio-Energetic Medicine**
1955 Lucile, Ste. D
Stockton, CA 95209
**Phone:** (209)473-4993        **Fax:** (209)473-4997
Michael J. Eakin, Contact

Program(s): Acupressure; Aromatherapy; Deep Tissue Massage; Energy Work; Massage Therapy; Qigong; Reflexology; Reiki; Thai Massage; Traditional Chinese Medicine.

**★ 3415 ★ Conscious Choice School of Massage and Integral Healing Arts**
698 Azalea
Redding, CA 96002
**Phone:** (530)224-0957
Robert Newman, Contact

Program(s): Acupressure; Ayurvedic Medicine; CranioSacral Therapy; Deep Tissue Massage; Energy Work; Hypnotherapy; Massage Therapy; Polarity Therapy; Reflexology; Reiki.

**★ 3416 ★ Curenter University**
11543 Olympic Blvd.
Los Angeles, CA 90064

**Phone:** (310)914-4116        **Fax:** (310)479-3376
Marlan Goodwin, Contact

Program(s): Biofeedback; Holistic Health; Honeopathy; Iridology.

**★ 3417 ★ Cypress Health Institute**
PO Box 2941
Santa Cruz, CA 95063
**Phone:** (831)476-2115
Larry Bernstein, Contact

Program(s): Acupressure; CranioSacral Therapy; Deep Tissue Massage; Holistic Health; Hypnotherapy; Massage Therapy; Polarity Therapy; Reflexology; Sports Massage; Swedish Massage; Thai Massage.

**★ 3418 ★ Dandelion Herbal Center**
4803 Greenwood Hts. Dr.
Kneeland, CA 95549
**Phone:** (707)442-8157
Jane Bothwell, Director

Program(s): Herbal Medicine.

**★ 3419 ★ Day Break Geriatric Massage Project**
19091 N 5th St.
216 Pleasant Hill Ave. N
Sebastopol, CA 95472
**Phone:** (707)829-2798        **Fax:** (707)829-2799
Felicity Doyle, Contact

Program(s): Geriatric Massage.

**★ 3420 ★ Desert Resorts School of Somatherapy**
13100 Palm Dr.
Desert Hot Springs, CA 92240
**Phone:** (760)329-1175        **Fax:** (760)329-5925
Ramona Moody French, Director

Program(s): Acupressure; Aromatherapy; CranioSacral Therapy; Deep Tissue Massage; Holistic Health; Manual Lymph Drainage; Massage Therapy; Polarity Therapy; Reflexology; Shiatsu; Sports Massage; Swedish Massage.

**★ 3421 ★ Desert Springs Therapy Center**
Banning Massage School
66-705 E 6th St.
Desert Hot Springs, CA 92240
**Phone:** (760)329-5066        **Fax:** (760)251-6206
**Email:** dstc@gnn.com
Charles Thomas, Director

Program(s): Deep Tissue Massage; Hydrotherapy; Massage Therapy; Sports Massage.

**★ 3422 ★ Diamond Light School of Massage and Healing Arts**
45 San Clemente Dr.
Corte Madera, CA 94925
**Phone:** (415)454-6651
Vajra Matusow, Director

Program(s): Acupressure; Energy Work; Hypnotherapy; Massage Therapy; Reflexology; Reiki; Swedish Massage.

**★ 3423 ★ Dongguk Royal University**
440 Shatto Pl.
Los Angeles, CA 90020
**Phone:** (213)487-0110        **Free:** 800-303-1800
**Fax:** (213)487-0527
David Burciaga, Contact

Program(s): Acupressure; Acupuncture; Herbal Medicine; Oriental Medicine; Qigong; Traditional Chinese Medicine.

**★ 3424 ★ Dry Creek Herb Farm and Learning Center**
13935 Dry Creek Rd.
Auburn, CA 95602

**Phone:** (530)878-2441 **Fax:** (530)878-0613
Shatoiya de la Tour, Director

**Program(s):** Aromatherapy; Ayurvedic Medicine; Energy Work; Herbal Medicine; Qigong; Traditional Chinese Medicine.


★ 3425 ★ **East West School of Herbology**
PO Box 712
Santa Cruz, CA 95061
**Free:** 800-717-5010 **Fax:** (831)336-4548
Jill Agnello, Contact

**Program(s):** Herbal Medicine.


★ 3426 ★ **Emperor's College of Traditional Oriental Medicine**
1807 Wilshire Blvd.
Santa Monica, CA 90403
**Phone:** (310)453-8300 **Fax:** (310)829-3838
**Email:** dsl@emperors.edu
**Website:** http://www.emperors.edu
Leah McMahan, Contact

**Program(s):** Acupressure; Acupuncture; Herbal Medicine; Massage Therapy; Oriental Medicine; Qigong; Reflexology; Reiki; Traditional Chinese Medicine.


★ 3427 ★ **Esalen Institute**
Hwy. 1
Big Sur, CA 93920
**Phone:** (408)667-3000

**Program(s):** Esalen Massage.


★ 3428 ★ **Evergreen Herb Garden and Learning Center**
PO Box 1445
Placerville, CA 95667
**Phone:** (916)626-9288 **Fax:** (916)626-9288
Candis Cantin Packard, Contact

**Program(s):** Ayurvedic Medicine; Herbal Medicine; Polarity Therapy.


★ 3429 ★ **Expanding Light at Ananda**
14618 Tyler Foote Rd.
Nevada City, CA 95959
**Free:** 800-346-5350 **Fax:** (530)478-7519
Richard McCord, Contact

**Program(s):** Yoga Teacher Training.


★ 3430 ★ **Feldenkrais Resources**
830 Bancroft Way, Ste. 112
Berkeley, CA 94710
**Phone:** (510)540-7600 **Fax:** (510)540-7683
**Email:** feldenres@aol.com
Carol Kress, Contact

**Program(s):** Feldenkrais.


★ 3431 ★ **Five Branches Institute of Traditional Chinese Medicine**
200 7th Ave.
Santa Cruz, CA 95062
**Phone:** (831)476-9424 **Fax:** (831)476-8928
**Email:** tcm@fivebranches.edu
**Website:** http://www.fivebranches.edu
Meredith Bigley, Contact

**Program(s):** Acupuncture; Herbal Medicine; Traditional Chinese Medicine.


★ 3432 ★ **Flower Essence Society**
PO Box 459
Nevada City, CA 95959
**Free:** 800-736-9222 **Fax:** (530)265-0584
**Email:** mail@flowersociety.org
**Website:** http://www.flowersociety.org
Patricia Kaminski, Director

**Program(s):** Flower Essences.


★ 3433 ★ **Foothills Massage School**
PO Box 826
North San Juan, CA 95960
**Phone:** (530)292-3123 **Fax:** (530)292-3123
Saria Farr, Contact

**Program(s):** Acupressure; Aromatherapy; Deep Tissue Massage; Energy Work; Herbal Medicine; Massage Therapy; Polarity Therapy; Reflexology; Shiatsu; Yoga Teacher Training.


★ 3434 ★ **Four Winds Seminars**
187 Hillside Dr.
Fairfax, CA 94930
**Phone:** (415)457-2079 **Fax:** (415)457-2079
**Email:** mfairbanks@igc.apc.org
Melissa Fairbanks, Director

**Program(s):** Homeopathy.


★ 3435 ★ **Friends Landing International Center for Conscious Living, Oakland**
419 48th St.
Oakland, CA 94609
Whitewind Swan Fisher, Contact

**Program(s):** Hypnotherapy.


★ 3436 ★ **Grof Transpersonal Training, Inc.**
20 Sunnyside, Ste. A314
Mill Valley, CA 94941
**Phone:** (415)383-8779 **Fax:** (415)383-0965
**Website:** http://www.holotropic.com
Cary Sparks, Director

**Program(s):** Breathwork.


★ 3437 ★ **Hahnemann College of Homeopathy**
80 Nicholl Ave.
Richmond, CA 94801
**Phone:** (510)232-2079 **Fax:** (510)412-9044
Debra Callahan, Contact

**Program(s):** Homeopathy.


★ 3438 ★ **Healing Arts Institute, Roseville**
112 Douglas Blvd.
Roseville, CA 95678
**Phone:** (916)782-1275 **Free:** 800-718-6824
**Fax:** (916)783-4258
Joyce Meredith, Contact

**Program(s):** Acupressure; Alexander Technique; Aromatherapy; Deep Tissue Massage; Massage Therapy; Reflexology; Reiki; Shiatsu; Soft Tisuue Release; Sports Massage; Swedish Massage.


★ 3439 ★ **Healing Hands School of Holistic Health**
125 W Mission, Ste. 212
Escondido, CA 92025
**Phone:** (760)746-9364 **Free:** 800-355-6463
Paula Curtiss, Director

**Program(s):** Acupressure; Aromatherapy; CranioSacral Therapy; Deep Tissue Massage; Herbal Medicine; Homeopathy; Holistic Health; Hypnotherapy; Massage Therapy; Reflexology; Reiki; Shiatsu; Sports Massage.


★ 3440 ★ **Heartwood Institute**
220 Harmony Ln.
Garberville, CA 95542
**Phone:** (707)923-5000 **Fax:** (707)923-5010
**Website:** http://www.heartwoodinstitute.com
Chela Burger, Director

**Program(s):** Acupressure; CranioSacral Therapy; Deep Tissue Massage; Energy Work; Holistic Health; Hypnotherapy; Massage Therapy; Neuromuscular Therapy; Oriental Medicine; Polarity Therapy; Shiatsu; Sports Massage; Swedish Massage; Traditional Chinese Medicine.


★ 3441 ★ **Hellerwork International LLC**
406 Berry St.
Mount Shasta, CA 96067
**Free:** 800-392-3900 **Fax:** (916)926-6839
**Website:** http://www.hellerwork.com
Joseph Heller, Contact

**Program(s):** Hellerwork; Structural Integration.


★ 3442 ★ **Hypnosis Clearing House**
3702 Mount Diablo Blvd.
Lafayette, CA 94549
**Phone:** (510)283-3941 **Fax:** (510)283-9044
**Email:** hch@hypnotherapytraining.com
**Website:** http://www.hypnotherapytraining.com
Holly Holmes-Meredith, Director

**Program(s):** Hypnotherapy.


★ 3443 ★ **Hypnosis Motivation Institute**
18607 Ventura Blvd., Ste. 310
Tarzana, CA 91356
**Phone:** (818)758-2745
Candace Coleman, Contact

**Program(s):** Hypnotherapy.


★ 3444 ★ **Hypnotherapy Training Institute**
4730 Alta Vista Ave.
Santa Rosa, CA 95404
**Phone:** (707)579-9023 **Free:** 800-256-6448
**Fax:** (707)578-1033
**Email:** hypno@sonic.net
**Website:** http://www.hypnoschool.com
Randal Churchill, Director

**Program(s):** Hypnotherapy.


★ 3445 ★ **Hypnotism Training Institute of Los Angeles**
700 S Central Ave.
Glendale, CA 91204
**Phone:** (818)242-1159 **Fax:** (818)247-9379
Gil Boyne, Director

**Program(s):** Hypnotherapy.


★ 3446 ★ **Inner Quest Awareness Center**
13924 Taft St., Ste. 3
Garden Grove, CA 92843
**Free:** 800-769-1230 **Fax:** (714)539-2977
Jeanne A. Neher-Schurz, Contact

**Program(s):** Hypnotherapy; Reiki.


★ 3447 ★ **Institute for Applied Iridology**
PO Box 301
Laguna Beach, CA 92652
**Free:** 888-886-8985 **Fax:** 888-886-8985
Harri Wolf, Contact

**Program(s):** Iridology.


★ 3448 ★ **Institute of Chinese Herbology**
3871 Piedmont Ave., Ste. 363
Oakland, CA 94611
**Phone:** (510)428-2061 **Fax:** (510)428-2061
Kenneth Morris, Director

**Program(s):** Herbal Medicine; Traditional Chinese Medicine.


★ 3449 ★ **Institute of Classical Homeopathy**
Fort Mason Center
San Francisco, CA 94123
**Phone:** (707)963-7796 **Fax:** (707)963-6131
Stephanie Bero, Contact

**Program(s):** Homeopathy.


★ 3450 ★ **Institute of Orthopedic Massage**
406 Berkeley Park Blvd.
Kensington, CA 94706

Phone: (510)524-8256          Fax: (510)524-8242
Thomas Hendrickson, Director
Program(s): Massage Therapy; Orthopedic Massage.


**★ 3451 ★ Institute of Professional**
**Practical Therapy**
1835 S La Cienega Blvd., Ste. 260
Los Angeles, CA 90035
Phone: (310)836-8811          Fax: (310)836-8857
Victor Dence, Contact
Program(s): Deep Tissue Massage; Massage Therapy.


**★ 3452 ★ Institute of Psycho-Structural**
**Balancing**
3767 Overland Ave., Ste. 103
Los Angeles, CA 90034
Phone: (310)815-3675          Fax: (310)815-3670
Website: http://www.ipsb.com
Eileen Hamsa Henry, Director
Program(s): Acupressure; Aromatherapy; CranioSacral Therapy; Energy Work; Massage Therapy; Polarity Therapy; Qigong; Reflexology; Sports Massage; Tai Chi.


**★ 3453 ★ Institute for the Study of**
**Somatic Education**
1158 Naples St.
San Francisco, CA 94112
Phone: (415)333-6644          Fax: (415)333-6644
Email: isse@aol.com
Paul Rubin, Director
Program(s): Feldenkrais; Somatic Education.


**★ 3454 ★ Internal Environment Institute**
11739 Washington Blvd.
Los Angeles, CA 90066
Phone: (310)572-6223          Fax: (310)572-6217
Conda J. Allred, Contact
Program(s): Colon Hydrotherapy.


**★ 3455 ★ International Association of**
**Infant Massage**
1891 Goodyear Ave., Ste. 622
Ventura, CA 93003
Phone: (805)644-8524          Free: 800-248-5432
Fax: (805)644-7699
Susan Campbell, Contact
Program(s): Infant Massage.


**★ 3456 ★ International College of**
**Homeopathy**
8306 Wilshire Blvd., Ste. 728
Beverly Hills, CA 90211
Phone: (310)645-0443          Fax: (310)645-1814
Email: registrar@qvius.edu
Cornella Franz, MD, Contact
Program(s): Energy Work; Homeopathy; Oriental Medicine.


**★ 3457 ★ International Professional**
**School of Bodywork**
1366 Hornblend St.
San Diego, CA 92109
Phone: (619)272-4142          Fax: (619)272-4772
Email: beingipsb@aol.com
Website: http://www.webcom.com/ipsb
Barbara Clark, Director
Program(s): Acupressure; Alexander Technique; CranioSacral Therapy; Feldenkrais; Herbal Medicine; Massage Therapy; Qigong; Shiatsu; Sports Massage.


**★ 3458 ★ International Sivananda Yoga**
**Vedanta Center**
14651 Ballantree Ln.
Grass Valley, CA 95949

Phone: (415)681-2731          Free: 800-469-9642
Fax: (415)681-5162
Email: swsita@ix.netcom.com
Website: http://www.sivananda.org
Swami Sitaramananda, Director
Program(s): Yoga Teacher Training.


**★ 3459 ★ Iyengar Yoga Institute**
2404 27th Ave.
San Francisco, CA 94116
Phone: (415)753-0909          Fax: (415)753-0913
Email: iyisf@sirius.com
Website: http://www.iyoga.com/iyisf
Janet MacLeod, Director
Program(s): Yoga Teacher Training.


**★ 3460 ★ Jin Shin Do Foundation for**
**Bodymind Acupressure**
1084G San Miguel Canyon Rd.
Watsonville, CA 95076
Phone: (831)763-7702          Fax: (831)763-1151
Iona Teeguarden, Director
Program(s): Acupressure; Jin Shin Do.


**★ 3461 ★ John F. Kennedy University**
Graduate School for Holistic Studies
12 Altarinda Rd.
Orinda, CA 94563
Phone: (925)254-0105          Fax: (925)254-3322
Website: http://www.jfku.edu
K. Sue Duncan, Contact
Program(s): Holistic Health.


**★ 3462 ★ Just for Your Health College**
**of Massage**
2075 Lincoln Ave., Ste. E
San Jose, CA 95125
Phone: (408)723-2131          Fax: (408)723-7389
Tina Garcia, Director
Program(s): Acupressure; Aromatherapy; Deep Tissue Massage; Energy Work; Homeopathy; Massage Therapy; Reflexology; Sports Massage; Tai Chi.


**★ 3463 ★ Kali Ray Tri Yoga Center**
PO Box 4287
Santa Cruz, CA 95063
Phone: (408)464-8100          Fax: (408)462-1945
Leela Vani, Contact
Program(s): Yoga Teacher Training.


**★ 3464 ★ Kate Jordan Seminars**
**Bodywork for the Childbearing Year**
8950 Villa La Jolla Dr., Ste. 2162
La Jolla, CA 92037
Phone: (619)436-0418          Free: 888-287-6860
Fax: (619)457-3615
Email: pregmassge@aol.com
Kathy Sartain, Director
Program(s): Pregnancy Massage; Postpartum Massage.


**★ 3465 ★ Kyung San University**
**USA School of Oriental Medicine**
8322 Garden Grove Blvd.
Garden Grove, CA 92844
Phone: (714)636-0337          Fax: (714)636-8459
Email: admin@kyungsan.edu
Eun Suk Lee, Contact
Program(s): Acupressure; Acupuncture; CranioSacral Therapy; Herbal Medicine; Oriental Medicine; Qigong; Reflexology; Shiatsu; Traditional Chinese Medicine.


**★ 3466 ★ Lake Tahoe Massage School**
1966 US Hwy 50
South Lake Tahoe, CA 96150
Phone: (530)544-1227
Jeannette Cunniff, Contact

Program(s): CranioSacral Therapy; Deep Tissue Massage; Massage Therapy; Medical Massage; Polarity Therapy; Reflexology; Reiki; Shiatsu; Sports Massage.


**★ 3467 ★ Life Chiropractic College West**
2005 Via Barrett
San Lorenzo, CA 94580
Free: 800-788-4476          Fax: (510)276-4893
Email: info@lifewest.edu
Website: http://www.lifewest.edu
Gerard W. Clum, Contact
Program(s): Chiropractic.


**★ 3468 ★ Linda Lack, Two-Snake**
**Studios**
1637 S La Cienega Blvd.
Los Angeles, CA 90035
Phone: (310)273-4797          Fax: (310)932-1441
Linda Lack, Contact
Program(s): Movement Therapy; Yoga Teacher Training; Yoga Therapy.


**★ 3469 ★ Los Angeles College of**
**Chiropractic**
16200 E Amber Valley Dr.
Whittier, CA 90609-1166
Phone: (562)947-8755          Free: 800-221-5222
Fax: (562)947-5724
Reed Phillips, PhD, Director
Program(s): Chiropractic.


**★ 3470 ★ Loving Hands Institute of**
**Healing Arts**
639 11th St.
Fortuna, CA 95540-2346
Phone: (707)725-9627          Fax: (707)725-2471
Dr. Rosalind Skyhawk Ojala, Director
Program(s): Acupressure; Deep Tissue Massage; Esalen Massage; Holistic Health; Lymphatic Massage; Massage Therapy; Reflexology; Swedish Massage; Trigger Point Therapy.


**★ 3471 ★ Lu Ross Academy of Health &**
**Beauty**
470 E Thompson Blvd.
Ventura, CA 93001
Phone: (805)643-5690
Chrys Huynh, Director
Program(s): Acupressure; Aromatherapy; CranioSacral Therapy; Energy Work; Herbal Medicine; Massage Therapy; Neuromuscular Therapy; Polarity Therapy; Qigong; Reflexology; Reiki; Shiatsu; Sports Massage.


**★ 3472 ★ Massage School of Santa**
**Monica**
1453 Third St. Promenade, Ste. 340
Santa Monica, CA 90401
Phone: (310)393-7461          Fax: (310)453-2386
Bernadette Gessner, Director
Program(s): Acupressure; Aromatherapy; CranioSacral Therapy; Energy Work; Massage Therapy; Polarity Therapy; Qigong; Reflexology; Shiatsu; Sports Massage; Swedish Massage.


**★ 3473 ★ Master Yoga Academy**
7592 Fay Ave.
La Jolla, CA 92037
Phone: (619)454-6978          Fax: (619)454-5541
Rama Berch, Director
Program(s): Yoga Teacher Training.


**★ 3474 ★ McKinnon Institute of**
**Professional Massage and Bodywork**
2940 Webster St.
Oakland, CA 94609-3407

**Phone:** (510)465-3488          **Fax:** (510)465-1533
Judith McKinnon, Director

**Program(s):** Acupressure; Anatomy and Physiology; CranioSacral Therapy; Deep Tissue Massage; Massage Therapy; On-Site Massage; Reflexology; Shiatsu; Sports Massage; Swedish Massage.

★ 3475 ★ **Meiji College of Oriental Medicine**
2550 Shattuck Ave.
Berkeley, CA 94704
**Phone:** (510)666-8248          **Fax:** (510)666-0111
Laura Pitre, Contact

**Program(s):** Acupuncture; Herbal Medicine; Oriental Medicine; Traditional Chinese Medicine.

★ 3476 ★ **Mendocino School of Holistic Massage and Advanced Healing Arts**
2680 Rd. B
Redwood Valley, CA 95470
**Phone:** (707)485-8197
**Email:** rammpack@pacific.net
Clark Ramm, Director

**Program(s):** Aromatherapy; Ayurvedic Medicine; Energy Work; Esalen Massage; Herbal Medicine; Holistic Health; Homeopathy; Hypnotherapy; Lymphatic Massage; Massage Therapy; Polarity Therapy; Rebirthing; Reflexology; Swedish Massage.

★ 3477 ★ **Meridian Institute**
99 Pacific St., Heritage Harbor Bldg. 375A
Monterey, CA 93940
**Phone:** (831)649-6684          **Fax:** (831)649-6688
Andy Seplow, Contact

**Program(s):** Acupuncture; Herbal Medicine; Massage Therapy; Traditional Chinese Medicine.

★ 3478 ★ **Mesa Institute**
150 N Felder
Orange, CA 92868
**Phone:** (714)937-4161          **Fax:** (714)937-6360
Chad Marta, Contact

**Program(s):** Acupressure; Aromatherapy; Ayurvedic Medicine; CranioSacral Therapy; Deep Tissue Massage; Energy Work; Holistic Health; Hypnotherapy; Massage Therapy; Polarity Therapy; Reflexology; Reiki; Shiatsu; Sports Massage.

★ 3479 ★ **Michael Scholes School of Aromatic Studies**
117 N Robertson Blvd.
Los Angeles, CA 90048
**Phone:** (310)276-1191          **Free:** 800-677-2368
**Fax:** (310)276-1156
**Email:** joanaroma@aol.com
Michael Scholes, Contact

**Program(s):** Aromatherapy; Energy Work.

★ 3480 ★ **Midwifery Institute of California**
3739 Balboa, Ste. 179
San Francisco, CA 94121
Shannon Ariton, Contact

**Program(s):** Midwifery.

★ 3481 ★ **Montebello Career College**
2465 W Whittier Blvd., Ste. 201
Montebello, CA 90640
**Phone:** (323)728-9636          **Fax:** (323)728-0952
Rosa Sanchez, Contact

**Program(s):** Massage Therapy.

★ 3482 ★ **Monterey Institute of Touch**
27820 Dorris Dr.
Carmel, CA 93923
**Phone:** (831)624-1006          **Fax:** (831)626-6916
**Email:** mit@redshift.com
Birgit Ball-Eisner, Contact

**Program(s):** Acupressure; Aromatherapy; CranioSacral Therapy; Massage Therapy; Polarity Therapy; Reflexology; Shiatsu; Sports Massage.

★ 3483 ★ **Monterey Peninsula College**
980 Fremont St.
Monterey, CA 93940
**Phone:** (831)646-4220          **Fax:** (831)645-1334
Dawn Sare, Contact

**Program(s):** Acupressure; Massage Therapy; Polarity Therapy; Refexology; Shiatsu; Sports Massage.

★ 3484 ★ **Mount Madonna Center**
445 Summit Rd.
Watsonville, CA 95076
**Phone:** (408)847-0406          **Fax:** (408)847-2683
**Email:** programs@mountmadonna.org
**Website:** http://www.mountmadonna.org
Gerald Friedberg, Director

**Program(s):** Ayurvedic Medicine; Yoga Teacher Training.

★ 3485 ★ **Movement Studies Institute**
1832 Second St.
Berkeley, CA 94710
**Free:** 800-342-3424          **Fax:** (510)548-4349
**Email:** info@movementstudies.com
Dr. Frank Wildman, Director

**Program(s):** Feldenkrais.

★ 3486 ★ **Mueller College of Holistic Studies**
4607 Park Blvd.
San Diego, CA 92116
**Phone:** (619)291-9811          **Fax:** (619)543-1113
**Email:** info@muellercollege.com
**Website:** http://www.muellercollege.com
Bill Mueller, Director

**Program(s):** Acupressure; Aromatherapy; Ayurvedic Medicine; CranioSacral Therapy; Herbal Medicine; Holistic Health; Massage Therapy; Oriental Medicine; Polarity Therapy; Qigong; Reflexology; Shiatsu; Traditional Chinese Medicine.

★ 3487 ★ **National Holistic Institute**
5900 Hollis St., Ste. J
Emeryville, CA 94608
**Phone:** (510)547-6442          **Free:** 800-315-3552
**Fax:** (510)547-6621
**Email:** nhi@nhimassage.com
**Website:** http://www.nhimassage.com
Nancy Seyfert, Director

**Program(s):** Holistic Health; Massage Therapy; Shiatsu; Sports Massage.

★ 3488 ★ **National Institute of Massage**
1150 E Palm Canyon Dr., Ste. 54
Palm Springs, CA 92264
**Phone:** (760)323-3535
Sharon Leeds, Contact

**Program(s):** Energy Work; Herbal Medicine; Massage Therapy; Polarity Therapy; Yoga Teacher Training.

★ 3489 ★ **Natural Healing Institute of Naturopathy, Inc.**
2146 Encinitas Blvd., Ste. 105
Encinitas, CA 92024
**Phone:** (760)943-8485          **Fax:** (760)943-9477
Patti Valentine, Contact

**Program(s):** Acupressure; Aromatherapy; Ayurvedic Medicine; Deep Tissue Massage; Energy Work; Herbal Medicine; Hypnotherapy; Massage Therapy; Naturopathic Medicine; Nutrition; Oriental Medicine; Reflexology; Shiatsu; Traditional Chinese Medicine.

★ 3490 ★ **New Life Institute of Massage Therapy**
1159 Hilltop Dr.
Redding, CA 96002
**Phone:** (530)222-1467          **Fax:** (530)222-3489
Shirley Latal, Contact

**Program(s):** CranioSacral Therapy; Massage Therapy; Myofascial Release; Reflexology.

★ 3491 ★ **Oakendell School of Massage and Healing Arts**
3585 Hawver Rd.
San Andreas, CA 95249
**Phone:** (209)754-0244          **Fax:** (209)754-1081
Steve Mertens, Contact

**Program(s):** Acupressure; Energy Work; Massage Therapy; Neuromuscular Therapy; Oriental Medicine; Qigong; Traditional Chinese Medicine.

★ 3492 ★ **Pacific Academy of Homeopathy**
1199 Sanchez St.
San Francisco, CA 94114
**Phone:** (415)458-8238          **Fax:** (415)695-8220
Richard Pitt, Contact

**Program(s):** Homeopathy.

★ 3493 ★ **Pacific College**
3160 Redhill Ave.
Costa Mesa, CA 92626
**Phone:** (714)662-4402          **Fax:** (714)662-1702
Betty Gross, Contact

**Program(s):** Acupressure; Aromatherapy; Massage Therapy; Reflexology; Shiatsu; Sports Massage.

★ 3494 ★ **Pacific College of Alternative Therapies**
19997 Stevens Creek Blvd., Ste. 2
Cupertino, CA 95014
**Phone:** (408)777-0102          **Fax:** (408)777-0188
**Email:** pcollege-atherapist@juno.com
Peter Hou, Director

**Program(s):** Acupressure; Massage Therapy; Qigong; Traditional Chinese Medicine; Tui Na.

★ 3495 ★ **Pacific College of Oriental Medicine**
7445 Mission Valley Rd., Ste. 105
San Diego, CA 92108
**Phone:** (619)574-6909          **Fax:** (619)574-6641
**Email:** jmiller@ormed.edu
**Website:** http://www.ormed.edu
Jack Miller, Contact

**Program(s):** Acupressure; Acupuncture; Energy Work; Herbal Medicine; Holistic Health; Massage Therapy; Oriental Medicine; Qigong; Reflexology; Shiatsu; Sports Massage; Traditional Chinese Medicine.

★ 3496 ★ **Pacific Institute for the Alexander Technique**
930 Alhambra Blvd., Ste. 270
Sacramento, CA 95816
**Phone:** (916)448-7424
Sherry Berjeron-Oliver, Contact

**Program(s):** Alexander Technique.

★ 3497 ★ **Pacific Institute of Aromatherapy**
PO Box 6723
San Rafael, CA 94903
**Phone:** (415)479-9121          **Fax:** (415)479-0119
Dr. Kurt Schnaubelt, Director

**Program(s):** Aromatherapy.

**★ 3498 ★ Pacific School of Herbal Medicine**
PO Box 2194
Berkeley, CA 94702
**Phone:** (510)685-4028
Adam Seller, Contact
**Program(s):** Aromatherapy; Ayurvedic Medicine; Herbal Medicine.

**★ 3499 ★ Pacific School of Massage & Healing Arts**
44800 Fish Rock Rd.
Gualala, CA 95445
**Phone:** (707)884-3138    **Fax:** (707)884-4106
**Email:** mitouer@mcn.org
Cheryl Mitouer, Director
**Program(s):** Massage Therapy; Transformational Bodywork.

**★ 3500 ★ Palmer College of Chiropractic West**
90 E Tasman Dr.
San Jose, CA 95134
**Phone:** (408)944-6000    **Free:** 800-442-4476
**Fax:** (408)944-6111
Peter A. Martin, Contact
**Program(s):** Chiropractic.

**★ 3501 ★ Palo Alto School of Hypnotherapy**
2443 Ash St., Ste. D
Palo Alto, CA 94306
**Phone:** (415)321-6419    **Free:** 800-774-9766
**Fax:** (650)941-2485
Josie Hadley, Contact
**Program(s):** Hypnotherapy; Qigong; Reiki.

**★ 3502 ★ Polarity Therapy Center of Marin**
PO Box 23
Tomales, CA 94971
**Phone:** (707)878-2278
Hanna Hammerli, Director
**Program(s):** Polarity Therapy.

**★ 3503 ★ Polarity Wellness Center West**
325 Shortt Rd.
Santa Rosa, CA 95405
**Phone:** (707)542-7966
Jan Milthaler, Director
**Program(s):** Polarity Therapy.

**★ 3504 ★ Quantum-Veritas International University Systems**
8306 Wilshire Blvd., Ste. 728
Beverly Hills, CA 90211
**Phone:** (310)645-0443    **Fax:** (310)645-1814
Cherie DeWonder, Contact
**Program(s):** Acupressure; Aromatherapy; Ayurvedic Medicine; CranioSacral Therapy; Deep Tissue Massage; Energy Work; Herbal Medicine; Kinesiology; Massage Therapy; Oriental Medicine; Polarity Therapy; Qigong; Reflexology; Shiatsu; Sports Massage; Traditional Chinese Medicine; Yoga Teacher Training.

**★ 3505 ★ Reese Movement Institute, Inc.**
2187 Newcastle
Cardiff, CA 92007
**Phone:** (760)436-9087    **Fax:** (760)436-9141
**Email:** rmiinc@aol.com
Mark Reese, Director
**Program(s):** Feldenkrais.

**★ 3506 ★ Reflexology Institute**
27636 Ynez Rd. L-7, Ste. 232
Temecula, CA 92591

**Phone:** (909)694-0225    **Fax:** (909)694-5910
Lynn Nelson, Contact
**Program(s):** Reflexology.

**★ 3507 ★ Reiki Center of Los Angeles**
16161 Ventura Blvd., Ste. 802
Encino, CA 91436
**Phone:** (818)881-5959    **Fax:** (818)881-1613
Joyce Morris, Contact
**Program(s):** Reiki.

**★ 3508 ★ reSource**
825 Bancroft Way
Berkeley, CA 94702
**Phone:** (510)433-7917    **Fax:** (510)841-3258
Gail Stewart, Director
**Program(s):** Deep Tissue Massage; Massage Therapy; Ortho-Bionomy; Trager.

**★ 3509 ★ Rosa Institute of Aromatherapy**
219 Carl St.
San Francisco, CA 94117-3804
**Phone:** (415)564-6785    **Fax:** (415)564-6799
Jeanne Rose, Contact
**Program(s):** Aromatherapy; Herbal Medicine.

**★ 3510 ★ Rosen Method: The Berkeley Center**
825 Bancroft Way
Berkeley, CA 94710
**Phone:** (510)845-6606    **Fax:** (510)845-8114
Abby Paige, Contact
**Program(s):** Rosen Method Bodywork.

**★ 3511 ★ Samra University of Oriental Medicine**
3000 S Robertson Blvd., 4th Flr.
Los Angeles, CA 90034
**Phone:** (310)202-6444    **Fax:** (310)202-6007
**Email:** admissions@samra.edu
**Website:** http://www.samra.edu
Kathryn P. White, PhD, Contact
**Program(s):** Acupressure; Acupuncture; Herbal Medicine; Oriental Medicine; Qigong; Traditional Chinese Medicine.

**★ 3512 ★ San Francisco School of Massage**
1327A Chestnut St.
San Francisco, CA 94123
**Phone:** (415)474-4600    **Fax:** (415)474-4601
Richard Bergess, Director
**Program(s):** Acupressure; Aromatherapy; Breema Bodywork; CranioSacral Therapy; Deep Tissue Massage; Esalen Massage; Lymphatic Massage; Massage Therapy; Reflexology; Reiki; Shiatsu; Sports Massage; Swedish Massage; Trigger Point Therapy.

**★ 3513 ★ Santa Barbara College of Oriental Medicine**
1919 State St., Ste. 204
Santa Barbara, CA 93101
**Phone:** (805)898-1180    **Fax:** (805)682-1864
**Email:** 76774.3507@compuserve.com
JoAnn Hickey, Contact
**Program(s):** Acupressure; Acupuncture; Chinese Herbal Medicine; Oriental Medicine; Qigong; Shiatsu; Traditional Chinese Medicine.

**★ 3514 ★ Santa Barbara Yoga Center**
32 E Micheltorena St.
Santa Barbara, CA 93101
**Phone:** (805)965-6045
Lais Da Silva, Contact
**Program(s):** Yoga Teacher Training.

**★ 3515 ★ School of Healing Arts**
1001 Garnet Ave., Ste. 200
San Diego, CA 92109
**Phone:** (619)581-9429    **Fax:** (619)490-2555
Seymour Koblin, Director
**Program(s):** Acupressure; Hypnotherapy; Holistic Health; Massage Therapy; Shiatsu.

**★ 3516 ★ School of Homeopathy**
2124 Kittredge St.
Berkeley, CA 94704
**Phone:** (510)649-0294    **Fax:** (510)649-1955
**Email:** mail@homeopathic.com
**Website:** http://www.homeopathic.com
Stuart Gracie, Contact
**Program(s):** Homeopathy.

**★ 3517 ★ School of Intuitive Massage and Healing**
503 Foxen Dr,
Santa Barbara, CA 93105
**Phone:** (805)687-2917    **Fax:** (805)563-0927
Anne Parks, Director
**Program(s):** Energy Work; Massage Therapy.

**★ 3518 ★ School of Shiatsu and Massage**
18424 Harbin Springs Rd.
PO Box 889
Middletown, CA 95461
**Phone:** (707)987-3801    **Fax:** (707)987-9638
**Email:** info@waba.edu
**Website:** http://www.waba.edu
Harold Dull, Director
**Program(s):** Acupressure; Massage Therapy; Shiatsu; Watsu Aquatic Bodywork.

**★ 3519 ★ Sebastopol Massage Center**
108 N Main, Ste. 5
Sebastopol, CA 95472
**Phone:** (707)823-3550
Patricia Oberg, Director
**Program(s):** Acupressure; CranioSacral Therapy; Energy Work; Esalen Massage; Massage Therapy; Ortho-Bionomy; Reflexology; Shiatsu; Swedish Massage.

**★ 3520 ★ South Bay Massage College**
3770 Highland Ave., Ste. 204
Manhattan Beach, CA 90266
**Phone:** (310)546-8774    **Fax:** (310)546-8775
Betsy Anderson, Contact
**Program(s):** Deep Tissue Massage; Massage Therapy; Refexology; Sports Massage.

**★ 3521 ★ South Baylo University**
1126 N Brookhurst St.
Anaheim, CA 92801
**Phone:** (714)533-1495    **Fax:** (714)533-6040
**Email:** ron@sbu.edu
**Website:** http://www.sbu.edu
Ronald Sokolsky, Director
**Program(s):** Acupuncture; Herbal Medicine; Qigong; Shiatsu; Traditional Chinese Medicine; Tui Na.

**★ 3522 ★ Southern California School of Massage**
12702 Magnolia Ave., Ste. 21
Riverside, CA 92503
**Phone:** (909)340-3336    **Fax:** (909)340-0154
Elizabeth Kelly, Contact
**Program(s):** Acupressure; Aromatherapy; Deep Tissue Massage; Energy Work; Holistic Health; Hypnotherapy; Massage Therapy; Polarity Therapy; Reflexology; Shiatsu; Sports Massage; Traditional Chinese Medicine.

## ★ 3523 ★ Taoist Institute
10630 Burbank Blvd.
North Hollywood, CA 91601
**Phone:** (818)760-4219
Carl Totton, Director

**Program(s):** Acupressure; Qigong; Tui Na.

## ★ 3524 ★ Therapeutic Learning Center
3636 N First St., Ste. 154
Fresno, CA 93727
**Phone:** (559)225-7772          **Fax:** (559)252-5313
Evangeline K. Hentrich, Contact

**Program(s):** Energy Work; Massage Therapy; Reflexology; Shiatsu; Swedish Massage.

## ★ 3525 ★ Touch for Health Kinesiology
11262 Washington Blvd.
Culver City, CA 90230
**Phone:** (310)313-5580          **Free:** 800-466-8342
**Fax:** (310)313-9319
Mark McCutcheon, Director

**Program(s):** Kinesiology; Touch for Health.

## ★ 3526 ★ Touch Therapy Institute
15720 Ventura Blvd., Ste. 101
Encino, CA 91436
**Phone:** (818)788-0824          **Fax:** (818)788-0875
**Website:** http://www.touchtherapyinstitute.com
Maria Grove, Director

**Program(s):** Acupressure; Alexander Technique; Anatomy and Physiology; Aromatherapy; Chair Massage; CPR/First Aid; CranioSacral Therapy; Energy Work; LomiLomi Massage; Lymphatic Massage; Massage Therapy; Myofascial Release; Pregnancy Massage; Qigong; Reflexology; Sports Massage; Swedish Massage; Therapeutic Touch; Trager.

## ★ 3527 ★ Touching for Health Center School of Professional Bodywork
628 Lincoln Ctr.
Stockton, CA 95207-2640
**Phone:** (209)474-9559          **Fax:** (209)474-9559
Roberta Baker, Director

**Program(s):** Acupressure; Aromatherapy; CranioSacral Therapy; Deep Tissue Massage; Manual Lymph Drainage; Massage Therapy; Myofascial Release; Polarity Therapy; Reflexology.

## ★ 3528 ★ TouchPro Institute of Chair Massage
584 Castro St., Ste. 555
San Francisco, CA 94114
**Free:** 800-999-5026          **Fax:** (415)621-1260
Douglas Hudson, Contact

**Program(s):** Chair Massage.

## ★ 3529 ★ Trager Institute
21 Locust Ave.
Mill Valley, CA 94941-2806
**Phone:** (415)388-2688          **Fax:** (415)388-2710
**Email:** admin@trager.com
Don Schwartz, PhD, Director

**Program(s):** Trager.

## ★ 3530 ★ Twin Lakes College of the Healing Arts
1210 Brommer St.
Santa Cruz, CA 95062
**Phone:** (831)476-2152
Becky Williams, Director

**Program(s):** Acupressure; Aromatherapy; Energy Work; Hypnotherapy; Massage Therapy; Polarity Therapy; Reflexology; Reiki; Shiatsu.

## ★ 3531 ★ United States Yoga Association
2159 Filbert St.
San Francisco, CA 94123
**Phone:** (415)931-9642          **Fax:** (415)921-6676
Sandy Wong, Contact

**Program(s):** Yoga Teacher Training.

## ★ 3532 ★ University of California, Los Angeles
**Primary Care Division**
**Nurse-Midwifery Education Program**
10833 LeConte Ave.
Los Angeles, CA 90099-4973
**Phone:** (310)794-4434          **Fax:** (310)206-3241
**Email:** mday@sonnet.ucla.edu
Mary Day, Contact

**Program(s):** Midwifery.

## ★ 3533 ★ University of California, San Diego
**Division of Graduate Nursing Education**
**Nurse-Midwifery Program**
9500 Gilman Dr.
La Jolla, CA 92093-0809
**Phone:** (619)543-5480          **Fax:** (619)543-7757
Lauren Hunter, Director

**Program(s):** Midwifery.

## ★ 3534 ★ University of Southern California
**Nurse-Midwifery Education Program**
1540 E Alcazar St.
CHP 222
Los Angeles, CA 90033
**Phone:** (323)442-2001          **Fax:** (323)442-2090
BJ Snell, Director

**Program(s):** Midwifery.

## ★ 3535 ★ Valley Hypnosis Center
3705 Sunnyside Dr.
Riverside, CA 92506
**Phone:** (909)781-0282
Sally Cernie, PhD, Contact

**Program(s):** Hypnotherapy; Pranic Healing; Reflexology; Reiki.

## ★ 3536 ★ Vitality Sciences Institute
70-A N El Camino Real
San Mateo, CA 94401-2866
**Phone:** (650)347-4565          **Fax:** (650)344-7783
Alicia Parnell, Contact

**Program(s):** Reposturing Dynamics.

## ★ 3537 ★ Vitality Training Center
243 N Hwy. 101, Ste. 5
Solana Beach, CA 92075
**Phone:** (619)259-9491          **Fax:** (619)259-2008
Annie Benefield, Director

**Program(s):** Acupressure; Aromatherapy; CranioSacral Therapy; Energy Work; Herbal Medicine; Holistic Health; Hypnotherapy; Massage Therapy; Neuromuscular Therapy; Reflexology; Reiki; Shiatsu; Sports Massage; Yoga Teacher Training.

## ★ 3538 ★ Wellness Holistic School of Massage
345 S E St.
Santa Rosa, CA 95404
**Phone:** (707)546-8115          **Free:** 800-939-6837
Virginia Romero, Director

**Program(s):** Energy Work; Esalen Massage; Kinesiology; Massage Therapy; Polarity Therapy; Reflexology; Swedish Massage; Touch for Health.

## ★ 3539 ★ West Pacific
434 N Lakeview Ave.
Anaheim, CA 92807
**Phone:** (714)998-8079          **Fax:** (714)998-8079
Joel Doti, Contact

**Program(s):** Deep Tissue Massage; Massage Therapy; Sports Massage.

## ★ 3540 ★ Western Institute of Neuromuscular Therapy
22981 Mill Creek Dr., Ste. A
Laguna Hills, CA 92653
**Phone:** (714)830-6151          **Fax:** (714)830-1729
Cynthia Ribeiro, Director

**Program(s):** Massage Therapy; Neuromuscular Therapy; Sports Massage.

## ★ 3541 ★ World School of Massage and Advanced Healing Arts
401 32nd Ave.
San Francisco, CA 94125
**Phone:** (415)221-2533          **Fax:** (415)221-0430
Patricia Cramer, Contact

**Program(s):** Aromatherapy; CranioSacral Therapy; Holistic Health; Massage Therapy; Reflexology; Vibrational Therapy.

## ★ 3542 ★ Wyrick Institute & Clinic
PO Box 99745
San Diego, CA 92169
**Phone:** (619)273-9764          **Fax:** (619)277-7358
Dana Wyrick, Director

**Program(s):** Manual Lymph Drainage.

## ★ 3543 ★ Yo San University of Traditional Chinese Medicine
1314 2nd St.
Santa Monica, CA 90401
**Phone:** (310)917-2202          **Fax:** (310)917-2203
**Email:** info@yosan.edu
**Website:** http://www.yosan.edu
Dr. Richard Hammerschlag, Director

**Program(s):** Acupuncture; Herbal Medicine; Lifestyle Counseling; Qigong; Traditional Chinese Medicine.

## ★ 3544 ★ Yoga Room
953-957 2nd St.
Encinitas, CA 92024
**Phone:** (619)753-1828          **Fax:** (619)753-4639
Peri Ness, Contact

**Program(s):** Yoga Teacher Training.

## ★ 3545 ★ Yoga Works, Inc.
1426 Montana Ave., 2nd Fl.
Santa Monica, CA 90403
**Phone:** (310)393-5150          **Fax:** (310)656-5892
Julie Jacobs, Contact

**Program(s):** Yoga Teacher Training.

## ★ 3546 ★ Zero Balancing Association
PO Box 1727
Capitola, CA 95010
**Phone:** (408)476-0665          **Fax:** (408)476-0665
**Email:** zbaoffice@aol.com
Fritz Smith, MD, Contact

**Program(s):** Zero Balancing.

### Colorado

## ★ 3547 ★ Academy of Natural Therapy
123 Elm Ave.
Eaton, CO 80615
**Phone:** (970)454-2224          **Fax:** (303)454-3147
**Email:** mongan@ibm.net
Dorothy Mongan, Director

**Program(s):** Acupressure; Herbal Medicine; Massage Therapy; Reflexology; Shiatsu.

**★ 3548 ★ Alexander Technique Institute - Colorado**
2545 Vine Pl.
Boulder, CO 80304
**Phone:** (303)449-4143
Colin Egan, Director
**Program(s):** Alexander Technique.


**★ 3549 ★ Ann Allen and Associates, Biofeedback and Stress Management**
1660 S Albion St.
Denver, CO 80222
**Phone:** (303)757-0508          **Fax:** (303)758-9203
Ann Allen, Contact
**Program(s):** Biofeedback.


**★ 3550 ★ Artemis Institute of Natural Therapies**
875 Alpine Ave., Ste. 5
Boulder, CO 80304
**Phone:** (303)443-9289          **Fax:** (303)443-6361
Peter J. Holmes, Director
**Program(s):** Aromatherapy; Herbal Medicine.


**★ 3551 ★ Association for Applied Psychophysiology and Biofeedback**
10200 W 44th Ave., Ste. 304
Wheat Ridge, CO 80033
**Phone:** (303)422-8436          **Fax:** (303)422-8894
Francine Butler, Contact
**Program(s):** Biofeedback.


**★ 3552 ★ BioSomatics**
PO Box 206
Grand Junction, CO 81502
**Phone:** (970)245-8903          **Fax:** (970)241-5653
Carol Welch, Contact
**Program(s):** CranioSacral Therapy; Neuromuscular Therapy; Somatic Education.


**★ 3553 ★ Boulder College of Massage Therapy**
6255 Longbow
Boulder, CO 80301
**Phone:** (303)530-2100          **Free:** 800-442-5131
**Fax:** (303)530-2204
Christopher Quinn, Contact
**Program(s):** Chair Massage; Hydrotherapy; Infant Massage; Integrative Massage; Massage Therapy; Orthopedic Massage; Polarity Therapy; Prenatal Massage; Reflexology; Shiatsu; Sports Massage; Swedish Massage.


**★ 3554 ★ Center of Advanced Therapeutics, Inc.**
1221 S Clarkson St., Ste. 412
Denver, CO 80210
**Phone:** (303)765-2201
Mary Uhl, Contact
**Program(s):** CranioSacral Therapy; Deep Tissue Massage; Massage Therapy.


**★ 3555 ★ Collinson School of Therapeutics & Massage**
2596 Palmer Park Blvd.
Colorado Springs, CO 80909
**Phone:** (719)473-0145
Dr. Torry Collinson, Contact
**Program(s):** Acupressure; Aromatherapy; CranioSacral Therapy; Massage Therapy; Reflexology; Reiki; Shiatsu.


**★ 3556 ★ Colorado Institute for Classical Homeopathy**
2299 Pearl St., Ste. 401
Boulder, CO 80302

**Phone:** (303)440-3717
Barbara Seideneck, Director
**Program(s):** Homeopathy.


**★ 3557 ★ Colorado Institute of Massage Therapy**
2601 E St. Vrain
Colorado Springs, CO 80909
**Phone:** (719)634-7486          **Fax:** (719)447-9198
**Website:** http://www.coimt.com
Greg Smith, Contact
**Program(s):** Acupressure; Fitness Therapy; Massage Therapy; Neuromuscular Therapy; Reflexology; Sports Massage.


**★ 3558 ★ Colorado School of Healing Arts**
7655 W Mississippi, Ste. 100
Lakewood, CO 80226
**Phone:** (303)986-2320
Chris Smith, Director
**Program(s):** Aromatherapy; CranioSacral Therapy; Herbal Medicine; Massage Therapy; Neuromuscular Therapy; Reflexology; Sports Massage.


**★ 3559 ★ Colorado School of Traditional Chinese Medicine**
1441 York St., Ste. 202
Denver, CO 80210
**Phone:** (303)329-6355          **Fax:** (303)388-8165
Dr. George H. Kitchie, Contact
**Program(s):** Acupuncture; Chinese Herbal Medicine; Qigong; Traditional Chinese Medicine.


**★ 3560 ★ Colorado Springs Academy of Therapeutic Massage**
3612 Galley, Ste. A
Colorado Springs, CO 80909
**Phone:** (719)597-0017          **Fax:** (719)597-6647
Dr. Daniel A. Sollee, Director
**Program(s):** Deep Tissue Massage; Massage Therapy; Neuromuscular Therapy; Sports Massage; Swedish Massage; Trigger Point Therapy.


**★ 3561 ★ Connecting Point School of Massage**
104 Society Dr.
Telluride, CO 81435
**Phone:** (970)728-6424
Sefra Maples, Contact
**Program(s):** Acupressure; Aromatherapy; Deep Tissue Massage; Massage Therapy; Reflexology; Shiatsu; Spa Therapies.


**★ 3562 ★ Cottonwood School of Massage Therapy**
2620 S Parker Rd., Ste. 300
Aurora, CO 80014
**Phone:** (303)745-7725          **Fax:** (303)751-1861
Jackie Otey, Contact
**Program(s):** Aromatherapy; CranioSacral Therapy; Energy Work; Massage Therapy; Polarity Therapy; Reflexology; Reiki; Shiatsu; Sports Massage.


**★ 3563 ★ Crestone Healing Arts Center**
1689 Columbine Overlook
Crestone, CO 81131
**Phone:** (719)256-4036
**Email:** retuta@crestonehac.com
Dan Retuta, Director
**Program(s):** Acupressure; Anatomy and Physiology; CPR/First Aid; Herbal Medicine; Integrated Massage; Massage Therapy; On-Site Massage; Prenatal Massage; Qigong; Reflexology; Shiatsu; Swedish Massage.


**★ 3564 ★ Day-Star Methpd of Yoga**
2565 S Meade St.
Denver, CO 80219
**Phone:** (303)934-6309
Susan Flanders, Contact
**Program(s):** Yoga Teacher Training.


**★ 3565 ★ Guild for Structural Integration**
3107 28th St.
PO Box 1559
Boulder, CO 80301
**Free:** 800-447-0150          **Fax:** (303)447-0108
**Email:** gsi@rolfguild.org
**Website:** http://www.rolfguild.org
Susan Melchior, Director
**Program(s):** Structural Integration.


**★ 3566 ★ Hahnemann Academy of North America**
PO Box 3024
Pagosa Springs, CO 81147
**Phone:** (970)731-9681
Robin Murphy, Director
**Program(s):** Homeopathy.


**★ 3567 ★ Institute of Taoist Education and Acupuncture, Inc.**
1321 5th St.
Boulder, CO 80302
**Phone:** (303)440-3492          **Fax:** (303)440-3492
Sandra L. Lillie, Contact
**Program(s):** Acupuncture.


**★ 3568 ★ Just for Health Enterprises, Inc.**
480 S Holly St.
Denver, CO 80246
**Phone:** (303)341-4384          **Fax:** (303)360-9118
Rachel Lord, Contact
**Program(s):** Acupressure; Anatomy and Physiology; Deep Tissue Massage; Energy Work Herbal Medicine; Massage Therapy; Reflexology.


**★ 3569 ★ Massage Therapy Institute of Colorado**
1441 York St., Ste. 301
Denver, CO 80206
**Phone:** (303)329-6345          **Fax:** (303)388-8165
Mark Manton, Director
**Program(s):** Acupressure; Alexander Technique; Aromatherapy; Ayurvedic Medicine; CranioSacral Therapy; Energy Work; Feldenkrais; Herbal Medicine; Homeopathy; Hypnotherapy; Massage Therapy; Neuromuscular Therapy; Polarity Therapy; Qigong; Reflexology; Reiki; Shiatsu; Sports Massage.


**★ 3570 ★ Modern Institute of Reflexology**
7043 W Colfax
Denver, CO 80215
**Phone:** (303)237-1530          **Fax:** (303)237-1606
Zachary K. Brinkerhoff, Contact
**Program(s):** Reflexology.


**★ 3571 ★ MountainHeart School of Bodywork and Transformational Therapy**
719 5th, Unit A
Denver, CO 80224
**Phone:** (970)349-0473          **Free:** 800-673-0539
**Fax:** (970)349-0473
Christine McLaughlin, Contact
**Program(s):** Acupressure; Energy Work; Massage Therapy; Neuromuscular Therapy; Oriental Medicine; Reflexology.

**★ 3572 ★ Polarity Center of Colorado**
1721 Redwood Ave.
Boulder, CO 80304-1118
**Phone:** (303)443-9847          **Fax:** (303)415-1839
John Chitty, Director
**Program(s):** CranioSacral Therapy; Polarity Therapy.


**★ 3573 ★ Qigong Research and Practice Center**
PO Box 1727
Nederland, CO 80466
**Phone:** (303)258-0971          **Fax:** (303)258-0971
Rebecca D. Cohen, Contact
**Program(s):** Energy Work, Qigong; Tai Chi.


**★ 3574 ★ Rocky Mountain Center for Botanical Studies**
2639 Spruce St.
PO Box 19254
Boulder, CO 80302
**Phone:** (303)442-6861          **Fax:** (303)442-6294
**Email:** rmcbs@indra.com
Feather Jones, Director
**Program(s):** Aromatherapy; Ayurvedic Medicine; Herbal Medicine; Traditional Chinese Medicine.


**★ 3575 ★ Rolf Institute of Structural Integration**
205 Canyon Blvd.
Boulder, CO 80302
**Phone:** (303)449-5903          **Free:** 800-530-8875
**Fax:** (303)449-5978
**Email:** rolfinst@aol.com
**Website:** http://www.rolf.org
Holly Hamilton, Director
**Program(s):** Structural Integration.


**★ 3576 ★ Ruseto College of Acupuncture and Chinese Medicine**
2900 Valmont Rd., Ste. E-1
Boulder, CO 80301
**Phone:** (303)449-1686
Pao-Chin R. Huang, Director
**Program(s):** Acupuncture; Herbal Medicine; Massage Therapy; Polarity Therapy; Qigong; Reflexology; Shiatsu; Traditional Chinese Medicine; Tui Na.


**★ 3577 ★ School of Natural Medicine**
PO Box 7369
Boulder, CO 80306-7369
**Phone:** (303)443-4882          **Fax:** (303)443-8276
**Email:** snm@purehealth.com
**Website:** http://www.purehealth.com
Dr. Farida Sharan, Director
**Program(s):** Energy Work; Herbal Medicine; Iridology; Naturopathy.


**★ 3578 ★ University of Colorado School of Nursing Nurse-Midwifery Option**
Health Sciences Center
4200 E 9th Ave., Box C288-14
Denver, CO 80262
**Phone:** (303)315-8654          **Fax:** (303)315-5666
**Email:** laraine.guyette@uchsc.edu
Laraine Guyette, PhD, Director
**Program(s):** Midwifery.


## Connecticut

**★ 3579 ★ Connecticut Center for Massage Therapy, Inc.**
25 Sylvan Rd. S
Westport, CT 06880
**Phone:** (203)221-7325          **Fax:** (203)221-0144
**Email:** info@ccmt.com
**Website:** http://www.ccmt.com
Susan Scoboria, Director

**Program(s):** Acupressure; Alexander Technique; Aromatherapy; CranioSacral Therapy; Energy Work; Feldenkrais; Massage Therapy; Neuromuscular Therapy; Polarity Therapy; Reflexology; Reiki; Shiatsu; Sports Massage.


**★ 3580 ★ Connecticut Center for Massage Therapy, Inc.**
75 Kitts Ln.
Newington, CT 06111
**Phone:** (860)667-1886          **Fax:** (860)667-2175
**Email:** info@ccmt.com
**Website:** http://www.ccmt.com
Wendy Dorsey, Director

**Program(s):** Acupressure; Energy Work; Massage Therapy; Meditation; Neuromuscular Therapy; Reflexology; Reiki; Shiatsu; Sports Massage.


**★ 3581 ★ Connecticut Institute for Herbal Studies**
87 Market Sq.
Newington, CT 06111
**Phone:** (860)666-5064          **Fax:** (860)666-5064
**Email:** laurachina@aol.com
Laura Mignosa, Director
**Program(s):** Herbal Medicine; Traditional Chinese Medicine.


**★ 3582 ★ QiGong Institute**
361 Post Rd. W
Westport, CT 06880
**Email:** akim.070972@aol.com
Dr. Richard M. Chin, Director
**Program(s):** Acupressure; CranioSacral Therapy; Energy Work; Herbal Medicine; Neuromuscular Therapy; Oriental Medicine; Polarity Therapy; Qigong; Reflexology; Shiatsu; Traditional Chinese Medicine.


**★ 3583 ★ Rosen Center East, LLC**
PO Box 5004
Westport, CT 06880
**Phone:** (203)319-1090          **Fax:** (203)319-0032
Sue Brenner, Director
**Program(s):** Rosen Method Bodywork.


**★ 3584 ★ School of Homeopathy-Devon, England**
82 E Pearl St.
New Haven, CT 06513
**Phone:** (203)624-8783          **Fax:** (203)624-8783
Betsy Levine, Contact
**Program(s):** Anatomy and Physiology; Homeopathy; Pathology and Disease.


**★ 3585 ★ University of Bridgeport College of Chiropractic**
75 Linden Ave.
Bridgeport, CT 06601
**Phone:** (203)576-4279          **Fax:** (203)576-4351
**Website:** http://www.bridgeport.edu/chiro/
Frank Zolli, Contact
**Program(s):** Chiropractic.


**★ 3586 ★ University of Bridgeport, College of Naturopathic Medicine**
60 Lafayette St.
Bridgeport, CT 06601
**Phone:** (203)576-4109          **Fax:** (203)576-4107
Miriam Madweb, Contact
**Program(s):** Acupuncture; Herbal Medicine; Homeopathy; Massage Therapy; Naturopathic Medicine; Nutrition.


**★ 3587 ★ Yale University School of Nursing**
100 Church St. S, Box 9740
New Haven, CT 06536-0740

**Phone:** (203)737-2344          **Fax:** (203)785-6455
Barbara Reif, Contact
**Program(s):** Midwifery.


## Delaware

**★ 3588 ★ Deep Muscle Therapy School**
5317 Limestone Rd.
Wilmington, DE 19808
**Phone:** (302)239-1613          **Fax:** (302)239-5195
Velda Martin, Contact
**Program(s):** Deep Tissue Massage; Massage Therapy.


**★ 3589 ★ Karen Carlson International Academy of Holistic Massage and Science**
PO Box 3940
Greenville, DE 19807
**Phone:** (302)777-7307
Marilue Hartman, Contact
**Program(s):** Acupressure; Biofeedback; Energy Work; Feldenkrais; Herbal Medicine; Homeopathy; Massage Therapy; Reflexology.


## District of Columbia

**★ 3590 ★ Focus on Healing Reflexology Center**
2808 Douglas St. NE
PO Box 26132
Washington, DC 20018
**Phone:** (301)779-8005          **Fax:** (301)779-8006
Njideka N. Olatunde, Director
**Program(s):** Reflexology.


**★ 3591 ★ Georgetown University, School of Nursing**
3700 Reservoir Rd. NW
Washington, DC 20007
**Phone:** (202)687-5041          **Fax:** (202)687-5553
Michele Havin, Contact
**Program(s):** Midwifery.


**★ 3592 ★ Institute for Ethical and Clinical Hypnosis**
2510 M St. NW
Washington, DC 20037
**Phone:** (202)331-1218          **Fax:** (202)659-9580
Masud Ansari, Contact
**Program(s):** Hypnotherapy.


**★ 3593 ★ Potomac Massage Training Institute**
4000 Albermarle St. NW 5th Fl.
Washington, DC 20016
**Phone:** (202)686-7046          **Fax:** (202)966-4579
Rose A. Gowdey, Director

**Program(s):** Alexander Technique; Aromatherapy; CranioSacral Therapy; Energy Work; Infant Massage; Massage Therapy; Myofascial Release; Neuromuscular Therapy; Polarity Therapy; Pregnancy Massage; Qigong; Reflexology; Reiki; Shiatsu; Sports Massage; Traditional Chinese Medicine.


## Florida

**★ 3594 ★ Academy of Chinese Healing Arts, Inc.**
505 S Orange Ave.
Sarasota, FL 34236
**Phone:** (941)955-4456          **Fax:** (941)330-1951
**Email:** acha@gte.net
Cynthia O'Donnell, Contact
**Program(s):** Acupressure; Acupuncture; Herbal Medicine; Homeopathy; Oriental Medicine; Qigong; Shiatsu; Traditional Chinese Medicine.

**★ 3595 ★ Academy for Five Element Acupuncture**
1170-A E Hallandale Beach Blvd.
Hallandale, FL 33009
**Phone:** (954)456-6336　　**Fax:** (954)456-3944
Isaac Goren, Director
**Program(s):** Acupuncture; Herbal Medicine.

**★ 3596 ★ Academy of Healing Arts, Massage and Facial Skin Care, Inc.**
3141 S Military Trail
Lake Worth, FL 33463
**Phone:** (561)965-5550　　**Fax:** (561)641-2603
Angela K. Artemik, Director
**Program(s):** Acupressure; Aromatherapy; Massage Therapy; Reflexology; Shiatsu.

**★ 3597 ★ Academy of Lymphatic Studies**
12651 W Sunrise Blvd.
Sunrise, FL 33323
**Phone:** (954)846-7855　　**Free:** 800-863-5935
**Fax:** (954)845-9207
Joachim E. Zuther, Director
**Program(s):** Complete Decongestive Physiotherapy; Manual Lymph Drainage.

**★ 3598 ★ Acupressure-Acupuncture Institute**
10506 N Kendall Dr.
Miami, FL 33176
**Phone:** (305)595-9500　　**Fax:** (305)595-2622
**Email:** aai@acupuncture.pair.com
Nancy Browne, Director
**Program(s):** Acupressure; Acupuncture; Herbal Medicine; Homeopathy; Massage Therapy; Oriental Medicine; Qigong; Reiki; Shiatsu; Traditional Chinese Medicine.

**★ 3599 ★ Alpha Institute of South Florida, Inc.**
904 Park Ave.
Lake Park, FL 33403
**Phone:** (561)845-1400　　**Fax:** (561)845-1360
Douglas C. Espie, Director
**Program(s):** Aromatherapy; CranioSacral Therapy; Deep Tissue Massage; Energy Work; Hypnotherapy; Massage Therapy; Oriental Medicine; Polarity Therapy; Reflexology; Reiki; Shiatsu; Skin Care.

**★ 3600 ★ Alpha School of Massage, Inc.**
4642 San Juan Ave.
Jacksonville, FL 32210
**Phone:** (904)389-9117　　**Fax:** (904)389-6496
Edward L. Driggers, Contact
**Program(s):** Acupressure; Aromatherapy; Energy Work; Herbal Medicine; Homeopathy; Massage Therapy; Neuromuscular Therapy; Reflexology; Reiki; Shiatsu; Sports Massage.

**★ 3601 ★ American Institute of Massage Therapy, Inc., Fort Lauderdale**
2101 N Federal Hwy.
Fort Lauderdale, FL 33301
**Phone:** (954)568-6200　　**Fax:** (954)568-6100
**Email:** info@aimt.com
**Website:** http://www.aimt.com
Lexa Allin Sutherland, Director
**Program(s):** Aromatherapy; Colon Hydrotherapy; CranioSacral Therapy; Massage Therapy; Neuromuscular Therapy; Reflexology; Sports Massage.

**★ 3602 ★ American Yoga Association**
PO Box 19986
Sarasota, FL 34276
**Phone:** (941)927-4977　　**Fax:** (941)921-9844
Patricia Rockwood, Director
**Program(s):** Yoga Teacher Training.

**★ 3603 ★ Atlantic Institute of Aromatherapy**
2514 W Kennedy Blvd.
Tampa, FL 33609
**Phone:** (813)265-2222　　**Fax:** (813)265-2222
Sylla Sheppard-Hanger, Director
**Program(s):** Aromatherapy.

**★ 3604 ★ Atlantic Institute of Oriental Medicine**
1057 SE 17th St.
Fort Lauderdale, FL 33316
**Phone:** (954)463-3888　　**Fax:** (954)463-3878
Edith Tonelli, Director
**Program(s):** Acupuncture; Herbal Medicine; Oriental Medicine; Traditional Chinese Medicine.

**★ 3605 ★ Bhakti Academe School of Intuitive Massage and Healing**
25400 US 19 N
Clearwater, FL 33763
**Phone:** (727)724-9727
Dale McNiff, Contact
**Program(s):** Bhakti Bodywork; Energy Work; Massage Therapy.

**★ 3606 ★ Biofeedback Therapist Training Institute**
1826 University Blvd. W
Jacksonville, FL 32217
**Phone:** (904)737-5821　　**Fax:** (904)730-3821
**Email:** hartje@aol.com
**Website:** http://www.hartje.com
Jack C. Hartje, PhD, Director
**Program(s):** Biofeedback.

**★ 3607 ★ Birth Buddies**
5329 Buggy Whip Dr. N
Jacksonville, FL 32257
**Phone:** (904)268-5629　　**Fax:** (904)363-6356
Susan Toffolon, Director
**Program(s):** Doula.

**★ 3608 ★ Boca Raton Institute**
5499 N Federal Hwy., Ste. A
Boca Raton, FL 33487
**Phone:** (561)241-8105　　**Fax:** (561)241-9789
Constance M. Gregg, Director
**Program(s):** Acupressure; Aromatherapy; CranioSacral Therapy; Massage Therapy; Neuromuscular Therapy; Polarity Therapy; Reflexology; Shiatsu.

**★ 3609 ★ Bonita Springs/Venice School of Massage Therapy**
10915 Bonita Beach Rd., Ste. 2121
Bonita Springs, FL 34135
**Phone:** (941)495-0714　　**Fax:** (941)498-7164
Fred Maehr, Director
**Program(s):** Aromatherapy; Colon Hydrotherapy; Herbal Medicine; Massage Therapy; Neuromuscular Therapy; Reflexology; Shiatsu; Spa Therapies.

**★ 3610 ★ The Bramham Institute**
1014 N Olive Ave.
West Palm Beach, FL 33401
**Free:** 800-575-0518　　**Fax:** (561)832-6642
Sara Eavenson, Director
**Program(s):** Aromatherapy; Connective Tissue Massage; Hydrotherapy; Manual Lymph Drainage; Reflexology; Spa Therapies.

**★ 3611 ★ Central Florida Hypnosis Institute**
9737 Fairway Cir.
Leesburg, FL 34788
**Phone:** (352)315-0555　　**Fax:** (352)315-0383
Earl J. Yawman, Director
**Program(s):** Hypnotherapy.

**★ 3612 ★ Classical Acupuncture Institute**
4237 Salisbury Rd., Ste. 108
Jacksonville, FL 32216
**Phone:** (904)296-0906
Debbie Rewis, Director
**Program(s):** Acupuncture.

**★ 3613 ★ CORE Institute School of Massage Therapy and Structural Bodywork**
223 W Carolina St.
Tallahassee, FL 32301
**Phone:** (850)222-8673　　**Fax:** (850)561-6160
**Email:** core@nettally.com
**Website:** http://www.coreinstitute.com
George Kousealeos, Director
**Program(s):** Massage Therapy; Myofascial Release.

**★ 3614 ★ Delphi Center for Midwifery Studies**
3102 W Cypress St., Ste. B
Tampa, FL 33607-5108
**Phone:** (813)873-7135　　**Fax:** (813)873-0274
**Email:** delphicntr@aol.com
Karin Kearns, Director
**Program(s):** Midwifery.

**★ 3615 ★ Educating Hands of School Massage**
120 SW 8th St.
Miami, FL 33130
**Phone:** (305)285-6991　　**Fax:** (305)857-0298
**Website:** http://massagetherapynetwork.com/edhand1.html
Kathy Ozzard, Director
**Program(s):** Massage Therapy.

**★ 3616 ★ Florida Academy of Massage**
8695 College Pkwy., Ste. 110
Fort Myers, FL 33919
**Phone:** (941)489-2282　　**Free:** 800-324-9543
**Fax:** (941)489-4065
Masud Ansari, Contact
**Program(s):** Massage Therapy.

**★ 3617 ★ Florida College of Natural Health**
8216 S Tamiami Trail
Sarasota, FL 34238
**Phone:** (941)966-7117　　**Free:** 800-966-7117
Prudence Sterling, Director
**Program(s):** Acupressure; Acupuncture; Aromatherapy; Herbal Medicine; Homeopathy; Massage Therapy; Neuromuscular Therapy; Polarity Therapy; Reflexology; Reiki; Shiatsu; Skin Care; Sports Massage; Traditional Chinese Medicine.

**★ 3618 ★ Florida College of Natural Health**
7925 NW 12th St., Ste. 201
Miami, FL 33126
**Phone:** (305)597-9599　　**Free:** 800-599-9599
**Fax:** (305)597-9110
Lucy Bonilla, Director
**Program(s):** Acupressure; Acupuncture; Aromatherapy; CranioSacral Therapy; Massage Therapy; Myofascial Release; Neuromuscular Therapy; Polarity Therapy; Reflexology; Shiatsu; Sports Massage.

**★ 3619 ★ Florida College of Natural Health**
887 E Altamonte Dr.
Altamonte Springs, FL 32701

Phone: (407)261-0319          Free: 800-393-7337
Fax: (407)261-0342
Thea Depinto, Director

Program(s): Acupressure; Acupuncture; Aromatherapy; CranioSacral Therapy; Energy Work; Massage Therapy; Neuromuscular Therapy; Reflexology; Shiatsu; Skin Care; Sports Massage; Swedish Massage.


★ **3620** ★ **Florida College of Natural Health, Pompano Beach**
2001 W Sample Rd., Ste. 100
Pompano Beach, FL 33064
Phone: (954)975-6400          Fax: (954)975-9633
Kristi Mollis, Director

Program(s): Acupuncture; Massage Therapy; Skin Care.


★ **3621** ★ **Florida Health Academy - Naples**
261 Ninth St. S
Naples, FL 34102
Phone: (941)263-9391          Fax: (941)263-8680
Clara E. McElroy, Director

Program(s): Acupuncture; Aromatherapy; Herbal Medicine; Massage Therapy; Skin Care; Traditional Chinese Medicine.


★ **3622** ★ **Florida Institute of Postural Integration**
5837 Mariner Dr.
Tampa, FL 33609
Phone: (813)286-2273          Fax: (813)287-2870
Joy K. Johnson, Director

Program(s): Acupressure; Deep Tissue Massage.


★ **3623** ★ **Florida Institute of Traditional Chinese Medicine**
5335 66th St. N
Saint Petersburg, FL 33709
Phone: (813)546-6565          Fax: (813)547-0703
Dr. Su Liang Ku, Director

Program(s): Acupuncture; Herbal Medicine; Traditional Chinese Medicine; Tui Na.


★ **3624** ★ **Florida School of Massage**
6421 SW 13th St.
Gainesville, FL 32608
Phone: (352)378-7891          Fax: (352)376-7218
Email: info@massageonline.com
Website: http://www.massageonline.com
Paul Davenport, Director

Program(s): Anatomy and Physiology; CPR/First Aid; Colon Hydrotherapy; Connective Tissue Massage; Hydrotherapy; Massage Therapy; Neuromuscular Therapy; Polarity Therapy; Reflexology; Shiatsu; Sports Massage; Structural Integration; Swedish Massage.


★ **3625** ★ **Florida School of Traditional Midwifery**
6501 SW 13 St.
PO Box 5505
Gainesville, FL 32608
Phone: (352)338-0766          Fax: (352)338-2013
Jana Borino, Director

Program(s): Midwifery.


★ **3626** ★ **Florida's Therapeutic Massage School**
1300 E Gadsden St.
Pensacola, FL 32501
Phone: (850)433-8212
Geraldine Vaurigaud, Director

Program(s): Acupressure; Aromatherapy; Herbal Medicine; Hydrotherapy; Massage Therapy; Neuromuscular Therapy; Oriental Medicine; Polarity Therapy; Reflexology; Shiatsu; Sports Massage.


★ **3627** ★ **HealthBuilders School of Therapeutic Massage Inc.**
2180 State Rd. A1A
Saint Augustine, FL 32084
Phone: (904)471-8828          Fax: (904)471-8838
Karen Peters, Director

Program(s): Aromatherapy; Deep Tissue Massage; Energy Work; Massage Therapy; Polarity Therapy; Reflexology; Reiki.


★ **3628** ★ **Holistic Health Services**
1551 S 1st St., Ste. 701
Jacksonville Beach, FL 32250
Phone: (904)246-6064          Fax: (904)247-1266
Gail Greenfield, Director

Program(s): Reiki.


★ **3629** ★ **Humanities Center Institute of Allied Health/School of Massage**
4045 Park Blvd.
Pinellas Park, FL 33781
Phone: (727)541-5200          Fax: (727)545-0053
Sherry L. Fears, Director

Program(s): Massage Therapy; Neuromuscular Therapy.


★ **3630** ★ **Integrated Health Care System**
PO Box 67153
Saint Petersburg, FL 33736
Phone: (813)367-3063          Fax: (813)367-3170
Shirley Begley, Director

Program(s): Energy Work; Guided Imagery; Holistic Nursing; Hypnotherapy; Therapeutic Touch.


★ **3631** ★ **International Institute of Reflexology**
5650 1st Ave. N
PO Box 12642
Saint Petersburg, FL 33710
Phone: (727)343-4811          Fax: (727)381-2807
Dwight C. Byers, Contact

Program(s): Reflexology.


★ **3632** ★ **Jacksonville School of Massage Therapy, Inc.**
5305 San Juan Ave.
Jacksonville, FL 32210
Phone: (904)389-3878
Earl F. Kennedy, PhD, Director

Program(s): Acupressure; Aromatherapy; Ayurvedic Medicine; Biofeedback; Colon Hydrotherapy; Massage Therapy; Polarity Therapy; Reflexology; Reiki; Shiatsu; Traditional Chinese Medicine.


★ **3633** ★ **National College of Oriental Medicine**
7100 Lake Ellenor Dr.
Orlando, FL 32806
Phone: (407)888-8689          Fax: (407)888-8211
Email: info@acupunctureschool.com
Lloyd Buss, MD, Contact

Program(s): Acupuncture; Herbal Medicine; Oriental Medicine; Traditional Chinese Medicine.


★ **3634** ★ **Omni Hypnosis Training Center**
830 N Woodland Blvd.
Deland, FL 32720
Phone: (904)738-9188          Fax: (904)736-7598
Email: omni@omnihypnosis.com
Website: http://www.omnihypnosis.com
Gerald F. Kein, Director

Program(s): Hypnotherapy.


★ **3635** ★ **Orlando Institute School of Massage Therapy, Inc.**
3385 S Hwy. 17-92, Ste. 221
Casselberry, FL 32707
Phone: (407)331-1101          Fax: (407)331-8331
Stacee Diehl, Director

Program(s): Aromatherapy; Massage Therapy; Polarity Therapy; Reflexology; Shiatsu.


★ **3636** ★ **Reiki Plus Institute**
707 Barcelona Rd.
Key Largo, FL 33037
Phone: (305)451-9881
David G. Jarrell, Director

Program(s): Energy Work; Reiki.


★ **3637** ★ **ReNew Life and Dotolo Institute School of Colon Hydrotherapy**
1007 N MacDill
Tampa, FL 33607
Phone: (813)871-3200          Fax: (813)877-2640
Suzanne M. Gray, Contact

Program(s): Colon Hydrotherapy.


★ **3638** ★ **Ridge Technical Center**
7700 State Rd. 544
Winter Haven, FL 33881
Phone: (941)299-2512          Fax: (941)419-3060
Steve Strodman, Director

Program(s): Massage Therapy.


★ **3639** ★ **Saint John Neuromuscular Pain Relief Institute**
10710 Seminole Blvd., Ste. 1
Seminole, FL 33778
Phone: (727)397-5525          Free: 888-668-4325
Fax: (727)397-5808
Paul St. John, Director

Program(s): Neuromuscular Therapy.


★ **3640** ★ **Sarasota School of Massage Therapy**
1970 Main St., 3rd Fl.
Sarasota, FL 34236
Phone: (941)957-0577          Fax: (941)957-1049
Michael Rosen-Pyros, Director

Program(s): Aromatherapy; CranioSacral Therapy; Massage Therapy; Neuromuscular Therapy; Polarity Therapy; Reflexology.


★ **3641** ★ **Seminar Network Intl., Inc. d/b/a SNI School of Massage and Allied Services**
518 N Federal Hwy.
Lake Worth, FL 33460
Phone: (561)582-5349          Free: 800-882-0903
Fax: (561)582-0807
Nancy Putzan, Director

Program(s): Colon Hydrotherapy; Massage Therapy.


★ **3642** ★ **Southeastern School of Neuromuscular and Massage Therapy, Inc.**
9088 Golfside Dr.
Jacksonville, FL 32256
Phone: (904)448-9499          Fax: (904)448-9270
Kyle C. Wright, Contact

Program(s): Acupressure; CranioSacral Therapy; Feldenkrais; Herbal Medicine; Homeopathy; Massage Therapy; Neuromuscular Therapy; Polarity Therapy; Reflexology; Reiki; Shiatsu.


★ **3643** ★ **University of Florida, Health Science Center**
653 W 8th St., Bldg 1, 2nd Flr.
Jacksonville, FL 32209-6561

Phone: (904)549-3245
Alice H. Poe, Director
**Program(s):** Midwifery.


★ 3644 ★ **University of Miami
School of Nursing**
5801 Red. Rd.
Coral Gables, FL 33124-3850
**Phone:** (305)284-6256
Virginia Crandall, Contact
**Program(s):** Midwifery.


★ 3645 ★ **The Upledger Institute**
11211 Prosperity Farms Rd., D-325
Palm Beach Gardens, FL 33410
**Phone:** (561)622-4334          **Free:** 800-233-5880
**Fax:** (561)622-4771
**Email:** upledger@upledger.com
Kevin Roberts, Director
**Program(s):** CranioSacral Therapy; Mechanical Link;
Visceral Manipulation; Zero Blancing.


★ 3646 ★ **Wood Hygienic Institute**
2220 E Irlo Bronson Hwy.
Kissimmee, FL 34744
**Phone:** (407)933-0009
**Program(s):** Colon Hydrotherapy; Massage Therapy.


★ 3647 ★ **Yoga Institute of Miami**
9350 S Dadeland Blvd., Ste. 207
Miami, FL 33156
**Phone:** (305)670-0558          **Fax:** (305)661-9943
Bobbi Goldin, Director
**Program(s):** Yoga Teacher Training.


### Georgia

★ 3648 ★ **Academy of Somatic Healing
Arts**
1924 Cliff Valley Way
Atlanta, GA 30329
**Phone:** (404)315-0394          **Fax:** (404)633-1270
Jim Gabriel, Director
**Program(s):** Massage Therapy; Neuromuscular Ther-
apy; Sports Massage.


★ 3649 ★ **Alexander Technique of
Atlanta**
4246 Peachtree Rd., Ste. 6
Atlanta, GA 30319
**Phone:** (770)454-1177
Ron Dennis, Director
**Program(s):** Alexander Technique.


★ 3650 ★ **Atlanta School of Massage**
2300 Peachford Rd., Ste. 3200
Atlanta, GA 30338
**Phone:** (770)454-7167          **Free:** 888-276-6277
**Fax:** (770)454-7367
**Program(s):** Acupressure; Aromatherapy; Deep Tissue Massage; Integrative Massage; Massage Therapy; Polarity Therapy; Reflexology; Shiatsu; Spa Therapies.


★ 3651 ★ **Capelli Learning Center**
2581 Piedmont Rd., Ste. C-1000
Atlanta, GA 30324
**Phone:** (404)261-5261          **Fax:** (404)261-5069
Deb Elkin, Contact
**Program(s):** Deep Tissue Massage; Massage Thera-
py; Qigong; Reflexology; Thai Massage; Traditional
Chinese Medicine.


★ 3652 ★ **Emory University,
Nell Hodgson Woodruff School of
Nursing**
Atlanta, GA 30322
**Phone:** (404)727-6961          **Fax:** (404)727-0536
L. Leush, Contact
**Program(s):** Midwifery.


★ 3653 ★ **Georgia Institute of
Therapeutic Massage, LLC**
2160 Centra Ave.
PO Box 3657
Augusta, GA 30904
**Phone:** (706)738-7695          **Fax:** (706)738-6232
Vicki N. Platt, Director
**Program(s):** Acupressure; Massage Therapy; Neuro-
muscular Therapy; Polarity Therapy; Reflexology;
Shiatsu; Sports Massage; Swedish Massage.


★ 3654 ★ **Lake Lanier School of
Massage**
400 Brenau Ave.
Gainesville, GA 30501
**Phone:** (770)287-0377          **Fax:** (770)536-7350
Sandra Easterbrooks, Contact
**Program(s):** Massage Therapy.


★ 3655 ★ **Life University, School of
Chiropractic**
1269 Barclay Cir.
Marietta, GA 30060
**Phone:** (770)426-2884          **Free:** 800-543-3345
**Fax:** (770)428-9886
Harry Harrison, Contact
**Program(s):** Chiropractic.


★ 3656 ★ **New Life Institute Inc., School
of Massage Excellence**
4330 Georgetown Sq., Ste. 500
Atlanta, GA 30338
**Phone:** (770)457-2021          **Fax:** (770)457-5614
Sandy Jones, Contact
**Program(s):** Massage Therapy.


★ 3657 ★ **Polarity Training Institute**
566 Pharr Rd.
Atlanta, GA 30305
**Phone:** (770)704-5170
Will Leichnitz, Contact
**Program(s):** Polarity Therapy.


### Hawaii

★ 3658 ★ **Aisen Shiatsu School**
1314 S King St., Ste. 601
Honolulu, HI 96814
**Phone:** (808)596-7354          **Fax:** (808)593-8282
Fumihiko Indei, Director
**Program(s):** Shiatsu.


★ 3659 ★ **Aloha Kaui Massage Workshop**
PO Box 622
Hanalei, HI 96714
**Phone:** (808)826-9990          **Fax:** (808)826-6180
Devaki Holman, Contact
**Program(s):** Massage Therapy.


★ 3660 ★ **American Institute of Massage
Therapy, Kailua**
407 Uluniu St., Ste. 204A
Kailua, HI 96734
**Phone:** (808)266-2468          **Fax:** (808)266-2460
Elizabeth Reveley, Contact
**Program(s):** Acupressure; Aromatherapy; CranioSa-
cral Therapy; Deep Tissue Massage; Energy Work;
Healing Touch; Hypnotherapy; Massage Therapy;
Reflexology.


★ 3661 ★ **American Viniyoga Institute**
PO Box 88
Makawao, HI 96768
**Phone:** (808)572-1414
Mary Lou Mellinger, Contact
**Program(s):** Yoga Teacher Training; Yoga Therapy.


★ 3662 ★ **Big Island Academy of
Massage, Inc.**
211 Kinoole St.
Hilo, HI 96720
**Phone:** (808)935-1405
Paul Rambo, Contact
**Program(s):** Acupressure; Aromatherapy; Deep Tis-
sue Massage; Energy Work; LomiLomi; Massage
Therapy; Polarity Therapy; Reflexology; Reiki; Shiat-
su; Sports Massage.


★ 3663 ★ **Hawaii College of Health
Sciences**
1750 Kalakuna Ave., Ste. 2404
Honolulu, HI 96826
**Phone:** (808)941-8223          **Fax:** (808)944-8343
Evelyn James, Contact
**Program(s):** Acupressure; CranioSacral Therapy;
Deep Tissue Massage; Herbal Medicine; Massage
Therapy; Polarity Therapy; Reflexology; Shiatsu; Tra-
ditional Chinese Medicine.


★ 3664 ★ **Hawaii College of Traditional
Oriental Medicine**
PO Box 457
Kula, HI 96790
**Phone:** (808)573-0899          **Fax:** (808)573-2450
**Program(s):** Acupressure; Acupuncture; Herbal Medi-
cine; Oriental Medicine; Qigong; Shiatsu; Traditional
Chinese Medicine.


★ 3665 ★ **Hawaiian Islands School of
Body Therapies**
78-6739 Alii Dr.
PO Box 390188
Kailua Kona, HI 96740
**Phone:** (808)322-0048          **Fax:** (808)322-4971
Peter Wind, Director
**Program(s):** Aromatherapy; CranioSacral Therapy;
Massage Therapy; Polarity Therapy; Reflexology; Re-
storative Treatment Therapy; Shiatsu.


★ 3666 ★ **Honolulu School of Massage,
Inc.**
1136 12th Ave., Ste. 240
Honolulu, HI 96816
**Phone:** (808)733-0000          **Fax:** (808)733-0045
**Email:** hsminc@msn.com
Gayle E. Volger, Director
**Program(s):** Applied Kinesiology; CranioSacral Ther-
apy; Deep Tissue Massage; Hydrotherapy; LomiLomi
Massage; Massage Therapy; Neuromuscular Thera-
py; Reflexology; Shiatsu; Sports Massage.


★ 3667 ★ **Institute of Clinical
Acupuncture and Oriental Medicine**
1270 Queen Emma St., Ste. 107
Honolulu, HI 96813
**Phone:** (808)521-2288          **Fax:** (808)521-2288
Catherine Low, Contact
**Program(s):** Acupuncture; Herbal Medicine; Oriental
Medicine; Traditional Chinese Medicine.


★ 3668 ★ **Maui Academy of the Healing
Arts**
1993 S Kihei Rd., Ste. 210
Kihei, HI 96753
**Phone:** (808)879-4266          **Fax:** (808)879-4484
**Email:** sancorp@maui.net
**Website:** http://www.maui.net/~sancorp/
John Sanderson, Director

**Program(s):** Acupressure; Esalen Massage; LomiLomi Massage; Lymphatic Massage; Massage Therapy; Reflexology; Shiatsu; Sports Massage; Swedish Massage; Thai Massage.

★ 3669 ★ **Pacific Center for Awareness and Bodywork**
7703 Koolau Rd.
PO Box 672
Kilauea, HI 96754
**Phone:** (808)828-6797          **Fax:** (808)828-6797
**Website:** http://www.oxford-intl.com/pacific
John Sanderson, Director

**Program(s):** Acupressure; Awareness Practices; Connective Bodywork; Hypnotherapy; Massage Therapy; Neuromuscular Therapy; Polarity Therapy; Reflexology; Structural Integration.

★ 3670 ★ **Tai Hsuan Foundation: College of Acupuncture and Herbal Medicine**
2600 S King St., Rm. 206
PO Box 11130
Honolulu, HI 96826
**Free:** 800-942-4788          **Fax:** (808)949-1005
**Email:** taihsuan@acupuncture-hi.com
**Website:** http://www.acupuncture-hi.com
Dr. Gayle Todoki, Contact

**Program(s):** Acupressure; Acupuncture; Herbal Medicine; Oriental Medicine; Qigong; Traditional Chinese Medicine.

★ 3671 ★ **Traditional Chinese Medical College of Hawaii**
PO Box 2288
Kamuela, HI 96743
**Phone:** (808)885-9226          **Fax:** (808)885-9226

**Program(s):** Acupuncture; Oriental Medicine; Traditional Chinese Medicine.

★ 3672 ★ **University of Health Sciences**
1778 Ala Moana Blvd., Ste. 1307
Honolulu, HI 96815
**Phone:** (808)951-8242          **Fax:** (808)951-8242
Lucy Han Lee, Contact

**Program(s):** Acupressure; Acupuncture; Herbal Medicine; Homeopathy; Iridology; Qigong; Reflexology; Shiatsu; Traditional Chinese Medicine.

## Idaho

★ 3673 ★ **Idaho Institute of Wholistic Studies**
1412 W Washington
Boise, ID 83702
**Phone:** (208)345-2704          **Fax:** (208)367-9242
Barbera Bashan, Director

**Program(s):** Acupressure; Massage Therapy; Shiatsu; Sports Massage; Traditional Chinese Medicine.

★ 3674 ★ **Idaho School of Massage Therapy**
5353 Franklin Rd.
Boise, ID 83705
**Phone:** (208)343-1847
Cindy J. Langston, Contact

**Program(s):** Connective Tissue Massage; Deep Tissue Massage; Massage Therapy; Relexology; Shiatsu; Sports Massage; Swedish Massage.

★ 3675 ★ **Moscow School of Massage**
S 600 Main
Moscow, ID 83843
**Phone:** (208)882-7867
Lisa O'Leary, Director

**Program(s):** Deep Tissue Massage; Massage Therapy; Oriental Medicine; Qigong.

## Illinois

★ 3676 ★ **Best Institute of Hypnosis**
832 16th Ave.
East Moline, IL 61244-2124
**Phone:** (309)755-2378          **Fax:** (309)755-1669
Kenn Geiger, Director

**Program(s):** Hypnotherapy.

★ 3677 ★ **Center for Therapeutic Massage and Wellness**
2704 Woodridge Rd.
Woodridge, IL 60517
**Phone:** (708)960-9053
Bea Stanton, Director

**Program(s):** CranioSacral Therapy; Energy Work; Massage Therapy; Qigong; Reflexology; Reiki; Sports Massage; Therapeutic Touch.

★ 3678 ★ **Chicago National College of Naprapathy**
3330 N Milwaukee Ave.
Chicago, IL 60641
**Phone:** (773)282-2686          **Fax:** (773)282-2688
Dr. Alexanne Osinski, Contact

**Program(s):** Naprapathy; Neuromuscular Therapy.

★ 3679 ★ **Chicago School of Massage Therapy**
2918 N Lincoln Ave.
Chicago, IL 60657
**Phone:** (773)477-9444          **Fax:** (773)477-7256
Jeff Marzano, Director

**Program(s):** Acupressure; Anatomy and Physiology; CranioSacral Therapy; Energy Work; Massage Therapy; Myofascial Release; Reflexology; Shiatsu; Sports Massage.

★ 3680 ★ **Edens Institute of Alternative Therapy**
212 N Park
Herrin, IL 62948
**Phone:** (618)942-8825
E. J. Engram, Director

**Program(s):** Massage Therapy.

★ 3681 ★ **Integrative Yoag Therapy**
1207 Lincoln Avee.
Galena, IL 61036
**Phone:** (815)777-6068          **Free:** 800-750-9642
**Fax:** (815)777-6629
Joseph LePage, Director

**Program(s):** Yoga Teacher Training.

★ 3682 ★ **International Thai Therapist Association, Inc.**
47 W Polk St., Ste. 100-329
Chicago, IL 60605
**Phone:** (773)792-4121          **Fax:** (773)326-6442
**Email:** itta@ix.netcom.com
Anthony B. James, PhD, Director

**Program(s):** Acupressure; Aromatherapy; Ayurvedic Medicine; CranioSacral Therapy; Energy Work; Herbal Medicine; Massage Therapy; Neuromuscular Therapy; Oriental Medicine; Qigong; Reflexology; Reiki; Shiatsu; Thai Massage; Traditional Chinese Medicine.

★ 3683 ★ **Kurashova Institute, Inc.**
PO Box 6246
Rock Island, IL 61201
**Phone:** (309)786-4888          **Fax:** (309)786-8687
Zhenya K. Wine, Director

**Program(s):** Massage Therapy; Neuromuscular Therapy; Russian Massage.

★ 3684 ★ **Leidecker Institute**
1901 N Roselle Rd., Ste. 800
Schaumburg, IL 60195
**Phone:** (847)844-1933
Lynsi Brule, Director

**Program(s):** Acupressure; Aromatherapy; Hypnotherapy; Reflexology; Reiki.

★ 3685 ★ **LifePath School of Massage Therapy**
7820 N University, Ste. 110
Peoria, IL 61614
**Free:** 888-254-3372          **Fax:** (309)693-7293
**Email:** rwasher@flink.com
Rhonda Washer, Director

**Program(s):** CranioSacral Therapy; Massage Therapy; Neuromuscular Therapy; Polarity Therapy; Reflexology; Shiatsu; Sports Massage; Swedish Massage.

★ 3686 ★ **Midwest Center for the Study of Oriental Medicine**
4334 N Hazel, Ste. 206
Chicago, IL 60613
**Phone:** (773)975-1295
William Dunbar, Director

**Program(s):** Acupressure; Acupuncture; Herbal Medicine; Oriental Medicine; Dtraditional Chinese Medicine.

★ 3687 ★ **National College of Chiropractic**
200 E Roosevelt Rd.
Lombard, IL 60148
**Phone:** (630)889-2000          **Free:** 800-826-6285
**Fax:** (630)889-6554
James F. Winterstein, Contact

**Program(s):** Acupuncture; Chiropractic.

★ 3688 ★ **Northern Prairie School of Therapeutic Massage and Bodywork, Inc.**
138 N Fair St.
Sycamore, IL 60178
**Phone:** (815)899-3382          **Fax:** (815)899-3381
Jeannette Vaupel, Director

**Program(s):** Acupressure; Aromatherapy; Ayurvedic Medicine; Biofeedback, CranioSacral Therapy; Energy Work; Herbal Medicine; Homeopathy; Hypnotherapy; Massage Therapy; Oriental Medicine; Polarity Therapy; Qigong; Reflexology, Reiki; Shiatsu; Traditional Chinese Medicine.

★ 3689 ★ **Ohashiatsu Chicago**
825 Chicago Ave.
Evanston, IL 60202
**Phone:** (847)864-1130          **Fax:** (847)733-9473
Matthew Sweigart, Director

**Program(s):** Acupressure; Shiatsu.

★ 3690 ★ **Pamela Arwine**
1701 Marguerite St.
Crystal Lake, IL 60014
**Phone:** (815)455-4502
Pamela Arwine, Director

**Program(s):** Hypnotherapy; Reiki.

★ 3691 ★ **University of Illinois, Chicago School of Nursing**
845 S Damen Ave.
Chicago, IL 60612
**Phone:** (312)996-7937
Janet Engstrom, Director

**Program(s):** Midwifery.

**★ 3692 ★ Urbana Center for the Alexander Technique**
508 W Washington St.
Urbana, IL 61801
**Phone:** (217)367-3172
Joan Murray, Director

**Program(s):** Alexander Technique.


**★ 3693 ★ Wellness and Massage Training Institute**
1051 Internationale Pkwy.
Woodridge, IL 60517
**Phone:** (630)325-3773
**Email:** info@wmti.com
**Website:** http://www.wmti.com
Raymond Miller, Director

**Program(s):** Aromatherapy; CranioSacral Therapy; Massage Therapy; Oriental Medicine; Ortho-Bionomy; Qigong; Reflexology; Shiatsu; Sports Massage; Traditional Chinese Medicine.


### Indiana

**★ 3694 ★ Academy of Reflexology and Health Therapy International**
8397 E 10th St.
Indianapolis, IN 46219-5330
**Phone:** (317)897-5111     **Fax:** (317)897-5115
E. James O'Donnell, Director

**Program(s):** Acupressure; Alexander Technique; Energy Work; Feldenkrais; Homeopathy; Massage Therapy; Polarity Therapy; Reflexology; Sports Massage.


**★ 3695 ★ Alexandria School of Scientific Therapeutics**
809 S Harrison St.
PO Box 287
Alexandria, IN 46001
**Phone:** (765)724-9152     **Fax:** (765)724-9156
Herbert L. Hobbs, Contact

**Program(s):** Acupressure; Aromatherapy; Ayurvedic Medicine; Deep Muscle Massage; Energy Work; Feldenkrais; Herbal Medicine; Homeopathy; Massage Therapy; Neuromuscular Therapy; Oriental Medicine; Polarity Therapy; Reflexology; Sports Massage; Swedish Massage; Shiatsu.


**★ 3696 ★ American Certified Massage School**
109 1/2 W Joliet St.
Crown Point, IN 46307
**Phone:** (219)661-9099     **Fax:** (219)661-8978
Gale Miller, Director

**Program(s):** Aromatherapy; Deep Tissue Massage; Massage Therapy; Reflexology; Sports Massage.


**★ 3697 ★ Dancing Feet Yoga Center, Inc.**
2501 Oriole Trl.
Long Beach, IN 46360
**Phone:** (219)872-9611     **Free:** 800-968-0694
**Fax:** (219)873-7612
Marsha Wenig, Director

**Program(s):** Yoga Teacher Training.


**★ 3698 ★ Indiana University, Purdue University, Indianapolis Massage Therapy Program**
620 N Union Dr., Rm. 102
Indianapolis, IN 46202
**Phone:** (317)274-2887     **Fax:** (317)274-2638
Janis Legendre, Contact

**Program(s):** Massage Therapy.


**★ 3699 ★ Ivy Tech State College**
3800 N Anthony Blvd.
Fort Wayne, IN 46805
**Phone:** (219)482-9171     **Fax:** (219)480-4149
Neal Davis, Director

**Program(s):** Massage Therapy.


**★ 3700 ★ Midwest Training Institute of Hypnosis**
2121 Engle Rd., Ste. 3A
Fort Wayne, IN 46809
**Phone:** (219)747-6774     **Fax:** (219)747-6774
Gisella Zukausky, Director

**Program(s):** Hypnotherapy.


### Iowa

**★ 3701 ★ Capri College, Davenport**
425 E 59th St.
Davenport, IA 52807
**Phone:** (319)388-6642
Heather McClanahan, Director

**Program(s):** Acupressure; Aromatherapy; Massage Therapy; Neuromuscular Therapy; Polarity Therapy; Reflexology; Reiki; Shiatsu; Sports Massage.


**★ 3702 ★ Capri College of Massage Therapy, Cedar Rapids**
315 2nd Ave. SE
PO Box 74912
Cedar Rapids, IA 52401
**Phone:** (319)364-1541
Joni Westphall, Director

**Program(s):** Acupressure; Aromatherapy; Deep Tissue Massage; Massage Therapy; Reflexology.


**★ 3703 ★ Carlson College of Massage Therapy**
11809 County Rd., X 28
Anamosa, IA 52205
**Phone:** (319)462-3402     **Fax:** (319)462-5990
Ruth A. Carlson, Director

**Program(s):** Aromatherapy; Energy Work; Herbal Medicine; Massage Therapy; Polarity Therapy; Reflexology; Shiatsu; Sports Massage.


**★ 3704 ★ Institute of Therapeutic Massage and Wellness**
516 W 35th St.
Davenport, IA 52806
**Phone:** (319)445-1055     **Fax:** (319)285-5201
Bonita Howes, Director

**Program(s):** Acupressure; Aromatherapy; CranioSacral Therapy; Ennergy Work; Massage Therapy; Neuromuscular Therapy; Polarity Therapy; Reflexology; Reiki; Shiatsu; Sports Massage; Yoga Teacher Training.


**★ 3705 ★ Maharishi University of Management**
College of Maharishi Vedic Medicine
Fairfield, IA 52557
**Phone:** (515)472-1110     **Fax:** (515)472-1179
**Email:** admissions@mum.edu
**Website:** http://www.mum.edu
Robert Schneider, MD, Contact

**Program(s):** Ayurvedic Medicine; Herbal Medicine; Maharishi Vedic Medicine.


**★ 3706 ★ Millenium College of Massage and Reflexology**
934 S 17th St.
Fort Dodge, IA 50501
**Phone:** (515)955-2296     **Fax:** (515)955-7709
Angie Eldridge, Contact

**Program(s):** Acupressure; Aromatherapy; CranioSacral Therapy; Massage Therapy; Reflexology.


**★ 3707 ★ MotherCare Doula Training**
244 S Walnut
West Union, IA 52175
**Phone:** (319)422-8833     **Free:** 800-648-3662
Debbie Young, Director

**Program(s):** Doula.


**★ 3708 ★ Palmer College of Chiropractic**
1000 Brady St.
Davenport, IA 52803
**Phone:** (319)884-5000     **Fax:** (319)884-5897
**Email:** pcadmit@palmer.edu
David B. Anderson, Director

**Program(s):** Chiropractic.


### Kansas

**★ 3709 ★ BMSI Institute**
8665 W 96th St., Ste. 300
Overland Park, KS 66212
**Phone:** (913)649-3322     **Fax:** (913)649-1010
Peggy Smith, Director

**Program(s):** Acupressure; Aromatherapy; CranioSacral Therapy; Energy Work; Massage Therapy; Polarity Therapy; Qigong; Reflexology; Reiki; Sports Massage; Traditional Chinese Medicine.


**★ 3710 ★ Frontier School of Midwifery and Family Nursing**
Hospital Hill
Hyden, KS 41749
Jeannette Woods, Director

**Program(s):** Midwifery.


**★ 3711 ★ Johnson County Community College**
9780 W 87th St.
Overland Park, KS 66212
**Phone:** (913)469-4422     **Fax:** (913)649-1050
Karen McDaniel, Director

**Program(s):** Aromatherapy; Cranial Sacral Therapy; Hydrotherapy; Massage Therapy; Reflexology.


**★ 3712 ★ Kansas College of Chinese Medicine**
9235 E Harry St., Bldg. 100, Ste. 1A
Wichita, KS 67207
**Phone:** (316)691-8822     **Fax:** (316)691-8868
Lawrence Scott, Director

**Program(s):** Acupressure; Acupuncture; Cranial Sacral Therapy; Deep Tissue Massage; Energy Work; Herbal Medicine; Massage Therapy; Oriental Medicine; Qigong; Shiatsu; Sports Massage; Traditional Chinese Medicine.


### Kentucky

**★ 3713 ★ Bluegrass Professional School of Massage Therapy**
501 Darby Creek, Ste. 14
Lexington, KY 40509
**Phone:** (606)264-1450     **Fax:** (606)264-1450
Terri Sloan, Director

**Program(s):** Acupressure; Aromatherapy; Deep Tissue Massage; Massage Therapy; Reflexology; Sports Massage.


**★ 3714 ★ Infinite Light Healing Studies Center, Inc.**
3509 W Dogwood Cir.
LaGrange, KY 40031
**Phone:** (502)454-0430     **Fax:** (502)241-8732
Laurelle Gaia, Director

**Program(s):** Energy Work; Reiki.


**★ 3715 ★ Louisville School of Massage**
7410 New LaGrange Rd.
Louisville, KY 40222
**Phone:** (502)429-5765     **Fax:** (502)429-8581
Brent C. Williams, Director

**Program(s):** Massage Therapy.

**★ 3716 ★ Sun Touch Massage School**
914 W Broadway
Mayfield, KY 42066
**Phone:** (502)247-8923      **Fax:** (502)247-6110
Marilyn Gossett, Director

**Program(s):** Aromatherapy; Deep Tissue Massage; Massage Therapy; Polarity Therapy; Qigong; Reflexology; Swedish Massage.

### Louisiana

**★ 3717 ★ Blue Cliff School of Therapeutic Massage, Lafayette**
103 Calco Blvd.
Lafayette, LA 70503
**Phone:** (318)269-0620      **Fax:** (318)269-0688
Claudette Hymel, Director

**Program(s):** CranioSacral Therapy; Massage Therapy; Neuromuscular Therapy; Shiatsu; Sports Massage.

**★ 3718 ★ Blue Cliff School of Therapeutic Massage and Oriental Bodywork**
1919 Veterans Blvd., Ste. 310
Kenner, LA 70062
**Phone:** (504)471-0294      **Fax:** (504)466-8514
**Email:** massage@ametro.net
J. Vernon Smith, PhD, Contact

**Program(s):** Acupressure; CranioSacral Therapy; Energy Work; Healing Touch; Massage Therapy; Neuromuscular Therapy; Oriental Medicine; Qigong; Reflexology; Shiatsu; Sports Massage; Traditional Chinese Medicine.

**★ 3719 ★ Blue Cliff School of Therapeutic Massage, Shreveport**
3823 Gilbret Dr., Ste. 103
Shreveport, LA 71104
**Phone:** (318)861-5959      **Fax:** (318)861-5957
Brenda Chadwick, Director

**Program(s):** Acupressure; CranioSacral Therapy; Deep Tissue Massage; Energy Work; Massage Therapy; Reflexology; Shiatsu.

**★ 3720 ★ Career Training Specialists**
Mid-City Plaza, 1611 Louisville Ave.
Monroe, LA 71201
**Phone:** (318)323-2889      **Fax:** (318)324-9883
Keith Hopkins, Director

**Program(s):** Aromatherapy; Deep Tissue Massage; Massage Therapy; Reflexology; Shiatsu.

**★ 3721 ★ Central Louisiana School of Therapeutic Massage**
2901 Hwy 28 E, Stes. C and D
Pineville, LA 71360
**Phone:** (318)449-1111      **Fax:** (318)445-5498
Andrea R. Martin, Director

**Program(s):** Acupressure; Deep Tissue Massage; Massage Therapy; Reflexology; Shiatsu.

**★ 3722 ★ Louisiana Institute of Massage Therapy**
1108 Lafitte St.
Lake Charles, LA 70601
**Phone:** (318)474-9435      **Fax:** (318)474-9432
**Email:** salvo.breaux@usaunwired.net
Susan Salvo, Director

**Program(s):** Hydrotherapy; Infant Massage; Massage Therapy; Pregnancy Massage; Reflexology; Sports Massage.

### Maine

**★ 3723 ★ Downeast School of Massage**
99 Moose Meadow Ln.
PO Box 24
Waldoboro, ME 04572
**Phone:** (207)832-5531      **Fax:** (207)832-0504
**Email:** dsm@midcoast.com
Nancy Dail, Director

**Program(s):** Massage Therapy; Shiatsu; Sports Massage.

**★ 3724 ★ Footloose, Inc., Professional Reflexology Training**
Egypt Rd.
PO Box 112
Alna, ME 04535
**Phone:** (207)586-6751      **Fax:** (207)586-6702
**Email:** footloos@gwi.net
Janet E. Stetser, Director

**Program(s):** Hypnotherapy; Reflexology.

**★ 3725 ★ New Hampshire Institute for Therapeutic Arts School for Massage Therapy**
39 Main St.
Bridgton, ME 04009
**Phone:** (207)647-3794
Patrick Cowan, Director

**Program(s):** Acupressure; Lymphatic Massage; Massage Therapy; Neuromuscular Therapy; Polarity Therapy; Reflexology; Sports Massage; Swedish Massage.

**★ 3726 ★ Polarity Realization Institute, Inc., Portland**
222 St. John St., Ste. 300
Portland, ME 04101
Nancy Risley, Director

**Program(s):** Aromatherapy; CranioSacral Therapy; Deep Tissue Massage; Energy Work; Massage Therapy; Polarity Therapy; Reflexology; Yoga Teacher Training.

### Manitoba

**★ 3727 ★ Professional Institute of Massage Therapy, Winnipeg**
570 Portage Ave.
Winnipeg, MB, Canada R3C 0G4
**Phone:** (204)775-1642      **Fax:** (204)775-1166
Sue Mamer, Contact

**Program(s):** Massage Therapy.

### Maryland

**★ 3728 ★ American Hypnosis Training Academy, Inc.**
8750 Georgia Ave., Ste. 125E
Silver Spring, MD 20910
**Phone:** (301)565-0103      **Free:** 800-343-9915
Ron Klein, Director

**Program(s):** Hypnotherapy.

**★ 3729 ★ Baltimore School of Massage**
6401 Dogwood Rd.
Baltimore, MD 21207
**Phone:** (410)944-8855      **Fax:** (410)944-8859
**Email:** registrar@bhhc.com
**Website:** http://www.bsom.com
Cindi Pridgen, Contact

**Program(s):** Massage Therapy.

**★ 3730 ★ Garrett Community College**
687 Mosser Rd.
Mc Henry, MD 21541
**Phone:** (301)387-3084      **Fax:** (301)387-3096
Carol Newman, Director

**Program(s):** Deep Tissue Massage; Massage Therapy.

**★ 3731 ★ Maryland Institute for Ericksonian Hypnosis and Psychotherapy**
6118 Park Heights Ave.
Baltimore, MD 21215
**Phone:** (410)358-1381      **Fax:** (410)358-5815
**Email:** mehyp@aol.com
Hillel Zeitlin, Director

**Program(s):** Hypnotherapy.

**★ 3732 ★ Maryland Institute of Traditional Chinese Medicine**
4641 Montgomery Ave., Ste. 400
Bethesda, MD 20814
**Phone:** (301)718-7373      **Fax:** (301)718-0735
**Website:** http://www.mitcm.org
Hee Junj Sunj, Director

**Program(s):** Acupuncture; Herbal Medicine; Qigong; Traditional Chinese Medicine.

**★ 3733 ★ Ohashiatsu Maryland**
8659 Baltimore National Pike
Ellicott, MD 21043
**Phone:** (410)313-8501      **Fax:** (410)313-8500
Hazel Chung, Director

**Program(s):** Shiatsu.

**★ 3734 ★ Polarity Center and Shamanic Studies**
9 Philadelphia Ave.
Takoma Park, MD 20912
Rose Diana Khalsa, Director

**Program(s):** CranioSacral Therapy; Energy Work; Polarity Therapy; Qigong; Reflexology; Yoga.

**★ 3735 ★ Traditional Acupuncture Institute**
American City Bldg.
10227 Wincopin Circle, Ste. 100
Columbia, MD 21044-3422
**Phone:** (301)596-6006
**Website:** http://www.acupuncture.com/TCMSchools/TAI1.htm

**Program(s):** Acupuncture; Traditional Chinese Medicine.

**★ 3736 ★ Unity Woods Yoga Center**
4853 Cordell Ave., Ste. PH9
Bethesda, MD 20814
**Phone:** (301)656-8992      **Fax:** (301)656-7792
John Schumacher, Director

**Program(s):** Yoga Teacher Training.

**★ 3737 ★ Yoga Center**
8950 Rte. 108, Ste. 114
Columbia, MD 21045
**Phone:** (410)720-4340      **Fax:** (410)461-4799
Bob Glickstein, Director

**Program(s):** Yoga Teacher Training.

### Massachusetts

**★ 3738 ★ Alexander Technique School of New England**
94 Lessey St.
Amherst, MA 01002
**Phone:** (413)253-2595
**Email:** mvine@netscape.com
Missy Vineyard, Director

**Program(s):** Alexander Technique.

**★ 3739 ★ Alexander Technique Training Center**
803 Boylston St.
Chestnut Hill, MA 02467
**Phone:** (617)734-6898

**Email:** kilroyr@tiac.net
Ruth Kilroy, Director

**Program(s):** Alexander Technique.


**★ 3740 ★ American School for Energy Therapies**
17 Spring St.
Watertown, MA 02472
**Phone:** (617)924-9150　　　**Free:** 800-875-6347
**Fax:** (617)924-2828
Douglas Jansenn, Director

**Program(s):** CranioSacral Therapy; Polarity Therapy.


**★ 3741 ★ Association of Labor Assistants and Childbirth Educators**
552 Massachusetts Ave.
Cambridge, MA 02139
**Free:** 888-222-5223　　　**Fax:** (617)441-3167
Jessica Porter, Director

**Program(s):** Childbirth Education; Doula.


**★ 3742 ★ Bach International Education Program**
100 Research Dr.
Wilmington, MA 01887
**Phone:** (978)988-3833　　　**Free:** 800-334-0843
**Fax:** (978)988-0233
Karen Zilinek, Director

**Program(s):** Flower Essences.


**★ 3743 ★ Bancroft School of Massage Therapy**
333 Shrewsbury St.
Worcester, MA 01604
**Phone:** (508)757-7923　　　**Fax:** (508)791-5930
**Email:** bsmttank@aol.com
Steven Tankanow, Director

**Program(s):** Massage Therapy.


**★ 3744 ★ Baystate Medical Center Nurse-Midwifery Education Program**
759 Chestnut St.
Springfield, MA 01199
**Phone:** (413)794-4448　　　**Fax:** (413)794-8770
Susan DeJoy, Director

**Program(s):** Midwifery.


**★ 3745 ★ BKS Iyengar Yoga Center of Greater Boston**
240A Elm St., Ste. 23
Somerville, MA 02144
**Phone:** (617)666-9551　　　**Fax:** (617)296-6194
Elizabeth Shields, Director

**Program(s):** Yoga Teacher Training.


**★ 3746 ★ Blazing Star Herbal School**
119 Pfersick Rd.
PO Box 6
Shelburne Falls, MA 01370
**Phone:** (413)625-6875　　　**Fax:** (413)625-6972
Gail Ulrich, Director

**Program(s):** Herbal Medicine; Plant Spirit.


**★ 3747 ★ Boston University, School of Public Health**
715 Albany St., Room A-207
Boston, MA 02118
**Phone:** (617)638-5012
Mary Barger, Director

**Program(s):** Midwifery.


**★ 3748 ★ Center for Traditional Medicine**
1770 Mass Ave., Ste. 624
Cambridge, MA 02140
**Phone:** (781)643-1918
**Email:** lekorn@wco.com

**Website:** http://www.halcyon.com/fwdp/medicine/tmp.html
Leslie Korn, PhD, Director

**Program(s):** CranioSacral Therapy; Energy Work; Herbal Medicine; Massage Therapy; Naturopathic Medicine; Polarity Therapy.


**★ 3749 ★ Center for Universal and Holistic Studies, Worchester**
3 Ruthaven Ave.
Worcester, MA 01606
**Phone:** (978)365-6104　　　**Fax:** (413)794-8770
Janice L. Lucht, Director

**Program(s):** Aromatherapy; Reflexology; Reiki.


**★ 3750 ★ Central Mass School of Massage and Therapy**
200 Main St.
Spencer, MA 01562
**Phone:** (508)885-0306　　　**Free:** 800-766-6572
Gregory St. Jacques, Director

**Program(s):** Acupressure; Aromatherapy, Deep Tissue Massage; Energy Work; Herbal Medicine; Massage Therapy; Meditation; Polarity Therapy; Reflexology; Reiki.


**★ 3751 ★ Certificate Program in Holistic Nursing**
PO Box 307
Shutesbury, MA 01072
**Phone:** (413)253-0443　　　**Fax:** (413)259-1034
**Email:** cphn@seedsandbridges.com
**Website:** http://www.seedsandbridges.com
Veda Andrus, Director

**Program(s):** Holistic Nursing.


**★ 3752 ★ Dimon School for the Alexander Technique**
15 Day St.
Cambridge, MA 02140
**Phone:** (617)876-3434
Ted Dimon, Director

**Program(s):** Alexander Technique.


**★ 3753 ★ Dovestar Institute**
120 Court St.
Plymouth, MA 02360
**Phone:** (508)830-0068　　　**Free:** 888-222-5603
**Fax:** (508)830-0288
Kamala Renner, Director

**Program(s):** Acupressure; Breathwork; Colon Hydrotherapy; Energy Work; Hypnotherapy; Kriya Massage; Massage Therapy; Qigong; Reflexology; Reiki; Shiatsu; Yoga Teacher Training.


**★ 3754 ★ East/West Institute of Alternative Medicine**
1972 Massachusetts Ave.
Cambridge, MA 02140
**Phone:** (617)876-4048　　　**Fax:** (617)497-4892
Erik Zutrau, Director

**Program(s):** Acupressure; Ayurvedic Medicine; Shiatsu; Traditional Chinese Medicine.


**★ 3755 ★ Ellen Evert Hopman Introduction to Botanical Medicine and Self Care**
PO Box 219
Amherst, MA 01004
**Phone:** (413)323-4494
Ellen Evert Hopman, Contact

**Program(s):** Aromatherapy; Herbal Medicine; Homeopathy.

**★ 3756 ★ Greater New England Academy of Hypnosis, Inc.**
PO Box 975
Andover, MA 01810
**Phone:** (978)474-4601　　　**Fax:** (978)474-4601
Alphonse M. Tatarunis, Director

**Program(s):** Hypnotherapy.


**★ 3757 ★ Greenfield Community College**
270 Main St.
PO Box 15
Greenfield, MA 01301
**Phone:** (413)775-1620　　　**Fax:** (413)774-2285
Laura Earl, Director

**Program(s):** Massage Therapy; Polarity Therapy; Reflexology; Shiatsu.


**★ 3758 ★ International Ayurvedic Medicine Institute, Inc.**
111 Elm St., Ste. 103-105
Worcester, MA 01609
**Phone:** (508)755-3744　　　**Fax:** (508)770-0618
**Email:** ayurveda@hotmail.com
Abbas Qutab, Director

**Program(s):** Ayurvedic Medicine.


**★ 3759 ★ Kripalu Center for Yoga and Health**
West St.
PO Box 793
Stockbridge, MA 01262
**Free:** 800-741-7353　　　**Fax:** (413)448-3384
**Website:** http://www.kripalu.org
John Willey, Director

**Program(s):** Holistic Health; Massage Therapy; Yoga Teacher Training.


**★ 3760 ★ Massage Institute of New England**
22 McGrath Hwy., Ste. 11
Somerville, MA 02143
**Phone:** (617)666-3700　　　**Fax:** (617)666-0109
Henry Corley, Director

**Program(s):** Energy Work; Massage Therapy; Neuromuscular Therapy; Sports Massage; Swedish Massage.


**★ 3761 ★ Muscular Therapy Institute**
122 Rindge Ave.
Cambridge, MA 02140
**Phone:** (617)576-1300　　　**Fax:** (617)864-8283
**Website:** http://www.mtti.com

**Program(s):** Massage Therapy.


**★ 3762 ★ New England School of Acupuncture**
30 Common St.
Watertown, MA 02472
**Phone:** (617)926-1788　　　**Fax:** (617)924-4167
**Website:** http://www.paris.maine.com/people/nesa
Daniel Seitz, Contact

**Program(s):** Acupuncture; Herbal Medicine; Oriental Medicine; Qigong; Traditional Chinese Medicine.


**★ 3763 ★ New England School of Homeopathy**
356 Middle St.
Amherst, MA 01002
**Phone:** (413)256-5949　　　**Fax:** (413)256-6223
**Email:** nesh@nesh.com
Dr. Amy Rothenberg, Contact

**Program(s):** Homeopathy.


**★ 3764 ★ New England School of Whole Health Education**
581 Boylston St., Ste. 506
Boston, MA 02216

**Phone:** (617)267-0516    **Fax:** (617)247-0896
Dr. Georgianna Donadio-McCormack, Director
**Program(s):** Holistic Health.

★ 3765 ★ **New England School of Whole Health Education, Dover**
60 Farm St.
Dover, MA 02030
**Phone:** (508)785-0309    **Fax:** (508)785-9743
Georgiana Donadio-McCormack, Director
**Program(s):** Holistic Health.

★ 3766 ★ **Phoenix Rising Yoga Therapy**
402 Park St.
PO Box 819
Housatonic, MA 01236
**Phone:** (413)274-3515    **Fax:** (413)274-6166
**Email:** moreinfo@pryt.com
**Website:** http://www.pryt.com
Becky McFarland, Contact
**Program(s):** Yoga Therapy.

★ 3767 ★ **Polarity Realization Institute**
126 High St.
Ipswich, MA 01938
**Phone:** (508)356-0980    **Fax:** (508)356-9818
**Email:** polaritytherapy@msn.com
Nancy Risley, Director
**Program(s):** Energy Work; Massage Therapy; Polarity Therapy.

★ 3768 ★ **Polarity Realization Institute, Inc., Plymouth**
59 Industrial Park Rd.
Plymouth, MA 02360
**Phone:** (978)356-0980    **Fax:** (978)356-9818
Nancy Risley, Director
**Program(s):** Aromatherapy, CranioSacral Therapy; Deep Tissue Massage; Energy Work; Massage Therapy; Polarity Therapy; Reflexology; Yoga Teacher Training.

★ 3769 ★ **School for Body-Mind Centering**
189 Pondview Dr.
Amherst, MA 01002-3230
**Phone:** (413)256-8615    **Fax:** (413)256-8239
Myra Avedon, Director
**Program(s):** Body-Mind Centering.

★ 3770 ★ **Yoga Therapy Center**
120A Westbourne Terrace
Brookline, MA 02446
**Phone:** (617)739-1146
Mukunda Stiles, Director
**Program(s):** Yoga Teacher Training.

## Michigan

★ 3771 ★ **Ann Arbor Institute of Massage Therapy**
2835 Carpenter Rd.
Ann Arbor, MI 48108
**Phone:** (734)677-4430    **Fax:** (734)677-4520
Jocelyn Granger, Director
**Program(s):** Massage Therapy; Neuromuscular Therapy; Shiatsu; Sports Massage.

★ 3772 ★ **Ann Arbor School of Massage and Bodywork**
1530 Northwood
Ann Arbor, MI 48103-4667
**Phone:** (734)662-1572    **Fax:** (734)662-2246
**Email:** luisa@umich.edu
Barry Ryder, Director
**Program(s):** Massage Therapy.

★ 3773 ★ **Blue Heron Academy of the Healing Arts and Sciences**
2020 Raybrook SE, Ste. 203
Grand Rapids, MI 49546
**Phone:** (616)285-9999    **Fax:** (616)956-7777
Gregory T. Lawton, Director
**Program(s):** Acupressure; CranioSacral Therapy; Herbal Medicine; Homeopathy; Massage Therapy; Naturopathic Medicine; Neuromuscular Therapy; Oriental Medicine; Qigong; Sports Massage; Tai Chi; Traditional Chinese Medicine.

★ 3774 ★ **Discovery Institute of Hypnotherapy**
6451 Belding Ave.
Fenwick, MI 48834
**Phone:** (616)761-3453    **Fax:** (616)761-3710
**Email:** discovery@ud/ager.net
Charles Kinney, Director
**Program(s):** Hypnotherapy.

★ 3775 ★ **Health Enrichment Center, Inc.**
1820 N Lapeer Rd.
Lapeer, MI 48446
**Phone:** (810)667-9453    **Fax:** (810)667-4095
**Email:** hec@tir.com
**Website:** http://www.healthenrichment.com
Sandy Fritz, Director
**Program(s):** Acupressure; CranioSacral Therapy; Massage Therapy; Polarity Therapy; Reflexology; Shiatsu.

★ 3776 ★ **Infinity International Institute of Hypnotherapy**
4110 Edgeland, Ste. 800
Royal Oak, MI 48073-2285
**Phone:** (248)549-5594    **Fax:** (248)549-5421
**Email:** aspencer@infinityinst.com
**Website:** http://www.infinityinst.com
Anne H. Spencer, PhD, Director
**Program(s):** Hypnotherapy; Reiki; Therapeutic Touch.

★ 3777 ★ **Institute of Natural Health Sciences**
43000 Nine Mile Rd.
Novi, MI 48375
**Phone:** (248)473-8522    **Fax:** (248)473-8141
C. Lois Grice, Director
**Program(s):** Herbal Medicine; Homeopathy.

★ 3778 ★ **Institute of Natural Therapies**
PO Box 222
Hancock, MI 49930
**Phone:** (906)482-2222
Hal Rudnianin, Director
**Program(s):** Acupressure; CranioSacral Therapy; Massage Therapy; Qigong; Traditional Chinese Medicine.

★ 3779 ★ **Institute of Transformational Hypnotherapy**
PO Box 1293
East Lansing, MI 48826
**Phone:** (517)374-6156
Robert Ranger, Director
**Program(s):** Hypnotherapy.

★ 3780 ★ **International Center for Reiki Training**
21421 Hilltop, Ste. 28
Southfield, MI 48034
**Free:** 800-332-8112    **Fax:** (810)948-8112
**Email:** reikicen@aol.com
**Website:** http://www.reiki.org
William Lee Rand, Contact
**Program(s):** Reiki.

★ 3781 ★ **Irene's Myomassology Institute, Inc.**
18911 Ten Mile
Southfield, MI 48075
**Phone:** (248)569-4263    **Fax:** (248)569-4261
Kathleen Grogan, Contact
**Program(s):** Aromatherapy; CranioSacral Therapy; Herbal Medicine; Massage Therapy; Myomassology; Prenatal Massage; Polarity Therapy; Qigong; Reflexology; Shiatsu; Sports Massage; Thai Massage.

★ 3782 ★ **Kalamazoo Center for the Healing Arts**
3715 W Main, Ste. 3
Kalamazoo, MI 49006-2842
**Phone:** (616)373-0910    **Fax:** (616)373-0271
**Email:** kchands@aol.com
Jim Herweg, Director
**Program(s):** Acupressure; CranioSacral Therapy; Massage Therapy; Polarity Therapy; Reflexology.

★ 3783 ★ **Michigan School of Myomassology**
3270 Greenfield Rd.
Berkley, MI 48072
**Phone:** (248)542-7228    **Fax:** (248)542-5830
Karrie Sladewski, Director
**Program(s):** Accupressure; Aromatherapy; CranioSacral Therapy; Energy Work; Massage Therapy; Myomassology; Neuromuscular Therapy; Polarity Therapy; Reflexology; Reiki; Shiatsu; Sports Massage.

★ 3784 ★ **Michigan School of Traditional Midwifery and Herbology**
PO Box 162
Mikado, MI 48745
**Phone:** (517)736-6583
Casey Makela, Director
**Program(s):** Herbal Medicine; Midwifery.

★ 3785 ★ **Naturopathic Institute of Therapies and Education**
1410 S Mission
Mount Pleasant, MI 48858
**Phone:** (517)773-1714    **Fax:** (517)775-7319
Beth Flaugher, Director
**Program(s):** Aromatherapy; CranioSacral Therapy; Energy Work; Flower Essences; Herbal Medicine; Homeopathy; Iridology; Massage Therapy; Naturopathic Medicine; Neuromuscular Therapy; Nutrition; Reflexology; Sports Massage; Traditional Chinese Medicine.

★ 3786 ★ **Polarity Center of Dearborn**
5824 Chase
Dearborn, MI 48126
**Phone:** (313)582-5034
John Bodary, Director
**Program(s):** CranioSacral Therapy; Polarity Therapy.

★ 3787 ★ **Polarity Therapy Program**
Lansing Community College
PO Box 40010
Lansing, MI 48901-7210
**Phone:** (517)887-1670
Sheila Cook, Director
**Program(s):** Polarity Therapy.

★ 3788 ★ **University of Michigan School of Nursing**
400 N Ingalls, Rm 3320
Ann Arbor, MI 48109-0482
**Phone:** (734)763-3710    **Fax:** (734)647-0351
Gloria Crothers, Director
**Program(s):** Midwifery.

★ 3789 ★ **Wellspring Institute School of Therapeutic Bodywork**
20312 Chalon St.
Saint Clair Shores, MI 48080
**Phone:** (810)772-8520
Sandra J. Todt, Director
**Program(s):** Acupressure; CranioSacral Therapy; Energy Work; Hypnotherapy; Massage Therapy; Polarity Therapy; Qigong; Reflexology; Shiatsu; Sports Massage; Therapeutic Touch.

★ 3790 ★ **Yogic Sciences Research Foundation**
1228 Daisy Ln.
East Lansing, MI 48823
**Phone:** (517)351-3056
Robert Eschbach, Director
**Program(s):** Yoga Teacher Training.

### Minnesota

★ 3791 ★ **Biofeedback Training and Treatment Center, Inc.**
7300 France Ave. S, Ste. 200
Edina, MN 55435
**Phone:** (612)893-9400     **Fax:** (612)893-0615
**Email:** pills@aol.com
Lilli Ann Jeffrey-Smith, PhD, Director
**Program(s):** Biofeedback.

★ 3792 ★ **BKS Iyengar Yoga Center**
2736 Lyndale Ave. S
Minneapolis, MN 55408
**Phone:** (612)872-8708     **Fax:** (612)872-1893
**Email:** chirh001@tc.umn.edu
Lee Sverkerson, Director
**Program(s):** Yoga Teacher Training.

★ 3793 ★ **Center for A Balanced Life, Inc.**
1535 Livingston Ave., Ste. 105
West Saint Paul, MN 55118-3411
**Phone:** (612)455-0473
Sister M. Janine Rajkowski, Director
**Program(s):** Acupressure; Massage Therapy; Polarity Therapy; Reflexology.

★ 3794 ★ **Hypnosis Research and Training Center**
1960 Cliff Lake Rd., Stes. 112-200
Eagan, MN 55122
**Phone:** (612)707-1898     **Fax:** (612)707-1898
Kevin Hogan, Director
**Program(s):** Hypnotherapy; Neuro-Linguistic Programming.

★ 3795 ★ **Lake Superior College**
2101 Trinity Rd.
Duluth, MN 55811
**Phone:** (218)733-5921     **Free:** 800-432-2884
Dave Burson, Director
**Program(s):** Massage Therapy.

★ 3796 ★ **Minneapolis School of Massage and Bodywork, Inc.**
85 22nd Ave. NE
Minneapolis, MN 55418
**Phone:** (612)788-8907     **Fax:** (612)788-8907
Joan Crawford-Dietsch, Director
**Program(s):** Deep Tissue Massage; Massage Therapy; Sports Massage.

★ 3797 ★ **Minnesota Center for Shiatsu Study**
1313 5th St. SE, Ste. 336
Minneapolis, MN 55414
**Phone:** (612)379-3565     **Fax:** (612)379-3568
**Email:** shiatsumn@aol.com
Cari Johnson Pelava, Director
**Program(s):** Shiatsu; Traditional Chinese Medicine.

★ 3798 ★ **Minnesota Institute of Acupuncture and Herbal Studies**
1821 University Ave. W, Ste. 278-S
Saint Paul, MN 55104
**Phone:** (612)603-0994     **Fax:** (612)603-0995
**Email:** miahs@millcomm.com
Page Purdy, Contact
**Program(s):** Acupuncture; Herbal Medicine; Oriental Medicine; Traditional Chinese Medicine.

★ 3799 ★ **Northern Lights School of Massage Therapy**
1313 SE 5th St., Ste. 209
Minneapolis, MN 55414
**Phone:** (612)379-3822     **Fax:** (612)379-5971
Deni Dantis, Director
**Program(s):** Massage Therapy.

★ 3800 ★ **Northwestern College of Chiropractic**
2501 W 84th St.
Bloomington, MN 55431
**Phone:** (612)888-4777     **Fax:** (612)888-6713
John F. Allenburg, Contact
**Program(s):** Acupressure; Acupuncture; Chiropractic.

★ 3801 ★ **Northwestern School of Homeopathy**
10700 Old County Rd. 15, Ste. 350
Plymouth, MN 55441
**Phone:** (612)794-6445     **Fax:** (612)525-9518
Eric Sommermann, Contact
**Program(s):** Homeopathy.

★ 3802 ★ **Sister Rosalind Gefre School of Professional Massage, Mankato**
165 W Lind Ct.
Mankato, MN 56001
**Phone:** (507)344-0220
**Program(s):** Deep Tissue Massage; Massage Therapy; Reflexology.

★ 3803 ★ **Sister Rosalind Gefre School of Professional Massage, Rochester**
300 Elton Hills Dr. NW
Rochester, MN 55901
**Phone:** (507)286-8608     **Fax:** (507)282-2893
Rolf Bollingberg, Director
**Program(s):** Deep Tissue Massage; Massage Therapy; Reflexology.

★ 3804 ★ **Sister Rosalind Gefre School of Professional Massage, Saint Paul**
400 Selby Ave., Ste. G
Saint Paul, MN 55102
**Phone:** (651)228-0960     **Fax:** (651)698-7436
Audry Handland, Director
**Program(s):** Acupressure; Chair Massage; CranioSacral Therapy; Massage Therapy; Neuromuscular Therapy; On-Site Massage; Reflexology; Sports Massage.

★ 3805 ★ **University of Minnesota Academic Health**
308 Harvard St. SE 6-101
Minneapolis, MN 55455
**Phone:** (612)624-9459     **Fax:** (612)624-3174
Mary Jo Krietzer, Director
**Program(s):** Midwifery.

### Mississippi

★ 3806 ★ **Blue Cliff School of Therapeutic Massage, Gulf Coast Campus**
942 E Beach Blvd.
Gulfport, MS 39507
**Phone:** (228)896-9727     **Fax:** (228)896-8659
Richard Lee Berry, Director
**Program(s):** Acupressure; CraanioSacral Therapy; Healing Touch; Massage Therapy; Neuromuscular Therapy; Reflexology; Shiatsu; Sports Massage.

★ 3807 ★ **Blue Cliff School of Therapeutic Massage, Jackson**
5120 Galaxie Dr.
Jackson, MS 39206
**Phone:** (601)362-3624     **Fax:** (601)362-3694
Dee A. Meux, Director
**Program(s):** Aromatherapy; CranioSacral Therapy; Deep Tissue Massage; Energy Work; Massage Therapy; Neuromuscular Therapy; Reflexology; Reiki; Shiatsu.

### Missouri

★ 3808 ★ **Cleveland Chiropractic College, Kansas City**
6401 Rockhill Rd.
Kansas City, MO 64131
**Phone:** (816)501-0100     **Fax:** (816)361-0272
Carl S. Cleveland, III, Contact
**Program(s):** Chiropractic.

★ 3809 ★ **Inochi Institute, Inc.**
70-D Grasso Plaza
Saint Louis, MO 63123
**Phone:** (314)544-9600     **Fax:** (314)631-0223
Thomas Duckworth, Director
**Program(s):** Acupressure; Acupuncture; Energy Work; Herbal Medicine; Homeopathy; Kototama Medicine; Massage Therapy; Naturopathic Medicine; Neuromuscular Therapy; Oriental Medicine; Shiatsu; Traditional Japanese Medicine.

★ 3810 ★ **Logan College of Chiropractic**
1851 Schoettler Rd.
PO Box 1065
Chesterfield, MO 63006-1065
**Phone:** (314)227-2100     **Free:** 800-533-9210
**Fax:** (314)207-2424
George A. Goodman, Contact
**Program(s):** Chiropractic.

★ 3811 ★ **Massage Therapy Institute of Missouri (MTIM)**
5 S 9th St., Ste. 202
Columbia, MO 65201
**Phone:** (573)875-7905     **Fax:** (573)443-7933
**Email:** eruvalca@digmo.org
Mirra Greenway, Director
**Program(s):** Deep Tissue Massage; Energy Work; Massage Therapy; Sports Massage; Swedish Massage.

★ 3812 ★ **Massage Therapy Training Institute, LLC**
9140 Ward Pkwy., Ste. 100
Kansas City, MO 64114
**Phone:** (816)523-9140
Terri Oglesby, Contact
**Program(s):** Aromatherapy; CranioSacral Therapy; Energy Work; Herbal Medicine; Massage Therapy; Myofascial Release; Neuromuscular Therapy; Polarity Therapy; Qigong; Reflexology; Shiatsu; Sports Massage; Therapeutic Touch; Trigger Point Therapy.

**★ 3813 ★ Professional Massage Training Center**
200 E Commercial
Springfield, MO 65803
Phone: (417)863-7682     Fax: (417)863-7652
Email: juliet@cland.net
Juliet Mee, Director
**Program(s):** Massage Therapy.

**★ 3814 ★ Saint Charles School of Massage Therapy**
2440 Executive Dr.
Saint Charles, MO 63301
Phone: (314)498-0777     Fax: (314)498-0708
Email: oasis@anet-stl.com
Website: http://www.britestar.net.oasis.com
Kathleen Crawford, Director
**Program(s):** Aromatherapy; CranioSacral Therapy; Massage Therapy; Polarity Therapy; Reflexology; Reiki; Shiatsu.

**★ 3815 ★ University of Missouri, Columbia**
**Sinclair School of Nursing**
Columbia, MO 65211
Phone: (573)882-0235     Fax: (573)884-4544
Nancy Johnson, Director
**Program(s):** Midwifery.

## Montana

**★ 3816 ★ Big Sky Somatic Institute**
1802 11th Ave., Ste. A
Helena, MT 59601
Phone: (406)442-8998
Ron Floyd, Director
**Program(s):** Acupressure; Energy Work; Herbal Medicine; Massage Therapy; Neuromuscular Therapy; Qigong; Shiatsu; Thai Massage; Traditional Chinese Medicine.

**★ 3817 ★ Rocky Mountain Herbal Institute**
305 2nd Ave. S
PO Box 579
Hot Springs, MT 59845
Phone: (406)741-3811
Email: rmhi@rmhiherbal.org
Website: http://www.rmhiherbal.org
Roger W. Wicke, PhD, Director
**Program(s):** Herbal Medicine; Traditional Chinese Medicine.

**★ 3818 ★ Starfire Massage School and Healing Center**
9819 Waldo Rd.
Missoula, MT 59808
Phone: (406)721-7519     Fax: (406)721-7519
Mary Marron, Director
**Program(s):** Acupressure; Energy Work; Hydrotherapy; Massage Therapy; Reiki; Shamanic Healing; Shiatsu; Sound Healing.

## Nebraska

**★ 3819 ★ Gateway College of Massage Therapy**
2607 Dakota Ave.
South Sioux City, NE 68776
Phone: (402)494-8390     Fax: (402)494-4561
Darrell J. Peck, PhD, Director
**Program(s):** Acupressure; CranioSacral Therapy; Massage Therapy; Neuromuscular Therapy; Reflexology; Sports Massage; Swedish Massage.

**★ 3820 ★ Myotherapy Institute**
6020 S 58th St.
Lincoln, NE 68516
Phone: (402)421-7410     Fax: (402)421-6736

**Program(s):** Hydrotherapy; Massage Therapy; Medical Massage; Spa Therapies.

**★ 3821 ★ Omaha School of Massage Therapy**
9748 Park Dr.
Omaha, NE 68127
Phone: (402)331-3694     Fax: (402)331-0280
Website: http://www.osmt.com
Ann Reuck, Director
**Program(s):** Acupressure; Aromatherapy; Energy Work; Massage Therapy; Reflexology; Sports Massage; Swedish Massage.

**★ 3822 ★ Universal Center of Healing Arts**
109 N 50th St.
Omaha, NE 68132
Phone: (402)556-4456     Fax: (402)561-0635
Patrick Davis, Director
**Program(s):** Acupressure; Aromatherapy; Ayurvedic Medicine; CranioSacral Therapy; Energy Work; Herbal Medicine; Massage Therapy; Neuromuscular Therapy; Oriental Medicine; Polarity Therapy; Qigong; Reflexology; Reiki; Shiatsu; Sports Massage; Tai Chi; Traditional Chinese Medicine; Yoga.

## Nevada

**★ 3823 ★ Aston-Patterning Training Center / A Continuing Education Service**
PO Box 3568
Incline Village, NV 89450
Phone: (702)831-8228
Judith Aston, Director
**Program(s):** Aston-Patterning Bodywork and Movement.

**★ 3824 ★ Dahan Institute of Massage Studies**
3430 E Tropicana, Ste. 62
Las Vegas, NV 89121
Phone: (702)434-1338     Fax: (702)434-3449
Serge Dahan, Director
**Program(s):** Acupressure; Aromatherapy; Massage Therapy; Polarity Therapy; Reflexology; Shiatsu; Sports Massage.

**★ 3825 ★ International BioMedical Research Institute**
6490 S McCarran Blvd., C-24
Reno, NV 89509
Phone: (702)827-1444     Fax: (702)827-2424
Edna Edsig, Director
**Program(s):** Herbal Medicine; Homeopathy.

**★ 3826 ★ Ralston School of Massage**
Washoe Med. Ctr.
77 Pringle Way
Reno, NV 89520-0109
Phone: (702)982-5450     Fax: (702)982-5452
Email: 2relax@intercomm.com
Robert H. Oliver, Director
**Program(s):** Massage Therapy.

## New Hampshire

**★ 3827 ★ Dovestar Institute**
50 Whitehall Rd.
Hooksett, NH 03106
Phone: (603)669-5104     Free: 888-222-5603
Fax: (603)625-1919
Kamala Renner, Director
**Program(s):** Acupressure; Colon Hydrotherapy; CranioSacral Therapy; Hypnotherapy; Kriya Massage; Qigong; Reflexology; Reiki; Shiatsu; Yoga Teacher Training.

**★ 3828 ★ New England Academy of Therapeutic Sciences**
402 Amherst St.
Nashua, NH 03063
Phone: (603)886-8433     Fax: (603)880-8654
Email: maureen@neats.com
Website: http://www.neats.com
Maureen J. Healy, Director
**Program(s):** Acupressure; Animal Therapy; CranioSacral Therapy; Equine Massage; Herbal Medicine; Homeopathy; Hypnotherapy; Massage Therapy; Neuromuscular Therapy; Polarity Therapy; Reflexology; Shiatsu; Swedish Massage; Traditional Chinese Medicine.

**★ 3829 ★ New Hampshire Institute for Therapeutic Arts School of Massage Therapy, Hudson**
153 Lowell Rd.
Hudson, NH 03051
Phone: (603)882-3022     Fax: (603)598-9101
Patrick Cowan, Contact
**Program(s):** Acupressure; Lymphatic Massage; Massage Therapy; Neuromuscular Therapy; Polarity Therapy; Reflexology; Sports Massage; Swedish Massage.

**★ 3830 ★ North Eastern Institute of Whole Health, Inc.**
22 Bridge St.
Manchester, NH 03101-1655
Phone: (603)623-5018     Fax: (603)641-5928
Dr. Douglas DuVerger, Director
**Program(s):** Acupressure; Anatomy and Physiology; Aromatherapy; Chair Massage; CPR/First Aid; CranioSacral Therapy; Esalen Therapy; Herbal Medicine; Hydrotherapy; Hypnotherapy; LomiLomi Massage; Lymphatic Massage; Massage Therapy; Neuromuscular Therapy; Oriental Medicine; Polarity Therapy; Pregnancy Massage; Qigong; Reflexology; Reiki; Shiatsu; Sports Massage; Traditional Chinese Medicine; Trigger Point Therapy.

## New Jersey

**★ 3831 ★ Academy of Massage Therapy**
401 S Van Brunt St.
Englewood, NJ 07631
Phone: (201)568-3220     Fax: (201)568-5181
Joanna Sechuk, Director
**Program(s):** Aromatherapy; Massage Therapy; Medical Massage; Qigong; Reflexology; Reiki; Shiatsu; Sports Massage;Thai Massage.

**★ 3832 ★ Academy of Natural Health Sciences**
102 Green St.
Woodbridge, NJ 07095
Phone: (732)634-2155     Fax: (732)634-2155
Frank Auriemma, Director
**Program(s):** Acupressure; Aromatherapy; Ayurvedic Medicine; Energy Work; Herbal Medicine; Holistic Health; Homeopathy; Hypnotherapy; Massage Therapy; Neuromuscular Therapy; Nutrition; Polarity Therapy; Reflexology; Reiki; Shiatsu; Sports Massage.

**★ 3833 ★ Academy of Professional Hypnosis**
1358 Burnet Ave.
Union, NJ 07083
Phone: (908)964-4417     Fax: (908)810-0255
Dr. John Gatto, Contact
**Program(s):** Hypnotherapy.

**★ 3834 ★ Body, Mind and Spirit Learning Alliance**
917-2 N Main St.
Toms River, NJ 08753
Phone: (908)349-7153
Dianne O'Brien, Director

**Program(s):** Aromatherapy; CranioSacral Therapy; Massage Therapy; Reflexology; Reiki; Shiatsu; Swedish Massage.

### ★ 3835 ★ Center for TransPersonal BodyMind Studies
51 Upland Ave.
Metuchen, NJ 08840
**Phone:** (732)548-8579
Joanne Rossi, Director

**Program(s):** Aromatherapy; Energy Work; Massage Therapy; Polarity Therapy; Somatic Psychology.

### ★ 3836 ★ Center for Universal and Holistic Studies, Paramus
PO Box 1306
Paramus, NJ 07653
**Phone:** (973)686-9700
Elaine Gordon, Director

**Program(s):** Energy Work; Reflexology.

### ★ 3837 ★ Classic Center for Health and Healing
25 Orchard St., Ste. 101
Denville, NJ 07834-2160
**Phone:** (973)627-4833
Zoe Elva Putnam, Director

**Program(s):** Therapeutic Touch.

### ★ 3838 ★ Five Elements School of Classical Homeopathy
115 Rte. 46, Bldg. D-29
Mountain Lakes, NJ 07046
**Phone:** (201)402-8510        **Fax:** (201)402-9753
Jane Cicchetti, Director

**Program(s):** Homeopathy.

### ★ 3839 ★ Garden State Center for Holistic Health Care
1203 Airport Rd.
Rte. 70 W
Lakewood, NJ 08701
**Phone:** (732)364-0882        **Fax:** (732)364-7096
Gloria Coppola, Director

**Program(s):** Acupressure; Aromatherapy; CranioSacral Therapy; Energy Work; Massage Therapy; Neuromuscular Therapy; Reiki; Swedish Massage; Thai Massage.

### ★ 3840 ★ Healing Hands Institute for Massage Therapy
41 Bergenline Ave.
Westwood, NJ 07675
**Phone:** (201)722-0099        **Fax:** (201)722-0690
**Email:** hhi@aol.com
Eva Carey, Contact

**Program(s):** Acupressure; Aromatherapy; Massage Therapy; Medical Massage; Reflexology; Reiki; Shiatsu; Sports Massage; Swedish Massage; Traditional Chinese Medicine.

### ★ 3841 ★ Healing Hands School of Massage
515 Whitehorse Pike
Haddon Heights, NJ 08035
**Phone:** (609)546-7471        **Fax:** (609)546-7491
Kristina Shaw, Director

**Program(s):** Acupressure; CranioSacral Therapy; Deep Tissue Massage; Herbal Medicine; Hydrotherapy; Massage Therapy; Myofascial Release; Neuromuscular Therapy; Polarity Therapy; Reflexology; Reiki; Shiatsu; Swedish Massage; Traditional Chinese Medicine.

### ★ 3842 ★ Health Choices Center for the Healing Arts
170 Township Line Rd., Bldg. B
Belle Mead, NJ 08502
**Phone:** (908)359-3995        **Fax:** (908)359-3902
Renate M. Novak, Director

**Program(s):** Acupressure; Aromatherapy; Massage Therapy; Neuromuscular Therapy; Polarity Therapy; Qigong; Reflexology; Reiki; Shiatsu.

### ★ 3843 ★ Herbal Therapeutics School of Botanical Medicine
PO Box 553
Broadway, NJ 08808
**Phone:** (908)835-0822        **Fax:** (908)835-0824
David Winston, Director

**Program(s):** Herbal Medicine.

### ★ 3844 ★ Institute of Hypnotherapy
10 Darby Ct.
Manalapan, NJ 07726
**Phone:** (732)446-5995
Jaime Feldman, Director

**Program(s):** Hypnotherapy; Neuro-Linguistic Programming.

### ★ 3845 ★ Institute for Therapeutic Massage, Inc.
125 Wanaque Ave.
Pompton Lakes, NJ 07442
**Phone:** (201)839-6131        **Fax:** (201)839-9878
Lisa Helbig, Director

**Program(s):** Aromatherapy; Chair Massage; Energy Work; Geriatric Medicine; Massage Therapy; Pregnancy Massage; Reflexology; Reiki; Sports Massage.

### ★ 3846 ★ Massage Therapy Center for Healing and Learning
4 Deerfield Pl.
Flanders, NJ 07836
**Phone:** (973)927-3151
Jack Hicks, Director

**Program(s):** CranioSacral Therapy; Deep Tissue Massage; Massage Therapy; Reflexology; Reiki.

### ★ 3847 ★ Morris Institute of Natural Therapeutics
3108 Rte. 10 W
Denville, NJ 07834
**Phone:** (201)989-8939        **Fax:** (201)989-5554
Vincent R. Iuppo, Director

**Program(s):** Acupressure; Applied Kinesiology; Aromatherapy; Chair Massage; CranioSacral Therapy; Manual Lymph Drainage; Massage Therapy; Neuromuscular Therapy; Reflexology; Shiatsu; Sports Massage.

### ★ 3848 ★ Mother Love, Doula Training
584 Echo Glen Ave.
River Vale, NJ 07675
**Phone:** (201)358-2703        **Fax:** (201)664-4405
Debra Pascali-Bonaro, Director

**Program(s):** Doula.

### ★ 3849 ★ New Jersey Institute of Reflexology
155 Franklin Ave.
Long Branch, NJ 07740-6616
**Free:** 888-722-6547
Mary Alice Arre, Director

**Program(s):** Reflexology.

### ★ 3850 ★ New Jersey Massage Training Center
3699 Rt. 46E
Parsippany, NJ 07054

**Phone:** (973)263-2229        **Fax:** (973)402-1222
Larry Heisler, Director

**Program(s):** Acupressure; Massage Therapy; Neuromuscular Therapy; Qigong; Reflexology; Shiatsu; Sports Massage; Swedish Massage; Yoga Teacher Training.

### ★ 3851 ★ Ocean County Vo-Tech
1299 Old Freehold Rd.
Toms River, NJ 08753
**Phone:** (732)349-8444
Sharon Spaziani, Director

**Program(s):** Deep Tissue Massage; Massage Therapy.

### ★ 3852 ★ Our Lady of Lourdes Institute of Wholistic Studies
900 Haddon Ave., Ste. 118
Collingswood, NJ 08108
**Phone:** (609)869-3134        **Fax:** (609)869-3129
Erika MacWilliams, Contact

**Program(s):** Aromatherapy; Ayurvedic Medicine; Feldenkrais; Guided Imagery; Massage Therapy; Reflexology; Reiki; Shiatsu; Sports Massage; Therapeutic Touch; Traditional Chinese Medicine; Yoga Teacher Training.

### ★ 3853 ★ School of Asian Healing Arts
Executive Mews G-38
1930 E Marlton Park
Cherry Hill, NJ 08003
**Phone:** (609)424-7501        **Fax:** (609)424-7379
Ruth Dalphin, Director

**Program(s):** Acupressure; Qigong; Reflexology; Reiki; Shiatsu; Thai Massage; Traditional Chinese Medicine; Yoga Teacher Training.

### ★ 3854 ★ Seashore Healing Arts Center
505 New Rd., Stes. 5 and 7
Somers Point, NJ 08244
**Phone:** (609)601-9272
Edward Smith, Director

**Program(s):** Acupressure; Deep Tissue Massage; Energy Work; Massage Therapy; Meditation; Polarity Therapy; Qigong; Reflexology; Reiki; Yoga.

### ★ 3855 ★ Somerset School of Massage Therapy
7 Cedar Grove Ln.
Somerset, NJ 08873
**Phone:** (732)356-0787        **Fax:** (732)469-3494
**Email:** ssmt@massagecareer.com
**Website:** http://www.massagecareer.com
Deborah Scarpitto, Contact

**Program(s):** Massage Therapy; Neuromuscular Therapy; Reflexology; Shiatsu.

### ★ 3856 ★ Studio Yoga
2 Green Village Rd., Rm. 301
PO Box 99
Madison, NJ 07940
**Phone:** (973)966-5311        **Fax:** (973)966-1477
Theresa Rowland, Director

**Program(s):** Yoga Teacher Training.

### ★ 3857 ★ Swedish American Massage Institute (SAMI)
120 Maple Ave.
Red Bank, NJ 07701
**Phone:** (908)530-1188        **Fax:** (908)530-1919
Sharyn Ross, Director

**Program(s):** Aromatherapy; Massage Therapy; Neuromuscular Therapy; On-Site Massage; Reflexology; Sports Massage; Swedish Massage.

**★ 3858 ★ Universal of Medicine and Dentistry of New Jersey**
**School of Health Related Professions**
65 Bergen St.
Newark, NJ 07107-3001
**Phone:** (973)972-4298
Elaine Diegmann, Director
**Program(s):** Midwifery.

**★ 3859 ★ Unlimited Potential**
PO Box 64
Roseland, NJ 07068
**Phone:** (973)325-0900          **Fax:** (973)403-9789
Roxanne Louise, Director
**Program(s):** Hypnotherapy; Reiki.

### New Mexico

**★ 3860 ★ Academy Institute of Vedic Studies**
1701 Santa Fe River Rd.
Santa Fe, NM 87501
**Phone:** (505)983-9385          **Fax:** (505)982-5807
Mira Foung, Director
**Program(s):** Ayurvedic Medicine.

**★ 3861 ★ Ayurvedic Institute**
11311 Menaul NE, Ste. A
PO Box 23445
Albuquerque, NM 87112
**Phone:** (505)291-9698          **Fax:** (505)294-7572
**Website:** http://www.ayurveda.com
Wynn Werner, Contact
**Program(s):** Anatomy and Physiology; Ayurvedic Medicine; Yoga.

**★ 3862 ★ Body-Mind Centering**
PO Box 4552
Taos, NM 87571
**Phone:** (505)758-1711          **Fax:** (505)751-0331
Ziji Beth Goren, Director
**Program(s):** Body-Mind Centering.

**★ 3863 ★ Crystal Mountain Apprenticeship in the Healing Arts**
118 Dartmouth SE
Albuquerque, NM 87106
**Phone:** (505)268-4411          **Free:** 800-967-5678
**Fax:** (505)268-4007
Rebecca Solomon, Director
**Program(s):** Anatomy and Physiology; Aromatherapy; CranioSacral Therapy; Energy Work; Esalen Massage; Herbal Medicine; Hydrotherapy; Kinesiology; LomiLomi Massage; Massage Therapy; Movement Education; Neuromuscular Therapy; Polarity Therapy; Reflexology; Shiatsu; Sports Massage; Traditional Chinese Medicine.

**★ 3864 ★ Eastern New Mexico School of Massage Therapy**
PO Box 2142
Clovis, NM 88101
**Phone:** (505)763-0551          **Fax:** (505)763-1405
Sue Pierce, Director
**Program(s):** CranioSacral Therapy; Energy Work; Herbal Medicine; Infant Massage; Manual Lymph Drainage; Massage Therapy; Polarity Therapy; Reflexology; Shiatsu.

**★ 3865 ★ International Institute of Chinese Medicine**
4884 La Junta del Alamo
PO Box 29988
Santa Fe, NM 87505
**Phone:** (505)473-5233          **Free:** 800-377-4561
**Fax:** (505)473-9279
**Email:** 102152.3463@compuserve.com

**Website:** http://www.thuntek.net/iicm
Dr. Michael Zeng, Contact
**Program(s):** Acupuncture; Oriental Medicine; Qigong; Traditional Chinese Medicine; Tui Na.

**★ 3866 ★ KRI**
Rt. 2 Box 4 Shady Lane
Espanola, NM 87532
**Phone:** (505)753-0423          **Fax:** (505)753-5982
Nam K. Khalsa, Director
**Program(s):** Yoga Teacher Training.

**★ 3867 ★ Maharishi College of Vedic Medicine**
2721 Arizona, St. NE
Albuquerque, NM 87110
**Phone:** (505)830-0435          **Fax:** (505)830-0538
**Email:** desmithmd@aol.com
D. Edwards Smith, MD, Contact
**Program(s):** Ayurvedic Medicine; Maharishi Vedic Medicine.

**★ 3868 ★ Medicine Wheel - A School of Holistic Therapies**
1243 W Apache
Farmington, NM 87401
**Free:** 888-327-1914          **Fax:** (505)327-2234
Randy Barnes, Director
**Program(s):** Acupressure; Aromatherapy; CranioSacral Therapy; Herbal Medicine; Holistic Health; Massage Therapy; Neuromuscular Therapy; Polarity Therapy; Qigong; Traditional Chinese Medicine; Tui Na.

**★ 3869 ★ Mesilla Valley School of Therapeutic Arts**
741 N Alameda, Ste. 15
PO Box 1227
Las Cruces, NM 88005
**Phone:** (505)527-1239
Wanita Thompson, Director
**Program(s):** Massage Therapy.

**★ 3870 ★ National College of Phytotherapy**
3030 Isleta Blvd. SW
Albuquerque, NM 87105
**Phone:** (505)452-3468          **Fax:** (505)452-3468
Teresa Merriken, Contact
**Program(s):** Herbal Medicine.

**★ 3871 ★ New Mexico Academy of Healing Arts**
501 Franklin Ave.
PO Box 932
Santa Fe, NM 87501
**Phone:** (505)982-6271          **Free:** 888-808-5188
**Fax:** (505)988-2621
**Website:** http://www.nmaha.com
Lorin Parrish, Director
**Program(s):** Aromatherapy; CranioSacral Therapy; Feldenkrais; Massage Therapy; Polarity Therapy; Reflexology; Shiatsu; Sports Massage; Swedish Massage.

**★ 3872 ★ New Mexico School of Natural Therapeutics**
202 Morningside SE
Albuquerque, NM 87108
**Phone:** (505)268-6870          **Free:** 800-654-1675
**Fax:** (505)268-0818
**Email:** jpendry@swcp.com
**Website:** http://www.nmsnt.org
Robert Stevens, Director
**Program(s):** Deep Tissue Massage; Flower Essences; Herbal Medicine; Massage Therapy; Polarity Therapy; Pregnancy Massage; Reflexology; Shiatsu; Sports Massage; Swedish Massage.

**★ 3873 ★ Rosen Method Center Southwest**
PO Box 344
Santa Fe, NM 87504
**Phone:** (505)982-7149          **Fax:** (505)254-7048
**Email:** sw.touch@ix.netcom.com
**Website:** http://www.mcn.org/b/rosen
Sandra Wooten, Director
**Program(s):** Rosen Method Bodywork.

**★ 3874 ★ Scherer Institute of Natural Healing**
935 Alto St.
Santa Fe, NM 87501
**Phone:** (505)982-8398          **Fax:** (505)982-1825
**Email:** tsi@rt66.com
**Website:** http://www.newmexiconet.com/scher.htm
Lonnie Howard, Director
**Program(s):** Aromatherapy; CarnioSacral Therapy; Energy Work; Herbal Medicine; Massage Therapy; Polarity Therapy; Reflexology; Shiatsu; Sports Massage.

**★ 3875 ★ Southwest Acupuncture College, Albuquerque**
4308 Carlisle NE, Ste. 205
Albuquerque, NM 87107
**Phone:** (505)888-8898
Skya Gardner Abbate, Director
**Program(s):** Acupuncture; Herbal Medicine; Oriental Medicine; Qigong; Shiatsu; Traditional Chinese Medicine.

**★ 3876 ★ Southwest Acupuncture College, Santa Fe**
2960 Rodeo Park Dr. W
Santa Fe, NM 87505
**Phone:** (505)438-8884          **Fax:** (505)438-8883
Skya Gardner Abbate, Director
**Program(s):** Acupuncture; Herbal Medicine; Oriental Medicine; Qigong; Traditional Chinese Medicine.

**★ 3877 ★ Taos School of Massage**
1021 Salazar
Taos, NM 87571
**Phone:** (505)758-2725
Eric Ritchie, Director
**Program(s):** Acupressure; Applied Kinesiology; Ayurvedic Medicine; Body-Mind Clearing; Energy Work; Massage Therapy; Neuromuscular Therapy; Qigong; Reflexology; Shiatsu; Sports Massage; Traditional Chinese Medicine.

**★ 3878 ★ Universal Therapeutic Massage Institute, Inc.**
3410 Aztec Rd. NE
Albuquerque, NM 87107
**Free:** 800-557-0020          **Fax:** (505)881-0749
Stacy Townsend, Contact
**Program(s):** CranioSacral Therapy; Massage Therapy; Myofascial Release; Neuromuscular Therapy; Polarity Therapy; Reflexology; Shiatsu; Sports Masssage; Traditional Chinese Medicine.

**★ 3879 ★ University of New Mexico College of Nursing**
Nursing/Pharmacy Bldg.
Albuquerque, NM 87131-1061
**Phone:** (505)272-1184
Barbara A. Overman, Director
**Program(s):** Midwifery.

**★ 3880 ★ Wellness Institute**
PO Box 2843
Taos, NM 87571
**Phone:** (505)776-1590          **Free:** 888-253-6331
**Email:** wellness@laplaza.taos.nm.us
Roger Gilchrist, Contact

**Program(s):** Polarity Therapy.


★ 3881 ★ **Westbrook University**
400 University Plaza
Aztec, NM 87410
**Phone:** (505)334-1115          **Free:** 800-447-6496
**Fax:** (505)334-7583
**Email:** admissions@cyberport.com
**Website:** http://www.westbrooku.edu
DeeAnne Greene, PhD, Contact

**Program(s):** Acupressure; Aromatherapy; Ayurvedic Medicine; Energy Work; Flower Essences; Herbal Medicine; Homeopathy; Midwifery; Naturopathic Medicine; Polarity Therapy; Reflexology.


★ 3882 ★ **White Mountain School of Applied Healing**
1204 Mechem, Ste. 10
Ruidoso, NM 88345
**Phone:** (505)258-3046
Pablo Falcon, Director

**Program(s):** Acupressure; Aromatherapy; Deep Tissue Massage; Energy Work; Manual Lymph Drainage; Massage Therapy; Reflexology; Reiki; Shiatsu.

## New York

★ 3883 ★ **Academy of Natural Healing**
40 W 72nd St., Ste. 117
New York, NY 10023
**Phone:** (212)724-8782          **Fax:** (212)724-2535
Lewis Harrison, Director

**Program(s):** Acupressure; Aromatherapy; CranioSacral Therapy; Energy Work; Herbal Medicine; Homeopathy; Polarity Therapy; Qigong; Reflexology; Shiatsu.


★ 3884 ★ **American Center for the Alexander Technique**
129 W 67th St.
New York, NY 10023
**Phone:** (212)799-0468          **Fax:** (212)799-0468
Barbara Kent, Director

**Program(s):** Alexander Technique.


★ 3885 ★ **American Taoist Healing Center**
396 Broadway, Ste. 502
New York, NY 10013-3500
**Phone:** (212)274-0999          **Fax:** (212)274-9879
Louise Di Bello, Contact

**Program(s):** Acupressure; Acupuncture; Qigong; Traditional Chinese Medicine.


★ 3886 ★ **Atlantic Academy of Classical Homeopathy**
399 6th Ave., Ste. 3D
Brooklyn, NY 11215
**Phone:** (718)768-3811
Gerald Gewiss, Director

**Program(s):** Homeopathy.


★ 3887 ★ **Ayurveda Holistic Center**
82 A0 Bayville Ave.
Bayville, NY 11709
**Phone:** (516)628-8200
**Email:** mail@ayurvedahc.com
**Website:** http://www.ayurvedahc.com
Swami Sada Shiva Tirtha, Contact

**Program(s):** Ayurvedic Medicine.


★ 3888 ★ **Barbara Brennan School of Healing**
PO Box 2005
East Hampton, NY 11937
**Phone:** (516)329-0951          **Fax:** (516)324-9745
**Website:** http://www.barbarabrennan.com
Kay Conboy, Contact

**Program(s):** Brennan Healing Science; Energy Work.


★ 3889 ★ **Biofeedback Training Associates**
255 W 98th St.
New York, NY 10025
**Phone:** (212)222-5665          **Fax:** (212)222-5667
**Email:** ac@inx.net
**Website:** http://www.biof.com/biofeedback.html
Dr. Philip Brotman, Director

**Program(s):** Biofeedback; Hypnotherapy; Neurofeedback.


★ 3890 ★ **Body Logic Institute**
295 W 11th St., Ste. 1F
New York, NY 10014
**Phone:** (212)633-2143          **Free:** 800-877-8429
**Fax:** (212)633-6190
Yamuna Zake, Contact

**Program(s):** Body Logic; Body Rolling.


★ 3891 ★ **Diana Kalfayan**
150 W 80th St., Apt. 6C
New York, NY 10024
**Phone:** (212)877-9626
Diana Kalfayan, Director

**Program(s):** Esoteric Healing; Polarity Therapy.


★ 3892 ★ **Finger Lakes School of Massage**
1251 Trumansburg Rd.
Ithaca, NY 14850
**Phone:** (607)272-9024          **Fax:** (607)272-4271
**Website:** http://www.flsm.com
Cindy Black, Director

**Program(s):** Aromatherapy; Energy Work; Massage Therapy; Neuromuscular Therapy; Polarity Therapy; Reflexology; Shiatsu; Sports Massage; Thai Massage; Trager.


★ 3893 ★ **Flynn's School of Herbology**
60 E 4th St.
New York, NY 10003
**Phone:** (212)677-8140
Arcus Flynn, Contact

**Program(s):** Herbal Medicine.


★ 3894 ★ **Hudson Valley School of Classical Homeopathy**
321 McKinstry Rd.
Gardiner, NY 12525
**Phone:** (914)255-6141          **Fax:** (914)255-6241
David Kramer, Director

**Program(s):** Homeopathy.


★ 3895 ★ **Hypnosis Institute**
139 Fulton St., Ste. 304
New York, NY 10038
**Phone:** (212)227-8643          **Fax:** (212)791-9517
**Email:** hypno1@interport.net
**Website:** http://www.infaith.com
Barry Seedman, PhD, Director

**Program(s):** Hypnotherapy; Reiki.


★ 3896 ★ **Institute for the Alexander Technique**
853 Broadway, Ste. 1007
New York, NY 10003
**Phone:** (212)529-3211
Thomas Lemens, Contact

**Program(s):** Alexander Technique.


★ 3897 ★ **Jivamukti Yoga Center**
404 Lafayette St., 3rd Flr.
New York, NY 10003
**Phone:** (212)353-0214          **Fax:** (212)995-1313
Adrienne Burke, Director

**Program(s):** Yoga Teacher Training.


★ 3898 ★ **Kundalini Yoga Center**
401 Layfayette St.
New York, NY 10003
**Phone:** (212)475-0212
**Email:** ravi@ziplink.net
**Website:** http://www.ziplink.net/~ravi
Ravi Singh, Director

**Program(s):** Yoga Teacher Training.


★ 3899 ★ **Kundalini Yoga East, Inc.**
873 Broadway, Ste. 614
New York, NY 10003
**Phone:** (212)995-0521
Sat Jivan Kaur Khalsa, Director

**Program(s):** Energy Work; Yoga Teacher Training.


★ 3900 ★ **Laura Norman Reflexology Training Center**
41 Park Ave., Ste. 8A
New York, NY 10016
**Phone:** (212)532-4404          **Fax:** (212)532-4504
Laura Norman, Director

**Program(s):** Reflexology.


★ 3901 ★ **Linden Tree Center for Holistic Health**
8 Noxon Rd.
Poughkeepsie, NY 12603-2926
**Phone:** (914)471-8000
Gary Seigel, Director

**Program(s):** CranioSacral Therapy; Polarity Therapy.


★ 3902 ★ **Long Island Reflexology Center**
14 E Broadway
Port Jefferson, NY 11777
**Phone:** (516)474-3137          **Fax:** (516)287-3127
Geraldine Brill, Director

**Program(s):** Reflexology; Therapeutic Touch.


★ 3903 ★ **Mathews School of the Alexander Technique**
74 MacDougal St.
New York, NY 10012
**Phone:** (212)473-3247          **Fax:** (212)473-0341
Troup Mathews, Director

**Program(s):** Alexander Technique.


★ 3904 ★ **Mercy College**
555 Broadway
Dobbs Ferry, NY 10522
**Phone:** (914)674-7401          **Fax:** (914)674-7374
Douglas McDaniel, Director

**Program(s):** Acupuncture; Oriental Medicine.


★ 3905 ★ **MotherMassage**
108 E 16th St., Ste. 401
New York, NY 10003
**Phone:** (212)533-3188          **Fax:** (212)533-3148
Elaine Stillerman, Contact

**Program(s):** Prenatal Massage; Postpartum Massage.


★ 3906 ★ **New Center College for Wholistic Health Education and Research**
6801 Jericho Tpk., Ste. 300
Syosset, NY 11791
**Phone:** (516)364-0808          **Fax:** (516)364-0989
Steven Schenkman, Contact

**Program(s):** Acupuncture; Herbal Medicine; Holistic Nursing; Massage Therapy; Oriental Medicine; Traditional Chinese Medicine.

**★ 3907 ★ New York Chiropractic College**
2360 SR 89
Seneca Falls, NY 13148-0800
**Phone:** (315)568-3000    **Fax:** (315)568-3015
**Email:** enrolnow@nycc.edu
**Website:** http://www.nycc.edu
Kenneth W. Padgett, Contact

**Program(s):** Chiropractic.

**★ 3908 ★ New York Institute of Massage**
4701 Transit Rd.
Williamsville, NY 14221
**Phone:** (716)633-0355    **Free:** 800-884-6946
**Fax:** (716)633-0213
Sharon Boyd, Director

**Program(s):** Massage Therapy.

**★ 3909 ★ New York Open Center**
83 Spring St.
New York, NY 10012
**Phone:** (212)274-1829    **Fax:** (212)226-4056
Lisa Schimski, Director

**Program(s):** Polarity Therapy; Reflexology; Yoga
Teacher Training.

**★ 3910 ★ New York University**
**Division of Nursing/School of Education**
50 W 4th St.
425 Shimkin Hall
New York, NY 10012
**Phone:** (212)998-5895
Patricia Burkhardt, Director

**Program(s):** Midwifery.

**★ 3911 ★ NLP Center of New York**
24 E 12th St., Ste. 402
New York, NY 10003
**Phone:** (212)647-0860    **Fax:** (212)509-2326
**Email:** nlp@earthlink.net
**Website:** http://www.nlptraining.com
Steven Leeds, Director

**Program(s):** Hypnotherapy; Neuro-Linguistic Programming.

**★ 3912 ★ Northeast School of Botanical**
**Medicine**
PO Box 6626
Ithaca, NY 14851
**Phone:** (607)564-1023

**Program(s):** Herbal Medicine.

**★ 3913 ★ Ohashi Institute**
12 W 27th St., 9th Flr.
New York, NY 10001
**Free:** 800-810-4190    **Fax:** (212)447-5819
**Email:** ohashiinst@aol.com
**Website:** http://www.ohashi.com

**Program(s):** Shiatsu.

**★ 3914 ★ Omega Institute for Holistic**
**Studies**
260 Lake Dr.
Rhinebeck, NY 12572
**Phone:** (914)266-4444    **Fax:** (914)266-4828
**Website:** http://omega-inst.org
Laurie Zollo, Director

**Program(s):** Energy Work; Healing Touch; Massage
Therapy; Mind-Body Medicine; Qigong; Reflexology;
Yoga Teacher Training.

**★ 3915 ★ Onondaga School of**
**Therapeutic Massage**
220 Walton St.
Syracuse, NY 13202
**Phone:** (315)424-1159    **Fax:** (315)424-0796
Jean Vatter, Director

**Program(s):** Massage Therapy.

**★ 3916 ★ Pacific College of Oriental**
**Medicine**
915 Broadway, 3rd Fl.
New York, NY 10010
**Phone:** (212)982-3456    **Free:** 800-729-3468
**Fax:** (212)982-6514
Jennifer Park, Contact

**Program(s):** Acupuncture; Oriental Medicine; Traditional Chinese Medicine.

**★ 3917 ★ R. J. Buckle Associates, LLC**
PO Box 868
Hunter, NY 12442
**Phone:** (518)263-4402    **Fax:** (518)263-4031
Jane Buckle, Director

**Program(s):** Aromatherapy.

**★ 3918 ★ Rainbow Reiki Center**
1330 Main St.
Ruby, NY 12475
**Phone:** (914)336-4609
Joyce Kaessinger, Director

**Program(s):** Reiki.

**★ 3919 ★ Reese Williams**
270 Lafayette St., Ste. 805
New York, NY 10012
**Phone:** (212)343-9382
Reese Williams, Director

**Program(s):** CranioSacral Therapy; Polarity Therapy.

**★ 3920 ★ Reflexhollogy - Science, Art**
**and Heart**
143-24 Poplar Ave.
Flushing, NY 11355
**Phone:** (718)961-2786
Holly Papa, Director

**Program(s):** Reflexology.

**★ 3921 ★ Rubenfeld Synergy Center**
115 Waverly Pl.
New York, NY 10011
**Free:** 800-747-6897    **Fax:** (212)254-1174
**Email:** rubenfeld@aol.com
Ilana Rubenfeld, Director

**Program(s):** Rubenfeld Synergy Method.

**★ 3922 ★ School of Homeopathy**
964 3rd Ave., 8th Flr.
New York, NY 10155-0003
**Phone:** (212)570-2576    **Fax:** (212)758-4079
**Email:** kathy@homeopathyschool.com
**Website:** http://www.homeopathyschool.com
Kathleen A. Lukas, Director

**Program(s):** Homeopathy.

**★ 3923 ★ Sivananda Yoga Ranch**
PO Box 195
Woodbourne, NY 12788
**Phone:** (914)436-6492    **Fax:** (914)434-1032
**Email:** yogaranch@sivananda.org
**Website:** http://www.sivananda.org/ranch.htm
**Program(s):** Yoga Teacher Training.

**★ 3924 ★ State University of New York**
**Health Science Center at Brooklyn**
450 Clarkson Ave., Box 1227
Brooklyn, NY 11203-2908
**Phone:** (718)270-7740    **Fax:** (718)270-7634
Liliana Montano, Director

**Program(s):** Midwifery.

**★ 3925 ★ State University of New York,**
**Stony Brook**
**School of Nursing**
Health Sciences Center
Stony Brook, NY 11794-8240
**Phone:** (516)444-2879    **Fax:** (516)444-6049
Linda Sacino, Director

**Program(s):** Midwifery.

**★ 3926 ★ Swedish Institute Inc.**
226 W 26th St., 5th Fl.
New York, NY 10001
**Phone:** (212)924-5900    **Fax:** (212)924-7600

**Program(s):** Acupressure; Acupuncture; Massage
Therapy; Oriental Medicine; Shiatsu.

**★ 3927 ★ Teleosis School of**
**Homeopathy**
61 W 62nd St.
New York, NY 10023
**Phone:** (212)707-8481    **Fax:** (212)707-8481
Kim Kalina, Director

**Program(s):** Homeopathy.

**★ 3928 ★ Traditional Reiki Network**
Fire No. 602, Case Hill Rd.
Treadwell, NY 13846-0262
**Phone:** (607)829-3702    **Fax:** (914)254-4835
Ellen Sokolow, Director

**Program(s):** Reiki.

**★ 3929 ★ Tri-State Institute of Traditional**
**Chinese Acupuncture**
80 8th Ave., Ste. 400
New York, NY 10024
**Phone:** (212)242-2255    **Fax:** (212)242-2920
Mark D. Seem, PhD, Contact

**Program(s):** Acupuncture; Herbal Medicine; Traditional Chinese Medicine.

**★ 3930 ★ Wise Woman Center**
416 Fishcreek
Saugerties, NY 12477
**Phone:** (914)246-8081    **Fax:** (914)246-8081
Susun S. Weed, Director

**Program(s):** Animal Therapy; Energy Work; Herbal
Medicine.

**★ 3931 ★ Woodstock Polarity Retreat**
**Center**
872 Buck Rd.
Stone Ridge, NY 12484
**Phone:** (914)687-4767    **Free:** 800-925-0159
**Fax:** (212)327-4049
**Email:** johnb310@aol.com
John Beaulieu, PhD, Director

**Program(s):** Polarity Therapy.

**★ 3932 ★ Yoga and Polarity Center**
32 Church St.
Malverne, NY 11565
**Phone:** (516)596-0397    **Fax:** (516)887-4747
Amy Bubser, Director

**Program(s):** Energy Work; Polarity Therapy; Reflexology; Yoga Teacher Training.

## North Carolina

**★ 3933 ★ Academy of Natural Therapies**
5 Piney View Estates
PO Box 9223
Marshall, NC 28753
**Phone:** (828)683-1737    **Fax:** (828)363-0265
Angela Plum, PhD, Director

**Program(s):** Acupressure; Aroomatherapy; CranioSacral Therapy; Polarity Therapy.

**★ 3934 ★ Asheville School of Massage**
729 Haywood Rd.
Asheville, NC 28806
**Phone:** (828)236-9977 **Fax:** (828)254-5613
Tracy McMahon, Director

**Program(s):** Acupressure; Aromatherapy; CranioSa-cral Therapy; Deep Tissue Massage; Energy Work; Manual Lymph Drainage; Massage Therapy; Polarity Therapy; Reflexology; Shiatsu; Yoga Teacher Training.

**★ 3935 ★ Body Therapy Institute**
300 S Wind Rd.
Siler City, NC 27344
**Phone:** (919)663-3111 **Free:** 888-500-4500
**Fax:** (919)663-0369
Rick Rosen, Director

**Program(s):** Massage Therapy.

**★ 3936 ★ Doula Training**
1007 W Lady Diana Ct.
Apex, NC 27502
**Phone:** (919)362-5517 **Fax:** (919)387-6273
Ann Tumblin, Director

**Program(s):** Doula.

**★ 3937 ★ East Carolina University School of Nursing**
Greenville, NC 27858
**Phone:** (919)328-4298
Nancy Moss, Director

**Program(s):** Midwifery.

**★ 3938 ★ G-Jo Institute**
PO Box 1460.
Columbus, NC 28722
**Phone:** (828)863-4660
Barbara Gail Watson, Director

**Program(s):** Acupressure; Reflexology.

**★ 3939 ★ Lighten Up Yoga Center**
60 Biltmore Ave.
Asheville, NC 28801
**Phone:** (828)254-7756 **Fax:** (828)254-3797
Alice Dawson, Director

**Program(s):** Yoga Teacher Training.

**★ 3940 ★ Listening Hands Polarity**
605 Jones Ferry Rd., EE2
Carrboro, NC 27510
**Phone:** (919)942-1819
Gabriella Tal, Director

**Program(s):** Polarity Therapy.

**★ 3941 ★ Natural Touch School of Massage Therapy, Greensboro**
4007 W Wendover
Greensboro, NC 27407
**Free:** 877-799-0060
Wanda Adkins, Director

**Program(s):** Acupressure; CranioSacral Therapy; Energy Work; Massage Therapy; Myofascial Release; Polarity Therapy; Shiatsu.

**★ 3942 ★ New Life Empowerment Center**
129 S Long St.
Salisbury, NC 28144
**Phone:** (704)633-2700 **Fax:** (704)633-2046
Thomas Hartman, Director

**Program(s):** Acupressure; Aromatherapy; Energy Work; Hypnotherapy; Qigong; Reflexology; Reiki.

**★ 3943 ★ North Carolina School of Natural Healing**
20 Battery Park Ave., Rm. 570
Asheville, NC 28801

**Phone:** (704)252-7096
Craig Ellis, Director

**Program(s):** Acupressure; Aromatherapy; CranioSa-cral Therapy; Energy Work; Herbal Medicine; Massage Therapy; Meditation; Polarity Therapy; Reiki; Shiatsu.

**★ 3944 ★ Professional Institute of Massage Therapy, Fargo**
4553 9th Ave. SW, Ste. 2
Fargo, NC 58103
**Phone:** (704)281-5078
Michael Stafford, Director

**Program(s):** Massage Therapy.

**★ 3945 ★ Southeastern School of Neuromuscular Massage Therapy of Charlotte, Inc.**
4 Woodlawn Green, Ste. 200
Charlotte, NC 28217
**Phone:** (704)527-4979 **Fax:** (704)527-3104
**Email:** massage@ch.mindspring.com
**Website:** http://www.se-massage.com
Kimberly Williams, Contact

**Program(s):** Massage Therapy; Neuromuscular Therapy.

**★ 3946 ★ Therapeutic Massage Training Institute**
726 E Blvd.
Charlotte, NC 28203
**Phone:** (704)338-9660 **Fax:** (704)523-4389
**Email:** asktmti@aol.com
Lynda L. Clay, Director

**Program(s):** Massage Therapy.

**★ 3947 ★ Tree of Life Polarity Center**
PO Box 281
Saxapahaw, NC 27340
**Phone:** (336)376-8186
Janice Durand, Director

**Program(s):** Energy Work; Polarity Therapy.

**★ 3948 ★ Wellness Training Center**
231 Erwin Hills Rd.
Asheville, NC 28806
**Phone:** (828)683-3369
Robert Luka, Director

**Program(s):** Hypnotherapy.

**★ 3949 ★ Whole You School of Massage and Bodywork**
143 Woodview Dr.
Rutherfordton, NC 28139
**Phone:** (828)287-0955 **Fax:** (828)287-0067
Kenneth Shew, Director

**Program(s):** Acupressure; Aromatherapy; CranioSa-cral Therapy; Deep Tissue Massage; Massage Therapy; Neuromuscular Therapy; Reflexology; Reiki.

### North Dakota

**★ 3950 ★ Sister Rosalind Gefre School of Professional Massage, Fargo**
McMerty Ctr., 619 7th St., Ste. L
Fargo, ND 58102
**Phone:** (701)297-5993

**Program(s):** Deep Tissue Massage; Massage Therapy; Reflexology.

### Nova Scotia

**★ 3951 ★ ICT Northumberland College**
1660 Hollis St., Ste. 301
Halifax, NS, Canada B3J 1V7
**Phone:** (902)425-2869 **Fax:** (902)425-2858
Dawn Schmidt, Contact

**Program(s):** Massage Therapy.

### Ohio

**★ 3952 ★ Alexander Technique of Cincinnati**
954 W Northbend Rd.
Cincinnati, OH 45224
**Phone:** (513)542-1010
Vivien Schapera, Director

**Program(s):** Alexander Technique.

**★ 3953 ★ Bhumi's Yoga and Wellness Center**
25068 Center Rideg Rd.
Cleveland, OH 44145
**Phone:** (440)899-9569 **Fax:** (440)899-9569
**Email:** healingbreath@mediaone.net
Harriet Russell, Director

**Program(s):** Acupressure; Energy Work; Meditation; Polarity Therapy; Reiki; Shiatsu; Yoga Teacher Training.

**★ 3954 ★ Case Western Reserve University**
**Frances Payne Bolton School of Nursing**
10900 Euclid Ave.
Cleveland, OH 44106-4904
**Phone:** (216)368-2532
Marcia Riegger, Director

**Program(s):** Midwifery.

**★ 3955 ★ Central Ohio School of Massage**
1120 Morse Rd., Ste. 250
Columbus, OH 43229
**Phone:** (614)841-1122 **Fax:** (614)841-0387
**Email:** admissions@cosm.org
**Website:** http://www.cosm.org

**Program(s):** Massage Therapy.

**★ 3956 ★ Cleveland School of Massage/ Advanced Bodywork Institute**
10683 Ravenna Rd.
Twinsburg, OH 44087
**Phone:** (330)405-1933
Jeff Kates, Director

**Program(s):** Aromatherapy; Deep Tissue Massage; Energy Work; Myofascial Release; Polarity Therapy; Reflexology; Swedish Massage.

**★ 3957 ★ Columbus Academy of Medical Massage**
3600 Main St.
Hilliard, OH 43026
**Phone:** (614)777-1161 **Fax:** (614)336-8478
Jennifer Hastings-Schunn, Contact

**Program(s):** Aromatherapy; Massage Therapy; Medical Massage; Myofascial Release; Trigger Point Therapy.

**★ 3958 ★ Columbus Polarity Therapy Institute**
170 W 5th Ave.
Columbus, OH 43201
**Phone:** (614)299-9438 **Fax:** (614)291-7252
Mary Jo Ruggieri, Director

**Program(s):** Acupressure; Aromatherapy; Ayurvedic Medicine; CranioSacral Therapy; Energy Work; Naturopathic Medicine; Polarity Therapy; Reflexology.

**★ 3959 ★ Cuyahoga Community College**
4250 Richmond Rd.
Highland Hills, OH 44122-6195
**Phone:** (216)987-2426 **Fax:** (216)987-2450
Sheila Batheja, Director

**Program(s):** Massage Therapy.

**★ 3960 ★ Healing Heart Herbals**
36254 McCumber Rd.
Rutland, OH 45775
**Phone:** (740)742-8901
Cindy Parker, Director

**Program(s):** Aromatherapy; Ayurvedic Medicine; Energy Work; Herbal Medicine; Homeopathy; Oriental Medicine; Polarity Therapy; Reflexology; Traditional Chinese Medicine.

**★ 3961 ★ Integrated Touch Therapy, Inc, for Animals**
7041 Zane Trail Rd.
Circleville, OH 43113
**Phone:** (740)474-6436 **Fax:** (740)474-2625
Patricia Whalen-Shaw, Director

**Program(s):** Acupressure; Animal Therapy; CranioSacral Therapy; Energy Work; Equine Massage; Herbal Medicine; Massage Therapy; Polarity Therapy.

**★ 3962 ★ International Academy for Reflexology Studies**
4759 Cornell Rd., Ste. D
Cincinnati, OH 45241
**Phone:** (513)489-9328 **Fax:** (513)489-9354
Marcia L. Aschendorf, Director

**Program(s):** Reflexology.

**★ 3963 ★ Massage Away, Inc, School of Therapy**
6685 Doubletree Ave.
Columbus, OH 43229
**Phone:** (614)825-6278 **Fax:** (614)825-6279
Gail Quinn, Director

**Program(s):** Massage Therapy.

**★ 3964 ★ National Institute of Massotherapy**
2110 Copley Rd.
Akron, OH 44320
**Phone:** (330)867-1996 **Fax:** (330)869-6422
Stephen Perkinson, Director

**Program(s):** Acupressure; CranioSacral Therapy; Massage Therapy; Neuromuscular Therapy; Polarity Therapy; Reflexology; Reiki; Shiatsu.

**★ 3965 ★ National Institute of Massotherapy, Garfield Heights**
12684 Rockside Rd.
Garfield Heights, OH 44125
**Phone:** (216)662-6955 **Fax:** (216)662-6980
Ewa Perkinson, Director

**Program(s):** Massage Therapy; Neuromuscular Therapy; Ortho-Bionomy; Polarity Therapy; Shiatsu.

**★ 3966 ★ Northwest Academy of Massotherapy**
1910 Indian Wood Circle, Ste. 301
Maumee, OH 43537
**Phone:** (419)893-6464
Eric Ritchie, Director

**Program(s):** Massage Therapy; Reflexology; Sports Massage.

**★ 3967 ★ Ohio Academy of Holistic Health, Inc.**
3033 Dayton-Xenia Rd.
Beavercreek, OH 45434
**Phone:** (937)427-0506 **Free:** 800-833-8122
**Fax:** (937)426-8883
Jedidiah Smith, Director

**Program(s):** Aromatherapy; Energy Work; Herbal Medicine; Hypnotherapy; Iridology; NeuroLinguistic Programming; Reflexology; Reiki; Touch for Health.

**★ 3968 ★ Ohio College of Massotherapy**
225 Heritage Woods Dr.
Akron, OH 44321
**Phone:** (330)665-1084 **Fax:** (330)665-5021
Ann K. Morrow, Contact

**Program(s):** Acupressure; Aromatherapy; CranioSacral Therapy; Massage Therapy; Myofascial Release; Neuromuscular Therapy; Reflexology; Sports Massage.

**★ 3969 ★ Ohio State University College of Nursing**
1585 Neil Ave.
Columbus, OH 43210-1289
**Phone:** (614)292-4041
Nancy K. Lowe, Director

**Program(s):** Midwifery.

**★ 3970 ★ Reflexology Science Institute**
1170 Old Henderson Rd., Ste. 206
Columbus, OH 43220
**Phone:** (614)457-5783 **Fax:** (614)442-0133
Eileen Motok, Director

**Program(s):** Acupressure; CranioSacral Therapy; Energy Work; Polarity Therapy; Reflexology; Reiki

**★ 3971 ★ Retha J. Martin School of Hypnotherapy**
5018 Mason Rd.
Berlin Heights, OH 44814
**Phone:** (419)433-2912
Retha J. Martin, Contact

**Program(s):** Energy Work; Hypnotherapy; Reiki.

**★ 3972 ★ SHI, Integrative Medical Massage School**
130 Cook Rd.
PO Box 474
Lebanon, OH 45036
**Phone:** (513)932-8712 **Fax:** (513)932-8180
Sharon L. Barnes, PhD, Director

**Program(s):** Alexander Technique; Biofeedback; CranioSacral Therapy; Energy Work; Feldenkrais; Massage Therapy; Medical Massage; Myofascial Release; Neuromuscular Therapy; Polarity Therapy; Somatic Education; Therapeutic Touch.

**★ 3973 ★ University of Cincinnati, College of Nursing and Health**
PO Box 210038
Cincinnati, OH 45221-0038
**Phone:** (513)558-5282
Mary Carol Akers, Director

**Program(s):** Midwifery.

**★ 3974 ★ Youngstown College of Massotherapy**
14 Highland Ave.
Struthers, OH 44471
**Phone:** (330)755-1406 **Fax:** (330)755-1605
Douglas M. Shodd, Sr., Contact

**Program(s):** Massage Therapy.

### Oklahoma

**★ 3975 ★ Massage Therapy Institute of Oklahoma**
9433 E 51st St., Ste. H
Tulsa, OK 74145
**Phone:** (918)622-6644 **Fax:** (918)622-3401
**Email:** mtio@swbell.net
Xerlan Geiser, Director

**Program(s):** Acupressure; Aromatherapy; CranioSacral Therapy; Massage Therapy; Oriental Medicine; Reflexology; Shiatsu; Sports Massage.

**★ 3976 ★ Oklahoma School of Natural Healing**
1660 E 71st, Ste. 2-O
Tulsa, OK 74136-5191
**Phone:** (918)496-9401 **Fax:** (918)496-4461
Dr. Robert L. Groves, Director

**Program(s):** Acupressure; CranioSacral Therapy; Energy Work; Herbal Medicine; Homeopathy; Massage Therapy; Naturopathic Medicine; Neuromuscular Therapy; Ortho-Bionomy; Polarity Therapy; Qigong; Reflexology; Reiki; Shiatsu; Sports Massage; Traditional Chinese Medicine.

**★ 3977 ★ Praxis College of Health Arts and Sciences**
808 NW 88
Oklahoma City, OK 73114
**Phone:** (405)949-2244 **Fax:** (405)946-7040
Andre F. Fountain, Director

**Program(s):** Acupressure; Acupuncture; Aromatherapy; CranioSacral Therapy; Energy Work; Herbal Medicine; Hydrotherapy; Massage Therapy; Oriental Medicine; Polarity Therapy; Qigong; Reflexology; Shiatsu; Sports Massage; Traditional Chinese Medicine.

### Ontario

**★ 3978 ★ Artemisia Institute for Botanical and Preventive Health Care Education**
PO Box 190
Jackson's Point, ON, Canada L0E 1L0
**Phone:** (905)722-1074
Christine E. DeVai, Contact

**Program(s):** Herbal Medicine.

**★ 3979 ★ British Institute of Homeopathy**
1445 St. Joseph Blvd.
Gloucester, ON, Canada K1C 7K9
**Phone:** (613)830-4759 **Free:** 800-579-4325
**Fax:** (613)830-9174
Patty Smith, Contact

**Program(s):** Animal Therapy; Herbal Medicine; Homeopathy; Midwifery; Naturopathic Medicine; Nutrition.

**★ 3980 ★ Canadian College of Massage and Hydrotherapy, Newmarket**
543 Timothy St.
Newmarket, ON, Canada L3Y 1R1
**Phone:** (905)853-5553 **Fax:** (905)853-5324
Kim Fountaine, Contact

**Program(s):** Acupuncture; Herbal Medicine; Humanistic Counseling; Hydrotherapy; Massage Therapy; Traditional Chinese Medicine.

**★ 3981 ★ Canadian College of Massage and Hydrotherapy, North York**
5160 Yonge St., Ste. 505
North York, ON, Canada M2N 6L7
**Phone:** (416)222-3586 **Fax:** (416)222-9424
Margaret Ward, Contact

**Program(s):** Acupuncture; Herbal Medicine; Humanistic Counseling; Hydrotherapy; Massage Therapy; Traditional Chinese Medicine.

**★ 3982 ★ Canadian College of Naturopathic Medicine**
2300 Yonge St., 18th Flr., Box 2431
Toronto, ON, Canada M4P 1E4
**Phone:** (416)486-8584 **Fax:** (416)484-6821
Catharine Shewell, Contact

**Program(s):** Acupuncture; Bodywork and Manipulation; Clinical Nutrition; Herbal Medicine; Homeopathy; Hydrotherapy; Naturopathic Medicine; Traditional Chinese Medicine.

★ **3983** ★ **Canadian Memorial Chiropractic College**
1900 Bayview Ave.
Toronto, ON, Canada M4G 3E6
**Phone:** (416)482-2340    **Fax:** (416)482-9745
Stefan Pallister, Contact
**Program(s):** Chiropractic.

★ **3984** ★ **D'Arcy Lane Institute, D'AL School of Equine Massage Therapy**
627 Maitland St.
London, ON, Canada N5Y 2V7
**Phone:** (519)673-4420    **Fax:** (519)673-0645
Marnie Byloo, Contact
**Program(s):** Animal Therapy; Equine Massage; Massage Therapy.

★ **3985** ★ **Esther Myers Yoga Studio**
390 Dupont St.
Toronto, ON, Canada M5R 1V9
**Phone:** (416)944-0838    **Fax:** (416)944-9151
Linda Cherney, Contact
**Program(s):** Yoga Teacher Training.

★ **3986** ★ **Homeopathic College of Canada**
280 Eglinton Ave. E
Toronto, ON, Canada M4P 1L4
**Phone:** (416)481-8816    **Fax:** (416)481-4444
Luba Plotkin, Contact
**Program(s):** Homeopathy.

★ **3987** ★ **ICT Kikkawa College**
1678 Bloor St. W
Toronto, ON, Canada M6P 1A9
**Phone:** (416)762-4857    **Fax:** (416)762-5733
**Program(s):** Massage Therapy.

★ **3988** ★ **Institute of Traditional Chinese Medicine**
368 Dupont St.
Toronto, ON, Canada M5R 1V9
**Phone:** (416)925-6752    **Fax:** (416)925-8920
David Lam, Contact
**Program(s):** Acupressure; Acupuncture; Herbal Medicine; Oriental Medicine; Qigong; Traditional Chinese Medicine.

★ **3989** ★ **Michener Institute for Applied Health Sciences**
222 St. Patrick St.
Toronto, ON, Canada M5T 1V4
**Phone:** (416)596-3177    **Fax:** (416)596-3180
Angi Gallupe, Contact
**Program(s):** Acupuncture; Traditional Chinese Medicine.

★ **3990** ★ **Reaching Your Potential**
11181 Yonge St., Room 141
Richmond Hill, ON, Canada L4S 1L2
**Phone:** (905)944-8867    **Fax:** (905)944-8869
Sher Smith, Contact
**Program(s):** CranioSacral Therapy; Polarity Therapy.

★ **3991** ★ **Shiatsu Academy of Tokyo**
320 Danforth Ave., Ste. 206
Toronto, ON, Canada M4K 1N8
**Phone:** (416)466-8780    **Fax:** (416)466-8719
Jan McClory, Contact
**Program(s):** Shiatsu.

★ **3992** ★ **Shiatsu School of Canada, Inc SSC Acupuncture Institute**
547 College St.
Toronto, ON, Canada M6G 1A9
**Phone:** (416)323-1818    **Free:** 800-263-1703
**Fax:** (416)323-1681
Euza Ierullo, Contact
**Program(s):** Acupuncture; Shiatsu.

★ **3993** ★ **Sutherland-Chan School and Teaching Clinic**
330 Dupont St., 4th Flr.
Toronto, ON, Canada M6R 1K4
**Phone:** (416)924-1107    **Fax:** (416)924-9413
Marion Bishop, Contact
**Program(s):** Massage Therapy.

★ **3994** ★ **Toronto School of Homeopathic Medicine**
17 Yorkville Ave., Ste. 200
Toronto, ON, Canada M4W 1L1
**Phone:** (416)966-2350    **Free:** 800-572-6001
**Fax:** (416)966-1724
Shobhna Kapoor, Contact
**Program(s):** Homeopathy.

## Oregon

★ **3995** ★ **American Herbal Institute**
3056 Lancaster Dr. NE
Salem, OR 97305
**Phone:** (503)364-7242
Constance Walker, Director
**Program(s):** Aromatherapy; Herbal Medicine; Hypnotherapy; Nutrition; Reflexology; Traditional Chinese Medicine.

★ **3996** ★ **Ashland Massage Institute**
PO Box 1233
Ashland, OR 97520
**Phone:** (541)482-5134
Beth Hoffman, Director
**Program(s):** Massage Therapy.

★ **3997** ★ **Australasian College of Herbal Studies**
530 1st St., Ste. A
PO Box 57
Lake Oswego, OR 97034
**Phone:** (503)635-6652    **Fax:** (503)636-0706
**Email:** achs@herbed.com
**Website:** http://www.herbed.com
Dorene Petersen, Contact
**Program(s):** Aromatherapy; Flower Essences; Herbal Medicine; Homeobotanical Therapy; Homeopathy; Iridology.

★ **3998** ★ **Birthingway Midwifery Center**
4620 N Maryland Ave.
Portland, OR 97217
**Phone:** (503)282-5729    **Fax:** (503)282-5729
Holly Scholles, Director
**Program(s):** Midwifery.

★ **3999** ★ **Cascade Institute of Massage and Body Therapies**
1250 Charnelton St.
Eugene, OR 97401
**Phone:** (541)687-8101    **Fax:** (541)687-0285
Wendy Doran, Contact
**Program(s):** Acupressure; Energy Work; Massage Therapy; Shiatsu; Swedish Massage.

★ **4000** ★ **East-West College of the Healing Arts**
4531 SE Belmont St.
Portland, OR 97215-1635
**Phone:** (503)231-1500    **Free:** 800-635-9141
**Fax:** (503)232-4087
**Email:** ewcha@aol.com
Richard Martin, Director
**Program(s):** Energy Work; Massage Therapy; Polarity Therapy; Shiatsu; Sports Massage.

★ **4001** ★ **Friends Landing International Centers for Conscious Living**
492 E 13th St., Ste. 101
Eugene, OR 97401
**Phone:** (541)484-6004    **Fax:** (541)741-1705
Whitewind Swan Fisher, Director
**Program(s):** Hypnotherapy.

★ **4002** ★ **International Loving Touch Foundation, Inc.**
PO Box 16374
Portland, OR 97292
**Phone:** (503)253-8482    **Fax:** (503)256-6753
Diana Moore, Director
**Program(s):** Infant Massage.

★ **4003** ★ **National College of Naturopathic Medicine**
049 SW Porter
Portland, OR 97201
**Phone:** (503)499-4343
Clyde Jensen, PhD, Contact
**Program(s):** Herbal Medicine; Homeopathy; Naturopathic Medicine; Oriental Medicine; Traditional Chinese Medicine.

★ **4004** ★ **Northwest Acupressure Institute**
966 Lorane Hwy.
Eugene, OR 97405
**Phone:** (503)345-2220
Kamala Quale, Director
**Program(s):** Acupressure; Jin Shin Do; Oriental Medicine; Qigong.

★ **4005** ★ **Northwest Center for Herbal Studies**
86437 Lorane Hwy.
Eugene, OR 97405
**Phone:** (541)484-6708
**Email:** herbs@ordata.com
Cherie Capps, Director
**Program(s):** Herbal Medicine.

★ **4006** ★ **Oregon Coast School of Massage**
1845 SW Hwy 101, Ste. 2
Lincoln City, OR 97367
**Phone:** (541)994-2728
Margaret Welch, Director
**Program(s):** Deep Tissue Massage; Energy Work; Massage Therapy; Shiatsu; Tai Chi.

★ **4007** ★ **Oregon College of Oriental Medicine**
10525 SE Cherry Blossom Dr.
Portland, OR 97216
**Phone:** (503)253-3443    **Fax:** (503)253-2701
**Email:** lpowell@teleport.com
**Website:** http://www.infinite.org/oregon.acupuncture
Linda Powell, Contact
**Program(s):** Acupressure; Acupuncture; Herbal Medicine; Oriental Medicine; Qigong; Shiatsu; Traditional Chinese Medicine.

★ **4008** ★ **Oregon Health Sciences University School of Nursing**
3181 SW Sam Jackson Park Rd.
Portland, OR 97210
**Phone:** (503)494-3114    **Fax:** (503)494-3878
Carol Howe, Director
**Program(s):** Midwifery.

**★ 4009 ★ Oregon School of Massage**
9500 SW Barbur Blvd., Ste. 100
Portland, OR 97219
**Phone:** (503)244-3420     **Free:** 800-844-3420
**Fax:** (503)244-1815
**Email:** osmlbg@teleport.com
Ray Siderius, Director
**Program(s):** Acupressure; Alexander Technique; CranioSacral Therapy; Energy Work; Massage Therapy; Neuromuscular Therapy; Oriental Medicine; Polarity Therapy; Reflexology; Reiki; Shiatsu; Traditional Chinese Medicine.

**★ 4010 ★ Oregon School of Massage, Salem**
440 Ferry St. NE
Salem, OR 97302-3605
**Phone:** (503)585-8912     **Free:** 800-844-3420
**Fax:** (503)585-0988
Lisa Barck Garofalo, Director
**Program(s):** Alexander Technique; Anatomy and Physiology; Energy Work; Kinesiology; Massage Therapy; Polarity Therapy; Reflexology; Reiki; Shiatsu; Sports Massage; Traditional Chinese Medicine.

**★ 4011 ★ Oregon School of Midwifery**
342 E 12th Ave.
Eugene, OR 97401
**Phone:** (541)338-9778     **Fax:** (541)338-9783
Daphne Singingtree, Director
**Program(s):** Midwifery.

**★ 4012 ★ Polarity Center of Salem**
1940 Breyman NE
Salem, OR 97301
**Phone:** (503)581-6512
Ann Watters, Contact
**Program(s):** Polarity Therapy.

**★ 4013 ★ Professional Course in Veterinary Homeopathy**
1283 Lincoln St.
Eugene, OR 97401
**Phone:** (541)342-7665     **Fax:** (541)344-5356
Susan Pitcairn, Director
**Program(s):** Animal Therapy; Homeopathy.

**★ 4014 ★ Sage Femme Midwifery School**
PO Box 91
O Brien, OR 97534
**Phone:** (541)596-2543     **Free:** 800-247-8422
**Fax:** (541)596-2543
Patricia Downing, Director
**Program(s):** Childbirth Education; Doula; Herbal Medicine; Homeopathy; Midwifery.

**★ 4015 ★ Western States Chiropractic College**
2900 NE 132nd St.
Portland, OR 97230
**Phone:** (503)251-5734     **Fax:** (503)251-5723
William Dallas, Contact
**Program(s):** Chiropractic.

## Pennsylvania

**★ 4016 ★ Academy of Medical Arts and Business**
2301 Academy Dr.
Harrisburg, PA 17112-1012
**Phone:** (717)545-4747     **Fax:** (717)901-9090
Gary Kay, Director
**Program(s):** Acupressure; Aromatherapy; CranioSacral Therapy; Deep Tissue Massage; Hypnotherapy; Massage Therapy; Prenatal Massage; Reflexology; Reiki; Shiatsu; Yoga Teacher Training.

**★ 4017 ★ Academy for Myofascial Trigger Point Therapy**
1312 E Carson St.
Pittsburgh, PA 15203
**Phone:** (412)481-2553     **Fax:** (412)481-3279
Joe Erdos, Director
**Program(s):** Trigger Point Therapy.

**★ 4018 ★ Alternative Conjunction Clinic and School of Massage Therapy**
716 State St.
Lemoyne, PA 17043
**Phone:** (717)737-6001     **Fax:** (717)737-6607
Melodie A. Adinolfi, Director
**Program(s):** Aromatherapy; Chair Massage; Esalen Massage; Massage Therapy; Neuromuscular Therapy; Russian Massage; Swedish Massage.

**★ 4019 ★ Berks Technical Institute**
2205 Ridgewood Dr.
Wyomissing, PA 19610
**Phone:** (610)372-1722     **Fax:** (610)376-4684
Tony Dooley, Director
**Program(s):** Massage Therapy; Swedish Massage.

**★ 4020 ★ Career Training Academy (Monroeville)**
Expo Mart
105 Mall Blvd., Ste. 300W
Monroeville, PA 15146
**Phone:** (412)372-3900     **Free:** 800-491-3470
**Fax:** (412)373-4262
**Email:** jreddy@careerta.com
**Website:** http://www.careerta.com
Maryagnes Luczak, Director
**Program(s):** Acupressure; Aromatherapy; Massage Therapy; Reflexology; Shiatsu; Sports Massage; Swedish Massage.

**★ 4021 ★ Career Training Academy (New Kensington)**
703 5th Ave.
New Kensington, PA 15068-6301
**Phone:** (724)337-1000     **Free:** 800-600-3470
**Fax:** (724)335-7140
John Reddy, Contact
**Program(s):** Acupressure; Aromatherapy; Massage Therapy; Reflexology; Shiatsu; Swedish Massage.

**★ 4022 ★ Center for Human Integration**
8400 Pine Rd.
Philadelphia, PA 19111
**Phone:** (215)742-3505     **Fax:** (215)742-3507
Kathy Schival, Director
**Program(s):** Acupressure; Aromatherapy; CranioSacral Therapy; Energy Work; Herbal Medicine; Hypnotherapy; Massage Therapy; Polarity Therapy; Reflexology; Reiki; Therapeutic Touch; Touch for Health; Zero Balancing.

**★ 4023 ★ Central Pennsylvania School of Massage, Inc.**
336 S Fraser St.
State College, PA 16801
**Phone:** (814)234-4900     **Fax:** (814)234-0440
Tom Broeren, Director
**Program(s):** Acupressure; Aromatherapy; Ayurvedic Medicine; Deep Tissue Massage; Energy Work; Geriatric Massage; Infant Massage; Massage Therapy; Oriental Medicine; Prenatal Massage; Qigong; Reflexology; Reiki; Shiatsu; Sports Massage; Traditional Chinese Medicine; Yoga Teacher Training.

**★ 4024 ★ East-West School of Massage Therapy**
504 Park Rd. N
Wyomissing, PA 19610
**Phone:** (610)375-7520     **Fax:** (610)375-7554
Elizabeth Brubaker, Director
**Program(s):** Acupressure; Aromatherapy; Energy Work; Massage Therapy; Polarity Therapy; Reflexology; Reiki; Shiatsu; Sports Massage.

**★ 4025 ★ Endless Mountain School of Shiatsu**
RR1, Box 1741
Factoryville, PA 18419
**Phone:** (570)942-4481     **Fax:** (570)942-6139
Samuel R. Kupetsky, Director
**Program(s):** Acupressure; Energy Work; Herbal Medicine; Oriental Medicine; Shiatsu; Traditional Chinese Medicine; Visualization.

**★ 4026 ★ Esthetic Training Institute**
702 Fountain Ave.
Lancaster, PA 17601
**Free:** 800-446-2260     **Fax:** (610)292-0299
Rose Ann Acuazzo-Linkens, Contact
**Program(s):** Aromatherapy; Massage Therapy; Reflexology; Reiki.

**★ 4027 ★ Feldenkrais Professional Training Programs**
59 Pebble Woods
Doylestown, PA 18901
**Phone:** (215)230-9208     **Fax:** (215)230-9086
David Zemach-Bersin, Director
**Program(s):** Feldenkrais.

**★ 4028 ★ Health Options Institute**
1410 Main St.
Northampton, PA 18067
**Phone:** (610)261-0880     **Fax:** (610)261-2964
Elizabeth Bieber, Director
**Program(s):** Acupressure; Aromatherapy; Deep Muscle Massage; Herbal Medicine; Massage Therapy; Neuromuscular Therapy; Reflexology; Reiki; Shiatsu.

**★ 4029 ★ Himalayan Institute**
RR 1, Box 400
Honesdale, PA 18431
**Phone:** (570)253-5551     **Free:** 800-822-4547
**Fax:** (570)253-9078
**Program(s):** Meditation; Yoga Teacher Training.

**★ 4030 ★ Institute of Midwifery, Women, and Health**
222 Hayward Hall, School House Lane and Henry Ave.
Philadelphia, PA 19144
**Phone:** (215)843-5775     **Fax:** (215)951-2526
Kate Siegrist, Director
**Program(s):** Midwifery.

**★ 4031 ★ International School of Shiatsu**
10 S Clinton St., Ste. 300
Doylestown, PA 18901
**Phone:** (215)340-9918     **Fax:** (215)340-9181
Megan Wilson, Director
**Program(s):** Acupressure; Shiatsu.

**★ 4032 ★ Lancaster School of Massage**
317 N Queen St.
Lancaster, PA 17603
**Phone:** (717)293-9698
Winona F. Bontrager, Director
**Program(s):** Connective Tissue Massage; CranioSacral Therapy; Massage Therapy; Neuromuscular Therapy; Polarity Therapy; Reflexology; Sports Massage; Swedish Massage.

**★ 4033 ★ Lehigh Valley Healing Arts Academy**
5412 Shimerville Rd.
Emmaus, PA 18049
**Phone:** (610)965-6165 **Fax:** (610)965-6165
Bonita A. Cassel-Beckwith, Director

**Program(s):** Acupressure; Alexander Technique; Aromatherapy; Ayurvedic Medicine; CranioSacral Therapy; Energy Work; Feldenkrais; Herbal Medicine; Homeopathy; Massage Therapy; Meditation; Polarity Therapy; Reflexology; Reiki; Shiatsu; Sports Massage; Therapeutic Touch; Traditional Chinese Medicine; Trager; Yoga.

**★ 4034 ★ Massage Arts and Sciences Center of Philadelphia**
1515 Locust St., 2nd Fl.
Philadelphia, PA 19102
**Phone:** (215)985-0674 **Fax:** (215)985-0175
Rosemarie Glaser, Director

**Program(s):** Massage Therapy; Reiki; Shiatsu; Sports Massage.

**★ 4035 ★ Meridian Shiatsu Institute**
998 Old Eagle School Rd., Ste. 1212
Wayne, PA 19087
**Phone:** (610)293-4030 **Fax:** (610)971-9860
**Email:** caroleepf@aol.com
Carolee Parker, Director

**Program(s):** Acupressure; Qigong; Reflexology; Reiki; Shiatsu; Traditional Chinese Medicine.

**★ 4036 ★ Mount Nittany Institute of Natural Health**
301 Shiloh Rd.
State College, PA 16801
**Phone:** (814)238-1121 **Fax:** (814)238-8145
Jennifer Welch, Director

**Program(s):** Acupressure; Anatomy and Physiology; Aromatherapy; Connective Tissue Massage; Energy Work; Herbal Medicine; Holistic Health; Massage Therapy; Neuromuscular Therapy; Polarity Therapy; Reflexology; Shiatsu; Sports Massage; Swedish Massage; Tai Chi; Yoga.

**★ 4037 ★ Myofascial Release Seminars**
222 W Lancaster Ave.
Paoli, PA 19301
**Free:** 800-327-2425 **Fax:** (610)644-1662
**Email:** fascia@erols.com
**Website:** http://www.vll.com/mfr/
Sandra Levengood, Director

**Program(s):** Myofascial Release.

**★ 4038 ★ Northeastern School of Medical Massage, Inc.**
2525 W Main, 2nd Flr.
Norristown, PA 19403
**Phone:** (610)631-5188
Constance J. Perry, Director

**Program(s):** Acupressure; Aromatherapy; Infant Massage; Massage Therapy; Medical Massage; Neuromuscular Therapy; Pregnancy Massage; Reflexology; Sports Massage; Swedish Massage.

**★ 4039 ★ Pennsylvania Institute of Massage Therapy**
93 SW End Blvd., Ste. 102
Quakertown, PA 18951-1150
**Phone:** (215)538-5339 **Fax:** (215)538-8896
Robert Tosh, Contact

**Program(s):** Animal Therapy; CPR/First Aid; Massage Therapy; Reflexology; Shiatsu; Tai Chi.

**★ 4040 ★ Pennsylvania School of Muscle Therapy, Ltd.**
994C Old Eagle School Rd., Ste. 1005
Wayne, PA 19087
**Phone:** (610)687-0888 **Fax:** (610)687-4726
**Email:** psmt@psmt.com
**Website:** http://www.psmt.com
MaryJo Myers, Contact

**Program(s):** Aromatherapy; Deep Muscle Massage; Massage Therapy; Qigong; Reflexology; Shiatsu; Sports Massage; Swedish Massage; Traditional Chinese Medicine.

**★ 4041 ★ Pittsburgh School of Massage Therapy**
10989 Frankstown Rd.
Pittsburgh, PA 15235
**Free:** 800-860-1114 **Fax:** (412)241-4933
**Email:** pghschmass@aol.com
Robert Jantsch, Director

**Program(s):** Acupressure; Alexander Technique; Aromatherapy; Energy Work; Massage Therapy; Neuromuscular Therapy; Reflexology; Shiatsu; Sports Massage; Swedish Massage.

**★ 4042 ★ Professional School of Massage**
131 E Maple Ave.
Langhorne, PA 19047
**Phone:** (215)750-0700
David Scott, Director

**Program(s):** Acupressure; Herbal Medicine; Massage Therapy; Polarity Therapy; Qigong; Reflexology; Reiki; Shiatsu.

**★ 4043 ★ A Rose Therapeutics**
352 E 6th Ave.
Conshohocken, PA 19428
**Phone:** (610)834-8140
Aura Rose, Director

**Program(s):** Acupressure; CranioSacral Therapy; Energy Work; Feldenkrais; Herbal Medicine; Hypnotherapy; Massage Therapy; Neuromuscular Therapy; Reflexology; Reiki; Shiatsu; Sports Massage; Swedish Massage; Yoga.

**★ 4044 ★ School of Body Therapies**
931 Langhorne-Yardley Rd.
Langhorne, PA 19047-1368
**Phone:** (215)752-7666 **Fax:** (215)752-1909
Lisa Barck Garofalo, Director

**Program(s):** Deep Muscle Massage; Massage Therapy; Thai Massage.

**★ 4045 ★ Somatic Institute, Pittsburgh**
8600 W Barkhurst Dr.
Pittsburgh, PA 15237
**Phone:** (412)366-5580 **Fax:** (412)367-1029
Kay Miller, Director

**Program(s):** Alexander Technique; Core Somatics; Feldenkrais; Somatic Education.

**★ 4046 ★ Unergi School of Holistic Therapy**
PO Box 335
Point Pleasant, PA 18950
**Phone:** (215)297-8006 **Fax:** (215)297-8199
Ute Arnold, Director

**Program(s):** Alexander Technique; Energy Work; Feldenkrais; Hypnotherapy; Unergi Integrated Therapy.

**★ 4047 ★ University of Pennsylvania School of Nursing**
420 Guardian Dr.
Philadelphia, PA 19104-6096
**Phone:** (215)898-4335
William McCool, Director

**Program(s):** Midwifery.

**★ 4048 ★ Valley Forge Institute of Muscle Therapy**
808 Valley Forge Rd.
Phoenixville, PA 19460
**Phone:** (610)935-3554
Thomas V. O'Ancona, Director

**Program(s):** Chair Massage; Neuromuscular Therapy; Polarity Therapy; Reflexology; Reiki; Sports Massage; Swedish Massage.

### Puerto Rico

**★ 4049 ★ University of Puerto Rico, Medical Sciences Campus**
PO Box 365067
San Juan, PR 00936
**Phone:** (787)759-6546 **Fax:** (787)759-6719
Irene G. dela Torre, Director

**Program(s):** Midwifery.

### Quebec

**★ 4050 ★ Canadian Academy of Homeopathy**
1173 Boul Mont Royal
Outremont, QC, Canada H2V 2H6
**Phone:** (514)279-6629 **Fax:** (514)279-0111
Francine Gauthier, Contact

**Program(s):** Homeopathy.

**★ 4051 ★ Centre Psycho-Corporel, Inc.**
675 Marguerite Bourgeoys
Quebec, QC, Canada G1S 3V8
**Phone:** (418)687-1165 **Fax:** (418)687-1166
Aline Dumas, Contact

**Program(s):** Acupressure; Kinesiology; Manual Lymph Drainage; Massage Therapy; Qigong; Reflexology; Shiatsu; Sports Massage; Swedish Massage.

**★ 4052 ★ Health Training Group**
3789 Hampton Ave.
Montreal, QC, Canada H4A 2K7
**Phone:** (514)485-6373
Howard Kiewe, Contact

**Program(s):** Polarity Therapy.

**★ 4053 ★ Polarity Associates of Montreal**
5535 Beaucort, Ste. 10
Montreal, QC, Canada H3W 2T7
**Phone:** (514)739-4673 **Fax:** (514)440-0251
Andrea Axt, Contact

**Program(s):** CranioSacral Therapy; Polarity Therapy.

**★ 4054 ★ Psychovisual Therapy Training**
7306 Sherbrooke W
Montreal, QC, Canada H4B 1R7
**Phone:** (514)489-6733 **Fax:** (514)485-3828
Bryan M. Knight, Contact

**Program(s):** Hypnotherapy; Psychovisual Therapy.

### Rhode Island

**★ 4055 ★ University of Rhode Island College of Nursing**
2 Heathman Rd.
Kingston, RI 02881
**Phone:** (401)874-5328 **Fax:** (401)874-2061
Holly Kennedy, Director

**Program(s):** Midwifery.

### Saskatchewan

**★ 4056 ★ Professional Institute of Massage Therapy, Saskatoon**
485 1st Ave. N
Saskatoon, SK, Canada S7K 1X5
**Phone:** (306)955-5833 **Fax:** (306)955-5864
Tracy Bazlak, Contact

Program(s): Massage Therapy.

## South Carolina

**★ 4057 ★ Charleston School of Massage, Inc.**
778 Folly Rd., Ste. 3
Charleston, SC 29412
**Phone:** (843)762-7727          **Fax:** (843)762-1392
Mark Hendler, Director

Program(s): Acupressure; Aromatherapy; Ayurvedic Medicine; Deep Tissue Massage; Energy Work; Herbal Medicine; Massage Therapy; Reflexology; Reiki; Shiatsu; Spa Therapies.

**★ 4058 ★ Dovestar Institute**
4C Northridge Dr.
Hilton Head Island, SC 29928
**Phone:** (803)342-3361          **Free:** 888-222-5603
**Fax:** (803)342-3639
Kamala Renner, Director

Program(s): Acupressure; Breathwork; Colon Hydrotherapy; Energy Work; Kriya Massage; Hypnotherapy; Massage Therapy; Qigong; Reflexology; Reiki; Shiatsu; Yoga Teacher Training.

**★ 4059 ★ Horry Georgetown Technical College**
743 Hemlock Ave.
Myrtle Beach, SC 29577
**Phone:** (843)477-0808          **Fax:** (843)477-0775
Lisa Aglietti, Director

Program(s): Massage Therapy.

**★ 4060 ★ Massage School of MTA, Inc.**
1901 Laurens Rd., Ste. H
Greenville, SC 29607
**Phone:** (864)232-9001
Kenn Elrod, Director

Program(s): Acupressure; Aromatherapy; CranioSacral Therapy; Deep Tissue Massage; Energy Work; Massage Therapy; Polarity Therapy; Reflexology; Reiki; Shiatsu.

**★ 4061 ★ Medical University of South Carolina**
**College of Nursing**
99 Jonathon Lucas St.
Charleston, SC 29403
**Phone:** (843)792-2051
Deborah Williamsom, Director

Program(s): Midwifery.

**★ 4062 ★ Sherman College of Straight Chiropractic**
2020 Springfield Rd.
Boiling Springs, SC 29316
**Phone:** (864)578-8770          **Fax:** (864)599-7145
Susan S. Newlin, Director

Program(s): Chiropractic.

**★ 4063 ★ Southeastern School of Neuromuscular and Massage Therapy, Inc.**
7000 N Pine St., Ste. 2B Pinewood Mall
Spartanburg, SC 29303
**Phone:** (864)591-1134          **Fax:** (864)582-7805
Janice Schuelke, Director

Program(s): Aromatherapy; Massage Therapy; Myofascial Release; Neuromuscular Therapy; Swedish Massage.

## South Dakota

**★ 4064 ★ Carrie's Kadesh and School of Massage**
112 E 3rd Ave.
Mitchell, SD 57301
**Phone:** (605)996-3916
Carrie Badker, Director

Program(s): Acupressure; Aromatherapy; Massage Therapy; Polarity Therapy; Reflexology; Sports Massage.

**★ 4065 ★ Scientific Massage Institute**
1523 1/2 Deadwood Ave.
Rapid City, SD 57702
**Phone:** (605)341-5402          **Fax:** (605)342-0554
Sandy Feist, Director

Program(s): Acupressure; Chair Massage; Infant Massage; Massage Therapy; Reflexology.

**★ 4066 ★ South Dakota School of Massage Therapy**
902 W 22nd St.
Sioux Falls, SD 57105
**Phone:** (605)334-4422          **Fax:** (605)334-4422
Robin Jensen, Director

Program(s): Acupressure; Anatomy and Physiology; Aromatherapy; Deep Tissue Massage; Hydrotherapy; Kinesiology; Massage Therapy; Qigong; Rebirthing; Reflexology; Shiatsu; Sports Massage; Swedish Massage; Yoga.

**★ 4067 ★ Stress Management Services, Inc.**
**Sioux Falls School of Massage Therapy**
317 S Cleveland Ave.
Sioux Falls, SD 57103
**Phone:** (605)330-0175
Kristie R. Knudtson, Director

Program(s): Massage Therapy.

## Tennessee

**★ 4068 ★ American Academy of Medical Hypnoanalysts**
5628 Murray Rd., Ste. 4
Memphis, TN 38119-3876
**Free:** 800-344-9766          **Fax:** (901)683-1224
David Leistikow, Director

Program(s): Hypnotherapy.

**★ 4069 ★ Cumberland Institute for Wellness Education**
500 Wilson Pike Circle, Ste. 121
PO Box 1527
Brentwood, TN 37027
**Phone:** (615)370-9794          **Fax:** (615)370-5869
Chad Porter, Director

Program(s): Acupressure; Aromatherapy; CranioSacral Therapy; Lymphatic Massage; Massage Therapy; Sports Massage.

**★ 4070 ★ Institute of Therapeutic Massage and Movement**
1161 Murfreesboro Rd., Ste. 405
Nashville, TN 37217
**Phone:** (615)360-8554
Angela Wood, Director

Program(s): Deep Tissue Massage; Massage Therapy.

**★ 4071 ★ Massage Institute of Memphis**
3445 Poplar, Ste. 4
Memphis, TN 38111
**Phone:** (901)324-4411          **Fax:** (901)324-4470
Karen E. Craig, Director

Program(s): Energy Work; Healing Touch; Massage Therapy; Reflexology; Sports Massage; Trigger Point Therapy.

**★ 4072 ★ Middle Tennessee Institute of Therapeutic Massage**
394 W Main St., Ste. A-15
Hendersonville, TN 37075
**Phone:** (615)826-9500          **Fax:** (615)826-9527
Shannon Dickson, Director

Program(s): Aromatherapy; CranioSacral Therapy; Massage Therapy; Neuromuscular Therapy; Polarity Therapy; Reflexology; Shiatsu; Sports Massage.

**★ 4073 ★ Natural Health Institute**
209 10th Ave. S, Ste. 212
Nashville, TN 37203
**Phone:** (615)242-6811          **Fax:** (615)242-6288
Angela Schlitt, Director

Program(s): Acupressure; Ayurvedic Medicine; Feldenkrais; Herbal Medicine; Hypnotherapy; Massage Therapy; Polarity Therapy; Reflexology; Reiki; Somatic Education.

**★ 4074 ★ Tennessee Institute of Healing Arts**
5779 Brainerd Rd.
Chattanooga, TN 37411
**Phone:** (423)892-9882          **Free:** 800-735-1910
**Fax:** (423)892-5006
**Email:** tiha@aol.com
Alan Jordan, Director

Program(s): Massage Therapy; Neuromuscular Therapy.

**★ 4075 ★ Tennessee School of Massage**
4726 Poplar, Ste. 4
Memphis, TN 38117
**Phone:** (901)767-8484
**Email:** relax@touchofhealth.com
**Website:** http://www.touchofhealth.com
Cissie Pryor, Director

Program(s): Acupressure; Aromatherapy; Hypnotherapy; Massage Therapy; Polarity Therapy; Reflexology; Shiatsu; Spa Therapies; Swedish Massage.

**★ 4076 ★ Vanderbilt University**
**School of Nursing**
102 Godchaux Hall
Nashville, TN 37240-0008
**Phone:** (615)322-3800
Barbara Petersen, Director

Program(s): Midwifery.

## Texas

**★ 4077 ★ Academy of Oriental Medicine - Austin**
2700 W Anderson Ln., Ste. 117
Austin, TX 78757
**Phone:** (512)454-1188          **Fax:** (512)454-7001
**Email:** info@aoma.edu
**Website:** http://www.aoma.edu
Stuart Watts, Director

Program(s): Acupressure; Acupuncture; Herbal Medicine; Jin Shin Do; Oriental Medicine; Qigong; Shiatsu; Tai Chi; Traditional Chinese Medicine, Tui Na.

**★ 4078 ★ American College of Acupuncture and Oriental Medicine**
9100 Park W Dr.
Houston, TX 77063
**Phone:** (713)780-9777          **Fax:** (713)781-5781
**Email:** 102657.1730@compuserve.com
**Website:** http://www.acaom.edu
Minmay Liang, Director

Program(s): Acupuncture; Herbal Medicine; Homeopathy; Oriental Medicine; Traditional Chinese Medicine.

**★ 4079 ★ Anne King's Hypnosis TRaining**
109 Smokey River N
Boerne, TX 78006
**Phone:** (830)537-5411 **Fax:** (830)537-5404
Anne King, Contact
**Program(s):** Hypnotherapy.

**★ 4080 ★ Asten Center of Natural Therapeutics**
797 N Grove Rd., Ste. 101
Richardson, TX 75081
**Phone:** (972)669-3245 **Fax:** (972)669-1191
Jill Townsend, Contact
**Program(s):** Massage Therapy; Polarity Therapy; Reflexology; Sports Massage; Swedish Massage; Trigger Point Therapy.

**★ 4081 ★ Austin School of Massage Therapy**
2600 W Stassney
Austin, TX 78745
**Phone:** (512)462-3005 **Free:** 800-276-2768
**Fax:** (512)462-3265
Bob Brock, Director
**Program(s):** Holistic Health; Massage Therapy; Neuromuscular Therapy; Polarity Therapy; Reflexology; Shiatsu.

**★ 4082 ★ Baylor College of Medicine**
6550 Fannin, Ste. 901
Houston, TX 77030
**Phone:** (713)798-7594 **Fax:** (713)798-3579
Betty Carter, Director
**Program(s):** Midwifery.

**★ 4083 ★ Beijing School of Acupuncture and Oriental Medicine**
4109 Cagle Dr., Ste. F
Fort Worth, TX 76107
**Phone:** (817)284-3037 **Fax:** (817)284-1047
Dr. Hadi Kareem, Contact
**Program(s):** Acupuncture; Oriental Medicine.

**★ 4084 ★ El Paso Community College**
100 W Rio Grande
El Paso, TX 79902
**Phone:** (915)831-4116 **Fax:** (915)831-4131
Marta de la Fuente, Director
**Program(s):** Massage Therapy; Reflexology.

**★ 4085 ★ El Paso School of Massage**
661 S Mesa Hills Dr., Ste. 100
El Paso, TX 79912
**Phone:** (915)833-2935 **Fax:** (915)833-3094
Hilda L. Chavez, Director
**Program(s):** Hydrotherapy; Massage Therapy; Neuromuscular Therapy; Swedish Massage.

**★ 4086 ★ European Massage Therapy Institute**
7220 Louis Pasteur, Ste. 140
San Antonio, TX 78229
**Phone:** (210)615-8207 **Fax:** (210)614-3732
Rosario Perez Garza, Director
**Program(s):** Aromatherapy; Manual Lymph Drainage; Massage Therapy; Postural Analysis; Reflexology.

**★ 4087 ★ Fort Worth School of Massage**
2929 Cleburne Rd.
Fort Worth, TX 76110
**Phone:** (817)923-9944 **Fax:** (817)923-9944
Joetta Payne, Director
**Program(s):** CranioSacral Therapy Massage Therapy; Reflexology; Reiki.

**★ 4088 ★ Giving Tree Cottage**
1808 S St.
Nacogdoches, TX 75964
**Phone:** (409)560-6299 **Fax:** (409)569-9400
Jo Harbison, Director
**Program(s):** Massage Therapy.

**★ 4089 ★ Greater Beaumont School of Massage**
229 Dowlen Rd., Ste. 15A
Beaumont, TX 77706
**Phone:** (409)866-8661 **Fax:** (409)866-4371
Jennifer Smith, Director
**Program(s):** Massage Therapy.

**★ 4090 ★ Hands On Therapy School of Massage**
1101 E 5th St.
Tyler, TX 75701
**Phone:** (903)535-7733 **Fax:** (903)535-7799
Jeannine Martin, Director
**Program(s):** Aromatherapy; Massage Therapy; Reflexology; Shiatsu; Swedish Massage; Deep Tissue Massage.

**★ 4091 ★ Healing Arts Institute, Lubbock**
5601 Aberdeen, Ste. G
Lubbock, TX 79414
**Phone:** (806)797-0034
Kay Nash, Director
**Program(s):** Aromatherapy; Deep Tissue Massage; Energy Work; Hydrotherapy; Massage Therapy; Polarity Therapy; Reflexology; Shiatsu.

**★ 4092 ★ Heartsong Hypnotherapy Training Center**
4314 W Lovers Ln.
PO Box 7972
Dallas, TX 75209
**Phone:** (214)358-3633 **Fax:** (214)352-1338
Bette Epstein, Director
**Program(s):** Aromatherapy; Biofeedback; Energy Work; Hypnotherapy; Reiki.

**★ 4093 ★ Hypnosis Institute of Houston**
13700 Veterans Memorial, Ste. 230
Houston, TX 77014
**Phone:** (281)587-1055 **Fax:** (281)379-3153
Gerald L. Schoonover, Director
**Program(s):** Hypnotherapy.

**★ 4094 ★ Institute of Natural Healing Sciences, Inc.**
4100 Felps Dr., Ste. E
Colleyville, TX 76034
**Phone:** (817)498-0716 **Free:** 800-448-4954
**Fax:** (817)281-1414
**Email:** hmmj@nkn.net
**Website:** http://www.body-mind-spirit.com
Hollis M. Morrow, Contact
**Program(s):** Acupressure; Chair Massage; CranioSacral Therapy; Massage Therapy; Polarity Therapy; Reflexology; Shiatsu; Sports Massage.

**★ 4095 ★ Lauterstein-Conway Massage School**
4701-B Burnet Rd.
Austin, TX 78756
**Phone:** (512)374-9222 **Free:** 800-474-0852
**Fax:** (512)374-9812
John Conway, Director
**Program(s):** Acupressure; CranioSacral Therapy; Energy Work; Massage Therapy; Reflexology; Shiatsu; Sports Massage; Swedish Massage; Zero Balancing.

**★ 4096 ★ Massage Therapy Clinic and School**
2045 Space Park Dr., Ste. 200
Houston, TX 77058
**Phone:** (281)333-0400 **Fax:** (281)333-9010
Charline L. Utley, Director
**Program(s):** Deep Tissue Massage; Energy Work; Massage Therapy; Polarity Therapy; Reflexology; Shiatsu; Swedish Massage.

**★ 4097 ★ Maternidad La Luz, the Birth Place**
1308 Magoffin
El Paso, TX 79901
**Phone:** (915)532-5895 **Fax:** (915)532-7127
Deborah Kalley, Director
**Program(s):** Midwifery.

**★ 4098 ★ Midland College Health Sciences Continuing Education**
3600 N Garfield
Midland, TX 79705
**Phone:** (915)685-6440
Norma Chavez, Director
**Program(s):** Massage Therapy.

**★ 4099 ★ Mind Body Naturopathic and Holistic Health Institute**
10911 W Ave.
San Antonio, TX 78213
**Phone:** (210)308-8888 **Fax:** (210)349-5679
Jeri C. Tiller, Contact
**Program(s):** Aromatherapy; Colon Hydrotherapy; Massage Therapy; Reflexology; Reiki; Yoga.

**★ 4100 ★ MRC School of Massage**
2990 Richmond, Ste. 142
Houston, TX 77098
**Phone:** (713)522-1423 **Fax:** (713)522-1446
Robert I. Garza, Director
**Program(s):** Massage Therapy; Swedish Massage.

**★ 4101 ★ Neuromuscular Concepts School of Massage**
8607 Wurzbach Rd., Bldg. Q, Ste. 101
San Antonio, TX 78240
**Phone:** (210)558-3148 **Fax:** (210)558-3114
Paul Frizzell, Director
**Program(s):** Acupressure; Aromatherapy; Ayurvedic Medicine; CranioSacral Therapy; Energy Work; Feldenkrais; Herbal Medicine; Homeopathy; Massage Therapy; Neuromuscular Therapy; Oriental Medicine; Polarity Therapy; Qigong; Reflexology; Reiki; Shiatsu; Sports Massage; Traditional Chinese Medicine; Yoga Teacher Training.

**★ 4102 ★ Parker College of Chiropractic**
2500 Walnut Hill Ln.
Dallas, TX 75229
**Phone:** (214)438-6932 **Free:** 800-438-6932
**Fax:** (214)357-3620
**Website:** http://www.parkercc.edu
Reba Sexton, Contact
**Program(s):** Chiropractic.

**★ 4103 ★ Parkland School of Nurse-Midwifery**
5201 Harry Hines Blvd., MS 6107A
Dallas, TX 75235
**Phone:** (214)590-2580
Mary C. Brucker, Director
**Program(s):** Midwifery.

**★ 4104 ★ PATH Foundation**
1006 Burning Tree
Kingwood, TX 77339

**Phone:** (281)358-3700        **Fax:** (281)359-5700
Ed R. Martin, PhD, Director
**Program(s):** Hypnotherapy.


★ 4105 ★ **Relax Station School of Massage Therapy**
1409 Kingwood Dr.
Kingwood, TX 77339
**Phone:** (281)358-0600        **Fax:** (281)358-4089
Allen Boxman, Director
**Program(s):** Acupressure; Aromatherapy; CranioSacral Therapy; Massage Therapy; Neuromuscular Therapy; Sports Massage.


★ 4106 ★ **Saint Phillip's College**
1801 Martin Luther King Blvd.
San Antonio, TX 78203
**Phone:** (210)531-4770        **Fax:** (210)531-4774
Barbara Witte-Howell, Director
**Program(s):** Massage Therapy.


★ 4107 ★ **School of Natural Therapy**
4309 N 10th, Stes. A, B, C
McAllen, TX 78504
**Phone:** (956)630-0928        **Fax:** (956)630-6103
Lorena Granados, Director
**Program(s):** Deep Tissue Massage; Massage Therapy; Reflexology.


★ 4108 ★ **South Texas Educational Center for Classical Homeopathy**
13526 George Rd., Ste. 101
San Antonio, TX 78230-3002
**Phone:** (210)493-0561        **Fax:** (210)492-8013
Sandra J. Perko, Director
**Program(s):** Clinical Nutrition; Herbal Medicine; Homeopathy.


★ 4109 ★ **Sterling Health Center**
15070 Beltwood Pkwy.
Dallas, TX 75244
**Phone:** (972)991-9293        **Fax:** (972)991-3292
Dianna Lee, Director
**Program(s):** Anatomy and Physiology; Aromatherapy; Chair Massage; Deep Tissue Massage; Manual Lymph Drainage; Massage Therapy; Myofascial Release; Pregnancy Massage; Reflexology; Shiatsu; Sports Massage; Trigger Point Therapy.


★ 4110 ★ **Texas Chiropractic College**
5912 Spencer Hwy.
Pasadena, TX 77505-1699
**Phone:** (281)487-1170        **Free:** 800-468-6839
**Fax:** (281)991-4871
**Email:** gabbygreen@ol.com
S.M. Elliott, Contact
**Program(s):** Chiropractic.


★ 4111 ★ **Texas College of Oriental Medicine, Inc.**
3917 Booth Calloway Rd.
Richland Hills, TX 76118
**Phone:** (817)595-2339        **Fax:** (817)284-1047
Hadi Kareem, Director
**Program(s):** Acupressure; Herbal Medicine; Oriental Medicine; Traditional Chinese Medicine.


★ 4112 ★ **Texas Healing Arts Institute, LLC, and School of Massage**
2704 Rio Grande, Ste. 11
Austin, TX 78705
**Phone:** (512)236-8424        **Fax:** (512)236-1040
Jo Bunny, Director
**Program(s):** CranioSacral Therapy; Deep Tissue Massage; Hydrotherapy; Massage Therapy; Myofascial Release; Reflexology; Shiatsu.


★ 4113 ★ **Texas Institute of Traditional Chinese Medicine**
4005 Manchaca Rd., Ste. 102
Austin, TX 78704
**Phone:** (512)444-8082        **Free:** 800-252-5088
**Fax:** (512)444-6345
**Email:** texastcm@texastcm.edu
**Website:** http://www.texastcm.edu
Kermit Heimann, Director
**Program(s):** Acupuncture; Herbal Medicine; Oriental Medicine; Qigong; Traditional Chinese Medicine.


★ 4114 ★ **Therapeutic Body Concepts**
6162 Wurzbach Rd.
San Antonio, TX 78238
**Phone:** (210)684-6563        **Fax:** (210)680-2782
Leon Gosset, Contact
**Program(s):** Massage Therapy.


★ 4115 ★ **University of North Texas**
PO Box 311337
Denton, TX 76203-1337
**Phone:** (940)565-2910        **Fax:** (940)565-2905
Michael Attekruse, Director
**Program(s):** Biofeedback; Mental Health Counseling.


★ 4116 ★ **University of Texas, El Paso/Texas Tech University**
4800 Alberta Ave.
El Paso, TX 79905
**Phone:** (915)545-6490
Carolyn Simmons, Director
**Program(s):** Midwifery.


★ 4117 ★ **University of Texas, Galveston School of Nursing**
1100 Mechanic
Galveston, TX 77555-1029
**Phone:** (409)772-8347        **Fax:** (409)772-3770
JoAnn Mahoney, Director
**Program(s):** Midwifery.


★ 4118 ★ **Wellness Skills, Inc., Dallas**
6102 E Mockingbird Ln., Ste. 401
Dallas, TX 75214-2620
**Phone:** (214)828-4000        **Fax:** (214)828-0065
Richard Nottingham, Director
**Program(s):** Aromatherapy; Massage Therapy; Polarity Therapy; Relexology; Shiatsu; Trigger Point Therapy.


★ 4119 ★ **Wellness Skills, Inc., Fort Worth**
6301 Airport Fwy., Ste. 200
Fort Worth, TX 76117-5360
**Phone:** (817)838-3800        **Fax:** (817)838-2933
Kelli Eager, Director
**Program(s):** Aromatherapy; Massage Therapy; Polarity Therapy; Reflexology; Shiatsu; Sports Massage; Trigger Point Therapy.


★ 4120 ★ **Winters School Inc.**
4625 SW Fwy., Ste. 142
Houston, TX 77027
**Phone:** (713)626-2200        **Fax:** (713)626-2230
Cari Denson West, Director
**Program(s):** Deep Tissue Massage; Massage Therapy; Polarity Therapy; Reflexology; Shiatsu.


★ 4121 ★ **Yoga Institute and Bookshop**
3830 Villanova St.
Houston, TX 77002-3640
**Free:** 800-524-6674
Lex Gillan, Director
**Program(s):** Yoga Teacher Training.


## Utah

★ 4122 ★ **Myotherapy College of Utah**
1174 E 2700 S, Ste. 19
Salt Lake City, UT 84106
**Phone:** (801)484-7624        **Fax:** (801)484-1928
Sheriden Black, Director
**Program(s):** Aromatherapy; CranioSacral Therapy; Deep Tissue Massage; Energy Work; Homeopathy; Massage Therapy; Polarity Therapy; Reflexology; Reiki; Shiatsu.


★ 4123 ★ **Ogden Institute of Massage Therapy**
3500 Harrison Blvd.
Ogden, UT 84403
**Phone:** (801)627-8227        **Fax:** (801)627-2228
Craig S. Anderson, Director
**Program(s):** CranioSacral Therapy; Deep Tissue Massage; Massage Therapy; Shiatsu.


★ 4124 ★ **School of Natural Healing**
25 W 200 S
PO Box 412
Springville, UT 84663
**Free:** 800-372-8255        **Fax:** (801)489-8341
**Email:** snh@qi3.com
**Website:** http://www.homestar.net/school
David W. Christopher, Director
**Program(s):** Herbal Medicine.


★ 4125 ★ **Sensory Development Institute**
1871 W Canyon View Dr.
Saint George, UT 84770
**Phone:** (435)652-9003        **Fax:** (435)652-8949
Pam Shelline, Director
**Program(s):** Aromatherapy; Energy Work; Massage Therapy; Oriental Medicine; Reflexology; Shiatsu; Spa Therapies.


★ 4126 ★ **University of Utah College of Nursing**
10 S 2000 E Front
Salt Lake City, UT 84112-5880
**Phone:** (801)581-8274        **Fax:** (801)581-4642
Marilyn Stewart, Director
**Program(s):** Midwifery.


★ 4127 ★ **Utah College of Massage Therapy**
25 S 300 E
Salt Lake City, UT 84111
**Free:** 800-617-3302        **Fax:** (801)521-3339
**Email:** info@ucmt.com
**Website:** http://www.ucmt.com
Norman Cohn, Director
**Program(s):** Acupressure; CranioSacral Therapy; Deep Tissue Massage; Feldenkrais; Injury Massage; Infant Massage; Massage Therapy; Qigong; Reflexology; Shiatsu; Russian Massage; Touch for Health; Trigger Point Therapy.


★ 4128 ★ **Utah College of Massage Therapy, Utah Valley Campus**
135 S State St., Ste. 12
Lindon, UT 84042
**Phone:** (801)796-0300        **Fax:** (801)796-0309
Karyn Grant, Director
**Program(s):** Acupressure; CranioSacral Therapy; Energy Work; Feldenkrais; Massage Therapy; Neuromuscular Therapy; Reflexology; Shiatsu; Sports Massage.


★ 4129 ★ **Utah College of Midwifery**
230 W 170 N
Orem, UT 84057
**Phone:** (801)764-9068        **Free:** 888-489-1238
Suzanne Smith, Director

**Program(s):** Childbirth Educator; Doula; Midwifery.

## Vermont

### ★ 4130 ★ Partner Earth Education Center
PO Box 298
Pawlet, VT 05761-0298
**Phone:** (802)325-2121    **Fax:** (802)325-2121
Pam Montgomery, Director

**Program(s):** Herbal Medicine; Plant Spirit Medicine.

### ★ 4131 ★ Sage Mountain Retreat Center and Botanical Sanctuary
PO Box 420
East Barre, VT 05649
**Phone:** (802)479-9825    **Fax:** (802)476-3722
Rosemary Gladstar, Director

**Program(s):** Herbal Medicine.

### ★ 4132 ★ Universal Institute of Healing Arts
RFD 3
Box 5285
Montpelier, VT 05602
**Phone:** (802)229-4844
Bob Onne, Director

**Program(s):** Acupressure; Deep Tissue Massage; Reflexology; Shiatsu.

### ★ 4133 ★ Vermont Institute of Massage Therapy
10 Cottage Grove Ave.
South Burlington, VT 05403
**Phone:** (802)862-1111    **Fax:** (802)660-3733
Kathleen Wright, Director

**Program(s):** Acupressure; Energy Work; Massage Therapy; Reflexology.

### ★ 4134 ★ Vermont School of Professional Massage
14 Merchant St.
Barre, VT 05641
**Phone:** (802)479-2340
Faeterri Silver, Director

**Program(s):** Massage Therapy.

## Virginia

### ★ 4135 ★ Alexander Technique Center of Washington DC
PO Box 449
McLean, VA 22101
**Phone:** (703)821-4277
Marian Goldberg, Director

**Program(s):** Alexander Technique.

### ★ 4136 ★ Applied Kinesthetic Studies School of Massage
692 Pine St.
Herndon, VA 20170
**Phone:** (703)464-0333    **Fax:** (703)464-5999
Katharine Hunter, Director

**Program(s):** Swedish Massage.

### ★ 4137 ★ Blue Ridge School of Massage and Yoga
201 S Main St.
Blacksburg, VA 24060
**Phone:** (540)552-2177
Colleen A. Kelly, Director

**Program(s):** Acupressure; Alexander Technique; Deep Tissue Massage; Energy Work; Massage Therapy; Meditation; Polarity Therapy; Qigong; Reflexology; Reiki; Shiatsu; Traditional Chinese Medicine; Yoga.

### ★ 4138 ★ Cayce/Reilly School of Massotherapy
215 67th St.
Virginia Beach, VA 23451
**Phone:** (757)437-7202    **Fax:** (757)428-0398
**Email:** are@are-cayce.com
**Website:** http://www.are-cayce.com
Dwight Zieman, Contact

**Program(s):** Acupressure; Alexander Technique; Aromatherapy; CranioSacral Therapy; Hypnotherapy; Massage Therapy; Neuromuscular Therapy; Reflexology; Reiki; Sports Massage.

### ★ 4139 ★ Eastern Institute of Hypnotherapy
PO Box 249
Goshen, VA 24439-0249
**Phone:** (540)997-0325    **Free:** 800-296-6463
**Fax:** (540)997-0324
**Email:** hyptrainer@aol.com
Allen S. Chips, Director

**Program(s):** Hypnotherapy; Neuro-Linguistic Programming.

### ★ 4140 ★ Eastern Institute of Reiki Therapy
**Transpersonal Reiki Institute**
956 Knob Rd.
PO Box 249
Goshen, VA 24439-0249
**Phone:** (540)997-0325    **Free:** 800-296-6463
**Fax:** (540)997-0324
**Email:** hyptrainer@aol.com
Dee Chips, Director

**Program(s):** Reiki.

### ★ 4141 ★ Equissage, Inc.
15715 Southern Cross Ln.
Round Hill, VA 20141
**Free:** 800-843-0224    **Fax:** (540)338-5569
Nelson R. Schreiber, Director

**Program(s):** Animal Therapy; Deep Tissue Massage; Equine Massage.

### ★ 4142 ★ Fuller School of Massage Therapy
3500 Virginia Beach Blvd.
Virginia Beach, VA 23452
**Phone:** (757)340-7132    **Fax:** (757)486-2192
Nancy Bender, Director

**Program(s):** Aromatherapy; CranioSacral Therapy; Herbal Medicine; Homeopathy; Massage Therapy; Polarity Therapy; Prenatal Massage; Qigong; Reflexology; Reiki; Shiatsu; Sports Massage.

### ★ 4143 ★ Institute for Integrated Therapies
3708 N Rosser St., Ste. 201
Alexandria, VA 22311
**Phone:** (703)931-8340    **Fax:** (703)931-8567
Margaret L. D'Urso, Director

**Program(s):** CranioSacral Therapy; Massage Therapy; Reflexology; Vibrational Therapy.

### ★ 4144 ★ National Center for Instruction of Homeopathy and Homeotherapeutics
National Center for Homeopathy Annual Summer School
801 N Fairfax St., Ste. 306
Alexandria, VA 22314
**Phone:** (703)548-7790    **Fax:** (703)548-7792
**Email:** nchinfo@igc.apc.org
**Website:** http://www.healthy.net
Stephen Messer, Contact

**Program(s):** Animal Therapy; Homeopathy.

### ★ 4145 ★ Natural Touch School of Massage Therapy
291 Park Ave.
Danville, VA 24541
**Phone:** (804)799-0060
Wanda Adkins, Director

**Program(s):** Acupressure; CranioSacral Therapy; Energy Work; Massage Therapy; Myofascial Release; Polarity Therapy; Shiatsu.

### ★ 4146 ★ Natural Touch School of Massage Therapy
1202 Main St.
Lynchburg, VA 24504
**Phone:** (804)845-3003
Wanda Adkins, Director

**Program(s):** Acupressure; CranioSacral Therapy; Energy Work; Massage Therapy; Myofascial Release; Polarity Therapy; Shiatsu.

### ★ 4147 ★ Piedmont School of Professional Massage
12712 Directors Loop
Woodbridge, VA 22192
**Phone:** (703)497-4437
Alan Coyne, Director

**Program(s):** Massage Therapy.

### ★ 4148 ★ Richmond Academy of Massage
2004 Bremo Rd., Ste. 102
Richmond, VA 23226
**Phone:** (804)282-5003    **Fax:** (804)288-7356
D.C. Ashburn, Director

**Program(s):** Massage Therapy.

### ★ 4149 ★ Satchidananda Ashram - Yogaville
Rt. 1, Box 1720
Buckingham, VA 23921
**Phone:** (804)969-3121    **Free:** 800-858-9642
**Fax:** (804)969-1303

**Program(s):** Yoga Teacher Training.

### ★ 4150 ★ Shenandoah University
1775 N Sector Ct.
Winchester, VA 22601
**Phone:** (540)678-4382    **Fax:** (540)665-5519
Juliana Fehr, Director

**Program(s):** Midwifery.

### ★ 4151 ★ Virginia Academy of Massage Therapy
5314 George Washington Memorial Hwy.
Yorktown, VA 23692
**Phone:** (757)872-0934    **Fax:** (757)898-0620
Barbara Marker, Director

**Program(s):** Acupressure; CranioSacral Therapy; Deep Tissue Massage; Energy Work; Hypnotherapy; Massage Therapy; Reflexology; Traditional Chinese Medicine.

### ★ 4152 ★ Virginia School for Alexander Technique
1021 Sheridan Ave.
Charlottesville, VA 22901
**Phone:** (804)977-7186
Daria T. Okugawa, Director

**Program(s):** Alexander Technique.

### ★ 4153 ★ Virginia School of Massage
2008 Morton Dr.
Charlottesville, VA 22903
**Phone:** (804)293-4031    **Fax:** (804)293-4190
**Email:** registrar@vasom.com
Sue Ellis Dyar, Contact

**Program(s):** Massage Therapy.

**★ 4154 ★ Virginia School of Massage, Blacksburg**
106B Southpark Dr.
Blacksburg, VA 24060
**Phone:** (804)293-4031          **Fax:** (804)293-4190
Lori Nicolaysen, Director
**Program(s):** Massage Therapy.

**★ 4155 ★ Virginia School of Massage, Winchester**
2820 Valley Ave.
Winchester, VA 22601
**Phone:** (804)293-4031          **Fax:** (804)293-4190
Lori Nicolaysen, Director
**Program(s):** Massage Therapy.

## Washington

**★ 4156 ★ Ashmead College, Everett**
2721 Wetmore Ave.
Everett, WA 98201
**Phone:** (425)339-2678          **Fax:** (425)258-2620
**Website:** http://www.ashmeadcollege.com
Cheryl France, Director
**Program(s):** Anatomy and Physiology; Aromatherapy; CPR/First Aid; Geriatric Massage; Hydrotherapy; Kinesiology; Massage Therapy; Pregnancy Massage; Spa Therapies; Sports Massage.

**★ 4157 ★ Ashmead College, Seattle**
7120 Woodlawn Ave. NE
Seattle, WA 98115
**Phone:** (206)527-0807          **Fax:** (206)527-1957
**Website:** http://www.ashmeadcollege.com
Marsha Aldinger, Director
**Program(s):** Anatomy and Physiology; Aromatherapy; First Aid/CPR; Geriatric Massage; Hydrotherapy; Kinesiology; Massage Therapy; Pregnancy Massage; Spa Therapies; Sports Massage.

**★ 4158 ★ Ashmead College, Tacoma Campus**
5005 Pacific Hwy. E, Ste. 20
Fife, WA 98424
**Phone:** (253)926-1435
**Website:** http://www.ashmeadcollege.com
Julie Currier, Director
**Program(s):** Anatomy and Physiology; Aromatherapy; CPR/First Aid; Geriatric Massage; Hydrotherapy; Kinesiology; Massage Therapy; Pregnancy Massage; Spa Therapies; Sports Massage.

**★ 4159 ★ Ayur-vedic Medicine, Yoga Therapy, UltraNutrition School**
819 NE 65th St.
Seattle, WA 98115
**Phone:** (206)729-9999          **Fax:** (206)729-0164
**Program(s):** Aromatherapy; Ayurvedic Medicine; Herbal Medicine; Naturopathic Medicine; Yoga Therapy.

**★ 4160 ★ Bastyr University**
14500 Juanita Dr. NE
Kenmore, WA 98028-4966
**Phone:** (425)823-1300          **Fax:** (425)823-6222
Sandra Lane, Director
**Program(s):** Acupuncture; Ayurvedic Medicine; Herbal Medicine; Homeopathy; Midwifery; Naturopathic Medicine; Nutrition; Qigong; Shiatsu; Traditional Chinese Medicine.

**★ 4161 ★ Bellevue Massage School**
16301 NE 8th St., Ste. 106
Bellevue, WA 98008
**Phone:** (425)641-3409          **Fax:** (425)641-3409
Elise Hockett, Director
**Program(s):** Deep Tissue Massage; Energy Work; Massage Therapy; Reflexology; Touch for Health.

**★ 4162 ★ BodyMind Academy**
1247 120th Ave. NE
Bellevue, WA 98005
**Phone:** (425)635-0145          **Fax:** (425)635-3588
Thomas J. Johnston, Director
**Program(s):** Breathwork; Hypnotherapy; Massage Therapy; Shiatsu.

**★ 4163 ★ BodyMind Energetics Institute**
15832 34th Ave. NE
Seattle, WA 98155
**Phone:** (206)361-4700
Reed Svadesh Johnson, Director
**Program(s):** Orgodynamics; Qigong; Shiatsu; Trager.

**★ 4164 ★ Brenneke School of Massage**
160 Roy St.
Seattle, WA 98109
**Phone:** (206)282-1233          **Fax:** (206)282-9183
Heida Brenneke, Director
**Program(s):** CranioSacral Therapy; Massage Therapy; Polarity Therapy; Relexology; Reiki; Shiatsu; Sports Massage.

**★ 4165 ★ Brian Utting School of Massage**
900 Thomas St.
Seattle, WA 98109
**Phone:** (206)292-8055          **Free:** 800-842-8731
**Fax:** (206)292-0113
Brian Utting, Director
**Program(s):** Connective Tissue Massage; Deep Tissue Massage; Hydrotherapy; Injury Treatment and Evaluation; Massage Therapy; Neuromuscular Therapy; Sports Massage.

**★ 4166 ★ Cedar Mountain Center for Massage, Inc.**
5601 NE St. John's Rd.
Vancouver, WA 98661
**Phone:** (360)696-2210          **Fax:** (360)696-0130
Sandra V. Hattan, Director
**Program(s):** Aromatherapy; Massage Therapy; Polarity Therapy; Reflexology; Shiatsu; Sports Massage.

**★ 4167 ★ Heartspring Transformation Trainings**
5404 Meridian Ave. N
Seattle, WA 98103
**Phone:** (206)547-4064
**Email:** byheart@wolfenet.com
Pamela Grace, Director
**Program(s):** Hypnotherapy; Reiki.

**★ 4168 ★ Inland Massage Institute**
111 E Magnesium Rd., Ste. F
Spokane, WA 99208
**Phone:** (509)465-3033          **Fax:** (509)326-1236
Sheryl L. Storro, Contact
**Program(s):** Massage Therapy; Swedish Massage.

**★ 4169 ★ Institute of Dynamic Aromatherapy**
2000 2nd Ave., Ste. 206
Seattle, WA 98121
**Phone:** (206)374-8773          **Free:** 800-260-7401
**Fax:** (206)374-9020
Jade Shutes, Director
**Program(s):** Aromatherapy; Herbal Medicine; Reflexology.

**★ 4170 ★ Institute for Therapeutic Learning**
9322 21st Ave. NW
Seattle, WA 98117
**Phone:** (206)783-1838
**Email:** jelias@sprynet.com

**Website:** http://www.home.sprynet.com/sprynet/jelias
Jack Elias, Director
**Program(s):** Energy Work; Hypnotherapy.

**★ 4171 ★ North American Institute of Neuro-Therapy**
117 E Louisa, Ste. 188
Seattle, WA 98102
**Phone:** (206)322-0633
Marilyn Michael, Director
**Program(s):** Neuro-Therapy.

**★ 4172 ★ Northwest Institute of Acupuncture and Oriental Medicine**
701 N 34th St., Ste 300
Seattle, WA 98103
**Phone:** (206)633-2419          **Fax:** (206)633-5578
**Email:** niaom@halcyon.com
**Website:** http://www.halcyon.com/niaom
Frederick O. Lanphear, PhD, Contact
**Program(s):** Acupuncture; Oriental Medicine; Traditional Chinese Medicine.

**★ 4173 ★ Peninsula College**
1502 E Lauridsen Blvd.
Port Angeles, WA 98362
**Phone:** (360)417-6569
Dona Smasal, Director
**Program(s):** Aromatherapy; Deep Muscle Massage; Energy Work; Massage Therapy; Oriental Medicine; Shiatsu.

**★ 4174 ★ Seattle Institute of Oriental Medicine**
916 NE 65th St., Ste. B
Seattle, WA 98115
**Phone:** (206)517-4541          **Fax:** (206)526-1932
**Email:** info@siom.com
**Website:** http://www.siom.com
Dan Bensky, Director
**Program(s):** Acupuncture; Oriental Medicine; Traditional Chinese Medicine.

**★ 4175 ★ Seattle Midwifery School**
2524 16th Ave. S, Room 300
Seattle, WA 98109
**Phone:** (206)322-8834
Melissa Hicks, Director
**Program(s):** Childbirth Education; Doula; Midwifery.

**★ 4176 ★ Soma Institute**
730 Klink
Buckley, WA 98321
**Phone:** (360)829-1025          **Fax:** (360)829-2805
Karen L. Bolesky, Director
**Program(s):** Soma Neuromuscular Integration.

**★ 4177 ★ Spectrum Center School of Massage**
12506 18th St. NE, Ste. 1
Lake Stevens, WA 98258
**Phone:** (425)334-5409
Barbara Collins, Director
**Program(s):** CranioSacral Therapy; Massage Therapy; Polarity Therapy; Sports Massage.

**★ 4178 ★ Tacoma Community College Alliance Hypnotherapy Professional Hypnosis Training**
30640 Pacific Hwy. S, Ste. E
Federal Way, WA 98003
**Phone:** (206)927-8888          **Fax:** (206)566-5020
Roy Hunter, Contact
**Program(s):** Hypnotherapy.

**★ 4179 ★ Tri City School of Massage**
26 E 3rd Ave.
Kennewick, WA 99336
**Phone:** (509)586-6434
Patty J. Kruschke, Director
**Program(s):** Massage Therapy.

**★ 4180 ★ University of Washington School of Nursing**
PO Box 357262
Seattle, WA 98195-7262
**Phone:** (206)543-8241
Aileen MacClaren, Director
**Program(s):** Midwifery.

**★ 4181 ★ Wellness Institute**
3716 274th Ave. SE
Issaquah, WA 98029
**Phone:** (425)391-9716  **Fax:** (425)391-9737
David Hartman, Director
**Program(s):** Breathwork; Energy Work; Hypnotherapy.

**★ 4182 ★ Yoga Centers**
2255 140th Ave. NE, Stes. E and F
Bellevue, WA 98005
**Phone:** (425)746-7476  **Fax:** (425)746-3961
Mona Renner, Director
**Program(s):** Aromatherapy; Energy Work; Yoga Teacher Training.

### West Virginia

**★ 4183 ★ Mountain State School of Massage**
3407 River Lane Dr.
PO Box 4487
Malden, WV 25306
**Phone:** (304)926-8822  **Fax:** (304)926-8837
Robert Rogers, Director
**Program(s):** Anatomy and Physiology; Chair Massage; Connective Tissue Massage; Hydrotherapy; Kinesiology; Massage Therapy; Neuromuscular Therapy; Polarity Therapy; Reflexology; Shiatsu; Sports Massage; Swedish Massage.

### Wisconsin

**★ 4184 ★ Blue Sky Educational Foundation, Professional School of Massage and Therapeutic Bodywork**
220 Oak St.
Grafton, WI 53024
**Phone:** (414)376-1011  **Fax:** (414)376-7707
Vicki Chossek, Director
**Program(s):** Massage Therapy.

**★ 4185 ★ Capri College Massage Therapy Program**
6414 Odana Rd.
Madison, WI 53719
**Phone:** (608)274-5390  **Fax:** (608)274-1215
**Program(s):** Acupressure; Aromatherapy; Massage Therapy; Reflexology; Reiki; Shiatsu; Swedish Massage.

**★ 4186 ★ Fox Valley School of Massage**
2003 N Meade St.
Appleton, WI 54914
**Phone:** (920)722-3271  **Fax:** (920)882-9412
Tom Finch, Director
**Program(s):** Aromatherapy; Massage Therapy; Neuromuscular Therapy; Polarity Therapy; Qigong; Reiki.

**★ 4187 ★ Institute for Wholistic Education**
33719 116th St.
Twin Lakes, WI 53181
**Phone:** (414)877-9396  **Fax:** (414)889-8591
Santosh Krinsky, Contact
**Program(s):** Ayurvedic Medicine.

**★ 4188 ★ Lakeside School of Massage Therapy**
1726 N 1st St., Ste. 100
Milwaukee, WI 53212
**Phone:** (414)372-4345  **Fax:** (414)372-5350
**Email:** lakeschool@aol.com
Claude Gagnon, Director
**Program(s):** Acupressure; Massage Therapy; Reflexology; Shiatsu.

**★ 4189 ★ Marquette University College of Nursing**
PO Box 1881
Milwaukee, WI 53201-1881
**Phone:** (414)288-3842
Leona Vandevusse, Director
**Program(s):** Midwifery.

**★ 4190 ★ Midwest Center for the Study of Oriental Medicine**
6226 Bankers Rd., Ste. 8
Racine, WI 53403
**Phone:** (414)554-2010  **Fax:** (414)554-7475
**Email:** dunbardoc@aol.com
Dr. William Dunbar, Contact
**Program(s):** Acupressure; Acupuncture; Herbal Medicine; Oriental Medicine; Traditional Chinese Medicine.

**★ 4191 ★ Milwaukee School of Massage**
830 E Chambers St.
Milwaukee, WI 53212
**Phone:** (414)347-1151
Wanda M. Beals, Director
**Program(s):** Acupressure; Ayurvedic Medicine; CranioSacral Therapy; Energy Work; Feldenkrais; Massage Therapy; Myofascial Release; Oriental Medicine; Reiki; Swedish Massage.

**★ 4192 ★ Saint Croix Center for the Healing Arts, Ltd.**
411 County Hwy UU
Hudson, WI 54016
**Phone:** (715)381-1402  **Fax:** (715)381-1502
June Motzer-Trollen, Director
**Program(s):** Acupressure; Aromatherapy; Massage Therapy; Reflexology; Sports Massage.

**★ 4193 ★ SpiriTouch Institute, Inc.**
6225 University
Madison, WI 53705
**Phone:** (608)236-9042  **Fax:** (608)236-9570
Lori Hellenbrand, Director
**Program(s):** Energy Work; Massage Therapy; Reiki.

**★ 4194 ★ Wisconsin Institute of Chinese Herbology**
6921 Mariner Dr.
Racine, WI 53406
**Phone:** (414)886-5858  **Fax:** (414)886-5858
**Email:** herbalstudies@aol.com
Arthur D. Shattuck, Director
**Program(s):** Animal Therapy; Herbal Medicine; Oriental Medicine; Traditional Chinese Medicine.

**★ 4195 ★ Wisconsin Institute of Natural Wellness**
6921 Mariner Dr.
Racine, WI 53406
**Phone:** (414)886-3344  **Fax:** (414)632-9533
Arthur D. Shattuck, Director
**Program(s):** Acupuncture; Massage Therapy; Reflexology; Reiki; Shiatsu; Tai Chi; Traditional Chinese Medicine.

# National & International Organizations

**★ 4196 ★ Academy of Upper Cervical Chiropractic Organizations (AUCCO)**
1637 Westbridge Dr., Unit H4
Fort Collins, CO 80526
**Website:** http://www.aucco.org/
**Desc:** Chiropractors and chiropractic organizations. Fosters and promotes information about atlas subluxation complex; disseminates information in order to preserve the science of upper cervical adjustment; provides resources and health tips **Pub:** Newsletter.Contains information of interest to members.

**★ 4197 ★ Accreditation Commission for Acupuncture and Oriental Medicine (ACAOM)**
7501 Greenway Ctr. Dr.
Greenbelt, MD 20770
**Phone:** (301)313-0868  **Fax:** (301)313-0869
**Email:** 73352.2467@compuserve.com
**Website:** http://www.ccaom.org
Dort Bigg, Exec. Dir.
**Fnded:** 1982. **Mem:** 45. **Desc:** Acts as an independent body to evaluate first professional master's degree and first professional master's level certificate and diploma programs in acupuncture and first professional master's degree and first professional master's level certificate and diploma programs in Oriental medicine with concentrations in both acupuncture and herbal therapy for a level of performance, integrity and quality that entitles them to the confidence of the educational community and the public they serve. Establishes accreditation criteria, arranges site visits, evaluates those programs that desire accredited status and publicly designates those programs that meet the criteria. **Pub:** *Accreditation Handbook.* Handbook. *Price:* $25. ● *Acupuncture and Oriental Medicine Accreditation,* semiannual. Newsletter. *Price:* Free. ● Brochure. ● Manuals. **Frmly:** (1998) National Accreditation Commission for Schools and Colleges of Acupuncture and Oriental Medicine.

**★ 4198 ★ Acupuncture Foundation of Canada Institute (AFC)**
2131 Lawarence Ave. E
Scarborough, ON, Canada M1R 5G4
**Phone:** (416)752-3988  **Fax:** (416)752-4398
**Email:** info@afcinstitute.ca
**Website:** http://www.afcinstitute.com
**Fnded:** 1974. **Mem:** 1,000. **Desc:** Promotes acupuncture's legimate place in health care by initiating and supporting research in acupuncture. **Pub:** Newsletter, periodic.

**★ 4199 ★ Acupuncture and Oriental Medicine Alliance**
14637 Starr Rd. SE
Olalla, WA 98359
**Phone:** (253)851-6896  **Fax:** (253)851-6883
**Website:** http://www.acuall.org/
Barbara Mitchell, Exec. Dir.
**Desc:** Dedicated to the advancement of acupuncture and Oriental medicine.

**★ 4200 ★ Alliance for Alternatives in Healthcare (AAH)**
PO Box 6279
Thousand Oaks, CA 91359-6279
**Phone:** (818)226-9829  **Fax:** (818)226-9820
**Email:** althlthins@aol.com
**Website:** http://www.alternativeinsurance.com
Steve Gorman, Pres.
**Fnded:** 1983. **Mem:** 1,500. **Desc:** Holistic physicians; employers; interested individuals. Seeks to enhance public recognition of holistic, homeopathic, naturopathic, chiropractic, and acupuncture treatments. (Hol-

istic medicine focuses on the treatment of the entire body, rather than on any one organ or system; homeopathic medicine treats diseases by administering minute quantities of a substance that would produce the disease's symptoms in a healthy person; naturopathic medicine avoids the use of surgery and drugs, focusing instead on natural agents, such as sunshine and fresh air, or on physical means, such as manipulation or acupuncture.) Encourages health insurance systems to cover holistic, homeopathic, and naturopathic treatments in their policies. Attends exhibitions to disseminate information on holistic, homeopathic, and naturopathic medicine to health care providers and the public. Offers group medical, dental, and vision plans to members. Manages network of holistic and natural providers who offer discounts to subscribers of the Holistic Health Network. **Pub:** *Natural Marketing News*, periodic. • *Press Releases*, periodic. **Frmly:** Alternative Health Insurance Services; (1989) Natural Marketing Association.

### ★ 4201 ★ American Academy of Acupuncture and Oriental Medicine (AAAOM)

1313 5th St. SE, Ste. 115
Minneapolis, MN 55414
**Website:** http://www.acuall.org/

**Desc:** Seeks to advance acupuncture and oriental medicine.

### ★ 4202 ★ American Academy of Alternative Medicine (AAAM)

c/o Dr. Alex Cougar
16126 E Warren, Box 24224
Detroit, MI 48224-0224
**Phone:** (313)882-0641          **Fax:** (313)882-0979
Dr. Alex Cougar, Contact

**Fnded:** 1984. **Mem:** 800. **Nat'l Groups:** 2. **Desc:** Advocates of alternative medicine. Promotes increased reliance on alternative treatments by professionals. Conducts research; sponsors training programs for health care professionals wishing to make use of alternative therapies. Conducts continuing education leading to American Board of Alternative Medicine Certification for members. **Pub:** *Restricted*, periodic. Newsletter. *Price:* Free for members.

### ★ 4203 ★ American Academy of Medical Acupuncture

4929 Wilshire Blvd., Ste. 428
Los Angeles, CA 90010
**Phone:** (323)937-5514          **Fax:** (323)937-0959
**Email:** jdowden@prodigy.net
**Website:** http://www.medicalacupuncture.org
C. James Dowden, Exec. Admin.

**Fnded:** 1987. **Mem:** 1,710. **State Groups:** 8. **Desc:** Professional society of physicians and osteopaths who utilize acupuncture in their practices. Provides ongoing training and information related to the Chinese practice of puncturing the body at specific points to cure disease or relieve pain. Offers educational and research programs. *Medical Acupuncture*, semiannual. Journal.

### ★ 4204 ★ American Acupuncture Association (AAA)

4262 Kissena Blvd.
Flushing, NY 11355
**Phone:** (718)886-4431          **Fax:** (718)463-0808
Dr. David P. J. Hung, Chm.

**Fnded:** 1972. **Mem:** 400. **Desc:** Physicians, nurses, acupuncturists, physical therapists, and herbologists. Promotes acceptance of acupuncture as a viable medical method. Works to legalize acupuncture on the state level. Offers continuing education course. Maintains speakers' bureau. Conducts lectures to educate public on acupuncture. **Pub:** *Journal of Chinese Acupuncture*, annual. Journal.

### ★ 4205 ★ American Association for Health Freedom

PO Box 458
Great Falls, VA 22066
**Phone:** (703)759-0662          **Free:** 800-230-2762
**Fax:** (703)759-6711
**Email:** aahf@healthfreedom.net
**Website:** http://www.healthfreedom.net
Candace Campbell, Exec. Dir.

**Fnded:** 1992. **Mem:** 500. **Desc:** Non-profit advocacy organization dedicated to promoting health care freedom and to protecting practitioners offering complementary and alternative therapies. **Pub:** *Directors Report*, monthly. Newsletter. *Price:* Free to members. **Frmly:** (2002) American Preventive Medical Association.

### ★ 4206 ★ American Association of Naturopathic Physicians (AANP)

8201 Greensboro Dr., Ste. 300
Mc Lean, VA 22102-3814
**Phone:** (703)610-9037          **Free:** 877-969-2267
**Fax:** (703)610-9005
**Email:** 74602.3715@compuserve.com
**Website:** http://www.naturopathic.org
Maria Bianchi, Exec. Dir.

**Fnded:** 1986. **Mem:** 1,300. **State Groups:** 29. **Desc:** Naturopathic physicians. Unites naturopathic physicians and represents their legislative interests; promotes high educational standards and uniform criteria for licensing; increases public awareness of naturopathic medicine. **Pub:** *AANP Quarterly Newsletter*, quarterly. Newsletter. *Price:* Included in membership fee. • *Journal of Naturopathic Medicine*. Journal.

### ★ 4207 ★ American Association of Oriental Medicine (AAOM)

433 Front St.
Catasauqua, PA 18032-2506
**Phone:** (610)266-1433          **Free:** 888-500-7999
**Fax:** (610)264-2768
**Email:** aaom1@aol.com
**Website:** http://www.aaom.org
David Molony, Exec. Dir.

**Fnded:** 1981. **Mem:** 1,300. **Reg. Groups:** 4. **State Groups:** 32. **Desc:** Professional acupuncturists and Oriental Medicine Practitioners. Seeks to: elevate the standards of education and practice of acupuncture and oriental medicine; establish laws governing acupuncture; provide a forum to share information on acupuncture techniques; increase public awareness of acupuncture; support research in the field. Conducts educational programs; compiles statistics. Operates speakers' bureau. **Pub:** *AAOM Membership Directory*, annual. Membership Directory. Contains listing of U.S. acupuncture and oriental medicine practitioners. *Price:* $12/copy. • *American Acupuncturist Newsletter*, semiannual. Newsletter. Contains political and educational news and information. • *American Acupuncturist Update*, quarterly. Newsletter. Contains political & educational news and info. **Frmly:** (1996) American Association for Acupuncture and Oriental Medicine.

### ★ 4208 ★ American Board of Alternative Medicine (ABAM)

c/o Dr. B. Alli
16126 E Warren
PO Box 24224
Detroit, MI 48224-0224
**Phone:** (313)882-0641
Dr. B. Alli, Contact

**Fnded:** 1994. **Mem:** 800. **Desc:** Practitioners of alternative medicine. Promotes increased use of alternative treatments including mind-body intervention, bioelectromagnetic therapy, and herbal medicines. Conducts research and educational programs; maintains hall of fame. **Pub:** *Newsletter of the American Board of Alternative Medicine*, periodic. Newsletter. *Price:* $120 for members only.

### ★ 4209 ★ American College of Orgonomy (ACO)

PO Box 490
Princeton, NJ 08542
**Phone:** (732)821-1144          **Fax:** (732)821-0174
**Email:** aco@orgonomy.org
**Website:** http://www.orgonomy.org
Gary A. Karpf, MD, Pres.

**Fnded:** 1968. **Mem:** 12. **Desc:** Physicians and social scientists seeking to promote and advance the science of orgonomy. (Orgonomy is derived from the theory formulated by Wilhelm Reich, M.D. "that all space is filled with a specific form of energy called orgone energy which accounts for life and living functions.") Provides training in medical orgonomy and character analysis for physicians. Sponsors training and research for physicians and scientists in orgone physics, orgone biology, and weather control. Holds laboratory workshops for physicians and scientists. Offers referral service. Conducts specialized education. **Pub:** *Journal of Orgonomy*, semiannual. Journal. Contains articles on scientific topics related to Orgonomy, sociopolitical and case studies. *Price:* $40/year in the U.S. and Canada; $45/year outside the U.S. and Canada, surface rate; $55/year outside the U.S. and Canada, airmail. • *Man in the Trap.* • *Orgonomic Medicine*.

### ★ 4210 ★ American CranioSacral Therapy Association (ACSTA)

c/o Upledger Institute
11211 Prosperity Farms Rd., Ste. D-325
Palm Beach Gardens, FL 33410
**Phone:** (561)622-4334          **Free:** 800-233-5880
**Fax:** (561)622-4771
**Email:** upledger@upledger.com
**Website:** http://www.acsta.com/

**Desc:** CranioSacral Therapy practitioners and proponents of the modality. Represents the CranioSacral Therapy profession; creates understanding and acceptance of CST within legislative, insurance, public, media, and medical arenas; supports educational and competency standards; monitors insurance and public policy.

### ★ 4211 ★ American Foundation for Alternative Health Care, Research and Development (AFAHCRD)

25 Landfield Ave.
Monticello, NY 12701
**Phone:** (914)794-8181          **Fax:** (914)794-5861
**Email:** efield@catskill.net
Edwin M. Field, Exec. Dir.

**Fnded:** 1978. **Desc:** Serves as an alternative health care information resource center. Compiles data. **Frmly:** (1985) American Foundation for Alternative Health Care.

### ★ 4212 ★ American Herbalists Guild (AHG)

1931 Gaddis Rd.
Canton, GA 30115
**Phone:** (770)751-6021          **Fax:** (770)751-7472
**Email:** ahgoffice@earthlink.net
**Website:** http://www.americanherbalistsguild.com
Steven H. Horne, Pres.

**Fnded:** 1989. **Mem:** 750. **State Groups:** 3. **Desc:** Promotes research and education in the field of herbal medicine. Works to establish high standards for the professional practice of herbalism. Provides a forum for the exchange of information in the field. **Pub:** *Directory of Herbal Education Programs. Price:* $7.95. • *The Herbalist*, quarterly. Newsletter. • *Recommended Reading List. Price:* $2.

### ★ 4213 ★ American Holistic Health Association

PO Box 17400
Anaheim, CA 92817
**Phone:** (714)779-6152
**Email:** ahha@healthy.net
**Website:** http://ahha.org
Ms. Suzan Walter, MBA, Pres.

**Fnded:** 1989. **Desc:** Seeks to further the understanding of holistic health care, a concept that stresses the integration of physical, mental, emotional, and spiritual concerns with environmental harmony.

★ **4214** ★ **American Holistic Medical Association (AHMA)**
6728 Old McLean Village Dr.
Mc Lean, VA 22101-8729
**Phone:** (703)556-9728          **Fax:** (703)556-8729
**Email:** info@holisticmedicine.org
**Website:** http://www.holisticmedicine.org
Larry Hulbert, Contact

**Fnded:** 1978. **Mem:** 700. **Reg. Groups:** 11. **Desc:** Licensed medical doctors, doctors of osteopathy, and students enrolled in medical or osteopathic programs who are interested in furthering the practice of holistic health care, a concept that stresses the integration of physical, mental, emotional, and spiritual concerns with environmental harmony. Medical education is provided in these areas through the association's conference. **Pub:** *AHMA Member Directory*, annual. Membership Directory. *Price:* available to members only. • *Members Brochures*. Brochures. • *National Referral Directory of Holistic Practitioners*. Directory. *Price:* $10. • *Newsletter to Members*. Newsletter.

★ **4215** ★ **American Holistic Nurses Association (AHNA)**
PO Box 2130
Flagstaff, AZ 86003-2130
**Phone:** (520)526-2196          **Free:** 800-278-2462
**Fax:** (520)526-2752
**Email:** ahna-flag@flaglink.com
**Website:** http://www.ahna.org
Doris Rager, Exec. Dir.

**Fnded:** 1981. **Mem:** 2,700. **State Groups:** 11. **Local Groups:** 63. **Desc:** The AHNA is a 501(c) (3) nonprofit educational organization whose membership is open to nurses and other individuals interested in holistically-oriented health care practices throughout the United States and the world. ASHNA supports the education of nurses, allied health practitioners, and the general public on health-related issues. The American Holistic Nurses' Association embraces nursing as a lifestyle and a profession and provides a means to create bonds within the nursing community. Because true healing comes from within, the AHNA recognizes that nurses must first heal themselves before they can facilitate the healing of others. **Pub:** *Beginnings*, bimonthly. Newsletter. Covers membership activities. Includes calendar of events, tape and book reviews, and regional reports. *Price:* Included in membership dues; $25/year for nonmembers. • *Come Home to the Heart of Nursing*. Brochure. • *Journal of Holistic Nursing*, quarterly. Journal. Presents academic and scholarly works from the field of holistic nursing practice; includes research news. *Price:* Included in membership dues; $28.80/year for nonmembers; $60/ year for institutions. • Also publishes membership directory.

★ **4216** ★ **American Holistic Veterinary Medical Association (AHVMA)**
2218 Old Emmorton Rd.
Bel Air, MD 21015
**Phone:** (410)569-0795          **Fax:** (410)569-2346
**Email:** ahvma82@cs.com
**Website:** http://www.ahvma.org
Dr. Carvel G. Tiekert, Exec. Dir.

**Fnded:** 1982. **Mem:** 1,000. **Desc:** Veterinarians and others interested in exploring alternative approaches in veterinary medicine, including clinical nutrition, homeopathy, and herbal medicine. **Pub:** Journal, quarterly. Includes association news and book reviews. *Price:* Included in membership dues. **Frmly:** (1985) American Veterinary Holistic Medical Association.

★ **4217** ★ **American Institute of Homeopathy (AIH)**
801 N Fairfax St., Ste. 306
Alexandria, VA 22314
**Phone:** 888-445-9988
**Email:** aih@homeopathyusa.org
**Website:** http://www.homeopathyusa.org
Bernardo A. Merizalde, MD, Contact

**Fnded:** 1844. **Mem:** 160. **Desc:** Professional society of medical doctors, osteopaths, and dentists practicing homeotherapeutics according to the three natural laws of cure propounded by German physician Samuel C. F. Hahnemann (1755-1843). Promotes research and quality homeopathic health care. **Pub:** *Homeopathy Notes*, monthly. Newsletter. • *Journal of the American Institute of Homeopathy*, quarterly. Journal. *Price:* $12/ each; $35/year (inside North America); $45/year (outside North America).

★ **4218** ★ **American Naprapathic Association (ANA)**
c/o Roy P. Krueger, D.N.
5913 W Montrose Ave.
Chicago, IL 60634
**Phone:** (773)685-6020
Roy P. Krueger, D.N., Corr. Sec.

**Fnded:** 1909. **Mem:** 300. **Desc:** Professional society of naprapathic physicians. (Naprapathy is the science and system of therapeutic manipulation of tissue structures that have become damaged due to stress and strain.) Promotes and publishes the principles of natural healing; seeks to further legislation and recognition of the system of treatment based on the belief that many functional disorders are caused by abnormal connective tissue and ligamentous changes and can be corrected by manipulation. Sponsors Naprapathic Education and Research Foundation. Conducts seminars and educational programs. Maintains speakers' bureau. **Pub:** *Back Pain*. • *Headache: A Warning*. • *Naprapathy: A Scientific Approach to Natural Healing*. • *The Three Facets of Naprapathy*. • *Voice of Naprapathy*. Booklet. Includes articles on nutrition and health topics. *Price:* Free. • *Why Manipulation?*. • Directory, periodic.

★ **4219** ★ **American Natural Hygiene Society (ANHS)**
PO Box 30630
Tampa, FL 33630
**Phone:** (813)855-6607          **Fax:** (813)855-8052
**Email:** anhs@anhs.org
**Website:** http://www.anhs.org
Lynn Grudnik, Exec. Dir.

**Fnded:** 1948. **Mem:** 6,500. **Desc:** Public health education organization dedicated to teaching and preserving a tradition of health freedom and independence. Promotes health maintenance through natural means such as natural foods, fresh air, pure water, sunshine, fasting, exercise, and rest. Emphasizes a lifestyle that encourages people to maximize their health by living in harmony with their physiological needs. Operates Natural Hygiene Press; maintains Herbert Shelton Library on fasting, natural hygiene, and related subjects. **Pub:** *Health Science*, quarterly. Journal. *Price:* Included in membership dues. • Also publishes and distributes books and tapes. **Frmly:** American Physiological and Natural Hygiene Society.

★ **4220** ★ **American Organization for Bodywork Therapies of Asia (AOBTA)**
1010 Haddonfield-Berlin Rd., STe 408
Voorhees, NJ 08043
**Phone:** (856)782-1616          **Fax:** (856)782-1653
**Email:** aobta@prodigy.net
**Website:** http://www.aobta.org
Angela Pflugfelder, OFC Mgr.

**Fnded:** 1984. **Mem:** 1,500. **Reg. Groups:** 3. **Desc:** Professional oriental bodyworkers and teachers; interested individuals. (Oriental bodywork is a form of massage which includes soft tissue and myofascial manipulation and techniques used in acupuncture.) Identifies qualified practitioners; serves as a legal entity representing members when dealing with the government, especially in terms of establishing professional status. Sets teaching standards for all styles of oriental bodywork including acupressure, five element shiatsu, macrobiotic shiatsu, nippon, and zen. Sponsors speakers' bureau; conducts educational programs. **Pub:** *AOBTA Directory*, annual. Membership Directory. Lists members of the association. • *PULSE Newsletter*, quarterly. Newsletter. **Frmly:** (1990) American Shiatsu Association; (1991) American Association of Oriental Healing Arts; (2001) American Oriental Bodywork Therapy Association.

★ **4221** ★ **American Podiatric Circulatory Society (APCS)**
c/o Dr. Stanley Goldstein
5704 18th Ave.
Brooklyn, NY 11204
**Phone:** (718)236-7952          **Fax:** (718)236-7953
**Email:** 72167.345@compuserve.com
**Website:** http://www.cmeonline.com/society/
Dr. Stanley Goldstein, Pres.

**Fnded:** 1979. **Mem:** 900. **Desc:** Podiatrists. Disseminates information on the Suffuse Osmotic Chemisorb Asphyxiation (SOCA) therapy, now known as the Tereno Method, devised by Dr. Isaac Tereno for treatment of geriatric patients suffering from arterial blockage in their limbs. (The Tereno Method uses vitamins to enrich the blood and enlarge subcutaneous capillaries and lymph vessels, thus creating an alternate circulatory network which bypasses blocked arteries. It is an alternative to major surgery and/or amputation in geriatric patients with poor circulation in their limbs.) Conducts research; maintains speakers' bureau. **Pub:** *American Podiatric Circulatory Society Bulletin*, quarterly. Bulletin. Contains case studies of patients treated using the Tereno Method.

★ **4222** ★ **American Polarity Therapy Association**
PO Box 19858
Boulder, CO 80308-2858
**Phone:** (303)545-2080          **Fax:** (303)545-2161
**Email:** hq@polaritytherapy.org
**Website:** http://www.polaritytherapy.org
E. Simmons, Exec. Dir.

**Fnded:** 1984. **Mem:** 1,200. **State Groups:** 6. **Desc:** Polarity therapy education. Dedicated to the advancement of polarity therapy. (Polarity therapy is a nondiagnostic holistic health system supplementing and supporting medical treatment. Polarity techniques include bodywork, diet, exercise and self awareness for health maintenance.) Develops and disseminates educational and support materials; registers practitioners; holds competitions. **Pub:** *Energy*, quarterly. Newsletter. • Books.

★ **4223** ★ **American Society of Alternative Therapists (ASAT)**
PO Box 703
Rockport, MA 01966
**Phone:** (978)281-4400          **Fax:** (978)282-1144
**Email:** asat@asat.org
**Website:** http://www.asat.org
Dr. Martin Hart, Pres.

**Fnded:** 1990. **Mem:** 1,700. **Desc:** CORE counselors. Seeks to advance CORE counseling training and services; promotes continuing professional development of members. Conducts educational programs to raise public awareness and acceptance of CORE counseling methods; sponsors training programs for CORE counselors; holds examinations and bestows CORE counseling certification upon qualified individuals; establishes and monitors CORE counseling guidelines.

★ **4224** ★ **Archaeus Project (AP)**
PO Box 7079
Kamuela, HI 96743
**Phone:** (808)887-1280          **Fax:** (808)885-9013
**Email:** fminfo@fivemtn.org
**Website:** http://www.fivemtn.org
Dennis Stillings, Dir.

**Fnded:** 1981. **Desc:** Business, medical, academic, and engineering professionals, scientists, psychologists, psi researchers, and interested others. Investigates the effects of ordinary and altered states of consciousness on conditions of health and disease; studies the relationships between the mind, body, and matter, and the implications of these relationships for medicine. Sponsors lecture series, seminars, and workshops; conducts cyberphysiology (science of self-regulation in physiology) research. **Pub:** *Healing Island*, quarterly. Journal. Contains items on health care, health care costs, and the integration of alternative with mainstream medicine, Hawaii as a health/healing destination. *Price:* Free on request at present. • *Project 2010.* Monograph. • *Tape Catalog.* Catalog.

**The Arlin J. Brown Information Center (TAJBIC)**
*See:* Entry 10114

**★ 4225 ★ Associated Bodywork and Massage Professionals (ABMP)**
1271 Sugarbush Dr.
Evergreen, CO 80439-9766
**Phone:** (303)674-8478        **Free:** 800-458-2267
**Fax:** 800-667-8260
**Email:** expectmore@abmp.com
**Website:** http://www.abmp.com
Katie Armitage, Exec. Dir.
**Fnded:** 1986. **Mem:** 38,000. **Nat'l Groups:** 1. **Desc:** Professional massage therapists and bodyworkers, sports massage therapists, skin care professionals, reflexologists, energy practitioners, etc.; massage therapy schools; affiliated organizations. Promotes massage and bodywork. Seeks to improve the image of massage therapy and bodywork, and to educate the public about its benefits. Fosters greater credibility and cooperation with the medical profession. Encourages ethical practices, high standards of professional conduct, and continuing education. Provides members with low-cost liability insurance coverage and product discounts. **Pub:** *ABMP Successful Business Handbook*, annual. Handbook. • *ABMP Touch Resource Guide.* Directory. • *Massage and Bodywork Magazine*, bimonthly. *Price:* $26 included in membership dues. • *Massage Marketplace*, annual. Directory. **Frmly:** (1988) Associated Professional Massage Therapists and Allied Health Practitioners International; (1990) Associated Professional Massage Therapists and Bodyworkers.

**★ 4226 ★ Association of Aromatherapists Southern Africa (AOASA)**
PO Box 23924
Claremont 7735, Republic of South Africa
**Phone:** 27 21 5317314
**Website:** http://www.naturalhealth.co.za/ASSOC/ass_201.html
**Desc:** Represents the professional interests of all its members nationally and internationally, as well as educational government level.

**Association for Dance Movement Therapy - United Kingdom (ADMTUK)**
*See:* Entry 20099

**★ 4227 ★ Australian Hypnotherapists' Association**
104/5 Karraabee Ave.
Tarban, NSW 2111, Australia
**Phone:** 61 2 94186730        **Fax:** 61 2 94890158
**Email:** query@dmtuk.demon.co.uk
**Website:** http://www.admt.org.uk
**Fnded:** 1949. **Mem:** 65. **State Groups:** 2. **Local Groups:** 1. **Lang(s):** English. **Desc:** Seeks to further the art of hypnotherapy and maintains a high level of standards and education for members. Lobbies health funds and the government for recognition; works to increase public awareness of hypnotherapy and its practitioners.

**Australian Music Therapy Association (AMTA)**
*See:* Entry 20105

**★ 4228 ★ Australian Society of Hypnosis**
Royal Talbot Hospital
Yarra Blvd.
Kew, VIC 3101, Australia
**Phone:** 61 3 94964548        **Fax:** 61 3 94964564
**Email:** hypnosis@alphalink.com.au
**Website:** http://www.austmta.org.au
**Fnded:** 1971. **Mem:** 1,000. **State Groups:** 6. **Lang(s):** English. **Desc:** Promotes training and research in hypnosis for health professionals in Australia.

**★ 4229 ★ Austrian Society of Acupuncture (ASA) (Osterreichische Gesellschaft fur Akupunktur — OGA)**
Kaiserin-Elisabeth Hospital
Huglgasse 1-3
A-1150 Vienna, Austria
**Phone:** 43 1 981045758        **Fax:** 43 1 981045759
**Email:** aku@kes.magwien.gv.at
**Website:** http://www.akupunktur.at/english/index.htm
**Fnded:** 1954. **Mem:** 2,147. **Lang(s):** Chinese, English, French, Italian. **Desc:** Promotes the acceptance of acupuncture as a recognized healing method in the western medical world. Works in conjunction with the World Health Organization to disseminate and standardize nomenclature. Offers training course.

**★ 4230 ★ Biofeedback Foundation of Europe (BFE)**
PO Box 75416
NL-1070 AK Amsterdam, Netherlands
**Phone:** 31 20 4422631        **Fax:** 31 20 4422632
**Email:** mail@bfe.org
**Website:** http://www.bfe.org
**Fnded:** 1996. **Lang(s):** Dutch, English. **Desc:** Health professionals and clinicians with an interest in biofeedback. Seeks to advance the study, teaching, and practice of biofeedback techniques. Conducts training and continuing professional development courses; serves as a clearinghouse on biofeedback. **Pub:** *Psychophysiology and Biofeedback Journal*, periodic. Journal.

**★ 4231 ★ British Acupuncture Association and Register (BAAR)**
22 Hockley rd.
Rayleigh M33 4RA, United Kingdom
**Phone:** 44 1268 742534
**Fnded:** 1962. **Mem:** 320. **Lang(s):** English. **Desc:** British acupuncturists. **Pub:** *BAAR Journal*, semiannual. Journal. • *Directory*, periodic. Directory. • Books, periodic. • Papers, periodic.

**★ 4232 ★ British Acupuncture Council**
63 Jeddo Rd.
London W12 9HQ, United Kingdom
**Phone:** 44 208 7350400        **Fax:** 44 208 7350404
**Email:** info@acupuncture.org.uk
**Website:** http://www.acupuncture.org.uk
**Fnded:** 1995. **Mem:** 2,000. **Lang(s):** English. **Desc:** Practitioners of acupuncture who have completed at least three year's training in traditional acupuncture and western medical sciences appropriate to the practice of acupuncture. Promotes the use of traditional Chinese acupuncture. Maintains standards of education, ethics, discipline, and practice to ensure the health and safety of the public. Encourages exchange of ideas among members. Disseminates information local practitioner members and accredited training courses. **Pub:** *BAcC News*, bimonthly. Newsletter. • *Register of Members*, semiannual. Membership Directory. **Frmly:** Traditional Acupuncture Society.

**★ 4233 ★ British Holistic Medical Association**
59 Landsdowne Place
East Sussex
Hove BN3 1FL, United Kingdom
**Phone:** 44 1273 725951        **Fax:** 44 1273 725951
**Email:** bhma@bhma.org
**Website:** http://www.bhma.org
**Fnded:** 1983. **Mem:** 800. **Desc:** Professional corporate/associate membership (for the lay public) nurse/student membership and overseas membership. To educate doctors and other healthcare professionals in the principles and practice of holistic medicine, to encourage research studies and publication of work carried out in the field of holistic medicine and to bring together holistic healthcare practitioners for mutual support and further personal and professional development. **Pub:** Newsletter, quarterly.

**★ 4234 ★ British Homeopathic Association**
15 Clerkenwell Close
London EC1R 0AA, United Kingdom
**Phone:** 44 2075 667800        **Fax:** 44 2075 667815
**Email:** info@trusthomeopathy.org
**Fnded:** 1902. **Mem:** 3,000. **Desc:** The Association is a registered charity supported by a membership of people who, being convinced of the efficacy of the homoeopathic system of medicine, give regular subscriptions or donations for its maintenance. Aims to support, extend and develop homoeopathy. Puts the general public in touch with homoeopathic doctors, veterinary surgeons and pharmacies. Also book publishers, maintaining in print a number of books on various aspects of homoeopathy as well as the magazine. **Pub:** *Health & Homoeopathy*, quarterly. Journal. • Books.

**★ 4235 ★ British Medical Acupuncture Society**
12 Marbury House
Higher Whitley
Warrington WA4 4QW, United Kingdom
**Phone:** 44 1925 730727        **Fax:** 44 1925 730492
**Email:** admin@medical-acupuncture.org.uk
**Website:** http://www.medical-acupuncture.co.uk
**Fnded:** 1980. **Mem:** 2,000. **Reg. Groups:** 11. **Desc:** Medically qualified practitioners. Concerned with the training of medical practitioners in acupuncture. Geographic listings of medically qualified practitioners of acupuncture. **Pub:** *Acupuncture in Medicine*, semiannual. Journal.

**★ 4236 ★ British Reflexology Association**
Monks Orchard
Whitbourne
Worcester WR6 5RB, United Kingdom
**Phone:** 44 1886 821207        **Fax:** 44 1886 822017
**Email:** bra@britreflex.co.uk
**Website:** http://www.britreflex.co.uk
**Fnded:** 1985. **Mem:** 750. **Lang(s):** English. **Desc:** Reflexology practitioners and students training to become reflexology practitioners. Representative body for persons practising the method of reflexology as a profession and for students training in the method. The official teaching body of the BRA is the Bayly School of Reflexology. **Pub:** *Footprints*, quarterly. Newsletter. • *Register of Members*, annual.

**★ 4237 ★ Canadian Association of Aromatherapists (CAA) (Federation Canadienne D'Aromatherapie — FCA)**
439 Wellington St. W, Ste. 5
Toronto, ON, Canada M5V 1E7
**Phone:** (416)591-0270        **Free:** 888-340-4445
**Fax:** (416)591-0273
**Fnded:** 1993. **Lang(s):** English, French. **Desc:** Aromatherapists and other individuals with an interest in aromatherapy. Fosters growth and high standards of education withing the aromatherapy profession. Gath-

ers and disseminates to consumers information about aromatherapy products and services; sponsors research and educational programs. **Pub:** *Aroma Scents Journal*, quarterly. Journal.


**★ 4238 ★ Canadian Massage Therapist Alliance (CMTA)**
365 Bloor St. E, Ste. 1807
Toronto, ON, Canada M4W 3L4
**Phone:** (416)968-2149          **Fax:** (416)968-6818
**Email:** cmta@collinscan.com
**Website:** http://www.cmta.ca
**Fnded:** 1991. **Mem:** 4,000. **Lang(s):** English. **Desc:** Alliance of provincial associations for massage therapists. Seeks to advance the practice of therapeutic massage; promotes professional development of members. **Pub:** *Hand in Hand*, semiannual. Newsletter.


**★ 4239 ★ Canadian Natural Health Association (CNHA)**
2219 Queen St. E Rear
Toronto, ON, Canada M4E 1E8
**Phone:** (416)686-7056
**Fnded:** 1960. **Mem:** 900. **Lang(s):** English. **Desc:** Holistic health care educators. Seeks to raise public awareness of holistic health care and the importance of a healthy lifestyle. Conducts educational programs; provides referral services; disseminates information on holistic health. **Pub:** *Natural Living Directory*, annual. Directory. • *Vegetarian Persuasion*. Book. textbooks and placemats. **Frmly:** (1995) Canadian Natural Hygiene Society.


**★ 4240 ★ Canadian Naturopathic Association (CNA)**
**(Association Canadienne de Naturopathie — ACN)**
1255 Sheppard Ave. E
North York, ON, Canada M2K 1E2
**Phone:** (416)496-8633          **Fax:** (416)496-8634
**Email:** info@naturopathicassoc.ca
**Website:** http://www.naturopathicassoc.ca
**Fnded:** 1953. **Mem:** 600. **Reg. Groups:** 6. **Lang(s):** English, French. **Desc:** Naturopathic medical practitioners. Promotes excellence in the practice of naturopathic medicine; encourages professional development of members. Gathers and disseminates information on naturopathic medicine; sponsors research and educational programs. **Pub:** *Vital Link*, quarterly. Newsletter.


**★ 4241 ★ Canadian Society for Homeopathy (CSH)**
87 Meadowlands Dr. W
Nepean, ON, Canada K2G 2R9
**Lang(s):** English, French. **Desc:** Homeopathic physicians and other individuals with an interest in homeopathy. Seeks to advance the study and practice of homeopathy; encourages ongoing professional development of members. Serves as a forum for the exchange of information among homeopathic physicians; sponsors research and educational programs.


**★ 4242 ★ Center for Attitudinal Healing (CAH)**
33 Buchanan Dr.
Sausalito, CA 94965
**Phone:** (415)331-6161          **Fax:** (415)331-4545
**Email:** cah@well.com
**Website:** http://www.healingcenter.org
Don Goewey, Exec. Dir.
**Fnded:** 1975. **Mem:** 12,000. **Desc:** Nonsectarian organization established to supplement traditional health care by offering free services in attitudinal healing for both children and adults with life-threatening illnesses, loss, or other crises. (The concept of attitudinal healing is based on the belief that it is possible to choose peace rather than conflict, and love rather than fear; the center defines health as inner peace and healing as the process of letting go of fear.) Offers support groups and arranges home and hospital visits for children, youth, and adults. Offers volunteer training program. Maintains speakers' bureau; conducts educational programs and charitable activities. **Pub:** *Advice to Doctors and Other Big People*. Book. • *Another Look at the Rainbow*. Book. • *Rainbow Connection*, 3/year. Newsletter. • *There is a Rainbow Behind Every Dark Cloud*. Book.


**★ 4243 ★ China Academy of Traditional Chinese Medicine**
18 Beixincang, Dongzhimennai
Beijing 100900, People's Republic of China
**Phone:** 852 10 446661


**★ 4244 ★ Citizens for Health**
1400 16th St. NW, Ste. 330
Washington, DC 20036-2222
**Free:** 800-357-2211
**Email:** cfh@citizens.org
**Website:** http://www.citizens.org
Susan Haeger, Pres. /CEO
**Fnded:** 1992. **Local Groups:** 150. **Desc:** Committed to protecting and expanding consumers natural health choices. Initiates and monitors legislation with the goal of ensuring access to health information and the freedom to choose from a broad range of health options. **Pub:** *Action Alert*, periodic. Bulletin. • *FAX Hotline*. • *The Natural Activist*, bimonthly. Newsletter. *Price:* Included in full member dues.


**★ 4245 ★ College of Phytotherapy**
Bucksteep Manor
Bodle St. Green
Hailsham BN27 4RJ, United Kingdom
**Phone:** 44 1323 834800      **Fax:** 44 1323 834801
**Email:** medherb@pavilion.co.uk.school
**Website:** http://www.geocities.com/HotSprings/Chalet/2436
**Fnded:** 1982. **Mem:** 500. **Desc:** Runs a training school for practitioners of phytotherapy (herbal medicine) incorporating a 4 year Bachelor of Science degree course, a 5-year BSC Degree Distance Learning Course, specially structured course for practising general practitioners, plus a one-year basic home study course. **Pub:** *British Journal of Phytotherapy*, semiannual. Journal. • *Training for a Career in Herbal Medicine*, annual. **Frmly:** (1999) School of Phytotherapy.


**★ 4246 ★ Committee for Freedom of Choice in Medicine (CFCM)**
1180 Walnut Ave.
Chula Vista, CA 91911
**Phone:** (619)429-8200          **Free:** 800-227-4473
**Fax:** (619)429-8004
**Email:** cfcm@americanbiologics.com
**Website:** http://www.americanbiologies.com
Robert W. Bradford, DSC, Founder/Pres.
**Fnded:** 1972. **Mem:** 30,000. **Local Groups:** 30. **Desc:** Purpose is to support freedom of choice for any therapy which shows clear evidence of efficacy and to prohibit the interference of government or any third party in the relationship between an informed patient and his or her physician. Activities include publishing information to keep members apprised of the latest developments in research and treatment, directing people with questions concerning alternative therapy to physicians in their areas, maintaining an information service for physicians interested in expanding their knowledge of metabolic/nutritional treatment, and providing educational exhibits for programs and seminars being conducted by various medical groups. Conducts research; compiles statistics on people with degenerative diseases who have been treated with metabolic therapy. Operates speakers' bureau. **Pub:** *Choice Magazine*, quarterly. Magazine. Includes science corner and heart, cancer, drug, and court watch sections. *Price:* Included in membership dues. • Audiotapes. • Books. • Brochures. • Pamphlets. • Reprints. •


Videos. **Frmly:** (1985) Committee for Freedom of Choice in Cancer Therapy.


**★ 4247 ★ Complementary Medicine Association (CMA)**
c/o Mary Wolken-Rodriguez
4649 E Malvern
Tucson, AZ 85711-4249
**Phone:** (602)323-6291          **Fax:** (602)323-0264
**Email:** compmeded@aol.com
Mary Wolken-Rodriguez, Exec. Off.
**Fnded:** 1990. **Mem:** 80. **Desc:** Provides education and supports cooperation between all medical disciplines. Fosters and teaches cost effective and more natural systems of medicine to professionals and the public. Focuses on homeopathic, acupuncture, herbal medicines, kinesiology and learning/memory improvement research and education. **Pub:** *Complementary Health*, annual. Journal. Holistic scientific publication.


**★ 4248 ★ Confederation of Complementary Health Association of South Africa (COCHASA)**
c/o Hugh St John Thomson
PO Box 2471
Clareinch 7740, Republic of South Africa
**Phone:** 27 83 4419407
**Email:** institute@kushido.co.za
**Desc:** Seeks to provide a consultative service to its member Associations. Promotes a wider understanding of complementary therapies to the public.


**★ 4249 ★ Council of Colleges of Acupuncture and Oriental Medicine (CCAOM)**
7501 Greenway Center Dr., Ste. 820
Greenbelt, MD 20770
**Phone:** (301)313-0868          **Fax:** (301)313-0869
**Email:** ccaom@compuserve.com
**Website:** http://www.ccaom.org
David Sale, Exec. Dir.
**Fnded:** 1982. **Mem:** 45. **Desc:** Acupuncture and oriental medicine colleges. Purposes are: to advance the status of acupuncture and oriental medicine through educational programs; to provide high-quality classroom and clinical instruction; to promote the improvement of research and teaching methods. **Pub:** Newsletter, annual. **Frmly:** (1992) National Council of Acupuncture Schools and Colleges.


**★ 4250 ★ Craniosacral Therapy Association of North America (CSTNA)**
710 Mountainview Pl.
Newmarket, ON, Canada L3Y 3P7
**Email:** info@craniosacraltherapy.org
**Website:** http://www.craniosacraltherapy.org
**Fnded:** 1998. **Desc:** Craniosacral therapists and students. Maintains high professional standards for practitioners, teachers, and students of biodynamic craniosacral therapy. Offers referral service. **Pub:** Membership Directory. • Newsletter, periodic.


**★ 4251 ★ Craniosacral Therapy Association of the UK**
Monomark House
27 Old Gloucester St.
London WC1N 3XX, United Kingdom
**Email:** info@craniosacral.co.uk
**Website:** http://www.craniosacral.co.uk
**Desc:** Craniosacral therapy practitioners in the United Kingdom. **Pub:** *The Fulcrum*, periodic. Journal.


**★ 4252 ★ Dinshah Health Society (DHS)**
PO Box 707
Malaga, NJ 08328-0707
**Phone:** (856)692-4686          **Fax:** (856)696-7890
**Email:** dinshahhealth@aol.com
**Website:** http://www.dinshahhealth.org/
Darius Dinshah, Pres.

**Fnded:** 1975. **Mem:** 3,794. **Desc:** Health professionals and other interested individuals who use and promote chromopathy as a therapy. Chromopathy, or color therapy, involves the use of projected colors of light to treat specific health problems. Seeks to stimulate interest in and knowledge of chromopathy and other lesser-known therapies. **Pub:** *Let There Be Light.* Book. *Price:* $15; $12. • Newsletter, 3-5/year.

**★ 4253 ★ East West Academy of Healing Arts (EWAHA)**
117 Topaz Way
San Francisco, CA 94108
**Phone:** (415)288-9400          **Fax:** (415)647-5745
**Email:** eastwestqi@aol.com
**Website:** http://www.eastwestqi.com
Dr. Effie Chow, Pres.

**Fnded:** 1973. **Desc:** Promotes holistic health, Qigong, and Oriental medicine. Sponsors educational and research programs; provides clinical services.

**★ 4254 ★ Faculty of Homeopathy**
15 Clerkenwell Close
London EC1R 0AA, United Kingdom
**Phone:** 44 20 75667800     **Fax:** 44 20 75667815
**Email:** info@trusthomeopathy.org
**Website:** http://www.trusthomeopathy.org
**Fnded:** 1950. **Mem:** 1,200. **Desc:** Professional body responsible for regulating the education, training and practice of homeopathy by medically qualified doctors, veterinary surgeons, dentists, pharmacists and other statutorily registered health care professionals. Accredited post-graduate training courses lead to the LFHom qualification and, for doctors and vets, medical/veterinary membership of the faculty. **Pub:** *British Homeopathic Journal*, quarterly. Journal.

**★ 4255 ★ Federation of Natural Medicine Users in North America**
c/o Christine Murphy
PO Box 237
Congers, NY 10920-0237
**Phone:** (845)268-2627          **Fax:** (845)268-2764
**Website:** http://fonmuna.org
Christine Murphy, Contact

**Fnded:** 1995. **Desc:** Supports and expands education and research into health care practices using an anthroposophical, or holistic approach. Liaison among health professionals. Studies groups in various geographical areas. Provides self-help instruction for lay people.

**★ 4256 ★ Flower Essence Society (FES)**
PO Box 459
Nevada City, CA 95959
**Phone:** (530)265-9163          **Free:** 800-736-9222
**Fax:** (530)265-0584
**Email:** mail@flowersociety.org
**Website:** http://www.flowersociety.org
Patricia A. Kaminski, Pres.

**Fnded:** 1979. **Mem:** 5,000. **Desc:** Project of Earth-Spirit Inc. Health centers, holistic health practitioners, and interested individuals. Seeks to increase public awareness of Nature and the evolving spiritual relationship between human beings and the earth. Promotes the use of flower essences as catalysts to health and important tools "for personal and planetary evolution." Seeks to establish a worldwide network among health practitioners and others using flower essences. Encourages intuitive and scientific investigation of the essences and the creation of a center for educational and research programs. Organizes introductory weekends and annual week-long intensives for professional and lay health practitioners. Sponsors lectures and research, educational, and experimental activities on topics concerning scientific and spiritual approaches to nature, preparation and use of flower essences, practical skills for flower essence practitioners, and recent developments in the field. Maintains library and referral service. Conducts seven-day professional training seminar and wildflower preservation and naturalist program. **Pub:** *Flower Essence Reper-*

*tory.* Books. *Price:* $19.95. • *Flower Essence Society–Members' Newsletter,* 1-2/year. Newsletter. Includes book reviews, calendar of events, and research updates. *Price:* Included in membership dues. • Also publishes informational flyer series. **AKA:** Earth-Spirit, Inc.

**★ 4257 ★ Fook Sang Acupuncture and Chinese Herbal Practitioners Association**
c/o Dr. Ac B.K. Lee
590 Wokingham Rd.
Earley
Reading RG6 7HN, United Kingdom
**Website:** http://www.fooksang.co.uk
**Desc:** Aims to further a genuine traditional Chinese Medical standards in the U.K.

**★ 4258 ★ Foundation for Advancement in Cancer Therapy (FACT)**
Box 1242, Old Chelsea Sta.
New York, NY 10113
**Phone:** (212)741-2790          **Fax:** (212)924-3634
**Website:** http://www.fact-ltd.org
Ruth Sackman, Pres.
**Fnded:** 1971. **Mem:** 2,500. **Reg. Groups:** 1. **Desc:** Believes that cancer is a symptom of imbalance in body chemistry; thus, to control the disease, not only must any tumors be destroyed, but the body must also be regenerated through the "total person approach" which emphasizes nutrition, detoxification, and mind-body cohesion. Asserts the right of the public to be informed of the "nontoxic biological" adjuncts and alternatives to surgery, chemotherapy, and radiotherapy, but cautions that patients be discriminating; disseminates information concerning only those preventive schemes and nontoxic therapies that have been verified as "safe" by long-term clinical tests. Does not intend to discredit traditional therapies, but to complement them; works cooperatively with established practitioners and instit utions. Seeks the elimination of carcinogens from the environment; supports cancer and nutrition research and compiles statistics; maintains speakers' bureau. **Pub:** *Cancer Forum*, bimonthly. Magazine. **Frmly:** (1988) Foundation for Alternative Cancer Therapies.

**★ 4259 ★ G-Jo Institute**
PO Box 1460
Columbus, NC 28722-1460
**Phone:** (828)863-4660
**Email:** office@g-jo.com
**Website:** http://www.g-jo.com
Michael Blate, Exec. Dir.
**Fnded:** 1977. **Mem:** 3,000. **Desc:** People interested in "self-health" techniques that are natural, require no drugs or medications, and are based on traditional Oriental healing philosophies, especially acupuncture and acupressure. Objective is to promote the use of self-health techniques. Makes available charts and teaching guides. Provides classes in self-health methods and natural (vegetarian) cooking. Conducts radio program and research on natural health and healing. Sponsors Vegetarian Gourmet Society. Institute derives name from G-Jo, the easiest form of acupressure. Publishes self-health reports.

**★ 4260 ★ General Council and Register of Naturopaths**
Goswell House
2 Goswel Rd.
Somerset BA16 0JG, United Kingdom
**Phone:** 44 1458 840072     **Fax:** 44 1458 840075
**Email:** admin@naturopathy.org.uk
**Website:** http://www.naturopathy.org.uk
**Fnded:** 1964. **Mem:** 325. **Desc:** Fully qualified naturopathic practitioners. Maintains educational, professional and ethical standards and the safe practice of naturopathy for the benefit and protection of the public. **Pub:** Membership Directory, annual.

**★ 4261 ★ German Association of Non-Medical Practitioners (Verband Deutscher Heilpraktiker)**
Ernst-Grote-Str. 13
D-30916 Isernhagen, Germany
**Phone:** 49 511 616980     **Fax:** 49 511 6169920
**Fnded:** 1963. **Mem:** 3,250. **Desc:** Promotes and protects the interests of non-medical health practitioners. Seeks to raise public awareness of holistic medicine.

**★ 4262 ★ Gerson Institute (GI)**
1572 Second Ave.
San Diego, CA 92101
**Phone:** (619)685-5353          **Free:** 888-4-GERSON
**Fax:** (619)685-5359
**Email:** mail@gerson.org
**Website:** http://www.gerson.org
Charlotte Gerson, Pres.

**Fnded:** 1977. **Mem:** 3,000. **Desc:** Individuals interested in health information. Purpose is to educate the public on nutritional health and to disseminate information about the Gerson therapy for healing. (The Gerson therapy was developed by Max Gerson, M.D., and seeks to prevent disease as well as to restore the natural healing mechanism in patients suffering from cancer and other degenerative diseases without the use of standard toxic therapies. Therapy includes a detoxification program to help the body eliminate toxins and waste materials that interfere with metabolism and healing and an intensive nutrition program.) Acts as consultant to operating physicians at hospital near Tijuana, Mexico; assists and trains physicians who want to learn the Gerson therapy. Presents lectures on health; conducts medical and nutritional research. **Pub:** *A Cancer Therapy - Results of 50 Cases.* Includes historical reviews and therapy details. *Price:* $25/year inside U.S.; $30/year outside U.S. • *Censored for Curing Cancer.* • *Healing Newsletter*, bimonthly. Newsletter. • Videos.

**★ 4263 ★ Health Optimizing Institute (HOI)**
PO Box 1233
Del Mar, CA 92014
**Phone:** (858)481-7751          **Fax:** (858)481-7751
**Email:** year2020vision@earthlink.net
Dr. Joseph Watson, Exec. Officer

**Fnded:** 1978. **Desc:** Disseminates information on holistic and alternative health therapies aimed at building the human immune system and reversing the aging process. Conducts research and training programs in energy medicine. **Pub:** *Chronicle of Holistic Health.* Journal. **Frmly:** National Center for the Exploration of Human Potential.

**★ 4264 ★ Herbal Association of South Africa (HAOSA)**
PO Box 1831, Escourt
Kwazulu 3310, Republic of South Africa
**Phone:** 27 33 2631227     **Fax:** 27 33 2631277
**Email:** jinxsnuf@futurest.co.za
**Website:** http://www.naturalhealth.co.za/ASSOC/ass_214.html
**Fnded:** 1991. **Desc:** Aims to provide an umbrella body. Provides an educational forum by teaching about herbs. Reduces the high cost of healthcare. Unites those interested in herbs.

**Holistic Dental Association (HDA)**
*See:* Entry 6530

**★ 4265 ★ Homeopathic Council for Research and Education (HCRE)**
c/o William Bergman, M.D.
37th St.
New York, NY 10016
**Phone:** (212)684-2290          **Fax:** (212)684-4694
**Email:** hda@frontier.net
**Website:** http://www.holisticdental.org
William Bergman, MD, Contact

**Fnded:** 1965. **Mem:** 5. **Desc:** Physicians and scholars united to encourage research and education in homeopathy. Endows and supervises homeopathic research and education.

★ **4266** ★ **Homeopathic Pharmacopoeia of the U.S.**
PO Box 2221
Southeastern, PA 19399-2221
**Phone:** (610)783-5124　　　**Fax:** (610)783-5180
John A. Borneman, III, Pres.

**Fnded:** 1980. **Mem:** 75. **Desc:** Prepares, publishes and distributes the Homeopathic Pharmacopoeia of the US. **Pub:** *Homeopathic Pharmacopoeia of the U.S.*.

★ **4267** ★ **Homeopaths Without Borders**
PO Box 570
Bolinas, CA 94924
**Phone:** (415)868-2950
**Email:** nkelly@igc.org
**Website:** http://www.homeopathy.org/

**Fnded:** NNas. **Mem:** soci,ate. **Desc:** Homeopaths working in other countries to improve health. **Pub:** *The American Homeopath*, annual. Journal. *Price:* 20 percent discount to members. • *NASH News*, quarterly. Newsletter.

★ **4268** ★ **Hygienic Community Network (HCN)**
c/o Helen Jean Story
PO Box 277
Boulder Creek, CA 95006-0277
**Phone:** (831)425-1292
Helen Jean Story, Newsletter Editor

**Fnded:** 1980. **Mem:** 100. **Reg. Groups:** 1. **Desc:** Individuals interested in gaining the healthful benefits of a lifestyle, known as natural hygiene, which includes: diets of mostly raw fruits, vegetables, nuts, and seeds; pursuit of fulfilling jobs and relationships; beneficial fasting; adequate rest, sunshine, and clean air and water; enjoyment of natural phenomena. Supports cooperative living and develops communities where natural hygiene is practiced; disseminates information on existing and proposed communities; provides networking services for individuals wishing to meet others with similar interests who are practicing natural hygiene. **Pub:** *Hygienic Community Network News*, bimonthly. Newsletter. Includes book reviews and letters from readers. *Price:* Included in membership dues.

★ **4269** ★ **Institute for Advanced Research in Asian Science and Medicine (IARASM)**
PO Box 555
Garden City, NY 11530
**Email:** admin@AJCM.org
Dr. John J. Kao, MD, Contact

**Fnded:** 1972. **Desc:** Purpose is to advance international understanding between Asia and the West in the areas of science, medical systems, and health care delivery. Serves as a clearinghouse for international scholarly efforts in the comparative study of science and medicine. Provides consulting services and mediation of scientific and biomedical exchange with Asian countries. Assists in generating innovative curricula in medical education; translates contemporary and classical Asian scientific and medical literature; provides training for medical professionals in acupuncture therapeutics. **Pub:** *American Journal of Chinese Medicine*, 3/year. Journal. Publishes original articles and essays related to traditional or ethnomedicine of all cultures. *Price:* $130 subscription price for 2001 vol. 29.

★ **4270** ★ **Institute for Complementary Medicine (ICM)**
PO Box 194
London SE16 7QZ, United Kingdom
**Phone:** 44 20 23775165　　**Fax:** 44 20 23775175
**Email:** icm@icmedicine.co.uk

**Website:** http://www.icmedicine.co.uk
**Fnded:** 1982. **Mem:** 6,000. **Lang(s):** English. **Desc:** Registered charity of individuals united to promote the practice of alternative medicine. Seeks to establish educational standards for practitioners and to establish ties between therapy groups, organizations, teachers, and practitioners. Cooperates with the British government to develop natural therapy curricula. Maintains British Register of Complementary Practitions. Conducts research; disseminates information. Advises groups establishing healing practices on legal, organizational, and practical matters. **Pub:** *Journal for Complementary Medicine*, semiannual. Journal. • *Newsletter*, quarterly. Newsletter. Supplement to journal.

★ **4271** ★ **Institute of Holistic Therapies**
PO Box 37
Scarborough YO11 1AR, United Kingdom
**Phone:** 44 1723 378573　　**Fax:** 44 1723 378573
**Email:** lnroche@talk21.com

**Fnded:** 1989. **Mem:** 1,200. **Nat'l Groups:** 1. **Desc:** Qualified holistic practitioners only. Provides indemnity and malpractice insurance cover and a register of all qualified professional holistic therapists who have satisfactorily completed a recognised study course worldwide.

★ **4272** ★ **International Acupuncture Institute**
301 Nathan Rd., Rm. 1304
Hong Kong, People's Republic of China
**Phone:** 852 27711066　　**Fax:** 852 23888836
**Fnded:** 1978. **Mem:** 700. **Nat'l Groups:** 2. **Lang(s):** Chinese, English. **Desc:** Acupuncturists and other health care professionals; individuals with an interest in acupuncture. Promotes effective practice of acupuncture; devises and maintains standards of practice. Conducts research and educational programs. **Pub:** *Clinical Acupuncture*. Book.

★ **4273** ★ **International Aromatherapy and Herb Association**
c/o Jeffrey Schiller
3541 W Acapulco Ln.
Phoenix, AZ 85053-4625
**Phone:** (602)938-4439
**Email:** jeffreys@aztec.asu.edu
**Website:** http://www.aztec.asu.edu/makingscents
Jeffrey Schiller, Pres.

**Fnded:** 1996. **Mem:** 300. **Desc:** People interested in aromatherapy, herbs and natural health. **Pub:** *Making Scents*, semiannual. Magazine. Includes article of interest, resource lists, and book and product reviews.

★ **4274** ★ **International Association for Dance Medicine and Science (IADMS)**
1214 University of Oregon
Department of Dance
Eugene, OR 97403-1214
**Fax:** (541)465-1763
**Email:** executivedirector@iadms.org
**Website:** http://www.iadms.org
Steven J. Chatfield, PhD, Exec. Dir.

**Fnded:** 1990. **Mem:** 600. **Desc:** Serves as a forum for reeducation, promotion of research and public services in the field of dance medicine and science. Committed to providing continuing education for the dance and medical communities as well as the public regarding appropriate training for dance. Offers educational programs. **Pub:** *The Dance Medicine/Science Bibliography*. Bibliography. Listing of all English language dance medicine articles (from 1975 to the present). *Price:* $45. • *IADMS Newsletter*, quarterly. Newsletter. Offers information of recent activities both within the organization and the dance medicine field in general. • *Journal of Dance Medicine/Science*, quarterly. Journal. Peer-reviewed medical journal.

★ **4275** ★ **International Association of Hygienic Physicians (IAHP)**
4620 Euclid Blvd.
Youngstown, OH 44512
**Phone:** (330)788-0526　　　**Fax:** (330)788-0093
**Email:** boar_mah@access-k12.org
**Website:** http://www.cisnet.com/iahp
Mark A. Huberman, Sec. -Treas.

**Fnded:** 1978. **Mem:** 45. **Desc:** Doctors of medicine, osteopathy, chiropractic, and naturopathy who specialize in the supervision of therapeutic fasting as part of a natural hygiene regimen. Promotes clinical advancement and ethical responsibility. Works for the health freedom of members. Provides certification for professionals and accreditation for schools and training programs; offers internship programs. Funds research. **Pub:** *IAHP Newsletter*, quarterly. Newsletter. Includes association news, bibliography, book reviews, case studies, Medical journal reviews, and reports from foreign countries. *Price:* Included in membership dues. **Frmly:** (1995) International Association of Professional Natural Hygienists.

★ **4276** ★ **International Association of Spiritual Psychiatry (IASP)**
Villa Alcedonia, 486, Chemin des Combattants
A.F.N
F-06140 Vence, France
**Phone:** 33 4 93585353　　　**Fax:** 33 4 93585363
**Email:** info@essence-euro.org
**Website:** essence-euro.org
**Fnded:** 1994. **Desc:** Integrates the spiritual dimension in medicine, psychology and psychiatry.

★ **4277** ★ **International College of Applied Kinesiology - U.S.A. (ICAK-U.S.A.)**
6405 Metcalf Ave., Ste. 503
Shawnee Mission, KS 66202-3929
**Phone:** (913)384-5336　　　**Fax:** (913)384-5112
**Email:** icak@dci-kansascity.com
**Website:** http://www.icakusa.com
Andria Dibbern, Membership Services

**Fnded:** 1975. **Mem:** 700. **Desc:** Promotes the science of applied kinesiology. Applied Kinesiology is the system of evaluating the structural, chemical, and mental aspect of human heath, involving muscle health, nutrition, manipulation, diet, acupressure, and exercise. Conducts educational programs, research programs, and training seminars. **Pub:** *Membership Directory*, annual. *Price:* $16/issue. **Frmly:** (2002) International College of Applied Kinesiology.

★ **4278** ★ **International Committee of Homeopathic Pharmacists (Comite International des Pharmaciens Homeopathiques — CIPH)**
c/o Emile Devey
Laboratories Boiron
Avenida Aldelaparra 27
Alcobendas
E-28100 Madrid, Spain
**Phone:** 349 1 6614615

**Fnded:** 1955. **Mem:** 73. **Lang(s):** English, French, German. **Desc:** Homeopathic pharmacists in 21 countries. **Pub:** *Annual Report.* • *Circular Letter*, semiannual. • *Draft of an International Homeopathic Pharmacopeia.*

★ **4279** ★ **International Federation of Aromatherapists**
182 Chiswick High Rd.
London W4 1PP, United Kingdom
**Phone:** 44 208 7422605　　**Fax:** 44 208 7422606
**Email:** i.f.a@ic24.net
**Website:** http://www.int-fed-aromatherapy.co.uk
**Fnded:** 1985. **Mem:** 2,000. **Reg. Groups:** 8. **Desc:** Professional aromatherapists, people with an interest in aromatherapy and complementary medicine. Represents and insures qualified aromatherapy practitioners. Acts as a watchdog for its registered members

and for the general public; keeps members up to date with new developments within the field of aromatherapy. **Pub:** *Aromatherapy Times*, quarterly. Newsletter.

★ **4280** ★ **International Federation of Associations of Defense in Phytotherapy, Research and Teaching (Federation internationale des Associations de defense, de recherche et d'enseignement de la phytotherapie — FIADREP)**
19, bd de Beausejour
F-75016 Paris, France
**Email:** sfpa@club-internet.fr
**Website:** perso.club-internet.fr/sfpa/

**Desc:** Carries out research on phytotherapy, aromatherapy or other natural medicinal techniques, biological or physical, for the improvement of health.

★ **4281** ★ **International Foundation of Oriental Medicine**
PO Box 640032
Flushing, NY 11364-0032
**Phone:** (718)886-4431          **Fax:** (718)463-0808
Dr. David P. J. Hung, Pres.

**Fnded:** 1989. **Desc:** Conducts research and public education programs on the use of oriental medicine (acupressure, acupuncture, chi-kong, and herbs). Offers fellowships and scholarships in oriental arts, medicine, and philosophy and Christian religion. Promotes East/West exchange. Conducts lectures and seminars; maintains speakers' bureau. Operates library and referral service. Plans to issue publications.

★ **4282** ★ **International Homeopathic Medical League**
134 Blvd. Leopold II
B-1080 Brussels, Belgium
**Phone:** 32 2 4140108          **Fax:** 32 2 4101600
**Email:** jimberex@cyclone.be
**Website:** http://www.lmhi.org.mx

**Fnded:** 1925. **Desc:** Creates links between homeopathic trained doctors, surgeons and pharmacists. Promotes scientific research.

★ **4283** ★ **International Institute for Bioenergetic Analysis (IIBA)**
155 Main St., Ste. 304
Brewster, NY 10509
**Phone:** (845)279-8474          **Fax:** (845)279-8402
**Email:** iibanet@aol.com
**Website:** http://www.bioenergetic-therapy.com
John Bustelos, Jr., Exec. Dir.

**Fnded:** 1956. **Mem:** 1,700. **Reg. Groups:** 50. **Desc:** Works to promote research and education in the fields of mental and physical health as they relate to biological energy processes. Areas of interest include: the role of muscle tension in emotional and physical illness, relationship of body structure and body movement, energy dynamics, disturbances in motility as a factor in illness, genetic factors, principles and methods of therapy, and growth and development of the child in response to patterns of child rearing. Conducts lectures, 1-day patient workshops, professional weekend workshops, seminars, and exercise classes. **Pub:** *Bioenergetic Analysis*, periodic. Journal. • Books. • Brochures. • Membership Directory, periodic. • Papers. **Frmly:** (1979) Institute for Bioenergetic Analysis.

★ **4284** ★ **International Institute of Reflexology**
5650 1st Ave. N
PO Box 12642
Saint Petersburg, FL 33733-2642
**Phone:** (727)343-4811          **Fax:** (727)381-2807
**Email:** ftreflex@concentric.net
**Website:** http://www.reflexology-usa.net/

**Desc:** Promotes the ancient art of reflexology, scientifically based on the premise that there are zones and reflex areas in the feet and hands which correspond to all glands, organs, parts and systems of the body.

★ **4285** ★ **International Iridology Practitioner's Association (IIPA)**
c/o Central Office
PO Box 3334
Escondido, CA 92033
**Free:** 888-682-2208          **Fax:** 888-682-2208
**Email:** iipacentraloffice@netzero.net
**Website:** http://www.iridologyassn.org
Ellen Tart-Jensen, Pres.

**Fnded:** 1982. **Mem:** 300. **Desc:** Organization for professional Iridologists who study the eye for indications of body stresses that may influence health. Offers members educational classes aned information, conventions, research and certification. **Pub:** *IIPA Insights*. Newsletter. • *The Iridology Review*, quarterly. Article. Presents research in Irigology. **Frmly:** (1999) National Iridology Reserach Association; (2002) International Iridology Research Association.

★ **4286** ★ **International Palmtherapy Association**
PO Box 7453
Van Nuys, CA 91409-7453
**Phone:** (661)944-4909
**Email:** info@palmtherapy.com
**Website:** http://www.palmtherapy.com

**Fnded:** 1995. **Desc:** Dedicated to the research of the "hand/mind connection". Palm therapy is the art and practice of "enhancing optimum potential, self-growth, fulfillment and success in all aspects of life through the massage stimulation of specific lines and areas of the hand". Offers seminars.

★ **4287** ★ **International Photodynamic Association (IPA)**
c/o Prof. Patrick Barron
Tokyo Medical University
International Medical Communications Center
6-7-1 Nishishinjuku
Shinjuku-ku
Tokyo 160, Japan
**Phone:** 81 3 33425315          **Fax:** 81 3 33425307
**Email:** imcc@tokyo-med.ac.jp
**Website:** http://www.sante.univ-nantes.fr/med/laser/ipa.html

**Fnded:** 1986. **Mem:** 300. **Lang(s):** English. **Desc:** Clinicians and scientists worldwide involved in photodynamic therapy and photodiagnosis. Promotes the study of diagnosis and treatment using light and sensitizers and disseminates information to the medical community and the general public. Provides training.

★ **4288** ★ **International Society of Professional Aromatherapists**
ISPA House,
82 Ashby Rd.
Hinckley LE10 1SN, United Kingdom
**Phone:** 44 1455 637987          **Fax:** 44 1455 890956
**Email:** lisabrown@ispa.demon.co.uk
**Website:** http://www.the-ispa.org

**Fnded:** 1990. **Mem:** 2,300. **Nat'l Groups:** 1. **Desc:** Various categories of membership, the main group of which has trained with or meet the high standards required by ISPA accredited schools. Only full membership, members are entitled to use the letter MISPA. To develop and stimulate high professional standards, through qualification and practice. Accredited schools across the country. Local practitioner lists and public hot-line service. **Pub:** *Aromatherapy World*, quarterly. Journal. Also publishes conference transcripts.

★ **4289** ★ **International Society for the Study of Subtle Energies and Energy Medicine**
c/o C. Penny Hiernu
11005 Ralston Rd., Ste. 100D
Arvada, CO 80004
**Phone:** (303)425-4625          **Fax:** (303)425-4685
**Email:** issseem@cs.com
**Website:** http://www.issseem.org
C. Penny Hiernu, Exec. Dir.

**Fnded:** 1989. **Mem:** 1,350. **Desc:** Individuals interested in the study of human capacities and the role of consciousness in Nature. Offers educational programs. **Pub:** *Bridges*, quarterly. Magazine. Written for Clinicians. **Price:** $50. • *Subtle Energies and Energy Medicine*, 3/year. Journal.

★ **4290** ★ **Israeli Association of Creative and Expressive Therapies (ICET)**
c/o Hava Kamerinsky
PO Box 49002
IL-91491 Jerusalem, Israel
**Phone:** 972 2 5817232          **Fax:** 972 2 5817232
**Email:** micnelso@isdn.net.il
**Website:** http://www.yahat.org

**Fnded:** 1971. **Mem:** 1,500. **Local Groups:** 4. **Lang(s):** Hebrew. **Desc:** Music, dance movement, and art therapists. Fosters public awareness of the use of art therapies in the treatment and prevention of various dysfunctions. Provides educational and growth opportunities for therapy professionals. Establishes training standards; conducts workshops and lectures; maintains placement service; offers childrens' services. **Pub:** *ICET Information Bulletin*, periodic. Bulletin. Includes yearly directory. • *Therapy Through Arts*, 2-3/year. • Brochure. Yearly calendar and diary including phone directory. **Frmly:** (1997) Israeli Association of Creative-Extensive Therapy.

★ **4291** ★ **Jin Shin Do Foundation for Bodymind Acupressure (JSDF)**
32012 Sage Rd.
Hemet, CA 92544
**Phone:** (831)763-7702          **Fax:** (831)763-1551
**Email:** erma@ktn.net
**Website:** http://www.jinshindo.org
Iona Marsaa Teeguarden, Dir.

**Fnded:** 1982. **Mem:** 2,000. **Desc:** A referral and educational organization of teachers and practitioners of the Jin Shin Do acupressure method. (Jin Shin Do acupressure integrates a traditional Japanese acupressure technique with classical Chinese acutheory, Taoist philosophy and Qigong breathing exercises, and Western psychology.) Outlines tension points associated with common physical problems and distressing feelings, and teaches points and exercises that help release physical and emotional tensions. Conducts continuing education classes, practicums, and workshops for students. **Pub:** *A Complete Guide to Acupressure*. Book. • *Acupressure News*, annual. Newsletter. General association information; claps catalog; product catalog. **Price:** $2.50. • *The Acupressure Way of Health: Jin Shin Do*. Book. • *Directory of Registered Practitioners and Authorized Teachers*, annual. Directory. Includes listing of authorized basic, intermediate, and advanced teachers. **Price:** $1. • *Fundamentals of Self-Acupressure*. Booklet. • *Joy of Feeling: Bodymind Acupressure*. Book. • *JSD Strange Flows Wall Chart*.

★ **4292** ★ **Lok Swasthya Parampara Samvardhan (LSPSS)**
Ayurbedic Trust Campus
Trichy Rd.
PO Box 7102
Ramanathapuram
Coimbatore 641 045, Tamil Nadu, India
**Phone:** 91 422 311095          **Fax:** 91 422 314953
**Email:** lspss@md3.vsnl.net.in

**Fnded:** 1985. **Mem:** 1,214. **Lang(s):** English, Hindi. **Desc:** Village healers, midwives, folk practitioners, and other individuals interested in traditional healing methods. Seeks to revitalize folk traditions in areas including: childcare, nutrition, and home remedies for common ailments. Encourages the integration of folk medicine and organized health care systems in India. Cultivates medicinal gardens, forests, and nurseries. Fosters communication among members; gathers and disseminates information. **Pub:** *LSPSS Newsletter*, quarterly. Newsletter.

### ★ 4293 ★ Massage Therapy Association

c/o Sandra Williams
PO Box 53320
Kenilworth 7745, Republic of South Africa
**Phone:** 27 21 6715313
**Email:** swilliams@mtasa.co.za
**Website:** http://www.naturalhealth.co.za/ASSOC/ass_204.html

**Fnded:** 1989. **Desc:** Aims to ensure professional educational and training standards. Regulates the registration of certified therapists. Provides continued educational programs for certified therapists. Creates better public awareness and understanding of the benefits of massage.

### ★ 4294 ★ Metamorphic Association

67 Ritherdon Rd.
London SW17 8QE, United Kingdom
**Phone:** 44 208 6725951      **Fax:** 44 208 6725951
**Email:** metatech1@compuserve.com
**Website:** http://www.geocities.com/~metam

**Fnded:** 1979. **Mem:** 200. **Lang(s):** French, German, Italian, Spanish. **Desc:** Promotion of good health and well-being through awareness, understanding and use of Metamorphic Technique in the UK and internationally, and to uphold standards and procedures and teaching the technique. **Pub:** *The Programme*, semiannual. Newsletter. Listing of practioners and teachers: details of courses and events, publication list.

### National Acupuncture Detoxification Association (NADA)

*See:* Entry 19311

### ★ 4295 ★ National Association of Alternative Medicines (NAAM)

PO Box 35189
Chicago, IL 60707-0189
**Phone:** (708)453-0080      **Fax:** (708)453-0083
**Email:** naam@rentamark.com
**Website:** http://www.rentamark.com/naam/
L. Stollen, Contact

**Fnded:** 1975. **Mem:** 65,532. **Nat'l Groups:** 1. **Desc:** Practitioners of alternative medical specialties. Seeks to increase members' public visibility and professional influence. Provides member education; also provides trademark licensing and product and service endorsement services to support members' activities. A major platform for professional advancement and knowledge. **Pub:** *NAAM Journal*, monthly. Journal. • Journal, monthly. Invites authors to submit articles in Word format via email. *Price:* for members. **AKA:** (2000) American Alternative Medicine Association.

### ★ 4296 ★ National Association for Holistic Aromatherapy

4509 Interlake Ave., N, No. 233
Seattle, WA 98103
**Phone:** (314)963-2071      **Free:** 888-ASK-NAHA
**Fax:** (206)547-2680
**Email:** info@naha.org
**Website:** http://www.naha.org/
Jade Shutes, Pres.

**Fnded:** 1990. **Mem:** 1,600. **Nat'l Groups:** 7. **Reg. Groups:** 30. **Desc:** Seeks to establish and promote the art and science of aromatherapy as a health care alternative. Works to elevate and maintain high standards of aromatherapy eduction. Works to raise public awareness of the benefits of aromatherapy. Fosters communication and exchange among members. Offers educational programs. Maintains speakers' bureau. **Pub:** *Aromatherapy Journal*, quarterly. Newsletter. *Price:* $35/year. • *Membership and Practitioner Directory*, annual.

### ★ 4297 ★ National Board for Certified Clinical Hypnotherapists (NBCCH)

1110 Fidler Ln., Ste. L1
Silver Spring, MD 20910
**Phone:** (301)608-0123      **Free:** 800-449-8144
**Fax:** (301)588-9535
**Email:** nbcch@natboard.com
**Website:** http://www.natboard.com/

**Fnded:** 1991. **Desc:** Dedicated to professionalizing the mental health specialty/sub-specialty of hypnotherapy, including addictions, counselors, marriage and family therapists, mental health counselors, pastoral counselors, psychiatric nurse, physicians, psychiatrists, psychologists, school counselors, and social workers; promotes standards for certification; sponsors educational activities; promotes public and professional awareness; sponsors scientific investigation into the uses of hypnotherapy. **Pub:** *Interlink*. Newsletter.

### ★ 4298 ★ National Center for Complementary and Alternative Medicine (NCCAM)

PO Box 7923
Gaithersburg, MD 20898
**Phone:** (301)519-3153      **Free:** 888-644-6226
**Fax:** (866)464-3616
**Email:** info@nccam.nih.gov
**Website:** http://nccam.nih.gov/
Stephen E. Straus, MD, Dir.

**Fnded:** 1992. **Desc:** Committed to exploring complementary and alternative healing practices, including but not limited to acupuncture, herbs, homeopathy, therapeutic massage, and traditional oriental medicine; trains CAM researchers; conducts biomedical research; disseminates information. Programs focus on evaluating the safety and efficacy of natural products, supporting pharmacological studies to determine potential interactive effects with standard treatment medications, evaluates CAM practices such as acupuncture and chiropractic. Acts as the NCCAM Clearinghouse. **Pub:** Newsletter.Features CAM updates, NIH research news, and information from the NCCAM.

### ★ 4299 ★ National Center for Homeopathy (NCH)

801 N Fairfax St., Ste. 306
Alexandria, VA 22314
**Phone:** (703)548-7790      **Free:** 877-624-0613
**Fax:** (703)548-7792
**Email:** info@homeopathic.org
**Website:** http://www.homeopathic.org
Sharon Stevenson, Exec., Contact

**Fnded:** 1974. **Mem:** 6,000. **Desc:** Comprises: National Center for Instruction in Homeopathy and Homeotherapeutics, and Homeopathic Information Service. Purposes are: to promote the art of healing according to the natural laws of cure from a strictly homeopathic standpoint; to facilitate the study of homeopathy by the medical and allied health professions; to implement the study of homeopathic philosophy and principles among laypersons; to fund scientific research in the field. Sponsors introductory courses in homeopathy to licensed health care practitioners and laypersons; maintains speakers' bureau and library. **Pub:** *Homeopathy Today*, monthly. Newsletter. Covers membership activities. Includes calendar of events, employment opportunity and new member listings, and book reviews. *Price:* $40 in U.S.; $55 outside U.S. • *Membership Directory & Homeopathic Resource Guide*, biennial. Directory. *Price:* $10. • Brochures. • Pamphlets. • Reprints. • Also distributes Homeopathic Household Kit.

### ★ 4300 ★ National Certification Board for Therapeutic Massage and Bodywork (NCBTMB)

c/o Christine D. Niero
8201 Greensboro Dr., Ste. 300
Mc Lean, VA 22102
**Phone:** (703)610-9015      **Free:** 800-296-0664
**Fax:** (703)610-9005

**Email:** info@ncbtmb.com
**Website:** http://www.ncbtmb.com/
Christine D. Niero, PhD, Exec. Dir.

**Desc:** Massage and bodywork practitioners. Formed to set standards of ethical and professional practice through a credible credentialing program.

### ★ 4301 ★ National Certification Commission for Acupuncture and Oriental Medicine

11 Canal Center Plaza, Ste. 300
Alexandria, VA 22314
**Phone:** (703)548-9004      **Fax:** (703)548-9079
**Email:** info@nccaom.org
**Website:** http://www.nccaom.org
Debra A. Duncan, PhD, Contact

**Fnded:** 1982. **Mem:** 10,200. **Desc:** National certification agency for practitioners of acupuncture, Chinese herbology, and Asian bodywork therapy in the United States. Establishes and maintains standards of competence for the safe and effective practice of Oriental medicine; to evaluate an applicant's qualifications in relation to these established standards through the administration of national board examinations; to certify practitioners who meet these standards. Acts as consultant to state agencies in regulation, certification, and licensing of the practice of acupuncture and Oriental medicine. of acupuncture and Oriental medicine. **Pub:** *The Diplomate*, periodic. Newsletter. • *NCCAOM Directory of Diplomates*, annual. Directory. **Frmly:** (1997) National Commission for the Certification of Acupuncturists; (1998) National Commission for the Certification of Acupuncture and Oriental Medicine.

### ★ 4302 ★ National Federation of Spiritual Healers

Old Manor Farm Studio
Church St.
Sunbury-On-Thames TW16 6RG, United Kingdom
**Phone:** 44 1932 783164      **Fax:** 44 1932 779648
**Email:** office@nfsh.org.uk
**Website:** http://www.nfsh.org.uk

**Desc:** Spiritual Healers. **Pub:** *Healing Today*, quarterly. Magazine.

### ★ 4303 ★ National Institute of Medical Herbalists

56 Longbrook St.
Exeter EX4 6AH, United Kingdom
**Phone:** 44 1392 426022      **Fax:** 44 1392 498963
**Email:** nimh@ukexeter.freeserve.co.uk
**Website:** http://www.nimh.org.uk

**Fnded:** 1864. **Mem:** 550. **Desc:** Practitioners of herbal medicine. **Pub:** *European Journal of Herbal Medicine*, 3/year. Journal. • *Register of Members*. Directory.

### ★ 4304 ★ North American College of Botanical Medicine

1116 Park Ave. SW
Albuquerque, NM 87102-2941
**Phone:** (505)873-8107      **Fax:** (505)873-4530
**Email:** phyto@swcp.com
**Website:** http://www.swcp.com/botanicalmedicine
Dick Brillault, Board Pres.

**Fnded:** 1996. **Desc:** Dedicated to providing herbal education by training herbalists and providing information for health care professionals and the community.

### ★ 4305 ★ North American Society of Homeopaths (NASH)

1122 E Pike St., No. 1122
Seattle, WA 98122
**Phone:** (206)720-7000      **Fax:** (206)248-1942
**Email:** nashinfo@aol.com
**Website:** http://www.homeopathy.org/

**Desc:** Professional practitioners. Dedicated to the development and maintenance of homeopathic practice standards in North America. Strives to develop and support a qualified and certified homeopathic profession, distinct from, and in cooperation with other medical professionals; promotes individual's rights to receive homeopathic care. Provides certification and maintains register of those certified. Promotes public awareness of homeopathy. **Pub:** *The American Homeopath.* Journal. • *NASH News.* Newsletter.


★ 4306 ★ **Norwegian Association for Classical Acupuncture (NFKA) (Norsk Forening for Klassisk Akupunktur)**
St. Olavsgt. 12
N-0165 Oslo, Norway
**Phone:** 47 22 988140                    **Fax:** 47 22 361853
**Email:** nfka@akupunktur.no
**Website:** http://www.akupunktur.no
**Fnded:** 1978. **Mem:** 250. **Nat'l Groups:** 1. **Lang(s):** English, Norwegian. **Desc:** Doctors, nurses, dentists, and physiotherapists; students. Encourages the practice of acupuncture in Norway. Operates training institute for members. Conducts educational programs. **Pub:** *DE Qi-Tidsskrift for Kinesisk Medisin,* 3/year. Journal. Includes information on acupuncture and Chinese medicine. • Brochure, periodic.


★ 4307 ★ **Ohashi Institute (OI)**
147 W 25th St., 8th Fl.
New York, NY 10001-7205
**Phone:** (646)486-1187          **Free:** 800-810-4190
**Fax:** (646)486-1409
**Email:** ohashiinst@aol.com
**Website:** http://www.ohashi.com/institut.html
Wataru Ohashi, Dir.
**Fnded:** 1974. **Nat'l Groups:** 30. **State Groups:** 4. **Desc:** Dedicated to the promotion and teaching of the Oriental healing arts, specifically Ohashiatsu - a method of bodywork that elevates traditional Japanese shiatsu to a more complete experience of self-development and healing to promote health of body, mind and spirit. Program focuses on expanding awareness of self and others through the use of exercise, meditation and touch techniques based on Oriental healing philosophies. Courses for both laypeople and professionals in beginning, intermediate, advanced and post-graduate Ohashiatsu are offered. Instructor certification program available. Operates programs in the United States, South America and Europe. **Pub:** *Ohashiatsu News.* Newsletter. **Frmly:** (1983) Shiatsu Education Center of America.


★ 4308 ★ **Physicians Association for Anthroposophical Medicine (PAAM)**
1923 Geddes Ave.
Ann Arbor, MI 48104
**Phone:** (734)930-9462          **Fax:** (734)662-1727
**Email:** paam@anthroposophy.org
**Website:** http://www.paam.net
Christian Wessling, MD, Pres.
**Fnded:** 1982. **Mem:** 70. **Nat'l Groups:** 1. **Desc:** Physicians promoting the use and learning of anthroposophical medicine. Sponsors educational programs. **Pub:** *Directory of Physicians,* biennial. Directory. *Price:* Free. • *PAAM Newsletter,* biennial. Newsletter.


★ 4309 ★ **The Radiance Technique International Association**
PO Box 40570
Saint Petersburg, FL 33743
**Phone:** (727)347-2106          **Free:** 888-878-7733
**Fax:** (727)347-2106
**Email:** trtia@aol.com
**Website:** http://www.trtia.org
Shoshanna Shay, Dir. Office Services
**Fnded:** 1980. **Desc:** Protects and preserves the science known as The Radiance Technique, an Authentic Reiki "science of universal energy which harmonizes and aligns the mind-body-spirit dynamic." Provides a network for those interested in The Radiance Technique. Maintains speakers' bureau. Compiles statistics and conducts research on the effectiveness of The Radiance Technique. Creates and promotes Radiant Peace Projects and sponsors the International Day of Radiant Peace on June 22 every year. **Pub:** *TRTIA Journal,* 3/year. Newsletter. *Price:* Included in membership dues. **Frmly:** (1980) American Reiki Association; (1987) American-International Reiki Association; (1997) Radiance Technique Association International; (1998) Radiance Technique and Peace Association International.


★ 4310 ★ **Reiki Alliance**
PO Box 41
Cataldo, ID 83810
**Phone:** (208)783-3535          **Fax:** (208)783-4848
**Email:** info@reikialliance.com
**Website:** http://www.reikialliance.com
Betty Didcoct, Acting Exec. Dir.
**Fnded:** 1983. **Mem:** 750. **Desc:** Teachers of Reiki, the Usui System of Reiki Healing. Supports teachers of the Usui System Of Reiki Healing in 40 countries. Promotes exchange among teachers and students; provides member referrals; supports workshops for additional teacher training. Sponsors annual Global Gathering. **Pub:** *Reiki Alliance Membership Newsletter,* 3/year. Newsletter. *Price:* Included in membership dues. • *Student Book.* Book.


★ 4311 ★ **Rolf Institute (RI)**
205 Canyon Blvd.
Boulder, CO 80302
**Phone:** (303)449-5903          **Free:** 800-530-8875
**Fax:** (303)449-5978
**Email:** info@rolf.org
**Website:** http://www.rolf.org
Lorraine Lombard, Contact
**Fnded:** 1971. **Mem:** 1,010. **Reg. Groups:** 14. **Desc:** Purposes are to: train and certify Rolfers and Movement Practitioners; serve the professional needs of members; inform the public about the benefits of Rolfing and Rolfing Movement Integration. (Rolfing is a technique devised by Dr. Ida P. Rolf, an American biochemist, for reordering the body to bring its major segments toward a vertical alignment.) Conducts research activities; maintains speakers' bureau. **Pub:** *Expressive Movement.* • *Healing Through Touch.* • *Ida Rolf Talks.* • *The Power of Balance.* • *Rolf Lines,* quarterly. *Price:* Only available to members of the Rolf Institute. • *Rolfing.* • *Rolfing and Physical Reality.* • *The Rolfing Experience.* • *Rolfing Stories of Personal Empowerment.* • Books. • Films. • Pamphlets. • Reprints. • Videos. **Frmly:** (1975) Ida P. Rolf Foundation for Structural Integration.


★ 4312 ★ **Scandinavian Association of Zone-Therapeutists (S.F.2.) (Skandinavisk Forening for Zoneterapeutes — S.F.2.)**
Krogholmgardsvej 50
DK-2950 Vedbaek, Denmark
**Phone:** 45 45890188          **Fax:** 45 45890188
**Fnded:** 1975. **Mem:** 500. **Lang(s):** Danish, English, German, Norwegian, Swedish. **Desc:** Zone therapy practitioners and students. (Zone therapy involves the division of the body into parts or zones. Certain zones are then studied and/or manipulated in order to maintain health or treat particular health problems.) Examines the impact of vitamins, minerals, and diet on health. Studies related therapeutic procedures. **Pub:** *Fodnoten.* Magazine. • *SFFF Medlemsblad,* periodic.


★ 4313 ★ **Society of Chiropractic Orthospinology**
8520 Hospital Dr.
Douglasville, GA 30134
**Phone:** (770)517-9921
**Email:** webmaster@orthospinology.org
**Website:** http://www.orthospinology.org/
Dr. Kirk Eriksen, Pres.
**Desc:** Doctors, student doctors, and patients. Promotes the Chiropractic approach for a healthy lifestyle, aims to increase understanding of the Orthospinology method. **Pub:** *Patient Brochure.* Brochure. *Price:* $2/psh, $10.


★ 4314 ★ **Society of Homeopaths**
4a Artizan Rd.
Northampton NN1 4HU, United Kingdom
**Phone:** 44 1604 621400          **Fax:** 44 1604 622622
**Email:** info@homeopathy-soh.org
**Website:** http://www.homeopathy-soh.org
**Fnded:** 1978. **Mem:** 2,706. **Desc:** Professional homeopaths on the Society's register. Aims to develop and maintain high standards for the practise of homeopathy and to promote public awareness of homeopathy. It also supports the establishment of education and training in homeopathy. **Pub:** *The Homoeopath Journal,* quarterly. Journal. • *Register of Professional Homoeopaths,* semiannual. • Newsletter, quarterly.


**Surfer's Medical Association**
*See:* Entry 2416


★ 4315 ★ **Touch for Health Kinesiology Association**
PO Box 392
New Carlisle, OH 45344-0392
**Phone:** (937)845-3404          **Free:** 800-466-8342
**Fax:** (937)845-3909
**Email:** admin@tfha.org
**Website:** http://www.tfhka.org
Gloria Godsey, Exec. Dir.
**Fnded:** 1974. **Mem:** 1,500. **Desc:** International network of independent instructors comprising laypersons, medical doctors, chiropractors, osteopaths, nurses, teachers, physical therapists, massage therapists, and other professionals. Promotes techniques for restoring natural energies and improving postural balance through muscle testing using applied kinesiology and acupressure points to improve muscle function and balance the body's energy. Stimulates trained professionals to utilize natural health care research techniques with laypeople and their associates, and disseminates information on research plans, methodology, and results of self-development programs in health care, both mental and physical. Increases the level of professional confidence and keeps interested instructors, trainers, laypeople, and those in the health care profession regularly and reliably informed on development in natural health care. Conducts research projects on Touch for Health methods and results. **Pub:** *Annual Meeting Journal,* annual. Journal. Compilation of papers presented at the annual meeting. *Price:* $30. • *Keeping in Touch,* quarterly. Newsletter. Includes coverage of research developments, book reviews, calendar of events tips for professionals, anecdotal reports, news of upcoming events. *Price:* $250 full page; $150 1/2 page; $75 1/4 page; $35 business card. • *Touch for Health Association Directory,* annual. Membership Directory. *Price:* $125 full page; $75 1/2 page; $50 1/4 page; $35 business card. • *Touch for Health Book.* Book. Reference manual. *Price:* $27.95. • *Touch for Health Folios. Price:* $24.95 full size; $19.95 pocket size. • *Touch for Health in Practice,* monthly. Newsletter. *Price:* Included w/ professional membership. • *Touch for Health Reference Chart. Price:* $34.95. **Frmly:** (1990) Touch for Health Foundation; (1993) Touch for Health Association of America; (1998) Touch for Health Association.


★ 4316 ★ **Upledger Institute (UI)**
11211 Prosperity Farms Rd., Ste. D-325
Palm Beach Gardens, FL 33410
**Phone:** (561)622-4771          **Free:** 800-233-5880
**Fax:** (561)622-4706
**Email:** upledger@upledger.com
**Website:** http://www.upledger.com
**Fnded:** 1985. **Desc:** Promotes complementary health care; provides educational and training courses to osteopathic physicians, medical doctors, dentists, nurses, doctors of Chiropractic, doctors of Oriental medicine, naturopathic physicians, psychiatric specialists, psychologists, physical therapists, occupational therapists, speech therapists, massage therapists, acupuncturists, and other professional bodyworkers. Maintains speakers bureau. **Pub:** *IAHP Connection.* Newsletter. • *UI UpDate.* Newsletter.

## ★ 4317 ★ Women's Association for Natural Medicinal Therapy

Private Mail Bag
Suva, Fiji
**Phone:** 679 315021        **Fax:** 679 315021
**Email:** wainimate@is.com.fj
**Fnded:** 1995. **Mem:** 30. **Lang(s):** English. **Desc:** Women practitioners of traditional medicine in Fiji, the Cook Islands, Naura, Kiribati, Tonga, Vanuatu, Papua New Guinea, the Solomon Islands, and Tahiti. Encourages: conservation of medicinal plants and their habitats; dissemination of information on traditional healing practices; communication among members; establishment of national traditional medicine associations.

## ★ 4318 ★ World Federation of Acupuncture-Moxibustion Societies (WFAS)

18 Beixincang
Beijing 100700, People's Republic of China
**Phone:** 852 10 64063648    **Fax:** 852 10 64013968
**Desc:** Promotes cooperation among acupuncture-moxibustion groups; develops the science of acupuncture-moxibustion.

## ★ 4319 ★ World Institute of Holistic Therapies

c/o Gabrielle Lesie
116 High St.
Ashland, OR 97520-0000
**Phone:** (541)552-9288      **Fax:** (541)552-9270
**Email:** admin@worldinstitute.net
**Website:** http://www.worldinstitute.net
Cheryl Rawson, Exec. Dir.
**Fnded:** 1997. **Mem:** 36. **Desc:** Seeks to implement a holistic approach for conscious living through education, research and service via a new understanding in consciousness, one which is reliant on the principle of self-responsibility. Implementation of this mission will be accomplished through the formation of partnerships with individuals and other organizations that work at the most advanced frontiers of education, research, healthcare and environmental health. Focused on creating a center of excellence for learning in areas that are key to our mission: experiential education, biological medicine, psychology of identity consciousness, and eco-development. By developing educational opportunities that promote a scientific understanding of the dynamic flow and interrelationship of all things, the institute desires to provide people with the tools to uplift their own lives, the lives of their families, the institutions that serve us, and by extension, the whole of humanity.

## ★ 4320 ★ Worldwide Aquatics Bodywork Association (WABA)

PO Box 889
Middletown, CA 95461
**Phone:** (707)987-3801      **Fax:** (707)987-9638
**Email:** info@waba.edu
**Website:** http://aspen.forest.net/waba/
**Desc:** Promotes the study, practice and teaching of Watsu and aquatic bodywork; maintains the Registry of the Worldwide Water Family.

## ★ 4321 ★ Zero Balancing Association (ZBA)

801 W Main St., Ste. 202
Charlottesville, VA 22903
**Phone:** (434)244-2458      **Fax:** (434)244-2645
**Email:** info@zerobalancing.com
**Website:** http://www.zerobalancing.com
**Fnded:** 1991. **Desc:** Promotes the teaching and practice of Zero-Balancing, the hands-on body/mind system designed to align body energy with the body's physical structure; strives to relieve physical and mental symptoms and improve quality of life. Offers educational courses. **Pub:** Articles.

## ★ 4322 ★ Zimbabwe National Traditional Healers Association (ZINATHA)

PO Box 116
Reliance House
Corner of Takcawira and Speke Ave.
Harare, Zimbabwe
**Phone:** 263 4 751902
**Fnded:** 1980. **Mem:** 45,000. **Desc:** Promotes public awareness of alternative medicine. Coordinates actions of the Ministry of Health of Zimbabwe and traditional healers. Disseminates information. **Pub:** *ZINATHA*. Booklet.

# Research Centers

## ★ 4323 ★ Columbia-Presbyterian Medical Center
### Richard and Hinda Rosenthal Center for Complementary and Alternative Medicine

Department of Rehabilitative Medicine
College of Physicians & Surgeons
Columbia University
630 W 168 St., Box 75
New York, NY 10032
**Phone:** (212)543-9542      **Fax:** (212)543-2845
**Website:** http://cpmcnet.columbia.edu/dept/rosenthal/
Fredi Kronenberg, PhD, Dir.
**Activities/Fields:** Complementary and alternative medicine, especially regarding effectiveness, safety and mechanisms of action. Research focuses on botanical medicine and traditional medicine systems.

## ★ 4324 ★ Columbia University
### Center for CAM Research in Aging

College of Physicians & Surgeons
630 W 168th St.
New York, NY 10032
**Phone:** (212)543-9542      **Fax:** (212)543-2845
**Website:** http://www.rosenthal.hs.columbia.edu
Fredi Kronenberg, PhD, Dir.
**Activities/Fields:** Dietary and herbal treatments in postmenopausal women.

## ★ 4325 ★ Duke University
### Duke Center for Integrative Medicine (DCIM)

DUMC Box 3022
Durham, NC 27710
**Phone:** (919)660-6801      **Free:** (866)313-0959
**Website:** http://dukehealth.org/health_services/integrative_medicine.asp
Tracy W. Gaudet, MD, Dir.
**Activities/Fields:** Integrative medicine, which combines the best of conventional Western medicine with mind-body-spirit approaches to health, and with complementary techniques (such as acupuncture and herbalism) that have proven efficacy.

## ★ 4326 ★ Hahnemannian Research Center, Inc.

18818 Teller Ave., Ste. 230
Irvine, CA 92612
**Phone:** (949)852-9038      **Fax:** (949)852-1353
**Email:** laiushshm@aol.com
**Website:** http://www.hahnemannian.com
Kattunilathu Oommen George, MD, Pres.
**Activities/Fields:** Homeopathic medicine and education, including biochemical analysis, micronutrition, Mother Tincture development, structural and degenerative studies, and deficiency detection (electromagnetic disturbances) with attention given to the emotional, mental, and physical aspects. **Pub:** *Hahnemannian Quarterly Publication*.

## Heart Disease Research Foundation
*See:* Entry 5098

## ★ 4327 ★ Holos Institutes of Health

5607 S 222nd Rd.
Fair Grove, MO 65648
**Phone:** (417)267-2900      **Fax:** (417)267-3102
**Email:** orme@normshealy.net
**Website:** http://www.rpbusa.org/hc2/index.asp
C. Norman Shealy, MD, Pres.
**Activities/Fields:** Clinical studies in holistic medicine with emphasis on neurochemical profiles and management of biochemical aspects of pain and stress. **Frmly:** Shealy Institutes of Health.

## ★ 4328 ★ Homeopathic Council for Research and Education

50 Park Ave.
New York, NY 10016
**Phone:** (212)684-2290      **Fax:** (212)684-4694
William Bergman, MD, Contact
**Activities/Fields:** Homeopathy, focusing on research and education.

## ★ 4329 ★ Institute of Noetic Sciences

PO Box 6007
Petaluma, CA 94955-6007
**Phone:** (707)775-3500      **Fax:** (707)781-7420
**Email:** schlitz@noetic.org
**Website:** http://www.noetic.org
Dr. Marilyn Schlitz, Res. Dir.
**Activities/Fields:** Nature and potential of the human mind and consciousness, particularly in the areas of exceptional human abilities, the mind/body link and healing, the role of intentionality, positive global change, and creative altruism. **Pub:** *Audiotapes, videotapes*. • *Connections*, 3/year. • *Noetic Sciences Book*. • *Noetic Sciences Review*, 3/year. • *Special reports*, periodically.

## ★ 4330 ★ Johns Hopkins University
### Center for Cancer Complementary Medicine

720 Rutland Ave.
Baltimore, MD 21205
**Website:** http://nccam.nih.gov/nccam/fi/research/desc.htmlcancer
Adrian S. Dobs, MD, Prin. Investigator
**Activities/Fields:** Complementary and alternative medicine (CAM) modalities for cancer.

## ★ 4331 ★ Kaiser Foundation Hospitals
### Oregon Center for Complementary and Alternative Medicine Research in Craniofacial Disorders

Center for Health Research
3800 N Interstate Ave.
Portland, OR 97227
**Phone:** (503)335-2400      **Fax:** (503)335-2424
**Email:** alex.white@kpchr.org
**Website:** http://www.kpchr.org/info/demo.htmloccam
B. Alexander White, DDS, Prin. Investigator
**Activities/Fields:** Potential, effectiveness, acceptability, effects on health care resource use, and psychosocial and other health outcomes associated with CAM practices for cranofacial disorders.

## ★ 4332 ★ Maharishi University of Management
### Center for Natural Medicine and Prevention

College of Maharishi Vedic Medicine
1000 N 4th St.
Fairfield, IA 52557
**Phone:** (641)472-1110      **Fax:** (641)472-1179
**Email:** rschneid@mum.edu
**Website:** http://www.mum.edu/cnmp/index.html
Robert H. Schneider, MD, Dir.
**Activities/Fields:** Prevention and treatment of major chronic illnesses. **Frmly:** Center for Health and Aging Studies.

**★ 4333 ★ Minneapolis Medical Research Foundation**
Center for Addiction and Alternative Medicine Research (CAAMR)
914 S 8th St., Ste. D917
Minneapolis, MN 55404
**Phone:** (612)347-7670 **Fax:** (612)337-7367
**Email:** clong@mmrf.org
**Website:** http://www.mmrf.org/research/addicton&alt_med/index.html
Thomas J. Kiresuk, PhD, Prin. Investigator

**Activities/Fields:** Complementary and alternative medicine treatments for addictions and their health and psychological complications.

**★ 4334 ★ Oregon Health and Science University**
Oregon Center for Complementary and Alternative Medicine Research in Neurological Disorders
3181 SW Sam Jackson Park Rd.
Portland, OR 97201
**Phone:** (503)494-9519 **Fax:** (503)494-9520
**Email:** orcamind@ohsn.edu
**Website:** http://www.ohsu.edu/orccamind
Barry S. Oken, MD, Prin. Investigator

**Activities/Fields:** The use of CAM therapies as treatments for neurodegenerative and demyelinating diseases.

**★ 4335 ★ Oregon State University**
Linus Pauling Institute (LPI)
571 Weniger Hall
Corvallis, OR 97331
**Phone:** (541)737-5078
**Website:** http://osu.orst.edu/dept/lpi/
Balz Frei, Dir.

**Activities/Fields:** Function and role of micronutrients, vitamins, and phytochemicals in promoting optimum health and preventing and treating disease; and the role of oxidative stress and antioxidants in human health and disease. **Pub:** *Newsletter*, semiannually.

**★ 4336 ★ Rocky Mountain Research Institute**
PO Box 190149
Boise, ID 83719
**Email:** farner@micron.net
**Website:** http://ufoinfo.com/organizations/usa_idaho.html

**Activities/Fields:** Anomalous experiences, unexplained phenomena, unidentified flying objects.

**★ 4337 ★ Rolf Institute of Structural Integration**
205 Canyon Blvd.
Boulder, CO 80302
**Phone:** (303)449-5903 **Free:** 800-530-8875
**Fax:** (303)449-5978
**Email:** rolfinst@rolf.org
**Website:** http://www.rolf.org
Gary Wolfe, Dir.

**Activities/Fields:** Rolfing (registered trademark) technique of connective tissue manipulation and its effect on integration of human physical structure and physical, emotional, and psychological functioning, including studies on human imbalance and its correction and/or improvement by a technique for reordering of the body to bring its major segments, head, shoulders, thorax, pelvis, and legs, toward a vertical alignment. **Pub:** *ROLF Lines.*

**★ 4338 ★ U.S. Department of Health and Human Services**
National Institutes of Health
National Center for Complementary and Alternative Medicine (NCCAM)
NIH 31
9000 Rockville Pike
Bldg. 31, Rm. 2B11
Bethesda, MD 20892-2182
**Phone:** (301)435-5042 **Fax:** (301)594-6757
**Email:** nccam@nccam.nih.gov
**Website:** http://nccam.nih.gov/
Stephen E. Straus, MD, Dir.

**Activities/Fields:** Conducts and supports basic and applied research and training and disseminates information on complementary and alternative medicine to practitioners and the public.

**★ 4339 ★ University of Arizona**
Center for Phytomedicine Research
College of Pharmacy
1703 E Mabel
PO Box 210207
Tucson, AZ 85721-0207
**Phone:** (520)626-6975 **Fax:** (520)626-2515
**Email:** ACPRx@pharmacy.arizona.edu
**Website:** http://nccam.nih.gov/nccam/fi/research/desc.htmlbot4
Barbara N. Timmermann, PhD, Prin. Investigator

**Activities/Fields:** Ginger, tumeric, and boswellia, widely used in Ayurvedic medicine for the treatment of inflammatory disease. Ayurveda, a medical system primarily practiced in India, includes diet and herbal remedies, while emphasizing the body, mind, and spirit in disease prevention and treatment. Studies include arthritis and other chronic inflammatory conditions, including respiratory diseases such as asthma. **Pub:** *The Leaf*, quarterly. Newsletter.

**★ 4340 ★ University of Arizona**
Pediatric Center for Complementary and Alternative Medicine
Department of Pediatrics
Health Sciences Center
1501 N Campbell
PO Box 245073
Tucson, AZ 85724-5073
**Phone:** (520)626-5170 **Fax:** (520)626-7176
**Email:** kjensen@peds.arizona.edu
**Website:** http://www.crc.arizona.edu
Fayez K. Ghishan, MD, Prin. Investigator

**Activities/Fields:** Integrative approaches in pediatrics to common pediatric problems, including recurrent abdominal pain, otitis media and cerebral palsy.

**★ 4341 ★ University of California, Los Angeles**
Center for Dietary Supplements Research: Botanicals
10945 LeConte Ave., Ste. 1401
Los Angeles, CA 90095-1406
**Website:** http://nccam.nih.gov/nccam/fi/research/desc.htmlbot3
David Heber, MD, Prin. Investigator

**Activities/Fields:** Explores potential mechanisms of action of yeast-fermented rice for cholesterol reduction; examines implications for heart disease prevention, green tea extract and soy for inhibition of tumor growth, St. John's wort, an herb used for relieving mild depression; assesses levels of bioactive compounds in several botanicals available as dietary supplements.

**★ 4342 ★ University of Illinois at Chicago**
Botanical Dietary Supplements for Women's Health
809 S Marshfield Ave.
Chicago, IL 60612
**Phone:** (312)413-9299 **Fax:** (312)413-5894
**Email:** norman@uic.edu
**Website:** http://nccam.nih.gov/fi/research/desc.htmlbot2
Norman R. Farnsworth, PhD, Dir.

**Activities/Fields:** Ten herbal supplements that have implications for benefit in women's health issues, including therapies for menopause.

**★ 4343 ★ University of Maryland**
Center for Alternative Medicine Research on Arthritis
Complementary Medicine Program
School of Medicine
2200 Kernan Dr.
Baltimore, MD 21207-6693
**Phone:** (410)448-6871 **Fax:** (410)448-6875
**Email:** bberman@compmed.ummc.umaryland.edu
**Website:** http://www.compmed.ummc.umaryland.edu
Brian M. Berman, MD, Prin. Investigator

**Activities/Fields:** The potential efficacy, safety, and cost-effectiveness of CAM therapies, including acupuncture treatment for osteoarthritis of the knee, mind/body therapies for fibromyalgia; electroacupuncture on persistent pain and inflammation; and a herbal combination with immunomodulatory properties.

**★ 4344 ★ University of Pennsylvania**
Specialized Center for Research in Hyperbaric Oxygen Therapy
3451 Walnut St., Rm. P221 (Franklin)
Philadelphia, PA 19104-6205
**Email:** sthan@mail.med.upenn.edu
**Website:** http://nccam.nih.gov/nccam/fi/research/desc.htmloxygen
Stephen R. Thom, MD, Prin. Investigator

**Activities/Fields:** Mechanisms of action, safety and clinical efficacy of hyperbaric oxygen therapy for head and neck tumors, and radiation injury.

**★ 4345 ★ University of Virginia**
Center for the Study of Complementary and Alternative Therapies (CSCAT)
West Complex, Ste. 6171
PO Box 801475
Charlottesville, VA 22908-1475
**Phone:** (434)924-0113 **Fax:** (434)243-9938
**Email:** cscat@virginia.edu
**Website:** http://www.nursing.virginia.edu/centers/cscat/
Ann Gill Taylor, Dir.

**Activities/Fields:** Complementary and alternative medicine, especially in treating pain.

**★ 4346 ★ World Research Foundation**
41 Bell Rock Plz.
Sedona, AZ 86351-8804
**Phone:** (520)284-3300 **Fax:** (520)284-3530
**Email:** info@wrf.org
**Website:** http://www.wrf.org
Steven Ross, PhD, Pres.

**Activities/Fields:** Encourages and supports scientific research to evaluate the phenomenon of healing as it occurs beyond the boundaries of traditional medicine. Projects at major universities funded by the Center have included the following: the existence of a measurable healing energy, the healing potential of lucid dreaming, the positive effects of self-help groups for persons suffering from catastrophic illness, the therapeutic effects of meditation and imagery as stress reducing factors in elementary school children, suggestion and psychic healing in human surgical patients, good humor and good health, and behavioral approaches to reduce pain and nausea of cancer treatments. **Pub:** *Research Report Series.* • *Research Reporter*, quarterly.

# Foundations & Other Funding Organizations

## Private Foundations

**Francis Families Foundation**
*See:* Entry 256

## Other Funding Organizations

**★ 4347 ★ American Society of Regional Anesthesia and Pain Medicine (ASRA)**
1910 Byrd Ave., No. 100
PO Box 11086
Richmond, VA 23230-1086
**Phone:** (804)282-0010   **Fax:** (804)282-0090
**Email:** asra@societyhq.com
**Website:** http://www.asra.com
James C. Eisenach, MD, Pres.
**Desc:** Physicians and research Ph.D.s. Conducts educational workshops. Sponsors annual refresher course. **Awards:** Gaston Labat Award (annual); Koller Research Grant; Pain Management Fellowship.

**★ 4348 ★ International Anesthesia Research Society (IARS)**
2 Summit Park Dr., Ste. 140
Cleveland, OH 44131-2571
**Phone:** (216)642-1124   **Fax:** (216)642-1127
**Email:** iarshq@iars.org
**Website:** http://www.iars.org
KC Wong, MD.PhD, Exec. Dir.
**Desc:** Anesthesiologists and other doctors of medicine and dentistry interested in the specialty of anesthesiology; associate members are registered nurses, physician assistants, and respiratory therapists. Fosters progress and research in all phases of anesthesiology. **Awards:** Ben Covino Research Award (biennial) research relating to the use of local anesthetics; Clinical Scholar Research Award (annual); Frontiers in Anesthesia Research Award (biennial).

**★ 4349 ★ International Trauma Anesthesia and Critical Care Society (ITACCS)**
PO Box 4826
Baltimore, MD 21211
**Phone:** (410)235-7697   **Fax:** (410)235-8084
**Email:** info@nwas.com
**Website:** http://www.trauma.itaccs.com
Christopher M. Grande, MD,MPH, Exec. Dir.
**Desc:** Healthcare professionals involved in trauma and critical care anesthesiology. Works to gain recognition for trauma anesthesiology as a discipline within anesthesiology and critical care medicine. Promotes cooperation and information sharing among healthcare professionals. Sponsors seminars and workshops; conducts research and educational programs; provides children's services; holds competitions; maintains speakers' bureau and placement service. **Awards:** ITACCS Research Award (annual) Application packet available.

**★ 4350 ★ Society of Cardiovascular Anesthesiologists (SCA)**
2209 Dickens Rd.
PO Box 11086
Richmond, VA 23230-1086
**Phone:** (804)282-0084   **Fax:** (804)282-0090
**Email:** sca@societyhq.com
**Website:** http://www.scahq.org
Heather A. Spiess, Chief Staff Exec.
**Desc:** Anesthesiologists who specialize in cardiovascular surgical conditions. Purpose is to further medical education of cardiovascular anesthesiologists. Establishes goals and objectives for education of trainees in cardiovascular anesthesia; promotes personnel exchange between the U.S. and other countries; reviews related literature; maintains workshops; conducts research competitions. Sponsors Anesthesia Grand Rounds: Case Presentations as a section of the annual meeting. **Awards:** Research Starter Grant (annual) for a SCA member.

**Society for Obstetric Anesthesia and Perinatology (SOAP)**
*See:* Entry 16592

# Medical & Allied Health Schools

## Nurse Anesthesia

*Listed below are nurse anesthesia educational programs accredited by the Council on Accreditation of Nurse Anesthesia Educational Programs, 222 S Prospect Ave., Park Ridge, IL 60068, (847)692-7050, http://www.aana.com/coa/.*

### Alabama

**★ 4351 ★ University of Alabama, Birmingham**
**Nurse Anesthesia Program**
Webb Bldg., Rm. 637
1530 3rd Ave. S
Birmingham, AL 35294
**Phone:** (205)934-3209   **Fax:** (205)934-3212
**Email:** williams@uab.edu
**Website:** http://www.uab.edu/dcdc/na/home.htm
Joe R. Williams, Director

### California

**★ 4352 ★ California State University, Fullerton**
**Department of Nursing**
**Kaiser Permanente School of Anesthesia**
100 S Los Robles, Ste. 550
Pasadena, CA 91188
**Phone:** (626)564-3000   **Fax:** (626)564-3099
**Email:** john.j.nagelhout@kp.org
**Website:** http://www.kpsan.org
John J. Nagelhout, Director

**★ 4353 ★ Samuel Merritt College**
**Program of Nurse Anesthesia**
435 Hawthorne Ave.
Oakland, CA 94609
**Phone:** (510)869-8926   **Fax:** (510)869-6677
**Email:** sfoster@samuelmerritt.edu
**Website:** http://www.samuelmerritt.edu
Scott D. Foster, Director

**★ 4354 ★ University of Southern California**
**Program of Nurse Anesthesia**
1540 Alcazar St., CHP 222
Los Angeles, CA 90089
**Phone:** (323)442-2012   **Fax:** (323)442-2090
**Email:** mgold@hsc.usc.edu
**Website:** http://www.usc.edu/hsc
Michele E. Gold, Director

### Connecticut

**★ 4355 ★ Central Connecticut State University**
**New Britain School of Nurse Anesthesia**
100 Grand St.
New Britain, CT 06050
**Phone:** (860)224-5612   **Fax:** (860)826-4992
**Email:** joancrna@aol.com
**Website:** http://www.biology.ccsu.edu/gradprograms.html
Joan H. Dobbins, Director

**★ 4356 ★ Hospital of St. Raphael**
**School of Nurse Anesthesia**
1423 Chapel St.
New Haven, CT 06511
**Phone:** (203)789-3351   **Fax:** (203)789-3352
**Email:** hsrsna@snet.net
**Website:** http://www.vaness.com/hsr/hsr.htm
Judy Thompson, Director

**★ 4357 ★ Southern Connecticut State University/Bridgeport Hospital**
**Nurse Anesthesia Program**
267 Grant St.
Bridgeport, CT 06610
**Phone:** (203)384-3280   **Fax:** (203)384-3855
**Email:** napbpthosp@aol.com

**Website:** http://www.bpthospnap.org
Diane M. Mericnyak, Director

## District of Columbia

**★ 4358 ★ Georgetown University**
**School of Nursing**
**Nurse Anesthesia Program**
Box 571107
3700 Reservoir Rd. NW
Washington, DC 20057
**Phone:** (202)687-4612          **Fax:** (202)687-5553
**Email:** jasinskd@georgetown.edu
**Website:** http://www.georgetown.edu
Donna M. Jasinski, Director

## Florida

**★ 4359 ★ Barry University**
**Master of Science Program in**
  **Anesthesiology**
11300 NE 2nd Ave.
Miami Shores, FL 33161
**Phone:** (305)899-3230          **Free:** 800-756-6000
**Fax:** (305)899-3366
**Email:** mrodriguez@mail.barry.edu
**Website:**          http://www2.barry.edu/vpaa-snhs/an-
esthe.htm
Dolores M. Gibbs, Director

**★ 4360 ★ Bay Medical Center**
**Gooding Institute of Nurse Anesthesia**
615 N Bonita Ave.
Panama City, FL 32401
**Phone:** (850)747-6918          **Free:** 800-422-2418
**Fax:** (850)747-6115
**Email:** gooding@baymedical.org
**Website:** http://www.baymedical.org
David R. Ely, Director

**★ 4361 ★ Florida Gulf Coast University**
**Norman R. Wolford School of Nurse**
  **Anesthesia**
PO Box 413012
Naples, FL 34101
**Phone:** (941)436-5370          **Fax:** (941)436-5639
**Email:** nrw@fgcu.edu
**Website:** http://www.fgcu.edu
Susan Campbell, Director

**★ 4362 ★ Florida International University**
**School of Nursing**
**Anesthesiology Nursing Program**
3000 NE 151 St.
North Miami, FL 33181
**Phone:** (305)919-5350          **Fax:** (305)919-5209
**Email:** mcdonoug@fiu.edu
**Website:** http://w3.fiu.edu/nursing/anesthesiology
John P. McDonough, Director

## Georgia

**★ 4363 ★ Medical College of Georgia**
**Nursing Anesthesia Program**
1120 15th St., EB-229
Augusta, GA 30912
**Phone:** (706)721-9558          **Fax:** (706)721-8206
**Email:** emonti@mail.mcg.edu
**Website:** http://www.mcg.edu
Elizabeth J. Monti, Director

## Illinois

**★ 4364 ★ Bradley University/Decatur**
  **Memorial Hospital**
**Nurse Anesthesia Program**
2300 N Edward St.
Decatur, IL 62526
**Phone:** (217)876-2578          **Fax:** (217)876-2587
**Email:** susang@dmhhs.org

**Website:** http://www.dmhhs.com
Sue M. Kiefer-Griffin, Director

**★ 4365 ★ Evanston Northwestern**
  **Healthcare/DePaul University**
**School of Anesthesia**
2650 Ridge Ave.
Evanston, IL 60201
**Phone:** (847)570-1959          **Fax:** (847)733-5392
**Email:** broche@enh.org
**Website:** http://www.advocatehealth.com/rhmcsa
Bernadette T. Roche, Director

**★ 4366 ★ Rush University**
**College of Nursing**
**Nurse Anesthesia Program**
600 S Paulina St., No. 1072B
Chicago, IL 60612
**Phone:** (312)942-7100          **Fax:** (312)942-3043
**Email:** mfaut-callahan@rushu.rush.edu
**Website:** http://www.rushu.rush.edu/nursing
Margaret Faut-Callahan, Director

**★ 4367 ★ Southern Illinois University,**
  **Edwardsville**
**School of Nursing**
**Anesthesia Nursing Specialization**
Campus Box 1066
Edwardsville, IL 62026-1066
**Phone:** (618)650-3906          **Free:** 800-234-4844
**Fax:** (618)650-3854
**Email:** wellis@siue.edu
**Website:** http://www.siue.edu
Wayne E. Ellis, Director

## Iowa

**★ 4368 ★ University of Iowa**
**College of Nursing**
**Anesthesia Nursing Program**
Rm. 6613 JCP, UIHC
200 Hawkins Dr.
Iowa City, IA 52242
**Phone:** (319)384-7354          **Free:** 800-553-4692
**Fax:** (319)384-7286
**Email:** e-s-thompson@uiowa.edu
**Website:** http://www.anesth.uiowa.edu/srna
Edward S. Thompson, Director

## Kansas

**★ 4369 ★ Newman University**
**Nurse Anesthesia Program**
3100 McCormick Ave., Ste. 214 ECK
Wichita, KS 67213
**Phone:** (316)942-4291          **Fax:** (316)942-4483
**Email:** chipasa@newmanu.edu
**Website:** http://www.newmanu.edu/gradnan.html
Anthony Chipas, Director

**★ 4370 ★ University of Kansas Medical**
  **Center**
**Program of Nurse Anesthesia Education**
3901 Rainbow Blvd.
Kansas City, KS 66160
**Phone:** (913)588-6612          **Fax:** (913)588-3334
**Email:** nanesthe@kumc.edu
**Website:** http://www2.kumc.edu/sah/nurseanesthesia
Carol G. Elliott, Chairman of the Board

## Kentucky

**★ 4371 ★ Trover Foundation/Murray State**
  **University**
**Program of Anesthesia**
435 N Kentucky Ave., Ste. A
Madisonville, KY 42431
**Phone:** (270)824-3460          **Fax:** (270)824-3469
**Email:** anesprog@trover.org

**Website:** http://www.crnaky.com
W. Gray McCall, Director

## Louisiana

**★ 4372 ★ Louisiana State University**
**Health Sciences Center**
**School of Nursing**
**Nurse Anesthesia Program**
1900 Gravier St.
Box G-4
New Orleans, LA 70112
**Phone:** (504)568-7505          **Fax:** (504)568-4136
**Email:** kwren@lsuhsc.edu
**Website:** http://nursing.lsuhsc.edu/sonweb/mn/crna
program/default.htm
Kathleen R. Wren, Director

## Maine

**★ 4373 ★ University of New England**
**School of Nurse Anesthesia**
716 Stevens Ave.
Portland, ME 04103
**Phone:** (207)797-7261          **Fax:** (207)797-7225
**Email:** ldeisering@une.edu
**Website:** http://www.une.edu
Leon F. Deisering, Director

## Maryland

**★ 4374 ★ Uniformed Services University**
  **of the Health Sciences**
**Graduate School of Nursing**
**Nurse Anesthesia Program**
1335 East-West Hwy., Ste. 9-700
Silver Spring, MD 20910
**Phone:** (301)295-0979          **Fax:** (301)295-1722
**Email:** paustin@usuhs.mil
**Website:** http://www.usuhs.mil
Lt. Col. Paul Austin, Director

**★ 4375 ★ U.S. Navy**
**Nurse Corps Anesthesia Program**
NSHS-Code ON1
8901 Wisconsin Ave.
Bethesda, MD 20889
**Phone:** (301)295-6091          **Fax:** (301)295-0827
**Email:** lheindel@nsh10.med.navy.mil
**Website:**   http://www-nshs.med.navy.mil/nncapwww/
nrsanes.htm
Louis Heindel, Director

## Massachusetts

**★ 4376 ★ Northeastern University/New**
  **England Medical Center**
**Nurse Anesthesia Program**
207 Robinson Hall
Boston, MA 02115
**Phone:** (617)373-7962          **Fax:** (617)373-8672
**Email:** st.alves@neu.edu
**Website:** http://www.neu.edu
Steve L. Alves, Director

## Michigan

**★ 4377 ★ Henry Ford Hospital/University**
  **of Detroit Mercy**
**Graduate Program of Nurse**
  **Anesthesiology**
Clara Ford Pavilion, Rm. 303
2799 W Grand Blvd.
Detroit, MI 48202
**Phone:** (313)916-2934          **Fax:** (313)916-2606
**Email:** schanes@hfhs.org
**Website:** http://ids.udmercy.edu/naprogram
Patrick J. Quinn, Director

**★ 4378 ★ Oakland University**
**Beaumont Graduate Program of Nurse**
**Anesthesia**
**(Beaumont Royal Oak and Troy)**
3601 W 13 Mile Rd.
Royal Oak, MI 48073
**Phone:** (248)551-8075          **Fax:** (248)551-8285
**Email:** kzaglaniczny@beaumont.edu
**Website:** http://www.beaumont.edu/crna
Karen L. Zaglaniczny, Director


**★ 4379 ★ University of Detroit Mercy**
**Graduate Program of Nurse**
**Anesthesiology**
St. Joseph Mercy Oakland
44405 Woodward Ave.
Pontiac, MI 48341
**Phone:** (248)858-6593          **Fax:** (248)859-6599
**Email:** doschm@trinity-health.org
**Website:** http://www.udmercy.edu/naprogram
Michael P. Dosch, Director


**★ 4380 ★ University of Michigan, Flint**
**Hurley Medical Center**
**Master of Science in Anesthesia Program**
Hurley Medical Center
1 Hurley Plaza
Flint, MI 48503
**Phone:** (810)257-9264          **Fax:** (810)760-0839
**Email:** dmcfarl1@hurleymc.com
**Website:** http://www.hurleymc.com/education/an-
esthes/index.htm
Francis Gerbasi, Director


**★ 4381 ★ Wayne State University**
**College of Pharmacy and Allied Health**
**   Professions**
**Nurse Anesthesia Program**
4201 St. Antoine, Rm. 2V-4
Detroit, MI 48201
**Phone:** (313)745-3610          **Fax:** (313)993-7729
**Email:** pworth@dmc.org
**Website:** http://wizard.pharm.wayne.edu/anesth
Prudentia Worth, Chairman of the Board


## Minnesota

**★ 4382 ★ Mayo School of Health**
**   Sciences**
**Master of Nurse Anesthesia Program**
1108 Siebens Bldg.
200 1st St. SW
Rochester, MN 55905
**Phone:** (507)284-8331          **Free:** 800-626-9041
**Fax:** (507)284-0656
**Email:** marienau.mary@mayo.edu
**Website:** http://www.mayo.edu/hrs/hrs_nam.htm
Mary E. Shirk Marienau, Director


**★ 4383 ★ Minneapolis School of**
**   Anesthesia**
6715 Minnetonka Blvd.
Saint Louis Park, MN 55426
**Phone:** (952)925-5222          **Fax:** (952)925-6004
**Email:** gombkoto.msa@worldnet.att.net
**Website:** http://www.nurseanesthesia.org
Rebecca L. Gombkoto, Director


**★ 4384 ★ Minneapolis VA School of**
**   Anesthesia**
1 Veterans Dr., 112A
Minneapolis, MN 55417
**Phone:** (612)725-2000          **Fax:** (612)970-5887
**Email:** fager003@umn.edu
Kathleen A. Fagerlund, Director


**★ 4385 ★ Saint Mary's University of**
**   Minnesota/Abbott Northwestern Hospital**
**Graduate Program in Nurse Anesthesia**
2500 Park Ave.
Minneapolis, MN 55404
**Phone:** (612)728-5133          **Fax:** (612)728-5167
**Email:** mmoody@smumn.edu
**Website:** http://www.smumn.edu
Merri L. Moody, Director


## Missouri

**★ 4386 ★ Southwest Missouri School of**
**   Anesthesia**
1235 E Cherokee
Springfield, MO 65804
**Phone:** (417)885-6890          **Fax:** (417)885-6895
**Email:** as14293@sprg.smhs.com
**Website:** http://www.smsu.edu/faculty/jmg230f/ronis/
naopen.html
William O. Kirk, Director


**★ 4387 ★ Truman Medical Center**
**School of Nurse Anesthesia**
2301 Holmes St.
Kansas City, MO 64108
**Phone:** (816)556-3216          **Fax:** (816)556-3963
**Email:** tmcanes@tmcmed.org
**Website:** http://www.trumanmed.org/crna
Mark Lipari, Director


**★ 4388 ★ Webster University**
**MS in Nurse Anesthesia**
470 E Lockwood Ave.
Saint Louis, MO 63119
**Phone:** (314)968-5916          **Fax:** (314)968-7194
**Email:** clarkga@webster.edu
**Website:** http://www.webster.edu
Gary D. Clark, Director


## Nebraska

**★ 4389 ★ Bryan LGH Medical Center/**
**   University of Kansas**
**School of Nurse Anesthesia**
1600 S 48 St.
Lincoln, NE 68506
**Phone:** (402)481-3135          **Free:** 800-742-7844
**Fax:** (402)481-8404
**Email:** jcuddeford@bryanlgh.org
**Website:** http://www.bryanlgh.org
James D. Cuddeford, Director


## New Jersey

**★ 4390 ★ University of Medicine and**
**   Dentistry of New Jersey**
**Our Lady of Lourdes Medical Center**
**Nurse Anesthesia Program**
1600 Haddon Ave.
Camden, NJ 08103
**Phone:** (856)757-3897          **Fax:** (856)968-2568
**Email:** roddend@lourdesnet.org
F. David Rodden, Director


## New York

**★ 4391 ★ Albany Medical College**
**Nurse Anesthesiology Program**
43 New Scotland Ave., MC-131
Albany, NY 12208
**Phone:** (518)262-4303          **Fax:** (518)262-5170
**Email:** amcnap@mail.amc.edu
**Website:** http://www.amc.edu/gradstu
Kathleen M. O'Donnell, Director


**★ 4392 ★ Columbia University**
**School of Nursing**
**Program in Nurse Anesthesia**
630 W 168th St.
New York, NY 10032
**Phone:** (212)305-4196          **Fax:** (212)305-6937
**Email:** tjl2@columbia.edu
**Website:** http://www.columbia.edu
Timothy J. Lehey, Director


**★ 4393 ★ State University of New York,**
**   Buffalo**
**School of Nursing**
**Nurse Anesthesia Program**
1116 Kimball Tower
3435 Main St.
Buffalo, NY 14214
**Phone:** (716)829-2410          **Fax:** (716)829-2021
**Email:** tobst@buffalo.edu
**Website:** http://nursing.buffalo.edu
Thomas E. Obst, Director


**★ 4394 ★ State University of New York,**
**   Health Science Center, Brooklyn**
**   (SUNY-HSCB)**
**Nurse Anesthesia with Kings County**
**   Hospital Center**
**Nurse Anesthesia with Harlem Hospital**
**   Center**
450 Clarkson Ave.
Box 22
Brooklyn, NY 11203
**Phone:** (212)939-3575          **Fax:** (212)939-3574
**Email:** varirao@netmail.hscbklyn.edu
**Website:** http://www.downstate.edu
Visitacion T. Arirao, Director


## North Carolina

**★ 4395 ★ Carolinas HealthCare System/**
**   University of North Carolina, Charlotte**
**Nurse Anesthesia Program**
PO Box 32861
Charlotte, NC 28232
**Phone:** (704)355-2375          **Fax:** (704)355-7263
**Email:** ymobley@carolinas.org
**Website:** http://www.carolinas.org/education
Jacqueline M. Hall, Director


**★ 4396 ★ Duke University**
**Nurse Anesthesia Program**
Box 3322 DUMC
Durham, NC 27710
**Phone:** (919)684-3786          **Free:** 877-415-3853
**Fax:** (919)681-8899
**Email:** mary.karlet@duke.edu
**Website:** http://www.nursing.duke.edu
Mary Karlet, Director


**★ 4397 ★ University of North Carolina,**
**   Greensboro**
**Raleigh School of Nurse Anesthesia**
23 Sunnybrook Rd., Ste. 163
Raleigh, NC 27610
**Phone:** (919)250-9740          **Fax:** (919)250-0348
**Email:** rsna@earthlink.net
**Website:** http://home.earthlink.net/~rsna
Nancy Bruton-Maree, Director


**★ 4398 ★ Wake Forest University Baptist**
**   Medical Center**
**The University of North Carolina,**
**   Greensboro**
**Nurse Anesthesia Program**
Medical Center Blvd.
Winston Salem, NC 27157
**Phone:** (336)716-1411          **Fax:** (336)716-1412
**Email:** vcbeane@wfubmc.edu

**Website:** http://www.wfubmc.edu
Sandra M. Ouellette, Director

## North Dakota

**★ 4399 ★ University of North Dakota**
**College of Nursing**
**Nurse Anesthesiology Program**
PO Box 9025
Grand Forks, ND 58202
**Phone:** (701)777-4509        **Fax:** (701)777-4096
**Email:** rick_brown@mail.und.nodak.edu
**Website:** http://www.und.nodak.edu/dept/nursing/an-esmstr.html
Rick Brown, Director

## Ohio

**★ 4400 ★ Case Western Reserve**
**University**
**Cleveland Clinic Foundation**
**Frances Payne Bolton School of Nursing**
**School of Nurse Anesthesia**
9500 Euclid Ave., E-31
Cleveland, OH 44195
**Phone:** (216)444-6547        **Free:** 800-223-2273
**Fax:** (216)444-9247
**Email:** blakelp@ccf.org
**Website:** http://fpb.cwru.edu/Program%20Areas/Right/NAMSN.htm
Paul R. Blakeley, Director

**★ 4401 ★ Case Western Reserve**
**University**
**Frances Payne Bolton School of Nursing**
**Program in Nurse Anesthesia**
10900 Euclid Ave.
Cleveland, OH 44106
**Phone:** (216)368-0221        **Free:** 800-825-2540
**Fax:** (216)368-3542
**Email:** jrk@po.cwru.edu
**Website:** http://fpb.cwru.edu
Jack R. Kless, Director

**★ 4402 ★ St. Elizabeth Health Center**
**School for Nurse Anesthetists, Inc.**
1044 Belmont Ave.
Youngstown, OH 44501
**Phone:** (330)480-3444        **Fax:** (330)480-5202
**Email:** brodgers@belpark.net
**Website:** http://www.belpark.net/crnaschool
Beverly A. Rodgers, Director

**★ 4403 ★ University of Akron**
**College of Nursing**
**Graduate Anesthesia Program**
209 Carroll St.
Akron, OH 44325
**Phone:** (330)972-5406        **Fax:** (330)972-6632
**Email:** barton@uakron.edu
**Website:** http://www.uakron.edu/nursing/academic/anesthesia.htm
Charles R. Barton, Director

**★ 4404 ★ University of Cincinnati**
**College of Nursing**
**Masters Program in Nurse Anesthesia**
PO Box 210038
Cincinnati, OH 45221
**Phone:** (513)558-5500        **Fax:** (513)558-7523
**Email:** wanda.wilson@uc.edu
**Website:** http://www.nursing@uc.edu
Wanda O. Wilson, Director

## Pennsylvania

**★ 4405 ★ Allegheny Valley Hospital/**
**LaRoche College**
**School of Nurse Anesthesia**
1301 Carlisle St.
Natrona Heights, PA 15065
**Phone:** (724)226-7013        **Fax:** (724)226-7199
**Email:** dadcrna@hotmail.com
**Website:**        http://nursing.auhs.edu/john_pages/napo.htm
Deborah A. Davison, Director

**★ 4406 ★ Hamot Medical Center**
**School of Anesthesia**
**Gannon University**
201 State St.
Erie, PA 16550
**Phone:** (814)877-2938        **Free:** 800-937-9133
**Fax:** (814)877-6070
**Email:** steve.anderson@hamot.org
**Website:** http://www.hamot.org
K. Stephen Anderson, Director

**★ 4407 ★ Lankenau Hospital**
**School of Anesthesia**
100 Lancaster Ave.
Wynnewood, PA 19096
**Phone:** (610)645-2145        **Fax:** (610)645-3411
**Email:** wildgustb@mlhs.org
**Website:**        http://www.nursing.villanova.edu/msn/gradstdy/anesth.htm
Bette M. Wildgust, Director

**★ 4408 ★ MCP Hahnemann University**
**Nurse Anesthesia Program**
245 N 15th St., MS 501
Philadelphia, PA 19102-1192
**Phone:** (215)762-4309        **Fax:** (215)762-1259
**Email:** booth@drexel.edu
**Website:**        http://nursing.mcphu.edu/sonbasics/napo.htm
Michael J. Booth, Director

**★ 4409 ★ Montgomery Hospital**
**Frank J. Tornetta School of Anesthesia**
1301 Powell St.
PO Box 992
Norristown, PA 19404
**Phone:** (610)270-2139        **Fax:** (610)270-2318
**Email:** philacrna@aol.com
Michael T. Kost, Director

**★ 4410 ★ Nazareth Hospital**
**School of Nurse Anesthesiology**
2601 Holme Ave.
Philadelphia, PA 19152
**Phone:** (215)335-6217        **Fax:** (215)335-6668
**Email:** jwoods@che-east.org
Joan E. Woods, Director

**★ 4411 ★ Pennsylvania Hospital**
**School of Nurse Anesthesia**
800 Spruce St.
Philadelphia, PA 19107
**Phone:** (215)829-3320        **Fax:** (215)829-8757
**Email:** phsa@pahosp.com
**Website:** http://www.med.upenn.edu/pahosp/pahpe/nurse_anesth/index.html
Kathleen Kinslow, Director

**★ 4412 ★ St. Francis Medical Center/**
**LaRoche College**
**School of Anesthesia**
400 45th St.
Pittsburgh, PA 15201
**Phone:** (412)622-4369        **Fax:** (412)688-3883
**Email:** loefflera@sfhs.edu

**Website:** http://www.sfhs.edu/library/schools/anesth
Arlene S. Loeffler, Director

**★ 4413 ★ University of Pittsburgh**
**School of Nursing**
**Nurse Anesthesia Program**
336 Victoria Bldg.
3500 Victoria St.
Pittsburgh, PA 15261
**Phone:** (412)624-4860        **Fax:** (412)383-7227
**Email:** napcrna@pitt.edu
**Website:** http://www.pitt.edu/~napcrna
John M. O'Donnell, Director

**★ 4414 ★ Westmoreland-Latrobe**
**Hospitals/LaRoche College**
**School of Anesthesia**
532 W Pittsburgh St.
Greensburg, PA 15601
**Phone:** (724)832-4144        **Fax:** (724)832-4164
**Email:** bighoward@aol.com
**Website:** http://www.laroche.edu/TOC/academic/academic.html
Howard F. Armour, Director

**★ 4415 ★ Wyoming Valley Health Care**
**System**
**University of Scranton**
**School of Nurse Anesthesia**
575 N River St.
Wilkes Barre, PA 18764
**Phone:** (570)552-7290        **Fax:** (570)552-7299
**Email:** eevanina@wvhcs.org
**Website:** http://www.scranton.edu/graduateschool
Eileen Evanina, Director

## Puerto Rico

**★ 4416 ★ Inter American University of**
**Puerto Rico**
**Master of Science in Anesthesia**
PO Box 4050
Arecibo, PR 00614
**Phone:** (787)878-5475        **Fax:** (787)881-3831
**Email:** imolina@arecibo.inter.edu
**Website:** http://www.arecibo.inter.edu
Ivan J. Molina, Director

**★ 4417 ★ University of Puerto Rico**
**School of Nursing**
**Nurse Anesthesia Program**
Medial Sciences Campus
PO Box 365067
San Juan, PR 00936
**Phone:** (787)758-2525        **Fax:** (787)281-0721
**Email:** mplaza@rcm.upr.edu
**Website:** http://www.rcm.upr.edu/pagenursing3.html
Crucita Mattei, Director

## Rhode Island

**★ 4418 ★ Memorial Hospital of Rhode**
**Island**
**School of Nurse Anesthesia**
111 Brewster St.
Pawtucket, RI 02860
**Phone:** (401)729-2485        **Fax:** (401)729-3476
**Email:** foster@ids.net
**Website:** http://www.mhri.org/anesth
Mark A. Foster, Director

**★ 4419 ★ Saint Joseph Hospital**
**School of Anesthesia for Nurses**
200 High Service Ave.
North Providence, RI 02904
**Phone:** (401)456-3639        **Fax:** (401)752-8140
**Email:** saintjoes@aol.com
**Website:** http://www.saintjosephri.com
Lucille S. Buono, Director

## South Carolina

**★ 4420 ★ Medical University of South Carolina**
**Anesthesia for Nurses Program**
165 Cannon St., Ste. 402
PO Box 250855
Charleston, SC 29425
**Phone:** (843)792-3785      **Fax:** (843)792-1984
**Email:** truverl@musc.edu
**Website:** http://www.musc.edu/afn
Lawrence H. Truver, Director

**★ 4421 ★ USC/PRMH**
**Graduate Program in Nurse Anesthesia**
15 Medical Park, Ste. 221
Columbia, SC 29203
**Phone:** (803)434-6344      **Fax:** (803)434-4099
**Email:** kwilliam@richmed.medpark.sc.edu
**Website:** http://www.med.sc.edu:88/mnuran.htm
Kristi H. Williams, Director

## South Dakota

**★ 4422 ★ Mount Marty College**
**Graduate Program in Nurse Anesthesiology**
3932 S Western Ave.
Sioux Falls, SD 57105
**Phone:** (605)322-8090      **Free:** 877-727-8672
**Fax:** (605)322-8095
**Email:** msna@mtmc.edu
**Website:** http://www.mtmc.edu/~ans
Larry L. Dahlen, Director

## Tennessee

**★ 4423 ★ Erlanger Health System/ University of Tennessee, Chattanooga**
**School of Nursing**
**Nurse Anesthesia Concentration**
615 McCallie Ave.
Chattanooga, TN 37403
**Phone:** (423)755-4750      **Fax:** (423)755-4668
**Email:** zacharra@erlanger.org
**Website:** http://www.utc.edu/~utcnurse/index.htm
Dana H. Wertenberger, Director

**★ 4424 ★ Middle Tennessee School of Anesthesia**
**Nurse Anesthesia Program**
PO Box 6414
Madison, TN 37116
**Phone:** (615)868-6503      **Fax:** (615)868-9885
**Email:** dean@mtsa.edu
**Website:** http://www.mtsa.edu
Mary E. DeVasher, Director

**★ 4425 ★ University of Tennessee**
**College of Nursing**
**Nurse Anesthesia Concentration**
1924 Alcoa Hwy.
Box U-109
Knoxville, TN 37920
**Phone:** (865)544-9222      **Fax:** (865)544-6852
**Email:** jpreston@mc.utmck.edu
**Website:** http://nightingale.con.utk.edu
John C. Preston, Director

**★ 4426 ★ University of Tennessee**
**Health Sciences Center**
**College of Nursing**
**Nurse Anesthesia Option**
877 Madison Ave.
Memphis, TN 38163
**Phone:** (901)448-6102      **Fax:** (901)448-4121
**Email:** lhill@utmem.edu
**Website:** http://www.utmem.edu/nursing
Linda Hill, Director

## Texas

**★ 4427 ★ Baylor College of Medicine**
**Graduate Program in Nurse Anesthesia**
6550 Fannin St., Ste. 1003
Houston, TX 77030
**Phone:** (713)873-2860      **Fax:** (713)873-2867
**Email:** jrwalker@bcm.tmc.edu
**Website:** http://www.bcm.tmc.edu/gpna
James R. Walker, Director

**★ 4428 ★ Texas Wesleyan University**
**Graduate Program of Nurse Anesthesia**
1201 Wesleyan St.
Fort Worth, TX 76105
**Phone:** (817)531-4406      **Fax:** (817)531-6508
**Email:** ksanders@txwes.edu
**Website:** http://www.txwesleyan.edu
Kay K. Sanders, Chairman of the Board

**★ 4429 ★ U.S. Army**
**Graduate Program in Anesthesia Nursing**
MCCS-HNE, Anesthesia Branch
2250 Stanley Rd., Ste. 214
San Antonio, TX 78234
**Phone:** (210)221-6905      **Fax:** (210)221-8114
**Email:** norma.garrett@amedd.army.mil
**Website:** http://www.dns.amedd.army.mil/crna
Normalynn Garrett, Director

**★ 4430 ★ University of Texas**
**Houston Health Science Center**
**School of Nursing**
**Nurse Anesthesia Division**
1100 Holcombe Blvd., Ste. 6, 150
Houston, TX 77030
**Phone:** (713)500-2159      **Fax:** (713)500-2171
**Email:** rlester@son1.nur.uth.tmc.edu
**Website:** http://son1.nur.uth.tmc.edu
Rodney C. Lester, Director

## Virginia

**★ 4431 ★ Old Dominion University**
**School of Nursing**
**Nurse Anesthesia Program**
Technology Bldg., Rm. 363
4608 Hampton Blvd.
Norfolk, VA 23529
**Phone:** (757)683-5068      **Free:** 800-572-2762
**Fax:** (757)683-5124
**Email:** joswaks@odu.edu
**Website:** http://web.odu.edu
Jill S. Detty Oswaks, Director

**★ 4432 ★ Virginia Commonwealth University**
**Department of Nurse Anesthesia**
PO Box 980226
Richmond, VA 23298
**Phone:** (804)828-9808      **Fax:** (804)828-0581
**Email:** mdfallac@hsc.vcu.edu
**Website:** http://views.vcu.edu/sahp/rngas
Michael D. Fallacaro, Chairman of the Board

## Washington

**★ 4433 ★ Gonzaga University**
**Sacred Heart Medical Center**
**Master of Anesthesiology Education Program**
101 W 8th Ave.
PO Box 2555
Spokane, WA 99220
**Phone:** (509)474-4971      **Fax:** (509)474-3113
**Email:** meyersmr@shmc.org
**Website:** http://www.gonzaga.edu/academic/Education/Masters/aci/aeindex.html
Margaret R. Meyers, Director

## West Virginia

**★ 4434 ★ Charleston Area Medical Center**
**School of Nurse Anesthesia**
3110 MacCorkle Ave. SE, Rm. 2041
Charleston, WV 25304
**Phone:** (304)388-9950      **Fax:** (304)388-9955
**Email:** nancy.tierney@camcare.com
**Website:** http://www.anesthesiaschool.org
Nancy L. Tierney, Director

## Wisconsin

**★ 4435 ★ Franciscan Skemp Healthcare**
**School of Anesthesia**
700 West Ave.
La Crosse, WI 54601
**Phone:** (608)785-0940      **Fax:** (608)791-9799
**Email:** jochman.barbara@mayo.edu
**Website:** http://perth.uwlax.edu/biology/graduate/crna.htm
Barbara J. Jochman, Director

---

# National & International Organizations

**★ 4436 ★ Aestheticians International Association (AIA)**
2611 N Belt Line, Ste. 140
Sunnyvale, TX 75182
**Phone:** (972)203-8530      **Free:** 877-968-7539
**Fax:** (972)226-2339
**Email:** aiathekey@aol.com
Douglas Preston, Pres.

**Fnded:** 1975. **Mem:** 600. **Desc:** Committed to raise standard of aesthetics with advancement of education and public awareness through legislation, educational institutes, certification, instructors, continuing education and to create a national standard for education.

**★ 4437 ★ American Academy of Anesthesiologist Assistants (AAAA)**
PO Box 81362
Wellesley, MA 02481-0004
**Phone:** 800-757-5858      **Fax:** (781)239-3259
**Website:** http://www.anesthetist.org
Sherri L. Oken, CAE, Assn. Mgr.

**Fnded:** 1975. **Mem:** 336. **Desc:** Active anesthesiologist assistants who have graduated from an accredited training program and full-time students currently enrolled in an accredited program. Establishes and maintains the standards of the profession. Fosters and encourages continuing education and research. Sponsors educational meetings for graduates and student anesthesiologist assistants. **Pub:** *The Anesthesia Record*, 5/year. Newsletter. • *Membership Directory*. Membership Directory.

**★ 4438 ★ American Association of Nurse Anesthetists (AANA)**
222 S Prospect Ave.
Park Ridge, IL 60068
**Phone:** (847)692-7050      **Fax:** (847)692-6968
**Email:** info@aana.com
**Website:** http://www.aana.com
Jeffery M. Beutler, Exec. Dir.

**Fnded:** 1931. **Mem:** 27,222. **State Groups:** 52. **Desc:** Active registered professional nurses who have successfully completed an accredited program in nurse anesthesia and passed a national examination for certification. Advances the art and science of anesthesiology; promotes research in anesthesia; develops educational standards and techniques for the administration of anesthesia. Sponsors continuing education; promotes biennial recertification. **Pub:** *AANA Journal*, bimonthly. Journal. Contains clinical, practical, theoretical, and research articles. Includes advertisers' index, and alphabetical inex by organization. *Price:* Included in membership dues; $24/year for nonmembers. • *AANA News Bulletin,* monthly. Bulletin. Contains legislative news, president's message, calendar of events, and employment listings. *Price:* Included in membership dues. • *American Association of Nurse Anesthetists List of Recognized Educational Programs,* semiannual. Arranged by state.

### ★ 4439 ★ American Board of Anesthesiology (ABA)

4101 Lake Boone Trail, Ste. 510
Raleigh, NC 27607-7506
**Phone:** (919)881-2570　　　**Fax:** (919)881-2575
**Website:** http://www.abanes.org
Stephen J. Thomas, MD, Pres.

**Fnded:** 1938. **Mem:** 15. **Desc:** Certification board which seeks to elevate and maintain the standards of the practice of anesthesiology and to establish criteria of fitness for the designation of a specialist in this field. Advises the Accreditation Council for Graduate Medical Education concerning training of individuals seeking certification. Arranges and conducts examinations to determine whether physicians who apply meet its standards; issues certificates to those who meet the required standards. **Pub:** *American Board of Anesthesiology–Booklet of Information,* annual. Booklet. Describes the examination system and the policies and regulations governing the board's examination and certification process. *Price:* Free.

### ★ 4440 ★ American Board of Peri Anesthesia Nursing Certification (ABPANC)

475 Riverside Dr., 6th Fl.
New York, NY 10115-0089
**Phone:** (212)367-4253　　　**Free:** 800-622-7262
**Fax:** (212)367-4256
**Email:** abpanc@proexam.org
**Website:** http://www.cpancapa.org
Bonnie Niebuhr, MS, RN, CAE, Exec. Dir.

**Fnded:** 1985. **Desc:** Administers examination to individuals wishing to attain perianesthesia nursing certification. **Pub:** *Certification Newsletter.* Newsletter. *Price:* Free.

### American College of Veterinary Anesthesiologists (ACVA)

*See:* Entry 20558

### American Dental Society of Anesthesiology (ADSA)

*See:* Entry 6445

### American Osteopathic College of Anesthesiologists (AOCA)

*See:* Entry 17001

### American Society for Advancement of Anesthesia and Sedation in Dentistry (ASAAD)

*See:* Entry 6452

### ★ 4441 ★ American Society of Anesthesia Technologists and Technicians (ASATT)

5800 Foxridge Dr., Ste. 115
Mission, KS 66202-2333
**Phone:** (913)262-2249　　　**Fax:** (913)262-0174
**Email:** asil@dir.net
**Website:** http://www.asatt.org
Frank Bistrom, Exec. Dir.

**Fnded:** 1989. **Mem:** 1,048. **Reg. Groups:** 7. **Desc:** Anesthesia technicians and technologists, medical technology students, and other individuals, organizations, and corporations with an interest in the field of anesthesiology. Promotes continuing professional development of members. Conducts continuing education programs for anesthesiology technicians and

technologists; represents members' interests at the national level in the United States; maintains certification program and develops standards of ethics and practice. **Pub:** *Sensor,* quarterly. Newsletter.

### ★ 4442 ★ American Society of Anesthesiologists (ASA)

520 N Northwest Hwy.
Park Ridge, IL 60068-2573
**Phone:** (847)825-5586　　　**Fax:** (847)825-1692
**Email:** mail@asahq.org
**Website:** http://www.asahq.org
Glenn W. Johnson, Exec. Dir.

**Fnded:** 1905. **Mem:** 36,000. **State Groups:** 50. **Desc:** Professional society of physicians specializing or interested in anesthesiology. Seeks "to develop and further the specialty of anesthesiology for the general elevation of the standards of medical practice." Encourages education, research, and scientific progress in anesthesiology. Conducts refresher courses and other postgraduate educational activities. Maintains placement service. **Pub:** *Anesthesiology,* monthly. Journal. *Price:* $223/year for individuals; $399/year for institutions. • *ASA Directory of Members,* annual. Membership Directory. • *ASA Newsletter,* monthly. Newsletter. Reports on the educational and scientific work of ASA. Contains calendar of events. *Price:* Included in membership dues; $25/year for nonmembers. **Frmly:** (1911) Long Island Society of Anesthetists; (1936) New York Society of Anesthetists; (1945) American Society of Anesthetists.

### ★ 4443 ★ American Society of Regional Anesthesia and Pain Medicine (ASRA)

1910 Byrd Ave., No. 100
PO Box 11086
Richmond, VA 23230-1086
**Phone:** (804)282-0010　　　**Fax:** (804)282-0090
**Email:** asra@societyhq.org
**Website:** http://www.asra.com
James C. Eisenach, MD, Pres.

**Fnded:** 1974. **Mem:** 8,000. **Desc:** Physicians and research Ph.D.s. Conducts educational workshops. Sponsors annual refresher course. **Pub:** *ASRA Newsletter,* quarterly. Newsletter. *Price:* Included in membership dues. • *Regional Anesthesia and Pain Medicine,* bimonthly, with annual supplement. Journal. *Price:* Included in membership dues. **Frmly:** (2002) American Society of Regional Anesthesia and Pain Practice.

### ★ 4444 ★ Anaesthetic Research Society (ARS)

Univ. Department of Anaesthesia & Intensive Care
Queen's Medical Centre
Nottingham NG7 2UH, United Kingdom
**Phone:** 44 115 9709229　　　**Fax:** 44 115 9700739
**Email:** ravi.mahajan@nottingham.ac.uk
**Website:** http://www.ars.ac.uk/

**Fnded:** 1958. **Mem:** 660. **Lang(s):** English. **Desc:** Facilitates the presentation of members' research in anesthesiology (clinical or experimental, completed or in progress). **Pub:** *Proceedings,* 3/year. Journal. Included in the *British Journal of Anaesthesia.*

### ★ 4445 ★ Asian and Oceania Society for Intravenous Anesthesia (AOSIA)

84 Queensbridge St.
Southbank, VIC 3006, Australia
**Phone:** 61 3 96820244　　　**Fax:** 61 3 96820288
**Email:** aosiva99@icms.com.au

**Fnded:** 1996. **Lang(s):** English, Japanese. **Desc:** Anesthesiologists. Promotes increased use of intravenous anesthetics; seeks to advance the study, teaching, and practice of anesthesiology. Facilitates exchange of information among members; sponsors research and continuing professional development programs.

### ★ 4446 ★ Asian Oceania Society of Regional Anesthesia (AOSRA)

Philippine Society of Anaesthesiologists
PMA Bldg.
Quezon City, Metro Manila, Philippines
**Phone:** 63 2 975852　　　**Fax:** 63 2 975852

**Lang(s):** English, Filipino. **Desc:** Anesthesiologists. Promotes increased use of regional anesthetics; seeks to advance anesthesiological study and practice. Serves as a clearinghouse on regional anesthesia; sponsors research and continuing professional development programs.

### ★ 4447 ★ Asian Society of Cardiothoracic Anaesthesia (ASCA)

c/o World Express
Singapore Society of Anaesthesiologists
114 Middle Rd., Ste. 05-01
Singapore 0718, Singapore
**Phone:** 65 3363875　　　**Fax:** 65 3397843

**Lang(s):** Chinese, English. **Desc:** Anesthesiologists specializing in cardiothoracic anesthesia. Seeks to advance the profession of cardiothoracic anesthesia; promotes continuing professional development among members. Serves as a forum for the exchange of information among members; sponsors research and training programs.

### ★ 4448 ★ Association of Anaesthetists of Great Britain and Ireland

9 Bedford Sq.
London WC1B 3RA, United Kingdom
**Phone:** 44 207 6311650　　　**Fax:** 44 207 6314352
**Email:** info@aagbi.org
**Website:** http://www.aagbi.org

**Fnded:** 1932. **Mem:** 7,000. **Lang(s):** English. **Desc:** Ordinary Members, Trainee Members and Associate Members. Aims to promote education and research in anaesthesia and to bring together as many members as is possible at the three annual meetings to disseminate relevant information both at home and abroad. Fosters research in anaesthesia and allied subjects; encourages collaborative ventures involving members; represents members' interests. **Pub:** *Anaesthesia,* monthly. Journal.

### ★ 4449 ★ Association of Cardiothoracic Anaesthetists

c/o Fiona Gibson
Department of Anaesthesia
Royal Hospitals Trust
Grosvenor Rd.
Belfast BT12 6BA, United Kingdom
**Phone:** 44 2890 230415　　　**Fax:** 44 2890 325725
**Email:** fmg@supanet.com
**Website:** http://www.acta.org.uk/

**Fnded:** 1984. **Mem:** 326. **Desc:** Consultants who are currently engaged in the practice of cardiothoracic anaesthesia. To further the development of the art and science of caring for patients undergoing heart and chest surgery. **Pub:** Articles. Produced in association with the British Journal of Intensive Care.

### ★ 4450 ★ Association of Paediatric Anaesthetists of Great Britain and Ireland (APA)

c/o Dr. G. H. Meakin
University Department of Anaesthesia
Royal Manchester Childrens Hospital
Manchester M30 9HF, United Kingdom
**Phone:** 44 161 7272291
**Email:** george.meakin@man.ac.uk
**Website:** http://www.apa-gbi.org

**Fnded:** 1973. **Mem:** 400. **Lang(s):** English. **Desc:** Pediatric anesthetists practicing in Great Britain and Ireland and outside the British Isles. Promotes the study of pediatric anesthesiology. Collects and disseminates information; conducts research; advises other professional bodies on matters pertaining to pediatric anesthesiology. **Pub:** *Paediatric Anaesthesia,* bimonthly. • *Yearbook.*

**★ 4451 ★ Association of University Anesthesiologists (AUA)**
520 N Northwest Hwy.
Park Ridge, IL 60068-2573
**Phone:** (847)825-5586      **Fax:** (847)825-5658
**Email:** aua@asahq.org
**Website:** http://www.auahq.org
Steven J. Baker, PhD, Sec.
**Fnded:** 1953. **Mem:** 700. **Desc:** Academic anesthesiologists from medical school faculties. Encourages members to pursue original investigations in the clinic and the laboratory; develops methods of teaching anesthesiology. **Pub:** Directory, annual. **Frmly:** (1990) Association of University Anesthetists.

**★ 4452 ★ Associazione Italiana di Anestesia Odonto-Stomatologica (AINOS)**
Colonia Servizi Italia
Via Altinate, 125
I-35121 Padova, Italy
**Phone:** 39 49 3766097      **Fax:** 39 49 8776917
**Email:** colonna.servizi@tim.it
**Fnded:** 1972. **Mem:** 60. **State Groups:** 1. **Lang(s):** Italian. **Desc:** Physicians concerned with dental anesthesiology. Sponsors educational and research programs. **Pub:** *Giornale di Anestesia Stomatologica*, semiannual. Magazine.

**★ 4453 ★ Australian Society of Anaesthetists (ASA)**
Ste. 603 Eastpoint Tower
Edgecliff, NSW 2027, Australia
**Phone:** 61 2 93274022      **Fax:** 61 2 93277666
**Email:** jbushell@fed.asa.org.au
**Website:** http://www.asa.org.au
**Fnded:** 1934. **Lang(s):** English. **Desc:** Anaesthetists and medical practitioners with an interest in anaesthesia. Represents members' interests and promotes public awareness of anaesthesia.

**★ 4454 ★ Canadian Anesthesiologists' Society (CAS) (Societe Canadienne des Anesthesiologistes — SCA)**
1 Eglinton Ave. E, Ste. 208
Toronto, ON, Canada M4P 3A1
**Phone:** (416)480-0602      **Fax:** (416)480-0320
**Email:** anesthesia@cas.ca
**Website:** http://www.cas.ca
**Fnded:** 1920. **Mem:** 2,250. **Nat'l Groups:** 10. **Local Groups:** 10. **Lang(s):** English, French. **Desc:** Professional anesthesiologists and students. Promotes the art and science of anesthesia in Canada. Advocates measures designed to improve health care in Canada and hospital standards regarding anesthesia. Works in conjunction with the Canadian Medical Association. Conducts discussion sessions, panels, refresher courses, and workshops. Maintains C.A.S. International Education Fund for aid to developing countries. **Pub:** *Canadian Journal of Anesthesia*, monthly. Journal. • *CAS Guidelines to the Practice of Anesthesia*, annual. Directory. • *CAS-SCA Newsletter*, quarterly. Newsletter. • *CJA Annual Meeting Supplement*, annual. Report. **Frmly:** (1924) Canadian Society of Anaesthetists; (1943) Anaesthesia Section of the Canadian Medical Association; (1998) Canadian Anaesthetists' Society.

**★ 4455 ★ Confederation of Latin American Societies of Anesthesiology (CLASA) (Confederacion Latinoamericana de Sociedades de Anestesiologia)**
c/o CLASA Admin. Office
Aranguren 1323 piso 3
1405 Buenos Aires, Argentina
**Phone:** 54 11 44312547      **Fax:** 54 11 44312463
**Email:** clasa@satlink.com
**Website:** http://www.clasa-anestesia.org
**Fnded:** 1962.

**★ 4456 ★ Council on Certification of Nurse Anesthetists (CCNA)**
222 S Prospect Ave.
Park Ridge, IL 60068
**Phone:** (847)692-7050      **Fax:** (847)692-7082
**Email:** chodson@aana.com
**Website:** http://www.catinc.com/clients/ccna.htm
Susan S. Caulk, Dir., Certification
**Fnded:** 1975. **Mem:** 11. **Desc:** Sets certification standards and policies; confers certification upon entry-level nurse anesthetists. Conducts research. Works within the framework of the American Association of Nurse Anesthetists.

**★ 4457 ★ Dannemiller Memorial Educational Foundation (DMEF)**
12500 Network Blvd., Ste. 101
San Antonio, TX 78249
**Phone:** (210)641-8311      **Free:** 800-328-2308
**Fax:** (210)641-8329
**Email:** editor@pain.com
**Website:** http://www.dannemiller.com
Alon P. Winnie, MD, Pres.
**Fnded:** 1971. **Mem:** 30. **Desc:** Conducts annual Anesthesia Review Course in June for M.D. anesthesiologists and in the fall for nurse anesthesiologists, and review course of current concepts in anesthesiology. Sponsors weekend anesthesia and pain management meetings. **Pub:** *AnalgesiaFile*, monthly. Journal. Contains abstracted articles monthly from leading journals on pain and pain management. *Price:* $225/year. • *Anesthesia File*, monthly. Journal. Contains abstracted articles on anesthesia. *Price:* $225/year. • *Progress In Anesthesiology*, monthly. Articles. *Price:* $295/year. **Frmly:** (1984) Society of Air Force Anesthesiologists.

**★ 4458 ★ European Society of Anesthesiologists (ESA)**
Av de Tervuren 32, bte 30
B-1040 Brussels, Belgium
**Phone:** 32 2 7433298      **Fax:** 32 2 7433290
**Email:** jpop.esa@euronet.be
**Website:** http://www.euroanesthesia.org/
**Fnded:** 1993. **Desc:** Provides continuous education and promotes organization, formation and improvement of qualifications of anesthetists in Europe.

**★ 4459 ★ European Society of Regional Anaesthesia (ESRA) (Societe Europeenne d'Anesthesie Loco-Regionale)**
Kempenlaan 12
B-2300 Turnhout, Belgium
**Phone:** 32 14 422773      **Fax:** 32 14 439284
**Email:** dionne@esraeurope.org
**Website:** http://www.esraeurope.org
**Fnded:** 1980. **Mem:** 2,200. **Reg. Groups:** 7. **Lang(s):** English, French. **Desc:** Doctors of medicine specializing in anesthesiology in 30 countries. Seeks to reduce the risks and heighten the effectiveness of anesthesia by improving techniques of anesthesiology. Provides professional training; conducts workshops and seminars. **Pub:** *International Monitor on Regional Anesthesia*, quarterly. • *Newsletter*, annual. Newsletter. • *Yearbook*.

**★ 4460 ★ French-Language Neuro-Anesthetic-Resuscitation Association (Association de Neuro-Anesthesie-Reanimation de Langue Francaise)**
12 rue de l'Ecole de Medicine
F-75100 Paris, France
**Lang(s):** English, French. **Desc:** Neurologists and anesthesiologists. Seeks to increase awareness of resuscitation techniques among members. Conducts training programs for members; serves as a clearinghouse on neuro-anesthetic resuscitation.

**★ 4461 ★ German Society of Anaesthesiology and Intensive Care Medicine (GSAIM) (Deutsche Gesellschaft fur Anaesthesiologie und Intensivmedizin — DGAI)**
Roritzstrasse 27
D-90419 Nuremberg, Germany
**Phone:** 49 911 933780      **Fax:** 49 911 3938195
**Email:** dgai@dgai-ev.de
**Website:** http://www.dgai-nuernberg.de
**Fnded:** 1953. **Mem:** 9,600. **Desc:** Promotes scientific advancement and high standards of practice in anesthesiology and intensive care medicine. **Pub:** *Anaesthesie, Intensivmedizin, Notfallmedizin, Schmerztherapie*, periodic. Journal. • *Anaesthesiologie und Intensivmedizin*, periodic. • *Der Anaesthesist*, periodic.

**★ 4462 ★ Indian Society of Anesthetists**
Parel
Bombay 400 012, India
**Fnded:** 1947.

**★ 4463 ★ International Anesthesia Research Society (IARS)**
2 Summit Park Dr., Ste. 140
Cleveland, OH 44131-2571
**Phone:** (216)642-1124      **Fax:** (216)642-1127
**Email:** iarshq@iars.org
**Website:** http://www.iars.org
KC Wong, MD,PhD, Exec. Dir.
**Fnded:** 1922. **Mem:** 15,000. **Desc:** Anesthesiologists and other doctors of medicine and dentistry interested in the specialty of anesthesiology; associate members are registered nurses, physician assistants, and respiratory therapists. Fosters progress and research in all phases of anesthesiology. **Pub:** *Anesthesia & Analgesia*, monthly. Journal. Contains research articles and clinical reports on anesthesia and anesthesia-related subjects. Includes book reviews and employment listings. *Price:* $120/year for members; $440/year for nonmember institutions.

**★ 4464 ★ International Federation of Dental Anesthesiology Societies (IFDAS)**
13 Corinna Chambers
Corinna St.
Woden, ACT 2606, Australia
**Phone:** 61 2 62822605      **Fax:** 61 2 62815321
**Email:** jameskg@ozenail.com.au
**Fnded:** 1982. **Nat'l Groups:** 14. **Lang(s):** English. **Desc:** Societies of dental and medical practitioners in 14 countries. Promotes and encourages the study and practice of improved methods for administering anesthesia, analgesia, and sedation in dentistry and its related branches. Works to bring the benefits of these methods to people throughout the world. Facilitates the international exchange of information, research, and technology in the field. **Pub:** *IFDAS Newsletter*, semiannual. Newsletter.

**★ 4465 ★ International Trauma Anesthesia and Critical Care Society (ITACCS)**
PO Box 4826
Baltimore, MD 21211
**Phone:** (410)235-7697      **Fax:** (410)235-8084
**Email:** info@nwas.com
**Website:** http://www.trauma.itaccs.com
Christopher M. Grande, MD,MPH, Exec. Dir.
**Fnded:** 1988. **Mem:** 2,000. **Desc:** Healthcare professionals involved in trauma and critical care anesthesiology. Works to gain recognition for trauma anesthesiology as a discipline within anesthesiology and critical care medicine. Promotes cooperation and information sharing among healthcare professionals. Sponsors seminars and workshops; conducts research and educational programs; provides children's services; holds competitions; maintains speakers' bureau and

placement service. **Pub:** *Textbook of Trauma Anesthesia and Critical Care*. Book. • *Trauma Care*, biennial. Magazine. *Price:* Free.

★ **4466** ★ **Israel Society of Anesthesiologists (ISA)**
c/o Dr. Daniel Geva, Head
Department of Anesthesiology
Kaplan Hospital
Rehovot, Israel
**Email:** president@isranest.org.il
**Website:** http://www.isranest.org.il
**Fnded:** 1952. **Mem:** 600. **Lang(s):** English. **Desc:** Specialists and residents in training in the field of anesthesiology. Promotes the profession of anesthesiology in Israel and works to enhance the status of its members. Develops professional guidelines and standards.

**Navy Anesthesia Society (NAS)**
*See:* Entry 13463

★ **4467** ★ **Scientific Society of Anaesthesiologists in Bulgaria**
St. G. Sofiski 1
BG-1431 Sofia, Bulgaria
**Phone:** 359 2 521046          **Fax:** 359 2 548038
**Email:** tempus@ns.medfac.acad.bg
**Website:**          http://www.geocities.com/Vienna/2209/nas.html
**Fnded:** 1970. **Mem:** 800. **Desc:** Fosters research in anaesthesiology.

★ **4468** ★ **Societe Francaise d'Anesthesie et de Reanimation (SFAR)**
74, rue Raynouard
F-75016 Paris, France
**Phone:** 33 1 45258225          **Fax:** 33 1 40503522
**Email:** sfar@invivo.edu
**Website:** http://www.sfar.org
**Fnded:** 1936. **Mem:** 4,125. **Lang(s):** French. Does not correspond in English. **Desc:** Anesthesiologists; interested others in France. Promotes scientific research and high standards of practice in the field. **Pub:** *Annales Francaises d'Anesthesie et de Reanimation*, monthly. Journal. • *Conferences d'Actuausation - Congres.*

**Society for the Advancement of Anaesthesia in Dentistry (SAAD)**
*See:* Entry 6590

★ **4469** ★ **Society of Cardiovascular Anesthesiologists (SCA)**
2209 Dickens Rd.
PO Box 11086
Richmond, VA 23230-1086
**Phone:** (804)282-0084          **Fax:** (804)282-0090
**Email:** sca@societyhq.com
**Website:** http://www.scahq.org
Heather A. Spiess, Chief Staff Exec.
**Fnded:** 1977. **Mem:** 6,000. **Desc:** Anesthesiologists who specialize in cardiovascular surgical conditions. Purpose is to further medical education of cardiovascular anesthesiologists. Establishes goals and objectives for education of trainees in cardiovascular anesthesia; promotes personnel exchange between the U.S. and other countries; reviews related literature; maintains workshops; conducts research competitions. Sponsors Anesthesia Grand Rounds: Case Presentations as a section of the annual meeting. **Pub:** *Anesthesia and Analgesia*, monthly. Journal. • *Society of Cardiovascular Anesthesiologists–Newsletter*, bimonthly. Newsletter. Contains discussions of major issues within the cardiovascular anesthesiology field and reviews of related literature being published. *Price:* Included in membership dues. • Also publishes monographs.

★ **4470** ★ **Society for Education in Anesthesia (SEA)**
520 N NE Hwy.
Park Ridge, IL 60068-2573
**Phone:** (847)825-5568          **Fax:** (847)825-5658
**Email:** sea@asahq.org
**Website:** http://www.seahq.org
Stewart Hinckley, Exec. Dir.
**Fnded:** 1984. **Desc:** Anesthesiology educators. Committed to improve skills in anesthesia education. Offers an online discussion forum. **Pub:** *Journal of Education in Perioperative Medicine*, quarterly. Journal. Provides educationally important material to perioperative physicians.

★ **4471** ★ **Society of Neurosurgical Anesthesia and Critical Care (SNACC)**
PO Box 11086
Richmond, VA 23230-1086
**Phone:** (804)673-9037          **Fax:** (804)282-0090
**Email:** snacc@societyhq.com
**Website:** http://www.snacc.org/
Daniel J. Cole, MD, Pres.
**Fnded:** 1973. **Mem:** 500. **Desc:** Neurosurgeons and anesthesiologists interested in the care of patients with neurological disorders. Sponsors continuing medical education and research concerning the care of neurosurgical patients. **Pub:** *Annuai Summary of Society Meeting Proceedings*, annual. Proceedings. • *Society Membership*, annual. • Newsletter, 3-4/year.

**Society for Obstetric Anesthesia and Perinatology (SOAP)**
*See:* Entry 16731

★ **4472** ★ **Society for Pediatric Anesthesia**
1910 Byrd Ave., Ste. 100
PO Box 11086
Richmond, VA 23230-1086
**Phone:** (804)282-9780          **Fax:** (804)282-0090
**Email:** spa@societyhq.com
**Website:** http://WWW.pedsanesthesia.org
Steven C. Hall, Pres.
**Desc:** Working to foster quality anesthesia and perioperative care, and to alleviate pain in children

★ **4473** ★ **World Federation of Societies of Anaesthesiologists (WFSA) (Federation Mondiale des Societes d'Anesthesiologistes)**
WFSA Office, Level 8
Imperial House, 15-19 Kingsway
London WC2B 6TH, United Kingdom
**Phone:** 44 20 78365652          **Fax:** 44 20 78365616
**Email:** wfsa@compuserve.com
**Fnded:** 1955. **Mem:** 86. **Lang(s):** English, French, German, Spanish. **Desc:** Societies of anesthesiologists. Objectives are to: promote research in anesthesiology; disseminate scientific information; encourage the establishment of safety measures including equipment standardization; recommend suitable standards for training in anesthesiology. Provides information regarding opportunities for postgraduate training and research. **Pub:** *WFSA Newsletter*, semiannual. Newsletter.

## Research Centers

★ **4474** ★ **American Society for the Advancement of Anesthesia in Dentistry**
6 E Union Ave.
Bound Brook, NJ 08805
**Phone:** (732)469-9050          **Fax:** (732)271-1985
Dr. David Crystal, Exec. Sec.

**Activities/Fields:** Anesthesia in dentistry, including the study of sedation and its relation to physiologic sleep and the use of sedatives in dentistry. **Pub:** *Pain Control in Dentistry Journal*, semiannually.

★ **4475** ★ **International Anesthesia Research Society**
2 Summit Park Dr., Ste. 140
Cleveland, OH 44131-2571
**Phone:** (216)642-1124          **Fax:** (216)642-1127
**Email:** iarshq@iars.org
**Website:** http://www.iars.org
Anne F. Maggiore, Exec. Dir.
**Activities/Fields:** Anesthesiology, focusing on progress and research in all phases of this subject. **Pub:** *Anesthesia and Analgesia*, monthly. Journal.

★ **4476** ★ **McGill University Anaesthesia Research Department**
McIntyre Medical Science Bldg.
3655 Drummond St.
Montreal, QC, Canada H3G 1Y6
**Phone:** (514)398-6001          **Fax:** (514)398-4376
**Email:** krnjevic@medcor.mcgill.ca
Dr. K. Krnjevic, Dir.
**Activities/Fields:** Physiology, neurochemistry, and pharmacology of synaptic mechanisms and effects of anoxia and anaesthetic drugs in the central nervous system.

★ **4477** ★ **State University of New York Health Science Center at Brooklyn Ambulatory Surgery Unit**
450 Clarkson Ave., Box 6
Brooklyn, NY 11203-2012
**Phone:** (718)780-1350          **Fax:** (718)780-1358
**Email:** twersky@pipeline.com
Rebecca S. Twersky, MD, Dir.
**Activities/Fields:** Pain assessment in the mentally-challenged patient undergoing ambulatory surgical procedures.

★ **4478** ★ **Thomas Jefferson University Malignant Hyperthermia Research Center**
8490 Gibbon
Department of Anesthesiology
Jefferson Medical College
111 S 11th St.
Philadelphia, PA 19107
**Phone:** (215)955-6161          **Fax:** (215)923-5507
**Email:** henry.rosenberg@mail.tju.edu
Dr. Henry Rosenberg, Dir.
**Activities/Fields:** Malignant hyperthermia, neuromuscular blocking agents, and general anesthetic agents. Studies focus on diagnosis of malignant hyperthermia susceptibility and basic research in mechanisms underlying malignant hyperthermia, anesthetic action, and drug mechanisms.

**U.S. Department of Health and Human Services**
**National Institute of Dental Research**
**Division of Intramural Research**
**Neurobiology and Anesthesiology Branch**
*See:* Entry 6624

★ **4479** ★ **University of Arizona Advanced Biotechnology Laboratory**
Department of Anesthesiology
1501 N Campbell
Tucson, AZ 85724-5114
**Phone:** (520)626-5605          **Fax:** (520)626-5596
**Email:** malan@u.arizona.edu
**Website:**          http://www.ahsc.arizona.edu/anesth/anes_res.shtml
Prof. T. Philip Malan, MD, Contact
**Activities/Fields:** Implementation of advanced technology to anesthesia, including utilization of computers for automation of monitoring and data collection,

development of improved anesthesia delivery and monitoring equipment, basic research and development of new monitoring parameters, and ergonomic approaches to anesthesia tasks. Pharmacologic research is also conducted with emphasis on molecular mechanisms of anesthetics. Pharmacologic clinical research is conducted in acute post-operative pain models in various post surgical patients, such as cardiothoracic, orthopedic, general surgery, gynecological, and ambulatory surgery, also studies investigational intraoperative medications. **Pub:** *Pain*, quarterly.

## Federal Government Agencies

**★ 4480 ★ U.S. Department of Transportation (FAA)**
Federal Aviation Administration
Associate Administrator for Regulation and Certification
Office of Aerospace Medicine
800 Independence Ave. SW
Washington, DC 20591
**Phone:** (202)366-4000
**Website:** http://www.cami.jccbi.gov/
Thomas A. Hart, Asst. Admin. for Reg. and Cert.

**Desc:** The Office is responsible for the medical certification of all airmen. It maintains the Civil Aeromedical Institute at the FAA Aeronautical Center in Oklahoma City.

## National & International Organizations

**★ 4481 ★ Aerospace Medical Association (AsMA)**
320 S Henry St.
Alexandria, VA 22314-3579
**Phone:** (703)739-2240          **Fax:** (703)739-9652
**Email:** rrayman@asma.org
**Website:** http://www.asma.org
Russell B. Rayman, MD, Exec. Dir.

**Fnded:** 1929. **Mem:** 3,300. **Desc:** Medical and scientific personnel engaged in clinical, operational, and research activities in aviation, space, and environmental medicine. Sponsors continuing professional education programs. **Pub:** *Aviation, Space, and Environmental Medicine*, monthly. Journal. Covers the medical aspects of survival in aviation, space, and undersea exploration. Includes annual index; book reviews; meetings calendar. *Price:* Included in membership dues; $140/year for nonmembers; $173/year foreign (agency discount available). • *Aviation, Space and Environmental Medicine*, annual. Membership Directory. • *Scientific Abstracts*, annual. **Frmly:** (1959) Aero Medical Association.

**★ 4482 ★ Airlines Medical Directors Association (AMDA)**
c/o Ralph G. Fennell, M.D.
United Airlines Medical
Denver International Airport
Denver, CO 80249-6363
**Phone:** (303)348-4300          **Fax:** (303)348-4338
Ralph G. Fennell, MD, Sec. Dir.

**Fnded:** 1946. **Mem:** 130. **Desc:** Physicians employed by, or consulting to, commerical airlines.

**★ 4483 ★ Civil Aviation Medical Association (CAMA)**
PO Box 23864
Oklahoma City, OK 73123-3864
**Phone:** (405)840-0199          **Fax:** (405)848-1053
**Email:** jmlharris@aol.com
**Website:** http://www.civilavmed.com
Robin Dodge, MD, Pres.

**Fnded:** 1948. **Mem:** 800. **Desc:** Aviation medical examiners, physicians who are pilots, aviation medical educators, flight instructors, fixed base operators, NASA physicians, and airline medical department physicians. Purposes are to: ascertain the basic mental and physical requirements of civil airmen and the proper methods for the physical assessment of airmen engaged in civil aviation; review continuously the scientific status of civil aviation medicine and advance and disseminate the information by which civil aviation medicine safeguards public safety; sponsor basic and advanced training in civil aviation medicine; foster international fellowship among members, allied medical and technical groups, and students of aviation medicine; unite the designated civil aviation medical examiners of the world into an effective medical body dedicated to the promotion and practice of aviation safety for the public benefit. Maintains speakers' bureau; compiles statistics. **Pub:** *FlightPhysician*, every other month. Newsletter. Covers membership activities. Contains meetings calendar and promotion of members. *Price:* $5/issue. **Frmly:** (1955) Airline Medical Examiners Association.

**★ 4484 ★ German Society for Aviation and Space Medicine (DGLRM) (Deutsche Gesellschaft fur Luft- und Raumfahrtmedizin)**
Konigswinter Strabe 522-524
D-53227 Bonn, Germany
**Phone:** 49 228 447528          **Fax:** 49 228 447707
**Email:** michael.reichert@dlr.de
**Website:** http://www.kp.dlr.de/DGLR
**Fnded:** 1963. **Mem:** 700. **Lang(s):** English, German. **Desc:** Scientists and physicians. Supports scientific work in the fields of aviation and space medicine. Conducts work group studies on ergonomics, the history of aviation medicine, and related subjects. Participates in the presentation of educational courses in aviation medicine for physicians. **Pub:** *Mitteilungen*, bimonthly.

**★ 4485 ★ National Association of Air Medical Communication Specialists (NAAMCS)**
PO Box 28
Otis Orchards, WA 99027-0028
**Free:** 877-396-2227
**Email:** shellsholl@aol.com
**Website:** http://www.naacs.org
Allan Adler, Pres.

**Fnded:** 1989. **Mem:** 300. **Desc:** Air medical communications specialists. Promotes professional advancement of members. Represents members at the national level; formulates standards of ethics and practice in air medical communications; sponsors educational and training programs. **Pub:** *NAACS Newsletter*, quarterly. Newsletter. • *NAACS Training Manual*. Manual.

**★ 4486 ★ Society of United States Air Force Flight Surgeons**
PO Box 35387
Brooks City-Base, TX 78235
**Phone:** (210)536-2844          **Fax:** (210)536-2017
**Email:** Robert.Yono@brooksaf.mil
**Website:** http://www.sousaffs.org
Col. Jay Neubauer, Sec.

**Fnded:** 1960. **Mem:** 500. **Desc:** Flight surgeons who are members of the Aerospace Medical Association and who are currently serving on active duty with or have retired from the United States Air Force, or are serving in the Air Force Reserve or Air National Guard. Fosters advancement of aerospace medicine throughout the Air Force and encourages the clinical, laboratory, flight line, and in-flight investigation of medical problems in Air Force flying, missile, and space operations. **Pub:** *Aircraft Mishap Investigation Handbook*. Handbook. • *Flight Surgeon's Checklist*. Book. • *Flightlines*, quarterly. Newsletter. *Price:* Included in membership dues; $15/year for nonmembers.

## Research Centers

**★ 4487 ★ Brandeis University**
Ashton Graybiel Spatial Orientation Lab
Mail Stop 033
415 South St.
Waltham, MA 02454
**Phone:** (781)736-2033          **Fax:** (781)736-2031
**Email:** lackner@brandeis.edu
James R. Lackner, Dir.

**Activities/Fields:** Human spatial orientation, effects of gravity on vestibulo-ocular reflex, the role of vestibular and cervical sensory and motor activity in hand movement control, oculomotor stability, and effects of different G levels. Also studies human sensorimotor adaptation to unusual force environments.

**★ 4488 ★ Columbia University**
Eye Radiation and Environmental Research Laboratory
Columbia-Presbyterian Medical Center
630 W 168th St., Rm. 212
New York, NY 10032-3784
**Phone:** (212)305-6748          **Fax:** (212)305-6749
**Email:** bvw1@columbia.edu
**Website:** http://cpmcnet.columbia.edu/dept/eye/rad
Dr. Basil Worgul, Dir.

**Activities/Fields:** Assessment of the eye lens following exposure to exogenous agents or systemically applied compounds; drugs suspected of cataractotoxicity or being tested for anticataractogenic potential, cellular mechanisms of radiation cataract, cataractogenesis, the effects of heavy particles on ocular tissue, and potential risks to the eyes of astronauts during extended manned flight in the hostile radiational environment of space. Also directing the Ukrainian/American Chernobyl ocular study. **Pub:** *Scientific papers*, bimonthly.

★ **4489** ★ **National Aeronautics and Space Administration**
**George C. Marshall Space Flight Center**
**Space Sciences Laboratory**
**Space Plasma Physics**
Mailcode ES83
Huntsville, AL 35812
**Phone:** (256)544-5339          **Fax:** (256)544-5244
**Email:** jim.spann@msfc.nasa.gov
**Website:** http://science.nasa.gov/ssl/pad/sppb/
James F. Spann, Jr., Contact
**Activities/Fields:** Physical processes that control the geospace plasma environment and its interaction with both banatural and man-made bodies in space. Emphases are on the plasma that originates in the ionosphere, and its heating in auroral light displays.

★ **4490** ★ **National Space Biomedical Research Institute (NSBRI)**
1 Baylor Plz., NA-425
Houston, TX 77030
**Phone:** (713)798-7412          **Fax:** (713)798-7413
**Email:** info@www.nsbri.org
**Website:** http://www.nsbri.org/
Bobby R. Alford, MD, Ch. /CEO
**Activities/Fields:** Prevention and solution of health problems related to long-duration space travel and prolonged exposure to microgravity. Byproducts of such research would be treatments for conditions such as osteoporosis, muscle wasting, shift-related sleep disorders and radiation-related conditions. The institute also is researching ways to deliver medical care on long-duration space travel through new technologies and remote-treatment advances.

★ **4491** ★ **New Jersey Specialized Center of Research and Training for Bioregenerative Life Support**
Foran Hall, Rm. 186
Rutgers University
59 Dudley Rd.
New Brunswick, NJ 08901-8520
**Phone:** (732)932-8978          **Fax:** (732)932-4882
**Email:** sauser@aesop.rutgers.edu
**Website:** http://nj-nscort.rutgers.edu
Dr. Harry W. Janes, Dir.
**Activities/Fields:** Problems of human life support associated with long duration space missions and lunar or Mars outposts.

★ **4492** ★ **U.S. Department of Defense**
**Air Force Materiel Command**
**Armstrong Laboratory**
**Division of Biodynamics and Biocommunications**
ATTN: AL/CFB
Wright Patterson AFB, OH 45433-7901
**Fax:** (513)255-2781
**Activities/Fields:** Conducts a multidisciplinary research and development program to protect man against mechanical force environments, provide him with the best protective equipment, and guarantee his full performance capability. The Division's program includes basic research, exploratory development, advanced development, and operational systems support in the areas of: noise, impact, acceleration, vibration, locomotion, microgravity, pilot performance, aircraft operations, communication effectiveness, aircrew protection, and emergency escape. Activities are carried out in these branches: Bioacoustics and Biocommunications, Vulnerability Assessment, Escape and Impact Protection, and Combined Stress.

★ **4493** ★ **U.S. Department of Defense**
**Air Force Materiel Command**
**Armstrong Laboratory**
**Division of Human Engineering**
2610 Seventh St., Bldg. 441
Wright Patterson AFB, OH 45433-7901
**Phone:** (937)255-5227          **Fax:** (937)656-7617
**Email:** ken.boff@wpafb.af.mil
Dr. Kenneth R. Boff, Chf. Scientist
**Activities/Fields:** Science and leading edge technology to define human capabilities, vulnerabilities, and effectiveness; train warriors; integrate operators and weapon systems; protect Air Force people; and sustain aerospace operations. **Pub:** *Proceedings.* • *Research Reports.*

★ **4494** ★ **U.S. Department of Defense**
**Air Force Materiel Command**
**Human Systems Center**
**Air Force School of Aerospace Medicine**
2602 Louis Bauer Dr.
USAFSAM
Brooks AFB, TX 78235
**Phone:** (210)536-3500          **Fax:** (210)536-2216
Col. Tom Travis, Comdr.
**Activities/Fields:** Science and technology divisions (Clinical Sciences, Crew Technology, and Radiation Sciences); operational support; and aeromedical education and training divisions (Education, Epidemiology, and Hyperbaric Medicine). Technical and Veterinary Sciences provide support. Products and services provided by the USAFSAM impact the USAF in crew protection and performance enhancement; occupational, safety and health by making sure appropriate standards are followed to protect the work force; and medical readiness in combat casualty care and aeromedical evacuation. **Pub:** *Technical Reports.*

★ **4495** ★ **U.S. Department of Defense**
**Army Medical Research and Materiel Command**
**Army Aeromedical Research Laboratory**
PO Box 620577
Fort Rucker, AL 36362-0577
**Phone:** (334)255-6907          **Fax:** (334)255-6067
**Email:** ssc@amedd.army.mil
**Website:** http://www.usaarl.army.mil
Col. Brian Campbell, Comdr., Contact
**Activities/Fields:** Health hazards of Army aviation, tactical combat vehicles, and selected weapon systems; assessing stress and fatigue in personnel operating these systems and developing countermeasures; and assisting in the development of criteria upon which to base standards for entry and retention in Army aviation specialties. Principal areas of interest include medical study of visual/auditory functions, man-machine integration, physiological responses to operational environments, impact of continuous operations on individual and crew performance, testing of aeromedical evacuation life support equipment, development of improved means of patient evacuation, and airworthiness.

★ **4496** ★ **U.S. Department of Transportation**
**Federal Aviation Administration**
**Civil Aeromedical Institute (CAMI)**
AAM-3
PO Box 25082
Oklahoma City, OK 73125-5060
**Phone:** (405)954-1000          **Fax:** (405)954-1010
**Email:** william_e_collins@mmacmail.jccbi.gov
**Website:** http://www.cami.jccbi.gov/
Dr. William E. Collins, Dir.
**Activities/Fields:** Civil aviation medicine directed toward preventing aircraft accidents and increasing survival rates associated with aircraft accidents. Studies are primarily in the fields of human factors, psychology, physiology, toxicology, cabin safety, restraint, ditching, and protective breathing equipment. Other areas of study include vision, human performance, and operator selection. Institute also conducts

programs in aircraft accident investigation; medical certification (more than 640,000 airmen); statistical studies from the airman data bank; occupational health; and medical education of physicians, pilots, flight inspectors, accident investigators, and flight attendants. flight attendants. **Pub:** *Aeromedical safety brochures.* • *Federal Air Surgeon's Medical Bulletin.* • *Office of Aviation Medicine reports.*

★ **4497** ★ **U.S. Department of Transportation**
**Federal Aviation Administration**
**Civil Aeromedical Institute**
**Aeromedical Research Division**
**(Toxicology and Accident Research Laboratory)**
6500 S MacArthur Blvd.
PO Box 25082
Oklahoma City, OK 73125-5066
**Phone:** (405)954-4866          **Fax:** (405)954-3705
**Email:** dennis_canfield@mmacmail.jccbi.gov
**Website:** http://www.cami.jccbi.gov
Dennis Canfield, Mgr.
**Activities/Fields:** Human factor safety in civilian aviation. Studies are concerned with medical evidence available from aircraft accidents, including the genesis of the injuries experienced in those accidents; and effects of toxicants that may be present in post-crash fires or that may be otherwise introduced into the aviation environment. **Pub:** *Office of Aviation Medicine Technical Reports.* **Frmly:** (1991) Aviation Pathology and Toxicology Laboratory.

★ **4498** ★ **U.S. Department of Transportation**
**Federal Aviation Administration**
**Civil Aeromedical Institute**
**Aeromedical Research Division**
Mail Code AAM-600
PO Box 25082
Oklahoma City, OK 73125-5066
**Phone:** (405)954-4808          **Fax:** (405)954-0130
**Email:** james.e.whinnery@faa.gov
**Website:** http://www.cami.jccbi.gov
Dr. James E. Whinnery, PhD, M, Mgr.
**Activities/Fields:** Provides the Federal Aviation Administration (FAA) and the Federal Air Surgeon with the capability to: resolve operational, regulatory, and administrative problems related to medical certification of pilots; define and optimize workload and performance in aviation-related activities; and improve protection and survival in hostile and adverse aspects of general and commercial aviation. Division comprises the Toxicology and Accident Research Laboratory, Protection and Survival Laboratory, and Data Processing and Analysis Team. **Pub:** *Proceedings.* • *Research Reports.*

★ **4499** ★ **U.S. Department of Transportation**
**Federal Aviation Administration**
**Civil Aeromedical Institute**
**Aeromedical Research Division**
**(Protection and Survival Laboratory)**
Mail Code AAM-630
6500 S MacArthur Blvd.
PO Box 25082
Oklahoma City, OK 73125
**Phone:** (405)954-5510          **Fax:** (405)954-4984
**Email:** van.gowdy@faa.gov
**Website:** http://www.cami.jccbi.gov/aam-600/630/600P&S-Lab.html
Van Gowdy, Mgr.
**Activities/Fields:** Problems concerning civil airmen and equipment in emergency conditions, such as function of seat/restraint/interior crash injury protection, emergency evacuation, flotation, and cabin safety. Principal areas of research interest are biomechanics of impact, human factors, and breathing equipment. Laboratory comprises the Biodynamics Research, and Cabin Safety Research units and Environ-

mental Physiology. **Pub:** *Memorandums.* • *Research reports.*

**★ 4500 ★ U.S. Department of Transportation**
**Federal Aviation Administration**
**Civil Aeromedical Institute**
**Human Resources Research Division**
Mail Code AAM-500
PO Box 25082
Oklahoma City, OK 73125
**Phone:** (405)954-4846     **Fax:** (405)954-4852
**Email:** david_schroeder@mmacmail.jccbi.gov
Dr. David J. Schroeder, Mgr.

**Activities/Fields:** Conducts an integrated program of applied field and laboratory performance research on organizational and human factors aspects of aviation work environments. Guidance for program development is obtained from the National Plan for Civil Aviation Human Factors, the FAA Strategic Plan, and senior agency management. Emphasis is placed on improving human performance through enhanced human machine/systems interfaces, equipment design, selection, training, opertating procedures, and business practices.

**★ 4501 ★ U.S. Department of Transportation**
**Federal Aviation Administration**
**Office of Aviation Medicine**
**Medical Specialities Division**
800 Independence Ave. SW
Washington, DC 20593
**Phone:** (202)267-8035     **Fax:** (202)493-5006
**Email:** nicholas.lomangino@faa.gov
Dr. Nicholas Lomangino, Mgr.

**Activities/Fields:** Program office for medical standards, certification policy, and aeromedical research and development. Principal area of research interest is clinical medicine. **Pub:** *Guidelines.* • *Newsletters.* • *Research Reports.*

**★ 4502 ★ Virginia Commonwealth University**
**Medical Informatics and Technology Applications Consortium (MITAC)**
1101 E Marshall St., Ste. 8017
PO Box 980480
Richmond, VA 23298-0480
**Phone:** (434)827-1020     **Fax:** (434)827-1029
**Email:** charles.doarn@vcu.edu
**Website:** http://www.meditac.com/
Charles R. Doarn, MBA, Exec. Dir.

**Activities/Fields:** Medical informatics and health care delivery systems that will revolutionize health care in space and on Earth.

# Chapter 7
# Biomedical Engineering

## Foundations & Other Funding Organizations

### Private Foundations

**★ 4503 ★ Whitaker Foundation**
1700 North Moore St., Ste. 2200
Arlington, VA 22209
**Phone:** (703)528-2430　　**Fax:** (703)528-2431
**Email:** info@whitaker.org
**Website:** http://www.whitaker.org
Peter Katona, President
**Fnded:** 1975. **Philosophy:** The foundation will spend all its assets, primarily in support of education and research programs in biomedical engineering, and then go out of business at the end of 2006. The Biomedical Engineering Research Grants program supports research projects that enable investigators to establish academic careers in biomedical engineering or a closely related field. ...the foundation's Graduate Fellowship program...is designed to support top students in their pursuit of a biomedical engineering-based doctorate. In 1999 the foundation merged its two major programs for building education infrastructure - the Leaderships Awards and Development Awards programs. The goal of the Leadership Development Awards program is to support major initiatives to enhance the field of biomedical engineering at research universities in the United States. Since 1992, the foundation's Special Opportunity's Awards program has encouraged innovations in biomedical engineering research and education program development. The goal of the foundation's Industrial Internship program is to support internships and cooperate with education programs that smooth the way from student life to company employment. The Teaching Materials Program, is designed to enhance the education of biomedical engineers through the development of quality teaching materials. The Biomedical Engineering Summer Internships Program (BESIP), a joint enterprise between the foundation and the National Institute of Health, pairs undergraduate biomedical engineering students with mentors at various NIH laboratories. The foundation supports conferences that enhance the field of biomedical engineering in a new and innovative way. This usually excludes the general support of a conference in an ongoing series. The foundation operates regional programs in the Harrisburg, PA, and Naples, FL, areas. 1999 Annual Report **Priorities:** *Education:* 8%. Supports graduate fellowships. *International:* 28%. Supports biomedical engineering research and other biomedical engineering programs. *Note:* Total contributions made in 1999. **Typ. Recipients:** Cancer, Children's Health/Hospitals, Clinics/Medical Centers, Eyes/Blindness, Geriatric Health, Heart, Hospices, Hospitals, Hospitals (University Affiliated), Medical Education, Medical Rehabilitation, Medical Research, Mental Health, Prenatal Health Issues, Preventive Medicine/Wellness Organizations, Public Health, Research/Studies Institutes, Respiratory, Speech & Hearing. **Geo. Dist:** for research, special opportunity, and other grant programs; Naples, FL, for regional programs; Harrisburg, PA, for

regional programs; for research and special opportunity programs.

## National & International Organizations

**★ 4504 ★ American Association of Electrodiagnostic Medicine (AAEM)**
421 1st Ave., SW, Ste. 300 East
Rochester, MN 55902
**Phone:** (507)288-0100　　**Fax:** (507)288-1225
**Email:** aaem@aaem.net
**Website:** http://www.aaem.net
Shirlyn A. Adkins, J.D., Exec. Dir.
**Fnded:** 1953. **Mem:** 4,414. **Desc:** M.D.'s and D.O.'s or equivalent foreign degrees who practice or are interested in electrodiagnostic medicine. Objective is to increase and extend knowledge of electromyography and electrodiagnostic medicine, and to improve patient care. **Pub:** *AAEM Case Reports*, periodic. Monograph. *Price:* $8 for members; $10 for nonmembers. • *AAEM Minimonographs*, 2-3/year. Monograph. *Price:* $10 for members; $15 for nonmembers. • *American Association of Electrodiagnostic Medicine–Membership Directory*, annual. Membership Directory. *Price:* Included in membership dues; $50 for nonmembers. • *Guidelines*, periodic. *Price:* $75 for members; $150 for nonmembers; $10 each, for individual chapters to members; $20 each, for individual chapters to nonmembers. • *Muscle & Nerve*, monthly. *Price:* Included in fellow/associate membership. • Also publishes course syllabi. **Frmly:** (1990) American Association of Electromyography and Electrodiagnosis.

**American Institute of Ultrasound in Medicine (AIUM)**
*See:* Entry 18109

**★ 4505 ★ American Lithotripsy Society (ALS)**
305 Second Ave., Ste. 200
Waltham, MA 02451
**Phone:** (781)895-9098　　**Fax:** (781)895-9088
**Email:** als@lithotripsy.org
**Website:** http://www.lithotripsy.org
Wesley E. Harrington, CAE, Contact
**Fnded:** 1987. **Mem:** 1,207. **Desc:** Promotes trade and public awareness of Lithotripsy. (Lithotripsy is a noninvasive procedure to treat kidney stones and gall stones.) Disseminates information; conducts educational programs, quality improvement and certification programs. **Pub:** *ALS Quarterly*, quarterly. Newsletter.

**American Registry of Diagnostic Medical Sonographers (ARDMS)**
*See:* Entry 18111

**American Society of Echocardiography (ASE)**
*See:* Entry 18114

**★ 4506 ★ American Society for Healthcare Engineering (ASHE)**
1 N Franklin, 27th Fl.
Chicago, IL 60606
**Phone:** (312)422-3800　　**Fax:** (312)422-4571
**Email:** ashe@aha.org
**Website:** http://www.ashe.org
**Desc:** Advocates for continual improvement in the health care engineering and facilities management professions. **Pub:** *Certified Healthcare Facility Manager Candidate Handbook.* Handbook.

**★ 4507 ★ Association for Applied Psychophysiology and Biofeedback (AAPB)**
10200 W 44th Ave., Ste. 304
Wheat Ridge, CO 80033
**Phone:** (303)422-8436　　**Free:** 800-477-8892
**Fax:** (303)422-8894
**Email:** fbutler@resourcecenter.com
**Website:** http://www.aapb.org
Francine Butler, PhD, Pres.
**Fnded:** 1969. **Mem:** 2,000. **State Groups:** 35. **Desc:** Persons interested in the "interrelationship of external feedback systems, states of consciousness, and the physiological mechanisms involved." Promotes rapid interchange of ideas and information among members. Offers Continuing Education Training Programs. Maintains numerous committees. **Pub:** *Applied Psychophysiology and Biofeedback*, quarterly. Journal. Study of physiological systems and social environmental health. • *Biofeedback News magazine*, quarterly. Newsletter. • *Proceedings of Annual Meeting.* Proceedings. **Frmly:** (1976) Biofeedback Research Society; (1988) Biofeedback Society of America.

**★ 4508 ★ Australian Federation for Medical and Biological Engineering**
Department of Electrical Engineering
University of Melbourne
Parkville, VIC 3052, Australia
**Fnded:** 1959.

**★ 4509 ★ Biomedical Engineering Association of Ireland (BEAI)**
c/o Mr. John McGivney, Chm.
Department of Medical Physics and Clinical Engineering
St. Luke's Hospital
Oaklands
Highfield Rd.
Dublin, Ireland
**Phone:** 353 1 4065382
**Email:** bjpwoa@indigo.ie
**Fnded:** 1990. **Nat'l Groups:** 1. **Reg. Groups:** 4. **Local Groups:** 6. **Lang(s):** English. **Desc:** Promotes

biomedical and clinical engineering in Ireland. **Pub:** *Spectrum*, quarterly.

### ★ 4510 ★ Board for Orthotist - Prosthetist Certification

c/o Dr. D.O. Fedder, CEO
506 W Fayette, Ste. 200
Baltimore, MD 21201-1715
**Phone:** (410)539-3910          **Free:** 877-776-2200
**Fax:** (410)706-0869
**Email:** info@bocusa.org
**Website:** http://www.bocusa.org
Dr. D.O. Fedder, CEO
**Fnded:** 1984. **Desc:** Certifies orthotists and prosthetists based on comprehensive performance and examinations. Also accredits orthotic and prosthetic facilities and maintains a registry of Orthotic Fitters and Mastectomy Fitters. **Pub:** *BOC Report*, quarterly. Newsletter. • *Candidate Handbook*, annual. Handbook.

### British Medical Ultrasound Society (BMUS)

*See:* Entry 18131

### ★ 4511 ★ Canadian Association of Prosthetists and Orthotists (Association Canadienne des Prothesistes et Orthesistes)

303-267 Edmonton St.
Winnipeg, MB, Canada R3C 1S2
**Phone:** (204)949-4972          **Fax:** (204)947-3627
**Email:** capo@mb.sympatico.ca
**Website:** http://www.pando.ca
**Lang(s):** English, French. **Desc:** Organizations and individuals engaged in the production and fitting of orthotic and prosthetic devices. Seeks to advance the science and practice of orthotics and prosthetics; facilitates professional development of members. Sponsors research and educational programs; serves as a clearinghouse on orthotics and prosthetics. **Pub:** *Alignment*, annual. Magazine.

### ★ 4512 ★ Chinese Mechanical Engineering Society (CMES)

Sanlihe Rd.
Beijing 100823, People's Republic of China
**Phone:** 852 10 68695319   **Fax:** 852 10 68533613

### ★ 4513 ★ Colombian Association of Bioengineering and Medical Electronics

Apdo Aereo 40253
Bucaramanga, Colombia
**Phone:** 57 7 6342225          **Fax:** 57 7 6437752
**Email:** ingelmed@bioingenieros.com

### ★ 4514 ★ International Association of Orthotists and Prosthetists (Union Internationale des Techniciens Orthopedistes — INTERBOR)

Rue de Laeken 67
1853 Strombeek
Brussels, Belgium
**Phone:** 32 2 2679544          **Fax:** 32 2 2679107
**Fnded:** 1958. **Mem:** 19. **Lang(s):** English, French, German. **Desc:** Organizations and individuals in 19 countries working to develop the science of orthotics and prosthetics. Conducts research and educational programs.

### ★ 4515 ★ International Federation for Medical and Biological Engineering (IFMBE) (Federation Internationale de Genie Medical et Biologique)

INSERM U455
Pavillon Riser, C.H.U. Purpan
Place Baylac
F-31059 Toulouse, France
**Phone:** 33 5 61778276          **Fax:** 33 5 61594636
**Email:** morucci@cict.fr
**Website:** http://www.who.int/ina-ngo/ngo/ngo066.htm
**Fnded:** 1959. **Lang(s):** English. **Desc:** Medical and biological engineers and others involved in the field. Encourages and fosters research in the field of medical and biological engineering. Promotes international cooperation; disseminates scientific information; cooperates with developing countries to encourage training of health personnel in maintenance and repair of laboratory and other equipment. **Pub:** *Medical and Biological Engineering and Computing*. Journal.

### International Society for Bioengineering and the Skin

*See:* Entry 6828

### ★ 4516 ★ International Society of Electrocardiology (ISE)

c/o Prof. Peter W. Macfarlane
University Department of Medical Cardiology
Royal Infirmary
10 Alexandra Parade
Glasgow G31 2ER, United Kingdom
**Phone:** 44 141 2114724          **Fax:** 44 141 5526114
**Email:** peter.w.macfarlane@clinmed.gla.ac.uk
**Website:** http://www.electrocardiology.sk
**Fnded:** 1994. **Mem:** 300. **Lang(s):** English. **Desc:** Researchers and physicians in 25 countries in cardiovascular physiology and pathology, cardiology, biomathematics, biophysics, and computer science who are interested in electrocardiology. Sponsors International Congress on Electrocardiology to develop professional programs. **Pub:** *Proceedings*, annual.

### International Society for Magnetic Resonance in Medicine

*See:* Entry 18146

### International Society for Prosthetics and Orthotics (ISPO) (Societe Internationale de Prothese et Orthese)

*See:* Entry 8006

### Japanese Society for Artificial Organs

*See:* Entry 20336

### ★ 4517 ★ National Institute of Electromedical Information (NIEI)

PO Box 4633
Bay Terrace, NY 11360-4633
**Phone:** (516)504-1423          **Fax:** (718)225-1041
**Email:** sniei@aol.com
**Website:** http://www.ispo.org
Stanley H. Kornhauser, PhD, Pres.
**Fnded:** 1984. **Mem:** 1,494. **Desc:** Health care practitioners, medical educators, research scientists, and electromedical device manufacturers. Disseminates information on research, case histories, new and proposed theories, and clinical applications of electromedicine to professionals, laypersons, federal agencies, U.S. industry, and universities. (Electromedicine deals with the application of diagnostic, monitoring and prosthetic electromedical devices used in research and clinical settings as well as the application of therapeutic electric currents in the prevention and treatment of diseases.) Supports the development of programs and materials for the preparation of those studying electromedicine; fosters the establishment of programs and creation of partnerships that provide resource-sharing networks and professional linkage among clinicians, researchers, colleges and universities, health care institutions, electromedical equipment manufacturers, and other scientific and educational organizations. Encourages exchange of information through an interdisciplinary forum between researchers and clinicians and advises and coordinates matters of mutual interest between members and other organizations. Enhances the career awareness of secondary or post-secondary students in the emerging fields of electromedical technology. Funds research and educational projects. Develops standards and certification systems for determining the efficacy of electromedical devices. Offers tutorials. Maintains consulting service and speakers' bureau; compiles statistics. **Pub:** *American Journal of Electromedicine included in Medical Electronics*, Temporarily Suspended. Journal. Includes case studies, original research documentation, interviews on state-of-the-art topics in electromedicine and product reports. • *National Institute of Electromedical Information–Membership Directory*, annual. Membership Directory. *Price:* Included in membership dues. • Books. • Bulletin, periodic. • Proceedings, periodic. • Also publishes book reviews and educational materials.

### ★ 4518 ★ National Institute for Rehabilitation Engineering (NIRE)

PO Box 1088
Hewitt, NJ 07421
**Phone:** (973)853-6585          **Free:** 800-736-2216
**Fax:** (973)832-2894
**Email:** nire@theoffice.net
**Website:** http://www.theoffice.net/nire
Donald Selwyn, Exec. VP
**Fnded:** 1967. **Desc:** Multidisciplinary research, training, and service organization providing custom-designed and custom-made tools and devices, along with intensive personal task-performance and driver training, to aid the handicapped person in becoming more self-sufficient and independent. Often an organization of "last resort" for permanently, severely, or multihandicapped persons, the NIRE is staffed by electronics engineers, physicists, psychologists, optometrists, and other volunteers who work as a team with the handicapped person. These specialists review the handicapped person's abilities, disabilities, and task-performance goals and are thus able to help advise, plan, and implement programs to increase the person's abilities to perform desired tasks, using a combination of methods involving different practitioners and disciplines. Staff members also adapt, modify, and construct equipment specially suited to the individual client's need. No handicapped person is denied the institute's services due to an inability to pay, and fees for others are based on each person's income and means. Conducts occasional seminars for the handicapped and for professionals serving the handicapped. Provides speakers and seminar participants for other agencies' programs. Compiles statistics. **Pub:** *Rehabilitation Newsletter*, quarterly. Newsletter. Features announcements of upcoming seminars. *Price:* Included in membership dues.

### North American Society of Pacing and Electrophysiology (NASPE)

*See:* Entry 5052

### Society of Computed Body Tomography and Magnetic Resonance (SCBT/MR)

*See:* Entry 18157

### Society for Psychophysiological Research (SPR)

*See:* Entry 12655

## Research Centers

### Arizona State University Biomedical Engineering Laboratories

*See:* Entry 4616

**★ 4519 ★ Brigham and Women's Hospital**
**Neuroimaging Analysis Center**
Department of Radiology
75 Francis St.
Boston, MA 02115
**Phone:** (617)732-7692 **Fax:** (617)582-6033
**Email:** kikinis@bwh.harvard.edu
**Website:** http://www.spl.harvard.edu
Ron Kikinis, MD, Prin. Investigator

**Activities/Fields:** Image processing and analysis techniques for basic and clinical neurosciences.

**★ 4520 ★ Carnegie Mellon University**
**Multidisciplinary Nuclear Magnetic Resonance Center for Biomedical Research**
4400 5th Ave.
Pittsburgh, PA 15213
**Phone:** (412)268-3395 **Fax:** (412)268-7083
**Email:** chienho@andrew.cmu.edu
**Website:** http://info.bio.cmu.edu/NMR-Center/
Chien Ho, PhD, Prin. Investigator

**Activities/Fields:** Methodologies for the acquisition of morphological, biochemical, and functional information in living animals using nuclear magnetic resonance imaging and spectroscopy.

**★ 4521 ★ Case Western Reserve University**
**Neural Engineering Center**
C.B. Bolton Bldg., Rm. 3510
Department of Biomedical Engineering
Cleveland, OH 44106
**Phone:** (216)368-2960 **Fax:** (216)368-4872
**Email:** dmdurand@po.cwru.edu
**Website:** http://nec.cwru.edu/content.htm
Dominique M. Durand, Dir.

**Activities/Fields:** Function of the nervous system, development of methods to restore damaged neurological function, and creation of artificial systems by integrating physical, chemical, mathematical and engineering tools.

**★ 4522 ★ Columbia University**
**Artificial Organs Research Laboratory**
Department of Chemical Engineering
814 Mudd Bldg., MC 4721
New York, NY 10027
**Phone:** (212)854-4448 **Fax:** (212)854-3054
**Email:** leonard@columbia.edu
**Website:** http://www.columbia.edu/~leonard
Prof. Edward F. Leonard, Dir.

**Activities/Fields:** Engineering and technical solutions for problems associated with extracorporeal circulation, cardiovascular implants, and artificial organs. Also studies blood-biomaterial interactions, extracorporeal immunotherapies, and photochemical reactions to transform cells and inactivate viruses.

**★ 4523 ★ Cornell University**
**Parallel Processing Resource for Biomedical Scientists**
Frank H.T. Rhodes Hall
Cornell Theory Center
Ithaca, NY 14853-3801
**Phone:** (607)254-8686 **Fax:** (607)254-8888
**Website:** http://www.tc.cornell.edu/reports/NIH/resource
Dr. Thomas F. Coleman, Prin. Investigator

**Activities/Fields:** Theoretical developments, the design of computational algorithms, and applications to biomedical problems, particularly protein structure determination and simulations of protein dynamics.

**Duke University**
**Center for Cellular and Biosurface Engineering (CBE)**
*See:* Entry 4816

**★ 4524 ★ Georgia Institute of Technology**
**Parker H. Petit Institute for Bioengineering and Bioscience**
315 Ferst Dr., Ste. 1104
Atlanta, GA 30332-0363
**Phone:** (404)894-2768 **Fax:** (404)894-2291
**Email:** robert.nerem@ibb.gatech.edu/flash_index.html
**Website:** http://www.ibb.gatech.edu
Prof. Robert M. Nerem, PhD, Dir.

**Activities/Fields:** Biomechanics research, including biaxial mechanical properties in tissue, biomechanical design, cardiovascular fluid mechanics, cellular engineering and non-invasive blood flow measurement; tissue engineering; and bioelectrical research, including electromagnetic systems for measuring the electrical properties of tissue, medical device/systems for diagnostic and therapeutic applications, and the applications of either air- or wire-coupled electromagnetic energy to stimulate biofunction; rehabilitation research, which entails developing orthotic devices for patients with lower body dysfunction, evaluating functional electrostimulation, and observance of the parvocellular division of the red nucleus for analyzing movement control; and computer applications research, which involves signal processing, image processing, and visualization, medical informatics, and simulation techniques to assist in making decisions regarding diagnostic and therapeutic strategies.

**★ 4525 ★ Georgia Tech/Emory Center for the Engineering of Living Tissues (GTEC)**
Parker H. Petit Institute for Bioengineering & Bioscience
315 Ferst Dr.
Atlanta, GA 30332-0363
**Phone:** (404)385-0216 **Fax:** (404)894-2291
**Email:** robert.nerem@ibb.gatech.edu
**Website:** http://www.gtec.gatech.edu
Dr. Robert M. Nerem, Dir.

**Activities/Fields:** Development of biological substitutes incorporating living cells and synthetic or natural materials to foster tissue regeneration and/or remodeling for the purpose of repair, replacement, or enhancement of tissue function. **Pub:** *Research reports.*

**★ 4526 ★ Illinois Institute of Technology**
**Pritzker Institute of Medical Engineering**
10 W 32nd St.
Chicago, IL 60616
**Phone:** (312)567-5324 **Fax:** (312)567-5707
**Email:** turitto@iit.edu
**Website:** http://www.iit.edu/~bme/
Dr. Vincent Turitto, Dir.

**Activities/Fields:** Cell and tissue engineering, neuroengineering, medical imaging and biomaterials. **Pub:** *Annual Report of Research.*

**★ 4527 ★ Illinois Institute of Technology**
**Research Laboratory in Human Biomechanics**
MMAE Department
10 W 32nd St.
Chicago, IL 60616-3793
**Phone:** (312)567-3179 **Fax:** (312)567-7230
**Email:** meade@iit.edu
Dr. Kevin Meade, Contact

**Activities/Fields:** Computer-aided biomechanical engineering and lower extremity neuromuscular engineering, including the use of force transducer arrays.

**★ 4528 ★ Johns Hopkins University**
**Middle Atlantic Mass Spectrometry Laboratory**
B-7 Biophysics Bldg.
725 N Wolfe St.
Baltimore, MD 21205
**Phone:** (410)955-3022 **Fax:** (410)955-3420
**Email:** rcotter@jhmi.edu

**Website:** http://www.med.jhu.edu/mams
Prof. Robert J. Cotter, Dir.

**Activities/Fields:** Kratos CONCEPT 1H high resolution mass spectrometer, a UV-laser desorption mass spectrometer and a Bio-Ion plasma desorption mass spectrometer as a collaborative resource for researchers from the University, from other academic institutions, or from industry and government laboratories who have need of special instrumentation and assistance in mass spectral measurement, sample preparation, chemical derivatization, and interpretation of spectra. The facility emphasizes analysis of ions of high mass (greater than 2,000 amu) and analysis of nonvolatile compounds. The high resolution mass spectrometer is equipped with an inhomogeneous high mass magnet and interfaced to a DS-90 data system, based upon the Data General Eclipse S-120 CPU with 256K MOS memory. The Laboratory also conducts in-house research focusing on the development of new instrumentation and instrumental techniques for mass spectral measurement.

**Johns Hopkins University**
**Vascular Bioengineering Laboratory**
*See:* Entry 5113

**★ 4529 ★ Joint Program in Biomedical Engineering**
University of Texas Southwestern Medical Center at Dallas
5323 Harry Hines Blvd., Rm. NA2-504
Dallas, TX 75390-9178
**Phone:** (214)648-1194 **Fax:** (214)648-1445
**Email:** bme@mednet.swmed.edu
**Website:** http://www.swmed.edu/home_pages/bme/index.html
Prof. Harold R. Garner, PhD, Contact

**Activities/Fields:** Biomedical engineering, including studies in molecular engineering, computational biology, magnetic resonance, gamma and ultrasound image analysis, orthopedics, human performance, biocompatible materials, biomechanics, artificial organs, biosensors, soft tissue biomechanics, neurological signal acquisition and analysis, recombinant DNA technology, human genome project and gene therapy. **Pub:** *BME Information Brochure.* • *BME Student Activity Reports.* • *Internship Brochure.*

**★ 4530 ★ Laval University**
**Laboratory of Experimental Tissue Engineering**
Hopital du Saint-Sacrement, Research Centre
1050 Chemin Ste.-Foy
Quebec, QC, Canada G1S 4L8
**Phone:** (418)682-7663 **Fax:** (418)682-8000
**Email:** Lucie.Germain@chg.ulaval.ca
**Website:** http://www.fmed.ulaval.ca/loex
Dr. Francois A. Auger, PhD, Dir.

**Activities/Fields:** Clinical and experimental human tissue engineering (blood vessel, skin, musculoskeletal, bronchial, ocular), including tissue transplantation and developing applications for living tissue equivalents such as percutaneous absorption, toxicology, and wound healing.

**Laval University**
**Saint-Francois-d'Assise Hospital Research Centre**
*See:* Entry 18400

**★ 4531 ★ Louisiana Tech University**
**Center for Biomedical Engineering and Rehabilitation Science**
PO Box 3185
Ruston, LA 71272
**Phone:** (318)257-4562 **Fax:** (318)255-4175
**Email:** cybers@coes.latech.edu
**Website:** http://www.cybers.latech.edu
Dr. Charles J. Robinson, Jr., Dir.

**Activities/Fields:** Studies conditions leading to disabilities (systems physiology), develops and applies technology to assist disabled people, and develops expert systems in systems physiology and rehabilitation services. **Frmly:** Center for Rehabilitation Science and Biomedical Engineering.

### ★ 4532 ★ Massachusetts Institute of Technology
**Biotechnology Resource Center for Research in Lasers and Medicine**
Bldg. 6, Rm. 014
NCRR
77 Massachusetts Ave.
Cambridge, MA 02139-4307
**Phone:** (617)253-5377 **Fax:** (617)253-4513
Dr. Ramachandra R. Dasari, Contact

**Activities/Fields:** Spectral diagnostics for tissue types, which can lead to real-time diagnosis of diseased tissue; and studies laser tissue damage and ablation, as a function of wavelength and the dependence on the optical and thermal properties of the tissue. Research includes development of the portable spectrometer for laser-induced fluorescence studies for use in a clinical setting and use of Raman spectroscopy techniques for diagnosing tissue characteristics.

**Massachusetts Institute of Technology**
**Center for Magnetic Resonance**
**Francis Bitter Magnet Laboratory**
*See:* Entry 18168

### ★ 4533 ★ Massachusetts Institute of Technology
**Eric P. and Evelyn E. Newman Laboratory for Biomechanics and Human Rehabilitation**
77 Massachusetts Ave., Rm. 3-146
Cambridge, MA 02139
**Phone:** (617)253-2277 **Fax:** (617)258-7018
**Email:** neville@mit.edu
**Website:** http://me.mit.edu/groups/hogan/
Prof. Neville Hogan, Dir.

**Activities/Fields:** Amputation prostheses, normal and pathological human neuromuscular systems, and diagnosis and therapy of muscular, skeletal, and joint malfunctions using an engineering approach. Studies include cybernetic limb and sensory prostheses, mobility aids for the blind, suppression of tremor, functional electrical stimulation, instrumentation for and kinematic studies of human movement, synovial joint mechanics, pathogenesis of osteoarthritis, biomechanics of the hip, knee, and ankle, musculoskeletal models for pathological diagnosis, and computer-aided surgical simulation. **Pub:** *Bibliography.* • *Excerpt from the Department of Mechanical Engineering Triennial Report.* **Frmly:** Laboratory for Human Mechanics and Rehabilitation.

**Massachusetts Institute of Technology**
**Laser Biomedical Research Center**
*See:* Entry 18169

### ★ 4534 ★ Mayo Biomedical Imaging Resource
Mayo Clinic
200 1st St. SW
Rochester, MN 55905
**Phone:** (507)284-4937 **Fax:** (507)284-1632
**Email:** rar@mayo.edu
**Website:** http://www.mayo.edu/bir
Richard A. Robb, PhD, Dir.

**Activities/Fields:** Provides expertise and technology related to biomedical imaging, scientific visualization, computer graphics, computer workstations, and computer networks. Through professional consultation, advanced software and hardware systems, and technical support, investigators use the Resource for ongoing research studies, ad hoc projects, feasibility testing, and/or development of applications and systems to be subsequently installed in the user's library.

Provides services in six major categories: consultation on biomedical imaging and scientific visualization problems, needs and applications; software packages (ANALYZE) for interactive display and quantitative analysis of multimodality, and multidimensional biomedical images; drop-in center containing several computer workstations connected to a powerful network providing image processing software and computer graphics hardware; hardware systems, including design and configuration of both standard and customized workstations for biomedical image processing; network support for connectivity to the Resource and/or within the investigative laboratory; and training and education in the use of Resource facilities and in biomedical imaging, scientific visualization and computer science.

**McGill University**
**McConnell Brain Imaging Centre**
*See:* Entry 14229

### ★ 4535 ★ McMaster University
**Centre for Electrophotonic Materials and Devices (CEMD)**
1280 Main St. W
Hamilton, ON, Canada L8S 4J7
**Phone:** (905)525-9140 **Fax:** (905)527-8409
**Email:** cemd@mcmaster.ca
**Website:** http://www.eng.mcmaster.ca/cemd/cemdhome.htm
Dr. David A. Thompson, Dir.

**Activities/Fields:** Neurosciences, cardiovascular system, mineralization, confocal microscopy, and analytical electron microscopy. Facility is used by many research groups.

**Medical College of Wisconsin**
**Biophysics Research Institute**
*See:* Entry 18170

### ★ 4536 ★ Milwaukee School of Engineering
**Electrical Engineering and Biomedical Science**
1025 N Broadway
Milwaukee, WI 53202-3109
**Phone:** (414)277-7331 **Fax:** (414)277-7465
**Email:** canino@msoe.edu
**Website:** http://www.biophysics.mcw.edu/
Prof. Vincent R. Canino, PhD, Dir.

**Activities/Fields:** Biomedical instrumentation systems, including the design and evaluation of extracorporeal perfusion instrumentation.

### ★ 4537 ★ National Association for Biomedical Research
818 Connecticut Ave. NW, Ste. 200
Washington, DC 20006
**Phone:** (202)857-0540 **Fax:** (202)659-1902
**Email:** info@nabr.org
**Website:** http://www.nabr.org
Frankie L. Trull, Pres.

**Activities/Fields:** Biomedical research, education, and testing, focusing on using laboratory animals for such purposes, monitors and attempts to infuence legislation and regulations on behalf of members dependent on laboratory animals for research and testing.

### ★ 4538 ★ National Institute for Rehabilitation Engineering
Box 1008
Hewitt, NJ 07421
**Phone:** (973)853-6585 **Free:** 800-736-2216
**Website:** http://www.theoffice.net/nire
Donald Selwyn, Dir.

**Activities/Fields:** Invention, design, construction, fitting, and servicing of special devices for individuals with any specific physical disability or combination of disabilities; time/motion analyses; job modification

engineering; task-performance mobility; driver training; computer software adapted for people with handicapping conditions. **Frmly:** Rehabilitation Engineering Institute.

### ★ 4539 ★ National Science Foundation
**Directorate for Engineering**
**Division of Bioengineering and Environmental Systems**
4201 Wilson Blvd., Rm. 565
Arlington, VA 22230
**Phone:** (703)292-7066 **Fax:** (703)292-9098
**Email:** bhamilton@nsf.gov
**Website:** http://www.eng.nsf.gov/bes
Bruce K. Hamilton, Div. Dir.

**Activities/Fields:** Critical engineering systems are those that are essential either because they significantly affect the economic viability and security needs of the nation, or because they are required for maintaining the public infrastructure. Major program areas include: biochemical and biomedical engineering; environmental engineering; research to aid people with disabilities. **Frmly:** (1993) Division of Biological and Environmental Systems; Division of Critical Engineering Systems.

### ★ 4540 ★ National Science Foundation
**Directorate for Engineering**
**Division of Bioengineering and Environmental Systems**
**Biochemical Engineering Program**
4201 Wilson Blvd., Rm. 565
Arlington, VA 22230
**Phone:** (703)292-8320 **Fax:** (703)292-9098
**Email:** fheineke@nsf.gov
Dr. Frederick Heineken, Prog. Dir.

**Activities/Fields:** Design and development of novel bioreactors, bioseparation systems, and the control of biochemical processes, as well as research aimed at improved utilization of biologically based resources. This includes support for programs in biochemical engineering fundamentals, biomass processing, and food process engineering.

### ★ 4541 ★ National Science Foundation
**Directorate of Engineering**
**Division of Bioengineering and Environmental Systems**
**Bioengineering and Aiding Persons with Disabilities Program**
4201 Wilson Blvd., Rm. 565
Arlington, VA 22230
**Phone:** (703)292-7943 **Fax:** (703)292-9098
**Email:** gdevey@nsf.gov
**Website:** http://www.eng.nsf.gov.bes/
Gilbert Devey, Prog. Dir.

**Activities/Fields:** Provides funding for fundamental and applied academic engineering research relevant to medical needs. To qualify for support, investigations should be directed toward engineering research associated with the characterization, restoration, or substitution of human structure, function, or control. Emphasis is on fundamental and applied research with a potential to produce medical-engineering technologies, especially those that could become medically valuable within 10 years. (Normally this medical-oriented research should have such a strong engineering component that direct clinical input to its activities is not required; however, clinicians may supply data or specimens necessary to conduct the engineering effort.). **Frmly:** Bioengineering and Research to Aid the Handicapped Program.

### ★ 4542 ★ New Jersey Institute of Technology
**Center for Biomedical Engineering**
323 Martin Luther King, Jr. Blvd.
Newark, NJ 07102
**Phone:** (973)596-3584 **Fax:** (973)596-5222
**Email:** kristol@njit.edu

**Website:** http://www.njit.edu/bme
David Kristol, Dir.
**Activities/Fields:** Design of prosthetic devices (including knee and hip joints), biosignal processing, heart rate variability studies, design and testing of prosthetic heart valves, rehabilitation engineering, modelling of the cardiovascular system, assessment of lower back pain, gait analysis, biomaterials engineering, tissue engineering, vision engineering, optimization of work performance, neuromuscular control mechanisms, functional MRI.

**★ 4543 ★ Northwestern University**
**Institute for Bioengineering and**
**Nanoscience in Advanced Medicine**
**(IBNAM)**
Tarry Bldg., Rm. 16-717
300 E Superior St.
Chicago, IL 60611
**Phone:** (312)503-0807          **Fax:** (312)503-2482
**Email:** ibnam@northwestern.edu
**Website:** http://www.ibnam.northwestern.edu/
Samuel I. Stupp, Dir.
**Activities/Fields:** Use of bioengineering and nanoscience in medicine, in such areas as self-assembly, tissue engineering, genomics, smart drug delivery, and other new technologies.

**★ 4544 ★ Oregon Health and Science**
**University**
**Vollum Institute**
3181 SW Sam Jackson Pk. Rd., L474
Portland, OR 97201-3098
**Phone:** (503)494-5453          **Fax:** (503)494-4590
**Email:** goodmanr@ohsu.edu
**Website:** http://www.ohsu.edu/vollum
Dr. Richard H. Goodman, Dir.
**Activities/Fields:** Molecular biology, protein chemistry, virology, and immunology of the endocrine system and brain and nervous system. Also conducts studies in electrophysiology and pharmacology. **Pub:** *Biennial Report.*

**Pennsylvania State University**
**Artificial Heart Research Project**
*See:* Entry 5132

**Polytechnical School of Montreal**
**Research Group in Biomechanics and**
**Biomaterials**
*See:* Entry 13702

**★ 4545 ★ Prosthetics Research Study**
675 S Lane St., Ste. 100
Seattle, WA 98104-2942
**Phone:** (206)903-8136          **Fax:** (206)903-8141
**Email:** dgsmith@u.washington.edu
**Website:** http://www.prs-research.org
Douglas G. Smith, MD, Dir.
**Activities/Fields:** Wound healing and limb viability, prosthesis research and development, mobility aids and artificial limbs, functional electrical physiological response, pain control, neuromuscular assist devices, electrical osteogenesis, mechanical engineering and automated fabrication of prosthetic components and mobility aids, and amputation surgery and post-surgical management.

**★ 4546 ★ Protein Engineering Network of**
**Centres of Excellence (PENCE)**
750 Heritage Medical Research Centre
University of Alberta
Edmonton, AB, Canada T6G 2S2
**Phone:** (780)492-8851          **Fax:** (780)492-6995
**Email:** info@pence.ca
**Website:** http://www.pence.ca
Steve Withers, CEO & Sci. Dir.
**Activities/Fields:** Research focuses on both discovery and development of proteins, peptides, glycopep-

tides and bioinformatics for applications as products or services for medical, veterinary and industry applications. **Pub:** *Pence News.* Newsletter.

**Radiation Oncology Research and**
**Development Center**
*See:* Entry 18171

**Rancho Rehabilitation Engineering**
**Program**
*See:* Entry 20199

**★ 4547 ★ Regenstrief Institute for Health**
**Care Research**
1050 Wishard Blvd.
Indianapolis, IN 46202
**Phone:** (317)630-7070          **Fax:** (317)630-2466
**Email:** cmcdonald@regenstrief.org
**Website:** http://www.regenstrief.org
Dr. Clement McDonald, Dir.
**Activities/Fields:** Health care, including use of computers in health care delivery, and use of engineering and computer techniques to improve medical diagnosis and therapy.

**★ 4548 ★ Rice University**
**Institute of Biosciences and**
**Bioengineering**
6100 Main St.
Houston, TX 77005-1892
**Phone:** (713)527-6034          **Fax:** (713)285-5154
**Email:** ibb@rice.edu
**Website:** http://www.bioc.rice.edu/Institute/IBB/
Dr. Larry V. McIntire, Ch.
**Activities/Fields:** Application of engineering skills to problems in biology and medicine, including cellular and tissue engineering, studies on circulation assistance devices, cardiovascular tissue mechanics, blood proteins, effects of physical forces on various components of blood, fluid mechanics and transport processes related to cardiovascular system, hematologic complications with prostheses, rheology, fluid mechanics of blood and blood flow, tissue culture reactor evaluation, biochemical reactor engineering, applications of artificial intelligence in bioreactor control and dynamics, plant cell bioreactors, bioseparation systems, and development of in vitro methods for studying cellular mechanisms of thrombosis and atherogenesis.

**★ 4549 ★ St. Francis Xavier University**
**Comparative Biomechanics Research**
**Laboratory**
Biology Department
PO Box 5000
Antigonish, NS, Canada B2G 2W5
**Phone:** (902)867-5116          **Fax:** (902)867-2368
**Email:** edemont@stfx.ca
**Website:** http://iago.stfx.ca/people/edemont/biomechanics-lab.html
M. Edwin DeMont, Dir.
**Activities/Fields:** Biological fluid dynamics and biomaterials.

**★ 4550 ★ Texas Health Research**
**Institute (THRI)**
6300 W Parker Rd., Ste. 100
Plano, TX 75093-8101
**Phone:** (972)981-3740          **Fax:** (972)981-3779
**Email:** tomfranklin@texashealth.org
**Website:** http://www.thri.org
Dr. Thomas D. Franklin, Jr., Pres. /CEO
**Activities/Fields:** Biomechanical testing/engineering, pre-clinical studies, minimally invasive technologies, clinical trials in general surgery, orthopedics/spine, oncology, interventional cardiology, urology, OB/Gyn, and internal medicine. **Frmly:** Institute for Spine and Biomedical Research.

**Texas Scottish Rite Hospital for Children**
**Research Department**
*See:* Entry 5814

**★ 4551 ★ Tulane University**
**Department of Orthopaedic Research**
Sch. of Medicine
1430 Tulane Ave., Box SL-32
New Orleans, LA 70112-2699
**Phone:** (504)588-2273          **Fax:** (504)584-2722
**Email:** scook2@tulane.edu
**Website:** http://www.tsrh.org
Stephen D. Cook, PhD, Dir.
**Activities/Fields:** Biomaterials, including study of the properties of porous materials and materials-bone interfaces; surface studies of tissue-implant interactions; and corrosion resistance analysis, especially degradation characteristics of materials in an in vivo environment. Conducts histological and microradiographic evaluations of bone and implant composites. **Frmly:** Biomaterials Laboratory.

**U.S. Department of Defense**
**Air Force Materiel Command**
**Armstrong Laboratory**
**Division of Biodynamics and**
**Biocommunications**
*See:* Entry 4492

**U.S. Department of Defense**
**Army Medical Research and Materiel**
**Command**
**Walter Reed Army Institute of Research**
**Biometrics Division**
*See:* Entry 13480

**★ 4552 ★ U.S. Department of Health and**
**Human Services**
**National Center for Research Resources**
**Biomedical Engineering and**
**Instrumentation Program**
NIH Bldg. 13, Rm. 3N17
9000 Rockville Pike
Bethesda, MD 20892
**Phone:** (301)496-4741          **Fax:** (301)496-6608
**Website:** http://www.nih.gov/od/ors/dbeps/index.htm
Dr. Henry Eden, Actg. Dir.
**Activities/Fields:** Supports NIH intramural scientists in applications of engineering, mathematics, physics, and the physical sciences to the solution of problems in biology and medicine through collaborations involving measurement, imaging, mathematical modeling, or design of specialized equipment; and construction, modification, maintenance, repair, or lease of scientific equipment.

**U.S. Department of Health and Human**
**Services**
**National Institute for Occupational Safety**
**and Health**
**Physical Sciences and Engineering**
**Division**
**Engineering Control Technology Branch**
*See:* Entry 16827

**★ 4553 ★ U.S. Department of Health and**
**Human Services**
**National Institute for Occupational Safety**
**and Health**
**Physical Sciences and Engineering**
**Division**
**Measurements Research Support Branch**
Robert A. Taft Laboratories
4676 Columbia Pkwy.
Cincinnati, OH 45226-1998
**Phone:** (513)841-4241          **Fax:** (513)841-4500
Paul Schlect, Chf.

**Activities/Fields:** Sampling and analytical chemistry measurements for industrial hygiene field investigations and other National Institute for Occupational Safety and Health activities; and provides field industrial hygiene measurement support, including research, to develop new sampling and analysis techniques. Branch comprised of sections for measurement, development, and support. **Pub:** *Analytical Methods Studies.*

**U.S. Department of Veterans Affairs Rehabilitation Research and Development Service**
**Center of Excellence for Limb Loss Prevention and Prosthetic Engineering**
*See:* Entry 8205

**★ 4554 ★ University of Akron**
**Institute for Biomedical Engineering Research**
Sidney L. Ste. Olson Research Center
260 S Forge St.
Akron, OH 44325-0302
**Phone:** (330)972-6650          **Fax:** (330)374-8834
**Email:** srittgers@uakron.edu
**Website:** http://www.biomed.uakron.edu
Dr. Stanley E. Rittgers, Dir.

**Activities/Fields:** Biomedical engineering, using and coordinating expertise and resources of biological, medical, engineering, and other scientific disciplines in greater Akron area for conducting research and promoting educational programs at the University, area hospitals, and the College of Medicine. **Pub:** *IBER Update Newsletter*, quarterly.

**★ 4555 ★ University of Arkansas at Little Rock**
**Biomedical Research Center**
College of Pharmacy, Slot 522-3
4301 W Markham
Little Rock, AR 72205
**Phone:** (501)686-6493          **Fax:** (501)686-6057
**Email:** compadrecesarm@wams.edu
Dr. Cesar Compadre, Dir.

**Activities/Fields:** Molecular modeling, including protein structure function relationships, toxicity modeling, and pharmocokinetic modeling; anatomical visualization, 3-D animation, and educational development. **Pub:** *Journals.*

**University of California, Irvine**
**Beckman Laser Institute and Medical Clinic**
*See:* Entry 18179

**University of California, Irvine**
**Laser Microbeam and Medical Program (LAMMP)**
*See:* Entry 18181

**★ 4556 ★ University of California, Los Angeles**
**Crump Institute for Molecular Imaging**
23-132-CHS
UCLA Sch. of Medicine
700 Westwood Plaza
Los Angeles, CA 90095-1770
**Phone:** (310)206-1798          **Fax:** (310)209-4655
**Email:** sgambhir@mednet.ucla.edu
**Website:** http://www.crump.ucla.edu/
Sanjiv Sam Gambhir, Dir.

**Activities/Fields:** Biological imaging technologies, including positron emmision tomography; autoradiographic images for in viro and in vitro assays of biochemical and biological process in tissue preparations; fluorescent microscopy to provide images of changing chemical environments in tissue and isolated cell preparations; and image based communication and educational systems using game strategies, expert systems, knowledge navigators, and personal computers.

**University of California, San Diego**
**Cartilage Tissue Engineering Laboratory**
*See:* Entry 13720

**★ 4557 ★ University of California, San Diego**
**Whitaker Institute of Biomedical Engineering**
SERF Rm. 228
MC 0427
9500 Gilman Dr.
La Jolla, CA 92093-0427
**Phone:** (858)822-2290          **Fax:** (858)822-1160
**Email:** tmatusov@ucsd.edu
**Website:** http://www-bioeng.ucsd.edu/wibe/
Dr. Shu Chien, Dir.

**Activities/Fields:** Biomedical engineering, emphasizing structure-function relationships in normal and pathological tissues and the development of biological substitutes to restore, maintain, or improve tissue functions. Tissue studies focus on the heart, blood, lung, kidney, liver, pancreas, muscle, bone, cartilage, tendon, ligament, skin, nerve, brain, retina, and cochlea. **Frmly:** Institute for Biomedical Engineering.

**University of California, San Francisco**
**Magnetic Resonance Laboratory**
*See:* Entry 4745

**University of California, San Francisco**
**Mass Spectrometry Facility**
*See:* Entry 4746

**★ 4558 ★ University of California, San Francisco**
**Resource for Biocomputing, Visualization, and Informatics**
Computer Graphics Laboratory
San Francisco, CA 94143-0446
**Phone:** (415)476-2299          **Fax:** (415)502-1755
**Email:** tef@cgl.ucsf.edu
**Website:** http://www.cgl.ucsf.edu/
Thomas E. Ferrin, PhD, Prin. Investigator

**Activities/Fields:** Genomic and molecular recognition problems. Research focuses on three key areas: sequence analysis and bioinformatics, structural informatics, and functional informatics.

**★ 4559 ★ University of Colorado**
**Clinical Mass Spectrometry Research Resource**
4200 E 9th Ave.
Denver, CO 80262
**Phone:** (303)315-7286          **Fax:** (303)315-0080
**Email:** paul.fennessey@uchsc.edu
**Website:** http://www.uchsc.edu
Dr. P.V. Fennessey, Co-Dir.

**Activities/Fields:** Clinical applications of mass spectrometry, including gas chromatograph mass spectrometry, high resolution mass spectrometry, bioactive substances, and application of fast atom bombardment mass spectrometry to biomolecules. Emphasizes methods for synthesis of internal standards for the quantitative analysis of bioactive molecules found in physiological fluids, identification of steroid profiles in patients with biochemical and pathological irregularities, and stable isotope studies for measuring the utilization of important metabolic intermediates in humans.

**★ 4560 ★ University of Florida**
**Center for Ambulatory Studies**
930 NW 8th Ave.
Gainesville, FL 32601
**Phone:** (352)375-0607          **Fax:** (352)375-6111
Dr. Mark Kane Goldstein, Dir.

**Activities/Fields:** Behavioral and biomedical engineering, including remote monitoring of ambulatory patients and behavioral aspects of chronically ill outpatients, precision measurement of health-related behaviors, and study of simulated breast with lumps for training in breast self-examination for cancer detection.

**★ 4561 ★ University of Illinois at Chicago**
**Research Resources Center**
Research Resources Center (M/C 937)
835 S Wolcott Ave.
Chicago, IL 60612-7341
**Phone:** (312)996-7600          **Fax:** (312)996-0539
**Email:** charlieb@uic.edu
**Website:** http://www.rrc.uic.edu/
Dr. C.E. Brown, Dir.,RRC-East

**Activities/Fields:** Electronic and mechanical instrumentation, biostatistics, micro and mini computer programming and databases, electron microscopy, confocal microscopy, raman microscopy, electron microprobe, nuclear magnetic resonance spectrometry, micro-imaging, mass spectrometry, X-ray crystallography, flow cytometry, and protein sequencing/peptide synthesis, DNA sequencing, bioinformatics, production and analysis of high-density DNA arrays using gene sets produced by the human genome project, and generation of transgenic and gene-targeted (knockout) mice. **Pub:** *Annual Users Report.*

**University of Michigan**
**Biomaterials Research Center**
*See:* Entry 6638

**University of Michigan**
**Orthopaedic Research Laboratories**
*See:* Entry 16961

**★ 4562 ★ University of Missouri—Columbia**
**John M. Dalton Cardiovascular Research Center**
Research Pk., Rm. 134
Columbia, MO 65211
**Phone:** (573)882-7586          **Fax:** (573)884-4232
**Email:** dalton@missouri.edu
**Website:** http://www.missouri.edu/~dalton/
Edward H. Blaine, PhD, Dir.

**Activities/Fields:** Multidisciplinary research in health science and related areas, emphasizing cardiovascular studies.

**★ 4563 ★ University of Montreal**
**Biomedical Modeling Research Group (BMRG)**
PO Box 6128, Downtown Sta.
Montreal, QC, Canada H3C 3J7
**Phone:** (514)343-4715          **Fax:** (514)343-6112
**Email:** roberge@igd.umontreal.ca
**Website:** http://www.umontreal.ca/
Fernard A. Roberge, Dir.

**Activities/Fields:** Computer simulation and mathematical modeling in cardiac electrophysiology, biomechanics of joints, and characterization of biological tissues by imaging.

**★ 4564 ★ University of Montreal**
**Institute of Biomedical Engineering**
Faculte de Medicine
PO Box 6128, Downtown Sta.
Montreal, QC, Canada H3C 3J7
**Phone:** (514)343-6357          **Fax:** (514)343-6112
**Email:** secretariat@igb.umontreal.ca
**Website:** http://www.igb.umontreal.ca

**Activities/Fields:** Cardiac electrophysiology, biomechanics, biomaterials, electrocardiology, biomedical modelling, neuromuscular physiology, medical imaging, medical instrumentati, and clinical engineering. **Pub:** *Annual Report.*

**★ 4565 ★ University of New Brunswick**
**Institute of Biomedical Engineering**
PO Box 4400
25 Dineen Dr.
Fredericton, NB, Canada E3B 5A3
**Phone:** (506)453-4966  **Fax:** (506)453-4827
**Email:** biomed@unb.ca
**Website:** http://www.unb.ca/biomed
Dr. Bernard Hudgins, Dir.

**Activities/Fields:** Interaction of man and modern technology, particularly in health care. Research focuses on developing electronic control systems for artificial limbs, bioelectric signal processing, modeling of human operators and muscle function, applications of electronic instrumentation in orthopedics, medical imaging, ergonomics, exercise physiology, and biomechanics. **Frmly:** Bio-Engineering Institute.

**University of Pennsylvania**
**Metabolic Magnetic Resonance Research**
  **and Computing Center**
*See:* Entry 18191

**★ 4566 ★ University of Pennsylvania**
**Ultrafast Optical Processes Laboratory**
231 S 34th St.
Philadelphia, PA 19104-6323
**Phone:** (215)898-8410  **Fax:** (215)898-0590
**Email:** hochstra@sas.upenn.edu
**Website:** http://rlbl.chem.upenn.edu
Prof. Robin M. Hochstrasser, PhD, Prin. Investigator

**Activities/Fields:** Development of methods for the investigation of rapid structural changes and ultrafast processes in proteins, enzymes, and nucleic acids.

**University of Quebec at Trois-Rivieres**
**Research Group in Membrane**
  **Biotechnology**
*See:* Entry 4862

**University of Rochester**
**Rochester Center for Biomedical**
  **Ultrasound**
*See:* Entry 18192

**★ 4567 ★ University of Texas at Austin**
**Biomedical Engineering Graduate**
  **Program**
Engineering Science Bldg., 610
Austin, TX 78712-1084
**Phone:** (512)471-3604  **Fax:** (512)471-0616
**Email:** kdiller@mail.utexas.edu
**Website:** http://www.bme.utexas.edu
Dr. Kenneth R. Diller, Dir.

**Activities/Fields:** Application of scientific and engineering knowledge to the solution of medical problems. Projects deal with molecular bioengineering, antibiotic synthesis, spectroscopic detection of early cancers, diagnostic applications of tissue fluorescence, image analysis by computer, cryopreservation of organs and tissues, quantitative thermographic imaging, electrosurgical safety, thrombosis on injured vessel and atherosclerotic surfaces and on polymeric biomaterials, pulsatile-flow cardiopulmonary bypass, chromatographic features of polar and nonpolar cardiac glycosides, hyperthermia in cancer therapy, effects of coenzyme Q-10 on cardiac function, biodegradable polymer implants for use in surgery, computer graphics analysis of sport biomechanics, rheology of synovial fluids, robotic surgical lasers, laser-tissue interaction, structure and function of hybrid proteins, and microvascular analysis of burn wounds.

**University of Texas at Austin**
**Laboratory for Artificial Neural Systems**
*See:* Entry 14460

**★ 4568 ★ University of Texas**
**Southwestern Medical Center at Dallas**
**Southwestern Biomedical Magnetic**
  **Resonance Facility**
Mary Nell & Ralph B. Rogers Magnetic
  Resonance Center
5801 Forest Park Rd.
Dallas, TX 75235-9085
**Phone:** (214)648-5886  **Fax:** (214)648-5881
**Email:** cmallo@mednet.swmed.edu
**Website:** http://www.swmed.edu/home_pages/rogersmr
Dr. Craig R. Malloy, Prin. Investigator

**Activities/Fields:** Development and refinement of the use of Nuclear Magnetic Resonance (NMR) isotopomer analysis for the investigation of intermediary metabolism in intact, functioning tissues, and application of these methods to current questions in metabolism; mathematical models to estimate the flux through different metabolic pathways using isotopomer analysis of NMR and/or mass spectroscopy data; techniques and agents for monitoring intercellular actions, particularly sodium, magnesium, and calcium, in perfused tissues and in vivo.

**University of Texas Southwestern Medical**
  **Center at Dallas**
**Southwestern Magnetic Resonance**
  **Facility**
**Mary Nell and Ralph B. Rogers Magnetic**
  **Resonance Center**
*See:* Entry 18194

**★ 4569 ★ University of Utah**
**Center for Engineering Design**
50 Central Campus Dr., Rm. 2202
Salt Lake City, UT 84112-9208
**Phone:** (801)581-6499  **Fax:** (801)581-5304
**Email:** s.jacobsen@ced.utah.edu
**Website:** http://www2.utsouthwestern.edu/rogersmr/
Dr. Stephen C. Jacobsen, Dir.

**Activities/Fields:** Robotic design and control, including teleoperated and entertainment robots; actuator technology; touch sensors; micro-electromechanical systems; biomechanics; bioengineering; rehabilitation research, including projects in artificial limb design; and micro pumps and fluid delivery systems. **Frmly:** Center for Biomedical Design.

**University of Utah**
**Dixon Laser Institute**
*See:* Entry 18195

**★ 4570 ★ University of Utah**
**Institute for Biomedical Engineering**
803 North 300 West, Ste. 180
Salt Lake City, UT 84103-1414
**Phone:** (801)581-6991  **Fax:** (801)323-1110
**Email:** dolsen@uahi.org
Dr. Don B. Olsen, Dir.

**Activities/Fields:** Design, development, and fabrication of cardiac assist devices, cardiac replacement devices with animal implantation and complete follow-up studies, basic physiologic and psychophysical studies of the effects of electrical stimulation in the scala tympani of deaf human volunteers, testing of new artificial kidneys, peritoneal access devices for peritoneal dialysis, drug metabolism in patients with end state renal disease, dialysis with high flux dialysers, research with chemical effect field transistors, research into the efficacy of insulin administered by intraperitoneal route, new access routers for peritoneal dialysis and peritoneal access routes for diabetes, artificial hearing and arms, implantation of a totally artificial heart in a human patient, and biomaterials research. Cooperates with Department of Biomedical Design for design and manufacture of compact hemodialysis machines and peritoneal access devices. **Pub:** *Institute for Biomedical Engineering–Some of its Projects–Some of its People.* • *Research Reports.*

**★ 4571 ★ University of Washington**
**Department of Bioengineering**
**Simulation Resource in Circulatory Mass**
  **Transport and Exchange Center**
Harris Hydraulics Laboratory
PO Box 357962
Seattle, WA 98195
**Phone:** (206)685-2005  **Fax:** (206)685-2651
**Email:** jbb@bioeng.washington.edu
**Website:** http://nsr.bioeng.washington.edu
James B. Bassingthwaights, Dir.

**Activities/Fields:** Logical structures for experiment design and analysis, including automating and fitting models to data, assessing the goodness-of-fit, choosing numerical approximations and, in some situations, the form of the model. Studies include estimates of conductances of capillary and cell membranes, volumes of distribution, and regional flows in organs; identification of receptor affinities and metabolic rates in intact organs via various tracer techniques; and development of an interactive simulation system that permits formulation of models without programming. Applications include: transport of hydrophilic molecules in microvasculature; simulation analysis for estimation of tracer uptake and depositionin cells, as indicators of regional blood flow and cellular function; use of fractals in describing heterogeneous systems, such as spatial and temporal flow variation.

**University of Washington**
**Diagnostic Imaging Sciences Center**
*See:* Entry 18196

**★ 4572 ★ University of Washington**
**Engineering Research Center for**
  **Engineered Biomaterials**
PO Box 351720
Seattle, WA 98195-1720
**Phone:** (206)616-8646  **Fax:** (206)616-9763
**Email:** ratner@uweb.engr.washington.edu
**Website:** http://www.uweb.engr.washington.edu
Dr. Buddy D. Ratner, Dir.

**Activities/Fields:** Exploitation of specific biological recognition mechanisms in order to develop a new generation of biomaterials for medical implants that will heal in the body in a facile, physiologically normal manner. **Pub:** *Journal of Undergraduate Research in Bioengineering.*

**★ 4573 ★ University of Washington**
**National ESCA and Surface Analysis**
  **Center for Biomedical Problems**
Departments of Bioengineering and
Chemical Engineering
PO Box 351750
Seattle, WA 98195-1750
**Phone:** (206)685-1229  **Fax:** (206)543-3778
**Email:** castner@nb.engr.washington.edu
**Website:** http://www.nb.engr.washington.edu
David G. Castner, PhD, Dir.

**Activities/Fields:** Surface analysis of biomaterial, polymer, and biological surfaces. Research directed toward integrating electron spectroscopy for chemical analytical tools for biomedical sciences. Provides ESCA and SIMS analysis of organic, metallic, and inorganic materials. Activities focus on understanding the nature of interactions that occur at biological interfaces such as tissue-body fluid, synthetic material-blood, and tooth-saliva. **Pub:** *Photoemissions Newsletter.*

**★ 4574 ★ University of Washington**
**Resource Facility for Population Kinetics**
Box 352255
Department of Bioengineering
Seattle, WA 98195-2255
**Phone:** (206)685-2009
**Email:** dmfoster@u.washington.edu
**Website:** http://tanami.rfpk.washington.edu
David M. Foster, PhD, Prin. Investigator

**Activities/Fields:** Application of computer modeling in biomedical research, focusing on compartmental population kinetics. Population kinetics is the methodology used to quantify intersubject variability in kinetic studies.

**Utah Artificial Heart Institute**
*See:* Entry 5207

**★ 4575 ★ Washington University in St. Louis**
**Biomedical Research Program**
Department of Internal Medicine, CB 8212
660 S Euclid
Saint Louis, MO 63110
**Phone:** (314)362-5300          **Fax:** (314)362-5306

**Email:** dolsen@uahi.org
David Kipnis, MD, Dir.
**Activities/Fields:** Allocates funds for exploratory and basic research and product development on the proteins, peptides, and other molecules regulating cellular communication and function. Facilitates the exchange of information between individual investigators in the Medical School and Monsanto's scientists.

**★ 4576 ★ Wayne State University**
**Bioengineering Center**
818 W Hancock St.
Detroit, MI 48202
**Phone:** (313)577-1344          **Fax:** (313)577-8333
**Email:** king@rrb.eng.wayne.edu
Dr. Albert I. King, Dir.

**Activities/Fields:** Automotive and aircraft safety, injury mechanisms, and spinal function, including lower back pain, orthopedic biomechanics, and head injury.

**★ 4577 ★ Wayne State University**
**Bioengineering Center**
**Gurdjian-Lissner Biomechanics Laboratory**
818 W Hancock St.
Detroit, MI 48202
**Phone:** (313)577-1344          **Fax:** (313)577-8333
**Email:** aa0003@wayne.edu
**Website:** http://www.ucomm.wayne.edu
Dr. Albert I. King, Dir.

**Activities/Fields:** Bioengineering sciences, including studies on head/neck injury mechanisms and prevention of such injuries.

# Chapter 8
# Biomedicine

## Federal Government Agencies

**★ 4578 ★ U.S. Department of Health and Human Services**
**National Institutes of Health (NIH)**
9000 Rockville Pike
Bethesda, MD 20892
**Phone:** (301)496-4000
**Website:** http://www.nih.gov/
Ruth L. Kirschstein, Acting Director
**Desc:** The National Institutes of Health supports biomedical and behavioral research domestically and abroad, conducts research in its own laboratories and clinics, trains promising young researchers, and promotes acquisition and distribution of medical knowledge. Research activities conducted or supported by NIH will determine the scope and direction of medical treatment and disease prevention in the future. The NIH is comprised of: National Institute on Aging; National Institute of Alcohol Abuse and Alcoholism; National Institute of Allergy and Infectious Diseases; National Institute of Arthritis and Musculoskeletal and Skin Diseases; National Institute of Cancer; National Institute of Child Health and Human Development; Clinical Center; National Institute on Deafness and Other Communication Disorders; National Institute of Dental and Craniofacial Research; National Institute of Diabetes, Digestive and Kidney Diseases; National Institute on Drug Abuse; National Institute of Environmental Health Sciences; Fogarty International Center; National Institute of General Medical Sciences; National Heart, Lung, and Blood Institute; National Human Genome Research Institute; National Library of Medicine; National Institute of Mental Health; National Institute of Neurological Disorders and Stroke; National Institute of Nursing Research; National Eye Institute; National Center for Research Resources; and the Center for Scientific Review.

**★ 4579 ★ U.S. Department of Health and Human Services**
**National Institutes of Health (NIH)**
**Fogarty International Center (FIC)**
9000 Rockville Pike
Bethesda, MD 20892
**Phone:** (301)496-2075        **Fax:** (301)594-1211
**Website:** http://www.nih.gov/fic/
Gerald T. Keusch, Director
**Desc:** The center is dedicated to advancing health of the people of the United States and other nations through international scientific cooperation. In pursuit of its mission, the Center fosters biomedical research partnership between U.S. scientists and foreign counterparts through grants, fellowships, and international agreements, and provides leadership in international science policy and research strategies.

**★ 4580 ★ U.S. Department of Health and Human Services**
**National Institutes of Health (NIH)**
**National Center for Research Resources (NCRR)**
9000 Rockville Pike
Bethesda, MD 20892
**Phone:** (301)435-0888
**Website:** http://www.ncrr.nih.gov/
Judith L. Vaitukaitis, MD, Director
**Desc:** The NCRR supports the development of technologies to enable sophisticated research; creates and supports a broad range of sophisticated multi-disciplinary research facilities for basic, clinical, and animal research; and supports development for minority-serving institutions which award doctoral degrees in health-related sciences. Programs include supporting biorepositories with companion web-based databases for a wide range of organisms.

**★ 4581 ★ U.S. Department of Health and Human Services**
**National Institutes of Health (NIH)**
**National Institute of General Medical Sciences (NIGMS)**
9000 Rockville Pike
Bethesda, MD 20892
**Phone:** (301)496-7301        **Fax:** (301)402-0156
**Website:** http://www.nih.gov/nigms/
Marvin Cassman, Director
**Desc:** NIGMS supports research and research training in basic biomedical sciences. Institute activities range from cell biology to genetics to pharmacology and systemic response to trauma and anesthesia.

## Foundations & Other Funding Organizations

### Private Foundations

**★ 4582 ★ Charles H. Revson Foundation**
55 East 59th St.
New York, NY 10022
**Phone:** (212)935-3340        **Fax:** (212)688-0633
**Email:** eevans@revsonfoundation.org
Eli Evans, President
**Fnded:** 1956. **Philosophy:** The foundation has four principal areas of interest: urban affairs with an emphasis on New York City; education; biomedical research policy; and Jewish education and philanthropy. Related to each of these interests are concerns for governmental accountability, the development of public leadership, the changing role of women, and the impact of modern communications on education. Many of the foundation grants are public-policy-oriented. Funds most often go to universities, such as City College of New York, Columbia University, and New York University; legal services organizations, such as Legal Aid Society of New York; national advocacy organizations, such as NAACP, Legal Defense Fund, and Children's Defense Fund; and biomedical research institutions, such as the National Academy of Sciences and Memorial Sloan-Kettering. Numerous grants have been awarded to the Children's Television Workshop and the Educational Broadcasting Corporation, the majority for productions about Jewish-related subjects. **Priorities:** *Arts & Humanities:* 14%. Supports public broadcasting and major support for history regarding the Holocaust and Jewish heritage. *Civic & Public Affairs:* 42%. Support public policy, womens affairs, Law & Justice, community and welfare to work. *Education:* 16%. Major support is in the form f fellowship, also supports international studies, public education, and legal education. *Environment:* 3%. Supports food distribution and the homeless. *International:* 12%. Supports biomedical research and adolescent health issues. *Note:* Total contributions made in 1999. **Typ. Recipients:** AIDS/HIV, Cancer, Clinics/Medical Centers, Medical Education, Medical Research. **Geo. Dist:** internationally; nationally; New York, NY.

**★ 4583 ★ Eleanor Naylor Dana Charitable Trust**
375 Park Ave., Ste. 3807
New York, NY 10152
**Phone:** (212)754-2890        **Fax:** (212)754-2892
**Fnded:** 1979. **Philosophy:** The trust gives funding priority in two areas: biomedical research, where it supports clinical investigation and "innovative projects designed to improve medical practice and prevent disease;" and the performing arts, "particularly those organizations which have an impact on the cultural climate of the nation." **Priorities:** *Arts & Humanities:* 42%. Supports performing arts. *Education:* 4%. Colleges and universities. *International:* 49%. Funds biomedical research, hospitals, and childrens health. *Note:* Total contributions made in fiscal 2000. **Typ. Recipients:** AIDS/HIV, Cancer, Children's Health/Hospitals, Clinics/Medical Centers, Diabetes, Eyes/Blindness, Family Planning, Heart, Hospitals, Hospitals (University Affiliated), Medical Education, Medical Research, Mental Health, Public Health, Transplant Networks/Donor Banks, Trauma Treatment. **Geo. Dist:** including the East Coast; New York, NY.

**★ 4584 ★ Helen Hay Whitney Foundation**
450 East 63rd St.
New York, NY 10021-7928
**Phone:** (212)751-8228        **Fax:** (212)688-6794
**Email:** hhwf@earthlink.net
**Website:** http://www.hhwf.org
Barbara Hugonnet, Administrative Director
**Fnded:** 1947. **Philosophy:** "The Helen Hay Whitney Foundation supports early postdoctoral training in all basic biomedical sciences. To attain its ultimate goal of increasing the number of imaginative, well-trained, and dedicated medical scientists, the foundation grants financial support of sufficient duration to help further the careers of young men and women engaged in biological or medical research." Residents of the United States, Canada, and Mexico, who hold M.D., Ph.D., or equivalent degrees are eligible to apply for

fellowships for beginning postdoctoral training in biomedical research. Also eligible are nonresidents training in the United States. Fellowships are normally for three years, with awards of $25,000 the first year, $27,000 the second year, and $29,000 the third year, as well as an annual allowance of $2,000 to defray research expenses. **Priorities:** *Education:* 50%.Primary focus is on medical education grants and fellowships. *Environment:* 5%. Supports general human services. *International:* 45% Supports universities and institutes for medical research fellowships. *Note:* Total contributions made in fiscal 2000. **Typ. Recipients:** Cancer, Children's Health/Hospitals, Hospitals, Medical Education, Medical Research, Research/Studies Institutes. **Geo. Dist:** North America.

**Howard Hughes Medical Institute**
*See:* Entry 362

**★ 4585 ★ James S. McDonnell Foundation**
1034 South Brentwood Boulevard, Ste. 1850
Saint Louis, MO 63117
**Phone:** (314)721-1532          **Fax:** (314)721-7421
**Email:** eesi@jsmF.org
**Website:** http://www.jsmf.org
Dr. Susan Fitzpatrick, Program Officer
**Fnded:** 1950. **Philosophy:** "The foundation's primary program interests are in biomedical and behavioral sciences, with over 90% of its annual grant awards supporting basic and applied research. Support for research, however, is provided primarily through foundation-initiated programs. Foundation-initiated programs are managed by advisory boards which assist in developing program guidelines, issue requests for proposals (RFPs), review submitted proposals and conduct program evaluation. In this way, the foundation is able to benefit from expert advice, fund work in targeted areas of interest, assure program applicants adequate peer review, and make specific funding decisions based on the relative merits of all proposals elicited by an RFP. Current foundation-initiated programs include: The McDonnell-Pew Program in Cognitive Neuroscience; Molecular Medicine in Cancer Research; Cognitive Studies for Educational Practice; The Initiative to Support Collaborative Research in Eastern Europe; and Cognitive Rehabilitation. The foundation's commitment to these programs severely limits funds available for other investigator-initiated research." 1997 Foundation Policies and Application Guidelines **Priorities:** *Civic & Public Affairs:* 46%. JSM Charitable Trust. *Education:* 33%. Supports universities. *International:* 16%. Funds biomedical and behavioral sciences research, and medical centers. *Note:* Contributions were made in 1998. **Typ. Recipients:** Cancer, Children's Health/Hospitals, Clinics/Medical Centers, Eyes/Blindness, Health Organizations, Hospitals, Medical Education, Medical Rehabilitation, Medical Research, Mental Health, Research/Studies Institutes. **Geo. Dist:** internationally; nationally.

**John D. and Catherine T. MacArthur Foundation**
*See:* Entry 12274

# National & International Organizations

**★ 4586 ★ American Association of Physicists in Medicine (AAPM)**
One Physics Ellipse
College Park, MD 20740-3846
**Phone:** (301)209-3350          **Fax:** (301)209-0862
**Email:** aapm@aapm.org
**Website:** http://www.aapm.org
Sal Trofi, Jr., Exec. Dir.
**Fnded:** 1958. **Mem:** 4,500. **Reg. Groups:** 20. **Desc:** Persons professionally engaged in application of phys-ics to medicine and biology in medical research and educational institutions; encourages interest and training in medical physics and related fields; promotes high professional standards; disseminates technical information. Maintains placement service. Conducts research programs. Member society of American Institute of Physics. **Pub:** *American Association of Physicists in Medicine–Membership Directory,* annual. Membership Directory. *Price:* Included in membership dues, Free. For members only. • *Medical Physics,* monthly. Journal. Contains articles broadly concerned with the relationship of human biology and medicine. *Price:* $390 for nonmembers; $430 library.

**★ 4587 ★ American College of Medical Physics**
11250 Roger Bacon Dr., Ste. 8
Reston, VA 20190-5202
**Phone:** (703)481-5001          **Fax:** (703)435-4390
**Email:** acmpwebmaster@radiationphysics.com
**Website:** http://www.acmp.org
Richard A. Guggolz, Exec. Dir.
**Fnded:** 1982. **Mem:** 450. **Reg. Groups:** 9. **Desc:** Covers socioeconomic aspects of practice, management issues, reimbursement, licensure, and practice standards. **Pub:** *Diagnostic Radiology.* Report. *Price:* $25 for nonmembers. • *Magnetic Resonance Imaging.* Report. *Price:* $25 for nonmembers. • *Mammography.* Report. *Price:* $25 for nonmembers. • *Medical Laser Systems.* Report. *Price:* $25 for nonmembers. • *Nuclear Medicine.* Report. *Price:* $25 for nonmembers. • *Radiation Oncology.* Report. *Price:* $25 for nonmembers. • Newsletter, 3-4/year.

**★ 4588 ★ Anatomical Society (AS) (Anatomische Gesellschaft — AG)**
c/o Wolfgang Kuhnel, M.D.
Institut fur Anatomie
Medizinische Universitat zu Lubeck
Ratzeburger Allee 160
D-23538 Lubeck, Germany
**Phone:** 49 451 5004030          **Fax:** 49 451 5004034
**Email:** kuchnel@anat.mu-luebeck.de
**Website:**          http://www.anat.mu-luebeck.de/anatpes.html
**Fnded:** 1886. **Mem:** 1,056. **Lang(s):** English, French, German. **Desc:** Anatomists, histochemists, histologists, biologists. **Pub:** *Annals of Anatomy.* Journal. • *Verhandlungen der Anatomischen Gesellschaft,* annual. Proceedings.

**★ 4589 ★ Anatomical Society of Great Britain and Ireland**
c/o Prof. J.P. Fraher
Department of Anatomy
University College
Cork, Ireland
**Phone:** 353 21 4902115          **Fax:** 353 21 4902246
**Email:** j.fraher@ucc.ie
**Website:** http://www.anatsoc.org.uk
**Fnded:** 1887. **Mem:** 650. **Lang(s):** English. **Desc:** Individuals involved in anatomical science. Promotes development and advancement in anatomy and related science through research and education. Offers program for graduate students. **Pub:** *Journal of Anatomy,* 12/year. Journal. Contains research information in the anatomical sciences.

**★ 4590 ★ Anatomical Society of Paris (Societe Anatomique de Paris)**
45, rue des Saints-Peres
F-75270 Paris, France
**Fax:** 33 1 42863366
**Fnded:** 1802. **Desc:** Promotes exchange between members on all subjects concerning anatomy; fosters studies on anatomy.

**★ 4591 ★ Anatomical Society of Southern Africa (ASSA) (Anatomiese Vereniging van Suider-Afrika)**
c/o Prof. H. B. Groenewald
Faculty of Veterinary Science
Private Bag X04
Onderstepoort 0110, Republic of South Africa
**Phone:** 27 12 5298247          **Fax:** 27 12 5298320
**Email:** hgroenew@op.up.acza
**Website:** http://www.satic.co.za/assa
**Fnded:** 1969. **Mem:** 200. **Lang(s):** Afrikaans, English. **Desc:** Individuals from 5 countries interested in the study of anatomy. Aims to: promote the study of anatomy; encourage anatomical research; represent anatomists of Southern Africa at the international level. Organizes seminars and workshops. Bestows awards. **Pub:** *Newsletter of the ASSA,* semiannual. Newsletter. • *Proceedings,* annual.

**★ 4592 ★ Argentine Society of Physiological Sciences (SACF) (Sociedad Argentina de Ciencias Fisiologicas)**
Solis 453
1078 Buenos Aires, Argentina
**Phone:** 54 1 3831110          **Fax:** 54 1 3810323
**Fnded:** 1950.

**★ 4593 ★ Asia and Oceania Federation of Nuclear Medicine and Biology (AOFNMB)**
Gazi University Medical Faculty
Department of Nuclear Medicine
Ergin Sokak 13-8 Mebusvleri
06580 Ankara, Turkey
**Phone:** 90 312 2229698          **Fax:** 90 312 2229698
**Lang(s):** English, Turkish. **Desc:** Health care professionals with an interest in nuclear medicine and biology. Seeks to advance the study, teaching, and practice of nuclear medicine; promotes ongoing professional development of members. Serves as a forum for the exchange of information among members; sponsors research and educational programs.

**Association of Biomedical Communication Directors (ABCD)**
*See:* Entry 12070

**★ 4594 ★ Association of Medical Physicists of India**
Bhabba Atomic Research Centre
Bombay 400 085, India
**Phone:** 91 22 556060          **Fax:** 91 5560750
**Fnded:** 1976.

**★ 4595 ★ Australian Biochemical Society**
PO Box 1600
Canberra, ACT, Australia
**Fax:** 61 7 473785
**Fnded:** 1955.

**★ 4596 ★ British Society for Antimicrobial Chemotherapy (BSAC)**
11 The Wharf
16 Bridge St.
Birmingham B1 2JS, United Kingdom
**Phone:** 44 121 6330410          **Fax:** 44 121 6434947
**Email:** tguest@bsac.org.uk
**Website:** http://www.bsac.org.uk
**Fnded:** 1971. **Mem:** 770. **Lang(s):** English. **Desc:** Individuals in 33 countries working in the field of antimicrobial chemotherapy. Furthers research and understanding of chemotherapy. **Pub:** *Journal of Antimicrobial Chemotherapy,* monthly. Journal.

**★ 4597 ★ Canadian Association for Clinical Microbiology and Infectious Diseases (CACMID)**
**(Association Canadienne de Microbiologie Clinique et des Maladies — ACMCM)**
c/o Darrel Cook
655 W 12th Ave.
Vancouver, BC, Canada V5Z 4R4
**Phone:** (604)660-6045      **Fax:** (604)660-6073
**Email:** darrel.cook@bccdc.hnet.bc.ca
**Website:** http://www.cacmid.ca
**Fnded:** 1980. **Mem:** 250. **Lang(s):** English, French. **Desc:** Microbiologists and other scientists and medical professionals engaged in the clinical study of infectious diseases. Seeks to advance the biological and medical sciences; promotes professional development of members. Serves as a clearinghouse on the clinical study of infectious diseases; facilitates exchange of information among members; conducts research and educational programs. **Pub:** *CACMID Contact*, quarterly. Newsletter.

**★ 4598 ★ Canadian Society of Diagnostic Medical Sonographers (CSDMS)**
PO Box 1220
Kemptville, ON, Canada K0G 1J0
**Phone:** (613)258-0855      **Free:** 888-273-6746
**Fax:** (613)258-0899
**Email:** csdms@sympatico.ca
**Website:** http://www.csdms.com
**Fnded:** 1981. **Mem:** 1,700. **Lang(s):** English. **Desc:** Ultrasound professionals from all specialty areas of Diagnostic Medical Ultrasound, as well as technical representatives, physicians, educators, and students. Fosters excellence in patient care and professional interaction and promotes the highest level of professional standards of practice for sonographers in Canada.

**★ 4599 ★ Chinese Association for Physiological Sciences**
42 Dongsixidajie
Beijing 100710, People's Republic of China

**★ 4600 ★ Danish Medical Society (Dansk Medicinsk Selskab — DMS)**
Kristianiagade 14
DK-2100 Copenhagen, Denmark
**Phone:** 45 35448407      **Fax:** 45 35448408
**Email:** cs@dadl.dk
**Website:** http://www.dms.dk
**Fnded:** 1919. **Desc:** Promotes Danish medical research and represents 92 Danish scientific societies in the field of biomedicine.

**★ 4601 ★ Danish Society for Medical Physics**
**(Dansk Selskab for Medicinsk Fysik — DSMF)**
Hobrovej 18-22
DK-9100 Alborg, Denmark
**Phone:** 45 99322891      **Fax:** 45 99322904
**Email:** jcarl@post8.tele.dk

**★ 4602 ★ European Federation for Experimental Morphology (EFEM)**
c/o Prof. Pierre Sprumont
Institut d'Anatomie de l'Universite
CH-1700 Fribourg, Switzerland
**Phone:** 41 26 3008450      **Fax:** 41 26 30009791
**Email:** pierre.sprumont@unifr.ch
**Fnded:** 1989. **Mem:** 21. **Desc:** European scientific societies and groups concerned with morphology, anatomy, and related fields. Promotes exchange and dissemination of information.

**★ 4603 ★ European Underwater and BaroMedical Society (EUBS)**
Benview
Prospect Ter.
Port Elphinstone
Inverurie AB51 3UN, United Kingdom
**Phone:** 44 1467 620408      **Fax:** 44 1467 620408
**Email:** secretary@eubs.org
**Website:** http://www.eubs.org
**Mem:** 390. **Lang(s):** English. **Desc:** Professionals and students interested in undersea medicine and related fields. Provides a forum for scientific communication among those interested in undersea medicine; encourages cooperation with related scientific disciplines. Strives to improve the safety of underwater activities by providing expert advice and educational programs; promotes undersea medicine. Holds workshops on topics concerning medical aspects of diving. **Pub:** *Long Term Neurological Consequences of Deep Diving.* • *Newsletter*, quarterly. Newsletter.

**★ 4604 ★ Foundation for Biomedical Research (FBR)**
818 Connecticut Ave. NW, Ste. 200
Washington, DC 20006
**Phone:** (202)457-0654      **Fax:** (202)457-0659
**Email:** info@fbresearch.org
**Website:** http://www.fbresearch.org
Ms. Frankie L. Trull, Pres.
**Fnded:** 1981. **Desc:** Individuals and organizations supporting humane animal research. Serves as public information and education program on what the foundation sees as the necessary and important role of laboratory animals in biomedical research and testing. Maintains speakers' bureau and public relations program. **Pub:** *Caring for Life*. Video. • *Fact vs. Myth.* Brochure. • *Foundation for Biomedical Research–Newsletter*, bimonthly. Newsletter. Includes foundation news and calendar of events. *Price:* Free. • *Hope!*. Film. • *Most Frequently Asked Questions About Animal Research*. Brochure. • *The New Research Environment*. Video. • *The Proud Achievements of Animal Research*. Brochure. • *Research Helping Animals*. Brochure. • *Science in Action*. Video. • *The Use of Animals in Biomedical Research and Testing*. • *Why I Should Stay Awake in Science Class*. Video.

**★ 4605 ★ Histochemical Society (HCS)**
c/o Dr. W.L. Stahl, Executive Director
Department Neurology, Box 356465
Univ. Washington Sch. Medicine
Seattle, WA 98195
**Phone:** (206)764-2088      **Fax:** (206)764-2164
**Email:** hcs@hcs.microscopy.com
**Website:** http://www.histochemicalsociety.org
Richard W. Burry, Pres.
**Fnded:** 1950. **Mem:** 550. **Desc:** Physicians and scientists who employ hisotchemical and cytochemical techniques in their research. **Pub:** *The Journal of Histochemistry and Cytochemistry*, monthly. Journal. • Newsletter, semiannual.

**★ 4606 ★ Howard Hughes Medical Institute (HHMI)**
4000 Jones Bridge Rd.
Chevy Chase, MD 20815-6789
**Phone:** (301)215-8500
**Email:** webmaster@hhmi.org
**Website:** http://www.hhmi.org
**Desc:** Works to help enhance biomedical science education at all levels. Conducts research.

**Institute for Laboratory Animal Research (ILAR)**
*See:* Entry 20624

**International Association of Biomedical Gerontology (IABG)**
*See:* Entry 2974

**★ 4607 ★ International Society for Biochemical Systematics (ISBS)**
Universiteitsplein 1
2610 Antwerp, Belgium
**Phone:** 32 3 8202248      **Fax:** 32 3 8202316
**Email:** yvdp@uia.ua.ac.be
**Website:** http://isbs-www.uia.ac.be/isbs/
**Fnded:** 1993. **Desc:** Promotes research and communication in the study of molecular aspects of systematics, from an evolutionary point of view and for phylogenetic comparison, covering micromolecules as well as macromolecules such as DNA and proteins.

**★ 4608 ★ International Union of Physiological Sciences (IUPS)**
83, bd de l'Hopital
F-75013 Paris, France
**Phone:** 33 1 42177537      **Fax:** 33 1 42177575
**Email:** schien@bioeng.ucsd.edu
**Website:** http://www.faseb.org/iups

**★ 4609 ★ Medical Research Society (MRS)**
c/o Dr. A. Chauldry
Renal Sec., Division of Medicine
Imperial College School of Medicine
Ducane Rd.
London W12 0NN, United Kingdom
**Phone:** 44 208 3832358      **Fax:** 44 208 3832062
**Email:** a.chauldry@ic.ac.uk
**Website:** http://www.medres.org
**Mem:** 1,300. **Lang(s):** English. **Desc:** Individuals engaged in basic and clinical medical research. Facilitates interdisciplinary exchange of information and provides a forum for data presentations by biomedical researchers. **Pub:** *Clinical Science*, monthly. • *Clinical Science Abstracts*, semiannual.

**★ 4610 ★ National Association for Biomedical Research (NABR)**
818 Connecticut Ave. NW, Ste. 200
Washington, DC 20006
**Phone:** (202)857-0540      **Fax:** (202)659-1902
**Email:** info@nabr.org
**Website:** http://www.nabr.org
Ms. Frankie L. Trull, Pres.
**Fnded:** 1979. **Mem:** 400. **Desc:** Universities, medical and veterinary schools, teaching hospitals, professional societies, voluntary health agencies, pharmaceutical companies and other research-related firms that use laboratory animals for biomedical research, education, and testing. Monitors and, when appropriate, attempts to influence legislation and regulations on behalf of members who are dependent on animals for biomedical research, education, and testing. **Pub:** *NABR Alert*, 6-10/year. Newsletter. Covers regulatory and legislative action related to the use of animals in biomedical research, research, and testing. *Price:* Included in membership dues. • *NABR Update*, 18-26/year. Bulletin. Covers national, state, and local regulatory and legislative activities affecting biomedical research. *Price:* Included in membership dues. • *National Association for BioMedical Research*. Annual Report. Describes the previous year's activities. *Price:* Included in membership dues.

**★ 4611 ★ Puerto Rico Society of Microbiologists (PRSM)**
PO Box 360175
San Juan, PR 00936-0175
**Phone:** (787)751-3057      **Fax:** (787)759-8559
**Email:** prsm40@hotmail.com
**Website:** http://www.asmusa.org/branch/brpr/objsmpr1b.htm
**Fnded:** 1957. **Desc:** Professionals in the field of microbiology. Aims to promote scientific interest in microbiology and to aid in the development and progress of professionals in the field. Organizes conferences, workshops, symposiums and conventions, sponsors student chapters. **Pub:** *PRSM-News*. Bulletin.

**Society of Biological Psychiatry (SBP)**
*See:* Entry 12643

★ **4612** ★ **W.M. Keck Foundation**
550 S Hope St., Ste. 2500
Los Angeles, CA 90071
**Phone:** (213)680-3833
**Email:** peterson.maggie@mayo.edu
**Website:** http://www.wmkeck.org
Robert A. Day, Pres.
**Fnded:** 1954. **Desc:** Works to support medical research, science, and engineering.

★ **4613** ★ **Yugoslav Association of Anatomists (YAA)**
**(Drustvo Anatoma Jugoslavije — DAJ)**
c/o Institute of Anatomy
Medical Faculty
Hajduk Veljkova 3
YU-21000 Novi Sad, Serbia
**Phone:** 381 21 615775          **Fax:** 381 21 624153
**Fnded:** 1956. **Mem:** 120. **Lang(s):** English, French, German, Russian, Serbian. **Desc:** Exchanges scientific information. Organizes courses in methodology. **Pub:** *Folia Anatomica*, semiannual. **Frmly:** (1994) Union of the Yugoslav Association of Anatomists.

# Research Centers

★ **4614** ★ **Albert Einstein Center for Synchrotron Biosciences**
Department of Biochemistry & Biophysics
Albert Einstein College of Medicine
Yeshiva University
1300 N Park Ave.
Bronx, NY 10461
**Phone:** (718)430-4136          **Fax:** (718)430-8819
**Email:** mrc@aecom.yu.edu
**Website:** http://www.aecom.yu.edu/home/csb/
Mark Chance, PhD, Dir.
**Activities/Fields:** Biological structure and function at the molecular level using synchrotron radiation, such as studies of protein and RNA folding, protein-protein interactions, structures of the active sites of metalloproteins, and macromolecular crystallography. **Pub:** *PRT Newsletter*. • *Technical Notes.* **Frmly:** Biostructures Participating Research Team.

★ **4615** ★ **American Type Culture Collection**
**Yeast Genetic Stock Center**
10801 University Blvd.
Manassas, VA 20110-2209
**Phone:** (703)365-2742
Shung-Chang Jong, PhD, Prin. Investigator
**Activities/Fields:** Improvement of the traditional collection of the yeast Saccharomyces cerevisiae.

★ **4616** ★ **Arizona State University Biomedical Engineering Laboratories**
College of Engineering
CBME Engineering Center, G-Wing, Rm. 202
Tempe, AZ 85287-9709
**Phone:** (480)965-3676          **Fax:** (480)727-7624
**Email:** guilbeau@asu.edu
Prof. Eric J. Guilbeau, Chm.
**Activities/Fields:** Biomechanics and bioinstrumentation, including medical devices, artificial organs, biosensors, analysis of motion, and nuclear imaging. Studies cardiovascular, biochemical, and physiological systems in relation to biomedical engineering. Conducts an industrial associate program, develops F.D.A. protocols, provides industrial development support, and offers continuing medical education. **Pub:** *Proceedings.* • *Transactions.*

★ **4617** ★ **Augusta Biomedical Research Corp.**
PO Box 3134
Augusta, GA 30914-3134
**Phone:** (706)823-2238          **Fax:** (706)823-3949
Delores (Dee) H. Vasquez, Exec. Dir.
**Activities/Fields:** Alzheimer's disease, strokes, cardiology, infectious diseases, gastroenterology, surgery, schizophrenia, neurology, mental health, substance abuse, and Parkinson's Disease.

**Baylor College of Medicine**
**Biochemical Genetics Laboratory**
*See:* Entry 8743

★ **4618** ★ **Baylor College of Medicine**
**Three-Dimensional Electron Microscopy of Macromolecules**
McLean Department of Biochemistry & Molecular Biology
1 Baylor Plz.
Houston, TX 77030
**Phone:** (713)798-6985          **Fax:** (713)798-1625
**Email:** wah@bcm.tmc.edu
**Website:** http://ncmi.bcm.tmc.edu
Wah Chiu, PhD, Prin. Investigator
**Activities/Fields:** Application of electron cryomicroscopy to the determination of three-dimensional structures of biological macromolecular assemblies at high resolution.

★ **4619** ★ **Baylor University**
**Baylor Research Institute**
3434 Live Oak St., No. 125
Dallas, TX 75204-6134
**Phone:** (214)820-2687          **Fax:** (214)820-4952
Brenda Russell, VP
**Activities/Fields:** Biomedicine, including digestive diseases, oncology, photobiology, organ transplants, muscle physiology, and metabolic diseases. **Pub:** *Baylor Proceedings*, quarterly. Proceedings.

★ **4620** ★ **Biomedical Research Foundation of Northwest Louisiana**
1505 Kings Hwy.
Shreveport, LA 71103
**Phone:** (318)675-4100          **Free:** 800-685-1152
**Fax:** (318)675-4120
**Email:** jsharp@biomed.org
**Website:** http://www.biomed.org
Jack Sharp, Pres.
**Activities/Fields:** Cardiovascular disease, neurobiology, stroke, medical imaging, medical information, and medical robotics development. **Pub:** *Annual report.* • *President's Report*, quarterly.

**Biomedical Research Institute**
*See:* Entry 11846

★ **4621** ★ **Boston Biomedical Research Institute (BBRI)**
64 Grove St.
Watertown, MA 02472-2829
**Phone:** (617)658-7700
**Email:** morgan@bbri.org
**Website:** http://www.bbri.org
Dr. Kathleen Morgan, Dir.
**Activities/Fields:** Biological and medical sciences, including fundamental biomedical studies on cell metabolism, developmental biology, gene regulation, recombinant DNA, monoclonal antibodies, intercellular matrix biology, muscle diseases, connective tissue diseases, and muscular dystrophy. **Pub:** *Messenger Newsletter*, semiannually. **Frmly:** Institute of Biological and Medical Sciences.

★ **4622** ★ **Boston University**
**Mass Spectrometry Resource for Biology and Medicine**
Departments of Biochemistry & Biophysics
School of Medicine
715 Albany St., R-806
Boston, MA 02118-2526
**Phone:** (617)638-6490          **Fax:** (617)638-6491
**Email:** cecmsms@bu.edu
**Website:** http://www.bumc.bu.edu/Departments/HomeMain.asp?DepartmentID=354
Catherine E. Costello, PhD, Prin. Investigator
**Activities/Fields:** High-sensitivity structural determination and analyses of biological compounds, especially glycoconjugates, oligosaccharides, and proteins; structure-activity studies related to proteins; structure-activity studies related to immunology, carcinogenesis, developmental biology, parasitology and infectious diseases, tissue implantation and rejection; biophysical properties of carbohydrates and glycoconjugates; carbohydrate and amino acid sequence determinations of glycoproteins and proteins; structure elucidation of unusual residues and posttranslational modifications; characterization of oligonucleotides and metal complexes such as imaging agents.

★ **4623** ★ **Brigham and Women's Hospital**
**Diagnostic Molecular Biology Laboratory**
75 Francis St.
Boston, MA 02115
**Phone:** (617)732-7446          **Fax:** (617)732-7449
**Email:** jsklar@rics.bwh.harvard.edu
Dr. Jeffrey Sklar, Dir.
**Activities/Fields:** Molecular biology, human genetics, and molecular oncology, including nucleic acid analysis for the diagnosis of cancer, inherited conditions, and infectious disorders.

★ **4624** ★ **Brigham and Women's Hospital**
**National Resource for Imaging Mass Spectrometry**
Laboratory of Cellular Physiology
221 Longwood Ave.
Boston, MA 02115
**Phone:** (617)732-7756          **Fax:** (617)732-4831
**Email:** cpl@harvard.edu
Claude Lechene, MD, Prin. Investigator
**Activities/Fields:** Use of stable isotopes and quantitative imaging mass spectrometry in biomedical research.

★ **4625** ★ **Brown University**
**International Health Institute**
Box G-B497
171 Meeting St.
Providence, RI 02912
**Phone:** (401)863-1186          **Fax:** (401)863-1243
**Email:** Stephen_McGarvey@brown.edu
**Website:** http://biomed.brown.edu/medicine_programs/IHI/
Stephen McGarvey, Dir.
**Activities/Fields:** Health problems of developing nations, including HIV/AIDS, cardiovascular disease, parasites and nutrition.

**Cancer Biotherapy Research Group (CBRG)**
*See:* Entry 10290

★ **4626** ★ **Case Western Reserve University**
**Program in Developmental Biology**
Department of Genetics, BRB 627
10900 Euclid Ave.
Cleveland, OH 44106-4955
**Phone:** (216)368-6417          **Fax:** (216)368-3432
**Email:** pjh3@po.cwru.edu

**Website:** http://www.cbrg.org
Peter Hart, Dir.

**Activities/Fields:** Developmental biology, genetics, neuroscience, molecular biology, regeneration, regulation of normal and neoplastic growth, biophysics, and biochemistry.

**Center for Biomedical Research**
*See:* Entry 18390

**★ 4627 ★ Center for Crystallographic Research**
Roswell Park Cancer Institute
Elm & Carlton Sts.
Buffalo, NY 14263
**Phone:** (716)845-3135     **Fax:** (716)845-8899
**Email:** sekwen.hui@roswellpark.org
Dr. Sek Wen Hui, Dir.

**Activities/Fields:** Conformational studies of nucleotides, peptides, and carbohydrates to determine interatomic arrangements in biological substances using nuclear magnetic resonance and electron spin resonance. Research is oriented to the field of cancer.

**★ 4628 ★ Center for Intelligent Biomedical Devices and Musculoskeletal Systems**
Brown Hall, Rm. 330A
Colorado School of Mines
1610 Illinois St.
Golden, CO 80401
**Phone:** (303)384-2032     **Fax:** (303)384-2212
**Email:** sjackson@mines.edu
**Website:** http://egweb.mines.edu/ibdms
Dr. Rahmat A. Shoureshi, Dir.

**Activities/Fields:** Advances in biomedical devices and musculoskeletal systems to enhance the quality of life for citizens with disabilities and reduce health care costs. Areas of interest include smart implants for hips and knees, enhanced mobility, and musculoskeletal systems stimulus.

**★ 4629 ★ City College of City University of New York**
**Center for the Study of the Cellular and Molecular Basis of Development**
City College Science Bldg., Rm. 501
138th St. & Convent Ave.
New York, NY 10031
**Phone:** (212)650-8300     **Fax:** (212)650-7989
**Email:** jerry@scisun.sci.ccny.cuny.edu
Dr. Jerry Guyden, Dir.

**Activities/Fields:** Molecular biology, including biomolecular structure and function, gene expression and regulation, cellular and organismic function, and neurobiology.

**★ 4630 ★ City of Hope**
**National Medical Center and Beckman Research Institute**
**Division of Biology**
1450 E Duarte Rd.
Duarte, CA 91010
**Phone:** (626)357-9711     **Fax:** (626)930-5486
**Website:** http://www.cityofhope.org
Gil Schwartzberg, Pres. /CEO

**Activities/Fields:** Molecular mechanisms of living systems. Research activities are carried out in Departments of Biology, Molecular Biochemistry, Molecular Genetics, and Theoretical Biology. Department of Biology focuses on dynamic and temporal properties of cell growth and proliferation as it is manifested in cultured cells and intact organisms, including cellular clocks, circadian rhythms, and chemical oscillators; mammalian genes and gene control mechanisms and defining the biological function of postreplication DNA modifications that occur in mammalian cells; the mechanisms of gene repression and its relationship to DNA replication time; the role of amino acid sequence in determining protein function and folding patterns; mammalian chromosome inactivation mechanisms; mutational generation and repair mechanisms; genetic imprinting; and embryonic stem cell biology. Department of Molecular Biochemistry studies the use of synthetic oligodeoxyribonucleotides in the study of human disease, including diagnosis of genetic disease and the analysis of bone marrow transplant patients; the role of genetically engineered antibodies for cancer therapy; the biological function of nucleic acids studied by chemical synthesis; genetic mechanisms of imprinting; and isolation and characterization of genes important to immune function and cancer. Department of Molecular Genetics examines gene expression sequence requirements in eukaryotic systems, diagnosis of viral diseases (including HIV and HCMV), biochemistry of RNA splicing, catalytic RNA function and applications in HIV infection and cancer, control of gene expression, isolation of biologically active pure insulin and insulin-like growth factor receptors, mitochondrial-nuclear interactions and mitochondrial biogenesis, and homologous DNA recombinations. Theoretical Biology examines origins of genetic information and patterns in coding regions of gene families.

**★ 4631 ★ City of Hope**
**National Medical Center and Beckman Research Institute**
**Division of Immunology**
1500 E Duarte Rd.
Duarte, CA 91010
**Phone:** (626)301-8164     **Fax:** (626)930-5300
**Email:** jmiser@coh.org
Dr. James Miser, Dir.

**Activities/Fields:** The Division is divided into five sections: Protein Chemistry, Immunobiology, Structural Biochemistry, Mass Spectrometry and NMR Spectroscopy. Sections collaborate on projects in cancer, virology, endocrinology, and immunology. Protein Chemistry Section research activities include development of sequencing strategies and structural studies on tumor markers, fibronectin, viral proteins, lymphokines, peptide hormones and neuroactive peptides. The Immunobiology Section studies the carcinoembryonic gene family, use of monoclonal antibodies in imaging and therapy of tumors, the transfer of antibody genes to tumor cells for enhanced immune response, regulation of the human interferon gene and production of a cytomegalovirus vaccine. The Structural Biochemistry Section performs active site stud ies on NAD enzymes and aromatase. The Mass Spectrometry Section analyzes peptides, protein glycoconjugates, and nucleotides using time of flight, magnetic sector, and quadruple mass spectrometers. A new NMR Section has been set up for solution phase determination of three dimensional structure of peptides and proteins.

**★ 4632 ★ Cleveland FES Center**
11000 Cedar Ave., Ste. 230
Cleveland, OH 44106-3052
**Phone:** (216)231-3257     **Free:** 800-666-2353
**Fax:** (216)231-3258
**Email:** info@fesc.org
**Website:** http://feswww.fes.cwru.edu/
P. Hunter Peckham, PhD, Dir.

**Activities/Fields:** Functional electrical stimulation (FES) in the restoration of muscle control or sensory function, particularly in the areas of lower and upper extremity deficits, scoliosis, spasticity, respiratory insufficiency, and bladder function. Studies focus on computer-controlled and implanted FES systems for paraplegic and quadriplegic users, persons with hemiplegia due to cerebral trauma or stroke, and persons with spinal cord injuries. **Pub:** *FES Update Newsletter*, semiannually. **Frmly:** Rehabilitation Engineering Center.

**★ 4633 ★ Columbia University**
**Biochemistry and Molecular Biophysics Laboratory**
630 W 168th St.
New York, NY 10032
**Phone:** (212)305-3669     **Fax:** (212)305-7932

**Email:** dih1@columbia.edu
**Website:** http://cpmcnet.columbia.edu/dept/gsas/biochem
Dr. David Hirsh, Chr.

**Activities/Fields:** Biochemistry, molecular biology, biophysics, and biochemical genetics, including X-ray diffraction studies of biological macromolecules, structure and function of membrane receptors and transport proteins, computer studies of protein and nucleic acid structure and function, NMR spectroscopy, neutron and electron diffraction, enzymology, regulation of transcription and translation in prokaryotic and eukaryotic cells, molecular virology, genomic and cDNA cloning in prokaryotes and eukaryotes, recombinant DNA technology, gene transfer and somatic-cell genetics, DNA sequencing, in vitro site-specific mutagenesis of cloned DNA, the role of oncogenes in neoplasia, control of gene expression in development, role of growth factors, regulation of oxygen transport by hemoglobin, hormonal regulation of ion transport, immunochemical properties of membrane antigens, structure and composition of synaptic components, metabolism of neurotransmitters, neurotoxic proteins and protein hormones, and chemical carcinogenesis.

**★ 4634 ★ Columbia University**
**Theoretical Simulation of Biological Systems**
Department of Chemistry, MC 3110
3000 Broadway
New York, NY 10027
**Phone:** (212)854-7606     **Fax:** (212)854-7454
**Email:** rich@chem.columbia.edu
**Website:** http://www.chem.columbia.edu/cbs/
Richard A. Friesner, PhD, Prin. Investigator

**Activities/Fields:** Algorithms, models, and software for simulation of biomolecular systems.

**★ 4635 ★ Connective Tissue Research Institute**
University City Science Center
3624 Market St.
Philadelphia, PA 19104-2614
**Phone:** (215)382-7840     **Fax:** (215)382-0056
**Email:** kefalide@mail.med.upenn.edu
Dr. Nicholas A. Kefalides, Dir.

**Activities/Fields:** Biochemistry, cell biology, immunology, and molecular biology of connective tissues, including characterization and study of basement membranes, blood vessels, cornea and lens capsule of the eye, and cell virus interaction. Research is applied toward problems in cardiovascular disease, kidney disease, ocular disease, and genetic disease.

**★ 4636 ★ Coriell Institute for Medical Research**
403 Haddon Ave.
Camden, NJ 08103
**Phone:** (856)757-4820     **Fax:** (856)964-0254
**Email:** dabeck@umdnj.edu
**Website:** http://cimr.umdnj.edu
David P. Beck, PhD, Pres.

**Activities/Fields:** Cell and molecular biology, microbiology, genetics, aging, cancer and cancer immunology, tumor virology, antibodies, genetic disorders, vascular disorders, infectious diseases and virus/chromosome relationships, environmental mutagenesis, and genetic probes. Studies utilization of cells grown in tissue culture for isolation and characterization of tumor cell antigens, viruses, genetic abnormalities, tumor viruses, and chromosomes. **Pub:** *Biennial Report.* • *Discover.* • *Newsletter*, quarterly.

**★ 4637 ★ Dalhousie University**
**Atlantic Research Centre**
5849 University Ave., Rm. C-304
Halifax, NS, Canada B3H 4H7
**Phone:** (902)494-6491     **Fax:** (902)494-1394
**Email:** david.byers@dal.ca
**Website:** http://www.medicine.dal.ca/arc/
Dr. David M. Byers, Dir.

**Activities/Fields:** Biochemistry and genetics, including human cytogenetics, human inherited metabolic diseases, biochemistry and metabolism in the developing brain, and lipid second messengers, signal transduction, and membrane metabolism in normal and diseased human cells in culture. Provides special biomedical services relating to the causes and prevention of mental handicap.

### ★ 4638 ★ Duke University
**Center for Emerging Cardiovascular Technologies (CECT)**
B237 Levine Science Research Center
PO Box 90295
Durham, NC 27708-0295
**Phone:** (919)660-5137 **Fax:** (919)684-8886
**Email:** mhr@acpub.duke.edu
**Website:** http://cect.egr.duke.edu
Olaf T. von Ramm, PhD, Dir.

**Activities/Fields:** Cardiovascular devices and technologies, including biosensors, implantable defibrillators, real-time 3-D ultrasound imaging equipment, custom integrated electronics, and systems design and simulation. Facilitates technology transfer and promotes interaction between engineering students and industrial investigators.

### ★ 4639 ★ Duke University
**Center for In Vivo Microscopy**
Department of Radiology
PO Box 3302
Durham, NC 27710
**Phone:** (919)684-7755 **Fax:** (919)684-7158
**Email:** gaj@orion.mc.duke.edu
**Website:** http://wwwcivm.mc.duke.edu
G. Allan Johnson, PhD, Dir.

**Activities/Fields:** Magnetic resonance microscopy, imaging of disease models, drug discovery and validation, pulmonary imaging toxicology testing and evaluation in live animals, and in vivo histology and microscopy.

### ★ 4640 ★ Eleanor Roosevelt Institute
1899 Gaylord St.
Denver, CO 80206
**Phone:** (303)336-5600 **Fax:** (303)333-8423
**Email:** davepatt@eri.uchsc.edu
**Website:** http://www-eri.uchsc.edu
David Patterson, PhD, Pres.

**Activities/Fields:** Biochemistry and mammalian genetics. Investigates human and other mammalian cell systems, biosynthetic pathways of purines and pyrimidines, biochemical structure and function of cell surface membranes, cytogenetics, cancer genetics, genetic biochemistry, mutagenesis, carcinogenesis, down syndrome, Lou Gehrig's disease (ALS) and arthritis. Results of studies applied to problems in malignancy, birth defects, and other diseases.

### ★ 4641 ★ Emory University
**Yerkes Regional Primate Research Center**
954 Gatewood Rd. NE
Atlanta, GA 30322
**Phone:** (404)727-7732 **Fax:** (404)727-3108
**Email:** gordon@rmy.emory.edu
**Website:** http://www.emory.edu/WHSC/YERKES/
Dr. Thomas P. Gordon, Interim Dir.

**Activities/Fields:** Primate studies, including neuroscience, psychobiology, microbioology and immunology, molecular medicine, and vision research. Specialty areas within the foregoing fields include drug abuse, aging, neurophysiology, neuroendocrinology, cardiovascular studies related to coronary disease, effects of drugs on behavior, social behavior, language capacities, in vitro fertilization, endocrine studies of reproductive cycles, diseases of nonhuman primates, infectious and degenerative diseases (including AIDS and retroviral immunodeficiency disorders) and vaccine development. **Frmly:** Yale Laboratories of Primate Biology.

### ★ 4642 ★ EPG Research Foundation, Inc.
111 E Shore Rd.
Manhasset, NY 11030-2922
**Phone:** (516)365-1288 **Fax:** (516)365-7522
**Email:** epglabs@igc.apc.org
Dr. J.L. Logan, Dir.

**Activities/Fields:** Molecular biology.

### ★ 4643 ★ Georgia State University
**Viral Immunology Center**
**National B Virus Resource Laboratory**
PO Box 4118
Atlanta, GA 30302-4118
**Phone:** (404)651-0808 **Fax:** (404)651-0814
**Email:** bvirus@gsu.edu
**Website:** http://www.gsu.edu/bvirus
Julia K. Hilliard, PhD, Dir.

**Activities/Fields:** B-virus infections, basic pathogenesis mechanisms of this and other neurotropic herpesviruses, control and prevention strategies. It provides rapid virological and serological analyses and collaborates in studies of Herpes virus simiae and B-virus infections in humans and nonhuman primates, particularly macaques. Also investigating new animal models of herpesvirus disease, antiviral testing and epidemiological analyses of alpha-herpes virus by biochemical, immunological and molecular biological approaches; development of recombinant reagents; identification of effective antiviral strategies and design of putative vaccines; elucidation of host-virus interactions during pathogenesis; collaborative identification and exploration of putative alpha-herpes viruses not previously described.

**H.L. Snyder Memorial Research Foundation**
*See:* Entry 10336

### ★ 4644 ★ Harvard University
**Laboratory for Cell and Molecular Biology**
Burl Bldg., 5th Fl.
Department of Medicine
New England Deaconess Hospital
185 Pilgrim Rd.
Boston, MA 02215
**Phone:** (617)632-9982 **Fax:** (617)632-9992
**Email:** lsmith@snyderrf.com
**Website:** http://www.snyderrf.org
Dr. Arthur J. Sytkowski, Dir.

**Activities/Fields:** Biology of blood cell production, control mechanisms involved in normal cell growth and development, and identification of factors responsible for malignant transformation and neoplastic or cancerous growth. Ongoing studies include identifying the structural and functional properties of the erythropoietin molecule and the mechanisms of interaction with its receptor on the cell surface, identifying the role of cellular oncogenes in blood cell growth and differentiation, characterizing erythropoietin early response genes, and investigating gene therapy and erythroid burst promoting activity. Studies have direct applications to clinical syndromes accompanied by disordered blood cell production, leukemia, lymphoma, and cancer.

### ★ 4645 ★ Helicon Foundation
4622 Santa Fe St.
San Diego, CA 92109
**Phone:** (858)272-3884 **Free:** 888-726-8698
**Fax:** (858)272-1621
**Email:** cathomas@ix.netcom.com
Dr. Charles A. Thomas, Jr., Pres.

**Activities/Fields:** Basic biological research in biochemistry, molecular biology, and genetics, including studies on oxidative damage to cellular DNA, structure of chromosomal telomeres, chromatin structure, and role of lipids in radical formation. Seeks to define the biochemical basis of disease prevention through antioxidant diagnostics.

### ★ 4646 ★ Hospital for Special Surgery
**Fannie E. Rippel Flow Cytometry Core Facility**
Belaire Bldg., Rm. 705
525 E 71st St.
New York, NY 10021
**Phone:** (212)606-1925 **Fax:** (212)717-1192
**Email:** merlins@hss.edu
**Website:** http://hss.hss.edu
Steven Merlin, Assoc. Dir.

**Activities/Fields:** Flow cytometry: multiparameter cell sorting and cellular analysis. **Pub:** *HSS Flow Core Newsletter.*

### ★ 4647 ★ Hospital for Special Surgery
**Research Division**
**Biomechanics and Biomaterials Section**
535 E 70th St.
New York, NY 10021
**Phone:** (212)606-1093 **Fax:** (212)606-1490
**Email:** wrightt@hss.edu
**Website:** http://www.hss.edu/
Timothy Wright, PhD, Sect. Hd.

**Activities/Fields:** Application of principles of mechanics and materials science in order to understand and treat orthopedic problems.

### ★ 4648 ★ Indiana University-Purdue University at Indianapolis
**Human Performance and Biomechanics Laboratory**
901 W New York St.
Indianapolis, IN 46202
**Phone:** (317)274-0608 **Fax:** (317)278-2041
**Email:** amikesky@iupui.edu
**Website:** http://www.indiana.edu/~rugs/ctrdir/hpmbl.html
Dr. Alan E. Mikesky, Dir.

**Activities/Fields:** Sports medicine and biomechanics.

### ★ 4649 ★ Indiana University-Purdue University at Indianapolis
**Oral Health Research Institute**
**Bioresearch Facility**
415 N Lansing St.
Indianapolis, IN 46202-2876
**Phone:** (317)274-1151 **Fax:** (317)274-5425
**Email:** jwarrick@iupui.edu
**Website:** http://www.iusd.iupui.edu/depts/OHRI/Bioresearch.htm
Janice M. Warrick, Dir.

**Activities/Fields:** Biomechanics, biomaterials, musculoskeletal research, polymers with therapeutic potential, and new dental restorative materials. **Frmly:** Biomechanics and Biomaterials Research Center.

### ★ 4650 ★ John L. McClellan Memorial Veterans' Hospital
**Research Office**
4300 W 7th St.
Little Rock, AR 72205
**Phone:** (501)257-4816 **Fax:** (501)257-4821
Philip A. Kern, MD, Dir.

**Activities/Fields:** Biomedicine, including studies of Histoplasmosis, the molecular biology of aging, molecular biology of tuberculosis and other mycobacterial diseases, molecular biology of diabetes, hyperthermia effects on tumors, anti-tumor drugs, nephrology. Also conducts clinical studies in cardiology, stroke, infectious diseases, prostate cancer, and aneurysms. Rehabilitation Research and Development, particularly research on falling in the elderly; and Health Services Research and Development Field Program for Mental Health, including schizophrenia management, stroke outcomes management, and protein-energy undernutrition among elderly patients.

**Johns Hopkins University**
**Biomechanics Research Laboratory**
*See:* Entry 16952

**Johns Hopkins University**
**Biomedical Instrumentation Laboratory**
*See:* Entry 2512


**★ 4651 ★ Johns Hopkins University**
**Biomedical Optics Laboratory**
Ross Research Bldg., Rm. 724
Department of Biomedical Engineering
Sch. of Medicine
720 Rutland Ave.
Baltimore, MD 21205
**Phone:** (410)614-2528          **Fax:** (410)955-0549
**Email:** skuo@bme.jhu.edu
**Website:** http://www.bme.jhu.edu/~skuo/Lab/
Scot C. Kuo, Prin. Investigator

**Activities/Fields:** Optical tools (optical tweezers, optical rheometry, video-enhanced optical microscopy,
fluorescence microscopy, digital image processing);
cell mechanics (non-invasive, real-time monitoring of
cell mechanics during chemotaxis, cell crawling, gran-
ule secretion, and mitosis); microtubule-based motility
(kinesin force generation, single-molecule assays,
genetic engineering, organelle transport, chromosome
movement); and collaborations (electromotility of outer
hair cells, chromosome movement, biological rheology, and mechanics of biological materials).


**★ 4652 ★ Johns Hopkins University**
**Polymeric Biomaterials Laboratory**
729 Ross Bldg.
Department of Biomedical Engineering
School of Medicine
Baltimore, MD 21205
**Phone:** (410)955-0075          **Fax:** (410)955-0549
**Email:** kleong@bme.jhu.edu
Dr. Kam W. Leong, Prin. Investigator

**Activities/Fields:** Application of synthetic and biological polymers to drug delivery, gene therapy, and tissue
engineering, particularly controlled delivery of cytokines and cytokine genes for cancer immunotherapy,
particulate HIV vaccine design, combinative gene and
drug therapy of cystic fibrosis; and synthesis of new
biodegradable poly(phosphoesters) for drug-carrier
and tissue scaffold applications.


**★ 4653 ★ Kansas State University**
**University Biochemistry Facility**
Willard Hall, Rm. 104
Department of Biochemistry
Manhattan, KS 66506-3702
**Phone:** (785)532-6121          **Fax:** (785)532-7278
**Email:** cxhedg@ksu.edu
**Website:** http://www.ksu.edu/bchem/
Dr. Charles Hedgcoth, Dept. Hd.

**Activities/Fields:** Biochemistry research, including
protein sequencing, peptide sequencing, and oligonu-
cleotide synthesis.


**Laval University**
**Molecular Microbiology and Protein**
  **Engineering Group**
*See:* Entry 9410


**★ 4654 ★ Louisiana State University**
**Pennington Biomedical Research Center**
6400 Perkins Rd.
Baton Rouge, LA 70808-4124
**Phone:** (225)763-2500          **Fax:** (225)763-2525
**Email:** rclevesq@rsvs.ulaval.ca
**Website:** http://www.pbrc.edu
Claude Bouchard, PhD, Exec. Dir.

**Activities/Fields:** Nutritional physiology and metabolism, molecular and cellular nutrition, nutrition and
behavior, nutritional epidemiology, neurobiology, taste
physiology, clinical physochlogy, biostatistics, and
metabolic studies. **Pub:** *Inside Pennington Newsletter.*
• *Pennington Nutrition Series.*


**★ 4655 ★ Mailman Research Center**
115 Mill St.
Belmont, MA 02478
**Phone:** (617)855-3227          **Fax:** (617)855-3670
**Email:** cohenb@mclean.harvard.edu
**Website:** http://www.McLeanHospital.org
Bruce M. Cohen, PhD, Pres.

**Activities/Fields:** Neuropharmacology, neurochemistry, neuropathology, molecular neurogenetics, neuro-
regeneration, and molecular neurobiology with emphasis on psychiatric neurosciences.


**★ 4656 ★ McGill University**
**Institute of Parasitology**
MacDonald Campus
21111 Lakeshore Rd.
Sainte Anne de Bellevue, QC, Canada H9X 3V9
**Phone:** (514)398-7722          **Fax:** (514)398-7857
**Email:** grad_sec@parasit.lan.mcgill.ca
**Website:** http://www.mcgill.ca/parasitology/
Dr. Roger Prichard, Dir.

**Activities/Fields:** Epidemiology, ecology, biochemistry, neurophysiology, immunology, population and
molecular genetics and molecular biology of parasites.
Research includes experimental studies on the relationships and interactions between parasite and host.
**Pub:** *Research Reports.* • *Scientific journals peer-
reviewed.*


**★ 4657 ★ McLaughlin Research Institute**
  **for Biomedical Sciences**
1520 23rd St. S
Great Falls, MT 59405-4900
**Phone:** (406)452-6208          **Fax:** (406)454-6019
**Email:** davec@po.mri.montana.edu
**Website:** http://www.montana.edu/wwwmri
Dr. George A. Carlson, Dir.

**Activities/Fields:** Genetics, immunogenetics, and
cancer immunology, including studies of mouse histocompatibility genes and antigens, immunoregulatory
gene family diversity and divergence, genetic basis of
susceptibility to transmissible neurodegenerative disease, and mitotic recombination in mammalian cells.
**Pub:** *Annual Report.* • *Newsletter,* 3/year.


**★ 4658 ★ Medical Research Foundation**
  **of Oregon**
1211 SW Salmon St., Ste. 200
Portland, OR 97205-2021
**Phone:** (503)228-1730          **Fax:** (503)228-9588
**Email:** muellerl@ohsu.edu
**Website:** http://www.ohsufoundation.org
Lori Mueller, Sr. VP. Fin. & Admin.

**Activities/Fields:** Biomedical research grants awarded to Oregon scientists for research done in Oregon.


**★ 4659 ★ Medical University of South**
  **Carolina**
**Marine Biomedicine and Environmental**
  **Sciences**
221 Ft. Johnson Rd.
Charleston, SC 29412
**Phone:** (843)762-5530          **Fax:** (843)762-5535
**Email:** lacyer@musc.edu
Dr. Eric R. Lacy, Dir.

**Activities/Fields:** Marine organisms and their cells as
models, particularly in toxicology, immunology, pathology, parasitology, and microbiology studies.


**★ 4660 ★ Michigan State University**
**Center for Biological Modeling**
502B Biochemistry Bldg.
East Lansing, MI 48824-1319
**Phone:** (517)432-9895          **Fax:** (517)353-9334
**Email:** cbm@msu.edu
**Website:** http://biomodel.msu.edu/
Robert I. Cukier, Dir.

**Activities/Fields:** Modeling of biological processes,
particularly protein folding, biomolecular catalysis, the
spread of disease, rational development of drugs, and
the evolution of organisms and molecules.


**★ 4661 ★ Mount Sinai School of**
  **Medicine of City University of New**
  **York**
**Brookdale Center for Molecular Biology**
1 Gustave Levy Plz., Box 1020
New York, NY 10029-6574
**Phone:** (212)241-4272          **Fax:** (212)860-9279
**Email:** paul.wassarman@mssm.edu
Dr. Paul Wassarman, Dir.

**Activities/Fields:** Molecular biology and medicine,
including molecular neurobiology; developmental molecular biology; receptor and channel structure, function, and regulation; hormone, oncogene, and growth
factor actions; the molecular and genetic basis of
disease; cytokine action; and control of gene transcription.


**★ 4662 ★ National Biomedical Research**
  **Foundation**
3900 Reservoir Rd. NW
Washington, DC 20007
**Phone:** (202)687-2121          **Fax:** (202)687-1662
**Email:** pirmail@nbrf.georgetown.edu
**Website:** http://pir.georgetown.edu
Dr. Cathy H. Wu, Dir.

**Activities/Fields:** Application of computers and electronic technology to medical research, including biomedical picture pattern analysis, biology, biochemistry,
origins of life, and computer technology. Specific
research projects include studies on automatic chromosome analysis, biomedical instrumentation, computer aid to medical diagnosis, and genetics, evolution, and function of proteins and nucleic acids. **Pub:**
*Computers in Biology and Medicine,* bimonthly. •
*Journal of Computer Languages,* quarterly. • *Journal
of Computerized Medical Imaging & Graphics,* bimonthly. • *Pattern Recognition Journal,* monthly.


**★ 4663 ★ National Science Foundation**
  **(NSF)**
**Directorate for Biological Sciences (BIO)**
**Division of Molecular and Cellular**
  **Biosciences**
**Ecological and Evolutionary Physiology**
  **Program (EEP)**
4201 Wilson Blvd.
Rm. 685
Arlington, VA 22230
**Phone:** (703)292-8421          **Fax:** (703)292-9153
**Email:** jhayes@nfs.gov
**Website:** http://www.nsf.gov/bio/ibn/ibnphysio.htmeep
Jack Hayes, Prog. Dir.

**Activities/Fields:** Ecological or evolutionary morphology, comparative physiology, physiological ecology,
and biomechanics of plants, animals, protists, fungi
and bacteria. **Frmly:** Regulatory Biology Program;
Physiological Processes Program.


**★ 4664 ★ National Science Foundation**
**Directorate for Biological Sciences**
**Division of Molecular and Cellular**
  **Biosciences**
**Microbial Genetics Program**
4201 Wilson Blvd., Rm. 655
Arlington, VA 22230
**Phone:** (703)292-8439          **Fax:** (703)292-9061
**Email:** pdennis@nsf.gov
**Website:** http://www.nsf.gov/bio/mcb/mcbgenet-
ics.htmmg
Patrick P. Dennis, Prog. Dir.

**Activities/Fields:** Supports research focused on the
organization, function, transmission, mutation, regulation, and recombination of genetic information of
microorganisms. Other topics supported include gene
evolution, genetics of microbial interactions with eukaryotic organisms, and genetics of microbial plasmids
and viruses.

### ★ 4665 ★ New York State Department of Health
**Wadsworth Center**
**Resource for the Visualization of Biological Complexity**
Empire State Plz.
Albany, NY 12201-0509
**Phone:** (518)474-7002          **Fax:** (518)486-2191
**Email:** joachim@wadsworth.org
**Website:** http://www.wadsworth.org/rvbc
Conly Rieder, PhD, Contact

**Activities/Fields:** Development of methods for the 3-D visualization of biological systems over a wide range of scales, from macromolecular assemblies to cells and tissues.

**New York University**
**Center for Neural Science**
*See:* Entry 14250

### ★ 4666 ★ Oklahoma Medical Research Foundation
825 NE 13th St.
Oklahoma City, OK 73104
**Phone:** (405)271-7210          **Free:** 800-522-0211
**Fax:** (405)271-3980
**Email:** Don-Capra@omrf.ouhsc.edu
**Website:** http://www.omrf.ouhsc.edu
J. Donald Capra, MD, Pres.

**Activities/Fields:** Arthritis and Immunology, including lupus, rheumatoid arthritis, and scleroderma; Cardiovascular Biology, including heart attack, blood diseases, stroke, and septic shock; Children's Diseases, including cancer, leukemia, genetic disorders, and cystic fibrosis; Clincial Pharmacology, including FDA drug trials for hypertension, cholesterol, asthma, and others; Development Biology, including genetic disorders, Down's syndrome, and obesity; Free Radical Biology and Aging, including Alzheimer's disease, Parkinson's disease, and stroke; Immunobiology and Cancer, including leukemia, Hogkins' disease, lymphoma, and breast cancer; Molecular and Cell Biology, including ALS, muscular dystrophy, multiple sclerosis, and new antibiotics; Molecular Immunogenetics, including diabetes, AIDS, and immune system disorders; and Protein Studies, including AIDS, HIV, diabetes, and ulcers. **Pub:** *Findings Newsletter.*

### ★ 4667 ★ Oklahoma Medical Research Foundation
**Crystallography Research Program**
825 NE 13th St.
Oklahoma City, OK 73104
**Phone:** (405)271-6673          **Fax:** (405)271-3980
**Email:** allen-edmundson@omrf.ouhsc.edu
**Website:** http://www.omrf.org/OMRF/Research/04/Program.asp
Allen B. Edmundson, PhD, Prog. Hd.

**Activities/Fields:** Structure and function of protein molecules.

### ★ 4668 ★ Oklahoma Medical Research Foundation
**Developmental Biology Research Program**
825 NE 13th St.
Oklahoma City, OK 73104
**Phone:** (405)271-6673          **Fax:** (405)271-3980
**Email:** ute-hochgeschwender@omrf.ouhsc.edu
**Website:** http://www.omrf.org/OMRF/Research/10/Program.asp
Ute Hochgeschwender, MD, Contact

**Activities/Fields:** Molecular basis of growth and differentiation, using the mouse as a model organism. Of particular interest are the processes of neural differentiation and brain development, as well as the tissue-specific regulation of gene expression and the relative stability of the genome to mutation and DNA recombination.

### ★ 4669 ★ Oklahoma Medical Research Foundation
**Protein Studies Program**
825 NE 13th St.
Oklahoma City, OK 73104
**Phone:** (405)271-7291          **Fax:** (405)271-7249
**Email:** jordan-tang@omrf.ouhsc.edu
Dr. Jordan Tang, Dir.

**Activities/Fields:** Alzheimer's Disease, especially regarding protein structure and function, including cloning, expression and mutagenesis of protease genes, mechanisms of proteases, proteolysis by lysosomal enzymes, and streptokinase interaction with plasminogen fibrinolysis.

### ★ 4670 ★ Oregon Health and Science University
**Division of Medical Informatics and Outcomes Research**
BICC
3181 SW Sam Jackson Pk. Rd.
Portland, OR 97201-3098
**Phone:** (503)494-4502          **Fax:** (503)494-4551
**Email:** hersh@ohsu.edu
**Website:** http://www.ohsu.edu/bicc-informatics/
Dr. William Hersh, Dir.

**Activities/Fields:** Medical informatics, including information retrieval, bioinformatics, clinician information needs, terminology, and electronic medical records; and outcomes research, including clinical epidemiology, health services research, and evidence-based medicine. **Frmly:** Biomedical Information Communication Center.

### ★ 4671 ★ Oregon Institute of Science and Medicine
2251 Dick George Rd.
Cave Junction, OR 97523-9622
**Phone:** (541)592-4142          **Fax:** (541)592-2597
**Email:** art@oism.org
**Website:** http://www.oism.org
Arthur B. Robinson, PhD, Pres.

**Activities/Fields:** Protein chemistry, molecular biology, nutrition and preventive medicine, and medical diagnostic techniques.

**Orentreich Foundation for the Advancement of Science, Inc.**
*See:* Entry 3063

### ★ 4672 ★ Pacific Northwest Research Institute
720 Broadway Ave.
Seattle, WA 98122
**Phone:** (206)726-1200          **Fax:** (206)726-1217
**Email:** rpr@uwashington.edu
**Website:** http://www.pnri.org
R. Paul Robertson, MD, CEO/Sci. Dir.

**Activities/Fields:** Medical sciences, including Type I and II diabetes, pancreas and islet transplantation, environmental biochemistry, membrane biochemistry, biochemical oncology, molecular epidemiology, and cell and molecular biology.

### ★ 4673 ★ Palo Alto Institute of Molecular Medicine
2462 Wyandotte St.
Mountain View, CA 94043
**Phone:** (650)694-1420          **Fax:** (650)694-7717
**Email:** paimm@netgate.net
**Website:** http://www.paimm.org
Dr. James W. Larrick, Dir.

**Activities/Fields:** Cellular and molecular biology, cancer, and immunoinflammatory diseases.

### ★ 4674 ★ Palo Alto Medical Foundation for Health Care, Research, and Education
795 El Camino Real
Palo Alto, CA 94301
**Phone:** (650)321-4121          **Fax:** (650)853-5702
**Website:** http://www.pamf.org
David Druker, MD, Pres./CEO

**Activities/Fields:** Basic and clinical biomedical research.

### ★ 4675 ★ Philadelphia Biomedical Research Institute
100 Ross & Royal Rds.
King of Prussia, PA 19406
**Phone:** (610)962-0615          **Fax:** (610)962-0614
**Email:** stohnishi@aol.com
**Website:** http://members.aol.com/stohnishi/phila_biomed/sickle.htm
S. Tsuyoshi Ohnishi, PhD, Dir.

**Activities/Fields:** Mechanisms, methods of diagnosis, and pharmacological treatment of membrane-linked diseases through investigation of structure-function relationship in normal and abnormal biological membranes. Studies focus on the nutritional means to manage sickle cell anemia. **Pub:** *Arzneimittel Forschung/Drug Research.* • *Brain Research.* • *Cancer Letters.* • *Free Radicals in Biology and Medicine.* • *Prostaglandins Leucotrienes and Essential Fatty Acids.*

### ★ 4676 ★ Picower Institute for Medical Research
350 Community Dr., 4th Fl.
Manhasset, NY 11030
**Phone:** (516)365-4200          **Fax:** (516)365-5090
**Email:** ejones@picower.edu
**Website:** http://www.picower.edu
Dr. Richard Bucala, VP/Sci. Dir.

**Activities/Fields:** Pathogenesis of diseases in order to discover the technology to treat them. Major areas of investigation include cancer, inflammation and infectious diseases including HIV, asthma and arthritis. **Pub:** *Molecular Medicine.*

### ★ 4677 ★ Public Health Research Institute
455 1st Ave.
New York, NY 10016
**Phone:** (212)578-0800          **Fax:** (212)578-0804
**Email:** lmw@phri.org
**Website:** http://www.phri.org
Lewis M. Weinstein, Pres.

**Activities/Fields:** Biomedical research with a focus on infectious diseases and public health issues. **Pub:** *Annual report.* • *Symposium proceedings.*

### ★ 4678 ★ Research Resource for Complex Physiologic Signals
Department of Medicine
Beth Israel Deaconess Medical Center
330 Brookline Ave.
Boston, MA 02215
**Phone:** (617)667-4267          **Fax:** (617)667-7268
**Email:** ary@astro.bidmc.harvard.edu
**Website:** http://www.physionet.org
Ary L. Goldberger, MD, Prin. Investigator

**Activities/Fields:** Complex physiologic signals.

**Rockefeller University**
**Laboratory of Cellular Physiology and Immunology**
*See:* Entry 3261

**Rockefeller University**
**Laboratory of Clinical Microbiology and Immunology**
*See:* Entry 3262

**★ 4679 ★ Rosenstiel Basic Medical Sciences Research Center**
Brandeis University
415 South St.
Waltham, MA 02454-9110
**Phone:** (781)736-2400     **Fax:** (781)736-2405
**Email:** petsko@brandeis.edu
**Website:** http://www.rose.brandeis.edu/
Dr. Gregory Petsko, Dir.

**Activities/Fields:** Genetics and molecular biology, biochemistry, structural biology, protein crytallography, microbiology, biophysics, and cellular immunology.


**★ 4680 ★ Rutgers University Bureau of Biological Research**
FAS Division of Life Science - Nelson Biological Laboratorie
604 Allison Rd.
Piscataway, NJ 08854-8082
**Phone:** (732)445-3972     **Fax:** (732)445-0644
**Email:** martin@biology.rutgers.edu
Charles Martin, Dir.

**Activities/Fields:** Neurobiology and physiology, cell and developmental biology, molecular biology, biomoleculer structure, biochemistry.


**★ 4681 ★ Rutgers University Cell and Cell Products Fermentation Facility**
Waksman Institute
190 Frelinghuysen Rd.
Piscataway, NJ 08855-8020
**Phone:** (732)445-2925     **Fax:** (732)445-5735
**Email:** callanan@mbcl.rutgers.edu
**Website:** http://waksman.rutgers.edu/ferment
Kenneth R. Callanan, Mgr.

**Activities/Fields:** Cell fermentation and production of primary and secondary metabolites such as recombinant proteins, hormones, enzymes, regulatory proteins, and antiviral, antibacterial, and antifungal compounds.


**★ 4682 ★ St. Louis University Institute for Molecular Virology**
3681 Park Ave.
Saint Louis, MO 63110
**Phone:** (314)577-8403     **Fax:** (314)577-8406
**Email:** green@slu.edu
Dr. Maurice Green, Chm.

**Activities/Fields:** Molecular biology, virology, cell biology, oncology, and AIDS, including structure and function of human viruses and mechanism of virus replication and cell transformation by ribonucleic and deoxyribose acid tumor viruses.


**★ 4683 ★ Salk Institute for Biological Studies**
PO Box 85800
San Diego, CA 92186-5800
**Phone:** (858)453-4100     **Fax:** (858)552-8285
**Email:** murphy@salk.edu
**Website:** http://www.salk.edu
Richard Murphy, Pres.

**Activities/Fields:** Cellular and molecular biology and neuroscience with particular emphasis on immunology, cancer, molecular genetics, tumor virology, reproductive biology, neurobiology, neuroendocrinology, growth control, prebiotic chemistry, and neurotransmitter/neuroreceptor structure and function; research aimed toward the discovery of cause, prevention, control, and cure of disease. **Pub:** *Newsletters.* • *Research Reports.*


**★ 4684 ★ San Francisco State University Center for Biomedical Laboratory Science**
1600 Holloway Ave.
San Francisco, CA 94132
**Phone:** (415)338-1696     **Fax:** (415)338-7747
**Email:** wbigler@sfsu.edu

**Website:** http://www.sfsu.edu/~cbls
Dr. William N. Bigler, Dir.

**Activities/Fields:** Clinical chemistry, immunology, microbiology, hematology, and virology. **Frmly:** Center for Advanced Medical Technology.


**★ 4685 ★ Scripps Research Institute Multiscale Modeling Tools for Structural Biology**
10550 N Torrey Pines Rd.
La Jolla, CA 92037
**Phone:** (858)784-8035     **Fax:** (858)784-8688
**Email:** brooks@scripps.edu
**Website:** http://mmtsb.scripps.edu
Dr. Charles L. Brooks, III, Prin. Investigator

**Activities/Fields:** Structural biology, focusing on the development of new and integrated approaches to multiscale modeling, especially large-scale assemblies of nucleic acids and proteins with nucleic acids; development of methods that combine lattice-based dynamic Monte Carlo and all atom molecular dynamics; the study of physical processes involved in and the development of models for the interactions associated with virus assembly; establishment of new tools for the combined treatment of crystallographic and low-resolution structural models from cryo-electron microscopy.


**★ 4686 ★ Sherbrooke University Centre for Study and Valorization of Microbial Diversity**
Departement de Biologie
Faculte des Sciences
2500, boul. de l'Universite
Sherbrooke, QC, Canada J1K 2R1
**Phone:** (819)821-8000     **Fax:** (819)821-8049
**Email:** rbrzezin@courrier.usherb.ca
**Website:** http://www.usherb.ca/SCES/BIO/microbio.html
Ryszard Brzezinski, PhD, Contact

**Activities/Fields:** Molecular biology and genetic engineering of actinomycetes, gene cloning and characterization, development of new cloning vectors. Studies on pathogenesis mechanisms of potato scab. Development of biocontrol agents against plant disease. Development of streptomyces strains for biotechnological product ion of enzymes (xylanase; glucanases, chitosanase). **Frmly:** Actinomycete Biology Research Group.


**★ 4687 ★ Sherbrooke University Fundamental Electrophysiology Research Group**
Departement de Physiologie et de Biophysique
Faculte de Medecine
3001 12th N
Sherbrooke, QC, Canada J1H 5N4
**Phone:** (819)564-5302     **Fax:** (819)564-5399
**Email:** dgirardi@courrier.usherb.ca
Marcel Daniel-Payet, Dir.

**Activities/Fields:** Excitation contraction coupling, involvement of ionic channels in the stimulus-secretion process, control of body fluid volumes, maturation of prenatal control of ventilation, function and regulation of ionic channels of sarcoplasmic reticulum in skeletal and cardiac muscles, physiopathology of cardiac electrical alterations, electrophysiological basis of normal and pathological automaticity, and ionic channels in airway smooth muscle.


**★ 4688 ★ Sierra Biomedical Research Corp.**
1000 Locust St.
Reno, NV 89502-2597
**Phone:** (775)328-1487     **Fax:** (775)328-1816
**Activities/Fields:** Biomedical and clinical research.


**★ 4689 ★ Southwest Foundation for Biomedical Research**
PO Box 760549
San Antonio, TX 78245-0549
**Phone:** (210)258-9400     **Fax:** (210)670-3301
**Email:** fledford@icarus.sfbr.org
**Website:** http://www.sfbr.org
Dr. Frank F. Ledford, Jr., Pres.

**Activities/Fields:** Arteriosclerosis, hypertension, cancer, pulmonary disease, aging, genetics, endocrinology, reproductive physiology, virology, neuropharmacology, behavioral science, and organic chemistry. **Pub:** *Annual Report.* • *Progress in Medical Research,* quarterly.


**Stanford University Beckman Center for Molecular and Genetic Medicine**
*See:* Entry 9430


**★ 4690 ★ Tampa Bay Research Institute**
10900 Roosevelt Blvd.
Saint Petersburg, FL 33716
**Phone:** (727)576-6675     **Fax:** (727)577-9862
**Email:** tbriat@aol.com
Dr. Akiko Tanaka, Pres.

**Activities/Fields:** Molecular genetics, virology, Hepatitis C, cellular biochemistry, AIDS, gene therapy, cytokines, and cancer. **Pub:** *Newsletter,* quarterly. **Frmly:** Showa University Research Institute.


**★ 4691 ★ Texas A&M University Institute of Biosciences and Technology**
2121 W Holcombe Blvd.
Houston, TX 77030-3303
**Phone:** (713)677-7777     **Fax:** (713)677-7725
**Email:** fbazer@cvm.tamu.edu
**Website:** http://www.tamu.edu/ibt/ibt.htm
Fuller W. Bazer, PhD, Dir.

**Activities/Fields:** Genome research, mammalian DNA and RNA viruses, eucaryotic gene expression, neurobiology, human nutrition, matrix biology, plant molecular biology, and cancer biology.


**★ 4692 ★ Thomas Jefferson University Daniel Baugh Institute**
Jefferson Alumni Hall
1020 Locust St.
Philadelphia, PA 19107
**Phone:** (215)503-7820     **Fax:** (215)923-3808
**Email:** james.schwaber@mail.tju.edu
Dr. James Schwaber, Dir.

**Activities/Fields:** Developmental biology; reproductive toxicology; biochemical, molecular and genetic mechanisms of birth defects; tissue and embryo culture, molecular biology, and cell biology.


**★ 4693 ★ Thomas Jefferson University Jefferson Institute of Molecular Medicine**
450 BLSB
233 S 10th St.
Philadelphia, PA 19107
**Phone:** (215)503-5785     **Fax:** (215)503-5788
**Email:** jouni.uitto@mail.tju.edu
Dr. Jouni Uitto, Dir.

**Activities/Fields:** Biochemistry and molecular medicine.


**U.S. Department of Defense Army Medical Research and Materiel Command Walter Reed Army Institute of Research Biochemistry Division**
*See:* Entry 13479

**U.S. Department of Defense**
**Army Medical Research and Materiel Command**
**Walter Reed Army Institute of Research**
**Department of Applied Biochemistry**
*See:* Entry 13481

---

**★ 4694 ★ U.S. Department of Health and Human Services**
**Food and Drug Administration**
**Center for Bilogics Evaluation and Research**
**Division of Bacterial Products**
1401 Rockville Pike (HFM-422)
Bethesda, MD 20892
**Phone:** (301)496-1014     **Fax:** (301)402-2776
**Website:** http://wrair-www.army.mil/divisions.htm
Dr. Richard Walker, MD, Dir.

**Activities/Fields:** Pathogenesis and prevention of medically important diseases due to bacteria and rickettsia. Emphasizes control of vaccines and immunotherapeutics. Conducts studies through the following laboratories: Mycobacteria, Pertussis, Enterics & Sexually Transmitted Diseases, Bacterial Polysaccharides, and Bacterial Toxins. **Pub:** *Annual Report.*

---

**★ 4695 ★ U.S. Department of Health and Human Services**
**Food and Drug Administration**
**Center for Bilogics Evaluation and Research**
**Division of Cellular and Gene Therapies**
1401 Rockville Pike, HFM-515
Rockville, MD 20852
**Phone:** (301)827-0680     **Fax:** (301)827-0449
**Website:** http://research.cber.fda.gov/dcgt.html
Philip D. Noguchi, MD, Actg. Dir.

**Activities/Fields:** Cell and developmental biology, immunology, and tumor biology.

---

**★ 4696 ★ U.S. Department of Health and Human Services**
**Food and Drug Administration**
**Center for Bilogics Evaluation and Research**
**Laboratory Cellular Immunology**
**(Division of Cellular and Gene Therapies)**
1401 Rockville Pike
Rockville, MD 20852-1448
**Phone:** (301)827-0452     **Fax:** (301)827-0449
Eda Bloom, PhD, Lab. Chf.

**Activities/Fields:** Regulation of lymphocyte activation and maturation at cellular and molecular levels, with emphasis on cytotoxic lymphocytes; roles of cytokines and cytokine-producing cells (lymphocytes and macrophages) in lymphocyte activation using models in vitro and invivo. **Pub:** *Proceedings. • Research Reports.*

---

**★ 4697 ★ U.S. Department of Health and Human Services**
**Food and Drug Administration**
**Center for Bilogics Evaluation and Research**
**Laboratory of Hemostasis**
1401 Rockville Pike
Rockville, MD 20852
**Phone:** (301)496-4833     **Fax:** (301)402-2780
**Email:** weinstein@cber.fda.gov
Mark Weinstein, PhD, Actg. Chf.

**Activities/Fields:** Characterization of proteins involved in hemostasis and thrombosis. Biochemical research includes receptor and binding studies, and analysis of protein structure and function. Principal research efforts include studies on factor VIII and von Willebrand factor.

---

**★ 4698 ★ U.S. Department of Health and Human Services**
**Food and Drug Administration**
**Center for Biologics Evaluation and Research**
1401 Rockville Pike
Rockville, MD 20852
**Phone:** (301)827-0370     **Fax:** (301)827-0440
**Website:** http://www.fda.gov/cber
Kathryn C. Zoon, Dir.

**Activities/Fields:** Ensures the safety, efficacy, potency, and purity of biological products intended for use in the treatment, prevention, or cure of human diseases. Reviews the safety and effectiveness of vaccines, blood products, diagnostic products, and other biological and biotechnology-derived human products. Supports active applied research programs and provides regulatory review of biological products. Investigates viral and bacterial vaccines, immunology, developmental biology, parasitic diseases, cytokines, growth factors, and AIDS and related diseases.

---

**★ 4699 ★ U.S. Department of Health and Human Services**
**Food and Drug Administration**
**Center for Biologics Evaluation and Research**
**Bone Marrow Growth Factors Staff**
9000 Rockville Pike
Bldg. 37, Rm. 5C25
Bethesda, MD 20892
**Phone:** (301)496-6968     **Fax:** (301)480-3256
Dov H. Pluznik, PhD, Actg. Chf.

**Activities/Fields:** Cellular and molecular mechanisms involved in the production of hematopoietic growth factors and the differentiation of hematopoietic cells.

---

**★ 4700 ★ U.S. Department of Health and Human Services**
**Food and Drug Administration**
**Center for Biologics Evaluation and Research**
**Division of Allergenic Products and Parasitology**
1401 Rockville Pike
CBER HFM-410
Rockville, MD 20852
**Phone:** (301)496-2893     **Fax:** (301)496-4684
**Email:** tebull@gandalf.cber.nih.gov
Dr. Thomas Bull, Research Chemist

**Activities/Fields:** Biophysics, NMR, and molecular dynamics simulations. **Pub:** *Annual report.* **Frmly:** (1993) Division of Biochemistry and Biophysics.

---

**★ 4701 ★ U.S. Department of Health and Human Services**
**Food and Drug Administration**
**Center for Biologics Evaluation and Research**
**Division of Cytokine Biology**
1401 Rockville Pike
Rockville, MD 20852
**Phone:** (301)827-1735     **Fax:** (301)402-1659
Dr. David Finbloom, Dir.

**Activities/Fields:** Cytokine and growth factor products. Studies interferons, interleukins, colony stimulating factors; and growth factors. Emphasizes immunology, molecular biology, protein chemistry, and AIDS. Activities are carried out through the following Laboratories: Cell Biology, Chemical Biology, and Cytokine Research. **Pub:** *Annual Report. • Proceedings. • Reports.*

---

**★ 4702 ★ U.S. Department of Health and Human Services**
**Food and Drug Administration**
**Center for Biologics Evaluation and Research**
**Division of Hematology**
**(Laboratory of Plasma Derivatives)**
1401 Rockville Pike
Rockville, MD 20852
**Phone:** (301)402-4634     **Fax:** (301)402-2780
Donald L. Tankersley, Chf.

**Activities/Fields:** Plasma volume expanders, immunoglobulins, and hepatitis B. Investigates thermally-induced albumin denaturation and thermal stabilization of albumin by saturated fatty acid anions; studies IgG dimer by electron microscopy and affinity chromatography; and conducts experiments to determine if the neutralization of hepatitis B virus infectivity could be achieved by formation of immune complexes with anti-HBs, which include antisera produced against a synthetic peptide of S region of the hepatitis B surface and antigen.

---

**★ 4703 ★ U.S. Department of Health and Human Services**
**Food and Drug Administration**
**Center for Biologics Evaluation and Research**
**Division of Hematology**
1401 Rockville Pike
Rockville, MD 20852
**Phone:** (301)496-4396     **Fax:** (301)402-2780
**Email:** weinstein@cber.fda.gov
Mark J. Weinstein, PhD, Dir.

**Activities/Fields:** Responsible for the safety, potency, purity, and efficacy of blood/plasma-derived/r-DNA biotechnology-derived therapeutic products. These include agents used in the management of clotting and bleeding disorders, immune deficiencies, hematologic malignancies, hypovolemia, anemia and related pathophysiologic states, and transplantation and autoimmune diseases. **Pub:** *Annual Report.*

---

**★ 4704 ★ U.S. Department of Health and Human Services**
**Food and Drug Administration**
**Center for Biologics Evaluation and Research**
**Division of Monoclonal Antibodies**
1401 Rockville Pike
HFM-555, NIH Bldg. 29B, Rm. 3NN-16
Rockville, MD 20852
**Phone:** (301)827-0850     **Fax:** (301)827-0852
**Email:** stein@cber.fda.gov
**Website:** http://www.fda.gov/cber
Kathryn E. Stein, PhD, Dir.

**Activities/Fields:** Monoclonal antibody structure and function; the regulation of antibody synthesis; the functions of radionuclide and toxin coupled monoclonal antibody therapeutics; and basic mechanisms involving the biology and physiology of cells involved in the immune system.

---

**★ 4705 ★ U.S. Department of Health and Human Services**
**Food and Drug Administration**
**Center for Biologics Evaluation and Research**
**Laboratory of Biophysics**
1401 Rockville Pike
Rockville, MD 20852-1448
**Phone:** (301)435-2035     **Fax:** (301)496-4684
**Email:** pastor@cber.fda.gov
Richard W. Pastor, PhD, Chf.

**Activities/Fields:** Development and application of high resolution NMR methods and light scattering for structural studies of biomacromolecules; development and application of computer modelling methods for studies of biomacromolecules; and characterization and development of adjuvants.

**★ 4706 ★ U.S. Department of Health and Human Services**
**Food and Drug Administration**
**Center for Biologics Evaluation and Research**
**Laboratory of Cell Biology-Cytokine**
1401 Rockville Pike
Rockville, MD 20852
**Phone:** (301)827-1735 **Fax:** (301)402-1659
David S. Finbloom, MD, Actg. Chf.

**Activities/Fields:** Characterization of new cytokines and growth factors, structure, functional relationship, and role in human growth. **Pub:** *Proceedings.* • *Research Reports.*

**★ 4707 ★ U.S. Department of Health and Human Services**
**Food and Drug Administration**
**Center for Biologics Evaluation and Research**
**Laboratory of Cell Viral Regulations**
FDA-CBER, HFM-541
Bldg. 29-A
Bethesda, MD 20892
**Phone:** (301)827-1806 **Fax:** (301)480-3256
**Email:** max@cber.fda.gov
Dr. Edward E. Max, Chf.

**Activities/Fields:** Regulation of immunoglobulin gene expression by cytokines and cell interactions focusing on the function of several immunoglobulin gene enhancers and the regulation of immunoglobulin isotype switching at the DNA level. Also focuses on the interaction of HIV with cells of the immune system centering on: the structural correlates of targets of neutralizing antibodies; and the activation of T cells by HIV through the T cell receptor and the surface molecules (other than CD4) that mediate viral entry into cells. **Frmly:** (2000) Laboratory of Cell Viral Regulation.

**★ 4708 ★ U.S. Department of Health and Human Services**
**Food and Drug Administration**
**Center for Biologics Evaluation and Research**
**Laboratory of Cellular Hematology**
1401 Rockville Pike, HFM-335
Rockville, MD 20852
**Phone:** (301)496-2577 **Fax:** (301)402-2780
**Email:** vostal@cber.fda.gov
Jaro Vostal, PhD, Acting Chief

**Activities/Fields:** Leukocytes, platelets, and signal transduction. Operates a hemoglobin and blood substitutes program. Principal area of research interest is blood cell physiology and platelet biochemistry, as related to transfusion. **Pub:** *Proceedings.* • *Reports.*

**★ 4709 ★ U.S. Department of Health and Human Services**
**Food and Drug Administration**
**Center for Biologics Evaluation and Research**
**Laboratory of Chemical Biology**
8800 Rockville Pike
Bethesda, MD 20892
**Phone:** (301)827-1777 **Fax:** (301)480-3256
Dr. Blair A. Fraser, Chf.

**Activities/Fields:** Biologically active peptides and proteins. Principal research efforts include isolation and structural analysis of novel neuropeptides, identification and isolation of precursor peptides, and identification of metabolic events responsible for post-translational protein processing. Conducts programs in regulation of membrane proteins and molecular pharmacology of signal transduction, developmental biology, and synthesis and use of modified oligodeoxyribonucleotides. Also develops methodologies and strategies for the microsequencing of proteins and the use of synthetic peptides.

**★ 4710 ★ U.S. Department of Health and Human Services**
**Food and Drug Administration**
**Center for Biologics Evaluation and Research**
**Laboratory of Cytokine Research**
29 Lincoln Dr.
Bethesda, MD 20892
**Phone:** (301)827-1720 **Fax:** (301)402-1659
David S. Finbloom, MD, Dir.

**Activities/Fields:** Structure and function of interferons and their receptors; identification and characterization of cytokines that modulate the function of monocytes and macrophages; mechanisms of interferon beta regulated gene expression; antitumor activities of cytokine or anticytokine receptor antibody toxin fusion proteins; and AIDS studies. **Pub:** *Proceedings.* • *Research Reports.*

**★ 4711 ★ U.S. Department of Health and Human Services**
**Food and Drug Administration**
**Center for Biologics Evaluation and Research**
**Laboratory of Developement Biology**
1401 Rockville Pike, HFM-515
Rockville, MD 20852-1448
**Phone:** (301)827-0462 **Fax:** (301)827-0449
Suzanne Epstein, MD, Chf.

**Activities/Fields:** Biology and developmental control of gene expression. Principal research efforts involve: identification of genetic elements that control the temporal and spatial expression of genes in *Drosophila*; elucidation of the role of homeobox genes in limb and organ development; and characterization of bone morphogenetic factors. **Pub:** *Proceedings.* • *Reports.* **Frmly:** Laboratory of Cellular and Molecular Biology.

**★ 4712 ★ U.S. Department of Health and Human Services**
**Food and Drug Administration**
**Center for Biologics Evaluation and Research**
**Laboratory of DNA Virus Research**
1401 Rockville Pike
Rockville, MD 20852
**Phone:** (301)827-0650 **Fax:** (301)496-1810
Dr. Andrew Lewis, Contact

**Activities/Fields:** Molecular biology of DNA viruses with emphasis on human herpesviruses and poxviruses. Focuses on gene expression, virus vectors, viral latency, viral replication, and immune responses. Conducts a program on the regulation of gene expression. **Pub:** *Proceedings.* • *Research Reports.*

**★ 4713 ★ U.S. Department of Health and Human Services**
**Food and Drug Administration**
**Center for Biologics Evaluation and Research**
**Laboratory of Hepatitis Viruses**
8800 Rockville Pike
Bethesda, MD 20892
**Phone:** (301)827-1880 **Fax:** (301)402-5585
**Email:** LABHR@HELIX.NIH.GOV
Dr. Stephen M. Feinstone, MD, Chf.

**Activities/Fields:** Molecular biology of the hepatitis A virus, emphasizing viral pathogenesis, replication, and antigenic structure. Supports a project on novel methods of producing hepatitis A vaccines. Operates a program focusing on non-A and non-B hepatitis, which includes hepatitis C virus and other yet to be identified hepatitis viruses.

**★ 4714 ★ U.S. Department of Health and Human Services**
**Food and Drug Administration**
**Center for Biologics Evaluation and Research**
**Laboratory of Immuno-Chemistry**
5510 Nicholson Ln.
Kensington, MD 20895
**Phone:** (301)594-6733
Walter Kuff, Contact

**Activities/Fields:** Chemical research involving the identification, structural elucidation, and quantitation of chemical constituents and impurities of vaccines and other biological products regulated by the Center. Laboratory is responsible for regulatory review of chemical aspects of biological products and for the testing of biological products to determine quantitatively the amounts of various preservatives, metals, stabilizers, adjuvants, chemical inactivators, nitrogen, and residual moisture present. Principal areas of research include inorganic and organic analysis; inductively coupled plasma emission and atomic absorption spectrometric aluminum analysis; residual moisture of freeze-dried biological products; and high-performance liquid chromatography of vaccine constituents. **Frmly:** Laboratory of Analytical Chemistry.

**★ 4715 ★ U.S. Department of Health and Human Services**
**Food and Drug Administration**
**Center for Biologics Evaluation and Research**
**Laboratory of Immunobiochemistry**
8800 Rockville Pike
Bethesda, MD 20892
**Phone:** (301)496-4357
Yuan L. Devries, PhD, Actg. Chf.

**Activities/Fields:** Characterization of allergenic extracts and the evaluation of the diagnostic and therapeutic safety and efficacy of allergenic extracts. Research program includes biochemical, biophysical, immunological, and molecular biology approaches to the characterization and human immune response to various allergens. Develops new methodologies, including using monoclonal antibodies and PCR techniques for the purification and characterization of allergens and HPLC or capillary electrophoresis. Evaluates the accuracy, precision, and sensitivity of allergen skin test procedures and defines potency of allergen extracts. **Frmly:** Laboratory of Allergy and Immunochemistry.

**★ 4716 ★ U.S. Department of Health and Human Services**
**Food and Drug Administration**
**Center for Biologics Evaluation and Research**
**Laboratory of Immunoregulation**
8800 Rockville Pike
Bethesda, MD 20892
**Phone:** (301)496-1870 **Fax:** (301)496-1810
**Email:** berkower@cber.fda.gov
Ira J. Berkower, MD,PhD, Chf.

**Activities/Fields:** Safety, efficacy, and potency of vaccines for human use including fundamental research into the immunogenicity of viral protein antigens. This includes antigen processing and presentation to antigen specific T cells; the mapping of a conserved neutralizing site that is shared across a broad spectrum of HIV-1 isolates, so antibodies to this site can neutralize diverse isolates; and novel vaccine constructs that assemble into particles for increased vaccine potency, while preserving the site in its native conformation.

## ★ 4717 ★ U.S. Department of Health and Human Services
**Food and Drug Administration**
**Center for Biologics Evaluation and Research**
**Laboratory of Molecular and Developemental Immunology**
29 Lincoln Dr.
NIH Bldg. 29-B
Bethesda, MD 20892-4555
**Phone:** (301)827-0717          **Fax:** (301)827-0852

**Activities/Fields:** Delineating the differences in the immune response to thymus-independent and thymus-dependent forms of polysaccharide antigens and the mechanism of signal transduction by thymus-independent antigens. Projects include: molecular analysis of monoclonal antibodies examining the roles of genetics and of the form of the antigen used for immunization. These studies have shown major differences in two sets of antibodies raised against bacterial levan in two different mouse strains in terms of fine specificity and immunoglobulin gene usage. Studies of two different forms of the meningococcal group C polysaccharide, the polysaccharide itself, and a polysaccharide-protein conjugate were used to examine the molecular consequences of altering the form of the vaccine on the subsequent antibody response. These studies have demonstrated that the polysaccharide-protein conjugate vaccine results in the development of antibodies with new specificities and of higher avidity than the polysaccharide, itself; employing a mutant strain of mice (*xid*) which is unresponsive to polysaccharide antigens to examine the role of a subpopulation of B lymphocytes, lacking in this strain, to examine the cellular requirements for mounting an immune response to polysaccharides; developing monoclonal antibodies to B lymphocytes; and examining signal transduction in B lymphocytes via polyclonal cross-linking of the Ig receptor. The last three studies will use subpopulations of B cells from normal mice as well as mice with the *xid* defect. Other studies involve the role of various adhesion molecular in the activation/waive CD8T cells.

## ★ 4718 ★ U.S. Department of Health and Human Services
**Food and Drug Administration**
**Center for Biologics Evaluation and Research**
**Laboratory of Molecular Immunology**
1401 Rockville Pike
Rockville, MD 20852-1448
**Phone:** (301)827-0450          **Fax:** (301)827-0449
Suzanne Epstein, PhD, Chf.

**Activities/Fields:** T- and B-cell immunity. Principal research efforts include: immune responses to viruses; T-cell and B-cell response to vaccine antigens; and B cell development and neoplasia. **Pub:** *Proceedings. • Research Reports.*

## ★ 4719 ★ U.S. Department of Health and Human Services
**Food and Drug Administration**
**Center for Biologics Evaluation and Research**
**Laboratory of Mycobacteria**
Bldg. 29, Rm. 502
29 Lincoln Dr.
Bethesda, MD 20892
**Phone:** (301)496-9559          **Fax:** (301)435-5675
**Email:** brennan@cber.fda.gov
Dr. Michael J. Brennan, PhD, Chf.

**Activities/Fields:** Development of novel vaccines for tuberculosis including research on DNA vaccines, immunopathogenesis of intracellular pathogens and bacterial adherene mechanisms. Areas of interest include molecular microbiology, immunology and bacterial pathogenesis. Regulatory duties include review of bacterial biologics including BCG vaccines and therapeutics, and skin test reagents.

## ★ 4720 ★ U.S. Department of Health and Human Services
**Food and Drug Administration**
**Center for Biologics Evaluation and Research**
**Laboratory of Pertussis**
8800 Rockville Pike
Bethesda, MD 20892
**Phone:** (301)402-3553          **Fax:** (301)402-2776
Drusilla Burns, PhD, Chf.

**Activities/Fields:** Regulation of bacterial vaccines (particularly pertussis vaccine). Initiates, directs, and participates in research on the immunochemistry of *Bordetella pertussis* and host parasite interactions in pertussis prerequisite to the development of improved pertussis vaccines and their control and clinical use. Activities involve biochemical, immunochemical, clinical, control testing, animal model, genetic, and serological studies. Serves as the World Health Organization Collaborating Center for Research on Pertussis Vaccines. Current research programs focus on the mechanisms by which *Bordetella pertussis* attaches to and infects susceptible tissues and the cellular components responsible for local and systemic symptoms of whooping cough. Continuing research studies involve isolation and characterization of virulence factors and development of in vitro and animal laboratory models to study diseases and evaluate potential immunogens. **Pub:** *Proceedings. • Research Reports.*

## ★ 4721 ★ U.S. Department of Health and Human Services
**Food and Drug Administration**
**Center for Biologics Evaluation and Research**
**Laboratory of Respiratory Viruses**
8800 Rockville Pike
Bethesda, MD 20892
**Free:** 888-463-6332
Roland A. Levandowski, MD, Actg. Chf.

**Activities/Fields:** Human respiratory viral diseases, including influenza viruses, respiratory syncytial viruses, parainfluenza viruses, and rhinoviruses. Techniques employed are intended to permit understanding of the biology of the individual agents through genomic evaluation as well as the biology of the individual agents through in vivo and in vitro studies of cellular and humoral immune parameters.

## ★ 4722 ★ U.S. Department of Health and Human Services
**Food and Drug Administration**
**Center for Biologics Evaluation and Research**
**Molecular Medical Genetics Staff**
1401 Rockville Pike
Rockville, MD 20852
**Phone:** (301)443-1544          **Fax:** (301)496-7027
Gerald Marti, Actg. Chf.

**Activities/Fields:** Molecular medical genetics.

## ★ 4723 ★ U.S. Department of Health and Human Services
**Food and Drug Administration**
**Center for Biologics Evaluation and Research**
**Molecular Tumor Biology Staff**
1401 Rockville Pike
Rockville, MD 20852
**Phone:** (301)827-0471          **Fax:** (301)827-0449
**Email:** puri@cber.fda.gov
Raj Puri, MD,PhD, Chf.

**Activities/Fields:** Biology of receptors on human tumor cells; mechanisms of lentivirus infection and expression; MRNA editing. **Pub:** *Documents. • Points to Consider.*

## ★ 4724 ★ U.S. Department of Health and Human Services
**Food and Drug Administration**
**Center for Biologics Evaluation and Research**
**Office of Therapeutics Research and Review**
1401 Rockville Pike
HFM-500
Rockville, MD 20851
**Phone:** (301)827-5098          **Fax:** (301)827-5395
**Email:** siegel@cber.fda.gov
**Website:** http://www.fda.gov/cber/therapies.htm
J. Siegel, Dir.

**Activities/Fields:** Development, manufacture, testing, and activities of therapeutic biological products including those related to AIDS and those prepared by genetic engineering and synthetic procedures. This is done in order to develop and maintain a scientific base for establishing standards designed to ensure the continued safety, purity, potency, and effectiveness of biological therapeutics products.

## ★ 4725 ★ U.S. Department of Health and Human Services
**Food and Drug Administration**
**Center for Biologics Evauluation and Research**
**Laboratory of Enteric and Sexually Transmitted Diseases**
8800 Rockville Pike
Bethesda, MD 20892
**Phone:** (301)496-1893          **Fax:** (301)402-2776
**Email:** kopecko@cber.fda.gov
**Website:** http://www.cber.fda.gov
Dennis Kopecko, PhD, Chf.

**Activities/Fields:** Genetic and molecular bases of enteric bacterial disease pathogenesis and the host's immune response to infection. Biochemical, immunological, molecular genetic and cell biology methods (including recombinant DNA, in vitro cell cultures, electron and fluorescent microscopy, video/confocal imaging, and molecular immunological technologies) and animal model systems that are employed to analyze the determinants of bacterial virulence, gene expression control mechanisms, and their functional nature in pathogenesis. Current molecular events being analyzed in detail include the prokaryotic and eukaryotic mechanisms involved in: bacterial invasion of mucosal epithelial cells, bacterial intracellular survival, cellular and molecular bases of specific protective immunity to infection, and global regulatory mechanisms involved in controlling virulence gene expression. **Pub:** *Proceedings. • Research Reports.*

**U.S. Department of Health and Human Services**
**National Cancer Institute**
**Laboratory of Biochemistry**
*See:* Entry 10476

**U.S. Department of Health and Human Services**
**National Cancer Institute**
**Laboratory of Biological Chemistry**
*See:* Entry 10477

**U.S. Department of Health and Human Services**
**National Cancer Institute**
**Laboratory of Cellular Carcinogenesis and Tumor Promotion**
*See:* Entry 10479

U.S. Department of Health and Human Services
National Cancer Institute
Laboratory of Experimental Carcinogenesis
*See:* Entry 10482

U.S. Department of Health and Human Services
National Cancer Institute
Laboratory of Human Carcinogenesis
*See:* Entry 10486

U.S. Department of Health and Human Services
National Cancer Institute
Laboratory of Mathematical Biology
*See:* Entry 10488

U.S. Department of Health and Human Services
National Cancer Institute
Laboratory of Medicinal Chemistry
*See:* Entry 10489

U.S. Department of Health and Human Services
National Cancer Institute
Laboratory of Molecular Biology
*See:* Entry 10490

U.S. Department of Health and Human Services
National Cancer Institute
Laboratory of Molecular Carcinogenesis
*See:* Entry 10491

U.S. Department of Health and Human Services
National Cancer Institute
Laboratory of Molecular Virology
*See:* Entry 10494

U.S. Department of Health and Human Services
National Cancer Institute
Laboratory of Tumor Cell Biology
*See:* Entry 10496

U.S. Department of Health and Human Services
National Cancer Institute
Laboratory of Tumor Immunology and Biology
Laboratory of Tumor Immunology and Biology
*See:* Entry 10497

U.S. Department of Health and Human Services
National Cancer Institute
Laboratory of Viral Carcinogenesis
*See:* Entry 10498

U.S. Department of Health and Human Services
National Eye Institute
Laboratory of Molecular and Developmental Biology
*See:* Entry 21154

U.S. Department of Health and Human Services
National Eye Institute
Laboratory of Retinal Cell and Molecular Biology
*See:* Entry 21155

U.S. Department of Health and Human Services
National Heart, Lung, and Blood Institute
Division of Intramural Research
Molecular Disease Branch
*See:* Entry 5159

U.S. Department of Health and Human Services
National Heart, Lung, and Blood Institute
Laboratory of Biochemical Genetics
*See:* Entry 5160

U.S. Department of Health and Human Services
National Heart, Lung, and Blood Institute
Laboratory of Biophysical Chemistry
*See:* Entry 5161

U.S. Department of Health and Human Services
National Heart, Lung, and Blood Institute (NHLBI)
Laboratory of Cell Biology (LCB)
*See:* Entry 5163

U.S. Department of Health and Human Services
National Heart, Lung, and Blood Institute
Laboratory of Cell Signaling
*See:* Entry 5164

U.S. Department of Health and Human Services
National Heart, Lung, and Blood Institute
Laboratory of Molecular Cardiology
*See:* Entry 5165

U.S. Department of Health and Human Services
National Institute on Aging
Biology of Aging Program
*See:* Entry 3072

U.S. Department of Health and Human Services
National Institute on Aging
Laboratory of Cellular and Molecular Biology
*See:* Entry 3080

U.S. Department of Health and Human Services
National Institute on Aging
Laboratory of Molecular Genetics
*See:* Entry 3082

U.S. Department of Health and Human Services
National Institute of Arthritis and Musculoskeletal and Skin Diseases
Intramural Research Program
Laboratory of Skin Biology
*See:* Entry 13716

**★ 4726 ★ U.S. Department of Health and Human Services**
**National Institute of Dental Research**
**Laboratory of Developmental Biology**
NIH Bldg. 30, Rm. 421
30 Convent Dr., MSC 4370
Bethesda, MD 20892-4370
**Phone:** (301)496-5974          **Fax:** (301)402-0897
**Email:** kenneth.yamada@nih.gov
**Website:** http://wwwdir.nidcr.nih.gov/dirweb/cdbrb/cdbrb.htm
Kenneth M. Yamada, Branch Chf.

**Activities/Fields:** Structure, function, and regulation of extracellular matrix molecules, their receptors, and other cell interaction systems. Research focuses on examining the functions and regulation of these systems in normal and abnormal development of craniofacial and other tissues; connective tissue remodeling; tumor metastasis and invasion; and other diseases and disorders involving extracellular molecules. Information on cell-matrix interaction mechanisms is applied to the development of biological and biochemical reagents for the understanding and therapy of oral and other diseases. **Frmly:** Developmental Biology and Anomalies Laboratory; (1997) Laboratory of Developmental Biology; (2000) National Institute of Dental Research; Craniofacial Developmental Biology and Regulation Branch.

U.S. Department of Health and Human Services
National Institute of Diabetes and Digestive and Kidney Diseases
Division of Intramural Research
Genetics and Biochemistry Branch
*See:* Entry 9442

**★ 4727 ★ U.S. Department of Health and Human Services**
**National Institute of Diabetes and Digestive and Kidney Diseases**
**Laboratory of Analytical Chemistry**
NIH Bldg. 8, Rm. B2A-17
9000 Rockville Pike
Bethesda, MD 20892
**Fax:** (301)402-1967
Edwin Becker, Actg. Chf.

**Activities/Fields:** Provides consultation and technical assistance to Institute scientists in the area of instrumental and chemical analysis, particularly related to experimental design and interpretation of spectra.

**★ 4728 ★ U.S. Department of Health and Human Services**
**National Institute of Diabetes and Digestive and Kidney Diseases**
**Laboratory of Bioorganic Chemistry**
NIH Bldg. 8A, Rm. B1A02
8 Center Dr. MSC 0810
Bethesda, MD 20892-0810
**Phone:** (301)496-2619          **Fax:** (301)402-0008
**Website:** http://www.niddk.nih.gov/intram/branchlb/lbc.htm
Kenneth L. Kirk, Chf.

**Activities/Fields:** Mission is to elucidate the mechanism of interaction of pharmacologically active substances with biological systems. Research is designed to develop new chemical agents as tools for the study of membrane and cytosol functions of cells. New mechanisms of action or metabolism of such agents are also investigated for their potential use as therapeutics. Emphasis is on development and application of modern techniques of organic chemistry for the synthesis, separation, and spectral investigation of these chemical agents and their interactions with macromolecules. The goal is to provide insights into the normal and pathologic function of biological systems and to delineate the metabolic formation, fate, and action of physiologically active agents such as amino acids, biogenic amines, cyclic nucleotides, hormones, neurotransmitters, and steroids. Studies include pharmacologically active agents such as natural products, central stimulants, depressants, tranquilizers, anxiolytics, and other therapeutic agents, toxins, carcinogens, and mutagens.


**★ 4729 ★ U.S. Department of Health and Human Services**
**National Institute of Diabetes and Digestive and Kidney Diseases**
**Laboratory of Cellular and Developmental Biology**
Bldg. 50 Room 3134
9000 Rockville Pike MSC 8028
Bethesda, MD 20892-8028
**Phone:** (301)496-6125 **Fax:** (301)496-5239
**Email:** jurrien@helix.nih.gov
Dr. Jurrien Dean, MD, Chf.

**Activities/Fields:** Endocrinology, including research on hormonal regulation of enzymes involved in chylomicron uptake and metabolism in adipose and mammary tissues, the influence of hormones on cellular development and metabolism, and the disposition of fat and metabolites in the cell as viewed from ultrastructural studies; nutritional biochemistry, including studies on the structural and functional aspects of dihydrofolic reductase and other enzymes involved in folic acid metabolism and the intermediary metabolism of lipids, carbohydrates, and amino acids in the small intestine; membrane regulation, including studies on the mechanism of action of hormones on adenylate cyclase and other membrane regulatory processes; and developmental biochemistry, including studies on the structure and function of chromatin and the regulation of gene function during development.


**★ 4730 ★ U.S. Department of Health and Human Services**
**National Institute of Diabetes and Digestive and Kidney Diseases**
**Laboratory of Chemical Biology**
NIH Bldg. 10, Rm. 9N307
10 Center Dr. MSC-1822
Bethesda, MD 20892-1822
**Phone:** (301)496-5408 **Fax:** (301)402-0101
**Email:** aschecht@helix.nih.gov
Dr. Alan N. Schechter, Chf.

**Activities/Fields:** Chemical biology, including protein chemistry; and molecular genetics, including sickle cell anemia and thassemia. Research focuses on the control of gene expression, folding of proteins, and therapy of genetic diseases.


**★ 4731 ★ U.S. Department of Health and Human Services**
**National Institute of Diabetes and Digestive and Kidney Diseases**
**Laboratory of Chemical Physics**
NIH Bldg. 5
15 Center Dr. MSC-0520
Bethesda, MD 20892-0520
**Phone:** (301)496-1024 **Fax:** (301)435-2413
William A. Eaton, Chf.

**Activities/Fields:** Application of modern physical techniques to the study of a wide range of biological problems. Much of the research involves the use of a variety of spectroscopic methods (e.g., nuclear and electron magnetic resonance, laser-Raman and resonance Raman spectroscopy), electric-field-induced dichroism, ultraviolet and visible microspectrophotometry, and time-resolved absorption spectroscopy with nanosecond lasers.


**★ 4732 ★ U.S. Department of Health and Human Services**
**National Institute of Diabetes and Digestive and Kidney Diseases**
**Laboratory of Molecular and Cellular Biology**
NIH Bldg. 8, Rm. 309
9000 Rockville Pike
Bethesda, MD 20892
**Phone:** (301)496-1490 **Fax:** (301)402-0053
Dr. Nancy G. Nossal, Chf.

**Activities/Fields:** Molecular and cellular biology. Principal areas of research interest include: replication and gene regulation; development of adenoassociated virus vectors for genetic engineering and gene therapy; endocrine regulation of mammary gland development and tumors; growth factors; and glucocorticoid hormones.


**U.S. Department of Health and Human Services**
**National Institute of Environmental Health Sciences**
**Division of Intramural Research**
**Laboratory of Molecular Biophysics**
*See:* Entry 8968


**★ 4733 ★ U.S. Department of Health and Human Services**
**National Institute of General Medical Sciences**
**Biophysics and Physiological Sciences Program**
45 Center Dr., MSC 6200
Bethesda, MD 20892-6200
**Phone:** (301)594-0828 **Fax:** (301)480-2004
**Email:** cassatj@nigms.nih.gov
**Website:** http://www.nigms.nih.gov
James Cassatt, Dir.

**Activities/Fields:** Works to further understanding of the structure and function of cells, cellular components, and the biological macromolecules that make up these components. Seeks to finds ways to prevent, treat, and cure diseases that result from disturbed or abnormal cellular activity. Maintains a Biophysics Branch and a Cell Biology Branch. **Frmly:** (2000) Biophysics and Physiological Sciences Program.


**★ 4734 ★ U.S. Department of Health and Human Services**
**National Institute of General Medical Sciences**
**Division of Cell Biology and Biophysics**
**Biophysics Branch**
45 Center Dr., MSC 6200
Bethesda, MD 20892-6200
**Phone:** (301)594-0828 **Fax:** (301)480-2004
Dr. Bert Shapiro, Dir.

**Activities/Fields:** Biophysics and bioengineering. Areas of emphasis in biophysical research include: the determination of the structures of proteins and nucleic acids; studies of the structural features that determine macromolecular conformation; the structural analysis of macromolecular interactions and of ligand-macromolecular interactions; the development of physical methodology for the analysis of molecular structure; and the development and use of theoretical methods to investigate biological systems. Bioengineering research interests include the development and refinement of instruments needed to conduct research in the areas described above. These instruments include: nuclear magnetic resonance spectroscopy, mass spectroscopy, and other forms of spectroscopy; x-ray and other scattering techniques; microscopy; and cell separation techniques. This area of research also includes the development of new bioanalytical methods and biomaterials.


**★ 4735 ★ U.S. Department of Health and Human Services**
**National Institute of General Medical Sciences**
**Division of Cell Biology and Biophysics**
**Cell Biology Branch**
45 Center Dr., MSC 6200
Bethesda, MD 20892-6200
**Phone:** (301)594-0828 **Fax:** (301)480-2004
James Cassatt, Div. Dir.

**Activities/Fields:** Molecular and biochemical activities of cells and subcellular components, as well as on the role of cellular dysfunction in disease. Emphasis is placed on research with applications to more than one cell type, model system, or disease state, as well as research that does not fall within the disease-oriented mission of another of the National Institutes of Health. Representative studies include those on: plasma and intracellular membranes, receptors, and signal transduction mechanisms; the structure and function of the cytoskeleton; cell motility; the regulation of protein and membrane synthesis and the activation of cell growth; subcellular organelles; cell division; and lipid biochemistry.


**U.S. Department of Health and Human Services**
**National Institute of Mental Health**
**Intramural Research Programs Division (Basic Research)**
**Cell Biology Laboratory**
*See:* Entry 12729


**U.S. Department of Health and Human Services**
**National Institute of Mental Health**
**Intramural Research Programs Division (Basic Research)**
**General and Comparative Biochemistry Laboratory**
*See:* Entry 12731


**U.S. Department of Health and Human Services**
**National Institute of Mental Health**
**Intramural Research Programs Division (Basic Research)**
**Molecular Biology Laboratory**
*See:* Entry 12732


**U.S. Department of Health and Human Services**
**National Institute of Neurological Disorders and Stroke**
**Division of Intramural Research (Basic Neurosciences Program)**
**Laboratory of Molecular and Cellular Neurobiology**
*See:* Entry 14302


**U.S. Department of Health and Human Services**
**National Institute of Neurological Disorders and Stroke**
**Division of Intramural Research (Basic Neurosciences Program)**
**Laboratory of Neurobiology**
*See:* Entry 14304

**U.S. Department of Health and Human Services**
**National Institute of Neurological Disorders and Stroke**
**Division of Intramural Research (Basic Neurosciences Program)**
**Laboratory of Neurophysiology**
*See:* Entry 14306

**U.S. Department of Health and Human Services**
**National Institute of Neurological Disorders and Stroke**
**Division of Intramural Research (Clinical Neurosciences Program)**
**Laboratory of Molecular Medicine and Neuroscience**
*See:* Entry 14312

**U.S. Department of Health and Human Services**
**National Institute for Occupational Safety and Health**
**Biomedical and Behavioral Science Division**
**Applied Biology Branch**
*See:* Entry 16822

**★ 4736 ★ U.S. Department of Health and Human Services**
**National Institutes of Health**
**National Center for Research Resources**
6705 Rockledge Dr., Ste. 5046
Bethesda, MD 20892-7965
**Phone:** (301)435-0888 **Fax:** (301)480-3558
**Email:** info@ncrr.nih.gov
**Website:** http://www.ncrr.nih.gov/
Dr. Judith Vaitukaitis, Dir.
**Activities/Fields:** Ensures that the essential tools, materials, and other research resources are readily available to the biomedical research community. Through grant programs, investigators across the nation have access to these technologies, instrumentation, specialized facilities, animal models and colonies (mammalian and nonmammalian), genetic stocks, and biomaterials such as cell lines, tissues, and organs. **Pub:** *Directories.* • *NCRR Reporter.* • *Reports.*

**★ 4737 ★ U.S. Department of Health and Human Services**
**National Institutes of Health**
**National Institute of Dental and Craniofacial Research**
**Division of Extramural Research**
**(Biomaterials, Biomimetics and Tissue Engineering Branch)**
Bldg. 45, Rm. 4AN-18A
45 Center Dr.
Bethesda, MD 20892-6402
**Phone:** (301)594-2427 **Fax:** (301)480-8318
**Email:** eleni.kousvelari@nih.gov
**Website:** http://www.nidcr.nih.gov/research/extramural/biomaterials.asp
Dr. Eleni Kousvelari, Dir.
**Activities/Fields:** Design, development and improvement of natural and novel synthetic biomaterials used in restoration, repair, and reconstruction of oral, dental and craniofacial tissues and organs.

**★ 4738 ★ University of Alberta**
**Alberta Peptide Institute**
728 Heritage Medical Research Centre
Edmonton, AB, Canada T6G 2S2
**Phone:** (780)492-2522 **Fax:** (780)492-1473
**Email:** bob.parker@ualberta.ca
**Website:** http://http://www.api.ualberta.ca/
J.M. Robert Parker, Mgr.

**Activities/Fields:** Peptide synthesis, analysis, and purification, amino acid analysis, sequencing, and mass spectrometry.

**★ 4739 ★ University of Alberta**
**Group in Protein Structure and Function**
Department of Biochemistry
4-74 Medical Sciences Bldg.
Edmonton, AB, Canada T6G 2H7
**Phone:** (780)492-0087 **Fax:** (780)492-0886
**Email:** brian.sykes@ualberta.ca
**Website:** http://www.pence.ualberta.ca/mrc/main.html
Dr. B.D. Sykes, Dir.
**Activities/Fields:** Protein structure and function.

**★ 4740 ★ University of Alberta**
**Molecular Biology of Membrane Proteins Research Group**
Department of Biochemistry
Edmonton, AB, Canada T6G 2H7
**Phone:** (780)492-4853 **Fax:** (780)492-0886
**Email:** bernard.lemire@ualberta.ca
**Website:** http://www.membranegroup.ualberta.ca
Dr. Marek Michalak, Dir.
**Activities/Fields:** Structure, function and biogenesis of biological membranes and subcellular compartments under normal and pathological conditions.

**University of Alberta**
**Surgical-Medical Research Institute**
*See:* Entry 19623

**★ 4741 ★ University of British Columbia**
**Biomedical Research Centre**
2222 Health Science Mall
Vancouver, BC, Canada V6T 1Z3
**Phone:** (604)822-7813 **Fax:** (604)822-7815
**Email:** john@brc.ubc.ca
**Website:** http://www.brc.ubc.ca/
Dr. John W. Schrader, Dir.
**Activities/Fields:** Structure and function of genes and proteins involved in regulation of the growth and differentiation of cells of the immune system, including growth factors or cytokines, their cell surface receptors, and the intracellular enzymes and other proteins that control cellular growth and function. Research activities lie in the general areas of immunology, cancer, ontogeny, and technology development. Uses gene targeting and transgenic animal techniques to develop novel models of human diseases, and analyzes mechanisms in lymphocyte development, tolerance, and autoimmunity.

**★ 4742 ★ University of California, Los Angeles**
**Biocybernetics Laboratory**
4531 Boelter Hall
Computer Science Department
Los Angeles, CA 90095-1596
**Phone:** (310)825-7482 **Fax:** (310)794-5057
**Email:** joed@cs.ucla.edu
**Website:** http://biocyb.cs.ucla.edu/
Prof. Joseph J. DiStefano, III, Dir.
**Activities/Fields:** Synergistic and methodologic interface between modeling and laboratory experimentation, with a focus on integrated approaches for solving complex biosystem problems from sparse biodata.

**★ 4743 ★ University of California, Los Angeles**
**UCLA-DOE Laboratory of Structural Biology and Molecular Medicine**
201 Boyer Hall, Box 951570
611 Young Dr. E
Los Angeles, CA 90095
**Phone:** (310)825-3754 **Fax:** (310)206-3914
**Email:** david@mbi.ucla.edu
**Website:** http://www.doe-mbi.ucla.edu
Dr. David Eisenberg, Dir.

**Activities/Fields:** Structural biology and nuclear medicine, including supporting fields of physics, engineering and radiopharmacology. **Frmly:** Laboratory of Nuclear Medicine and Radiation Biology; Laboratory of Biomedical and Environmental Sciences.

**★ 4744 ★ University of California, San Francisco**
**Bio-organic Biomedical Mass Spectrometry Resource**
521 Parnassus, Rm. 1124S
San Francisco, CA 94143-0446
**Phone:** (415)476-5641 **Fax:** (415)476-0688
**Email:** alb@itsa.ucsf.edu
**Website:** http://donatello.ucsf.edu
Prof. Alma L. Burlingame, PhD, Prin. Investigator
**Activities/Fields:** Mass spectrometric techniques for sequencing peptides and structural characterization of modified proteins and glycoconjugates.

**★ 4745 ★ University of California, San Francisco**
**Magnetic Resonance Laboratory**
Department of Pharmaceutical Chemistry
513 Parnassus Ave.
San Francisco, CA 94143-0446
**Phone:** (415)476-4378 **Fax:** (415)476-0688
**Email:** james@picasso.ucsf.edu
**Website:** http://picasso.ucsf.edu/
Prof. T.L. James, Contact

**Activities/Fields:** Theory and practice of nuclear magnetic resonance and computer modeling studies of proteins and nucleic acids. Performs quantitative determinations of molecular structure in noncrystalline environments using nuclear Overhauser effects and complete relaxation matrix calculations.

**★ 4746 ★ University of California, San Francisco**
**Mass Spectrometry Facility**
Department of Pharmaceutical Chemistry
San Francisco, CA 94143
**Phone:** (415)476-5641 **Fax:** (415)502-1655
**Email:** alb@itsa.ucsf.edu
**Website:** http://donatello.ucsf.edu/
Prof. Alma L. Burlingame, PhD, Dir.

**Activities/Fields:** Molecular identification problems in human health and disease and biological chemistry, including studies in chemical and biochemical structure and mechanism. Conducts investigations of the structure of covalently modified informational biopolymers, drug metabolism, chemical carcinogenesis, signal transduction, proteins in cancer biology, irreversible inhibitors of cytochrome P-450, various genetic diseases, and membrane-bound glycoproteins, such as acetylcholine receptor and esterase, and scrapie glycoprotein. Develops techniques of computerized mass spectrometry. **Pub:** *Annual Report.*

**★ 4747 ★ University of Chicago**
**BioCARS: A Synchrotron Structural Biology Resource**
5640 S Ellis
Chicago, IL 60637
**Phone:** (773)702-2116 **Fax:** (773)702-0439
**Email:** moffat@cars.uchicago.edu
**Website:** http://cars9.uchicago.edu/biocars/
Keith Moffat, PhD, Prin. Investigator

**Activities/Fields:** Crystallographic studies of viruses, ribosomes and other complexes with very large unit cells; studies of microcrystals; time-resolved crystallography; and scattering from less-ordered biological systems. In all cases, the goal is to understand basic biological processes in structural terms, a goal fundamental to the pharmaceutical and biotechnology industries as well as to basic science.

**★ 4748 ★ University of Chicago**
**EM Core Facility for Biological Research**
920 E 58th St.
Chicago, IL 60637
**Phone:** (773)702-1650  **Fax:** (773)834-1094
**Email:** ewillia@midway.uchicago.edu
**Website:** http://gingi.uchicago.edu
Dr. Edward Williamson, Tech. Dir.

**Activities/Fields:** Biomedical research, including cell biology and molecular imaging.


**★ 4749 ★ University of Chicago**
**Lipoprotein Study Unit**
MC 5041
5841 S Maryland Ave.
Chicago, IL 60637-5041
**Phone:** (773)702-1775  **Fax:** (773)702-4534
**Email:** ascanu@medicine.bsd.uchicago.edu
Dr. Angelo M. Scanu, Dir.

**Activities/Fields:** Atherosclerotic cardiovascular disease, genetics of lipoprotein disorders, and structure and function of lipoproteins.


**★ 4750 ★ University of Connecticut**
**Health Center**
**National Resource for Cell Analysis and Modeling**
Center for Biomedical Imaging Technology
Farmington, CT 06030-1507
**Email:** les@volt.uchc.edu
**Website:** http://www.nrcam.uchc.edu
Leslie M. Loew, PhD, Prin. Investigator

**Activities/Fields:** Modeling of cell physiological processes in the context of the actual 3-D structure of individual cells.


**★ 4751 ★ University of Hawaii at Manoa**
**Kewalo Marine Laboratory**
41 Ahui St.
Honolulu, HI 96813
**Phone:** (808)539-7300  **Fax:** (808)599-4817
**Website:** http://www.kewalo.hawaii.edu/
Dr. Michael G. Hadfield, Dir.

**Activities/Fields:** Marine biology, including developmental, cellular and molecular biology; and symbiosis and microbiology using marine organisms as experimental models.


**★ 4752 ★ University of Hawaii at Manoa**
**Pacific Biomedical Research Center**
1993 East-West Rd.
Honolulu, HI 96822
**Phone:** (808)956-7401  **Fax:** (808)956-4768
**Email:** director@pbrc.hawaii.edu
**Website:** http://www.pbrc.hawaii.edu
Dr. Martin D. Rayner, Interim Dir.

**Activities/Fields:** Cell biology, neuro-behavioral biology, molecular biology, matrix pathobiology, biotechnology, Hawaiian evolutionary and conservation biology, molecular endocrinology, retrovirology (HIV and HTLV-1), infectious diseases, and native Hawaiian health research.


**★ 4753 ★ University of Illinois at Chicago**
**Laboratory for Molecular Biology**
MC 567
Department of Biological Science
900 S Ashland
Chicago, IL 60607-7020
**Phone:** (312)996-0716  **Fax:** (312)413-2691
**Email:** damorris@uic.edu
**Website:** http://www.uic.edu/depts/bios/lmb
Don Morrison, Coord.

**Activities/Fields:** Regulatory mechanisms involving signal transduction pathways and eukaryotic developmental systems.


**★ 4754 ★ University of Illinois at Urbana-Champaign**
**Resource for Macromolecular Modeling and Bioinformatics**
3147 Beckman Institute
405 N Mathews Ave.
Urbana, IL 61801
**Phone:** (217)244-1604  **Fax:** (217)244-6078
**Email:** kschulte@ks.uiuc.edu
**Website:** http://www.ks.uiuc.edu/
Klaus J. Schulten, PhD, Prin. Investigator

**Activities/Fields:** Structure and function of biopolymers and biopolymer aggregates by theoretical and computational means and investigation of genomes from different origins.


**★ 4755 ★ University of Iowa**
**Flow Cytometry Facility**
48 EMRB
College of Medicine
Iowa City, IA 52242
**Phone:** (319)335-8103  **Fax:** (319)335-8049
Justin Fishbaugh, Tech. Dir.

**Activities/Fields:** Cytometry research in the biomedical sciences, including cell biology, cancer biology, immunology, neurology, hepatology, pathology, tumor biology, and genetics.


**★ 4756 ★ University of Iowa**
**Hybridoma Facility**
EMRB
238 Eckstein Medical Research Bldg.
College of Medicine
Iowa City, IA 52242-1101
**Phone:** (319)335-8004  **Fax:** (319)335-6718
**Email:** charles-lovig@uiowa.edu
Dr. Charles Lovig, Contact

**Activities/Fields:** Provides monoclonal antibodies, tissue cultures, and reagents for cell cultures to individual investigators for their research.


**★ 4757 ★ University of Iowa**
**Molecular Analysis Facility**
355 EMRB
Iowa City, IA 52242
**Phone:** (319)353-5489  **Fax:** (319)335-7925
**Email:** lynn-teesch@uiowa.edu
**Website:** http://www.medicine.uiowa.edu/maf/
Lynn M. Teesch, Dir.

**Activities/Fields:** Proteins and peptides, focusing on amino acid composition and sequence, HPLC separations, and equilibrium and kinetic solution spectroscopy, GC-MS, LC-MS, Maldi-Tof MS. **Frmly:** Protein Structure Facility; GC/MC Facility.


**★ 4758 ★ University of Kansas**
**Biochemical Research Service Laboratory**
Department of Chemistry
1251 Wescoe Hall Dr.
Lawrence, KS 66045
**Phone:** (785)864-4166  **Fax:** (785)864-5396
**Email:** altermam@kuhub.cc.ukans.edu
**Website:** http://anylresc.idl.ukans.edu/BRSL
Mike Alterman, Dir.

**Activities/Fields:** Primarily a service facility, the Laboratory cultures large quantities of microorganisms, purifies and characterizes enzymes and other biological materials, immobilizes proteins, performs amino acid analyses, bio-mass spectrometry, protein sequence analyses, analytical and preparative HPLC, peptide synthesis, and automated DNA sequencing. **Frmly:** Enzyme Laboratory.


**★ 4759 ★ University of Kansas**
**Center for Drug Delivery Research**
Higuchi Biosciences Center
2095 Constant Ave.
Lawrence, KS 66047-2535
**Phone:** (785)864-5158  **Fax:** (785)749-7393

**Website:** http://hbc.ukans.edu
Roger Rajenski, PhD, Acting Dir.

**Activities/Fields:** Basic and applied research on chemically-driven drug delivery systems; physiochemical and biological factors that affect delivery systems; and unstable and insoluble drugs such as anticancer agents, peptides, and proteins.


**★ 4760 ★ University of Kansas**
**Higuchi Biosciences Center**
**Center for Biomedical Research**
2099 Constant Ave.
Lawrence, KS 66047-2535
**Phone:** (785)864-7339  **Fax:** (785)864-3578
**Email:** emichaelis@ku.edu
**Website:** http://www.hbc.ukans.edu
Dr. Elias K. Michaelis, Dir.

**Activities/Fields:** Integration of various aspects of drug design currently directed at several specific diseases such as epilepsy, cancer, heart and lung disease, and various mental disorders. Conducts biomedical and chemical projects in neurotransmitter receptors, ion transport mechanisms, phase transport kinetics, metabolism as a barrier to drug delivery, and development of highly sensitive bioanalytical techniques. **Frmly:** Center for Drug Design.


**★ 4761 ★ University of Manitoba**
**Manitoba Institute of Cell Biology**
675 McDermot Ave.
Winnipeg, MB, Canada R3E 0V9
**Phone:** (204)787-2155  **Fax:** (204)787-2190
**Email:** lestera@ms.umanitoba.ca
**Website:** http://www.umanitoba.ca/institutes/manitoba_institute_cell_biology/

**Activities/Fields:** Molecular mechanisms of cancer and other diseases, through cell biology, genomics, molecular biology, biochemistry, experimental chemotherapy, and tumor immunology.


**★ 4762 ★ University of Maryland**
**Graduate Program in Molecular and Cell Biology**
Microbiology Bldg.
College Park, MD 20742
**Phone:** (301)405-8422  **Fax:** (301)314-9921
**Email:** ia1@umail.umd.edu
**Website:** http://www.life.umd.edu/grad/mocb/index.html
Dr. Ibrahim Z. Ades, Prog. Dir.

**Activities/Fields:** Molecular genetics, cell biology, regulation of gene expression, molecular virology and immunology, membrane biochemistry, photoregulation, cell mobility, signal transduction, host-parasite interactions, transport channels, protein and enzyme and function, and neural processes.


**★ 4763 ★ University of Michigan**
**Biochemical Engineering Laboratory**
3324 H.H. Dow Bldg.
Department of Chemical Engineering
Ann Arbor, MI 48109-2136
**Phone:** (734)763-5659  **Fax:** (734)763-0459
**Email:** hywang@engin.umich.edu
Dr. Henry Y. Wang, Dir.

**Activities/Fields:** Biochemistry and biochemical engineering, including cell culture engineering and scale-up of genetically engineered microbial products and their bioseparation.


**★ 4764 ★ University of Minnesota**
**Hormel Institute**
801 16th Ave. NE
Austin, MN 55912
**Phone:** (507)433-8804  **Fax:** (507)437-9606
**Email:** hoschmid@smig.net
**Website:** http://www.smig.net/hi
Dr. Harald H.O. Schmid, Exec. Dir.

**Activities/Fields:** Biochemistry, bio-organic chemistry, biophysics, cell biology, and molecular biology relating to biological membranes and cellular signal transduction. Topics include membrane assembly and packing properties, regulation of lipolytic enzymes, and the role of membrane lipids in heart disease and cancer. **Pub:** *Annual Report*.


**★ 4765 ★ University of Minnesota**
**Institute of Medical Biotechnology**
7-121 Basic Science & Biomedical Engineering
  Bldg., Box 609
420 Delaware St. SE
Minneapolis, MN 55455
**Phone:** (612)624-7116     **Fax:** (612)625-1121
**Email:** hoffm003@tc.umn.edu
**Website:** http://www.med.umn.edu/imb
William Hoffman, Contact

**Activities/Fields:** The application of engineering principles to advance human health and well-being. **Frmly:** Biomedical Engineering Center.


**★ 4766 ★ University of Minnesota**
**Minnesota Molecular and Cellular**
  **Therapeutics Facility**
1900 Fitch Ave.
Saint Paul, MN 55108
**Phone:** (612)624-8700     **Fax:** (612)624-1777
**Email:** john.s.coleman-1@to.umn.edu
**Website:** http://www.ahc.umn.edu/mmct/
John S. Coleman, Dir.

**Activities/Fields:** Gene therapy, cell therapy (which involves the purification, expansion and genetic modification of blood and bone marrow cells), biotherapeutics, and educational issues.


**★ 4767 ★ University of Missouri**
**Mutant Mouse Regional Resource Center**
Laboratory Animal Medicine
Harlan Sprague Dawley, Inc.
298 S Carroll Rd.
Indianapolis, IN 46229
**Phone:** (317)894-7521     **Fax:** (317)894-4473
**Email:** rjrussell@harlan.com
Robert J. Russell, DVM, Prin. Investigator

**Activities/Fields:** Cryobiology focusing on improving methods for cryopreservation and banking of mouse spermatozoa and ovarian tissue; health monitoring, focusing on developing novel antemortem techniques for detection of microbial pathogens.


**★ 4768 ★ University of Montreal**
**Membrane Transport Research Group**
PO Box 6128, Downtown Sta.
Montreal, QC, Canada H3C 3J7
**Phone:** (514)343-7924     **Fax:** (514)343-7146
Remy Sauve, PhD, Dir.

**Activities/Fields:** Transport of ions, sugars, and amino acids in renal, intestinal and endothelial cells, including ionic permeability of cellular membranes of epithelia, molecular biology of transporters, computer simulation of atomic models, transport energetics, cell ultrastructure and transport, and cell primary cultures.


**★ 4769 ★ University of Nevada, Reno**
**Natural Products Lab**
Department of Biochemistry, Mail Stop 330
Reno, NV 89557
**Phone:** (775)784-4107     **Fax:** (775)784-1419
**Email:** ronp@cabnr.unr.edu
Dr. Ronald S. Pardini, Dir.

**Activities/Fields:** Cancer, biochemical pharmacology, and oxidative stress, including investigations of biochemical mechanisms of antitumor drugs and evaluations of the role of oxidative stress in the anticancer activity of drugs.


**★ 4770 ★ University of Notre Dame**
**Lobund Laboratory**
Notre Dame, IN 46556
**Phone:** (219)631-7564     **Fax:** (219)631-8583

**Email:** morris.pollard.3@nd.edu
Dr. Morris Pollard, Dir.

**Activities/Fields:** Research on prostate cancer including the development and use of model systems to study nutrition and endocrine manipulations for prevention and treatment of the disease; metastasis and angiogenesis.


**★ 4771 ★ University of Pennsylvania**
**Eldridge Reeves Johnson Foundation**
1005 Stellar-Chance Bldg.
Department of Biochemistry & Biophysics
University of Pennsylvania Medical Center
Philadelphia, PA 19104-6059
**Phone:** (215)898-8699     **Fax:** (215)573-2235
**Email:** dutton@mail.med.upenn.edu
**Website:** http://www.uphs.upenn.edu/~biocbiop/jf/
jf.html
P. Leslie Dutton, Dir.

**Activities/Fields:** Biochemical and biophysical aspects of medicine and biology.


**★ 4772 ★ University of Pennsylvania**
**William Pepper Laboratory**
Hospital of University of Pennsylvania
Philadelphia, PA 19104
**Phone:** (215)662-3435     **Fax:** (215)349-5090
**Email:** donaldyo@mail.med.upenn.edu
Donald S. Young, MD, Dir.

**Activities/Fields:** Microbiology, immunology, clinical chemistry, hematology, toxicology, therapeutic drug monitoring characterization and specificity of blood group, characterization and specificity of blood group antibodies, clinical correlation of disturbances of endocrine metabolism, coagulation disorders, and clinical enzymology. Conducts complete histocompatability evaluations, blood component therapy, therapeutic plasma exchange, therapeutic red cell exchange procedures, tumor receptor-site studies, as well as basic research in cancer biology, endocrine biochemistry, and membrane biology.


**★ 4773 ★ University of Rochester**
**Resource for the Study of Neural Models**
  **of Behavior**
734 Computer Science Department
Rochester, NY 14627-0226
**Phone:** (716)275-3772     **Fax:** (716)461-2018
**Email:** dana@cs.rochester.edu
**Website:** http://www.cs.rochester.edu/research/brain
Dana H. Ballard, PhD, Prin. Investigator

**Activities/Fields:** Monitoring and simulation of behavior in conjunction with relevant neural parameters to extend the capability to monitor behavior in natural situations. Under development are equipment to measure eye movements in freely moving head situations; devices for measuring kinematic state, such as arm and hand movements; devices for producing whole-body accelerations; and anthropomorphic devices to simulate experiments and develop experimental protocols.


**University of Southern California**
**Center for Craniofacial Molecular Biology**
*See:* Entry 6651


**★ 4774 ★ University of Southern**
  **California**
**Laboratory for Developmental Genetics**
School of Dentistry
University Park
925 W 34th St., DEN 4264
Los Angeles, CA 90089-0641
**Phone:** (213)740-1400     **Fax:** (213)740-7650
**Email:** tjaskoll@hsc.usc.edu
**Website:**     http://www.usc.edu/hsc/dental/ccmb/index.html
Dr. Tina Jaskoll, Co-Dir.

**Activities/Fields:** Cellular, molecular, and developmental biology issues associated with craniofacial and

salivary gland development, with an emphasis on functional genomics of craniofacial genetics.


**★ 4775 ★ University of Tennessee**
**Medical Center at Knoxville**
Graduate Sch. of Medicine
1924 Alcoa Hwy.
Knoxville, TN 37920
**Phone:** (865)544-9290     **Fax:** (865)544-6819
**Email:** mcaudle@mc.utmck.edu
**Website:** http://www.utmedicalcenter.org
Dr. Michael R. Caudle, Dean

**Activities/Fields:** Hematology, oncology, and the molecular processes of disease, including cellular and humoral immunity, colon cancer and colitis, cytogenetics, experimental and comparative pathology, platelet function, immunobiology, and membrane transport.


**★ 4776 ★ University of Tennessee**
**Molecular Resource Center**
Coleman Bldg., 2nd Fl., A205
956 Court Ave.
Memphis, TN 38163
**Phone:** (901)448-6191     **Fax:** (901)448-8229
**Email:** mdokter@utmem.edu
Dr. Michael Dokter, Dir.

**Activities/Fields:** Function and regulation of genes. Conducts experiments with gene replication and with isolation and manipulation of genetic components, with applications to cancer. Studies include cloning, mapping, probing, and sequencing of genes. **Pub:** *Annual Report*.


**★ 4777 ★ University of Texas at Austin**
**Biochemical Institute**
WEL 5.266, A5300
Austin, TX 78712
**Phone:** (512)471-1105     **Fax:** (512)471-8696
**Email:** m.hackert@mail.utexas.edu
**Website:** http://neon.cm.utexas.edu/bioinst/
Dr. Marvin L. Hackert, Dir.

**Activities/Fields:** Drug metabolism, mechanism and regulation of protein synthesis, structure, function, and regulation of enzymes and other proteins, nutritional aspects of human disease, and cloning, sequencing, and site specific mutagenesis of genes, their regulation, and repair. **Frmly:** Clayton Foundation Biochemical Institute.


**★ 4778 ★ University of Texas at Dallas**
**Molecular and Cell Biology Program**
Mail Stop FO3.1
PO Box 830688
Richardson, TX 75083-0688
**Phone:** (972)883-2500     **Fax:** (972)883-2409
**Email:** sgoodmn@utdallas.edu
**Website:** http://www.utdallas.edu/
Dr. Steven R. Goodman, Interim Prog. Hd.

**Activities/Fields:** Biochemistry, macromolecular physical chemistry, microbial and molecular genetics, and cell biology. **Pub:** *Research Reports*.


**★ 4779 ★ University of Texas—Houston**
  **Health Science Center**
**Houston Biomaterials Research Center**
6516 M.D. Anderson Blvd., Rm. 4.109
Houston, TX 77030-3402
**Phone:** (713)500-4191     **Fax:** (713)500-4372
**Email:** biomaterials@mail.db.uth.tmc.edu
**Website:** http://www.db.uth.tmc.edu/Biomaterials/default.htm
John M. Powers, PhD, Dir.

**Activities/Fields:** Biological, clinical, mechanical, chemical, and physical properties of biomaterials for dental, orthopaedic, craniofacial and other applications.

## ★ 4780 ★ University of Texas Medical Branch at Galveston
### Marine Biomedical Institute
301 University Blvd.
Galveston, TX 77555-1069
**Phone:** (409)772-2103          **Fax:** (409)772-4687
**Email:** wdwillis@utmb.edu
**Website:** http://www2.utmb.edu/mbi/
Dr. William D. Willis, Jr., Dir.
**Activities/Fields:** Studies on problems in comparative neurobiology, marine medicine and biology, and biophysics. **Pub:** *Bulletin.* • *Project Reports.*

## ★ 4781 ★ University of Texas Medical Branch at Galveston
### Sealy Center for Molecular Science
5.104 Medical Research Bldg., Rte. 1068
301 University Blvd.
Galveston, TX 77555-1068
**Phone:** (409)772-3367          **Fax:** (409)772-6334
**Email:** lpipper@utmb.edu
**Website:** http://www.scms.utmb.edu
Dr. E. Brad Thompson, Interim Dir.
**Activities/Fields:** Molecular biology and biochemistry. Specialized research includes eukaryotic DNA repair, HIV molecular biology, molecular toxicology and oncology, transcription regulation, signal transduction steroids and apoptosis. **Pub:** *Departmental Newsletter*, semiannually.

## ★ 4782 ★ University of Texas Southwestern Medical Center at Dallas
### Center for Biomedical Inventions (CBI)
6000 Harry Hines Blvd.
Dallas, TX 75390-9185
**Phone:** (214)648-1408          **Fax:** (214)648-4156
**Email:** thomas.kodadek@utsouthwestern.edu
**Website:** http://cbi.swmed.edu/
Thomas J. Kodadek, Contact
**Activities/Fields:** Biomedicine, particularly relating to the diagnosis and treatment of cancer and heart disease. Research focuses on chemical synthesis, tissue culture, molecular biology, computation, robotics, and instrument construction.

## ★ 4783 ★ University of Virginia
### Center for Cell Signaling
Health Science Center
PO Box 800577
Charlottesville, VA 22908
**Phone:** (434)924-1235          **Fax:** (434)924-1236
**Email:** signals@virginia.edu
**Website:** http://hsc.virginia.edu/signals/
Dr. David L. Brautigan, PhD, Dir.
**Activities/Fields:** Molecular biology of cellular signaling processes, including membranes, receptors, transduction, genome-level signals, and molecular structure. **Frmly:** Markey Center.

## ★ 4784 ★ University of Washington
### Center on Human Development and Disability
PO Box 357920
Seattle, WA 98195-7920
**Phone:** (206)543-2832          **Fax:** (206)543-3417
**Email:** chdd@u.washington.edu
**Website:** http://depts.washington.edu/chdd
Michael J. Guralnick, PhD, Dir.
**Activities/Fields:** Biomedical and behavioral research of human development, including studies in developmental biology, perinatal biology, neurological sciences, psychology, psychiatry, speech and hearing sciences, social work, nursing, and special education. **Pub:** *Outlook*, quarterly. **Frmly:** Child Development and Mental Retardation Center.

## ★ 4785 ★ University of Wisconsin—Milwaukee
### Marine and Freshwater Biomedical Sciences Center
600 E Greenfield Ave.
PO Box 413
Milwaukee, WI 53201
**Phone:** (414)229-5853          **Fax:** (414)229-5427
**Email:** petering@uwm.edu
**Website:** http://www.uwm.edu/Dept/MFB
Dr. David Petering, Dir.
**Activities/Fields:** Aquatic models in biomedicine and comparative toxicology. Studies transformation and metabolism of toxic organic chemicals and metals and investigates genetic, neurobehavioral, and immunological responses of organisms to such chemicals. **Pub:** *Annual report.*

## ★ 4786 ★ W.M. Keck Center for Computational Biology
6100 S Main St.
Houston, TX 77005
**Phone:** (713)348-4752          **Fax:** (713)348-4659
**Email:** keckcenter@bioc.rice.edu
**Website:** http://www.bioc.rice.edu/keck
George N. Phillips, Co-Dir.
**Activities/Fields:** Biological research, including chemistry and molecular biology of DNA binding, molecular genetics of inborn errors of metabolism, electron crystallography and tomography of macromolecular assemblies, DNA sequence information and human disease, computational neuroscience, parallel computation and language, high resolution NMR spectroscopy of macromolecular structure and dynamics, computation in molecular genetics, computation in image reconstruction and biofluid mechanics, structure and metabolism of lipoproteins, rapid kinetics of hemeprotein-ligand reactions, structure and function of electron transport proteins, nicotinic synaptic transmission in the central nervous system, X-ray crystallography, molecular dynamics of proteins and nucleic acids, a tomic structures and functions of proteins, artificial intelligence, and design and analysis of algorithms. **Pub:** *Keck Center Newsletter.*

## ★ 4787 ★ Wake Forest University
### Lipid Analytic Laboratory
Gray Bldg., Rm. 2063
School of Medicine
Medical Center Blvd.
Winston Salem, NC 27157-1072
**Email:** rstclair@wfubmc.edu
**Website:** http://www.wfubmc.edu/or/core31.html
Richard W. St. Clair, PhD, Lab. Dir.
**Activities/Fields:** Provision of standardized plasma lipid and lipoprotein analyses for clinical and research purposes.

## ★ 4788 ★ Washington University in St. Louis
### Resource for Biomedical and Bio-organic Mass Spectrometry
1 Brookings Dr.
Saint Louis, MO 63130
**Phone:** (314)935-4814          **Fax:** (314)935-7484
**Email:** mgross@wuchem.wustl.edu
**Website:** http://wunmr.wustl.edu/~msf
Michael L. Gross, PhD, Prin. Investigator
**Activities/Fields:** Instrument and method development of mass spectrometry; structure determination of peptides, proteins, carcinogen-modified DNA fragments, and lipids; stable isotope tracer and complex lipids.

## ★ 4789 ★ Webb-Waring Institute for Cancer, Aging, and Antioxidant Research
Box C-321
4200 E 9th Ave.
Denver, CO 80262
**Phone:** (303)315-8231          **Fax:** (303)315-8541
**Email:** john.repine@uchsc.edu
**Website:** http://www.uchsc.edu/sm/waring/webpages/
John E. Repine, MD, Pres. /Dir.
**Activities/Fields:** Role of oxygen radicals in health and diseases, oxidants and antioxidants, air pollution, basic immunology, biochemistry, genetics, cell biology, pathology, and physiology. **Pub:** *Annual Report.* Newsletter. **Frmly:** Webb-Waring Institute for Biomedical Research.

## ★ 4790 ★ Whitehead Institute for Biomedical Research
9 Cambridge Center
Cambridge, MA 02142
**Phone:** (617)258-5000          **Fax:** (617)258-6294
**Email:** info@wi.mit.edu
**Website:** http://www.wi.mit.edu/home.html
Dr. Susan Lindquist, Dir.
**Activities/Fields:** Cancer, genomics, infectious disease, developmental and cell biology, structural biology, and molecular medicine. **Pub:** *BiologyWeek Newsletter*, weekly. • *Director's Report*, biennially. • *Discovery*, quarterly. • *Research summaries*, annually.

## ★ 4791 ★ Wistar Institute
3601 Spruce St.
Philadelphia, PA 19104
**Phone:** (215)898-7325          **Fax:** (215)573-2097
**Email:** buck@wistar.upenn.edu
**Website:** http://www.wistar.upenn.edu
Clayton A. Buck, PhD, Actg. Dir. /CEO
**Activities/Fields:** Virology and immunology using a molecular-based approach primarily to cancer as well as virus-induced diseases, degenerative diseases such as Alzheimer's and autoimmune diseases including multiple sclerosis, rheumatoid arthritis, lupus, scleroderma, and phemphigo. Specific areas of research include structural biology emphasizing the structure of viruses and the interaction of a variety of ligands to cell surface receptors; tumor biology emphasizing early embryonic development, including the development of the immune and cardiovascular systems; molecular genetics, focusing on suppressor genes and oncogenes in leukemias, lymphomas, childhood cancers, melanomas, breast carcinomas, bladder carcinomas, and tumors of the gastrointestinal tract; and tumor immunology, particularly emphasizing on gene therapy and immune therapy. **Pub:** *Newsletters.* • *Scientific report*, annually. • *Wistar Symposia.* **Frmly:** Wistar Institute of Anatomy and Biology.

# Chapter 9
# Biotechnology

## Foundations & Other Funding Organizations

### Other Funding Organizations

**★ 4792 ★ American Society for Laser Medicine and Surgery (ASLMS)**
2404 Stewart Sq.
Wausau, WI 54401
**Phone:** (715)845-9283        **Fax:** (715)848-2493
**Email:** information@aslms.org
**Website:** http://www.aslms.org
Richard O. Gregory, MD, Sec.

**Desc:** Physicians, physicists, and other scientists; nurses, dentists, podiatrists, veterinarians, and other paramedical personnel; technicians and commercial representatives concerned with the medical applications of lasers. Facilitates exchange of information concerning lasers. **Awards:** Grant.

## National & International Organizations

**★ 4793 ★ Accreditation Review Committee on Education in Surgical Technology (ARC-ST)**
c/o Paul Price, CST/CFA, MBA
7108-C S Alton Way
Centennial, CO 80112-2106
**Phone:** (303)694-9262        **Fax:** (303)741-3655
**Email:** acollinsworth@ast.org
**Website:** http://www.arcst.org
Paul Price, Exec. Dir.

**Fnded:** 1974. **Mem:** 317. **Desc:** Reviews accreditation applications of surgical techology programs in hospitals, community colleges, technical schools, and universities and makes recommendations to the Commission on Accreditation of Allied Health Education Programs. Collaborates with American College of Surgeons, American Hospital Association, and the Association of Surgical Technologists. **Pub:** *Surgical Technology: A Growing Career.* Brochure. Contains information on careers in surgical technology, educational requirements, and a list of accredited programs. *Price:* Free (first copy); $1/each additional copy. **Frmly:** (1987) Joint Review Committee on Education for the Surgical Technologist; (1990) Accreditation Review Committee for Educational Programs in Surgical Technology.

**★ 4794 ★ Advanced Medical Technology Association (AdvaMed)**
1200 G St. NW, Ste. 400
Washington, DC 20005-3814
**Phone:** (202)783-8700        **Fax:** (202)783-8750
**Email:** info@advamed.org
**Website:** http://www.advamed.org
Mary Plock, VP Pub. Affairs

**Fnded:** 1974. **Mem:** 800. **Desc:** Represents domestic (including U.S. territories and possessions) manufacturers of medical devices, diagnostic products, and healthcare information systems. Develops programs and activities on economic, technical, medical, and scientific matters affecting the industry. Gathers and disseminates information concerning the United States and international developments in legislative, regulatory, scientific or standards-making areas. Conducts scientific and educational seminars and programs. **Pub:** *Health Industry Manufacturers Association–Directory,* annual. Directory. Covers issues facing the health industry. *Price:* Free. For members only. • *In Brief,* monthly. *Price:* Free. For members only. • Manuals. • Proceedings. • Reports. • Also publishes a catalogue. **Frmly:** (2001) Health Industry Manufacturers Association.

**★ 4795 ★ American Society for Healthcare Central Service Professionals (ASHCSP)**
c/o American Hospital Association
1 N Franklin, No. 2800
Chicago, IL 60606
**Phone:** (312)422-3750        **Fax:** (312)422-4572
**Email:** pcostello@aha.org
**Website:** http://www.ashcsp.org
Patti Costello, Exec. Dir.

**Fnded:** 1967. **Mem:** 1,000. **Reg. Groups:** 9. **Local Groups:** 48. **Desc:** Managers, directors, technicians and supervisors of central service-supply distribution and sterile processing of medical devices and instrumentation. Certification, education and training. **Pub:** *Healthcare Central Service,* bimonthly. Newsletter. *Price:* available to members only. • Also publishes technical materials and training manuals. **Frmly:** (1987) American Society for Hospital Central Service Personnel.

**★ 4796 ★ Association of Industrial Laser Users (AILU)**
100 Ock St.
Abingdon OX14 5DH, United Kingdom
**Phone:** 44 1235 539595        **Fax:** 44 1235 550499
**Email:** admin@ailu.org.uk
**Website:** http://www.ailu.org.uk

**Fnded:** 1995. **Mem:** 270. **Desc:** Aims to foster co-operation and collaboration on non-competitive technical matters and provide a forum and mechanisms for sharing experience and expertise. Represents and promotes the interests of industrial laser users. Disseminates professional and other information to members. Promotes the best practice in the industrial applications of lasers in materials processing and allied technologies. Supports the maintenance and improvement of standards of safety and performance in the industrial user of lasers.

**★ 4797 ★ Australasian Society for Ultrasound in Medicine**
2/181 High St.
Willoughby, NSW 2068, Australia
**Phone:** 61 2 99587655        **Fax:** 61 2 99588002
**Email:** asum@asum.com.au
**Website:** http://www.asum.com.au

**Fnded:** 1975. **Mem:** 2,400. **Desc:** Doctors, scientists, sonographers, trainee sonographers/radiographers and corporations in ultrasound field. **Pub:** *Australasian Society for Ultrasound in Medicine,* quarterly. Bulletin.

**★ 4798 ★ Canadian Association of Electroneurophysiology Technologists (Association Canadienne des Technologues en Electroneurophysiologie)**
St. Boniface
409 Tache Ave.
Winnipeg, MB, Canada R2H 2A6
**Phone:** (204)737-6350        **Fax:** (204)737-6656
**Email:** caet@canada.com
**Website:** http://www.caet.org

**Lang(s):** English, French. **Desc:** Medical technologists specializing in electroneurophysiology. Promotes professional advancement of members; works to advance the practice of electroneurophysiology. Represents members' interests; conducts continuing professional development courses.

**★ 4799 ★ Danish Association of Medical Imaging (Danske Radiologers Organisation — DRO)**
Department of Radiology, Sonderborg Sygehus
DK-6400 Sonderborg, Denmark
**Phone:** 45 74430311
**Fnded:** 1921.

**Electrophysiological Technologists' Association (EPTA)**
*See:* Entry 13986

**★ 4800 ★ European Biosafety Association (EBSA)**
Dreefstr 19
B-1880 Kapelle-op-den-Bos, Belgium
**Phone:** 32 1 5713189        **Fax:** 32 1 5711037
**Email:** mdc@net4all.be
**Website:** http://www.ebsa.be/

**Fnded:** 1996. **Desc:** Promotes biosafety as a scientific discipline, supports emerging legislation and standards in the area of biological safety, biotechnology, transport and associated activities.

**★ 4801 ★ European Chinese Society for Clinical Magnetic Resonance (ECSCMR)**
c/o Prof. Dr. Juergen Hennig
Rontgendiagnostik Hugstetterstr. 55
D-79106 Freiburg, Germany

**Phone:** 49 761 2703836    **Fax:** 49 761 2703831
**Email:** hennig@nz11.ukl.uni-freiburg.de

**Fnded:** 1991. **Desc:** Fosters exchange of information between Europe and China on the application of magnetic resonance tomography.

★ 4802 ★ **European Society for Artificial Organs (ESAO)**
c/o Prof. Jean Maria Wojcicki
Institute of Biocybernetics and Biomedical Engineering P.A.S
Trojedena 4
P-02-109 Warsaw, Poland
**Phone:** 48 22 6582875      **Fax:** 48 22 6597030
**Email:** jan.wojcicki@ibib.waw.pl
**Website:** http://www.esao.donau-uni.ac.at

**Fnded:** 1974. **Mem:** 450. **Lang(s):** English. **Desc:** Associations and individuals concerned with advancement in the creation of artificial organs. Promotes research. **Pub:** *International Journal of Artificial Organs*, monthly. Journal. Includes congress proceedings. • *Life Systems*, quarterly. Also publishes modifications.

★ 4803 ★ **European Society for Computing and Technology in Anaesthesia and Intensive Care (ESCTAIC)**
c/o Lutz Krummereich
Draegerwerk AG
Moislinger Allee 53-55
D-23542 Lubeck, Germany
**Fax:** 49 451 8822796
**Email:** lutz.krummereich@draeger.com
**Website:** http://www.eur.nl/fgg/anest/esctaic/

**Fnded:** 1989. **Mem:** 200. **Desc:** Fosters interchange of ideas among individuals as well as manufacturers in the field of computing and technology in anesthesia and intensive care medicine. Promotes exploration and innovation in medical technology.

★ 4804 ★ **European Society for Magnetic Resonance in Medicine and Biology (ESMRMB)**
Neutorgasse 9/2A
A-1010 Vienna, Austria
**Phone:** 43 1 5351306       **Fax:** 43 1 5357041
**Email:** office@esmrmb.org
**Website:** http://www.esmrmb.org

**Mem:** 500. **Lang(s):** English, German. **Desc:** Physicians, engineers, and scientists with an interest in the medical applications of magnetic resonance (MR) technologies. Promotes advancement of MR technologies and seeks to increase and improve their use by the medical profession. Conducts educational and training programs for physicians wishing to make use of MR; sponsors MR research and development programs; serves as a clearinghouse on MR technologies and their medical applications. **Pub:** *MAGMA*, periodic. Journal.

★ 4805 ★ **International Society for Plastination (ISP)**
c/o R.W. Henry
University of Tennessee
College of Veterinary Medicine
2407 River Dr.
Knoxville, TN 37996
**Fax:** (865)974-5640
**Email:** rhenry@utk.edu
Robert W. Henry, Treas.

**Fnded:** 1984. **Mem:** 200. **Desc:** Anatomists, pathologists, and technologists. Seeks to share information about plastination, a means of infiltrating biological specimens with curable polymers. **Pub:** *Journal of the International Society for Plastination*, semiannual. Journal. *Price:* $20/issue.

★ 4806 ★ **International Society of Technology Assessment in Health Care (ISTAHC)**
PO Box 1390
Montreal, QC, Canada H3B 3L2
**Phone:** (514)844-3033       **Fax:** (514)844-3823
**Email:** gtombs@istahc.org
**Website:** http://www.istahc.org/en/welcome.html

**Fnded:** 1985. **Desc:** Aims to lead the world in partnering for research and education on the clinical, economic and social implications of health technologies.

★ 4807 ★ **Japanese Society of Medical Imaging Technology**
c/o Quantum
YU Bldg., 3F
3-19-6 Hongou
Bunkyou-ku
Tokyo 113-0033, Japan
**Phone:** 81 3 56841636       **Fax:** 81 3 56841650
**Email:** qyp06453@nifty.ne.jp
**Website:** http://www.jamit.jp/index.html

**Desc:** Fosters the advancement of medical imaging technology. **Pub:** *Medical Imaging Technology*, bi-monthly. Journal.

★ 4808 ★ **Latin American Federation of Societies of Ultrasound in Medicine and Biology**
Av Dr. Eneas C Aguiar 255
050403-001 Sao Paulo, Brazil
**Phone:** 55 11 30648015       **Fax:** 55 11 8817358
**Email:** gcerri@hcnet.usp.br
**Website:** http://www.flaus.org

★ 4809 ★ **Society of Diagnostic Medical Sonography (SDMS)**
2745 N Dallas Pky., No. 350
Plano, TX 75093-4706
**Phone:** (972)239-7367       **Free:** 800-229-9506
**Fax:** (972)239-7378
**Email:** alysdale@sdms.org
**Website:** http://www.sdms.org
Kevin Evans, Pres.

**Fnded:** 1970. **Mem:** 11,000. **Reg. Groups:** 7. **State Groups:** 50. **Local Groups:** 40. **Desc:** Works to advance and educate its members and the medical community in the science of diagnostic medical sonography, to advance the science of ultrasound technology and to establish and maintain high standards of education and training. **Pub:** *Journal of Diagnostic Medical Sonography*, biennial. Journal. • *National Certification Examination Rewiew.* • *News Wave*, quarterly. • *SDMS Annual Conference Videotapes.* Videos. • *Sonography Benchmark Survey Annual Income.* Survey. • Books. **Frmly:** (1980) American Society of Ultrasound Technical Specialists.

★ 4810 ★ **Unione Nazionale Industrie Dentarie Italiane (UNDI)**
Via Tamburini 2
I-20123 Milan, Italy
**Phone:** 39 2 467510       **Fax:** 39 2 461330
**Email:** unidi@unidi.it
**Website:** http://www.unidi.it/unidi.htm

**Fnded:** 1969. **Mem:** 135. **Lang(s):** English, French, Italian. **Desc:** Companies manufacturing dental equipment and supplies. Establishes international standards and technical harmonization for dental equipment. Represents members' interests before government bodies, international agencies, and the public. Maintains liaison with organizations representing dentists, dental technicians, and dental supply dealers and distributors. Compiles statistics. **Pub:** *Unidipress*, bi-monthly. Magazine.

★ 4811 ★ **World Federation for Ultrasound in Medicine and Biology**
Dept. of Ultrasound, Herlev Hospital, University of Copenhag
DK-2730 Herlev, Denmark
**Phone:** 45 44884704       **Fax:** 45 44948090
**Email:** soha@herlevhosp.dk
**Website:** www.who.int/ina-ngo/ngo/ngo164.htm

**Fnded:** 1969. **Desc:** Promotes research in the field by international cooperation; disseminates scientific information on education programs internationally.

# Research Centers

**Boston University Neuromuscular Research Center Design Laboratory**
*See:* Entry 14152

★ 4812 ★ **Carnegie Mellon University High Performance Computing for Biomedical Research**
Mellon Institute Bldg.
4400 5th Ave.
Pittsburgh, PA 15213
**Phone:** (412)268-4960       **Fax:** (412)268-5832
**Email:** roskies@psc.edu
**Website:** http://www.psc.edu/biomed/biomed.html
Ralph Z. Roskies, PhD, Prin. Investigator

**Activities/Fields:** Biomedical computer programs for access to high-performance computing resources; bioinformatics, structural biology, computational genomics and proteomics, computational neuroscience, computational pathology, and scientific visualization.

★ 4813 ★ **Center for Advanced Biotechnology and Medicine**
679 Hoes Ln.
Piscataway, NJ 08854-5638
**Phone:** (732)235-5300       **Fax:** (732)235-5318
**Email:** cabm@umdnj.edu
**Website:** http://www.cabm.rutgers.edu
Prof. Aaron J. Shatkin, PhD, Dir.

**Activities/Fields:** Cell and developmental biology, molecular pharmacology, molecular genetics, and structural biology. Collaborates with biopharmaceutical firms in New Jersey on technology transfer and research and development.

★ 4814 ★ **Center for Biotechnology**
Psychology A Bldg., 3rd Fl.
State University of New York at Stony Brook
Stony Brook, NY 11794-2580
**Phone:** (631)632-8521       **Fax:** (631)632-8577
**Email:** clinton.rubin@sunysb.edu
**Website:** http://www.biotech.sunysb.edu
Clinton T. Rubin, PhD, Dir.

**Activities/Fields:** Supports biomedical research in New York, and facilitates collaborations between small businesses and the research community within the state. Conducts sponsored research projects in biochemistry, immunology, microbiology, pharmacology, and chemistry.

★ 4815 ★ **Dartmouth College Electron Paramagnetic Resonance Center for the Study of Viable Systems**
Department of Radiology
Medical School
7785 Vail, Rm. 702
Hanover, NH 03755
**Phone:** (603)650-1955       **Fax:** (603)650-1717
**Email:** harold.swartz@dartmouth.edu
**Website:** http://www.dartmouth.edu/~eprctr/
Harold M. Swartz, MD, Prin. Investigator

**Activities/Fields:** Development and application of techniques that make it feasible to carry out well-resolved EPR spectroscopy in fully functional living systems, especially living animals (with or without anesthesia) but also viable cells.

**★ 4816 ★ Duke University**
**Center for Cellular and Biosurface**
**Engineering (CBE)**
Box 90281
Durham, NC 27708
**Phone:** (919)660-5452 **Fax:** (919)684-4488
**Email:** dkatz@acpub.duke.edu
**Website:** http://bme-www.mc.duke.edu/Research/
Cellsurf/
David F. Katz, PhD, Dir.

**Activities/Fields:** Biotechnology, especially protein engineering, cellular engineering, and biosurface engineering.

**★ 4817 ★ Emory-Georgia Tech**
**Biomedical Technology Research**
**Center**
Institute for Bioengineering and Bioscience
Georgia Institute of Technology
315 Ferst Dr., Ste. 1126
Atlanta, GA 30332-0535
**Phone:** (404)894-6228 **Fax:** (404)894-4243
**Email:** ajit.yioganathan@bme.gatech.edu
**Website:** http://www.ibb.gatech.edu
Prof. Ajit P. Yoganathan, Co-Dir.

**Activities/Fields:** Cardiovascular mechanics, corneal mechanics, medical imaging, biomedical artificial intelligence, biomedical instrumentation, vascular biology, tissue engineering, telemedicine. **Pub:** *Newsletter*, 3/ year.

**★ 4818 ★ Johns Hopkins University**
**Sensory Communication and**
**Microsystems Laboratory**
223 Latrobe Hall
3400 N Charles St.
Baltimore, MD 21218-2686
**Phone:** (410)516-8361 **Fax:** (410)516-8313
**Email:** andreou@jhu.edu
**Website:** http://olympus.ece.jhu.edu/
Andreas G. Andreou, Gp. Ldr.

**Activities/Fields:** Sensory microsystems performing tasks such as vision and audition. Research focuses on new technologies and devices, mixed analog/digital circuits, architecture, and algorithms.

**Laval University**
**Laboratory of Experimental Tissue**
**Engineering**
*See:* Entry 4530

**Lawrence Berkeley National Laboratory**
**Center for Functional Imaging**
*See:* Entry 18166

**★ 4819 ★ Lawrence Berkeley National**
**Laboratory**
**National Tritium Labelling Facility (NTLF)**
Mail Stop 75-123
1 Cyclotron Rd.
Berkeley, CA 94720
**Phone:** (510)486-4373 **Fax:** (510)486-4877
**Email:** dewemmer@lbl.gov
**Website:** http://www.lbl.gov/LBL-Programs/NTLF.html
David E. Wemmer, Dir.

**Activities/Fields:** Provides specialty equipment and professional assistance for biomedical researchers to produce very high specific activity tritiated compounds, with high radiochemical purity. Labeling is achieved via one of the major tritiation techniques: hydrogenation, dehalogenation, methylation, hydride reduction, or exchange. Research projects range from the improvement of tritium labeling techniques to the understanding of ligand-protein interactions. Recent works include the development of highly tritiated hydride

reducing agents such as LiEt3BT and LiA1T4, the production of very high specific activity tritomethyl iodide, the tritium NMR study of glucose metabolism in red blood cells, and the NMR investigation of the binding maltose to a 40kD protein. **Pub:** *Newsletter*, occasionally.

**★ 4820 ★ Lawrence Livermore National**
**Laboratory**
**Resource for Biomedical Accelerator**
**Mass Spectrometry**
7000 E Ave.
PO Box 808, L-452
Livermore, CA 94551-0808
**Phone:** (925)423-8152 **Fax:** (925)422-2282
**Email:** turteltaub2@llnl.gov
**Website:** http://www.llnl.gov/bioams/
Kenneth W. Turteltaub, PhD, Prin. Investigator

**Activities/Fields:** New methods and instrumentation for the use of accelerator mass spectrometry in biomedical research.

**★ 4821 ★ Massachusetts General**
**Hospital**
**Center for Functional Neuroimaging**
**Technologies**
149 13th St., Rm. 2301
Charlestown, MA 02129
**Phone:** (617)724-7139 **Fax:** (617)726-7422
**Email:** bruce@nmr.mgh.harvard.edu
**Website:** http://www.nmr.mgh.harvard.edu/CFNT
Bruce R. Rosen, MD, Prin. Investigator

**Activities/Fields:** Understanding of the human brain in health and disease through the development and dissemination of innovative multimodal magnetic resonance based neuroimaging techniques and technologies.

**★ 4822 ★ McGill University**
**Artificial Cells and Organs Research**
**Centre**
3655 Drummond St.
Montreal, QC, Canada H3G 1Y6
**Phone:** (514)398-3512 **Fax:** (514)398-4983
**Email:** artcell@med.mcgill.ca
**Website:** http://www.medicine.mcgill.ca/artcell/
Prof. T.M.S. Chang, Dir.

**Activities/Fields:** Interdisciplinary research using biotechnology, biochemistry, chemical engineering, medicine, enzyme engineering, and chemistry on projects concerning artificial cells, blood substitutes from crosslinked hemoglobin and encapsulated hemoglobin, oral therapy for kidney failure, detoxifier, immobilized enzymes, cells, including genetically engineered cells, hemoperfusion, microencapsulation, nanoencapsulation, enzyme replacement therapy, drug carriers, and biomaterials. **Pub:** *Artificial Cells, Blood Substitutes and Immobilization Biotechnology.* Journal. • *International Journal.* Journal.

**★ 4823 ★ Medical College of Georgia**
**Center for Clinical Investigation**
1521 Pope Ave., FF-1001
Augusta, GA 30912-3152
**Phone:** (706)721-2131
**Website:** http://www.mcg.edu/Research/core/Cinvestigation.htm
Anthony L. Mulloy, PhD, Dir.

**Activities/Fields:** Pharmaceutical agents and medical devices.

**★ 4824 ★ Medical Technology and**
**Practice Patterns Institute, Inc.**
4733 Bethesda Ave., Ste. 510
Bethesda, MD 20814
**Phone:** (301)652-4005 **Fax:** (301)652-8335
**Email:** inquiry@mtppi.org
**Website:** http://www.mtppi.org
Dennis J. Cotter, Pres.

**Activities/Fields:** New and emerging health-care technologies and their implications for local, national, and international policy. Research efforts fall into three broad areas: Health Services Research, encompassing patient outcomes, pharmacoeconomics, quality-of-life assessments, and cost-effectiveness analyses; International Activities, including conducting surveys of health technology assessment activities worldwide technology assessment modeling, and sponsorship of workshops and seminars on health policy issues; and Special Programs, encompassing health-facility planning, vaccine research and development, and educational outreach. Technologies studied include magnetic resonance imaging, extracorporeal shockwave lithotripsy, endocardial electrical stimulation, implantable cardiac defibrillators, percutaneous transluminal coronary angioplasty, percutaneous lithotripsy, heart transplantation, ambulatory blood pressure monitoring, total parenteral nutrition, liver transplantation, bone marrow transplantation, and dialysis treatment for end-stage renal disease. **Pub:** *Diagnostic Imaging and Child Abuse.* • *Direct and Indirect Costs of Diabetes.* • *Implications of NAFTA for Trade in Health Care Technology.* • *Rational Use of Health Technologies.* • *Reports on various health technologies.*

**★ 4825 ★ Northwestern University**
**Center for Biotechnology**
1801 Maple Ave.
Evanston, IL 60201-3155
**Phone:** (847)467-1454 **Fax:** (847)467-2180
**Email:** l-wainright@nwu.edu
**Website:** http://www.nucb.nwu.edu
Alicia Loffler, Dir.

**Activities/Fields:** Cooperates with industry on issues of national and international significance. **Pub:** *Biotechnology News*, quarterly.

**Northwestern University**
**Multipurpose Arthritis and**
**Musculoskeletal Diseases Center**
*See:* Entry 3061

**★ 4826 ★ Oklahoma State University**
**Microbiology and Molecular Genetics**
307 Life Sciences East
Stillwater, OK 74078-9947
**Phone:** (405)744-6243 **Fax:** (405)744-6790
**Email:** nirmal@okstate.edu
**Website:** http://microbiology.okstate.edu
Moses Vijayakumar, PhD, Dept. Hd.

**Activities/Fields:** Production and characterization of hybridomas and monoclonal antibodies and production of polyclonal antiserum. **Frmly:** Hybridoma Center for Agricultural and Biological Sciences.

**★ 4827 ★ Pennsylvania State University**
**Resource on Medical Ultrasonic**
**Transducer Technology**
231 Hallowell Bldg.
Center for Medical Ultrasonic Transducer
Engineering
University Park, PA 16802
**Phone:** (814)865-1407 **Fax:** (814)863-0490
**Email:** kksbio@engr.psu.edu
**Website:** http://bioeng.psu.edu/nih_transducer.html
K. Kirk Shung, PhD, Prin. Investigator

**Activities/Fields:** High frequency ultrasonic transducers/arrays for applications in medicine and biology that include ophthalmology, dermatology, and vascular surgery. **Pub:** *Proceedings.*

**★ 4828 ★ Riverside Research Institute**
156 William St., 9th Fl.
New York, NY 10038-2609
**Phone:** (212)502-1750 **Fax:** (212)502-1742
**Website:** http://www.rri-usa.org

**Activities/Fields:** Biomedical ultrasound, electromagnetic scattering and interactions, photonic systems, signal processing, image processing, radar, military systems, and computer modeling of physical processes in ultrasound and electromagneticism.

## ★ 4829 ★ Rockefeller University
**National Resource for Mass Spectrometry of Biological Macro-Molecules**
1230 York Ave.
New York, NY 10021
**Phone:** (212)327-8849　　　**Fax:** (212)327-7547
**Email:** chait@rockvax.rockefeller.edu
Dr. Brian T. Chait, Dir.

**Activities/Fields:** Application of mass spectrometry to biomedical problems.

## ★ 4830 ★ Stanford University
**Center for Advanced Magnetic Resonance Technology**
Lucas Magnetic Resonance Spectroscopy & Imaging Center
Schools of Medicine & Engineering
Stanford, CA 94305-5488
**Phone:** (650)723-7577　　　**Fax:** (650)723-5795
**Email:** gary@s-word.stanford.edu
**Website:** http://www-radiology.stanford.edu/research/RR.html
Gary H. Glover, PhD, Prin. Investigator

**Activities/Fields:** Development of innovative magnetic resonance techniques for fundamental anatomic, physiologic, and pathophysiologic studies involving animals and humans. Core technology development encompasses these five areas: reconstruction methods, imaging of brain activation, MR spectroscopy and multinuclear imaging, cardiovascular structure and function, and interventional imaging methods.

**Stanford University**
**Image Guidance Laboratories (IGL)**
*See:* Entry 19621

## ★ 4831 ★ Stanford University
**National Biocomputation Center**
701 Welch Rd., Ste. 1128
Palo Alto, CA 94304
**Phone:** (650)498-6978　　　**Fax:** (650)498-5626
**Email:** kevin@biocomp.stanford.edu
**Website:** http://biocomp.stanford.edu/introtop.html
Stephen Schendel, MD,DDS, Dir.

**Activities/Fields:** 3D imaging, visualization, and simulation.

## ★ 4832 ★ State University of New York at Buffalo
**Center for Assistive Technology (CAT)**
515 Kimball Tower
Buffalo, NY 14214-3079
**Phone:** (716)829-3141　　　**Free:** 800-828-2281
**Fax:** (716)829-3217
**Email:** kbeaver@acsu.buffalo.edu
**Website:** http://cat.buffalo.edu/
Dr. William C. Mann, Dir.

**Activities/Fields:** Assistive devices for persons with disabilities.

## ★ 4833 ★ State University of New York at Buffalo
**Center for Positron Emission Tomography**
105 Parker Hall
Buffalo, NY 14214-3007
**Phone:** (716)838-5889　　　**Fax:** (716)838-4918
**Email:** bob@nucmed.buffalo.edu
**Website:** http://www.nucmed.buffalo.edu/cpethm.htm
Dr. Robert E. Ackerhalt, Dir.

**Activities/Fields:** Neurology, oncology, and cardiology, focusing on the use of Positron Emission Tomography (PET).

## ★ 4834 ★ Taconic Farms Inc.
**Mutant Mouse Regional Resource Center**
273 Hover Ave.
Germantown, NY 12526
**Phone:** (518)537-5200　　　**Fax:** (518)537-7287
**Email:** jgei@taconic.com
James G. Geistfeld, DVM, Prin. Investigator

**Activities/Fields:** Value of microarray technology for mutant phenotyping of mice.

**U.S. Department of Defense**
**Air Force Materiel Command**
**Armstrong Laboratory**
**Division of Human Engineering**
*See:* Entry 4493

**U.S. Department of Defense**
**Air Force Materiel Command**
**Human Systems Center**
**Air Force School of Aerospace Medicine**
*See:* Entry 4494

**U.S. Department of Energy**
**Department of Energy Program Offices—Environment, Safety and Health**
**Office of Biological and Environmental Research**
**((Medical Sciences Division)**
**Genome Instrumentation Research Program)**
*See:* Entry 9439

## ★ 4835 ★ U.S. Department of Energy
**Department of Energy Program Offices—Environment, Safety and Health**
**Office of Biological and Environmental Research**
**((Medical Sciences Division)**
**Computational Biology Program)**
19901 Germantown Rd., SC-73
Germantown, MD 20874-1290
**Phone:** (301)903-9009
**Email:** roland.hirsch@science.doe.gov
**Website:** http://www.sc.doe.gov/production/ober/msd_compbio.html
Roland Hirsch, Prog. Mgr.

**Activities/Fields:** Computational molecular biology.

## ★ 4836 ★ U.S. Department of Energy
**Department of Energy Program Offices—Environment, Safety and Health**
**Office of Biological and Environmental Research**
**((Medical Sciences Division)**
**Laser Medicine Research Program)**
19901 Germantown Rd., SC-73
Germantown, MD 20874-1290
**Phone:** (301)903-3268
**Email:** dean.cole@science.doe.gov
**Website:** http://www.sc.doe.gov/production/ober/msd_laser.html
Dean A. Cole, PhD, Prog. Mgr.

**Activities/Fields:** Laser applications for non-invasive medicine.

## ★ 4837 ★ U.S. Department of Energy
**Department of Energy Program Offices—Environment, Safety and Health**
**Office of Biological and Environmental Research**
**((Medical Sciences Division)**
**Structural Biology Research Program)**
19901 Germantown Rd., SC-73
Germantown, MD 20874-1290
**Phone:** (301)903-9009
**Email:** roland.hirsch@science.doe.gov
**Website:** http://www.sc.doe.gov/production/ober/msd_struct_bio.html
Roland F. Hirsch, PhD, Prog. Mgr.

**Activities/Fields:** Structural biology techniques aimed at determining three-dimensional structure of important proteins, nucleic acids, and other biological materials.

## ★ 4838 ★ U.S. Department of Energy
**Department of Energy Program Offices—Environment, Safety and Health**
**Office of Biological and Environmental Research**
**((Medical Sciences Division)**
**Advanced Imaging Instrumentation Research Program)**
19901 Germantown Rd., SC-73
Germantown, MD 20874-1290
**Phone:** (301)903-3268
**Email:** dean.cole@science.doe.gov
**Website:** http://www.sc.doe.gov/production/ober/msd_med_image.html
Dean A. Cole, Prog. Mgr.

**Activities/Fields:** PET, single photon emission computing tomograph, magnetic resonance imaging, and magnetoencephalography; study of neurochemical status of the brain in patients with neurodegenerative diseases, substance abuse, and for improved confidence in management of disease such as cancer (diagnosis, design and planning treatment, and monitoring course of therapy); strives to make nuclear imaging more compatible to current and advancing future molecular medicine needs such as imaging gene expression and monitoring gene therapy.

**U.S. Department of Energy**
**Department of Energy Program Offices—Environment, Safety and Health**
**Office of Biological and Environmental Research**
**((Medical Sciences Division)**
**Molecular Nuclear Medicine)**
*See:* Entry 18174

## ★ 4839 ★ U.S. Department of Energy
**Department of Energy Program Offices—Fossil Energy**
**Office of Biological and Environmental Research**
**(Medical Sciences Division)**
19901 Germantown Rd., SC-73
Germantown, MD 20874-1290
**Phone:** (301)903-3213　　　**Fax:** (301)903-0567
**Email:** michael.viola@science.doe.gov
**Website:** http://www.sc.doe.gov/production/ober/msd_top.html
Michael Viola, MD, Dir.

**Activities/Fields:** Strives to develop beneficial applications of nuclear and other energy-related technologies for medical diagnosis and treatment of patient's problems.

## ★ 4840 ★ U.S. Department of Health and Human Services
**National Center for Research Resources**
**Biomedical Technology Program**
1 Rockledge Centre, Rm. 6030
6705 Rockledge Rd., MSC 7965
Bethesda, MD 20892-7965
**Phone:** (301)435-0772　　　**Fax:** (301)480-3659
Dr. Michael Marron, Dir.

**Activities/Fields:** Physical sciences, mathematics, engineering, and computer sciences; biology; and medicine. Its purpose is to support and develop biomedically relevant technologies to be utilized by health scientists in solving biomedical and clinical research problems. Such technologies include mass spectrometers, high voltage electron microscopes, and nuclear magnetic and electron spin resonance spectrometers. BTP provides grants and contracts for establishing, maintaining, and developing these resources and for adapting technological capabilities developed in the commercial sector for use by the biomedical community. Support is currently provided in three main areas: computer resources; instruments and materials for studying biomolecular and cellular structure and function; and biomedical engineering and technology resources.

**★ 4841 ★ U.S. Department of Health and Human Services**
**National Institutes of Health**
**National Center for Biotechnology Information**
Bldg. 38A, 8-N-805
8600 Rockville Pike
Bethesda, MD 20894
**Phone:** (301)496-2475          **Fax:** (301)480-9241
**Email:** info@ncbi.nlm.nih.gov
Dr. David J. Lipman, MD, Dir.

**Activities/Fields:** Supports and develops biotechnology databases. Operates GenInfo Backbone Database.

**★ 4842 ★ U.S. Department of Health and Human Services**
**National Institutes of Health**
**National Institute of Environmental Health Sciences**
**Laboratory of Structural Biology**
**(Macromolecular Structure Group)**
PO Box 12233
Research Triangle Park, NC 27709
**Phone:** (919)541-1017          **Fax:** (919)316-4617
**Email:** hall4@niehs.nih.gov
**Website:** http://dir.niehs.nih.gov/dirlsb/hall_home.html
Traci Hall, Prin. Investigator

**Activities/Fields:** Structural biology, primarily x-ray crystallography, to study overlapping areas of embryonic development, cell signaling, and RNA-protein interactions.

**★ 4843 ★ U.S. Department of Health and Human Services**
**National Institutes of Health**
**National Institute of Environmental Health Sciences**
**Laboratory of Structural Biology**
**(Computational Chemistry/Molecular Modeling Group)**
PO Box 12233
Research Triangle Park, NC 27709
**Phone:** (919)541-3198          **Fax:** (919)541-7880
**Email:** darden@niehs.nih.gov
**Website:** http://dir.niehs.nih.gov/dirlsb/cchome.htm
Tom Darden, PhD, Prin. Investigator

**Activities/Fields:** Understanding structural, mutational and sequence data generated using graphics, energy minimization, simulations, relative free energy, and homology-structure; provides current molecular modeling methodology. **Pub:** *Papers.*

**★ 4844 ★ U.S. Department of Health and Human Services**
**National Institutes of Health (NIH)**
**National Institute of Neurological Disorders and Stroke**
**Division of Intramural Research (Advanced MRI Section)**
Bldg. 10, Rm. B1D108
10 Center Dr., MSC 1065
Bethesda, MD 20892-1065
**Phone:** (301)402-1981          **Fax:** (301)402-3216
**Email:** jhd@helix.nih.gov
**Website:** http://www.ninds.nih.gov/about_ninds/labs/106.htm
Jeff H. Duyn, PhD, Investigator

**Activities/Fields:** Mechanisms behind MRI contrast, exploring avenues to manipulate contrast, and optimizing MRI data acquisition and analysis to achieve optimum sensitivity, resolution, reliability, and accuracy.

**U.S. Department of Veterans Affairs**
**Rehabilitation Research and Development Service**
**Center for Restoring Function through Electrical Stimulation (FES)**
*See:* Entry 8206

**★ 4845 ★ University of Alabama at Birmingham**
**Center for Nuclear Imaging Research (CNIR)**
School of Medicine
Center for NMR Research and Development
CNIR 106
Birmingham, AL 35294-4470
**Phone:** (205)934-9450          **Fax:** (205)934-7367
**Email:** ferry@uab.edu
**Website:** http://www.cnir.uab.edu/cnir.htm
Gerald M. Pohost, MD, Dir.

**Activities/Fields:** Application of clinical magnetic resonance methods to biological systems.

**★ 4846 ★ University of Arizona**
**Center for Gamma-Ray Imaging**
Department of Radiology
Arizona Health Sciences Center
PO Box 245067
Tucson, AZ 85724
**Phone:** (520)626-6815          **Fax:** (520)626-2892
**Email:** barrett@radiology.arizona.edu
**Website:** http://gamma.radiology.arizona.edu
Harrison H. Barrett, PhD, Prin. Investigator

**Activities/Fields:** Gamma-ray imaging instruments with dramatically improved spatial and temporal resolution for use in research in functional genomics, cardiovascular disease, cognitive neuroscience, breast cancer, and surgical tumor detection.

**★ 4847 ★ University of Arkansas at Little Rock**
**Particle Accelerator Lab**
Physics Department
2801 S University Ave.
Little Rock, AR 72204
**Phone:** (501)569-3275          **Fax:** (501)569-3314
**Email:** aarollefson@ualr.edu
**Website:** http://www.physics.ualr.edu
Dr. Andre Rollefson, Contact

**Activities/Fields:** Fast-neutron radiobiology with cultured cells.

**★ 4848 ★ University of British Columbia**
**Biotechnology Laboratory**
Wesbrook Bldg., Rm. 237
6174 University Blvd.
Vancouver, BC, Canada V6T 1Z3
**Phone:** (604)822-4838          **Fax:** (604)822-2114
**Email:** dcrowe@cmmt.ubc.ca
**Website:** http://www.biotech.ubc.ca
Dr. Philip Hieter, Dir.

**Activities/Fields:** Molecular genetics as related to forest, plant, and animal biology and medicine. Interests include process engineering and fermentation studies. **Frmly:** Molecular Genetics Centre.

**★ 4849 ★ University of California, San Diego**
**Resource for Solid-State Nuclear Magnetic Resonance of Proteins**
Department of Chemistry & Biochemistry
9500 Gilman Dr., 0307
La Jolla, CA 92093-0307
**Phone:** (858)822-4820          **Fax:** (858)822-4821
**Email:** sopella@ucsd.edu
**Website:**          http://chem-faculty.ucsd.edu/opella/resource
Stanley J. Opella, PhD, Prin. Investigator

**Activities/Fields:** Development and application of solid-state Nuclear Magnetic Resonance (NMR) spectroscopy for structure determination of peptides and proteins.

**★ 4850 ★ University of California, San Diego**
**San Diego Supercomputer Center**
**National Biomedical Computation Resource**
9500 Gilman Dr.
La Jolla, CA 92093-0505
**Phone:** (858)534-5079          **Fax:** (858)822-0948
**Email:** parzberg@sdsc.edu
**Website:** http://nbcr.sdsc.edu
Peter W. Arzberger, PhD, Prin. Investigator

**Activities/Fields:** Advanced computational technology, particularly the integration of computational and visualization tools in a transparent, advanced computing environment to enable better access to distributed data, computational resource and instruments; development and deployment of advanced computational tools for modeling, data query, linking of data resources, 3-D image processing, and interactive visualization.

**★ 4851 ★ University of Connecticut Health Center**
**Center for Biomedical Imaging Technology (CBIT)**
263 Farmington Ave.
Farmington, CT 06030-1507
**Phone:** (860)679-1452
**Website:** http://www.cbit.uchc.edu/
Leslie M. Loew, PhD, Dir.

**Activities/Fields:** Diagnostic and cell biological imaging, optoelectronic design, and computer/imaging science.

**★ 4852 ★ University of Florida**
**Interdisciplinary Center for Biotechnology Research (ICBR)**
PO Box 110580
South Newell Dr.
Gainesville, FL 32611-0580
**Phone:** (352)392-8408          **Fax:** (352)392-8598
**Email:** schuster@biotech.ufl.edu
Dr. Sheldon M. Schuster, Dir.

**Activities/Fields:** Biotechnology, including flow cytometric analysis, DNA sequencing, hybridoma technologies, protein microisolation, peptide synthesis, electron microscopy, biological computing, and genetics and reproductive analyses. Research activities include biotechnologies for ecological, evolutionary, and conservation sciences.

**University of Illinois at Chicago**
**Center for Pharmaceutical Biotechnology**
*See:* Entry 17389

**★ 4853 ★ University of Illinois at Urbana-Champaign**
**Electron Paramagnetic Resonance Research Center**
190 Medical Sciences Bldg.
College of Medicine
506 S Mathews Ave.
Urbana, IL 61801
**Phone:** (217)244-1186          **Fax:** (217)333-8868
**Email:** ierc@uiuc.edu
**Website:** http://ierc.scs.uiuc.edu
R. Linn Belford, PhD, Dir.

**Activities/Fields:** Free radicals and metal ion centers, especially in biological systems; characterization of metalloproteins; development and evaluation of S-band (2-4 GHz) ESE, high-frequency (e.g. 94GHz) EPR, and low-frequency DNP spectrometry; EPR study of paramagnetic contrast agents for magnetic resonance imaging (MRI); research in EPR and ENDOR theory; dynamics in biomolecules; protein folding and unfolding. **Pub:** *EPR Newsletter.*

### ★ 4854 ★ University of Kentucky
**Tobacco and Health Research Institute (THRI)**
Cooper & University Drs.
Lexington, KY 40546-0236
**Phone:** (859)257-5798　　**Fax:** (859)323-1077
**Email:** mdavies@pop.uky.edu
**Website:** http://www.uky.edu/RGS/THRI/
Maelor Davies, Dir.

**Activities/Fields:** Application of biotechnology for the development of new crops based on the tobacco plant and the investigation of animal physiology related to the use of tobacco products.

### ★ 4855 ★ University of Maryland
**Biotechnology Institute**
**Medical Biotechnology Center**
725 W Lombard St.
Baltimore, MD 21201
**Phone:** (410)706-8181　　**Fax:** (410)706-8184
**Email:** lederer@umbi.umd.edu
**Website:** http://www.umbi.umd.edu/~mbc/
W. Jonathon Lederer, MD, Dir.

**Activities/Fields:** Bioengineering, optical biology, biosensing, neurobiology, genetics molecular and cellular signalling, molecular cardiology, biology of aging, cellular biophysics, muscle biology, protein structure and function.

### ★ 4856 ★ University of Maryland at
**Baltimore**
**Center for Fluorescence Spectroscopy**
School of Medicine
725 W Lombard St.
Baltimore, MD 21201
**Phone:** (410)706-8409　　**Fax:** (410)706-8408
**Email:** cfs@cfs.umbi.umd.edu
**Website:** http://cfs.umbi.umd.edu/cfs
Joseph R. Lakowicz, PhD, Prin. Investigator

**Activities/Fields:** Fluorescence spectroscopy and its applications to the biological and medical sciences.

### ★ 4857 ★ University of Maryland at
**College Park**
**Public Health Informatics Research Laboratory (PHI)**
Department of Health Education
Valley Dr., Ste. 2387
College Park, MD 20742-2611
**Phone:** (301)405-2522　　**Fax:** (301)405-1654
**Email:** rg14@umail.umd.edu
**Website:** http://www.phi.umd.edu
Robert S. Gold, PhD, Dir.

**Activities/Fields:** Improvement of the health of populations through the appropriate use of technology.

**University of Michigan**
**Division of Nuclear Medicine**
*See:* Entry 18188

### ★ 4858 ★ University of Minnesota
**Center for Magnetic Resonance Research**
**Nuclear Magnetic Resonance Imaging and Localized Spectroscopy**
2021 6th St. SE
Minneapolis, MN 55455
**Phone:** (612)626-9591　　**Fax:** (612)626-2004
**Email:** kamil@cmrr.umn.edu
**Website:** http://www.cmrr.umn.edu
Kamil Ugurbil, PhD, Prin. Investigator

**Activities/Fields:** Development of high-resolution and high-contrast anatomic images of the human brain; functional images of the human brain for sensory and cognitive tasks; localized spectroscopy in humans;

adiabatic pulses for imaging and multinuclear spectroscopy; and improved methods for chemical shift imaging, functional imaging, and single voxel localized spectroscopy.

**University of Minnesota**
**Institute of Medical Biotechnology**
*See:* Entry 4765

### ★ 4859 ★ University of North Carolina at
**Chapel Hill**
**Interactive Graphics for Molecular Studies and Microscopy**
Sitterson Hall, CB 3175
Chapel Hill, NC 27599-3175
**Phone:** (919)962-1701　　**Fax:** (919)962-1799
**Email:** taylorr@cs.unc.edu
**Website:** http://www.cs.unc.edu/research/nano
Dr. Russell M. Taylor, II, Prin. Investigator

**Activities/Fields:** The development of instruments and interfaces in scanned-probe microscopy so that individual macromolecules, viruses, and cells can be imaged, their properties can be measured, and they can be physically modified.

### ★ 4860 ★ University of Pennsylvania
**Resource for Magnetic Resonance Research and Optical Research**
B1, Stellar-Chance Laboratories
Department of Radiology
422 Curie Blvd.
Philadelphia, PA 19104-6100
**Phone:** (215)898-9357　　**Fax:** (215)573-2113
**Email:** jack@mail.mmrrcc.upenn.edu
**Website:** http://www.mmrrcc.upenn.edu
John S. Leigh, PhD, Prin. Investigator

**Activities/Fields:** Instrumentation, methodologies, and data analysis for in vivo monitoring of specific metabolites in localized regions of tissues and organs in humans, utilizing multinuclear magnetic resonance spectroscopy; and novel spectral functional and perfusion imaging techniques.

### ★ 4861 ★ University of Pittsburgh
**McGowan Institute for Regenerative Medicine (MIRM)**
409 Center for Biotechnology & Bioengineering
300 Technology Dr.
Pittsburgh, PA 15219-3112
**Phone:** (412)383-9998　　**Fax:** (412)383-9460
**Email:** mirm@pitt.edu
**Website:** http://www.mirm.pitt.edu/contact.htm
Alan J. Russell, PhD, Dir.

**Activities/Fields:** Tissue engineering, cellular therapies, biosurgery, and artificial and biohybrid organ devices.

### ★ 4862 ★ University of Quebec at Trois-
**Rivieres**
**Research Group in Membrane Biotechnology**
PO Box 500
Trois-Rivieres, QC, Canada G9A 5H7
**Phone:** (819)376-5052　　**Fax:** (819)376-5084
**Email:** claude_gicquaud@uqtr.uquebec.ca
Claude Gicquaud, Dir.

**Activities/Fields:** Fundamental research on the use of artificial membrane systems applied to biophysical and medical problems. Research includes the study of cytoskeleton-membrane interactions, pharmacological use of liposomes, and physiochemical basis of membrane interactions with physiologically active substances.

### ★ 4863 ★ University of Rochester
**Center for Future Health (CFH)**
PO Box CFH
601 Elmwood Ave.
Rochester, NY 14627-0231

**Phone:** (716)273-1507　　**Fax:** (716)273-2981
**Email:** futurehealth@futurehealth.rochester.edu
**Website:** http://www.centerforfuturehealth.org
Prof. Philippe M. Fauchet, Dir.

**Activities/Fields:** System of affordable, easy to use and integrated smart health tools for use by consumers in their homes, including technologies for aging well, healthy skin, pathogen detection and health care support for developing nations and underserved communities.

### ★ 4864 ★ University of Southern
**California**
**Biomedical Simulations Resource**
Department of Biomedical Engineering
School of Engineering, OHE 500
3650 McClintock Ave.
Los Angeles, CA 90089-1451
**Phone:** (213)740-0342　　**Fax:** (213)740-0343
**Email:** vzm@bmsr.usc.edu
**Website:** http://bmsr.usc.edu
Vasilis Z. Marmarelis, PhD, Prin. Investigator

**Activities/Fields:** Development of modeling methodologies for nonlinear and nonstationary dynamic systems, sparse-data systems, and biological control systems. Application areas include sensory and neuronal systems, pharmacodynamics, and cardiorespiratory control.

**University of Tennessee**
**Molecular Resource Center**
*See:* Entry 4776

### ★ 4865 ★ University of Texas at Austin
**Center for Biotechnology**
WEL, 4.260C
Austin, TX 78712-1159
**Phone:** (512)471-3279　　**Fax:** (512)471-8696
**Email:** bkitto@mail.utexas.edu
Barrie Kitto, PhD, Dir.

**Activities/Fields:** Biotechnology.

### ★ 4866 ★ University of Texas Health
**Science Center at San Antonio**
**Institute for Biotechnology**
15355 Lambda
San Antonio, TX 78245-3207
**Phone:** (210)567-7000　　**Fax:** (210)567-7277
**Email:** hottle@uthscsa.edu
**Website:** http://www.molecularmedicine.uthscsa.edu
Dr. Wen-Hwa Lee, Dir. /Ch.

**Activities/Fields:** Biotechnology and molecular medicine.

### ★ 4867 ★ University of Utah
**Center for Cell Signaling (CCS)**
421 Wakara Way, Ste. 360
Salt Lake City, UT 84108
**Phone:** (801)585-9704　　**Fax:** (801)585-6354
**Email:** nbernshaw@hnu.pharm.utah.edu
**Website:** http://hnu.pharm.utah.edu/CCS/
Glenn D. Prestwich, PhD, Dir.

**Activities/Fields:** Molecular mechanisms by which cells communicate in normal conditions and in disease states, in efforts to develop new technologies important to the treatment of cancer, allergy, asthma and inflammation.

**University of Virginia**
**Surgical Therapeutic Advancement Center (STAC)**
*See:* Entry 19630

### ★ 4868 ★ University of Waterloo
**BioTechnology Research Centre**
200 University Ave. W
Waterloo, ON, Canada N2L 3G1
**Phone:** (519)888-4567　　**Fax:** (519)746-4979

**Email:** rllegge@engmail.uwaterloo.ca
**Website:** http://www.uwaterloo.ca
Dr. R.L. Legge, Exec. Dir.

**Activities/Fields:** Fundamental and applied R&D, including research in molecular biology, genetics, cell culture, biochemistry, bioorganic and natural products chemistry, enyzmology, molecular modeling, bioreactor and bioprocess development, bioseparations engineering and environmental biotechnology.

**★ 4869 ★ Very Low Frequency Electron Paramagnetic Resonance Imaging for In Vivo Physiology**
Department of Radiation/Cell Oncology, MC1105
University of Chicago
5841 S Maryland Ave.
Chicago, IL 60637
**Phone:** (773)702-6871  **Fax:** (773)702-5940
**Email:** h-halpern@uchicago.edu
Howard J. Halpern, MD, Prin. Investigator
**Activities/Fields:** Development of instrumentation, analysis techniques, spin probes and spin traps, and methodologies for imaging physiologically relevant aspects of tissue fluids, including high-resolution oxygen maps, with very low frequency electron paramagnetic resonance imaging.

**★ 4870 ★ Wake Forest University Center for Medical Ultrasound (CMU)**
School of Medicine
Medical Center Blvd.
Winston Salem, NC 27157
**Phone:** (336)716-4505  **Fax:** (336)716-2447
**Email:** cmu@wfubmc.edu
**Website:** http://www.wfubmc.edu/research/med_ultra.html
Dr. Frederick W. Kremkau, Dir.

**Activities/Fields:** Application of ultrasound in medical diagnosis and therapy for better patient care.

**★ 4871 ★ Yeshiva University Analytical Imaging Facility**
Albert Einstein College of Medicine
Resnick Campus
1300 Morris Park Ave.
Bronx, NY 10461
**Phone:** (718)430-3547
**Email:** macaluso@aecom.yu.edu
**Website:** http://www.aecom.yu.edu/aif/welcome.htm
Dr. John Condeelis, Sci. Dir.

**Activities/Fields:** Analytical imaging for medical studies.

# Federal Government Agencies

★ **4872** ★ **U.S. Department of Health and Human Services**
**Centers for Disease Control and Prevention**
**National Center on Birth Defects and Developmental Disabilities**
1600 Clifton Rd. NE
Atlanta, GA 30333
**Phone:** (404)639-3311
**Website:** http://www.cdc.gov/ncbddd/

# Foundations & Other Funding Organizations

## Other Funding Organizations

★ **4873** ★ **Cleft Palate Foundation**
104 S Estes Dr., Ste. 204
Chapel Hill, NC 27514-2866
**Phone:** (919)933-9044          **Free:** 800-242-5338
**Fax:** (919)933-9604
**Email:** cleftline@aol.com
**Website:** http://www.cleftline.org
Nancy C. Smythe, Exec. Dir.

**Desc:** Enhances the quality of life for individuals with facial birth defects through education, research support, and facilitation of family-centered care. Provides research programs and information services. **Awards:** Parent-Patient Leadership Award (annual) outstanding contribution by individual or parent affected by facial birth defects.

★ **4874** ★ **March of Dimes Birth Defects Foundation (MDBDF)**
1275 Mamaroneck Ave.
White Plains, NY 10605
**Phone:** (914)428-7100          **Free:** 888-663-4637
**Fax:** (914)428-8203
**Website:** http://www.modimes.org/publicaffairs/contact.cfm
Dr. Jennifer L. Howse, Pres.

**Desc:** Founded by President Franklin D. Roosevelt as the National Foundation for Infantile Paralysis. Promotes prevention of birth defects by focusing on maternal and child health issues including low birthweight, infant mortality, prenatal care, and maternal substance abuse. Offers public and professional health education and community service programs to improve maternal and newborn health. Works with other national and local organizations to initiate and implement community programs of prenatal care education and service. Operates Campaign for Healthier Babies to support research and educational programs. Develops and distributes educational materials for health professionals and the public. **Awards:** Grant to hospitals and universities for clinical research; grant for professionals concerned with prevention of birth defects; grant for improved perinatal and genetic services; monetary for promising young scientists and medical students.

# National & International Organizations

★ **4875** ★ **American Cleft Palate-Craniofacial Association (ACPA)**
104 S Estes Dr., Ste. 204
Chapel Hill, NC 27514-2866
**Phone:** (919)933-9044          **Fax:** (919)933-9604
**Email:** cleftline@aol.com
**Website:** http://www.cleftline.org
Nancy Smythe, Exec. Dir.

**Fnded:** 1943. **Mem:** 2,700. **Desc:** Physicians, dentists, speech pathologists, audiologists, psychologists, nurses and others surgeons actively engaged in the care of individuals with cleft lip and palate and associated craniofacial anomalies. Works to extend and improve the understanding of the scientific and clinical problems involved in the habilitation of patients with cleft lip and palate, and to stimulate professional and public interest in the field. Conducts educational programs. **Pub:** *American Cleft Palate-Craniofacial Association Membership and Team Directory*, annual. Membership Directory. *Price:* available to members only. • *American Cleft Palate-Craniofacial Association Newsletter*, quarterly. Newsletter. *Price:* Included in membership dues. • *Cleft Palate-Craniofacial Journal*, bimonthly. Journal. Includes research reports, book reviews, and commentaries. *Price:* Included in membership dues; $110 for nonmembers; $145 for institutions. **Frmly:** American Association for Cleft Palate Rehabilitation; (1949) American Academy of Cleft Palate Prosthesis; (1988) American Cleft Palate Association.

★ **4876** ★ **Association for Spina Bifida and Hydrocephalus (ASBAH)**
ASBAH House
42 Park Rd.
Peterborough PE1 2UQ, United Kingdom
**Phone:** 44 1733 555988          **Fax:** 44 1733 555985
**Email:** postmaster@asbah.org
**Website:** http://www.asbah.org

**Fnded:** 1966. **Nat'l Groups:** 1. **Reg. Groups:** 4. **Desc:** Provides help and information to individuals/ families with spina bifida and/or hydrocephalus in England, Wales and Northern Ireland; trained advisers visit families; team of specialist advisers in continence, education, mobility etc. Organises study days for professionals and families. Produces factsheets and magazines. **Pub:** *LINK*, bimonthly.

★ **4877** ★ **Avenues, National Support Group for Arthrogryposis Multiplex Congenita**
c/o Mary Anne Schmidt
PO Box 5093
Sonora, CA 95370
**Phone:** (209)928-3688          **Free:** 888-SONNET-1
**Fax:** (209)533-9778
**Email:** avenues@sonnet.com
**Website:** http://www.sonnet.com/avenues/
Mary Anne Schmidt, Dir.

**Fnded:** 1980. **Mem:** 1,200. **Desc:** Individuals with arthrogryposis multiplex congenita (AMC), their families and friends, and interested professionals. (AMC, a birth defect, is a muscle and/or nerve syndrome affecting some or all of the body's limbs.) Purpose is to share positive attitudes and selfhelp ideas for the handicapped and for all who deal with them. **Pub:** *Avenues*, semiannual. Newsletter. Lists doctors and families interested in corresponding with others about arthrogryposis. *Price:* Included in membership dues; $10 annual donation requested for members in U.S.; $15 annual donation requested for members outside U.S. • Audiotapes. • Bibliography. • Pamphlet.*Price:* $1. • Also a $3.00 Resource Packet for Doctors, Therapists, Pen Pals Families, Clinics, Support Groups.

★ **4878** ★ **Beckwith-Wiedemann Support Network (BWSN)**
2711 Colony Rd.
Ann Arbor, MI 48104
**Phone:** (734)973-0263          **Free:** 800-837-2976
**Fax:** (734)973-9721
**Email:** a800bwsn@aol.com
**Website:** http://www.beckwith-wiedemann.org
Susan Fettes, Pres.

**Fnded:** 1989. **Mem:** 500. **Desc:** Patients with Beckwith-Wiedemann Syndrome and their families; health care professionals; interested others. Works to provide information and peer support to individuals and families affected by Beckwith-Wiedemann Syndrome (BWS). (BWS is a congenital growth-related disorder. Patients are at risk for developing hypoglycemia and various tumors.) Seeks to increase public and professional awareness of BWS. Encourages research on the cause, early detection, and treatment of BWS as well as Simpson Golabi-Belomel Syndrome. **Pub:** *Beckwith Wiedeman Support Network Newsletter*, 3/ year. Newsletter. • *Family Directory for Parent Members*. Directory. • *What Is Beckwith-Wiedemann Syndrome*. Brochure.

★ **4879** ★ **Birth Defect Research for Children**
930 Woodcock Rd., Ste. 225
Orlando, FL 32803
**Phone:** (407)895-0802          **Fax:** (407)895-0824
**Email:** abdc@birthdefects.org
**Website:** http://www.birthdefects.org
Betty Mekdeci, Exec. Dir.

**Fnded:** 1982. **Desc:** Parents, health professionals, educators, members of Congress, hospitals, libraries, organizations and services for the handicapped, and individuals united to prevent birth defects, especially those associated with drugs, chemicals, radiation, and other environmental substances. Provides parents, educators, and professionals in medical- and health-related fields with information on birth defects and research in prosthetics. Acts as a support group for those afflicted with birth defects and offers help in adjusting to the problems faced by individuals with physical malformations. Seeks to inform the medical community and the public about the risk involved with prenatal environmental exposures. Conducts studies and compiles statistics. Monitors and takes part in legislative activities; sponsors petitions. Sponsors National Birth Defect Registry and parent match-up service. Accesses data from world medical literature. **Pub:** *Association of Birth Defect Children–Newsletter*, quarterly. Provides information on environmental causes of birth defects and services for the handicapped. *Price:* Donation requested. • *Birth Defects News*, quarterly. Newsletter. Includes parent-to-parent column and a birth defects registry. *Price:* Free with membership. • *Why My Child?*. Videos. **Frmly:** (1982) Association of Benedictin Children; (2000) Association of Birth Defect Children.

### ★ 4880 ★ Cleft Lip and Palate Association (CLPA)

235-237 Finchley Rd., 3rd Fl.
London NW3 6LS, United Kingdom
**Phone:** 44 20 74310033     **Fax:** 44 20 74318881
**Email:** info@clapa.com
**Website:** http://www.clapa.mcmail.com/
**Fnded:** 1979. **Reg. Groups:** 60. **Lang(s):** English. **Desc:** Local groups comprising parents of children with cleft lips or palates and health care professionals. Seeks to improve treatment of cleft lips and palates; promotes an improved quality of life for children with cleft lips and palates. Provides support to children with cleft lips and palates and their parents; supports research into the causes and treatment of cleft lips and palates; conducts educational programs; undertakes fundraising campaigns. Maintains specialist service for parents having difficulty feeding children with cleft lips or palates. **Pub:** Pamphlets.

### ★ 4881 ★ Cleft Palate Foundation

104 S Estes Dr., Ste. 204
Chapel Hill, NC 27514-2866
**Phone:** (919)933-9044     **Free:** 800-242-5338
**Fax:** (919)933-9604
**Email:** cleftline@aol.com
**Website:** http://www.cleftline.org
Nancy C. Smythe, Exec. Dir.
**Fnded:** 1973. **Desc:** Enhances the quality of life for individuals with facial birth defects through education, research support, and facilitation of family-centered care. Provides research programs and information services. **Pub:** *Cleft Lip and Cleft Palate: The First Four Years*. Booklet. *Price:* $2.00. • *Cleft Lip and Cleft Palate - The School-Aged Child*. Booklet. *Price:* $2.00. • *For Parents of Newborn Babies with Cleft Lip/Palate*. Brochure. *Price:* $.25. • *The Genetics of Cleft Lip and Palate: Information for Families*. Booklet. *Price:* $2.00. • *Information About Choosing a Cleft Palate or Craniofacial Team*. *Price:* Free. • *Information About Crouzon's Disease*. *Price:* Free. • *Information About Dental Care*. *Price:* Free. • *Information About Financial Assistance*. *Price:* Free. • *Information About Pierre Robin Malformation Sequence*. *Price:* Free. • *Information About Submucous Cleft Palate*. *Price:* Free. • *Information About Teacher Collins Syndrome*. *Price:* Free. • *Information About Treatment for Adults with Cleft Lip and Palate*. *Price:* Free. • *Information for the Teenager Born with a Cleft Lip and/or Palate*. Booklet. *Price:* 2.00. **Frmly:** (2000) American Cleft Palate Educational Foundation.

### ★ 4882 ★ Cornelia de Lange Syndrome Foundation (CdLSF)

302 W Main St., No. 100
Avon, CT 06001
**Phone:** (860)676-8166     **Free:** 800-223-8355
**Fax:** (860)676-8337
**Email:** info@cdlsusa.org

**Website:** http://www.cdlsusa.org
Julie Mairano, Exec. Dir.
**Fnded:** 1977. **Mem:** 5,000. **Desc:** Cornelia de Lange Syndrome is a rare birth defect thought to be genetic in origin. A child with this syndrome develops mentally and physically, at a slower rate. The CDLS foundation seeks to ensure early and accurate diagnosis of the syndrome and to enable families, friends, and professionals to make informed decisions and plans for the affected person. Provides updates on the medical aspects of CdLS and responds to correspondences and members' inquiries on an individual basis. Support research programs. **Pub:** *CdLS Foundation - Album*, periodic. Yearbook. Lists families and professionals interested in providing mutual support. *Price:* $25. • *Facing the Challenges: A Parent's Guide to CdLS*. Book. • *Facts about Cornelia de Lange Syndrome*. Pamphlet. • *Reaching Out*, bimonthly. Newsletter. Provides articles of general interest dealing with the complexities of raising a handicapped child. Includes medical column. • Videos. **Frmly:** (1981) Cornelia de Lange Parents Group.

### FACES: The National Craniofacial Association

*See:* Entry 7986

### ★ 4883 ★ Forward Face

317 E 34th St.. Ste. 901A
New York, NY 10016
**Phone:** (212)684-5860     **Free:** 800-FWD-FACE
**Fax:** (212)684-5864
**Email:** faces@faces-cranio.org
**Website:** http://www.forwardface.org/
Pam D'Elia, Admin. Coor.
**Fnded:** 1978. **Mem:** 900. **State Groups:** 1. **Desc:** Individuals with craniofacial disorders, their families and friends, and health care professionals. Provides medical, psychological, and financial support services. Facilitates communication and cooperation between patients and health care professionals; operates referral service. Offers workshops; conducts networking activities and children's services; Also includes a support group, Inner Faces, specifically for teenagers and young adults; activities include communications workshops theatre productions and social functions. Operates family assistance fund to assist families with expenses not covered by insurance, such as lodging and transportation. **Pub:** *Face Facts*. Videos. • *Forward Face Newsletter*, quarterly. Videos. *Price:* Included in membership. • *Forward Face Newsletter*, quarterly. Newsletter. *Price:* $20/year. • *My Face*, book about a child with Mobius Syndrome.

### ★ 4884 ★ Freeman-Sheldon Parent Support Group (FSPSG)

509 E Northmont Way
Salt Lake City, UT 84103-3324
**Phone:** (801)364-7060
**Email:** fspsg@aol.com
**Website:** http://www.fspsg.org
Joyce Dolcourt, Exec. Dir.
**Fnded:** 1982. **Mem:** 150. **Desc:** Families affected by Freeman-Sheldon Syndrome; interested health professionals. (Freeman-Sheldon Syndrome, also known as Whistling Face Syndrome and Cranio-Carpo-Tarsal Dysplasia, is a disorder characterized by a flat, stiff, immobile face with excessively bulging cheeks, resembling that seen when whistling; retarded growth, flexion contraction of the fingers and thumbs, walking difficulties, and speech impairment may also be experienced. The syndrome is believed to be transmitted genetically.) Compiles information on the growth and development of individuals with Freeman-Sheldon Syndrome; disseminates information for parents of afflicted children. Operates referral services; promotes medical research. **Pub:** *FSPSG Newsletter*, annual. Newsletter. Updates members on research and news. • Also publishes brochures. Bibliography of Medical Literature on Freeman-Sheldon syndrome.

### ★ 4885 ★ International Federation of Teratology Societies (IFTS)

Department of Anatomy & Developmental Biology
St. George's Hospital
Medical School
University of London
London SW17 0RE, United Kingdom
**Phone:** 44 208 725830     **Fax:** 44 208 6727098
**Email:** ifts@sghms.ac.uk
**Website:** http://www.ifts-atlas.org
**Fnded:** 1983. **Mem:** 2,600. **Reg. Groups:** 4. **Lang(s):** English. **Desc:** Individuals from the European Teratology Society, Teratology Society, Japanese Teratology Society, and Australian Teratology Society. Fosters international cooperation, increased understanding, and a greater interest in the global aspects of teratology. (Teratology is the study of congenital malformations and serious deviations from normal characteristics.) Encourages information exchange and collaboration with health and charitable agencies. Provides education to organizations and individuals interested in prevention and treatment of birth defects. Supports research in the area of teratology.

### ★ 4886 ★ Irish Association for Spina Bifida and Hydrocephalus (IASBH)

Old Nangor Rd.
Clandalkin
Dublin 22, Ireland
**Phone:** 353 1 4572329     **Fax:** 353 1 4572328
**Lang(s):** English, Irish. **Desc:** Individuals and organizations. Seeks to improve the quality of life of people with spina bifida or hydrocephalus and their families. Makes available support and services; conducts educational and advocacy campaigns.

### ★ 4887 ★ IVH Parents (IVHP)

PO Box 56-1111
Miami, FL 33256-1111
**Phone:** (305)232-0381     **Fax:** (305)232-9890
Ronnie Londner, Dir.
**Fnded:** 1984. **Mem:** 400. **Desc:** Parents of children with intraventricular hemorrhage; health care professionals. (Intraventricular hemorrhage is an intracerebral hemorrhage that can occur in an infant after premature or traumatic birth. Potential effects are hydrocephalus, cerebral palsy, sensory loss, seizures, mental retardation, and multiple handicaps.) Provides support services including information on development needs of IVH children. Conducts follow-ups; maintains speakers' bureau. Compiles statistics. **Pub:** *IVH Parents Newsletter*, periodic. Newsletter.

### ★ 4888 ★ March of Dimes Birth Defects Foundation (MDBDF)

1275 Mamaroneck Ave.
White Plains, NY 10605
**Phone:** (914)428-7100     **Free:** 888-663-4637
**Fax:** (914)428-8203
**Website:** http://www.modimes.org/publicaffairs/contact.cfm
Dr. Jennifer L. Howse, Pres.
**Fnded:** 1938. **Reg. Groups:** 3. **State Groups:** 60. **Desc:** Founded by President Franklin D. Roosevelt as the National Foundation for Infantile Paralysis. Promotes prevention of birth defects by focusing on maternal and child health issues including low birthweight, infant mortality, prenatal care, and maternal substance abuse. Offers public and professional health education and community service programs to improve maternal and newborn health. Works with other national and local organizations to initiate and implement community programs of prenatal care education and service. Operates Campaign for Healthier Babies to support research and educational programs. Develops and distributes educational materials for health professionals and the public. **Frmly:** (1958) National Foundation for Infantile Paralysis; (1979) National Foundation - March of Dimes.

### National Disability Sports Alliance (NDSA)

*See:* Entry 14074

**★ 4889 ★ Nevus Network**
c/o The Congenital Nevus Support Group
PO Box 305
West Salem, OH 44287
**Phone:** (419)853-4525
**Email:** info@nevusnetwork.org
**Website:** http://www.nevusnetwork.org
BJ Bett, Co-Founder

**Fnded:** 1983. **Mem:** 900. **Reg. Groups:** 6. **Desc:** Works to support people with a large congenital nevus (large brown birth marks). Offers pen pals and information. **Pub:** *Nevus Network News*, periodic. Newsletter. *Price:* None. • Brochure.

**★ 4890 ★ Organization of Teratology Information Services**
1501 N Campbell
Arizona Poison and Drug Information Center, Rm. 1156
Tucson, AZ 85724
**Phone:** (520)626-3410       **Free:** 888-285-3410
**Fax:** (520)626-5115
**Email:** bdefects@ucsd.edu
**Website:** http://www.otispregnancy.org
Dee Quinn, Pres.

**Fnded:** 1990. **Mem:** 60. **State Groups:** 23. **Desc:** Provides information on teratology. Teratology is the study of agents used during pregnancy and their potential effects on the developing baby. **Pub:** *Fact Sheets*, annual. Report. Sixteen different fact sheets available on website.

**★ 4891 ★ Prader-Willi Syndrome Association (U.S.A.) (PWSAUSA)**
5700 Midnight Pass Rd., Ste. 6
Sarasota, FL 34242
**Phone:** (941)312-0400       **Free:** 800-926-4797
**Fax:** (941)312-0142
**Email:** national@pwsausa.org
**Website:** http://www.pwsausa.org
Janalee Heinemann, Exec. Dir.

**Fnded:** 1975. **Mem:** 3,000. **Nat'l Groups:** 1. **State Groups:** 34. **Desc:** Parents, physicians, educators, dieticians, group homes, and others interested in the Prader-Willi Syndrome, the most common known genetic cause of morbid obesity in children. (The significant manifestations of the syndrome are obesity, short stature, lack of muscle tone, hypogonadism, and central nervous system performance dysfunction.) Works to provide a forum for communication about the syndrome, particularly the means to cope with it; to promote research and the establishment of treatment facilities. **Pub:** *Gathered View*, bimonthly. Newsletter. Provides information on education, learning problems, and new resources for individuals with PWS. Includes book reviews and research updates. *Price:* Included in membership dues. • *Management of Prader-Willi Syndrome*. Book. • Handbooks.For parents. • Also publishes information packets and produces videos. **Frmly:** (1977) Prader-Willi Syndrome Parents and Friends; (1992) Prader-Willi Syndrome Association; (1998) Prader-Willi Syndrome Association U.S.A; (2002) PWSA USA.

**★ 4892 ★ Pull-Thru Network (PTN)**
2312 Savoy St.
Hoover, AL 35226-1528
**Phone:** (205)978-2930
**Email:** pullthru@bellsouth.net
**Website:** http://www.pullthrough.org/
Bonnie McElroy, Pres.

**Fnded:** 1988. **Mem:** 550. **Desc:** Families, individuals, and professionals dedicated to children born with congenital defects of the lower intestine. Provides support to parents of children who've had or will have a "pull-through" type of surgery to correct a congenital defect such as imperforate anus, or Hirsch sprung's disease, or any other conditions which may require an ostomy or cause bladder or bowel incontinence. Conducts educational programs. Affiliated with the United Ostomy Association. **Pub:** *Pull-Thru Network News*, quarterly. Newsletter.

**Reach Ireland (RI)**
*See:* Entry 5748

**★ 4893 ★ Rubinstein-Taybi Parent Group U.S.A. (RTSPG)**
PO Box 146
Smith Center, KS 66967
**Phone:** (785)697-2989       **Free:** 888-447-2989
**Fax:** (785)697-2985
**Email:** lbaxter@ruraltel.net
**Website:** http://www.rubinstein-taybi.org
Lorrie Baxter, Coord.

**Fnded:** 1984. **Mem:** 380. **Desc:** Families with children diagnosed with Rubinstein-Taybi Syndrome. Provides information and support. **Pub:** *Rubinstein-Taybi Syndrome*. Brochure. **AKA:** RTS Parent Group U.S.A.

**★ 4894 ★ Scottish Spina Bifida Association (SSBA)**
190 Queensferry Rd.
Edinburgh EH4 2BW, United Kingdom
**Phone:** 44 131 3320743       **Fax:** 44 131 3433651
**Email:** gail@ssba.org.uk
**Website:** http://www.ssba.org.uk

**Fnded:** 1965. **Mem:** 3,000. **Reg. Groups:** 5. **Local Groups:** 4. **Desc:** Seeks to increase public awareness and understanding of individuals with Spina Bifida/Hydrocephalus and allied disorders. Aims to secure provision for their special needs and those of their families.

**★ 4895 ★ Society for Research into Hydrocephalus and Spina Bifida (SRHSB)**
11 Linwood Grove
Darlington
Durham DL3 8DP, United Kingdom
**Phone:** 44 1325 465033       **Fax:** 44 1325 465033
**Email:** maureensrhsb@btinternet.com
**Website:** http://www.demon.co.uk/charities/srhsb

**Fnded:** 1957. **Mem:** 284. **Lang(s):** English. **Desc:** Nursing, psychology, social work, scientific, and medical professionals from 29 countries with a common interest in hydrocephalus (an abnormal accumulation of fluid in the cranium) and spina bifida (a defect in the closing of the bony spinal canal). Object is to advance education and research on hydrocephalus and spina bifida. Brings together members to aid them in their endeavors to prevent, cure, and alleviate the conditions. **Pub:** *Zeitschrift fur Kinder Chirurgie*, annual. Journal.

**★ 4896 ★ Spina Bifida Association of America (SBAA)**
4590 MacArthur Blvd. NW, Ste. 250
Washington, DC 20007-4226
**Phone:** (202)944-3285       **Free:** 800-621-3141
**Fax:** (202)944-3295
**Email:** sbaa@sbaa.org
**Website:** http://www.sbaa.org
Cindy Brownstein, CEO

**Fnded:** 1972. **Mem:** 6,000. **Local Groups:** 75. **Desc:** Individuals with spina bifida; their parents, relatives, and friends; concerned professionals. (Spina bifida, or "open spine," is the second most common disabling birth defect and results in muscle weakness or paralysis and incontinence. Its cause is unknown and there is no complete cure.) Purposes are to: develop an information service of materials relating to spina bifida; conduct research into the causes of the birth defect; improve vocational training of individuals with spina bifida; monitor development of legislation applying to disabled persons. Promotes public awareness and action through national media; provides referral services; participates in appropriate legislative activities; holds seminars on scientific, social, medical, and educational programs. Provides training of competent personnel to aid in the treatment, care, education, adjustment, and rehabilitation of individuals with spina bifida. **Pub:** *Insights*, bimonthly. Booklets. • *Spina Bifida Insights*, bimonthly. Newsletter. Reports on the developments in medicine, education, and legislation

affecting the problems and needs of persons with spina bifida. *Price:* Included in membership dues; $25/year for nonmembers; $40/year for professionals; $50/year outside U.S. • Pamphlets. • Reports.

**Sturge-Weber Foundation (SWF)**
*See:* Entry 14121

**United Cerebral Palsy Associations (UCP)**
*See:* Entry 14127

# Research Centers

**★ 4897 ★ Lancaster Cleft Palate Clinic**
223 N Lime St.
Lancaster, PA 17602
**Phone:** (717)396-7415       **Fax:** (717)396-7409
**Email:** relong@lha.org
**Website:** http://www.ucp.org
Dr. Ross E. Long, Jr., Dir.

**Activities/Fields:** Plastic surgery, dentistry, orthodontics, prosthodontics, craniofacial morphology, speech, hearing, otolaryngology, genetics, and behavioral science, particularly in regard to children with craniofacial anomalies. Conducts interdisciplinary study of problems of oral/facial growth, orthognathic surgery, and communicative disorders. **Frmly:** H.K. Cooper Clinic.

**★ 4898 ★ University of Florida Craniofacial Center**
JHMHC
PO Box 100424
Gainesville, FL 32610-0424
**Phone:** (352)846-0801       **Fax:** (352)846-1539
**Email:** williams@dental.ufl.edu
Dr. W.N. Williams, Dir.

**Activities/Fields:** Studies the efficacy of specific surgical, prosthetic, and health-related professional management and therapy procedures in the early treatment of cleft palate and related craniofacial anomalies; prevention of communicative disorders in children from birth to three years; relationship between craniofacial abnormalities, speech, and hearing disorders; studies on craniofacial, cleft lip, and palate surgery; facial growth and disfigurement; psychological effects of craniofacial disfigurement; and the efficacy of a coordinated, interdisciplinary, team approach in health care delivery. Maintains records on clinical research and graduate or professional education within the three colleges. **Pub:** *Communicative Disorders Related to Cleft Lip and Palate*.

**★ 4899 ★ University of Illinois at Chicago Craniofacial Center**
811 S Paulina, 1st Fl.
Chicago, IL 60612-7308
**Phone:** (312)996-7546       **Fax:** (312)413-1157
**Email:** dreisber@uic.edu
Dr. David J. Reisberg, Dir.

**Activities/Fields:** Craniofacial biology, growth, and genetics, including mechanisms of cleft palate and psychological and speech development of children with cleft palate and other craniofacial anamolies. **Pub:** *Journal articles*. Journal.

**★ 4900 ★ University of Iowa Birth Defects and Genetic Disorders Unit**
Pediatrics, 440 EMRB
Iowa City, IA 52242
**Phone:** (319)335-6898
**Email:** val-sheffield@uiowa.edu
Val Sheffield, Dir.

**Activities/Fields:** Causes, prevention, and treatment of birth defects and genetic disorders. Coordinates University clinical service programs and related educational programs throughout the state of Iowa with afflicted individuals. Service and research fields include biochemical and molecular genetics, teratology, dysmorphology, genetic counseling, management of inborn errors of metabolism, epidemiology of birth defects and genetic screening, and neuromuscular disorders.

**★ 4901 ★ University of Iowa**
**Cleft Palate Research Center**
Otolaryngology, 21200 PFP
200 Hawkins Dr.
Iowa City, IA 52242

**Phone:** (319)356-2292    **Fax:** (319)356-6739
**Email:** michael-karnell@uiowa.edu
Michael P. Karnell, Contact

**Activities/Fields:** Cleft lip and palate and related disorders. Research is focused on maxillofacial growth, surgery, speech pathology, speech physiology, and neuropsychology.

**★ 4902 ★ University of Pittsburgh**
**Cleft Palate-Craniofacial Center**
Sch. of Dental Medicine
317 Salk Hall

3501 Terrace St.
Pittsburgh, PA 15261
**Phone:** (412)648-8400    **Free:** 800-408-7390
**Fax:** (412)648-8404
**Website:** http://www.cpc.pitt.edu
Dr. Michael Buckley, Dir.

**Activities/Fields:** Cleft palate, cleft lip, and craniofacial anomalies, including interdisciplinary, basic, clinical, genetic, embryological, and teratology studies. Also studies ear diseases, velopharyngeal valving, laryngeal characteristics and motor control for speech, computer reconstruction of nasal capsule, and anatomy of pharyngeal walls.

## Foundations & Other Funding Organizations

### Other Funding Organizations

★ **4903** ★ **American Burn Association (ABA)**
c/o National Headquarters Office
625 N Michigan Ave., Ste. 1530
Chicago, IL 60611
**Phone:** (312)642-9260    **Free:** 800-548-2876
**Fax:** (312)642-9130
**Email:** info@ameriburn.org
**Website:** http://www.ameriburn.org
Jeffrey R. Saffle, MD, Pres.
**Desc:** Physicians, nurses, physical therapists, occupational therapists, dietitians, biomedical engineers, social service workers, and researchers interested in the care of burn injuries. Objective is the improvement of the care and treatment of burns, which includes a program of prevention of burn injuries. Sponsors visiting professorship, education, and awards. **Awards:** Burn Prevention Award for contributions having worldwide, nationwide, or statewide impact; contributions at a local level serving as a model prevention effort; collection and reporting of epidemiological data; or for individuals who have shaped the careers of others; Carl A. Moyer Resident Award for the best paper submitted by a medical doctor who has not yet completed his/her formal training; Curtis P. Artz Distinguished Service Award (annual) for a nonphysician member of the ABA for his/her outstanding contributions in the burn field; Education Exchange Program for OT's, PT's, RN's, and other nonphysician individuals to visit another (or other) burn center; Everett Idris Evans Memorial Lecture Award for an outstanding scientist in the burn field outside the U.S.; Harvey Stuart Allen Distinguished Service Award for an outstanding U.S. scientist for his/her contributions in the burn field; International Association of Fire Fighters Burn Foundation Research Grant for burn-injury related research; Presidents Continuing Education Grant for an ABA member other than a physician who has made significant contributions to the care of burned patients; Robert A. Lindberg Award for the best scientific paper submitted by a nonphysician; Travelling Fellowship Award (annual) for a physician or postdoctoral fellow who has given evidence of a continuing interest and productivity in the field of burn care, teaching, and/or research; Visiting Professor Program for a physician, educator, or specialist to visit a specified school, hospital, or community and present his/her expertise in the burn field.

## National & International Organizations

★ **4904** ★ **American Burn Association (ABA)**
c/o National Headquarters Office
625 N Michigan Ave., Ste. 1530
Chicago, IL 60611
**Phone:** (312)642-9260    **Free:** 800-548-2876
**Fax:** (312)642-9130
**Email:** info@ameriburn.org
**Website:** http://www.ameriburn.org
Jeffrey R. Saffle, MD, Pres.
**Fnded:** 1967. **Mem:** 3,500. **Desc:** Physicians, nurses, physical therapists, occupational therapists, dietitians, biomedical engineers, social service workers, and researchers interested in the care of burn injuries. Objective is the improvement of the care and treatment of burns, which includes a program of prevention of burn injuries. Sponsors visiting professorship, education, and awards. **Pub:** *American Burn Association–Book of Abstracts*, annual. Journal. *Price:* Included in membership dues; $15/copy for nonmembers. • *American Burn Association–Membership Directory*, annual. Directory. *Price:* Included in membership dues. • *Burn Care Services in North America*, annual. Directory. Lists specialized burn care facilities in the United States and Canada. *Price:* Included in membership dues; $50/copy for nonmembers. • *Journal of Burn Care and Rehabilitation*, bimonthly. Journal. Covers burn injuries and their treatment. Includes a list of employment opportunities, research reports, and statistics. *Price:* Included in membership dues; $35/year for nonmembers; $52/year for institutions.

★ **4905** ★ **British Burn Association**
BBA Secretariat
PO Box 74
Morpeth NE65 8YT, United Kingdom
**Phone:** 44 1670 788475    **Fax:** 44 1670 788475

★ **4906** ★ **Burns United Support Groups (BUSG)**
PO Box 36416
Detroit, MI 48236
**Phone:** (313)881-5577    **Fax:** (313)417-8702
**Email:** burnsunited@hotmail.com
Donna Schneck, Exec. Officer
**Fnded:** 1986. **Mem:** 150. **Nat'l Groups:** 2. **Reg. Groups:** 4. **State Groups:** 4. **Local Groups:** 3. **Desc:** Burn survivors and their families. Provides support services and information on burn care and prevention. Conducts educational programs and childrens' services. Operates speakers' bureau.

**Canadian Association of Burn Nurses (CABN)**
*See:* Entry 15677

★ **4907** ★ **Canadian Burn Survivors Association (BSA)**
c/o Ross Tilley Burn Centre
Sunnybrook & Women's College Health Centre
247 Willow St.
Truro, NS, Canada B2N 5A3
**Website:** http://cburnsa.netfirms.com
**Lang(s):** English, French. **Desc:** People who have suffered burns. Seeks to improve the quality of life of burn survivors. Facilitates communication among members; makes available support and services to burn survivors.

★ **4908** ★ **European Burns Association (EBA)**
Akademisch Ziekenhius Sint-Pieter
Katholiek Universiteit
3000 B-Leuven, Belgium

★ **4909** ★ **International Society for Burn Injuries (ISBI)**
c/o Naoki Aikawa, M.D.
Keio University Hospital
35 Shinanomachi
Shinjuku-Ku
Tokyo 160-8582, Japan
**Fax:** 81 3 32269877
**Fnded:** 1965. **Mem:** 1,820. **Lang(s):** English. **Desc:** Physicians, surgeons, nurses, scientists, and other interested medical and non-medical personnel who are engaged in the care and research of burns. Seeks to disseminate knowledge and stimulate prevention in the field of burns. Promotes and coordinates scientific, clinical, and social research in burns; promotes first aid, nursing, and other types of education in all phases of burn care. **Pub:** *BURNS*, 8/year. Journal. • Membership Directory, annual.

★ **4910** ★ **National Burn Victim Foundation (NBVF)**
PO Box 409
Basking Ridge, NJ 07920
**Phone:** (908)953-9091    **Fax:** (908)953-9099
**Email:** natlbvf@nac.net
Harry J. Gaynor, Exec. Dir.
**Fnded:** 1974. **Nat'l Groups:** 1. **Reg. Groups:** 2. **State Groups:** 1. **Desc:** Supporters are physicians specializing in burn treatment and care, fire services prevention personnel, nurses, communications experts, health and chemical industry representatives, and others interested in burn treatment and care. Maintains 24-hour emergency burn referral service. Conducts medical emergency burn care seminars and workshops for physicians, nurses, EMTs, and emergency rescue personnel. Operates Medical Disaster Response System, which utilizes private helicopters for transporting medical teams to disaster sites where large numbers of survivors have been tramatized. Collects burn data from New Jersey hospitals daily. Program currently provides direct professional services in New Jersey and information and referral services nationally. Offers consultation and evaluation services to the Division of Youth and Family Services

and law enforcement agencies in cases involving suspected child abuse or neglect by burning. Presents burn awareness and prevention programs to schools, civic organizations, and day-care centers. Maintains speakers' bureau; conducts specialized education, children's services, and research programs; compiles statistics. **Pub:** *Burn Awareness.* Pamphlets. • *Child Abuse? Think Again.* Video. *Price:* $125. • *Disaster Medical Response.* Video. *Price:* $29.95. • *General Burn Awareness.* Video. • *Training Professionals - Child Abuse/Neglect Investigation.* Video. • Also publishes The Use of Forensics in the Investgation of Burn Injuries.

### ★ 4911 ★ National Institute for Burn Medicine (NIBM)

PO Box 15138
Ann Arbor, MI 48106-5138
**Phone:** (734)769-9000          **Fax:** (734)769-9009
Claudella A. Jones, Dir.

**Fnded:** 1968. **Desc:** Participants are dedicated to preventing burn injuries; improving the survival rate of and developing the quality of life for burn victims. Provides consultation for development of specialized burn care facilities; prevention programs and materials; education, information, and statistics in burn treatment and care. Maintains International Burn Library containing over 35,000 citations. **Pub:** Books. • Brochures. • Films. • Also publishes poster. **Frmly:** (1968) American Burn Research Corporation; (1971) Institute for Burn Medicine.

### ★ 4912 ★ Phoenix Society for Burn Survivors (PSBS)

2153 Wealthy St. SE, No. 215
East Grand Rapids, MI 49506
**Phone:** (616)458-2773          **Free:** 800-888-2876
**Fax:** (616)458-2831
**Email:** info@phoenix-society.org
**Website:** http://www.phoenix-society.org
Amy Acton, RN, Exec. Dir.

**Fnded:** 1977. **Mem:** 7,500. **Local Groups:** 340. **Desc:** Selfhelp service organization for burn survivors and their families. Works to ease the psychosocial adjustment of severely burned and disfigured persons during and after hospitalization so they may return to normal and satisfactory lives within their communities. Former burn survivors work as volunteers on a one-to-one basis with other burn survivors and their families. Offers a training program for volunteers; seeks to educate the public about the nature and problems of disfigurement; discourages concealment of disfigurement, which the society believes compounds the difficulty of adjustment; conducts research on psychological ramifications of burn disfigurement and disseminates information on burns and trauma and their treatment. Conducts school programs for burned children returning to classes. Maintains speakers' bureau and contains books on burn recovery, films, and videocassettes. **Pub:** *Audiovisual Materials on Burns, Disfigurement, and Related Subjects*, annual. List of audiovisual materials; includes educational and inspirational materials on coping with burns and disfigurement. *Price:* $10. • *Bibliographic References–Burns in Children*, annual. Bibliography. Lists reading material for the education and inspiration of parents, siblings, and professionals involved wiht burned children. *Price:* $5. • *Coping Strategies for Burn Survivors and Their Families.* • *Guidelines for Burn Volunteers.* • *Phoenix Society Newsletter*, quarterly. Newsletter. Provides news items on burn prevention, cosmetology for burn survivors, and other topics of interest; includes member news and book reviews. *Price:* Included in membership dues; $4/year for nonmembers; $10 outside U.S. **Frmly:** (1991) Phoenix Center.

### Shriners Hospitals for Children

*See:* Entry 11509

---

## Research Centers

### ★ 4913 ★ Shriners Burns Institute

815 Market St.
Galveston, TX 77550-2725
**Phone:** (409)770-6731          **Fax:** (409)770-6919

**Email:** dherndon@sbi.utmb.edu
**Website:** http://www.shrinershq.org/Hospitals/
David N. Herndon, MD, Ch.

**Activities/Fields:** Thermal injuries, wound healing, and scar formation, including treatment of burned children, cardiopulmonary complications, microcirculatory changes, nutritional and metabolic status, epidemiology and ideology of burn injuries, host responsiveness to secondary infections, lung injuries, and long term outcomes.

### ★ 4914 ★ University of Cincinnati Shriners Hospitals for Children— Cincinnati

3229 Burnet Ave.
Cincinnati, OH 45229-3095
**Phone:** (513)872-6206          **Fax:** (513)872-6999
Glenn D. Warden, MD, Dir.

**Activities/Fields:** Burns, including nutrition, infection, coverage (autografts/allografts), conversion (topical antimicrobials), pain, scar formation, and care and treatment of children who have suffered from thermal injuries and resulting problems. **Frmly:** Shriners Burns Institute.

### ★ 4915 ★ University of Michigan Trauma Burn Center

1500 E Medical Center Dr.
Ann Arbor, MI 48109-0033
**Phone:** (734)936-9666          **Fax:** (734)936-9657
Dr. Paul Ta Heri, Div. Ch.

**Activities/Fields:** Clinical research, standards review, and vaccine and plasma preparation to combat growth of gram negative organisms in burns. **Pub:** *International Bibliography on Burns.*

## Federal Government Agencies

**★ 4916 ★ U.S. Department of Health and Human Services**
**National Institutes of Health (NIH)**
**National Heart, Lung, and Blood Institute (NHLBI)**
9000 Rockville Pike
Bethesda, MD 20892
**Phone:** (301)496-2411    **Fax:** (301)402-0818
**Website:** http://www.nhlbi.nih.gov
Claude J.M. Lenfant, MD, Director
**Desc:** NHLBI provides leadership for a national program in diseases of the heart, blood vessels, blood, lungs; sleep disorders; and blood resources. It conducts, fosters, and supports an integrated and coordinated program of basic research, clinical investigations and trials, and observational studies.

## Foundations & Other Funding Organizations

### Private Foundations

**★ 4917 ★ Bugher Foundation**
PO Box 555
Barneveld, NY 13304
**Phone:** (212)896-2580    **Fax:** (212)896-2580
**Email:** dau@daniel-adams.com
Don Adams, Trustee
**Fnded:** 1961. **Philosophy:** The foundation is dedicated to cardiovascular disease research. **Priorities:** *Education:* 23% Supports universities, schools, and medical edu. *International:* 77%. Supports American Heart Association, blood centers, and cardiovascular research. *Note:* Total contributions were made in fiscal 2000. **Typ. Recipients:** Cancer, Emergency/Ambulance Services, Heart, Medical Education, Medical Research, Single-Disease Health Associations, Transplant Networks/Donor Banks. **Geo. Dist:** nationally.

**E. L. Wiegand Foundation**
*See:* Entry 188

**Fannie E. Rippel Foundation**
*See:* Entry 2889

**★ 4918 ★ Harry S. Moss Heart Trust**
PO Box 830241
Bank of America, 19th Floor
Dallas, TX 75283-0242
**Phone:** (214)209-1965
**Email:** rippel@gti.net
**Website:** http://www.fdncenter.org/grantmaker/rippel
Dan Kelly, Trust Officer & Vice President

**Fnded:** 1973. **Philosophy:** The trust provides funds for research, equipment, and buildings for the prevention and cure of heart disease, primarily in Dallas County, TX. **Priorities:** *Environment:* 5%. Supports Young Men's Christian AssociationAs. *International:* 95%. Supports medical research, heart, medical centers, and emergency/ambulance services. *Note:* Contributions made in fiscal 1998. **Typ. Recipients:** Children's Health/Hospitals, Clinics/Medical Centers, Health Organizations, Heart, Hospitals, Hospitals (University Affiliated), Medical Education, Medical Research, Nursing Services, People with Disabilities, Single-Disease Health Associations. **Geo. Dist:** Dallas, TX.

**★ 4919 ★ Nora Eccles Treadwell Foundation**
241 Joaquin Ave.
San Leandro, CA 94577
**Phone:** (415)775-2879
Patricia Canepa, President & Director
**Fnded:** 1962. **Philosophy:** The foundation's principal concerns are medical research, primarily in the areas of cardiovascular disease, diabetes, and arthritis. Currently, its major priority is the Nora Eccles Treadwell Cardiovascular Research and Training Institute at the University of Utah's Medical Center. **Priorities:** *International:* 100%. Supports medical research, primarily cardiovascular, arthritis, and diabetes. Major grant to the University of Utah. *Note:* Total contributions made in 1998. **Typ. Recipients:** Arthritis, Children's Health/Hospitals, Diabetes, Emergency/Ambulance Services, Family Planning, Health Funds, Health Organizations, Health-General, Heart, Hospitals, Hospitals (University Affiliated), Medical Education, Medical Research, Mental Health, People with Disabilities, Prenatal Health Issues, Single-Disease Health Associations. **Geo. Dist:** CA; UT.

**Park Foundation**
*See:* Entry 10052

**★ 4920 ★ Paul Ogle Foundation**
323 East Court Ave.
Box 946
Jeffersonville, IN 47130
**Phone:** (812)282-7566    **Fax:** (812)284-5519
**Email:** rlanum@stites.com
Robert Lanum, Secretary/Managing Director
**Fnded:** 1979. **Philosophy:** The Paul Ogle Foundation focuses on capital improvement projects and one-time projects that fall within the mission and current priorities of the foundation. Scholarship funding goes to colleges in Indiana and Kentucky. Social services, such as youth welfare organizations, are a priority. **Priorities:** *Arts & Humanities:* 8%. Supports historical societies, libraries, and arts funds. *Civic & Public Affairs:* 16%. Supports community foundations, urban parks, zoos, and municipalities. *Education:* 45%. Primarily gives to colleges, universities, and schools. *Environment:* 22%. Funds youth clubs, scouting, and the United Way. *International:* 2%. Funds American Red Cross. *Religion:* 4%. Supports a science center.

*Note:* Total contributions made in 1999. **Typ. Recipients:** Clinics/Medical Centers, Domestic Violence, Emergency/Ambulance Services, Heart, Medical Rehabilitation, People with Disabilities. **Geo. Dist:** IN, Clark County; IN, Floyd County; IN, Harrison County; IN, Scott County; IN, Switzerland County; IN, Washington County.

**Ray C. Fish Foundation**
*See:* Entry 608

### Corporate Foundations

**AEGON U.S.A. Charitable Foundation**
*See:* Entry 800

**Alaska Airlines, Inc.**
*See:* Entry 809

**Allianz Life Insurance Co. of North America**
*See:* Entry 817

**FBW Foundation**
*See:* Entry 7878

**★ 4921 ★ Gordon V. and Helen C. Smith Foundation**
8716 Crider Brook Way
Potomac, MD 20854
**Phone:** (301)469-8597    **Fax:** (301)974-1248
**Email:** donna.hartman@alaskaair.com
**Website:** http://www.allianzlife.com
Gordon Smith, Contact

**Priorities:** *Arts & Humanities:* 1%. *Education:* 52%. Funds higher education. *Environment:* 6%. YMCA receives funding. *Note:* Total contributions made in 1999. **Typ. Recipients:** Heart.

**Warren Alpert Foundation**
*See:* Entry 11470

### Other Funding Organizations

**★ 4922 ★ American College of Angiology (ACA)**
295 Northern Blvd., Ste. 104
Great Neck, NY 11021-4701
**Phone:** (516)466-4055    **Fax:** (516)466-4099
**Email:** aca@collegeofangiology.org
**Website:** http://www.collegeofangiology.org
H. E. Shaftel, MD, Meeting Chm.

**Desc:** Scientists from 27 countries interested in the field of vascular medicine and surgery and dedicated to scientific advancement and continued education in angiology (the study of the circulatory, or vascular system). Seeks to: define, represent, and foster the growth and development of the specialty practice of angiology; improve patient care by advising physicians on recent developments in the field; provide a common forum for the exchange of ideas, technical research, and clinical experiences. Conducts continuing medical education programs. Disseminates original research findings related to cerebrovascular, cardiovascular, and peripheral vascular diseases, diagnostic methods, therapeutic procedures, clinical and laboratory research, and case reports. Holds clinical, diagnostic, and therapeutic symposia and seminars. **Awards:** Young Investigators Award (annual).

### ★ **4923** ★ **American College of Cardiology (ACC)**
9111 Old Georgetown Rd.
Bethesda, MD 20814-1699
**Phone:** (301)897-5400　　　**Free:** 800-253-4636
**Fax:** (301)897-9745
**Email:** exec@acc.org
**Website:** http://www.acc.org
Christine W. McEntee, CEO
**Desc:** Professional society of physicians, surgeons, and scientists specializing in cardiology (heart) and cardiovascular (circulatory) diseases. Operates Heart House Learning Center. Maintains numerous committees. **Awards:** ACC/Bristol-Myers Squibb Affiliate Travel Awards (annual) bestowed to 20 Affiliate-In-Training members of the American College of Cardiology to attend the American College of Cardiology annual scientific session; ACC/Merck Adult Cardiology Research Fellowship Awards bestowed to 6 cardiology trainees enrolled in adult cardiology fellowship training to support advanced research fellowship training in adult cardiology.

### ★ **4924** ★ **American College of Chest Physicians (ACCP)**
3300 Dundee Rd.
Northbrook, IL 60062
**Phone:** (847)498-1400　　　**Free:** 800-343-ACCP
**Fax:** (847)498-5460
**Email:** accp@chestnet.org
**Website:** http://www.chestnet.org
Alvin Lever, Exec. VP/CEO
**Desc:** Professional society of physicians and surgeons specializing in diseases of the chest (heart and lungs). Promotes undergraduate and postgraduate medical education and research in the field. Sponsors forums. Maintains placement service; conducts educational programs. **Awards:** Grant; recognition; scholarship.

### ★ **4925** ★ **American Society of Echocardiography (ASE)**
1500 Sunday Dr., Ste. 102
Raleigh, NC 27607
**Phone:** (919)787-5181　　　**Fax:** (919)787-4916
**Email:** rbarry@asecho.org
**Website:** http://www.asecho.org
Robin L. Barry, Exec. Dir.
**Desc:** Physicians and sonographers specializing in ultrasound heart imaging and diagnosis. Promotes excellence in the ultrasonic examination of the heart and assists in establishing standards for education of physicians and cardiac-sonographers in echocardiography. Sponsors educational activities including distribution of self-testing materials, continuing education calendar, and annual scientific sessions. Maintains liaison with governmental agencies and other professional groups. **Awards:** Outcomes Research Grants (annual); Research Awards (annual).

### ★ **4926** ★ **American Society of Extra-Corporeal Technology (AmSECT)**
503 Carlisle Dr. No. 125
Herndon, VA 20170-4838
**Phone:** (703)435-8556　　　**Fax:** (703)435-0056
**Email:** gcate@amsect.org
**Website:** http://www.amsect.org
George M. Cate, Exec. Dir.
**Desc:** Perfusionists, technologists, doctors, nurses, and others actively employed and using the applied skills relating to the practice of extracorporeal technology (involving heart-lung machines); student members. Disseminates information necessary to the proper practice of the technology. Conducts programs in continuing education and professional-public liaison and hands-on workshops. Maintains placement service. **Awards:** Recognition (annual); Research Grant Award (annual); scholarship.

### ★ **4927** ★ **American Society of Nuclear Cardiology (ASNC)**
9111 Old Georgetown Rd.
Bethesda, MD 20814
**Phone:** (301)493-2360　　　**Fax:** (301)493-2376
**Email:** admin@asnc.org
**Website:** http://www.asnc.org
Steven D. Carter, Exec. Dir.
**Desc:** Physicians, scientists, technologist, biomedical engineers and health care workers. Seeks to foster optimal delivery of nuclear cardiology services and promote research. Provides continuing medical education opportunities; establishes guidelines and standards for training and practice; provides information on licensure requirements. **Awards:** ASNC/Amersham Clinical Research in Nuclear Cardiology (annual).

**Donald W. Reynolds Foundation**
*See:* Entry 2898

**North American Society for Cardiac Imaging (NASCI)**
*See:* Entry 18098

### ★ **4928** ★ **Phlebology Society of America (PSA)**
c/o Denise M. Rossignol, Exec. Dir.
5 Daremy Ct.
Nesconset, NY 11767-1547
**Phone:** (631)366-1429　　　**Fax:** (631)366-3609
**Email:** denisemrossignol@cs.com
**Website:** http://www.nasci.org
Dr. John B. Chang, Bd. Chm.
**Desc:** Physicians and scientists with an interest in phlebitis and other diseases of the vascular system. Seeks to advance the diagnosis and treatment of peripheral vascular disease. Serves as a certifying board for professional phlebologists; functions as a clearinghouse on phlebology; facilitates exchange of information among members. Conducts educational programs. **Awards:** Young Investigator Award (annual) presentation and originality of research.

### ★ **4929** ★ **Pulmonary Hypertension Association (PHA)**
850 Sligo Ave., No. 800
Silver Spring, MD 20910
**Phone:** 800-748-7274　　　**Fax:** (301)565-3994
**Email:** pha@phassociation.org
**Website:** http://www.phassociation.org
Rino Aldrighetti, Exec. Dir.
**Desc:** Patients with pulmonary hypertension (PH) and primary pulmonary hypertension (PPH); families and physicians of patients; researchers. Provides fellowship and educational support for members and the public on PH and PPH, including current research and findings, early detection, resource organizations, organ transplantation, and support networks. Conducts support group meetings. Funds medical research. **Awards:** Outstanding Physician Award (biennial); Outstanding Volunteer Award (biennial); Research Fellowships (annual) proposal.

**Society of Cardiovascular Anesthesiologists (SCA)**
*See:* Entry 4350

**Society of Cardiovascular and Interventional Radiology (SCVIR)**
*See:* Entry 18100

**Society for Clinical Vascular Surgery**
*See:* Entry 19453

**Society of Geriatric Cardiology**
*See:* Entry 2904

# Medical & Allied Health Schools

## Perfusion

*The following perfusion training programs are accredited by the Commission on Accreditation of Allied Health Education Programs, 35 E Wacker Dr., Ste. 1970, Chicago, IL 60601-2208, (312)553-9355, http://www.caahep.org/. For information on careers in this field, contact the American Society of Extra-Corporeal Technology, 503 Carlisle Dr., Ste. 125, Herndon, VA 20170, (703)435-8556, http://www.amsect.org/.*

### Arizona

### ★ **4930** ★ **University of Arizona Department of Cardiothoracic Surgery Perfusion Sciences**
1501 N Campbell Ave., Rm. 4402
Tucson, AZ 85724
**Phone:** (520)626-6339　　　**Fax:** (520)626-4042
**Email:** dflarson@u.arizona.edu
**Website:** http://www.sgcard.org
Douglas Larson, PhD, Contact

### Connecticut

### ★ **4931** ★ **Quinnipiac College Cardiovascular Perfusion Program**
Hamden, CT 06518
**Phone:** (203)288-5251　　　**Fax:** (203)281-8706
**Email:** msmith@quinnipiac.edu
**Website:** http://www.quinnipiac.edu
Michael Smith, PhD, Contact

### District of Columbia

### ★ **4932** ★ **Walter Reed Army Medical Center Cardiovascular Physician Assistant / Perfusion Training Program**
6825 16th St. NW, Bldg. 2, Rm. 4655
Washington, DC 20307-5001
**Phone:** (202)782-4865　　　**Fax:** (202)782-8253
**Email:** mogletree@vs.wramc.amedd.army.mil
James M. Ogletree, Contact

### Florida

### ★ **4933** ★ **Barry University Cardiovascular Perfusion Program**
11300 NE 2nd Ave.
Miami Shores, FL 33161-6695
**Phone:** (305)899-3214　　　**Fax:** (305)899-3845
**Email:** jfreed@buaxpl.barry.edu
**Website:** http://www.barry.edu/snhs/cvp/cvp1/html
Jason Freed, Contact

### Illinois

### ★ **4934** ★ **Rush University College of Health Sciences School of Perfusion Technology**
1653 W Congress Pkwy.
Chicago, IL 60612
**Phone:** (312)942-2305　　　**Fax:** (312)942-4048
**Email:** mdjuric@rush.edu
**Website:** http://www.rushu.rush.edu/perfusion/
Michael Djuric, Contact

## Iowa

**★ 4935 ★ University of Iowa**
**Department of Surgery CT**
**Perfusion Technology Education Program**
1601 JCP
Iowa City, IA 52242
**Phone:** (319)356-8496　　**Fax:** (319)353-7174
**Email:** jean-fobian@uiowa.edu
**Website:** http://www.surgery.uiowa.edu/surgery/ptep/
Scott D. Niles, Director

## Maryland

**★ 4936 ★ Johns Hopkins Hospital**
**School of Perfusion Science**
600 N Wolfe St. / 814 Blalock
Baltimore, MD 21287-4814
**Phone:** (410)955-5168　　**Fax:** (410)955-4163
**Email:** retemad@welchlink.welch.jhu.edu
**Website:** http://www.med/jhu.edu/perfusion/
Roshi Etemad-Moghadam, CCP, Director

## Massachusetts

**★ 4937 ★ Northeastern University**
**Bouve College of Pharmacy and Health**
**Sciences**
**Perfusion Technology Program**
360 Huntington Ave.
Boston, MA 02115
**Phone:** (617)373-3666　　**Fax:** (617)373-2968
**Email:** p.plunkett@nunet.neu.edu
**Website:** http://www.neu.edu/bouvegrad/perf-tech.html
Patrick Plunkett, EdD, Contact

## Nebraska

**★ 4938 ★ University of Nebraska Medical**
**Center**
**Division of Clinical Perfusion Education**
600 S 42nd St.
Omaha, NE 68198-5155
**Phone:** (402)559-7227　　**Fax:** (402)559-6455
**Email:** astammer@unmc.edu
**Website:** http://www.unmc.edu/cpe/
Al Stammers, CCP, Contact

## New Jersey

**★ 4939 ★ Cooper Health System**
**Center for Allied Health**
**School of Perfusion**
1 Cooper Plaza
Box 217
Camden, NJ 08103
**Phone:** (609)342-3277　　**Fax:** (609)584-1833
**Email:** brownstein-lou@cooperhealth.edu
Louis Brownstein, CCP, Contact

## New York

**★ 4940 ★ State University of New York**
**Health Science Center, Syracuse**
**Cardiovascular Perfusion Program**
750 E Adams St.
Syracuse, NY 13210
**Phone:** (315)464-6933　　**Fax:** (315)464-6914
**Email:** searlesb@vax.cs.hscsyr.edu
**Website:** http://www.upstate.edu/chp/
Bruce Searles, CCP, Contact

## Ohio

**★ 4941 ★ Christ Hospital**
**School of Perfusion Science**
2139 Auburn Ave.
Cincinnati, OH 45219
**Phone:** (513)585-1106　　**Fax:** (513)585-3241
**Email:** warmutcr@healthall.com

**Website:** http://www.health-alliance.com/perfusion/
Craig Warmuth, CCP, Contact

**★ 4942 ★ Cleveland Clinic Foundation**
**School of Perfusion**
G-33 One Clinic Center
9500 Euclid Ave.
Cleveland, OH 44195-5001
**Phone:** (216)444-3895　　**Fax:** (216)444-2725
**Email:** moyers@cesmtp.ccf.org
**Website:** http://www.ccf.org/ed/ahcardp.htm
Carolyn Moyers, CCP, Contact

**★ 4943 ★ Ohio State University**
**School of Allied Medical Professions**
**Division of Circulation Technology**
1583 Perry St.
Columbus, OH 43210
**Phone:** (614)292-7261　　**Fax:** (614)292-0210
**Email:** beckley.1@osu.edu
**Website:** http://circ-tech.amp.ohio-state.edu/
Philip Beckley, PhD, Contact

## Oregon

**★ 4944 ★ Saint Vincent Hospital and**
**Medical Center**
**Heart Institute**
**Perfusion Training Program**
9205 SW Barnes Rd.
Portland, OR 97225
**Phone:** (503)297-1419　　**Fax:** (503)291-2488
**Email:** gregory_meiling@phsor.org
**Website:** http://www.phsor.org/oregon/
Gregory Meiling, CCP, Contact

## Pennsylvania

**★ 4945 ★ Allegheny University of the**
**Health Sciences Center**
**City Program in Cardiovascular Perfusion**
**Technology**
Broad and Vine Sts.
Philadelphia, PA 19102-1192
**Phone:** (215)762-7895　　**Fax:** (215)246-5347
**Email:** stroud@auhs.edu
**Website:** http://www.auhs.edu/shp/shpprogs/cardiop-erf.html
Robert Stroud, CCP, Contact
**Frmly:** Allegheny University of the Health Sciences

**★ 4946 ★ Duquesne University**
**John G. Rangos School of Health**
**Sciences**
**Department of Perfusion Technology**
215 Health Science Bldg.
Pittsburgh, PA 15282
**Phone:** (412)396-5555　　**Fax:** (412)396-5554
**Email:** dantonio@duq2.cc.duq.edu
**Website:** http://www.duq.edu/healthsciences/perf/perfhome.html
Joyce D'Antonio, PhD, Contact

**★ 4947 ★ Pennsylvania State University**
**Milton S. Hershey Medical Center**
**CV Perfusion Technology Training**
**Program**
PO Box 850
Hershey, PA 17033
**Phone:** (717)531-8550　　**Fax:** (717)531-4017
**Email:** dwilliam@nursing.vmi.psghs.edu
Dennis R. Williams, CCP, Contact

**★ 4948 ★ University of Pittsburgh**
**Medical Center**
**Shadyside Hospital**
**School of Cardiovascular Perfusion**
5230 Centre Ave.
Pittsburgh, PA 15232

**Phone:** (412)623-2482　　**Fax:** (412)623-1091
**Email:** sborecky@carlow.edu
**Website:** http://www.upmc.edu/Shadyside/default.htm
Robert Rush, CCP, Contact

## South Carolina

**★ 4949 ★ Medical University of South**
**Carolina**
**College of Health Professions**
**ECT Educational Program**
101 Doughty St., 2nd Fl., Rm. 206
Charleston, SC 29401
**Phone:** (843)792-2298　　**Fax:** (843)792-4417
**Email:** suttonr@musc.edu
**Website:** http://www.musc.edu/chp-clin/ect/ect.htm
Robin Sutton, CCP, Contact

## Tennessee

**★ 4950 ★ Vanderbilt University**
**Department of CV Surgery**
**Perfusion Training Program**
Vanderbilt Clinic, Ste. 2986 TVC
Nashville, TN 37232-5734
**Phone:** (615)343-9195　　**Fax:** (615)343-9194
**Email:** James.Ramsey@mcmail.Vanderbilt.Edu
**Website:** http://www.mc.Vanderbilt.Edu/cvpt/
James J. Ramsey, CCP, Contact

## Texas

**★ 4951 ★ Texas Heart Institute**
**Cardiovascular Perfusion Program**
PO Box 20345
MC1-224
Houston, TX 77225
**Phone:** (713)791-4026　　**Fax:** (713)791-4993
**Email:** tstafford@biost1.thi.tmc.edu
**Website:** http://www.tmc.edu/thi/perfuse.html
Raymond McInnis, CCP, Contact

## Wisconsin

**★ 4952 ★ Milwaukee School of**
**Engineering**
**Biomedical Engineering Program**
1025 N Broadway
Milwaukee, WI 53202-3109
**Phone:** (414)277-7209　　**Fax:** (414)277-7465
**Email:** hietpas@msoe.edu
**Website:** http://www.msoe.edu/eecs/be/
Matthew J. Hietpas, CCP, Contact

---

# National & International
# Organizations

**Academy of Veterinary Cardiology (AVC)**
*See:* Entry 20528

**★ 4953 ★ Albanian Society for**
**Cardiology**
c/o University Hospital Centre
Dibra St. 370
Tirana, Albania
**Phone:** 355 42 65154
**Email:** drspit@icc.al.eu.org
**Fnded:** 1994. **Mem:** 106. **Desc:** Cardiologists in
Albania. Fosters research of cardiac diseases. **Pub:**
Journal, quarterly.

**★ 4954 ★ Alliance of Cardiovascular**
**Professionals**
4456 Corporation Ln., No. 120
Virginia Beach, VA 23462
**Phone:** (757)497-1225　　**Fax:** (757)497-0010
**Email:** seanmce@aol.com

**Website:** http://www.acp-online.org/
Peggy McElgunn, Exec. Dir.

**Fnded:** 1967. **Mem:** 3,200. **Desc:** Dedicated to meeting educational needs, developing programs to meet those needs, and providing a structure to offer the cardiovascular and pulmonary technology professional a key to the future as a valuable member of the medical team. Seeks advancement for members through communication and education. Provides coordinated programs to orient the newer professional to his field and continuing educational opportunities for technologist personnel. Has established guidelines for educational programs in the hospital and university setting. Works with educators and physicians to provide basic, advanced, and in-service programs for technologists. Sponsors registration and certification programs which provide technology professionals with further opportunity to clarify their level of expertise. Compiles statistics. **Pub:** *ACP Membership Directory*, annual. Membership Directory. Arranged alphabetically; includes field specialty, geographical location, and chapter affiliation. *Price:* Included in membership dues; $25/year for nonmembers. • *Beat Goes On.* • *CP Digest*, bimonthly. Newsletter. Includes employment opportunity listings, legislative reports, and new member information. *Price:* Included in membership dues; $35/year for nonmembers. • *Heart to Heart.* • *Pulmonary News*, quarterly. • *Strategies.* • Books. • Monographs. **Frmly:** (1980) National Society of Cardiopulmonary Technologists; (1986) National Society for Cardiopulmonary Technology; (1988) National Alliance of Cardiovascular Technologists; (1989) American Cardiology Technologists Association; (1998) American Society of Cardiovascular Professionals/Society for Cardiovascular Management.


★ **4955** ★ **American Association of Cardiovascular and Pulmonary Rehabilitation (AACVPR)**
401 N Michigan Ave., Ste. 2200
Chicago, IL 60611-4267
**Phone:** (312)321-5146          **Fax:** (312)245-1085
**Email:** aacvpr@tmahq.com
**Website:** http://www.aacvpr.org
Susan M. Rees, Exec. Dir.

**Fnded:** 1985. **Mem:** 3,000. **Desc:** Allied health professionals involved in the field of cardiovascular and pulmonary rehabilitation. Fosters the improvement of clinical practice in CVPR; promotes scientific CVPR research; seeks the advancement of CVPR education for health care professionals and the public. **Pub:** *AACVPR Directory*, annual. Directory. • *Directory of Cardiovascular and Pulmonary Rehabilitation Programs*, annual. Directory. • *Journal of Cardiopulmonary Rehabilitation*, bimonthly. Journal. Provides theoretical and practical information on cardiovascular and pulmonary rehabilitation. Includes reviews and calendar of events. *Price:* Included in membership dues; $120/year for nonmembers. • *News and Views of AACVPR*, monthly. Newsletter.


**American Association for Thoracic Surgery (AATS)**
*See:* Entry 19473


★ **4956** ★ **American Board of Cardiovascular Perfusion (ABCP)**
207 N 25th Ave.
Hattiesburg, MS 39401
**Phone:** (601)582-2227          **Fax:** (601)582-2271
**Email:** abcp@abcp.org
**Website:** http://www.abcp.org
Drs. Mark and Beth Richmond, Exec. Dirs.

**Fnded:** 1975. **Mem:** 3,400. **Desc:** Certified clinical perfusionists. Seeks to protect the public through the establishment and maintenance of standards in the field. Has established qualifications for examination and procedures for recertification. Administers annual board examinations.


★ **4957** ★ **American College of Angiology (ACA)**
295 Northern Blvd., Ste. 104
Great Neck, NY 11021-4701
**Phone:** (516)466-4055          **Fax:** (516)466-4099
**Email:** aca@collegeofangiology.org
**Website:** http://www.collegeofangiology.org
H. E. Shaftel, MD, Meeting Chm.

**Fnded:** 1959. **Mem:** 1,700. **Desc:** Scientists from 27 countries interested in the field of vascular medicine and surgery and dedicated to scientific advancement and continued education in angiology (the study of the circulatory, or vascular system). Seeks to: define, represent, and foster the growth and development of the specialty practice of angiology; improve patient care by advising physicians on recent developments in the field; provide a common forum for the exchange of ideas, technical research, and clinical experiences. Conducts continuing medical education programs. Disseminates original research findings related to cerebrovascular, cardiovascular, and peripheral vascular diseases, diagnostic methods, therapeutic procedures, clinical and laboratory research, and case reports. Holds clinical, diagnostic, and therapeutic symposia and seminars. **Pub:** *Angiology*, bimonthly. Journal.


★ **4958** ★ **American College of Cardiology (ACC)**
9111 Old Georgetown Rd.
Bethesda, MD 20814-1699
**Phone:** (301)897-5400          **Free:** 800-253-4636
**Fax:** (301)897-9745
**Email:** exec@acc.org
**Website:** http://www.acc.org
Christine W. McEntee, CEO

**Fnded:** 1949. **Mem:** 26,000. **State Groups:** 37. **Desc:** Professional society of physicians, surgeons, and scientists specializing in cardiology (heart) and cardiovascular (circulatory) diseases. Operates Heart House Learning Center. Maintains numerous committees. **Pub:** *ACC Current Journal Review*, bimonthly. Journal. Provides abstracts and reviews of pertinent clinical articles. *Price:* Included in membership dues; $105 for individuals; $185 for institutions; $60 for interns. • *ACCEL*, monthly. Journal. On audiocassette. Contains 15 to 20 interviews with leaders in the field of cardiovascular medicine. *Price:* $165/year for members; $200/year for nonmembers. • *Affiliates in Training*, bimonthly. Newsletter. Provides information of the association pertinent to the Affiliate-In-Training category. Includes list of employment opportunities. *Price:* Included in membership dues; $20/year for nonmembers. • *Cardiology*, monthly. Newsletter. Contains information on clincal cardiology practice. Covers health care issues, legislative and socioeconomic activities, and education opportunities. *Price:* Included in membership dues; $59/year. • *Journal of the American College of Cardiology*, monthly. Journal. Covers original clinical and experimental papers on cardiovascular disease featuring reports on medical and surgical therapy, and other subjects. *Price:* Included in membership dues; $152/year for nonmember individuals; $236/year for institutions; $92/year for interns, residents, health professionals. • Also publishes self-study materials.


**American College of Cardiovascular Administrators (ACCA)**
*See:* Entry 9692


★ **4959** ★ **American College of Chest Physicians (ACCP)**
3300 Dundee Rd.
Northbrook, IL 60062
**Phone:** (847)498-1400          **Free:** 800-343-ACCP
**Fax:** (847)498-5460
**Email:** accp@chestnet.org
**Website:** http://www.chestnet.org
Alvin Lever, Exec. VP/CEO

**Fnded:** 1935. **Mem:** 15,000. **Desc:** Professional society of physicians and surgeons specializing in diseases of the chest (heart and lungs). Promotes

undergraduate and postgraduate medical education and research in the field. Sponsors forums. Maintains placement service; conducts educational programs. **Pub:** *American College of Chest Physicians Membership Directory*, annual. Membership Directory. Arranged geographically and by specialty. *Price:* Included in membership dues. • *Chest: The Pulmonary and Critical Care Journal*, monthly. Journal. Presents clinical investigations and case reports in cardiopulmonary medical and surgical specialties. Contains author and subject indexes. *Price:* Included in membership dues; $132/year for nonmembers; $162/year for institutions. • Books. • Brochures.On smoking and health, bronchitis, and asthma. • Also publishes self-teaching series on pulmonary and critical care medicine.


★ **4960** ★ **American Heart Association (AHA)**
7272 Greenville Ave.
Dallas, TX 75231-4596
**Phone:** (214)373-6300          **Free:** 800-242-USA1
**Fax:** (214)987-4334
**Website:** http://www.americanheart.org
M. Cass Wheeler, CEO

**Fnded:** 1924. **Mem:** 26,000. **Reg. Groups:** 15. **State Groups:** 56. **Desc:** Physicians, scientists, and laypersons. Supports research, education, and community service programs with the objective of reducing premature death and disability from cardiovascular diseases and stroke; coordinates the efforts of physicians, nurses, health professionals, and others engaged in the fight against heart and circulatory disease. Financed entirely by voluntary contributions of the public, principally during the Heart Campaign held in February. **Pub:** *Arteriosclerosis, Thrombosis, and Vascular Biology*, monthly. Journal. Contains findings of basic and clinical research related to vascular biology and related topics. *Price:* $227/year for individuals; $363/year for institutions. • *Circulation*, weekly. Journal. Covers clinical research, including clinical studies and trials, and advances in cardiovascular medicine. *Price:* $223/year for individuals; $396/year for institutions. • *Circulation Research*, biweekly. Journal. Covers basic cardiovascular research in the areas of biology, biochemistry, biophysics, microbiology, cellular biology, genetics, molecular biology. *Price:* $267/year for individuals; $487/year for institutions. • *Currents in Emergency Cardiac Care*, quarterly. Newsletter. Offers scientific information about ideas, development, and trends in emergency cardiac care; published in conjunction with the Citizen CPR Foundation. *Price:* Free. • *Hypertension*, monthly. Journal. Reports clinical and laboratory investigations in blood pressure regulation and pathophysiological mechanisms underlying the hypertensive diseases. *Price:* $213/year for individuals; $302/year for institutions. • *Stroke–A Journal of Cerebral Circulation*, monthly. Journal. Provides information on the prevention, diagnosis, treatment, and rehabilitation of cerebrovascular disease. *Price:* $213/year for individuals; $299/year for institutions.


**American Society of Echocardiography (ASE)**
*See:* Entry 18114


★ **4961** ★ **American Society of Extra-Corporeal Technology (AmSECT)**
503 Carlisle Dr. No. 125
Herndon, VA 20170-4838
**Phone:** (703)435-8556          **Fax:** (703)435-0056
**Email:** gcate@amsect.org
**Website:** http://www.amsect.org
George M. Cate, Exec. Dir.

**Fnded:** 1964. **Mem:** 3,000. **Reg. Groups:** 11. **Desc:** Perfusionists, technologists, doctors, nurses, and others actively employed and using the applied skills relating to the practice of extracorporeal technology (involving heart-lung machines); student members. Disseminates information necessary to the proper practice of the technology. Conducts programs in continuing education and professional-public liaison and hands-on workshops. Maintains placement service. **Pub:** *AMSECT Today*, 11/year. Magazine. Includes calendar of events, reading and employment opportunities lists, and reports of regional events. *Price:* Included in membership dues; $55/year for nonmembers. • *Journal of Extra-Corporeal Technology*, quarterly. Journal. Covers dialysis, hemodynamics, organs and tissues , oxygenation, and research. Includes book reviews, case studies and membership directory. *Price:* Included in membership dues; $70/year for nonmembers. • Also publishes self-study modules and monographs. **Frmly:** (1968) American Society of Extracorporeal Circulation Technicians.

### ★ 4962 ★ American Society of Hypertension (ASH)
515 Madison Ave., Ste. 1212
New York, NY 10022
**Phone:** (212)644-0650 **Fax:** (212)644-0658
**Email:** ash@ash-us.org
**Website:** http://www.ash-us.org
Torry Mark Sansone, Exec. Dir.

**Fnded:** 1985. **Mem:** 4,000. **Desc:** To organize and conduct educational activities designed to promote and encourage the development, advancement and exchange of scientific information in all aspects of research, diagnosis and treatment of hypertension and related cardiovascular diseases. **Pub:** *American Journal of Hypertension*, monthly. Journal. A peer-review, available in print or online. *Price:* $120. • *ASH Membership Directory*. Membership Directory.

### ★ 4963 ★ American Society of Nuclear Cardiology (ASNC)
9111 Old Georgetown Rd.
Bethesda, MD 20814
**Phone:** (301)493-2360 **Fax:** (301)493-2376
**Email:** admin@asnc.org
**Website:** http://www.asnc.org
Steven D. Carter, Exec. Dir.

**Fnded:** 1993. **Mem:** 4,100. **Reg. Groups:** 28. **Desc:** Physicians, scientists, technologist, biomedical engineers and health care workers. Seeks to foster optimal delivery of nuclear cardiology services and promote research. Provides continuing medical education opportunities; establishes guidelines and standards for training and practice; provides information on licensure requirements. **Pub:** *Journal of Nuclear Cardiology*, bimonthly. Journal. • Membership Directory, biennial.

### ★ 4964 ★ Armenian Society of Cardiology
Institute of Cardiology
5 P Sevak Sts.
375044 Yerevan, Armenia
**Phone:** 374 2 288550 **Fax:** 374 2 288895
**Email:** sgrigor@ipia.sci.com
**Mem:** 56. **Desc:** Promotes the study of cardiology in Armenia.

### ★ 4965 ★ ASEAN Cardiologists' Federation
Indonesia Heart Association
Rumah Sakit Jantung, Harapan Kita
Jalan Jend
S Parman, Kav. 87
Jakarta, Indonesia
**Lang(s):** English, Indonesian. **Desc:** Cardiologists and health care facilities. Seeks to advance the study, teaching, and practice of cardiology; promotes professional development of cardiologists. Functions as a clearinghouse on cardiology; conducts continuing professional education courses.

### ★ 4966 ★ Asian Pacific Society of Atherosclerosis and Vascular Disease
c/o Department of Endocrinology
Singapore General Hospital
Outram Rd.
Singapore 169608, Singapore
**Phone:** 65 3214654 **Fax:** 65 2273576
**Email:** ce_tan@sgh.gov.sg
**Lang(s):** Chinese, English. **Desc:** Physicians and other health care personnel with an interest in atherosclerosis. Seeks to advance the prevention, diagnosis, and treatment of atherosclerosis; promotes continuing professional development of members. Gathers and disseminates information on atherosclerosis and related diseases; sponsors research and educational programs. **Frmly:** (2000) Asian Pacific Athersclerosis Society.

### ★ 4967 ★ Asian-Pacific Society of Atherosclerosis and Vascular Diseases (APSAVD)
Jen-Ai Rd. 9F-3, No. 33, Section 4
Taipei 106, Taiwan
**Phone:** 886 2 7762260
**Lang(s):** Chinese, English. **Desc:** Physicians and other health care personnel with an interest in atherosclerosis and vascular diseases. Seeks to advance the prevention, diagnosis, and treatment of atherosclerosis; promotes continuing professional development of members. Gathers and disseminates information on atherosclerosis and related diseases; sponsors research and educational programs.

### ★ 4968 ★ Asian-Pacific Society of Cardiology (APSC)
Seoul National University Hospital, Rm. 9603
28 Yunkun-Dong
Chongno-ku
Seoul 110 744, Republic of Korea
**Phone:** 82 2 7602262 **Fax:** 82 2 7438694
**Lang(s):** English, Korean. **Desc:** Cardiologists and other health care professionals and scientists with an interest in cardiology. Seeks to advance cardiological study, teaching, and practice. Serves as a forum for the exchange of information among members; sponsors research programs and continuing professional development courses.

### Asian-Pacific Society of Cardiovascular and Interventional Radiology (APSCIR)
*See:* Entry 18123

### Asian Society of Cardiothoracic Anaesthesia (ASCA)
*See:* Entry 4447

### Asian Society for Cardiovascular Surgery (ASCS)
*See:* Entry 19509

### ★ 4969 ★ Asian Vascular Society (AVS)
Kangnam St. Mary's Hospital
Catholic University Medical College
505 Panp'o-dong
Soch'o-gu
Seoul 137-701, Republic of Korea
**Lang(s):** English, Korean. **Desc:** Physicians and surgeons specializing in the vascular system. Seeks to advance the prevention, diagnosis, and treatment of vascular diseases; promotes development of improved vascular surgical techniques. Facilitates exchange of information among members; sponsors research and continuing professional development programs.

### ★ 4970 ★ Association of Black Cardiologists (ABC)
6849-B2 Peachtree Dunwoody Rd.
Atlanta, GA 30328
**Phone:** (678)302-4222 **Free:** 800-753-9222
**Fax:** (678)302-4223
**Email:** abcardio@abcardio.org
**Website:** http://www.abcardio.org
B. Waine Kong, PhD,JD, CEO
**Fnded:** 1974. **Mem:** 800. **Desc:** Physicians and other health professionals interested in lowering mortality and morbidity resulting from cardiovascular diseases. Seeks to improve prevention and treatment of cardiovascular diseases. Conducts educational and research programs; maintains speakers' bureau. **Pub:** *ABC*, quarterly. Newsletter. *Price:* Free. • *The Digest of Urban Cardiology*, periodic. Journal.

### ★ 4971 ★ Association of Cardiologists of Bosnia & Herzegovina
Udruzenje Kardiologa BIH
Klinica za bolesti srca I reumatizam
Ul Bolnicka 25
Sarajevo, Bosnia-Hercegovina
**Phone:** 387 71 524093 **Fax:** 387 71 524093
**Email:** cardreum@bih.net.ba
**Mem:** 107. **Desc:** Promotes the study of cardiology in Bosnia & Herzegovina. **Pub:** Book. Contains abstracts of papers. • Papers.

### Association of Cardiothoracic Anaesthetists
*See:* Entry 4449

### Association for European Paediatric Cardiology (AEPC)
*See:* Entry 5624

### Association of Physician Assistants in Cardiovascular Surgery (APACVS)
*See:* Entry 19516

### ★ 4972 ★ Association of Professors of Cardiology (APC)
9111 Old Georgetown Rd.
Bethesda, MD 20814-1699
**Phone:** (301)493-2330 **Fax:** (301)897-9745
**Email:** sthayer@cardiologyprofessors.org
**Website:** http://www.cardiologyprofessors.org
Susan C. Thayer, Contact

**Fnded:** 1990. **Mem:** 115. **Desc:** Directors or acting directors of divisions of cardiology in accredited medical schools in the U.S. and Puerto Rico. Conducts educational and scientific programs with respect to cardiology.

### Association for Research in Vascular Surgery (ARVS) (Association de Recherche en Chirurgie Vasculaire — ARCV)
*See:* Entry 19518

### ★ 4973 ★ Austrian Society of Cardiology
p.A. Universitatsklinik fur Innere Medizin II
Abteilung fur Kardiologie
Wahringer Gurtel 18-20
AT-1090 Vienna, Austria
**Phone:** 43 1 404004616 **Fax:** 43 1 4081148
**Email:** office@atcardio.at
**Website:** http://www.atcardio.at
**Mem:** 1,016. **Desc:** Promotes the study of cardiology in Austria.

### ★ 4974 ★ Belgian Society of Cardiology
Elyzeese-Veldenstraat
43 rue des Champs Elysees
B-1050 Brussels, Belgium
**Email:** gillebe@uia.ua
**Website:** http://www.bscardio.be
**Fnded:** 1936. **Mem:** 350. **Desc:** Promotes the study of cardiology in Belgium. **Pub:** *ActaCardiologica*. Journal.

## ★ 4975 ★ Belorussian Scientific Society of Cardiologists (BSSC)

Belorussian Research Institute of Cardiology
110 Luxembourg St.
220036 Minsk, Belarus
**Phone:** 375 172 567634  **Fax:** 375 172 567634
**Email:** pharm@bcsmi.minsk.by

**Mem:** 50. **Desc:** Promotes the study of cardiology in Belarus, including instrumental investigation methods on cardiology, coronary heart disease, and drug therapy and nonmedicamentous treatment of arterial hypertension. **Pub:** Reports.

## ★ 4976 ★ British Heart Foundation (BHF)

14 Fitzhardinge St.
London W1H 6DH, United Kingdom
**Phone:** 44 207 9350185  **Fax:** 44 207 4865820
**Email:** internet@bhf.org.uk
**Website:** http://www.bhf.org.uk

**Fnded:** 1961. **Reg. Groups:** 9. **Local Groups:** 430. **Lang(s):** English. **Desc:** Funds research into the causes and prevention diagnosis and treatment of cardiovascular disease. Sponsors postgraduate medical education; distributes fellowships and research funds. Organizes symposia, and workshops for health care and research professionals. Provides cardiac equipment for hospitals and ambulance services. Supports heart patients through rehabilitation programmes, heart support groups and BHF nurses. Conducts fundraising events. Compiles statistics. **Pub:** *BHF Heart News*, bimonthly. Newsletter. Magazine for heart patients.

## ★ 4977 ★ British Microcirculation Society (BMS)

c/o Department of Bioengineering
Imperial College
London SW7 2BY, United Kingdom
**Phone:** 44 171 5945172  **Fax:** 44 171 5945177
**Email:** m.j.lever@ic.ac.uk
**Website:** http://www.microcirculation.org.uk

**Fnded:** 1963. **Mem:** 220. **Lang(s):** English. **Desc:** Individuals interested in the study of microcirculation and endothelium. Conducts clinical and scientific research.

## ★ 4978 ★ Bulgarian Society of Cardiology

National Center of Cardiovascular Diseases
65 Mico Papo St.
BG-1309 Sofia, Bulgaria
**Phone:** 359 2 223134  **Fax:** 359 2 223128
**Email:** bulcardsoc@yahoo.com

**Mem:** 116. **Desc:** Promotes the study of cardiology in Bulgaria. **Pub:** *Bulgarian Cardiology*. Journal. Contains abstracts in Bulgarian and English.

## ★ 4979 ★ Canadian Adult Congential Heart Network

c/o BB&C Association Management Services
191 The West Mall, Ste. 1105
Etobicoke, ON, Canada M9C 5K8
**Phone:** (416)340-4752  **Fax:** (416)340-5014
**Email:** gwebb77452@aol.com
**Website:** http://www.cachnet.org

**Fnded:** 1992. **Mem:** 86. **Reg. Groups:** 15. **Lang(s):** English, French. **Desc:** Represents the interests of Canadian adults who were born with heart defects. Encourages efforts to educate the public on the problems and treatment of heart disease. Works as a support network for congenital heart patients. **Pub:** *CACH News*, quarterly. Newsletter.

## ★ 4980 ★ Canadian Association of Cardiac Rehabilitation (CACR)

1390 Taylor Ave.
Winnipeg, MB, Canada R3M 3V8
**Phone:** (204)488-5854  **Fax:** (204)488-4819
**Email:** mthomas@cacr.ca

**Website:** http://www.cacr.ca/

**Desc:** Promotes leadership in clinical practice, research and advocacy in cardiac disease prevention and rehabilitation in order to improve and maintain the cardiovascular health of Canadians. **Pub:** Newsletter. Contains information about cardiac rehabilitation and related topics. • Membership Directory, annual.

## ★ 4981 ★ Canadian Association of Cardio-Pulmonary Technologists (CACPT)

PO Box 848, Sta. A
Toronto, ON, Canada M5W 1G3
**Phone:** (416)670-1190
**Email:** cacpt@hotmail.com
**Website:** http://cacpt.ca

**Fnded:** 1970. **Mem:** 240. **Lang(s):** English, French. **Desc:** Medical technologists specializing in cardiopulmonary practice. Promotes professional advancement of members. Supports cardio-pulmonary research; conducts continuing professional education programs. **Pub:** *CP-Update*, quarterly. Newsletter.

## ★ 4982 ★ Canadian Cardiovascular Society (CCS) (Societe Canadienne de Cardiologie — SCC)

222 Queen St., Ste. 1403
Ottawa, ON, Canada K1P 5V9
**Phone:** (613)569-3407  **Fax:** (613)569-6574
**Email:** ccsinfo@ccs.ca
**Website:** http://www.ccs.ca

**Fnded:** 1946. **Mem:** 1,150. **Lang(s):** English, French. **Desc:** Physicians, surgeons, and scientists practicing or conducting research in cardiology and related fields. Works to advance the cardiovascular health and care of Canadians through leadership on professional development, advocacy, and the promotion, dissemination of research. **Pub:** *Abstract Program*, annual. **Frmly:** (1962) Canadian Heart Association.

## ★ 4983 ★ Canadian Coalition for High Blood Pressure Prevention and Control (Coalition Canadienne pour la Prevention et le Controle de l'Hypertension Arterielle)

Heart Health and Exercise Laboratory
Centre for Activity and Ageing, Rm. 208A
1490 Richmond St. N
London, ON, Canada N6G 2M3
**Phone:** (519)661-1610  **Fax:** (519)661-1635
**Email:** petrella@julian.uwo.ca
**Website:** http://www.canadianbpcoalition.org

**Lang(s):** English, French. **Desc:** Individuals with high blood pressure; health care professionals with an interest in hypertension. Seeks to advance the diagnosis and treatment of high blood pressure. Sponsors research; conducts educational programs; serves as a clearinghouse on hypertension and its treatment.

## Canadian Council of Cardiovascular Nurses (CCCN) (Conseil Canadien des Infirmieres en Nursing Cardiovasculaire — CCINC)

*See:* Entry 15685

## ★ 4984 ★ Canadian Hypertension Society (CHS) (Societe Canadienne d'Hypertension Arterielle — SCHA)

c/o IRCM
110, Ave. des Pins W
Montreal, QC, Canada H2W 1R7
**Phone:** (514)987-5802  **Fax:** (514)987-5804
**Email:** chs@ircm.qc.ca
**Website:** http://www.chs.md

**Lang(s):** English, French. **Desc:** Health care professionals and other individuals with an interest in hypertension. Seeks to advance the prevention, diag-

nosis, and treatment of high blood pressure. Conducts educational programs to raise public awareness of hypertension prevention; sponsors research and continuing professional development programs.

## ★ 4985 ★ Canadian Physiotherapy Cardio-respiratory Society (CPCRS)

300-3 Raymond St.
Ottawa, ON, Canada K1R 1A3
**Phone:** (613)569-6411  **Fax:** (613)569-8860
**Website:** http://www.lung.ca/physio/index.html

**Lang(s):** English. **Desc:** Promotes cardio-pulmonary research. Administers Canadian Lung Association research funds.

## ★ 4986 ★ Canadian Society of Atherosclerosis, Thrombosis and Vascular Biology (CSATVB)

Centre des Maladies Lipidiques, Bureau S-102
CHUQ pavillon CHUL
2705 Blvd. Laurier
Ste.-Foy, QC, Canada G1V 4G2
**Email:** mrichard@mcmaster.ca
**Website:** http://www3.sympatico.ca/csatvb/

**Lang(s):** English, French. **Desc:** Canadian scientists and physicians specializing in atherosclerosis, thrombosis and vascular biology. Promotes in Canada the advancement of science, research, and teaching related to the fields of atherosclerosis, thrombosis and vascular biology.

## ★ 4987 ★ Canadian Society of Cardiology Technologists (CSCT) (Societe Canadienne des Technologistes en Cardiologie — SCTC)

PO Box 3121
Winnipeg, MB, Canada R3C 4E6
**Email:** csct@technologist.com
**Website:** http://www.csct.ca

**Lang(s):** English, French. **Desc:** Cardiology technologists. Seeks to advance the practice of cardiology; promotes professional development of members. Facilitates exchange of information among members; sponsors research and educational programs.

## ★ 4988 ★ Cardiac Arrhythmias Research and Education Foundation (CARE)

2082 Michelson Dr., No. 301
Irvine, CA 92612
**Phone:** (949)752-2273  **Free:** 800-404-9500
**Email:** care@longqt.org
**Website:** http://www.longqt.org/

**Desc:** Dedicated to research and education about cardiac arrhythmias that cause sudden death.

## ★ 4989 ★ Cardiac Society of Australia and New Zealand

145 Macquarie St
Sydney, NSW 2000, Australia
**Phone:** 61 2 274461  **Fax:** 61 2 231320
**Fnded:** 1951.

## ★ 4990 ★ Cardiovascular Credentialing International (CCI)

4456 Corporation Ln., Ste. 120
Virginia Beach, VA 23462
**Phone:** (757)497-3380  **Free:** 800-326-0268
**Fax:** (757)497-3491
**Email:** ccij@widowmaker.com
**Website:** http://www.cci-online.org/
Randy Christian, Exec. Dir.

**Fnded:** 1988. **Mem:** 26,000. **Desc:** Cardiovascular technologists involved in the allied health professions. Conducts testing of allied health professionals throughout the U.S. and Canada. Provides study guides and reliability and validity testing. Compiles statistics. **Pub:** *Pulse*, quarterly. Newsletter. For Level II registered cardiovascular technologists. *Price:* Included in membership dues; $25/year for nonmembers. • Directory, biennial. **Frmly:** (1984) National Board for Cardiopulmonary Credentialing; (1986) National Board for Cardiovascular and Pulmonary Credentialing; (1991) Cardiovascular Credentialing International/Board of Cardiovascular Technology.


### ★ 4991 ★ Cardiovascular and Interventional Radiological Society of Europe (CIRSE)
Bellerivestr. 42
CH-8008 Zurich, Switzerland
**Phone:** 41 1 3849330          **Fax:** 41 1 3849339
**Email:** office@cirse.org
**Website:** http://www.cirse.org

**Fnded:** 1985. **Mem:** 1,350. **Lang(s):** English, French, German, Italian. **Desc:** Cardiologists, radiologists, and other health care personnel with an interest in cardiology and interventional radiology. Seeks to advance cardiological and radiological study, teaching, and practice. Sponsors continuing professional development courses for members; serves as a clearinghouse on cardiology and interventional radiology. **Pub:** *Cardio Vacular and Interventional Radiology*. Newsletter.


### ★ 4992 ★ Carers Northern Ireland
11 Lower Crescent
Belfast BT7 1NR, United Kingdom
**Phone:** 44 28 90439843          **Fax:** 44 28 90329299
**Email:** info@carersni.org
**Website:** http://www.carersni.org

**Lang(s):** English. **Desc:** Individuals and organizations involved in caring. Seeks to raise the awareness of the needs of carers. Works with all levels of government and society to inform, support and advise.


### Children's Heart Association for Support and Education (CHASE)
*See:* Entry 5659


### Children's HeartLink (CHL)
*See:* Entry 5660


### ★ 4993 ★ Chilean Society of Cardiology and Cardiovascular Surgery (Sociedad Chilena de Cardiologia y Cirugia Cardiovascular)
Esmeralda 678
Santiago, Chile
**Email:** info@childrensheartlink.org
**Website:** http://www.childrensheartlink.org
**Fnded:** 1949.


### ★ 4994 ★ Colombian Society of Cardiology (Sociedad Colombiana de Cardiologia)
Apdo Aereo 1875
Santa Fe de Bogota, Colombia
**Phone:** 57 1 2191388          **Fax:** 57 1 2191399
**Fnded:** 1950.


### ★ 4995 ★ Coronary Club (CC)
9500 Euclid Ave.
Mailcode EE-37
Cleveland, OH 44195
**Fax:** (216)444-9385
Kathryn E. Ryan-Muldoon, Adm. Asst.

**Fnded:** 1969. **Mem:** 9,000. **Desc:** Heart patients, doctors, nurses, therapists, educators, and other health professionals involved in cardiac care. **Pub:** *Heartline*, monthly. Newsletter. Covers heart care and rehabilitation. Includes surgery, medication, diet, exercise, depression, stress management, and new research developments. *Price:* $29/year.


### ★ 4996 ★ Council on Arteriosclerosis, Thrombosis and Vascular Biology of the American Heart Association
c/o Henry Ginsberg, MD, FAHA
Prof. of Medicine
Columbia University College Phys/Surg
630 W 168th St. Department Med
New York, NY 10032-3702
**Phone:** (212)305-9562          **Fax:** (212)305-3212
**Email:** hng1@columbia.edu
**Website:** http://www.americanheart.org/presenter.jhtml?identifier=1201
Henry Ginsberg, MD, Chairperson

**Fnded:** 1946. **Mem:** 1,014. **Desc:** Professional society of physicians and others interested in cardiovascular diseases, especially arteriosclerosis (hardening of the arteries). **Pub:** *Arteriosclerosis and Thrombosis - A Journal of Vascular Biology*, bimonthly. Journal. • Newsletter, semiannual. **Frmly:** (1959) American Society for the Study of Arteriosclerosis; (1997) Council on Arteriosclerosis of the American Heart Association.


### ★ 4997 ★ Croatian Cardiac Society
c/o University Hospital Sestre Milosrdnice
Division of Cardiology
Department of Int. Medicine
Vinogradska 29
10000 Zagreb, Croatia
**Phone:** 385 1 3768286          **Fax:** 385 1 3768286
**Email:** mihatov@mef.hr

**Mem:** 203. **Desc:** Promotes the study of cardiology in Croatia, including congestive heart failure and secondary prevention of coronary heart disease.


### ★ 4998 ★ Cyprus Society of Cardiology
PO Box 27010
Lefkosia
Nicosia CY-1641, Cyprus
**Phone:** 357 2 377888          **Fax:** 357 2 377275
**Email:** papeli@cytanet.com.cy

**Desc:** Promotes the study of cardiology in Cyprus, including coronary risk factors, desirable cholesterol levels in adults, and guidelines on hypertension. **Pub:** *Prevention of Coronary Heart Disease in Clinical Cardiology Practice*. Journal.


### ★ 4999 ★ Czech Society of Cardiology
Faculty Hospital
FN U. Sv. Anny
Pekarska 53
CZ-656 91 Brno, Czech Republic
**Phone:** 42 5 43182508          **Fax:** 42 5 43184231
**Email:** cks@telecom.cz

**Fnded:** 1999. **Mem:** 364. **Desc:** Promotes the study of cardiology in the Czech Republic, including diagnosis and treatment of heart valve diseases, heart failure, hypertension, acute myocardial infarction and angina pectoris, chronic forms of ischemic heart disease, cerebral vascular accidents, arrhythmias, coronary heart disease and complications, pulmonary embolism, and infective endocarditis, as well as pacemaker and antiarrhythmic device implantation, coronarography, and stress tests. **Pub:** *Cor et Vasa*, 10/year. Journal. • *Kardio*. Newsletter. Copies are included in the Journal Cor et Vasa.


### ★ 5000 ★ Danish Society of Cardiology
Hauser Plads 10, 2nd Fl.
DK-1127 Copenhagen, Denmark
**Phone:** 45 65412691          **Fax:** 45 33917964
**Email:** dcs@dadlnet.dk
**Website:** http://www.cardio.dk

**Fnded:** 1960. **Mem:** 812. **Desc:** Promotes the study of cardiology in Denmark, including acute coronary syndrome, antithrombotic treatment in cardiovascular diseases, cardiac rehabilitation, cardiac risk in non-cardiac surgery, heart failure, driving and heart disease, dyslipidaemia and heart disease, ischaemic heart disease and stress tests, pulmonary embolism, stable angina pectoris, valvular heart disease, heart catheterization, coronary angiography and angioplasty, and pacemakers and implantable defibrillators. **Pub:** *Cardiologisk Forum*, quarterly. Journal. • Newsletter, quarterly.


### ★ 5001 ★ Donald W. Reynolds Foundation
1701 Village Center Cir.
Las Vegas, NV 89134
**Phone:** (702)804-6000          **Fax:** (702)804-6099
**Email:** generalquestions@dwrf.org
**Website:** http://www.dwreynolds.org

**Desc:** Works to provide support for cardiovascular clinical research and aging and quality of life programs.


### ★ 5002 ★ Egyptian Society of Cardiology
Egyptian Heart House
9 El-Saraya St.
Dokki
Giza EG-12311, Egypt
**Phone:** 20 2 3381308          **Fax:** 20 2 3381309
**Email:** esc@idsc1.gov.eg

**Fnded:** 1951. **Mem:** 739. **Desc:** Promotes the study of cardiology in Egypt, including diagnosis and management of hypertension, and management of coronary heart disease. **Pub:** *Egyptian Heart*, 3/year. Journal. • *Pediatric Cardiology*, semiannual. Newsletter.


### ★ 5003 ★ Estonian Cardiac Society (Eesti Kardioloogide Selts)
Puusepa Str. 8
EE-51014 Tartu, Estonia
**Phone:** 372 7 448109          **Fax:** 372 7 448106

**Fnded:** 1963. **Mem:** 203. **Lang(s):** English. **Desc:** Physicians and scientists interested in the field of cardiology.


### ★ 5004 ★ European Society of Cardiology
c/o The European Heart House
2035 Route des Colles
Les Templiers
Boite Postale 179
F-06903 Sophia Antipolis cedex, France
**Phone:** 33 4 92947600          **Fax:** 33 4 92947601
**Email:** webmaster@escardio.org
**Website:** http://www.escardio.org/

**Fnded:** 1950. **Mem:** 40,000. **Nat'l Groups:** 47. **Lang(s):** English, French. **Desc:** Cardiologists. Seeks to "improve the quality of life of the European population by reducing the impact of cardiovascular disease." Fosters interdisciplinary research and cooperation to advance the practice of cardiology; facilitates exchange of information among members and between members and individuals working in related fields; conducts public education programs. Serves as a clearinghouse on cardiovascular diseases and their prevention and treatment. **Pub:** *Cardiovascular Research*, monthly. Journal. • *European Heart Journal*, biweekly. Journal.


### European Society for Cardiovascular Surgery (ESCVS) (Societe Europeenne de Chirurgie Cardiovasculaire)
*See:* Entry 19547


### ★ 5005 ★ European Society for Microcirculation (ESM)
Department of Physiology
Freie Universitat Berlin
Arnimallee 22
D-14195 Berlin, Germany
**Phone:** 49 30 84 451632          **Fax:** 49 30 84451634
**Email:** pries@zedat.fu-berlin.de
**Website:** http://www.medizin.fu-berlin.de/esm

**Fnded:** 1960. **Mem:** 386. **Lang(s):** English. **Desc:** Individuals from 27 countries involved in education, clinical medicine, and the pharmaceutical industry interested in the study of microcirculation. (Microcirculation is the flow of blood and other tissue fluids into

small vessels.) Coordinates research among participating laboratories in areas directly affecting the
development, application, and promotion of microcirculation methods that will benefit health care. **Pub:**
*European Society for Microcirculation*, periodic. Directory. • *Journal of Vascular Research*, bimonthly.
Journal. • *Newsletter*, periodic. Newsletter.

### ★ 5006 ★ European Society for Noninvasive Cardiology

c/o Cardiology Department
UZ Gasthuisberg O/N
Herestraat 49
B-3000 Leuven, Belgium
**Phone:** 32 16 345840          **Fax:** 32 16 345846
**Fnded:** 1979. **Mem:** 250. **Reg. Groups:** 3. **Desc:**
Promotes noninvasive cardiology.

### ★ 5007 ★ European Society for Noninvasive Cardiovascular Dynamics (ESNICVD)

Institute of Physiology
Faculty of Medicine
Zaloska 4
SLO-1100 Ljubljana, Slovenia
**Phone:** 386 1 5437500          **Fax:** 386 1 5437501
**Email:** esnicvd@mf.uni-lj.si
**Website:** http://www2.mf.uni-lj.si/~esnicvd_
**Fnded:** 1960. **Mem:** 86. **Lang(s):** English. **Desc:**
Scientists and professionals in 17 countries active in
fields such as biology, cardiology, physiology, sports
science, hydraulics, and physics who seek better
knowledge of the cardiovascular system. Promotes
the exchange of ideas in noninvasive cardiovascular
research. Fosters the study of cardiovascular function
from a mechanical point of reference to gain knowledge applicable to medical practice and technical
disciplines. Works to standardize methods used to
study the mechanical activity of the cardiovascular
system. **Pub:** *Bibliotheca Cardiologica*, periodic. •
*Cardiovascular*, annual. Newsletter. Includes information on conferences, working groups, and ESNICVD. •
*Proceedings of Congress*, biennial. **Frmly:** (1970)
European Society for Ballistocardiographic Research;
(1978) European Society for Ballistocardiography and
Cardiovascular Dynamics.

### European Society for Vascular Surgery (ESVS)

*See:* Entry 19554

### ★ 5008 ★ Finnish Cardiac Society (FCS) (Suomen Kardiologinen Seura — SKS)

PO Box 50
FIN-00621 Helsinki, Finland
**Phone:** 358 9 75275238          **Fax:** 358 9 75275233
**Email:** fcs@fimnet.fi
**Website:** http://www.esvs.org
**Fnded:** 1967. **Mem:** 685. **Lang(s):** English, Finnish,
Swedish. **Desc:** Physicians practicing in Finland.
Encourages contact between cardiology specialists
and doctors interested in the field. Organizes educa-
tional courses. **Pub:** *Sydanaani (Cardiac Sound)*,
periodic. Newsletter.

### ★ 5009 ★ French Society of Cardiology

15 rue Cels
F-75014 Paris, France
**Phone:** 33 1 43223333          **Fax:** 33 1 43226361
**Email:** contact@cardio-sfc.org
**Website:** http://www.webcardio.com/main.asp
**Mem:** 1,873. **Desc:** Promotes the study of cardiology
in France.

### ★ 5010 ★ Georgian Society of Cardiology

Institute of Cardiology
2 Gudamakari St.
380092 Tbilisi, Georgia
**Phone:** 995 32 607535          **Fax:** 995 32 605373
**Email:** drugmonc@access.sanet.ge

**Mem:** 96. **Desc:** Promotes the study of cardiology in
Georgia.

### ★ 5011 ★ German Cardiac Society

Goethestrasse 38
DE-40237 Dusseldorf, Germany
**Phone:** 49 211 6006920          **Fax:** 49 211 60069210
**Email:** info@dgkardio.de
**Website:** http://www.dgkardio.de
**Fnded:** 1927. **Mem:** 4,025. **Desc:** Promotes the study
of cardiology in Germany. **Pub:** *Basic Research in
Cardiology*, bimonthly. Journal. • *Cardio News*, month-
ly. Journal. • *Zeitschrift fur Kardiologie*, monthly.
Journal.

### ★ 5012 ★ Heart Disease Research Foundation (HDRF)

50 Court St.
Brooklyn, NY 11201
**Phone:** (718)649-6210
Dr. Yoshiaki Omura, MD, Dir., Med. Research
**Fnded:** 1962. **Desc:** Promotes research aimed at the
prevention, early diagnosis, and treatment of cardiovascular disease and related medico-social problems.
Supports and conducts research, both basic and
clinical, in the early diagnosis, prevention, and treatment of cardiovascular diseases using a multidisciplinary approach. Studies include the effects of acupuncture and electrotherapeutics on blood chemistry and
the cardiovascular system, the clinical applications of
these methods, and the noninvasive early diagnostic
methods of cardiovascular diseases. Sponsors postgraduate continuing medical educational courses for
physicians, dentists, and medical researchers. Conducts public education programs on the heart and
heart disease. Answers questions from the public and
professionals; supplies available educational information on cardiovascular diseases and research.

### ★ 5013 ★ Hellenic Cardiological Society

6 Potamianou St.
GR-115 28 Athens, Greece
**Phone:** 30 1 7221633          **Fax:** 30 1 7226139
**Email:** hcs@eexi.gr
**Website:** http://www.hcs.gr
**Fnded:** 1927. **Mem:** 1,633. **Desc:** Promotes the study
of cardiology in Greece, including electrophysiologic
studies and ablation techniques, pacemakers and
defibrillators, echocardiography, cardiac MRI, nuclear
cardiology procedures and applications, exercise
stress tests, and cardiac rehabilitation. **Pub:** *Hellenic
Journal of Cardiology*. Journal. Contains articles on
aspects of cardiovascular disease.

### ★ 5014 ★ HHT Foundation International

PO Box 8087
New Haven, CT 06530
**Free:** 800-448-6389
**Email:** hhtinfor@hht.com
**Website:** http://www.hht.org
Rita Van Bergeijk, Pres.
**Fnded:** 1991. **Mem:** 300. **Reg. Groups:** 3. **State
Groups:** 3. **Desc:** Patients and their families; physi-
cians, counselors, and health administrators; interested others. Promotes research into the treatment,
causes, and cure of hereditary hemmorrhagic telangiectasia (HHT), also known as Osler-Weber-Rendu
Syndrome. A rare genetic blood vessel disorder, HHT
causes malformations of arteries and veins; hemor-
rhaging from the nose and intestine is also common.
Malformations in the lungs cause shortness of breath,
stroke, and brain abscess. Provides information exchange. Raises funds for research and patient service
programs. Sponsors support groups. **Pub:** *HHT Newsletter*, quarterly. Newsletter. • *Our Blood Vessels*.
Pamphlet. • Brochures. • Newsletter, semiannual.

### ★ 5015 ★ Hungarian Society of Cardiology (HSC) (Magyar Kardiologusok Tarsasaga — MKT)

Chazar A. u. 19 1/3
PO Box 24
HU-1406 Budapest, Hungary
**Phone:** 36 1 4610665          **Fax:** 36 1 4610665
**Email:** mkt@mail.matav.hu
**Website:** http://www.medicine.iif.hu/MKT/
**Fnded:** 1955. **Mem:** 1,200. **Local Groups:** 17.
**Lang(s):** English, Hungarian. **Desc:** Cardiologists and
other medical specialists. Promotes development of
cardiology; facilitates scientific exchanges of information among members. Monitors standards in cardiology training programs; provides cardiologists with ethical advice. Conducts educational, research, and public
service programs. **Pub:** *Cardiologia Hungarica*, quarterly. Journal.

### ★ 5016 ★ Icelandic Cardiac Society (ICS) (Hjartasjukdomafelag Islenskra Laekna — HIL)

Department of Medicine
Division of Cardiology
Landspitalinn 101
PO Box 10
IS-121 Reykjavik, Iceland
**Phone:** 354 1 5601000          **Fax:** 354 1 5601287
**Email:** ragnarda@rsp.is
**Fnded:** 1968. **Mem:** 33. **Nat'l Groups:** 1. **Lang(s):**
Danish, English, Finnish, Icelandic, Norwegian, Swed-
ish. **Desc:** Physicians and scientists interested in the
field of cardiology.

### ★ 5017 ★ Implanted Defibrilator Association of Scotland (IDAS)

6 Argyll St.
Brechin
Angus
Brechin DD9 6JL, United Kingdom
**Phone:** 44 1356 622554
**Email:** peisoslater@themail.co.uk
**Fnded:** 1994. **Mem:** 104. **Reg. Groups:** 4. **Lang(s):**
English. **Desc:** Individuals with implanted defibrilating
devices and their families. Promotes and improved
quality of life for people with implanted defibrilators.
Sponsors support groups for members; advocates on
behalf of members before medical organizations and
the public; conducts educational programs; partici-
pates in charitable activities. **Pub:** *Vital Spark*, quarterly. Newsletter.

### ★ 5018 ★ Inter-American Society of Cardiology (ISC) (Sociedad Interamericana de Cardiologia)

Instituto Nacional de Cardiologia
Calle Jaun Bardiano 1
14080 Mexico City, DF, Mexico
**Phone:** 52 5 5732911          **Fax:** 52 5 5730994
**Fnded:** 1944. **Lang(s):** English, French, Portuguese,
Spanish. **Desc:** National societies of cardiology from
the Americas; medical doctors; individuals who have
made outstanding contributions in the cardiovascular
and allied fields. Purpose is to unite members for the
development and advancement of cardiology and
related fields, particularly by promoting the association
of physicians, surgeons, and scientists with cardiovascular specialties. Fosters cooperation and exchange of
information, medical specialists, and scientists at
national, regional, and world levels; provides advice to
governments seeking counsel. Sponsors exchange
programs. **Pub:** *News Bulletin*, periodic. Bulletin.

### ★ 5019 ★ InterAmerican Heart Foundation (IAHF)

7272 Greenville Ave.
Dallas, TX 75231-4596
**Phone:** (214)706-1218          **Fax:** (214)373-0268
**Email:** beatrizc@ix.netcom.com
Javier Valenzuela, PhD, Office Coordinator

**Fnded:** 1992. **Mem:** 31. **Desc:** The InterAmerican Heart Program was created in September, 1992 under the auspices of the International Society and Federation of Cardiology with the support of the American Heart Association, the InterAmerican Society of Cardiology and heart foundations and societies throughout the American continent. **Pub:** *Heart of the Americas*, quarterly. Newsletter. *Price:* Free. **Frmly:** International Cardiology Foundation; (1998) Interamerican Heart Cardiology Foundation.


**★ 5020 ★ International Atherosclerosis Society (IAS)**
6550 Fannin, Ste. 1211
Houston, TX 77030-2704
**Phone:** (713)797-0401　　　**Fax:** (713)797-8853
**Email:** info@athero.org
**Website:** http://www.athero.org
Ann S. Jackson, Exec. Dir.

**Fnded:** 1979. **Mem:** 9,500. **Nat'l Groups:** 36. **Desc:** Scientists and other professionals involved in research in the field of atherosclerosis; corporations and firms supporting aims of the IAS. Promotes the advancement of science, research, and teaching in the field of atherosclerosis throughout the world. (Atherosclerosis is a form of arteriosclerosis characterized by the deposition of fatty substances in and fibrosis of the inner layer of the arteries.) Advocates an interdisciplinary approach to the study of atherosclerosis and related diseases. Facilitates international communication and exchange of knowledge among scientists in the field. Assists in the organization of exchange visits among scientists at various research centers. Fosters and encourages young researchers by arranging contacts, and offering travel support to world gatherings in the field. Coordinates activities in atherosclerosis research. **Pub:** *Proceedings of Symposia*, triennial. Proceedings. • *Roster of Member Societies*. • Newsletter, semiannual.


**★ 5021 ★ International Bundle Branch Block Association (IBBBA)**
6631 W 83rd St.
Los Angeles, CA 90045-2899
**Phone:** (310)670-9132
Rita Kurtz Lewis, Exec. Dir.

**Fnded:** 1979. **Desc:** Individuals with bundle branch block (BBB), concerned professionals, and laypersons. (BBB is a rare heart condition caused by an "electrical malfunction".) Objectives are: to increase public awareness of BBB; to disseminate information on the disease; to answer inquiries of members; to serve as a forum for sharing information and experiences; to maintain a bank of information to aid professional research on BBB. Compiles statistics. Plans to conduct specialized education and research programs. **Pub:** *Heartbeat*, quarterly. Provides professional replies to readers' medical questions, reprints from other publications, and names and addresses of members. *Price:* Included in membership dues.


**★ 5022 ★ International Cardiac Doppler Society (ICDS)**
Viamonte 1336, Piso 9, Of 52/53
1053 Buenos Aires, Argentina
**Phone:** 54 11 43749911　　　**Fax:** 54 11 43749911
**Email:** sppi@movi.com.ar


**★ 5023 ★ International College of Angiology**
5 Daremy Ct.
Nesconset, NY 11767-1547
**Phone:** (631)366-1429　　　**Fax:** (631)366-3609
**Email:** denisemrossignol@cs.com
**Fnded:** 1958. **Desc:** Dedicated to advancement and education in angiology, the study of the circulatory and vascular system. **Pub:** *International Journal of Angiology*, quarterly. Journal. Promotes multi-disciplinary approaches to all aspects of vascular disease.


**★ 5024 ★ International Society for Adult Congenital Cardiac Disease**
c/o Pamela D. Sproul
9111 Old Georgetown Rd.
Bethesda, MD 20814-1616
**Phone:** (919)787-5181　　　**Fax:** (919)787-4916
**Email:** isaccd@olsonmgmt.com

**Fnded:** 1992. **Mem:** 200. **Desc:** Seeks to achieve and promote execellence in the care of adolescents and adults with contgenital cardiac disease. **Pub:** *ISACCD Update*, quarterly. Newsletter.


**★ 5025 ★ International Society of Cardiovascular Pharmacotherapy (ISCP)**
Austin Hospital
University of Melbourne
Melbourne, VIC 3084, Australia


**★ 5026 ★ International Society for Cardiovascular Surgery (ISCVS)**
13 Elm St.
Manchester, MA 01944-1314
**Phone:** (978)526-8330　　　**Fax:** (978)526-7521
**Email:** iscvs@prri.com
William T. Maloney, Exec. Dir.

**Fnded:** 1951. **Mem:** 2,500. **Desc:** Encourages exchange and cooperation between cardiovascular specialists. Promotes discussion of ideas pertinent to the cardiovascular disease field and stimulates investigation and study of cardiovascular diseases. **Pub:** *Cardiovascular Surgery*, bimonthly. Journal. **Frmly:** (1983) International Cardiovascular Society.


**International Society of Electrocardiology (ISE)**
*See:* Entry 4516


**International Society for Heart and Lung Transplantation (ISHLT)**
*See:* Entry 20334


**★ 5027 ★ International Society for Heart Research**
c/o Division of Cardiology, ACB 3rd Fl.
Department of Medicine
University of Louisville Health Science Center
550 S Jackson
Louisville, KY 40292
**Phone:** (502)852-1837　　　**Fax:** (502)852-6474
**Email:** rbolli@louisville.edu
**Website:** http://www.ishrworld.org
Dr. Roberto Bolli, MD, Sec. Gen.

**Fnded:** 1967. **Mem:** 2,000. **Desc:** Professionals and investigators in the field of experimental cardiology united to foster multidisciplinary approaches for finding solutions to the problems of heart disease. Conducts research in cardiac metabolism. **Pub:** *Advances in Myocardiology*. Journal. • *Journal of Molecular and Cellular Cardiology*, monthly. Journal. **Frmly:** International Society for Cardiovascular Research.


**★ 5028 ★ International Society of Hypertension (ISH)**
GPO Box X2213
Perth, WA 6847, Australia
**Phone:** 61 8 92240258　　　**Fax:** 61 8 92240246
**Email:** judyr@cyllene.uwa.edu.au

**Fnded:** 1966. **Desc:** Promotes the advancement of scientific knowledge in all aspects of research in hypertension and connected cardiovascular diseases.


**★ 5029 ★ International Society for Minimally Invasive Cardiac Surgery (ISMICS)**
13 Elm St.
Manchester, MA 01944
**Phone:** (978)526-0330　　　**Fax:** (978)526-4018
**Email:** ismics@prri.com


**Website:** http://www.ismics.org
Aurelie M. Alger, JD, Asst. Dir.

**Fnded:** 1997. **Mem:** 550. **Desc:** Concerned with patient outcomes, techniques, and progressive development of less invasive forms of heart surgery. **Pub:** *The Heart Surgery Forum*. Journal.


**★ 5030 ★ International Society of Non-invasive Cardiology (ISCN)**
Herestr 49
3000 Leuven, Belgium
**Phone:** 32 1 6345844　　　**Fax:** 32 1 6345840
**Email:** Andre.Aubert@med.kuleuven.ac.be

**Fnded:** 1980. **Desc:** Promotes research on the heart and the circulation by non-invasive means.


**★ 5031 ★ Intersocietal Commission for the Accreditation of Vascular Laboratories (ICAVL)**
8840 Stanfod Blvd., Ste. 4900
Columbia, MD 21045-5852
**Phone:** (410)872-0100　　　**Fax:** (410)872-0030
**Email:** morales@intersocietal.org
**Website:** http://www.icavl.org
Sandra Katanick, Exec. Dir.

**Fnded:** 1994. **Desc:** Establishes industry standards. **Frmly:** (2000) Intersocietal Commission for the Accreditation of Vascular Laboratories.


**★ 5032 ★ Irish Cardiac Society**
University College Hospital
Newcastle Rd.
Galway, Ireland
**Phone:** 353 91 524222　　　**Fax:** 353 91 527197
**Email:** kieran-daly@bsi.ie

**Mem:** 135. **Desc:** Promotes the study of cardiology in Ireland.


**★ 5033 ★ Israel Heart Society**
Twin Towers 2, Rm. 1322
35 Jabotinsky Str.
IL-52511 Ramat Gan, Israel
**Phone:** 972 3 6122577　　　**Fax:** 972 3 6122588
**Email:** ihs@israel-heart.org.il
**Website:** http://www.israel-heart.org.il

**Mem:** 497. **Desc:** Promotes the study of cardiology in Israel. **Pub:** *Journal of the Israel Heart Society*. Includes review articles and abstracts.


**★ 5034 ★ Italian Federation of Cardiology**
c/o Cardio Thoracic Department
Universita degliStudi di Pisa
Via Paradisa 2
IT-56124 Pisa, Italy
**Phone:** 39 50 542929　　　**Fax:** 39 50 542947
**Email:** fedcard@docline.it

**Mem:** 5,506. **Desc:** Promotes the study of cardiology in Italy. **Pub:** *The Italian Heart Journal*.


**★ 5035 ★ Japanese Society of Hypertension (JSH)**
c/o Business Center for Academic Societies Japan
5-16-9 Honkomagome
Bunkyo-ku
Tokyo 113-8622, Japan
**Phone:** 81 3 58145810　　　**Fax:** 81 3 58145825

**Fnded:** 1978. **Mem:** 2,450. **Desc:** Studies the causes and prevention of hypertension. **Pub:** *Hypertension Research - Clinical and Experimental*, periodic. Journal. • Newsletter, semiannual.


**★ 5036 ★ Korean Vascular Surgical Society (KVSS)**
Kangnam St. Mary's Hospital
Catholic University Medical College
505 Panp'o-dong

Soch'o-gu
Seoul 137-701, Republic of Korea
**Lang(s):** English, Korean. **Desc:** Physicians and surgeons specializing in the vascular system. Seeks to advance the prevention, diagnosis, and treatment of vascular diseases; promotes development of improved vascular surgical techniques. Facilitates exchange of information among members; sponsors research and continuing professional development programs.

### ★ 5037 ★ Latin American Society for Interventional Cardiology (SOLACI) (Sociedad Latinoamericana de Cardiologia Intervencionista)

A Alsina 2653, Piso 2H
1090 Buenos Aires, Argentina
**Phone:** 54 11 49547173　　**Fax:** 54 1 49547173
**Email:** solaci@satlink.com
**Website:** http://www.solaci.cl
**Fnded:** 1995. **Desc:** Seeks to improve and develop the practice of cardiovascular interventions in Latin America.

### ★ 5038 ★ Latvian Society of Cardiology

Latvia Center of Cardiology
13 Pilsonu iela
LV-1002 Riga, Latvia
**Phone:** 371 7 613915　　**Fax:** 371 7 613915
**Email:** cardio@mailbox.riga.lv
**Mem:** 280.

### ★ 5039 ★ Lebanese Society of Cardiology

PO Box 6301
Beirut, Lebanon
**Phone:** 961 1 653414　　**Fax:** 961 1 653411
**Email:** orca@cyberia.net.lb
**Mem:** 207. **Desc:** Promotes the study of cardiology in Lebanon. **Pub:** *The Lebanese Medical Journal.* • Newsletter, monthly.

### ★ 5040 ★ Lithuanian Society of Cardiology

Department of Cardiology
Vilnius University Hospital
Santariskiu Klinikos
Santariskiu 2
LT-2021 Vilnius, Lithuania
**Phone:** 370 2 365200　　**Fax:** 370 2 365211
**Email:** cardio@cardio.lt
**Mem:** 401. **Desc:** Promotes the study of cardiology in Lithuania. **Pub:** *Lithuanian Journal of Cardiology*, 2-4/yr. Published jointly with the Institut of Cardiology. • *Seminars in Cardiology*, quarterly. Journal. Published jointly with the Lithuanian Heart Association.

### ★ 5041 ★ Mended Hearts (MH)

7272 Greenville Ave.
Dallas, TX 75231-4596
**Phone:** (214)706-1442　　**Free:** 800-242-8721
**Fax:** (214)706-5231
**Email:** info@mendedhearts.org
**Website:** http://www.mendedhearts.org
Cathy Clapp, Exec. Dir.
**Fnded:** 1951. **Mem:** 25,000. **Local Groups:** 200. **Desc:** Persons who have heart disease; their families and friends. Works to: provide advice, encouragement, and services to heart disease patients and to their families; establish programs of assistance to surgeons, physicians, and hospitals. Conducts and assists in research programs designed to benefit heart patients. **Pub:** *Heartbeat*, quarterly. Magazine. **Frmly:** (1955) Mended Hearts Club.

### Michael E. DeBakey International Surgical Society (MEDISS)

*See:* Entry 19578

### ★ 5042 ★ Microcirculatory Society (MCS)

Department of Veterinary and Biomedical Sciences
University of Missouri
Columbia, MO 65211
**Phone:** (573)882-7012
**Email:** gore@u.arizona.edu
**Website:** http://microcirc.org/
Dr. Robert W. Gore, Contact
**Fnded:** 1955. **Mem:** 450. **Desc:** Encourages the exchange and dissemination of information on microcirculation. **Pub:** *Microcirculatory Society Directory*, annual. Membership Directory. • *Microcirculatory Society Newsletter*, 3/year. Newsletter.

### ★ 5043 ★ Moldavian Society of Cardiology

Moldavian Research Institute of Preventive & Clinical Medici
Cardiology Clinic
N Testemitsanu str. 20
MD-2025 Chisinau, Moldova
**Phone:** 373 2 727511　　**Fax:** 373 2 739586
**Email:** mpopovici@madnet.md
**Mem:** 78. **Desc:** Promotes the study of cardiology in Moldavia.

### ★ 5044 ★ Moroccan Society of Cardiology

BP 1326
Rabat, Morocco
**Phone:** 212 767 1549　　**Fax:** 212 767 3232
**Email:** bcardio@arcnet.com.net.ma
**Mem:** 218. **Desc:** Promotes the study of cardiology in Morroco. **Pub:** *Bulletin de la societe marocaine de cardiology.* Journal.

### ★ 5045 ★ National Association of Vascular Access Networks (NAVAN)

PMB 205
11417 S 700 E
Draper, UT 84020-9131
**Phone:** (801)576-1824　　**Free:** 888-576-2826
**Fax:** (801)553-9137
**Email:** Nava@navanet.org
**Website:** http://www.navannet.org
Mary Lea Nations, Exec. Dir.
**Fnded:** 1988. **Mem:** 850. **Local Groups:** 10. **Desc:** Physicians, pharmacists, nurses, and manufacturers involved in the care and management of patients with vascular access devices. Seeks to advance the effectiveness of vascular access devices; promotes professional development of members. Serves as a network linking members; conducts educational programs. **Pub:** *JVAD*, periodic. Journal.

### National Heart Council (NHC)

*See:* Entry 8595

### ★ 5046 ★ National Heart Savers Association (NHSA)

9140 W Dodge Rd.
Omaha, NE 68114
**Phone:** (402)398-1993　　**Fax:** (402)398-1994
**Email:** nhsa@aol.com
**Website:** http://www.heartsavers.org
Phil Sokolof, Pres.
**Fnded:** 1985. **Desc:** Promotes cardiac health care by informing the public of the dangers of a high-cholesterol diet. Conducts public cholesterol screening program; secured congressional designation of September as National Cholesterol Education Month. Has been successful in persuading major food processing and fast food restaurants companies to stop using palm and coconut oil, lard, and beef tallow, which are high in saturated fats, as ingredients in prepared foods. Promotes nutrition education in public schools and lobbies for more healthful school lunches. **Pub:** Books. • Pamphlets.

### ★ 5047 ★ National Hypertension Association (NHA)

324 E 30th St.
New York, NY 10016
**Phone:** (212)889-3557　　**Fax:** (212)447-7032
**Website:** http://www.nathypertension.org
William M. Manger, MD, Chm.
**Fnded:** 1977. **Desc:** Physicians, medical researchers, and business professionals dedicated to the prevention of the complications of hypertension. Seeks to combat hypertension by developing, directing, and implementing effective programs to educate physicians and the public about the severe, life-threatening dangers of this health disorder. Conducts research on the cause of hypertension through basic laboratory studies. Provides the public with basic information on hypertension; conducts hypertension and hypercholesterol detection programs. Offers medical consulting to those found to have high blood pressure or hypercholesterolemia. Develops educational materials and participates in radio and television programs. **Pub:** *Clinical and Experimental Pheochromocytoma.* Book. • *High Blood Pressure and What You Can Do About It*, annual. Pamphlet. *Price:* $1. • *News Report*, annual. Newsletter. • *100 Questions and Answers About Hypertension.* Book. *Price:* $14.95. • Also publishes medical journal periodicals.

### ★ 5048 ★ National Institute of Hypertension Studies - Institute of Hypertension School of Research (NIHS)

PO Box 02006
Detroit, MI 48202
**Fax:** (313)872-0505
Dr. H. R. Lockett, Exec. Dir.
**Fnded:** 1975. **Desc:** Purposes are: to help find causes of and to help prevent essential hypertension; to educate people concerning essential hypertension; to diagnose, counsel, and refer afflicted individuals for treatment and follow-up activities; to conduct research on hypertension and to extend that research into the areas of crime and drug addiction and psychosocial and occupational stress. Sponsors hypertension detection clinics. Offers youth leadership courses. Compiles statistics and disseminates educational materials. Conducts research programs on psychosocial and occupational stress which offer diplomas to those completing the programs; survey project with Pharmaceutical Research and Manufacturers of America; also conducts research on drugs and hypertension. **Pub:** *IHS 1992 Report*, annual. Research report on causes of essential hypertension. • *OHRST Assessment Report Series*, annual. • *Pharmaceutical Research and Manufacturers of America.* • Magazine, periodic. **Frmly:** (1971) Institute of Hypertension Studies; (1981) Institute of Hypertension Studies - Institute of Hypertension School of Research.

### ★ 5049 ★ Netherlands Society of Cardiology (NSC) (Nederlandse Vereniging voor Cardiologie — NVVC)

PO Box 19192
NL-3501 DD Utrecht, Netherlands
**Phone:** 31 30 2345000　　**Fax:** 31 30 2345002
**Email:** bureau@nvvc.nl
**Fnded:** 1934. **Mem:** 950. **Desc:** Promotes the profession of cardiology, cardiological research, and cardiac care in the Netherlands. Defends the professional interests of members. **Pub:** *Cardiologie*, monthly. Journal. **Frmly:** (1999) Dutch Society of Cardiology.

### ★ 5050 ★ Nordic Federation of Heart and Lung Associations (NHL) (Nordiska Hjart and Lungsjukas Forbund)

Kampementsgatan 14
S-115 38 Stockholm, Sweden
**Phone:** 46 8 6626882
**Email:** info@heartlung.org
**Website:** http://www.heartlung.org

Fnded: 1948. Mem: 150,000. Reg. Groups: 126. Lang(s): Danish, Finnish, Icelandic, Norwegian, Swedish. Desc: Lung and heart disease specialists in 5 countries. Addresses medical issues in the context of social welfare. Engages in political activities; operates vocational and training centers. Pub: *BM-Bladet*, monthly. • *Silmu*, monthly. • *Status*, monthly. • *Trygd og Arbeid*, monthly.

### ★ 5051 ★ North American Society for Cardiac Imaging (NASCI)

930 Edgecliff Way
Redwood City, CA 94061
Phone: (650)216-6621     Fax: (650)556-1678
Email: info@nasci.org
Website: http://www.nasci.org
Joan Oefner, CAE, Exec. Dir.

Fnded: 1973. Mem: 350. Desc: Approved individuals engaged in the practice and advancement of cardiac and vascular imaging are active members; medical students, other individuals, and corporations with an interest in cardiac imaging are sponsors. Seeks to advance the practice of cardiac imaging and to develop improved medical imaging technologies. Serves as a forum for the exchange of information among individuals and corporations with an interest in cardiac imaging; sponsors educational programs; maintains NASCI Research and Education Fund. Pub: *International Journal of Cardiovascular Imaging*, bimonthly. Journal. • *NASCI Membership Directory*, annual. Directory.

### ★ 5052 ★ North American Society of Pacing and Electrophysiology (NASPE)

Six Strathmore Rd.
Natick, MA 01760-2499
Phone: (508)647-0100     Fax: (508)647-0124
Email: info@naspe.org
Website: http://www.naspe.org
James H. Youngblood, CEO

Fnded: 1979. Mem: 3,200. Desc: Physicians, scientists, and allied professionals throughout the world dedicated to the study and management or cardiac arrhythmias; to improve the care of patients by promoting research, education and training, and providing leadership towards optimal health care policies and standards. Pub: *Journal of Cardiovascular Electrophysiology*, monthly. Journal. • *NASPE News*, 5/year. Newsletter. Covers membership activities. Includes calendar of events and information updates. • *North American Society of Pacing and Electrophysiology Annual Scientific Session Program*. • *PACE: The Journal of Pacing and Clinical Electrophysiology*, monthly. Journal. • Brochure. • Membership Directory, annual. Includes geographic index.

### ★ 5053 ★ Norwegian Society of Cardiology

University Hospital of Trondheim
Department of Medicine, Cardiology
Regionsykehuset i Trondheim
N-7006 Trondheim, Norway
Phone: 47 73868514     Fax: 47 73867966
Email: rune.wiseth@medisin.ntnu.no

Mem: 206. Desc: Promotes the study of cardiology in Norway. Pub: Journal, quarterly.

### ★ 5054 ★ Peruvian Heart Association (PHA)

100 S Greenleaf Ave.
Gurnee, IL 60031-3378
Phone: (847)249-2111     Free: 800-367-7378
Fax: (847)249-2772
Email: milalatin@aol.com
Luis Vasquez, MD, Intl. Dir.

Fnded: 1967. Mem: 400. Reg. Groups: 6. Desc: Peruvian physicians, nurses, and other health care professionals specializing in cardiology who are devoted to research, training, teaching, and patient care. Offers continuing education courses for Peruvian physicians, enabling them to fulfill coursework required by Peruvian law for continuance of medical practice. Provides community health care information to residents of Lima, Peru concerning heart attacks, high blood pressure, cholesterol, diabetes, diet, and exercise. Conducts programs in conjunction with the American College of Cardiology and the American Heart Association, providing printed information and speakers on health care. Also provides information to U.S. doctors who wish to study and assist with Peruvian health care.

### ★ 5055 ★ Phlebology Society of America (PSA)

c/o Denise M. Rossignol, Exec. Dir.
5 Daremy Ct.
Nesconset, NY 11767-1547
Phone: (631)366-1429     Fax: (631)366-3609
Email: denisemrossignol@cs.com
Dr. John B. Chang, Bd. Chm.

Fnded: 1962. Mem: 300. Desc: Physicians and scientists with an interest in phlebitis and other diseases of the vascular system. Seeks to advance the diagnosis and treatment of peripheral vascular disease. Serves as a certifying board for professional phlebologists; functions as a clearinghouse on phlebology; facilitates exchange of information among members. Conducts educational programs. Pub: *International Journal of Angiology*, quarterly. Journal.

### ★ 5056 ★ Polish Cardiac Society

ul. Niemodlinska 33
PL-04-635 Warsaw, Poland
Phone: 48 228156553     Fax: 48 226133806
Email: aninko@yahoo.com
Website: http://www.ptkardio.pl

Mem: 2,300. Desc: Promotes the study of cardiology in Poland. Pub: *Polish Heart Journal*.

### ★ 5057 ★ Portuguese Society of Cardiology

Campo Grande 28-13
1700 Lisbon, Portugal
Phone: 351 21 7970685     Fax: 351 21 7931095
Email: secretariado@mail.spc.pt
Website: http://www.spc.pt

Fnded: 1949. Mem: 573. Desc: Promotes the study of cardiology in Portugal, including coronary heart disease prevention in clinical practice, and cardiovascular prevention in the elderly. Pub: *Boletim da Sociedade Portuguesa de Cardiologia*, monthly. Newsletter. • *Portuguese Journal of Cardiology*, monthly.

### ★ 5058 ★ Pulmonary Hypertension Association (PHA)

850 Sligo Ave., No. 800
Silver Spring, MD 20910
Phone: 800-748-7274     Fax: (301)565-3994
Email: pha@phassociation.org
Website: http://www.phassociation.org
Rino Aldrighetti, Exec. Dir.

Fnded: 1990. Mem: 4,100. Local Groups: 85. Desc: Patients with pulmonary hypertension (PH) and primary pulmonary hypertension (PPH); families and physicians of patients; researchers. Provides fellowship and educational support for members and the public on PH and PPH, including current research and findings, early detection, resource organizations, organ transplantation, and support networks. Conducts support group meetings. Funds medical research Pub: *Pathlight*, quarterly. Newsletter. • *Patients Guide to Pulmonary Hypertension, 2nd Ed.*. Book. *Price:* $25. • *Persistent Voices*, semiannual. • *PHA News*, biweekly. Newsletter. Electronic newsletter. *Price:* Free. Frmly: (1998) United Patients Association for Pulmonary Hypertension.

### ★ 5059 ★ Raynaud's and Scleroderma Association (RSAT)

112 Crewe Rd.
Alsager
Stoke-On-Trent ST7 2JA, United Kingdom
Phone: 44 1270 872776     Fax: 44 1270 883556
Email: webmaster@raynauds.demon.co.uk
Website: http://www.raynauds.demon.co.uk

Fnded: 1982. Mem: 8,000. Nat'l Groups: 1. Reg. Groups: 4. Lang(s): English. Desc: Individuals afflicted with Raynaud's Disease or scleroderma; concerned medical professionals. Raynaud's Disease is marked by interruption of blood flow to the extremities, primarily the toes and fingers but can include the ears and nose, due to spasmodic contraction of small blood vessels; in severe cases this phenomenon is often noted in individual suffering from scleroderma, which affects the blood vessels, immune system and connective tissue. Encourages better communication among doctors and patients and provides mutual support among those with the condition. Strives to heighten public awareness on Raynaud's Disease and scleroderma. Conducts fundraising activities to help finance research. Pub: *Raynaud's Association Newsletter*, quarterly. Newsletter. • Books, periodic. • Handbooks, periodic. Frmly: (1990) Raynaud's Association Trust.

### ★ 5060 ★ Romanian Society of Cardiology (SRC) (Societatea de Cardiologie — SC)

Cardiology Department
Fundeni Hospital
258 Fundeni Way
R-72435 Bucharest, Romania
Phone: 40 1 2402224     Fax: 40 1 2402224
Email: rs.cardio@fx.ro
Website: http://www.rscardio.ro

Fnded: 1947. Mem: 250. Nat'l Groups: 3. Lang(s): English, Romanian. Desc: Cardiologists. Promotes investigation into cardiovascular diseases. Areas of research include: clinical physiopathology; epidemiology; physiopathology; prophylaxy; therapeutics. Maintains educational programs. Pub: *Romanian Heart Journal*, quarterly. Frmly: (1991) Society of Cardiology.

### Scandinavian Association for Thoracic Surgery (SATS) (Nordisk Thoraxkirurgisk Forening — NTF)

See: Entry 19593

### ★ 5061 ★ Scandinavian Society for Research in CardioThoracic Surgery (SSRCTS)

c/o J. Michael Hasenkam
Department of Cardiothoracic and Vascular Surgery
Skyjby Sygehus
Aarhus University Hospital
DK-8200 Arhus, Denmark
Phone: 45 89 495480     Fax: 45 89 496016
Email: hasenkam@iekf.au.dk
Website: http://www.scandinavian-ats.org

Desc: Cardiothoracic surgeons, students, and researchers. Provides a forum for young researchers to present their work.

### ★ 5062 ★ Slovak Society of Cardiology

Krasnou horkoul
SK-83348 Bratislava, Slovakia
Phone: 42 1 759320400     Fax: 42 1 754788742
Email: hatala@susch.sk
Website: http://www.escardio.org/society/natsoc/slovakia.htm

Lang(s): English, Slovak. Desc: Cardiologists and other health care professionals with an interest in the human heart and its diseases. Seeks to enhance the professional standing and skill of members; represents members' interests before government agencies and the public.

### ★ 5063 ★ Slovenian Society of Cardiology

University Medical Centre
Clinic of Cardiology

Zaloska 7
SLO-1000 Ljubljana, Slovenia
**Phone:** 386 1 2317057　　　**Fax:** 386 1 2317057
**Email:** mfkenda@mf.uni.lj.si
**Website:** http://www.kclj.si/org/ssc
**Mem:** 141. **Desc:** Promotes the study of cardiology in Slovenia. **Pub:** *Newsletter of the Slovenian Society of Cardiology*, semiannual.

★ **5064** ★ **Societe Francaise d'Angeiologie (SFA)**
145, rue de la Pompe
F-75116 Paris, France
**Phone:** 33 1 47551433　　　**Fax:** 33 1 47272147
**Email:** micazang@noos.fr
**Website:** http://www.sfa-online.com/pri.htm
**Fnded:** 1947. **Mem:** 400. **Lang(s):** English, French. **Desc:** Individuals in France interested in angiology (the study of blood vessels and lymphatics). **Pub:** *Angeiologie*, bimonthly. Journal.

★ **5065** ★ **Society for Cardiac Angiography and Interventions (SCA&I)**
9111 Old Georgetown Rd.
Bethesda, MD 20814
**Phone:** (301)581-3450　　　**Free:** 800-992-7224
**Fax:** (301)581-3408
**Email:** info@scai.org
**Website:** http://www.scai.org
Norm Linsky, Exec. Dir.
**Fnded:** 1978. **Mem:** 2,000. **Desc:** Angiographers united to foster excellence in the field of cardiac catheterization, especially coronary arteriography and interventional angiography. (Angiography involves injecting substances opaque to radiation into blood vessels so that diagnostic X-rays of those blood vessels may be made.) Conducts clinical research. **Pub:** *Catheterization and Cardiovascular Interventions*, monthly. Journal. • *News Highlights*, quarterly. Newsletter. Includes calender of events and committee reports. *Price:* Free.

★ **5066** ★ **Society for Cardiological Science and Technology**
c/o Dept. of Cardiology
Ayr Hospital
Dalmellinton Rd.
Ayr KA6 6DX, United Kingdom
**Phone:** 44 116 2563888　　　**Fax:** 44 116 2314751
**Email:** egt@ulth.northy.nhs.uk
**Website:** http://www.scst.org.uk
**Fnded:** 1948. **Mem:** 1,000. **Reg. Groups:** 3. **Desc:** Persons whom the Council of the Society consider to be qualified to practice cardiography, technical cardiology and allied subjects. Aims to advance for the public benefit the science and practice of cardiography, technical cardiology and allied subjects by the promotion of improved standards of education and training and of research work therein and by making the results of such study and research available to practitioners and the general public. **Pub:** *SCST Update*, monthly.

★ **5067** ★ **Society of Cardiothoracic Surgeons of Great Britain and Ireland**
35-43 Lincoln's Inn Fields
London WC2A 3PN, United Kingdom
**Phone:** 44 207 8696893　　　**Fax:** 44 207 8696890
**Email:** sctsadmin@scts.org
**Website:** http://www.scts.org
**Fnded:** 1933. **Mem:** 519. **Desc:** Cardiac and thoracic surgeons. Concerned with the study of cardiothoracic disease. **Pub:** Bulletin, semiannual.

**Society of Cardiovascular Anesthesiologists (SCA)**
*See:* Entry 4469

**Society of Cardiovascular and Interventional Radiology (SCVIR)**
*See:* Entry 18155

★ **5068** ★ **Society for Cardiovascular Magnetic Resonance (SCMR)**
c/o Tom Sims
19 Mantua Rd.
Mount Royal, NJ 08061
**Phone:** (856)423-7222　　　**Fax:** (856)423-3420
**Email:** hq@scmr.org
**Website:** http://www.scmr.org
Tom Sims, Exec. Dir.
**Fnded:** 1994. **Mem:** 550. **Desc:** Physicians and scientists with an interest in cardiovascular magnetic resonance imaging are members; physiciansin-training and doctoral candidates with an interest in the field are associates; medical technologists with at least two years of experience in cardiovascular magnetic resonance are technologist members; nonscientific professionals employed by companies engaged in magnetic resonance imaging are industrial members. Seeks to advance the practice of cardiovascular magnetic resonance; works to improve study and teaching in the field. Facilitates exchange of information among members and between members and physicians and scientists working in related fields. Conducts educational programs in the application of magnetic resonance imaging to cardiovascular conditions. Serves as a clearinghouse on cardiovascular magnetic resonance imaging; sets equipment standards; conducts multicenter trials to develop cardiovascular magnetic resonance imaging methods, clinical applications, and practice standards. **Pub:** *Journal for Cardiovascular Magnetic Resonance*, quarterly. Journal.

**Society of Geriatric Cardiology**
*See:* Entry 3034

★ **5069** ★ **Society of Invasive Cardiovascular Professionals (SICP)**
c/o HMP Communications, LLC
83 General Warren Blvd., No. 100
Malvern, PA 19355-1245
**Phone:** (610)688-8220　　　**Free:** 800-237-7285
**Fax:** (610)688-8050
**Email:** sicphelp@voicnet.com
**Website:** http://www.sicp.com
Tina Thomas, Association Liason
**Fnded:** 1992. **Mem:** 700. **Desc:** Cardiac catheterization laboratory personnel. Supports the highest quality of patient care. Serves as a forum for exchange of information among members. Defines core curricula for cardiovascular professionals; makes available educational opportunities to members; establishes standards of ethics and practice for the field. Facilitates cardiovascular research. **Pub:** *Cath-Lab Digest*, monthly. Journal. *Price:* Free with membership. • *Journal of Invasive Cardiology*, monthly. Journal.

**Society of Thoracic Radiology (STR)**
*See:* Entry 18161

**Society of Thoracic Surgeons (STS)**
*See:* Entry 19603

★ **5070** ★ **Society for Vascular Medicine and Biology (SVMB)**
c/o Judy Regensteiner, Ph.D.
13 Elm St.
Manchester, MA 01944-1314
**Phone:** (978)526-8330　　　**Fax:** (978)526-4018
**Email:** svmb@prri.com
**Website:** http://www.svmb.org
Judy Regensteiner, PhD, Chair, Membership/Credentials Committee
**Fnded:** 1989. **Mem:** 270. **Desc:** Individuals with a professional interest in vascular medicine, surgery, or nursing are members; individuals in approved training programs are associates; individuals who have dem-

onstrated leadership in vascular medicine teaching, practice, or research are fellows. Promotes advancement in the disciplines of vascular medicine and vascular biology. Provides consultation and advice to educational institutions, government agencies, and health care policy makers. Facilitates formation of vascular medicine training programs; promotes establishment of Centers of Excellence for the diagnosis and treatment of vascular diseases. Promulgates standards for postgraduate continuing medical education curricula. **Pub:** *Vascular Medicine*, quarterly. Journal. • *Vascular Medicine Directory*, periodic. Directory.

**Society for Vascular Nursing (SVN)**
*See:* Entry 15778

**Society for Vascular Surgery (SVS)**
*See:* Entry 19606

★ **5071** ★ **Society of Vascular Technology (SVT)**
4601 Presidents Dr., Ste. 260
Lanham, MD 20706-4831
**Phone:** (301)459-7550　　　**Fax:** (301)459-5651
**Email:** info@svtnet.org
**Website:** http://www.svtnet.org
Suzanne Stone, Exec. Dir.
**Fnded:** 1977. **Mem:** 4,300. **Local Groups:** 29. **Desc:** Vascular technologists and others in the field of noninvasive vascular technology. (Noninvasive vascular technology is a highly technical and specialized method of monitoring the blood flow in arms and legs and veins and arteries away from the heart in order to better diagnose disease and blood clots.) Seeks to establish an information clearinghouse providing reference and assistance in matters relating to noninvasive vascular technology; facilitate cooperation among noninvasive vascular facilities and other health professions; provide continuing education for individuals in the field. **Pub:** *Glossary of Terms*. *Price:* $10 for members; $20 for nonmembers. • *Journal of Vascular Technology*, quarterly. Journal. *Price:* Included in membership dues; $80/year for nonmembers; $105/year (outside the U.S. and Canada). • *Medicare Compliance Manual*. Handbook. *Price:* $250 for members; $350 for nonmembers. • *Patient Education Pamphlets*. Pamphlets. Covers peripheral arterial, venous, and cerebrovascular diseases. • *Referenced Study Outline*. *Price:* $10 for members; $15 for nonmembers. • *Spectrum*, bimonthly. Newsletter. *Price:* Included in membership dues; $35/year for nonmembers in the U.S. and Canada; $40/year overseas. • *Vascular Registry Review*. Two-volume (three-ring binder) set. *Price:* $75 for members; $100 for nonmembers. • Brochures. • Videos. • Also publishes information kits. **Frmly:** (1988) Society of Non-Invasive Vascular Technology.

★ **5072** ★ **Spanish Society of Cardiology**
Nuestra Senora de Guadalupe, 5-7
28028 Madrid, Spain
**Phone:** 34 91 7242370　　　**Fax:** 34 91 7242371
**Email:** sec@secardiologia.es
**Website:** http://www.secardiologia.es
**Mem:** 2,179. **Desc:** Promotes the study of cardiology in Spain. **Pub:** Journal. • Newsletter.

★ **5073** ★ **Stroke Network**
PO Box 492
Abingdon, MD 21009
**Website:** http://www.strokenetwork.org
**Desc:** Stroke survivors and caregivers. Promotes stroke awareness, provides support to stroke survivors, offers information for those suffering physical problems such as Central Pain and emotional scars. Offers Web Casts, private chat rooms, bookstore. **Pub:** Newsletter, monthly.

**★ 5074 ★ Sudden Arrythmia Death Syndromes Foundation (SADS)**
508 E South Temple, Ste. 20
Salt Lake City, UT 84102-1013
**Phone:** (801)531-0937    **Free:** 800-STO-PSAD
**Fax:** (801)531-0945
**Email:** sads@sads.org
**Website:** http://www.sads.org
Lynne Godfrey, Prg. Dir.

**Fnded:** 1991. **Mem:** 29,000. **Reg. Groups:** 4. **Desc:** Seeks to identify, help diagnose and help treat children and young adults who are genetically predisposed to sudden death by cardia arrhythmias. Supports patients, families and physicians dealing with Long QT Syndrome (LQTS) and other sudden death syndromes; educates medical personnel and the public about cardiac arrhythmias; supports genetic research; offers genealogical research and family notification services; links individuals with similar concerns for support; establishes support groups. **Pub:** *Acquired Long QT Syndrome*. Brochure. • *Heart to Hearth*, semiannual. Newsletter. • *Inherited Long QT Syndrome*. Brochure.

**★ 5075 ★ Swedish Society of Cardiology**
Karolinska Hospital
Department of Cardiology
SE-171 76 Stockholm, Sweden
**Phone:** 46 8 5177871    **Fax:** 46 8 333962
**Email:** lennart.bergfeldt@medks.ki.se
**Website:** http://www.svls.se

**Mem:** 1,171. **Desc:** Promotes the study of cardiology in Sweden.

**★ 5076 ★ Swiss Society of Cardiology**
Schwarztorstrasse 18
CH-3007 Bern, Switzerland
**Phone:** 41 31 3888090    **Fax:** 41 31 3888098
**Email:** info@swisscardio.com
**Website:** http://www.swisscardio.com

**Fnded:** 1949. **Mem:** 490. **Desc:** Promotes the study of cardiology in Switzerland, including heart failure and pacemakers. **Pub:** *Kardiovaskulare Medizin/Medecine Cardiovasculare*, 8/year. Journal. • Newsletter, 3/year.

**★ 5077 ★ Tunisian Society of Cardiology and Cardiovascular Surgery**
BP 30
El Omrane
TN-1005 Tunis, Tunisia
**Phone:** 216 1 563181    **Fax:** 216 1 563181
**Mem:** 96. **Desc:** Promotes the study of cardiology in Tunisia.

**★ 5078 ★ Turkish Society of Cardiology (TSC)**
**(Turk Kardiyoloji Dernegi — TKD)**
Ortaklar Caddesi 4/7, Aksu apt.
Mecidiyekoy
TR-80290 Istanbul, Turkey
**Phone:** 90 212 2884455    **Fax:** 90 212 2884433
**Email:** tkd@ixir.com
**Website:** http://www.tkd.org.tr

**Fnded:** 1963. **Mem:** 700. **Nat'l Groups:** 9. **Lang(s):** English, Turkish. **Desc:** Cardiologists and specialists in related fields. Promotes increased public and professional awareness of cardiovascular diseases. Encourages and funds cardiological research; gathers and disseminates information to members. Offers postgraduate course in cardiology. Has conducted survey on heart disease and risk factors. **Pub:** *Archives of the Turkish Society of Cardiology*, monthly. Journal. Contains research work, reviews, and case reports. English summaries available. • *Congress Supplement for Abstracts*, annual. • Directory, biennial.

**★ 5079 ★ Ukrainian Society of Cardiology**
Institute of Cardiology
5 Narodnoje Opolchenje St.
252151 Kiev, Ukraine
**Phone:** 380 44 2776622    **Fax:** 380 44 2774209
**Email:** alex@cardio.pp.kiev.ua
**Website:** http://www.rql.kiev.ua/cardio_j

**Mem:** 91. **Desc:** Promotes the study of cardiology in Ukraine. **Pub:** *Ukrainian Journal of Cardiology*, bimonthly.

**★ 5080 ★ Velo-Cardio-Facial Syndrome (VCFS)**
c/o Dr. Robert J. Shprintzen
Upstate Medical University
University Hospital
708 Jacobsen Hall (CDU)
750 E Adams St.
Syracuse, NY 13210
**Phone:** (315)464-6590    **Fax:** (315)464-6593
**Email:** vcfsef@mail.upstate.edu
**Website:** http://www.vcfsef.org
Dr. Robert J. Shprintzen, Exec. Dir.

**Mem:** 1,300. **Desc:** Committed to educating the lay and professional public, offers family programs, provides parent-to-parent networking; promotes the diagnosis and treatment of individuals with VCF; distributes educational materials about Velo-Cardio-Facial (also known as Shprintzen Syndrome, DiGeorge Sequence, and Catch 22); and distributes questionnaire regarding the medical diagnosis and management of individuals with this disorder. **Pub:** Newsletter, periodic.

**★ 5081 ★ World Heart Federation**
5, avenue du Mail
CH-1205 Geneva, Switzerland
**Phone:** 41 22 8070300    **Fax:** 41 22 8070339
**Email:** admin@worldheart.org
**Website:** http://www.worldheart.org

**Fnded:** 1978. **Mem:** 167. **Nat'l Groups:** 144. **Reg. Groups:** 8. **Lang(s):** English, French, German, Spanish. **Desc:** Promotes international study, prevention, and treatment of cardiovascular diseases; encourages, coordinates, and assists the development of educational and scientific programs focusing on cardiovascular problems. Seeks to help people achieve a longer and better life through prevention and control of heart disease and stroke, with a focus on low and middle income countries. **Pub:** *Heartbeat*, quarterly. **Frmly:** (1999) International Society and Federation of Cardiology.

**★ 5082 ★ Yugoslav Society of Cardiology**
Institut of Cardiovascular Diseases
Clinic of Cardiology
Institutski put N4
YU-21204 Sremska Kamenica, Yugoslavia
**Phone:** 381 21 613286    **Fax:** 381 21 622881
**Email:** ukj@eunet.yu

**Fnded:** 1955. **Mem:** 330. **Desc:** Promotes the study of cardiology in Yugoslavia. **Pub:** *Cardiology*, quarterly. Journal. • *Hypertension*, quarterly. Journal.

# Research Centers

**★ 5083 ★ Arizona Heart Institute**
2632 N 20th St.
Phoenix, AZ 85006
**Phone:** (602)266-2200    **Free:** 800-835-2920
**Fax:** (602)240-5862
**Email:** information@azheart.com
**Website:** http://www.azheart.com
Robert K. Strumpf, MD, Dir. of Interventional Cardiology

**Activities/Fields:** Ambulatory cardiovascular drugs, including medications for hypertension, angina pectoris, cholesterol reduction, congestive heart failure, and peripheral vascular occlusive disease. Also investigates cardiovascular diagnostic testing procedures and nonpharmacological interventions. **Pub:** *Newsletter*, quarterly.

**Baylor College of Medicine Center for Cell and Gene Therapy**
*See:* Entry 9372

**★ 5084 ★ Baylor College of Medicine DeBakey Heart Center**
Texas Medical Center
One Baylor Plz.
Houston, TX 77030
**Phone:** (713)798-8600    **Fax:** (713)793-1192
**Email:** mdebakey@bcm.tmc.ed
**Website:** http://www.debakeyheartcenter.com
Dr. Michael E. DeBakey, Chancellor

**Activities/Fields:** Atherosclerosis with an emphasis on lipoprotein structure and function and cholesterol metabolism; cardiovascular studies on calcium metabolism, fatty acid metabolism, and cellular ultrastructure; cardiology and cardiovascular surgery, including therapeutic intervention in heart failure, ischemic cardiomyopathy, and role of complement in myocardial infarction; transplantation; and hypertension studies that focus on aldosteronerenin ratio antihypertensive agents. Community outreach studies include control of blood pressure, diabetes, and diet modification. **Pub:** *The DeBakey Health Letter*. **Frmly:** Cardiovascular Research and Training Center; National Heart and Blood Vessel Research and Demonstration Center.

**★ 5085 ★ Cardiothoracic Education and Research Institute**
792-A Foothill Blvd., pmb119
San Luis Obispo, CA 93405
**Phone:** (805)220-3585    **Fax:** (805)220-2793
**Email:** karen@amainc.com
Karen Morgan, Contact

**Activities/Fields:** Cardiothoracic surgery.

**★ 5086 ★ Center for Cardiovascular Biomaterials (CCB)**
Department of Biomedical Engineering
Case Western Reserve University
10900 Euclid Ave.
Cleveland, OH 44106-7207
**Phone:** (216)368-3005    **Fax:** (216)368-4969
**Email:** rxm4@po.cwru.edu
**Website:** http://www.case.cwru.edu/research/inter.html
Roger Marchant, Dir.

**Activities/Fields:** Biomaterials, tissue engineering and biomimetic nanotechnologies for use in cardiovascular implants and drug delivery. Services include nanoscale analysis, blood and tissue biocompatibility evaluations.

**★ 5087 ★ Charles R. Drew University of Medicine and Science**
**Hypertension Research Center**
1621 E 120th St., MP 11
Los Angeles, CA 90059
**Phone:** (310)668-3177    **Fax:** (323)563-4924
**Email:** haward@cdrew.edu
Harry Ward, MD, Dir.

**Activities/Fields:** Epidemiology, causes, and treatment of high blood pressure in blacks. Analyzes twin studies to assess genetic and environmental factors in blood pressure variations. Conducts cross-cultural studies in Barbados and Nigeria.

**★ 5088 ★ Children's Heart and Health Institute of Texas**
PO Box 3966
Corpus Christi, TX 78463
**Phone:** (361)887-4505    **Fax:** (361)887-0539
Laura Berlanga, CEO

**Activities/Fields:** Pediatric cardiology. Projects include investigations of the prevalence of developmental disabilities and heart disease risk factors in various counties, coronary disease among Hispanic children, arterial sclerotic heart disease, hypertension, and prevention.

### ★ 5089 ★ Cornell University
**Division of Hypertension**
New York Hospital-Cornell Medical Center
520 E 70th St.
New York, NY 10021
**Phone:** (212)746-2210          **Fax:** (212)746-8277
**Email:** paugust@med.cornell.edu
Phyllis August, MD, Ch.

**Activities/Fields:** Research into causation, diagnosis, and treatment of hypertension and related disorders of the heart, kidneys, and adrenal glands. Research also includes pathogenesis and treatment of heart attacks, congestive heart failure, renal failure, and stroke. **Frmly:** Hypertension and Cardiovascular Center.

### ★ 5090 ★ Creighton University
**Cardiac Center**
3006 Webster St.
Omaha, NE 68131
**Phone:** (402)280-4566          **Fax:** (402)280-4938
**Email:** smm@cardiac.creighton.edu
Dr. Mohiuddin, Med. Dir.

**Activities/Fields:** Cardiology, including drug research, medical care, valvular diseases, invasive and noninvasive treatment techniques, electrocardiogram tests, pacemakers, implants, and ventricular assist devices.

**Duke University**
**Center for Emerging Cardiovascular**
**Technologies (CECT)**
*See:* Entry 4638

**Duke University**
**Pediatric Cardiac Catheterization**
**Laboratory**
*See:* Entry 5791

### ★ 5091 ★ Emory University
**Cardiac Catheterization Laboratory**
1364 Clifton Rd. NE, Ste. C430
Atlanta, GA 30322
**Phone:** (404)712-7034          **Free:** 800-434-3278
**Fax:** (404)727-3377
**Email:** olaug001@mc.duke.edu
**Website:** http://cect.egr.duke.edu
Jane C. Wilson, Mgr. Invasive Cardiology

**Activities/Fields:** Cardiovascular hemodynamics and coronary circulation.

### ★ 5092 ★ Falor Division of Surgical Research
Summa Health System/Akron City Hospital
525 E Market St.
Akron, OH 44309
**Phone:** (330)375-3693          **Fax:** (330)375-4648
**Email:** schmidts@summa-health.org
Dr. Steven Schmidt, Dir.

**Activities/Fields:** Vascular cells, focusing on cell and molecular biology, hyperplasia, and wound healing. **Frmly:** Vascular Research Laboratory.

### ★ 5093 ★ Framingham Heart Study
5 Thurber St.
Framingham, MA 01702
**Phone:** (508)935-3400          **Fax:** (508)626-1262
**Email:** sandra@fram.nhlbi.nih.gov
**Website:** http://www.nhlbi.nih.gov/about/framingham/index.html
Daniel Levy, MD, Dir.

**Activities/Fields:** Constitutional and conditioning factors in atherosclerotic, hypertensive, and cardiovascular diseases based on a long-term study of a section of the population of Framingham, Massachusetts. There were 5209 men and women who originally participated in the study, begun in 1948, and subsequent studies have focused on 5124 descendents and spouses of descendents in the second generation. One hundred families of its third and fourth generations are also under study.

### ★ 5094 ★ George Washington University
**Lipid Research Clinic**
908 New Hampshire Ave. NW, Ste. 500
Washington, DC 20037
**Phone:** (202)872-3700          **Fax:** (202)659-8627
Judith Hsia, Dir.

**Activities/Fields:** Clinical trials of cholesterol and prevention of heart disease, including cholesterol lowering food and fibers, products, and medication. Also studies cholesterol lowering in senior citizens and trials of postmenopausal hormone replacement and heart disease risk factors in women.

### ★ 5095 ★ Gladstone Institute of Cardiovascular Disease
San Francisco General Hospital
PO Box 419100
San Francisco, CA 94141-9100
**Phone:** (415)826-7500          **Fax:** (415)285-5632
**Email:** rmahley@gladstone.ucsf.edu
**Website:** http://gladstone.ucsf.edu
Robert W. Mahley, MD, Dir.

**Activities/Fields:** Lipoprotein metabolism and biochemistry, cell biology and arterial wall metabolism, molecular biology, and clinical nutrition and metabolism, including studies of the molecular structures of various liproteins and their function in transporting blood cholesterol, the relationship of diet to cholesterol levels, and the role of platelets and white blood cells in thrombosis and atherosclerosis. **Pub:** *Gladstone Focus Newsletter*. Newsletter. • *SPIN*.

### ★ 5096 ★ Good Samaritan Hospital
**Heart Institute**
1225 Wilshire Blvd.
Los Angeles, CA 90017-2395
**Phone:** (213)977-4040          **Fax:** (213)977-4107
**Email:** rkloner@goodsam.org
Dr. Robert A. Kloner, Dir.

**Activities/Fields:** Myocardial biochemistry, myocardial infarction, effects of toxins on the heart, clinical hypertension trials, and lipid trials. **Pub:** *Scientific and clinical papers*.

### ★ 5097 ★ Harvard Thorndike Laboratory
330 Brookline Ave.
Boston, MA 02215
**Phone:** (617)667-3020          **Fax:** (617)667-1615
**Email:** jnorris@caregroup.harvard.edu
Dr. James P. Morgan, Dir.

**Activities/Fields:** Effects of drugs and disease on cardiac hypertrophy and failure; cardiovascular effects of drug abuse. Specific areas of research include cardiac and vasculary pharmacology, physiology, and biochemistry.

### ★ 5098 ★ Heart Disease Research Foundation
50 Court St.
Brooklyn, NY 11201
**Phone:** (718)649-6210          **Fax:** (718)649-6210
Dr. Yoshiaki Omura, Dir. of Med. Res.

**Activities/Fields:** Early diagnosis, prevention, and treatment of cardiovascular diseases and related medical and social problems. Studies include the effects of acupuncture and electro-therapeutics on blood chemistry and the cardiovascular system and clinical approaches of these methods directed toward the treatment of abnormal brain circulation and blood pressure and lower extremity circulatory disturbances.

### ★ 5099 ★ Heart Institute of Spokane
122 W 7th Ave., Ste. 230
Spokane, WA 99204-2340
**Phone:** (509)625-3020          **Fax:** (509)625-3025
**Email:** ktuttle@this.org
**Website:** http://www.this.org
Katherine R. Tuttle, MD, Dir.

**Activities/Fields:** Heart and vascular diseases. **Pub:** *Newsletter*.

### ★ 5100 ★ Heart Research Foundation of Sacramento
3900 J St.
Sacramento, CA 95819
**Phone:** (916)456-3365          **Fax:** (916)452-7579
**Email:** rjfrank@pol.net
Patti Gantenbein, Exec. Dir.

**Activities/Fields:** Clinical and pathological studies of atherosclerosis, experimental cardiovascular pharmaceutical testing, and coronary, myocardial, and conduction system morphology. **Pub:** *Newsletter*, semiannually.

### ★ 5101 ★ Heart and Stroke Foundation of British Columbia and Yukon
1212 W Broadway
Vancouver, BC, Canada V6H 3V2
**Phone:** (604)736-4404          **Fax:** (604)736-8732
**Email:** info@hsf.ca
**Website:** http://www.bc.heartandstroke.ca
Bobbe Wood, Exec. Dir.

**Activities/Fields:** Provides research support in the form of personnel awards and grants-in-aid for studies on heart disease and stroke. Fellowships provide salary support for young scientists just beginning a career in research. Grants-in-aid finance research projects of an experienced and salaried professional or university faculty member, paying for such things as equipment, expendables (glassware and chemicals), and technical assistance. A limited number of Heart and Stroke Foundation research traineeships are available to highly qualified graduate students enrolled in a PhD program and who are undertaking full-time research training in the cardiovascular or cerebrovascular fields. **Pub:** *Pacesetter Newsletter*, quarterly. • *Research Annual Report*.

### ★ 5102 ★ Heart and Stroke Foundation of Canada
222 Queen St., Ste. 1402
Ottawa, ON, Canada K1P 5V9
**Phone:** (613)569-4361          **Fax:** (613)569-3278
**Email:** jgee@hsf.ca
**Website:** http://www.hsf.ca/research
Jennifer Gee, Acting Assoc. Dir.

**Activities/Fields:** Provides grants for research in cardiovascular and cerebrovascular diseases, particularly the elucidation of fundamental laws and the development of materials, devices, systems, or methods useful in treating stroke, heart attack, hypertension, and effects of smoking. **Frmly:** Canadian Heart and Stroke Foundation.

### ★ 5103 ★ Heart and Stroke Foundation of Newfoundland and Labrador
169-173 Water St.
PO Box 5819
Saint John's, NF, Canada A1C 5X3
**Phone:** (709)753-8521          **Free:** 888-473-4636
**Fax:** (709)753-3117
**Website:** http://www.hsf.ca/prov/newfoundland.htm
Stephen Browne, Exec. Dir.

**Activities/Fields:** Causes of and cures for cardiovascular and cerebrovascular disease.

### ★ 5104 ★ Heart and Stroke Foundation of Nova Scotia
5523 Spring Garden Rd., Ste. 204
Halifax, NS, Canada B3J 3T1
**Phone:** (902)423-7530          **Fax:** (902)492-1464

**Website:** http://ww2.heartandstroke.ca/
J.E. Fraser, Exec. Dir.

**Activities/Fields:** Cardiovascular and cerebrovascular basic and clinical research, including educational and behavioral science approaches to cardiovascular health. **Pub:** *Research Directory.* **Frmly:** Nova Scotia Heart Foundation.

### ★ 5105 ★ Heineman Medical Research
PO Box 32861
Charlotte, NC 28232-2861
**Phone:** (704)355-3200　　　　**Fax:** (704)355-1435
**Website:** http://www.heineman.org
Francis Robicsek, MD, Pres.

**Activities/Fields:** Diseases of heart, lungs, and great vessels, with special interest in organ preservation, electrophysiology, and laser applications to arrhythmias and vascular diseases. **Pub:** *Bulletin of Cardiopulmonary Disease.* • *Heineman Report.*

### ★ 5106 ★ Hope Heart Institute
1124 Columbia St., Ste. 120
Seattle, WA 98104-2046
**Phone:** (206)903-2001　　　　**Fax:** (206)903-2144
**Email:** ksnow@hopeheart.org
**Website:** http://www.hopeheart.org
Kristin Snow, Contact

**Activities/Fields:** Prevention and treatment of heart and blood vessel disease. The institute has three research divisions: Basic Sciences, Translational Sciences, and Community Public Health. Basic Sciences is primarily vascular biology and includes cellular and molecular biology, as well as histology. Translational Sciences include cardiovascular gene therapy and tissue engineering, as well as cardioneurology. Community Public Health includes general public education on heart disease through educational research in multicultural settings. Major research projects include understanding angiogenesis (the growth of new blood vessels), extracellular matrix deposition (the formation of atherosclerotics plaques), new techniques for repair of myocardio infarction, and education research in underserved communities. **Pub:** *Brochures, booklets and videos.* • *Hope Health Letter.* • *Newsletter.*

### ★ 5107 ★ House Ear Institute
2100 W 3rd St.
Los Angeles, CA 90057
**Phone:** (213)483-4431　　　　**Fax:** (213)483-8789
**Email:** webmaster@hei.org
**Website:** http://www.hei.org
James D. Boswell, CEO

**Activities/Fields:** Cause, treatment, and prevention of hearing and balance disorders, including investigations on cochlear implants and auditory prostheses, electrophysiology, electron microscopy, anatomy, cellular and molecular biology, and psychoacoustics. **Pub:** *Annual Report.* • *The Review,* 3/year. **Frmly:** Ear Research Institute.

### ★ 5108 ★ Indiana University-Purdue University at Indianapolis Hypertension Research Center
541 Clinical Dr., Rm. 423
Indianapolis, IN 46202-5111
**Phone:** (317)274-8153　　　　**Fax:** (317)278-0673
**Email:** mweinbe@iupui.edu
Dr. Myron H. Weinberger, Dir.

**Activities/Fields:** Hypertension, including a broad-based, multidisciplinary research program of clinical studies involving genetics of hypertension, pathophysiology of hypertension with plasma renin suppression, role of renin and aldosterone in toxemia of pregnancy, causes of childhood hypertension, and role of renin and aldosterone in heart failure. Also studies myocardial metabolism and cyclic AMP system in spontaneously hypertensive rats, role of sympathetic nervous system in human experimental forms of hypertension, control of renin release in vitro and of renal sodium handling, role of sodium in blood pressure, sodium restriction in the treatment of hypertension, and role of

calcium and potassium in blood pressure. **Frmly:** Specialized Center for Research in Hypertension.

### ★ 5109 ★ Institute for Clinical Research, Inc.
PO Box 29545
Washington, DC 20017-0745
**Phone:** (202)462-6820　　　　**Fax:** (202)462-2006
Steven Singh, Chm.

**Activities/Fields:** Hypertension, cardiology, infectious diseases, and oncology.

### Johns Hopkins Bayview Medical Center General Clinical Research Center
*See:* Entry 3054

### ★ 5110 ★ Johns Hopkins University Cardiac Bioelectric Systems Laboratory
Traylor Research Bldg., 7th Fl.
Department of Biomedical Engineering
School of Medicine
720 Rutland Ave.
Baltimore, MD 21205
**Phone:** (410)955-9603　　　　**Fax:** (410)955-0549
**Email:** ltung@bme.jhu.edu
**Website:** http://www.bme.jhu.edu/~ltung/CBS_Lab/
Leslie Tung, PhD, Dir.

**Activities/Fields:** Electrical properties of the heart, in particular as they relate at the cellular and multicellular levels to defibrillation and arrhythmia.

### ★ 5111 ★ Johns Hopkins University Center for Computational Medicine and Biology Computational Modeling Group
Department of Biomedical Engineering
School of Medicine
720 Rutland Ave.
Baltimore, MD 21205
**Phone:** (410)614-6685　　　　**Fax:** (410)614-8796
**Email:** ccmb@bme.jhu.edu
**Website:** http://www.cmbl.jhu.edu/
Prof. Raimond L. Winslow, Dir.

**Activities/Fields:** Understanding the origins of cardiac arrhythmias through the use of biophysically detailed computer models.

### ★ 5112 ★ Johns Hopkins University Lipid Research Atherosclerosis Unit
550 North Broadway, Ste. 308
Baltimore, MD 21205
**Phone:** (410)955-3198　　　　**Fax:** (410)955-1276
**Email:** pkwitero@jhmi.edu
Dr. Peter Kwiterovich, Contact

**Activities/Fields:** Lipids, lipoproteins, apolipoproteins, atherosclerosis, genetics, coronary artery diseases, and basic serum proteins.

### ★ 5113 ★ Johns Hopkins University Vascular Bioengineering Laboratory
Department of Biomedical Engineering
School of Medicine
720 Rutland Ave.
619 Traylor
Baltimore, MD 21205
**Phone:** (410)614-2951　　　　**Fax:** (410)614-8796
**Email:** ralevria@bme.jhu.edu
**Website:** http://www.bme.jhu.edu/~thuang/lab/lab.html
B. Rita Alevriadou, PhD, Prin. Investigator

**Activities/Fields:** Fluid mechanics; thrombosis/atherosclerosis; vascular cell biology; and cell and tissue engineering.

### ★ 5114 ★ Krannert Institute of Cardiology
1800 N Capitol Ave.
Indianapolis, IN 46202

**Phone:** (317)962-0500　　　　**Fax:** (317)962-0501
**Email:** dzipes@iupui.edu
Douglas Zipes, Dir.

**Activities/Fields:** Electrophysiology, cardiac membrane biology, echocardiography, vascular biology, exercise physiology, and cardiovascular transgenics. **Pub:** *Cardiology in Review,* bimonthly. • *Contemporary Treatments in Cardiology,* quarterly. • *Journal of Cardiovascular Electrophysiology,* monthly.

### ★ 5115 ★ Laval University Hopital Laval Cardiopulmonary Institute
2725 Chemin Ste. Foy
Sainte Foy, QC, Canada G1V 4G5
**Phone:** (418)656-4760　　　　**Fax:** (418)656-4509
**Email:** denis.richard@phs.ulaval.ca
Denis Richard, PhD, Dir.

**Activities/Fields:** All major fields of cardiopulmonary diseases, and obesity and energetic metabolism. **Pub:** *Publications and Absracts (200/year).*

### ★ 5116 ★ Laval University Medical Research Centre Lipid Research Centre
2705 Blvd. Laurier, TR-93
Sainte Foy, QC, Canada G1V 4G2
**Phone:** (418)654-2244　　　　**Fax:** (418)654-2714
**Email:** pierre.julien@crchul.ulaval.ca
**Website:** http://www.crchul.ulaval.ca/crchul/fr/default.asp
Pierre Julien, PhD, Dir.

**Activities/Fields:** Pharmacological studies on hypolipidemic agents, lipoproteins, apoproteins, LDL receptors, lipoprotein lipase and hepatic lipase activity, abdominal and visceral obesity, metabolism and genetic polymorphism, nutritional studies on polysaturated and omega fatty acids, and epidemiology of ischemic heart disease in the region of Quebec City.

### Loyola University Chicago Heart Transplant and Heart Failure Program
*See:* Entry 20350

### ★ 5117 ★ Masonic Medical Research Laboratory (MMRL)
2150 Bleecker St.
Utica, NY 13501
**Phone:** (315)735-2217　　　　**Fax:** (315)735-5648
**Email:** ca@mmrl.edu
**Website:** http://www.mmrl.edu
Dr. Charles Antzelevitch, Exec. Dir.

**Activities/Fields:** Ischemic heart disease, cardiac arrhythmias, forms of sudden cardiac death known as idiopathic ventricular fibrillation or the Brugada Syndrome death as well as the cellular basis for the different waves found in the electrocardiogram and molecular biology.

### ★ 5118 ★ MCP Hahnemann University of the Health Sciences Cardiothoracic Surgery Department
Broad & Vine Sts.
Philadelphia, PA 19102
**Phone:** (215)762-4955　　　　**Fax:** (215)762-1858
**Email:** wechsla@wpo.auhs.edu
**Website:** http://www.hearthospital.org
Andrew Wechsler, MD, Chm.

**Activities/Fields:** Diseases of the heart and great vessels, including studies in myocardial metabolism, physioloy, electrophysiology, cardiac surgery, echocardiography, pharmacology, and nuclear cardiology. Initiates research in causes, diagnosis, and treatment of cardiac and pulmonary disease.

**★ 5119 ★ MCP Hahnemann University of the Health Sciences**
**Institute for Cardiovascular Research**
Allegheny General Hospital
320 E North Ave.
Pittsburgh, PA 15212
**Phone:** (412)359-8255
**Website:** http://www.mcphu.edu/institutes/instcardi-o.html
Stephen F. Vatner, MD, Dir.
**Activities/Fields:** Cardiovascular disease.


**★ 5120 ★ Medical College of Georgia**
**Vascular Biology Center (VBC)**
1120 15th St.
Augusta, GA 30912-2500
**Phone:** (706)721-6338          **Fax:** (706)721-9799
**Email:** jcatrava@mail.mcg.edu
**Website:** http://www.mcg.edu/Centers/VBC
John D. Catravas, PhD, Dir.
**Activities/Fields:** Cellular and integrated vascular function under normal and pathologic conditions in order to elucidate specific homeostatic vascular functions, as well as the pathogenesis, diagnosis and treatment of vascular disease. **Pub:** *Vascular Pharmacology*, monthly.


**Medical University of South Carolina**
**Molecular Morphology and Imaging Core**
*See:* Entry 12219


**★ 5121 ★ Miami Heart Research Institute**
801 Arthur Godfrey Rd., 5th Fl.
Miami Beach, FL 33140
**Phone:** (305)674-3020          **Fax:** (305)535-3642
**Email:** mhri@miamiheartresearch.org
**Website:** http://www.miamiheartresearch.org
Kathleen DuCasse, CEO
**Activities/Fields:** Cardiovascular disease, including tracking genetic cardiovascular abnormalities, sudden cardiac death, emergency response resuscitation techniques, stress reduction techniques as well as hypertension and cholesterol studies. **Pub:** *Heartbeats Newsletter*.


**★ 5122 ★ Midwest Heart Research Foundation**
2340 Highland Ave., Ste. 310
Lombard, IL 60148
**Phone:** (630)932-2165          **Fax:** (630)268-9609
**Email:** lbarr@midwestheart.com
Lawrence A. Barr, MD, Med. Dir.
**Activities/Fields:** Cardiovascular medicine clinical research. **Pub:** *Medical Journal.* • *Proceedings.*


**★ 5123 ★ Minneapolis Heart Institute Foundation**
920 E 28th St., Ste. 100
Minneapolis, MN 55407-1139
**Phone:** (612)863-3833          **Free:** 877-800-2729
**Fax:** (612)863-3801
**Website:** http://www.mplsheartfoundation.org/
Ford Watson Bell, DVM, Pres.
**Activities/Fields:** Clinical cardiovascular studies with emphasis on cardiac death in the young.


**Minneapolis Vascular Institute**
*See:* Entry 8760


**★ 5124 ★ New England Medical Center Hospitals, Inc.**
**Center for Cardiovascular Health Services Research**
New England Medical Center, Box 63
750 Washington St.
Boston, MA 02111
**Phone:** (617)636-5009          **Fax:** (617)636-8023

**Email:** hselker@lifespan.org
Harry P. Selker, MD, Contact
**Activities/Fields:** Cardiovascular health services, particularly in the development and testing of predictive instruments for acute cardiac ischemia, thrombolytic therapy, and the use of cardiac care units in hospitals.


**★ 5125 ★ Northeastern University**
**Center for Cardiovascular Targeting**
205 Mugar Life Sciences Bldg.
Department of Pharmaceutical Sciences
Boston, MA 02115
**Phone:** (617)373-4203          **Fax:** (617)373-3663
**Email:** b.khaw@nunet.neu.edu
**Website:** http://www.neu.edu/top/research3.html
Ban-An Khaw, PhD, Dir.
**Activities/Fields:** In vivo targeting of myriad cardiovascular-related health problems, such as atherosclerotic lesions, myocardial necrosis, brain infarction and various tumors.


**★ 5126 ★ Ohio State University**
**Dorothy M. Davis Heart and Lung Research Institute**
473 W 12th Ave.
Columbus, OH 43210-1252
**Phone:** (614)247-7766          **Fax:** (614)247-7799
**Email:** HLRI@medctr.osu.edu
**Website:** http://heartlung.osu.edu
Mark D. Wewers, MD, Interim Dir.
**Activities/Fields:** Development of novel strategies to cure patients affected with heart and lung diseases and to prevent such diseases from developing in individuals at risk.


**★ 5127 ★ Oklahoma Medical Research Foundation**
**Cardiovascular Biology Research Program**
825 NE 13th St.
Oklahoma City, OK 73104
**Phone:** (405)271-7048          **Free:** 800-522-0211
**Fax:** (405)271-3137
**Email:** jdonald-capra@omrf.ouhsc.edu
**Website:** http://www.omrf.ouhsc.edu/OMRF/Research/15/Program.asp
J. Donald Capra, MD, Pres.
**Activities/Fields:** Cardiovascular disease, especially blood clotting and inflammatory aspects of vascular diseases; structure determination of blood coagulation enzymes and design of inhibitors; regulation of inflammation by the coagulation system and the impact of inflammation on coagulation; mechanisms by which autoimmune diseases modulate blood coagulation and vascular function; septic shock; and the mechanisms of leukocyte binding to vascular endothelium. Gene deletion and transgenic approaches are designed to identify targets for therapeutic intervention.


**★ 5128 ★ Oklahoma Medical Research Foundation**
**Lipid and Lipoprotein Laboratory**
825 NE 13th St.
Oklahoma City, OK 73104
**Phone:** (405)271-7703          **Fax:** (405)271-8575
**Email:** hamptonk@omrf.ouhsc.edu
Dr. Petar Alaupovic, PhD, Contact
**Activities/Fields:** Chemistry and metabolism of plasma lipid transport, pathophysiology and treatment of dyslipoproteinemias, and model systems of atherosclerosis, including studies on the chemistry and interaction of lipoprotein particles, formation and lipolytic degradation of lipoprotein particles, dietary and drug treatment of dyslipoproteinemias, and determination of apolipoprotein profiles in dyslipoproteinemias.


**★ 5129 ★ Oregon Health and Science University**
**Heart Research Center**
3181 SW Sam Jackson Pk. Rd., L-464
Portland, OR 97201-3098
**Phone:** (503)494-2382          **Fax:** (503)494-4352
**Email:** thornbur@ohsu.edu
**Website:** http://www.ohsu.edu/chrc/
Kent L. Thornburg, PhD, Dir.
**Activities/Fields:** Broad-based heart research, including the link between fetal heart development and adult heart disease. **Pub:** *Heart Developments*, periodically. Newsletter. • *Heart Sounds*, semiannually.


**★ 5130 ★ Ottawa Heart Institute Research Corp.**
40 Ruskin St.
Ottawa, ON, Canada K1Y 4W7
**Phone:** (613)761-5000          **Fax:** (613)761-5323
**Email:** jirvine@ottawaheart.ca
**Website:** http://www.ottawaheart.ca
D. Joe Irvine, Pres.
**Activities/Fields:** Cardiac diseases, emphasizing arteriosclerosis research and dyslipidemia, hypertension, cell and molecular biology of the heart, vascular biology, pharmacology, medical devices, artificial hearts, clinical trials and prevention and rehabilitation.


**★ 5131 ★ Pacific Vascular Research Foundation**
3627 Sacramento St.
San Francisco, CA 94118
**Phone:** (415)771-3541          **Fax:** (415)771-3902
**Email:** pvrfsf@aol.com
Donald C. McFerren, Dir.
**Activities/Fields:** Issues related to vascular health.


**★ 5132 ★ Pennsylvania State University**
**Artificial Heart Research Project**
Milton S Hershey Medical Center
500 University Dr.
Hershey, PA 17033
**Phone:** (717)531-4494          **Fax:** (717)531-4464
**Email:** grosenberg@psu.edu
**Website:** http://www.hmc.psu.edu
Gerson Rosenberg, PhD, Dir.
**Activities/Fields:** Development of an implantable, long-term, motor-driven left ventricular assist pump, an implantable, pneumatically-driven total artificial heart, and an implantable, motor-driven electric artificial heart, including all aspects of design of implantable blood pumps, implantable energy convertors, bench testing and evaluation, and animal implantation studies.


**★ 5133 ★ Pennsylvania State University**
**Vascular Health Interventions Laboratory**
315 Health & Human Development Bldg. E
Department of Biobehavioral Health
University Park, PA 16802
**Phone:** (814)863-0176          **Fax:** (814)863-7525
**Email:** sgw2@psu.edu
**Website:** http://bbh.hhdev.psu.edu/labs/westlab/
Sheila G. West, PhD, Dir.
**Activities/Fields:** Effects of dietary changes and nutritional supplements designed to promote normal function of the vascular endothelium.


**★ 5134 ★ Rees-Stealy Research Foundation**
2001 4th Ave.
San Diego, CA 92101
**Phone:** (858)235-8744          **Fax:** (858)235-8745
**Email:** md1os@aol.com
Dr. H.D. Peabody, Jr., Dir.
**Activities/Fields:** Basic cardiac research involving cardio myocyte contractility studies. Research includes the analysis of recording heart cell function, utilizing the video camera technique of living motion

using electronic devices for computer transfer, heart cell preparation, and cell culture.

**Rockefeller University**
**Laboratory of Biochemical Genetics and Metabolism**
*See:* Entry 9423

**★ 5135 ★ Rocky Mountain Clinical Research, Inc.**
29 Rogers Ct.
Golden, CO 80401-6515
**Phone:** (303)279-1550          **Fax:** (303)278-2602
**Email:** gailrmcr@aol.com
Gail Danhour, Exec. Dir.

**Activities/Fields:** Medical research, clinical drug trials, and the development of new diagnostic techniques. **Frmly:** Rocky Mountain Heart Research Institute Inc.; Rocky Mountain Assoc., Inc.

**★ 5136 ★ Rush University**
**Rush Heart Institute**
Rush-Presbyterian-St. Luke's Medical Center
1725 W Harrison, Ste. 1159
Chicago, IL 60612
**Phone:** (312)563-2230          **Free:** 800-942-4144
**Fax:** (312)733-1221
**Email:** rusheart@rush.edu
**Website:**          http://www.rush.edu/patients/heart/index.html
Dr. James E. Calvin, Dir. of Cardiology

**Activities/Fields:** Medical cardiovascular research, including cardiac and vascular physiology and cardiovascular surgery, including open heart procedures and major aortic replacement surgery.

**★ 5137 ★ St. Boniface General Hospital Research Centre**
351 Tache Ave.
Winnipeg, MB, Canada R2H 2A6
**Phone:** (204)235-3206          **Fax:** (204)235-0793
**Email:** admin_office@sbrc.umanitoba.ca
**Website:** http://www.sbrc.umanitoba.ca/
Dr. John Foerster, Res. Dir.

**Activities/Fields:** Cardiovascular sciences, magnetic resonance imaging and spectroscopy, and the degenerative disorders associated with aging, such as senile dementias.

**★ 5138 ★ St. Francis Hospital (Brookville, NY)**
**DeMatteis Center for Education and Research**
Northern Blvd.
Brookville, NY 11545
**Phone:** (516)629-2000          **Fax:** (516)629-2113
**Email:** yadon@earthlink.net
**Website:** http://www.stfrancisheartcenter.com
Dr. Yadon Arad, Dir.

**Activities/Fields:** Heart studies, focusing on drugs and diet in reversing coronary heart disease; lipid metabolism; diabetes; steroid hormones.

**★ 5139 ★ San Francisco Heart Institute**
1900 Sullivan Ave.
Daly City, CA 94015
**Phone:** (650)991-6358          **Fax:** (650)755-7315
**Email:** rshaw@chw.edu
**Website:** http://www.sfhi.com
Richard E. Shaw, PhD, Dir. Res. & Oper.

**Activities/Fields:** Analysis of success, complications, and long-term outcome of coronary angioplasty and cardiac surgery; technological advances applied to angioplasty, including new dilatation balloons, lasers, and coronary stents; transdermal therapies in treatment of hypertension; and atherectomy (rotational and directional) research.

**Southwest Foundation for Biomedical Research**
**Genetics Core Laboratory**
*See:* Entry 9429

**★ 5140 ★ Stanford University**
**Stanford Cardiac Rehabilitation Program**
780 Welch Rd., Ste. 106
Palo Alto, CA 94304-5735
**Phone:** (650)723-6463          **Fax:** (650)723-6798
**Email:** scole@darwin.sfbr.org
**Website:** http://www.sfbr.org
Robert F. DeBusk, MD, Dir.

**Activities/Fields:** Recovery from heart attack and coronary heart surgery, systems to facilitate risk factor modification in healthy individuals and patients with heart disease, and systems to enhance the cost-effectiveness of care provided to patients with heart disease. Coordinates random clinical trials in Kaiser foundation hospitals.

**★ 5141 ★ Temple University**
**Sol Sherry Thrombosis Research Center**
Old Medical School
3400 N Broad St., Rm. 300
Philadelphia, PA 19140
**Phone:** (215)707-4418          **Fax:** (215)707-2783
**Email:** colmanr@vm.temple.edu
**Website:** http://www.temple.edu/SSTRC/
Robert W. Colman, MD, Dir.

**Activities/Fields:** Thrombotic hemorrhage disorders, biochemistry and molecular biology of blood coagulation, platelet structure and function, and vascular biology and angiogeneses. Clinical studies are conducted. Core laboratories are established for cell culture, monoclonal antibody production, and molecular modeling.

**★ 5142 ★ Texas A&M University**
**Cardiovascular Research Institute**
114 TAMU
College of Medicine
College Station, TX 77843-1114
**Phone:** (979)845-7491          **Fax:** (979)862-4638
**Email:** gam@tamu.edu
**Website:** http://mphywww.tamu.edu/cvri.html
Dr. Gerald A. Meininger, Dir.

**Activities/Fields:** Applies high technology to analysis of normal and diseased microscopic blood vessels, including studies on bloodflow in both normal and diseased states, basic control and exchange processes in microcirculation, role of microcirculation in hypertension, edema, stroke, and diabetes, computer analysis of microscopic images, cellular and molecular bases of endothelial and vascular smooth muscle functions, and pathobiology of inflammation and ischemic injury. **Frmly:** Microcirculation Research Institute.

**★ 5143 ★ Texas Heart Institute**
PO Box 20345
Houston, TX 77225-0345
**Phone:** (713)791-4011          **Fax:** (713)791-3089
**Email:** his@heart.thi.tmc.edu
**Website:** http://www.texasheart.org
Denton A. Cooley, MD, Pres.

**Activities/Fields:** Diseases of the heart and cardiovascular system. Specific areas of study include cardiovascular surgery, including coronary artery bypass surgery, valve replacement, transplantation, and mechanical circulatory support and replacement/assist devices; invasive and non-invasive cardiology, including gene therapy, and molecular biochemistry; cardiovascular anesthesiology and pathology; and biostatistics and epidemiology. **Pub:** *Texas Heart Institute Journal*, quarterly.

**★ 5144 ★ Thomas Jefferson University**
**Ischemia-Shock Research Center**
Department of Physiology
1020 Locust St.
Philadelphia, PA 19107
**Phone:** (215)503-7760          **Fax:** (215)503-2073
**Email:** allan.m.lefer@mail.tju.edu
Dr. Allan M. Lefer, Dir.

**Activities/Fields:** Myocardial, splanchnic, and cerebral ischemia and circulatory shock, particularly pathophysiology and therapeutics. Promotes collaborative research among members, facilitates basic science and joint research efforts, and provides research opportunities to fellows.

**★ 5145 ★ Tulane University**
**Tulane Center for Cardiovascular Health**
1430 Tulane Ave., Box SL 29
New Orleans, LA 70112
**Phone:** (504)585-7197          **Fax:** (504)585-7194
**Email:** berenson@mailhost.tcs.tulane.edu
**Website:** http://www.tmc.tulane.edu/cardiohealth/
Gerald S. Berenson, MD, Dir.

**Activities/Fields:** Cardiovascular disease risk factors in children and young adults, including a descriptive epidemiology study (Bogalusa Heart Study), laboratory investigations on the mechanisms of arteriosclerosis, structural studies of proteoglycans, and health education and promotion in elementary school children (Health Ahead/Heart Smart).

**★ 5146 ★ U.S. Department of Health and Human Services**
**National Heart, Lung, and Blood Institute**
NIH Bldg. 31, Rm. 5A52
31 Center Dr. MSC 2486
Bethesda, MD 20892-2486
**Phone:** (301)496-5166          **Fax:** (301)402-0818
**Email:** lenfant@nhlbi.nih.gov
**Website:** http://www.nhlbi.nih.gov/
Claude Lenfant, Dir.

**Activities/Fields:** Responsible for a national program of research leading to the prevention and treatment of heart, lung, and blood diseases. The scope of the Institute's effort encompasses all forms of heart and vascular disease (except the consequences of cerebrovascular disease), most forms of pulmonary disease (except cancers), sleep disorders, many blood diseases (including sickle cell disease), and the utilization of blood resources. Research scope is primarily basic and clinical but also includes applied research and clinical trials as well as demonstration and education research. The Institute plans and directs research in the development, trial, and evaluation of drugs and devices relating to the prevention and treatment of these diseases and the rehabilitation of patients suffering from them; conducts studies into the clinical uses of blood and all aspects of the management of blood resources and supports training in basic and clinical research programs relating to heart, blood vessel, blood, and lung disease; conducts educational activities (including collection and dissemination of educational materials), with emphasis on prevention, for health professionals and the public and maintains relationships with various institutions, agencies, and organizations working in these areas; and awards pre- and postdoctoral fellowships and training grants to develop adequate research investigators. The NHLBI program also includes support for Specialized Centers of Research (SCORs), which are research units within institutions focusing on studies of a specific disease or group of diseases and the Women's Health Initiative, a multicenter observational study and clinical trail. Principal components of the Institute include divisions of: Blood Diseases and Resources, Epidemiology and Clinical Applications, Extramural Affairs, Heart and Vascular Diseases, Intramural Research, Lung Diseases.

**★ 5147 ★ U.S. Department of Health and Human Services**
**National Heart, Lung, and Blood Institute**
**Division of Epidemiology and Clinical Applications**
2 Rockledge Centre
6701 Rockledge Dr. MSC 7938
Bethesda, MD 20892-7938
**Phone:** (301)435-0422     **Fax:** (301)480-1864
**Email:** savagep@nhlbi.nih.gov
Dr. Peter Savage, MD, Dir.

**Activities/Fields:** Epidemiological studies, clinical trials, basic and applied behavioral research, demonstration and education research, and projects for disease prevention and health promotion in heart, vascular, pulmonary, and blood diseases and blood resources. It maintains surveillance over developments in its program area and assesses the national need for research on the prevention, diagnosis, and treatment of these diseases by maintaining the necessary scientific management capability to foster and guide an effective attack upon them. Activities are carried out in the Clinical Applications and Prevention Program and Epidemiology and Biometry Program.

**★ 5148 ★ U.S. Department of Health and Human Services**
**National Heart, Lung, and Blood Institute**
**Division of Epidemiology and Clinical Applications**
**Clinical Applications and Prevention Program**
2 Rockledge Centre
6701 Rockledge Dr. MSC 7936
Bethesda, MD 20892-7936
**Phone:** (301)435-0414     **Fax:** (301)480-1669
Dr. Denise Simons-Morton, Actg. Dir.

**Activities/Fields:** Supports clinical trials, demonstration and educational research, basic and applied behavioral research, and projects for the prevention of cardiovascular, lung, and blood diseases as well as therapeutic measures. Principal areas of research are preventive medicine, nutrition, behavioral medicine, cardiology, and community demonstration and education projects. **Pub:** *Proceedings.* • *Research Reports.*

**★ 5149 ★ U.S. Department of Health and Human Services**
**National Heart, Lung, and Blood Institute**
**Division of Extramural Affairs**
6701 Rockledge Dr. MSC 7924, Ste. 7100
Bethesda, MD 20892-7924
**Phone:** (301)435-0260     **Fax:** (301)480-4754
Dr. Deborah Beebe, Dir.

**Activities/Fields:** Responsible for advising the Director of the Institute on research contract, grant, and research training program policies. It represents the Institute on overall NIH committees on extramural program policy, oversees compliance with such policy within NHLBI, and coordinates the Institute's research grant and research training and development programs with the National Heart, Lung, and Blood Advisory Council. Division also provides grant and contract management and processing services to the Institute's program divisions; and supplies initial scientific merit review of applications and proposals for project grants, program project and center grants, research training and development grants, and research contracts for the Institute.

**★ 5150 ★ U.S. Department of Health and Human Services**
**National Heart, Lung, and Blood Institute**
**Division of Heart and Vascular Diseases**
Two Rockledge Centre, Ste. 9044
6701 Rockledge Dr. MSC 7940
Bethesda, MD 20892-7940
**Phone:** (301)435-0466     **Fax:** (301)480-1336
**Email:** mockrins@nhlbi.nih.gov

**Website:** http://www.nhlbi.nih.gov/about/dhvd/index.htm
Dr. Stephen Mockrin, Dir.

**Activities/Fields:** Control of heart and vascular diseases. Major areas of investigat ion include arrythmias, congenital and infectious diseases, heart failure, ischemic heart disease, interventional cardiology, bioengineering, atherosclerosis, hypertension, vascular biology, vascular medicine, cardiovascular homeostasis and bionutrition, and molecular genetics and medicine. **Pub:** *Monographs.*

**★ 5151 ★ U.S. Department of Health and Human Services**
**National Heart, Lung, and Blood Institute**
**Division of Heart and Vascular Diseases**
**Heart Research Program**
**(Bioengineering Research Group)**
2 Rockledge Center
6701 Rockledge Dr., Rm. 9178
Bethesda, MD 20892-7940
**Phone:** (301)435-0513     **Fax:** (301)480-1336
**Email:** jw53F@nih.gov
**Website:** http://www.nih.gov
John T. Watson, PhD, Chf.

**Activities/Fields:** Mechanical circulatory support, biomaterials (blood-material interactions), and diagnostic and therapeutic devices, as well as technolgy transfer through Small Business Innovation Research Grants.

**★ 5152 ★ U.S. Department of Health and Human Services**
**National Heart, Lung, and Blood Institute**
**Division of Heart and Vascular Diseases**
**Heart Research Program**
**(Arrhythmia Research Program)**
2 Rockledge Ctr., Ste. 9192
6701 Rockledge Dr., MSC 7940
Bethesda, MD 20892-7940
**Phone:** (301)435-0504     **Fax:** (301)480-1454
**Email:** ps48j@nih.gov
**Website:** http://www.nhlbi.nih/gov/personal/laura/nhlbi/extlocal.html
Peter M. Spooner, PhD, Contact

**Activities/Fields:** Administers research grants and implements new research programs in the basic medical sciences as related to cardiology, physiology, anatomy, pharmacology, biochemistry, and bioengineering as they relate to cause and prevention of cardiac arrhythmias, sudden cardiac death, and cardiac ischemia. **Frmly:** (2000) Arrythmia Research Program.

**★ 5153 ★ U.S. Department of Health and Human Services**
**National Heart, Lung, and Blood Institute**
**Division of Heart and Vascular Diseases**
**Heart Research Program**
Two Rockledge Centre
6701 Rockledge Dr., MSC 7940
Bethesda, MD 20892-7940
**Phone:** (301)435-0494     **Fax:** (301)480-7971
**Email:** fakundingj@nhlbi.nih.gov
Dr. John Fakunding, PhD, Dir., Heart Research Prog.

**Activities/Fields:** Heart function; normal and abnormal mechanisms of heart action; advanced diagnostic methods; and therapies for cardiac and vascular disorders. Research includes studies on myocardial infarction (MI); angina pectoris; arrhythmias; cardiac resuscitation; quantification of infarct size; heart muscle changes during ischemia; effectiveness of thrombolytic therapy in patients with acute MI; effects of coronary bypass grafts on morbidity and mortality in chronic coronary heart disease patients with stable angina pectoris; the effects of PTCA in patients with coronary disease; prototype cardiovascular devices for partial or total replacement of heart function; and development of devices and techniques for noninvasive detection and measurement of arteriosclerotic plaques within the carotid, coronary, and larger arteries of the limbs. Principal components are the following Scientific Research Groups: Arrythias, Congenital and Infectious Diseases, Heart Failure, Ischemic Heart Disease, Bioengineering, Interventional Cardiology, and Research Training and Development.

**★ 5154 ★ U.S. Department of Health and Human Services**
**National Heart, Lung, and Blood Institute**
**Division of Heart and Vascular Diseases**
**Heart Research Training and Development Group**
2 Rockledge Ctr., Ste. 9044
6701 Rockledge Dr., MSC 7940
Bethesda, MD 20892-7940
**Phone:** (301)435-0535     **Fax:** (301)480-1454
**Email:** mc63a@nih.gov
Beth Schucker, Trng. Ldr.

**Activities/Fields:** Administers training grants, fellowships, and career program awards to individuals and academic institutions for research training relating to cardiovascular disease.

**★ 5155 ★ U.S. Department of Health and Human Services**
**National Heart, Lung, and Blood Institute**
**Division of Heart and Vascular Diseases**
**Specialized Centers of Research in Coronary and Peripheral Vascular Disease, Heart Failure, and Congenital Heart**
2 Rockledge Ctr.
6701 Rockledge Dr.
Bethesda, MD 20892
**Phone:** (301)435-0466     **Fax:** (301)480-7971
Dr. Stephen Mockrin, Dir.

**Activities/Fields:** Supports cardiac and vascular disease research through grants.

**★ 5156 ★ U.S. Department of Health and Human Services**
**National Heart, Lung, and Blood Institute**
**Division of Heart and Vascular Diseases**
**Vascular Research Program**
Two Rockledge Center, Ste. 10198
6701 Rockledge Dr., MSC 7956
Bethesda, MD 20892-7956
**Phone:** (301)435-0545     **Fax:** (301)480-2849
**Email:** ss90g@nih.gov
**Website:** http://www.nhlbi.nih.gov/about/dhvd/index.htm
Sonia I. Skarlatos, PhD, Dir.

**Activities/Fields:** Arteriosclerosis, lipid metabolism, hypertension, vascular biology and medicine, and molecular genetics and medicine. This includes support for: research grants; Specialized Centers of Research (SCORs) in arteriosclerosis and hypertension; and nonhuman primate resources to facilitate study of disease states. Principal areas of research interest are: fundamental and metabolic research relating to the etiology, pathogenesis, and prevention of atherosclerosis; etiology, pathogenesis, and prevention of coronary artery and peripheral vascular arteriosclerosis; causes, development, complication, and prevention of cerebrovascular diseases that affect the vessels of the head and neck; the relationship of lipids and lipoproteins to coronary heart disease; and causes, mechanisms of development, treatment, and prevention of hypertension.

**★ 5157 ★ U.S. Department of Health and Human Services**
**National Heart, Lung, and Blood Institute**
**Division of Intramural Research**
**Cardiology Branch**
NIH Bldg. 10, Rm 7B-14
10 Center Dr. MSC 1650
Bethesda, MD 20892
**Phone:** (301)496-5817     **Fax:** (301)402-0888
**Email:** finkelt@nih.gov
Dr. Toren Finkel, III, Chf.

**Activities/Fields:** Clinical and basic research efforts, including: studies into the genetic causes and pathophysiologic mechanisms responsible for hypertrophic cardiomyopathy; development of approaches to revascularize the ischemic heart, including the promotion of angiogenesis; studies into pathogenesis and treatment of coronary artery disease and of myocardial iscemia secondary to microvascular disease; elucidation of the mechanisms responsible for Syndrome X (chest pain in the presence of normal coronary arteries); elucidation of the molecular mechanisms responsible for restenosis; development of gene therapy for the treatment of restenosis and atherosclerosis; studies of vascular effects of estrogen and anti-estrogen therapies; and the development of techniques to detect stunned and hibernating myocardium and the elucidation of responsible mechanisms.

**★ 5158 ★ U.S. Department of Health and Human Services**
**National Heart, Lung, and Blood Institute**
**Division of Intramural Research**
**Molecular Disease Branch**
**(Experimental Atherosclerosis Section)**
NIH Bldg. 10, Rm. 5N113
10 Center Dr., MSC 1422
Bethesda, MD 20892-1422
**Phone:** (301)496-4826
Howard S. Kruth, MD, Chf.

**Activities/Fields:** Atherosclerosis.

**★ 5159 ★ U.S. Department of Health and Human Services**
**National Heart, Lung, and Blood Institute**
**Division of Intramural Research**
**Molecular Disease Branch**
NIH Bldg. 10, Rm. 7N115
10 Center Dr., MSC 1666
Bethesda, MD 20892-1666
**Phone:** (301)496-5095     **Fax:** (301)402-0190
Dr. H. Bryan Brewer, Chf.

**Activities/Fields:** Elucidation of the molecular mechanisms involved in lipid transport and metabolism in normal individuals and patients with disorders of lipid metabolism and atherosclerosis. Biochemical studies involve protein chemistry, immunology, tissue culture, molecular biology, and enzymology. Clinical research focuses on the effects of drugs and therapeutic diets on dyslipoproteinemia and on kinetic analysis of the metabolic defects in patients with these diseases.

**★ 5160 ★ U.S. Department of Health and Human Services**
**National Heart, Lung, and Blood Institute**
**Laboratory of Biochemical Genetics**
NIH Bldg. 36, Rm. 1C-06
9000 Rockville Pike MSC 4036
Bethesda, MD 20892
**Phone:** (301)496-2401     **Fax:** (301)402-0270
**Email:** marshall@codon.nih.gov
Dr. Marshall Nirenberg, PhD, Chf.

**Activities/Fields:** Molecular Biology and Macromolecules. The Molecular Biology Section studies basic problems in molecular biology and biochemistry, particularly those that pertain to the development of the nervous system. Current research focuses on elucidating mechanisms that regulate gene expression using recombinant DNA techniques; and on cyclic nucleotides, ion channels, and cell recognition. The Macromolecules Section studies cellular control in *Escherichia coli.* Areas of interest include: the control of the synthesis and metabolism of cyclic AMP in bacterial cells; the regulation of expression of the gene for adenylate cyclase as well as the factors that regulate enzyme activity, using biological and recombinant DNA approaches; and analyses of structure, function, and repression mechanisms involving the *E. coli* cycle AMO receptor protein.

**★ 5161 ★ U.S. Department of Health and Human Services**
**National Heart, Lung, and Blood Institute**
**Laboratory of Biophysical Chemistry**
NIH Bldg. 50, Rm. 3403
50 South Dr.
Bethesda, MD 20892-1676
**Phone:** (301)496-2135     **Fax:** (301)402-3404
**Email:** jafer@helix.nih.gov
Dr. James Ferretti, Chf.

**Activities/Fields:** Physical and chemical properties of molecules with a view to elucidating their biochemical functions. Specialties are nuclear magnetic resonance, mass spectrometry, computational chemistry, chromatography, and laboratory computer techniques. A special concern is the development of new techniques and their application to problems of current interest.

**★ 5162 ★ U.S. Department of Health and Human Services**
**National Heart, Lung, and Blood Institute**
**Laboratory of Cardiac Energetics**
NIH Bldg. 10, Rm. B1D 416
10 Center Dr. MSC 1061
Bethesda, MD 20892
**Phone:** (301)496-3658     **Fax:** (301)402-2389
**Email:** RSB@ZEUS.NHLBI.NIH.GOV
Dr. Robert Balaban, Chf.

**Activities/Fields:** Cardiology, nuclear magnetic resonance imaging/spectrography, cardiac energetics, and optical spectroscopy.

**★ 5163 ★ U.S. Department of Health and Human Services**
**National Heart, Lung, and Blood Institute (NHLBI)**
**Laboratory of Cell Biology (LCB)**
NIH Bldg. 50, Rm. 2517
9000 Rockville Pike
Bethesda, MD 20892
**Phone:** (301)496-1616     **Fax:** (301)402-1519
**Email:** edk@nih.gov
Edward Korn, PhD, Chf.

**Activities/Fields:** Structure/function studies of the regulation of non-muscle class II, and class I myosins by heavy and light chain phosphorylation in vitro and in vivo. The role of class II and class I myosins in vivo, particularly in the cellular slime mold Dictyostelium discoideum, for example, cytokinesis, differentiation and development, phagocytosis, motility and chemotaxis.

**★ 5164 ★ U.S. Department of Health and Human Services**
**National Heart, Lung, and Blood Institute**
**Laboratory of Cell Signaling**
NIH Bldg. 50, Rm. 3523
9000 Rockville Pike
Bethesda, MD 20892
**Phone:** (301)496-9646     **Fax:** (301)480-0357
**Email:** sgrhee@nih.gov
Dr. Sue Rhee, Chf.

**Activities/Fields:** Cell signaling in relation to the human heart, lung, and blood interaction.

**★ 5165 ★ U.S. Department of Health and Human Services**
**National Heart, Lung, and Blood Institute**
**Laboratory of Molecular Cardiology**
NIH Bldg. 10, Rm. 8N-202
10 Center Dr. MSC 1762
Bethesda, MD 20892
**Phone:** (301)496-1865     **Fax:** (301)402-1542
**Email:** adelster@nhlbi.nih.gov
Dr. Robert S. Adelstein, Chf.

**Activities/Fields:** Regulation function and expression of the contractile proteins in muscle and nonmuscle cells. The role of calcium, calmodulin, and phosphorylation in regulating actin-myosin interaction is of particular interest. Projects include studies of the mechanism by which phosphorylation alters contractile activity in smooth muscle and nonmuscle cells, regulation of contractile protein expression in cultured smooth muscle cells, and cloning the genes for selected contractile proteins. Current interest is the role these proteins and their genes play in cellular development, differentiation, and tumorigenicity.

**★ 5166 ★ U.S. Department of Health and Human Services**
**National Heart, Lung, and Blood Institute**
**Specialized Centers of Research on Arteriosclerosis**
2 Rockledge Center, Ste. 10193
MSC 79516
6701 Rockledge Dr.
Bethesda, MD 20892-7956
**Phone:** (301)435-0550     **Fax:** (301)480-2858
**Email:** wassefm@nih.gov
Dr. Momtaz Wassef, Dir.

**Activities/Fields:** Hyperlipidemia and vascular diseases, including animal and tissue studies and other basic laboratory investigations. The research goal is to expedite development and application of new knowledge essential to improved diagnosis, treatment, and prevention of these disorders. **Frmly:** (2000) Specialized Centers of Research on Ateriosclerosis.

**★ 5167 ★ U.S. Department of Health and Human Services**
**National Heart, Lung, and Blood Institute**
**Specialized Centers of Research on Ischemic Heart Disease**
National Heart, Lung, and Blood Inst.
6701 Rockledge Dr., MSC 7940
Bethesda, MD 20892
**Phone:** (301)435-0505     **Fax:** (301)480-1454
**Email:** jf46f@nih.gov
Dr. John Fakunding, Contact

**Activities/Fields:** Myocardial infarction, angina pectoris, heart rhythm disturbances, heart failure, and emergency and rehabilitation techniques and procedures. The research goal is to expedite development and application of new knowledge essential for improved diagnosis, treatment, and prevention of these disorders.

**U.S. Department of Health and Human Services**
**National Institute on Aging**
**Laboratory of Cardiovascular Science**
*See:* Entry 3078

**U.S. Department of Health and Human Services**
**National Institute on Aging**
**Laboratory of Cardiovascular Science**
**Membrane Biology Section**
*See:* Entry 3079

**U.S. Department of Health and Human Services**
**National Institutes of Health (NIH)**
**National Institute on Aging**
**Intramural Research Programs**
**(Cardiac Function Unit)**
*See:* Entry 3093

**U.S. Department of Health and Human Services**
**National Institutes of Health**
**National Institute of Environmental Health Sciences**
**Division of Extramural Research and Training**
**(Organs and Systems Toxicology Branch)**
*See:* Entry 14325

**U.S. Department of Health and Human Services**
**National Institutes of Health (NIH)**
**National Institute of Neurological Disorders and Stroke**
**Division of Intramural Research (Clinical Neurocardiology Section)**
*See:* Entry 14376


**★ 5168 ★ University of Arizona**
**Sarver Heart Center**
Arizona Health Science Center
1501 N Campbell Ave.
Tucson, AZ 85724-5037
**Phone:** (520)626-2000          **Free:** 800-665-2328
**Fax:** (520)626-0967
**Email:** gaewy@aol.com
**Website:** http://www.heart.arizona.edu
Dr. Gordon A. Ewy, Dir.

**Activities/Fields:** Multidisciplinary studies of the heart, including basic, preclinical and clinical research. Basic research focuses on cell growth and development, including genetics, biochemistry, and molecular biology; preclinical research focuses on the microvascular, pharmacologic, and physiologic aspects of heart disease; and clinical research focuses on new drugs, techniques, devices, and interventions. Specific areas of study include cardiac elecrtrical instability, molecular biology and genetics, end-stage heart disease (including heart and lung transplantation and the use of mechanical assist devices and the artificial heart), atherosclerotic heart and vascular disease, detection and diagnosis of cardiovascular disorders, congenital heart disorders, microvascular and vascular disorders, heart disease prevention, cardiovascular diseases specific to Hispanics and Native Americans, and cardiovascular diseases in women and the elderly. **Pub:** *Newsletter.*


**★ 5169 ★ University of British Columbia**
**Atherosclerosis Specialty Laboratory**
St. Paul's Hospital
1081 Burrard St., Rm. B-180-1081
Vancouver, BC, Canada V6Z 1Y6
**Phone:** (604)806-8591          **Fax:** (604)806-8590
**Email:** jshill@interchange.ubc.ca
**Website:** http://www.healthyheart.org
Dr. John S. Hill, Dir.

**Activities/Fields:** Lipids and lipoproteins, lipoprotein metabolism, inherited disorders of lipoprotein metabolism, the enzymes lecithin, cholesterol acyltransferase (LCAT), hepatic lipase (HL), and lipoprotein lipase (LPL); the relationship of genetic polymorphisms and coronary artery disease. Conducts clinical research trials. **Frmly:** Lipid and Lipoprotein Research Laboratory.


**★ 5170 ★ University of British Columbia**
**McDonald Research Laboratories**
St. Paul's Hospital
1081 Burrard St.
Vancouver, BC, Canada V6Z 1Y6
**Phone:** (604)682-2344          **Fax:** (604)806-8135
**Email:** jmcmanus@mrl.ubc.ca
**Website:** http://www.providencehealthcare.org
Dr. Michael O'Shaughnessy, Dir.

**Activities/Fields:** Pulmonary, cardiovascular and critical care research, including studies of asthma, chronic obstructive pulmonary disease, and acute lung injury. Areas of study include latent viral infections in the heart, pathology, biochemistry, molecular biology, physiology, immunology, structure and ultrastructure, and toxicology. Cardiovascular research includes studies on inflammatory diseases of the heart and blood vessels, viral injury, persistence and trafficking, cardiac myocyte metabolism, injury and repair, and vascular wall biology. **Pub:** *Annual Report.*


**★ 5171 ★ University of Calgary**
**Cardiovascular Research Group**
Health Science Centre
Faculty of Medicine
3330 Hospital Dr. NW
Calgary, AB, Canada T2N 4N1
**Phone:** (403)220-4532          **Fax:** (403)220-4532
**Email:** terkeurs@ucalgary.ca
**Website:** http://www.cvr.ucalgary.ca
Dr. Henk J. Keurs, Contact

**Activities/Fields:** Clinical and basic cardiac electrophysiology, cardiac mechanics, and heart failure. Research thrusts include: ion channels, electrophysiology, and arrhythmias, focusing on cardiovascular electrophysiology of cardiac and smooth muscle under physiological and pathophysiological conditions; electrical-mechanical coupling, cardiovascular mechanics, and congestive heart failure, emphasizing electrical-mechanical coupling and cardiovascular mechanics under physiological and pathophysiological conditions; and ischemia and interventional cardiology, focusing on coronary ischemia and reperfusion.


**★ 5172 ★ University of California at Berkeley**
**Cholesterol, Genetics and Heart Disease Institute**
1875 S Grant St., Ste. 700
San Mateo, CA 94402
**Phone:** (650)372-1960          **Free:** 800-HEART-89
**Fax:** (650)372-1948
**Email:** superko@berkeleyhartlab.com
Dr. Robert Superko, Dir.

**Activities/Fields:** Atherosclerosis and lipidology. **Frmly:** Center for Progressive Atherosclerosis Management.


**★ 5173 ★ University of California, Los Angeles**
**Ahmanson/UCLA Adult Congenital Heart Disease Center**
Center for the Health Sciences, Rm. 47-123
Departments of Medicine, Pediatrics & Surgery
UCLA School of Medicine
650 Charles E Young Dr. S
Los Angeles, CA 90095-1679
**Phone:** (310)825-2019          **Fax:** (310)206-9133
**Email:** achdc@mednet.ucla.edu
**Website:** http://www.cardiology.med.ucla.edu/achdc
John S. Child, MD, Dir.

**Activities/Fields:** Congenital heart disease in adults.


**★ 5174 ★ University of California, Los Angeles**
**Cardiovascular Research Laboratory**
MRLB, Rm. 3645
675 Charles E Young Dr. S
Los Angeles, CA 90095-1760
**Phone:** (310)825-2554          **Fax:** (310)206-5777
**Email:** jweiss@mednet.ucla.edu
**Website:** http://www.heartlab.mednet.ucla.edu
Dr. James N. Weiss, Dir.

**Activities/Fields:** Cellular and subcellular mechanisms of cardiovascular physiology, including ultrastructure, electrophysiology, mechanics, biochemistry, molecular biology, and molecular genetics.


**★ 5175 ★ University of California, San Diego**
**Specialized Center of Research in Molecular Medicine and Atherosclerosis**
MC 0682
Department of Medicine
9500 Gilman Dr.
La Jolla, CA 92093-0682
**Phone:** (858)534-0569          **Fax:** (858)534-2005
Dr. Joseph L. Witztam, Dir.

**Activities/Fields:** Arteriosclerosis and atherogenesis, including studies of lipoprotein metabolism, oxidation of low density lipoprotein molecules, and molecular basis of arteriosclerosis.


**★ 5176 ★ University of California, San Francisco**
**Cardiovascular Research Institute**
**Intravascular Ultrasound Laboratory**
1347 Moffitt Hospital
505 Parnassus Ave.
San Francisco, CA 94143-0130
**Phone:** (415)476-1614          **Fax:** (415)476-1020
**Email:** ports@medicine.ucsf.edu
**Website:** http://cardiology.ucsf.edu/clinical/ivus
Thomas Ports, MD, Co-Dir.

**Activities/Fields:** Use of catheter-based ultrasound devices to examine coronary physiology.


**★ 5177 ★ University of California, San Francisco**
**Vascular Research Laboratory**
Cardiology Division, 134
San Francisco, CA 94143
**Free:** 800-827-3478
**Email:** chou@medicine.ucsf.edu
**Website:** http://cardiology.ucsf.edu/research/vascular/
Tony Chou, MD, Contact

**Activities/Fields:** Determinants of vascular tone and its role in the genesis of atherosclerotic disease, specifically the effects of sex steroid hormones on the conductance and resistance arterial vasculature in coronary, pulmonary, and systemic circulation.


**★ 5178 ★ University of Cincinnati**
**Cardio-Vascular Laboratory**
University Hospital
234 Goodman Ave.
Cincinnati, OH 45267-0756
**Phone:** (513)584-5148          **Fax:** (513)584-3515
**Email:** adkinsb@healthall.com
Wm. Brian Adkins, Contact

**Activities/Fields:** Computerized vascular research, including ultrasound, instrumentation, and pharmaceutical research.


**★ 5179 ★ University of Cincinnati**
**Cardiovascular Research and Education Center**
231 Albert B. Sabin Way
Cincinnati, OH 45267-0542
**Phone:** (513)558-4721          **Fax:** (513)558-3116
**Email:** jerald.dorn@uc.edu
Dr. Jerald W. Dorn, II, Dir.

**Activities/Fields:** Cardiology and drug device clinical trials.


**★ 5180 ★ University of Connecticut Health Center**
**Center for Vascular Biology (CVB)**
Academic Research Bldg., E5052
Department of Physiology
263 Farmington Ave.
Farmington, CT 06030-3501
**Phone:** (860)679-4128          **Fax:** (860)679-1201
**Email:** hla@nso2.uchc.edu
**Website:** http://cvb.uchc.edu/
Timothy Hla, PhD, Prin. Investigator

**Activities/Fields:** Molecular mechanisms of blood vessels in normal physiological conditions and in disease. Research focuses on tumor angiogenesis, signal transduction in endothelial cells, vascular proteomics, post-transcriptional gene expression, vascular developmental biology and cell invasion and metastasis.


**★ 5181 ★ University of Houston**
**Institute for Cardiovascular Studies**
SR2, Rm. 460
4800 Calhoun
Houston, TX 77204-5515
**Phone:** (713)743-1218          **Fax:** (713)743-1232
**Email:** jandhyala@uh.edu
Dr. B.S. Jandhyala, Dir.

**Activities/Fields:** Cardiovascular research, including central and peripheral control of the cardiovascular system and renal functions; pharmacology of compounds affecting cardiovascular function, ischemia-reperfusion injury; oxygen free radicals; anti-oxidants; organ protection; hypertension in obesity; and insulin resistance.

### ★ 5182 ★ University of Iowa
### Iowa Cardiovascular Center
616 MRC
College of Medicine
Iowa City, IA 52242-1182
**Phone:** (319)335-8588 **Fax:** (319)335-6969
**Email:** francois-abboud@uiowa.edu
Prof. Francois M. Abboud, Dir.

**Activities/Fields:** Coronary and vascular disease, hypertension, lipid arteriosclerosis, the regulation of circulation in pathological states, neurovascular control, clinical management of lipid disorders, lipoproteins, cerebral blood vessels, occupational and immunologic lung disease, cystic fibrosis, and cardiovascular research training program.

### ★ 5183 ★ University of Iowa
### Lipid Research Clinic
Westlawn, 2191
Department of Internal Medicine/Preventive
 Medicine
Iowa City, IA 52242
**Phone:** (319)335-8201 **Free:** 800-887-6917
**Fax:** (319)335-6671
**Email:** helmut-schrott@mail.pmeh.uiowa.edu
**Website:** http://www.uiowa.edu/%7evpr/research/organize/lipid.htm
Helmut G. Schrott, MD, Dir.

**Activities/Fields:** Lipids, including the relationship of cholesterol and other blood lipids to heart disease. Conducts studies on cholesterol reducing effects of lipid lowering drugs. Also studies community cholesterol screening and educational programs for physicians. Awarded a clinical lipid disorders treatment program. Other activities include studies in post-menopausal women (PEPI Trial and HRS Trial) and diabetes studies (DCCT Trial).

### ★ 5184 ★ University of Kentucky
### Gill Heart Institute (GHI)
Kentucky Clinic, Rm. L543
Division of Cardiovascular Medicine
740 S Limestone St.
Lexington, KY 40536-0284
**Phone:** (859)323-5479 **Fax:** (859)323-6475
**Website:** http://www.mc.uky.edu/ghi/
William T. Abraham, MD, Dir.

**Activities/Fields:** Atherosclerosis, coronary artery disease and heart failure, especially the mechanisms causing acute onset of these diseases.

### ★ 5185 ★ University of Kentucky
### Sanders-Brown Center on Aging
### Stroke Program
101 Sanders-Brown Bldg.
800 S Limestone St.
Lexington, KY 40536-0230
**Phone:** (859)257-5560 **Fax:** (859)257-8990
**Email:** swillia@uky.edu
**Website:** http://www.mc.uky.edu/stroke
Dr. L. Creed Pettigrew, Dir.

**Activities/Fields:** Role of vitamins in stroke prevention and treatment of aphasia and related disorders; use of proteolysis in cerebral ischemia and apolipoprotein E in neuronal cell death.

### ★ 5186 ★ University of Maryland
### Claude D. Pepper Older Americans
### Independence Center (UM-OAIC)
VA Medical Center, GRECC 18
10 N Greene St.
Baltimore, MD 21201
**Phone:** (410)605-7185 **Fax:** (410)705-7913

**Email:** apgoldbe@umaryland.edu
**Website:** http://gerontology.umaryland.edu/pepper.html
Andrew P. Goldberg, MD, Prin. Investigator

**Activities/Fields:** Effects of aggressive risk factor modification in the treatment of disability in older patients with claudication due to peripheral arterial disease (PAD) or congestive heart failure (CHF). The center conducts clinical trials to improve functional independence, reduce cardiovascular risk factors and enrich the lifestyle of such patients. There are also investigations in the pathophysiology and mechanisms by which exercise and diet rehabilitation collectively improve muscular, cardiovascular and metabolic function in older patients with PAD and CHF.

### ★ 5187 ★ University of Michigan
### Division of Cardiology
3910 Taubman Center
1500 E Medical Center Dr.
Ann Arbor, MI 48109-0366
**Phone:** (734)936-5275 **Fax:** (734)764-4119
**Email:** keagle@umich.edu
Kim Eagle, MD, Interim Ch.

**Activities/Fields:** Diagnosis, treatment, and prevention of cardiovascular disease, including new therapeutic approaches to patients with heart failure and development of digital coronary and left ventricular angiography and digital echocardiography, myocardial reperfusion with thrombolytic agents and acute PTCA, and electrophysiology with emphasis on catheter ablation techniques. Also studies molecular biology of myocardial proteins and vascular adhesion molecules as well as new approaches to gene transfer into specific vascular beds.

### ★ 5188 ★ University of Michigan
### Hypertension Division
Department of Internal Medicine
3918 Taubman Center
1500 E Medical Center Dr.
Ann Arbor, MI 48109-0356
**Phone:** (734)936-4790 **Fax:** (734)936-8898
**Email:** aweder@umich.edu
**Website:** http://www.med.umich.edu/intmed/hypertension
Dr. Alan B. Weder, Div. Ch.

**Activities/Fields:** Hypertension and hyperlipidemia, including pathophysiology of various forms of human hypertension, epidemiology, mechanism of action of drugs, and improvement of health care delivery.

### University of Michigan
### Thoracic Surgery Research Lab
*See:* Entry 19628

### ★ 5189 ★ University of Minnesota
### Experimental Surgical Services
### Laboratories
MMC 220
420 Delaware St. SE
Minneapolis, MN 55455
**Phone:** (612)625-5914 **Fax:** (612)626-6949
**Email:** bianc001@tc.umn.edu
**Website:** http://www.ess-umn.com
Richard Bianco, Dir.

**Activities/Fields:** Cardiovascular surgery devices and techniques. **Frmly:** Cardiovascular Surgical Research Laboratories.

### ★ 5190 ★ University of Missouri—
### Columbia
### Division of Cardiothoracic Surgery
Medical Science Bldg., MA 312
Sch. of Medicine
1 Hospital Dr.
Columbia, MO 65212
**Phone:** (573)882-6954 **Fax:** (573)884-0437
**Email:** curtisj@health.missouri.edu
**Website:** http://www.surgery.missouri.edu
Dr. Jack Curtis, Hd.

**Activities/Fields:** Cardiac physiology and cardiothoracic surgery. **Pub:** *Manuscripts, abstracts and presentations,* annually.

### University of Missouri—Columbia
### John M. Dalton Cardiovascular Research
### Center
*See:* Entry 4562

### ★ 5191 ★ University of Montreal
### Clinical Research Institute of Montreal
### Multidisciplinary Research Group on
### Hypertension
110 Pine Ave. W
Montreal, QC, Canada H2W 1R7
**Phone:** (514)987-5528 **Fax:** (514)987-5602
**Email:** schiffe@ircm.qc.ca
**Website:** http://www.missouri.edu/~dalton/
Dr. Ernesto L. Schiffrin, Dir.

**Activities/Fields:** Biochemistry; molecular biology; cellular physiology; pharmacology and clinical and experimental pathophysiology of hypertension, with an emphasis on the renin-angiotensin system, the neurobiology of hypertension, and the biology of blood vessels and the heart and kidney; the role of vasoactive peptides, particularly angiotensin, endothelin, and the role of endothelium; the effects of antihypertensive treatment on blood vessels of hypertensive patients; and the biochemical, molecular, and genetic determinants of elevated blood pressure and cardiac development and hypertrophy.

### ★ 5192 ★ University of Montreal
### Montreal Heart Institute
### Research Centre
5000 Belanger St.
Montreal, QC, Canada H1T 1C8
**Phone:** (514)376-3330 **Fax:** (514)593-2540
**Email:** nattel@icm.umontreal.ca
**Website:** http://www.icm-mhi.org/english/default.asp
Dr. Stanley Nattel, Dir.

**Activities/Fields:** Cardiovascular physiology, pharmacology, molecular biology, and electrophysiology. Develops visualization techniques such as quantitative angiography, numerical angiography, and videodensitometry in echocardiography and nuclear medicine. **Pub:** *Annual Report.*

### University of Oklahoma Health Sciences
### Center
### Center for American Indian Health
### Research
*See:* Entry 2710

### ★ 5193 ★ University of Ottawa
### Heart Institute
40 Ruskin St.
Ottawa, ON, Canada K1Y 4W7
**Phone:** (613)761-4905 **Fax:** (613)761-5281
**Email:** aaffairs@ottawaheart.ca
**Website:** http://www.ottawaheart.ca/
Dr. Wilbert Keon, Dir. Gen.

**Activities/Fields:** All aspects of heart disease, including hypertension, cardiovascular devices, genetics of cardiovascular diseases, vascular biology, arrythmia, cardiac surgery, cardiac anesthesia, and prevention and rehabilitation. **Pub:** *Annual report.*

### ★ 5194 ★ University of Rochester
### Aab Institute of Biomedical Sciences
### Center for Cardiovascular Research
School of Medicine & Dentistry
601 Elmwood Ave., Box 679
Rochester, NY 14642
**Phone:** (716)273-1947 **Fax:** (716)473-1573
**Email:** bradford_berk@urmc.rochester.edu
**Website:** http://www.urmc.rochester.edu/Aab/Cardio.htm
Bradford C. Berk, MD, Dir.

**Activities/Fields:** Pathophysiology of cardiovascular disease. Research focuses on vascular biology; developmental biology; ischemic injury, molecular pharmacology and signal transduction; and genetics of cardiovascular disease.

### ★ 5195 ★ University of Southern California
**Cardiovascular Care Research**
1200 N State St., Rm. 8350
PO Box 305
Los Angeles, CA 90033
**Phone:** (323)226-7116				**Fax:** (323)226-7458
**Email:** jhaywood@hsc.usc.edu
Dr. L. Julian Haywood, Dir.

**Activities/Fields:** Clinical pathophysiology and management of myocardial infarction and other cardiovascular disorders, rhythm disturbances of the heart, computer-based monitoring techniques, vectorcardiography, and related investigations of electrophysiology, with emphasis on noninvasive methods, the use of radioisotopes in nuclear cardiology, and other radiological techniques. **Frmly:** Coronary Care Research.

### ★ 5196 ★ University of Tennessee
**Division of Cardiovascular Diseases**
951 Court Ave.
Memphis, TN 38163
**Phone:** (901)448-5759				**Fax:** (901)448-8084
**Email:** ktweber@utmem.edu
Dr. Karl T. Weber, Dir.

**Activities/Fields:** Cardiovascular system in health and disease, including investigations of hypertension, hemodynamics, echocardiographs, estrogen replacement, and cardiovascular pharmacology.

### ★ 5197 ★ University of Texas Medical Branch at Galveston
**Cardiovascular/Thoracic Surgery**
6.120 John Scaly Annex
301 University Blvd.
Galveston, TX 77555-0528
**Phone:** (409)772-1203				**Fax:** (409)772-1421
**Email:** vconti@utmb.edu
Dr. Vincent R. Conti, Dir.

**Activities/Fields:** Myocardial metabolism with ischemia using the isolated working rat heart and isolated cardiac mitochondria. Also conducts laboratory and clinical studies of the physiologic effects of cardiopulmonary bypass.

### ★ 5198 ★ University of Texas Southwestern Medical Center at Dallas
**Cardiology Division**
5323 Harry Hines Blvd., Rm. NB11.200
Dallas, TX 75390-8573
**Phone:** (214)648-1400				**Fax:** (214)648-1450
**Website:** http://www.swmed.edu/home_pages/cardiology/index.html
John D. Rutherford, MD, Interim Ch.

**Activities/Fields:** Cardiology, including molecular biology of the cardiovascular system, clinical and basic studies of heart disease, and clinical and basic studies of congestive heart failure.

**University of Texas Southwestern Medical Center at Dallas**
**Center for Biomedical Inventions (CBI)**
*See:* Entry 4782

### ★ 5199 ★ University of Toronto
**Centre for Cardiovascular Research**
Toronto General Hospital
200 Elizabeth St.
Toronto, ON, Canada M5G 2C4
**Phone:** (416)340-4790				**Fax:** (416)340-5985
**Email:** msole@torhosp.toronto.on.ca
**Website:** http://cbi.swmed.edu/
Michael J. Sole, MD, Dir.

---

**Activities/Fields:** Atherosclerotic cardiovascular disease, myocardial hypertrophy and failure, and arrhythmias and sudden death.

**University of Toronto**
**Centre for Cardiovascular Research**
**Cardiac Gene Unit**
*See:* Entry 9521

### ★ 5200 ★ University of Utah
**Cardiovascular Genetic Research Clinic**
410 Chipeta Way, Rm. 161
Salt Lake City, UT 84108
**Phone:** (801)581-3888				**Fax:** (801)581-6862
**Email:** barbara@ucng.med.utah.edu
**Website:** http://www.tcgu.med.utoronto.ca
Steven C. Hunt, PhD, Co-Dir.

**Activities/Fields:** Cardiovascular genetics, focusing on the correlations between environment, genetics, and the incidence of early heart disease.

### ★ 5201 ★ University of Utah
**Nora Eccles Harrison Cardiovascular Research and Training Institute (CVRTI)**
95 South 2000 East Back
Salt Lake City, UT 84112-5000
**Phone:** (801)581-8183				**Fax:** (801)581-3128
**Email:** info@cvrti.utah.edu
**Website:** http://www.cvrti.utah.edu/
Dr. Rob MacLeod, Co-Dir.

**Activities/Fields:** Cardiac electrophysiology, with investigative expertise ranging from the molecular/cellular level to the whole heart. Two other areas of cellular research are intracellular PH regulation and excitation-contraction coupling in cardiac cells.

### ★ 5202 ★ University of Virginia
**Cardiovascular Research Center (CVRC)**
MR-4 Bldg., 6th Fl.
University of Virginia Health System, Box 801394
Charlottesville, VA 22908
**Phone:** (434)924-5092
**Website:** http://hsc.virginia.edu/medicine/inter-dis/cvrc
Brian R. Duling, PhD, Dir.

**Activities/Fields:** Cardiovascular disease.

### ★ 5203 ★ University of Virginia
**Molecular Biomechanics Laboratory**
Box 800759
Department of Biomedical Engineering
Charlottesville, VA 22901
**Phone:** (434)243-2740				**Fax:** (434)982-3870
**Email:** whg2n@virginia.edu
**Website:** http://yakko.bme.virginia.edu/lab/
Prof. William H.O. Guilford, PhD, Dir.

**Activities/Fields:** Molecular mechanisms by which cells move, and the application of this knowledge to the understanding and treatment of cardiovascular disease.

**University of Virginia**
**Vascular Medicine and Preventive Cardiology Unit**
*See:* Entry 17853

### ★ 5204 ★ University of Washington
**National Simulation Resource for Circulatory Transport and Exchange**
Box 357962
Department of Bioengineering
Seattle, WA 98195-7962
**Phone:** (206)685-2005				**Fax:** (206)685-2651
**Email:** jbb@bioeng.washington.edu
**Website:** http://nsr.bioeng.washington.edu
James B. Bassingthwaighte, MD, Prin. Investigator

---

**Activities/Fields:** Estimates of conductances of capillary and cell membranes, volumes of distributions, and regional flows.

### ★ 5205 ★ University of Wisconsin— Madison
**Biodynamics Laboratory**
2000 Observatory Dr., Rm. 1149
Madison, WI 53706
**Phone:** (608)263-6308				**Fax:** (608)262-1656
**Email:** gcartee@education.wisc.edu
Dr. Greg Cartee, Dir.

**Activities/Fields:** Mechanisms associated with the response and adaptation of humans and animals to exercise and environmental stress, focusing on cardiorespiratory and musculoskeletal systems.

### ★ 5206 ★ University of Wisconsin— Madison
**Cardiovascular Research Center (CVRC)**
5710 Medical Sciences Center
1300 University Ave.
Madison, WI 53706
**Phone:** (608)263-2266				**Fax:** (608)265-8745
**Email:** uwcvrc@cardiovascres.wisc.edu
**Website:** http://www.cardiovascres.wisc.edu/
Richard L. Moss, PhD, Dir.

**Activities/Fields:** Diagnosis and treatment of diseases of the heart and blood vessels.

### ★ 5207 ★ Utah Artificial Heart Institute
803 North 300 West St., Rm. 304 W
Salt Lake City, UT 84103-1414
**Phone:** (801)323-1122				**Fax:** (801)323-1110
**Email:** dolsen@uahi.org
Dr. Don B. Olsen, Pres.

**Activities/Fields:** Cardiac replacement, cardiac assist devices, and artificial organs, including investigations into acute and chronic ventricular assist and total replacement, cardiac valves, total artificial hearts (pneumatic, electrohydraulic, and electromechanical), and associated pathophysiology. Experiments concern the introduction of such devices in sheep and calves.

### ★ 5208 ★ Vanderbilt University
**Autonomic Dysfunction Center**
AA-3228 Medical Center N
Nashville, TN 37232-2195
**Phone:** (615)343-6499				**Fax:** (615)343-8649
**Email:** david.robertson@mcmail.vanderbilt.edu
**Website:** http://www.mc.vanderbilt.edu/gcrc/adc
Dr. David Robertson, Dir.

**Activities/Fields:** Pathophysiology of autonomic disorders and orthostatic hypotension, including dopamine-B-hydroxylase deficiency, a syndrome characterized by congenital absence of norepinephrine and epinephrine, and norepinephrine transporter deficiency. Other areas of research focus on therapeutic modalities for the management of orthostatic intolerance and tachycardia, Shy-Drager syndrome, multiple system atrophy, and baroreflex failure in human subjects.

### ★ 5209 ★ Victoria Heart Institute Foundation (VHIF)
315-1900 Richmond Ave.
Victoria, BC, Canada V8R 4R2
**Phone:** (250)595-1884				**Fax:** (250)595-5367
**Email:** vhif@vhif.org
**Website:** http://www.vhif.org/html/about_vhif.htm
Dr. W. Peter Klinke, Dir.

**Activities/Fields:** Cardiovascular disease.

**★ 5210 ★ Wake Forest University**
**Hypertension and Vascular Disease**
**Center**
Baptist Medical Center
Janeway Clinical Sciences Bldg., 5th Fl.
Winston Salem, NC 27157-1032
**Phone:** (336)716-9623　　　**Free:** 800-277-8839
**Fax:** (336)716-6644
**Email:** cferrari@wfubme.edu
**Website:** http://www.wfubmc.edu/hypertension
Dr. Carlos Ferrario, Dir.
**Activities/Fields:** Hypertension and cardiovascular
disease. Activities include a clinical hypertension drug
trial to treat high blood pressure on individuals 70
years or older and two clinical hypertension drug trials
to treat high blood pressure on individuals 21 years or
older. **Frmly:** Hypertension Center.


**★ 5211 ★ Washington University in St.**
**Louis**
**Atherosclerosis, Nutrition, and Lipid**
**Research Division**
660 S Euclid Ave., Campus Box 8046
Saint Louis, MO 63110
**Phone:** (314)362-7038　　　**Fax:** (314)747-4477
**Email:** semenkov@im.wustl.edu
Clay F. Semenkovich, MD, Assoc. Dir.
**Activities/Fields:** Atherosclerosis and lipid disorders,
including research on genetic lipid disorders, atherogenesis and the roles of growth factors, cytokines, and
chemically modified oxidized lipoproteins. Uses chemical, molecular, biologic, immunologic and cell culture
techniques for studies of lipogenesis, lipoprotein structure and function. Performs clinical trials to determine
optimum diagnostic and treatment modalities for dyslipoproteinemias. **Frmly:** Lipid Research Center.


# State & Regional
# Organizations


## Heart

*State affiliates of the American Heart Association
are listed below. The Association's national center
is located at 7272 Greenville Ave., Dallas, TX
75231,　　　　(800)AHA-USA1,　　　　http://
www.americanheart.org/.*


### Alabama

**★ 5212 ★ American Heart Association**
**Southeast Affiliate**
**Birmingham Chapter**
1449 Medical Park Dr.
Birmingham, AL 35213
**Phone:** (205)510-1500　　　**Fax:** (205)510-1501
**Website:** http://www.americanheart.org/al


**★ 5213 ★ American Heart Association**
**Southeast Affiliate**
**Dothan Chapter**
1152 W Main St.
Dothan, AL 36301
**Phone:** (334)794-4570　　　**Fax:** (334)677-4488


**★ 5214 ★ American Heart Association**
**Southeast Affiliate**
**Huntsville Chapter**
605 Davis Cir., Bldg. 10, Ste. 26
Huntsville, AL 35801
**Phone:** (256)536-0400　　　**Fax:** (256)535-9631

**★ 5215 ★ American Heart Association**
**Southeast Affiliate**
**Mobile Chapter**
900 Western America Cir., Ste. 209
Mobile, AL 36609
**Phone:** (251)461-4000　　　**Fax:** (251)461-4001


**★ 5216 ★ American Heart Association**
**Southeast Affiliate**
**Montgomery Chapter**
448 S Lawrence St.
Montgomery, AL 36104
**Phone:** (334)832-4400　　　**Fax:** (334)832-4900


**★ 5217 ★ American Heart Association**
**Southeast Affiliate**
**Sheffield Chapter**
501 N Montgomery Ave., Rm. 305
Sheffield, AL 35660
**Phone:** (256)381-4042　　　**Fax:** (256)381-4092


**★ 5218 ★ American Heart Association**
**Southeast Affiliate**
**Tuscaloosa Chapter**
2901 7th St.
Tuscaloosa, AL 35401
**Phone:** (205)752-5521　　　**Fax:** (205)758-7775


### Alaska

**★ 5219 ★ American Heart Association**
**Northwest Affiliate**
**Anchorage Chapter**
1057 W Fireweed Ln., Ste. 100
Anchorage, AK 99503
**Phone:** (907)263-2044　　　**Free:** 888-276-0858
**Fax:** (907)263-2045
**Website:** http://www.americanheart.org/ak
Craig Harpel, Vice President
Peggy Spittler, Director


### Arizona

**★ 5220 ★ American Heart Association**
**Desert/Mountain Affiliate**
**Phoenix Chapter**
2929 S 48th St.
Tempe, AZ 85282
**Phone:** (602)414-5353　　　**Fax:** (602)414-5355


**★ 5221 ★ American Heart Association**
**Desert/Mountain Affiliate**
**Tucson Chapter**
5325 E Pima Rd.
Tucson, AZ 85712
**Phone:** (520)795-1403　　　**Fax:** (520)795-1426


**★ 5222 ★ American Heart Association**
**Desert/Mountain Affiliate**
**Williams Chapter**
117 W Rte. 66, Ste. 155
Williams, AZ 86046
**Phone:** (520)635-0368　　　**Fax:** (520)635-4800


### Arkansas

**★ 5223 ★ American Heart Association**
**Heartland Affiliate**
**Fayetteville Chapter**
92 W Sunbridge
Fayetteville, AR 72703
**Phone:** (501)442-6540　　　**Fax:** (501)442-4580

**★ 5224 ★ American Heart Association**
**Heartland Affiliate**
**Jonesboro Chapter**
2512 S Culberhouse, Ste. E
Jonesboro, AR 72401
**Phone:** (870)931-3070　　　**Fax:** (870)930-9046


**★ 5225 ★ American Heart Association**
**Heartland Affiliate**
**Little Rock Chapter**
909 W 2nd St.
Little Rock, AR 72203
**Phone:** (501)375-9148　　　**Fax:** (501)375-9066
**Website:** http://www.americanheart.org/ar


### California

**★ 5226 ★ American Heart Association**
**Western States Affiliate**
**Bakersfield Division**
404 Truxtun Ave.
Bakersfield, CA 93301
**Phone:** (661)327-1173　　　**Fax:** (661)323-6981
**Website:** http://www.heartsource.org


**★ 5227 ★ American Heart Association**
**Western States Affiliate**
**Chico Division**
1372 Longfellow Ave.
Chico, CA 95926
**Phone:** (530)342-4247　　　**Fax:** (530)345-4072
**Website:** http://www.heartsource.org


**★ 5228 ★ American Heart Association**
**Western States Affiliate**
**East Bay Division**
11200 Golf Links Rd.
Oakland, CA 94605
**Phone:** (510)632-9606　　　**Fax:** (510)635-5848
**Website:** http://www.heartsource.org


**★ 5229 ★ American Heart Association**
**Western States Affiliate**
**Eureka Division**
1400 N Dutton Ave., Ste. 20
Santa Rosa, CA 95401
**Phone:** (707)542-1992　　　**Fax:** (510)576-7377
**Website:** http://www.heartsource.org


**★ 5230 ★ American Heart Association**
**Western States Affiliate**
**Fresno Division**
1495 W Shaw Ave.
Fresno, CA 93711
**Phone:** (559)224-8215　　　**Fax:** (559)228-8115
**Website:** http://www.heartsource.org


**★ 5231 ★ American Heart Association**
**Western States Affiliate**
**Inland Empire Division**
1003 E Cooley Dr., Ste. 102
Colton, CA 92324
**Phone:** (909)424-1670　　　**Fax:** (909)825-2484
**Website:** http://www.heartsource.org


**★ 5232 ★ American Heart Association**
**Western States Affiliate**
**Los Angeles County Division**
1055 Wilshire Blvd., Ste. 900
Los Angeles, CA 90017
**Phone:** (213)580-1408　　　**Free:** 800-AHA-USA1
**Fax:** (213)580-1461
**Email:** caroll@heart.org
**Website:** http://www.heartsource.org
Carol Lugo, Exec Director

★ 5233 ★ **American Heart Association**
**Western States Affiliate**
**Merced Division**
PO Box 1325
Merced, CA 95341
**Phone:** (209)723-2974 **Fax:** (209)228-8115
**Website:** http://www.heartsource.org

★ 5234 ★ **American Heart Association**
**Western States Affiliate**
**Monterey Peninsula Division**
1514 Moffett St., Ste. A
Salinas, CA 93905
**Phone:** (831)757-6221 **Fax:** (831)757-6355
**Website:** http://www.heartsource.org

★ 5235 ★ **American Heart Association**
**Western States Affiliate**
**North Bay Division**
1400 N Dutton Ave., Ste. 20
Santa Rosa, CA 95401
**Phone:** (707)542-1992 **Fax:** (707)576-7377
**Website:** http://www.heartsource.org

★ 5236 ★ **American Heart Association**
**Western States Affiliate**
**Orange County Division**
4600 Campus Dr.
Irvine, CA 92612
**Phone:** (949)856-3555 **Fax:** (949)856-3364
**Website:** http://www.heartsource.org

★ 5237 ★ **American Heart Association**
**Western States Affiliate**
**Palm Desert Division**
74-020 Alessandro, Ste. A
Palm Desert, CA 92260
**Phone:** (760)346-8109 **Fax:** (760)773-0766
**Website:** http://www.heartsource.org

★ 5238 ★ **American Heart Association**
**Western States Affiliate**
**Sacramento Division**
2007 O St.
Sacramento, CA 95814
**Phone:** (916)446-6505 **Fax:** (916)443-2865
**Website:** http://www.heartsource.org

★ 5239 ★ **American Heart Association**
**Western States Affiliate**
**Salinas Division**
1514 Moffett St.
Salinas, CA 93905
**Phone:** (831)757-6221 **Fax:** (831)757-6355
**Website:** http://www.heartsource.org

★ 5240 ★ **American Heart Association**
**Western States Affiliate**
**San Diego Division**
3640 5th Ave.
San Diego, CA 92103
**Phone:** (619)291-7454 **Fax:** (619)291-9454
**Website:** http://www.heartsource.org

★ 5241 ★ **American Heart Association**
**Western States Affiliate**
**San Francisco Division**
120 Montgomery St., Ste. 1650
San Francisco, CA 94104
**Phone:** (415)433-2273 **Fax:** (415)228-8402
**Email:** howards@heart.org
**Website:** http://www.heartsource.org
Howard Shiflett, Exec Director

★ 5242 ★ **American Heart Association**
**Western States Affiliate**
**San Joaquin County Division**
1495 W Shaw Ave.
Fresno, CA 93711
**Phone:** (559)224-8215 **Fax:** (559)228-8115
**Website:** http://www.heartsource.org

★ 5243 ★ **American Heart Association**
**Western States Affiliate**
**San Jose Division**
1 Almaden Blvd., Ste. 500
San Jose, CA 95113
**Phone:** (408)977-4950 **Fax:** (408)977-4959
**Website:** http://www.heartsource.org

★ 5244 ★ **American Heart Association**
**Western States Affiliate**
**San Luis Obispo Division**
1371 Pacific St.
San Luis Obispo, CA 93401
**Phone:** (805)544-1505 **Fax:** (805)549-9627
**Website:** http://www.heartsource.org

★ 5245 ★ **American Heart Association**
**Western States Affiliate**
**San Mateo Division**
1710 Gilbreth Rd., Ste. 100
Burlingame, CA 94010
**Phone:** (650)259-6700 **Fax:** (650)259-6890
**Website:** http://www.heartsource.org

★ 5246 ★ **American Heart Association**
**Western States Affiliate**
**Santa Barbara Division**
212 W Figueroa St.
Santa Barbara, CA 93101
**Phone:** (805)963-8862 **Fax:** (805)963-8866
**Website:** http://www.heartsource.org

★ 5247 ★ **American Heart Association**
**Western States Affiliate**
**Stockton Division**
1212 W Robinhood Dr., Ste. 5-D
Stockton, CA 95207
**Phone:** (209)477-2683 **Fax:** (209)477-1271
**Email:** todd@heart.org
**Website:** http://www.heartsource.org
Tod Davis, Exec Director

★ 5248 ★ **American Heart Association**
**Western States Affiliate**
**Ventura Division**
333 Lantana St., Ste. 265
Camarillo, CA 93010
**Phone:** (805)445-7050 **Fax:** (805)445-9882
**Email:** kathys@heart.org
**Website:** http://www.heartsource.org
Kathy Shoemate, Exec Director
**Remarks:** Serves the cities of Ventura, Ojai, Oxnard, Port Hueneme, Camarillo, Somis, Moorpark, Simi Valley, Newbury Park, Thousand Oaks, Westlake Village, and Agoura.

## Colorado

★ 5249 ★ **American Heart Association**
**Desert/Mountain Affiliate**
**Boulder Chapter**
3135 23rd St.
Boulder, CO 80304
**Phone:** (303)673-0292 **Fax:** (303)673-0249

★ 5250 ★ **American Heart Association**
**Desert/Mountain Affiliate**
**Colorado Springs Chapter**
415 N Tejon, Ste. 201
Colorado Springs, CO 80903

**Phone:** (719)635-7688 **Fax:** (719)635-3606

★ 5251 ★ **American Heart Association**
**Desert/Mountain Affiliate**
**Denver Chapter**
1280 S Parker Rd.
Denver, CO 80231
**Phone:** (303)369-5433 **Free:** 800-242-8721
**Fax:** (303)369-8087

★ 5252 ★ **American Heart Association**
**Desert/Mountain Affiliate**
**Grand Junction Chapter**
123 N 7th St.
Grand Junction, CO 81501
**Phone:** (970)241-4577 **Fax:** (970)241-4637

★ 5253 ★ **American Heart Association**
**Desert/Mountain Affiliate**
**Pueblo Chapter**
720 N Main St., Ste. 440
Pueblo, CO 81003
**Phone:** (719)583-9388 **Fax:** (719)583-4247

## Connecticut

★ 5254 ★ **American Heart Association**
**Connecticut Affiliate**
5 Brookside Dr.
PO Box 5022
Wallingford, CT 06492
**Phone:** (203)294-0088 **Fax:** (203)294-3577
**Website:** http://www.americanheart.org/ct

## Delaware

★ 5255 ★ **American Heart Association**
**Pennsylvania-Delaware Affiliate**
**Kent County Chapter**
1151 Walker Rd., Ste. 202
Dover, DE 19904
**Phone:** (302)734-9321 **Fax:** (302)734-5571

★ 5256 ★ **American Heart Association**
**Pennsylvania-Delaware Affiliate**
**New Castle County Chapter**
1096 Old Churchmans Rd.
Newark, DE 19713
**Phone:** (302)633-0200 **Fax:** (302)633-3964

★ 5257 ★ **American Heart Association**
**Pennsylvania-Delaware Affiliate**
**Sussex County Chapter**
Georgetown Professional Park, Ste. 201A
Georgetown, DE 19947
**Phone:** (302)856-7386 **Fax:** (302)856-2828

## Florida

★ 5258 ★ **American Heart Association**
**Boca Raton Chapter**
500 NE Spanish River Blvd., Ste. 22
Boca Raton, FL 33431
**Phone:** (561)394-0170 **Fax:** (561)391-8669

★ 5259 ★ **American Heart Association**
**Bonita Springs Chapter**
28441 Bonita Crossings Blvd.
Bonita Springs, FL 34135
**Phone:** (941)498-9288 **Fax:** (941)498-9188

★ 5260 ★ **American Heart Association**
**Ft. Lauderdale Chapter**
1751 W Cypress Creek Rd.
Fort Lauderdale, FL 33309
**Phone:** (954)772-8100 **Fax:** (954)491-3511

**★ 5261 ★ American Heart Association**
**Ft. Walton Beach Chapter**
222 Hospital Dr. NE
Fort Walton Beach, FL 32548
**Phone:** (850)243-9715          **Fax:** (850)664-7976

**★ 5262 ★ American Heart Association**
**Gainesville Chapter**
210 NW 75th Dr., Ste. 1
Gainesville, FL 32607
**Phone:** (352)333-3244          **Fax:** (352)333-3254

**★ 5263 ★ American Heart Association**
**Jacksonville Chapter**
5851 St. Augustine Rd.
Jacksonville, FL 32207
**Phone:** (904)739-0197          **Fax:** (904)739-0012

**★ 5264 ★ American Heart Association**
**Lakeland Chapter**
1545 Lakeland Hills Blvd.
Lakeland, FL 33805
**Phone:** (863)686-8421          **Fax:** (863)683-4667

**★ 5265 ★ American Heart Association**
**Melbourne Chapter**
2800 Aurora Rd., Ste. I
Melbourne, FL 32935
**Phone:** (321)255-3557          **Fax:** (321)255-7810

**★ 5266 ★ American Heart Association**
**Miami Chapter**
2600 SW 3rd Ave., Ste. 900
Miami, FL 33129
**Phone:** (305)856-1449          **Fax:** (305)860-6780

**★ 5267 ★ American Heart Association**
**New Port Richey Chapter**
7137 Congress St.
PO Box 2251
New Port Richey, FL 34656-2251
**Phone:** (727)848-8924          **Fax:** (727)842-5931

**★ 5268 ★ American Heart Association**
**Orlando Chapter**
237 East Marks St.
Orlando, FL 32803
**Phone:** (407)843-1330          **Fax:** (407)423-9415

**★ 5269 ★ American Heart Association**
**Ormond Beach Chapter**
555 W Granada Blvd., Ste. A-1
Ormond Beach, FL 32174
**Phone:** (386)676-0001          **Fax:** (386)676-0204

**★ 5270 ★ American Heart Association**
**Panama City Chapter**
2697 Jenks Ave.
Panama City, FL 32405
**Phone:** (850)769-3070          **Fax:** (850)872-9133

**★ 5271 ★ American Heart Association**
**Pensacola Chapter**
4400 Bayou Blvd., Ste. 49-A
Pensacola, FL 32503
**Phone:** (850)473-0411          **Fax:** (850)473-2993

**★ 5272 ★ American Heart Association**
**Saint Petersburg Chapter**
9900 9th St. N
PO Box 21203
Saint Petersburg, FL 33742-1203
**Phone:** (727)570-8610     **Fax:** (727)570-8519
**Website:** http://www.americanheart.org/fl

**★ 5273 ★ American Heart Association**
**Sarasota Chapter**
2975 Bee Ridge Rd., Ste. B
Sarasota, FL 34239
**Phone:** (941)927-4997          **Fax:** (941)927-1427

**★ 5274 ★ American Heart Association**
**Stuart Chapter**
1111 S Federal Hwy., Ste. 110
Stuart, FL 34994
**Phone:** (561)286-1966          **Fax:** (561)220-2605

**★ 5275 ★ American Heart Association**
**Tallahassee Chapter**
1304 E 6th Ave.
Tallahassee, FL 32303
**Phone:** (850)878-3885          **Fax:** (850)942-2803

**★ 5276 ★ American Heart Association**
**Tampa Chapter**
1411 N Westshore Blvd., Ste. 216
Tampa, FL 33607
**Phone:** (813)289-6003          **Fax:** (813)289-4351

**★ 5277 ★ American Heart Association**
**West Palm Beach Chapter**
1301 S Olive Ave.
West Palm Beach, FL 33401
**Phone:** (561)655-8155          **Fax:** (561)832-6014

## Georgia

**★ 5278 ★ American Heart Association**
**Southeast Affiliate**
**Albany Chapter**
1512 Gillionville Rd., Ste. 6
Albany, GA 31707
**Phone:** (912)883-5858          **Fax:** (912)883-5999

**★ 5279 ★ American Heart Association**
**Southeast Affiliate**
**Athens Chapter**
1353 Jennings Mill Rd., Ste. A
Bogart, GA 30622
**Phone:** (706)549-0939          **Fax:** (706)549-3141

**★ 5280 ★ American Heart Association**
**Southeast Affiliate**
**Augusta Chapter**
246 Davis Rd., Ste. E
Augusta, GA 30907
**Phone:** (706)855-5005          **Fax:** (706)855-5101

**★ 5281 ★ American Heart Association**
**Southeast Affiliate**
**Brunswick Chapter**
1614 Union St.
Brunswick, GA 31520
**Phone:** (912)264-5466          **Fax:** (912)264-1931

**★ 5282 ★ American Heart Association**
**Southeast Affiliate**
**Columbus Chapter**
1300 Wynnton Rd., Ste. 108
Columbus, GA 31906
**Phone:** (706)324-0173          **Fax:** (706)324-0174

**★ 5283 ★ American Heart Association**
**Southeast Affiliate**
**Macon Chapter**
3312 Northside Dr., Ste. 140-A
Macon, GA 31210
**Phone:** (478)405-3200          **Fax:** (478)405-3201

**★ 5284 ★ American Heart Association**
**Southeast Affiliate**
**Marietta Chapter**
1101 Northchase Pkwy., Ste. 1
Marietta, GA 30067
**Phone:** (678)385-2000          **Fax:** (678)385-2001
**Website:** http://www.americanheart.org/ga

**★ 5285 ★ American Heart Association**
**Southeast Affiliate**
**Metro Atlanta Chapter**
1101 Northchase Pkwy., Ste. 1
Marietta, GA 30067
**Phone:** (770)952-1316          **Fax:** (770)952-2208

**★ 5286 ★ American Heart Association**
**Southeast Affiliate**
**Savannah Chapter**
7505 Waters Ave., Ste. C7
Savannah, GA 31406
**Phone:** (912)355-0233          **Fax:** (912)355-0234

**★ 5287 ★ American Heart Association**
**Southeast Affiliate**
**Valdosta Chapter**
305 University Dr., Ste. 1
Valdosta, GA 31602
**Phone:** (229)247-1550          **Fax:** (229)241-8323

## Hawaii

**★ 5288 ★ American Heart Association**
**East Hawaii Chapter**
400 Hualani St., Ste. 15
Hilo, HI 96720
**Phone:** (808)961-2825          **Fax:** (808)961-2827

**★ 5289 ★ American Heart Association**
**Kauai Chapter**
4303-C3 Rice St.
Lihue, HI 96766
**Phone:** (808)245-7311          **Fax:** (808)245-7311

**★ 5290 ★ American Heart Association**
**Maui Chapter**
J. Walter Cameron Center
95 Mahalani St., No. 13
Wailuku, HI 96793
**Phone:** (808)244-7185          **Fax:** (808)242-1857

**★ 5291 ★ American Heart Association**
**Oahu Chapter**
245 N Kukui St., Ste. 204
Honolulu, HI 96817
**Phone:** (808)538-7021

**★ 5292 ★ American Heart Association**
**West Hawaii Chapter**
74-5588 Pawai Pl., Bldg. H
Kailua Kona, HI 96740
**Phone:** (808)329-0783          **Fax:** (808)329-0784

## Idaho

**★ 5293 ★ American Heart Association**
**Northwest Affiliate**
**Greater Treasure Valley, Idaho/Oregon**
270 S Orchard, Ste. B
Boise, ID 83705
**Phone:** (208)384-5066          **Free:** 800-589-4204
**Fax:** (208)336-5867
**Email:** jrobinso@heart.org
**Website:** http://www.americanheart.org/idmt
Mary T. MacConnell, Vice President
Julie Robinson, Director

## Illinois

**★ 5294 ★ American Heart Association**
**Midwest Affiliate**
**Chicago Chapter**
208 S LaSalle St., Ste. 900
Chicago, IL 60604
**Phone:** (312)346-4675          **Fax:** (312)346-8236
**Email:** kwest2@heart.org
**Website:** http://www.americanheart.org/il/Chicago

**★ 5295 ★ American Heart Association**
**Midwest Affiliate**
**Rockford Chapter**
5192 Harrison Ave.
Rockford, IL 61108
**Phone:** (815)397-6112          **Free:** 800-694-8618
**Fax:** (815)397-5024

**★ 5296 ★ American Heart Association**
**Midwest Affiliate**
**Springfield Chapter**
2524 Farragut Dr., Ste. A
Springfield, IL 62704
**Phone:** (217)698-3838          **Free:** 800-252-8511
**Fax:** (217)698-4585
**Website:** http://www.americanheart.org/il

**★ 5297 ★ American Heart Association**
**Midwest Affiliate**
**Westmont Chapter**
801 N Cass Ave., Ste. 200
Westmont, IL 60559
**Phone:** (630)789-9222          **Fax:** (630)789-9235

## Indiana

**★ 5298 ★ American Heart Association**
**Midwest Affiliate**
**Evansville Chapter**
233 SE 3rd St.
Evansville, IN 47713
**Phone:** (812)424-4464          **Free:** 800-966-7113
**Fax:** (812)424-4467

**★ 5299 ★ American Heart Association**
**Midwest Affiliate**
**Indianapolis Chapter**
8645 Guion Rd., Ste. H
PO Box 681550
Indianapolis, IN 46268
**Phone:** (317)876-4850          **Free:** 800-229-1503
**Fax:** (317)876-4859
**Website:** http://www.americanheart.org/in

**★ 5300 ★ American Heart Association**
**Midwest Affiliate**
**Mishawaka Chapter**
2410 N Grape Rd., Ste. 5A
Mishawaka, IN 46545
**Phone:** (219)258-4018          **Free:** 800-966-4572
**Fax:** (219)256-6687

## Iowa

**★ 5301 ★ American Heart Association**
**Heartland Affiliate**
**Cedar Rapids Chapter**
3741 Center Point Rd. NE
Cedar Rapids, IA 52402
**Phone:** (319)378-1763

**★ 5302 ★ American Heart Association**
**Heartland Affiliate**
**Council Bluffs Chapter**
Edwards Professional Center
715 Harmony St., Ste. 101
Council Bluffs, IA 51503

**Phone:** (712)322-4755

**★ 5303 ★ American Heart Association**
**Heartland Affiliate**
**Davenport Chapter**
1606 Brady St., Ste. 213
Davenport, IA 52803
**Phone:** (563)323-4321

**★ 5304 ★ American Heart Association**
**Heartland Affiliate**
**Des Moines Chapter**
1111 9th St., Ste. 280
Des Moines, IA 50314
**Phone:** (515)244-3278          **Fax:** (515)244-5164
**Website:** http://www.americanheart.org/ia

**★ 5305 ★ American Heart Association**
**Heartland Affiliate**
**Mason City Chapter**
Westside Office Bldg.
1312-4th St. SW, No. 123
Mason City, IA 50401
**Phone:** (641)424-0256

**★ 5306 ★ American Heart Association**
**Heartland Affiliate**
**Sioux City Chapter**
Benson Bldg., Ste. 621
705 Douglas
Sioux City, IA 51101
**Phone:** (712)255-4798

**★ 5307 ★ American Heart Association**
**Heartland Affiliate**
**Waterloo Chapter**
1825 Logan Ave., No. 331
Waterloo, IA 50703
**Phone:** (641)235-3912

## Kansas

**★ 5308 ★ American Heart Association**
**Heartland Affiliate**
**Kansas City Chapter**
6800 W 93rd St.
Overland Park, KS 66212
**Phone:** (913)648-6727          **Fax:** (913)648-0423

**★ 5309 ★ American Heart Association**
**Heartland Affiliate**
**Topeka Chapter**
5375 SW 7th St.
Topeka, KS 66606
**Phone:** (785)272-7056          **Free:** 800-284-3979
**Fax:** (785)272-2425
**Email:** mmclaugh@heart.org
**Website:** http://www.americanheart.org/ks

**★ 5310 ★ American Heart Association**
**Heartland Affiliate**
**Wichita Chapter**
2100 E Douglas
Wichita, KS 67214
**Phone:** (316)265-4238          **Fax:** (316)265-1390

## Kentucky

**★ 5311 ★ American Heart Association**
**Kentucky Affiliate**
**Central Kentucky Chapter**
2201 Regency Rd., Ste. 401
Lexington, KY 40503-2339
**Phone:** (859)278-1632          **Fax:** (859)278-6236
**Remarks:** Serves Anderson, Bourbon, Clark, Fayette, Jessamine, Mercer, Scott, and Woodford counties.

**★ 5312 ★ American Heart Association**
**Kentucky Affiliate**
**Eastern Kentucky Chapter**
333 Guthrie St., Ste. 207
Louisville, KY 40202
**Phone:** (502)587-8641          **Free:** 800-AHA-USA1
**Fax:** (502)585-7001
**Remarks:** Serves Bullitt, Jefferson, Oldham and Shelby counties.

**★ 5313 ★ American Heart Association**
**Kentucky Affiliate**
**Southcentral Kentucky Chapter**
1212 Ashley Circle, Ste. 1
Bowling Green, KY 42104
**Phone:** 800-AHA-USA1          **Fax:** (270)842-8931

**★ 5314 ★ American Heart Association**
**Kentucky Affiliate**
**Southwestern Kentucky Chapter**
222 Kentucky Ave., Ste. 4
Paducah, KY 42003
**Phone:** 800-AHA-USA1          **Fax:** (270)442-3730

**★ 5315 ★ American Heart Association**
**Kentucky Affiliate**
**Western Kentucky Chapter**
318 St. Elizabeth St.
Owensboro, KY 42301
**Phone:** 800-AHA-USA1          **Fax:** (270)683-2149

## Louisiana

**★ 5316 ★ American Heart Association**
**Southeast Affiliate**
**Alexandria Chapter**
2304 S MacArthur Dr., Ste. F
Alexandria, LA 71301
**Phone:** (318)443-7522          **Fax:** (318)443-2679

**★ 5317 ★ American Heart Association**
**Southeast Affiliate**
**Baton Rouge Chapter**
4962 Florida Blvd., Ste. 402
Baton Rouge, LA 70806
**Phone:** (225)248-7700          **Fax:** (225)248-7701

**★ 5318 ★ American Heart Association**
**Southeast Affiliate**
**Houma Chapter**
220 Progressive Blvd.
Houma, LA 70360
**Phone:** (985)851-3479          **Fax:** (985)580-2844

**★ 5319 ★ American Heart Association**
**Southeast Affiliate**
**Lafayette Chapter**
312 Guilbeau Rd., Ste. 6C
Lafayette, LA 70506
**Phone:** (337)988-2212          **Fax:** (337)988-2214

**★ 5320 ★ American Heart Association**
**Southeast Affiliate**
**Lake Charles Chapter**
1 Lakeside Plaza, Ste. 808
Lake Charles, LA 70601
**Phone:** (337)439-4050          **Fax:** (337)430-0305

**★ 5321 ★ American Heart Association**
**Southeast Affiliate**
**New Orleans Chapter**
105 Campus Dr. E
PO Box 159
Destrehan, LA 70047
**Phone:** (504)456-7224          **Free:** 800-242-8721
**Fax:** (985)764-8712

Website: http://www.americanheart.org/la

## Maine

**★ 5322 ★ American Heart Association**
**New England Affiliate**
**Maine Chapter**
343 Gorham Rd.
South Portland, ME 04106
Phone: (207)879-5700          Free: 800-937-0944
Fax: (207)879-5918

## Maryland

**★ 5323 ★ American Heart Association**
**Baltimore Chapter**
415 N Charles St.
Baltimore, MD 21201
Phone: (410)685-7074          Free: 800-242-8721
Fax: (410)539-5049
Website: http://www.americanheart.org/md

## Massachusetts

**★ 5324 ★ American Heart Association**
**New England Affiliate**
**Framingham Chapter**
20 Speen St.
Framingham, MA 01701
Phone: (508)620-1700          Free: 800-662-1701
Fax: (508)620-6157
Email: webmaster@ahama.org
Website: http://www.americanheart.org/ma

**★ 5325 ★ American Heart Association**
**New England Affiliate**
**South Yarmouth Chapter**
2 White's Path
South Yarmouth, MA 02664
Phone: (508)760-6818          Fax: (508)760-6824

**★ 5326 ★ American Heart Association**
**New England Affiliate**
**West Springfield Chapter**
1111 Elm St., Ste. 9A
West Springfield, MA 01089
Phone: (413)827-0400          Fax: (413)827-9390

## Michigan

**★ 5327 ★ American Heart Association**
**Midwest Affiliate**
**Grand Rapids Chapter**
The Lakeview Bldg.
3940 Peninsular Dr. SE, Ste. 180
Grand Rapids, MI 49546-6107
Phone: (616)285-1888          Free: 800-968-1040
Fax: (616)285-1895
Email: ahami.gr@greatid.com
Lisa Bennett, Vice President

**★ 5328 ★ American Heart Association**
**Midwest Affiliate**
**Okemos Chapter**
2140 University Park, Ste. 210
Okemos, MI 48864
Phone: (517)349-3102          Fax: (517)349-3240

**★ 5329 ★ American Heart Association**
**Midwest Affiliate**
**Saginaw Chapter**
3875 Bay Rd.. Ste. 1-N
Saginaw, MI 48603
Phone: (989)792-6400          Free: 800-968-2422
Fax: (989)792-6556

**★ 5330 ★ American Heart Association**
**Midwest Affiliate**
**Southfield Chapter**
24445 Northwestern Hwy., Ste. 100
Southfield, MI 48075
Phone: (248)827-4214          Fax: (248)827-4234

## Minnesota

**★ 5331 ★ American Heart Association**
**Northland Affiliate**
**Central Minnesota Chapter**
110 S 2nd St., Ste. 305
Waite Park, MN 56387-1367
Phone: (320)255-9930          Fax: (320)255-9808

**★ 5332 ★ American Heart Association**
**Northland Affiliate**
**Duluth Chapter**
401 W Michigan St.
Duluth, MN 55802
Phone: (218)727-7297          Fax: (218)727-0621

**★ 5333 ★ American Heart Association**
**Northland Affiliate**
**Minneapolis Chapter**
4701 W 77th St.
Minneapolis, MN 55435
Phone: (952)835-3300          Fax: (952)835-5828
Email: hmail@ahamn.attmail.com
Website: http://www.americanheart.org/mn

**★ 5334 ★ American Heart Association**
**Northland Affiliate**
**Northwest Minnesota Chapter**
220 W Washington
Fergus Falls, MN 56537
Phone: (218)739-3329          Fax: (218)739-3320

**★ 5335 ★ American Heart Association**
**Northland Affiliate**
**Southeast Minnesota Chapter**
1500 1st Ave. NE, Ste. 200
Rochester, MN 55906
Phone: (507)288-6749          Fax: (507)288-9287

**★ 5336 ★ American Heart Association**
**Northland Affiliate**
**Southwest Minnesota Chapter**
Northwestern Chapter Bldg., No. 205
209 S 2nd St.
Mankato, MN 56001
Phone: (507)345-8206          Fax: (507)345-8202

## Mississippi

**★ 5337 ★ American Heart Association**
**Southeast Affiliate**
**Biloxi Chapter**
2320 14th St., Ste. 110
Gulfport, MS 39501
Phone: (228)864-1629          Fax: (228)864-4856

**★ 5338 ★ American Heart Association**
**Southeast Affiliate**
**Greenwood Chapter**
227 W Market, Ste. 8
Greenwood, MS 38930
Phone: (662)455-5877          Fax: (662)451-5810

**★ 5339 ★ American Heart Association**
**Southeast Affiliate**
**Hattiesburg Chapter**
609 Corinee St., Ste. B-1
Hattiesburg, MS 39401
Phone: (601)583-0108          Fax: (601)582-0496

**★ 5340 ★ American Heart Association**
**Southeast Affiliate**
**Jackson Chapter**
4830 McWillie Cir.
Jackson, MS 39206
Phone: (601)321-1200          Fax: (601)321-1201
Website: http://www.americanheart.org/ms
Teresa Humphrey, Director

## Missouri

**★ 5341 ★ American Heart Association**
**Heartland Affiliate**
**Columbia Office**
2600 I-70 Dr. NW
Columbia, MO 65201
Phone: (573)446-3000          Fax: (573)445-6243
Email: hmail@ahamo.attmail.com
Website: http://www.americanheart.org/mo

**★ 5342 ★ American Heart Association**
**Heartland Affiliate**
**Greater St. Louis Division**
4643 Lindell Blvd.
Saint Louis, MO 63108
Phone: (314)367-3383          Fax: (314)367-8605
Email: hmail@ahamo.attmail.com
Website: http://www.americanheart.org/mo

**★ 5343 ★ American Heart Association**
**Heartland Affiliate**
**Springfield Chapter**
2446 E Madrid
Springfield, MO 65804
Phone: (417)881-1121          Fax: (417)881-8972

## Montana

**★ 5344 ★ American Heart Association of**
**Idaho/Montana**
**Northwest Affiliate**
**Central Montana Chapter**
600 Central Plaza, Ste. 304
Great Falls, MT 59401
Phone: (406)452-2362          Free: 800-592-7821
Fax: (406)452-0899
Email: aingerso@heart.org
Alice Ingersoll, Director

**★ 5345 ★ American Heart Association of**
**Idaho/Montana**
**Northwest Affiliate**
**Eastern Montana Chapter**
2812 1st Ave. N, Rm. 216
Billings, MT 59101
Phone: (406)256-3855          Fax: (406)256-3728
Email: deckhard@heart.org
Dawn Eckhardt, Director

**★ 5346 ★ American Heart Association of**
**Idaho/Montana**
**Northwest Affiliate**
**Northwest Montana Chapter**
PO Box 1236
Condon, MT 59826
Phone: (406)754-3015          Fax: (406)754-3015
Email: jwheeler@heart.org
Jabet Wheeler, Director

## Nebraska

**★ 5347 ★ American Heart Association**
**Heartland Affiliate**
**Lincoln Chapter**
1550 S 70th St., Ste. 100
Lincoln, NE 68506
Phone: (402)489-5115          Fax: (402)489-6949
Website: http://www.americanheart.org/ne

**★ 5348 ★ American Heart Association**
**Heartland Affiliate**
**Omaha Chapter**
10100 J St., Ste. A
Omaha, NE 68127
**Phone:** (402)346-0771          **Fax:** (402)346-1717
**Website:** http://www.americanheart.org/ne

## Nevada

**★ 5349 ★ American Heart Association**
**Western States Affiliate**
**Clark County/Laughlin Division**
6370 W Flamingo, Ste. 1
Las Vegas, NV 89103
**Phone:** (702)367-1366          **Fax:** (702)367-1975
**Email:** vickis@heart.org
**Website:** http://www.heartsource.org
Vicki K. Sylvia, Exec Director

**★ 5350 ★ American Heart Association**
**Western States Affiliate**
**Reno Division**
1281 Terminal Way, Ste. 111
Reno, NV 89502
**Phone:** (775)322-7065          **Fax:** (775)322-8959
**Website:** http://www.heartsource.org

## New Hampshire

**★ 5351 ★ American Heart Association**
**New England Affiliate**
**New Hampshire Chapter**
20 Merrimack St., Ste. 1
Manchester, NH 03101
**Phone:** (603)669-5833          **Free:** 888-907-6933
**Fax:** (603)669-6745

## New Jersey

**★ 5352 ★ American Heart Association**
**Heritage Affiliate**
**Central New Jersey Chapter**
2550 U.S. Hwy. 1
North Brunswick, NJ 08902
**Phone:** (732)821-2610          **Fax:** (732)821-2736
**Website:** http://www.americanheart.org/nj

**★ 5353 ★ American Heart Association**
**Heritage Affiliate**
**Northern New Jersey Chapter**
1 Bleeker St.
Millburn, NJ 07041
**Phone:** (973)376-3636          **Fax:** (973)912-9570

**★ 5354 ★ American Heart Association**
**Heritage Affiliate**
**Southern New Jersey Chapter**
600 S White Horse Pike
Audubon, NJ 08106
**Phone:** (856)546-5600          **Fax:** (856)546-0861

## New Mexico

**★ 5355 ★ American Heart Association**
**Desert/Mountain Affiliate**
**Albuquerque Chapter**
6100 Pan American Fwy. NE, No. 345
Albuquerque, NM 87109
**Phone:** (505)823-8700          **Fax:** (505)823-8701

## New York

**★ 5356 ★ American Heart Association**
**Heritage Affiliate**
**Long Island Region**
125 E Bethpage Rd.
Plainview, NY 11803
**Phone:** (516)777-8447          **Fax:** (516)370-1060

**★ 5357 ★ American Heart Association**
**New York State Affiliate**
**Central Region**
120 Lomond Ct.
Utica, NY 13502
**Phone:** (315)797-8906          **Fax:** (315)732-6563

**★ 5358 ★ American Heart Association**
**New York State Affiliate**
**Dutchess County Region**
301 Manchester Rd., Ste. 105
Poughkeepsie, NY 12603
**Phone:** (845)485-4703          **Fax:** (845)486-9950

**★ 5359 ★ American Heart Association**
**New York State Affiliate**
**Genesee Valley Region**
2113 Chili Ave.
Rochester, NY 14624
**Phone:** (716)426-4050          **Fax:** (716)426-1312

**★ 5360 ★ American Heart Association**
**New York State Affiliate**
**Mid-State Region**
59 Court St., 4th Fl.
Binghamton, NY 13903
**Phone:** (607)723-0208          **Fax:** (607)724-1875

**★ 5361 ★ American Heart Association**
**New York State Affiliate**
**New York City Region**
122 E 42nd St., 18th Fl.
New York, NY 10168
**Phone:** (212)878-5900          **Fax:** (212)878-5960
**Email:** ccendoma@heart.org
**Website:** http://www.americanheart.org/nyc

**★ 5362 ★ American Heart Association**
**New York State Affiliate**
**Northeastern Region**
440 New Karner Rd.
Albany, NY 12205
**Phone:** (518)869-1961          **Fax:** (518)869-8180

**★ 5363 ★ American Heart Association**
**New York State Affiliate**
**Northern Region**
PO Box 155
Watertown, NY 13601
**Phone:** (315)641-1000          **Fax:** (315)641-1098

**★ 5364 ★ American Heart Association**
**New York State Affiliate**
**Orange-Rockland-Sullivan Regional**
**Chapter**
Good Samaritan Hospital
255 Lafayette Ave.
Suffern, NY 10901
**Phone:** (845)369-1320          **Fax:** (845)369-3801

**★ 5365 ★ American Heart Association**
**New York State Affiliate**
**Southern Tier Region**
PO Box 1461
Corning, NY 14830
**Phone:** (315)641-1000          **Fax:** (315)641-1098

**★ 5366 ★ American Heart Association**
**New York State Affiliate**
**Upstate Region**
5575 Thompson Rd.
Syracuse, NY 13214
**Phone:** (315)446-8334          **Fax:** (315)446-6986

**★ 5367 ★ American Heart Association**
**New York State Affiliate**
**Westchester/Putnam Region**
3020 Westchester Ave.
Purchase, NY 10577
**Phone:** (914)694-6464          **Fax:** (914)694-1285

**★ 5368 ★ American Heart Association**
**New York State Affiliate**
**Western/Southwestern Region**
25 Hazelwood Dr., Ste. 116
Amherst, NY 14228-2220
**Phone:** (716)564-1100          **Fax:** (716)564-1101

## North Carolina

**★ 5369 ★ American Heart Association**
**North Carolina Affiliate**
**Charlotte Chapter**
1229 Greenwood Cliff, Ste. 109
Charlotte, NC 28204
**Phone:** (704)374-0632          **Fax:** (704)374-0634
**Website:** http://www.americanheart.org/nc

**★ 5370 ★ American Heart Association**
**North Carolina Affiliate**
**Eastern North Carolina Chapter**
3131 RDU Center Dr., Ste. 100
Morrisville, NC 27560
**Phone:** (919)463-8300          **Fax:** (919)463-8392

**★ 5371 ★ American Heart Association**
**North Carolina Affiliate**
**Greater Greensboro Chapter**
202 CentrePort Dr., No. 100
Greensboro, NC 27409
**Phone:** (336)668-0167          **Fax:** (336)668-8241

**★ 5372 ★ American Heart Association**
**North Carolina Affiliate**
**Greenville Chapter**
3015 S Memorial Dr., Ste. A
Greenville, NC 27834
**Phone:** (252)355-1112          **Fax:** (252)355-1375
**Website:** http://www.americanheart.org/nc

## North Dakota

**★ 5373 ★ American Heart Association**
**Northland Affiliate**
**Greater Fargo Area Chapter**
712 51st SW St.
Fargo, ND 58103
**Phone:** (701)277-5029          **Fax:** (701)277-5029

**★ 5374 ★ American Heart Association**
**Northland Affiliate**
**Jamestown Chapter**
1005 12 Ave. SE
Jamestown, ND 58401
**Phone:** (701)252-5122          **Free:** 800-437-9710
**Fax:** (701)251-2092
**Remarks:** Serves eastern North Dakota and South
Dakota.

**★ 5375 ★ American Heart Association**
**Northland Affiliate**
**West North Dakota Chapter**
1305 12 St. SW
Minot, ND 58701
**Phone:** (701)838-4635          **Free:** 800-437-9710
**Fax:** (701)838-4635

## Ohio

**★ 5376 ★ American Heart Association**
**Ohio Affiliate**
**Akron Metro Chapter**
1236 Weathervane, Ste. 300C
Akron, OH 44313
**Phone:** (330)867-9987 **Fax:** (330)867-3460
**Website:** http://www.americanheart.org/oh

**★ 5377 ★ American Heart Association**
**Ohio Affiliate**
**Cincinnati Metro Chapter**
2936 Vernon Pl.
Cincinnati, OH 45219
**Phone:** (513)281-4048 **Fax:** (513)281-1433
**Website:** http://www.americanheart.org/oh
Amy Howe, Director

**★ 5378 ★ American Heart Association**
**Ohio Affiliate**
**Cleveland Metro Chapter**
1689 E 115th St.
Cleveland, OH 44106
**Phone:** (216)791-7500 **Fax:** (216)791-5202
**Website:** http://www.americanheart.org/oh

**★ 5379 ★ American Heart Association**
**Ohio Affiliate**
**Columbus Metro**
5455 N High St.
Columbus, OH 43214
**Phone:** (614)848-6676 **Free:** 800-282-0291
**Fax:** (614)848-4227
**Remarks:** Covering Franklin and Delaware counties.

**★ 5380 ★ American Heart Association**
**Ohio Affiliate**
**Miami Valley Division**
24 N Jefferson St., 3rd Fl.
Dayton, OH 45402
**Phone:** (937)224-3571 **Fax:** (937)224-0926
**Website:** http://www.americanheart.org/oh

**★ 5381 ★ American Heart Association**
**Ohio Affiliate**
**Northwestern Ohio Chapter**
5164 Monroe St., Ste. 201
Toledo, OH 43623
**Free:** 800-AHA-USA1 **Fax:** (419)841-8745
**Website:** http://www.americanheart.org/oh

**★ 5382 ★ American Heart Association**
**Ohio Affiliate**
**Stark County Division**
4916 Hills & Dales Rd.
Canton, OH 44708
**Phone:** (330)478-8383 **Fax:** (330)478-8681
**Website:** http://www.americanheart.org/oh

**★ 5383 ★ American Heart Association**
**Ohio Affiliate**
**Youngstown Metro Chapter**
840 Southwestern Run
Youngstown, OH 44514
**Phone:** (330)965-9230 **Fax:** (330)965-9233
**Website:** http://www.americanheart.org/oh

## Oklahoma

**★ 5384 ★ American Heart Association**
**Heartland Affiliate**
**Oklahoma City Chapter**
5700 N Portland, Ste. 203
Oklahoma City, OK 73112
**Phone:** (405)942-2444 **Fax:** (405)942-6616
**Website:** http://www.americanheart.org/ok

**★ 5385 ★ American Heart Association**
**Heartland Affiliate**
**Tulsa Chapter**
2227 Skelly Dr., Ste. 100-S
Tulsa, OK 74105
**Phone:** (918)747-8254 **Free:** 888-242-0280
**Fax:** (918)745-2043

## Oregon

**★ 5386 ★ American Heart Association**
**Northwest Affiliate**
**Central Oregon Chapter**
440 Charnelton St., No. 3
Eugene, OR 97401
**Phone:** (541)344-6345 **Fax:** (541)344-9289
**Website:** http://www.americanheart.org/or
Karen Young, Director

**★ 5387 ★ American Heart Association**
**Northwest Affiliate**
**Portland/Southwest Washington Chapter**
1425 NE Irving, No. 100
Portland, OR 97232
**Phone:** (503)233-0100 **Free:** 800-452-9445
**Fax:** (503)233-4464
**Website:** http://www.americanheart.org/or

**★ 5388 ★ American Heart Association**
**Northwest Affiliate**
**Salem Chapter**
PO Box 6015
Salem, OR 97304
**Phone:** (503)364-5400 **Fax:** (503)364-6200
**Remarks:** Serves Marion, Polk, and Yamhill counties.

**★ 5389 ★ American Heart Association**
**Northwest Affiliate**
**Southern Oregon Chapter**
10 Crater Lake Ave., Ste. 10
Medford, OR 97504
**Phone:** (541)799-2709 **Fax:** (541)734-3809
**Website:** http://www.americanheart.org/or
Janice Watson, Director

## Pennsylvania

**★ 5390 ★ American Heart Association**
**Pennsylvania-Delaware Affiliate**
**Altoona Chapter**
Bldg. D, Ste. 101
501 Howard Ave.
Altoona, PA 16601
**Phone:** (814)949-3160 **Fax:** (814)949-0540

**★ 5391 ★ American Heart Association**
**Pennsylvania-Delaware Affiliate**
**Berks Chapter**
40 Berkshire Ct.
Wyomissing, PA 19610
**Phone:** (610)376-8001 **Fax:** (610)376-3008

**★ 5392 ★ American Heart Association**
**Pennsylvania-Delaware Affiliate**
**Bethlehem Chapter**
212 E Broad St.
Bethlehem, PA 18018
**Phone:** (610)867-0583 **Fax:** (610)867-7218

**★ 5393 ★ American Heart Association**
**Pennsylvania-Delaware Affiliate**
**Capital Region Chapter**
1517 Cedar Cliff Dr.
Camp Hill, PA 17001
**Phone:** (717)730-4080 **Fax:** (717)730-6725
**Email:** pda@heart.org

**★ 5394 ★ American Heart Association**
**Pennsylvania-Delaware Affiliate**
**Chambersburg Chapter**
225 E King St.
Chambersburg, PA 17201
**Phone:** (717)263-2870

**★ 5395 ★ American Heart Association**
**Pennsylvania-Delaware Affiliate**
**Clearfield Chapter**
440 Front St.
Clearfield, PA 16830
**Phone:** (814)765-7579

**★ 5396 ★ American Heart Association**
**Pennsylvania-Delaware Affiliate**
**Conshohocken Chapter**
625 W Ridge Pike, Bldg. A, Ste. 100
Conshohocken, PA 19428
**Phone:** (610)940-9540 **Fax:** (610)940-9541
**Remarks:** Covers Bucks, Chester, Delaware, Montgomery, and Philadelphia counties.

**★ 5397 ★ American Heart Association**
**Pennsylvania-Delaware Affiliate**
**Erie Chapter**
823 Filmore Ave.
Erie, PA 16505
**Phone:** (814)836-0013 **Fax:** (814)836-9213

**★ 5398 ★ American Heart Association**
**Pennsylvania-Delaware Affiliate**
**Greensburg Chapter**
615 S Main St.
Greensburg, PA 15601
**Phone:** (724)837-5468 **Fax:** (724)837-2037

**★ 5399 ★ American Heart Association**
**Pennsylvania-Delaware Affiliate**
**Hermitage Chapter**
59 N Crescent Dr.
Hermitage, PA 16148
**Phone:** (724)983-1055 **Fax:** (724)346-3706

**★ 5400 ★ American Heart Association**
**Pennsylvania-Delaware Affiliate**
**Johnstown Chapter**
400 Luray Ave.
Johnstown, PA 15904
**Phone:** (814)266-8905 **Fax:** (814)269-3134

**★ 5401 ★ American Heart Association**
**Pennsylvania-Delaware Affiliate**
**Kulpmont Chapter**
1020 Ash St.
Kulpmont, PA 17834
**Phone:** (570)373-1093

**★ 5402 ★ American Heart Association**
**Pennsylvania-Delaware Affiliate**
**Lancaster Chapter**
610 Community Way
Lancaster, PA 17603
**Phone:** (717)393-0725 **Free:** 800-264-2785
**Fax:** (717)393-0731

**★ 5403 ★ American Heart Association**
**Pennsylvania-Delaware Affiliate**
**Lebanon Chapter**
335 S 8th St.
Lebanon, PA 17042
**Phone:** (717)273-0463 **Fax:** (717)273-8616

**★ 5404 ★ American Heart Association**
**Pennsylvania-Delaware Affiliate**
**Luzerne Chapter**
71 N Franklin St.
Wilkes-Barre, PA 18701
**Phone:** (570)822-6247          **Fax:** (570)823-9538

**★ 5405 ★ American Heart Association**
**Pennsylvania-Delaware Affiliate**
**Pittsburgh Chapter**
10 Duff Rd., Ste. 304
Pittsburgh, PA 15235
**Phone:** (412)243-5393          **Fax:** (412)243-5497

**★ 5406 ★ American Heart Association**
**Pennsylvania-Delaware Affiliate**
**Scranton Chapter**
730 Pittston Ave.
Scranton, PA 18505
**Phone:** (570)342-8374          **Fax:** (570)969-4122

**★ 5407 ★ American Heart Association**
**Pennsylvania-Delaware Affiliate**
**Uniontown Chapter**
7829 National Pike, Ste. 2
Uniontown, PA 15401
**Phone:** (724)437-2798          **Fax:** (724)437-5536

**★ 5408 ★ American Heart Association**
**Pennsylvania-Delaware Affiliate**
**Venango/Clarion County Chapter**
174 E Bissell Ave.
Oil City, PA 16301
**Phone:** (814)676-2445          **Fax:** (814)677-5469

**★ 5409 ★ American Heart Association**
**Pennsylvania-Delaware Affiliate**
**Warren Chapter**
185 Hospital Dr.
Warren, PA 16365
**Phone:** (814)723-4860          **Fax:** (814)723-4860

**★ 5410 ★ American Heart Association**
**Pennsylvania-Delaware Affiliate**
**Williamsport Chapter**
1704 Warren Ave.
Williamsport, PA 17701
**Phone:** (570)322-4733          **Fax:** (570)322-0435

**★ 5411 ★ American Heart Association**
**Pennsylvania-Delaware Affiliate**
**York Chapter**
Cape Horn Plaza, Ste. B2
2997 Cape Horn Rd.
Red Lion, PA 17356
**Phone:** (717)246-9661          **Fax:** (717)246-9578

## Puerto Rico

**★ 5412 ★ American Heart Association**
**San Juan Chapter**
554 Cabo Alverio St.
San Juan, PR 00918
**Phone:** (787)751-6595          **Fax:** (787)250-0281

## Rhode Island

**★ 5413 ★ American Heart Association**
**Rhode Island Affiliate**
275 Westminster St., Ste. 100
Providence, RI 02903
**Phone:** (401)274-4544          **Fax:** (401)274-3332
**Website:** http://www.americanheart.org/ri

## South Carolina

**★ 5414 ★ American Heart Association**
**South Carolina Affiliate**
**Charleston Chapter**
409 King St., Ste. 300
Charleston, SC 29403
**Phone:** (843)853-1597          **Fax:** (843)853-2498
**Website:** http://www.americanheart.org/sc

**★ 5415 ★ American Heart Association**
**South Carolina Affiliate**
**Columbia Chapter**
400 Percival Rd.
PO Box 6604
Columbia, SC 29260
**Phone:** (803)738-9540          **Fax:** (803)787-0804
**Website:** http://www.americanheart.org/sc

**★ 5416 ★ American Heart Association**
**South Carolina Affiliate**
**Florence Chapter**
181 E Evans St., Ste. 204 BTC-009
Florence, SC 29506
**Phone:** (843)665-0985          **Fax:** (843)665-1855

**★ 5417 ★ American Heart Association**
**South Carolina Affiliate**
**Myrtle Beach Chapter**
1506 Gumm Plaza
Hwy. 501
Myrtle Beach, SC 29577
**Phone:** (843)626-3939          **Fax:** (843)626-2856

**★ 5418 ★ American Heart Association**
**South Carolina Affiliate**
**Upstate South Carolina/Western North**
**  Carolina Chapter**
310B Bennett Center Dr.
Greer, SC 29650
**Phone:** (864)801-9550          **Fax:** (864)801-3589

## South Dakota

**★ 5419 ★ American Heart Association**
**Northland Affiliate**
**Greater Sioux Falls Area Chapter**
218 S Main Ave., Ste. 200
Sioux Falls, SD 57104
**Phone:** (605)743-5194          **Fax:** (605)743-5194

**★ 5420 ★ American Heart Association**
**Northland Affiliate**
**West South Dakota Chapter**
22161 New Underwood Rd.
New Underwood, SD 57761
**Free:** 800-437-9710

## Tennessee

**★ 5421 ★ American Heart Association**
**Southeast Affiliate**
**Chattanooga Chapter**
519 E 4th St.
Chattanooga, TN 37403
**Phone:** (423)265-3466          **Fax:** (423)267-5508

**★ 5422 ★ American Heart Association**
**Southeast Affiliate**
**Johnson City Chapter**
208 Sunset Dr., Ste. 521
Johnson City, TN 37604
**Phone:** (423)282-5388

**★ 5423 ★ American Heart Association**
**Southeast Affiliate**
**Knoxville Chapter**
4708 Papermill Dr.
Knoxville, TN 37909
**Phone:** (865)588-7646          **Fax:** (865)584-4109

**★ 5424 ★ American Heart Association**
**Southeast Affiliate**
**Memphis Chapter**
11 S Orleans
Memphis, TN 38103
**Phone:** (901)572-4200          **Fax:** (901)572-4201

**★ 5425 ★ American Heart Association**
**Southeast Affiliate**
**Nashville Chapter**
1818 Patterson St.
Nashville, TN 37203
**Phone:** (615)340-4100          **Fax:** (615)340-4101
**Website:** http://www.americanheart.org/tn

## Texas

**★ 5426 ★ American Heart Association**
**Arkansas Affiliate**
**Texarkana Chapter**
McKnight Center
4150 McKnight Rd.
Texarkana, TX 75503
**Phone:** (903)832-2477          **Fax:** (903)838-6006

**★ 5427 ★ American Heart Association**
**Texas Affiliate**
**Abilene Chapter**
149 N Willis, No. 10
Abilene, TX 79603
**Phone:** (915)627-0070          **Fax:** (915)627-0071

**★ 5428 ★ American Heart Association**
**Texas Affiliate**
**Amarillo Chapter**
6605 I-40 West, Bldg. A-6
Amarillo, TX 79106
**Phone:** (806)457-0090          **Fax:** (806)457-0099

**★ 5429 ★ American Heart Association**
**Texas Affiliate**
**Austin Chapter**
1700 Rutherford Ln.
Austin, TX 78754
**Phone:** (512)433-4000          **Fax:** (512)433-4200
**Website:** http://www.americanheart.org/tx

**★ 5430 ★ American Heart Association**
**Texas Affiliate**
**Beaumont Chapter**
5675 Eastex Fwy., Ste. 3
Beaumont, TX 77706
**Phone:** (409)980-8800          **Fax:** (409)980-8808

**★ 5431 ★ American Heart Association**
**Texas Affiliate**
**Bryan Chapter**
3833 S Texas Ave., No. 216
Bryan, TX 77802
**Phone:** (979)268-0068          **Fax:** (979)268-0070

**★ 5432 ★ American Heart Association**
**Texas Affiliate**
**Corpus Christi Chapter**
500 N Shoreline Blvd., Ste. 203 N
Corpus Christi, TX 78471
**Phone:** (361)692-0606          **Fax:** (361)692-0607

**★ 5433 ★ American Heart Association**
**Texas Affiliate**
**Dallas Area Chapter**
1615 Stemmons Fwy.
Dallas, TX 75207
**Phone:** (214)748-7212　　　　**Fax:** (214)748-1307

**★ 5434 ★ American Heart Association**
**Texas Affiliate**
**El Paso Chapter**
233 Mesa Hills Dr.
El Paso, TX 79912
**Phone:** (915)833-1231　　　　**Fax:** (915)581-0423

**★ 5435 ★ American Heart Association**
**Texas Affiliate**
**Fort Worth Chapter**
2401 Scott Ave.
Fort Worth, TX 76103
**Phone:** (817)315-5000　　　　**Fax:** (817)315-5220

**★ 5436 ★ American Heart Association**
**Texas Affiliate**
**Harlingen Chapter**
712 Morgan Blvd., Ste. 102
Harlingen, TX 78550
**Phone:** (956)425-3924　　　　**Fax:** (956)412-0139

**★ 5437 ★ American Heart Association**
**Texas Affiliate**
**Houston Chapter**
2626 S Loop W, Ste. 510
Houston, TX 77054
**Phone:** (713)610-5000　　　　**Fax:** (713)610-5200

**★ 5438 ★ American Heart Association**
**Texas Affiliate**
**Longview Chapter**
1125 Judson Rd., No. 150
Longview, TX 75601
**Phone:** (903)323-8800　　　　**Fax:** (903)323-8808

**★ 5439 ★ American Heart Association**
**Texas Affiliate**
**Lubbock Chapter**
4630 50th St., Ste. 400
Lubbock, TX 79414
**Phone:** (806)762-6599　　　　**Fax:** (806)762-6598

**★ 5440 ★ American Heart Association**
**Texas Affiliate**
**Midland Chapter**
3205 W Cuthbert, A-8
Midland, TX 79701
**Phone:** (915)520-7041　　　　**Fax:** (915)520-5714

**★ 5441 ★ American Heart Association**
**Texas Affiliate**
**San Angelo Chapter**
3135 Executive Dr.
San Angelo, TX 76904
**Phone:** (915)223-2345　　　　**Fax:** (915)223-2211

**★ 5442 ★ American Heart Association**
**Texas Affiliate**
**Tyler Chapter**
5604 Old Bullard Rd., Ste. 106
Tyler, TX 75703
**Phone:** (903)324-1444　　　　**Fax:** (903)324-1443

**★ 5443 ★ American Heart Association**
**Texas Affiliate**
**Waco Chapter**
6801 Sanger, Ste. 102
Waco, TX 76710

**Phone:** (254)299-0880　　　　**Fax:** (254)299-0881

**★ 5444 ★ American Heart Association**
**Texas Affiliate**
**Wichita Falls Chapter**
811 6th St., Ste. 160
Wichita Falls, TX 76301
**Phone:** (940)397-0700　　　　**Fax:** (940)397-0707

## Utah

**★ 5445 ★ American Heart Association**
**Western States Affiliate**
**Utah Chapter**
1937 South 300 West, Ste. 120
Salt Lake City, UT 84115
**Phone:** (801)484-3838　　　　**Fax:** (801)484-4448
**Website:** http://www.heartsource.org

## Vermont

**★ 5446 ★ American Heart Association**
**Vermont Affiliate**
**PO Box 485**
434 Hurricane Ln.
Williston, VT 05495
**Phone:** (802)878-7700　　　　**Free:** 800-639-6024
**Fax:** (802)878-7850

## Virginia

**★ 5447 ★ American Heart Association**
**Virginia Affiliate**
**Central Virginia Chapter**
3025 Berkmar Dr.
Charlottesville, VA 22901
**Phone:** (434)973-5072　　　　**Fax:** (434)973-1784

**★ 5448 ★ American Heart Association**
**Virginia Affiliate**
**Greater Washington DC Regional Chapter**
7203 Poplar St.
Annandale, VA 22003
**Phone:** (703)941-8500　　　　**Fax:** (703)914-3795

**★ 5449 ★ American Heart Association**
**Virginia Affiliate**
**Richmond Chapter**
4217 Park Pl. Ct.
Glen Allen, VA 23060
**Phone:** (804)747-8334　　　　**Fax:** (804)965-6421
**Website:** http://www.americanheart.org/va

**★ 5450 ★ American Heart Association**
**Virginia Affiliate**
**Tidewater Chapter**
360 Southport Cir., Ste. 104
Virginia Beach, VA 23452
**Phone:** (757)671-8636　　　　**Fax:** (757)456-0486

**★ 5451 ★ American Heart Association**
**Virginia Affiliate**
**Western Virginia Chapter**
4504 Starkey Rd. SW, No. 115
Roanoke, VA 24014
**Phone:** (540)989-2810　　　　**Fax:** (540)772-4243

## Washington

**★ 5452 ★ American Heart Association**
**Northwest Affiliate**
**Greater Pierce County Region**
1101 S Fawcett, Ste. 100
Tacoma, WA 98402
**Phone:** (253)272-7854　　　　**Fax:** (253)627-1035
**Website:** http://www.americanheart.org/wa

**★ 5453 ★ American Heart Association**
**Northwest Affiliate**
**Greater Thurston County Chapter**
505 4th Ave. W, Ste. D
Olympia, WA 98501
**Phone:** (360)236-8136　　　　**Fax:** (360)236-8137

**★ 5454 ★ American Heart Association**
**Northwest Affiliate**
**Inland Northwest Chapter**
140 S Arthur Ave., Ste. 610
Spokane, WA 99202
**Phone:** (509)536-1500　　　　**Free:** 800-536-1314
**Fax:** (509)536-1515
**Website:** http://www.americanheart.org/wa
**Remarks:** Also serves Idaho.

**★ 5455 ★ American Heart Association**
**Northwest Affiliate**
**King County Chapter**
155 NE 100th St., Ste. 306
Seattle, WA 98125
**Phone:** (206)525-7665　　　　**Free:** 888-440-2328
**Fax:** (206)525-7645
**Website:** http://www.americanheart.org/wa

**★ 5456 ★ American Heart Association**
**Northwest Affiliate**
**Tri-Cities Chapter**
805 S Auburn
Kennewick, WA 99336
**Phone:** (509)582-9001　　　　**Fax:** (509)582-6676
**Remarks:** Also serves north-central Oregon.

## West Virginia

**★ 5457 ★ American Heart Association**
**West Virginia Affiliate**
**Charleston Chapter**
4510-C Pennsylvania Ave.
PO Box 12110
Charleston, WV 25302
**Phone:** (304)965-7998　　　　**Fax:** (304)965-7992
**Remarks:** Also serves Ohio.

**★ 5458 ★ American Heart Association**
**West Virginia Affiliate**
**Wheeling Chapter**
McLain Bldg., Rm. 206
40 12th St.
Wheeling, WV 26003
**Phone:** (304)233-1525　　　　**Fax:** (304)233-2075

## Wisconsin

**★ 5459 ★ American Heart Association**
**Northland Affiliate**
**Greater Milwaukee Chapter**
795 N Van Buren St.
Milwaukee, WI 53202
**Phone:** (414)271-9999　　　　**Free:** 800-242-8721
**Fax:** (414)271-3299
**Email:** ahawi@execpc.com
**Website:** http://www.americanheart.org/wi
**Telecom. Serv:** TDD: (414)271-0450.

**★ 5460 ★ American Heart Association**
**Northland Affiliate**
**Northcentral Wisconsin Division**
903 Grand Ave. C6
Rothschild, WI 54474
**Phone:** (715)359-4278　　　　**Fax:** (715)359-7285

**★ 5461 ★ American Heart Association**
**Northland Affiliate**
**Northeast Wisconsin Division**
2149 Velp Ave.
Green Bay, WI 54303
**Phone:** (920)662-2268          **Fax:** (920)662-2273

**★ 5462 ★ American Heart Association**
**Northland Affiliate**
**Northwest Wisconsin Division**
800 Wisconsin St., Ste. 312
Eau Claire, WI 54703
**Phone:** (715)834-1108          **Fax:** (715)834-1401

**★ 5463 ★ American Heart Association**
**Northland Affiliate**
**Southcentral Wisconsin Division**
2850 Dairy Dr., Ste. 300
Madison, WI 53718
**Phone:** (608)221-8866          **Fax:** (608)221-9233

**★ 5464 ★ American Heart Association**
**Northland Affiliate**
**Southwest Wisconsin Division**
400 La Crosse St.
La Crosse, WI 54601
**Phone:** (608)784-4020          **Fax:** (608)782-8553

# Chapter 13
# Child Abuse & Family Violence

## Foundations & Other Funding Organizations

### Private Foundations

**★ 5465 ★ Carthage Foundation**
One Oxford Centre
301 Grant St., Ste. 3900
Pittsburgh, PA 15219-6401
**Phone:** (412)392-2900          **Fax:** (412)392-2922
**Website:** http://www.scaife.com
Michael Gleba, Treasurer
**Fnded:** 1964. **Philosophy:** The foundation's primary interests include national and international organizations that deal with public policy issues. **Priorities:** *Arts & Humanities:* 2%. Primary support for accuracy in media. *Civic & Public Affairs:* (Public Policy) 67%. Major grant to the Free Congress Research and Education Foundation. *Education:* 11%. Public policy education. *Environment:* 1%. Funds social services and substance abuse prevention. *International:* 1%. Supports the Institute for Health Freedom. *Note:* Total contributions made in 1998. **Typ. Recipients:** Domestic Violence, Health Policy/Cost Containment, Public Health, Substance Abuse. **Geo. Dist:** no restrictions.

**CTW Foundation, Inc.**
*See:* Entry 11377

**★ 5466 ★ F. B. Heron Foundation**
100 Broadway, 17th Floor
New York, NY 10005
**Phone:** (212)649-5613
**Website:** http://www.heronfdn.org
Sharon King, Secretary & Treasurer
**Fnded:** 1992. **Priorities:** *Civic & Public Affairs:* 54%. Funds housing, minority and urban affairs, economic development, and community foundations. *Education:* 22%. Supports educational funds and scholarships. *Environment:* 6%. Supports shelters, food banks, and services for children. *International:* 10%. Supports healthcare institutes and foundations. *Note:* Total contributions made in 1999. **Typ. Recipients:** AIDS/HIV, Domestic Violence, Emergency/Ambulance Services, Home-Care Services, Research/Studies Institutes, Substance Abuse.

**Geraldine R. Dodge Foundation**
*See:* Entry 289

**Hartford Courant Foundation**
*See:* Entry 11689

**Kelly Gene Cook, Sr. Charitable Foundation**
*See:* Entry 449

**★ 5467 ★ Lannan Foundation**
313 Read St.
Santa Fe, NM 87501-2628
**Phone:** (505)986-8160          **Fax:** (505)986-8195
**Email:** jo@lannan.org
**Website:** http://www.lannan.org
Frank Lawler, Director
**Fnded:** 1950. **Philosophy:** The Foundation gives in the following areas: the arts, literature, indigenous communities and special project. "(The) art program is designed to further the careers of emerging and under-recognized artists, foster serious criticism and discussion of contemporary art, and to bring new, experimental and sometimes controversial works of arts to a wide audience." "(The literary program supports) the creation of literature written originally in the English language and to develop a wider audience for contemporary prose and poetry." The foundation gives out literary awards and grants. "(The indigenous communities program is) dedicated to benefiting rural Native Americans who suffer from racial and cultural discrimination, lack of education and economic opportunities, in adequate health care and widespread poverty." **Priorities:** *Arts & Humanities:* 54%. Focus on museums, literary arts, and arts funds. *Civic & Public Affairs:* 15%. Funds organizations dealing with Native American issues and law/justice. *Education:* 24%. Native American colleges and universities. *Environment:* 1%. *Note:* Total contributions made in 1999. **Typ. Recipients:** Domestic Violence, Hospitals, Medical Rehabilitation.

**Lois U. Horvitz Foundation**
*See:* Entry 474

**★ 5468 ★ Lyndhurst Foundation**
517 East Fifth St.
Chattanooga, TN 37403-1826
**Phone:** (423)756-0767          **Fax:** (423)756-0770
**Website:** http://www.lyndhurstfoundation.org
Jack Murrah, President
**Fnded:** 1938. **Philosophy:** Through the end of the century, the foundation intends to focus upon a number of activities. In Chattanooga, the foundation will focus on: continued development of the Tennessee Riverpark; redevelopment of the Southside as a live-and-work urban neighborhood with a zero-emissions industrial park; facilitation of historic preservation; stimulation of downtown housing development; strengthening of the city's arts and cultural life; protection and enhancement of the community's natural environment; the reform of the community's elementary and secondary public schools; the continued development of improved housing opportunities for people of modest means; and innovations in social service programs that provide genuine progress against social problems and genuine enhancement of community strengths. In the South, the foundation will focus on: continued development of the Center for Documentary Studies at Duke University, a center supporting responsible involvement in the world by encouraging photographers, filmmakers, writers, scholars, teachers, and students to work by direct observation, to participate in the lives of individuals and communities, and to render these lives in works of artistic, literary, and social value; support of individuals providing significant contributions within various fields of interest (through the Lyndhurst Prize program); continued evolution of a significant education reform initiative in rural Alabama; and protection and enhancement of the natural environment of the Southern Appalachian region. Most of the foundation's grants are distributed solely at the foundation's initiative. This means that, in most categories, the foundation does not seek or fund uninvited requests. For instance, within the field of education, the foundation has made a commitment extending through the end of the century to support certain reform initiatives within the city of Chattanooga and in rural Alabama. Within two categories, however, the foundation is open to requests. These are in the fields of arts and culture within the Chattanooga area, and environmental improvement throughout the six-state region (Tennessee, North Carolina, South Carolina, Georgia, Alabama, and Mississippi) that defines the Southeast. Strong preference is given to programs that focus on the Southern Appalachian region. **Priorities:** *Arts & Humanities:* 8%. Arts organizations within Chattanooga. *Civic & Public Affairs:* 54%. Includes organizations concerned with the revitalization of Chattanooga. *Education:* 24%. Major support for an education reform initiative and a primary school. *Environment:* 2%. Community services. *International:* 1%. Supports health centers. *Note:* Total contributions made in 2000. **Typ. Recipients:** Child Abuse, Clinics/Medical Centers, Mental Health, Sexual Abuse, Substance Abuse. **Geo. Dist:** Southeastern USA; Chattanooga, TN.

**Mary Stuart Rogers Foundation**
*See:* Entry 5560

**★ 5469 ★ Powell Foundation**
2121 San Felipe, Ste. 110
Houston, TX 77019
**Phone:** (713)523-7557          **Fax:** (713)523-7553
**Email:** nanpmoore@aol.com
**Website:** www.powellfoundation.org
Nancy Moore, Manager & Trustee
**Fnded:** 1967. **Priorities:** *Arts & Humanities:* 13%. Supports theater, museums, ballet, opera, symphony and art festivals. *Civic & Public Affairs:* 2%. Funds philanthropy and community programs. *Education:* 66%. Educational programs, schools, academies, colleges, and universities receive funding. *International:* 10%. Funds the American Red Cross, health associations, medical research, and planned parenthood. *Note:* Total contributions made in 2000. **Typ. Recipients:** Adolescent Health Issues, AIDS/HIV, Child Abuse, Clinics/Medical Centers, Emergency/Ambulance Services, Eyes/Blindness, Family Planning, Hospitals (University Affiliated), Mental Health, Public Health, Research/Studies Institutes, Single-Disease Health Associations, Speech & Hearing, Substance Abuse. **Geo. Dist:** TX, Harris County; TX, Travis County; TX, Walker County.

**R. J. Maclellan Charitable Trust**
*See:* Entry 12275

**Ross Foundation**
*See:* Entry 644

**Samuel Rubin Foundation**
*See:* Entry 657

**William Penn Foundation**
*See:* Entry 773

## Corporate Foundations

**Appleton Papers Inc.**
*See:* Entry 843

**ARCO Foundation**
*See:* Entry 846

**★ 5470 ★ BankAtlantic Foundation**
1750 East Sunrise Boulevard
Fort Lauderdale, FL 33304-3013
**Phone:** (954)760-5458
**Email:** dkolb@appletonpapers.com
**Website:** http://www.bankatlantic.com/communityinvestment/bafoundation.asp
Shelley Levan, Executive Director
**Fnded:** 1994. **Priorities:** *Arts & Humanities:* 29%. Supports fine arts, libraries, museums, and music. *Civic & Public Affairs:* 37%. Supports urban/community affairs, housing, civil rights, legal affairs, and community foundations. *Education:* 22%. Supports continuing studies, literacy programs, and higher education. *Environment:* 10%. Supports child and youth services, elder care, and human services. *International:* 1%. Supports prenatal health, children's health, and hearing & deaf services. *Religion:* 1%. Funds science museums. *Note:* Total contributions made in 2000. **Typ. Recipients:** AIDS/HIV, Domestic Violence, Emergency/Ambulance Services, People with Disabilities, Prenatal Health Issues. **Geo. Dist:** FL, Southern Florida.

**★ 5471 ★ Best Buy Children's Foundation**
c/o Community Relations Department
PO Box 9312
Minneapolis, MN 55440-9312
**Phone:** (952)947-2000
**Website:** http://www.bestbuy.com/About/CommunityRelations/ChildrensFoundation.asp
Richard Schulze, Chairman, Director
**Fnded:** 1995. **Priorities:** *Arts & Humanities:* Less than 1%. Gives to libraries and community arts. *Civic & Public Affairs:* 4%. Supports women's affairs and civic groups. *Education:* 28%. Funds alternative schools, community involvement in schools, Junior Achievement, colleges, and universities. *Environment:* 67%. Supports child and family services, youth organizations, scouts, senior services, domestic violence services, and shelters. *Note:* Total contributions made in fiscal 2001. **Typ. Recipients:** Sexual Abuse.

**★ 5472 ★ The Boeing Co. Charitable Trust**
PO Box 3707 MS 11-83
Seattle, WA 98124
**Phone:** (206)655-1131          **Fax:** (206)655-2000
**Website:** http://www.boeing.com/companyoffices/aboutus/community/guidelines.htm
Antoinette Bailey, Vice President, Community Relations
**Fnded:** 1964. **Priorities:** *Arts & Humanities:* 18%. Supports arts, music, drama, and dance. Especially interested in projects that explore the relationships between art, science, and technology. Contributions include grants for capital campaigns, performance scholarships and outreach programs, and one-time special grants. *Civic & Public Affairs:* 7%. Includes environmental grants. Funds initiatives concerned with long-term community growth, sustainable economic

development, affordable housing, and free enterprise. Also interested in projects that aid communities and the environment at the same time. Contributions generally support capital campaigns, seed money for new programs that address community needs and priorities, and one-time grants for equipment purchases or special projects. *Education:* 41%. Supports K-12 and higher education. K-12 support focuses on schools with an emphasis on high academic standards, commitment to improving student achievement, effective school-to-work strategies, and the Tech Prep program. Higher education grants support engineering, business, technology, math, and selected science education; faculty preparation and development; collaborative academic programs; curriculum development; laboratory equipment that directly supports learning and academic performance; scholarships; and minority and women's programs. Two-year colleges are supported through the Tech Prep program. Favors innovative proposals in the following areas: aviation maintenance, manufacturing and engineering technologies, information technology, telecommunications/networks, business technologies or disciplines, electronics, machine tool maintenance, machine shop technology, quality assurance, and evaluation (learning assessment). The company recognizes excellence in higher education teaching with the annual Boeing Outstanding Educator Award. *International:* 34%. Includes human service organizations and United Way. Supports agencies that ease mental and physical suffering, addiction or substance abuse, and family problems. Funds basic needs for housing and nutrition, boys and girls clubs, and programs for the homeless. *Note:* Total contributions made in 2000. **Typ. Recipients:** Clinics/Medical Centers, Domestic Violence, Emergency/Ambulance Services, Hospices, Mental Health, People with Disabilities, Substance Abuse. **Geo. Dist:** headquarters and operating communities where Boeing employees work and reside; national.

**Chicago Sun-Times Charity Trust**
*See:* Entry 936

**Copolymer Foundation**
*See:* Entry 13520

**★ 5473 ★ Gulfstream Aerospace Corp.**
PO Box 2206
MIS D-03
Savannah, GA 31402
**Phone:** (912)965-4212          **Fax:** (912)965-7178
**Email:** tracy.jaynes@gulfaero.com
**Website:** http://www.gulfaero.com
Tracy Jaynes, Community Administrator
**Fnded:** 1990. **Typ. Recipients:** Domestic Violence, Hospices. **Geo. Dist:** headquarters and operating communities; national organizations.

**Hunt Corp.**
*See:* Entry 11696

**MGIC Investment Corp.**
*See:* Entry 1240

**National Life Group**
*See:* Entry 1257

**The Oklahoman Foundation**
*See:* Entry 1286

**Oshkosh Truck Foundation**
*See:* Entry 10067

**Pieper Power Foundation, Inc.**
*See:* Entry 5586

**★ 5474 ★ R.R. Donnelley & Sons Co.**
77 West Wacker Dr.
Chicago, IL 60601-1696
**Phone:** (312)326-8102          **Fax:** (312)326-8262
**Email:** susan.levy@rrd.com
**Website:** http://www.rrdonnelley.com/public/community/
Susan Levy, Vice President
**Priorities:** *Arts & Humanities:* 10% to 15%. Interests include museums, libraries, and literary and performing arts. Matches employee gifts to cultural institutions. *Civic & Public Affairs:* About 10%. Supports better government groups, and conservation and environmental projects. Other interests include civil rights and economic development. Main focus of national giving is public policy organizations. *Education:* 20% to 25%. Emphasis is on higher education, especially independent college funds and educational institutions located in operating communities. Precollegiate education is also of interest. Matches employee gifts to higher and secondary education and provides scholarships for employees' children. *Environment:* 55% to 60%. Company contributes to organizations serving operating locations, including united funds and groups concerned with youth, the disabled, and minorities. *Voluntarism:* The company sponsors the Donnelley Dollars for Doers program, which provides grants to organizations for which Donnelley employees or retirees volunteer. Grant amounts are based on the number of hours donated by the employee or retiree, to a maximum of $500 per employee and $5,000 to any one organization. *Note:* Total contributions made in 1999. Donations are given either as special purpose grants, to support initiatives that require defined funds to launch or develop a major program, or as general operating grants, for ongoing assistance to local organizations. An overall company priority is organizations which promote the written word, including libraries and literary organizations. **Typ. Recipients:** Domestic Violence, Hospitals, Mental Health, People with Disabilities. **Geo. Dist:** principally near operating locations and to national organizations.

**The Reebok Human Rights Foundation**
*See:* Entry 1346

**Spang & Co. Charitable Trust**
*See:* Entry 5588

**★ 5475 ★ Star Tribune Foundation**
Minneapolis, MN 55415
**Phone:** (612)673-7314          **Fax:** (612)673-7020
**Email:** geri.noonan@reebok.com
Sandra Fleitman, Foundation Coordinator
**Priorities:** *Arts & Humanities:* 29%. Support goes to major organizations that form the core of the cultural community, primarily in the Twin Cities. Also funds smaller organizations that have demonstrated promise or community interest. Recipients include theaters, orchestral and music groups, the visual arts, and organizations concerned with literature and writing. *Civic & Public Affairs:* 20%. Funds organizations concerned with neighborhood development, both socially and economically. Also supports programs that help people understand world issues and that encourage people to participate in important civc issues. Sponsors an employee matching gifts program for civic and cultural organizations that have a company employee on the governing board. *Education:* 9%. Emphasis is on the preeminent institutions and on writing-related programs that also enlighten social consciousness. Support is directed to organizations concerned with the First Amendment and to policy issues in journalism and communications, and to professional education programs. Recipients include: journalism education programs, particularly for minorities; the Minnesota Newspaper Foundation, conferences concerned with newspapers, reports, and editors; and groups interested in Libel and freedom of the press. *Environment:* 32%. A majority of giving supports social services. Funds organizations which assist people to move from dependence to self-reliance; in particular, those organizations which help create opportunities, aid self-reliance, assist people to meet

basic needs, and respond to current and future needs. Supports local United Way chapter in the headquarters area; a portion of this funding is in matching gifts. Also supports organizations concerned with adolescents, youth groups, teen pregnancy and parenting. Aids emergency services such as food distribution and matches employee gifts to the Emergency Food Shelf. *Religion:* 6%. Funds a science museum. *Note:* Total contributions in fiscal 1998. **Typ. Recipients:** Domestic Violence, Family Planning, Medical Rehabilitation, People with Disabilities, Substance Abuse. **Geo. Dist:** Minneapolis-St. Paul, MN. **Frmly:** Cowles Media Foundation.

**Stonecutter Foundation**
*See:* Entry 1413

**UST Inc.**
*See:* Entry 1471

**★ 5476 ★ Xerox Foundation**
PO Box 1600
800 Long Ridge Rd.
Stamford, CT 06904
**Phone:** (203)968-3445　　　**Fax:** (203)968-4312
**Email:** mminton@usthq.com
**Website:** http://www.ustshareholder.com
Joseph Cahalan, Vice President

**Priorities:** *Education:* 34%. Emphasis is on higher education. Makes large grants to colleges and universities located in communities where company has facilities. Interests include science, technology, and minority education. Also sponsors employee matching gifts. *Note:* Total foundation contributions made in 2000. **Typ. Recipients:** Domestic Violence, Health Policy/Cost Containment, People with Disabilities, Substance Abuse. **Geo. Dist:** nationally, with emphasis on operating locations.

# National & International Organizations

**★ 5477 ★ Family Therapy Network (FTN)**
7705 13th St. NW
Washington, DC 20012
**Phone:** (202)829-2452　　　**Fax:** (202)726-7983
**Email:** info@psychnetworker.org
Richard Simon, Dir.

**Fnded:** 1976. **Mem:** 65,000. **Desc:** Promotes the exchange of ideas and information among psychotherapists. **Pub:** *Family Therapy Networker*, bimonthly. Magazine. Contains case studies, calendar of events, listing of employment opportunities, and book and movie reviews. **Price:** $24/year for individuals; $30 outside U.S.

**Global Alliance for Women's Health**
*See:* Entry 2130

**★ 5478 ★ Life Works Institute (LWI)**
14622 Ventura Blvd., No. 800
Sherman Oaks, CA 91403-3600
**Phone:** (818)386-9100　　　**Fax:** (818)386-9102
**Email:** lifeworks@lifeonnet.org
**Website:** http://lifeonnet.org/lifeworks.htm
Sanford Holst, Exec. Dir.

**Fnded:** 1996. **Desc:** Works to raise public awareness of life improvement and develop the belief that something can be done to make lives better. Develops and provides educational material and charitable services through others, and directly to the public, to begin improving people's lives. **Pub:** Newsletter. • Brochure.

**National Committee for the Prevention of Elder Abuse (NCPEA)**
*See:* Entry 3009

# Research Centers

**Georgia Southern University Center for Rural Health and Research**
*See:* Entry 17981

**Legacy Clinical Research and Technology Center**
*See:* Entry 5801

**★ 5479 ★ U.S. Department of Health and Human Services**
**Administration for Children and Families**
**National Center on Child Abuse and Neglect**
330 C St., SW
Washington, DC 20447
**Phone:** (703)385-7565　　　**Free:** 800-FYI-3366
**Fax:** (703)385-3206
**Email:** nccanch@calib.com
**Website:** http://www.calib.com/nccanch
Candy Hughes, Proj. Dir.

**Activities/Fields:** Conducts research; collects, analyzes, and disseminates information; provides assistance to states and communities in developing programs and activities related to the prevention, identification, and treatment of child abuse and neglect; and coordinates Federal efforts to combat child maltreatment.

# State & Regional Organizations

## Domestic Violence

*The following are state affiliates of the National Coalition Against Domestic Violence, PO Box 18749, Denver, CO 80218, (303)839-1852, http:// www.ncadv.org/.*

### Alabama

**★ 5480 ★ Alabama Coalition Against Domestic Violence**
PO Box 4762
Montgomery, AL 36101
**Free:** 800-650-6522
**Website:** http://www.acadv.org

### Alaska

**★ 5481 ★ Alaska Network on Domestic Violence and Sexual Assault**
130 Seward St., Rm. 209
Juneau, AK 99801
**Phone:** (907)586-3650　　　**Fax:** (907)463-4493
**Website:** http://www.andvsa.org

### Arizona

**★ 5482 ★ Arizona Coalition Against Domestic Violence**
100 W Camelback Rd., Ste. 109
Phoenix, AZ 85013
**Phone:** (602)279-2900　　　**Fax:** (602)279-2980
**Email:** acadv@azcadv.org
**Website:** http://www.azacadv.org

### Arkansas

**★ 5483 ★ Arkansas Coalition Against Domestic Violence**
1 Sheriff Ln., Ste. C
North Little Rock, AR 72114
**Phone:** (501)812-0571　　　**Fax:** (501)812-0578
**Email:** ssigmon@arkansas.net

### California

**★ 5484 ★ Coalition to End Domestic and Sexual Violence**
2064 Eastman Ave., Ste. 104
Ventura, CA 93003
**Phone:** (805)654-8141　　　**Free:** 800-300-2181
**Fax:** (805)654-1264
**Website:** http://www.thecoalition.org/index.html
**Crisis Phone(s):** 24-hour hotline: (805) 656-1111.

**★ 5485 ★ Statewide California Coalition for Battered Women**
3711 Long Beach Blvd., Ste. 718
Long Beach, CA 90807
**Phone:** (562)981-1202　　　**Free:** 888-SCCBW-52
**Fax:** (562)981-3202
**Email:** sccbw@sccbw.org
**Website:** http://www.sccbw.org

### Colorado

**★ 5486 ★ Colorado Domestic Violence Coalition**
PO Box 18902
Denver, CO 80218
**Phone:** (303)831-9632　　　**Free:** 888-778-7091
**Fax:** (303)832-7067
**Email:** ccadv@ix.netcom.com
**Website:** http://www.psynet.net/ccadv

### Delaware

**★ 5487 ★ Delaware Coalition Against Domestic Violence**
PO Box 847
Wilmington, DE 19899
**Phone:** (302)658-2958　　　**Fax:** (302)658-5049
**Crisis Phone(s):** 24-hour bilingual line: (888) 522-2571.

### District of Columbia

**★ 5488 ★ District of Columbia Coalition Against Domestic Violence**
513 U St., NW
Washington, DC 20001
**Phone:** (202)783-5332　　　**Fax:** (202)387-5684
**Website:** http://www.dccadv.org

**★ 5489 ★ My Sister's Place**
PO Box 29596
Washington, DC 20017
**Phone:** (202)529-5261
**Crisis Phone(s):** 24-hour hotline: (202) 529-5991.

### Florida

**★ 5490 ★ Florida Coalition Against Domestic Violence**
308 E Park Ave.
Tallahassee, FL 32301
**Phone:** (850)425-2749　　　**Free:** 800-500-1119
**Fax:** (850)425-3091

### Georgia

**★ 5491 ★ Georgia Advocates for Battered Women and Children**
250 Georgia Ave. SE, Ste. 308
Atlanta, GA 30312
**Phone:** (404)524-3847　　　**Free:** 800-334-2836
**Fax:** (404)524-5959

## Hawaii

**★ 5492 ★ Hawaii State Coalition Against Domestic Violence**
716 Umi St., No. 210
Honolulu, HI 96819
**Phone:** (808)832-9316     **Fax:** (808)841-6028
**Email:** hscadv@pixi.com

## Idaho

**★ 5493 ★ Idaho Coalition Against Sexual and Domestic Violence**
815 Park Blvd., Ste. 140
Boise, ID 83712
**Phone:** (208)384-0419     **Free:** 888-293-6118
**Fax:** (208)331-0687
**Email:** domvio@micron.net

## Illinois

**★ 5494 ★ Friends of Battered Women and Their Children**
PO Box 5185
Evanston, IL 60204
**Phone:** (773)274-5232     **Fax:** (773)274-2214
**Email:** info@afriendsplace.org
**Website:** http://www.afriendsplace.org
**Crisis Phone(s):** (800) 603-HELP.

**★ 5495 ★ Illinois Coalition Against Domestic Violence**
801 S 11th St.
Springfield, IL 62703
**Phone:** (217)789-2830     **Fax:** (217)789-1939
**Email:** ilcadv@springnet1.com

**★ 5496 ★ Life Span**
PO Box 445
Des Plaines, IL 60016
**Phone:** (847)824-0382     **Fax:** (847)824-5311
**Email:** life-span@life-span.org
**Website:** http://www.life-span.org
**Crisis Phone(s):** 24-hour line: (847) 824-4454.

## Indiana

**★ 5497 ★ Indiana Coalition Against Domestic Violence**
2511 E 46th St., Ste. 3
Indianapolis, IN 46205
**Phone:** (317)543-3908     **Free:** 800-332-7385
**Fax:** (317)377-7050
**Website:** http://www.violenceresource.org

## Iowa

**★ 5498 ★ Iowa Coalition Against Domestic Violence**
2603 Bell Ave., Ste. 100
Des Moines, IA 50321
**Phone:** (515)244-8028     **Free:** 800-942-0333
**Fax:** (515)244-7417

## Kansas

**★ 5499 ★ Kansas Coalition Against Sexual and Domestic Violence**
820 SE Quincy, Ste. 600
Topeka, KS 66612
**Phone:** (785)232-9784     **Fax:** (785)232-9937
**Crisis Phone(s):** state-wide hotline: (888) END-ABUSE.

## Kentucky

**★ 5500 ★ Kentucky Domestic Violence Association**
PO Box 356
Frankfort, KY 40602
**Phone:** (502)875-4132     **Fax:** (502)875-4268

## Louisiana

**★ 5501 ★ Louisiana Coalition Against Domestic Violence**
PO Box 77308
Baton Rouge, LA 70879-7308
**Phone:** (225)752-1296     **Fax:** (225)751-8927

## Maine

**★ 5502 ★ Maine Coalition to End Domestic Violence**
128 Main St.
Bangor, ME 04401
**Phone:** (207)941-1194     **Fax:** (207)941-2327

## Maryland

**★ 5503 ★ Maryland Network Against Domestic Violence**
6911 Laurel Bowie Rd., Ste. 309
Bowie, MD 20715
**Phone:** (301)352-4574     **Free:** 800-MD-HELPS
**Fax:** (301)809-0422

## Massachusetts

**★ 5504 ★ Massachusetts Coalition Against Sexual Assault and Domestic Violence**
Jane Doe Inc.
14 Beacon St., Ste. 507
Boston, MA 02108
**Phone:** (617)248-0922     **Fax:** (617)248-0902
**Website:** http://www.besafe.org

## Michigan

**★ 5505 ★ Bay County Women's Center**
PO Box 1458
Bay City, MI 48706
**Phone:** (517)686-4551     **Free:** 800-834-2098
**Fax:** (517)686-0906
**Crisis Phone(s):** 24-hour line: (517) 265-6776.

## Minnesota

**★ 5506 ★ Minnesota Coalition for Battered Women**
450 N Syndicate St., Ste. 122
Saint Paul, MN 55104
**Phone:** (651)646-6177     **Fax:** (651)646-1527
**Email:** mcbw@pclink.com
**Website:** http://members.tripod.com/~DAWN-1/MCBW/index.html
**Crisis Phone(s):** (651) 646-0994.

## Mississippi

**★ 5507 ★ Mississippi State Coalition Against Domestic Violence**
PO Box 4703
Jackson, MS 39296-4703
**Phone:** (601)981-9196     **Free:** 800-898-3234
**Fax:** (601)981-2501
**Email:** mcadv@misnet.com

## Missouri

**★ 5508 ★ Missouri Coalition Against Domestic Violence**
415 E McCarty St.
Jefferson City, MO 65101
**Phone:** (573)634-4161     **Fax:** (573)636-3728

**★ 5509 ★ Women's Support and Community Services**
2838 Olive St.
Saint Louis, MO 63103
**Phone:** (314)531-9100
**Crisis Phone(s):** (314) 531-2003.

## Montana

**★ 5510 ★ Crisis Line**
PO Box 6644
Great Falls, MT 59406
**Phone:** (406)453-HELP     **Free:** 888-587-0199

**★ 5511 ★ Montana Coalition Against Domestic and Sexual Violence**
PO Box 633
Helena, MT 59624
**Phone:** (406)443-7794     **Fax:** (406)443-7818
**Website:** http://www.mt.net/~mcadsv

## Nebraska

**★ 5512 ★ Nebraska Domestic Violence and Sexual Assault Coalition**
825 M St., Ste. 404
Lincoln, NE 68508-2253
**Phone:** (402)476-6256     **Free:** 800-876-6238
**Fax:** (402)476-6806
**Website:** http://www.ndvsac.org

## Nevada

**★ 5513 ★ Nevada Network Against Domestic Violence**
100 W Grove, Ste. 315
Reno, NV 89509
**Phone:** (775)828-1115     **Free:** 800-500-1556
**Fax:** (775)828-9991

**★ 5514 ★ SAFE House**
18 Sunrise Dr., Ste. G-70
Henderson, NV 89014
**Phone:** (702)451-4203     **Fax:** (702)451-4302
**Email:** safe@intermind.net

## New Hampshire

**★ 5515 ★ New Hampshire Coalition Against Domestic and Sexual Violence**
PO Box 353
Concord, NH 03302-0353
**Phone:** (603)224-8893     **Free:** 800-852-3388
**Fax:** (603)228-6096
**Website:** http://www.mhcadsv.org
**Crisis Phone(s):** outside of New Hampshire: (603) 225-9000.

## New Jersey

**★ 5516 ★ New Jersey Coalition for Battered Women**
2620 Whitehorse/Hamilton Sq. Rd.
Trenton, NJ 08690
**Phone:** (609)584-8107     **Free:** 800-224-0211
**Fax:** (609)584-9750
**Crisis Phone(s):** For battered lesbians: (800) 224-0211.

★ **5517 ★ Strengthen Our Sisters**
PO Box U
Hewitt, NJ 07421
**Email:** ssisters@warwick.net
**Crisis Phone(s):** 24-hour line: (973) 728-0007.

### New Mexico

★ **5518 ★ New Mexico State Coalition Against Domestic Violence**
PO Box 25266
Albuquerque, NM 87125
**Phone:** (505)246-9240  **Fax:** (505)246-9434
**Email:** nmcadv@nmcadv.org
**Website:** http://www.nmcadv.org/dv/
**Alt. Contact:** Legal helpline: (800) 773-3645.

### New York

★ **5519 ★ New York State Coalition Against Domestic Violence**
79 Central Ave.
Albany, NY 12206
**Phone:** (518)432-4864  **Free:** 800-942-6906
**Fax:** (518)463-3155

### North Carolina

★ **5520 ★ North Carolina Coalition Against Domestic Violence**
115 Market St.
Durham, NC 27701
**Phone:** (919)956-9124  **Fax:** (919)682-1449

### North Dakota

★ **5521 ★ North Dakota Council on Abused Women's Services**
State Networking Office
418 E Rosser Ave., Ste. 320
Bismarck, ND 58501
**Phone:** (701)255-6240  **Free:** 800-472-2911
**Fax:** (701)255-1904
**Website:** http://www.btigate.com/~endabuse

### Ohio

★ **5522 ★ Ohio Domestic Violence Network**
4041 N High St., Ste. 400
Columbus, OH 43214
**Phone:** (614)784-0023  **Free:** 800-934-9840
**Fax:** (614)784-0033
**Website:** http://www.ohiodvnetwork.org

### Oklahoma

★ **5523 ★ Oklahoma Coalition Against Domestic Violence and Sexual Assault**
2525 NW Expressway, Ste. 208
Oklahoma City, OK 73116
**Phone:** (405)848-1815  **Free:** 800-522-9054
**Fax:** (405)848-3469
**Website:** http://www.ocadvsa.org/

### Oregon

★ **5524 ★ Oregon Coalition Against Domestic and Sexual Violence**
520 NW Davis, Ste. 310
Portland, OR 97209
**Phone:** (503)223-7411  **Free:** 800-622-3782
**Fax:** (503)223-7490

### Pennsylvania

★ **5525 ★ Laurel House**
PO Box 764
Norristown, PA 19404
**Fax:** (610)275-4018

**Email:** LaurelHaus@aol.com
**Website:** http://www.libertynet.org/laurelh
**Crisis Phone(s):** (800) 642-3150.

★ **5526 ★ Pennsylvania Coalition Against Domestic Violence**
**National Resource Center on Domestic Violence**
6440 Flank Dr., Ste. 1300
Harrisburg, PA 17112-2778
**Phone:** (717)545-6400  **Free:** 800-932-4632
**Fax:** (717)545-9456

★ **5527 ★ Pennsylvania Coalition Against Rape**
125 N Enola Dr.
Enola, PA 17025
**Phone:** (717)728-9740  **Free:** 800-692-7445
**Fax:** (717)728-9781
**Email:** Stop@pcar.org
**Website:** http://www.pcar.org
**Crisis Phone(s):** (800) 692-7445.

★ **5528 ★ Women's Center of Montgomery County**
101 Washington Ln., Ste. WC-1
Jenkintown, PA 19046
**Website:** http://www.wcmontco.org
**Crisis Phone(s):** 24-hour hotline: (800) 773-2424.

### Rhode Island

★ **5529 ★ Rhode Island Council Against Domestic Violence**
422 Post Rd., Ste. 202
Warwick, RI 02888
**Phone:** (401)467-9940  **Free:** 800-494-8100
**Fax:** (401)467-9943

### South Carolina

★ **5530 ★ South Carolina Coalition Against Domestic Violence and Sexual Assault**
PO Box 7776
Columbia, SC 29202-7776
**Phone:** (803)256-2900  **Free:** 800-260-9293
**Fax:** (803)256-1030

### South Dakota

★ **5531 ★ South Dakota Coalition Against Domestic Violence and Sexual Assault**
PO Box 141
Pierre, SD 57501
**Phone:** (605)945-0869  **Free:** 800-572-9196
**Fax:** (605)945-0870

### Tennessee

★ **5532 ★ Tennessee Task Force Against Domestic Violence**
PO Box 120972
Nashville, TN 37212
**Phone:** (615)386-9406  **Free:** 800-356-6767
**Fax:** (615)383-2967
**Website:** http://www.citysearch.com/nas/ttfadv

### Texas

★ **5533 ★ Families in Crisis, Inc.**
PO Box 25
Killeen, TX 76540
**Phone:** (254)634-1184  **Free:** 888-799-SAFE
**Website:** http://www.familiesincrisis.net

★ **5534 ★ Texas Council on Family Violence**
PO Box 161810
Austin, TX 78716
**Phone:** (512)794-1133  **Free:** 800-525-1978
**Fax:** (512)794-1199
**Website:** http://www.ndvh.org

### Utah

★ **5535 ★ Domestic Violence Advisory Council**
120 North 200 West
Salt Lake City, UT 84103
**Phone:** (801)538-4100  **Free:** 800-897-LINK
**Fax:** (801)538-3993

### Vermont

★ **5536 ★ Vermont Network Against Domestic Violence and Sexual Assault**
PO Box 405
Montpelier, VT 05601
**Phone:** (802)223-1302  **Fax:** (802)223-6943
**Email:** vnadvsa@sover.net
**Website:** http://www.vnadvsa.together.com

### Virginia

★ **5537 ★ Virginians Family Violence and Sexual Assault Hotline**
2850 Sandy Bay Rd., Ste. 101
Williamsburg, VA 23185
**Phone:** (757)221-0990  **Free:** 800-838-VADV
**Fax:** (757)229-1553
**Website:** http://www.rtk.net/vadv/

### Washington

★ **5538 ★ Washington State Coalition Against Domestic Violence**
8645 Martin Way NE, Ste. 103
Lacey, WA 98516
**Phone:** (360)407-0756  **Fax:** (360)407-0761
**Email:** wscadv@cco.net

### West Virginia

★ **5539 ★ West Virginia Coalition Against Domestic Violence**
Elk Office Ctr.
4710 Chimney Dr., Ste. A
Charleston, WV 25302
**Phone:** (304)965-3552  **Fax:** (304)965-3572
**Website:** http://www.wvcadv.org

### Wisconsin

★ **5540 ★ Manitowoc Domestic Violence Center**
PO Box 1142
Manitowoc, WI 54220
**Phone:** (920)684-5770
**Website:** http://www.lakeshorebizdir.com/dvc.htm

★ **5541 ★ Wisconsin Coalition Against Domestic Violence**
1400 E Washington Ave., Ste. 232
Madison, WI 53703
**Phone:** (608)255-0539  **Fax:** (608)255-3560

### Wyoming

★ **5542 ★ Wyoming Coalition Against Domestic Violence and Sexual Assault**
PO Box 236
Laramie, WY 82073
**Phone:** (307)755-5481  **Free:** 800-990-3877
**Fax:** (307)755-5482
**Website:** http://www.bcn.com/wcadvsa

# Chapter 14
# Child Health

## Federal Government Agencies

**★ 5543 ★ U.S. Department of Health and Human Services**
**National Institutes of Health (NIH)**
**National Institute of Child Health and Human Development (NICHD)**
9000 Rockville Pike
Bethesda, MD 20892
**Phone:** (301)496-5133 **Fax:** (301)402-1104
**Website:** http://www.nichd.nih.gov/
Duane F. Alexander, MD, Director
**Desc:** The Institute conducts and supports biomedical and behavioral research on child health and maternal health; sudden infant death syndrome (SIDS); pediatric, maternal, and adolescent AIDS; the reproductive process; problems of human development; mental retardation and developmental disabilities; family structure; and the dynamics of human population.

## Foundations & Other Funding Organizations

### Private Foundations

**★ 5544 ★ Amateur Athletic Foundation of Los Angeles**
c/o Grants Program
2141 West Adams Boulevard
Los Angeles, CA 90018
**Phone:** (323)730-4600 **Fax:** (323)730-9637
**Email:** info@aafla.org
**Website:** http://www.aafla.org
Carmen Zimmerle, Executive Assistant
**Fnded:** 1984. **Philosophy:** The Amateur Athletic Foundation's mission is to promote and enhance youth sports in Southern California and to increase the knowledge of sports and its impact on people's lives. The Foundation grants awards to youth sports organizations within the eight southern most counties of CA and conducts youth sports and coaching education programs. The current objectives of the foundation's board of directors encourage grant making to organizations that provide ongoing, structured youth programs combining the essential elements of teaching, learning, and competition. **Priorities:** *Civic & Public Affairs:* 10%. Major support for a community center. *Environment:* 90%. Funds youth athletic programs and equipment. *Note:* Total contributions made in 2000. **Typ. Recipients:** Children's Health/Hospitals, Clinics/Medical Centers, People with Disabilities. **Geo. Dist:** CA, Imperial County; CA, Los Angeles County; CA, Orange County; CA, Riverside County; CA, San Bernadino County; CA, San Diego County; CA, Santa Barbara County; CA, Ventura County.

**★ 5545 ★ Annie E. Casey Foundation**
701 Saint Paul St.
Baltimore, MD 21202
**Phone:** (410)547-6624 **Fax:** (410)223-2956
**Website:** http://www.aecf.org
Ralph Smith, Vice President
**Fnded:** 1948. **Philosophy:** "The Annie E. Casey Foundation is a private charitable organization dedicated to helping build better futures for disadvantaged children in the United States. The primary mission of the Foundation is to foster public policies, human service reforms, and community supports that more effectively meet the needs of today's vulnerable children and families. In pursuit of this goal, the Foundation makes grants that help states, cities, and neighborhoods fashion more innovative, cost-effective responses to these needs." **Priorities:** *Civic & Public Affairs:* 36%. Focus on Baltimore. *Education:* 6%. Public schools and education reform, emphasis on urban areas. *Environment:* 52%. Supports social services programs and the Casey family services program. *International:* 6%. Health care and mental health. *Note:* Total contributions made in 1999. **Typ. Recipients:** Children's Health/Hospitals, Clinics/Medical Centers, Family Planning, Health Organizations, Health Policy/Cost Containment, Hospitals, Medical Education, Mental Health, Nutrition, People with Disabilities, Prenatal Health Issues, Preventive Medicine/Wellness Organizations, Public Health, Substance Abuse. **Geo. Dist:** nationally.

**Anschutz Family Foundation**
*See:* Entry 46

**Assisi Foundation of Memphis**
*See:* Entry 11687

**★ 5546 ★ Atlantic Foundation of New York**
125 Park Ave., 21st Floor
New York, NY 10017
**Phone:** (212)922-0350 **Fax:** (212)922-0360
**Website:** http://www.anschutzfamilyfoundation.org
Joel Fleishman, Secretary, Treasurer & Director
**Fnded:** 1990. **Priorities:** *Arts & Humanities:* 5%. Gives to libraries and public broadcasting. *Civic & Public Affairs:* 17%. Supports women's affairs, public policy organizations, nonprofit management, law and justice. *Education:* 58%. Supports colleges, universities, medical education, and various education programs. *Environment:* 20%. Supports child welfare, and family and senior services. *Note:* Total contributions made in 2000. **Typ. Recipients:** Adolescent Health Issues. **Geo. Dist:** national.

**Benson and Edith Ford Fund**
*See:* Entry 11368

**The California Endowment**
*See:* Entry 102

**★ 5547 ★ California Wellness Foundation**
6320 Canoga Ave., Ste. 1700
Woodland Hills, CA 91367
**Phone:** (818)593-6600 **Fax:** (818)593-6614
**Email:** phinz@calendow.org
**Website:** http://www.tcwf.org
Gary Yates, President
**Fnded:** 1991. **Typ. Recipients:** Children's Health/Hospitals, Clinics/Medical Centers, Family Planning, Geriatric Health, Health Organizations, Hospitals, Medical Education, Medical Research, Public Health, Trauma Treatment.

**★ 5548 ★ Carnegie Corp. of New York**
437 Madison Ave.
New York, NY 10022
**Phone:** (212)371-3200 **Fax:** (212)753-0395
**Website:** http://www.carnegie.org
Kathleen Whittemore, Secretary
**Fnded:** 1938. **Philosophy:** The corporation's charter states that funds are to be used to promote "the advancement and diffusion of knowledge and understanding among the people of the United States." Its Charter was later amended to permit the use of funds for the same purposes in certain countries that are or were members of the British overseas Commonwealth. The corporation makes grants into the following program areas: education, international peace and security, international development, and democracy. A major goal of the education program's goal is rebuild the public confidence in education. To accomplish this goal the corporation will focus on early childhood education, urban school reform, and higher education. The International Peace and Security program builds on previous activities of the Corporation. The program will have three major focuses: non-proliferation of weapons, Russia and other Post Soviet States, and New Dimensions of Security. The International Development program will not accept unsolicited proposals until after October 1999. The following themes define the Program: strengthening African universities, enhancing women's opportunities in higher education and revitalizing public libraries. The corporation has devoted grants to improving the effectiveness of government, increasing public understanding of social issues, and encouraging active participation. **Priorities:** *Arts & Humanities:* 6%. Public Broadcasting Service. *Civic & Public Affairs:* 15%. Supports public policy and human rights programs; libraries. *Education:* 29%. Program development and improvement and science education. *Environment:* 22%. Supports national youth and adolescent programs. *Note:* Total contributions made in fiscal 1999. **Typ. Recipients:** Adolescent Health Issues, Child Abuse, Children's Health/Hospitals, Clinics/Medical Centers, Family Planning, Health Organizations, Health Policy/Cost Containment, Medical Education, Medical Research, Mental Health, Prenatal Health Issues, Public Health, Substance Abuse. **Geo. Dist:** internationally, especially to countries that are or have been members of the British commonwealth.

**Carrie Estelle Doheny Foundation**
*See:* Entry 108

## ★ 5549 ★ Charles H. Hood Foundation, Inc.

95 Berkeley St., Rm. 201
Boston, MA 02116
**Phone:** (617)695-9439　　**Fax:** (617)423-4619
**Email:** doheny@dohenyfoundation.org
**Website:** http://www.dohenyfoundation.org
Raymond Considine, Secretary & Executive Director
**Fnded:** 1942. **Philosophy:** "The Charles H. Hood Foundation is interested in supporting projects concerned with child health in New England. Emphasis is on the initiation and furtherance of medical research which will help to diminish health problems affecting large numbers of children. The Foundation funds productive research efforts undertaken by junior faculty in medically oriented tax exempt institutions in the six New England states. It undertakes no research on its own. The intent of the award is to support initial independent investigations, provide the opportunity to demonstrate creativity, and assist in the transition to other sources of research funding." *Charles H. Hood Foundation Application Guidelines* **Priorities:** *International:* 100%. Support given to hospitals and medical centers. *Note:* Total contributions made in 2000. **Typ. Recipients:** Adolescent Health Issues, Cancer, Children's Health/Hospitals, Clinics/Medical Centers, Diabetes, Eyes/Blindness, Hospitals, Hospitals (University Affiliated), Medical Research, Medical Training, Nutrition, Prenatal Health Issues, Public Health. **Geo. Dist:** CT; ME; MA; NH; RI; VT.

## Conrad N. Hilton Foundation
*See:* Entry 144

## David, Helen, and Marian Woodward Fund-Atlanta
*See:* Entry 11378

## ★ 5550 ★ David and Lucile Packard Foundation

300 Second St., Ste. 200
Los Altos, CA 94022
**Phone:** (650)948-7658　　**Fax:** (650)948-5793
**Email:** cnhf@hiltonfoundation.org
**Website:** http://www.packfound.org
Richard Schlosberg, III, President, Chief Executive Officer
**Fnded:** 1964. **Philosophy:** The foundation makes grants in the following categories: science; conservation; population; children, arts; and community and special areas that include organizational effectiveness and philanthropy. Current initiatives include childcare center technology and health-care access, quality, and insurance for low-income children; land, marine, and energy conservation will also receive support. **Priorities:** *Arts & Humanities:* 3%. Focus on cultural facilities and arts education. *Civic & Public Affairs:* 15%. Primarily to organizations concerned with population issues, reproductive rights, and family planning. *Environment:* 17%. Supports the Center for the Future of Children program and community programs. *Religion:* 17%. Supports ocean science, fellowships for science and engineering, historically black colleges and universities, and tribal scholars. *Note:* Total contributions made in 1998. **Typ. Recipients:** Children's Health/Hospitals, Clinics/Medical Centers, Emergency/Ambulance Services, Family Planning, Health Organizations, Health Policy/Cost Containment, Heart, Hospitals, Long-Term Care, Medical Education, Medical Research, Nursing Services, Nutrition, People with Disabilities, Prenatal Health Issues, Preventive Medicine/Wellness Organizations, Public Health, Research/Studies Institutes. **Geo. Dist:** internationally; nationally; CA; Monterey County; CA, San Mateo County; CA, Santa Clara County; CA, Santa Cruz County.

## Duke Endowment
*See:* Entry 183

## Dyson Foundation
*See:* Entry 186

## E. J. Grassmann Trust
*See:* Entry 11382

## ★ 5551 ★ E. K. and Lillian F. Bishop Foundation

c/o Bank of America, Trustee
701 5th Ave., Floor 47
Seattle, WA 98104
**Phone:** (206)749-2004　　**Fax:** (206)749-2990
**Email:** thomas.nevers@azbar.org
**Website:** http://www.dyson.org
Tom Nevers, Grants Manager
**Fnded:** 1971. **Philosophy:** "The E.K. and Lillian F. Bishop Foundation promotes the welfare of young people through grants to qualified organizations. The Foundation supports a wide range of charitable, cultural, educational and recreational programs. Inspirational experiences such as opportunities to explore the arts, to participate in sports and in wholesome group activities are considered to be of special importance. Some of the projects supported by the Foundation include a youth employment center, community cultural and athletic events, special medical equipment and treatment centers for young people. The Awards Committee looks for projects that focus on prevention of problems and those that seek innovative solutions to youth-oriented problems. Enlisting community support for a project is also encouraged." *Foundation Guidelines.* **Priorities:** *Arts & Humanities:* 4%. Funds cultural enrichment programs. *Civic & Public Affairs:* 12%. Supports employment assistance, city government, and fire departments. *Education:* 8%. Supports educational programs, colleges and universities. *Environment:* 70%. Funds social service organizations, youth activities, and athletics. *International:* 4%. Gives to hospitals and clinics. *Note:* Total contributions made in fiscal 2000. **Typ. Recipients:** Children's Health/Hospitals, Clinics/Medical Centers, Domestic Violence, Emergency/Ambulance Services, Eyes/Blindness, Family Planning, Health Funds, Heart, Hospitals, Medical Research, Nursing Services, Research/Studies Institutes, Single-Disease Health Associations, Substance Abuse, Trauma Treatment. **Geo. Dist:** WA; WA, Grays Harbor County.

## E. L. Wiegand Foundation
*See:* Entry 188

## Edna McConnell Clark Foundation
*See:* Entry 196

## Elizabeth Morse Genius Charitable Trust
*See:* Entry 10043

## F. R. Bigelow Foundation
*See:* Entry 233

## Flinn Foundation
*See:* Entry 241

## Florence V. Burden Foundation
*See:* Entry 243

## Ford Family Foundation
*See:* Entry 246

## Forrest C. Lattner Foundation
*See:* Entry 250

## ★ 5552 ★ Foundation for Child Development

145 East 32nd St.
14th Floor
New York, NY 10016-6055
**Phone:** (212)213-8337　　**Fax:** (212)213-5897
**Email:** info@flinn.org
**Website:** http://www.ffcd.org
Claudia Conner, Grants Associate
**Fnded:** 1900. **Philosophy:** The foundation is "dedicated to the principle that all families should have the social and material resources to raise their children to be healthy, educated, and productive members of their communities. The Foundation seeks to understand children, particularly the disadvantaged, and to promote their well-being. We believe that families, schools, nonprofit organizations, businesses, and government at all levels share complementary responsibilities in the critical task of raising new generations. "Seeking to achieve its goals, the Foundation supports: basic and policy-relevant research about the factors that promote and support the optimal development of children and adolescents; policy analysis, advocacy, services, and public education to enhance the discussion and adoption of social policies that support families in their important child-raising responsibilities; leadership development activities linked to the programmatic focus of the foundation. "The Foundation believes that by integrating these approaches, FCD will strengthen its effectiveness in achieving its mission." *Foundation Mission Statement* **Priorities:** *Arts & Humanities:* 7% Supports museum, film and video, and public broadcasting. *Civic & Public Affairs:* 31%. Supports public policy, philanthropic organizations, economic policy, urban and rural affairs. *Education:* 24%. Supports social science education, leadership training, preschool education, colleges and universities, and technical education. *Environment:* 15%. Supports day care, family services, and child welfare. *International:* 17%. Funds childrens health, and nutrition, and medical rehabilitation. *Religion:* 1%. Supports scientific centers and institution and scientific organizations. *Note:* Total contributions made in fiscal 1999. **Typ. Recipients:** Child Abuse, Children's Health/Hospitals, Domestic Violence, Family Planning, Geriatric Health, Health Funds, Hospitals, Medical Education, Medical Rehabilitation, Medical Research, Mental Health, Nutrition, People with Disabilities, Public Health, Research/Studies Institutes. **Geo. Dist:** nationally.

## ★ 5553 ★ Foundation for Seacoast Health

PO Box 4606
Portsmouth, NH 03802-4606
**Phone:** (603)433-3008　　**Fax:** (603)433-2036
**Email:** ffsh@nh.ultranet.com
**Website:** http://www.nh.ultranet.com/~ffsh
Susan Bunting, President
**Fnded:** 1984. **Philosophy:** The Foundation for Seacoast Health supports Seacoast area nonprofit organizations and scholarships for students pursuing health-related fields of study. The foundation has recently shifted in hopes of "narrowing the funding focus and concentrating on fewer, more comprehensive programs, assisting the most successful foundation-funded programs in becoming financially independent; concentrating resources on improving health care delivery systems, rather than on particular services; and focusing on prevention rather than intervention through a gradual shift in funding from the elderly and adolescent populations to the earlier childhood years, focusing on the child's health in relation to the family unit." Although the foundation has concentrated on health care for the elderly and adolescents in the past, it feels that as a whole, health care funding should begin supporting programs aimed at young children in order to encourage a healthier population for the future. "The Foundation for Seacoast Health will continue to focus its resources on programs which have a prevention orientation and which address the systemic issues of health care access and utilization. Believing that the future of our community rests with our children, our top priority will be programs which promote the health of infants, children, and adolescents." *Annual Report* **Priorities:** *Civic & Public Affairs:* 6%. *Education:* 8%. For health-related scholarships. *Environment:* 34%. Supports Families First and community child care centers. *International:* 52%. Supports health-related initatives through major grants programs, including the infant/child/adolescent program, the health promotion program, the women's health initiative, medical financial assistance, and the discretionary fund. *Note:* Total contributions made in 1998. **Typ. Recipients:** Adolescent Health Issues,

AIDS/HIV, Cancer, Children's Health/Hospitals, Clinics/Medical Centers, Diabetes, Domestic Violence, Emergency/Ambulance Services, Family Planning, Geriatric Health, Health Funds, Health Organizations, Health Policy/Cost Containment, Health-General, Home-Care Services, Hospices, Hospitals, Medical Rehabilitation, Mental Health, Nursing Services, People with Disabilities, Prenatal Health Issues, Preventive Medicine/Wellness Organizations, Public Health, Sexual Abuse, Single-Disease Health Associations, Substance Abuse, Trauma Treatment. **Geo. Dist:** Eliot, ME; Kittery, ME; York, ME; Greenland, NH; New Castle, NH; Newington, NH; North Hampton, NH; Portsmouth, NH; Rye, NH.


**The Frances L. and Edwin L. Cummings Memorial Fund**
*See:* Entry 254


**★ 5554 ★ Frederick P. and Sandra P. Rose Foundation**
200 Madison Ave., 5th Floor
New York, NY 10016
**Phone:** (212)210-6666
Sandra Rose, President & Director

**Fnded:** 1982. **Priorities:** *Arts & Humanities:* 27%. Funds libraries, art museums, and the performing arts. *Civic & Public Affairs:* 3%. Supports voters organizations, community parks, and public safety forces. *Education:* 10%. Gives to colleges, universities, and music education. *Environment:* Less than 1%. *International:* Less than 1%. *Religion:* 42%. Provides major support to the American Museum of Natural History. *Note:* Total contributions made in fiscal 2000. **Typ. Recipients:** Children's Health/Hospitals, Clinics/Medical Centers, Health Organizations, People with Disabilities. **Geo. Dist:** NY.


**★ 5555 ★ The Hall Family Foundation**
PO Box 419580
Mail Drop 323
Kansas City, MO 64141-6580
**Phone:** (816)274-8516          **Fax:** (816)274-8547
William Hall, President

**Fnded:** 1993. **Philosophy:** "The Hall Family Foundation is a private philanthropic organization dedicated to enhancing the quality of human life. Programs that enrich the community, help people and promote excellence are considered to be of prime importance. The Foundation views its critical function as that of a catalyst. It seeks to be responsive to programs that are innovative, yet strive to create permanent solutions to community needs in the greater Kansas City area." "The Hall Family Foundation concentrates its philanthropic efforts on five areas of interest in the greater Kansas City area:" "Education: In a continuing tradition of concern for youth, the Foundation has an interest in programs that enhance or promote excellence in elementary, secondary and higher education. Programs which address the educational needs of urban school children, and efforts and initiatives targeting systemic educational reform are a high priority." "Children, Youth and Families: The Foundation has a strong interest in improving the lives of children, youth and families. The Foundation values programs which help prevent family violence, improve child well-being, expand youth services and respond to families' physical and emotional health needs." "The Arts: The Foundation considers programs which encourage excellence in the community's major performing and visual arts organizations. The Foundation is interested in programs that enhance quality, strengthen management, broaden existing funding bases and increase audience development." "Community Development: The Foundation is interested in programs and initiatives which help prevent or overcome blight and deterioration of the central city and its neighborhoods. Redevelopment projects which help to stabilize these areas are a high priority." "Additional Interests: Included in this category is Foundation support of community-wide efforts that seek to provide long-term solutions to local issues of high priority." 1997 Guidelines and Procedures for Grant Applicants **Priorities:** *Arts & Humanities:* 44%.Supports perform-

ing arts, art centers, and museums. *Civic & Public Affairs:* 10%. Supports community development initiatives. *Education:* 13%. Supports education centers, colleges and universities, and provides scholarships. *Environment:* 9%. Funds children, youth and family services. *International:* 5%. *Religion:* 10%. *Note:* Five-year summary of contributions supplied by foundation. **Typ. Recipients:** Child Health, Children's Health/Hospitals, Clinics/Medical Centers, Domestic Violence, Health Organizations, Home-Care Services, Hospitals, Hospitals (University Affiliated), Medical Rehabilitation, Mental Health, Public Health, Sexual Abuse, Substance Abuse. **Geo. Dist:** Kansas City, MO, metropolitan area.


**Harris and Eliza Kempner Fund**
*See:* Entry 320


**★ 5556 ★ Heckscher Foundation for Children**
17 East 47th St.
New York, NY 10017
**Phone:** (212)371-7775          **Fax:** (212)371-7787
Virginia Sloane, President

**Fnded:** 1921. **Philosophy:** The foundation promotes the health and general welfare of children and makes grants in a number of different areas within this framework. The general welfare of children is interpreted broadly to include child care, recreation, and exposure of children to the arts. Needy and orphaned children are a special concern of the foundation, evidenced by support for adoption services, children's homes, distribution of clothing and other essentials for needy children, and the provision of gifts at Christmas. **Priorities:** *Arts & Humanities:* 21%. Supports music, ballet, historic preservation, dance, theater, children's museum. *Civic & Public Affairs:* 19%. Supports botanical gardens/parks, safety, community foundation, women's affairs, and inner-city development. *Education:* 10%. Supports colleges, pre-school education, scholarship, arts school. *Environment:* 31%. Supports homes, shelter/homeless, youth organizations, community center, camps, Young Women's Christian Association, Young Men's Christian Association, and family planning services. *International:* 5%. Supports hospital and children's health. *Note:* Total contributions made in 1998. **Typ. Recipients:** Adolescent Health Issues, AIDS/HIV, Cancer, Children's Health/Hospitals, Clinics/Medical Centers, Emergency/Ambulance Services, Family Planning, Health Organizations, Hospitals, Medical Education, Medical Rehabilitation, Medical Research, Mental Health, Nursing Services, People with Disabilities, Preventive Medicine/Wellness Organizations, Single-Disease Health Associations, Speech & Hearing, Substance Abuse, Transplant Networks/Donor Banks. **Geo. Dist:** New York, NY.


**Jack N. and Lilyan Mandel Foundation**
*See:* Entry 8539


**John R. McCune Charitable Trust**
*See:* Entry 11400


**Joseph B. Whitehead Foundation**
*See:* Entry 436


**★ 5557 ★ Lee and Ramona Bass Foundation**
309 Main St.
Fort Worth, TX 76102
**Phone:** (817)336-0494          **Fax:** (817)332-2176
**Email:** fdns@woodruff.org
**Website:** http://www.sidrichardson.org/lrbf.htm
Valleau Wilkie, Jr., Executive Director

**Fnded:** 1993. **Philosophy:** The foundation typically considers funding in the following areas: schools, colleges, and universities within Texas, with emphasis placed upon faculty development and liberal arts programs; community programs and projects, particularly related to the arts and the environment, such as

museums, zoos, and educational/research institutions; and national and regional conservation programs. **Priorities:** *Arts & Humanities:* 4%. *Civic & Public Affairs:* 19%. Supports zoos. *Education:* 43%. Major suppport for All Saints Episcopal School in Fort Worth, Texas. *Note:* Total contributions made in 1998. **Typ. Recipients:** Children's Health/Hospitals, Medical Research. **Geo. Dist:** no restrictions.


**Louise H. and David S. Ingalls Foundation**
*See:* Entry 482


**Louise Manoogian Simone Foundation**
*See:* Entry 483


**Mars Foundation**
*See:* Entry 507


**★ 5558 ★ Marshall L. and Perrine D. McCune Charitable Foundation**
345 E Alameda St.
Santa Fe, NM 87501-2229
**Phone:** (505)983-8300          **Fax:** (505)983-7887
**Email:** fsowers@swcp.com
**Website:** http://www.nmmccune.org
Frances Sowers, Associate Director

**Fnded:** 1988. **Typ. Recipients:** AIDS/HIV, Children's Health/Hospitals, Clinics/Medical Centers, Diabetes, Hospices, Hospitals, Nursing Services, Prenatal Health Issues, Preventive Medicine/Wellness Organizations, Public Health, Sexual Abuse. **Geo. Dist:** NM.


**Mary Ranken Jordan and Ettie A. Jordan Charitable Foundation**
*See:* Entry 514


**★ 5559 ★ Mary Reynolds Babcock Foundation**
2522 Reynolda Rd.
Winston-Salem, NC 27106-5123
**Phone:** (336)748-9222          **Fax:** (336)777-0095
**Email:** info@mrbf.org
**Website:** http://www.mrbf.org
Gayle Williams, Executive Director

**Fnded:** 1953. **Philosophy:** The Babcock Foundation concentrates on assisting people in the South to build communities that nurture people, encourage enterprise, bridge differences, foster fairness, and promote civility. The foundation places special emphasis on strategies that increase communities' commitment, sense of responsibility, and capacity toward three ends: assuring the well-being of children, youth, and families; bridging the faultlines of race and class; and protecting and investing in human and natural resources for the long term. "In particular, we seek to have impact in areas where poverty prevails or race divides." The foundation will invest in organizations, individuals, and communities through three grantmaking programs: Organizational Development Program, for 75-100 local, statewide, and regional organizations over five years; Community Problem Solving, a program of intensive work with coalitions of organizations in 10-15 communities in the Southeast; and Grassroots Leadership Development. **Priorities:** *Arts & Humanities:* 17%. Supports historic preservation. *Civic & Public Affairs:* 69%. Primary support for economic development, nonprofit management, urban and community affairs, housing, employment and job training women's affairs and philanthropic. *Education:* 3%. Focus on education reform, colleges and universities, public education, and literacy. *Environment:* 6%. Supports community services, youth and family services, food banks and emergency relief. *International:* 1%. *Note:* Total contributions made in 2000. **Typ. Recipients:** Emergency/Ambulance Services, Family Planning, Health Organizations, Hospitals, Nutrition. **Geo. Dist:** Southeastern United States.

## ★ 5560 ★ Mary Stuart Rogers Foundation
Care of Stockton & Sadler
PO Box 3153
Modesto, CA 95353
**Phone:** (626)523-6416          **Fax:** (626)523-2315
**Email:** msroger1@pacebell.net

**Fnded:** 1985. **Priorities:** *Education:* 60%. Funds colleges, universities, schools, and religious education. *Environment:* 3%. Funds family services. *International:* 3%. Supports children's health. *Note:* Total contributions made in 2000. **Typ. Recipients:** Cancer, Children's Health/Hospitals, Diabetes, Domestic Violence, Eyes/Blindness, Health Organizations, Heart, Hospitals, Medical Research, People with Disabilities, Public Health, Single-Disease Health Associations. **Geo. Dist:** CA.

## Max Factor Family Foundation
*See:* Entry 2891

## ★ 5561 ★ Monterey Fund
c/o Bear, Stearns & Co.
1 Metrotech Center N, 9th Fl.
Brooklyn, NY 11201
**Phone:** (347)643-4590
Gilbert Sherman, Contact

**Fnded:** 1967. **Typ. Recipients:** Cancer, Children's Health/Hospitals, Clinics/Medical Centers, Hospitals, Medical Education, People with Disabilities, Prenatal Health Issues, Public Health, Single-Disease Health Associations. **Geo. Dist:** New York, NY, metropolitan area.

## Nathan Cummings Foundation
*See:* Entry 18215

## Oberkotter Foundation
*See:* Entry 13857

## Robert Stewart and Helen Pfeiffer Odell Fund
*See:* Entry 632

## Sabbah Family Foundation
*See:* Entry 10053

## ★ 5562 ★ St. Giles Foundation
420 Lexington Ave., Ste. 32329
New York, NY 10170
**Phone:** (212)338-9001
**Email:** George_Nofer@SHSL.com
**Website:** http://www.ncf.org
Richard Arkwright, President

**Fnded:** 1979. **Philosophy:** The St. Giles Foundation has a special interest in medical science. It also funds hospitals and child services. **Priorities:** *Education:* 5%. Special education and student aid. *International:* 63%. Mainly supporting children's health, hospitals, and medical research. *Religion:* 32%. Funds medical sciences. *Note:* Contributions made in fiscal 1999. **Typ. Recipients:** AIDS/HIV, Cancer, Children's Health/Hospitals, Clinics/Medical Centers, Health-General, Hospitals, Medical Education, Medical Rehabilitation, Medical Research, Mental Health, People with Disabilities, Prenatal Health Issues. **Geo. Dist:** NY.

## Sidney J. Weinberg, Jr. Foundation
*See:* Entry 11413

## Skillman Foundation
*See:* Entry 683

## Statler Foundation
*See:* Entry 11415

## Strauss Foundation
*See:* Entry 708

## ★ 5563 ★ Taconic Foundation
60 Wall St., 46th Fl.
New York, NY 10260-0060
**Phone:** (212)648-9673          **Fax:** (212)648-5082
**Email:** reginald.middleton@firstunion.com
**Website:** http://www.skillman.org
Hildy Simmons, Managing Director

**Fnded:** 1958. **Philosophy:** The foundation continues the Curriers' commitment to equal opportunity. Currently, it emphasizes programs related to housing opportunity, youth employment, economic development, and youth. The foundation's interests in housing and associated aspects of land use stem from Stephen Currier, who organized Urban America just three years before he died. He created this organization from the remnants of the old American Planning and Civic Association and the American Council to Improve Our Neighborhoods. Urban America merged with the Urban Coalition in the spring of 1970 to become the National Urban Coalition. Urban Coalition. **Priorities:** *Civic & Public Affairs:* 64%. Funds civic and community organizations focusing on housing opportunities, economic development and housing services. *Education:* 15%. Supports after-school education, education funds. *Environment:* 19%. Supports youth programs and services. *Note:* Total contributions made in 1999. **Typ. Recipients:** Children's Health/Hospitals, Family Planning. **Geo. Dist:** nationally; New York, NY.

## Thomas and Agnes Carvel Foundation
*See:* Entry 722

## ★ 5564 ★ Thomas J. Watson Foundation
293 South Main St.
Providence, RI 02903
**Phone:** (401)274-1952          **Fax:** (401)274-1954
**Email:** WatsonFoundation@Brown.edu
**Website:** http://www.WatsonFellowship.org
Norv Brasch, Executive Director

**Fnded:** 1961. **Philosophy:** In 1968, in recognition of Mr. and Mrs. Watson's interests in education and world affairs, their children decided that a fellowship program should constitute the major activity of the foundation. The Watson Fellowship Program, administered in cooperation with 49 private colleges and universities throughout the United States, enables outstanding college graduates to engage in a year of independent study and travel abroad following graduation. **Priorities:** *Arts & Humanities:* 5%. Funds museums and literary associations. *Education:* 3% Supports religious school and the Watson Fellowship Program. *International:* 2%. Funds AIDS coalition. *Note:* Total contributions made in fiscal 1998. **Typ. Recipients:** AIDS/HIV, Children's Health/Hospitals. **Geo. Dist:** nationally.

## Turner Foundation
*See:* Entry 733

## ★ 5565 ★ Turrell Fund
21 Van Vleck St.
Montclair, NJ 07042-2358
**Phone:** (973)783-9358          **Fax:** (973)783-9283
**Email:** turrell@bellatlantic.net
**Website:** http://www.fdncenter.org/grantmaker/turrell
Dr. E. Williams, Executive Director & Secretary

**Fnded:** 1935. **Philosophy:** The Turrell Fund's principal interest is supporting organizations that help youth, with emphasis on needy youngsters. "Our purpose is to support activities that will contribute to the development of young persons from families which could not afford these services without help." These activities may be educational, vocational, recreational, and corrective; or they may be programs to provide care for the child. Programs to make such activities available to handicapped children are also eligible. Primary consideration is given to children age twelve or younger. The fund makes grants in the following

program areas: Educational Programs, with emphasis on day care centers, day nurseries, elementary and intermediate schools, libraries, and museums; Social Support Services, with emphasis on children's aid and adoption services, community centers, family centers, neighborhood youth centers, and neighborhood organizations; Youth Activities, with emphasis on boys and girls clubs, boys and girls scouts, camps, and YM-YWCAs. **Priorities:** *Arts & Humanities:* 1%. Supports arts programs. *Civic & Public Affairs:* 5%. Supports foundations and councils. *Education:* 38%. Primary support for elementary and secondary education. *Environment:* 45%. Supports youth organizations, child welfare, adoption services, community centers, family services, day care centers, and neighborhood organizations. *International:* 9%. Funds single disease health associations. *Note:* Total contributions made in 1998. **Typ. Recipients:** Adolescent Health Issues, AIDS/HIV, Children's Health/Hospitals, Clinics/Medical Centers, Family Planning, Hospitals, Medical Education, Medical Rehabilitation, People with Disabilities, Preventive Medicine/Wellness Organizations, Research/Studies Institutes, Substance Abuse. **Geo. Dist:** NJ, Essex County; NJ, Hudson County; NJ, Passaic County; NJ, Union County; VT.

## Valley Foundation
*See:* Entry 734

## Van Houten Memorial Fund (Edward W. and Stella C.)
*See:* Entry 735

## ★ 5566 ★ Victoria Foundation
40 South Fullerton Ave.
Montclair, NJ 07042
**Phone:** (973)783-4450          **Fax:** (973)783-6664
**Email:** catherinemcfarland@victoriafoundation.org
**Website:** http://www.valley.org
Catherine McFarland, Secretary & Executive Officer

**Fnded:** 1924. **Philosophy:** "At its 75th anniversary, the foundation's desire to help individuals in need reach their potential remains its core value. Whether providing emergency coal for needy families, treating rheumatic fever in children or helping Newark, NJ, become a shining City on the Hill, Victoria has worked to create greater access and opportunities for people and to improve the quality of life in the communities in which they live. Today, the foundation's efforts center on educational, urban development, and youth and family initiatives predominantly in Newark, NJ, as well as pressing environmental issues throughout the state. The foundation has grown from granting $2,000 in 1924 to approving more than $11 million in grants during 1999." 1999 Annual Report **Priorities:** *Arts & Humanities:* 10%. supports performing art center, public broadcasting, orchestra. *Civic & Public Affairs:* 27%. Supports libraries, public policy organizations, parks, job training, community foundations and housing initiatives. *Environment:* 13%. Supports food banks, family planning, scouting, community centers, YWCA. *Note:* Total contributions made in 1999. **Typ. Recipients:** Children's Health/Hospitals, Clinics/Medical Centers, Family Planning, Medical Education, People with Disabilities, Research/Studies Institutes, Substance Abuse. **Geo. Dist:** Newark, NJ.

## Vira I. Heinz Endowment
*See:* Entry 737

## ★ 5567 ★ William T. Grant Foundation
570 Lexington, 18th Floor
New York, NY 10022-6837
**Phone:** (212)752-0071          **Fax:** (212)752-1398
**Email:** info@wtgrantfdn.org
**Website:** http://fdncenter.org/grantmaker/wtgrant/
Nancy Rivera, Contact

**Fnded:** 1936. **Philosophy:** "The William T. Grant Foundation's mission is to support research studies relevant to the healthy psychological and social development of children and youth. It pursues this goal primarily through its Major Grants program by supporting of research in medical or social-behavioral scientific disciplines. Major Grants are awarded for basic research, program evaluations, policy analyses, communications research/dissemination projects; and capacity building activities. The Foundation supports a variety of studies whose goals are to understand and prevent some of the major problems of children and youth, to facilitate successful child and adolescent development, and to assure optimal preparation for the transition to adulthood. The Foundation is especially interested in interdisciplinary research." "Additionally, through the Youth Service Grants program, a limited number of relatively small one-time grants are made annually in support of small-scale research, training or service projects within the program interests of the Foundation. Preference for the service programs is given to projects that adopt a comprehensive approach to serving the youth of the New York Metropolitan area." **Priorities:** *Education:* (Faculty Scholars Program) 13%. Supports promising post-doctoral scholars from different disciplines, whose research deepens and broadens the knowledge base in areas that contribute to the foundation's mission. *Environment:* (Youth Service Grants) 5%. Supports programs that actively engage young people in the New York Tri-state area, and enable them to reach their full potential. *Note:* Total contributions made in 2000. **Typ. Recipients:** Adolescent Health Issues, AIDS/HIV, Cancer, Child Abuse, Children's Health/Hospitals, Clinics/Medical Centers, Family Planning, Hospitals, Medical Education, Medical Research, Mental Health, Prenatal Health Issues, Research/Studies Institutes, Respiratory. **Geo. Dist:** internationally, for major grants; nationally, for major grants; CT, youth services grants; NJ, youth services grants; NY, youth services grants.

## Corporate Foundations

**★ 5568 ★ Ace Hardware Foundation**
2200 Kensington Court
Oak Brook, IL 60523-2100
**Phone:** (630)990-6444          **Fax:** (630)990-1742
**Email:** pthom@memo.acehardware.com
**Website:** http://www.acehardware.com/about/community/community.asp
Paula Erickson, Manager, Corporate Communication and Pub

**Priorities:** *International:* 100%. Corporate sponsorship includes funding to The Children's Miracle Network. Through the foundation, funding is given to The American Red Cross. **Typ. Recipients:** Children's Health/Hospitals, Emergency/Ambulance Services. **Geo. Dist:** nationally.

**Aetna Foundation**
*See:* Entry 801

**Alabama Power Foundation**
*See:* Entry 808

**Ameren Corp. Charitable Trust**
*See:* Entry 821

**American Snuff Co. Charitable Trust**
*See:* Entry 827

**Amon G. Carter Star Telegram Employees Fund**
*See:* Entry 834

**★ 5569 ★ AOL Time Warner Foundation**
75 Rockefeller Plaza, 4th Floor
New York, NY 10019
**Phone:** (212)484-8720
**Email:** aoltwfoundation@aol.com
**Website:** http://aoltwfoundation.org
Kirsten Powers, Contact

**Priorities:** *Civic & Public Affairs:* 24%. Primary support for community affairs. *Education:* 64%. Supports

primary and secondary education, education associations, and special education. *Environment:* 3%. Supports social welfare groups, the elderly, and youth organizations. *International:* 7%. Funds single-disease health associations. *Religion:* 1%. Supports a science museum. *Note:* Total contributions made in 1999. **Typ. Recipients:** Cancer, Children's Health/Hospitals, Health Organizations, Health-General, Medical Education, People with Disabilities, Public Health. **AKA:** AOL Foundation. **Geo. Dist:** nationally. **Frmly:** Time Warner Foundation.

**ARCO Foundation**
*See:* Entry 846

**★ 5570 ★ Avery Dennison Foundation**
150 North Orange Grove Boulevard
Pasadena, CA 91103
**Phone:** (626)304-2000          **Fax:** (626)577-9587
Joyce Reid, Director, Corporate Programs

**Priorities:** *Arts & Humanities:* 33%. Supports museums and performing arts centers. *Education:* 56%. Supports educational funds and foundations. *Environment:* 4%. Funds Boy Scouts. *Note:* Total foundation giving in 2000. **Typ. Recipients:** Children's Health/Hospitals, Health-General. **Geo. Dist:** headquarters and operating communities.

**Bandai Foundation**
*See:* Entry 11694

**Barclays Capital**
*See:* Entry 871

**Binney & Smith Inc.**
*See:* Entry 887

**Boler Co. Foundation**
*See:* Entry 10061

**Burlington Resources Foundation**
*See:* Entry 11424

**Caring Foundation**
*See:* Entry 917

**Chicago Sun-Times Charity Trust**
*See:* Entry 936

**CIGNA Foundation**
*See:* Entry 940

**Citizens Bank-Flint**
*See:* Entry 945

**Comdisco Foundation**
*See:* Entry 956

**Copolymer Foundation**
*See:* Entry 13520

**★ 5571 ★ Crown Books Foundation**
1899 L St. NW, 9th Floor
Washington, DC 20036
**Phone:** (202)293-4500
**Email:** deborah.veney-robinson@cigna.com
**Website:** http://www.cbclientsfirst.com
Elliot Arditti, Contact

**Fnded:** 1988. **Priorities:** *Arts & Humanities:* 9%. Supports public broadcasting. *Civic & Public Affairs:* 19%. Supports employment/job training. *Education:* 51%. Supports faculty development, literacy, scholarship, and universities. *Environment:* 2%. Supports youth programs, community service organizations,

and child welfare. *International:* 10%. Supports AIDS and single-disease health association. *Note:* Total contributions made in 1997. **Typ. Recipients:** AIDS/HIV, Cancer, Child Abuse, Children's Health/Hospitals, Health-General, Heart, Hospitals, Kidney, Medical Education, Medical Research, People with Disabilities, Single-Disease Health Associations. **Geo. Dist:** nationally.

**CSR America Companies Foundation**
*See:* Entry 10063

**D.B. Reinhart Family Foundation**
*See:* Entry 985

**Ecolab Foundation**
*See:* Entry 8548

**Equitable Resources, Inc.**
*See:* Entry 1030

**F.K. Bemis Family Foundation**
*See:* Entry 1036

**★ 5572 ★ Franklin Electric, Edward J. Schaefer, and T. W. Kehoe Charitable and Educational Foundation**
400 E Spring St.
Bluffton, IN 46714
**Phone:** (219)824-2900          **Fax:** (219)827-5530
**Email:** corp@BemisMfg.com
**Website:** http://www.eqt.com/about_EQT/Community.asp
Gary Merritt, Finance Manager

**Priorities:** *Arts & Humanities:* 2%. Funds arts councils and museums. *Civic & Public Affairs:* 16%. Supports a park, chamber of commerce, and festivals. *Education:* 2%. Provides scholarships. *Environment:* 59%. Supports community centers, youth organizations, and the United Way. *International:* 1%. Supports health centers and single-disease health organizations. *Religion:* 19%. Supports a science center. *Note:* Total contributions made in 1999. **Typ. Recipients:** Cancer, Children's Health/Hospitals, Hospitals, Multiple Sclerosis. **Geo. Dist:** Bluffton, IN, including surrounding area.

**GenCorp Foundation**
*See:* Entry 1078

**Genesis Foundation**
*See:* Entry 10065

**★ 5573 ★ Gerber Foundation**
4747 W 48th St., Ste. 153
Fremont, MI 49412
**Phone:** (231)924-3175          **Fax:** (231)924-7906
**Email:** bgetz@ncisd.net
**Website:** http://www.gerberfoundation.org
Barbara Getz, Executive Director

**Priorities:** *Arts & Humanities:* 2%. *Civic & Public Affairs:* 7%. Supports minority and legal affairs, and local initiatives. *Education:* 22%. Supports programs which promote responsible parenting, beginning at young ages and extending to adulthood. Supports formal and informal instruction in such areas as parenting skills, infant and young child care, nutrition and development training, child abuse prevention, school readiness and early school success, and avoidance of too-early child bearing. Funds health research at accredited colleges and universities. Scholarship grants are occasionally made to institutions to support students pursuing degrees for future careers in fields related to these areas. *Environment:* 19%. Funds programs that ensure access to health and human services by infants and young children across all spectra of American society. *International:* 30%. Supports teaching hospitals, and independent research institutions for research projects in the areas of nutrition, health, and development of infants and young children. Priority is given to projects which have the potential of resulting in publication of findings with broad applicability for the public good. *Religion:* 23%. Supports accredited colleges and universities, teaching hospitals, and independent research institutions for research projects in the areas of nutrition, health, and development of infants and young children. Priority is given to projects which have the potential of resulting in publication of findings with broad applicability for the public good. *Note:* Total contributions made in 2000. **Typ. Recipients:** AIDS/HIV, Arthritis, Cancer, Child Abuse, Children's Health/Hospitals, Clinics/Medical Centers, Diabetes, Domestic Violence, Eyes/Blindness, Health Organizations, Health Policy/Cost Containment, Health-General, Heart, Hospices, Hospitals, Medical Education, Medical Rehabilitation, Medical Research, Medical Training, Mental Health, Nursing Services, Nutrition, People with Disabilities, Prenatal Health Issues, Preventive Medicine/Wellness Organizations, Public Health, Speech & Hearing. **Geo. Dist:** nationally.

★ **5574 ★ Griffith Laboratories Foundation**
1 Griffith Ctr.
Alsip, IL 60803
**Phone:** (708)371-0900          **Fax:** (708)371-4783
Joseph Maslick, Chief Financial Officer

**Priorities:** *Environment:* 6%. Children's groups and Special Olympics. *Note:* Total contributions made in fiscal 1999. **Typ. Recipients:** Children's Health/Hospitals, Multiple Sclerosis, Single-Disease Health Associations.

★ **5575 ★ Harley-Davidson Foundation**
3700 West Juneau Ave.
Milwaukee, WI 53208
**Phone:** (414)343-4001
Mary Martiny, Manager

**Fnded:** 1993. **Priorities:** *Arts & Humanities:* 17%. Supports public broadcasting, performing arts programs, and museums. *Civic & Public Affairs:* 18%. Supports community foundations, development, and housing. *Education:* 10%. Funds universities, colleges, and educational programs. *Environment:* 43%. Primarily funds the United Way and youth organizations. *International:* 10%. Supports single-disease associations and hospitals. *Religion:* 1%. Funds a science center. *Note:* Total foundation contributions made in 2000. **Typ. Recipients:** Cancer, Children's Health/Hospitals, Clinics/Medical Centers, Diabetes, Emergency/Ambulance Services, Family Planning, Health Organizations, Mental Health, Public Health, Single-Disease Health Associations, Substance Abuse. **Geo. Dist:** AL, headquarters and operating communities; MO; PA, headquarters and operating communities; WI, headquarters and operating communities.

**Hasbro Charitable Trust Inc.**
*See:* Entry 1123

**High Meadow Foundation**
*See:* Entry 1128

**Hoffer Foundation**
*See:* Entry 11439

★ **5576 ★ Hofmann Foundation**
PO Box 907
Concord, CA 94520-4912
**Phone:** (925)682-4830          **Fax:** (925)682-0126
**Email:** hofferpl@inil.com
**Website:** http://www.hasbro.org
Nick Rossi, General Counsel

**Fnded:** 1963. **Priorities:** *Arts & Humanities:* 1%. Most funding supports theatre, public broadcasting, symphonies, and museums. *Civic & Public Affairs:* 3%. Funding includes support for juveniles, crisis centers, food banks, animal rescue, and legal issues. Religious

welfare also receives support. *Education:* 35%. Supports a variety of institutions, ranging from high schools and elementary schools to colleges and universities, that demonstrate a profound desire to challenge and improve the hearts and minds of their students. *Environment:* 32%. Support includes Boys and Girls Clubs, Little Leagues and the Make-A-Wish Foundation. *International:* 1%. Supports the local medical and health community as well as single-disease health associations including cancer, AIDS, paralysis and heart disease. *Note:* Total contributions made in 1999. **Typ. Recipients:** AIDS/HIV, Cancer, Children's Health/Hospitals, Clinics/Medical Centers, Diabetes, Domestic Violence, Emergency/Ambulance Services, Health Organizations, Heart, Heart, Hospices, Hospitals, Medical Education, Medical Research, People with Disabilities, Preventive Medicine/Wellness Organizations, Public Health, Respiratory, Single-Disease Health Associations. **Geo. Dist:** CA, Bay Area organizations only.

**HON Industries Charitable Foundation**
*See:* Entry 11440

**Hunt Corp.**
*See:* Entry 11696

★ **5577 ★ Kupferberg Foundation**
131-38 Sanford Ave.
Flushing, NY 11352
**Phone:** (718)461-7000
**Email:** cheryl_walmsley@Hunt-Corp.com
**Website:** http://www.hunt-corp.com
Jack Kupferberg, Purchasing Agent

**Fnded:** 1961. **Priorities:** *Arts & Humanities:* 19%. *Civic & Public Affairs:* 1%. *Education:* 17%. *Environment:* 16%. *International:* 17%. *Note:* Total contributions made in fiscal 1998. **Typ. Recipients:** Cancer, Children's Health/Hospitals, Clinics/Medical Centers, Emergency/Ambulance Services, Eyes/Blindness, Geriatric Health, Health Funds, Health Organizations, Hospitals, Hospitals (University Affiliated), Mental Health, Nursing Services, People with Disabilities, Single-Disease Health Associations, Substance Abuse. **Geo. Dist:** Queens, NY.

★ **5578 ★ Laclede Gas Charitable Trust**
720 Olive St., Ste. 1528
Saint Louis, MO 63101
**Phone:** (314)342-0503          **Fax:** (314)421-1979
Mary Kullman, Secretary, Charitable Contributions

**Priorities:** *Arts & Humanities:* 8%. Supports arts councils, music, and the performing arts. *Civic & Public Affairs:* 13%. Supports community development, housing, parks, and clubs. *Education:* 11%. Supports colleges and universities, schools, and education prgs. *Environment:* 64%. Major support for the United Way; also funds youth organizations and serves for the disabled and disadvantaged. *International:* 2%. Funds single-disease health associations. *Religion:* 1%. Funds a science center. *Note:* Total foundation contributions in fiscal 2000. **Typ. Recipients:** Children's Health/Hospitals, Hospitals, Mental Health, People with Disabilities, Prenatal Health Issues, Respiratory. **Geo. Dist:** MO, St. Louis area.

★ **5579 ★ Land O'Lakes Foundation**
PO Box 64150
Saint Paul, MN 55164-0150
**Phone:** (651)481-2212          **Fax:** (651)481-2000
**Email:** bbbass@landolakes.com
**Website:** http://foundation.landolakes.com
Bonnie Bassett, Executive Director

**Priorities:** *Arts & Humanities:* 10%. Supports quality artistic endeavors that enhance the cultural environment in communities with significant numbers of employees or members. *Civic & Public Affairs:* 21%. Supports organizations active in addressing and solving community problems, and programs that work toward the preservation and wise use of water and soil resources between the environment, agriculture, and global food needs. Rural and general agricultural

programs also receive special consideration. *Education:* 42%. Supports programs that reflect the business and membership interests of the company, such as agriculture, business, economic, and cooperative education programs, and programs designed to develop knowledge and leadership skills in rural youth. Matches employee gifts to colleges and universities. *Environment:* 27%. Primarily supports the United Way and hunger relief organizations. *Voluntarism:* Supports a Dollars for Doers program, which provides cash donations to organizations where employees volunteer. At many company plants and offices, Community Involvement Councils organize and coordinate community activities for employees. The company also supports Expanding Community and Horizon Outreach for Seniors (ECHOS), a volunteer program for company retirees. *Note:* Total foundation contributions made in 2000. **Typ. Recipients:** Children's Health/Hospitals, Clinics/Medical Centers, Domestic Violence, Emergency/Ambulance Services, Geriatric Health, People with Disabilities. **Geo. Dist:** CA; ID; IA; MN; MT; NE; ND; OR; PA; SD; WA; WI.

**Leviton Foundation New York**
*See:* Entry 1202

**LG&E Energy Foundation**
*See:* Entry 8551

★ **5580 ★ M&T Charitable Foundation**
1 M&T Plaza, 6th Floor
Buffalo, NY 14240
**Phone:** (716)842-5110          **Fax:** (716)848-7318
**Email:** hleviton@leviton.com
Debbie Pringle, Charitable Contributions Coordinator

**Fnded:** 1994. **Priorities:** *Arts & Humanities:* 17%. Supports historic preservation, museums, arts centers, the theater, orchestra, and performing arts. *Civic & Public Affairs:* 23%. Funds community development, job training, housing, zoos, and parks. *Education:* 36%. Major grant to the Westminster Community School; supports K-12 education, colleges and universities. *Environment:* 17%. Major support for the United Way; also funds youth services, shelters, and family agencies. *International:* 4%. *Note:* Total foundation contributions made in 1999. **Typ. Recipients:** Cancer, Children's Health/Hospitals, Health Organizations, Hospitals, Medical Research, People with Disabilities, Public Health, Single-Disease Health Associations. **Geo. Dist:** headquarters and operating communities.

★ **5581 ★ MDU Resources Foundation**
PO Box 5650
Bismarck, ND 58506-5650
**Phone:** (701)222-7828          **Fax:** (701)222-7607
**Email:** benzw@mduresources.com
Robert Wood, President

**Priorities:** *Arts & Humanities:* 3%. Funds museums, historic preservation. *Civic & Public Affairs:* 14%. Funds civic parks, ethnic organizations, zoological society. *Education:* 18%. Supports schools, funds scholarships for higher education. *Environment:* 35%. Funds food banks, scouts, recreation, youth issues. *International:* 27%. Funds Red Cross, medical foundations, health centers. *Note:* Total contributions made in 1999. **Typ. Recipients:** Alzheimers Disease, Children's Health/Hospitals, Clinics/Medical Centers, Domestic Violence, Emergency/Ambulance Services, Eyes/Blindness, Health Organizations, Health Policy/Cost Containment, Health-General, Hospitals, Long-Term Care, Medical Education, Medical Rehabilitation, Mental Health, People with Disabilities, Public Health, Research/Studies Institutes. **Geo. Dist:** near operating locations.

★ **5582 ★ Mid-American Foundation**
4700 Westown Parkway, Ste. 303
West Des Moines, IA 50266
**Phone:** (515)244-3600
Joe Pierce, President

**Priorities:** *Arts & Humanities:* 11%. Supports art museums, art festivals, performing arts, libraries, history organizations, and public broadcasting. *Civic & Public Affairs:* 20%. Funds minority affairs, civic centers, zoos, law & justice, and economic and urban development. *Education:* 15%. Supports a Jewish academy, scholarship funds, minority education, and universities. *Environment:* 23%. Supports the United Way, family services, family planning, youth organizations, and sports and recreation. *International:* 17%. Supports alternative medicine, pediatric disease and mental health organizations, and national single-disease associations. *Note:* Total contributions made in 2000. **Typ. Recipients:** Cancer, Children's Health/Hospitals, Diabetes, Emergency/Ambulance Services, Eyes/Blindness, Family Planning, Health-General, Heart, Multiple Sclerosis, People with Disabilities, Prenatal Health Issues. **Geo. Dist:** headquarters and operating communities.

## Mitsubishi Electric America Foundation
*See:* Entry 1246

## ★ 5583 ★ NEC Foundation of America
8 Corporate Center Dr.
Melville, NY 11747-3112
**Phone:** (631)753-7444          **Fax:** (631)753-7096
**Email:** clarks@ccgate.ml.nec.com
**Website:** http://www.nec.com/company/foundation
Ms. Sylvia Clark, Executive Director

**Fnded:** 1991. **Priorities:** *Civic & Public Affairs:* 13%. Funds a video center for public educational, artistic, and nonprofit use; and the American Youth Policy Forum. *Education:* 53%. Focus is on education for youth with disabilities, science and technology at the secondary level, and education councils. *Environment:* 14%. Gives to organizations that provide services to the disabled through the use of technology. *Religion:* 20%. Supports science museums and space science education. *Note:* Total foundation contributions made in fiscal 2000. **Typ. Recipients:** Children's Health/Hospitals, Eyes/Blindness, Medical Rehabilitation, Medical Research, People with Disabilities, Single-Disease Health Associations. **Geo. Dist:** nationally.

## ★ 5584 ★ Nissan Foundation
PO Box 191
Gardena, CA 90248-0191
**Phone:** (310)771-3161
**Website:** http://www.nissandriven.com/insidenissan/corporateoutreach/

**Fnded:** 1992. **Priorities:** *Arts & Humanities:* 11%. Supports a symphony association. *Civic & Public Affairs:* 11%. Gives to women's affairs and economic development organizations. *Education:* 13%. Funds The Accelerated School. *Environment:* 33%. Supports youth organizations and community centers that promote youth safety and community development. *International:* 16%. Supports public health centers and charities. *Note:* Total foundation contributions made in fiscal 2000. **Typ. Recipients:** Adolescent Health Issues, Children's Health/Hospitals, Clinics/Medical Centers, Health Funds, Health Organizations. **Geo. Dist:** Los Angeles, CA, South Central LA.

## The Oklahoman Foundation
*See:* Entry 1286

## ★ 5585 ★ OMNOVA Solutions Foundation
175 Ghent Rd.
Fairlawn, OH 44333-3300
**Phone:** (330)869-4000          **Fax:** (330)869-4345
**Email:** lbrown@oklahoman.com
Gregory Troy, Director

**Fnded:** 1999. **Priorities:** *Arts & Humanities:* 5%. Provides limited support to arts and cultural institutes and activities that offer opportunities to enrich the lives of employees and communities. *Civic & Public Affairs:* 27%. Supports urban affairs, crime prevention and safety, and community awareness. *Education:* 46%. Supports schools K-12, reading and economic literacy programs, teacher development initiatives, parental involvement, and adult literacy programs. *Environment:* 18%. Primary support to the United Way; also

funds disaster relief programs, human services, and youth organizations. *International:* 2%. Funds hospitals. *Religion:* 2%. Funds science museums. *Note:* Total contributions made in fiscal 2000. **Typ. Recipients:** Children's Health/Hospitals, Emergency/Ambulance Services.

## ★ 5586 ★ Pieper Power Foundation, Inc.
5070 North 35th St.
Milwaukee, WI 53209-5302
**Phone:** (414)462-7700          **Fax:** (414)462-3589
Barbara Jones, Executive Secretary

**Priorities:** *Arts & Humanities:* 5%. Funds art museums, orchestras, opera, theater, children's arts programs, arts councils, historical societies, and libraries. *Civic & Public Affairs:* 14%. Supports and affordable housing, community development, trade associations, public policy, nonprofit management/services, and community parks/playgrounds. *Education:* 21%. Supports construction and technical education, colleges, literacy initiatives, and Junior Achievement. *Environment:* 52%. Primarily supports the United Way and the Milwaukee County Council. Also gives to food banks, domestic violence prevention, and youth organizations, including scouting, Boys and Girls Clubs, YMCA/YWCA, and Big Brothers/Big Sisters. *International:* 8%. Gives to national single-disease health organizations and medical centers. *Note:* Total contributions made in 2000. **Typ. Recipients:** Children's Health/Hospitals, Clinics/Medical Centers, Domestic Violence, Emergency/Ambulance Services, Family Planning, Heart, Multiple Sclerosis, People with Disabilities, Research/Studies Institutes, Single-Disease Health Associations, Speech & Hearing. **Geo. Dist:** Milwaukee, WI.

## The Reebok Human Rights Foundation
*See:* Entry 1346

## ★ 5587 ★ Reliant Energy Foundation
PO Box 4567
Houston, TX 77210-4567
**Phone:** (713)207-5155          **Fax:** (713)207-0207
**Email:** cathy.guy@reliantenergy.com
**Website:** http://www.reliantenergy.com/company/community/
Robert Gibbs, Director, Corporate Community Relations

**Fnded:** 1997. **Priorities:** *Arts & Humanities:* About 2%. *Civic & Public Affairs:* 65%. Supports community festivals; organizational programs, foundations, local rodeo, parks, city beautification, Junior Archievement, and neighborhood centers. *Education:* About 13%. Funds scholarships to schools of medicine; college funds, and universities. *Environment:* 20%. Provides support to child advocates, scouting, Habitat for Humanity, Special Olympics, United Way, and food banks. *International:* Less than 1%. *Note:* Total contributions made in 1998. **Typ. Recipients:** Cancer, Children's Health/Hospitals, Diabetes, Emergency/Ambulance Services, Health Organizations, Heart, Hospitals, Medical Education, Medical Research, Mental Health, People with Disabilities, Single-Disease Health Associations, Substance Abuse. **Geo. Dist:** headquarters and operating communities. **Frmly:** Houston Industries, Inc.

## ★ 5588 ★ Spang & Co. Charitable Trust
PO Box 751
Butler, PA 16003-0751
**Phone:** (724)287-8781
K. McKnight, Contact

**Priorities:** *Arts & Humanities:* 16%. Supports libraries, theaters, music, symphony, public broadcasting, and opera. *Civic & Public Affairs:* 22%. Supports safety, zoos, community foundations and development, and fire departments. *Education:* 15%. Supports private schools and educational funds. *Environment:* 21%. Supports United Way, scouts, animal protection, senior services, and camps. *International:* 26%. Funds hospitals, medical institutes, and single-disease associations. *Note:* Total foundation contributions made in 2000. **Typ. Recipients:** Cancer, Children's Health/

Hospitals, Clinics/Medical Centers, Domestic Violence, Eyes/Blindness, Heart, Hospitals, Hospitals (University Affiliated), Kidney, Medical Education, Medical Research, Nursing Services, People with Disabilities, Single-Disease Health Associations. **Geo. Dist:** PA.

## Sprint Foundation
*See:* Entry 10069

## Sprint/United Telephone
*See:* Entry 1403

## Susquehanna-Pfaltzgraff Foundation
*See:* Entry 1421

## Sverdrup Corp. Charitable Trust
*See:* Entry 1422

## ★ 5589 ★ Synetic Foundation
PO Box 616
Fairlawn, NJ 07410
**Phone:** (201)701-3400
**Website:** http://www.sprint.com
Richard Clark, Chief Operating Officer

**Fnded:** 1991. **Priorities:** *Civic & Public Affairs:* 10%. Funds community services. *Education:* 7%. Supports schools. *Environment:* 13%. Supports programs for youth and family services. *International:* 70%. Supports public health issues and children's health. *Note:* Total contributions made in fiscal 2000. **Typ. Recipients:** Adolescent Health Issues, AIDS/HIV, Alzheimers Disease, Cancer, Children's Health/Hospitals, Clinics/Medical Centers, Family Planning, Health Organizations, Health Policy/Cost Containment, Health-General, Hospitals, Medical Research, Public Health. **Geo. Dist:** NJ. **Frmly:** Medco Containment Services Foundation.

## ★ 5590 ★ Truland Foundation
3330 Washington Blvd., 7th Fl.
Arlington, VA 22201
**Phone:** (703)524-4900
Robert Truland, President & Chief Executive Officer

**Fnded:** 1954. **Priorities:** *Arts & Humanities:* 54%. Funds museums. *Civic & Public Affairs:* 4%. Funds civic programs. *Education:* 7%. Funds primary schools, universities. *International:* 35%. Funds health foundations and groups. *Note:* Total contributions made in fiscal 2000. **Typ. Recipients:** Cancer, Children's Health/Hospitals, Health-General, Hospices, Hospitals, Hospitals (University Affiliated), Mental Health, People with Disabilities, Public Health.

## UPS Foundation
*See:* Entry 1466

## USAA Foundation, A Charitable Trust
*See:* Entry 1468

## ★ 5591 ★ Wolfe Associates, Inc.
34 South Third St.
Columbus, OH 43215
**Phone:** (614)461-5211          **Fax:** (614)461-5225
**Email:** comrel@dispatch.com
**Website:** http://www.dispatch.com
Sherry Lewis, Contact

**Fnded:** 1973. **Priorities:** *Arts & Humanities:* 7%. Grants made to organizations which perform and promote public appreciation of music, drama and dance, and those institutions which provide public access to the visual arts; institutions, such as museums, libraries, and historical societies dedicated to the preservation of and providing public access to the political, social and cultural heritage of the United States; and programs dedicated to arts and humanities, history, language, and literature. *Civic & Public*

*Affairs:* 7%. Supports programs dedicated to improving quality of life operating communities and programs promoting minority opportunities. *Education:* 33%. Contributions are designed to provide opportunities for advanced study to those unable to procure funds. Scholarship grants are not made directly to individuals, but to the endowment of chaired professorships at colleges and universities; public and private institutions of higher learning which offer students of high scholastic achievement the opportunity to pursue their studies, and programs dedicated to adult continuing education, adult literacy, and special education are given high priority. *Environment:* 25%. Supports organizations and groups providing social services to children, families, and the elderly, who through misfortune, disability, or other adversity, are deprived of basic living needs. Supports United Way. *International:* 26%. Funds groups organized on a statewide/national basis, as well as local chapters, committed to research in and treatment of a variety of catastrophic diseases; hospitals and healthcare institutions dedicated to delivering quality health care services to the communities they serve; programs dedicated to mental health, health education, substance abuse, public health and medical care. *Note:* Total foundation contributions made in fiscal 2000. **Typ. Recipients:** Cancer, Children's Health/Hospitals, Clinics/Medical Centers, Emergency/Ambulance Services, Family Planning, Health Funds, Health-General, Heart, Hospices, Hospitals, Long-Term Care, Medical Rehabilitation, Medical Research, People with Disabilities, Single-Disease Health Associations. **Geo. Dist:** OH, Central Ohio and other areas in which the corporate donors have a substantial presence.

**Yellow Corp. Foundation**
*See:* Entry 1516

## Other Funding Organizations

**American Action Fund for Blind Children and Adults (AAFBCA)**
*See:* Entry 20803

**★ 5592 ★ American Guild for Infant Survival (AGIS)**
301 Eastwood Cir., Ste. 200
Virginia Beach, VA 23454-4014
**Phone:** (757)463-3845
**Email:** afgisinc@ivilliage.com
**Website:** http://www.actionfund.org
Scott Hessek, Pres.

**Desc:** Works to reduce infant mortality, especially Sudden Infant Death Syndrome. Develops low-tech innovations to reduce infant mortality, such as the AFGIS test, which scores risk categories of infants and fetuses. Promotes the home monitoring program. Conducts educational and research programs. Compiles statistics. Maintains speakers' bureau. Offers children's services. **Awards:** Grant (annual) for research.

**Association for Child Psychoanalysis (ACP)**
*See:* Entry 12289

**Batten Disease Support and Research Association (BDSRA)**
*See:* Entry 13867

**★ 5593 ★ Children's Brain Tumor Foundation (CBTF)**
274 Madison Ave., No. 1301
New York, NY 10016
**Phone:** (212)448-9494          **Free:** (866)CBT-HOPE
**Fax:** (212)448-1022
**Email:** info@cbtf.org
**Website:** http://www.cbtf.org
Judy Hurley, Exec. Dir.

**Desc:** Works to improve the outlook for children with brain and spinal cord tumors. Raises funds for research; provides counseling, education and support services for families and survivors. **Awards:** Fellowship for young physicians studying pediatric neuro-oncology; grant for research scientists.

**★ 5594 ★ Children's PKU Network (CPN)**
3790 Via De La Valle, Ste. 120
Del Mar, CA 92014-4248
**Phone:** (858)509-0767          **Free:** 800-377-6677
**Fax:** (858)509-0768
**Email:** pkunetwork@aol.com
**Website:** http://www.pkunetwork.org
Cindy Neptune, Exec. Dir.

**Desc:** Works to address the special needs of all people involved in the treatment of Phenylketonuria (PKU), a genetic metabolic disease whereby the body is unable to process the amino acid phenyalanine. Networks families and individuals with each other; provides discount dietary aids; offers financial assistance and support groups; provides crisis intervention; advocates mandatory guidelines for insurance carriers to cover expenses of medical food treatment of PKU individuals; conducts fundraisers; endows research benefiting PKU and other metabolic disorders. **Awards:** Children's PKU Network Annual Scholarship (annual) students with PKU.

**Cystic Fibrosis Foundation (CFF)**
*See:* Entry 9275

**International Rett Syndrome Association (IRSA)**
*See:* Entry 9281

**International Society of Psychiatric Mental Health Nurses (ISPN)**
*See:* Entry 14925

**★ 5595 ★ Klingenstein Third Generation Foundation**
787 Seventh Ave., 6th Fl.
New York, NY 10019-6016
**Phone:** (212)492-6179          **Fax:** (212)492-7007
**Email:** sally@ktgf.org
**Website:** http://www.ktgf.org/
Sally Klingenstein, Exec. Dir.

**Desc:** Works to support intervention and referral, prevention, and public education and training relating to childhood and adolescent depression and Attention Deficit Disorder. **Awards:** Grant.

**★ 5596 ★ National Association of Child Care Professionals**
c/o Sherry Workman
PO Box 90723
Austin, TX 78709-0723
**Phone:** (512)301-5557          **Free:** 800-537-1118
**Fax:** (512)301-5080
**Email:** admin@naccp.org
**Website:** http://www.naccp.org
Sherry Workman, Exec. Dir.

**Desc:** Child care supervisors and individuals involved in decision making at a child care facility. Offers networking opportunities and support services to child care professionals. Dedicated to the professional development of child care directors. Conducts educational programs. **Awards:** National Child Care Director of the Year Award (annual) recipient for exceptional contributions to the child care industry.

**★ 5597 ★ National Child Care Association (NCCA)**
1016 Rosser St.
Conyers, GA 30012
**Phone:** (770)922-8198          **Free:** 800-543-7161
**Fax:** (770)388-7772
**Email:** nccallw@mindspring.com

**Website:** http://www.nccanet.org
Lynn White, Exec. Dir.

**Desc:** Works to promote and safeguard the interest of quality child care in the United States. Focuses on licensed, private providers of child care and preschool services. Conducts lobbying activities; offers casualty insurance programs; conducts educational and research programs; provides networking opportunities. **Awards:** National Early Childhood Program Accreditation; scholarship.

**National Children's Eye Care Foundation (NCECF)**
*See:* Entry 20819

**Pediatric AIDS Foundation**
*See:* Entry 11706

**Pediatric Endocrinology Nursing Society (PENS)**
*See:* Entry 8664

**Pediatric Orthopaedic Society of North America (POSNA)**
*See:* Entry 16906

**Society for Maternal Fetal Medicine (SMFM)**
*See:* Entry 16590

**Society of Pediatric Nurses (SPN)**
*See:* Entry 14940

**★ 5598 ★ Society for Physician Assistants in Pediatrics (SPAP)**
950 N Washington St.
Alexandria, VA 22314-1552
**Free:** 800-596-4398          **Fax:** (703)684-1924
**Email:** jrv1007@aol.com
**Website:** http://www.geocities.com/spap_peds1
Tom Moreno, Membership Coor.

**Desc:** Designed to gather and disseminate information affecting the practice of pediatric physician assistants, collect demographic data to share within the profession or with other organizations, assist in developing guidelines for physician assistant utilization in clinical settings, and to enhance the relationship with the American Academy of Pediatrics. **Awards:** Scholarship (annual) PA student with documented interest in pediatric practice.

**★ 5599 ★ Williams Syndrome Association (WSA)**
PO Box 297
Clawson, MI 48017-0297
**Phone:** (248)541-3630          **Fax:** (248)541-3631
**Email:** tmonkaba@aol.com
**Website:** http://www.williams-syndrome.org
Terry Monkaba, Exec. Dir.

**Desc:** Individuals with Williams Syndrome and their families; medical and health care professionals; educators. (Williams Syndrome is characterized by similar facial features, low birth weight, heart disorders, hearing sensitivity, talkative personality, mild to severe learning disabilities, and developmental delays.) Provides support and assistance to families with a WS child. Conducts networking in the medical, scientific, educational, and professional communities for referral and study of newly-diagnosed WS individuals. Encourages medical behavior and supports research into all aspects of the syndrome. Compiles statistics. **Awards:** Chloe Reisig Music Scholarship (annual) for interest and ability in music and financial need; monetary; Research Grant (periodic).

**Yes I Can Foundation for Exceptional Children**
*See:* Entry 7897

---

# National & International Organizations

## ★ 5600 ★ Action Health - Nigeria (AHI)
PO Box 803
Yaba Post Office
Lagos, Lagos, Nigeria
**Phone:** 234 1 7743745     **Fax:** 234 1 1861166
**Email:** ahi@linkserve.com.ng
**Website:** http://www.cec.sped.org

**Fnded:** 1989. **Lang(s):** English. **Desc:** Individuals interested in the health and well-being of Nigerian youth. Promotes increased availability of health and social services for youth; works to improve public understanding of reproductive health and related issues. Conducts educational programs for youth; sponsors reproductive health clinics. **Pub:** *Growing Up,* periodic. Newsletter.

## Advisory Council for Children with Impaired Hearing
*See:* Entry 5968

## ★ 5601 ★ Allergy and Asthma Network/ Mothers of Asthmatics (AAN/MA)
2751 Prosperity Ave., Ste. 150
Fairfax, VA 22031
**Phone:** (703)641-9595     **Free:** 800-878-4403
**Fax:** (703)573-7794
**Email:** aanma@aol.com
**Website:** http://www.aanma.org
Nancy Sander, Pres.

**Fnded:** 1985. **Mem:** 6,000. **Desc:** Professional associations, physicians, patients, parents, and educators. Dedicated to the education and support of people with allergies and asthma. Nonprofit patient education organization dedicated to people with allergies and asthma. Members include individuals, parents, physicians, patients, educators and professional associations. Resources include monthly newsletter books, quarterly magazines, videos, pamphlets on asthma and allergies. **Pub:** *Allergy & Asthma Health*, quarterly. Magazine. Provides in-depth coverage of allergy and asthma issues from leading medical and consumer experts. Includes a mini-magazine for kids. *Price:* $15. • *Breathing Easy with Day Care.* • *Consumer Update on Asthma.* • *I'm a Meter Reader.* Video. • *MA Report*, monthly. Newsletter. Provides patients and families of children with asthma and allergies with coping strategies, medical information, product reviews & how to articles. *Price:* $25/year. • *So You Have Asthma Too!.* Book. **Frmly:** (1991) Mothers of Asthmatics; (1993) National Allergy and Asthma Network.

## ★ 5602 ★ ALSAC - St. Jude Children's Research Hospital
501 St. Jude Pl.
Memphis, TN 38105
**Phone:** (901)578-2000     **Free:** 800-USS-JUDE
**Fax:** (901)523-6658
**Email:** info@stjude.org
**Website:** http://www2.stjude.org/
Richard C. Shadyac, Exec. Dir.

**Fnded:** 1957. **Mem:** 2,000. **Reg. Groups:** 8. **Local Groups:** 60. **Desc:** Fundraising organization maintaining St. Jude Children's Research Hospital and laboratories in Memphis, TN. Conducts research and children's services and provides patient care in children's catastrophic diseases. Incorporated as American Lebanese Syrian Associated Charities, ALSAC was organized through the auspices of Danny Thomas, television and theatre personality. **Pub:** *ALSAC News*, quarterly. Tabloid informing members of St. Jude Hospital activities and ALSAC fundraising programs.

Covers regional news. *Price:* Included in membership dues. • *Partners in Hope*, quarterly. Tabloid providing human interest stories and news of St. Jude Hospital activities. *Price:* Available to donors only. **Frmly:** (1972) Aiding Leukemia Stricken American Children.

## ★ 5603 ★ Ambulatory Pediatric Association (APA)
6728 Old McLean Village Dr.
Mc Lean, VA 22101
**Phone:** (703)556-9222     **Fax:** (703)556-8729
**Email:** info@ambpeds.org
**Website:** http://www.ambpeds.org
Marge Degnon, Exec. Dir.

**Fnded:** 1960. **Mem:** 2,000. **Reg. Groups:** 10. **Desc:** Health care providers interested in the care of children in ambulatory care facilities, particularly directors of outpatient departments in private, university, and other teaching hospitals and those engaged in public health work or private practice. Aims to improve methods of care of children. Studies methods of research and the teaching of outpatient care. Conducts collaborative research; compiles statistics; presents annual scientific program. **Pub:** *Ambulatory Pediatric Association–Membership Directory*, biennial. Membership Directory. • *Ambulatory Pediatric Association–Newsletter*, 3/year. Newsletter. Includes book reviews, calendar of events, listing of employment opportunities, research reports, and statistics. • *Ambulatory Pediatrics, (The Journal of the Ambulatory Pediatric Assn.)*, 6/year. • Also publishes abstracts of scientific papers. **Frmly:** (1967) Association for Ambulatory Pediatric Services.

## ★ 5604 ★ American Academy of Child and Adolescent Psychiatry (AACAP)
3615 Wisconsin Ave. NW
Washington, DC 20016-3007
**Phone:** (202)966-7300     **Free:** 800-333-7636
**Fax:** (202)966-2891
**Email:** executive@aacap.org
**Website:** http://www.aacap.org
Virginia Q. Anthony, Exec. Dir.

**Fnded:** 1953. **Mem:** 6,500. **Reg. Groups:** 57. **Desc:** Professional society of degreed physicians who have completed an additional five years of residency in child and adolescent psychiatry. Seeks to stimulate and advance medical contributions to the knowledge and treatment of psychiatric illnesses of children and adolescents. **Pub:** *AACAP News*, bimonthly. Newsletter. Includes listing of employment opportunities, research updates, and statistics. *Price:* Included in membership dues. • *Journal of the AACAP*, monthly. Journal. • Bulletin, periodic. • Catalog. • Manuals. • Membership Directory, periodic. **Frmly:** (1986) American Academy of Child Psychiatry.

## ★ 5605 ★ American Academy of Pediatric Dentistry (AAPD)
211 E Chicago Ave., Ste. 700
Chicago, IL 60611-2663
**Phone:** (312)337-2169     **Fax:** (312)337-6329
**Email:** gsandoval@aapd.org
**Website:** http://www.aapd.org
Dr. John Rutkauskas, Exec. Dir.

**Fnded:** 1947. **Mem:** 4,500. **Reg. Groups:** 45. **Desc:** Professional society of dentists whose practice is limited to children; teachers and researchers in pediatric dentistry. Seeks to advance the specialty of pediatric dentistry through practice, education, and research. Sponsors graduate student pediatric dentistry award program. **Pub:** *American Academy of Pediatric Dentistry–Membership Roster*, annual. Membership Directory. • *American Academy of Pediatric Dentistry–Today*, bimonthly. Newsletter. Includes employment listings, meetings calendar, research updates, and obituaries. *Price:* Included in membership dues. • *Pediatric Dentistry*, bimonthly. Journal. Includes employment listings and conference proceedings. *Price:* Included in membership dues; $50/year for nonmembers; $65/year for institutions. • Pamphlets. **Frmly:** (1984) American Academy of Pedodontics.

## ★ 5606 ★ American Academy of Pediatrics (AAP)
141 Northwest Point Blvd.
Elk Grove Village, IL 60007-1098
**Phone:** (847)434-4000     **Fax:** (847)434-8000
**Email:** kidsdocs@aap.org
**Website:** http://www.aap.org
Louis Z. Cooper, MD, Pres.

**Fnded:** 1930. **Mem:** 55,000. **State Groups:** 66. **Desc:** Professional medical society of pediatricians and pediatric subspecialists. Operates small member library of books and journals on pediatric medicine, office practice, and child health care policy. Maintains 42 committees, councils, and tasks forces including: Accident and Poison Prevention; Early Childhood, Adoption and Dependent Care; Infectious Diseases. Operates 47 sections. Sponsors Pediatrics Review and Education Program (PREP), a self-assessment, continuing education program for practicing pediatricians. **Pub:** *AAP News*, monthly. Newspaper. Covers the social, economic, and professional aspects of pediatric care. Includes association news and chapter news. *Price:* Included in membership dues; $40/year for nonmembers. • *Fellowship List*, annual. • *Pediatrics*, monthly. Journal. Includes employment listings. *Price:* $110/year for individuals; $180/year for institutions; $70/year for students; $70/nurses. • *Pediatrics in Review*, monthly. Journal. Contains review articles and abstracts. Subscribers are eligible for Category/Continuing Medical Education credit. *Price:* $130/year for members; $165/year for nonmembers and institutions. • Also publishes professional manuals and patient education materials.

## ★ 5607 ★ American Association for Pediatric Ophthalmology and Strabismus
PO Box 193832
San Francisco, CA 94119
**Phone:** (415)561-8505     **Fax:** (415)561-8531
**Email:** rblocker@acs.bu.edu
**Website:** http://med-aapos.bu.edu/
Sue A. Brown, Admin.

**Fnded:** 1974. **Mem:** 844. **Desc:** Ophthalmologists who limit their practice largely to children. Encourages quality eye care for children by establishing high ethical standards of practice, supporting educational training programs for pediatric ophthalmologists, and promoting basic research in children's eye diseases. Conducts research programs. **Pub:** Journal, bimonthly. • Membership Directory, annual. **Frmly:** (1978) American Association of Pediatric Ophthalmology.

## ★ 5608 ★ American Board of Pediatric Dentistry (ABPD)
1193 Woodgate Dr.
Carmel, IN 46033
**Phone:** (317)573-0877     **Fax:** (317)846-7235
**Email:** drjrroche@cs.com
**Website:** http://www.abpd.org
James R. Roche, D.D.S., Exec. Sec. -Treas.

**Fnded:** 1940. **Mem:** 1,222. **Desc:** Certification board whose purpose is to investigate the qualifications of, administer examinations to, and certify as diplomates, dentists specializing in the care of children. Sponsored by American Academy of Pediatric Dentistry. **Pub:** *Directory of Diplomates*, biennial. Directory. Lists all board certified pediatric dentists. *Price:* $28. **Frmly:** (1986) American Board of Pedodontics.

## ★ 5609 ★ American Board of Pediatrics (ABP)
111 Silver Cedar Ct.
Chapel Hill, NC 27514
**Phone:** (919)929-0461     **Fax:** (919)929-9255
**Email:** abpeds@abpeds.org
**Website:** http://www.abp.org
James A. Stockman, MD, Pres.

**Fnded:** 1933. **Mem:** 250. **Desc:** Certification board to establish qualifications, conduct examinations, and certify as diplomates those whom the board finds qualified as specialists in pediatrics. **Pub:** *American Board of Pediatrics–Booklet of Information*, annual.

Booklet. Outlines requirements for admission to certifying examinations; includes details of examinations. *Price:* Free. • *American Board of Pediatrics–Informal Newsletter to Members*, periodic. Newsletter. • *American Board of Pediatrics–Newsletter for Diplomates*, annual. Newsletter. *Price:* Free. • *Newsletter to Pediatric Training Program Directors*. Newsletter. *Price:* Free.

## American College of Foot and Ankle Pediatrics (ACFAP)
*See:* Entry 17706

## ★ 5610 ★ American College of Osteopathic Pediatricians (ACOP)
5550 Friendship Blvd., Ste. 300
Chevy Chase, MD 20815-7201
**Phone:** (301)968-4180      **Fax:** (301)968-4199
**Website:** http://www.acopeds.org
Kristen Sokolowski, Contact

**Fnded:** 1940. **Mem:** 365. **Desc:** Osteopathic physicians who have received or are receiving advanced training in pediatrics and who are specializing in pediatric practice. **Pub:** *ACOP Pulse*, quarterly. Newsletter. Reports on new regulations and sources of information in the field of osteopathic pediatrics. *Price:* $10/year. • Membership Directory, annual.

## American Foundation for Maternal and Child Health (AFMCH)
*See:* Entry 16645

## ★ 5611 ★ American Guild for Infant Survival (AGIS)
301 Eastwood Cir., Ste. 200
Virginia Beach, VA 23454-4014
**Phone:** (757)463-3845
**Email:** afgisinc@ivilliage.com
Scott Hessek, Pres.

**Fnded:** 1972. **Mem:** 170. **Nat'l Groups:** 1. **Reg. Groups:** 1. **Local Groups:** 2. **Desc:** Works to reduce infant mortality, especially Sudden Infant Death Syndrome. Develops low-tech innovations to reduce infant mortality, such as the AFGIS test, which scores risk categories of infants and fetuses. Promotes the home monitoring program. Conducts educational and research programs. Compiles statistics. Maintains speakers' bureau. Offers children's services. **Pub:** *The Baby and Family Newspaper*, semiannual. Newspaper. • Brochures. • Directory. **AKA:** American Forces Guild for Infant Survival; Tidewater Guild for Infant Survival, Inc.

## American Osteopathic Board of Pediatrics (AOBP)
*See:* Entry 17000

## ★ 5612 ★ American Pediatric Society (APS)
3400 Research Forest Dr., Ste. B7
The Woodlands, TX 77381-4259
**Phone:** (281)419-0052      **Fax:** (281)419-0082
**Email:** info@aps-spr.org
**Website:** http://www.aps-spr.org
Kathy A. Cannon, Assoc. Exec. Dir.

**Fnded:** 1888. **Mem:** 1,400. **Desc:** Professional academic society of M.D. educators and researchers interested in the study of children and their diseases, prevention of illness, and promotion of health in childhood. Maintains archives. **Pub:** *Pediatric Research*, monthly. Journal. • *Program and Abstracts of Annual Meeting*.

## American Pediatric Surgical Association (APSA)
*See:* Entry 19486

## ★ 5613 ★ American Society for Adolescent Psychiatry (ASAP)
PO Box 570218
Dallas, TX 75357-0218
**Phone:** (972)686-6166      **Fax:** (972)613-5532
**Email:** info@adolpsych.org
**Website:** http://www.adolpsych.org
Sidney H. Weissman, MD, Pres.

**Fnded:** 1967. **Mem:** 800. **Reg. Groups:** 20. **Desc:** Qualified psychiatrists concerned with the behavior of adolescents. Provides for the exchange of psychiatric knowledge; encourages the development of adequate standards and training facilities; stimulates research in the psychopathology and treatment of adolescents. Consults with national organizations interested in the welfare of youth and adolescence. **Pub:** *Adolescent Psychiatry*, annual. Journal. Contains articles and case studies on adolescent psychiatry. • *American Society for Adolescent Psychiatry–Newsletter*, quarterly. Newsletter. Includes society news, calendar of events, and research updates. *Price:* Included in membership dues; $10/year for nonmembers. • *ASAP Membership Directory*, biennial. Membership Directory. • *Journal of Youth and Adolescence*, bimonthly. Journal.

## American Society of Dentistry for Children (ASDC)
*See:* Entry 6454

## ★ 5614 ★ American Society of Pediatric Hematology/Oncology (ASPHO)
4700 W Lake Ave.
Glenview, IL 60025-1485
**Phone:** (847)375-4716      **Fax:** (847)375-6316
**Email:** info@aspho.org
**Website:** http://www.aspho.org
George Buchanan, MD, Pres.

**Fnded:** 1981. **Mem:** 750. **Desc:** Active members are: physicians who have served residencies in pediatrics and fellowships in pediatric hematology/oncology; specialists in allied disciplines including surgery, pathology, radiology, pedodontics, and psychiatry; physicians trained in hematology or oncology of adults who are interested in the treatment of blood diseases and cancer in children; individuals holding doctoral degrees who are involved in research relevant to the field. Affiliated members are: nurses and physician assistants and others working with children with cancer, sickle cell disease, thalassemia, hemophilia, and other hematological disorders; psychologists, social workers, research scientists, and others interested in comprehensive care or research in the field. Purpose is to promote the knowledge, understanding, and management of disorders of the blood and of cancer in children. Seeks improvements in the total care of children with these diseases through the fostering of education and all relevant clinical and basic research. Provides a forum for the exchange of ideas on issues in the field. Cooperates with other societies concerned with the field. **Pub:** *ASPH/O News*, bimonthly. Newsletter. News of the society, members, committees, etc. • *Directory of Members*, annual. Membership Directory. • *Journal of Pediatric Hematology/Oncology*, bimonthly. Journal.

## American Society of Pediatric Nephrology
*See:* Entry 20877

## ★ 5615 ★ American Society of Pediatric Neuroradiology
c/o A. James Barkovich, Md
2210 Midwest Rd., Ste. 207
Oak Brook, IL 60523-8205
**Phone:** (630)574-0220      **Fax:** (630)574-0661
**Email:** info@asnr.org
**Website:** http://www.asnr.org
James Gantenberg, CHE, Exec. Dir.

**Desc:** Promotes the profession of pediatric neuroradiology.

## ★ 5616 ★ American Sudden Infant Death Syndrome Institute (ASIDSI)
2480 Windy Hill Rd., Ste. 380
Marietta, GA 30067
**Phone:** (770)612-1030      **Free:** 800-232-SIDS
**Fax:** (770)612-8277
**Email:** prevent@sids.org
**Website:** http://www.sids.org
Dr. Betty McEntire, Exec. Dir.

**Fnded:** 1983. **Reg. Groups:** 1. **Desc:** Participants include health care professionals, researchers, and laypeople concerned about sudden infant death syndrome (SIDS); families who have lost babies to SIDS. Works to identify the cause and cure of SIDS. Promotes infant health through research, clinical services, education, and support for SIDS families. Conducts research on siblings of SIDS babies; sponsors research programs seeking the cause and cure of SIDS. Conducts seminars for health care professionals and laypeople; maintains speakers' bureau. **Pub:** Brochures. • Also publishes research results. **AKA:** American SIDS Institute.

## ★ 5617 ★ Argentin Society of Pediatrics (Sociedad Argentina de Pediatria)
Coronel Diaz 1971
1425 Buenos Aires, Argentina
**Phone:** 54 1 8242063
**Fnded:** 1911.

## ★ 5618 ★ ASEAN Pediatric Federation
Academy of Medicine
Singapore Paediatric Society
Chapter of Physicians
16 College Rd., No. 01-01
Singapore 169854, Singapore
**Phone:** 65 2238968      **Fax:** 65 2255155
**Lang(s):** Chinese, English. **Desc:** Pediatrists and other health care professionals with an interest in pediatrics. Seeks to advance pediatric study, teaching, and practice. Facilitates exchange of information among members; sponsors continuing professional development courses.

## Asian Association of Pediatric Surgeons (AAPS)
*See:* Entry 19506

## ★ 5619 ★ Asian Pan-Pacific Society for Paediatric Gastroenterology and Nutrition
Department of Pediatrics
Juntendo University School of Medicine
2-1-1 Hongo
Bunkyō-ku
Tokyo 113, Japan
**Lang(s):** English, Japanese. **Desc:** Pediatric gastroenterologists and nutritionists. Seeks to advance the study, teaching, and practice of pediatric gastroenterology and nutrition. Functions as a clearinghouse on pediatric gastroenterology and nutrition; sponsors research and educational programs.

## ★ 5620 ★ Association for Child Psychoanalysis (ACP)
PO Box 253
Ramsey, NJ 07446
**Phone:** (201)825-3138      **Fax:** (201)825-3138
**Email:** childanalysis@compuserve.com
**Website:** http://www.westnet.com/acp/
Erna Furman, Pres.

**Fnded:** 1965. **Mem:** 650. **Desc:** Child psychoanalysts united to provide a forum for discussion and dissemination of information in their field. Conducts national and international scientific meetings. **Pub:** *Abstracts*, triennial. • *Association for Child Psychoanalysis–Newsletter*, semiannual. Newsletter. Covers child analysis methods, child psychoanalysis training, and the treatment and education of children throughout the world. *Price:* Included in membership dues. • *Member-*

*ship Roster*, biennial. **Frmly:** (1971) American Association for Child Psychoanalysis.

**★ 5621 ★ Association for Child Psychology and Psychiatry (ACPP)**
Child Clinical Psychology Service, Mary Sheridan Centre for
Child Health
405 Kerrington Rd.
London SE11 4QW, United Kingdom
**Phone:** 44 207 4141400    **Fax:** 44 207 4037081
**Website:** http://www.acpp.org.uk/

**Fnded:** 1956. **Mem:** 2,750. **Nat'l Groups:** 15. **Lang(s):** English. **Desc:** Professionals working in the field of child mental health. Encourages dissemination of scientific research and information. **Pub:** *Child Psychology and Psychiatry Review*, quarterly. • *Journal of Child Psychology and Psychiatry*, 8/year. Journal.

**★ 5622 ★ Association of Child Psychotherapists (ACP)**
120 W Heath Rd.
London NW3 7TU, United Kingdom
**Phone:** 44 181 4581609    **Fax:** 44 181 4581482
**Email:** acp@dial.pipex.com

**Fnded:** 1949. **Mem:** 597. **Desc:** Safeguards the interests of psychotherapists and fosters the exchange of information on the treatments of psychological disturbances of behavior, thinking, and feeling. Provides a forum for discussion. **Pub:** *Journal of Child Psychotherapy*, 3/year. Journal. • Bulletin, monthly.

**★ 5623 ★ Association of Children's Prosthetic-Orthotic Clinics (ACPOC)**
6300 N River Rd., No. 727
Rosemont, IL 60018-4226
**Phone:** (847)698-1637    **Fax:** (847)823-0536
**Email:** king@aaos.org
**Website:** http://www.acpoc.org
Sheril B. King, Society Dir

**Fnded:** 1980. **Mem:** 450. **Desc:** Prosthetic-orthotic clinics for children. Promotes the exchange of information concerning children's prosthetic-orthotic devices. Fosters cooperative research development and evaluative efforts among member clinics. Seeks to improve care in member clinics. **Pub:** Newsletter, quarterly.

**★ 5624 ★ Association for European Paediatric Cardiology (AEPC)**
c/o Dr. Ingrid Oberhansli-Weiss
Hopital Cantonal Universitaire de Geneve
Paediatric Cardiology Unit
6, rue Willy Donze
CH-1211 Geneva, Switzerland
**Phone:** 41 22 3824583    **Fax:** 41 22 3824546
**Email:** secr@aepc.org
**Website:** http://www.aepc.org

**Fnded:** 1963. **Mem:** 620. **Lang(s):** English, French. **Desc:** Physicians specializing in pediatric cardiology. Seeks to advance pediatric cardiological study, teaching, and practice. Serves as a clearinghouse on pediatric cardiology; conducts research and continuing professional development programs, and courses in pediatric cardiology.

**Association of the Handicapped Children of Romania**
*See:* Entry 7926

**★ 5625 ★ Association of Maternal and Child Health Programs (AMCHP)**
1220 19th St. NW, Ste. 801
Washington, DC 20036
**Phone:** (202)775-0436    **Fax:** (202)775-0061
**Email:** info@amchp.org
**Website:** http://www.amchp.org
Stephanie Cook-McDaniel, Proj. Mgr.

**Fnded:** 1944. **Mem:** 450. **Desc:** Individuals responsible for or involved in the Administration of state and territorial maternal and child health programs and programs for children with special health care needs. Seeks to: inform public and private sector decision makers of the health care needs of mothers and children; develop and recommend maternal and child health policies and programs; develop coalitions with other interested organizations. Promotes exchange of ideas and experiences among members; studies and reports on the health of and services for mothers and children; develops models and standards for and provides technical assistance to maternal and child health programs. **Pub:** *Abstinence Education in the States: Implementation of the 1996 Abstinence Education Law*. • *AMCHP Updates*, bimonthly. Newsletter. *Price:* Included in membership dues. • *Caring for Mothers and Children: A Report of a Survey of 1987 State MCH Program Activities*. • *Dedicated to Care for Children: A Report on States Use of OBRA 1986 Earmarked Title V Funds*. • *Home Visiting: An Effective Strategy for Improving the Health of Mothers and Children*. • *The Impact of the State Child Health Insurance Program (CHIP) on Title V Children with Special Health Care Needs Programs*. • *Smoking Cessation Makes Cents: The Cost-Effectiveness of Tobacco Interventions*. • Magazines. • Proceedings. • Reports. • Also publishes cost-based reimbursement studies and health care reform studies. **Frmly:** Association of State and Territorial Maternal and Child Health and Crippled Children's Directors.

**★ 5626 ★ Association of Medical School Pediatric Department Chairs (AMSPDC)**
c/o Jean Bartholomew
111 Silver Cedar Ct.
Chapel Hill, NC 27514-1651
**Phone:** (919)942-1993    **Fax:** (919)929-9255
**Email:** jbartholomew@abpeds.org
M. Douglas Jones, MD, Sec. -Treas.

**Fnded:** 1961. **Mem:** 147. **Desc:** Chairmen of the department of pediatrics of each accredited medical school in the United States and Canada. Fosters education and research in the field of child health and human development. Is cooperating with other national pediatric groups to consider problems of pediatric education, research, and care. **Pub:** *AMSPDC Membership List*, annual.

**Association of Nursery Training Colleges**
*See:* Entry 15665

**Association of Paediatric Anaesthetists of Great Britain and Ireland (APA)**
*See:* Entry 4450

**★ 5627 ★ Association for Pediatric Education in Europe (APEE)**
Pl Amelie-Raba-Leon
F-33076 Bordeaux, France
**Fax:** 33 5 56796038
**Email:** Claude.Billeaud@atsneonata.u-bordeaux2.Fr
**Website:** http://www.atinternet.com/apee/

**Fnded:** 1970. **Desc:** Fosters research and advances in pediatric education.

**★ 5628 ★ Association of Pediatric Oncology Nurses (APON)**
4700 W Lake Ave.
Glenview, IL 60025-1485
**Phone:** (847)375-4724    **Fax:** 877-734-8755
**Email:** info@apon.org
**Website:** http://www.apon.org/
CJ Hutto, RNCPON, Pres.

**Fnded:** 1973. **Mem:** 2,000. **Reg. Groups:** 37. **Desc:** Scientific and educational association seeking to establish lines of communication among nurses caring for children and adolescents with cancer. Encourages updating of literature and development of standards of care for children with cancer. Plans annual conference. **Pub:** *APON Counts*, quarterly. Newsletter. • *Journal of Pediatric Oncology Nursing*, bimonthly. • *Nursing Care of the Child With Cancer*.

**Association of Pediatric Oncology Social Workers (APOSW)**
*See:* Entry 19077

**★ 5629 ★ Association of Pediatric Program Directors (APPD)**
6728 McLean Village Dr.
Mc Lean, VA 22101
**Phone:** (703)556-9222    **Fax:** (703)556-8729
**Email:** info@appd.org
**Website:** http://www.appd.org
Laura E. Degnon, Exec. Dir.

**Fnded:** 1984. **Mem:** 1,024. **Desc:** Directors of accredited pediatric residency programs. Seeks to advance the study, teaching, and practice of pediatrics. Facilitates communication and cooperation among members; supports research in clinical medicine as it relates to resident education.

**★ 5630 ★ Association for Research of Childhood Cancer (AROCC)**
PO Box 251
Buffalo, NY 14225-0251
**Phone:** (716)681-4433
**Email:** odonnell@msn.com
**Website:** http://www.arocc.org
Ann O'Donnell, Pres.

**Fnded:** 1971. **Mem:** 1,000. **Reg. Groups:** 2. **Desc:** Parents who have lost children to various pediatric cancers; persons supporting cancer research. Seeks to fund the expansion and continuation of research in pediatric cancer centers and to provide seed money for pilot projects in cancer research. Offers support to parents of children with cancer. Bestows research and clinical investigation grants; offers research and medical student fellowships. **Pub:** *AROCC–Newsletter*, quarterly. Newsletter. Contains book reviews; donations list; memorial list. • *Parent/Child Handbook*.

**★ 5631 ★ Association of SIDS and Infant Mortality Programs**
c/o MNSID Center, Children's Hospitals and Clinics
2525 Chicago Ave. So.
Minneapolis, MN 55404
**Phone:** (612)813-6285    **Fax:** (612)813-7344
**Email:** kathyfountain@adph.state.al.us
**Website:** http://www.asip1.org
Kathleen Fernbach, Contact

**Fnded:** 1987. **Mem:** 110. **Desc:** Health and human services professionals who provide support services to those affected by Sudden Infant Death Syndrome (SIDS). Represents SIDS information and counseling services at the national, state, and international levels. Acts as an advocate for continued developmental and expansion of SIDS and bereavement services. Organizes activities which promote professional growth, develops practice standards and links together practitioners working with SIDS families. Supports research. **Pub:** *SIDs and Sleeping Position: Counseling Implications*, annual. Newsletter. • *Standards of Service*. **Frmly:** (1998) Association for SIDS Program Professionals.

**Association of Workers for Children with Emotional and Behavioural Difficulties**
*See:* Entry 12410

**★ 5632 ★ Ataxia Telangiectasia Children's Project**
668 S Military Tr.
Deerfield Beach, FL 33442
**Email:** info@atcp.org
**Website:** http://www.atcp.org/mission_of_the_a.htm

**Fnded:** 1993. **Desc:** Supports laboratory research to accelerate the discovery of a cure or possible therapies for Ataxia Telangiectasia; develops and maintains international registry of A-T patients; supports and oversees clinical center and information clearinghouse; maintains a tissue/cell bank; develops quantitative endpoints for measuring the rate and severity of the symptoms of A-T.

★ **5633** ★ **Athletics and Entertainers for Kids**

3337 Colorado St.
Long Beach, CA 90814
**Phone:** (562)438-5905          **Free:** 800-933-KIDS
**Fax:** (562)438-9175
**Website:** http://www.aefk.org
Elise Kim, Exec. Dir.

**Fnded:** 1986. **State Groups:** 5. **Desc:** Participants include individuals and corporations concerned about children with catastrophic illnesses, particularly AIDS. Seeks to bring hope to seriously ill children. Provides services to children and their families including: counseling and referral services; community outings; educational rallies. Provides AIDS education and awareness programs and presentations. Conducts hospital and charitable programs; provides placement and children's services. Sponsored by Athletes and Entertainers for Kids. **Pub:** *Financial Report*, annual. Report. • *Heros*, quarterly. Newsletter. **Frmly:** (1998) Ryan White National Teen Education Program.

★ **5634** ★ **Australian College of Pediatrics (ACP)**

34 Gatehouse Str
Parkville, VIC 3052, Australia
**Phone:** 61 3 93474310          **Fax:** 61 93472120
**Email:** acp@cryptic.rch.unimelb.edu.au
**Fnded:** 1956.

**Blind Children's Fund (BCF)**
*See:* Entry 20904

★ **5635** ★ **British Association of Paediatric Surgeons (BAPS)**

c/o Royal College of Surgeons of England
35-43 Lincoln's Innfields
London WC2A 3PN, United Kingdom
**Phone:** 44 207 8696915     **Fax:** 44 171 8696919
**Email:** adminsec@baps.org.uk
**Website:** http://www.baps.org.uk

**Fnded:** 1953. **Mem:** 700. **Lang(s):** English. **Desc:** Pedriatric surgeons, consultants, and trainees. Works to improve the techniques of study, practice, and research in pediatric surgery; fosters professional relations among pediatric surgeons. Sponsors training program. **Pub:** *Journal of Pediatric Surgery*, periodic.

★ **5636** ★ **Bulgarian Pediatric Association**

Katedra po Pediatria
D.Nestorov 11
BG-1431 Sofia, Bulgaria
**Phone:** 359 2 541289          **Fax:** 359 2 521650
**Email:** pediatr@internet-bg.net

**Fnded:** 1961. **Mem:** 960. **Reg. Groups:** 20. **Lang(s):** English. **Desc:** Fosters research in pediatrics, including Immunological, diabetological, neonatological, oncochematology, cardiological and neurological. **Pub:** *Pediatria*, quarterly. Journal. Discusses scientific and practical problems in pediatrics. **Frmly:** Scientific Society of Pediatrics.

★ **5637** ★ **Canadian Association for Adolescent Health (CAAH) (Association canadienne pour la sante des adolescents — ACSA)**

Sainte-Justine Hospital
3175 Cote Ste-Catherine, 7th Fl., 2nd Block
Montreal, QC, Canada H3T 1C5
**Phone:** (514)345-9959          **Fax:** (514)345-4778
**Email:** acsacaah@microtec.ca
**Website:** http://www.acsa-caah.ca/

**Fnded:** 1993. **Mem:** 900. **Desc:** Professionals, students, community workers and organizations. Promotes health, education and well-being of adolescents in Canada at the regional and national level; provides self-advocacy among adolescents or serves as an

advocate for adolescent health issues. **Pub:** *Pro-Teen*. Contains articles of scientific events, description of programs, news, research summaries, clinical facts, original articles, and a section on ethics.

★ **5638** ★ **Canadian Association for Child Neurology (CACN) (Association Canadienne de Neurologie Pediatrique — ACNP)**

c/o Canadian Congress of Neurological Sciences
PO Box 5456, Station A.
Calgary, AB, Canada T2H 1X8
**Phone:** (403)229-9544          **Fax:** (403)229-1661
**Email:** brains@ccns.org
**Website:** http://www.ccns.org/cacnpage.htm

**Fnded:** 1991. **Mem:** 110. **Lang(s):** English, French. **Desc:** Neurologists with an interest in neurological disorders in children. Seeks to advance the practice of child neurology; promotes professional development of members. Serves as a clearinghouse on child neurology; conducts continuing professional education courses; provides support and assistance to research projects. **Pub:** *Canadian Journal of Neurological Sciences*, quarterly. Journal. Contains papers from all branches of neuroscience.

★ **5639** ★ **Canadian Association of Paediatric Surgeons (CAPS) (Association Canadienne de la Chirurgie Pediatrique — ACCP)**

c/o Hopital Sainte-Justine
3175 Ste. Catherine Rd.
Montreal, QC, Canada H3T 1C5
**Phone:** (514)345-4688          **Fax:** (514)345-4964
**Email:** salam.yazbeck@videotron.ca
**Website:** http://www.caps.ca

**Lang(s):** English, French. **Desc:** Pediatric surgeons and other health care professionals with an interest in the field. Seeks to advance the practice of pediatric surgery; promotes professional development of members. Facilitates communication and cooperation among members; makes available continuing professional education courses.

★ **5640** ★ **Canadian Association of Pediatric Nurses (CAPN)**

c/o Montreal Children's Hospital
2300, rue Tupper
Montreal, QC, Canada H3H 1P3
**Phone:** (514)934-8466          **Fax:** (514)934-4355
**Email:** info@children.com
**Website:** http://www.mcgill.ca/mch

**Lang(s):** English, French. **Desc:** Nurses specializing in pediatrics. Promotes professional development of members; seeks to advance the practice of pediatric nursing. Encourages exchange of information among members; makes available continuing professional education courses.

★ **5641** ★ **Canadian Association of Pediatric Surgeons (CAPS)**

c/o Dr. Salam Yazbeck
Hopital Ste. Justine
3175 Cote Ste. Catherine
Montreal, QC, Canada H3T 1C5
**Phone:** (514)345-4688          **Fax:** (514)345-4964
**Email:** salam.yazbeck@videotron.ca
**Website:** http://www.caps.ca

**Fnded:** 1968. **Mem:** 120. **Lang(s):** English, French. **Desc:** Pediatric surgeons and other health care professionals with an interest in pediatric surgery. Seeks to advance the practice of pediatric surgery; works to improve diagnostic, treatment, and research techniques in the field. Facilitates exchange of information among members; conducts research and educational programs. **Pub:** *Capsule*, quarterly. Newsletter.

★ **5642** ★ **Canadian Association of Psychoanalytic Child Therapists**

42 Brookmount Rd.
Toronto, ON, Canada M4L 3N2
**Phone:** (416)690-5464          **Fax:** (416)690-2746
**Email:** capct@interlog.com
**Website:** http://www.interlog.com/~capct/

**Mem:** 65. **Lang(s):** English, French. **Desc:** Child therapists specializing in psychoanalysis. Promotes use of psychoanalysis in child therapy; encourages professional advancement of members. Serves as a forum for the exchange of information among members; conducts continuing professional development courses.

**Canadian Association for School Health (CASH)**
*See:* Entry 2021

★ **5643** ★ **Canadian Child Care Federation (CCCF) (Federation Canadienne des Services de Garde a l'Enfance — FCSGE)**

201-383 Parkdale Ave.
Ottawa, ON, Canada K1Y 4R4
**Phone:** (613)729-1412          **Free:** 800-858-1412
**Email:** cfc@cfc-efc.ca
**Website:** http://www.cfc-efc.ca/cccf

**Fnded:** 1986. **Mem:** 8,000. **Lang(s):** English, French. **Desc:** Child care services and their employees. Promotes increased availability and improved quality of child care services. Provides support and services to members; serves as a clearinghouse on child care; conducts continuing professional development courses for child care personnel.

★ **5644** ★ **Canadian Foundation for the Study of Infant Deaths (CFSID)**

586 Eglinton Ave. E, Ste. 308
Toronto, ON, Canada M4P 1P2
**Phone:** (416)488-3860          **Free:** 800-END-SIDS
**Fax:** (416)488-3864
**Email:** sidsinfo@sidscanada.org
**Website:** http://www.sidscanada.org

**Fnded:** 1973. **Mem:** 125. **Local Groups:** 10. **Lang(s):** English, French. **Desc:** Health care providers, families who have lost a child to sudden infant death syndrome, and other individuals with an interest in SIDS. Provides emotional support to families that have experienced the loss of a child to SIDS. Operates network of support groups; serves as a clearinghouse on SIDS and grief; provides educational programs for general public; conducts fundraising activities benefitting SIDS research projects. **Pub:** *Baby's Breath*, quarterly. Newsletter.

★ **5645** ★ **Canadian Institute of Child Health (CICH) (Institut Canadien de la Sante Infantile — ICSI)**

384 Bank St., Ste. 300
Ottawa, ON, Canada K2P 1Y4
**Phone:** (613)230-8838          **Fax:** (613)230-6654
**Email:** cich@cich.ca
**Website:** http://www.cich.ca

**Fnded:** 1977. **Mem:** 600. **Lang(s):** English, French. **Desc:** Health care providers and other individuals and organizations with an interest in child health. Promotes increased access to quality health services for all children. Serves as a clearinghouse on child health, health services, and related topics; sponsors educational and advocacy activities in areas including children's health, pregnancy, and childbirth.

★ **5646** ★ **Canadian Paediatric Society (CPS) (Societe Canadienne de Pediatrie — SCP)**

100-2204 Walkley Rd.
Ottawa, ON, Canada K1G 4G8
**Phone:** (613)526-9397          **Fax:** (613)526-3332

**Email:** info@csp.ca
**Website:** http://www.cps.ca
**Fnded:** 1922. **Mem:** 1,954. **Lang(s):** English, French. **Desc:** Professional organization of pediatricians serving on committees and sections focusing on adolescent medicine, bioethics, drug therapy, hazardous substances, fetus and newborns, Indian and Inuit health, infectious disease and immunization, injury prevention, paediatric practice, nutrition, and psychological paediatrics. Provides services to Canadian children and to its membership. Serves as an advocate on issues relating to child health and welfare. Provides continuing education for the maintenance of competence of its members. Establishes Canadian standards/guidelines for paediatric care and practice, and promotes the interest of pediatricians. **Pub:** *Clinical Practice Guidelines*, periodic. Paper. • *CPS News*, bimonthly. Newsletter. • *Paediatrics & Child Health*, bimonthly. Journal. • *Well Beings*. Book. • *Your Child's Best Shot: A Parent's Guide to Vaccination*. Book. • Reports. **Frmly:** (1951) Canadian Society for the Study of Diseases of Children.

### ★ 5647 ★ Canadian Society for Mucopolysaccharide and Related Diseases

PO Box 64714
Unionville, ON, Canada L3R 0M9
**Phone:** (905)479-8701      **Free:** 800-667-1846
**Fax:** (905)479-8701
**Email:** lori@mpssociety.ca
**Website:** http://www.mpssociety.ca
**Fnded:** 1984. **Lang(s):** English. **Desc:** Families whose children are affected with lysosomal storage diseases, and other interested individuals. Works to increase public awareness of lysosomal storage diseases. Raises funds for research; provides support for affected families. **Pub:** *The Connection*, quarterly. Newsletter.

### ★ 5648 ★ Candlelighters Childhood Cancer Foundation (CCCF)

3910 Warner St.
Kensington, MD 20895
**Phone:** (301)962-3520      **Free:** 800-366-2223
**Fax:** (301)962-3521
**Email:** info@candlelighters.org
**Website:** http://www.candlelighters.org
Ruth Hoffman, Exec. Dir.
**Fnded:** 1970. **Mem:** 50,000. **Nat'l Groups:** 1. **Local Groups:** 400. **Desc:** Educates, supports, serves and advocates for children and adolescents with cancer, their family members, survivors of childhood cancer, and professionals who work with them. Coordinates a network of more than 400 peer support groups and contacts for parents of children/adolescents with cancer. Offers newsletters, other publications, literature and searches. Makes referrals to volunteers who can assist with health insurance problems, second opinions, and employment issues. Local groups offer meetings at which parents share information and emotional support and hear speakers. Referrals for parent-to-parent visitation, transportation, blood or wig banks, speakers' bureaus, meetings for young people, and bereavement groups. Named for the Chinese proverb, "It is better to light one candle than to curse the darkness." **Pub:** *Bone Marrow Transplant Guide*. Handbook. *Price:* $7.50; Free to families with children with cancer. • *CCCF Bibliography and Resource Guide*, annual. Bibliography. Annotated reviews of books, articles, pamphlets, and videos. *Price:* $5 in U.S.; $8 in Canada and Mexico; $12 all other countries; Free to families with children with cancer. • *CCCF Quarterly Newsletter*, quarterly. Newsletter. Articles, poetry, and reviews pertaining to living with and treating childhood cancer. *Price:* Free-families and health/education professionals. • *Educating the Child with Cancer*. Handbook. *Price:* $7.50; Free to families with children with cancer. • *Know before You Go, The Childhood Cancer Journey*. Handbook. • *The Phoenix*, periodic. Newsletter. For adult survivors of childhood cancer. • *You are not Alone, A Sourcebook for Support Groups for Families of Children with Cancer*. Handbook. • Also publishes basic family

library, publications list, guide to the Americans with Disabilities Act, camp list, and wish fulfillment organizations list. **Frmly:** (1984) Candlelighters Foundation.

### ★ 5649 ★ Child Care Action Campaign (CCAC)

330 7th Ave., 17th Fl.
New York, NY 10001
**Phone:** (212)239-0138      **Fax:** (212)268-6515
**Email:** info@childcareaction.org
**Website:** http://www.childcareaction.org
Elinor Guggenheimer, Founder
**Fnded:** 1983. **Mem:** 3,500. **Desc:** Individuals and organizations interested and active in child care; corporations and financial institutions; labor organizations; editors of leading magazines; leaders in government and representatives of civic organizations. Purposes are to alert the country to the problems of and need for child care services; prepare and disseminate information responsive to inquiries resulting from publicity; analyze existing services and identify gaps; work directly with communities to stimulate the development of local task forces and long-range plans for improved and coordinated services. Promotes development of language skills in child care settings. Has worked to help make liability insurance available for child care providers. **Pub:** *An Employer's Guide to Child Care Consultants*. Focuses on the reasons for using a child care consultant, services that consultants can offer, and how to choose the child care consultant for you. *Price:* $10 for members; $15 for nonmembers. • *Building Links: Developer Initiatives for Financing Child Care*. Covers financing alternatives for child care and examines the ways in which communities have begun to involve real estate developers in child care. *Price:* $15 for members; $25 for nonmembers. • *Child Care ActioNews*, bimonthly. Newsletter. Covers innovations in the field of child care for working parents. Includes calendar of events, legislative update, and resource information. *Price:* Included in membership dues. • *Investing in the Future: Child Care Financing Options for the Public and Private Sectors*. Highlights successful financing models, including grants and loans, bank reinvestment strategies, community initiatives, bonds and pension funds. *Price:* $15 for members; $25 for nonmembers. • *Not Too Small to Care: Small Businesses and Child Care*. Profiles 29 small businesses that have implemented child care benefits: on-or-near-site child care centers, employee subsidies, and parental leave. *Price:* $15 for members; $25 for nonmembers. • *Where They Stand: A Digest of Organizational Policies on Child Care and Education*. Provides a guide to 45 national organizations' policy positions on quality child care, early childhood education, and education reform. *Price:* $15 for members; $25 for nonmembers. • Also publishes resource guides for parents who need help finding appropriate child care services.

### ★ 5650 ★ Child Health Association (CHA)

PO Box 366
Rosny Park, TAS 7018, Australia
**Phone:** 61 3 62314765      **Fax:** 61 3 62314749
**Fnded:** 1917. **Mem:** 400. **State Groups:** 34. **Lang(s):** English. **Desc:** Network of parent groups who work with and for the family, child, and youth health service in Tasmania, Australia. Aims to support parents and enhance the health and wellbeing of children and families. Offers friendship and support; provides information and resources; actively participates and advocates within health services organizations; sponsors pram walking groups, nutrition programs, and playgroups; conducts fundraising for children's items.

### ★ 5651 ★ Child Health Foundation (ICHF)

10630 Little Patuxat Pkwy., Ste. 126
Columbia, MD 21044
**Phone:** (301)596-4514      **Fax:** (410)992-5641
**Email:** chf@erols.com
**Website:** http://www.childhealthfoundation.org
Rosario P. Davison, Dir. of Admin.
**Fnded:** 1985. **Desc:** Addresses significant health issues of children and families, primarily in developing

countries and medically underserved populations in the U.S. Focuses on diarrheal diseases, related social and medical problems of malnutrition, and poverty. Develops and encourages use of simple, low-cost technologies. Conducts health programs in research training in oral rehydration therapies, nutrition, breastfeeding and other lowcost approaches to better health. Operates programs to strengthen research capabilities of institutions in developing countries to enable them to develop and perform research on diseases most prevalent in their own countries. Conducts educational training programs and workshops for: volunteers in disease prevention and simple treatments effective in rural and urban areas. Conducts charitable activities; maintains speakers' bureau. **Pub:** *Cereal-Based Oral Rehydration Therapy Symposium Proceedings*. Journal. • *Child Health Foundation Newsletter*, quarterly. Newsletter. Includes research summaries and foundation information. • *Food-based Oral Rehydration Therapy Report*. • *Proper Nutrition and Hygiene*. • *Training Manual for Treatment and Prevention of Childhood Diarrhea with Oral Rehydration Therapy*. • Annual Report. **Frmly:** International Child Health Foundation; (1994) International Child Health Foundation.

### ★ 5652 ★ Child Life Council (CLC)

11820 Parklawn Dr., Ste. 202
Rockville, MD 20852-2529
**Phone:** (301)881-7090      **Free:** 800-CLC-4515
**Fax:** (301)881-7092
**Email:** clcstaff@childlife.org
**Website:** http://www.childlife.org
Deborah E. Brouse, Exec. Dir.
**Fnded:** 1982. **Mem:** 2,200. **Desc:** Professional organization representing child life personnel, patient activities specialists, and students in the field. Promotes psychological well-being and optimum development of children, adolescents, and their families in health care settings. Works to minimize the stress and anxiety of illness and hospitalization. Addresses professional issues such as program standards, competencies, and core curriculum. Provides resources and conducts research and educational programs. Offers a Job Bank Service listing employment openings. **Pub:** *Child Life Council Bulletin*, quarterly. Bulletin. • *Child Life Programs*, biennial. Directory. • *Making Ethical Decisions in Child Life Practice*. • *Official Documents of the Child Life Council*. • *Program Review Guidelines*. • *Psychosocial Care of Children in Hospitals: A Clinical Practice Manual*. **Frmly:** (1975) Child Life Specialist Committee; (1979) Child Life Activity Study Section; (1982) Child Life Task Force.

### ★ 5653 ★ Child Neurology Society (CNS)

1000 West County Rd. E, Ste. 126
Saint Paul, MN 55112-6966
**Phone:** (651)486-9447      **Fax:** (651)486-9436
**Email:** nationaloffice@childneurologysociety.org
Mary Currey, Exec. Dir.
**Fnded:** 1971. **Mem:** 1,287. **Desc:** Neurologists certified by the American Board of Psychiatry and Neurology and specializing in child neurology; individuals eligible for the certifying examination and those who have made significant contributions to the field of child neurology; individuals enrolled in approved child neurology training programs. To advance child neurology by establishing a scientific forum for professionals in the field; to define areas of pediatric neurological practices and to make known these procedures among professionals and medical students. Promotes interest in the field of child neurology among medical students. Advertises positions available in pediatric neurology. **Pub:** *Annals of Neurology*, monthly. Journal. • Booklets.

### Childhood Cancer Foundation - Candlelighters Canada
*See:* Entry 10148

### Children and Adults With Attention Deficit/Hyperactivity Disorder (CHADD)
*See:* Entry 13976

## ★ 5654 ★ Children of the Night (CN)

**Children of Alcoholics Foundation (COAF)**
*See:* Entry 19266

---

### ★ 5654 ★ Children of the Night (CN)
14530 Sylvan St.
Van Nuys, CA 91411
**Phone:** (818)908-4474          **Free:** 800-551-1300
**Fax:** (818)908-1468
**Email:** cotnll@aol.com
**Website:** http://www.childrenofthenight.org
Dr. Lois Lee, Pres.

**Fnded:** 1979. **Desc:** Provides assistance to children between the ages of 11-17 who are sexually abused and are forced to prostitute on the streets. Children of the night's goal is to mainstream street children into the larger society. Operates a 24-hour toll-free hotline, a street program which travels throughout the Western Region of the United States, and a 24-bed shelter home that also features a private school approved by the California Department of Education. **Pub:** Brochures.

### ★ 5655 ★ Children of Russia
4117 Kahala Ave.
Honolulu, HI 96816
**Phone:** (808)737-5248          **Fax:** (808)737-7806
**Email:** nowen@lava.net
**Website:** http://www.leahi.net/russia

**Fnded:** 2000. **Desc:** Advocates for the children of Russia. Current projects include the collection of art supplies for classes at a children's oncology center; provides a program of social rehabilitation for children suffering from tuberculosis.

### ★ 5656 ★ Children's Blood Foundation (CBF)
333 E 38th, Room 830
New York, NY 10016
**Phone:** (212)297-4336          **Fax:** (212)297-4340
**Email:** info@childrensbloodfoundation.org
**Website:** http://www.childrensbloodfoundation.org
William J. Horan, Exec. Dir.

**Fnded:** 1952. **Reg. Groups:** 1. **Desc:** Seeks to raise funds to combat diseases of the blood in children, such as leukemia, hemophilia, thalassemia (Cooley's anemia), childhood cancers, sickle cell, and other anemias and diseases of the immune system, and AIDS. Supports a total patient care center in the New York Hospital-Cornell Medical Center, which includes diagnostic and treatment clinics, progressive research laboratories, and intensive training of physicians in the specialty of pediatric hematology/oncology. Also sponsors specialized social events.

**Children's Brain Tumor Foundation (CBTF)**
*See:* Entry 10149

**Children's Craniofacial Association (CCA)**
*See:* Entry 7953

### ★ 5657 ★ Children's Healthcare Is a Legal Duty (CHILD)
PO Box 2604
Sioux City, IA 51106
**Phone:** (712)948-3500          **Fax:** (712)948-3704
**Email:** childinc@netins.net
**Website:** http://www.childrenshealthcare.org
Dr. Rita Swan, Pres.

**Fnded:** 1983. **Mem:** 450. **Desc:** Advocate for the provision of healthcare for all children; opposes child abuse and neglect related to religion or cultural tradition. **Pub:** *CHILD, Inc. Newsletter*, quarterly. Newsletter. *Price:* Included in membership dues; $25/year for nonmembers. • *Children, Medicine, Religion and the Law.* Reprint. *Price:* $5. • *Cry, the Beloved Children.* Booklet. *Price:* $2. **AKA:** CHILD, Inc.

### ★ 5658 ★ Children's Health Fund
317 E 64th St.
New York, NY 10021
**Phone:** (212)535-9400          **Fax:** (212)535-7488
**Email:** lseim@chfund.org
**Website:** http://www.childrenshealthfund.org
Irwin Redlener, MD, Pres.

**Fnded:** 1987. **Desc:** Supports pediatric programs for children who are homeless, poor, or have no other access to medical care. Maintains Children's Health Projects in urban and rural areas throughout the United States. Provides mobile medical units in order to bring health care to underserved children.

### ★ 5659 ★ Children's Heart Association for Support and Education (CHASE)
Hospital for Sick Children
Cardiac Clinic
Division of Cardiology
Toronto, ON, Canada M5G 1X8
**Phone:** (416)410-2427
**Website:** http://www.angelfire.com/on/chase

**Fnded:** 1983. **Mem:** 550. **Lang(s):** English, French. **Desc:** Parents of children with congential heart defects. Works to improve the quality of life of children with cardiological problems and their families. Maintains network of support groups for members; encourages exchange of information among members and between members and cardiologists; conducts social and educational activities; works to increase public awareness of pediatric cardiology. Provides support and assistance to the Hospital for Sick Children's Division of Pediatric Cardiology. **Pub:** *Straight from the Heart*, monthly. Newsletter.

### ★ 5660 ★ Children's HeartLink (CHL)
5075 Arcadia Ave.
Minneapolis, MN 55436-2306
**Phone:** (612)928-4860          **Fax:** (612)928-4859
**Email:** info@childrensheartlink.org
**Website:** http://www.childrensheartlink.org
Claudia Liebrecht, Pres.

**Fnded:** 1969. **Reg. Groups:** 1. **Desc:** Medical charity and service agency. Advocates the prevention and treatment of heart disease in needy children throughout the world; helps selected developing countries expand and improve their cardiac services for children. Provides: treatment for needy children with heart disease; support for rheumatic fever prevention programs; education and training opportunities for foreign physicians, nurses, and other medical professionals; technical advice and problem-solving assistance; medical equipment and supplies. Organizes fund-raising events. **Pub:** *Heartbeat*, 3/year. Newsletter. *Price:* Free. **Frmly:** (1994) Children's Heart Fund.

### ★ 5661 ★ Children's Hospice International (CHI)
901 N Pitt St., No. 230
Alexandria, VA 22314
**Phone:** (703)684-0330          **Free:** 800-24-CHILD
**Fax:** (703)684-0226
**Email:** chiorg@aol.com
**Website:** http://www.chionline.org
Ann Armstrong Dailey, Founding Dir.

**Fnded:** 1983. **Mem:** 700. **Desc:** Physicians, nurses, teachers, social workers, clergy, psychologists, art and music occupational therapists, volunteers, and students who work or are interested in hospice programs. Objectives are to: promote hospice support through pediatric care facilities; encourage the inclusion of children in existing and developing hospices and home care programs; include hospice perspectives in all areas of pediatric care and education. Supports health care agencies that engage in the treatment of terminally ill children and their families. Disseminates information concerning support groups and research, education, and training programs. Children's hospice care involves an interdisciplinary team of physicians, social workers, nurses, clergy, therapists, teachers and trained volunteers; parents act as primary caregivers. **Pub:** *Approaching Grief*. Pamphlet. • *Children's Hospice/Home Care*. Manual. • *Children's*

*Hospice International–Newsletter*, quarterly. Newsletter. Contains calendar of events and list of resources. *Price:* Included in membership dues; $20/year for nonmembers. • *Home Care for Seriously Ill Children: A Manual for Parents*. Manual. • *Palliative Pain and Symptom Management for Children and Adolescents*. • *The Psychological Aspects of Pain and Symptom Management.* • Audiotapes. • Videos.

### ★ 5662 ★ Children's Medical Ministries (CMM)
PO Box 3382
Crofton, MD 21114
**Phone:** (301)261-3211          **Fax:** (301)721-4647
**Email:** childmed@olg.com
**Website:** http://www.childmed.org/

**Fnded:** 1988. **Mem:** 700. **Desc:** Committed to serving the poor and needy children by offering health care, nutritional support, and dental care.

### ★ 5663 ★ Children's Organ Transplant Association (COTA)
2501 COTA Dr.
Bloomington, IN 47403
**Phone:** (812)336-8872          **Free:** 800-366-2682
**Fax:** (812)336-8885
**Email:** jennifer@cota.org
**Website:** http://www.cota.org/
Richard E. Lofgren, Pres.

**Fnded:** 1986. **Mem:** 550. **Desc:** Dedicated to ensuring that no U.S. child is ever denied a life-saving transplant, or access to a transplant waiting list, due solely to lack of funds; promotes organ donations and provides public education on all aspects of the organ donation process. **Pub:** *Life-Giving Report*, quarterly. Newsletter.

### ★ 5664 ★ Christina Noble Foundation - Vietnam (CNF)
38 Tu Xuong
District 3
PO Box 1289, Post Office Center
Ho Chi Minh City, Vietnam
**Phone:** 84 8 222276          **Fax:** 84 8 90784
**Email:** info@cncf.org
**Website:** http://www.cncf.org

**Fnded:** 1991. **Desc:** Individuals interested in child health. Seeks to improve the quality of life of children in Vietnam. Makes available primary health care services; conducts nutrition programs; sponsors educational and vocational training programs. Maintains center for abandoned children.

### ★ 5665 ★ Clayton Fund
c/o Cycle News
2201 Cherry Ave.
Long Beach, CA 90806
**Phone:** (714)216-4513
**Website:** http://www.usmarshalls.org/injured.html
Charlene Slack, Contact

**Desc:** Strives to fund programs related to children, the environment, family planning, education, agriculture, arts and culture.

**Coeliac Society of the United Kingdom (CSUK)**
*See:* Entry 9111

**Colombian Institute of Pediatric Oncology (Instituto Colombiano de Oncologia Pediatrica)**
*See:* Entry 10152

### ★ 5666 ★ Confederation of European Specialists in Pediatrics (CESP)
Pediatric Intensive Care Unit
Laarbeeklaan 101
B-1090 Brussels, Belgium
**Phone:** 32 2 4775172          **Fax:** 32 2 4775179

**Email:** pedrtj@az.vub.ac.be
**Website:** http://www.uems.be

**Fnded:** 1959. **Mem:** 70. **Nat'l Groups:** 12. **Lang(s):** English, French. **Desc:** Representatives of professional associations of member nations of the European Union and SEFTA countries. Purpose is to coordinate the practice of and training in pediatric medicine within the EEC; promotes development of the European Academy of Pediatrics. **Pub:** *Report of Annual Meeting.* • Newsletter, quarterly.

### ★ 5667 ★ Council for Professional Recognition
2460 16th St. NW
Washington, DC 20009-3575
**Phone:** (202)265-9090        **Free:** 800-424-4310
**Fax:** (202)265-9161
**Email:** webmaster@cdacouncil.org
**Website:** http://www.cdacouncil.org
Dr. Carol Brunson Day, Pres. and CEO

**Fnded:** 1985. **Desc:** Promotes availability of quality child care through the Child Development Associate National Credentialing Program. Credentials are awarded to family child care, center-based infant/toddler and preschool caregivers, and home visitors. Offers annual training program, the CDA Professional Preparation Program. **Pub:** *Council News and Views,* 3/year. Newsletter. • *Essentials.* • *Improving Child Care Through the Child Development Associate Program.* Book. **AKA:** CDA National Credentialing Program. **Frmly:** (1987) Child Development Associate National Credentialing Program; (1999) Council for Early Childhood Professional Recognition.

### ★ 5668 ★ Craniosynostosis and Positional Plagiocephaly Support (CAPPS)
c/o Jennifer Pitchke
6905 Xandu Ct.
Fredericksburg, VA 22407-2580
**Free:** 877-686-2277
**Email:** cappsorg@aol.com
**Website:** http://caps2000.org.cnchost.com/
Jennifer Pitchke, Pres. /Dir.

**Fnded:** 1999. **Desc:** Provides support and information to families with children suffering from craniosynostosis and positional plagiocephaly. Committed to increasing awareness through education, and to ensure proper diagnosis and appropriate treatment for children afflicted with these conditions.

### ★ 5669 ★ CVSA USA/Canada
3585 Cedar Hill Rd. NW
Canal Winchester, OH 43110
**Phone:** (614)837-2586        **Fax:** (614)837-2586
**Email:** waitesd@cvsaonline.org
**Website:** http://www.cvsaonline.org
Debra Waites, Exec. Dir.

**Fnded:** 1993. **Mem:** 700. **Reg. Groups:** 11. **Desc:** Individuals suffering from Cyclic Vomiting Syndrome (CVS), their families, and interested medical professionals. CVS is a rare disorder that usually affects children ages 3-7, and is characterized by recurrent, prolonged attacks of unexplained nausea and vomiting. Promotes medical research on CVS, and seeks to raise public awareness about CVS. Encourages support and information exchange among members. Acts as an information clearinghouse. **Pub:** Newsletter, semiannual. *Price:* Available to members only. **Frmly:** (1999) Cyclic Vomiting Syndrome Association.

### Cystinosis Foundation (CF)
*See:* Entry 9318

### ★ 5670 ★ Daycare Trust (NCCCDCT)
21 St. George's Rd.
London SE1 6ES, United Kingdom
**Phone:** 44 207 78403350   **Fax:** 44 207 78403355
**Email:** info@daycaretrust.org.uk
**Website:** http://www.daycaretrust.org.uk

**Fnded:** 1986. **Lang(s):** English. **Desc:** Promotes the development of quality, affordable, accessible, and equitable child care. Works to improve child care nationwide through: dissemination of information; negotiations with politicians, administrators, and trade unions; and cooperation with other voluntary organizations having similar goals. Provides free childcare information to parents. **Pub:** *Checkout Childcare.* • *Childcare Now,* quarterly. Magazine. • *Childwise,* periodic. Pamphlet. • *Daycare Trust,* periodic. Pamphlet. • *The Family-Friendly Employer: Examples from Europe.* • *Reaching First Base.* Refugees' access to series for children. • Videos. **Frmly:** (2000) National Childcare Campaign/Daycare Trust.

### Dysautonomia Foundation
*See:* Entry 13984

### ★ 5671 ★ Dyspraxia Association of Ireland
Capri
5 Blackglen Ct.
Sandyford
Dublin, Ireland
**Email:** dys212@aol.com
**Website:** http://indigo.ie/~dyspraxi/

**Fnded:** 1995. **Lang(s):** English. **Desc:** Parents of children with dyspraxia. Seeks to raise awareness of dyspraxia in Ireland and to create a better understanding of the difficulties children and parents face. Ensures adequate professional and medical resources are available to parents; provides information and a support network; works to improve diagnostic services.

### ★ 5672 ★ Erb's Palsy Association of Ireland
Canrawer
Oughterard, Galway, Ireland
**Phone:** 353 91 552623
**Email:** info@erbspalsy.ie
**Website:** http://www.erbspalsy.ie
**Mem:** 125. **Lang(s):** English. **Desc:** Parents of children born with Erb's Palsy. Seeks to raise awareness of and provide information on Erb's Palsy, a childbirth injury causing temporary and sometimes permanent paralysis in the arm.

### European Academy of Childhood Disability (EACD)
*See:* Entry 7983

### European Association of Multidisciplinary Practice in Child, Adolescent and Family Mental Health
(Association Europeene de Pratiques Multidisciplinaires en Sante Mentale de l'Enfant, l'Adolescent et de la Familie)
*See:* Entry 12465

### ★ 5673 ★ European Association for Nutrition and Child Development Studies
(Association Europeene pour l'Etude de l'Alimentation et du Developpement de l'Enfant)
Hopital Trousseau
26 avenue Dr. Arnold Netter
F-75012 Paris, France
**Phone:** 33 1 43461390        **Fax:** 33 1 43467800
**Email:** henri.szliwowski@ulb.ac.be

**Lang(s):** English, French. **Desc:** Physicians, nutritionists, and other individuals with an interest in nutrition and child development. Promotes increased understanding of the role played by nutrition in child development. Serves as a forum for the exchange of information among members; conducts public education courses to raise awareness of the importance of nutrition to health child development; sponsors research programs.

### European Association for Studies on Nutrition and Child Development (ADE)
(Association Europeenne pour l'Etude de l'Alimentation et du Developpement de l'Enfant — ADE)
*See:* Entry 16476

### ★ 5674 ★ European Blue Cross Youth Association (EBY)
Stenkullavn 3
61160 Nykoping, Sweden
**Phone:** 46 155 266206        **Fax:** 36 155 266206
**Email:** ulrika_hagen@hotmail.com

**Fnded:** 1979. **Mem:** 5. **Nat'l Groups:** 5. **Lang(s):** English. **Desc:** National societies in Germany, Great Britain, Norway, Sweden, and Switzerland representing 12,000 individuals. Purpose is to enhance cooperation among groups working with young people with substance abuse problems. Sponsors seminars, educational programs, camp sessions, student trips, and youth exchange programs.

### ★ 5675 ★ European Board of Pediatrics (EBP)
Laarbeeklaan 101
B-1090 Brussels, Belgium
**Phone:** 32 2 4775179        **Fax:** 32 2 4775172
**Email:** pedrtj@az.vub.ac.be

**Fnded:** 1994. **Desc:** Promotes education of European pediatricians, tries to improve the quality of pediatric care.

### European Federation of Child Neurology Societies (EFCNS)
*See:* Entry 13996

### European Pediatric Neurology Society
*See:* Entry 14000

### European Pediatric Orthopedic Society (EPOS)
*See:* Entry 16929

### ★ 5676 ★ European Society of Child and Adolescent Psychiatry (ESCAP)
(Societe Europeene de Psychiatrie de l'Enfant et de l'Adolescent — SEPEA)
c/o Prof. H. van Engeland
Academisch Ziekenhuis Utrecht
Kinder en Jeugdpsychiatrie
Postbus 85500
NL-3508 GA Utrecht, Netherlands
**Phone:** 31 30 2506362        **Fax:** 31 30 2505444
**Email:** h.vanengeland@psych.azu.nl

**Fnded:** 1954. **Mem:** 28. **Lang(s):** English, French, German. **Desc:** National societies. **Pub:** *European Child and Adolescent Psychiatry,* quarterly. Journal.

### European Society for Developmental Pharmacology (ESDP)
*See:* Entry 17338

### European Society of Paediatric Gastroenterology, Hepatology and Nutrition (ESPGHAN)
*See:* Entry 9122

### ★ 5677 ★ European Society of Paediatric Otorhinolaryngology
2 Via Belpoggio
I-34123 Trieste, Italy
**Phone:** 39 40 304798
**Email:** fiorfior@tin.it

**Website:** http://www.eur.nl/fgg/kno/ACTIF/espo.htm
**Fnded:** 1997. **Mem:** 250. **Lang(s):** English, French, German, Italian. **Desc:** Pediatric otorhinolaryngologists. Promotes the advancement of pediatric otorhinolaryngology (ORL), the prevention and control of disorders of the ear, nose, and throat. Conducts research and disseminates information. **Pub:** Newsletter, semiannual.

**European Society of Paediatric Radiology (ESPR)**
*See:* Entry 18141

**★ 5678 ★ European Society for Pediatric Endocrinology (ESPE)**
c/o Dr. Martin Savage
Division of Paediatric Endocrinology
St. Bartholomew's Hospital
London EC1A 7BE, United Kingdom
**Phone:** 44 207 6018468     **Fax:** 44 207 2622743
**Email:** secretariat@europe.org
**Website:** http://www.eurospe.org
**Fnded:** 1961. **Mem:** 450. **Lang(s):** English. **Desc:** Pediatricians, medical practitioners, and scientific staff in 28 countries involved in research and clinical practice of pediatric endocrinology. Promotes discussion and collaboration in the field. Operates summer school for pediatric endocrinologists in training. **Pub:** *Hormone Research*, monthly. • *Membership Directory*, annual. • *Program of Annual Meeting*, annual.

**★ 5679 ★ European Society of Pediatric and Neonatal Intensive Care (ESPNIC)**
78, rue de General Leclerc
F-94275 Bicetre, France
**Phone:** 33 1 45213205     **Fax:** 33 1 45212255
**Email:** d.devictor@bct.ap-hop-paris.fr
**Fnded:** 1986. **Desc:** Stimulates pediatric and neonatal intensive care through promotion of activities, fostering research and education.

**★ 5680 ★ European Society for Pediatric Nephrology (ESPN)**
c/o Prof. Jochen Ehrich
Children's Hospital
Hanover Medical School
Carl Neuberg Str. 1
D-30625 Hannover, Germany
**Phone:** 49 5115323212     **Fax:** 49 5115323911
**Email:** kindernephrologie@mh-hannover.de
**Website:** http://www.uwcm.ac.uk/uwcm/ch/espn/
**Fnded:** 1967. **Mem:** 320. **Lang(s):** English. **Desc:** Pediatricians and medical scientists in 26 countries involved in pediatric nephrology. Promotes knowledge of and research on childhood renal disease. Coordinates international studies and disseminates information on pediatric nephrology. **Pub:** *Abstract of Communications*, annual. • *News Letter*, semiannual. • *Pediatric Nephrology*. Journal.

**European Society of Pediatric Otorhinolaryngology (ESPO)**
*See:* Entry 2099

**European Union of Paediatric Surgical Associations (EUPSA)**
*See:* Entry 19555

**★ 5681 ★ Every Child by Two**
c/o Amy Pisani
666 11th St., NW, Ste. 202
Washington, DC 20001-4542
**Phone:** (202)783-7034     **Fax:** (202)783-7042
**Email:** info@ecbt.org
**Website:** http://www.ecbt.org
Amy Pisani, Exec. Dir.
**Fnded:** 1981. **Desc:** Campaigns for early immunization. Visit health departments, hospitals, and schools nationwide to promote timely immunizations. Works to

raise awareness and foster a systematic way to ensure the health of all America's children. Targets community leaders of service organizations for assistance. Compiles statistics. Sponsors educational programs and children's services. **Pub:** *Every Child By Two*, quarterly. Newsletter.

**Fathers Network (NFN)**
*See:* Entry 6883

**★ 5682 ★ Federation of Families for Children's Mental Health (FFCMH)**
1101 King St., Ste. 420
Alexandria, VA 22314
**Phone:** (703)684-7710     **Fax:** (703)836-1040
**Email:** ffcmh@ffcmh.org
**Website:** http://www.ffcmh.org
Gail B. Daniels, Pres.
**Fnded:** 1987. **Mem:** 6,300. **Nat'l Groups:** 122. **Desc:** Parents, children, and mental health and related professionals. Seeks to ensure the rights to full citizenship, support, and access to services for children and youth with mental disorders and their families. Provides leadership in the field of children's mental health care and services; works to address the needs of children and youth with emotional, behavioral, and mental disorders. Gathers and disseminates information on mental illness and mental health care and services; conducts educational and training programs; makes available support, referral, and transition services to children and youth with mental disorders and their families. Maintains speakers' bureau. **Pub:** *Claiming Children*, quarterly. Newsletter.

**Foundation for the Children's Oncology Group (NCCF)**
*See:* Entry 10170

**★ 5683 ★ Fundacion Antidrogas de El Salvador**
71 S Ave. and Olympic Ave. No. 3718
Colonia Step.
San Salvador, El Salvador
**Phone:** 503 982233     **Fax:** 503 234873
**Email:** fundasalva@ejje.com
**Website:** http://www.fundasalva.org.sv
**Fnded:** 1989. **Mem:** 50. **Lang(s):** Spanish. **Desc:** Works to prevent substance abuse among at-risk children and youths. Conducts activities for at-risk youths in urban areas; makes available services for young people attempting to quit abusing substances.

**★ 5684 ★ Gift from the Heart Foundation**
2653 N Narragansett
Chicago, IL 60639
**Phone:** (773)237-4800     **Fax:** (773)237-1221
**Email:** giftheart@att.net
**Website:** http://www.giftfromtheheart.org
Krystyna B. Pasek, Pres.
**Fnded:** 1988. **Nat'l Groups:** 1. **Local Groups:** 1. **Desc:** Works to assist seriously ill children around the world by obtaining information regarding medical care. Provides food, lodging, transportation, and interpreters for children and their accompanying parents. Purchases rehabilitation equipment. Provides charitable programs and various social activities. **Pub:** *Gift From the Heart Foundation*, triennial. Brochure. Regular charitable organization's pamphlet. *Price:* Free. • *Gift from the Heart Foundation's Newletter*, semiannual. Newsletter. **Frmly:** (1992) Dar Serca.

**★ 5685 ★ Girls and Boys Town**
c/o Father Val. J. Peter
Boys Town Center
Boys Town, NE 68010
**Free:** 800-448-3000
**Website:** http://www.girlsandboystown.org/hotline/index.htm
Father Val J. Peter, Contact

**Desc:** Provides a 24-hour hotline available to children and parents.

**★ 5686 ★ Hospital Organization of Pedagogues in Europe (HOPE)**
100 Knightlow Rd.
Harborne
Birmingham B17 8QA, United Kingdom
**Phone:** 44 121 4291561     **Fax:** 44 121 4291561
**Email:** cogels@pedi.ucl.ac.be
**Website:** http://www.connect-to-hope.org
**Fnded:** 1988. **Mem:** 350. **Desc:** Aims to establish the rights of children in hospitals to receive an appropriate education to their individual needs, in a suitable adapted environment. Ensures the continuity of this education during convalescent.

**★ 5687 ★ Human Growth Foundation (HGF)**
997 Glen Cove Ave.
Glen Head, NY 11545-1584
**Free:** 800-451-6434     **Fax:** (516)671-0455
**Email:** hgf1@hgfound.org
**Website:** http://www.hgfound.org/
Patricia D. Costa, Exec. Dir.
**Fnded:** 1965. **Mem:** 1,000. **Nat'l Groups:** 30. **Desc:** Families of children with physical growth problems and interested persons united to help medical science better understand the process of growth. Distributes money for basic and clinical growth research. Disseminates informative literature and presents educational programs to families and physicians. **Pub:** *Fourth Friday*, quarterly. Newsletter. • *Growth Series*. Brochure. **Frmly:** (1971) Human Growth.

**Indian Association of Paediatric Surgeons (IAPS)**
*See:* Entry 19560

**★ 5688 ★ Interamerican Association of Pediatric Otolaryngology (IAPO)**
c/o Dr. Eavey
243 Charles St.
Boston, MA 02114-3002
**Email:** santoshjk@yahoo.com
Dr. Eavey, Contact
**Fnded:** 1996. **Mem:** 2,000. **Desc:** Pediatric Otolaryngologists.

**★ 5689 ★ International Academy for Child Brain Development (IACBD)**
8801 Stenton Ave.
Glenside, PA 19038
**Phone:** (215)233-2050     **Fax:** (215)233-1530
**Email:** institutes@iahp.org
**Website:** http://www.iahp.org
Neil Harvey, PhD, Sec.
**Fnded:** 1985. **Desc:** Professionals from a variety of disciplines including physicians, psychologists, and anthropologists, who are interested in the physical and psychological processes involved in child brain development. Seeks to gain recognition for the study of child brain development as a discipline in itself and establish criteria for the certification of child brain developmentalists. Provides a forum for presentation of scholarly works in the field; offers courses in child-brain development; conducts field research and prepares reports of results. **Pub:** *The In-Report*, quarterly. Journal.

**★ 5690 ★ International Association for Adolescent Health (IAAH)**
c/o Section Medecine de l'Adoescence
Hopital Sainte-Justine
3175 Cote Ste.-Catherine
Montreal, QC, Canada H3T 1C5
**Fax:** (514)345-4778
**Email:** president@iaah.org
**Website:** http://www.iaah.org/files/iaah.htm

**Fnded:** 1987. **Mem:** 330. **Desc:** Aims to foster wider understanding of the importance of youth health in each region of the world; to encourage interaction and co-operation between youth and non-youth and between organizations and individuals on youth health issues.

### ★ 5691 ★ International Association for Child and Adolescent Psychiatry and Allied Professions (IACAPAP)

PO Box 207900
New Haven, CT 06520-7900
**Phone:** (203)785-5759          **Fax:** (203)785-7402
**Email:** donald.cohen@yale.edu
**Website:** http://www.iacapap.org
Donald J. Cohen, MD, Pres.

**Fnded:** 1948. **Mem:** 50. **Nat'l Groups:** 50. **Desc:** National societies; others in the field of child and adolescent psychiatry and allied professions. Promotes collaboration among related professions including pediatrics, psychology, public health, social work, education, nursing, and others involved in research and practice in the field of child and adolescent psychiatry. **Pub:** *IACAPAP Newsletter*, quarterly. Newsletter. • Monograph, semiannual. **AKA:** Association Internationale de Psychiatrie de l'Enfant et de l'Adolescent et des Professions Associees. **Frmly:** (1978) International Association for Child Psychiatry and Allied Professions.

### International Association for Gastrointestinal Motility in Children (GIMIC)

*See:* Entry 9134

### ★ 5692 ★ International Association of Infant Massage (IAIM)

1891 Goodyear Ave., Ste. 622
Ventura, CA 93003
**Phone:** (805)644-8524          **Free:** 800-248-5432
**Fax:** (805)644-7699
**Email:** iaim4us@aol.com
**Website:** http://www.iaim-us.com
Susan Campbell, Business Admin.

**Fnded:** 1981. **Mem:** 3,000. **Nat'l Groups:** 1. **Desc:** Parents, caregivers. Works to promote nurturing touch, positive interactive contact, and communication through massage. Trains and certifies individuals to teach parents and caregivers to massage their babies. **Pub:** *Tender Loving Care*, semiannual. Newsletter.

### International Association for Maternal and Neonatal Health (IAMENEH)

*See:* Entry 16687

### International Association of Paediatric Dentistry (IAPD)

*See:* Entry 6547

### ★ 5693 ★ International Child Care - Canada (ICC)

2476 Argentia Rd. Ste. 113
Mississauga, ON, Canada L5N 6M1
**Phone:** (905)821-6318          **Free:** 888-72-CHILD
**Fax:** (905)821-6319
**Email:** canada@intlchildcare.org
**Website:** http://www.gospelcom.net/icc/
**Fnded:** 1966. **Lang(s):** English, French. **Desc:** Health care personnel. Promotes global availability of community-based health care, with emphasis on the prevention of tuberculosis, maternal and child health, and provision of primary health care services. Cooperates with local administrative bodies to strengthen public health programs in the Dominican Republic and Haiti. Conducts primary health care and immunization services. Sponsors health care training courses for people living in underserved areas.

### International Chiropractic Pediatric Association (ICPA)

*See:* Entry 5935

### International Federation of Hard of Hearing Young People (IFHOHYP)

*See:* Entry 6059

### ★ 5694 ★ International Federation of Infantile and Juvenile Gynecology (IFIJG)
### (Federation Internationale de Gynecologie Infantile et Juvenile — FIGIJ)

c/o George Creatsas
9 Kanari St.
GR-106 71 Athens, Greece
**Phone:** 30 1 7286353          **Fax:** 30 1 7233330
**Email:** geocze@azetaieio.uooc.gz

**Fnded:** 1972. **Mem:** 3,850. **Nat'l Groups:** 40. **Lang(s):** English, French, German. **Desc:** Gynecologists and pediatricians in 43 countries. Promotes the diagnosis and treatment of gynecological problems during childhood and adolescence. Maintains the FIGO Joint Committee for the Study of Gynecological Problems in Childhood and Adolescence. **Pub:** *Gynecologie*, periodic. Magazine. • *Pediatric and Adolescent Gynecology*, periodic. Newsletter.

### ★ 5695 ★ International Nanny Association (INA)

Membership Services Office
900 Haddon Ave., Ste. 438
Collingswood, NJ 08108-2101
**Phone:** (856)858-0808          **Free:** 800-297-1477
**Fax:** (856)858-2519
**Email:** ina@nanny.org
**Website:** http://www.nanny.org
Pat Cascio, Pres.

**Fnded:** 1985. **Mem:** 700. **Nat'l Groups:** 1. **Desc:** An educational association for nannies and those who educate, place, employ, and support professional in-home child care. Membership is open to those who are directly involved with the in-home child care profession, including nannies, nanny employers, nanny placement agency owners (and staff), nanny educators, and providers of special services related to the nanny profession. **Pub:** *A Nanny for Your Family.* Brochure. *Price:* $0.30/each for members; $0.40/each for nonmembers. • *Beyond Peanut Butter and Jelly.* *Price:* $19.95 + 4.95 shipping. • *Directory of Nanny Placement Agencies, Training Programs and Special Services*, annual. Directory. *Price:* $19.95/year. • *Family and Nanny Agreement. Price:* $50. • *INA Vision.* Newsletter. *Price:* Included in membership dues. • *Recommended Competencies for the Education of Nurses.* • *Recommended Practices for Nannies.* • *Recommended Practices for Nanny Placement Agencies.* • *So You Want to Be a Nanny.* Brochure. *Price:* $0.30/each for members; $0.40/each for nonmembers.

### ★ 5696 ★ International Paediatric Pathology Association

c/o Dr. A.J. Bourne
Women's and Children's Hospital
North Adelaide, SA 5006, Australia
**Phone:** 61 8 81617318          **Fax:** 61 8 81617022
**Email:** bournet@wch.sa.gov.au

**Fnded:** 1976. **Mem:** 700. **Reg. Groups:** 5. **Desc:** Works throughout the world to facilitate increased knowledge of diseases of the embryo, fetus, infant, and child.

### ★ 5697 ★ International Pediatric Endosurgery Group (IPEG)

2716 Ocean Park Blvd., Ste. 3000
Santa Monica, CA 90405
**Phone:** (310)314-2536          **Fax:** (310)314-2589
**Email:** admin@ipeg.org
**Website:** http://www.ipeg.org

**Desc:** Doctors, surgeons, pediatricians, and those in the medical field. Present materials and articles keeping up to date on pediatric endosurgery and endoscopy, offer open forum for discussions and ideas, and extend support.

### ★ 5698 ★ International Pediatric Nephrology (IPNA)

c/o F. Bruder Stapleton, MD
Children's Hospital and Regional Medical Center
CH-65
4800 Sand Point Way, NU
Seattle, WA 98105
**Phone:** (206)526-2150          **Fax:** (206)527-3836
**Email:** bstaplet@u.washington.edu
F. Bruner Stapleton, MD, Treas.

**Fnded:** 1973. **Mem:** 1,752. **Reg. Groups:** 7. **Desc:** Specialists in children's kidney disease. Purpose is to promote communication and disseminate information among pediatric nephrologists. Maintains training facilities. **Pub:** *Pediatric Nephrology*, monthly. Journal. Peer review journal, peer reviewed original research, clinical data. *Price:* Included with membership dues. • *Proceedings*, triennial. Book.

### ★ 5699 ★ International Rett Syndrome Association (IRSA)

9121 Piscataway Rd.
Clinton, MD 20735
**Phone:** (301)856-3334          **Free:** 800-818-RETT
**Fax:** (301)856-3336
**Email:** irsa@rettsyndrome.org
**Website:** http://www.rettsyndrome.org
Kathy Hunter, Pres.

**Fnded:** 1985. **Mem:** 2,000. **State Groups:** 20. **Desc:** Parents of children with Rett Syndrome; interested professionals and supporters. (A child afflicted with Rett Syndrome, which strikes only females, seems normal until 7 to 18 months of age, when autistic-like withdrawal sets in; though this symptom eases in time, higher brain functions continue to deteriorate, leading to severe retardation. The child also loses purposeful use of her hands, wringing them in a constant "hand-washing" movement in front of the face or chest. The syndrome is named for Dr. Andreas Rett, of Vienna, Austria, who described it in 1966. The cause of Rett Syndrome has been traced to a defective gene, called the MeCP2 on the X chromosome.) Provides support to parents; encourages research; collects and disseminates information. Assists in identifying syndrome victims; conducts activities aimed at the prevention, treatment, and eventual eradication of Rett Syndrome. **Pub:** *Educational and Therapeutic Intervention in Rett Syndrome.* Journal. Explores a variety of treatment strategies & learning approaches, decisions about placement and/or inclusion in classrooms. *Price:* $5 members; $10 non-members. • *International Rett Syndrome Association–Newsletter*, quarterly. Newsletter. *Price:* Included in membership dues. • *Orthopedic Problems in Rett Syndrome.* • *The Parent Idea Book.* • *Rett Sydrome: A Physician's Approach.* Video. • *Rett Syndrome: A Closer Look.* Video. • *Rett Syndrome: A Conversation with Families.* Video. • *Rett Syndrome: A Therapeutic Approach.* Video. • *Rett Syndrome Handbook. Price:* $15 members; $29.95 nonmembers. • *Understanding Rett Syndrome.* • *What is Rett Syndrome.* **Frmly:** (1985) International Rett's Syndrome Association.

### International School Psychology Association

*See:* Entry 12525

### ★ 5700 ★ International Society for Adolescent Psychiatry

150 E 58th St., No. 31
New York, NY 10155-0002
**Phone:** (718)892-4868
**Email:** rlandy7257@aol.com
**Website:** http://www.ispaweb.org/
Rosalie Landy, Admin. Dir.

**Fnded:** 1985. **Mem:** 500. **Desc:** Psychiatrists, psychologists, psychoanalysts, social workers, sociologists, pediatricians, educators, and health care professionals involved in the treatment of adolescents. Seeks to advance treatment of psychiatric illnesses of adolescents. Maintains research and educational programs. **Pub:** *International Annals of Adolescent Psychiatry*, triennial. Monograph. *Price:* Included in membership dues. • Newsletter, 3/year. *Price:* Included in membership dues.


★ 5701 ★ **International Society for Child and Adolescent Injury Prevention (ISCAIP)**
c/o Child Accident Prevention Trust
18-20 Farringdon Ln.
London EC1R 3AU, United Kingdom
**Email:** iscaip@capt.demon.co.uk
**Website:** http://www.iscaip.org/

**Fnded:** 1993. **Desc:** Persons with interest or involvement in prevention of childhood and adolescent injuries. Promotes reduction and severity of injury to children and adolescents; provides multi-disciplinary forum; provides advocacy at national and international levels; fosters national injury prevention initiatives; disseminates research findings and funding opportunities; proposes policy on international basis. **Pub:** *Injury Prevention.* Journal. • Newsletter. Contains information about professional meetings, specialists, and research.


★ 5702 ★ **International Society for Pediatric and Adolescent Diabetes (ISPAD)**
c/o Dr. Knut Dahl-Jorgensen
Ulleval University Hospital
Department of Paediatrics
N-0407 Oslo, Norway
**Phone:** 47 23015577        **Fax:** 47 22894204
**Email:** knut.dahl-jorgensen@ioks.uio.no
**Website:** http://www.ispad.org

**Fnded:** 1974. **Mem:** 700. **Lang(s):** Dutch, English, Finnish, Japanese, Norwegian. **Desc:** Health professionals worldwide who study and treat juvenile diabetes. Promotes improvements in research and clinical care of children and adolescents with diabetes.


★ 5703 ★ **International Society of Pediatric Oncology (SIOP) (Societe Internationale d'Oncologie Pediatrique — SIOP)**
c/o IMEDEX
Bruistensingel 360
PO Box 3283
NL-5203 DG Hertogenbosch, Netherlands
**Phone:** 31 73 6462929
**Email:** imedex@pi.net
**Website:** http://www.siopbrain.org/

**Fnded:** 1969. **Mem:** 955. **Lang(s):** English. **Desc:** Pediatric oncologists, pediatric surgeons involved in oncology, pathologists, radiotherapists, researchers, and others interested in malignant tumors in children. Purpose is to promote research, treatment, and clinical review of cancerous growths in children. Facilitates collaboration and exchange of information among members and others in the field. Organizes and participates in controlled therapeutic trials. **Pub:** *Medical and Pediatric Oncology*, monthly. Journal. • *SIOP Newsletter*, semiannual. Newsletter. • Brochure, periodic.


★ 5704 ★ **International Society of Psychiatric Mental Health Nurses (ISPN)**
1211 Locust St.
Philadelphia, PA 19107
**Phone:** (215)545-2843        **Free:** 800-826-2950
**Fax:** (215)545-8107
**Email:** ispn@nursecominc.com
**Website:** http://www.ispn-psych.org
Kenneth Cleveland, Acct. Exec.

**Fnded:** 1999. **Mem:** 900. **Local Groups:** 25. **Desc:** Psychiatric and mental health nurses. Seeks to advance the study, teaching, and practice of psychiatric and mental health nursing. Represents members' professional and economic interests. **Pub:** *Archives of Psychiatric Nursing*, quarterly. Journal. *Price:* $43/year for nonmembers; included in membership dues. • *ISPN Connections*, 3/year. Newsletter. *Price:* Included in membership dues; $20 for nonmembers. • *Journal of Child and Adolescent Psychiatric Nursing*, quarterly. Journal. *Price:* Included in membership dues; $43 for nonmembers. **Frmly:** (1992) Advocates for Child Psychiatric Nursing; (1999) Association of Child and Adolescent Psychiatric Nurses.


**IVH Parents (IVHP)**
*See:* Entry 4887


**John Tracy Clinic**
*See:* Entry 6066


**Juvenile Diabetes Foundation of Australia (JDFA)**
*See:* Entry 8712


★ 5705 ★ **Juvenile Diabetes Foundation in Israel (JDFI) (Haagudah LeSukereth Neurim Beyisrael)**
10 Blvd. Rothschild
IL-66881 Tel Aviv, Israel
**Phone:** 972 3 5160171        **Fax:** 972 3 5100724
**Email:** jdf_il@netvision.net.il
**Website:** http://www.johntracyclinic.org

**Fnded:** 1981. **Mem:** 2,000. **Lang(s):** English, Hebrew. **Desc:** Strives to improve the situation of children and young adults with Juvenile diabetes in Israel. Conducts fundraising activities and research programs. **Pub:** *Ad-Kan*, semiannual. • *Update*, semiannual. • Newsletter, quarterly.


**Juvenile Diabetes Research Foundation**
*See:* Entry 8713


**Juvenile Diabetes Research Foundation - Hellas**
*See:* Entry 8714


★ 5706 ★ **Juvenile Diabetes Research Foundation International (JDFI)**
120 Wall St.
New York, NY 10005-4001
**Phone:** (212)785-9500        **Free:** 800-533-CURE
**Fax:** (212)785-9595
**Email:** info@jdfcure.org
**Website:** http://www.jdrf.org
Peter Van Etten, Pres.

**Fnded:** 1970. **Mem:** 40,000. **Reg. Groups:** 114. **Desc:** World's leading nonprofit, nongovernmental funder of diabetes research. Mission is to find a cure for diabetes and its complications through the support of research. Sponsors international workshops and conferences for biomedical researchers. Individual chapters offer support groups and other activities for families affected by diabetes. **Pub:** *Countdown*, quarterly. Magazine. Covers diabetes treatment and research. *Price:* $25/year. • Also publishes pamphlets and brochures for diabetics, families, medical personnel, and teachers; produces videotapes. **Frmly:** (1983) Juvenile Diabetes Foundation.


★ 5707 ★ **Juvenile Scleroderma Network (JSDN)**
1204 W 13th St.
San Pedro, CA 90731
**Phone:** (310)519-9511
**Email:** outreachjsdn@aol.com
**Website:** http://www.sclero.org
Kathy Gaither, Contact

**Desc:** Children afflicted with scleroderma, parents and families, doctors. Provide online support, pen-pal programs, information, facts and literature.


★ 5708 ★ **Keren-Or, Inc. (K-OI)**
350 7th Ave., Rm. 200
New York, NY 10001
**Phone:** (212)279-4070        **Fax:** (212)279-4043
**Email:** info@keren-or.org
**Website:** http://www.keren-or.org/
Albert Hornblass, MD, Pres.

**Fnded:** 1956. **Desc:** Maintains the Keren-Or Center for Multi-Disabled Blind Children in Jerusalem for rehabilitation and training which houses more than 70 children and young adults. Funds acquired through public contributions and Israeli government funding. **Pub:** *InSights*, quarterly. Newsletter. **Frmly:** (1987) Jerusalem Institutions for the Blind.


★ 5709 ★ **Kiribati Family Health Association**
c/o Mrs. Katikova Amon
Bedio Hospital
PO Box 509
Tarawa, Kiribati
**Phone:** 686 28749        **Fax:** 686 28728

**Fnded:** 1992. **Mem:** 56. **Desc:** Promotes family planning and general health care. Offers health education programs for new mothers.


★ 5710 ★ **Klingenstein Third Generation Foundation**
787 Seventh Ave., 6th Fl.
New York, NY 10019-6016
**Phone:** (212)492-6179        **Fax:** (212)492-7007
**Email:** sally@ktgf.org
**Website:** http://www.ktgf.org/
Sally Klingenstein, Exec. Dir.

**Desc:** Works to support intervention and referral, prevention, and public education and training relating to childhood and adolescent depression and Attention Deficit Disorder.


**Latin American Society for Pediatric Gastroenterology and Nutrition (Sociedad Latinoamericana de Gastroenterologia Pediatrica y Nutricion — SLAGPN)**
*See:* Entry 9143


★ 5711 ★ **MAGIC Foundation for Children's Growth (MAGIC)**
c/o Mary Andrews
1327 N Harlem Ave.
Oak Park, IL 60302
**Phone:** (708)383-0808        **Free:** 800-3MA-GIC3
**Fax:** (708)383-0899
**Email:** mary@magicfoundation.org
**Website:** http://www.magicfoundation.org
Mary Andrews, Exec. Dir.

**Fnded:** 1989. **Mem:** 10,000. **Local Groups:** 16. **Desc:** Provides support and assistance to families of children with physical growth related disorders. Sponsors educational programs, family networking, and Pen Pal for the Kids service. Maintains speakers' bureau **Pub:** *MAGIC Touch*, quarterly. Newsletter. *Price:* Free with membership. • Brochures. **Frmly:** Major Aspects of Growth in Children Foundation.


**Maternity Alliance - England (MA)**
*See:* Entry 16700


★ 5712 ★ **Medical Officers of Schools Association**
21 St. Botorpa's Rd.
Sevenoaks TN13 3AQ, United Kingdom
**Phone:** 44 1732 459255        **Fax:** 44 1732 750586
**Email:** info@maternityalliance.org.uk
**Website:** http://www.mosa.org.uk

**Fnded:** 1884. **Mem:** 440. **Desc:** School doctors and doctors with an interest in the health of the school child. To represent school doctors and those doctors with an interest in the health of the school child; to provide an advisory service for members, and non-members, on any aspect of school medicine. **Pub:** *Handbook of School Health*, quarterly. Handbook. • Newsletter, quarterly. • Report, annual.

**★ 5713 ★ MSUD Family Support Group (MSUDFSG)**
82 Ravine Rd.
Powell, OH 43065
**Phone:** (740)548-4475
**Email:** msud-support@juno.com
**Website:** http://www.msud-support.org
Sandra Bulcher, Contact

**Fnded:** 1982. **Desc:** Those affected by Maple Syrup Urine Disease (MSUD) and their families; health care professionals. (Maple Syrup Urine Disease usually occurs in infancy and is characterized by a strong odor of the urine, loss of sucking reflex, general list-lessness, episodes of rigidity, and high-pitched crying. If undiagnosed, the condition can progress to seizures, coma and death. Symptoms sometimes do not occur for several months.) Gathers and distributes information on MSUD. Seeks to strengthen the liaison between families and health care professionals. Encourages increased research and newborn screening for MSUD. Sponsors education programs. **Pub:** Brochure. • Newsletter, semiannual. *Price:* $10. • Also publishes information packet. **Frmly:** Families with Maple Syrup Urine Disease.

**★ 5714 ★ National Association of Child Care Professionals**
c/o Sherry Workman
PO Box 90723
Austin, TX 78709-0723
**Phone:** (512)301-5557     **Free:** 800-537-1118
**Fax:** (512)301-5080
**Email:** admin@naccp.org
**Website:** http://www.naccp.org
Sherry Workman, Exec. Dir.

**Fnded:** 1984. **Mem:** 2,662. **State Groups:** 4. **Desc:** Child care supervisors and individuals involved in decision making at a child care facility. Offers networking opportunities and support services to child care professionals. Dedicated to the professional development of child care directors. Conducts educational programs. **Pub:** *Caring for Your Children*, quarterly. Newsletter. Contains information for parents. *Price:* Free. For members only; $39 nonmembers. • *Professional Connections*, bimonthly. Newsletter. Contains management information for directors. • *Team Work*, bimonthly. Newsletter. Directed toward staff members. • Directory.Contains contact information for other child care professionals. • Management Tools of the Trade-Personnel resource management forms specific to child care industry.

**★ 5715 ★ National Association of Child Care Resource and Referral Agencies (NACCRRA)**
1319 F St. NW, Ste. 500
Washington, DC 20004-1106
**Phone:** (202)393-5501     **Fax:** (202)393-1109
**Email:** info@naccrra.org
**Website:** http://www.naccrra.net/
Yasmina Vinci, Exec. Dir.

**Fnded:** 1987. **Mem:** 750. **Reg. Groups:** 8. **State Groups:** 32. **Local Groups:** 600. **Desc:** Network of community-based child care resource and referral programs that promote a diverse, high quality child care system with parental choice that is accessible to all families. National leadership to build such a system; promotes growth and development of quality resource and referral services.

**★ 5716 ★ National Association of Children's Hospitals and Related Institutions (NACHRI)**
401 Wythe St.
Alexandria, VA 22314
**Phone:** (703)684-1355     **Fax:** (703)684-1589
**Website:** http://www.childrenshospitals.net
Louise Baldwin, Contact

**Fnded:** 1968. **Mem:** 149. **Desc:** Children's hospitals and related institutions whose programs are clinical (as opposed to social or custodial). Purposes are: to promote the quality of child health care through the dissemination of information and the promotion of research and education programs related to such care; to participate in related charitable, scientific, and educational endeavors. Conducts surveys and research; disseminates information; maintains computerized services. Compiles statistics. **Pub:** *Childrens Hospitals Today*, quarterly. Magazine.

**National Association of Pediatric Nurse Practitioners (NAPNAP)**
*See:* Entry 15735

**★ 5717 ★ National Association of Psychiatric Treatment Centers for Children (NAPTCC)**
1025 Connecticut Ave. NW, Ste. 1012
Washington, DC 20036
**Phone:** (202)857-9735     **Fax:** (202)362-5145
**Email:** naptcc@aol.com
**Website:** http://www.napnap.org
Joy Midman, Exec. Dir.

**Fnded:** 1983. **Mem:** 80. **Desc:** Treatment centers and programs for children and adolescents with or at risk of serious emotional or behavioral disorders, providing a full array of mental health and related services including residential treatment, partial hospitalization, outpatient treatment, therapeutic foster care, group homes, independent living programs, in-home treatment, intensive case management, and accredited education, special education, and alternative education programs. **Pub:** *Friday Facts*, weekly. • *Member Facilities*, annual. Directory. • Brochures.Contains informational material.

**★ 5718 ★ National Association for Sick Child Daycare (NASCD)**
c/o Hugs & Kisses
1716 5 Ave. N
Birmingham, AL 35203
**Phone:** (205)324-8447     **Fax:** (205)324-8050
**Email:** jackiestewart@nascd.com
**Website:** http://www.nascd.com
Stewart Jacklyn, President

**Fnded:** 1979. **Mem:** 75. **Desc:** Works to promote the establishment of sick child daycare programs nationwide. Conducts educational programs; compiles statistics. **Pub:** *Survey of Sick Child Care Facilities*, quarterly. Newsletter. *Price:* $50 facility; $260 directory; $75 conference synopsis. • Brochure.

**★ 5719 ★ National Association for Support of Parents of Children with Stomas**
c/o John Malcolm, Pres.
51 Anderson Dr.
Valley View Park
Darvel KA17 ODE, United Kingdom
**Phone:** 44 1563 322024
**Email:** john@stoma.freeserve.co.uk

**Fnded:** 1988. **Mem:** 650. **Lang(s):** English. **Desc:** Parents of children suffering from serious bladder and bowel disorders. Provides an information service for parents on the practical day-to-day management of all aspects of coping with a child who has undergone a colostomy, ileostomy, or urostomy and provides advice on the incontinence often encountered with bowel and bladder problems.

**★ 5720 ★ National Center for Education in Maternal and Child Health (NCEMCH)**
2000 15th St. N, Ste. 701
Arlington, VA 22201-2617
**Phone:** (703)524-7802     **Fax:** (703)524-9335
**Email:** info@ncemch.org
**Website:** http://www.ncemch.org

**Fnded:** 1982. **Desc:** Multidisciplinary staff in such diverse fields as pediatrics, public health, law, public policy, social work, psychology, behavioral health, nutrition, nursing, child development, education, communications, library science, and systems technology. Work with a broad range of public and private organizations to develop comprehensive program initiatives to advance the health of children and families. **Frmly:** (2000) Association of Teachers of Maternal and Child Health.

**★ 5721 ★ National Center for Tobacco-Free Kids**
1707 L St., NW, Ste. 800
Washington, DC 20036
**Phone:** (202)296-5469     **Fax:** (202)296-5427
**Email:** info@tobaccofreekids.org
**Website:** http://www.tobaccofreekids.org

**Desc:** People interested in helping keep kids tobacco-free. Fights to protect America's kids from tobacco. Information forum, sponsors Federal initiatives.

**National Center for Youth with Disabilities**
*See:* Entry 8038

**National Certification Board of Pediatric Nurse Practitioners and Nurses (NCBPNP/N)**
*See:* Entry 15745

**★ 5722 ★ National Child Care Association (NCCA)**
1016 Rosser St.
Conyers, GA 30012
**Phone:** (770)922-8198     **Free:** 800-543-7161
**Fax:** (770)388-7772
**Email:** nccallw@mindspring.com
**Website:** http://www.nccanet.org
Lynn White, Exec. Dir.

**Fnded:** 1987. **Mem:** 7,000. **State Groups:** 25. **Desc:** Works to promote and safeguard the interest of quality child care in the United States. Focuses on licensed, private providers of child care and preschool services. Conducts lobbying activities; offers casualty insurance programs; conducts educational and research programs; provides networking opportunities. **Pub:** *National Focus*, quarterly. Newsletter. • *Professional Development Video Series*. Videos.

**★ 5723 ★ National Childminding Association (NCMA)**
8 Masons Hill
Bromley BR2 9EY, United Kingdom
**Phone:** 44 208 4646164     **Fax:** 44 208 2906834
**Email:** info@ncma.org.uk
**Website:** http://www.ncma.org.uk

**Fnded:** 1977. **Mem:** 50,000. **Local Groups:** 1000. **Lang(s):** English. **Desc:** Child care professionals, parents, and interested individuals. Promotes quality day care, recreation, and education for young children and seeks to advance the education of child care professionals. Offers seminars; conducts research. **Pub:** *Who Minds?*, quarterly. Magazine. • Pamphlets, periodic.

**★ 5724 ★ National Children's Eye Care Foundation (NCECF)**
c/o American Association for Pediatric Ophthalmology and Strabismus

PO Box 193832
San Francisco, CA 94119-3832
**Phone:** (415)561-8505          **Fax:** (415)561-8531
**Email:** aapos@aao.org
**Website:** http://med-aapos.bu.edu
Suzanne C. Beauchamp, Admin.

**Fnded:** 1970. **Desc:** Seeks to optimize the quality of life of infants, children, and families by fostering normal development and protection of vision through promoting programs of prevention, detection, treatment, research and education. **Pub:** Annual Report, annual. • Brochures. **Frmly:** (1982) Children's Eye Care Foundation.


★ 5725 ★ **National Coalition for Campus Children's Centers**

119 Schindler Education Center
University of Northern Iowa
Cedar Falls, IA 50614
**Phone:** (319)273-3113          **Free:** 800-813-8207
**Fax:** (319)273-3109
**Email:** ncccc@uni.edu
**Website:** http://www.campuschildren.org
Bridget Davis, Coord.

**Fnded:** 1980. **Mem:** 450. **Reg. Groups:** 4. **Desc:** Promotes child care centers on college campuses and provides information on organizing and operating these centers. Believes that campus child care programs should be an integral part of higher education systems and should provide safe and healthy environments for children, developmentally sound educational programs, and services to both parents and campus programs. **Pub:** Bibliographies. • Books. • Brochure. • Newsletter, 3/year. • Also compiles list of campus child care centers. **Frmly:** (1997) National Coalition for Campus Child Care; (1998) National Coalition for Children's Centers.


★ 5726 ★ **National Council of Voluntary Child Care Organisations**

Unit 4, Pride Court
80-82 White Lion St.
London N1 9PF, United Kingdom
**Phone:** 44 20 78333319          **Fax:** 44 20 78338637
**Email:** office@ncvcco.org
**Website:** http://www.ncvcco.org

**Fnded:** 1942. **Mem:** 108. **Reg. Groups:** 8. **Lang(s):** English. **Desc:** Voluntary organisations providing child care or supporting child care work throughout England. Aims to be an independent, identifiable member-led organisation maintaining the distinctive voice of voluntary child care; promotes and sustains the voluntary sector's contribution to the provision of services for children and families. **Pub:** *Magnet*, monthly. Bulletin. • *Outlook*, quarterly. Newsletter.


★ 5727 ★ **National Healthy Mothers, Healthy Babies Coalition**

121 N Washington St., Ste. 300
Alexandria, VA 22314
**Phone:** (703)836-6110          **Fax:** (703)836-3470
**Email:** info@hmhb.org
**Website:** http://www.hmhb.org
Anita Boles, Exec. Dir.

**Fnded:** 1981. **Mem:** 110. **Nat'l Groups:** 110. **State Groups:** 21. **Local Groups:** 30. **Desc:** Coalition of national and state organizations concerned with maternal and child health. Serves as a network through which members share ideas and information regarding issues such as prenatal care, nutrition for pregnant women, and infant mortality. **Pub:** *Healthy Mothers, Healthy Babies Newsletter*, quarterly. Newsletter. *Price:* Free. • *IEAC News*, quarterly. Newsletter. *Price:* Free. • *Power News*, quarterly. *Price:* Free. **Frmly:** (1999) Healthy Mothers, Healthy Babies.


★ 5728 ★ **National Maternal and Child Health Clearinghouse (NMCHC)**

5600 Fishers Ln.
Rockville, MD 20857
**Phone:** (703)356-1964          **Free:** 888-275-4772
**Fax:** (703)821-2098

**Email:** ask@hrsa.gov
**Website:** http://www.ask.hrsa.gov/
Kristin C. Moyer, Project Dir.

**Fnded:** 1983. **Desc:** Federal, state, and local agencies; voluntary organizations; health professionals; consumers. Collects, and disseminates information on maternal and child health, including perinatal health; prenatal care; infant, child, and adolescent health; immunization; newborn screening; oral health; emergency medical services for children; health and safety in child care; lead poisoning prevention; violence and injury prevention; children with special health needs; family support and family-centered care; maternal and child health programs and services; human genetics, nutrition, and pregnancy care. Human Services, Health Resources and Services Administration, and Maternal and Child Health Bureau. **Pub:** *Maternal and Child Health Publicaitons Catalog*, annual. Catalog. Lists approximatley 350 volumes and ordering information. *Price:* Free. • *Maternal and Child Health Thesaurus, Second Edition.* • *Reaching Out: A Directory of National Organizations Related to Maternal and Child Health.* Directories. • *The Surgeon General's Workshop on Self-Help and Public Health.* Proceedings. • Approximately 350 active volumes; most written for professionals.


**National MPS Society**
*See:* Entry 8723


★ 5729 ★ **National Network for Youth (NNY)**

1319 F St. NW, 4th Fl.
Washington, DC 20004
**Phone:** (202)783-7949          **Fax:** (202)783-7955
**Email:** mail@nn4youth.org
**Website:** http://www.nn4youth.org
Brenda Russell, Contact

**Fnded:** 1974. **Mem:** 850. **Reg. Groups:** 10. **State Groups:** 35. **Local Groups:** 400. **Desc:** Works to ensure that young people can be safe and grow up to lead healthy and productive lives. engages in public education efforts, promotes youth/adult partnerships, and strives to strengthen staff and community-based organization capacity to provide effective programs and services to youth in high-risk situations. Training and technical assistance is provided in a variety of areas including professional development of youth workers, youth leadership, peer education, HIV/AIDS and substance abuse prevention, grant writing, and community and youth development. The National Network for Youth is a sponsoring member of the Council on Accreditation of Services for Families and Children. **Pub:** *CYD Journal*, quarterly. Journal. Serves as an international voice to promote a holistic view of youth and community development. *Price:* $29. • *Doing What We Do Best: Guide to Replication of an Independent Living Project.* Outlines ways to develop a successful independent living program; includes project definition, implementation procedures, local reports, resources. *Price:* $3 for members; $4 for nonmembers. • *Helping Them Do Their Best: Guide to Using Volunteers in Runaway Centers.* Describes the benefits and essential components of a successful volunteer program; includes volunteer profile and innovative program models. *Price:* $3 for members; $4 for nonmembers. • *Network News*, quarterly. Provides updates on youth issues from a national perspective; features columns written by youth, an issues forum, legislative updates, and resources. *Price:* Free to members; $30/year for nonmembers. • *Policy Reporter*, quarterly. Newsletter. Reports on and analyzes current legislation, federal policy, and court decisions that impact services to youth. *Price:* Included in membership dues; $30/year for nonmembers. • Newsletters.Two newsletters emailed to members. *Price:* For members. **AKA:** National Network.


★ 5730 ★ **National Resource Center for Health and Safety in Child Care (NRCHSCC)**

c/o UCHSC at Fitzsimons
Campus Mail Stop F 541

PO Box 6508
Aurora, CO 80045-0508
**Phone:** (303)724-0665          **Free:** 800-598-KIDS
**Fax:** (303)724-0960
**Email:** natl.child.res.ctr.@uchsc.edu
**Website:** http://nrc.uchsc.edu
Marilyn Krajicek, Ed.D,, Exec. Dir.

**Fnded:** 1992. **State Groups:** 50. **Desc:** Seeks to enhance the quality of child care by supporting state and local health departments, child care regulatory agencies, child care providers, and parents in their effort to promote health and safety in child care. Provides information services and training and technical assistance. **Pub:** Bibliographies. • Brochure.


★ 5731 ★ **National Reye's Syndrome Foundation (NRSF)**

426 N Lewis
PO Box 829
Bryan, OH 43506
**Phone:** (419)636-2679          **Free:** 800-233-7393
**Fax:** (419)636-9897
**Email:** nrsf@reyessyndrome.org
Susan Landversicht, Dir. of Dev.

**Fnded:** 1974. **Mem:** 5,000. **Reg. Groups:** 6. **State Groups:** 47. **Local Groups:** 148. **Desc:** Families of children who have had Reye's Syndrome; doctors, scientists, nurses, and other health professionals and concerned individuals. (Reye's Syndrome is a disease affecting the liver and brain. Cause and cure unknown, its mortality rate is over 57 percent. Death may occur within a few hours after onset.) Aims to disseminate information to the public and the medical community and to raise and provide funds for research into the cause, treatment, cure, and prevention of the disease through research grants to individual scientists. Gives support and guidance to families experiencing Reye's Syndrome; assists federal and state agencies in obtaining data on Reye's cases; encourages governmental funding of research. Promotes service through a resource clearinghouse, support groups, and referral services. Promotes awareness via lay-oriented literature, information services, professional training, lay/professional slide presentations, and emergency room posters. Sponsors National Reye's Syndrome Month in September. Compiles statistics; maintains speakers' bureau. **Pub:** *National Reye's Syndrome Foundation–In the News*, semiannual. Newsletter. *Price:* Included in membership dues.


★ 5732 ★ **National School-Age Care Alliance (NSACA)**

1131 Washington St.
Boston, MA 02124
**Phone:** (617)298-5012          **Fax:** (617)298-5022
**Email:** staff@nsaca.org
**Website:** http://www.nsaca.org
Linda Sisson, Exec. Dir.

**Fnded:** 1981. **Mem:** 8,000. **Reg. Groups:** 5. **Local Groups:** 35. **Desc:** Professional providers of day care services for school age children outside of school hours. Seeks to advance the profession of school-age child care. Provides support and services to members including coalition building, networking, and group rates for video licensing. **Pub:** *Caring, Stimulating, Responsive.* Brochure. • *NSACA News*, quarterly. Newsletter.


★ 5733 ★ **National SIDS/Infant Death Resource Center (NSIDRC)**

2070 Chain Bridge, Ste. 450
Vienna, VA 22182-2536
**Phone:** (703)821-8955          **Free:** (866)866-7437
**Fax:** (703)821-2098
**Email:** sids@circlesolutions.com
**Website:** http://www.sidscenter.org
Olivia Cowdrill, Proj. Dir.

**Fnded:** 1980. **Desc:** Funded by Maternal and Child Health Bureau, Health Resources and Services Administration, U.S. Department of Health and Human Services, National SIDS/Infant Death Resource Center. Provides resources, referrals, and technical assistance to SIDS families, public health and other professionals, and the general public. **Pub:** *Fact Sheets.* • *Information Exchange*, periodic. Newsletter. Includes list of resources, calendar of events, and national, state and legislative news. • *Table of SIDS Deaths and Mortality Rates*, annual. • Bibliographies, annual. Research bibliographies. • Also publishes fact sheets and educational publications. **Frmly:** (1991) National Sudden Infant Death Syndrome Clearinghouse.

**National Tay-Sachs and Allied Diseases Association (NTSAD)**
*See:* Entry 8726

**★ 5734 ★ National Vaccine Information Center**
421-E Church St.
Vienna, VA 22180
**Phone:** (703)938-3783          **Free:** 800-909-SHOT
**Fax:** (703)938-5768
**Email:** info@909shot.com
**Website:** http://www.909shot.com
Kathryn Williams, Contact
**Fnded:** 1982. **Mem:** 40,000. **Desc:** Parents of children who have had reactions to or been injured by vaccines; individuals interested in working to reform the vaccine system. Disseminates information concerning vaccines to parents and doctors in order to assure safer administration of vaccines. Promotes the development of safer vaccines. Refers parents of vaccine-injured children to doctors, lawyers, and other parents for support services. Maintains speakers' bureau; compiles statistics. **Pub:** *The Compensation System and How It Works.* • *Law Firm Directory.* Directory. • *The Vaccine Reaction*, quarterly. **AKA:** Dissatisfied Parents Together.

**★ 5735 ★ New Zealand Child Care Association**
**(Te Tari Puna Ora o Aotearoa)**
PO Box 11-863
Wellington, New Zealand
**Phone:** 64 4 4734672          **Fax:** 64 4 4737295
**Email:** rose.cole@nzchildcare.ac.nz
**Website:** http://www.nzchildcare.ac.nz
**Fnded:** 1963. **Mem:** 1,000. **Reg. Groups:** 17. **Desc:** Promotes and supports accessibility to quality child care in New Zealand. **Pub:** *Itirearea*, semimonthly. Newsletter. Also publishes texts concerned with parent education, student texts, and general information on childcare.

**★ 5736 ★ NIPPA-The Early Years Organisation (NIPPA)**
6c Wildflower Way
Apollo Rd.
Belfast, United Kingdom
**Phone:** 44 2890 662825          **Fax:** 44 2890 381270
**Email:** mail@nippa.org
**Fnded:** 1965. **Mem:** 960. **Local Groups:** 19. **Lang(s):** English, Irish. **Desc:** Promotes the availability of child care facilities for women with children under 5 years of age. Fosters children's educational and physical development. **Pub:** *NIPPA Network*, quarterly. Newsletter. • Annual Report. • Books.

**★ 5737 ★ North American Society for Pediatric Gastroenterology, Hepatology and Nutrition (NASPGHAN)**
PO Box 6
Flourtown, PA 19031
**Phone:** (215)233-0808          **Fax:** (215)233-3939
**Email:** naspghan@naspghan.org
**Website:** http://www.naspghan.org
Margaret Stallings, Exec. Dir.
**Fnded:** 1970. **Mem:** 350. **Desc:** Mission is to be a world leader in advancing the science and clinical practice of Pediatric Gastroenterology, Hepatology and Nutrition in health and disease. Strives to improve the care of infants, children and adolescents with digestive disorders by promoting advances in clinical care, research and education. Pediatric gastroenterol-

ogists specialize in the care of children with chronic abdominal pain, diarrhea, constipation, vomiting, bleeding from the GI tract, inflammatory bowel disease, liver diseases, diseases of the pancreas, poor weight gain and nutritional problems. Objectives include: improving the digestive health and nutrition of children worldwide and particularly in North America; fostering dialogue and research on pertinent issues that impact the pediatric gastroenterology patient and their family; providing opportunities for clinicians and researchers to gain knowledge of the scientific advances in the field; and disseminating scientific information in order to improve clinical outcomes and advance the practice of the field. **Pub:** *NASPGN Membership Directory*, annual. Membership Directory. • *Newsletter of the NASPGN*, 4-6/year. Newsletter. **Frmly:** (1988) North American Society for Pediatric Gastroenterology.

**Norwegian Association for Children and Adults with Minimal Brain Dysfunction (ADHD)**
**(MBD-foreningen)**
*See:* Entry 6891

**★ 5738 ★ Our Youths Foundation (OYF)**
**(Fundacion Nuestros Jovenes — FNJ)**
Baron de Carondelet 641 Y Villaengua
Quito, Ecuador
**Phone:** 593 2 247250          **Fax:** 593 2 443964
**Email:** gerencia@uio.satnet.net
**Website:**                                                       http://
www.fundacionnuestrosjovenes.org.ec
**Fnded:** 1982. **Mem:** 400. **Lang(s):** English, French, German, Spanish. **Desc:** Works to provide assistance to young substance abusers in Ecuador. Conducts drug awareness programs and offers medical and psychological assistance for young abusers. Investigates the extent and severity of illicit drug use in Ecuador and disseminates information to increase public awareness of the causes and effects of drug trafficking; VIH-SIDA prevention in high-risk groups and other health and educational projects. **Pub:** *Sin Limites*, bimonthly. Magazine. Contains analysis of adolescents' problems and prevention.

**★ 5739 ★ Papua New Guinea Paediatric Society (PNGPS)**
Medical Faculty
PO Box 5623
Boroko, Papua New Guinea
**Phone:** 675 3248461          **Fax:** 675 3254935
**Fnded:** 1974. **Mem:** 30. **Lang(s):** English. **Desc:** Formulates practices and procedures in pediatic medicine in Papua New Guinea; advises the government on health policy; facilitates information exchange in the field; advises on undergraduate and postgraduate curricula in regards to child health. **Pub:** *Standard Treatment for Common Illnesses of Children in Papua New Guinea*, periodic. Handbook. Contains information on the management of commonly present pediatric problems.

**★ 5740 ★ Parents at Work (PAW)**
45 Beech St., 5th Fl.
London EC2Y 8AD, United Kingdom
**Phone:** 44 20 76283565          **Fax:** 44 20 76283591
**Email:** info@parentsatwork.org.uk
**Website:** http://www.parentsatwork.org.uk
**Fnded:** 1985. **Mem:** 1,500. **Lang(s):** English. **Desc:** Campaign to improve quality of life for all working parents and their children. Lobbies employers and policy makers for improvement of childcare facilities. Provides working parents with childcare information. **Pub:** *Balanced Lives*, quarterly. Newsletter. • *Waving Not Drowning*. Newsletter. Features information for parents of disabled children who work or want to work. **Frmly:** (1994) Working Mothers Association.

**★ 5741 ★ Pediatric AIDS Foundation**
2950 31st St., Ste. 125
Santa Monica, CA 90405-3037
**Phone:** (310)314-1459          **Fax:** (310)314-1469
**Email:** info@pedAIDS.org
**Website:** http://www.pedaids.org
Kate Carr, CEO
**Fnded:** 1988. **Desc:** Confronts medical problems unique to children infected with HIV/AIDS, and focuses on finding medical answers that will bring hope. Identifies and funds critically needed pediatric AIDS research worldwide. Provides funds to hospitals around the country which serve children with HIV/AIDS through an Emergency Assistance Program. Encourages students to enter the field of pediatric AIDS through a Student Intern Award Program. Develops and distributes national Parent Education Program for parents of elementary and pre-school age children. **Pub:** Annual Report.

**★ 5742 ★ Pediatric Digestion and Motility Disorders Society (PEDS)**
PO Box 1360
Buffalo, NY 14203-1360
**Phone:** (716)852-2857
**Email:** pedskids@aol.com
**Website:** http://www.the-art-dept.com/peds.htm
**Desc:** Volunteers. Work towards finding cures. Host events to fund research. Promote public awareness.

**Pediatric Endocrinology Nursing Society (PENS)**
*See:* Entry 15766

**★ 5743 ★ Pediatric Orthopaedic Society of North America (POSNA)**
6300 N River Rd., Ste. 727
Rosemont, IL 60018-4226
**Phone:** (847)698-1692          **Fax:** (847)823-0536
**Email:** goldberg@aaos.org
**Website:** http://www.posna.org
Sharon Goldberg, Exec. Dir.
**Fnded:** 1983. **Mem:** 800. **Desc:** Pediatric orthopedic surgeons. Purpose is to provide continuing education to members. Conducts tutorial programs. **Pub:** *Newsletter*, quarterly. Bulletin. **Price:** available to members only. • Membership Directory, annual.

**★ 5744 ★ Pediatric Pharmacy Advocacy Group (PPAG)**
9866 W Victoria Dr.
Littleton, CO 80128
**Phone:** (720)981-7356          **Fax:** (720)981-7357
**Email:** hankw@ppag.org
**Website:** http://www.ppag.org
**Desc:** Dedicated to safe and effective medication use to improve the lives of children by being a primary resource for drug therapy.

**★ 5745 ★ Polish Paediatric Pathology Society**
**(Polski Towarzystwo Patologii Dzieciecej)**
Aleja Dzieci Polskich 20
PL-04736 Warsaw, Poland
**Phone:** 48 22 8151971          **Fax:** 48 22 8151971
**Email:** ptpd@cxd.wow.pl
**Fnded:** 1996. **Mem:** 50. **Lang(s):** English, Polish. **Desc:** Pediatric pathologists. Seeks to advance the science and practice of pediatric pathology. Facilitates integration of scientific developments in the field; conducts continuing medical education programs. **Pub:** *Annals of Diagnostic Paediatric Pathology*, quarterly. Journal.

**★ 5746 ★ Puerto Rico Association of Pediatric Surgeons**
PO Box 10426
Caparra Hts. Station
San Juan, PR 00922-0426

**Phone:** (787)777-3535　　**Fax:** (787)720-6103
**Email:** titolugo@coqui.net
**Website:** http://home.coqui.net/titolugo/praps.htm
**Fnded:** 1997. **Desc:** General pediatric surgeons. Strives to improve the care of newborns, infants, children, adolescent and young adults with surgically related diseases. Provides educational forum, research and teaching of surgery, consults and recommends programs and policy statements.

★ 5747 ★ **REACH: Association for Children with Hand or Arm Deficiency**
25 High St.
Wellingborough NN8 4JZ, United Kingdom
**Phone:** 44 1933274126　　**Fax:** 44 7721929583
**Email:** reach@reach.org.uk
**Website:** http://www.reach.org.uk
**Fnded:** 1978. **Mem:** 1,200. **Desc:** Aims to offer support to families of children with upper limb deficiency.

★ 5748 ★ **Reach Ireland (RI)**
Fair Stream
Hedge Rd.
Garristown
Dublin, Ireland
**Phone:** 353 1 8354953　　**Fax:** 353 1 8427788
**Website:** http://www.reach.org.uk
**Fnded:** 1990. **Mem:** 230. **Nat'l Groups:** 1. **Lang(s):** English, Irish. **Desc:** Individuals and organizations. Seeks to improve the quality of life of children with limb deficiencies and their families. Makes available support and services; conducts educational and advocacy campaigns. **Pub:** *Within Reach*, quarterly. Magazine.

★ 5749 ★ **Reach Out for Youth with Ileitis and Colitis**
84 Northgate Cir.
Melville, NY 11747-3042
**Phone:** (631)293-3102　　**Fax:** (631)293-3102
**Email:** reachoutforyouth@reachoutforyouth.org
**Website:** http://www.reachoutforyouth.org
Susan Spellman, Exec. Dir.
**Fnded:** 1979. **Desc:** Works to provide support groups for families whose children have Inflammatory Bowel Disease (IBD). Provides educational and emotional support to patients and families; conducts fund-raising events; promotes research into the cause and treatment of IBD. **Pub:** *The Inner Circle*, quarterly. Newsletter. **Price:** Free. • *The Inside Story*. Brochure.

**Retinoblastoma Society (RS)**
*See:* Entry 21064

★ 5750 ★ **Royal College of Paediatrics and Child Health**
50 Hallam St.
London W1W 6DE, United Kingdom
**Phone:** 44 207 3075600　　**Fax:** 44 207 3075601
**Email:** enquiries@rcpch.ac.uk
**Website:** http://www.rcpch.ac.uk
**Fnded:** 1928. **Mem:** 3,751. **Desc:** Consultant paediatricians, community child health doctors, trainee paediatricians, research workers, general practitioners and other medical specialists who work with children. Aims to advance the understanding, treatment and prevention of disease in childhood, to further the study of child health and to promote excellence in paediatric practice. **Frmly:** (1996) British Paediatric Association.

**Royal Institute for Deaf and Blind Children (RIDBC)**
*See:* Entry 6102

★ 5751 ★ **Sargent Cancer Care for Children (SCCC)**
Mercantile Chambers
5th Fl, 53 Bothwell St.
Glasgow G2 6TS, United Kingdom

**Phone:** 44 1415 725700　　**Fax:** 44 1415 725701
**Email:** online@ridbc.org.au
**Website:** http://www.ridbc.org.au
**Fnded:** 1969. **Lang(s):** English. **Desc:** Health care professionals and other individuals working with children with cancer. Seeks to improve the quality of life of children with cancer; promotes advancement of cancer diagnosis and treatment techniques. Provides support and assistance to families of children with cancer; makes available children's services; conducts educational programs; participates in charitable activities. **Pub:** Brochures. • Annual Report.

**Scandinavian Association of Paediatric Surgeons (SCAPS)**
**(Nordisk Barnkirurgisk Forening — NBF)**
*See:* Entry 19591

★ 5752 ★ **Scottish Out of School Care Network (SOSCN)**
6th Fl., Fleming House
134 Renfrew St.
Glasgow G3 6ST, United Kingdom
**Phone:** 44 141 3311301　　**Fax:** 44 141 3321206
**Email:** info@soscn.org
**Website:** http://www.soscn.org
**Fnded:** 1991. **Mem:** 400. **Nat'l Groups:** 1. **Reg. Groups:** 30. **Local Groups:** 600. **Lang(s):** English. **Desc:** Organizations and agencies engaged in out-of-school child care. Promotes increased availability of affordable, quality child care. Establishes partnerships among members and between members and other organizations pursuing similar goals. Works to increase awareness of child care issues. Conducts research; makes available information about children's services; compiles statistics. **Pub:** *Connections*, quarterly. Newsletter.

**Shriners Hospitals for Children**
*See:* Entry 11509

★ 5753 ★ **SIDS Alliance (SIDSA)**
1314 Bedford Ave., Ste. 210
Baltimore, MD 21208
**Phone:** (410)653-8226　　**Free:** 800-221-SIDS
**Fax:** (410)653-8709
**Email:** info@sidsalliance.org
**Website:** http://www.sidsalliance.org/
Judith S. Jacobson, Exec. VP
**Fnded:** 1991. **Local Groups:** 50. **Desc:** Unites concerned citizens, health professionals, and parents who have lost a child to sudden infant death syndrome (SIDS), a condition commonly known as "crib death" that accounts for about 6000 infant deaths annually in the United States. (Deaths of this type usually occur at night and during the cold weather months among apparently healthy infants generally under 6 months of age.) Although the common causes and methods of prevention have yet to be determined, recent research findings suggest an increased risk of SIDS for infants sleeping on the stomach, sleeping on soft bedding, exposed to smoke, or overheated. Serves as a central source of medical and scientific information about SIDS. Works to eliminate SIDS through research; Assists bereaved parents who have lost a child to SIDS; seeks to make the public aware of SIDS and related issues. **Pub:** *Synopsis*, periodic. Newsletter.

★ 5754 ★ **Slovak Society of Pediatrics**
c/o Children's Hospital
1 Children's Clinic
Limbova 1
SK-833 40 Bratislava, Slovakia
**Phone:** 42 2 54774511　　**Fax:** 42 2 54774511
**Email:** benedek@fmed.uniba.sk
**Mem:** 2,000. **Lang(s):** English, Slovak. **Desc:** Pediatricians and other health care professionals with an interest in child health. Promotes proper pediatric medical care; represents members' interests. **Pub:** *Detsky Lekar*, quarterly. Journal. Contains information regarding pediatric problems of primary care.

★ 5755 ★ **Society for Adolescent Medicine (SAM)**
1916 NW Copper Oaks Circle
Blue Springs, MO 64015
**Fax:** (816)224-8009
**Email:** cirwin@itsa.ucsf.edu
**Website:** http://www.adolescenthealth.org
Charles E. Irwin, Jr., Pres.
**Fnded:** 1968. **Mem:** 1,300. **Reg. Groups:** 18. **Desc:** Physicians, psychologists, social workers, psychiatrists, nurses, and other health care professionals. Goals are: to improve the quality of health care for adolescents; to encourage the investigation of normal growth and development during adolescence and of those diseases that affect adolescents; to stimulate the creation of health services for adolescents; to increase communication among health care professionals who care for adolescents; to foster and improve the quality of training of those individuals providing health care to adolescents. Seeks to: offer opportunities for discussion of teaching, research, and other common problems, through which coordinated efforts can be made toward their solution; publish and disseminate information related to adolescent medicine; identify, investigate, and list opportunities for careers in adolescent medicine; help plan and coordinate professional educational programs in the health care of the adolescent. Conducts research programs. **Pub:** *Journal of Adolescent Health*, monthly. Journal. Peer-reviewed scientific journal of articles on study results of the anthropology, biochemistry, endocrinology, physiology and psychology. *Price:* Included in membership dues; $199/year for nonmembers; $475/year for institutions.

★ 5756 ★ **Society for Developmental and Behavioral Pediatrics (SDBP)**
c/o Noreen M. Spota
19 Station Ln.
Philadelphia, PA 19118-2939
**Phone:** (215)248-9168　　**Fax:** (215)248-1981
**Email:** admin@sdbp.org
**Website:** http://www.sdbp.org
Noreen M. Spota, Admin. Dir.
**Fnded:** 1982. **Mem:** 720. **Reg. Groups:** 2. **State Groups:** 2. **Desc:** Pediatricians, child psychologists, and other allied health care professionals. Seeks to improve the health care of infants, children, and adolescents by promoting research and scholarly instruction in the area of developmental-behavioral pediatrics. **Pub:** *Journal of Developmental and Behavioral Pediatrics*, bimonthly. Journal. Includes original scientific articles, book and journal article reviews, commentaries, and letters to the editor. *Price:* Included in membership dues; $221/year for nonmembers. **Frmly:** Society for Behavioral Pediatrics.

★ 5757 ★ **Society of Nursery Nursing (SNN)**
40 Archdale Rd.
East Dulwich
London SE22 9HJ, United Kingdom
**Phone:** 44 208 6930555　　**Fax:** 44 208 6930555
**Email:** snn@totalise.co.uk
**Fnded:** 1991. **Mem:** 1,500. **Reg. Groups:** 5. **Local Groups:** 3. **Lang(s):** English. **Desc:** Nursing managers, nursing administrators and nurses, nursery teachers, school nurses, nannies, and other workers and employers with an interest in the education, health and welfare of children from birth to five years of age. Seeks to establish professional standards and a uniform code of ethics within the field; works to enhance the professional standing of members. Gathers and disseminates information to inform legislative debate concerning child health issues. Conducts examinations and educational programs and maintains speakers' bureau. **Pub:** *Nursery Nursing Administrator*, quarterly. Newsletter. **Frmly:** (2000) Society of Nursery Nursing Administrators.

**Society for Pediatric Anesthesia**
*See:* Entry 4472

**★ 5758 ★ Society for Pediatric Dermatology (SPD)**
c/o Pat Fraser, Admin.
5422 N Bernard
Chicago, IL 60625
**Phone:** (773)583-9780          **Fax:** (773)583-9765
**Email:** patrici107@aol.com
**Website:** http://www.pedsderm.net
Pat Fraser, Admin.
**Fnded:** 1975. **Mem:** 500. **Desc:** Pediatricians, dermatologists, pediatric or dermatologic house officers, manufacturers of children's skin products, and researchers in biomedicine with studies in pediatric dermatology. Conducts research programs. **Pub:** *Society for Pediatric Dermatology–Newsletter*, quarterly. Newsletter. Reviews current publications in the field of pediatric dermatology; includes reviews in the areas of allergy and immunology, genetics and syndromes. *Price:* Included in membership dues.

**Society of Pediatric Nurses (SPN)**
*See:* Entry 15775

**Society for Pediatric Pathology**
*See:* Entry 17151

**Society for Pediatric Psychology (SPP)**
*See:* Entry 12649

**Society for Pediatric Radiology (SPR)**
*See:* Entry 18159

**★ 5759 ★ Society for Pediatric Research (SPR)**
3400 Research Forest Dr., Ste. B7
The Woodlands, TX 77381
**Phone:** (281)419-0052          **Fax:** (281)419-0082
**Email:** info@aps-spr.org
**Website:** http://www.aps-spr.org
Debbie Anagnostelis, Exec. Dir.
**Fnded:** 1929. **Mem:** 2,400. **Desc:** Physicians and scientists under age 46 who are engaged in research in diseases of infancy and childhood; those over age 46 are senior members. **Pub:** *Pediatric Research*, monthly. Journal. Includes calendar of events, obituaries, and abstracts. *Price:* $85/year. **Frmly:** (1932) Eastern Society for Pediatric Research.

**★ 5760 ★ Society for Pediatric Urology (SPU)**
Section of Urology, MC 4056
University of Chicago
5844 S Maryland Ave.
Chicago, IL 60637
**Phone:** (773)702-6150          **Fax:** (773)702-8702
**Website:** http://www.spu.org
Stephen Koff, Pres.
**Fnded:** 1941. **Mem:** 300. **Local Groups:** 45. **Desc:** Medical doctors who are specialists in urology (relating to the genito-urinary tract in health and disease) and who have a special interest in the field of childhood urological problems. Seeks to encourage the study, improve the practice, elevate the standards, and further the advancement of pediatric urology. Conducts educational programs. **Pub:** *Dialogues in Pediatric Urology*, monthly. Magazine. *Price:* $32. • *Pedictric Urology*, monthly. Newsletter. *Price:* Included in membership dues. • Audiotapes. • Books. • Pamphlets. • Videos.

**★ 5761 ★ Society for Physician Assistants in Pediatrics (SPAP)**
950 N Washington St.
Alexandria, VA 22314-1552
**Free:** 800-596-4398          **Fax:** (703)684-1924
**Email:** jrv1007@aol.com
**Website:** http://www.geocities.com/spap_peds1
Tom Moreno, Membership Coor.
**Fnded:** 1994. **Mem:** 250. **Desc:** Designed to gather and disseminate information affecting the practice of pediatric physician assistants, collect demographic data to share within the profession or with other organizations, assist in developing guidelines for physician assistant utilization in clinical settings, and to enhance the relationship with the American Academy of Pediatrics. **Pub:** *Physician Assistants in Pediatrics*, quarterly. Newsletter.

**Society of Professors of Child and Adolescent Psychiatry (SPCAP)**
*See:* Entry 12653

**★ 5762 ★ South African Association of Paediatric Surgeons (SAAPS) (Suid-Afrikaanse Vereniging van Kinderchirurge — SAVK)**
c/o Prof. H. Rode
Department of Paediatric Surgery
Red Cross War Memorial Children's Hospital
Rondebosch 7700, Republic of South Africa
**Phone:** 27 21 6585339          **Fax:** 27 21 6856632
**Email:** hrode@ich.uct.ac.za
**Fnded:** 1975. **Mem:** 50. **Lang(s):** Afrikaans, English. **Desc:** Pediatric surgeons in South Africa. Promotes research, training, and clinical services in pediatric surgery. Grants postgraduate fellowships. Conducts educational programs; compiles statistics.

**★ 5763 ★ STEPS: National Association for Children with Lower Limb Abnormalities**
c/o Ms. Sue Banton
Lower Ground Floor, Lymm Court
11 Eagle Brow
Lymm WA13 0LP, United Kingdom
**Phone:** 44 671 7170045          **Fax:** 44 671 7170044
**Email:** info@steps-charity.org.uk
**Website:** http://www.steps-charity.org.uk
**Fnded:** 1980. **Mem:** 2,000. **Reg. Groups:** 15. **Desc:** Provides information and support for families of children with lower limb abnormalities. Objectives are to put families in touch with one another, develops a network of local contacts providing support, help and advise and to gather and exchange information with parents and health professionals.

**Stop Teen-Age Addiction to Tobacco (STAT)**
*See:* Entry 18930

**★ 5764 ★ StopSIDS.org**
1673 Rte. 9, Ste. 2
Clifton Park, NY 12065
**Free:** 888-521-9499
**Email:** info@stopsids.org
**Website:** http://www.stopsids.org/
Dr. Tracey Mulhall, Co-Founder
**Fnded:** 2000. **Desc:** Committed to research and education in order to end sudden infant death syndrome (SIDS) and other infant deaths; promotes health in babies and children through chiropractic-atlas correction and other healthy lifestyle choices. **Pub:** *The Best-Kept Secret to Raising a Healthy Child...and the Possible Prevention of Sudden Infant Death Syndrome (SIDS)*. Book.

**★ 5765 ★ Sudden Infant Death Syndrome Alliance**
1314 Bedford Ave., Ste. 210
Baltimore, MD 21208
**Phone:** (410)653-8226          **Fax:** (410)653-8709
**Email:** info@sidalliance.org
**Website:** http://www.sialliance.org
**Fnded:** 1987. **Desc:** Working to unite parents and friends of SIDS victims with medical, business and civic groups concerned about the health of America's babies and to provide education and advocacy opportunities.

**★ 5766 ★ Taiwan Pediatric Association (TPA)**
10-1F, No. 69, Hang-Chow S Rd
Sec. 1
Taipei 10022, Taiwan
**Phone:** 886 2 23516446          **Fax:** 886 2 23516448
**Email:** pediatr@pediatr.org.tw
**Website:** http://www.pediatr.org.tw/main.htm
**Fnded:** 1960. **Mem:** 2,600. **Lang(s):** Chinese, English. **Desc:** Pediatricians and others working in the field of pediatric medicine in 6 countries. Promotes the health and welfare of infants, children, and adolescents. Encourages research and teaching in the field; sponsors educational and scientific programs. Facilitates information exchange. **Pub:** *Acta Paediatrica Sinica*, bimonthly. Journal. • *Members' Directory*, triennial. • *Supplement*, semiannual. For the purpose of continuing medical education. **Frmly:** (2000) Chinese Taipei Pediatric Association.

**★ 5767 ★ Think First Foundation: National Injury Prevention Program**
5550 Meadowbrook Dr., Ste. 110
Rolling Meadows, IL 60008
**Phone:** (847)290-8600          **Free:** 800-THI-NK56
**Fax:** (847)290-9005
**Email:** thinkfirst@thinkfirst.org
**Website:** http://www.thinkfirst.org
Bill Biebuyck, CEO
**Fnded:** 1986. **State Groups:** 20. **Local Groups:** 200. **Desc:** Works to educate young people about personal vulnerability and the consequences of risk taking behavior. Our goal is to prevent permanent brain, spinal cord, and other traumatic injuries. Conducts school-based educational programs, reinforcement activities, general public education and public policy initiatives. **Pub:** *Prevention Pages*, quarterly. Newsletter. • *Think First for Kids Curriculum Packet*. Instructional materials for children in grads 1-3. *Price:* $249. **Frmly:** (2000) Think First Foundation: National Injury Prevention Programs.

**★ 5768 ★ Toxoplasmosis Trust (TTT)**
Edgebrook House
13 E Feltes Ave.
Edinburgh EH4, United Kingdom
**Phone:** 44 131 3325589
**Email:** info@toxo.org.uk
**Fnded:** 1989. **Mem:** 5,000. **Lang(s):** English. **Desc:** Aims to raise awareness of toxoplasmosis among health professionals and the general public. (Toxoplasmosis is a parasitic infection, which, if caught during pregnancy, can cause damage to the unborn baby.) Provides information and support to those affected by or concerned about taxoplasmosis. **Pub:** *Toxoplasmosis and Lambing: How to Avoid an Unnecessary Risk*. • *Toxoplasmosis in Pregnancy: Avoid Unnecessary Risk*. • *Toxoplasmosis: Information for People with HIV and AIDS*. • *Toxoplasmosis: The Facts*. Videos. • *The Toxoplasmosis Trust Trust Update*, periodic. Magazine. • *Toxopliasmosis & Your Pet Cat*. • Newsletter, semiannual. • Reports. • Papers.

**★ 5769 ★ Union of Middle Eastern and Mediterranean Pediatric Societies (UMEMPS) (Union des Societes de Pediatrie du Moyen-Orient et de la Mediterranee — USPMOM)**
c/o Prof. T. Thomaidis
Milioni 6
GR-106 73 Athens, Greece
**Phone:** 30 1 3615168          **Fax:** 30 1 3615168
**Website:** http://www.medistatweb.com/societies/u-memps
**Fnded:** 1966. **Mem:** 23. **Nat'l Groups:** 23. **Reg. Groups:** 1. **Lang(s):** English, French. **Desc:** National societies of pediatricians and pediatric surgeons.

## ★ 5770 ★ Wellstart International
4062 1st Ave.
San Diego, CA 92103-2045
**Phone:** (619)295-5192
**Email:** info@wellstart.org
**Website:** http://www.wellstart.org/
Audrey Naylor, CEO

**Desc:** Seeks to advance the knowledge, skills, and ability of breastfeeding to health care providers in order to promote, protect, and support infant and maternal health and nutrition from conception through the completion of weaning.

## ★ 5771 ★ World Association for Infant Mental Health (WAIMH)
Kellogg Center, Rm. 4
East Lansing, MI 48824-1022
**Phone:** (517)432-3793          **Fax:** (517)432-3694
**Email:** waimh@pilot.msu.edu
**Website:** http://www.msu.edu/user/waimh
Hiram E. Fitzgerald, Exec. Dir.

**Fnded.** 1992. **Mem:** 850. **Reg. Groups:** 19. **Desc:** Child development specialists, child psychiatrists, child psychoanalysts, infant care workers, linguists, nurses, obstetricians, pediatricians, psychologists, and social workers. Works to further research and understanding of mental development and disorders in children from conception through age 3. Promotes studies on the conditions affecting the mental health of infants, their parents, and other caregivers; explores mental development during infancy and its subsequent effects on psychopathological development. Advocates international multidisciplinary discussions of research and intervention in infant psychiatry within the framework of the total life cycle. Facilitates communication and exchange of information and theories; fosters discussion of questions, problems, and issues in infant mental health. **Pub:** *Infant Mental Health Journal*, quarterly. Journal. *Price:* $37.50 for members; $50 for members outside the U.S.; $154 for Institutions; $75 for USA non members. • *The Signal*, bimonthly. Newsletter. *Price:* $99 for Non members outside the USA.

## World Federation of Associations of Pediatric Surgeons
*See:* Entry 19610

## ★ 5772 ★ Youth Development Coalition
3080 N Lincoln
Chicago, IL 60657
**Free:** 800-231-6946          **Fax:** (312)929-5150
**Email:** 1800hithome@horizonsd.org
**Website:** http://www.bakersfield.org/ydc
Nancy Eschbach, Contact

**Desc:** Provides assistance to youth and families in crisis situations.

## Zero to Three: National Center for Infants, Toddlers and Families
*See:* Entry 10000

# Research Centers

## American Academy of Pediatrics Division of Health Policy Research
*See:* Entry 9767

## ★ 5773 ★ American Sudden Infant Death Syndrome Institute
2480 Windy Hill Rd., Ste. 380
Marietta, GA 30067
**Phone:** (770)612-1030          **Free:** 800-232-SIDS
**Fax:** (770)612-8277
**Email:** prevent@sids.org
**Website:** http://www.sids.org
Alfred Steinschneider, MD, Pres.

**Activities/Fields:** Sudden Infant Death Syndrome (SIDS), commonly known as crib death, including the search for abnormalities in SIDS victims, study of normal and abnormal infant control mechanisms, pregnancy-related factors, identification of infants at risk, effectiveness of preventive measures, effect of SIDS on families, and effect of preventive measures on families. **Pub:** *Towards an Understanding of SIDS.*

## Association for Research of Childhood Cancer
*See:* Entry 10273

## Autism Research Institute
*See:* Entry 12680

## Barbara Davis Center for Childhood Diabetes
*See:* Entry 8742

## ★ 5774 ★ Baylor College of Medicine Children's Nutrition Research Center
1100 Bates St.
Houston, TX 77030
**Phone:** (713)798-7971          **Fax:** (713)798-7098
**Email:** cnrc@bcm.tmc.edu
**Website:** http://www.bcm.tmc.edu/cnrc
Dr. Dennis M. Bier, Dir.

**Activities/Fields:** Nutrition of infants, children, and pregnant and lactating women. Reseach also focuses on nutrient-gene interactions, and cell, developmental, and plant biology. **Frmly:** Child Health Research Center.

## ★ 5775 ★ Baylor College of Medicine General Clinical Research Center
MC 1-3420
Texas Children's and The Methodist Hospital
TXWT 10041
Houston, TX 77030
**Phone:** (832)826-1079          **Fax:** (832)825-1061
**Email:** dbier@bcm.tmc.edu
Dr. Dennis M. Bier, Prog. Dir.

**Activities/Fields:** Cardiology, endocrinology, gastroenterology, genetics, infectious diseases, pulmonary system, pharmacology, immunology, hematology, rheumatology, and renal disease, including studies on ventricular dysrhythmias, hypopituitarism, bile acid metabolism, argininemia, HIV, and renal tubular acidosis.

## ★ 5776 ★ Baylor College of Medicine Meyer Center for Developmental Pediatrics
MC 3-2335
Texas Children's Hospital Feigin Center
6621 Fannin St.
Houston, TX 77030
**Phone:** (713)824-3400          **Fax:** (713)825-3399
Dr. Gregory Miller, Contact

**Activities/Fields:** Developmentally disabled, developmental pediatrics, learning disabilities, low-birth-weight infants, maternal medications, cytomegalo inclusion virus, congenital rubella syndrome, neonatal intracranial hemorrhage, outcome prematurity, and attention deficit/hyperactivity disorder. **Frmly:** Child Development Clinics.

## British Columbia Children's Hospital Children's and Women's Health Centre of British Columbia
*See:* Entry 10287

## ★ 5777 ★ Brooklyn College of City University of New York Infant Study Center
Department of Psychology
2900 Bedford Ave.
Brooklyn, NY 11210
**Phone:** (718)951-5033          **Fax:** (718)951-4825
**Email:** louiseh@brooklyn.cuny.edu
**Website:** http://depthome.brooklyn.cuny.edu/psych/infant
Dr. Louise Hainline, Dir.

**Activities/Fields:** Human vision and normal and abnormal visual development; visual development in infancy, including studies of acuity, pattern perception, color vision, eye movement control, and perception of complex events; behavioral studies of visual attention and use of information in medical images in adults. Assessment procedures utilize photo-refraction methods, visual-evoked response techniques, and electrophysiological studies of dyslexia.

## ★ 5778 ★ Canadian Institute of Child Health (CICH)
384 Bank St., Ste. 300
Ottawa, ON, Canada K2P 1Y4
**Phone:** (613)230-8838          **Fax:** (613)230-6654
**Email:** cich@cich.ca
**Website:** http://www.cich.ca
The Hon. Judith Erola, Ch.

**Activities/Fields:** Improving the health and well-being of children and youth in Canada. The objectives to accomplish this vision include monitoring the health and well-being of children and youth; improving the health and well-being of mothers and infants; creating safe, supportive, nurturing environments for children; and encouraging cooperation between consumers, professionals, industry and government agencies to ensure a better life for Canadian children. **Pub:** *Annual Report.* • *Child Health Newsletter*, quarterly. • *The Health of Canada's Children: A CICH Profile.* • *Our Promise to Children.*

## Cancer Research Laboratory
*See:* Entry 10297

## Center for Human Nutrition, Inc.
*See:* Entry 9163

## ★ 5779 ★ Child Health Research Center
Newborn Medicine
Children's Hospital
300 Longwood Ave.
Boston, MA 02115
**Phone:** (617)355-6366          **Fax:** (617)355-7677
**Email:** merton.bernfield@tch.harvard.edu
Dr. Merton Bernfield, Co-Dir.

**Activities/Fields:** Child health, particularly developmental biology.

## Children's Heart and Health Institute of Texas
*See:* Entry 5088

## ★ 5780 ★ Children's Hospital of Alabama Southeast Child Safety Institute
1600 7th Ave. S
Birmingham, AL 35233
**Phone:** (205)939-9720          **Fax:** (205)939-9245
**Email:** bill.king@chsys.org
Dr. Bill King, Dir.

**Activities/Fields:** Poisonings, including studies on prescription drug ingestions in preschool age children, research on adolescent parasuicides, and epidemiology of childhood trauma. Provides statewide poison control. **Pub:** *Poison Bulletin*, quarterly.

**★ 5781 ★ Children's Hospital and Health Center**
**Center for Pediatric Clinical Research**
3020 Children's Way, MC 5105
San Diego, CA 92123-4282
**Phone:** (858)966-8047          **Fax:** (858)966-8048
**Email:** jyoung@chsd.org
**Website:** http://www.chsd.org/body.cfm?id=494
Joan Young, Contact

**Activities/Fields:** Pharmaceuticals and medical devices for children.

**★ 5782 ★ Children's Hospital Medical Center**
**General Clinical Research Center**
3333 Burnet Ave.
Cincinnati, OH 45229-3039
**Phone:** (513)636-4273          **Fax:** (513)636-4695
**Email:** andrea.smirh@chmcc.org
**Website:** http://www.cincinnatichildrens.org/reseach/research_cores/genral_clinical_research_ce nter/default.htm
Andrea Smith, Mgr.

**Activities/Fields:** Pediatrics, including studies of congenital and acquired diseases of the gastrointestinal tract, pancreas, and liver, cholestatic liver disease, hepatic storage diseases, and cystic fibrosis. Other studies include growth, diabetes mellitus, hypertension, child and adult bone disease (including rickets and osteoporosis), and insulin sensitivity.

**★ 5783 ★ Children's Hospital Oakland Research Institute (CHORI)**
5700 Martin Luther King Jr. Way
Oakland, CA 94609
**Phone:** (510)450-7600          **Fax:** (510)450-7910
**Email:** blubin@chori.org
**Website:** http://www.chori.org
Dr. Bertram Lubin, Dir. of Med. Res.

**Activities/Fields:** Biomedical sciences, especially pediatric diseases but also cancer, cardiovascular disease, and aging. **Pub:** *Research News*, quarterly.

**★ 5784 ★ Children's Hospital of Philadelphia**
**General Clinical Research Center**
Abramson Research Center
34th St. and Civic Ctr., Blvd., Rm. 1202
Philadelphia, PA 19104
**Phone:** (215)590-2017          **Fax:** (215)590-2025
**Email:** starr@email.chop.edu
**Website:** http://stokes.chop.edu
Dr. Stuart E. Starr, MD, Prog. Dir.

**Activities/Fields:** Biomedicine, allergy and immunology, cardiology, diabetes endocrinology, gastroenterology, gene therapy, genetics, hematology, infectious disease, metabolism, neonatology, neurology, nutrition, and oncology.

**★ 5785 ★ Children's Hospital of Pittsburgh**
**General Clinical Research Center**
3705 5th Ave.
Pittsburgh, PA 15213
**Phone:** (412)692-6565          **Fax:** (412)692-6783
Dr. Silva Arslanian, MD, Dir.

**Activities/Fields:** Biomedicine, allergy and immunology, endocrinology, hematology and oncology, infectious disease, metabolism, nutrition, otolaryngology, pulmonology, pharmacology, transplantation surgery, gastroenterology, and diabetes mellitus.

**★ 5786 ★ Children's Hospital Research Center**
3020 Children's Way, MC 5074
San Diego, CA 92123
**Phone:** (858)576-5934          **Fax:** (858)495-8589
Matthew Niedzwiecki, Interim Dir.

**Activities/Fields:** Causes and prevention of childhood diseases, including studies in diagnostic techniques and methods, neurosciences, autism, language development, sudden infant death syndrome, and industrial technology.

**★ 5787 ★ Children's Hospital Research Foundation**
3333 Burnet Ave.
Cincinnati, OH 45229-3039
**Phone:** (513)636-4588          **Fax:** (513)636-0345
**Email:** thomas.boat@chmcc.org
**Website:** http://www.chmcc.org/chrf.html
Thomas F. Boat, MD, Dir.

**Activities/Fields:** Development biology, molecular and cell biology, biochemistry, physiology, microbiology, pathology, and clinical investigations of infancy and childhood, and animal models of childhood illnesses. Research activities are carried out in the divisions of adolescent medicine, allergy/immunology, general pediatrics, development biology, cardiology, molecular cardiovascular biology, clinical pharmacology, critical care medicine, emergency medicine, endocrinology, gastroenterology, hematology-oncology, experimental hematology, human genetics, immunobiology, infectious disease, developmental disabilities, molecular cardiovascular biology, neonatology, nephrology, neurology, pathology, child psychology, child psychiatry, pulmonary biology, pulmonary medicine, radiology, rheumatology, surgery, health policy and clinical effectiveness; the veterinary services division provides care and maintenance of laboratory animals.

**Children's Oncology Group**
**Research Data Center**
*See:* Entry 10310

**★ 5788 ★ Children's Research Institute (Columbus, OH)**
700 Children's Dr.
Columbus, OH 43205
**Phone:** (614)722-2700          **Fax:** (614)722-2716
**Email:** pjohnson@chi.osu.edu
**Website:** http://www.childrenscolumbus.org
Phil Johnson, Pres.

**Activities/Fields:** Molecular retrovirology, gene transfer, molecular genetics, vaccine development, vascular and cellular biology, children's cancer chemotherapy, cancer immunology, gastroenterology, infectious diseases, pathology, surgery, virology, metabolic disorders, cystic fibrosis, pulmonology, pharmacology/toxicology, cardiology, neonatology, pediatrics, and clinical problems of infancy and childhood. **Pub:** *Annual Report.* **Frmly:** Children's Hospital Research Foundation.

**★ 5789 ★ Cornell University**
**General Clinical Research Center— Children**
525 E 68th St., Rm. M-627B
New York, NY 10021-4885
**Phone:** (212)746-3450          **Fax:** (212)746-0300
**Email:** minew@med.cornell.edu
**Website:** http://www.tc.faa.gov
Dr. Maria I. New, MD, Prog. Dir.

**Activities/Fields:** Major areas of investigation include cardiology, endocrinology, genetic diseases, hematology, infectious diseases, metabolism, and neurology.

**Cornell University**
**Laboratory of Pediatric Critical Care**
*See:* Entry 17356

**Duke University**
**Children's Environmental Health Initiative (CEHI)**
*See:* Entry 8938

**★ 5790 ★ Duke University**
**Division of Pediatric Hematology Oncology**
PO Box 2916
Durham, NC 27710
**Phone:** (919)684-3401          **Fax:** (919)681-7950
**Email:** rosof001@mc.duke.edu
**Website:** http://www.env.duke.edu/cehi/about/about.htm
Dr. Philip Rosoff, Div. Ch.

**Activities/Fields:** Clinical trials of new cancer therapies for children. Special interests include neuro-oncology and bone marrow transplantation. **Frmly:** Pediatric Oncology Consortium.

**★ 5791 ★ Duke University**
**Pediatric Cardiac Catheterization Laboratory**
Pediatric Cardiology
DUMC 3090
Medical Center, Rm. 7607 DHN
Durham, NC 27710
**Phone:** (919)684-3574          **Fax:** (919)681-5903
**Email:** olaug001@mc.duke.edu
Dr. Martin P. O'Laughlin, Dir.

**Activities/Fields:** Pediatric cardiology, including development of catheter-delivered devices to treat congenital heart disease.

**★ 5792 ★ Duke University**
**Pediatric Rheumatoid Clinic**
Duke Medical Center, Box 3212
Durham, NC 27710
**Phone:** (919)684-6575          **Fax:** (919)684-6616
**Email:** kredi002@mc.duke.edu
Dr. Deborah Kredich, Contact

**Activities/Fields:** Clinical and laboratory pediatric rheumatology and immunology. **Frmly:** Arthritis Pediatric Research Center.

**★ 5793 ★ Florida State University**
**Center for Prevention and Early Intervention**
1339 E Lafayette St.
Tallahassee, FL 32301-4770
**Phone:** (850)922-1302          **Fax:** (850)922-1352
**Email:** mgraham@mailer.fsu.edu
**Website:** http://www.cpeip.fsu.edu
Dr. Mimi A. Graham, Dir.

**Activities/Fields:** Child care, infant mental health, teen parents, violence prevention.

**★ 5794 ★ Hospital for Sick Children**
**Research Institute**
555 University Ave.
Toronto, ON, Canada M5G 1X8
**Phone:** (416)813-8138          **Fax:** (416)813-5085
**Email:** showe@sickkids.ca
**Website:** http://www.sickkids.on.ca/
Stuart D. Howe, PhD, Contact

**Activities/Fields:** Understanding, prevention, treatment and care of children's diseases.

**★ 5795 ★ Howard University**
**Child Development Center**
Department of Pediatrics and Child Health
College of Medicine
525 Bryant St. NW, Ste.100
PO Box 19
Washington, DC 20059
**Phone:** (202)806-6973          **Fax:** (202)806-7940
Sheila J. Moseend, Dir.

**Activities/Fields:** Child development and handicapping conditions of childhood, including interdisciplinary studies in pediatrics, neurology, genetics, psychology, speech pathology, and infant development.

**Indiana University**
**Herman B. Wells Center for Pediatric Research**
*See:* Entry 10347

**Indiana University-Purdue University at Indianapolis**
**Cystic Fibrosis and Pediatric Pulmonary Clinic**
*See:* Entry 9398

★ 5796 ★ **Indiana University-Purdue University at Indianapolis**
**Riley Child and Adolescent Psychiatry Clinic**
702 Barnhill Dr., Rm. 3701
Indianapolis, IN 46202-5200
**Phone:** (317)278-3473     **Fax:** (317)278-3762
**Email:** cmcdougl@iupui.edu
**Website:** http://www.iupui.edu/~wellsctr/
Christopher J. McDougle, MD, Dir.
**Activities/Fields:** Clinical phenomenology, neurobiology and psychopharmacology of autistic and related pervasive developmental disorders, obsessive-compulsive and chronic tic disorders, attention-deficit and other disruptive behavior disorders, and mood disorders. **Frmly:** Riley Child Guidance Clinic.

**Institutes for Achievement of Human Potential**
*See:* Entry 14208

★ 5797 ★ **Johns Hopkins University**
**Center for Adolescent Health Promotion and Disease Prevention**
Bloomberg School of Public Health
2007 E Monument St.
Baltimore, MD 21205
**Phone:** (410)614-3953     **Fax:** (410)614-3956
**Email:** calexand@jhsph.edu
**Website:** http://www.jhsph.edu/hao/cah/ceninfo.htm
Dr. Cheryl Alexander, Dir.
**Activities/Fields:** Health needs of adolescents, including developmental transitions which serve as opportunities for community-based health promotion interventions; interventions to modify risk-taking behaviors; interventions which involve the family, school, and community settings; and dissemination of adolescent health information to practitioners and policy makers.

★ 5798 ★ **Johns Hopkins University**
**Child Health Research Center**
600 N Wolfe St., CMSC 2-116
Baltimore, MD 21287
**Phone:** (410)955-5976     **Fax:** (410)955-9850
**Email:** gdover@jhmi.edu
Dr. George Dover, Dir.
**Activities/Fields:** Applies molecular biology techniques to the diagnosis, treatment, and prevention of genetic and acquired hematologic disorders in children. Activities focus on developing techniques to analyze genes and gene products, especially those required for normal development.

★ 5799 ★ **Johns Hopkins University**
**National Policy Center for Children with Special Health Care Needs (CSHCN)**
Department of Population & Family Health Sciences
School of Public Health
624 N Broadway
Baltimore, MD 21205
**Phone:** (410)614-5553
**Email:** cshcn@jhsph.edu
**Website:** http://www.jhsph.edu/centers/cshcn/
Janis Lambert Connallon, Contact

**Activities/Fields:** Systems of care for children with special health care needs and their families. **Pub:** *Fact sheets.*

**Kennedy Krieger Institute**
*See:* Entry 20194

★ 5800 ★ **La Rabida Children's Hospital and Research Center**
E 65th St. at Lake Michigan
Chicago, IL 60649
**Phone:** (773)363-6700     **Fax:** (773)363-7160
**Email:** info@larabida.org
**Website:** http://www.larabida.org
Edem Ekwo, MD, Dir.
**Activities/Fields:** Economic, educational, cultural, and medical effects of childhood chronic illness and disability on families and society. Areas of research include patterns of health care financing, medically complex children, community-based service systems, and the nature of family constellations, including the tracking of child development in family contexts, and intervention studies.

★ 5801 ★ **Legacy Clinical Research and Technology Center**
1225 NE 2nd Ave.
Portland, OR 97208-3950
**Phone:** (503)413-2491     **Fax:** (503)413-4942
**Email:** tmelarag@lhs.org
**Website:** http://www.legacyhealth.org
Dr. Anthony J. Melaragno, Ch. of Res.
**Activities/Fields:** Cardiology, biomechanics, neonatalogy, trauma, burns, infectious diseases, neurobiology, pediatric/adult diabetes, ophthalmology, neurology, transplantation, neuromuscular physiology, neurootology. **Frmly:** Emanuel Research Center.

**Louisiana State University in Shreveport**
**Genetics Section of Pediatrics**
*See:* Entry 9412

★ 5802 ★ **Massachusetts General Hospital for Children**
**Pediatric Pulmonary Unit**
55 Fruit St., VBKBA 015
Boston, MA 02114
**Phone:** (617)726-5576
**Email:** tthurm@lsumc.edu
**Website:** http://www.mgh.harvard.edu/children/dept/medical/pulmonary.html
Daniel Shannon, MD, Contact
**Activities/Fields:** Sudden infant death, the role of mast cells and eosinophils in asthma and the regulation of lung development.

★ 5803 ★ **McGill University**
**Montreal Children's Hospital Research Institute**
2300 Tupper St.
Montreal, QC, Canada H3H 1P3
**Phone:** (514)934-4300     **Fax:** (514)934-4331
Roy Gravel, Dir.
**Activities/Fields:** Basic, clinical,and epidemiologic research into various disorders affecting infants and children, including diabetes, prematurity cystic fibrosis, abnormal growth, learning disabilities, hyperactivity, and genetic diseases.

**Medical College of Georgia**
**Georgia Prevention Institute (GPI)**
*See:* Entry 2542

**Medical University of South Carolina**
**Department of Pediatrics**
**Division of Genetics and Developmental Pediatrics**
**The Vince Moseley Center**
*See:* Entry 8191

★ 5804 ★ **Miami Children's Hospital Research Institute**
3196 SW 62nd Ave.
Miami, FL 33155
**Phone:** (305)663-5811     **Free:** 800-533-1792
**Fax:** (305)663-2461
**Email:** fima.lishitz@mch.com
**Website:** http://www.mch.com
Christian Patrick, MD, Dir.
**Activities/Fields:** Genetic vectoring, nutrition, hematology/oncology, immunology, forensic DNA identity, cardiac surgery, critical care physiology, nephrology. **Pub:** *International Journal of Pediatrics.*

**Mid-Missouri Mental Health Center**
*See:* Entry 12699

★ 5805 ★ **Pediatric Clinical Trials International**
555 S 18th St., Ste. 6E
Columbus, OH 43205
**Phone:** (614)722-4453     **Fax:** (614)722-2662
**Email:** wentzelg@pedcti.com
**Website:** http://www.pedcti.com
Belinda Pinyerd, PhD, Dir.,Oper.
**Activities/Fields:** Childhood illnesses, pharmacology, metabolic and infectious diseases, drug metabolism in children, and endocrine disorders of children. **Frmly:** Children's Hospital Clinical Studies Center.

**Pediatric Oncology Group**
*See:* Entry 10399

★ 5806 ★ **Pennsylvania State University**
**Children's Eating Laboratory (CEL)**
S-110 Henderson Bldg.
University Park, PA 16802
**Phone:** (814)863-9972     **Fax:** (814)865-7307
**Email:** llb15@psu.edu
**Website:** http://www.psu.edu/dept/kidseatinglab/
Dr. Leann L. Birch, Dir.
**Activities/Fields:** Development of children's eating behaviors, including food preferences, food selection, and regulation of meal size.

**Pittsburgh Adolescent Alcohol Research Center (PAARC)**
*See:* Entry 19359

★ 5807 ★ **Research Institute of The Hospital for Sick Children**
555 University Ave.
Toronto, ON, Canada M5G 1X8
**Phone:** (416)813-6350     **Fax:** (416)813-4931
**Email:** buchwald@sickkids.on.ca
**Website:** http://www.sickkids.on.ca
Dr. Manuel Buchwald, Dir.
**Activities/Fields:** Basic and clinical research focused on improving, understanding, preventing, treating and curing children's diseases. Six disciplinary research programs: genetics and genomic biology; structural biology and biochemistry; cell biology; developmental biology; integrative biology; population health sciences. Six interdisciplinary research programs: brain and behavior; cancer and blood; cardiovascular; infection, immunity, injury and repair; lung biology; metabolism. Interdisciplinary research groups focused on specific challenges: cystic fibrosis, lung gene therapy. **Pub:** *Annual Report.*

**★ 5808 ★ Rush University**
**Pediatric Critical Care Research Center**
Rush-Presbyterian-St. Luke's Medical Center
1653 W Congress Pky.
Chicago, IL 60612
**Phone:** (312)942-6194     **Fax:** (312)942-4370
**Email:** sbarnes2@rpslsnc.edu
Dr. Steven Barnes, Res. Dir.

**Activities/Fields:** Pediatric patients, analgesia (for pain relief), sedation, broncholitis, neonatal tetanus in Nigeria.

**★ 5809 ★ St. Jude Children's Research Hospital**
332 N Lauderdale
Memphis, TN 38105-2794
**Phone:** (901)495-3300     **Fax:** (901)525-2720
**Email:** info@stjude.org
**Website:** http://www2.stjude.org
Arthur W. Nienhuis, MD, Dir.

**Activities/Fields:** Pediatric studies in hematology, oncology, infectious diseases, neurology, cardiopulmonary diseases, diagnostic imaging, pharmacokinetics, psychology, and pathology; biomedical studies in biochemistry, immunology, pharmacology, virology and molecular biology, tumor cell biology, experimental oncology, genetics, biostatistics, structural biology, surgery and developmental neurobiology. **Pub:** *Annual Report.* • *Scientific Report,* semiannually. • *St Jude Rounds Newsletter for Pediatricians,* quarterly.

**Shriners Hospital for Children (St. Louis, MO)**
**Center for Metabolic Bone Disease and Molecular Research**
*See:* Entry 8764

**★ 5810 ★ Southwest SIDS Research Institute, Inc.**
100 Medical Dr.
Lake Jackson, TX 77566-5674
**Phone:** (409)297-4411     **Free:** 800-245-SIDS
**Email:** swsids@sat.net
**Website:** http://www.swsids.hicd.com
Judith A. Henslee, Exec. Dir.

**Activities/Fields:** Sudden Infant Death Sydrome (SIDS). **Pub:** *Medical articles and abstracts.*

**★ 5811 ★ State University of New York Health Science Center at Brooklyn**
**Child Psychiatry Research Program**
451 Clarkson Ave., Box 32
Brooklyn, NY 11203
**Phone:** (718)270-1430     **Fax:** (718)245-2517
Dr. Lenora Engle, Dir.

**Activities/Fields:** Behavioral and physiological investigation of development and pathology. Projects include observations of mother-child interaction during infancy and later stages, the objective study of children with behavior disorders, autism, minimal brain damage, and mental retardation. Focuses on psychological, physiological, and neurological phenomena.

**★ 5812 ★ State University of New York Health Science Center at Brooklyn**
**Infant and Child Behavior Laboratory**
450 Clarkson Ave., Box 1203
Brooklyn, NY 11203
**Phone:** (718)270-2598     **Fax:** (718)270-3910
**Email:** jhittelman@downstate.edu
Dr. Joan Hittelman, Exec. Dir. /CEO

**Activities/Fields:** Infant development, including evaluation of various methods of eye protection in jaundiced newborn infants undergoing phototherapy with respect to behavioral, physiological, and biochemical parameters; studies of the contribution of the neonate's sex to the parent-child interaction, particularly with respect to neonatal eye contact and maternal attitudes toward the baby; and follow-up of high risk infants (infants born weighing less than 1000 grams and infants exposed to the HIV virus).

**★ 5813 ★ Temple University**
**Motor Development Laboratory**
PO BOx 2840
Philadelphia, PA 19122-0840
**Phone:** (215)204-1960
Dr. Marcella V. Ridenour, Dir.

**Activities/Fields:** Motor development of infants and young children, including studies on safety of toys, juvenile furniture, cribs, strollers, walkers, high chairs, tricycles and wheeled toys, and playgrounds. Performs biomechanics analysis of infants and young children and evaluations of toys and play equipment through the use of motion pictures.

**★ 5814 ★ Texas Scottish Rite Hospital for Children**
**Research Department**
2222 Welborn St.
Dallas, TX 75219
**Phone:** (214)559-7877     **Fax:** (214)559-7872
**Email:** richb@tsrh.org
**Website:** http://www.tsrh.org
Richard H. Browne, PhD, Res. Prog. Admn.

**Activities/Fields:** Treatment of children with orthopedic and neuromuscular disorders. Primary areas of focus are bioengineering and orthopedic biomechanics, including Ilizarov fixators, spine mechanics, spinal implants design and evaluation, and physical properties of bone; and neurophysiology, including gait analysis and muscle strength assessment. Also conducts drug research, studies of innovative care, and application of new technology.

**U.S. Department of Health and Human Services**
**National Center for Infectious Diseases**
**Division of Bacterial and Mycotic Diseases**
**Childhood and Respirtory Diseases Branch**
*See:* Entry 11889

**U.S. Department of Health and Human Services**
**National Institute of Allergy and Infectious Diseases**
**Division of Acquired Immunodeficiency Syndrome (AIDS)**
**Pediatric Project Team**
*See:* Entry 11910

**U.S. Department of Health and Human Services**
**National Institute of Allergy and Infectious Diseases**
**Division of Acquired Immunodeficiency Syndrome (AIDS)**
**Therapeutics Research Program**
**(Pediatric Medicine Branch)**
*See:* Entry 11913

**U.S. Department of Health and Human Services**
**National Institute of Mental Health**
**Division of Clinical and Treatment Research**
**Child and Adolescent Disorders Research Branch**
*See:* Entry 12718

**U.S. Department of Health and Human Services**
**National Institute of Mental Health**
**Intramural Research Programs Division (Clinical Research)**
**Child Psychiatry Branch**
*See:* Entry 12734

**U.S. Department of Health and Human Services**
**National Institutes of Health**
**National Cancer Institute**
**Division of Clinical Sciences**
**((HIV and AIDS Malignancy Branch — HAMB)**
**Pediatric HIV Working Group — PHWG)**
*See:* Entry 10562

**U.S. Department of Health and Human Services**
**National Institutes of Health**
**National Institute of Child Health and Human Development**
**Division of Intramural Research**
**((Division of Epidemiology, Statistics and Prevention Research)**
**Biometry and Mathematical Statistics Branch)**
*See:* Entry 17830

**U.S. Department of Health and Human Services**
**National Institutes of Health**
**National Institute of Child Health and Human Development**
**Division of Intramural Research**
**(Division of Epidemiology, Statistics and Prevention Research)**
*See:* Entry 9065

**U.S. Department of Health and Human Services**
**National Institutes of Health**
**National Institute of Child Health and Human Development**
**Division of Intramural Research**
**(Pediatric and Reproductive Endocrinology Branch)**
*See:* Entry 8785

**U.S. Department of Health and Human Services**
**National Institutes of Health**
**National Institute of Diabetes and Digestive and Kidney Diseases**
**Division of Diabetes, Endocrinology, and Metabolic Diseases**
**(Type 2 Diabetes in the Pediatric Population Program)**
*See:* Entry 8789

**U.S. Department of Health and Human Services**
**National Institutes of Health**
**National Institute of Diabetes and Digestive and Kidney Diseases**
**Pediatric Nephrology Programs**
*See:* Entry 9179

**U.S. Department of Health and Human Services**
**National Institutes of Health**
**National Institute of Environmental Health Sciences**
**Division of Extramural Research and Training**
**(Centers for Children's Environmental Health and Disease Prevention)**
*See:* Entry 17832

**U.S. Department of Health and Human Services**
**National Institutes of Health**
**National Institute of Mental Health**
**Pediatrics and Developmental Neuropsychiatry Branch**
*See:* Entry 12750

**University of Alabama at Birmingham**
**UAB Civitan International Research Center**
*See:* Entry 8207

**★ 5815 ★ University of Alberta**
**Perinatal Research Centre (PRC)**
220 HMRC
Edmonton, AB, Canada T6G 2S2
**Phone:** (780)492-2765          **Fax:** (780)492-1308
**Email:** david.olson@ualberta.ca
**Website:** http://www.ualberta.ca/PERINATAL/
David Olson, Dir.
**Activities/Fields:** Causes and cures of perinatal illness.

**University of Arizona**
**Pediatric Center for Complementary and Alternative Medicine**
*See:* Entry 4340

**★ 5816 ★ University of British Columbia**
**Centre for Community Health and Health Evaluation Research**
4480 Oak St., Rm. L-408
Vancouver, BC, Canada V6H 3V4
**Phone:** (604)875-3570          **Fax:** (604)875-3569
**Email:** childhealth@sunnyhill.bc.ca
**Website:** http://www.bcricwh.bc.ca/child-health
Dr. Robert Armstrong, Co-Dir.
**Activities/Fields:** Factors that influence and support the healthy development of children and youth and the use and development of scientific methods to measure the effectiveness of health policy, practices, and technologies.

**University of California, Davis**
**Gastroenterology and Nutrition Center**
*See:* Entry 9183

**★ 5817 ★ University of California, San Francisco**
**General Clinical Research Center— Children**
Box 0105
M679 Moffitt Hospital
San Francisco, CA 94143
**Phone:** (415)476-2865          **Fax:** (415)476-3466
**Email:** warad@peds.ucsf.edu
**Website:** http://www.ucdmc.ucdavis.edu
Diane W. Wara, MD, Prog. Dir.
**Activities/Fields:** Major areas of investigation include adolescent medicine, biochemistry, endocrinology, genetic diseases, immunology, neonatology, nephrology, nutrition, oncology, pediatric AIDS, pharmacology and radiation therapy.

**University of California, Santa Barbara**
**Autism Research Center**
*See:* Entry 14407

**★ 5818 ★ University of Cincinnati**
**Institute for Health Policy and Health Services Research**
**Child Policy Research Center**
Children's Hospital Medical Center
3333 Burnet Ave., TCHRF 7523
Cincinnati, OH 45229
**Phone:** (513)636-0180          **Fax:** (513)636-0171
**Email:** diehd0@chmcc.org
**Website:** http://www.chsc-chmc.uc.edu
Dr. Edward F. Donovan, Dir.
**Activities/Fields:** Children's well-being in regards to health issues, services, and outcomes. **Frmly:** Child Health Statistics Center.

**★ 5819 ★ University of Colorado**
**General Clinical Research Center— Pediatric**
The Children's Hospital
1056 E 19th Ave., Box B-218
Denver, CO 80218
**Phone:** (303)837-2957          **Fax:** (303)764-8407
**Email:** sokol.ronald@tchden.org
**Website:** http://www.uchsc.edu/ctrsinst/pedgcrc/ped-index.htm
Ronald J. Sokol, MD, Prog. Dir.
**Activities/Fields:** Developmental behavior, diabetes mellitus, gastroenterology, genetics, hematology, immunology, infectious disease, metabolism, neonatology, neurology, nephrology, nutrition, and pulmonary physiology.

**University of Connecticut**
**A.J. Pappanikou Center for Developmental Disabilities**
*See:* Entry 8213

**★ 5820 ★ University of Florida**
**Institute for Child Health Policy**
5700 SW 34th St., Ste. 323
Gainesville, FL 32608-5367
**Phone:** (352)392-5904          **Fax:** (352)392-8822
**Email:** saf@ichp.edu
**Website:** http://www.ichp.edu
Steve A. Freedman, PhD, Exec. Dir.
**Activities/Fields:** Child health policy and family and child health care delivery issues, including development of an equitable and comprehensive child health policy model for states; development of case management programs for children with special health care needs; development of health care financing strategies, including school enrollment-based health insurance; and comprehensive program development and health services research and evaluation. **Pub:** *Developmental Screening and Family-Centered Care Module.* • *Florida Children's Medical Services Five Year Plan.* • *Maternal and Child Health Thesaurus.* • *Special Care.* • *Special Children.* • *SSI Handbook.* • *SSI Liaison Newsletter.* • *SSInsights.* • *Think! A Forum for Ideas on Child Health Policy Newsletter.*

**★ 5821 ★ University of Illinois at Chicago**
**Psychiatric Institute**
1601 W Taylor St.
Chicago, IL 60612
**Phone:** (312)355-1659          **Fax:** (312)996-7658
**Email:** ealtman@psych.uic.edu
**Website:** http://www.psych.uic.edu/research/ctso
Dr. Edward Altman, Contact
**Activities/Fields:** Psychological and biological factors associated with schizophrenia and major depression and mania, drug trials, brain imaging (PET, MRI, EEG, and ERP), genetic vulnerability, and neurotransmitter receptor studies. Prior to assignment to a research protocol, patients may undergo a drug-free washout period lasting from 3 to 14 days. **Frmly:** Illinois State Psychiatric Institute; Metropolitan Child and Adolescent Services/Psychiatric Institute; Psychiatric Clinical Research Center.

**★ 5822 ★ University of Iowa**
**Child Health Research Center**
Department of Pediatrics
Iowa City, IA 52242
**Phone:** (319)356-0469          **Fax:** (319)356-4855
**Email:** frank-morriss@uiowa.edu
Dr. Frank H. Morriss, Jr., Dir.
**Activities/Fields:** Pediatrics, particularly developmental molecular biology. Activities emphasize the identification and localization of genes on the human genome, investigations of the mechanisms used by specific genes to regulate the synthesis and timing of gene products, and a study on the effects of gene products on the structure and function of developing tissues.

**★ 5823 ★ University of Iowa**
**National Maternal and Child Health Resource Center**
Law, 406 BLB
Iowa City, IA 52242
**Phone:** (319)335-9073          **Fax:** (319)335-9098
**Email:** josephine-gittler@uiowa.edu
**Website:** http://www.uiowa.edu/~vpr/research/organize/maternal.htm
Josephine Gittler, Co-Dir.
**Activities/Fields:** Organization and financing of maternal and child health services, children in the legal system, and public policy in these areas.

**★ 5824 ★ University of Kansas**
**Child and Family Research Center**
4001 Dole Ctr.
Lawrence, KS 66045
**Phone:** (785)864-0528          **Fax:** (785)864-5202
Dr. Dale Walker, Dir.
**Activities/Fields:** Processes of social-emotional development and learning in children, early receptive and expressive language development, early intervention, and parent-infant interaction in normal and high-risk infants. **Frmly:** Infant Research Laboratory.

**University of Kentucky**
**Children's Cancer Study Group**
*See:* Entry 10602

**University of Louisville**
**Child Evaluation Center**
*See:* Entry 8222

**★ 5825 ★ University of Maryland**
**Pediatric Sleep Disorder Center**
22 S Greene St., Rm. N5W67
Baltimore, MD 21201
**Phone:** (410)328-3363          **Fax:** (410)328-0645
**Email:** mfgree0@pop.uky.edu
Catherine Currey, Dir.
**Activities/Fields:** Sudden Infant Death Syndrome (SIDS), including efforts to detect abnormalities present before or at death, correlation of data from clinical evaluation of infants at risk (especially those suffering from apnea or cyanosis), development of animal models to test hypotheses about the etiology of SIDS, examination of tissues from infants who have died from SIDS and other illnesses, animal studies to determine the relationship of specific tissue abnormalities to cause of death, and the psychological effect of infant death on family members. **Frmly:** Sudden Infant Death Syndrome Institute.

**★ 5826 ★ University of Miami**
**Mailman Center for Child Development**
School of Medicine
1601 NW 12th Ave.
Miami, FL 33136
**Phone:** (305)243-6801          **Fax:** (305)243-5978
**Email:** rgarcia@peds.med.miami.edu
**Website:** http://pediatrics.med.miami.edu
F. Daniel Armstrong, PhD, Dir.
**Activities/Fields:** Developmental disabilities, genetic disorders, sensory disorders, and child behavior and development, including prevention and intervention strategies. **Pub:** *Annual Report*.


**University of Michigan**
**Pediatric Surgery Research Laboratories**
*See:* Entry 19627


**★ 5827 ★ University of Minnesota**
**KDWB Variety Family Center**
University Gateway/McNamara Alumni Center
200 Oak St. SE, Ste. 160
Minneapolis, MN 55455-2002
**Phone:** (612)626-3087          **Free:** 800-276-8642
**Fax:** (612)624-0097
**Email:** kdwb-var@umn.edu
**Website:** http://www.allaboutkids.umn.edu
Peggy Mann Rinehart, Exec. Dir.
**Activities/Fields:** Family dynamics and resiliency; self-regulation abilities; physical, emotional, psychological and social health and well-being for children and youth at risk, especially children and youth with disabilities. **Pub:** *Health Issues*. **Frmly:** Institute for Health and Disability; Center for Children with Chronic Illness and Disability.


**★ 5828 ★ University of Nebraska Medical**
**Center**
**Munroe-Meyer Institute**
985450 Nebraska Medical Center
Omaha, NE 68198-5450
**Phone:** (402)559-6400          **Free:** 800-65-MEYER
**Fax:** (402)559-5737
**Email:** mleibowi@unmc.edu
**Website:** http://www.unmc.edu/mmi/
Dr. Bruce Buehler, Dir.
**Activities/Fields:** Problems and needs of children and adults (medical, genetic, or behavioral), including interdisciplinary studies on congenital disorders, dentistry, infant development, language and cognitive disorders, behavioral disorders, and sensory/motor development. Subject populations include families receiving service at the Institute, infants, preschoolers, adolescents, and adults with developmental disabilities. **Pub:** *Annual Report*. **Frmly:** Meyer Rehabilitation Institute.


**University of North Carolina at**
**Greensboro**
**Institute for Health, Science, and Society**
**(IHSS)**
*See:* Entry 3112


**★ 5829 ★ University of Rochester**
**Strong Children's Research Center**
Medical Center
601 Elmwood Ave.
PO Box 777
Rochester, NY 14642
**Phone:** (716)275-0414          **Fax:** (716)271-7512
**Email:** scrc@urmc.rochester.edu
**Website:** http://www.urmc.rochester.edu/scrc
Richard A. Insel, MD, Dir.
**Activities/Fields:** Pediatrics. **Pub:** *Newsletter*, quarterly.


**★ 5830 ★ University of South Florida**
**Lawton and Rhea Chiles Center for**
**Healthy Mothers and Babies**
College of Public Health
13201 Bruce B. Downs Blvd., MDC 56
Tampa, FL 33612-3805
**Phone:** (813)974-8888          **Free:** 877-724-2359
**Fax:** (813)974-8889
**Email:** llanders@hsc.usf.edu
**Website:** http://www.chilescenter.org
Dr. Stanley N. Graven, Dir.
**Activities/Fields:** Pregnancy, infancy, and childhood up to age five. The goal is to determine the most effective strategies, programs and systems for reducing illness and death among mothers and babies, and promoting a healthy, productive lifestyle.


**★ 5831 ★ University of South Florida**
**Research and Training Center for**
**Children's Mental Health**
Florida Mental Health Institute
13301 Bruce B. Downs Blvd.
Tampa, FL 33612-3899
**Phone:** (813)974-4661          **Fax:** (813)974-6257
**Email:** friedman@hal.fmhi.usf.edu
**Website:** http://www.rtckids.fmhi.usf.edu
Robert M. Friedman, PhD, Exec. Dir.
**Activities/Fields:** Children and adolescents with emotional disturbances, focusing on characteristics and development; factors associated with successful transition to adulthood; the relationship between functional abilities and successful employment, residential, educational, and social outcomes; identification and evaluation of model programs to assist transition from school to work; efficacy and cost-effectiveness of alternatives to residential treatment; and financing options, incentives, and disincentives for community and home-treatment.


**University of Tennessee**
**Center of Excellence in Pediatric**
**Pharmacokinetics and Therapeutics**
*See:* Entry 17401


**University of Tennessee**
**Children's Mental Health Services**
**Research Center**
*See:* Entry 12775


**University of Tennessee, Knoxville**
**Children's Mental Health Services**
**Research Center**
*See:* Entry 12776


**★ 5832 ★ University of Texas Medical**
**Branch at Galveston**
**Child Health Research Center (CHRC)**
Department of Pediatrics
301 University Blvd.
Galveston, TX 77555-0351
**Phone:** (409)772-1751          **Fax:** (409)772-1761
**Email:** lstanbe@utmb.edu
**Website:** http://utcmhsrc.csw.utk.edu/
Dr. Lawrence Stanberry, Chm.
**Activities/Fields:** Pediatrics, focusing on applying research in developmental immunology, improving health, and combatting childhhod diseases. **Pub:** *The Growth Chart*, biennially.


**★ 5833 ★ University of Texas**
**Southwestern Medical Center at Dallas**
**Sleep Disorders Center for Children**
Children's Medical Center of Dallas
1935 Motor St.
Dallas, TX 75235-7794
**Phone:** (214)456-2793          **Fax:** (214)456-8740
Dr. John Herman, Dir.
**Activities/Fields:** Studies infants with respiratory problems, children with obstructive sleep apnea, and

excessive daytime sleepiness (narcolepsy). Conducts studies of vigilance and related visual evoked potentials.


**★ 5834 ★ University of Washington**
**Center for Child Environmental Health**
**Risks Research (CHC)**
Department of Environmental Health
4225 Roosevelt Way NE, No. 100
Seattle, WA 98105-6099
**Phone:** (206)616-3523          **Fax:** (206)616-4875
**Email:** chc@u.washington.edu
**Website:** http://depts.washington.edu/chc/
Thomas Burbacher, PhD, Dep. Dir.
**Activities/Fields:** Children's susceptibility to pesticides and the ways pesticides affect normal development and learning.


**★ 5835 ★ University of Washington**
**Child Health Institute (CHI)**
146 N Canal St., Ste. 300
Seattle, WA 98103-8652
**Phone:** (206)616-9410          **Fax:** (206)543-5318
**Email:** chiorg@u.washington.edu
**Website:** http://depts.washington.edu/chiorg/
Dimitri Christakis, Co-Dir.
**Activities/Fields:** Access, cost-effectiveness, quality and outcomes of health care for children.


**★ 5836 ★ University of Washington**
**Fetal Alcohol and Drug Unit**
Department of Psychiatry & Behavioral Sciences
180 Nickerson St., Ste. 309
Seattle, WA 98109
**Phone:** (206)543-7155          **Fax:** (206)685-2903
**Email:** astreiss@u.washington.edu
**Website:**          http://depts.washington.edu/fadu/content.html
Prof. Ann P. Streissguth, PhD, Dir.
**Activities/Fields:** Prevention, intervention and treatment of Fetal Alcohol Syndrome (FAS) and Fetal Alcohol Effects (FAE).


**★ 5837 ★ University of Washington**
**Pediatric Epilepsy Research Center**
**(PERC)**
HSB RR 705A
Box 356470
1959 NE Pacific Ave.
Seattle, WA 98195-6470
**Phone:** (206)221-5364          **Fax:** (206)221-5721
**Email:** perc@u.washington.edu
**Website:** http://depts.washington.edu/perc/
Philip Schwarzkroin, PhD, Dir.
**Activities/Fields:** Prevention, control, and cure of pediatric epilepsy.


**University of Wisconsin—Madison**
**Pediatric Pulmonary Center**
*See:* Entry 9526


**Vanderbilt University**
**John F. Kennedy Center for Research on**
**Human Development**
*See:* Entry 6911


**★ 5838 ★ W.M. Krogman Center for**
**Research in Child Growth and**
**Development**
University of Pennsylvania
4019 St. Irving
Philadelphia, PA 19104-6003
**Phone:** (215)898-1470          **Fax:** (215)898-5243
**Email:** childquest@eudoramail.com
**Website:** http://www.vanderbilt.edu/kennedy
Dr. Solomon H. Katz, Dir.
**Activities/Fields:** Obesity, nutrition, and other health and mental disorders, epidemiology of high blood

pressure in adolescents, neuropsychological development, developmental disorders, hypertension, and subclinical lead intoxication and other trace element studies in children. Also establishes norms of physical growth and development of Philadelphia and international children from birth to 17 years of age, including norms for head, face, and jaws (cephalometric and roentgenographic cephalometric), body (height, weight, somatometric size, and proportion of trunk and limbs), and maturation levels (via X-ray films and hand and knee), applied to clinical problems in medicine and dentistry. **Frmly:** Philadelphia Center for Research in Child Growth and Development.

★ 5839 ★ **Wayne State University**
**Institute of Maternal and Child Health**
　　**(IMCH)**
Department of Community Medicine
4201 St. Antoine, No. 9D UHC
Detroit, MI 48201
**Phone:** (313)577-1033
**Email:** aa2266@wayne.edu
**Website:** http://www.med.wayne.edu/communitymedicine/imch.htm
Dr. John B. Waller, Ch.
**Activities/Fields:** Maternal and child health.

★ 5840 ★ **Yale University**
**Child Health Research Center**
Department of Pediatrics
PO Box 208081
New Haven, CT 06520
**Phone:** (203)737-5970　　　**Fax:** (203)737-5972
**Email:** margaret.hostetter@yale.edu
Margaret K. Hostetter, MD, Dir.
**Activities/Fields:** Cellular and molecular biological studies of normal development and the ability of the fetus and child to adapt to environmental or genetic influences.

★ 5841 ★ **Yale University**
**General Clinical Research Center—**
　　**Children**
Department of Pediatrics
Yale New Haven Hospital
20 York St.
7-4 S Pavililion
New Haven, CT 06504
**Phone:** (203)785-4648　　　**Fax:** (203)737-1998
**Email:** william.tamborlane@yale.edu
**Website:** http://info.med.yale.edu/crc/welcome.html
Dr. William V. Tamborlane, Jr., Prog. Dir.
**Activities/Fields:** Major areas of investigation include anesthesiology, cardiology, endocrinology, gastrointestinal disorders, genetic diseases, infectious diseases, mineral and bone metabolism, neonatology, neurology, psychiatry and pulmonary diseases.

**Yale University**
**Pediatric Cystic Fibrosis Research Center**
*See:* Entry 9533

★ 5842 ★ **Yeshiva University**
**Preventive Intervention Research Center**
　　**for Child Health**
1300 Morris Park Ave.
Bronx, NY 10461
**Phone:** (718)918-4390　　　**Fax:** (718)918-4388
**Email:** rstein@aecom.yu.edu
Ruth E.K. Stein, MD, Dir.
**Activities/Fields:** Children with serious ongoing health problems (infancy through adolescence) and their families and the effect of parental illness on children. Activities include preventive interventions for children with asthma and HIV/AIDS, secondary analyses of large scale data sets on childhood disability, measurement development on chronic conditions, functional status and social support. Also studies the social support of minority mothers of chronically ill youngsters, epidemiology and consequences of serious ongoing health conditions, psychological and

social adaptation among children with juvenile rheumatoid arthritis.

★ 5843 ★ **Zero to Three/National Center**
　　**for Infants, Toddlers and Families**
2000 M St. NW, Ste. 200
Washington, DC 20036
**Phone:** (202)638-1144　　　**Fax:** (202)638-0851
**Email:** 0to3@zerotothree.org
**Website:** http://www.zerotothree.org
Matthew E. Melmed, Exec. Dir.
**Activities/Fields:** Parent informational needs (conducted through survey and focus groups) and development of a diagnostic classification system for mental health and development disorders of infants and young children.

# State Government Agencies

## Maternal & Child Health

★ 5844 ★ **Alabama Department of Public**
　　**Health**
**Family Health Services Bureau**
RSA Tower
201 Monroe St. Ste 1350
PO Box 303017
Montgomery, AL 36104
**Phone:** (334)206-5661　　　**Fax:** (334)206-2950
**Email:** webmaster@www.alapubhealth.org
**Website:** http://www.alapubhealth.org

★ 5845 ★ **Alaska Department of Health**
　　**and Social Services**
**Public Health Division**
**Maternal and Child Family Health Section**
3601 C St., Ste. 934
PO Box 240249
Anchorage, AK 99524-0249
**Phone:** (907)269-3400　　　**Free:** 800-799-7570
**Fax:** (907)269-3465
**Email:** pam_muth@health.state.ak.us
**Website:** http://www.hss.state.ak.us/dph/mcfh/SectionMCFH.htm

★ 5846 ★ **Arizona Department of Health**
　　**Services**
**Family Health and Community Services**
　　**Division**
**Women and Children's Health Office**
2927 N35th Ave, Ste. 300
Phoenix, AZ 85017
**Phone:** (602)364-1400　　　**Fax:** (602)364-1494
**Website:** http://www.hs.state.az.us/cfhs/owch/

★ 5847 ★ **California Health and Welfare**
　　**Agency**
**Health Services Department**
**Maternal and Child Health Branch**
714 P St., Rm. 750
Sacramento, CA 95814
**Phone:** (916)657-1347
**Website:** http://www.dhs.cahwnet.gov/org/pcfh/mchb/mchbindex.htm

★ 5848 ★ **Colorado Public Health and**
　　**Environment Department**
**Health Office**
**Division of Prevention and Intervention**
　　**Services for Children and Youth**
4300 Cherry Creek Dr. S A-4
Denver, CO 80246
**Phone:** (303)692-2310
**Website:** http://www.cdphe.state.co.us/fc/fchom.asp

★ 5849 ★ **Connecticut Department of**
　　**Public Health**
**Community Health Bureau**
**Child Adolescent Health Division**
Hartford, CT
**Phone:** (860)509-8066　　　**Fax:** (860)509-7720
**Email:** webmaster.dph@po.state.ct.us
**Website:** http://www.state.ct.us/dph/BCH/Family%20Health/HPFamHS.html
Beth Weinstein, M.P.H., Contact

★ 5850 ★ **Delaware Department of Health**
　　**and Social Services**
**Public Health Division**
**Family Health Services**
Jesse Cooper Bldg.
417 Federal St.
PO Box 637
Dover, DE 19903
**Phone:** (302)739-4787　　　**Fax:** (302)739-6653
**Email:** dhssinfo@state.de.us
**Website:** http://www.state.de.us/dhss/dph/chca/fhs_index.html

★ 5851 ★ **District of Columbia**
　　**Department of Health**
**Office of Maternal and Child Health**
825 N Capitol St. NE, 3rd Fl.
Washington, DC 20002
**Phone:** (202)442-5925　　　**Fax:** (202)442-4947
**Website:** http://www.dchealth.com/mch

★ 5852 ★ **Georgia Department of**
　　**Community Health**
**Division of Medical Assistance**
**Maternal and Child Health Division**
2 Peachtree St. NW
Atlanta, GA 30303
**Phone:** (404)656-4507
**Website:** http://www.communityhealth.state.ga.us/

★ 5853 ★ **Hawaii Department of Health**
**Health Resources Administration**
**Family Health Services Division**
**Maternal and Child Health Branch**
741 Sunset Ave.
Honolulu, HI 96816
**Phone:** (808)733-9022　　　**Fax:** (808)733-9068
**Website:** http://www.state.hi.us/health/about/resources.html
Momi Kamau, Director

★ 5854 ★ **Idaho Department of Health**
　　**and Welfare**
**Health Division**
**Maternal and Child Health Bureau**
PO Box 83720
707 N Armitage Pl.
Boise, ID 83704-0825
**Phone:** (208)327-8595　　　**Fax:** (208)334-6581
**Website:** http://www2.state.id.us/dhw/hwgd_www/contentlist.htmlHealth

★ 5855 ★ **Indiana Department of Health**
**Maternal and Child Health Services**
　　**Division**
2 N Meridian
Indianapolis, IN 46204
**Phone:** (317)233-1262　　　**Fax:** (317)233-1299
**Email:** jganser@isdh.state.in.us
**Website:** http://www.state.in.us/isdh/programs/mch/index2.htm
Judith A. Ganser, MD, Director

**★ 5856 ★ Iowa Department of Public Health**
**Family and Community Health Division**
**Maternal and Child Health Section**
Lucas State Office Bldg., 3rd Fl.
321 E 12th St.
Des Moines, IA 50319-0075
**Phone:** (515)242-6388          **Fax:** (515)242-6384
**Email:** webmaster@idph.state.ia.us
**Website:** http://idph.state.ia.us/fch/fam_serv/mhs.htm
Janet L. Peterson, Contact


**★ 5857 ★ Kansas Department of Health and Environment**
**Health Division**
**Family Health Bureau**
1000 SW Jackson St., Ste. 220
Topeka, KS 66612-1274
**Phone:** (785)291-3368        **Fax:** (785)296-6553
**Email:** lkenney@kdhe.state.ks.us
**Website:** http://www.kdhe.state.ks.us/bcyf/index.html
Linda Kenney, Director


**★ 5858 ★ Kentucky Health Services Cabinet**
**Health Services Department**
**Maternal and Child Health Services Division**
275 E Main St.
Frankfort, KY 40621
**Phone:** (502)564-9538         **Fax:** (502)564-7091
**Website:** http://chs.state.ky.us/


**★ 5859 ★ Louisiana Department of Health and Hospitals**
**Public Health Office**
**Health Services Programs**
**Maternal and Child Health Section**
325 Loyola Ave.
PO Box 60630
New Orleans, LA 70160
**Phone:** (504)568-5073         **Fax:** (504)568-8162
**Email:** ophwebmaster@dhhmail.dhh.state.la.us
**Website:** http://www.dhh.state.la.us/OPH/mch.htm


**★ 5860 ★ Maine Department of Human Services**
**Health Bureau**
**Maternal and Child Health Division**
11 State House Station
157 Capitol St.
Augusta, ME 04333
**Phone:** (207)287-8016
**Email:** Cheryl.M.DiCara@state.me.us
**Website:** http://janus.state.me.us/dhs/boh/
Marcie Sanders, Contact


**★ 5861 ★ Massachusetts Executive Office of Health and Human Services**
**Public Health Department**
**Family Health Services Division**
250 Washington St. 5th Floor
Boston, MA 02108-4619
**Phone:** (617)624-6060         **Fax:** (617)624-6062
**Website:** http://www.state.ma.us/dph/bfch/index.htm
Sally Fogerty, Contact


**★ 5862 ★ Minnesota Department of Health**
**Maternal and Child Health Section**
717 Delaware St. SE
PO Box 64975
Minneapolis, MN 55414
**Phone:** (651)281-9888
**Email:** fh@kids.health.state.mn.us
**Website:** http://www.health.state.mn.us/divs/fh/fh.html


**★ 5863 ★ Mississippi Department of Health**
**Health Services Bureau**
**WIC Services**
570 E Woodrow Wilson Blvd.
PO Box 1700
Jackson, MS 39215
**Phone:** (601)576-7100          **Fax:** (601)576-7070
**Email:** cjordan@msdh.state.ms.us
**Website:** http://www.msdh.state.ms.us/osho/fldsvcs/Centrllk.htm
Curtis Jordan, Contact


**★ 5864 ★ Missouri Department of Health**
**Maternal, Child and Family Health Division**
930 Wildwood
PO Box 570
Jefferson City, MO 65102
**Phone:** (573)751-8394          **Fax:** (573)751-6041
**Email:** info@mail.health.state.mo.us
**Website:** http://www.health.state.mo.us/AbouttheDepartment/DS9.html


**★ 5865 ★ Montana Department of Public Health and Human Services**
**Child and Family Services Division**
1400 Broadway
PO Box 8005
Helena, MT 59604-8005
**Phone:** (406)444-5900          **Fax:** (406)444-5956
**Email:** cfsd@state.mt.us
**Website:** http://www.dphhs.state.mt.us/divisions/cfs/cfs.htm
Chuck Hunter, Director


**★ 5866 ★ Nebraska Department of Health and Human Services**
**Health Promotion and Disease Prevention**
**Office of Family Health**
301 Centennial Mall S
PO Box 95044
Lincoln, NE 68509-5044
**Phone:** (402)471-2907
**Email:** family.health@hhs.state.ne.us
**Website:** http://www.hhs.state.ne.us/hpe/hpeindex.htm
Paula Eurek, Director


**★ 5867 ★ Nevada Department of Human Resources**
**Health Division**
**Family Health Service**
505 E King St.
Carson City, NV 89701
**Phone:** (775)684-4285
**Website:** http://health2k.state.nv.us/BFHS/index.htm


**★ 5868 ★ New Hampshire Department of Health and Human Services**
**Public Health Services Division**
**Maternal and Child Health Bureau**
129 Pleasant St.
Concord, NH 03301-6527
**Phone:** (603)271-4517          **Fax:** (603)271-3827
**Website:** http://www.dhhs.state.nh.us/


**★ 5869 ★ New Jersey Department of Health**
**Family Health Services Division**
**Maternal and Child Health Services**
E State St.
PO Box 364
Trenton, NJ 08625-0364
**Phone:** (609)292-4043          **Fax:** (609)292-9599
**Email:** cfa@doh.state.nj.us
**Website:** http://www.state.nj.us/health/fhs/chshome.htm
Celeste Andriot Wood, Director


**★ 5870 ★ New Mexico Department of Health**
**Public Health Division**
**Maternal and Child Health Bureau**
1190 St. Francis Dr.
Santa Fe, NM 87502-6110
**Phone:** (505)476-8586          **Free:** 877-696-1472
**Fax:** (505)476-8512
**Website:** http://www.health.state.nm.us/


**★ 5871 ★ North Carolina Department of Health, and Human Services**
**Public Health Division**
**Women's and Children's Health**
1916 Mail Service Ctr.
Raleigh, NC 27699-1916
**Phone:** (919)715-7937          **Fax:** (919)715-3925
**Email:** WCH.Info@ncmail.net
**Website:** http://wch.dhhs.state.nc.us/


**★ 5872 ★ North Dakota Department of Health**
**Preventive Health Section**
**Maternal and Child Health Division**
600 E Boulevard Ave.
Bismarck, ND 58505-0200
**Phone:** (701)328-2493          **Fax:** (701)328-1412
**Email:** sanseth@state.nd.us
**Website:** http://www.health.state.nd.us/ndhd/prevent/mch/
Sandra Anseth, Director


**★ 5873 ★ Oklahoma Department of Health**
**Personal Health Services**
**Maternal and Child Health Services**
1000 NE 10th St., Rm. 506
Oklahoma City, OK 73117
**Phone:** (405)271-4477
**Website:** http://www.health.state.ok.us/PROGRAM/mchs/index.html


**★ 5874 ★ Oregon Department of Human Resources**
**Health Division**
**Child and Family Health Center**
Portland State Office Bldg.
800 NE Oregon St.
Portland, OR 97232
**Phone:** (503)731-4000
**Email:** ohd.info@state.or.us
**Website:** http://www.ohd.hr.state.or.us/ccfh/welcome.htm


**★ 5875 ★ Rhode Island Department of Health**
**Family Health Office**
3 Capitol Hill, Rm. 302
Providence, RI 02908
**Phone:** (401)222-2312          **Free:** 800-942-7434
**Fax:** (401)222-1442
**Email:** library@health.state.ri.us
**Website:** http://www.health.state.ri.us/yhd07.htm


**★ 5876 ★ South Carolina Department of Health and Environmental Control**
**Health Services Office**
**Maternal and Child Health Bureau**
2600 Bull St.
PO Box 101106
Columbia, SC 29211-0106
**Phone:** (803)898-0773
**Email:** kyleja@dhec.state.sc.us
**Website:** http://www.scdhec.net/hs/mch/mch.htm

## ★ 5877 ★ South Dakota Department of Health
**Maternal and Child Health Program**
615 E Fourth St.
Pierre, SD 57501-1700
**Phone:** (605)773-3737          **Free:** 800-738-2301
**Email:** DOH.INFO@state.sd.us
**Website:**          http://www.state.sd.us/doh/Famhlth/index.htm


## ★ 5878 ★ Tennessee Department of Health
**Health Services Bureau**
**Maternal and Children's Health Section**
Cordell Hull Bldg., 5th Fl.
425 5th Ave. North
Nashville, TN 37247-0101
**Phone:** (615)741-7353          **Fax:** (615)741-1063
**Email:** DDenton@mail.state.tn.us
**Website:** http://www.state.tn.us/health/


## ★ 5879 ★ Vermont Agency of Human Services
**Health Department**
**Maternal and Child Health Bureau**
1193 North Ave, Ste. 1
Burlington, VT 05401-2749
**Phone:** (802)863-7323          **Fax:** (802)863-7571
**Website:** http://www.state.vt.us/health/
Jan Campbell, Contact


## ★ 5880 ★ Virginia Office of Health and Human Resources
**Health Department**
**Women and Infants Health Division**
1500 E Main St., Rm. 132
Richmond, VA 23219
**Phone:** (804)786-5420          **Free:** 888-942-3663
**Website:** http://www.vahealth.org/wic/


## ★ 5881 ★ Washington Department of Health
**Community and Family Health Services Division**
New Market Industrial Campus
Bldg. 10
PO Box 47835
Olympia, WA 98504-7835
**Phone:** (360)236-3505
**Email:** glenda.moore@doh.wa.gov
**Website:**          http://www.doh.wa.gov/Org/org.htmCommunity


## ★ 5882 ★ West Virginia Department of Health and Human Resources
**Public Health Bureau**
**Bureau for Children and Families**
350 Capitol St.
Room 730
Charleston, WV 25305-3711

**Email:** michaelpack@wvdhhr.org
**Website:** http://www.wvdhhr.org/bcf/
Fred Boothe, Contact


## ★ 5883 ★ Wisconsin Department of Health and Family Services
**Division of Public Health**
**Family Health Program**
**Maternal and Child Health Section**
1 W Wilson St.
PO Box 2659
Madison, WI 53702
**Phone:** (608)267-3561          **Free:** 800-722-2295
**Email:** uttecsm@dhfs.state.wi.us
**Website:**          http://www.dhfs.state.wi.us/aboutdhfs/dph/dph.htm
Susan Uttech, Contact


## ★ 5884 ★ Wyoming Department of Health
**Public Health Division**
**Maternal and Child Health Services**
Hathaway Bldg., 4th Fl.
Cheyenne, WY 82002
**Phone:** (307)777-6004          **Fax:** (307)777-3617
**Email:** pshera@state.wy.us
**Website:** http://wdhfs.state.wy.us/dcfh/
Jimm Murray, Contact

# Chapter 15
# Chiropractic

## Foundations & Other Funding Organizations

### Other Funding Organizations

**★ 5885 ★ American Chiropractic Association (ACA)**
1701 Clarendon Blvd.
Arlington, VA 22209
**Phone:** (703)276-8800 **Free:** 800-986-4636
**Fax:** (703)243-2593
**Email:** memberinfo@amerchiro.org
**Website:** http://www.amerchiro.org
Garrett F. Cuneo, HCD, Exec. VP
**Desc:** Enhances the philosophy, science, and art of chiropractic, and the professional welfare of individuals in the field. Promotes legislation defining chiropractic health care and improves the public's awareness and utilization of chiropractic. Conducts chiropractic survey and statistical study; maintains library. Sponsors Correct Posture Week in May and Spinal Health Month in October. Chiropractic colleges have student ACA groups. **Awards:** Scholarship (periodic) to students at chiropractic colleges.

**★ 5886 ★ American College of Chiropractic Orthopedists (ACCO)**
c/o Dr. Jesse Rothenberger
1030 Broadway, Ste. 101
El Centro, CA 92243
**Phone:** (760)370-9106
**Website:** http://www.accoweb.org
Dr. Jesse Rothenberger, Pres.
**Desc:** Certified (426) and noncertified (304) chiropractic orthopedists; students enrolled in a postgraduate chiropractic orthopedic program (100). Seeks to establish and maintain optimal educational and clinical standards within the field of chiropractic orthopedics. Sponsors educational programs. **Awards:** F. Maynard Lipe Scholarship (annual); recognition.

**★ 5887 ★ Association of Chiropractic Colleges (ACC)**
c/o David S. O'Bryon
4424 Montgomery Ave., Ste. 102
Bethesda, MD 20814
**Phone:** (301)652-5066 **Fax:** (301)913-9146
**Email:** Info@ChiroColleges.org
**Website:** http://www.chirocolleges.org
David S. O'Bryon, CAE, Exec. Dir.
**Desc:** Presidents of chiropractic colleges that are members of the Council on Chiropractic Education. Objective is to provide a cooperative base that assists members in the search for and promotion of the practices and concepts most effective in the academic and continuing education of doctors of chiropractic. Serves as a clearinghouse for information related to opportunities and advancement in research as they affect chiropractic education and health care. Seeks to enhance services to the consumer of chiropractic education and to the public. **Awards:** Student Scholarships in Chiropractic (annual).

**★ 5888 ★ Foundation for Chiropractic Education and Research (FCER)**
704 E 4th St.
Des Moines, IA 50309
**Phone:** (515)282-3347 **Free:** 800-622-6309
**Fax:** (515)282-3347
**Email:** fcernow@aol.com
**Website:** http://www.fcer.org
DeAnna L. Beck, Dir.
**Desc:** Chiropractors and laymen. Provides funding for scientific research and research training that will "enhance the knowledge and practice of chiropractic as a conservative approach to health care restoration, maintenance, and disease prevention." **Awards:** Fellowship for postdoctorate students; grant for research in clinical science; grant for dissertations in biomechanics and public health.

## Medical & Allied Health Schools

### Chiropractic

*Listed below are programs and institutions accredited by The Council on Chiropractic Education, 804 N 85th Way, Scottsdale, AZ 85258, (480)443-8877. Information on chiropractic as a career is available from the American Chiropractic Association, 1701 Clarendon Blvd., Arlington, VA 22209, (800)986-4636, http://www.amerchiro.org.*

#### California

**★ 5889 ★ Cleveland Chiropractic College, Los Angeles**
590 N Vermont Ave.
Los Angeles, CA 90004
**Phone:** (323)660-6166 **Free:** 800-466-2252
**Fax:** (323)906-2090
**Email:** givradm@cleveland.edu
**Website:** http://www.clevelandchiropractic.edu

**★ 5890 ★ Life Chiropractic College, West**
25001 Industrial Blvd.
Hayward, CA 94545
**Phone:** (510)780-4500 **Free:** 800-788-4476
**Fax:** (510)780-4515
**Email:** gclum@LifeWest.edu
**Website:** http://www.lifewest.edu
Gerard W. Clum, President

**★ 5891 ★ Palmer College of Chiropractic, West**
90 E Tasman Dr.
San Jose, CA 95134
**Phone:** (408)944-6005 **Free:** 800-442-4476
**Fax:** (408)944-6111
**Email:** riekeman_g@palmer.edu
**Website:** http://www.palmer.edu
Guy Riekeman, President

**★ 5892 ★ Southern California University of Health Sciences**
**Los Angeles College of Chiropractic**
16200 E Amber Valley Dr.
PO Box 1166
Whittier, CA 90609-1166
**Phone:** (562)902-3330 **Free:** 800-221-5222
**Fax:** (562)947-7863
**Email:** reedphillips@scuhs.edu
**Website:** http://www.scuhs.edu
Reed B. Phillips, PhD, President

#### Connecticut

**★ 5893 ★ University of Bridgeport College of Chiropractic**
75 Linden Ave.
Bridgeport, CT 06601
**Phone:** (203)576-4278 **Free:** 888-822-4476
**Fax:** (203)576-4483
**Email:** frank.zolli@snet.net
**Website:** http://www.bridgeport.edu/chiro
Frank A. Zolli, Contact

#### Georgia

**★ 5894 ★ Life University College of Chiropractic**
1269 Barclay Circle
Marietta, GA 30060
**Phone:** (770)424-0554 **Free:** 800-543-3202
**Fax:** (770)429-4819
**Email:** drsid@life.edu
**Website:** http://www.life.edu
Sid E. Williams, President

#### Illinois

**★ 5895 ★ National University of Health Sciences**
**College of Professional Studies**
**Doctor of Chiropractic Degree Program**
200 E Roosevelt Rd.
Lombard, IL 60148-4583
**Phone:** (630)889-6604 **Free:** 800-826-6285
**Fax:** (630)889-6600
**Email:** jwinterstein@nuhs.edu
**Website:** http://www.nuhs.edu
James F. Winterstein, President

#### Iowa

**★ 5896 ★ Palmer College of Chiropractic**
1000 Brady St.
Davenport, IA 52803
**Phone:** (563)884-5621 **Free:** 800-722-2586
**Fax:** (563)884-5409

**Email:** riekeman_g@palmer.edu
**Website:** http://www.palmer.edu

## Minnesota

**★ 5897 ★ Northwestern Health Sciences University**
**Northwestern College of Chiropractic**
2501 W 84th St.
Bloomington, MN 55431
**Phone:** (952)885-5410          **Free:** 800-888-4777
**Fax:** (952)886-7583
**Email:** njohnson@nwhealth.edu
**Website:** http://www.nwhealth.edu
Alfred D. Traina, President

## Missouri

**★ 5898 ★ Cleveland Chiropractic College, Kansas City**
6401 Rockhill Rd.
Kansas City, MO 64131
**Phone:** (816)501-0100          **Free:** 800-467-2252
**Fax:** (816)361-0272
**Email:** drcsciii@cleveland.edu
**Website:** http://www.clevelandchiropractic.edu
Carl S. Cleveland, III, President

**★ 5899 ★ Logan College of Chiropractic**
1851 Schoettler Rd.
PO Box 1065
Chesterfield, MO 63006-1065
**Phone:** (636)227-2100          **Free:** 800-782-3344
**Fax:** (636)207-2420
**Email:** goodman@logan.edu
**Website:** http://www.logan.edu
George A. Goodman, President

## New York

**★ 5900 ★ New York Chiropractic College**
2360 State Rd. 89
PO Box 800
Seneca Falls, NY 13148-0800
**Phone:** (315)568-3100          **Free:** 800-234-6922
**Fax:** (315)568-3012
**Email:** fnicchi@nycc.edu
**Website:** http://www.nycc.edu
Frank Nicchi, President

## Ontario

**★ 5901 ★ Canadian Memorial Chiropractic College**
1900 Bayview Ave.
Toronto, ON, Canada M4G 3E6
**Phone:** (416)482-2340          **Fax:** (416)482-9745
**Website:** http://www.cmcc.ca
Jean A. Moss, President

## Oregon

**★ 5902 ★ Western States Chiropractic College**
2900 NE 132nd Ave.
Portland, OR 97230
**Phone:** (503)251-5712          **Free:** 800-641-5641
**Fax:** (503)251-2817
**Email:** whdallas@wschiro.edu
**Website:** http://www.wschiro.edu
William H. Dallas, President

## Quebec

**★ 5903 ★ University of Quebec, Trois Rivieres**
**Chiropractic Program**
CP 500
Trois Rivieres, QC, Canada G9A 5H7
**Phone:** (819)376-5186          **Fax:** (819)376-5204
**Email:** andre_m_gonthier@uqtr.uquebec.ca
Dr. Andre-Marie Gonthier, Director

## South Carolina

**★ 5904 ★ Sherman College of Straight Chiropractic**
2020 Springfield Rd.
PO Box 1452
Spartanburg, SC 29304
**Phone:** (864)578-8770          **Free:** 800-849-8771
**Fax:** (864)599-7145
**Email:** jhardee@sherman.edu
**Website:** http://www.sherman.edu
Jerry L. Hardee, President

## Texas

**★ 5905 ★ Parker College of Chiropractic**
2500 Walnut Hill Ln., Ste. 100E
Dallas, TX 75229-5668
**Phone:** (214)902-3470          **Free:** 800-438-6932
**Fax:** (214)352-6603
**Email:** president@parkercc.edu
**Website:** http://www.parkercc.edu
Fabrizio Mancini, President

**★ 5906 ★ Texas Chiropractic College**
5912 Spencer Hwy.
Pasadena, TX 77505-1699
**Phone:** (281)487-1170          **Free:** 800-468-6839
**Fax:** (281)487-0329
**Email:** smelliott@txchiro.edu
**Website:** http://www.txchiro.edu
Shelby M. Elliott, President

# National & International Organizations

**★ 5907 ★ American Chiropractic Association (ACA)**
1701 Clarendon Blvd.
Arlington, VA 22209
**Phone:** (703)276-8800          **Free:** 800-986-4636
**Fax:** (703)243-2593
**Email:** memberinfo@amerchiro.org
**Website:** http://www.amerchiro.org
Garrett F. Cuneo, HCD, Exec. VP
**Fnded:** 1930. **Mem:** 18,000. **Desc:** Enhances the philosophy, science, and art of chiropractic, and the professional welfare of individuals in the field. Promotes legislation defining chiropractic health care and improves the public's awareness and utilization of chiropractic. Conducts chiropractic survey and statistical study; maintains library. Sponsors Correct Posture Week in May and Spinal Health Month in October. Chiropractic colleges have student ACA groups. **Pub:** *ACA/Today*, monthly. Newsletter. Covers the issues facing the profession and the association. *Price:* Included in membership dues. • *American Chiropractic Association Membership Directory*, annual. Directory. • *Journal of the American Chiropractic Association*, monthly. Journal. Provides information on the progress of chiropractic procedures and research, and developments in other fields of interest to chiropractors. *Price:* Included in membership dues; $3/year for student members; $80/year for nonmembers; $150/year for international members. **Frmly:** (1963) National Chiropractic Association.

**★ 5908 ★ American Chiropractic Association - Council on Sports Injuries and Physical Fitness (ACA)**
303 Beach Dr.
Annapolis, MD 21403
**Phone:** (410)990-1112          **Free:** 800-593-3222
**Fax:** (410)990-1134
**Website:** http://www.acasc.org
Tim Ray, Pres.
**Desc:** Active chiropractors. Promotes the treatment of athletes; works closely with athletic organizations and health professionals to promote better understanding of chiropractic care as valuable in athletic training and treatment.

**★ 5909 ★ American Chiropractic College of Radiology (ACCR)**
PO Box 1151
Lombard, IL 60148
**Phone:** (630)372-7260
**Email:** dacbr219@hotmail.com
**Website:** http://www.accr.org/
J. Todd Knudsen, Sec. /Treas.
**Desc:** Seeks to educate the chiropractic and health care communities.

**★ 5910 ★ American Chiropractic Registry of Radiologic Technologists (ACRRT)**
2330 Gull Rd.
Kalamazoo, MI 49048
**Phone:** (616)343-6666          **Fax:** (616)343-7236
Dr. Edward Maurer, Exec. VP
**Fnded:** 1982. **Mem:** 2,000. **Desc:** Chiropractic assistants and radiologic technologists employed in chiropractic offices. Educates the general public concerning the importance of having highly skilled radiologic technologists (those who administer X-rays) in chiropractic offices. Serves as a national certifying agency for individuals in the field; maintains registry of certified chiropractic radiologic technologists. **Pub:** *Wavelengths*, bimonthly. Newsletter.

**★ 5911 ★ American College of Chiropractic Consultants (ACCC)**
1720 Washington Rd., Ste. 201
Pittsburgh, PA 15241
**Fax:** (412)833-6320
**Email:** willtell@usaor.net
**Website:** http://www.accc-chiro.com/
William Tellin, DC, Pres.
**Fnded:** 1980. **Desc:** Independent contractors providing advisory consulting services to insurance carriers and health care organizations, and other entities sponsoring chiropractic benefits. Promotes adherence to high standards of ethics and practice among chiropractors. Establishes chiropractic standards and conducts certification examinations; sponsors continuing professional development courses for chiropractors.

**American College of Chiropractic Orthopedists (ACCO)**
*See:* Entry 16911

**American Society of Podiatrists and Chiropractors (ASPC)**
*See:* Entry 17715

**★ 5912 ★ Anglo-European College of Chiropractic (AECC)**
13-15 Parkwood Rd.
Bournemouth BH5 2DF, United Kingdom
**Phone:** 44 1202 436200          **Fax:** 44 1202 436312
**Email:** aecc@aecc.ac.uk
**Website:** http://www.aecc.ac.uk
**Fnded:** 1965. **Mem:** 25. **Lang(s):** English. **Desc:** Chiropractic practitioners, educators, and students. Seeks to advance the study, teaching, and practice of chiropractic. Facilitates communication among members; sponsors research and educational programs. **Pub:** Newsletter, semiannual.

**★ 5913 ★ Association of Chiropractic Colleges (ACC)**
c/o David S. O'Bryon
4424 Montgomery Ave., Ste. 102
Bethesda, MD 20814
**Phone:** (301)652-5066          **Fax:** (301)913-9146
**Email:** Info@ChiroColleges.org
**Website:** http://www.chirocolleges.org
David S. O'Bryon, CAE, Exec. Dir.

**Fnded:** 1977. **Mem:** 18. **Desc:** Presidents of chiropractic colleges that are members of the Council on Chiropractic Education. Objective is to provide a cooperative base that assists members in the search for and promotion of the practices and concepts most effective in the academic and continuing education of doctors of chiropractic. Serves as a clearinghouse for information related to opportunities and advancement in research as they affect chiropractic education and health care. Seeks to enhance services to the consumer of chiropractic education and to the public. **Pub:** *Journal of Chiropractic Education*, quarterly. Journal. **Frmly:** (1985) Association of Chiropractic College Presidents.

★ **5914** ★ **Association for the History of Chiropractic (AHC)**
c/o Alana Callender
1000 Brady St.
Davenport, IA 52803
**Phone:** (563)884-5855          **Fax:** (563)884-5616
**Email:** callender_a@palmer.edu
**Website:** http://chirohistory.com
Alana Callender, Exec. Dir.

**Fnded:** 1980. **Mem:** 340. **Nat'l Groups:** 2. **Desc:** Chiropractors, students, educators, and writers; chiropractic colleges; organizations. Researches and records the history of the chiropractic profession and disseminates information on the subject. Maintains speakers' bureau. **Pub:** *AHC Bulletin*, quarterly. Newsletter. *Price:* Included in membership dues. • *Association for the History of Chiropractic Membership Directory*, periodic. Membership Directory. Includes association bylaws. *Price:* available to members only. • *Chiropractic History: The Archives and Journal of the Association of the History of Chiropractic*, semiannual. Magazine. Includes association news. Index available. *Price:* Included in membership dues; $24 for nonmembers. • *Style Manual for Authors.* Manual.

★ **5915** ★ **Blair Chiropractic Society**
c/o Todd A. Hubbard, D.C.
610 Plaza Dr., Ste. 2
Sycamore, IL 60178
**Free:** 877-732-6300
**Email:** hubchiro@tbcnet.com
**Website:** http://www.blairchiropracticsoc.org
Todd A. Hubbard, D.C., Contact

**Desc:** For practitioners using the Blair method of upper cervical chiropractic.

★ **5916** ★ **British Chiropractic Association**
Blagrave House
17 Blagrave St.
Reading RG1 1QB, United Kingdom
**Phone:** 44 118 9505950      **Fax:** 44 118 9588946
**Email:** enquiries@chriropractic-uk.co.uk
**Website:** http://www.chiropractic-uk.co.uk
**Fnded:** 1925. **Mem:** 860. **Desc:** Complementary medicine practitioners/chiropractors. Concerned with treatment of spinal disorders by specialised manipulative techniques. **Pub:** *Contact*, quarterly. • *In Touch*, monthly. Newsletter.

★ **5917** ★ **Canadian Chiropractic Association (CCA)**
**(Association Chiropratique Canadienne — ACC)**
1396 Eglinton Ave. W
Toronto, ON, Canada M6C 2E4
**Phone:** (416)781-5656      **Fax:** (416)781-7344
**Email:** querry@ccachino.org
**Website:** http://www.ccachiro.org
**Lang(s):** English, French. **Desc:** Chiropractors. Promotes excellence in the study, teaching, and practice of chiropractic. Sponsors continuing professional education courses for members; conducts promotional activities.

★ **5918** ★ **Canadian Chiropractic Examining Board (CCE B)**
1144 29th Ave. NE, Ste. 103
Calgary, AB, Canada T2E 7P1
**Phone:** (403)230-5997          **Fax:** (403)230-3221
**Email:** drlawson@cceb.ca
**Website:** http://www.cceb.ca
**Fnded:** 1962. **Lang(s):** English, French. **Desc:** Chiropractic practitioners and educators. Promotes excellence in the practice of chiropractic. Conducts examinations and bestows certification upon chiropractic practitioners; develops standards of practice for chiropractors.

★ **5919** ★ **Canadian Chiropractic Protective Association (CCPA)**
**(L'Association de Protection Chiropratique Canadienne)**
1396 Eglinton Ave. W
Toronto, ON, Canada M6C 2E4
**Phone:** (416)785-4570          **Fax:** (416)781-7344
**Email:** query@ccachiro.org
**Website:** http://www.ccachiro.org
**Lang(s):** English, French. **Desc:** Chiropractors. Promotes professional advancement of members; seeks to increase public awareness of chiropractic. Conducts promotional and educational programs.

★ **5920** ★ **ChiroFeed International**
300 Vine St., Ste. 18
Seattle, WA 98121
**Phone:** (206)448-2004
**Email:** julianemes@reachone.com
**Website:** http://www.chirofeed.org
**Fnded:** 1998. **Desc:** Chiropractors. Provide chiropractic exams and care to underprivileged people.

★ **5921** ★ **Chiropractic Association of South Africa (CASA)**
**(Chiropraktiese Vereniging van Suid-Afrika)**
PO Box 706
Bethlehem 9700, Republic of South Africa
**Phone:** 27 58 3034571      **Fax:** 27 58 3091480
**Email:** rve@nnet.co.za
**Website:** http://www.chiropractic.co.za
**Fnded:** 1970. **Mem:** 140. **Nat'l Groups:** 1. **Reg. Groups:** 4. **State Groups:** 1. **Local Groups:** 4. **Lang(s):** Afrikaans, English. **Desc:** Seeks to: heighten public awareness of the chiropractic system of therapy; improve medical insurance coverage of such treatment. Offers training curricula; conducts periodic seminars. **Pub:** *Newswire*, periodic. Newsletter. • *Inter-Association Newsletter*, periodic. Newsletter. Membership.

★ **5922** ★ **Congress of Chiropractic State Associations (COCSA)**
PO Box 2054
Lexington, SC 29071
**Phone:** (803)356-6809          **Fax:** (803)356-6826
**Email:** cocsa@sc.rr.com
**Website:** http://www.cocsa.org
Janet Jordan, Exec. Dir.
**Fnded:** 1968. **Mem:** 69. **Nat'l Groups:** 8. **Reg. Groups:** 5. **State Groups:** 54. **Desc:** State chiropractic associations. Seeks to "provide an apolitical forum for the promotion and advancement of the chiropractic profession." Works to advance the study, teaching, and practice of chiropractic and natural health; serves as a clearinghouse on problems facing the chiropractic profession; provides support and services to members. **Pub:** *Congress Connection*, quarterly. Newsletter.

★ **5923** ★ **Council on Chiropractic Education (CCE)**
8049 N 85th Way
Scottsdale, AZ 85258-4321
**Phone:** (480)443-8877          **Fax:** (480)483-7333

**Email:** cce@cce-usa.org
**Website:** http://www.cce-usa.org
Vincent Lucido, Pres.
**Fnded:** 1971. **Mem:** 16. **Desc:** Advocates high standards in chiropractic education; establishes criteria of institutional excellence for educating chiropractic physicians; acts as national accrediting agency for chiropractic colleges. Conducts workshops for college teams, consultants, and chiropractic college staffs. **Pub:** *CCE Board of Directors*, annual. • *Educational Standards for Chiropractic Colleges*, semiannual. • Newsletter, periodic. • Also publishes pamphlets, news releases, and lists of institutions conforming to its standards and policies.

★ **5924** ★ **Council on Chiropractic Orthopedics (CCO)**
472 E 1930 N
Orem, UT 84097-2234
**Email:** docrussell@aol.com
**Website:** http://www.ccodc.org
Roger A. Russell, Pres.
**Fnded:** 1967. **Mem:** 750. **Desc:** Licensed doctors of chiropractic who have completed 360 hours of postgraduate courses in orthopedics (690); chiropractic physicians with an interest in orthopedics (60). Objectives are: to assist in the advancement of chiropractic as a science and healing art; to protect the welfare and interests of members; to encourage and maintain the highest standards of moral and ethical conduct; to romote research; to encourage the standardization of terminology; to disseminate information; to encourage the teaching of chiropractic orthopedics at all levels. Reviews and revises postgraduate courses in chiropractic. Fosters seminars and courses in personal, athletic, and industrial injuries; provides consulting. Maintains American Board Board of Chiropractic Orthopedists which serves as an examining body for certification. Certified orthopedists comprise the Academy of Chiropractic Orthopedists. A division of the American Chiropractic Association. **Pub:** *Orthopedic Briefs*, bimonthly. • Brochure. • Directory, annual.

★ **5925** ★ **Council on Chiropractic Physiological Therapeutics and Rehabilitation (CCPT)**
c/o Donald Fedoryk
2035 Brooks Blvd.
Hillsborough, NJ 08844
**Phone:** (908)722-9075          **Fax:** (908)722-1144
**Website:** http://www.ccptr.org/
Donald Fedoryk, DC, Sec. -Treas.
**Fnded:** 1920. **Mem:** 200. **Desc:** Chiropractors who use physiotherapy in their practice and are dedicated to furthering the extended use of physiotherapy in the chiropractic field. Plans to provide a diplomate or certification program. **Pub:** *Physiotherapy Briefs*, periodic. **Frmly:** (1985) American Council on Chiropractic Physiotherapy.

★ **5926** ★ **European Chiropractors' Union (ECU)**
c/o Mrs. A. Kemp
9 Cross Deep Gardens
Twickenham TW1 4QZ, United Kingdom
**Phone:** 44 181 8912546      **Fax:** 44 181 7442902
**Fnded:** 1932. **Mem:** 2,300. **Nat'l Groups:** 16. **Lang(s):** English. **Desc:** National associations (16) representing 2200 chiropractors; interested others (25). Promotes the development of chiropractic medicine and colleges through legal, educational, and research activities; maintains standards for chiropractic education in Europe. Works to foster unity among European chiropractors' associations. Provides research funds. **Pub:** *European Chiropractors' Union Directory*, annual. Directory. • *European Journal of Chiropractic*, quarterly. Journal.

★ **5927** ★ **European Council on Chiropractic Education**
8, chemin de Tison
F-86000 Poitiers, France

**Phone:** 33 5 49415825

---

**★ 5928 ★ European Federation of Pro Chiropractic Associations (EFPC)**
Frederikkevej 2A
Hellerup
DK-2900 Copenhagen, Denmark
**Phone:** 45 39 400540          **Fax:** 45 39 400540
**Email:** etogalt@get2net.dk
**Website:** http://www.efpc.org
**Desc:** Promotes chiropractic in Europe to allow all people access, if needed, to chiropractic care. **Pub:** Newsletter, periodic.

---

**★ 5929 ★ Federation of Chiropractic Licensing Boards (FCLB)**
901 54th Ave., Ste. 101
Greeley, CO 80634-4400
**Phone:** (970)356-3500          **Fax:** (970)356-3599
**Email:** fclb@fclb.org
**Website:** http://www.fclb.org
Wayne C. Wolfson, Pres.
**Fnded:** 1926. **Desc:** Dedicated to protecting the public promoting excellence in chiropractic regulation. **Pub:** *Chiropractic Licensure and Practice Statistics*, annual. Directory.

---

**★ 5930 ★ Federation of Straight Chiropractors and Organizations (FSCO)**
2276 Wassergass Rd.
Hellertown, PA 18055
**Phone:** (610)838-3030          **Free:** 800-521-9856
**Fax:** (610)838-3031
**Email:** fsco@straightchiropractic.com
**Website:** http://www.straightchiropractic.com
Dr. Richard Plummer, Chm.
**Fnded:** 1978. **Mem:** 600. **State Groups:** 5. **Desc:** Individuals and organizations in the chiropractic field. Promotes the practice of straight (traditional) chiropractic. Conducts lobbying and educational programs. **Pub:** *FSCO Insider*, bimonthly. Reports on current organization news and professional information. • *President's Update*, bimonthly. **Frmly:** Federation of Straight Chiropractic Organizations.

---

**★ 5931 ★ Flying Chiropractors Association (FCA)**
2001 Bridgeway St.
Sausalito, CA 94965
**Phone:** (415)332-4304
Dr. Dwight A. Shaneyfelt, Contact
**Fnded:** 1968. **Mem:** 300. **Reg. Groups:** 9. **Desc:** Flying chiropractic physicians. Objectives are to: promote fellowship; seek designation as aviation medical examiners (doctors who examine pilots for their licensure); promote aviation safety. Conducts seminars. **Pub:** *D.C. Flyer*, quarterly.

---

**★ 5932 ★ Foundation for the Advancement of Chiropractic Tenets and Science (FACTS)**
c/o International Chiropractors Association
1110 N Glebe Rd., Ste. 1000
Arlington, VA 22201
**Phone:** (703)528-5000          **Free:** 800-423-4690
**Fax:** (703)528-5023
**Email:** chiro@chiropractic.org
**Website:** http://www.chiropractic.org
Ronald Hendrickson, Exec. Dir.
**Fnded:** 1972. **Desc:** Dedicated to the improvement of human health through understanding and development of new chiropractic information. Offers financial aid for education and research programs in colleges and independent institutions; supports chiropractic research program at University of Colorado in Boulder. Has conducted extensive survey of the chiropractic profession for the federal government. Is approved by the National Institutes of Health of the U.S. Public Health Service. **Pub:** *Chiropractic Health Care*. **Frmly:** International Chiropractors Research Foundation.

---

**★ 5933 ★ Foundation for Chiropractic Education and Research (FCER)**
704 E 4th St.
Des Moines, IA 50309
**Phone:** (515)282-3347          **Free:** 800-622-6309
**Fax:** (515)282-3347
**Email:** fcernow@aol.com
**Website:** http://www.fcer.org
DeAnna L. Beck, Dir.
**Fnded:** 1944. **Mem:** 3,000. **Desc:** Chiropractors and laymen. Provides funding for scientific research and research training that will "enhance the knowledge and practice of chiropractic as a conservative approach to health care restoration, maintenance, and disease prevention." **Pub:** *Chiropractic Healthways Newsletter*, bimonthly. Newsletter. Promotes health and fitness. Includes research updates. • *Foundation for Chiropractic Education and Research–Advance*, quarterly. Magazine. Foundation activities newsletter. *Price:* Free. • Also publishes pamphlets. **Frmly:** (1958) Chiropractic Research Foundation; (1967) Foundation for Accredited Chiropractic Education.

---

**★ 5934 ★ Gonstead Clinical Studies Society**
2778 Cumberland Blvd., No. 230
Smyrna, GA 30080
**Free:** 888-556-4277          **Fax:** 888-556-4277
**Email:** gcsschiro@aol.com
**Website:** http://www.gonstead.com
**Desc:** Promotes awareness of the Gonstead System of chiropractic and its record of safety and effectiveness in correcting vertebral subluxation.

---

**★ 5935 ★ International Chiropractic Pediatric Association (ICPA)**
5295 Hwy. 78, Ste. D362
Stone Mountain, GA 30087-3414
**Phone:** (770)565-2360          **Free:** 800-670-KIDS
**Fax:** (770)736-1651
**Email:** info@icpa4kids.com
**Fnded:** 1996. **Mem:** 1,200. **Desc:** Chirpractors and chiropractic students with an interest in the treatment of pediatric patients. Seeks to advance the study, teaching, and practice of pediatric chiropractic; promotes continuing professional development of members. Serves as a clearinghouse on pediatric health; sponsors research and educational programs; formulates standards of practice for pediatric chiropractic and conducts certification examinations. **Pub:** Newsletter, bimonthly.

---

**★ 5936 ★ International Chiropractors Association (ICA)**
1110 N Glebe Rd., Ste. 1000
Arlington, VA 22201
**Phone:** (703)528-5000          **Free:** 800-423-4690
**Fax:** (703)528-5023
**Email:** chiro@chiropractic.org
**Website:** http://www.chiropractic.org/
Ronald Hendrickson, Exec. Dir.
**Fnded:** 1926. **Mem:** 6,000. **Desc:** Professional society of chiropractors, chiropractic educators, students, and laypersons. Sponsors professional development programs and practice management seminars. **Pub:** *Congressional Directory*, annual. Directory. • *ICA Today*, bimonthly. Newsletter. Covers membership and association activities; includes legislative information and research updates. *Price:* Included in membership dues. • *International Chiropractors Association Membership Directory*, annual. Directory. • *International Review of Chiropractic*, bimonthly. • Also publishes materials on patient education. **Frmly:** (1941) Chiropractic Health Bureau.

---

**★ 5937 ★ Japanese Chiropractic Association (JCA)**
IK Bldg.
6-20-11 Shinbashi
Minato-ku
Tokyo 105-0004, Japan
**Phone:** 81 3 54010961          **Fax:** 81 3 54010956
**Fnded:** 1961. **Mem:** 170. **Desc:** Promotes the use of chiropractic therapy in Japan. Maintains and upholds standards of conduct of members. Conducts educational programs.

---

**★ 5938 ★ National Board of Chiropractic Examiners (NBCE)**
901 54th Ave.
Greeley, CO 80634
**Phone:** (970)356-9100
**Email:** nbce@nbce.org
**Website:** http://www.nbce.org
**Fnded:** 1963. **Desc:** Develops, administers and scores examinations taken by applicants for chiropractic licensure by experienced practitioners seeking reciprocity, endorsement or relicensure. **Pub:** *NBCE Journal*. Journal.

---

**★ 5939 ★ National Board of Forensic Chiropractors (NBOFC)**
601 S Mill St.
PO Box 356
Manning, SC 29102
**Phone:** (803)435-5078          **Fax:** (803)435-8096
**Email:** omyback@gte.net
**Website:** http://www.forensicexaminers.org/
**Desc:** Association of examiners, scientists and professionals dedicated to orderly analysis, investigation and examination to obtain the truth, then provide expert opinion. **Pub:** Newsletter.

---

**★ 5940 ★ National Upper Cervical Chiropractic Association (NUCCA)**
c/o Dennis P. Allen
121 W Locust St., Ste. 208
Davenport, IA 52803
**Phone:** (319)322-7486          **Fax:** (319)322-0628
**Website:** http://www.nucca.org
Dr. Robert Goodman, Pres.
**Desc:** Promotes chiropractic, especially the NUCCA technique; seeks to improve the art of chiropractic; promotes education; sponsors studies.

---

**★ 5941 ★ Parker Chiropractic Resource Foundation (PCRF)**
2619 Electronic LN, Ste 206
Dallas, TX 75220-1226
Chance Parker, Pres.
**Fnded:** 1951. **Mem:** 30,000. **Desc:** Doctors of chiropractic. Seeks to keep the chiropractic profession abreast of new developments, practices, and procedures concerning the administration of health care. **Pub:** *Share*, monthly. Magazine. **Frmly:** (1987) Parker Chiropractic Research Foundation.

---

**★ 5942 ★ Women's Auxiliary of the ICA (WAICA)**
1110 N Glebe Rd., Ste. 1000
Arlington, VA 22201
**Phone:** (703)528-5000          **Fax:** (703)528-5023
Robert Braile, Pres.
**Fnded:** 1951. **Mem:** 500. **Desc:** Women chiropractors; wives, daughters, and mothers of chiropractors who are members of the International Chiropractors Association. Promotes and educates the public about chiropractice. Grants scholarships to chiropractic students. Supports charitable programs. **Pub:** *Membership Roster*, biennial. Membership Directory. • Newsletter, quarterly.

**★ 5943 ★ World Federation of Chiropractic (WFC)**
3080 Yonge St., Ste. 5065
Toronto, ON, Canada M4N 3N1
**Phone:** (416)484-9978     **Fax:** (416)484-9665
**Website:** http://www.wfc.org
**Fnded:** 1988. **Desc:** Chiropractors, colleges, corporations, and national associations of chiropractors in over 60 countries. Represents the chiropractic profession internationally. Provides information and assistance in the fields of chiropractic and world health. Promotes uniformly high standards of chiropractic education, research, and practice. **Pub:** Membership Directory.

## Research Centers

**★ 5944 ★ Consortial Center for Chiropractic Research**
741 Brady St.
Davenport, IA 52803
**Phone:** (319)884-5162     **Fax:** (319)884-5227
**Email:** info@c3r.org
**Website:** http://www.c3r.org
William C. Meeker, VP,Res.
**Activities/Fields:** Potential effectiveness and validity of chiropractic health care.

**★ 5945 ★ Foundation for Chiropractic Education and Research**
1330 Beacon St., Ste. 315
Brookline, MA 02446-3202
**Phone:** (617)734-3397     **Free:** 888-690-1378
**Fax:** (617)734-0989
**Email:** rosnerfcer@aol.com
**Website:** http://www.fcer.org
Anthony Rosner, PhD, Dir.,Res. & Educ.
**Activities/Fields:** Chiropractic medicine. Research areas include biomechanical studies of the spine and related soft tissue structures; the relationship between spine and body functions; the effects of manipulation upon various body functions; clinical traits of spinal manipulation; the effectiveness of manipulation for various conditions; reliability of various chiropractic analytical and diagnostic procedures; the various instrumentations used in chiropractic; and surveys of utilization of chiropractic treatment and epidemiological and sociological studies. **Pub:** *Chiropractic Healthways Pamphlet Series.* • *This Week in Chiropractic Advance.*

**★ 5946 ★ Northwestern Health Sciences University**
**Wolfe-Harris Center for Clinical Studies**
2501 W 84th St.
Bloomington, MN 55431
**Phone:** (952)888-4777     **Free:** 800-888-4777
**Fax:** (952)888-1957

**Email:** csawyer@nwhealth.edu
**Website:** http://www.nwhealth.edu/nwchiro/research/face.html
Charles E. Sawyer, VP
**Activities/Fields:** Chiropractic clinical research, including ambulatory health care.

**★ 5947 ★ Precision Chiropractic Research Society**
3462 Windsor Ct.
Costa Mesa, CA 92626
**Phone:** (714)641-4700
A.C. Fulkerson, Pres.
**Activities/Fields:** Spinal problems and treatment, including an investigation of the relationship between the cure for headaches and spinal adjustment. Also studies Duchennne muscular dystrophy.

**★ 5948 ★ Sacro Occipital Research Society International**
PO Box 6067
Leawood, KS 66206
**Free:** 888-245-1011     **Fax:** (913)341-7685
**Email:** cbinyon@kc.rr.com
**Website:** http://www.sorsi.com
Candice Binyon, Contact
**Activities/Fields:** Chiropractic studies, focusing on the sacro occipital area of the brain.

<h1 align="center">Chapter 16<br>Communicative Disorders</h1>

## Federal Government Agencies

**★ 5949 ★ U.S. Department of Health and Human Services**
**National Institutes of Health (NIH)**
**National Institute on Deafness and Other Communication Disorders (NIDCD)**
9000 Rockville Pike
Bethesda, MD 20892
**Phone:** (301)496-7243
**Website:** http://www.nidcd.nih.gov
James F. Battey, Jr., Director

**Desc:** NIDCD conducts and supports biomedical and behavioral research and research training on normal mechanisms as well as diseases and disorders of hearing, balance, smell, taste, voice, speech, and language through a deiversity of research performed in its own laboratories; a program of research grants, individual and institutional research training awards, career development awards, center grants, and contracts to public and private research institutions and organizations.

## Foundations & Other Funding Organizations

### Private Foundations

**Joseph Meyerhoff Fund**
*See:* Entry 11402

**Oberkotter Foundation**
*See:* Entry 13857

**Robert W. Wilson Foundation**
*See:* Entry 13519

**★ 5950 ★ Rockefeller Brothers Fund, Inc.**
437 Madison Ave., 37th Floor
New York, NY 10022-7001
**Phone:** (212)812-4200          **Fax:** (212)812-4299
**Email:** rock@rbf.org
**Website:** http://www.rbf.org
Benjamin Shute, Jr., Secretary

**Fnded:** 1940. **Philosophy:** "The fund seeks to achieve its major objective of improving the well-being of all people through support of efforts in the United States and abroad that contribute ideas, develop leaders, and encourage institutions in the transition to global interdependence and that counter world trends of resource depletion, militarization, protectionism, and isolation which now threaten to move humankind everywhere further away from cooperation, trade and economic growth, arms restraint, and conservation." In order to achieve these goals, the fund makes grants in eight general areas. *One World Nonprofit Sector* The second of the fund's initiatives seeks to promote the health and vitality of the nonprofit sector, both nationally and internationally. The fund promotes the growth of philanthropy, encourages greater accountability within the nonprofit sector, and fosters increased understanding of the sector and its roles in society. *Education* Its goal is to strengthen the number and quality of teachers in public education in the United States and, in particular, to encourage minorities to enter the teaching profession. To this end, the fund awards fellowships to minority teaching students at 25 participating colleges and universities. *New York City* The Fund is committed to strengthening and enhancing civil society by supporting efforts to build civic engagement and capacity in communities. *Special Concerns* South Africa "Seeks to improvr the quality and accessibility of basic education for children and adults in South Africa, in the areas of early childhood development, lower primary learning, and adult basic education and training." Arts and Culture "Primary focus is to create access with the goal of building greater understanding and appreciation of the art forms or cultural activities served by applicant organizations." Health "Suppoorts projects involving research and education in the field of human health." The program includes the Charles E. Culpeper Biomedical Pilot Initiative and the Charles E. Culpeper Scholarship Medicine Science program. 1999 Annual Report. The Fund also supports the Ramon Magsaysay Award Foundation, which grants the Ramon Magsaysay Awards, named after the former president of the Philippines, that were established by the trustees of the Fund in the late 1950s, and the Pocantico Programs which provide public access to the Pocantico Historic Area, the heart of the Rockefeller family estate in Westchester County, New York, and were established when the Fund leased the area from the National Trust for Historic Preservation in 1991. **Priorities:** *Arts & Humanities:* 13%. Funds museums, theater, and cultural activities. *Civic & Public Affairs:* 35%. Grants given to the Nonprofit Sector and New York City. *Education:* 35%. Supports programs and educational scholarships that attempt to enhance the quality of education by enhancing the quality of the professionals in the education field. *International:* 1%. Supports medical research. *Note:* Total contributions made in 1999. **Typ. Recipients:** Speech & Hearing. **Geo. Dist:** internationally; nationally; New York, NY.

**★ 5951 ★ Samuel M. Soref and Helene K. Soref Foundation**
123 S Broad St.
Philadelphia, PA 19109-1199
**Phone:** (954)467-5131
Michael Krofton, Administrator

**Fnded:** 1983. **Philosophy:** The foundation primarily grants major contributions to large, select Jewish organizations. **Priorities:** *Civic & Public Affairs:* 3%. Supports ethnic organizations. *Education:* 42%. Supports Jewish educational institutions and Judaic programs in non-Jewish schools, and universities. *Environment:* 8%. Suports homes, shelters, food banks, and senior services. *International:* 1%. *Note:* Total contributions made in 1999. **Typ. Recipients:** Children's Health/Hospitals, Emergency/Ambulance Services, Health Organizations, Hospitals, Long-Term Care, Medical Education, People with Disabilities, Speech & Hearing. **Geo. Dist:** CA; FL.

### Corporate Foundations

**Binney & Smith Inc.**
*See:* Entry 887

**Wachtell, Lipton, Rosen & Katz Foundation**
*See:* Entry 2894

### Other Funding Organizations

**★ 5952 ★ Alexander Graham Bell Association for the Deaf (AGBAD)**
3417 Volta Pl. NW
Washington, DC 20007
**Phone:** (202)337-5220          **Fax:** (202)337-8314
**Email:** cfisk@agbell.org
**Website:** http://www.agbell.org
K. Todd Houston, PhD, Exec. Dir.

**Desc:** Teachers of the hearing impaired, speech-language pathologists and audiologists, physicians, parents of hearing impaired children, oral deaf adults, and others interested in the problems of the hearing impaired; affiliate members are organized groups of parents of deaf children and coordinators of state and provincial chapters. Works to: promote the teaching of speech, lipreading, and use of residual hearing to the deaf; encourage research on deafness; assist schools and agencies working for better educational facilities for deaf and oral hearing impaired children. Conducts workshops and educational programs. Compiles statistics. Maintains speakers' bureau. Serves as information center and maintains library on speech and hearing. Operates charitable program, biographical archives, museum, and placement service. **Awards:** Recognition; scholarship (annual) for oral deaf students.

**★ 5953 ★ American Auditory Society (AAS)**
512 E Canterbury Ln.
Phoenix, AZ 85022
**Phone:** (602)789-0755          **Fax:** (602)942-1486
**Email:** amaudsoc@aol.com
**Website:** http://www.amauditorysoc.org
Wayne J. Staab, PhD, Sec. -Treas.

**Desc:** Audiologists, otolaryngologists, scientists, hearing aid industry professionals, and educators of hearing impaired people; individuals involved in industries serving hearing impaired people, including the amplification systems industry. Works to increase knowledge and understanding of: the ear, hearing, and balance; disorders of the ear, hearing, and balance; prevention of these disorders; habilitation and rehabilitation of individuals with hearing and balance dyofunction. **Awards:** Carhart Memorial Lecturer (annual) for contribution to goals of the society; Lifetime Achievement Award (periodic) for contributions to the discipline of hearing.

**★ 5954 ★ Children of Deaf Adults (CODA)**
Box 30715
Santa Barbara, CA 93130
**Phone:** (805)682-0997          **Fax:** (617)789-3801
**Email:** coda@coda-international.org
**Website:** http://www.coda-international.org
Millie Brother, Founder

**Desc:** Hearing children of deaf parents who are interested in sharing experiences with others of similar backgrounds. Provides information to professional organizations, libraries, community agencies, researchers, and other interested persons. Acts upon issues regarding deafness; provides support to deaf parent/hearing child families. Serves as clearinghouse for deaf parent/hearing children families. **Awards:** Millie Brother Scholarship (annual).

**★ 5955 ★ Cochlear Implant Association**
5335 Wisconsin Ave. NW, Ste. 440
Washington, DC 20015-2052
**Phone:** (202)895-2781          **Fax:** (202)895-2782
**Email:** info@cici.org
**Website:** http://www.cici.org
Peg Williams, PhD, Exec. Dir.

**Desc:** Cochlear implant users, candidates for cochlear implant, and their families and friends; health care professionals. Provides support services including advocacy for the hearing impaired. Promotes improved cochlear implant technology and research on hearing impairment. Serves as an information clearinghouse. Conducts educational programs and childrens' services; operates speakers' bureau. **Awards:** Dr. Bill House (biennial) child who overcomes his/her hearing loss and shows good response to cochlear implant.

**★ 5956 ★ Deafness Research Foundation (DRF)**
1050 17th St.NW, Ste701
Washington, DC 20036
**Phone:** (202)289-5850          **Free:** 800-829-5934
**Fax:** (202)293-1805
**Email:** drf@drf.org
**Website:** http://www.drf.org
Kromeklia Bryant, Off. Mgr.

**Desc:** Participates in the National Temporal Bone and Balance Pathology Resource Registry Program of the National Institute on Deafness and Other Communication Disorders. Approximately 1000 physicians and other professionals in ear medicine and research and 52 medical societies underwrite the foundation's fundraising costs through membership in the Centurions of the Deafness Research Foundation; approximately 300 other interested individuals raise funds through membership in the Deafness Research Foundation Alliance. **Awards:** Otologic Fellowship (annual) for third-year medical students to allow research for one year; Otologic Research Grant (annual) for 1-3 years of support to promising new research projects related to hearing disorders and ear diseases.

**★ 5957 ★ HIKE Fund**
c/o Shirley R. Terrill
10115 Cherry Hill Pl.
Spring Hill, FL 34608-7116
**Phone:** (352)688-2579          **Fax:** (352)688-2579
**Email:** ceterrilli@aol.com
**Website:**      http://www.missouriiojd.org/MO-HIKE/HIKE.htm
Dr. Albert L. Howe, Pres.

**Desc:** Supported by the International Order of Job's Daughters. Works for complete equality and integration of the hearing impaired in society. Provides support and information services. Provides hearing devices for children (up to the age of 20) with financial need. **Awards:** The HIKE Fund (monthly).

**★ 5958 ★ National Association of the Deaf (NAD)**
814 Thayer Ave., Ste. 250
Silver Spring, MD 20910-4500
**Phone:** (301)587-1788          **Fax:** (301)587-1791
**Email:** nadinfo@nad.org
**Website:** http://www.nad.org
Nancy J. Bloch, Exec. Dir.

**Desc:** Safeguards accessibility and civil rights of America's deaf population in areas of education, employment, healthcare, and telecommunications. **Awards:** Stokoe Scholarship (annual) for deaf graduate student pursuing studies in field related to sign language or the deaf community.

**★ 5959 ★ Registry of Interpreters for the Deaf (RID)**
333 Commerce St.
Alexandria, VA 22314
**Phone:** (703)838-0030          **Fax:** (703)838-0454
**Email:** admin@rid.org
**Website:** http://www.rid.org
Clay Nettles, Exec. Dir.

**Desc:** Advocates sign language and oral interpreters. programs. Maintains 34 committees. Compiles statistics. **Awards:** Elizabeth Benson Scholarship (annual) Desc: For a student member who has completed at least one semester of a related program.

**★ 5960 ★ Speak Easy International Foundation (SEIF)**
233 Concord Dr.
Paramus, NJ 07652
**Phone:** (201)262-0895          **Fax:** (201)262-0895
**Email:** bob-antoinette@worldnet.att.net
**Website:** http://members.tripod.com/speakeasynj/
Antoinette Gathman, Exec. Dir.

**Desc:** Support group and information source for individuals with a speech dysfluency (stuttering). Seeks to instill confidence in stutterers and reinforce fluency in their speech. Educates public, families, and friends on the problems of speech dysfluent individuals. **Awards:** Scholarship (periodic).

**★ 5961 ★ Stuttering Foundation of America (SFA)**
3100 Walnut Grove Rd., Ste. 603
PO Box 11749
Memphis, TN 38111-0749
**Phone:** (901)452-7343          **Free:** 800-992-9392
**Fax:** (901)452-3931
**Email:** stutter@vantek.net
**Website:** http://www.stutteringhelp.org
Jane Fraser, Pres.

**Desc:** Provides comprehensive materials, including videotapes, books and brochures, on stuttering to both the public and professionals. Seeks to bring together speech pathologists concerned with the prevention and treatment of stuttering. Provides referrals to speech-language pathologists specializing in stuttering. Provides support for research into the causes of stuttering. **Awards:** SFA Award for Excellence in Reporting (annual).

**★ 5962 ★ Voice Foundation (VF)**
1721 Pine St.
Philadelphia, PA 19103
**Phone:** (215)735-7999          **Fax:** (215)735-9293
**Email:** voicefound@onrampcom.com
**Website:** http://www.voicefoundation.org
Robert T. Sataloff, MD, Chm. of the Board

**Desc:** Sponsors research and education on the causes, prevention, and treatment of voice disorders. Sponsors educational programs. Holds fundraising events. **Awards:** Grant; recognition; scholarship.

# National & International Organizations

**★ 5963 ★ Academy of Aphasia (AA)**
c/o Luci Varian
East Bay Institute for Research and Education
150 Muir Rd. 126-S
Martinez, CA 94553
**Phone:** (925)372-2670          **Fax:** (925)372-2553
**Email:** contact@academyofaphasia.org
**Website:** http://www.academyofaphasia.org
Alan Bandler, Esq., Pres.

**Fnded:** 1962. **Mem:** 189. **Desc:** Neurologists, psychologists, linguists, speech pathologists, and others specializing in aphasia (impairment of language caused by focal brain damage). Seeks to encourage research and promote communication among the scientific disciplines that can contribute to the understanding of aphasia.

**★ 5964 ★ Academy of Dispensing Audiologists (ADA)**
3008 Millwood Ave.
Columbia, SC 29205
**Phone:** (803)252-5646          **Free:** 800-445-8629
**Fax:** (803)765-0860
**Email:** info@audiologist.org
**Website:** http://www.audiologist.org
Robert D. Manning, Pres.

**Fnded:** 1977. **Mem:** 525. **Desc:** Individuals with graduate degrees in audiology who dispense hearing aids as part of a rehabilitative practice. Fosters and supports professional dispensing of hearing aids by qualified audiologists; encourages audiology training programs to include pertinent aspects of hearing aid dispensing in their curriculums; conducts seminars on the business aspects of the hearing aid industry. **Pub:** *ADA Feedback*, quarterly. Newsletter. Includes book reviews and new members listing. *Price:* Free. • *ADA Membership Directory*, annual. Membership Directory. Arranged alphabetically and geographically. *Price:* Included in membership dues.

**★ 5965 ★ Academy of Rehabilitative Audiology (ARA)**
c/o Frances Laven
PO Box 26532
Minneapolis, MN 55426
**Phone:** (952)920-0484          **Fax:** (952)920-6098
**Email:** ara@incnet.com
**Website:** http://www.audrehab.org
Barbara Parker, PhD, Pres.

**Fnded:** 1966. **Mem:** 400. **Nat'l Groups:** 1. **Desc:** Individuals who hold graduate degrees in audiology, language, or speech pathology, education of the deaf, or allied fields, and who have at least two years of post-degree involvement in rehabilitative or educational programs for the hearing impaired. Provides a forum for exchange of ideas in audiology; fosters professional education, research, and interest in programs for hearing handicapped persons. Maintains speakers' bureau. **Pub:** *ARA Membership Directory*, annual. Membership Directory. • *Journal of the Academy of Rehabilitative Audiology*, annual. Journal. *Price:* $25/year. • *Monograph of Academy of Rehabilitative Audiology*, quinquennial. *Price:* $20.

**★ 5966 ★ Acoustic Neuroma Association (ANA)**
600 Peachtree Pkwy., No. 108
Cumming, GA 30041
**Phone:** (770)205-8211          **Fax:** (770)205-0239
**Email:** anausa@aol.com
**Website:** http://www.anausa.org
Lois White, Exec. Dir.

**Fnded:** 1981. **Mem:** 5,000. **Reg. Groups:** 42. **State Groups:** 42. **Local Groups:** 42. **Desc:** Provides information and support to patients who have been diagnosed with or experienced an acoustic neuroma or other benign problem affecting the cranial nerves.

The association also furnishes information on patient rehabilitation to physicians and health care personnel, promotes research on acoustic neuroma, thus promoting early diagnosis and successful treatment. **Pub:** *A Glimpse of the Brain.* Booklet. • *Acoustic Neuroma, Basic Overview,* quarterly. Booklet. • *The Acoustic Neuroma Experience 1988/Member Surey.* Booklet. • *ANA Notes.* Newsletter. • *Diagnosis Acoustic Neuroma: What Next?.* Booklet. • *Eye Care after Acoustic Neuroma Surgery.* Booklet. • *Facial Nerve and Acoustic Neuroma: Possible Damage and Rehabilitation.* Booklet. • *Headache Following Acoustic Neuroma.* Booklet. • *Improving Balance Following Treatment for AN.* Booklet. • Newsletter, quarterly. Newsletter covering advances in the treatment of acoustic neuroma, patient letters, support group information. *Price:* Included in membership dues. • Booklets.

**★ 5967 ★ ADARA**
PO Box 727
Lusby, MD 20657
**Phone:** (410)495-8440          **Fax:** (410)495-8442
**Email:** adaraorgn@aol.com
**Website:** http://www.adara.org
Sherri Gallagher, Natl. Off. Coord.

**Fnded:** 1966. **Mem:** 600. **State Groups:** 12. **Desc:** Psychiatrists, mental health counselors, students, teachers, researchers, rehabilitation facility personnel, interpreters, speech therapists, social workers, doctors, and rehabilitation counselors who serve deaf and deaf-blind persons. Promotes the development and expansion of quality services to deaf and hard-of-hearing persons. Strives to bring about a better understanding of deaf, hard-of-hearing, and deaf-blind people as a whole by encouraging students, professionals, and laymen to develop more than a superficial understanding of the needs and problems of this group, especially the problems related to communication techniques needed to work effectively with deaf, hard-of-hearing, and deaf-blind persons in human services or a rehabilitation setting. Encourages scientific research of the needs and problems engendered by deafness. Promotes and develops recruitment and training of professional workers with deaf, hard-of-hearing, and deaf-blind persons. Sponsors a professional publication for the promotion of inter- and intradisciplinary communication among professionals concerned with deaf adults and others interested in such activities. Cooperates with other organizations in promoting and encouraging legislation pertinent to the development of professional services and facilities for deaf, hard-of-hearing, and deaf-blind persons. **Pub:** *ADARA Update,* quarterly. Newsletter. Includes membership activities information, research reports, and list of employment opportunities. *Price:* Included in membership dues. • *JADARA: A Journal for Professionals Networking for Excellence in Service Delivery with Individuals who are Deaf or Hard of Hearing,* 3/year. Journal. Provides research findings and information on new ideas within the field. Includes reviews of current literature. *Price:* Included in membership dues; $55/year for nonmembers in U.S.; $65/year for nonmembers outside U.S. • Monographs. **Frmly:** American Deafness and Rehabilitation Association.

**★ 5968 ★ Advisory Council for Children with Impaired Hearing**
137 Blackburn Rd.
Blackburn, VIC 3130, Australia
**Phone:** 61 3 98771300          **Fax:** 61 3 98771922
**Email:** moreinfo@edumail.vic.gov.au
**Website:** http://www.accih.vic.edu.au

**Fnded:** 1968. **Lang(s):** English. **Desc:** Individuals with a specific interest in the field of hearing impairment, and/or early childhood development. Seeks to maximize the opportunity for deaf children to develop oral skills. Maintains an early intervention center and unit within a school setting.

**★ 5969 ★ Advocates for Communication Technology for Deaf/Blind People (ACT)**
1498M Reisterstown Rd.
PMB 289
Baltimore, MD 21208
**Phone:** (410)381-3377          **Fax:** (410)381-6838
Sheryl Cooper, Co. Pres.

**Fnded:** 1987. **Desc:** Seeks to enhance the quality of communication for deaf and blind people through improved technology. Provides communication technology to persons unable to afford it.

**★ 5970 ★ AFASIC - Overcoming Speech Impairments**
50 - 52 Great Sutton St.
London EC1V 0DJ, United Kingdom
**Phone:** 44 20 74909410          **Fax:** 44 20 72512834
**Email:** info@afasic.org.uk
**Website:** http://www.afasic.org.uk/

**Fnded:** 1968. **Mem:** 2,300. **Local Groups:** 30. **Lang(s):** English. **Desc:** Promotes the interests of young people with speech and/or language difficulties. Seeks to enhance understanding of speech and language disorders and improve educational and employment opportunities for young adults with such disorders. Offers advice and support for parents of individuals with speech and language disorders. Conducts research on children's language development. Organizes art/drama weekends, activity weeks, international symposia, national seminars, and workshops. Maintains speakers' bureau; compiles statistics. **Pub:** *Annual Review,* annual. • *Newsletter,* 3/year, always January, May, and September. Newsletter.

**★ 5971 ★ Alexander Graham Bell Association for the Deaf (AGBAD)**
3417 Volta Pl. NW
Washington, DC 20007
**Phone:** (202)337-5220          **Fax:** (202)337-8314
**Email:** cfisk@agbell.org
**Website:** http://www.agbell.org
K. Todd Houston, PhD, Exec. Dir.

**Fnded:** 1890. **Mem:** 5,000. **State Groups:** 17. **Local Groups:** 110. **Desc:** Teachers of the hearing impaired, speech-language pathologists and audiologists, physicians, parents of hearing impaired children, oral deaf adults, and others interested in the problems of the hearing impaired; affiliate members are organized groups of parents of deaf children and coordinators of state and provincial chapters. Works to: promote the teaching of speech, lipreading, and use of residual hearing to the deaf; encourage research on deafness; assist schools and agencies working for better educational facilities for deaf and oral hearing impaired children. Conducts workshops and educational programs. Compiles statistics. Maintains speakers' bureau. Serves as information center and maintains library on speech and hearing. Operates charitable program, biographical archives, museum, and placement service. **Pub:** *Alexander Graham Bell Association for the Deaf–Our Kids Magazine,* 2-3/year. Newsletter. For parents of hearing impaired children. *Price:* Included in membership dues. • *Children's Corner.* • *Newsounds,* 10/year. Membership activities newsletter. Includes chapter news and calendar of events. *Price:* Included in membership dues. • *OK Kids.* • *Volta Review,* bimonthly. Professional journal covering issues related to hearing impairment for teachers of the hearing impaired. *Price:* Included in membership dues; $35/year for institutions. • Also publishes bibliographies, teachers' and clinicians' textbooks, lipreading books, and references; produces audiovisuals. **Frmly:** (1948) American Association to Promote the Teaching of Speech to the Deaf; (1953) Volta Speech Association for the Deaf.

**★ 5972 ★ All-Russian Society of the Deaf (ARFD)**
**(Vserossiiskoe Obshchestvo Glukhikh — VOG)**
ulitsa 1905-goda 10A
123022 Moscow, Russia

**Phone:** 7 95 2556704          **Fax:** 7 95 2522381
**Fnded:** 1926. **Mem:** 120,985. **Reg. Groups:** 74. **Local Groups:** 75. **Lang(s):** Russian. **Desc:** Protects the rights and interests of citizens with hearing problems. Promotes social rehabilitation and full participation in society. Coordinates the activities of governmental organizations providing for the deaf and hearing-impaired; conducts courses in sign language and computer use for hearing-impaired individuals. Operates 62 production associations, which make consumer and light industrial goods. **Frmly:** (1991) All-Union Society of the Deaf; (1993) All-Russian Society of the Deaf.

**★ 5973 ★ American Academy of Audiology (AAA)**
8300 Greensboro Dr., Ste. 750
Mc Lean, VA 22102
**Phone:** (703)790-8466          **Free:** 800-AAA-2336
**Fax:** (703)790-8631
**Email:** mail@audiology.org
**Website:** http://www.audiology.org
Angela Leavenbruck, EdD, Pres.

**Fnded:** 1988. **Mem:** 7,600. **Nat'l Groups:** 1. **Desc:** Professionals in the field of audiology. Seeks to "enhance the ability of our members to achieve career and practice objectives through professional development." Conducts research and educational programs; sponsors public education campaigns to raise awareness of hearing disorders and audiological services. **Pub:** *Audiology Today,* bimonthly. Magazine. • *Journal of the American Academy of Audiology: Audiology Today,* 10/year. Journal.

**American Academy of Otolaryngic Allergy Foundation (AAOA)**
*See:* Entry 3189

**American Academy of Otolaryngology - Head and Neck Surgery (AAO-HNS)**
*See:* Entry 19465

**★ 5974 ★ American Auditory Society (AAS)**
512 E Canterbury Ln.
Phoenix, AZ 85022
**Phone:** (602)789-0755          **Fax:** (602)942-1486
**Email:** amaudsoc@aol.com
**Website:** http://www.amauditorysoc.org
Wayne J. Staab, PhD, Sec. -Treas.

**Fnded:** 1973. **Mem:** 2,000. **Desc:** Audiologists, otolaryngologists, scientists, hearing aid industry professionals, and educators of hearing impaired people; individuals involved in industries serving hearing impaired people, including the amplification systems industry. Works to increase knowledge and understanding of: the ear, hearing, and balance; disorders of the ear, hearing, and balance; prevention of these disorders; habilitation and rehabilitation of individuals with hearing and balance dysfunction. **Pub:** *The Bulletin of the AAS,* 3/year. Newsletter. • *Ear and Hearing,* bimonthly. Journal. Includes periodic supplements. • *Peer Reviewed Clinical Research Publication. Price:* $77 in U.S. personal; $112 outside U.S. personal; $145 in U.S. institution; $180 outside U.S. institution. **Frmly:** (1982) American Audiology Society.

**★ 5975 ★ American Board of Otolaryngology (ABO)**
3050 Post Oak Blvd. Ste.1700
Houston, TX 77056
**Phone:** (713)850-0399          **Fax:** (713)850-1104
**Email:** czw@aboto.org
**Website:** http://www.aboto.org
Gerald B. Healy, MD, Exec. VP

**Fnded:** 1924. **Desc:** Purposes are to: elevate standards of practice in otolaryngology (the medical specialty dealing with ear, nose, throat, head, and neck surgery); hold examinations and certify qualified otolaryngologists; advance the cause of the field. Conducts annual in-training, written and oral examinations. **Pub:** Newsletter, semiannual.

★ 5976 ★ **American Hearing Impaired Hockey Association (AHIHA)**
1143 W Lake St.
Chicago, IL 60607
**Phone:** (312)226-5880  **Fax:** (312)829-2250
Stan Mikita, Pres.

**Fnded:** 1973. **Mem:** 80. **Desc:** Hearing impaired boys and men, aged 5 to 26, who wish to play ice hockey. Seeks to develop members' skills and self-confidence, both as hockey players and as individuals, through participation in the annual Stan Mikita Hockey School for the Hearing Impaired. **Pub:** *Locker Room Briefs*. Newsletter.

★ 5977 ★ **American Hearing Research Foundation (AHRF)**
55 E Washington St., Ste. 2022
Chicago, IL 60602
**Phone:** (312)726-9670  **Fax:** (312)726-9695
**Email:** blederer@american-hearing.org
**Website:** http://www.american-hearing.org/
William L. Lederer, Exec. Dir.

**Fnded:** 1956. **Mem:** 1,585. **Desc:** Works to encourage and support medical research, education, and public information concerning deafness and other hearing disorders. Produces scientific exhibits and film exhibits for professional and public audiences. **Pub:** *American Hearing Research Foundation Newsletter*, 3/year. Newsletter. Reviews developments in hearing research and education. *Price:* Free. • *Hearing Health*. Brochure. • *Progress Report*, semiannual. Report. • Also publishes research papers.

★ 5978 ★ **American Institute for Stuttering Treatment and Professional Training**
c/o Catherine Montgomery
27 W 20th St., Ste. 1203
New York, NY 10011-3707
**Phone:** (212)633-6400  **Free:** 877-378-8883
**Fax:** (212)220-3922
**Email:** ais@stutteringtreatment.org
**Website:** http://www.stutteringtreatment.org
Catherine Montgomery, Exec. Dir.

**Fnded:** 1995. **Desc:** Facility offers both intensive and non-intensive treatment options for people of all ages who stutter, while also providing clinical training to both new and established speech-language pathologists. **Frmly:** (1998) Total Immersion Fluency Training.

★ 5979 ★ **American Laryngological Association (ALA)**
c/o Robert H. Ossoff, D.M.D., M.D.
Medical Ctr. North
Vanderbilt University Medical Ctr.
S-100 MCN
Nashville, TN 37232-2559
**Phone:** (615)322-6326  **Fax:** (615)343-7604
**Email:** robert.ossoff@mcmail.vanderbilt.edu
**Website:** http://www.alahns.org
Stanley M. Shapshay, MD, Pres.

**Fnded:** 1879. **Mem:** 232. **Desc:** Professional medical society of otorhinolaryngologists (specialists in ear, nose, and throat diseases). Works to advance research in medicine and surgery, with emphasis on the upper aerodigestive tract. **Pub:** *Transactions*, annual.

★ 5980 ★ **American Laryngological, Rhinological and Otological Society (ALROS)**
c/o Boy's Town National Research Hosp.
555 N 30th St.
Omaha, NE 68131
**Phone:** (402)346-5500  **Fax:** (402)346-5300
**Email:** info@triological.org
**Website:** http://www.triological.org/
Gerald B. Healy, MD, Pres.

**Fnded:** 1896. **Mem:** 1,300. **Reg. Groups:** 4. **Desc:** Professional society of medical specialists dealing with the ear, nose, and throat. **Pub:** *Laryngoscope*, monthly. Journal. Covers annual meeting; includes membership list. *Price:* Included in membership dues. • *The Laryngoscope Journal*, monthly. **AKA:** Triological Society.

★ 5981 ★ **American Neurotology Society (ANS)**
c/o Paul Lambert, MD, Chairman
Medical University of South Carolina
Box 250582
Charleston, SC 29425
**Phone:** (843)792-7161  **Fax:** (843)792-0546
**Email:** lambert@muse.edu
**Website:** http://itsa.ucsf.edu/~ajo/ANS/ANS.html
Stephen G. Harner, MD, Pres.

**Fnded:** 1965. **Mem:** 500. **Desc:** Physicians and audiologists interested in the diagnosis and treatment of hearing and balance disorders. Promotes education and research in the field of neurotology. **Pub:** Directory, annual. Published in conjunction with American Academy of Otolaryngology - Head and Neck Surgery. **Frmly:** (1965) ENG Study Group.

★ 5982 ★ **American Otological Society (AOS)**
2720 Tartan Way
Springfield, IL 62707
**Phone:** (217)483-6966  **Fax:** (217)483-6966
**Email:** segossard@aol.com
Dr. Horst R. Konrad, Sec. -Treas.

**Fnded:** 1868. **Mem:** 285. **Desc:** Otologists and contributors to the advancement of otology. Encourages study and research in otology (the science of the ear and its diseases). Objectives are to advance and promote medical and surgical otology, including the rehabilitation of the hearing impaired, and to encourage and promote research in otology and related disciplines. Maintains research fund for advanced studies of otosclerosis. **Pub:** *Otology & Neurotology*. Journal.

★ 5983 ★ **American Rhinologic Society (ARS)**
c/o Marvin P. Fried, MD
Montefiore Medical Center Department of Otolaryngology
3400 Bainbridge Ave.
3rd Fl. MAP
Bronx, NY 10467
**Phone:** (718)675-6262  **Free:** 888-520-9585
**Fax:** (718)675-6260
**Email:** info@american-rhinologic.org
**Website:** http://www.american-rhinologic.org
Marvin P. Fried, Sec.

**Fnded:** 1954. **Mem:** 1,087. **Desc:** Physicians who are diplomates of the American Board of Otolaryngology, the American Board of Plastic Surgery, and other boards and who have had additional training and interest in the study of medical and surgical rhinology. Works to advance knowledge of rhinology (branch of medicine that relates to the nose and its diseases) internationally through short, frequent teaching courses at universities in conjunction with their faculties. Conducts research in nasal physiology, rhinomanometry, and anatomy. **Pub:** *American Journal of Rhinology*, bimonthly. Journal. • Membership Directory, biennial. • Newsletter, 4-5/year.

★ 5984 ★ **American Society for Deaf Children (ASDC)**
PO Box 3355
Gettysburg, PA 17325
**Phone:** (717)334-7922  **Free:** 800-942-ASDC
**Fax:** (717)334-8808
**Email:** asdc@deafchildren.org
**Website:** http://www.deafchildren.org/
Dr. Cheron Mayhall, Pres.

**Fnded:** 1965. **Mem:** 1,300. **Local Groups:** 93. **Desc:** Parents of deaf and hard of hearing children; researchers, professionals, and others interested in the welfare of deaf and hard of hearing children and their families. Seeks to provide parent-to-parent support to help improve the education, recreation, health, and employment opportunities of deaf and hard of hearing children and youth. Promotes "total communication" as a way of life for deaf and hard of hearing children and their families. Assists other organizations in locating parents for seminars, workshops, and learning sessions regarding parental needs and the education of deaf and hard of hearing children. Provides speakers for meetings, seminars, and conventions. **Pub:** *The Endeavor*, quarterly. Newsletter. *Price:* Included in membership dues. **Frmly:** (1984) International Association of Parents of the Deaf.

★ 5985 ★ **American Speech Language Hearing Association**
10801 Rockville Pike
Rockville, MD 20852
**Free:** 800-638-8255  **Fax:** (301)897-7355
**Email:** actioncenter@asha.org
**Website:** http://www.asha.org
Frederick Samphor, Exec. Dir.

**Fnded:** 1919. **Desc:** Consumers of speech, language, and hearing services and their families. Provides educational and referral information on speech, language, and hearing disabilities. **Pub:** Pamphlets.Covers a wide range of communication disorders and development of speech, language, and hearing in children. **Frmly:** (1922) American Association for the Hard of Hearing; (1935) American Federation of Organizations for the Hard of Hearing; (1946) American Society for the Hard of Hearing; (1966) American Hearing Society; (1974) National Association of Hearing and Speech Agencies; (1999) National Association for Hearing and Speech Action.

★ 5986 ★ **American Tinnitus Association (ATA)**
PO Box 5
Portland, OR 97207-0005
**Phone:** (503)248-9985  **Free:** 800-634-8978
**Fax:** (503)248-0024
**Email:** Tinnitus@ata.org
**Website:** http://www.ata.org
Cheryl McGinnis, Exec. Dir.

**Fnded:** 1971. **Mem:** 18,000. **Nat'l Groups:** 115. **State Groups:** 1. **Desc:** Dedicated to tinnitus research and educating patients, and professionals through conferences, books, brochures, videos and the quarterly journal Tinnitus Today. ATA is the national champion of tinnitus awareness, prevention and treatment. Under its guiding principles - Education, Advocacy, Research and Support - the ATA offers prevention programs in schools, uges governmental and private organizations to support hearing conservation, funds the nation's brightest researchers and facilitates self-help groups around the country. **Pub:** *Coping With the Stress of Tinnitus*. Brochure. • *If You Have Tinnitus - The First Steps To Take*. Brochure. • *Information About Tinnitus*. Brochure. • *Noise - Its Effects on Hearing and Tinnitus*. Brochure. • *Tinnitus Bibliography*. Bibliography. • *Tinnitus Family Information*. Brochure. • *Tinnitus Today*, quarterly, March, July, September, December. Newsletter. Includes book reviews, calendar of events, research updates, and statistics. *Price:* $25/year. • *Understanding Tinnitus - Advice for Family and Friends*. Brochure.

★ 5987 ★ **Anne Sullivan Foundation for Deafblind**
40 Lower Drumcondra Rd.
Dublin 9, Ireland
**Phone:** 353 1 8300562  **Fax:** 353 1 8300562
**Fnded:** 1989. **Desc:** Irish national agency formed to help people who are both deaf and blind, and particularly those who are also low-functioning. Operates a residential center, a home for life, for young congenital deaf and blind people. Provides outreach services to other agencies.

**★ 5988 ★ Arab Federation of Organizations for the Deaf (AFOD)**
PO Box 4230
Damascus, Syrian Arab Republic
**Phone:** 963 11 2217401   **Fax:** 963 11 3320652
**Fnded:** 1972. **Lang(s):** Arabic, English. **Desc:** Organizations providing support and services to people with hearing impairment. Seeks to improve the quality of life of people with hearing impairment and their families. Coordinates members' activities; advocates on behalf of people with impaired hearing.

**★ 5989 ★ Asia Pacific Deaf Sports Confederation (APDSC)**
PO Box 416
Mount Ommaney, QLD 4074, Australia
**Fax:** 63 3 92226536
**Website:** http://www.geocities.com/deafsportsap
**Lang(s):** English. **Desc:** Sports programs for people with impaired hearing; hearing impaired athletes. Promotes increased participation in athletics by people with impaired hearing. Facilitates communication and cooperation among members; sponsors competitions.

**Assistance Dogs International (ADI)**
*See:* Entry 20885

**★ 5990 ★ Association of the Deaf in Israel (ADI) (Agudat Hachershim Beisrael)**
Helen Keller Center
13 Yad Lebanim Blvd.
PO Box 9001
61090 Tel Aviv, Israel
**Phone:** 972 3 303355   **Fax:** 972 3 396419
**Email:** w1@zak.co.il
**Website:** http://www.adionline.org
**Mem:** 2,200. **Lang(s):** English, Hebrew. **Desc:** Works toward the cultural, social, and professional rehabilitation of the deaf in Israel. **Pub:** *Mabat Shelanu*, quarterly. Magazine.

**★ 5991 ★ Association of Late-Deafened Adults (ALDA)**
1131 Lake St.
Oak Park, IL 60301-1001
**Free:** 877-348-7537   **Fax:** 877-348-7537
**Email:** gottabekk@aol.com
**Website:** http://www.alda.org
Karen Krull, Pres.
**Fnded:** 1987. **Mem:** 1,500. **Reg. Groups:** 25. **Desc:** People who have become deaf adventitiously and rely on visual systems to communicate effectively. Provides information, support, and social opportunities through selfhelp groups, general membership meetings, and social events. Advocates for the needs of late-deafened people. Conducts and participates in surveys, workshops, and seminars on late-deafness. Maintains speakers' bureau and biographical archives. **Pub:** *ALDA News*, quarterly. Newsletter. Includes pen pal section. *Price:* Included in membership dues. • *Proceedings of ALDAcon*. Monograph.

**★ 5992 ★ Association of Medical Professionals with Hearing Losses**
c/o Danielle N. Rastetter
3709 Waterbridge Ln.
Miamisburg, OH 45342-6728
**Email:** drastet@attglobal.net
**Website:** http://www.amphl.org
Danielle N. Rastetter, Pres.
**Fnded:** 1999. **Desc:** Provides information, promotes advocacy and mentorship. Creates a network for individuals with hearing losses interested in or working in health care fields.

**★ 5993 ★ Association for Research in Otolaryngology (ARO)**
c/o Susan Whitehouse
19 Mantua Rd.
Mount Royal, NJ 08061
**Phone:** (856)423-0041   **Fax:** (856)423-3420
**Email:** headquarters@aro.org
**Website:** http://www.aro.org
Susan Whitehouse, Exec. Dir.
**Fnded:** 1973. **Mem:** 2,000. **Desc:** Medical professionals, scientists, and researchers with an interest in otolaryngology. Promotes increased understanding of basic science and clinical practice associated with hearing, speech, balance, the senses of taste and smell, and diseases of the head and neck. Conducts educational programs; facilitates exchange of information among members. **Pub:** *Journal of the Association for Research in Otolaryngology (JARO)*, quarterly. Journal. • *Membership Directory*, annual. Directory. Contains membership information.

**★ 5994 ★ Association of Teachers of Lipreading to Adults**
PO Box 56
Hanley
Stoke-On-Trent ST2 9RE, United Kingdom
**Fax:** 44 870 7062916
**Email:** atla@lipreading.org.uk
**Website:** http://www.lipreading.org.uk
**Fnded:** 1975. **Mem:** 340. **Desc:** To promote understanding of the needs of people with an acquired hearing loss. To advance the awareness of the benefits of lipreading and other communication skills in the rehabilitation of people with an acquired hearing loss. **Pub:** *Catchword*, semiannual. Magazine.

**★ 5995 ★ Australian Association of the Deaf (AAD)**
149 Castlereagh St., Ste. 513
Sydney, NSW 2000, Australia
**Phone:** 61 2 92863944   **Fax:** 61 2 92863955
**Email:** aad@aad.org.au
**Website:** http://www.aad.org.au
**Fnded:** 1986. **State Groups:** 6. **Lang(s):** English. **Desc:** Deaf people who use Australian Sign Language (Auslan). Educates the Deaf community about their basic rights and obligations under the law and promotes public awareness about issues relating to deafness. **Pub:** *AAD Outlook*, quarterly. Magazine. • *Lookout*. Bulletin.

**★ 5996 ★ Australian Deaf Sports Federation (ADSF)**
101-117 Wellington Parade South
East Melbourne, VIC 3002, Australia
**Phone:** 61 3 96502524   **Fax:** 61 3 96542868
**Email:** dsa@deafsports.org.au
**Website:** http://www.deafsports.org.au
**Fnded:** 1954. **Lang(s):** English. **Desc:** Encourages an increased level and standard of sports participation and performance for all Deaf Australians.

**★ 5997 ★ Autism Treatment Services of Canada (ATSC)**
404 94th Ave. SE
Calgary, AB, Canada T2J 0E8
**Phone:** (403)253-6961   **Fax:** (403)253-6974
**Email:** atsc@autism.ca
**Website:** http://www.autism.ca
**Lang(s):** English, French. **Desc:** Organizations providing treatment services to people with autism and their families. Seeks to advance the treatment of autism. Serves as a clearinghouse on the treatment of autism; provides support and services to people with autism and their families; conducts research and educational programs.

**★ 5998 ★ Better Hearing Australia (BHA)**
5 High St.
Prahran, VIC 3181, Australia
**Phone:** 61 3 95101577   **Fax:** 61 3 95106076

**Email:** bhavic@betterhearing.org.au
**Website:** http://www.betterhearing.org.au
**Fnded:** 1940. **Mem:** 3,000. **Local Groups:** 18. **Desc:** Adults with acquired deafness. Works toward the rehabilitation of the deaf; represents the hearing impaired before government. Provides hearing education and rehabilitation activities. **Pub:** *Better Hearing*, quarterly.

**★ 5999 ★ Better Hearing Institute (BHI)**
515 King St., Ste. 420
Alexandria, VA 22314
**Phone:** (703)684-3391   **Free:** 800-EAR-WELL
**Fax:** (703)684-6048
**Email:** mail@betterhearing.org
**Website:** http://www.betterhearing.org
John T. Olive, Jr., Exec. Dir.
**Fnded:** 1973. **Desc:** Professionals and others dedicated to helping persons with impaired hearing. Purpose is to inform the public about the nature of hearing loss and the available medical, surgical, rehabilitative, and amplification help. Methods of communication used include television and radio public service announcements, films, speakers' bureaus, booklets, editorial publicity, and exhibits. Produces general information and education kits of communication tools. Maintains telephone service that provides information on hearing loss and help to callers from anywhere in the United States and Canada. **Pub:** Pamphlets.

**★ 6000 ★ British Association of Audiological Physicians**
c/o Dr. Ros Davies
National Hospital for Neurology & Neurosurgery
Queen's Square
London WC1N 3BG, United Kingdom
**Phone:** 44 207 8373611   **Fax:** 44 207 8298775
**Email:** info@baap.org.uk
**Website:** http://www.baap.org.uk/
**Fnded:** 1977. **Mem:** 40. **Desc:** Consultant physicians practising in audiology. Concerned with the diagnosis and care/management of adults and children suffering from disorders of balance and hearing; the promotion of education (postgraduate) and standards of medical practice.

**British Association of Otorhinolaryngologists - Head and Neck Surgeons**
*See:* Entry 19529

**★ 6001 ★ British Association of Teachers of the Deaf**
21 The Haystacks
High Wycombe
Buckinghamshire HP13 6PY, United Kingdom
**Phone:** 44 1494 464190   **Fax:** 44 1494 464190
**Email:** secretary@batod.org.uk
**Website:** http://www.batod.org.uk
**Fnded:** 1976. **Mem:** 1,700. **Reg. Groups:** 7. **Local Groups:** 7. **Desc:** Qualified teachers of the deaf; Associate membership available to persons not qualified as teachers of the deaf. Represents the interests of all teachers of the hearing-impaired in Britain. It exists to promote the education of all hearing impaired persons and to promote and safeguard the interests and status of all teachers of the hearing-impaired. **Pub:** *Association Magazine*, 5/year. Magazine. • *The Journal of the British Association of Teachers of the Deaf-Deafness and Education International*, 3/year. Journal. Also publishes booklets and leaflets relating to the education of deaf people.

**★ 6002 ★ British Deaf Association**
1-3 Worship St.
London EC2A 2AB, United Kingdom
**Phone:** 44 207 5883520   **Fax:** 44 207 5883527
**Email:** helpline@bda.org.uk
**Website:** http://www.bda.org.uk
**Fnded:** 1890. **Mem:** 6,500. **Desc:** Mainly profoundly deaf people who use sign language as their means of

communication. Aims to serve and protect the deaf community. **Pub:** *British Deaf News*, monthly.


★ **6003** ★ **British Deaf Sports Council**
7A Bridge St.
Otley LS21 1BQ, United Kingdom
**Phone:** 44 1943 850214      **Fax:** 44 1943 850828
**Fnded:** 1930. **Mem:** 4,500. **Desc:** Deaf people interested in sport. **Pub:** *READS - Record of Effort and Achievement of Deaf Sportspeople*, 3/year. • Yearbook.


★ **6004** ★ **British Society of Audiology**
80 Brighton Rd.
Reading RG6 1PS, United Kingdom
**Phone:** 44 118 9660622      **Fax:** 44 118 9351915
**Email:** ann@b-s-a.demon.co.uk
**Website:** http://www.b-s-a.demon.co.uk
**Fnded:** 1968. **Mem:** 1,400. **Desc:** Anyone with an interest in audiology. To promote the science of audiology (i.e. the study of hearing and balance) and the diagnosis, alleviation and prevention of hearing and balance impairment. The advancement of education in audiology and the furtherance of research in audiology and the publication of the results of such research. **Pub:** *BSA News*, 3/year. • *Journal of Audiology*, bimonthly. Journal.


★ **6005** ★ **British Society of Hearing Aid Audiologists**
9 Lukins Dr.
Great Dunmow
Essex CM6 1XQ, United Kingdom
**Phone:** 44 1371 876623      **Fax:** 44 1371 876623
**Email:** secretary@bshaa.com
**Website:** http://www.bshaa.com
**Fnded:** 1957. **Mem:** 700. **Desc:** Educational and trade association for private hearing aid dispensers. Promotion of ethical standards through training, examination and codes of practice. **Pub:** *BSHAA News*, quarterly. Newsletter. **Frmly:** BSHAA.


★ **6006** ★ **British Stammering Association**
15 Old Ford Rd.
Bethnal Green
London E2 9PJ, United Kingdom
**Phone:** 44 181 9831003      **Fax:** 44 181 9833591
**Email:** mail@stammering.org
**Website:** http://www.stammering.org
**Fnded:** 1978. **Mem:** 1,600. **Lang(s):** English. **Desc:** Self-help organization aimed at assisting individuals with stammering speech patterns. Conducts free information and advice service for all stammerers and parents/teachers with stammering children. Operates facilities and activities for members. Projects on early referral to speech therapy for dysfunctional children, and stammering pupils project. **Pub:** *Annual Report*. • *Speaking Out*, quarterly. • Pamphlets, periodic. Offers guidance to stutterers.


★ **6007** ★ **British Tinnitus Association**
4th Fl., White Bldg.
Fitzalan Square
Sheffield S1 2 AZ, United Kingdom
**Phone:** 44 114 2796600      **Fax:** 44 114 2796222
**Email:** equiries@tinnitus.org.uk
**Website:** http://www.tinnitus.org.uk
**Fnded:** 1979. **Mem:** 9,000. **Reg. Groups:** 80. **Desc:** Individual Members or via a network of 80 local self-help groups and contacts. Offers information about tinnitus and helps to found and implement self-help groups to provide mutual support and varying degrees of counselling. BTA campaigns for better services for people with tinnitus and for more tinnitus clinics. A national conference is held annually. **Pub:** *BTA Information Pack*. Journal. • *QUIET*, quarterly.


★ **6008** ★ **Canadian Apheresis Group (CAG)**
**(Groupe Canadien d' Apherese — GCA)**
435 St. Laurent Blvd., Ste. 199
Ottawa, ON, Canada K1K 2Z8
**Phone:** (613)748-9613      **Fax:** (613)748-6392
**Email:** cag@magi.com
**Fnded:** 1980. **Lang(s):** English, French. **Desc:** Apheresis practitioners. Seeks to advance the study and practice of apheresis. Conducts research and educational programs.


★ **6009** ★ **Canadian Association of the Deaf (CAD)**
203-251 Bank St.
Ottawa, ON, Canada K2P 1X3
**Phone:** (613)565-2882      **Fax:** (613)565-1207
**Email:** cad@cad.ca
**Website:** http://www.cad.ca
**Fnded:** 1940. **Mem:** 44. **Lang(s):** English, French. **Desc:** Regional and local organizations for the deaf. Promotes interests of the deaf through advocacy; provides educational and support facilities. Maintains speakers' bureau; conducts research; compiles statistics. **Pub:** *CAD Chat*, 10/year. Newsletter.


★ **6010** ★ **Canadian Association for People Who Stutter (CAPS)**
575 32nd Ave., No. 408
Lachine, QC, Canada H8T 1Y2
**Phone:** (514)637-2893
**Email:** dblock@videotron.ca
**Website:** http://www.caps.webcon.net
**Lang(s):** English. **Desc:** Individuals who stutter and self-help groups for people who stutter. Provides coordination for a national network of autonomous Canadian self-help groups that serve people who stutter and their families. Works closely with speech professionals and treatment centers; seeks to increase public awareness and acceptance of people who stutter. **Pub:** Newsletter, quarterly.


★ **6011** ★ **Canadian Association of Speech-Language Pathologists and Audiologists**
**(Association Canadienne des Orthophonistes et Audiologistes)**
200 Elgin, Ste. 401
Ottawa, ON, Canada K2P 1L5
**Phone:** (613)567-9968      **Fax:** (613)567-2859
**Email:** caslpa@caslpa.ca
**Website:** http://www.caslpa.ca
**Fnded:** 1964. **Mem:** 4,300. **Lang(s):** English, French. **Desc:** Audiologists, speech and language pathologists, and other individuals with an interest in speech and hearing. Seeks to increase availability and effectiveness of treatment programs for people with communication disabilities. Makes available programs and services for people with speech and language disorders; conducts continuing professional development courses for members. **Pub:** *Journal of Speech-Language Pathology and Audiology*. Journal.


★ **6012** ★ **Canadian Cultural Society of The Deaf (CCSD)**
House 144, 11337 - 61 Ave.
Edmonton, AB, Canada T6H 1M3
**Phone:** (780)436-2599      **Free:** 800-855-0511
**Fax:** (780)430-9489
**Email:** ccsd@connect.ab.ca
**Website:** http://www.ccsdeaf.com
**Fnded:** 1970. **Desc:** Deaf and hard of hearing people. Promotes the use of American Sign Language (ASL) and Langue des Signes Quebecois (LSQ). Promotes fellowship in the deaf community and deaf culture. Encourages new and developing forms of creativity, research, participation, and interests in the arts, humanities, and social sciences. Promotes improved understanding between deaf and hearing populations. Advocates for progress in literacy at all levels and promotes bilingual bicultural education of deaf chil-

dren. **Pub:** *Canadian Dictionary of ASL*. Book. • *Deaf People Are Like You But....* Manual.


★ **6013** ★ **Canadian Deaf Sports Association (CDSA)**
**(Association des Sports des Sourds du Canada — ASSC)**
4545 ave. Pierre du coubertin
CP 1000, succ. M
Montreal, QC, Canada H1V 3R2
**Phone:** (514)252-3069      **Free:** 800-855-0511
**Fax:** (514)252-3213
**Email:** office@assc-cdsa.com
**Website:** http://www.assc-cdsa.com
**Lang(s):** English, French. **Desc:** Individuals with impaired hearing who participate in athletics; sports organizations. Promotes increased participation in athletics by people with impaired hearing. Organizes athletic leagues and competitions for people with impaired hearing.


★ **6014** ★ **Canadian Deafblind and Rubella Association (CDBRA)**
350 Brandt Ave.
Brantford, ON, Canada N3T 3J9
**Phone:** (519)759-0729      **Fax:** (519)754-5400
**Email:** cdbra.nat@sympatico.ca
**Website:** http://www.cdbra.ca
**Fnded:** 1975. **Mem:** 400. **Lang(s):** English, French. **Desc:** Deafblind individuals and their families; volunteer service providers. Seeks to ensure availability of services to enable deafblind individuals to participate in society to the fullest of their capabilities. Provides lifelong intervention and educational services; conducts training programs for individuals wishing to work with the deafblind. Sponsors advocacy campaigns on behalf of deafblind individuals; facilitates cooperation between government agencies and programs assisting the deafblind. **Pub:** *Intervention*, semiannual. Magazine. • Brochure.


★ **6015** ★ **Canadian Hard of Hearing Association (CHHA)**
2435 Holly Ln., Ste. 205
Ottawa, ON, Canada K1V 7P2
**Phone:** (613)526-1584      **Free:** 800-263-8068
**Fax:** (613)526-4718
**Email:** chhanational@chha.ca
**Website:** http://www.chha.ca
**Fnded:** 1982. **Mem:** 2,100. **Lang(s):** English, French. **Desc:** Individuals with or without hearing impairments. Seeks to raise public awareness of issues of concern to members; promotes full integration into society of people with hearing loss. Identifies and works to remove barriers to full social and economic participation by people with hearing impairments; conducts educational programs. **Pub:** *Listen*, quarterly. Magazine.


★ **6016** ★ **Canadian Hearing Society (CHS)**
**(La Societe Canadienne de l'Ouie)**
271 Spadina Rd.
Toronto, ON, Canada M5R 2V3
**Phone:** (416)964-9595      **Fax:** (416)928-2525
**Email:** info@chs.ca
**Website:** http://www.chs.ca
**Fnded:** 1940. **Lang(s):** English, French. **Desc:** Those who are deaf or experience hearing loss, and their families; health care and other professionals; and educators. Provides services that enhance the independence of deaf, deafened, and hard of hearing people and encourages the prevention of hearing loss. **Pub:** *Vibes*, quarterly. Magazine.


★ **6017** ★ **Child Aid**
2902 SW Fairmount Blvd.
Portland, OR 97201
**Phone:** (503)223-3008      **Free:** 888-881-8241
**Fax:** (503)295-3042
**Email:** childaid@attbi.com

Website: http://www.child-aid.org
David Roy, Dir. Development

**Fnded:** 1988. **Desc:** Individuals who volunteer to aid hearing impaired children in Mexico and Guatemala. Promotes increased access to audiological aids and services among Mexican, Guatemalan, and Turkish children. Provides audiological and educational services to indigent children with impaired hearing; provides funds and assistance to organizations pursuing similar goals; conducts fundraising programs; recruits and trains volunteers. Supports literacy, education and health programs in Latin America. **Frmly:** (2001) SoundAid.

### ★ 6018 ★ Children of Deaf Adults (CODA)

Box 30715
Santa Barbara, CA 93130
**Phone:** (805)682-0997    **Fax:** (617)789-3801
**Email:** coda@coda-international.org
**Website:** http://www.coda-international.org
Millie Brother, Founder

**Fnded:** 1983. **Mem:** 500. **Desc:** Hearing children of deaf parents who are interested in sharing experiences with others of similar backgrounds. Provides information to professional organizations, libraries, community agencies, researchers, and other interested persons. Acts upon issues regarding deafness; provides support to deaf parent/hearing child families. Serves as clearinghouse for deaf parent/hearing children families. **Pub:** *CODA Connection*, quarterly. Newsletter. For the adult hearing children of deaf parents. Reports on national and international meetings and resources. Includes association news. *Price:* Included in membership dues. • *Hearing Children/ Deaf Parents.* Bibliography. • *Proceedings from Annual Conferences.* Proceedings.

### ★ 6019 ★ Cochlear Implant Association

5335 Wisconsin Ave. NW, Ste. 440
Washington, DC 20015-2052
**Phone:** (202)895-2781    **Fax:** (202)895-2782
**Email:** info@cici.org
**Website:** http://www.cici.org
Peg Williams, PhD, Exec. Dir.

**Fnded:** 1981. **Mem:** 1,500. **Local Groups:** 38. **Desc:** Cochlear implant users, candidates for cochlear implant, and their families and friends; health care professionals. Provides support services including advocacy for the hearing impaired. Promotes improved cochlear implant technology and research on hearing impairment. Serves as an information clearinghouse. Conducts educational programs and childrens' services; operates speakers' bureau. **Pub:** *Contact*, quarterly. Magazine. Covers current research, legislation, insurance issues, association activities, and coping advice. *Price:* Included in membership dues.

### ★ 6020 ★ Commonwealth Society for the Deaf (CSD)

Sound Seekers
34 Buckingham Palace Rd.
London SW1W 0RE, United Kingdom
**Phone:** 44 20 72335700    **Fax:** 44 20 72335800
**Email:** sound.seekers@btinternet.com
**Website:** http://www.sound-seekers.org.uk

**Fnded:** 1959. **Mem:** 102. **Lang(s):** English. **Desc:** Works for the deaf, especially children, in developing Commonwealth countries. In conjunction with governmental and voluntary organizations, deploys working parties of ENT Surgeons/Audiologists who are volunteers; trains technicians to support audiologists, and to maintain and repair electronic equipment; provides equipment for use by schools for the deaf. Conducts research into the prevention of deafness and compiles statistics on such research; has studied the incidence and causes of deafness in Gambia, Nigeria, and Botswana. Maintains contact with and disseminates information about schools, societies, and government councils for the deaf throughout the Commonwealth. **Pub:** *Newsletter*, annual. Newsletter. Provides information documents to supporters. • *Sound Seekers*

*Zutomation Leaflet*, periodic. Brochure. • Annual Report, annual.

### ★ 6021 ★ Compulsive Stutterers Anonymous (CSA)

3138 Overhulse Rd. NW Apt. 147
Olympia, WA 98502-3856

**Fnded:** 1989. **Local Groups:** 6. **Desc:** Men and women with the problem of compulsive stuttering. Uses an adaptation of the 12-step program used by Alcoholics Anonymous World Services. Encourages members to share their experiences and maintain personal contact with others at meetings and on the telephone. Encourages members to combine a program of professional speech therapy with spiritual principles of recovery. Provides sponsors to encourage individual members in their recovery and in developing a speech plan with the goal of gaining greater freedom in speaking.

### ★ 6022 ★ Conference of Educational Administrators of Schools and Programs for the Deaf (CEASD)

c/o Joseph P. Finnegan, Jr.
PO Box 1778
Saint Augustine, FL 32085-1778
**Phone:** (904)810-5200    **Fax:** (904)810-5525
**Email:** email@ceasd.org
**Website:** http://www.ceasd.org
Joseph P. Finnegan, Jr., Exec. Dir.

**Fnded:** 1868. **Mem:** 355. **Desc:** Executive heads of public, private, and denominational schools for the deaf in the U.S. and Canada. Coordinates research on the problems of deafness. Compiles statistics on pupils, teachers, and programs from schools for the deaf. **Pub:** *American Annals of the Deaf*, 5/year. • Newsletter, bimonthly. **Frmly:** Association of Superintendents and Principals of American Schools for the Deaf; (1980) Conference of Executives of American Schools for the Deaf; (2000) Conference of Eduactional Administrators Serving the Deaf.

### ★ 6023 ★ Convention of American Instructors of the Deaf (CAID)

PO Box 377
Bedford, TX 76095-0377
**Phone:** (817)354-8414
**Email:** caid@swbell.net
Dr. Liz O'Brien, Pres.

**Fnded:** 1850. **Mem:** 1,200. **Desc:** Professional organization of teachers, administrators, and professionals in allied fields related to education of the deaf and hard-of-hearing. Objectives are: to provide opportunities for a free interchange of views concerning methods and means of educating the deaf and hard-of-hearing; to promote such education by the publication of reports, essays, and other information; to develop more effective methods of teaching deaf and hard-of-hearing children. **Pub:** *American Annals of the Deaf*, quarterly. Journal. Includes scholarly articles on deafness. *Price:* Included in membership dues; $77/ year for nonmembers. • *News 'N' Notes*, quarterly. Newsletter. Includes articles on education of the deaf and organization activities. *Price:* Free. For members only. • *Reference Issue of the American Annals of the Deaf.* Directory. • Proceedings. **AKA:** American Instructors of the Deaf.

### ★ 6024 ★ Council for the Advancement of Communication with Deaf People

Durham University Science Park
Block 4
Stockton Rd.
Durham DH1 3UZ, United Kingdom
**Phone:** 44 191 3831155    **Fax:** 44 191 3837914
**Email:** durham@cacdp.demon.co.uk
**Website:** http://www.cacdp.demon.co.uk

**Fnded:** 1982. **Mem:** 1,000. **Desc:** Aims to improve communication between deaf and hearing people by the development of curricula and examinations in communication skills. Offers certification in British Sign

Language, Lipspeaking. Communicating with Deafblind people and Deaf Awareness, and carries out the selection, training, monitering and registration of examiners. **Pub:** *CACDP Directory*, annual. Book. • *CACDP Standard Newsletter*, quarterly. Newsletter.

### ★ 6025 ★ Council on Education of the Deaf (CED)

c/o Department of Administration; Gallaudet University
800 Florida Ave. NE
Washington, DC 20002-3695
**Phone:** (202)651-5525    **Fax:** (202)651-5749
**Email:** roz.rosen@gallaudet.edu
**Website:** http://www.deafed.net
Roz Rosen, Ed.D., Exec. Dir.

**Fnded:** 1930. **Nat'l Groups:** 6. **Desc:** Representatives from the Alexander Graham Bell Association for the Deaf, the Conference of Educational Administrators Serving the Deaf, the Convention of American Instructors of the Deaf, Association of College Educators; Deaf and Hard of Hearing, National Association of the Deaf and The American Society for Deaf Children. Certifies teachers and accredits university teacher training programs specializing in deaf education and the related. Seeks to improve educational opportunities for deaf and hard of hearing children through cooperation in publication practices, liaison with lay and peripheral groups, teacher certification, public information, and research. Provides certification programs for educators and professionals. Establishes, evaluates, accredits, and maintains certification standards for teacher education programs. **Pub:** *Certification Standards Document.* • *Standards for Evaluation of Programs.*

### ★ 6026 ★ Danish Deaf Association

Postboks 704
Rantzausgade 60, 1
DK-2200 Copenhagen, Denmark
**Phone:** 45 35240910    **Fax:** 45 35240920
**Email:** lf@deaf.dk
**Website:** http://www.deaf.dk

**Fnded:** 1935. **Mem:** 2,000. **Local Groups:** 17. **Lang(s):** Danish, English. **Desc:** People with hearing impairments, their families, and health care and speech and hearing professionals. Works to improve the quality of life of people with impaired hearing. Works to insure that the legal and economic rights of people with hearing impairments are respected. Conducts research and educational programs on sign language and other means of nonverbal communication. Serves as a liaison with other national and international associations with similar aims. Assists members in obtaining assistive technologies including text telephones, alarm services, and TTD messages. **Pub:** *Dovebladet*, monthly. Magazine. **Frmly:** (2000) National Association for the Deaf in Denmark.

### DB-Link
*See:* Entry 20940

### ★ 6027 ★ Deaf-Blind Association

600 Nicholson St.
North Fitzroy, VIC 3068, Australia
**Phone:** 61 3 94821155    **Fax:** 61 3 94862092
**Email:** dba@internex.net.au
**Website:** http://www.dba.asn.au

**Fnded:** 1967. **Lang(s):** English. **Desc:** Deafblind people and their families. Represent the interests of people with a multi-sensory impairment; provides community support for them and their families; provides short term care and long term accommodation and respite care; educates the public about multi-sensory impairment; supports the rubella immunization campaign; offers an information resource about deafblindness; acts as a catalyst for the provision of services to the group of people it represents. Operates group homes for children and adults; provides respite care and counseling; provides community education and awareness.

**★ 6028 ★ Deaf Education Through Listening and Talking (DELTA)**
PO Box 20
Haverhill CB9 7BD, United Kingdom
**Phone:** 44 1440 783689      **Fax:** 44 1440 783689
**Email:** delta@connevans.com
**Website:** http://www.connevans.com/delta

**Fnded:** 1980. **Mem:** 800. **Reg. Groups:** 6. **Lang(s):** English. **Desc:** Parents and teachers of children with hearing impairment; adults with hearing impairment. Promotes development of natural and effective spoken language among children with profound hearing impairment. Advocates use of the natural aural approach in teaching children with profound hearing impairment to use spoken language. Conducts workshops for teachers and families of children with profound hearing impairment; makes available teaching resources; sponsors research; provides children's services. **Pub:** *Chat*, semiannual. Newsletter. • *Chatting*, quarterly. Newsletter. • *Deaf Children*. Handbook. • *Deaf Children Talking*. Book. A guide for parents. • *Guide to the Natural Aural Approach*. Handbook. **Frmly:** (1995) National Aural Group.

**★ 6029 ★ Deaf-REACH**
3521 12th St. NE
Washington, DC 20017
**Phone:** (202)832-6681      **Fax:** (202)832-8454
**Email:** info@deafreach.org
**Website:** http://www.deaf-reach.org/otis.html
Patrick M. Gleason, Pres.

**Fnded:** 1972. **Desc:** Committed to maximizing the self-sufficiency of deaf people needing special services by providing referral, education, advocacy, counseling, and housing. Seeks to establish residential homes and provide psychological, physical, spiritual, and social aid to deaf persons with mental and emotional problems. Operates Otis House and Kearny House, group homes for mentally ill deaf persons, designed to help meet the residents' emotional and social needs and teach them independent living skills. Administers the Community Housing for the Hearing Impaired Program which also provides a group home. Offers in-take, referral, housing placement assistance, and personal counseling; provides day-programs for learning disabled, deaf adults. Works in community advocacy for the mentally ill hearing impaired. **Pub:** Annual Report.*Price:* Free. • Brochure. • Newsletter, quarterly. **Frmly:** (1990) National Health Care Foundation for the Deaf.

**★ 6030 ★ Deaf Women United (DWU)**
PO Box 92028
Washington, DC 20090
**Website:** http://www.dwu.org/

**Fnded:** 1985. **Desc:** Promotes opportunity for deaf women in the areas of deaf culture, politics, employment and education, social activities and networking. Provides tools, information and training in organizational management, personal growth and empowerment; assists in setting up a home office which becomes a clearinghouse of resource information; maintains mentoring system. **Pub:** Newsletter, quarterly.

**★ 6031 ★ Deafblind International (Dbl)**
c/o SENSE International
11-13 Clifton Terrace
London N4 3SR, United Kingdom
**Phone:** 44 20 72727774      **Fax:** 44 20 72726012
**Email:** dbi@sense.org.uk
**Website:** http://www.deafblindinternational.org

**Fnded:** 1976. **Mem:** 1,000. **Lang(s):** English. **Desc:** Serves as a network for deaf-blind people, their families, and professionals with an interest in their well-being. Seeks to develop public awareness of the needs and potential of deaf-blind people. Conducts charitable and educational programs. **Pub:** *DBI Review*, semiannual. Journal. **Frmly:** International Association for the Education of Deafblind People.

**★ 6032 ★ Deafblind UK**
100 Bridge St.
Peterborough PE1 1DY, United Kingdom
**Phone:** 44 1733 358100      **Fax:** 44 1733 358356
**Email:** info@deafblinduk.org.uk
**Website:** http://www.deafblinduk.org.uk

**Fnded:** 1928. **Mem:** 2,030. **Local Groups:** 24. **Lang(s):** English. **Desc:** Deafblind persons. Helps alleviate the isolation felt by those with dual sensory loss. Negotiates with government to secure better services and facilities for individuals with visual and hearing impairments. Conducts public service programs. Offers advice and financial consultation and some housing assistance. Organizes conferences, seminars, and communication courses. **Pub:** *The Rainbow*, quarterly. Available in large print, Braille, Moon, and cassette versions. • *Snippets*, weekly. Newspaper. Available in Braille, Moon, large print, and disk.

**★ 6033 ★ Deafness Research Foundation (DRF)**
1050 17th St.NW, Ste701
Washington, DC 20036
**Phone:** (202)289-5850      **Free:** 800-829-5934
**Fax:** (202)293-1805
**Email:** drf@drf.org
**Website:** http://www.drf.org
Kromeklia Bryant, Off. Mgr.

**Fnded:** 1958. **Mem:** 2,000. **Desc:** Participates in the National Temporal Bone and Balance Pathology Resource Registry Program of the National Institute on Deafness and Other Communication Disorders. Approximately 1000 physicians and other professionals in ear medicine and research and 52 medical societies underwrite the foundation's fundraising costs through membership in the Centurions of the Deafness Research Foundation; approximately 300 other interested individuals raise funds through membership in the Deafness Research Foundation Alliance. **Pub:** *Deafness Research Foundation Annual Report*. Annual Report. *Price:* Free. • *Hear Today, Tomorrow May Be Only Silence*. Brochure. *Price:* Free. • *The Hearing Advocate*, 3/year. Newsletter. Covers current developments in deafness research; includes foundation news. *Price:* Free. • *Noise Can Be Harmful to Your Health*. Brochure. *Price:* Free. • *Otitis Media: Just an Ear Infection?*. Brochure. *Price:* Free. • *You and the Latest in Ear Research*. Brochure. *Price:* Free. • Booklets. • Brochures.

**★ 6034 ★ Dogs for the Deaf (DFD)**
10175 Wheeler Rd.
Central Point, OR 97502
**Phone:** (541)826-9220      **Free:** 800-990-DOGS
**Fax:** (541)826-6696
**Email:** info@dogsforthedeaf.org
**Website:** http://www.dogsforthedeaf.org
Robin Dickson, CEO/Pres.

**Fnded:** 1977. **Mem:** 30,000. **Desc:** Trains hearing dogs to alert deaf persons to certain sounds. Dogs are chosen from pet adoption shelters and assigned on the basis of a prioritized waiting list. They undergo four to five months of training during which they are taught to alert their masters to the sounds of alarm clocks, smoke alarms, doorbells, oven timers, crying babies, and telephones. Deaf or severely hearing impaired persons are eligible to be recipients if they are old enough to assume responsibility for the care of the dog. When assigned, a trainer and the dog travel to the recipient's home for a week to teach the dog and recipient to work together. Costs of dog selection, veterinary care, housing, training, and placement are covered; recipients make a donation only if able. Trains individuals to be certified audio canine trainers. Has appeared on local and national television programs to present the hearing ear dog training process and the results of dog placement. **Pub:** *Canine Listener*, quarterly. Provides information on the Hearing Ear Dog Program for the deaf; includes profiles of dogs and owners. *Price:* Free.

**★ 6035 ★ Dutch Deafship (Dovenschap)**
PO Box 323
NL-3500 AH Utrecht, Netherlands
**Fax:** 31 30 29700030
**Email:** info@dovenschap.nl
**Website:** http://www.dovenschap.nl

**Fnded:** 1995. **Lang(s):** Dutch. **Desc:** Umbrella organization of associations for the hearing impaired. Encourages the emancipation and participation of the hearing impaired in society; disseminates information. Represents member organizations before government agencies and institutions; coordinates contact between members; works with other organizations concerned with the welfare of the deaf. **Frmly:** (1997) Dutch DeafAssociation.

**★ 6036 ★ Dutch Parents Organization of Hearing and Speech Impaired Children (FOSS)**
**(Federaties van Ouders van Slechthorende- en Spraakgestoorde)**
De Molen SgA
Postbus 14
NL-3990 DA Houten, Netherlands
**Phone:** 31 30 2340663      **Fax:** 31 30 6360689

**Fnded:** 1973. **Mem:** 40. **Lang(s):** Dutch. **Desc:** Institutions and organizations representing the parents of 4500 children in the Netherlands concerned with the welfare of hearing and speech impaired children. Works to insure the provision of quality education for the hearing and speech impaired; assists in diagnosis; provides moral support to the parents of hearing or speech impaired children; disseminates information. Sponsors competitions; maintains speakers' bureau. **Pub:** *FOSSTAAL*, quarterly. Journal. • *Hearing and Speech Impaired Children*. • *Not an Easy Way to Go*. Video.

**★ 6037 ★ Ear Foundation (EF)**
1817 Patterson St.
Nashville, TN 37203
**Phone:** (615)284-7807      **Fax:** (615)284-7935
**Email:** earfound@earfoundation.org
**Website:** http://www.theearfound.com
Joseph DiBartolomeo, MD, Dir.

**Fnded:** 1980. **Desc:** Benefactors dedicated to advance medical knowledge concerning ear diseases and to encourage public understanding of such disorders. Offers professional and public education programs; research directed towards Eustachian tube disorders, ear diseases, and related disorders such as hearing loss, tinnitus, and vertigo. **Pub:** Brochures. • Monographs. • Newsletter, periodic. • Video.Describes ear surgery and the treatment of hearing loss.

**★ 6038 ★ Educational Audiology Association (EAA)**
4319 Ehrlich Rd.
Tampa, FL 33624
**Free:** 800-460-7322      **Fax:** (813)968-3597
**Email:** eaa@l-tgraye.com
**Website:** http://www.edaud.org
Lois Kostroski, Exec. Dir.

**Mem:** 1,020. **Desc:** Audiologists and others with an interest in the field. Promotes advancement in the field of audiology and its educational applications. Conducts educational programs. **Pub:** *EAA Newsletter*, quarterly. Newsletter. • Journal, annual. Includes membership directory. **Frmly:** (1998) Educational Audiology Society.

**★ 6039 ★ European Association of Hearing Aid Audiologists**
16 Av General Jourdan
B-6220 Fleurus, Belgium
**Fnded:** 1968.

**★ 6040 ★ European Laryngological Society (ELS)**
c/o Prof. M. Remacle
University Hospital of Mont-Godinne
ENT Department
B-5530 Yvoir, Belgium
**Phone:** 32 81 422111  **Fax:** 32 81 423023
**Email:** remacle@orlo.ucl.ac.be
**Website:** http://www.md.ucl.ac.be/els
**Fnded:** 1995. **Mem:** 200. **Lang(s):** Dutch, English, French, German. **Desc:** Physicians and researchers working in the field of laryngology. Promotes increased understanding of diseases of the neck and their treatments. Conducts research and continuing professional education programs. **Pub:** *European Archives of Otorhinolaryngology*, monthly. Journal.

**★ 6041 ★ European Rhinologic Society (ERS)**
c/o Dr. K. Ingels
Dept of Otorhinolaryngology
Ph. Van Leydenlan 15
NL-6525 EX Nijmegen, Netherlands
**Phone:** 31 24 3614450  **Fax:** 31 24 3540251
**Email:** k.ingels@kno.azn.nl
**Website:** http://www.azn.nl/ent/ers
**Fnded:** 1963. **Mem:** 700. **Lang(s):** English. **Desc:** Rhinosurgeons and otolaryngologists in 42 countries. Offers education and research in clinical, allergological, and immunological rhinology; provides training in functional and aesthetic rhinosurgery. Holds courses. **Pub:** *Rhinology*, quarterly. Journal.

**★ 6042 ★ European Union of the Deaf (EUD)**
rue Franklinstraat 110
B-1000 Brussels, Belgium
**Phone:** 32 2 7357218  **Fax:** 32 2 7355354
**Email:** info@eudnet.org
**Website:** http://www.eudnet.org
**Fnded:** 1985. **Desc:** Coordination of activities on a pan-European level, which includes dissemination of information, policy development, advice, lobbying and promoting use of the indigenous sign languages of Europe and recognition of the deaf culture.

**★ 6043 ★ Friends: The Association of Young People Who Stutter**
1220 Rosita Rd.
Pacifica, CA 94044-4223
**Phone:** (650)355-0215
**Email:** jtahlbach@aol.com
**Website:** http://www.friendswhostutter.org
John Ahlbach, Contact
**Fnded:** 1998. **Desc:** Children and teenagers who stutter; family members of young people who stutter; professionals working with people who stutter. Seeks to create a network of love and support for members; promotes increased self-esteem among young people who stutter. Facilitates communication among members. **Pub:** *Reaching Out*, 9/year. Journal.

**★ 6044 ★ Hear Center (HEAR)**
301 E Del Mar Blvd.
Pasadena, CA 91101
**Phone:** (626)796-2016  **Fax:** (626)796-2320
**Email:** auditory@mindspring.com
**Website:** http://www.hearcenter.org
Josephine F. Wilson, MA, Exec. Dir.
**Fnded:** 1954. **Desc:** Auditory and verbal program designed to help hearing impaired children, infants, and adults lead normal and productive lives. Seeks to develop auditory techniques to aid people who have communication problems due to deafness. Primary objectives include early identification of hearing loss in infants and children and early amplification. Operates a program involving: binaural hearing aids where appropriate; continuous exposure to sound; development of auditory perception; wide-range amplification; environmental stimulation. Provides services in: diagnosis and audiological evaluation; hearing aid evaluation and trial use; development of listening skills and

articulation; speech therapy; hearing aid dispensing; parent counseling. **Pub:** *Conquering Childhood Deafness*. Book. • *Effectiveness of Early Detection and Auditory Stimulation on the Speech and Language of Hearing Impaired Children.* • *Hear: A Four Letter Word.* Book. • *HEAR Center Proceedings*, periodic. Proceedings. • *The Listener*, quarterly. Newsletter. Covers topics of interest to the hearing and speech impaired community, as well as services and activities of the center. *Price:* Free. **Frmly:** (1975) Hearing Education Through Auditory Research Foundation.

**★ 6045 ★ Hear Now (HN)**
6700 Washington Ave. S
Eden Prairie, MN 55344-3405
**Phone:** (303)695-7797  **Free:** 800-648-HEAR
**Fax:** (303)695-7789
**Email:** jostelter@aol.com
Joanita Stelter, PR Officer
**Fnded:** 1988. **Desc:** Provides hearing aids for very low income hard of hearing individuals of all ages. Offers financial and fund raising assistance for hard of hearing and deaf individuals who need cochlear implants. Collects broken and used hearing aids through its HEAR-O Recycling Program to support assistance programs. **Pub:** Newsletter, quarterly. Includes news about current projects and reports on those who have requested or received help from Hear Now. *Price:* Free. • Also publishes information packet.

**★ 6046 ★ Hearing Concern**
7/11 Armstrong Rd.
London W3 7JL, United Kingdom
**Phone:** 44 181 7429151  **Fax:** 44 181 7429043
**Email:** info@hearingconcern.org.uk
**Website:** http://www.hearingconcern.org.uk
**Fnded:** 1947. **Mem:** 3,000. **Reg. Groups:** 180. **Lang(s):** English, Welsh. **Desc:** Seeks to help overcome the frustration, isolation, and loneliness experienced by millions of people in the UK who have a hearing loss. Country's leading provider of advice and support of campaigns on behalf of its client group. Promotes awareness of the communication needs of deaf and hard of hearing people. **Pub:** *Hearing Concern*, quarterly. Magazine. • *Talkabout*. Magazine. Magazine of youth section. **Frmly:** Hearing Concern, British Association of the Hard of Hearing; (1993) British Association of the Hard of Hearing.

**★ 6047 ★ Hearing Education and Awareness for Rockers (HEAR)**
PO Box 460847
San Francisco, CA 94146-0847
**Phone:** (415)773-9590  **Fax:** (415)409-5683
**Email:** hear@hearnet.com
**Website:** http://www.hearnet.com
Kathy Peck, Exec. Dir.
**Fnded:** 1988. **Desc:** Musicians, music industry professionals, and music lovers. Seeks to prevent hearing loss and Tinnitus by promoting public awareness regarding the dangers of over amplified music and noise. Promotes the use of hearing protection and enhancement devices, especially among young people. Produces public service announcements recording artists, school programs, distributes ear protection and information at music events, conducts free hearing screening programs and provides hearing information and resources and H.E.A.R. Affiliate referrals via HEARNET.COM. **Pub:** *Can't Hear You Knocking.* Video. *Price:* $39.95. • *HEAR Information Packet. Price:* $10.

**Helen Keller National Center for Deaf-Blind Youths and Adults (HKNC)**
*See:* Entry 20973

**★ 6048 ★ HIKE Fund**
c/o Shirley R. Terrill
10115 Cherry Hill Pl.
Spring Hill, FL 34608-7116
**Phone:** (352)688-2579  **Fax:** (352)688-2579
**Email:** ceterrilli@aol.com

**Website:** http://www.missouriiojd.org/MO-HIKE/HIKE.htm
Dr. Albert L. Howe, Pres.
**Fnded:** 1985. **Mem:** 14. **Nat'l Groups:** 36. **Desc:** Supported by the International Order of Job's Daughters. Works for complete equality and integration of the hearing impaired in society. Provides support and information services. Provides hearing devices for children (up to the age of 20) with financial need. **AKA:** Hearing Impaired Kids Endowment Fund.

**★ 6049 ★ Hong Kong Association for the Deaf**
Duke of Windsor Social Service Bldg. No. 903
15 Hennesy Rd., Wanchai
Hong Kong, People's Republic of China
**Phone:** 852 25278969  **Fax:** 852 25293316
**Email:** ho@deaf.org.hk
**Website:** http://www.deaf.org.hk
**Lang(s):** Chinese, English. **Desc:** Individuals with impaired hearing; others with an interest in the well-being of people with impaired hearing. Seeks to improve the quality of life, and insure the full integration into society, of people with impaired hearing. Facilitates communication and cooperation among members; makes available therapeutic and other services to people with impaired hearing.

**★ 6050 ★ Hong Kong Society for the Deaf (HKS.D)**
Duke of Windsor Social Service Bldg., Rm. 903
15 Hennessy Rd.
Hong Kong, People's Republic of China
**Phone:** 852 25278969  **Fax:** 852 25293316
**Email:** ho@deaf.org.hk
**Website:** http://www.deaf.org.hk
**Fnded:** 1968. **Mem:** 3,900. **Lang(s):** Chinese, English. **Desc:** Seeks to undertake projects of publicity, education, recreation, counseling, clinical, audio logical and medical services for the hearing impaired: and to assist or cooperate with any institutions, organizations or individuals to improve the services for the hearing impaired to work towards improving the educational standards for the hearing impaired, to provide scholarship and special equipment for the hearing impaired as well as to provide guidance for the parents of hearing-impaired children to inform the public about the problems and needs of hearing impaired, to give necessary information to hearing-impaired persons and their families about institutions and services available to them, and to exchange information among institutions serving the hearing impaired. **Pub:** Newsletter, monthly.

**★ 6051 ★ House Ear Institute (HEI)**
2100 W 3rd St.
Los Angeles, CA 90057
**Phone:** (213)483-4431  **Fax:** (213)483-8789
**Email:** webmaster@hei.org
**Website:** http://www.hei.org
James Boswell, CEO
**Fnded:** 1946. **Desc:** Develops conceptual and technically feasible approaches to resolving hearing and balance disorders through applied research. Conducts research on subjects including hearing aids, auditory implants, aging ear, brain mapping, nearoanatomy, infant hearing diagnosis, and acoustic tumor. Offers seminars and classes for senior residents and practicing physicians. Operates children's center to serve profoundly deaf children and their families. Maintains library of 2700 volumes and 180 journal titles on otology. Sponsors videotape seminars and conducts courses on the use of hearing devices and how to evaluate hearing disorders. Provides a support group for parents. Compiles statistics; offers children's services; maintains speakers' bureau, library, and museum. **Pub:** *Housecalls*, semiannual. Magazine. News magazine. • Annual Report. • Manuals. • Monographs. • Papers. **Frmly:** (1972) Los Angeles Foundation of Otology; (1981) Ear Research Institute.

## ★ 6052 ★ I CAN

4 Dyer's Bldg.s
Holborn
London EC1N 2QP, United Kingdom
**Phone:** 44 870 104066      **Fax:** 44 870 104067
**Email:** info@ican.org.uk
**Website:** http://www.ican.org.uk
**Fnded:** 1888. **Lang(s):** English. **Desc:** National educational charity for children with speech and language difficulties. Services include three residential schools, an early years program, mainstream support language resources in secondary schools, and a national training program for professionals. **Pub:** *Annual Report*, annual. • *Communicate!*, semiannual. Newsletter.

## International Association of Audio Information Services (IAAIS)

*See:* Entry 20981

## ★ 6053 ★ International Association of Laryngectomees (IAL)

8900 Thornton Rd.
Box 99311
Stockton, CA 95209
**Free:** (866)425-3678        **Fax:** (209)472-0516
**Email:** ial@larynxlink.com
**Website:** http://www.larynxlink.com
Jack Henslee, Exec. Dir.
**Fnded:** 1952. **Nat'l Groups:** 275. **Desc:** Persons who have had their larynx removed; physicians, surgeons, speech therapists, rehabilitation experts, nurses, and others interested in the rehabilitation of laryngectomees. Encourages exchange of ideas and methods for training and teaching of alaryngeal methods of communication. Fosters recognized standards for the rehabilitation of laryngectomees. Maintains the Voice Rehabilitation Institute for training teachers of alaryngeal voice and the Lost Chord Clubs. Organizes support groups for laryngectomes and their families. **Pub:** *IAL News*, 3/year. Newsletter. *Price:* Free. • Directory, annual. • Films.Provides information on first aid and post-laryngectomy speech. • Pamphlets.Provides information on laryngectomees, esophageal voice, and rehabilitation.

## ★ 6054 ★ International Association of Logopedics and Phoniatrics (IALP)

c/o Prof. Dolores Battle
141 South Ln.
Orchard Park, NY 14127
**Phone:** (716)878-6210        **Fax:** (716)878-6234
**Email:** battlede@buffalostate.edu
**Website:** http://www.ldc.lu.se/logopedi/IALP
Prof. Eva Soder Palm, Pres.
**Fnded:** 1924. **Mem:** 450. **Nat'l Groups:** 59. **Desc:** Phoniatricians (voice disorder specialists), logopedists (speech-language defect therapists), and audiologists (hearing specialists) from 59 affiliated societies in 38 countries. Fosters and conducts scientific study of disorders in human communication. **Pub:** *Folia Phoniatrica et Logopaedica*, quarterly. Journal. • *Folia Phoniatrica et Logopedica*, quarterly. Journal. Professional scientific journal. • *IALP Directory*, triennial. Directory.

## ★ 6055 ★ International Association of Physicians in Audiology (IAPA)

c/o Prof. Dr. K. Schorn
ENT - University Hospital
Kinikum Grosshadern
Marchinoninistrasse15
D-81377 Munich, Germany
**Website:** http://www.barajas.vanaga.es/iapa/
**Fnded:** 1980. **Mem:** 200. **Lang(s):** English. **Desc:** Practitioners of medical audiology in 35 countries. Promotes the field of medical audiology and practitioners' interests worldwide. **Pub:** *Journal of Audiological Medicine*, 3/year. Journal.

## ★ 6056 ★ International Committee of Sports for the Deaf (CISS)

814 Thayer Ave., Ste. 350
Silver Spring, MD 20910
**Fax:** (301)650-6595
**Email:** info@ciss.org
**Website:** http://www.ciss.org
Dr. Donalda K. Ammons, Sec. Gen.
**Fnded:** 1924. **Mem:** 77. **Reg. Groups:** 4. **Desc:** National athletic organizations for the deaf. Provides an international sports competition for the deaf patterned after the International Olympic Games. Promotes and develops physical education and the practice of sports among the deaf. Encourages friendly relations between countries with programs in silent sports and countries without programs for deaf athletes. Holds Summer World Games and Winter Games alternately at 2-year intervals for competitors with hearing loss of 55 decibels or more. The committee is recognized by the International Olympic Committee. **Pub:** *Bulletin*, quarterly. Magazine. *Price:* $20/year. • *Handbook*, periodic. **AKA:** (2000) Deaf Olympics.

## ★ 6057 ★ International Dyslexia Association (IDA)

8600 LaSalle Rd.
Chester Bldg., Ste. 382
Baltimore, MD 21286-2044
**Phone:** (410)296-0232        **Free:** 800-ABCD-123
**Fax:** (410)321-5069
**Email:** info@interdys.org
**Website:** http://www.interdys.org
J. Thomas Viall, Exec. Dir.
**Fnded:** 1949. **Mem:** 13,000. **Nat'l Groups:** 44. **Desc:** Offers free information to the public and referrals for diagnosis and treatment. Professionals in the fields of neurology, pediatrics, psychiatry, education, social work, and psychology; parents; other persons interested in the study, treatment, and prevention of the problems of specific language disability, often called developmental dyslexia or simply dyslexia. Provides a focal point for activities and ideas generated in various fields as they relate to problems of language development and learning. IDA is founded in memory of Dr. Samuel T. Orton, a pioneer in the field of dyslexia. Disseminates materials. Offers support groups. **Pub:** *Annals of Dyslexia*, annual. Peer-reviewed journal with current research on dyslexia. *Price:* Free with membership; $17. • *Orton Emeritus Series*. Monographs. Series 12 of 26 published. • *Perspectives*, quarterly. Magazine. • Also issues reprints of papers. **Frmly:** (1981) Orton Society; (1998) Orton Dyslexia Society.

## ★ 6058 ★ International Federation of Hard of Hearing People (IFHOH)

PO Box 13
Abbots Langley WD5 0RQ, United Kingdom
**Phone:** 44 1923 264584      **Fax:** 44 1923 261635
**Email:** c_shaw@compuserve.com
**Website:** http://www.ifhoh.org
**Fnded:** 1977. **Mem:** 40. **Lang(s):** English. **Desc:** National organizations for individuals with acquired deafness representing 24 countries. Objectives are to: improve the standards of technical and social provisions for the hearing impaired; increase the understanding of the problems and needs of the hard of hearing; stimulate research into hearing impairment and the development of facilities for the hearing impaired; improve communication between the hard of hearing and among organizations for the hearing impaired. Coordinates the work of member organizations. Cooperates with governments and organizations for the prevention and cure of hearing impairments. Collects research data, public relations materials, and technical aids. **Pub:** *Congress and Symposia Proceedings*, quadrennial. Proceedings. • *Congress Report*. Report. • *IFHOH Journal*, 3/year. Journal. • *Working for the Hard of Hearing Within the IFHOH*. Brochure. **Frmly:** International Federation of the Hard of Hearing.

## ★ 6059 ★ International Federation of Hard of Hearing Young People (IFHOHYP)

c/o Vanessa Mogliosi
Via Oriola 12
I-38100 Trento, Italy
**Phone:** 39 461 236966      **Fax:** 39 461 236966
**Email:** nivane@tin.it
**Fnded:** 1968. **Mem:** 15. **Lang(s):** English, German. **Desc:** National organizations; hearing impaired individuals under the age of 30 living in countries where no organizations for the hearing impaired exist. Encourages friendship between individuals of different nationalities. Objectives are to: increase understanding of the problems and needs of the hard of hearing; improve self-confidence of young hearing impaired people. Supervises annual summer camps. **Pub:** *The Ear Talking*, quarterly. Magazine. • *IFHOHYP Annual Report*, annual. Annual Report. • *IFHOHYP Newsletter*, quarterly. Newsletter. **Frmly:** (1994) International Committee of Hard of Hearing Young People.

## ★ 6060 ★ International Federation of Oto-Rhino-Laryngological Societies (IFOS) (Federation Internationale des Societes Oto-Rhino-Laryngologiques)

148 Lee Ave.
Toronto, ON, Canada M4E 2P3
**Phone:** (416)690-3472        **Fax:** (416)690-2199
**Email:** peter.alberti@utoronto.ca
**Website:** http://www.ifosworld.org
**Fnded:** 1965. **Mem:** 105. **Reg. Groups:** 6. **Lang(s):** English, French, German, Japanese, Spanish. **Desc:** National (105) and international otorhinolaryngological societies (12) in 140 countries. Promotes the advancement of otorhinolaryngology (ORL), the prevention and control of diseases and disorders of the ear, nose, and throat, and the training of otorhinolaryngologists. Participates, as an affiliate to the World Health Organization, in the Worldwide Prevention Action on Hearing Impairment. Encourages international cooperation between otorhinolaryngologists and members. Plans to establish a museum. Sponsors film and video competitions. **Pub:** *IFOS Newsletter*, quarterly. Newsletter. • Films, periodic. • Reports, periodic. • Videos, periodic.

## ★ 6061 ★ International Hearing Dog (IHDI)

5901 E 89th Ave.
Henderson, CO 80640
**Phone:** (303)287-3277        **Fax:** (303)287-3425
**Email:** ihdi@aol.com
**Website:** http://www.ihdi.org/
Martha A. Foss, Pres.
**Fnded:** 1979. **Desc:** An independent organization formed to train and place dogs, free of cost, with the deaf. Hearing dogs are trained to alert the hearing impaired to important sounds that occur in the owners' environment, such as a door knock or bell, a baby crying, a smoke alarm, an alarm clock, a telephone, a security buzzer, and other sounds which might indicate danger. Presents public awareness demonstrations. **Pub:** *Paws for Silence*, 3/year. Newsletter. Reports on the group's current activities and includes stories about hearing dog recipients. *Price:* Free. **Frmly:** (1981) Hearing Dogs.

## ★ 6062 ★ International Hearing Society (IHS)

16880 Middlebelt Rd.
Livonia, MI 48154-3367
**Phone:** (734)522-7200        **Free:** 800-521-5247
**Fax:** (734)522-0200
**Email:** rclowers@ihsinfo.org
**Website:** http://www.ihsinfo.org/
Robin Clowers, BC-HIS, Exec. Dir.
**Fnded:** 1951. **Mem:** 3,000. **State Groups:** 54. **Desc:** Hearing aid specialists who test hearing for the selection, adaptation, fitting, adjusting, servicing, and sale of hearing aids. Members counsel the hearing impaired and instruct them in care and use of hearing aids. Activities include: administration of a qualification

**Fnded:** 1908. **Mem:** 755. **Nat'l Groups:** 32. **Desc:** Members are involved in all branches of speech and drama work - schools, colleges of further education and universities. They work in the professional and amateur theatre as producers, directors and coaches. Some are involved with the disabled whilst. others teach communication and presentation skills in the business world. The Society aims to uphold a high standard of teaching and support those working in the field. Each region has a representative who is responsible for promoting the work of the Society. A Conference is held in London in February and during August in another region. **Pub:** *Speech and Drama*, semiannual. Magazine. • Newsletter, 3/year, for members.

**Society of University Otolaryngologists - Head and Neck Surgeons (SUO-HNS)**
*See:* Entry 19604

**★ 6111 ★ Speak Easy (SE)**
95 Evergreen Ave.
Saint John's, NB, Canada E2N 1H4
**Phone:** (506)696-6799        **Fax:** (506)696-6799
**Email:** info@speakeasycanada.com
**Fnded:** 1984. **Mem:** 1,000. **Lang(s):** English. **Desc:** People who stutter, parents of children who stutter, and health professionals with an interest in speech. Promotes public awareness of stuttering. Provides support and assistance to members; conducts educational programs; sponsors charitable initiatives. **Pub:** *Speaking Out*, monthly. Newsletter. • Brochure, periodic.

**★ 6112 ★ Speak Easy International Foundation (SEIF)**
233 Concord Dr.
Paramus, NJ 07652
**Phone:** (201)262-0895        **Fax:** (201)262-0895
**Email:** bob-antoinette@worldnet.att.net
**Website:** http://members.tripod.com/speakeasynj/
Antoinette Gathman, Exec. Dir.
**Fnded:** 1977. **State Groups:** 8. **Local Groups:** 1. **Desc:** Support group and information source for individuals with a speech dysfluency (stuttering). Seeks to instill confidence in stutterers and reinforce fluency in their speech. Educates public, families, and friends on the problems of speech dysfluent individuals. **Pub:** *Speak Easy Newsletter*, quarterly. Newsletter. Contains activities of selfhelp groups, research reports on stuttering; convention schedules. *Price:* $25/year. • *Why Can't We Talk*. Video. Theatre-piece on stuttering. ng. *Price:* $129.95 institution; $25 individuals.

**★ 6113 ★ Speakability**
1 Royal St.
London SE1 7LL, United Kingdom
**Phone:** 44 207 2619572      **Fax:** 44 207 9289542
**Email:** speakability@speakability.org.uk
**Website:** http://www.speakability.org.uk
**Fnded:** 1980. **Mem:** 1,500. **Lang(s):** English. **Desc:** People with dysphasia (acquired language disorder), their friends and families, professionals working in the field. Works to raise awareness and understanding of dysphasia, offers help and advice through booklets and telephone helpline, membership scheme and newsletter, lectures and conferences. Professional backup and advocacy. Presses for improved provision of services; local branches, and self help groups are being developed across the country. **Pub:** *Dysphasia Matters: A Medical Teaching Pack*. Includes video and lecture packs. • *How to Help*. Booklets. • *Speaking Up*, quarterly. Newsletter. • *Talking About Dysphasia*. Audiotapes. **Frmly:** (2001) Action for Dysphasic Adults.

**★ 6114 ★ Speech Pathology Australia**
2nd Floor, 11-19 Bank Place
Melbourne, VIC 3000, Australia
**Phone:** 61 3 96424899      **Fax:** 61 3 96424922
**Email:** office@speechpathologyaustralia.org.au
**Website:** http://www.speechpathologyaustralia.org.au

**Fnded:** 1949. **Mem:** 2,950. **Lang(s):** English. **Desc:** Speech pathologists working in private practice, hospitals, rehabilitation centers, education centers, and with agencies for specific disabilities. Represents and promotes the professional interests of speech pathologists in Australia. Lobbies government on behalf of members and their clients for improved services and facilities; works with the media to provide information on communication disorders; and sets professional standards for its members.

**★ 6115 ★ Standing Liaison Committee of EU Speech and Language Therapists and Logopedists (Comite Permanent de Liaison des Orthophonistes-Logopedes de l'UE — CPLOL)**
2, rue des Deux Gares
F-75010 Paris, France
**Phone:** 33 1 40356375      **Fax:** 33 1 40374142
**Email:** cplol@hotmail.com
**Website:** http://www.cplol.org
**Fnded:** 1988. **Mem:** 21. **Desc:** Speech and language therapists in the European Union. Promotes high standards of conduct for members; equivalence of qualifications; harmonization of legislation relating to the profession and of initial training; exchange of scientific knowledge and research in the fields of logopedics.

**★ 6116 ★ Stuttering Foundation of America (SFA)**
3100 Walnut Grove Rd., Ste. 603
PO Box 11749
Memphis, TN 38111-0749
**Phone:** (901)452-7343        **Free:** 800-992-9392
**Fax:** (901)452-3931
**Email:** stutter@vantek.net
**Website:** http://www.stutteringhelp.org
Jane Fraser, Pres.
**Fnded:** 1947. **Desc:** Provides comprehensive materials, including videotapes, books and brochures, on stuttering to both the public and professionals. Seeks to bring together speech pathologists concerned with the prevention and treatment of stuttering. Provides referrals to speech-language pathologists specializing in stuttering. Provides support for research into the causes of stuttering. **Pub:** *Advice to Those Who Stutter*. Book. • *The Child Who Stutters: To the Health Care Provider*. • *The Child Who Stutters: To the Pediatrician, 2nd Ed.*. • *Do You Stutter: A Guide for Teens, 3rd Ed.*. • *If Your Child Stutters: A Guide for Parents, 5th Ed.*. • *The School-Age Child Who Stutters: Working Effectively with Attitudes and Emotions*. • *Self Therapy for the Stutterer, 10th Ed.*. • *SFA Newsletter*, quarterly. Newsletter. Contains SFA activities and information on stuttering. *Price:* Free. • *Sometimes I Just Stutter*. • *Stuttering and Your Child: Questions and Answers, 3rd Ed.*. **Frmly:** (1991) Speech Foundation of America.

**★ 6117 ★ Swedish National Association of the Deaf (SDR)**
Magnus Ladulas
Gatan 63
S-118 27 Stockholm, Sweden
**Phone:** 46 8 4421461        **Fax:** 46 8 4421499
**Email:** sdr@sdrf.se
**Website:** http://www.sdrf.se
**Fnded:** 1922. **Mem:** 6,000. **Nat'l Groups:** 1. **Reg. Groups:** 3. **State Groups:** 1. **Local Groups:** 48. **Lang(s):** English, Swedish. **Desc:** Deaf people, their families, and health care and speech and hearing professionals. Works to improve the quality of life of people with impaired hearing. Works to insure that the legal and economic rights of people with hearing impairments are respected. Conducts research and educational programs on sign language and other means of nonverbal communication. Serves as a liaison with other national and international associations with similar aims. Assists members in obtaining assistive technologies including text telephones, alarm

services, and TTD messages. **Pub:** *Dovtidningen*, monthly. Magazine.

**★ 6118 ★ Swiss Association of Logopedics and Communication Disorders (SALCD)**
Feldeggstrasse 69
CH-8008 Zurich, Switzerland
**Phone:** 41 1 3882690        **Fax:** 41 1 3882695
**Email:** sekr@salogopaedie.ch
**Website:** http://www.salogopaedie.ch
**Fnded:** 1942. **Mem:** 1,250. **State Groups:** 1250. **Lang(s):** English, French, German, Italian. **Desc:** Speech and hearing professionals and other individuals in related fields. Seeks to advance the study, understanding, and treatment of communications disorders. Conducts research and educational programs. **Pub:** *Mitglieder - Bulletin*, quarterly. Bulletin.

**★ 6119 ★ TDI**
8630 Fenton St., Ste. 604
Silver Spring, MD 20910-3803
**Phone:** (301)589-3006        **Fax:** (301)589-3797
**Email:** ExecDir@tdi-online.org
**Website:** http://www.tdi-online.org
Claude Stout, Exec. Dir.
**Fnded:** 1968. **Mem:** 55,000. **Desc:** Hearing impaired individuals and their families, and organizations participating in telecommunications over regular telephone lines through special equipment. Promotes equal access to telecommunications and media for individuals who are deaf, late-deafened, hard of hearing, or deaf-blind. Strives to constantly improve technology and accessibility for all who rely on visual telecommunications. Advocate for standards and compatibility for all telecommunication devices. Promotes closed captioning on television, cable, and the Internet. Seeks to extend the installation of text telephones (TTYs) in public buildings, railroads, airlines, bus terminals, and other places where they can be of service to the hearing impaired. Sells International TTY Logo Decals to the public. **Pub:** *Emergency Acess Evaluation Kit*. Manual. Contains emergency personnel training for use of TTY's and dealing with deaf and hard of hearing callers. *Price:* $35. • *GA-SK Newsletter*, quarterly. Newsletter. • *National Directory of TTY Numbers*, annual. Directory. • *Using Your TTY/TDD Videotape*. *Price:* $34.95. **Frmly:** (1980) Teletypewriters for the Deaf; (2000) Telecommunications for the Deaf, Inc.

**★ 6120 ★ TRIPOD**
1727 W Burbank Blvd.
Burbank, CA 91506
**Phone:** (818)972-2080        **Free:** 800-2-TRIPOD
**Fax:** (818)972-2090
**Email:** info@tripod.org
**Website:** http://www.tripod.org
Debra Leavitt, Office Mgr.
**Fnded:** 1983. **Desc:** Established a private/public partnership with Burbank Unified School District to assist individuals who are deaf or hard of hearing. Offers educational programs. **Pub:** *Language Says It All*. Videos. • *We Can Do Anything*. Video.

**★ 6121 ★ Union of the Deaf in Bulgaria**
12-14 Denkooglu St.
BG-1000 Sofia, Bulgaria
**Phone:** 359 2 9804778        **Fax:** 359 2 9801696
**Email:** sgb@i-n.net
**Fnded:** 1934. **Mem:** 8,800. **Desc:** Promotes and protects members' cultural, educational, and social interests. **Pub:** *Tishina*, semimonthly. Newspaper. Reflects the problems of the deaf in Bulgaria and worldwide.

**★ 6122 ★ U.S. Deaf Cycling Association (USDCA)**
247 Jack London Ct.
Pittsburg, CA 94565-3661
**Phone:** (510)471-9011        **Fax:** (510)471-6064
**Email:** skedsmo@earthlink.net

**Website:** http://home.earthlink.net/~skedsmo/usdca.htm
Bobby Skedsmo, Pres.

**Fnded:** 1975. **Mem:** 27. **Reg. Groups:** 5. **Desc:** Promotes recreational and competitive cycling among the deaf and hearing impaired in the U.S. Conducts educational programs; sponsors competitions. **Pub:** *Breakaway*, 3/year. Newsletter. *Price:* $1.

---

### ★ 6123 ★ United States Deaf Ski and Snowboard Association (USDSSA)

c/o Robert Lewis
9408 Inglewood Ct.
Frederick, MD 21701-7688
**Email:** rlewis@usdssa.org
**Website:** http://www.usdssa.org/
Robert Lewis, Pres.

**Fnded:** 1968. **Mem:** 350. **Reg. Groups:** 8. **Desc:** Promotes recreational and competitive skiing among the deaf and hearing impaired in the U.S. Provides deaf skiers with benefits, activities, and opportunities that will increase their enjoyment of the sport. Encourages ski racing among the deaf and sponsors national and regional races for deaf skiers, including the U.S.A. National Deaf Alpine and Nordic Ski Championships. Assists in the selection, organization, and training of the United States Deaf Ski Teams for international competition such as the World Winter Games for the Deaf. Presents awards; maintains hall of fame; offers children's services. **Pub:** Newsletter, 3/year. *Price:* available to members only.

---

### ★ 6124 ★ USA Deaf Sports Federation (USADSF)

3607 Washington Blvd., No. 4
Ogden, UT 84403-1761
**Phone:** (801)393-7916          **Fax:** (801)393-2263
**Email:** homeoffice@usadsf.org
**Website:** http://www.usadsf.org
Valerie Kinney, Admin. Asst.

**Fnded:** 1945. **Mem:** 4,000. **Nat'l Groups:** 20. **Reg. Groups:** 8. **State Groups:** 50. **Local Groups:** 200. **Desc:** Provides year-round training to athletes and coordinates athletic competition in a variety of sports at the state, regional, national, and international level. **Pub:** *Deaf Sports Review*, annual. Magazine. • *USADSF Bulletin*, quarterly. Bulletin. **Frmly:** (1999) American Athletic Association for the Deaf.

---

### ★ 6125 ★ Vestibular Disorders Association (VEDA)

PO Box 4467
Portland, OR 97208-4467
**Phone:** (503)229-7705          **Free:** 800-837-8428
**Fax:** (503)229-8064
**Email:** veda@vestibular.org
**Website:** http://www.vestibular.org
Jerry Underwood, Exec. Off.

**Fnded:** 1983. **Mem:** 4,000. **Local Groups:** 115. **Desc:** Individuals suffering from vestibular disorders, their families and friends, and health care professionals. (Vestibular disorders are characterized by persistent dizziness or vertigo which often indicates a problem in the inner ear.) Provides support services including information and referrals; encourages public education about vestibular disorders and their effects. **Pub:** *Balancing Act, 2nd Ed.*. Book. *Price:* $15. • *BPPV: What You Need to Know*. Book. *Price:* $24.95 softbound; $34.95 hardbound. • *Getting Better*. Video. Closed caption VHS tape. *Price:* $25. • *Managing Your Symptoms*. Videos. Closed caption VHS tape. *Price:* $25. • *Meniere's Disease: What You Need to Know*. Book. *Price:* $24.95 softbound; $34.95 hardbound. • *On the Level*, quarterly. Newsletter. Includes coping tips, health-related items, reviews, and association news. *Price:* Included in membership dues. • *Stories and Strategies: Coping with Vestibular Disorders*. Booklet. • *VEDA Low-Salt Cookbook*. Book. *Price:* $17. • Audiotapes. • Bibliographies. • Pamphlets. • Reports. **Frmly:** (1989) Dizziness and Balance Disorders Association.

---

### ★ 6126 ★ Voice Foundation (VF)

1721 Pine St.
Philadelphia, PA 19103
**Phone:** (215)735-7999          **Fax:** (215)735-9293
**Email:** voicefound@onrampcom.com
**Website:** http://www.voicefoundation.org
Robert T. Sataloff, MD, Chm. of the Board

**Fnded:** 1969. **Mem:** 450. **Desc:** Sponsors research and education on the causes, prevention, and treatment of voice disorders. Sponsors educational programs. Holds fundraising events. **Pub:** *Journal of Voice*, quarterly. Journal. *Price:* $99/year for individuals; $126/year for individuals outside U.S.; $98/year for libraries/institutions; $112/year for libraries/institutions outside U.S. • *Voice Foundation Newsletter*, 3-4/year. Newsletter. *Price:* Included in membership dues. • Videos.

---

### ★ 6127 ★ World Federation of the Deaf (WFD)

PO Box 65
SF-00401 Helsinki, Finland
**Phone:** 358 9 5803572          **Fax:** 358 9 5803573
**Email:** info@wfdnews.org
**Website:** http://www.wfdnews.org

**Fnded:** 1951. **Mem:** 120. **Nat'l Groups:** 120. **Reg. Groups:** 8. **Lang(s):** English. **Desc:** Ordinary members are National associations of the deaf that are legally constituted and represent in the widest sense the deaf in their country; other members are national or international associations, societies, and bodies for and of the deaf; health, educational, social, and similar establishments that accept the aims of the federation; professionals interested in deafness and related subjects; persons performing special tasks connected with the aims of the federation; parents and friends of the deaf. Represents the worldwide deaf community in international forums such as the United Nations. Makes policy statements and recommendations. Coordinates research and other projects with the deaf community; conducts surveys. Has established a network of experts on deafness and related issues. Promotes the use of national sign language as the first language of deaf people. **Pub:** *WFD News*, 3/year. Journal. • *WFD Survey of Deaf People in the Developing World*. Report.

---

## Research Centers

### ★ 6128 ★ Abilene Christian University Voice Institute of West Texas

Box 28058
Abilene, TX 79699-8048
**Phone:** (915)674-2074          **Fax:** (915)674-2552
**Email:** ashbyj@nicanor.acu.edu
**Website:** http://www.acu.edu/academics/voiceinstitute/
Jon Ashby, PhD, Co-Dir.

**Activities/Fields:** Human voice, and evaluation, diagnosis, and treatment of voice disorders.

---

### ★ 6129 ★ Adelphi University Hy Weinberg Center for Communication Disorders

PO Box 701
Garden City, NY 11530-4299
**Phone:** (516)877-4850          **Free:** 800-233-5744
**Fax:** (516)877-4783
**Email:** soman@adelphi.edu
Dr. Bonnie Soman, Dir.

**Activities/Fields:** Speech-language pathology and audiology, and speech and hearing disorders.

---

### ★ 6130 ★ American Hearing Research Foundation

55 E Washington St., Ste. 2022
Chicago, IL 60602
**Phone:** (312)726-9670          **Fax:** (312)726-9695

---

**Email:** blederer@american-hearing.org
William L. Lederer, Contact

**Activities/Fields:** Deafness and hearing disorders, focusing on medical research, education, and public information.

---

### ★ 6131 ★ Association for Research in Otolaryngology, Inc. (ARO)

19 Mantua Rd.
Mount Royal, NJ 08061
**Phone:** (856)423-0041          **Fax:** (856)423-3420
**Email:** headquarters@aro.org
**Website:** http://www.aro.org
Tom Sims, Exec. Dir.

**Activities/Fields:** Basic science and clinical problems associated with hearing, speech, the sense of balance, smell, taste, and diseases of the head and neck. **Pub:** *ARO News*, semiannually. Newsletter. • *Book of Abstracts*, annually. Book. • *JARO Journal of the Association for Research in Otolaryngology*, quarterly.

---

### ★ 6132 ★ Baylor College of Medicine Stuttering Center and Speech Motor Control Laboratory

6501 Fannin St., Ste. NB302
Houston, TX 77030
**Phone:** (713)798-7415          **Fax:** (713)798-6417
**Email:** davidr@bcm.tmc.edu
Dr. David Rosenfield, Dir.

**Activities/Fields:** Speech motor control system, including stuttering, voice problems, motor control, and digital signal and acoustic processing. **Pub:** *Annual Report*. • *Neuro/Speech Newsletter*.

---

### ★ 6133 ★ Boston University Hearing Research Center (HRC)

Department of Biomedical Engineering
44 Cummington St.
Boston, MA 02215
**Phone:** (617)353-4342          **Fax:** (617)353-6766
**Email:** colburn@bu.edu
**Website:** http://www.bu.edu/hrc/
H. Steven Colburn, PhD, Dir.

**Activities/Fields:** Auditory processing in order to understand hearing in both normal and impaired auditory systems. Research focuses on anatomical studies of the cochlea and brainstem, measurements of mechanical properties of cochlear structures, single-unit and multi-unit recordings up to the level of the inferior colliculus, and measurements of auditory evoked potentials and otoacoustic emissions, as well as measurements of hearing abilities of human listeners with and without hearing impairments.

---

### ★ 6134 ★ Boys Town National Research Hospital Center for Hereditary Communication Disorders

555 N 30th St.
Omaha, NE 68131
**Phone:** (402)498-6556          **Free:** 800-320-1171
**Fax:** (402)498-6331
William J. Kimberling, Dir.

**Activities/Fields:** Genetic communication disorders, with emphasis on hearing loss, including Usher Syndrome, recessive non-syndromic hearing loss, dominant progressive hearing loss, branchio-oto-renal syndrome, and hypopigmentation and hearing loss.

---

### ★ 6135 ★ Brooklyn College of City University of New York Speech and Hearing Center

Boylan Hall, Rm. 4400
Brooklyn, NY 11210
**Phone:** (718)951-5186          **Fax:** (718)951-4363
**Email:** pbottino@brooklyn.cuny.edu
Patti Bottino, Contact

**Activities/Fields:** Normal communications and communication disorders, including studies of speech, language, and hearing.

**★ 6136 ★ Central Institute for the Deaf**
4560 Clayton Ave.
Saint Louis, MO 63110
**Phone:** (314)977-0000   **Fax:** (314)977-0025
**Email:** nielsen@cid.wustl.edu
**Website:** http://www.cid.wustl.edu
Donald W. Nielsen, Dir.
**Activities/Fields:** Auditory communication and its disorders, including studies of hearing function, auditory physiology, sensory neuroscience, auditory biophysics and biomechanics, effects of noise, and regeneration in the auditory nervous system. Also performs clinical studies of speech and linguistics, communication in infants and the elderly, characteristics of deaf speech, evaluation of cochlear implants in children, aural rehabilitation, psychosocial therapy, and audiology. Also engineers, designs, and evaluates instruments to evaluate and/or assist the deaf and the hard-of-hearing, and develops multimedia network communication systems with special applications for the deaf community.

**★ 6137 ★ Central Institute for the Deaf**
**Center for Childhood Deafness and Adult**
**Aural Rehabilitation**
909 S Taylor Ave.
Saint Louis, MO 63110
**Phone:** (314)977-0156   **Fax:** (314)977-0024
**Email:** geers@cid.wustl.edu
**Website:** http://www.cid.wustl.edu/research/ccdaar/intro.htm
Ann E. Geers, PhD, Hd.
**Activities/Fields:** Problems confronted by hearing-impaired children and adults, including education, use of sensory aids, speech and language acquisition, and communication development, improved telecommunications for the hearing impaired, and the effects of noise on hearing.

**★ 6138 ★ Central Institute for the Deaf**
**Fay and Carl Simons Center for Biology**
**of Hearing and Deafness**
4560 Clayton Ave.
Saint Louis, MO 63110
**Phone:** (314)977-0260   **Fax:** (314)977-0030
**Email:** rbaird@cid.wustl.edu
**Website:** http://www.cid.wustl.edu/research/fcscbhd/intro.htm
Richard Baird, PhD, Dir.
**Activities/Fields:** Sensory loss and recovery in the inner ear, with a particular emphasis on increasing understanding of the cellular and molecular mechanisms that may lead to sensory rescue, repair or regeneration. Ongoing research includes studies of inner ear development; age-related, noise-induced, and drug-induced hearing loss; cell proliferation, migraton, and differentiation; neuronal innervation; and auditory and vestibular function.

**★ 6139 ★ Cleveland Hearing and Speech**
**Center**
11206 Euclid Ave.
Cleveland, OH 44106
**Phone:** (216)231-8787   **Fax:** (216)231-7141
**Email:** bphenri@chsc.org
**Website:** http://www.chsc.org
Bernard P. Henri, PhD, Exec. Dir.
**Activities/Fields:** Speech, language, and hearing disorders; speech production in patients with Parkinson's Disease; and managed care, financial incentives and clinical decision making. **Frmly:** Cleveland Association for the Hard of Hearing.

**★ 6140 ★ Colorado Neurological Institute**
**CNI Rocky Mountain Cochlear Implant**
**Center**
799 E Hampden Ave., Ste. 510
Englewood, CO 80110
**Phone:** (303)788-7880   **Fax:** (303)788-7884
**Email:** jbriles@thecni.org
**Website:** http://thecni.org/hearing/
Dr. David C. Kelsall, Dir.
**Activities/Fields:** Cochlear implant devices.

**★ 6141 ★ Deafness Research Foundation**
1050 17th St. NW, Ste. 701
Washington, DC 20036
**Phone:** (202)289-5850   **Free:** 800-829-5934
**Fax:** (202)293-1805
**Email:** drf@drf.org
**Website:** http://www.drf.org
Susan M. Greco, Exec. Dir.
**Activities/Fields:** Causes and treatment of deafness and other serious ear disorders, including studies of implants, deafness in the young and the elderly, middle ear infections, Meniere's disease, tinnitus (ringing in the ears), excessive noise, hair cell regeneration, genetics, and otoacoustic emissions. **Pub:** *The Hearing Health Advocate*, quarterly. • *The Research News*.

**★ 6142 ★ Ear Research Foundation**
1961 Floyd St.
Sarasota, FL 34239-2909
**Phone:** (941)366-1148   **Fax:** (941)365-2269
**Email:** erf@family-net.org
**Website:** http://www.earsinus.org/frame_intro.htm
Dr. Herbert Silverstein, Pres.
**Activities/Fields:** Meniere's disease, acoustic neuroma, benign positional vertigo, laser-assisted otological surgery for inner- and middle-ear disorders, cholesteatoma in children, cochlear implants, and vestibular rehabilitation.

**★ 6143 ★ Eaton-Peabody Laboratory of**
**Auditory Physiology**
Massachusetts Eye & Ear Infirmary
243 Charles St.
Boston, MA 02114
**Phone:** (617)573-3745   **Fax:** (617)720-4408
M. Charles Liberman, PhD, Dir.
**Activities/Fields:** Vertebrate auditory system and auditory information processing, including feedback control systems in normal and pathologic hearing. Approaches include anatomical, physiological, functional imaging, pharmacological, chemical and molecular biological studies of animal models as well as human subjects.

**★ 6144 ★ Harvard University**
**Center for Health Communication**
Harvard School of Public Health
677 Huntington Ave.
Boston, MA 02115
**Phone:** (617)432-1038   **Fax:** (617)731-8184
**Email:** tmendoza@hsph.harvard.edu
**Website:** http://www.hsph.harvard.edu/chc
Jay A. Winsten, PhD, Dir.
**Activities/Fields:** Contributions of mass communication to healthy behavior changes and policy. **Pub:** *World Health News*.

**★ 6145 ★ Haskins Laboratories**
270 Crown St.
New Haven, CT 06511
**Phone:** (203)865-6163   **Fax:** (203)865-8963
**Email:** haskins@haskins.yale.edu
**Website:** http://www.haskins.yale.edu
Dr. Carol A. Fowler, Pres.
**Activities/Fields:** Speech production and perception by humans and computers, motor control, and reading.

**★ 6146 ★ Hollins Communications**
**Research Institute**
PO Box 9737
Roanoke, VA 24020-1737
**Phone:** (540)265-5650   **Fax:** (540)265-0386
**Email:** adm-hcri@rbnet.com
**Website:** http://www.stuttering.org
Ronald L. Webster, PhD, Dir.
**Activities/Fields:** Basic features of stuttering, behaviorally-based stuttering therapy, and variables that modify speech fluency in people who stutter and fluent speakers.

**★ 6147 ★ Houston Ear Research**
**Foundation**
7737 Southwest Fwy., Ste. 630
Houston, TX 77074
**Phone:** (713)771-9966   **Free:** 800-843-0807
**Fax:** (713)771-0546
**Email:** jangil@hern.org
Jan Gilden, Exec. Dir.
**Activities/Fields:** Aims to improve health care and education for deaf and hearing-impaired children. Provides funds for follow-up testing for recipients of cochlear implants. **Pub:** *Newsletter*, annually.

**★ 6148 ★ Indiana University-Purdue**
**University at Indianapolis**
**De Vault Otologic Research Laboratory**
Riley 044
Indianapolis, IN 46202-4949
**Phone:** (317)274-4915   **Fax:** (317)274-4949
**Email:** kkirk@iupui.edu
**Website:** http://www.indiana.edu/~rugs/ctrdir/dvorl.html
Karen Iler Kirk, Dir.
**Activities/Fields:** Benefit of different sensory aids to hearing-impaired children, specifically changes in speech production, speech perception, language, cognitive skills after cochlear implants.

**★ 6149 ★ International Center for**
**Hearing and Speech Research**
52 Lomb Memorial Dr.
Rochester, NY 14623
**Phone:** (716)475-6403   **Fax:** (716)475-6677
**Email:** rxf1389@ritvax.isc.rit.edu
Dr. Robert Frisina, Sr., Dir.
**Activities/Fields:** Prevention, early detection, diagnosis, and treatment of people with hearing and speech impairments.

**★ 6150 ★ Johns Hopkins University**
**Center for Laryngeal and Voice Disorders**
Department of Otolaryngology-Head & Neck Surgery
601 N Caroline St.
Baltimore, MD 21287
**Phone:** (410)955-1654
**Website:** http://www.med.jhu.edu/voice/
Paul W. Flint, MD, Dir.
**Activities/Fields:** Diagnostic and therapeutic protocols for laryngeal and voice disorders.

**★ 6151 ★ Johns Hopkins University**
**Research and Training Center for Hearing**
**and Balance**
**Auditory Anatomy and Physiology**
**Laboratory**
Traylor Bldg., Rm. 510
School of Medicine
720 Rutland Ave.
Baltimore, MD 21205
**Phone:** (410)955-4543   **Fax:** (410)614-4748
**Email:** dryugo@bme.jhu.edu
**Website:** http://www.bme.jhu.edu/labs/chb/labs/ap_aud.html
David K. Ryugo, Prin. Investigator
**Activities/Fields:** Identified cell populations, their synaptic connections, and revealing features of their signaling capabilities.

**★ 6152 ★ Johns Hopkins University**
**Research and Training Center for Hearing**
**and Balance**
**Auditory Neurophysiology Laboratory**
Ross Research Bldg., Rm. 424
Department of Biomedical Engineering
Sch. of Medicine
720 Rutland Ave.
Baltimore, MD 21205
**Phone:** (410)614-4547          **Fax:** (410)614-9599
**Email:** xwang@bme.jhu.edu
**Website:** http://www.bme.jhu.edu/~xwang/lab.html
Xiaoqin Wang, PhD, Prin. Investigator
**Activities/Fields:** Auditory neurophysiology.


**★ 6153 ★ Johns Hopkins University**
**Research and Training Center for Hearing**
**and Balance**
**Neural Encoding Laboratory**
505 Traylor Bldg.
Sch. of Medicine
720 Rutland Ave.
Baltimore, MD 21205
**Phone:** (410)955-3162          **Fax:** (410)955-1299
**Email:** eyoung@bme.jhu.edu
**Website:** http://www.bme.jhu.edu/labs/chb/labs/neural_enc.html
Eric D. Young, PhD, Prin. Investigator
**Activities/Fields:** Representation and processing of complex stimuli in the auditory system.


**★ 6154 ★ Kent State University**
**Speech and Hearing Clinic**
A104 Music & Speech Bldg.
Kent, OH 44242
**Phone:** (330)672-2672          **Fax:** (330)672-2643
**Email:** csommer@kent. edu
**Website:** http://dept.kent.edu/sp&a/clinic/clinic.html
Carol Sommer, Contact
**Activities/Fields:** Speech pathology and audiology, including staff specialties in infant, children's, and adult languages, stuttering, phonology, aural rehabilitation, and hearing aids.


**★ 6155 ★ Louisiana State University**
**Kresge Hearing Research Laboratory of**
**the South**
533 Bolivar St., 5th Fl.
New Orleans, LA 70112
**Phone:** (504)568-4785          **Fax:** (504)568-4460
**Email:** cberli@lsuhsc.edu
**Website:** http://www.kresgelab.org
Dr. Charles I. Berlin, Dir.
**Activities/Fields:** Auditory research, pharmacology, anatomy, psychophysics, molecular genetics, and audiology, including studies on cochlear implants, auditory evoked potentials, ultra-high frequency hearing, effects of hearing impairments on brain structure, temporal order in hearing, auditory processing of frequency-varying signals, perceptual skills in learning-disabled children, speech perception, cochlear emissions, auditory neuropathy, and the role of chemical elements in hearing. **Frmly:** Communication Sciences Laboratory.


**★ 6156 ★ Loyola University Chicago**
**Parmly Hearing Institute**
6525 N Sheridan Rd.
Chicago, IL 60626
**Phone:** (773)508-2710          **Fax:** (773)508-2719
**Email:** rfay@luc.edu
**Website:** http://www.parmly.luc.edu
Dr. Richard R. Fay, Dir.
**Activities/Fields:** Psychophysics, physiology, and anatomy of audition and investigation of sensory/perceptual processes, including studies on relations among sense/organ action, anatomy and physiology of afferent nervous system, cerebral sensory mechanisms, psychophysical characteristics of auditory system, application of theory of signal detectability to psychophysics, and detection and recognition of audi-

tory signals in noise. **Pub:** *Parmly Hearing Institute Annual Report.*


**Medical University of South Carolina**
**Department of Pediatrics**
**Division of Genetics and Developmental**
**Pediatrics**
**The Vince Moseley Center**
*See:* Entry 8191


**★ 6157 ★ Midwest Ear Institute, Inc.**
2940 Baltimore Ave., Ste. 300
Kansas City, MO 64108-3405
**Phone:** (816)751-2570          **Fax:** (816)751-4616
**Email:** tstohs@mei-kc.org
**Website:** http://www.mei-kc.org
Teresa Stohs, Exec. Dir.
**Activities/Fields:** Auditory prostheses.


**★ 6158 ★ New York Foundation for**
**Otologic Research**
920 Park Ave.
New York, NY 10028
**Phone:** (212)988-3100          **Fax:** (212)517-8699
**Email:** mideardoc@aol.com
Dr. Alan Austin Scheer, Dir.
**Activities/Fields:** Unsolved hearing problems, including otosclerosis, nerve deafness, Menieres disease, and other associated problems of dizziness and head noises. Analyzes electrical patterns of sound conduction and studies conduction of sound through the skin and dental nerves.


**★ 6159 ★ Ohio State University**
**Division of Otologic Research**
4331 University Hospitals Clinic
456 W 10th Ave.
Columbus, OH 43210
**Phone:** (614)293-8103          **Fax:** (614)293-5506
**Email:** demaria.2@osu.edu
Dr. Thomas F. DeMaria, Dir.
**Activities/Fields:** Otology, including animal models for otitis media, acoustic trauma, morphological studies on the inner ear, and immunologic investigations of the middle and inner ear. Also studies the development of animal models for studying middle ear infection using microbiological, immunologic, morphologic and molecular biological methods, temporal bone histopathology (human and animal), electron microscopy of auditory and vestibular systems, pathogenesis of otitis media, and sensory transduction mechanism. **Frmly:** Ear Research Group.


**★ 6160 ★ Oregon Health and Science**
**University**
**Oregon Hearing Research Center**
3181 SW Sam Jackson Pk. Rd.
Portland, OR 97201-3098
**Phone:** (503)494-8032          **Free:** 800-222-6478
**Fax:** (503)494-5656
**Website:** http://www.ohsu.edu/ohrc/
Alfred L. Nuttall, PhD, Dir.
**Activities/Fields:** Hearing problems, including clinical studies of ototoxicity, vestibular physiology, noise damage, anatomy of the ear, tinnitus, and interactions between various insults to the ear, through a multiple attack utilizing electrophysiological measures, behavioral measures, histological evaluations, and human psychophysics. **Frmly:** Kresge Hearing Research Laboratory.


**★ 6161 ★ Plattsburgh State University of**
**New York**
**Auditory Research Laboratory**
107 Beaumont Hall
101 Broad St.
Plattsburgh, NY 12901
**Phone:** (518)564-7701          **Fax:** (518)564-3175
**Email:** roger.hamernik@plattsburgh.edu

**Website:** http://www.plattsburgh.edu/arl/
Dr. Roger P. Hamernik, Dir.
**Activities/Fields:** Pathology of hearing associated with noise, drugs, congenital birth defects, and disease processes.


**★ 6162 ★ Queens College of City**
**University of New York**
**Augmentative Communication Center**
Linguistics & Communication Disorders Department
65-30 Kissena Blvd.
Flushing, NY 11367-1597
**Phone:** (718)997-2940          **Fax:** (718)997-2935
**Email:** arlene_kraat@qc.edu
Dr. Arlene Kraat, Dir.
**Activities/Fields:** Severe speech and language disabilities, including treatment methods of augmentative and alternative communication (AAC) modes. AAC enhances communication through the use of signs, symbolic gestures, language boards, and computerized communication devices.


**★ 6163 ★ Queens College of City**
**University of New York**
**Speech and Hearing Center**
Gertz Bldg.
65-30 Kissena Blvd.
Flushing, NY 11367-1597
**Phone:** (718)997-2930          **Fax:** (718)997-2935
Dr. Joel Stark, Dir.
**Activities/Fields:** Communicative disorders in children and adults, focusing on testing and treatment.


**★ 6164 ★ State University of New York**
**at Buffalo**
**Center for Hearing and Deafness**
215 Parker Hall
435 Main St.
Buffalo, NY 14214
**Phone:** (716)829-2001          **Fax:** (716)829-2980
**Email:** salvi@buffalo.edu
**Website:** http://wings.buffalo.edu/faculty/research/chd/
Dr. Richard J. Salvi, Hd.
**Activities/Fields:** Restoring the hearing of the deaf, hearing loss due to loud noises, medication, or age, middle ear infections in children, hearing loss in infants. Studies include hair cell regeneration, drug therapy and ototoxic drugs, noise-induced hearing loss, middle ear disease, infant hearing assessment, auditory plasticity, mechanical transduction, age-related hearing loss, and central auditory processing.


**★ 6165 ★ State University of New York**
**at Buffalo**
**Hearing Research Laboratory**
215 Parker Hall
Buffalo, NY 14214
**Phone:** (716)829-2001          **Fax:** (716)829-2980
**Email:** salvi@buffalo.edu
**Website:** http://wings.buffalo.edu/faculty/research/chd
Dr. Richard J. Salvi, Co-Dir.
**Activities/Fields:** Hearing, including effects of noise, effects of ototoxic drugs, and basic auditory processes. **Pub:** *J. Acoustical Society of America*, 3/year.


**★ 6166 ★ State University of New York**
**at Buffalo**
**Speech-Language and Hearing Clinic**
50 Biomedical Education Bldg.
3435 Main St.
Buffalo, NY 14214
**Phone:** (716)829-3980          **Fax:** (716)829-3974
**Email:** srobert@acsu.buffalo.edu
Susan T. Roberts, Dir.
**Activities/Fields:** Audiology, speech and hearing sciences, speech/language pathology, speech perception and acoustics, and augmentative communication. **Pub:** *Journal of Speech and Hearing Disorders.* • *Journal of Speech/Hearing Research.*

**★ 6167 ★ State University of New York College at Fredonia**
**Youngerman Center for Communications Disorders**
Thompson Hall
Fredonia, NY 14063
**Phone:** (716)673-3202          **Fax:** (716)673-3235
**Email:** michele.notte@fredonia.edu
**Website:** http://www.fredonia.edu/department/speechpathology/newspeech/speechhomepage.html
Dr. Michele T. Notte, Dir.
**Activities/Fields:** Community clinic and student training center for speech/language pathology and audiology. Provides facilities and data for faculty engaged in research projects in the areas of audiology, voice and speech science, and language.

**★ 6168 ★ State University of New York Health Science Center at Brooklyn**
**Research Unit on Communicative Processes**
450 Clarkson Ave., Box 88
Brooklyn, NY 11203
**Phone:** (718)270-3078          **Fax:** (718)270-3017
Dr. Norbert Freedman, Dir.
**Activities/Fields:** Communicative issues in psychiatric treatment, including doctor-patient interaction, the clinical interview, the psychotherapeutic interview, and the psychoanalytic interview. Objective studies of communicative behavior are also conducted through analysis of language, kinesics, and cognitive processes.

**★ 6169 ★ Temple University**
**Section of Audiology and Auditory Research**
Kresge W Bldg., Rm. 302
3440 N Broad St.
Philadelphia, PA 19140
**Phone:** (215)707-3661          **Fax:** (215)707-8079
**Activities/Fields:** Psychological and physiological acoustics, clinical research in audiology, clinical and basic research in evoked potentials, auditory and vestibular functioning, and human and animal experimentation in otology.

**★ 6170 ★ Tennessee Center for the Study and Treatment of Dyslexia**
Middle Tennessee State University
200 N Baird Ln.
PO Box 397
Murfreesboro, TN 37132
**Phone:** (615)494-8880          **Fax:** (615)494-8881
**Email:** dyslexia@mtsu.edu
**Website:** http://www.mtsu.edu/~dyslexia
Diane J. Sawyer, PhD, Dir.
**Activities/Fields:** Dyslexia, focusing on diagnostic services and monitoring the progress of students with dyslexia who are receiving intervention in their schools.

**U.S. Department of Health and Human Services**
**Centers for Disease Control and Prevention**
**National Institute for Occupational Safety and Health**
**National Occupational Research Agenda (Hearing Loss)**
*See:* Entry 16814

**★ 6171 ★ U.S. Department of Health and Human Services**
**National Institute on Deafness and Other Communication Disorders**
NIH Bldg. 31, Rm. 3C02
31 Center Dr.
Bethesda, MD 20892-2320
**Phone:** (301)402-0900          **Fax:** (301)402-1590

**Email:** jrf3@cdc.gov
**Website:** http://www.cdc.gov/niosh/nrhear.html
Dr. James F. Buttey, Dir.
**Activities/Fields:** Biomedical and behavioral research and research training on normal processes and disorders of hearing, balance, smell, taste, voice, speech, and language, including hearing and deafness, hearing loss, hearing impairment, tinnitus, presbycusis, Waardenburg syndrome, Usher syndrome, dizziness, Meniere's disease, vestibular system, smell and taste disorders, voice disorders, spasmodic dysphonia, vocal cord paralysis, stuttering, speech disorders, language disorders, and aphasia.

**★ 6172 ★ U.S. Department of Health and Human Services**
**National Institute on Deafness and Other Communication Disorders**
**Division Extramural Activities**
31 Center Dr., MSC 2320
Bethesda, MD 20892
**Phone:** (301)496-8693          **Fax:** (301)402-6250
**Website:** http://www.nided.nih.gov/about/org/der.htm
Robert A. Dobie, MD, Dir.
**Activities/Fields:** Communication sciences and disorders. **Frmly:** (2000) Division of Extramural Activities.

**★ 6173 ★ U.S. Department of Health and Human Services**
**National Institute on Deafness and Other Communication Disorders**
**Division of Human Communications**
Executive Plaza S, Rm. 400C
6120 Executive Blvd.
MSC 7180
Bethesda, MD 20892-7180
**Phone:** (301)496-5061          **Fax:** (301)402-6251
**Website:** http://www.nidcd.nih.gov/about/org/der.htm
Judith Cooper, Chf.,Sci. Prog. Br.
**Activities/Fields:** Administers grants, contracts, and national research service awards for extramural research on hearing, balance, smell, taste, voice, speech, and language. Areas of research interest include diagnosis, treatment, and prevention of communication disorders, including the prevention and early diagnosis of hearing impairments that may result from exposure to noise or ototoxic drugs; the causes and treatment of tinnitus; the normal function of the central nervous system and the relationship of the taste, smell, and touch senses to the early detection of systemic disease; disorders such as stuttering, misarticulation, delayed language development, and phonatory disorders. disorders. **Frmly:** Communicative and Neurosensory Disorders Division.

**★ 6174 ★ U.S. Department of Health and Human Services**
**National Institute on Deafness and Other Communication Disorders**
**Division of Intramural Research**
50 South Dr., Rm. 4-4140
Bethesda, MD 20892
**Phone:** (301)496-6530          **Fax:** (301)402-2324
**Email:** wenthold@nidcd.nih.gov
**Website:** http://www.nidcd.nih.gov/intram/intram.htm
Dr. Robert J. Wenthold, PhD, Contact
**Activities/Fields:** Genetic and immune pathogenesis of head and neck neoplasms affecting human communication.

**★ 6175 ★ U.S. Department of Health and Human Services**
**National Institute on Deafness and Other Communication Disorders**
**Division of Intramural Research**
**Audiology Unit**
NIH Bldg. 10, Rm. 5C-306
9000 Rockville Pk.
Bethesda, MD 20892
**Phone:** (301)496-5368          **Fax:** (301)402-0409

**Email:** shotland@nidcd.nih.gov
**Website:** http://www.nih.gov/nidcd/
Lawrence L. Shotland, PhD, Chf.
**Activities/Fields:** Hearing and auditory function in various genetic, immunologic, or acquired conditions, including type 2 neurofibromatosis, Waardenburg syndrome, inherited metabolic degenerative disorders and non-syndromic hereditary hearing loss, and von-Hippel Lindau disease.

**★ 6176 ★ U.S. Department of Health and Human Services**
**National Institute on Deafness and Other Communication Disorders**
**Division of Intramural Research**
**Voice and Speech Section**
NIH Bldg. 10, Rm. 5D38
10 Center Dr., MSC 1416
Bethesda, MD 20892-1416
**Phone:** (301)496-9365          **Fax:** (301)480-0803
Christy L. Ludlow, PhD, Chf.
**Activities/Fields:** Speech and voice studies, including the neurophysiological and biomechanical bases of normal speech and voice production, pathophysiology of idiopathic speech and voice disorders such as spasmodic dysphonia and stuttering, and medical and surgical approaches to treatment of these disorders. Investigates sensorimotor regulation of the laryngeal musculature; motion and electromyographic analyses of laryngeal functioning during speech, respiration, and swallowing; magnetic and electrical stimulation of the central and peripheral laryngeal nervous system; and new treatment approaches including botulinum toxin, medication trials in patients with stuttering disorders, and phonosurgery for voice disorders. **Pub:** *Research Reports.*

**U.S. Department of Veterans Affairs**
**Veterans Health Administration**
**Office of Research and Development**
**Rehabilitation and Development Service**
**(Center for Rehabilitative Auditory Research)**
*See:* Entry 13513

**★ 6177 ★ University of Alabama**
**Speech and Hearing Center**
Department of Communicative Disorders, Box 870242
Tuscaloosa, AL 35487-0242
**Phone:** (205)348-7131          **Fax:** (205)348-1845
**Email:** gculton@cd.as.ua.edu
**Website:** http://www.as.ua.edu/comdis/
Dr. Gerald L. Culton, Chm.
**Activities/Fields:** Communication disorders, including clinical studies associated with graduate training in speech-language pathology and audiology.

**★ 6178 ★ University of Alabama at Birmingham**
**Speech and Hearing Sciences Department**
Bishop Bldg. 101
1530 3rd Ave. S
Birmingham, AL 35294-2030
**Phone:** (205)934-4814          **Fax:** (205)934-0402
**Email:** adamsl@uab.edu
Dr. Larry Adams, Hd.
**Activities/Fields:** Physiology, aerodynamics, acoustics, and perception of speech. Activities focus on basic physiology and acoustic studies of normal and abnormal speech learning. Experimental populations include hearing impaired, foreign dialect, and oral surgical patients. Specific research includes studies of temporomandibular joint functions and disorders, second-language speech acquisition, deaf speech, and neurogenic communication disorders. **Pub:** *Biocommunication Research Reports*, periodically.

**University of Alabama at Birmingham**
**UAB Civitan International Research**
**Center**
*See:* Entry 8207


**★ 6179 ★ University of Arkansas**
**Rehabilitation Research and Training**
**Center for Persons Who Are Deaf or**
**Hard of Hearing**
4601 W Markham
Little Rock, AR 72205
**Phone:** (501)686-9691          **Fax:** (501)686-9698
**Email:** DWatson@uark.edu
**Website:** http://www.uark.edu/depts/rehabres
Dr. Douglas Watson, Dir.

**Activities/Fields:** Improvement of vocational rehabilitation of individuals who are deaf or hard of hearing, focusing on improving career preparation, entry, retention, and advancement of these individuals in the workplace. **Frmly:** Research & Training Center on Deafness & Hearing Impairment.


**★ 6180 ★ University of British Columbia**
**Institute of Hearing Accessibility**
**Research (IHEAR)**
5804 Fairview Ave.
Vancouver, BC, Canada V6T 1Z3
**Phone:** (604)822-9474          **Fax:** (604)822-6569
**Email:** kathy@audiospeech.ubc.ca
Dr. M. Kathleen Pichora-Fuller, Dir.

**Activities/Fields:** Problems facing hard-of-hearing people, in order to find appropriate solutions to these problems and to promote hearing accessibility.


**★ 6181 ★ University of Colorado at**
**Boulder**
**Speech, Language, and Hearing Center**
Campus Box 409
Boulder, CO 80309
**Phone:** (303)492-5375
Susan M. Moore, Dir.

**Activities/Fields:** Evaluation and treatment of speech, language, learning, and hearing disorders. **Frmly:** Communication Disorders Clinic.


**★ 6182 ★ University of Iowa**
**Cochlear Implant Clinical Research**
**Center**
Otolaryngology, 21200 PFP
Iowa City, IA 52242
**Phone:** (319)356-2173          **Fax:** (319)356-3967
**Email:** bruce-gantz@uiowa.edu
**Website:** http://www.uiowa.edu/~vpr/research/organize/cochlear.htm
Bruce J. Gantz, Dir.

**Activities/Fields:** Cochlear implants in deaf children and adults. Research areas include audiology, psychophysics, aural rehabilitation, psychology, electrophysiology, speech production, and music.


**★ 6183 ★ University of Iowa**
**National Center for Voice and Speech**
250 Hawkins Dr.
Iowa City, IA 52242
**Phone:** (319)335-6600          **Fax:** (319)335-8851
**Email:** ingo-titze@uiowa.edu
**Website:** http://www.ncvs.org
Ingo R. Titze, Dir.

**Activities/Fields:** Protection, rehabilitation, and enhancement of voice and speech, including biomechanic and neurological investigations of the voice and speech mechanisms; normal, pathological and highly trained voices, and surgical techniques for correcting voice disorders.


**★ 6184 ★ University of Maine**
**Albert D. Conley Speech and Hearing**
**Center**
5724 Dunn Hall
Orono, ME 04469
**Phone:** (207)581-2006          **Fax:** (207)581-2060
**Email:** mboyd@maine.edu
**Website:** http://www.umaine.edu/comscidis/
Dr. Nancy E. Hall, Contact

**Activities/Fields:** Vocal development, speech and language disorders of adults and children, including aphasia, voice disorders, acquisition of language by children, stuttering, articulation disorders, apraxia, and interpersonal skills in clinical processes.


**★ 6185 ★ University of Memphis**
**Center for Research Initiatives and**
**Strategies for the Communicatively**
**Impaired (CRISCI)**
807 Jefferson Ave.
Memphis, TN 38105
**Phone:** (901)678-5800          **Fax:** (901)525-1282
**Email:** mmendel@memphis.edu
Maurice I. Mendel, Dir.

**Activities/Fields:** Speech and hearing, especially high technology applications to habilitation and rehabilitation of the communicatively impaired. Contributes to master's and doctoral programs in speech and hearing sciences. **Pub:** *Reports.*


**★ 6186 ★ University of Miami**
**Ear Institute**
PO Box 016960
Miami, FL 33101-6960
**Phone:** (305)243-4641          **Fax:** (305)243-5552
**Email:** ftelisch@med.miami.edu
Dr. Fred. F. Telischi, Dir.

**Activities/Fields:** Diseases of the ear and other communication disorders, with emphasis on implantable hearing aids and cochlear implants.


**★ 6187 ★ University of Michigan**
**Kresge Hearing Research Institute**
1301 E Ann St., Rm. 5032
Ann Arbor, MI 48109-0506
**Phone:** (734)764-8110          **Fax:** (734)764-0014
**Email:** carolet@umich.edu
**Website:** http://www.med.umich.edu/khri/
Dr. Jochen Schacht, Dir.

**Activities/Fields:** Auditory physiology and pathology, including studies on the reception, coding and processing of complex speech signals by the auditory system, transduction processes of the inner ear, cochlear blood flow and inner ear metabolism, development of cochlear prostheses and appropriate speech processor schemes, immune mediated hearing loss, the effects of age and environmental stress factors on hearing, biochemistry and motility of hair cells, afferent and efferent transmitters of the inner ear, psychophysics of hearing in normal individuals, immunology and immune systems related to squamous cell carcinoma, mechanisms of sound, localization, molecular biology and genetics of the inner ear, and human genetics (limkage studies).


**★ 6188 ★ University of Michigan**
**Kresge Hearing Research Institute**
**Auditory Anatomy Laboratory**
1301 E Ann St.
Ann Arbor, MI 48109-0506
**Phone:** (734)763-0060          **Fax:** (734)764-0014
**Email:** shuler@umich.edu
**Website:** http://www.khri.med.umich.edu/research/altschuler_lab/index.htm
Dr. Richard Altschuler, Dir.

**Activities/Fields:** Protective mechanisms to develop molecular interventions to reduce acquired deafness, such as from noise or ototoxic drugs; central auditory pathways, neurotransmitters, receptors and channels in normal function, how they change as a consequence of deafness and interventions to restore

hearing; evaluate the risks of new otologic treatments and devices, including the cochlear prosthesis. **Frmly:** Otopathology Laboratory.


**★ 6189 ★ University of Michigan**
**Kresge Hearing Research Institute**
**Auditory Prosthesis Animal**
**Psychophysics Laboratory**
PO Box 0506
Ann Arbor, MI 48109-0506
**Phone:** (734)763-2292          **Fax:** (734)764-0014
Dr. Bryan Pfingst, Dir.

**Activities/Fields:** Restoration of hearing in profoundly deaf persons. Studies the processing of speech in the brain and encoding of speech in the auditory system, and uses hearing tests with rhesus monkeys, humans, and other animals to design and develop bionic ear implants, also called cochlear prostheses.


**★ 6190 ★ University of Michigan**
**Kresge Hearing Research Institute**
**Biochemistry Laboratory**
1301 E Ann St.
Ann Arbor, MI 48109-0506
**Phone:** (734)763-3572          **Fax:** (734)764-0014
**Email:** schacht@umich.edu
**Website:** http://www.med.umich.edu/khri/biochem/
Dr. Jochen Schacht, Dir.

**Activities/Fields:** Cellular and molecular mechanisms of hearing and deafness. Investigates the normal biochemical events that occur in cells of the inner ear when hearing and that are impaired in hearing disorders such as those induced by noise and certain drugs. Studies methods for ameliorating hearing loss.


**★ 6191 ★ University of Michigan**
**Kresge Hearing Research Institute**
**Electrophysiology Laboratory**
1301 E Ann St.
Ann Arbor, MI 48109-0506
**Phone:** (734)764-8110          **Fax:** (734)764-0014
**Email:** ddolan@umich.edu
David F. Dolan, PhD, Dir.

**Activities/Fields:** Electrical responses to sound in the inner ear. Studies the response of individual receptor cells, or hair cells, of one ear while the other ear is acoustically or electrically stimulated. Also investigates the relationship between hearing loss and hair cell loss.


**★ 6192 ★ University of Michigan**
**Kresge Hearing Research Institute**
**Pharmacology Laboratory**
1301 E Ann St.
Ann Arbor, MI 48109-0506
**Phone:** (734)764-8111          **Fax:** (734)764-0014
**Email:** sbledsoe@umich.edu
Dr. Sanford Bledsoe, Contact

**Activities/Fields:** Studies the chemical substances (transmitters), used in intercellular communication which mediate the transduction and encoding of sounds from the inner ear to the auditory structures of the brain. Also studies auditory physiology, psychophysics, molecular biology and genetics, clinical investigations of auditory function.


**★ 6193 ★ University of Montreal**
**Acoustics Group**
Faculte de Medecine
Ecole d'Orthophonie et d'Audiologie
PO Box 6128, Downtown Sta.
Montreal, QC, Canada H3C 3J7
**Phone:** (514)343-7301          **Fax:** (514)343-5740
**Email:** louise.getty@umontreal.ca
Louise Getty, Dir.

**Activities/Fields:** Noise and its effect on health and safety, effects of occupational hearing loss, occupational and psychosocial rehabilitation of individuals with hearing loss, audiological rehabilitation of individuals with acquired hearing loss, noise as a nuisance, cultural aspects of acquired hearing loss, and sound warning signal recognition in industrial rooms.

**★ 6194 ★ University of Nebraska—Lincoln**
**Barkley Memorial Center**
Barkley Center, Rm. 301
Lincoln, NE 68583-0738
**Phone:** (402)472-5496          **Fax:** (402)472-7697
**Email:** ereiners1@unl.edu
**Website:** http://www.unl.edu/barkley
John Bernthal, Dir.

**Activities/Fields:** Communication deficiency and disorder research, including study of brain stem audiometry; fluency, motor speech disorders, phonological, acquisition of sign language, speech perception, language and learning disorders; behavioral impairment; hearing impairment; behavioral disorders and children with behavioral disorders; school violence; augmentative and alternative communication; and use of paraprofessionals in special education.

**★ 6195 ★ University of Oklahoma**
**Keys Speech and Hearing Center**
825 Northeast 14th St.
PO Box 26901
Oklahoma City, OK 73104
**Phone:** (405)271-4214          **Fax:** (405)271-3360
**Email:** richard-talbott@ouhsc.edu
Dr. Richard Talbott, Dept. Chm.

**Activities/Fields:** Loudness and acoustic reflex, temporal integration and acoustic reflex, critical bands measured with pulsation pattern psychophysical technique, sensory scaling, absolute thresholds for frequency modulated signals, bone conduction vibrator calibration, bone conduction speech audiometry, intelligibility of distorted speech, electrocochleography, brain stem auditory-evoked responses, acoustic correlates of abnormal vocal quality, aerodynamics of voice production, phonemic and morphologic studies of language of the communicatively impaired, and assessment of receptive and expressive language abilities.

**University of Quebec at Montreal**
**Cognitive Neuroscience Centre**
*See:* Entry 14456

**★ 6196 ★ University of Texas at Dallas**
**Callier Center for Communication Disorders**
1966 Inwood Rd.
Dallas, TX 75235-7298
**Phone:** (214)905-3000          **Fax:** (214)905-3022
**Email:** roeser@callier.utdallas.edu
**Website:** http://www.callier.utdallas.edu/
Dr. Ross J. Roeser, Dir.

**Activities/Fields:** Behavioral, electrophysiological, and anatomical studies of audition; behavioral and electrophysiological studies of normal and disordered speech production and perception; evoked potential and brain mapping; the linguistic and cognitive abilities of persons with aphasia and other neurogenic speech and language impairments; language development of children with chronic otitis media; development and assessment of communicative abilities in children with multiple handicaps; vibrotactile aids; and aural rehabilitation.

**★ 6197 ★ University of Texas**
**Southwestern Medical Center at Dallas**
**Division of Communicative and Vestibular Disorders**
Department of Otolaryngology-Head and Neck Surgery
5323 Harry Hines Blvd.
Dallas, TX 75390-9035
**Phone:** (214)648-2018          **Fax:** (214)648-9122
**Email:** ashoup@mednet.swmed.edu
**Website:** http://www.swmed.edu
Angela Shoup, PhD, Contact

**Activities/Fields:** Dizziness, vertigo, gait and balance disorders, inner ear fluid disorders, auditory perception, and auditory neurophysiology. **Frmly:** Audiovestibular Laboratory.

**★ 6198 ★ University of Tulsa**
**Mary K. Chapman Center for Communicative Disorders**
600 S College Ave.
Tulsa, OK 74104-3189
**Phone:** (918)631-2903          **Fax:** (918)631-3668
**Email:** karen-patterson@utulsa.edu
**Website:** http://www.utulsa.edu/
Karen Patterson, PhD, Contact

**Activities/Fields:** Communication disorders, including laryngectomy and speech, and language and hearing problems. Also conducts aid tests.

**★ 6199 ★ University of Virginia**
**Communication Disorders Program**
Colony Plz.
Speech Language Hearing Center
2205 Fountain Ave., Ste. 202
Charlottesville, VA 22903
**Phone:** (434)924-6351          **Fax:** (434)924-4621
**Email:** rrr7w@virginia.edu
Dr. Randall Robbey, Dir.

**Activities/Fields:** Speech and language pathology, audiology, early detection in infant speech/language/hearing disorders, education of the deaf, and speech and hearing science, including computer applications to communications disorders treatment. Supervises doctoral research in these fields and sponsors meetings of interest to speech and language pathologists, audiologists, and educators of the hearing impaired. **Frmly:** Speech and Hearing Center.

**★ 6200 ★ University of Washington**
**Developmental Speech Physiology Laboratory**
Department of Speech & Hearing Sciences, Box 354875
1417 NE 42nd St.
Seattle, WA 98105-6246
**Phone:** (206)616-5273          **Fax:** (206)543-1093
**Email:** camoore@u.washington.edu
**Website:** http://faculty.washington.edu/spchphys/
Prof. Christopher A. Moore, PhD, Contact

**Activities/Fields:** Development of articulatory, laryngeal, and respiratory coordination for speech and other oromotor behaviors, including chewing and sucking.

**★ 6201 ★ University of Washington**
**Virginia Merrill Bloedel Hearing Research Center**
Box 357923
CHDD Bldg., CD176
Seattle, WA 98195-7923
**Phone:** (206)685-2962          **Fax:** (206)616-1828
**Email:** bloedel@u.washington.edu
**Website:** http://depts.washington.edu/hearing/
Dr. George Gates, Contact

**Activities/Fields:** Hearing, hearing loss, and related communication disorders.

**★ 6202 ★ University of Wisconsin**
**Auditory Physiology Research Laboratory**
625 Waisman Ctr.
Madison, WI 53706
**Phone:** (608)263-5928          **Fax:** (608)265-4103
**Email:** brugge@physiology.wisc.edu
**Website:** http://www.physiology.wisc.edu/aud/
Dr. John F. Brugge, Contact

**Activities/Fields:** Auditory research at the systems, cellular, and molecular levels.

**★ 6203 ★ University of Wisconsin—Madison**
**Hearing Development Research Laboratory (HDRL)**
573 Waisman Center
1500 Highland Ave.
Madison, WI 53705-2280
**Phone:** (608)263-3270          **Fax:** (608)263-2918
**Email:** wightman@waisman.wisc.edu
**Website:** http://www.waisman.wisc.edu/~wightman/
Frederic Wightman, Dir.

**Activities/Fields:** Mechanisms and processes of human hearing.

**University of Wisconsin—Madison**
**Trace Research and Development Center**
*See:* Entry 8230

**★ 6204 ★ Vanderbilt Bill Wilkerson Center**
1114 19th Ave. S
Nashville, TN 37212
**Phone:** (615)936-5000          **Fax:** (615)936-5013
**Email:** d.wesley.grantham@vanderbilt.edu
**Website:** http://www.mc.vanderbilt.edu/VanderbiltBill-WilkersonCenter/hearing.htm
Dr. Fred H. Bess, Dir.

**Activities/Fields:** Hearing science, speech science, and language science, including psychoacoustics, speech perception and production, and child language acquisition and development. Conducts clinical studies of communication disorders dealing with hearing, speech, and language in children and adults, and child language development and its assessment. **Pub:** *Annual Report.* • *Research Report.*

**★ 6205 ★ Vanderbilt University**
**Vanderbilt Bill Wilkerson Center for Otolaryngology and Communication Sciences (VBWC)**
1301 22nd Ave. S, No. 2900
Nashville, TN 37232
**Phone:** (615)343-7267          **Fax:** (615)322-9725
**Email:** robert.ossoff@mcmail.vanderbilt.edu
**Website:** http://www.mc.vanderbilt.edu/VanderbiltBill-WilkersonCenter/
Robert H. Ossoff, Dir.

**Activities/Fields:** Otolaryngological, communicative and related diseases and disorders. **Pub:** *Research report*, annually.

**★ 6206 ★ Virginia Lions Hearing Foundation and Research Center, Inc.**
University of Virginia Health System
PO Box 800477
Charlottesville, VA 22908-0477
**Phone:** (434)296-5466          **Free:** 800-251-3627
**Fax:** (434)243-6732
**Email:** grb8b@virginia.edu
**Website:** http://www.lions24b.org/VLHF/
Gwynn Berkowitz, Admin.

**Activities/Fields:** Cochlear implants, newborn hearing screening, implantable hearing aids, hair cell regeneration in the cochlea, ototoxicity (drug damage), noise damage, electrical stimulation of auditory nerves. **Pub:** *Eardrum Update*, quarterly.

**★ 6207 ★ Yeshiva University**
**Institute of Communication Disorders**
c/o Montefiore Medical Center
Department ENT, 3rd Fl., Green Pavillion
3400 Bainbridge Ave.
Bronx, NY 10467
**Phone:** (718)920-2991          **Fax:** (718)405-9014
**Email:** ruben@aecom.yu.edu
Robert J. Ruben, MD, Chm.

**Activities/Fields:** Communicative disorders, including hearing, listening, voice, speech, and language studies; molecular developmental biology; molecular genetics; the synergy of culture and disease; morbidity;

genetic studies; and genetics of communication disorders.

## Foundations & Other Funding Organizations

### Private Foundations

**Arthur Vining Davis Foundations**
*See:* Entry 54

**Eugene B. Casey Foundation**
*See:* Entry 224

**Perkins-Prothro Foundation**
*See:* Entry 583

## Medical & Allied Health Schools

### Mortuary Science

*The following colleges and programs in funeral service education and mortuary science are accredited by the American Board of Funeral Service Education, 38 Florida Ave., Portland, ME 04103, (207) 878-6530, http://www.abfse.org/.*

### Alabama

★ **6208** ★ **Bishop State Community College**
**Funeral Service Education Program**
1365 Dr. Martin Luther King Jr. Ave.
Mobile, AL 36603-5362
**Phone:** (334)405-4400      **Fax:** (334)405-4427
**Email:** wthompson@bscc.cc.al.us
**Website:** http://www.bscc.cc.al.us/
William Thompson, Director

★ **6209** ★ **Jefferson State Community College**
**Funeral Service Education Program**
2601 Carson Rd.
Birmingham, AL 35215
**Phone:** (205)856-7844      **Fax:** (205)856-8518
**Website:** http://www.jscc.cc.al.us
Dr. William Counce, Director

### Arizona

★ **6210** ★ **Mesa Community College**
**Mortuary Science Program**
Williams Ed. Ctr.
7440 E Tahoe Ave.
Mesa, AZ 85212-0908
**Phone:** (480)988-8501      **Fax:** (480)988-8520
**Email:** tom.taggart@mcmail.maricopa.edu
**Website:** http://www.mc.maricopa.edu/academic/mort_sci
Dr. Thomas R. Taggart, Director

### Arkansas

★ **6211** ★ **Arkansas State University Mountain Home**
**Funeral Service Program**
1600 S College St.
Mountain Home, AR 72653
**Phone:** (870)508-6100      **Fax:** (870)508-6283
**Email:** rschofield@brook.asumh.edu
**Website:** http://www.asumh.edu/funeral.htm
Ron Schofield, Director

★ **6212** ★ **University of Arkansas Community College at Hope**
**Funeral Service Program**
PO Box 140
Hope, AR 71802-0140
**Phone:** (870)722-8206      **Fax:** (870)777-5957
**Email:** Kdavis@mail.uacch.cc.ar.us
Karen Davis, Director

### California

★ **6213** ★ **Cypress College**
**Mortuary Science Department**
9200 Valley View St.
Cypress, CA 90630
**Phone:** (714)484-7279      **Fax:** (714)527-2175
**Email:** mortsci@cypress.cc.ca.us
**Website:** http://www.cypress.cc.ca.us
Douglas Metz, Director

★ **6214** ★ **San Francisco College of Mortuary Science**
1598 Dolores St. (at 29th St.)
San Francisco, CA 94110
**Phone:** (415)824-1313      **Fax:** (415)824-1390
**Email:** jtsfcms@ix.netcom.com
**Website:** http://www.sfcms.org/
Jacquelyn Taylor, President

### Colorado

★ **6215** ★ **Arapahoe Community College**
**Mortuary Science Program**
PO Box 9002
Littleton, CO 80160-9002
**Phone:** (303)797-5954
**Email:** mgaidies@arapahoe.edu
**Website:** http://www.arapahoe.edu/Programs/Mortuary/
Martha L. Gaidies, Chairman of the Board

### Connecticut

★ **6216** ★ **Briarwood College**
**Mortuary Science Program**
2279 Mt. Vernon Rd.
Southington, CT 06489
**Phone:** (860)628-4751      **Free:** 800-952-2444
**Fax:** (860)628-6444
**Email:** laskowskib@briarwood.edu
**Website:** http://www.briarwood.edu
Bernard Laskowski, Director

### District of Columbia

★ **6217** ★ **University of the District of Columbia**
**Van Ness Campus**
**Mortuary Science Department**
4200 Connecticut Ave. NW
MB4407
Washington, DC 20008
**Phone:** (202)274-5858
Courtney Terry, Director

### Florida

★ **6218** ★ **Lynn University**
**Institute for Funeral Service Education**
3601 N Military Trail
Boca Raton, FL 33431-9990
**Phone:** (561)237-7020      **Free:** 800-544-8035
**Fax:** (561)237-7023
**Email:** mpiasecki@lynn.edu
**Website:** http://www.lynn.edu
Marcela Plasecki, Contact

★ **6219** ★ **Miami-Dade Community College**
**W.L. Philbrick School of Funeral Sciences**
11380 NW 27th Ave.
Miami, FL 33167
**Phone:** (305)237-1245      **Fax:** (305)237-8195
**Email:** rcovert@mdcc.edu
**Website:** http://www.mdcc.edu
Ralph Covert, Director

★ **6220** ★ **Saint Petersburg Junior College**
**Funeral Services Program**
PO Box 13489
Saint Petersburg, FL 33733-3489
**Phone:** (727)341-3781      **Fax:** (727)341-3770
**Email:** davisk@email.spjc.cc.fl.us
**Website:** http://www.spjc.cc.fl.us
Kevin Davis, Director

## Georgia

**★ 6221 ★ Gupton-Jones College of Funeral Service**
5141 Snapfinger Woods Dr.
Decatur, GA 30035-4022
**Phone:** (770)593-2257    **Free:** 800-848-5352
**Fax:** (770)593-1891
**Email:** gjcfs@mindspring.com
**Website:** http://www.gupton-jones.edu/
Patty S. Hutchinson, President

## Illinois

**★ 6222 ★ Carl Sandburg College Mortuary Science Program**
2400 Tom L. Wilson Blvd. Lake Storey Rd.
Galesburg, IL 61401-9576
**Phone:** (309)341-0831    **Fax:** (309)341-1040
**Email:** tkrause@csc.cc.il.us
**Website:** http://www.csc.cc.il.us/html/mortuary_science.html
Tim Krause, Contact

**★ 6223 ★ Malcolm X College Department of Mortuary Science**
1900 W Van Buren St.
Chicago, IL 60612
**Fax:** (312)850-7453
**Email:** alwilliams@ccc.edu
**Website:** http://www.ccc.edu/malcolmx/home/htm
Alta L. Williams, Director

**★ 6224 ★ Southern Illinois University Mortuary Science and Funeral Service**
ASA-MC6615
Carbondale, IL 62901-6615
**Phone:** (618)453-7214    **Fax:** (618)453-7020
**Email:** cgriffit@siu.edu
**Website:** http://www.siu.edu/~hcp/msfs/mshome.html
Cydney Griffith, Director

**★ 6225 ★ Worsham College of Mortuary Science**
495 Northgate Pkwy.
Wheeling, IL 60090-2646
**Phone:** (847)808-8444    **Fax:** (847)808-8493
**Email:** soulfillet@aol.com
**Website:** http://www.worshamcollege.com
Stephanie J. Kann, Director

## Indiana

**★ 6226 ★ Mid-America College of Funeral Service**
3111 Hamburg Pike
Jeffersonville, IN 47130
**Phone:** (812)288-8878    **Free:** 800-221-6158
**Fax:** (812)288-5942
**Email:** macfs@mindspring.com
**Website:** http://www.mid-america.edu
John R. Braboy, President

**★ 6227 ★ Vincennes University Funeral Service Education Program**
1002 N 1st St.
Vincennes, IN 47591
**Phone:** (812)888-5469    **Fax:** (812)888-4550
**Email:** jalsobro@indian.vinu.edu
**Website:** http://www.vinu.edu
John Alsobrooks, Chairman of the Board

## Kansas

**★ 6228 ★ Kansas City Kansas Community College Mortuary Science Department**
7250 State Ave.
Kansas City, KS 66112
**Phone:** (913)596-9607    **Fax:** (913)596-9606

**Email:** wwright@toto.net
**Website:** http://www.kckcc.edu
Wiley Wright, Contact

## Louisiana

**★ 6229 ★ Delgado Community College Department of Funeral Service Education**
City Park Campus
615 City Park Ave.
New Orleans, LA 70119-4399
**Phone:** (504)483-4014    **Fax:** (504)483-4609
**Email:** jbodet@dcc.edu
**Website:** http://www.dcc.edu
Janice Bodet, Director

## Maryland

**★ 6230 ★ Community College of Baltimore County, Catonsville Campus Mortuary Science Program**
800 S Rolling Rd.
Baltimore, MD 21228
**Phone:** (410)455-4162    **Fax:** (410)719-6547
**Email:** jdoe151@aol.com
**Website:** http://www.ccbc.cc.md.us
William C. Gonce, Chairman of the Board

## Massachusetts

**★ 6231 ★ Funeral Institute of the North East, LLC**
77 University Ave.
Westwood, MA 02090
**Phone:** (781)461-9080    **Fax:** (781)461-8787
**Email:** lynlou@tiac.net
**Website:** http://www.fine-ne.com
Louis Misantone, President

**★ 6232 ★ Mount Ida College New England Institute of Funeral Service Education**
777 Dedham St.
Newton Centre, MA 02459
**Phone:** (617)928-4711    **Fax:** (617)928-4713
**Email:** bcarter12@aol.com
**Website:** http://www.mountida.edu
Bill Carter, Director

## Michigan

**★ 6233 ★ Wayne State University Department of Mortuary Science**
5439 Woodward Ave.
Detroit, MI 48202
**Phone:** (313)577-2050    **Fax:** (313)577-4456
**Email:** mmwilli@wayne.edu
**Website:** http://mortuarysciencewayne.org
Michael Wilk, Director

## Minnesota

**★ 6234 ★ University of Minnesota Program of Mortuary Science**
MMC 740
420 Delaware St. SE
Minneapolis, MN 55455
**Phone:** (612)624-6464    **Fax:** (612)626-4163
**Email:** mpl@umn.edu
**Website:** http://www1.umn.edu/mortsci/g-index.htm
Michael LuBrant, Director

## Mississippi

**★ 6235 ★ East Mississippi Community College Funeral Service Technology**
PO Box 158
Scooba, MS 39358
**Phone:** (662)476-5101    **Fax:** (662)476-8822
**Email:** dmullins@emcc.cc.ms.us

**Website:** http://www.emcc.cc.ms.us
Don Webb, Director

**★ 6236 ★ Holmes Community College Funeral Services Technology**
412 W Ridgeland Ave.
Ridgeland, MS 39157
**Phone:** (601)605-3323    **Fax:** (601)605-3410
**Email:** bdepriest@holmes.cc.ms.us
**Website:** http://www.holmes.cc.ms.us/fst/index.html
Bill W. DePriest, Director

**★ 6237 ★ Mississippi Gulf Coast Community College Funeral Service Technology**
PO Box 548
Perkinston, MS 39573
**Phone:** (601)528-8909    **Fax:** (601)528-8422
**Email:** michael.normansr@mgccc.cc.ms.us
**Website:** http://www.mgccc.cc.ms.us
Michael Norman, Contact

**★ 6238 ★ Northwest Mississippi Community College Funeral Service Technology Program**
Desoto Center
5197 WE Ross Pkwy.
Southaven, MS 38671
**Phone:** (662)280-6120    **Fax:** (662)280-6161
**Email:** jmitchell@nwcc.cc.ms.us
**Website:** http://www.nwcc.cc.ms.us/
John M. Mitchell, Director

## Missouri

**★ 6239 ★ Saint Louis Community College at Forest Park Department of Funeral Service Education**
5600 Oakland Ave.
Saint Louis, MO 63110
**Phone:** (314)644-9327    **Fax:** (314)644-9752
**Email:** skoosmann@stlcc.cc.mo.us
**Website:** http://www.stlcc.cc.mo.us
Steven B. Koosmann, Director

## New Jersey

**★ 6240 ★ Mercer County Community College Funeral Service Curriculum**
1200 Old Trenton Rd.
PO Box B
Trenton, NJ 08690
**Phone:** (609)586-3472    **Fax:** (609)586-5602
**Email:** smithr@mccc.edu
**Website:** http://www.mccc.edu
Robert C. Smith III, Director

## New York

**★ 6241 ★ American Academy McAllister Institute of Funeral Service, Inc.**
450 W 56th St.
New York, NY 10019
**Phone:** (212)757-1190    **Fax:** (212)765-5923
**Email:** aamifs@aol.com
**Website:** http://members.aol.com/aamifs/main.html
Meg Dunn, President

**★ 6242 ★ Hudson Valley Community College Mortuary Science Department**
80 Vandenburgh Ave.
Troy, NY 12180
**Phone:** (518)629-7113    **Fax:** (518)266-8025
**Email:** reinhela@hvcc.edu
**Website:** http://www.hvcc.edu
D. Elaine Reinhard, Chairman of the Board



Encyclopedia of Medical Organizations and Agencies, 13th Edition

**★ 6243 ★ Nassau Community College**
**Mortuary Science Department**
1 Education Dr.
Bldg. 111
Garden City, NY 11530-6793
**Phone:** (516)572-7277      **Fax:** (516)572-0626
**Email:** lieblaj@sunynassau.edu
**Website:** http://www.sunynassau.edu
John M. Lieblang, Chairman of the Board

**★ 6244 ★ Simmons Institute of Funeral**
**Service**
1828 South Ave.
Syracuse, NY 13207
**Phone:** (315)475-5142      **Fax:** (315)475-3817
**Email:** mcwightman20@aol.com
**Website:** http://www.simmonsinstitute.com
Maurice C. Wightman, President

**★ 6245 ★ State University of New York**
**College of Technology at Canton**
**Mortuary Science Program**
Canton, NY 13617
**Phone:** (315)386-7110      **Fax:** (315)386-7959
**Email:** walch@canton.edu
**Website:** http://www.canton.edu
Barry Walch, Contact

### North Carolina

**★ 6246 ★ Fayetteville Technical**
**Community College**
**Funeral Service Education Department**
PO Box 35236
Fayetteville, NC 28303
**Phone:** (910)678-8301      **Fax:** (910)484-6600
**Email:** landonm@ftccmail.faytech.cc.nc.us
**Website:** http://atlas.faytech.cc.nc.us
Michael Landon, Chairman of the Board

### Ohio

**★ 6247 ★ Cincinnati College of Mortuary**
**Science**
645 W N Bend Rd.
Cincinnati, OH 45224-1462
**Phone:** (513)761-2020      **Free:** 888-377-8433
**Fax:** (513)761-3333
**Email:** dflory@ccms.edu
**Website:** http://www.ccms.edu
Dan Flory, President

### Oklahoma

**★ 6248 ★ University of Central Oklahoma**
**Department of Funeral Service Education**
Edmond, OK 73034-5209
**Phone:** (405)974-5192      **Fax:** (405)974-3848
**Email:** kcurl@ucok.edu
**Website:** http://204.154.117.119
Kenneth Curl, Chairman of the Board

### Oregon

**★ 6249 ★ Mount Hood Community**
**College**
**Department of Funeral Service Education**
26000 SE Stark St.
Gresham, OR 97030
**Phone:** (503)491-6941      **Fax:** (503)491-6050
**Email:** malcomw@mhcc.cc.or.us
**Website:** http://mhcc.cc.or.us/programs/sci/funeral/
main.htm
William Malcolm, Director

### Pennsylvania

**★ 6250 ★ Northampton Community**
**College**
**Department of Funeral Service Education**
3835 Green Pond Rd.
Bethlehem, PA 18017
**Phone:** (610)861-5388      **Fax:** (610)861-4581
**Email:** jlunsford@northampton.edu
**Website:** http://www.Northampton.edu
John Lunsford, Director

**★ 6251 ★ Pittsburgh Institute of Mortuary**
**Science**
5808 Baum Blvd.
Pittsburgh, PA 15206
**Phone:** (412)362-8500      **Fax:** (412)362-1684
**Email:** pims5808@aol.com
**Website:** http://www.p-i-m-s.com
Eugene C. Ogrodnik, President

### South Carolina

**★ 6252 ★ Piedmont Technical College**
PO Drawer 1467
Emerald Rd.
Greenwood, SC 29648-1467
**Phone:** (864)941-8690      **Fax:** (864)941-8711
**Email:** vessels_g@piedmont.tec.sc.us
**Website:** http://www.piedmont.tec.sc.us
Gloria Walker Vessels, Contact

### Tennessee

**★ 6253 ★ John A. Gupton College**
1616 Church St.
Nashville, TN 37203
**Phone:** (615)327-3927      **Fax:** (615)321-4518
**Email:** spann@guptoncollege.com
**Website:** http://www.gupton.college.com
B. Steven Spann, President

### Texas

**★ 6254 ★ Amarillo College**
**Mortuary Science Program**
PO Box 447
Amarillo, TX 79178-0001
**Phone:** (806)371-5188
**Email:** altieri-jc@actx.edu
**Website:** http://www.actx.edu/schedules/degrees/
degr42.htm
Jason Altieri, Director

**★ 6255 ★ Commonwealth Institute of**
**Funeral Service**
415 Barren Springs
Houston, TX 77090
**Phone:** (281)873-0262      **Fax:** (281)873-5232
**Email:** gposton@pdq.net
**Website:** http://www.commonwealthinst.org/
George Poston, President

**★ 6256 ★ Dallas Institute of Funeral**
**Service**
3909 S Buckner Blvd.
Dallas, TX 75227
**Phone:** (214)388-5466      **Free:** 800-235-5444
**Fax:** (214)388-0316
**Email:** difs@mindspring.com
**Website:** http://www.dallasinstitute.edu
James Shoemake, President

**★ 6257 ★ San Antonio College**
**Mortuary Science Program**
1300 San Pedro Ave.
NTC 124
San Antonio, TX 78212-4299
**Phone:** (210)733-2905      **Fax:** (210)733-2907
**Email:** fegonzal@accd.edu

**Website:** http://www.accd.edu/sac/mortuary/
home.html
Felix Gonzales, Contact

### Virginia

**★ 6258 ★ John Tyler Community College**
**Funeral Service Program**
Chester, VA 23831
**Phone:** (804)796-4119      **Fax:** (804)796-4362
Rick Fikon, Contact

### Wisconsin

**★ 6259 ★ Milwaukee Area Technical**
**College**
**West Campus**
**Funeral Service Department**
1200 S 71st St.
West Allis, WI 53214
**Phone:** (414)456-5500      **Fax:** (414)456-5360
**Email:** augustij@matc.edu
**Website:** http://matc.edu
James Augustine, Contact

# National & International
# Organizations

**★ 6260 ★ Alcor Life Extension**
**Foundation (ALEF)**
7895 E Acoma Dr., Ste. 110
Scottsdale, AZ 85260-6916
**Phone:** (480)905-1906      **Fax:** (480)922-9027
**Email:** info@alcor.org
**Website:** http://www.alcor.org
Jennifer Chapman, Membership Admin.

**Fnded:** 1972. **Mem:** 555. **Reg. Groups:** 10. **Desc:**
Individuals who have made anatomical donation for
purpose of being cryonically suspended. Seeks to
extend lives of Alcor members; currently 47 members
in suspension. **Pub:** *ALCOR: Reaching for Tomorrow*,
quarterly. Magazine. Covers cryonics, life extension,
and immortality. *Price:* $35/year; $25/year in Canada
and Mexico; $30/year in all other countries. • *Cryonics:
Reaching for Tomorrow*, biennial. Booklet. Covers
cryonics, life extension, and immortality. *Price:* $8.95/
year in the U.S.; $20/year in Canada and Mexico; $25/
year overseas. • Brochures. **AKA:** Alcor Foundation.

**★ 6261 ★ American Cryonics Society**
**(ACS)**
PO Box 1509
Cupertino, CA 95015
**Phone:** (650)254-2001      **Free:** 800-523-2001
**Fax:** (408)253-0444
**Email:** cryonics@americancryonics.org
**Website:** http://pweb.jps.net/~cryonics/contact
Edgar Swark, Pres.

**Fnded:** 1969. **Mem:** 500. **Desc:** Individuals interested
in life extension through cryonics (the practice of
freezing a clinically dead human in hopes of bringing
the person back to life when resuscitation or reconstruction is possible). Promotes education and provides information about cryonic suspension, suspended animation, and low-temperature medicine. Enables
individuals to arrange for their own cryonic suspension. Sponsors research into suspended animation,
life extension sciences, and low temperature medicine. Conducts programs to freeze tissue samples
from endangered species for possible future cloning.
Maintains library; operates speakers' bureau; conducts charitable programs. **Pub:** *American Cryonics*,
semiannual. Journal. Synopsis of research, national
news and editorials affecting cryonics field. • *American
Cryonics News*, bimonthly. Newsletter. Covers cryonics and life extension. Includes calendar of events and
research reports. *Price:* Included in membership dues;
$35/year for nonmembers. • *The Immortalist*, monthly.
Contains articles on cryonics, health, aging research,

and science. **Frmly:** (1985) Bay Area Cryonics Society.

### ★ 6262 ★ American Foundation for Suicide Prevention

120 Wall St., Fl. 22
New York, NY 10005-4001
**Phone:** (212)363-3500      **Free:** 888-333-AFSP
**Fax:** (212)363-6237
**Email:** inquiry@afsp.org
**Website:** http://www.afsp.org
Robert Gebbia, Exec. Dir.
**Fnded:** 1987. **Mem:** 1,500. **Reg. Groups:** 12. **Desc:** Medical professionals, community leaders, and suicide survivors. Provides funding for research on the causes and prevention of suicide. Trains professionals in the treatment of suicidal individuals; offers support programs for suicide survivors. **Pub:** *Lifesavers*, quarterly. Newsletter. *Price:* Included with membership dues. **Frmly:** (1998) Maryland Suicide Foundation.

### ★ 6263 ★ Americans for Better Care of the Dying

4125 Albemarle St. NW, Ste. 210
Washington, DC 20016
**Phone:** (202)895-9485      **Fax:** (202)895-9484
**Email:** info@abcd-caring.org
**Website:** http://www.abcd-caring.org
Joanne Lynn, Pres.
**Fnded:** 1997. **Mem:** 500. **Desc:** Strives to improve the experience of the last phase of life for all Americans. Advocates the interests of patients and families. Works to improve communication between providers and patients.

### Association of SIDS and Infant Mortality Programs
*See:* Entry 5631

### ★ 6264 ★ European Association for Palliative Care (EAPC)

Instituto Nazional dei Tumori
Via Venezian 1
I-20133 Milan, Italy
**Phone:** 39 2 23902792      **Fax:** 39 2 70600462
**Email:** eapc@institutomori.mi.it
**Website:** http://www.eapcnet.org
**Fnded:** 1990. **Desc:** Specialists in palliative care and hospice services. Promotes palliative care to health authorities and other agencies. **Pub:** *European Journal of Palliative Care*, periodic. Journal.

### ★ 6265 ★ Heartbeat

2015 Devon St.
Colorado Springs, CO 80909
**Phone:** (719)596-2575
**Email:** archlj@msn.com
LaRita Archibald, Founder
**Fnded:** 1980. **Desc:** Persons who have lost a loved one due to suicide. Provides an atmosphere whereby grieving participants receive support, understanding, direction, and encouragement from those who have successfully resolved their grief. Offers "postvention" education program aimed at preventing the suicide of survivors. Maintains speakers' bureau. **Pub:** *Forming Heartbeat Chapters*. Manual. **Frmly:** Heartbeat/Survivors After Suicide.

### ★ 6266 ★ Hospice Education Institute (HEI)

3 Unity Sq.
PO Box 98
Machiasport, ME 04655-0098
**Phone:** (207)255-8800      **Free:** 800-331-1620
**Fax:** (207)255-8008
**Email:** hospiceall@aol.com
**Website:** http://www.hospiceworld.org
Michal Galazka, Exec. Dir.
**Fnded:** 1985. **Desc:** Provides educational and informational services to health professionals and the public on subjects such as hospice and palliative care, death and dying, and bereavement counseling. Encourages educational exchange among hospice and palliative care professionals and volunteers. Offers advice and support to persons working to open local hospice programs. Organizes continuing education seminars on hospice care throughout the U.S. and abroad. **Pub:** *Notes on Symptom Control in Hospice and Palliative Care*. Book. *Price:* $28.95. • Booklets.

### ★ 6267 ★ National Committee on the Treatment of Intractable Pain (NCTIP)

c/o Wayne Coy, Jr.
Cohn and Marks
1920 N St. NW, Ste. 300
Washington, DC 20036
**Phone:** (202)452-4836      **Fax:** (202)293-4827
Wayne Coy, Jr., Pres.
**Fnded:** 1977. **Mem:** 3,500. **Desc:** Individuals promoting education and research into more effective methods of pain prevention and control with the coordinated help of professionals in the medical, legal, bioethical, psychological, and religious fields. Endorses the British hospice concept of care of the dying, which allows the dying person to remain among family, friends, community, and skilled professionals and provides constant, effective medical and psychological support for pain control. Advocates legalization of heroin for medical purposes. Plans to sponsor speakers' bureau. **Pub:** *Newsletter of the National Committee on the Treatment of Intractable Pain*, annual. Newsletter. Covers concern generated by the use of medication to relieve intractable pain caused by cancer, specifically the effort to legalize heroin. *Price:* Free. • Monographs. • Reports. **Frmly:** (1977) American Intractable Pain Foundation.

### ★ 6268 ★ National Council for Hospice and Specialist Palliative Care Services

34-44 Britannia St.
London WC1X 9JG, United Kingdom
**Phone:** 44 207 5208299      **Fax:** 44 207 5208298
**Email:** enquiries@hospice-spc-council.org.uk
**Website:** http://www.hospice-spc-council.org.uk
**Fnded:** 1991. **Mem:** 35. **Reg. Groups:** 15. **Desc:** Members are nominated by national charities and professional organisations or elected by regional hospice and palliative care units. To represent the views and interests of hospice and palliative care services to ministers, civil servants, MPs, the media and statutory and other agencies. To provide advice to hospice and specialist palliative care services in their relations with health authorities, local authorities and other agencies. **Pub:** *Information Exchange*, quarterly. Newsletter. • Papers.

### ★ 6269 ★ National Hospice and Palliative Care Organization

1700 Diagonal Rd., Ste. 625
Alexandria, VA 22314-2848
**Phone:** (703)837-1500      **Free:** 800-658-8898
**Fax:** (703)837-1233
**Email:** info@nhpco.org
**Website:** http://www.nhpco.org
Karen A. Davie, Pres.
**Fnded:** 1978. **Mem:** 5,000. **State Groups:** 48. **Local Groups:** 2400. **Desc:** Hospice organizations and individuals interested in the promotion of the hospice concept and program of care. (Hospice is a concept of caring for the terminally ill and their families which enables the patient to live as fully as possible, makes the entire family the unit of care, and centers the caring process in the home whenever appropriate. Inpatient facilities are available for those unable to be cared for at home.) Promotes standards of care in program planning and implementation; monitors health care legislation and regulation relevant to hospice care. Sponsors professional liaison and peer group networking. Collects data for the purpose of demonstrating definitive national trends in the hospice movement; encourages recognized medical and other health teaching institutions to provide instruction in hospice care of terminally ill patients and their families.

Compiles statistics. Conducts educational and training programs in numerous aspects of hospice care for administrators and care-givers. Maintains nonlending library of hospice-related books. Operates helpline to assist public in identifying hospice programs in their area. **Frmly:** (2000) National Hospice Organization.

### ★ 6270 ★ National Prison Hospice Association (NPHA)

PO Box 3769
Boulder, CO 80307
**Phone:** (303)544-5923      **Fax:** (303)444-2824
**Email:** npha@npha.org
**Website:** http://www.npha.org/
Fleet Maull, Founder/Dir.
**Fnded:** 1991. **Reg. Groups:** 4. **Desc:** Promotes hospice care for terminally ill inmates and those facing the prospect of dying in prison. Hospice is a comfort-oriented care that allows seriously ill and dying patients to die with dignity and humanity with as little pain as possible. **Pub:** *NPHA News*, annual. Newsletter. *Price:* Free.

### ★ 6271 ★ Pen-Parents

c/o Maribeth Wilder Doerr
PO Box 8738
Reno, NV 89507-8738
**Phone:** (702)826-7332      **Fax:** (702)852-2069
**Email:** penparents@penparents.org
M.A. Melissa Swanson, Exec. Dir.
**Fnded:** 1988. **Mem:** 725. **Desc:** Parents who have experienced pregnancy loss or the death of a child through adulthood. Provides support to those parents who may not have access to traditional support group meetings, for those who may feel uncomfortable participating in a group setting, and for those who need additional support through correspondence (the group feels that writing can be a powerful release for feelings, and that sharing these thoughts with someone who has also experienced death of their children can be very healing). **Pub:** *HeartSongs*, quarterly. Newsletter. *Price:* $15/year; $20/year foreign parents; $25/year professionals. • *PAILS of Hope*, bimonthly. Newsletter. Focus is supporting parents contemplating or experiencing pregnancy after infertility and/or pregnancy/infant loss. *Price:* $15 for parents in the U.S.; $20 for parents outside the U.S.; $25 for professionals and support groups.

### ★ 6272 ★ Ray of Hope (ROH)

PO Box 2323
Iowa City, IA 52244
**Phone:** (319)337-9890      **Fax:** (319)337-9890
**Email:** rayofhopeinc@juno.com
E. Betsy Ross, Exec. Dir.
**Fnded:** 1977. **Mem:** 25. **Nat'l Groups:** 10. **Reg. Groups:** 13. **State Groups:** 2. **Local Groups:** 1. **Desc:** Selfhelp organization offering support for coping with sucide, loss, and grief. Organizes suicide survivor support groups. Offers training courses and consultation on bereavement and suicide postvention. Telephone counseling (pre-arranged). **Pub:** *After Suicide: A Unique Grief Process*. Booklet. *Price:* $5.95 plus $1.50 first book, and .25 each addition. • *Life After Suicide: A Ray of Hope for Those Left Behind*. Book. Guide for suicide survivor's bereavement process. *Price:* $27.95 plus $3 postage and .50 each additional book. • *Survivorship After Suicide*. Video. *Price:* $75 postage included.

## Research Centers

### ★ 6273 ★ Center for Thanatology Research

391 Atlantic Ave.
Brooklyn, NY 11217-1701
**Phone:** (718)858-3026      **Fax:** (718)852-1846
**Email:** rhalporn@pipeline.com
**Website:** http://www.thanatology.org
Roberta Halporn, Dir.

**Activities/Fields:** Aging, dying, death, bereavement, and gravestone studies. **Pub:** *Advances in Thanatology.* • *Archives of the Foundation of Thanatology.*

# State Government Agencies

## Funeral Service Examining Boards

**★ 6274 ★ Alaska Division of Occupational Licensing**
**Mortuary Science Section**
PO Box 110806
Juneau, AK 99811-0806
**Phone:** (907)465-2695          **Fax:** (907)465-2974
**Email:** p.j._gingras@dced.state.ak.us
**Website:** http://www.dced.state.ak.us/occ/pmor.htm
P. J. Gingras, Contact

**★ 6275 ★ Arizona State Board of Funeral Directors and Embalmers**
1400 W Washington, Ste. 230
Phoenix, AZ 85007
**Phone:** (602)542-3095          **Fax:** (602)542-3095
**Website:** http://www.mmimarketing.com/afda/statebrd.htm
Rudy Thomas, Director

**★ 6276 ★ Arkansas State Board of Embalmers and Funeral Directors**
101 E Capitol, Ste. 113
Little Rock, AR 72201
**Phone:** (501)682-0574          **Fax:** (501)682-0575
**Email:** fdemb@mail.state.ar.us
**Website:** http://www.state.ar.us/fdemb/
Rachel McGrew, Contact

**★ 6277 ★ Board of Embalmers and Funeral Directors of Ohio**
77 S High St., 16th Fl.
Columbus, OH 43266-0313
**Phone:** (614)466-4252          **Fax:** (614)728-6825
**Website:** http://www.state.oh.us/fun

**★ 6278 ★ California Department of Consumer Affairs**
**Cemetery and Funeral Bureau**
400 R St.
Sacramento, CA 95814
**Phone:** (916)322-7737          **Free:** 800-952-5210
**Website:** http://www.dca.ca.gov/cemetery/

**★ 6279 ★ Colorado Funeral Service Board**
7583 E Araphahoe Ct., No. 2100
Englewood, CO 80112-1361
**Phone:** (303)694-4728          **Fax:** (303)694-4869
**Email:** mail@cofda.org
**Website:** http://www.cofda.org/
Scott Moser, MSP, Contact

**★ 6280 ★ Delaware State Board of Funeral Services**
Cannon Bldg., Ste. 203
861 Silver Lake Blvd.
Dover, DE 19904-2467
**Phone:** (302)744-4506          **Fax:** (302)739-2711
**Email:** smiccio@state.de.us
**Website:** http://professionallicensing.state.de.us/boards/funeralservices/index.shtml
Susan Miccio, Contact

**★ 6281 ★ District of Columbia Board of Funeral Directors**
**Occupational and Professional Licensing Administration**
**DC Board of Funeral Directors**
941 North Capitol St. NE
Washington, DC 20002
**Phone:** (202)442-4461          **Fax:** (202)442-8390
**Website:** http://dcra.dc.gov/about/index_bpla_funeral.shtm

**★ 6282 ★ Florida Board of Funeral Directors and Embalmers**
1940 N Monroe St., Ste. 426
Tallahassee, FL 32399-0754
**Phone:** (904)488-8690          **Fax:** (904)922-2918
**Website:** http://www.state.fl.us/dbpr/prof/fd_index.shtml
Sherry Landrum, Director

**★ 6283 ★ Georgia State Examining Boards**
237 Coliseum Dr.
Macon, GA 31217-3858
**Phone:** (478)207-1460
**Website:** http://www.sos.state.ga.us/ebd/
Mollie Fleeman, Director

**★ 6284 ★ Hawaii Department of Health**
**Sanitation Branch**
591 Ala Moana
Honolulu, HI 96813
**Phone:** (808)586-4700          **Fax:** (808)586-4729
**Website:** http://www.state.hi.us/health/eh/sanitation/index.htm

**★ 6285 ★ Idaho Occupational Licensing Bureau**
Owyhee Plaza
1109 Main St., Ste. 220
Boise, ID 83702
**Phone:** (208)334-3233          **Fax:** (208)334-3945
**Email:** ibol@ibol.state.id.us
**Website:** http://www2.state.id.us/ibol/
Rayola Jacobson, Contact

**★ 6286 ★ Illinois Department of Professional Regulation**
**Professional Services Section**
320 W Washington St.
Springfield, IL 62786
**Phone:** (217)785-0800          **Fax:** (217)782-7645
**Website:** http://www.dpr.state.il.us

**★ 6287 ★ Indiana Funeral Service Board**
302 W Washington, Rm. E034
Indianapolis, IN 46204-2700
**Phone:** (317)232-2980          **Fax:** (317)232-2312
**Website:** http://www.state.in.us/pla/funeral/index.html

**★ 6288 ★ Iowa Board of Mortuary Science**
**Iowa Department of Public Health**
Lucas State Office Bldg., 5th Fl.
321 E 12th St.
Des Moines, IA 50319-0075
**Phone:** (515)281-4287          **Fax:** (515)281-3121
**Email:** mbledsoe@idph.state.ia.us
**Website:** http://www.iowaccess.org/idph_pl/mortuary/index.html

**★ 6289 ★ Kansas State Board of Mortuary Arts**
700 SW Jackson, Ste. 904
Topeka, KS 66603-3733
**Phone:** (785)296-3980          **Fax:** (785)296-0891
**Email:** boma1@ink.org
**Website:** http://www.ink.org/public/ksbma/

**★ 6290 ★ Kentucky State Board of Embalmers & Funeral Directors**
7025 W Hwy. 22, Ste. 7
PO Box 324
Crestwood, KY 40014
**Phone:** (502)241-3918

**★ 6291 ★ Louisiana State Board of Embalmers & Funeral Directors**
3500 N Causeway Blvd., Ste. 1232
Metairie, LA 70002
**Phone:** (504)838-5109          **Fax:** (504)838-5112
**Email:** labefd@ix.netcom.com
**Website:** http://www.dhh.state.la.us/boards.htm
Dawn Scardino, Director

**★ 6292 ★ Maine Board of Funeral Service**
35 State House Station
Augusta, ME 04333-0035
**Phone:** (207)624-8623          **Fax:** (207)624-8637
**Email:** elaine.m.thibodeau@state.me.us
**Website:** http://www.state.me.us/pfr/olr/categories/cat19.htm
Elaine M. Thibodeau, Contact

**★ 6293 ★ Maryland State Board of Morticians**
**Department of Health and Mental Hygiene**
4201 Patterson Ave.
Room 315
Baltimore, MD 21215
**Phone:** (410)764-4792          **Fax:** (410)358-6571
**Email:** groninge@dhmh.state.md.us
**Website:** http://www.dhmh.state.md.us/bom/
Elizabeth Groninger, Contact

**★ 6294 ★ Massachusetts Board of Funeral Service**
239 Causeway St., Ste. 500
Boston, MA 02114
**Phone:** (617)727-1718          **Fax:** (617)727-2197
**Email:** kim.m.scully@state.ma.us
**Website:** http://www.state.ma.us/reg/boards/em/default.htm
Kim Scully, Contact

**★ 6295 ★ Michigan Department of Commerce**
**Board of Examiners in Mortuary Science**
PO Box 30004
Lansing, MI 48909
**Phone:** (517)373-1820          **Fax:** (517)373-2129
**Email:** bcsinfo@michigan.gov
**Website:** http://www.michigan.gov/cis/

**★ 6296 ★ Minnesota Mortuary Science Section**
121 E 7th Pl., Ste. 400
PO Box 64975
Saint Paul, MN 55164-0975
**Phone:** (651)282-3829          **Fax:** (651)282-3839
**Email:** david.benke@health.state.mn.us
**Website:** http://www.health.state.mn.us/divs/hpsc/mortsci/mortsci.htm
David Benke, Contact

**★ 6297 ★ Mississippi State Board of Funeral Service**
7 Riverbend Place, Ste. A
Flowood, MS 39208
**Phone:** (601)932-1973          **Fax:** (601)932-1901
**Email:** funeral_board@msbfs.state.ms.us
**Website:** http://www.msfuneralboard.com/
Dolores K. Kenney, Director

**★ 6298 ★ Missouri State Board of Funeral Directors & Embalmers**
3605 Missouri Blvd.
PO Box 423
Jefferson City, MO 65102
**Phone:** (573)751-0813 **Fax:** (573)751-1155
**Email:** embalmer@mail.state.mo.us
**Website:** http://www.ecodev.state.mo.us/pr/embalm/
Patricia A. Handly, Director

**★ 6299 ★ Montana Board of Funeral Service**
301 S Park, 4th Fl.
PO Box 200513
Helena, MT 59620-0513
**Phone:** (406)841-2393
**Email:** compolfnr@mt.gov
**Website:** http://commerce.state.mt.us/LICENSE/pol/pol_boards/fnr_board/board_page.htm
Cheryl Smith, Contact

**★ 6300 ★ Nebraska Department of Health and Human Services Credentialing Division**
301 Centennial Mall South 3rd Flr.
PO Box 94986
Lincoln, NE 68509-4986
**Phone:** (402)471-2115 **Fax:** (402)471-3577
**Email:** Marie.McClatchey@hhss.state.ne.us
**Website:** http://www.hhs.state.ne.us/crl/crlindex.htm
Mary McClatchey, Contact

**★ 6301 ★ Nevada State Board of Funeral Directors and Embalmers**
4894 Lone Mountain Rd. Ste. 186
Las Vegas, NV 89130
**Phone:** (702)646-6860
**Website:** http://www.state.nv.us/funeral/

**★ 6302 ★ New Hampshire Board of Registration of Funeral Directors and Embalmers**
Health and Welfare Bldg.
6 Hazen Dr.
Concord, NH 03301-6527
**Phone:** (603)271-4648 **Fax:** (603)271-3447
**Email:** funeralbd@dhhs.state.nh.us
**Website:** http://webster.state.nh.us/funeral/
Robert J. Diluzio, Sr., Director

**★ 6303 ★ New Jersey State Board of Mortuary Science**
Board of Mortuary Science
PO Box 45009
Newark, NJ 07101
**Phone:** (973)504-6425
**Email:** askconsumeraffairs@smtp.lps.state.nj.us
**Website:** http://www.state.nj.us/lps/ca/nonmed.htmmort7
Paul Brush, Director

**★ 6304 ★ New Mexico State Board of Thanatopractice**
2055 Pacheco St., Ste. 400
Santa Fe, NM 87504
**Phone:** (505)476-7090 **Fax:** (505)476-7095
**Email:** FuneralBoard@state.nm.us
**Website:** http://www.rld.state.nm.us/b&c/thanato/index.htm

**★ 6305 ★ New York State Department of Health**
Funeral Directing Bureau
Empire State Plaza
Corning Tower
Albany, NY 12237-0681
**Phone:** (518)474-7354
**Website:** http://www.health.state.ny.us
Claudia Hutton, Director

**★ 6306 ★ North Carolina Board of Mortuary Science**
2321 Crabtree Blvd., Ste. 100
PO Box 27368
Raleigh, NC 27611-7368
**Phone:** (919)733-9380 **Free:** 800-862-0636
**Fax:** (919)733-8271
**Email:** aritter@ncbms.org
**Website:** http://www.ncbms.org/
Andrew Ritter, Director

**★ 6307 ★ North Dakota Board of Funeral Service**
PO Box 633
Devils Lake, ND 58301
**Phone:** (701)662-2511
**Website:** http://www.governor.state.nd.us/boards/boards-query.asp?Board_ID=42
Rodger E. Haugen, Contact
**Frmly:** North Dakota Board of Embalmers.

**★ 6308 ★ Oklahoma State Board of Embalmers and Funeral Directors**
4545 N Lincoln Blvd., Ste. 175
Oklahoma City, OK 73105
**Phone:** (405)522-1790 **Fax:** (405)522-1797
**Email:** info@okfuneral.com
**Website:** http://www.state.ok.us/~embalm/index.htm
Terry McEnany, Director

**★ 6309 ★ Oregon State Mortuary and Cemetery Board**
State Office Bldg., Ste. 430
800 NE Oregon St., Box 19
Portland, OR 97232-2162
**Phone:** (503)731-4040 **Fax:** (503)731-4494
**Website:** http://bluebook.state.or.us/state/executive/Mortuary_Cemetary/mortuary_cemetary_home.htm
Carla G. Knapp, Contact

**★ 6310 ★ Pennsylvania State Board of Funeral and Funeral Directors**
PO Box 2649
Harrisburg, PA 17105-2649
**Phone:** (717)783-3397 **Fax:** (717)783-7769
**Email:** funeral@pados.dos.state.pa.us
**Website:** http://www.nfda.org/careers/licensing/pa.html

**★ 6311 ★ Rhode Island Division of Professional Regulation**
State Health Department
3 Capital Hill, Rm. 104
Providence, RI 02908
**Phone:** (401)222-6015 **Fax:** (401)222-1272
**Email:** DonW@doh.state.ri.us
**Website:** http://www.health.state.ri.us/hsr/professions_reg.htm
Donald C. Williams, Contact

**★ 6312 ★ South Carolina State Board of Funeral Service**
Department of Labor, Licensing & Regulation
Koger Office Park
Kingstree Bldg.
110 Centerview Dr., Ste. 104
PO Box 11329
Columbia, SC 29211
**Phone:** (803)896-4496 **Fax:** (803)896-4484
**Email:** bryantr@mail.llr.state.sc.us
**Website:** http://www.llr.state.sc.us/POL/Funeral/Default.htm
Dwight Hayes, Contact

**★ 6313 ★ South Dakota State Board of Funeral Service**
135 E Illinois
PO Box 214
Spearfish, SD 57783
**Phone:** (605)642-1600 **Fax:** (605)642-1756
**Email:** proflic@rushmore.com
**Website:** http://www.state.sd.us/dcr/funeral/funhom.htm
Carol Tellinghuisen, Contact

**★ 6314 ★ Tennessee Board of Funeral Directors and Embalmers**
Davy Crockett Tower
500 James Robertson Pkwy., 2nd Fl.
Nashville, TN 37243-1149
**Phone:** (615)741-5062 **Fax:** (615)532-1903
**Email:** bteague@mail.state.tn.us
Arthur Giles, Director

**★ 6315 ★ Texas Funeral Service Commission**
510 S Congress, Ste. 206
PO Box 12217
Austin, TX 78704-7222
**Phone:** (512)936-2474 **Free:** 888-667-4881
**Email:** general@tfsc.state.tx.us
**Website:** http://www.tfsc.state.tx.us/

**★ 6316 ★ Utah Department of Professional Licensing**
160 E 300 S
PO Box 146701
Salt Lake City, UT 84114-6701
**Phone:** (801)530-6628 **Fax:** (801)530-6511
**Email:** gbowen@br.state.ut.us
**Website:** http://www.commerce.state.ut.us/dopl/dopl1.htm
Gary Bowen, Director

**★ 6317 ★ Vermont Board of Funeral Service**
Office of Professional Regulation
109 State St.
Montpelier, VT 05609-1106
**Phone:** (802)828-3228 **Fax:** (802)828-2496
**Email:** dbacon@sec.state.vt.us
**Website:** http://www.vtprofessionals.org/funeral/
Judith Churchill, Contact

**★ 6318 ★ Virginia Board of Funeral Directors**
Department of Health Professions
6606 W Broad St., 4th Fl.
Richmond, VA 23230-1717
**Phone:** (804)662-9907 **Free:** 800-533-1560
**Fax:** (804)662-9523
**Email:** fanbd@dhp.state.va.us
**Website:** http://www.dhp.state.va.us/fun/default.htm
Elizabeth Y. Tisdale, Contact

**★ 6319 ★ Washington Funeral and Cemetary Office**
Business & Professional Divisions
PO Box 9012
Olympia, WA 98507-9012
**Phone:** (360)664-1555 **Fax:** (360)586-4414
**Email:** Funerals@dol.wa.gov
**Website:** http://www.wa.gov/dol/bpd/funfront.htm

**★ 6320 ★ West Virginia Board of Funeral Directors and Embalmers**
179 Summers St., Ste. 305
Charleston, WV 25301
**Phone:** (304)558-0302
**Email:** perryle@wvnvm.wvnet.edu
**Website:** http://www.state.wv.us/bep/lmi/license/LICOCCMS.HTMfuneral

**★ 6321 ★ Wisconsin Funeral Directors Examining Board**
**Department of Regulation and Licensing**
1400 E Washington Ave.
PO Box 8935
Madison, WI 53708-8935
**Phone:** (608)266-5511
**Email:** dorl@drl.state.wi.us
**Website:** http://www.drl.state.wi.us/Regulation/applicant_information/dod278.html

**★ 6322 ★ Wyoming State Board of Embalming**
2020 Carey Ave., Ste. 201
Cheyenne, WY 82002
**Phone:** (307)777-7788    **Fax:** (307)777-3508
**Email:** vskora@state.wy.us
**Website:** http://www.state.wy.us/governor/boards/bdlist.html
Veronica Skoranski, Contact

# Chapter 18
# Dentistry



## Federal Government Agencies

★ 6323 ★ **U.S. Department of Health and Human Services**
**National Institutes of Health (NIH)**
**National Institute of Dental and Craniofacial Research (NIDR)**
9000 Rockville Pike
Bethesda, MD 20892
**Phone:** (301)496-4261
**Website:** http://www.nidr.nih.gov/
Lawrence A. Tabak, Director
**Desc:** The Institute supports and conducts clinical and laboratory research into the causes, prevention, diagnosis, and treatment of oral diseases and conditions.

## Foundations & Other Funding Organizations

### Private Foundations

**Beazley Foundation**
*See:* Entry 68

### Corporate Foundations

**Wm. Jr. Wrigley Co. Foundation**
*See:* Entry 1511

### Other Funding Organizations

★ 6324 ★ **Academy of Osseointegration**
85 W Algonquin Rd., Ste. 550
Arlington Heights, IL 60005-4460
**Phone:** (847)439-1919          **Free:** 800-656-7736
**Fax:** (847)439-1569
**Email:** academy@osseo.org
**Website:** http://www.osseo.org
Kevin P. Smith, Exec. Dir.
**Desc:** Works for the advancement of osseointegration among dentists, physicians and related professionals. Conducts research and educational programs; disseminates information to the public and medical agencies; provides a forum for interdisciplinary discussions. **Awards:** Osseointegration Foundation Implant Research Grant (annual); Osseointegration Foundation Patient Care Grants.

★ 6325 ★ **Alpha Omega International Dental Fraternity**
500 Commonwealth Dr.
Warrendale, PA 15086
**Phone:** (724)778-3419          **Free:** 800-MRS-TINT
**Fax:** (724)772-8349

**Email:** headquarters@ao.org
**Website:** http://www.ao.org/
Stephanie Block, Exec. Dir.
**Desc:** Professional fraternity - dentistry. Encourages fraternalism and monitors discrimination in dental schools. Maintains the Alpha Omega Foundation, which sends funds to dental schools in Israel and the U.S. Holds continuing education seminars. **Awards:** Grant for post-graduate dental students; recognition (annual) for students with superior scholastic standing.

★ 6326 ★ **American Academy of Esthetic Dentistry (AAED)**
401 N Michigan Ave.
Chicago, IL 60611
**Phone:** (312)321-5121          **Fax:** (312)673-6952
**Email:** aaed@sba.com
**Website:** http://www.estheticacademy.org/
Frank M. Spear, DDS, Pres.
**Desc:** Dentists seeking to advance the art and science of esthetic dentistry (dentistry concerned with restorative procedures of natural teeth). **Awards:** AAED Research Grant.

★ 6327 ★ **American Academy of Fixed Prosthodontics (AAFP)**
PO Box 1409
Bodega Bay, CA 94923-1409
**Phone:** (707)875-3040          **Free:** 800-785-9188
**Fax:** (707)875-2927
**Email:** secaafp@worldnet.att.net
**Website:** http://www.prosthodontics.org/aafp
Dr. Robert S. Staffanou, Sec.
**Desc:** Dentists. Provides 2-day professional continuing education course in the specialty of fixed prosthodontics. **Awards:** Stanley D. Tylman (annual) bestowed upon six graduate students for outstanding research in fixed prosthodontics.

★ 6328 ★ **American Academy of the History of Dentistry (AAHD)**
c/o Aletha A. Kowitz
100 S Vail Ave.
Arlington Heights, IL 60005-1866
**Phone:** (847)670-7561
Aletha A. Kowitz, Sec. -Treas.
**Desc:** Seeks to stimulate interest, study, and research in the history of dentistry and promote the teaching of dental history. **Awards:** Bremner Award (annual) for dental students only.

★ 6329 ★ **American Academy of Oral and Maxillofacial Radiology (AAOMR)**
PO Box 55722
Jackson, MS 39296
**Phone:** (601)984-6060          **Fax:** (601)984-6086
**Email:** mocarroll@sod.umsmed.edu
**Website:** http://www.aaomr.org
Dr. M. Kevin O Carroll, Exec. Dir.
**Desc:** Dentists and other professionals who specialize in oral and maxillofacial rediology in clinical practice,

teaching or research. Serves as authoritative body on radiation hygiene and hazards for the American Dental Association. **Awards:** Albert G. Richards Graduate Student Research Grant (annual) applied research in radiology; Charles R. Morris Student Research Award (annual); Howard R. Raper Oral and Maxillofacial Radiology Award (annual) academic achievement in graduate studies and potential for a career in academia.; Howard R. Raper Oral and Maxillofacial Radiology Award (annual) for senior dental students for achievement in oral and maxillofacial radiology; Radiology Centennial Scholarship (annual) performance during first year of graduate study; Student Award for senior dental students for achievement in oral and maxillofacial radiology; William H. Rollins Award (annual) basic research in radiology; William H. Rollins Graduate Student Research Grant (annual) academic achievement in graduate studies and potential for a career in academia.

★ 6330 ★ **American Association for Dental Research (AADR)**
1619 Duke St.
Alexandria, VA 22314-3406
**Phone:** (703)548-0066          **Fax:** (703)548-1883
**Email:** research@iadr.com
**Website:** http://www.dentalresearch.org
Eli Schwarz, DDS, Exec. Dir.
**Desc:** A division of the International Association for Dental Research. Dentists, researchers, dental schools, and dental products manufacturing companies. Seeks to promote better dental health and research activities. Presents current research information at annual meeting. Sponsors competitions; sponsors seminars. **Awards:** Distinguished Scientist Award (triennial) Outstanding scientific achievement; Research Fellowship (annual).

★ 6331 ★ **American Association of Oral and Maxillofacial Surgeons (AAOMS)**
9700 W Bryn Mawr Ave.
Rosemont, IL 60018-5701
**Phone:** (847)678-6200          **Free:** 800-822-6637
**Fax:** (847)678-6286
**Email:** inquiries@aaoms.org
**Website:** http://www.aaoms.org
Dr. Robert Rinaldi, Asst. Exec. Dir.
**Desc:** Dentists specializing in disease diagnosis and surgical, adjunctive, and esthetic treatment of diseases, injuries, and defects of the oral and maxillofacial region (jaw deformities, dental implants, infections, and oral cancer). **Awards:** Committeeman of the Year (annual); Distinguished Service Award; fellowship (annual) bestows $25,000 for research; fellowship bestows $30,000 for clinical surgery; Foundation Fellowship bestows $23,000 for one year; grant (annual) bestows two research grants of $35,000; monetary (annual) bestows up to five research awards of $1,000 each; recognition (annual) for research.

**★ 6332 ★ American Society of Master Dental Technologists (ASMDT)**
PO Box 640248
Oakland Gardens, NY 11364
**Phone:** (718)347-1239          **Fax:** (718)347-3113
**Email:** info@asmdt.com
**Website:** http://www.asmdt.com
Sue Heppenheimer, Exec. Sec.

**Desc:** Dental lab technicians. Dedicated to the upgrading of dental technology. Seeks to provide educational resources such as texts, instructors, and guidance for technicians interested in becoming master dental technologists. Conducts associate and master level courses in conjunction with New York University School of Dentistry, Dept. of Continuing Education. **Awards:** Irving Sutla Award (annual) for best tooth carving; NGS (Northeastern Grathological Society) Award (annual) for best student in courses.

**American Society of Maxillofacial Surgeons (ASMS)**
*See:* Entry 19444

**★ 6333 ★ Hispanic Dental Association**
188 W Randolph St., Ste. 1811
Chicago, IL 60601
**Phone:** (312)577-4013          **Free:** 800-852-7921
**Fax:** (312)577-4013
**Email:** hdassoc@aol.com
**Website:** http://www.hdassoc.org
Sandy Reed, Exec. Dir.

**Desc:** Provides leadership and represents professionals who share a common commitment to improve the oral health of the Hispanic community. **Awards:** HDA Foundation for entry-level dental school students.

**★ 6334 ★ International Association for Dental Research (IADR)**
1619 Duke St.
Alexandria, VA 22314
**Phone:** (703)548-0066          **Fax:** (703)548-1883
**Email:** research@iadr.com
**Website:** http://www.dentalresearch.org
Eli Schwarz, DDS, Exec. Dir.

**Desc:** Individuals engaged or interested in advancing research in the various aspects of dental and related sciences. **Awards:** Edward H. Hatton Award for winners of Junior Investigators competition; H. Trendley Dean Memorial Award for research in epidemiology and public health; Young Investigator Award for basic research in all dental research disciplines.

**★ 6335 ★ International College of Prosthodontists**
PO Box 99119
San Diego, CA 92169-1119
**Phone:** (858)270-1814
**Email:** res-inc@msn.com
**Website:** http://www.icp-org.com
Eben Yancy, Exec. Dir.

**Desc:** Prosthodontists. **Awards:** Young Prosthodontists Award (biennial).

**★ 6336 ★ National Association of Dental Assistants (NADA)**
900 S Washington St., No. G-13
Falls Church, VA 22046
**Phone:** (703)237-8616          **Fax:** (703)533-1153
R. Ludeman, Dir.

**Desc:** Professional dental auxiliaries. Seeks to: bring added stature and purpose to the profession through continuing education; make available to dental assistants the special benefits normally limited to members of specialized professional and fraternal groups. **Awards:** Scholarship (annual).

**★ 6337 ★ National Dental Association (NDA)**
3517 16th St., NW
Washington, DC 20010

**Phone:** (202)588-1697          **Fax:** (202)588-1244
**Email:** admin@ndaonline.org
**Website:** http://www.ndaonline.org
Dr. Gregory A. Stoute, Pres.

**Desc:** Professional society for dentists. Aims to provide quality dental care to the unserved and underserved public and promote knowledge of the art and science of dentistry. Advocates the inclusion of dental care services in health care programs on local, state, and national levels. Fosters the integration of minority dental health care providers in the profession, and promotes dentistry as a viable career for minorities through support programs. Conducts research programs. Group is distinct from the former name of the American Dental Association. **Awards:** Recognition; scholarship bestowed to minorities for dentistry careers.

**★ 6338 ★ National Dental Hygienists' Association (NDHA)**
c/o Barbara Seldon, Trustee
28315 Kalong Cir. W
Southfield, MI 48034
Darchelle Strickland, Pres.

**Desc:** Minority dental hygienists. To cultivate and promote the art and science of dental hygiene and to enhance the professional image of dental hygienists. Attempts to meet the needs of society through educational, political, and social activities while giving the minority dental hygienist a voice in shaping the profession. Encourages cooperation and mutual support among minority professionals. Seeks to increase opportunities for continuing education and employment in the field of dental hygiene. Works to improve individual and community dental health. Sponsors annual seminar, fundraising events, and scholarship programs; participates in career orientation programs; counsels and assists students applying for or enrolled in dental hygiene programs. Maintains liaison with American Dental Hygienists' Association. **Awards:** NDHA Scholarship (annual) for an African American individual.

**★ 6339 ★ Oral Health America**
410 N Michigan Ave., Ste. 352
Chicago, IL 60611-4211
**Phone:** (312)836-9900          **Free:** 800-523-3438
**Fax:** (312)836-9986
**Email:** liz@oralhealthamerica.org
**Website:** http://www.oralhealthamerica.org
Robert J. Klaus, Pres. & CEO

**Desc:** Funds dental education, research, and service programs. Operates speakers' bureau. **Awards:** Dental Education Fellowship (annual) for dental teacher training; Dental Laboratory Technology Scholarship (annual) for dental laboratory technology; grant for research and dental health projects; Hillenbrand Fellowship in Oral Health Policy (biennial) for dental administrator; Minority Dental Student Scholarship (annual) for minority dental students.

**★ 6340 ★ Sigma Phi Alpha**
University of Texas, Health Science Center
   Houston, Dental B
PO Box 20068
Houston, TX 77225
**Phone:** (713)500-4085
Patricia Campbell, Treas.

**Desc:** Honorary society, dental hygiene. **Awards:** Scholarship bestowed to individuals in dental hygiene; Sigma Phi Alpha Award (annual) for dental hygiene students in their final semester.

**★ 6341 ★ Society for Occlusal Studies (SOS)**
c/o Dr. Bernard Williams
4601 W 109th St., Ste. 225
Overland Park, KS 66211-1314
**Fax:** (913)941-4832
Dr. Bernard Williams, Pres.

**Desc:** Dentists and laboratory technicians who have completed the society's continuing education course in occlusion (bringing opposing surfaces of the teeth of the two jaws into contact). Promotes effective occlusal treatment. Conducts Principles of Occlusion Seminar, Advanced Restorative Seminar, laboratory technician program, and practice management program. **Awards:** Scholarship for paper presented on occlusion.

**★ 6342 ★ Xi Psi Phi**
c/o Dr. Keith W. Dickey
1623 Washington Ave., No. 300
Alton, IL 62002
**Phone:** (618)463-1889
**Email:** xipsiphi@hotmail.com
**Website:** http://www.xipsiphi.org
Dr. Keith W. Dickey, Sec. -Treas.

**Desc:** Professional dental fraternity - dentistry. Maintains Hall of Fame. Conducts educational programs. **Awards:** Reagan Scholarship (annual).

# Medical & Allied Health Schools

## Dentistry

*The following dental schools are accredited by the Commission on Dental Accreditation of the American Dental Association (ADA). For information on all dental programs, including advanced dental education, dental hygiene, dental assistant, and dental laboratory technician, contact the ADA at 211 E Chicago Ave., Chicago, IL 60611, (312)440-2500, http://www.ada.org/.*

### Alabama

**★ 6343 ★ University of Alabama, Birmingham School of Dentistry**
1919 7th Ave. S
Birmingham, AL 35294
**Phone:** (205)934-4720          **Fax:** (205)934-9283
**Website:** http://www.dental.uab.edu
Dr. Mary Lynne Capilouto, Director

### California

**★ 6344 ★ Loma Linda University School of Dentistry**
Loma Linda, CA 92350
**Phone:** (909)558-1200          **Free:** 800-422-4558
**Fax:** (714)824-4211
**Website:** http://www.llu.edu/llu/dentistry
Dr. Charles J. Goodacre, Director

**★ 6345 ★ University of California, Los Angeles School of Dentistry**
Center for the Health Sciences
10833 Leconte Ave., Rm. 53-038
Los Angeles, CA 90095-1668
**Phone:** (310)825-7354          **Fax:** (310)206-5539
**Website:** http://www.dent.ucla.edu
Dr. No-Hee Park, Director

**★ 6346 ★ University of California, San Francisco School of Dentistry**
513 Parnassus Ave., S-630
San Francisco, CA 94143
**Phone:** (415)476-1323          **Fax:** (415)476-4226
**Website:** http://www.ucsf.edu
Dr. Charles Bertolami, Director

**★ 6347 ★ University of the Pacific**
**School of Dentistry**
2155 Webster St.
San Francisco, CA 94115
**Phone:** (415)929-6400     **Fax:** (415)929-6654
**Website:** http://www.dental.uop.edu
Dr. Arthur A. Dugoni, Director

**★ 6348 ★ University of Southern California**
**School of Dentistry**
University Park, MC-0641, Rm. 203
Los Angeles, CA 90089-0641
**Phone:** (213)740-2800     **Fax:** (213)740-3607
**Website:** http://www.usc.edu/hsc/dental
Dr. Harold Slavkin, Director

### Colorado

**★ 6349 ★ University of Colorado Medical Center**
**School of Dentistry**
4200 E 9th Ave.
Box C-284
Denver, CO 80262
**Phone:** (303)315-8752     **Fax:** (303)315-8773
**Website:** http://www.uchsc.edu/sd/sd
Dr. Howard M. Landesman, Director

### Connecticut

**★ 6350 ★ University of Connecticut**
**School of Dental Medicine**
263 Farmington Ave.
Farmington, CT 06032-5332
**Phone:** (203)679-2808     **Fax:** (203)679-1330
**Website:** http://sdm.uchc.edu
Dr. Peter J. Robinson, Director

### District of Columbia

**★ 6351 ★ Howard University**
**College of Dentistry**
600 W St. NW
Washington, DC 20059
**Phone:** (202)806-0440     **Fax:** (202)806-0354
**Website:** http://www.howard.edu
Dr. Charles Sanders, Director

### Florida

**★ 6352 ★ Nova Southeastern University**
**College of Dental Medicine**
3200 S University Dr.
Fort Lauderdale, FL 33328
**Phone:** (954)262-7319     **Fax:** (954)262-1782
**Website:** http://www.nova.edu/cwis/centers/hpd/dental
Dr. Robert Uchin, Director

**★ 6353 ★ University of Florida**
**College of Dentistry**
PO Box 100405
Gainesville, FL 32610-0405
**Phone:** (352)392-2911     **Fax:** (352)392-3070
**Website:** http://www.dental.ufl.edu
Dr. Frank A. Catalanotto, Director

### Georgia

**★ 6354 ★ Medical College of Georgia**
**School of Dentistry**
1459 Laney Walker Blvd.
Augusta, GA 30912-0200
**Phone:** (706)721-3587     **Fax:** (706)721-6276
**Website:** http://www.mcg.edu/SOD
Dr. Brad J. Potter, Director

### Illinois

**★ 6355 ★ Southern Illinois University**
**School of Dental Medicine**
Bldg. 273/2300
2800 College Ave.
Alton, IL 62002
**Phone:** (618)474-7170     **Fax:** (618)474-7150
**Website:** http://www.siue.edu/DMSCH
Dr. Patrick Ferrillo, Jr., Director

**★ 6356 ★ University of Illinois, Chicago**
**College of Dentistry**
801 S Paulina St.
Chicago, IL 60612
**Phone:** (312)996-7520     **Fax:** (312)996-1022
**Website:** http://dentistry.uic.edu
Dr. Bruce S. Graham, Director

### Indiana

**★ 6357 ★ Indiana University**
**School of Dentistry**
1121 W Michigan St.
Indianapolis, IN 46202
**Phone:** (317)274-7957     **Fax:** (317)274-2419
**Website:** http://www.iusd.iupui.edu
Dr. Lawrence Goldblatt, Director

### Iowa

**★ 6358 ★ University of Iowa**
**College of Dentistry**
Dental Bldg.
Iowa City, IA 52242
**Phone:** (319)335-9650     **Fax:** (319)335-7155
**Website:** http://www.uiowa.edu/homepage/academics
Dr. David Johnsen, Director

### Kentucky

**★ 6359 ★ University of Kentucky**
**College of Dentistry**
Medical Center
800 Rose St.
Lexington, KY 40536-0084
**Phone:** (606)233-5850     **Fax:** (606)258-1042
**Website:** www.mc.uky.edu/Dentistry
Dr. Leon A. Assael, Director

**★ 6360 ★ University of Louisville**
**School of Dentistry**
Health Sciences Center
Louisville, KY 40202
**Phone:** (502)588-5293     **Fax:** (502)588-7163
**Website:** http://www.dental.louisville.edu/dental
Dr. John N. Williams, Director

### Louisiana

**★ 6361 ★ Louisiana State University**
**School of Dentistry**
1100 Florida Ave., Bldg. 101
New Orleans, LA 70119
**Phone:** (504)619-8700
**Website:** http://www.lsusd.lsumc.edu
Dr. Eric J. Hovland, Contact

### Maryland

**★ 6362 ★ University of Maryland**
**Baltimore College of Dental Surgery**
666 W Baltimore St., Rm. 4-A-11
Baltimore, MD 21201
**Phone:** (410)706-7461     **Fax:** (410)706-0406
**Website:** http://www.dental.umaryland.edu
Dr. Richard Ranney, Director

### Massachusetts

**★ 6363 ★ Boston University**
**Henry M. Goldman School of Dental Medicine**
100 E Newton St.
Boston, MA 02118
**Phone:** (617)638-4700     **Fax:** (617)638-4490
**Website:** http://dentalschool.bu.edu
Dr. Spencer N. Frankl, Director

**★ 6364 ★ Harvard University**
**School of Dental Medicine**
188 Longwood Ave.
Boston, MA 02115
**Phone:** (617)432-1405     **Fax:** (617)432-4266
**Website:** http://www.hsdm.med.harvard.edu
Dr. R. Bruce Donoff, Director

**★ 6365 ★ Tufts University**
**School of Dental Medicine**
1 Kneeland St.
Boston, MA 02111
**Phone:** (617)636-7000     **Fax:** (617)636-0309
**Website:** http://www.tufts.edu/dental
Dr. Lonnie H. Norris, Director

### Michigan

**★ 6366 ★ University of Detroit Mercy**
**School of Dentistry**
8200 W Outer Dr.
PO Box 98
Detroit, MI 48219-0900
**Phone:** (313)446-1800     **Free:** 800-635-5020
**Fax:** (313)446-1839
Dr. H. Robert Steiman, Director

**★ 6367 ★ University of Michigan**
**School of Dentistry**
1234 Dental Bldg.
Ann Arbor, MI 48109-1078
**Phone:** (734)763-6933     **Fax:** (313)747-4024
**Website:** http://www.dent.umich.edu
Dr. William E. Kotowicz, Director

### Minnesota

**★ 6368 ★ University of Minnesota**
**School of Dentistry**
515 SE Delaware St.
Minneapolis, MN 55455
**Phone:** (612)625-9982     **Fax:** (612)626-2654
**Website:** http://www.umn.edu/dental
Dr. Peter Polverini, Director

### Mississippi

**★ 6369 ★ University of Mississippi**
**School of Dentistry**
Medical Center
2500 N State St.
Jackson, MS 39216-4505
**Phone:** (601)984-6028
**Website:** http://www.dentistry.umc.edu
Dr. Willie J. Hill, Director

### Missouri

**★ 6370 ★ University of Missouri, Kansas City**
**School of Dentistry**
650 E 25th St.
Kansas City, MO 64108
**Phone:** (816)235-2100     **Fax:** (816)235-2157
**Website:** http://www.umkc.edu/dentistry
Dr. Michael J. Reed, Director

## Nebraska

**★ 6371 ★ Creighton University**
**School of Dentistry**
2500 California St.
Omaha, NE 68178
**Phone:** (402)280-5060          **Fax:** (402)280-5094
**Website:** http://cudental.creighton.edu
Dr. Wayne W. Barkmeier, Director

**★ 6372 ★ University of Nebraska Medical Center**
**College of Dentistry**
Medical Center
40th and Holdrege Sts.
Lincoln, NE 68583-0740
**Phone:** (402)472-1363          **Free:** 800-626-8431
**Fax:** (402)472-6681
**Website:** http://www.unmc.edu/dentistry
Dr. John Reinhardt, Director

## New Jersey

**★ 6373 ★ University of Medicine and Dentistry of New Jersey**
**Dental School**
110 Bergen St.
Newark, NJ 07103-2425
**Website:** http://www.umdnj.edu
Dr. Cecile Feldman, Director

## New York

**★ 6374 ★ Columbia University**
**School of Dental and Oral Surgery**
630 W 168th St.
New York, NY 10032
**Phone:** (212)305-2500          **Fax:** (212)305-7134
**Website:** http://cpmcnet.columbia.edu/dept/dental
Dr. Ira B. Lamster, Director

**★ 6375 ★ New York University**
**College of Dentistry**
345 E 24th St.
New York, NY 10010
**Phone:** (212)998-9800          **Fax:** (212)995-4080
**Website:** http://www.nyu.edu/Dental
Dr. Michael C. Alfano, Director

**★ 6376 ★ State University of New York, Buffalo**
**School of Dental Medicine**
325 Squire Hall
Buffalo, NY 14214
**Phone:** (716)829-2836          **Fax:** (716)829-2387
**Website:** http://www.sdm.buffalo.edu
Dr. Richard N. Buchanan, Director

**★ 6377 ★ State University of New York, Stony Brook**
**School of Dental Medicine**
Rockland Hall
Stony Brook, NY 11794-8700
**Phone:** (516)632-8950          **Fax:** (516)632-9105
**Website:** http://www.informatics.sunysb.edu/dental
Dr. Barry R. Rifkin, Director

## North Carolina

**★ 6378 ★ University of North Carolina, Chapel Hill**
**School of Dentistry**
104 Brauer Hall, 211-H
Chapel Hill, NC 27599-7450
**Phone:** (919)966-1161          **Fax:** (919)966-4049
**Website:** http://www.dent.unc.edu
Dr. John W. Stamm, Director

## Ohio

**★ 6379 ★ Case Western Reserve University**
**School of Dentistry**
2123 Abington Rd.
Cleveland, OH 44106
**Phone:** (216)368-3200          **Fax:** (216)368-3204
**Website:** http://www.cwru.edu/dental/casewebsite
Dr. Jerold Goldberg, Director

**★ 6380 ★ Ohio State University**
**College of Dentistry**
305 W 12th Ave.
Columbus, OH 43210
**Phone:** (614)292-9755          **Fax:** (614)292-7619
**Website:** www.dent.ohio-state.edu
Dr. Jan E. Kronmiller, Director

## Oklahoma

**★ 6381 ★ University of Oklahoma**
**College of Dentistry**
PO Box 26901
Oklahoma City, OK 73190
**Phone:** (405)271-5444          **Fax:** (405)271-3423
**Email:** dentistry@ouhsc.edu
**Website:** http://dentistry.ouhsc.edu
Dr. Stephen K. Young, Director

## Oregon

**★ 6382 ★ Oregon Health Sciences University**
**School of Dentistry, Sam Jackson Pk.**
611 SW Campus Dr.
Portland, OR 97201
**Phone:** (503)494-8801          **Fax:** (503)494-8801
**Website:** http://www.ohsu.edu/sod-A
Dr. Sharon P. Turner, Director

## Pennsylvania

**★ 6383 ★ Temple University**
**School of Dentistry**
3223 N Broad St.
Philadelphia, PA 19140
**Phone:** (215)221-2803          **Fax:** (215)221-2802
**Website:** http://www.temple.edu
Dr. Martin F. Tansy, Director

**★ 6384 ★ University of Pennsylvania**
**School of Dental Medicine**
4001 W Spruce St.
Philadelphia, PA 19104
**Phone:** (215)898-8961          **Fax:** (215)898-5243
**Website:** http://www.dental.upenn.edu
Dr. Raymond Fonseca, Director

**★ 6385 ★ University of Pittsburgh**
**School of Dental Medicine**
3501 Terrace St.
Pittsburgh, PA 15261
**Phone:** (412)648-8900          **Fax:** (412)648-8219
**Website:** http://www.dental.pitt.edu
Dr. Thomas Braun, Director

## Puerto Rico

**★ 6386 ★ University of Puerto Rico**
**School of Dentistry**
Medical Sciences Campus
PO Box 365067
San Juan, PR 00936-5067
**Phone:** (787)758-2525          **Fax:** (787)751-0990
Dr. Fernadndo Haddock, Director

## South Carolina

**★ 6387 ★ Medical University of South Carolina**
**College of Dental Medicine**
171 Ashley Ave.
Charleston, SC 29425
**Phone:** (803)792-3811          **Fax:** (803)792-0390
**Website:** http://www2.musc.edu/dentistry/dental.html
Dr. Richard De Champlain, Director

## Tennessee

**★ 6388 ★ Meharry Medical College**
**School of Dentistry**
1005 Dr. D.B. Todd Blvd.
Nashville, TN 37208
**Phone:** (615)327-6207          **Fax:** (615)327-6213
Dr. William B. Butler, Director

**★ 6389 ★ University of Tennessee, Memphis**
**College of Dentistry**
875 Union Ave.
Memphis, TN 38163
**Phone:** (901)448-6204          **Free:** 800-788-0040
**Fax:** (901)448-7104
**Website:** http://www.utmem.edu/dentistry
Dr. William F. Slagle, Director

## Texas

**★ 6390 ★ Texas A&M University**
**Baylor College of Dentistry**
3302 Gaston Ave.
Dallas, TX 75246
**Phone:** (214)828-8100          **Fax:** (214)828-8496
**Website:** http://www.tambcd.edu
Dr. James Cole, Director

**★ 6391 ★ University of Texas Health Science Center, Houston**
**Dental Branch**
6516 John Freeman Ave.
Houston, TX 77030
**Phone:** (713)792-4021          **Fax:** (713)792-4189
**Website:** http://www.db.uth.tmc.edu
Dr. Ronald Johnson, Director

**★ 6392 ★ University of Texas Health Science Center, San Antonio**
**Dental School**
7703 Floyd Curl Dr.
San Antonio, TX 78284-7914
**Phone:** (512)567-3160          **Fax:** (512)567-6721
**Website:** http://www.dental.uthscsa.edu
Dr. Kenneth L. Kalkwarf, Director

## Virginia

**★ 6393 ★ Virginia Commonwealth University**
**School of Dentistry**
PO Box 980566
Richmond, VA 23298-0566
**Phone:** (804)828-9196          **Fax:** (804)371-6072
**Website:** http://www.dentistry.vcu.edu
Dr. Ronald J. Hunt, Jr., Director

## Washington

**★ 6394 ★ University of Washington**
**School of Dentistry**
Health Sciences Bldg., Room D-322
PO Box 356365
Seattle, WA 98195
**Phone:** (206)543-5840          **Fax:** (206)616-2612
**Website:** http://www.dental.washington.edu
Dr. James C. Steiner, Director

## West Virginia

**★ 6395 ★ West Virginia University
School of Dentistry**
The Medical Ctr.
PO Box 9400
Morgantown, WV 26506-9400
**Phone:** (304)293-3511  **Fax:** (304)293-2859
Dr. James J. Koelbl, Director

## Wisconsin

**★ 6396 ★ Marquette University
School of Dentistry**
PO Box 1881
Milwaukee, WI 53201
**Phone:** (414)288-3532  **Fax:** (414)288-6505
**Website:** http://www.dental.mu.edu
Dr. William K. Lobb, Director

# National & International
# Organizations

**★ 6397 ★ Academy of Dental Materials
(ADM)**
WVU School of Dentistry
HSC North
Morgantown, WV 26506-9403
**Phone:** (304)293-2859  **Fax:** (304)293-4719
**Email:** mbagby@hsc.wvu.edu
**Website:** http://www.academydentalmaterials.org
Mike Bagby, Treas.
**Fnded:** 1940. **Mem:** 300. **Desc:** Active members are licensed dentists, members of academic institutions, industrial employees, and individuals active or interested in dental materials. Coordinates activities relating to the use of dental materials. **Pub:** *ADM Newsletter*, 3/year. Newsletter. • *Dental Materials*, bimonthly. Journal. Covers scientific research. *Price:* Included in membership dues; $195 for nonmembers. • *Transactions of the Academy of Dental Materials.* • Directory, periodic. **Frmly:** (1983) American Academy for Plastics Research in Dentistry.

**★ 6398 ★ Academy of Dental Sleep
Medicine**
10592 Perry Hwy., No. 220
Wexford, PA 15090-9244
**Phone:** (724)935-0836  **Fax:** (724)935-0383
**Email:** execdirector@dentalsleepmed.org
**Website:** http://www.dentalsleepmed.org
Mary Beth Rogers, Exec. Dir.
**Fnded:** 1991. **Mem:** 500. **Desc:** Dentists, physicians, and PhD's active in sleep disorder medicine. Seeks to improve the treatment of patients with sleep disorders through the involvement of dental practicioners and use of oral appliances in overall therapy and to enhance the lives of people suffering form sleep disorders. Supports research in application of dental appliances in the treatment of sleep disorders, such as snoring and sleep apnea; conducts educational and certification programs; establishes dental treatment protocol; disseminates information on sleep disorder treatment; facilitates the exchange of information; operates the SDDS Resource Center. **Pub:** *ADSM Dialogue*, quarterly. Newsletter.

**★ 6399 ★ Academy of Dentistry
International (ADI)**
PO Box 307
Hicksville, OH 43526
**Phone:** (419)542-0101
**Email:** rramus@bright.net
**Website:** http://www.adint.org
Robert L. Ramus, DDS, Exec. Dir.
**Fnded:** 1974. **Mem:** 2,400. **Nat'l Groups:** 55. **Reg. Groups:** 10. **State Groups:** 4. **Desc:** Dentists; membership by invitation only. Works to further dentistry and the prevention of dental diseases worldwide. Disseminates and promotes the exchange of scientific information and fosters research. **Pub:** *International Communicator*, semiannual. Newsletter. *Price:* Included in membership dues. • *Roster of ADI*, periodic.

**★ 6400 ★ Academy of General Dentistry
(AGD)**
211 E Chicago Ave., Ste. 900
Chicago, IL 60611
**Phone:** (312)440-4300  **Free:** 888-243-3368
**Fax:** (312)440-0559
**Email:** agddented@agd.org
**Website:** http://www.agd.org
Harold E. Donnell, Jr., Exec. Dir.
**Fnded:** 1952. **Mem:** 37,000. **Reg. Groups:** 20. **State Groups:** 62. **Local Groups:** 35. **Desc:** Seeks to serve the needs and represent the interest of general dentists. Fosters their dentists'continued proficiency through quality continuing dental education. **Pub:** *AGD Impact*, 11/year. Magazine. Covers issues, legislation, and trends that affect the practice and role of dentistry in the health care community. *Price:* Included in membership dues; $25/year for nonmembers. • *Dentalnotes*, quarterly. Newsletter. Provides information on the latest dental issues and trends; intended for the national media and to be displayed in dentists' reception areas. *Price:* $20 /year for members; $40 / year for nonmembers. • *General Dentistry*, bimonthly. Journal. Provides research and clinical reports for the continuing education of general dentists. Contains advertisers' index, book reviews, and quizzes. *Price:* Included in membership dues; $30/year for nonmembers.

**★ 6401 ★ Academy for Implants and
Transplants (AIT)**
PO Box 223
Springfield, VA 22150
**Phone:** (703)451-0001  **Fax:** (703)451-0004
Anthony J. Viscido, D.D.S., Sec. -Treas.
**Fnded:** 1972. **Mem:** 180. **Reg. Groups:** 15. **Desc:** Dentists united to: motivate and assist men and women in the general practice of dentistry in the field of implants and transplants; encourage and promote the art and science of implant and transplant dentistry; assist in research in this and allied fields. Conducts seminars; teaches implantology. **Pub:** *Implant Update*, quarterly. Newsletter. Discusses developments in the field of implant and transplant dentistry. *Price:* Included in membership dues. • Journal, periodic.

**★ 6402 ★ Academy of Laser Dentistry**
PO Box 8667
Coral Springs, FL 33075
**Phone:** (954)346-3776  **Fax:** (954)757-2598
**Email:** memberservices@laserdentistry.org
**Website:** http://www.laserdentistry.org
Gail S. Siminovsky, Exec. Dir.
**Fnded:** 1993. **Mem:** 600. **Nat'l Groups:** 3. **Desc:** Dentists, hygienists, dental academicians and researchers, and corporate laser and laser accessory dental vendors. Promotes clinical education, research, and development of standards and guidelines for the safe and ethical use of dental laser technology. Conducts educational programs. Provides certification. **Pub:** *Wavelengths*, quarterly. Journal. Clinical case studies, industry and academy news. *Price:* Included in membership.

**★ 6403 ★ Academy of Operative
Dentistry (AOD)**
PO Box 991
Midway, UT 84049
**Phone:** (435)654-0794
Dr. Ebb A. Berry, III, Pres.
**Fnded:** 1972. **Mem:** 1,000. **Desc:** Dentists and persons in allied industries. Seeks to ensure quality in all of operative dentistry, teaching, service, research. **Pub:** *Membership Roster*, periodic. • *Operative Dentistry*, 6/year.

**★ 6404 ★ Academy of Oral Dynamics
(AOD)**
8919 Sudley Rd.
Manassas, VA 20110
**Phone:** (703)368-8527  **Fax:** (703)331-0356
Dr. E. Paul Byrne, Sec.
**Fnded:** 1950. **Mem:** 75. **Desc:** Professional society of dentists. Promotes the study of oral dynamics, especially as it applies to the use of natural teeth in restoring and maintaining a healthy, functioning mouth; disseminates information gained through research. Conducts educational programs. **Frmly:** (1950) International Academy of Oral Dynamics.

**★ 6405 ★ Academy of Osseointegration**
85 W Algonquin Rd., Ste. 550
Arlington Heights, IL 60005-4460
**Phone:** (847)439-1919  **Free:** 800-656-7736
**Fax:** (847)439-1569
**Email:** academy@osseo.org
**Website:** http://www.osseo.org
Kevin P. Smith, Exec. Dir.
**Fnded:** 1987. **Mem:** 4,200. **Desc:** Works for the advancement of osseointegration among dentists, physicians and related professionals. Conducts research and educational programs; disseminates information to the public and medical agencies; provides a forum for interdisciplinary discussions. **Pub:** *Academy News*, bimonthly. Newsletter. • *International Journal of Oral & Maxillofacial Implants*, bimonthly. Journal. Includes current information related to the management of patients utilizing implant modalities. *Price:* $118 in U.S.; $158 outside U.S.

**★ 6406 ★ Alliance of the American
Dental Association (AADA)**
211 E Chicago Ave., 5th Fl.
Chicago, IL 60611
**Phone:** (312)440-2865  **Free:** 800-621-8099
**Fax:** (312)440-2587
**Email:** allianceada@mindspring.com
**Website:** http://www.allianceADA.org
Sheila Duda, Exec. Dir.
**Fnded:** 1955. **Mem:** 12,000. **Nat'l Groups:** 1. **State Groups:** 32. **Local Groups:** 160. **Desc:** Spouses of dentists. Promotes public dental health and creates public awareness of dentistry. Conducts preventive dental health education programs and assists organized dentistry in encouraging state and national legislation that benefits the public and dentistry. Maintains legislative projects and leadership skill development. **Pub:** *Key*, quarterly. Newsletter. **Frmly:** Auxiliary to the American Dental Association; (1982) Women's Auxiliary to the American Dental Association.

**★ 6407 ★ Alpha Omega International
Dental Fraternity**
500 Commonwealth Dr.
Warrendale, PA 15086
**Phone:** (724)778-3419  **Free:** 800-MRS-TINT
**Fax:** (724)772-8349
**Email:** headquarters@ao.org
**Website:** http://www.ao.org/
Stephanie Block, Exec. Dir.
**Fnded:** 1907. **Mem:** 15,000. **Local Groups:** 125. **Desc:** Professional fraternity - dentistry. Encourages fraternalism and monitors discrimination in dental schools. Maintains the Alpha Omega Foundation, which sends funds to dental schools in Israel and the U.S. Holds continuing education seminars. **Pub:** *Alpha Omegan*, quarterly. • *AO Today*, quarterly. Newsletter. Provides information on dental education in the United States and Israel. *Price:* Included in membership dues.

**★ 6408 ★ American Academy of
Cosmetic Dentistry (AACD)**
2810 Walton Commons W, Ste. 200
Madison, WI 53718
**Phone:** (608)222-8583  **Free:** 800-543-9220
**Fax:** (608)222-9540
**Email:** info@aacd.com

**Website:** http://www.aacd.com
Kenneth L. Zakariasen, DDS, Contact
**Fnded:** 1984. **Mem:** 4,300. **Desc:** Cosmetic dentists. Seeks to advance the study, teaching, and practice of cosmetic dentistry. Facilitates exchange of information among members; conducts educational programs.

## ★ 6409 ★ American Academy of Craniofacial Pain (AACP)

520 W Pipeline Rd.
Hurst, TX 76053-4924
**Phone:** (817)282-1501    **Free:** 800-322-8651
**Fax:** (817)282-8012
**Email:** central@aacfp.org
**Website:** http://www.aacfp.org
Cordelia Mason, Exec. Sec.
**Fnded:** 1985. **Mem:** 525. **Desc:** Health Care Practitioners who treat head, facial, and neck pain. Functions as a referral service for patients suffering from head, facial, and neck pain worldwide. Plans to establish computerized medical procedures and insurance database. **Pub:** *Membership List*, periodic.

## ★ 6410 ★ American Academy of Dental Group Practice (AADGP)

2525 E Arizona Biltmore Cir., Ste. 127
Phoenix, AZ 85016
**Phone:** (602)381-1185    **Fax:** (602)381-1093
**Email:** info@aadgp.org
**Website:** http://www.aadgp.org
Dr. Hugh Norsted, Pres.
**Fnded:** 1973. **Mem:** 2,000. **Nat'l Groups:** 1. **Desc:** Active dentists and dental group practices. Purpose is to improve the level of dental service provided by members through exchanging and expanding of ideas and techniques for patient treatment and practice administration. Promotes group practice and research; accumulates and disseminates information; seeks to achieve the proper recognition for the aims and goals of group practice. Helps support an accreditation program as a system of voluntary peer review. **Pub:** *AADGP Contact*, quarterly. Newsletter. • Membership Directory, biennial.

## ★ 6411 ★ American Academy of Dental Practice Administration (AADPA)

c/o Kathleen Uebel
1063 Whippoorwill Ln.
Palatine, IL 60067-7064
**Phone:** (847)934-4404    **Fax:** (847)934-4410
**Email:** aadpa@aol.com
**Website:** http://www.aadpa.org
Kathleen S. Uebel, Exec. Ed.
**Fnded:** 1956. **Mem:** 250. **Desc:** Professional society of dentists interested in efficient administration of dental practice. Offers educational programs. **Pub:** *American Academy of Dental Practice Administration–Communicator*, 3/year. Newsletter. *Price:* Free. For members only. • *American Academy of Dental Practice Administration–Roster*, annual. *Price:* For members only. • *Essay Tapes*, annual.

## ★ 6412 ★ American Academy of Esthetic Dentistry (AAED)

401 N Michigan Ave.
Chicago, IL 60611
**Phone:** (312)321-5121    **Fax:** (312)673-6952
**Email:** aaed@sba.com
**Website:** http://www.estheticacademy.org/
Frank M. Spear, DDS, Pres.
**Fnded:** 1975. **Mem:** 138. **Desc:** Dentists seeking to advance the art and science of esthetic dentistry (dentistry concerned with restorative procedures of natural teeth). **Pub:** *Journal of Esthetic Dentistry*. Journal. • *Journal of Pasthetic Dentistry*. Journal. *Price:* $105.50.

## ★ 6413 ★ American Academy of Fixed Prosthodontics (AAFP)

PO Box 1409
Bodega Bay, CA 94923-1409

**Phone:** (707)875-3040    **Free:** 800-785-9188
**Fax:** (707)875-2927
**Email:** secaafp@worldnet.att.net
**Website:** http://www.prosthodontics.org/aafp
Dr. Robert S. Staffanou, Sec.
**Fnded:** 1951. **Mem:** 606. **Desc:** Dentists. Provides 2-day professional continuing education course in the specialty of fixed prosthodontics. **Pub:** *American Academy of Fixed Prosthodontics Newsletter*, semiannual. Newsletter. *Price:* Included in membership dues. • *Journal of Prosthetic Dentistry*, monthly. Journal. • *Meeting Program/Directory*, annual. Directory. **Frmly:** (1991) American Academy of Crown and Bridge Prosthodontics.

## ★ 6414 ★ American Academy of Gnathologic Orthopedics (AAGO)

2651 Oak Grove Rd.
Walnut Creek, CA 94598
**Free:** 800-510-AAGO    **Fax:** (925)676-7678
**Website:** http://www.aago.com
John Rothchild, D.D.S., Exec. Dir.
**Fnded:** 1970. **Mem:** 700. **Nat'l Groups:** 1. **Reg. Groups:** 9. **State Groups:** 16. **Desc:** Dentists dealing with the prevention or correction of malocclusion and bony misformation of the jaw and face. Conducts activities in the fields of maxillofacial orthopedics/orthodontics and preventative and corrective orthodontics. **Pub:** *American Academy of Gnathologic Orthopedics–Journal*, quarterly. Journal. Includes scientific articles and case reports on orthodontic treatment. *Price:* $80 plus postage in U.S.; $85 Canada; $100 foreign. • *American Academy of Gnathologic Orthopedics–Membership Roster*, annual. Membership Directory. *Price:* Included in membership dues. • Articles.On the Crozat Method.

## ★ 6415 ★ American Academy of Gold Foil Operators (AAGFO)

17922 Tallgrass Ct.
Noblesville, IN 46060
**Phone:** (317)867-3011    **Fax:** (317)867-3011
**Email:** piperon@earthlink.net
**Website:** http://www.goldfoil.org
Dr. Ronald K. Harris, Sec. -Treas.
**Fnded:** 1952. **Mem:** 285. **Desc:** Dentists who perform restorative procedures utilizing gold foil, cast gold, and the rubber dam. Formulates and applies new ideas for research on gold restorations and the rubber dam; encourages members of the dental profession and research institutions in the armed forces, government, dental schools, and private enterprise to study gold restorations and rubber dam procedures. Presents chair demonstrations at dental schools. **Pub:** *Gold Leaf*, semiannual. • *Journal of Operative Dentistry*, bimonthly. Journal. • *Roster*, biennial. • Also prepares slides, charts, models, and written materials.

## ★ 6416 ★ American Academy of the History of Dentistry (AAHD)

c/o Aletha A. Kowitz
100 S Vail Ave.
Arlington Heights, IL 60005-1866
**Phone:** (847)670-7561
Aletha A. Kowitz, Sec. -Treas.
**Fnded:** 1951. **Mem:** 450. **Desc:** Seeks to stimulate interest, study, and research in the history of dentistry and promote the teaching of dental history. **Pub:** *Journal of the History of Dentistry*, 3/year. Journal. Includes articles on the history of dentistry, book reviews, and 5yr cumulative index. *Price:* $55/year.

## ★ 6417 ★ American Academy of Implant Dentistry (AAID)

211 E Chicago Ave., Ste. 750
Chicago, IL 60611
**Phone:** (312)335-1550    **Free:** 877-335-2243
**Fax:** (312)335-9090
**Email:** aaid@aaid-implant.org
**Website:** http://www.aaid-implant.org
J. Vincent Shuck, Exec. Dir.

**Fnded:** 1952. **Mem:** 2,200. **Reg. Groups:** 4. **Desc:** Dedicated to furthering scientific research and development in the field of implantology. **Pub:** *AAIDNEWS*, quarterly. Newsletter. Includes news and calendar updates of Academy events. *Price:* Free to members. • *American Academy of Implant Dentistry*, annual. Directory. Arranged geographically and alphabetically. *Price:* Free to members. • *Journal of Oral Implantology*, bimonthly. Journal. Contains original manuscripts, clinical presentations, research annotations, and educational reports pertinent to dental studies. *Price:* Included in membership dues; $75/year for nonmembers; $100/year for libraries, corporations, and institutes. **Frmly:** American Academy of Implant Dentures.

## ★ 6418 ★ American Academy of Implant Prosthodontics (AAIP)

760 Whitehall Way
Roswell, GA 30076
**Phone:** (770)594-8380    **Fax:** (770)998-9924
**Email:** drmfaganjr@mindspring.com
Dr. Maurice Fagan, Jr., Contact
**Fnded:** 1980. **Mem:** 300. **Nat'l Groups:** 1. **Desc:** Experts in dental implantology; dental school professors. Encourages continuing education, advancement, and research in implant dentistry; believes that prosthodontics and implantology education and research should take place in academic institutions. Promotes the surgical insertion of dental transplants and the design and insertion of prosthodontic devices to replace missing teeth. Emphasizes research on the construction and maintenance of fixed and removable prostheses. Conducts continuing education courses in conjunction with dental schools. Maintains speakers' bureau and small library. **Pub:** *The Dental Implant - Clinical and Biological Response of Oral Tissues.* • *Implant Prosthodontics - Surgical and Prosthetic Techniques for Dental Implants.* • Membership Directory, periodic. • Newsletter, 3/year.

## ★ 6419 ★ American Academy of Maxillofacial Prosthetics (AAMP)

c/o Dr. Thomas Cowper
9360 Winchester Valley
Chesterland, OH 44026
**Phone:** (216)444-2084    **Fax:** (216)445-6360
**Email:** rjacob@mail.mdanderson.org
**Website:** http://www.maxillofacialprosth.org/maxillofacial/
Dr. Thomas Cowper, Exec. Sec. -Treas.
**Fnded:** 1953. **Mem:** 148. **Desc:** Dentists specializing in maxillofacial prosthetics. **Pub:** *Journal of Prosthetic Dentistry*, monthly. Journal.

## American Academy of Oral and Maxillofacial Pathology (AAOMP)

*See:* Entry 17123

## ★ 6420 ★ American Academy of Oral and Maxillofacial Radiology (AAOMR)

PO Box 55722
Jackson, MS 39296
**Phone:** (601)984-6060    **Fax:** (601)984-6086
**Email:** mocarroll@sod.umsmed.edu
**Website:** http://www.aaomr.org
Dr. M. Kevin O Carroll, Exec. Dir.
**Fnded:** 1949. **Mem:** 400. **Nat'l Groups:** 1. **Desc:** Dentists and other professionals who specialize in oral and maxillofacial radiology in clinical practice, teaching or research. Serves as authoritative body on radiation hygiene and hazards for the American Dental Association. **Pub:** *AAOMR Newsletter*, quarterly. Newsletter. Features news, president's messages, & announcements. *Price:* Free. • *Oral and Maxillofacial Radiology Section of Oral Surgery, Oral Medicine, Oral Pathology, Oral Radiology, and Endodontics*, monthly. Journal. *Price:* Included in active membership dues; $45 for corporate, associate, affiliate, student, and Life members. • *Roster of Membership*, annual. **Frmly:** (1951) American Academy of Oral Roentgenology; (1967) American Academy of Dental Radiology.

**★ 6421 ★ American Academy of Oral Medicine (AAOM)**
2910 Lightfoot Dr.
Baltimore, MD 21209
**Phone:** (410)602-8585
**Email:** info@AAOM.com
**Website:** http://www.aaom.com
Joyce Caplan, Exec. Sec.

**Fnded:** 1946. **Mem:** 800. **Reg. Groups:** 4. **Desc:** Dental educators, specialists, general dentists, and physicians interested in the study of the oral health care of medically compromised patients and the nonsurgical management of medically related diseases and disorders affecting the maxillofacial region. Promotes an improved quality of life for people with oral and maxillofacial diseases and disorders; fosters better scientific understanding between the fields of dentistry and medicine. Maintains speakers' bureau; offers continuing education lectures and seminars. **Pub:** *AAOM/OTOD*, quarterly. Newsletter. • *The Clinician's Guide to Oral Health in Geriatric Patients.* Monograph. • *The Clinician's Guide to the Treatment of the Medically-Complex Dental Patient.* Monograph. • *The Clinician's Guide to Treatment of Common Oral Conditions*, every 3-5 years. Monograph. *Price:* $11.95. • *The Clinician's Guide to Treatment of HIV-infected Patients*, periodic. Monograph. *Price:* Included in membership dues; $12/year for nonmembers. • *Diagnosis and Treatment of Chronic Orofacial Pain.* Monograph. • *Oral Surgery, Oral Medicine, Oral Pathology, Oral Radiology and Endodontics.* Journal.

**★ 6422 ★ American Academy of Orofacial Pain (AAOP)**
19 Mantua Rd.
Mount Royal, NJ 08061
**Phone:** (856)423-3629          **Fax:** (856)423-3420
**Email:** aaopco@talley.com
**Website:** http://www.aaop.org
Steven G. Messing, Pres.

**Fnded:** 1975. **Mem:** 330. **Desc:** Medical and dental doctors. Seeks to further knowledge of Orofacial Pain and Temporomandibular Disorders. Maintains patient referral program. **Pub:** *Journal of Orofacial Pain*, quarterly. Journal. • *Orofacial Pain: Guidelines for Classification, Assessment, and Management.* • *Temporomandibular Disorders: Guidelines for Classification, Assessment, and Management.* **Frmly:** (1979) American Academy of Craniomandibular Orthopedics; (1992) American Academy of Craniomandibular Disorders.

**★ 6423 ★ American Academy of Orthodontics for the General Practitioner (AAOGP)**
9701 Wesley St., Ste. 202
Greenville, TX 75402
**Free:** 800-634-2027          **Fax:** 888-634-2028
**Website:** http://www.academygportho.com/
Cynthia Bordelon, Dir.

**Fnded:** 1959. **Mem:** 250. **Reg. Groups:** 2. **State Groups:** 5. **Desc:** Licensed dentists. Provides dentists in general practice with an organization through which they can augment their basic knowledge and training in orthodontics. Offers continuing education courses for dentists and auxiliary personnel; sponsors seminars. Provides facilities and audiovisual material for its affiliated study clubs. **Pub:** *American Academy of Orthodontics for the General Practitioner—Continuing Education*, annual. Brochure. Lists AAOGP-sponsored continuing education courses, seminars, and meetings for the coming year. *Price:* Free. • *International Journal of Orthodontics*, semiannual. Journal.

**American Academy of Pediatric Dentistry (AAPD)**
*See:* Entry 5605

**★ 6424 ★ American Academy of Periodontology (AAP)**
737 N Michigan Ave., Ste. 800
Chicago, IL 60611-2615
**Phone:** (312)787-5518          **Fax:** (312)787-3670
**Email:** aapsite@perio.org
**Website:** http://www.perio.org
Alice DeForest, Exec. Dir.

**Fnded:** 1914. **Mem:** 7,500. **Desc:** Professional society of dentists specializing in the prevention, diagnosis, and treatment of diseases affecting the gums and supporting structures of the teeth and in the placement and maintenance of dental implants. **Pub:** *AAP News*, bimonthly. Newsletter. • *Annals of Periodontology*, annual. Journal. • *Directory of Members*, annual. • *Journal of Periodontology*, monthly. Journal.

**★ 6425 ★ American Academy of Restorative Dentistry (AARD)**
985 Fuller Rd.
Colorado Springs, CO 80920
**Phone:** (719)633-1060          **Fax:** (719)593-7926
**Website:** http://www.aard-dental-video.org/
John H. Martin, D.D.S., Pres.

**Fnded:** 1928. **Mem:** 285. **Desc:** Professional society of dentists practicing restorative dentistry, and educators interested in dentistry as it applies to treatment of the natural teeth to restore and maintain a healthy functioning mouth as part of a healthy body. **Pub:** *Journal of Prosthetic Dentistry*, periodic. Journal. • *Roster*, annual. **Frmly:** (1928) American Society of Dental Ceramics.

**★ 6426 ★ American Association of Dental Examiners (AADE)**
211 E Chicago Ave., Ste. 760
Chicago, IL 60611
**Phone:** (312)440-7464          **Fax:** (312)440-3525
**Email:** info@aadexam.org
**Website:** http://www.aadexam.org
Dr. Jerome c. Scales, Pres.

**Fnded:** 1883. **Mem:** 850. **Desc:** Present and past members of state dental examining boards and board administrators. To assist member agencies with problems related to state dental board examinations and licensure, and enforcement of the state dental practice act. Conducts research; compiles statistics. **Pub:** *American Association of Dental Examiners Bulletin*, quarterly, 3-4/year. Newsletter. *Price:* Available to members and related organizations. • *Proceedings*, annual. **Frmly:** National Association of Dental Examiners.

**★ 6427 ★ American Association for Dental Research (AADR)**
1619 Duke St.
Alexandria, VA 22314-3406
**Phone:** (703)548-0066          **Fax:** (703)548-1883
**Email:** research@iadr.com
**Website:** http://www.dentalresearch.org
Eli Schwarz, DDS, Exec. Dir.

**Fnded:** 1972. **Mem:** 5,000. **Reg. Groups:** 40. **Desc:** A division of the International Association for Dental Research. Dentists, researchers, dental schools, and dental products manufacturing companies. Seeks to promote better dental health and research activities. Presents current research information at annual meeting. Sponsors competitions; sponsors seminars. **Pub:** *AADReports*, quarterly. Newsletter. Association and professional newsletter for dental researchers. Includes calendar of events. *Price:* Included in membership dues. • *Advances in Dental Research*, periodic. • *Journal of Dental Research*, monthly, 16/year. Journal. Provides information on all sciences relevant to dentistry and to the oral cavity and associated structures in health and disease. *Price:* $70/year for members; $20/year for student members; $350/year in U.S.; $360/year outside U.S.

**★ 6428 ★ American Association of Endodontists (AAE)**
211 E Chicago Ave., Ste. 1100
Chicago, IL 60611-2691
**Phone:** (312)266-7255          **Free:** 800-872-3636
**Fax:** (312)266-9867
**Email:** info@aae.org
**Website:** http://www.aae.org
Dr. Samuel O. Dorn, Pres.

**Fnded:** 1943. **Mem:** 5,800. **Desc:** Endodontic specialists and other interested professionals. (Endodontics is a branch of dentistry that deals with the soft tissues inside the tooth.) Seeks to promote the exchange of ideas, to stimulate research, and to encourage the highest standard of quality care in the practice of endodontics. **Pub:** *Appropriateness of Care and Quality Assurance Guidelines.* • *Communique*, quarterly. Newsletter. • *Endodontics: Collegues for Excellence*, semiannual. Newsletter. • *Glossary: Contemporary Terminology for Endodontics.* • *Journal of Endodontics*, monthly. Journal. • *Membership Roster*, annual. • *Tooth Pain Guide*. Brochure. • *Your Guide to Cracked Teeth*. Brochure. • *Your Guide to Endodontic Retreatment*. Brochure. • *Your Guide to Endodontic Surgery*. Brochure. • *Your Guide to Endodontic Treatment*. Brochure. • *Your Guide to Traumatic Dental Injuries*. Brochure. • Brochure. • Brochure.

**★ 6429 ★ American Association for Functional Orthodontics (AAFO)**
106 S Kent St.
Winchester, VA 22601
**Phone:** (540)662-2200          **Free:** 800-441-3850
**Fax:** (540)665-8910
**Email:** info@aafo.org
**Website:** http://www.aafo.org
Dr. Craig C. Stoner, Co-Founder

**★ 6430 ★ American Association of Oral and Maxillofacial Surgeons (AAOMS)**
9700 W Bryn Mawr Ave.
Rosemont, IL 60018-5701
**Phone:** (847)678-6200          **Free:** 800-822-6637
**Fax:** (847)678-6286
**Email:** inquiries@aaoms.org
**Website:** http://www.aaoms.org
Dr. Robert Rinaldi, Asst. Exec. Dir.

**Fnded:** 1918. **Mem:** 6,100. **Reg. Groups:** 9. **State Groups:** 53. **Desc:** Dentists specializing in disease diagnosis and surgical, adjunctive, and esthetic treatment of diseases, injuries, and defects of the oral and maxillofacial region (jaw deformities, dental implants, infections, and oral cancer). **Pub:** *AAOMS Digest*, bimonthly. Newsletter. Contains association news and events. • *AAOMS Directory*, annual. Directory. • *AAOMS Forum*, quarterly. • *Journal of Oral Maxillofacial Surgery*, monthly. Journal. • *Office Anesthesia Evaluation Manual.* Manual. • *Report of Annual Meeting.* Report. • *Surgical Update*, 3/year. • Annual Report. **Frmly:** (1944) American Society of Exodontists; (1977) American Society of Oral Surgeons.

**★ 6431 ★ American Association of Orthodontists (AAO)**
401 N Lindbergh Blvd.
Saint Louis, MO 63141-7816
**Phone:** (314)993-1700          **Free:** 800-424-2841
**Fax:** (314)997-1745
**Email:** info@aaortho.org
**Website:** http://www.aaortho.org
Richard B. Myers, Pres.

**Fnded:** 1901. **Mem:** 13,000. **Nat'l Groups:** 1. **Reg. Groups:** 8. **State Groups:** 54. **Desc:** Professional society of orthodontists. To advance the art and science of orthodontics through continuing education, encouragement of research and cooperation with other health groups. Maintains museum. **Pub:** *AAO Bulletin*, bimonthly. Newsletter. Includes meetings schedules. *Price:* Included in membership dues. • *American Association of Orthodontists Membership Directory*, biennial. Membership Directory. *Price:* $55 for members; $110 for nonmembers. • *American Journal of Orthodontics and Dentofacial Orthopedics*, monthly. Journal. *Price:* Included in membership dues. • Pamphlets. • Also publishes administration guide kits. **Frmly:** American Society of Orthodontists.

**American Association of Public Health Dentistry (AAPHD)**
*See:* Entry 17913


**★ 6432 ★ American Association of Women Dentists (AAWD)**
645 N Michigan Ave., No. 800
Chicago, IL 60611
**Phone:** (312)280-9296 **Free:** 800-920-2293
**Fax:** (312)280-9893
**Email:** info@womendentists.org
**Website:** http://www.womendentists.org
Marti DeGraaf, CEO
**Fnded:** 1921. **Reg. Groups:** 17. **Desc:** Dental students or dentists who is interested in dentistry and advancing women in dentistry. AAWD dedicates itself to enhancing and promoting unique participation and leadership for women in organized dentistry. **Pub:** *AAWD Membership Directory,* annual. Directory. • *The Chronicle,* quarterly. Newsletter. Includes member activities at the local and national level, scientific and technical news, upcoming events and a list of various jobs. *Price:* Included in membership dues; $30/year for nonmembers. **Frmly:** (1978) Association of American Women Dentists.


**American Board of Dental Public Health (ABDPH)**
*See:* Entry 17915


**★ 6433 ★ American Board of Endodontics (ABE)**
211 E Chicago Ave., Ste. 1100
Chicago, IL 60611-2691
**Phone:** (312)266-7255 **Free:** 800-872-3636
**Fax:** (312)266-9867
**Email:** info@aae.org
**Website:** http://www.aae.org/ABE1.html
Dr. Jeffrey W. Hutter, Pres.
**Desc:** Dentists who have successfully completed study and training in an advanced endodontics education program that is accredited by the Commission on Dental Accreditation of the American Dental Association . Primary objective is to protect the public by raising the standards of endodontic practice and requiring candidates for diplomate status to show strong evidence of specialized skills and knowledge in endodontics. Administers examinations and certifies dentists who successfully complete the examinations. **Pub:** *Membership Roster,* annual. Published in conjunction with American Association of Endodontists.


**American Board of Oral and Maxillofacial Pathology**
*See:* Entry 17126


**American Board of Oral and Maxillofacial Surgery (ABOMS)**
*See:* Entry 19477


**★ 6434 ★ American Board of Orthodontics (ABO)**
401 N Lindbergh Blvd., Ste. 308
Saint Louis, MO 63141
**Phone:** (314)432-6130 **Fax:** (314)432-8170
**Email:** amboard@earthlink.net
**Website:** http://www.americanboardortho.com
R. Don James, Pres.
**Fnded:** 1929. **Nat'l Groups:** 1. **Reg. Groups:** 8. **Desc:** Certification board to investigate the qualifications of, administer examinations to, and certify as diplomats dentists specializing in orthodontics (prevention and correction of irregularities and faulty positions of the teeth). Sponsored by the American Association of Orthodontists. **Frmly:** (1938) American Board of Orthodontia.


**American Board of Pediatric Dentistry (ABPD)**
*See:* Entry 5608


**★ 6435 ★ American Board of Periodontology (ABP)**
4157 Mountain Rd.
PBN 249
Pasadena, MD 21122
**Fax:** (410)437-4021
**Email:** abperio@msn.com
**Website:** http://www.perio.org/amboard
Dr. Gerald Bowers, Contact
**Fnded:** 1939. **Mem:** 1,400. **Desc:** Conducts examinations to determine the qualifications and competence of periodontists who voluntarily apply for certification as diplomates in the field of periodontology. Maintains registry of holders of diplomate certificates.


**★ 6436 ★ American Board of Prosthodontics (ABP)**
c/o Dr. Thomas D. Taylor
211 E Chicago Ave., Ste. 1000
Chicago, IL 60611
**Phone:** (312)573-1260 **Fax:** (312)573-1257
**Email:** dc_atl@bellsouth.net
**Website:** http://www.prosthodontics.org
Dr. Thomas D. Taylor, Exec. Dir.
**Desc:** Seeks to advance the science and art of prosthodontics by encouraging its study and improving its practice. Certifies dentists who specialize in the field of fixed, removable, and maxillofacial prosthodontics. Approved by the American Dental Association and the Council on Dental Education.


**★ 6437 ★ American Central European Dental Institute (ACEDI)**
60 Federal St.
Boston, MA 02110-2510
**Phone:** (617)423-6165 **Fax:** (617)426-0006
**Email:** info@watkinosorio.com
Dr. Arnold Watkin, Chm.
**Fnded:** 1991. **Mem:** 2. **Desc:** Dentists and others serving in capacities related to the dental profession. Seeks to advance standards in the profession of dentistry. Conducts educational programs; maintains speakers' bureau. **Pub:** *ACEDI,* annual. Newsletter.


**★ 6438 ★ American College of Dentists (ACD)**
839-J Quince Orchard Blvd.
Gaithersburg, MD 20878-1614
**Phone:** (301)977-3223 **Fax:** (301)977-3330
**Email:** info@facd.org
**Website:** http://www.facd.org
Dr. Stephen A. Ralls, Exec. Dir.
**Fnded:** 1920. **Mem:** 7,000. **Reg. Groups:** 8. **Local Groups:** 46. **Desc:** Dentists and others serving in capacities related to the dental profession. Seeks to advance the standards of the profession of dentistry. Conducts educational and research programs. Maintains speakers' bureau and charitable programs. **Pub:** *American College of Dentists News and Views,* quarterly. Newsletter. *Price:* Included in membership dues. • *Journal of the American College of Dentists,* quarterly. Journal. Includes news and reserach reports. *Price:* Included in membership dues; $40/year for nonmembers.


**American College of Oral and Maxillofacial Surgeons (ACOMS)**
*See:* Entry 19483


**★ 6439 ★ American College of Prosthodontists (ACP)**
211 E Chicago Ave., Ste. 1000
Chicago, IL 60611-2616
**Phone:** (312)573-1260 **Free:** 800-378-1260
**Fax:** (312)573-1257
**Email:** acp@prosthodontics.org


**Website:** http://www.prosthodontics.org
Edward J. Cronin, Jr., Exec. Dir.
**Fnded:** 1970. **Mem:** 2,800. **Reg. Groups:** 40. **Desc:** Dentists specializing in prosthetics who are either board certified, board eligible, or under training in approved graduate or residency programs. Seeks to improve prosthodontic treatment for patients by encouraging educational activities designed to bring new ideas, techniques, and research into clinical practice. Sponsors annual prosthodontic research competition. **Pub:** *Journal of Prosthodontics,* quarterly. Journal. • *Journal of Prosthodontics–Clinical Journal.* Articles. • Newsletter, 4/year. ACP Messenger–Membership Newsletter. *Price:* Included in membership dues. • Also publishes study guide.


**★ 6440 ★ American Dental Assistants Association (ADAA)**
203 N LaSalle St., Ste. 1320
Chicago, IL 60601-1225
**Phone:** (312)541-1550 **Fax:** (312)541-1496
**Email:** adaa1@aol.com
**Website:** http://www.dentalassistant.org
Lawrence H. Sepin, Exec. Dir.
**Fnded:** 1923. **Mem:** 16,000. **State Groups:** 50. **Local Groups:** 175. **Desc:** Individuals employed as dental assistants in dental offices, clinics, hospitals, or institutions; instructors of dental assistants; dental students. Sponsors workshops and seminars; maintains governmental liaison. Offers group insurance; maintains scholarship trust fund. Dental Assisting National Board examines members who are candidates for title of Certified Dental Assistant. **Pub:** *The Dental Assistant,* bimonthly. Journal. Features articles pertaining to dental assisting. *Price:* $20/yr. for nonmembers. • Also publishes educational materials.


**★ 6441 ★ American Dental Association (ADA)**
211 E Chicago Ave.
Chicago, IL 60611
**Phone:** (312)440-2500 **Fax:** (312)440-2800
**Email:** adahf@ada.org
**Website:** http://www.ada.org
James Branson, Exec. Dir.
**Fnded:** 1859. **Mem:** 144,510. **State Groups:** 54. **Local Groups:** 535. **Desc:** Professional society of dentists. Encourages the improvement of the health of the public and promotes the art and science of dentistry in matters of legislation and regulations. Inspects and accredits dental schools and schools for dental hygienists, assistants, and laboratory technicians. Conducts research programs at ADA Health Foundation Research Institute. Produces most of the dental health education material used in the U.S. Sponsors National Children's Dental Health Month. Compiles statistics on personnel, practice, and dental care needs and attitudes of patients with regard to dental health. Sponsors 13 councils. **Pub:** *ADA News,* biweekly. *Price:* $55 for nonmembers. • *Journal of the American Dental Association,* monthly. Journal. *Price:* $100 for nonmembers. **Frmly:** (1922) National Dental Association.


**★ 6442 ★ American Dental Education Association**
1625 Massachusetts Ave. NW, Ste. 600
Washington, DC 20036-2212
**Phone:** (202)667-9433 **Fax:** (202)667-0642
**Email:** adea@adea.org
**Website:** http://www.adea.org/
Prof. Pamela Zarkowski, Pres.
**Fnded:** 1923. **Mem:** 3,600. **Desc:** Individuals interested in dental education; schools of dentistry, graduate dentistry, and dental auxiliary education in the U.S., Canada, and Puerto Rico; affiliated institutions of the federal government. To promote better teaching and education in dentistry and dental research and to facilitate exchange of ideas among dental educators. Sponsors meetings, conferences, and workshops; conducts surveys, studies, and special projects and publishes their results. Maintains 37 sections representing teaching and administrative areas of dentistry.

*Pub: Admission Requirements of United States and Canadian Dental Schools*, annual. Catalog. Helps students decide on a career in dentistry, and explains how to go about it. *Price:* $25. • *Bulletin of Dental Education*, monthly. Newsletter. • *Directory of Institutional Members*, annual. Directory. • *Journal of Dental Education*, monthly. Journal. • *Opportunities for Minority Students in U.S. Dental Schools*, annual. Catalog. *Price:* $10. • *Proceedings*, annual. *Price:* $10. **Frmly:** (2000) American Association Dental Schools.

**★ 6443 ★ American Dental Hygienists' Association (ADHA)**
444 N Michigan Ave., Ste. 3400
Chicago, IL 60611
**Phone:** (312)440-8911 **Free:** 800-243-ADHA
**Fax:** (312)440-8929
**Email:** exec.office@adha.net
**Website:** http://www.adha.org
Stanley B. Peck, Exec. Dir.

**Fnded:** 1923. **Mem:** 35,000. **Nat'l Groups:** 1. **Reg. Groups:** 12. **State Groups:** 53. **Local Groups:** 360. **Desc:** Professional organization of licensed dental hygienists possessing a degree or certificate in dental hygiene granted by an accredited school of dental hygiene. Makes available scholarships, research grants, and continuing education programs. Maintains accrediting service through the American Dental Association's Commission on Dental Accreditation. Compiles statistics. **Pub:** *American Dental Hygienists' Association Access*, 10/year. Magazine. Covers current dental hygiene topics, regulatory and legislative developments, and association news. Includes membership profiles. *Price:* Included in membership dues; $30/year for nonmembers. • *Journal of Dental Hygiene*, quarterly. Journal. Includes association news, book reviews, abstracts, government news, and information on research and new products. *Price:* Included in membership dues; $40/year for nonmembers.

**★ 6444 ★ American Dental Interfraternity Council (ADIC)**
c/o Alpha Omega Fraternity
505 Couch Ave., Ste. 130
Baltimore, MD 21208
**Fax:** (314)822-3085
Dr. RCharles D. Fuszner, D.M.D, Exec. Sec.

**Fnded:** 1923. **Mem:** 4. **Desc:** Federation of professional dental Greek letter societies. Promotes good public relations.

**★ 6445 ★ American Dental Society of Anesthesiology (ADSA)**
211 E Chicago Ave., Ste. 780
Chicago, IL 60611
**Phone:** (312)664-8270 **Free:** 800-722-7788
**Fax:** (312)642-9713
**Email:** adsahome@cs.com
**Website:** http://www.adsahome.org
Jeffrey D. Bennett, DMD, Pres.

**Fnded:** 1953. **Mem:** 3,200. **State Groups:** 21. **Desc:** Dentists and physicians. Encourages study and progress in dental anesthesiology. **Pub:** *ADSA Directory*, annual. Directory. • *ADSA Pulse*, bimonthly. Newsletter. Includes society news, calendar of events, and research updates. *Price:* Included in membership dues; $5/year for nonmembers. • *Anesthesia Progress*, bimonthly. *Price:* $30/year for members; $35/year for nonmembers; $55/year for institutions.

**★ 6446 ★ American Dental Society of Europe (ADSE)**
c/o Paul O'Neilly
5A Oriental Rd.
Woking GU22 7AH, United Kingdom
**Phone:** 44 171 6374518 **Fax:** 44 171 6291869
**Email:** lloydsearson@compuserve.com

**Fnded:** 1873. **Mem:** 250. **Lang(s):** English. **Desc:** Graduates of North American schools of dentistry who practice in Europe. Seeks the interchange of dental information and the advancement of the profession.

Offers scholarship for European dentists to study in the United States.

**★ 6447 ★ American Endodontic Society (AES)**
1321 N Harbor Blvd., No. 201
Fullerton, CA 92835
**Phone:** (714)870-5590 **Fax:** (714)526-2818
**Email:** amendsoc@aol.com
**Website:** http://www.aesoc.com
Dr. Ramon Werts, Exec. Dir.

**Fnded:** 1969. **Mem:** 10,000. **Desc:** Dentists united to promote and provide educational and scientific information on simplified root canal therapy for the general practitioner. Conducts research programs. **Pub:** *American Endodontic Society Newsletter*, quarterly. Newsletter. Contains society news, member profiles, and instructional articles. • *Hotline*, periodic.

**★ 6448 ★ American Equilibration Society (AES)**
8726 N Ferris Ave.
Morton Grove, IL 60053
**Phone:** (847)965-2888 **Fax:** (847)965-4888
**Email:** aesdental@sprynet.com
**Website:** http://www.occlusion-tmj.org/
Dr. Lawrence Rd. Huber, Pres.

**Fnded:** 1955. **Mem:** 1,100. **Desc:** Dentists, orthodontists, oral surgeons, and physicians interested in study and proficiency in the diagnosis and treatment of occlusal and temporomandibular joint disorders. Bestows Student Recognition Certificates annually to outstanding graduating students. **Pub:** *American Equilibration Society Newsletter*, 3/year. Newsletter. *Price:* Included in membership dues. • *Roster*, annual. • *TMJ Update*, bimonthly. *Price:* Included in membership dues.

**★ 6449 ★ American Institute of Oral Biology (AIOB)**
PO Box 7184
Loma Linda, CA 92354-7184
**Phone:** (909)558-4671 **Fax:** (909)558-0285
**Email:** jbarrientos@sd.llu.edu
**Website:** http://www.aiob.org
June J. Barrientos, Exec. Sec.

**Fnded:** 1943. **Mem:** 150. **Desc:** Dental and medical health professionals united for continuing education. Conducts lectures. **Pub:** *AIOB Proceedings Manual*, annual. *Price:* $75.

**★ 6450 ★ American Orthodontic Society (AOS)**
11884 Greenville Ave., No. 112
Dallas, TX 75243-3537
**Phone:** (972)234-4000 **Free:** 800-448-1601
**Fax:** (972)234-4290
**Email:** tchapman@orthodontic.com
Tom Chapman, Exec. Dir.

**Fnded:** 1974. **Mem:** 1,900. **Desc:** General and pediatric dentists. Objectives are: to make orthodontic information readily available to any ethical dentist; to zealously protect the right of members to pursue orthodontic knowledge; to keep a watchful eye on third party services and government programs. Offers courses in orthodontic techniques. Conducts educational programs. **Pub:** *American Orthodontic Society Newsletter*, quarterly. Newsletter. Provides information on the society's seminars and conventions and news of interest to members. *Price:* Included in membership dues. • *American Orthodontic Society Technique Directory*, biennial. Membership Directory. Lists members by city and state; includes the type of orthodontic technique used by listee. *Price:* $150. • Brochures.

**★ 6451 ★ American Prosthodontic Society (APS)**
426 Hudson St.
PO Box 552
Hackensack, NJ 07602-0522

**Phone:** (201)440-8144 **Free:** 877-499-3500
**Fax:** (201)440-7963
**Email:** aps@prostho.com
**Website:** http://www.prostho.com
Dr. Alan C. Keyes, D.D.S., Exec. Dir.

**Fnded:** 1928. **Mem:** 800. **Desc:** Dentists interested in the discipline of prosthodontics (the art and science of replacing missing teeth and supporting structures). **Pub:** *Journal of Prosthetic Dentistry*, monthly. Journal. Published in conjunction with 21 other prosthodonic organizations. *Price:* Included in membership dues.

**★ 6452 ★ American Society for Advancement of Anesthesia and Sedation in Dentistry (ASAAD)**
6 East Union Ave.
Bound Brook, NJ 08805
**Phone:** (732)469-9050 **Fax:** (732)271-1985
**Email:** info@sedation4dentists.com
**Website:** http://www.sedation4dentists.com
Dr. David Crystal, Contact

**Fnded:** 1925. **Mem:** 200. **Desc:** Dentists and physicians interested in dental anesthesia. Studies new anesthetics and chemicals; researches pain control methods. Organized and sponsored international congresses on modern pain control in dentistry in Latin America, Europe, and Japan. Advances education opportunities for dentists using sedation and anesthesia. Maintains speakers' bureau. **Pub:** *Modern Anesthesia in Dentistry*. Book. • *Modern Dental Anesthesia*. Book. • *Modern Pain Control*, biennial. • *Pain Control in Dentistry*, semiannual. Journal. Covers and promotes the use of dental anesthesia. *Price:* Included in membership dues. • *Transcripts*, semiannual. **Frmly:** (1975) American Society for Advancement of General Anesthesia in Dentistry; (2001) American Society for Advancement of Anesthesia in Dentistry.

**★ 6453 ★ American Society for Dental Aesthetics (ASDA)**
14497 Dale Mabry Hwy., No. 205N
Tampa, FL 33618
**Phone:** (813)264-2772 **Free:** 800-454-ASDA
**Fax:** (813)755-3263
**Email:** info@asdatoday.com
**Website:** http://www.asdatoday.com
Irwin Smigel, DDS, Pres.

**Fnded:** 1978. **Mem:** 175. **Desc:** Accredited dentists practicing aesthetic concepts in dentistry, including porcelain lamination (a technique where porcelain veneer is chemically fused to teeth to lengthen them, close spaces, or recontour the entire mouth). Dentists must have 5 years experience and submit 5 "before and after" photos of their work in aesthetic dentistry to qualify for membership. Promotes development, research, and teaching of aesthetic concepts in dentistry. Although centered in New York City, the group promotes expansion of aesthetic dentistry concepts in other states and abroad. Sponsors educational programs on tooth and crown repair, aesthetic fillings, orthodontics, periodontics, implantology, and other topics. **Pub:** *ASDA Today*, semiannual. Journal.

**★ 6454 ★ American Society of Dentistry for Children (ASDC)**
211 E Chicago Ave., Ste. 710
Chicago, IL 60611-2663
**Phone:** (312)943-1244 **Fax:** (312)943-5341
**Email:** asdckids@aol.com
**Website:** http://asdckids.org
Carol Teuscher, Asst. Exec. Dir.

**Fnded:** 1927. **Mem:** 3,000. **State Groups:** 50. **Desc:** General practitioners and specialists interested in dentistry for children. Conducts specialized education and research programs. **Pub:** *ASDC News*, quarterly. Newsletter. Contains news about children's dental health concerns. Includes scientific references and governmental activities related to children's health. *Price:* Included in membership dues. • *Directory of the Membership of the American Society of Dentistry for Children*. Membership Directory. • *Journal of Dentistry for Children*, bimonthly. Journal.

**★ 6455 ★ American Society of Forensic Odontology (ASFO)**
c/o Dr. Susan Rivera
11 Tiffany Pl.
Saratoga Springs, NY 12866-9050
**Phone:** (518)584-2342          **Fax:** (518)584-9706
**Email:** skrivera@global2000.net
**Website:** http://www.asfo.org
Susan Rivera, Contact
**Fnded:** 1970. **Mem:** 1,013. **Reg. Groups:** 1. **Desc:** Individuals interested in furthering the field of forensic dentistry. Conducts research and specialized education programs. Maintains library. **Pub:** *The Manual of Forensic Odontology, Third Edition.* Book. • Membership Directory, annual. • Newsletter, 3/year.

**★ 6456 ★ American Society of Master Dental Technologists (ASMDT)**
PO Box 640248
Oakland Gardens, NY 11364
**Phone:** (718)347-1239          **Fax:** (718)347-3113
**Email:** info@asmdt.com
**Website:** http://www.asmdt.com
Sue Heppenheimer, Exec. Sec.
**Fnded:** 1976. **Mem:** 125. **Desc:** Dental lab technicians. Dedicated to the upgrading of dental technology. Seeks to provide educational resources such as texts, instructors, and guidance for technicians interested in becoming master dental technologists. Conducts associate and master level courses in conjunction with New York University School of Dentistry, Dept. of Continuing Education.

**American Society of Maxillofacial Surgeons (ASMS)**
*See:* Entry 19497

**★ 6457 ★ American Society for the Study of Orthodontics (ASSO)**
70-15 164th St.
Flushing, NY 11365
**Phone:** (718)591-6411          **Fax:** (718)591-5424
**Email:** admin@maxface.org
**Website:** http://www.maxface.org
Dr. Milton Bloch, Pres.
**Fnded:** 1945. **Mem:** 100. **Desc:** Members of the American Dental Association or other societies, with special interest in orthodontics but not limited to those who practice in the field. Purposes are to: preserve the highest ideals in orthodontics and in dentistry; encourage and assist the diffusion of orthodontic knowledge to all dentists who include orthodontics as an integral part of their health service or limit their practice to orthodontics; institute an intensive program of fundamental and advanced studies and guidance for its members in theoretical, didactic, and applied orthodontics; encourage the orthodontic departments of university dental schools to provide both short and extended courses in orthodontics; to establish discussion and clinical study groups throughout the U.S. Conducts lectures, panel discussions, postgraduate seminars, table clinics, and consultation service. **Pub:** *ASSO Newsletter*, quarterly. Newsletter. • *International Journal of Orthodontics*, 3/year. Journal. **Frmly:** (1962) New York Society for the Study of Orthodontics.

**★ 6458 ★ American Student Dental Association (ASDA)**
211 E Chicago Ave., Ste. 1160
Chicago, IL 60611
**Phone:** (312)440-2795          **Free:** 800-621-8099
**Fax:** (312)440-2820
**Email:** asda@asdanet.org
**Website:** http://www.asdanet.org/
Cindy Kennedy, Exec. Dir.
**Fnded:** 1971. **Mem:** 15,000. **Local Groups:** 54. **Desc:** Predoctoral and postdoctoral dental students organized to improve the quality of dental education and to promote the accessibility of oral health care. Additional membership categories include predental, postdoctoral, international and associate. Represents dental students before legislative bodies, organizations, and associations that affect dental students. Disseminates information to dental students. Sponsors advocacy program and "externships" inc luding Washington National Helath Policy, Chicago Administrative, State Governm ent Affairs, and Research. **Pub:** *ASDA Handbook*, annual. Handbook. Contains annual reference volumes, with information on applying to dental school, financial aid, membership benefits, post-doctoral opportunities. Price: $25 in U.S.; $40 outside U.S. • *ASDA News*, monthly. • *Dentistry*, quarterly. • Also publishes a series of guides to postgraduate programs in dentistry and reprints of National Board Examinations. **Frmly:** (1971) Student American Dental Association.

**★ 6459 ★ Asia Pacific Endodontic Confederation (APEC)**
c/o Dr. Seung-Jong Lee
169 Cruz St., Mandaluyong
Manila, Metro Manila, Philippines
**Fax:** 82 2 3137575
**Website:** http://www.hku.hk/consden/apec
**Lang(s):** Chinese, English. **Desc:** Endodontists. Seeks to advance the study, teaching, and practice of endodontia. Serves as a forum for the exchange of information among members; sponsors research and continuing professional development programs.

**★ 6460 ★ Asia-Pacific Implantology Center**
Rm. 704 Takshing House
20 Des Voeux Rd.
Hong Kong, People's Republic of China
**Phone:** 852 25225571          **Fax:** 852 25243557
**Website:** http://www.implantcentre.com
**Desc:** Dental and medical practitioners. Dedicated to the advancement of oral implantology in the Asia-Pacific region. Provides practicing clinicians with opportunities for professional education and training, as well as clinical facilities services for oral implant treatment. Fully equipped with educational, teaching, and clinical facilities.

**★ 6461 ★ Asia Pacific Society of Periodontology (APSP)**
741-1 Hannam, 2-Dong
Yongsan-gu
Seoul 140-212, Republic of Korea
**Phone:** 82 2 7926114          **Fax:** 82 2 7926116
**Email:** shsen@smc.samsung.co.kr
**Lang(s):** English, Korean. **Desc:** Periondontists. Seeks to advance the study, teaching, and practice of periodontology. Facilitates communication among members; sponsors research and continuing professional development programs.

**★ 6462 ★ Asian Academy of Aesthetic Dentistry (AAAD)**
268 Orchard Rd. 05-02
Singapore 238856, Singapore
**Phone:** 65 7343162          **Fax:** 65 7321979
**Email:** singdent@singnet.com.sg
**Fnded:** 1990. **Lang(s):** Chinese, English. **Desc:** Dentists practicing aesthetic dentistry. Seeks to advance the study, teaching, and practice of aesthetic dentistry. Gathers and disseminates information on aesthetic dentistry; sponsors research and Continuing professional development programs. **Pub:** *Asian Journal of Aesthetic Dentistry*, annual. Journal.

**★ 6463 ★ Asian Academy of Preventive Dentistry (AAPD)**
Fukuoka Dental College
Department of Preventive Dentistry
2-15-1 Tamura
Sawara-ku
Fukuoka 814-01, Japan
**Phone:** 81 92 8014011          **Fax:** 81 92 8014909
**Email:** sakaio1@college.fdcnet.ac.jp
**Lang(s):** English, Japanese. **Desc:** Dentists with an interest in preventive dentistry. Seeks to advance the study, teaching, and practice of preventive dentistry. Gathers and disseminates information on preventive dentistry; sponsors research and continuing professional development programs.

**★ 6464 ★ Asian Oral Implant Academy (AOIA)**
268 Orchard Rd. 05-07
Singapore 0923, Singapore
**Phone:** 65 7343162          **Fax:** 65 7321979
**Lang(s):** Chinese, English. **Desc:** Dentists specializing in oral implantology. Seeks to advance the practice of oral implantology. Facilitates communication and cooperation among members; conducts continuing professional development programs.

**★ 6465 ★ Asian Pacific Dental Federation/Asian Pacific Regional Organisation (APDF/APRO)**
242 Tanjong Katong Rd.
Singapore 437030, Singapore
**Phone:** 65 3453125          **Fax:** 65 3442116
**Email:** bibi@pacific.net.sg
**Fnded:** 1955. **Mem:** 23. **Lang(s):** English. **Desc:** National dental associations in Australia, Bangladesh, Guam, Hong Kong, India, Figi, Jordan, Macau, Papua New Guines, Saudi Arabia, Indonesia, Japan, Malaysia, Mongolia, Myanmar, Nepal, New Zealand, Pakistan, Philippines, Republic of Korea, Singapore, Sri Lanka, Taiwan, and Thailand. Works to improve dental and general health in the Asia Pacific region. Encourages education and research links between national dental associations. **Pub:** *APDF/APRO Technical Report*, periodic. • *Dentistry in the Asian Pacific Region*, periodic.

**★ 6466 ★ Association of Canadian Faculties of Dentistry (ACFD) (Association des Facultes Dentaires du Canada — AFDC)**
100 Bronson St.
Ottawa, ON, Canada K1R 6G8
**Phone:** (613)237-6505          **Fax:** (613)236-8386
**Email:** director@acfd.ca
**Website:** http://www.acfd.ca
**Lang(s):** English, French. **Desc:** Dental school faculties. Promotes improvement of dental education; seeks to advance the teaching, study, and practice of dentistry. Conducts research and educational programs; facilitates exchange of information among members.

**★ 6467 ★ Association Dentaire Francaise (ADF)**
c/o Michel Chabre
7, rue Mariotte
F-75017 Paris, France
**Phone:** 33 1 58221710          **Fax:** 33 1 58221740
**Email:** adf@adf.asso.fr
**Website:** http://www.adf.asso.fr
**Fnded:** 1970. **Mem:** 33,000. **Lang(s):** French. **Desc:** Federation of dental associations in France. Promotes and defends the dental profession; works for the evaluation and standardization of dental products. Organizes an annual conference for continuing education. **Pub:** *Les Cahiers de F A.D.F*, quarterly. Journal.

**★ 6468 ★ Association of Dental Dealers in Europe (ADDE)**
Moosstrasse 2
PO Box 29
CH-3073 Bern, Switzerland
**Phone:** 41 31 9527892          **Fax:** 41 31 9527683
**Email:** uwanner@swissonline.ch
**Mem:** 16. **Lang(s):** English, French, German, Italian. **Desc:** Manufacturers of dental equipment and supplies. Promotes growth and development of members' businesses; seeks to advance dental technologies.

Represents members' interests before labor, industrial, and professional organizations, government agencies, and the public; sponsors research and development programs. **Pub:** *Economic Survey 2000 on the European Dental Trade*, annual. Survey.


**★ 6469 ★ Association for Dental Education in Europe (ADEE)**
Malmo University
Carl Gustafs vag 34
S-21421 Malmo, Sweden
**Phone:** 46 40 6658410     **Fax:** 46 40 6658549
**Email:** adee@od.mah.se
**Website:** http://tmk.odont.ku.dk/adee
**Fnded:** 1975. **Mem:** 85. **Lang(s):** English. **Desc:** Teachers of dentistry. Objectives are: to further dental education in Europe; to evaluate the goals and methods of dental education; to assess training programs for teachers; to promote ties among dentistry teachers. Holds lectures, seminars, and working discussion groups in conjunction with annual meeting. **Pub:** Proceedings, annual.


**★ 6470 ★ Association of Dental Hospitals of the UK**
Birmingham Dental Hospital
Birmingham B4 6NN, United Kingdom
**Phone:** 44 121 2368611     **Fax:** 44 121 2372750
**Fnded:** 1952. **Mem:** 32. **Desc:** Open only to representatives of Dental Hospitals and Schools. .


**Association of German Dental Manufacturers (Verband der Deutschen Dental-Industrie — VDDI)**
*See:* Entry 9958


**★ 6471 ★ Association of Managed Care Dentists (AMCD)**
1223 Wilshire Blvd., Ste. 483
Santa Monica, CA 90403
**Phone:** (310)453-3439     **Free:** 800-864-6848
**Fax:** (310)453-7895
**Email:** jmaguire@dentalgroup.com
**Website:** http://www.amcd.org
John Maguire, DDS, Contact
**Desc:** Dentists participating in managed dental care programs. Seeks to advance the provision of managed dental care. Serves as liaison linking members with government agencies and dental plan administrators; sponsors educational programs. **Pub:** *News Flash*, periodic. Newsletter. **Frmly:** (2000) Association of Managed Care Providers.


**Association of State and Territorial Dental Directors (ASTDD)**
*See:* Entry 9715


**Associazione Italiana di Anestesia Odonto-Stomatologica (AINOS)**
*See:* Entry 4452


**★ 6472 ★ Australasian Society of Oral Medicine and Toxicology (ASOMAT)**
PO Box A860
Sydney, NSW 2000, Australia
**Phone:** 61 2 98671111     **Fax:** 61 2 92832230
**Email:** asomat@asomat.com
**Website:** http://www.asomat.com
**Lang(s):** English. **Desc:** Medical professionals working in the fields of oral medicine and toxicology. Promotes "concepts of "Bio-Compatible Dentistry" which are supported by scientific, peer reviewed research. Serves as a clearinghouse on research in oral medicine, toxicology, and natural therapies.


**★ 6473 ★ Australian Dental Association (ADA)**
75 Lithgow St.
Saint Leonards, NSW 2065, Australia
**Phone:** 61 2 99064412     **Fax:** 61 2 99064917
**Email:** adainc@ada.org.au
**Website:** http://www.ada.org.au
**Fnded:** 1928. **Mem:** 7,500. **State Groups:** 7. **Lang(s):** English. **Desc:** Dentists, specialists, and dental students. Represents dentists' interests nationally and internationally. Seeks to improve the dental health of the community. Sponsors educational and research programs; cosponsors the Australian Dental Research Fund. **Pub:** *ADA News Bulletin*, 11/year. • *Australian Dental Journal*, quarterly. • *Facts and Figures - Australian Dentistry*, annual. • Directory, biennial.


**★ 6474 ★ Australian Society of Orthodontists**
Private Bag No. 1
Darlinghurst, NSW 2010, Australia
**Phone:** 61 2 93316920     **Fax:** 61 2 93317296
**Email:** aso@pcasyd.com
**Website:** http://www.aso.org.au/
**Fnded:** 1927.


**★ 6475 ★ Bangladesh Dental Society**
PO Box 4168
Dhaka 1000, Bangladesh
**Phone:** 880 2 802500     **Fax:** 880 2 863797
**Fnded:** 1977. **Mem:** 800. **Lang(s):** Bangla, English. **Desc:** Dental surgeons. Promotes prevention, treatment, and reduction of oral and dental disease. Works to improve the standard of dental practice and to enhance the professional standing of members. Conducts charitable, educational, and children's programs. **Pub:** *Bangladesh Dental Journal*, quarterly. Journal.


**★ 6476 ★ Barbados Dental Association (BDA)**
PO Box 95
Bridgetown, Barbados
**Phone:** (246)228-6488     **Fax:** (246)228-6488
**Fnded:** 1965. **Mem:** 34. **Local Groups:** 1. **Lang(s):** English. **Desc:** Promotes dentistry and the interests of dental professionals in Barbados; works to improve the dental and general health of the public. Conducts educational programs at schools. Offers competitions for school children to foster dental health awareness.


**★ 6477 ★ Bermuda Dental Association (BDA)**
c/o Dr. Laidlaw Fraser-Smith
PO Box 3059
Hamilton HM NX, Bermuda
**Phone:** (441)295-2452     **Fax:** (441)292-7678
**Email:** bdadental@ibl.bm
**Website:** http://www.bermudadental.bm/
**Mem:** 25. **Lang(s):** English. **Desc:** Dentists in Bermuda. Promotes dentistry; represents members' interests. Sponsors study club.


**British Association of Dental Nurses**
*See:* Entry 15674


**★ 6478 ★ British Association of Prosthetists and Orthotists (BAPO)**
Sir James Clark Bldg.
Abbey Mills Business Centre
Paisley PA1 1TJ, United Kingdom
**Phone:** 44 141 5617217     **Fax:** 44 141 5617218
**Email:** admin@bapo.com
**Website:** http://www.bapo.com
**Lang(s):** English. **Desc:** Orthotists and prosthetists. Seeks to "protect the prosthetic and orthotic profession with regard to its status and interests." Encourages high standards of ethics and practice among


members; conducts continuing professional education and training programs; serves as a clearinghouse on orthotics and prosthetics; provides advice and assistance to members. **Pub:** *BAPOMAG*, periodic. Magazine.


**★ 6479 ★ British Dental Association (BDA)**
64 Wimpole St.
London W1G 8YS, United Kingdom
**Phone:** 44 207 9350875     **Fax:** 44 207 4875232
**Email:** enquiries@bda-dentistry.org.uk
**Website:** http://www.bda-dentistry.org.uk
**Fnded:** 1880. **Mem:** 20,000. **Reg. Groups:** 21. **Local Groups:** 130. **Lang(s):** English. **Desc:** Professional association and trade union for dental surgeons in the United Kingdom. Promotes dentistry and the provision of dental services to the public. Represents members' interests individually and collectively before the government. **Pub:** *BDA News*, monthly. Newsletter. • *British Dental Journal*, bimonthly. Journal.


**British Dental Practice Managers Association**
*See:* Entry 9722


**British Dental Trade Association (BDTA)**
*See:* Entry 9962


**★ 6480 ★ British Fluoridation Society**
5th Fl., Dental School
University of Liverpool
PO Box 147, Pembroke Pl.
Liverpool L69 3GN, United Kingdom
**Phone:** 44 151 7065216     **Fax:** 44 151 7065845
**Email:** bfs@liv.ac.uk
**Website:** http://www.liv.ac.uk/bfs
**Fnded:** 1969. **Desc:** Promotes fluoridation of the water supplies to improve dental health and reduce health inequalities.


**★ 6481 ★ British Orthodontic Society**
c/o BOS Office
291 Grays Inn Rd.
London WC1X 8QJ, United Kingdom
**Phone:** 44 207 8372193     **Fax:** 44 207 8372193
**Website:** http://www.bos.org.uk
**Fnded:** 1994. **Mem:** 1,600. **Desc:** Persons interested in orthodontics eligible for membership. Members (normally resident in the UK), honorary members, life members, international members, associate members, retired members, laboratory and trades members. Concerned with the promotion of the study and practice of orthodontics. Orthodontics is a speciality of dentistry and involves the treatment of abnormalities of jaw size and dental arch relationship and irregularities of tooth position. **Pub:** *BOS Newsletter*, 3/year. Newsletter. • *British Journal of Orthodontics*, quarterly. Journal.


**★ 6482 ★ British Society for Dental and Maxillofacial Radiology**
Department of Dental Radiology
University of Bristol Dental School & Hospital
Lower Mardlen St.
Bristol BS1 2LY, United Kingdom
**Phone:** 44 113 2336209     **Fax:** 44 113 2336165
**Email:** j.luker@bristol.ac.uk
**Website:** http://www.bsdmfr.org.uk
**Mem:** 150. **Desc:** Dental radiologists. Offers educational and public service programs. Conducts research. **Pub:** Newsletter, semiannual.


**★ 6483 ★ British Society for Dental Research (BSDR)**
c/o Prof. Colin Robinson
Division of Oral Biology
Leeds Dental Institute

Clarendon Way
Leeds LS2 9LU, United Kingdom
**Phone:** 44 113 2336159　　**Fax:** 44 113 2336158
**Website:** http://www.umds.ac.uk/dental/bsdr/

**Lang(s):** English. **Desc:** Individuals engaged in all aspects of dental research. Seeks to "advance research and increase knowledge for the improvement of oral health worldwide." Provides support and assistance to the oral health research community; facilitates dissemination of new research findings. Conducts continuing professional development programs for members. Works closely with international public health and dental organizations.

**British Society of Medical and Dental Hypnosis**
*See:* Entry 11668

**★ 6484 ★ British Society of Periodontology**
44 Pool Rd.
Hartley Wintney
Hook RG27 8RD, United Kingdom
**Phone:** 44 1252 843598　　**Fax:** 44 1252 844018
**Email:** bspadmin@btinternet.com
**Website:** http://www.bsperio.org

**Fnded:** 1949. **Mem:** 800. **Desc:** Members are dental surgeons. To promote for the benefit of the public the art and science of dentistry and in particular the art and science of periodontology. **Pub:** *Journal of Clinical Periodontology*, monthly. Journal.

**★ 6485 ★ British Society for the Study of Prosthetic Dentistry**
University Dental School and Hospital
Wilton, Cork, Ireland
**Phone:** 353 21 4901141　　**Fax:** 353 21 4345737
**Email:** finbarrallen@hotmail.com
**Website:** http://www.derweb.co.uk/bsspd

**Fnded:** 1953. **Mem:** 390. **Desc:** Ordinary and Honorary Members. Ordinary membership shall be available to those dentists, doctors or scientists who profess an interest in prosthetic dentistry and shall be by election. Established to advance education in prosthetic dentistry for the benefit of the public. **Pub:** *BSSPD Proceedings*, annual. Proceedings.

**★ 6486 ★ Canadian Academy of Denturism (CAD)**
2 Athabascan Ave., Ste. 200
Sherwood Park, AB, Canada T8A 4E3
**Phone:** (780)467-5541　　**Fax:** (780)467-9263

**Mem:** 90. **Lang(s):** English, French. **Desc:** Dentists and related health professionals. Promotes advancement in the study and practice of denturism. Conducts continuing professional education programs. Sponsors research. **Pub:** *Academy Report*, annual. Journal.

**★ 6487 ★ Canadian Academy of Endodontics (CAE)**
**(Academie Canadienne d'Endodontie — ACE)**
Dentue colorado
Univ. of Saskatchewan
105 Wiggins Rd.
Saskatoon, SK, Canada S7N 5E4
**Phone:** (306)966-5089　　**Fax:** (306)966-5018
**Email:** teplitsky@skyfox.usask.la
**Website:** http://www.caendo.ca/default.htm

**Fnded:** 1965. **Mem:** 200. **Lang(s):** English, French. **Desc:** Member dentists of the Canadian Dental Association or other Canadian national dental associations who have been graduated for at least 3 years or have earned recognition by graduate or postgraduate training, teaching, or research. Works to maintain and improve public health through the advancement of endodontics. Sponsors competitions and bestows awards; maintains speakers' bureau; compiles statistics. **Pub:** *Roster*, annual. • Newsletter, 2-3/year.

**★ 6488 ★ Canadian Academy of Periodontology (CAP)**
**(Academie Canadienne de Parodotologie)**
1815 Alta Vista Dr., Unit 105
Ottawa, ON, Canada K1G 3Y6
**Phone:** (613)523-9800　　**Fax:** (613)523-1968
**Email:** central-office@cap-acp.ca
**Website:** http://www.cap-acp.ca

**Mem:** 300. **Lang(s):** English, French. **Desc:** Periodontologists, educators, and students. Promotes advancement in the practice and teaching of periodontology. Conducts continuing professional education courses for members. Maintains speakers' bureau. **Pub:** *CAPsule*, 3/year. Newsletter. • Directory, annual.

**★ 6489 ★ Canadian Association for Dental Research (CADR)**
**(Association Canadienne de Recherches Dentaires — ACRD)**
Univ. of Alberta
45 University Campus NW
Edmonton, AB, Canada T6G 2N8
**Phone:** (403)491-1624

**Lang(s):** English, French. **Desc:** Dentists, dental schools, and dental research facilities. Seeks to advance the practice of dentistry. Sponsors dental research projects; conducts continuing professional education courses.

**★ 6490 ★ Canadian Association of Orthodontists (CAO)**
**(Association Canadienne des Orthodontistes — ACO)**
2175 Sheppard Ave. E, Ste. 310
North York, ON, Canada M2J 1W8
**Phone:** (416)491-3186　　**Fax:** (416)491-1670
**Email:** cao@taylorenterprises.com
**Website:** http://www.cao-aco.org

**Lang(s):** English, French. **Desc:** Orthodontists. Promotes excellence in the practice of orthodonture. Conducts continuing professional development courses for members.

**★ 6491 ★ Canadian Association of Public Health Dentistry**
**(L'Association Canadienne des Dentistes en Sante Communautaire)**
44 Peel Centre Dr., Ste. 102
Brampton, ON, Canada L6T 4B5
**Phone:** (905)791-7800　　**Fax:** (905)791-2697
**Email:** otchered@region.peel.on.ca
**Website:** http://www.caphd-acsdp.org

**Lang(s):** English, French. **Desc:** Public health dentists. Seeks to advance the practice of public health dentistry; encourages continuing professional development of members. Sponsors research and educational programs.

**★ 6492 ★ Canadian Dental Assistants Association (CDAA)**
1750 Courtwood Cres.
Ste. 208
Ottawa, ON, Canada K2C 2B5
**Phone:** (613)521-5495　　**Fax:** (613)521-5572
**Email:** info@cdaa.ca
**Website:** http://www.cdaa.ca

**Reg. Groups:** 10. **Lang(s):** English. **Desc:** Dental assistants in Canada. Fosters opportunities for growth in the field in of dental assisting and represents members' interests.

**★ 6493 ★ Canadian Dental Association (CDA)**
**(Association Dentair Canadienne — ADC)**
1815 Alta Vista Dr.
Ottawa, ON, Canada K1G 3Y6
**Phone:** (613)523-1770　　**Free:** 800-267-6354
**Fax:** (613)523-7736
**Email:** reception@cda-adc.ca

**Website:** http://www.cda-adc.ca

**Lang(s):** English, French. **Desc:** Dentists. Seeks to advance the profession of dentistry. Facilitates exchange of information among members; sponsors continuing professional education courses.

**★ 6494 ★ Canadian Dental Hygienists' Association (CDHA)**
96 Centerpointe Dr.
Ottawa, ON, Canada K2G 6B1
**Phone:** (613)224-5515　　**Fax:** (613)224-7283
**Email:** info@cdha.ca

**Lang(s):** English, French. **Desc:** Dental hygienists. Promotes development of standards of ethics and practice in the field of dental hygiene; facilitates professional advancement of members. Provides dental hygiene services to previously underserved populations; conducts educational programs.

**★ 6495 ★ Canadian Dental Protective Association (CDPA)**
2175 Sheppard Ave. E
Ste. 310
Toronto, ON, Canada M2J 1W8
**Phone:** (416)491-5932　　**Free:** 800-876-2372
**Fax:** (416)491-1670
**Email:** cdpa@taylorenterprises.com
**Website:** http://www.cdpa.com

**Lang(s):** English. **Desc:** Dentists in Canada. Cares for the risk management needs of its members. Sponsors legal benefits insurance plan for members and their families.

**★ 6496 ★ Ceska Stomatologi Komora**
Jecna 3
CZ-120 00 Prague 2, Czech Republic
**Phone:** 42 2 24918611　　**Fax:** 42 2 24917372
**Email:** csk@dent.cz

**Desc:** Represents dentists' interests.

**★ 6497 ★ Christian Dental Society (CDS)**
PO Box 296
Sumner, IA 50674
**Phone:** (563)578-8843　　**Free:** 800-CDS-SENT
**Fax:** (563)578-8843
**Email:** cdssent@sbt.net
**Website:** http://www.christiandental.org
Jim Jespersen, DDS, contact

**Fnded:** 1962. **Mem:** 900. **Desc:** Encourages dentists to donate their professional services to Christian schools, clinics, and hospitals. Members also supply materials and equipment to missions. Maintains speakers' bureau. **Pub:** *CDS News Update*, monthly. Newsletter. • *CDS Newsletter*, quarterly. Newsletter. • *Portable Mission Dentistry*. **Frmly:** (1962) Presbyterian Missionary Committee.

**Christian Medical and Dental Society of Canada (CMDS)**
*See:* Entry 2055

**★ 6498 ★ Clinical Dental Technicians Association**
7 The Studios
The Row
Longfield
New Ash Green
Longfield DA3 8JL, United Kingdom
**Phone:** 44 1474 879430　　**Fax:** 44 1474 872086
**Email:** cdta@btinternet.com
**Website:** http://www.cmdsemas.ca

**Fnded:** 1950. **Mem:** 115. **Desc:** Dental technicians seeking legal status in the United Kingdom to train and qualify to make and fit dentures directly with the public under Act of Parliament. **Pub:** *The Denturist*, monthly. Newsletter. **Frmly:** Association for Denture Prosthesis.

**★ 6499 ★ College of Diplomates of the American Board of Orthodontics (CDABO)**
427 Kenwood Ave.
Delmar, NY 12054
**Phone:** (518)439-0981          **Fax:** (518)439-0980
**Email:** 105673.1513@compuserve.com
**Website:** http://www.cdabo.org/
Elizabeth Matterson, Exec. Dir.

**Mem:** 1,726. **Desc:** Members are diplomates of the American Board of Orthodontics who pass qualifying examinations. Promotes self-evaluation and ongoing professional improvement among orthodontists. Conducts seminars. **Pub:** *The Diplomate*, semiannual. Newsletter. *Price:* For members only.

**★ 6500 ★ Commonwealth Dental Association (CDA)**
64 Wimpole St.
London W1G 8YS, United Kingdom
**Phone:** 44 20 72293931     **Fax:** 44 20 76812758
**Email:** juliacampion@cdauk.com
**Website:** http://www.cdauk.com

**Fnded:** 1991. **Mem:** 44. **Lang(s):** English. **Desc:** Local dental associations. Serves as a forum for discussion of matters of interest to members; works to coordinate members' activities. Promotes dental hygiene and oral health. Develops primary preventive dental strategies; conducts training programs for dental health workers; provides technical support to members in implementing programs. Holds educational courses. **Pub:** *CDA News*, semiannual. Newsletter.

**★ 6501 ★ Confederation of Dental Employers (CODE)**
c/o CODE Office
Penroses
Bodmin St.
Holsworthy EX22 6EB, United Kingdom
**Phone:** 44 1409 254354   **Fax:** 44 1409 254364
**Email:** info@codeuk.com
**Website:** http://www.codeuk.com

**Fnded:** 1978. **Mem:** 450. **Lang(s):** English. **Desc:** Owners of dental practices. Promotes success of dental businesses; seeks to advance the profession of dentistry. Develops codes of business ethics and standards of professional practice for members; conducts research and advises members on business issues including taxation, business management, and the law. Implements discount care schemes for promotional use by members. **Pub:** *CODE of Practice*, quarterly. Newsletter.

**★ 6502 ★ Consejo Gerneal de Colegios de Odontologos y Estomatologos de Espana**
Alcala 79-2do
E-28009 Madrid, Spain
**Phone:** 34 1 914264410     **Fax:** 34 1 915770639
**Email:** consejo@infomed.es
**Desc:** Represents the dental profession in Spain.

**★ 6503 ★ Croatian Dental Society**
Avenija Gojka Suska 6
CT-10040 Zagreb, Croatia
**Phone:** 385 1 2903565      **Fax:** 385 1 2864250
**Email:** hsd@kbd.hr
**Website:** http://www.kbd.hr/hsd
**Mem:** 2,800. **Desc:** Dentists and others with an interest in providing dental care in Croatia. Represents members' interests.

**★ 6504 ★ Danish Dental Association (DDA)**
**(Dansk Tandlaegeforening — DTF)**
Amaliegade 17
Postboks 143
DK-1256 Copenhagen, Denmark
**Phone:** 45 70257711          **Fax:** 45 33151637
**Email:** dtfnet@dtf-dk.dk

**Website:** http://www.dtf-dk.dk
**Fnded:** 1873. **Mem:** 6,000. **Reg. Groups:** 11. **Lang(s):** Danish, English. **Desc:** Danish dentists. Represents members' interests; promotes dental health care in Denmark. Offers postgraduate training. Maintains placement services; compiles statistics. **Pub:** *Tandlaegebladet*, 18/year. Journal. Provides scientific information.

**Danish Dental Manufacturers**
*See:* Entry 9963

**★ 6505 ★ Delta Dental Plans Association (DDPA)**
1515 W 22nd St., No. 1200
Oak Brook, IL 60523
**Phone:** (630)574-6001          **Fax:** (630)574-6999
**Email:** cs@ddpa.org
**Website:** http://www.deltadental.com
Kim Volk, Pres.

**Fnded:** 1965. **Mem:** 30. **Desc:** Active state dental service corporations; state dental societies; foreign dental service plans. Seeks to increase the availability of dental service to the public by assisting and coordinating the activities of dental service corporations and helping them in the development of dental care programs for application to multistate and national accounts. A dental service corporation (or dental service plan) refers to a nonprofit corporation organized by the dental profession to provide prepaid dental care coverage to the public on a group basis. Maintains speakers' bureau; conducts specialized education programs; compiles statistics. Holds marketing, management, financial, and educational workshops, seminars, and conferences. **Pub:** *The Communicator*, quarterly. Newsletter. Covers members news. • *Legal Briefs*, quarterly. Newsletter. Covers legislative issues. • Also publishes educational and promotional literature. **Frmly:** National Association of Dental Service Plans.

**★ 6506 ★ Delta Sigma Delta**
296 15th Ave.
Nekoosa, WI 54457
**Phone:** (715)325-6320          **Free:** 800-335-8744
**Fax:** (715)325-3057
**Email:** supremescribe@deltsig.com
**Website:** http://www.deltsig.com
Dr. John H. Prey, Supreme Scribe

**Fnded:** 1882. **Mem:** 29,000. **Nat'l Groups:** 10. **State Groups:** 35. **Local Groups:** 34. **Desc:** Professional fraternity - dentistry. Maintains museum; offers educational programs. **Pub:** *Alumni Directory*, quadrennial. Directory. • *Desmos*, quarterly. Magazine. Includes chapter news, scientific articles, and announcements. *Price:* Free to members.

**DENIP**
*See:* Entry 9964

**★ 6507 ★ Dental Assisting National Board (DANB)**
676 N St. Clair, Ste. 1880
Chicago, IL 60611
**Phone:** (312)642-3368          **Free:** 800-FOR-DANB
**Fax:** (312)642-1475
**Email:** danbmail@danb.org
**Website:** http://www.danb.org
Diane Owen, Chair

**Fnded:** 1948. **Desc:** Certifying agency that administers examinations to dental assistants. **Frmly:** Certifying Board of the American Dental Assistants Association.

**★ 6508 ★ Dental Association of Russia**
34 New Arbat St., Of. 201
121099 Moscow, Russia
**Phone:** 7 95 2053918          **Fax:** 7 95 2053918
**Email:** sadovski@dentist.ru
**Website:** http://www.dentist.ru

**Desc:** Represents the dental profession in Russia.

**★ 6509 ★ Dental Association of Thailand (DAT)**
71 Ladprao 95
Wangtonglhang
Bangkok 10310, Thailand
**Phone:** 66 2 5394748          **Fax:** 66 2 5141100
**Email:** thaident@asiaaccess.net.th
**Website:** http://www.welcome.to/thaidental

**Fnded:** 1947. **Mem:** 5,500. **Lang(s):** English, Thai. **Desc:** Licensed dentists. Promotes dental health and the advancement of the profession. **Pub:** *Dental Association of Thailand*, bimonthly. Journal. With English abstracts. • *News Letter of the Dental Association of Thailand*, periodic.

**★ 6510 ★ Dental Association of Zimbabwe**
PO Box 3303
Harare, Zimbabwe
**Phone:** 263 4 861639          **Fax:** 263 4 707300
**Mem:** 80. **Reg. Groups:** 2. **Lang(s):** English. **Desc:** Dentists and others working in the field of dentistry. Promotes dental health and the efficient practice of dentistry. Works to enhance the professional standing of members. **Pub:** Newsletter, periodic.

**★ 6511 ★ Dental Group Management Association (DGMA)**
PO Box 42036
Phoenix, AZ 85080
**Phone:** (623)465-5691
**Email:** dreid@dentfirst.com
**Website:** http://www.dgma.org

**Fnded:** 1951. **Mem:** 200. **Reg. Groups:** 2. **Desc:** Dental group business managers and others interested in group practice management. **Pub:** *DGMA Communicator*, bimonthly. Newsletter. Includes job listings and membership profiles. *Price:* Free. • Newsletter, semimonthly. • Also publishes articles and books.

**★ 6512 ★ Dental Health International (DHI)**
847 S Milledge Ave.
Athens, GA 30605
**Phone:** (706)546-1716          **Fax:** (706)546-1715
**Email:** bsdds@earthlink.com
Barry Simmons, D.D.S., Pres.

**Fnded:** 1973. **Desc:** Dentists, dental hygienists, dental technicians, and the International Association of Dental Students. Purposes are to promote dental health programs in developing countries; to provide general dental care using portable modular dental units in areas without electricity or water. Utilizes minimal fee structure to support projects; professionals in the field of dentistry donate their services for a period of 3 months. Volunteer dentists and dental technicians collect permanent non-obsolete dental equipment in their local areas and rendevous with the equipment in the host country and assist with the installation of it. Serves "pro-United States" countries.

**★ 6513 ★ Dental Laboratories Association (DLA)**
44-46 Wollaton Rd.
Nottingham NG9 2NR, United Kingdom
**Phone:** 44 115 9254888     **Fax:** 44 115 9254800
**Email:** dental.laboratories@btinternet.com
**Website:** http://www.dla.org.uk

**Fnded:** 1961. **Mem:** 1,000. **Lang(s):** English. **Desc:** Seeks to advance the study, teaching, and practice of dentistry and the dental sciences. Represents members' commercial and professional interests; facilitates communication and cooperation among members; sponsors research and educational programs. **Pub:** *Dental Laboratory*, monthly. Magazine.

★ **6514** ★ **Denturist Association of Canada**
PO Box 46114, RPO Westdale
Winnipeg, MB, Canada R3R 3S3
**Phone:** (204)897-9092　　　**Fax:** (204)895-9595
**Email:** dentcda@mb.sympatico.ca
**Website:** http://www.denturist.org
**Fnded:** 1971. **Mem:** 1,800. **Lang(s):** English, French. **Desc:** Professional denturists, denturist students, and educators. Seeks to advance the profession of denturism and to establish educational standards in the field. Formulates standards of ethics and practice; represents members' interests before legislative bodies and the public; facilitates exchange of information among members; monitors advancements in the field of denturism. **Pub:** *Journal of Canadian Denturism*, quarterly. Journal.

★ **6515** ★ **European Association of Dental Graphology (Association Dentologique Europeene de Graphologues)**
Ave. Vandersmissen 27
B-1040 Brussels, Belgium
**Phone:** 32 2 7713645
**Lang(s):** English, French. **Desc:** Dental graphologists. Promotes adherence to high standards of ethics and practice by members. Establishes standards for dental graphology certification; sponsors continuing professional development courses.

★ **6516** ★ **European Organization for Caries Research (ORCA) (Organisme Europeen de Recherche sur la Carie — ORCA)**
c/o Prof. Lutz Stoesser
University of Jena
Preventive Dentistry
Nordhauser Str. 78
D-99089 Erfurt, Germany
**Phone:** 49 361 7411205　　　**Fax:** 49 361 7411105
**Email:** stoesser@zmkh.ef.uni-jena.de
**Website:** http://www.orca-caries-research.org
**Fnded:** 1953. **Mem:** 333. **Lang(s):** English. **Desc:** Scientists and organizations in 24 countries engaged in research on dental caries. Promotes research on dental caries and evaluates research findings. Establishes contact among organizations and individuals involved in similar research. **Pub:** *Caries Research*, bimonthly.

★ **6517** ★ **European Orthodontic Society (EOS)**
49 Hallam St., Flat 20
London W1W 6JN, United Kingdom
**Phone:** 44 20 79352795　　　**Fax:** 44 20 73230410
**Email:** eoslondon@compuserve.com
**Fnded:** 1907. **Mem:** 2,700. **Lang(s):** English. **Desc:** Orthodontists in 78 countries promoting the science of orthodontics. **Pub:** *European Journal of Orthodontics*, bimonthly. Journal. **Frmly:** (1935) European Orthodontia Society.

★ **6518** ★ **European Prosthodontic Association (EPA)**
Eastman Dental Hospital
256 Grays Inn Rd.
London WC1X 8LD, United Kingdom
**Phone:** 44 20 79151073　　　**Fax:** 44 20 79151246
**Email:** r.welfare@eastman.ucl.ac.uk
**Website:** http://www.eastman.ucl.ac.uk/~epa
**Fnded:** 1978. **Mem:** 528. **Lang(s):** English. **Desc:** Prosthodontists. Seeks to advance the profession of dentistry; promotes continuing professional development of members. Serves as a forum for the exchange of information among European prosthodontists; sponsors research and educational programs.

★ **6519** ★ **European Regional Organization of the International Dental Federation (ERO)**
Postfach 41 01 68
D-50861 Cologne, Germany
**Phone:** 49 2204 427698　　　**Fax:** 49 2204 205316
**Email:** m.bader@bzaek.de
**Fnded:** 1955. **Mem:** 34. **Lang(s):** English, French, German. **Desc:** National dental associations in Europe belonging to the International Dental Federation. Works to establish common professional and health policies in European nations. Provides for the exchange of information; fosters cooperation among members. **Pub:** *ERO Circular Letter*, quarterly. Newsletter.

★ **6520** ★ **European Society for Dental Ergonomics (ESDE)**
Kliniekstraat 9
B-3500 Hasselt, Belgium
**Phone:** 32 89412010　　　**Fax:** 32 11272248
**Email:** hpk@zahn-net.de
**Website:** http://www.esde.org
**Fnded:** 1987. **Mem:** 80. **Desc:** Promotes the collection, analysis, following up, publication and archiving of scientific knowledge concerning dental ergonomics and dental practice.

★ **6521** ★ **European Society for Dental Ergonomics (ESDE)**
BP 162
F-67500 Haguenau, France
**Phone:** 33 3 88937007　　　**Fax:** 33 3 88936366
**Email:** hpk.rickling@zahnmedizin-online.de
**Fnded:** 1987. **Desc:** Analyzes, processes, publishes and files all existing information in the field of dental ergonomics and administration.

★ **6522** ★ **European Union of Clinicians in Implant Dentistry (EUCID)**
Rue Leon Mignon 21
4000 Liege, Belgium
**Phone:** 32 4 2210654　　　**Fax:** 32 4 2237556
**Fnded:** 1989. **Desc:** supports clinical and statistical studies and their application in the odonto-stomatological practice; provides information of patients and of the concerned bodies

★ **6523** ★ **Faculty of Dental Surgery (FDS)**
c/o The Royal College of Surgeons of England
35-43 Lincoln's Inn Fields
London WC2A 3PE, United Kingdom
**Phone:** 44 20 78696810　　　**Fax:** 44 20 78696816
**Email:** fds@rcseng.ac.uk
**Website:** http://www.rcseng.ac.uk/fds
**Fnded:** 1947. **Mem:** 2,500.

★ **6524** ★ **FDI World Dental Federation**
13 chemin du levant
l'Avant Centre
F-01210 Ferney, France
**Phone:** 33 4 50405050　　　**Fax:** 33 4 50405555
**Email:** worldental@fdi.org.uk
**Website:** http://www.fdi.org.uk
**Fnded:** 1900. **Mem:** 650,000. **Nat'l Groups:** 129. **Reg. Groups:** 5. **Lang(s):** French, German, Spanish. **Desc:** National Dental Associates and individual dentists worldwide. A federation of National Dental Association and individual member dentists with the aim of helping to promote oral health worldwide. **Pub:** *Community Dental Health*, quarterly. Magazine. • *The European Journal of Prosthodontics and Restorative Dentistry*, quarterly. Journal. • *FDI World*, bimonthly. Magazine. • *International Dental Journal*, bimonthly. Magazine.

**Federation of the European Dental Industry (Federation de l'Industrie Dentaire en Europe — FIDE)**
*See:* Entry 9967

★ **6525** ★ **Flying Dentists Association (FDA)**
PO Box 189
Buena Park, CA 90621
**Phone:** (714)994-1212
**Email:** flydentist@earthlink.net
**Website:** http://www.flyingdentists.org/
Winnie Houston, Contact
**Fnded:** 1960. **Mem:** 500. **Reg. Groups:** 4. **Desc:** Members of the American Dental Association who have an active aircraft pilot's license. Many members make use of private air travel in conducting their dental practice. **Pub:** *Flight Watch*, monthly.

★ **6526** ★ **Friends of the National Institute of Dental and Craniofacial Research**
1555 Connecticut Ave. NW
Ste. 200
Washington, DC 20036
**Phone:** (202)483-1057　　　**Fax:** (202)462-9043
**Email:** alec@fnider.org
**Website:** http://www.fnidcr.org
Keith Krueger, CAE, Exec. Officer
**Fnded:** 1998. **Mem:** 250. **Desc:** Individuals, institutions, and corporations with an interest in dental research. Believes dental, oral and craniofacial health are of critical importance to the well-being of society. **Pub:** *Online Update!*, monthly. Newsletter. • *Update!*, semiannual. Newsletter.

★ **6527** ★ **General Dental Council**
c/o Antony Townsend, Chief Exec.
37 Wimpole St.
London W1G 8DQ, United Kingdom
**Phone:** 44 207 8873800　　　**Fax:** 44 207 2243294
**Email:** information@gdc-uk.org
**Website:** http://www.gdc-uk.org
**Fnded:** 1956. **Mem:** 50. **Desc:** President (a registered dentist elected by the Council), 6 lay members appointed by The Queen on the advice of her Privy Council, 18 elected members (registered dentists), 17 nominated members (registered dentists nominated by dental authorities), 1. elected dental auxiliary, 4 Chief Dental Officers (ex officio), 3 members appointed by the General Medical Council. Maintains register of dentists; promotes high standards of dental education at all its stages and of professional conduct among dentists, and certain functions in relation to sick dentists. **Pub:** *Dentists Register*, annual. • *Minutes of Meeting of the Council and Professional Conduct Committee*, annual. Proceedings. • *Roles of Dental Auxiliaries*, annual.

★ **6528** ★ **German Dental Association (BundeszahnArztekammer-BZAK)**
Kassenzahnarztliche
Bundesrereinigung
Universitatsstr. 73
D-73 Koln, Germany
**Phone:** 49 30 400050　　　**Fax:** 49 30 40005200
**Email:** post@kzbv.de
**Website:** http://www.kzbv.de
**Fnded:** 1953. **State Groups:** 17. **Desc:** Promotes the dental sciences in Germany and represents German dentistry internationally. Promotes dental education and continuing education. Represents the interests of members to authorities, associations, and the public. Promotes quality assurance, is ethical body. **Pub:** *Zahnarztlidie Mi*, bimonthly. Journal. Contains professional and scientific papers and political statements on dentistry. **Frmly:** National Association of German Dentists; Bundesverband der Deutschen Zahnarzte.

**★ 6529 ★ Hispanic Dental Association**
188 W Randolph St., Ste. 1811
Chicago, IL 60601
**Phone:** (312)577-4013        **Free:** 800-852-7921
**Fax:** (312)577-4013
**Email:** hdassoc@aol.com
**Website:** http://www.hdassoc.org
Sandy Reed, Exec. Dir.
**Fnded:** 1990. **Mem:** 1,950. **Reg. Groups:** 20. **Desc:**
Provides leadership and represents professionals who
share a common commitment to improve the oral
health of the Hispanic community. **Pub:** *HDA News &
Reports*, quarterly. Newsletter.

**★ 6530 ★ Holistic Dental Association**
**(HDA)**
c/o Dr. Paul Plowman
PO Box 5007
Durango, CO 81301
**Phone:** (970)259-1091        **Fax:** (970)259-1091
**Email:** hda@frontier.net
**Website:** http://www.holisticdental.org
Dr. Dick Shepard, Exec. Dir.
**Fnded:** 1980. **Mem:** 200. **Desc:** Dentists, chiropractors, dental hygienists, physical therapists, and medical doctors. Goals are: to provide a holistic approach
to better dental care for patients; to expand techniques, medications, and philosophies that pertain to
extractions, anesthetics, fillings, crowns, and orthodontics. Encourages use of homeopathic medications,
acupuncture, cranial osteopathy, nutritional techniques, and physical therapy in treating patients in
addition to conventional treatments. Sponsors training
and educational seminars. **Pub:** *Communicator*, quarterly. Newsletter. Includes calendar of events and
research updates. *Price:* Included in membership
dues. **Frmly:** Holistic Dental Association International.

**★ 6531 ★ Hong Kong Association of**
**Dental Surgery Assistants (HKADSA)**
c/o Ms. M.A. Crosswaite
Tutor DSA's Office
Department of Conservative Dentistry, 6/F
Prince Philip Dental Hospital
34 Hospital Rd.
Hong Kong, People's Republic of China
**Phone:** 852 28590325        **Fax:** 852 25470164
**Fnded:** 1987. **Mem:** 120. **Lang(s):** Putonghua. **Desc:**
Dental surgery assistants and trainees. Promotes the
study and practice of dental surgery assistance; seeks
to further the professional development of members.
Serves as a clearinghouse on dental surgery assistance. Facilitates exchange of information among
members; conducts educational and continuing professional development courses; sponsors social activities; maintains speakers' bureau. **Pub:** Newsletter,
monthly.

**★ 6532 ★ Hong Kong Dental Association**
8/F Duke of Windsor Social Service Bldg.
15 Hennesey Rd.
Hong Kong, People's Republic of China
**Phone:** 852 25285327        **Fax:** 852 25290755
**Email:** hkda@hkda.org
**Website:** http://www.hkda.org
**Fnded:** 1950. **Mem:** 1,200. **Lang(s):** Chinese, English. **Desc:** Dentists, orthodontists, and others with an
interest in the provision of dental care in Hong Kong.
Promotes the welfare of the dental profession; encourages continuing professional education of members.
Represents members' interests before government
agencies and the public. Conducts research to advance dental practice; disseminates information to
encourage public dental health maintenance. Maintains liaison with other dental organizations worldwide.
Operates speakers' bureau; sponsors competitions;
compiles statistics. **Pub:** *Hong Kong Dental Association Newsletter*, monthly. Newsletter. • *Hong Kong
Dental Association Yearbook*, annual. Yearbook.

**★ 6533 ★ Hong Kong Dental Hygienists'**
**Association (HKDHA)**
GPO Box 706
Centralital Rd.
Hong Kong, People's Republic of China
**Phone:** 852 28590299        **Fax:** 852 28587874
**Fnded:** 1981. **Mem:** 60. **Lang(s):** Chinese, English.
**Desc:** Dental hygienists and students of dental hy-
giene. Promotes the study and practice of dental
hygiene. Represents the dental hygiene profession;
serves as a clearinghouse for government agencies
and public and private organizations with an interest in
dental hygiene. Conducts educational programs. **Pub:**
*HKDHA Newsletter*, quarterly. Newsletter.

**★ 6534 ★ Hong Kong Society of Oral**
**Implantology**
Takshing House, Rm. 704
20 Des Voeux Rd.
Central
Hong Kong, People's Republic of China
**Phone:** 852 25225571        **Fax:** 852 25243557
**Email:** hksoi@netvigator.com
**Website:** http://www.oralimplant.org.hk
**Fnded:** 1995. **Mem:** 100. **Lang(s):** Chinese, English.
**Desc:** Registered dental and medical practitioners;
dental and medical students. Seeks to advance the
practice of oral implantology; promotes professional
development of members. Establishes standards of
professional conduct and practice; conducts research,
educational, and continuing professional development
courses; makes available to members technical and
other assistance. **Pub:** *Newsletter of the Hong Kong
Society of Oral Implantology*, quarterly. Newsletter.

**★ 6535 ★ Icelandic Dental Association**
**(Tannlaeknafelag Islands — TFI)**
Sidumuli 35
PO Box 8596
IS-128 Reykjavik, Iceland
**Phone:** 354 1 5750500        **Fax:** 354 1 5750501
**Email:** tannsi@tannsi.is
**Website:** http://www.tannsi.is
**Fnded:** 1927. **Mem:** 308. **Local Groups:** 4. **Lang(s):**
English, Swedish. **Desc:** Professional association of
active and retired dentists. Conducts charitable activi-
ties; provides emergency dental assistance. Conducts
educational programs. **Pub:** *Journal of Dentistry*,
annual. Journal. • *Newsletter*, monthly. Newsletter.

**INDENT, Dutch Dental Association**
*See:* Entry 9977

**★ 6536 ★ Independent Association of**
**German Dentists**
**(Freier Verband Deutscher Zahnarzte)**
Mallwitzstr. 16
D-53177 Bonn, Germany
**Phone:** 49 228 85570        **Fax:** 49 228 340671
**Email:** info@fvdz.de
**Website:** http://www.fvdz.de
**Fnded:** 1955. **Mem:** 24,000. **Nat'l Groups:** 1. **Reg.
Groups:** 60. **State Groups:** 17. **Lang(s):** English.
**Desc:** Represents and promotes the professional
interests of German dentists. **Pub:** *Der Freie Zahnarzt*,
monthly. Magazine. Informs members of relevant
politics, science, technologies, and service supplies of
the association.

**★ 6537 ★ Indian Dental Association (IDA)**
c/o Dr. V.M. Veerabahu
83 Dewan Bahadur Rd.
R S Puram
Coimbatore 641 002, Tamil Nadu, India
**Phone:** 91 422 453684        **Fax:** 91 442 449555
**Fnded:** 1945. **Mem:** 9,000. **State Groups:** 22. **Local
Groups:** 176. **Lang(s):** English. **Desc:** Dental surgeons; dental students. Promotes the dental profession and educates the public concerning the contributions of dental professionals. Offers educational and
public service programs; conducts research programs.

**Pub:** *Journal of IDA*, monthly. Journal. • Directory,
annual.

**★ 6538 ★ Indian Dental Association**
**U.S.A.**
3540 82nd St.
Jackson Heights, NY 11372
**Phone:** (718)639-0192        **Fax:** (718)639-8122
Dr. Parikh Amrish, Pres.
**Fnded:** 1983. **Mem:** 345. **State Groups:** 5. **Desc:**
Dentists in the U.S. who are of Asian-Indian descent.
Seeks to further the professional education of mem-
bers. Conducts social events. **Pub:** *IDA Newsletter*,
monthly. Newsletter.

**★ 6539 ★ International Academy of**
**Myodontics (IAM)**
c/o Dr. Harry Cooperman D.D.S.
777 Ferry Rd. P-6
Doylestown, PA 18901
**Phone:** (215)345-1149        **Fax:** (215)609-2588
**Email:** myodont@comcat.com
**Website:** http://www.comcat.com/~myodont/
Harry N. Cooperman, D.D.S., Pres.
**Fnded:** 1970. **Mem:** 1,100. **Reg. Groups:** 2. **Desc:**
Dentists who specialize in the treatment of head and
neck syndromes that cause dental or oral malfunction.
Works with physicians and dentists in the field of
myodontics, especially those working on the treatment
of Cooperman-Muira Syndrome, also known as uvula-
tongue malposture syndrome.

**★ 6540 ★ International Academy of Oral**
**Medicine and Toxicology (IAOMT)**
PO Box 608531
Orlando, FL 32860-8531
**Phone:** (407)298-2450        **Fax:** (407)298-3075
**Email:** mziff@iaomt.org
**Website:** http://www.iaomt.org
Michael F. Ziff, D.D.S., Exec. Dir.
**Fnded:** 1984. **Mem:** 1,000. **Nat'l Groups:** 11. **Desc:**
Dentists, physicians, and medical scientists. Encour-
ages, sponsors, and disseminates scientific research
on the biocompatibility of materials used in dentistry.
Offers educational programs; maintains speakers'
bureau. **Pub:** *Bio-Probe Newsletter*, bimonthly. Newsletter. Review of scientific literature and legislative
activities. *Price:* Included in membership dues. • *IN
VIVO*, quarterly. Newsletter. Available to members
only. *Price:* Included in membership dues. • Membership Directory.Indexed alphabetically and geographically.

**★ 6541 ★ International Academy for**
**Sports Dentistry (IASD)**
118 Faye St.
Farmersville, IL 62533
**Phone:** (217)227-3431        **Free:** 800-273-1788
**Email:** iasdsportsdentistry@cillnet.com
**Website:** http://www.acadsportsdent.org/
Susan D. Ferry, Exec. Sec.
**Fnded:** 1983. **Mem:** 750. **Nat'l Groups:** 1. **Desc:**
Dentists, dental students, physicians, athletic trainers,
and others interested in the study and prevention of
dental injuries incurred during sports participation.
Purpose is to foster research, development, and
education in all sciences related to sports dentistry
and its relationship to the body as a whole. Encourages utilization of this knowledge in promoting better
approaches to the prevention and treatment of athletic
injuries and oral disease. Facilitates the exchange of
ideas and experience among members. **Pub:** *ASD
Newsletter*, 2-3/year. Newsletter. Provides information
on the use of craniofacial protection such as helmets,
mouthguards, and faceguards. *Price:* Included in
membership dues. **Frmly:** (2002) Academy for Sports
Dentistry.

### ★ 6542 ★ International Association for Dental Research (IADR)

1619 Duke St.
Alexandria, VA 22314
**Phone:** (703)548-0066    **Fax:** (703)548-1883
**Email:** research@iadr.com
**Website:** http://www.dentalresearch.org
Eli Schwarz, DDS, Exec. Dir.

**Fnded:** 1920. **Mem:** 10,000. **Desc:** Individuals engaged or interested in advancing research in the various aspects of dental and related sciences. **Pub:** *Abstracts, A Special Issue of Journal of Dental Research*, quarterly. Journal. • *Advances in Dental Research*, periodic. Journal. Covers developments in dental research and the chemistry, biology, and function of the oral cavity. Also includes conference proceedings. • *Critical Reviews in Oral Biology and Medicine*, quarterly. • *IADReports*, 5/year. Newsletter. Includes calender of events. *Price:* Included in membership dues. • *Journal of Dental Research*, monthly. Journal. Disseminates new information and knowledge on all sciences relevant to dentistry, the oral cavity, and associated structures in health and disease.

### ★ 6543 ★ International Association of Dental Students (IADS)

c/o FDI World Dental Federation
7 Carlisle St.
London W1V 5RG, United Kingdom
**Phone:** 44 171 9357852    **Fax:** 44 171 4860183
**Email:** elizabethreilly@fdi.org.uk
**Website:** http://www.iads.ndirect.co.uk

**Fnded:** 1951. **Mem:** 52. **Nat'l Groups:** 47. **Local Groups:** 5. **Lang(s):** English. **Desc:** Coordinating body between National Association of Dental students. Association members in 52 countries. Promotes international contact among dental students; facilitates exchange of students between member countries; develops international programs. Organises annual concerts. Conducts competitions. **Pub:** *ADS Newsletter*, semiannual. Newsletter. • *IADS Exchange Guide*. Manual.

### ★ 6544 ★ International Association of Dental Traumatology

20 Tagensvej
DK-2200 Copenhagen, Denmark
**Phone:** 45 35457565    **Fax:** 45 35457506

**Fnded:** 1989. **Desc:** Furthers clinical, experimental research in dental traumatology; promotes integrated education and treatment in dental trauma; fosters public awareness for the purpose of prevention of dental trauma.

### International Association for Disability and Oral Health (IADH)

*See:* Entry 8001

### International Association of Oral and Maxillofacial Surgeons (IAOMS)

*See:* Entry 19563

### ★ 6545 ★ International Association of Oral Pathologists (IAOP)

Eastman Dental Institute for Oral Health Care Sciences
University College London
256 Gray's Inn Rd.
London WC1X 8LD, United Kingdom
**Phone:** 44 20 79151000    **Fax:** 44 20 79151039
**Email:** academic@eastman.ucl.ac.uk
**Website:** http://www.eastman.ucl.ac.uk

**Fnded:** 1976. **Mem:** 380. **Lang(s):** English. **Desc:** Dentists who have had postgraduate instruction in pathology. Seeks to advance the science of oral pathology; works to foster international cooperation in the field. **Pub:** *Journal of Oral Pathology and Medicine*, 10/year. Journal. • *Membership List*, periodic.

### ★ 6546 ★ International Association of Orthodontics (IAO)

c/o Detlef B. Moore
735 N Water St., Ste. 617
Milwaukee, WI 53202
**Phone:** (414)272-2757    **Free:** 800-447-8770
**Fax:** (414)272-2754
**Email:** worldheadquarters@iaortho.org
**Website:** http://www.iaortho.org
Detlef B. Moore, Exec. Dir.

**Fnded:** 1961. **Mem:** 3,050. **Reg. Groups:** 15. **Local Groups:** 80. **Desc:** Dentists. Promotes the study and dissemination of information on the cause, control, treatment, and prevention of malocclusion of the teeth; facilitates exchange of ideas and experiences, based on a biomechanical approach, between the various fields of dentistry related to orthodontics. **Pub:** *IAO Straight Talk*, quarterly. Newsletter. Provides information on membership activities. *Price:* Included in membership dues; $15/year for nonmembers. • *International Association of Orthodontics–Directory of Members*, annual. Directory. *Price:* Included in membership dues; $75 for nonmembers. • *International Journal of Orthodontics*, quarterly. Journal. Contains clinical articles on orthodontics, self-assessment, troubleshooting, and new products. *Price:* $40/year. **Frmly:** International Academy of Orthodontics.

### ★ 6547 ★ International Association of Paediatric Dentistry (IAPD)

c/o FDI World Dental Federation
123 Gray's Inn Rd.
London WC1X 8WD, United Kingdom
**Phone:** 44 20 79051251    **Fax:** 44 20 79051285
**Email:** iapd@fdi.org.uk
**Website:** http://www.iapd.org.uk

**Fnded:** 1969. **Mem:** 700. **Lang(s):** English, French. **Desc:** Dentists, dental and medical libraries, bookshops, and research institutions in 36 countries. Encourages research and foster progress in the field of children's dental health. Provides a forum for the exchange of information concerning children's dentistry worldwide. **Pub:** *International Journal of Paediatric Dentistry.*, quarterly. Journal. • *Newsletter*, semiannual. Newsletter.

### ★ 6548 ★ International College of Dentists (ICD)

51 Monroe St., Ste. 1400
Rockville, MD 20850-2408
**Phone:** (301)251-8861    **Fax:** (301)738-9143
**Email:** reg-sg@icd.org
**Website:** http://www.icd.org
Victor J. Lanctis, Pres.

**Fnded:** 1928. **Mem:** 9,200. **Desc:** Dentists who have made outstanding contributions to the profession. Acclaims meritorious service to dentistry; fosters growth and diffusion of dental information; upholds high standards in dental education. Supports the Dental Career Option Seminar for Students. Promotes continuing education through the International Clinicians Program. Operates charitable programs. **Pub:** *Globe*, annual. Journal. • *Key*, annual. Magazine. • *Keynotes*, semiannual. Newsletter. • *Roster*, periodic.

### ★ 6549 ★ International College of Prosthodontists

PO Box 99119
San Diego, CA 92169-1119
**Phone:** (858)270-1814
**Email:** res-inc@msn.com
**Website:** http://www.icp-org.com
Eben Yancy, Exec. Dir.

**Mem:** 750. **Desc:** Prosthodontists.

### ★ 6550 ★ International Congress of Oral Implantologists (ICOI)

248 Lorraine Ave., 3rd Fl.
Upper Montclair, NJ 07043
**Phone:** (973)783-6300    **Free:** 800-442-0525
**Fax:** (973)783-1175
**Email:** icoi@dentalimplants.com

**Website:** http://www.dentalimplants.com
R. Craig Johnson, Exec. Dir.

**Fnded:** 1975. **Mem:** 6,000. **Desc:** Dentists and oral surgeons dedicated to the teaching of and research in oral implantology (branch of dentistry dealing with dental implants placed into or on top of the jaw bone). Offers fellowship and course certification programs. Compiles statistics and maintains registry of current research in the field. Sponsors classes, seminars, and workshops at universities, hospitals, and societies worldwide. Provides consultation and patient information/referral services. **Pub:** *ICOI News*, quarterly. Newsletter. *Price:* Included in membership dues. • *Implant Dentistry*, quarterly. Journal. Includes scientific manuscripts, new product reports, membership updates, and calendar of seminars. *Price:* Included in membership dues; $76 for nonmembers; $95 for nonmembers outside U.S. • *Membership Directory*, annual. **Frmly:** (1976) International College of Oral Implantologists.

### ★ 6551 ★ International Dental Health Foundation (IDHF)

2414 Black Cap Ln., Ste. L-1
Reston, VA 20191
**Phone:** (703)860-9244    **Free:** 800-368-3396
**Fax:** (703)860-9245
**Email:** idhf@aol.com
**Website:** http://members.aol.com/idhf/
Patricia L. Cartwright, Exec. Dir.

**Fnded:** 1981. **Mem:** 450. **Desc:** Dentists, dental hygienists, and other dental professionals. Advocates a method of treating periodontal disease that de-emphasizes cleaning and surgery and instead concentrates on eliminating the disease-causing bacteria. **Pub:** *Annotations*, bimonthly. Newsletter. *Price:* Included in membership dues. • *Seminar Brochures*. Brochures.

### International Federation of Dental Anesthesiology Societies (IFDAS)

*See:* Entry 4464

### ★ 6552 ★ International Federation of Denturists

PO Box 46132
Westdale, MB, Canada R3R 3S3
**Phone:** (204)897-9092    **Fax:** (204)895-9595
**Email:** hansentg@mb.sympatico.ca
**Website:** http://www.international-denturist.org

**Fnded:** 1985. **Mem:** 8,000. **Nat'l Groups:** 8. **Desc:** International voice of denturism; facilitates communication among member nations; promotes denturism and legislation for denturism throughout the world.

### ★ 6553 ★ International French-Speaking Association for Odontological Research (Association Internationale Francophone de Recherche Odontologique)

Faculte d'Odontologie de Reims
2 rue du General Koenig
F-51100 Reims, France
**Phone:** 33 3 26053450    **Fax:** 33 3 26053480

**Lang(s):** English, French. **Desc:** Odontologists and ondontology researchers. Seeks to advance odontological research, study, and practice. Serves as a clearinghouse on developments in odontology; sponsors educational and continuing professional development programs.

### ★ 6554 ★ International Group for Scientific Research in Stomatology and Odontology (GIRSO) (Groupement International pour la Recherche Scientifique en Stomatologie et Odontologie)

c/o Corporation Prof. R. Rodembourg
Faculte de Medecine ULB
Rte. de Lennik 808/621
B-1070 Brussels, Belgium

**Phone:** 32 2 5556361      **Fax:** 32 2 5556361
**Fnded:** 1957. **Mem:** 100. **Lang(s):** English, French, German, Italian. **Desc:** Physicians and dentists doing basic research in stomatology (the science dealing with the treatment of the mouth and its diseases). Encourages exchange of material, documentation, and visits. **Pub:** *Bulletin*, quarterly. Bulletin.


★ **6555** ★ **International Ontological Aid -
France (IOA)
(Aide Ontologique Internationale — AOI)**
115 rue Lamarcq
F-75018 Paris, France
**Phone:** 33 1 42265290      **Fax:** 33 1 42250792
**Lang(s):** English, French. **Desc:** Dentists and dental organizations. Seeks to increase access to dental health care in underpriveleged areas worldwide. Develops dental services at rural hospitals; makes available dental care; supports local dental health centers through provision of equipment and supplies, technical expertise, and voluntary assistance. Conducts educational and training programs for indigenous dental care providers.


★ **6556** ★ **International Ontological Aid -
Vietnam (IOA)
(Aide Ontologique Internationale — AOI)**
19/30 Tran Binh Trong
P5 Binh Thanh
Ho Chi Minh City, Vietnam
**Phone:** 84 8 940797      **Fax:** 84 8 940797
**Lang(s):** English, French, Vietnamese. **Desc:** Dentists and dental organizations. Seeks to increase access to dental health care in underpriveleged areas of Vietnam. Develops dental services at rural hospitals; makes available dental care; supports local dental health centers through provision of equipment and supplies, technical expertise, and voluntary assistance. Conducts educational and training programs for indigenous dental care providers.


★ **6557** ★ **International Organization for
Forensic Odonto-Stomatology (IOFOS)**
c/o Eddy De Valck, B.D.S.
Parklaan 10
B-1852 Beigem, Belgium
**Phone:** 32 2 2690642
**Fnded:** 1973. **Mem:** 1,500. **Nat'l Groups:** 30. **Lang(s):** English. **Desc:** National professional societies active in the field of forensic odonto-stomatology. Promotes forensic dentistry worldwide. Fosters cooperation among members; collects and disseminates information and ideas on forensic dentistry. Compiles statistics. Supports educational and research programs. **Pub:** *Forensic Odontology, Its Scope and History*. Book. Out of Print, but obtainable through co. Pres. • *International Journal of Forensic Odonto-Homatology*. Journal. • *IOFOS Newsletter*, 3/year. Newsletter. • *The Journal of Forensic Odonto-Stomatology*, semiannual. **Frmly:** (1981) International Society of Forensic Odonto-Stomatology.


★ **6558** ★ **International Society of
Computerized Denisty (ISCD)**
c/o Dr. Bernd Reiss
Bendestorfer Strasse 5
D-21244 Buchholz, Germany
**Phone:** 49 4181 39773      **Fax:** 49 4181 39557
**Email:** wiedhahn@dgcz.org
**Website:** http://www.iscd.de
**Fnded:** 1996. **Mem:** 2,500. **Lang(s):** English. **Desc:** Membership includes national societies of computerized dentistry from countries around the world and individual dentists from countries where no national society exists. Promotes the use of computer-supported methods in odontology. Initiates and supports research in practical dentistry involving the use of computerized methods; assists members in dealing with other dental institutions, corporations, and government authorities; offers members continuing and specialized training; cooperates with other internation-

al institutions to further the exchange of knowledge and research. **Pub:** *International Journal of Computerized Dentistry*, quarterly. Journal.


★ **6559** ★ **Japanese Society of
Conservative Dentistry**
c/o Kouku Hoken Kyoukai
Domagome TS Bldg.
1-43-9 Komagome
Toshimaku
Tokyo 170-0003, Japan
**Phone:** 81 3 39478891      **Fax:** 81 3 39478341
**Email:** gakkai8@kokuhoken.or.jp
**Mem:** 4,553. **Desc:** Specialists from all dental schools in Japan, individual dentists in private practice or hospitals. Areas of research interests include application of laser endodontics and immunological studies of periodontal diseases. **Pub:** *Japanese Journal of Conservative Dentistry*, bimonthly. Journal. Includes articles concerning operative dentistry, endodontics, and periodontics.


★ **6560** ★ **Latin American Odontological
Federation (FOLA)
(Federacion Odontologica
Latinoamericana)**
Riobamba 373 - 2D
1025 Buenos Aires, Argentina
**Phone:** 54 11 43722135
**Email:** fola@infovia.com.ar
**Website:** http://www.folaoral.org
**Fnded:** 1917.


★ **6561** ★ **National Association of Dental
Assistants (NADA)**
900 S Washington St., No. G-13
Falls Church, VA 22046
**Phone:** (703)237-8616      **Fax:** (703)533-1153
R. Ludeman, Dir.
**Fnded:** 1974. **Mem:** 6,000. **Desc:** Professional dental auxiliaries. Seeks to: bring added stature and purpose to the profession through continuing education; make available to dental assistants the special benefits normally limited to members of specialized professional and fraternal groups. **Pub:** *Communication in the Workplace*. • *Dental Assistant Salary Survey*, biennial. Survey. • *The Explorer*, monthly. Newsletter. Includes job exchange. *Price:* Included in membership dues; $20/year for nonmembers. • *Infection Control*. • *Mercury Poisoning*. • *Radiology*.


★ **6562** ★ **National Association of Dental
Laboratories (NADL)**
1530 Metropolitan Blvd.
Tallahassee, FL 32308
**Phone:** (850)222-0053      **Free:** 800-950-1150
**Fax:** (850)222-0053
**Email:** nadl@nadl.org
**Website:** http://www.nadl.org
Bennett E. Napier, CAE, Exec. Dir.
**Fnded:** 1951. **Mem:** 2,900. **State Groups:** 45. **Desc:** Represents 2900 commercial dental laboratories, manufacturers/suppliers and educators serving the dental profession. Develops criteria for ethical dental laboratories. Offers business and personal insurance programs, Hazardous Materials Training Program, and an infectious disease prevention training program, business management and technical education programs. Compiles statistics; maintains speakers' bureau and museum; conducts educational and charitable programs and sponsors annual DentalTech Expo. **Pub:** *The Journal of Dental Technology*, 10/year. Magazine. *Price:* $40 for members; $50 for members outside U.S. • *Leadership Newsletter*, periodic. Newsletter. • *Managing for Profit*. Book. • *NADL*, quarterly. Newsletter. *Price:* for members. • *Who's Who in the Dental Laboratory Industry*, annual. Directory. • Also publishes standardized accounting system and makes available videotapes. **Frmly:** National Association of Certified Dental Laboratories.

★ **6563** ★ **National Association of Dental
Plans (NADP)**
8111 Lyndon B. Johnson Fwy., Ste. 935
Dallas, TX 75251-1347
**Phone:** (972)458-6998      **Fax:** (972)458-2258
**Email:** info@nadp.org
**Website:** http://www.nadp.org
Evelyn F. Ireland, CAE, Exec. Dir. /Pres.
**Fnded:** 1989. **Desc:** Dental HMO, PPO's and dental referral plans with Associate members that provide dental indemnity and dental practice management companies. Strives to improve consumer access to affordable quality dental care.


★ **6564** ★ **National Association of Public
Health Service Dentists
(Bundesverband der Zahnarzte des
Offentlichen Gesundheitsdienstes)**
Bergstr. 11
D-37308 Heiligenstadt, Germany
**Phone:** 49 551 61140      **Fax:** 49 551 61140
**Fnded:** 1954. **Mem:** 420. **Nat'l Groups:** 1. **Reg. Groups:** 15. **Lang(s):** English, French, German, Spanish. **Desc:** Safeguards the interests of public health service dentists and promotes their continuing education. Also promotes the prevention of oral diseases, especially in children. **Pub:** *Zahnaerztlicher Gesundheitsdienst*, quarterly, always last week of March, June, September, and December. Magazine.


★ **6565** ★ **National Association of
Seventh-Day Adventist Dentists
(NASDAD)**
c/o Judson Klooster
PO Box 101
Loma Linda, CA 92354
**Phone:** (909)558-8187      **Fax:** (909)558-0209
**Email:** nasdad@sd.llu.edu
Judson Klooster, Exec. Dir.
**Fnded:** 1944. **Mem:** 600. **Reg. Groups:** 11. **Desc:** Promotes the interests and businesses of dentists who are Seventh Day Adventists. **Pub:** *News*, quarterly. • *SDA Dentist*, annual.


★ **6566** ★ **National Board for Certification
of Dental Laboratories (CDL)**
1530 Metropolitan Blvd.
Tallahassee, FL 32308
**Phone:** (850)205-5626      **Free:** 800-950-1150
**Fax:** (850)222-0053
**Email:** nadl@nadl.org
**Website:** http://www.nadl.org/html/cdl.html
Bennett E. Napier, Exec. Dir.
**Fnded:** 1979. **Mem:** 600. **Desc:** Certified dental laboratories, including commercial, private, and dental or dental technology schools. Purpose is the certification and recognition of dental laboratories that demonstrate and document compliance with standards set by the industry for laboratory facilities, technical resources, safety, prevention of cross-contamination, and competence of personnel. **Pub:** *Certified Mail*, periodic. Newsletter. • Directory, semiannual.


★ **6567** ★ **National Board for Certification
in Dental Technology**
c/o National Association of Dental Laboratories
1530 Metropoliton
Tallahassee, FL 32308
**Phone:** (850)205-5626      **Free:** 800-950-1150
**Fax:** (850)222-0053
**Email:** nadl@nadl.org
**Website:** http://www.nadl.org
Richard Harrell, Nat'l Pres.
**Fnded:** 1958. **Mem:** 10,000. **Desc:** Certifies dental technicians with formal education in dental technology and a minimum of three years' experience who have passed written and practical exams administered by the NBC. Provides continuing education to certificants and recognizes competent dental technicians. Also certifies dental laboratories that meet published standards for personnel, facility and infection control

practice. **Pub:** *Who's Who in the Dental Laboratory Industry*, annual. Directory. Published in conjunction with the National Association of Dental Laboratories. *Price:* $45.

### ★ 6568 ★ National Dental Assistants Association (NDAA)

c/o Robert Johns
3517 16th St. NW
Washington, DC 20010
**Phone:** (202)588-1697     **Fax:** (202)588-1244
**Email:** admin@ndaonline.org
**Website:** http://www.ndaonline.org
Joseph Gay, Pres.

**Mem:** 500. **Desc:** An auxiliary of the National Dental Association. Works to encourage education and certification among dental assistants. Conducts clinics and workshops to further the education of members. Bestows annual Humanitarian Award; offers scholarships. **Pub:** *NDAA Journal*, annual. Journal.

### ★ 6569 ★ National Dental Association (NDA)

3517 16th St., NW
Washington, DC 20010
**Phone:** (202)588-1697     **Fax:** (202)588-1244
**Email:** admin@ndaonline.org
**Website:** http://www.ndaonline.org
Dr. Gregory A. Stoute, Pres.

**Fnded:** 1913. **Mem:** 7,000. **Reg. Groups:** 6. **State Groups:** 15. **Local Groups:** 48. **Desc:** Professional society for dentists. Aims to provide quality dental care to the unserved and underserved public and promote knowledge of the art and science of dentistry. Advocates the inclusion of dental care services in health care programs on local, state, and national levels. Fosters the integration of minority dental health care providers in the profession, and promotes dentistry as a viable career for minorities through support programs. Conducts research programs. Group is distinct from the former name of the American Dental Association. **Pub:** *Flossline*, bimonthly. Contains educational news. *Price:* Included in membership dues. • *NDA Journal*, quarterly. Journal. **Frmly:** (1932) Interstate Dental Association.

### ★ 6570 ★ National Dental Hygienists' Association (NDHA)

c/o Barbara Seldon, Trustee
28315 Kalong Cir. W
Southfield, MI 48034
Darchelle Strickland, Pres.

**Fnded:** 1932. **Mem:** 100. **State Groups:** 10. **Desc:** Minority dental hygienists. To cultivate and promote the art and science of dental hygiene and to enhance the professional image of dental hygienists. Attempts to meet the needs of society through educational, political, and social activities while giving the minority dental hygienist a voice in shaping the profession. Encourages cooperation and mutual support among minority professionals. Seeks to increase opportunities for continuing education and employment in the field of dental hygiene. Works to improve individual and community dental health. Sponsors annual seminar, fundraising events, and scholarship programs; participates in career orientation programs; counsels and assists students applying for or enrolled in dental hygiene programs. Maintains liaison with American Dental Hygienists' Association. **Pub:** *The Lore*, quarterly. Newsletter. Information relative to NDHA and Dental Hygiene Activities.

### ★ 6571 ★ National Denturist Association (NDA)

PO Box 618
Poulsbo, WA 98370-0618
**Phone:** (360)779-5326
**Email:** wandaa@tscnet.com
Dr. James Davis, Exec. Dir.

**Fnded:** 1975. **Mem:** 350. **Reg. Groups:** 8. **State Groups:** 22. **Desc:** Denturists and other dental professionals. Promotes recognition and authorization of the

profession of denturism. Conducts research regarding law pertaining to the dental profession and to the profession and practice of denturism. Offers seminars for continuing education requirements. Compiles statistics. Provides political action counseling and organizing guidance. **Pub:** *NDA Denturist News*, quarterly. Newsletter. Contains educational and business management articles and political reports. Includes new product information and legal news. *Price:* Included in membership or free upon request.

### National Foundation of Dentistry for the Handicapped (NFDH)

*See:* Entry 8044

### ★ 6572 ★ National Institute of Dental and Craniofacial Research (NIDCR)

45 Center Dr., MSC-6400
Bethesda, MD 20892-2190
**Phone:** (301)496-4261     **Fax:** (301)402-2185
**Email:** nidcrinfo@mail.nih.gov
**Website:** http://www.nidr.nih.gov/
Harold C. Slavkin, DDS, Dir.

**Desc:** Promotes general health by improving oral, dental and craniofacial health.

### ★ 6573 ★ National Oral Health Information Clearinghouse (NOHIC)

1 NOHIC Way
Bethesda, MD 20892-3500
**Phone:** (301)402-7364     **Fax:** (301)907-8830
**Email:** nohic@nidcr.nih.gov
**Website:** http://www.nohic.nidcr.nih.gov
Patricia Sheridan, Project Officer

**Fnded:** 1994. **Desc:** Serves as resource for patients, health professionals, and the public seeking information on the oral health of special care patients, including people with genetic or systemic disorders that compromise oral health, people whose medical treatment causes oral problems, and people with mental or physical disabilities that make good oral hygiene practices difficult. Collects and maintains an online database on oral health and special care issues. **Pub:** *Chemotherapy and Your Mouth*. Brochure. *Price:* Free. • *Diabetes and Periodontal Disease: A Guide for Patients*. Brochure. *Price:* Free. • *Radiation Treatment and Your Mouth*, annual. Brochure. *Price:* Free. • *Temporomandibular Disorders*. Brochure. *Price:* Free. • Also distributes other publications on special care topics, oral health care, oral cancer, smokeless tobacco, dry mouth, and oral complications of cancer treatment.

### ★ 6574 ★ New Zealand Dental Association (NZDA)

PO Box 28084
Auckland 5, New Zealand
**Phone:** 64 9 5242778     **Fax:** 64 9 5205256
**Email:** nzdainfo@nzda.org.nz
**Website:** http://www.nzda.org.nz

**Fnded:** 1905. **Mem:** 1,500. **Local Groups:** 15. **Lang(s):** English. **Desc:** Registered dental practitioners in New Zealand. Promotes improved dental health through the increased availability of dental and allied services. Collects and disseminates data on topics including AIDS, infection control, and oral health costs. **Pub:** *Membership Booklet of the New Zealand Dental Association*, annual. Directory. • *New Zealand Dental Journal*, quarterly. Journal. • *NZDA News*, bimonthly. Newsletter.

### ★ 6575 ★ New Zealand Dental Therapists Association

c/o Kathryn Holdaway
203 Lovedale Rd.
Hastings
Hawkes Bay, New Zealand
**Phone:** 64 6 8787504     **Fax:** 64 6 8787504
**Email:** nzdta@ihug.co.nz
**Website:** http://webnz.com/nzdta

**Fnded:** 1921. **Mem:** 400. **Nat'l Groups:** 1. **Reg. Groups:** 4. **Local Groups:** 18. **Lang(s):** English. **Desc:** Women dental therapists of New Zealand. Promotes the professional interests of members. Works to ensure the provision of dental services to children and adults in New Zealand. Establishes industry standards. **Pub:** *Dental Therapist Journal*, annual. Journal.

### ★ 6576 ★ Omicron Kappa Upsilon (OKU)

University of Nebraska Medical Center
College of Dentistry
40th & Holdgege St.
Lincoln, NE 68583-0740
**Phone:** (402)472-1339     **Fax:** (402)472-5290
**Email:** j.delahanty@umdnj.edu
**Website:** http://www.oku.org
Jan John, Corr. Sec.

**Fnded:** 1914. **Mem:** 17,500. **Desc:** Honorary society of men and women in the field of dentistry. **Pub:** Bulletin, annual.

### ★ 6577 ★ Oral Health America

410 N Michigan Ave., Ste. 352
Chicago, IL 60611-4211
**Phone:** (312)836-9900     **Free:** 800-523-3438
**Fax:** (312)836-9986
**Email:** liz@oralhealthamerica.org
**Website:** http://www.oralhealthamerica.org
Robert J. Klaus, Pres. & CEO

**Fnded:** 1955. **Desc:** Funds dental education, research, and service programs. Operates speakers' bureau. **Pub:** *Advocate*, quarterly. Newsletters. • *Programs and Priorities*, periodic. • Annual Report. **Frmly:** (1963) Fund for Dental Education; (1973) American Fund for Dental Education; (1998) American Fund for Dental Health.

### ★ 6578 ★ Organization for Safety and Asepsis Procedures (OSAP)

PO Box 6297
Annapolis, MD 21401
**Phone:** (410)571-0003     **Free:** 800-298-6727
**Fax:** (410)571-0028
**Email:** osap@clark.net
**Website:** http://www.osap.org

**Fnded:** 1984. **Desc:** Academicians, health care practitioners and dental industry representatives. Works to maximize problem solving of difficult dental infection control issues. **Pub:** Newsletter, quarterly.

### ★ 6579 ★ Orthodontic Education and Research Foundation (OERF)

3320 Rutger St.
Saint Louis, MO 63104-1008
**Phone:** (314)577-8189     **Fax:** (314)268-5673
Joe Mellion, Exec. Dir.

**Fnded:** 1957. **Mem:** 500. **Desc:** Orthodontists. Promotes research; conducts continuing education programs, seminars, and clinical and professional training. **Pub:** *OERF Journal*, annual. Proceedings. Includes new members listing. *Price:* Included in membership dues. • *OERF Newsletter*, annual. Newsletter.

### ★ 6580 ★ Osterreichisches Nationalkomitee der FDI

c/o Bundeskurie Zahnarzte der Osterreichischen Arztekammer
Weihburggasse 9/3/22
A-1011 Vienna, Austria
**Phone:** 43 1 512512662     **Fax:** 43 1 512512667
**Email:** w.doneus@lion.cc
**Website:** http://www.vienna.to/oggg

**Desc:** Represents the dental profession in Austria.

### ★ 6581 ★ Pancyprian Dental Association (PDA)

14 Thason
Rita Ct., 5th Fl.

Off. 501
Nicosia, Cyprus
**Phone:** 357 2 316812          **Fax:** 357 2 316937
**Fnded:** 1968. **Mem:** 440. **Local Groups:** 4. **Lang(s):**
English, Greek. **Desc:** Dentists concerned with the
dental health of the Cyprian populace. Conducts
educational and public service programs. **Pub:** *Dental
Tribune*, quarterly. Magazine.

**★ 6582 ★ Pierre Fauchard Academy
    (PFA)**
c/o Dr. Richard Kozal
PO Box 80330
Las Vegas, NV 89180-0330
**Phone:** (702)651-5013          **Free:** 800-232-0099
**Fax:** (702)651-5537
**Email:** rkozal@aol.com
**Website:** http://www.fauchard.org
Dr. Richard A. Kozal, Sec. -Treas.
**Fnded:** 1936. **Mem:** 6,000. **Reg. Groups:** 10. **State
Groups:** 50. **Local Groups:** 5. **Desc:** Dentists "of
high standards and leadership" who are nominated to
the academy by state or section chairmen. Objectives
are to educate dentists by providing literature on
developments and opinions in dentistry; promote
continuing education for all members of the dental
profession; facilitate the exchange of knowledge
among dentists; foster contact between dentistry leaders and those who seek advice on scientific, technical,
or economic subjects; encourage advancement of
professional and scientific standards; further the improvement of oral health of the public through prevention, therapy, and restoration; emphasize professional
responsibility to the public. Sponsors annual Memorial
Lecture honoring a past leader of dentistry. The
academy is named for Pierre Fauchard (1678-1761), a
French dentist who pioneered modern dental practice
and dental education. **Pub:** *Dental Abstracts*, quarterly. *Price:* $22/year. • *Dental World*, bimonthly. News-
letter. Includes member news, meeting announcements, abstracts, book reviews, and editorials. •
*Leadership Manual of the PFA*. Manual. • *Legacy, The
Dental Profession*. Book. • *The Life and Times of
Pierre Fauchard*. Book. • Membership Directory.

**★ 6583 ★ Portuguese Society of
    Stomatology and Dental Medicine
    (PSSDM)**
**(Sociedade Portugesa de Estomatolgia
    Emedicina Dentaria — SPEMD)**
Rua Prof. Fernando de Fonseca, 10A
Esc. 7
P-1600 Lisbon, Portugal
**Phone:** 351 217 520056      **Fax:** 351 217 520057
**Email:** mail@spemd.pt
**Website:** http://www.spemd.pt
**Fnded:** 1919. **Mem:** 2,200. **Local Groups:** 3.
**Lang(s):** English, Portuguese. **Desc:** Stomatologists,
dentists, and oral and maxillofacial surgeons in Portu-
gal. Promotes research in all disciplines of oral
medicine. Sponsors community dental hygiene pro-
grams. Establishes standards and qualifications for
oral medicine specialists. Represents' members interests; operates legal defense fund for members. Monitors the manufacture of dental materials in Portugal.
Promotes continuing education programs for members. **Pub:** *Revista Portuguese de Estomatologia e
Cirurgia Maxilofacial*, quarterly. Journal. Journal of
dentistry and maxillofacial surgery. • *Stoma*, quarterly.

**★ 6584 ★ Royal Australasian College of
    Dental Surgeons**
64 Castlereagh St.
Sydney, NSW 2000, Australia
**Phone:** 61 2 92323800        **Fax:** 61 2 92218108
**Email:** registrar@racds.org
**Website:** http://www.racds.org
**Fnded:** 1965. **Mem:** 1,200. **Reg. Groups:** 9. **Lang(s):**
English. **Desc:** Dental surgeons. Promotes continuing
professional development of members. Serves as a
clearinghouse on dental surgical techniques and tech-
nologies; conducts educational programs for dental
surgeons. Assists in the formulation of standards for

dental surgical training and practice. Maintains muse-
um. **Pub:** *Annals*, semiannual. Journal. • *Lecture
Notes in Anatomy*, semiannual. • *Lecture Notes in
Histology*. • *Lecture Notes in Microbiology*. • *Lecture
Notes in Pathology*. • *Lecture Notes in Physiology*. •
*Presidential Letter*, periodic. Newsletter.

**Royal College of Surgeons of England
    (RCS Eng)**
*See:* Entry 19590

**★ 6585 ★ Scientific Society of
    Stomatology**
Katedra po Protetichna Stomatologia
Department of Prosthetic Dentistry
1 G.Sofiiski str.
BG-1431 Sofia, Bulgaria
**Phone:** 359 2 542669          **Fax:** 359 2 9520559
**Email:** mitredoc@dentist.bg
**Website:** http://www.rcseng.ac.uk
**Fnded:** 1952. **Mem:** 104. **Nat'l Groups:** 1. **Reg.
Groups:** 2. **State Groups:** 2. **Local Groups:** 15.
**Lang(s):** English. **Desc:** Fosters research in all dis-
eases of the mouth. **Pub:** *Stomatologia - Sofia BG*,
semiannual. Journal.

**★ 6586 ★ Sigma Phi Alpha**
University of Texas, Health Science Center
    Houston, Dental B
PO Box 20068
Houston, TX 77225
**Phone:** (713)500-4085
Patricia Campbell, Treas.
**Fnded:** 1958. **Mem:** 9,000. **Local Groups:** 163.
**Desc:** Honorary society, dental hygiene. **Pub:** *Sigma
Phi Alpha*, annual. Newsletter. **AKA:** National Dental
Hygiene Honor Society.

**★ 6587 ★ Singapore Dental Association
    (SDA)**
2 College Rd.
Singapore 169850, Singapore
**Phone:** 65 2239343          **Fax:** 65 2247967
**Email:** sda@pacific.net.sg
**Website:** http://www.sda.org.sg
**Desc:** Promotes the art and science of dentistry.
Represents the interests of the dental profession.
Upholds high ethical standards and professional con-
duct. Encourages study and research in the field of
dental science and related subjects.

**★ 6588 ★ Slovak Chamber of Dentists**
Fibichova 14
SK-821 05 Bratislava, Slovakia
**Phone:** 421 2 43410517      **Fax:** 421 2 43413198
**Email:** skzl@skzl.sk
**Website:** http://www.skzl.sk
**Desc:** Represents the dental profession in Slovakia.

**★ 6589 ★ Slovenian Dental Association
    (SDA)**
Komenskega 4
SLO-1000 Ljubljana, Slovenia
**Phone:** 386 1 2317868        **Fax:** 386 1 2301955
**Email:** katarina.jovanovic@quest.ames.si
**Fnded:** 1945. **Mem:** 350. **State Groups:** 1. **Lang(s):**
English, German. **Desc:** Dentists and others interest-
ed in promoting and maintaining good dental health.
Conducts educational programs; makes available chil-
dren's services. **Pub:** *Informator*, periodic. Bulletin.

**★ 6590 ★ Society for the Advancement
    of Anaesthesia in Dentistry (SAAD)**
51 Wimpole St.
London W1A 8YH, United Kingdom
**Phone:** 44 207 9351656      **Fax:** 44 1246 208729
**Website:** http://www.saaduk.org
**Fnded:** 1957. **Mem:** 2,100. **Desc:** Dentists and physi-
cians interested in dental anesthesia. Seeks to ad-

vance pain and anxiety control in dentistry. Offers
courses on intravenous techniques and relative analgesia. **Pub:** *Dental Sedation and Anaesthesia*. Book. •
*SAAD Digest*, quarterly.

**Society of Medical-Dental Management
    Consultants (SMD)**
*See:* Entry 9995

**★ 6591 ★ Society for Occlusal Studies
    (SOS)**
c/o Dr. Bernard Williams
4601 W 109th St. Ste. 225
Overland Park, KS 66211
**Fax:** (816)941-4832
**Email:** chuck@smdmc.org
**Website:** http://www.smdmc.org
Dr. Bernard Williams, Pres.
**Fnded:** 1964. **Mem:** 800. **Local Groups:** 95. **Desc:**
Dentists and laboratory technicians who have completed the society's continuing education course in
occlusion (bringing opposing surfaces of the teeth of
the two jaws into contact). Promotes effective occlusal
treatment. Conducts Principles of Occlusion Seminar,
Advanced Restorative Seminar, laboratory technician
program, and practice management program. **Pub:**
*Roster*, annual. • *SOS Newsletter*, quarterly. Newsletter. Covers developments in the treatment and diagnosis of temporomandibular joint dysfunction and principles of occlusion instrumentation. *Price:* Included in
membership dues.

**★ 6592 ★ South African Dental
    Association (SADA)**
Private Bag 1
Houghton
Gauteng 2041, Republic of South Africa
**Phone:** 27 11 4845288        **Fax:** 27 11 6425718
**Email:** info@sada.co.za
**Website:** http://www.edoc.co.za/sadanet/index.html
**Fnded:** 1922. **Mem:** 3,083. **Reg. Groups:** 11.
**Lang(s):** Afrikaans, English. **Desc:** Practicing and
retired dentists. Represents the dental profession in
South Africa. Promotes research and investigation into
dentistry and allied sciences. Sponsors National Den-
tal Health Week in South Africa. **Pub:** *South African
Dental Journal*, monthly. Journal. Includes original
scientific articles and general dental material. **Frmly:**
(1998) Dental Association of South Africa.

**★ 6593 ★ Special Care Dentistry**
211 E Chicago Ave., 5th Fl.
Chicago, IL 60611-9361
**Phone:** (312)440-2660          **Fax:** (312)440-2824
**Email:** specialcaredent@yahoo.com
**Website:** http://www.foscod.org
James J. Balija, CAE, Exec. Dir.
**Fnded:** 1987. **Mem:** 1,600. **Nat'l Groups:** 3. **Desc:**
Dentists, hygienists, and lay public interested in spe-
cial care dentistry. Seeks to improve the quality of oral
health for persons with special needs; offers fellow-
ships in hospital care dentistry, geriatric care dentistry,
and disability care dentistry. Conducts educational
programs. **Pub:** *Oral Facial Emergencies*. Book. • *Oral
Medicine in Hospital Practice*. Book. • *Special Care in
Dentistry*, bimonthly. Journal. Features information of
practice and patient care, trends, policy changes, and
calendar of events. **Frmly:** (2001) Federation of
Special Care Organizations in Dentistry.

**★ 6594 ★ Stomatological Society of
    Greece**
17 Kallirroes St.
GR-117 43 Athens, Greece
**Phone:** 30 1 9214325          **Fax:** 30 1 9214204
**Email:** stomsoc@otenet.gr
**Website:** http://www.mednet.gr/stomsoc
**Fnded:** 1937. **Mem:** 600. **Lang(s):** English, Greek.
**Desc:** Dentists. Promotes dentistry in Greece. Pro-
vides members with the latest technological informa-

tion. **Pub:** *Stomatologia*, quarterly. Journal. Includes English summaries.

★ **6595** ★ **Swedish Dental Association (SDA)**
**(Sveriges Tandlakarforbund — STF)**
PO Box 1217
S-111 82 Stockholm, Sweden
**Phone:** 46 8 6661500          **Fax:** 46 8 6625842
**Email:** info@tandlabarforbundet.se
**Website:** http://www.tandlakarforbundet.se/eng
**Fnded:** 1908. **Mem:** 9,000. **Lang(s):** English, Swedish. **Desc:** Union of dentists in Sweden. Offers over 200 continuing dental education courses annually. **Pub:** *Swedish Dental Journal*, bimonthly. Journal. • *Tandlakartidningen*, 18/year. Journal.

**Swedish Dental Trade Association**
**(Foreningen Svensk Dentalhandel — FSD)**
*See:* Entry 9997

**Union of American Physicians and**
**Dentists (UAPD)**
*See:* Entry 2429

★ **6596** ★ **World Federation of**
**Orthodontists (WFO)**
401 N Lindbergh Blvd.
Saint Louis, MO 63141-7816
**Phone:** (314)993-1700          **Fax:** (314)993-5208
**Email:** ldupont@wfo.org
**Website:** http://www.wfo.org/index.html
Lorraine DuPont, Exec. Sec.
**Fnded:** 1995. **Mem:** 6,219. **Desc:** Orthodontic specialists. Encourages high standards in orthodontics and promotes research in the field. **Pub:** *WFO Gazette*, semiannual. Newspaper.

★ **6597** ★ **Xi Psi Phi**
c/o Dr. Keith W. Dickey
1623 Washington Ave., No. 300
Alton, IL 62002
**Phone:** (618)463-1889
**Email:** xipsiphi@hotmail.com
**Website:** http://www.xipsiphi.org
Dr. Keith W. Dickey, Sec. -Treas.
**Fnded:** 1889. **Mem:** 19,000. **Local Groups:** 22. **Desc:** Professional dental fraternity - dentistry. Maintains Hall of Fame. Conducts educational programs. **Pub:** *Quarterly*, quarterly. *Price:* $8.

## Research Centers

★ **6598** ★ **American Association for**
**Dental Research**
1619 Duke St.
Alexandria, VA 22314
**Phone:** (703)548-0066          **Fax:** (703)548-1883
**Email:** research@iadr.com
**Website:** http://www.dentalresearch.org
Dr. Eli Schwarz, Exec. Dir.
**Activities/Fields:** Promotes the advancement of multidisciplinary research of the oral cavity, the adjacent structures, and their relation to the body as a whole. American Association for Dental Research (AADR) supports research fellows and trainees. **Pub:** *AADR Newsletter*. • *Advances in Dental Research*, occasionally. • *Critical Reviews in Oral Biology and Medicine*, bimonthly. • *Journal of Dental Research*, monthly. • *Special Care in Dentistry*, bimonthly.

**American Society for the Advancement of**
**Anesthesia in Dentistry**
*See:* Entry 4474

★ **6599** ★ **American Society for the**
**Study of Orthodontics**
5012 Clearview Pkwy.
Flushing, NY 11364-1041
**Phone:** (718)224-8898
Dr. Milton Bloch, Pres.
**Activities/Fields:** Theoretical, didactic, and applied orthodontics.

★ **6600** ★ **Bureau of Legal Dentistry**
**(BLD)**
146 2355 East Mall
Vancouver, BC, Canada V6T 1Z4
**Phone:** (604)822-8822          **Fax:** (604)822-8884
**Email:** boldlab@unixg.ubc.ca
**Website:** http://www.boldlab.org/
Dr. David Sweet, Dir.
**Activities/Fields:** Dental DNA, including the recovery of DNA from teeth, oral structures and bones; bite mark wound healing; etc.

★ **6601** ★ **Canadian Institute of Health**
**Research**
**Group in Matrix Dynamics**
Medical Science Bldg.
University of Toronto
239 Fitzgerald Bldg.
150 College St.
Toronto, ON, Canada M5S 3E2
**Phone:** (416)978-6681          **Fax:** (416)978-5956
**Email:** christopher.mcculloch@utoronto.ca
**Website:** http://www.cihrmatrix.ca/indexhtml.html
Christopher A. McCulloch, Dir.
**Activities/Fields:** Structure and function of periodontal tissues (tooth supporting apparatus), regulation of cell activity, and relationships to periodontal disease and tooth implants.

★ **6602** ★ **Case Western Reserve**
**University**
**Bolton-Brush Growth Study Center**
Bolton Dental Bldg.
School of Dentistry
2123 Abington Rd.
Cleveland, OH 44106-4905
**Phone:** (216)368-6715          **Fax:** (216)368-3204
**Email:** dean@lucifer.cwru.edu
**Website:** http://www.cwru.edu/dental/bbgsc/home-page.html
Dr. B. Holly Broadbent, Jr., Dir.
**Activities/Fields:** Investigations into the growth and development of dentition, face and cranium, and roentgenographic studies of the epiphyses of the human body. Conducts an ongoing study of longitudinal cephalometric radiographs and dental casts.

★ **6603** ★ **Clinical Research Foundation**
212 Church Ave., Ste. A
Chula Vista, CA 91910-2703
**Phone:** (858)420-8696          **Free:** 800-900-0489
**Fax:** (858)420-6915
Naomi Tanaka, Exec. Dir.
**Activities/Fields:** Head, neck and temporomandibular joint (TMJ) diagnosis, treatment and management; anatomy, radiography, and other therapies; restorative dentistry. **Pub:** *TMD and Restorative Dentistry*.

★ **6604** ★ **Craniofacial Center**
1847 Old York Rd.
Abington, PA 19001
**Phone:** (215)657-7788          **Fax:** (215)657-5483
Dr. Neil Gottehrer, Dir.
**Activities/Fields:** Clinical research on dental implants, including type of implant, longevity, and coatings used on implants.

★ **6605** ★ **The Forsyth Institute**
140 Fenway
Boston, MA 02115-3799
**Phone:** (617)262-5200          **Fax:** (617)262-4021
**Email:** dpdepaola@forsyth.org
**Website:** http://www.forsyth.org
Dr. Dominick P. DePaola, Pres. /CEO
**Activities/Fields:** Physical, biomedical, and clinical sciences pertinent to field of oral biology. Seeks to obtain a better understanding of normal and diseased structures of the oral cavity and its related parts, including bioadhesion, molecular genetics, immunology, biomineralization, clinical trials, cytokine biology, periodontology, electron microscopy, nutrition, and craniofacial growth and development. Conducts research into the cause, cure and prevention of dental caries, periodontal diseases, oral cancer, oral and facial deformities and oral manifestations of other diseases.

★ **6606** ★ **Indiana University-Purdue**
**University at Indianapolis**
**Oral Health Research Institute**
415 N Lansing St.
Indianapolis, IN 46202-2876
**Phone:** (317)274-8822          **Fax:** (317)274-5425
**Email:** dzero@iupui.edu
**Website:** http://134.68.72.125/depts/ohri/default.htm
Domenick Zero, DDS, Dir.
**Activities/Fields:** Etiology, early detection, and prevention of dental caries and periodontal disease; biocompatibility of dental materials. Investigates preventive measures concentrated on fluorides and antimicrobial agents, including a wide variety of in vitro test procedures, research on a number of animal models for determining safety and therapeutic potential, and human clinical investigations of safety and efficacy.

**Indiana University-Purdue University at**
**Indianapolis**
**Oral Health Research Institute**
**Bioresearch Facility**
*See:* Entry 4649

★ **6607** ★ **International Association for**
**Dental Research**
**Craniofacial Biology Group**
Department of Biomedical Sciences
Baylor College of Dentistry
3302 Gaston Ave.
Dallas, TX 75246
**Phone:** (214)828-8277          **Fax:** (214)828-8951
**Email:** pdechow@tambcd.edu
**Website:** http://www.craniofacialbiology.com
Dr. Paul C. Dechow, Contact
**Activities/Fields:** Craniofacial biology, including anthropology, teratology, pharmacology, orthodontics, pedodontics, genetics, cellular biology, anatomy, pediatrics, and neurology. **Pub:** *Newsletter*, semiannually.

★ **6608** ★ **Laval University**
**Research Group in Oral Ecology**
Pavillon de Medecine Dentair
Quebec, QC, Canada G1K 7P4
**Phone:** (418)656-5985          **Fax:** (418)656-2861
**Email:** greb@greb.ulaval.ca
**Website:** http://www.greb.ulaval.ca
Daniel Grenier, Info. Off.
**Activities/Fields:** Studies the biological equilibrium between host and microorganism, including prevention of microbial diseases of the mouth, early identification of high-risk subjects, and outcome predictions of elaborate and frequently expensive curative treatments.

★ **6609** ★ **New York University**
**David B. Kriser Dental Center**
345 E 24th St.
New York, NY 10010
**Phone:** (212)998-9800
**Email:** louis.terracio@nyu.edu

**Website:** http://www.nyu.edu/dental
Dr. Louis Terracio, Dir.

**Activities/Fields:** Dentistry, dental history, and allied health sciences. **Pub:** *Newsletter*, 3/year.


**★ 6610 ★ Ohio State University**
**George C. Paffenbarger Dental Research**
  **Laboratory**
Postle Hall
College of Dentistry
305 W 12th Ave.
Columbus, OH 43210
**Phone:** (614)292-0880      **Fax:** (614)292-9422
**Email:** rosenstiel.1@osu.edu
**Website:** http://www.dent.ohio-state.edu
Dr. S.F. Rosenstiel, Dir.

**Activities/Fields:** Dental bio-materials engineering. Currently studying dental polymers, maxillo-facial polymer synthesis, and optical properties of esthetic biomaterials.


**★ 6611 ★ Oral and Maxillofacial Surgery**
  **Foundation**
9700 W Bryn Mawr Ave.
Rosemont, IL 60018-5701
**Phone:** (847)678-6200      **Free:** 800-822-6637
**Fax:** (847)678-6286
**Email:** omsf@aaoms.org
**Website:** http://www.omsfoundation.org
Dr. James F. Kelly, Exec. Dir.

**Activities/Fields:** Oral and maxillofacial surgery focusing on providing fellowships and grants to both residents and investigators and financial support of other special projects and activities. **Pub:** *American Association of Maxillofacial Surgeons Today.* • *Foundation Insight.* Newsletter. • *Journal of Oral and Maxillofacial Surgery.*


**★ 6612 ★ Orthodontic Education and**
  **Research Foundation**
3320 Rutger
Saint Louis, MO 63104
**Phone:** (314)577-8189      **Fax:** (314)268-5673
**Email:** moscalb@slu.edu
Becky Moscal, Contact

**Activities/Fields:** Orthodontics, focusing on research and education.


**★ 6613 ★ State University of New York**
  **at Buffalo**
**Center for Dental Studies**
250 Squire Hall
School of Dental Medicine
Buffalo, NY 14214
**Phone:** (716)829-3848      **Fax:** (716)837-7623
**Email:** ciancio@buffalo.edu
**Website:**      http://www.sdm.buffalo.edu/
dept.asp?dept=CDS
Dr. Sebastian G. Ciancio, Dir.

**Activities/Fields:** Dental research, including new product evaluation.


**★ 6614 ★ State University of New York**
  **at Buffalo**
**Center for Oral Health Research**
Foster Hall
Buffalo, NY 14214
**Phone:** (716)829-2854      **Fax:** (716)829-2387
**Email:** rjgenco@acsu.buffalo.edu
**Website:** http://research.sdm.buffalo.edu
Dr. Robert J. Genco, Chm. /Dir.

**Activities/Fields:** Laboratory, clinical, and epidemiological investigations of periodontal disease, particularly the etiology, risk factors pathogenesis, and management of this and other chronic bacterial infections; Specific areas of study include microbiology, host response mechanisms, clinical analysis, risk factors, and the development of genetic probes, novel antibiotics, and growth factors as they apply to periodontal diseases. Periodontal disease as a factor in poor diabetic control, cardiovascular disease, respiratory disease and other systemic conditions is also under investigation. **Pub:** *Contemporary Periodontics.* **Frmly:** Periodontal Disease Research Center; Comprehensive Oral Health Research Center of Discovery.


**★ 6615 ★ State University of New York**
  **at Buffalo**
**Periodontal Disease Clinical Research**
  **Center**
Foster Hall, Rm. 120
Buffalo, NY 14260
**Phone:** (716)829-2853      **Fax:** (716)829-2387
**Email:** rigenco@buffalo.edu
**Website:** http://www.sdm.buffalo.edu/research/cent_
per.html
Dr. Robert J. Genco, Dir.

**Activities/Fields:** Periodontal disease.


**★ 6616 ★ U.S. Department of Health and**
  **Human Services**
**National Institute of Dental Research**
**Division of Epidemiology and Oral**
  **Disease Prevention**
45 Center Dr., MSC 6401, RM. 4A5-13D
5333 Westbard Ave., Rm. 528
Bethesda, MD 20892-6401
**Phone:** (301)594-7651      **Fax:** (301)480-8322
Dr. L. Jackson Brown, Dir.

**Activities/Fields:** Descriptive and analytical epidemiologic studies of the etiology, distribution, and trends in dental caries, periodontal diseases, and other oral diseases and disorders. Program's Disease Prevention and Health Promotion Branch manages activities involving health promotion research and application. Research is supported both through intramural projects and research and development contracts. **Pub:** *NIDR's Annual Report.* • *Symposia proceedings.*


**★ 6617 ★ U.S. Department of Health and**
  **Human Services**
**National Institute of Dental Research**
**Division of Extramural Research**
Natcher Bldg.
45 Center Dr., MSC-6402
Bethesda, MD 20892-2904
**Phone:** (301)480-8303      **Fax:** (301)480-8318
**Email:** george.hausch@nih.gov
**Website:** http://www.nidcr.nih.gov
H. George Hausch, Dir., Division of Extramural Acts.

**Activities/Fields:** Administers grant and contract funds for research and training research manpower. Support is provided for investigations ranging from basic laboratory studies on the causes of oral disorders to clinical trials of new therapies or means of disease prevention.


**★ 6618 ★ U.S. Department of Health and**
  **Human Services**
**National Institute of Dental Research**
**Division of Extramural Research**
**Chronic Disabling Diseases Program**
Natcher Bldg.
45 Center Dr., MSC 6402
Bethesda, MD 20892-6402
**Phone:** (301)594-4836      **Fax:** (301)480-8318
**Website:** http://www.nih.gov
Dr. Kenneth A. Gruber, Chief, Chronic Diseases Branch

**Activities/Fields:** Acquired chronic and disabling conditions of the craniofacial region, as well as this areas normal physiology. This includes, but is not limited to, osteoporosis and other bone diseases, autoimmune conditions, temporomandibular disorders, orofacial pain, normal physiology and pathological conditions of the salivary gland. **Frmly:** Craniofacial Anomalies Pain Control, and Behavioral Research Branch.


**★ 6619 ★ U.S. Department of Health and**
  **Human Services**
**National Institute of Dental Research**
**Division of Extramural Research**
**Grants Management Section**
45 Center Dr., Rm. 4AS-55
Bethesda, MD 20892
**Phone:** (301)594-4800      **Fax:** (301)480-8301

**Activities/Fields:** Supports extramural research through grant and contract awards.


**★ 6620 ★ U.S. Department of Health and**
  **Human Services**
**National Institute of Dental Research**
**Division of Extramural Research**
**Oral Soft Tissue Diseases and AIDS**
  **Program**
45 Center Dr., MSC 6402
Bethesda, MD 20892-6402
**Phone:** (301)594-5500      **Fax:** (301)480-8318
Ann Sandberg, Dir. of Basic and Translational Scis.

**Activities/Fields:** Etiology, diagnosis, treatment, and prevention of oral soft tissue diseases and disorders and AIDS as related to oral health.


**★ 6621 ★ U.S. Department of Health and**
  **Human Services**
**National Institute of Dental Research**
**Division of Extramural Research**
**Periodontal Disease Program**
Bldg. 45, Ste. 4AN-18
Bethesda, MD 20892-6402
**Phone:** (301)594-2421      **Fax:** (301)480-8318
**Email:** dennis.mangan@nih.gov
**Website:** http://www.nidcr.nih.gov
Dr. Dennis Mangan, Chf., Infectious Disease Immunity Branch

**Activities/Fields:** Support of research on the microbiology and immunology of oral infectious diseases.


**★ 6622 ★ U.S. Department of Health and**
  **Human Services**
**National Institute of Dental Research**
**Division of Extramural Research**
**Salivary Glands and Oral Biology**
  **Program**
NIH 4S
45 Center Dr.
Bethesda, MD 20892
**Phone:** (301)594-5500
Gerassimos Roussos, Dir.

**Activities/Fields:** Development, structure, function, and diseases of the salivary glands in an attempt to determine the influence of salivary constituents on oral health.


**★ 6623 ★ U.S. Department of Health and**
  **Human Services**
**National Institute of Dental Research**
**Division of Intramural Research**
**Bone Research Branch**
NIH Bldg. 30, Rm. 228
30 Convent Dr., MSC 4320
Bethesda, MD 20892-4320
**Phone:** (301)496-4563      **Fax:** (301)402-0824
**Email:** probey@dir.nidcr.nih.gov
**Website:** http://csbd.nider.nih.gov
Pamela Gehron Robey, Chf.

**Activities/Fields:** Basic and clinical mineralized tissue research. **Pub:** *Research Reports.*

**★ 6624 ★ U.S. Department of Health and Human Services**
**National Institute of Dental Research**
**Division of Intramural Research**
**Neurobiology and Anesthesiology Branch**
NIH Bldg. 49, Rm. IA-04
10 Center Dr.
Bethesda, MD 20892
**Phone:** (301)496-6804          **Fax:** (301)402-0667
**Email:** rdionne@dir.nidcr.nih.gov
Raymond A. Dionne, PhD, Chf.

**Activities/Fields:** Oral-facial sensation, emphasizing mechanisms of pain and the development of new methods for controlling pain in humans. Branch sections utilize anatomical, physiological, behavioral, pharmacological, and psychophysical techniques to study neural function as it relates to the processing of sensory signals about the threat of tissue-damaging stimulation. **Frmly:** Neurobiology and Anesthesiology Branch.


**U.S. Department of Health and Human Services**
**National Institute of Dental Research**
**Laboratory of Developmental Biology**
*See:* Entry 4726


**★ 6625 ★ U.S. Department of Health and Human Services**
**National Institute of Dental Research**
**Laboratory of Microbial Ecology**
NIH Bldg. 30, Rm. 316
9000 Rockville Pike
Bethesda, MD 20892
**Phone:** (301)496-2232          **Fax:** (301)402-0396
**Email:** kenneth.yamada@nih.gov
**Website:** http://wwwdir.nidcr.nih.gov/dirweb/cdbrb/cdbrb.htm

**Activities/Fields:** Microbial ecology.


**★ 6626 ★ U.S. Department of Health and Human Services**
**National Institute of Dental Research**
**Office of Extramural Program Review**
**Basic Sciences Review Branch**
6001 Exec. Blvd., Rm. 3158
Bethesda, MD 20892
**Phone:** (301)443-2620          **Fax:** (301)443-0538
Kursheed Asghar, Chf.

**Activities/Fields:** Coordinates initial scientific review of applications for center research grants, small research grants, conference grants, institutional training grants, short-term grants, and fellowship grants.


**U.S. Department of Health and Human Services**
**National Institutes of Health**
**National Institute of Dental and Craniofacial Research**
*See:* Entry 17831


**★ 6627 ★ U.S. Department of Health and Human Services**
**National Institutes of Health**
**National Institute of Dental and Craniofacial Research**
**Division of Extramural Research**
**(Office of Clinical, Behavioral and Health Promotion Research)**
Bldg. 45, Rm. 4AN-24B
45 Center Dr.
Bethesda, MD 20892-6402
**Phone:** (301)594-2089          **Fax:** (301)480-8318
**Email:** norman.braveman@nih.gov
**Website:** http://www.nidcr.nih.gov/research/extramural/behavior.asd
Norman S. Braveman, PhD, Actg. Dir.

**Activities/Fields:** Development, evaluation and implementation of interventions to prevent or treat craniofacial, dental and oral diseases and disorders; assess behavioral and economic processes influencing health care delivery; researches alternative and complementary medicine; aims to improve end-of-life care.


**★ 6628 ★ U.S. Department of Health and Human Services**
**National Institutes of Health**
**National Institute of Dental and Craniofacial Research**
**Division of Extramural Research**
**(Clinical Trials Program)**
Bldg. 45, Rm. 4AN-24B
45 Center Dr.
Bethesda, MD 20892-6402
**Phone:** (301)594-2089          **Fax:** (301)480-8318
**Website:** http://www.nidcr.nih.gov/research/CTP/clinical_trials.asp
Norman S. Braveman, PhD, Actg. Dir.

**Activities/Fields:** Testing of interventions to prevent, inhibit, or reverse dental and craniofacial diseases and conditions; aims to promote and maintain oral health, using molecular biology, genetics, immunology and imaging.


**U.S. Department of Health and Human Services**
**National Institutes of Health**
**National Institute of Dental and Craniofacial Research**
**Division of Intramural Research**
**(Craniofacial Epidemiology and Genetics Branch)**
*See:* Entry 9067


**★ 6629 ★ U.S. Department of Health and Human Services**
**National Institutes of Health**
**National Institute of Dental and Craniofacial Research**
**Division of Intramural Research**
Bldg. 30, Rm. 132
30 Convent Dr., MSC 4326
Bethesda, MD 20892-4326
**Phone:** (301)496-1483          **Fax:** (301)402-1512
**Email:** henning.birkedal-hansen@nih.gov
**Website:** http://wwwdir.nidcr.nih.gov/dirweb/dirhome.asp
Henning Birkedal-Hansen, DDS, Dir.

**Activities/Fields:** Investigates biochemistry, structure, function and development of bone, teeth, salivary glands and connective tissues; studies role of bacteria and viruses in oral disease; genetic disorders and tumors of the oral cavity; cause and treatment of acute and chronic pain; development of new methods to diagnose oral diseases.


**★ 6630 ★ University of Alabama at Birmingham**
**Center for Research in Oral Biology**
845 S 19th St., BBRB 258/5
Birmingham, AL 35294-2170
**Phone:** (205)934-3470          **Fax:** (205)934-9256
**Email:** suemich@uab.edu
Dr. Suzanne M. Michalek, Dir.

**Activities/Fields:** Oral biology, mucosal immunology, and connective tissue biochemistry. **Frmly:** Institute of Dental Research.


**★ 6631 ★ University of California, Los Angeles**
**Dental Research Institute**
Center for Health Science
PO Box 951668
Los Angeles, CA 90095-1668
**Phone:** (310)206-6063          **Fax:** (310)794-7734
**Email:** npark@dent.ucla.edu
**Website:** http://www.dent.ucla.edu/
Dr. No-Hee Park, Dir.

**Activities/Fields:** Oral cancer, molecular oncology, viral oncology, molecular mechanisms of periodontal diseases, ultrastructure and cell biology, dental implantology, TMJ disorders and orofacial pain, neuroimmunology, molecular immunology, AIDS/HIV immunology, pain control/pharmacology, biomaterials, and wound repair/keloid tissue formation mechanisms. Also conducts clinical dental science studies. **Pub:** *International Journal of Oral Biology*, quarterly. • *UCLA Dental Research Annual Report.*


**University of Florida**
**Claude D. Pepper Center for Research on Oral Health in Aging**
*See:* Entry 3103


**★ 6632 ★ University of Florida**
**Periodontal Disease Research Center**
JHMHC
PO Box 100442
Gainesville, FL 32610-0442
**Phone:** (352)392-4377          **Fax:** (352)392-2361
**Email:** mheft@dental.ufl.edu
Dr. William P. McArthur, Dir.

**Activities/Fields:** Microbial etiology of destructive periodontal diseases, antibiotic therapy in the treatment of periodontal diseases, mechanisms of bacterial attachment to teeth, bacterial virulence factors in periodontal diseases, and immune response to bacterial antigens. Evaluates risk factors for periodontal disease. Studies statistical models for progression of periodontal disease. Specializes in clinical trials.


**★ 6633 ★ University of Illinois at Chicago**
**Center for Molecular Biology of Oral Diseases**
MC 860
801 S Paulina
Chicago, IL 60612-7213
**Phone:** (312)996-6118          **Fax:** (312)413-1604
**Website:** http://www.uic.edu/UI-Service/programs/UIC131.html
Dr. Donald A. Chambers, Dir.

**Activities/Fields:** Molecular biological approaches to pathobiology, including the molecular biology of cell proliferation and differentiation, the molecular basis of hematology, immunobiology and the inflammatory response, and mechanisms of host-microbial interaction.


**★ 6634 ★ University of Iowa**
**Center for Clinical Studies**
College of Dentistry
Iowa City, IA 52242
**Phone:** (319)335-7414          **Fax:** (319)335-8895
**Email:** chris-white@uiowa.edu
Dr. James S. Wefel, Dir.

**Activities/Fields:** Oral health, including disease processes (caries, periodontal disease, and oral lesions), restorative materials, and preventive techniques and agents.


**★ 6635 ★ University of Iowa**
**Dows Institute for Dental Research**
Dental Science Bldg.
Iowa City, IA 52242
**Phone:** (319)335-7388          **Fax:** (319)335-8895
**Email:** chris-white@uiowa.edu
**Website:** http://dentistry.vh.org/dows.html
Dr. Christopher A. Squier, Assoc. Dean, Res.

**Activities/Fields:** Normal and pathological development and ultrastructure of oral soft tissues, cariology, oral microbiology, implant biomaterials and bone. Center for Clinical Studies performs research and testing of new oral health materials, products, and treatment modalities in normal and special populations. Provides supportive environment for investigations contributing to the goal of achieving the maintenance of sound dental health through elimination of major oral diseases.

**University of Maryland**
**Center for the Study of Human**
**Performance in Dentistry**
*See:* Entry 16839

**★ 6636 ★ University of Medicine and**
**Dentistry of New Jersey**
**Dental Research Center**
University Heights
185 S Orange Ave.
MSB-C-636
Newark, NJ 07103-2400
**Phone:** (973)972-3728     **Fax:** (973)972-0045
**Email:** finedh@umdnj.edu
Dr. Daniel H. Fine, Dir.

**Activities/Fields:** Host-bacterial interactions in infectious diseases, such as periodontal diseases, mucositis, colitis, cloning of virulence genes that enable attachment and penetration of noxious substances; mucus-drug interaction; synthesis, cotranslational, and posttranslational processing of mucus glycoproteins; sulfation; proteoglycans; and intergrins.

**University of Michigan**
**Antiviral Laboratory**
*See:* Entry 17396

**★ 6637 ★ University of Michigan**
**Bacteriology Laboratory**
3209 Sch. of Dentistry
1101 N University Ave.
Ann Arbor, MI 48109
**Phone:** (734)764-8386     **Fax:** (734)764-2110
**Email:** wloesche@umich.edu
**Website:** http://loeschelabs.dent.umich.edu
Walter J. Loesche, PhD, Dir.

**Activities/Fields:** Oral bacteria and its role in human tooth decay and periodontal disease. Current studies focus on the development of diagnostic indicators of anaerobic infections in periodontal disease, the treatment of anaerobic infections, and the connection between good dental health, xerostomia, swallowing, cardiovascular disease, and aspiration pneumonia in senior citizens.

**★ 6638 ★ University of Michigan**
**Biomaterials Research Center**
Department of Biologic & Materials Science
Sch. of Dentistry
1011 N University Ave.
Ann Arbor, MI 48109-1078
**Phone:** (734)763-9339     **Fax:** (734)647-5293
**Email:** wjobrien@umich.edu
Dr. William J. O'Brien, Dir.

**Activities/Fields:** Develops elastomers for dental prostheses and denture liners, polymerceramic composites for dental restorations, and advanced ceramics for crowns and bridges. Also establishes biocompatibility of dental materials. **Frmly:** Specialized Materials Science Research Center.

**★ 6639 ★ University of Michigan**
**Clinical Research Laboratories**
1324 Sch. of Dentistry
1011 N University Ave.
Ann Arbor, MI 48109
**Phone:** (734)764-9148     **Fax:** (734)936-0374
**Email:** homlay@umich.edu
Dr. Hom-Lay Wang, Dir.

**Activities/Fields:** Etiology of periodontal diseases, focusing on preventive and surgical methods; determining risk factors to predict and treat periodontal disease; assessment of the effectiveness of specific factors and materials in the regeneration of tissues lost

through disease; and assessment of implant materials for optimal osseous integration.

**★ 6640 ★ University of Michigan**
**Electrodiagnostic and Electromyographic**
**Laboratory**
1565 Kuehnle
Ann Arbor, MI 48103
**Phone:** (734)763-3367
**Email:** sew@umich.edu
Dr. Sven E. Widmalm, Dir.

**Activities/Fields:** Etiology and treatment of functional disturbances of the masticatory system, including disturbances of the muscles and joints of mastication.

**★ 6641 ★ University of Michigan**
**Immunology Laboratory**
4208 Sch. of Dentistry
1011 N University Ave.
Ann Arbor, MI 48109
**Phone:** (734)647-3912     **Fax:** (734)764-2425
**Email:** lopatin@umich.edu
Dennis E. Lopatin, Dir.

**Activities/Fields:** Aspects of the interactions between the oral microbial flora and the immune system. Studies address humoral immunity to specific oral microorganisms; cellular networks involved in the responses to different classes of antigens; oral factors that create risk for the development of a variety of diseases and negative health consequences such as caries, periodontal disease, aspiration pneumonia, cardiovascular disease, and immunochemical reagents for the identification of specific microorganisms in dental plaque.

**★ 6642 ★ University of Michigan**
**Prosthodontic Research Laboratory**
1011 N University Ave., Rm. 1064
Ann Arbor, MI 48109-1078
**Phone:** (734)763-5280     **Fax:** (734)763-3453
**Email:** merrm@umich.edu
Prof. Michael Razzoog, Dir.

**Activities/Fields:** Measures wear of prosthodontic devices and conducts serial and longitudinal biopsies of bone.

**★ 6643 ★ University of Minnesota**
**Dental Research Institute**
18-104 Moos Tower
515 Delaware St. SE
Minneapolis, MN 55455
**Phone:** (612)626-3349     **Fax:** (612)626-7017
**Email:** dri@tc.umn.edu
**Website:** http://www.umn.edu/dri/
Dr. Charles F. Schachtele, Dir.

**Activities/Fields:** Coordinates research and training proposals, pilot projects funding, space and equipment maintenance, and research faculty recruitment and development.

**★ 6644 ★ University of Minnesota**
**Minnesota Dental Research Center for**
**Biomaterials and Biomechanics**
16-212 Moos Health Sciences Tower
Sch. of Dentistry
515 Delaware St. SE
Minneapolis, MN 55455
**Phone:** (612)625-9636     **Fax:** (612)626-1484
**Email:** dougl001@tc.umn.edu
**Website:** http://web.dent.umn.edu
Dr. William Douglas, Dir.

**Activities/Fields:** Conducts research on the density dependent growth of dental and other bacterial plaques; neural pathways and electronic anaesthesia; and the development of simulated dental wear, including lubrication and friction of dental wear structures, toothbrush biomechanics, and the fracture toughness of dental hard tissues. Program missions include investigation of new evaluative technologies in biomechanics, service evaluation of biomaterials, and the

clinical measurement of anatomic change in oral structures.

**★ 6645 ★ University of Minnesota**
**Minnesota Oral Health Clinical Research**
**Center**
17-116 Moos Health Sciences Tower
School of Dentistry
Minneapolis, MN 55455
**Phone:** (612)626-5722     **Fax:** (612)626-2651
**Email:** bpihls@umn.edu
Dr. Bruce L. Pihlstrom, Contact

**Activities/Fields:** Dentistry, including materials and restorative sciences, oral facial pain and neuroscience, and caries and periodontal disease. **Pub:** *Newsletter.*

**★ 6646 ★ University of Missouri—Kansas**
**City**
**Dental Research Program**
650 E 25th St.
Kansas City, MO 64108
**Phone:** (816)235-2200     **Free:** 800-887-4447
**Fax:** (816)235-2157
Karen B. Williams, Coord., Grants Admin.

**Activities/Fields:** Biochemistry, dental biomaterials, radiology, analgesics, and pathology, related to dentistry. Clinical programs include study of anomalies of oral region, hard and soft tissues, prosthodontics, occlusion, durapatite particles, prostaglandins and analgesic inflammation, orthodontics, pedodontics, oral diagnosis, periodontics, bone physiology, dental caries, and related pathoses. **Pub:** *Explorer*, quarterly.

**★ 6647 ★ University of North Carolina at**
**Chapel Hill**
**Dental Research Center**
CB 7450
Chapel Hill, NC 27599-7450
**Phone:** (919)966-1538     **Fax:** (919)966-3683
**Email:** pat_flood@dentistry.unc.edu
**Website:** http://www.dent.unc.edu/research/drc
Dr. Patrick Flood, Dir.

**Activities/Fields:** Oral health problems organized into several primary areas: biomaterials research, growth mechanisms, hemostasis research, mechanisms of mineralization, neural mechanisms, biology of extracellular matrices, viral properties and host-pathogen interaction in oral biology, involving both basic and clinical research. Studies problems in oral health related to growth, development, and function of craniofacial region.

**★ 6648 ★ University of Pennsylvania**
**Research Center in Oral Biology**
4010 Locust Walk
Philadelphia, PA 19104-6002
**Phone:** (215)898-8994     **Fax:** (215)573-2324
**Email:** jrosen@biochem.dental.upenn.edu
Dr. Joel Rosenbloom, Dir.

**Activities/Fields:** Oral health, including team studies on biochemistry of connective and hard tissues, analyses of structural and functional constituents of oral microbes, and immunobiology of oral tissues and investigation of plaque formation and effect on periodontal tissues. **Pub:** *COHR Newsletter.* **Frmly:** Center for Oral Health Research.

**★ 6649 ★ University of Rochester**
**Aab Institute of Biomedical Sciences**
**Center for Oral Biology**
Medical Center
601 Elmwood Ave.
PO Box 611
Rochester, NY 14642-8611
**Phone:** (716)275-3441     **Fax:** (716)506-0190
**Email:** james_melvin@URMC.Rochester.edu
**Website:**     http://www.urmc.rochester.edu/aab/oral-bio2/index.html
Dr. James E. Melvin, Interim Dir.

**Activities/Fields:** Saliva glucosyltransferase interactions on surfaces, polysaccharide metabolism by oral bacteria, base production in dental plaque, regulation of mucous cell secretion, basic and applied microbial physiology, interaction of infectious eukaryotic microorganisms with host defense systems, mechanisms and regulation of fluid and electrolyte secretion, genetic engineering of bacteria and regulation of bacterial gene expression, and biosynthesis, structure, function of mucin-glycoproteins, craniofacial development, transgenic and gene-targeted miue, and role of O-glycosylation in oro-pharyngeal development.

★ 6650 ★ **University of Rochester Eastman Dental Center**
Department of Dentistry
625 Elmwood Ave.
Rochester, NY 14620
**Phone:** (716)275-5001          **Fax:** (716)256-3154
**Email:** meyc@troi.cc.rochester.edu
**Website:** http://www.urmc.rochester.edu/dentistry
Cyril Meyerowitz, DDS, Dir.
**Activities/Fields:** Oral diseases, including dental caries, periodontal disease, craniofacial disorders, oral pain and health behavior.

★ 6651 ★ **University of Southern California**
**Center for Craniofacial Molecular Biology**
School of Dentistry
2250 Alcazar St., CSA 1003
Los Angeles, CA 90033
**Phone:** (323)442-3170          **Fax:** (323)442-2981
**Email:** emiranda@hsc.usc.edu
**Website:** http://www.usc.edu/hsc/dental/ccmb/index.html
Dr. Charles F. Shuler, Dir.
**Activities/Fields:** Craniofacial molecular biology, including cleft palate, congenital malformations, myogenesis, and taste and biotechnologies.

**University of Southern California**
**Laboratory for Developmental Genetics**
*See:* Entry 4774

★ 6652 ★ **University of Washington**
**Research Center in Oral Biology**
B-530 HSB, Box 357480
1959 NE Pacific St.
Seattle, WA 98195-7480
**Phone:** (206)543-5599          **Fax:** (206)685-8024
**Email:** ccohr@u.washington.edu
Dr. Beverly Dale-Crunk, Dir.
**Activities/Fields:** Wound healing and tissue regeneration at the molecular and genetic levels and genetic regulation of cell growth and synthetic activities. **Pub:** *Annual Report.*

★ 6653 ★ **Virginia Commonwealth University**
**Clinical Research Center for Periodontal Diseases**
521 N 11th St.
PO Box 980566
Richmond, VA 23298-0566
**Phone:** (434)828-9185          **Fax:** (434)828-5787
**Email:** haschenk@vcu.edu
Dr. Harvey A. Schenkein, Dir.
**Activities/Fields:** Periodontal diseases, including bacteriology, immunology, and genetics, to determine causative bacteria and the mechanism and role of genetic factors and host response in pathogenesis in order to devise improved preventive and therapeutic methods.

# State Government Agencies

## Dental Boards

★ 6654 ★ **Alaska State Board of Dental Examiners**
PO Box 110806
Juneau, AK 99811-0806
**Phone:** (907)465-2542          **Fax:** (907)465-2974
**Email:** wanda_fleming@dced.state.ak.us
**Website:** http://www.dced.state.ak.us/occ/pden.htm
Ms. Wanda Fleming, Contact

★ 6655 ★ **Arkansas State Board of Dental Examiners**
101 E Capitol, Ste. 111
Little Rock, AR 72201
**Phone:** (501)682-2085          **Fax:** (501)682-3543
**Email:** judith.rickard@mail.state.ar.us
**Website:** http://www.asbde.org
Ms. Judith Rickard, Director

★ 6656 ★ **Board of Dental Examiners, Inc.**
**North East Regional Board of Dental Examiners, Inc. (NERB)**
8484 Georgia Ave., Ste. 900
Silver Spring, MD 20910
**Phone:** (301)563-3300          **Fax:** (301)563-3307
**Website:** http://www.nerb.org/
Jack Feldesman, Director

★ 6657 ★ **Central Regional Dental Testing Service, Inc.**
**CRDTS**
1725 SW Gage Blvd.
Topeka, KS 66604-3333
**Phone:** (785)273-0380          **Fax:** (785)273-5015
**Email:** info@crdts.org
**Website:** http://www.crdts.org/
Ted Carter, Director

★ 6658 ★ **Colorado State Board of Dental Examiners**
1560 Broadway, Ste. 1310
Denver, CO 80202
**Phone:** (303)894-7758          **Fax:** (303)894-7764
**Email:** Dental@dora.state.co.us
**Website:** http://www.dora.state.co.us/dental
Karen Brumley, Director

★ 6659 ★ **Florida Board of Dentistry**
4042 Bald Cypress Way, Bin A13
Tallahassee, FL 32399-1721
**Phone:** (850)245-4333          **Fax:** (850)921-5389
**Email:** Sue_Foster@doh.state.fl.us
**Website:** http://www9.myflorida.com/mqa/dentistry/dn_home.html
Sue Foster, Director

★ 6660 ★ **Georgia Board of Dentistry**
237 Coliseum Dr.
Macon, GA 31217-3858
**Phone:** (478)207-1680
**Email:** tathomas@sos.state.ga.us
**Website:** http://www.sos.state.ga.us/plb/dentistry/
Tachunta Thomas, Director

★ 6661 ★ **Hawaii State Board of Dental Examiners**
1010 Richards St.
PO Box 3469
DCCA-PVL
ATTN: DENTAL
Honolulu, HI 96801
**Phone:** (808)586-3000
**Email:** dental@dcca.state.hi.us

**Website:** http://www.state.hi.us/dcca/pvl/areas_dentist.html
Mr. James Kobashigawa, Director

★ 6662 ★ **Idaho State Board of Dentistry**
708 1/2 W Franklin St.
PO Box 83720
Boise, ID 83720-0021
**Phone:** (208)334-2369          **Fax:** (208)334-3247
**Email:** smiller@isbd.state.id.us
**Website:** http://www2.state.id.us/isbd/
Michael Sheeley, Director

★ 6663 ★ **Indiana State Board of Dentistry**
**Health Professions Bureau**
402 W Washington, Rm. W041
Indianapolis, IN 46204
**Phone:** (317)234-2057          **Fax:** (317)233-4236
**Email:** stansinsin@hpb.state.in.us
**Website:** http://www.in.gov/hpb/boards/isbd/
Rosendo L. Tansinsin, Director

★ 6664 ★ **Iowa Board of Dental Examiners**
400 SW 8th St., Ste. D
Des Moines, IA 50309-4687
**Phone:** (515)281-5157          **Fax:** (515)281-7969
**Email:** ibde@bon.state.ia.us
**Website:** http://www.iowaccess.org/dentalboard/
Mrs. Constance L. Price, Director

★ 6665 ★ **Kentucky Board of Dentistry**
10101 Linn Station Rd., Ste. 540
Louisville, KY 40223
**Phone:** (502)423-0573          **Fax:** (502)423-1239
**Website:** http://dentistry.state.ky.us/
Mr. Gary Munsie, Director

★ 6666 ★ **Louisiana State Board of Dentistry**
365 Canal St., Ste. 2680
New Orleans, LA 70130
**Phone:** (504)568-8574          **Fax:** (504)568-8598
**Email:** bogden@lsbd.org
**Website:** http://www.lsbd.org/
C. Barry Ogden, Esq., Director

★ 6667 ★ **Maine Board of Dental Examiners**
143 State House Station
Two Bangor St.
Augusta, ME 04333-0143
**Phone:** (207)287-3333          **Fax:** (207)287-8140
**Email:** anita.c.merrow@state.me.us
**Website:** http://www.licenseverification.com/medental/
Anita C. Merrow, Contact

★ 6668 ★ **Maryland State Board of Dental Examiners**
Benjamin Rush Bldg.
Spring Grove State Hospital
55 Wade Ave.
Baltimore, MD 21228
**Phone:** (410)402-8501          **Fax:** (410)402-8505
**Website:** www.dhmh.state.md.us/dental/
Kim Mayer, Director

★ 6669 ★ **Massachusetts Board of Registration in Dentistry**
239 Causeway St., Ste. 500
Boston, MA 02114
**Phone:** (617)727-3074          **Fax:** (617)727-2197
**Email:** REG.Webmaster@state.ma.us
**Website:** http://www.state.ma.us/reg/boards/dn/default.htm
Patricia Ramsay, Director

**★ 6670 ★ Michigan Board of Dentistry**
**Department of Consumer/Industry Services**
PO Box 30670
Lansing, MI 48909
**Phone:** (517)335-0918     **Fax:** (517)373-2179
**Email:** bhserinfo@cis.state.mi.us
**Website:** http://www.cis.state.mi.us/bhser/lic/boards/bdden.htm

**★ 6671 ★ Mississippi State Board of Dental Examiners**
600 E Amite St.
Jackson, MS 39201-2801
**Phone:** (601)944-9622     **Fax:** (601)944-9624
**Email:** dental@msbde.state.ms.us
**Website:** http://www.msbde.state.ms.us/
Ms. Leah Diane Howell, Director

**★ 6672 ★ Missouri Dental Board**
3605 Missouri Blvd.
PO Box 1367
Jefferson City, MO 65102
**Phone:** (573)751-0040     **Fax:** (573)751-8216
**Email:** dental@mail.state.mo.us
**Website:** http://www.ecodev.state.mo.us/pr/
Sharlene Rimiller, Director

**★ 6673 ★ Montana Board of Dentistry**
301 S Park, 4th Fl.
PO Box 200513
Helena, MT 59620-0513
**Phone:** (406)841-2390     **Fax:** (406)841-2305
**Email:** dlibsdden@state.mt.us
**Website:** http://www.discoveringmontana.com/dli/bsd/license/bsd_boards/den_board/board_page.htm
Ms. Sharon McCullough, Director

**★ 6674 ★ Nebraska Board of Examiners in Dentistry**
**Credentialing Division**
PO Box 94986
301 Centennial Mall South, 3rd Fl.
Lincoln, NE 68509-4986
**Phone:** (402)471-2115     **Fax:** (402)471-3577
**Email:** Marie.Mcclatchey@hhss.state.ne.us
**Website:** http://www.hhs.state.ne.us/crl/crlindex.htm
Ms. Helen Meeks, Director

**★ 6675 ★ Nevada Board of Dental Examiners**
2295-B Renaissance Dr.
Las Vegas, NV 89119
**Phone:** (702)486-7044     **Free:** 800-337-3926
**Fax:** (702)486-7046
**Email:** nsbde@govmail.state.nv.us
**Website:** http://www.nvdentalboard.org/
Ms. VaLonne S. Harmon, Director

**★ 6676 ★ New Hampshire Board of Dental Examiners**
2 Industrial Park Dr.
Concord, NH 03301-8520
**Phone:** (603)271-4561     **Fax:** (603)271-6702
**Website:** http://webster.state.nh.us/dental/
Dr. Raymond J. Jarvis, Secretary

**★ 6677 ★ New Jersey State Board of Dentistry**
124 Halsey St.
PO Box 45005
Newark, NJ 07101
**Phone:** (973)504-6405     **Fax:** (973)273-8075
**Email:** askconsumeraffairs@dca.lps.state.nj.us
**Website:** http://www.state.nj.us/lps/ca/medical.htmden3
Kevin Earle, Exec Director

**★ 6678 ★ New Mexico Board of Dental Health Care**
2055 Pacheco St., Ste. 400
Santa Fe, NM 87504
**Phone:** (505)476-7125     **Fax:** (505)476-7126
**Email:** Cynthia.Salazar@state.nm.us
**Website:** http://www.rld.state.nm.us/b&c/dental/index.htm
Ms. Cynthia Salazar, Contact

**★ 6679 ★ New York State Education Dept**
**Office of the Professions**
**Board of Dentistry**
Office of the Professions
State Education Bldg., 2nd Fl.
89 Washington Ave.
Albany, NY 12234
**Phone:** (518)474-3817     **Fax:** (518)473-6995
**Email:** dentbd@mail.nysed.gov
**Website:** http://www.op.nysed.gov/dent.htm

**★ 6680 ★ North Carolina State Board of Dental Examiners**
15100 Weston Pkwy., Ste. 101
Cary, NC 27513
**Phone:** (919)678-8223     **Fax:** (919)678-8472
**Email:** info@ncdentalboard.org
**Website:** http://www.ncdentalboard.org
David D. Cashwell, Director

**★ 6681 ★ North Dakota State Board of Dental Examiners**
PO Box 7246
Bismarck, ND 58507-7246
**Phone:** (701)258-8600     **Fax:** (701)224-9824
**Email:** ndsbde@aptnd.com
**Website:** http://www.nddentalboard.org/
Dr. Wayne Mattern, DDS, Director

**★ 6682 ★ Ohio State Dental Board**
77 S High St.
Columbus, OH 43266-0306
**Phone:** (614)466-2580     **Fax:** (614)752-8995
**Website:** http://www.state.oh.us/den/
Lili C. Reitz, Esq., Director

**★ 6683 ★ Oklahoma Board of Dentistry**
201 NE 23th Terrace Ste. 2
Oklahoma City, OK 73105
**Phone:** (405)524-9037     **Fax:** (405)524-2223
**Email:** dentist@oklaosf.state.ok.us
**Website:** http://www.state.ok.us/~dentist/
Ms. Linda Campbell, CPM, Director

**★ 6684 ★ Oregon Board of Dentistry**
1515 SW 5th Ave., Ste. 602
Portland, OR 97201-5451
**Phone:** (503)229-5520     **Fax:** (503)229-6606
**Email:** information@oregondentistry.org
**Website:** http://www.oregondentistry.org/
Ms. Jo Ann L. Bones, Director

**★ 6685 ★ Pennsylvania State Board of Dentistry**
PO Box 2649
Harrisburg, PA 17105-2649
**Phone:** (717)783-7162     **Fax:** (717)787-7769
**Email:** dentistr@pados.state.pa.us
**Website:** http://www.dos.state.pa.us/bpoa/cwp/view.asp?a=1104&q=432687
Lisa M. Burns, Director

**★ 6686 ★ Rhode Island State Board of Examiners in Dentistry**
3 Capitol Hill , Rm. 404
Providence, RI 02908
**Phone:** (401)222-2151     **Fax:** (401)222-1272
**Email:** GailG@doh.state.ri.us

**Website:** http://www.health.state.ri.us/hsr/dental.htm
Gail Giuliano, Contact

**★ 6687 ★ South Carolina State Board of Dentistry**
PO Box 11329
Kingstree Bldg.
110 Centerview Dr.
Columbia, SC 29211
**Phone:** (803)896-4599     **Fax:** (803)896-4596
**Email:** joness@mail.llr.state.sc.us
**Website:** http://www.llr.state.sc.us/POL/Dentistry/Default.htm
Mr. Rion Alvey, Contact

**★ 6688 ★ South Dakota State Board of Dentistry**
PO Box 1037
Pierre, SD 57501-1037
**Phone:** (605)224-1282     **Fax:** (605)224-7426
**Email:** sdsbd@dtgnet.com
**Website:** http://www.state.sd.us/dcr/dentistry/denthom.htm
Mr. Steve Willard, Secretary

**★ 6689 ★ Southern Regional Testing Agency, Inc.**
**SRTA**
303 34th St., Ste. 7
Virginia Beach, VA 23451
**Phone:** (757)428-1003     **Fax:** (757)437-4507
**Website:** http://www.srta.org/

**★ 6690 ★ State of California Department of Consumer Affairs**
**Dental Board of California**
1432 Howe Ave., Ste. 85B
Sacramento, CA 95825
**Phone:** (916)263-2300     **Fax:** (916)263-2140
**Website:** http://www.dca.ca.gov/r_r/dentalbd.htm

**★ 6691 ★ Tennessee Board of Dentistry**
425 5th Ave. N
Cordell Hull Bldg., 1st Fl.
Nashville, TN 37247-1010
**Phone:** (615)532-5073     **Free:** 888-310-4650
**Fax:** (615)532-5369
**Website:** http://170.142.76.180/bmf-bin/BMFprofgen.pl
Denise Moran, Director

**★ 6692 ★ Texas State Board of Dental Examiners**
333 Guadalupe, Ste. 800, Tower 3
Austin, TX 78701
**Phone:** (512)463-6400     **Free:** 800-821-3205
**Fax:** (512)463-7452
**Email:** webmaster@tsbde.state.tx.us
**Website:** http://www.tsbde.state.tx.us/Default.htm
Jeffry Hill, Director

**★ 6693 ★ Utah Board of Dentists and Dental Hygienists**
**Division of Occupational and Professional Licencing**
160 E 300 South
PO Box 146741
Salt Lake City, UT 84114
**Phone:** (801)530-6628     **Free:** (866)275-3675
**Fax:** (801)530-6511
**Email:** dtjones@br.state.ut.us
**Website:** http://www.dopl.utah.gov/

**★ 6694 ★ Vermont Board of Dental Examiners**
26 Terrace St., Drawer 09
Montpelier, VT 05609-1106
**Phone:** (802)828-2390     **Fax:** (802)828-2465

**Website:** http://www.nerb.org/stateboards.htm
Diane W. Lafaille, Secretary

★ **6695** ★ **Virgin Islands Board of Dental Examiners**
Roy Lester Schneider Hospital
48 Sugar Estate
St Thomas, VI 00802
**Phone:** (340)774-0117 **Fax:** (340)777-4001
**Email:** webmaster@usvi.org
**Website:** http://www.usvi.org/health/

★ **6696** ★ **Virginia Board of Dentistry**
6606 W Broad St., 4th Fl.
Richmond, VA 23230-1717
**Phone:** (804)662-9906 **Free:** 800-533-1560
**Fax:** (804)662-7246
**Email:** denbd@dhp.state.va.us
**Website:** http://www.dhp.state.va.us/dentistry/default.htm
Ms. Sandra Reen, Director

★ **6697** ★ **Washington Dental Health Care**
Health Professions Quality Assurance Commission
1112 SE Quince St.
PO Box 47860
Olympia, WA 98504-7860
**Phone:** (360)236-4700 **Fax:** (360)236-4818
**Email:** hpqa.csc@doh.wa.gov
**Website:** https://www2.wa.gov/doh/hpqa-licensing/HPS3/Dental/default.htm
Ms. Lisa Anderson, Contact

★ **6698** ★ **West Virginia Board of Dental Examiners**
PO Drawer 1459
Beckley, WV 25802-1459
**Phone:** (304)252-8266 **Fax:** (304)252-2779
**Email:** perryle@wvnvm.wvnet.edu
**Website:** http://www.state.wv.us/bep/lmi/license/LICOCCMS.HTMdentist

★ **6699** ★ **Western Regional Examining Board (WREB)**
9201 N 25 Ave, Ste. 185
Phoenix, AZ 85021
**Phone:** (602)944-3315 **Fax:** (602)371-8131
**Email:** generalinfo@wreb.org
**Website:** http://www.wreb.org/

★ **6700** ★ **Wisconsin Dentistry Examining Board**
Department of Regulation and Licensing
1400 E Washington Ave.
PO Box 8935
Madison, WI 53708-8935
**Phone:** (608)261-7083 **Fax:** (608)267-0644
**Email:** web@drl.state.wi.us
**Website:** http://badger.state.wi.us/agencies/drl/Regulation/applicant_information/dod087.html

## Dental Health

★ **6701** ★ **Arizona Department of Health Services**
Family Health and Community Services Division
Oral Health Office
1740 W Adams Room 10
Phoenix, AZ 85007
**Phone:** (602)542-1866 **Fax:** (602)542-2936
**Website:** http://www.hs.state.az.us/cfhs/ooh/

★ **6702** ★ **California Health and Welfare Agency**
Health Services Department
Chronic Disease and Injury Control Branch
Office of Oral Health
601 N 7th St., MS-725
PO Box 942732
Sacramento, CA 94234-7320
**Phone:** (916)322-4933 **Fax:** (916)324-7764
**Website:** http://www.dhs.ca.gov/ps/cdic/cdcb/Medicine/OralHealth/index.htm

★ **6703** ★ **Connecticut Department of Public Health**
Community Health Bureau
Oral Health Program
410 Capitol Ave.
PO Box 340308
Hartford, CT 06134-0308
**Phone:** (860)509-7655 **Fax:** (860)509-7717
**Email:** webmaster.dph@po.state.ct.us
**Website:** http://www.state.ct.us/dph/BCH/HPBCH.HTML
Dr. Ardell Wilson, Director

★ **6704** ★ **Delaware Department of Health and Social Services**
Public Health Division
Community Health Care Access Section
Dental Health Program
Jesse Cooper Bldg.
Federal & Water St.
PO Box 637
Dover, DE 19903
**Phone:** (302)739-4787 **Fax:** (302)739-6653
**Email:** dhssinfo@state.de.us
**Website:** http://www.state.de.us/dhss/dph/chca/hsd_dental.htm

★ **6705** ★ **Georgia Department of Human Resources**
Public Health Division
Oral Health Section
2 Peachtree St. NW
Atlanta, GA 30303-3186
**Phone:** (404)657-2571 **Fax:** (404)657-2715
**Email:** GDPHINFO@dhr.state.ga.us
**Website:** http://www.ph.dhr.state.ga.us/programs/oral/index.shtml

★ **6706** ★ **Hawaii Department of Health**
Health Resources Administration
Dental Health Division
Lanakila Health Ctr.
1700 Lanakila Ave.
Honolulu, HI 96817
**Phone:** (808)832-5700 **Fax:** (808)832-5722
**Email:** mhkgreer@mail.health.state.hi.us
**Website:** http://www.state.hi.us/health/resource/dental/index.html
Mark Greer, DMD, Director

★ **6707** ★ **Idaho Department of Health and Welfare**
Division of Health
Health Promotions Bureau
Oral Health Program
Pete T. Cenarrusa Bldg. 1st Fl. W
450 W State St.
PO Box 83720
Boise, ID 83720-0036
**Phone:** (208)334-5964 **Free:** 800-926-2588
**Fax:** (208)334-6573
**Email:** garzac@idhw.state.id.us
**Website:** http://www2.state.id.us/dhw/hwgd_www/contentlist.htmlHealth
Catarina Garza, Contact

★ **6708** ★ **Illinois Department of Public Health**
Office of Health and Wellness
Division of Oral Health
535 W Jefferson St., 2nd Fl.
Springfield, IL 62761
**Phone:** (217)782-4977 **Fax:** (217)782-3987
**Email:** mailus@idph.state.il.us
**Website:** http://www.idph.state.il.us/HealthWellness/oralhlth/home.htm

★ **6709** ★ **Iowa Department of Public Health**
Family and Community Health Division
Dental Health Bureau
Lucas State Office Bldg.
321 E 12th St.
Des Moines, IA 50319-0075
**Phone:** (515)281-3733 **Fax:** (515)281-4958
**Email:** webmaster@idph.state.ia.us
**Website:** http://www.idph.state.ia.us/fch/dh.htm
Stephen C. Gleason, Director

★ **6710** ★ **Kansas Department of Health and Environment**
Health Division
Local and Rural Health Systems Bureau
Dental Program
1000 SW Jackson, Ste. 340
Topeka, KS 66612-1365
**Phone:** (785)296-1200 **Fax:** (785)368-1231
**Email:** rmorriss@kdhe.state.ks.us
**Website:** http://www.kdhe.state.ks.us/olrh/
Richard Morrissey, Director

★ **6711** ★ **Kentucky Health Services Cabinet**
Public Health Department
Maternal and Child Health Services Division
Oral Health Program
275 E Main St.
Frankfort, KY 40621
**Phone:** (502)564-3246 **Fax:** (502)564-6533
**Website:** http://publichealth.state.ky.us/dental.htm
Dr. James Curtis Cecil, III, Director

★ **6712** ★ **Louisiana Department of Health and Hospitals**
Office of Public Health
Maternal and Child Health Division
Oral Health Section
1100 Florida Ave. Box 510
New Orleans, LA 70119
**Phone:** (504)670-2738 **Fax:** (504)670-2746
**Email:** koertlin@dhh.state.la.us
**Website:** http://www.dhh.state.la.us/OPH/mch.htm
Karen M. Oertling, RDH, Director

★ **6713** ★ **Maine Department of Human Services**
Community and Family Health Division
Oral Health Program
11 State House Station
Key Plaza
286 Water St.
Augusta, ME 04333
**Phone:** (207)287-3267 **Fax:** (207)287-9058
**Email:** Judith.a.feinstein@state.me.us
**Website:** http://www.state.me.us/dhs/bohdcfh/odh/index2.htm
Judith Feinstein, Director

**★ 6714 ★ Massachusetts Department of Public Health**
**Bureau of Family and Community Health**
**Office of Oral Health**
250 Washington St., 5th Fl.
Boston, MA 02108-4619
**Phone:** (617)624-5943        **Fax:** (617)624-6062
**Email:** mary.foley@state.ma.us
**Website:** http://www.state.ma.us/dph/bfch/ooh/index.htm
Mary E. Foley, RDH, Director

**★ 6715 ★ Michigan Community Health Department**
**Child and Family Services Bureau**
**Oral Health Program**
3423 N Martin Luther King, Jr. Blvd.
PO Box 30195
Lansing, MI 48909
**Phone:** (517)335-9371        **Fax:** (517)335-8560
**Email:** tallmanjac@state.mi.us
**Website:** http://www.mdch.state.mi.us/dch/clcf/fch_12.asp
Jackie Tallman, Contact

**★ 6716 ★ Missouri Department of Health**
**Maternal, Child, and Family Health Division**
**Dental Health Bureau**
930 Wildwood
PO Box 570
Jefferson City, MO 65102
**Phone:** (573)751-6247        **Fax:** (573)751-6041
**Email:** info@mail.health.state.mo.us
**Website:** http://www.health.state.mo.us/AbouttheDepartment/DS9.htmldental

**★ 6717 ★ Nebraska Department of Health and Human Services**
**Health Promotion and Disease Prevention**
**Dental Health Division**
301 Centennial Mall S, 3rd Fl.
PO Box 95007
Lincoln, NE 68509-5007
**Phone:** (402)471-0166        **Fax:** (402)471-0820
**Email:** kim.mcfarland@hhss.state.ne.us
**Website:** http://www.hhs.state.ne.us/deh/dehindex.htm
Kim McFarland, Contact

**★ 6718 ★ New Hampshire Department of Health and Human Services**
**Public Health Services Division**
**Board of Dental Examiners**
2 Industrial Park Dr.
Concord, NH 03301-8520
**Phone:** (603)271-4561        **Fax:** (603)271-6702
**Website:** http://webster.state.nh.us/dental/
Raymond J. Jarvis, Director

**★ 6719 ★ North Carolina Department of Health, and Human Services**
**Public Health Division**
**Community Health Division**
**Oral Health**
1910 Mail Service Ctr.
Raleigh, NC 27699-1910
**Phone:** (919)733-3853        **Fax:** (919)733-4688
**Email:** rick.mumford@ncmail.net
**Website:** http://www.communityhealth.dhhs.state.nc.us/dental/
Rick Mumford, Director

**★ 6720 ★ Ohio Department of Health**
**Family and Community Health Services Division**
**Oral Health Services Bureau**
246 N High St.
PO Box 118
Columbus, OH 43216-0118
**Phone:** (614)466-4180        **Fax:** (614)564-2421
**Email:** BOHS@gw.odh.state.oh.us
**Website:** http://www.odh.state.oh.us/ODHPrograms/ORAL/Oral1.htm
Mark D. Siegal, D.D.S., Director

**★ 6721 ★ Oklahoma State Department of Health**
**Personal Health Services**
**Dental Health Service**
1000 NE 10th St.
Room 712
Oklahoma City, OK 73117
**Phone:** (405)271-5502        **Fax:** (405)271-3431
**Website:** http://www.health.state.ok.us/PROGRAM/dental/index.html

**★ 6722 ★ Oregon Department of Human Resources**
**Health Division**
**Dental Health Section**
Portland State Office Bldg.
800 NE Oregon St.
Portland, OR 97232
**Phone:** (503)731-4021        **Fax:** (503)731-4091
**Email:** h.whitney.payne@state.or.us
**Website:** http://www.ohd.hr.state.or.us/dental/welcome.htm
H. Whitney Payne, DDS, Director

**★ 6723 ★ Pennsylvania Department of Health**
**Chronic Diseases and Injury Prevention Bureau**
**Oral Health Program**
Health and Welfare Bldg.
PO Box 90
Harrisburg, PA 17108
**Phone:** (717)783-1760        **Fax:** (717)783-5498
**Email:** ngardner@state.pa.us
**Website:** http://www.ohd.hr.state.or.us/dental/welcome.htm
Neil Gardner, DDS, Director

**★ 6724 ★ Rhode Island Department of Health**
**Dental Health Division**
3 Capitol Hill, Rm 408
Providence, RI 02908
**Phone:** (401)222-1171        **Fax:** (401)222-4415
**Email:** MaureenR@doh.state.ri.us
**Website:** http://www.healthri.org/disease/primarycare/oralhealth/home.htm

**★ 6725 ★ South Dakota Department of Health**
**Health Promotion Division**
**Dental Program**
600 E Capitol
Pierre, SD 57501-2536
**Phone:** (605)773-3361        **Free:** 800-738-2301
**Fax:** (605)773-5509
**Email:** DOH.INFO@state.sd.us
**Website:** http://www.state.sd.us/doh/Disease2/index.htm

**★ 6726 ★ Tennessee Department of Health**
**Oral Health Services Division**
Cordell Hull Bldg., 5th Fl.
425 5th Ave. N
Nashville, TN 37247
**Phone:** (615)741-7213        **Fax:** (615)741-1063
**Email:** Diane.Denton@state.tn.us
**Website:** http://www2.state.tn.us/health/oralhealth/
Diane Denton, Contact

**★ 6727 ★ Texas Department of Health**
**Dental Health Bureau**
1100 W 49th St.
Austin, TX 78756-3199
**Phone:** (512)458-7323        **Fax:** (512)458-7358
**Email:** dental@tdh.state.tx.us
**Website:** http://www.tdh.state.tx.us/dental/default.htm
Jerry Felkner, DDS, Director

**★ 6728 ★ Virgin Islands Department of Health**
**Dental Health Services**
St. Thomas Hospital
48 Sugar Estate
Charlotte Amalie, VI 00802
**Phone:** (340)774-0117        **Fax:** (340)777-4001
**Website:** http://www.usvi.org/health/index.html

**★ 6729 ★ Virginia Office of Health and Human Resources**
**Health Department**
**Dental Health Division**
1500 E Main St.
Rm. 136
Richmond, VA 23219
**Phone:** (804)786-3556        **Fax:** (804)371-4004
**Email:** kday@vdh.state.va.us
**Website:** http://www.vahealth.org/teeth/index.htm
Karen C. Day, DDS, Director

**★ 6730 ★ West Virginia Department of Health and Human Resources**
**Public Health Bureau**
**Maternal and Child Health Office**
**Oral Health Division**
350 Capitol St.
Charleston, WV 25301-3712
**Phone:** (304)558-1117        **Fax:** (304)558-2183
**Website:** http://www.wvdhhr.org/bph/maternal.htm
Kay Medley, Contact

**★ 6731 ★ Wisconsin Department of Health and Family Services**
**Health Division**
**Public Health Bureau**
**Oral Health Program**
1 W Wilson St.
PO Box 2659
Madison, WI 53707-2659
**Phone:** (608)266-5152        **Fax:** (608)267-2832
**Email:** lemaywr@dhfs.state.wi.us
**Website:** http://www.dhfs.state.wi.us/health/Oral_Health/
Dr. Warren LeMay, Director

**★ 6732 ★ Wyoming Department of Health**
**Public Health Division**
**Dental Health Services**
Hathaway Bldg., 4th Fl.
Cheyenne, WY 82002
**Phone:** (307)777-7945        **Fax:** (307)777-3617
**Email:** cmeyer@state.wy.us
**Website:** http://wdhfs.state.wy.us/dcfh/
Charlie Meyer, Director

# State & Regional Organizations

## Dentistry

*The following are constituent societies of the American Dental Association, 211 E Chicago Ave., Chicago, IL 60611, (312)440-2500, http://www.ada.org/.*

### Alabama

**★ 6733 ★ Alabama Dental Association**
836 Washington Ave.
Montgomery, AL 36104-3839
**Phone:** (334)265-1684    **Free:** 800-489-2532
**Fax:** (334)262-6218
**Email:** concactus@aldaonline.org
**Website:** http://www.aldaonline.org
Wayne McMahon, Exec Director
Wayne McMahan, Exec Director

### Alaska

**★ 6734 ★ Alaska Dental Society**
9170 Jewel Lake Rd., Ste. 203
Anchorage, AK 99502-5381
**Phone:** (907)563-3003    **Fax:** (907)563-3009
**Email:** akdental@alaska.net
**Website:** http://www.akdental.org
Martha Reinbold, Exec Director

### Arizona

**★ 6735 ★ Arizona Dental Association**
4131 N 36th St.
Phoenix, AZ 85018-4761
**Phone:** (602)957-4777    **Fax:** (602)957-1342
**Email:** azda@azda.org
**Website:** http://www.azda.org
Rick Murray, Exec Director
Greg McFarland, Exec Director

### Arkansas

**★ 6736 ★ Arkansas State Dental Association**
2501 Crestwood Dr., Ste. 205
North Little Rock, AR 72116-7613
**Phone:** (501)771-7650    **Fax:** (501)771-1016
**Email:** asda@aristotle.net
**Website:** http://www.dental-asda.org
Billy Tarpley, Exec Director

### California

**★ 6737 ★ California Dental Association**
1201 "K" St., 14th Fl.
Sacramento, CA 95814
**Phone:** (916)443-0505    **Free:** 800-736-8702
**Fax:** (916)443-2943
**Email:** info@cda.org
**Website:** http://www.cda.org
Dr. Dennis Kalebjian, President
Timothy Comstock, Exec Director

### Colorado

**★ 6738 ★ Colorado Dental Association**
3690 S Yosemite, Ste. 100
Denver, CO 80237-1808
**Phone:** (303)740-6900    **Fax:** (303)740-7989
**Email:** info@cdaonline.org
**Website:** http://www.cdaonline.org
Gary J. Cummins, Exec Director
Jim Towle, Exec Director

### Connecticut

**★ 6739 ★ Connecticut State Dental Association**
62 Russ St.
Hartford, CT 06106-1522
**Phone:** (860)278-5550    **Fax:** (860)244-8287
**Email:** noel@csda.com
**Website:** http://www.csda.com
Noel Bishop, Exec Director

### Delaware

**★ 6740 ★ Delaware State Dental Society**
Christiana Executive Campus
200 Continental Dr., Ste. 111
Newark, DE 19713
**Phone:** (302)368-7634    **Fax:** (302)368-7669
**Email:** dsds@delanet.com
**Website:** http://www.dedental.com
Betty Dencler, Exec Director
Margaret Novak, Exec Director

### District of Columbia

**★ 6741 ★ District of Columbia Dental Society**
502 C St. NE
Washington, DC 20002-5810
**Phone:** (202)547-7613    **Fax:** (202)546-1482
**Email:** cbrown@cdental.org
**Website:** http://www.dcdental.org
C. Jay Brown, Exec Director

### Florida

**★ 6742 ★ Florida Dental Association**
1111 E Tennessee St., Ste. 102
Tallahassee, FL 32308-6913
**Phone:** (850)681-3629    **Fax:** (850)561-0504
**Email:** dbuker@floridadental.org
**Website:** http://www.floridadental.org
Daniel J. Buker, Exec Director

### Georgia

**★ 6743 ★ Georgia Dental Association**
Bldg. 17, Ste. 200
7000 Peachtree Dunwoody Rd. NE
Atlanta, GA 30328-1655
**Phone:** (404)636-7553    **Fax:** (404)633-3943
**Email:** phillips@gadental.org
**Website:** http://www.gadental.org
Martha Phillips, Exec Director

### Hawaii

**★ 6744 ★ Hawaii Dental Association**
1345 S Beretania St., Ste. 301
Honolulu, HI 96814-1821
**Phone:** (808)593-7956    **Fax:** (808)593-7636
**Email:** hda@hawaiidentalassociation.net
**Website:** http://www.hawaiidentalassociation.net
Loren Liebling, Contact

### Idaho

**★ 6745 ★ Idaho State Dental Association**
1220 W Hays St.
Boise, ID 83702-5315
**Phone:** (208)343-7543    **Fax:** (208)343-0775
**Email:** isda@mindspring.com
**Website:** http://www.isdaweb.com
A. Jerry Davis, Exec Director

### Illinois

**★ 6746 ★ Illinois State Dental Society**
PO Box 376
Springfield, IL 62705
**Phone:** (217)525-1406    **Fax:** (217)525-8872
**Email:** rrechner@isds.org
**Website:** http://www.isds.org
Robert Rechner, Exec Director

### Indiana

**★ 6747 ★ Indiana Dental Association**
PO Box 2467
Indianapolis, IN 46206-2467
**Phone:** (317)634-2610    **Fax:** (317)634-2612
**Email:** dbush@indental.org
**Website:** http://www.indental.org
Douglas M. Bush, Exec Director

### Iowa

**★ 6748 ★ Iowa Dental Association**
505 5th Ave., Ste. 333
Des Moines, IA 50309-2379
**Phone:** (515)282-7250    **Fax:** (515)828-7256
**Email:** info@iowadental.org
**Website:** http://www.iowadental.org
Lawrence F. Carl, Exec Director
Robert W. Harpster, Contact

### Kansas

**★ 6749 ★ Kansas Dental Association**
5200 SW Huntoon St.
Topeka, KS 66604-2398
**Phone:** (785)272-7360    **Fax:** (785)272-2301
**Email:** kevin@ksdental.org
**Website:** http://www.ksdental.org
Dr. Kevin J. Robertson, Exec Director

### Kentucky

**★ 6750 ★ Kentucky Dental Association**
1940 Princeton Dr.
Louisville, KY 40205-1838
**Phone:** (502)459-5373    **Fax:** (502)458-5915
**Email:** porter_mike@msn.com
**Website:** http://www.kyda.org
Michael R. Porter, Exec Director

### Louisiana

**★ 6751 ★ Louisiana Dental Association**
7833 Office Park Blvd.
Baton Rouge, LA 70809-7604
**Phone:** (225)926-1986    **Fax:** (225)926-1886
**Email:** info@ladental.org
**Website:** http://www.ladental.org
Dr. Mark S. Chaney, President
Ward Blackwell, Exec Director

### Maine

**★ 6752 ★ Maine Dental Association**
PO Box 215
Manchester, ME 04351-0215
**Phone:** (207)622-7900    **Fax:** (207)622-6210
**Email:** info@medental.org
**Website:** http://www.medental.org
Frances Miliano, Exec Director

### Maryland

**★ 6753 ★ Maryland State Dental Association**
6410 Dobbin Rd., Ste. F
Columbia, MD 21045-4774
**Phone:** (410)964-2880    **Free:** 800-766-2880
**Fax:** (410)964-0583
**Email:** elza@msda.com
**Website:** http://www.msda.com
David Williams, President
Elza Harrison, Exec Director

## Massachusetts

**★ 6754 ★ Massachusetts Dental Society**
2 Willow St., Ste. 200
Southborough, MA 01745-1027
**Phone:** (508)480-9797          **Fax:** (508)480-0002
**Email:** madental@massdental.org
**Website:** http://www.massdental.org
Dr. Rene Bousquet, President
Dr. James B. Bramson, Exec Director

## Michigan

**★ 6755 ★ Michigan Dental Association**
230 N Washington Sq., Ste. 208
Lansing, MI 48933-1312
**Phone:** (517)372-9070          **Fax:** (517)372-0008
**Email:** mda@michigandental.org
**Website:** http://www.michigandental.org
Gerri Cherney, Exec Director

## Minnesota

**★ 6756 ★ Minnesota Dental Association**
2236 Marshall Ave.
Saint Paul, MN 55104-5758
**Phone:** (651)646-7454          **Fax:** (651)646-8246
**Email:** info@mndental.org
**Website:** http://www.mndental.org
Richard Diercks, Exec Director

## Mississippi

**★ 6757 ★ Mississippi Dental Association**
2630 Ridgewood Rd.
Jackson, MS 39216-4903
**Phone:** (601)982-0442          **Fax:** (601)366-3050
**Email:** connie@msdental.org
**Website:** http://www.msdental.org
Connie Lane, Exec Director

## Missouri

**★ 6758 ★ Missouri Dental Association**
230 W McCarty St.
PO Box 1707
Jefferson City, MO 65102-1707
**Phone:** (573)634-3436          **Fax:** (573)635-0764
**Email:** jake@modental.org
**Website:** http://www.modental.org
Dr. Jacob J. Lippert, Exec Director

## Montana

**★ 6759 ★ Montana Dental Association**
17 ½ S Last Chance Gulch
Helena, MT 59601
**Phone:** (406)443-2061          **Fax:** (406)443-1546
**Email:** mda@mt.net
**Website:** http://www.mtdental.com
Mary McCue, Exec Director

## Nevada

**★ 6760 ★ Nevada Dental Association**
6889 W Charleston Blvd., Ste. B
Las Vegas, NV 89117-1600
**Phone:** (702)255-4211          **Fax:** (702)255-3302
**Email:** nda@nvda.net
**Website:** http://www.nvda.org
Maury Astley, Exec Director

## New Hampshire

**★ 6761 ★ New Hampshire Dental Society**
PO Box 2229
Concord, NH 03302-2229
**Phone:** (603)225-5961          **Fax:** (603)226-4880
**Email:** nhds@nhdental.com
**Website:** http://www.nhdental.com
Henry Dougherty, Exec Director

## New Jersey

**★ 6762 ★ New Jersey Dental Association**
1 Dental Plaza
PO Box 6020
North Brunswick, NJ 08902-6020
**Phone:** (732)821-9400          **Fax:** (732)821-1082
**Email:** ddavis@njda.org
**Website:** http://www.njda.org
Ms. Ricky Dibofsky, Contact
Arthur Meisel, Exec Director

## New Mexico

**★ 6763 ★ New Mexico Dental Association**
3736 Eubank Blvd. NE, Ste. D-2
Albuquerque, NM 87111-3556
**Phone:** (505)294-1368          **Fax:** (505)294-9958
**Email:** kcravens@nmdental.org
**Website:** http://www.newmexicodental.org
Kent Cravens, Exec Director
Rick Murray, Exec Director

## New York

**★ 6764 ★ New York State Dental Association**
121 State St., 4th Fl.
Albany, NY 12207-1622
**Phone:** (518)465-0044          **Free:** 800-255-2100
**Fax:** (518)465-3219
**Email:** info@nysdental.org
**Website:** http://www.nysdental.org
Roy Lasky, Exec Director

## North Carolina

**★ 6765 ★ North Carolina Dental Society**
PO Box 4099
Cary, NC 27519-4099
**Phone:** (919)677-1396          **Free:** 800-662-8754
**Fax:** (919)677-1397
**Email:** ncds@ncdental.org
**Website:** http://www.ncdental.org
Faye K. Marley, Contact

## North Dakota

**★ 6766 ★ North Dakota Dental Association**
PO Box 1332
Bismarck, ND 58502-1332
**Phone:** (701)223-8870          **Fax:** (701)223-0855
**Email:** ndda@olsoncichy.com
**Website:** http://www.nddental.com
Joseph J. Cichy, Exec Director

## Ohio

**★ 6767 ★ Ohio Dental Association**
1370 Dublin Rd.
Columbus, OH 43215-1009
**Phone:** (614)486-2700          **Fax:** (614)486-0381
**Email:** dentist@oda.org
**Website:** http://www.oda.org
David J. Owsiany, Exec Director
Nancy C. Quinn, Contact

## Oklahoma

**★ 6768 ★ Oklahoma Dental Association**
629 NW Grand Blvd., Ste. A
Oklahoma City, OK 73118-6032
**Phone:** (405)848-8873          **Fax:** (405)848-8875
**Email:** odjessic@swbell.net
**Website:** http://www.okdentassoc.org
Stephen Glenn, Exec Director
Bob D. Berry, Exec Director

## Oregon

**★ 6769 ★ Oregon Dental Association**
17898 SW McEwan Rd.
Portland, OR 97224-7798
**Phone:** (503)620-3230          **Fax:** (503)620-4169
**Email:** info@oregondental.org
**Website:** http://www.oregondental.org
William E. Zep, Exec Director
William E. Zepp, Exec Director

## Pennsylvania

**★ 6770 ★ Pennsylvania Dental Association**
PO Box 3341
Harrisburg, PA 17105-3341
**Phone:** (717)234-5941          **Free:** 800-223-0016
**Fax:** (717)232-7169
**Email:** ckc@padental.org
**Website:** http://www.padental.org
Camille Kostelac-Cherry, Exec Director

## Puerto Rico

**★ 6771 ★ Colegio de Cirujanos Dentistas de Puerto Rico**
Avenida Domenech 200
Hato Rey, PR 00918
**Phone:** (787)764-1969          **Fax:** (787)763-6335
Myrna Cruz-Garay, Exec Director

## Rhode Island

**★ 6772 ★ Rhode Island Dental Association**
200 Centerville Rd.
Warwick, RI 02886-0204
**Phone:** (401)732-6833          **Fax:** (401)732-9351
**Email:** info@ridental.com
**Website:** http://www.ridental.com
Valerie Donnelly, Exec Director

## South Carolina

**★ 6773 ★ South Carolina Dental Association**
120 Stonemark Ln.
Columbia, SC 29210-3841
**Phone:** (803)750-2277          **Fax:** (803)750-1644
**Email:** zomh@scda.org
**Website:** http://www.scda.org
Hal Zom, Exec Director
Hal Zorn, Exec Director

## South Dakota

**★ 6774 ★ South Dakota Dental Association**
711 E Wells Ave., Ste. 240
PO Box 1194
Pierre, SD 57501-1194
**Phone:** (605)224-9133          **Fax:** (605)224-9168
**Email:** info@sddental.org
**Website:** http://www.sddental.org
Paul Knecht, Exec Director

## Tennessee

**★ 6775 ★ Tennessee Dental Association**
2104 Sunset Pl.
PO Box 120188
Nashville, TN 37212-4917
**Phone:** (615)383-8962          **Fax:** (615)383-0214
**Email:** tda@tenndental.org
**Website:** http://www.tenndental.org
David S. Horvat, Exec Director

### Texas

**★ 6776 ★ Texas Dental Association**
1946 S Interstate Hwy. 35, Ste. 400
Austin, TX 78704
**Phone:** (512)443-3675    **Fax:** (512)443-3031
**Email:** amsimmons@tda.org
**Website:** http://www.tda.org
Mary Kay Linn, Exec Director

### Utah

**★ 6777 ★ Utah Dental Association**
1151 East 3900 South, Ste. B160
Salt Lake City, UT 84124-1216
**Phone:** (801)261-5315    **Fax:** (801)261-1235
**Email:** uda@uda.org
Monte Thompson, Exec Director

### Vermont

**★ 6778 ★ Vermont State Dental Society**
100 Dorset St., Ste. 18
South Burlington, VT 05403-6241
**Phone:** (802)864-0115    **Fax:** (802)864-0116
**Email:** ptaylorvt@aol.com
**Website:** http://www.vsds.org
Peter Taylor, Exec Director

### Virgin Islands

**★ 6779 ★ Virgin Islands Dental Association**
Medical Arts Complex, Ste. 10
Saint Thomas, VI 00802
**Phone:** (340)777-5950    **Fax:** (340)775-4172
**Email:** jawdocvi@netscape.net
Dr. Horace Griffith, President

### Virginia

**★ 6780 ★ Virginia Dental Association**
7525 Staples Mill Rd.
Richmond, VA 23228
**Phone:** (804)261-1610    **Fax:** (804)261-1660
**Email:** dickinson@vadental.org
**Website:** http://www.vadental.org
Dr. Terry D. Dickinson, Exec Director

### Washington

**★ 6781 ★ Washington State Dental Association**
2033 6th Ave., Ste. 333
Seattle, WA 98121
**Phone:** (206)448-1914    **Fax:** (206)443-9266
**Email:** wsda@wsda.org
**Website:** http://www.wsda.org
Stephen A. Hardymon, Exec Director

### West Virginia

**★ 6782 ★ West Virginia Dental Association**
2003 Quarrier St.
Charleston, WV 25311-2212
**Phone:** (304)344-5246    **Fax:** (304)344-5316
**Email:** wvrds@aol.com
Richard D. Stevens, Exec Director

### Wisconsin

**★ 6783 ★ Wisconsin Dental Association**
111 E Wisconsin Ave., Ste. 1300
Milwaukee, WI 53202-4815
**Phone:** (414)276-4520    **Fax:** (414)276-8431
**Email:** dmcguire@wda.org
**Website:** http://www.wda.org
Dennis McGuire, Exec Director

### Wyoming

**★ 6784 ★ Wyoming Dental Association**
502 S 4th St.
Laramie, WY 82070-3704
**Phone:** (307)755-4009    **Fax:** (307)745-8009
**Email:** keefeo2000@yahoo.com
**Website:** http://www.medicinebow.org/wyodental
Diane O'Keefe, Exec Director
Marvin Cronberg, Exec Director

## Federal Government Agencies

**U.S. Department of Health and Human Services**
**National Institutes of Health (NIH)**
**National Institute of Arthritis and Musculoskeletal and Skin Diseases (NIAMS)**
*See:* Entry 13518

## Foundations & Other Funding Organizations

### Private Foundations

**Carl J. Herzog Foundation**
*See:* Entry 105

### Other Funding Organizations

**★ 6785 ★ American Skin Association (ASA)**
346 Park Ave. S
New York, NY 10010
**Phone:** (212)889-4858     **Free:** 800-499-SKIN
**Fax:** (212)889-4959
**Email:** info@skinassn.org
**Website:** http://www.skinassn.org
Joyce Weidler, Mng. Dir.
**Desc:** Supports research on all skin diseases. Promotes public education on prevention and treatment of skin disorders. Created School Skin Health Education Program, K-12, with the New York Academy of Medicine. **Awards:** Categorical Research (annual) for dermatologi research on psoriasis, lupus, melanoma/skin cancer, vitiligo, childhood diseases/disfigurement and inflammatory diseases; Dermatitis Award (annual) for original research; Psoriasis Award (annual) for original research; Research Scholar Awards (annual) for dermatological investigation; Vitiligo Award (annual) for original research.

**Dystrophic Epidermolysis Bullosa Research Association of America (DEBRA)**
*See:* Entry 9278

**★ 6786 ★ Foundation for Ichthyosis and Related Skin Types (FIRST)**
650 N Cannon Ave., Ste. 17
Lansdale, PA 19446
**Phone:** (215)631-1411     **Free:** 800-545-3286
**Fax:** (215)631-1413
**Email:** info@scalyskin.org
**Website:** http://www.scalyskin.org
Jean R. Pickford, Exec. Dir.
**Desc:** Dedicated to helping persons affected with ichthyosis, a rare genetic skin disease characterized by dry, cracked, scaling and thickened skin, and related diseases. **Awards:** Dermatology Foundation (annual).

**★ 6787 ★ National Rosacea Society**
800 S Northwest Hwy., Ste. 200
Barrington, IL 60010
**Free:** 800-NO-BLUSH     **Fax:** (847)382-5567
**Email:** rosaceas@aol.com
**Website:** http://www.rosacea.org
**Desc:** Provides information, care, and treatment of rosacea. Operates a Physician Referral Service. **Awards:** Research Grants Program.

**Skin Cancer Foundation (SCF)**
*See:* Entry 10091

## National & International Organizations

**★ 6788 ★ African Association of Dermatology (AAD)**
Rabito Clinic
PO Box 7286
Accra, Ghana
**Phone:** 233 21 774526     **Fax:** 233 21 777465
**Email:** info@skincancer.org
**Website:** http://www.skincancer.org
**Lang(s):** English. **Desc:** Dermatologists. Seeks to advance the study and practice of dermatology; encourages continuing professional development of members. Serves as a forum for the exchange of information among members; conducts educational programs.

**★ 6789 ★ American Academy of Dermatology (AAD)**
PO Box 4014
Schaumburg, IL 60168-4014
**Phone:** (847)330-0230     **Fax:** (847)330-0050
**Email:** memsrv@aad.org
**Website:** http://www.aad.org
Thomas P. Conway, Exec. Dir.
**Fnded:** 1938. **Mem:** 14,000. **Desc:** Professional society of medical doctors specializing in skin diseases. Provides educational opportunities through meetings and publications. Provides support to members' practices. Promotes dermatologists as experts in treating skin, hair, and nail conditions. Maintains liaison with Congress, Federal agencies, State legislatures and State agencies. **Pub:** *Derm Coding Consult*, quarterly. • *Dermatology Insights*, quarterly. Magazine. • *Dermatology World*, monthly. • *Dialogues in Dermatology*, monthly. Audiotapes. • *Journal of the American Academy of Dermatology*, monthly. Journal.

Scientific journal. **Frmly:** American Academy of Dermatology and Syphilology.

**★ 6790 ★ American Board of Dermatology (ABD)**
Henry Ford Health System
1 Ford Pl.
Detroit, MI 48202-3450
**Phone:** (313)874-1088     **Fax:** (313)872-3221
**Email:** abderm@hfhs.org
**Website:** http://www.abderm.org
Antoinette F. Hood, MD, Exec. Dir.
**Fnded:** 1932. **Mem:** 15. **Desc:** Examining and certifying body. Seeks to assure provision of competent care for patients with cutaneous diseases, via capable board representation. Establishes requirements of postdoctoral training. Creates and conducts annual comprehensive examination to determine the competence of physicians who meet the requirements for examination by the board. Issues appropriate certificate to those who satisfactorily complete examination. Member of American Board of Medical Specialties . **Pub:** *Booklet of Information*, annual. Describes requirements for certification. *Price:* Free.

**American College of Veterinary Dermatology (ACVD)**
*See:* Entry 20559

**★ 6791 ★ American Hair Loss Council (AHLC)**
401 N Michigan Ave.
Chicago, IL 60611-4212
**Phone:** (312)321-5128     **Free:** 888-873-9719
**Fax:** (312)245-1080
**Email:** membership@ahlc.org
**Website:** http://www.ahlc.org
Russell Bodnar, Exec. Dir.
**Fnded:** 1985. **Mem:** 420. **Desc:** Dermatologists, plastic surgeons, cosmetologists, barbers, and interested others. Provides nonbiased information regarding treatments for hair loss in both men and women. Facilitates communication and information exchange between professionals in different areas of specialization. Conducts educational programs; compiles statistics. **Pub:** *AHLC News*, quarterly. Brochures. A newsletter for members only (association & industry news). *Price:* Free for members.

**American Osteopathic College of Dermatology (AOCD)**
*See:* Entry 17002

**★ 6792 ★ American Skin Association (ASA)**
346 Park Ave. S
New York, NY 10010
**Phone:** (212)889-4858     **Free:** 800-499-SKIN
**Fax:** (212)889-4959
**Email:** info@skinassn.org

**Website:** http://www.skinassn.org
Joyce Weidler, Mng. Dir.
**Fnded:** 1987. **Mem:** 200. **Desc:** Supports research on all skin diseases. Promotes public education on prevention and treatment of skin disorders. Created School Skin Health Education Program, K-12, with the New York Academy of Medicine. **Pub:** *Childhood Skin Diseases.* Brochure. • *Healthy Skin and Gardening.* Brochure. • *Melanoma.* Brochure. • *Outdoor Sports and Your Skin.* Brochure. • *Skin Facts,* quarterly. Newsletter. • *The Sun, Your Skin, and Your Health.* Brochure. • *Your Newborn's Skin and the Sun.* Brochure.

**American Society for Dermatologic Surgery (ASDS)**
*See:* Entry 19492

### ★ 6793 ★ American Society of Dermatology (ASD)
2721 Capital Ave.
Sacramento, CA 95816-6004
**Phone:** (916)446-5054          **Fax:** (916)446-0500
**Email:** asds@neton-line.com
**Website:** http://www.asd.org
M. John Hanni, Jr., C, Exec. Dir.
**Desc:** Dermatologists. Committed to make dermatology care available to everyone in the U.S.

### ★ 6794 ★ American Society of Dermatopathology (ASDP)
930 E Woodfield Rd.
Schaumburg, IL 60173-4927
**Phone:** (847)330-9830          **Fax:** (847)330-1135
**Email:** info@asdp.org
**Website:** http://www.asdp.org
Leah McCrackin, Acct. Mgr.
**Fnded:** 1962. **Mem:** 998. **Desc:** Seeks to: improve the quality of dermatopathology (the study of abnormal skin conditions, especially the structural and functional changes produced by disease); aid in the dissemination of information; encourage continuing education and research. **Pub:** *Journal of Cutaneous Pathology,* 10/year. Journal. • Membership Directory, annual.

**American Society of Podiatric Dermatology (ASPD)**
*See:* Entry 17712

### ★ 6795 ★ Argentinian Association of Dermatology (AAD) (Asociacion Argentina de Dermatologia — AAD)
Mexico 1720
1100 Buenos Aires, Argentina
**Phone:** 54 1 3812737          **Fax:** 54 1 3812737
**Email:** info@aad.org.ar
**Website:** http://www.aad.org.ar
**Fnded:** 1907. **Mem:** 950. **Reg. Groups:** 5. **State Groups:** 14. **Local Groups:** 6. **Lang(s):** English, Spanish. **Desc:** Dermatologists in Argentina. Bestows awards; provides educational programs. **Pub:** *Indice General,* periodic. Contains dermatological articles. • *Journal of Argentine Dermatology.* Journal. • *Revista Argentina de Dermatologia,* quarterly. Includes summary in English.

### ★ 6796 ★ Asian Dermatological Association
c/o The Federation of Medical Societies of Honk Kong
Duke of Windsor Social Service Bldg., 4th Fl.,
  Hennessy Rd.
Hong Kong, People's Republic of China
**Phone:** 852 25278898          **Fax:** 852 28650345
**Email:** fms@hkstar.com
**Website:** http://www.medicine.org.hk
**Lang(s):** Chinese, English. **Desc:** Dermatologists and medical students with an interest in dermatology.

Seeks to advance the study, teaching, and practice of dermatology. Facilitates exchange of information among members; sponsors research and educational programs.

### ★ 6797 ★ Association of French-Speaking Dermatologists (AFSD) (Association des Dermatologistes Francophone — ADF)
Hopital de Grenoble (Dermatologie)
Boite Postale 217
F-38043 Grenoble Cedex, France
**Phone:** 33 4 76765508          **Fax:** 33 4 76765558
**Email:** pamblard@chu-grenoble.fr
**Lang(s):** English, French. **Desc:** Dermatologists and dermatology students and educators. Seeks to advance the study, teaching, and practice of dermatology. Establishes standards for dermatological certification and practice; sponsors continuing professional development courses.

### ★ 6798 ★ Association Pour La Lutte Contre Le Psoriasis (APLCP)
Contre Le Psoriasis
1 allee dee stade
95610 Eragny, France
**Phone:** 33 1 34641768          **Fax:** 33 1 30374581
**Email:** michelle.corvest@wanadoo.fr
**Fnded:** 1983. **Mem:** 1,400. **Nat'l Groups:** 1. **Reg. Groups:** 12. **Lang(s):** English. **Desc:** National psoriasis organizations. Acts as advisory, consulting, and coordinating body for member groups implementing medical, social, and psychological research into psoriasis. Seeks to influence related social legislation and to collect all available information on psoriasis. Promotes public awareness of psoriasis and works to remove the social stigma associated with skin conditions. **Pub:** *IFPA Newsletter,* quarterly. Newsletter.

### ★ 6799 ★ Association for Psoriasis
Strubervoska 2941
CZ-14 100 Prague, Czech Republic
**Phone:** 42 2 71761056          **Fax:** 42 2 71761056
**Fnded:** 1990. **Mem:** 880. **Reg. Groups:** 5. **Desc:** People with psoriasis and their families, health care providers, and others interested in dermatology. Promotes improved quality of life for people with psoriasis.

### ★ 6800 ★ Australasian College of Dermatologists
136 Pittwater Rd.
Gladesville, NSW 2111, Australia
**Phone:** 61 2 98796177          **Fax:** 61 2 98161174
**Fnded:** 1966. **Desc:** Aims to train dermatologists and to promote dermatology.

### ★ 6801 ★ Belgian Royal Society of Dermatology and Venerology (BSD) (Societe Royale Belge de Dermatologie et Venerologie)
c/o Dr. J. De Weert
Department of Dermatology
University Hospital
B-9000 Gent, Belgium
**Phone:** 32 9 2402287          **Fax:** 32 9 2404996
**Fnded:** 1901. **Mem:** 600. **Lang(s):** Dutch, English, French. **Desc:** Dermatologists and other scientists interested in dermatology. Conducts biennial postgraduate course. **Pub:** *Dermatology,* 10/year.

### ★ 6802 ★ Brazilian Society of Dermatology (SBD)
CP 389
20001-970 Rio de Janeiro, Brazil
**Phone:** 55 21 2536747
**Fnded:** 1912.

### ★ 6803 ★ British Association of Dermatologists (BAD)
19 Fitzroy Sq.
London W1T 6EH, United Kingdom
**Phone:** 44 207 3830266          **Fax:** 44 207 3885263
**Email:** admin@bad.org.uk
**Website:** http://www.bad.org.uk
**Fnded:** 1921. **Mem:** 946. **Nat'l Groups:** 6. **Lang(s):** English. **Desc:** Medical professionals united to further the knowledge and teaching of dermatology. Promotes the interests of members and their patients. Conducts medical and scientific research; disseminates information. **Pub:** *British Journal of Dermatology,* monthly. Journal. Also publishes results of research projects.

### ★ 6804 ★ British Association of Skin Camouflage
c/o Resources for Business
PO Box 202
South Park Rd.
Macclesfield SK1 16FP, United Kingdom
**Phone:** 44 162 5267880          **Fax:** 44 162 5267879
**Email:** elizabethallen@compuserve.com
**Fnded:** 1986. **Mem:** 100. **Desc:** Trains professionals. Encourages and supports members. Informs and provides remedial camouflage service for patients.

### ★ 6805 ★ Bulgarian Dermatological Society (BDS) (Balgarsko Dermatologichno Drujestvo — BDD)
Georgi Sofiisky St. 1
BG-1431 Sofia, Bulgaria
**Phone:** 359 2 9522774          **Fax:** 359 2 9522774
**Email:** tsankn@medfac.acad.bg
**Website:** http://www.ilds.org/memsocs/bulgariandermatologicalsociety.shtml
Dr. N. Tsankov, Sec.
**Fnded:** 1923. **Mem:** 400. **Reg. Groups:** 1. **Local Groups:** 7. **Lang(s):** Bulgarian, English, French. **Desc:** Dermatologists and individuals interested in furthering the development of dermatology in Bulgaria. Coordinates efforts in combatting the spread of skin and venereal diseases. Furthers post-graduate education. Conducts educational and research programs. **Pub:** *Dermatologia i Venerologia Bulgaran,* quarterly. Journal. • Books. • Monographs.

### ★ 6806 ★ Canadian Dermatology Association (CDA)
774 Echo Dr., Ste. 521
Ottawa, ON, Canada K1S 5N8
**Phone:** (613)730-6262          **Fax:** (613)730-8262
**Email:** cda@dermatology.ca
**Website:** http://www.dermatology.ca
**Fnded:** 1925. **Mem:** 600. **Lang(s):** English, French. **Desc:** Certified dermatologists and related professionals interested in the professional advancement of dermatology. Promotes continuing education programs in dermatology. Provides public education program on skin cancer prevention. Holds an annual National Sun Awareness Week. Recognizes sun protection products. **Pub:** *Canadian Dermatology Association Bulletin,* 3/year. Bulletin. Contains Association news for members. • *Journal of Cutaneous Medicine and Surgery,* quarterly. Journal. • Directory, annual.

### ★ 6807 ★ Canadian Psoriasis Foundation (CPF)
100A-824 Meath St.
Ottawa, ON, Canada K1Z 6E8
**Phone:** (613)728-4000          **Fax:** (613)728-8913
**Email:** cpf-fcp@psoriasis.ca
**Fnded:** 1983. **Mem:** 1,200. **Lang(s):** English, French. **Desc:** People with psoriasis and their families; health care providers with an interest in dermatology. Promotes an improved quality of life for people with psoriasis; seeks advancement in the prevention and treatment of psoriasis and related disorders. Maintains support groups; conducts research and educational

programs. **Pub:** *CPF Newsletter*, 3/year. Newsletter. • Brochure.

★ **6808** ★ **Danish Dermatological Society (DDS)**
**(Dansk Dermatologisk Selskab — DDS)**
Bispebjerg Hospital
Department of Dermatology D
Bispebjerg Bakke 23
DK-2400 Copenhagen NV, Denmark
**Phone:** 45 35313107　　　**Fax:** 45 35313113
**Fnded:** 1899. **Mem:** 295. **Lang(s):** English, German. **Desc:** Dermatologists in Denmark, Norway, and Sweden. Promotes advances in dermatology and venereology. Offers courses for members.

★ **6809** ★ **DEBRA Ireland**
Carmichael House Centre
Brunswick St.
Dublin 7, Ireland
**Phone:** 353 1 8725192　　　**Fax:** 353 1 8735737
**Email:** info@debraireland.org
**Website:** http://homepage.eircom.net/~debraireland/
**Lang(s):** English, Irish. **Desc:** Individuals and organizations. Seeks to improve the quality of life of people with EB and their families. Makes available specialist care; conducts educational programs for health care personnel and the public.

★ **6810** ★ **Dermatological Society of Malaysia (DSM)**
**(Persatuan Dermatologi Malaysia — PDM)**
c/o Department of Dermatology
Hospital Kuala Lumpur
Jalan Pahang
50586 Kuala Lumpur, Malaysia
**Phone:** 60 3 26155251　　　**Fax:** 60 3 26985927
**Email:** dermal@tm.net.my
**Website:** http://www.dermatology.org.my
**Fnded:** 1976. **Mem:** 104. **Lang(s):** English. **Desc:** Dermatologists and other practitioners interested in dermatology. Promotes the research and development of dermatological medicine in Malaysia. Organizes scientific seminars and congresses. **Pub:** *Malaysian Journal of Dermatology*, annual. Journal.

★ **6811** ★ **Dermatological Society of Singapore (DSS)**
c/o National Skin Centre
1 Mandalay Rd.
Singapore 308205, Singapore
**Phone:** 65 2534455　　　**Fax:** 65 2533255
**Fnded:** 1972. **Mem:** 96. **Lang(s):** English. **Desc:** Dermatologists in Singapore. Holds clinico-pathological sessions and other academic meetings for dermatologists. Maintains research fund. **Pub:** *Proceedings of Dermatological Society of Singapore*, annual. Journal.

★ **6812** ★ **Dermatology Foundation (DF)**
1560 Sherman Ave., Ste. 870
Evanston, IL 60201-4802
**Phone:** (847)728-2256　　　**Fax:** (847)328-0509
**Email:** info@dermfnd.org
**Website:** http://www.dermfnd.org/
Sandra Rahn Benz, Exec. Dir.
**Fnded:** 1964. **Mem:** 3,300. **Desc:** Members of national and regional dermatological societies; board-certified dermatologists. Raises funds for the control of skin diseases through research, improved education, and better patient care. Stimulates interest of graduate physicians in academic dermatology. Supports basic and clinical investigations. **Pub:** *Dermatology Focus*, quarterly. Newsletter. Covers membership activities. Includes research articles and lists recipients of foundation awards, fellowships, and grants. • *Progress in Dermatology*, quarterly. Bulletin. Bulletin containing research reports. *Price:* Included in membership dues. • *Stewardship Report*. Annual Report. *Price:* Free.

**Dermatology Nurses' Association (DNA)**
*See:* Entry 15704

★ **6813** ★ **Dystrophic Epidermolysis Bullosa Research Association of America (DEBRA)**
5 W 36th St., No. 404
New York, NY 10018
**Phone:** (212)868-1573　　　**Fax:** (212)863-9296
**Email:** mrivera@debra.org
**Website:** http://www.debra.org
Martin Hassner, Exec. Dir.
**Fnded:** 1979. **Mem:** 5,000. **Desc:** People with Epidermolysis Bullosa and their families; other interested individuals. (Epidermolysis Bullosa represents a group of inherited disorders of the skin characterized by formation of blisters resulting from the most minimal trauma.) To raise funds to promote and support research into the cause, nature, and treatment of EB in all its forms; to relieve the physical and mental distress of victims by providing practical advice, guidance, support, and other assistance. Distributes educational material to the public and medical professionals. Works for federal funding for biomedical research of EB and related disorders. Offers children's services; conducts educational programs. conducts educational programs. **Pub:** *EB Currents*, semiannual. **AKA:** DEBRA of America.

★ **6814** ★ **European Society of Contact Dermatitis (ESCD)**
Department of Occupational and Social Medicine
Ruprecht-Karls-University Heidelberg
Thibaustrasse 3
D-69115 Heidelberg, Germany
**Phone:** 49 6221 568751　　　**Fax:** 49 6221 565584
**Website:** http://www.dermis.net/org/escd/index.htm
**Lang(s):** English, German. **Desc:** Dermatologists and other health care professionals and medical researchers with an interest in contact dermatitis and other environmental and occupational skin diseases. Seeks to advance the prevention, diagnosis, and treatment of environmental and occupational dermatological disorders. Facilitates exchanger of information among members; stimulates dermatological research; serves as a clearinghouse on contact dermatitis and related disorders; sponsors educational programs. **Pub:** *Contact Dermatitis*, periodic. Journal. • Newsletter, periodic.

★ **6815** ★ **European Society for Dermatological Research (ESDR)**
Department of Dermatology
HUG
Rue Micheli du Crest 24
CH-1211 Geneva 14, Switzerland
**Phone:** 41 22 3729694　　　**Fax:** 41 22 37279695
**Email:** office@esdr.ch
**Website:** http://www.esdr.org/
**Fnded:** 1974. **Mem:** 800. **Reg. Groups:** 33. **Desc:** Promotes dermatological research in Europe.

★ **6816** ★ **Finnish Dermatological Society (FDS)**
**(Suomen Ihotautilaakariyhdistys Ry)**
Department of Dermatology
PO Box 160
FIN-00029 Hyks, Finland
**Phone:** 358 9 471961639　　　**Fax:** 358 9 94716561
**Fnded:** 1916. **Mem:** 278. **Lang(s):** English, Finnish. **Desc:** Professional organization for dermatologists in Finland. Conducts educational programs. **Pub:** *Skinfo*, 4-6/year. Newsletter.

★ **6817** ★ **Foundation for Ichthyosis and Related Skin Types (FIRST)**
650 N Cannon Ave., Ste. 17
Lansdale, PA 19446
**Phone:** (215)631-1411　　　**Free:** 800-545-3286
**Fax:** (215)631-1413
**Email:** info@scalyskin.org

**Website:** http://www.scalyskin.org
Jean R. Pickford, Exec. Dir.
**Fnded:** 1981. **Mem:** 3,300. **Reg. Groups:** 10. **Desc:** Dedicated to helping persons affected with ichthyosis, a rare genetic skin disease characterized by dry, cracked, scaling and thickened skin, and related diseases. **Pub:** *A Handbook for Teachers of Children with Ichthyosis*. Handbook. Tool for parents to help make the transition to the school environment for children with ichthyosis. *Price:* $5. • *Butterflies: The Children of Ichthyosis*. Video. • *Ichthyosis: An Overview*. *Price:* Free. For members only; $1 for nonmembers; Free for members. • *Ichthyosis Focus*, quarterly. Newsletter. Features medical news, tips for day-to-day coping, and correspondence column for members who would like to exchange letters. *Price:* Free. For members only. • *Ichthyosis: The Genetics of Its Inheritance*. Booklet. Description of the genetic inheritance patterns for the different forms of ichthyosis. *Price:* Free. For members only; $1 for nonmembers; Free, available to members only. • *Release The Butterfly: A Handbook for Parents and Caregivers of Children with Ichthyosis*. Handbook. Covers care, medication, therapy, and nutrition for child with ichthyosis. *Price:* $5. **Frmly:** (1986) National Ichthyosis Foundation.

★ **6818** ★ **German Dermatological Society (GRS)**
**(Deutsche Dermatologische Gesellschaft — DDG)**
c/o Prof. Dr. Gernot Rassner
Department of Dermatclogy
Univ. of Tuebingen
Liebermeisterstr. 25
D-72076 Tuebingen, Germany
**Phone:** 49 2151 523850　　　**Fax:** 49 7071 295113
**Website:** http://www.derma.de
**Fnded:** 1888. **Mem:** 1,800. **Lang(s):** English, German. **Desc:** Individuals united to promote dermatology. Conducts educational and research programs. **Pub:** *Der Hautarzt*, periodic.

★ **6819** ★ **Hellenic Association of Dermatology and Venereology**
5 I. Dragoumi St.
GR-161 21 Athens, Greece
**Phone:** 30 1 7239611　　　**Fax:** 30 1 7211122
**Email:** info@edae.gr
**Website:** http://www.edae.gr/index.html
**Mem:** 600. **Lang(s):** English, Greek. **Desc:** Offers awards; Conducts educational programs; compiles statistics. Maintains museum. **Pub:** *Hellenic Dermato-Venereological Review*, quarterly. **Frmly:** (2000) Hellenic Society of Dermatology and Venereology.

★ **6820** ★ **Hong Kong Society of Dermatology and Venereology (HKSD)**
c/o Social Hygiene Service
Sai Ying Pun Jockey Club Clinic, 3rd Fl.
Queen's Rd. W
Hong Kong, People's Republic of China
**Phone:** 852 25409804　　　**Fax:** 852 25409804
**Email:** lychong@cuhk.edu.hk
**Website:** http://www.medicine.org.hk/hksdv/
**Fnded:** 1983. **Mem:** 150. **Lang(s):** English. **Desc:** Dermatologists and physicians in Hong Kong. Stimulates interest in dermatology; promotes exchange and cooperation among members; encourages discussions to address problems in the field. Inspires high standards of dermatological care. Fosters international contacts; disseminates information.

★ **6821** ★ **Hungarian Dermatological Society (HDS)**
**(Magyar Dermatologiai Tarsulat — MDT)**
c/o Prof. Janos Hunydi
Department of Dermatology
Medical School of Debrecen
H-4012 Debrecen, Hungary
**Phone:** 36 62 442204　　　**Fax:** 36 62 414632
**Email:** hunyadi@jaghar.dote.hu

**Fnded:** 1928. **Mem:** 500. **Local Groups:** 3. **Lang(s):** English, Hungarian. **Desc:** Promotes dermatological practice and research. Monitors progress in the field of dermatology. Participates in international forums. **Pub:** *Borgyogyaszati es Venerologiai Szemle*, bimonthly. Journal. Accepts English and German papers. Contains English abstracts. • *Progress of Dermatology and Venereology*. Yearbook.

★ 6822 ★ **Ibero-Latin American College of Dermatology (ILACD)**
**(Colegio Ibero-Latino-Americano de Dermatologia — CILAD)**
Av. Callao 852, Piso 2
1023 Buenos Aires, Argentina
**Phone:** 54 11 49590392      **Fax:** 54 11 48117581
**Fnded:** 1948. **Mem:** 2,210. **Lang(s):** Portuguese, Spanish. **Desc:** Iberian or Latin American doctors in 29 countries working in various fields related to dermatology including mycology (the study of fungi), venereology (the study of sexually transmitted diseases), the treatment of leprosy, dermatologic surgery, and criosurgery. Seeks to foster a working relationship between Ibero-Latin American specialists and those in other countries. **Pub:** *Boletin del CILAD*, quarterly. Bulletin. Contains information about the activities of the college. • *Ciladerma*, bimonthly. Magazine. • *Medicina Cutanea Ibero-Latino-Americana*, bimonthly. • Directory, periodic. • Monographs, periodic.

★ 6823 ★ **Institute of Trichologists (IT)**
20/22 Queensberry Place
London SW7 2D2, United Kingdom
**Phone:** 44 171 4917253      **Fax:** 44 1329 835363
**Fnded:** 1902. **Mem:** 240. **Lang(s):** English. **Desc:** Promotes study, research, and application in the treatment and care of human scalp and hair. Provides scientific training of individuals qualified to advise and offer treatment of hair and scalp disorders and serves as an examining body for students of trichology. Provides centers for clinical study. Maintains Scalp and Hair Hospital where students conduct clinical observations and gain practical experience. Bestows awards; sponsors charitable program; maintains speakers' bureau. **Pub:** *Membership Directory*, annual. Membership Directory. • *Monograph*, periodic. • *Update*, 3/year. Journal. • Newsletter, 3/year.

★ 6824 ★ **International Academy of Cosmetic Dermatology**
c/o Timothy C. Flynn, Md
1430 Tulane Ave., Ste. Sl73
New Orleans, LA 70112-2699
**Phone:** (504)588-5114      **Fax:** (504)587-7382
**Website:** http://www.dermato.med.br/iacd/
Larry Millikan, MD, Sec. Treas.
**Desc:** Cosmetic dermatologists.

★ 6825 ★ **International Contact Dermatitis Research Group (ICDRG)**
Clos Chapelle aux Champs 30
B-1200 Brussels, Belgium
**Phone:** 32 2 7643334      **Fax:** 32 2 7643324
**Email:** lachapelle@dpro.ucl.ac.be
**Website:** http://www.med.nagoya-u.ac.jp/Environ-derm/icdrg.htm
**Fnded:** 1967. **Desc:** Encourages research into skin problems related to the environment.

★ 6826 ★ **International Federation of Psoriasis Associations (IFPA)**
6600 SW 92nd, Ste. 300
Portland, OR 97223-7195
**Phone:** (503)244-7404      **Free:** 800-723-9166
**Fax:** (503)245-0626
**Email:** getinfo@npfusa.org
**Website:** http://www.psoriasis.org
**Fnded:** 1968. **Mem:** 37,000. **Desc:** Individuals suffering from psoriasis, or psoriatic arthritis, their families and friends. Supports research at various university research centers. Facilitates communication through pen pal programs, group sessions, and other activities. Testifies annually to Congress for psoriasis research. Provides literature to schools and libraries; works with the media to disseminate information on psoriasis. Compiles physician directory. Sponsors regional educational symposia. Established and maintains a public tissue bank for gene research in psoriasis and psoriatic arthritis. **Pub:** *National Psoriasis Foundation–Annual Report*. Annual Report. *Price:* Included in membership dues. • *National Psoriasis Foundation–Bulletin*, bimonthly. Newsletter. Covers psoriasis treatment and research. Includes doctor's question and answer column. *Price:* Included in membership dues. • *National Psoriasis Foundation–Psoriasis Rsource*, 3/year. *Price:* Included in membership dues. • *Psoriasis Forum*, quarterly. Newsletter. Published for medical professionals. *Price:* Included in dues. • Brochures. • Pamphlets. **Frmly:** (2000) National Psoriasis Foundation.

★ 6827 ★ **International League of Dermatological Societies (ILDS)**
PO Box 35069
Sarasota, FL 34242
**Phone:** (941)346-1226      **Fax:** (941)927-1936
**Email:** mtgmgr@gte.net
**Website:** http://www.ilds.org/
Barbara Nichols, Admin. Officer
**Fnded:** 1957. **Mem:** 102. **Nat'l Groups:** 102. **Desc:** Works to stimulate cooperation between dermatology societies and encourage worldwide advancement of the profession. Promotes personal and professional relations among the dermatologists of the world. Provides educational programs; represents dermatology in commissions and health organizations. **Pub:** Directory, annual. • Newsletter, quarterly.

**International Oculoplastic Society (IOSI)**
*See:* Entry 20992

★ 6828 ★ **International Society for Bioengineering and the Skin**
c/o Prof. Humbert
Dermatology - CHU St. Jacques
25000 Besancon, France
**Fax:** 33 38 1218279
**Email:** randy.wickett@uc.edu
**Website:** http://pharmacy.uc.edu/isbs
**Fnded:** 1993. **Mem:** 120. **Lang(s):** English. **Desc:** Promotes development of instrumentation and standardized methods for measuring the properties of skin. Develops techniques and instruments for diagnosis and treatment of skin diseases; promotes the study and development of synthetic materials for skin grafting and as dressings for wounds. **Pub:** *Skin Research and Technology*, quarterly. Journal.

★ 6829 ★ **International Society for Dermatologic Surgery (ISDS)**
930 N Meacham R.
Schaumburg, IL 60173
**Phone:** (847)330-9830      **Fax:** (847)330-1135
**Email:** info@isdswordl.org
**Website:** http://www.isdsworld.org
Cathy Powers, Exec. Dir.
**Fnded:** 1976. **Mem:** 1,200. **Desc:** Dermatologists, otolaryngologists, plastic surgeons, and skin surgery specialists. Goals are to: promote high standards of patient care; provide for continuing education and research in dermatologic surgery; encourage public interest in the field. Provides a forum for the exchange of ideas and methodology in dermatologic surgery and related basic sciences. **Pub:** Directory, annual.

★ 6830 ★ **International Society of Dermatology (ISD)**
930 E Woodfield Rd.
Schaumburg, IL 60173
**Phone:** (847)330-9830      **Fax:** (847)330-1135
**Email:** info@IntSocDermatol.org
**Website:** http://www.intsocdermatol.org
Coleman Jacobson, MD, Pres.
**Fnded:** 1957. **Mem:** 2,000. **Desc:** Dermatologists and general physicians. Promotes interest, education, and research in dermatology. **Pub:** *International Journal of Dermatology*, monthly. Journal. **Frmly:** (1984) International Society of Tropical Dermatology; (1997) International Society of Dermatology: Tropical, Geographic, and Ecologic.

★ 6831 ★ **International Society of Dermatology: Tropical, Geographic, and Ecological Colombia**
c/o Torello M. Lotti, MD, Sec.Gen
Department of Dermatology
University of Florence
23, Via Dante Alighieri
51016 Montecatini Terme, Italy
**Phone:** 39 572 767957      **Fax:** 39 572 772328
**Email:** tlotti@italway.it
**Fnded:** 1960. **Mem:** 3,000. **Desc:** Promotes the study of dermatology. Concerned with the education and tracking of skin diseases. **Pub:** *International Journal of Dermatology*, 10/year. Journal. Practical dematology for practicioners all over the world.

★ 6832 ★ **Jordanian Psoriasis Association**
PO Box 184 194
Amman, Jordan
**Phone:** 962 6 5601554      **Fax:** 962 6 5688100
**Email:** dssh@nets.com.jo
**Fnded:** 1991. **Mem:** 85. **Reg. Groups:** 2. **Lang(s):** English, German. **Desc:** Offers support to individuals suffering from psoriasis. Seeks to create awareness of psoriasis and new treatment methods.

★ 6833 ★ **Mexican Academy of Dermatology (MAD)**
**(Academia Mexicana de Dermatologia — AMD)**
c/o Dr. Javier Ruiz-Avila
Georgia 114-503
Colonia Napoles
03810 Mexico City, DF, Mexico
**Phone:** 52 56 822545      **Fax:** 52 56 828963
**Email:** jraderma@yahoo.com
**Website:** http://www.amd.org.mx
**Fnded:** 1952. **Mem:** 300. **Nat'l Groups:** 1. **Reg. Groups:** 3. **Lang(s):** English, Spanish. **Desc:** Provides continuing medical education programs to members. Offers support to dermatology residents. **Pub:** *Dermatologia-Revista Mexicana*, monthly. Journal.

★ 6834 ★ **National Alopecia Areata Foundation (NAAF)**
PO Box 150760
San Rafael, CA 94915-0760
**Phone:** (415)472-3780      **Fax:** (415)472-5343
**Email:** info@naaf.org
**Website:** http://www.naaf.org
Vicki Kalabokes, CEO
**Fnded:** 1981. **Mem:** 56,000. **Nat'l Groups:** 65. **Reg. Groups:** 4. **State Groups:** 6. **Local Groups:** 2. **Desc:** Individuals concerned about alopecia areata, a disease causing partial scalp hair loss, total scalp hair loss (alopecia totalis), or total loss of body hair (alopecia universalis); cause and cure are unknown and the course of the disease is unpredictable. Objectives are to: develop public awareness of the disease; provide a support network; raise funds for research; keep patients medically informed with explanations about AA and the latest treatments. Maintains medical advisory board; operates information booth at meetings of the American Academy of Dermatology. **Pub:** *National Alopecia Areata Foundation Newsletter*, quarterly. Newsletter. Covers treatment, research, and developments. Includes wig and cosmetic tips. *Price:* Included with donation of $35 or more. • Also publishes medical description of AA and assorted brochures.

**★ 6835 ★ National Eczema Association for Science and Education**
6600 SW 92nd Ave., Ste. 230
Portland, OR 97223
**Phone:** (503)228-4430     **Free:** 800-818-7546
**Fax:** (503)224-3363
**Email:** info@nationaleczema.org
**Website:** http://www.nationaleczema.org
Melodie Silverwolf, Off. Mgr.

**Fnded:** 1988. **Mem:** 10,000. **Desc:** Works to raise awareness of the inflammatory condition of the skin called eczema. Provides patient & provider education materials. Supports research. **Pub:** *The Advocate*, quarterly. Newsletter. Contains eczema related news & letters from patients and family members. *Price:* Donations accepted. • Brochures. • Videos. **Frmly:** (1997) Eczema Association for Science and Education.

**★ 6836 ★ National Eczema Society (NES)**
Hill House
Highgate Hill
London N19 5NA, United Kingdom
**Phone:** 44 207 2813553     **Fax:** 44 207 2816395
**Website:** http://www.eczema.org/

**Fnded:** 1975. **Lang(s):** English. **Desc:** People with eczema, dermatitis, and sensitive skin. Seeks to improve the quality of life of people with eczema; promotes advancement of the diagnosis and treatment of eczema and related disorders. Conducts Skin Information Days to raise public awareness of eczema; raises funds to support dermatological research; represents the interests of people with eczema before pertinent government agencies and health care organizations. **Pub:** *Exchange*, quarterly. Journal.

**National Institute of Arthritis and Musculoskeletal and Skin Diseases Information Clearinghouse**
*See:* Entry 13635

**★ 6837 ★ National Psoriasis Foundation/ USA (NPF)**
6600 SW 92nd Ave., Ste. 300
Portland, OR 97223
**Phone:** (503)244-7404     **Free:** 800-723-9166
**Fax:** (503)245-0626
**Email:** getinfo@npfusa.org
**Website:** http://www.psoriasis.org

**Fnded:** 1968. **Desc:** People who have psoriasis and psoriatic arthritis, their family members, friends, physicians, nurses, researchers and corporations. Untied to improve the quality of life for people who have psoriasis and psoriatic arthritis to educate the public about psoriasis and to support research. **Pub:** *Psoriasis Forum*. Newsletter. Features reports on new and updated psoriasis treatments, new drug approvals, and insurance problems.

**★ 6838 ★ National Rosacea Society**
800 S Northwest Hwy., Ste. 200
Barrington, IL 60010
**Free:** 800-NO-BLUSH     **Fax:** (847)382-5567
**Email:** rosaceas@aol.com
**Website:** http://www.rosacea.org

**Desc:** Provides information, care, and treatment of rosacea. Operates a Physician Referral Service. **Pub:** Newsletter.

**★ 6839 ★ National Vitiligo Foundation**
611 S Fleishel Ave.
Tyler, TX 75701-2013
**Phone:** (903)531-0074     **Fax:** (903)525-1234
**Email:** vtiligo@ballistic.com
**Website:** http://www.vitiligofoundation.org
Shannon Hearron, Exec. Dir.

**Fnded:** 1985. **Mem:** 25,000. **Reg. Groups:** 11. **Desc:** Doctors and patients; contributors and supporters. Provides information and counseling to vitiligo patients and their families. (Vitiligo is a skin disease which destroys pigment cells causing smooth, white-colored patches of skin.) Seeks to increase awareness and concern for the vitiligo patient. Raises funds for scientific and clinical research on the cause, treatment, and cure of vitiligo. **Pub:** *Handbook for Patients.* • *Handbook for Physicians.* • *Handbook for Schools.* • *Vitiligo*, semiannual. Newsletter. • Brochures.

**★ 6840 ★ Netherlands Society for Dermatology and Venereology (Nederlandse Vereniging voor Dermatologie en Venereologie — NVDV)**
c/o Dr. J.C.J.M. Veraart
Postbus 8552
NL-3503 RN Utrecht, Netherlands
**Phone:** 31 30 2474695     **Fax:** 31 30 2474439
**Email:** nvdv@vvaa.nl

**Fnded:** 1896. **Mem:** 500. **Desc:** Physicians and interested individuals. Promotes the study of dermatology and venereal infection and treatment. **Pub:** *Nederlands Tydschrift Voor Dermatologie en Veneredogie*, 8/year. Magazine. **Frmly:** (1999) Dutch Association for Dermatology and Venereology.

**★ 6841 ★ North American Clinical Dermatologic Society (NACDS)**
c/o John W. White, Jr., M.D.
Mayo Clinic
4500 San Pablo Rd. S
Jacksonville, FL 32224
**Phone:** (904)953-2303     **Fax:** (904)953-2590
**Email:** white.john@mayo.edu
**Website:** http://www.nacds.com
John W. White, Jr.,MD, Sec. Gen.

**Fnded:** 1959. **Mem:** 210. **Desc:** Dermatologists practicing primarily in the U.S. and Canada and leaders of dermatology throughout the world. Promotes the interchange of information and research. **Pub:** *Program*, annual.

**★ 6842 ★ Pacific Dermatologic Association (PDA)**
930 E Woodfield Rd.
Schaumburg, IL 60173-6016
**Phone:** (847)330-9830     **Fax:** (847)330-1135
**Email:** alkayne@washington.edu
**Website:** http://www.pacificderm.org
William D.R. Shellow, MD, Pres.

**Fnded:** 1948. **Mem:** 1,200. **Reg. Groups:** 1. **Desc:** Dermatologists united to provide opportunities for exchange of information and advancement of knowledge of dermatology and syphilology among physicians within the Pacific Rim. Conducts specialized education programs; sponsors competitions. **Pub:** *Transactions*, annual. • Membership Directory, triennial.

**★ 6843 ★ Psoriasis Association (PA)**
16 Musgrave St.
Kirra, QLD 4225, Australia
**Phone:** 61 7 55991166     **Fax:** 61 7 55991166
**Email:** info@psoriasus.org.au
**Website:** http://www.psoriasus.org.au

**Fnded:** 1983. **Mem:** 4,000. **Lang(s):** English. **Desc:** People with psoriasis. Seeks to improve the quality of life of people with psoriasis. Serves as a clearinghouse on psoriasis and its treatment; sponsors fundraising activities; makes available counseling services; maintains support group network for people with psoriasis. **Pub:** *Members' Circular*, bimonthly. Newsletter.

**★ 6844 ★ Psoriasis Association of New Zealand (PANZI)**
PO Box 44-007
Lower Hutt, New Zealand
**Phone:** 64 4 5687139     **Fax:** 64 4 5650422
**Email:** psoriasis@xtra.co.nz

**Fnded:** 1994. **Mem:** 400. **Reg. Groups:** 4. **Lang(s):** English. **Desc:** People with psoriasis. Seeks to improve the quality of life of people with psoriasis; promotes improved understanding of psoriasis and its treatment. Serves as a clearinghouse on psoriasis; assists people with psoriasis in locating support groups and services; sponsors educational programs for health care providers and the public. Holds two yearly national psoriasis awareness campaigns. **Pub:** *Psoriasis Association of New Zealand*. Brochure.

**Psoriatric Arthropathy Alliance (PAA)**
*See:* Entry 13654

**★ 6845 ★ Scleroderma Support Group (SSG)**
224 Thompson St., No. 198
Hendersonville, NC 28792-2806
**Phone:** (704)892-5297     **Fax:** (704)893-2427
**Email:** scleroderma@juno.com
**Website:** http://www.angelfire.com/ri/scleroderma
Clara K. Ihlbrock, Pres.

**Fnded:** 1989. **Mem:** 1,000. **Nat'l Groups:** 1. **State Groups:** 2. **Desc:** Scleroderma patients and interested individuals. Serves as a support group for patients; provides information; raises funds for research; holds medical meetings and rap sessions.

**Skin Cancer Foundation (SCF)**
*See:* Entry 10249

**★ 6846 ★ Society of Dermatology Physician Assistants (SDPA)**
6218 E 78th Pl.
Tulsa, OK 74136
**Phone:** (918)523-1992     **Fax:** (918)523-1920
**Email:** monroejo@swbell.net
**Website:** http://www.pacifier.com/~jomonroe
Mary Monroe, Exec. Sec.

**Fnded:** 1993. **Mem:** 400. **Nat'l Groups:** 1. **Desc:** Physician assistants who are employed in or have an interest in the practice of dermatology. Seeks to advance the practice of dermatology physician assistants supervised by dermatologists; promotes continuing professional development of members. Acts as liaison between members and the American Academy of Dermatology; educates physicians and the public regarding the role of members in the practice of dermatology; assists in the training of dermatology physician assistants and students. Maintains writers' bureau. **Pub:** Newsletter, periodic. *Price:* for members only. **AKA:** (1995) Physician Assistants in Dermatology.

**★ 6847 ★ Society for Investigative Dermatology (SID)**
c/o Angela Welsh
820 W Superior Ave., Ste. 340
Cleveland, OH 44113-1800
**Phone:** (216)579-9300     **Fax:** (216)579-9333
**Email:** sid@sidnet.org
**Website:** http://www.sidnet.org
Angela Welsh, Admin. Dir.

**Fnded:** 1937. **Mem:** 2,300. **Desc:** Professional society promoting research in dermatology and allied subjects. **Pub:** *Journal of Investigative Dermatology*, monthly. Journal.

**Society for Pediatric Dermatology (SPD)**
*See:* Entry 5758

**★ 6848 ★ Swedish Society for Dermatology and Venereology**
c/o Anders Strand
Department of Dermatology
University Hospital
SE-75185 Uppsala, Sweden
**Phone:** 46 18 6115095     **Fax:** 46 18 662680
**Email:** anders.strand@wedsci.uu.se
**Website:** http://www.pedsderm.net

**Fnded:** 1901. **Mem:** 450. **Lang(s):** English. **Desc:** Dermatologists in Sweden. Represents members' interests. **Pub:** *Forum for Nordic Dermatu-Venereology*, quarterly. Newsletter.

## Research Centers

**★ 6849 ★ Dystrophic Epidermolysis Bullosa Research Association of America**
301 E 57th St., 3rd Fl.
New York, NY 10022
**Phone:** (212)715-1583     **Fax:** (212)715-1507
**Email:** jcampbell21@nyc.rr.com
**Website:** http://www.debra.org
Jean P. Campbell, Exec. Dir.

**Activities/Fields:** Epidermolysis Bullosa patients and their families. (Epidermolysis Bullosa represents a group of inherited disorders of the skin characterized by formation of blisters resulting from the most minimal trauma.). **Pub:** *EB Current*, 3/year.

**★ 6850 ★ Fulton Skin Institute**
13372 Newport Ave., Ste. I
Tustin, CA 92780
**Phone:** (714)665-1966     **Fax:** (714)730-0275
**Email:** fultonskin@earthlink.net
Dr. James E. Fulton, Jr., Contact

**Activities/Fields:** Cosmetic surgery, aggravating factors, and pathogenesis and treatment of acne.

**★ 6851 ★ Indiana University-Purdue University at Indianapolis**
**Hackney Dermatology Research Laboratory**
975 W Walnut St., Rm. 349
Indianapolis, IN 46202
**Phone:** (317)274-7115     **Fax:** (317)278-2815
**Email:** dspanda@iupui.edu
Dan F. Spandau, Dir.

**Activities/Fields:** Skin diseases, including skin cancer and psoriasis and the genetic changes that occur with these conditions. Wound healing and the aging of skin are also studied.

**★ 6852 ★ Massachusetts General Hospital**
**Harvard Cutaneous Biology Research Center**
Massachusetts General Hospital East, Bldg. 149
Charlestown, MA 02129
**Phone:** (617)726-4425     **Fax:** (617)724-9394

**Email:** jparrish@cbrc2.mgh.harvard.edu
Dr. John Parrish, Dir.

**Activities/Fields:** Dermatology, including photobiology of skin, including photoimmunology, photoaging, free radical biology and photoprotection; pigment cell biology; growth and differentiation of epidermis, hair and nails, and keratin biochemistry; immunology, allergy, inflammation, and modifiers of host response; physical properties of skin, including water content, percutaneous transport of chemicals, and optical properties; physiology and pharmacology of the skin; and biology of dermis and dermal-epidermal junction and their constituents.

**★ 6853 ★ National Psoriasis Foundation**
6600 SW 92nd, Ste. 300
Portland, OR 97223
**Phone:** (503)244-7404     **Free:** 800-723-9166
**Fax:** (503)245-0626
**Email:** getinfo@npfusa.org
**Website:** http://www.psoriasis.org
Gail M. Zimmerman, Pres. /CEO

**Activities/Fields:** Psoriasis, including investigations into causes, treatment, and cure of this dermatological disease. Provides funds to researchers. Recruits volunteers for FDA-approved clinical studies. Searches for three-generation families whose living members are affected by psoriasis, and refers them to the National Psoriasis Tissue Bank. Disseminates authoritative scientific information about psoriasis to psoriatics, physicians, and other concerned persons. **Pub:** *Annual report.* • *Psoriasis Bulletin*, bimonthly. • *Psoriasis Resource*, 3/year.

**★ 6854 ★ Rockefeller University**
**Laboratory for Investigative Dermatology**
1230 York Ave.
New York, NY 10021-6399
**Phone:** (212)327-8091     **Fax:** (212)327-8232
**Email:** kruegej@rockvax.rockfeller.edu
James G. Krueger, MD, Contact

**Activities/Fields:** A variety of skin conditions, including the biology of epithelial cells and the study of psoriasis.

**★ 6855 ★ U.S. Department of Health and Human Services**
**Centers for Disease Control and Prevention**
**National Institute for Occupational Safety and Health**
**National Occupational Research Agenda (Allergic and Irritant Dermatitis)**
PO Box 538707
Cincinnati, OH 45253
**Phone:** (513)841-4503     **Free:** 800-356-4676
**Fax:** (513)841-4483

**Email:** bdtl@cdc.gov
**Website:** http://www.cdc.gov/niosh/nrderm.html
Boris Lushniak, Med. Officer

**Activities/Fields:** Identify the prevalence, causes, exposure assessment methods, and early biologic markers of occupational skin diseases.

**★ 6856 ★ U.S. Department of Health and Human Services**
**National Cancer Institute**
**Division of Clinical Sciences**
**Dermatology Branch**
37 Convent Dr.
Bldg. 10, Rm. 12N238
Bethesda, MD 20892
**Phone:** (301)496-2481     **Fax:** (301)496-5370
**Email:** skatz@boy-s.nih.gov
**Website:** http://www-dcs.nci.nih.gov/branches/dermatology/index.html
Stephen L. Katz, Chief

**Activities/Fields:** Etiology, diagnosis, and treatment of inflammatory and malignant diseases involving the skin and the host's response to these diseases.

**★ 6857 ★ U.S. Department of Health and Human Services**
**National Institute of Arthritis and Musculoskeletal and Skin Diseases**
**Extramural Activities Program**
**Skin Diseases Branch**
Bldg. 45, Rm. 5AS25L
45 Center Dr.
Bethesda, MD 20892-6500
**Phone:** (301)594-5017     **Fax:** (301)480-4543
**Email:** moshella@ep.niams.nih.gov
Alan N. Moshell, MD, Dir.

**Activities/Fields:** Structure, function, and physiology of skin as well as on the causes and improved treatment of a wide variety of skin diseases, including psoriasis, lupus, eczema, vitiligo, bullous skin diseases, acne, and ichthyosis.

**★ 6858 ★ University of California, San Francisco**
**Dermatology Drug Research Unit**
Box 1212
515 Spruce
San Francisco, CA 94118
**Phone:** (415)476-4701     **Fax:** (415)502-4126
**Email:** jxmkoo@orca.ucsf.edu
John Koo, MD, Dir.

**Activities/Fields:** Conducts clinical testing of new or existing pharmacologic agents used in the treatment of skin disorders and develops protocols for drug testing. Areas of interest include phototherapy, psoriasis, and psychodermatology.

# Chapter 20
# Developmental Disabilities



## Federal Government Agencies

**U.S. Department of Health and Human Services**
**Centers for Disease Control and Prevention**
**National Center on Birth Defects and Developmental Disabilities**
*See:* Entry 4872

## Foundations & Other Funding Organizations

### Private Foundations

★ **6859** ★ **Edith L. Trees Charitable Trust**
620 Liberty Ave.
Pittsburgh, PA 15222-2705
**Phone:** (412)471-1751 **Fax:** (412)471-8117
**Website:** http://www.cdc.gov/ncbddd/
J. Eagan, III, Trust Officer
**Fnded:** 1976. **Philosophy:** The Edith L. Trees Charitable Trust provides support to organizations that serve mentally retarded children. Generally, the trust focuses its efforts in three categories–social services, education, and civic causes. The trust's social service funding supports Associations for Retarded Citizens (ARCs), community service organizations, and community centers. The trust's contributions to education fund schools and special/gifted education, and its civic funds support philanthropic organizations. **Priorities:** *Arts & Humanities:* 6%. Funds theater arts and fine arts. *Civic & Public Affairs:* 20%. Funds employment/job training services and community affairs. *Education:* 8%. Funds special education and vocational training for the mentally retarded. *Environment:* 51%. Supports services for disabled and mentally retarded children and adults; funds boys and girls clubs and camps. *International:* 15%. Supports children's hospital and rehabilitation centers. *Note:* Total contributions made in 1998. **Typ. Recipients:** Children's Health/Hospitals, Clinics/Medical Centers, Eyes/Blindness, Health Organizations, Health Policy/Cost Containment, Health-General, Hospitals (University Affiliated), Medical Rehabilitation, Mental Health, People with Disabilities, Public Health, Single-Disease Health Associations. **Geo. Dist:** Pittsburgh, PA.

★ **6860** ★ **John Merck Fund**
11 Beacon St., Ste. 1230
Boston, MA 02108
**Phone:** (617)723-2932 **Fax:** (617)523-6029
**Email:** info@jmfund.org
Ms. Ruth Hennig, Executive Director
**Fnded:** 1970. **Philosophy:** The fund makes grants in the following fields: developmental disabilities, to medical teaching hospitals for research in connection with developmental disabilities in children; the environment, to encourage preservation of productive farmland in Vermont, and to address global problems relating to climate change and the dangers of synthetic chemicals; reproductive health, to support access to women's reproductive health care in the U.S.; international human rights; and disarmament, for promoting nonproliferation of nuclear weapons; and job opportunities in the northeast U.S. "The Fund endeavors to assist outstanding individuals working on promising projects in organizations that may have difficulty attracting funds; favors grants for pilot projects that have potential for widespread application; supports advocacy, including litigation, to establish precedents the Fund considers to be in the public interest; concentrates on smaller organizations, including start-ups; favors matching grants." The foundation has recently begun to focus on economic opportunities and to support job creation projects. **Priorities:** *Civic & Public Affairs:* 37%. Supports law & justice, public policy, economic development, philanthropic organizations, rural affairs, womens affairs, and employment/job training. *Education:* 10%. Supports medical education, technical education, and universities. *Environment:* 3%. Supports family planning services. *International:* 5%. Supports medical research, reproductive health issues, and public health. *Note:* Total contributions made in 1998. **Typ. Recipients:** Adolescent Health Issues, Cancer, Children's Health/Hospitals, Emergency/Ambulance Services, Family Planning, Geriatric Health, Health Funds, Health Organizations, Health-General, Medical Education, Medical Research, Mental Health, People with Disabilities, Prenatal Health Issues, Public Health, Respiratory, Single-Disease Health Associations. **Geo. Dist:** nationally; VT.

★ **6861** ★ **Joseph P. Kennedy, Jr. Foundation**
1325 G St., Northwest, Ste. 500
Washington, DC 20005-4709
**Phone:** (202)393-1250 **Fax:** (202)824-0351
**Email:** sswenson@specialolympics.org
**Website:** http://www.familyvillage.wisc.edu/jpkf/
Dr. Sue Swenson, Executive Director
**Fnded:** 1946. **Philosophy:** "The Joseph P. Kennedy, Jr. Foundation believes that persons with mental retardation have the ability to live, learn, work, recreate, and worship like everyone else. We recognize that people with mental retardation may need assistance to do these things." "We believe that families of people with mental retardation, especially families of children with mental retardation, benefit from support and information to successfully include their family member in the everyday activities of their community." The foundation maintains two firm objectives: to seek the prevention of mental retardation by identifying its causes and to improve the means by which society deals with its citizens with mental retardation. To accomplish these objectives, the foundation has traditionally used its funds and influence in those areas in which a "multiplier effect" could be achieved. This is accomplished in these ways: "1. Enhance the quality of life of persons with mental retardation and their families." "2. Provide seed funding to capitalize on Federal and/or State or Local spending on behalf of persons with mental retardation and their families by funding initiatives that evolve beyond where existing programs are going, and do not duplicate public efforts." "3. Increase professional and public awareness of the needs of persons with mental retardation and their families." "4. Work to reduce the incidence of mental retardation." The foundation supports a variety of demonstration programs in newly-defined areas in the field of mental retardation with the hope that the programs will be replicable on a wide scale to benefit persons with mental retardation and their families. Another major area of concern is teen pregnancy. Because a significant cause of mental retardation is prematurity and low birth weight among the newborn babies of adolescents, the foundation developed a values-based curriculum, "A Community of Caring," for use in programs for pregnant teens in clinics, hospitals, agencies, or schools. The program is currently being implemented to address pregnancy prevention and examine other high-risk behavior by youth. The foundation is also concerned with the development of public policy relating to mental retardation, and funds a number of programs to raise public consciousness regarding rights, capabilities, and needs of persons with mental retardation. The foundation sponsors a Public Policy Leadership Program for professionals in mental retardation and participates in a variety of national and international meetings dealing with mental retardation and disability issues. The foundation also reports that it is decreasing activity in the sciences and focusing more upon projects which help integrate persons with mental retardation into community life, as well as on projects which empower persons with mental retardation. Programs focusing on family support; health care and oral health; and self advocacy will be highlighted in future funding priorities. **Priorities:** *Civic & Public Affairs:* 30%. Supports public policy groups that deal with the disabled. *Education:* 9%. Primarily for special education and job training projects. *Environment:* 23%. Focus on programs for people with disabilities. *International:* 35%. Supports hospitals, people with disabilities and health organizations. *Note:* Total contributions made in fiscal 1998. **Typ. Recipients:** Children's Health/Hospitals, Clinics/Medical Centers, Family Planning, Health Policy/Cost Containment, Hospitals, Medical Education, Medical Research, Medical Training, Mental Health, People with Disabilities, Prenatal Health Issues, Preventive Medicine/Wellness Organizations, Substance Abuse. **Geo. Dist:** nationally.

### Other Funding Organizations

★ **6862** ★ **Association for the Help of Retarded Children**
200 Park Ave. S, 4th Fl.
New York, NY 10003
**Phone:** (212)780-2690 **Fax:** (212)777-5893
**Email:** sbstein@ahrcnyc.org
**Website:** http://www.ahrcnyc.org
Shirley Berenstein, Dir.
**Desc:** Developmentally disabled children and adults; their families; interested individuals. Provides support

services, training programs, clinics, schools, and residential facilities to the developmentally disabled. **Awards:** Scholarship (annual).


### ★ 6863 ★ Attention Deficit Information Network (ADIN)

c/o Moira Munns
475 Hillside Ave.
Needham, MA 02494
**Phone:** (781)455-9895          **Fax:** (781)444-5466
**Email:** adin@gis.net
**Website:** http://www.addinfonetwork.com

**Desc:** People with Attention Deficit Disorders (ADD), their families, and other individuals with an interest in ADD. Promotes improved quality of life for people with ADD. Works to expand home, school, and work-based strategies for aiding people with ADD; advocates for improved responsiveness to the needs of people with ADD by schools, businesses, and organizations. Provides support and information to families of people with ADD; conducts educational programs; maintains speakers' bureau. **Awards:** AD-IN Scholarship (annual).


### ★ 6864 ★ NADD - An Association for Persons with Developmental Disabilities and Mental Health Needs

c/o Robert Fletcher
132 Fair St.
Kingston, NY 12401-4802
**Phone:** (845)331-4336          **Free:** 800-331-5362
**Fax:** (845)331-4569
**Email:** thenadd@aol.com
**Website:** http://www.thenadd.org
Dr. Robert Fletcher, Dir.

**Desc:** People with developmental disabilities and mental health care needs; mental health professionals; other interested individuals. Promotes public and professional interest in developmental disability; seeks to improve access to mental health care. Supports research programs; facilitates exchange of information among mental health professionals and consumers; conducts advocacy to insure implementation of effective public mental health policies and legislation. Holds educational programs; maintains speakers' bureau. **Awards:** Menolacino Award (annual); Merck Award (annual).


### ★ 6865 ★ National Alliance for Autism Research (NAAR)

99 Wall St., Research Park
Princeton, NJ 08540
**Phone:** (609)430-9160          **Free:** 888-777-NAAR
**Fax:** (609)430-9163
**Email:** naar@naar.org
**Website:** http://www.naar.org
Karen Margulis London, Pres.

**Desc:** Dedicated to finding the causes, prevention, effective treatment and, ultimately, cure of the autism spectrum disorders. **Awards:** NAAR Autism Research (annual).


## National & International Organizations


### ★ 6866 ★ American Association on Mental Retardation (AAMR)

444 N Capitol St. NW, Ste. 846
Washington, DC 20001-1512
**Phone:** (202)387-1968          **Free:** 800-424-3688
**Fax:** (202)387-2193
**Email:** dcroser@aamr.org
**Website:** http://www.aamr.org
Ms. M. Doreen Croser, Exec. Dir.

**Fnded:** 1876. **Mem:** 9,500. **Reg. Groups:** 9. **State Groups:** 40. **Desc:** Physicians, educators, administrators, social workers, psychologists, psychiatrists, students, and others interested in the general welfare of persons with mental retardation and the study of the cause, treatment, and prevention of mental retardation. Maintains 17 divisions and subdivisions. **Pub:** *American Journal of Mental Retardation*, bimonthly. Journal. Research in the Biological Sciences. *Price:* $175. • *Innovations: A Research to Practice Series*, 3/year. • *Mental Retardation*, bimonthly. Journal. Contains a journal of policy, practices, and perspectives. *Price:* 149. • *Mental Retardation: Definition, Classification, and Systems of Supports*. Manual. Contains terminology and classification in mental retardation. • *News and Notes*, bimonthly. • Monograph. • Also publishes testing materials. **Frmly:** (1906) Association of Medical Officers of American Institutions of Idiotic and Feebleminded Children; (1933) American Association for the Study of the Feebleminded; (1987) American Association on Mental Deficiency.


### ★ 6867 ★ Asperger Syndrome Association of Ireland (ASPIRE)

85 Woodley Park
Kilmacud
Dublin 14, Ireland
**Phone:** 353 1 2871122
**Email:** aspire@indigo.ie
**Website:** http://www.aspire-irl.com

**Lang(s):** English, Irish. **Desc:** People with Asperger's syndrome and their families; health care providers and other individuals providing support and services to people with Asperger's syndrome. Seeks to improve the quality of life of people with Asperger's syndrome. Functions as a support network for people with Asperger's syndrome and their families; facilitates research projects.


### ★ 6868 ★ Association for the Advancement of Blind and Retarded (AABR)

PO Box 560247
College Point, NY 11356
**Phone:** (718)321-3800          **Fax:** (718)321-8688
**Email:** blm@aabr.org
**Website:** http://aabr.org
Glesner C. Jones, Pres.

**Fnded:** 1955. **Desc:** Community groups and individuals interested in multi-handicapped blind and severely retarded adults. Operates 19 group residences providing intermediate care and individual residential alternative facilities for blind and retarded adults; two treatment centers for blind, multi-handicapped, and severely retarded adults; NYS approved special education program for autistic children from pre-school to school age. Provides information and referral services. **Pub:** *AABR Newsletter*, 3/year. Newsletter. Contains donor update letter. *Price:* Free. **Frmly:** (1974) Association for Advancement of Blind Children.


### ★ 6869 ★ Association for the Help of Retarded Children

200 Park Ave. S, 4th Fl.
New York, NY 10003
**Phone:** (212)780-2690          **Fax:** (212)777-5893
**Email:** sbstein@ahrcnyc.org
**Website:** http://www.ahrcnyc.org
Shirley Berenstein, Dir.

**Fnded:** 1949. **Mem:** 12,000. **Desc:** Developmentally disabled children and adults; their families; interested individuals. Provides support services, training programs, clinics, schools, and residential facilities to the developmentally disabled. **Pub:** *The Chronicle*, monthly. Newsletter.


### ★ 6870 ★ Autism-Europe

Ave. E Van Becelaere 26b, Bte 21
B-1170 Brussels, Belgium
**Phone:** 32 2 6757505          **Fax:** 32 2 6757270
**Email:** autisme.europe@arcadis.be
**Website:** http://www.autismeurope.arc.be

**Fnded:** 1982. **Mem:** 40. **Lang(s):** English, French. **Desc:** National and regional associations of parents of children with autism in 21 European countries. Seeks to improve the lives of those whose existence is affected by autism. Works to advance research on the causes of autism and its prevention and treatment; ensures effective liaison between various associations, governments, European and international exchange programs involved with autism; works to provide a charter of rights for people with autism. **Pub:** *LINK*. Journal.


### ★ 6871 ★ Autism Independent UK

199-205 Blandford Ave.
Kettering NN16 9AT, United Kingdom
**Phone:** 44 1536 523274          **Fax:** 44 1536 523274
**Email:** autism@autism.com
**Website:** http://www.autismuk.com/

**Fnded:** 1987. **Mem:** 4,000. **Lang(s):** English. **Desc:** Individuals with autism and their families. Seeks to increase awareness of autism; promotes development of improved diagnosis and treatment of people with autism. Works to improve the quality of life of people with autism. Serves as a nonmedical information center on autism and its treatment; sponsors research and educational programs; provides support and services to people with autism and their families. Maintains Diagnosis and Assessment Resource Centre, where interested individuals can access information on autism and its treatment. Collaborates with county agencies in the development of public health policies impacting people with autism. **Frmly:** (2000) Society of the Austically Handicapped.


### ★ 6872 ★ Autism Society of Canada (ASC) (Societe Canadienne de l'Autisme — SCA)

PO Box 65
Orangeville, ON, Canada L9W 2Z5
**Phone:** (519)942-8720          **Free:** (866)874-3334
**Fax:** (519)942-3566
**Website:** http://autismsocietycanada.ca

**Lang(s):** English, French. **Desc:** People with autism and their families; health care professionals, educators, therapists, and others working with people with autism. Promotes advancement in the diagnosis and treatment of autism; seeks to improve the quality of life of people with autism and their families. Provides support and services to people with autism and their families; serves as a clearinghouse on autism and its diagnosis and treatment; conducts educational programs.


### ★ 6873 ★ Autistic Association - Singapore

Blk 381, Clementi Ave. 5, No. 01-398
Singapore 120381, Singapore
**Phone:** 65 7746649          **Fax:** 65 7746957
**Email:** autism@signet.com.sg

**Lang(s):** English. **Desc:** Parents, caregivers, and professionals who are concerned with autism in Singapore. Works to assist people with autism, their parents and caregivers, and professionals involved in the field of autism. Provides resources, training, and information about autism.


### ★ 6874 ★ British Dyslexia Association

98 London Rd.
Reading RG1 5AU, United Kingdom
**Phone:** 44 118 9668271          **Fax:** 44 118 9351927
**Email:** admin@bda-dyslexia.demon.co.uk
**Website:** http://www.bda-dyslexia.org.uk/

**Fnded:** 1970. **Mem:** 10,000. **Local Groups:** 100. **Desc:** Acts as an umbrella organization for dyslexia in the UK.


### ★ 6875 ★ British Institute of Learning Disabilities

Wolverhampton Rd.
Kidderminster DY10 3PP, United Kingdom
**Phone:** 44 1562 850251          **Fax:** 44 1562 851970
**Email:** bild@bild.demon.co.uk
**Website:** http://www.bild.org.uk

**Fnded:** 1972. **Mem:** 2,000. **Desc:** Works towards improving the quality of life of people with learning disabilities, by the promotion and provision of education and training; information; research; books and journals. **Pub:** *British Journal of Learning Disabilities*, quarterly. Journal. • *Current Awareness Service*, monthly. • *Journal of Applied Research in Intellectual Disability*, quarterly. Journal. • *Learning Disability Bulletin*, quarterly. Bulletin.

**★ 6876 ★ Canadian Coalition for the Prevention of Developmental Disabilities (CCPDD)**
384 Banks St. Ste. 300
Ottawa, ON, Canada K2P 1Y4
**Phone:** (613)230-8838 **Fax:** (613)230-6654
**Email:** cich@cich.ca
**Website:** http://www.cich.ca

**Lang(s):** English, French. **Desc:** Health care professionals and other individuals with an interest in developmental disabilities. Seeks to advance understanding of the causes and prevention of developmental disabilities. Facilitates interdisciplinary exchange of information among scientists and medical professionals studying developmental disabilities; sponsors research and educational programs.

**★ 6877 ★ Canadian Dyslexia Association (CDA)**
**(Association Canadienne de la Dyslexie)**
290, avenue Picton Ave.
Ottawa, ON, Canada K1Z 8P8
**Phone:** (613)722-2699 **Fax:** (613)722-7881
**Email:** cda@ottawa.com
**Website:** http://www.dyslexiaassociation.ca

**Lang(s):** English, French. **Desc:** Promotes awareness of dyslexia and seeks to develop and implement specialized methods to improve the quality of life for Canadian s who have dyslexia.

**Chromosone 9P Network (9P)**
*See:* Entry 9310

**Coffin-Lowry Syndrome Foundation**
*See:* Entry 9312

**★ 6878 ★ Council for the Registration of Schools Teaching Dyslexic Pupils (CRESTED)**
Greygarth
Littleworth
Winchcombe
Cheltenham GL54 5BT, United Kingdom
**Phone:** 44 1242 604852 **Fax:** 44 1242 604852
**Email:** crested@crested.org.uk
**Website:** http://clsfoundation.tripod.com

**Fnded:** 1989. **Desc:** Offers guidance to parents seeking a school for their dyslexic child, providing a list of schools approved for their dyslexia provision. **Pub:** Directory, semiannual.

**Developmental Disabilities Nurses Association**
*See:* Entry 15705

**Down Syndrome Ireland (DSI)**
*See:* Entry 9320

**★ 6879 ★ Down's Syndrome Association (DSA)**
155 Mitcham Rd.
London SW17 9PG, United Kingdom
**Phone:** 44 208 6824001 **Fax:** 44 208 6824012
**Email:** info@downs-syndrome.org.uk
**Website:** http://www.dsa-uk.com

**Fnded:** 1970. **Mem:** 12,000. **Lang(s):** English. **Desc:** Provides information, advice, and support in England, Wales, and Northern Ireland on Down's Syndrome.

Does this through its information service and helpline, regional offices, and parent-led local branches. Works toward creating the conditions whereby individuals with Down's Syndrome can receive necessary medical, educational, social, and financial support to develop to their full potential. **Pub:** Newsletter, quarterly. Contains information contributed by members and research updates.

**★ 6880 ★ Dyslexia Institute**
133 Gresham Rd.
Staines TW18 2AJ, United Kingdom
**Phone:** 44 1784 463851 **Fax:** 44 1784 460747
**Email:** info@dyslexia-inst.org.uk
**Website:** http://www.dyslexia-inst.org.uk

**Fnded:** 1972. **Reg. Groups:** 25. **Desc:** Specializes in the development of individuals involved in the field of dyslexia; increases networking opportunities; broadens the sphere of influence, develops and maintains links with other bodies at all levels. **Pub:** *As We See It*, 3/year. Newsletter. • *Dyslexia Review*, 3/year. Journal. • *National DI Fee Guidelines*. • *Understanding Dyslexia*. Video. Contains practical advice and information including a guide for teachers and a guide for parents. Also publishes leaflets.

**★ 6881 ★ Egyptian Autistic Society**
9, Rd. 215
Degla
Maadi
Cairo, Egypt
**Phone:** 20 2 5199033 **Fax:** 20 2 5197055

**Lang(s):** English. **Desc:** Families with autistic children in Egypt. Works to increase awareness and understanding of autism. Provides a social club, workshops, summer camp, various forms of therapy; support groups, and training.

**★ 6882 ★ European Dyslexia Association - International Organization for Specific Learning Disabilities (EDA)**
46, av. de Port Royal des Champs
F-78320 Le Mesnil-Saint-Denis, France
**Phone:** 33 5 34619252

**Fnded:** 1987.

**★ 6883 ★ Fathers Network (NFN)**
16120 NE 8th St.
Bellevue, WA 98008-3937
**Phone:** (425)747-4004
**Email:** jmay@fathersnetwork.org
**Website:** http://www.fathersnetwork.org

**Desc:** Fathers and families raising children with special health care needs and developmental disabilities. Advocates for and provides resources and support to all men who have children with special needs. Developed national and statewide databases, support and mentoring programs, workshops and videos. **Pub:** Videos.

**★ 6884 ★ Glenkirk**
3504 Commercial Ave.
Northbrook, IL 60062
**Phone:** (847)272-5111 **Fax:** (847)272-7350
**Email:** info@glenkirk.org
**Website:** http://www.glenkirk.org

**Desc:** Advocacy for, and support and service to empower individuals with developmental disabilities in order for them to participate fully in all areas of life, including day and residential services.

**★ 6885 ★ International Association for the Scientific Study of Intellectual Disabilities (IASSID)**
c/o Association De Villepinte
28 Re De L'eglise
F-93420 Villepinte, France
**Phone:** 33 1 43851206 **Fax:** 33 1 49361154
**Email:** iassidoffice@aol.com
**Website:** http://www.iassid.org

**Fnded:** 1964. **Nat'l Groups:** 50. **Reg. Groups:** 1. **Lang(s):** English, French, Spanish. **Desc:** National associations representing 15,000 scientists and clinicians in 40 countries working in the field of intellectual disabilities. Encourages research in the field of intellectual disabilities, including its causes, prevention, diagnosis, evaluation, therapy, and rehabilitation, management, education, and social inclusion. **Pub:** *IASSID*, biennial. Newsletter. • *JIDR - Journal of Intellectual Disability Research*. Journal. • Proceedings, quadrennial. Printed in specialized journals. **Frmly:** (1995) International Association for the Scientific Study of Mental Deficiency.

**★ 6886 ★ Logan Community Resources**
PO Box 1049
1235 N Eddy St.
South Bend, IN 46624
**Website:** http://logancenter.org

**Desc:** Individuals, families, volunteers, neighbors, employers, donors. Strives to create opportunities for persons with developmental disabilities. Offers person directed planning.

**★ 6887 ★ NADD - An Association for Persons with Developmental Disabilities and Mental Health Needs**
c/o Robert Fletcher
132 Fair St.
Kingston, NY 12401-4802
**Phone:** (845)331-4336 **Free:** 800-331-5362
**Fax:** (845)331-4569
**Email:** thenadd@aol.com
**Website:** http://www.thenadd.org
Dr. Robert Fletcher, Dir.

**Fnded:** 1983. **Mem:** 1,300. **State Groups:** 6. **Desc:** People with developmental disabilities and mental health care needs; mental health professionals; other interested individuals. Promotes public and professional interest in developmental disability; seeks to improve access to mental health care. Supports research programs; facilitates exchange of information among mental health professionals and consumers; conducts advocacy to insure implementation of effective public mental health policies and legislation. Holds educational programs; maintains speakers' bureau. **Pub:** *NADD Bulletin*, bimonthly. Journal. • Also publishes books, audio tapes, video tapes, and training materials. **Frmly:** (1997) National Association for the Dually Diagnosed.

**★ 6888 ★ National Association for Adults with Special Learning Needs (NAASLN)**
c/o CEA
4380 Forbes Blvd.
Lanham, MD 20706
**Free:** 800-496-9222
**Website:** http://www.naasln.org/
Richard J. Cooper, PhD, Treasurer

**Fnded:** 1989. **Mem:** 350. **Desc:** Works to organize and promote a coalition of individuals interested in educating adults with special learning needs. Fosters development and implementation of educational programs for adults. Promotes unification of adult education professionals. Encourages research and dissemination of information on adult education. Acts as a forum for the exchange of information on adult education. Seeks to unify adults with special learning needs. Bestows annual NAASLN Distinguished Services Award.

**National Association of County Behavioral Health Directors (NACBHD)**
*See:* Entry 12569

**National Down's Syndrome Association (NDSA)**
*See:* Entry 9348

**National Fragile X Foundation (NFXF)**
*See:* Entry 9351

**★ 6889 ★ National Parent Network on Disabilities (NPND)**
1130 17th St., NW, Ste. 400
Washington, DC 20007
**Phone:** (202)463-2299          **Fax:** (202)463-9403
**Email:** npnd@mindspring.com
**Website:** http://www.npnd.org
**Desc:** Families caring for people with special health care needs and developmental disabilities. Dedicated to empowering parents. Sponsors relays, leadership exchanges, weekly newsletter, legislative updates. **Pub:** *Friday Facts*, weekly. Newsletter.

**★ 6890 ★ New Zealand Association for the Scientific Study of Mental Deficiency (NZASSMD)**
PO Box 19099
Wellington, New Zealand
**Phone:** 64 6 8774296
**Email:** mgahreus@xtra.co.uz
**Fnded:** 1980. **Lang(s):** English. **Desc:** Promotes research on intellectual disability. Unites professionals working in the field and facilitates data exchange; disseminates information. Establishes standards for practice and ethics. Monitors relevant legislation. **Pub:** *Australia and New Zealand Journal of Developmental Disability*, periodic. • Magazine, periodic.

**★ 6891 ★ Norwegian Association for Children and Adults with Minimal Brain Dysfunction (ADHD) (MBD-foreningen)**
Alexandragarden
Arnstein Arnebergsv 30
N-1366 Lysaker, Norway
**Phone:** 47 67583757          **Fax:** 47 67583747
**Email:** mbd-for@online.no
**Website:** http://www.mbd.no
**Fnded:** 1979. **Mem:** 5,000. **Reg. Groups:** 18. **Local Groups:** 18. **Lang(s):** English, Norwegian. **Desc:** Parents of children with ADHD - Attention Deficit/Hyperactivity Disorder; health personnel. Acts as support group. **Pub:** *Artikkelsamling om MBD*. Book. • *Ett Oyeblikk, Noe Barm / Volksne Med ADHD*, quarterly, always March, June, July, and December. Brochure. • *Sta Pa*, quarterly, always March, June, September, and December. Magazine. • *Sta Pa Temanummer om ADHD 1998*.

**Option Institute and Fellowship (OIF)**
*See:* Entry 12603

**★ 6892 ★ Parents and Professionals and Autism Northern Ireland (PAPA)**
Graham House
Knockbracken Healthcare Park
Saintfield Rd.
Belfast BT8 8BH, United Kingdom
**Phone:** 44 28 90401729     **Fax:** 44 28 90403467
**Email:** info@papa-ni.freeserve.co.uk
**Website:** http://www.option.org
**Fnded:** 1989. **Local Groups:** 13. **Lang(s):** English. **Desc:** Parents of autistic children and professionals that are concerned with autism in Northern Ireland. Seeks to ensure that people within the autistic spectrum and their caregivers have access to appropriate services, enabling people with autism to be valued members of their community. Provides resources, information, and advice on autism; encourages research and training; works in partnership with a range of voluntary, private, and statutory agencies; works to increase public awareness of autism. **Pub:** *Contact*, semiannual. Newsletter.

**★ 6893 ★ Rural Institute**
52 Corbin Hall
University of Montana
Missoula, MT 59812
**Phone:** (406)243-5467          **Free:** 800-732-0323
**Fax:** (406)243-4730
**Email:** muarid@selway.umt.edu
**Website:** http://ruralinstitute.umt.edu/
**Desc:** Devoted to supporting the independence, productivity, and inclusion into the community of persons with developmental disabilities and their families.

**★ 6894 ★ Scottish Society for Autism**
Head Office
Hilton House
Alloa Business Park
Whins Rd.
Alloa FK10 3SA, United Kingdom
**Phone:** 44 1259 720044     **Fax:** 44 1259 720051
**Website:** http://www.autism-in-scotland.org.uk
**Mem:** 600. **Local Groups:** 8. **Lang(s):** English. **Desc:** Families affected by autism, Asperger syndrome, or related communication disorders, as well as professionals and caregivers in the field. Works to deliver a comprehensive range of expertise in care, support, and education for people with autism, their families, and caregivers in Scotland. Operates community houses, respite care centers, and schools; provides family support visits and other community support services.

**★ 6895 ★ Special Olympics (SOI)**
1325 G St., NW, Ste. 500
Washington, DC 20005
**Phone:** (202)628-3630          **Free:** 800-700-8585
**Fax:** (202)824-0200
**Email:** info@specialolympics.org
**Website:** http://www.specialolympics.org/
Timothy P. Shriver, Pres. and CEO
**Fnded:** 1968. **Mem:** 1,200,000. **Desc:** International year-round program of sports training and competition for individuals with mental retardation. More than one million athletes in over 150 countries train and compete in 26 Olympic-type summer and winter sports. Founded in 1968 by Eunice Kennedy Shriver, Special Olympics provides people with mental retardation continuing opportunities to develop fitness, demonstrate courage, and experience joy as they participate in the sharing of gifts and friendship with other athletes, their families and the community. There is no cost to participate. **Pub:** *Spirit*, quarterly. Magazine. • *Update*, monthly. • Also publishes informational brochures, guides, instructional manual, and list of state programs.

**★ 6896 ★ UK Sports Association for People with Learning Disabilities**
Ground Fl.
Leroy House
436 Essex Rd.
London N1 3QP, United Kingdom
**Phone:** 44 207 3541030     **Fax:** 44 20 735425930
**Email:** office@uksapld.freeserve.co.uk
**Fnded:** 1980. **Reg. Groups:** 4. **Desc:** Develops lins with governing bodies of sports. Supports regional associations in developing sporting and recreational opportunities for people with learning disabilities. **Pub:** *Bulletin*, quarterly. Newsletter. Features information on sport and learning disability.

## Research Centers

**★ 6897 ★ American Association on Mental Retardation**
444 North Capitol St. NW, Ste. 846
Washington, DC 20001-1512
**Phone:** (202)387-1968          **Free:** 800-424-3688
**Fax:** (202)387-2193
**Website:** http://www.aamr.org/index.shtml
M. Doreen Croser, Exec. Dir.
**Activities/Fields:** Mental retardation, including studies on programmatic aspects of service to persons with mental retardation in residential facilities and community-based settings. Prevention, behavioral, family support, employment, education and health are other areas of research and programmatic concern. **Pub:** *American Journal on Mental Retardation*, bimonthly. • *Mental Retardation*, bimonthly. • *Monographs*. • *News & Notes*, bimonthly.

**★ 6898 ★ Baylor College of Medicine Mental Retardation Research Center**
Mail Stop BCM 225
1 Baylor Plaza, T809
Houston, TX 77030
**Phone:** (713)798-7353          **Fax:** (713)798-8704
**Email:** hzoghbi@bcm.tmc.edu
**Website:** http://mrrc.bcm.tmc.edu
Huda Y. Zoghbi, MD, Dir.
**Activities/Fields:** Mental retardation and its prevention. Research includes Rett syndrome, epilepsy, Angelman and Prader-Willi syndrome, gene therapy, human X chromosome, cytomegalovirus infection, group b streptococci, chondrodysplasia punctata, and spinocerebellar ataxia, Fragile X Syndrome, Aicardi Syndrome, HIV infection, metabolic disorders, Incontinentia Pigmenti, Williams Syndrome, Retinal degeneration and neuropathies.

**★ 6899 ★ Cincinnati Center for Developmental Disorders**
Pavilion Bldg.
3333 Burnet Ave.
Cincinnati, OH 45229-3039
**Phone:** (513)636-4626          **Fax:** (513)636-7361
Dr. Sonya Oppenheimer, Dir.
**Activities/Fields:** Prevention, early detection, and improved methods of therapy and management of developmental disabilities. Also studies genetics, learning disabilities, and birth defects. **Pub:** *Developments, Newsletter*, quarterly.

**Columbia-Presbyterian Medical Center Gertrude H. Sergievsky Center**
*See:* Entry 14178

**★ 6900 ★ Institute for Community Inclusion**
Children's Hospital
300 Longwood Ave.
Boston, MA 02115
**Phone:** (617)355-6506          **Fax:** (617)355-7940
**Email:** kiernanw@a1.tch.harvard.edu
**Website:** http://www.childrenshospital.org/ici
William E. Kiernan, PhD, Dir.
**Activities/Fields:** Etiology of mental retardation, the impact of AIDS in adult populations, the development of employment opportunities for people with disabilities using natural supports, the development of supports for infants at risk, development of a managed care design for children with complex medical needs served in community settings, and clinical investigation of issues of autism and related behavior in community settings. **Pub:** *Institute Briefs*.

**★ 6901 ★ Louisiana State University Human Development Center**
Sch. of Allied Health Professions
1100 Florida Ave., Bldg. 138
New Orleans, LA 70119-2799
**Phone:** (504)942-8200          **Fax:** (504)942-8305
**Email:** rcrow@lsuhsc.edu
Robert E. Crow, PhD, Dir.
**Activities/Fields:** Developmental disabilities, including educational technology, curriculum research, and integrated basic and applied behavioral interventions. Operates as a University Affiliated Program for interdisciplinary training, research, and dissemination.

**★ 6902 ★ Northwest Woodhaven Center Inc.**
2900 Southampton Rd.
Philadelphia, PA 19154
**Phone:** (215)671-5001 **Fax:** (215)671-7522
Michael Barton, MD, VP

**Activities/Fields:** Treatment effectiveness, program evaluation, clinical treatment research (medications and behavior modification), and policy research in mental retardation at Woodhaven Center, a University-operated residential program for mentally retarded persons. **Pub:** *Evaluation and Research Technical Report Series.*

**★ 6903 ★ Ohio State University Nisonger Center for Mental Retardation and Developmental Disabilities**
1581 Dodd Dr.
Columbus, OH 43210-1257
**Phone:** (614)292-8365 **Fax:** (614)292-3727
**Email:** reiss.7@osu.edu
Steven Reiss, PhD, Dir.

**Activities/Fields:** Developmental disabilities, psychometric assessment, rehabilitation engineering, psychopathology, psychopharmacology, adults and aging, and family studies. Special attention given to applied research related to mental retardation and development and implementation of training programs to prepare professional personnel to work with the developmentally disabled. Provides early childhood classes for developmentally disabled preschoolers and offers information services to clients, students, staff, and faculty.

**★ 6904 ★ University of California, Los Angeles Mental Retardation Research Center**
Neuropsychiatric Institute & Hospital
760 Westwood Plz., 68-177 NPI
Los Angeles, CA 90024-1759
**Phone:** (310)825-5189 **Fax:** (310)206-5061
**Email:** jdevellis@mednet.ucla.edu
**Website:** http://www.mrrc.npi.ucla.edu/mrr/page1.html
Dr. Jean de Vellis, Dir.

**Activities/Fields:** Mental retardation and related aspects of human development, including interdisciplinary basic and clinical studies on problems in developmental biology, human genetics, neurobiochemistry, neurophysiology, and sociobehavioral categories. Collaborates with other institutes, schools, and departments at the University. **Pub:** *Annual Report.*

**★ 6905 ★ University of Chicago Joseph P. Kennedy, Jr., Mental Retardation Research Center**
MC 5058
Wyler Children's Hospital
5841 S Maryland Ave.
Chicago, IL 60637-5058
**Phone:** (773)702-6428 **Fax:** (773)702-9234
**Email:** n-schwartz@uchicago.edu
**Website:** http://peds-www.bsd.uchicago.edu/sections/Kennedy/index.html
Dr. Nancy B. Schwartz, Dir.

**Activities/Fields:** Mental retardation, emphasizing membrane glycoconjugate structure and synthesis, lysosomes (inborn errors of metabolism), regulation of enzymatic action, protein chemistry, chemistry and metabolism of sphingolipids and other lipids and lipoprotein complexes, carbohydrate chemistry, biology of biochemistry of the extracellular matrix (normal development and inborn errors), collagen gene structure and expression, DNA sequence studies, DNA methylation and chromatin structure, recombinant DNA technology, cell-free translation and transcription in differentiating eukaryotic cells, regulation of gene expression and mRNA regulation during embryonic development, regulation of catecholamine neurotransmitter biosynthesis and secretion, signal transduction pathways in neuronal systems, opioid actions during embryogenesis and opioid signal transduction, musca-

rinic receptor signal transduction pathways in differentiating neurons, proteoglycan participation in CNS histomorphogenesis, glia phenotypes and the role of protein kinases, electron microscope visualization of specific gene products in differentiating nervous system and cartilage (use of monoclonal antibodies), neurotransmitter receptor structure and function, mechanisms of synapse formation, neurobiology and neuropathology of dopaminergic pathways, regulation of myelination (oligodendrocyte neurobiology), isolation and tissue culture of specialized cells (oligodendrocytes, neurononal aggregates, neuroblastoma x neuron hybrids, chromaffin cells, and chondrocytes), neuroanatomical mapping, mitochondrial function and dysfunction, and neurological, genetic, biological, biochemical, and embryological studies.

**★ 6906 ★ University of Colorado B.F. Stolinsky Research Laboratories**
4200 E 9th Ave., Campus Box C233
Denver, CO 80262
**Phone:** (303)315-7301 **Fax:** (303)315-8080
Stephen I. Goodman, MD, Dir.

**Activities/Fields:** Biochemical genetics and nutrition. The Laboratories are federally designated as a center for research in mental retardation or related aspects of human development.

**★ 6907 ★ University of Kansas Mental Retardation Research Center (MRRC)**
University of Kansas Medical Center
3901 Rainbow Blvd.
Kansas City, KS 66160-7336
**Phone:** (913)588-5970 **Fax:** (913)588-5677
**Email:** pcheney@kumc.edu
**Website:** http://www2.kumc.edu/mrrc
Dr. Paul D. Cheney, Dir.

**Activities/Fields:** Fundamental problems of mental retardation and developmental disabilties, including molecular biology and physiology of pregnancy, neuroendocrinology, fetal development, impaired fetal and infant development, infant language, cognitive development, prenatal and postnatal risk factors, developmental neurobiology and neuroplasticity. Conducts animal models studies concerning pregnancy, early developmental processes, and neurobiological mechanisms involved in motor and sensory functions of the brain and neuropathology of AIDS.

**★ 6908 ★ University of Kansas Mental Retardation Research Center Institute for Life Span Studies Parsons Research Center**
PO Box 738
Parsons, KS 67357-0738
**Phone:** (316)421-6550 **Fax:** (316)421-0954
**Email:** ksaunders@parsons.lsi.ukans.edu
**Website:** http://www.parsons.lsi.ukans.edu/lsiparsons
Dr. Kathryn Saunders, Dir.

**Activities/Fields:** Experimental analysis of cognitive functions, including discrimination, classification, and representation skills among retarded persons; language and communication behavior, including social, and symbolic behaviors of severely retarded persons; and analysis and treatment of chronic aberrant behavior, behavioral pharmacology, and reading. **Pub:** *Parsons Research Center Reports.*

**★ 6909 ★ University of Miami Center on Aging and Disabilities**
1400 NW 10th Ave., Ste. 601
Miami, FL 33136
**Phone:** (305)243-6397 **Fax:** (305)243-4804
**Email:** pbloom@med.miami.edu
Patricia Bloom, Dir.

**Activities/Fields:** Future care planning for adults with developmental disabilities; pet therapy.

**★ 6910 ★ University of Michigan Center for Human Growth and Development**
300 N Ingalls Bldg., 10th Level
Ann Arbor, MI 48109-0406
**Phone:** (734)764-2443 **Fax:** (734)936-9288
**Email:** blozoff@umich.edu
**Website:** http://www.umich.edu/~chgdwww/
Dr. Betsy Lozoff, Dir.

**Activities/Fields:** Human growth and development through childhood and adolescence, including interdisciplinary studies on normal and abnormal behavioral, physical, and mental development, focusing especially on the challenges to children who grow up in adverse conditions. **Pub:** *Biennial Report.* • *Craniofacial Growth Monograph Series*, annually.

**University of Washington Center on Human Development and Disability**
*See:* Entry 4784

**★ 6911 ★ Vanderbilt University John F. Kennedy Center for Research on Human Development**
Box 40
230 Appleton Place
Peabody College
Nashville, TN 37203-5701
**Phone:** (615)322-8240 **Fax:** (615)322-8236
**Email:** elaine.bush@mcmail.vanderbilt.edu
**Website:** http://www.vanderbilt.edu/kennedy
Elaine Sanders-Bush, PhD, Contact

**Activities/Fields:** Behavioral, biomedical, and educational aspects of mental retardation and other disabilities and child development, including cognitive strategies, social and communicative processes, neural development, neural plasticity. Investigates cognitive modifiability, computer applications to facilitate thinking and learning, normal and abnormal nervous system maturation, perceptual and locomotor behavior, self-injurious behavior, language and social development, development of aggressive behavior, early education of mentally retarded and economically disadvantaged children. **Pub:** *Kennedy Center News*, quarterly. • *Research Project Brochures.* • *TOT Talk*, semiannually.

**★ 6912 ★ Waisman Center**
University of Wisconsin—Madison
1500 Highland Ave.
Madison, WI 53705
**Phone:** (608)263-5910 **Fax:** (608)263-0529
**Email:** mseltzer@waisman.wisc.edu
**Website:** http://www.waisman.wisc.edu
Marsha Mailick Seltzer, PhD, Actg. Dir.

**Activities/Fields:** Individuals with developmental disabilities, including noncompromised infants, children, and adults, as well as nonhuman subjects. Studies focus on genetics, molecular biology, neurochemistry, sensory and perceptual processes, neurophysiology, communication processes, development intervention processes, and biological, behavioral, and social processes across the lifespan. Divided into the following units: Molecular and Genetic Sciences Unit, Sensory and Cognitive Processes Unit, Communication Processes Unit, Social and Affective Processes Unit. **Pub:** *Waisman Center Interactions*, annually. **Frmly:** Harry A. Waisman Center.

**★ 6913 ★ Windsor Regional Hospital Ozad Institute for Developmental Disabilities**
3901 Connaught Ave.
Windsor, ON, Canada N9C 4H4
**Phone:** (519)257-5219 **Fax:** (519)257-5212
**Email:** rccneuro@mnsi.net
John Strang, PhD, Dir.

**Activities/Fields:** Developmental disabilities in children, focusing on applied neuropsychological research, autism and related disorders, and developmental handicap research.

★ 6914 ★ **Yeshiva University**
**Rose F. Kennedy Center for Research in**
**Mental Retardation and Developmental**
**Disabilities**
Albert Einstein College of Medicine
1410 Pelham Pky. S
Bronx, NY 10461
**Phone:** (718)430-2511　　　**Fax:** (718)881-8821
**Email:** dfaber@aecom.yu.edu
Dr. Donald S. Faber, Dir.
**Activities/Fields:** Mental retardation and other forms of aberrant human development, including biomedical, behavioral, educational, and social studies.

# State Government Agencies

## Developmental Disabilities

★ 6915 ★ **Alabama Department of Mental**
**Health and Mental Retardation**
RSA Union
100 N Union St., Ste. 518
Montgomery, AL 36130-1410
**Phone:** (334)242-3147　　　**Fax:** (334)242-0684
**Website:** http://www.mh.state.al.us/
Kathy E. Sawyer, Director

★ 6916 ★ **Alaska Department of Health**
**and Social Services**
**Mental Health and Developmental**
**Disabilities Division**
350 Main St., Ste. 217
PO Box 110620
Juneau, AK 99811-0620
**Phone:** (907)465-3370　　　**Free:** 800-465-4828
**Fax:** (907)465-2668
**Email:** DMHDD_Webmaster@health.state.ak.us
**Website:** http://www.hss.state.ak.us/dmhdd/
Leonard Abel, Contact
Karl Brimner, Director

★ 6917 ★ **Arkansas Department of**
**Human Services**
**Developmental Disabilities Services**
**Division**
Donaghey Plaza N
PO Box 1437, Slot N503
Little Rock, AR 72203-1437
**Phone:** (501)682-8665　　　**Fax:** (501)682-8380
**Website:** http://www.state.ar.us/dhs/ddds/index.html
David Fray, Director

★ 6918 ★ **California Health and Welfare**
**Agency**
**Developmental Services Department**
PO Box 944202
Sacramento, CA 94244-2020
**Phone:** (916)654-1690　　　**Fax:** (916)654-2167
**Email:** ddsweb@dds.ca.gov
**Website:** http://www.dds.cahwnet.gov

★ 6919 ★ **Colorado Department of**
**Human Services**
**Developmental Disabilities Division**
3824 W Princeton Cir.
Denver, CO 80236
**Phone:** (303)866-7450　　　**Fax:** (303)866-7470
**Website:** http://www.cdhs.state.co.us/ohr/dds/DDS_center.html
Kerry O. Stern, Director

★ 6920 ★ **Connecticut Department of**
**Mental Retardation**
460 Capitol Ave.
Hartford, CT 06106
**Phone:** (860)418-6000　　　**Fax:** (860)418-6001
**Email:** dmrct.co@po.state.ct.us
**Website:** http://www.dmr.state.ct.us/
Peter H. O'Meara, Director

★ 6921 ★ **Delaware Department of Health**
**and Social Services**
**Mental Retardation Division**
Jesse Cooper Bldg.
417 Federal St.
Dover, DE 19901
**Phone:** (302)739-4452　　　**Fax:** (302)739-6652
**Email:** dhssinfo@state.de.us
**Website:**　　　http://www.state.de.us/dhss/dmr/dmrhome.htm
Marianne Smith, Director

★ 6922 ★ **Indiana Family and Social**
**Services Administration**
**Disability, Aging and Rehabilitative**
**Services Division**
**Developmental Disability Services Bureau**
402 W Washington St.
PO Box 7083
Indianapolis, IN 46207-7083
**Phone:** (317)232-7842　　　**Free:** 800-545-2320
**Fax:** (317)233-2320
**Website:**　　　http://www.state.in.us/fssa/servicedisabl/ddars/bdds.html

★ 6923 ★ **Iowa Department of Human**
**Services**
**Mental Health, Mental Retardation and**
**Developmental Disabilities Division**
Department of Human Services
1305 E Walnut
Des Moines, IA 50319-0114
**Phone:** (515)281-8472　　　**Fax:** (515)281-8512
**Email:** jchesni@dhs.state.ia.us
**Website:** http://www.dhs.state.ia.us/mhdd/
Jim Chesnik, Contact

★ 6924 ★ **Louisiana Department of**
**Health and Hospitals**
**Citizens with Developmental Disabilities**
**Office**
1201 Capitol Access Rd.
PO Box 3117
Baton Rouge, LA 70821-3117
**Phone:** (225)342-0095　　　**Fax:** (225)342-8823
**Email:** Webmaster@dhh.state.la.us
**Website:** http://www.dhh.state.la.us/OCDD/index.htm
Raymond A. Jetson, Secretary

★ 6925 ★ **Maryland Department of Health**
**and Mental Hygiene**
**Developmental Disabilities Administration**
201 W Preston St., 4th Fl.
Baltimore, MD 21201
**Phone:** (410)767-5600　　　**Fax:** (410)767-6489
**Email:** ddaweb@dhmh.state.md.us
**Website:** http://www.dhmh.state.md.us/dda_md/
Diane K. Coughlin, Director

★ 6926 ★ **Massachusetts Executive**
**Office of Health and Human Services**
**Mental Retardation Services Department**
500 Harrison Ave.
Boston, MA 02118
**Phone:** (617)727-5608　　　**Fax:** (617)624-7577
**Email:** info@dmr.state.ma.us
**Website:** http://www.dmr.state.ma.us/

★ 6927 ★ **Michigan Community Health**
**Department**
**Behavioral Health Services**
**Developmental Disabilities Council**
Lewis Cass Bldg.
Lansing, MI 48913
**Phone:** (517)334-6123　　　**Fax:** (517)334-7353
**Email:** vanhornr@michigan.gov
**Website:** http://www.michigan.gov/mdch/

★ 6928 ★ **Minnesota Department of**
**Human Services**
**Health and Continuing Care Strategies**
**Developmental Disabilities Division**
444 Lafayette Rd. N
Saint Paul, MN 55155
**Phone:** (651)296-3933　　　**Fax:** (651)297-4692
**Email:** dhs.webmaster@state.mn.us
**Website:**　　　http://www.dhs.state.mn.us/contcare/default.htm

★ 6929 ★ **Mississippi Department of**
**Mental Health**
**Mental Retardation Bureau**
1101 Robert E Lee Bldg.
239 N Lamar St.
Jackson, MS 39201
**Phone:** (601)359-1288　　　**Fax:** (601)359-6295
**Email:** kfeisel@msdmh.org
**Website:** http://www.dmh.state.ms.us/
Albert R. Hendrix, PhD, Director

★ 6930 ★ **Montana Department of Public**
**Health and Human Services**
**Disability Services Division**
111 N Sanders
PO Box 4210
Helena, MT 59604-4210
**Phone:** (406)444-2590　　　**Free:** 877-296-1197
**Fax:** (406)444-3632
**Email:** jmathews@state.mt.gov
**Website:** http://www.dphhs.state.mt.us/divisions/dsd/dsd.htm
Joe Mathews, Director

★ 6931 ★ **New Jersey Department of**
**Human Services**
**Developmental Disabilities Division**
50 E State St.
PO Box 726
Trenton, NJ 08625-0726
**Phone:** (609)292-3742　　　**Free:** 800-832-9173
**Fax:** (609)292-6610
**Email:** dmhsmail@dhs.state.nj.us
**Website:**　　　http://www.state.nj.us/humanservices/dhspwd1.html
James W. Smith, Director

★ 6932 ★ **North Carolina Department of**
**Health and Human Services**
**Mental Health, Developmental Disabilities**
**and Substance Abuse Services**
**Division**
**Developmental Disabilities Services**
3006 Mail Service Ctr.
325 N Salisbury
Raleigh, NC 27699-3006
**Phone:** (919)733-3654　　　**Fax:** (919)733-9455
**Email:** contactdmh@ncmail.net
**Website:** http://www.dhhs.state.nc.us/mhddsas/
Stan Slawinski, PhD, Director

★ 6933 ★ **North Dakota Department of**
**Human Services**
**Disability Services**
600 S Second St.
Bismarck, ND 58504-5729
**Phone:** (701)328-8930　　　**Free:** 800-755-8529
**Fax:** (701)328-8969

**Email:** dhsds@state.nd.us
**Website:** http://lnotes.state.nd.us/dhs/dhsweb.nsf/ServicePages/DisabilityServices

★ **6934** ★ **Oklahoma Department of Human Services**
**Developmental Disability Services Division**
2400 N Lincoln Blvd.
PO Box 25352
Oklahoma City, OK 73125
**Phone:** (405)521-6267  **Fax:** (405)522-3037
**Email:** James.Nicholson@okdhs.org
**Website:** http://www.okdhs.org/ddsd/
Jim Nicholson, Director

★ **6935** ★ **Oregon Department of Human Resources**
**Mental Health and Developmental Disabilities Services Division**
**Developmental Disabilities Services Office**
2575 Bittern St. NE
Salem, OR 97309
**Phone:** (503)945-9774  **Fax:** (503)373-7274
**Email:** dhrinfo@state.or.us
**Website:** http://oddsweb.mhd.hr.state.or.us/

★ **6936** ★ **Pennsylvania Department of Public Welfare**
**Mental Retardation Office**
PO Box 2675
Health & Welfare Bldg., Rm. 512
Harrisburg, PA 17105-2675
**Phone:** (717)787-3700  **Fax:** (717)772-2062
**Website:** http://www.dpw.state.pa.us/omr/dpwmr.asp

★ **6937** ★ **Rhode Island Department of Mental Health, Retardation and Hospitals**
**Developmental Disabilities Division**
14 Harrington Rd.
Cranston, RI 02920
**Phone:** (401)462-3234  **Fax:** (401)462-6636
**Email:** lkahn@mhrh.state.ri.us
**Website:** http://www.mhrh.state.ri.us/developmental_disabilities.htm
Lynda D. Kahn, Director

★ **6938** ★ **South Carolina Department of Disabilities and Special Needs**
3440 Harden St. Ext.
PO Box 4706
Columbia, SC 29240
**Phone:** (803)898-9600  **Free:** 888-376-4636
**Fax:** (803)898-9653
**Email:** DDSNweb@ddsn.state.sc.us
**Website:** http://www.state.sc.us/ddsn
Stan Butkus, Director

★ **6939** ★ **Tennessee Department of Mental Health and Mental Retardation**
**Mental Retardation Services Division**
425 Fifth Ave. N
Cordell Hull Bldg.
Nashville, TN 37243
**Phone:** (615)532-6500  **Fax:** (615)532-6514
**Email:** martha.robinson@state.tn.us
**Website:** http://www.state.tn.us/mental/
Elizabeth Rukeyser, Director

★ **6940** ★ **Texas Department of Mental Health and Mental Retardation**
**Mental Retardation Facilities Division**
909 W 45th St.
PO Box 12668
Austin, TX 78711-2668
**Phone:** (512)454-3761  **Free:** 800-252-8154
**Fax:** (512)206-4560
**Email:** Webmaster@mhmr.state.tx.us

**Website:** http://www.mhmr.state.tx.us/
Karen F. Hale, Director

★ **6941** ★ **Vermont Agency of Human Services**
**Developmental and Mental Health Services Department**
**Mental Retardation Programs Division**
Weeks Bldg.
103 S Main St.
Waterbury, VT 05671-1601
**Phone:** (802)241-2610  **Fax:** (802)241-1129
**Email:** webmaster@ddmhs.state.vt.us
**Website:** http://www.state.vt.us/dmh
Susan W. Besio, PhD, Contact

★ **6942** ★ **Virginia Office of Health and Human Resources**
**Mental Health, Retardation and Substance Abuse Services Department**
**Mental Retardation Division**
PO Box 1797
Richmond, VA 23218
**Phone:** (804)371-3921  **Free:** 800-451-5544
**Fax:** (804)371-6638
**Email:** bbrenzovich@dmhmrsas.state.va.us
**Website:** http://www.dmhmrsas.state.va.us/
James Reinhard, MD, Contact

★ **6943** ★ **Wyoming Department of Health**
**Developmental Disabilities Division**
Herschler Bldg., 1st Fl. W
122 W 25th St.
Cheyenne, WY 82002
**Phone:** (307)777-7115  **Fax:** (307)777-6047
**Email:** ddmail@state.wy.us
**Website:** http://ddd.state.wy.us/
Robert T. Clabby, II, Director

# State & Regional Organizations

## Mental Retardation

*Listed below are state offices of The Arc (1010 Wayne Ave., Ste. 650, Silver Spring, MD 20910; (301)565-3842, http://www.thearc.org/), a national organization on mental retardation.*

### Alabama

★ **6944** ★ **The Arc of Alabama**
300 S Hull St.
Montgomery, AL 36104
**Phone:** (334)262-7688
**Website:** http://www.arcalabama.org

★ **6945** ★ **The Arc of Athens-Limestone**
427 Rogers St.
Athens, AL 35611
**Phone:** (256)232-0366

★ **6946** ★ **The Arc of Autauga and Western Elmore Counties**
926 Selma Hwy.
Prattville, AL 36067
**Phone:** (334)365-4054

★ **6947** ★ **The Arc of Baldwin County, Inc.**
PO Box 400
Loxley, AL 36551
**Phone:** (334)964-4451

★ **6948** ★ **The Arc of Blount County**
615 Fairground Ave.
PO Box 210
Oneonta, AL 35121
**Phone:** (205)625-3552

★ **6949** ★ **The Arc of Calhoun and Cleburne Counties**
PO Box 1848
Anniston, AL 36202
**Phone:** (256)236-2857

★ **6950** ★ **The Arc of Clarke County**
PO Box 100
Jackson, AL 36545
**Phone:** (334)246-3000

★ **6951** ★ **The Arc of Cullman County**
95 County Rd. 1218
Vinemont, AL 35179
**Phone:** (205)739-1161

★ **6952** ★ **The Arc of Dale County**
717 W Main St.
Daleville, AL 36322
**Phone:** (334)255-3831

★ **6953** ★ **The Arc of DeKalb County**
201 Grand Ave. S
Fort Payne, AL 35967
**Phone:** (205)845-0165

★ **6954** ★ **The Arc of Dothan/Houston Counties**
7 Harrington Ln.
Dothan, AL 36305
**Phone:** (334)792-0002

★ **6955** ★ **The Arc of Eastern Elmore County**
PO Box 847
Wetumpka, AL 36092
**Phone:** (334)514-0708

★ **6956** ★ **The Arc of Etowah County**
PO Box 1172
Gadsden, AL 35902
**Phone:** (256)547-6800

★ **6957** ★ **The Arc of Fayette/Lamar**
1428 S Temple Ave.
Fayette, AL 35555
**Phone:** (205)932-8642

★ **6958** ★ **The Arc of Franklin County**
Red Bay, AL 35582
**Phone:** (256)356-8855

★ **6959** ★ **The Arc of Geneva County**
Rte. 1, Box 102
Coffee Springs, AL 36318

★ **6960** ★ **The Arc of Jackson County**
180 Mack Morris Dr.
Scottsboro, AL 35769
**Phone:** (256)259-1603

★ **6961** ★ **The Arc of Jefferson County**
215 21st Ave. S
Birmingham, AL 35205
**Phone:** (205)323-6383

**★ 6962 ★ The Arc of Lawrence County**
23343 State Hwy. 33
Courtland, AL 35618
**Phone:** (256)974-0496

**★ 6963 ★ The Arc of Madison County**
1100 Washington St.
Huntsville, AL 35801
**Phone:** (256)536-1035

**★ 6964 ★ The Arc of Marshall County**
5104 Porter Harvey Dr.
Guntersville, AL 35976
**Phone:** (256)582-5009

**★ 6965 ★ The Arc of Montgomery**
527 Buckingham Dr.
Montgomery, AL 36116
**Phone:** (334)281-6938
**Website:** http://www.mindspring.com/%7Emarc1
Lee Conner, Exec Director

**★ 6966 ★ The Arc of Morgan County**
401 14th St. SE, Bldg. 4E
Decatur, AL 35601
**Phone:** (256)355-6192

**★ 6967 ★ The Arc of North Talladega County**
PO Box 853
Talladega, AL 35160
**Phone:** (205)362-8064

**★ 6968 ★ The Arc of Randolph County**
PO Box 127
Roanoke, AL 36274
**Phone:** (334)863-8991

**★ 6969 ★ The Arc of St. Clair County**
282 Chula Vista Dr.
Pell City, AL 35125-6293
**Phone:** (205)884-2680

**★ 6970 ★ The Arc of Shelby County**
1960-H Chandalar Dr.
Pelham, AL 35124-4323
**Phone:** (205)664-9313

**★ 6971 ★ The Arc of South Talladega County**
PO Box 360
Sylacauga, AL 35150
**Phone:** (205)245-2323

**★ 6972 ★ The Arc of The Chattahoochee Valley**
PO Box 416
Valley, AL 36854
**Phone:** (205)644-2277

**★ 6973 ★ The Arc of The Shoals**
PO Box 501
Tuscumbia, AL 35674
**Phone:** (256)383-1472

**★ 6974 ★ The Arc of Tuscaloosa County**
PO Box 40246
Tuscaloosa, AL 35403
**Phone:** (205)556-4900
**Email:** bcarroll@dbtech.net
**Website:** http://www.dbtech.net/arc
Barbara Carroll, Exec Director

**★ 6975 ★ The Arc of Walker County**
910 Oak Hill Rd.
Jasper, AL 35504
**Phone:** (205)387-0562

**★ 6976 ★ The Arc of Winston County**
145 County Hwy. 76
Haleyville, AL 35565
**Phone:** (205)486-2178

**★ 6977 ★ Mobile Association for Retarded Citizens, Inc. (MARC)**
2424 Gordon Smith Dr.
Mobile, AL 36617
**Phone:** (251)479-7409   **Fax:** (251)473-7649
**Email:** jzoghby@mobilecan.org
**Website:** http://www.mobilearc.org
Jeffrey Zoghby, Exec Director

## Alaska

**★ 6978 ★ The Arc of Anchorage**
2211 Arca Dr.
Anchorage, AK 99508
**Phone:** (907)277-6677
**Website:** http://www.arc-anchorage.org

## Arizona

**★ 6979 ★ The Arc of Arizona**
5610 S Central Ave.
Phoenix, AZ 85040
**Phone:** (602)243-1787
**Email:** arcofarizona@aol.com
**Website:** http://www.arcarizona.org

**★ 6980 ★ The Arc of Cottonwood**
3165 Calle Del Montana
Sedona, AZ 86336

**★ 6981 ★ The Arc of Douglas**
PO Box 252
Douglas, AZ 85608
**Phone:** (520)364-7473

**★ 6982 ★ The Arc of Gila County**
PO Box 1262
Globe, AZ 85502
**Phone:** (520)425-6053

**★ 6983 ★ The Arc of Graham County**
PO Box 870
Safford, AZ 85548
**Phone:** (520)428-7968

**★ 6984 ★ The Arc of Mesa**
924 N Country Club
Mesa, AZ 85201
**Phone:** (602)969-3800

**★ 6985 ★ The Arc of Mohave County**
2090 Airway
Kingman, AZ 86401
**Phone:** (520)757-3988

**★ 6986 ★ The Arc of Northeastern Pinal County**
PO Box 535
Kearny, AZ 85237
**Phone:** (520)363-5581

**★ 6987 ★ The Arc of the Prescott Area**
PO Box 11784
Prescott, AZ 86301
**Phone:** (520)749-3197

**★ 6988 ★ The Arc of Santa Cruz County**
PO Box 972
Nogales, AZ 85628

**★ 6989 ★ The Arc of Sierra Huachuca**
120 N 6th St.
Sierra Vista, AZ 85635
**Phone:** (520)458-4611

**★ 6990 ★ The Arc of Tempe**
PO Box 26014
Tempe, AZ 85285-6014
**Phone:** (602)966-8536

**★ 6991 ★ The Arc of Tucson, Inc.**
PO Box 44324
Tucson, AZ 85733
**Phone:** (520)570-1295
**Website:** http://www.arcoftucson.org

**★ 6992 ★ The Arc of Yuma County**
256 S 2nd Ave., Ste. A
Yuma, AZ 85364
**Phone:** (928)783-1588

**★ 6993 ★ Chandler/Gilbert Arc**
3434 N San Marcos Pl.
Chandler, AZ 85224
**Phone:** (480)892-9422
**Website:** http://www.cgarc.org

**★ 6994 ★ Early Intervention Infant Toddler Program, Inc.**
413 E Florence Blvd.
Casa Grande, AZ 85222-4122
**Phone:** (520)836-7939

**★ 6995 ★ Parents and Friends**
3818 W Rose Ln.
Phoenix, AZ 85019

**★ 6996 ★ The Peaks Arc**
604 W Havasupai Rd.
Flagstaff, AZ 86001

## Arkansas

**★ 6997 ★ The Arc of Arkansas**
2004 S Main St.
Little Rock, AR 72206-1597
**Phone:** (501)375-7770
**Website:** http://www.arcark.org

**★ 6998 ★ The Arc of Nevada County**
PO Box 480
Prescott, AR 71857
**Phone:** (870)887-6675

**★ 6999 ★ The Arc of Randolph County**
PO Box 425
Pocahontas, AR 72455-2114

**★ 7000 ★ The Arc of Sebastian County**
121 N 6th St.
Fort Smith, AR 72901
**Phone:** (501)783-5529

**★ 7001 ★ The Arc of Sevier County**
PO Box 246
De Queen, AR 71832
**Phone:** (870)642-6077

## California

**★ 7002 ★ Alpha Resource Center of Santa Barbara**
4501 Cathedral Oaks Rd.
Santa Barbara, CA 93110
**Phone:** (805)683-2145

**★ 7003 ★ The Arc of Alameda County**
575 Independent Rd.
Oakland, CA 94621-3721
**Phone:** (510)639-4680
**Website:** http://www.arc-alameda.com

**★ 7004 ★ The Arc of Amador and Calaveras Counties**
75 Academy Dr.
Sutter Creek, CA 95685
**Phone:** (209)267-5978

**★ 7005 ★ The Arc of Bakersfield**
2240 S Union Ave.
Bakersfield, CA 93307
**Phone:** (661)834-2272
**Website:** http://www.barc-inc.org

**★ 7006 ★ The Arc of Butte County**
PO Box 3697
Chico, CA 95927-3697
**Phone:** (916)891-5866

**★ 7007 ★ Arc California**
1225 8th St., Ste. 590
Sacramento, CA 95814-2213
**Phone:** (916)552-6619
**Email:** arcgary@quiknet.com

**★ 7008 ★ The Arc of El Dorado County**
175 Placerville Dr., Ste. W
Placerville, CA 95667

**★ 7009 ★ The Arc of Fresno**
5755 E Fountain Way
Fresno, CA 93727
**Phone:** (559)291-0611
**Website:** http://www.arcfresno.org

**★ 7010 ★ The Arc of Imperial Valley**
502 E Main St.
PO Box 1828
El Centro, CA 92243
**Phone:** (760)352-0180
**Email:** arcinfo@arciv.org
**Website:** http://www.arciv.org

**★ 7011 ★ The Arc of Orange County**
225 W Carl Karcher Way
Anaheim, CA 92801
**Phone:** (714)744-5301

**★ 7012 ★ The Arc of Riverside**
8138 Mar Vista Ct.
Riverside, CA 92504
**Phone:** (909)688-5141
**Email:** ArcRiverCA@aol.com
**Website:** http://www.arcriversideca.org

**★ 7013 ★ The Arc of the San Bernardino Area**
796 E 6th St.
San Bernardino, CA 92410
**Phone:** (909)884-6484

**★ 7014 ★ The Arc of San Diego**
9575 Aero Dr.
San Diego, CA 92123
**Email:** info@arc-sd.com
**Website:** http://www.arc-sd.com

**★ 7015 ★ The Arc of San Francisco**
1500 Howard St.
San Francisco, CA 94103
**Phone:** (415)255-7200
**Website:** http://www.thearcsanfrancisco.org

**★ 7016 ★ The Arc of Santa Maria Valley**
PO Box 1037
Santa Maria, CA 93456
**Phone:** (805)922-7381
**Email:** kirkspry@vtc-sm.org
**Website:** http://www.vtc-sm.org

**★ 7017 ★ The Arc of Solano**
PO Box 4119
Vallejo, CA 94590
**Phone:** (707)552-2935

**★ 7018 ★ The Arc of Sonoma County Advocacy Resource Center**
PO Box 219
Santa Rosa, CA 95402
**Phone:** (707)578-5454

**★ 7019 ★ The Arc of South Bay**
1735 W Rosecrans Ave.
Gardena, CA 90249
**Phone:** (310)532-6333
**Website:** http://www.lafn.org/community/arcsobay

**★ 7020 ★ The Arc of Southeast Los Angeles County**
12049 S Woodruff Ave.
Downey, CA 90241-5669
**Phone:** (562)803-4606
**Email:** info@arcselac.org
**Website:** http://www.arcselac.org

**★ 7021 ★ The Arc of Taft**
204 Van Buren St.
Taft, CA 93268
**Phone:** (661)763-1532

**★ 7022 ★ The Arc of Ventura County**
5103 Walker St.
Ventura, CA 93003
**Phone:** (805)650-8611

**★ 7023 ★ Casa De Esperanza**
12000 Denholm Dr.
El Monte, CA 91732
**Phone:** (626)444-8943

**★ 7024 ★ Contra Costa Association for Retarded Citizens**
1340 Arnold Dr., Ste. 127
Martinez, CA 94553
**Phone:** (925)370-1818
**Email:** arcofcc@aol.com
**Website:** http://www.contracostaarc.com

**★ 7025 ★ Life Options, Vocational and Resource Center (LOVARC)**
123 N D St.
Lompoc, CA 93436-6911
**Phone:** (805)735-3428
**Website:** http://www.lovarc.com

**★ 7026 ★ OPARC**
8939 Vernon St., Ste. L
Montclair, CA 91763
**Phone:** (909)985-3116
**Website:** http://www.oparc.com

## Colorado

**★ 7027 ★ The Arc of Adams County**
8805 Fox Dr., Ste. 100
Denver, CO 80260-6828
**Phone:** (303)428-0310

**★ 7028 ★ The Arc of Arapahoe and Douglas Counties**
7600 E Arapahoe Rd., No. 101
Englewood, CO 80112
**Phone:** (303)220-9228
**Website:** http://www.arc-arapahoe-douglas.org

**★ 7029 ★ The Arc of Aurora**
14111 E Alameda Ave.
Aurora, CO 80012-2509
**Phone:** (303)344-5390

**★ 7030 ★ The Arc of Colorado**
777 Grant St., Ste. 303
Denver, CO 80203
**Phone:** (303)864-9334

**★ 7031 ★ The Arc of Colorado**
777 Grant St., Ste. 303
Denver, CO 80203
**Phone:** (303)864-9334

**★ 7032 ★ The Arc of Denver, Inc.**
899 Logan St., No. 311
Denver, CO 80203
**Phone:** (303)831-7733

**★ 7033 ★ The Arc in Jefferson County**
8725 W 14th Ave., No. 100
Lakewood, CO 80215
**Phone:** (303)232-1338
**Email:** info@arcjc.org
**Website:** http://www.arcjc.org

**★ 7034 ★ The Arc of Lake County**
PO Box 317
Leadville, CO 80461
**Phone:** (719)486-3239

**★ 7035 ★ The Arc of Mesa County**
PO Box 2292
Grand Junction, CO 81501
**Phone:** (970)245-5775

**★ 7036 ★ The Arc of the Pikes Peak Region**
12 N Meade Ave.
Colorado Springs, CO 80909
**Phone:** (719)633-4601

**★ 7037 ★ The Arc of Pueblo**
2705 Vinewood
Pueblo, CO 81005
**Phone:** (719)545-5845
**Website:** http://www.arcofpueblo.org

**★ 7038 ★ The Arc of Weld County**
1025 9th Ave., Ste. 313
Greeley, CO 80631
**Phone:** (970)353-5219

**★ 7039 ★ Association for Community Living in Boulder County, Inc.**
6897 Paiute Ave., No. 6
Longmont, CO 80503
**Phone:** (303)652-3000
**Email:** info@aclboulder.org
**Website:** http://www.aclboulder.org

## Connecticut

**★ 7040 ★ The Arc of Connecticut**
1030 New Britain Ave., Ste. 102
West Hartford, CT 06110
**Phone:** (860)953-8335

**★ 7041 ★ The Arc of Greater Enfield**
75 Hazard Ave., Unit E
Enfield, CT 06082
**Phone:** (860)763-5411

**★ 7042 ★ The Arc of New London County**
PO Box 361
Gales Ferry, CT 06335
**Phone:** (860)464-6302

**★ 7043 ★ The Arc of Plainville**
PO Box 12
Plainville, CT 06062
**Phone:** (860)747-1560

**★ 7044 ★ The Arc of Quinebaug Valley**
PO Box 398
Putnam, CT 06260
**Phone:** (860)928-1951

**★ 7045 ★ The Arc of Southington, Inc.**
201 W Main St.
Plantsville, CT 06479
**Phone:** (860)628-9220
**Email:** advocacy@arcsouthington.org
**Website:** http://www.arcsouthington.org

**★ 7046 ★ The Arc of Waterbury**
1929 E Main St.
Waterbury, CT 06705-1894
**Phone:** (203)575-0707

**★ 7047 ★ Central Connecticut Arc, Inc.**
1 Hartford Sq.
New Britain, CT 06052
**Phone:** (860)229-6665
**Email:** aruwet@ccarc.com
**Website:** http://www.ccarc.com
Anne L. Ruwet, Exec Director

**★ 7048 ★ Farmington Valley Arc, Inc.**
225 Commerce Dr.
PO Box 1099
Canton, CT 06019-1099
**Phone:** (860)693-6662
**Email:** favarh@connix.com
**Website:** http://www.connix.com/%7Efavarh

**★ 7049 ★ Friends of New Milford, Inc.**
283 Chestnutland Rd.
New Milford, CT 06776
**Phone:** (860)355-5343

**★ 7050 ★ Litchfield County Association for Retarded Citizens, Inc. (LARC)**
84-R Main St.
Torrington, CT 06790
**Phone:** (860)485-9364
**Website:** http://www.litchfieldarc.org

**★ 7051 ★ Lower Valley Association for Retarded and Handicapped, Inc.**
1 Hartford Ave.
Old Saybrook, CT 06475
**Phone:** (860)399-7431

**★ 7052 ★ Marc Community Resources, Ltd.**
12 Fairview St.
Portland, CT 06480
**Phone:** (860)342-0700

**★ 7053 ★ MARC, Inc. of Manchester**
376R W Middle Tpke.
Manchester, CT 06040
**Phone:** (860)645-5718
**Email:** lprytko@marcct.org
**Website:** http://www.marcct.org
Laurie Prytko, Exec Director

**★ 7054 ★ The Meriden-Wallingford Society for the Handicapped, Inc.**
223-226 Cook Ave.
Meriden, CT 06450
**Phone:** (860)237-9975

**★ 7055 ★ Options Unlimited, Inc.**
584 W Hill Rd.
Winsted, CT 06098
**Phone:** (860)738-1410

**★ 7056 ★ Sarah, Inc.**
246 Gooselane., Ste. 101
Guilford, CT 06437
**Phone:** (203)458-4040
**Website:** http://www.sarah-inc.org

**★ 7057 ★ Sarah Seneca**
11 Park Dr., Ste. 1
Branford, CT 06405
**Phone:** (203)315-3770

**★ 7058 ★ Sarah Tuxis Residential Services, Inc.**
45 Boston St.
Guilford, CT 06437
**Phone:** (203)458-8532
**Email:** Tuxis@cshore.com
**Website:** http://www.sarah-tuxis.org

**★ 7059 ★ STAR, Inc.**
182 Wolfpit Ave.
Norwalk, CT 06851
**Phone:** (203)846-9581

**★ 7060 ★ Tri-County Arc**
65 Route 66 E
Columbia, CT 06237
**Phone:** (860)228-2070

**★ 7061 ★ WeCAHR**
211 Main St.
Danbury, CT 06810
**Phone:** (203)792-3540

## Delaware

**★ 7062 ★ The Arc of Delaware**
1016 Centre Rd., Ste. 1
Wilmington, DE 19805
**Phone:** (302)996-9400

## District of Columbia

**★ 7063 ★ District of Columbia Arc**
900 Varnum St. NE
Washington, DC 20017
**Phone:** (202)636-2950

## Florida

**★ 7064 ★ The Arc of Alachua County, Inc.**
3303 NW 83rd St.
Gainesville, FL 32606-6227
**Phone:** (352)334-4060
**Email:** dvanslooten@arcalachua.org
**Website:** http://www.arcalachua.org

**★ 7065 ★ The Arc of Bradford County**
PO Box 1026
Starke, FL 32091-1026
**Phone:** (904)964-7699

**★ 7066 ★ The Arc of Brevard, Inc.**
1694 Cedar St.
Rockledge, FL 32955
**Phone:** (407)690-3436
**Email:** fr4arc@arc-brevard.org
**Website:** http://www.arc-brevard.org

**★ 7067 ★ The Arc of Charlotte County, Inc.**
PO Box 3569
Port Charlotte, FL 33949
**Phone:** (941)627-8771
**Email:** cc_arc@geocities.com
**Website:** http://www.geocities.com/heartland/hills/4840/

**★ 7068 ★ The Arc of Desoto**
PO Box 787
Nocatee, FL 34268
**Phone:** (863)494-2328

**★ 7069 ★ The Arc of Escambia County**
3916 N 10th Ave.
Pensacola, FL 32503
**Phone:** (850)434-2638
**Website:** http://www.arc-escambia.org

**★ 7070 ★ The Arc of Flagler**
3510 S Ocean Shore Blvd.
Flagler Beach, FL 32136-4105

**★ 7071 ★ Arc/Florida**
411 E College Ave.
Tallahassee, FL 32301
**Phone:** (850)921-0460
**Email:** arcfl@supernet.net
**Website:** http://www.arcflorida.org

**★ 7072 ★ The Arc of the Glades Area**
4250 NW 16th St.
Belle Glade, FL 33430
**Phone:** (561)996-9583

**★ 7073 ★ The Arc of the Gulf**
303 Peters St.
Port Saint Joe, FL 32456
**Phone:** (904)229-6327

**★ 7074 ★ The Arc of Indian River**
1375 16th Ave.
Vero Beach, FL 32960
**Phone:** (561)562-6854

**★ 7075 ★ The Arc of Jackson County**
2944 Pennsylvania Ave., Ste. A
Marianna, FL 32448
**Phone:** (850)594-3901

**★ 7076 ★ The Arc of Jacksonville**
1050 N Davis St.
Jacksonville, FL 32209
**Phone:** (904)355-0155

**★ 7077 ★ The Arc of the Keys, Inc.**
PO Box 9285
Tavernier, FL 33070
**Phone:** (305)517-9508

**★ 7078 ★ The Arc of Lee County**
2570 Hanson St.
Fort Myers, FL 33901
**Phone:** (941)334-6285

**★ 7079 ★ The Arc of Levy County**
PO Box 86
Otter Creek, FL 32683
**Phone:** (352)486-4293

**★ 7080 ★ The Arc of Madison-Jefferson**
100 Commerce Dr.
PO Box 912
Madison, FL 32341
**Phone:** (850)973-4614

**★ 7081 ★ The Arc of Marion County**
2800 SE Maricamp Rd.
Ocala, FL 34471
**Phone:** (352)620-7460

**★ 7082 ★ The Arc of Nassau County**
PO Box 999
Yulee, FL 32097
**Phone:** (904)225-9355

**★ 7083 ★ The Arc of Nature Coast**
5283 Neff Lake Rd.
Brooksville, FL 34601
**Phone:** (352)544-2322
**Email:** thearc@thearc-naturecoast.org
**Website:** http://www.thearc-naturecoast.org

**★ 7084 ★ The Arc of Palm Beach County**
1201 Australian Ave.
Riviera Beach, FL 33404
**Phone:** (561)842-3213
**Website:** http://www.arcpbc.org

**★ 7085 ★ The Arc of Putnam County, Inc.**
1209 Westover Dr.
Palatka, FL 32177
**Phone:** (904)325-2249

**★ 7086 ★ The Arc of the Ridge Area**
120 E College Dr.
Avon Park, FL 33825
**Phone:** (863)452-1295

**★ 7087 ★ The Arc of St. Johns County**
2101 Arc Dr.
Saint Augustine, FL 32095
**Phone:** (904)824-7249    **Fax:** (904)824-8063
**Website:** http://www.arcsj.org

**★ 7088 ★ The Arc of St. Lucie County, Inc.**
PO Box 1016
Fort Pierce, FL 34954-1016
**Phone:** (561)465-5499

**★ 7089 ★ The Arc of Santa Rosa**
409 Dixie Rd.
Milton, FL 32570
**Phone:** (850)623-9320

**★ 7090 ★ The Arc of South Florida**
5555 Biscayne Blvd.
Miami, FL 33137-2656
**Phone:** (305)759-8500
**Website:** http://www.miamivr.com/arc

**★ 7091 ★ The Arc of Taylor County**
c/o Leon Advocacy and Resource Center
1589 Metropolitan Blvd.
Tallahassee, FL 32308
**Phone:** (850)422-0355
**Email:** larc@nettally.com
**Website:** http://www.leonarc.org

**★ 7092 ★ The Arc of Volusia County**
PO Box 9658
Daytona Beach, FL 32120
**Phone:** (904)274-4736

**★ 7093 ★ The Arc of Walton County**
1408 State Hwy. 83
PO Box 813
Defuniak Springs, FL 32435
**Phone:** (850)892-5013

**★ 7094 ★ The Arc of Washington-Holmes Counties, Inc.**
1335 South Blvd.
Chipley, FL 32428
**Phone:** (850)638-7517

**★ 7095 ★ The Center for Independence, Inc.**
5532 Auld Ln.
Holiday, FL 34690
**Phone:** (727)943-2019
**Email:** emile@marlowe.net
**Website:** http://www.thecenterforindependence.com
**Frmly:** The Association for Retarded Citizens/Pasco, Inc.

**★ 7096 ★ Comprehensive Community Services, Inc.**
511 Gold Kist Ave.
PO Drawer L
Live Oak, FL 32064
**Phone:** (904)362-7143

**★ 7097 ★ Gadsden Association Rehabilitation Center**
600 S Adams St.
Quincy, FL 32351
**Phone:** (850)627-9058

**★ 7098 ★ Horizons of Okaloosa County, Inc.**
PO Box 2350
Fort Walton Beach, FL 32549
**Phone:** (850)863-1530
**Email:** horizons@emeraldcoast.com
**Website:** http://www.horizons.nu

**★ 7099 ★ Manosota Arc, Inc.**
PO Box 9292
Bradenton, FL 34206-9292

**Phone:** (941)752-2976

**★ 7100 ★ Osceola Association for Retarded Citizens**
310 N Clyde Ave.
Kissimmee, FL 34741
**Phone:** (407)847-6016

**★ 7101 ★ Pyramid, Inc.**
345 S Magnolia Dr., Ste. B-11
Tallahassee, FL 32301
**Phone:** (850)671-1690

**★ 7102 ★ Scarc**
213 W McCollum Ave.
Bushnell, FL 33513
**Phone:** (352)793-5156

**★ 7103 ★ Sunrise Arc of Lake County, Inc.**
12340 County Rd. 44
Leesburg, FL 34788
**Phone:** (352)357-3486
**Email:** sunrisearc@aol.com
**Website:** http://www.sunrisearc.org

**★ 7104 ★ UPARC**
1501 N Belcher Rd., Ste. 249
Clearwater, FL 33765
**Phone:** (727)799-3330

## Georgia

**★ 7105 ★ The Arc of the Habersham Area**
1068 Twin River Rd.
Demorest, GA 30535

**★ 7106 ★ The Arc of Irwin County**
PO Box 614
Ocilla, GA 31774

**★ 7107 ★ The Arc of Macon**
4664 Sheraton Dr.
Macon, GA 31210-1322
**Phone:** (912)477-7764

**★ 7108 ★ The Arc of Newnan-Coweta**
61 Hospital Rd.
Newnan, GA 30263
**Phone:** (770)253-1189

**★ 7109 ★ The Arc of Stephens County**
4331 Ledan
Gainesville, GA 30506

**★ 7110 ★ The Arc of Walker County**
PO Box 438
LaFayette, GA 30728
**Phone:** (706)638-1669

**★ 7111 ★ The Coastal Arc**
1211 Eisenhower Dr.
Savannah, GA 31416
**Phone:** (912)355-7633

**★ 7112 ★ The Georgia Arc Network, Inc.**
1996 Cliff Valley Way, Ste. 102
Atlanta, GA 30329
**Phone:** (404)634-5512
**Email:** Tomquery@worldnet.att.net
**Website:** http://www.arcga.org

**★ 7113 ★ Hart County Association of Retarded Citizens, Inc.**
PO Box 706
Hartwell, GA 30643

## Hawaii

**★ 7114 ★ The Arc in Hawaii**
3989 Diamond Head Rd.
Honolulu, HI 96816-4413
**Phone:** (808)737-7995
**Email:** arc-hi@aloha.com

**★ 7115 ★ The Arc of Hilo**
1099 Waianuenue Ave.
Hilo, HI 96720
**Phone:** (808)935-7644

**★ 7116 ★ The Arc of Kauai**
3201 Akahi St.
Lihue, HI 96766
**Phone:** (808)245-4132

**★ 7117 ★ The Arc of Kona**
PO Box 127
Kealakekua, HI 96750
**Phone:** (808)323-2626

**★ 7118 ★ The Arc of Maui**
95 Mahalani St., Cameron Ctr.
Wailuku, HI 96793
**Phone:** (808)242-5781

## Idaho

**★ 7119 ★ The Arc of Eastern Idaho**
PO Box 1545
Idaho Falls, ID 83403

**★ 7120 ★ The Arc of Idaho, Inc.**
PO Box 1016
Boise, ID 83701
**Phone:** (208)343-5583

## Illinois

**★ 7121 ★ Access Services of Northern Illinois**
7399 Forest Hills Rd.
Loves Park, IL 61111
**Phone:** (815)282-8835
**Email:** info@AccessNI.com
**Website:** http://www.accessni.com

**★ 7122 ★ Ada S. McKinley Community Services, Inc.**
725 S Wells St.
Chicago, IL 60607
**Phone:** (312)554-0600

**★ 7123 ★ Advocates Network of Kane and Kendall Counties**
1736 W State St.
Geneva, IL 60134
**Phone:** (630)232-7661

**★ 7124 ★ The Arc of Adams County**
1824 Maine
Quincy, IL 62301
**Phone:** (217)224-8328

**★ 7125 ★ The Arc of Glenkirk**
3504 Commercial Ave.
Northbrook, IL 60062
**Phone:** (847)272-5111
**Website:** http://www.glenkirk.org

**★ 7126 ★ The Arc of Illinois**
1820 Ridge Rd., No. 300
Homewood, IL 60430
**Phone:** (708)206-1930
**Email:** tony@thearcofil.org
**Website:** http://www.thearcofil.org

**★ 7127 ★ The Arc of Iroquois County**
700 E Elm St.
Watseka, IL 60970
**Phone:** (815)432-6191
**Email:** info@thearcirq.org
**Website:** http://www.thearcirq.org

**★ 7128 ★ The Arc of Lee County**
500 Anchor Rd.
Dixon, IL 61021
**Phone:** (815)288-6691

**★ 7129 ★ The Arc of McLean County MARC**
1606 Hunt Dr.
Normal, IL 61761-2192
**Phone:** (309)451-8888 **Fax:** (309)451-8989
**Website:** http://www.marcofillinois.org

**★ 7130 ★ The Arc of Park Lawn**
10833 S Laporte Ave.
Oak Lawn, IL 60453
**Phone:** (708)425-3344

**★ 7131 ★ The Arc of Rock Island County**
4016 9th St.
Rock Island, IL 61201
**Phone:** (309)786-6474
**Email:** arcricIL@arcric.org
**Website:** http://www.arcric.org

**★ 7132 ★ The Arc of Winnebago, Boone, and Ogle Counties**
400 N 1st St.
Rockford, IL 61107-3978
**Phone:** (815)965-3455 **Fax:** (815)965-3673
**Website:** http://www.thearcofwinn-boone.org

**★ 7133 ★ Aspire**
9901 Derby Ln.
Westchester, IL 60154
**Phone:** (708)547-3550

**★ 7134 ★ Association for the Developmentally Disabled in Woodford County**
200 Moody St.
Eureka, IL 61530

**★ 7135 ★ Association for Individual Development**
309 W New Indian Trail Ct.
Aurora, IL 60506
**Phone:** (630)844-5040

**★ 7136 ★ Bethphage**
220 N LaFayette
Macomb, IL 61455
**Phone:** (309)837-5506

**★ 7137 ★ Blue Island Citizens for Developmental Disabilities**
2155 Broadway
Blue Island, IL 60406
**Phone:** (708)389-6578

**★ 7138 ★ Chicago Association for Retarded Citizens (CARC)**
8 S Michigan Ave., No. 1700
Chicago, IL 60603
**Phone:** (312)346-6230
**Website:** http://www.chgoarc.org

**★ 7139 ★ Community Support Services, Inc.**
7575 S Kostner
Chicago, IL 60652
**Phone:** (773)884-1000
**Email:** css@communitysupportservices.org
**Website:** http://www.communitysupportservices.org

**★ 7140 ★ Community Support Services Inc.**
9021 Ogden Ave.
Brookfield, IL 60513
**Phone:** (708)354-4547

**★ 7141 ★ Futures Unlimited, Inc.**
210 E Torrance Ave.
Pontiac, IL 61764
**Phone:** (815)842-1122

**★ 7142 ★ Gateway Services, Inc.**
406 S Gosse Blvd.
Princeton, IL 61356
**Phone:** (815)875-4548

**★ 7143 ★ Helping Hand Rehabilitation Center**
9649 W 55th St.
Countryside, IL 60525
**Phone:** (708)352-3580

**★ 7144 ★ Kane Kendall Case Coordination Services**
179 Oswalt Ave.
Batavia, IL 60510
**Phone:** (630)879-2277

**★ 7145 ★ The Lambs Farm, Inc.**
14245 W Rockland Rd.
Libertyville, IL 60048
**Phone:** (847)362-4636

**★ 7146 ★ LARC, An Association for Retarded Citizens**
19043 Wentworth Ave.
PO Box 77
Lansing, IL 60438
**Phone:** (708)474-1540 **Fax:** (708)474-1586
**Email:** LARCLansng@aol.com
**Website:** http://www.thetimesonline.com/org/larc/

**★ 7147 ★ Malcolm Eaton Enterprises**
570 W Lamm Rd.
Freeport, IL 61032
**Phone:** (815)235-7181

**★ 7148 ★ Marklund**
290 Town Center
Glendale Heights, IL 60139
**Phone:** (630)529-2018

**★ 7149 ★ New Hope Association, Inc.**
1624 E 154th St.
Dolton, IL 60419
**Phone:** (708)841-1071

★ **7150** ★ **Oak-Leyden Developmental Services**
411 W Chicago Ave.
Oak Park, IL 60302
**Phone:** (708)524-1050

★ **7151** ★ **Occupational Development Center**
1201 E Bell St., Ste. A
Bloomington, IL 61701
**Phone:** (309)820-0723

★ **7152** ★ **Options and Advocacy for McHenry County**
333 Commerce Dr., Ste. 800
Crystal Lake, IL 60014-3598
**Phone:** (815)477-4720

★ **7153** ★ **Pathway Services Unlimited, Inc.**
1201 S Main St.
PO Box 400
Jacksonville, IL 62651
**Phone:** (217)479-2300

★ **7154** ★ **Peoria Association for Retarded Citizens, Inc.**
PO Box 3418
Peoria, IL 61612
**Phone:** (309)691-3800
**Email:** peoriaarc@yahoo.com
**Website:** http://www.peoriaarc.org

★ **7155** ★ **Seguin Retarded Citizens Association**
6223 W Ogden Ave.
Berwyn, IL 60402
**Phone:** (708)788-5777

★ **7156** ★ **Seguin Services, Inc.**
3100 S Central Ave.
Cicero, IL 60804
**Phone:** (708)863-3803    **Fax:** (708)863-3863
**Website:** http://www.seguin.org

★ **7157** ★ **South Chicago Parents and Friends of Retarded Children**
10241 S Commercial Ave.
Chicago, IL 60617
**Phone:** (773)734-2222

★ **7158** ★ **Southern Illinois Case Coordination Services, Inc.**
519 S Locust
PO Box 588
Centralia, IL 62801
**Phone:** (618)532-4300

★ **7159** ★ **SouthStar Services**
1005 W End Ave.
Chicago Heights, IL 60411
**Phone:** (708)755-8030

★ **7160** ★ **Springfield Association for Retarded Citizens (SPARC)**
232 Bruns Ln.
Springfield, IL 62702
**Phone:** (217)793-2100
**Email:** inquire@springfieldsparc.org
**Website:** http://www.spfldsparc.org

★ **7161** ★ **Suburban Access**
925 W 175th St., 3rd Fl.
Homewood, IL 60430
**Phone:** (708)799-9190

★ **7162** ★ **Trinity Services of Will County**
100 N Gougar Rd.
Joliet, IL 60432
**Phone:** (815)485-6197

★ **7163** ★ **Victor C. Neumann Association**
5547 N Bavenswood
Chicago, IL 60640
**Phone:** (773)769-4313

★ **7164** ★ **Western Illinois Service Coordination, Inc.**
1117 E Jackson St.
Macomb, IL 61455
**Phone:** (309)833-1621

### Indiana

★ **7165** ★ **ADEC—Resources for Independence**
PO Box 398
Bristol, IN 46507
**Phone:** (219)848-7451
**Email:** options@adecinc.com
**Website:** http://www.adecinc.com
**Remarks:** Serves Elkhart County.

★ **7166** ★ **The Arc of Bartholomew County**
PO Box 411
Columbus, IN 47202
**Phone:** (812)372-0610

★ **7167** ★ **The Arc of Boone County**
900 W Main
Lebanon, IN 46052
**Phone:** (765)482-6815
**Email:** bcarc@aol.com
**Website:** http://www.in-motion.net/~arc/

★ **7168** ★ **The Arc of Brown County**
PO Box 411
Columbus, IN 47202
**Phone:** (812)372-0610

★ **7169** ★ **The Arc of Carroll County**
35 N Washington St.
Delphi, IN 46923

★ **7170** ★ **The Arc of Dearborn County**
1030 Fairview
Lawrenceburg, IN 47025

★ **7171** ★ **The Arc of Decatur County Inc.**
PO Box 411
Columbus, IN 47202
**Phone:** (812)372-0610

★ **7172** ★ **The Arc of Evansville**
PO Box 4089
Evansville, IN 47724-0089
**Phone:** (812)428-4500
**Website:** http://www.evansvillearc.org

★ **7173** ★ **The Arc of Hancock County**
PO Box 93
Greenfield, IN 46140
**Phone:** (317)462-3727

★ **7174** ★ **The Arc of Indiana**
22 E Washington, Ste. 210
Indianapolis, IN 46204
**Phone:** (317)977-2375    **Free:** 800-382-9100
**Fax:** (317)977-2385
**Email:** arcin@in.net

**Website:** http://www.arcind.org

★ **7175** ★ **The Arc of Jackson County, Inc.**
PO Box 411
Columbus, IN 47202
**Phone:** (812)372-0610

★ **7176** ★ **The Arc of Owen County**
RR 7, Box 296
Spencer, IN 47460

★ **7177** ★ **The Arc of Tippecanoe County**
PO Box 6449
Lafayette, IN 47904
**Phone:** (765)423-5531

★ **7178** ★ **The Arc of Vigo County**
89 Cherry St.
Terre Haute, IN 47807
**Phone:** (812)232-4112

★ **7179** ★ **Association for Retarded Citizens of Wabash County**
PO Box 400
Wabash, IN 46992
**Phone:** (219)563-8411

★ **7180** ★ **Benton County Association for Retarded Citizens**
PO Box 12
Fowler, IN 47944

★ **7181** ★ **Bi-County Services of Adams and Wells Counties**
425 E Harrison Rd.
Bluffton, IN 46714
**Phone:** (219)824-1253
**Email:** info@adifferentlight.com
**Website:** http://www.bi-countyservices.com

★ **7182** ★ **Blue River Services, Inc.**
1365 Highway 135 NW
Corydon, IN 47112
**Phone:** (812)738-2408
**Website:** http://www.brsinc.org
**Remarks:** Serves Crawford, Harrison, and Washington counties.

★ **7183** ★ **Carey Services, Inc.**
2724 S Carey St.
Marion, IN 46953
**Phone:** (765)668-8961
**Email:** info@careyservices.com
**Website:** http://www.careyservices.com
**Remarks:** Serves Blackford and Grant counties.

★ **7184** ★ **Clinton County Association for Retarded Citizens**
5780 S County Rd. 250 E
Frankfort, IN 46041-8698
**Phone:** (765)659-6380

★ **7185** ★ **Davies-Martin Rehabilitation Services**
PO Box 249
Linton, IN 47441
**Phone:** (812)847-2231

★ **7186** ★ **Dubois County Association for Retarded Citizens**
1250 Justin St.
Jasper, IN 47546
**Phone:** (812)367-6111

**★ 7187 ★ Easter Seals Arc of Northeast Indiana, Inc.**
2542 Thompson Ave.
Fort Wayne, IN 46807
**Phone:** (219)456-4534
**Website:** http://www.esarc.org
Stephen L. Hinkle, President
**Remarks:** Serves Allen, Dekalb, Huntington and Steuben counties.

**★ 7188 ★ Fountain County Association for Retarded Citizens**
1500 E State Rd. 32
Veedersburg, IN 47987

**★ 7189 ★ Green Acres Inc.**
PO Box 1252
Richmond, IN 47375-1252
**Phone:** (765)966-0502
**Email:** wccrc@GACenter.org
**Website:** http://www.gacenter.org
Dan Stewart, CEO & Pres

**★ 7190 ★ Greene County Area Rehabilitation Center**
c/o Four Rivers Resource Services
PO Box 249
Linton, IN 47441
**Phone:** (812)847-2231
**Email:** fourrivers@frrs.org
**Website:** http://www.frrs.org

**★ 7191 ★ Hopewell Center, Madison County**
PO Box 3150
Anderson, IN 46018
**Phone:** (765)642-0201

**★ 7192 ★ Jayland Association for Retarded Citizens**
1104 S Massachusetts Ave.
Portland, IN 47371

**★ 7193 ★ Jefferson Switzerland Association for Retarded Citizens**
3355 N State Rte. 7
Madison, IN 47250

**★ 7194 ★ Jennings County Association for Retarded Citizens**
PO Box 411
Columbus, IN 47202
**Phone:** (812)372-0610

**★ 7195 ★ Johnson County Association for Retarded Citizens**
PO Box 216
Franklin, IN 46131
**Phone:** (317)738-5500

**★ 7196 ★ Knox County Association for Retarded Citizens**
2830 E ARC Ave.
Vincennes, IN 47591
**Phone:** (812)886-4312
**Website:** http://www.knoxcountyarc.com

**★ 7197 ★ Lake County Association for the Retarded**
2650 W 35th Ave.
Gary, IN 46408
**Phone:** (219)884-9441

**★ 7198 ★ Landmark Services, Inc.**
531 N Central Ave., Ste. 3
Connersville, IN 47331-2019

**Phone:** (765)825-3626

**★ 7199 ★ Lawrence County Association for Retarded Citizens**
PO Box 393
Bedford, IN 47421
**Phone:** (812)279-3229

**★ 7200 ★ Marshall-Starke Development Center**
1901 Pidco Dr.
Plymouth, IN 46563
**Phone:** (219)936-9400
**Remarks:** Serves Fulton, Marshall, and Starke counties.

**★ 7201 ★ Noble Arc of Central Indiana**
7701 E 21st St.
Indianapolis, IN 46219
**Phone:** (317)375-2700
**Website:** http://www.nobleofindiana.org
**Remarks:** Serves Hamilton, Howard, Marion, Shelby, and Tipton counties.

**★ 7202 ★ Noble County Association for Retarded Citizens**
506 S Orange St.
Albion, IN 46701
**Phone:** (219)636-2155

**★ 7203 ★ Opportunity Enterprises, Porter County**
PO Box 1206
Valparaiso, IN 46384
**Phone:** (219)464-9621

**★ 7204 ★ Parke County Association for Retarded Citizens**
PO Box 170
Rockville, IN 47872
**Phone:** (765)569-2076

**★ 7205 ★ Passages, Inc.**
PO Box 1005
Columbia City, IN 46725
**Phone:** (219)244-7688
**Email:** passages@whitleynet.org
**Website:** http://www.passagesinc.org

**★ 7206 ★ Pike County Area Rehabilitation Center**
PO Box 535
Petersburg, IN 47567
**Phone:** (812)354-6560

**★ 7207 ★ Posey County Association for Retarded Citizens**
609 Short St.
New Harmony, IN 47631

**★ 7208 ★ Rush County Association for Retarded Citizens**
814 W 11th St.
Rushville, IN 46173
**Phone:** (765)932-2961

**★ 7209 ★ Spencer County Association for Retarded Citizens**
PO Box 11
Dale, IN 47523
**Website:** http://www.spencercountyarc.org

**★ 7210 ★ Stone Belt Arc, Inc.**
2815 E 10th St.
Bloomington, IN 47408

**Phone:** (812)332-2168
**Email:** sbcarc@bloomington.in.us
**Website:** http://www.stonebelt.org
**Remarks:** Serves Monroe County.

**★ 7211 ★ Sullivan County Area Rehabilitation Center**
c/o Four Rivers Resource Services
PO Box 249
Linton, IN 47441
**Phone:** (812)847-2231
**Email:** fourrivers@frrs.org
**Website:** http://www.frrs.org

**★ 7212 ★ Sycamore Services, Inc.**
1001 Sycamore Ln.
PO Box 369
Danville, IN 46122
**Phone:** (317)745-4715          **Fax:** (317)745-8271
**Email:** info@sycamoreservices.com
**Website:** http://www.sycamoreservices.com
**Remarks:** Serves Hendricks County.

**★ 7213 ★ Woodlawn Center of Cass and Pulaski Counties**
1416 Woodlawn Ave.
Logansport, IN 46947
**Phone:** (219)753-4104

## Iowa

**★ 7214 ★ The Arc of Allamakee County**
1270 Hwy. 9
Lansing, IA 52151

**★ 7215 ★ The Arc of Appanoose County**
700 N Main
Centerville, IA 52544

**★ 7216 ★ The Arc of Black Hawk County**
2518 Pleasant Dr.
Cedar Falls, IA 50613

**★ 7217 ★ The Arc of Buchanan County**
308 2nd St. SW
Independence, IA 50644
**Phone:** (319)334-2508

**★ 7218 ★ The Arc of Cedar County**
795 195th St.
Mechanicsville, IA 52306

**★ 7219 ★ The Arc of Chickasaw County**
1826 Jasper Ave.
New Hampton, IA 50659

**★ 7220 ★ The Arc of Delaware County**
1841 210th Ave.
Manchester, IA 52057

**★ 7221 ★ The Arc of the Dubuque Area**
3475 Windsor Ave.
Dubuque, IA 52001
**Phone:** (319)556-1785

**★ 7222 ★ The Arc of East Central Iowa**
214 1st St. SW
Cedar Rapids, IA 52404
**Phone:** (319)365-0487

**★ 7223 ★ The Arc of Grundy County**
105 Clark St.
Reinbeck, IA 50669

**★ 7224 ★ The Arc of Hamilton County**
702 Laura Ln.
Webster City, IA 50595

**★ 7225 ★ The Arc of Hardin County**
PO Box 336
Hubbard, IA 50122

**★ 7226 ★ The Arc of Henry County**
2444 Nebraska Ave.
New London, IA 52645

**★ 7227 ★ The Arc of Iowa**
715 E Locust
Des Moines, IA 50309-1915
**Phone:** (515)283-2358

**★ 7228 ★ The Arc of Iowa County**
503 Henry St.
Williamsburg, IA 52361

**★ 7229 ★ The Arc of Jackson County**
14065 407th Ave.
Bellevue, IA 52031

**★ 7230 ★ The Arc of Jefferson and Nearby Counties**
PO Box 71
Richland, IA 52585

**★ 7231 ★ The Arc of Johnson County**
1700 1st Ave., Ste. 16
Iowa City, IA 52240
**Phone:** (319)351-5017
**Email:** Arcofjc@mcleodusa.net
**Website:** http://www.jccn.iowa-city.ia.us/%7Ethearcjc/

**★ 7232 ★ The Arc of Lee County**
1102 Morgan
Keokuk, IA 52632

**★ 7233 ★ The Arc of Lucas County**
Rte. 1, Box 333
Chariton, IA 50049

**★ 7234 ★ The Arc of Muscatine County**
PO Box 251
Muscatine, IA 52761

**★ 7235 ★ The Arc of North Central Iowa**
Box 168
Mason City, IA 50402-0168

**★ 7236 ★ The Arc of Sac County**
2580 350th St.
PO Box 128
Wall Lake, IA 51466-0128

**★ 7237 ★ The Arc of Scott County**
729 21st St.
Bettendorf, IA 52722

**★ 7238 ★ The Arc of Story County**
PO Box 5004
Ames, IA 50010-5004
**Phone:** (515)232-9330

**★ 7239 ★ The Arc of Tama County**
231 W 3rd St.
Tama, IA 52339

**★ 7240 ★ The Arc of Washington County**
2240 Larch Ave.
Washington, IA 52353

**★ 7241 ★ The Arc of Wayne County**
PO Box 37
Promise City, IA 52583-0037

**★ 7242 ★ The Arc of Winneshiek County**
738 Ridge Rd.
Decorah, IA 52101

**★ 7243 ★ The Arc of Woodbury County**
3001 Malloy Rd.
Sioux City, IA 51103

## Kansas

**★ 7244 ★ The Arc of Anderson County**
105 Park Plaza N, Apt. 9
Garnett, KS 66032

**★ 7245 ★ The Arc of Atchison County**
1201 S 7th
Atchison, KS 66002

**★ 7246 ★ The Arc of Bourbon County**
PO Box 802
Fort Scott, KS 66701

**★ 7247 ★ The Arc of Butler County**
2375 W Central Ave.
El Dorado, KS 67042-3208

**★ 7248 ★ The Arc of Central Plains**
Box 163
Hays, KS 67601
**Phone:** (785)628-6512

**★ 7249 ★ The Arc of Cheyenne-Rawlins Counties**
RR 1, Box 16B
Atwood, KS 67730

**★ 7250 ★ The Arc of Cloud County**
503 E 6th
Concordia, KS 66901

**★ 7251 ★ The Arc of Douglas County**
2518 Ridge Ct., Rm. 238
Lawrence, KS 66046
**Phone:** (785)749-0121
**Email:** thearcdc@grapevine.net
**Website:** http://www.grapevine.net/~thearcdc/

**★ 7252 ★ The Arc of Leavenworth County**
217A Delaware
Leavenworth, KS 66048
**Phone:** (913)651-6464

**★ 7253 ★ The Arc of Marshall County**
1150 11th Rd.
Marysville, KS 66508

**★ 7254 ★ The Arc of Mitchell County**
Rte. 1, Box 13
Beloit, KS 67420

**★ 7255 ★ The Arc of Northwest Kansas**
Rte. 2, Box 7
Norton, KS 67654

**★ 7256 ★ The Arc of Russell County**
647 E 5th St., No. 261
PO Box 371
Russell, KS 67665
**Phone:** (785)483-3742

**★ 7257 ★ The Arc of Saline County**
PO Box 362
Salina, KS 67401

**★ 7258 ★ The Arc of Sedgwick County, Inc.**
2919 W 2nd St.
Wichita, KS 67212
**Phone:** (316)943-1191
**Website:** http://www.arc-sedgwickcounty.org

**★ 7259 ★ The Arc of Solomon Valley**
507 S Madison
Plainville, KS 67663

**★ 7260 ★ The Arc of Topeka**
2701 Randolph
Topeka, KS 66611
**Phone:** (785)232-0597

**★ 7261 ★ The Arc of Wabaunsee County**
6 Cedar N
Eskridge, KS 66423

## Kentucky

**★ 7262 ★ The Arc of Barren County**
PO Box 205
Glasgow, KY 42142
**Phone:** (270)651-3357

**★ 7263 ★ The Arc of the Bluegrass, Inc.**
898 Georgetown St.
Lexington, KY 40511
**Phone:** (859)233-1483     **Fax:** (859)231-9695
**Email:** ellerbrk@mis.net
**Website:** http://www.arcbluegrass.com

**★ 7264 ★ The Arc of Kentucky**
833 E Main St.
Frankfort, KY 40601
**Phone:** (502)875-5225
**Website:** http://www.arcofky.org

**★ 7265 ★ The Arc of Lake Cumberland**
PO Box 1377
Somerset, KY 42501

**★ 7266 ★ The Arc of Logan County**
443 Hopkinsville Rd.
Russellville, KY 42276

**★ 7267 ★ The Arc of Madison County, Inc.**
PO Box 161
Berea, KY 40403

**★ 7268 ★ The Arc of Owensboro, Inc.**
PO Box 1833
Owensboro, KY 42302
**Phone:** (502)685-2976

**★ 7269 ★ Breckenridge County Educational Association for the Handicapped**
Hardinsburg, KY 40143-9802

**★ 7270 ★ Citizen Advocacy Program of Northern Kentucky**
426 Hallam Ave.
Erlanger, KY 41018
**Phone:** (606)491-3344

**★ 7271 ★ Frankfort Habilitation, Inc.**
Rte. 7. U.S. Hwy. 127 S
Frankfort, KY 40601
**Phone:** (502)227-9529

**★ 7272 ★ Hardin County Arc and Handicapped**
PO Box 2013
Elizabethtown, KY 42702
**Phone:** (502)737-1140

**★ 7273 ★ Hugh E. Sandefur Training Center**
801 S Main St.
PO Box 714
Henderson, KY 42419-0714
**Phone:** (502)827-2401

**★ 7274 ★ J. U. Kevil Foundation, Inc.**
PO Box 345
Mayfield, KY 42066

**★ 7275 ★ The Point/Arc of Northern Kentucky**
104 Pike St.
Covington, KY 41011
**Phone:** (859)491-9191

### Louisiana

**★ 7276 ★ The Arc of Baton Rouge**
8326 Kelwood Ave.
Baton Rouge, LA 70806
**Phone:** (225)927-0855　　　**Fax:** (225)924-3935
**Website:** http://www.arcbatonrouge.org

**★ 7277 ★ The Arc of Beauregard**
PO Box 13
Deridder, LA 70634
**Phone:** (337)462-2513

**★ 7278 ★ The Arc of Caddo-Bossier**
351 Jordan St.
Shreveport, LA 71101
**Phone:** (318)221-8392　　　**Fax:** (318)221-4262
**Website:** http://www.cbarc.org
**Alt. Contact:** Adult services can be contacted at 5320 Greenwood Rd., Shreveport, LA 71109; phone (318) 631-9501; fax (318) 631-9583.

**★ 7279 ★ The Arc of Calcasieu**
4100 J Bennett Johnston Ave.
Lake Charles, LA 70615
**Phone:** (337)433-3620
**Email:** hstroud@thecarc.com
**Website:** http://www.thecarc.com
Howard Stroud, Exec Director

**★ 7280 ★ The Arc of DeSoto**
1528 Old Jefferson Hwy.
PO Drawer 1238
Mansfield, LA 71052
**Phone:** (318)872-3255

**★ 7281 ★ The Arc of Donaldsonville**
PO Box 624
Donaldsonville, LA 70346
**Phone:** (504)473-4516

**★ 7282 ★ The Arc of Evangeline**
PO Box 677
Ville Platte, LA 70586
**Phone:** (318)363-5553

**★ 7283 ★ The Arc of Greater New Orleans**
5700 Loyola Ave.
New Orleans, LA 70115
**Phone:** (504)897-0134
**Email:** arcgnolee@juno.com
**Website:** http://www.arcgno.org

**★ 7284 ★ The Arc of Iberia**
PO Box 9610
New Iberia, LA 70562-9610
**Phone:** (318)364-7215

**★ 7285 ★ The Arc of Iberville**
PO Box 201
Plaquemine, LA 70765-0201
**Phone:** (225)687-4062

**★ 7286 ★ The Arc of Jackson Parish**
123 Gansville Rd.
Jonesboro, LA 71251

**★ 7287 ★ The Arc of Lafayette**
303 New Hope Rd.
Lafayette, LA 70506
**Phone:** (318)984-6110

**★ 7288 ★ The Arc of Lafourche**
PO Box 269
Thibodaux, LA 70302
**Phone:** (504)447-6214

**★ 7289 ★ The Arc of Livingston**
10494 Florida Blvd.
Walker, LA 70785
**Phone:** (504)664-7384

**★ 7290 ★ The Arc of Louisiana**
PO Box 65129
Baton Rouge, LA 70896-5129
**Phone:** (225)383-1033

**★ 7291 ★ The Arc of Morehouse**
10650 Lucy Hudson
Bastrop, LA 71220
**Phone:** (318)283-2338

**★ 7292 ★ The Arc of North Webster**
PO Box 351
Sarepta, LA 71071-0351
**Phone:** (318)847-4356

**★ 7293 ★ The Arc of Rapides**
3136 Cotton Wright Dr.
Alexandria, LA 71301
**Phone:** (318)445-5287

**★ 7294 ★ The Arc of Sabine**
545 W San Antonio
PO Box 1150
Many, LA 71449
**Phone:** (318)256-2025

**★ 7295 ★ The Arc of St. Charles, Inc.**
PO Box 455
Boutte, LA 70039-0455
**Phone:** (504)785-0971

**★ 7296 ★ The Arc of St. James**
Rte. 1, Box 924
Vacherie, LA 70090
**Phone:** (504)265-7910

**★ 7297 ★ The Arc of St. John**
101 Bamboo Rd.
Laplace, LA 70068
**Phone:** (504)652-8003

**★ 7298 ★ The Arc of St. Martin**
500 Lelia St.
PO Box 128
Saint Martinville, LA 70582
**Phone:** (337)394-4928

**★ 7299 ★ The Arc of St. Mary**
PO Box 3
Centerville, LA 70522
**Phone:** (318)836-9445

**★ 7300 ★ The Arc of St. Tammany**
1541 St. Ann Pl.
Slidell, LA 70460
**Phone:** (504)641-0197

**★ 7301 ★ The Arc of Terrebonne**
1 McCord Rd.
Houma, LA 70363
**Phone:** (504)876-4465
**Email:** TARC@cajun.net
**Website:** http://www.terrebonnearc.org

**★ 7302 ★ The Arc of Vermilion**
809 S Severin St.
Erath, LA 70533

**★ 7303 ★ Assumption Arc**
PO Drawer 1040
Napoleonville, LA 70390
**Phone:** (504)369-2907

**★ 7304 ★ Community Opportunities of East Ascension**
1122 SE Ascension Complex Blvd.
Gonzales, LA 70737
**Phone:** (225)621-2000　　　**Fax:** (225)621-2022
**Email:** jrr12@eatel.net
**Website:** http://www.homestead.com/coea
Mark Thomas, Exec Director

**★ 7305 ★ Minden Association for Retarded Citizens**
PO Box 423
Minden, LA 71058
**Phone:** (318)377-4774

**★ 7306 ★ TARC**
201 E Church St.
Hammond, LA 70401
**Phone:** (504)345-8811
**Email:** tarc@tarc-hammond.com
**Website:** http://www.tarc-hammond.com

### Maine

**★ 7307 ★ The Arc of Central Aroostook**
26 Lombart St
PO Box 1245
Presque Isle, ME 04769
**Phone:** (207)764-0134

**★ 7308 ★ The Arc of Green Valley**
PO Box 127
Island Falls, ME 04747
**Phone:** (207)463-2156

★ **7309** ★ **The Arc of Northern Aroostook**
459 Main St.
Van Buren, ME 04785
**Phone:** (207)868-5203

★ **7310** ★ **The Arc of Oxford County**
85 Lincoln Ave.
Rumford, ME 04276
**Phone:** (207)369-0141

★ **7311** ★ **The Arc of Sebasticook Farms**
PO Box 65
Saint Albans, ME 04971
**Phone:** (207)938-4615

★ **7312** ★ **The Arc/Waban Projects, Inc.**
RR 1, Box 2405
Sanford, ME 04073
**Phone:** (207)324-7955

★ **7313** ★ **Coastal Workshop**
35 Limerock St.
PO Box 637
Camden, ME 04843
**Phone:** (207)236-6008

★ **7314** ★ **Community Living Association**
45 School St.
Houlton, ME 04730
**Phone:** (207)532-9446

★ **7315** ★ **Community Partners, Inc.**
PO Box 363
Biddeford, ME 04005
**Phone:** (207)282-7113

★ **7316** ★ **Downeast Horizons, Inc.**
RFD 1, Box 2042
Bar Harbor, ME 04609
**Phone:** (207)288-4234

★ **7317** ★ **Independence Arc**
PO Box 642
Brunswick, ME 04011
**Phone:** (207)725-4371

★ **7318** ★ **Kathadin Friends Inc.**
1024 Central St., Ste. A
Millinocket, ME 04462-2111
**Phone:** (207)723-9466

★ **7319** ★ **Ken-A-Set Arc**
PO Box 334
Waterville, ME 04903
**Phone:** (207)872-6484

★ **7320** ★ **Landmark Human Resources**
PO Box 178
Bridgton, ME 04009
**Phone:** (207)647-8396

★ **7321** ★ **Life Enrichment Advancing People Inc.**
36 ½ High St.
PO Box 979
Farmington, ME 04938
**Phone:** (207)778-3443

★ **7322** ★ **Maine Independent Living Services Inc.**
475 Western Ave., Ste. 13
Augusta, ME 04330
**Phone:** (207)326-1115

★ **7323** ★ **Pathways, Inc. Arc**
PO Box 1267
Auburn, ME 04210

★ **7324** ★ **Work First Inc.**
PO Box 86
Farmington, ME 04938
**Phone:** (207)778-3200

## Maryland

★ **7325** ★ **The Arc of Anne Arundel County, Inc.**
931 Spa Rd.
Annapolis, MD 21401
**Phone:** (410)269-1883
**Website:** http://www.arcofannearundel.org
Kate Rollason, Exec Director

★ **7326** ★ **The Arc of Baltimore**
7215 York Rd.
Baltimore, MD 21212
**Phone:** (410)296-2272
**Website:** http://www.arcofbaltimore.org

★ **7327** ★ **The Arc of Carroll County**
180 Kriders Church Rd.
Westminster, MD 21158
**Phone:** (410)848-4124

★ **7328** ★ **The Arc of Frederick County, Inc.**
620-A Research Dr.
Frederick, MD 21703-8619
**Phone:** (301)693-0909  **Fax:** (301)695-6454
**Email:** info@arcfc.org
**Website:** http://www.arcfc.org

★ **7329** ★ **The Arc of Howard County, Inc.**
11735 Homewood Rd.
Ellicott City, MD 21042
**Phone:** (410)730-0638
**Website:** http://www.archoward.org

★ **7330** ★ **The Arc of Maryland, Inc.**
49 Old Solomon's Island Rd., Ste. 205
Annapolis, MD 21401
**Phone:** (410)571-9320  **Fax:** (410)974-6021
**Email:** info@thearcmd.org
**Website:** http://www.thearcmd.org

★ **7331** ★ **The Arc of Montgomery County, Inc.**
11600 Nebel St.
Rockville, MD 20852
**Phone:** (301)984-5777
**Email:** info@arcmontmd.org
**Website:** http://www.arcmontmd.org

★ **7332** ★ **The Arc of the Northern Chesapeake Region**
PO Box 610
Aberdeen, MD 21001
**Phone:** (410)836-7177
**Website:** http://www.arcncr.org

★ **7333** ★ **The Arc of Prince George's County**
1401 McCormick Dr.
Largo, MD 20774
**Phone:** (301)925-7050  **Fax:** (301)925-4387
**Email:** info@thearcofpgc.org
**Website:** http://www.thearcofpgc.org

★ **7334** ★ **The Arc of Southern Maryland**
PO Box 1860
Prince Frederick, MD 20678
**Phone:** (410)535-2413
**Email:** arcadmin@arcsomd.org
**Website:** http://www.arcsomd.org

★ **7335** ★ **The Arc of Talbot County**
PO Box 776
Easton, MD 21601
**Phone:** (410)820-5151

★ **7336** ★ **The Arc of Washington County**
820 Florida Ave.
Hagerstown, MD 21740
**Phone:** (301)733-3550

★ **7337** ★ **The Arc of Worcester**
PO Box 126
Newark, MD 21841
**Phone:** (410)632-2382

## Massachusetts

★ **7338** ★ **Advocacy Resource Center of Greater New Bedford**
412 B County St.
New Bedford, MA 02740
**Phone:** (508)996-8551

★ **7339** ★ **The Arc of the Brockton Area**
1250 W Chestnut St.
Brockton, MA 02301
**Phone:** (508)583-8030

★ **7340** ★ **The Arc of Cape Cod**
PO Box 428
Hyannis, MA 02601
**Phone:** (508)790-3667

★ **7341** ★ **The Arc of East Middlesex (EMARC)**
20 Gould St.
Reading, MA 01867-2927
**Phone:** (781)245-5262
**Email:** info@theemarc.org
**Website:** http://www.theemarc.org
Jo Ann Simons, Exec Director

★ **7342** ★ **The Arc of Greater Fall River**
PO Box 1943
Fall River, MA 02722
**Phone:** (508)679-0001

★ **7343** ★ **The Arc of Greater Lawrence**
1 Parker St.
Lawrence, MA 01843
**Phone:** (978)975-8587
**Website:** http://www.classinc.org/arc_page.htm

★ **7344** ★ **The Arc of Greater Plymouth**
4 Main St.
Kingston, MA 02364
**Phone:** (781)585-1310
**Website:** http://www.thearcofgp.com

★ **7345** ★ **The Arc of Greater Waltham**
56 Chestnut St.
Waltham, MA 02453
**Phone:** (781)899-1344

★ **7346** ★ **Arc Massachusetts**
217 South St.
Waltham, MA 02453
**Phone:** (781)891-6270
**Email:** arcmass@gis.net

**Website:** http://www.arcmass.org

★ **7347** ★ **The Arc of North Central, Inc.**
564 Main St.
Fitchburg, MA 01420
**Phone:** (978)343-8852          **Fax:** (978)343-8852
**Email:** info@arcofnorthcentral.org
**Website:** http://arcofnorthcentral.org

★ **7348** ★ **The Arc of Northern Bristol County**
5 Bank St.
Attleboro, MA 02703
**Phone:** (508)226-1445
**Website:** http://www.arcnbc.org

★ **7349** ★ **The Arc of Northern Essex**
4 Summer St., Rm 6
Haverhill, MA 01830
**Phone:** (508)373-0552

★ **7350** ★ **The Arc of South Norfolk County**
789 Clapboardtree St.
Westwood, MA 02090
**Phone:** (617)762-4001
**Website:** http://www.sncarc.org

★ **7351** ★ **The Arc of Southern Worcester County**
14 Mechanic St.
Box 66
Southbridge, MA 01550
**Phone:** (508)764-4085

★ **7352** ★ **Berkshire County Arc, Inc.**
395 South St.
Pittsfield, MA 01201
**Phone:** (413)499-4241
**Email:** bcarc@netconnx.net
**Website:** http://www.bcarc.org

★ **7353** ★ **Charles River Arc**
49 E Militia Hits
Needham, MA 02492-0002
**Phone:** (781)444-4347          **Fax:** (781)444-5146
**Email:** familysupport@crarc.org
**Website:** http://www.crarc.org

★ **7354** ★ **Greater Boston Arc**
1505 Commonwealth Ave.
Boston, MA 02135-3605
**Phone:** (617)783-3900
**Email:** gbarc1@msn.com
**Website:** http://www.gbarc.org

★ **7355** ★ **Minute Man Arc for Human Services, Inc.**
1269 Main St.
West Concord, MA 01742
**Phone:** (978)371-1543          **Fax:** (978)287-0468
**Email:** MMAHS@aol.com
**Website:** http://www.minutemanarc.org

★ **7356** ★ **North Shore Arc**
64 Holten St.
Danvers, MA 01923
**Phone:** (978)762-4878

★ **7357** ★ **South Shore ARC**
371 River St.
North Weymouth, MA 02191
**Phone:** (781)335-3023
**Email:** info@southshorearc.org
**Website:** http://www.southshorearc.org

★ **7358** ★ **The United Arc of Franklin and Hampshire Counties**
111 Summer St.
Greenfield, MA 01301
**Phone:** (413)774-5558
**Email:** arc@crocker.com

## Michigan

★ **7359** ★ **The Arc of Allegan**
219 Hubbard St.
Allegan, MI 49010
**Phone:** (616)673-8841

★ **7360** ★ **The Arc of Arenac Area**
PO Box 805
Standish, MI 48658

★ **7361** ★ **The Arc of Arro/Berrien County**
515 Ship St., Ste. 209
Saint Joseph, MI 49085
**Phone:** (616)429-8166

★ **7362** ★ **The Arc of Bay County**
709 Columbus Ave.
Bay City, MI 48708
**Phone:** (517)893-1346

★ **7363** ★ **The Arc of Benzie County**
11721 Maple Rd.
Beulah, MI 49617

★ **7364** ★ **The Arc of Calhoun County**
368 Capital Ave. NE
Battle Creek, MI 49017
**Phone:** (616)966-2575

★ **7365** ★ **The Arc of Charlevoix-Emmet**
6149 E Jordan Rd.
Ellsworth, MI 49729

★ **7366** ★ **The Arc of Copper County**
114 1st Centennial Heights
Calumet, MI 49913

★ **7367** ★ **The Arc of Delta County**
PO Box 651
Escanaba, MI 49829
**Phone:** (906)786-9212

★ **7368** ★ **The Arc of Detroit**
51 W Hancock
Detroit, MI 48201
**Phone:** (313)831-0202

★ **7369** ★ **The Arc, Downriver**
4212 13th St.
Wyandotte, MI 48192
**Phone:** (313)283-0710

★ **7370** ★ **The Arc of Genesee County**
G-5069 Van Slyke Rd.
Flint, MI 48507
**Phone:** (313)238-2140

★ **7371** ★ **The Arc of Gogebic County**
127 E Mary
PO Box 45
Bessemer, MI 49911

★ **7372** ★ **The Arc of the Grand Traverse Area**
PO Box 204
Traverse City, MI 49685-0204
**Phone:** (231)941-0560

★ **7373** ★ **The Arc of Gratiot County**
7205 N McClelland Rd.
Breckenridge, MI 48615-9504

★ **7374** ★ **The Arc of Grosse Point/ Harper Woods**
621 Washington
Grosse Pointe Park, MI 48230
**Email:** LKel584817@aol.com
**Website:** http://www.geocities.com/thearcgrossepointeharperwoods
Laura Kellett, Contact

★ **7375** ★ **The Arc of Ionia County**
5827 N Orleans Rd.
Orleans, MI 48865
**Phone:** (616)761-3151

★ **7376** ★ **The Arc of Iosco**
5589 Schaefer Rd.
Oscoda, MI 48750

★ **7377** ★ **The Arc of Isabella**
PO Box 171
Mount Pleasant, MI 48804
**Phone:** (517)772-8081

★ **7378** ★ **The Arc of Kent County**
1331 Lake Dr. SE, No. 2
Grand Rapids, MI 49506
**Phone:** (616)459-3339

★ **7379** ★ **The Arc of Lenawee**
PO Box 291
Adrian, MI 49221

★ **7380** ★ **The Arc of Livingston**
3075 E Grand River
Howell, MI 48843
**Phone:** (517)546-1228

★ **7381** ★ **The Arc of Manistee**
481 Bryant Ave.
Manistee, MI 49660

★ **7382** ★ **The Arc Michigan**
1325 S Washington Ave.
Lansing, MI 48910
**Phone:** (517)487-5426          **Free:** 800-292-7851
**Fax:** (517)487-0303
**Website:** http://www.arcmi.org
Eric Roberts, Exec Director

★ **7383** ★ **The Arc of Midland**
220 W Main St., No. 14
Midland, MI 48640
**Phone:** (989)631-4439          **Fax:** (989)832-5528
**Email:** arcadmin@thearcofmidland.org
**Website:** http://www.thearcofmidland.org

★ **7384** ★ **The Arc of Monroe County**
752 S Monroe St., Ste. B
Monroe, MI 48161-1453
**Phone:** (734)241-5881

★ **7385** ★ **The Arc of Montcalm**
PO Box 1011
Stanton, MI 48888

**★ 7386 ★ The Arc of Muskegon**
1145 E Wesley Ave.
Muskegon, MI 49442-2197
**Phone:** (231)777-2006
**Email:** arcmusk@i2k.com
**Website:** http://community.mlive.com/cc/arc-muskeg-on

**★ 7387 ★ The Arc of Newaygo County**
37 E Main St.
Fremont, MI 49412
**Phone:** (616)924-5840

**★ 7388 ★ The Arc of Northwest Wayne County**
26049 5 Mile Rd.
Redford, MI 48239
**Phone:** (313)532-7915  **Fax:** (313)532-7488
**Email:** ArcNW@aol.com
**Website:** http://comnet.org/arcnw

**★ 7389 ★ The Arc of Oakland County**
1641 W Big Beaver Rd.
Troy, MI 48084-3501
**Phone:** (248)816-1900
**Email:** tfk@thearcoakland.org
**Website:** http://www.thearcoakland.org
Thomas F. Kendziorski, Exec Director

**★ 7390 ★ The Arc of Oceana**
PO Box 121
Shelby, MI 49455

**★ 7391 ★ The Arc of Ogemaw County**
117 Somerset Terrace
Roscommon, MI 48653

**★ 7392 ★ The Arc of St. Clair County**
1033 26th St.
Port Huron, MI 48060
**Phone:** (313)982-3261

**★ 7393 ★ The Arc of Sanilac**
1155 Shabbona Rd.
Snover, MI 48472

**★ 7394 ★ The Arc Services**
310 Johnson St., Ste. 165
Saginaw, MI 48601
**Phone:** (517)752-6104

**★ 7395 ★ The Arc Services of Macomb, Inc.**
44050 N Gratiot Ave.
Clinton Township, MI 48036-1308
**Phone:** (810)469-1600
**Email:** arcmc@tir.com
**Website:** http://comnet.org/local/orgs/arc/index.html

**★ 7396 ★ The Arc of Shiawassee**
1905 W 21
Owosso, MI 48867
**Phone:** (517)723-7377
**Email:** arcshia@shianet.org
**Website:** http://www.angelfire.com/mi/arcshia

**★ 7397 ★ The Arc of Tuscola County**
2266 W Caro Rd.
Caro, MI 48723

**★ 7398 ★ The Arc of Van Buren**
65651 43 Hwy.
Bangor, MI 49013
**Phone:** (616)427-7247

**★ 7399 ★ The Arc of Western Wayne County**
2257 S Wayne Rd.
Westland, MI 48186
**Phone:** (734)729-9100  **Fax:** (734)729-9695
**Email:** thearcww@tir.com
**Website:** http://comnet.org/arcww

**★ 7400 ★ The Association for Community Advocacy**
1100 N Main St., No. 205
Ann Arbor, MI 48104
**Phone:** (734)662-1256

**★ 7401 ★ Association for Macomb-Oakland Regional Center**
8080 Huntington Ridge Ct.
Washington Township, MI 48094

**★ 7402 ★ Community Advocates for Persons with Developmental Disabilities**
814 S Westnedge
Kalamazoo, MI 49008-1162
**Phone:** (616)342-9801
**Email:** commadvoc@worldnet.att.net
**Website:** http://www.communityadvocates.org
George Martin, CEO & Pres

**★ 7403 ★ Parents and Advocates for Wayne Community Services**
28623 W Chicago
Livonia, MI 48150

**★ 7404 ★ Tri-County Community Advocates for People with Developmental Disabilities, Inc.**
921 N Washington Ave.
Lansing, MI 48906-5137
**Phone:** (517)484-3068

### Minnesota

**★ 7405 ★ The Arc of Alexandria**
107 Donna Ave.
Alexandria, MN 56308
**Phone:** (320)762-2015

**★ 7406 ★ The Arc of Anoka, Ramsey, and Suburban Counties**
1526 E 122nd St.
Burnsville, MN 55337-6804
**Phone:** (952)890-3057

**★ 7407 ★ The Arc of Blue Earth/Nicollet Counties**
2113 Excalibur Rd.
North Mankato, MN 56003
**Phone:** (507)345-1542

**★ 7408 ★ The Arc of Brown County**
Box 641
New Ulm, MN 56073
**Phone:** (507)354-7445

**★ 7409 ★ The Arc of Central Minnesota**
6112 322nd St.
Saint Cloud, MN 56303
**Phone:** (320)240-9550

**★ 7410 ★ The Arc of Clay County**
Townsite Ctr., Rm. 141
810 4th Ave. S
Moorhead, MN 56560
**Phone:** (218)233-5949

**★ 7411 ★ The Arc of Crow Wing County**
2881 44th St. NW
Pine River, MN 56474
**Phone:** (218)587-5259

**★ 7412 ★ The Arc of Fergus Falls**
PO Box 1032
Fergus Falls, MN 56537

**★ 7413 ★ The Arc of Freeborn County**
407 E William St.
Albert Lea, MN 56007-2964
**Phone:** (507)377-3469

**★ 7414 ★ The Arc of the Headwaters**
522 Beltrami Ave., Ste. 108
Bemidji, MN 56601
**Phone:** (218)759-0097

**★ 7415 ★ The Arc of Hennepin-Carver**
4301 Hwy 7, No. 140
Minneapolis, MN 55416
**Phone:** (952)920-0855
**Website:** http://www.archennepincarver.org

**★ 7416 ★ The Arc of Kandiyohi County**
201 SW 4th St., No. 12
Willmar, MN 56201-0801
**Phone:** (320)231-1777

**★ 7417 ★ The Arc of LeSueur County**
812 Central Ave. S
New Prague, MN 56071

**★ 7418 ★ Arc Minnesota**
770 Transfer Rd., Ste. 26
Saint Paul, MN 55114-1422
**Phone:** (651)523-0823
**Email:** arcminn@mtn.org
**Website:** http://www.arcminnesota.com

**★ 7419 ★ The Arc of Mower County**
709 N Main St.
Austin, MN 55912
**Phone:** (507)433-8994

**★ 7420 ★ The Arc of Norman County**
209 Jamison Dr.
Ada, MN 56510

**★ 7421 ★ The Arc of Northland**
201 Ordean Bldg., Ste. 201
424 W Superior
Duluth, MN 55802
**Phone:** (218)726-4725

**★ 7422 ★ The Arc of Range**
309 7th St. S
Virginia, MN 55792
**Phone:** (218)741-2928

**★ 7423 ★ The Arc of Rice County**
12 6th St. NW
Faribault, MN 55021

**★ 7424 ★ The Arc of St. Cloud**
PO Box 251
Saint Cloud, MN 56302
**Phone:** (320)251-7272

**★ 7425 ★ The Arc of Southeastern Minnesota**
903 W Center, No. 140
Rochester, MN 55902

**Phone:** (507)287-2032

★ **7426** ★ **The Arc of Southwestern Minnesota**
1271 76th Ave.
Sherburn, MN 56171
**Phone:** (507)764-6894

★ **7427** ★ **The Arc of Stevens County**
Rte. 2, Box 200
Morris, MN 56267

★ **7428** ★ **The Arc of Wadena County**
513 2nd St. SW
Wadena, MN 56482

★ **7429** ★ **The Arc of Waseca County**
601 16th Ave. NE
Waseca, MN 56093
**Phone:** (612)758-2615

★ **7430** ★ **The Arc of Western Stearns**
34934 Queensfield Rd.
Sauk Centre, MN 56378

## Mississippi

★ **7431** ★ **The Arc of Adams County**
PO Box 275
Natchez, MS 39121-0275
**Phone:** (601)442-2264

★ **7432** ★ **The Arc of Biloxi**
771 Water St.
Biloxi, MS 39530
**Phone:** (228)374-1200

★ **7433** ★ **The Arc of Clay County**
PO Box 613
West Point, MS 39773

★ **7434** ★ **The Arc of Forrest County**
PO Box 18800
Hattiesburg, MS 39404-8800

★ **7435** ★ **The Arc of Itawamba County**
Rte. 3, Box 184A
Fulton, MS 38843

★ **7436** ★ **The Arc of Jones County**
PO Box 1233
Laurel, MS 39441
**Phone:** (601)426-2944

★ **7437** ★ **The Arc of Mississippi**
7 Lakeland Cir., Ste. 600
Jackson, MS 39216
**Phone:** (601)982-1180
**Website:** http://www.arcms.org

★ **7438** ★ **The Arc of Pearl River**
PO Box 1816
Picayune, MS 39466

★ **7439** ★ **The Arc of Tishomingo County**
1133 County Rd. 992
Iuka, MS 38852
**Phone:** (662)423-4517

★ **7440** ★ **The Arc of Warren County**
100 Smokey Ln.
Vicksburg, MS 39180
**Phone:** (601)638-2761

★ **7441** ★ **The Arc of Washington County**
136 S Poplar St.
PO Box 1733
Greenville, MS 38702-1733
**Phone:** (662)332-3271

★ **7442** ★ **The Arc of West Jackson County**
1904 Government St.
Ocean Springs, MS 39564
**Phone:** (228)872-2939

★ **7443** ★ **Gulf Coast Society for Retarded Citizens**
PO Box 6651
Gulfport, MS 39506
**Phone:** (601)868-9755

★ **7444** ★ **North Mississippi Special Needs Arc**
403 S Commerce St.
Ripley, MS 38663
**Phone:** (662)837-9883

★ **7445** ★ **Tri County Arc**
PO Box 1084
Summit, MS 39666
**Phone:** (601)276-3603

## Missouri

★ **7446** ★ **The Arc of Clay and Platte Counties, Inc.**
7400 C N Oak Traffic Way
Gladstone, MO 64118
**Phone:** (816)436-3009

★ **7447** ★ **The Arc of Eastern Jackson County**
704 E 121 St.
Kansas City, MO 64146

★ **7448** ★ **The Arc of the Ozarks**
1501 E Pythian
Springfield, MO 65802
**Phone:** (417)864-7887
**Website:** http://www.thearcoftheozarks.org

★ **7449** ★ **The Arc of Stoddard County**
PO Box 444
Dexter, MO 63841
**Phone:** (573)624-8525

★ **7450** ★ **St. Louis Arc**
1816 Lackland Hill Pkwy., No. 200
Saint Louis, MO 63146
**Phone:** (314)569-2211      **Fax:** (314)569-0778
**Website:** http://www.slarc.org

## Montana

★ **7451** ★ **Rocky Mountain Arc**
207 S Montana St.
Butte, MT 59701

★ **7452** ★ **Yellowstone Arc**
602 18th St. W
Billings, MT 59102

## Nebraska

★ **7453** ★ **The Arc of Adams/Clay Counties**
414 E 6th St.
Hastings, NE 68901
**Phone:** (402)463-5797

★ **7454** ★ **The Arc of Buffalo County**
2022 Ave. A, Ste. 17
Kearney, NE 68847
**Phone:** (308)237-4343

★ **7455** ★ **The Arc of Butler County**
328 S 4th St.
David City, NE 68632

★ **7456** ★ **The Arc of Central Nebraska**
720 W Stolley Park Rd.
Grand Island, NE 68801

★ **7457** ★ **The Arc of Cheyenne County**
1544 King
Sidney, NE 69162

★ **7458** ★ **The Arc of Colfax County**
935 Rd. 6
Schuyler, NE 68661-7160

★ **7459** ★ **The Arc of Custer**
PO Box 34
Broken Bow, NE 68822
**Phone:** (308)872-6067

★ **7460** ★ **The Arc of Elkhorn Valley**
800 Cornhusker Dr.
West Point, NE 68788

★ **7461** ★ **The Arc of Hamilton/Merrick Counties**
915 P St.
Aurora, NE 68818
**Phone:** (402)694-3519

★ **7462** ★ **The Arc of Lincoln-Lancaster County**
1101 Arapahoe, Ste. 5
Lincoln, NE 68502
**Phone:** (402)421-8866
**Website:** http://www.lincolnne.com/nonprofit.arc

★ **7463** ★ **The Arc of Nebraska**
1672 Van Dorn St.
Lincoln, NE 68502
**Phone:** (402)475-4407      **Free:** 800-666-7907
**Website:** http://www.arc-nebraska.org

★ **7464** ★ **The Arc of Norfolk**
PO Box 32
Norfolk, NE 68702
**Phone:** (402)379-1160

★ **7465** ★ **The Arc, North Central**
1310 Sheridan Pl.
Grand Island, NE 68803

★ **7466** ★ **The Arc of Platte County**
Rte. 2, Box 62
Genoa, NE 68640
**Phone:** (402)993-2489

★ **7467** ★ **The Arc of Sarpy**
3222 Chad St.
Bellevue, NE 68123
**Phone:** (402)291-8494

★ **7468** ★ **The Arc of Saunders**
1550 N Linder
Wahoo, NE 68066

★ 7469 ★ **The Arc of Seward**
255 N 7th
Staplehurst, NE 68439


★ 7470 ★ **The Arc, South Central**
11557 RD 740
Holdrege, NE 68949


★ 7471 ★ **The Arc, Southeast**
2423 R St.
Auburn, NE 68305


★ 7472 ★ **The Arc, Southwest**
RR3, Box 7621
Culbertson, NE 69024
**Phone:** (308)278-2788


★ 7473 ★ **The Ollie Webb Center**
1941 S 42nd St., Ste. 122
Omaha, NE 68105-2942
**Phone:** (402)346-5220


## Nevada

★ 7474 ★ **The Arc of Churchill County**
PO Box 1641
Fallon, NV 89407
**Phone:** (775)423-4760


★ 7475 ★ **The Arc of Ormsby**
PO Box 491
Carson City, NV 89702
**Phone:** (702)882-8520


★ 7476 ★ **The Arc of Washoe**
790 Sutro St.
Reno, NV 89512
**Phone:** (775)333-9272


★ 7477 ★ **Opportunity Village Arc**
6300 W Oakey Blvd.
Las Vegas, NV 89146
**Phone:** (702)259-3707
**Website:** http://www.opportunityvillage.org


## New Hampshire

★ 7478 ★ **The Arc of Greater Manchester**
PO Box 3363
Manchester, NH 03105-3363


★ 7479 ★ **Concord Regional Arc, Inc.**
PO Box 1173
Concord, NH 03302


★ 7480 ★ **Salem Arc, Inc.**
8 Centerville Dr.
Salem, NH 03079
**Phone:** (603)893-9889


## New Jersey

★ 7481 ★ **The Arc
Ocean County Chapter**
815 Cedar Bridge Ave.
Lakewood, NJ 08701
**Phone:** (732)363-3335


★ 7482 ★ **The Arc
Warren County Chapter**
319 W Washington Ave.
Washington, NJ 07882
**Phone:** (908)689-7525


★ 7483 ★ **The Arc of Atlantic County**
101 Shore Rd.
Somers Point, NJ 08244
**Phone:** (609)926-0800


★ 7484 ★ **The Arc of Bergen and
Passaic Counties, Inc.**
223 Moore St.
Hackensack, NJ 07601
**Phone:** (201)343-0322
**Email:** ArcBP@aol.com
**Website:** http://www.arcbergenpassaic.org


★ 7485 ★ **The Arc of Burlington**
1 Underwood Ct., Unit 2
Delran, NJ 08075
**Phone:** (856)764-9494
**Email:** info@arcofburlington.org
**Website:** http://www.arcofburlington.org


★ 7486 ★ **The Arc of Camden**
215 W White Horse Pike
Berlin, NJ 08009
**Phone:** (856)767-3650


★ 7487 ★ **The Arc of Cape May County,
Inc.**
922 Rte. 47
PO Box 255
South Dennis, NJ 08245
**Phone:** (609)861-7100
**Email:** support@arcofcapemay.org
**Website:** http://www.arcofcapemay.org
Jean McCarthy, President


★ 7488 ★ **The Arc of Cumberland**
1680 W Sherman Ave.
Vineland, NJ 08360
**Phone:** (609)691-9138
**Website:** http://www.arccumberland.org


★ 7489 ★ **The Arc of Essex**
7 Regent St.
Livingston, NJ 07039
**Phone:** (973)535-1181
**Website:** http://www.arcessex.org


★ 7490 ★ **The Arc of Gloucester**
1555 Gateway Blvd.
Woodbury, NJ 08096
**Phone:** (856)848-8648


★ 7491 ★ **The Arc of Hunterdon County**
1322 State Route 31 N, Ste. 5
Annandale, NJ 08801
**Phone:** (908)730-7827
**Website:** http://www.archunterdon.org


★ 7492 ★ **The Arc/Mercer, Inc.**
231 Lawrenceville Rd.
Lawrenceville, NJ 08648
**Phone:** (609)278-1211
**Email:** arcmercer@aol.com
**Website:** http://www.arcmercer.org


★ 7493 ★ **The Arc of Middlesex County**
32 Ford Ave., 2nd Fl.
Milltown, NJ 08850
**Phone:** (732)247-8155
**Email:** arcmc@arc-middlesex.org
**Website:** http://www.arc-middlesex.org


★ 7494 ★ **The Arc of Monmouth County**
1158 Wayside Rd.
Tinton Falls, NJ 07712
**Phone:** (732)493-1919
**Email:** arcmon@superlink.net
**Website:** http://www.arcofmonmouth.org


★ 7495 ★ **The Arc of Morris County**
PO Box 123
Morris Plains, NJ 07950-0123
**Phone:** (973)326-9750


★ 7496 ★ **The Arc of New Jersey**
985 Livingston Ave.
North Brunswick, NJ 08902
**Phone:** (732)246-2525    **Fax:** (732)214-1834
**Email:** info@arcnj.org
**Website:** http://www.arcnj.org
Thomas Baffuto, Exec Director


★ 7497 ★ **The Arc of Salem**
150 Salem-Woodstown Rd.
PO Box 5
Salem, NJ 08079
**Phone:** (609)935-3600


★ 7498 ★ **The Arc of Somerset County**
141 S Main St.
Manville, NJ 08835
**Phone:** (908)725-8544
**Email:** ArcOffice@TheArcOfSomerset.org
**Website:** http://www.thearcofsomerset.org


★ 7499 ★ **The Arc of Sussex**
11 U.S. Rte. 206., Ste. 100
Augusta, NJ 07822
**Phone:** (973)383-7442
**Website:** http://www.scarc.org


★ 7500 ★ **The Arc of Union County, Inc.**
1225 South Ave.
Plainfield, NJ 07062
**Phone:** (908)754-5910
**Email:** info@arcunion.org
**Website:** http://www.arcunion.org


## New Mexico

★ 7501 ★ **The Arc of Artesia**
1504 W Dallas Ave.
Artesia, NM 88210
**Phone:** (505)746-4811


★ 7502 ★ **The Arc of Cibola County**
1405 Dona
Grants, NM 87020


★ 7503 ★ **The Arc of Curry County**
2118 Carolina
Box 1835
Clovis, NM 88101


★ 7504 ★ **The Arc of Las Cruces**
2225 E Griggs Ave.
Las Cruces, NM 88001
**Phone:** (505)525-3811


★ 7505 ★ **The Arc of Luna County**
2020 S Columbus Rd.
Deming, NM 88030


★ 7506 ★ **The Arc of New Mexico**
3655 Carlisle NE
Albuquerque, NM 87110-5564
**Phone:** (505)883-4630    **Free:** 800-358-6493
**Fax:** (505)883-5564
**Email:** arcnm@arcnm.com
**Website:** http://www.arcnm.com

**★ 7507 ★ The Arc of Otero County**
873 Wright Ave.
Alamogordo, NM 88310
**Phone:** (505)437-0919

**★ 7508 ★ The Arc of Roswell**
712 N Lea
Roswell, NM 88201

**★ 7509 ★ The Arc of Santa Fe**
945 Vuelta del Sur
Santa Fe, NM 87505

**★ 7510 ★ The Arc of Taos County**
7421 NDCBU
Taos, NM 87571
**Phone:** (505)758-4274

**★ 7511 ★ The Arc of Thriftown, Inc.**
200 W Broadway
Farmington, NM 87401
**Phone:** (505)325-8998

**★ 7512 ★ ARCA**
11300 Lomas Blvd. NE
Albuquerque, NM 87112
**Phone:** (505)332-6700
**Website:** http://www.arc-a.org
Elaine Solimon, Exec Director

### New York

**★ 7513 ★ The Arc of Onondaga**
600 S Wilbur Ave.
Syracuse, NY 13204
**Phone:** (315)476-7441
**Email:** tonipaglia@aol.com
**Website:** http://www.arcon.org
Toni Paglia, Contact

**★ 7514 ★ The Arc of Ontario**
3071 County Complex Dr.
Canandaigua, NY 14424
**Phone:** (716)394-7500
**Email:** contact@ontarioarc.org
**Website:** http://www.ontarioarc.org

**★ 7515 ★ The Arc of Orleans County**
PO Box 439
Albion, NY 14411-0439
**Phone:** (716)589-5516
**Email:** dcolquhoun@arcoforleans.com
**Website:** http://www.arcoforleans.org
Donald Colquhoun, Exec Director

**★ 7516 ★ The Arc of Otsego County**
35 Academy St.
PO Box 490
Oneonta, NY 13820
**Phone:** (607)432-8595

**★ 7517 ★ The Arc of Schuyler County**
203 12th St.
Watkins Glen, NY 14891
**Phone:** (607)535-6934
**Email:** manager@arcofschuyler.org
**Website:** http://www.schuylerarc.com

**★ 7518 ★ The Arc of Seneca-Cayuga**
1083 Waterloo Geneva Rd.
Waterloo, NY 13165
**Phone:** (315)539-5067
**Email:** mail@sencayarc.org
**Website:** http://www.sencayarc.org
Kevin M. Smith, Exec Director

**★ 7519 ★ The Arc of Westchester**
74 Westmoreland Ave.
White Plains, NY 10606
**Phone:** (914)428-8330
**Website:** http://www.westchesterarc.org

**★ 7520 ★ Heritage Centers**
**Erie County Chapter**
101 Oak St.
Buffalo, NY 14203
**Phone:** (716)856-4201
**Website:** http://www.heritagecenters.org

**★ 7521 ★ Herkimer Area Resource Center**
333 S Main St.
PO Box 271
Herkimer, NY 13350
**Phone:** (315)866-8339

**★ 7522 ★ Livingston-Wyoming Association for Retarded Citizens**
18 Main St.
Mount Morris, NY 14510
**Phone:** (716)658-2828

**★ 7523 ★ NYSArc**
393 Delaware Ave.
Delmar, NY 12054
**Phone:** (518)439-8311      **Fax:** (518)439-1893
**Email:** nysarc@nysarc.org
**Website:** http://www.nysarc.org

**★ 7524 ★ NYSARC, Inc.**
**Chautauqua County Chapter**
880 E 2nd St.
Jamestown, NY 14701
**Phone:** (716)483-2344

**★ 7525 ★ NYSARC, Inc.**
**Delaware County Chapter**
RR 1, Box 67A
Walton, NY 13856
**Phone:** (607)865-7126

**★ 7526 ★ NYSARC, Inc.**
**Essex County Chapter**
7 St. Patricks Pl.
Port Henry, NY 12974
**Phone:** (518)546-3381

**★ 7527 ★ NYSARC, Inc.**
**Franklin County Chapter**
12 Mohawk St.
Tupper Lake, NY 12986
**Phone:** (518)359-3351

**★ 7528 ★ NYSARC, Inc.**
**Monroe County Chapter**
1000 Elmwood Ave.
Rochester, NY 14620
**Phone:** (716)271-0660
**Website:** http://www.arcmonroe.org

**★ 7529 ★ NYSARC, Inc.**
**Montgomery County Chapter**
Rte. 55
PO Box 639
Amsterdam, NY 12010
**Phone:** (518)842-5080

**★ 7530 ★ NYSARC, Inc.**
**Oneida-Lewis Chapter**
245 Genesee St.
Utica, NY 13501
**Phone:** (315)738-1366

**Website:** http://www.thearcolc.org

**★ 7531 ★ NYSARC, Inc.**
**Steuben Chapter**
6838 Industrial Park Rd.
Bath, NY 14810-8315
**Phone:** (607)776-4146
**Email:** steubenarc1@infoblvd.net
**Website:** http://www.steubenarc.com

**★ 7532 ★ NYSARC, Inc.**
**Yates County Chapter**
235 North Ave.
Penn Yan, NY 14527
**Phone:** (315)536-7447

### North Carolina

**★ 7533 ★ The Arc of Alamance County, Inc.**
PO Box 1275
Burlington, NC 27215
**Phone:** (336)438-2040
**Email:** thearcal@netpath.net
**Website:** http://www.netpath.net/%7Ethearcal/

**★ 7534 ★ The Arc of Beaufort County Inc.**
1534 W 5th St.
Washington, NC 27889
**Phone:** (252)946-0151

**★ 7535 ★ The Arc of Brunswick County**
PO Box 806
Supply, NC 28462

**★ 7536 ★ The Arc of Buncombe County**
PO Box 1365
Asheville, NC 28802
**Phone:** (704)253-1255

**★ 7537 ★ The Arc of Cabarrus County**
PO Box 1367
Concord, NC 28026-1367
**Phone:** (704)788-1616
**Email:** arccabarrus@ctc.net
**Website:** http://www.arcnc.org/cabarrus

**★ 7538 ★ The Arc of Cherokee-Clay Inc.**
PO Box 156
Murphy, NC 28906
**Phone:** (828)837-7874

**★ 7539 ★ The Arc of Craven County**
PO Box 12211
New Bern, NC 28562

**★ 7540 ★ The Arc of Cumberland County**
3623 Sycamore Dairy Rd.
Fayetteville, NC 28303
**Phone:** (910)867-2141
**Email:** ArcCumberland@aol.com
**Website:** http://www.disabilityresourcecenter.net

**★ 7541 ★ The Arc of Davidson County**
6 Vance Circle
Lexington, NC 27292
**Phone:** (704)246-2842

**★ 7542 ★ The Arc of Durham County**
3500 Westgate Dr., Ste 303
Durham, NC 27707
**Phone:** (919)493-8141
**Email:** thearcdc@mindspring.com
**Website:** http://www.arcnc.org/durham

**★ 7543 ★ The Arc of Forsyth County**
4265 Brownsboro Rd., Ste. 100
Winston-Salem, NC 27106-3425
**Phone:** (336)759-9619

**★ 7544 ★ The Arc of Greensboro, Inc.**
207-M S Westgate Dr.
Greensboro, NC 27407
**Phone:** (336)373-1076

**★ 7545 ★ The Arc of Halifax County**
PO Box 921
Littleton, NC 27850
**Phone:** (919)445-3378

**★ 7546 ★ The Arc of Harnett County**
PO Box 42
Buies Creek, NC 27506

**★ 7547 ★ The Arc of Haywood County, Inc.**
PO Box 832
Waynesville, NC 28786

**★ 7548 ★ The Arc of High Point**
153 E Bellevue Dr.
High Point, NC 27265
**Phone:** (336)883-0650
**Website:** http://www.arc-of-hp.com

**★ 7549 ★ The Arc of Iredell County**
328 Grant Rd.
Statesville, NC 28677
**Phone:** (704)873-2101

**★ 7550 ★ The Arc of Jackson County**
1262 Locust Creek Rd.
Sylva, NC 28779

**★ 7551 ★ The Arc of Lee County**
PO Box 4941
Sanford, NC 27331
**Phone:** (919)718-9122

**★ 7552 ★ The Arc of Lenoir County**
PO Box 1677
Kinston, NC 28503
**Phone:** (252)522-2814

**★ 7553 ★ The Arc of Lincoln County**
227 E Water St.
Lincolnton, NC 28092

**★ 7554 ★ The Arc of Mecklenburg County, Inc.**
5601 Executive Center Dr., No. 106
Charlotte, NC 28212
**Phone:** (704)535-4289
**Website:** http://www.homestead.com/arcmeck

**★ 7555 ★ The Arc of Montgomery County**
694 Horseshoe Bend Rd.
Troy, NC 27371
**Phone:** (910)428-4298

**★ 7556 ★ The Arc of Moore County**
PO Box 773
Southern Pines, NC 28387
**Phone:** 800-909-9272

**★ 7557 ★ The Arc of North Carolina**
4200 Six Forks Rd.
Raleigh, NC 27609

**Phone:** (919)782-4632    **Free:** 800-662-8706
**Fax:** (919)782-4634
**Email:** Rsewell108@aol.com
**Website:** http://www.arcnc.org

**★ 7558 ★ The Arc of Onslow Advocacy for Special Needs**
201 Taylor Notion Rd.
Cape Carteret, NC 28584
**Phone:** (252)393-4414

**★ 7559 ★ The Arc of Orange County**
PO Box 2594
Chapel Hill, NC 27515-2594
**Phone:** (919)942-5119
**Website:** http://www.arcoforange.org

**★ 7560 ★ The Arc of Person County**
PO Box 1182
Roxboro, NC 27573-1182

**★ 7561 ★ The Arc of Pitt County**
609-A Country Club Dr.
Greenville, NC 27834-6210
**Phone:** (919)756-1056

**★ 7562 ★ The Arc of Robeson County**
116 W 8th St.
Lumberton, NC 28359

**★ 7563 ★ The Arc of Rockingham County**
568 Glovenia St.
Eden, NC 27288

**★ 7564 ★ The Arc of Rocky Mount**
1230 Beal St.
Rocky Mount, NC 27804

**★ 7565 ★ The Arc of Rowan County**
1918 W Innes St.
Salisbury, NC 28144
**Phone:** (704)637-1521

**★ 7566 ★ The Arc of Stanly County**
PO Box 2448
Albemarle, NC 28002-2448
**Phone:** (704)983-3911
**Website:** http://www.arcofstanlync.org

**★ 7567 ★ The Arc of Stokes County**
221 Whispering Creek Dr.
King, NC 27021
**Phone:** (910)773-4166

**★ 7568 ★ The Arc of Surry County**
Rte. 1, Box 528
Dobson, NC 27017

**★ 7569 ★ The Arc of Union County**
102 E Franklin St.
Monroe, NC 28112
**Phone:** (704)283-1537

**★ 7570 ★ The Arc of Vance County**
2550 Flemingtown Rd.
Henderson, NC 27536

**★ 7571 ★ The Arc of Wake County, Inc.**
401 Oberlin Rd., Ste. 225
Raleigh, NC 27605
**Phone:** (919)832-2660

**★ 7572 ★ The Arc of Wilson County**
PO Box 3943
Wilson, NC 27895-3943
**Phone:** (252)237-8266

**★ 7573 ★ The Arc of Yadkin County**
PO Box 233
East Bend, NC 27018

**★ 7574 ★ Columbus Arc, Inc.**
777 Vinson Blvd.
Whiteville, NC 28472

**★ 7575 ★ Davie County Arc, Inc.**
PO Box 291
Mocksville, NC 27028

**★ 7576 ★ Gaston County Arc, Inc.**
200 E Franklin Blvd.
Gastonia, NC 28052
**Phone:** (704)861-1036

**★ 7577 ★ Scotland County Association for Retarded Citizens**
1028 Elizabeth Dr.
Laurinburg, NC 28352

## North Dakota

**★ 7578 ★ The Arc of Barnes County**
141 2nd St. NE
Valley City, ND 58072

**★ 7579 ★ The Arc of Bismarck**
1211 Park Ave.
Bismarck, ND 58504
**Phone:** (701)222-1854

**★ 7580 ★ The Arc of Cass County**
2533 S University Dr.
PO Box 6461
Fargo, ND 58109-6461
**Phone:** (701)293-8191
**Email:** arccassnd@aol.com
**Website:** http://www.arccassnd.com

**★ 7581 ★ The Arc of Little Missouri**
608 1st St. NW
Bowman, ND 58623

**★ 7582 ★ The Arc of North Dakota, Inc.**
c/o The Arc, Upper Valley
PO Box 12420
Grand Forks, ND 58208-2420
**Phone:** (701)772-6191    **Free:** 877-250-2022

**★ 7583 ★ The Arc of Stutsman County, Inc.**
PO Box 1646
Jamestown, ND 58401

**★ 7584 ★ The Arc, Upper Valley, Inc.**
2500 Demers Ave.
PO Box 12420
Grand Forks, ND 58208-2420
**Phone:** (701)772-6191    **Free:** 877-250-2022
**Website:** http://www.thearcuppervalley.com

**★ 7585 ★ Dickinson Area Arc, Inc.**
PO Box 1421
Dickinson, ND 58601
**Phone:** (701)264-7828

## Ohio

★ 7586 ★ **The Arc of Allen County**
546 S Collett
Lima, OH 45805
**Phone:** (419)225-6285

★ 7587 ★ **The Arc of Ashtabula County**
1120 Rte. 167
Jefferson, OH 44047

★ 7588 ★ **The Arc of Auglaize County**
428 W Haven Dr.
New Bremen, OH 45869
**Phone:** (419)629-2419

★ 7589 ★ **The Arc of Butler County**
5645 Liberty Fairfield Rd.
Hamilton, OH 45011
**Phone:** (513)863-3735

★ 7590 ★ **The Arc of Clark County**
PO Box 3011
Springfield, OH 45501
**Phone:** (513)323-3755

★ 7591 ★ **The Arc of Clermont/Brown Counties**
1075 Ohio Pike
Withamsville, OH 45245
**Phone:** (513)752-4330
**Email:** thearccb@aol.com
**Website:** http://www.thearc-cb.org

★ 7592 ★ **The Arc of Erie County**
The Kaleidoscope Ctr.
4405 Galloway Rd., No. 112
Sandusky, OH 44870
**Phone:** (419)625-9677
**Email:** arc@arcoferiecounty.linkohio.com
**Website:** http://arcoferiecounty.linkohio.com

★ 7593 ★ **The Arc of Geauga, Inc.**
12843 Opalocka
Chesterland, OH 44026

★ 7594 ★ **The Arc of Hamilton County**
1821 Summit Rd., No. 30
Cincinnati, OH 45237-2187
**Phone:** (513)821-2113

★ 7595 ★ **The Arc of Knox County**
600 N Fay St.
Mount Vernon, OH 43050

★ 7596 ★ **The Arc of Licking County**
175 S William St.
Newark, OH 43055
**Phone:** (740)345-9793

★ 7597 ★ **The Arc of Lucas County**
1 Stranahan Sq., No. 540
Toledo, OH 43604
**Phone:** (419)242-9587

★ 7598 ★ **The Arc of Mercer County**
372 E Main
PO Box 413
Saint Henry, OH 45883

★ 7599 ★ **The Arc of Miami County**
204 E Franklin St.
Troy, OH 45373
**Phone:** (513)339-6222

★ 7600 ★ **The Arc of Ohio**
1335 Dublin Rd., Ste. 205C
Columbus, OH 43212
**Phone:** (614)487-4720          **Free:** 800-875-2723
**Fax:** (614)487-4725
**Email:** TheArcOhio@aol.com
**Website:** http://www.thearcofohio.org
Gary Tonks, Exec Director

★ 7601 ★ **The Arc of Ottawa County**
1 Stranahan Sq., No. 540
Toledo, OH 43604-1900

★ 7602 ★ **The Arc of Shelby County**
PO Box 925
Sidney, OH 45365

★ 7603 ★ **The Arc of Stark County**
Belden Village Tower
4450 Belden Village St. NW, No. 503
Canton, OH 44718-2564
**Phone:** (330)492-5225

★ 7604 ★ **The Arc of Summit and Portage Counties**
90 N Prospect St.
Akron, OH 44304
**Phone:** (330)374-1594
**Email:** ArcSCPC@worldnet.att.net
**Website:** http://www.arcsummitportage.org

★ 7605 ★ **The Arc of Warren County**
3023 Ash Ct.
Mason, OH 45040
**Phone:** (513)763-2879

★ 7606 ★ **The Arc of Washington County**
PO Box 1003
Marietta, OH 45750

★ 7607 ★ **The Arc of Wood County**
PO Box 264
Bowling Green, OH 43402
**Phone:** (419)353-1099

★ 7608 ★ **Center for Mental Retardation**
1621 Euclid Ave., Ste. 802
Cleveland, OH 44115-2107
**Phone:** (216)621-4504

★ 7609 ★ **Mahoning County Council for Retarded Citizens**
3024 Center Rd., Rte. 224
Poland, OH 44514
**Phone:** (330)707-1134

★ 7610 ★ **Society for the Handicapped of Medina County**
4283 Paradise Rd.
Seville, OH 44273
**Phone:** (330)725-7041

## Oklahoma

★ 7611 ★ **The Arc of Edmond**
PO Box 268
Edmond, OK 73083
**Phone:** (405)341-7132

★ 7612 ★ **The Arc of Oklahoma**
2442 N Walnut Ave., Ste. D
Oklahoma City, OK 73105
**Phone:** (405)528-1525

★ 7613 ★ **Homelife Association**
PO Box 35903
Tulsa, OK 74153-0903
**Phone:** (918)745-1114

★ 7614 ★ **Tulsa Advocates for the Rights of Citizens with Developmental Disabilities**
16 E 16th St., Ste. 405
Tulsa, OK 74119
**Phone:** (918)582-8272

## Oregon

★ 7615 ★ **The Arc of Benton County**
Plaza 9 Shopping Ctr.
1885 NW 9th St.
Corvallis, OR 97330
**Phone:** (541)753-1711
**Email:** info@arcbenton.org
**Website:** http://www.arcbenton.org
Karin Frederick, Exec Director

★ 7616 ★ **The Arc of Douglas County**
PO Box 694
Roseburg, OR 97470
**Phone:** (541)672-5208

★ 7617 ★ **The Arc of Eastern Oregon**
PO Box 1393
Ontario, OR 97914
**Phone:** (541)889-2651

★ 7618 ★ **The Arc of Jackson County**
PO Box 1485
Medford, OR 97501
**Phone:** (541)779-4520

★ 7619 ★ **The Arc of Josephine County**
PO Box 54
Grants Pass, OR 97526
**Phone:** (541)479-0301

★ 7620 ★ **The Arc of Lane County**
2710 Taylor
Eugene, OR 97403
**Phone:** (541)343-5256
**Website:** http://www.arclane.org

★ 7621 ★ **The Arc of Linn County**
PO Box 577
Lebanon, OR 97355
**Phone:** (541)259-5528

★ 7622 ★ **The Arc of Marion County**
PO Box 12474
Salem, OR 97309
**Phone:** (503)581-3451

★ 7623 ★ **The Arc of Multnomah County**
619 SW 11th Ave., Ste. 234
Portland, OR 97205-2692
**Phone:** (503)223-7279
**Website:** http://www.thearcmult.org

★ 7624 ★ **The Arc of Oregon**
1745 State St.
Salem, OR 97301
**Phone:** (503)581-2726          **Free:** 877-581-2726
**Fax:** (503)363-7168
**Email:** arcoforg@CallAtg.com
**Website:** http://www.open.org/arcoforg

★ 7625 ★ **The Arc of Polk**
9990 Oak Hill Rd.
Independence, OR 97351

**★ 7626 ★ The Arc of Tillamook County**
2410 5th St.
PO Box 416
Tillamook, OR 97141

**★ 7627 ★ The Arc of Umatilla County**
215 W Orchard Ave.
Hermiston, OR 97838-1738
**Phone:** (541)567-7615

**★ 7628 ★ The Arc of Washington County**
PO Box 5778
Aloha, OR 97006-5778
**Phone:** (503)649-6110

**★ 7629 ★ Central Oregon Arc, Inc.**
2050 Bluebird Ln.
Bend, OR 97701

**★ 7630 ★ Jackson County Family
Consortium**
2535 Griffin Creek Rd.
Medford, OR 97501-4219

**★ 7631 ★ Residential Assistance
Program**
2050 NE Bluebird Ct.
Bend, OR 97701
**Phone:** (541)388-3060

**★ 7632 ★ Share House, Inc.**
3761 Kinciad St.
Eugene, OR 97405
**Phone:** (541)485-4330

**★ 7633 ★ Specialized Housing, Inc.**
5319 SW Westgate Dr., No. 124
Portland, OR 97221
**Phone:** (503)292-5066

### Pennsylvania

**★ 7634 ★ Achieva**
711 Bingham St.
Pittsburgh, PA 15203
**Phone:** (412)995-5000      **Free:** 888-272-7229
**Fax:** (412)995-5001
**Email:** contact@achieva.info
**Website:** http://www.achieva.info
**Frmly:** Arc Allegheny.

**★ 7635 ★ The Arc of Adams County**
17 Rice Ave.
PO Box 551
Biglerville, PA 17307
**Phone:** (717)677-8487

**★ 7636 ★ The Arc of Beaver County**
Beaver Valley Professional Bldg., No. 103
1260 N Broadhead Rd.
Monaca, PA 15061
**Phone:** (724)775-1602

**★ 7637 ★ The Arc of Berks County**
1829 New Holland Rd., Ste. 9
Reading, PA 19607-2228
**Phone:** (610)603-0227

**★ 7638 ★ The Arc of Blair County**
431 Jackson Ave.
Altoona, PA 16602
**Phone:** (814)946-1011

**★ 7639 ★ The Arc of Bucks County, Inc.**
PO Box 755
Newtown, PA 18940-0755
**Phone:** (215)295-3848

**★ 7640 ★ The Arc of Butler County**
100 N Washington St.
Butler, PA 16001
**Phone:** (724)282-1500

**★ 7641 ★ The Arc of Cambria County**
960 Bedford St.
Johnstown, PA 15902
**Phone:** (814)535-1511

**★ 7642 ★ The Arc of Centre County**
1840 N Atherton St.
State College, PA 16803
**Phone:** (814)238-1444
**Website:** http://centreconnect.org/arc

**★ 7643 ★ The Arc of Chester County**
900 Lawrence Dr.
West Chester, PA 19380
**Phone:** (610)696-8090      **Fax:** (610)696-8300
**Email:** info@arcofchestercounty.org
**Website:** http://www.arcofchestercounty.org
Diane Carey, Exec Director

**★ 7644 ★ The Arc of Crawford County**
222 Chestnut St.
Meadville, PA 16335
**Phone:** (814)724-7346

**★ 7645 ★ The Arc of Cumberland/Perry
Counties**
117 N Hanover St.
PO Box 386
Carlisle, PA 17013
**Phone:** (717)249-2611

**★ 7646 ★ The Arc of Dauphin and
Lebanon Counties**
4309 Linglestown Rd., Ste. 114E
Harrisburg, PA 17112
**Phone:** (717)540-5800
**Email:** arcofdc@paonline.com
**Website:** http://www.arcofdc.org

**★ 7647 ★ The Arc of Elk County**
507 Arch St.
Saint Marys, PA 15857
**Phone:** (814)834-7851

**★ 7648 ★ The Arc of Erie County**
18 Hess Ave.
Erie, PA 16507
**Phone:** (814)452-4865

**★ 7649 ★ The Arc of Fayette County**
80 Old New Salem Rd.
Uniontown, PA 15401
**Phone:** (724)438-9042

**★ 7650 ★ The Arc of Franklin/Fulton**
Financial Trust Bldg., Ste. 218
Chambersburg, PA 17201
**Phone:** (717)264-4390

**★ 7651 ★ The Arc of Indiana County**
720 Church St.
Indiana, PA 15701
**Phone:** (724)349-8230

**★ 7652 ★ The Arc of Jefferson County**
RD 2, Box 513
Brockway, PA 15824

**★ 7653 ★ The Arc of Juniata County**
22 Cross St.
Mifflintown, PA 17059
**Phone:** (717)436-8827

**★ 7654 ★ The Arc of Lackawanna
County**
115 Meadow Ave.
Scranton, PA 18508
**Phone:** (570)346-4010
**Email:** arclacka@intergrafix.net
**Website:** http://www.geocities.com/Heartland/Acres/
6855/homepagearc.html

**★ 7655 ★ The Arc of Lancaster County**
630 Janet Ave.
Lancaster, PA 17601
**Phone:** (717)394-5251

**★ 7656 ★ The Arc of Lehigh and
Northampton Counties Inc.**
1036 N Godfrey St.
Allentown, PA 18103
**Phone:** (610)434-8076
**Email:** thearc@ptd.net
**Website:** http://www.arcofl-n.org

**★ 7657 ★ The Arc of Luzerne County**
New Bridge Ctr.
480 Pierce St., Ste. 307
Kingston, PA 18704
**Phone:** (570)714-6320

**★ 7658 ★ The Arc of Lycoming County**
329 ½ Stanton St.
Williamsport, PA 17701
**Phone:** (570)326-6997

**★ 7659 ★ The Arc of Mercer County**
850 Hermitage Rd.
PO Box 1069
Hermitage, PA 16148
**Phone:** (724)981-2950
**Email:** shassel@mercerarc.org
**Website:** http://www.nauticom.net/www/mcar/

**★ 7660 ★ The Arc of Montgomery
County**
Continental Plaza
1010 W 9th Ave.
King of Prussia, PA 19406
**Phone:** (610)265-4700
**Email:** owensmj@aol.com
**Website:** http://marcpa.org

**★ 7661 ★ The Arc of Northumberland
County**
622 W Walnut St.
Shamokin, PA 17872
**Phone:** (570)648-2871

**★ 7662 ★ The Arc—Pennsylvania**
Bldg. No. 2, Ste. 221
2001 N Front St.
Harrisburg, PA 17102
**Phone:** (717)234-2621
**Website:** http://www.thearcpa.org

**★ 7663 ★ The Arc of Philadelphia**
2350 W Westmoreland St.
Philadelphia, PA 19140
**Phone:** (215)229-4550
**Email:** info@arcpddc.org

**Website:** http://www.arcpddc.org

★ **7664** ★ **The Arc of Pike County**
c/o Pike Area Agency on Aging
150 Pike County Blvd.
Hawley, PA 18428
**Phone:** (570)686-3656

★ **7665** ★ **The Arc of Schuylkill County**
143 Steins Rd.
Ashland, PA 17921

★ **7666** ★ **The Arc of Warren/Forest Counties**
PO Box 244
Warren, PA 16365
**Phone:** (814)723-8531

★ **7667** ★ **The Arc of Washington County**
PO Box 385
Meadow Lands, PA 15347
**Phone:** (724)222-6960
**Website:** http://www.thearcofwashpa.com

★ **7668** ★ **The Arc of Wayne County**
PO Box 1121
Honesdale, PA 18431

★ **7669** ★ **The Arc of Westmoreland**
Donohoe Rd.
RD 12, Box 227
Greensburg, PA 15601
**Phone:** (724)837-8159

★ **7670** ★ **The Arc of Wyoming County**
86 E Tioga St.
PO Box 338
Tunkhannock, PA 18657
**Phone:** (570)836-4001

★ **7671** ★ **The Arc of York County**
1803 Mount Rose Ave., Ste. C1
York, PA 17403
**Phone:** (717)846-6589

★ **7672** ★ **Greene Arc, Inc.**
RD 2, Box 107
Prosperity, PA 15329
**Phone:** (724)627-5511

★ **7673** ★ **PARC**
**Armstrong County Chapter**
309 Market St.
Kittanning, PA 16201
**Phone:** (724)545-3426

## Rhode Island

★ **7674** ★ **The Arc of Bristol County**
PO Box 711
Bristol, RI 02809
**Phone:** (401)253-5900

★ **7675** ★ **The Arc/Down Syndrome Society of Rhode Island**
99 Bald Hill Rd.
Cranston, RI 02920
**Phone:** (401)463-5751

★ **7676** ★ **The Arc of Greater Providence**
220 Woonasquatucket Ave.
North Providence, RI 02911
**Phone:** (401)353-7000

★ **7677** ★ **The Arc of Newport County**
PO Box 4390
Middletown, RI 02842
**Phone:** (401)846-4600

★ **7678** ★ **The Arc of Northern Rhode Island**
320 Main St.
Woonsocket, RI 02895
**Phone:** (401)765-3700

★ **7679** ★ **The Arc of South County**
24 Salt Pond Rd., Bldg G3
Wakefield, RI 02879
**Phone:** (401)789-4386

★ **7680** ★ **Cranston Arc, Inc.**
905 Pontiac Ave.
Cranston, RI 02920
**Phone:** (401)941-1112
**Website:** http://www.cranstonarc.org

★ **7681** ★ **Rhode Island Arc**
99 Bald Hill Rd.
Cranston, RI 02920
**Phone:** (401)463-9191

★ **7682** ★ **Rhode Island Arc Blackstone Valley Chapter**
115 Manton St.
Pawtucket, RI 02861
**Phone:** (401)727-0150
**Email:** contact@bvcriarc.org
**Website:** http://www.bvcriarc.org

★ **7683** ★ **Rhode Island Arc Kent County Chapter**
3445 Post Rd.
Warwick, RI 02886
**Phone:** (401)739-2700
**Website:** http://www.kentcountyarc.org

★ **7684** ★ **Rhode Island Arc Westerly Chariho Chapter**
93 Airport Rd.
Westerly, RI 02891
**Phone:** (401)596-2091
**Email:** info@oleancenter.org
**Website:** http://www.oleancenter.org

## South Carolina

★ **7685** ★ **The Arc of Anderson**
1105 Hanover Rd.
Anderson, SC 29621

★ **7686** ★ **The Arc of Cherokee County**
PO Box 397
Gaffney, SC 29342

★ **7687** ★ **The Arc of Horry County**
PO Box 1628
250 Victory Ln.
Conway, SC 29526
**Phone:** (843)347-0261

★ **7688** ★ **The Arc of the Midlands**
PO Box 8707
Columbia, SC 29202
**Phone:** (803)935-5266

★ **7689** ★ **The Arc of Pickens County**
PO Box 1308
Easley, SC 29641
**Phone:** (864)859-5416

★ **7690** ★ **The Arc of South Carolina**
PO Box 8707
Columbia, SC 29202
**Phone:** (803)935-5266        **Free:** (866)300-9331
**Email:** TheARCSC@arcsc.org
**Website:** http://www.arcsc.org

## South Dakota

★ **7691** ★ **The Arc of Brown County**
13084 385th Ave.
Aberdeen, SD 57401

★ **7692** ★ **The Arc of Grant County**
310 W 6th Ave.
Milbank, SD 57252

★ **7693** ★ **The Arc of Kampeska**
710 2nd St. NE
Watertown, SD 57201

★ **7694** ★ **The Arc of Lake County**
Box 450
Madison, SD 57042

★ **7695** ★ **The Arc of Lyman-Brule**
HCR 69, Box 42
Chamberlain, SD 57325

★ **7696** ★ **The Arc of Mid-Dakota**
RR 1, Box 215
Cavour, SD 57324

★ **7697** ★ **The Arc of Oahe Chapter**
PO Box 503
Pierre, SD 57501
**Phone:** (605)224-4501

★ **7698** ★ **The Arc of South Dakota**
708 SW 7th
PO Box 450
Pierre, SD 57501-0220
**Phone:** (605)224-8211

★ **7699** ★ **East Central Arc**
1800 Ohio Dr.
Brookings, SD 57006

★ **7700** ★ **Sioux Arc**
2308 S 1st Ave.
Sioux Falls, SD 57105

## Tennessee

★ **7701** ★ **Advocacy and Resources Corp.**
453 Gould Dr.
Cookeville, TN 38506
**Phone:** (931)432-5981
**Email:** arc@arcdiversified.com
**Website:** http://www.arcdiversified.com
**Frmly:** The Arc of Putnam County.

★ **7702** ★ **The Arc of Anderson County**
PO Box 4823
Oak Ridge, TN 37831-4823
**Phone:** (865)481-0550

★ **7703** ★ **The Arc of Claiborne County**
Box 538
Tazewell, TN 37879
**Phone:** (423)626-6757

★ **7704** ★ **The Arc of Coffee-Moore County**
PO Box 1146
Tullahoma, TN 37388-1146
**Phone:** (931)759-4344

★ **7705** ★ **The Arc of Cumberland County**
PO Box 389
Crossville, TN 38557
**Phone:** (931)456-0206

★ **7706** ★ **The Arc of Davidson County**
1207 17th Ave. S, No. 100
Nashville, TN 37212
**Phone:** (615)321-5699

★ **7707** ★ **The Arc of Hamblen County**
PO Box 1793
Morristown, TN 37813
**Phone:** (423)581-1092

★ **7708** ★ **The Arc of Hamilton County, Inc.**
4613 Brainerd Rd.
Chattanooga, TN 37411
**Phone:** (423)624-6887
**Email:** arc@hamilton.theinbox.org
**Website:** http://www.geocities.com/localarc2001

★ **7709** ★ **The Arc of Hickman County**
571 Hurricane Branch Rd.
Pleasantville, TN 37147
**Phone:** (931)729-9625

★ **7710** ★ **The Arc of Knox County**
3000 N Central
Knoxville, TN 37914
**Phone:** (423)524-1311

★ **7711** ★ **The Arc of Lincoln County**
73 Prospect Rd.
Fayetteville, TN 37334
**Phone:** (931)433-7333

★ **7712** ★ **The Arc of Marshall County**
715 Fairlane Dr.
Lewisburg, TN 37091
**Phone:** (931)359-3125

★ **7713** ★ **The Arc of Montgomery County**
PO Box 2145
Clarksville, TN 37042
**Phone:** (931)905-0900

★ **7714** ★ **The Arc of Obion County**
4301 Mt. Zion Rd.
Union City, TN 38261
**Phone:** (901)885-5323

★ **7715** ★ **The Arc of Sullivan County**
400 Shelby St.
Box 100, People Pl.
Bristol, TN 37620
**Phone:** (423)652-1899

★ **7716** ★ **The Arc of Tennessee**
44 Vantage Way, Ste. 550
Nashville, TN 37228
**Phone:** (615)248-5878　　**Free:** 800-835-7077
**Email:** arctn@worldnet.att.net
**Website:** http://www.thearctn.org

★ **7717** ★ **The Arc of Warren County**
71 Flood Rd.
McMinnville, TN 37110
**Phone:** (931)668-3710

★ **7718** ★ **The Arc of Washington County**
2700 S Roan St., Ste. 300B
Johnson City, TN 37601
**Phone:** (423)928-9362

★ **7719** ★ **The Arc of Wayne County**
RR 1, Box 282-D
Collinwood, TN 38450

★ **7720** ★ **The Arc of Williamson County**
129 W Fowlkes St., Ste. 151
Franklin, TN 37064
**Phone:** (615)790-5815

★ **7721** ★ **Mid-South Arc**
3485 Poplar Ave., No. 225
Memphis, TN 38111
**Phone:** (901)327-2473

## Texas

★ **7722** ★ **The Arc**
PO Box 1484
Alvin, TX 77512
**Phone:** (281)388-1161

★ **7723** ★ **The Arc of Anderson and Cherokee Counties**
Rte. 8, Box 129
Jacksonville, TX 75766
**Phone:** (903)586-6150

★ **7724** ★ **The Arc of the Bay Area**
2704 Northern
League City, TX 77573
**Phone:** (281)484-7447

★ **7725** ★ **The Arc of Baytown**
5416 Shepard Rd.
PO Box 1085
Baytown, TX 77521

★ **7726** ★ **The Arc of Bell County**
PO Box 311
Temple, TX 76503

★ **7727** ★ **The Arc of the Big Country**
1021 Wolf Rd.
Abilene, TX 79602
**Phone:** (915)793-3500

★ **7728** ★ **The Arc of Bluebonnet Circle**
PO Box 1842
Brenham, TX 77833
**Phone:** (409)836-1002

★ **7729** ★ **The Arc of Brown County**
PO Box 1201
Brownwood, TX 76801
**Phone:** (915)543-5822

★ **7730** ★ **The Arc of Bryan-College Station**
2518 Dartmouth
College Station, TX 77840
**Phone:** (409)693-0812

★ **7731** ★ **The Arc of Calhoun County**
11 Pecan Dr.
Port Lavaca, TX 77979

**Phone:** (512)552-9403

★ **7732** ★ **The Arc of the Capital Area**
2818 San Gabriel
Austin, TX 78705
**Phone:** (512)476-7044　　**Fax:** (512)476-9054
**Email:** info@arcofthecapitalarea.org
**Website:** http://www.arcofthecapitalarea.org

★ **7733** ★ **The Arc of Cypress Creek**
PO Box 11123
Spring, TX 77391-1123
**Phone:** (281)376-7072

★ **7734** ★ **The Arc of Dallas**
2114 Anson Rd.
Dallas, TX 75235
**Phone:** (214)634-9810
**Email:** info@arcdallas.org
**Website:** http://www.arcdallas.org

★ **7735** ★ **The Arc of Denton County**
PO Box 1279
Denton, TX 76202
**Phone:** (972)436-8471

★ **7736** ★ **The Arc of East Texas**
Rte. 9, Box 1900
Lufkin, TX 75901
**Phone:** (409)632-7944

★ **7737** ★ **The Arc of Ector County**
PO Box 13023
Odessa, TX 79768-3023
**Phone:** (915)362-2702

★ **7738** ★ **The Arc of El Campo**
PO Box 227
El Campo, TX 77437

★ **7739** ★ **The Arc of Fort Bend County**
3660 Glen Lakes Dr.
Missouri City, TX 77459
**Phone:** (281)499-2234
**Website:** http://www.arcoffortbend.org

★ **7740** ★ **The Arc of Gillespie County**
PO Box 770
Fredericksburg, TX 78624
**Phone:** (830)997-7163

★ **7741** ★ **The Arc of Greater Corpus Christi**
PO Box 72713
Corpus Christi, TX 78472-0713
**Phone:** (512)886-6900

★ **7742** ★ **The Arc of Greater Houston**
PO Box 924168
Houston, TX 77292-4168
**Phone:** (713)957-1600

★ **7743** ★ **The Arc of Greater Tarrant County**
259 Bailey Ave., Ste. A
Fort Worth, TX 76107
**Phone:** (817)877-1474

★ **7744** ★ **The Arc of Gregg County**
PO Box 522
Longview, TX 75606
**Phone:** (903)753-8773

**★ 7745 ★ The Arc of Hopkins County**
PO Box 1215
Sulphur Springs, TX 75482

**★ 7746 ★ The Arc of Howard County**
514 Westover Rd.
Big Spring, TX 79720
**Phone:** (915)264-5095

**★ 7747 ★ The Arc of Hunt County**
2603 Templeton St.
Greenville, TX 75401
**Phone:** (903)454-9170

**★ 7748 ★ The Arc of Katy**
PO Box 1106
Katy, TX 77492-1106

**★ 7749 ★ The Arc of Kerrville**
4800 Goat Creek Rd.
Kerrville, TX 78028

**★ 7750 ★ The Arc of Madison-Leon County**
Rte. 2, Box 162
Midway, TX 75852

**★ 7751 ★ The Arc of Marshall**
PO Box 24
Marshall, TX 75671

**★ 7752 ★ The Arc of Matagorda County**
4101 Holly Glen
Bay City, TX 77414
**Phone:** (409)245-6318

**★ 7753 ★ The Arc of McLennan County**
PO Box 3367
Waco, TX 76707
**Phone:** (254)756-7491

**★ 7754 ★ The Arc of Midland**
2701 N "A" St.
Midland, TX 79705
**Phone:** (915)498-8590
**Email:** brose@arcmidlandtx.org
**Website:** http://www.arcmidlandtx.org
Robert K. Rose, Exec Director

**★ 7755 ★ The Arc of Milam**
1705 Pakus St.
Rockdale, TX 76567

**★ 7756 ★ The Arc of Northeast Tarrant County**
PO Box 14455
Fort Worth, TX 76117
**Phone:** (817)834-7700

**★ 7757 ★ The Arc of Panola County**
102 N Shelby
Carthage, TX 75633
**Phone:** (903)693-4230

**★ 7758 ★ The Arc of Plano**
PO Box 260727
Plano, TX 75026
**Phone:** (972)682-9044

**★ 7759 ★ The Arc of Potter and Randall Counties**
202 S Louisiana
Amarillo, TX 79106
**Phone:** (806)372-5699

**★ 7760 ★ The Arc of San Angelo**
PO Box 1922
San Angelo, TX 76902
**Phone:** (915)655-3205

**★ 7761 ★ The Arc of San Antonio**
13430 West Ave.
San Antonio, TX 78216
**Phone:** (210)490-4300

**★ 7762 ★ The Arc of Scurry County**
PO Box 105
Snyder, TX 79550
**Phone:** (915)573-5610

**★ 7763 ★ The Arc of Spring Branch/ Memorial**
9524 Kempwood
Houston, TX 77080
**Phone:** (713)460-4274

**★ 7764 ★ The Arc of Texas**
1600 W 38th St., Ste. 200
Austin, TX 78731
**Phone:** (512)454-6694  **Free:** 800-252-9729
**Fax:** (512)454-4956
**Email:** secretary@thearcoftexas.org
**Website:** http://www.thearcoftexas.org

**★ 7765 ★ The Arc of Texoma**
223 N Walnut
Sherman, TX 75090
**Phone:** (903)892-6102

**★ 7766 ★ The Arc of Tyler**
810 Vine Heights
Tyler, TX 75701
**Phone:** (903)597-0995

**★ 7767 ★ The Arc of Wharton**
1017 ½ Alabama Rd.
Wharton, TX 77488
**Phone:** (409)282-9200

**★ 7768 ★ The Arc of Wichita County**
3307 Buchanan
Wichita Falls, TX 76308
**Phone:** (940)692-2303

## Utah

**★ 7769 ★ The Arc of Cache**
426 East 500 South
River Heights, UT 84321

**★ 7770 ★ The Arc of Davis County**
811 South 500 West, No. 105
Bountiful, UT 84010

**★ 7771 ★ The Arc of Morgan County**
PO Box 597
Morgan, UT 84050

**★ 7772 ★ The Arc of Salt Lake**
2595 East 3300 South, Ste. 360
Salt Lake City, UT 84109
**Phone:** (801)412-3798

**★ 7773 ★ The Arc of Utah**
455 East 400 South, Ste. 202
Salt Lake City, UT 84111
**Phone:** (801)364-5060
**Email:** Arcutah@burgoyne.com

**★ 7774 ★ The Arc of Utah County**
687 West 1800 North
Provo, UT 84604

**★ 7775 ★ The Arc of Washington County**
334 W Tabernacle, Unit H
Saint George, UT 84770
**Phone:** (801)673-5251

## Virginia

**★ 7776 ★ The Arc of Augusta**
1025 Fairfax Ave.
PO Box 102
Waynesboro, VA 22980
**Phone:** (540)943-1618

**★ 7777 ★ The Arc of the Blue Ridge**
PO Box 1401
Culpeper, VA 22701
**Phone:** (540)439-3505

**★ 7778 ★ The Arc of Central Virginia**
1508 Bedford Ave.
Lynchburg, VA 24504
**Phone:** (804)845-4071

**★ 7779 ★ The Arc of the Eastern Shore**
PO Box 626
Exmore, VA 23350
**Phone:** (757)442-3933

**★ 7780 ★ The Arc of Greater Prince William/Insight, Inc.**
13505 Hillendale Dr.
Woodbridge, VA 22193
**Phone:** (703)670-4800
**Email:** info@arcgpw.org
**Website:** http://www.arcgpw.org

**★ 7781 ★ The Arc of Greater Williamsburg**
202D Packets Ct.
Williamsburg, VA 23185
**Phone:** (757)229-3535

**★ 7782 ★ The Arc of Halifax**
PO Box 36
South Boston, VA 24592

**★ 7783 ★ The Arc of Hanover County**
PO Box 91
Ashland, VA 23005
**Phone:** (804)798-2400

**★ 7784 ★ The Arc of Harrisonburg/ Rockingham County**
1000 S High St.
Harrisonburg, VA 22801
**Phone:** (540)434-2469  **Fax:** (540)433-7759
**Email:** michaels@hrarc.org
**Website:** http://www.hrarc.org

**★ 7785 ★ The Arc of Lenowisco**
PO Box 1794
Gate City, VA 24251

**★ 7786 ★ The Arc of Loudoun County (LARC)**
PO Box 243
Leesburg, VA 20178
**Phone:** (703)777-1939
**Website:** http://www.loudoun-arc.org
Nancy Kysela, Director

**★ 7787 ★ The Arc of Mecklenburg**
515 N Lunenburg Ave.
South Hill, VA 23970

**★ 7788 ★ The Arc of Northern**
**Shenandoah Valley**
PO Box 3263
Winchester, VA 22604
**Phone:** (540)665-0461

**★ 7789 ★ The Arc of Northern Virginia**
100 N Washington St., No. 234
Falls Church, VA 22046
**Phone:** (703)532-3214
**Email:** info@thearcofnova.org
**Website:** http://www.arcofnova.org

**★ 7790 ★ The Arc of Petersburg**
114 N Union St., Ste. B
PO Box 2085
Petersburg, VA 23804
**Phone:** (804)732-0685

**★ 7791 ★ The Arc of the Piedmont**
509 Park St.
Charlottesville, VA 22902
**Phone:** (434)977-4002   **Free:** 800-732-9507
**Fax:** (434)977-7964
**Email:** thearc@cstone.net
**Website:** http://www.avenue.org/arc

**★ 7792 ★ The Arc of Rappahannock, Inc.**
701 Westwood Office Park
Fredericksburg, VA 22401
**Phone:** (540)899-3789   **Fax:** (540)370-0179
**Email:** arc_r@msn.com
**Website:** http://www.arcvap.org

**★ 7793 ★ The Arc of the Richmond Area**
1901 Westwood Ave.
Richmond, VA 23227
**Phone:** (804)358-1874

**★ 7794 ★ The Arc of Roanoke**
3355 Shenandoan Ave. NW
PO Box 6220
Roanoke, VA 24017
**Phone:** (540)342-9624

**★ 7795 ★ The Arc of Rockbridge**
PO Box 657
Lexington, VA 24450
**Phone:** (540)348-5510

**★ 7796 ★ The Arc of Smyth County**
221 Look Ave.
Marion, VA 24354
**Phone:** (540)783-6801

**★ 7797 ★ The Arc of Twin Galax County**
PO Box 202
Woodlawn, VA 24381

**★ 7798 ★ The Arc of Virginia**
2025 E Main St., Ste. 120
Richmond, VA 23223
**Phone:** (804)649-8481   **Fax:** (804)649-3585
**Email:** tstokes@arcofva.org
**Website:** http://www.arcofva.org
Teja Stokes, Exec Director

**★ 7799 ★ The Arc of the Virginia**
**Peninsula**
51 Battle Rd.
Hampton, VA 23666
**Phone:** (757)896-6461

**Website:** http://www.arcvap.org

**★ 7800 ★ The Arc of Warren County**
PO Box 1473
Front Royal, VA 22630-1473
**Phone:** (540)631-9092

**★ 7801 ★ The Beach Arc**
PO Box 8063
Virginia Beach, VA 23450
**Phone:** (757)340-5998
**Website:** http://groups.hamptonroads.com/BeachArc/

**★ 7802 ★ Danville Association for**
**Retarded Citizens, Inc.**
7180 U.S. Hwy. N 29
Blairs, VA 24527
**Phone:** (804)836-3272

## Washington

**★ 7803 ★ The Arc of Clark County**
9415 NE Fourth Plain Rd.
PO Box 2608
Vancouver, WA 98668-2608
**Phone:** (360)254-1562   **Fax:** (360)896-7382
**Email:** thearc@arcofclarkcounty.org
**Website:** http://www.arcofclarkcounty.org

**★ 7804 ★ The Arc of Cowlitz Valley**
1410 8th Ave., No. 15
Longview, WA 98632-3807
**Phone:** (360)425-5494
**Website:** http://www.cowlitzarc.org

**★ 7805 ★ The Arc of King County**
10550 Lake City Way NE, Ste. A
Seattle, WA 98125-7752
**Phone:** (206)364-6337
**Email:** inforef@arcofkingcounty.org
**Website:** http://www.arcofkingcounty.org

**★ 7806 ★ The Arc of Kitsap and**
**Jefferson Counties**
3243 N Perry Ave.
Bremerton, WA 98310
**Phone:** (360)377-3473

**★ 7807 ★ The Arc of the Olympic**
**Peninsula**
PO Box 2092
Port Angeles, WA 98362
**Phone:** (360)457-1301

**★ 7808 ★ The Arc of Snohomish County**
1615 California Ave.
Everett, WA 98201
**Phone:** (425)258-2459

**★ 7809 ★ The Arc of Spokane**
127 W Boone Ave.
Spokane, WA 99201
**Phone:** (509)328-6326
**Website:** http://www.arc-spokane.org

**★ 7810 ★ The Arc of the Tri-Cities**
761 Williams Blvd.
Richland, WA 99352
**Phone:** (509)946-5157

**★ 7811 ★ The Arc of Washington State**
1703 E State Ave. NE
Olympia, WA 98506
**Phone:** (360)357-5596   **Free:** 888-754-8798
**Email:** info@arcwa.org
**Website:** http://www.arcwa.org

**★ 7812 ★ The Arc of Whatcom, Skagit,**
**and Island Counties**
1111 Cornwall, No. 205
Bellingham, WA 98225
**Phone:** (360)715-0170

## West Virginia

**★ 7813 ★ The Arc of Harrison County**
PO Box 764
Clarksburg, WV 26301
**Phone:** (304)624-9114

**★ 7814 ★ The Arc of Kanawha Putnam**
1021 Quarrier St., Ste. 200
Charleston, WV 25301
**Phone:** (304)344-3403

**★ 7815 ★ The Arc of Marion County**
309 Cleveland Ave., Ste 101
Fairmont, WV 26554
**Phone:** (304)366-3213

**★ 7816 ★ The Arc of Ohio County**
439 Warwood Ave.
Wheeling, WV 26003
**Phone:** (304)277-1466

**★ 7817 ★ The Arc of Wood County**
521 Market St.
Box 17
Parkersburg, WV 26101
**Phone:** (304)422-3151   **Fax:** (304)422-1025
**Email:** arcwd@wirefire.com
**Website:** http://www.arcwd.org

**★ 7818 ★ Bridges, Inc.**
201 Walnut St., Ste. 207
Morgantown, WV 26505
**Phone:** (304)296-3092

## Wisconsin

**★ 7819 ★ The Arc of Barron County**
103 E Sawyer St.
Rice Lake, WI 54868

**★ 7820 ★ The Arc of Columbia County**
711 E Cook St.
Portage, WI 53901
**Phone:** (608)742-9204

**★ 7821 ★ The Arc Consumer Council**
c/o Nan Upright-Sexton
7519 W Oklahoma Ave.
Milwaukee, WI 53219

**★ 7822 ★ The Arc of Dane County**
1320 Mendota St., Ste. 111A
Madison, WI 53714
**Phone:** (608)257-9738
**Email:** arcdane@chorus.net
**Website:** http://www.arcdanecounty.org
Ken Hobbs, Exec Director

**★ 7823 ★ The Arc of Dunn County, Inc.**
390 Red Cedar St., Ste. G
Menomonie, WI 54751-2265
**Phone:** (715)235-7373

**★ 7824 ★ The Arc of Eau Claire**
513 S Barstow St.
Eau Claire, WI 54701
**Phone:** (715)834-7204

★ **7825** ★ **The Arc of Fond Du Lac County**
500 N Park Ave.
Fond Du Lac, WI 54935
**Phone:** (920)923-3810

★ **7826** ★ **The Arc of Juneau County**
8978 County Rd. M
New Lisbon, WI 53950

★ **7827** ★ **The Arc of Kenosha County, Inc.**
c/o Kenosha Achievement Center
1218 79th St.
Kenosha, WI 53144

★ **7828** ★ **The Arc of Langlade County**
N2437 Sunnyside Rd.
Antigo, WI 54409
**Phone:** (715)627-7458

★ **7829** ★ **The Arc of Lincoln County**
11012 Koffke Dr.
Merrill, WI 54452
**Phone:** (715)453-4939

★ **7830** ★ **The Arc of Marinette Area**
2528 Gilbert St.
Marinette, WI 54143

★ **7831** ★ **The Arc of Monroe County**
509 Jefferson Ave.
Sparta, WI 54656-2118
**Phone:** (608)269-6157

★ **7832** ★ **The Arc of Neenah-Menasha**
375 Winnebago Ave.
Menasha, WI 54952
**Phone:** (920)725-0943

★ **7833** ★ **The Arc of Outagamie County**
633 W Wisconsin Ave.
Appleton, WI 54911
**Phone:** (920)731-9831

★ **7834** ★ **The Arc of Ozaukee County**
11649 N Lake Shore Dr.
Mequon, WI 53092
**Website:** http://www.ocarc.org

★ **7835** ★ **The Arc of Racine County, Inc.**
818 6th St.
Racine, WI 53403
**Phone:** (414)634-6303

★ **7836** ★ **The Arc of Richland County**
284425 Coop Wood Rd.
Richland Center, WI 53581

★ **7837** ★ **The Arc of Washington County**
916 Chestnut St.
West Bend, WI 53095

★ **7838** ★ **The Arc of Waupaca County**
45 20th St.
Clintonville, WI 54929

★ **7839** ★ **The Arc of Western Racine County**
26509 Ketterhagen Rd.
Burlington, WI 53105

★ **7840** ★ **The Arc—Wisconsin**
600 Williamson St.
Madison, WI 53703
**Phone:** (608)251-9272

★ **7841** ★ **Green County Arc, Inc.**
1615 22 ½ Ave.
Monroe, WI 53566

## Wyoming

★ **7842** ★ **The Arc, Diversified Services Inc.**
PO Box EE
Torrington, WY 82240
**Phone:** (307)532-5911

★ **7843** ★ **The Arc of Lander/Riverton**
PO Box 213
Lander, WY 82520
**Phone:** (307)335-8801

★ **7844** ★ **The Arc of Laramie County**
PO Box 1812
Cheyenne, WY 82003
**Phone:** (307)632-1209
**Website:** http://www.arcoflaramiecounty.org

★ **7845** ★ **The Arc, Magic City Enterprises Inc.**
1780 Westland Rd.
Cheyenne, WY 82001
**Phone:** (307)637-8869

★ **7846** ★ **The Arc of Natrona County**
PO Box 393
Casper, WY 82602
**Phone:** (307)577-4913

★ **7847** ★ **The Arc Regional Services**
1150 N 3rd St.
Laramie, WY 82070
**Phone:** (307)742-6641

★ **7848** ★ **The Arc of Sheridan County**
PO Box 1028
Sheridan, WY 82801
**Phone:** (307)672-8665

★ **7849** ★ **The Arc of Uinta and Lincoln Counties**
528 Country Rd., Ste. 7
Evanston, WY 82930
**Phone:** (307)789-7679
**Email:** thearc@vcn.com
**Website:** http://www.geocities.com/thearcuinta/home.html
Cathy Frame, Exec Director

★ **7850** ★ **The Arc of Weston County Children's Center**
104 Stampede
Newcastle, WY 82701
**Phone:** (307)746-4560

★ **7851** ★ **The Arc of Wyoming**
318 W 'B' St.
PO Box 2161
Casper, WY 82602
**Phone:** (307)237-9110   **Free:** 800-801-0569
**Fax:** (307)577-4014
**Email:** arc-wy@home.com
**Website:** http://www.arcofwyoming.org

★ **7852** ★ **Child Development Center**
PO Box 7237
Sheridan, WY 82801
**Phone:** (307)672-6610

★ **7853** ★ **Child Development Center of Natrona County**
2020 E 12th St.
Casper, WY 82601
**Phone:** (307)235-5097

★ **7854** ★ **Children's Resource Center/ Special Touch Preschool Inc.**
PO Box 1191
Powell, WY 82435
**Phone:** (307)754-2864

★ **7855** ★ **The Learning Center**
PO Box 342
Pinedale, WY 82941
**Phone:** (307)733-3791

★ **7856** ★ **Lincoln-Uinta Child Development Association**
PO Box 570
Mountain View, WY 82939
**Phone:** (307)782-6601

★ **7857** ★ **Sweetwater County Child Development Center**
821 Norton Ave.
Rock Springs, WY 82901
**Phone:** (307)352-6600

# Chapter 21
# Disabilities

## Federal Government Agencies

★ 7858 ★ **Architectural and Transportation Barriers Compliance Board**
1331 F St. NW, Ste. 1000
Washington, DC 20004-1111
**Phone:** (202)272-5434
**Website:** http://www.access-board.gov
**Desc:** The Board was established to investigate and examine alternative approaches to the architectural, transportation, and attitudinal barriers confronting disabled persons; determine what measures are being taken by federal, state, and local governments and by other public and private agencies to eliminate those barriers; and promote the use of the International Accessibility Symbol in all public facilities that meet the standards prescribed by the Administrator of the General Services Administration Board. **AKA:** Access Board.

★ 7859 ★ **Interagency Committee on Employment of People With Disabilities**
Equal Employment Opportunity Commission
Federal Sector Programs
1801 L St., NW, Rm. 5238
Washington, DC 20507
**Phone:** (202)663-4560　　　　**Fax:** (202)376-6219
**Desc:** Seeks to identify and eliminate barriers standing in the way of full social and vocational opportunities for physically handicapped, mentally retarded, and mentally restored persons; promotes employment opportunities for the physically and mentally handicapped. **Alt. Contact:** (202)663-4593 (TDD).

★ 7860 ★ **National Council on Disability**
1331 F St. NW, Ste. 1050
Washington, DC 20004
**Phone:** (202)272-2004
**Website:** http://www.ncd.gov
**Desc:** The Council reviews all laws, programs, and policies of the federal government that affect individuals with disabilities. The Council then makes recommendations to the President, Congress, and federal agencies on these issues. In addition, the Council is studying the availability of health insurance coverage for persons with disabilities and sponsors conferences for families caring for the disabled. **Alt. Contact:** (202)272-2074 (TDD).

★ 7861 ★ **U.S. Department of Education Office of Special Education and Rehabilitative Services (OSERS)**
400 Maryland Ave. SW
Washington, DC 20202
**Free:** 800-USA-LEARN
**Website:** http://www.ed.gov/
**Desc:** The Office of Special Education and Rehabilitative Services provides leadership to ensure that people with disabilities have services, resources, and equal opportunities to learn, work, and live as fully-integrated, contributing members of society. OSERS supports programs that serve millions of disabled children, youth, and adults and that impact on the lives of the nation's 49 million citizens with disabilities. It coordinates the activities of the Office of Special Education Programs, which works to help states provide quality educational opportunities and early-intervention services to help students with disabilities achieve their goals. OSERS' Rehabilitation Services Administration, among other efforts, supports state vocational rehabilitation programs that give disabled people the education, job training, and job placement services they need to gain meaningful employment. OSERS' National Institute on Disability and Rehabilitation Research supports research and technological programs that are crafting blueprints for a barrier-free, inclusive society.

★ 7862 ★ **U.S. Department of Health and Human Services**
**Administration for Children and Families (ACF)**
**Administration on Developmental Disabilities (ADD)**
370 L'Enfant Promenade SW
Washington, DC 20447
**Phone:** (202)690-6590
**Website:** http://www.acf.hhs.gov/programs/add/
**Desc:** The Administration on Developmental Disabilities (ADD) supports and encourages provision of quality services to persons with developmental disabilities; assists States in increasing the independence, productivity, and community inclusion of all persons with developmental disabilities, through the design and implementation of a comprehensive and continuing State plan; administers the State developmental disabilities councils, the Protection and Advocacy Grant Program, and the discretionary grant programs.

★ 7863 ★ **U.S. Department of Veterans Affairs**
**Veterans Benefits Administration**
**Vocational Rehabilitation Service**
810 Vermont Ave. NW
Washington, DC 20420
**Phone:** (202)273-4800
**Website:** http://www.va.gov/
Joseph Thompson, Under Secretary for Benefits
**Desc:** The Vocational Rehabilitation Service is responsible for outreach, motivation, evaluation, counseling, training, employment, and other rehabilitation services to disabled veterans; evaluation, counseling, and miscellaneous services to veterans and service persons and other VA education programs; evaluation, counseling, education and miscellaneous services to sons, daughters and spouses of totally and permanently disabled veterans and to surviving orphans, widows, or widowers of certain deceased veterans, including rehabilitation services to to certain handicapped dependents,; affirmative action activities; and vocational training and rehabilitation to children with spina bifida who are children of Vietnam veterans.

**U.S. Library of Congress**
**National Library Service for the Blind and Physically Handicapped**
*See:* Entry 11998

## Foundations & Other Funding Organizations

### <u>Private Foundations</u>

**Allegheny Foundation**
*See:* Entry 10039

**Amateur Athletic Foundation of Los Angeles**
*See:* Entry 5544

★ 7864 ★ **Ann Jackson Family Foundation**
PO Box 5580
Santa Barbara, CA 93150
**Phone:** (805)969-2258　　　　**Fax:** (805)969-0315
**Email:** info@aafla.org
**Website:** http://www.aafla.org
**Fnded:** 1978. **Philosophy:** The Ann Jackson Family Foundation gives to charities and services which "foster religious, charitable, educational, and scientific purposes and to organizations which promote the prevention of cruelty to children and animals." **Priorities:** *Arts & Humanities:* 13%. Historic preservation and art museums. *Civic & Public Affairs:* 11%. Botanic and zoological gardens, and community foundations. *Education:* 28%. Secondary schools. *Environment:* 22%. Youth and family services. *International:* 14%. A Mental health associations, hospitals, and health centers. *Note:* Total contributions made in fiscal 1999. **Typ. Recipients:** Cancer, Clinics/Medical Centers, Emergency/Ambulance Services, Eyes/Blindness, Family Planning, Family Planning, Geriatric Health, Health Organizations, Heart, Hospitals, Medical Rehabilitation, Medical Research, Mental Health, Multiple Sclerosis, Nursing Services, People with Disabilities, Prenatal Health Issues, Respiratory, Substance Abuse. **Geo. Dist:** Santa Barbara, CA, and surrounding areas.

**Christian A. Johnson Endeavor Foundation**
*See:* Entry 20801

**★ 7865 ★ Conn Memorial Foundation, Inc.**
2910 West Bay to Bay Boulevard, Ste. 200
Tampa, FL 33629
**Phone:** (813)282-4922     **Fax:** (813)282-8542
**Website:** http://www.edlead.org
Fran Powers, Director of Services
**Fnded:** 1954. **Philosophy:** The Foundation "exists for the purpose of providing leadership, direction and funding assistance to tax-exempt and nonprofit youth and family organizations." The Foundation's primary interests are children, youth, and family programs; education, human service, and emergency/disaster relief; and program capital support and agency expansion. The foundation reports that scholarship assistance will be made available to foundation funded agencies whose clients seek education beyond high school. **Priorities:** *Arts & Humanities:* About 4%. *Civic & Public Affairs:* About 10%. Urban community affairs, aquariums, and African American affairs. *Education:* 5%. *Environment:* 47%. Youth organizations, community service, and child abuse counseling programs. *International:* 4%. *Note:* Total contributions made in fiscal 1997. **Typ. Recipients:** AIDS/HIV, Cancer, Child Abuse, Children's Health/Hospitals, Clinics/Medical Centers, Health Organizations, People with Disabilities, Research/Studies Institutes, Substance Abuse. **Geo. Dist:** FL, Hillsborough and Pinellas counties.


**D and DF Foundation**
*See:* Entry 10042


**DeWitt Wallace-Reader's Digest Fund**
*See:* Entry 166


**★ 7866 ★ Duffield Family Foundation**
2223 Santa Clara Ave., Ste. B
Alameda, CA 94501
**Phone:** (510)337-8989     **Fax:** (510)337-8988
**Email:** info@maddiesfund.org
**Website:** http://www.maddiesfund.org
Rich Avanzino, President
**Fnded:** 1995. **Philosophy:** The foundation primarily supports programs for domestic animal welfare that promote humane education, adoption and rescue, medical assistance and emergency care, quality of life, spaying and neutering, and human/animal interaction. **Priorities:** *Arts & Humanities:* 6%. A museum received funding. *Civic & Public Affairs:* 1%. Support went to the Oakland Zoo. *Education:* 1%. Gives to animal-related educational programs. *Environment:* 92%. Emphasis on humane societies and animal welfare causes. *Note:* Total contributions made in fiscal 1998. **Typ. Recipients:** Cancer, Child Abuse, Children's Health/Hospitals, People with Disabilities. **Geo. Dist:** CA.


**★ 7867 ★ Earhart Foundation**
2200 Green Rd., Ste. H
Ann Arbor, MI 48105
**Phone:** (734)761-8592
David Kennedy, President
**Fnded:** 1929. **Philosophy:** The foundation initially centered its grant making on charitable, religious, and educational purposes. Emphasis was also placed on the social sciences and the humanities. Currently, the foundation directs a majority of its funding to fellowship research grants to individuals from established institutions pursuing endeavors of their own choice. Designated graduate students, scholars, and research principals are considered for support. Three program areas have been established for awards: The H. B. Earhart Fellowships are awarded to graduate students ready to embark upon careers in college or university teaching or in research. Graduate students are nominated by faculty sponsors, and applications for this program are not accepted. The Fellowship Research Grants Program is open to individuals who have established themselves professionally and who are affiliated with educational or research institutions. The effort funded should lead to the advancement of knowledge through teaching, lecturing, and publication. Earhart Foundation grants are occasionally awarded to "publicly supported" educational and research organizations qualified for private foundation support. However, resources allotted to this program have been reduced as the foundation concentrates more funding on individual research grants. **Priorities:** *Civic & Public Affairs:* 33%. Funds economic research and public policy. *Education:* 55% Supports colleges, universities, and educational programs. *Note:* Total contributions made in 1998. **Typ. Recipients:** People with Disabilities.


**★ 7868 ★ Elinor Patterson Baker Foundation**
c/o Putnam Trust Co.
10 Mason St.
Greenwich, CT 06830
**Phone:** (203)869-3000     **Fax:** (203)869-7412
**Email:** apanoli@bankofny.com
Anne Panoli, Foundation Administrator
**Fnded:** 1984. **Philosophy:** "The Elinor Patterson Baker Foundation makes grants for the general charitable purposes of organizations that fulfill the aims, principles, goals, and purposes of The Humane Society of the United States." **Priorities:** *Arts & Humanities:* 1%. *Civic & Public Affairs:* 1%. *Education:* 1%. *Environment:* 88%. Supports animal welfare organizations. *Note:* Total contributions made in fiscal 1999. **Typ. Recipients:** Clinics/Medical Centers, People with Disabilities. **Geo. Dist:** nationally and to U.S.-based international organizations.


**★ 7869 ★ First Fruit**
14 Corporate Plz.
Newport Beach, CA 92660
**Phone:** (949)720-3774     **Fax:** (949)760-5349
**Email:** info@firstfruit.org
**Website:** http://www.firstfruit.org
Robert Martin, Executive Director
**Fnded:** 1976. **Philosophy:** The foundation's main interests are religion and education. Religious support varies from prison fellowships to a variety of religious affiliations and beliefs. Usually, religious gifts have international interests. Educational support is mainly centered on giving to seminaries with a worldwide scope. The foundation supports other areas of philanthropy only if it involves religious activities or international concerns. **Priorities:** *Environment:* 12%. *Note:* Total contributions made in 1998. **Typ. Recipients:** People with Disabilities. **Geo. Dist:** internationally.


**Frederick P. and Sandra P. Rose Foundation**
*See:* Entry 5554


**Harriet Ford Dickenson Foundation**
*See:* Entry 18209


**★ 7870 ★ Hugh and Hazel Darling Foundation**
520 S Grand Ave. 7th Floor
Los Angeles, CA 90071
**Phone:** (213)683-5200     **Fax:** (213)627-7795
Richard Stack, Trustee
**Fnded:** 1988. **Philosophy:** The Hugh and Hazel Darling Foundation supports the advancement of education in California, with primary emphasis on legal education and education programs calculated to impart a better understanding and appreciation of our legal system through its support of educational institutions. Due to multi-year pledges, funds for new projects are limited. "We've made multi-year commitments to what we believe to be worthwhile projects, so that limits our ability to commit new funds," explained Richard L. Stack, trustee of the foundation. **Priorities:** *Education:* 100%. **Typ. Recipients:** People with Disabilities, Speech & Hearing. **Geo. Dist:** CA.


**Jack N. and Lilyan Mandel Foundation**
*See:* Entry 8539


**JM Foundation**
*See:* Entry 411


**★ 7871 ★ Kern Foundation Trust**
50 S LsSalle St., Fl. B3
Chicago, IL 60675
**Phone:** (312)557-2703     **Fax:** (312)444-4122
**Email:** dgr@ntrs.com
Dale Rudy, Contact
**Fnded:** 1959. **Philosophy:** The Kern Foundation Trust's aim is to support "the dissemination of the theosophical philosophy as broadly as possible, in a non-proselytizing, non-propagandizing manner." **Priorities:** *Education:* 5%. *Note:* Total contributions made in 1998. **Typ. Recipients:** People with Disabilities. **Geo. Dist:** CA; IL.


**Lilly Endowment**
*See:* Entry 18213


**★ 7872 ★ Louise Taft Semple Foundation**
425 Walnut St.
Cincinnati, OH 45202
**Phone:** (513)381-2838     **Fax:** (513)381-0205
**Website:** http://www.lilly.com/about/community/foundation/endowment.html
Eileen Heyob, Contact
**Fnded:** 1941. **Philosophy:** The Louise Taft Semple Foundation makes most of its grants in the areas of the arts, humanities, education, and social services. Social service funding favors united funds, homes, youth organizations, and community centers. Educational support goes to private and public school systems, university legal education, and religious learning. In the arts, support favors art funds, museums, and opera. **Priorities:** *Arts & Humanities:* 33%. Primary support for Aronoff Performing Arts Center, arts funds, ballet, music, opera, and public broadcasting. *Civic & Public Affairs:* 11%. Focus on a zoological society, women's affairs, legal aid, and towns/municipalities. *Education:* 29%. Support for primary and secondary education, faculty development, arts education, and schs. *Environment:* 20%. Supports United Way, YMCA, scouting, and youth programs. *International:* 6%. Supports children's health and speech & hearing. *Note:* Total contributions made in 2000. **Typ. Recipients:** Children's Health/Hospitals, Medical Rehabilitation, People with Disabilities, Preventive Medicine/Wellness Organizations, Speech & Hearing, Substance Abuse, Substance Abuse. **Geo. Dist:** OH, Hamilton County; Cincinnati, OH.


**Marion O. and Maximilian E. Hoffman Foundation**
*See:* Entry 505


**Mary Duke Biddle Foundation**
*See:* Entry 511


**Mary Ranken Jordan and Ettie A. Jordan Charitable Foundation**
*See:* Entry 514


**Monterey Fund**
*See:* Entry 5561


**Moody Foundation**
*See:* Entry 551


**★ 7873 ★ Needmor Fund**
2305 Canyon Boulevard Ste. 101
Boulder, CO 80302
**Phone:** (303)449-5801
**Website:** http://www.moodyf.org
Mr. Charles Shuford, Executive Director
**Fnded:** 1956. **Philosophy:** "The primary goal of the Needmor Fund is to empower those individuals whose basic rights to justice and opportunity are systemati-

cally ignored or denied. We have identified community organizing as a highly effective process through which such people may learn to take control of their lives and change those conditions which adversely affect them." "We look for grassroots, community-based organizations whose members are committed to maintaining the energy of the group; whose leadership is developed from within; which are capable of determining the major problems facing their community; and, finally, which can formulate and implement effective strategic plans. We recognize the problem faced will vary from group to group, and do not specify certain areas of concern–only that the process of defining and implementing solutions is community controlled and truly empowering to each member of the group." Grants are made from the Broad Common Pool, which funds nationwide; and from the Toledo Common Pool, which supports only Toledo organizations. The fund allocates a number of donor-suggested grants, reflecting the interests of the Stranahan family. Donor-suggested grants cannot be applied for and thus are not represented in the figures and analysis in this report. **Priorities:** *Civic & Public Affairs:* 47%. Supports employment, Gay/Lesbian issues, public policy. *Education:* 4%. Supports public education, education funds and religious education. *Environment:* 35%. Supports family planning, family services, scouting, and food distribution programs. *International:* 1%.Funds public health. *Note:* Total contributions made in 1999. **Typ. Recipients:** People with Disabilities, Public Health. **Geo. Dist:** nationally; Toledo, OH, and surrounding area.

### Norcross Wildlife Foundation
*See:* Entry 562

### Paul Ogle Foundation
*See:* Entry 4920

### Robert W. Wilson Foundation
*See:* Entry 13519

### Rockefeller Family Fund
*See:* Entry 17870

### St. Giles Foundation
*See:* Entry 5562

### Schwartz Foundation
*See:* Entry 667

### Wayne and Gladys Valley Foundation
*See:* Entry 753

### William and Mary Greve Foundation
*See:* Entry 10058

### ★ 7874 ★ Winthrop Rockefeller Foundation
308 East Eighth St.
Little Rock, AR 72202-3999
**Phone:** (501)376-6854          **Fax:** (501)374-4797
**Email:** williamary@msn.com
**Website:** http://www.wrockefellerfoundation.org
Dr. Sybil Hampton, President
**Fnded:** 1973. **Philosophy:** The underlying goal of the Winthrop Rockefeller Foundation is to improve the quality of life in Arkansas by creating an environment that makes development and improvement possible. Mr. Rockefeller believed economic conditions in Arkansas would improve only through the creation of opportunity within the state. To support economic development, the foundation has chosen to focus on strengthening local economies; providing access to capital, management, and technical assistance for small businesses; strengthening agriculture; developing leadership; supporting organizations that can improve the economic status of Arkansas; and improving the economic status of women and minorities.

Enhancing the effectiveness of citizens and the institutions serving them is viewed as a method for improving the quality of life in Arkansas. In the area of civic affairs, the foundation supports efforts to improve the effectiveness of government and private service providers; to focus attention on and promote discussion of public policy issues; to identify and develop leaders at the state, local, and institutional levels; and to improve civic opportunities for minority and disadvantaged citizens. Improving the quality of education is another major focus. The foundation has made a long-term commitment to eliminate educational barriers by supporting efforts to restructure schools, encourage parental involvement, increase minority participation, and identify issues and problems. The foundation also supports organizations promoting literacy. The foundation achieves its charitable purposes through several types of support. Major grants are made primarily in the areas of economic development, civic affairs, and education. Community incentive grants of up to $10,000 are available for special assistance to community-based organizations for general operating support, construction funds, or equipment purchases. To be eligible for a community incentive grant, an organization must serve a minority or disadvantaged population, and must not be a previous grantee of the foundation. Mini-grants of up to $2,000 are made at the discretion of the foundation president for technical assistance, organizational development, or program planning. Such grants also are made to educators. The foundation may directly invest its capital in projects related to its goals. These investments can be in the form of low-interest loans, equity, or other financing mechanisms. The foundation often develops initiatives to address an area of concern, particularly in education, and supports or initiates in-house public policy projects focusing on important issues in economic development, civic affairs, or education. Other goals are to strengthen the capacity of local communities to break the cycle of poverty by supporting local economic development, and nurture strong leadership through the development of community-based organizations. **Priorities:** *Arts & Humanities:* 10%. Funds historical groups, museums, and performing arts. *Civic & Public Affairs:* 64%. Funds community development, economic interests, community services, and empoloyment. *Education:* 20%. Supports public schools and higher education. *Environment:* 1%. *International:* 2%. *Note:* Total contributions made in 1998. **Typ. Recipients:** AIDS/HIV, Medical Education, People with Disabilities. **Geo. Dist:** AR.

## Corporate Foundations

### ABC Foundation
*See:* Entry 795

### Advanced Micro Devices, Inc.
*See:* Entry 799

### AGL Resources Inc.
*See:* Entry 803

### Allianz Life Insurance Co. of North America
*See:* Entry 817

### Ameren Corp. Charitable Trust
*See:* Entry 821

### Appleton Papers Inc.
*See:* Entry 843

### Aristech Foundation
*See:* Entry 848

### ★ 7875 ★ ASARCO Foundation
180 Maiden Lane
New York, NY 10038
**Phone:** (212)510-1813          **Fax:** (212)510-1835

**Email:** dkolb@appletonpapers.com
**Website:** http://www.appletonpapers.com
Kevin McCaffrey, Secretary
**Fnded:** 1956. **Priorities:** *Arts & Humanities:* 37%. Supports public broadcasting. *Civic & Public Affairs:* 2%. Funds fire fighter/police organizations and civic organizations. *Education:* 21%. Majority of funding supports higher education. Also funds science and technology education and private secondary schools through grants and matching gifts. *Environment:* 10%. Supports the United Way. *International:* 5%. Funds hospitals and public health organizations. *Note:* Total contributions made in 1999. **Typ. Recipients:** Cancer, Hospices, People with Disabilities. **Geo. Dist:** headquarters and operating communities.

### ★ 7876 ★ Bank One Foundation
1 Bank One Plaza, Ste. 0308
Chicago, IL 60670
**Phone:** (312)732-8052          **Fax:** (312)732-2437
James Donovan, Treasurer
**Priorities:** *Arts & Humanities:* 3%. Contributes to a variety of arts organizations in the Chicago area, including music, theater, museums, and libraries. *Civic & Public Affairs:* 14%. Supports civic organizations concerned with better government; economic and housing development; crime, justice, and law; environment and ecology; race and ethnic relations; and improvement of the public sector. Prefers to fund specific projects/programs and favors programs that promote self-sufficiency. Also supports organizations that reinforce Chicago's reputation as a world-class city and have active employee involvement. *Education:* 12%. Education support is primarily disbursed through matching gifts and general support for colleges and universities. *Environment:* 68%. Major support to the United Way/Crusade of Mercy as principal means of addressing a broad variety of social welfare needs. *International:* 1%. Supports hospitals and medical centers. *Religion:* 1%. Supports science museums, natural history museums, and planetariums. *Note:* Total foundation contributions made in 1999. **Typ. Recipients:** Children's Health/Hospitals, Clinics/Medical Centers, Hospitals, People with Disabilities. **Geo. Dist:** Chicago, IL.

### BankAtlantic Foundation
*See:* Entry 5470

### Bausch & Lomb Foundation, Inc.
*See:* Entry 14914

### The Boeing Co. Charitable Trust
*See:* Entry 5472

### California Bank & Trust
*See:* Entry 912

### Central Newspapers Foundation
*See:* Entry 10062

### Chicago Sun-Times Charity Trust
*See:* Entry 936

### Citigroup Foundation
*See:* Entry 11426

### Citizens Bank-Flint
*See:* Entry 945

### CNA Foundation
*See:* Entry 950

### ★ 7877 ★ CNF Transportation, Inc.
3240 Hillview Ave.
Palo Alto, CA 94304
**Phone:** (650)494-2900          **Fax:** (650)813-0158

**Email:** pdudek@hollingerintl.com
**Website:** http://www.cnf.com
Chris Kidwell, Vice President, Corporate Benefits

**Priorities:** *Civic & Public Affairs:* Supports organizations involved in the community and public well-being similar to United Way. *Education:* Supports scholarship programs. **Typ. Recipients:** People with Disabilities. **Geo. Dist:** nationally, with an emphasis on areas where company operates.


**Domino's Pizza Inc.**
*See:* Entry 10064


**Dow Jones Foundation**
*See:* Entry 11429


**E.L. Craig Foundation**
*See:* Entry 1012


**Equitable Resources, Inc.**
*See:* Entry 1030


**Fabri-Kal Foundation**
*See:* Entry 1037


★ **7878** ★ **FBW Foundation**
8403 Colesville Rd., No. 900
Silver Spring, MD 20910-4704
**Phone:** (301)273-6000
**Email:** len.doherty@dowjones.com
**Website:** http://www.eqt.com/about_EQT/Community.asp
**Fnded:** 1994. **Priorities:** *Arts & Humanities:* 4%. Gives to opera, theater, arts centers, choral groups, and museums. *Civic & Public Affairs:* 8%. Funds affordable housing programs, city councils, and an aquarium. *Education:* 25%. Supports colleges, universities, business education, parochial schools, reading programs, scholarship funds, and public schools. *Environment:* 29%. Supports local United Way offices, youth activities, senior services, food distribution, animal welfare organizations, services for the disabled, family services, and child welfare organizations. *International:* 33%. Funds wellness programs, hospitals and medical centers, single-disease health associations, and hospice programs. *Note:* Total contributions made in fiscal 2001. **Typ. Recipients:** Alzheimers Disease, Cancer, Clinics/Medical Centers, Heart, Hospices, People with Disabilities, Preventive Medicine/Wellness Organizations. **Geo. Dist:** MD; VA; Washington, WA; WV.


★ **7879** ★ **Foundation of the Litton Industries**
21240 Burbank Blvd.
Woodland Hills, CA 91367-6675
**Phone:** (818)598-2003　　**Fax:** (818)598-3315
Lynne Brickner, President

**Priorities:** *Arts & Humanities:* 22%. Interests include community television, music, museums, and the performing arts. *Civic & Public Affairs:* 7%. Interests include law, ethics, and minorities. *Education:* 24%. Emphasis on math, engineering, and science. Supports universities and public and private schools at the elementary and secondary levels. Also supports minorities and students with military ties. *Environment:* 45%. Supports the United Way and organizations for children and youth. *Note:* Above percentages reflect 1999 foundation priorities only. The company also operates a scholarship program for higher education. **Typ. Recipients:** People with Disabilities. **Geo. Dist:** nationally; Los Angeles, CA, national and and regional appeals centered in metropolitan area.


**FPL Group Foundation, Inc.**
*See:* Entry 1067


★ **7880** ★ **Frontier Corp. Educational Fund**
3441 W Henrietta Rd.
Rochester, NY 14623
**Phone:** (716)777-7702　　**Fax:** (716)546-7898
**Email:** pgrover@frontiercorp.com
**Website:** http://www.fpl.com
Pat Grover, Contact

**Priorities:** *Education:* 100%. Supports scholarships. *Voluntarism:* Company supports the Genesee Chapter of the Telephone Pioneers. **Typ. Recipients:** People with Disabilities. **Geo. Dist:** company's service areas.


**Gannett Foundation**
*See:* Entry 12281


**Genesis Foundation**
*See:* Entry 10065


**Hasbro Children's Foundation**
*See:* Entry 11435


**Hershey Foods Corp.**
*See:* Entry 11437


**Household International Inc.**
*See:* Entry 1132


★ **7881** ★ **International Multifoods Charitable Foundation**
110 Cheshire Ln., Ste. 300
Minnetonka, MN 55305-1060
**Phone:** (952)594-3568　　**Fax:** (952)594-3304
**Email:** dmfunk@household.com
**Website:** http://www.household.com
Karen Anderson, Foundation Administrator

**Priorities:** *Arts & Humanities:* 3% to 5%. Supports art groups with strong touring companies and educational outreach in company communities. *Civic & Public Affairs:* 3% to 5%. Funds programs involving youth leadership, community involvement, and urban affairs. *Education:* 30% to 35%. Recipients include educational institutions and associations that prepare youth to become responsible adults. Also sponsors an employee matching gift program. *Environment:* 50% to 60%. Funding supports the United Way and independent programs throughout the country. Also funds organizations that target the problems of hunger and nutrition among youth. Special Funding grants focus on organizations that meet the needs of youth in selected operating locations. Employee committees solicit proposals from local nonprofits, and financial contributions are leveraged with employee volunteers. *Voluntarism:* Company donates to nonprofit organizations where employees volunteer through its Employee Volunteer Bonus program. Additionally, the company sponsors the Employee Board Member Bonus where employees serve on nonprofit boards. **Typ. Recipients:** Diabetes, Medical Education, People with Disabilities, Substance Abuse. **Geo. Dist:** Major principally near operating locations and to national organizations; Minneapolis, MN; St. Paul, MN.


**J.D. Edwards Foundation**
*See:* Entry 1154


★ **7882** ★ **Kiewit Companies Foundation**
1000 Kiewit Plaza
Omaha, NE 68131-3374
**Phone:** (402)271-2950　　**Fax:** (402)943-1302
**Email:** mike.faust@kiewit.com
**Website:** http://www.kiewit.com
Michael Faust, Foundation Administrator

**Fnded:** 1963. **Priorities:** *Arts & Humanities:* 5%. Funds art museums, symphonies, and a children's museum. *Civic & Public Affairs:* 49%. Supports business and free enterprise, housing and community development, civil rights, and women's affairs. *Education:* 32%. Majority of education funds are provided to

colleges and universities. Other interests include private precollege education, education funds, economic education, university athletic programs, and higher education in engineering. *Environment:* 8%. Primarily supports united funds in operating areas. Also supports youth organizations, religious welfare, and family planning. *International:* 2%. Supports single-disease health organizations and children's hospitals. *Note:* Total contributions made in 2000. Figures based on partial grants list. **Typ. Recipients:** Arthritis, Clinics/Medical Centers, Health Organizations, People with Disabilities. **Geo. Dist:** operating locations; Omaha, NE.


**Laclede Gas Charitable Trust**
*See:* Entry 5578


**Mallinckrodt Inc.**
*See:* Entry 11449


★ **7883** ★ **Marriott International Inc.**
1 Marriott Dr.
Washington, DC 20058
**Phone:** (301)380-7430　　**Fax:** (301)380-2843
**Email:** judi.hadfield@marriot.com
**Website:** http://www.mallincrodt.com
Judi Hadfield, Vice President Community Relations & Cor

**Priorities:** *Arts & Humanities:* 5% to 10%. Supports the performing arts, arts organizations, public broadcasting, and historic preservation in headquarters area or programs which are national in scope. *Civic & Public Affairs:* 10% to 15%. Grants disbursed primarily in headquarters area. Interests are professional and tradeorganizations, urban and community affairs, cultural diversity, and minority affairs. *Education:* About 30%. Most contributions are made at the university level, supporting schools where company actively recruits, with interest in the hospitality industry. Contributions at the secondary level are national in scope and promote cultural diversity or serve minority or disadvantaged students. *International:* About 50%. Primarily supports the United Way in operating communities. The remaining funds support health and human service organizations in headquarters community and select national organizations, with focus on people with disabilities and hunger relief. **Typ. Recipients:** Health Funds, Health Organizations, People with Disabilities, Single-Disease Health Associations. **Geo. Dist:** organizations near headquarters and some national organizations.


★ **7884** ★ **Maytag Corp. Foundation**
403 W 4th St. N
PO Box 39
Newton, IA 50208
**Phone:** (515)787-6357　　**Fax:** (515)787-8676
**Website:** http://www.maytag.com/mths/our_company/default.jsp?partner=none
Janis Cooper, Director, Foundation Programs

**Priorities:** *Arts & Humanities:* 9%. Supports community-wide arts and culture. Grants go to historical organizations, music, museums, and public broadcasting. *Civic & Public Affairs:* 15%. Supports organizations concerned with business and free enterprise. Interest is in community betterment and public service. Supports innovative community problem solving and community development. *Education:* 44%. Major support is given to colleges through college funds and the foundation's gift-matching plan. Direct student aid is given through scholarships and career education awards to the children of U.S. employees. Supports school-to-work training and technical skills. *Environment:* 30%. Supports United Way, YMCA, recreation, and community centers. *International:* 1%. Supports medical centers. *Note:* Total foundation contributions made in 2000. **Typ. Recipients:** People with Disabilities. **Geo. Dist:** Galesburg, IL; Herrin, IL; Newton, IA; Clarence, MO; Jefferson City, MO; Bow, NH; North Canton, OH; Quakertown, PA; Williston, SC; Cleveland, TN; Jackson, TN; El Paso, TX; Burlington, VT; Williston, VT.

**Mellon Financial Corp.**
*See:* Entry 1232

**Mid-American Foundation**
*See:* Entry 5582

**Mitsubishi Electric America Foundation**
*See:* Entry 1246

**National Fuel Gas Co.**
*See:* Entry 11454

**NEC Foundation of America**
*See:* Entry 5583

**North American Royalties Foundation**
*See:* Entry 11456

**Northern Indiana Public Service Co.**
*See:* Entry 1276

**Public Service Electric & Gas Foundation**
*See:* Entry 8553

**Questar Corp.**
*See:* Entry 1340

**R.R. Donnelley & Sons Co.**
*See:* Entry 5474

**Robbins and Myers Foundation**
*See:* Entry 8554

**Scripps Howard Foundation**
*See:* Entry 8555

**Sentry Insurance Foundation Inc.**
*See:* Entry 1382

**Solo Cup Foundation**
*See:* Entry 1397

**Southern New England Telephone Co.**
*See:* Entry 11463

**Star Tribune Foundation**
*See:* Entry 5475

**Sunoco Inc.**
*See:* Entry 11465

**★ 7885 ★ SuperValu Foundation**
PO Box 990
Minneapolis, MN 55440
**Phone:** (612)828-4000          **Fax:** (952)828-4838
**Email:** cottingham@scripps.com
**Website:**      http://www.supervalu.com/community/comm_main.html
Frank O'Keefe, Vice President, Assistant Treasurer
**Fnded:** 1993. **Priorities:** *Arts & Humanities:* 3%. Funds arts councils, children's art programs, theaters, art museums and centers, and orchestras. *Civic & Public Affairs:* 4%. Gives to citizen's leagues, ethnic organizations, cities, zoos and parks, chambers of commerce, and job training. *Education:* 21%. Supports business, political, and cooperative education programs; programs designed to build knowledge and leadership skills of youth; and urban projects relating to the employability of youth. *Environment:* 54%. Supports the United Way in the headquarters area; organizations providing assistance to minority, physically challenged, disabled, and disadvantaged per-

sons; and hunger relief efforts. Also supports organizations and programs aimed at promotion of nutrition and organizations established to educate and train people to enter the workforce. *International:* 18%. Primarily supports single-disease health associations. *Note:* Total foundation contributions made in fiscal 2000. **Typ. Recipients:** Arthritis, Cancer, Health-General, People with Disabilities, Single-Disease Health Associations, Substance Abuse. **Geo. Dist:** organizations in the company's general service area; Minneapolis-St. Paul, MN.

**Torchmark Corp.**
*See:* Entry 1443

**Toro Foundation**
*See:* Entry 10070

**Tribune New York Foundation**
*See:* Entry 1446

**Valspar Foundation**
*See:* Entry 1474

**Varian Medical Systems, Inc.**
*See:* Entry 1477

**Wells Fargo Bank Nebraska, N.A.**
*See:* Entry 1496

**Wells Fargo Foundation**
*See:* Entry 1497

**Woodward Governor Co. Charitable Trust**
*See:* Entry 11473

**Xerox Foundation**
*See:* Entry 5476

**Zenith Electronics Corp.**
*See:* Entry 11474

## Other Funding Organizations

**★ 7886 ★ Ambucs Resource Center**
3315 North Main St.
High Point, NC 27265
**Phone:** (336)869-2166          **Fax:** (336)887-8451
**Email:** ambucs@ambucs.com
**Website:** http://www.ambucs.com
**Desc:** Dedicated to creating independence and opportunities for people with disabilities. Conducts service projects designed to give children with disabilities their first set of wheels. **Awards:** AMBUCS Scholars (annual) for PT, OT, Speech or Audiology students in junior year or higher.

**★ 7887 ★ American Association of People with Disabilities (AAPD)**
1819 H St. NW, Ste. 330
Washington, DC 20006
**Phone:** (202)457-0046          **Free:** 800-840-8844
**Fax:** (202)457-0473
**Email:** aapd@aol.com
**Website:** http://www.aapd-dc.org
Helena Berger, Chief Operating Officer
**Desc:** Promotes economic and political empowerment of persons with disabilities; educating businesses and general public about disability issues. **Awards:** Paul G Heane/AAPD Leadership Awards (annual) for leadership achievements that show a positive impact on the community of people with disabilities or within their area of disability interest.

**★ 7888 ★ Christopher Reeve Paralysis Foundation**
500 Morris Ave.
Springfield, NJ 07081
**Phone:** (973)379-2690          **Free:** 800-225-0292
**Fax:** (973)912-9433
**Website:** http://www.christopherreeve.org
David R. Landrey, Chair/Exec. Committee
**Desc:** Seeks to encourage and support research to find a cure for paralysis caused by spinal cord injury and other central nervous system disorders. **Awards:** Grant to research laboratories and individuals for postgraduate study; grant to physicians and scientists conducting research on the spinal cord and central nervous system.

**★ 7889 ★ Foundation for Science and Disability (FSD)**
236 Grand St.
Morgantown, WV 26505-7509
**Phone:** (304)293-5201          **Fax:** (304)293-6363
**Email:** ekeller@wvu.edu
E. C. Keller, Jr., Treas.
**Desc:** Disabled scientists and interested individuals. Offers consultation and advice concerning problems faced by persons with disabilities in scientific fields. **Awards:** Disabled Graduate Students in Science (annual) for U.S. graduate students with disabilities.

**Gazette International Networking Institute (GINI)**
*See:* Entry 12003

**★ 7890 ★ Life Sharing Foundation**
S Sandisfield Rd.
Great Barrington, MA 01230
**Phone:** (413)229-2600          **Fax:** (413)455-2992
**Email:** gini_intl@msn.com
**Website:** http://www.post-polio.org
Allan Baer, Pres.
**Desc:** Seeks to enhance the independence of disabled individuals by providing financial support and other support to families who share their homes w/ people w/disabilities. **Awards:** Scholarship.

**★ 7891 ★ National AMBUCS**
PO Box 5127
High Point, NC 27262
**Phone:** (336)869-2166          **Fax:** (336)887-8451
**Email:** ambucs@ambucs.com
**Website:** http://www.ambucs.com
J. Joseph Copeland, Exec. Dir.
**Desc:** Dedicated to creating opportunities for independence for people with disabilities. Performs community service; provides physically challenged children with tricycles that can be operated by hand, foot or both: operates the Living Endowment Fund. **Awards:** Scholarships for Therapists (annual) for students majoring in occupational, physical, therapy, speech pathology, hearing audiology.

**★ 7892 ★ National Amputee Golf Association (NAGA)**
11 Walnut Hill Rd.
Amherst, NH 03031-1713
**Free:** 800-633-6242
**Email:** info@nagagolf.org
**Website:** http://www.nagagolf.org
Bob Wilson, Dir.
**Desc:** Individuals who have lost a hand, foot, or a combination thereof at a major joint. Purpose is to promote the mental and physical rehabilitation of amputees through the sport of golf. Conducts first swing program for therapists. Organizes local, regional, national, and international tournaments. Compiles statistics. **Awards:** Recognition; scholarship bestowed to college students demonstrating financial need.

**★ 7893 ★ National Network for the Disabled**
c/o Linda Walls
PO Box 3574
Gardena, CA 90247-7274
**Phone:** (310)638-5717    **Fax:** (310)638-5986
Linda Walls, Founder-Pres.

**Desc:** Provides support, companionship, and networking opportunities for elderly individuals and parents of disabled children. Conducts research. Sponsors education on such topics as assertiveness, resources, and medical options. Provides transportation and emergency services, including a food program through which meals are delivered to homes. Conducts special events for parents and children, including picnics and field trips; special programs on nutrition and accessible travel with groups. **Awards:** Scholarship.

**★ 7894 ★ National Service Dog Center (NSDC)**
c/o Delta Society
289 Perimeter Rd. E
Renton, WA 98055
**Phone:** (425)226-7357    **Fax:** (425)235-1076
**Email:** info@deltasociety.org
**Website:** http://www.deltasociety.org
Tamara Whitehall, Contact

**Desc:** A joint program of the American Humane Association and the Delta Society. Provides a national service dog education, advocacy and referral service. Promotes the health benefits of service animals for people with disabilities. **Awards:** Service Animals of the Year (annual) for outstanding work by animals trained to help people with disabilities.

**★ 7895 ★ Society for Disability Studies**
c/o Carol J. Gill, PhD
University of Illinois at Chicago, MC626
Department of Disability and Human Development
1640 W Roosevelt Rd., No. 236
Chicago, IL 60608-6904
**Phone:** (312)996-4664
**Email:** cg16@uic.edu
**Website:** http://www.uic.edu/orgs/sds/
Carol J. Gill, PhD, Exec. Officer

**Desc:** Social scientists and scholars studying the problems of disabled people in society. Strives to develop theoretical and practical knowledge about disability and promotes equal participation in society for individuals with disabilities. **Awards:** Irving Kenneth Zola Emerging Scholar Award (annual); recognition.

**★ 7896 ★ Vocational Evaluation and Work Adjustment Association (VEWAA)**
PO Box 26273
Colorado Springs, CO 80936
**Phone:** (719)380-1412    **Fax:** (719)638-6153
**Email:** sjctcm@aol.com
**Website:** http://www.vewaa.org
Robin Cook, Pres.

**Desc:** A division of the National Rehabilitation Association (see separate entry). Specialists in vocational evaluation and work adjustment whose goals are to improve and advance the field and to promote high ethical practices through training and research. Conducts educational programs at state, regional, and national levels. Works with other organizations to develop a certification program for vocational evaluators and work adjustment personnel. Keeps legislators informed of the needs of persons with disabilities; promotes adequate funding of state and federal programs benefiting persons with disabilities. Disseminates employment information to members. **Awards:** Grant to members for small research projects; Paul R. Hoffman Service Award.

**★ 7897 ★ Yes I Can Foundation for Exceptional Children**
1110 N Glebe Rd., Ste. 300
Arlington, VA 22201-5704

**Phone:** (703)264-3660    **Free:** 800-224-6830
**Fax:** (703)264-9494
**Email:** service@cec.sped.org
**Website:** http://www.cec.sped.org
Trudy Kerr, Sr. Exec. Asst.

**Desc:** The Council for Exceptional Children. Advocates for quality education for all individuals with physical disabilities, multiple disabilities, and special health care needs served in schools, hospitals, or home settings. The council also advocates for gifted and talented children and youth. Operates the ERIC Clearinghouse on Disabilities and Gifted Education, and the National Clearinghouse for Professions in Special Education. Develops programs to help teachers, administrators, and related services professionals improve their practice. **Awards:** Business Award (annual); Clarissa Hug Teacher of the Year (annual); Elizabeth Wetzel Scholarship (annual); J.E. Wallace Wallin Special Education Lifetime Achievement (annual); Joan Wald Baaken Award (annual); Outstanding Leadership (annual); Outstanding Public Service Award (annual); Special Education Research (annual).

# National & International Organizations

**★ 7898 ★ Access Technology Association**
3612 Bent Branch Ct.
Falls Church, VA 22041
**Phone:** (703)941-4329    **Fax:** (703)941-4329
Dr. William T. Tobin, Exec. Dir.

**Fnded:** 1990. **Desc:** Provides forum and national clearinghouse on a variety of issues related to the disabled. Represents manufacturers and suppliers of assistive devices for the disabled.

**★ 7899 ★ Achilles Track Club (ATC)**
42 W 38th St., 4th Fl.
New York, NY 10018-6210
**Phone:** (212)354-0300    **Fax:** (212)354-3978
**Email:** achillesclub@aol.com
**Website:** http://www.achillestrackclub.org/
James M. Benson, Pres.

**Fnded:** 1982. **Mem:** 3,400. **Nat'l Groups:** 43. **Local Groups:** 40. **Desc:** Disabled runners; volunteer coaches. (Membership, though drawn primarily from New York City, also includes international members who are coached by mail.) Purpose is to encourage people with all types of disabilities to participate in running, and to improve the self-image of the disabled and demonstrate that they are energetic and capable people. Encourages the disabled to be aerobically fit and to run in competitions beside the able-bodied. Stresses that no previous athletic experience is necessary, just a desire to improve fitness with regular training. Conducts childrens' programs. Maintains speakers' bureau. Group is named for the mythical Greek hero whose disability was a vulnerable heel on an otherwise invincible body. **Pub:** *The Achilles Heel and Kid's Bits*, 3/year. Newsletter.

**★ 7900 ★ ACROD**
33 Thesiger Ct.
Acrod House
Deakin, ACT 2600, Australia
**Phone:** 61 2 62824333    **Fax:** 61 2 62813488
**Email:** acrodnat@acrod.org.au
**Website:** http://www.acrod.org.au

**Fnded:** 1962. **Mem:** 550. **State Groups:** 8. **Desc:** National industry association for disability services. Seeks to promote the development of quality services and life opportunities for Australians with disabilities. **Pub:** *ACROD Newsletter*, bimonthly. Newsletter. • *Discussion Papers*. Papers.

**★ 7901 ★ Action on Disability and Development (ADD)**
Vallis House
57 Vallis Rd.
Frome BA11 3EG, United Kingdom
**Phone:** 44 1373 473064    **Fax:** 44 1373 452075
**Email:** info@add.org.uk
**Website:** http://www.add.org.uk

**Fnded:** 1985. **Lang(s):** English. **Desc:** Development organizations. Seeks to increase participation by people with disabilities in the development process. Conducts educational and training courses to enhance the income-generation potential of people with disabilities; supports inclusion of people with disabilities in community rehabilitation initiatives.

**★ 7902 ★ Adaptive Sports Association**
PO Box 1884
Durango, CO 81302
**Phone:** (970)259-0374    **Fax:** (970)259-2175
**Email:** asa@frontier.net
**Website:** http://www.asadurango.org
Timothy S. Kroes, Exec. Dir.

**Fnded:** 1983. **Mem:** 420. **Desc:** Provides ski lessons to people with disabilities. Also offers summer sports opportunities to individuals with disabilities including river rafting, kayaking, canoeing, hiking, and fishing. **Pub:** *Membership Newsletter*, quarterly. Newsletter. • Newsletter, quarterly. *Price:* $30. **Frmly:** (1995) Durango/Purgatory Adaptive Sports Association.

**★ 7903 ★ Adventures in Movement for the Handicapped (AIM)**
945 Danbury Rd.
Dayton, OH 45420
**Phone:** (937)294-4611    **Free:** 800-332-8210
**Fax:** (937)294-3783
**Email:** aimkids@siscom.net
Dr. Jo A. Geiger, Exec. Dir.

**Fnded:** 1958. **Mem:** 4,000. **Desc:** Organizes activities for people with physical challenges. **Pub:** *Adventures in Movement*. Book. • Brochure. **Frmly:** (1969) DANCE, Inc.

**★ 7904 ★ African Rehabilitation Institute (ARI)**
Batanai Gardens
1st St.
PO Box 4056
Harare, Zimbabwe
**Fax:** 263 4 731089

**Lang(s):** English. **Desc:** Government agencies, organizations, and individuals with an interest in the social and economic integration of people with disabilities. Seeks to improve the quality of life of people with disabilities. Develops model public policies governing accessibility and other issues impacting people with disabilities; provides technical assistance to rehabilitation programs; serves as a clearinghouse on disability and legislation protecting the rights of people with disabilities.

**★ 7905 ★ Agape Center**
c/o Japan Church World Service
2-10-14 Komatsubara
Zama-shi
Kanagawa 228-0002, Japan
**Phone:** 81 46 2547111    **Fax:** 81 46 2552915
**Email:** agape@mb.infoweb.ne.jp

**Fnded:** 1980. **Lang(s):** English, Japanese. **Desc:** Works to improve the living conditions of people with disabilities throughout Asia. Conducts social work, rehabilitation, and vocational training programs. Sends Japanese social workers to assist in programs for people with disabilities overseas; distributes equipment to facilities for people with disabilities. **Frmly:** (1998) Agape Workshop for the Disabled.

**★ 7906 ★ All-Russian Society for Disabled**
Vdalzova 11
117415 Moscow, Russia
**Phone:** 7 95 9350064          **Fax:** 7 95 9350064
**Email:** vol@relcom.ru

**Fnded:** 1988. **Mem:** 2500,000. **Reg. Groups:** 80. **Lang(s):** Russian. **Desc:** Promotes the interests of disabled people. **Pub:** *Nadedgda*, monthly. Newspaper. Also publishes 23 other magazines and newspapers all over the Russia.

**★ 7907 ★ Ambucs Resource Center**
3315 North Main St.
High Point, NC 27265
**Phone:** (336)869-2166          **Fax:** (336)887-8451
**Email:** ambucs@ambucs.com
**Website:** http://www.ambucs.com

**Fnded:** 1922. **Mem:** 5,600. **Desc:** Dedicated to creating independence and opportunities for people with disabilities. Conducts service projects designed to give children with disabilities their first set of wheels. **Pub:** *AMBUC Magazine*, quarterly. Magazine.

**★ 7908 ★ American Academy of Disability Evaluating Physicians (AADEP)**
150 N Wacker Dr., Ste. 1420
Chicago, IL 60606-1605
**Phone:** (312)658-1171          **Free:** 800-456-6095
**Fax:** (312)658-1175
**Website:** http://www.aadep.org
Sandra L. Yost, Exec. Dir.

**Fnded:** 1987. **Mem:** 1,300. **Desc:** Physicians. Seeks to provide graduate and continuing medical education programs to qualify doctors of medicine and doctors of osteopathy to meet the needs of the public in the practice of the medical science of disability evaluation as well as disability consultation. Works to develop educational programs and training programs in disability evaluation and disability consultation for health care professionals. Fosters and develops the medical science of disability evaluation. Sponsors research programs. Establishes standards for physicians in the practice of disability evaluation and disability consultation. **Pub:** *AADEP Membership Directory*, annual. Directory. *Price:* $100. • *AADEP News*, quarterly. Newsletter. • *Disability*, quarterly. Journal. Papers pertaining to information useful to physicians' disability arena. *Price:* Free. For members only; $80 /year for nonmembers.

**★ 7909 ★ American Academy of Orthotists and Prosthetists (AAOP)**
526 King St., Ste. 201
Alexandria, VA 22314
**Phone:** (703)836-0788          **Fax:** (703)836-0737
**Email:** academy@oandp.com
**Website:** http://www.oandp.org
Gary Lamb, Pres.

**Fnded:** 1970. **Mem:** 2,100. **Reg. Groups:** 15. **Desc:** Professional practitioners certified by the American Board for Certification in Orthotics and Prosthetics. Dedicated to the advancement of the profession and the improvement of patient care. Provides continuing education designed to increase professional competence of the individual practitioner. **Pub:** *Academician*, monthly. Newsletter. • *Journal of Prosthetics and Orthotics*, quarterly. Journal. Scientific, research articles on latest products, fitting techniques and patient care regimens. • *JPO Selected Readings*. • Handbooks. • Manuals. • Also publishes home study videos.

**★ 7910 ★ American Amputee Foundation (AAF)**
Box 250218, Hillcrest Sta.
Little Rock, AR 72225
**Phone:** (501)666-2523          **Fax:** (501)666-8367
**Email:** cjwaiden@hotmail.com
C.J. Waiden, Exec. Dir. /CEO

**Fnded:** 1975. **Nat'l Groups:** 1. **State Groups:** 13. **Local Groups:** 2. **Desc:** Provides information and referral service to new amputees and their families to aid them in their adjustment to amputation. Sponsors programs and resources on state-of-the-art prosthetics, coalition building, and self-help life care planning services to those with catastrophic injury. on a very limited basis, aid in buying the first limb for amputees who qualify. Sponsors programs on state-of-the-art prosthetics, coalition building, and selfhelp. **Pub:** *National Resource Directory*, biennial. Directory. • Books. Provides information on self-help methods.

**★ 7911 ★ American Association of People with Disabilities (AAPD)**
1819 H St. NW, Ste. 330
Washington, DC 20006
**Phone:** (202)457-0046          **Free:** 800-840-8844
**Fax:** (202)457-0473
**Email:** aapd@aol.com
**Website:** http://www.aapd-dc.org
Helena Berger, Chief Operating Officer

**Fnded:** 1995. **Mem:** 28,000. **Nat'l Groups:** 1. **Desc:** Promotes economic and political empowerment of persons with disabilities; educating businesses and general public about disability issues. **Pub:** *AAPD News*, quarterly. Newsletter.

**★ 7912 ★ American Board for Certification in Orthotics and Prosthetics (ABC)**
330 John Carlyle St., Ste. 210
Alexandria, VA 22314
**Phone:** (703)836-7114          **Fax:** (703)836-0838
**Email:** lhoxie@opoffice.org
**Website:** http://www.opoffice.org/frameindex.htm
Lance O. Hoxie, Exec. Dir.

**Fnded:** 1948. **Mem:** 5,400. **Desc:** Certification board to establish qualifications, conduct examinations, and certify individuals (4200) and facilities (1200) whom board standards deem qualified to practice orthotics and prosthetics (the science of making and fitting artificial limbs and braces). **Pub:** *Mark of Merit*, bimonthly. Newsletter. • *O&P Almanac*, monthly. Magazine. • *Practice Analysis Report On the Scope of Practice in Prosthetics and Orthotics.*. Report. • *Registry of Board-Credentialed Orthotic and Prosthetic Professionals and Facilities*, annual. Directory. Contains lists all certified orthotists & prosthetists, registered technicians, and accredited facilities. *Price:* $20 for libraries; $75 for general public.

**★ 7913 ★ American Disability Association**
2201 Sixth Ave. South
Birmingham, AL 35233
**Phone:** (205)328-9090          **Fax:** (205)251-7417
**Email:** adanet@adanet.org
**Website:** http://www.adanet.org
William J. Freeman, Pres.

**Fnded:** 1991. **Mem:** 60,000. **Reg. Groups:** 20. **State Groups:** 40. **Desc:** Serves as a support group for individuals with disabilities. Provides exchange of information on disability issues. Makes available children's services, educational and research programs, and charitable services. **Pub:** *Journal of the American Disability Association*, monthly. Journal. *Price:* Free.

**American Disabled for Attendant Program Today (ADAPT)**
*See:* Entry 2921

**★ 7914 ★ American Society of Handicapped Physicians (ASHP)**
3424 S Culpepper Ct.
Springfield, MO 65804
**Phone:** (417)881-1570          **Fax:** (417)887-9830
**Email:** national@adapt.org
**Website:** http://www.adapt.org/
Jericho Peden, Contact

**Fnded:** 1981. **Mem:** 1,200. **Desc:** Handicapped physicians and others concerned with the problems faced by handicapped physicians. Acts as a forum to address the needs of physically disabled physicians. Works against discrimination of the handicapped and serves as a support group and legal and career counselor. Disseminates information about resources for handicapped physicians. Plans to offer rehabilitation services. Maintains speakers' bureau and placement service; compiles statistics; offers specialized education. Founded by the late Spencer B. Lewis, M.D. and Terry Winkler, M.D. **Pub:** *American Society of Handicapped Physicians–SYNAPSE*, quarterly. Includes book reviews and research updates. *Price:* Free. • Directory, annual.

**★ 7915 ★ American Wheelchair Bowling Association (AWBA)**
2912 Country Woods Ln.
Palm Harbor, FL 34683-6412
**Phone:** (727)734-0023
**Email:** bowiawba@juno.com
**Website:** http://www.awba.org/
Earle Annis, Exec. Sec. -Treas.

**Fnded:** 1962. **Mem:** 600. **Reg. Groups:** 12. **Desc:** Male and female athletes with permanent disabilities who are confined to wheelchairs. To organize and promote wheelchair bowling and regulate rules. Provides information about wheelchair bowling. Conducts state and national wheelchair bowling tournaments. Maintains hall of fame and museum; compiles statistics. **Pub:** *The 11th Frame*, bimonthly. • *Wheelchair Bowling*. Book.

**★ 7916 ★ Americans With Disabilities Act (ADA)**
10765 SW 104 St.
Miami, FL 33176
**Phone:** (305)271-0012          **Fax:** (305)273-1221
**Email:** ergobobl@aol.com
**Website:** http://www.rehabserv.com
Robert L. Lessne, PhD, Contact

**Fnded:** 1990. **Mem:** 100. **Desc:** Individuals and organizations united to ensure compliance with the Americans With Disabilities Act of 1992. Compiles statistics; sponsors competitions; maintains speakers' bureau; and operates a museum with cones for visually impaired individuals. **Pub:** *ADA Compliance Kit*. Booklet. *Price:* $100. • *ADA Compliance Sourcebook*.

**★ 7917 ★ Amity Goodwill Industries (AGI)**
225 King William St.
Hamilton, ON, Canada L8R 1B1
**Phone:** (905)526-8481          **Fax:** (905)526-9342
**Email:** amity@amity.on.ca
**Website:** http://www.amity.on.ca

**Lang(s):** English, French. **Desc:** Individuals with disabilities. Promotes employment and full participation in society by members. Operates businesses providing employment to people with disabilities; provides support and services to industries employing people with disabilities.

**★ 7918 ★ Amputees in Motion, International (AIM)**
PO Box 2703
Escondido, CA 92033
**Phone:** (619)454-9300
**Website:** http://www.usinter.net/wasa/sandiego1.html
John Murphy, Pres.

**Fnded:** 1973. **Mem:** 80. **Desc:** Amputees and their families. Helps amputees of any age reestablish an active and satisfying life through visitation program and civic, social, and recreational participation. Attempts to prove that losing a limb doesn't mean losing the ability to participate in physical activities. Works with physicians, physical therapists, prosthetists, and others as part of the amputee rehabilitation team. Makes available sporting and social activities. Provides speakers who talk before professional and civic organizations regarding amputees. **Pub:** *Amputees in Motion Newsletter*, 3/year. Newsletter. Includes membership meeting information. *Price:* Free. **Frmly:** (2000) Amputees in Motion.

### ★ 7919 ★ Arab Disabled Confederation (ADC)

88 Kasr El-Eini St., Apt. 52
Cairo, Egypt
**Phone:** 20 2 3489367    **Fax:** 20 2 714394
**Lang(s):** Arabic, English. **Desc:** People with disabilities and organizations serving the disabled. Seeks to improve the quality of life and legal status of people with disabilities. Provides support and services to people with disabilities and their families; lobbies for legislation expanding the human and civil rights of the disabled.

### ★ 7920 ★ L'Arche Australia (AA)

PO Box 1326
Woden, ACT 2606, Australia
**Phone:** 61 2 62952627    **Fax:** 61 2 62952627
**Fnded:** 1989. **Mem:** 9. **Local Groups:** 3. **Lang(s):** English. **Desc:** Individuals and corporate members. Advocates a holistic approach to human development through the establishment of L'Arche communities for intellectually disabled individuals in neighborhood homes. Promotes a Christian perspective in L'Arche communities in Australia and abroad. **Pub:** *L'Arche Australia Newsletter*, quarterly. Provides news of Australian L'Arche communities. • *Letters of L'Arche*, quarterly. Journal. Includes articles about life in L'Arche communities and issues concerning persons with intellectual disabilities.

### ★ 7921 ★ Assistance Dogs of America (ADAI)

8806 State Rte. 64
Swanton, OH 43558
**Phone:** (419)825-3622    **Fax:** (419)825-3710
**Email:** adaifacili@aol.com
**Website:** http://www.adai.org
Chris Diefenthaler, Prog. Dir.
**Fnded:** 1984. **Mem:** 3,000. **Desc:** Promotes increased independence for people with disabilities. Locates, trains, and places highly skilled service and therapy dogs with disabled adults and children. **Pub:** *Hearts in Harness*, 3/year. Newsletter. **Frmly:** (1989) Guide Dogs for the Handicapped, Inc.

### ★ 7922 ★ Association of Adult Day Support Programs (AADSP)

9735 80th Ave.
Edmonton, AB, Canada T6E 1S8
**Phone:** (780)434-4747    **Fax:** (780)433-3758
**Email:** aadsp@tnc.com
**Fnded:** 1979. **Mem:** 160. **Desc:** Educational and recreational programs for adults with disabilities living in non-institutional settings. Promotes an improved quality of life for adults with disabilities that prevent them from participating in mainstream recreational activities. Facilitates communication and cooperation among members; provides educational and recreational programs to adults with disabilities.

### ★ 7923 ★ Association of Central African Centres for the Handicapped (ACACH)

Boite Postale 51
Butare, Rwanda
**Phone:** 250 82020
**Lang(s):** English, French. **Desc:** Organizations providing services to people with disabilities. Seeks to improve the quality of life of people with disabilities and their families. Coordinates provision of services to people with disabilities in central Africa; facilitates cooperation, communication, and exchange among members.

### Association of Children's Prosthetic-Orthotic Clinics (ACPOC)
*See:* Entry 5623

### ★ 7924 ★ Association Congolaise des Personnes Handicapees

BP 242
Kinshasa, Republic of the Congo
**Email:** king@aaos.org
**Website:** http://www.acpoc.org
**Fnded:** 1981. **Mem:** 150. **Local Groups:** 4. **Lang(s):** French. Does not correspond in English. **Desc:** Association of mentally or physically disabled persons, their families, and concerned individuals. Promotes equal opportunity and participation for the disabled. Provides children's services. **Frmly:** (1999) Association Zairoise des Handicapes.

### ★ 7925 ★ Association of Disabled Professionals (ADP)

BCM ADP
London WC1N 3XX, United Kingdom
**Phone:** 44 208 7785008    **Fax:** 44 208 7782599
**Email:** assdisprof@aol.com
**Website:** http://www.adp.org.uk
**Fnded:** 1971. **Mem:** 230. **Lang(s):** English. **Desc:** Professionals and students with disabilities. Offers advice and information especially on employment issues. Provides means to disabled professionals and those in managerial positions to network and offer advice and support. Maintains liaisons with government authorities. **Pub:** *ADP Quarterly*, quarterly.

### ★ 7926 ★ Association of the Handicapped Children of Romania

Str. Gral Haralambie 36, Sector 4
Bucharest, Romania
**Phone:** 40 1 3371875    **Fax:** 40 1 3371875
**Email:** aschfr@ant.ro
**Fnded:** 1990. **Mem:** 2,500. **Reg. Groups:** 7. **Lang(s):** English, Romanian. **Desc:** Promotes improved quality of life for children with physical disabilities in Romania. Conducts educational and instructional programs for children with physical handicaps and their teachers and family members; makes available physical therapy and other treatment programs. **Pub:** *Informative Bulletin*, semiannual. Newsletter.

### ★ 7927 ★ Association for Higher Education Access and Disability (AHEAD)

Newman House
86 St.
Stephens Green 2, Dublin, Ireland
**Phone:** 353 1 4752386    **Fax:** 353 1 4752387
**Email:** ahead@iol.ie
**Website:** http://www.ahead.ie
**Fnded:** 1989. **Mem:** 70. **Lang(s):** English, Irish. **Desc:** Individuals and organizations. Promotes increased access to higher education for people with disabilities. Lobbies for more stringent statutes mandating accessibility of educational institutions; represents the interests of people with disabilities before institutions of higher education.

### ★ 7928 ★ Association on Higher Education and Disability (AHEAD)

University of Massachusetts Boston
100 Morrissey Blvd.
Boston, MA 02125-3393
**Phone:** (617)287-3880    **Fax:** (617)287-3881
**Email:** stephan.smith@umb.edu
**Website:** http://www.ahead.org
Stephan J. Smith, Exec. Dir.
**Fnded:** 1977. **Mem:** 2,000. **Desc:** Individuals interested in promoting the equal rights and opportunities of disabled postsecondary students, staff, faculty, and graduates. Provides an exchange of communication for those professionally involved with disabled students; collects, evaluates, and disseminates informa-

tion; encourages and supports legislation for the benefit of disabled students. Conducts surveys on issues pertinent to college students with disabilities; offers resource referral system and employment exchange for positions in disability student services. Conducts research programs; compiles statistics. **Pub:** *ALERT*, quarterly. Newsletter. • *Journal of Postsecondary Education & Disability*. Journal. • Membership Directory, ongoing. **AKA:** AHEAD.

### Association of Maternal and Child Health Programs (AMCHP)
*See:* Entry 5625

### Association of Rehabilitation Programs in Computer Technology (ARPCT)
*See:* Entry 20104

### ★ 7929 ★ Association for Research and Training on Integration in Europe (ARTI) (Association de Recherche et Formation pour l'Insertion — ARFI)

38, rue de Fontenay
F-94130 Nogent-sur-Marne, France
**Phone:** 33 1 48733207    **Fax:** 33 1 43943249
**Email:** jsarfaty@free.fr
**Website:** http://www.arfie.org
**Fnded:** 1987. **Mem:** 15. **Lang(s):** English, French. **Desc:** Promotes and conducts multidisciplinary research on the incorporation of disabled persons into mainstream society and other issues impacting the disabled. Organizes reflection groups. Interacts with related associations elsewhere in Europe. Conducts research and educational programs.

### ★ 7930 ★ Association for Support of Social and Community Integration (ASSCI) (Espaco t)

Centro Comercial Capitolio-lojs 5, 22e23
Av. Franca n0 256
P-4050 Porto, Portugal
**Phone:** 351 22 8302432    **Fax:** 351 22 8305593
**Email:** espacot@espacot.pt
**Website:** http://www.espacot.pt
**Fnded:** 1994. **Mem:** 396. **Lang(s):** English, Portuguese. **Desc:** Individuals and organizations working with people with disabilities. Promotes integration of people with disabilities into mainstream society. Conducts programs in the arts, martial arts, theater, and language to better equip people with disabilities for integration into society. Makes available counseling, support, and services to people with disabilities and to people suffering from addictions, psychological disorders, and health problems. **Pub:** *Contacto*, semiannual. Magazine.

### ★ 7931 ★ Associazione la Nostra Famiglia (LNF)

Via don Luigi Monza 1
I-22037 Ponte Lambro, Italy
**Phone:** 39 31 625111    **Fax:** 39 31 625243
**Email:** info@pl.lnf.it
**Website:** http://www.lanostrafamiglia.it/
**Fnded:** 1947. **Mem:** 150. **Lang(s):** English, Italian. **Desc:** Association, based on evangelical principles, devoted to the social and physical rehabilitation of disabled children and young adults. Particular emphasis is placed on individuals with physical neuromotor and sensorial dysfunctions. Maintains more than 30 rehabilitation centers throughout Italy; also operates work centers and family homes providing social and educational training. Manages developing cooperation projects in Sudan, Brazil, and Ecuador and collaborates with projects in China and Palestina. Offers training and continuing education courses to specialists in the field. Sponsors seminars; maintains the Eugenio Medea Scientific Institute for hospitalization and treatment. Conducts research; compiles statistics. Maintains a clinic. **Pub:** *Notiziario d'Informazione*,

quarterly. Newsletter. • *SAGGI-Child Development and Disabilities*, bimonthly. Journal. Scientific magazine.

**★ 7932 ★ Australian Quadriplegic Association (AQA)**
1 Jennifer St.
Little Bay, NSW 2036, Australia
**Phone:** 61 2 96618855    **Fax:** 61 2 96619598
**Email:** aqa@aqa.org.au
**Website:** http://www.aqa.com.au
**Fnded:** 1967. **Lang(s):** English. **Desc:** People with severe physical disabilities and their families. Seeks to enable people with severe physical disabilities to achieve maximum independence through a rehabilitation perspective in all its services. Provides community support and counseling, peer support, advocacy, and disability awareness training. **Pub:** *QUAD WRANGLE*, quarterly. Journal.

**★ 7933 ★ Bellwoods Centres for Community Living (BCCL)**
300 Shaw St.
Toronto, ON, Canada M6J 2X2
**Phone:** (416)530-1448    **Fax:** (416)536-8189
**Lang(s):** English, French. **Desc:** Community living centers serving adults with physical disabilities. Seeks to improve the quality of life of individuals with physical disabilities residing in community living facilities. Provides support and services to increase the self-reliance of people with physical disabilities; facilitates communication and cooperation among members.

**Board for Orthotist - Prosthetist Certification**
*See:* Entry 4510

**★ 7934 ★ British Amputee and Les Autres Sports Association**
30, Greaves Close
Arnold
Nottingham NG5 6RS, United Kingdom
**Phone:** 44 115 9260220    **Fax:** 44 115 9260220
**Email:** info@bocusa.org
**Website:** http://www.bocusa.org
**Fnded:** 1980. **Mem:** 250. **Desc:** Promotes sports among amputees and Les Autres. **Pub:** Newsletter, quarterly. Contains general sports news for and about members. **Frmly:** (1999) British Amputee Association.

**★ 7935 ★ British Columbia Wheelchair Sports Association**
1367 W Broadway, Ste. 224
Vancouver, BC, Canada V6H 4A9
**Phone:** (604)737-3090    **Free:** 877-737-3090
**Fax:** (604)737-6043
**Email:** info@bcwheelchairsports.com
**Website:** http://www.bcwheelchairsports.com
**Fnded:** 1967. **Mem:** 800. **Reg. Groups:** 5. **Local Groups:** 5. **Lang(s):** English, French. **Desc:** Assists wheelchair sport development through advocacy, marketing, and providing information and resources. Works in close partnership with community groups and agencies to ensure that there are opportunities for participation. Supports participation froma recreational to elite level in a wide variety of sports. **Pub:** *The Newswheel*, 3/year. Newsletter. **Frmly:** (1996) Canadian Wheelchair Sports Association.

**★ 7936 ★ British Council of Disabled People (BCODP)**
Litchurch Plaza
Litchurch Ln.
Derby DE24 8AA, United Kingdom
**Phone:** 44 1332 295551    **Fax:** 44 1332 295580
**Email:** general@bcodp.org.uk
**Website:** http://www.bcodp.org.uk
**Fnded:** 1981. **Mem:** 140. **Reg. Groups:** 123. **Desc:** Organizations controlled by disabled people and individual membership is now available to all disabled people and their supporters. The national umbrella organisation representing groups controlled by disabled people. Current concern is to secure anti-discrimination legislation. Has begun a 3-year group development programme to actively support the growth of regional organisations controlled by disabled people. **Pub:** *Amazons*. Newsletter. • *Personal Assistance Users Newsletter*. Newsletter. • *Update*, monthly. Newsletter. **Frmly:** (1999) British Council of Organisations of Disabled People.

**★ 7937 ★ British Disabled Water Ski Association**
c/o Tony Edge National Centre
Heron Lake
Staines TW19 6HW, United Kingdom
**Phone:** 44 1784 483664    **Fax:** 44 1784 482747
**Website:** http://www.bdwsa.org
**Fnded:** 1979. **Reg. Groups:** 4. **Desc:** Disabled full members and able-bodied helpers associate members. Teaches people with a disability to water ski and trains drivers, observers and instructors.

**★ 7938 ★ British Wheelchair Sports Foundation**
Guttmann Rd.
Stoke Mandeville HP21 9PP, United Kingdom
**Phone:** 44 1296 395995    **Fax:** 44 1296 424171
**Email:** enquiries@britishwheelchairsports.org
**Website:** http://www.britishwheelchairsports.org
**Fnded:** 1952. **Mem:** 2,500. **Desc:** Promotes wheelchair sports. **Pub:** *Annuae Handbook*, quarterly. Newsletter.

**★ 7939 ★ Canadian Amputee Sports Association (Association Canadienne des Sports pour Amputes)**
217 Holmes Ave.
Willowdale, ON, Canada M2N 4M9
**Phone:** (416)222-8625    **Fax:** (416)229-6547
**Email:** ampsport@interlog.com
**Website:** http://www.interlog.com/~ampsport/can_amputee.html
**Lang(s):** English, French. **Desc:** Amputees and other individuals with an interest in sports for people with disabilities. Seeks to increase the availability of sports programs for amputees. Conducts athletic and other recreational programs.

**★ 7940 ★ Canadian Association for Disabled Skiing (CADS) (Association Canadienne des Sports pour Skieurs Handicapes — ACSSH)**
PO Box 307
Kimberly, BC, Canada V1A 2Y9
**Phone:** (250)427-7712    **Fax:** (250)427-7715
**Email:** info@disabledskiing.ca
**Website:** http://www.disabledskiing.ca
**Fnded:** 1976. **Mem:** 3,000. **Nat'l Groups:** 10. **Lang(s):** English, French. **Desc:** People with disabilities. Promotes participation in skiing by members. Provides skiing opportunities for people with disabilities.

**★ 7941 ★ Canadian Association of Independent Living Centers (CAILC)**
1004-350 Sparks St.
Ottawa, ON, Canada K1R 7S8
**Phone:** (613)563-2581    **Fax:** (613)235-4497
**Email:** cailc@magma.ca
**Website:** http://www.cailc.ca
**Lang(s):** English, French. **Desc:** Promotes and fosters the development of Independent Living Resource Centres in Canada. Fosters full integration of people with disabilities into society.

**Canadian Association of Prosthetists and Orthotists (Association Canadienne des Prothesistes et Orthesistes)**
*See:* Entry 4511

**★ 7942 ★ Canadian Cerebral Palsy Sports Association (CCPSA)**
1600 James Naismith Dr., 607A
Gloucester, ON, Canada K1B 5N4
**Phone:** (613)748-5725    **Fax:** (613)748-5899
**Email:** ccpsa@cyberas.ca
**Website:** http://www.ccpsa.ca
**Fnded:** 1985. **Mem:** 2,000. **Reg. Groups:** 7. **Lang(s):** English, French. **Desc:** Individuals with cerebral palsy and their families; volunteer officials and organizers. Promotes participation in competitive sports, such as boccia, cycling, athletics, and powerlifting by people with cerebral palsy. Conducts training programs; sponsors competitions. **Pub:** *Canadian Cerebral Palsy Sports Association*. Brochure.

**★ 7943 ★ Canadian Foundation for Physically Disabled Persons (CFPDP)**
731 Runnymede Rd.
Toronto, ON, Canada M6N 3V7
**Phone:** (416)760-7351    **Fax:** (416)760-9405
**Email:** whynot@sympatico.ca
**Website:** http://www3.sympatico.ca/whynot/
**Fnded:** 1987. **Lang(s):** English. **Desc:** Works to bring public attention to the needs and accomplishments of people with physical disabilities. Creates public awareness in public, business, and government on issues of housing, employment, education, accessibility, sports and recreation, and research. Provides financial assistance to organizations that share concerns for adults with physical disabilities.

**★ 7944 ★ Canadian Paralympic Committee (CPC) (Comite Paralympique du Canada — CPC)**
1400-85 Albert St.
Ottawa, ON, Canada K1P 6A4
**Phone:** (613)569-4333    **Fax:** (613)569-2777
**Email:** karenmc@magma.ca
**Website:** http://www.paralympic.ca
**Lang(s):** English, French. **Desc:** Athletic organizations providing sporting opportunities to people with paralysis and amputees. Seeks to improve the quality of life and fitness of people with paralysis and amputees. Assists in the foundation of local paralympic organizations; sponsors competitions and recreational events.

**★ 7945 ★ Canadian Paraplegic Association (CPA)**
230-1101 Prince of Wales Dr.
Ottawa, ON, Canada K2C 3W7
**Phone:** (613)723-1033    **Free:** 800-720-4933
**Fax:** (613)723-1060
**Email:** info@canparaplegic.org
**Website:** http://www.canparaplegic.org
**Fnded:** 1945. **Lang(s):** English, French. **Desc:** To assist persons with spinal cord injuries and other physical disabilities to achieve independence, self-reliance and full community participation. **Pub:** *Caliper*, quarterly. Journal.

**★ 7946 ★ Canadian Special Olympics (CSO)**
40 St. Clair Ave. E, Ste. 209
Toronto, ON, Canada M4V 1M2
**Phone:** (416)927-9050    **Free:** 877-291-7404
**Fax:** (416)927-8475
**Email:** solympic@inforamp.net
**Website:** http://www.cso.on.ca
**Fnded:** 1969. **Mem:** 30. **Lang(s):** English, French. **Desc:** Provides sport training and competition for people with a mental disability at local, provincial,

national and international levels. Conducts research, provides coach training. **Pub:** *Canadian Special Olympics.* Brochure. • *Canadian Special Olympics National Office Bulletin,* semiannual. Newsletter. • *Canadian Special Olympics National Team.* Brochure.

★ 7947 ★ **Canine Companions for Independence (CCI)**
PO Box 446
Santa Rosa, CA 95402-0446
**Phone:** (707)577-1700 **Free:** 800-572-2275
**Fax:** (707)577-1712
**Email:** info@caninecompanions.org
**Website:** http://www.caninecompanions.org/
Mr. Corey Hudson, Exec. Dir.

**Fnded:** 1975. **Nat'l Groups:** 1. **Reg. Groups:** 5. **State Groups:** 3. **Desc:** Provides to people with disabilities, specially-bred and trained dogs enabling them to lead more personally fulfilling and socially productive lives. Believes that human attendant care is reduced with the aid these dogs provide. Provides four types of Canine Companions: Hearing Dogs trained to alert the hearing-impaired to sounds such as the doorbell, smoke alarm, or a baby's cry; skilled companion dogs used for children and adults with disabilities, people with developmental disabilities, or anywhere the supervision of a third party is required; Service Dogs trained to provide physical assistance, such as retrieving dropped objects, operating elevator buttons and light switches, and pulling wheelchairs and Facility dogs placed with professionals in facilities where interaction with a dog will be beneficial to the mental or physical health of those in their care. Works to expand services to aid more persons with disabilities. Sponsors puppy raising programs where puppies are placed and raised in volunteer homes for 13 months; advanced training takes about 6-8 months to master over 60 required working commands. Conducts ongoing research in canine breeding, training, and nutrition. **Pub:** *Canine Companion Courier,* quarterly. Newsletter. *Price:* Free. • Annual Report. • Brochures. • Manuals.

★ 7948 ★ **Center on Human Policy (CHP)**
Syracuse University
School of Education
805 S Crouse Ave.
Syracuse, NY 13244-2280
**Phone:** (315)443-3851 **Free:** 800-894-0826
**Fax:** (315)443-4338
**Email:** thechp@sued.syr.edu
**Website:** http://soeweb.syr.edu/thechp
Steven Taylor, PhD, Dir.

**Fnded:** 1971. **Desc:** Consumers and students; parents of persons with disabilities; human services administrators and staff members; professionals in psychology, special education, rehabilitation, sociology, law, social work, and planning. Goal is to promote the inclusion of persons with severe disabilities into the mainstream of society. Disseminates information to families, human services professionals, and others on laws, regulations, and programs affecting children and adults with disabilities, focusing on those with developmental disabilities. Provides speakers to professional gatherings and parents' groups. Documents outstanding community living and educational programs and assists in creating exemplary services. Evaluates public policies to determine their impact on people with disabilities. Participates in public forums, legislative hearings, national conventions, and other community events involving issues relating to people with disabilities. Operates National Resource Center on Supported Living and Choice for people with developmental disabilities. Offers technical assistance, consultation, and training on service system issues to local, regional, state, and national organizations and agencies. Conducts research related to community inclusion.

★ 7949 ★ **Cerebral Palsy International Sports and Recreation Association (CP-ISRA)**
Postbus 16
NL-6666 ZG Heteren, Netherlands
**Phone:** 31 26 4722593 **Fax:** 31 26 4723914
**Email:** cpisra_nl@hotmail.com
**Website:** http://surf.to/cpisra

**Fnded:** 1978. **Mem:** 60. **Lang(s):** English. **Desc:** Organizations in 60 countries interested in sports and recreation for the cerebral palsied. Provides greater opportunities for the cerebral palsied to participate in a wide variety of sports and recreational activities. Assists members in developing sports and recreation programs through demonstrations, courses, films, and seminars; provides means for communication and dissemination of information among members. **Pub:** *Classification and Sport Rules Manual.* Manual. • *Classification Video.* Video. • *News,* semiannual. Newsletter.

★ 7950 ★ **Cerebral Palsy Ireland (CPI)**
Kiltartan House
Forster St.
Galway 4, Ireland
**Phone:** 353 91 566686 **Fax:** 353 1 2694983
**Fnded:** 1951. **Local Groups:** 20. **Lang(s):** English. **Desc:** Works to provide therapy, training, and vocational education programs for children and adults with cerebral palsy and other physical dissabilities.

★ 7951 ★ **Challenged Conquistadors**
c/o Shaun Best
Rt2 Box 32
Hampton, AR 71744
**Phone:** (870)798-4558
**Email:** shaun_best_2000@yahoo.com
**Website:** http://www.geocities.com/shaun_best_2000/personalpageblue.html
Shaun Best, Pres. & Founder

**Fnded:** 1993. **Mem:** 10,000. **Local Groups:** 1. **Desc:** Works to increase self preservation, reduce dependency, and eradicate negative stereotypes, myths, and stigmas. Targets active, positive, challenged role models to show others that success is obtainable. Reinforces individual empowerment and capabilities to reveal the talents inherent in all challenged individuals and reap rewards as opposed to the "stagnation and destruction that many social programs have achieved." Offers educational and research programs.

★ 7952 ★ **Cheshire Foundation in Ireland (CFI)**
1-4 Adelaide Rd.
Glasthule
Dublin 4, Ireland
**Phone:** 353 1 2804879 **Fax:** 353 1 2804954
**Email:** info@cheshire-foundation.ie
**Website:** http://www.cheshire-foundation.ie

**Lang(s):** English, Irish. **Desc:** Individuals and organizations. Seeks to improve the quality of life of people with disabilities. Provides housing and support and services to people with disabilities and their families.

★ 7953 ★ **Children's Craniofacial Association (CCA)**
13140 Coit Rd., Ste. 307
Dallas, TX 75240
**Phone:** (214)570-9099 **Free:** 800-535-3643
**Fax:** (972)566-8489
**Email:** contactCCA@ccakids.com
**Website:** http://www.ccakids.com
Charlene Smith, Exec. Dir.

**Fnded:** 1989. **Desc:** Participants include craniofacial surgeons and others wishing to aid individuals with craniofacial deformities. Promotes increased awareness of craniofacial deformities and their treatment among health care professionals and the public. Provides financial assistance to craniofacially deformed patients for costs related to treatment such as food, travel and lodging. Functions as a networking and referral service for patients. Makes referrals to qualified centers. Conducts craniofacial family workshops. **Pub:** Booklets. Provides information on craniofacial conditions and their treatment. • Films. • Videos. • Also publishes materials for health care professionals, government officials, and parents of craniofacially deformed children. **Frmly:** (1992) International Craniofacial Foundations.

★ 7954 ★ **Christian Council on Persons with Disabilities (CCPD)**
7120 W Dove Ct.
Milwaukee, WI 53223
**Phone:** (414)357-6672
**Email:** info@ccpd.org
**Website:** http://www.ccpd.org/

**Desc:** Christian disability advocacy organization promoting the spiritual well-being of people with physical, mental or emotional disabilities. **Pub:** *CCPD News,* quarterly. Newsletter. Contains information in the field of Christian disability ministry and developments in the U.S. and worldwide.

★ 7955 ★ **Christian Overcomers (CO)**
c/o Debbie Neillyh
PO Box 2007
Garfield, NJ 07026
**Phone:** (973)253-2343 **Fax:** (973)253-2351
**Website:** http://www.gracechurchweb.org/missions/missionaries/overcomers.htm
Debbie Neilley, Exec. Dir.

**Fnded:** 1977. **Desc:** Individuals with physical disabilities and volunteers. Provides holistic physical and spiritual guidance to help members live with their disabilities. Sponsors camp program that provides Bible study, worship, recreational and social activities, and encourages "commitment to Jesus Christ and each other." Functions as a resource for local groups that wish to conduct activities including athletic events, outings, dinners, and other socially oriented educational programs for physically disabled individuals. Maintains speakers' bureau. Provides volunteer training. **Pub:** *Library Catalog,* annual. Catalog. • *The Overcomer,* quarterly. Newsletter. • Brochure.

★ 7956 ★ **Christian Record Services (CRS)**
1300 King St. E, Ste. 119
Oshawa, ON, Canada L1H 8N9
**Phone:** (905)436-6938 **Fax:** (905)436-7102
**Email:** crs-ncb@oix.com
**Website:** http://www.christianrecord.org

**Fnded:** 1899. **Lang(s):** English, French. **Desc:** Volunteers. Seeks to "enrich the lives of blind, deaf, and physically handicapped individuals." Provides services including reading, braille materials and personal visitations to people with physical disabilities. Maintains National Camps for the Blind; conducts educational programs to raise public awareness on meeting the needs of blind people. **Pub:** *NCB News,* annual. Newsletter. • Brochure.

★ 7957 ★ **Clearinghouse on Disability Information (CDI)**
Office of Special Educ. and Rehabilitative Services
Switzer Bldg., Rm. 3132
Washington, DC 20202-2524
**Phone:** (202)205-8241 **Fax:** (202)401-2608
**Website:** http://www.health.gov/nhic/NHICScripts/Entry.cfm?RCode=hR0035
Carolyn Corlett, Tech. Asst.

**Fnded:** 1973. **Desc:** Responds to inquiries on topics concerning federally-funded programs serving disabled persons and federal legislation affecting the disabled community. Researches and documents information providers serving the handicapped. Makes resource referrals. **Pub:** *Pocket Guide to Federal Help for Individuals With Disabilities.* **Frmly:** (1989) Clearinghouse on the Handicapped.

**★ 7958 ★ Coalition for Education and Self-help Training Advocates (C'esta)**
c/o John-Paul LeBlanc
52 Faith Ln.
PO Box 6368
Manchester, NH 03108-6368
**Phone:** (603)627-5656 **Fax:** (603)679-4693
John-Paul LeBlanc, Pres. -Dir.

**Fnded:** 1993. **Desc:** Disabled individuals, their families, and advocates. Provides public, educational, and information services. Strives to help increase independent skills regardless of disability. **Pub:** Newsletter, monthly. *Price:* Free. • Journal, annual. *Price:* Free.

**Council of State Administrators of Vocational Rehabilitation (CSAVR)**
*See:* Entry 20121

**★ 7959 ★ Dateable International**
7830 Wisconsin Ave.
Bethesda, MD 20814
**Phone:** (301)656-8723 **Fax:** (301)657-4327
**Email:** robert@dateable.org
**Website:** http://www.dateable.org
Robert S. Watson, MSW, Exec. Dir.

**Fnded:** 1982. **Mem:** 600. **Local Groups:** 1. **Desc:** Purpose is to bring together persons with disabilities for love and friendship. Provides individual counseling and support network. **Pub:** *DateLine*, annual, 3-4/year. Newsletter. *Price:* Free. **Frmly:** (1994) Handicap Introductions; (1997) Date-Able/HI.

**DB-Link**
*See:* Entry 20940

**★ 7960 ★ Disability Alliance**
Universal House
89-94 Wentworth St.
London E1 7SA, United Kingdom
**Phone:** 44 20 72478776 **Fax:** 44 20 72478765
**Email:** office.da@dial.pipex.com
**Website:** http://www.disabilityalliance.org

**Fnded:** 1974. **Mem:** 350. **Desc:** Statutory and voluntary organizations with an interest in disability and poverty. Campaigns for the introduction of a Comprehensive Disability Income schedule, and operates a Rights Advice telephone line on 0171-247-8763 for free information on disability benefits. **Pub:** *AA Guide and Checklist.* Handbook. • *Disability Rights Handbook*, annual. Handbook. • *OLA Guide and Checklist.* Handbook. • Bulletin, 3/year. **Frmly:** (1999) Disability Alliance Education and Research Association.

**★ 7961 ★ Disability Central**
PO Box 8612
Long Beach, CA 90808-0612
**Website:** http://www.disabilitycentral.com

**Desc:** People with disabilities. Promote disability awareness. Provide information and resources.

**★ 7962 ★ Disability Federation of Ireland (DFI)**
2 Sandyford Office Park
Blackthorn Ave.
Dublin 18, Ireland
**Phone:** 353 1 2959344 **Fax:** 353 1 2959346
**Email:** info@disability-federation.ie
**Website:** http://ireland.iol.ie/~dfi/
**Fnded:** 1960. **Mem:** 73. **Lang(s):** English, Irish. **Desc:** Voluntary and nonstatutory agencies providing support services to people with disabilities. Seeks to increase the availability and quality of services for people with disabilities; promotes development of the full potential of all people. Provides support and assistance to members; facilitates communication and networking among members; develops training programs for people providing services to people with disabilities; serves as a liaison linking members with public agencies responsible for statutes affecting people with disabilities. Makes available resource

services; sponsors research and educational programs; conducts lobbying activities. **Pub:** *DFI Newsletter*, monthly. Newsletter. • *Disability Federation of Ireland Directory*, annual. Directory.

**★ 7963 ★ Disability Resources**
c/o Avery Klauber
4 Glatter Ln.
Centereach, NY 11720-1032
**Phone:** (631)585-0290 **Fax:** (631)585-0290
**Email:** pubs@disabilityresources.org
**Website:** http://www.disabilityresources.org
Avery Klauber, Exec. Dir.

**Fnded:** 1993. **Desc:** Works to promote and improve awareness, availability and accessibility of information to help people with disabilities to live independently. Advises libraries, independent living centers, rehabilitation professionals, hospitals, health and social service organizations, and consumers of resources and publications concerning independent living. **Pub:** *Disability Information at Your Fingertips, 3rd Ed..* Book. *Price:* $10. • *Disability Resources Monthly (DRM)*, monthly. Newsletter. Reports on and reviews resources for independent living. *Price:* $33/year.

**★ 7964 ★ Disability Rights Center (DRC)**
PO Box 2007
Augusta, ME 04338-2007
**Phone:** (207)626-2774 **Free:** 800-452-1948
**Fax:** (207)621-1419
**Email:** advocate@drcme.org
**Website:** http://www.drcme.org
Kim Moody, Exec. Dir.

**Fnded:** 1976. **Desc:** Public interest research group committed to educating society about the disability rights movement. Objectives are to inform the public, political activists, consumer activists, advocates, and students on the disability movement. Major current projects are disability photo project, capital ADAPT and using media effectively. Through its activities, the center seeks to involve as many disabled citizens as possible in processes that directly affect their lives, to work closely with other disability-related, consumer-based advocacy groups, and to educate the public in the legitimate demands and needs of the disabled. Through its activites, the center seeks to involve as many disabled citizens as possible in processes that directly affect their lives, to work closely wiht other disability-related, consumer-based advocacy groups, and to educate the public in the legitimate demands and needs of the disabled. Compiles statistics.

**★ 7965 ★ Disability Rights Education and Defense Fund (DREDF)**
2212 6th St.
Berkeley, CA 94710
**Phone:** (510)644-2555 **Fax:** (510)841-8645
**Email:** dredf@dredf.org
**Website:** http://www.dredf.org/
Beverly Bertaina, Pres.

**Fnded:** 1979. **Desc:** Dedicated to the principle that people with disabilities have the right to lead full and integrated lives, with the freedom of choice and dignity. Seeks to educate the public and policymakers in order to further the civil rights and liberties of people with disabilities. Educational activities include: training state and local government officials, attorneys, and judges on disability rights compliance requirements such as the Americans with Disabilities Act; preparing materials pertaining to the right of children with disabilities to a free and appropriate public education. Houses the Disability Rights Clinical Legal Education Program which educates law students about disability rights laws and represents people with disabilites who have experienced unlawful discrimination. Provides technical assistance. **Pub:** *Disability Rights News*, quarterly. • *Explanation of the Contents of the ADA.* Book. *Price:* $118. • Manuals.

**★ 7966 ★ Disability Scotland (DS)**
5 Shandwick Pl.
Edinburgh EH2 4RG, United Kingdom
**Phone:** 44 131 2298632 **Fax:** 44 131 2295168

**Email:** ccurry@disabilityscotland.org.uk
**Website:** http://www.disabilityscotland.org.uk
**Fnded:** 1982. **Mem:** 200. **Lang(s):** English. **Desc:** Individuals and organizations. Promotes legal and social equality for people with disabilities. Represents the interests of people with disabilities before government agencies, medical organizations, and the public; cooperates with public officials to draft policies encouraging the full inclusion of people with disabilities in society. Participates in charitable activities. **Pub:** *Disability News*, quarterly. Newsletter. • Journal, periodic.

**★ 7967 ★ Disability Sport - England (DSE)**
Unit 4G
784-788 High Rd.
Tottenham
London N17 0DA, United Kingdom
**Phone:** 44 208 8014466 **Fax:** 44 208 8016644
**Email:** info@dse.org.uk
**Website:** http://www.disabilitysport.org.uk
**Fnded:** 1961. **Mem:** 50,000. **Reg. Groups:** 10. **Desc:** Provides opportunities for persons with any kind of disability to enjoy and compete in physical recreation and sport. Promotes the benefits of physical fitness and encourages people with disabilities to participate in the organization and development of sports at all levels. Supports local clubs and groups in their provision of recreational and sporting opportunities. Educates the public, the sporting world, and the media of the sporting abilities and achievements of people with disabilities. Organizes 12 national championships and more than 200 regional events for persons with disabilities. **Pub:** *Info Pack.* Newsletter. • *Newsletter*, periodic. Newsletter. • Brochures, periodic. **Frmly:** British Sports Association for the Disabled.

**★ 7968 ★ Disabled and Alone/Life Services for the Handicapped**
c/o Roslyn Brilliant
352 Park Ave. S, 11th Fl.
New York, NY 10010
**Phone:** (212)532-6740 **Free:** 800-995-0066
**Fax:** (212)532-3588
**Email:** disabledandalone@aol.com
**Website:** http://www.disabledandalone.org
Roslyn Brilliant, Exec. Dir.

**Fnded:** 1988. **Mem:** 30. **Desc:** Helps families plan for the time when they will not be able to care for their disabled children. Provides services for disabled people whose families have left assets for their care. Conducts educational programs on lifetime planning for families with a disabled member. Maintains speakers' bureau. **Pub:** *How to be a Friend to the Handicapped.* Book. *Price:* $50 for a prepaid shipment of 10 books; $6.95 for 1 book including postage. • *Lifelines*, 3/year. Newsletter. Provides information about "lifetime care" (future care) planning for a person with a disability. *Price:* Free. • Also publishes brochures, prospectus, articles about "lifetime care" (future care) planning for a person with a disability. **Frmly:** (2000) Life Services for the Handicapped.

**★ 7969 ★ Disabled Drivers' Association - England (DDA)**
Ashwellthorpe
Norwich NR16 1EX, United Kingdom
**Phone:** 44 1508 489449 **Fax:** 44 1508 488173
**Email:** ddahq@aol.com
**Website:** http://www.dda.org.uk
**Fnded:** 1948. **Mem:** 26,500. **Local Groups:** 34. **Desc:** Available to all disabilities and also able bodied members. Offers advice and information, benefits and concessions with RAC and most ferry companies. Local and national campaigns.

**★ 7970 ★ Disabled Drivers' Association - Ireland (DDA)**
Ballindine, Mayo, Ireland
**Phone:** 353 1 9464054 **Fax:** 353 1 9464336
**Email:** ability@iol.ie
**Website:** http://www.iol.ie/~ability

**Fnded:** 1970. **Mem:** 4,500. **Reg. Groups:** 1. **Lang(s):** English, Irish, Russian. **Desc:** Individuals and organizations. Promotes improve mobility for people with disabilities. Lobbies to safeguard the right of people with disabilities to obtain drivers' licenses; conducts educational and training programs. **Pub:** *Steering Wheel*, annual. Magazine. Contains general interest information.

### ★ 7971 ★ Disabled Living Foundation
380-384 Harrow Rd.
London W9 2HU, United Kingdom
**Phone:** 44 207 2896111   **Fax:** 44 207 2662922
**Email:** advice@dlf.org.uk
**Website:** http://www.dlf.org.uk
**Fnded:** 1977. **Desc:** Provides impartial information on disability equipment for daily living.

### ★ 7972 ★ Disabled People's Association (DPA)
150 A Pandun Gardens
No. 02-00 Day Care Center
Singapore 609342, Singapore
**Phone:** 65 8991220   **Fax:** 65 8991232
**Email:** dpa@dpa.org.sg
**Website:** http://www.dpa.org.sg
**Fnded:** 1986. **Mem:** 200. **Nat'l Groups:** 4. **Lang(s):** French, Malagasy. **Desc:** Physically, mentally, and sensorially disabled persons, their families, and other supporters. To empower disabled people to promote the changing of negative attitudes towards disability, advocacy and struggle for the equalization of opportunities in education, access to buildnga, information and documentation and income generation. All projects come under RRICCH - Resource and Research, Information Communications Centre of the Handicapped. Public education and awareness, disability groups, development and running of disability database - Enablenet - globally accessible through Internet. **Pub:** *Integrator*, quarterly. Newspaper. Contains news regarding disability issues locally, regionally and internationally.

### ★ 7973 ★ Disabled Peoples Finance Trust of Kenya (DPFTK)
PO Box 67641
Nairobi, Kenya
**Phone:** 254 2 568305   **Fax:** 254 2 330170
**Fnded:** 1982. **Mem:** 2,000. **Nat'l Groups:** 1. **Reg. Groups:** 10. **State Groups:** 2. **Local Groups:** 4. **Lang(s):** English, Swahili. **Desc:** Mentally or physically disabled persons and their families united to promote the rights of the disabled. Conducts research; compiles statistics; sponsors competitions. Operates placement services. Distributes publications of affiliated organizations. Maintains speakers' bureau. **Pub:** Newsletter, quarterly.

### ★ 7974 ★ Disabled Peoples' International - Canada (DPI)
101-7 Evergreen
Winnipeg, MB, Canada R3L 2T3
**Phone:** (204)287-8010   **Fax:** (204)453-1367
**Email:** dpi@dpi.org
**Website:** http://www.dpi.org
**Fnded:** 1981. **Mem:** 160. **Nat'l Groups:** 160. **Reg. Groups:** 5. **Lang(s):** English, French, Spanish. **Desc:** National organizations of physically or mentally disabled persons, their parents, and other advocates. Promotes equal opportunity and full participation of disabled people in all aspects of society as a matter of justice rather than charity and based on the principle of integration. Encourages unity among members and mutual cooperation, assistance, and understanding among all people. Is particularly concerned with developing organizations of disabled persons in the Third World and in developing selfhelp efforts in these countries. **Pub:** *Disability International*, quarterly. Magazine.

### ★ 7975 ★ Disabled People's International - Jamaica (Organizacion Mundial de Peronas Impedidas)
PO Box 220
Liguarea
Kingston 6, Jamaica
**Phone:** (876)931-6155   **Fax:** (876)924-6766
**Website:** http://www.dpi.org
**Desc:** Promotes the interests of disabled individuals in Jamaica. **Pub:** *Statement on Equalization of Opportunities.* • *Vox Nostra.*

### ★ 7976 ★ Disabled Persons Assembly (DPA)
PO Box 27524
Wellington, New Zealand
**Phone:** 64 4 8019100   **Fax:** 64 4 8019565
**Email:** gen@dpa.org.nz
**Website:** http://www.dpa.org.nz
**Fnded:** 1983. **Mem:** 1,700. **Reg. Groups:** 20. **Lang(s):** English. **Desc:** People with disabilities, their families, and others with an interest in the rights of people with disabilities. Works to ensure that people with disabilities are considered in the formation of public policy; advocates to expand the rights of people with disabilities. **Pub:** *Able Update*, quarterly. Magazine. • *Blueprint for Change.* • *Guide to Access Legislation.* • Annual Report, annual. • Manual. Covers DPA policies. DPA Bites (all available on website).

### ★ 7977 ★ Disabled Sports USA
451 Hungerford Dr., Ste. 100
Rockville, MD 20850
**Phone:** (301)217-0960   **Fax:** (301)217-0968
**Email:** dsusa@dsusa.org
**Website:** http://www.dsusa.org
Kirk M. Bauer, Exec. Dir.
**Fnded:** 1967. **Mem:** 20,000. **Reg. Groups:** 7. **Local Groups:** 86. **Desc:** Promotes sports and recreation opportunities for individuals with physical disabilities. Provides direct services to people with mobility impairments, including amputations, paraplegia, quadriplegia, spinal cord injuries, stroke, head injuries, cerebral palsy, polio, muscular dystrophy, multiple sclerosis, arthrogryposis, birth defects, neuromuscular disabilities, and visual impairments. Offers and sanctions recreational winter and summer programs, including learn-to-ski, learn-to-sail, and learn-to-race clinics, competitive alpine and nordic skiing, archery, basketball, cycling, lawnbowling, shooting, swimming, table tennis, track and field, volleyball, sailing, and weightlifting. Conducts special programs for children, women, and veterans with disabilities. Offers training and certification of adaptive fitness and adaptive ski instructors. Sponsors U.S. Disabled Ski Team, U.S. Amputee Summer Sports Team, and U.S. Disabled Sports Team. Maintains hall of fame. **Pub:** *Adaptive Ski Teaching Methods*, every 3/months. Newsletter. In two volumes. • *Aerobics for Amputees.* Video. • *Aerobics for Cerebral Palsy.* Video. • *Aerobics for Paraplegia.* Video. • *Aerobics for Quadriplegia.* Video. • *Disabled Children in Physical Education: Learning Through Movement.* Handbook. Overview of proper adapted physical education programs for disabled children. *Price:* $14.95. • *Fitness Programming and Physical Disabilities.* Manual. • *Manual for Adaptive Fitness Instructors.* Manual. • *Manual for Adaptive Ski Instructors.* Manual. • *Strengthen Flexibility Exercises for All Types of Disabilities.* Video. **Frmly:** (1972) National Amputee Skiers Association; (1977) National Inconvenienced Sportsmen's Association; (1989) National Handicapped Sports and Recreation Association; (1998) National Handicapped Sports.

### ★ 7978 ★ Disabled Women Union
Dachniy Ave. 7-5-23
Saint Petersburg, Russia
**Phone:** 7 812 1572937   **Fax:** 7 812 1572937
**Fnded:** 1990. **Mem:** 130. **Desc:** Disabled women. Promotes the interests of disabled women in Russia.

Conducts charitable programs. **Frmly:** Disabled Women Foundation.

### ★ 7979 ★ Disabled Women's Network Canada
PO Box 22003
Downtonw PO
Brandon, MB, Canada R7A 6Y9
**Phone:** (204)726-1406   **Fax:** (204)726-1409
**Email:** dawnca@canada.com
**Website:** http://www.dawncanada.net
**Fnded:** 1985. **Mem:** 300. **Lang(s):** English, French. **Desc:** Women with disabilities, organizations concerned with disability issues, and non-disabled supporters. A feminist organization that recognizes and addresses issues of concern to women with disabilities such as: poverty; employment equity; violence against women; parenting; health; access to services; and education. Provides information regarding issues of concern to disabled women, women's organizations, and the government. Allows women with disabilities the opportunity to participate in the women's movement. Cooperates with other groups involved in the quest for social justice nationally and internationally. Offers role models to girls with disabilities. Participates in research. **Pub:** *Beating the Odds: Violence and Women with Disabilities.* Book. • *Different Therefore Unequal: Employment and Women with Disabilities.* Book. • *Meeting Our Needs: An Access Manual for Transition Houses.* Book. • *New Reproductive Technologies.* Book. • *The Only Parent in the Neighbourhood: Mothering and Women with Disabilities.* Book. • *Thriving*, quarterly. Newsletter. • *Who Do We Think We Are?: Self-Image and Women with Disabilities.* Book.

### ★ 7980 ★ Disabled Womyn's Educational Project
PO Box 8773
Madison, WI 53708-8773
**Phone:** (608)256-8883   **Fax:** (608)256-8883
**Email:** catherine-odette@juno.com
Catherine Odette, Exec. Officer
**Fnded:** 1988. **Desc:** Lesbians with disabilities. Promotes members' interests. Supports legislation sensitive to members' needs. Maintains speakers' bureau. **Pub:** *Building Community Through Access.* • *Dykes, Disability, and Stuff*, quarterly. Newsletter. Available in the format of audiocassette, braille, DOS diskette, large print, modem transfer, audio tape. • *Dykes, Disability & Stuff*, quarterly. Newsletter. *Price:* $25/year. • *The Time for Access is Now.*

### ★ 7981 ★ Dutch Council of the Chronically Ill and Disabled (DCD) (Federatie Nederlandse Gehandicaptenraad)
Postbus 169
NL-3500 AD Utrecht, Netherlands
**Phone:** 31 30 2916600   **Fax:** 31 30 2970111
**Email:** bureau@cg-raad.nl
**Website:** http://www.cg-raad.nl
**Fnded:** 1977. **Mem:** 75. **Lang(s):** Dutch, English. **Desc:** Physically handicapped individuals, their families, and affiliated organizations. Works for equality and full participation and opportunity for the disabled. Seeks to influence public policy toward the disabled in areas of: financial, social, technical, and infrastructural provisions; employment and volunteer work; education and educational services. Conducts educational programs. **Pub:** *Aan Zet*, monthly. • *Gehandicaptenraad Nieuws*, bimonthly. Newsletter. • *Norms and Values as a Handicap.* • Books, periodic.

### ★ 7982 ★ Easter Seals National Headquarters
230 W Monroe, Ste. 1800
Chicago, IL 60606
**Phone:** (312)726-6200   **Free:** 800-221-6827
**Fax:** (312)726-1494
**Email:** info@easter-seals.org

**Website:** http://www.easter-seals.org
James E. Williams, Jr., Pres. /CEO
**Fnded:** 1919. **Mem:** 420. **Nat'l Groups:** 2. **State Groups:** 52. **Desc:** Provides services for children and adults with disabilities or special needs, and supports their families. Primary services include: medial rehabilitation, early intervention, physical therapy, occupational therapy, speech and hearing therapy, job therapy and employment, inclusive childcare, adult day services, camping and recreation. **Pub:** *Publications.* Catalog. **Frmly:** (1998) National Easter Seal Society.

**Erb's Palsy Association of Ireland**
*See:* Entry 5672

**★ 7983 ★ European Academy of Childhood Disability (EACD)**
Rte de Lennik 808
B-1070 Brussels, Belgium
**Phone:** 32 2 5553942      **Fax:** 32 2 5553429
**Email:** henri.szliwowski@ulb.ac.be
**Website:** http://www.erbspalsy.ie
**Fnded:** 1989.

**★ 7984 ★ European Action of the Handicapped (AEH) (Europaische Aktion der Behinderten)**
Wurzerstr. 4A
D-53175 Bonn, Germany
**Phone:** 49 228 820930      **Fax:** 49 228 8209346
**Email:** aeh.europe@t-online.de
**Fnded:** 1979. **Mem:** 19. **Lang(s):** English, French, German. **Desc:** Promotes the interests of disabled individuals throughout Europe. Advocates that disabled people can lead self-determining lives. Supports equal opportunity for all types of disabled people. Supports vocational and social integration of disabled people. **Pub:** *Information Newsletter*, 2-3/year. Contains information about social policy of the EU-member states and the European development in the social sector.

**★ 7985 ★ Extensions for Independence (EI)**
555 Saturn Blvd., B-368
San Diego, CA 92154
**Phone:** (619)423-7709      **Free:** (866)632-7149
**Fax:** (619)423-7709
**Email:** info@mouthstick.net
**Website:** http://www.mouthstick.net
Arthur Heyer, Pres.
**Fnded:** 1976. **Desc:** Develops, manufactures, and markets vocational equipment for the physically handicapped. Promotes improvements in design, materials, production, and quality of products while maintaining affordable prices. Products include the Multi-Tip Telescoping H-A Modular Mouthstick which enables individuals to talk and swallow while drawing, turning pages, loading and unloading computer software, and performing other tasks.

**★ 7986 ★ FACES: The National Craniofacial Association**
PO Box 11082
Chattanooga, TN 37401
**Phone:** (423)266-1632      **Free:** 800-332-2373
**Fax:** (423)267-3124
**Email:** faces@faces-cranio.org
**Website:** http://www.faces-cranio.org
Lynne G. Mayfield, Pres.
**Fnded:** 1969. **Desc:** Provides financial assistance for travel expenses to individuals with severe facial deformities resulting from congenital defects or accidents. Provides a resource file of available treatment centers, support groups, and general information concerning severe facial deformities. Is currently involved in an extensive fundraising campaign in order to increase awareness of the organization and to broaden its base of support. **Pub:** *FACES*, quarterly. Newsletter. Provides information and support for craniofacially handicapped persons. Includes updates on

clients and medical updates. *Price:* Free. ● *FACES Brochure.* Brochure. Provides information on the organization. ● *So Brightly Within.* Video. *Price:* $20 donation. **Frmly:** (1977) Debbie Fox Foundation for Treatment of Cranio-Facial Deformities; (1985) Debbie Fox Foundation; (1998) National Association for the Craniofacially Handicapped.

**★ 7987 ★ Family Resource Center on Disabilities (FRCD)**
c/o Charlotte Des Jardins
20 E Jackson Blvd., Rm. 300
Chicago, IL 60604
**Phone:** (312)939-3513      **Free:** 800-952-4199
**Fax:** (312)939-7297
**Email:** frcdptiil@ameritech.net
Charlotte Des Jardins, Exec. Dr
**Fnded:** 1969. **Desc:** Parents, professionals, and volunteers seeking to improve services for all children with disabilities. Originally organized as a result of the 1969 Illinois law mandating the education of all children with disabilities, FRCD operates as a coalition to inform and activate parents. Provides information and referral services, individualized support services for low-income Chicago families, transition services, and special education rights training. **Pub:** *How to Get Services by Being Assertive.* Manual. *Price:* $10 plus shipping and handling. ● *How to Organize an Effective Parent/Advocacy Group and Move Bureaucracies.* Manual. *Price:* $10 plus shipping and handling. ● *Rehabilitation Act Manual.* Manual. *Price:* $25 plus shipping and handling. ● Also publishes pamphlets. **Frmly:** Coordinating Council for Handicapped Children.

**★ 7988 ★ Foundation for Science and Disability (FSD)**
236 Grand St.
Morgantown, WV 26505-7509
**Phone:** (304)293-5201      **Fax:** (304)293-6363
**Email:** ekeller@wvu.edu
E. C. Keller, Jr., Treas.
**Fnded:** 1978. **Mem:** 206. **Nat'l Groups:** 1. **Desc:** Disabled scientists and interested individuals. Offers consultation and advice concerning problems faced by persons with disabilities in scientific fields. **Pub:** *The Abled Disabled in Science*, periodic. Book. ● *Newsletter of FSD*, semiannual. Newsletter. *Price:* available to members only. **Frmly:** (1993) Foundation for Science and the Handicapped; (2002) Foundation for Science and Disability Department of Biology.

**★ 7989 ★ Gazette International Networking Institute (GINI)**
4207 Lindell Blvd., No. 110
Saint Louis, MO 63108-2915
**Phone:** (314)534-0475      **Fax:** (314)534-5070
**Email:** gini_intl@msn.com
**Website:** http://www.post-polio.org
Joan L. Headley, Dir.
**Fnded:** 1958. **Mem:** 6,500. **Desc:** Polio survivors, ventilator users, other individuals with neuromuscular diseases, health care personnel, insurance agencies, government agencies, independent living centers, and interested others. Works to inform, encourage, dignify, and sustain people with disabilities. Seeks to create a communications network to provide information on issues related to disabilities. Serves as clearinghouse for information on polio, ventilators, neuromuscular diseases, and independent living. Sponsors seminars. Coordinates International Polio Network and International Ventilator Users Network. **Pub:** *Handbook on the Late Effects of Poliomyelitis for Physicians and Survivors.* Handbook. *Price:* $18.50/copy. ● *IUUN Resource Directory*, annual. Directory. *Price:* $5/copy. ● *IVUN News*, semiannual. Newsletter. Includes information for those interested in home mechanical ventilation. *Price:* $17/year. ● *Polio Network News*, quarterly. Contains information about the late effects of polio and topics related to disability. *Price:* $20/year for institutions/individuals. ● *Post Polio Directory*, annual. Directory. Lists self-identified clinics, health professionals, and support groups knowledgeable about the

late effects of polio. *Price:* $5/copy for individuals. ● *Rehabilitation Gazette*, semiannual. Journal. Written by persons with disabilities. *Price:* $12. ● *Rehabilitation into Independent Living.* **Frmly:** (1983) Rehabilitation Gazette.

**★ 7990 ★ Goodwill Industries International (GII)**
9200 Rockville Pike
Bethesda, MD 20814
**Phone:** (240)333-5200
**Email:** contactus@goodwill.org
**Website:** http://www.goodwill.org
George W. Kessinger, Pres. & CEO
**Fnded:** 1902. **Mem:** 226. **Reg. Groups:** 7. **State Groups:** 12. **Desc:** Federation of Goodwill Industries organizations across North America and the world are concerned primarily with providing employment, training, evaluation, counseling, placement, job training, and other vocational rehabilitation services and opportunities for individual growth for people with disabilities and other special needs. Member Goodwill Industries organizations collect donated goods and sell them in Goodwill retail stores as a means of providing employment and generating income. Conducts seminars and training programs; compiles statistics. **Pub:** *Corporate Brochure*, annual. Brochure. ● *Internal Membership Directory*, annual. Membership Directory. ● *Working!*, quarterly. Magazine. ● Annual Report. ● Also publishes promotional materials. **Frmly:** (1910) Morgan Memorial and Cooperative Industries and Stores; (1946) National Association of Goodwill Industries; (1994) Goodwill Industries of America.

**★ 7991 ★ Goodwill Industries of Venezuela (Industrias Venezolanas de Buena Voluntad)**
S abana Grande
Apartado 50074
Caracas 1050-A, Venezuela
**Phone:** 58 2 9444555      **Fax:** 58 2 9444815
**Email:** buenavoluntadivbv@hotmail.com
**Website:** http://www.goodwill.org
**Fnded:** 1964. **Lang(s):** English, Spanish. **Desc:** Provides vocational training, employment, and rehabilitation services to people with disabilities. Promotes economic and social self-sufficiency for people with disabilities; maintains social worker visitation program.

**★ 7992 ★ Goodwill Industries Volunteer Services (GIVS)**
c/o Goodwill Industries International Inc.
9200 Rockville Pike
Bethesda, MD 20814
**Phone:** (301)530-6500      **Free:** 800-664-6577
**Fax:** (301)530-1516
**Email:** contactus@goodwill.org
**Website:** http://www.goodwill.org
**Fnded:** 1933. **Mem:** 3,000. **Nat'l Groups:** 1. **Local Groups:** 71. **Desc:** Persons interested in volunteer work in programs serving people with disabilities or other barriers to employment. Supports the efforts of national and local Goodwill Industries International, Inc., programs through volunteer services. Programs vary according to local needs and include such activities as direct program services, fundraising, and public relations. **Pub:** *Giving*, quarterly. Directory. ● *Goodwill Volunteer Services Directory*, annual. Manual. ● *Goodwill Volunteer Services Handbook*, annual. ● Annual Report, annual. **Frmly:** National Auxiliary of Goodwill Industries; National Women's Auxiliary to the Goodwill Industries.

**★ 7993 ★ Great Britain Wheelchair Basketball Association**
104 London Rd.
Chatteris PE16 6SF, United Kingdom
**Phone:** 44 1354 695560      **Fax:** 44 1354 695752
**Email:** s.spilka@gbwba.org.uk
**Website:** http://www.gbwba.org.uk

**Fnded:** 1981. **Mem:** 800. **Reg. Groups:** 10. **Desc:** Persons with a physical (lower limb) disability. Develops and promotes wheelchair basketball in the UK. Administers the national leagues and non-league clubs to enhance, through sport, the lives and lifestyles of physically disabled people. Administers and runs national teams, senior men's, juniors and women. **Pub:** *GBWBA Handbook*, annual. Handbook. • *GBWBA Newsletter*, quarterly. Newsletter.

### ★ 7994 ★ Handicap International - France (HI)

14, ave. Berthelot
F-69361 Lyon Cedex 07, France
**Phone:** 33 7 8697979　　　**Fax:** 33 7 8697994
**Email:** handicap-international@infonie.fr
**Website:** http://www.handicap-international.org
**Fnded:** 1982. **Mem:** 56,000. **Lang(s):** English, French, Portuguese, Spanish. **Desc:** Works for the rehabilitation of physically disabled persons in Third World countries. Trains local technicians in appropriate technologies to create small prosthetics and physical rehabilitation units. Offers charitable programs. **Pub:** *L'Enfant Handicape et Village*. Book. • *Operations Handicap International*, quarterly. • Books. Contains translations of text from other languages. **Frmly:** Operation Handicap Internationale.

### ★ 7995 ★ Handicapped Scuba Association (HSA)

1104 El. Prado
San Clemente, CA 92672-4637
**Phone:** (949)498-4540　　　**Fax:** (949)498-6128
**Email:** hsa@hsascuba.com
**Website:** http://www.hsascuba.com
Jim Gatacre, Pres.
**Fnded:** 1975. **Mem:** 2,000. **Nat'l Groups:** 34. **Reg. Groups:** 30. **State Groups:** 50. **Desc:** Individuals with handicaps and interested others. Purpose is to advance and promote scuba diving among the handicapped. Seeks to enhance the self-image of handicapped divers by emphasizing their abilities rather than their disabilities. Stresses the importance of education and safety procedures in diving; maintains training agency for handicapped divers. Offers training and certification worldwide for scuba diving instructors in teaching the handicapped. Holds monthly diving excursion and lectures, and conducts four diving vacations per year. Offers instructor referrals worldwide. **Pub:** *Freedom in Depth*. Film. • *Getting Down Scuba News*, annual. *Price:* $20. • *Instructor Training Manual*. Manual. • *To Fly in Freedom*. Film. • Also is producing a film about the association with the Cousteau Society. To fly in freedom IS with Cousteau.

### ★ 7996 ★ Handidactis

146 Haslam St.
Toronto, ON, Canada M1N 3N7
**Phone:** (416)267-5939　　　**Fax:** (416)267-8183
**Email:** handidac@idirect.com
**Website:** http://pages.infinit.net/handidac
**Fnded:** 1986. **Lang(s):** English, French. **Desc:** Promotes awareness of the needs of people with disabilities among employers and service providers. Seeks to ensure full integration of workplaces with employees with disabilities while maintaining excellence in custom service. Conducts customized cross-disability awareness training programs; sponsors educational courses. Develops and delivers site audits to remove work-place barriers.

### HEATH Resource Center (GWHRC)

*See:* Entry 12086

### ★ 7997 ★ Independence Dogs

146 State Line Rd.
Chadds Ford, PA 19317
**Phone:** (610)358-2723　　　**Fax:** (610)358-5314
**Email:** idi@independencedogs.org
**Website:** http://www.independencedogs.org
M. Jean King, Founder & Pres.

**Fnded:** 1984. **Desc:** Professional staff of 10 assisted by 70 volunteers who train service dogs for the mobility impaired. The use of these well trained dogs teamed up with a handicapped partner makes more independent living possible. Maintains speaker's bureau. **Pub:** *Knoll News is Good News*, annual. Newsletter. Features calendar.

### ★ 7998 ★ Independent Living Centre

St. Loyes Foundation
Topsham Rd.
Exeter EX2 6EP, United Kingdom
**Phone:** 44 1392 286239　　　**Fax:** 44 1392 286239
**Fnded:** 1986. **Lang(s):** English. **Desc:** Provides a permanent exhibition and demonstration centre of equipment for people of all ages with a variety of needs and disabilities providing information to their families, carers, health professionals, students and the general public. **Pub:** Brochure.

### ★ 7999 ★ Indian Olympic Association

Jawahar Lal Nehru Stadium
New Delhi 110 003, Delhi, India
**Phone:** 91 11 4366950　　　**Fax:** 91 11 4365953
**Email:** ioa@nde.vsnl.net.in
**Desc:** Amateur sports associations. Promotes the Asian games and Afro-Asian games movement.

### ★ 8000 ★ Inspiration Ministries (CLH)

PO Box 948
Corner State Rd. 67 and County F
Walworth, WI 53184-0948
**Phone:** (262)275-6131　　　**Fax:** (262)275-3355
**Email:** tschnake@inspirationministries.org
**Website:** http://www.inspirationministries.org
Tim Schnake, VP Resident Services
**Fnded:** 1948. **Mem:** 90. **Desc:** Seeks to provide fully accessible, permanent residence with attendant care in room and board facility for physically disabled adults. Conducts summer camping program for disabled persons and retreat opportunities for groups. **Pub:** *Seasons*, quarterly. Newsletter. *Price:* Free. **Frmly:** (2001) Christian League for the Handicapped.

### ★ 8001 ★ International Association for Disability and Oral Health (IADH)

c/o Dr. Jan Andersson-Norinder
Mun-H-Center
Odontologen
Medicinaregatan 12 A
413 90 Goteborg, Sweden
**Phone:** 46 31 7952952　　　**Fax:** 46 31 7951800
**Email:** jan.andersson-norinder@vgregion.se
**Website:** http://www.iadh.org
**Lang(s):** English. **Desc:** Promotes oral health care for people with disabilities.

### ★ 8002 ★ International Association for Handicapped Divers

Hazelaarlaan 47
1775 EE Middenmeer, Switzerland
**Phone:** 31 227 503631　　　**Fax:** 31 227 503729
**Email:** iahdnl@hotmail.com
**Website:** http://www.duik.net/info/iand.htm
**Fnded:** 1993. **Mem:** 500. **Lang(s):** English, Swedish. **Desc:** Scuba diving instructors, divemasters, and underwater assistants trained to meet the specific needs of divers with physical handicaps. Encourages divers with disabilities to assume a role of leadership in diving. Promotes participation in diving by people with disabilities as a means to better physical fitness and increased self-esteem. Conducts training programs for divemasters, instructors, and assistants wishing to work with people with disabilities. **Pub:** Newsletter, quarterly. Contains member information.

### ★ 8003 ★ International Cerebral Palsy Society (ICPS)

19 St. Mary's Grove
London W4 3LL, United Kingdom

**Phone:** 44 208 9946386　　　**Fax:** 44 208 7478528
**Email:** a.loring@easynet.co.uk
**Website:** http://www.icps.org.uk
**Fnded:** 1969. **Mem:** 317. **Lang(s):** English. **Desc:** Professionals, parents, handicapped persons, and organizations in 60 countries. Seeks to stimulate research in cerebral palsy and promote related improvements and developments in early diagnosis, methods of treatment, and appropriate teaching and rehabilitation programs. Acts as the international coordinating organization for collection, distribution, and exchange of specialized information on cerebral palsy. Disseminates information about: architectural design for the handicapped; operation and equipment of a mobile visiting aid unit; aids and appliances; how to obtain entry visas for handicapped children emigrating with their families; medical matters; sex education; research on integration; publications for parents; alternative forms of physiotherapy; employment opportunities. Offers consulting services and referrals. **Pub:** *Bulletin*, 3/year. Bulletin.

### ★ 8004 ★ International Council for Education of People with Visual Impairment (ICEVI)

37 Jesselton Crescent
10450 Penang, Malaysia
**Phone:** 60 4 369933　　　**Fax:** 60 4 369357
**Email:** brohier@pc.jaring.my
**Website:** http://www.icevi.org
**Fnded:** 1952. **Reg. Groups:** 8. **Lang(s):** English, Spanish. **Desc:** Teachers and educators of the visually handicapped and other interested persons. Advocates education of the visually handicapped worldwide; works to improve existing facilities through training programs for teachers, refresher courses, and provision of teaching materials. Offers assistance for professional training. Conducts teacher training courses in developing countries. **Pub:** *The Educator*, semiannual. Journal. • *International Resource Directory*. Book. **Frmly:** International Council for Education of the Visually Handicapped; (1972) International Conference of Educators of Blind Youth.

### ★ 8005 ★ International Federation of Persons with Physical Disabilities (Federation Internationale des Personnes Handicapees Physiques)

Beethovenallee 56-58
D-53173 Bonn, Germany
**Phone:** 49 228 9564130　　　**Fax:** 49 228 9564132
**Email:** fimitic@t-online.de
**Website:** http://www.fimitic.org
**Fnded:** 1953. **Mem:** 5000,000. **Lang(s):** English, French, German. **Desc:** National organizations in 28 countries united to promote physical and vocational rehabilitation and full employment for the disabled. Seeks to foster international cooperation in the development of rehabilitation services; sponsors the International Day of the Disabled. Holds seminars. Acts as clearinghouse. **Pub:** *Congress Reports*. • *Nouvelles*, quarterly. Bulletin. **Frmly:** (2000) International Federation of Disabled Workers and Civilan Handicapped.

### International French-Speaking Association of Paraplegic Therapy Groups (AFIGAP) (Association Francophone Internationale des Groupes d'Animation de la Paraplegie — AFIGAP)

*See:* Entry 20141

### International Friendly Circle of the Blind (IFCB)

*See:* Entry 20990

**★ 8006 ★ International Society for Prosthetics and Orthotics (ISPO) (Societe Internationale de Prothese et Orthese)**
Borgervaenget 5
DK-2100 Copenhagen, Denmark
**Phone:** 45 39207260        **Fax:** 45 39207501
**Email:** webmaster@i-s-p-o.org
**Website:** http://www.ispo.org
**Fnded:** 1970. **Mem:** 2,700. **Nat'l Groups:** 28. **Lang(s):** English. **Desc:** Medical and paramedical professionals in 83 countries interested in prosthetics, orthotics, and other fields of rehabilitation engineering. Promotes improvements in the care of people with neuromuscular and skeletal impairments. Serves as nonpolitical coordinating and advisory organization on prosthetics, orthotics, rehabilitation engineering, and other matters related to the neuromuscular and skeletal system. Promotes and guides programs in research, development, and evaluation regarding prosthetics and orthotics. Fosters quality practice and develops standards for nomenclature, device design, techniques, processes, and patient care. Sponsors exhibits, conferences, regional and international courses, seminars, and symposia; supports education and training in the field. **Pub:** *Directory of Films in Prosthetics and Orthotics.* Directory. • *Prosthetics and Orthotics International,* 3/year. Journal. • *Standards for Lower-Limb Prostheses.* • Proceedings.

**★ 8007 ★ International Sports Organisation for the Disabled (ISOD) (Federation Internationale de Sport pour Handicapes)**
c/o Alan Dean
353 Ontario St.
Newmarket, ON, Canada L3Y 2K2
**Phone:** (905)898-3661        **Fax:** (905)895-5527
**Fnded:** 1963. **Mem:** 52. **Lang(s):** English, French, German, Spanish. **Desc:** National federations in countries concerned with development of sports for the disabled. Encourages international cooperation among national organizations in the field of sports for the disabled; coordinates international activities of members. Sponsors training and education seminars and world championship Olympic games for the physically handicapped. **Pub:** *Circular,* semiannual. Newsletter. • *ISOD Handbook,* periodic.

**★ 8008 ★ International Stoke Mandeville Wheelchair Sports Federation (ISMWSF)**
Olympic Village
Guttmann Rd.
Aylesbury HP21 9PP, United Kingdom
**Phone:** 44 1296 436179        **Fax:** 44 1296 436484
**Email:** info@wsw.org.uk
**Website:** http://www.wsw.org.uk
**Fnded:** 1952. **Mem:** 80. **Desc:** National organizations concerned with development of sport for paralyzed and other disabled individuals. Promotes sports activities and competitions to foster self-confidence in disabled individuals. **Pub:** Newsletter, 3/year. **Frmly:** (1991) International Stoke Mandeville Games Federation.

**★ 8009 ★ Irish Wheelchair Association (IWA)**
Aras Chuchulainn
Blackheath Dr.
Clontarf
Dublin 3, Ireland
**Phone:** 353 1 8338241        **Fax:** 353 1 8333873
**Email:** info@iwa.ie
**Website:** http://www.iwa.ie
**Fnded:** 1960. **Mem:** 11,000. **Reg. Groups:** 5. **Lang(s):** English, Irish. **Desc:** Individuals and organizations. Seeks to improve the social, economic, and legal status of people with disabilities. Makes available support and services; conducts educational and advocacy campaigns. **Pub:** Magazine, quarterly.

**★ 8010 ★ Italian Association of Friends of Raoul Follereau (IAFRF) (Associazione Italiana Amici di Raoul Follereau — AIFO)**
Via Borselli 4-6
I-40135 Bologna, Italy
**Phone:** 39 51 433402        **Fax:** 39 51 434046
**Email:** info@aifo.it
**Website:** http://www.aifo.it
**Fnded:** 1961. **Lang(s):** English, French, Portuguese. **Desc:** Promotes increased availability of medical services and assistance for people with disabilities in developing areas worldwide. Provides medical supplies and equipment to development projects; makes available technical assistance to health and rehabilitation services. Conducts educational and training programs to enhance local administrative capabilities and ensure sustainability and autonomy of health services. Sponsors educational campaigns to raise public awareness in Italy of global health and development issues. **Pub:** *Amici dei Lebbrosi,* monthly. Magazine. • *Quaderni di Cooperazione Sanitaria,* periodic. Report. • Books.

**★ 8011 ★ Japanese Association on Disability and Handicap**
Nishiwaseda Sekiguchi Bldg. 4F
2-15-10 Nishiwaseda
Shinjuku-ku
Tokyo 169-0051, Japan
**Phone:** 81 3 52852601        **Fax:** 81 3 52852603
**Email:** webmaster@nginet.or.jp
**Desc:** Seeks to protect the human rights of individuals with disabilities in Japan.

**★ 8012 ★ Job Accommodation Network (JAN)**
WVU PO Box 6080
Morgantown, WV 26506-6080
**Phone:** (304)293-7186        **Free:** 800-526-7234
**Fax:** (304)293-5407
**Email:** jan@jan.icdi.wvu.edu
**Website:** http://www.jan.wvu.edu
D.J. Hendricks, Proj. Mgr.
**Fnded:** 1984. **Desc:** A service of U.S. Department of Labor's Office of Disability Employment Policy. An international toll-free consulting service that provides information about job accommodation and the employability of people with functional limitations. Calls are answered by consultants who understand the functional limitations associated with disabilities and who have instant access to the most comprehensive and up-to-date information about accommodation methods, devices, and strategies.

**★ 8013 ★ Joint Council for the Physically and Mentally Disabled - Hong Kong**
Duke of Windsor Social Service Bldg., 12/F
15 Hennessy Rd.
Hong Kong, People's Republic of China
**Phone:** 852 28642931        **Fax:** 852 28642962
**Email:** rh@hkcss.org.hk
**Fnded:** 1964. **Mem:** 118. **Lang(s):** Chinese, English. **Desc:** Organizations representing people with disabilities; interested individuals. Seeks to improve the quality of life of people with disabilities. Provides consulting to government agencies formulating legislation affecting people with disabilities; coordinates activities of members organizations and agencies. Conducts research and educational programs; participates in charitable activities; sponsors competitions. **Pub:** *Hong Kong Access Guide for Disabled Visitors,* periodic. Directory. • Brochure. • Reports.

**★ 8014 ★ Just One Break (JOB)**
120 Wall St.
New York, NY 10005
**Phone:** (212)785-7300        **Fax:** (212)785-4513
**Email:** justonebreak@interactive.net
**Website:** http://www.justonebreak.org/
Kathryn Croft, Exec. Dir.
**Fnded:** 1947. **Desc:** Employment service for people with disabilities. Works to place job-ready people with disabilities into competitive employment. Concentrates efforts in New York, New Jersey, and Connecticut, but advises companies nationwide. Offers placement services, employment counseling, skills evaluation, college recruitment, a summer intern program, and an annual jobs fair. Conducts on-site Americans with Disabilities Act accessibility studies and advisory assistance for human resources managers to help them ease the transition of people with disabilities into their workforce. **Pub:** *Informational Brochure.* Brochure. • Annual Report, annual.

**★ 8015 ★ KDWB Variety Family Center**
University of Minnesota Gateway
200 Oak St. SE, Ste. 160
Minneapolis, MN 55455-2002
**Phone:** (612)626-3087        **Free:** 800-276-8642
**Fax:** (612)624-0997
**Email:** kdwb-var@unm.edu
**Website:** http://www.allaboutkids.umn.edu/kdwbvfc/index.htm
Elizabeth Latts, Resource Coordinator
**Desc:** Provides family-centered services that promote physical, emotional, psychological and social health and well-being for children and youth at risk, including children and youth with disabilities. **Pub:** *Health Issues,* periodic. Newsletter. • Report, periodic. • Monograph, periodic.

**★ 8016 ★ Korea Polio Foundation (KPF) (Chung Nip Hwe Gwan — CNHG)**
c/o ChungNip Center
16-3 Gueui-Dong
KwangJin-Ku
Seoul 143-200, Republic of Korea
**Phone:** 82 2 4661237        **Fax:** 82 2 4542144
**Fnded:** 1965. **Mem:** 13,000. **Lang(s):** English, Japanese, Korean. **Desc:** Handicapped individuals and others in the Republic of Korea. Fosters the physical and mental development of the disabled. Strives to: increase awareness of the needs of the handicapped; promote and protect the rights of the disabled. Offers educational, vocational, and medical counseling and assistance. Cooperates with firms in sponsoring employment programs for the handicapped. Organizes collective living for the disabled; maintains specialized developmental camps. Operates the Institute of Sports Science for the Disabled. Sponsors athletic competitions; participates in the Paralympics (an athletic competition modeled after the Olympic Games and adapted to the handicapped). Distributes medical braces and supports for needy disabled individuals. Communicates concerns to government authorities; campaigns for adaptive transportation for the disabled. Holds classes and seminars. Operates the Institute of Physical and Mental Disability. Conducts research and surveys. Bestows awards. **Pub:** *Chung Nip Hwe Gwan Bulletin,* periodic. Bulletin. • *Chung Nip Newsletter,* periodic. Also publishes research reports, dissertations, and surveys.

**★ 8017 ★ Kuwait Society for the Handicapped (KSH)**
PO Box 6832
Hawalli 32043, Kuwait
**Phone:** 965 2631277        **Fax:** 965 2642630
**Email:** feedback@kshkw.com
**Website:** http://www.kshkw.com
**Fnded:** 1971. **Mem:** 250. **Local Groups:** 2. **Lang(s):** Arabic, English. **Desc:** Individuals dedicated to the care of the handicapped in Kuwait. Provides physical and psychological care for children who have not been accepted by other institutions; offers financial and moral support to the families of handicapped individuals; works to inform the public on the causes of handicaps. Conducts research. **Pub:** Magazine, quarterly. • Booklet, quinquennial. Also publishes pamphlets and offers posters and greeting cards.

## ★ 8018 ★ Latin American Society of Paraplegia (SLAP)

Triunvirato 5237, Dto G
Buenos Aires, Argentina
**Fax:** 54 1 45429338
**Email:** monisanchez@conmed.com.ar

## ★ 8019 ★ Learning Disabilities Association of Canada (LDAC) (Troubles d'Apprentissage - Association Canadienne)

323 Chapel St., Ste. 200
Ottawa, ON, Canada K1N 7Z2
**Phone:** (613)238-5721          **Fax:** (613)235-5391
**Email:** information@ldac-taac.ca
**Website:** http://www.ldac-taac.ca
**Fnded:** 1963. **Mem:** 10,000. **State Groups:** 12. **Local Groups:** 150. **Lang(s):** English, French. **Desc:** Parents of children with learning disabilities and individuals with learning disabilities; educators and administrators, psychologists, language experts, lawyers, and health care professionals. Works to advance the education, social development, legal rights, and general well-being of individuals with learning disabilities. Encourages early recognition, diagnosis, and treatment of individuals with learning disabilities. Develops educational, social, recreational, and career-oriented programs and promotes legislation, research, and training of personnel in the field. Initiates programs to increase public awareness and understanding of learning disabilities. Acts as an advocate for individuals before government and other agencies; develops parent support services to maximize parental involvement. **Pub:** *National*, quarterly. • Handbooks, periodic. • Papers, periodic. **Frmly:** (1986) Canadian Association for Children and Adults with Learning Disabilities.

## Lemko Housing Organization (LHO)

*See:* Entry 2989

## ★ 8020 ★ Leonard Cheshire International

30 Millbank
London SW1P 4QD, United Kingdom
**Phone:** 44 171 8028200          **Fax:** 44 171 8028275
**Email:** info@london.leonard-chesire.org.uk
**Website:** http://www.leonard-cheshire.org
**Fnded:** 1948. **Mem:** 14. **Nat'l Groups:** 50. **Reg. Groups:** 9. **Local Groups:** 250. **Lang(s):** English, French, Spanish. **Desc:** Locally operated programs for people with disabilities and their families in 54 countries. Seeks to improve the quality of life of people with disabilities. Maintains rehabilitation centers, skills training centers, support for employment and education programs, independent living programs, community-based support and residential services. **Pub:** *COMPASS*, quarterly. Magazine. Contains news, featurs, and letters about Cheshire services. • *The Leonard Cheshire International*, periodic. Directory. • Handbooks. • Videos.

## ★ 8021 ★ Life Sharing Foundation

S Sandisfield Rd.
Great Barrington, MA 01230
**Phone:** (413)229-2600          **Fax:** (413)455-2992
Allan Baer, Pres.
**Fnded:** 1989. **Desc:** Seeks to enhance the independence of disabled individuals by providing financial support and other support to families who share their homes w/people w/disabilities. **Pub:** Brochures. • Newsletter, quarterly. **AKA:** Cadmus Lifesharing Association.

## ★ 8022 ★ Limbless Association

Rehabilitation Centre
Roehampton Ln.
London SW15 5PR, United Kingdom
**Phone:** 44 20 87881777     **Fax:** 44 20 87883444
**Email:** membership@limbless.association.org
**Website:** http://www.limbless-association.org
**Fnded:** 1983. **Mem:** 1,500. **Reg. Groups:** 4. **Lang(s):** English. **Desc:** Provides information and advice to people who have had amputations or who have been born without upper or lower limbs. Through a nationwide network of volunteer representatives who are all amputees themselves, offers support and encouragement to prospective amputees, carers, and those already trying to come to terms with limb loss or deficiency. **Pub:** *Step Forward*, quarterly. Magazine.

## ★ 8023 ★ Mainstream

6930 Carroll Ave., Ste. 240
Takoma Park, MD 20912
**Phone:** (301)891-8777          **Fax:** (301)891-8778
**Email:** info@mainstreaminc.org
David Pichette, Exec. Dir.
**Fnded:** 1975. **Desc:** Offers services and products to increase employment opportunities for people with disabilities. Assists companies and organizations in their efforts to "mainstream" people with disabilities into employment. Operates Project LINK (linking individuals with disabilities with competitive employment), which helps place job-ready disabled applicants in the Dallas, TX and Washington, DC areas. Provides in-house training; conducts workshops, seminars and annual conference. Promotes job assistance throughout website. **Pub:** *Informational Brochure*, periodic. Brochure. Provides informational material. • *Mainstream Magazine*, quarterly. Magazine. • Annual Report, annual.

## Medicare Rights Center

*See:* Entry 2994

## ★ 8024 ★ Mobility International USA (MIUSA)

PO Box 10767
Eugene, OR 97440
**Phone:** (541)343-1284          **Fax:** (541)343-6812
**Email:** info@miusa.org
**Website:** http://www.miusa.org
Susan Sygall, Exec. Dir.
**Fnded:** 1981. **Mem:** 300. **Desc:** Strives to empower people with disabilities through international exchange opportunities. Organizes international exchange programs annually. Provides information on the range of international exchange opportunities available including work, study, research, and volunteering. Also provides information to international exchange organizations on accessibility, homestays, recruiting and inclusion in international development programs. **Pub:** *A World Awaits You: A Journal of Success of People with Disabilities in International Exchange*. Journal. *Price:* Free. • *A World of Options: A Guide to International Educational Exchange, Community Service, and Travel for Persons with Disabilities*. Book. *Price:* $35/individuals; $45/organizations. • *All Abroad!*. Video. Available with or without audio description and with captions. For People with Disabilities Interested in International Exchange. *Price:* $40 for members; $49 for nonmembers. • *Building Bridges: A Manual on Including People w/Disabilities in International Exchange Programs*. Manual. *Price:* $20. • *Building Bridges: A Training Video on Including People w/Disabilities in International Exchange Programs*. Video. Available with captions and with or without audio description. *Price:* $40 for members; $49 for nonmembers. • *Emerging Leaders*. Video. Available with or without captions. *Price:* $40 for members; $49 for nonmembers. • *Home Is in the Heart: Recruiting and Accommodating Persons with Disabilities into the Homestay Experience*. Video. Available with captions. *Price:* $40 for members; $49 for nonmembers. • *Loud, Proud and Passionate*. Video. Available with captions. *Price:* $40 for members; $49 for nonmembers. • *Loud, Proud and Passionate Including Women with Disabilities in International Development Programs*, quarterly. Book. Available with captions. *Price:* $18 for members; $25 for nonmembers. • *Over the Rainbow*, quarterly. Newsletter. Also available on audio cassette. *Price:* Included in membership dues; $35/year for individual. • *Sustainable Transport*, semiannual. Available upon request. **Frmly:** (1989) Haitian Development Fund.

## ★ 8025 ★ National Ability Center (NAC)

PO Box 682799
Park City, UT 84068
**Phone:** (435)649-3991          **Fax:** (435)658-3992
**Email:** nac@xmission.com
**Website:** http://www.nationalabilitycenter.org/
Meeche White, Exec. Dir.
**Fnded:** 1985. **Mem:** 250. **Nat'l Groups:** 2. **State Groups:** 4. **Desc:** People with disabilities and their families. Promotes the development of lifetime skills for persons with disabilities and their families; works to increase the self-esteem of people with disabilities. Sponsors affordable sports and recreational activities, including clcying, challenge course, houseback riding, and river rafting, for members. **Pub:** *Ability Bulletin*, quarterly. Newsletter.

## ★ 8026 ★ National Accessible Apartment Clearinghouse (NAAC)

201 N Union St., No. 200
Alexandria, VA 22314
**Free:** 800-421-1221          **Fax:** (703)518-6191
**Email:** clearinghouse@naahq.org
**Website:** http://www.forrent.com/naac/
**Desc:** Dedicated to providing an effective means to connect individuals with disabilities with apartments designed for an individual's particular needs.

## ★ 8027 ★ National AMBUCS

PO Box 5127
High Point, NC 27262
**Phone:** (336)869-2166          **Fax:** (336)887-8451
**Email:** ambucs@ambucs.com
**Website:** http://www.ambucs.com
J. Joseph Copeland, Exec. Dir.
**Fnded:** 1927. **Mem:** 5,600. **Reg. Groups:** 6. **Local Groups:** 145. **Desc:** Dedicated to creating opportunities for independence for people with disabilities. Performs community service; provides physically challenged children with tricycles that can be operated by hand, foot or both; operates the Living Endowment Fund. **Pub:** *AMBUCS*, quarterly. Magazine. **Frmly:** American Business Clubs Spastic Paralysis Fund.

## ★ 8028 ★ National Amputation Foundation (NAF)

40 Church St.
Malverne, NY 11565
**Phone:** (516)887-3600          **Fax:** (516)887-3667
**Email:** amps76@aol.com
**Website:** http://www.nationalamputation.org
Donald A. Sioss, Exec. Sec.
**Fnded:** 1919. **Mem:** 2,500. **Desc:** Veterans with service-connected amputation. Assists all amputees, including nonveterans, in employment, social, and mental rehabilitation. Provides services, including legal counsel, vocational guidance and placement, social activities, liaison with other groups, and psychological aid. Sponsors Amp-to-Amp program arranging for amputees who have returned to a normal life to visit new amputees. **Pub:** *The Amp*, bimonthly. Newsletter.

## ★ 8029 ★ National Amputee Golf Association (NAGA)

11 Walnut Hill Rd.
Amherst, NH 03031-1713
**Free:** 800-633-6242
**Email:** info@nagagolf.org
**Website:** http://www.nagagolf.org
Bob Wilson, Dir.
**Fnded:** 1955. **Mem:** 3,700. **Reg. Groups:** 3. **State Groups:** 6. **Desc:** Individuals who have lost a hand, foot, or a combination thereof at a major joint. Purpose is to promote the mental and physical rehabilitation of amputees through the sport of golf. Conducts first swing program for therapists. Organizes local, regional, national, and international tournaments. Compiles statistics. **Pub:** *Amputee Golfer Magazine*, annual. Magazine. *Price:* Included in membership dues; $5 to nonmembers in the U.S.; $7.50 to nonmembers outside the U.S. • Newsletter, semiannual, spring and fall. *Price:* Included in membership dues.

**★ 8030 ★ National Association of Advisory Officers for Special Educational Needs**
Princes St.
Tunbridge Wells TN2 4SL, United Kingdom
**Phone:** 44 1892 534034 **Fax:** 44 1799 521257
**Email:** diana.robinson@btclick.com

**Desc:** Advisory officers for special education. **Frmly:** (2000) National Association of Advisor Officers for Special Education.

**★ 8031 ★ National Association of Disability Examiners (NADE)**
PO Box 243
Raleigh, NC 27602
**Phone:** (919)212-3222 **Free:** 800-443-9359
**Fax:** (919)212-3155
**Website:** http://www.nade.org/
Jeff Price, Pres.

**Fnded:** 1963. **Mem:** 2,373. **Reg. Groups:** 7. **Local Groups:** 56. **Desc:** Disability claims examiners, attorneys, and physicians involved in determining the eligibility of applicants for social security benefits based on disability. Purpose is to foster, promote, and participate in activities designed to improve the documentation of applications for disability insurance benefits and the evaluation of medical and/or vocational information obtained in connection with such applications. Provides for the exchange of technical information, ideas, and philosophies. **Pub:** *NADE Advocate*, bimonthly. Newsletter. Includes listings of newly-certified examiners. *Price:* Included in membership dues. • *Nationwide Report*, quarterly. • Directory, annual.

**National Association of Multicultural Rehabilitation Concerns (NAMRC)**
*See:* Entry 20146

**★ 8032 ★ National Association of the Physically Handicapped (NAPH)**
1375 Dewitt Dr.
Akron, OH 44313
**Free:** 800-743-5008
**Email:** trumanjm@aol.com
**Website:** http://www.naph.net
Jerry Snyder, Pres.

**Fnded:** 1958. **Mem:** 700. **Nat'l Groups:** 1. **State Groups:** 1. **Local Groups:** 13. **Desc:** Physically handicapped persons; associate members are non-handicapped. Seeks to advance the social, economic, and physical welfare of the physically handicapped. Promotes involvement of the physically handicapped in the planning and administration of all programs in their interest. Sponsors fundraising activities. **Pub:** *NAPH National Newsletter*, quarterly. Newsletter. *Price:* $12/year for nonmembers. • Brochure.

**★ 8033 ★ National Association of Protection and Advocacy Systems (NAPAS)**
900 2nd St. NE, Ste. 211
Washington, DC 20002
**Phone:** (202)408-9514 **Fax:** (202)408-9520
**Email:** napas@earthlink.net
**Website:** http://www.protectionandadvocacy.com/napas12.htm
Curtis L. Decker, Exec. Dir.

**Fnded:** 1978. **Mem:** 96. **Reg. Groups:** 5. **State Groups:** 96. **Desc:** Executive directors and designees of state or territorial Developmental Disability, Mentally Ill Protection and Advocacy Systems, and Client Assistance Programs. Furthers the human, civil, and legal rights of persons with disabilities; advances the interests of protection and advocacy systems; facilitates coordination and mutual support among such systems and enhance their capacity to provide optimal services. Offers professional training; collects data. **Pub:** *NAPAS Newsletter*, periodic. Newsletter. • *State Protection and Advocacy Agencies*, annual. Directory. • Manuals. • Reports.

**National Association of Rehabilitation Support Staff (NARSS)**
*See:* Entry 20150

**National Association of Service Providers in Private Rehabilitation (NASPPR)**
*See:* Entry 20151

**★ 8034 ★ National Association of Societies for the Care of the Handicapped (NASCOH)**
PO Box UA 504
Union Ave.
Harare, Zimbabwe
**Phone:** 263 4 724678 **Fax:** 263 4 724678
**Email:** nascoh@zol.co.zw
**Website:** http://www.geocities.com/nascoh

**Fnded:** 1969. **Mem:** 52. **Desc:** Offers social and medical services to physically handicapped individuals. Conducts educational and informational programs. Acts as an advocate for the rights of the disabled. Co-ordinates the activities of societies working with and for people with disabilities. **Pub:** *NASCOH News*, quarterly. Magazine.

**★ 8035 ★ National Association for Special Educational Needs (NASEN)**
Nasen House
4/5 Amber Business Village
Amber Close
Amington
Tamworth B77 4RP, United Kingdom
**Phone:** 44 1827 311500 **Fax:** 44 1827 313005
**Email:** welcome@nasen.org.uk
**Website:** http://www.nasen.org.uk

**Fnded:** 1992. **Mem:** 11,000. **Reg. Groups:** 50. **Desc:** Mainly teachers and other practitioners in special education, also lectures in further and higher education, LEA staff, HMI and those from the caring professions. Promotes the development of children and young people with special educational needs, wherever they are located, and supports those who work with them. It has a trading company: NASEN Enterprises Ltd. from which a comprehensive list of publications and details of course and conferences may be obtained. **Pub:** *British Journal of Special Education and Support for Learning*, quarterly. Journal. • Magazine, 3/year.

**★ 8036 ★ National Association of Swimming Clubs for the Handicapped**
c/o The Willows
Mayles Lane
Wickham
Hampshire PO17 5ND, United Kingdom
**Phone:** 44 1329 833689

**Fnded:** 1966. **Mem:** 12,120. **Desc:** All ages with any disabilities. Aims to encourage disabled youngsters and adults to participate in swimming. Registered charity organization 247772.

**★ 8037 ★ National Center for Disability Services (NCDS)**
201 I.U. Willets Rd.
Albertson, NY 11507
**Phone:** (516)465-1470 **Fax:** (516)746-3298
**Email:** ecortez@ncds.org
**Website:** http://www.ncds.org
Edmund L. Cortez, Pres.

**Fnded:** 1952. **Desc:** Serves as a center providing educational, vocational, rehabilitation, and research opportunities for persons with disabilities. Work is conducted through the following: Abilities Health and Rehabilitation Services, a New York state licensed diagnostic and treatment center which offers comprehensive outpatient programs in physical therapy, occupational therapy, speech therapy, and psychological services; Career and Employment Institute, which evaluates, trains, and counsels more than 600 adults with disabilities each year, with the goal of productive competitive employment; Henry Viscardi School,

which conducts early childhood, elementary, and secondary programs, as well as adult and continuing education programs; Research and Training Institute, which conducts research on the education, employment, and career development of persons with disabilities, and holds seminars and workshops for rehabilitation services professionals. Maintains library and speakers' bureau; compiles statistics; offers placement service; conducts research and educational programs. **Frmly:** (1991) Human Resources Center.

**★ 8038 ★ National Center for Youth with Disabilities**
University of Minnesota - Box 721
420 Delaware St. SE
Minneapolis, MN 55455-0392
**Phone:** (612)626-2825 **Free:** 800-333-6293
**Fax:** (612)626-2134
Nancy Okinow, MSW, Exec. Dir.

**Fnded:** 1985. **Desc:** Information and resource center that strives to raise awareness of the needs of adolescents with chronic illnesses and disabilities. Develops activities and programs. **Pub:** *Connections*. Newspaper. Highlights critical issues relating to youth with chronic illnesses and disabilities. Provides a forum for the exchange of information. • *Cydline Reviews*. • *Teenagers at Risk*. • Bulletins.

**★ 8039 ★ National Council of Disabled Peoples International in Pakistan (NCDPIP)**
c/o Saluhuddin Malik
34 Sadar Bazar
Ghulam Mohammed Abad
Faisalabad, Pakistan
**Phone:** 92 41 680434 **Fax:** 92 41 695094
**Email:** dpipak@fsd.comsats.net.pk

**Fnded:** 1982. **Mem:** 125. **Nat'l Groups:** 1. **Reg. Groups:** 4. **Lang(s):** English, Urdu. **Desc:** Mentally and physically handicapped individuals, their families, and other supporters. Works for equality in participation and opportunity for the disabled. Acts as an umbrella organization registered with the Social Welfare Dept. for guidance and councilling to the provincial chapters for education and rehabilitation of disabled person in need throughout the country.

**★ 8040 ★ National Council of Disabled Persons of Zimbabwe (NCDPZ)**
PO Box 1952
Bulawayo, Zimbabwe
**Phone:** 263 9 74426 **Fax:** 263 9 68023
**Email:** ncd@telconet.co.za

**Fnded:** 1975. **Mem:** 500,000. **Reg. Groups:** 45. **Local Groups:** 71. **Lang(s):** English. **Desc:** Encourages unity of disabled persons in Zimbabwe. Promotes the interests of the disabled. Disseminates information. Continues to lobby for the implementation of our 1992 Disability Act, which our organization championed. **Pub:** *Disability Rights Up*, quarterly. Magazine. • *Program Report*, monthly. • Newsletter.

**★ 8041 ★ National Council on Independent Living (NCIL)**
1916 Wilson Blvd., Ste. 209
Arlington, VA 22201
**Phone:** (703)525-3406 **Fax:** (703)525-3409
**Email:** ncil@ncil.org
**Website:** http://www.ncil.org
Anne-Marie Hughey, Dir.

**Fnded:** 1982. **Mem:** 380. **Local Groups:** 80. **Desc:** Independent living centers, organizations that provide support to independent living centers, and individuals. (Independent living centers offer programs to assist disabled individuals, including help in locating housing and finding appropriate personal care assistance, peer counseling, and independent living skills training.) Encourages the integration of people with disabilities into society; promotes independent lifestyles and decision-making for people with disabilities; works to strengthen independent living centers. Offers technical assistance and encourages cooperation among independent living centers. Seeks to develop leadership skills among people with disabilities; works to increase public awareness of the rights and needs of disabled individuals. Provides information and referral service; sponsors Peer Technical Assistance Network. Maintains speakers' bureau and placement service. **Pub:** *NCIL Newsletter*, quarterly. Newsletter. • *President's Bulletin*, monthly. Bulletin. **Frmly:** (1985) National Coalition of Independent Living Programs.

### ★ 8042 ★ National Council on Intellectual Disability (NCID)

51 Tenant St., Unit 7
Fyshwick, ACT 2609, Australia
**Phone:** 61 6 6280868     **Fax:** 61 2 62964488
**Email:** nicd@dice.org.au
**Website:** http://www.dice.org.au
**Fnded:** 1953. **Mem:** 400. **Lang(s):** English. **Desc:** Organizations in Australia representing 25,000 individuals involved in the study of or the provision of services to individuals with intellectual disabilities. Works to: ensure that the best services are provided to the intellectually disabled and their families; eliminate discrimination against and establish equality for the developmentally disabled. Acts as a liaison between member organizations and government authorities; lobbies public officials. Seeks the establishment of free public education in adapted environments when necessary, the provision of free health care, the establishment of freedom in the choice of an occupation, the granting of voting rights, and the equal participation by intellectually disabled in poli cy development and management of related service organizations. Monitors and proposes modifications to relevant legislation. Works for the establishment of regional authorities on intellectual disability which will monitor research on intellectual disability and services for the intellectually disabled. Sponsors training programs and seminars; offers courses. Maintains the Australian Institute on Intellectual Disability. **Pub:** *Interaction*, 5/year. Journal. • *Library Catalogue*, periodic. • Monographs, periodic. **Frmly:** (1957) Australian Council of Organizations for Subnormal Children; (1971) Australian Council for the Mentally Retarded; (1984) Australian Association for the Mentally Retarded; (1988) AAMR - National Association on Intellectual Disability.

### ★ 8043 ★ National Cristina Foundation (NCF)

500 W Putnam Ave.
Greenwich, CT 06830
**Phone:** (203)863-9100     **Fax:** (203)863-9230
**Email:** ncf@cristina.org
**Website:** http://www.cristina.org
Yvette Marrin, PhD, Pres.
**Fnded:** 1985. **Desc:** Looks for donations of commercially obsolete computer equipment, software, and audio/visual equipment from the business community, the government sector, and the public; redistributes this technology to partner organizations that maintain programs for persons with special needs, such as the disabled, the disadvantaged, and students at risk of school failure. Conducts public awareness campaigns; accepts donations.

### National Education for Assistance Dog Services (NEADS)
*See:* Entry 6085

### ★ 8044 ★ National Foundation of Dentistry for the Handicapped (NFDH)

1800 15th St., Unit 100
Denver, CO 80202
**Phone:** (303)534-5360     **Fax:** (303)534-5290
**Email:** fleviton@nfdh.org
**Website:** http://www.nfdh.org
Larry Coffee, D.D.S., Pres.
**Fnded:** 1974. **State Groups:** 29. **Desc:** Promotes preventive dentistry for handicapped individuals in order to reduce dental disease. Sponsors Campaign of Concern and Donated Dental Services program, which enlists the cooperation of members of the dental profession, special education personnel, disabled individuals and their parents, counselors, and civic organizations in helping developmentally disabled people enjoy good dental health. These programs currently serves 23,841 people in 29 states. Conducts preventive health education through in-service training for members of participating special education schools, sheltered workshops, day centers, and group/nursing homes; teaches handicapped individuals how to maintain their own oral hygiene and provides them with dental supplies; evaluates the oral health status of each participant; suggests dentists who will accept handicapped patients if such a referral is desired. Sponsors Donated Dental Services Programs, which match indigent, elderly, and handicapped individuals with volunteer dentists. Operates a portable dental treatment system for the homebound, nursing home residents, and the developmentally disabled that is currently in use in Denver, CO, Newark, NJ, and Chicago, IL; has assisted in developing similar programs in Detroit, MI and Houston, TX. **Pub:** *Guidelines for Dental Programs in Institutions for Developmentally Disabled Persons.* • *Guidelines for Using Fluorides Among Handicapped Persons.* • *Special Smiles*, periodic. • Annual Report. • Also distributes audiovisual and written materials on dentistry for the handicapped.

### ★ 8045 ★ National Information Center for Children and Youth with Disabilities (NICHCY)

PO Box 1492
Washington, DC 20013-1492
**Phone:** (202)884-8200     **Free:** 800-695-0285
**Fax:** (202)884-8441
**Email:** nichcy@aed.org
**Website:** http://www.nichcy.org
Suzanne Ripley, Dir.
**Fnded:** 1970. **Desc:** Provides information to assist parents, educators, care-givers, advocates, and others in helping children and youth with disabilities participate as fully possible in school, at home, and in the community. Provides personal responses to specific questions, referrals to other organizations/sources of help, prepared information packets, and technical assistance to parent and professional groups. **Pub:** *Disability Fact Sheet*, annual. • *News Digest*, periodic. Newsletter. Addresses current issues affecting individuals concerned with handicapped children and youth with disabilities. *Price:* Free. • *Parent Guide.* • *State Resource Sheet*, annual. • *Transition Summary.* • Booklets. • Papers. **Frmly:** National Information Center for the Handicapped; National Special Education Information Center; (1982) Parents Campaign for Handicapped Children and Youth; (1987) National Information Center for Handicapped Children and Youth; (1991) National Information Center for Children and Youth with Handicaps.

### National Institute for Rehabilitation Engineering (NIRE)
*See:* Entry 4518

### ★ 8046 ★ National League of the Blind and Disabled (NLBD)

2 Tenterden Rd.
London N17 8BE, United Kingdom
**Phone:** 44 181 8086030     **Fax:** 44 181 8853235
**Email:** nire@theoffice.net
**Website:** http://www.theoffice.net/nire
**Fnded:** 1893. **Mem:** 2,371. **Reg. Groups:** 3. **State Groups:** 4. **Local Groups:** 50. **Desc:** Blind, partially sighted and seeing disabled people 16 years of age and over. Represents, negotiates, campaigns for provisions of equality of resources and services for people with disabilities in education, rehabilitation, training, employment and benefits by the State and local authorities. **Pub:** *Advocate*, quarterly. Magazine.

### ★ 8047 ★ National Network for the Disabled

c/o Linda Walls
PO Box 3574
Gardena, CA 90247-7274
**Phone:** (310)638-5717     **Fax:** (310)638-5986
Linda Walls, Founder-Pres.
**Fnded:** 1980. **Mem:** 11,000. **Desc:** Provides support, companionship, and networking opportunities for elderly individuals and parents of disabled children. Conducts research. Sponsors education on such topics as assertiveness, resources, and medical options. Provides transportation and emergency services, including a food program through which meals are delivered to homes. Conducts special events for parents and children, including picnics and field trips; special programs on nutrition and accessible travel with groups. **Pub:** Brochure, monthly. • Newsletter, monthly. **Frmly:** Parent Networking Program.

### ★ 8048 ★ National Odd Shoe Exchange (NOSE)

3200 North Delaware St.
Chandler, AZ 85225-1100
**Phone:** (480)892-3484     **Fax:** (480)892-3568
**Website:** http://www.angelfire.com/in2/oddshoes/
John A. Schwiesow, Exec. Dir.
**Fnded:** 1943. **Desc:** Provides new single shoes to amputees and pairs of different sizes to people with feet of significantly different sizes due to disease, injury, and genetic disorders. **Frmly:** (1972) National Odd Shoe Foundation; (1993) Ruth Rubin Feldman National Odd Shoe Exchange 1943-1983.

### ★ 8049 ★ National Organization on Disability (NOD)

910 16th St. NW, Ste. 600
Washington, DC 20006
**Phone:** (202)293-5960     **Fax:** (202)293-7999
**Email:** ability@nod.org
**Website:** http://www.nod.org
Brewster Thackeray, Dir. Communications
**Fnded:** 1982. **State Groups:** 50. **Local Groups:** 4500. **Desc:** Works to promote the full and equal participation of people with disabilities in all aspects of life. **Frmly:** (1993) World Committee on Disability.

### ★ 8050 ★ National Orthotic and Prosthetic Research Institute (NOPRI)

PO Box 491
Lenox Hill
New York, NY 10021
Ralph Florio, Pres.
**Fnded:** 1969. **Mem:** 10. **Desc:** Retired male and female nurses. Trains high school dropouts to work with aluminum by fabricating it into canes, crutches, and walkers, which are then distributed to needy persons free of charge. Once they are accustomed to working with aluminum, trainees are placed with a company that produces aluminum products.

### ★ 8051 ★ National Specialized Equestrian Training Centre (NSETC)

Bri Chualann Equestrian Centre
Old Connaught Ave.
Bray, Wicklow, Ireland
**Phone:** 353 1 2720704     **Fax:** 353 1 2720708
**Lang(s):** English, Irish. **Desc:** Individuals and organizations. Promotes increased participation in athletics by people with disabilities. Sponsors horseback riding and other equestrian activities for people with disabilities.

### National Therapeutic Recreation Society (NTRS)
*See:* Entry 20160

**★ 8052 ★ National Union of Disabled Persons of Uganda (NUDPU)**
PO Box 8567
Kampala, Uganda
**Phone:** 256 41 540179    **Fax:** 256 41 540178
**Email:** nudipu@starcom.co.ug
**Website:** http://www.nrpa.org/branches/ntrs.htm
**Fnded:** 1987. **Mem:** 45. **Nat'l Groups:** 8. **Reg. Groups:** 48. **Lang(s):** English. **Desc:** People with disabilities and their families; health care personnel and other people working with individuals with disabilities. Seeks to improve the quality of life of people with disabilities; promotes advancement of assistive technologies and therapeutic methods. Provides support and services to people with disabilities and their families; conducts lobbying and advocacy activities; sponsors training programs. **Pub:** *NUDPU News*, semiannual. Newsletter.

**★ 8053 ★ National Wheelchair Basketball Association (NWBA)**
110 Seaton Bldg.
Lexington, KY 40506-0219
**Phone:** (859)257-1623    **Fax:** (859)258-1090
**Email:** info@nwba.org
**Website:** http://www.nwba.org/
Stan Labanowich, PhD, Commissioner
**Fnded:** 1949. **Mem:** 185. **Desc:** Wheelchair basketball teams comprised of individuals with severe permanent physical disabilities of the lower extremities. Seeks to provide opportunities on a national basis for the physically disabled to participate in the sport of wheelchair basketball, with its adjunct psychological, social, and emotional benefits, and to maintain a high level of competition through continuing refinement and standardization of playing rules and officiating. Sponsors sectional and regional tournaments leading up to the National Wheelchair Basketball Tournament. Maintains hall of fame; compiles statistics; participates in charitable activities. **Pub:** *National Wheelchair Basketball Tournament Program*, annual. • *Rules and Case Book*, annual. • *Standings and Statistics*, 10/year. • Directory, annual. Conference officers, team representatives names & addresses. • Newsletter, 12/year.

**★ 8054 ★ National Wheelchair Softball Association (NWSA)**
1616 Todd Ct.
Hastings, MN 55033
**Phone:** (612)437-1792    **Fax:** (612)437-3889
**Email:** ecmjon@mediaone.net
**Website:** http://www.wheelchairsoftball.com
Jon Speake, Commissioner
**Fnded:** 1976. **Mem:** 24. **Desc:** Teams that are active in wheelchair softball competitions. Acts as governing agency for the promotion, interpretation, standardization, and continued growth of wheelchair softball. Coordinates efforts of member teams and encourages formation of new teams; protects the interests of members and enforces existing rules and regulations established by member teams. Conducts seminars on wheelchair softball and wheelchair sports; sponsors tournaments. Maintains hall of fame and compiles statistics.

**★ 8055 ★ Netherlands Institute of Care and Welfare**
Catharijnesingel 47
Postbus 19152
NL-3501 DD Utrecht, Netherlands
**Phone:** 30 2306311    **Fax:** 30 2319641
**Website:** http://www.nizw.nl
**Lang(s):** Dutch, English, French, German. **Desc:** Health professionals and institutions providing care to people with disabilities. Promotes an improved quality of life for people with disabilities. Represents members' interests; conducts research and educational programs.

**★ 8056 ★ Networking Project for Young Adults with Disabilities (NPDWG)**
c/o YWCA of City of New York
650 Lexington Ave.
New York, NY 10022
**Phone:** (212)735-4500    **Fax:** (212)755-3362
**Email:** kstruve@ywcanyc.org
**Website:** http://www.ywcanyc.org
Ken Struve, Dir.
**Fnded:** 1984. **Desc:** A project of the Young Women's Christian Association of New York City. Purpose is to increase the educational, social, and career aspirations of adolescents with disabilities by linking them to successful, disabled role models. Provides support groups; offers advocacy training, pre-employment skills development, and one-to-one mentoring. Organizes visits to the role model's workplace. Currently operates in the New York City area and is providing technical assistance to facilitate replication at several sites throughout the country. **Pub:** *Replication Manual*. Manual. • Books.

**★ 8057 ★ NISH**
2235 Cedar Ln.
Vienna, VA 22182-5200
**Phone:** (703)560-6800    **Fax:** (703)698-0124
**Email:** info@nish.org
**Website:** http://www.nish.org
Patricia Szervo, Chair
**Fnded:** 1974. **Mem:** 550. **Reg. Groups:** 6. **Desc:** Provides employment opportunities for people with severe disabilities under the Javits-Wagner O'Day Act. Promotes their placement into competitive industry. Conducts research and development to identify to the government commodities and services which are feasible for production and/or performance by work centers. (Work centers are nonprofit agencies that provide rehabilitative, training, and vocational services for persons with severe disabilities.) Provides training and technical assistance in the form of industrial engineering, production planning, quality control, inventory management, cost analysis, procurement, and contract administration. Acts as a liaison between work centers and the federal government. **Pub:** *NISH News*, monthly. Newsletter. Reports on work centers employing persons with severe disabilities, and legislation and regulations affecting these centers. *Price:* Free to participants of the J-W O'Day Program. • Annual Report. *Price:* Free. • Brochure. **Frmly:** (1991) National Industries for the Severely Handicapped.

**★ 8058 ★ Nordic Cooperation on Disability (Nordiska Samarbetsorganet for Handikappfragor — NSH)**
Box 510
S-162 15 Vallingby, Sweden
**Phone:** 46 8 6201890    **Fax:** 46 8 7392400
**Email:** nsh@nsh.se
**Website:** http://www.nsh.se
**Fnded:** 1980. **Mem:** 5. **Lang(s):** Danish, English, Finnish, Norwegian, Swedish. **Desc:** Governmental organization for Denmark, Finland, Iceland, Norway, and Sweden. Initiates, organizes, and expedites cooperation among Nordic countries on efforts concerning disability and rehabilitation.

**★ 8059 ★ North American Riding for the Handicapped Association (NARHA)**
PO Box 33150
Denver, CO 80233
**Phone:** (303)452-1212    **Free:** 800-369-7433
**Fax:** (303)252-4610
**Email:** narha@narha.org
**Website:** http://www.narha.org
William J. Scebbi, Exec. Dir.
**Fnded:** 1969. **Mem:** 3,700. **Reg. Groups:** 11. **Local Groups:** 500. **Desc:** Individuals and riding centers. Provides therapeutic riding for individuals with disabilities with good safety and proper care; offers appropriate training and certification for instructors working with the disabled. Provides educational programs. **Pub:** *AHA News*, 3/year. Newsletter. • *CAN Hoof-*

beats, 3/year. Newsletter. • *EFMHA News*, 3/year. Newsletter. • *NARHA Guide*, annual. Directory. Included in membership dues. • *NARHA News*, 8/year. *Price:* Included in membership. • *NARHA Strides*, quarterly. Magazine. *Price:* Included in membership.

**★ 8060 ★ Norwegian Dyslexia Association (NDA) (Norsk Dysleksiforbundet i Norge — DIN)**
Postboks 8731 Youngstorget
N-0028 Oslo, Norway
**Phone:** 47 22334275    **Fax:** 47 22429554
**Email:** post@dyslekskiforbundet.no
**Fnded:** 1976. **Mem:** 5,000. **Local Groups:** 40. **Lang(s):** English, Norwegian. **Desc:** Individuals with dyslexia and their parents; organizations. Acts as a support group. **Pub:** *Dyslektikeren*, bimonthly.

**★ 8061 ★ Norwegian Federation of Organisations of Disabled People (NFODP) (Funksjonshemmeds Fellesorganisasjon — FFO)**
Sandakerveien 99
PO Box 4568
Nydalen
N-0404 Oslo, Norway
**Phone:** 47 2 2799100    **Fax:** 47 2 2799198
**Email:** info@ffo.no
**Website:** http://www.ffo.no
**Fnded:** 1950. **Mem:** 61. **Reg. Groups:** 19. **Local Groups:** 60. **Lang(s):** Norwegian. **Desc:** Organizations of disabled persons representing 250,000 individuals in Norway. Works for social integration and equality for disabled people; cooperates with the Norwegian Agency for International Development to ensure that aid also reaches the disabled. Serves as liaison between members and government; maintains contact with similar organizations abroad. **Pub:** *FFO's Ukeseddel*, weekly. Newsletter. • *Funksjonshemmedi i Europa*. Also issues press releases. **Frmly:** Norwegian League of Handicap Organizations.

**★ 8062 ★ Odamist Humanitarian Rehabilitation Centre (OHRC)**
Tekhron 12
Dushanbe, Tajikistan
**Phone:** 7 3772 216582
**Fnded:** 1996. **Mem:** 15. **Lang(s):** English, Russian. **Desc:** Medical, nursing, and rehabilitation centers providing services to disabled veterans and other people with disabilities. Seeks to improve the quality of life of people with disabilities; promotes advancement of treatment and rehabilitation techniques. Facilitates communication and cooperation among members; sponsors educational and training programs.

**★ 8063 ★ One-Arm Dove Hunt Association (OADH)**
Box 582
Olney, TX 76374
**Email:** 1armjack@brazosnet.com
Jack R. Northrup, Co-Founder
**Fnded:** 1972. **Mem:** 550. **Desc:** Hand or arm amputees who enjoy the sport of shotgun shooting; interested nonamputees. Works to help amputees accept their handicap and to provide fellowship and shooting competitions. Activities include dove hunts, One-Arm Tales, One-Arm Talent, pool Tournament, golf tournament, horshoe tournament, and dove dinner. **Pub:** Newsletter, annual.

**★ 8064 ★ The One Shoe Crew (TOSC)**
9328 Aizenberg Cir.
Elk Grove, CA 95624
**Phone:** (916)685-8746    **Fax:** (916)685-8746
Janice Piercy, Mgr.
**Fnded:** 1986. **Mem:** 2,500. **Desc:** Service for adults or teens whose feet have stopped growing. Finds cost-

sharing partners for people who wear only one shoe or those who wear shoes of different sizes on each foot. (Clients include individuals with mismatched feet, amputees, people wearing a brace on one foot, and anyone with a one-sided foot problem who still wears one regular shoe.) Matches shoe size, width, needs, preferences, and approximate age of clients seeking partners. Many thousands of new, unused shoes and over 3,000 pairs of mismatched shoes (same shoe, different size) are available free to clients; shipping must be prepaid. Clients indicate the general shoe style they prefer. All services are free for U.S. Veterans.

### ★ 8065 ★ Opportunity Plus
PO Box 35481
Charlotte, NC 28235
**Phone:** (704)376-4735　　**Fax:** (704)376-4738
**Email:** info@opportunity-plus.org
**Website:** http://www.opportunity-plus.org
Dallas R. Bolan, Exec. Dir.
**Fnded:** 1979. **Mem:** 1,100. **Reg. Groups:** 5. **Desc:** Works with the physically disabled community by providing the opportunity to be independent through mentoring, training, and employment programs, and by educating the community at large through information, referral, and networking. **Pub:** *Mentor Newsletter*, quarterly. Newsletter. Includes client updates, resources, and legislative updates. **AKA:** (2002) Learning How. **Frmly:** (1987) Handicapped Organized Women; (1988) HOW.

### ★ 8066 ★ Overcoming Mobility Barriers International (OMBI)
1022 S 41st St.
Omaha, NE 68105-8108
**Phone:** (402)342-5731　　**Fax:** (402)342-5731
Kay E. Neil, Exec. Dir.
**Fnded:** 1979. **Mem:** 104. **Desc:** Government officials, service consumers and providers, and other persons interested in removing mobility barriers for elderly, handicapped, and disadvantaged persons. Advises and works in conjunction with other groups and government agencies to establish safety standards for special equipment used in retrofitting vehicles and works to retrain drivers in the use of nonconventional driving controls. Addresses such problems as possible allocation of fuel to social service agencies and others working in nontransit areas. **Pub:** *A Positive Approach*, quarterly. Newsletter. Includes calendar of events. *Price:* Included in membership dues.

### P.R.I.D.E. Foundation - Promote Real Independence for the Disabled and Elderly (P.R.I.D.E.)
*See:* Entry 20166

### ★ 8067 ★ Paws With a Cause (PWC)
4646 S Division
Wayland, MI 49348
**Phone:** (616)877-7297　　**Free:** 800-253-PAWS
**Fax:** (616)877-0248
**Email:** paws@ionline.com
**Website:** http://www.pawswithacause.org
Antoinette Joni Sapp, CEO
**Fnded:** 1979. **Nat'l Groups:** 37. **Reg. Groups:** 2. **Desc:** Trains Assistance Dogs nationally for people with disabilities and provides lifetime team support which encourages independence. Promotes awareness through education. **Pub:** *Dogs for Dignity*, quarterly. Newsletter. **Frmly:** (1988) Ears for the Deaf.

### ★ 8068 ★ People-to-People Committee on Disability (PPCOD)
PO Box 42692
Washington, DC 20015
**Phone:** (703)535-6011　　**Fax:** (703)535-6011
**Email:** ngvb09b@prodigy.com
**Website:** http://www.ppcd.org/
David Waugh, Chm.

**Fnded:** 1956. **Mem:** 250. **Desc:** Individuals concerned about the circumstances of disabled people throughout the world. Disseminates information; acts as consultant in promoting exchange activities; coordinates special assistance projects in developing countries. Compiles statistics. **Pub:** Newsletter, quarterly. • Also publishes reports and surveys. **Frmly:** (1994) People-to-People Committee for the Handicapped.

### ★ 8069 ★ Perceptions, Inc. (PI)
1400 Broadway 5th Fl.
New York, NY 10018
**Phone:** (212)944-7717　　**Fax:** (212)719-5609
**Website:** http://www.perceptions-inc.com/
Rene Nieva, Pres.
**Fnded:** 1978. **Desc:** Parents, professionals, schools, and libraries are subscribers. Publishes a newsletter that serves as an information source for parents wishing to develop expertise in meeting the educational, social, and emotional needs of their learning-disabled children. Holds seminars and workshops for parents and professionals. Maintains speakers' bureau. **Pub:** *Annual Index*. Directory. • Manual. Provides instructions on clothing and grooming.

### ★ 8070 ★ Physically Handicapped Welfare Association
Joseph d'Argent Aven
Rose Hill, Mauritius
**Phone:** 230 4644845　　**Fax:** 230 4650549
**Fnded:** 1960. **Mem:** 150. **Desc:** Aims to improve the lives of physically challenged people in Mauritius. Operates rehabilitation center. **Frmly:** (1981) Cripple Welfare Association.

### ★ 8071 ★ Polio Fellowship of Ireland (PFI)
Park House Vocational and Residential Training Center
Stillorgan Grove
Stillorgan
Dublin, Ireland
**Phone:** 353 1 2888366　　**Fax:** 353 1 2836128
**Email:** parkhouse@rehab.ie
**Fnded:** 1949. **Lang(s):** English, Irish. **Desc:** Seeks to improve the quality of life of people who have physical disabilities, including polio, and mental health learning difficulties. Provides day activities, training, and residential accommodation.

### ★ 8072 ★ Private Voluntary Organizations (PVO)
191 Constant Spring Rd.
PO Box 2818
Kingston 8, Jamaica
**Phone:** (876)931-4584　　**Fax:** (876)969-5721
**Email:** prov@jol.com
**Fnded:** 1982. **Lang(s):** English. **Desc:** Health care personnel and other trained individuals. Promotes improved health care and increased economic and social opportunities for people with disabilities. Provides services including medical assessment, parent training, vision screening, educational testing and placement. Conducts public awareness, parent support, early intervention, and home-based intervention programs.

### REACH: Association for Children with Hand or Arm Deficiency
*See:* Entry 5747

### Reach Ireland (RI)
*See:* Entry 5748

### ★ 8073 ★ Research and Training Center on Independent Living (RTCIL)
University of Kansas
4089 Dole
RTC on Independent Living

1000 Sunnyside Ave.
Lawrence, KS 66045
**Phone:** (785)864-4095　　**Fax:** (785)864-5063
**Email:** rtcil@ku.edu
**Website:** http://www.rtcil.org
Dr. James Budde, Dir.
**Fnded:** 1980. **Mem:** 180. **Desc:** U.S. independent living centers helping individuals with severe disabilities lead independent lives. Works to: identify attributes of successful self-help support groups; develop and test instruments to assess social support levels within self-help support groups; implement and evaluate intervention strategies for accurate and positive portrayals of people with disabilities by the media; deter unlawful parking in handicapped-designated parking spaces and enhance public awareness of issues related to disability and independent living; establish accreditation standards to evaluate ILC programs, services, and management. Has developed: Personal Attendant Care Management Training model in seven states to increase the ability of consumers to manage attendants an d reduce management problems and institutionalization; program to assist ILC consumers in identifying personal goals and initiating behavioral changes to attain them. Provides direct training and technical assistance to individuals, ILCs, state agencies, and consumers' groups; university courses, and presentations. Places an emphasis on the needs of underserved populations, including the mentally ill, patients with brain injuries, minorities, the elderly, and persons living in rural areas. **Pub:** *Catalogue of Publications*, annual. Lists publications available from the center; includes abstracts. • *Guidelines for Reporting and Writing About People with Disabilities*. • Manuals. • Monographs.

### ★ 8074 ★ Responsible Hospitality Institute (RHI)
World Trade Center
1250 Sixth Ave., Ste. 217
San Diego, CA 92101
**Phone:** (619)234-0007　　**Fax:** (619)234-0319
**Email:** jim@hospitalityweb.org
**Website:** http://www.hospitalityweb.org/rhi
James Peters, Dir.
**Fnded:** 1983. **Mem:** 300. **Local Groups:** 1. **Desc:** Individuals from the U.S., Canada, New Zealand, and Australia concerned with: accessibility of restaurants and other hospitality businesses to disabled persons; responsible operation of establishments selling alcoholic beverages. Presently Inactive. **Pub:** *Hospitality Insighter*, monthly. Newsletter. *Price:* $60. • *Networker*. **Frmly:** Intermission.

### ★ 8075 ★ Restricted Growth Association
PO Box 4744
Dorchester DT2 9FA, United Kingdom
**Phone:** 44 1308 898445
**Email:** rga1@talk21.com
**Website:** http://www.rgaonline.org.uk
**Fnded:** 1970. **Mem:** 650. **Lang(s):** English. **Desc:** Open to persons with restricted growth, families with a child with restricted growth, health professionals, and other interested persons. Aims to help reduce the distress and disadvantages of persons of restricted growth by trying to reduce social barriers, improve the quality of life and enhance their role in society. Offers counseling training, family support, medical information and other practical help. Regional co-ordinators. **Pub:** *RGA Information Magazine*, semiannual. Magazine. • *RGA News*, quarterly. Newsletter. • *Walking Through Leaves: Autobiography of William Shakespeare*.

### ★ 8076 ★ Riding for the Disabled Association - Ireland (RDAI)
c/o Rathlinn
Templecarrig Lower
Delgany, Wicklow, Ireland
**Phone:** 353 1 2876498　　**Fax:** 353 1 2876503
**Fnded:** 1969. **Mem:** 85. **Nat'l Groups:** 85. **Lang(s):** English, Irish. **Desc:** Equestrian coaches and enthusiasts. Promotes increased participation in equestrian

activities among people with disabilities. Sponsors horseback riding programs for people with disabilities.

**★ 8077 ★ Royal Association for Disability and Rehabilitation (RADAR)**
12 City Forum
250 City Rd.
London EC1V 8AF, United Kingdom
**Phone:** 44 207 2503222     **Fax:** 44 171 2500212
**Email:** radar@radar.org.uk
**Website:** http://www.radar.org.uk

**Fnded:** 1977. **Mem:** 500. **Desc:** Represents the rights and interests of disabled individuals in the United Kingdom. Strives to improve educational, health, and social services for disabled people and stresses their full integration and participation in community life. Seeks to eliminate barriers that impose restrictions on disabled people. Provides advice. UK Secretariat of Rehabilitation International. **Pub:** *Holiday Guides*, annual. • Bulletin, monthly. • Pamphlets.

**★ 8078 ★ Scope**
6 Market Rd.
London N7 9PW, United Kingdom
**Phone:** 44 20 76197100
**Email:** information@scope.org.uk
**Website:** http://www.scope.org.uk

**Lang(s):** English. **Desc:** People with cerebral palsy, their families, and carers in England and Wales. Promotes equality for disabled people. Provides residential, job help, and education services for people with cerebral palsy; carries out research into issues affecting disabled people. **Pub:** *Disability Now*, monthly. Newspaper.

**★ 8079 ★ Scottish Sports Association for Disabled People**
Fife Sports Institute
Viewfield Rd.
Glenrothes KY6 2RB, United Kingdom
**Phone:** 44 1592 415700     **Fax:** 44 1592 415710
**Desc:** Promotes sports for the disabled in Scotland.

**Shriners Hospitals for Children**
*See:* Entry 11509

**★ 8080 ★ Siblings for Significant Change (SSC)**
350 5th Ave., Ste.627
New York, NY 10118
**Phone:** (212)420-0776     **Free:** 800-841-8251
**Fax:** (212)643-1244
**Email:** gerriscfu@aol.com
**Website:** http://www.specialcitizens.com
Gerri Zatlow, Dir.

**Fnded:** 1982. **Mem:** 75. **Desc:** Siblings of disabled individuals; parents, educators, social workers, medical professionals, and researchers interested in siblings of disabled individuals. Provides peer support, legal assistance, and psychological counseling to siblings of the handicapped. Coordinates social activities for families with handicapped members and works on projects and audiovisual programs designed to increase national awareness of the difficulties faced by families of disabled individuals. Maintains speakers' bureau. Division of Special Citizens Futures Unlimited, a New York state organization that offers ongoing programs for autistic and autistic-like adults. **Pub:** *Directory of Sibling Related Services*. Directory. • Journal, semiannual. • Newsletter, periodic.

**★ 8081 ★ Ski for Light**
1455 W Lake St.
Minneapolis, MN 55408
**Phone:** (612)827-3232     **Fax:** (612)779-0211
**Email:** info@sfl.org
**Website:** http://www.sfl.org
Nancy McKinney, Pres.

**Fnded:** 1975. **Nat'l Groups:** 1. **Reg. Groups:** 10. **Desc:** Dedicated to encouraging and assisting inter-

ested groups in conducting cross-country skiing programs and other health sports activities for visually impaired and other physically disabled people. Brings together disabled and nondisabled people from throughout the U.S., Canada, Norway, and other countries. The group is modeled after the Knight's Race (Ridderrennet) in Norway, which has been held annually since 1964 with international participation. Sponsors physically demanding health sports events throughout the year in North America including the Ski for Light International Program. Maintains speakers' bureau. Maintains speakers' bureau. **Pub:** *SFL Bulletin*, quarterly. Bulletin. Contains organizational news. *Price:* Free. • *Ski for Light Even Journal*. Journal. **Frmly:** (1980) Ski for Light; (1983) HEALTHsports, Inc.

**★ 8082 ★ Societe Logique (SL)**
3250 Saint Joseph Blvd. E
Montreal, QC, Canada H1Y 3G2
**Phone:** (514)522-8284     **Fax:** (514)522-2659
**Email:** soclog@connectmmic.net

**Fnded:** 1981. **Mem:** 50. **Lang(s):** English, French. **Desc:** Architects interested in barrier-free design. Promotes erection of buildings accessible to people with physical disabilities. Serves as a clearinghouse on barrier-free architecture; provides consulting services to members; conducts educational programs; maintains speakers' bureau.

**★ 8083 ★ Society for Accessible Travel for the Handicapped (SATH)**
347 5th Ave., Ste. 610
New York, NY 10016
**Phone:** (212)447-7284     **Fax:** (212)725-8253
**Email:** sathtravel@aol.com
**Website:** http://www.sath.org
Laurel VanHorn, Exec. Dir.

**Fnded:** 1976. **Mem:** 2,500. **Desc:** Travel professionals, consumers with disabilities, other individuals and corporations supporting this mission. Strives to raise awareness of needs of all travelers with disabilities, remove physical and attitudinal barriers to free access and expand travel opportunities in the United States and abroad. Operates speaker's bureau. library. Compiles statistics on the potential travel market of various handicapped groups and their locations. **Pub:** *Open World*, quarterly. Magazine. Contains articles on travel and related matters of interest to all handicapped persons. *Price:* Included in membership dues; $13/year plus shipping and handling; $24/2 years plus shipping and handling; $30/3 years plus shipping and handling. • *The Travel Related Industries Accessibility Guide, 1996*. • Information sheets on matter related to travel. The travel related Industries Accessibility Guide.

**★ 8084 ★ Society for Disability Studies**
c/o Carol J. Gill, PhD
University of Illinois at Chicago, MC626
Department of Disability and Human Development
1640 W Roosevelt Rd., No. 236
Chicago, IL 60608-6904
**Phone:** (312)996-4664
**Email:** cg16@uic.edu
**Website:** http://www.uic.edu/orgs/sds/
Carol J. Gill, PhD, Exec. Officer

**Fnded:** 1986. **Mem:** 300. **Desc:** Social scientists and scholars studying the problems of disabled people in society. Strives to develop theoretical and practical knowledge about disability and promotes equal participation in society for individuals with disabilities. **Pub:** *Annual Proceedings*, annual. *Price:* $25.

**★ 8085 ★ Society of Homes for the Handicapped (SHH)**
G/F 2A Po On Rd.
Cronin Garden
Shamshuipo
Hong Kong, People's Republic of China
**Phone:** 852 227454214     **Fax:** 852 227864097
**Email:** fhs@fuhong.org

**Website:** http://www.fuhong.org

**Fnded:** 1977. **Mem:** 210. **Lang(s):** English. **Desc:** Works to integrate mentally and physically disabled individuals, as well as those who have recovered from mental illnesses, into Hong Kong society. Instructs family members on care for the disabled; operates residential homes and day care centers. Conducts courses for handicapped individuals; trains volunteers to work with the disabled. Provides vocational assessment and employment opportunities for the disabled. Offers social work services to families with disabled members. Organizes community educational programs for a better understanding and positive attitude towards persons with disabilities. **Pub:** *SHH Annual Report*, annual. Annual Report. • *SHH NEWS*, quarterly. Newsletter. SHH News and activities.

**Society of Teachers of Speech and Drama**
*See:* Entry 6110

**★ 8086 ★ Southern Africa Federation of the Disabled (SAFOD)**
19, Lobengula St.
PO Box 2247
Bulawayo, Zimbabwe
**Phone:** 263 9 69356     **Fax:** 263 9 74398
**Email:** safod@telconet.co.zw
**Website:** http://www.stsd.org.uk

**Fnded:** 1986. **Mem:** 10. **Lang(s):** English. **Desc:** Seeks to defend the rights of disabled people. Provides a forum for discussion among disabled persons. **Pub:** *Disability Frontline & CBR News*, quarterly. Newsletter. Includes focusing on disability issues and activities within the region.

**★ 8087 ★ Southern African Association for Learning and Educational Difficulties (SAALED)**
PO Box 2404
Clareinch 7740, Republic of South Africa
**Phone:** 27 21 7626306     **Fax:** 27 21 7626306
**Email:** info@saaled.org.za
**Website:** http://www.saaled.org.za

**Fnded:** 1973. **Mem:** 300. **Reg. Groups:** 4. **Local Groups:** 5. **Lang(s):** Afrikaans, English. **Desc:** Education professionals, associates, and parents. Works to influence official policy and improve educational facilities and practices for anyone with learning difficulties. Promotes interdisciplinary and interracial cooperation. Conducts community projects and charitable programs. **Pub:** *SAALED Newsletter*, semiannual. Newsletter. **Frmly:** (1992) Southern African Association for Learning and Educational Disabilities.

**★ 8088 ★ Special Olympics Albania**
c/o Koco Gaba
RR Mine Peza
Pall 254/1/9
SHK 1/9
Tirana, Albania
**Fax:** 352 42 40964
**Email:** sabian@icc.al.eu.org

**Desc:** Offers support and training for disabled individuals in Albania who wish to participate in athletic competitions.

**★ 8089 ★ Special Olympics Andorra**
c/o Escola Meritxell
dels Barrers 10
Santa Coloma, Andorra
**Phone:** 376 821731     **Fax:** 376 860540
**Email:** eensdm@mypic.ad

**Desc:** Offers support and training for disabled individuals in Andorra who wish to participate in athletic competitions.

**★ 8090 ★ Special Olympics Argentina**
c/o Pia Soldatti
Nueva Olimpiada Especial Argentina

Almirante Onofre Betbeder
1252 Buenos Aires, Argentina
**Phone:** 54 11 48961413  **Fax:** 54 11 1544275117
**Email:** info@olimpiadaespecial.org.ar
**Desc:** Offers support and training for disabled individuals in Argentina who wish to participate in athletic competitions.


★ **8091** ★ **Special Olympics Armenia**
c/o Mr. Gavrush Mnatsakanyan, Pres.
Ministry of Education
43/65 Horenatsi St.
375018 Yerevan, Armenia
**Phone:** 374 2576967          **Fax:** 372 2541511
**Desc:** Offers support and training for disabled individuals participating in athletic competitions.


★ **8092** ★ **Special Olympics Australia**
c/o Rex Langthorne
PO Box 712
Glebe, NSW 2037, Australia
**Phone:** 61 2 95526188     **Fax:** 61 2 95523848
**Desc:** Offers support and training for disabled individuals in Australia who wish to participate in athletic competitions.


★ **8093** ★ **Special Olympics Austria**
c/o Marc Angelini
Zangtalerstrasse 64
8570 Voitsberg, Austria
**Phone:** 43 36 8723358      **Fax:** 43 31 44339410
**Email:** soo-graz@specialolympics.at
**Desc:** Offers support and training for disabled individuals in Austria who wish to participate in athletic competitions.


★ **8094** ★ **Special Olympics Azerbaijan**
c/o Mr. Shahin Aliyev, Pres.
46/50 U. Hadjibayov Str, Apr. 3-4
370010 Baku, Azerbaijan
**Phone:** 994 12 988170      **Fax:** 994 12 985525
**Website:** http://www.specialolympics.org/program_locations/
**Desc:** Offers support and training for disabled individuals participating in athletic competitions.


★ **8095** ★ **Special Olympics Bangladesh**
c/o Ms. Sanchita Begum
Sharif Mansion, 4th Fl.
56-57 Motijheel C/A
GPO Box 829
Dhaka 1000, Bangladesh
**Phone:** 880 2 233383      **Fax:** 880 2 8912085
**Email:** sobangla@bdmail.com
**Desc:** Offers support and training for disabled individuals in Bangladesh who wish to participate in athletic competitions.


★ **8096** ★ **Special Olympics Belarus**
c/o Mr. Valentin Shukh, Pres.
K. Libknehta, 68-906
220036 Minsk, Belarus
**Phone:** 375 17 2226584     **Fax:** 375 17 2862573
**Email:** olcom@user.unibel.by
**Website:** http://www.specialolympics.org/program_locations/
**Desc:** Offers support and training for disabled individuals participating in athletic competitions.


★ **8097** ★ **Special Olympics Benin**
c/o Marie Jeanne Dagnon-Yalo
BP 0912
Cotonou, Benin
**Phone:** 229 323650          **Fax:** 229 312535
**Desc:** Offers support and training for disabled individuals in Benin who wish to participate in athletic competitions.


★ **8098** ★ **Special Olympics Bolivia**
c/o Henry Jordan
Juan Manuel Loza 1776
Condominio San Andres
Bloque 1 Depto. 1B
Miaflores
La Paz, Bolivia
**Phone:** 591 2 227808
**Email:** paola2311@yahoo.com
**Desc:** Offers support and training for disabled individuals in Bolivia who wish to participate in athletic competitions.


★ **8099** ★ **Special Olympics Bosnia & Herzegovina**
c/o Ministry of Social Policy
A.B. Slimica 4
Sarajevo, Bosnia-Hercegovina
**Phone:** 387 71616433          **Fax:** 387 71648828
**Desc:** Offers support and training for disabled individuals in Bosnia & Herzegovina who wish to participate in athletic competitions.


★ **8100** ★ **Special Olympics Botswana**
c/o Botswana Council for the Disabled
Private Bag 459
Gaborone, Botswana
**Phone:** 267 373599          **Fax:** 267 311784
**Email:** bcd@info.bw
**Desc:** Offers support and training for disabled individuals in Botswana who wish to participate in athletic competitions.


★ **8101** ★ **Special Olympics Brazil**
c/o Dieter Fanta
Rua Ulysses Pedroso de Oliveira Filho, N 321
13270-420 Valinhos, SP, Brazil
**Phone:** 55 19 38693161
**Email:** aoebr@valinhos.correionet.com.br
**Website:** http://www.olimpiadasespeciais.com.br
**Desc:** Offers support and training for disabled individuals in Brazil who wish to participate in athletic competitions.


★ **8102** ★ **Special Olympics Bulgaria**
c/o Nikolay Dagorov
23, Rozhen Blvd.
BG-1040 Sofia, Bulgaria
**Phone:** 359 2 372145          **Fax:** 359 2 387592
**Email:** solympics-bg@hotmail.com
**Desc:** Offers support and training for disabled individuals in Bulgaria who wish to participate in athletic competitions.


★ **8103** ★ **Special Olympics Burkina Faso**
c/o Alexandre Yougbare
BP 4411
Ouagadougou 01, Burkina Faso
**Phone:** 226 314978          **Fax:** 226 320134
**Desc:** Offers support and training for disabled individuals in Burkina Faso who wish to participate in athletic competitions.


★ **8104** ★ **Special Olympics Cameroon**
c/o Mbarga Panda Simon
PO Box 6991
Yaounde, Cameroon
**Phone:** 237 216650          **Fax:** 237 221873
**Desc:** Offers support and training for disabled individuals in Cameroon who wish to participate in athletic competitions.


★ **8105** ★ **Special Olympics Chad**
c/o Doubrain Ngabaye
BP 4398
N'Djamena, Chad
**Phone:** 235 514038          **Fax:** 235 516677
**Desc:** Offers support and training for disabled individuals in Chad who wish to participate in athletic competitions.


★ **8106** ★ **Special Olympics China**
c/o Yong Zhi Jun
44 Beichizi St.
Dongcheng District
Beijing 100006, People's Republic of China
**Phone:** 86 10 65139719     **Fax:** 86 10 65139722
**Email:** sochn@263.net
**Desc:** Offers support and training for disabled individuals in China who wish to participate in athletic competitions.


★ **8107** ★ **Special Olympics Colombia**
c/o D. Alejandro Escallon
Carrera 13-A, No. 8734
Bogota, D.E., Colombia
**Phone:** 57 1 2182122          **Fax:** 57 1 6163859
**Email:** aescallo@impsat.net.co
**Desc:** Offers support and training for disabled individuals in Colombia who wish to participate in athletic competitions.


★ **8108** ★ **Special Olympics Costa Rica**
c/o Carlos Valverde
Apartado 7232
San Jose 1000, Costa Rica
**Phone:** 506 2267458          **Fax:** 506 2273101
**Email:** lauravalverde@usa.net
**Desc:** Offers support and training for disabled individuals in Costa Rica who wish to participate in athletic competitions.


★ **8109** ★ **Special Olympics Croatia**
c/o Verica Paulic
Trg Sportova 11, Rm. 30A
10000 Zagreb, Croatia
**Phone:** 385 1 3650214          **Fax:** 385 1 3091119
**Email:** igor.paulic@zg.tel.hr
**Desc:** Offers support and training for disabled individuals in Croatia who wish to participate in athletic competitions.


★ **8110** ★ **Special Olympics Cuba**
c/o Luis Gomez Gutierrez
17 y 0 Vedado
Havana, Cuba
**Phone:** 53 7 322452          **Fax:** 53 7 553105
**Email:** cdmined@ceniai.inf.cu
**Desc:** Offers support and training for disabled individuals in Cuba who wish to participate in athletic competitions.


★ **8111** ★ **Special Olympics Cyprus**
c/o Andreas Hadjivasiliou
20 Ionos St. Engomini
PO Box 3931
Nicosia 1687, Cyprus
**Phone:** 357 2 662984          **Fax:** 357 2 664986
**Email:** megalemo@cytanet.com.cy
**Desc:** Offers support and training for disabled individuals in Cyprus who wish to participate in athletic competitions.


★ **8112** ★ **Special Olympics Czech Republic**
c/o Martina Stredova
Ricni 6
CS-11800 Prague, Czech Republic
**Phone:** 42 2 535338
**Email:** kurznet@vol.cz
**Desc:** Offers support and training for disabled individuals in Czech Republic who wish to participate in athletic competitions.

★ 8113 ★ **Special Olympics Denmark**
c/o Dansk Handicap, Idraets-Forbund
Idraettens Hus-Brondby Stadion 20
DK-2605 Brondby, Denmark
**Phone:** 45 43262455    **Fax:** 45 43262470
**Email:** handicapidraet@dhif.dk
**Desc:** Offers support and training for disabled individuals in Denmark who wish to participate in athletic competitions.

★ 8114 ★ **Special Olympics Dominican Republic**
c/o Vicenta Peignand
Apartado de Coreos 1054
Santo Domingo, Dominican Republic
**Phone:** (809)688-6444    **Fax:** (809)688-1566
**Email:** dirladr@tricom.net
**Desc:** Offers support and training for disabled individuals in Dominican Republic who wish to participate in athletic competitions.

★ 8115 ★ **Special Olympics Ecuador**
c/o Hector Cueva Jimenez
Calle Berlin 158 y Ave. 9 de Octubre
Oficina 014 - 1er piso
Quito, Ecuador
**Phone:** 593 2 550818    **Fax:** 593 2 562759
**Email:** olimpes@hotmail.com
**Desc:** Offers support and training for disabled individuals in Ecuador who wish to participate in athletic competitions.

★ 8116 ★ **Special Olympics El Salvador**
c/o Hector Hugo Matasol
Palacio de los Deportes
Indes 2o Nivel, Salon 3
San Salvador, El Salvador
**Phone:** 503 2715693    **Fax:** 503 2711208
**Desc:** Offers support and training for disabled individuals in El Salvador who wish to participate in athletic competitions.

★ 8117 ★ **Special Olympics Estonia**
c/o Toomas Hendrick lives
Amrop International
Kaupmehe 8
EE-10114 Tallinn, Estonia
**Phone:** 372 2 6403155    **Fax:** 372 2 6558361
**Email:** meeli.hunt@amrop.com
**Desc:** Offers support and training for disabled individuals in Estonia who wish to participate in athletic competitions.

★ 8118 ★ **Special Olympics Finland**
c/o Finnish Sports Federation for Persons with Intellectual Disabilities
Radio Katu 20, 5.KRS
SF-00093 Slu, Finland
**Phone:** 358 9 8776868    **Fax:** 358 9 8776869
**Email:** eija.kangas-virtanen@kolumbus.fi
**Desc:** Offers support and training for disabled individuals in Finland who wish to participate in athletic competitions.

★ 8119 ★ **Special Olympics France**
c/o Bruno Grob
182 rue Raymond Losserand
F-75014 Paris, France
**Phone:** 33 1 44126011    **Fax:** 33 1 44126019
**Desc:** Offers support and training for disabled individuals in France who wish to participate in athletic competitions.

★ 8120 ★ **Special Olympics Gabon**
c/o Daoveda Leocadie
BP 18349
Libreville, Gabon
**Phone:** 241 244980    **Fax:** 241 705658

**Desc:** Offers support and training for disabled individuals in Gabon who wish to participate in athletic competitions.

★ 8121 ★ **Special Olympics Gambia**
c/o Alieu Y. Cham
PO Box 2554
Serekunda, Gambia
**Phone:** 220 228601    **Fax:** 220 227861
**Email:** acham.baes@ganet.gm
**Desc:** Offers support and training for disabled individuals in Gambia who wish to participate in athletic competitions.

★ 8122 ★ **Special Olympics Georgia**
c/o Rcheulishrili Vaxtang
Apart 49, Chavchardnadze
380072 Tbilisi, Georgia
**Phone:** 995 32 331827    **Fax:** 995 32 970076
**Email:** ketosi@mailexcite.com
**Desc:** Offers support and training for disabled individuals in Georgia who wish to participate in athletic competitions.

★ 8123 ★ **Special Olympics Germany**
c/o Institut fur Sportwissenschaften der Universitat
Judenbuhl Western Euroweg, 11
D-97082 Wurzburg, Germany
**Phone:** 49 931 86010    **Fax:** 49 931 84390
**Email:** special_olympics@mail.uni-wuerzburg.de
**Desc:** Offers support and training for disabled individuals in Germany who wish to participate in athletic competitions.

★ 8124 ★ **Special Olympics Ghana**
c/o National Sports Council
PO Box 1272
Accra, Ghana
**Phone:** 233 21 674369    **Fax:** 233 21 669562
**Email:** eessifie@accra.vra.com
**Desc:** Offers support and training for disabled individuals in Ghana who wish to participate in athletic competitions.

★ 8125 ★ **Special Olympics Greece**
c/o Epirotiki Bldg.
87 Akti Miaouli
GR-185 38 Piraeus, Greece
**Phone:** 30 1 6068956    **Fax:** 30 1 6068955
**Email:** spolimpicsgr@mail.com
**Desc:** Offers support and training for disabled individuals in Greece who wish to participate in athletic competitions.

★ 8126 ★ **Special Olympics Honduras (Olimpiadas Especiales de Hondras)**
c/o Ana de Galeano
Estadio de Beisbol
Complejo Deportivo Jose Simon Azcona
Tegucigalpa, Honduras
**Phone:** 504 2356405    **Fax:** 504 2356405
**Email:** oliesphonduras@sigmanet.hn
**Desc:** Offers support and training for disabled individuals in Honduras who wish to participate in athletic competitions.

★ 8127 ★ **Special Olympics Hungary (Magyar Specialis Olimpia Eyesulet)**
c/o Janos Wisinger
Istvanmezei ut. 1-3
H-1146 Budapest, Hungary
**Phone:** 36 1 2522236    **Fax:** 36 1 9995563
**Email:** hunolimp@nograd.net
**Desc:** Offers support and training for disabled individuals in Hungary who wish to participate in athletic competitions.

★ 8128 ★ **Special Olympics Iceland**
c/o Sveinn Aki Ludviksson
Throttamidstodin Laugardal
IS-104 Reykjavik, Iceland
**Phone:** 354 5686301    **Fax:** 354 5686315
**Email:** annak@toto.is
**Desc:** Offers support and training for disabled individuals in Iceland who wish to participate in athletic competitions.

★ 8129 ★ **Special Olympics India**
c/o J.A. Benji Benjamin
106 Church St.
Lingarajapuram
St. Thomas Town
Bangalore 560 084, India
**Phone:** 91 80 5461379    **Fax:** 91 80 5478382
**Email:** benji_sivus@usa.net
**Desc:** Offers support and training for disabled individuals in India who wish to participate in athletic competitions.

★ 8130 ★ **Special Olympics Italy**
c/o Alessandro Palazzotti
via di Decima 40
I-00144 Rome, Italy
**Phone:** 39 6 52246486    **Fax:** 39 6 5295062
**Email:** specialolympics@inwind.it
**Website:** http://www.specialolympics.it
**Desc:** Offers support and training for disabled individuals in Italy who wish to participate in athletic competitions.

★ 8131 ★ **Special Olympics Japan**
c/o Fukujiro Shiroki
Viale Bld. 3F
1-24 Kamitori-cho
Kumamoto 860-0845, Japan
**Phone:** 81 96 3524000    **Fax:** 81 96 3521820
**Email:** so-jpn@fa2.so-net.ne.jp
**Website:** http://www.specialolympics-nippon.gr.jp/
**Desc:** Offers support and training for disabled individuals in Japan who wish to participate in athletic competitions.

★ 8132 ★ **Special Olympics Kazakhstan**
Furmanova Str. 50, of. 412
480004 Almaty, Kazakhstan
**Phone:** 7 3272 332979    **Fax:** 7 3272 332979
**Email:** specialkaz@asdc.kz
**Website:** http://www.sok.nursat.kz
**Fnded:** 1991. **Mem:** 6,500. **Nat'l Groups:** 1. **Reg. Groups:** 14. **State Groups:** 1. **Local Groups:** 73. **Lang(s):** Russian. **Desc:** Individuals and organizations. Promotes the Special Olympics in Kazakhstan. Works to advance the social rehabilitation of people with mental retardation. **Pub:** *The Target*, quarterly. Newsletter.

★ 8133 ★ **Special Olympics Kenya**
c/o Joe N. Mutua
PO Box 70483
Nairobi, Kenya
**Phone:** 254 2 725836    **Fax:** 254 2 336885
**Email:** kitololo@africaonline.co.ke
**Desc:** Offers support and training for disabled individuals in Kenya who wish to participate in athletic competitions.

★ 8134 ★ **Special Olympics Korea**
c/o Jung-Hoon Lee
288-1 Hagye-Dong
Nowon-gu
Seoul 139-231, Republic of Korea
**Phone:** 82 2 9727630    **Fax:** 82 2 9784287
**Email:** hoon6910@chollian.net
**Desc:** Offers support and training for disabled individuals in Korea who wish to participate in athletic competitions.

**★ 8135 ★ Special Olympics Latvia**
c/o Dzidra Kupca
LV-1001 Riga, Latvia
**Phone:** 371 2 7376244     **Fax:** 371 2 7376759
**Email:** eglons@lmuza.lv
**Desc:** Offers support and training for disabled individuals in Latvia who wish to participate in athletic competitions.

**★ 8136 ★ Special Olympics Lesotho**
c/o Lesotho Society of Mentally Handicapped
   Persons
PO Box 9204
Maseru 100, Lesotho
**Phone:** 266 320407     **Fax:** 266 322462
**Email:** lsmhp@lesoff.co.za
**Desc:** Offers support and training for disabled individuals in Lesotho who wish to participate in athletic competitions.

**★ 8137 ★ Special Olympics Malawi**
c/o Sports Council Malawi
Box 452
Blantyre, Malawi
**Phone:** 265 675084     **Fax:** 265 675110
**Email:** mmathias@malawi.net
**Desc:** Offers support and training for disabled individuals in Malawi who wish to participate in athletic competitions.

**★ 8138 ★ Special Olympics Malaysia**
c/o Joan Lai
PO Box 10462
Kota Kinabalu
88805 Sabah, Malaysia
**Phone:** 60 88 223221     **Fax:** 60 88 244672
**Email:** scngo@pop.jaring.my
**Desc:** Offers support and training for disabled individuals in Malaysia who wish to participate in athletic competitions.

**★ 8139 ★ Special Olympics Malta**
c/o Paul Micallef
New York Bldg., Ste. 9
Qawra Rd.
Qawra, Malta
**Phone:** 356 570326     **Fax:** 356 570326
**Email:** paul@novanet.net.mt
**Desc:** Offers support and training for disabled individuals in Malta who wish to participate in athletic competitions.

**★ 8140 ★ Special Olympics Moldova**
c/o Nicolai Barbieru
ul. Pushkina, 26
277024 Kishinev, Moldova
**Phone:** 373 2 244479     **Fax:** 373 2 227707
**Desc:** Offers support and training for disabled individuals in Moldova who wish to participate in athletic competitions.

**★ 8141 ★ Special Olympics Nepal**
c/o Dr. Jyoti Sherchan
Kamalpokhari
PO Box 12189
Kathmandu, Nepal
**Phone:** 977 1 424736     **Fax:** 977 1 425774
**Email:** sonepal@ccsl.com.np
**Desc:** Offers support and training for disabled individuals in Nepal who wish to participate in athletic competitions.

**★ 8142 ★ Special Olympics Netherlands**
c/o Netherlands Sports Federation for Citizens with
   Intellectual Handicaps
Regulierenring 2b
Postbus 200
NL-3980 Bunnik, Netherlands
**Phone:** 31 30 6597310     **Fax:** 31 30 6597373

**Email:** info@nsg-son.nl
**Desc:** Offers support and training for disabled individuals in Netherlands who wish to participate in athletic competitions.

**★ 8143 ★ Special Olympics New Zealand**
c/o Chris Hooper
Epuni
PO Box 45041
Lower Hutt, New Zealand
**Phone:** 64 4 5693474     **Fax:** 64 4 5701067
**Email:** nzspec@clear.net.nz
**Desc:** Offers support and training for disabled individuals in New Zealand who wish to participate in athletic competitions.

**★ 8144 ★ Special Olympics Norway**
c/o IPU-Utvalget
Serviceboks 1, Ulleval I Stadion
N-0840 Oslo, Norway
**Phone:** 47 21029000     **Fax:** 47 21029481
**Email:** goril.hansen@nif.idrett.no
**Desc:** Offers support and training for disabled individuals in Norway who wish to participate in athletic competitions.

**★ 8145 ★ Special Olympics Pakistan**
c/o Parveen Ali
Defence Housing Society, Phase II
7-B 4th Central Ln.
Karachi, Pakistan
**Phone:** 92 21 5887260     **Fax:** 92 21 7725753
**Email:** pali@alephx.org
**Desc:** Offers support and training for disabled individuals in Pakistan who wish to participate in athletic competitions.

**★ 8146 ★ Special Olympics Panama**
**(Olimpiadas Especiales de Panama)**
c/o Yolanda Eleta de Varela
Apartado Postal 394
Ancon
Panama City, Panama
**Phone:** 507 2288224
**Email:** olimesp@sinfo.net
**Desc:** Offers support and training for disabled individuals in Panama who wish to participate in athletic competitions.

**★ 8147 ★ Special Olympics Paraguay**
**(Olimpiadas Especiales de Paraguay)**
c/o Irma Cuevas de Cabezudo
Rca. de Colombia 1112
Asuncion, Paraguay
**Phone:** 595 21 491493     **Fax:** 595 21 494314
**Email:** cabezudo@rieder.net
**Desc:** Offers support and training for disabled individuals in Paraguay who wish to participate in athletic competitions.

**★ 8148 ★ Special Olympics Peru**
**(Olimpiadas Especiales de Peru)**
c/o Aldo Barbieri
Ave. Prolongacion Ricardo
Palma 1391, LaAurora
Miraflores
Lima 18, Peru
**Phone:** 51 14 470780     **Fax:** 51 14 473360
**Email:** olimpiadasespecialesperu@ddm.com.pe
**Desc:** Offers support and training for disabled individuals in Peru who wish to participate in athletic competitions.

**★ 8149 ★ Special Olympics Philippines**
c/o Nicanor Jorge
4 Lands St., Vasra Village
Quezon City, Metro Manila, Philippines
**Phone:** 63 2 9288448     **Fax:** 63 2 9295707
**Email:** best@pacific.net.ph

**Desc:** Offers support and training for disabled individuals in Philippines who wish to participate in athletic competitions.

**★ 8150 ★ Special Olympics Poland**
c/o Katerina Niemczycka
ul. Wilcza 38a p. 15
PL-00-679 Warsaw, Poland
**Phone:** 48 2 26270758     **Fax:** 48 2 26218418
**Email:** olimpiad@polbox.com
**Website:** http://www.olimpiadyspecjalne.pl
**Desc:** Offers support and training for disabled individuals in Poland who wish to participate in athletic competitions.

**★ 8151 ★ Special Olympics Portugal**
c/o Liga Portuguesa dos Deficientes Motores
Rua do Sitio do Casalinho da Ajuda
P-1349012 Lisbon, Portugal
**Phone:** 351 1 213626608     **Fax:** 351 1 3648639
**Email:** lj.lpdm.crs@mail.telepac.pt
**Desc:** Offers support and training for disabled individuals in Portugal who wish to participate in athletic competitions.

**★ 8152 ★ Special Olympics Romania**
c/o Federatia Romana a Sportului Pentru
   Handicapati
Ministerul Tineretului si Sportului
str. Vasile Conte, n. 16
Sector 2
R-70139 Bucharest, Romania
**Phone:** 40 1 2122719
**Email:** maria_milea2000@k.ro
**Desc:** Offers support and training for disabled individuals in Romania who wish to participate in athletic competitions.

**★ 8153 ★ Special Olympics Russia**
c/o Dr. Andrei Pavlov, Pres.
5, Sadovniki Str.
115487 Moscow, Russia
**Phone:** 7 95 1120047     **Fax:** 7 95 1122321
**Email:** specialolympica@euro.ru
**Website:** http://specialolympics.euro.ru
**Desc:** Offers support and training for disabled individuals participating in athletic competitions.

**★ 8154 ★ Special Olympics Singapore**
c/o Robin Chua
Blk. 2, No. 01-65, St. George's Rd.
Singapore 322-002, Singapore
**Phone:** 65 2933182     **Fax:** 65 2938497
**Email:** sosinga@mbox4.singnet.com.sg
**Desc:** Offers support and training for disabled individuals in Singapore who wish to participate in athletic competitions.

**★ 8155 ★ Special Olympics Slovakia**
c/o Eva Lysicanova
Nabr.arm.gen. L.'Svobu 1
811 02 Bratislava, Slovakia
**Phone:** 421 7 50225390     **Fax:** 421 7 54416398
**Email:** shso@ba.psg.sk
**Website:** http://www.shso.sk
**Desc:** Offers support and training for disabled individuals in Slovakia who wish to participate in athletic competitions.

**★ 8156 ★ Special Olympics Slovenia**
c/o Marijan Lacen
Samova 9/2o
SLO-1000 Ljubljana, Slovenia
**Phone:** 386 61 613617     **Fax:** 386 61 1362406
**Email:** info@zveza-sozitje.si
**Desc:** Offers support and training for disabled individuals in Slovenia who wish to participate in athletic competitions.

**★ 8157 ★ Special Olympics South Africa**
c/o Dr. Francois Jacobsz
Halfway House
PO Box 3818
Gauteng 1685, Republic of South Africa
**Phone:** 27 11 8055969 **Fax:** 27 11 8058081
**Email:** sosa@iafrica.com
**Desc:** Offers support and training for disabled individuals in South Africa who wish to participate in athletic competitions.

**★ 8158 ★ Special Olympics Spain**
c/o Francesc Martinez de Foix
Consell de Cent, 391, 2o 2a, Izq.
E-08009 Barcelona, Spain
**Phone:** 34 93 4874000 **Fax:** 34 93 4576003
**Email:** solympic@solympic.ictnet.es
**Website:** http://www.dyr.es/org/specialolympics
**Desc:** Offers support and training for disabled individuals in Spain who wish to participate in athletic competitions.

**★ 8159 ★ Special Olympics Sweden**
c/o Victor Wahlstrom
Graddvagen 12
S-640 45 Kvicksund, Sweden
**Phone:** 46 278 626064 **Fax:** 46 278 24456
**Email:** peter_bjork@telia.com
**Desc:** Offers support and training for disabled individuals in Sweden who wish to participate in athletic competitions.

**★ 8160 ★ Special Olympics Switzerland**
c/o Christian Lohr
Route u Petit-Moncor 17/19
Case postale 788
CH-1701 Fribourg, Switzerland
**Phone:** 41 37 264020045 **Fax:** 41 37 264020046
**Email:** specialolympics@compuserve.com
**Desc:** Offers support and training for disabled individuals in Switzerland who wish to participate in athletic competitions.

**★ 8161 ★ Special Olympics Tajikistan**
c/o Ms. Baikarim Tutenov, Pres.
Prospekt Dostyk, 38
Room 713A
734000 Almaty, Tajikistan
**Phone:** 7 327 2 638341 **Fax:** 7 327 2 332979
**Email:** specialkaz@asdc.kz
**Website:** http://www.specialolympics.org/program_locations/
**Desc:** Offers support and training for disabled individuals participating in athletic competitions.

**★ 8162 ★ Special Olympics Tanzania**
c/o Claude Njimba
PO Box 1949
Dar es Salaam, United Republic of Tanzania
**Phone:** 255 51 183082 **Fax:** 255 51 112054
**Desc:** Offers support and training for disabled individuals in Tanzania who wish to participate in athletic competitions.

**★ 8163 ★ Special Olympics Thailand**
c/o Rachaniwan Bulakul
339 Soi Pipat, Silom Rd.
Bangrak
Bangkok 10500, Thailand
**Phone:** 66 2 2666708 **Fax:** 66 2 2381149
**Email:** sothai@inet.co.th
**Desc:** Offers support and training for disabled individuals in Thailand who wish to participate in athletic competitions.

**★ 8164 ★ Special Olympics Turkmenistan**
c/o Mr. Bairam Seitlikov, Chair
PO Box 191

Krugozoi Main Post Office
744000 Ashgabat, Turkmenistan
**Email:** adji@online.tm
**Fnded:** 1990. **Mem:** 2,045. **Nat'l Groups:** 1. **Reg. Groups:** 5. **Lang(s):** English. **Desc:** Offers support and training for disabled individuals participating in athletic competitions.

**★ 8165 ★ Special Olympics Uganda**
c/o Edward Babumba
PO Box 5444
Kampala, Uganda
**Phone:** 256 41 267640 **Fax:** 256 41 345047
**Email:** souline@swiftuganda.com
**Desc:** Offers support and training for disabled individuals in Uganda who wish to participate in athletic competitions.

**★ 8166 ★ Special Olympics Ukraine**
c/o Mr. Konstantyn Slynavchuk, Pres.
20/6 Serpova St.
115-03115 Kiev, Ukraine
**Phone:** 380 44 444145 **Fax:** 380 44 4448200
**Desc:** Offers support and training for disabled individuals participating in athletic competitions.

**★ 8167 ★ Special Olympics Uruguay (Olimpiadas Especiales de Uruguay)**
c/o Alcides Abarno
Av. Brasil 2377, Depto. 1001
Montevideo, Uruguay
**Phone:** 598 2 7071007 **Fax:** 598 2 9021126
**Desc:** Offers support and training for disabled individuals in Uruguay who wish to participate in athletic competitions.

**★ 8168 ★ Special Olympics Uzbekistan**
c/o Mr. Adisman Dmitriv
Furkata 14
Tchilazarskij Rayon
700003 Tashkent, Uzbekistan
**Phone:** 998 712 451618 **Fax:** 998 712 459609
**Email:** adaminova@uz.peacecorps.gov
**Website:** http://www.specialolympics.org/program_locations/
**Desc:** Offers support and training for disabled individuals participating in athletic competitions.

**★ 8169 ★ Special Olympics Venezuela (Olimpiadas Especiales de Venezuela)**
c/o Evelyn Guiralt
Residence Sans Souci, Edificio El Aman
Piso 12, Apart. 122
Avenida Solano Lopez Chacaito
Caracas 1050, Venezuela
**Phone:** 58 2 2618530 **Fax:** 58 2 9528390
**Desc:** Offers support and training for disabled individuals in Venezuela who wish to participate in athletic competitions.

**★ 8170 ★ Special Olympics Zambia**
c/o Jumali Nkhama
PO Box 31202
Lusaka, Zambia
**Phone:** 260 1 281529 **Fax:** 260 1 223645
**Desc:** Offers support and training for disabled individuals in Zambia who wish to participate in athletic competitions.

**★ 8171 ★ Special Olympics Zimbabwe**
c/o Bonny Woodman
Greendale
PO Box GD 143
Harare, Zimbabwe
**Phone:** 263 4 499701 **Fax:** 263 4 499701
**Email:** sozim@id.co.zw
**Desc:** Offers support and training for disabled individuals in Zimbabwe who wish to participate in athletic competitions.

**★ 8172 ★ Special Recreation for disABLED International (SRDI)**
701 Oaknoll Dr.
Iowa City, IA 52246
**Phone:** (319)466-3192
**Email:** john-nesbitt@uiowa.edu
**Website:** http://www.jccniowa.org/~recdsabl
John A. Nesbitt, EdD, Pres. /CEO

**Fnded:** 1978. **Desc:** Seeks to serve and advocate special and therapeutic play and recreation for infants, children, youth, adults, and seniors throughout the world. Services include advisory and consultation, awards, employment information, professional education, public education, publishing, research, resource information and referral, technical assistance on programs and management methods, and an international library. Does international service work to: collect and disseminate international information on special recreation services for disabled persons, special recreation programs, and personnel training; conduct, provide, and support international exchange of technical, professional, and general information on special recreation for the disabled; cooperate with both governmental and voluntary organizations on national and international levels. Maintains Pioneers in Special Recreation Hall of Fame. Offers career guidance and placement service. Maintains speakers' bureau; compiles statistics. **Pub:** *Camping/Outdoor Recreation, National Institute on Camping for DisABLED*. Monograph. • *Community-Based Special Recreation, National Institute on New Models of Community-Based Special Recreation for DisABLED*. Monograph. • *Deaf-Blind, National Institute on Play and Recreation for Deaf-Blind*. Monograph. • *Health-PE-Recreation, World Seminar on Special Recreation, World Congress of the International Council on Health, Physical Education, Recreation and Dance*. Monograph. • *Mental Health, World Seminar on Special Recreation, World Congress of the World Federation for Mental Health, Manila, Philippines*. Monograph. **Frmly:** (1998) Special Recreation for Disabled.

**STEPS: National Association for Children with Lower Limb Abnormalities**
*See:* Entry 5763

**★ 8173 ★ Support Dogs (SD)**
9510 Page Ave.
Saint Louis, MO 63132
**Phone:** (314)423-1988 **Fax:** (314)423-5564
**Email:** info@supportdogs.org
**Website:** http://www.supportdogs.org
Joan Pace, Exec. Dir.

**Fnded:** 1981. **Mem:** 15,000. **Desc:** Helps people with special needs achieve greater independence and improve the quality of their lives by providing them with professionally trained dogs. Breeding program produces Golden Retrievers, Labradors, German Shepherds, and selected crossbreeds. Dogs are pre-matched and custom trained for each individual and assist their owners with tasks such as: opening mall and house doors; pulling wheelchairs long distances and up ramps; loading wheelchairs into vehicles; retreiving a dropped or distant object; bringing the phone and operating an emergency assistance switch; rising to high counters to assist with business transactions. **Pub:** *Support Dog News*, quarterly. Newsletter. Contains education about service dogs. **Price:** Free. **Frmly:** Support Dogs for the Handicapped.

**Swedish Association of Neurologically Disabled (Neurologiskt Handikappades Riksforbund — NHR)**
*See:* Entry 14122

**★ 8174 ★ Swimming/Natation Canada**
2197 Riverside Dr., Ste. 700
Ottawa, ON, Canada K1H 7X3
**Phone:** (613)260-1348 **Fax:** (613)260-0804
**Email:** natloffice@swimming.ca
**Website:** http://www.swimming.ca

**Fnded:** 1909. **Mem:** 83,604. **Lang(s):** English, French. **Desc:** Promotes swimming as a recreational and competitive activity for Canadians, including persons with a disability. Conducts educational and training programs; sponsors competitions. Seeks to provide opportunities for every individual in the sport to reach his/her maximum potential in fitness and excellence. **Frmly:** Canadian Wheelchair Swimming Association.

★ **8175** ★ **TASH (TASH)**
29 W Susquehanna Ave., Ste. 210
Baltimore, MD 21204
**Phone:** (410)828-8274　　**Fax:** (410)828-6706
**Email:** nweiss@tash.org
**Website:** http://www.tash.org
Nancy Weiss, Exec. Dir.
**Fnded:** 1973. **Mem:** 6,300. **Reg. Groups:** 2. **State Groups:** 35. **Desc:** Teachers, therapists, parents, administrators, university faculty, lawyers, and advocates involved in all areas of service to people with severe disabilities. Seeks to ensure an autonomous, dignified lifestyle for all people with severe disabilities; advocates quality education, from birth through adulthood, for disabled individuals. Disseminates updated information on solutions to problems, research findings, trends, and practices relevant to people with severe disabilities. Provides information and referral service. **Pub:** *JASH*, quarterly. Journal. *Price:* Included in membership dues. • *TASH Connections*, monthly. Magazine. **Frmly:** (1984) The Association for the Severely Handicapped; (2000) Association for Persons with Severe Handicaps.

**Uganda Association for the Mentally Handicapped (UAMH)**
*See:* Entry 12664

★ **8176** ★ **Union of Disabled People in Bulgaria**
Hristo Belchev 21
BG-1000 Sofia, Bulgaria
**Phone:** 359 2 9867070　　**Fax:** 359 2 9863986
**Fnded:** 1989. **Mem:** 30,000. **Desc:** Defends the interests of disabled persons. **Pub:** *Bulletin*, monthly. • *Kurazh*, periodic.

★ **8177** ★ **United Amputee Services Association**
c/o Jim Moore, Dir.
PO Box 4277
Winter Park, FL 32793
**Phone:** (407)678-2920　　**Fax:** (407)678-2203
**Email:** unitedamp@aol.com
**Website:** http://www.oandp.com/resources/organizations/uasa/index.htm
Kathy Hogan, Office Mgr.
**Fnded:** 1980. **Mem:** 400. **Desc:** Provides support and education to amputees and their families. **Pub:** *A Survivor's Guide for the Recent Amputee.* Booklet. Provides pertinent information regarding amputation. *Price:* $5 shipping and handling. • *Amputee Review*, quarterly. Newsletter.

★ **8178** ★ **Viet Nam Assistance for the Handicapped (VNAH)**
27 Dang Taf Dist. I
Ho Chi Minh City, Vietnam
**Phone:** 84 8 8480320　　**Fax:** 84 8 8480512
**Email:** vnah2@hcm.vnn.vn
**Website:** http://vnah-hev.org
**Fnded:** 1992. **Lang(s):** English, Vietnamese. **Desc:** Organizations and individuals concerned about the status of people with disabilities. Seeks to fully integrate people with disabilities into economic and social life. Provides support and services to people with disabilities and their families.

★ **8179** ★ **VSA arts**
1300 Connecticut Ave. NW, 700
Washington, DC 20036
**Phone:** (202)628-2800　　**Free:** 800-933-VSA1
**Fax:** (202)737-0725
**Email:** info@vsarts.org
**Website:** http://www.vsarts.org
Johanna Bentwood, Information Specialist
**Fnded:** 1974. **Nat'l Groups:** 87. **State Groups:** 47. **Desc:** An international Organization that promotes educational and lifelong learning opportunities through the arts for people of all abilities. Ambassador Jean Kennedy Smith founded the Organization in 1974 as an affiliate of The John F. Kennedy Center for the Performing Arts based on the concept that "the arts belong to all of us, and that everyone without exception must have equal opportunity to participate in, learn from, and enjoy the arts". The United States Congress has designated VSA arts as the coordinating Organization for arts programming for children and youth with disabilities. The Organization's educational programs use alternative curricula and teaching strategies designed to promote optimal learning experiences in a fully inclusive environment, providing youth and adults with an artistic means of self-expression, creating self-confidence and teaching marketable skills while fostering communication and independence. Offers comprehensive programs in literary, performing, and visual arts, in collaboration with local educational agencies, cultural institutions, institutions of higher education, arts agencies, disability Associations, and health and rehabilitation Organizations in 49 states and DC, and in more than 60 countries worldwide. Programs have served over 5 million people. **Pub:** *The Creative Spirit*, quarterly. Newsletter. • Also publishes manuals and guides and makes available videotapes. **Frmly:** (2000) Very Special Arts.

★ **8180** ★ **Wheelchair Motorcycle Association (WMA)**
101 Torrey St.
Brockton, MA 02301
**Phone:** (508)583-8614
Dr. Eli Factor, Pres.
**Fnded:** 1975. **Mem:** 1,000. **Local Groups:** 1. **Desc:** Handicapped persons confined to wheelchairs interested in rediscovering the outdoors; institutional and individual supporters. Researches, develops, and tests off-road vehicles for quadriplegics and other severely handicapped persons. Has audiovisual program showing the use of cycles by the handicapped. **Pub:** *Climb for Independence*, quarterly. Newsletter. *Price:* Included in membership dues.

★ **8181** ★ **Wheelchair Sports, USA (WSUSA)**
3595 E Fountain Blvd., Ste. L-1
Colorado Springs, CO 80910
**Phone:** (719)574-1150　　**Fax:** (719)574-9840
**Email:** wsusa@aol.com
**Website:** http://www.wsusa.org
Patricia Shepherd, Exec. Dir.
**Fnded:** 1958. **Mem:** 4,000. **Reg. Groups:** 14. **Desc:** Men and women athletes with significant permanent neuromuscular-skeletal disability (spinal cord disorder, poliomyelitis, or amputation) who compete in various amateur sports events in wheelchairs. Members compete in regional events and in the annual National Wheelchair Games, which include competitions in track and field (including pentathlon), swimming, archery, shooting, fencing, table tennis, weightlifting, basketball, and rugby. Compiles statistics; maintains hall of fame and speakers' bureau. competition. Compiles statistics; maintains hall of fame and speakers' bureau. **Pub:** *Constitution and By-Laws*, biennial. Newsletter. *Price:* $10 for 4 issues; $17 for 8 issues. • *WSUSA Newsletter*, quarterly. Newsletter. *Price:* $10/year. • Also publishes rule books. **Frmly:** (1994) National Wheelchair Athletic Association.

★ **8182** ★ **Winged Fellowship Trust**
Angel House
20-32 Pentonville Rd.
London N1 9XD, United Kingdom
**Phone:** 44 207 8332594　　**Fax:** 44 207 2780370
**Email:** admin@wft.org.uk
**Website:** http://www.wft.org.uk
**Fnded:** 1963. **Reg. Groups:** 5. **Lang(s):** English. **Desc:** Volunteers required to provide respite care for physically disabled persons in England. Organizes holidays for disabled individuals at five regional centers operated by the Trust. **Pub:** *Volunteer Information Brochure*, annual. Brochure. Includes descriptions of facilities and application form.

★ **8183** ★ **World Institute on Disability (WID)**
510 16th St., Ste. 100
Oakland, CA 94612-1500
**Phone:** (510)763-4100　　**Fax:** (510)763-4109
**Email:** webpoobah@wid.org
**Website:** http://www.wid.org
Deborah Kaplan, Exec. Dir.
**Fnded:** 1983. **Desc:** International public policy center that conducts research on disability issues and overcoming obstacles to independent living for all people with disabilities. **Pub:** *An Independent Living Approach to Disability Policy Studies*. Report. *Price:* $17.50. • *The Cost of Program Models Providing Personal Assistance Services for Independent Living*. *Price:* $6. • *Ethical Issues in Disability and Rehabilitation: A Report on an International Conference*. Report. *Price:* $5. • *Executive Summary of Attending to America*. Video. *Price:* $5. • *Personal Assistance Service: People with Disabilities Forging Public Policy*.

★ **8184** ★ **Yad Sarah**
Yad Sarah House
Kiryat Weinberg
124 Herzl Blvd.
IL-956187 Jerusalem, Israel
**Phone:** 972 2 6444444　　**Fax:** 972 2 6444423
**Email:** info@yadsarah.org.il
**Website:** http://www.yadsarah.org.il
**Fnded:** 1976. **Nat'l Groups:** 90. **Lang(s):** Dutch, English, French, German, Hebrew, Portuguese, Spanish. **Desc:** Provides volunteer home care services and supplemental care for the handicapped, sick, and elderly in Israel so that they may live at home with their families without need for hospitalization or institutionalization. Lends medical equipment for no fee and assists disabled tourists. **Pub:** *Health News*, semiannual. Newsletter.

★ **8185** ★ **Yes I Can Foundation for Exceptional Children**
1110 N Glebe Rd., Ste. 300
Arlington, VA 22201-5704
**Phone:** (703)264-3660　　**Free:** 800-224-6830
**Fax:** (703)264-9494
**Email:** service@cec.sped.org
**Website:** http://www.cec.sped.org
Trudy Kerr, Sr. Exec. Asst.
**Fnded:** 1922. **Mem:** 50,000. **State Groups:** 51. **Desc:** The Council for Exceptional Children. Advocates for quality education for all individuals with physical disabilities, multiple disabilities, and special health care needs served in schools, hospitals, or home settings. The council also advocates for gifted and talented children and youth. Operates the ERIC Clearinghouse on Disabilities and Gifted Education, and the National Clearinghouse for Professions in Special Education. Develops programs to help teachers, administrators, and related services professionals improve their practice. **Pub:** *DPHD Newsletter*, quarterly. Newsletter. Covers information regarding the education of individuals with physical disabilities and health impairments. *Price:* Included in membership dues. • *Exceptional Child Education Resources*, quarterly. Journal. Includes abstracts of book, nonprint media, and journal literature. • *Exceptional Children*, quarterly. Journal. Covers special education and research. *Price:* $58/year for nonmembers. • *Teaching Excep-*

*tional Children*, bimonthly. Magazine. Includes classroom-oriented information about instructional methods, materials, and techniques for students of all ages with special needs. *Price:* $58/year for nonmembers. • Audiotapes. • Books. • Films. • Videos. **Frmly:** (1968) Association of Educators for Homebound and Hospitalized Children; (1979) Division on Physically Handicapped, Homebound and Hospitalized; (1993) Division for Physically Handicapped; (2002) Foundation for Exceptional Children.

**★ 8186 ★ Zambia National Association of Disabled Women (ZNADW)**
PO Box 36450
Lusaka, Zambia
**Lang(s):** English. **Desc:** Women with disabilities and organizations providing support and services to people with disabilities and their families. Promotes full integration into society of women with disabilities. Monitors the human rights status of people with disabilities and publicizes abuses; conducts advocacy activities.

# Research Centers

**★ 8187 ★ Baylor College of Medicine**
**Center for Research on Women with**
**Disabilities (CROWD)**
3440 Richmond Ave., Ste. B
Houston, TX 77046
**Phone:** (713)960-0505        **Free:** 800-442-7693
**Fax:** (713)961-3555
**Email:** crowd@bcm.tmc.edu
**Website:** http://www.bcm.tmc.edu/crowd/
Margaret A. Nosek, PhD, Dir.
**Activities/Fields:** Specific problems effecting women with disabilities, particularly such issues as health, aging, civil rights, abuse, and independent living.

**★ 8188 ★ Center on State Systems and**
**Employment**
Institute for Community Inclusion
Children's Hospital
300 Longwood Ave.
Boston, MA 02115
**Phone:** (617)355-6506        **Fax:** (617)739-5853
**Email:** ici@tch.harvard.edu
**Website:** http://www.childrenshospital.org/ici/rrtc
William E. Kiernan, PhD, Dir.
**Activities/Fields:** How state agencies provide employment supports to people with disabilities and access to postsecondary education. **Frmly:** Center on Promoting Employment.

**★ 8189 ★ Dyslexia Research Institute**
5746 Centerville Rd.
Tallahassee, FL 32308-2899
**Phone:** (850)893-2216        **Fax:** (850)893-2440
**Email:** dri@talstar.com
**Website:** http://www.dyslexia-add.org
Dr. Patricia K. Hardman, Dir.
**Activities/Fields:** Dyslexia and attention deficit disorders, including educational techniques, teacher training, diagnostic procedures, biochemistry, allergies, and links alcoholism and eye movement.

**Georgia Institute of Technology**
**Center for Assistive Technology and**
**Environmental Access (CATEA)**
*See:* Entry 20191

**★ 8190 ★ Matheny Institute for Research**
**in Developmental Disabilities**
Matheny School & Hospital
PO Box 339
Peapack, NJ 07977
**Phone:** (908)234-0011        **Fax:** (908)234-0963
**Email:** research@matheny.org

**Website:** http://www.matheny.org/about/ab_ias.html
Kenneth Robey, PhD, Dir.
**Activities/Fields:** Neurodevelopmental disorders such as cerebral palsy, spina bifida, muscular dystrophy, and Lesch-Nyhan Disease; and the improvement of the lives of those with developmental disabilities.
**Pub:** *Matheny Bulletin*, quarterly.

**★ 8191 ★ Medical University of South**
**Carolina**
**Department of Pediatrics**
**Division of Genetics and Developmental**
**Pediatrics**
**The Vince Moseley Center**
135 Rutledge Ave., 395
Charleston, SC 29425
**Phone:** (843)876-1516        **Fax:** (843)876-1518
**Email:** pais@musc.edu
Dr. G. Shashida Pai, Dir.
**Activities/Fields:** Genetic disorders and diseases; learning problems and communication disorders research, including attention deficit disorder, spina bifida, autism, chronic disease and adjustment. **Frmly:** Vince Moseley Center for Children with Developmental Disabilities.

**★ 8192 ★ Miami Jewish Home and**
**Hospital for the Aged**
**Stein Gerontological Institute, Inc.**
5200 NE 2nd Ave.
Miami, FL 33137-2706
**Phone:** (305)762-1465        **Free:** 800-322-7881
**Fax:** (305)762-1445
Dr. Bernie Roos, Dir.
**Activities/Fields:** Promotes greater independence for the disabled through technology.

**★ 8193 ★ Minot State University**
**North Dakota Center for Persons with**
**Disabilities (NDCPD)**
500 University Ave. W
Minot, ND 58707
**Phone:** (701)858-3580        **Free:** 800-233-1737
**Fax:** (701)858-3483
**Email:** ndcpd@farside.cc.misu.nodak.edu
**Website:** http://www.ndcpd.org
Dr. M. Bryce Fifield, Exec. Dir.
**Activities/Fields:** Independence, productivity, integration, and inclusion of people who have disabilities.

**National Science Foundation**
**Directorate of Engineering**
**Division of Bioengineering and**
**Environmental Systems**
**Bioengineering and Aiding Persons with**
**Disabilities Program**
*See:* Entry 4541

**★ 8194 ★ New York Medical College**
**Westchester Institute for Human**
**Development (WIHD)**
Westchester County Medical Center
Valhalla, NY 10595
**Phone:** (914)493-8204        **Fax:** (914)493-1973
**Email:** ansley_bacon@nymc.edu
**Website:** http://www.nymc.edu/wihd/
Ansley Bacon, PhD, Dir.
**Activities/Fields:** Enhancement of the quality of life of individuals with or at risk for, disabilities and their families.

**★ 8195 ★ New York State Institute for**
**Basic Research in Developmental**
**Disabilities**
1050 Forest Hill Rd.
Staten Island, NY 10314-6330
**Phone:** (718)494-0600        **Fax:** (718)494-0833
W. Ted Brown, MD, Interim Dir.

**Activities/Fields:** Molecular biology and developmental biochemistry of human development, developmental disabilities, and clinical, behavioral, and developmental psychology of mental retardation, including neuroimmunology, membrane biochemistry, lipid biochemistry, neurotransmitter physiology and pathology, inborn errors of metabolism, blood-brain barrier, and persistent, latent, and unconventional viruses. Focuses on the causes and prevention of developmental disabilities, autism, aging and Alzheimer's disease, Down's syndrome, fragile X syndrome, fetal alcohol syndrome, neurodegenerative diseases, pediatric AIDS and neuroinfectious diseases, environmental neurotoxicology (including alcohol, lead, aluminum, and cocaine), prevention (including vaccines, diagnostic tests, and early intervention), and treatment (including drug evaluation). **Pub:** *Annual Report*.

**★ 8196 ★ Oregon Health and Science**
**University**
**Child Development and Rehabilitation**
**Center (CDRC)**
PO Box 574
Portland, OR 97207
**Phone:** (503)494-8364        **Fax:** (503)494-6868
**Email:** oidd@ohsu.edu
**Website:** http://www.ohsu.edu/cdrc/
Gloria Krahn, PhD, Exec. Dir.
**Activities/Fields:** Empowerment of individuals with developmental disabilities to improve the quality of their lives by developing, enhancing and sustaining culturally sensitive areas of support systems which function across the entire life span and include all domains of daily life.

**★ 8197 ★ Packard Children's Hospital at**
**Stanford**
**Rehabilitation Technology Center**
1010 Corporation Way
Palo Alto, CA 94303
**Phone:** (650)237-9200        **Fax:** (650)237-9204
**Email:** ve.hzo@lpch.stanford.edu
**Website:** http://www-med.stanford.edu/lpch/rec/
Hugh O'Neill, Actg. Dir.
**Activities/Fields:** Rehabilitation technology, emphasizing speech aids, prosthetics, orthotics, seating, mobility, and worksite accommodation for people with disabilities.

**Prosthetics Research Study**
*See:* Entry 4545

**Rehabilitation Research and Training**
**Center on Aging With a Disability**
*See:* Entry 3066

**★ 8198 ★ Research and Development**
**Institute**
PO Box 351
Sycamore, IL 60178-2738
**Phone:** (815)895-3078        **Fax:** (815)895-2448
**Email:** gkapper@niu.edu
**Website:** http://www.agingwithdisability.org
Dr. Gaylen G. Kapperman, Dir.
**Activities/Fields:** Rehabilitation and education for disabled persons, with emphasis on blindness and visual impairment.

**★ 8199 ★ Research and Training Center**
**on Managed Care and Disability (RTC-**
**MC&D)**
6858 Old Dominion Dr., Ste. 250
McLean, VA 22101
**Phone:** (703)448-6155        **Fax:** (703)442-9015
**Website:** http://www.cessi.net/contracts/dps/nrhrc_rtcmed.html
Bonnie O'Day, PhD, Contact
**Activities/Fields:** Delivery of quality health care to people with disabilities, particularly the impact of alternative managed care arrangements on the provi-

sion of acute care services for working-age people with disabilities.

**State University of New York at Buffalo**
**Center for Assistive Technology (CAT)**
*See:* Entry 4832

★ 8200 ★ **U.S. Department of Health and Human Services**
**National Center for Health Statistics**
**Office of Vital and Health Statistics Systems**
**Health Interview Statistics Division**
**(Illness and Disability Statistics Branch)**
6525 Belcrest Rd.
Hyattsville, MD 20782
**Phone:** (301)458-4004          **Fax:** (301)458-4035
**Email:** bzg5@cdc.gov
**Website:** http://www.cdc.gov
Dr. Jane F. Gentleman, PhD, Contact

**Activities/Fields:** Responsible for maintaining, analyzing, and preparing reports from National Health Interview Survey data. Areas of interest include estimates on illness and disability, use of health care services, and other health-related topics. **Pub:** *Series #10 National Health Interview Survey.*

★ 8201 ★ **U.S. Department of Health and Human Services**
**Office of Family, Community and Long-Term Care Policy**
**Division of Disability, Aging and Long-Term Care Policy**
200 Independence Ave. SW, Rm. 424E
Washington, DC 20201
**Phone:** (202)690-6443          **Fax:** (202)690-7733
**Email:** daltcp2@hhs.gov
**Website:** http://aspe.HHS.gov/daltcp/home.htm
Brenda Veazey, Staff Asst.

**Activities/Fields:** Financing, organization, and delivery of services to chronically impaired populations; informs the Department's policy development process. Recent work has centered on the needs of the impaired elderly, employment of working age adults with disabilities, and mentally disabled. Research areas include population characteristics, quality of care, home and community based services, disability issues, and data needs. **Pub:** *Reports.* • *Working papers.* **Frmly:** (2001) Office of Family, Community and Long-Term Care Policy; Division of Disability, Aging and Long-Term Care Policy.

★ 8202 ★ **U.S. Department of Health and Human Services**
**Research and Training Center on Rural Disabilities**
Univ. of Montana
52 Corbin Hall
Missoula, MT 59812-7056
**Phone:** (406)243-5467          **Fax:** (406)243-2349
Dr. Tom Seekins, Dir.

**Activities/Fields:** Employment and vocational rehabilitation service needs of people with disabilities in rural areas; intervention development to improve employment outcomes; self-employment and economic development models; rural independent living; improvement of transportation, health care, housing, and accessibility; rural models for prevention of secondary disabilities; disability legislation and American Indian Tribes; and alternative models of delivery of rural rehabilitation services. **Pub:** *Newsletter.*

★ 8203 ★ **U.S. Department of Veterans Affairs**
**Rehabilitation Research and Development Service**
**Center for Anabolic Therapies in Spinal Cord Injury**
VA Medical Center, Rm. 1E-02
130 W Kingsbridge Rd.
Bronx, NY 10468
**Phone:** (718)584-9000          **Fax:** (718)733-5291
**Email:** wabauman@earthlink.net
**Website:** http://www.vard.org/cent/bronx.htm
William A. Bauman, MD, Dir.

**Activities/Fields:** Use of anabolic steroids and other pharmaceuticals to treat secondary disabilities of spinal cord injury.

★ 8204 ★ **U.S. Department of Veterans Affairs**
**Rehabilitation Research and Development Service**
**Center of Excellence on Geriatric Rehabilitation**
1670 Clairmont Rd. (151R)
Decatur, GA 30033
**Phone:** (404)728-5064          **Fax:** (404)728-4837
**Email:** horace.denney@med.va.gov
**Website:** http://www.varrd.emory.edu/
Ronald A. Schuchard, PhD, Dir.

**Activities/Fields:** Improvement in the function, independence, and quality of life of veterans aging with disabilities and those acquiring disabilities as they age. The center focuses on vision rehabilitation research, environment and behavior research, physical performance and function research, and research that highlights the interaction among these areas. Research is directed towards understanding the mechanisms underlying impairments and disabilities, and applying this understanding to the design, testing, and evaluation of creative, rehabilitative interventions.

★ 8205 ★ **U.S. Department of Veterans Affairs**
**Rehabilitation Research and Development Service**
**Center of Excellence for Limb Loss Prevention and Prosthetic Engineering**
Seattle VAMC
1660 S Columbian Way, MS 151
Seattle, WA 98108
**Phone:** (206)764-2962          **Fax:** (206)764-2127
**Email:** bsangeor@u.washington.edu
**Website:** http://rehab.research.seattle.med.va.gov/
Bruce J. Sangeorzan, MD, Dir.

**Activities/Fields:** Prosthetics and amputation. Research focuses on preservation of the lower limb and its function, understanding deformities that lead to ulceration, the role of prophylactic correction of the deformity, and the role of protective footwear.

★ 8206 ★ **U.S. Department of Veterans Affairs**
**Rehabilitation Research and Development Service**
**Center for Restoring Function through Electrical Stimulation (FES)**
11000 Cedar Ave., Ste. 230
Cleveland, OH 44106-3052
**Phone:** (216)231-3257          **Free:** 800-666-2353
**Fax:** (216)231-3258
**Email:** info@fes.org
**Website:** http://feswww.fes.cwru.edu/
P. Hunter Peckham, PhD, Dir.

**Activities/Fields:** Restoration of function for persons with paralysis through functional electrical stimulation (FES) systems that improve health, productivity, and quality of life. **Pub:** *Newsletter.*

**U.S. Department of Veterans Affairs**
**Veterans Health Administration**
**Office of Research and Development**
**Rehabilitation and Development Service**
**(Center for Mobility)**
*See:* Entry 13514

**U.S. Department of Veterans Affairs**
**Veterans Health Administration**
**Office of Research and Development**
**Rehabilitation and Development Service**
**(Center for Healthy Aging with Disabilities)**
*See:* Entry 13515

**U.S. Department of Veterans Affairs**
**Veterans Health Administration**
**Office of Research and Development**
**Rehabilitation and Development Service**
**(Center for Functional Electric Stimulation)**
*See:* Entry 13516

★ 8207 ★ **University of Alabama at Birmingham**
**UAB Civitan International Research Center**
1719 6th Ave. S
Birmingham, AL 35294-0021
**Phone:** (205)934-8900          **Fax:** (205)975-6330
**Email:** info@civmail.circ.uab.edu
**Website:** http://www.circ.uab.edu
Dr. Sharon Ramey, Dir.

**Activities/Fields:** Stress in families with a handicapped child, parents' perception of temperament of handicapped and nonhandicapped infants, and developmentally disabled individuals and their families. Projects include studies of the memory function of children who are mentally retarded, the relationship between cognitive development and increasing auditory impairment of people with Down's syndrome, Head Start Program research, a Patient Outcomes Research Team, and the effects of therapeutic positioning on functional activities. **Frmly:** Sparks Center.

★ 8208 ★ **University of Alaska Anchorage**
**Center for Human Development**
2210 ARCA Dr.
Anchorage, AK 99508
**Phone:** (907)272-8270          **Fax:** (907)274-4802
**Email:** info@alaskachd.org
**Website:** http://www.alaskachd.org
Karen Ward, Dir.

**Activities/Fields:** Improvement in the lives of the disabled.

★ 8209 ★ **University of Alberta**
**Steadward Centre for Personal and Physical Achievement**
W1-67 Van Vliet Centre
Edmonton, AB, Canada T6G 2H9
**Phone:** (780)492-3182          **Fax:** (780)492-7161
**Email:** info@steadwardcentre.org
**Website:** http://www.steadwardcentre.org
Dr. Robert D. Steadward, Dir.

**Activities/Fields:** Fitness, sport training and conditioning, and motor performance for adults with disabilities. **Frmly:** Rick Hansen Centre.

★ 8210 ★ **University of Arkansas at Little Rock**
**Partners for Inclusive Communities**
Center on Developmental Disabilities
2001 Pershing Cir., Ste. 300
North Little Rock, AR 72114
**Phone:** (501)682-9900          **Free:** 800-831-4827
**Fax:** (501)682-9901

**Email:** swansonmarke@uams.edu
Mark E. Swanson, MD, Dir.

**Activities/Fields:** Improvement in the life of individuals with disabilities and families of children with disabilities to fully and meaningfully participate in community life. **Frmly:** Center for Research on Teaching and Learning.


**★ 8211 ★ University of California, Davis**
**M.I.N.D. (Medical Investigation of Neurodevelopmental Disorders) Institute**
UC Davis Medical Center
4860 Y St., Rm. 3020
Sacramento, CA 95817
**Free:** 888-883-0961  **Fax:** (916)734-5153
**Email:** dgamaral@ucdavis.edu
**Website:** http://mindinstitute.ucdmc.ucdavis.edu
David G. Amaral, PhD, Res. Dir.

**Activities/Fields:** Neurodevelopmental disorders in children and adults, including autism and autism spectrum disorders; pervasive developmental disorder; cerebral palsy; Fragile X Syndrome; Tourette's Syndrome; mental retardation; attention deficit hyperactivity disorder; dyslexia; and other learning, developmental delay, and communication disorders.


**★ 8212 ★ University of California, San Francisco**
**Disability Statistics Center**
Institute for Health & Aging
3333 California St., Ste. 340
Campus Mail Box 0646
San Francisco, CA 94118
**Phone:** (415)502-5205  **Fax:** (415)502-5208
**Email:** lplante@itsa.ucsf.edu
**Website:** http://dsc.ucsf.edu/
Mitchell P. LaPlante, PhD, Dir.

**Activities/Fields:** Production and dissemination of statistical information on disability and the status of people with disabilities in society and the establishment and monitoring of indicators on how conditions are changing to meet their health, housing, economic and social needs. **Pub:** *Disability Statistics Abstracts.* • *Disability Statistics Reports.*


**★ 8213 ★ University of Connecticut**
**A.J. Pappanikou Center for Developmental Disabilities**
263 Farmington Ave., MC 6222
Farmington, CT 06030-6222
**Phone:** (860)679-1500  **Fax:** (860)679-1571
**Email:** bruder@nso1.uchc.edu
**Website:** http://www.uconnced.org
Mary Beth Bruder, PhD, Dir.

**Activities/Fields:** Developmental disabilities across the life span, psychosocial developmental needs mainly of children with disabilities, best practices in early intervention, learning opportunities for children in natural environments, assistive technology, employment, health services; addresses needs of persons with disabilities across academic and community settings, focuses on life span. **Pub:** *Monographs.* **Frmly:** Research and Training Center for Pediatric Rehabilitation; Pediatric Research and Training Center.


**★ 8214 ★ University of Delaware**
**Center for Disabilities Studies**
166 Graham Hall
Academy St.
Newark, DE 19716-7355
**Phone:** (302)831-6974  **Fax:** (302)831-4690
**Email:** mgm@udel.edu
**Website:** http://www.udel.edu/chep/cds
Michael Gamel-McCormick, PhD, Dir.

**Activities/Fields:** Enhancement of the lives of disabled individuals and their families through research, education, and service in the areas of prevention and intervention. **Pub:** *Annual report.* • *delAWARE.*


**★ 8215 ★ University of Georgia**
**Institute on Human Development and Disability (IHDD)**
Rivers Crossing Bldg.
College of Family & Consumer Science
850 College Station Rd.
Athens, GA 30602-4806
**Phone:** (706)542-3457  **Fax:** (706)542-4815
**Email:** ihddweb@uap.uga.edu
**Website:** http://www.uap.uga.edu
Zolinda Stoneman, PhD, Dir.

**Activities/Fields:** Improvement of the quality of life for people with disabilities and their families. **Pub:** *Newsletter.*


**★ 8216 ★ University of Hawaii at Manoa**
**Center on Disability Studies**
1776 University Ave., UA 4-6
Honolulu, HI 96822
**Phone:** (808)956-5011  **Fax:** (808)956-7878
**Email:** juana@hawaii.edu
**Website:** http://www.cds.hawaii.edu
Robert A. Stodden, PhD, Exec. Dir.

**Activities/Fields:** Improvement in the quality of life, inclusion, and empowerment of all persons with disabilities and their families.


**★ 8217 ★ University of Idaho**
**Center on Disabilities and Human Development (CDHD)**
129 W 3rd St.
Moscow, ID 83843
**Phone:** (208)885-3559  **Fax:** (208)885-3628
**Email:** jfodor@uidaho.edu
**Website:** http://www.ets.uidaho.edu/cdhd/
Julie Fodor, Interim Dir.

**Activities/Fields:** Improvement of the quality of life for people with developmental disabilities across the age span by promoting their independence, productivity, and participation in integrated community settings.


**★ 8218 ★ University of Illinois at Chicago**
**Center on Emergent Disability**
Department of Disability & Human Development, MC 626
College of Health & Human Development Sciences
1640 W Roosevelt Rd.
Chicago, IL 60608
**Phone:** (312)413-1977  **Fax:** (312)413-4098
**Email:** Gfujiura@uic.edu
**Website:** http://www.uic.edu/depts/idhd/ced
Glenn T. Fujiura, PhD, Coord.

**Activities/Fields:** Impact of major health, social, and economic trends on the manifestation of disability in America.


**★ 8219 ★ University of Illinois at Chicago**
**Center on Health Promotion for Persons with Disabilities (CHP)**
Department of Disability & Human Development
College of Applied Health Sciences
1919 W Taylor St., Rm. 560
Chicago, IL 60612-7249
**Phone:** (312)413-9651
**Email:** dhd@uic.edu
**Website:** http://www.uic.edu/depts/idhd/chp.htm
Prof. James Rimmer, PhD, Dir.

**Activities/Fields:** Effects of exercise and health promotion on persons with stroke, diabetes, arthritis, spinal cord injury, and Down syndrome.


**★ 8220 ★ University of Illinois at Chicago**
**Chicago Center for Disability Research**
Department of Disability & Human Development
College of Health & Human Development Sciences
1640 W Roosevelt Rd.
Chicago, IL 60608
**Phone:** (312)355-0550
**Email:** cg16@uic.edu
Carol J. Gill, PhD, Dir.

**Activities/Fields:** Disabilities.


**★ 8221 ★ University of Kansas**
**University Affiliated Program for Developmental Disabilities**
1052 Dole Center
Lawrence, KS 66045
**Phone:** (785)864-4950  **Fax:** (785)864-5338
**Email:** schroede@kuhub.cc.ukans.edu
**Website:** http://www.lsi.ukans.edu/uap/uap.htm
Steve Schroeder, PhD, Dir.

**Activities/Fields:** Improvement in the lives of persons with disabilities who live in metropolitan and rural eastern Kansas.


**★ 8222 ★ University of Louisville**
**Child Evaluation Center**
571 S Floyd, Ste. 100
Louisville, KY 40202-3828
**Phone:** (502)852-5331  **Fax:** (502)852-0955
Joseph Herst, MD, Dir.

**Activities/Fields:** Developmentally disabled and handicapped children in Kentucky. Clinical research is conducted in support of the following clinical, evaluative, and consultative service programs: diagnosis and evaluation, learning disorders, genetics and dysmorphology, genetics testing, education and counseling, genetics laboratory, community clinics and outreach, hyperactive child treatment, infant therapy, behavior modification, diagnostic teaching, pastoral counseling, and cytogenetics laboratory.


**University of Miami**
**Mailman Center for Child Development**
*See:* Entry 5826


**University of Montana**
**Research and Training Center on Rural Rehabilitation Services**
*See:* Entry 20211


**★ 8223 ★ University of Montana**
**Rural Institute: Center for Excellence in Developmental Disabilities Education, Research, and Service**
52 N Corbin Hall
Missoula, MT 59812
**Phone:** (406)243-5467  **Free:** 800-732-0323
**Fax:** (406)243-4730
**Email:** rtvogels@selway.umt.edu
**Website:** http://www.ruralinstitute.umt.edu
R. Timm Vogelsberg, Dir.

**Activities/Fields:** Human resources and technical services for rural Americans with disabilities. Studies encompass the areas of employment, housing, transportation, health promotion, secondary conditions, special education, social work, guidance and counseling, physical medicine and rehabilitation, mechanical and rehabilitation engineering, business management, sociology, interpersonal communication, and psychology. **Pub:** *Child Care Plus.* • *Common Threads Newsletter.* • *Research Reports.* • *The Rural Exchange.* • *Transition Topics.* **Frmly:** Institute for Human Resources in Rural America; University Affiliated Rural Institute on Disabilities.


**★ 8224 ★ University of New Hampshire**
**Institute on Disability (IOD)**
7 Leavitt Ln., Ste. 101
Durham, NH 03824-3522
**Phone:** (603)862-4320  **Fax:** (603)862-0555
**Email:** institute.disability@unh.edu
**Website:** http://www.iod.unh.edu/
Dr. Jan Nisbet, Dir.

**Activities/Fields:** Needs of individuals with severe disabilities. **Pub:** *Newsletters.*

**★ 8225 ★ University of Rochester**
**Strong Center for Developmental**
**Disabilities (SCDD)**
PO Box 14627
Rochester, NY 14627-0140
**Phone:** (716)275-4031     **Fax:** (716)275-9492
**Email:** scdd@cc.urmc.rochester.edu
**Website:** http://www.urmc.rochester.edu/strong/scdd
Philip W. Davidson, PhD, Exec. Dir.
**Activities/Fields:** Inclusion of persons with developmental disabilities in their communities and the maximization of their potential for leading independent and productive lives.

**★ 8226 ★ University of South Carolina**
**Center for Disability Resources**
Department of Pediatrics
School of Medicine
Columbia, SC 29208-0001
**Phone:** (803)935-5248     **Fax:** (803)935-5059
**Website:** http://www.cdd.sc.edu
Richard R. Ferrante, PhD, Exec. Dir.
**Activities/Fields:** Causation and prevention of developmental disabilities and the delivery of family centered approaches for assisting people with developmental disabilities.

**★ 8227 ★ University of Tennessee**
**Boling Center for Developmental**
**Disabilities (BCDD)**
711 Jefferson
Memphis, TN 38105
**Phone:** (901)448-6511     **Free:** 888-572-2249
**Fax:** (901)448-7097
**Email:** fpalmer@utmem.edu
**Website:** http://www.utmem.edu/bcdd
Frederick B. Palmer, MD, Dir.
**Activities/Fields:** Independence, productivity, integration, and inclusion of individuals with disabilities and their families in the community. **Pub:** *newsletter.*

**★ 8228 ★ University of Vermont**
**Center on Disability and Community**
**Inclusion**
101 Cherry St., Ste. 450
Burlington, VT 05401-4439
**Phone:** (802)656-4031     **Fax:** (802)656-1357
**Email:** ccloning@zoo.uvm.edu
**Website:** http://www.uvm.edu/~uapvt/
Chigee Cloninger, Exec. Dir.
**Activities/Fields:** Independence, inclusion, participation, and personal choice of individuals with disabilities of all ages in all environments.

**★ 8229 ★ University of Washington**
**Center for Disability Policy and Research**
**(CDPR)**
Department of Health Services, Box 358852
School of Public Health & Community Medicine
146 N Canal St., Ste. 313
Seattle, WA 98103-8652
**Phone:** (206)685-7260     **Fax:** (206)616-3135
**Email:** cdpr@u.washington.edu
**Website:** http://depts.washington.edu/cdpr/
Donald Patrick, Co-Dir.
**Activities/Fields:** Disablement process and disabling conditions, the health needs of people with disabilities, the personal, and the delivery of health and human services to people with disabilities and their families. **Pub:** *Reports.*

**★ 8230 ★ University of Wisconsin—**
**Madison**
**Trace Research and Development Center**
5901 Research Pk. Blvd.
Madison, WI 53719-1252
**Phone:** (608)262-6966     **Fax:** (608)262-8848
**Email:** info@trace.wisc.edu
**Website:** http://www.trace.wisc.edu
Dr. Gregg Vanderheiden, Dir.
**Activities/Fields:** How to make standard information technologies and telecommunications systems more accessible and usable by people with disabilites. **Pub:** *Annual Report.* • *Trace Resourcebook Series.* **Frmly:** Cerebral Palsy Communication Group.

**★ 8231 ★ University of Wisconsin—Stout**
**Research and Training Center on**
**Community Rehabilitation Programs to**
**Improve Employment Outcomes**
Stout Vocational Rehabilitation Institute
College of Human Development
Menomonie, WI 54751
**Phone:** (715)232-1389     **Fax:** (715)232-2251
**Email:** menz@uwstout.edu
**Website:** http://www.rtc.uwstout.edu
Dr. Fredrick E. Menz, Dir.
**Activities/Fields:** Improvement of community-based rehabilitation through vocational transition of people with disabilities from community-based rehabilitation programs into competitive employment.

**★ 8232 ★ University of Wyoming**
**Wyoming Institute for Disabilities (WIND)**
PO Box 4298
Laramie, WY 82071-4298
**Phone:** (307)766-2761
**Email:** wind.uw@uwyo.edu
**Website:** http://wind.uwyo.edu
Keith A. Miller, PhD, Exec. Dir.
**Activities/Fields:** Disabilities, particularly in the area of developmental disabilities.

**★ 8233 ★ Utah State University**
**Center for Persons with Disabilities**
6800 Old Main Hill
Logan, UT 84322-6800
**Phone:** (435)797-1981     **Free:** (866)284-2821
**Fax:** (435)797-3944
**Email:** s_rule@cpd2.usu.edu
**Website:** http://www.cpd.usu.edu
Dr. Sarah Rule, Dir.
**Activities/Fields:** Developmental disabilities including biomedical research, systems change, assistive technologies, video production, and distance education. **Pub:** *Annual report.* • *CPD News.* • *Parent Newsletter.*

**Vanderbilt University**
**John F. Kennedy Center for Research on**
**Human Development**
*See:* Entry 6911

**Virginia Commonwealth University**
**Rehabilitation Research and Training**
**Center on Workplace Supports**
*See:* Entry 16852

**★ 8234 ★ Virginia Commonwealth**
**University**
**Virginia Institute for Developmental**
**Disabilities (VIDD)**
700 E Franklin St., 10th Fl.
PO Box 843020
Richmond, VA 23284-3020
**Phone:** (434)828-3876     **Fax:** (434)828-0042
**Email:** forelove@saturn.vcu.edu
**Website:** http://www.vcu.edu/vidd
Fred P. Orelove, PhD, Exec. Dir.
**Activities/Fields:** Independence, productivity, integration, and inclusion of individuals with developmental disabilities.

# State & Regional Organizations

## Disabilities

*Listed below are intermediary affiliates of the National Easter Seal Society, 230 W Monroe St., Ste. 1800, Chicago, IL 60606, (312)726-6200, http://www.easter-seals.org/.*

### Alabama

**★ 8235 ★ Easter Seals Alabama**
6005-A E Shirley Ln.
Montgomery, AL 36117
**Phone:** (334)395-4489     **Free:** 800-388-7325
**Fax:** (334)395-4492
**Email:** bcaven@aleaster-seals.org
**Website:** http://www.al.easter-seals.org
Barry F. Cavan, President
**Program(s):** Easter Seal Rehabilitation Centers; Janice Capilouto Center for the Deaf; Easter Seal Opportunity Center; Camp Civitan; Camp ASCCA; Achievement Center; and support services.

**★ 8236 ★ Easter Seals Birmingham Area**
200 Beacon Pkwy. W
Birmingham, AL 35209
**Phone:** (205)942-6277     **Fax:** (205)945-4906
**Email:** jwebster@easterbham.org
Johnny Webster, Exec Director
**Program(s):** Job training and employment services; school-aged children; and support services.

**★ 8237 ★ Easter Seals Central Alabama**
2125 E South Blvd.
Montgomery, AL 36116-2454
**Phone:** (334)288-0240     **Fax:** (334)288-7171
**Email:** easterseals@worldnet.att.net
**Website:** http://www.eastersealsmontgomery.com
Barry F. Cavan, President
**Program(s):** Continuing education; early intervention; job training and employment services; and medical rehabilitation and health services.

**★ 8238 ★ Easter Seals West Alabama**
1110 6th Ave. E
Tuscaloosa, AL 35401
**Phone:** (205)759-1211     **Fax:** (205)349-1162
**Email:** eswa@eastersealswestal.org
**Website:** http://www.easter-seals.org/tuscaloosa
Barry F. Cavan, President
**Program(s):** Job training and employment services; medical rehabilitation and health services; and support services.

**★ 8239 ★ Goodwill Easter Seals of the**
**Gulf Coast**
2448 Gordon Smith Dr.
Mobile, AL 36617
**Phone:** (334)471-1581     **Free:** 800-411-0068
**Fax:** (334)476-4303
**Email:** frank@gesgc.org
**Website:** http://www.goodwill-easterseals.org
Barry F. Cavan, President
**Program(s):** Camping and recreation; early education and care; early intervention; job training and employment services; school-aged children; and support services.

### Alaska

**★ 8240 ★ Easter Seals Alaska**
126 W 15th Ave.
Anchorage, AK 99501
**Phone:** (907)277-7325     **Fax:** (907)272-7325

**Email:** eseals@gci.net
Vilma Gutierrez-Osborne, CEO & Pres
Colette Michaelson, Contact
**Program(s):** Ketchikan Thrift Store; camping and recreation; continuing education; medical rehabilitation and health services; school-aged children; and support services.

## Arizona

### ★ 8241 ★ Easter Seals Arizona
903 N 2nd St.
Phoenix, AZ 85004-1996
**Phone:** (602)252-6061          **Free:** 800-626-6061
**Fax:** (602)252-6065
**Email:** bpatchett@azseals.org
**Website:** http://www.azseals.org
Michael T. Fitzgerald, CEO & Pres
**Program(s):** Adult and senior services; camping and recreation; continuing education; early education and care; early intervention; job training and employment services; medical rehabilitation and health services; school-aged children; and support services.

### ★ 8242 ★ Easter Seals Arizona
### Tucson Office
5740 E 22nd St.
Tucson, AZ 85711
**Phone:** (520)745-5222          **Fax:** (520)745-9030
Michael T. Fitzgerald, President
Jim Neville, Mgr
**Program(s):** Camping and recreation; continuing education; early education and care; early intervention; job training and employment services; medical rehabilitation and health services; school-aged children; and support services.

### ★ 8243 ★ Easter Seals Arizona
### Yuma Office
661 E 32nd St., Ste. A
Yuma, AZ 85364
**Phone:** (520)726-6800          **Fax:** (520)726-1690
**Email:** azseals@msn.com
Michael T. Fitzgerald, CEO & Pres
**Program(s):** Continuing education; early education and care; early intervention; job training and employment services; medical rehabilitation and health services; and school-aged children.

## Arkansas

### ★ 8244 ★ Easter Seals Arkansas
3920 Woodland Heights Rd.
Little Rock, AR 72212-2495
**Phone:** (501)227-3600          **Free:** 877-533-3600
**Fax:** (501)227-3658
**Email:** mail@ar.easter-seals.org
**Website:** http://www.arkeasterseals.org
Sharon Moone-Jochums, CEO & Pres
**Program(s):** Easter Seal Work Center; NISH Project; Butler House; Rehabilitation Center; camping and recreation; early education and care; early intervention; medical rehabilitation and health services; school-laged children; and support services.

## California

### ★ 8245 ★ Easter Seals
### Southern California Hollywood Office
6515 Sunset Blvd., 4th Fl.
Los Angeles, CA 90028
**Phone:** (323)442-2424          **Fax:** (323)462-1515
**Email:** sylvia.wolf@essc.org
**Website:** http://www.essc.org
Mark Whitley, Contact
Guadalupe Trevizo, Director

### ★ 8246 ★ Easter Seals
### Superior California Yuba City Center
144 Gibson Rd.
PO Box 266
Yuba City, CA 95992-0266
**Phone:** (916)673-4585          **Fax:** (916)673-4328
**Email:** info@easterseals.com
**Website:** http://www.easterseals.com
Gary Kasai, CEO & Pres

### ★ 8247 ★ Easter Seals Bay Area
### Contra Costa and Solano County
###   Programs
1870 Arnold Industrial Pl., Ste. 1025
Concord, CA 94520
**Phone:** (510)689-1777          **Fax:** (510)689-2220
**Email:** sgerdtz@esba.org
**Website:** http://www.esba.org
Michael Pelfini, CEO & Pres
**Program(s):** Early intervention.

### ★ 8248 ★ Easter Seals Bay Area
### Tri-Valley Campus
7425 Larkdale Ave.
Dublin, CA 94568
**Phone:** (925)828-8857          **Fax:** (925)828-5245
**Email:** rhalog@esba.org
**Website:** http://www.esba.org
Dr. Michael Pelfini, CEO & Pres
**Program(s):** School-aged children.

### ★ 8249 ★ Easter Seals Central California
9010 Soquel Dr.
Aptos, CA 95003-4002
**Phone:** (831)684-2166          **Fax:** (831)685-6055
**Email:** dalvarez@es-cc.org
**Website:** http://www.es-cc.org
Bruce Hinman, CEO
**Program(s):** Camp Harmon; early education and care; early intervention; medical rehabilitation and health services; school-aged children; and support services.

### ★ 8250 ★ Easter Seals Central California
### Fresno Office
1685 E St., Ste. 101
Fresno, CA 93706
**Phone:** (559)264-7113          **Fax:** (559)264-8305
**Email:** twalker@theworks.com
**Website:** http://www.es-cc.org
Bruce Hinman, CEO
Ruth Hutchison, Vice President
**Program(s):** Early education and care; early intervention; medical rehabilitation and health services; school-aged children; and support services.

### ★ 8251 ★ Easter Seals Central California
### Marina Office
445 Reservation Rd., Ste. A
Marina, CA 93933-3301
**Phone:** (831)883-3010          **Fax:** (831)883-3013
**Email:** scook@earthlink.com
**Website:** http://www.es-cc.org
Bruce Hinman, CEO
**Program(s):** Camping and recreation; early education and care; medical rehabilitation and health services; residential and housing services; school-aged children; and support services.

### ★ 8252 ★ Easter Seals Northern
### California
3289 Edgewood Rd.
Eureka, CA 95502-0109
**Phone:** (707)445-3106
**Email:** emorgan@northcoast.com
**Website:** http://www.esncal.org
Jackie K. Reinhardt, CEO & Pres
Eddie Morgan, Mgr

**Program(s):** Adult and senior services; camping and recreation; continuing education; early education and care; early intervention; medical rehabilitation and health services; school-aged children; and support services.

### ★ 8253 ★ Easter Seals Northern
### California
1074 East Ave., Ste. A-1
Chico, CA 95973
**Phone:** (530)894-0205          **Fax:** (530)894-0206
**Email:** jschifferens@ca-no.easter-seals.org
**Website:** http://www.esncal.org
Jackie K. Reinhardt, CEO & Pres
John Schifferns, Mgr
**Program(s):** Adult and senior services; continuing education; early education and care; early intervention; medical rehabilitation and health services; school-aged children; and support services.

### ★ 8254 ★ Easter Seals Northern
### California
### Lakeport Office
501 B Main St.
Lakeport, CA 95453
**Phone:** (707)263-3949          **Fax:** (707)263-3985
**Email:** mborjon@ca-no.easter-seals.org
**Website:** http://www.esncal.org
Jackie K. Reinhardt, CEO & Pres
**Program(s):** Continuing education; early education and care; early intervention; medical rehabilitation and health services; school-aged children; and support services.

### ★ 8255 ★ Easter Seals Northern
### California
### Novato Office
20 Pimentel Ct., Ste. A1
Novato, CA 94949
**Phone:** (415)382-7450          **Fax:** (415)382-6052
**Email:** jreinhardt@ca-no.easter-seals.org
**Website:** http://www.esncal.org
Jackie K. Reinhardt, CEO & Pres
**Program(s):** Camping and recreation; continuing education; early education and care; early intervention; medical rehabilitation and health services; school-aged children; and support services.

### ★ 8256 ★ Easter Seals Northern
### California
### Rohnert Park Office
5440 State Farm Dr.
Rohnert Park, CA 94928
**Phone:** (707)584-1443          **Fax:** (707)584-3438
**Email:** skreuzer@ca-no.easter-seals.org
**Website:** http://www.esncal.org
Jackie K. Reinhardt, CEO & Pres
Susanne Kreuzer, Vice President
**Program(s):** Camping and recreation; continuing education; early education and care; early intervention; medical rehabilitation and health services; school-aged children; and support services.

### ★ 8257 ★ Easter Seals Southern
### California
### Alhambra Office
3055 W Valley Blvd.
Alhambra, CA 91803
**Phone:** (626)281-9404          **Fax:** (626)457-2868
**Email:** lupe.trevizoreinoso@essc.org
**Website:** http://www.essc.org
Guadalupe Trevizo, Director
**Program(s):** Adult and senior services; and support services.

**★ 8258 ★ Easter Seals Southern California**
**Escondido Office**
1035 E Valley Pkwy.
Escondido, CA 92025
**Phone:** (760)737-3990     **Fax:** (760)432-8549
**Email:** debbie.ball@essc.org
**Website:** http://www.essc.org
Debbie Ball, Director

**Program(s):** Adult and senior services; camping and recreation; and medical rehabilitation and health services.

**★ 8259 ★ Easter Seals Southern California**
**Inland Counties Program**
241 E 9th St.
San Bernardino, CA 92410-4408
**Phone:** (909)888-4125     **Fax:** (909)884-5741
**Email:** debbie.ball@essc.org
**Website:** http://www.essc.org
Mark Whitley, CEO
Debbie Davies, Director

**Program(s):** Adult and senior services; camping and recreation; school-aged children; and support services.

**★ 8260 ★ Easter Seals Southern California**
**Inland County Region**
**Rancho Cucamonga Office**
8560 Vinyard Ave., Ste. 201
Rancho Cucamonga, CA 91730
**Phone:** (909)481-5324     **Fax:** (909)481-5140
**Email:** debbie.ball@essc.org
**Website:** http://www.essc.org
Debbie Davies, Director

**Program(s):** Camping and recreation; school-aged children.

**★ 8261 ★ Easter Seals Southern California**
**Inland County Region**
**Victorville Office**
14360 St. Andrews Ave., No. 7
Victorville, CA 92392
**Phone:** (760)952-0018     **Fax:** (760)952-0059
**Email:** debbie.ball@essc.org
**Website:** http://www.essc.org
Debbie Davies, Director

**Program(s):** Adult and senior services; camping and recreation; school-aged children.

**★ 8262 ★ Easter Seals Southern California**
**Los Angeles Office**
4727 Wilshire Blvd., Ste. 210
Los Angeles, CA 90010
**Phone:** (323)954-3770     **Fax:** (323)954-3775
**Email:** lupe.trevizoreinoso@essc.org
**Website:** http://www.essc.org
Guadalupe Trevizo, Director

**Program(s):** Adult and senior services.

**★ 8263 ★ Easter Seals Southern California**
**North-Central Los Angeles County Programs**
315 Arden, Ste. 2
Glendale, CA 91203
**Phone:** (818)551-0128     **Fax:** (818)551-9846
**Email:** lupe.trevizoreinoso@essc.org
**Website:** http://www.essc.org
Guadalupe Trevizo, Director

**Program(s):** Adult and senior services.

**★ 8264 ★ Easter Seals Southern California**
**North Los Angeles County**
1146 Commerce Center Dr.
Lancaster, CA 93534
**Phone:** (661)723-3414     **Fax:** (661)729-3318
**Email:** paula.pompa.craven@essc.org
**Website:** http://www.essc.org
Christine Edgeworth, Director

**Program(s):** Adult and senior services; job training and employment services; and support services.

**★ 8265 ★ Easter Seals Southern California**
**North Los Angeles County Programs**
25115 Ave. Stanford, Ste. B-122
Valencia, CA 91355
**Phone:** (661)257-8558     **Fax:** (661)257-8110
**Email:** christine.edgeworth@essc.org
**Website:** http://www.essc.org
Christine Edgeworth, Director

**Program(s):** Adult and senior services; camping and recreation; job training and employment services; school-aged children; and support services.

**★ 8266 ★ Easter Seals Southern California**
**Orange County Programs**
1661 N Raymond Ave., Ste. 100
Anaheim, CA 92801
**Phone:** (714)441-3070     **Fax:** (714)441-3477
**Email:** kathleen.kolenda@essc.org
**Website:** http://www.essc.org
Mark Whitley, CEO
Kathleen Kolenda, Director

**Program(s):** Adult and senior services; camping and recreation; medical rehabilitation and health services; and school-aged children.

**★ 8267 ★ Easter Seals Southern California**
**Pasadena Office**
100 N Hill Ave., Ste. 100
Pasadena, CA 91106
**Phone:** (626)793-7700     **Fax:** (626)793-8244
Mark Whitley, CEO
Guadalupe Trevizo, Director

**Program(s):** Adult and senior services.

**★ 8268 ★ Easter Seals Southern California**
**Riverside**
1450 University Ave., Ste. F2
Riverside, CA 92507
**Phone:** (909)248-4873     **Fax:** (909)248-4487
**Email:** debbie.ball@essc.org
**Website:** http://www.essc.org
Mark S. Whitley, CEO

**Program(s):** Adult and senior services.

**★ 8269 ★ Easter Seals Southern California**
**Santa Ana Office**
1801 E Edinger Ave., Ste. 190
Santa Ana, CA 92705-4734
**Phone:** (714)834-1111     **Fax:** (714)834-1128
**Email:** infor@essc.org
**Website:** http://www.essc.org
Mark Whitley, President

**Program(s):** Early education and care; and support services.

**★ 8270 ★ Easter Seals Southern California**
**South San Diego County Programs**
101 E 30th St., Unit C
National City, CA 91950
**Phone:** (619)336-0630     **Fax:** (619)336-0697

**Email:** debbie.ball@essc.org
**Website:** http://www.essc.org
Mark Whitley, CEO
Laura Orcutt, Director

**Program(s):** Adult and senior services; and camping and recreation.

**★ 8271 ★ Easter Seals Southern California**
**Southwest Programs**
**Torrance Office**
3625 Del Amo Blvd., Ste. 120
Torrance, CA 90503
**Phone:** (310)542-2148     **Fax:** (310)542-0048
**Email:** dee.prescott@essc.org
**Website:** http://www.essc.org
Mark S. Whitley, CEO & Pres
Dee Prescott, Director

**Program(s):** Adult and senior services; and school-aged children.

**★ 8272 ★ Easter Seals Southern California**
**Van Nuys Office**
16946 Sherman Way, Ste. 100
Van Nuys, CA 91406
**Phone:** (818)996-9902     **Fax:** (818)996-1606
**Email:** carlene.holden@essc.org
**Website:** http://www.essc.org
Christine Edgeworth, Director
Carlene Holden, Vice President

**Program(s):** Adult and senior services; and support services.

**★ 8273 ★ Easter Seals Southern California**
**West Los Angeles County**
6133 Bristol Pkwy., Ste. 200
Culver City, CA 90230
**Phone:** (310)641-4884     **Fax:** (310)641-4883
**Email:** dee.prescott@essc.org
**Website:** http://www.essc.org
Mark Whitley, CEO
Dee Prescott, Director

**Program(s):** Adult and senior services; and job training and employment services.

**★ 8274 ★ Easter Seals Southern California**
**Whittier Office**
13601 Whittier Blvd., Ste. 100
Whittier, CA 90605
**Phone:** (562)698-8229     **Fax:** (562)698-8499
**Email:** kathleen.kolenda@essc.org
**Website:** http://www.essc.org
Kathleen Kolenda, Director

**Program(s):** Adult and senior services.

**★ 8275 ★ Easter Seals Superior California**
3205 Hurley Way
Sacramento, CA 95864-3898
**Phone:** (916)485-6711     **Fax:** (916)485-2653
**Email:** info@eastersealsca.com
**Website:** http://www.eastersealsca.com
Gary Kasai, CEO & Pres

**Program(s):** Adult and senior services; early intervention; job training and employment services; medical rehabilitation and health services; and support services.

**★ 8276 ★ Easter Seals Tri-Counties, California**
4251 S Higuera St., Ste. 101
San Luis Obispo, CA 93401
**Phone:** (805)543-4122     **Fax:** (805)692-5330
**Email:** easter@fix.net
Janet Napier, Exec Director

**Program(s):** Early education and care; and support services.

**★ 8277 ★ Easter Seals, Tri-Counties California**
**Ventura Office**
10730 Henderson Rd.
Ventura, CA 93004-1898
**Phone:** (805)647-1141        **Fax:** (805)647-1148
**Email:** lholzinger@ca-tr.easter-seals.org
**Website:** http://www.ca-tr.easter-seals.org
Janet V. Napier, Exec Director
**Program(s):** Continuing education; early education and care; early intervention; medical rehabilitation and health services; school-aged children; and support services.

## Colorado

**★ 8278 ★ Easter Seals Colorado**
5755 W Alameda Ave.
Lakewood, CO 80226-3500
**Phone:** (303)233-1666        **Free:** 800-875-4732
**Fax:** (303)233-1028
**Email:** escinfo@cess.org
**Website:** http://www.eastersealsco.org
Lynn Robinson, CEO & Pres
**Program(s):** Camping and recreation; medical rehabilitation and health services; and support services.

**★ 8279 ★ Easter Seals Southern Colorado**
310 E Abriendo Ave.
Pueblo, CO 81004
**Phone:** (719)265-2604        **Free:** 800-332-7019
**Email:** nwhittemore@ssfcu.org
**Website:** http://www.co-so.easter-seals.org
Nancy Whittemore, Director
**Program(s):** Camping and recreation; job training and employment services; and support services.

**★ 8280 ★ Easter Seals Southern Colorado**
**Colorado Springs Office**
225 S Academy Blvd., Ste. 104
Colorado Springs, CO 80910-2768
**Phone:** (719)574-9002        **Fax:** (719)574-1330
**Email:** jschmidt@easter-sealssc.org
**Website:** http://www.co-so.easter-seals.org
John Schmidt, President
**Program(s):** Camping and recreation; medical rehabilitation and health services; school-aged children; and support services.

## Connecticut

**★ 8281 ★ Easter Seals**
**Greater Hartford Rehabilitation Center**
100 Deerfield Rd.
Windsor, CT 06095-4207
**Phone:** (860)714-9500        **Fax:** (860)714-8979
**Email:** agouse@stfranciscare.org
**Website:** http://www.stfranciscare.org
Allen S. Gouse, PhD, Exec Director

**★ 8282 ★ Easter Seals Connecticut**
85 Jones St.
Hebron, CT 06248
**Phone:** (860)228-9438        **Free:** 800-874-7687
**Fax:** (860)228-9670
**Email:** johnq@eastersealsofct.org
**Website:** http://www.ct.easter-seals.org
John R. Quinn, President
**Program(s):** Camping and recreation; and support services.

**★ 8283 ★ Easter Seals Norwalk**
14 Strawberry Hill Ave.
Norwalk, CT 06855

**Phone:** (203)838-7231        **Fax:** (203)838-7283
**Email:** bto3norwalk@snet.net
**Website:** http://www.eastersealsofct.org
John R. Quinn, President
**Program(s):** Job training and employment services; school-aged children.

**★ 8284 ★ Easter Seals Waterbury**
22 Tompkins St.
Waterbury, CT 06708-1496
**Phone:** (203)754-5141        **Fax:** (203)757-1198
**Email:** rvitale@eswct.com
**Website:** http://www.eswct.com
Francis N. Deblasio, President
**Program(s):** Early education and care; early intervention; and medical rehabilitation and health services.

## Delaware

**★ 8285 ★ Easter Seals Delaware and Maryland's Eastern Shore**
New Castle County
61 Corporate Circle
New Castle, DE 19720-2405
**Phone:** (302)324-4444        **Free:** 800-677-3800
**Fax:** (302)324-4441
**Email:** wja@nc.esdel.org
**Website:** http://www.de.easter-seals.org
Sandra J. Tuttle, President
William J. Adami, Vice President
**Program(s):** Adult and senior services; early intervention; job training and employment services; medical rehabilitation and health services; and support services.

## District of Columbia

**★ 8286 ★ Easter Seals Mid-Atlantic**
**The Children's Center**
2800 13th St. NW
Washington, DC 20009-5399
**Phone:** (202)387-4434        **Fax:** (202)462-7379
**Email:** shedgepeth@eseal.org
**Website:** http://www.eseal.org
Tracey Smith, Director
Sharon Hedgepeth, Director
**Program(s):** Continuing education; early education and care; early intervention; medical rehabilitation and health services; and support services.

## Florida

**★ 8287 ★ Easter Seals Broward County**
6951 W Sunrise Blvd.
Plantation, FL 33313
**Phone:** (954)792-8772        **Fax:** (954)791-8275
**Email:** bdausman@esbc-fl.easter-seals.org
Rebecca C. Dausman, Exec Director
**Program(s):** Continuing education; early education and care; early intervention; job training and employment services; medical rehabilitation and health services; school-aged children; and support services.

**★ 8288 ★ Easter Seals Florida**
1040 Woodcock Rd., Ste. 215
Orlando, FL 32803
**Phone:** (407)896-7881        **Free:** 877-257-3257
**Fax:** (407)896-8422
**Email:** info@fl.easter-seals.org
**Website:** http://www.fl.easter-seals.org
Robert J. Griggs, President
Sue Ventura, Vice President

**★ 8289 ★ Easter Seals Florida**
1300 Executive Center Dr., Ste. 201
Tallahassee, FL 32301
**Phone:** (850)222-4606        **Fax:** (850)222-4615
**Email:** rgriggs@fl.easter-seals.org
**Website:** http://www.fl.easter-seals.org
Robert J. Griggs, CEO

**★ 8290 ★ Easter Seals Florida**
**Central Florida Region**
1040 Woodcock Rd., Ste. 215
Orlando, FL 32803
**Phone:** (407)896-7881        **Fax:** (407)896-8422
**Email:** jnasser@fl.easter-seals.org
**Website:** http://www.fl.easter-seals.org
Robert J. Griggs, President

**★ 8291 ★ Easter Seals Florida**
**East Coast Region**
**Melbourne Office**
3661 S Babcock St.
Melbourne, FL 32901-8221
**Phone:** (321)723-4474        **Fax:** (321)676-3843
**Email:** gedwards@fl.easter-seals.org
**Website:** http://www.fl.easter-seals.org
Gail Edwards, Exec Director

**★ 8292 ★ Easter Seals Florida**
**Keys Region**
5220 College Rd.
Key West, FL 33040
**Phone:** (305)294-1089        **Fax:** (305)296-1530
**Email:** mmurphy@fl.easter-seals.org
**Website:** http://www.fl.easter-seals.org
Bob Griggs, CEO & Pres
Jonathan Weinshank, Director
**Program(s):** Early education and care; early intervention; and medical rehabilitation and health services.

**★ 8293 ★ Easter Seals Florida**
**Palm Beach/Martin Region**
**Martin County Regional Office**
1700 SE Monterey Rd.
Stuart, FL 34996-4109
**Phone:** (561)286-4444        **Fax:** (561)286-4643
**Email:** kbarnes@fl.easter-seals.org
**Website:** http://www.fl.easter-seals.org
Kendra Barnes, Director

**★ 8294 ★ Easter Seals Florida**
**West Coast Region**
7402 N 56th St., Ste. 906
Tampa, FL 33617
**Phone:** (813)988-7633        **Fax:** (813)914-0403
**Email:** garmstrong@fl.easter-seals.org
**Website:** http://www.fl.easter-seals.org
Robert J. Griggs, President
Gracy McLeary, Exec Director
**Program(s):** Early education and care; early intervention; medical rehabilitation and health services; and support services.

**★ 8295 ★ Easter Seals Miami-Dade**
1475 NW 14th Ave.
Miami, FL 33125-1692
**Phone:** (305)325-0470        **Fax:** (305)325-0578
**Email:** essdade@aol.com
Joan Bornstein, President

**★ 8296 ★ Easter Seals North Florida**
910 Myers Park Dr.
Tallahassee, FL 32301-4586
**Phone:** (850)222-4465        **Fax:** (850)222-4468
**Email:** enorthflorida@aol.com
**Website:** http://www.freenet.tlh.fl.us/EasterSeals/tal-lyes.htm
Christine Hall, President
**Program(s):** Early intervention; job training and employment services; and support services.

**★ 8297 ★ Easter Seals Volusia and Flagler Counties Florida**
1219 Dunn Ave.
Daytona Beach, FL 32120
**Phone:** (386)255-4568        **Free:** 877-255-4568
**Fax:** (386)258-7677
**Email:** info@fl.vf.easter-seals.org

**Website:** http://www.fl.vf.easter-seals.org
Lynn Sinnott, CEO & Pres

**Program(s):** Camping and recreation; continuing education; early education and care; early intervention; medical rehabilitation and health services; school-aged children; and support services.

## Georgia

### ★ 8298 ★ Easter Seals East Georgia
1500 Wrightsboro Rd.
Augusta, GA 30904-2441
**Phone:** (706)667-9695          **Free:** (866)667-9695
**Fax:** (706)667-8831
**Email:** info@esega.org
**Website:** http://www.ga-ea.easter-seals.org
Sheila Thomas, Exec Director

**Program(s):** Job training and employment services; and support services.

### ★ 8299 ★ Easter Seals East Georgia
PO Box 1836
Thomson, GA 30824
**Phone:** (706)595-2212
**Email:** info@esega.org
**Website:** http://www.ga-ea.easter-seals.org
Sheila Thomas, Exec Director

**Program(s):** Job training and employment services.

### ★ 8300 ★ Easter Seals Middle Georgia
602 Kellam Rd.
Dublin, GA 31021
**Phone:** (478)275-8850          **Fax:** (478)275-8852
**Email:** ehooks@ga-mi.easterseals.org
Eloyce Hooks, Exec Director

**Program(s):** Job training and employment services; school-aged children; and support services.

### ★ 8301 ★ Easter Seals North Georgia
Prado North, Ste. 100
5600 Roswell Rd.
Atlanta, GA 30342
**Phone:** (404)943-1070          **Fax:** (404)943-0890
**Email:** info@ga-no.easter-seals.org
**Website:** http://www.ga-no.easter-seals.org
Donna Davidson, CEO & Pres

### ★ 8302 ★ Easter Seals Southern Georgia
1906 Palmyra Rd.
Albany, GA 31701-1598
**Phone:** (229)439-7061          **Free:** 800-365-4583
**Fax:** (229)435-6278
**Email:** benglish@swga-easterseals.org
**Website:** http://www.swga-easterseals.org
Beth English, Exec Director

**Program(s):** Adult and senior services; camping and recreation; early education and care; job training and employment services; residential and housing services; school-aged children; and support services.

### ★ 8303 ★ Easter Seals West Georgia
2515 Double Churches Rd.
Columbus, GA 31909
**Phone:** (706)660-1144          **Fax:** (706)660-1146
**Email:** easter-sealscolsga@mchsi.com
Barry F. Cavan, President
Sharon Borger, Exec Director

**Program(s):** Camping and recreation; early education and care; early intervention; job training and employment services; medical rehabilitation and health services; school-aged children; and support services.

## Hawaii

### ★ 8304 ★ Easter Seals Hawaii
710 Green St.
Honolulu, HI 96813-2119
**Phone:** (808)536-1015          **Fax:** (808)536-3765
**Email:** info@eastersealshawaii.org

**Website:** http://www.eastersealshawaii.org
John F. Howell, CEO & Pres

**Program(s):** Adult and senior services; camping and recreation; continuing education; early education and care; early intervention; school-aged children; and support services.

## Illinois

### ★ 8305 ★ Easter Seals Central Illinois
2715 N 27th St.
Decatur, IL 62526
**Phone:** (217)429-1052          **Free:** 800-500-7325
**Fax:** (217)423-7605
**Email:** jankel@easterseals-ci.org
**Website:** http://www.easterseals-ci.org
Janet Kelscheimer, President

**Program(s):** Camping and recreation; early education and care; early intervention; job training and employment services; medical rehabilitation and health services; school-aged children; and support services.

### ★ 8306 ★ Easter Seals of LaSalle and Bureau Counties
1013 Adams St.
Ottawa, IL 61350-4399
**Phone:** (815)434-0857          **Fax:** (815)434-2260
Leslie D. Ziel, Contact

**Program(s):** Camping and recreation; continuing education; early education and care; early intervention; medical rehabilitation and health services; school-aged children; and support services.

### ★ 8307 ★ Easter Seals Metro. Chicago
14 E Jackson Blvd., 9th Fl.
Chicago, IL 60604-2212
**Phone:** (312)939-5115          **Fax:** (312)939-0283
**Email:** essmc@eastersealchicago.org
**Website:** http://www.eastersealchicago.org
F. Timothy Muri, CEO & Pres

**Program(s):** Camping and recreation; medical rehabilitation and health services; and support services.

### ★ 8308 ★ Easter Seals Mid-Eastern Illinois
1137 E 5000 North Rd.
Bourbonnais, IL 60914
**Phone:** (815)932-0623          **Fax:** (815)932-2577
**Email:** eskkk@main.keynet.net
**Website:** http://www.easterseals-kankakee.org
Jackie Havener, Exec Director

**Program(s):** Camping and recreation; early education and care; early intervention; and medical rehabilitation and health services.

### ★ 8309 ★ Easter Seals Moline, Illinois
1504 13th Ave.
Moline, IL 61265-3196
**Phone:** (309)762-9552          **Fax:** (309)762-9610
George McDaniel, Exec Director

**Program(s):** Camping and recreation; and medical rehabilitation and health services.

### ★ 8310 ★ Easter Seals Southwestern Illinois
602 E 3rd St.
Alton, IL 62002
**Phone:** (618)462-7325          **Fax:** (618)462-8170
**Website:** http://www.mo.easter-seals.org
Craig A. Byrd, CEO & Pres

**Program(s):** Camping and recreation; and early education and care.

### ★ 8311 ★ Easter Seals Will-Grundy Counties
735 Essington, Ste. 103
Joliet, IL 60435-2830
**Phone:** (815)773-9362          **Fax:** (815)773-9365
**Email:** dcondotti@il-wg.easter-seals.org

**Website:** http://www.il-wg.easter-seals.org
Debra Condotti, President

## Indiana

### ★ 8312 ★ Bridgepointe Goodwill Industries and Easter Seals, Inc.
1329 Applegate Ln.
Clarksville, IN 47129-9610
**Phone:** (812)283-7908          **Free:** 800-660-3355
**Fax:** (812)283-6248
**Email:** cmarshall@bridgepointe.org
Caren Marshall, Exec Director

**Program(s):** Camping and recreation; early education and care; early intervention; job training and employment services; medical rehabilitation and health services; school-aged children; and support services.

### ★ 8313 ★ Easter Seals ARC of Northeast Indiana
2542 Thompson Ave.
Fort Wayne, IN 46807
**Phone:** (260)456-4534          **Free:** 800-234-7811
**Fax:** (260)745-5200
**Email:** shinkle@arc-nei.org
**Website:** http://www.esarc.org
Steve Hinkle, CEO

**Program(s):** Camping and recreation; continuing education; early education and care.

### ★ 8314 ★ Easter Seals Committee Wayne & Union Counties
Centerville, IN 47330-0086
**Phone:** (317)855-2482          **Fax:** (317)855-2482
**Email:** easterseals@juno.com
Patricia Bowers, Exec Director

**Program(s):** Camping and recreation; school-aged children; and support services.

### ★ 8315 ★ Easter Seals Crossroads, Bartholomew County
4251 S 600 E
Columbus, IN 47203
**Phone:** (812)579-5790          **Fax:** (812)579-5790
**Email:** debbies@iquest.net
Deborah Siefker, Exec Director

**Program(s):** Camping, recreation, and support services.

## Iowa

### ★ 8316 ★ Easter Seals Iowa
401 NE 66th Ave.
Des Moines, IA 50313
**Phone:** (515)289-1933          **Fax:** (515)289-1281
**Email:** info@eastersealsia.org
Donna Elbrecht, CEO & Pres

**Program(s):** Camping and recreation; early education and care; job training and employment services; medical rehabilitation and health services; school-aged children; and support services.

## Kansas

### ★ 8317 ★ Easter Seals Kansas
3636 N Oliver
Wichita, KS 67220
**Phone:** (316)744-9291          **Fax:** (316)744-1428
**Website:** http://www.goodwilleastersealsks.org
Marie Mareda, President

**Program(s):** Job training and employment services; and support services.

## Kentucky

### ★ 8318 ★ Easter Seals Kentucky
9810 Bluegrass Pkwy.
Louisville, KY 40299-1906
**Phone:** (502)584-9781          **Fax:** (502)589-2409
**Email:** bls@loueaster.org

**Website:** http://www.loueaster.org
Susan Eisenback, Exec Director
**Program(s):** Early intervention, medical rehabilitation, and health services.

★ **8319** ★ **Easter Seals of Northern Kentucky**
31 Spiral Dr.
Florence, KY 41042
**Phone:** (859)491-1171     **Fax:** (859)491-8132
**Email:** vickie@nkeaster.org
Margaret Baker-Wernersbach, Exec Director
**Program(s):** Medical rehabilitation and health services.

★ **8320** ★ **Easter Seals West Kentucky**
2229 Mildred St.
Paducah, KY 42001
**Phone:** (270)444-9687     **Free:** (866)673-3565
**Fax:** (270)444-0655
**Email:** info@ky-ws.easter-seals.org
**Website:** http://www.ky-ws.easter-seals.org
Kenneth R. Lucas, President
**Program(s):** Adult and senior services; continuing education; early education and care; early intervention; job training and employment services; medical rehabilitation and health services; school-aged children; and support services.

## Louisiana

★ **8321** ★ **Easter Seals Louisiana Covington Office**
600 N Hwy. 190, Ste. 213
Covington, LA 70433
**Phone:** (504)892-7604     **Fax:** (504)892-5735
**Email:** escasmgt9@compsurf.com
Daniel H. Underwood, CEO
**Program(s):** Camping and recreation; early education and care; early intervention; medical rehabilitation and health services; school-aged children; and support services.

★ **8322** ★ **Easter Seals Louisiana Monroe Office**
1900 N 18th St., Ste. 203B
Monroe, LA 71201
**Phone:** (318)322-4788     **Fax:** (318)322-1549
**Email:** esldeltaproject@aol.com
Joan Oursler, Contact
**Program(s):** Camping and recreation; continuing education; early education and care; early intervention; medical rehabilitation and health services; school-aged children; and support services.

★ **8323** ★ **Easter Seals Louisiana New Orleans Office**
305 Baronne St., Ste. 400
New Orleans, LA 70112-1617
**Phone:** (504)523-7325     **Free:** 800-695-7325
**Fax:** (504)523-3465
**Email:** essla@aol.com
Daniel H. Underwood, CEO & Pres
**Program(s):** Camping and recreation; early education and care; early intervention; school-aged children; and support services.

★ **8324** ★ **Easter Seals Louisiana Shreveport Office**
900 Pierremont Rd., Ste. 220
PO Box 6105
Shreveport, LA 71106
**Phone:** (318)868-5840     **Fax:** (318)868-3612
**Email:** esshreveport@aol.com
Daniel H. Underwood, CEO & Pres
Gordon Grafton, Vice President
**Program(s):** Camping and recreation; early education and care; early intervention; medical rehabilitation and health services; school-aged children; and support services.

## Maryland

★ **8325** ★ **Easter Seals Mid-Atlantic**
4041 Powder Mill Rd., Ste. 100
Beltsville, MD 20705
**Phone:** (301)931-8700     **Free:** 800-862-1377
**Fax:** (301)931-8690
**Email:** lreeves@eseal.org
**Website:** http://www.eseal.org
Lisa Reeves, CEO & Pres
**Remarks:** Serves Washington DC, Maryland, northern Virginia, south-central Pennsylvania, and eastern West Virginia.

★ **8326** ★ **Easter Seals Salisbury**
1915 N Salisbury Blvd.
Salisbury, MD 21801
**Phone:** (410)546-2894     **Fax:** (410)546-4913
**Email:** ncotter@gt.esdel.org
**Website:** http://www.de.easter-seals.org
Sandra J. Tuttle, President
**Program(s):** Early intervention, medical rehabilitation and health services, and support services.

## Massachusetts

★ **8327** ★ **Easter Seals Massachusetts**
Denholm Bldg.
484 Main St.
Worcester, MA 01608-1817
**Phone:** (508)757-2756     **Free:** 800-244-2756
**Fax:** (508)831-9768
**Email:** maryd@eastersealsma.org
**Website:** http://www.eastersealsma.org
Kirk N. Joslin, CEO & Pres
**Program(s):** Camping and recreation; continuing education; early education and care; job training and employment services; medical rehabilitation and health services; school-aged children; and support services.

## Michigan

★ **8328** ★ **Easter Seals Southeastern Michigan**
21111 Haggerty Rd.
Novi, MI 48375
**Phone:** (248)447-4711     **Fax:** (248)372-7472
John R. Cocciolone, CEO & Pres
Valerie Pearson, Director

★ **8329** ★ **Easter Seals Genesee County**
1420 W 3rd Ave.
Flint, MI 48504-4897
**Phone:** (810)238-0475     **Fax:** (810)238-9270
**Email:** eslily@intouchmi.com
Elliott C. Fauster, Exec Director
**Program(s):** Camping and recreation; medical rehabilitation and health services; school-aged children; and support services.

★ **8330** ★ **Easter Seals Michigan**
4065 Saladin Dr. SE
Grand Rapids, MI 49546-6299
**Phone:** (616)942-2081     **Free:** 800-292-2729
**Fax:** (616)942-5932
**Email:** essofmich@aol.com
**Website:** http://www.mi-ws.easter-seals.org
David Lankford, Contact
Kathy Hayden, Contact
**Program(s):** Adult and senior services; camping and recreation; early education and care; early intervention; job training and employment services; medical rehabilitation and health services; school-aged children; and support services.

★ **8331** ★ **Easter Seals Michigan East Central Region**
804 S Hamilton
Saginaw, MI 48602-1516

**Phone:** (517)797-0880     **Free:** 800-292-2729
**Fax:** (517)797-0888
**Email:** esofmi@aol.com
**Website:** http://www.mi-ws.easter-seals.org
Julie S. Dorsey, Director
**Program(s):** Adult and senior services; camping and recreation; early education and care; job training and employment services; medical rehabilitation and health services; school-aged children; and support services.

★ **8332** ★ **Easter Seals Michigan Northwestern Region**
109 S Union, Ste. 209
Traverse City, MI 49684
**Phone:** (231)941-1271     **Fax:** (231)941-1990
**Email:** essofmich@aol.com
**Website:** http://www.mi-ws.easter-seals.org
Robert Dean, CEO & Pres
Betty Reynolds-Maciejewski, Director
**Program(s):** Camping and recreation; continuing education; early education and care; early intervention; job training and employment services; medical rehabilitation and health services; school-aged children; and support services.

★ **8333** ★ **Easter Seals Michigan Upper Peninsula Region**
104 Coles Dr., Ste. A
Marquette, MI 49855-4059
**Phone:** (906)228-5816     **Free:** 800-292-2729
**Fax:** (906)228-6199
**Email:** esofupmich@aol.com
Karen Taylor, Director
Nancy A. Bell, Director
**Program(s):** Early education and care; medical rehabilitation and health services; school-aged children; and support services.

★ **8334** ★ **Easter Seals Southeastern Michigan**
22150 W 9 Mile Rd.
Southfield, MI 48034
**Phone:** (248)386-9600     **Free:** 800-757-3257
**Fax:** (248)386-9604
**Email:** jcocciolne@essmichigan.org
**Website:** http://www.essmichigan.org
Mr. John R. Cocciolone, CEO & Pres

## Minnesota

★ **8335** ★ **Easter Seals Minnesota Rochester Office**
660 37th St. NW
Rochester, MN 55901
**Phone:** (507)287-8699     **Fax:** (507)281-3749
Michael Wirth-Davis, CEO & Pres

★ **8336** ★ **Easter Seals Minnesota St. Paul Office**
2543 Como Ave.
Saint Paul, MN 55108-1298
**Phone:** (651)646-2591     **Free:** 800-669-6719
**Fax:** (651)646-0302
**Email:** kmatter@goodwilleasterseals.org
**Website:** http://www.goodwilleasterseals.org
Michael Wirth-Davis, President
**Program(s):** Job training and employment services; and support services.

★ **8337** ★ **Easter Seals Minnesota Waite Park Office**
50 S 2nd St.
Waite Park, MN 56387
**Phone:** (320)654-9527     **Fax:** (320)654-9542
Michael Wirth-Davis, CEO & Pres
**Program(s):** Job training and employment services; and support services.

**★ 8338 ★ Easter Seals Minnesota**
**Willmar Office**
2424 1st St. S
Willmar, MN 56201
**Phone:** (320)214-9238     **Fax:** (320)214-9140
Michael Wirth-Davis, CEO & Pres
**Program(s):** Job training and employment services; and support services.

## Missouri

**★ 8339 ★ Easter Seals Greater Kansas City**
908 NE 116th Terrace
Kansas City, MO 64155
**Phone:** (816)734-7068     **Fax:** (816)734-7068
**Email:** kkroh@mo.easter-seals.org
**Website:** http://www.mo.easter-seals.org
Craig A Byrd, CEO & Pres
**Program(s):** Camping and recreation; early education and care; job training and employment services; medical rehabilitation and health services; school-aged children; and support services.

**★ 8340 ★ Easter Seals Missouri**
5025 Northrup Ave., Ste. 110
Saint Louis, MO 63110-2050
**Phone:** (314)664-5025     **Free:** 800-664-5025
**Fax:** (314)664-4838
**Email:** pat@easterseals-mo.org
**Website:** http://www.mo.easter-seals.org
Craig A. Byrd, CEO & Pres
**Program(s):** Support services.

**★ 8341 ★ Easter Seals Southwest Missouri**
2200 E Sunshine, Ste. 103
Springfield, MO 65804
**Phone:** (417)882-6500     **Fax:** (417)882-0230
**Email:** clawless@mo.easter-seals.org
**Website:** http://www.mo.easter-seals.org
Christine Lawless, Director
**Program(s):** Camping and recreation; early education and care; early intervention; school-aged children; and support services.

## Montana

**★ 8342 ★ Easter Seals Northern Rocky Mountains**
4400 Central Ave.
Great Falls, MT 59405-1695
**Phone:** (406)761-3680     **Free:** 800-771-2153
**Fax:** (406)761-5110
**Email:** michelleb@esgw.org
**Website:** http://www.goodwill.org/localweb/greatfalls/
Michelle Belknap, CEO
Sally Cerny, President
**Remarks:** Serves Idaho, Montana, and Wyoming.

## Nebraska

**★ 8343 ★ Easter Seals Nebraska**
2727 W 2nd, Ste. 471
Hastings, NE 68901
**Phone:** (402)462-3031     **Free:** 800-471-6425
**Fax:** (402)462-2040
**Email:** bkoehler@ne.easter-seals.org
**Website:** http://www.ne.easter-seals.org
Karen Ginder, President
**Program(s):** Job training and employment services.

## Nevada

**★ 8344 ★ Easter Seals Nevada**
6100 Neil Rd., Ste. 201
Reno, NV 89511
**Phone:** (775)322-6555     **Fax:** (775)834-5933
**Email:** info@eastersealsnv.org
Donald Stromquist, President

**Program(s):** Adult and senior services; camping and recreation; job training and employment services; residential and housing services; school-aged children; and support services.

## New Hampshire

**★ 8345 ★ Easter Seals Lancaster**
525 Prospect St.
Lancaster, NH 03584
**Phone:** (603)788-0911
**Email:** essofny@aol.com
**Website:** http://www.nh.easter-seals.org
Larry Gammon, CEO & Pres
**Program(s):** Residential and housing services; and school-aged children.

**★ 8346 ★ Easter Seals New Hampshire**
390 Union Ave.
Laconia, NH 03246
**Phone:** (603)524-8552     **Fax:** (603)524-8566
**Email:** essofny@aol.com
**Website:** http://www.nh.easter-seals.org
Larry Gammon, CEO & Pres
**Program(s):** Adult and senior services; and job training and employment services.

**★ 8347 ★ Easter Seals New Hampshire**
**Claremont Office**
54 Pleasant St.
Claremont, NH 03743
**Phone:** (603)543-3795
**Email:** essofny@aol.com
**Website:** http://www.nh.easter-seals.org
Larry Gammon, CEO & Pres
**Program(s):** Job training and employment services.

**★ 8348 ★ Easter Seals New Hampshire**
**Concord Office**
2 Industrial Dr.
Concord, NH 03301
**Phone:** (603)226-3791     **Fax:** (603)226-2540
**Email:** essofny@aol.com
**Website:** http://www.nh.easter-seals.org
Larry Gammon, CEO & Pres
**Program(s):** Adult and senior services; early education and care; early intervention; and support services.

**★ 8349 ★ Easter Seals New Hampshire**
**Derry Office**
44 Birch St.
Derry, NH 03038
**Phone:** (603)432-1945     **Fax:** (603)434-2134
**Email:** essofny@aol.com
**Website:** http://www.nh.easter-seals.org
Larry Gammon, CEO & Pres
**Program(s):** Early intervention.

**★ 8350 ★ Easter Seals New Hampshire**
**Keene Office**
12 Kingsbury St.
Keene, NH 03431
**Phone:** (603)355-1067     **Fax:** (603)358-3947
**Email:** essofny@aol.com
**Website:** http://www.nh.easter-seals.org
Larry Gammon, CEO & Pres
**Program(s):** Early education and care; job training and employment services; and school-aged children.

**★ 8351 ★ Easter Seals New Hampshire**
**Manchester Office**
555 Auburn St.
Manchester, NH 03103
**Phone:** (603)623-8863     **Fax:** (603)621-3461
**Email:** mail@eseals.org
**Website:** http://www.nh.easter-seals.org
Larry Gammon, CEO & Pres
Christine McMahon, Contact

**Program(s):** Adult and senior services; camping and recreation; continuing education; early education and care; early intervention; job training and employment services; medical rehabilitation and health services; residential and housing services; school-aged children; and support services.

**★ 8352 ★ Easter Seals New Hampshire**
**Portsmouth Office**
147 Congress St., Ste. A
Portsmouth, NH 03801
**Phone:** (603)431-7242     **Fax:** (603)427-2895
**Email:** essofny@aol.com
**Website:** http://www.nh.easter-seals.org
Larry Gammon, CEO & Pres
**Program(s):** Early education and care; job training and employment services; and school-aged children.

**★ 8353 ★ Easter Seals Plymouth**
1000 Texas Hill Rd.
Plymouth, NH 03264
**Phone:** (603)968-4467
**Email:** essofny@aol.com
**Website:** http://www.nh.easter-seals.org
Larry Gammon, CEO & Pres
**Program(s):** Residential and housing services.

**★ 8354 ★ Easter Seals Rumney**
1849 Rumney Rd.
Rumney, NH 03266
**Phone:** (603)786-2510
**Email:** essofny@aol.com
**Website:** http://www.nh.easter-seals.org
Larry Gammon, CEO & Pres
**Program(s):** Residential and housing services.

## New Jersey

**★ 8355 ★ Easter Seals New Jersey**
1 Kimberly Rd.
East Brunswick, NJ 08816
**Phone:** (732)257-6662     **Free:** 800-468-0027
**Fax:** (732)257-7373
**Email:** mschneier@nj.easter-seals.org
**Website:** http://www.eastersealsnj.org
Brian J. Fitzgerald, CEO & Pres
Helen Drobnis, Director
**Program(s):** Adult and senior services; camping and recreation; job training and employment services; medical rehabilitation and health services; residential and housing services; and support services.

## New Mexico

**★ 8356 ★ Easter Seals New Mexico**
2819 Richmond Dr. NE
Albuquerque, NM 87107-1918
**Phone:** (505)888-3811     **Free:** 800-279-5261
**Fax:** (505)888-0490
**Email:** esnm1@aol.com
**Website:** http://www.nm.easter-seals.org
Marlis Hadley, CEO & Pres
**Program(s):** Camping and recreation; continuing education; early education and care; school-aged children; and support services.

## New York

**★ 8357 ★ Easter Seals Monroe County**
349 W Commercial St., Ste. 1350
East Rochester, NY 14445-2402
**Phone:** (585)264-9550     **Fax:** (585)264-9547
**Email:** fighttowin@aol.com
**Website:** http://www.eastersealsny.com
Larry Gammon, President
**Program(s):** Residential and housing services.

**★ 8358 ★ Easter Seals New York**
**Albany Office**
230 Washington Ave. Ext.
Albany, NY 12203
**Phone:** (518)456-4880      **Free:** 800-727-8785
**Fax:** (518)456-5094
**Email:** fighttowin@aol.com
**Website:** http://www.eastersealsny.com
Larry Gammon, President
Ms. Chris McMahon, COO

**Program(s):** Camping and recreation; early education and care; medical rehabilitation and health services.

**★ 8359 ★ Easter Seals New York**
**New York City Chapter**
300 Park Ave., 17th Fl.
New York, NY 10022
**Phone:** (212)572-6227      **Free:** 800-727-8785
**Fax:** (212)705-4210
**Email:** jkohomban@ny.easter-seals.org
**Website:** http://www.eastersealsny.com
Larry Gammon, President

**Program(s):** Camping and recreation; and support services.

## North Carolina

**★ 8360 ★ Easter Seals North Carolina**
2315 Myron Dr.
Raleigh, NC 27607-3399
**Free:** 800-662-7119      **Fax:** (919)782-5486
**Email:** info@esnc.easter-seals.org
**Website:** http://www.nc.easter-seals.org
Adele R. Foschia, CEO

**Program(s):** Camping and recreation; continuing education; early education and care; early intervention; job training and employment services; medical rehabilitation and health services; school-aged children; and support services.

## North Dakota

**★ 8361 ★ Easter Seals/Goodwill North Dakota**
**Fargo Office**
15 S 21st St.
Fargo, ND 58103-9376
**Phone:** (701)237-9908
Gordon Hauge, CEO & Pres
Cindy Gabbert, Contact

**Program(s):** Continuing education; early education and care; early intervention; job training and employment services; medical rehabilitation and health services; school-aged children; and support services.

**★ 8362 ★ Easter Seals/Goodwill North Dakota**
**Mandan Office**
211 Collins Ave.
Mandan, ND 58554-7206
**Phone:** (701)663-6828      **Fax:** (701)663-6859
**Email:** kodioak@btigate.com
Gordon Hauge, Contact
Cindy Sheldon, Contact

**Program(s):** Continuing education; early education and care; early intervention; job training and employment services; medical rehabilitation and health services; school-aged children; and support services.

**★ 8363 ★ Easter Seals/Goodwill North Dakota**
**Minot Office**
800 12th Ave. SW
Minot, ND 58702-1801
**Phone:** (701)838-0669      **Fax:** (701)838-5998
Gordon Hauge, CEO & Pres
Theresa Gochanour, Director

**Program(s):** Continuing education; early education and care; early intervention; job training and employment services; medical rehabilitation and health services; school-aged children; and support services.

**★ 8364 ★ Easter Seals North Dakota**
2125 Sims
Dickinson, ND 58601
**Phone:** (701)264-1060      **Free:** (866)895-1587
**Fax:** (701)264-1099
**Email:** kodiak@btigate.com
Gordon Hauge, CEO & Pres

**Program(s):** Continuing education; early education and care; early intervention; job training and employment services; school-aged children; and support services.

**★ 8365 ★ Easter Seals North Dakota**
**Grand Forks Office**
1811 DeMers Ave.
Grand Forks, ND 58208
**Phone:** (701)772-0704      **Fax:** (701)772-0336
**Email:** kodioak@btigate.com
Gordon Hauge, CEO & Pres
Laurie Forsberg, Contact

**Program(s):** Continuing education; early education and care; early intervention; job training and employment services; medical rehabilitation and health services; school-aged children; and support services.

**★ 8366 ★ Easter Seals North Dakota**
**Jamestown Office**
713 10th St. SE
Jamestown, ND 58402
**Phone:** (701)251-1446      **Fax:** (701)252-9527
**Email:** kodioak@btigate.com
Gordon Hauge, Contact
Rose Greer, Contact

**Program(s):** Continuing education; early education and care; early intervention; job training and employment services; medical rehabilitation and health services; school-aged children; and support services.

## Ohio

**★ 8367 ★ Easter Seals Central and Southeast Ohio, Inc.**
**Central Ohio Office**
565 Children's Dr. W
Columbus, OH 43205-0166
**Phone:** (614)228-5523      **Free:** 800-860-5523
**Fax:** (614)228-8249
**Email:** kzuckerman@easterseals-cseohio.org
**Website:** http://www.oh-cn.easter-seals.org
Karin Zuckerman, CEO & Pres

**Program(s):** Adult and senior services; camping and recreation; early education and care; early intervention; medical rehabilitation and health services; and support services.

**★ 8368 ★ Easter Seals Central and Southeast Ohio, Inc.**
**River Cities Office**
609 Putnam St.
Marietta, OH 45750-0031
**Phone:** (740)374-8876      **Fax:** (740)374-4501
**Website:** http://www.oh-cn.easter-seals.org
Karin A. Zuckerman, CEO & Pres
Steve Parks, Mgr

**Program(s):** Camping and recreation; early intervention; medical rehabilitation and health services; schoolaged children; and support services.

**★ 8369 ★ Easter Seals Central and Southeast Ohio, Inc.**
**Shawnee Regional Office**
810 E Main St.
PO Box 354
Chillicothe, OH 45601
**Phone:** (740)773-1273      **Fax:** (740)773-0936
**Email:** abouilli@easterseals-cseohio.org
**Website:** http://www.oh-cn.easter-seals.org
Karin A. Zuckerman, President
Alexis Bouillon, Mgr

**Program(s):** Adult and senior services; camping and recreation; medical rehabilitation and health services; and support services.

**★ 8370 ★ Easter Seals Northeast Ohio**
**Akron Office**
3085 W Market St., Ste. 124
Akron, OH 44333-3363
**Phone:** (330)836-9741      **Fax:** (330)836-4967
**Website:** http://www.eastersealsneo.org
Sheila M. Dunn, CEO & Pres
Greg Tesniarz, Director

**Program(s):** Early education and care; early intervention; medical rehabilitation and health services; school-aged children; and support services.

**★ 8371 ★ Easter Seals Northeast Ohio**
**Canton Office**
3996 Fulton Dr. NW
Canton, OH 44718-3051
**Phone:** (330)649-9374      **Fax:** (330)649-9376
**Email:** linda@eastersealsneo.org
**Website:** http://www.eastersealsneo.org
Sheila M. Dunn, CEO & Pres
Greg Tesniarz, Director

**Program(s):** Camping and recreation; continuing education; early education and care; early intervention; medical rehabilitation and health services; and support services.

**★ 8372 ★ Easter Seals Northeast Ohio**
**Cleveland Office**
1929-A E Royalton Rd.
Cleveland, OH 44147
**Phone:** (440)838-0990      **Free:** 800-437-3288
**Fax:** (440)838-8440
**Email:** sdunn@eastersealsneo.org
**Website:** http://www.eastersealsneo.org
Sheila M. Dunn, CEO & Pres

**Program(s):** Camping and recreation; early education and care; early intervention; medical rehabilitation and health services; school-aged children; and support services.

**★ 8373 ★ Easter Seals Northeast Ohio**
**Lakewood Office**
14701 Detroit Ave., Ste. 252
Lakewood, OH 44107
**Phone:** (216)228-5170      **Fax:** (216)228-1018
**Website:** http://www.eastersealsneo.org
Sheila M. Dunn, CEO & Pres

**★ 8374 ★ Easter Seals Northeast Ohio**
**University Heights Office**
2175 Taylor
University Heights, OH 44118
**Phone:** 888-325-8532      **Fax:** (440)838-8440
**Email:** spowers@easter-sealsneo.org
Sheila M. Dunn, CEO

**★ 8375 ★ Easter Seals Northeast Ohio**
**Willoughby Office**
37415 Euclid Ave.
Willoughby, OH 44094
**Phone:** (440)953-2627      **Fax:** (440)953-2627
**Website:** http://www.eastersealsneo.org
Sheila M. Dunn, CEO & Pres

**Program(s):** Early intervention.

**★ 8376 ★ Easter Seals Northwestern Ohio**
**Ashland Office**
516 Claremont Ave.
Ashland, OH 44805
**Phone:** (419)281-5368      **Fax:** (419)289-8741
**Email:** jlambert@eastersealsnwohio.org
**Website:** http://www.eastersealsnwohio.org
Margaret Halter, Contact

**Program(s):** Adult and senior services; camping and recreation; early education and care; school-aged children; and support services.

### ★ 8377 ★ Easter Seals Northwestern Ohio
**Fremont Office**
309 Garrison St.
Fremont, OH 43420
**Phone:** (419)332-5921
**Email:** lgonzales@eastersealsnwohio.org
**Website:** http://www.eastersealsnwohio.org
Lori Gonzales, Contact

**Program(s):** Camping and recreation; continuing education; early education and care; early intervention; medical rehabilitation and health services; school-aged children; and support services.

### ★ 8378 ★ Easter Seals Northwestern Ohio
**Lorain Office**
1909 N Ridge Rd., Bldg. 6
Lorain, OH 44055-3344
**Phone:** (440)277-7337          **Fax:** (440)277-7339
**Email:** kwalter@eastersealsnwohio.org
**Website:** http://www.eastersealsnwohio.org
Kevin Walter, Exec Director

**Program(s):** Adult and senior services; camping and recreation; continuing education; early education and care; early intervention; medical rehabilitation and health services; school-aged children; and support services.

### ★ 8379 ★ Easter Seals Northwestern Ohio
**Norwalk Office**
226 State Rte. 61 E
Norwalk, OH 44857
**Phone:** (419)668-6791          **Fax:** (419)663-4529
**Email:** kwalter@eastersealsnwohio.org
**Website:** http://www.eastersealsnwohio.org
Philomena Fisher, Contact

**Program(s):** Adult and senior services; camping and recreation; continuing education; early education and care; school-aged children; and support services.

### ★ 8380 ★ Easter Seals Northwestern Ohio
**Sandusky Office**
Sandusky Plaza
1044 Cleveland Rd.
Sandusky, OH 44870
**Phone:** (419)626-8447          **Fax:** (419)627-9063
**Website:** http://www.eastersealsnwohio.org
Kevin Walter, Contact

**Program(s):** Camping and recreation; continuing education; early education and care; early intervention; medical rehabilitation and health services; school-aged children; and support services.

### ★ 8381 ★ Easter Seals Northwestern Ohio
**Toledo Office**
435 S Hawley St., Ste. A
Toledo, OH 43609
**Phone:** (419)241-2600          **Fax:** (419)241-5046
**Email:** kwalter@eastersealsnwohio.org
**Website:** http://www.eastersealsnwohio.org
Diana Harmon, Director
Lori Conti, Contact

**Program(s):** Camping and recreation; continuing education; early education and care; medical rehabilitation and health services; school-aged children; and support services.

### ★ 8382 ★ Easter Seals St. Clairsville
330 Fox-Shannon Pl.
Saint Clairsville, OH 43950
**Phone:** (740)695-5979          **Fax:** (740)695-6764

**Email:** mhon@wv.easter-seals.org
**Website:** http://www.wv.easter-seals.org
Martha Hon, CEO & Pres

**Program(s):** Early intervention; medical rehabilitation and health services; and school-aged children.

### ★ 8383 ★ Easter Seals Southwestern Ohio
**Cincinnati Office**
231 Clark Rd.
Cincinnati, OH 45215
**Phone:** (513)821-9890          **Free:** 800-288-1123
**Fax:** (513)821-9895
**Email:** twatson@oh-sw.easter-seals.org
**Website:** http://www.oh-sw.easter-seals.org
Tammy Watson, CEO & Pres

**Program(s):** Adult and senior services; continuing education; early education and care; early intervention; medical rehabilitation and health services; school-aged children; and support services.

### ★ 8384 ★ Easter Seals Trumbull County
155 S Park Ave.
Warren, OH 44481
**Phone:** (330)399-1001          **Fax:** (330)339-4001
**Email:** easterseals@cisnet.com
**Website:** http://www.oh-ya.easter-seals.org
Kenan J. Sklener, CEO

**Program(s):** Adult and senior services; early education and care; early intervention; medical rehabilitation and health services; and support services.

### ★ 8385 ★ Easter Seals West Central Ohio
**Lima Office**
3123 W Elm St.
Lima, OH 45805-2478
**Phone:** (419)222-7047          **Fax:** (419)222-9303
**Email:** k.oglesbee@goodwilldayton.org
**Website:** http://wwww.oh-wc.easter-seals.org
Amy Luttrell, President
Karen Oglesbee, Mgr

**Program(s):** Camping and recreation; early education and care; school-aged children; and support services.

### ★ 8386 ★ Easter Seals Youngstown Area
299 Edwards St.
Youngstown, OH 44502-1599
**Phone:** (330)743-1168          **Fax:** (330)743-1616
**Email:** eastersealsceo@cisnet.com
**Website:** http://www.oh-ya.easter-seals.org
Kenan J. Sklener, CEO

**Program(s):** Adult and senior services; early education and care; early intervention; medical rehabilitation and health services; school-aged children; and support services.

## Oklahoma

### ★ 8387 ★ Easter Seals Oklahoma
**Oklahoma City Office**
2100 NW 63rd. St.
Oklahoma City, OK 73116
**Phone:** (405)848-2525          **Fax:** (405)842-9704
**Email:** easok@ilinkusa.net
Patricia Filer, CEO & Pres

**Program(s):** Adult and senior services; camping and recreation; early education and care; medical rehabilitation and health services; school-aged children; and support services.

### ★ 8388 ★ Easter Seals Oklahoma
**Tulsa Office**
2738 E 51st St., Ste. 130
Tulsa, OK 74105
**Phone:** (918)743-2311          **Fax:** (918)749-8510
Pat Filer, CEO & Pres

**Program(s):** Medical rehabilitation and health services.

## Oregon

### ★ 8389 ★ Easter Seals
**Medford Office**
Medford, OR 97501
**Phone:** (541)842-2199          **Fax:** (541)842-2199
**Email:** medford@or.easter-seals.org
**Website:** http://www.or.easter-seals.org
Diane Mathews, Director

**Program(s):** Camping and recreation; school-aged children; and support services.

### ★ 8390 ★ Easter Seals Oregon
**Eugene Center**
3575 Donald St.
Eugene, OR 97405
**Phone:** (541)344-2247          **Free:** 800-244-5289
**Fax:** (541)344-7082
**Email:** eugene@or.easter-seals.org
**Website:** http://www.or.easter-seals.org
Jane Welch, Director

**Program(s):** Camping and recreation; continuing education; medical rehabilitation and health services; and support services.

### ★ 8391 ★ Easter Seals Oregon
**Portland Office**
5757 SW Macadam Ave.
Portland, OR 97201-3797
**Phone:** (503)228-5108          **Free:** 800-556-6020
**Fax:** (503)228-1352
**Email:** info@or.easter-seals.org
**Website:** http://www.or.easter-seals.org
Bob Baker, Vice President

**Program(s):** Camping and recreation; medical rehabilitation and health services; school-aged children; and support services.

## Pennsylvania

### ★ 8392 ★ Easter Seals Central Pennsylvania
**Altoona Office**
501 Valley View Blvd.
Altoona, PA 16602
**Phone:** (814)941-1613          **Free:** 888-463-3039
**Fax:** (814)944-6500
**Email:** jhanlin@homenursingagency.com
**Website:** http://www.homenursingagency.com/east-seal.htm
Jeanne Hanlin, Contact

**Program(s):** Camping and recreation; continuing education; early education and care; early intervention; job training and employment services; medical rehabilitation and health services; school-aged children; and support services.

### ★ 8393 ★ Easter Seals Central Pennsylvania
**State College Office**
1300 S Allen St.
State College, PA 16801
**Phone:** (814)941-1613          **Free:** 888-463-3093
**Fax:** (814)238-3721
**Email:** bwallen@homenursingagency.com
**Website:** http://www.homenursingagency.com/east-seal.htm
Bill Wallen, Director
Carol McEwen, Director

**Program(s):** Camping and recreation; early education and care; and job training and employment services.

### ★ 8394 ★ Easter Seals Eastern Pennsylvania
1503 N Cedar Crest Blvd., Ste. 317
Allentown, PA 18104
**Phone:** (610)289-0114          **Fax:** (610)289-4282
**Email:** lindalm@easter-sealseasternpa.org
**Website:** http://www.easter-sealseasternpa.org
Linda LaMona, CEO & Pres

★ 8395 ★ **Easter Seals Eastern
Pennsylvania**
**Berks/Schuylkill Division**
1040 Liggett Ave.
Reading, PA 19611
**Phone:** (610)775-1431  **Fax:** (610)796-1954
**Email:** essbks@voicenet.com
**Website:** http://www.easter-sealseasternpa.com
Linda LaMona, CEO & Pres

**Program(s):** Camping and recreation; early intervention; medical rehabilitation and health services; school-aged children; and support services.


★ 8396 ★ **Easter Seals Eastern
Pennsylvania**
**Lehigh Valley Division**
2200 Industrial Dr.
Bethlehem, PA 18017-2198
**Phone:** (610)866-8092  **Fax:** (610)866-3450
**Website:** http://www.easter-sealseasternpa.com
Barbara C. Carlson, Contact

**Program(s):** Camping and recreation; early education and care; early intervention; medical rehabilitation and health services; school-aged children; and support services.


★ 8397 ★ **Easter Seals Eastern
Pennsylvania**
**Lehighton Site**
325 Alum St.
Lehighton, PA 18235
**Phone:** (610)379-9160  **Fax:** (610)379-9162
**Website:** http://www.easter-sealseasternpa.com
Linda LaMona, CEO & Pres

**Program(s):** Camping and recreation; early education and care; early intervention; medical rehabilitation and health services; and school-aged children.


★ 8398 ★ **Easter Seals Eastern
Pennsylvania**
**Pocono Division**
109 Seven Bridge Rd.
East Stroudsburg, PA 18301-9100
**Phone:** (570)421-1254  **Fax:** (570)424-2346
**Email:** nancylt@easterseals-easternpa.org
**Website:** http://www.easterseals-easternpa.org
Linda LaMona, CEO & Pres

**Program(s):** Early intervention.


★ 8399 ★ **Easter Seals Franklin and
Adams Counties**
34 Rd.side Ave.
Waynesboro, PA 17268
**Phone:** (717)762-5315  **Fax:** (717)762-0362
**Email:** easter-w@cvn.net
Robert S. Hoover, President

**Program(s):** Early education and care; early intervention; medical rehabilitation and health services; and support services.


★ 8400 ★ **Easter Seals Franklin & Adams
Counties**
55 Hamilton Rd.
Chambersburg, PA 17201-6432
**Phone:** (717)264-7578  **Fax:** (717)264-1309
**Email:** easter-w@cvn.net
**Website:** http://www.gettysburg.edu/project/sl/health/
easter.html
Robert S. Hoover, President

**Program(s):** Early education and care; early intervention; medical rehabilitation and health services; school-aged children; and support services.


★ 8401 ★ **Easter Seals South Central
Pennsylvania**
**York Office**
2201 S Queen St.
York, PA 17402-4695
**Phone:** (717)741-3891  **Free:** 888-273-7351
**Fax:** (717)741-5359
**Email:** dnoel3@aol.com
**Website:** http://www.visiteasterseals.org
Debbie Noel, President


★ 8402 ★ **Easter Seals Southeastern
Pennsylvania**
**Bucks County Office**
2400 Trenton Rd.
Levittown, PA 19056
**Phone:** (215)945-7200  **Fax:** (215)945-4073
**Email:** philaess@liberynet.org
**Website:** http://www.easterseals-sepa.org
Carl Webster, Exec Director

**Program(s):** Camping and recreation; continuing education; early education and care; early intervention; medical rehabilitation and health services; school-aged children; and support services.


★ 8403 ★ **Easter Seals Southeastern
Pennsylvania**
**Chester County Office**
797 E Lancaster Ave., Ste. 2
Downingtown, PA 19335
**Phone:** (610)873-3990  **Fax:** (610)873-3992
**Email:** dkeiths@easterseals-sepa.org
**Website:** http://www.easterseals-sepa.org
Carl Webster, Exec Director

**Program(s):** Camping and recreation; continuing education; early education and care; early intervention; job training and employment services; medical rehabilitation and health services; school-aged children; and support services.


★ 8404 ★ **Easter Seals Southeastern
Pennsylvania**
**Delaware County Office**
468 N Middletown Rd.
Media, PA 19063
**Phone:** (610)565-2353  **Fax:** (610)565-5256
**Email:** philaess@libertynet.org
**Website:** http://www.easterseals-sepa.org
Jan Wright, Director

**Program(s):** Camping and recreation; continuing education; early education and care; early intervention; medical rehabilitation and health services; and support services.


★ 8405 ★ **Easter Seals Southeastern
Pennsylvania**
**Montgomery County Office**
1161 Forty Foot Rd.
Kulpsville, PA 19443
**Phone:** (215)368-7000  **Fax:** (215)368-1199
**Email:** philaess@libertynet.org
**Website:** http://www.easterseals-sepa.org
Carl Webster, Exec Director

**Program(s):** Camping and recreation; continuing education; early education and care; early intervention; medical rehabilitation and health services; school-aged children; and support services.


★ 8406 ★ **Easter Seals Southeastern
Pennsylvania**
**Philadelphia County Office**
3975 Conshohocken Ave.
Philadelphia, PA 19131-5484
**Phone:** (215)879-1000  **Fax:** (215)879-8424
**Email:** philaess@libertynet.org
Mr. Carl Webster, CEO & Pres
John Podgajny, Director

**Program(s):** Camping and recreation; continuing education; early education and care; medical rehabilitation and health services; school-aged children; and support services.


★ 8407 ★ **Easter Seals Western
Pennsylvania**
**Cambria-Somerset Division**
232 Walnut St.
Johnstown, PA 15901
**Phone:** (814)535-5508  **Fax:** (814)536-4943
**Website:** http://www.pa-ws.easter-seals.org
Lawrence P. Rager, Jr., CEO & Pres

**Program(s):** Early intervention; medical rehabilitation and health services; and support services.


★ 8408 ★ **Easter Seals Western
Pennsylvania**
**Cambria/Somerset Office**
571 Main St.
Somerset, PA 15501
**Phone:** (814)445-4834
**Website:** http://www.pa-ws.easter-seals.org
Lawrence P. Rager, Jr., CEO & Pres

**Program(s):** Medical rehabilitation and health services.


★ 8409 ★ **Easter Seals Western
Pennsylvania**
**Clarion/Jefferson Division**
103 N Gilpin St.
Punxsutawney, PA 15767
**Phone:** (814)938-6750  **Fax:** (814)938-9083
**Website:** http://www.pa-ws.easter-seals.org
Peg Swarm, Contact

**Program(s):** Early education and care; and job training and employment services.


★ 8410 ★ **Easter Seals Western
Pennsylvania**
**Fayette Division**
141 Oakland Ave.
Uniontown, PA 15401
**Phone:** (724)437-4047  **Fax:** (724)437-5485
Lawrence P. Rager, Jr., CEO & Pres

**Program(s):** Camping and recreation; medical rehabilitation and health services; and support services.


★ 8411 ★ **Easter Seals Western
Pennsylvania**
**Fayette Division**
c/o Greensboro Head Start
7 Glassworks Rd.
Greensboro, PA 15338
**Phone:** (724)437-4047  **Fax:** (724)437-5485
**Website:** http://www.pa-ws.easter-seals.org
Lawrence P. Rager, Jr., CEO & Pres

**Program(s):** Early education and care; and medical rehabilitation and health services.


★ 8412 ★ **Easter Seals Western
Pennsylvania**
**Pittsburgh Office**
632 Fort Duquesne Blvd.
Pittsburgh, PA 15222
**Phone:** (412)281-7244  **Free:** 800-587-3257
**Fax:** (412)281-9333
**Email:** toutrich@pa-ws.easter-seals.org
**Website:** http://www.pa-ws.easter-seals.org
Lawrence P. Rager, Jr., CEO & Pres
Tina L. Outrich, Vice President

**Program(s):** Adult and senior services; continuing education; early education and care; job training and employment services; medical rehabilitation and health services; school-aged children; and support services.


★ 8413 ★ **Easter Seals Western
Pennsylvania**
**Venago Division**
200 12th St.
Franklin, PA 16323-0231
**Phone:** (814)437-3071  **Fax:** (814)432-2269

**Email:** easterseals2@usachoice.net
**Website:** http://www.pa-ws.easter-seals.org
Lawrence P. Rager, Jr., CEO & Pres
Diana Griffith, Director
**Program(s):** Camping and recreation; early intervention; residential and housing services; and support services.

## Puerto Rico

### ★ 8414 ★ Easter Seals Puerto Rico
Calle Universidad 500
Urbanizacion Perez Morris
Hato Rey
San Juan, PR 00918
**Phone:** (787)767-6710          **Fax:** (787)758-0950
**Email:** nmorales@serpr.org
**Website:** http://www.pr.easter-seals.org
Mrs. Nilda M. Morales, Exec Director
**Program(s):** Adult and senior services; camping and recreation; early intervention; and residential and housing services.

## South Carolina

### ★ 8415 ★ Easter Seals South Carolina Anderson County Office
1104 Ella St.
Anderson, SC 29621
**Phone:** (864)225-1371          **Fax:** (864)225-2943
**Email:** essand@carol.net
**Website:** http://www.sc.easter-seals.org
Cecilia Page, Contact
**Program(s):** Early education and care; and support services.

### ★ 8416 ★ Easter Seals South Carolina Georgetown County Office
614 S Hazard St.
Georgetown, SC 29442
**Phone:** (843)546-2212          **Fax:** (843)545-5251
**Email:** eastergt@ftc.net
**Website:** http://www.sc.easter-seals.org
Richard S. Carter, CEO
**Program(s):** Support services.

### ★ 8417 ★ Easter Seals South Carolina Greenville County Office
1122 Rutherford Rd.
Greenville, SC 29609
**Phone:** (864)232-4185          **Fax:** (864)232-8161
**Website:** http://www.sc.easter-seals.org
Richard S. Carter, CEO
**Program(s):** Support services.

### ★ 8418 ★ Easter Seals South Carolina Greenwood County Office
118 W Alexander Ave.
Greenwood, SC 29648
**Phone:** (864)229-5428          **Fax:** (864)942-0553
**Website:** http://www.sc.easter-seals.org
Richard S. Carter, CEO
**Program(s):** Support services.

### ★ 8419 ★ Easter Seals South Carolina Pee Dee Office
119 S McQueen St.
Florence, SC 29501
**Phone:** (803)661-6909          **Fax:** (803)661-6905
**Website:** http://www.sc.easter-seals.org
Richard S. Carter, CEO
**Remarks:** Serves Darlington and Florence counties.
**Program(s):** Job training, employment services, and support services.

### ★ 8420 ★ Easter Seals South Carolina Spartanburg County
1004 S Pine St.
Spartanburg, SC 29302

**Phone:** (864)582-8050          **Fax:** (864)582-1156
**Website:** http://www.sc.easter-seals.org
Connie Rollins, Director
**Program(s):** Support services.

### ★ 8421 ★ Easter Seals South Carolina State Headquarters
3020 Farrow Rd.
Columbia, SC 29203-7099
**Phone:** (803)256-0735          **Free:** 800-951-4090
**Fax:** (803)765-9765
**Email:** tskelton@eastersc.org
**Website:** http://www.sc.easter-seals.org
Richard S Carter, CEO
**Program(s):** Support services.

### ★ 8422 ★ Easter Seals South Carolina Trident Office
4500 Leeds Ave., Ste. 202B
Charleston, SC 29405
**Phone:** (843)308-7391          **Fax:** (843)308-7392
**Email:** eastersc@scsn.net
**Website:** http://www.sc.easter-seals.org
Robyn Linnen, Contact
**Remarks:** Serves Berkley, Charleston, and Dorchester counties. **Program(s):** Support services.

## South Dakota

### ★ 8423 ★ Easter Seals South Dakota Eastern Regional Office
3801 S Western Ave., Ste. 106
Sioux Falls, SD 57105
**Phone:** (605)339-6969          **Fax:** (605)977-0640
**Email:** tanderson@sd.easter-seals.org
**Website:** http://www.essd.org
Ms. Pat Miller, CEO & Pres
Martin Hagemann, Contact
**Program(s):** Early education and care; school-aged children; and support services.

### ★ 8424 ★ Easter Seals South Dakota Pierre Office
1351 N Harrison Ave.
Pierre, SD 57501-2373
**Phone:** (605)224-5879          **Free:** 800-592-1852
**Fax:** (605)224-1033
**Email:** administrator@sd.easter-seals.org
**Website:** www.essd.org
Ms. Pat Miller, Contact
**Program(s):** Camping and recreation.

### ★ 8425 ★ Easter Seals South Dakota Western Regional Office
919 Main St., Ste. 203
Rapid City, SD 57702
**Phone:** (605)348-6459          **Fax:** (605)348-6459
**Email:** administrator@sd.easter-seals.org
**Website:** www.essd.org
Ms. Pat Miller, Contact
Ms. Lori Schreiner, Director
**Program(s):** Early education and care; school-aged children; and support services.

## Tennessee

### ★ 8426 ★ Easter Seals Tennessee
2001 Woodmont Blvd.
Nashville, TN 37215
**Phone:** (615)292-6640          **Free:** 800-264-0078
**Fax:** (615)292-7206
**Email:** kroder@eastersealstn.com
**Website:** http://www.tn-easter-seals.org
Jayne Perkins, CEO & Pres
Ms. Kathleen Roder, Contact
**Program(s):** Continuing education; medical rehabilitation and health services; school-aged children; and support services.

## Texas

### ★ 8427 ★ Easter Seals Central Texas
919 W 28-1/2 St.
Austin, TX 78705-3595
**Phone:** (512)478-2581          **Fax:** (512)476-1638
**Email:** smiller@eastersealstx.com
**Website:** http://www.eastersealstx.com
Sharon R. Miller, CEO & Pres
**Program(s):** Camping and recreation; early education and care; early intervention; job training and employment services; medical rehabilitation and health services; school-aged children; and support services.

### ★ 8428 ★ Easter Seals of Greater Dallas
3820 W Northwest Hwy., Ste. 100
Dallas, TX 75220
**Phone:** (972)394-8900          **Free:** 800-580-4718
**Fax:** (972)366-4209
**Email:** info@easterseals.com
**Website:** http://www.easterseals.com
Elizabeth Hart, CEO & Pres
**Program(s):** Medical rehabilitation and health services; and support services.

### ★ 8429 ★ Easter Seals Greater Northwest Texas
2100 Cicle Dr.
Fort Worth, TX 76119-8130
**Phone:** (817)536-8693          **Free:** 888-288-8324
**Fax:** (817)536-5214
**Email:** mail@easterseals-fw.org
**Website:** http://www.tx-nw.easter-seals.org
Ms. Francy Kragle, President
**Program(s):** Early intervention; medical rehabilitation and health services; and support services.

### ★ 8430 ★ Easter Seals Permian Basin
620 N Alleghany
Odessa, TX 79761
**Phone:** (915)332-8244          **Free:** 800-583-2404
**Fax:** (915)580-7428
**Email:** rehab@nwol.net
Tom Snoddy, Exec Director
**Program(s):** Early education and care; medical rehabilitation and health services; and support services.

### ★ 8431 ★ Easter Seals Rio Grande Valley Harlingen Office
1514 S 77 Sunshine Strip, Ste. 4
Harlingen, TX 78550
**Phone:** (956)423-9171          **Fax:** (956)423-7457
**Email:** prosenlund@easterseals-rgv.org
**Website:** http://www.easterseals-rgv.org
Deborah A. Paganelli, Exec Director
**Program(s):** Early intervention; medical rehabilitation and health services; and support services.

### ★ 8432 ★ Easter Seals Rio Grande Valley McAllen Office
1217 Houston St.
McAllen, TX 78501
**Phone:** (956)631-9171          **Free:** 800-728-5491
**Fax:** (956)631-7566
**Email:** prosenlund@easterseals-rgv.org
**Website:** http://www.easterseals-rgv.org
Deborah A. Paganelli, Exec Director
**Program(s):** Early education and care; early intervention; medical rehabilitation and health services; school-aged children; and support services.

### ★ 8433 ★ Easter Seals San Antonio
2203 Babcock Rd.
San Antonio, TX 78229-4498
**Phone:** (210)614-3911          **Fax:** (210)616-0443
Linda H. Tapia, Exec Director

**Program(s):** Medical rehabilitation and health services.

**★ 8434 ★ Easter Seals Texarkana, Texas**
1315 Walnut St.
Texarkana, TX 75501-4489
**Phone:** (903)794-2705        **Fax:** (903)793-1203
**Email:** temple@txk.com
Jerry Bedwell, President

**Program(s):** Adult and senior services; continuing education; early education and care; early intervention; medical rehabilitation and health services; school-aged children; and support services.

## Utah

**★ 8435 ★ Easter Seals Utah**
**Salt Lake City Office**
638 E Wilmington Ave.
Salt Lake City, UT 84106-1491
**Phone:** (801)486-3778        **Free:** 800-388-1991
**Fax:** (801)486-3123
**Email:** rstarley@easterealsutah.org
**Website:** http://www.ut.easter-seals.org
Richard O. Starley, President

**Program(s):** Adult and senior services; camping and recreation; early education and care; job training and employment services; school-aged children; and support services.

## Vermont

**★ 8436 ★ Easter Seals Rutland**
195 Stratton Rd.
Rutland, VT 05702
**Phone:** (802)775-4882
**Email:** mjohnso@eseals.org
**Website:** http://www.nh.easter-seals.org
Larry Gammon, CEO & Pres

**Program(s):** Residential and housing services; and school-aged children.

**★ 8437 ★ Easter Seals Vermont**
641 Comstock Rd., Ste. 1
Berlin, VT 05602
**Phone:** (802)223-4744        **Fax:** (802)229-0848
**Email:** mjohnso@eseals.org
**Website:** http://www.nh.easter-seals.org
Larry Gammon, CEO & Pres

**Program(s):** Early education and care; and school-aged children.

## Virginia

**★ 8438 ★ Easter Seals Central Virginia**
9291 Laurel Grove Rd., Ste. 2
Mechanicsville, VA 23116-2969
**Phone:** (804)746-1007        **Fax:** (804)746-9214
**Email:** essoc@aol.com
**Website:** http://www.va.easter-seals.org
Edward J. Hamilton, President
Jewel Cooke, Director

**Program(s):** Adult and senior services; and support services.

**★ 8439 ★ Easter Seals Northern Virginia**
6319 Castle Pl., Ste. A
Falls Church, VA 22044-1907
**Phone:** (703)538-4480        **Fax:** (703)237-0249
**Email:** jcooke@va.easter-seals.org
**Website:** http://www.va.easter-seals.org
Edward J. Hamilton, PhD, CEO & Pres

**Program(s):** Camping, recreation, and support services.

**★ 8440 ★ Easter Seals Virginia**
201 E Main St.
Salem, VA 24153
**Phone:** (540)777-7325        **Free:** 800-365-1656
**Fax:** (540)777-2194

**Email:** info@va.easter-seals.org
**Website:** http://www.va.easter-seals.org
Edward J. Hamilton, PhD, CEO & Pres

**Program(s):** Early intervention and support services.

## Washington

**★ 8441 ★ Easter Seals Washington**
1740 NE Riddell Rd., Ste. 315
Bremerton, WA 98310-3870
**Phone:** (360)373-2502        **Fax:** (360)373-5620
**Email:** spritchard@seals.org
**Website:** http://www.seals.org
Garry Wyckoff, CEO
Glenn LeDuc, Director

**Program(s):** Adult and senior services; job training and employment services.

**★ 8442 ★ Easter Seals Washington**
**State Office**
521 2nd Ave. W
Seattle, WA 98119-5998
**Phone:** (206)281-5700        **Fax:** (206)281-5700
**Email:** esw@seals.org
**Website:** http://www.seals.org
Gary Wyckoff, Contact
Cathy Bisaillon, Vice President

**Program(s):** Adult and senior services; camping and recreation; continuing education; early education and care; early intervention; job training and employment services; medical rehabilitation and health services; school-aged children; and support services.

## West Virginia

**★ 8443 ★ Easter Seals West Virginia**
1305 National Rd.
Wheeling, WV 26003-5780
**Phone:** (304)242-1390        **Free:** 800-677-1390
**Fax:** (304)243-5880
**Email:** mhon@wv-easter-seals.org
**Website:** http://www.wv.easter-seals.org
Martha Hon, CEO & Pres

**Program(s):** Camping and recreation; early education and care; early intervention; medical rehabilitation and health services; school-aged children; and support services.

## Wisconsin

**★ 8444 ★ Easter Seals Southeastern**
**Wisconsin**
3090 N 53rd St.
Milwaukee, WI 53210-1699
**Phone:** (414)449-4444        **Fax:** (414)449-4447
**Email:** tbiondo@wi-se.easter-seals.org
**Website:** http://www.wi-se.easter-seals.org
Tim Biondo, Exec Director

**Program(s):** Adult and senior services; camping and recreation; continuing education; early education and care; early intervention; medical rehabilitation and health services; school-aged children; and support services.

**★ 8445 ★ Easter Seals Wisconsin**
101 Nob Hill Rd., Ste. 301
Madison, WI 53713-3969
**Phone:** (608)277-8288        **Free:** 800-422-2324
**Fax:** (608)277-8333
**Email:** tpaprock@wi-easterseals.org
**Website:** www.wi-easterseals.org
Christine Fessler, CEO & Pres

**Program(s):** Camping and recreation; continuing education; early education and care; job training and employment services; school-aged children; and support services.

## Dyslexia

*State chapters of the International Dyslexia Association are listed below. The national office is located at*

*8600 LaSalle Rd., Chester Bldg., Ste. 382, Baltimore, MD 21286-2044. Additional information can be obtained by calling the national office at (800) ABCD-123, or by consulting their web site at http://www.interdys.org/.*

## Arizona

**★ 8446 ★ International Dyslexia**
**Association**
**Arizona Branch**
PO Box 6284
Scottsdale, AZ 85261-6284
**Phone:** (480)941-0308
**Website:** http://www.dyslexia-az.org
Dawn Gutierrez, President

**Remarks:** Also serves parts of Nevada.

## British Columbia

**★ 8447 ★ International Dyslexia**
**Association**
**British Columbia Branch**
1260 Hornby St., Ste. 104
Vancouver, BC, Canada V6Z 1W2
**Phone:** (604)669-5811        **Fax:** (604)669-5161
**Email:** idabcb@infoserve.net
Fran Thompson, President

**Remarks:** Also serves Alberta, Northwest Territories, Saskatchewan, and Yukon Territory.

## California

**★ 8448 ★ International Dyslexia**
**Association**
**Central California Branch**
4594 Michigan Ave.
Fresno, CA 93703
**Phone:** (559)251-9385        **Fax:** (559)252-1216
**Email:** dyslexias@attbi.com
**Website:** http://communitycalendar.centralvalley.com/566
Joy Moody, President

**Remarks:** Also serves parts of Nevada.

**★ 8449 ★ International Dyslexia**
**Association**
**Inland Empire Branch**
PO Box 6701
San Bernardino, CA 92412
**Phone:** (909)686-9837
**Website:** http://www.dyslexia-ca.org
Sandy Marzullo, President

**Remarks:** Also serves parts of Nevada.

**★ 8450 ★ International Dyslexia**
**Association**
**Los Angeles Branch**
4379 Tujunga Blvd.
Studio City, CA 91604
**Phone:** (818)506-8866
Barbara Shaub, President

**★ 8451 ★ International Dyslexia**
**Association**
**Northern California Branch**
PO Box 2618
Menlo Park, CA 94026
**Phone:** (650)328-7667        **Fax:** (650)325-3041
**Email:** cushen@itsa.ucsf.edu
**Website:** http://www.dyslexia-ncbida.org
Heidi Renner, President

**★ 8452 ★ International Dyslexia**
**Association**
**Orange County Branch**
1801 E Parkcourt Pl., Bldg. D, Ste. 101
Santa Ana, CA 92701
**Phone:** (714)564-0777        **Fax:** (714)564-0770

**Email:** info@dyslexiaoc.org
**Website:** http://www.dyslexiaoc.org
Joanne Sellers, President


★ **8453** ★ **International Dyslexia Association**
**San Diego Branch**
2515 Camino del Rio Dr., Ste. 111
San Diego, CA 92108
**Phone:** (619)295-3722
**Email:** pph@tfb.com
**Website:** http://www.dyslexiasd.org
Jose Cruz, President


## Colorado

★ **8454** ★ **International Dyslexia Association**
**Rocky Mountain Branch**
PO Box 3598
Boulder, CO 80307
**Phone:** (303)721-9425
Holly Graves, President
**Remarks:** Serves Colorado, Utah, and Wyoming.


## Florida

★ **8455** ★ **International Dyslexia Association**
**Florida Branch**
4141 Bayshore Blvd., Ste. 1701
Tampa, FL 33611
**Phone:** (813)281-3148
Sylvia O. Richardson, President
**Remarks:** Also serves Puerto Rico.


## Georgia

★ **8456** ★ **International Dyslexia Association**
**Georgia Branch**
1951 Greystone Rd. NW
Atlanta, GA 30318
**Phone:** (404)256-1232
**Email:** rdavis@schenck.org
**Website:** http://www.schenck.org
Rosalie Davis, President
**Remarks:** Also serves Alabama.


## Hawaii

★ **8457** ★ **International Dyslexia Association**
**Hawaii Branch**
PO Box 61610
Honolulu, HI 96839-1610
**Phone:** (808)538-7007　　　　**Fax:** (808)566-6837
**Email:** info@HIBIDA.org
**Website:** http://www.HIBIDA.org
Ron Yoshimoto, President
**Remarks:** Also serves American Samoa.


## Illinois

★ **8458** ★ **International Dyslexia Association**
**Illinois Branch**
751 Roosevelt Rd., Ste. 301
Glen Ellyn, IL 60137
**Phone:** (630)469-6900　　　　**Fax:** (630)469-6810
**Email:** ilbranch_ida@ameritech.net
Sue Grisko, President
**Remarks:** Also serves Missouri.


## Indiana

★ **8459** ★ **International Dyslexia Association**
**Indiana Branch**
1100 W 42nd St., Ste. 385
Indianapolis, IN 46208
**Phone:** (317)926-1450　　　　**Fax:** (317)927-9285
**Email:** inbofida@hotmail.com
Wayne LaMade, President


## Iowa

★ **8460** ★ **International Dyslexia Association**
**Iowa Branch**
1030 5th Ave., Ste. 1450
Cedar Rapids, IA 52403
**Phone:** (319)551-2851　　　　**Fax:** (319)365-1038
**Email:** sue_ida_ia@yahoo.com
Pat McGuire, President


## Louisiana

★ **8461** ★ **International Dyslexia Association**
**Louisiana Branch**
410 N Hazel
Hammond, LA 70401
**Phone:** (504)876-0034　　　　**Free:** 888-323-0332
**Fax:** (504)448-4423
Carolyn Blackwood, President
**Remarks:** Also serves Missouri.


## Maryland

★ **8462** ★ **International Dyslexia Association**
**Maryland Branch**
PO Box 792
Brooklandville, MD 21022
**Phone:** (410)825-2881
Jean-Fryer Schedler, President


## Massachusetts

★ **8463** ★ **International Dyslexia Association**
**Massachusetts Branch**
PO Box 662
Lincoln, MA 01773
Mary Ann Bonneau, President
**Remarks:** Serves Maine, New Hampshire, Vermont, Massachusetts, Rhode Island, Connecticut, and eastern Canada.


## Michigan

★ **8464** ★ **International Dyslexia Association**
**Michigan Branch**
4050 Waverly Pl.
Ann Arbor, MI 48105
**Phone:** (734)663-9884
**Email:** postmaster@idamib.org
**Website:** http://www.idamib.org
Sally Burden, President


## Minnesota

★ **8465** ★ **International Dyslexia Association**
**Upper Midwest Branch**
PMB 159
5021 Vernon Ave.
Minneapolis, MN 55436
**Phone:** (651)450-7589
Sarah Sevcik, President
**Remarks:** Also serves North Dakota, South Dakota, and Manitoba, Canada.


## Missouri

★ **8466** ★ **International Dyslexia Association**
**Kansas/Western Missouri Branch**
7713 Quail Ridge Ct.
Parkville, MO 64152
**Phone:** (816)587-3240
**Email:** wolfden@jc.net
Lorrie Wolf, President
**Remarks:** Also serves Oklahoma.


## Nebraska

★ **8467** ★ **International Dyslexia Association**
**Nebraska Branch**
6111 S 32nd St.
Lincoln, NE 68516
**Phone:** (402)434-6434
**Email:** gcarlson@lps.org
**Website:** http://www.lps.org
Gwelda Carlson, President


## New Hampshire

★ **8468** ★ **International Dyslexia Association**
**New Hampshire Branch**
PO Box 3724
Concord, NH 03302
**Phone:** (603)229-7355
Mike Angwin, President


## New Jersey

★ **8469** ★ **International Dyslexia Association**
**New Jersey Branch**
PO Box 32
Long Valley, NJ 07853
**Phone:** (908)879-0466　　　　**Fax:** (908)879-0466
David Katz, President


## New Mexico

★ **8470** ★ **International Dyslexia Association**
**Southwest Branch**
PO Box 25891
Albuquerque, NM 87125
**Phone:** (505)255-8234　　　　**Fax:** (505)262-8547
**Email:** swida84@hotmail.com
Mary Gilroy, President


## New York

★ **8471** ★ **International Dyslexia Association**
**Buffalo Branch**
c/o Gow School
Emory Rd.
South Wales, NY 14139
**Phone:** (716)687-2030
**Email:** bufida@gow.org
Kathy Rose, President
**Remarks:** Also serves Ontario, Canada.


★ **8472** ★ **International Dyslexia Association**
**New York Branch**
71 W 23rd St., Ste. 1527
New York, NY 10010
**Phone:** (212)691-1930　　　　**Fax:** (212)633-1620
**Email:** info@nybida.org
**Website:** http://www.nybida.org
Judith R. Birsh, President

★ 8473 ★ **International Dyslexia Association**
**Suffolk Branch**
728 Route 25A
Northport, NY 11768
**Phone:** (631)423-7834        **Fax:** (631)423-7834
**Email:** ckent@optonline.net
Carol Kent, President

## North Carolina

★ 8474 ★ **International Dyslexia Association**
**North Carolina Branch**
184-D2 Mountain Club Dr.
Vilas, NC 28692
**Phone:** (252)243-8843
**Email:** tommcd@boone.net
Tom McDonough, President

## Ohio

★ 8475 ★ **International Dyslexia Association**
**Central Ohio Branch**
PO Box 16216
Columbus, OH 43216-6216
**Phone:** (614)899-5711
**Email:** abc@columbus.rr.com
Cameron James, President

★ 8476 ★ **International Dyslexia Association**
**Northern Ohio Branch**
34750 Ada Dr.
Solon, OH 44139-5808
**Phone:** (216)556-0883
Karen Lieberman, President

★ 8477 ★ **International Dyslexia Association**
**Ohio Valley Branch**
317 E 5th St.
Cincinnati, OH 45202
**Phone:** (513)651-4747
Carol Greiser, President
**Remarks:** Serves Ohio and Kentucky.

## Oregon

★ 8478 ★ **International Dyslexia Association**
**Oregon Branch**
PO Box 3677
Portland, OR 97208-3677
**Phone:** (503)228-4455        **Free:** 800-530-2234
**Fax:** (503)228-3152
**Email:** orbida@aracnet.com
**Website:** http://www.aracnet.com/~orbida/
Betsy Ramsey, President

## Pennsylvania

★ 8479 ★ **International Dyslexia Association**
**Philadelphia Branch**
PO Box 251
Bryn Mawr, PA 19010
**Phone:** (610)527-1548        **Fax:** (610)527-5011
**Email:** dyslexia@libertynet.org
**Website:** http://www.gpbida.org
Marianne Cook, President
**Remarks:** Also serves Delaware.

## South Carolina

★ 8480 ★ **International Dyslexia Association**
**South Carolina Branch**
1500 Hallbrook Dr.
Columbia, SC 29209
**Phone:** (803)772-8065
**Email:** a.s.lawrence@worldnet.att.net
Amy Lawrence, President

## Tennessee

★ 8481 ★ **International Dyslexia Association**
**Tennessee Branch**
6525 Brownlee Dr.
Nashville, TN 37205
**Free:** 877-TENN-IDA
Susan Smartt, President
**Remarks:** Also serves Kentucky.

## Texas

★ 8482 ★ **International Dyslexia Association**
**Austin Branch**
Del Valle Junior High School
5500 Ross St.
Del Valle, TX 78617
**Phone:** (512)452-7658
**Website:** http://home.austin.rr.com/aabida/
Sharon Roberts, President

★ 8483 ★ **International Dyslexia Association**
**Dallas Branch**
13140 Coit Rd., Ste. 320
LB 120
Dallas, TX 75240
**Phone:** (972)233-9107        **Fax:** (972)490-4219
Leigh Miller, President
**Remarks:** Also serves Arkansas and Oklahoma.

★ 8484 ★ **International Dyslexia Association**
**Houston Branch**
PO Box 540504
Houston, TX 77254-0504
**Phone:** (713)529-1975
**Email:** cwills@briarwoodschool.org
Carole Wills, President

## Virginia

★ 8485 ★ **International Dyslexia Association**
**DC Capital Branch**
4914 Reservoir Heights Ave.
Alexandria, VA 22311
**Phone:** (703)827-9019
Ruth Tifford, President
**Remarks:** Serves Washington DC and parts of Maryland, Virginia, and West Virginia.

★ 8486 ★ **International Dyslexia Association**
**Virginia Branch**
PO Box 23226
Richmond, VA 23226
**Free:** 800-988-8336
**Email:** vbida@hotmail.com
Rebecca Hurrell Aldred, President
**Remarks:** Also serves West Virginia.

## Washington

★ 8487 ★ **International Dyslexia Association**
**Washington State Branch**
PO Box 7192
Seattle, WA 98133
**Phone:** (206)382-1020
**Website:** http://www.wabida.org
Pat Morton, President
**Remarks:** Also serves Alaska, Idaho, and Montana.

## Wisconsin

★ 8488 ★ **International Dyslexia Association**
**Wisconsin Branch**
2002 N Cambridge Ave.
Milwaukee, WI 53202
**Phone:** (414)299-0551
**Email:** lorej@nconnect.net
**Website:** http://www.wis-dys.org
Jan Lorenzen, President

## Learning Disabilities

*Listed below are state offices of the Learning Disabilities Association of America, 4156 Library Rd., Pittsburgh, PA 15234-1349, (412)341-1515, http://www.ldanatl.org/.*

## Alabama

★ 8489 ★ **Learning Disabilities Association of Alabama**
PO Box 11588
Montgomery, AL 36111
**Phone:** (334)277-9151
**Email:** alabama@ldaal.org
**Website:** http://www.ldaal.org

## Arizona

★ 8490 ★ **Learning Disabilities Association of Arizona**
13106 W Limewood Ave.
Sun City West, AZ 85375
**Phone:** (623)975-4551
**Email:** dcrawford_1@msn.com
**Website:** http://www.ldanatl.org/Affiliates/Az/welcome.htm

## Arkansas

★ 8491 ★ **Learning Disabilities Association of Arkansas**
7509 Cantrell, Ste. 103C
Little Rock, AR 72207
**Phone:** (501)666-8777        **Fax:** (501)666-4070
**Website:** http://www.ldaarkansas.org

## California

★ 8492 ★ **Learning Disabilities Association of California**
PO Box 601067
Sacramento, CA 95860-1067
**Phone:** (916)725-7881        **Free:** (866)532-6322
**Fax:** (916)725-8786
**Email:** office@ldaca.org
**Website:** http://www.ldaca.org

★ 8493 ★ **Learning Disabilities Association San Diego**
3550 Kearny Villa Rd., Ste. 222
San Diego, CA 92123
**Phone:** (858)467-9158        **Fax:** (858)467-1333
**Website:** http://www.LDASanDiego.org/

**★ 8494 ★ Sacramento Learning Disabilities Association**
PO Box 276645
Sacramento, CA 95827
**Phone:** (530)672-3145
**Website:** http://www.SacramentoLDA.org/

## Colorado

**★ 8495 ★ Learning Disabilities Association of Colorado**
4500 E Iliff Ave.
Denver, CO 80222
**Phone:** (303)894-0992        **Fax:** (303)830-1645
**Email:** info@ldacolorado.com
**Website:** http://www.ldacolorado.com

## Connecticut

**★ 8496 ★ Learning Disabilities Association of Connecticut**
999 Asylum Ave.
Hartford, CT 06105
**Phone:** (860)560-1711        **Fax:** (860)560-1750
**Email:** ldact@juno.com
**Website:** http://www.ldanatl.org/Affiliates/CT/LDAof-Connecticut.html

## Florida

**★ 8497 ★ Learning Disabilities Association of Florida**
331 E Henry St.
Punta Gorda, FL 33950
**Phone:** (941)637-8957        **Fax:** (941)637-0617
**Email:** ldaf00@sunline.net
**Website:** http://www.ldafl.org/
**Frmly:** Florida ACLD.

## Georgia

**★ 8498 ★ Learning Disabilities Association of Georgia**
PO Box 1337
Roswell, GA 30077
**Phone:** (678)461-4471        **Fax:** (678)461-4472
**Email:** services@ldag.org
**Website:** http://www.ldag.org/

## Hawaii

**★ 8499 ★ Learning Disabilities Association of Hawaii**
200 N Vineyard Blvd., Ste. 310
Honolulu, HI 96817
**Phone:** (808)536-9684        **Free:** 800-533-9684
**Fax:** (808)537-6780
**Email:** ldah@gte.net
**Website:** http://www.ldanatl.org/Hawaii/ldah.html

## Illinois

**★ 8500 ★ Learning Disabilities Association of Illinois**
10101 S Roberts Rd., Ste. 106
Palos Hills, IL 60465
**Phone:** (708)430-7532        **Fax:** (708)430-7592
**Email:** JanetLerner@juno.com
**Website:** http://www.ldanatl.org/Affiliates/IL/index.htm
Bev Johns, President

## Indiana

**★ 8501 ★ Learning Disabilities Association of Indiana**
PO Box 20584
Indianapolis, IN 46220
**Free:** 800-284-2519
**Email:** bluhrig@inct.net
**Website:** http://www.inct.net/~bluhrig/

## Kansas

**★ 8502 ★ Learning Disabilities Association of Kansas**
PO Box 4424
Topeka, KS 66604
**Phone:** (913)272-0033
**Website:** http://www.ldakansas.org/

## Kentucky

**★ 8503 ★ Learning Disabilities Association of Kentucky**
2210 Goldsmith Lane, No. 222
Louisville, KY 40218
**Phone:** (502)473-1256        **Free:** 877-587-1256
**Fax:** (502)473-4695
**Email:** LDAofKY@aol.com
**Website:** http://www.ldaofky.org/

## Maine

**★ 8504 ★ Learning Disabilities Association of Maine**
PO Box 67
Oakland, ME 04963
**Phone:** (207)465-7700        **Fax:** (207)873-4146
**Email:** ldame@ldame.org
**Website:** http://www.ldame.org/

## Maryland

**★ 8505 ★ Learning Disabilities Association of Maryland**
PO Box 526
Bowie, MD 20718-0526
**Free:** 800-673-6777        **Fax:** (410)337-3702
**Website:** http://www.ldanatl.org/Affiliates/MD/md.htm

## Massachusetts

**★ 8506 ★ Learning Disabilities Association of Massachusetts**
1275 Main St.
Waltham, MA 02451
**Phone:** (781)891-5009        **Fax:** (781)647-5141
**Website:** http://www.ldam.org/

## Michigan

**★ 8507 ★ Learning Disabilities Association of Michigan**
200 Museum Dr., Ste. 101
Lansing, MI 48933
**Phone:** (517)485-8160

## Mississippi

**★ 8508 ★ Learning Disabilities Association of Mississippi**
PO Box 4477
4080 Old Canton Rd.
Jackson, MS 39216
**Phone:** (601)362-1667        **Fax:** (601)362-9180
**Email:** ldams@bellsouth.net
**Website:** http://www.ldams.org

## Missouri

**★ 8509 ★ Learning Disabilities Association of Missouri**
PO Box 3303
1942 E Meadowmere, No. 104
Springfield, MO 65808
**Phone:** (417)864-5110        **Fax:** (417)864-7290
**Email:** ldamo@cland.net
**Website:** http://www.ldamo.org

**★ 8510 ★ Learning Disabilities Association of the Ozarks**
PO Box 4362
Springfield, MO 65808
**Phone:** (417)882-2008
**Website:**        http://www.ldaozarks.com/HOME_PAGEx.html

**★ 8511 ★ St. Louis Learning Disabilities Association**
10702 Manchester, Ste. 7
Saint Louis, MO 63122
**Phone:** (314)966-3088        **Fax:** (314)966-1806
**Email:** stloulda@mindspring.com
**Website:** http://www.ldastl.org/

## Nebraska

**★ 8512 ★ Learning Disabilities Association of Nebraska**
PO Box 6464
Omaha, NE 68106

## New Jersey

**★ 8513 ★ Learning Disabilities Association of New Jersey**
PO Box 401
Old Bridge, NJ 08857-0401
**Phone:** (732)360-0399

## New Mexico

**★ 8514 ★ Learning Disabilities Association of New Mexico**
6301 Menaul Blvd. NE, No. 556
Albuquerque, NM 87110-3323
**Phone:** (505)821-2545
**Email:** bp@peavler.com
**Website:** http://www.vivanewmexico.com/nmlda/

## New York

**★ 8515 ★ Learning Disabilities Association of Central New York**
722 W Manlius St.
East Syracuse, NY 13057
**Phone:** (315)432-0665        **Free:** 800-253-2269
**Fax:** (315)431-0606
**Email:** LDACNY@LDACNY.org
**Website:** http://www.ldacny.org

**★ 8516 ★ Learning Disabilities Association of the Genesee Valley**
339 East Ave.
Rochester, NY 14604
**Phone:** (716)263-3323
**Website:** http://www.ldagvi.org/

**★ 8517 ★ Learning Disabilities Association of the Mohawk Valley**
401 Columbia St.
Utica, NY 13502-3413
**Phone:** (315)797-1253        **Fax:** (315)797-4006
**Website:** http://www.ldalearningcenter.org/

**★ 8518 ★ Learning Disabilities Association of Nassau and Suffolk**
PO Box 461
Massapequa Park, NY 11762
**Phone:** (631)242-8943
**Email:** info@ldans.org
**Website:** http://www.ldans.org/

**★ 8519 ★ Learning Disabilities Association of New York**
27 W 20th St., Ste. 303
New York, NY 10011
**Phone:** (212)645-6730        **Fax:** (212)924-8896

**★ 8520 ★ Learning Disabilities Association of New York City**
27 W 20th St., Ste. 303
New York, NY 10011
**Phone:** (212)645-6730    **Fax:** (212)924-8896
**Website:** http://www.learningdisabilitynyc.org

**★ 8521 ★ Learning Disabilities Association of New York City, Inc.**
27 W 20th St., Ste. 303
New York, NY 10011
**Phone:** (212)645-6730    **Fax:** (212)924-8896
**Email:** helplineldanyc@earthlink.net

**★ 8522 ★ Learning Disabilities Association of Western New York**
2555 Elmwood Ave.
Kenmore, NY 14217
**Phone:** (716)874-7200    **Fax:** (716)874-7205
**Email:** LDAofWNY@aol.com
**Website:** http://members.aol.com/ldaofwny/home.html

## North Carolina

**★ 8523 ★ Learning Disabilities Association of North Carolina**
PO Box 3542
Chapel Hill, NC 27515-3542
**Phone:** (919)493-5362    **Fax:** (919)489-0788
**Email:** ldanc@mindspring.com
**Website:** http://www.ldanc.org/

## Oklahoma

**★ 8524 ★ Learning Disabilities Association of Oklahoma**
PO Box 1134
Jenks, OK 74037
**Free:** 800-532-6365
**Email:** ldao@fullnet.net

## Pennsylvania

**★ 8525 ★ Learning Disabilities Association of America**
4156 Library Rd.
Pittsburgh, PA 15234-1349
**Phone:** (412)341-1515    **Fax:** (412)344-0224
**Email:** info@ldaamerica.org
**Website:** http://www.ldaamerica.org

**★ 8526 ★ Learning Disabilities Association of Pennsylvania**
Toomey Bldg., Box 208
Uwchland, PA 19480
**Phone:** (610)458-8193

**★ 8527 ★ Learning Disabilities Association of Pennsylvania**
Toomey Bldg., Box 208
Uwchland, PA 19480
**Phone:** (610)458-8193
Anna Mary McHugh, President
Lynn Reinhold, Vice President

## Rhode Island

**★ 8528 ★ Rhode Island Learning Disabilities Association**
PO Box 8128
Cranston, RI 02920
**Email:** lindixx@email.com
**Website:** http://www.worldville.com/lifestyles/ldari/

## South Dakota

**★ 8529 ★ Learning Disabilities Association of South Dakota**
PO Box 9760
Rapid City, SD 57709
**Phone:** (605)342-4320    **Free:** 888-388-5553
**Email:** dthom@rapidnet.com
**Website:** http://ldasd.rapidnet.com/

## Texas

**★ 8530 ★ Learning Disabilities Association of Texas**
1011 W 31st St.
Austin, TX 78705
**Phone:** (512)458-8234    **Free:** 800-604-7500
**Fax:** (512)458-3826
**Email:** LDATexas@cs.com
**Website:** http://ourworld.compuserve.com/homepages/LDAT/

## Utah

**★ 8531 ★ Learning Disabilities Association of Utah**
309 East 100 South, Ste. 2
PO Box 651052
Salt Lake City, UT 84165-1052
**Phone:** (801)363-6320    **Fax:** (801)363-6332

**Email:** LDAU@ldau.org
**Website:** http://www.ldau.org/

## Vermont

**★ 8532 ★ Learning Disabilities Association of Vermont**
PO Box 1041
Manchester Center, VT 05255
**Phone:** (802)362-3127    **Fax:** (802)362-3128

## Virginia

**★ 8533 ★ Learning Disabilities Association of Virginia**
Randolph Towers, No. 505
4100 N 9th St.
Arlington, VA 22203
**Phone:** (703)243-2614    **Fax:** (703)243-0894
**Email:** info@ldavirginia.org
**Website:** http://www.ldavirginia.org/index.html

## Washington

**★ 8534 ★ Learning Disabilities Association of Washington**
7819 159th Pl., NE
Redmond, WA 98052
**Phone:** (425)882-0820    **Fax:** (425)861-4642
**Email:** info@ldawa.org
**Website:** http://www.ldawa.org

## West Virginia

**★ 8535 ★ West Virginia Learning Disabilities Association, Inc.**
4726 Teays Valley Rd.
Scott Depot, WV 25560
**Phone:** (304)755-0347
**Email:** wvlda@hotmail.com
**Frmly:** Learning Disabilities Association of West Virginia.

## Wisconsin

**★ 8536 ★ Learning Disabilities Association of Wisconsin**
1446 Baytree Ln.
Neenah, WI 54956
**Phone:** (920)720-5755    **Free:** 888-590-4141
**Email:** ldawisconsin@hotmail.com
**Website:** http://www.njsd.org/lda

# Chapter 22
# Emergency Medicine

## Foundations & Other Funding Organizations

### Private Foundations

**★ 8537 ★ Camille and Henry Dreyfus Foundation**
555 Madison Ave., Ste. 1305
New York, NY 10022-3301
**Phone:** (212)753-1760 **Fax:** (212)593-2256
**Email:** admin@drefus.org
**Website:** http://www.dreyfus.org
Dr. Robert Lichter, Executive Director
**Fnded:** 1946. **Philosophy:** The foundation's goal is to "advance the science of chemistry, chemical engineering, and related sciences as a means of improving human relations and circumstances around the world." To reflect this philosophy, the foundation offers funding through seven programs: Camille Dreyfus Teacher-Scholar Awards, Henry Dreyfus Teacher-Scholar Awards, New Faculty Awards, Faculty Start-up Grants for Undergraduate Institutions, Scholar/Fellow Program for Undergraduate Institutions, Special Grant Program in the Chemical Sciences, and the Postdoctoral Program in Environmental Science. The Camille Dreyfus Teacher-Scholar Awards Program focuses primarily on individual research attainment and promise, with the expectation that the nominee will demonstrate a commitment to education as well; the Henry Dreyfus Teacher-Scholar Awards Program stresses teaching, mentorship, and the nominee's accomplishments as a role model for undergraduates planning careers in the chemical sciences. The Camille and Henry Dreyfus New Faculty Award Program offers starter grants in research for newly appointed faculty members at graduate institutions just prior to their first year of teaching. Candidates are nominated by their respective institutions, and each institution is limited to one nomination. The Camille and Henry Dreyfus Faculty Start-up Grants for Undergraduate Institutions began in 1993. The program aims to provide funding for new faculty members in the chemical sciences at the start of their research and teaching activities. An unrestricted grant of $12,500 is awarded in September of the year the new faculty member formally begins the first year appointment, in order to encourage new faculty to begin the teaching-research interplay as early as possible in their careers. The Special Grant Program in Chemical Sciences supports innovative ways to advance the chemical sciences, primarily by enhancement of academic curricula and of presentation of chemistry to the public. The Scholar/Fellow Program for Undergraduate Institutions aims to encourage teaching and research in undergraduate colleges. The program is designed to attract talented Ph.D. recipients to careers in undergraduate education and to recognize outstanding research accomplishments or potential among established undergraduate faculty. The Postdoctoral Program in Environmental Chemistry was established in 1996. This program encourages experts in the field of environmental science to submit proposals for the training of Ph.D. chemists and chemical engineers in research

activities related to chemistry and the environment. This award is granted annually to five institutions and the total of the each grant is $90,0000. **Priorities:** *Education:* 100%. Support directed toward the chemical sciences. The foundation focuses its funding on established award programs in colleges and universities. *Note:* Total contributions made in 2000. **Typ. Recipients:** Emergency/Ambulance Services, Medical Research. **Geo. Dist:** nationally.

**★ 8538 ★ Cannon Foundation**
57 Union St. South
Concord, NC 28025-0548
**Phone:** (704)786-8216
Dan Gray, Executive Director
**Fnded:** 1996. **Typ. Recipients:** AIDS/HIV, Emergency/Ambulance Services, Hospitals, Mental Health. **Geo. Dist:** NC.

**Chisholm Foundation**
*See:* Entry 125

**Elizabeth Morse Genius Charitable Trust**
*See:* Entry 10043

**F. B. Heron Foundation**
*See:* Entry 5466

**Frances and Benjamin Benenson Foundation**
*See:* Entry 253

**★ 8539 ★ Jack N. and Lilyan Mandel Foundation**
2829 Euclid Ave.
Cleveland, OH 44115
**Phone:** (216)875-6500
**Website:** http://www.heronfdn.org
Jack Mandel, Trustee
**Fnded:** 1963. **Priorities:** *Arts & Humanities:* Less than 1%. *Civic & Public Affairs:* 93%. Major support for Mandel Supporting Foundations. *Education:* 1%. *Environment:* Less than 1%. *International:* Less than 1%. *Note:* Total contributions made in 1999. **Typ. Recipients:** AIDS/HIV, Alzheimers Disease, Children's Health/Hospitals, Clinics/Medical Centers, Diabetes, Emergency/Ambulance Services, Eyes/Blindness, Geriatric Health, Heart, Multiple Sclerosis, People with Disabilities, Public Health, Single-Disease Health Associations. **Geo. Dist:** OH.

**★ 8540 ★ James L. Stamps Foundation**
2000 E Fourth St., Ste. 230
Santa Ana, CA 92705
**Phone:** (714)568-9740 **Fax:** (714)568-9754
Delores Boutault, Manager
**Fnded:** 1963. **Philosophy:** The Stamps Foundation primarily supports Christian religious organizations and Christian-based education. Churches, fellowships, and conferences along with seminaries and bible

schools account for most of the foundation's interests. Support to social services is based on a religious outlook. **Priorities:** *Arts & Humanities:* 10%. Funds libraries. *Civic & Public Affairs:* 1%. Supports outreach centers. *Education:* 46%. Primary support for Christian colleges and universities and scholarships. *Environment:* 6%. Supports camps, seniorior citizen organizations and food banks. *Note:* Total contributions made in 1999. **Typ. Recipients:** Clinics/Medical Centers, Emergency/Ambulance Services, Public Health. **Geo. Dist:** CA, Southern California.

**★ 8541 ★ Jeffris Family Foundation**
PO Box 650
Janesville, WI 53547-0650
**Phone:** (608)757-1039 **Fax:** (608)754-7248
Thomas Jeffris, President & Director
**Fnded:** 1977. **Philosophy:** The foundation typically supports historic preservation projects and community and urban affairs programs. **Priorities:** *Arts & Humanities:* 47%. Supports historic preservation and historical societies. *Civic & Public Affairs:* 53%. Municipalities are funded. *Note:* Total contributions made in 2000. **Typ. Recipients:** Emergency/Ambulance Services. **Geo. Dist:** WI.

**★ 8542 ★ Joyce Foundation**
3 First National Plaza
70 West Madison St., Ste. 2750
Chicago, IL 60602
**Phone:** (312)782-2464 **Fax:** (312)782-4160
**Email:** info@joycefdn.org
**Website:** http://www.joycefdn.org
Ellen Alberding, President
**Fnded:** 1948. **Philosophy:** "The Joyce Foundation supports efforts to protect the natural environment of the Great Lakes to reduce poverty and nonviolence in the region, and to ensure that its people have access to good schools, decent jobs, and a diverse and thriving culture." It is especially interested in improving public policies, because public systems such as education and welfare directly affect the lives of so many people, and because public policies help shape private sector decisions about jobs, the environment, and the health of our communities. To ensure that public policies truly reflect public rather than private interests, the foundation supports efforts to reform the system of financing election campaigns. 1998 Annual Report. **Priorities:** *Arts & Humanities:* 3%. Supports museums, theater, and music organizations. *Civic & Public Affairs:* 37%. Funds employment, policies to prevent gun violence, and money and poli tics initiatives. *Education:* 26%. Supports organizations promoting education reform, minority education, and colleges and universities. *Note:* Total contributions made in 1999. **Typ. Recipients:** Emergency/Ambulance Services, Health Policy/Cost Containment, Medical Education. **Geo. Dist:** IL; Chicago, IL; IN; IA; MI; MN; OH; WI.

**★ 8543 ★ Kreielsheimer Foundation**
10 Harrison St., Ste. 302
Seattle, WA 98109

**Phone:** (206)284-7461          **Fax:** (206)442-7911
Donald Johnson, Trustee

**Fnded:** 1979. **Philosophy:** Trustees of the foundation are authorized to fund a wide range of organizations, with preference given to cultural and educational institutions. "While Mr. and Mrs. Kreielsheimer were very conscious of the need for financial support for many social programs, they elected that the bulk of the foundation funds be distributed to cultural and educational institutions and programs." The foundation looks for programs with value to their community and the possibility of wider future support. and the possibility of wider future support. **Priorities:** *Arts & Humanities:* About 85%. Supports theaters, opera, symphonies, museums, ballet, and arts associations. *Education:* 11%. Emphasis on arts education. *Religion:* 4%. Grant to Pacific Science Center. *Note:* Total contributions made in fiscal 1997. **Typ. Recipients:** Emergency/ Ambulance Services. **Geo. Dist:** AK; WA.

**Lincy Foundation**
*See:* Entry 470

**Maurice Amado Foundation**
*See:* Entry 520

**Powell Foundation**
*See:* Entry 5469

**Robert W. Wilson Foundation**
*See:* Entry 13519

**Teagle Foundation**
*See:* Entry 716

**★ 8544 ★ Town Creek Foundation**
PO Box 159
Oxford, MD 21654
**Phone:** (410)226-5315          **Fax:** (410)226-5468
**Email:** towncrk@dmv.com
**Website:** http://www.towncreekfdn.org
Christine Shelton, Executive Director

**Fnded:** 1981. **Philosophy:** The Town Creek Foundation makes grants in the areas of conservation and the environment, public broadcasting, and the search for a peaceful and democratic society. Funding is also available for the improvement of economic and social conditions in Talbot County, Maryland, and its communities. The foundation no longer supports international efforts. Primary focus is on organizations dedicated to action and advocacy. **Priorities:** *Arts & Humanities:* 4%. Supports public broadcasting. *Civic & Public Affairs:* 7%. Supports public policy organizations, social research, and Talbot County organizations. *Education:* 3%. Supports education funds. *Note:* Total contributions made in 1999. **Typ. Recipients:** Emergency/Ambulance Services, Public Health, Respiratory. **Geo. Dist:** nationally; statewide or large regions; MD.

## Corporate Foundations

**Ameren Corp. Charitable Trust**
*See:* Entry 821

**★ 8545 ★ American Standard Foundation**
One Centennial Ave.
Piscataway, NJ 08855-6820
**Phone:** (732)980-6000          **Fax:** (732)980-6121
**Email:** ocowan@ameren.com
**Website:** http://www.ameren.com

**Priorities:** *Civic & Public Affairs:* 10%. Supports and employment and economic policy, affordable housing, and legal foundations. *Education:* 10%. Funds scholarship, fellowship, and an education foundation. *Environment:* 72%. Primarily supports the United Way. *Note:* Total contributions made in 1999. **Typ. Recipients:** Emergency/Ambulance Services. **Geo. Dist:** headquarters and operating communities.

**★ 8546 ★ Ameritech Foundation**
30 South Wacker Dr., 34th Floor
Chicago, IL 60606
**Phone:** (312)750-5037
Michael Kuhlin, Senior Director, Corporate
    Contributions

**Fnded:** 1984. **Priorities:** *Arts & Humanities:* 10%. Priority is given to: projects and programs that are rich in cultural diversity, provide broad educational experiences and enhance the economic vitality where Ameritech has a significant business presence; exhibits, events and performances on a selected and limited basis, and all with a strong educational component; and title sponsorships. *Civic & Public Affairs:* 36%. Priority is given to: projects which stimulate urban renewal in partnership with key civic and community leaders and organizations; initiatives which address crime prevention and safety issues; programs that address environmental issues where company's outputs impact community needs and interest–e.g., recycling phone directories, cable, computer, telecommuting; projects which advance diversity, affirmative action and equal employment access; and a limited number of public policy organizations that address telecommunications, economic development, and regulation. *Education:* 38%. Higher education priorities are: staffing and programs that advance state-of-the-art telecommunications technologies and their applications on campuses; faculty training programs for utilizing technology in the classroom; research, training and innovative applications of communications technologies; public policy that contributes to the understanding of communications and technology; and programs for colleges to attract and retain minority faculty and students. Elementary and secondary education priorities are: reading and economic literacy programs as basic educational needs; programs that help school administrators and teachers understand the use of telecommunications technologies; initiatives which encourage professional development for teachers to incorporate communications technologies into the classroom; programs that recognize and reward teachers who apply telecommunications technologies in teaching and learning; and alliances among schools to introduce new telecommunications technologies where it would otherwise be unaffordable. *Environment:* 8%. *International:* 27%. Majority of funding goes to United Ways in operating locations. Among other health and human service agencies, priority is given to: human service organizations that work collaboratively with educational and/or health institutions on clearly defined community needs; nonprofits that help seniors, the disabled and other health-related groups for programs that enhance the quality of life through the deployment of advanced telecommunications technologies; disaster relief efforts on a case-by-case basis; Special Olympics; and hospitals in limited, targeted, and proactive ways, to advance innovative uses of telecommunications technologies in measurable ways other health care providers can benefit from or emulate. *Religion:* 7%. *Note:* Total contributions in 1998. **Typ. Recipients:** Emergency/Ambulance Services, Medical Rehabilitation, People with Disabilities. **Geo. Dist:** headquarters and operating communities; IL; IN; MI; MO; OH; WI.

**Aristech Foundation**
*See:* Entry 848

**BankAtlantic Foundation**
*See:* Entry 5470

**Bassett Furniture Industries Foundation**
*See:* Entry 875

**Bechtel Foundation**
*See:* Entry 10059

**Binney & Smith Inc.**
*See:* Entry 887

**The Boeing Co. Charitable Trust**
*See:* Entry 5472

**★ 8547 ★ Boise Cascade Corp.**
1111 West Jefferson St.
PO Box 50
Boise, ID 83728-0001
**Phone:** (208)384-7673          **Fax:** (208)384-7224
**Email:** mvoden@binney-smith.com
**Website:** http://www.bc.com
Connie Weaver, Manager,Community Relations

**Typ. Recipients:** Emergency/Ambulance Services, Hospitals, Substance Abuse. **Geo. Dist:** headquarters and operating communities.

**CCB Foundation**
*See:* Entry 923

**Circuit City Foundation**
*See:* Entry 943

**Citigroup Foundation**
*See:* Entry 11426

**Corning Inc. Foundation**
*See:* Entry 11427

**★ 8548 ★ Ecolab Foundation**
370 North Wabasha St.
Saint Paul, MN 55102
**Phone:** (651)293-2658          **Fax:** (651)225-3123
**Website:**  http://www.corning.com/inside_corning/
foundation.asp
Lois West Duffy, Director, Community & Public Relations

**Priorities:** *Arts & Humanities:* (Arts & Culture) 15%. Supports major performing arts groups, mid-size arts organizations, museums, and theaters. *Civic & Public Affairs:* (Civic & Community Development) 13%. Contributions are set aside to fund community relations task forces and contingencies. Funds community service organizations, community foundations, leadership development, and family services. Ecolab also donates products in cases of national disaster through disaster relief organizations. *Education:* (Youth & Education) 38%. Supports programs for at-risk youth, teacher grants, and colleges and universities. *Environment:* (Community-based Contributions) 30%. Provides contributionss to the United Way and to health and human services organizations in Ecolab communities. *Voluntarism:* Employees volunteer as classroom speakers and with Business/Education Partnership. Company also provides technical assistance and coordinates volunteer projects for two weekends of the United Way's Week of Caring, Volunteer Fair, and provides contributions to nonprofit organizations to reward employee volunteers. *Note:* Contributions analysis provided by foundation in 2001. **Typ. Recipients:** AIDS/HIV, Cancer, Children's Health/Hospitals, Clinics/Medical Centers, Emergency/Ambulance Services, Family Planning, Hospitals, Long-Term Care, Medical Rehabilitation, Nutrition, People with Disabilities, Public Health, Speech & Hearing, Substance Abuse. **Geo. Dist:** areas where company has a major presence, and large numbers of employees live and work; St. Paul, MN.

**★ 8549 ★ Edward D. Jones & Co. Foundation**
12555 Manchester Rd.
Saint Louis, MO 63131
**Phone:** (314)515-2000          **Fax:** (314)515-3269
John Bachmann, Chairman

**Fnded:** 1992. **Priorities:** *Education:* 57%. Supports colleges and universities. *Environment:* 29%. Supports the United Way. *Note:* Total contributions made in 2000. **Typ. Recipients:** Emergency/Ambulance Services. **Geo. Dist:** Claremont, CA; St. Louis, MO.

**Ethyl Corp.**
*See:* Entry 1032

**FPL Group Foundation, Inc.**
*See:* Entry 1067

★ **8550** ★ **Goldman Sachs Foundation**
375 Park Ave., Ste. 1002
New York, NY 10152
**Phone:** (212)902-5402
**Email:** John_Kitchens@fpl.com
**Website:** http://www.fpl.com
Stephanie Bell-Rose, President

**Priorities:** *Civic & Public Affairs:* 1%. Funds the National Urban League. *Education:* 65%. Supports higher education, education to develop minority leaders, and provides scholarships and fellowships. *Voluntarism:* The company encourages employee volunteerism through its Community TeamWorks program, which allows employees to spend a day working at a charitable organization of their choice while receiving full salary. *Note:* Total contributions made in fiscal 2000. **Typ. Recipients:** Emergency/Ambulance Services, Hospitals, Hospitals (University Affiliated), Medical Education. **Geo. Dist:** nationally and internationally.

**Harley-Davidson Foundation**
*See:* Entry 5575

**Hewlett-Packard Co. Foundation**
*See:* Entry 1127

**Hickory Tech Corp. Foundation**
*See:* Entry 11438

**IBP Foundation**
*See:* Entry 11441

**Landmark Communications Foundation**
*See:* Entry 1196

★ **8551** ★ **LG&E Energy Foundation**
PO Box 32030
Louisville, KY 40232
**Phone:** (502)627-2000
**Email:** Lhyatt@Lcimedia.com
**Website:** http://www.hp.com/go/grants
Shauna Cole, Grants Administrator

**Fnded:** 1994. **Priorities:** *Arts & Humanities:* 9%. Supports music, dance, arts funds, and libraries. *Civic & Public Affairs:* 2%. Funds youth leadership programs, zoos, and housing. *Education:* 43%. Supports colleges and universities, scholarships funds, and special programs in pre-college education. *Environment:* 38%. Major support to the United Way; also funds social service programs for children, YMCA, and community organizations. *International:* 2%. Funds the Children's Hospital Foundation. *Religion:* 3%. Funds a science center and science education. *Note:* Total foundation contributions in 1999. **Typ. Recipients:** Children's Health/Hospitals, Emergency/Ambulance Services, Geriatric Health. **Geo. Dist:** headquarters and operating communities; Louisville, KY.

★ **8552** ★ **MacMillan Bloedel Foundation**
c/o MacMillan Bloedel Packaging Inc.
PO Box 336
Pine Hill, AL 36769
**Phone:** (334)963-4391      **Fax:** (334)963-2762
**Email:** rcraig@mbpi.com
Lynn Jonakin, President

**Fnded:** 1989. **Priorities:** *Arts & Humanities:* 2%. Giving to the theater, library, and an arts institute. *Civic & Public Affairs:* 10%. Supports festivals and city foundations. *Education:* 76%. Supports literacy programs for children and adults, public education, and science and math education. *Environment:* 5%. Sup-

ports community programs. *International:* 2%. Supports health organizations and single-disease health associations. *Note:* Total contributions made in 1999. **Typ. Recipients:** Emergency/Ambulance Services, Heart, Home-Care Services. **Geo. Dist:** headquarters area only.

**MDU Resources Foundation**
*See:* Entry 5581

**Mid-American Foundation**
*See:* Entry 5582

**Monroe Auto Equipment Co. Foundation**
*See:* Entry 10066

**OMNOVA Solutions Foundation**
*See:* Entry 5585

★ **8553** ★ **Public Service Electric & Gas Foundation**
80 Park Plaza, Mail Code T-10
Newark, NJ 07101
**Phone:** (973)430-5867
**Email:** benzw@mduresources.com
Maria Pinho, President

**Priorities:** *Arts & Humanities:* 1%. Funds cultural programs in urban communities. *Civic & Public Affairs:* 29%. Focuses on economic development, urban improvement projects, and the environment. *Education:* 34%. Primarily supports higher education, including minority education, educational funds, capital campaigns. *Environment:* 11%. Supports youth organizations and children's issues, particularly programs that target the at-risk population. Also funds United Way. *International:* 21%. Supports hospitals and health organizations. *Religion:* 3%. *Note:* Total foundation contributions made in 1999. **Typ. Recipients:** Emergency/Ambulance Services, Hospitals, People with Disabilities, Substance Abuse. **Geo. Dist:** nationally for education grants; primarily in service area.

**Publix Supermarkets Charities**
*See:* Entry 11462

★ **8554** ★ **Robbins and Myers Foundation**
1400 Kettering Tower
Dayton, OH 45423
**Phone:** (937)222-2610
**Website:** http://www.publix.com/comm_involvement.htm
Gerald Connelly, President & Chief Executive Officer

**Priorities:** *Arts & Humanities:* 21%. Supports dance, music, historic preservation, and art institutes. *Civic & Public Affairs:* 10%. Supports civic organizations, and community foundations. *Education:* 43%. Supports schools, colleges, and scholarships. *Environment:* 26%. Primarily supports United Way. *Note:* Total contributions made in 1999. **Typ. Recipients:** Alzheimers Disease, Cancer, Emergency/Ambulance Services, Health Organizations, Hospices, People with Disabilities, Sexual Abuse. **Geo. Dist:** headquarters and operating communities; OH.

★ **8555** ★ **Scripps Howard Foundation**
312 Walnut St.
PO Box 5380
Cincinnati, OH 45201
**Phone:** (513)977-3035      **Fax:** (513)977-3800
**Email:** cottingham@scripps.com
**Website:** http://www.scripps.com/foundation
Patty Cottingham, Executive Director

**Priorities:** *Civic & Public Affairs:* 38%. The Fund supports various charitable organizations that improve the quality of life in operating areas through the Community Fund and the Greater Cincinnati Fund. Supports educational institutions that produce potential employees, readers or viewers; or that promote strong community conscience and encourage alterna-

tives in education. Social welfare organizations which make significant contributions to the disadvantaged are supported, including the United Way, the Salvation Army, food banks, and scouting and Big Brothers. Supports civic organizations that promote leadership, community involvement, good government, sound public policy, free speech or journalism. Company also awards grants up to $1,000 to qualifying organizations where employees volunteer, and encourages employees to become involved in the communities where they live and work. *Education:* 21%. Awards scholarships, fellowships, and internships to full-time students preparing for careers in journalism. Preference is given to students with continuing interest and work in the field of journalism, prior recipients, and students residing in or attending schools located in communities served by company operations. The Robert P. Scripps Graphic Arts Grant is awarded to graphic arts majors who, in the opinion of college authorities, have the potential for becoming newspaper production administrators. Also provides grants to organizations that promote literacy, and matches employee gifts to educational institutions. *Note:* Total contributions made in 2001. **Typ. Recipients:** Emergency/Ambulance Services, Geriatric Health, People with Disabilities, Prenatal Health Issues, Preventive Medicine/Wellness Organizations, Substance Abuse. **Geo. Dist:** nationally, with emphasis on operating locations; particularly Greater Cincinnati, OH; OH, operating locations; Cincinnati, OH, metropolitan area.

**Sprint/United Telephone**
*See:* Entry 1403

★ **8556** ★ **Taco Bell Foundation**
17901 Von Karman Ave., MD 1207
Irvine, CA 92614
**Phone:** (949)863-3970      **Fax:** (949)863-2246
**Email:** lgannon@tacobell.com
**Website:** http://www.tacobell.com/ourcompany/index.htm
Laurie Gannon, Manager, Public Affairs

**Fnded:** 1993. **Priorities:** *Environment:* 100%. **Typ. Recipients:** Emergency/Ambulance Services, Health Organizations. **Geo. Dist:** CA, Southern California.

★ **8557** ★ **Tektronix Foundation**
PO Box 500, M.S 55-715
Beaverton, OR 97077
**Phone:** (503)627-6972      **Fax:** (503)685-4017
Patty Larkins, Executive Director

**Priorities:** *Arts & Humanities:* 17%. Majority supports arts outreach programs, which combine arts and education. Also supports Oregon arts groups, with an emphasis on Portland. Matches gifts to art and culture. *Civic & Public Affairs:* 15%. Supports the Portland Metro Zoo and minority and employment programs. *Education:* 41%. Major support is awarded to colleges and universities emphasizing technical, business, and computer science education. Also supports K-12 education, focusing on math, physical sciences, and supplementary programs. Matches gifts to education, and provides scholarships for employees' children. *Environment:* 27%. Majority supports the United Way; also funds youth organizations. *Note:* Total contributions in 2000. **Typ. Recipients:** Emergency/Ambulance Services, Hospitals. **Geo. Dist:** OR, Northwestern Oregon; WA, Southwestern Washington.

★ **8558** ★ **Telcordia Technologies**
445 South St., Room 1H342G
Morristown, NJ 07960
**Phone:** (973)829-2177      **Fax:** (973)829-2159
Ron Reichmann, Manager, Corporate Contributions

**Fnded:** 1984. **Priorities:** *Arts & Humanities:* About 10%. Supports arts associations. *Civic & Public Affairs:* 10% to 15%. Includes grants to professional and trade associations. *Education:* Approximately 50%. Focus is on colleges and universities. *International:* About 25%. Primarily supports the United Way, hospitals, and emergency services. **Typ. Recipients:** Emergency/Ambulance Services, Hospitals. **Geo. Dist:** headquarters area only.

**Thomasville Furniture Industries Foundation**
*See:* Entry 1435

**The Timken Co. Charitable Trust**
*See:* Entry 1438

**Toro Foundation**
*See:* Entry 10070

**★ 8559 ★ Valero Energy Corp.**
1 Valero Pl.
San Antonio, TX 78212
**Phone:** (210)370-2000     **Fax:** (210)370-2327
**Email:** vholder@thomasville.com
**Website:** http://www.valero.com/
Mary Brown, Sr. Vice Pres., Corporate Communications
**Typ. Recipients:** Emergency/Ambulance Services.
**Geo. Dist:** headquarters and operating communities.

**Wolverine World Wide Foundation**
*See:* Entry 1512

## Other Funding Organizations

**★ 8560 ★ American College of Osteopathic Emergency Physicians (ACOEP)**
142 E Ontario St., Ste. 550
Chicago, IL 60611
**Phone:** (312)587-3709     **Free:** 800-521-3709
**Fax:** (312)587-9951
**Email:** jwachtler@acoep.org
**Website:** http://www.acoep.org
Janice Wachtler, Exec. Dir.
**Desc:** Provides and evaluates postdoctoral and continuing education for osteopathic emergency physicians; encourages and implements the training of emergency physicians; promotes the coordination of community emergency care facilities and personnel. Sponsors Emergency Medicine CME Program for Accreditation. Conducts research and educational programs. Maintains speakers' bureau. **Awards:** Fellowship; Resident Research Award (annual).

**★ 8561 ★ Emergency Nurses Association (ENA)**
915 Lee St.
Des Plaines, IL 60016
**Phone:** 800-900-9659     **Free:** 800-243-8362
**Fax:** (847)460-4001
**Email:** gvelianoff@ena.org
**Website:** http://www.ena.org
George Velianoff, CEO
**Desc:** Registered nurses, licensed practical nurses, and licensed vocational nurses; emergency medical technicians or nurses and members of allied health fields engaged or interested in emergency patient care. Objectives are: to promote emergency nursing and to establish standards in the field; to work with other health-related organizations toward the improvement of emergency care; to serve as a resource for emergency nursing education and research. Seeks to identify and address emergency nursing issues. Disseminates educational and research information in the field. Sponsors: Emergency Nursing Core Curriculum; Standards of Emergency Nursing Practice; Emergency Nursing Pediatric Course; Trauma Nursing Core Course; Concepts in Advanced Trauma Nursing Course. **Awards:** Grant (annual); recognition (annual) for contributions of members; scholarship (annual).

**★ 8562 ★ National EMS Pilots Association (NEMSPA)**
526 King St., Ste. 415
Alexandria, VA 22314
**Phone:** (703)836-8930     **Fax:** (703)836-8920
**Email:** dmancuso@nemspa.org

**Website:** http://www.nemspa.org
Dawn Mancuso, Account Exec.
**Desc:** Pilots in the air medical industry and interested individuals. Works to help the air medical industry prosper safely and enhance the delivery of health care. Facilitates the exchange of information; evaluates new equipment; conducts educational programs; monitors governmental organizations; supports research; offers legal assistance. **Awards:** EMS Pilot of the Year (annual).

# National & International Organizations

**★ 8563 ★ AirLifeLine (ALL)**
50 Fullerton Ct., Ste. 200
Sacramento, CA 95825
**Phone:** (916)641-7800     **Free:** 877-AIR-LIFE
**Fax:** (916)641-0600
**Email:** staff@airlifeline.org
**Website:** http://www.airlifeline.org
Randall R. Quast, CEO
**Fnded:** 1978. **Mem:** 1,120. **Nat'l Groups:** 1. **Desc:** Voluntary association of pilots who donate their time, skills, fuel, and aircraft to fly medical missions. Provides free air transportation for financially needy patients who require specialized treatment at medical facilities far from their homes. **Pub:** *Pilot and Patient*, quarterly. Newsletter. Includes Victory Roll, a list of volunteer pilots who have flown medical missions and stories of patients. *Price:* Free. • *Skylines*, 3/year. Newsletter. Provides information on the program and on aviation in general. • Membership Directory, 3/year.

**★ 8564 ★ Ambulance Service Association**
Friars House, 2nd Fl.
157-168 Blackfriars Rd.
London SE1 8EU, United Kingdom
**Phone:** 44 20 79289620     **Fax:** 44 20 79289502
**Email:** richard@bizuk.com
**Website:** http://www.ambex.co.uk
**Fnded:** 1948. **Reg. Groups:** 6. **Desc:** Ambulance services in the United Kingdom. Promotes members' interests. Fosters collaboration and sharing of best practices among members. **Pub:** *ASA News*, bimonthly. Magazine. **Frmly:** Association of Chief Ambulance Officers.

**★ 8565 ★ American Academy of Emergency Medicine (AAEM)**
c/o Kay Whalen
611 E Wells St.
Milwaukee, WI 53202-3816
**Phone:** (414)276-7390     **Free:** 800-884-AAEM
**Fax:** (414)276-3349
**Email:** info@aaem.org
**Website:** http://www.aaem.org
Kay Whalen, Dir.
**Fnded:** 1993. **Mem:** 3,000. **State Groups:** 5. **Desc:** Board certified physicians specializing in emergency medicine or pediatric emergency medicine; medical students and residents. Promotes "unencumbered access to quality emergency care provided by a specialist in emergency medicine" for every individual. Seeks to advance the study and profession of emergency medicine. Represents members economic and professional interests; supports growth of medical residency and graduate medical education programs; works to create a professional and legal environment conducive to the delivery of quality emergency medical care. **Pub:** *Common Sense*, bimonthly. Newsletter. • *Official Journal: Journal of Emergency Medicine.* Journal.

**★ 8566 ★ American Ambulance Association (AAA)**
1255 23rd NW
PO Box 18218
Washington, DC 20037

**Phone:** (703)610-9018     **Free:** 800-523-4447
**Fax:** (703)610-9025
**Email:** questions@the-aaa.org
**Website:** http://www.the-aaa.org
Steve Haracznak, Exec. VP
**Fnded:** 1977. **Mem:** 830. **Desc:** Private suppliers of ambulance service. Purposes are: to aid in developing private enterprise pre-hospital emergency medical treatment and medical transportation services as a viable cost-effective alternative to publicly-operated services; to promote improved patient care; to develop efficient medical transportation at a reasonable cost; to improve personnel and equipment standards; to work with organizations offering medical transportation; to encourage high standards of ethics and conduct. Acts as an information clearinghouse; informs members of developments in the industry. Offers advice on federal statutes and regulations related to the medical transportation industry, such as insurance and antitrust regulations. Holds four regional seminars per year on topics such as training requirements, insurance systems, medicare reimbursement, and local, state, and federal legislation and regulations. Conducts quarterly emergency medical services management seminar. **Pub:** *Ambulance Industry Journal*, quarterly. Journal. Includes book reviews and legislative reports. *Price:* Free to members; $25 for nonmembers. **Frmly:** (1978) Ambulance and Medical Service Association of America.

**★ 8567 ★ American Association of Women Emergency Physicians (AAWEP)**
3020 Legacy Dr., No. 100-200
Plano, TX 75023
**Phone:** (972)208-4543     **Fax:** (972)208-4544
**Email:** info@aawep.org
John Walker, Exec. Dir.
**Fnded:** 1983. **Mem:** 400. **Desc:** Women engaged in the practice of emergency medicine. Promotes professional advancement of members. Provides support and guidance to female emergency physicians; conducts leadership skills development programs for female emergency physicians, residents, and medical students. Maintains speakers' bureau. **Pub:** *Epic Quarterly Newsletter*, periodic. Directory. • Newsletter, periodic.

**★ 8568 ★ American Board of Emergency Medicine (ABEM)**
3000 Coolidge Rd.
East Lansing, MI 48823-6319
**Phone:** (517)332-4800     **Fax:** (517)332-2234
**Email:** abem@abem.org
**Website:** http://www.abem.org
Mary Ann Reinhart, PhD, Contact
**Fnded:** 1976. **Desc:** Seeks to: improve the quality of emergency medical care; establish and maintain high standards of excellence in the specialty of emergency medicine and its approved subspecialties; improve medical education and facilities for training emergency physicians and subspecialist in approved ABEM subspecialties; evaluate specialists in emergency medicine and subspecialist in approved ABEM subspecialties applying for certification and recertification; serve the public, subcertification physicians, hospitals, and medical schools by furnishing lists of those diplomats certified by ABEM. **Pub:** *ABEM Annual Report*, annual. Annual Report. Includes summary of current year's events and activities, volunteers, and exam statistics. • *ABEM Policies and Procedures*, annual. Booklet. *Price:* Free. • *ABEMemo*, semiannual. Newsletter. For diplomates and organizations associated with ABEM.

**★ 8569 ★ American College of Emergency Physicians (ACEP)**
1125 Executive Cir.
Irving, TX 75038-2522
**Phone:** (972)550-0911     **Free:** 800-798-1822
**Fax:** (972)580-2816
**Email:** info@acep.org
**Website:** http://www.acep.org
Dr. Colin C. Rorrie, Jr., Exec. Dir.

**Fnded:** 1968. **Mem:** 20,438. **State Groups:** 53. **Desc:** Physicians who devote a significant portion of their professional time to emergency medicine. Aim is to provide a unifying direction of purpose in the field, which is a new medical specialty. Encourages training of emergency physicians, with the aim of improving emergency department care in hospitals; conducts continuing education programs for emergency physicians and other healthcare personnel. Provides information regarding the practice of emergency medicine. Compiles statistics. **Pub:** *ACEP News*, monthly. Newsletter. Discusses socioeconomic issues affecting emergency medicine. *Price:* Included in membership dues; $20/year for nonmembers. • *Annals of Emergency Medicine*, monthly. Journal. Covers emergency medicine and emergency health services. Includes abstracts of emergency medical literature, book reviews, and calendar of events. *Price:* Included in membership dues. • *Foresight*, quarterly. Newsletter. Covers emergency medicine risk management. • *Physicians Evaluation and Education Review.* • Also publishes a homestudy series, and reference manuals on diagnosis and procedure coding, quality assurance, independent contractor status, EMS medical direction, working with managed care plans, patient transfer, risk management, developing and negotiating contracts, and advanced pediatric life support.

**American College of Osteopathic Emergency Physicians (ACOEP)**
*See:* Entry 16989

**American Osteopathic Board of Emergency Medicine (AOBEM)**
*See:* Entry 16998

### ★ 8570 ★ American Trauma Society (ATS)
8903 Presidential Pky., Ste. 512
Upper Marlboro, MD 20772
**Phone:** (301)420-4189 **Free:** 800-556-7890
**Fax:** (301)420-0617
**Email:** info@amtrauma.org
**Website:** http://www.amtrauma.org
John W. Ashworth, III, Exec. VP/COO

**Fnded:** 1968. **Mem:** 3,000. **State Groups:** 22. **Desc:** Physicians, nurses, EMT personnel, other healthcare professionals, institutions, corporations, and interested individuals. Seeks to: prevent trauma situations; improve trauma care through professional and paraprofessional education; educate the public through campaigns and dissemination of information. **Pub:** *Promotional Media Resource Catalog.* Catalog. • *Traumagram Newsletter*, 4/year. Newsletter. Includes prevention activities, news on the annual meeting, and legislative and research updates. *Price:* Included in membership dues for institutions. • *TraumaView Newsletter.* Newsletter. *Price:* Included in membership dues.

### ★ 8571 ★ Association of Air Medical Services (AAMS)
526 King St., Ste. 415
Alexandria, VA 22314-3143
**Phone:** (703)836-8732 **Fax:** (703)836-8920
**Email:** information@aams.org
**Website:** http://www.aams.org
Dawn Mancuso, CAE, Exec. Dir.

**Fnded:** 1980. **Mem:** 400. **Desc:** Air medical transport providers; manufacturers and distributors of air medical transport equipment. Objective is to provide quality medical care during rapid air transport. Seeks to develop standards for aircraft configuration, minimum professional and educational requirements for personnel on board, medical and communications equipment, and operations. **Pub:** *Air Medical Journal*, bimonthly. Magazine. Published in conjunction with several other Associations. *Price:* Included in membership dues. • *Membership Directory*, annual. • AAMS *News & Views Newsletter* Monthly Member-only faxed newsletter. **Frmly:** (1988) American Society of Hospital-Based Emergency Air Medical Services.

### ★ 8572 ★ Australasian College for Emergency Medicine (ACEM)
17 Grattan St.
Carlton, VIC 3053, Australia
**Phone:** 61 3 96633800 **Fax:** 61 3 96638013
**Email:** admin@acem.org.au
**Website:** http://www.acem.org.au

**Fnded:** 1984. **Mem:** 510. **Reg. Groups:** 6. **Lang(s):** English. **Desc:** Provides the training and examination of specialist emergency physicians. **Pub:** *Emergency Medicine*, quarterly. Journal. Peer-reviewed scientific journal.

### ★ 8573 ★ British Association for Accident and Emergency Medicine
c/o Royal College of Surgeons of England
35-43 Lincoln's Inn Fields
London WC2A 3PN, United Kingdom
**Phone:** 44 207 8319405 **Fax:** 44 207 4050318
**Email:** baem1@compuserve.com
**Website:** http://www.baem.org.uk

**Fnded:** 1967. **Mem:** 1,156. **Desc:** Membership of the British Association for Accident and Emergency Medicine is available to any registered medical practitioner who has an interest in Accident and Emergency Medicine. Concerned with the development of the specialty of Accident and Emergency Medicine and, in particular, to achieve a minimum of one Accident and Emergency Consultant in every major Accident and Emergency Department. It has a network of Regional Representatives who are available to advise Districts on the establishment of Accident and Emergency Consultant posts, staffing issues, design of Accident and Emergency Departments, etc. **Pub:** *Journal of Accident & Emergency Medicine*, bimonthly. Journal.

### ★ 8574 ★ British Association for Immediate Care (BASICS)
Turret House, Turret Ln.
Ipswich IP4 1DL, United Kingdom
**Phone:** 44 870 1654999 **Fax:** 44 870 1654949
**Email:** admin@basics.org.uk
**Website:** http://www.basics.org.uk

**Fnded:** 1977. **Mem:** 2,500. **Local Groups:** 87. **Desc:** Medical practitioners and non-medical practitioners (e.g., ambulance, nurse, emergency planning personnel) involved in pre-hospital immediate medical care. Aims to foster co-operation between existing Immediate Care Schemes and to encourage and aid the formation and extension of schemes in the UK; to develop and strengthen co-operation between all services in dealing with emergencies and to encourage and assist research into all aspects of pre-hospital immediate medical care and accident prevention. **Pub:** Newsletter, 3/year.

### ★ 8575 ★ Canadian Association of Emergency Physicians (Association Canadienne des Medecins d'Urgence)
1785 Alta Vista Dr., Ste. 104
Ottawa, ON, Canada K1G 3Y6
**Phone:** (613)523-3343 **Free:** 800-643-1158
**Fax:** (613)523-0190
**Email:** admin@caep.ca
**Website:** http://www.caep.ca

**Fnded:** 1978. **Mem:** 1,500. **Lang(s):** English, French. **Desc:** National, voluntary, charitable organization dedicated to excellence in providing emergency health care. Promotes education for health professionals involved in emergency health care as well as providing leadership in the advancement of knowledge through research in emergency medicine. **Pub:** *Canadian Journal of Emergency Medicine*, quarterly. Journal.

### ★ 8576 ★ Canadian Confederation of Ambulance Service Associations (CCASA)
PO Box 129
Rodney, ON, Canada N0L 2C0
**Phone:** (519)785-0318 **Fax:** (519)785-2002

**Email:** oaoa@mco.net
**Website:** http://www.educom.on.ca/ccasa/

**Lang(s):** English. **Desc:** Ambulance operators in Canada. Works to improve the standard of emergency prehospital care for Canadians.

### ★ 8577 ★ ComCARE Alliance
888 17th St., NW, 12th Fl.
Washington, DC 20006
**Phone:** (202)429-0574 **Fax:** (202)296-2962
**Email:** info@comcare.org
**Website:** http://www.comcare.org
Patrick Halley, Outreach Coord.

**Fnded:** 1998. **Mem:** 80. **Desc:** Emergency doctors and nurses, state and local public safety officials, departments of transportation, citizen organizations, wireless transportation and technology companies committed to improving emergency communications and response. **Pub:** *ComCARE Insider*, monthly. Newsletter.

### ★ 8578 ★ Doctors for Disaster Preparedness (DDP)
1601 N Tucson Blvd Ste. 9
Tucson, AZ 85716
**Phone:** (520)325-2680 **Fax:** (520)326-3529
**Website:** http://www.oism.org/ddp
Jane Orient, MD, Pres.

**Fnded:** 1982. **Mem:** 200. **Desc:** Doctors, health professionals, medical students and interested individuals. Prepares physicians, health professionals, personnel, and the public for medical response in the case of natural or human-caused disaster. Seeks to prevent human suffering and death resulting from any catastrophe. Believes that "there is no disaster so great - including nuclear war - that the medical profession is not obliged to care for the survivors." Promotes accurate risk assessment. Supports civil defense measures; maintains no position on specific military or foreign policy measures, weapons systems, or arms control. Sponsors lectures for health professionals, government leaders, and the public concerning disaster preparedness. Compiles statistics; maintains speakers' bureau. **Pub:** *Civil Defense Perspectives*, bimonthly. Newsletter. *Price:* Included in membership dues. • *Doctors for Disaster Preparedness Newsletter*, bimonthly. Newsletter. *Price:* Included in membership fees. • Reprints.Consists of literature related to disaster preparedness.

### ★ 8579 ★ Emergency Medicine Foundation (EMF)
PO Box 619911
Dallas, TX 75261-9911
**Phone:** (972)550-0911 **Fax:** (972)580-2816
**Email:** emf@acep.org
**Website:** http://www.acep.org
Colin C. Rorrie, Jr., CAE Exec. Dir.

**Fnded:** 1972. **Desc:** Board of trustees is composed of representatives of American College of Emergency Physicians, Emergency Medicine Residents' Association, Emergency Nurses Association, Society for Academic Emergency Medicine . To promote and provide improved education and research in the field of emergency medicine in order to improve the availability and quality of emergency medical treatment. Conducts research programs. Funds hypothesis-based emergency medical research. **Pub:** *Scope*, semiannual. Newsletter. Donor newsletter that includes research funding information.

### ★ 8580 ★ Emergency Medicine Residents' Association (EMRA)
1125 Executive Cir.
Irving, TX 75038-2522
**Phone:** (972)550-0920 **Free:** 800-798-1822
**Fax:** (972)580-2829
**Email:** lmcdonald@emra.org
**Website:** http://www.emra.org
Liz McDonald, Exec. Dir.

**Fnded:** 1974. **Mem:** 4,500. **Desc:** Physicians enrolled in emergency medicine residency training programs;

medical students. Purposes are to provide a unified voice for emergency medicine residents and encourage high standards in training and education for emergency physicians. Encourages research to improve emergency medicine education; promotes community, state, and national representation for emergency medicine in organized and academic medicine. **Pub:** *Career Development Guide.* • *EM Resident*, bimonthly. Newsletter. Focuses on issues such as residency issues, utilization of emergency department services, and educational opportunities. *Price:* Included in membership dues. • *Emergency Medicine in Focus: A Handbook for Medical Students and Prospective Residents.* Handbook. • *EMRA Job Catalog*, annual. Catalog. • *Outpatient Guide to Antibiotics.*

**Emergency Nurses Association (ENA)**
*See:* Entry 15706

### ★ 8581 ★ International Cytokine Society (ICS)
Biotech Park, Ste. 9
1021 15th St.
Augusta, GA 30901
**Phone:** (706)722-7511          **Fax:** (706)722-7515
**Email:** maps@csranet.com
**Website:** http://bioinformatics.weizmann.ac.il/cytokine/
Dr. Sherwood M. Reichard, Exec. Mgr.
**Fnded:** 1978. **Mem:** 700. **Desc:** Physicians and scientists associated with universities; private, industrial, and government institutes; hospital clinics; and the pharmaceutical industry. Promotes research into and awareness of the health importance of shock and trauma; fosters the dissemination and application of information in these fields; provides a forum for the multidisciplinary integration of current and basic clinical knowledge and concepts in the study of shock and trauma. **Pub:** *Advances in Shock Research.* Book. • *American Society for Photobiology–Directory and Constitution*, biennial. Directory. • *Cytokine*, monthly. Journal. • *Directory and Constitution*, biennial. Directory. • Newsletter, quarterly. **Frmly:** (2001) Shock Society.

### ★ 8582 ★ International Rescue and Emergency Care Association (IRECA)
PO Box 13527
Charleston, SC 29422-3527
**Free:** 800-221-3435
**Email:** goodneiss@msn.com
**Website:** http://www.ireca.org
Randy Tanner, Pres.
**Fnded:** 1948. **Mem:** 3,000. **Local Groups:** 500. **Desc:** Organized volunteers and paid industrial rescue and emergency squads, ambulance and first aid crews, fire departments, military personnel, and other units equipped with rescue equipment and emergency care supplies which can be carried in mobile units; county, state, and other associations and individuals interested in rescue and emergency patient care. To cooperate in, foster, and conduct research designed to advance the science and art of rescue and emergency care and to encourage standardization of practice and equipment. Sponsors seminars. **Pub:** *International Rescuer*, quarterly. • Also publishes and endorses the publication of emergency care and rescue training information. **Frmly:** (1978) International Rescue and First Aid Association.

### ★ 8583 ★ International Society of Disaster Medicine (ISDM) (Societe Internationale de Medecine de Catastrophe — SIMC)
Case Postale 133
Jussy
CH-1254 Geneva, Switzerland
**Phone:** 41 22 7591312          **Fax:** 41 22 7590550
**Fnded:** 1975. **Mem:** 500. **Reg. Groups:** 8. **Lang(s):** Arabic, English, French, Spanish. **Desc:** Physicians in 42 countries who promote study and advancement in the field of disaster medicine. Conducts symposia and

research programs; organizes scientific commissions. **Pub:** Proceedings, 5/year.

### ★ 8584 ★ Irish Association of the Sovereign Military Order of Malta (IASMOM)
St. John's House
32 Clyde Rd.
Dublin 4, Ireland
**Phone:** 353 1 6684891          **Fax:** 353 1 6685288
**Email:** smom@indigo.ie
**Website:** http://www.orderofmalta.ie
**Fnded:** 1934. **Mem:** 4,000. **Nat'l Groups:** 1. **Reg. Groups:** 6. **Local Groups:** 80. **Lang(s):** English, Irish. **Desc:** Volunteers committed to serving those in need. Seeks to increase the availability of emergency services. Operates ambulance corps.

### ★ 8585 ★ Miracle Flights for Kids
2756 N Green Valley Pkwy., No. 115
Green Valley, NV 89014-2120
**Phone:** (702)261-0494          **Free:** 800-FLY-1711
**Fax:** (702)261-0497
**Email:** info@miracleflights.org
**Website:** http://www.miracleflights.org
Ann McGee, Pres.
**Fnded:** 1985. **Mem:** 500. **Desc:** Provides free air transportation to families who are unable to get to medical treatment centers far from home. **Pub:** Newsletter, quarterly. Includes safety and pilot news, flight updates, fundraising news, news about flights. *Price:* Free. **Frmly:** (1998) The Angel Planes.

### ★ 8586 ★ National Association of Emergency Medical Technicians (NAEMT)
408 Monroe St.
Clinton, MS 39056-4210
**Phone:** (601)924-7744          **Free:** 800-34-NAEMT
**Fax:** (601)924-7325
**Email:** president@naemt.org
**Website:** http://www.naemt.org
Nathan Williams, Pres.
**Fnded:** 1975. **Mem:** 5,000. **State Groups:** 24. **Desc:** Nationally registered or state certified emergency medical technicians (EMTs) and EMT-paramedics. Promotes the professional status of EMTs and national acceptance of a uniform standard of recognition for their skills; encourages constant upgrading of these skills and EMT qualifications and educational requirements; engages in scientific research related to the care and transportation of the sick and injured; supports the establishment of emergency medical services systems. Sponsors insurance, credit card, and member loan programs. Maintains placement services. **Pub:** *NAEMT News*, bimonthly. Newsletter. *Price:* Free. For members only.

### ★ 8587 ★ National Association of EMS Educators (NAEMSE)
c/o J. Freel
700 N Bell Ave., Ste. 260
Carnegie, PA 15106-4310
**Phone:** (412)429-9550          **Fax:** (412)429-9554
**Email:** naemse@naemse.org
**Website:** http://www.naemse.org
Joann Freel, Exec. Dir.
**Fnded:** 1996. **Mem:** 2,038. **Desc:** Promotes EMS education, develops and delivers educational resources, and advocates research and life long learning. **Pub:** *Domain3*, quarterly. Journal. Features teaching tips, current research, an educator's toolbox. • *Educator Update*, bimonthly. Magazine.

### ★ 8588 ★ National Association of EMS Physicians (NAEMSP)
PO Box 15945281
Lenexa, KS 66285
**Phone:** (913)492-5858          **Free:** 800-228-3677
**Fax:** (913)541-0156
**Email:** info-naemsp@goamp.com

**Website:** http://www.naemsp.org
Dede Gish-Panjada, Exec. Dir.
**Fnded:** 1983. **Mem:** 1,480. **Desc:** Medical directors responsible for emergency medical services (EMS) programs throughout the United States; other physicians and nonphysicians dedicated to out-of-hospital emergency care. (Most physicians within this organization are medically-legally responsible for the provision of out-of-hospital emergency care.) Strives to foster excellence and provide medical leadership so that all individuals and communities receive quality out-of-hospital emergency medical services. Works to develop guidelines and strategies to reduce and prevent discomfort, disability, and death in the community; define roles, responsibilities, authority, and accountability of EMS physicians; promote communication and cooperation among EMS professionals; define the unique body of medical knowledge of prehospital and disaster medicine; promote cost-effective programs and interventions that optimize patient outcomes; advocate or initiate public policy for optimal emergency medical care; encourage and support quality EMS research. Provides forums for definition and debate of EMS issues. Encourages and promotes career development, career longevity, and professional well-being of EMS professionals. Defines and promotes ethical principles in the delivery of out-of-hospital emergency care. **Pub:** *EMS Medical Directors' Handbook.* Handbook. • *NAEMSP Newsletter*, bimonthly. Newsletter. • *Prehospital Emergency Care*, quarterly. Journal. • *Prehospital Systems and Medical Oversight.* Book. • *Quality Management in Prehospital Care.* Book.

### ★ 8589 ★ National Association of Private Ambulance Services
21 Bassenhally Rd.
Whittlesey
Peterborough PE7 1RN, United Kingdom
**Phone:** 44 1733 350916          **Free:** 44 8000929112
**Fax:** 44 1733 350916
**Email:** pas@ambulanceservice.co.uk
**Website:** http://www.ambulanceservice.co.uk
**Fnded:** 1992. **Mem:** 41. **Reg. Groups:** 41. **Desc:** Provides self-regulation for private and professional ambulance service throughout the U.K and Ireland.

**National Association of State EMS Directors (NASEMSD)**
*See:* Entry 9753

### ★ 8590 ★ National Council of State Emergency Medical Services Training Coordinators (NCSEMSTC)
111 Park Pl.
Falls Church, VA 22046
**Phone:** (703)538-1794          **Fax:** (703)241-5603
**Email:** chairman@ncsemstc.org
**Website:** http://www.ncsemstc.org
Liza K. Burrill, Chair, Exec. Committee
**Fnded:** 1977. **Mem:** 159. **Reg. Groups:** 9. **Desc:** Individuals employed by state-level emergency medical services agencies who are responsible for coordination or supervision of EMS training programs. Promotes the responsible movement of emergency medical technicians (EMTs) throughout the nation through standardization of policies related, but not limited to, curriculum, certification, recertification, revocation, and reciprocity; seeks to further develop the public recognition and trust of the emergency medical technician as a health care professional. **Pub:** *Membership List*, annual. Membership Directory.

**National Emergency Equipment Dealers Association (NEEDA)**
*See:* Entry 9990

### ★ 8591 ★ National Emergency Medicine Association (NEMA)
306 W Joppa Rd.
Baltimore, MD 21204-4048

**Phone:** (410)494-0300 **Free:** 800-332-NEMA
**Fax:** (410)494-0725
**Email:** info@nmahealth.org
**Website:** http://www.nemahealth.org
Howard H. Farrington, Pres.

**Fnded:** 1982. **Mem:** 5,000. **Desc:** Seeks to prevent trauma and improve emergency medical care nationwide. Concerned with: promoting lifestyles that reduce the likelihood of trauma; educating the public on how to help a trauma victim before emergency personnel arrive; ensuring that trained emergency personnel have the necessary resources to effectively do their jobs; promoting effective treatment and care of trauma victims at hospitals and trauma centers; ensuring the availability of proper services and facilities to the recovering trauma victim. Provides The Heart of the Matter, an educational radio program, to more than 250 radio stations nationwide. Maintains speakers' bureau; offers grants; provides direct-mail program focusing on heart disease prevention. **Pub:** *A Guide to the Emergency Room.* • *Heart of the Matter.* • *Heartlines*, quarterly. Newsletter. • *How to Survive Trauma.*

**★ 8592 ★ National Emergency Number Association (NENA)**
422 Beecher Rd.
Columbus, OH 43230-1797
**Free:** 800-332-3911 **Fax:** (614)933-0911
**Email:** jgoerke@austin.rr.com
**Website:** http://www.nena9-1-1.org/
James D. Goerke, Interm Exec. Dir.

**Fnded:** 1982. **Mem:** 7,500. **Local Groups:** 46. **Desc:** Fosters the technical advancement, availability, and implementation of a universal emergency telephone number system. Promotes research, planning, training, and education. **Pub:** *Connections*, quarterly. Newsletter. Devoted to regional information. • *NENA News*, quarterly. Magazine. Covers many issues of the association.

**★ 8593 ★ National EMS Pilots Association (NEMSPA)**
526 King St., Ste. 415
Alexandria, VA 22314
**Phone:** (703)836-8930 **Fax:** (703)836-8920
**Email:** dmancuso@nemspa.org
**Website:** http://www.nemspa.org
Dawn Mancuso, Account Exec.

**Fnded:** 1988. **Mem:** 250. **Desc:** Pilots in the air medical industry and interested individuals. Works to help the air medical industry prosper safely and enhance the delivery of health care. Facilitates the exchange of information; evaluates new equipment; conducts educational programs; monitors governmental organizations; supports research; offers legal assistance. **Pub:** *Air Medical Journal*, bimonthly. Magazine. • *AirNet*, quarterly. Newsletter.

**★ 8594 ★ National Flight Paramedics Association (NFPA)**
383 F St.
Salt Lake City, UT 84103
**Free:** 800-381-NFPA **Fax:** (801)534-0434
**Email:** jpburkejr@aol.com
**Website:** http://www.nfpa.rotor.com
Pat Petersen, Account Exec.

**Fnded:** 1986. **Mem:** 850. **State Groups:** 2. **Desc:** Flight paramedics. Promotes education, professionalism, and communication within the emergency medical service community. **Pub:** *Air Medical Journal*, semimonthly. Journal. • *Flight Paramedic News*, quarterly. Newsletter.

**★ 8595 ★ National Heart Council (NHC)**
306 W Joppa Rd.
Baltimore, MD 21204
**Phone:** (410)494-0300 **Fax:** (410)494-0725
**Email:** info@nemahealth.org
**Website:** http://www.nemahealth.org/heartcouncil.html
Howard H. Farrington, Pres.

**Fnded:** 1982. **Desc:** A project of the National Emergency Medicine Association. Seeks to further advances made in the field of emergency medicine, particularly as related to heart trauma. Awards grants to organizations and individuals for the purpose of conducting research, meetings, or other activities that gather and disseminate information on traumatic medicine, particularly cardiac disorders. **Pub:** *Heart Research Newsletter*, quarterly. Newsletter. • Also publishes guides, reports, and brochures; plans to produce videotapes on first aid for household accidents, heart attacks, and choking. **Frmly:** (1994) National Heart Research.

**★ 8596 ★ National Registry of Emergency Medical Technicians (NREMT)**
Rocco V. Morando Bldg.
PO Box 29233
6610 Bush Blvd.
Columbus, OH 43229
**Phone:** (614)888-4484 **Fax:** (614)888-8920
**Email:** nremtwebofc@attmail.com
**Website:** http://www.nremt.org
Howard A. Werman, MD, Chairman

**Fnded:** 1970. **Mem:** 170,000. **Desc:** Promotes the improved delivery of emergency medical services by: assisting in the development and evaluation of educational programs to train emergency medical technicians; establishing qualifications for eligibility to apply for registration; preparing and conducting examinations designed to assure the competency of emergency medical technicians and paramedics; establishing a system for biennial registration; establishing procedures for revocation of certificates of registration for cause; maintaining a directory of registered emergency medical technicians. **Pub:** Newsletter, quarterly. **Frmly:** (1973) Registry of Emergency Medical Technicians - Ambulance.

**★ 8597 ★ Professional Aeromedical Transport Association (PATA)**
4627 Beverly Blvd.
Los Angeles, CA 90004
**Free:** 800-541-7517 **Fax:** (323)463-0433
Jim McNeal, Pres.

**Fnded:** 1986. **Mem:** 200. **Desc:** Firms that provide air ambulance service, primarily by means of fixed-wing aircraft; suppliers to the industry; individuals interested in the field. Goals are to standardize operations and services, improve patient care, and educate members and the public. Provides a network for locating providers of professional aeromedical services. Conducts scientific programs. **Pub:** Newsletter, quarterly.

**★ 8598 ★ Residency Review Committee for Emergency Medicine (RRCEM)**
515 N State St., Ste. 2000
Chicago, IL 60610
**Phone:** (312)464-5404 **Fax:** (312)464-4098
**Website:** http://www.acgme.org
Dr. Larry Sulton, Dir.

**Fnded:** 1982. **Mem:** 12. **Desc:** Representatives from the American College of Emergency Physicians, the American Board of Emergency Medicine, Council on Medical Education of the American Medical Association, and the Emergency Medicine Residents' Association. Accredits residency training programs in emergency medicine. **Pub:** *Directory of Graduate Medical Education Programs*, annual. Directory.

**★ 8599 ★ Society for Academic Emergency Medicine (SAEM)**
901 N Washington Ave.
Lansing, MI 48906-5137
**Phone:** (517)485-5484 **Fax:** (517)485-0801
**Email:** saem@saem.org
**Website:** http://www.saem.org
Marcus L. Martin, MD, Pres.

**Fnded:** 1989. **Mem:** 5,000. **Desc:** Physicians teaching emergency medicine, emergency medicine residents, and nonphysicians teaching emergency care. Purposes are: to educate teachers of emergency medicine and encourage its development as an academic discipline; to apply sound educational principles, thus improving the quality of teaching in the field; to promote research in educational methods and clinical procedures. Provides a forum for the exchange of ideas and information. Promotes improved emergency patient care through more direct involvement of teachers and consumers in the needs assessment, planning, and implementation of projects and programs. Sponsors educational workshops; conducts lectures. **Pub:** *Academic Emergency Medicine*, monthly. Journal. • *SAEM Newsletter*, bimonthly. Newsletter. Promotes research and education in emergency medicine. *Price:* Included in membership dues.

**★ 8600 ★ Society of Critical Care Medicine (SCCM)**
701 Lee St., Ste. 200
Des Plaines, IL 60016
**Phone:** (847)827-6869 **Fax:** (847)827-6886
**Email:** info@sccm.org
**Website:** http://www.sccm.org
David Julian Martin, CEO/Exec. VP

**Fnded:** 1970. **Mem:** 9,100. **Reg. Groups:** 14. **Desc:** Physicians, nurses, scientists, technicians, respiratory therapists, engineers, pharmacists, and physicians assistants involved in the field of critical care medicine. Purposes are: to improve care for acute life-threatening illnesses and injuries; to promote development of optimal care facilities; to guarantee high educational standards in critical care medicine. SCCM has initiated self-assessment testing program in an effort to establish core curriculum and assist physicians in self-evaluation. SCCM established American College of Critical Care Medicine in 1988. **Pub:** *Critical Care Medicine*, monthly. Journal. *Price:* $130 for nonmembers. • *Educational and Scientific Symposium Syllabus*, annual. Proceedings. Compilation of proceedings of annual meeting. • *FORUM*, quarterly. Newsletter. Membership newsletter. • *New Horizons: The Science and Practice of Acute Medicine*, quarterly, February, May, August, November. Journal. *Price:* $105 for nonmembers.

**★ 8601 ★ Society of Emergency Medicine Physician Assistants (SEMPA)**
950 N Washington St.
Alexandria, VA 22314-1552
**Phone:** (703)519-7334 **Fax:** (703)684-1924
**Email:** info@sempa.org
**Website:** http://www.sempa.org
Tom Moreno, Exec. Dir.

**Fnded:** 1990. **Mem:** 700. **Nat'l Groups:** 1. **Reg. Groups:** 6. **Desc:** Works to collect demographic data to share with the PA profession and other agencies; strives to devise a more standardized approach to credentialing the development and granting of clinical privileges. Seeks to enhance the EM PAs ability to provide the best quality patient care. **Pub:** *SEMPA News*, quarterly. Newsletter.

**★ 8602 ★ Union of Estonian Emergency Medical Services (Eesti Kiirabi Liit)**
Riia 18
EE-51010 Tartu, Estonia
**Phone:** 372 7 408805 **Fax:** 372 7 408809
**Email:** ekliit@pb.uninet.ee
**Website:** http://www.kiirabi.ee

**Fnded:** 1992. **Mem:** 1,118. **Reg. Groups:** 50. **Lang(s):** Estonian. **Desc:** Organizations and individuals providing emergency medical services; members of other medical specialty associations. Assists members in clarifying their rights and responsibilities under the present Estonian healthcare system. Represents the interests of EMS providers. Participates in training for EMS providers. Certifies emergency healthcare providers. Provides first aid training to the public. **Frmly:** Estonian First Medical Aid Association.

# Research Centers

**★ 8603 ★ Center for Emergency Medicine of Western Pennsylvania**
230 McKee Pl., Ste. 500
Pittsburgh, PA 15213
**Phone:** (412)647-5300      **Fax:** (412)647-4670
**Email:** lenartdl@msx.upmc.edu
**Website:** http://www.centerem.com
Dr. James J. Menegazzi, Res. Dir.
**Activities/Fields:** Systems, therapy, and techniques involved in the delivery of emergency care, including monitoring and evaluation of field care, personnel training and performance, and patient outcome. Sample projects include study of resuscitation from cardiac arrest, endobronchial drug delivery, pediatric ventilation alternatives, surgical versus percutaneous cricothyrotomy, techniques used for the transport of the seriously ill or injured, and alternative methods of emergency airway management, including transillumination methods of intubation and translaryngeal jet ventilation.

**★ 8604 ★ Disaster Relief and Emergency Medical Services Project (DREAMS)**
3139 TAMU
459 Blocker Bldg.
College Station, TX 77843-3139
**Phone:** (979)458-1135      **Fax:** (979)862-3983
**Email:** joan@academy.tamu.edu
**Website:** http://academy.tamu.edu/dreams/
Joan F. Tatge, Contact
**Activities/Fields:** Enhancement of emergency medical care, particularly in remote areas where medical attention is not readily available through the use of emerging medical, scientific and telecommunications technologies.

**★ 8605 ★ Institute of Critical Care Medicine**
1695 N Sunrise Way, Bldg. 3
Palm Springs, CA 92262
**Phone:** (760)323-6867      **Fax:** (760)323-6167
**Email:** weilm@aol.com
**Website:** http://www.911research.org
Dr. Max Harry Weil, Pres.
**Activities/Fields:** Critically ill patients, especially those in coronary care, intensive care, concentrated care, post anaesthesia recovery, and emergency services, suffering from heart attacks, accidents, postsurgical complications, overwhelming infections, blood loss, trauma, central nervous system injury, circulatory shock, burns, and shock from a variety of causes. Interdisciplinary studies focus on critical care medicine, automation of bedside equipment, computer application to bedside medicine, hospital environment, cardiopulmonary resuscitation, physiological instrumentation, and ethical studies of patient care. **Pub:** *Newsletters.*

**★ 8606 ★ Loyola University Chicago Burn and Shock Trauma Institute**
Bldg. 110, 4th Fl.
Loyola University Medical Center
Maywood, IL 60153
**Phone:** (708)327-2400      **Fax:** (708)327-2813
**Email:** rgamell@luc.edu
**Website:** http://www.lumc.edu/burnshock
Richard L. Gamelli, MD, Dir.
**Activities/Fields:** Body responses to injury and post-injury sequelae of infection, metabolic change, alteration in host defense, and wound healing. Clinical research in care and management of injury victims, injury analysis and prevention, etiology, epidemiology, cost, rehabilitation, and outcome of trauma.

**★ 8607 ★ Memorial University of Newfoundland Centre for Offshore and Remote Medicine (MEDICOR)**
Health Science Centre
Saint John's, NF, Canada A1B 3V6
**Phone:** (709)737-6433      **Fax:** (709)737-6746
**Email:** ddecker@mun.ca
Dale Decker, Hyperbaric Diving Spec.
**Activities/Fields:** Petroleum related offshore health and safety, telemedicine and teleconferencing, hypermedic medicine, occupational medicine, and hypothermia, survival, immersion suits, hyperbaric medicine, and marine research.

**★ 8608 ★ R.A. Cowley Shock Trauma Center**
University of Maryland Shock Trauma Center
22 S Greene St.
Baltimore, MD 21201-1595
**Phone:** (410)328-3774      **Fax:** (410)328-8664
**Email:** jashworth@stc1.4mmc.umaryland.edu
John W. Ashworth, III, Contact
**Activities/Fields:** Clinical research on resuscitation and treatment of critically ill and severely injured. Crash injury research studies focus on automotive safety and design based on in-depth engineering analysis of automotive crashes. Emerging technologies such as telemedicine initiatives, blood substitute studies, and biomechanics and clinical aspects of orthopedic injuries are also explored.

**★ 8609 ★ Trauma Foundation**
San Francisco General Hospital, Bldg. 1, Rm. 300
San Francisco, CA 94110
**Phone:** (415)821-8209      **Fax:** (415)282-2563
**Email:** tf@tf.org
**Website:** http://www.tf.org
Andrew McGuire, Exec. Dir.
**Activities/Fields:** Injury and violence prevention, public policy, and epidemiology, including epidemiology of traumatic injuries and health policy research on such issues as fire-safe cigarettes, motorcycle helmets, burn injury prevention, violence prevention, handgun control, and alcohol policy. **Pub:** *Newsletter.* • *Policy papers, briefs, factsheets.*

**★ 8610 ★ University of Arizona Arizona Emergency Medicine Research Center (AEMRC)**
Box 245057
1501 N Campbell Ave.
Tucson, AZ 85724-5057
**Phone:** (520)626-6312      **Fax:** (520)626-2455
**Email:** harvey@aemrc.arizona.edu
**Website:** http://www.aemrc.arizona.edu
Harvey W. Meislin, MD, Dir.
**Activities/Fields:** Prevention of injuries. Specific areas of research include epidemiology of acute medical and traumatic problems, epidemiology and prevention of injury, pathophysiology of acute illness and injury, characteristics and performance of prehospital emergency medical care systems, and outcome research relating to injuries and traumatic deaths.

**★ 8611 ★ University of Calgary Injury Research Unit**
3330 Hospital Dr. NW
Calgary, AB, Canada T2N 2A1
**Phone:** (403)531-3383      **Fax:** (403)283-2805
**Email:** vppanlil@ucalgary.ca
Prof. Vladimir P. Panlilio, Contact
**Activities/Fields:** Conducts multidisciplinary contract studies of motor vehicle accidents. Specific projects include the study of injuries in accidents involving light trucks, vans, and passenger cars; pedestrian injury; protection of children with handicaps in motor vehicles; effectiveness of child car seats; injury scoring; and air cushion restraint systems. **Pub:** *Proceedings of the Canadian Multidisciplinary Road Safety Conferences.* **Frmly:** Multidisciplinary Accident Investigation Unit.

**University of California, San Diego Division of Pulmonary and Critical Care Medicine**
*See:* Entry 18770

**University of Iowa Injury Prevention Research Center**
*See:* Entry 17841

**★ 8612 ★ University of Maryland at Baltimore National Study Center for Trauma and Emergency Medical Systems**
School of Medicine
701 W Pratt St., 5th Fl.
Baltimore, MD 21201-1023
**Phone:** (410)328-5085      **Fax:** (410)328-3699
**Email:** cmack003@umaryland.edu
**Website:** http://nsc.umaryland.edu
Colin F. Mackenzie, MD, Dir.
**Activities/Fields:** Trauma, emergency medicine, and emergency medical systems.

**★ 8613 ★ University of Pittsburgh Safar Center for Resuscitation Research**
3434 5th Ave.
Pittsburgh, PA 15260
**Phone:** (412)383-1900      **Fax:** (412)624-0943
**Email:** kochanekpm@anes.upmc.edu
**Website:** http://www.safar.pitt.edu
Patrick M. Kochanek, MD, Dir.
**Activities/Fields:** Traumatic brain injury and mechanisms of secondary injury, cardiopulmonary arrest and resuscitation, disaster medicine, and suspended animation. **Pub:** *Annual Report.* **Frmly:** Resuscitation Research Center.

**★ 8614 ★ West Virginia University Center for Rural Emergency Medicine (CREM)**
Robert C. Byrd Health Sciences Center
1299 Pineview Dr.
PO Box 9151
Morgantown, WV 26506-9151
**Phone:** (304)293-6682      **Fax:** (304)293-0265
**Email:** jwilliams@hfc.wvu.edu
**Website:** http://www.hsc.wvu.edu/som/crem/
Dr. Janet M. Williams, Dir.
**Activities/Fields:** Delivery and efficacy of emergency medical care in rural areas, including the etiologies and risk factors associated with emergency care visits and the reduction of morbidity and mortality in rural areas.

**★ 8615 ★ West Virginia University West Virginia Poison Center**
3110 MacCorkle Ave. SE
Charleston, WV 25304
**Phone:** (304)347-1212      **Fax:** (304)348-9560
**Website:** http://www.hsc.wvu.edu/charleston/wvpc/
Elizabeth J. Scharman, Dir.
**Activities/Fields:** Demographics of poison victims and epidemiology of poisoning. Research is conducted in support of the Center's service program in poison prevention and management.

# State Government Agencies

## Emergency Medical Services

**★ 8616 ★ Alaska Department of Health and Social Services**
**Public Health Division**
**Community Health and Emergency Medical Services Section**
410 Willoughby St., Rm. 109
PO Box 110616
Juneau, AK 99811-0616
**Phone:** (907)465-3027    **Fax:** (907)465-4101
**Email:** Mark_Johnson@health.state.ak.us
**Website:** http://www.chems.alaska.gov/
Mark S. Johnson, Director


**★ 8617 ★ Arizona Department of Health Services**
**Office of Emergency Medical Services**
1651 E Morten
Phoenix, AZ 85020
**Phone:** (602)861-0708    **Free:** 800-200-8523
**Fax:** (602)861-9812
**Email:** jcrume@hs.state.az.us
**Website:** http://www.hs.state.az.us/bems/index.htm
Judi Crume, RN,PhD, Director


**★ 8618 ★ Connecticut Department of Public Health**
**Emergency Medical Services Office**
410 Capitol Ave.
PO Box 340308
Hartford, CT 06134-0308
**Phone:** (860)509-7975    **Fax:** (860)509-7987
**Email:** webmaster.dph@po.state.ct.us
**Website:** http://www.state.ct.us/dph/DPH_Main/About_DPH/oems/oems.htm
Mark C. N. Libby, R.N., Director


**★ 8619 ★ DOH/Office of Emergency Health and Medical Services**
**Emergency Health and Medical Services**
825 N Capitol St., NE, Rm. 4177
Washington, DC 20002
**Phone:** (202)442-9111    **Fax:** (202)442-4812
**Website:** http://www.dchealth.com/ehms/welcome.htm


**★ 8620 ★ Florida Department of Health**
**Bureau of Emergency Medical Services**
4052 Esplanade Way, 3rd Fl.
Tallahassee, FL 32311-1738
**Phone:** (850)245-4440    **Fax:** (850)921-8162
**Email:** EMSCHR@doh.state.fl.us
**Website:** http://www.doh.state.fl.us/workforce/ems1/index.html
Charles Bement, Director


**★ 8621 ★ Georgia Department of Human Resources**
**Division of Public Health**
**Office of Emergency Medical Services**
Skyland Ctr., Lower Level
2600 Skyland Dr.
Atlanta, GA 30319
**Phone:** (404)679-0547    **Fax:** (404)679-0526
**Email:** gdphinfo@dhr.state.ga.us
**Website:** http://www.ph.dhr.state.ga.us/programs/ems/index.shtml
R. Keith Wages, Director


**★ 8622 ★ Guam Office of Emergency Medical Services**
**Department of Public Health and Social Services**
PO Box 2816
Agana, GU 96932
**Phone:** (671)735-7303    **Fax:** (671)734-5910
Christine Gyulavics-Reyes, Director


**★ 8623 ★ Hawaii Board of Osteopathic Examiners**
**Department of Commerce & Consumer Affairs**
DCCA-PVL
PO Box 3469
Honolulu, HI 96801
**Phone:** (808)586-2698    **Fax:** (808)586-2874
**Website:** http://www.state.hi.us/dcca/pvl/areas_medical.html


**★ 8624 ★ Hawaii State Department of Health**
**Emergency Medical Services & Injury Prevention System**
3627 Kilauea Ave., Rm. 102
Honolulu, HI 96816-2317
**Phone:** (808)733-9210    **Fax:** (808)733-8332
**Email:** emss@camhmis.health.state.hi.us
**Website:** http://www.hawaii.gov/health/resource/ems/
Donna Maiava, Director


**★ 8625 ★ Idaho Department of Health and Welfare**
**Emergency Medical Services Bureau**
3092 Elder St.
Boise, ID 83705
**Phone:** (208)334-4000    **Free:** 800-926-2588
**Fax:** (208)334-4015
**Email:** IdahoEMS@idhw.state.id.us
**Website:** http://www2.state.id.us/dhw/ems/home.htm
Dia Gainor, Director


**★ 8626 ★ Illinois Department of Public Health**
**Emergency Medical Services Division**
525 W Jefferson St.
Springfield, IL 62761
**Phone:** (217)785-2080    **Fax:** (217)785-0253
**Email:** info@ilems.com
**Website:** http://www.ilems.com/
Leslee Stein-Spencer, Director


**★ 8627 ★ Indiana Emergency Medical Services Commission**
302 W Washington, Rm. E208 IGCS
Indianapolis, IN 46204-2258
**Phone:** (317)232-3980    **Fax:** (317)232-3895
**Email:** mgarvey@sema.state.in.us
**Website:** http://www.state.in.us/sema/ems.html


**★ 8628 ★ Iowa Department of Public Health**
**Emergency Medical Services**
401 SW 7th St., Ste. D
Des Moines, IA 50309
**Phone:** (515)281-3239    **Free:** 800-728-3367
**Fax:** (515)281-4958
**Website:** http://idph.state.ia.us/pa/ems/default.htm
Timothy D. Peterson, MD, Director


**★ 8629 ★ Kansas Board of Emergency Medical Services**
109 SW 6th Ave.
Topeka, KS 66603-3826
**Phone:** (785)296-7296    **Fax:** (785)296-6212
**Email:** emsdl@ink.org
**Website:** http://www.ksbems.org/
David Lake, Contact


**★ 8630 ★ Kentucky Department for Public Health**
**Division of Adult and Child Health**
**Emergency Medical Services Branch**
275 E Main St., HS1E-F
Frankfort, KY 40621-0001
**Phone:** (502)564-8963    **Fax:** (502)564-4687
**Email:** kbems@mail.state.ky.us
**Website:** http://www.kbems.org/
Brian Bishop, Director


**★ 8631 ★ Louisiana Department of Health and Hospitals**
**Public Health Services Office**
**Emergency Medical Services Bureau**
1201 Capitol Access Rd.
PO Box 94215
Baton Rouge, LA 70804
**Phone:** (225)342-4881    **Fax:** (225)342-4419
**Website:** http://www.dhh.state.la.us/OPH/ems.htm
Nancy Bourgeois, Director


**★ 8632 ★ Maine Emergency Medical Services**
16 Edison Dr.
Augusta, ME 04330
**Phone:** (207)287-3953    **Fax:** (207)287-6251
**Email:** Maine.EMS@state.me.us
**Website:** http://www.state.me.us/dps/ems/
Jay Bradshaw, Director


**★ 8633 ★ Maryland Institute for Emergency Medical Services Systems**
653 W Pratt St.
Baltimore, MD 21201-1536
**Phone:** (410)706-5074    **Fax:** (410)706-4768
**Email:** jbrown@miemss.org
**Website:** http://miemss.umaryland.edu/Home.htm
Robert Bass, MD, Director


**★ 8634 ★ Massachusetts Department of Public Health**
**Office of Emergency Medical Services**
56 Roland St.
Boston, MA 02129
**Phone:** (617)284-8300    **Fax:** (617)284-8350
**Website:** http://www.state.ma.us/dph/oems/oems.htm
Louise Goyette, Director


**★ 8635 ★ Michigan Department of Public Health**
**Emergency Medical Services Division**
525 W Ottawa St.
PO Box 30664
Lansing, MI 48909
**Phone:** (517)241-3020
**Email:** johnfhubin@michigan.gov
**Website:** http://www.cis.state.mi.us/bhs/ems/home.htm
John Hubinger, Director


**★ 8636 ★ Minnesota Emergency Medical Services Regulatory Board**
**Emergency Medical Services Section**
University Park Plaza
2829 University Ave. SE, Ste. 310
Minneapolis, MN 55414-3250
**Phone:** (612)627-6000    **Fax:** (612)627-5442
**Email:** EMSRB.Webmaster@state.mn.us
**Website:** http://www.emsrb.state.mn.us
Mary Hedges, Director


**★ 8637 ★ Mississippi State Department of Health**
**Emergency Medical Services**
570 E Woodrow Wilson, Annex Bldg 3rd Fl.
Jackson, MS 39215-1700
**Phone:** (601)576-7366    **Fax:** (601)576-7373

**Website:** http://www.msdh.state.ms.us/ems/index.htm
Jim Craig, Director

★ **8638** ★ **Missouri Department of Health**
**Emergency Medical Services Bureau**
PO Box 570
912 Wildwood
Jefferson City, MO 65109
**Phone:** (573)751-6356　　　**Fax:** (573)751-6348
**Email:** info@mail.health.state.mo.us
**Website:** http://www.health.state.mo.us/EMS/index.html
Steve Hise, DIR, Contact

★ **8639** ★ **Montana Department of Health**
**and Environmental Sciences**
**Emergency Medical Services Bureau**
Cogswell Bldg., Rm.C204
1400 Broadway
PO Box 202951
Helena, MT 59620
**Phone:** (406)444-3895　　　**Fax:** (406)444-1814
**Email:** jdetienne@state.mt.us
**Website:** http://www.dphhs.state.mt.us/hpsd/pubheal/healsafe/ems/index.htm
Ken Leighton-Boster, Director

★ **8640** ★ **Nebraska Division of**
**Emergency Medical Services**
301 Centennial Mall S, 3rd Fl.
PO Box 95007
Lincoln, NE 68509-5007
**Phone:** (402)471-3578　　　**Fax:** (402)471-6446
**Email:** Doug.Fuller@hhss.state.ne.us
**Website:** http://www.hhs.state.ne.us/ems/emsindex.htm
Doug Fuller, Contact

★ **8641** ★ **New Hampshire Bureau of**
**Emergency Medical Services**
10 Hazen Dr.
Concord, NH 03305-0003
**Phone:** (603)271-4568　　　**Fax:** (603)271-4567
**Email:** sprentiss@safety.state.nh.us
**Website:** http://webster.state.nh.us/safety/ems/
Suzanne Prentiss, Director

★ **8642** ★ **North Carolina Office of**
**Emergency Medical Services**
701 Barbour Dr.
Raleigh, NC 27603-2008
**Phone:** (919)855-3935　　　**Fax:** (919)733-7021
**Email:** drexdal.pratt@ncmail.net
**Website:** http://facility-services.state.nc.us/EMS/ems.htm
Drexdal Pratt, Director

★ **8643** ★ **North Dakota Department of**
**Health**
**Emergency Health Services Division**
600 E Boulevard Ave.
Bismarck, ND 58505-0200
**Phone:** (701)328-2388　　　**Fax:** (701)328-1890
**Email:** dehs@state.nd.us
**Website:** http://www.health.state.nd.us/ndhd/resource/dehs/dehs.htm
Timothy W. Wiedrich, Director

★ **8644** ★ **Ohio Department of Public**
**Safety**
**Division of Emergency Medical Services**
1970 W Broad St.
PO Box 182073
Columbus, OH 43218-2073

**Phone:** (614)466-9447　　　**Free:** 800-233-0785
**Fax:** (614)466-9461
**Email:** ltiberi@dps.state.oh.us
**Website:** http://www.state.oh.us/odps/division/ems/ems_local/default.htm
Laura Ludwig Tiberi, Director

★ **8645** ★ **Oklahoma State Department of**
**Health**
**Emergency Medical Services**
1000 NE 10th St., Rm. 1104
Oklahoma City, OK 73117
**Phone:** (405)271-4027　　　**Fax:** (405)271-3442
**Email:** webmaster@health.state.ok.us
**Website:** http://www.health.state.ok.us/program/ems/index.html
Eddie Manley, Director

★ **8646** ★ **Oregon Department of Human**
**Resources**
**Emergency Medical Services and**
**Systems**
800 NE Oregon St., Ste. 607
Portland State Office Bldg.
Portland, OR 97232
**Phone:** (503)731-4011　　　**Fax:** (503)731-4077
**Email:** j.chin@state.or.us
**Website:** http://www.ohd.hr.state.or.us/ems/welcome.htm
Jonathan Chin, Director

★ **8647** ★ **Pennsylvania Division of**
**Emergency Medical Services**
Health and Welfare Bldg., Rm. 1033
PO Box 90
Harrisburg, PA 17108
**Phone:** (717)787-8741　　　**Fax:** (717)772-0910
**Email:** ptrimble@health.state.pa.us
**Website:** http://www.health.state.pa.us/HPA/EMS/DEFAULT.HTM
Margaret E. Trimble, Director

★ **8648** ★ **Rhode Island Department of**
**Health**
**Emergency Medical Services Division**
3 Capitol Hill, Rm. 404
Providence, RI 02908-5097
**Phone:** (401)222-2231　　　**Fax:** (401)222-6548
**Email:** peterl@doh.state.ri.us
**Website:** http://www.health.state.ri.us
Peter Leary, Director

★ **8649** ★ **South Dakota Department of**
**Health**
**Emergency Medical Services Program**
600 E Capitol
Pierre, SD 57501-2536
**Phone:** (605)773-4031　　　**Free:** 800-738-2301
**Fax:** (605)773-5904
**Email:** bob.graff@state.sd.us
**Website:** http://www.state.sd.us/doh/EMS/index.htm
Robert Graff, Director

★ **8650** ★ **Tennessee Department of**
**Health**
**Manpower and Facilities Bureau**
**Emergency Medical Services Division**
Cordell Hull Bldg., 1st Fl.
425 Fifth Ave. N
Nashville, TN 37247-0701
**Phone:** (615)741-2584　　　**Free:** 888-310-4650
**Fax:** (615)741-4217
**Email:** DDenton@mail.state.tn.us
**Website:** www2.state.tn.us/health/ems/
Joseph B. Phillips, Director

★ **8651** ★ **Texas Department of Health**
**Bureau of Emergency Management**
**EMS Services**
1100 49th St.
Austin, TX 78756-3199
**Phone:** (512)834-6700　　　**Fax:** (512)834-6736
**Email:** emsinfo@tdh.state.tx.us
**Website:** http://www.tdh.state.tx.us/hcqs/ems/emshome.htm
Jim Arnold, Director

★ **8652** ★ **Vermont Department of Health**
**Emergency Medical Services Division**
108 Cherry St.
PO Box 70
Burlington, VT 05402-0070
**Phone:** (802)863-7310　　　**Free:** 800-244-0911
**Fax:** (802)863-7577
**Email:** vtems@vdh.state.vt.us
**Website:** http://www.state.vt.us/health/ems/
W. Dan Manz, Director

★ **8653** ★ **Virginia State Department of**
**Health**
**Emergency Medical Services Division**
1538 E Parham Rd.
Richmond, VA 23228
**Phone:** (804)371-3500　　　**Free:** 800-523-6019
**Fax:** (804)371-3543
**Email:** gbrown@vdh.state.va.us
**Website:** http://www.vdh.state.va.us/oems/index.asp
Gary Brown, Director

★ **8654** ★ **Washington Department of**
**Health**
**Office of Emergency Medical and Trauma**
**Prevention**
1112 Quince St.
PO Box 47853
Olympia, WA 98504-7853
**Phone:** (360)705-6700　　　**Free:** 800-525-0127
**Fax:** (360)705-6706
**Email:** marquita.schlender@doh.wa.gov
**Website:** http://www.doh.wa.gov/hsqa/emtp/default.htm

★ **8655** ★ **Wisconsin Division of Health**
**Emergency Medical Services**
1 W Wilson St.
Madison, WI 53702
**Phone:** (608)266-1865　　　**Fax:** (608)261-6392
**Email:** webmaildph@dhfs.state.wi.us
**Website:** http://www.dhfs.state.wi.us/DPH_EMSIP/index.htm
Jon Morgan, Contact

★ **8656** ★ **Wyoming State**
**Preventative Health and Safety Division**
**Emergency Medical Services Program**
Hathaway Bldg. 4th Floor
Cheyenne, WY 82002
**Phone:** (307)777-7955　　　**Free:** 888-228-8996
**Fax:** (307)777-5639
**Email:** EMSWebmaster@state.wy.us
**Website:** http://wdhfs.state.wy.us/ems/
Jimm Murray, Contact

# Chapter 23
# Endocrinology & Metabolism

## Federal Government Agencies

**★ 8657 ★ U.S. Department of Health and Human Services**
**National Institutes of Health (NIH)**
**National Institute of Diabetes, Digestive and Kidney Diseases (NIDDK)**
9000 Rockville Pike
Bethesda, MD 20892
**Phone:** (301)496-3583
**Website:** http://www.niddk.nih.gov/
Allen M. Spiegel, Director

**Desc:** The Institute conducts, fosters, and supports basic and clinical research into the causes, prevention, diagnosis, and treatment of diabetes, endocrine and metabolic diseases, digestive diseases and nutrition, kidney and urologic diseases, and blood diseases. It provides research grants and individual and institutional research training awards, and conducts and supports epidemiological and clinical studies on selected populations in the United States.

## Foundations & Other Funding Organizations

### Private Foundations

**Dale J. Bellamah Foundation**
*See:* Entry 155

**Nora Eccles Treadwell Foundation**
*See:* Entry 4919

**Robert G. Cabell III and Maude Morgan Cabell Foundation**
*See:* Entry 624

**Robert J. Kleberg, Jr. and Helen C. Kleberg Foundation**
*See:* Entry 625

**Willard T. C. Johnson Foundation**
*See:* Entry 761

### Corporate Foundations

**American Snuff Co. Charitable Trust**
*See:* Entry 827

**Eli Lilly Foundation**
*See:* Entry 1022

**International Multifoods Charitable Foundation**
*See:* Entry 7881

**John Wiley & Sons, Inc.**
*See:* Entry 1171

**Mitsubishi Electric America Foundation**
*See:* Entry 1246

**Riggs Bank NA**
*See:* Entry 1355

## Other Funding Organizations

**★ 8658 ★ American Diabetes Association (ADA)**
1701 N Beauregard St.
Alexandria, VA 22311
**Phone:** (703)549-1500          **Free:** 800-DIABETES
**Fax:** (703)836-7439
**Email:** customerservice@diabetes.org
**Website:** http://www.diabetes.org
John H. Graham, IV, CEO

**Desc:** Physicians, laypersons, and health professionals interested in diabetes mellitus. Promotes research, information and advocacy to find a prevention and cure for diabetes and to improve the lives of all people with diabetes. Promotes public awareness of diabetes as a serious disease. Conducts educational programs and provides information to people with diabetes and the health professionals who care for them. Administers research grants. **Awards:** Career Development Award (semiannual) for promising new investigators who hold an assistant professor or justified equivalent academic position within his/her institution. The award supports salary and the research project; Clinical Research Grant (semiannual) for investigators whose studies directly involve humans and focus on human subjects in which the effect of a change in the individual's external or internal environment is evaluated; Lions SightFirst Retinopathy Research Award (annual) for clinical or applied research in diabetic retinopathy; Medical Student Diabetes Research Fellowships (annual) for medical students to conduct a 3-6 month diabetes research project. The applicant must have a qualified sponsor; Mentor-Based Postdoctoral Fellowships (annual) for established diabetes investigators to provide stipend support of postdoctoral fellows who will train with them in diabetes research; Research Award (semiannual) for investigators who are conducting studies in diabetes research.

**Children's PKU Network (CPN)**
*See:* Entry 5594

**Cystinosis Foundation (CF)**
*See:* Entry 9276

**★ 8659 ★ Gluten Intolerance Group of North America (GIGNA)**
15110 10th Ave., SW
Ste. A
Seattle, WA 98116-1820
**Phone:** (206)246-6652          **Fax:** (206)246-6531
**Email:** info@gluten.net
**Website:** http://www.gluten.net
Cynthia Kupper, CRD, CDE, Exec. Dir.

**Desc:** Persons with gluten-sensitive enteropathy (celiac sprue) or dermatitis herpetiformis, family members, physicians, dietitians, and celiac sprue societies. (Gluten is a protein found in wheat, rye, oats, and barley. Gluten-sensitive enteropathy is an inherited disorder characterized by gluten-related destruction of the small intestine. Symptoms include diarrhea, weight loss, fatigue, and anemia.) Works to educate patients, health care personnel, and the public; to offer psychological support to celiac sprue patients and their families in dealing with the adjustment and nutritional limitations of the disease; to conduct research into the causes. Promotes practical application in specific food research, such as recipe development and information on gluten content of products. Offers children's services and group and individual counseling. **Awards:** Campership (annual); Membership (annual).

**★ 8660 ★ Juvenile Diabetes Research Foundation International (JDFI)**
120 Wall St.
New York, NY 10005-4001
**Phone:** (212)785-9500          **Free:** 800-533-CURE
**Fax:** (212)785-9595
**Email:** info@jdfcure.org
**Website:** http://www.jdrf.org
Peter Van Etten, Pres.

**Desc:** World's leading nonprofit, nongovernmental funder of diabetes research. Mission is to find a cure for diabetes and its complications through the support of research. Sponsors international workshops and conferences for biomedical researchers. Individual chapters offer support groups and other activities for families affected by diabetes. **Awards:** Fellowship for research; grant; recognition (annual) for scientific and humanitarian achievements, and for public service.

**★ 8661 ★ National Gaucher Foundation (NGF)**
5410 Edson Ln., Ste. 260
Rockville, MD 20852
**Phone:** (301)816-1515          **Free:** 800-GAU-CHER
**Fax:** (301)816-1516
**Email:** ngf@gaucherdisease.org
**Website:** http://www.gaucherdisease.org
Rhonda P. Buyers, Exec. Dir.

**Desc:** Persons with Gaucher Disease; interested medical professionals and individuals. Gaucher Disease, one of the most common inherited metabolic disorders, is caused by an enzyme deficiency which renders the body unable to break down and dispose of complex lipids (fat-like substances). These lipids accumulate in the spleen, liver, and bone marrow, causing enlargement of the organs and intermittent pain of varying severity. Gaucher is treatable through enzyme replacement therapy. (The disease is named for Phillippe C.E. Gaucher, a French physician who described it in 1882.) One in 10 Jews of E. European descent is a carrier and one in 450 has Gaucher Disease. Sponsors direct funding of and support for research and clinical programs at medical centers in the U.S. and abroad to develop a cure and/or treatment for Gaucher Disease. Seeks to help persons with the disorder by providing them the opportunity to share experiences and feelings on a confidential, personal basis. Disseminates technical and nontechnical information concerning the disease. Advocates increased screening for carriers and availability of prenatal diagnosis for families at risk. **Awards:** Grant.

★ 8662 ★ **National Niemann Pick Disease Foundation (NPD)**
c/o Barb Vorpahl
415 Madison Ave.
PO Box 49
Fort Atkinson, WI 53538
**Phone:** (920)563-0930          **Free:** 877-287-3672
**Fax:** (920)563-0931
**Email:** webmaster@nnpdf.org
**Website:** http://www.nnpdf.org
Barb Vorpahl, Chm.

**Desc:** Parents, medical and educational professionals, and friends. Works to promote medical research on Niemann-Pick Disease (NPD), a disorder which prevents metabolizing of the sphingomyelin lipid or cholesterol. Provides medical and educational information; offers support to families of children with NPD; facilitates genetic counseling for parents; supports legislation that affects patients and families with NPD; sponsors medical research. **Awards:** Grant for research of Niemann Pick Disease.

★ 8663 ★ **Oxalosis and Hyperoxaluria Foundation (OHF)**
5718 Holly Hills
Saint Louis, MO 63109
**Phone:** (314)351-2177          **Free:** 888-721-2432
**Fax:** (314)481-6368
**Email:** execdirector@ohf.org
**Website:** http://www.ohf.org
Shirley Schirmer, Natl. Sec.

**Desc:** Individuals affected by oxalosis and hyperoxaluria; health care professionals. Hyperoxaluria is a metabolic disease affecting the kidneys. Oxalosis occurs when calcium crystals have deposited elsewhere in the body, often the eyes, bones, and joints. Provides support services and information regarding the conditions and their affects. Encourages research. Operates referral service. **Awards:** Grant (annual) for hyperoxaluria and oxalosis researchers.

★ 8664 ★ **Pediatric Endocrinology Nursing Society (PENS)**
PO Box 2933
Gaithersburg, MD 20886-2933
**Website:** http://www.pens.org

**Desc:** Pediatric endocrine nurses. Promotes professional responsibility, accountability, ethics and respect; dedicated to the advancement of the art and science of pediatric endocrine nursing; establishes and maintains standards of practice; enhances nursing research, clinical expertise and recognition of excellence in nursing. **Awards:** Academic Education Scholarships for nursing academic programs (BSN, MSN, PhD); Continuing Education Scholarships to assist members attending PENS annual conference; Manual Chapter Author Grant provides financial support to active members authoring an original or revised chapter for the manual; Poster Presentation Grant for materials necessary to create a poster presentation for the PENS annual conference; Research grants to support pediatric endocrinology nursing research projects.

**Preventive Cardiovascular Nurses Association (PCNA)**
*See:* Entry 14938

★ 8665 ★ **Purine Research Society**
c/o Tahma Metz
5424 Beech Ave.
Bethesda, MD 20814-1730
**Phone:** (301)530-0354          **Fax:** (301)564-9597
**Email:** purine@erols.com
**Website:** http://www2.dgsys.com/~purine/
Tahma Metz, Exec. Dir.

**Desc:** Dedicated to funding research and treatment of diseases resulting from errors in purine metabolism, specifically purine autism, the largest single subgroup of autism. As with other metabolic diseases, purine disorders are caused by a defective gene that results in the production of an enzyme with too little or too much catalytic activity. Purine metabolic diseases include gout, Lesch-Nyhan syndrome, purine autism, ADA deficiency and others. We are supporting research to find the defective enzyme(s) responsible for purine overproduction in purine autism, particularly, and to find effective screening and treatment methods, including newborn screening, so that symptoms will never occur. **Awards:** Grant.

# National & International Organizations

★ 8666 ★ **Albinism World Alliance (AWA)**
PO Box 959
East Hampstead, NH 03826-0959
**Free:** 800-473-2310          **Fax:** (603)887-2310
**Email:** webmaster@albinism.org
**Website:** http://www.albinism.org/awa.html
Janice L. Knuth, Co-Chair

**Fnded:** 1992. **Desc:** Albinism support groups in 15 countries. (Albinism is an inherited metabolic disorder that results in reduced pigment in the hair, eyes, and/or skin of those it affects; people with albinism also have impaired eye function including decreased visual acuity, involuntary eye movements, and increased sensitivity to light.) Fosters communication among albinism support groups, and promotes development of albinism support groups worldwide. Disseminates information.

★ 8667 ★ **American Association of Clinical Endocrinologists (AACE)**
1000 Riverside Ave., Ste. 205
Jacksonville, FL 32204
**Phone:** (904)353-7878          **Fax:** (904)353-8185
**Email:** djones@aace.com
**Website:** http://www.aace.com
Donald C. Jones, CEO

**Fnded:** 1991. **Mem:** 4,000. **Desc:** Clinical endocrinologists and physicians with special education in diabetes, osteoporosis, thyroid illness, lipid-cholesterol problems, reproductive disorders, obesity and nutrition. Seeks to enhance the practice of clinical endocrinology. **Pub:** *Endocrine Practice*, bimonthly. Journal. Features peer reviewed scientific articles on clinical endocrinology. • *The First Messenger*, bimonthly. Newsletter.

★ 8668 ★ **American Association of Diabetes Educators (AADE)**
100 W Monroe, Ste. 400
Chicago, IL 60603-1901
**Phone:** (312)424-2426          **Free:** 800-338-3633
**Fax:** (312)424-2427
**Email:** aade@aadenet.org
**Website:** http://www.aadenet.org
Judy Neel, Exec. Dir.

**Fnded:** 1973. **Mem:** 10,000. **Local Groups:** 105. **Desc:** Nurses, dietitians, social workers, physicians, pharmacists, podiatrists, and others involved in teaching diabetes self-management to diabetics. Purposes are to: provide educational opportunities for the professional growth and development of members; to promote the development of quality diabetes education for the diabetic consumer; to foster communication and cooperation among individuals and organiza-

tions involved in diabetes patient education. Offers continuing education programs for diabetes educators. **Pub:** *AADE FYI*, quarterly. Newsletter. Includes calendar of events, and articles on diabetes education and practice. *Price:* Included in membership dues. • *AADE Member Resource Guide*, annual. Membership Directory. • *Core Curriculum for Diabetes Education.* • *The Diabetes Educator*, bimonthly. Journal. Contains original articles from all disciplines regarding diabetes and diabetes patient education. Includes advertisers index and book reviews. *Price:* Included in membership dues; $45/year for nonmembers. • Also publishes position statements and various guidelines for diabetes education.

★ 8669 ★ **American Diabetes Association (ADA)**
1701 N Beauregard St.
Alexandria, VA 22311
**Phone:** (703)549-1500          **Free:** 800-DIABETES
**Fax:** (703)836-7439
**Email:** customerservice@diabetes.org
**Website:** http://www.diabetes.org
John H. Graham, IV, CEO

**Fnded:** 1940. **Mem:** 280,000. **State Groups:** 53. **Local Groups:** 800. **Desc:** Physicians, laypersons, and health professionals interested in diabetes mellitus. Promotes research, information and advocacy to find a prevention and cure for diabetes and to improve the lives of all people with diabetes. Promotes public awareness of diabetes as a serious disease. Conducts educational programs and provides information to people with diabetes and the health professionals who care for them. Administers research grants. **Pub:** *Clinical Diabetes*, bimonthly. Newsletter. Provides current scientific information about diabetes and its treatment to the primary care provider. *Price:* $15/year member; $30/year nonmember; $40/year institution. • *Diabetes*, monthly. Contains original research papers on the physiology and pathophysiology of diabetes mellitus and related disorders. *Price:* $75/year members; $135/year nonmembers; $200/year institution. • *Diabetes Care*, monthly. Journal. Covers original clinical research and commentaries primarily directed toward improving the medical management of people with diabetes mellitus. *Price:* $75/year members; $100/year nonmembers; $150/year institution. • *Diabetes Forecast*, monthly. Magazine. Healthy life styles magazine for people with diabetes. Provides in fo. about diabetes, self-care exercise, diet, travel, and personal development. *Price:* Included in membership dues. • *Diabetes Reviews*, quarterly. Journal. Provides comprehensive reviews of basic science and clinical issues in diabetes. *Price:* $45/year for members; $85/year for nonmembers; $125/year for institutions. • *Diabetes Spectrum: From Research to Practice*, quarterly. Journal. *Price:* Included in membership dues; $30/uear member; $45/year nonmember. • Videos. • Publishes a catalog of publications available.

★ 8670 ★ **American Porphyria Foundation (APF)**
PO Box 22712
Houston, TX 77227
**Phone:** (713)266-9617          **Fax:** (713)871-1788
**Email:** porphyrus@juno.com
**Website:** http://www.enterprise.net/apf
Desiree H. Lyon, Exec. Dir.

**Fnded:** 1981. **Mem:** 1,900. **Desc:** Persons interested in advancing awareness and treatment of the porphyrias; affected patients. Porphyria is a class of seven rare (and usually inherited) metabolic disorders of varying severity affecting the nervous system or the skin. It is characterized by a deficiency of an enzyme used in making heme (a ring-shaped molecule called a porphyrin), which in turn is used in making hemoglobin. One of porphyria's recurrent though not requisite symptoms is purple-red urine. The foundation's purposes are to: provide financial support for researchers in porphyria; improve the diagnosis and treatment of porphyria through educational programs; locate porphyria patients. Maintains a lending library of videotapes, papers, and pamphlets. **Pub:** *American Porphyria Foundation–Newsletter*, quarterly. Newsletter.

Contains educational information. *Price:* Included in membership dues. • Pamphlets. • Also compiles list of physicians with experience in treating porphyria.

---

**★ 8671 ★ American Prostate Society**
PO Box 870
Hanover, MD 21076
**Phone:** (410)859-3735 **Free:** 800-308-1106
**Fax:** (410)850-0818
**Email:** ameripros@mindspring.org
**Website:** http://www.ameripros.org
Claude Gerard, Chm.

**Fnded:** 1991. **Mem:** 51,000. **Nat'l Groups:** 1. **Local Groups:** 1. **Desc:** Works to increase the public's awareness of prostate disease. Encourages men to get annual exams. Aids hospitals and other health care facilities that are dedicated exclusively to detection and treatment of prostate disease. Sponsors Prostate Awareness Week. Conducts speakers' bureau. Sponsors educational programs. **Pub:** *Update*, quarterly. Newsletter. Review and special reports on developments in prostate disease. *Price:* Free. • Brochures, annual.

**★ 8672 ★ American Thyroid Association (ATA)**
PO Box 1836
Falls Church, VA 22041-1836
**Phone:** (703)998-8890 **Fax:** (703)998-8891
**Email:** admin@thyroid.org
**Website:** http://www.thyroid.org
Barbara Smith, Exec. Dir.

**Fnded:** 1923. **Mem:** 650. **Desc:** Internists, surgeons, pathologists, radiologists, and research workers interested in the thyroid gland and its diseases. **Pub:** *Thyroid*, periodic. Journal. • Membership Directory, annual. **Frmly:** (1948) American Association for the Study of Goiter; (1961) American Goiter Association.

**★ 8673 ★ Argentine Society of Endocrinology and Metabolism (Sociedad Argentina de Endocrinologia y Metabolismo)**
Diaz Velez 3889
Buenos Aires, Argentina
**Fnded:** 1941.

**★ 8674 ★ ASEAN Federation of Endocrine Societies**
Philippine Diabetes Association
Unit 25 Facilities Center
Shaw Blvd.
Mandaluyong City, Philippines
**Lang(s):** English, Filipino. **Desc:** Endocrinologists and health care facilities. Seeks to advance the study and practice of endocrinology. Facilitates exchange of information among members; conducts continuing professional development courses.

**★ 8675 ★ Asian and Oceania Thyroid Association (AOTA)**
Department of Internal Medicine
Asian Medical Center
University of Ulsan College of Medicine
388-1 Poongnap-dong, Sonpa-gu
Seoul 138-736, Republic of Korea
**Phone:** 82 2 30103911 **Fax:** 82 2 30106962
**Email:** imahn@aota.or.kr
**Website:** http://aota.or.kr
**Lang(s):** English, Japanese. **Desc:** Endocrinologists and other medical professionals and scientists with an interest in the thyroid gland. Seeks to advance the understanding of the thyroid gland and its functions; works to improve the diagnosis and treatment of thyroid diseases. Gathers and disseminates endocrinological information pertaining to the thyroid gland; sponsors researcha and continuing professional development programs.

**★ 8676 ★ Association for Glycogen Storage Disease**
1 Cridlands
Lydiard St. Lawrence
Taunton TA4 3RZ, United Kingdom
**Phone:** 44 161 9807303 **Fax:** 44 161 2263813
**Email:** president@agsd.org.uk
**Website:** http://www.agsd.org.uk
**Mem:** 150. **Desc:** Provides contacts and support for all persons with Glycogen Storage Disease. Encourages the provision of Specialist Centres for the diagnosis, monitoring and treatment of GSD affected persons, both children and adults. Provides a focus for scientific, educational and charitable activities concerning GSD. Encourages the formation and interaction of GSD families and professionals around the world.

**★ 8677 ★ Association for Glycogen Storage Disease (AGSD)**
PO Box 896
Durant, IA 52747
**Phone:** (563)785-6038 **Fax:** (563)785-6038
**Website:** http://www.agsdus.org
Hollie Swain, Pres.

**Fnded:** 1979. **Mem:** 400. **Desc:** Individuals afflicted with glycogen storage disease; families of GSD sufferers; health care professionals. (GSD is a hereditary condition characterized by a lack of or deficiency in any of the enzymes used by the body to break down glycogen, resulting in hypoglycemia and related disorders, and requiring diet modifications and frequent or continual feeding, and in extreme cases resulting in death.) Acts as a forum for the discussion of GSD, its treatment, and the problems faced by parents raising children with GSD. Disseminates medical information; fosters communication between the families of GSD patients and health care professionals. Conducts fundraising drive. Aids members in obtaining equipment necessary for home care of GSD patients; provides referral services for individuals seeking GSD treatment facilities. **Pub:** *Could Someone You Know be Affected?*. Brochures. *Price:* Free. • *Parent Handbook*. Book. *Price:* $10. • *The Ray*, quarterly. Newsletter. *Price:* Free.

**★ 8678 ★ Association of Program Directors in Endocrinology, Diabetes and Metabolism**
4350 East West Highway, Ste. 500
Bethesda, MD 20814
**Phone:** (301)941-0243 **Fax:** (301)941-0259
**Email:** nchill@endo-society.org
**Website:** http://www.apdem.org
Nancy Chill, Association Mgr.

**Fnded:** 1996. **Mem:** 160. **Desc:** Founded to benefit and aid the education, research and patient care missions of subspecialty training programs in endocrinology, diabetes and metabolism. Supports new initiative in educational and public research and patient care. **Frmly:** (2002) Association of Program Directors in Endocrinology and Metabolism.

**★ 8679 ★ Bahrain Diabetic Association**
PO Box 29080
Bahrain, Bahrain
**Phone:** 973 9602422 **Fax:** 973 400488
**Email:** fzurba@batelco.com.bh
**Desc:** Individuals in Bahrain with diabetes. Seeks to assist and inform diabetic individuals. Furthers public understanding of diabetes by disseminating information.

**★ 8680 ★ British Diabetic Association**
5th FL., Charles House
148/9 Great Charles St.
Queensway
Birmingham W1M 0BD, United Kingdom
**Phone:** 44 121 2008080 **Fax:** 44 121 2008081
**Email:** info@bda.uk.com
**Website:** http://www.bda.uk.com

**Fnded:** 1934. **Mem:** 190,000. **Reg. Groups:** 450. **Lang(s):** English. **Desc:** Open to everyone. Life and annual subscription rates. Provides help and advice to everyone living with diabetes and those who care for them. Represents people with diabetes on matters affecting the individual. Supports diabetes research; assists diabetes associations and medical professionals in Bulgaria, Russia, and Ukraine. **Pub:** *Balance*, bimonthly. Magazines. • *Diabetes Update*, periodic. Report. • *Diabetic Medicine*, monthly. Newsletter.

**★ 8681 ★ Bulgarian Society of Endocrinology**
Bolnitsa po Endokrinologia
Dame Gruev 6
BG-1303 Sofia, Bulgaria
**Phone:** 359 2 9871497 **Fax:** 359 2 9874145
**Email:** dimitar@medicalnet-bg.org
**Fnded:** 1973. **Mem:** 170. **Nat'l Groups:** 1. **Reg. Groups:** 3. **State Groups:** 1. **Local Groups:** 3. **Lang(s):** English. **Desc:** Fosters research in endocrinology. **Pub:** *Journal of Endocrinology: Endocrinologia*, quarterly. Journal. **Frmly:** (1997) Scientific Society of Endocrinology.

**★ 8682 ★ Canadian Association of Centers for the Management of Hereditary Metabolic Diseases (Association Canadienne des Centres de Traitement pour les Malades Metaboliques Hereditaires)**
c/o Winnipeg Children's Hospital
820 Sherbrook St.
Winnipeg, MB, Canada R3A 1R9
**Phone:** (204)787-2494 **Fax:** (204)787-1419
**Email:** cgroenberg@hsc.mb.ca
**Lang(s):** English, French. **Desc:** Medical centers specializing in the treatment of people with hereditary metabolic disorders. Seeks to advance the diagnosis and treatment of hereditary metabolic disorders. Facilitates exchange of information among members; serves as a clearinghouse on hereditary metabolic disorders.

**★ 8683 ★ Canadian Chronic Prostatitis Research Foundation**
PO Box 4123, Stn. E
Ottawa, ON, Canada K1S 5B2
**Email:** prostatitis@prostatitiscanada.ca
**Website:** http://www.prostatitiscanada.org
**Fnded:** 1998. **Mem:** 200. **Lang(s):** English. **Desc:** Canadian sufferers of chronic prostatitis and their families. Promotes research into the causes, treatments, and cures of persistent inflammation of the prostate gland. Works to educate Canadian men and their physicians and to raise funds for the dissemination of information regarding chronic prostatitis.

**★ 8684 ★ Canadian Diabetes Association (CDA) (Association Canadienne du Diabete — ACD)**
15 Toronto St., Ste. 800
Toronto, ON, Canada M5C 2E3
**Phone:** (416)363-3373 **Free:** 800-BAN-TING
**Fax:** (416)363-3393
**Email:** info@diabetes.ca
**Website:** http://www.diabetes.ca
**Lang(s):** English, French. **Desc:** People with diabetes and their families; health care professionals with an interest in diabetes. Seeks to advance the prevention, diagnosis, and treatment of diabetes. Provides support and services to people with diabetes and their families; sponsors research and educational programs.

**★ 8685 ★ Canadian Diabetes Association - Diabetes Educator Section**
15 Toronto St., Ste. 800
Toronto, ON, Canada M5C 2E3

**Phone:** (416)363-0177　　**Free:** 800-226-8464
**Fax:** (416)363-7465
**Email:** info@diabetes.ca
**Website:** http://www.diabetes.ca

**Fnded:** 1973. **Mem:** 2,200. **Local Groups:** 43. **Lang(s):** English, French. **Desc:** Health professionals with an interest in diabetes. Seeks to advance the prevention and management of diabetes. Conducts research and educational programs. **Pub:** *Canadian Journal of Diabetes Care*, quarterly. Journal. • *Diabetes Quarterly*, quarterly. Newsletter.


### ★ 8686 ★ Canadian Hemochromatosis Society (CHS)

272-7000 Minoru Blvd.
Richmond, BC, Canada V6Y 3Z5
**Phone:** (604)279-7135　　**Fax:** (604)279-7138
**Email:** office@cdnhemochromatosis.ca
**Website:** http://www.cdnhemochromatosis.ca

**Fnded:** 1982. **Mem:** 794. **Lang(s):** English, French. **Desc:** People with hemochromatosis and their families; health care providers with an interest in metabolic and genetic disorders. Promotes early diagnosis, and treatment of hemochromatosis. Operates national support group network; conducts fundraising activities benefiting medical research. Conducts educational programs to raise awareness of hemochromatosis. **Pub:** *Among Ourselves*, biennial. Newsletter. Provides information about hemochromatosis and the activities of the society. Information packages; "The Bronze Killer" (book).


### ★ 8687 ★ Canadian Porphyria Foundation

PO Box 1206
Neepawa, MB, Canada R0J 1H0
**Phone:** (204)476-2800　　**Fax:** (204)476-2800
**Email:** porphyria@cpf-inc.ca
**Website:** http://www.cpf-inc.ca

**Lang(s):** English. **Desc:** Porphyria patients and their families. Works to improve the quality of life for people affected by prophyria. **Pub:** *A Guide to Porphyria*. Booklet. • Newsletter, semiannual.


### ★ 8688 ★ Canadian Society of Endocrinology and Metabolism (CSEM) (Societe Canadienne d'Endocrinologie et Metabolisme — SCEM)

Lady Davis Institute Rm 602
3755 Cote St. Cahterine Rd.
Montreal, QC, Canada H3T 1E2
**Phone:** (514)340-8222　　**Fax:** (514)340-7502
**Email:** lenore.beitel@mcgill.ca
**Website:** http://ww2.mcgill.ca/csem

**Lang(s):** English, French. **Desc:** Endocrinologists and other health care professionals with an interest in metabolism. Seeks to advance the study of metabolism and the practice of endocrinology; promotes ongoing professional development of members. Serves as a forum for the exchange of information among members; sponsors research and educational programs.


### Canadian Society for Mucopolysaccharide and Related Diseases

*See:* Entry 5647


### ★ 8689 ★ Coeliac Society of Ireland

4 North Brunswick
Dublin, Ireland
**Email:** lori@mpssociety.ca
**Website:** http://www.mpssociety.ca

**Fnded:** 1970. **Mem:** 2,500. **Reg. Groups:** 8. **State Groups:** 1. **Desc:** Promotes, safeguards, and protects the interests of our members in relation to coeliac disease. Produces a list of gluten free foods, information leaflets, and cook books.


### ★ 8690 ★ Diabetes Exercise and Sports Association (DESA)

PO Box 1935
Litchfield Park, AZ 85340
**Phone:** (623)535-4593　　**Free:** 800-898-4322
**Fax:** (623)535-4741
**Email:** desa@diabetes-exercise.org
**Website:** http://www.diabetes-exercise.org
Paula Harper, RN, CDE, Pres.

**Fnded:** 1985. **Mem:** 3,500. **Reg. Groups:** 12. **Desc:** Individuals with diabetes and healthcare professionals. Promotes the participation of individuals with diabetes in sports activities. Provides a network and support group for athletes with diabetes. Conducts educational programs to increase self care skills for individuals with diabetes and counseling skills for healthcare professionals. Offers blood sugar screenings; sponsors volunteer services and speakers' bureau. Conducts children's services. **Pub:** *Challenge*, quarterly. Newsletter. Educational with inspiring stories of success with diabetes and exercise. *Price:* Free for members. • *Get Ready-Get Set-Go*. Pamphlet.


### ★ 8691 ★ Diabetes Federation of Ireland

76 Lower Gardiner St.
Dublin 1, Ireland
**Phone:** 353 1 8363022　　**Fax:** 353 1 8365182
**Email:** diabetestfederation@diabetesireland.ie
**Website:** http://www.diabetesireland.ie

**Fnded:** 1967. **Mem:** 4,000. **Local Groups:** 21. **Desc:** Represents people with diabetes. Provides information, creates awareness encourages research and ongoing support of people with diabetes. **Pub:** *Identity*, quarterly. Magazine. Contains diabetes information.


### ★ 8692 ★ Diabetes Research Institute Foundation (DRIF)

3440 Hollywood Blvd.
Hollywood, FL 33021
**Phone:** (954)964-4040　　**Free:** 800-321-3437
**Fax:** (954)964-7036
**Email:** info@drif.org
**Website:** http://www.drinet.org
Robert A. Pearlman, Exec. VP

**Fnded:** 1971. **Mem:** 10,000. **Reg. Groups:** 2. **Desc:** Works to improve the quality of life for individuals with diabetes and to find a cure for diabetes. Acts as an information clearinghouse. Offers referral services. Fosters research on diabetes. Conducts educational programs; maintains speakers' bureau. Compiles statistics. **Pub:** *Focus*, 3/year. Newsletter. Covers foundation events, research news, and donor profiles.


### ★ 8693 ★ Endocrine Fellows Foundation

2950 31st St., Ste. 354
Santa Monica, CA 90405
**Phone:** 877-877-6515
**Email:** endofellowsfnd@cs.com
**Website:** http://www.endocrinefellows.org
Marilyn Fishman, Exec. Dir.

**Fnded:** 1990. **Desc:** Endocrine fellows. Providing support to endocrine fellows in education, research grant funding and career guidance. Also, works to provide both fellows and endocrinology professionals with cutting-edge research results on developments in the fields of endocrinology, metabolism and diabetology.


### ★ 8694 ★ Endocrine Society (ES)

4350 East West Hwy., Ste. 500
Bethesda, MD 20814-4426
**Phone:** (301)941-0200　　**Fax:** (301)941-0259
**Email:** endostaff@endo-society.org
**Website:** http://www.endo-society.org
Scott Hunt, Exec. Dir.

**Fnded:** 1915. **Mem:** 8,000. **Desc:** Promotes excellence in research, education, and clinical practice in endocrinology and related disciplines. Maintains placement service. **Pub:** *Endocrine News*, bimonthly. Newsletter. Includes calendar of events and listing of honors and awards recipients; legislative issues and clinical practice column. *Price:* Included in member-

ship dues. • *Endocrine Reviews*, bimonthly. Journal. Covers clinical and experimental endocrinology; readers are encouraged to suggest prospective authors and to submit their own manuscripts. *Price:* $50 /year for members in U.S.; $115 /year for nonmembers in U.S.; $195 /year for institutions in U.S.; $85 for those in training in U.S. • *Endocrinology*, monthly. Journal. Covers current biomedical research for basic scientists. *Price:* $95/year for members in U.S.; $195 /year for nonmembers in U.S.; $410/year for institutions in U.S.; $125/year for those in training in U.S. • *Journal of Clinical Endocrinology and Metabolism*, monthly. Journal. Provides current information on the clinical applications of endocrine research for internists, pediatricians, and practicing obstetricians. *Price:* $85/year for members in U.S.; $180 /year for nonmembers in U.S.; $310/year for institutions in U.S.; $110/year for those in training in U.S. • *Molecular Endocrinology*, monthly. Journal. Covers the molecular mechanisms of cellular regulation and hormone action. *Price:* $80/year for members in U.S.; $175 /year for nonmembers in U.S.; $295/year for institutions in U.S.; $110/year for those in training in U.S. **Frmly:** Association for Study of Internal Secretions.


### ★ 8695 ★ Endocrine Society of Australia (ESA)

Institute of Reproduction and Development
Monash University
Clayton, VIC 3168, Australia
**Phone:** 61 3 95503571　　**Fax:** 61 3 95503584
**Email:** gail.risbridge@med.monash.edu.au

**Fnded:** 1958.


### ★ 8696 ★ European Association for the Study of Diabetes (EASD)

c/o
Merowingerstr, 29
D-40223 Dusseldorf, Germany
**Phone:** 49 211 316738　　**Fax:** 49 211 3190987
**Email:** easd@uni-duesseldorf.de
**Website:** http://www.easd.org

**Fnded:** 1964. **Mem:** 5,500. **Lang(s):** English. **Desc:** Individuals and firms in over 100 countries. Promotes research into the disease of diabetes. Sponsors postgraduate education courses. **Pub:** *Diabetologia*, periodic. Journal. Scientific medical journal, containing diabetic research. • *Membership List*, triennial.


### ★ 8697 ★ European Federation of Endocrine Societies (EFES)

29, rue Soeur Bouvier
F- 69322 Lyon, France
**Phone:** 33 4 72385848　　**Fax:** 33 4 78256168
**Email:** forest@lyon151.inserm.fr
**Website:** http://www.unige.ch/efes/

**Fnded:** 1984.


### ★ 8698 ★ European Federation of Endocrine Societies

c/o J.A.H. Wass
Endocrine Unit
Radcliffe Infirmary
Woodstock Rd.
Oxford OX2 6HE, United Kingdom
**Phone:** 44 1865 742348　　**Fax:** 44 1865 227621
**Email:** john.wass@noc.anglox.nhs.uk

**Desc:** Promotes endocrinology in Europe. Seeks to advance research and education in endocrinology. Organizes postgraduate courses.


### ★ 8699 ★ European Study Group on Lysosomal Diseases (ESGLD)

c/o Professor B. Winchester
Institute of Child Health, University of London
Biochemistry, Endocrinology and Metabolism Unit
30 Guilford St.
London WC1N 1EH, United Kingdom
**Phone:** 44 207 2429789　　**Fax:** 44 207 8310488
**Email:** b.byth@ich.vcl.ac.uk
**Website:** http://www.ich.ucl.ac.uk/

**Fnded:** 1978. **Mem:** 90. **Lang(s):** English. **Desc:** Laboratories in 22 countries conducting research on lysosomal storage diseases. (Lysosomal storage diseases are hereditary disorders, resulting from defects in lysosomal enzymes or membrane components, characterized by accumulation of partially digested metabolites in tissues and excretion in urine.) Promotes research; encourages exchange of ideas and personnel among member laboratories. **Pub:** *Lysosome Newsletter*, biennial. Newsletter. • *Register of Laboratories*, biennial.

### ★ 8700 ★ FOD Family Support Group
c/o Deb Lee Gould
805 Montrose Dr.
Greensboro, NC 27410
**Phone:** (336)547-8682
**Email:** deb@fodsupport.org
**Website:** http://www.fodsupport.org
Deb Lee Gould, Dir.

**Fnded:** 1991. **Mem:** 1,100. **Desc:** Seeks to provide emotional and practical support and medical information for families confronting fatty oxidation disorders (FOD), as well as interested professionals. **Pub:** *FOD Communication Network*, semiannual. Newsletter. Contains medical and pharmaceutical updates, family stories, questions and answers. Also available in hardcopy. *Price:* Free. **Frmly:** MCAD Family Support Group.

### ★ 8701 ★ French Diabetes Association (FDA)
### (Association Francaise des Diabetiques — AFD)
58, rue Alexandre Dumas
F-75544 Paris, France
**Phone:** 33 1 40092425    **Fax:** 33 1 40092030
**Email:** afdsiege@aoos.fr
**Website:** http://www.afd.asso.fr
**Fnded:** 1938. **Mem:** 30,000. **Reg. Groups:** 130. **Local Groups:** 130. **Lang(s):** English, French. **Desc:** Individuals with diabetes in France. Works to inform, assist, and defend diabetics. Furthers public understanding of diabetes by disseminating information to the public and medical specialists. **Pub:** *Equilibre*, quarterly. Magazine. • *Medical and Informations sur le Diabete*, periodic.

### ★ 8702 ★ French-Language Association for the Study of Diabetes and Metabolic Disorders
### (Association de Langue Francaise pour l'Etude du Diabete et des Maladies Metaboliques — ALFEDIAM)
58, rue Alexandre Dumas
F-75011 Paris, France
**Phone:** 33 1 40098907    **Fax:** 33 1 40092914
**Email:** alfediam@magic.fr
**Website:** http://www.alfediam.org
**Fnded:** 1954. **Mem:** 1,100. **Lang(s):** English, French. **Desc:** Health care professionals and researchers with an interest in diabetes and other metabolic disorders. Seeks to advance the prevention, diagnosis, and treatment of metabolic disorders. Provides support and services to people with diabetes and their families; serves as a clearinghouse on research on metabolic disorders; sponsors research and continuing professional development programs. **Pub:** *Diabetes and Metabolism*, bimonthly. Magazine.

### French-Speaking Association of Surgical Endocrinology (FSASE)
### (Association Francophone de Chirurgie Enocrinienne — AFCE)
*See:* Entry 19557

### ★ 8703 ★ Gaucher's Association (GA)
c/o Exec.Dir.
25 W Cottages
London NW6 1RJ, United Kingdom

**Phone:** 44 207 4331121
**Email:** office@gauchersassociation.org.uk
**Website:** http://www.gaucher.org.uk

**Fnded:** 1991. **Lang(s):** English. **Desc:** Individuals with Gaucher's disease. (Gaucher's disease is a genetic disorder resulting in enzyme deficiency, producing symptoms including anemia, fatigue, bone pain and degeneration, easy bruising, and a tendency to bleed. The rare Type 2 and Type 3 forms of Gaucher's disease can also cause various neurological problems.) Seeks to improve the quality of life of people with Gaucher's disease; encourages medical research on the diagnosis, prevention, and treatment of the disease. Serves as a support group for people with Gaucher's disease; works to increase the availability of enzyme treatments; facilitates contact among the families of people with Gaucher's disease in the UK.

### ★ 8704 ★ Graves' Disease Foundation
PO Box 1969
Brevard, NC 28712-1969
**Phone:** (828)877-5251    **Fax:** (828)885-7122
**Email:** ngdf@citcom.net
**Website:** http://www.ngdf.org
Nancy H. Patterson, PhD, Exec. Dir.

**Fnded:** 1990. **Mem:** 1,400. **State Groups:** 19. **Local Groups:** 25. **Desc:** People with Graves' disease; families of those affected; physicians and other professionals. Facilitates establishments of support groups for members in all states. Fosters public awareness and education on the causes, effects, and treatment of Grave's disease, a result of hyperthyroidism (the excess production by the body of thyroxine and triiodothyronine) in which the thyroid gland may be slightly enlarged, and symptoms such as a rapid heartbeat, eye problems, weight loss, or fatigue may occur. Participates in research on Graves' disease. **Pub:** Bulletin, periodic. • Newsletter, quarterly. **AKA:** National Graves' Disease Foundation.

### ★ 8705 ★ HELP - Institute for Body Chemistry (HELP)
PO Box 1338
Bryn Mawr, PA 19010
**Email:** ekrimmel2@earthlink.net
**Website:** http://home.earthlink.net/~ekrimmel2
Edward & Patricia Krimmel, Dirs.

**Fnded:** 1979. **Mem:** 2,500. **Desc:** Health professionals and interested individuals. Promotes public awareness of body chemistry problems within the context of general health. Seeks to collect, verify, and distribute information related to body chemistry especially hypoglycemia (low blood sugar), Celiac Disease, and cholesterol management. Conducts seminars regarding nutrition, exercise, life style, and emotional stability. Develops support groups and encourages communication among members. **Pub:** *Advocate*. Newsletter. Includes information on body chemistry, nutrition, and related medical research. • *Cholesterol Control Handbook and Cookbook.* • *Low Blood Sugar Cookbook.* • *Low Blood Sugar Handbook.* • *Vital Health Facts and Composition of Foods.*

### ★ 8706 ★ Hemochromatosis Foundation (HF)
c/o Margit A. Krikker, MD
PO Box 8569
Albany, NY 12208-0569
**Phone:** (518)489-0972    **Fax:** (518)489-0227
**Website:** http://www.hemochromatosis.org
Margit A. Krikker, MD, Med. Dir.

**Fnded:** 1982. **Mem:** 4,000. **Reg. Groups:** 8. **State Groups:** 6. **Local Groups:** 4. **Desc:** Physicians and other individuals concerned with hereditary hemochromatosis. (Hereditary hemochromatosis is a disorder of iron metabolism in which dietary iron absorption exceeds body needs. If not diagnosed and treated, the accumulating iron may result in one or more complications: liver enlargement, heart irregularities and failure, diabetes and other hormonal deficiencies, arthritis, and early death.) Seeks to increase public and professional awareness of hereditary hemochromatosis and of the hazards of supplemental iron. Encourages

routine use of screening tests by physicians, conducts screening studies of apparently healthy blood donors. Assists public, patients, families, and physicians with HH diagnosis, treatment, and genetic counseling and in forming regional support networks. Sponsors periodic teaching day for physicians and patients and their families. Conducts research programs. Plans to establish a central registry of persons with the disorder. **Pub:** *Family Teaching Conference 1992 at Cleveland Clinic.* Video. • *Hemochromatosis Awareness: A Quarterly Update on Hereditary and Acquired Iron-Overload.* Newsletter. Includes calendar of events and information on available services. *Price:* Free. • Booklets. **Frmly:** (1992) Hemochromatosis Research Foundation.

### ★ 8707 ★ Indian Society of Nephrology (ISN)
c/o Department of Nephrology
Sir Ganga Ram Hospital
Rajinder Nagar
New Delhi 110 060, Delhi, India
**Phone:** 91 11 5758660    **Fax:** 91 11 5812727
**Email:** dsrana@bol.net.in

**Fnded:** 1970. **Mem:** 732. **Desc:** Physicians specializing in nephrology. Fosters professional development of members.

### ★ 8708 ★ International Diabetes Federation (IDF)
### (Federation Internationale du Diabete — FID)
1, rue Defacqz
B-1000 Brussels, Belgium
**Phone:** 32 2 5385511    **Fax:** 32 2 5385114
**Email:** idf@idf.org
**Website:** http://www.idf.org
**Fnded:** 1949. **Mem:** 1,100. **Nat'l Groups:** 156. **Reg. Groups:** 7. **Lang(s):** English, French, Spanish. **Desc:** National diabetes associations; diabetes sections of national academies; endocrinology, metabolic, and diabetes societies; diabetes supplies companies are supporting members; association represents over one million individuals through its national associations. Objectives are: to improve the quality of life in the global diabetic community; to promote the exchange of information; to improve standards of treatment; to develop educational methods designed to patients a better understanding of there disease; to educate the public in the early recognition of the disease and the importance of its medically supervised treatment; to encourage medical, scientific, and socioeconomic research. Maintains liaison with the World Health Organization. Compiles statistics. Provides educational grants through the IDF Educational Foundation. **Pub:** *Diabetes Voice*, quarterly. Journal. • *The Economics of Diabetes & Diabetes Care: Costing Diabetes, the cause for Prevention.* • *IDF Bulletin*, quarterly. Journal. • *IDF Diabetes Voice*, 3/year. • *Triennial Report.*

### ★ 8709 ★ International Society of Endocrinology (ISE)
c/o Prof. Lesley H. Rees
51-53 St. Bartholomew's Hospital
Bartholomew Close
London EC1A 7BE, United Kingdom
**Phone:** 44 207 6064012    **Fax:** 44 207 7964676
**Email:** l.h.rees@mds.ac.uk
**Website:** http://www.jingo.com/ise/
**Fnded:** 1966. **Mem:** 53. **Desc:** Federation of national endocrinology societies with 15,000 individual members. Disseminates information on endocrinology and facilitates collaboration between national endocrinological societies and persons interested in the field. **Pub:** *Abstracts of Congresses*, annual. Newsletter. • *Symposia Abstracts*, periodic.

### International Society on Metabolic Eye Disease (ISMED)
*See:* Entry 20999

### ★ 8710 ★ Iron Overload Diseases Association (IOD)

433 Westwind Dr.
North Palm Beach, FL 33408-5123
**Phone:** (561)840-8512　　　**Fax:** (561)842-9881
**Email:** iod@ironoverload.org
**Website:** http://www.ironoverload.org
Roberta Crawford, Pres.

**Fnded:** 1981. **Mem:** 8,000. **Reg. Groups:** 4. **Desc:** Physicians and patients. Purposes are to: serve hemochromatosis patients and families; encourage research and public information; press for earlier diagnosis and more effective treatment. (Hemochromatosis is a genetic condition of iron overload in which excess iron damages organs and tissues, producing varying late-stage symptoms including liver cirrhosis, diabetes, heart failure, arthritis, and skin pigmentation, leading to death unless diagnosed early and treated adequately.) Specific plans are: to organize chapters and to develop a public relations plan, television interviews, and press releases; to sponsor screening programs and patient referral service; prepare diagnosis sheets for doctors and medical schools. Current emphasis is on alerting the public to the dangers of excess iron, since the disease is more prevalent than previously believed, and most susceptible individuals are unaware of the hazard. Authorities believe that five in 1000 carry both genes and that one in eight carries a single gene. Acts as a clearinghouse for doctors to call on for research materials and plans to establish a toll-free number for the public. Sponsors fundraising program. Is also in the process of setting up an index of laboratory research in progress. Conducts programs; compiles statistics; maintains speakers' bureau; conducts research programs. **Pub:** *Ironic Blood*, bimonthly. Newsletter. Information on iron overload. *Price:* Free. • *Overload: An Ironic Disease.* Booklet.

### ★ 8711 ★ Joslin Diabetes Center (JDC)

One Joslin Pl.
Boston, MA 02215
**Phone:** (617)732-2400　　　**Free:** 800-JOSLIN-1
**Fax:** (617)732-2562
**Email:** stephen.mally@joslin.harvard.edu
**Website:** http://www.joslin.org
Stephen M. Mally, Pres.

**Fnded:** 1898. **Desc:** An internationally recognized diabetes treatment, research and education institution affiliated with Harvard Medical School. Clinical programs include the Diabetes Outpatient Intensive Treatment (DO IT) Program, a three and a half day program designed to instruct and empower people with diabetes to better manage the disease. Other clinical services include internal medicine/endocrinology, ophthalmology, nephrology, pediatric endocrinology, pregnancy, mental health, nutrition and exercise physiology. The center also has affiliated treatment facilities in the Boston area and at prestigious hospitals from Florida to Washington state. Offers a disease management program as well as educational programs for health professionals, patients and corporations. **Pub:** *Joslin Magazine*, quarterly. Magazine. Provides information on diet, education, and research; also covers the activities of the center. *Price:* Included in membership dues. • Report, annual. • Newsletter. • Books. • Videos. **Frmly:** (1981) Joslin Diabetes Foundation.

### ★ 8712 ★ Juvenile Diabetes Foundation of Australia (JDFA)

48 Atchison St., Level 1
Leonards, NSW 2065, Australia
**Phone:** 61 2 996600400　　　**Fax:** 61 2 996600172
**Email:** jdfa@jdfa.org.au

**Fnded:** 1982. **Nat'l Groups:** 16. **Desc:** Aims to find a cure for diabetes and its complications, raise funds for research and educational programs. **Pub:** *Update*, quarterly. Magazine.

### Juvenile Diabetes Foundation in Israel (JDFI)
### (Haagudah LeSukereth Neurim Beyisrael)

*See:* Entry 5705

### ★ 8713 ★ Juvenile Diabetes Research Foundation

7100 Woodbine Ave., Ste. 311
Markham, ON, Canada L3R 5J2
**Phone:** (905)944-8700　　　**Free:** 877-CUR-EJDF
**Fax:** (905)944-0800
**Email:** general@jdfc.ca
**Website:** http://www.jdfc.ca

**Fnded:** 1974. **Desc:** Aims to raise funds for research into the cure for diabetes and educational programs.

### ★ 8714 ★ Juvenile Diabetes Research Foundation - Hellas

PO Box 17177
GR-10024 Athens, Greece
**Phone:** 30 1 7796660　　　**Fax:** 30 1 3627777
**Fnded:** 1983. **Mem:** 1,300. **Desc:** Offers financial support (grants) to diabetes research scholarships to young investigators.

### Juvenile Diabetes Research Foundation International (JDFI)

*See:* Entry 5706

### ★ 8715 ★ Latin American Thoracic Association (ALAT)
### (Asociacion Latinoamericana del Torax)

Rua Botucatu 740, 3o andar
04023-062 Sao Paulo, Brazil
**Phone:** 55 11 5756847
**Email:** josejardim@pneumo.epm.br
**Website:** http://alat.brz.net
**Fnded:** 1996. **Desc:** Supports the development of thoracic medicine in Latin America.

### ★ 8716 ★ Latin American Thyroid Society (LATS)

Departamento de Fmsiologia e Biofmsica
ICB-USP
05508-900 Sao Paulo, Brazil
**Phone:** 55 11 8187365　　　**Fax:** 55 11 8187285
**Email:** acbianco@usp.br
**Website:** http://www.lats.org
**Fnded:** 1974.

### ★ 8717 ★ National Adrenal Diseases Foundation (NADF)

505 Northern Blvd., Ste. 200
Great Neck, NY 11021
**Phone:** (516)487-4992
**Email:** nadfmail@aol.com
**Website:** http://www.medhelp.org/www/nadf.htm

**Fnded:** 1985. **Mem:** 1,300. **Local Groups:** 19. **Desc:** Individuals with adrenal diseases, especially Addison's disease, and their families; physicians. Seeks to provide a national selfhelp network for educational and emotional support for patients and their families. **Pub:** *NADF News*, quarterly. Newsletter. *Price:* $25/year. • Also publishes educational materials. **Frmly:** (1991) National Addison's Disease Foundation.

### ★ 8718 ★ National Center for the Study of Wilson's Disease (NCSWD)

10 W 66th St.
New York, NY 10023
**Phone:** (212)496-6558　　　**Fax:** (212)496-6711
**Email:** info@msgiinteractive.com
Carl H. Nacht, MD, Pres.

**Fnded:** 1971. **Mem:** 9. **Desc:** Performs and supports research concerning hereditary diseases of metal metabolism, in particular Wilson's disease and Menkes' disease. Seeks to increase doctors' awareness of these diseases. (Wilson's disease, named for S.A.K. Wilson, who discovered the disease and published his findings in 1912, is caused by a genetic defect that permits excessive amounts of copper to accumulate in the liver and brain. The disease is fatal if untreated, but, if detected early enough, can be completely suppressed.) Encompasses research, diagnostic, and treatment center for Wilson's disease. Compiles statistics. **Pub:** *What is Wilson's Disease?*. Brochure. • *Wilson's Disease, 1st Ed. 1984; 2nd Ed in preparation.* Monograph. **Frmly:** Foundation for the Study of Wilson's Disease.

### ★ 8719 ★ National Gaucher Foundation (NGF)

5410 Edson Ln., Ste. 260
Rockville, MD 20852
**Phone:** (301)816-1515　　　**Free:** 800-GAU-CHER
**Fax:** (301)816-1516
**Email:** ngf@gaucherdisease.org
**Website:** http://www.gaucherdisease.org
Rhonda P. Buyers, Exec. Dir.

**Fnded:** 1984. **Mem:** 1,000. **Reg. Groups:** 2. **Local Groups:** 2. **Desc:** Persons with Gaucher Disease; interested medical professionals and individuals. Gaucher Disease, one of the most common inherited metabolic disorders, is caused by an enzyme deficiency which renders the body unable to break down and dispose of complex lipids (fat-like substances). These lipids accumulate in the spleen, liver, and bone marrow, causing enlargement of the organs and intermittent pain of varying severity. Gaucher is treatable through enzyme replacement therapy. (The disease is named for Phillippe C.E. Gaucher, a French physician who described it in 1882.) One in 10 Jews of E. European descent is a carrier and one in 450 has Gaucher Disease. Sponsors direct funding of and support for research and clinical programs at medical centers in the U.S. and abroad to develop a cure and/or treatment for Gaucher Disease. Seeks to help persons with the disorder by providing them the opportunity to share experiences and feelings on a confidential, personal basis. Disseminates technical and nontechnical information concerning the disease. Advocates increased screening for carriers and availability of prenatal diagnosis for families at risk. **Pub:** *Gaucher Disease Newsletter*, quarterly. Newsletter. Includes index, reprints of recent literature, legislative reports, and medical questions and answers. *Price:* $35/year.

### ★ 8720 ★ National Hormone and Pituitary Program (NHPP)

Harbor - UCLA Medical Ctr.
1000 W Carson St.
Torrance, CA 90509
**Phone:** (310)222-3537　　　**Fax:** (310)222-3432
**Email:** parlow@humc.edu
**Website:** http://www.humc.edu/hormones
Dr. A.F. Parlow, Scientific Officer

**Fnded:** 1963. **Desc:** The agency collects human pituitary glands obtained through autopsies and extracts from them human growth hormone (hGH), human follicle stimulating hormone (hFSH), human luteinizing hormone (hLH), human adrenocorticotrophic hormone (ACTH), human thyroid stimulating hormone (hTSH), human prolactin, and beta-lipotropin. These and similar hormones of rat, ovine, bovine, porcine, and monkey origin are distributed to doctors in research centers for research in endocrinology. Promotes basic studies with all pituitary hormones and seeks to make these available to investigators. **Frmly:** (1983) National Pituitary Agency.

### ★ 8721 ★ National Hypoglycemia Association (NHA)

PO Box 120
Ridgewood, NJ 07451
**Phone:** (201)670-1189
Lenore L. Cohen, Founder & Dir.

**Fnded:** 1982. **Desc:** Hypoglycemics and health professionals who provide educational, informational, and support services to individuals with hypoglycemia and their families. (Hypoglycemia is a deficiency in the blood sugar level that deprives the central nervous system of glucose needed to function normally.) Maintains speakers' bureau; organizes support groups. Provides professional referrals, consultations, and evaluations for individuals with hypoglycemia and related conditions. **Pub:** *Hypoglyeemia-This Is What*

*It's All About.* Booklets. • *National Hypoglycemia Association–Booklet.* Contains information on hypoglycemia for patients, families, doctors, and the public. Includes research reports on all aspects of Hypoglycemia. *Price:* $5 includes postage and handling.


## ★ 8722 ★ National Lymphedema Network

1611 Telegraph Ave., Ste. 1111
Oakland, CA 94612
**Phone:** 800-541-3259        **Fax:** (510)208-3110
**Email:** nln@lymphnet.org
**Website:** http://www.lymphnet.org
Saskia R.J. Thiadens, R.N., Pres.
**Fnded:** 1988. **Mem:** 2,800. **Desc:** Persons with lymphedema and their families, health care professionals. Provides education and support to patients, health care professionals and the general public by disseminating information on the prevention and management of primary and secondary lymphedema. Also support research into the causes and possible alternative treatments for this often incapacitating condition. Offers referral service to medical facilities, helps locate support groups and sponsors research and educational programs. **Pub:** *NLN Newsletter,* quarterly. Newsletter. Features cutting-edge medical articles, features, and resource listings. • *Resource Guide.* Contains list of treatment centers, health care professionals and sup pliers, Support Groups, PenPals, and updates on professional training courses.


## ★ 8723 ★ National MPS Society

102 Aspen Dr.
Downingtown, PA 19335
**Phone:** (610)942-0100        **Fax:** (610)942-7188
**Email:** info@mpssociety.org
**Website:** http://www.mpssociety.org
Barbara Wedehase, Exec. Dir.
**Fnded:** 1974. **Mem:** 800. **Reg. Groups:** 9. **Desc:** Professionals and families devoted to educating the public and discovering and aiding families of MPS and ML children. Mucopolysaccharidoses (MPS) and mucolipidoses (ML) are extremely rare hereditary diseases caused by particular enzyme deficiencies and range in severity from strictly bone and joint involvement to massive complications in all organ systems. Helps to facilitate diagnosis and treatment through referrals to doctors and hospitals. Maintains parent referral service to direct families with newly diagnosed MPS and ML children to other members. **Pub:** *Courage,* quarterly. Newsletter. • *Ethan's Feeling Switch.* Book. *Price:* $5. • *Hunter.* Booklet. *Price:* $1. • *Hurler.* Booklet. *Price:* $1. • *I-Cell.* Booklet. • *Management Anesthesia.* Booklet. • *Maroteaux-Lamy.* Booklet. *Price:* $1. • *Morquio.* Booklet. *Price:* $1. • *Sanfilippo.* Booklet. • *Sly.* Booklet. **Frmly:** (1975) Parents for MPS; (1985) MPS Society.


## ★ 8724 ★ National Niemann Pick Disease Foundation (NPD)

c/o Barb Vorpahl
415 Madison Ave.
PO Box 49
Fort Atkinson, WI 53538
**Phone:** (920)563-0930        **Free:** 877-287-3672
**Fax:** (920)563-0931
**Email:** webmaster@nnpdf.org
**Website:** http://www.nnpdf.org
Barb Vorpahl, Chm.
**Fnded:** 1992. **Mem:** 4,500. **Desc:** Parents, medical and educational professionals, and friends. Works to promote medical research on Niemann-Pick Disease (NPD), a disorder which prevents metabolizing of the sphingomyelin lipid or cholesterol. Provides medical and educational information; offers support to families of children with NPD; facilitates genetic counseling for parents; supports legislation that affects patients and families with NPD; sponsors medical research. **Pub:** *Niemann-Pick Newsletter,* quarterly. Newsletter. *Price:* Free. • Directory.


## ★ 8725 ★ National Organization for Albinism and Hypopigmentation (NOAH)

PO Box 959
East Hampstead, NH 03826-0959
**Free:** 800-473-2310        **Fax:** (603)887-2310
**Email:** noah@albinism.org
**Website:** http://www.albinism.org
Charla McMillan, Pres.
**Fnded:** 1982. **Mem:** 1,000. **Reg. Groups:** 40. **State Groups:** 21. **Desc:** Individuals with albinism and their familes; health care professionals; others interested in learning more about albinism. (Albinism is an inherited metabolic disorder that results in reduced pigment in the hair, eyes, and/or skin of those it affects; people with albinism also have impaired eye function including decreased visual acuity, involuntary eye movements, and increased sensitivity to light.) Seeks to educate teachers, health care professionals, and the public about albinism. Provides support to individuals with albinism and their families. Encourages research on the cause, results, and management of the disorder. **Pub:** *NOAH Information Bulletin,* periodic. Bulletin. Provides information on various aspects of albinism. • *NOAH News,* semiannual. • *The Student with Albinism in the Regular Classroom.* Book.


## ★ 8726 ★ National Tay-Sachs and Allied Diseases Association (NTSAD)

2001 Beacon St., Ste. 204
Boston, MA 02135
**Phone:** (617)277-4463        **Free:** 800-906-8723
**Fax:** (617)277-0134
**Email:** ntsad-boston@att.net
**Website:** http://www.ntsad.org
Jayne C. Gershkowitz, Exec. Dir.
**Fnded:** 1956. **Mem:** 5,000. **State Groups:** 6. **Desc:** Supports educational, prevention, family service, and research programs concerning Tay-Sachs and allied degenerative lysosomal and leukodystrophy and neurological diseases occurring in infants, children, and adults. Provides educational literature on Tay-Sachs and allied diseases; serves as a referral agency for the layperson and professional on all aspects of Tay-Sachs and related diseases; promotes mass screening programs and appropriate legislation locally and nationally. Sponsors International Laboratory Quality Control and Reference Sample Center for TSD laboratories. Offers support groups and services for parents of children with Tay-Sachs and related diseases, grandparents and extended family members. Compiles statistics; operates speakers' bureau. **Pub:** *Breakthrough,* semiannual. Newsletter. • *Home Care Manual.* Manual. *Price:* $3 includes shipping and handling. • *Lay-Onset Tay-Sachs.* Information sheet. *Price:* Free. • *Lifeline,* quarterly. Newsletter. Distributed to affected families only. • *National Tay-Sachs and Allied Diseases Association–Breakthrough,* semiannual. Newsletter. • *What Is Canavan Disease?.* • *What Is Tay-Sachs Disease?.* • Also makes available brochures and educational materials. **Frmly:** (1966) National Tay-Sachs Association.


## ★ 8727 ★ Netherlands Society for Endocrinology (Nederlandse Vereniging voor Endocrinologie — NVE)

c/o D. Braat
Department of Gynaecology and Obstetrics
St. Radboudziekenhuis
Geert Grooteplein Zuid 14
NL-6500 HB Nijmegen, Netherlands
**Phone:** 31 24 3610398        **Fax:** 31 24 3541194
**Fnded:** 1947. **Mem:** 500. **Desc:** Fosters research and clinical practice in endocrinology.


## ★ 8728 ★ Norwegian Diabetes Association (NDF) (Norges Diabetesforbund)

Postboks 6442
Etterstad
N-0605 Oslo, Norway
**Phone:** 47 23 051800        **Fax:** 47 23 051801
**Email:** norges.diabetesforbund@online.no
**Fnded:** 1948. **Mem:** 29,000. **Nat'l Groups:** 5. **Reg. Groups:** 19. **Local Groups:** 150. **Lang(s):** English. **Desc:** Diabetics and their families; health personnel. Acts as support group. Disseminates information on availability of insulin, diabetes products, and health care. Lobbies the government to incorporate diabetes treatment into national health care plans and to provide free insulin, syringes, and urine and blood glucose strips. Provides research and medical services. Offers educational courses; conducts camps; maintains youth club. **Pub:** *Diabetikeren,* bimonthly. Magazine. Features educational material. Includes Annual medical supplement. • Booklets.


## ★ 8729 ★ Organic Acidemia Association (OAA)

c/o Kathy Stagni
13210 35th Ave N
Plymouth, MN 55441-2227
**Phone:** (763)559-1797        **Fax:** (763)694-0017
**Email:** oaanews@aol.com
**Website:** http://www.oaanews.org
Kathy Stagni, Exec. Dir.
**Fnded:** 1982. **Mem:** 800. **Desc:** Dietitians, researchers, and geneticists; clinics; parents and relatives of children suffering from organic acidemia disorders. (Organic acidemia is a class of genetic metabolic disorders that lead to cellular enzyme deficiencies and require restricted diets.) Fosters communication among parents and professionals; acts as support group. **Pub:** *Organic Acidemia Association Newsletter,* 3/year. Newsletter. *Price:* $25/year domestic; $35/year international.


## ★ 8730 ★ Oxalosis and Hyperoxaluria Foundation (OHF)

5718 Holly Hills
Saint Louis, MO 63109
**Phone:** (314)351-2177        **Free:** 888-721-2432
**Fax:** (314)481-6368
**Email:** execdirector@ohf.org
**Website:** http://www.ohf.org
Shirley Schirmer, Natl. Sec.
**Fnded:** 1989. **Mem:** 900. **Desc:** Individuals affected by oxalosis and hyperoxaluria; health care professionals. Hyperoxaluria is a metabolic disease affecting the kidneys. Oxalosis occurs when calcium crystals have deposited elsewhere in the body, often the eyes, bones, and joints. Provides support services and information regarding the conditions and their affects. Encourages research. Operates referral service. **Pub:** *In Touch,* 3/year. Newsletter. • *Understanding Hyperoxaluria and Oxalosis.* Brochure.


## ★ 8731 ★ Parents of Galactosemic Children (PGC)

885 Del Sol St.
Sparks, NV 89436
**Phone:** (775)626-0885
**Email:** mesameadow@aol.com
**Website:** http://www.galactosemia.org
Evelyn A. Rice, Pres.
**Fnded:** 1985. **Mem:** 1,200. **Nat'l Groups:** 1. **Desc:** Parents of children born with galactosemia. (Children with galactosemia are missing an enzyme in all body cells that breaks galactose into gulcose, possibly causing jaundice, an enlarged liver, cataracts, kidney failure, and brain damage.) Works to obtain financial support for galactosemia research professionals. Offers support, educational programs, and other information to galactosemic families and interested professionals. Seeks ways for children and adults with galactosemia to live their lives to their fullest potential. **Pub:** Newsletter, semiannual.


**Pediatric Endocrinology Nursing Society (PENS)**
*See:* Entry 15766

**Prader-Willi Syndrome Association (U.S.A.) (PWSAUSA)**
*See:* Entry 4891

★ 8732 ★ **Purine Research Society**
c/o Tahma Metz
5424 Beech Ave.
Bethesda, MD 20814-1730
**Phone:** (301)530-0354 **Fax:** (301)564-9597
**Email:** purine@erols.com
**Website:** http://www2.dgsys.com/~purine/
Tahma Metz, Exec. Dir.

**Fnded:** 1986. **Desc:** Dedicated to funding research and treatment of diseases resulting from errors in purine metabolism, specifically purine autism, the largest single subgroup of autism. As with other metabolic diseases, purine disorders are caused by a defective gene that results in the production of an enzyme with too little or too much catalytic activity. Purine metabolic diseases include gout, Lesch-Nyhan syndrome, purine autism, ADA deficiency and others. We are supporting research to find the defective enzyme(s) responsible for purine overproduction in purine autism, particularly, and to find effective screening and treatment methods, including newborn screening, so that symptoms will never occur. **Pub:** Brochure. *Price:* Free. • Bulletin. **Frmly:** (1995) Purine 24, Inc.

**Sjogren's Syndrome Foundation (SSF)**
*See:* Entry 13665

★ 8733 ★ **Sociedad Chilena de Endocrinologia y Metabolismo**
Casilla 166, Correo 55
Santiago, Chile
**Phone:** 56 2 3412909 **Fax:** 56 2 3512909
**Email:** ssf@sjorgrens.org
**Website:** http://www.sjogrens.com
**Fnded:** 1961.

★ 8734 ★ **Society for Behavioral Neuroendocrinology (SBN)**
University of Virginia
Department of Biology
Gilmer Hall
Charlottesville, VA 22903
**Website:** http://www.sbn.org
Michael Baum, Pres.

**Desc:** Promotes the field of neuroendocrinology. **Pub:** *Hormones and Behavior.* Journal. *Price:* Electronic version $75 paper version; $50 paper version for student members.

★ 8735 ★ **Society for Endocrinology**
17/18 The Courtyard
Woodlands
Bradley Stole
Bristol BS32 4NQ, United Kingdom
**Phone:** 44 1454 642210 **Fax:** 44 1454 642222
**Email:** info@endocrinology.org
**Website:** http://www.endocrinology.org
**Fnded:** 1939. **Mem:** 2,000. **Desc:** Clinicians and scientists working within the field of hormones and hormone related disease. Undertakes scientific/medical publishing, conferences (including commercial exhibitions) and training courses. **Pub:** *Endocrine-Related Cancer*, quarterly. Journal. • *European Journal of Endocrinology*, monthly. Journal. • *Journal of Endocrinology*, monthly. Journal. • *Journal of Molecular Endocrinology*, bimonthly. Journal.

★ 8736 ★ **Society for Mucopolysaccharide Diseases (MPS)**
46 Woodside Rd.
Amersham HP6 6RU, United Kingdom
**Phone:** 44 1494 434156 **Fax:** 44 1494 434252
**Email:** mps@mpssociety.co.uk
**Website:** http://www.mpssociety.co.uk

**Fnded:** 1982. **Mem:** 1,000. **Nat'l Groups:** 24. **Reg. Groups:** 12. **Lang(s):** English, French, German. **Desc:** Acts as a support group for families of children worldwide afflicted with Mucopolysaccharide Diseases. (MPS diseases, known individually as Hurler, Scheie, Hunter, Sanfilippo, Morquio, Maroteaux-Lamy, and Sly, and associated diseases called mucolipidosis, Fucosidosis, and Sialic Acid Disease, are genetic diseases. Children born with MPS are unable to produce certain enzymes necessary for appropriate metabolism to take place; consequently complex sugars become stored in connective tissues, causing progressive damage, including physical and mental handicaps. In most cases, MPS patients die before reaching adulthood.) Encourages public awareness of MPS diseases and the international transmission of medical knowledge and techniques. Raises funds to further MPS research and arranges for MPS families to assist in research such as carrier testing and biochemical diagnosis. Accepts donations to provide individual advocacy for MPS families. Sponsors research program on the natural history of MPS and the psychosocial problems of MPS children. **Pub:** *Conference Reports*, annual. Report. • Newsletter, quarterly. • Report, annual.

**Society for Reproductive Endocrinology and Infertility**
*See:* Entry 18378

★ 8737 ★ **Society for the Study of Inborn Errors of Metabolism (SSIEM)**
c/o Department of Child Health
University Hospital of Wales
Heath Park
Cardiff
South Glamorgan S1O 2TH, United Kingdom
**Phone:** 44 29 2074 6322 **Fax:** 44 29 2074 6322
**Email:** malcolmheron@msn.com
**Website:** http://www.ssiem.org.uk
**Fnded:** 1962. **Mem:** 800. **Lang(s):** English. **Desc:** Biochemists, dietitians, pediatricians, pathologists, geneticists, and interested individuals in 41 countries. Purpose is to foster study of inherited metabolic disease diagnosis and treatment. Promotes exchange of ideas through meetings and publications. **Pub:** *Journal of Inherited Metabolic Diseases*, quarterly. Journal. • *Membership Handbook*, periodic. • Pamphlets. • Proceedings.

★ 8738 ★ **Thyroid Foundation of America**
Ruth Sleeper Hall, RSL 350
40 Parkman St.
Boston, MA 02114
**Phone:** (617)726-8500 **Free:** 800-832-8321
**Fax:** (617)726-4136
**Email:** info@allthyroid.org
**Website:** http://www.allthyroid.org
Dr. Lawrence C. Wood, Pres.

**Fnded:** 1985. **Mem:** 4,500. **Reg. Groups:** 1. **State Groups:** 2. **Local Groups:** 1. **Desc:** Individuals with thyroid conditions; health professionals. Provides education and support for thyroid patients and health professionals; promotes public awareness of thyroid problems. Conducts educational programs. Operates referral service. **Pub:** *The Bridge*, quarterly. Newsletter. Reports on current research, articles of interest to individuals with thyroid disorders. *Price:* Included in membership dues. • Brochures.

★ 8739 ★ **Wilson's Disease Association (WDA)**
4 Navaho Dr.
Brookfield, CT 06804
**Phone:** (203)775-9666 **Free:** 800-399-0266
**Fax:** (203)775-9666
**Email:** hasellner@worldnet.att.net
**Website:** http://www.wilsonsdisease.org
H. Ascher Sellner, Pres.

**Fnded:** 1979. **Mem:** 1,000. **Nat'l Groups:** 1. **Local Groups:** 2. **Desc:** Patients of Wilson's disease relatives and friends of patients; physicians and other health care professionals. (Wilson's disease, named for S.A.K. Wilson, a pioneer in the study of the disease, is a genetic nervous disorder in which excessive amounts of copper collect in the liver, brain, and kidneys.) Purpose is to promote and sponsor research regarding the cause, treatment, cure, and prevention of Wilson's and related diseases. Stresses the importance of public awareness, early diagnosis, and treatment. Provides financial aid and moral support to needy individuals and organizations sharing the association's goals; serves as liaison among members and cooperating organizations. Collects and disseminates information to members and the public concerning developments, current research, and legislation in the field; acts as clearinghouse. **Pub:** *The Copper Connection*, quarterly. Newsletter. Includes research reports, member profiles, and book reviews. • *Wilson's Disease Association–Membership Directory*, annual. Membership Directory. *Price:* Included in membership dues. • *Wilson's Disease: Questions & Answers.* Brochures. • Also publishes many other brochures on various aspects of Wilson's disease.

★ 8740 ★ **Women in Endocrinology (WE)**
c/o Ursula Kaiser, MD
Endocrine-Hypertension Division
Brigham and Women's Hospital
221 Longwood Ave.
Boston, MA 02115
**Email:** ukaiser@partners.org
**Website:** http://www.women-in-endo.org/Pages/index.shtml
Ursula Kaiser, MD, Sec. -Treas.

**Desc:** Women employed in the field of endocrinology; female endocrinology students and residents. Promotes "professional development and advancement of women in the field of endocrinology." Facilitates exchange of information among members; conducts educational programs.

## Research Centers

★ 8741 ★ **Aoki Diabetes Research Institute**
1935 Stockton Blvd.
Sacramento, CA 95816
**Phone:** (916)455-2374 **Fax:** (916)455-3734
Thomas T. Aoki, MD, Dir. of Res.

**Activities/Fields:** Metabolic diseases, including diabetes mellitus. Current projects include clinical investigations in the treatment of Type I and II diabetic patients.

★ 8742 ★ **Barbara Davis Center for Childhood Diabetes**
4200 E 9th Ave., Box B140
Denver, CO 80262
**Phone:** (303)315-8796 **Fax:** (303)315-4124
**Email:** marian.rewers@uchsc.edu
**Website:** http://www.uchsc.edu/misc/diabetes/bdc.html
Dr. Marian J. Rewers, Clin. Dir.

**Activities/Fields:** Diabetes in children and young adults, including immunogenetics, islet cell development and transplantation, complications, and clinical trials of prevention and new treatments in type 1 diabetes and type 2 diabetes in children. **Pub:** *Research papers.*

★ 8743 ★ **Baylor College of Medicine Biochemical Genetics Laboratory**
1 Baylor Plz., Rm. T530
Houston, TX 77030
**Phone:** (713)798-4982 **Free:** 800-246-2436
**Fax:** (713)798-8937
**Email:** bioc@bcm.tmc.edu
**Website:** http://www.bcmgeneticlabs.org
William E. O'Brien, PhD, Dir.

**Activities/Fields:** Diagnosing and monitoring patients with inborn errors of metabolism.

**Carcinoid Cancer Foundation, Inc.**
*See:* Entry 10300

**★ 8744 ★ Case Western Reserve University**
**Center for Inherited Disorders of Energy Metabolism (CIDEM)**
Department of Pediatrics, Rm. 4010
Rainbow Babies and Childrens Hospital
11100 Euclid Ave.
Cleveland, OH 44106-6004
**Phone:** (216)844-1286     **Fax:** (216)844-8005
**Email:** cidem@po.cwru.edu
**Website:** http://www.cwru.edu/med/CIDEM/cidem.htm
Dr. Douglas Kerr, Dir.

**Activities/Fields:** Defects of human energy metabolism, focusing on diagnosis and management. Emphasis is on disorders of pyruvate fatty acid oxidation, and mitochondrial function, including pyruvate metabolism, oxidative phosphorylation, and fatty acid oxidation.

**Center for Biological Timing**
*See:* Entry 14168

**★ 8745 ★ Columbia-Presbyterian Medical Center**
**Naomi Berrie Diabetes Center**
1150 St. Nicholas Ave.
New York, NY 10032
**Phone:** (212)304-5494     **Fax:** (212)304-5493
**Email:** diabetes@columbia.edu
**Website:** http://cpmcnet.columbia.edu/dept/diabetes
Robin S. Goland, MD, Dir.

**Activities/Fields:** Biologic basis of diabetes, the prevention of Type 1 and Type 2 diabetes and diabetic complications.

**★ 8746 ★ Dartmouth College**
**Biomedical NMR Research Center**
Department of Radiology, HB 7786
Dartmouth Medical School
Hanover, NH 03755
**Phone:** (603)650-1677     **Fax:** (603)650-1717
**Email:** Jeffrey.F.Dunn@dartmouth.edu
**Website:** http://www.dartmouth.edu/www/dms/nmrbrl/body.htm
Dr. Jeff Dunn, Dir.

**Activities/Fields:** Metabolic disorders, especially those disorders linked to hypoxia and oxygen utilization.

**★ 8747 ★ Deaconess Billings Clinic**
**Research Division**
1500 Poly Dr., Ste. 103
Billings, MT 59102
**Phone:** (406)255-8470     **Free:** 800-996-2663
**Fax:** (406)255-8479
**Email:** research@billingsclinic.org
**Website:** http://www.billingsclinic.com/frontpage/default.htm
Howard R. Knapp, MD, Exec. Dir.

**Activities/Fields:** Regulation of bone remodeling, arthritis, hormone replacement therapy, infectious diseases in man, hepatitis-C, diabetes, pneumonia, hypertension, and hyperlipidemia.

**★ 8748 ★ Diabetes Education and Research Center**
Franklin Medical Bldg.
829 Spruce St., Ste. 302
Philadelphia, PA 19107
**Phone:** (215)829-3426     **Fax:** (215)829-5807
**Email:** webmaster@diabeteseducationandresearchcenter.org
**Website:** http://www.diabeteseducationandresearchcenter.org
Dr. Theodore G. Duncan, Dir.

**Activities/Fields:** Diabetes, including the effects of oral diabetic medication, hypertension as an indicator of diabetes, and drug trials.

**★ 8749 ★ Garfield G. Duncan Research Foundation, Inc.**
829 Spruce St.
Philadelphia, PA 19107-5752
**Phone:** (215)829-3426     **Fax:** (215)829-5807
**Website:** http://www.diabeteseducationandresearchcenter.org
Dr. Theodore G. Duncan, Dir.

**Activities/Fields:** Diabetes.

**★ 8750 ★ Hauptman-Woodward Medical Research Institute, Inc.**
73 High St.
Buffalo, NY 14203-1196
**Phone:** (716)856-9600     **Fax:** (716)852-6086
**Email:** hauptman@hwi.buffalo.edu
**Website:** http://www.hwi.buffalo.edu
Herbert A. Hauptman, PhD, Pres.

**Activities/Fields:** Molecular endocrinology to determine molecular structures of biologically important small and macromolecular compounds, to correlate the structures with their biological activities, and to elucidate the mechanism of hormone biosynthesis. Also has programs in space- and ground-based crystal growth and phasing methods in macromolecular structure determination. Specific interests include structural biology and molecular endocrinology. molecular level. **Pub:** *Structures Newsletter,* quarterly. **Frmly:** Medical Foundation of Buffalo Inc.

**★ 8751 ★ Indiana University-Purdue University at Indianapolis**
**Diabetes Research and Training Center**
250 University Blvd., Ste. 122
Indianapolis, IN 46202
**Phone:** (317)630-6375     **Fax:** (317)278-0900
**Website:** http://www.indiana.edu/~rugs/ctrdir/drtc.html
Dr. David G. Marrerro, Dir.

**Activities/Fields:** Diabetes mellitus treatment and prevention.

**Indiana University-Purdue University at Indianapolis**
**Mead Johnson Mass Spectrometry Laboratory**
*See:* Entry 16513

**★ 8752 ★ Institute for Metabolic Research**
3508 Market St., Ste. 420
Philadelphia, PA 19104
**Phone:** (215)222-1818     **Fax:** (215)222-5325
**Email:** drmpcohen@AOL.com
**Website:** http://www.indiana.edu/~rugs/ctrdir/mjmsl.html
Dr. Margo P. Cohen, Dir.

**Activities/Fields:** Metabolic effects, diagnosis, and management of diabetes mellitus and other metabolic diseases. Studies include the biochemistry and metabolism of glomerular and retinal microvascular basement membranes; role of polyol pathway in complications of diabetes; structure/function effects of non-enzymatic glycosylation of proteins; measurement of glycohemoglobin and glycoalbumin in biologic samples by immunologic methods; identification and purification of islet cell antigens.

**★ 8753 ★ Johns Hopkins University**
**Office of Psychohormonal Research**
1235 E Monument St., Ste. LL20
Baltimore, MD 21202
**Phone:** (410)955-3740

**Email:** jmoney@mail.jhmi.edu
Dr. John Money, Dir.

**Activities/Fields:** Longitudinal psychohormonal research studies of patients with diverse endocrine, genital, and sexological syndromes, related to clinical psychoendocrinology, clinical sexology, gender identity/role (G-I/R), abuse-dwarfism (Kaspar Hauser syndrome), and Munchausen syndrome by proxy.

**★ 8754 ★ Joslin Diabetes Center**
1 Joslin Pl.
Boston, MA 02215
**Phone:** (617)732-2400     **Fax:** (617)732-2487
**Website:** http://www.joslin.harvard.edu/
Dr. C. Ronald Kahn, Pres.

**Activities/Fields:** Diabetes mellitus, including investigations on chemical composition of basement membrane, physiological control of glucose metabolism, neonatal and fetal growth and metabolism, cellular and molecular mechanisms of insulin action, vascular cell biology, ultrastructure of beta cell, pancreatic islets, muscle perfusion, experimental diabetes in animals, immunologic aspects of diabetes, diabetic eye disease, and epidemiology of diabetes. Conducts clinical studies of early stages of diabetic state, treatment, and prevention of diabetes and its complications, especially of a vascular nature, with emphasis on diabetic retinopathy. **Pub:** *Annual Report.* • *Joslin Magazine,* quarterly.

**★ 8755 ★ Laval University**
**Medical Research Centre**
**Diabetes Research Group**
2705 Blvd. Laurier
Sainte Foy, QC, Canada G1V 4G2
**Phone:** (418)654-2741     **Fax:** (418)654-2792
**Email:** andre.nadeau@crchul.ulaval.ca
Andre Nadeau, Dir.

**Activities/Fields:** The relationship between physical activity and diabetes, and the identification of factors responsible for the increased level of cardiac mortality in diabetes patients. Participation in clinical trials on new therapeutic agents for diabetes mellitus.

**★ 8756 ★ Laval University**
**Medical Research Centre**
**Oncology and Molecular Endocrinology Research Center**
2705 Blvd. Laurier
Sainte Foy, QC, Canada G1V 4G2
**Phone:** (418)654-2296     **Fax:** (418)654-2761
**Email:** fernand.labrie@crchul.ulaval.ca
**Website:** http://www.crchul.ulaval.ca
Dr. Fernand Labrie, Dir.

**Activities/Fields:** Prostate and other hormone-sensitive cancers, strategies for early screening for prostate cancer, mechanisms regulating C-19 steroid formation by adrenal glands, characterization of effects of steroid sex hormones, adrenal hormone effects on brain dopaminergic systems, molecular mechanisms responsible for the expression of genes in specific tissues and their extinction in others, cloning and characterization of enzymes implicated in steroidogenesis, hormonal control of growth factors, polyamine biosynthesis in human breast cancer, and regulation of the expression of enzymes involved in steroidogenesis in placenta and adrenal glands. **Pub:** *Scientific (400/year).* **Frmly:** Molecular Endocrinology Research Group.

**Laval University**
**Saint-Francois-d'Assise Hospital Research Centre**
**Reproductive Endocrinology Unit**
*See:* Entry 18401

## ★ 8757 ★ Massachusetts General Hospital
**Reproductive Endocrine Unit**
Bulfinch Bldg., Ste. 051
Fruit St.
Boston, MA 02114
**Phone:** (617)724-5309     **Fax:** (617)726-9330
**Email:** sluss.patrick@mgh.harvard.edu
**Website:** http://www.go-testing.com
William F. Crowley, MD, Ch.

**Activities/Fields:** Reproductive endocrinology, focusing on local regulators of gonadal physiology and characterization and regulation of posttransitional processing of inhibin subunits using a variety of techniques, including protein purification and characterization and molecular biology.

## ★ 8758 ★ Massachusetts General Hospital Diabetes Center
50 Staniford St., Ste. 340
Boston, MA 02114-2517
**Phone:** (617)726-1847     **Fax:** (617)726-1871
**Email:** nathan@gcrc.mgh.harvard.edu
Dr. David M. Nathan, Prin. Investigator

**Activities/Fields:** Diabetes research, including clinical trials.

## Massachusetts Institute of Technology
**Laboratory of Neuroendocrine Regulation**
*See:* Entry 14226

## ★ 8759 ★ McGill University
**McGill Centre for Endocrine Studies**
Fraser Labs., Rm. M3-15
Royal Victoria Hospital
687 Pine Ave. W
Montreal, QC, Canada H3A 1A1
**Phone:** (514)842-1231     **Fax:** (514)849-3681
**Email:** patel@rvhmed.lan.mcgill.ca
Dr. Yogesh C. Patel, Dir.

**Activities/Fields:** Endocrinology; molecular biology of peptide hormones and their receptors; molecular pharmacology of G protein coupled receptors; proliferative and anti-proliferative cell signaling; apoptosis; neuropeptides in brain, gut, pancreas, and immune system; peptide hormones and development; prostaglandins and metabolites of arachedonic acid.

## ★ 8760 ★ Minneapolis Vascular Institute
4570 W 77th St.
Edina, MN 55435
**Phone:** (952)897-9877     **Fax:** (952)832-5597
**Email:** ruthe@surgicalconsultantpa.com
Ruth K. Edwards, Exec. Dir.

**Activities/Fields:** Peripheral vascular disease and diabetic revasculization.

## ★ 8761 ★ National Center for the Study of Wilson's Disease
432 W 58th St., Ste. 614
New York, NY 10019
**Phone:** (212)523-8717     **Fax:** (212)523-8708
I. Herbert Scheinberg, MD, Contact

**Activities/Fields:** Wilson's disease and Menkes' disease, focusing on the genetic control of copper balance and the biochemical regulatory mechanism that prevents the lethal copper deficiency of Menkes' disease and lethal copper toxicity of Wilson's disease.

## ★ 8762 ★ Northwestern University
**Center for Endocrinology, Metabolism and Molecular Medicine**
15-755 Tarry
303 Chicago Ave.
Chicago, IL 60611
**Phone:** (312)503-2902     **Fax:** (312)908-9032
**Email:** a_dunaif@northwestern.edu
**Website:** http://www.endocrine.nwu.edu/
Dr. Andrea Dunaif, Ch.

**Activities/Fields:** Endocrinology, metabolism, and nutrition, including diabetes, growth hormones, obesity and hypertension, and catecholamines.

## Rockefeller University
**Laboratory of the Biology of Addictive Diseases**
*See:* Entry 19360

## ★ 8763 ★ Rockefeller University
**Laboratory of Human Behavior and Metabolism**
Rockefeller University Hospital
1230 York Ave., Box 181
New York, NY 10021-6399
**Phone:** (212)327-8426     **Fax:** (212)327-7150
**Email:** hirsch@rockefeller.edu
**Website:** http://www.rockefeller.edu
Prof. Jules Hirsch, MD, Hd.

**Activities/Fields:** The biology of weight regulation changes in systematic energetics which result from weight changes.

## Rockefeller University
**Laboratory of Metabolism-Pharmacology**
*See:* Entry 17370

## Rockefeller University
**Laboratory of Neuroendocrinology**
*See:* Entry 14266

## ★ 8764 ★ Shriners Hospital for Children (St. Louis, MO)
**Center for Metabolic Bone Disease and Molecular Research**
2001 S Lindbergh Blvd.
Saint Louis, MO 63131-3597
**Phone:** (314)432-3600     **Fax:** (314)872-7844
**Email:** mwhyte@shrinenet.org
Michael P. Whyte, MD, Med. Dir.

**Activities/Fields:** Metabolic bone diseases and skeletal dysplasias in children, including evaluation of potential medical therapies and analysis of inheritance factors. **Frmly:** Metabolic Research Unit.

## ★ 8765 ★ Texas A&M University
**Laboratory for Protein and Amino Acid Analysis**
Kleberg Center, Rm. 212
Department of Animal Science
College Station, TX 77843-2471
**Phone:** (979)845-5064     **Fax:** (979)845-5292
Dr. Guoyao Wu, Hd.

**Activities/Fields:** Analysis of amino acids and how they relate to various biochemical systems in fetal and neonatal systems, including Arginine metabolism and its crucial role in nitric oxide synthesis.

## ★ 8766 ★ Tulane University Health Sciences Center
**U.S.-Japan Biomedical Research Laboratories**
F. Edward Herbert Research Center, Bldg. 30
3705 Main St.
Belle Chasse, LA 70037-3001
**Phone:** (504)394-7199     **Fax:** (504)394-7169
**Email:** arimura@tulane.edu
Dr. Akira Arimura, Dir.

**Activities/Fields:** Neuroendocrinology and neuroscience, particularly in the areas of neuropeptides and immune-neuroendocrine interactions. **Pub:** *Neuroendocrinology*, 10/year. • *Neuroscience*, 10/year.

## U.S. Department of Health and Human Services
**National Cancer Institute**
**Division of Clinical Sciences**
**Intramural Research Program (Metabolism Branch)**
*See:* Entry 10468

## U.S. Department of Health and Human Services
**National Heart, Lung, and Blood Institute**
**Division of Intramural Research**
**Molecular Disease Branch**
*See:* Entry 5159

## ★ 8767 ★ U.S. Department of Health and Human Services
**National Heart, Lung, and Blood Institute**
**Laboratory of Kidney and Electrolyte Metabolism**
NIH Bldg. 10, Rm. 6N260
10 Center Dr., MSC 1603
Bethesda, MD 20892
**Phone:** (301)496-3187     **Fax:** (301)402-1443
**Email:** maurice_burg@nih.gov
Dr. Maurice B. Burg, Chf.

**Activities/Fields:** Mechanism and regulation (hormonal and otherwise) of a variety of transport processes in systems, including the intact kidney, isolated perfused segments of renal tubules, and epithelial cell cultures. Emphasis is on electrophysiology, quantitative microscopy, nuclear magnetic resonance, and intermediary metabolism as related to transport. **Pub:** *Proceedings*.

## ★ 8768 ★ U.S. Department of Health and Human Services
**National Institute of Diabetes and Digestive and Kidney Diseases (NIDDK)**
NIH Bldg. 31
31 Center Dr. MSC 2560
Bethesda, MD 20892-2560
**Phone:** (301)496-5877     **Fax:** (301)402-2125
**Email:** spiegela@extra.niddk.nih.gov
**Website:** http://www.niddk.nih.gov
Allen Spiegel, MD, Dir.

**Activities/Fields:** Serious diseases affecting public health. The Institute supports clinical research on the diseases of internal medicine and related subspecialty fields as well as in many basic science disciplines. Institute activities include both intramural programs, which are carried out in the Institute's laboratory and clinical facilities on the NIH campus in Bethesda, MD and Phoenix, AZ; and extramural programs, which are supported by NIDDK and carried out at universities, private and public research facilities, and hospital-based clinical research centers. The Institute's Intramural Research Division encompasses the broad spectrum of metabolic diseases such as diabetes and other inborn errors of metabolism, endocrine disorders, mineral metabolism, digestive diseases, nutrition, urology and renal disease, and hematology. Basic research includes studies in biochemistry; nutrition; pathology; histochemistry; chemistry; physical, chemical, and molecular biology; pharmacology; and toxicology. NIDDK extramural research is organized in four divisions: Diabetes, Endocrinology, and Metabolic Diseases; Digestive Diseases and Nutrition; Kidney, Urologic, and Hematologic Diseases; and Extramural Activities. Mechanisms of NIDDK support for extramural programs include investigator-initiated grants, program project and center grants, and career development and training awards. The Institute also supports research and development projects and large-scale clinical trials through contracts.

**★ 8769 ★ U.S. Department of Health and Human Services**
**National Institute of Diabetes and Digestive and Kidney Diseases**
**Clinical Nutrition Research Units Program**
6707 Democracy Blvd.
MSC 5450
Bethesda, MD 20892-5450
**Phone:** (301)594-8883        **Fax:** (301)480-8300
**Email:** vh16h@nih.gov
Dr. Van S. Hubbard, Prog. Dir.

**Activities/Fields:** Integrated array of research, educational, and service activities focused on human nutrition in health and disease. Each unit serves as the focal point for an interdisciplinary approach to clinical nutrition research and for the stimulation of research in areas such as improved nutritional support of acutely and chronically ill persons, assessment of nutritional status, effects of disease states on nutrient needs, and effects of changes in nutritional status on disease. Funding for the CNRU program is provided through core center grants, which provide funds for: core resources such as cell culture, immunoassay, biostatistics, or other central research service facilities; pilot/feasibility projects, which support new investigators or investigators from other fields who wish to pursue new and innovative ideas to a point where they can compete for independent support; program enrichment funds to provide for small conferences or symposia and special consultants for the center; and a new investigator position. An existing base of high-quality nutrition-related research is a requirement for the establishment of a CNRU. Due to a restriction in the number of core center grants that can be made, investigator-initiated proposals are accepted only in response to a request for applications announced in the NIH Guide for Grants and Contracts.

**★ 8770 ★ U.S. Department of Health and Human Services**
**National Institute of Diabetes and Digestive and Kidney Diseases**
**Division of Diabetes, Endocrinology, and Metabolic Diseases**
NIH Bldg. 31, Rm. 9A16
31 Center Dr. MSC 2560
Bethesda, MD 20892-2560
**Phone:** (301)496-7349        **Fax:** (301)480-6792
**Email:** jf58s@nih.gov
**Website:**        http://www.niddk.nih.gov/fund/divisions/dem/demintro.htm
Judith Fradkin, MD, Dir.

**Activities/Fields:** Diabetes mellitus (both insulin dependent and noninsulin dependent diabetes); endocrinological diseases and disorders; and metabolic diseases, including research on the etiology, pathogenesis, and treatment of acquired or inborn errors of metabolism and cystic fibrosis. Support for basic and clinical biomedical research as well as epidemiologic and behavioral studies and clinical trials is provided through investigator-initiated research grants, new investigator awards, program project and center grants, and cooperative agreements. The Division also supports research fellowships, training grants, and a variety of career development awards as well as a limited number of resource and research and development contracts; and provides leadership in coordinating activities relating to diabetes and cystic fibrosis throughout the National Institutes of Health and various other federal agencies. Division's main branches are the Diabetes Programs Branch and the Endocrine and Metabolic Diseases Research Programs Branch.

**U.S. Department of Health and Human Services**
**National Institute of Diabetes and Digestive and Kidney Diseases**
**Division of Diabetes, Endocrinology, and Metabolic Diseases**
**Cystic Fibrosis Research Program**
*See:* Entry 9441

**★ 8771 ★ U.S. Department of Health and Human Services**
**National Institute of Diabetes and Digestive and Kidney Diseases**
**Division of Diabetes, Endocrinology, and Metabolic Diseases**
**Diabetes Center Program**
6707 Democracy Blvd. MSC 5460
Room 685
Bethesda, MD 20892-5460
**Phone:** (301)594-8803        **Fax:** (301)480-3503
**Email:** McKeonC@extra.niddk.nih.gov
**Website:** http://www.niddk.nih.gov/fund/program/a-el-ist.htmcystic
Dr. Sanford A. Garfield, Prog. Dir.

**Activities/Fields:** Administers two types of center awards: the Diabetes-Endocrinology Research Centers (DERC) and the Diabetes Research and Training Centers (DRTC). The DERC is exclusively oriented toward biomedical research goals, while the DRTCs include training and translation components in addition to biomedical research. An existing base of high-quality diabetes-related research is a primary requirement for establishment of either type of center. Through shared resources (core facilities), both types of center grants provide a mechanism for integrating, coordinating, and fostering the interdisciplinary cooperation of a group of established investigators conducting programs of active high quality research in diabetes and related endocrine and metabolic disorders.

**★ 8772 ★ U.S. Department of Health and Human Services**
**National Institute of Diabetes and Digestive and Kidney Diseases**
**Division of Diabetes, Endocrinology, and Metabolic Diseases**
**Diabetes Clinical Trials Program**
6707 Democracy Blvd.
Bethesda, MD 20892
**Phone:** (301)594-8803        **Fax:** (301)402-6271
**Email:** garfields@extra.niddk.nih.gov
**Website:**        http://www.niddk.nih.gov/patient/dpp/dpp.htm
Sanford Garfield, PhD, Sr.Adv. for Biometry and Behavioral Sci.

**Activities/Fields:** Supports a multicenter randomized clinical trial to determine whether interventions in high risk individuals can prevent the onset of type-2 diabetes. Participating in this study are 25 medical centers, a data coordinating center, and other supporting institutions that provide centralized technical and biochemical services. A group of expert consultants which is independent of the trial and external to the Institute continually reviews all operational aspects of the trial and provides policy advice to the Institute regarding the conduct of the study.

**★ 8773 ★ U.S. Department of Health and Human Services**
**National Institute of Diabetes and Digestive and Kidney Diseases**
**Division of Diabetes, Endocrinology, and Metabolic Diseases**
**Diabetes Research Section**
6707 Democracy Blvd.
Bethesda, MD 20892-2560
**Phone:** (301)594-8808        **Fax:** (301)480-3503
Dr. Judith Fradkin, Dir.

**Activities/Fields:** Provides grant support for investigator-initiated studies covering a wide range of fundamental and clinical studies related to the etiology, pathogenesis, prevention, diagnosis, treatment, and cure of diabetes mellitus and its complications. Specific areas of research interest encompass the structure/function of the pancreatic hormones and related peptides and enzymes; carbohydrate, lipid, and protein metabolism; and nutritional interrelationships, including obesity. Other areas of research support include the genetic nature of diabetes and identification of specific markers that characterize individuals predisposed to diabetes; studies to assess immunologic, infectious, and environmental factors as they relate to diabetes; and studies related to nutrition, metabolic regulation, and hormone synthesis/secretion/action with respect to the pathobiology of diabetes mellitus and its sequelae. Program also provides support for studies related to pancreas and islet transportation, automated insulin delivery systems and glucose sensors, the psychosocial and behavioral aspects of diabetes, the epidemiology of diabetes, and diabetes-related conferences.

**★ 8774 ★ U.S. Department of Health and Human Services**
**National Institute of Diabetes and Digestive Kidney Diseases**
**Division of Diabetes, Endocrinology, and Metabolic Diseases**
**Endocrinology and Metabolic Diseases Research Programs Branch**
45 Center Dr. MSC 6600
Bethesda, MD 20892-2560
**Phone:** (301)594-7567        **Fax:** (301)480-3503
**Email:** fradkinj@ep.niddk.nih.gov
Dr. Judith Fradkin, Chf.

**Activities/Fields:** Componets are Cystic Fibrosis Research Program, Endocrinology Research Programs Section, Bone and Mineral Research Program, Metabolism and Structural Biology Research Program, Metabolic Diseases and Gene Therapy Research Program, Pituitary and Neuroendocrinology Research Program, and Growth Factors Research Program.

**★ 8775 ★ U.S. Department of Health and Human Services**
**National Institute of Diabetes and Digestive and Kidney Diseases**
**Division of Diabetes, Endocrinology, and Metabolic Diseases**
**Endocrinology Research Section**
45 Center Dr. MSC 6600
Bethesda, MD 20892-6600
**Phone:** (301)594-8819        **Fax:** (301)480-3503
Dr. Ronald N. Margolis, Chf.

**Activities/Fields:** Supports (through research grants) investigator-initiated basic and clinical studies of normal and abnormal function of the pituitary, thyroid, parathyroid, adrenal, pineal, and thymus glands. Studies of the mode of action of hormones, their biosynthesis, secretion, and metabolism as well as their binding to protein carriers, subsequent release, and the kinetics of binding represent a major component of the Program. A substantial portion of the Program is devoted to structure/function studies of the hypothalamic releasing factors as they affect endocrine function as well as the physiology and pathophysiology of bone disease. In addition, studies of somatomedin and somatostatin and their effects on other hormones are supported, as is research on substances with hormone-like action such as prostaglandins and the brain peptides.

**★ 8776 ★ U.S. Department of Health and Human Services**
**National Institute of Diabetes and Digestive and Kidney Diseases**
**Division of Diabetes, Endocrinology, and Metabolic Diseases**
**National Diabetes Data Group**
45 Center Dr. MSC 5460
Bethesda, MD 20892-5460
**Phone:** (301)594-8801        **Fax:** (301)480-3503

**Activities/Fields:** Serves as the major federal focus for the collection, analysis, and dissemination of data on diabetes and its complications. Drawing upon the expertise of the research, medical, and lay communities, the Data Group initiates efforts to: define the data needed to address the scientific and public health issues in diabetes; foster and coordinate the collection of these data from multiple sources; promote the timely availability of reliable data to pertinent scientific, medical, and public organizations; modify data reporting systems to identify and categorize more appropriately the medical and socio-economic impact of diabetes; and promote the standardization of data collection and terminology in clinical and epidemiologic research. In addition, the NDDG staff works closely with members of the scientific community to stimulate development of new investigator-initiated research programs in diabetes epidemiology.

## ★ 8777 ★ U.S. Department of Health and Human Services
National Institute of Diabetes and Digestive and Kidney Diseases
Division of Diabetes, Endocrinology, and Metabolic Diseases
**Research Career Development Program**
45 Center Dr. MSC 6600
Bethesda, MD 20892-6600
**Phone:** (301)594-8819          **Fax:** (301)480-3503
Dr. Ron Margolis, Dir.

**Activities/Fields:** Administers a variety of research training and career development awards that span the full range of research programs falling within the Division. Prospective applicants are encouraged to contact the Research Career Development Program office regarding any questions about eligibility or provisions of the awards and to obtain current instructions for preparing applications. The available awards include National Research Service Awards, Physician Scientist Award, Clinical Investigator Award, and Research Career Development Award.

## ★ 8778 ★ U.S. Department of Health and Human Services
National Institute of Diabetes and Digestive and Kidney Diseases
Division of Diabetes, Endocrinology, and Metabolic Diseases
**Special Program Branch**
6707 Democracy Blvd.
Bethesda, MD 20892
**Phone:** (301)594-7692          **Fax:** (301)480-3503
James Hyde, PhD, Contact

**Activities/Fields:** Responsible for all of the Division-related research career development and training awards. These include individual and institutional National Research Service Awards (NRSA), Physician Scientist Awards (PSA), Clinical Investigator Awards (CIA), and Research Career Development Awards (RCDA). Branch components include the National Diabetes Data Group, Research Career Development Program; and the Special Programs Branch.

## ★ 8779 ★ U.S. Department of Health and Human Services
National Institute of Diabetes and Digestive and Kidney Diseases
Division of Digestive Diseases and Nutrition
**Obesity and Eating Disorders Program**
6707 Democracy Blvd.
Bethesda, MD 20892-5450
**Phone:** (301)594-8880          **Fax:** (301)480-8300
**Email:** sy29f@nih.gov
Dr. Susan Yanovski, Dir.

**Activities/Fields:** Biomedical and behavioral aspects of obesity, anorexia nervosa, bulimia, and other eating disorders. Goals are to establish a clear understanding of the etiology, prevention, and treatment of these multifaceted conditions. Studies focus on the physiological, metabolic, psychological, and genetic factors that affect food choices, food intake, eating behavior, appetite, and satiety; the effects of taste, smell, and gastric and humoral (including neurotransmitters) response in association with dietary intake and subsequent behavior; the physiologic and metabolic consequences of weight loss or weight gain; the effect of mild exercise on appetite and weight control; and individual variabilities in energy utilization and thermogenesis. The program also encourages investigations on the dietary determinants of the growth and control of adipocyte size and number; the responsiveness of the adipocyte to various metabolic and pharmacologic stimuli; the prevention of obesity and other eating disorders; improved methods of assessing body composition; examination of health risk factors associated with specific degrees of obesity or body composition; and determining the effect of exercise on body composition.

## ★ 8780 ★ U.S. Department of Health and Human Services
National Institute of Diabetes and Digestive and Kidney Diseases
Division of Digestive Diseases and Nutrition
**Pancreas Program**
Room 671, MSC 5450
6707 Democracy Blvd.
Bethesda, MD 20892
**Phone:** (301)594-8871          **Fax:** (301)480-8300
**Website:** http://www.niddk.nih.gov/fund/programs/mrlist.htmpancreas
Dr. Jose Serrano, PhD, Dir.

**Activities/Fields:** Structure, function, and diseases (excluding cancer and cystic fibrosis) of the exocrine pancreas. Areas of research interest include: hormonal and neural regulation of electrolyte, fluid, and enzyme secretion; receptors for secretagogs; stimulus-secretion coupling mechanisms; gut-islet-acinar interrelations; organization and expression of pancreatic genes; protein synthesis and export; tissue injury, repair, and regeneration; physiology and pathology of trophic responses; neural innervention; transcapillary solute and fluid exchange; pancreatic tissue culture and storage, and preservation; imaging of the pancreas; pancreatic insufficiency; and acute and chronic pancreatitis and relevant experimental models.

## ★ 8781 ★ U.S. Department of Health and Human Services
National Institute of Diabetes and Digestive and Kidney Diseases
Division of Extramural Activities
6707 Democracy Dr., Rm. 715
MSC 5452
Bethesda, MD 20892-5452
**Phone:** (301)594-8834          **Fax:** (301)480-3505
**Email:** hammond2@extra.niddk.nih.gov
**Website:** http://www.niddk.nih.gov/funds/divisions/dea/deaintro.htm
Dr. Robert Hammond, Dir.

**Activities/Fields:** Serves as the service organization to the rest of the extramural division and is comprised of three branches: the review branch which reviews research grant applications; the grants management branch which prepares and issues grant awards; and the contracts and acquisition management branch which prepares and issues contracts.

## ★ 8782 ★ U.S. Department of Health and Human Services
National Institute of Diabetes and Digestive and Kidney Diseases
Division of Intramural Research
NIH Bldg. 10, Rm. 9M222
9000 Rockville Pike
Bethesda, MD 20892-1818
**Phone:** (301)496-4128          **Fax:** (301)496-9943
**Email:** marving@intra.niddk.nih.gov
Dr. Marvin C. Gershengorn, MD, Sci. Dir.

**Activities/Fields:** Metabolic diseases such as diabetes, other inborn errors of metabolism, endocrine disorders, mineral metabolism, digestive diseases, nutrition, urology and renal disease, and hematology. Basic research includes studies in biochemistry; nutrition; pathology; histochemistry; chemistry; physical, chemical, and molecular biology; pharmacology; and toxicology. Division comprises branches for: Clinical Endocrinology; Clinical Hematology; Diabetes; Digestive Diseases; Genetics and Biochemistry; Mathematical Research; Metabolic Diseases; Molecular, Cellular, and Nutritional Endocrinology; and Pediatric Metabolism; the Phoenix Epidemiology and Clinical Research Branch; and numerous laboratories.

## ★ 8783 ★ U.S. Department of Health and Human Services
National Institute of Diabetes and Digestive and Kidney Diseases
Division of Intramural Research
**Metabolic Diseases Branch**
NIH Bldg. 10 /Rm. 9C-101
9000 Rockville Pike
Bethesda, MD 20892-1802
**Phone:** (301)496-5051          **Fax:** (301)496-0200
Dr. Stephen Marx, Actg. Chf.

**Activities/Fields:** Physiology and nature of metabolic diseases and disorders, with emphasis on the physiology, biochemistry, and mechanism of action of hormones controlling calcium metabolism. Investigations are directed at hormone-receptor interactions, regulation and characterization of adenylate cyclase, and cellular responses to hormones, particularly parathyroid hormone, calcitonin, and parathyroid related peptide. The clinical program involves studies of patients with disorders of mineral metabolism, including familial hyperparathyroid syndromes and patients with multiple endocrine neoplasia type I, hereditary resistance to parathyroid hormone or to calciferols. Patients with hyperparathyroidism are evaluated with arte riography, selective thyroid venous cath eterization, and radioimmunoassays for parathyroid hormone and cyclic AMP in plasma and/or urine. Excised parathyroid tissue is used for in vitro studies gene characterization and on control of hormone secretion.

## ★ 8784 ★ U.S. Department of Health and Human Services
National Institute of Diabetes and Digestive and Kidney Diseases
Division of Intramural Research
**Molecular, Cellular, and Nutritional Endocrinology Branch**
NIH Bldg. 10, Rm. 8D14
9000 Rockville Pike
Bethesda, MD 20892
**Phone:** (301)496-1540          **Fax:** (301)496-1649

**Activities/Fields:** Neuroendocrinology; experimental diabetes, metabolism, and nutrition; and growth and development. Research in neuroendocrinology includes basic and clinical investigations on the regulation of hypothalamic, pituitary, and placental polypeptide hormones. Studies in experimental diabetes, metabolism, and nutrition include investigation of the structure, function, and biosynthesis of integral membrane proteins involved in the hormonal regulation of carbohydrate and lipid metabolism; studies on the molecular and cellular basis of hormone action; and studies on the influence of altered metabolic and nutritional states on cellular function and its regulation by hormones. In the area of growth and development, Branch seeks to understand the mechanisms by which hormonal, nutritional, and cellular factors interact to regulate cell growth in different physiological states (e.g., fetal/embryonic development, post-natal growth, wound repair, neural cell growth, and maintenance), and how these controlled processes become deranged in pathological states involving excessive or inadequate cell growth (e.g., intrauterine growth retardation, dwarfism, neoplasia, atherosclerosis, diabetic retinopathy). The biosynthesis and action of polypeptide hormones/growth factors and their regulation is studied in appropriate model systems (e.g., cell cultures established from human subjects and animals) using state-of-the-art techniques of molecular and cell biology. Special emphasis is given to interactions between different cell types and their products, regulation of tissue responsiveness to growth factors, and alternative expression of growth factor genes resulting in novel peptides with biological functions not directly related to cell growth.

**U.S. Department of Health and Human Services**
**National Institute of Diabetes and Digestive and Kidney Diseases**
**Laboratory of Cellular and Developmental Biology**
*See:* Entry 4729

**U.S. Department of Health and Human Services**
**National Institute of Mental Health**
**Intramural Research Programs Division (Clinical Research)**
**Clinical Neuroendocrinology Branch**
*See:* Entry 12735

**★ 8785 ★ U.S. Department of Health and Human Services**
**National Institutes of Health**
**National Institute of Child Health and Human Development**
**Division of Intramural Research (Pediatric and Reproductive Endocrinology Branch)**
Bldg. 10, Rm. 9D42
10 Center Dr., MSC 1583
Bethesda, MD 20892-1583
**Phone:** (301)496-5800     **Fax:** (301)402-0884
**Email:** chrousog@mail.nih.gov
**Website:** http://preb.nichd.nih.gov/
Dr. George Chrousos, Ch.

**Activities/Fields:** Pediatric and reproductive endocrinology and metabolism, especially physiology and pathophysiology of growth, development, metabolic, immune, and reproductive functions and study of major neurohormonal systems, hypothalamic-pituitary-adrenal (HPA) and -gonadal (HPG) axes and autonomic nervous system, that sub-serve these functions.

**★ 8786 ★ U.S. Department of Health and Human Services**
**National Institutes of Health**
**National Institute of Diabetes and Digestive and Kidney Diseases**
**Division of Diabetes, Endocrinology, and Metabolic Diseases (Endocrine Pancreas Program)**
MSC-5460
6707 Democracy Blvd., Rm. 697
Bethesda, MD 20892-5460
**Phone:** (301)594-8802     **Fax:** (301)480-3503
**Email:** laughlinm@extra.niddk.nih.gov
**Website:** http://www.niddk.nih.gov/fund/program/A-Elist.htmendo
Maren Laughlin, PhD, Dir.

**Activities/Fields:** Endocrine cells (alpha, beta, delta, etc.) of the pancreas and the islets.

**★ 8787 ★ U.S. Department of Health and Human Services**
**National Institutes of Health**
**National Institute of Diabetes and Digestive and Kidney Diseases**
**Division of Diabetes, Endocrinology, and Metabolic Diseases (Cytoarchitecture and Matrix Research Program)**
2 Democracy Plz., Rm. 6105
Bethesda, MD 20892
**Phone:** (301)594-8811
**Email:** satos@extra.niddk.nih.gov
**Website:** http://www.niddk.nih.gov/fund/program/A-Elist.htmAIDS
Sheryl Sato, PhD, Dir.

**Activities/Fields:** Properties and functions of intracellular and extracellular, filamentous suprastructures that are involved in hormone signaling and endocrine and metabolic disorders.

**★ 8788 ★ U.S. Department of Health and Human Services**
**National Institutes of Health**
**National Institute of Diabetes and Digestive and Kidney Diseases**
**Division of Diabetes, Endocrinology, and Metabolic Diseases (Transcriptional Regulation of Metabolic Pathways Program)**
2 Democracy Pl., Rm. 6105
Bethesda, MD 20892
**Phone:** (301)594-8811
**Email:** satos@extra.niddk.nih.gov
**Website:** http://www.niddk.nih.gov/program/S-Zlist.htmTRMP
Sheryl Sato, PhD, Dir.

**Activities/Fields:** Understanding the significance of gene regulation to control of metabolism. Specific areas of support include (1) identifying and characterizing transcription factors and cis-acting regulatory elements in DNA using structural and functional approaches; (2) identifying mechanisms whereby signal transduction pathways elicit changes in gene expression; and (3) identifying the molecular response to environmental cues including hormonal stimulation, nutrients, development, and stress.

**★ 8789 ★ U.S. Department of Health and Human Services**
**National Institutes of Health**
**National Institute of Diabetes and Digestive and Kidney Diseases**
**Division of Diabetes, Endocrinology, and Metabolic Diseases (Type 2 Diabetes in the Pediatric Population Program)**
2 Democracy Pl., Rm. 699
Bethesda, MD 20892
**Phone:** (301)594-0021
**Email:** linderb@extra.niddk.nih.gov
**Website:** http://www.niddk.nih.gov/fund/program/S-Zlist.htm
Barbara Linder, MD, Dir.

**Activities/Fields:** Pathophysiology, prevention, and treatment of Type 2 diabetes in children.

**★ 8790 ★ U.S. Department of Health and Human Services**
**National Institutes of Health**
**National Institute of Diabetes and Digestive and Kidney Diseases**
**Division of Diabetes, Endocrinology, and Metabolic Diseases (Therapeutic Approaches to Diabetes Mellitus Program)**
MSC 5460
6707 Democracy Blvd., Rm. 6101
Bethesda, MD 20892-5460
**Phone:** (301)594-8802     **Fax:** (301)480-3503
**Email:** laughlinm@extra.niddk.nih.gov
**Website:** http://www.niddk.nih.gov/fund/program/S-Zlist.htm
Maren Laughlin, PhD, Dir.

**Activities/Fields:** Therapeutic approaches to achieving euglycemia. Specific areas of support include (1) studies on drug development; (2) transplantation of pancreas or pancreatic endocrine cells (islets or beta cells); (3) glucose sensors (including their combination with insulin delivery systems to provide a closed-loop system); (4) cellular therapy, (including gene therapy approaches) that is being proposed to treat or prevent either type 1 or type 2 diabetes; (5) studies in cell culture to bioengineer or genetically manipulate cells to produce an insulin secreting cell or a glucose-responsive insulin secreting cell for the eventual treatment of diabetes; and (6) creation of animal models for therapeutic trials.

**★ 8791 ★ U.S. Department of Health and Human Services**
**National Institutes of Health**
**National Institute of Diabetes and Digestive and Kidney Diseases**
**Division of Diabetes, Endocrinology, and Metabolic Diseases (Thyroid Research Program)**
2 Democracy Pl., Rm. 699
Bethesda, MD 20892
**Phone:** (301)594-0021
**Email:** linderb@extra.niddk.nih.gov
**Website:** http://www.niddk.nih.gov/fund/program/S-Zlist.htm
Barbara Linder, PhD, Dir.

**Activities/Fields:** Normal thyroid physiology and no-nautoimmune thyroid disease including thyroid neoplasia. Specific areas of support include (1) physiologic regulation of the expression, processing, and secretion of thyroid hormones; (2) dysfunctional regulation of thyroid hormones that results in disease; (3) studies of the etiology, pathogenesis, diagnosis, and therapy of thyroid disorders; (4) studies on the deiodinase enzymes that convert inactive thyroid hormone to active thyroid hormone; and (5) studies on neural cells that are targets of regulation by and feedback to the thyroid.

**★ 8792 ★ U.S. Department of Health and Human Services**
**National Institutes of Health**
**National Institute of Diabetes and Digestive and Kidney Diseases**
**Division of Diabetes, Endocrinology, and Metabolic Diseases (Steroid Metabolism Program)**
MSC 5460
2 Democracy Pl., Rm. 603
Bethesda, MD 20892-5460
**Phone:** (301)451-9871     **Fax:** (301)480-3503
**Email:** mt270t@nih.gov
**Website:** http://www.niddk.nih.gov/fund/program/S-Zlist.htm
Mehrdah Tondraui, PhD, Dir.

**Activities/Fields:** Biochemistry, molecular biology, genetics, metabolism, and biological function of steroids and similar molecules derived from cholesterol, including sex steroids and other hormones (glucocorticoids, mineralocorticoids), retinoids, cardiac glycosides, prostaglandins, eicosanoids, and bile acids. Specific areas of support include (1) structure and reaction mechanisms of enzymes and enzyme-substrate complexes in steroidogenesis and steroid interconversion pathways; (2) cholesterol activation for steroidogenesis, including cholesterol esterase and intramitochondrial translocation of cholesterol; (3) structure, function, and reaction mechanism of the p450 class of enzymes; (4) estrogens and androgens in development; and (5) structure and function of the mitochondrial cytochromes.

**★ 8793 ★ U.S. Department of Health and Human Services**
**National Institutes of Health**
**National Institute of Diabetes and Digestive and Kidney Diseases**
**Division of Diabetes, Endocrinology, and Metabolic Diseases (Reproductive Endocrinology Program)**
2 Democracy Pl., Rm. 699
Bethesda, MD 20892
**Phone:** (301)594-0021
**Email:** linderb@extra.niddk.nih.gov
**Website:** http://www.niddk.nih.gov/program/M-Rlist.htmreproendo
Barbara Linder, MD, Dir.

**Activities/Fields:** Structure and function of gonadotropins including LH, FSH, and hCG and their receptors. Specific areas of support include (1) oligosaccharide modification and its effects on gonadotropin function; (2) metabolic responses of target tissue (e.g., prostate); (3) studies on the interaction of gonadotropins with their receptors; (4) physiological effects of the hormones (e.g., menopause, age at onset of menstruation); and (5) development and study of analogs of gonadotropins.


★ 8794 ★ **U.S. Department of Health and Human Services**
**National Institutes of Health**
**National Institute of Diabetes and Digestive and Kidney Diseases**
**Division of Diabetes, Endocrinology, and Metabolic Diseases**
**(Protein Trafficking/Secretion/Processing Research Program)**
2 Democracy Pl., Rm. 6101
Bethesda, MD 20892
**Phone:** (301)594-7689          **Fax:** (301)435-6047
**Email:** haftc@extra.niddk.nih.gov
**Website:** http://www.niddk.nih.gov/fund/program/M-Rlist.htm
Carol Sato, PhD, Dir.

**Activities/Fields:** Understanding the mechanisms accounting for the fate of proteins after initial translation. Specific areas of support include (1) protein folding; (2) post-translational modifications and the enzymes that catalyze them; (3) movement of proteins in vesicles from endoplasmic reticulum (ER) through the golgi and endosomes and their ultimate secretion; (4) mechanisms that account for vesicle formation (pinching-off) and vesicle fusion, which are paramount to understanding trafficking; (5) movement of proteins in the direction opposite of secretion, including endocytosis and retrograde transport; (6) proteins and small molecules that regulate protein trafficking; and (7) proteasomes, ubiquitin conjugation, and the N-end rule.


★ 8795 ★ **U.S. Department of Health and Human Services**
**National Institutes of Health**
**National Institute of Diabetes and Digestive and Kidney Diseases**
**Division of Diabetes, Endocrinology, and Metabolic Diseases**
**(Regulation of Energy Balance and Body Composition Program)**
MSC 5460
6707 Democracy Blvd., Rm. 693
Bethesda, MD 20892-5460
**Phone:** (301)594-8816          **Fax:** (301)480-3503
**Email:** smithp@.extra.niddk.nih.gov
**Website:** http://www.niddk.nih.gov/fund/program/M-Rlist.htm
Philip Smith, PhD, Sr. Adv.

**Activities/Fields:** Regulation of body composition by the hypothalamus and circulating factors. Specific areas of support include (1) endocrinology of body composition including interactions between nutrition, exercise, and anabolic hormones; (2) neuropeptides and their receptors involved in regulatory pathways controlling feeding behavior, satiety, and energy expenditure; (3) interactions between hypothalamic-pituitary-adrenal axis and peripheral metabolic signals (e.g., insulin, leptin, glucocorticoids); (4) hormones and cytokines involved in wasting syndromes (cancer); (5) endocrine regulation of energy balance via uncoupling proteins; and (6) hypothalamic integration of peripheral endocrine and metabolic signals.


★ 8796 ★ **U.S. Department of Health and Human Services**
**National Institutes of Health**
**National Institute of Diabetes and Digestive and Kidney Diseases**
**Division of Diabetes, Endocrinology, and Metabolic Diseases**
**(Protein Metabolism Program)**
MSC 5460
6707 Democracy Blvd., Rm. 6101
Bethesda, MD 20892-5460
**Phone:** (301)594-8802          **Fax:** (301)480-3503

**Email:** laughlinm@.extra.niddk.nih.gov
**Website:** http://www.niddk.nih.gov/fund/program/M-Rlist.htm
Maren Laughlin, PhD, Dir.

**Activities/Fields:** Basic and clinical studies of protein, peptide, and amino acid metabolism, as well as studies of purified protein structure, kinetics, function, and enzyme reaction mechanism, including hormone regulation, effects of diet and exercise, and the pathology associated with metabolic diseases. Specific areas of support include (1) studies of flux or regulation of total protein synthesis and turnover in health and disease, including investigations of the specific enzymes of protein and amino acid metabolism; (2) amino acid and peptide membrane transport; (3) uptake, metabolism, and synthesis of specific amino acids; (4) regulation of urea production and nitrogen balance; (5) role of cofactors, vitamins, and minerals in metabolism and enzyme action; and (6) structure of specific classes of enzymes (redox, phosphate transfer, etc.) elucidated by x-ray, NMR, or electron microscopy.


★ 8797 ★ **U.S. Department of Health and Human Services**
**National Institutes of Health**
**National Institute of Diabetes and Digestive and Kidney Diseases**
**Division of Diabetes, Endocrinology, and Metabolic Diseases**
**(Minority Health Program)**
6707 Democracy Blvd.
Bethesda, MD 20892
**Phone:** (301)496-4000
**Email:** agodoal@extra.niddk.nih.gov
**Website:** http://www.niddk.nih.gov/fund/program/M-Rlist.htmmhp
Lawrence Y. Agodoa, MD, Dir.

**Activities/Fields:** Disease that disproportionately affect minority populations, especially pathogenesis mechanisms, risk factors, and potential treatments for renal disease and hypertension, kidney disease of diabetes, and hemoglobinopathies such as sickle cell disease.


★ 8798 ★ **U.S. Department of Health and Human Services**
**National Institutes of Health**
**National Institute of Diabetes and Digestive and Kidney Diseases**
**Division of Diabetes, Endocrinology, and Metabolic Diseases**
**(Neuroendocrinology Program)**
MSC 5460
2 Democracy Pl., Rm. 6105
Bethesda, MD 20892
**Phone:** (301)594-8811          **Fax:** (301)480-3503
**Email:** satos@extra.niddk.nih.gov
**Website:** http://www.niddk.nih.gov/program/M-Rlist.htmneuroendo
Sheryl Sato, PhD, Dir.

**Activities/Fields:** Neuropeptides of the hypothalamus. Specific areas of research support include (1) physiological response to stress through the hypothalamic-pituitary-adrenal axis; (2) neuropeptides and neuropeptide receptor signalling pathways; (3) gene regulation in the hypothalamus and pituitary gland; (4) diseases of the pituitary including neoplasia; (5) hypopituitary dwarfism; (6) identification and characterization of novel hypothalamic or pituitary hormones; (7) tissue specific and developmental expression of pituitary and hypothalamic genes; (8) pituitary hormone receptors and actions on target tissues (eg., GH IGF-1 axis); (9) neuropeptide receptors in diagnosis and treatment of disease; and (10) neuroendocrine-immune interactions.


★ 8799 ★ **U.S. Department of Health and Human Services**
**National Institutes of Health**
**National Institute of Diabetes and Digestive and Kidney Diseases**
**Division of Diabetes, Endocrinology, and Metabolic Diseases**
**(Lipid Metabolism Program)**
MSC 5460
6707 Democracy Blvd., Rm. 6101
Bethesda, MD 20892-5460
**Phone:** (301)594-8802          **Fax:** (301)480-3503
**Email:** laughlinm@.extra.niddk.nih.gov
**Website:** http://www.niddk.nih.gov/fund/program/F-Llist.htm
Maren Laughlin, PhD, Dir.

**Activities/Fields:** Basic and clinical studies of the metabolism of fatty acid, triacylglycerols, cholesterol, and related molecules, which will lead to the development of effective treatments for diabetes, obesity, hypertriglyceridemia, hypercholesterolemia, burn injury, sepsis, and other metabolic diseases. Specific areas of support include (1) flux and regulation of oxidation, storage, and remodeling of dietary lipids in health and disease, and effects of diet and exercise; (2) regulation of lipid esterification, hormone-sensitive lipases, and phospholipid metabolism; (3) membrane transport and movement of lipids within the cell, or between organs (binding proteins, carnitine transferases); (4) lipid-protein interactions; (5) metabolism of bioactive lipids and their precursors; and (6) lipid peroxidation, especially associated with disease.


★ 8800 ★ **U.S. Department of Health and Human Services**
**National Institutes of Health**
**National Institute of Diabetes and Digestive and Kidney Diseases**
**Division of Diabetes, Endocrinology, and Metabolic Diseases**
**(Insulin Resistance Program)**
MSC 5460
6707 Democracy Blvd., Rm. 6101
Bethesda, MD 20892-5460
**Phone:** (301)594-8802          **Fax:** (301)480-3503
**Email:** laughinm@extra.niddk.nih.gov
**Website:** http://www.niddk.nih.gov/program/F-Llist.htminsulin
Maren Laughlin, PhD, Dir.

**Activities/Fields:** Role of insulin resistance in the pathogenesis of type 2 diabetes mellitus; relationship between insulin resistance and obesity; relationship between insulin resistance and physical activity; new methods to measure peripheral insulin resistance; molecular basis of decreased sensitivity to insulin; insulin receptor desensitization; uncoupling of receptor activation to downstream events; and animal models of insulin resistance.


★ 8801 ★ **U.S. Department of Health and Human Services**
**National Institutes of Health**
**National Institute of Diabetes and Digestive and Kidney Diseases**
**Division of Diabetes, Endocrinology, and Metabolic Diseases**
**(Insulin Receptor/Structure/Function/Action Program)**
MSC 5460
2 Democracy Pl., Rm. 607
Bethesda, MD 20892-5460
**Phone:** (301)594-8817          **Fax:** (301)480-6047
**Email:** abrahamk@extra.niddk.nih.gov
**Website:** http://www.niddk.nih.gov/program/F-Llist.htminsulinRSFA
Kristin Abraham, PhD, Dir.

**Activities/Fields:** Structure, function, and action of the insulin receptor, including molecular analysis of ligand binding to receptor; activation of tyrosine kinase; subsequent insulin receptor function in signal transduction by serving as a platform for the attachment of downstream signaling molecules involved in insulin action; and the Insulin Receptor Signaling proteins ((IRS)-1,2,3,4) and other proteins containing Src Homology Domains (e.g., Sh(2)).

**★ 8802 ★ U.S. Department of Health and Human Services**
**National Institutes of Health**
**National Institute of Diabetes and Digestive and Kidney Diseases**
**Division of Diabetes, Endocrinology, and Metabolic Diseases**
**(Hypoglycemia Program)**
MSC 5460
2 Democracy Pl., Rm. 699
Bethesda, MD 20892
**Phone:** (301)594-0021       **Fax:** (301)480-3503
**Email:** linder@extra.niddk.nih.gov
**Website:** http://www.niddk.nih.gov/fund/program/F-Llist.htm
Barbara Linder, PhD, Dir.

**Activities/Fields:** Pathogenesis, prevention, treatment, and sequelae of hypoglycemia (low blood glucose) in both type 1 and type 2 diabetes.

**★ 8803 ★ U.S. Department of Health and Human Services**
**National Institutes of Health**
**National Institute of Diabetes and Digestive and Kidney Diseases**
**Division of Diabetes, Endocrinology, and Metabolic Diseases**
**(Inborn Errors of Metabolism Program)**
MS 5460
6707 Democracy Blvd., Rm. 6103
Bethesda, MD 20892-5460
**Phone:** (301)594-8810       **Fax:** (301)480-3503
**Email:** mckeonc@extra.niddk.nih.gov
**Website:** http://www.niddk.nih.gov/fund/program/F-Llist.htm
Catherine McKeon, PhD, Sr. Adv.

**Activities/Fields:** Pathophysiology and treatment of genetic metabolic diseases; including studies of etiology, pathogenesis, prevention, diagnosis, pathophysiology, and treatment of these diseases; characterization of the genes, gene defects, and regulatory alterations that underlie causes of these diseases; studies of the mutant enzyme and its effect on the structure and function of the protein; development of animal models for genetic disease; development of dietary, pharmacologic, and enzyme replacement therapies; and development of stem cell transplantation, both prenatally and postnatally, as a treatment for metabolic diseases.

**★ 8804 ★ U.S. Department of Health and Human Services**
**National Institutes of Health**
**National Institute of Diabetes and Digestive and Kidney Diseases**
**Division of Diabetes, Endocrinology, and Metabolic Diseases**
**(Growth Factor/Receptor/Structure/Function Program)**
MSC 5460
6707 Democracy Blvd., Rm. 693
Bethesda, MD 20892-5460
**Phone:** (301)594-8816       **Fax:** (301)480-3503
**Email:** smithp@extra.niddk.nih.gov
**Website:** http://www.niddk.nih.gov/fund/program/F-Llist.htm
Philip Smith, PhD, Dir.

**Activities/Fields:** Growth factors and cytokines and their receptors, binding proteins, and inhibitors. Specific areas of support include regulation of expression of growth factors and their receptors in endocrine cells and tissues; structure/function studies; role of growth factors in endocrine tumor progression; identification of genes that are downstream targets of growth factor receptor activation; modulation of growth factor action by binding proteins; autocrine and paracrine actions of

growth factors and cytokines to regulate cell/tissue growth and function.

**★ 8805 ★ U.S. Department of Health and Human Services**
**National Institutes of Health**
**National Institute of Diabetes and Digestive and Kidney Diseases**
**Division of Diabetes, Endocrinology, and Metabolic Diseases**
**(Glucose Metabolism Program)**
MSC-5460
6707 Democracy Blvd., Rm. 6101
Bethesda, MD 20892-5460
**Phone:** (301)594-8802       **Fax:** (301)480-3503
**Email:** laughlinm@extra.niddk.nih.gov
**Website:** http://www.niddk.nih.gov/fund/program/F-Llist.htm
Maren Laughlin, PhD, Dir.

**Activities/Fields:** Glucose and glycogen metabolism; development of effective treatments for diabetes, glycogen storage disease, obesity, burn injury, sepsis and trauma, and other metabolic diseases.

**★ 8806 ★ U.S. Department of Health and Human Services**
**National Institutes of Health**
**National Institute of Diabetes and Digestive and Kidney Diseases**
**Division of Diabetes, Endocrinology, and Metabolic Diseases**
**(Glucose Transport Program)**
DEM 2605
6707 Democracy Blvd., Rm. 6101
Bethesda, MD 20892
**Phone:** (301)594-7689       **Fax:** (301)453-6047
**Email:** laughlinm@extra.niddk.nih.gov
**Website:** http://www.niddk.nih.gov/fund/program/F-Llist.htm
Carol Haft, PhD, Dir.

**Activities/Fields:** Glucose transport in health and disease, especially as relating to glucose homeostasis in diabetes and obesity.

**★ 8807 ★ U.S. Department of Health and Human Services**
**National Institutes of Health**
**National Institute of Diabetes and Digestive and Kidney Diseases**
**Division of Diabetes, Endocrinology, and Metabolic Diseases**
**(G-Protein Coupled Receptors Program)**
MSC-5460
2 Democracy Plz., Rm. 607
Bethesda, MD 20892
**Phone:** (301)594-8817       **Fax:** (301)435-6047
**Email:** abrahamk@extra.niddk.nih.gov
**Website:** http://www.niddk.nih.gov/program/F-Llist.htmg-Protein
Kristin Abraham, PhD, Dir.

**Activities/Fields:** Studies on the G-protein coupled receptor superfamily, particularly cell surface, or seven transmembrane domain (7-TM), receptors coupled to GTP-binding ("G")-proteins for signal transduction; receptor structure; receptor down-regulation; role(s) of mutated receptors in disease; coupling of signaling through the receptor to other membrane-bound effectors or regulators such as adenylyl cyclase, ion channels, protein phosphatases or kinases, and other receptors.

**★ 8808 ★ U.S. Department of Health and Human Services**
**National Institutes of Health**
**National Institute of Diabetes and Digestive and Kidney Diseases**
**Division of Digestive Diseases and Nutrition**
**(Nutrient Metabolism Program)**
MSC 5450
6707 Democracy Blvd., Rm. 663
Bethesda, MD 20892-5450
**Phone:** (301)594-8884       **Fax:** (301)480-8300
**Email:** maym@extra.niddk.nih.gov
**Website:** http://www.niddk.nih.gov/fund/program/M-RLlist.htm
Michael Ken May, PhD, Dir.

**Activities/Fields:** Basic and clinical studies related to the requirement, bioavailability, and metabolism of nutrients and other dietary components at the organ, cellular, and subcellular levels in normal and diseased states. Areas of research include the understanding of physiologic function and mechanism of action/interaction of nutrients within the body; nutrient influence on gene regulation and expression; metabolism and function of nutrient antioxidants; effects of environment, heredity, stress, drug use, toxicants, and physical activity on problems of nutrient imbalance and nutrient requirements in health and disease; and specific metabolic considerations relating to alternative forms of nutrient delivery and use, such as total parenteral nutrition. Also supports research to improve methods of assessing nutritional status in health and disease.

**★ 8809 ★ U.S. Department of Health and Human Services**
**National Institutes of Health**
**National Institute of Diabetes and Digestive and Kidney Diseases**
**Division of Digestive Diseases and Nutrition**
**(Obesity/Nutrition Research Centers)**
MSC 5461
2 Democracy Pl., Rm. 631
45 Center Dr.
Bethesda, MD 20892-5461
**Phone:** (301)594-8822       **Fax:** (301)480-3768
**Email:** hubbardv@extra.niddk.nih.gov
**Website:** http://www.niddk.nih.gov/program/A-El-ist.htmCNRU
Van S. Hubbard, MD, Dir.

**Activities/Fields:** Biomedical research in obesity and nutrition; develop new knowledge concerning the development, treatment, and prevention of obesity and eating disorders; understand control and modulation of energy metabolism; understand and treat disorders associated with abnormalities of energy balance and weight management such as in anorexia nervosa, AIDS, and cancer.

**U.S. Department of Health and Human Services**
**National Institutes of Health**
**National Institute of Diabetes and Digestive and Kidney Diseases**
**Division of Digestive Diseases and Nutrition**
**(Gastrointestinal Neuroendocrinology Research Program)**
*See:* Entry 9175

**★ 8810 ★ U.S. Department of Health and Human Services**
**National Institutes of Health**
**National Institute of Environmental Health Sciences**
**Laboratory of Signal Transduction**
**(Molecular Endocrinology Group)**
PO Box 12233
Research Triangle Park, NC 27709

**Phone:** (919)541-1564   **Fax:** (919)541-1367
**Email:** cidlowsk1@niehs.nih.gov
**Website:** http://dir.niehs.nih.gov/dirlst/groups/cidlowski.htm
Dr. John Cidlowski, Hd.
**Activities/Fields:** Mechanisms and control of apoptosis; glucocorticord receptors; orphan receptors.


**★ 8811 ★ U.S. Department of Health and Human Services**
**National Institutes of Health**
**National Institute of Mental Health**
**Experimental Therapeutics Branch**
**(Behavioral Endocrinology Branch)**
MSC 1276
Bldg. 10, Rm. 3N238
Bethesda, MD 20892-1380
**Phone:** (301)496-4588   **Fax:** (301)496-9576
**Email:** nimhinfo@nih.gov
**Website:** http://intramural.nimh.nih.gov/research/beb/index2.htm
David R. Rubinow, MD, Ch.
**Activities/Fields:** Impact of reproductive endocrine function on the brain, including mood, cerebral blood flow, immune function, cognition, circadian function, signal transduction effectors, and response to stressors.


**U.S. Department of Health and Human Services**
**National Institutes of Health**
**National Institute of Mental Health**
**Experimental Therapeutics Branch**
**(Section on Neuroendocrine Immunology and Behavior)**
*See:* Entry 14340


**U.S. Department of Health and Human Services**
**National Institutes of Health**
**National Institute of Mental Health**
**Experimental Therapeutics Branch**
**(Clinical Neuroendocrinology Branch)**
*See:* Entry 14341


**★ 8812 ★ U.S. Department of Health and Human Services**
**National Institutes of Health**
**National Institute of Mental Health**
**Section on Pharmacology**
Bldg. 10, Rm. 2D57
9000 Rockville Pike
Bethesda, MD 20892
**Phone:** (301)496-0160
**Email:** saavedrj@irp.nimh.nih.org
**Website:** http://intramural.nimh.nih.gov/research/sop/
Juan Saavedra, Ch.
**Activities/Fields:** Effects of drugs and hormones on the central regulation of endocrine, autonomous and immune functions; biological rhythms; cerebral blood flow.


**★ 8813 ★ University of Alberta**
**Muttart Diabetes Research and Training Centre**
458 Heritage Medical Research
Edmonton, AB, Canada T6G 2S2
**Phone:** (780)492-6855   **Fax:** (780)492-4666
A. Rabinovitch, MD, Co-Dir.
**Activities/Fields:** Causes, treatment, and prevention of diabetes mellitus in humans and experimental animals. Provides core research laboratory support services. **Pub:** *Annual Reports.*


**★ 8814 ★ University of Calgary**
**Diabetes and Endocrine Research Group**
Health Science Centre, Rm. 2501
3330 Hospital Dr. NW
Calgary, AB, Canada T2N 4N1
**Phone:** (403)220-2261   **Fax:** (403)210-8113
**Email:** vsimpson@ucalgary.ca
Dr. D.C.W. Lau, Dir.
**Activities/Fields:** Cause, cure and prevention of type I and type II diabetes and obesity from molecular, cellular and clinical approaches. Participates in national and international collaborative research projects.


**★ 8815 ★ University of California, San Francisco**
**Center for Reproductive Sciences**
505 Parnassus Ave., HSW 1656
San Francisco, CA 94143-0556
**Phone:** (415)476-4295   **Fax:** (415)502-7866
**Email:** taylor@obgyn.ucsf.edu
Dr. Robert N. Taylor, Dir.
**Activities/Fields:** Hormonal regulation of reproductive events at the subcellular, cellular, tissular, and organismic levels. Research projects utilize a variety of species, including domestic and laboratory animals, subhuman primates, and humans. Conducts a multifaceted investigative and training program directed toward studies of the hypothalamic/pituitary/gonadal/target tissue axis and the endocrinologic physiology of pregnancy. **Frmly:** Reproductive Endocrinology Center.


**★ 8816 ★ University of California, San Francisco**
**Hormone Research Institute**
513 Parnassus Ave.
PO Box 0534
San Francisco, CA 94143-0534
**Phone:** (415)476-1683   **Fax:** (415)476-1660
**Email:** jbluest@diabetes.ucsf.edu
Dr. Jeffrey Bluestone, Dir.
**Activities/Fields:** Hormone receptors, gene regulation in endocrine tissue, mechanisms of regulated secretion, glutamic acid decarboxylase in juvenile diabetes, the immunology of Type 1 diabetes, and the development of the endocrine pancreas.


**★ 8817 ★ University of Chicago**
**Diabetes Research and Training Center**
MC 1027
5841 S Maryland Ave.
Chicago, IL 60637
**Phone:** (773)702-6217   **Fax:** (773)834-0486
Dr. Donald Steiner, Dir.
**Activities/Fields:** Etiology and pathogenesis of diabetes mellitus and improvement of care of diabetic patients, including studies on isolation and properties of proinsulin, proglucagon and amylin, isolation and characterization of beta cell plasma membranes, regulation of insulin biosynthesis and secretion, hyperlipidemia in diabetes, tissue culture of islet cells and cell tumors, mechanism of enzymatic conversion of proinsulin to insulin, insulin binding, degradation and action, particularly involving glucose transporters in various cells, serum proinsulin and C-peptide levels in normal and diabetic subjects, including studies of insulin of secretion and metabolism. Encourages new endeavors and provides a framework and stimulus for additional collaborative research programs among investigators of different disciplines and backgrounds. Conducts studies into the genetic basis of diabetes and alterations in gene expression in diabetes. Works to define the role of ion channels in insulin secretion.


**★ 8818 ★ University of Iowa**
**Diabetes and Endocrinology Research Center**
3E19 VA Hospital
Iowa City, IA 52240
**Phone:** (319)339-7147   **Fax:** (319)339-7025
**Email:** rbar@icva.gov
**Website:** http://uiderc.icva.gov
Robert S. Bar, MD, Dir.
**Activities/Fields:** Mechanism of action of insulin and related hormones at the cellular level and eucaryotic gene regulation.


**★ 8819 ★ University of Iowa**
**Epidemiology of Diabetes Intervention and Complications Study**
316 GH
Iowa City, IA 52242
**Phone:** (319)356-4878   **Fax:** (319)356-3564
**Email:** william-sivitz@uiowa.edu
**Website:** http://www.uiowa.edu/~vpr/research/organize/edics.htm
Wm. Sivitz, MD, Co-Dir.
**Activities/Fields:** Progression of diabetes and the effect of treatment on patients. **Frmly:** Diabetes Research and Programs.


**★ 8820 ★ University of Kentucky**
**Metabolic Research Group (MRG)**
919 S Limestone St.
Lexington, KY 40536-9841
**Phone:** (859)257-4058   **Fax:** (859)257-8410
**Email:** rlposk0@pop.uky.edu
**Website:** http://www.mc.uky.edu/nutritionresearch/Default.htm
James W. Anderson, MD, Dir.
**Activities/Fields:** Metabolic diseases, including diabetes, obesity, atherosclerosis, and high cholesterol.


**★ 8821 ★ University of Manitoba**
**Diabetes Research and Treatment Centre (DRTC)**
Health Sciences Centre, Rm. GB409
820 Sherbrook St.
Room GB409
Winnipeg, MB, Canada R3A 1R9
**Phone:** (204)787-3381   **Fax:** (204)787-3279
**Email:** aangel@hsc.mb.ca
**Website:** http://www.umanitoba.ca/outreach/drtc/
Dr. Aubie Angel, Pres.
**Activities/Fields:** Diabetes, its treatment and awareness; health promotion, disease prevention.


**★ 8822 ★ University of Maryland**
**Obesity and Diabetes Research Center**
Sch. of Medicine
10 S Pine St., Rm. 6-00MSTF
Baltimore, MD 21201
**Phone:** (410)706-3168   **Fax:** (410)706-7540
**Email:** bchansen@aol.com
Dr. Barbara Hansen, Dir.
**Activities/Fields:** Basic and applied research focusing on the mechanisms underlying the metabolic and endocrine disorders associated with obesity, diabetes and aging. Also studies hypertriglyceridemia, low HDL-cholesterol, hypertension, nephropathy, neuropathy, retinopathy and therapeutic agents for treatment of diabetes.


**University of Massachusetts at Amherst**
**Center for Neuroendocrine Studies (CNS)**
*See:* Entry 14429


**★ 8823 ★ University of Massachusetts at Worcester**
**Diabetes-Endocrinology Research Center**
Medical School
373 Plantation St., Ste. 218
Worcester, MA 01605
**Phone:** (508)856-3800   **Fax:** (508)856-4093
**Email:** aldo.rossini@umassmed.edu
**Website:** http://www.umass.edu/cns/
Dr. Aldo A. Rossini, Dir.
**Activities/Fields:** Diabetes, including autoimmunity of diabetic rats (Biobreeding/Worcester variety), renin secretion of kidney, lipid metabolism, lipid and growth

factor receptors, neurotensin calcium metabolism and bone disease steroid action, and steroid receptors. **Pub:** *Annual Report.* • *Highlights.*

**★ 8824 ★ University of Miami**
**Diabetes Research Institute**
School of Medicine
PO Box 016960
Miami, FL 33136
**Phone:** (305)243-6913      **Fax:** (305)243-4404
**Email:** ricordi@miami.edu
**Website:** http://www.drinet.org
Camillo Ricordi, MD, Sci. Dir.

**Activities/Fields:** Etiology, pathogenesis, and treatment of diabetes mellitus, emphasizing the cure of diabetes through biological replacement strategies, particularly the study of the immunoregulatory defects that result in the destruction of the pancreatic beta cell as well as the transplantation of (allogeneic and/or xenogeneic) pancreatic islets cells in insulin-deficient diabetic animals and humans. Clinical investigations include new intervention studies to prevent progression of latent insulin-dependent diabetes to clinical diseases, and studies of new insulin analogues and evaluation of procedures to quantify high standards for care of patients with diabetes in community-based studies.

**★ 8825 ★ University of Michigan**
**Diabetes Research and Training Center**
1331 E Ann St.
Box 0580, Rm. 5111
Ann Arbor, MI 48109-0580
**Phone:** (734)936-5504      **Fax:** (734)936-9240
**Email:** wherman@umich.edu
William H. Herman, MD, Dir.

**Activities/Fields:** Diabetes, including studies on thematic foci of islet hormone secretion and action and complications of diabetes. **Pub:** *MDRTC Newsletter.*

**★ 8826 ★ University of Missouri—**
**Columbia**
**Cosmopolitan International Diabetes**
**Center**
Columbia, MO 65212
**Phone:** (573)882-3818      **Fax:** (573)884-4609
Dr. David W. Gardner, Interim Dir.

**Activities/Fields:** Hormonal control of lipolysis, glycosylated proteins, and the effect of diabetic control on vascular complications of diabetes.

**★ 8827 ★ University of Nebraska Medical**
**Center**
**Molecular Reproductive Endocrinology**
**Laboratory**
Department of Obstetrics & Gynecology
Olson Center for Women's Health
600 S 42nd St.
Omaha, NE 68198-4515
**Phone:** (402)559-6163
**Website:** http://www.unmc.edu/Olson/research/labmre.htm
Shyamal K. Roy, PhD, Dir.

**Activities/Fields:** How preantral follicular growth is regulated by the orchestrated actions of pituitary gonadotropins and intraovarian peptide growth factors.

**★ 8828 ★ University of Pennsylvania**
**Center for Molecular Studies in Digestive**
**and Liver Disease**
Clinical Research Bldg., Ste. 600
School of Medicine
Philadelphia, PA 19104-6140
**Phone:** (215)573-4264      **Fax:** (215)573-2024
**Email:** anil2@mail.med.upenn.edu
**Website:** http://www.uphs.upenn.edu/moleculr/
Dr. Anil K. Rustgi, Dir.

**Activities/Fields:** Digestive biology, pathobiology, and therapy, specifically the molecular controls of cellular growth and differentiation in digestive organs.

**★ 8829 ★ University of Pennsylvania**
**Diabetes Research Center**
501 Stemmler Hall
36th & Hamilton Walk
Philadelphia, PA 19104-6015
**Phone:** (215)898-4365      **Fax:** (215)898-2178
**Email:** Pharaoh@mail.med.upenn.edu
Mitchell Lazar, Contact

**Activities/Fields:** Diabetes. Conducts basic studies on both pancreatic islet cell function and insulin action; evaluates new methods to detect and measure early signs of diabetes affecting the nervous systems, the retina, the vascular system, the heart, and the kidney; performs controlled clinical trials of new diets, drugs, and insulin-administration techniques; defines the nature of genetic susceptibility to diabetes; studies factors that increase the risk of complications in diabetes; and reevaluates the long-term benefits of kidney and pancreas transplants in diabetics. The Center is organized in two components: Core Basic Research Facilities, which supply investigators with special equipment and support, and the Clinical Center for Diabetes Research and Education, which provides the opportunity to perform controlled studies on volunteer ambulatory diabetic patients.

**★ 8830 ★ University of Southern**
**California**
**Research Center for Alcoholic Liver and**
**Pancreatic Diseases**
MMR 4th Fl.
1333 San Pablo St.
Los Angeles, CA 90089-9141
**Phone:** (323)442-3121      **Fax:** (323)442-3126
**Email:** htsukamo@hsc.usc.edu
**Website:** http://www.usc.edu/schools/medicine/research/alcohol_center/
Hide Tsukamoto, PhD, Dir.

**Activities/Fields:** How alcohol and secondary risk factors cross-interact to determine an individual's predisposition toward liver and pancreatic diseases. **Pub:** *Newsletter.* • *Papers.*

**★ 8831 ★ University of Virginia**
**Nephrology Clinical Research Center**
**(NCRC)**
UVA Health System, No. 133
Charlottesville, VA 22908
**Phone:** (434)924-5820      **Fax:** (434)924-1979
**Email:** lbr@virginia.edu
**Website:** http://www.med.virginia.edu/internal/nephrology/ncrc.html
Lori Ratliff, Admin. Dir.

**Activities/Fields:** Kidney disease and related problems, like hypertension and diabetes; mild to severe renal (kidney) insufficiency; end stage renal disease and related problems, like anemia and hyperparathyroidism; and polycystic kidney disease. **Pub:** *Newsletter.*

**★ 8832 ★ University of Washington**
**Diabetes Endocrinology Research Center**
DVA Puget Sound Health Care System
1660 S Columbian Way
PO 358285
Seattle, WA 98108
**Phone:** (206)764-2688      **Fax:** (206)764-2693
**Email:** jpp@u.washington.edu
**Website:** http://depts.washington.edu/diabetes/
Jerry P. Palmer, MD, Dir.

**Activities/Fields:** Diabetes Mellitus and its complications. Provides biomedical research facilities and services that are not readily available to individual investigators, including light and electron microscopy, recruitment of patient volunteers, radioimmunoassays, skin fibroblast and other cultures. Supports investigators in the field through a pilot and feasability program.

**★ 8833 ★ University of Wisconsin—**
**Madison**
**Radioimmunoassay Laboratory**
Veterinary Medicine
2015 Linden Dr. W, Rm. 4426
Madison, WI 53706-1102
**Phone:** (608)263-4908      **Fax:** (608)263-6748
**Email:** armstroj@svm.vetmed.wisc.edu
**Website:** http://www.vetmed.wisc.edu/research/radioimmunoassay
Prof. Mark S. Brownfield, Dir.

**Activities/Fields:** Performs peptide iodinations and radioimmunoassay tests of endocrinologic samples, including antiserum development and immunocytochemistry, with the potential for development of peptide and protein hormone antisera and purification and labeling of antisera.

**Vanderbilt University**
**Clinical Nutrition Research Unit**
See: Entry 16528

**★ 8834 ★ Vanderbilt University**
**Diabetes Research and Training Center**
707 Light Hall
Vanderbilt University Medical Center
Nashville, TN 37232-0615
**Phone:** (615)322-7004      **Fax:** (615)322-7236
**Email:** daryl.granner@mcmail.vanderbilt.edu
**Website:** http://www.vanderbilt.edu/vumc/centers/drtc
Dr. Daryl K. Granner, Contact

**Activities/Fields:** Diabetes and diabetes treatment.

**Vanderbilt University**
**Energy Balance Laboratory**
See: Entry 19211

**★ 8835 ★ Washington University in St.**
**Louis**
**Diabetes Research and Training Center**
660 S Euclid Ave., CB 8127
Saint Louis, MO 63110
**Phone:** (314)362-8680      **Fax:** (314)747-2692
**Email:** apermutt@im.wustl.edu
**Website:** http://www.medicine.wustl.edu/drtc
M. Alan Permutt, Dir.

**Activities/Fields:** Diabetes research, including the causes of diabetes, insulin action, growth factors, and diabetic complications. Promotes biomedical and psychosocial studies of diabetes mellitus by operating core facilities to support established investigators. Core facilities include the Clinical Research Facility, where a patient registry of 500 diabetic patients undergoes clinical evaluation and is available for clinical studies; Radioimmunoassay Facility, which provides assays of insulin and conducts hormone studies; Mass Spectrometry Facility, supporting analytic and metabolic studies requiring mass spectrometry techniques; Animal and Transgenic Core Facility; Morphology Facility; Training and Translation Facility with an Education Center specialized in training professionals for diabetic patient care; Molecular Biology Facility; and Human Pancreatic Islet Facility, which provides human islets for NIH-funded projects.

**★ 8836 ★ Whittier Institute for Diabetes**
9894 Genesee Ave., Ste. 316
La Jolla, CA 92037
**Phone:** (858)450-1280      **Fax:** (858)626-5680
**Email:** hodginsr@whittier.org
**Website:** http://www.whittier.org
John Engle, Pres. /CEO

**Activities/Fields:** Diabetes and endocrinology research, including islet transplantation, CNS and pituitary function, reproductive biology, growth factor biochemistry, and angiogenesis.

**★ 8837 ★ Yeshiva University**
**Diabetes Research and Training Center**
Albert Einstein College of Medicine
1300 Morris Park Ave.
Bronx, NY 10461
**Phone:** (718)430-2908      **Fax:** (718)430-8557
**Email:** diabetes@aecom.yu.edu
**Website:** http://medicine.aecom.yu.edu/diabetes/
DC.htm
Norman Fleischer, MD, Dir.
**Activities/Fields:** Development and assessment of interventions focused on both primary and secondary prevention of complications of diabetes. Evaluation of innovative health professional educational materials and research instruments. **Pub:** *Books, papers, education materials.*

## State & Regional Organizations

### Diabetes

*State affiliates of the American Diabetes Association are listed below. The national service center is located at 1701 N Beauregard St., Alexandria, VA 22311, (800)DIABETES, http://www.diabetes.org/.*

#### Alabama

**★ 8838 ★ American Diabetes Association**
200 Office Park Dr., Ste. 303
Birmingham, AL 35223
**Phone:** (205)870-5172      **Free:** 800-824-7891
**Website:** http://www.diabetes.org/adaal

#### Alaska

**★ 8839 ★ American Diabetes Association**
**Alaska Area**
801 W Fireweed, Ste. 103
Anchorage, AK 99503
**Phone:** (907)272-1424      **Free:** 800-DIABETES
**Fax:** (907)272-1428
**Website:** http://www.diabetes.org/adaak

#### Arizona

**★ 8840 ★ American Diabetes Association**
**Arizona Affiliate**
8125 N 23rd Ave., Ste. 222
Phoenix, AZ 85021-4961
**Phone:** (602)861-4731      **Free:** 800-342-2383
**Fax:** (602)995-1344
**Website:** http://www.diabetes.org/adaaz

#### Arkansas

**★ 8841 ★ American Diabetes Association**
**Arkansas Affiliate**
212 Natural Resources Dr.
Little Rock, AR 72205
**Phone:** (501)221-7444      **Free:** 888-DIABETES
**Fax:** (501)221-3138
**Email:** nbaxter@diabetes.org
**Website:** http://www.diabetes.org/adaar/

#### Connecticut

**★ 8842 ★ American Diabetes Association**
**Connecticut Information Center**
300 Research Pkwy.
Meriden, CT 06450
**Phone:** (203)639-0385      **Free:** 888-DIABETES
**Website:** http://www.diabetes.org/adact

#### Delaware

**★ 8843 ★ American Diabetes Association**
**Delaware Information Center**
Community Services Bldg.
100 W 10th St., Ste. 1002
Wilmington, DE 19801
**Phone:** (302)656-0030      **Fax:** (302)656-7331
**Website:** http://www.diabetes.org/main/application/
commercewf

#### District of Columbia

**★ 8844 ★ American Diabetes Association**
**- Washington, D.C. Metro Area**
1211 Connecticut Ave. NW, Ste. 204
Washington, DC 20036
**Phone:** (202)331-8303      **Free:** 800—DIABETES
**Fax:** (202)331-1402
**Website:** http://www.diabetes.org/adadc

#### Florida

**★ 8845 ★ American Diabetes Association**
**Florida Information Center**
1101 N Lake Destiny Rd., Ste. 415
Maitland, FL 32751
**Phone:** (407)660-1926      **Free:** 800-741-5698
**Fax:** (407)660-1080
**Website:** http://www.diabetes.org/adafl

#### Georgia

**★ 8846 ★ American Diabetes Association**
1 Corporate Sq., Ste. 120
Atlanta, GA 30329
**Phone:** (404)320-7100      **Free:** 800-342-2383
**Fax:** (404)320-0025
**Website:** http://www.diabetes.org/adaga

**★ 8847 ★ American Diabetes Association**
**Greater Augusta, Georgia/Aiken, South**
**Carolina Area**
326 Greene St.
Augusta, GA 30901
**Phone:** (706)828-0420      **Free:** 800-433-7061
**Website:** http://www.diabetes.org

#### Idaho

**★ 8848 ★ American Diabetes Association**
1111 S Orchard, Ste. 234
Boise, ID 83705
**Phone:** (208)342-2774      **Free:** 888-DIABETES
**Fax:** (208)345-9334
**Email:** tsutton@diabetes.org
**Website:** http://www.diabetes.org/adaid
**Remarks:** Serving Southern Idaho.

#### Illinois

**★ 8849 ★ American Diabetes Association**
**Greater Illinois Are**
2580 Federal Dr., Ste. 403
Decatur, IL 62526
**Phone:** (217)875-9011      **Free:** 800-445-1667
**Fax:** (217)875-6849
**Website:** http://www.diabetes.org/adadil

#### Indiana

**★ 8850 ★ American Diabetes Association**
**Indiana Information Center**
7363 E 21st St.
Indianapolis, IN 46219
**Phone:** (317)352-9226      **Free:** 800-228-2897
**Fax:** (317)357-4288
**Website:** http://www.diabetes.org/adain

#### Iowa

**★ 8851 ★ American Diabetes Association**
**Mid-American Region**
6200 Aurora Ave., Ste. 504W
Des Moines, IA 50322
**Phone:** (515)276-2237      **Free:** 888-DIABETES
**Fax:** (515)276-2662
**Website:** http://www.diabetes.org
**Remarks:** Serving Iowa, Nebraska, and South Dakota.

#### Kansas

**★ 8852 ★ American Diabetes Association**
**Kansas Area Office**
837 S Hillside St.
Wichita, KS 67211-3005
**Phone:** (316)684-6091      **Free:** 800-676-4065
**Website:** http://www.diabetes.org/adaks

#### Kentucky

**★ 8853 ★ American Diabetes Association**
**Kentucky Information Center**
Watterson City Office Park
1941 Bishop Ln., Ste. 110
Louisville, KY 40218
**Phone:** (502)452-6072      **Free:** 888-DIABETES
**Fax:** (502)452-2705
**Website:** http://www.diabetes.org/adaky

#### Maine

**★ 8854 ★ American Diabetes Association**
**Maine Affiliate, Inc.**
10 Bangor St., Ste. F
PO Box 2208
Augusta, ME 04330
**Phone:** (207)623-2232      **Free:** 800-870-8000
**Website:** http://www.diabetes.org/adame

#### Michigan

**★ 8855 ★ American Diabetes Association**
**Michigan Affiliate**
30600 Telegraph Rd., Ste. 2255
Bingham Farms, MI 48025
**Phone:** (810)433-3830      **Free:** 800-525-9292
**Website:** http://www.diabetes.org/adami

#### Minnesota

**★ 8856 ★ American Diabetes Association**
**Minnesota Area, Great Lakes Region**
715 Florida Ave. S, Ste. 307
Minneapolis, MN 55426
**Phone:** (763)593-5333      **Free:** 800-342-2383
**Fax:** (763)593-1520
**Website:** http://www.diabetes.org/adamn

#### Missouri

**★ 8857 ★ American Diabetes Association**
**Regional Office**
1316 Parkade Blvd.
Columbia, MO 65203
**Phone:** (573)443-8611      **Free:** 800-404-2873
**Fax:** (314)875-2152
**Email:** pbixler@diabetes.org
**Website:** http://www.diabetes.org/missouri

#### Nevada

**★ 8858 ★ American Diabetes Association**
**Nevada Information Center**
2785 E Desert Inn Rd., Ste. 140
Las Vegas, NV 89121
**Phone:** (702)369-9995      **Free:** 800-800-4232
**Website:** http://www.diabetes.org/adanv

## New Hampshire

**★ 8859 ★ American Diabetes Association**
**New Hampshire Information Center**
249 Canal St.
Manchester, NH 03101
**Phone:** (603)627-9579     **Free:** 888-DIA-BETES
**Website:** http://www.diabetes.org/adanh

## New Jersey

**★ 8860 ★ American Diabetes Association**
**New Jersey Office**
19 Schoolhouse Rd.
Somerset, NJ 08873-1235
**Phone:** (732)469-7979     **Free:** 888-DIABETES
**Website:** http://www.diabetes.org/adanj

## New Mexico

**★ 8861 ★ American Diabetes Association**
**New Mexico Area Office**
525 San Pedro NE, Ste. 101
Albuquerque, NM 87108
**Phone:** (505)266-5716     **Free:** 800-DIABETES
**Fax:** (505)268-4533
**Website:** http://www.diabetes.org/adanm

## North Carolina

**★ 8862 ★ American Diabetes Association**
**North Carolina Information Center**
2 Hanover Sq.
434 Fayetteville St. Mall, Ste. 1600
Raleigh, NC 27601
**Phone:** (919)743-5400     **Free:** 800-682-9692
**Fax:** (919)743-5430
**Website:** http://www.diabetes.org

## North Dakota

**★ 8863 ★ American Diabetes Association**
**North Dakota/Northern Minnesota**
315 N 4th St.
Grand Forks, ND 58203
**Phone:** (701)746-4427     **Free:** 800-666-6709
**Fax:** (701)746-9337
**Email:** ghand@diabetes.org
**Website:** http://www.diabetes.org

## Ohio

**★ 8864 ★ American Diabetes Association**
**Central Ohio Area**
937 N High St.
Worthington, OH 43085
**Phone:** (614)436-1917     **Free:** 888-DIABETES
**Fax:** (614)436-6351
**Website:** http://www.diabetes.org/

## Oregon

**★ 8865 ★ American Diabetes Association**
**Oregon Information Center**
380 SE Spokane St., Ste. 110
Portland, OR 97202
**Phone:** (503)736-2770     **Free:** 888-342-2383
**Fax:** (503)736-2774
**Website:** http://www.diabetes.org/adaor

## South Carolina

**★ 8866 ★ American Diabetes**
**Association—South Carolina**
2711 Middleburg Dr., Ste. 205
Kittrell Ctr.
Columbia, SC 29204
**Phone:** (803)799-4246     **Free:** 800-DIABETES
**Fax:** (803)799-5792
**Email:** lbundrick@diabetes.org
**Website:** http://www.diabetes.org/adasc

## Tennessee

**★ 8867 ★ American Diabetes Association**
**Middle Tennessee Area**
4205 Hillsboro Rd., Ste. 200
Nashville, TN 37215-3339
**Phone:** (615)298-3066     **Free:** 800-DIABETES
**Fax:** (615)292-5357
**Website:** http://www.diabetes.org/adatn

## Texas

**★ 8868 ★ American Diabetes Association**
**Texas Information Center**
**South Central Region**
4425 W Airport Freeway, Ste. 130
Irving, TX 75062
**Phone:** (972)255-6900     **Fax:** (972)255-7900

## Utah

**★ 8869 ★ American Diabetes Association**
**Serving Utah**
250 E 300 S, Ste. 110
Salt Lake City, UT 84111
**Phone:** (801)363-3024     **Free:** 888-DIABETES
**Email:** gburns@diabetes.org
**Website:** http://www.diabetes.org/adaut

## Vermont

**★ 8870 ★ American Diabetes Association**
**Vermont Information Center**
77 Hegeman Dr.
Colchester, VT 05446
**Phone:** (802)654-7716     **Free:** 888-DIABETES
**Fax:** (802)654-7657
**Email:** tdanto@diabetes.org
**Website:** http://www.diabetes.org
**Remarks:** Serving Vermont.

## Virginia

**★ 8871 ★ American Diabetes Association**
**National Office**
1701 N Beauregard St.
Alexandria, VA 22311
**Phone:** (703)549-1500     **Free:** 800-232-3472
**Fax:** (703)836-7439
**Email:** customerservice@diabetes.org
**Website:** http://www.diabetes.org

## West Virginia

**★ 8872 ★ American Diabetes Association**
**West Virginia Information Center**
1221-A Ohio Ave.
Dunbar, WV 25064
**Phone:** (304)768-2596     **Free:** 800-DIABETES
**Website:** http://www.diabetes.org/adawv

## Wisconsin

**★ 8873 ★ American Diabetes Association**
**Wisconsin Information Center**
2323 N Mayfair Rd., No. 502
Wauwatosa, WI 53226
**Phone:** (414)778-5500     **Free:** 888-DIABETES
**Website:** http://www.diabetes.org/adawi

## Wyoming

**★ 8874 ★ American Diabetes Association**
**Wyoming Area**
330 S Center St.
Casper, WY 82601
**Phone:** (307)232-0322     **Free:** (866)877-4232
**Fax:** (307)232-0321
**Email:** nvreeland@diabetes.org
**Website:** http://www.diabetes.org

# Chapter 24

# Environmental Health & Medicine

## Federal Government Agencies

### ★ 8875 ★ Environmental Protection Agency (EPA)
1200 Pennsylvania Ave., NW
Washington, DC 20460-0001
**Free:** 888-372-8255
**Website:** http://www.epa.gov/
Christine Todd Whitman, Dir of Admin
**Desc:** The EPA functions to protect human health and to safeguard the natural environment in cooperation with state and local governments. Its mission is to control and abate pollution in the areas of air, water, solid waste, pesticides, radiation, and toxic substances.

### ★ 8876 ★ U.S. Department of Energy
Office of the Environment, Safety, and Health
1000 Independence Ave. SW
Washington, DC 20585
**Phone:** (202)586-5000          **Fax:** (202)586-0956
**Website:** http://www.doe.gov/
Steven C. Cary, Acting Assistant Secretary
**Desc:** Provides independent oversight of departmental execution of environmental, occupational safety and health, and nuclear/nonnuclear safety and security laws, regulations, and policies; ensures that departmental programs are in compliance with environmental, health, and nuclear/nonnuclear safety protection plans, regulations, and procedures; exercises independent review and approval of environmental impact statements prepared within the Department; and carries out the legal functions of the nuclear safety civil penalty and criminal referral activities.

### ★ 8877 ★ U.S. Department of Health and Human Services
Agency for Toxic Substances and Disease Registry
1600 Clifton Rd. NE
Atlanta, GA 30333
**Phone:** (404)639-0700
**Website:** http://www.atsdr.cdc.gov
Jeffrey Koplan, Administrator
**Desc:** The Agency's mission is to prevent exposure and adverse health effects and diminished quality of life associated with exposure to hazardous substances from waste sites, unplanned releases, and other sources of pollution present in the environment.

### ★ 8878 ★ U.S. Department of Health and Human Services
Centers for Disease Control and Prevention
National Center for Environmental Health
1600 Clifton Rd. NE
Atlanta, GA 30333
**Phone:** (404)639-3311          **Fax:** (404)488-7015
**Website:** http://www.cdc.gov/nceh/default.htm
Richard J. Jackson, MD, Director
**Desc:** The Center administers national programs that promote a healthy environment and prevent premature death and avoidable illness and disability caused by non-infectious, non-occupational, environmental and related factors.

### ★ 8879 ★ U.S. Department of Health and Human Services
National Institutes of Health (NIH)
National Institute of Environmental Health Sciences (NIEHS)
PO Box 12233
Research Triangle Park, NC 27709
**Phone:** (919)541-3211
**Website:** http://www.niehs.nih.gov/
**Desc:** NIEHS seeks to reduce the burden of human illness and dysfunction by understanding the elements of environmental exposures, human susceptibility, and time and how these elements interrelate. The mission is achieved through multidisciplinary biomedical research programs, prevention and intervention efforts, and communication strategies that encompass training, education, technology transfer, and community outreach.

## Foundations & Other Funding Organizations

### Other Funding Organizations

### ★ 8880 ★ Association of Occupational and Environmental Clinics (AOEC)
1010 Vermont Ave. NW, Ste. 513
Washington, DC 20005-1503
**Phone:** (202)347-4976          **Fax:** (202)347-4950
**Email:** aoec@aoec.org
**Website:** http://www.aoec.org
Katherine H. Kirkland, Exec. Dir.
**Desc:** Seeks to enhance the practice of occupational and environmental medicine. Shares information. Provides educational and research programs. **Awards:** Grant.

### ★ 8881 ★ Delta Society (DS)
289 Perimeter Rd. E
Renton, WA 98055-1329
**Phone:** (425)226-7357          **Fax:** (425)235-1076
**Email:** info@deltasociety.org
**Website:** http://www.deltasociety.org
Linda M. Hines, Pres. /CEO
**Desc:** Doctors, nurses, veterinarians, therapists, nursing home personnel, animal trainers and breeders, pet owners, academicians, and students of gerontology, psychology, therapeutic recreation, and other health fields. Assesses the role of animal companions in society and the effect of human-animal interaction on the mental and physical well-being of people. Seeks to establish an interdisciplinary approach to studying human-animal interactions, and to increase awareness of these interactions among health and social care professionals. Provides training to for persons seeking to establish and maintain programs that involve animals in animal-assisted activities/therapy. Operates National Service Dog Center serving people with disabilities in conjunction with the American Humane Association; and Pet Partners, a national registration for volunteers and animals involved in programs. Creating Service Dog Education System to train trainers of service dogs. Distributes information on research, programs, and legislation concerning human-animal relationships. Maintains collection of article reprints. **Awards:** Delta Society Beyond Limits Service and Therapy Animals Awards (annual); Harris Sweatt Travel Grant (annual).

### ★ 8882 ★ Society of Environmental Toxicology and Chemistry (SETAC)
1010 N 12th Ave.
Pensacola, FL 32501-3367
**Phone:** (850)469-1500          **Free:** 888-899-2088
**Fax:** (850)469-9778
**Email:** setac@setac.org
**Website:** http://www.setac.org
Rodney Parrish, Exec. Dir.
**Desc:** Professionals in the fields of chemistry, toxicology, biology, and ecology; atmospheric, health, and earth sciences; and environmental engineering. Promotes the use of multidisciplinary approaches to examine the impacts of chemicals and technology on the environment. Strives to balance the interests of academia, business, and government. Conducts workshops and symposia on research topics of interest to members. **Awards:** Exceptional Service Award (annual) to an individual who has performed long-term, exceptionally high quality service for SETAC; Founders Award (annual) for outstanding career with clearly identifiable contributions in the environmental sciences consistent with the goals of SETAC; Rachel Carson Award (periodic) for substantially increasing public awareness and understanding of critical environmental issues; SETAC-ABC Laboratories Environmental Education Award (annual) for individuals, organizations, or corporations making significant contributions to environmental education; SETAC - Procter & Gamble Pre-Doctoral Fellowship (annual) for pursuit of a Ph.D. degree in environmental toxicology, chemistry, or related disciplines; SETAC/Roy F. Weston Award (annual) for individuals under the age of 35, selection based on the significance of contribution of published papers to the field of environmental chemistry; SETAC/ Taylor Francis Award (annual) for pre- or postdoctoral scholars conducting research in an area related to environmental toxicology, chemistry or ecological risk assessment.

# Medical & Allied Health Schools

## Environmental Health

*The following institutions offer undergraduate and graduate environmental health programs accredited by the National Environmental Health Association, 720 S Colorado Blvd., South Tower, Ste. 970, Denver, CO 80246-1925, (303)756-9090, http://www.neha.org/.*

### California

**★ 8883 ★ California State University, Fresno**
**Health Science Department**
Box 38
Fresno, CA 93740-0038
**Phone:** (559)278-4747      **Fax:** (559)278-4179
**Email:** sdonohue@csufresno.edu
**Website:** http://www.csufresno.edu/schoolofhealth/school.html
Sandra Donohue, Contact

**★ 8884 ★ California State University, Northridge**
**College of Health and Human Development**
**Department of Environmental and Occupational Health**
1811 Nordhoff St.
Northridge, CA 91330-8285
**Phone:** (818)677-4719      **Fax:** (818)677-2045
**Email:** peter.bellin@csun1.csun.edu
**Website:** http://www.csun.edu/~vchsc00b/Program.html
Peter Bellin, PhD, Contact

### Colorado

**★ 8885 ★ Colorado State University**
**Department of Environmental Health**
Fort Collins, CO 80523-1676
**Phone:** (970)491-6074      **Fax:** (970)491-2940
**Email:** ehinfo@colostate.edu
**Website:** http://www.bernardino.colostate.edu/enhealth
John S. Reif, Contact

### Georgia

**★ 8886 ★ University of Georgia**
**College of Agricultural and Environmental Sciences**
**Environmental Health Science**
206 Environmental Health Bldg.
Athens, GA 30602-2102
**Phone:** (706)542-2454      **Fax:** (706)542-7472
**Email:** jwfisher@arches.uga.edu
**Website:** http://www.uga.edu/~ehs
Jeff Fisher, PhD, Contact

### Idaho

**★ 8887 ★ Boise State University**
**College of Health Sciences**
**Environmental Health Program**
1910 University Dr.
M/S 1835
Boise, ID 83725
**Phone:** (208)426-3795      **Fax:** (208)426-2199
**Email:** gshook@boisestate.edu
**Website:** http://hs.boisestate.edu/envhlth
Gary Shook, MD, Contact

### Illinois

**★ 8888 ★ Illinois State University**
**Environmental Health Program**
**Department of Health Sciences**
Campus Box 5220
Normal, IL 61790-5220
**Phone:** (309)438-7121      **Fax:** (309)438-2450
**Email:** tbierma@ilstu.edu
**Website:** http://www.cast.ilstu.edu/hsc/EnHealth/Eh-home.htm
Thomas J. Bierma, Contact

**★ 8889 ★ University of Illinois, Springfield**
**Department of Environmental Studies**
PO Box 19243
Springfield, IL 62794-9243
**Email:** lafollette.sharron@uis.edu
Sharron LaFollette, PhD, Contact

### Indiana

**★ 8890 ★ Indiana State University**
**Environmental Health Program**
**School of Health and Human Performance**
Health and Human Performance Bldg., Rm. B-83
Terre Haute, IN 47809
**Phone:** (812)237-3079      **Fax:** (812)237-4338
**Email:** hselieze@scifac.indstate.edu
**Website:** http://web.indstate.edu/hlthsfty/eh/eh.htm
Eliezer Bermudez, PhD, Contact

### Kentucky

**★ 8891 ★ Eastern Kentucky University**
**Department of Environmental Health Sciences**
521 Lancaster Ave.
Richmond, KY 40475-3102
**Phone:** (606)622-1939
**Email:** carolyn.harvey@eku.edu
**Website:** http://www.environmentalhealth.eku.edu
Carolyn H. Harvey, PhD, Contact

### Maryland

**★ 8892 ★ Salisbury State University**
**Environmental Health Program**
Salisbury, MD 21801
**Phone:** (410)543-6499      **Fax:** (410)548-3318
**Email:** eavenso@ssu.edu
**Website:** http://www.ssu.edu/schools/Henson/Dept.html
Elicia A. Venso, PhD, Contact

### Missouri

**★ 8893 ★ Missouri Southern University**
**Environmental Health Program**
3950 E Newman Rd.
Joplin, MO 64801-1595
**Phone:** (417)625-9765      **Fax:** (417)625-3169
**Email:** fletcher-m@mail.mssc.edu
**Website:** http://www.mssc.edu/biology/home.htm
Michael Fletcher, Contact

### New Jersey

**★ 8894 ★ Richard Stockton College of New Jersey**
**Public Health Program**
**Environmental Health Track**
PO Box 195
Pomona, NJ 08240-0195
**Phone:** (609)652-4395      **Fax:** (609)652-4858
**Email:** Bruce.DeLussa@Stockton.Edu
**Website:** http://loki.stockton.edu/~calamide/phealth.htm
Bruce DeLussa, Contact

### New Mexico

**★ 8895 ★ New Mexico State University**
**Department of Health Sciences**
**Environmental Health Program**
Las Cruces, NM 88005
**Phone:** (505)646-8194      **Fax:** (505)646-4343
**Email:** sarnold@nmsu.edu
Stephen D. Arnold, PhD, Contact

### North Carolina

**★ 8896 ★ East Carolina University**
**Department of Environmental Health Sciences, Safety, and Technology**
**School of Industry and Technology**
Bldg. 310
Greenville, NC 27858-4353
**Phone:** (252)328-4249      **Fax:** (919)328-0380
**Email:** spraud@mail.ecu.edu
**Website:** http://www.ecu.edu/ehlt
Daniel D. Sprau, PhD, Contact

### Ohio

**★ 8897 ★ Bowling Green University**
**College of Health and Human Services**
**Environmental Health Program**
214 Health Center
Bowling Green, OH 43403-0280
**Phone:** (419)372-7774      **Fax:** (419)372-2897
**Email:** Silverma@bgnet.bgsu.edu
**Website:** http://www.bgsu.edu/departments/envh/envh-hp.htm
Gary Silverman, Contact

**★ 8898 ★ Ohio University**
**Environmental Health Science Program**
**School of Health Sciences**
416 The Tower
Athens, OH 45701-2979
**Phone:** (740)593-1223      **Fax:** (740)593-0555
**Email:** morrone@ohiou.edu
**Website:** http://cscwww.cats.ohiou.edu/healthsciences/envrhlth.htm
Michele Morrone, PhD, Contact

**★ 8899 ★ Wright State University**
**Institute for Environmental Quality**
3640 Colonel Glenn Hwy.
Dayton, OH 45435
**Phone:** (937)775-2201      **Fax:** (937)775-4997
**Email:** allen.burton@wright.edu
**Website:** http://www.wright.edu/academics/ieq
G. Allen Burton, Jr., P, Contact

### Oregon

**★ 8900 ★ Oregon State University**
**College of Health and Human Performance**
**Department of Public Health**
**Environmental Health and Safety Program**
310 Waldo Hall
Corvallis, OR 97331-6406
**Phone:** (541)737-3833      **Fax:** (541)737-4001
**Email:** cathy.neuman@orst.edu
**Website:** http://www.orst.edu/dept/HHP/PH/ph_undergrad.html
Catherine Neumann, PhD, Contact

### Pennsylvania

**★ 8901 ★ Indiana University of Pennsylvania**
**Department of Biology**
**Environmental Health Program**
315 Weyandt Hall
Indiana, PA 15705
**Phone:** (724)357-4898      **Fax:** (724)357-5700

**Email:** tsimmons@grove.iup.edu
Tom Simmons, PhD, Contact

### Tennessee

**★ 8902 ★ East Tennessee State University**
**Environmental Health Department**
PO Box 70682
Johnson City, TN 37614-0682
**Phone:** (423)439-7633          **Fax:** (423)439-5238
**Email:** philsche@etsu.edu
**Website:** http://www.etsu-TN.edu/cpah/environ.htm
Phil Scheuerman, PhD, Contact

### Washington

**★ 8903 ★ University of Washington**
**School of Public Health and Community Medicine**
**Environmental Health Department**
PO Box 357234
Seattle, WA 98195-7234
**Phone:** (206)543-4207          **Fax:** (206)616-2651
**Email:** ctreser@u.washington.edu
**Website:** http://depts.washington.edu/envhlth
Charles D. Treser, Contact

### Wisconsin

**★ 8904 ★ University of Wisconsin, Eau Claire**
**Environmental and Public Health**
**Division of Allied Health Professions**
**Environmental and Public Health Program**
School of Arts and Sciences
Eau Claire, WI 54702-4004
**Phone:** (715)836-2628          **Fax:** (715)836-3379
**Email:** nelsonr@uwec.edu
**Website:** http://www.uwec.edu/academic/ah/enph
Robert Nelson, PhD, Contact

## National & International Organizations

**★ 8905 ★ American Academy of Environmental Medicine (AAEM)**
7701 E Kellogg Dr. Ste. 625
Wichita, KS 67207-1705
**Phone:** (316)684-5500          **Fax:** (316)684-5709
**Email:** aaem@swbell.net
**Website:** http://www.aaem.com
Bobbie Hinshaw, Exec. Dir.

**Fnded:** 1965. **Mem:** 400. **Desc:** Physicians, and others interested in the clinical aspect of environmental medicine. Supports physicians and other professionals in serving the public through education about the interactions between humans and their environment. **Pub:** AAEM Directory, annual. Directory. Price: $50/copy for nonmembers. • Environmental Physician, quarterly. Newsletter. • Journal of Nutritional and Environmental Medicine, quarterly. Journal. **Frmly:** (1984) Society for Clinical Ecology.

**★ 8906 ★ American Academy of Sanitarians (AAS)**
c/o Gary Noonan
3815 Stonebriar Ct.
Duluth, GA 30097
**Fax:** (770)488-7335
Gary Noonan, contact

**Fnded:** 1966. **Mem:** 400. **Desc:** Legally registered sanitarians who possess at least a master's degree in public health, environmental health sciences, or environmental management. Purpose is to improve the environmental health status of humanity through certification of those sanitarians who have helped or who are helping to achieve this long-range goal. **Pub:**

Register of Professional Sanitarians, quinquennial. • Roster of Diplomates, annual. • Newsletter, semiannual. **Frmly:** American Intersociety Academy for Certification of Sanitarians.

**★ 8907 ★ American Institute of Biomedical Climatology (AIBC)**
1050 Eagle Rd.
Newtown, PA 18940-2818
**Phone:** (215)968-4483
**Email:** info@aibc.cc
**Website:** http://www.aibc.cc
George W. King, Sec. -Treas.

**Fnded:** 1958. **Mem:** 45. **Desc:** Meteorologists, biologists, epidemiologists, physicians, atmospheric physicists, engineers, architects, physiologists, climatologists, and other professionals interested in investigating the influence of the outdoor and indoor environment on the health and diseases of man. Areas of interest include: global warming, indoor and outdoor air pollution, biological effects of electromagnetic fields, power lines, cell phones and cell towers, and beneficial and detrimental effects of climate and weather on health. **Pub:** AIBC News Med-Clime Currents. Newsletter. Contains news concerning new publications and research studies. Available via member contributions. Price: Included in membership dues. • Membership List. Available to members only. • Also publishes scientific papers. **Frmly:** (1988) American Institute of Medical Climatology.

**Association of Occupational and Environmental Clinics (AOEC)**
See: Entry 16761

**★ 8908 ★ Association of Port Health Authorities**
Dutton House
46 Church St.
Runcorn WA7 1LL, United Kingdom
**Phone:** 44 8707 444505          **Fax:** 44 1928 581596
**Email:** apha@cieh.org.uk
**Website:** http://www.aoec.org

**Fnded:** 1899. **Mem:** 65. **Lang(s):** English. **Desc:** Local authorities, port health authorities in the United Kingdom, Ireland and the Channel Islands. Promoting the health and safety of seafarers, discussing issues on imported food, environmental health etc with central government, EU organisations etc. **Pub:** Lookout Newsletter, monthly. Newsletter. • Port Health Handbook. Handbook.

**★ 8909 ★ Center Perzent**
PO Box 27
Karakalpakstan
12 Nukus 742012, Uzbekistan
**Phone:** 998 61 2223417          **Fax:** 998 61 2222794
**Email:** perzent@online.ru
**Website:** http://www.perzent.org

**Fnded:** 1992. **Mem:** 1,000. **Lang(s):** English, Uzbekistani. **Desc:** Environment and health professionals. Seeks to research the impact of environmental degradation on reproductive health; encourages improvement of the status of women and children in the Aral Sea region of the former Soviet Union. Conducts environmental mitigation programs around the Aral Sea, which has suffered a collapse due to overuse as a source of water for agricultural irrigation; seeks to raise public awareness of public health issues arising from the demise of the Aral Sea. **Pub:** Perzent, monthly. Bulletin.

**★ 8910 ★ Chartered Institute of Environmental Health**
Chadwick Court
15 Hatfields
London SE1 8DJ, United Kingdom
**Phone:** 44 207 9286006          **Fax:** 44 207 8275866
**Email:** cieh@cieh.org.uk
**Website:** http://www.cieh.org.uk/

**Fnded:** 1883. **Mem:** 9,400. **Desc:** The majority of its members are employed by local government to enforce a wide range of legislation on issues such as food safety, pollution, housing standards, safety at work and to educate the public on matters of hygiene and safety. An increasing. number of its members are working in the commercial sector either for individual companies or as private environmental health consultants. Responsible for the training and professional development of over 8000 environmental health officers. Its primary objective is the promotion of environmental health and the dissemination of knowledge about environmental health issues. The CIEH represents the views of its members on environmental and public health issus and is independent of central and local government. **Pub:** Environmental Health, monthly. Journal. • Environmental Health News, weekly. • Food Forum, quarterly. • Health and Housing Insight, quarterly. • Pollution Control Bulletin, quarterly. Bulletin. **Frmly:** Institution of Environmental Health Offices.

**Clayton Fund**
See: Entry 5665

**★ 8911 ★ Environmental Health Accreditation Council (EHAC)**
c/o National Environmental Health Association
720 S Colorado Blvd., Ste. 970
S Tower
Denver, CO 80246
**Phone:** (303)756-9090          **Fax:** (303)691-9490
**Email:** becky.roland@juno.com
**Website:** http://www.nea.org
Gary Smith, PhD, Contact

**Fnded:** 1969. **Mem:** 28. **Desc:** Purposes are: to establish a system for accreditation of environmental health curricula and related procedures; to accredit and carry out other responsibilities as may be essential to the accreditation of academic programs leading to baccalaureate and graduate degrees in environmental health. Assumes responsibility for all functions, related records, and correspondence pertaining to accreditation of environmental health curricula. Renders advice and counsel to institutions in the development of curricula and the conduct of educational programs in the environmental health sciences. Acts as clearinghouse for reports and information pertaining to the environmental health accreditation process and activities. **Frmly:** National Accreditation Council for Environmental Health Curricula; (1993) National Accreditation Council for Environmental Health Science and Protection; (1998) National Environmental Health Science and Protection Accreditation Council.

**★ 8912 ★ European Institute of Environmental Medicine**
GR-162 32 Athens, Greece
**Phone:** 30 1 7628460          **Fax:** 30 1 7628675
**Email:** eiec@athens.com

**Lang(s):** English, Greek. **Desc:** Scientists and researchers. Promotes interdisciplinary study of environmental issues. Facilitates collaboration among environmental scientists and researchers worldwide; conducts research and educational programs.

**★ 8913 ★ Human Ecology Action League (HEAL)**
PO Box 29629
Atlanta, GA 30359
**Phone:** (404)248-1898          **Fax:** (404)248-0162
**Email:** HEALNatnl@aol.com
**Website:** http://members.aol.com/HEALNatnl
Muriel A. Dando, Pres.

**Fnded:** 1977. **Mem:** 10,000. **Nat'l Groups:** 1. **Local Groups:** 50. **Desc:** Individuals and organizations interested in the study of human ecology and multiple chemical sensitivities, specifically how human health may be affected by synthetic and natural substances in the environment. Objectives are: to collect and disseminate information on human ecology and ecological illness to persons suffering from such illness, and to government agencies, scientists, and health care professionals; to raise public awareness about potential dangers from substances in the environment. **Pub:** *Chemicals and Health.* Brochure. • *Electomagnetic Fields: Investigations into the Biological Activity of Low Frequency Electromagnetic Fields.* • *Fragrance and Health.* Book. *Price:* $12 members in the U.S.; $15 members in Canada; $20 members in other countries. • *Hospitality Directory,* periodic. Directory. Lists environmentally safe lodgings in the United States for allergic and chemical-sensitive travelers; arranged by state. *Price:* $10/copy for members; $20/copy for nonmembers. • *Human Ecologist,* quarterly. Journal. Includes association news, book and video reviews, environmental health tips for children, and pesticide update. *Price:* Included in membership dues; $26/year for low-income Individuals; $20 in Canada; $38 international. • *Multiple Chemical Sensitivities and the Americans with Disabilities Act: A Guide to Accommodation.* • *Perspectives on Pesticides.* • *Selected Bibliography: Chemicals and Health.* Bibliography. • *Selected Bibliography: Perspectives on Pesticides and Human Health 1983-1993.* Bibliography. • *Service List/Back Issue Guide,* periodic.

★ 8914 ★ **International Association of Medicine and Biology of Environment (IAMBE)**
**(Association Internationale de Medecine et de Biologie de l'Environnement — AIMBE)**
115, rue de la Pompe
F-75116 Paris, France
**Phone:** 33 1 45534504          **Fax:** 33 1 45534175
**Email:** aimbe.world@online.fe
**Fnded:** 1971. **Lang(s):** English, French, Spanish. **Desc:** Individuals, associations, and firms in 72 countries concerned with ecological medicine and biology. Purpose is to study the adaptation of mankind to the environment and to study and treat sicknesses resulting from this adaptation. Examines natural cycles and balances; promotes research in ecological medicine and biology and corollary sciences; collects and disseminates information concerning the protection of mankind and the environment. Facilitates contacts with persons who deal professionally with problems related to the protection of humans and their surroundings. Organizes symposia and congresses; conducts courses and seminars.

★ 8915 ★ **International Board of Environmental Medicine (IBEM)**
65 Wehrle Dr.
Buffalo, NY 14225
**Phone:** (716)837-1320          **Fax:** (716)833-2244
**Website:** http://www.medical-library.net
Dr. Kalpana Patel, Pres.
**Fnded:** 1988. **Mem:** 110. **Desc:** An accrediting agency for physicians and osteopaths working in related environmental professions. Examines licensed practitioners, facilities, and relevant training programs. Offers programs to evaluate qualifications of healthcare professionals, their training programs, and those facilities offering special types of treatment. Plans and supervises accrediting examinations. **Pub:** *Register of the International Board of Environmental Medicine,* annual. Directory. Contains names of diplomates. *Price:* $25.

★ 8916 ★ **International Commission on Biological Effects of Noise (ICBEN)**
Department of Psychology
University of Sydney
Sydney, NSW 2006, Australia
**Phone:** 61 2 93512859          **Fax:** 61 2 93512603
**Email:** soamesj@psychvax.psych.su.oz.au
**Website:** http://www.icben.org
**Fnded:** 1973. **Desc:** Encourages international cooperation in the study of the biological effects of noise; promotes communication among research scientists, governmental agencies, industrial workers and managers, and other parties and entities concerned with noise effects.

**International Contact Dermatitis Research Group (ICDRG)**
*See:* Entry 6825

★ 8917 ★ **International Programme on Chemical Safety (IPCS)**
**(Programme International sur la Securite des Substances Chimiques — PISSC)**
c/o World Health Organization
Ave. Appia
CH-1211 Geneva 27, Switzerland
**Phone:** 41 22 7913590          **Fax:** 41 22 7914848
**Email:** lpcsmail@who.int
**Website:** http://www.med.nagoya-u.ac.jp/Environderm/icdrg.htm
**Fnded:** 1980. **Mem:** 33. **Lang(s):** English, French. **Desc:** States belonging to the World Health Organization, the International Labour Organization, and the United Nations Environment Programme. Evaluates the health risks posed to humans and the environment by exposure to chemicals. Proposes methods and guidelines for measuring chemical exposure and for assessing health risks. Encourages the use and improvement of methods for laboratory testing and epidemiological studies. Provides guidelines on safe levels of chemical exposure through daily intake of food additives and pesticide and veterinary drug residues. Disseminates information regarding diagnosis and treatment of chemical poisoning; promotes international cooperation in dealing with chemical emergencies. Seeks to enhance the sci entific basis for health risk assessment for determination of chemical hazards controls. Conducts training courses on subjects such as ecotoxicology, clinical toxicology, the detection of mutagenesis, and occupational hazards and human reproduction; coordinates international research programs; maintains expert advisory groups and offers advisory services for technical cooperation in regulation and control of chemicals. Organizes symposia and workshops on chemical safety. **Pub:** *Environmental Health Criteria Document,* 15/year. • *Health and Safety Guides,* 20/year. • *IPCS Newsletter,* 2-3/year. Newsletter. • *Poison Information Monographs,* periodic. • *Technical Document on Food Additives and on Pesticide Residues,* periodic.

★ 8918 ★ **Latin American Association of Environmental Mutagens, Carcinogens and Teratogens (ALAMCTA)**
**(Asociacion Latinoamericana de Mutagenesis, Carcinogenesis y Teratogenesis Ambiental)**
Depto de Patologia, Faculdade de Medicina, UNESP, 18
618-000 Botucatu, Brazil
**Phone:** 55 14 8212116
**Email:** lribeiro@fmb.unesp.br
**Website:** http://www.iaems.nl/alamcta.htm
**Fnded:** 1980. **Desc:** Fosters scientific cooperation among Latin American researchers; supports research projects.

★ 8919 ★ **National Association of Physicians for the Environment (NAPE)**
1643 Prince St.
Alexandria, VA 22314-2818
**Phone:** (301)571-9791          **Fax:** (301)530-8910
**Email:** nape@napenet.org
John T. Grupenhoff, PhD, Exec. VP
**Fnded:** 1993. **Mem:** 34. **Desc:** Physicians, medical and environmental organizations, and coporations. Promotes improved understanding of the impacts of environmental pollutants on the organs, systems, and disease processes of the human body. Strives to enlist physicians in the campaign to protect biological diversity; encourages institution of more stringent pollution control programs. Works to involve the medical professions in pollution control. Conducts educational programs for physicians. **Pub:** *NAPE Fact Sheet.* Brochure. • Annual Report. • Newsletter, periodic.

★ 8920 ★ **National Center for Environmental Health Strategies (NCEHS)**
c/o Mary Lamielle, Dir.
1100 Rural Ave.
Voorhees, NJ 08043
**Phone:** (856)429-5358
**Email:** ncehs@ncehs.org
**Website:** http://www.ncehs.org/
Mary Lamielle, Dir. & Pres.
**Fnded:** 1986. **Mem:** 2,000. **Desc:** Persons with environmental illnesses, including those with chemical sensitivity disorders; medical, legal, and scientific professionals; government agencies; environmentalists; interested others. Promotes public awareness of health problems caused by chemical and environmental pollutants, focusing on chemical sensitivity disorders. Testifies before government agencies on behalf of persons with such health problems. Encourages the development and implementation of programs and policies aimed at assisting victims of pollutants and preventing future public health problems. Conducts educational programs and research. Gathers information and compiles statistics on indoor and outdoor pollutants, less-toxic products, pesticides, natural foods, and environmental disabilities, including alternative employment, workplace accommodations, social security disability and workmen's compensation, and housing. Maintains speakers' bureau. Provides advocacy and technical, referral, and children's services. Acts as a clearinghouse. **Pub:** *Chemical Sensitivity: A Report to the New Jersey Department of Health.* • *The Delicate Balance,* quarterly. Newsletter. Covers issues related to indoor contaminants, outdoor toxins, legislative and policy updates, research summaries, information on consumer products. *Price:* Included in membership dues; $15/year for nonmembers. • Also publishes reports, bibliographies, information packets, and books. **Frmly:** (1989) Environmental Health Association of New Jersey.

★ 8921 ★ **National Conference of Local Environmental Health Administrators (NCLEHA)**
c/o University of Washington
Department of Environmental Health
PO Box 357234
Seattle, WA 98195-7234
**Phone:** (206)543-4207          **Fax:** (206)616-2651
**Email:** ctresen@u.washington.edu
**Website:** http://depts.washington.edu/clehaweb/
Elwin Coll, Sec.
**Fnded:** 1939. **Mem:** 220. **Desc:** Professional environmental health personnel engaged in or officially concerned with municipal (city, county, or district) environmental health administration or teaching of environmental health. Promotes improvement and greater use of science and practice of environmental health in community life. **Pub:** Newsletter, quarterly. **Frmly:** (1969) Conference of Municipal Public Health Engineers; (1981) Conference of Local Environmental Health Administrators.

★ 8922 ★ **National Environmental Health Association (NEHA)**
720 S Colorado Blvd., Ste. 970, S Tower
Denver, CO 80246-1925
**Phone:** (303)756-9090          **Fax:** (303)691-9490
**Email:** staff@neha.org
**Website:** http://www.neha.org
Nelson E. Fabian, Exec. Dir. & CEO
**Fnded:** 1937. **Mem:** 5,100. **Nat'l Groups:** 3. **Reg. Groups:** 10. **State Groups:** 50. **Local Groups:** 3. **Desc:** Represents all professionals in environmental health and protection, including Registered Sanitarians, Registered Environmental Health Specialists, Registered Environmental Technicians, Certified Environmental Health Technicians, Registered Hazardous Substances Professionals and Registered Hazardous Substances Specialists. NEHA's mission is to advance the environmental health and protection profession for the purpose of providing a healthful environment for all. Educational materials, publications, credentials and meetings are available to NEHA members and

non-member professionals who strive to improve the environment. **Pub:** *Food Environment News Digest*, 3/year. Magazine. Contains information relevant to food professionals. *Price:* $10 members; $17 non-members. • *Journal of Environmental Health*, 10/year. Journal. *Price:* $90. • *National Environmental Health Association–Membership Directory*, annual. Membership Directory. **Frmly:** (1937) California Association of Sanitarians; (1970) National Association of Sanitarians.

**National Foundation for the Chemically Hypersensitive (NFCH)**
*See:* Entry 3224

**★ 8923 ★ NSF International**
PO BOX 130140
Ann Arbor, MI 48113-0140
**Phone:** (734)769-8010 **Free:** 877-867-3435
**Fax:** (734)769-0109
**Email:** info@nsf.org
**Website:** http://www.nsf.org
**Fnded:** 1944. **Desc:** Specializes in the areas of public health and environmental quality focusing on water quality, food safety, indoor air health and the environment. Develops standards, operates product certification and listings programs for products that meet or exceed public health safety standards. Maintains a worldwide network of auditors who conduct unannounced inspections of manufacturer facilities to ensure compliance and to protect the integrity of the NSF Certification Mark. Provides special research and testing services to industry, government, and foundations. **Pub:** *Bottled Water and Packaged Ice*, periodic. • *Class II Biohazard Cabinetry*, periodic. Book. • *Drinking Water Additives-Health Effects*, periodic. • *Drinking Water Treatment Units and Related Products, Components, and Materials*, periodic. • *Environmental Management Systems Standards and Guidance Documents*. • *Food Equipment and Related Products, Components, and Materials*, periodic. • *Plastics Piping Components and Related Materials*, periodic. • *Swimming Pools, Spas, and Hot Tubs*, periodic. • *Wastewater Treatment Units and Related Products and Components*, periodic. • Also publishes educational material. **Frmly:** (1993) National Sanitation Foundation.

**★ 8924 ★ Occupational and Environmental Diseases Association (OEDA)**
Mitre House
66 Abbey Rd.
Bush Hill Park
Enfield EN1 2QH, United Kingdom
**Phone:** 44 208 3608490
**Website:** http://www.oeda.demon.co.uk
**Fnded:** 1995. **Desc:** Asbestos is still responsible for much of our work. **Frmly:** (1978) Society for the Prevention of Asbestosis and Industrial Diseases.

**Occupational and Environmental Medical Association of Canada (OEMAC)**
*See:* Entry 16782

**★ 8925 ★ Population and Environment Society of China (PESC)**
PO Box A-1
No. 14 E Chang'An St.
Beijing 100741, People's Republic of China
**Phone:** 86 10 5121005 **Fax:** 86 10 5121005
**Email:** oemac@esc.net
**Website:** http://www.oemac.org
**Fnded:** 1992. **Lang(s):** Chinese, English. **Desc:** Promotes scientific research and increased public awareness of population control and environmental protection issues. Provides information and technical assistance to government bodies.

**★ 8926 ★ Reproductive Toxicology Center (RTC)**
7831 Woodmont Ave., Ste. 375
Bethesda, MD 20814-6054
**Phone:** (301)620-8690 **Fax:** (301)740-7498
**Email:** reprotox@reprotox.org
**Website:** http://reprotox.org
Anthony R. Scialli, MD, Dir.
**Fnded:** 1981. **Desc:** Works to gather and disseminate information on the effects of the chemical and physical environment on human fertility, pregnancy, and fetal development. Provides subscribers with information from the most relevant articles in the field.

**★ 8927 ★ Royal Environmental Health Institute of Scotland**
3 Manor Place
Edinburgh EH3 7DH, United Kingdom
**Phone:** 44 131 2256999 **Fax:** 44 131 2253993
**Email:** rehis@rehis.org.uk
**Website:** http://www.royal-environmental-health.org.uk
**Fnded:** 1983. **Mem:** 1,100. **Reg. Groups:** 2. **Desc:** Persons interested or engaged in any aspect of environmental health. **Pub:** *Environmental Health Scotland*, quarterly. Journal. Environmental Health Scotland.

**★ 8928 ★ Self-Help Association for the Electrically Sensitive (Selbsthilfeverein fuer Elektrosensible)**
Gesundheitshaus
Dachauerstr. 90
D-80335 Munich, Germany
**Phone:** 49 89 23337501
**Fnded:** 1989. **Mem:** 230. **Lang(s):** German. **Desc:** Individuals suffering from electrical hypersensitivity in Germany (electrical hypersensitivity is brought on from overexposure to electrical and magnetic fields emitted by appliances, particularly television sets, computers and mobile phones). Supports afflicted individuals and works to stop the spread of these conditions; works to insure recognition of these maladies by insurance companies and government agencies; promotes research into the causes and cure of electrical hypersensitivity.

**Society for Occupational and Environmental Health (SOEH)**
*See:* Entry 16784

**Society of Toxicologic Pathologists (STP)**
*See:* Entry 17152

**★ 8929 ★ Swedish Association for the Electrosensitive**
Box 6023
S-102 31 Stockholm, Sweden
**Fax:** 46 8 7128948
**Email:** info@feb.se
**Website:** http://www.feb.se
**Fnded:** 1987. **Mem:** 2,000. **Lang(s):** English, Swedish. **Desc:** Individuals suffering from electrical oversensitivity or electrical hypersensitivity in Sweden (electrical oversensitivity and hypersensitivity are brought on from overexposure to electrical and magnetic fields emitted by appliances, particularly television sets and video display terminals). Supports afflicted individuals and works to stop the spread of these conditions; works to insure recognition of these maladies by insurance companies and government agencies; promotes research into the causes and cure of electrical over- and hypersensitivity. Organizes grass roots groups. **Pub:** *Ljusglimten*, quarterly. Magazine. **Frmly:** (1998) Swedish Association for the Electrically and VDT Injured.

**★ 8930 ★ Victims of Asbestos and Industrial Disease (VAID)**
547 Victoria Ave.
Windsor, ON, Canada N9A 4N1
**Phone:** (519)973-4800 **Free:** 800-565-3185
**Fax:** (519)973-1906
**Fnded:** 1986. **Mem:** 500. **Lang(s):** English, French. **Desc:** Individuals with asbestos-related illness and other industrial diseases. Promotes improved quality of life for members. Makes available medical, social, and legal services to victims of asbestos-related diseases and other industrial illnesses.

**★ 8931 ★ Voluntary Protection Programs Participants' Association (VPPPA)**
7600 E Leesburg Pike, Ste. 440
Falls Church, VA 22043
**Phone:** (703)761-1146 **Fax:** (703)761-1148
**Email:** administration@vpppa.org
**Website:** http://www.vpppa.org
**Mem:** 450. **Desc:** Companies participating in voluntary protection programs and other workplace environmental protection, health, and safety programs. Promotes cooperation between labor, management, and government agencies to insure safe and environmentally sustainable workplaces. Works closely with federal environmental and safety agencies to develop and implement cooperative programs; provides information on environmental health and workplace safety to congressional committees considering legislation.

**★ 8932 ★ World Research Foundation (WRF)**
41 Bell Rock Plz.
Sedona, AZ 86351-8804
**Phone:** (520)284-3300 **Fax:** (520)284-3530
**Email:** info@wrf.org
**Website:** http://www.wrf.org
Steven A. Ross, Pres.
**Fnded:** 1980. **Desc:** Informs the public of the latest developments in health and environmental issues. Provides health care professionals and the public with information on health tools and technologies currently available outside the U.S. but which have been overlooked or are unavailable in the U.S. Acts as a depository of public information. **Pub:** *World Research News*, quarterly. Newsletter. • Journal, quarterly. Contains traditional and nontraditional international health news. *Price:* $20. • Proceedings, annual. • Reports.

# Research Centers

**★ 8933 ★ Arizona Health Services Department**
**Public Health Services**
**Epidemiology and Disease Control**
**Environmental Health Office**
3815 N Black Canyon Hwy.
Phoenix, AZ 85015
**Phone:** (602)230-5808 **Fax:** (602)230-5959
**Email:** lbland@hs.state.az.us
**Website:** http://www.hs.state.az.us
Lee A. Bland, Bur. Ch.
**Activities/Fields:** Environmental health.

**★ 8934 ★ Arizona Health Services Department**
**Public Health Services**
**State Laboratory Services**
**Environmental and Analytical Chemistry Office**
1520 W Adams
Phoenix, AZ 85007-2698
**Phone:** (602)542-6108 **Fax:** (602)364-0281
**Email:** padler@hs.state.az.us
Patricia Adler, Mgr.

**Activities/Fields:** Environmental and analytical chemistry.

**★ 8935 ★ Arizona Health Services Department**
**Public Health Services**
**State Laboratory Services**
**Office of Public Health Microbiology**
1520 W Adams
Phoenix, AZ 85007-2698
**Phone:** (602)542-6128          **Fax:** (602)542-0760
**Email:** wslanta@hs.state.az.us
William Slanta, Contact

**Activities/Fields:** Microbiology and environmental microbiology. **Frmly:** Environmental and Clinical Microbiology Office.

**★ 8936 ★ Colorado State University**
**Institute for Rural Environmental Health**
College of Veterinary Medicine & Biomedical Sciences
Fort Collins, CO 80523-1601
**Phone:** (970)491-7051          **Fax:** (970)491-2250
**Email:** cvmbsweb@colostate.edu
**Website:** http://www.cvmbs.colostate.edu/cvmbs/reh.html
Dr. John Reif, Dir.

**Activities/Fields:** Environmental toxicology, hazardous waste disposal, environmental epidemiology, health risk assessment, comparative human and animal health, and occupational health.

**★ 8937 ★ Columbia University**
**Center for Environmental Health in Northern Manhattan**
School of Public Health
701 W 168th St.
New York, NY 10032
**Phone:** (212)305-1996          **Fax:** (212)305-5328
**Email:** RPS1@columbia.edu
**Website:** http://www.niehs.nih.gov/centers/center/colctr.htm
Regina M. Santella, PhD, Dir.

**Activities/Fields:** Diseases due to, or exacerbated by, hazardous urban ecosystems, particularly neurotoxicology and neurodegenerative diseases; pulmonary disorders, especially asthma; and cancer. The neighborhoods of Northern Manhattan (Harlem and Washington Heights) typify this problem in that their outdoor and indoor environments provide excessive opportunity for exposure to air pollutants and allergens, lead, asbestos, and indoor residues of insecticides.

**★ 8938 ★ Duke University**
**Children's Environmental Health Initiative (CEHI)**
Box 90328
Nicholas School of the Environment & Earth Sciences
Durham, NC 27708-0328
**Phone:** (919)613-8088          **Free:** (866)264-7891
**Fax:** (919)684-8741
**Email:** cehi@env.duke.edu
**Website:** http://www.env.duke.edu/cehi/about/about.htm
Marie Lynn Miranda, PhD, Dir.

**Activities/Fields:** Environmental threats facing children today.

**★ 8939 ★ Environmental Health Service**
Rancho Los Amigos Med. Center
Med. Science Bldg., Rm. 51
7601 E Imperial Hwy.
Downey, CA 90242
**Phone:** (562)401-7561          **Fax:** (562)803-6883
**Email:** hgong@dhs.co.la.ca.us
Dr. Henry Gong, Jr., Contact

**Activities/Fields:** Drug studies of patients with asthma or COPD; air pollution, including effects of ozone on healthy subjects and patients with mild asthma; physiological and cellular responses to acute exposures to ozone, sulfur dioxide, nitrogen dioxide, carbon monoxide, and particulates; health effects of acid aerosols; pharmaceutical drugs; and development of field study programs, including in-home method for self-testing and lung function performance using research quality instrumentation and personal computers, and documentation of typical hourly and daily activity to assess potential effects of air pollution on those activities.

**★ 8940 ★ Environmental and Occupational Health Sciences Institute (EOHSI)**
170 Frelinghuysen Rd.
Piscataway, NJ 08854
**Phone:** (732)445-0200          **Fax:** (732)455-0131
**Email:** info@eohsi.rutgers.edu
**Website:** http://www.eohsi.rutgers.edu
Brian T. Buckley, PhD, Exec. Dir.

**Activities/Fields:** Toxicology, public education and risk communication, occupational health, exposure measurement and assessment, environmental health, and environmental policy. Studies the basic mechanisms by which environmental exposures harm the body, investigates methods for measuring and reducing exposure and improving health including clinical evaluation of individuals potentially affected adversely by environmental agents, and develops and analyzes ways to communicate information. **Pub:** EOHSI Newsletter.

**★ 8941 ★ Environmental and Occupational Health Sciences Institute**
**Ozone Research Center**
170 Frelinghuysen Rd.
PO Box 1179
Piscataway, NJ 08854
**Phone:** (732)445-0200
**Email:** panosg@fidelio.rutgers.edu
**Website:** http://www.ccl.rutgers.edu/orc/index.html
Dr. Panos G. Georgopoulos, Dir.

**Activities/Fields:** Causes, dynamics, and effects of photochemical air pollution (smog), focusing on issues and air quality problems affecting the Northeastern United States and in particular New Jersey, especially the enhancement of the scientific understanding of photochemical air pollution and associated human exposures and health effects and to provide the necessary scientific rationale for developing and implementing efficient air quality management strategies.

**★ 8942 ★ Environmental Protection Agency**
**Office of Research and Development**
**Office of Health and Environmental Assessment**
**Human Health Assessment Group**
Mail Code 6103
401 M St., SW
Washington, DC 20460
**Phone:** (202)260-5898          **Fax:** (202)260-9766
Robert Brenner, Dir.

**Activities/Fields:** Health assessments for carcinogens, genotoxic agents, and reproductive and developmental toxicants as encountered in environmental exposure scenarios. **Pub:** Proceedings.

**★ 8943 ★ Harvard University**
**Center for Health and the Global Environment**
Harvard Medical School
333 Longwood Ave., No. 640
Boston, MA 02115
**Phone:** (617)432-0493          **Fax:** (617)432-2595
**Email:** chge@hms.harvard.edu
**Website:** http://www.med.harvard.edu/chge
Eric Chivian, MD, Dir.

**Activities/Fields:** Human health consequences of global environmental change and the protection of the environment.

**★ 8944 ★ Harvard University**
**Kresge Center for Environmental Health**
665 Huntington Ave.
Boston, MA 02115
**Phone:** (617)432-1272          **Fax:** (617)277-2382
**Email:** brain@hsph.harvard.edu
**Website:** http://www.hsph.harvard.edu/kresge
Prof. Joseph D. Brain, Dir.

**Activities/Fields:** Environmental health, including interdisciplinary studies on effects and control of air pollutants, occupational health and medicine, environmental and respiratory physiology, radiation biology, toxicology and air sampling, exposure/dose assessment, water microbiology, and personnel protection. Serves as a focus for envi activities within the School. **Pub:** Annual Report.

**★ 8945 ★ Health Effects Institute (HEI)**
Charlestown Navy Yard
120 2nd Ave.
Boston, MA 02129-4533
**Phone:** (617)886-9330          **Fax:** (617)886-9335
**Email:** dgreenbaum@healtheffects.org
**Website:** http://www.healtheffects.org/index.html
Daniel S. Greenbaum, Pres.

**Activities/Fields:** Health effects of pollutants from motor vehicles and from other sources in the environment. **Pub:** Research reports. • Special reports. • Annual report. • Newsletter, quarterly.

**Health Research, Inc.**
*See:* Entry 17983

**★ 8946 ★ Johns Hopkins University**
**Center in Urban Environmental Health**
Department of Environmental Health Sciences
School of Hygiene & Public Health Sciences
615 N Wolfe St.
Baltimore, MD 21205
**Phone:** (410)955-3720          **Fax:** (410)955-9334
**Email:** jgroopma@jhsph.edu
**Website:** http://www.niehs.nih.gov/centers/center/jhpctr.htm
John Groopman, PhD, Dir.

**Activities/Fields:** Identification of environmental exposures and susceptibility factors that alone or together increase the risk of illness for people living in urban environments and to use these findings to develop prevention strategies to improve public health.

**Johns Hopkins University**
**Education and Research Center for Occupational Safety and Health**
*See:* Entry 16792

**★ 8947 ★ Massachusetts Institute of Technology**
**Environmental Health Sciences Center**
77 Massachusetts Ave., 16-743B
Cambridge, MA 02139
**Phone:** (617)258-7813          **Fax:** (617)253-8099
**Email:** lsamson@mit.edu
**Website:** http://www.niehs.nih.gov/centers/center/mitctr.htm
Leona D. Samson, PhD, Dir.

**Activities/Fields:** Causes and mechanisms of genetic changes that lead to human disease. The center's primary hypothesis is that a significant fraction of the point mutations and other genetic changes in the human body are caused by exposure to environmental chemicals or radiation.

**★ 8948 ★ McGill University**
**Centre for Indigenous Peoples' Nutrition**
**    and Environment (CINE)**
21,111 Lakeshore Rd.
Sainte Anne de Bellevue, QC, Canada H9X 3V9
**Phone:** (514)398-7544          **Fax:** (514)398-1020
**Email:** cine@cine.mcgill.ca
**Website:** http://www.cine.mcgill.ca/
Dr. Timothy Johns, Dir.

**Activities/Fields:** Integrity of the traditional food systems of the Aboriginal peoples of Canada, particularly
food selection in relation to environment and culture,
determination of nutrient and contaminant content in
traditional foods and how food use relates to nutrition
and health. **Pub:** *Reports.* • *Newsletters.* • *Videos.* •
*Posters.*


**★ 8949 ★ New York University**
**Institute of Environmental Medicine**
550 1st Ave.
New York, NY 10016
**Phone:** (212)263-5280          **Fax:** (212)263-2838
**Email:** costam@env.med.nyu.edu
Max Costa, PhD, Dir.

**Activities/Fields:** Toxicology, chemical carcinogenesis, radiation carcinogenesis and dosimetry, respiratory disease and aerosol physiology, environmental
pollution and ecology, epidemiology, and biostatistics
and biomathematics, including studies on skin, bladder, and lung cancer from environmental sources,
environmental hazards to which industrial and community populations are exposed, industrial and environmental health hazards and means for their control, and
sources of human exposures to radiation. **Pub:** *Annual
Report.* **Frmly:** Institute of Industrial Medicine.


**★ 8950 ★ Nova Scotia Environmental**
**    Health Centre**
PO Box 2130
Fall River, NS, Canada B2T 1K6
**Phone:** (902)860-0057          **Fax:** (902)860-2046
**Email:** nsehc@dal.ca
**Website:** http://www.nsehc.com/
Dr. Roy Fox, Dir.

**Activities/Fields:** Environmentally-triggered sensitivities, causes, and treatment.


**★ 8951 ★ NYCAMH**
Bassett Healthcare
1 Atwell Rd.
Cooperstown, NY 13326
**Phone:** (607)547-6023          **Free:** 800-343-7527
**Fax:** (607)547-6087
**Email:** jmay@lakenet.org
**Website:** http://www.nycamh.com
John J. May, MD, Dir.

**Activities/Fields:** Studies barn dusts, mites, health
needs of agricultural workers in New York, dosimetry
on farms, agricultural lung hazards, farm machinery
safety, and migrant health. **Pub:** *FARMSAFE: Focus
on Agricultural Health.* Video. • *How Safe Are Your
Farm Tractors?.* • *Respiratory Hazards in the Farm
Environment.* • *Using Personal Protective Equipment
on the Farm.* • *What You Should Know About Using
Dust/Mist Masks on the Farm.* **Frmly:** New York
Center for Agricultural Medicine and Health.


**★ 8952 ★ Oregon State University**
**Environmental Health Sciences Center**
1011 ALS
Corvallis, OR 97331-7302
**Phone:** (541)737-8820          **Fax:** (541)737-4371
**Email:** mosbaugd@ucs.orst.edu
**Website:** http://www.ehsc.orst.edu
Dale Mosbaugh, PhD, Interim Dir.

**Activities/Fields:** Provides and stimulates coordinated multidisciplinary research to assess the impact of
environmental chemicals on human health and to
predict associated short- and long-term effects. Specific research draws upon capabilities of faculty, staff,
and graduate students in chemistry, biochemistry,

agricultural chemistry, biology, food science, fisheries
and wildlife, veterinary medicine, pharmacology, toxicology, immunology, and statistics. Focal areas include toxicology of environmental chemicals and naturally occurring toxins, cellular and biochemical toxicology, carcinogenesis of environmental chemicals,
mechanisms of toxicity, genetic toxicology, immunotoxicology, mass spectrometry, statistical studies, and
analysis of enumerative data related to environmental
health research.


**★ 8953 ★ Simon Fraser University**
**Environmental Physiology Unit**
Sch. of Kinesiology
8888 University Dr.
Burnaby, BC, Canada V5A 1S6
**Phone:** (604)291-3782          **Fax:** (604)291-3040
**Email:** ablaber@sfu.ca
**Website:** http://www.sfu.ca/epu
Andrew P. Blaber, Dir.

**Activities/Fields:** Professional divers response to
carbon dioxide and nitrogn narcosis, models of thermoregulatory control, altitude acclimation, decompression sickness, astronaut EVA decompression protocols, health hazard appraisal, design and performance
evaluation of underwater breathing apparatus, hyperbaric oxygen toxicity, evaluation of personal flotation
devices, hypothermia protection, environmental testing of equipment, and pressure testing of diving
equipment.


**★ 8954 ★ South Carolina Health and**
**    Environmental Control Department**
**Health Services Division**
**Bureau of Environmental Health**
2600 Bull St.
Columbia, SC 29201
**Phone:** (803)896-0646          **Fax:** (803)896-0645
**Email:** hatfierl@columb72.dhec.state.sc.us
**Website:** http://www.scdhec.net
Richard L. Hatfield, Dir.

**Activities/Fields:** Environmental pollution and its effects.


**★ 8955 ★ Texas A&M University**
**Center for Environmental and Rural**
**    Health (CERH)**
Department of Veterinary Physiology &
    Pharmacology
College Station, TX 77843-4466
**Phone:** (979)845-5993          **Fax:** (979)862-4929
**Email:** kramos@cvm.tamu.edu
**Website:**     http://www.niehs.nih.gov/centers/center/
tam-ctr.htm
Kenneth Ramos, PhD, Dir.

**Activities/Fields:** Impact of environmental factors on
human health and disease in rural communities. **Pub:**
*Annual report.*


**Thomas Jefferson University**
**Occupational and Environmental Health**
**    Sciences Division**
*See:* Entry 17375


**★ 8956 ★ Tulane University**
**Environmental Health Sciences Research**
**    Laboratory**
1440 Canal St., Ste. 2100
New Orleans, LA 70112
**Phone:** (504)588-5374          **Fax:** (504)584-1726
**Email:** assafa@tulane.edu
**Website:** http://www.sph.tulane.edu
Dr. Assaf Abdelghani, Dir.

**Activities/Fields:** Air and water pollution abatement,
water quality evaluation and control, environmental
health management, bacterial and mammalian cell
mutagenesis, vector control, toxicology, and occupational safety and health, including interdisciplinary
studies of toxic effects of pesticides on the environment, biological and physical-chemical treatment of

industrial waste, fumigation with air contaminants,
environmental toxicology, industrial hygiene, and
heavy metal, hazardous waste management, and
related studies.


**U.S. Department of Defense**
**Army Medical Research and Materiel**
**    Command**
**Army Research Institute of Environmental**
**    Medicine**
*See:* Entry 13474


**U.S. Department of Defense**
**Army Medical Research and Materiel**
**    Command**
**Army Research Institute of Environmental**
**    Medicine**
**Thermal and Mountain Medicine Division**
*See:* Entry 13477


**★ 8957 ★ U.S. Department of Health and**
**    Human Services**
**Agency for Toxic Substances and**
**    Disease Registry**
1600 Clifton Rd., NE
Mail Stop E-28
Atlanta, GA 30333
**Phone:** (404)498-0004          **Fax:** (404)498-0086
**Email:** RY52@cdc.gov
**Website:** http://www.atsdr.cdc.gov
Dr. Henry Falk, Asst. Admin.

**Activities/Fields:** Epidemiologic studies on human
health effects related to hazardous substance exposure, emphasizing substance-specific research on
priority hazardous substances. Comprises Division of
Health Studies, Division of Toxicology, Division of
Health Assessment and Consultation, and Division of
Health Education. **Pub:** *Biennial Report.* • *Health
assessments.* • *Proceedings.* • *Research reports.* •
*Toxicological profiles.*


**★ 8958 ★ U.S. Department of Health and**
**    Human Services**
**Centers for Disease Control and**
**    Prevention**
**National Center for Environmental Health**
4770 Buford Hwy. NE (MS F-29)
Chamblee, GA 30341-3724
**Phone:** (770)488-7000          **Fax:** (770)488-7015
**Email:** rxj4@cdc.gov
**Website:** http://www.cdc.gov/nceh/default.htm
Richard J. Jackson, MD, Dir.

**Activities/Fields:** Administers national programs that
promote a healthy environment and prevent premature
death and avoidable illness and disability caused by
non-infectious, non-occupational, environmental, and
related factors. The Center is to be reorganized into
divisions on Birth Defects and Pediatric Genetics,
Childhood Development Disabilities and Health Environmental Hazards and Health Effects, and Laboratory
Sciences.


**U.S. Department of Health and Human**
**    Services**
**Centers for Disease Control and**
**    Prevention—National Institute for**
**    Occupational Safety and Health**
**National Farm Medicine Center**
**Midwest Center for Agricultural Disease**
**    and Injury Research, Education, and**
**    Prevention**
*See:* Entry 16819

## ★ 8959 ★ U.S. Department of Health and Human Services
**National Center for Environmental Health**
**Birth Defects and Developmental**
**Disabilities Division**
**Health Studies Branch**
4770 Buford Hwy, NE, F34
Chamblee, GA 30341-3724
**Phone:** (770)488-7366          **Fax:** (770)488-7361
**Email:** gpo1@cec.gov
**Website:** http://www.cdc.gov/ncbddd/default.htm
Dr. Colleen Boyle, Asst. Dir.

**Activities/Fields:** Surveillance research, intervention methods, and technical consultations leading to the design, conduct, analysis, and evaluation of epidemiologic studies of adverse reproductive outcomes (i.e., birth defects, developmental disabilities, genetic abnormalities, mental retardation, and spontaneous abortion). Activities include population-based surveillance, use of case-control methods, and randomized controlled trails. In addition, cooperative agreements with states have been developed in an effort to increase the Division's research capacity into prevention effectiveness. **Pub:** *Proceedings.* • *Research Reports.*

## ★ 8960 ★ U.S. Department of Health and Human Services
**National Center for Environmental Health**
**Environmental Hazards and Health**
**Effects Division**
1600 Clifton Rd. M.S E-19
Atlanta, GA 30333
**Phone:** (404)498-1300          **Fax:** (404)498-1313
**Email:** mam7@cdc.gov
Dr. Michael McGeehin, Dir.

**Activities/Fields:** Environmental public health problems and their prevention. Specific areas of interest include toxic chemicals, natural environmental hazards, environmentally-induced disease, international environmental health, and indoor air pollution.

## ★ 8961 ★ U.S. Department of Health and Human Services
**National Center for Environmental Health**
**Environmental Hazards and Health**
**Effects Division**
**Health Studies Branch**
1600 Clifton Rd. NE
MS-E23
Atlanta, GA 30333
**Phone:** (404)498-1340          **Fax:** (404)498-1355
**Email:** chr1@cdc.gov
**Website:** http://www.cdc.gov/nech/hsb
Carol Rubin, DVM, Chf.

**Activities/Fields:** Epidemiologic studies on environmental exposure and health effects. Also studies the epidemiology of natural disasters. This includes planning, implementing, and reporting epidemiologic research and providing technical assistance and assessment of risk from environmental hazards such as toxic chemicals, waste disposal, indoor air pollution, passive smoking, controlled substance analogs, and natural and man-made disasters.

## ★ 8962 ★ U.S. Department of Health and Human Services
**National Center for Environmental Health**
**Environmental Health Laboratory**
**Sciences Division**
CDC
4770 Buford Hwy.
Chamblee, GA 30341-3724
**Phone:** (770)488-7950          **Fax:** (770)488-4839
**Email:** ejs1@cdc.gov
**Website:** http://www.cdc.gov/nceh/dls/default.htm
Dr. Eric J. Sampson, Dir.

**Activities/Fields:** Chronic disease and toxicant exposure. Laboratory methods development accounts for most of the activities related to problem definition in chronic disease. These activities include developing laboratory methods in cardiovascular disease, cancer, genetic markers of certain chronic diseases, and biomedical indices of nutritional status. To improve problem definition in toxicant exposure, Division is developing new and improving existing laboratory methods for detecting and measuring: body burdens of hazardous substances and their metabolites; and early stages of organ damage (using biochemical markers for organ-specific dysfunction). Services, including advice, assistance, and information, are available to state and local public health authorities, federal agencies, international organizations, academic, international, and private laboratories, and professional organizations in support of laboratory science in the fields of environmental health and non-infectious chronic diseases. The Division also collaborates with other CDC organizations as appropriate. Its consists of the Toxicology Branch, Clinical Biochemistry Branch, Nutritional Biochemistry Branch, Special Activities Branch, and Molecular Biology Branch. **Pub:** *Proceedings.*

## ★ 8963 ★ U.S. Department of Health and Human Services
**National Institute of Environmental Health**
**Sciences**
MD B2-01
PO Box 12233
Research Triangle Park, NC 27709
**Phone:** (919)541-3201          **Fax:** (919)541-2260
**Email:** olden@niehs.nih.gov
**Website:** http://www.niehs.nih.gov
Dr. Kenneth Olden, Dir.

**Activities/Fields:** Conducts environmental health sciences research and supports research through its extramural and intramural programs. The Institute's Extramural Research and Training Division supports research within educational institutions, research institutes, and other public and private nonprofit organizations through individual grants, contracts, and Research Career Development Awards. Programs emphasize studies that provide information essential to an understanding of the way in which human health is adversely affected by environmental factors. Grant programs include support for Environmental Health Science Centers, Marine and Freshwater Biomedical Science Centers, Children's Environmental Health Centers, and research manpower development programs, as well as the Superfund Basic Research Program, a university-based program of basic research supported by NIEHS as part of the 1986 Superfund Amendments and Reauthorization Act. This Program combines basic research in the fields of ecology, engineering, and hydrogeology into a core program of biomedical research to provide a broader and more detailed body of scientific information to be used in decision-making related to the management of hazardous substances. In addition to the Basic Research Program, the Institute supports a model worker training program for workers involved in hazardous waste cleanup and emergency response. **Pub:** *Environmental Health Perspectives*, monthly. Journal.

## ★ 8964 ★ U.S. Department of Health and Human Services
**National Institute of Environmental Health**
**Sciences**
**Division of Environmental Carcinogenesis**
**Experimental Carcinogenesis and**
**Mutagenesis Laboratory**
PO Box 12233
Research Triangle Park, NC 27709
**Phone:** (919)541-4141          **Fax:** (919)541-1460
**Email:** tennant@niehs.nih.gov
**Website:** http://www.niehs.nih.gov/diredmp/home.htm
Dr. Raymond Tennant, Chf.

**Activities/Fields:** Central role played by genetic and epigenetic events in the processes of carcinogenesis. Seeks to; understand the involvement of specific gene mutations and epigenetic events in cancer development; understand the role of chemicals and other environmental factors in the induction of cancer; derive insights into relationships between mutagenicity, chemical structure, and mechanisms of mutagenesis and carcinogenesis; and minimize the risks to human health by improving the ability to rapidly identify, classify, or quantitate the effects of potential mutagens and carcinogens.

## ★ 8965 ★ U.S. Department of Health and Human Services
**National Institute of Environmental Health**
**Sciences**
**Division of Extramural Research and**
**Training**
PO Box 12233
Research Triangle Park, NC 27709
**Phone:** (919)541-7723          **Fax:** (919)541-2843
**Email:** SASSAMAN@NIEHS.NIH.GOV
**Website:** http://www.niehs.nih.gov/dert/home.htm
Anne P. Sassaman, PhD, Dir.

**Activities/Fields:** Consequences of the exposure of humans and other biological systems to potentially toxic or harmful agents in the environment. Investigators at colleges, universities, and research foundations are supported through individual research grants, program project grants, and other support mechanisms. Research activities focus on the ways in which human health is adversely affected by chemical, physical, and other environmental factors. This involves: characterization of environmental health hazards; research on biological responses to environmental health hazards; applied toxicological research and testing; biometry and risk estimation; and resource and manpower development. (Research and training may span one, several, or all program areas.) The extramural program also includes support for Environmental Health Sciences Centers and for Marine and Freshwater Biomedical Science Centers. Environmental Health Sciences Centers serve as national focal points and resources for research and manpower development in health problems related to air, water, and food pollution; occupational and industrial neighborhood health and safety; heavy metal toxicity; agricultural chemical hazards; and the relationships of environment to cancer, birth defects, behavioral anomalies, respiratory and cardiovascular diseases, and diseases of other organs. Marine and Freshwater Biomedical Science Centers provide core support to foster multidisciplinary research on marine and fresh-water organisms in the study of mechanisms of toxicity of environmental agents and as models for human diseases and disorders resulting from exposure to environmental toxicants.

## ★ 8966 ★ U.S. Department of Health and Human Services
**National Institute of Environmental Health**
**Sciences**
**Division of Intramural Research**
PO Box 12233
Research Triangle Park, NC 27709
**Phone:** (919)541-3205          **Fax:** (919)541-4214
**Email:** lutzb@niehs.nih.gov
Dr. Lutz Birnbaumer, Actg. Sci. Dir.

**Activities/Fields:** Plans and conducts the Institute's basic laboratory and clinical research, which encompasses the environmental areas of medicine, biology, pharmacology, neurosciences and pulmonary pathobiology, chemistry, toxicology, genetics, and biophysics. Plans and conducts a program of toxicology and carcinogenesis studies to establish and characterize the toxicity of chemicals and other environmental agents, and to develop, validate, and evaluate such methods. Plans and conducts basic and applied research related to environmental health in the areas of risk assessment, statistics, biomathematics, and epidemiology. Ensures optimal utilization of available resources in the attainment of Institute objectives. Evaluates research efforts and establishes intramural priorities. Integrates ongoing and new research activities into the division structure. Collaborates with other NIH institutes, divisions and programs. Maintains an active association with peer groups in other federal agencies, academic and private institutions, and international organizations with similar environmental health research interests, and disseminates research results. Provides advice to the Institute Director and staff on matters of scientific interest. Comprises The Environmental Biology Program, The Environmental Diseases and Medicine Program, and The Environmental Toxicology Program.

**★ 8967 ★ U.S. Department of Health and Human Services**
**National Institute of Environmental Health Sciences**
**Division of Intramural Research**
**Environmental Toxicology Program**
PO Box 12233, MD A3-02
Research Triangle Park, NC 27709
**Phone:** (919)541-3802　　**Fax:** (919)541-3647
**Email:** portier@niehs.nih.gov
**Website:** http://dir.niehs.nih.gov/diretp/
Dr. Christopher J. Portier, Actg. Dir.

**Activities/Fields:** Environmental toxicology.

**★ 8968 ★ U.S. Department of Health and Human Services**
**National Institute of Environmental Health Sciences**
**Division of Intramural Research**
**Laboratory of Molecular Biophysics**
PO Box 12233
Research Triangle Park, NC 27709
**Phone:** (919)541-4575　　**Fax:** (919)541-5750
**Email:** CHIGNELL@NIEHS.NIH.GOV
Dr. Colin F. Chignell, Chf.

**Activities/Fields:** Spectroscopic methods to monitor the molecular interactions that occur between environmental agents and biological systems; develop, improve, and utilize analytical methodology for specified chemical agents; and conduct biochemical, physical, organic, and bio-organic studies of environmental agents and their conversion products, with emphasis on biomechanism elucidation.

**★ 8969 ★ U.S. Department of Health and Human Services**
**National Institute of Environmental Health Sciences**
**Division of Intramural Researh**
**Laboratory of Pulmonary Pathobiology**
Niehs Mail Drop A2-09
PO Box 12233
Research Triangle Park, NC 27709
**Phone:** (919)541-3540　　**Fax:** (919)541-4133
**Email:** Nettesheim@Niehs.nih.gov
**Website:** http://dir.niehs.nih.gov/dirlppon
Dr. Paul Nettesheim, Chf.

**Activities/Fields:** Elucidate biochemical and molecular mechanisms of differentiation of airway epithelium; elucidate the role of growth factors in regulation of growth of normal and neoplastically transformed airway cells; explore pathogenetic mechanisms of inflammatory processes of the lung, particularly the cellular and biochemical basis of fibrogenesis; and elucidate the mechanisms of regulation of surfactant biosynthesis.

**★ 8970 ★ U.S. Department of Health and Human Services**
**National Institute of Environmental Health Sciences**
**Environmental Toxicology Program**
**Toxicology Branch**
Mail Drop A3-02
Research Triangle Park, NC 27709
**Phone:** (919)541-7992　　**Fax:** (919)541-3647
**Email:** portier@niehs.nih.gov
Dr. Christopher Portier, Dir.

**Activities/Fields:** Activities are carried out in five work groups; the Chemical Dispositon Group studies the absorption, distribution,metabolism, and excretion of a range of chemicals to provide information useful in the design and interpretation of chemical toxicity and carcinogenicity activities; the Developmental and Reproductive Toxicology Group provides an in-house

research program, consultation to program toxicologists on the design of special studies, and participation with National Institute for Occupational Safety and Health and National Center for Toxicological Research personnel in the organization, coordination, and long-range planning of the National Toxicology Program's reproductive and developmental toxicology program (in-house research activities include evaluating the reproductive toxicity of environmental and industrial chemicals, providing data on the toxic potential and mechanism of chemicals, and enhancing the development of new and more appropriate testing systems); the Immunologic Toxicology Group selects, refines, and validates a panel of immunology and host resistance procedures to define immunotoxicity and correlating changes in immune function with alterations in host resistance; and the Inhalation Toxicology Group conducts studies on compounds that enter the body primarily by inhalation; and works toward the technologic advancement of gas-vapor inhalation methodologies/facilities. (Further information on a fifth group, the Metal Toxicology Group, was not available for this edition. In addition, the Biochemical Toxicology Group that was previously listed in this Directory no longer exists.).

**U.S. Department of Health and Human Services**
**National Institutes of Health (NIH)**
**National Cancer Institute (NCI)**
**Division of Basic Sciences**
**((Laboratory of Biosystems and Cancer) Cancer and Aging Section)**
*See:* Entry 10511

**U.S. Department of Health and Human Services**
**National Institutes of Health**
**National Cancer Institute**
**Division of Basic Sciences**
**(Laboratory of Biosystems and Cancer)**
*See:* Entry 10512

**U.S. Department of Health and Human Services**
**National Institutes of Health**
**National Institute of Dental and Craniofacial Research**
**Division of Intramural Research**
**(Molecular and Genetic Epidemiology Section)**
*See:* Entry 9066

**U.S. Department of Health and Human Services**
**National Institutes of Health**
**National Institute of Environmental Health Sciences**
**Division of Extramural Research and Training**
**(Centers for Children's Environmental Health and Disease Prevention)**
*See:* Entry 17832

**U.S. Department of Health and Human Services**
**National Institutes of Health**
**National Institute of Environmental Health Sciences**
**Division of Extramural Research and Training**
**(Chemical Exposures and Molecular Biology Branch)**
*See:* Entry 9073

**★ 8971 ★ U.S. Department of Health and Human Services**
**National Institutes of Health**
**National Institute of Environmental Health Sciences**
**Environmental Genome Project**
PO Box 12233
Research Triangle Park, NC 27709
**Phone:** (919)541-3345
**Email:** barnes@niehs.nih.gov
**Website:** http://www.niehs.nih.gov/envgenom/home.htm
Martha I. Barnes, Contact

**Activities/Fields:** Understanding the impact and interaction of environmental exposures on human health and disease.

**U.S. Department of Health and Human Services**
**National Institutes of Health**
**National Institute of Environmental Health Sciences**
**Environmental Genomic SNP Database Platform**
*See:* Entry 9475

**U.S. Department of Health and Human Services**
**National Institutes of Health**
**National Institute of Environmental Health Sciences**
**Laboratory of Molecular Carcinogenesis (Molecular and Genetic Epidemiology)**
*See:* Entry 10573

**U.S. Department of Health and Human Services**
**National Institutes of Health**
**National Institute of Environmental Health Sciences**
**Laboratory of Molecular Carcinogenesis (Cell Adhesion and Migration)**
*See:* Entry 9476

**★ 8972 ★ U.S. Department of Health and Human Services**
**National Institutes of Health**
**National Institute of Environmental Health Sciences**
**Laboratory of Structural Biology**
M/D F3-02
PO Box 12233
Research Triangle Park, NC 27709
**Phone:** (919)541-3198　　**Fax:** (919)541-7880
**Email:** london@niehs.nih.gov
**Website:** http://dir.niehs.nih.gov/dirlsb/
Robert E. London, Prin. Inv.

**Activities/Fields:** Provides insights into biological processes that impact human environmental health, including signal transduction processes, nucleic acid transactions, gene expression and protein translation and modification. Investigates relationship between atomic level structures of macromolecules and their biochemical properties, their abilities to interact with other macromolecules and with substrates, and their functions in vivo (requiring highly integrated approach wherein x-ray crystallography, nuclear magnetic resonance, mass spectroscopy and computational chemistry are combined with biochemical and genetic approaches).

**U.S. Department of Health and Human Services**
**National Institutes of Health**
**National Institute of Mental Health**
**Experimental Therapeutics Branch**
**(Section on Clinical and Experimental Neurospychology)**
*See:* Entry 14332


**★ 8973 ★ U.S. Department of Transportation**
**Coast Guard**
**Office of Health and Safety**
**Safety and Environmental Health Division**
Coast Headquarters Bldg.
2100 2nd St. SW
Washington, DC 20593
**Phone:** (202)267-1883　　**Fax:** (202)267-4355
**Email:** nimhinfo@nih.gov
**Website:** http://lbc.nimh.nih.gov/research.html
Al Kotz, Chf.

**Activities/Fields:** Responsible for all internal mishap prevention, environmental health, and occupational health within the Coast Guard, including aircraft crashes, vessel collisions, fires, explosions, and chemical exposures.


**U.S. Department of Veterans Affairs**
**Veterans Health Administration**
**Office of Research and Development**
**Medical Research Service**
**(Environmental Hazards Research Center )**
*See:* Entry 13507


**Universities Associated for Research and Education in Pathology, Inc.**
*See:* Entry 17160


**★ 8974 ★ University of Arizona**
**Southwest Environmental Health Sciences Center (SWEHSC)**
Center for Toxicology
College of Pharmacy
1703 E Mabel St.
Tucson, AZ 85721
**Phone:** (520)626-4488　　**Fax:** (520)626-2466
**Email:** liebler@pharmacy.arizona.edu
**Website:** http://www.niehs.nih.gov/centers/center/az-ctr.htm
Daniel Liebler, PhD, Dir.

**Activities/Fields:** Health effects of environmental agents on living organisms. Activity has been grouped into five research cores: cellular processing of chemicals, cell injury, and environmental carcinogenesis and prevention.


**★ 8975 ★ University of California, Berkeley**
**Environmental Health Sciences Center**
School of Public Health
Berkeley, CA 94720-7360
**Phone:** (510)642-8770　　**Fax:** (510)642-5815
**Email:** martynts@uclink4.berkeley.edu
**Website:** http://www.niehs.nih.gov/centers/center/ucb-ctr.htm
Prof. Martyn T. Smith, PhD, Dir.

**Activities/Fields:** DNA damage and its consequences for health, as well as the causes, mechanisms, and prevention of DNA damage and cancer.


**★ 8976 ★ University of California, Davis**
**Center for Environmental Health Sciences (CEHS)**
1 Shields Ave.
Davis, CA 95616
**Phone:** (530)752-2732　　**Fax:** (530)752-3394
**Email:** rlmorrison@ucdavis.edu

**Website:** http://www.envtox.ucdavis.edu/cehs/
Dr. Fumio Matsumura, Dir.

**Activities/Fields:** Effects of the environment on human health, including human epidemiology, target organ toxicity, biomarkers of exposure, and effects and mechanisms of toxics. **Pub:** *Annual report.*


**★ 8977 ★ University of California, Davis**
**Center for Health and the Environment**
Old Davis Rd.
1 Shields Ave.
Davis, CA 95616
**Phone:** (530)752-1340　　**Fax:** (530)752-5300
**Email:** pahunter@ucdavis.edu
**Website:** http://iteh.ucdavis.edu
Dr. Kent E. Pinkerton, Dir.

**Activities/Fields:** Coordinates interdisciplinary research on biomedical and toxicological problems related to exposure to chemical, physical, and biological toxic agents or to ionizing radiation. Seeks to determine basic mechanisms of toxic effects and to predict human health hazards from continual exposure to realistic levels of toxic substances in the environment or in the workplace. **Pub:** *Annual Research Report.* **Frmly:** Institute of Toxicology and Environmental Health.


**★ 8978 ★ University of California, Irvine**
**Air Pollution Health Effects Laboratory**
Department of Community & Environmental Medicine
Irvine, CA 92697-1825
**Phone:** (949)824-5860　　**Fax:** (949)824-4763
**Email:** rfphalen@uci.edu
Dr. Robert F. Phalen, Dir.

**Activities/Fields:** Lung development and defenses, particle deposition in the lungs, inhalation exposure to oxidant, fine particulate and acidic aerosol mixtures, inhalation exposure methodology, and environmental and occupational inhalation toxicology, emphasizing particle plus gas mixtures. Also develops and validates mathematical models of inhaled particle deposition. **Pub:** *Research Reports,* quarterly.


**University of California, Los Angeles**
**California Education and Research Center-Southern**
*See:* Entry 16835


**★ 8979 ★ University of Cincinnati**
**Center for Environmental Genetics (CEG)**
Department of Environmental Health
College of Medicine
3223 Eden Ave.
Cincinnati, OH 45267-0056
**Phone:** (513)558-3625　　**Fax:** (513)558-4617
**Email:** marshall.anderson@uc.edu
**Website:** http://www.niehs.nih.gov/centers/center/cin-ctr.htm
Marshall W. Anderson, PhD, Dir.

**Activities/Fields:** Environmental health sciences, with a focus on the interaction between genes and the environment, especially the impact of genetic diversity on the response of the individual to toxic environmental agents.


**★ 8980 ★ University of Connecticut**
**Center for Environmental Health**
Department of Animal Science
College of Agriculture & Natural Resources
3636 Horsebarn Rd., Box U-39
Storrs, CT 06269-4039
**Phone:** (860)486-6073　　**Fax:** (860)486-5067
**Email:** ihart@canr.uconn.edu
**Website:** http://www.sp.uconn.edu/~an226vc/index.html
Dr. Ian C. Hart, Dir.

**Activities/Fields:** Interdisciplinary studies of environmental health problems of concern to Connecticut, emphasizing carcinogenesis, pesticides, epidemiology and biostatistics, and genetic biomonitoring.


**★ 8981 ★ University of Connecticut**
**Health Center**
**Waterborne Disease Center**
School of Dental Medicine
263 Farmington Ave.
Farmington, CT 06030-3705
**Phone:** (860)679-2622　　**Fax:** (860)679-2910
**Email:** drrossomando@waterbornediseases.org
**Website:** http://www.waterbornediseases.org
Edward Rossomando, DDS, Dir.

**Activities/Fields:** Global and national health problems caused by waterborne diseases.


**★ 8982 ★ University of Florida**
**Center for Environmental and Human Toxicology**
College of Veterinary Medicine
PO Box 110885
Gainesville, FL 32611-0885
**Phone:** (352)392-4700　　**Fax:** (352)392-4707
**Email:** smr@ufl.edu
**Website:** http://www.floridatox.org
Dr. Stephen M. Roberts, Dir.

**Activities/Fields:** Environmental and human toxicology.


**★ 8983 ★ University of Iowa**
**Center for Health Effects of Environmental Contamination (CHEEC)**
100 Oakdale Campus, Rm. N202 OH
Iowa City, IA 52242-5000
**Phone:** (319)335-4550　　**Fax:** (319)335-4077
**Email:** peter_weyer@uiowa.edu
**Website:** http://www.cheec.uiowa.edu
Peter Weyer, PhD, Dir.

**Activities/Fields:** Fate and transport of toxic substances in the environment, radon and indoor air contaminants, nonpoint source chemical contamination of water supplies, and epidemiologic studies that relate the occurrence of diseases to contaminant exposure. **Pub:** *Annual Report.* • *Newsletter.* • *Technical Report.*


**★ 8984 ★ University of Iowa**
**Center for International Rural and Environmental Health (CIREH)**
120 IREH Bldg.
100 Oakdale Campus
Iowa City, IA 52242-5000
**Phone:** (319)335-4541　　**Fax:** (319)353-4225
**Email:** robin-ungar@uiowa.edu
**Website:** http://www.public-health.uiowa.edu/cireh
Dr. Thomas Cook, Dir.

**Activities/Fields:** Occupational, environmental and public health topics, particularly issues connected to rural and agricultural populations. epidemiology and care models, and the history of medicine science and public health.


**★ 8985 ★ University of Iowa**
**Environmental Health Sciences Research Center (EHSRC)**
124 Agricultural Medical Research Facility
Department of Preventive Medicine & Environmental Health
Oakdale Campus
Iowa City, IA 52242
**Phone:** (319)335-4189　　**Fax:** (319)335-4225
**Email:** james-merchant@uiowa.edu
**Website:** http://www.niehs.nih.gov/centers/center/iowa-ctr.htm
James A. Merchant, MD, Dir.

**Activities/Fields:** Agricultural and rural environmental exposures and their effects on health, particularly environmental cancer, pulmonary biology, occupational health, and environmental assessment and control. **Pub:** *EHSRC Newsletter,* 3/year.

**University of Iowa
Institute for Rural and Environmental
   Health**
*See:* Entry 16838

**University of Iowa
State Hygienic Laboratory**
*See:* Entry 18011

**University of Manitoba
Health, Leisure, and Human Performance
   Research Institute (HLHP)**
*See:* Entry 19202

**★ 8986 ★ University of Massachusetts at
   Amherst
Northeast Regional Environmental Public
   Health Center (NREPHC)**
Morrill Science Center I, N233
Department of Environmental Health Sciences
School of Public Health & Health Sciences
639 N Pleasant St.
Amherst, MA 01003-9298
**Phone:** (413)545-3164
**Email:** edwardc@schoolph.umass.edu
**Website:**   http://www.umass.edu/sphhs/centers/
nrephc.html
Edward J. Calabrese, Contact

**Activities/Fields:** Environmental health, focusing on
regional issues of national importance, namely the
analysis, assessment, and remediation of contaminated soils and groundwater; and the biological effects of
low levels of exposure.

**★ 8987 ★ University of Miami
Toxicology Laboratory**
Bldg. B
12500 SW 152 St.
Miami, FL 33177-1411
**Phone:** (305)232-7020        **Fax:** (305)232-7461
**Email:** hchipw@aol.com
Chip Walls, Lab. Mgr.

**Activities/Fields:** Pesticides, air pollutants, carcinogens, and chemicals, with emphasis on biological,
agricultural, and environmental samples. **Frmly:** Pesticide Residue, Toxic Waste and Basic Research
Analytical Laboratory.

**★ 8988 ★ University of Minnesota
Center for Environment and Health Policy**
Box 807
Mayo Memorial Bldg.
420 Delaware St. SE
Minneapolis, MN 55455
**Phone:** (612)626-4244        **Fax:** (612)626-0650
**Email:** ksexton@mail.eoh.umn.edu
Ken Sexton, Dir.

**Activities/Fields:** Center promotes the use of environmental, biological, and social science knowledge in
the development of public policies relevant to environmental agents and their effects on the health of
people. Center's focus is on applying existing scientific
data to analyze environmental risks while considering
economic, social, and political implications. Programmatic areas of the Center include risk analysis, risk
communication, economic analysis, and legal/regula-
tory affairs.

**★ 8989 ★ University of Mississippi
Research Institute of Pharmaceutical
   Sciences
Environmental Toxicology Research
   Program (ETRP)**
University, MS 38677
**Phone:** (662)915-5759        **Fax:** (662)915-1285
**Website:**   http://www.olemiss.edu/depts/pharmacolo-
gy/etrp/index.html
**Activities/Fields:** Identification and resolution of prob-
lems related to environmental health issues.

**★ 8990 ★ University of New Mexico
Environmental Health Sciences
   Developmental Center**
Pulmonary, Allergy & Critical Care
Internal Medicine, 5-ACC
Albuquerque, NM 87131-5271
**Phone:** (505)272-4289        **Fax:** (505)272-8700
**Email:** pmoseley@salud.unm.edu
**Website:**   http://www.niehs.nih.gov/centers/center/
unm-ctr.htm
Pope Moseley, MD, Dir.

**Activities/Fields:** Environmental respiratory disease
in Native Americans. The issues of importance to the
center are inhalation exposures and toxicology, environmental signaling, human genetics, epidemiology,
and community outreach on respiratory health issues.

**University of North Alabama
Occupational and Environmental Health
   Laboratory**
*See:* Entry 16843

**★ 8991 ★ University of North Carolina at
   Chapel Hill
Center for Environmental Medicine and
   Lung Biology**
CB 7310
104 Mason Farm Rd.
Chapel Hill, NC 27599-7310
**Phone:** (919)962-0126        **Fax:** (919)966-9863
**Email:** pwspar@med.unc.edu
**Website:**        http://www.med.unc.edu/envlung/
welcome1.htm
Philip A. Bromberg, MD, Dir.

**Activities/Fields:** Environmental impacts on human
health, including effects of inhaled agents on the
respiratory system in diseased and healthy human
subjects and on human cell lines and basic and clinical
studies in environmental health sciences.

**★ 8992 ★ University of Pennsylvania
Institute for Environmental Medicine**
1 John Morgan Bldg.
3620 Hamilton Walk
Philadelphia, PA 19104-6068
**Phone:** (215)898-9100        **Fax:** (215)898-0868
**Email:** abf@mail.med.upenn.edu
**Website:** http://www.med.upenn.edu/~ifem
Dr. Aron B. Fisher, Dir.

**Activities/Fields:** Cellular and molecular biology of
lung function with special emphasis on the lung
surfactant system, undersea physiology, physiological
and toxic effects of oxygen, isobaric gas counterdiffu-
sion, and hyperbaric oxygen therapy. **Pub:** *Research
Reports.*

**University of Quebec at Montreal
Centre for Study of Biological
   Interactions Between Environment and
   Health**
*See:* Entry 16845

**★ 8993 ★ University of Rochester
Environmental Health Sciences Center**
Medical Center
601 Elmwood Ave.
Rochester, NY 14642
**Phone:** (716)275-1963        **Fax:** (716)256-2591
**Email:** deborah_slechta@urmc.rochester.edu
**Website:** http://www.niehs.nih.gov/centers/center/roc-
ctr.htm
Deborah Cory-Slechta, PhD, Dir.

**Activities/Fields:** Understanding of the mechanisms
whereby exposures to environmental and occupational agents contribute to human disease and dysfunction. The center operates four research cores. The
Neurotoxicology Core focuses on the extent to which
toxicants act as risk factors for diseases and dysfunctions of the nervous system, particularly on the
interaction between environmental factors and genetic

predisposition. The Pulmonary Toxicology Core addresses mechanisms of lung injury and how these are
modulated by underlying disease processes. The
Protein Modulators of Toxicity Core focuses on the
biologically active proteins that critically regulate molecules in normal cells as molecular mechanisms of
toxicity. The Osteotoxicology Core addresses the
impact of environmental and occupational agents on
mineralized tissue, in particular the role of lead in
caries in children, and the extent to which lead
exposure serves as a risk factor for osteoporosis and
related skeletal diseases associated with advanced
aging.

**★ 8994 ★ University of Southern
   California
Environmental Health Sciences Center
   (SCEHSC)**
Bldg. CHP 236
School of Medicine
1540 Alcazar St.
Los Angeles, CA 90033
**Phone:** (323)442-1096        **Fax:** (323)442-3272
**Email:** jpeters@hsc.usc.edu
**Website:**   http://www.niehs.nih.gov/centers/center/
usc-ctr.htm
John Peters, MD, Dir.

**Activities/Fields:** Effects of the environment on human health and how personal factors modify response, especially with regard to multiethnic populations of California and the Pacific Rim.

**★ 8995 ★ University of Texas
M.D. Anderson Cancer Center
Center for Research on Environmental
   Disease (CRED)**
Science Park Research Division
Park Rd. 1C
PO Box 389
Smithville, TX 78957
**Phone:** (512)237-9444        **Fax:** (512)237-2990
**Email:** jdigiovanni@sprd1.mdacc.tmc.edu
**Website:** http://www.niehs.nih.gov/centers/center/uts-
ctr.htm
John DiGiovanni, PhD, Dir.

**Activities/Fields:** Mechanisms by which environmental factors may cause or influence human disease and
methods for early detection, prevention, and control of
environmentally related diseases. **Pub:** *Annual report.*
• *Newsletter.*

**★ 8996 ★ University of Texas Medical
   Branch at Galveston
Center in Environmental Toxicology**
5.138 MR Bldg.
Sealy Center for Molecular Science
Department of Human Biological Genetics &
   Chemistry
301 University Blvd.
Galveston, TX 77555-1071
**Phone:** (409)772-2179        **Fax:** (409)772-1790
**Email:** rslloyd@utmb.edu
**Website:** http://www.niehs.nih.gov/centers/center/utg-
ctr.htm
R. Stephen Lloyd, PhD, Dir.

**Activities/Fields:** Effects of environmental factors on
the health of a local community, particularly the
molecular and cellular factors that influence the onset
and severity of asthma, and asthma's relationship to
environmental toxicants. **Pub:** *Annual report.*

**University of Utah
Rocky Mountain Center for Occupational
   and Environmental Health**
*See:* Entry 16848

**★ 8997 ★ University of Victoria
Centre for Environmental Health**
PO Box 1700, STN CSC
Victoria, BC, Canada V8W 2Y2

**Phone:** (250)472-4071  **Fax:** (250)472-4075
**Email:** bkoop@uvic.ca
**Website:** http://web.uvic.ca/ceh/index.html
Dr. Barry Glickman, Dir.

**Activities/Fields:** Impact and influence of the environment on genetic organization and expression, and the consequences of this impact upon the health and genetic integrity of individuals, populations, and species.

**University of Washington**
**Center for Child Environmental Health**
**Risks Research (CHC)**
*See:* Entry 5834

★ **8998** ★ **University of Washington**
**Institute for Risk Analysis and Risk**
**Communication (IRARC)**
Department of Environmental Health
School of Public Health & Community Medicine
4225 Roosevelt Way NE, No. 100
Seattle, WA 98105-6099
**Phone:** (206)543-9394
**Email:** irarc@u.washington.edu
**Website:** http://depts.washington.edu/irarc/
Ruth Woods, Admin. Dir.

**Activities/Fields:** Biological risk caused by chemicals.

★ **8999** ★ **University of Washington**
**Northwest Center for Particulate Matter**
**and Health**
Department of Environmental Health, Box 354803
Seattle, WA 98195-4803
**Phone:** (206)543-2026  **Fax:** (206)685-3990
**Email:** jkoenig@u.washington.edu
**Website:** http://depts.washington.edu/pmcenter/
Jane Q. Koenig, PhD, Dir.

**Activities/Fields:** Effects on human health of particulate air pollution. **Pub:** *Papers.* • *Reports,* annually.

★ **9000** ★ **University of Wisconsin—**
**Madison**
**Molecular and Environmental Toxicology**
**Center**
Enzyme Institute, Rm. 290
1710 University Ave.
Madison, WI 53705
**Phone:** (608)263-5557  **Fax:** (608)262-5245
**Email:** jefcoate@facstaff.wisc.edu
**Website:** http://www.niehs.nih.gov/center/center/madctr.htm
Prof. Colin R. Jedcoate, PhD, Dir.

**Activities/Fields:** Toxicology and problems related to presence of potentially hazardous synthetic and naturally occurring chemicals in the environment, e.g. heavy metals, chlorinated hydrocarbons, pesticides, mycotoxins, and food-borne toxins, including identification, quantification, and toxicologic studies of such chemicals. **Pub:** *Newsletter,* occasionally. **Frmly:** Environmental Toxicology Center.

**Vanderbilt University**
**Vanderbilt Addiction Center (VAC)**
*See:* Entry 9527

★ **9001** ★ **Wayne State University**
**C.S. Mott Center for Human Growth and**
**Development**
275 E Hancock St.
Detroit, MI 48201
**Phone:** (313)577-1337  **Fax:** (313)577-8554
**Email:** rsokol@moore.med.wayne.edu
**Website:** http://www.mc.vanderbilt.edu/addiction/
Dr. Robert J. Sokol, Dir.

**Activities/Fields:** Human growth and development, including causative factors, identification, prevention, and remedy of birth defects. Uses mechanical, chemical, and hormonal devices as well as acceptable

social, psychological, ethical, and moral approaches. Identifies environmental pollutants, drugs, infections, and other teratogens responsible for increasing incidence of birth defects and studies the relationships between environmental deterioration, dwindling natural resources, population density, and quality of human existence. Develops and implements population controls. **Pub:** *Annual Report.*

**West Virginia University**
**Institute of Occupational and**
**Environmental Health**
*See:* Entry 16853

# State Government Agencies

## Environmental Health

★ **9002** ★ **Alaska Department of**
**Environmental Conservation**
**Environmental Health Division**
555 Cordova St.
Anchorage, AK 99501
**Phone:** (907)269-7500  **Fax:** (907)269-7600
**Email:** Kristin_Ryan@envircon.state.ak.us
**Website:** http://www.state.ak.us/dec/deh/
Kristin Ryan, Contact

★ **9003** ★ **Arizona Department of Health**
**Services**
**Disease Control Services Bureau**
**Environmental Health Office**
3815 N Black Canyon Hwy.
Phoenix, AZ 85015
**Phone:** (602)230-5948  **Fax:** (602)230-5933
**Email:** whumble@hs.state.az.us
**Website:** http://www.hs.state.az.us/phs/oeh/index.htm

★ **9004** ★ **California Health and Human**
**Services Agency**
**Department of Health Services**
**Division of Environmental and**
**Occupational Disease Control**
1515 Clay St., Ste. 1700
Oakland, CA 94612
**Phone:** (510)622-4500  **Fax:** (510)622-4505
**Email:** mlee@dhs.ca.gov
**Website:** http://www.dhs.ca.gov/ps/deodc/

★ **9005** ★ **Colorado Public Health and**
**Environment Department**
**Environment Office**
4300 Cherry Creek Dr. S
Denver, CO 80246-1530
**Phone:** (303)692-2035  **Fax:** (303)782-4969
**Email:** cdphe.information@state.co.us
**Website:** http://www.cdphe.state.co.us/environ.asp

★ **9006** ★ **Delaware Department of Health**
**and Social Services**
**Public Health Division**
**Health Systems Protection Branch**
Jesse Cooper Bldg.
Federal & Water St.
PO Box 637
Dover, DE 19903-0637
**Phone:** (302)739-4731  **Fax:** (302)739-3839
**Email:** dhssinfo@state.de.us
**Website:** http://www.state.de.us/dhss/dph/hsp.htm
Kevin E. Charles, Director

★ **9007** ★ **Florida Department of Health**
**Health Program Office**
**Environmental Health Services Office**
4052 Bald Cypress Way, Bin No. A08
Tallahassee, FL 32399-1709
**Phone:** (850)245-4250
**Email:** EnvironmentalHealth@doh.state.fl.us
**Website:** http://www.doh.state.fl.us/

★ **9008** ★ **Georgia Department of Human**
**Resources**
**Public Health Division**
**Environmental Health Section**
2 Peachtree St. NW
Atlanta, GA 30303-3186
**Phone:** (404)657-6534  **Fax:** (404)657-2715
**Email:** gdphinfo@dhr.state.ga.us
**Website:** http://www.ph.dhr.state.ga.us/programs/environmental/index.shtml

★ **9009** ★ **Hawaii Department of Health**
**Environmental Health Administration**
919 Ala Moana Blvd.
Honolulu, HI 96814
**Phone:** (808)586-4424  **Fax:** (808)586-4444
**Website:** http://www.state.hi.us/health/about/enviro.html
Gary Gill, Director

★ **9010** ★ **Idaho Department of Health**
**and Welfare**
**Health Division**
**Bureau of Environmental Health and**
**Safety**
PO Box 83720
450 W State St.
Boise, ID 83720-0036
**Phone:** (208)334-0606  **Fax:** (208)334-6581
**Email:** behs@idhw.state.id.us
**Website:** http://www2.state.id.us/dhw/BEHS/index.htm
Maura Mack, PhD, Director

★ **9011** ★ **Illinois Department of Public**
**Health**
**Health Protection Office**
**Environmental Health Division**
535 W Jefferson St.
Springfield, IL 62761
**Phone:** (217)782-4977  **Fax:** (217)782-3987
**Email:** mailus@idph.state.il.us
**Website:** http://www.idph.state.il.us/envhealth/ehhome.htm
John R. Lumpkin, MD, Director

★ **9012** ★ **Kansas Department of Health**
**and Environment**
**Environment Division**
1000 SW Jackson, Ste. 420
Topeka, KS 66612-1367
**Phone:** (785)296-1535  **Fax:** (785)296-8464
**Email:** rhammers@kdhe.state.ks.us
**Website:** http://www.kdhe.state.ks.us/environment/index.html
Ronald Hammerschmidt, PhD, Director

★ **9013** ★ **Louisiana Department of**
**Health and Hospitals**
**Public Health Office**
**Center for Environmental Health**
6867 Bluebonnet Rd.
Baton Rouge, LA 70810
**Phone:** (225)763-3590  **Fax:** (225)763-5552
**Email:** cnenweb@dhh.state.la.us
**Website:** http://www.oph.dhh.state.la.us/
Bobby Savoie, Director

**★ 9014 ★ Maine Department of Human Services**
**Health Bureau**
**Disease Control Division**
**Environmental Health Unit**
11 State House Station
286 Water St.
Augusta, ME 04333
**Phone:** (207)287-3201        **Fax:** (207)287-9058
**Email:** Philip.W.Haines@state.me.us
**Website:** http://janus.state.me.us/dhs/boh/index.htm
Philip W. Haines, Contact

**★ 9015 ★ Maryland Department of Health and Mental Hygiene**
**Environmental Health Office**
201 W Preston St., 3rd Floor
Baltimore, MD 21210
**Phone:** (410)767-6941        **Fax:** (410)333-7392
**Email:** matique@dhmh.state.md.us
**Website:** http://mdpublichealth.org/oeh/index.html
Mahboobuddin M. Atique, MBBS, Director

**★ 9016 ★ Massachusetts Executive Office of Health and Human Services**
**Public Health Department**
**Bureau of Environmental Health Assessment**
250 Washington St., 7th Fl.
Boston, MA 02108
**Phone:** (617)624-5757        **Fax:** (617)624-5777
**Email:** dph.info@state.ma.us
**Website:** http://www.state.ma.us/dph/beha/beha.htm
Suzanne K. Condon, Director

**★ 9017 ★ Minnesota Department of Health**
**Health Protection Bureau**
**Environmental Health in Minnesota**
PO Box 64975
Saint Paul, MN 55164-0975
**Phone:** (651)215-5800
**Email:** ehweb@health.state.mn.us
**Website:** http://www.health.state.mn.us/divs/eh/index.html

**★ 9018 ★ Mississippi Department of Health**
**General Environmental Services**
PO Box 1700
Jackson, MS 39215
**Phone:** (601)576-7690        **Fax:** (601)576-7632
**Email:** lstrayer@msdh.state.ms.us
**Website:** http://www.msdh.state.ms.us/sanitation/index.htm
Lydia Strayer, Contact

**★ 9019 ★ New Jersey Department of Health and Senior Services**
**Consumer and Environmental Health Services**
PO Box 369
Trenton, NJ 08625-0369
**Phone:** (609)588-3120        **Fax:** (609)588-7431
**Email:** james.brownlee@doh.state.nj.us
**Website:** http://www.state.nj.us/health/eoh/cehsweb/
James A. Brownlee, Director

**★ 9020 ★ New Mexico Department of Environment**
Harold S Runnels Bldg
1190 St. Francis Dr.
Santa Fe, NM 87505-4182
**Phone:** (505)827-2855        **Free:** 800-219-6157
**Fax:** (505)827-2836
**Email:** Peter_Maggiore@nmenv.state.nm.us
**Website:** http://www.nmenv.state.nm.us/
Peter Maggiore, Director

**★ 9021 ★ North Dakota Department of Health**
**Environmental Health Section**
1200 Missouri Ave.
PO Box 5520
Bismarck, ND 58506-5520
**Phone:** (701)328-5150        **Fax:** (701)328-5200
**Email:** dglatt@state.nd.us
**Website:** http://www.health.state.nd.us/ndhd/environ/
Dave Glatt, Director

**★ 9022 ★ Oklahoma Department of Health**
**Health Promotion and Policy Analysis**
**Environmental Health Education**
1000 NE 10th St., Rm. 1106
Oklahoma City, OK 73117
**Phone:** (405)271-3950        **Fax:** (405)271-3431
**Email:** sharonkt@ionet.net
**Website:** http://www.health.state.ok.us/PROGRAM/envhlth/index.html
Sharon Montgomery, Director

**★ 9023 ★ Oregon Department of Human Resources**
**Health Division**
**Environment and Health Systems Office**
Portland State Office Bldg., Ste. 640
800 NE Oregon St.
Portland, OR 97232
**Phone:** (503)731-4009        **Fax:** (503)731-3184
**Email:** thomas.w.johnson@state.or.us
**Website:** http://www.ohd.hr.state.or.us/cehs/welcome.htm
Thomas W. Johnson, Director

**★ 9024 ★ Rhode Island Department of Health**
**Environmental Health Services Office**
235 Promenade St.
Providence, RI 02908-5767
**Phone:** (401)222-6800        **Fax:** (401)222-6953
**Email:** tepstein@dem.state.ri.us
**Website:** http://www.state.ri.us/dem/
Jan H. Reitsma, Director

**★ 9025 ★ South Carolina Department of Health and Environmental Control**
**Health Services Office**
**Environmental Health Bureau**
2600 Bull St.
Columbia, SC 29201
**Phone:** (803)896-0647
**Email:** sheridwd@columb72.dhec.state.sc.us
**Website:** http://www.scdhec.net/hs/envhlth/envhlth.htm
Wally Sheridan, Contact

**★ 9026 ★ Texas Department of Health**
**Environmental Health Bureau**
1100 W 49th St.
Austin, TX 78756-3199
**Phone:** (512)834-6640        **Fax:** (512)834-6707
**Email:** claren.kotrla@tdh.state.tx.us
**Website:** http://www.tdh.state.tx.us/beh/default.htm
Claren Kotrla, Director

**★ 9027 ★ Washington Department of Health**
**Environmental Health Programs**
PO Box 47820
Olympia, WA 98504-7820
**Phone:** (360)236-3000        **Free:** 800-525-0127
**Fax:** (360)236-2250
**Email:** teresa.lohr@doh.wa.gov
**Website:** http://www.doh.wa.gov/ehp/default.htm
Teresa Lohr, Contact

**★ 9028 ★ West Virginia Department of Health and Human Resources**
**Public Health Bureau**
**Environmental Health Services Office**
815 Quarrier St., Ste. 418
Charleston, WV 25301-2616
**Phone:** (304)558-2981        **Fax:** (304)558-1291
**Email:** delzey@wvdhhr.org
**Website:** http://www.wvdhhr.org/oehs/
Barbara S. Taylor, Director

**★ 9029 ★ Wyoming Department of Agriculture**
**Consumer Health Services**
2219 Carey Ave.
Cheyenne, WY 82002-0100
**Phone:** (307)777-7321        **Fax:** (307)777-6593
**Email:** lleis@state.wy.us
**Website:** http://wyagric.state.wy.us/CHS/chs.html
Laurie Leis, Director

# Chapter 25
# Epidemiology

## Federal Government Agencies

★ **9030** ★ **U.S. Department of Health and Human Services**
**Centers for Disease Control and Prevention**
**Epidemiology Program Office**
1600 Clifton Rd. NE
Atlanta, GA 30333
**Phone:** (404)639-3311
**Website:** http://www.cdc.gov/

## Foundations & Other Funding Organizations

### Other Funding Organizations

**International Society of Neurovirology**
*See:* Entry 13874

## National & International Organizations

★ **9031** ★ **American College of Epidemiology (ACE)**
1500 Sunday Dr., Ste. 102
Raleigh, NC 27607
**Phone:** (919)787-5181      **Fax:** (919)787-4916
**Email:** info@acepidemiology.org
**Website:** http://www.acepidemiology.org
Peter Kralka, Exec. Dir.

**Fnded:** 1979. **Mem:** 850. **Desc:** Medical professionals involved in the field of epidemiology. (Epidemiology is the study of the causes of human disease and the pattern of disease in human populations.) Promotes education in the practice of epidemiology and maintains professional standards in the field. Relates epidemiological issues to public policy. **Pub:** *Annals of Epidemiology*, monthly. • Newsletter, quarterly.

★ **9032** ★ **Association of French Language Epidemiologists (AFLE)**
**(Association des Epidemiologistes de Langue Francaise — ADELF)**
INSERM U 88
Hopital Nationale de Saint Maurice
14, rue du Val d'Osne
F-94410 Saint Maurice, France
**Phone:** 33 1 45183850    **Fax:** 33 1 45183889
**Email:** adelf@st_maurice.inserm.fr
**Fnded:** 1976. **Mem:** 510. **Lang(s):** French. **Desc:** Epidemiologists, doctors, surgeons, veterinarians, bi-

ologists, medical and social science educators, and public health planners. Facilitates communication among epidemiologists. Develops and provides information on epidemiological methods. Promotes epidemiological research. **Pub:** *ADELF-Info*, bimonthly. Newsletter.

**Association for Professionals in Infection Control and Epidemiology (APIC)**
*See:* Entry 11741

★ **9033** ★ **Canadian Bacterial Diseases Network (CBDN)**
Heritage Medical Research Bldg. - Rm. 282
3330 Hospital Dr. NW
Calgary, AB, Canada T2N 4N1
**Phone:** (403)220-2562    **Fax:** (403)283-5241
**Email:** woods@acs.ucalgary.ca
**Website:** http://www.cbdn.ca
**Fnded:** 1989. **Mem:** 50. **Lang(s):** English. **Desc:** Canadian researchers from 15 universities whose focus is on bacterial diseases that affect humans, animals, fish, plants and the environment. Seeks to advance scientific knowledge and enhance Canada's economic competitiveness through networking, excellence in fundamental research on bacterial diseases and collaboration with industry through a virtual research network.

★ **9034** ★ **Council of State and Territorial Epidemiologists (CSTE)**
2872 Woodcock Blvd., No. 303
Atlanta, GA 30341-4015
**Phone:** (770)458-3811    **Fax:** (770)458-8516
**Email:** dknutson@cste.org
**Website:** http://www.cste.org
Donna Knutson, Exec. Dir.
**Fnded:** 1951. **Mem:** 435. **Reg. Groups:** 4. **Desc:** State epidemiologists. Works to establish closer working relationships among members; consults with and advises appropriate disciplines in other health agencies; provides technical advice and assistance to the Association of State and Territorial Health Officials; works closely with Centers for Disease Control on epidemiology, surveillance, and prevention activities. **Pub:** *CSTE Update*, quarterly. Newsletter. • *Minutes to State and Territorial Epidemiologists.* **Frmly:** (1986) Conference of State and Territorial Epidemiologists.

★ **9035** ★ **European Society for Emerging Infections (ESEI)**
Rue Bruyns 2
B-1120 Brussels, Belgium
**Phone:** 32 2 2644048    **Fax:** 32 2 2644044
**Email:** jan.clement@msw.smd.be
**Fnded:** 1997. **Desc:** Determines infections affecting animals or humans which have emerged or are appearing with new, altered properties.

★ **9036** ★ **Indian Association of Parasitologists**
110 Chittaranjan Av
Calcutta 700 012, India

★ **9037** ★ **International Clinical Epidemiology Network (INCLEN)**
3600 Market St., Ste. 380
Philadelphia, PA 19104-2644
**Phone:** (215)222-7700    **Fax:** (215)222-7741
**Email:** inclen@inclen.org
**Website:** http://www.inclen.org/
**Desc:** Physicians, statisticians, social scientists. Seeks to improve the health of individuals; promotes clinical practice, research and medical education. **Pub:** Brochure.

★ **9038** ★ **International Committee on Food Microbiology and Hygiene**
Rolighedsvej 30
DK-1958 Frederikshavn, Denmark
**Fax:** 45 35283214
**Email:** mg@kvl.dk
**Fnded:** 1953. **Desc:** Aims at improving the control of diseases of microbial etiology transmitted by foods and of food spoilage.

★ **9039** ★ **International Epidemiological Association (IEA)**
c/o Dr. Haroutune Armenian
111 Market Pl., Ste. 840
Baltimore, MD 21202
**Phone:** (410)223-1625    **Fax:** (410)223-1620
**Email:** htelljoh@jhsph.edu
**Website:** http://www.dundee.ac.uk/iea/
Dr. Haroutune Armenian, Contact
**Fnded:** 1950. **Mem:** 2,250. **Desc:** Individuals interested in epidemiology (science dealing with incidence, distribution, and control of disease in populations). Studies methods and applications of disease control, clinical medicine, and health services. Conducts seminars and workshops. Encourages epidemiologic research. **Pub:** *Dictionary of Epidemiology.* • *International Journal of Epidemiology*, bimonthly. Journal. • Manuals. • Membership Directory, triennial. • Monographs.

**Nordic Association for Psychiatric Epidemiology (NAPE)**
*See:* Entry 12596

★ **9040** ★ **Organization for Co-Ordination and Co-Operation in the Control of Endemic Diseases (OCCGE)**
**(Organisation de Coordination et de Cooperation pour la Lutte Contre Grandes Endemies — OCCGE)**
BP 153
Bobo-Dioulasso 1, Burkina Faso
**Phone:** 226 970101    **Fax:** 226 970099

**Email:** occgoas@fasonet.bf
**Fnded:** 1960. **Mem:** 8. **Lang(s):** French. Does not correspond in English. **Desc:** Doctors and scientists. Organizes, coordinates, supports, and evaluates programs aimed at controlling and eradicating major endemic and epidemic diseases within member states and in West Africa. Seeks achievements in applied medical research, investigations, missions, and operational actions in West Africa; promotes professional training of administrators; disseminates research information on epidemics and the methods and means of combatting them. Cooperates with the World Health Organization. Promotes educational program. Involved in Epidemioly and Management Formation Project. **Pub:** *Bulletin Bibliographique*, quarterly. • *OCCGE Informations*, 3/year. • *Profil OCCGE.*

★ **9041** ★ **Scandinavian Society for Parasitology**
Jaegersborg Alle 1D
DK- 2920 Charlottenlund, Denmark
**Phone:** 45 77327743          **Fax:** 45 77327733
**Email:** mvj@bilharziasis.dk
**Fnded:** 1967.

★ **9042** ★ **Society for Epidemiologic Research (SER)**
c/o Joseph L. Lyon
Department of Family & Preventive Medicine
50 N Medical Dr., 1C26
Salt Lake City, UT 84132
**Phone:** (801)581-7234          **Fax:** (801)585-9805
**Email:** jlyon@dfpm.utah.edu
**Website:** http://www.epiresearch.org/
Dr. Joseph L. Lyon, Sec. -Treas.
**Fnded:** 1967. **Mem:** 3,000. **Desc:** Epidemiologists, researchers, public health administrators, educators, mathematicians, statisticians, and others interested in epidemiological research. To stimulate scientific interest in and promote the exchange of information about epidemiological research. **Pub:** *American Journal of Epidemiology*, bimonthly. Journal. Includes research reports and reviews, computer programs for epidemiologists, and annual meeting abstracts. *Price:* $190/year. • *Society for Epidemiologic Research–Membership Directory*, every 3-5 years. Membership Directory. • *Society for Epidemiologic Research–Newsletter*, semiannual. Newsletter.

★ **9043** ★ **Society for Healthcare Epidemiology of America**
19 Mantua Rd.
Mount Royal, NJ 08061
**Phone:** (856)423-0087          **Fax:** (856)423-3420
**Email:** sheahq@talley.com
**Website:** http://www.shea-online.org
Stephanie Dickinson, Exec. Dir.
**Fnded:** 1981. **Mem:** 1,100. **Desc:** Fosters the development and application of the science of healthcare epidemiology, broadly defined as any activity designed to study and/or improve outcomes in any type of healthcare institution or setting. **Pub:** *Infection Control and Hospital Epidemiology*, monthly. Journal. **Frmly:** Society of Hospital Epidemiologists of America; (2000) Society of Healthcare Epidemiologists of America.

★ **9044** ★ **South American Commission for the Control of Foot-and-Mouth Disease (COSALFA)**
**(Comision Sudamericana para la Lucha contra la Febre Aftosa)**
Caixa de Postal 589
20001-970 Rio de Janeiro, Brazil
**Phone:** 55 21 6713128          **Fax:** 55 21 6712387
**Email:** vsaraiva@panaftosa.ops-oms.org
**Fnded:** 1973.

---

# Research Centers

**AIDS Research Consortium of Atlanta, Inc.**
*See:* Entry 11843

★ **9045** ★ **Arizona Disease Control Research Commission**
1616 W Adams, Ste. B-25
Phoenix, AZ 85007
**Phone:** (602)542-1028          **Fax:** (602)542-6380
**Email:** adcrc1@getnet.com
**Website:** http://www.aidsresearchatlanta.org
Dawn C. Schroeder, Exec. Dir.
**Activities/Fields:** Medical, behavioral, preventive and health policy.

★ **9046** ★ **Arizona Health Services Department**
**Public Health Services**
**Bureau of Epidemiology and Disease Control**
**Office of Infectious Disease Services Office**
3815 N Black Canyon Hwy.
Phoenix, AZ 85015
**Phone:** (602)230-5820          **Fax:** (602)230-5818
**Email:** vvaz@hs.state.az.us
Victorio J. Vaz, PhD, Ch.
**Activities/Fields:** Infectious diseases.

★ **9047** ★ **Arizona Health Services Department**
**Public Health Services**
**Epidemiology and Disease Control**
3815 N Black Canyon Hwy.
Phoenix, AZ 85015
**Phone:** (602)230-5808          **Fax:** (602)230-5959
**Email:** lbland@hs.state.az.us
**Website:** http://www.hs.state.az.us
Lee A. Bland, Bur. Ch.
**Activities/Fields:** Epidemiology and disease control.

★ **9048** ★ **Arizona Health Services Department**
**Public Health Services**
**Epidemiology and Disease Control**
**Chronic Disease Epidemiology Office**
2700 N 3rd St.
Phoenix, AZ 85004
**Phone:** (602)542-7333          **Fax:** (602)364-0082
**Email:** rporter@hs.state.az.us
Richard Porter, Ch.
**Activities/Fields:** Chronic disease.

★ **9049** ★ **Brigham and Women's Hospital**
**Channing Laboratory**
181 Longwood Ave.
Boston, MA 02115-5804
**Phone:** (617)525-2270          **Fax:** (617)731-1541
**Email:** dennis_kasper@hms.harvard.edu
**Website:** http://www.channing.harvard.edu
Dr. Dennis Kasper, Dir.
**Activities/Fields:** Infectious diseases and population-based medicine.

**Dana-Farber Cancer Institute**
**Department of Biostatistical Science**
*See:* Entry 10319

★ **9050** ★ **Johns Hopkins University**
**Center for Epidemiology and Policy**
615 N Wolfe St., Ste. W6041
Baltimore, MD 21205

---

**Phone:** (410)614-4714          **Fax:** (410)955-0863
**Email:** lgordis@jhsph.edu
**Website:** http://www.med.jhu.edu/cep/
Dr. Jonathan M. Samet, Co-Dir.
**Activities/Fields:** Use of epidemiologic evidence in the development of public policy.

★ **9051** ★ **Johns Hopkins University Welch Center for Prevention, Epidemiology, and Clinical Research**
2024 E Monument St., Ste. 2-600
Baltimore, MD 21205-2223
**Phone:** (410)955-6953          **Fax:** (410)955-0476
**Email:** npowe@jhmi.edu
**Website:** http://www.med.jhu.edu/welchcenter/
Neil R. Powe, MD, Dir.
**Activities/Fields:** Etiology of disease and disability in populations, through observational epidemiology, randomized controlled trials, and effectiveness outcomes research. Also responsible for the generation and dissemination of knowledge required for prevention of disease and disability.

★ **9052** ★ **Kaiser Permanente Medical Care Program**
**Division of Research**
3505 Broadway
Oakland, CA 94611-5714
**Phone:** (510)450-2000          **Fax:** (510)450-2073
**Email:** jvs@dor.kaiser.org
**Website:** http://www.dor.kaiser.org
Dr. Joseph V. Selby, Dir.
**Activities/Fields:** Epidemiology, biometrics and biostatistics, technology assessment, health services research, and health education research and evaluation. Supports clinical research in medical centers.

**Kansas City AIDS Research Consortium**
*See:* Entry 11861

★ **9053** ★ **Laval University**
**Saint-Sacrement Hospital Research Centre**
**Unite de Recherche en Sante des Populations**
**Centre hospitalier affilie universitaire de Que et Universite Laval**
1050 Chemin Ste-Foy
Quebec, QC, Canada G1S 4L8
**Phone:** (418)682-7390          **Fax:** (418)682-7949
**Email:** jocelyne.moisan@pha.ulaval.ca
Jocelyne Moisan, Dir.
**Activities/Fields:** Population health research, cancer, infectious diseases, environmental and work related diseases, drug utilisation; biostatistics, and mathematical modelling. Research programs include: clinical trials, cohort and case-control studies.

★ **9054** ★ **Metro Health Medical Center**
**Department of Epidemiology and Biostatistics**
**Human Genetic Analysis Resource**
2500 MetroHealth Dr.
Cleveland, OH 44109
**Phone:** (216)778-3863          **Fax:** (216)778-3280
**Email:** rce@darvin.cwru.edu
**Website:** http://darwin.cwru.edu/index.html
Robert Elston, PhD, Dir.
**Activities/Fields:** Identification and chromosome mapping of genes involved in common diseases that may be primarily environmentally-influenced, as well as the genes underlying rarer monogenic diseases with much smaller environmental influence. Research focuses on theoretical development of statistical methods for analysis of family data, especially to detect and identify genetic components that underlie disease susceptibility. **Pub:** *SAGE Advice.* Newsletter.

**★ 9055 ★ National Disease Research Interchange**
1880 John F. Kennedy Blvd., 6th Fl.
Philadelphia, PA 19103
**Phone:** (215)557-7361     **Free:** 800-222-6374
**Fax:** (215)557-7154
**Email:** lducat@primenet.com
**Website:** http://www.ndri.com
Lee Ducat, Pres.

**Activities/Fields:** Procurement, preservation, and distribution of over 100 types of human tissues and organs for medical research. Also coordinates retrieval of pancreatic tissue for the clinical trials of islet cell transplants, a treatment being investigated for insulin-dependent diabetics. **Pub:** *Annual Report.* • *Interchange Newsletter.*

**★ 9056 ★ New York Blood Center, Inc.**
**Lindsley F. Kimball Research Institute**
310 E 67th St.
New York, NY 10021
**Phone:** (212)570-3034     **Fax:** (212)570-3195
**Website:** http://www.nybloodcenter.org
Robert L. Jones, MD, Pres.

**Activities/Fields:** Immunogenetics and immunohematology, epidemiology and virology of AIDS and hepatitis viruses, molecular and cell biology of red blood cells and developing erythroid cells, platelet interactions with coagulation proteins, human genetics, and hematopoietic growth factors. Performs studies of plasma proteins and seeks to develop new plasma derivatives for therapeutic use.

**★ 9057 ★ Society for Epidemiologic Research**
Department of Family & Preventive Medicine
50 N Medical Dr., 1C26
Salt Lake City, UT 84132
**Phone:** (801)581-7234     **Fax:** (801)585-9805
**Email:** jlyon@dfpm.utah.edu
Dr. Joseph L. Lyon, Treas.

**Activities/Fields:** Epidemiology, focusing on research and education. **Pub:** *American Journal of Epidemiology.*

**★ 9058 ★ U.S. Department of Health and Human Services**
**Agency for Toxic Substances and Disease Registry**
**Division of Health Studies**
1600 Clifton Rd., NE
Mail Stop E-31
Atlanta, GA 30333
**Phone:** (404)498-0105     **Fax:** (404)498-0077
G. David Williamson, Dir.

**Activities/Fields:** Epidemiology and other human health studies, evaluating the relationship between exposure to hazardous substances at waste sites and adverse health effects. Conducts health studies, surveillance programs, and registries. Subsidiary branches include Health Investigations Branch, Epidemiology and Surveillance Branch, and Exposure and Disease Registry Branch. Maintains National Exposure Registry and Emergency Event Surveillance System databases.

**★ 9059 ★ U.S. Department of Health and Human Services**
**Centers for Disease Control and Prevention**
**Epidemiology Program Office**
Bldg. 1, Rm. 5009
1600 Clifton Rd., NE
Atlanta, GA 30333
**Phone:** (404)639-3661     **Fax:** (404)639-4088
**Email:** sbtl@cdc.gov
**Website:** http://www.cdc.gov/epo/index.htm
Stephen B. Thacker, Dir.

**Activities/Fields:** Public health surveillance, epidemiologic training and research, and consultation in statistical and epidemiologic methods. **Pub:** *MMWR*

*Annual Summary.* • *MMWR Surveillance Summaries.* • *Morbidity and Mortality Weekly Report.* • *Recommendations and Reports.*

**★ 9060 ★ U.S. Department of Health and Human Services**
**Centers for Disease Control and Prevention**
**Epidemiology Program Office**
**Division of Prevention Research and Analytic Methods**
4770 Buford Hwy.
M.S K-73
Atlanta, GA 30341
**Phone:** (770)488-8188     **Fax:** (770)488-8461
Stephanie Zaza, Dir.

**Activities/Fields:** Methods for assessing the effectiveness of prevention strategies.

**★ 9061 ★ U.S. Department of Health and Human Services**
**Food and Drug Administration**
**Center for Drug Evaluation and Research**
**Office of Epidemiology and Biostatistics**
**(Surveillance and Data Processing Branch)**
Mail Code HFD-737
5600 Fishers Ln.
Rockville, MD 20857
**Phone:** (301)443-6414
George Armstrong, Jr., Chf.

**Activities/Fields:** Receives, processes, and maintains data for the Adverse Drug and Biological Product Reaction Database, a compilation of data from adverse reaction reports submitted to the Food and Drug Administration primarily by drug manufacturers, physicians, pharmacists, other health professionals, and consumers. These data are used by the Epidemiology and Surveillance Division to generate alerts and to monitor and support special studies on adverse reactions to drugs and biological products. Also maintains the Drug Quality Reporting System, a drug product defect monitoring system. Receives, processes, and maintains data chiefly from pharmacists in hospital, nursing home, and retail practice. **Pub:** *DQRS Annual Review.* • *Drug Utilization Annual Review.*

**★ 9062 ★ U.S. Department of Health and Human Services**
**Food and Drug Administration**
**Center for Drug Evaluation and Research**
**Office of Epidemiology and Biostatistics**
Mail Code HFD-700
5600 Fishers Ln., Rm. 15B45
Rockville, MD 20857
**Phone:** (301)827-3209     **Fax:** (301)480-2825
Dr. Robert O'Neill, Chf.

**Activities/Fields:** Provides statistical and computational support for the Center for Drug Evaluation and Research. Areas of interest are statistics and drug safety, efficacy and quality.

**★ 9063 ★ U.S. Department of Health and Human Services**
**Food and Drug Administration**
**Center for Drug Evaluation and Research**
**Office of Epidemiology and Biostatistics**
**(Statistical Evaluation and Research Branch)**
Mail Code HFD-713
5600 Fishers Ln., Rm. 18B45
Rockville, MD 20857
**Phone:** (301)443-4594     **Fax:** (301)443-9279
Dr. Satya D. Dubey, Chf.

**Activities/Fields:** Clinical trials for assessing the efficacy and safety of pharmaceuticals; and conducts research in statistical methodologies involving applications of computers in improving review, evaluation, and research methods.

**U.S. Department of Health and Human Services**
**National Cancer Institute**
**Division of Cancer Control and Population Sciences**
**Extramural Epidemiology and Genetics Program**
*See:* Entry 10440

**U.S. Department of Health and Human Services**
**National Cancer Institute**
**Division of Cancer Epidemiology and Genetics**
**Epidemiology and Biostatistics Program**
*See:* Entry 10442

**U.S. Department of Health and Human Services**
**National Center for Infectious Diseases**
**Division of Parasitic Diseases**
**Epidemiology Branch**
**(Parasitic Diseases Section)**
*See:* Entry 11893

**U.S. Department of Health and Human Services**
**National Heart, Lung, and Blood Institute**
**Division of Epidemiology and Clinical Applications**
*See:* Entry 5147

**U.S. Department of Health and Human Services**
**National Institute on Aging**
**Epidemiology, Demography, and Biometry Program**
*See:* Entry 3074

**★ 9064 ★ U.S. Department of Health and Human Services**
**National Institute of Allergy and Infectious Diseases**
**Division of Acquired Immunodeficiency Syndrome (AIDS)**
**Basic Science Program**
**(Epidemiology Branch)**
6700 B. Rockledge Dr., Rm. 4255
Bethesda, MD 20892
**Phone:** (301)402-0135     **Fax:** (301)402-3211
**Email:** cwilliams@niaid.nih.gov
**Website:** http://www.nia.nih.gov/research/intramural/edb
Dr. Carolyn Williams, Contact

**Activities/Fields:** Coordinates population-based research that will advance the understanding of the biology and clinical course of HIV infection. Serves as a foundation for advancing treatment and prevention.

**U.S. Department of Health and Human Services**
**National Institute of Dental Research**
**Division of Epidemiology and Oral Disease Prevention**
*See:* Entry 6616

**U.S. Department of Health and Human Services**
**National Institute of Mental Health**
**Epidemiology and Services Research Division**
*See:* Entry 12722

**U.S. Department of Health and Human Services**
**National Institute of Mental Health**
**Epidemiology and Services Research Division**
**Epidemiology and Psychopathology Research Branch**
*See:* Entry 12723

**U.S. Department of Health and Human Services**
**National Institute of Neurological Disorders and Stroke**
**Division of Intramural Research (Basic Neurosciences Program)**
**Neuroepidemiology Branch**
*See:* Entry 14307

**U.S. Department of Health and Human Services**
**National Institute for Occupational Safety and Health**
**Surveillance, Hazard Evaluations, and Field Studies Division**
**Industrywide Studies Branch**
*See:* Entry 16832

**U.S. Department of Health and Human Services**
**National Institutes of Health**
**National Eye Institute**
**Intramural Research**
**(Division of Epidemiology and Clinical Research)**
*See:* Entry 21163

**U.S. Department of Health and Human Services**
**National Institutes of Health**
**National Institute of Child Health and Human Development**
**Division of Intramural Research**
**((Division of Epidemiology, Statistics and Prevention Research)**
**Biometry and Mathematical Statistics Branch)**
*See:* Entry 17830

**★ 9065 ★ U.S. Department of Health and Human Services**
**National Institutes of Health**
**National Institute of Child Health and Human Development**
**Division of Intramural Research**
**(Division of Epidemiology, Statistics and Prevention Research)**
6100 Bldg., Rm. 7B05
MSC 7510
Bethesda, MD 20892-7510
**Phone:** (301)496-5064 **Fax:** (301)402-2084
**Email:** mk90h@nih.gov
**Website:** http://www.nichd.nih.gov/about/despr/despr.htm
Mark A. Klebanoff, MD, Dir.
**Activities/Fields:** Epidemiologic, behavioral and biometric studies relating to reproductive, maternal, and child health, particularly reproductive processes, pregnancy, infant mortality and morbidity, child growth and development, clinical trials, vaccinology, and community-based interventions designed to promote healthful behaviors.

**★ 9066 ★ U.S. Department of Health and Human Services**
**National Institutes of Health**
**National Institute of Dental and Craniofacial Research**
**Division of Intramural Research (Molecular and Genetic Epidemiology Section)**
Bldg. 45, Rm. 4AS-43G
45 Center Dr., MSC 6401
Bethesda, MD 20892-6401
**Phone:** (301)594-4830 **Fax:** (301)480-8327
**Email:** sd31d@nih.gov
**Website:** http://wwwdir.nidcr.nih.gov/dirweb/cegb/scott.asp
Dr. Scott R. Diehl, Contact
**Activities/Fields:** Basic causes of oral and craniofacial disorders, involving environmental risk factors such as smoking, drinking, and genetics. Research is focused on cleft lip and palate, Kartagener syndrome, early onset periodontitis, oral cancers, and nasopharyngeal carcinoma.

**★ 9067 ★ U.S. Department of Health and Human Services**
**National Institutes of Health**
**National Institute of Dental and Craniofacial Research**
**Division of Intramural Research (Craniofacial Epidemiology and Genetics Branch)**
Bldg. 30
30 Convent Dr., MSC 4326
Bethesda, MD 20892-4326
**Phone:** (301)496-1483 **Fax:** (301)402-1512
**Email:** henning.birkedal-hansen@nih.gov
**Website:** http://wwwdir.nidcr.nih.gov/dirweb/cegb/cegb.asp
Henning Birkedal-Hansen, DDS, Actg. Ch.
**Activities/Fields:** Seeks to improve and promote dental, oral and craniofacial health through epidemiology and health promotion.

**★ 9068 ★ U.S. Department of Health and Human Services**
**National Institutes of Health**
**National Institute of Diabetes and Digestive and Kidney Diseases**
**Division of Diabetes, Endocrinology, and Metabolic Diseases**
**(Epidemiology Type 2 Diabetes Research Program)**
MSC-5460
6707 Democracy Blvd., Rm. 695
Bethesda, MD 20892-5460
**Phone:** (301)594-8801 **Fax:** (301)480-3503
**Email:** harrisa@extra.niddk.nih.gov
**Website:** http://www.niddk.nih.gov/fund/program/A-Elist.htmepidT2
Maureen Harris, PhD, Dir.
**Activities/Fields:** Distribution and determinants of Type 2 diabetes, gestational diabetes, and complications of diabetes in populations, including community-based groups and large patient populations.

**★ 9069 ★ U.S. Department of Health and Human Services**
**National Institutes of Health**
**National Institute of Diabetes and Digestive and Kidney Diseases**
**Division of Diabetes, Endocrinology, and Metabolic Diseases**
**(Epidemiology Type 1 Diabetes Research Program)**
MSC-5460
6707 Democracy Blvd., Rm. 695
Bethesda, MD 20892-5460
**Phone:** (301)594-8801 **Fax:** (301)480-3503
**Email:** harrism@extra.niddk.nih.gov
**Website:** http://www.niddk.nih.gov/fund/program/a-elist.htmepidt1
Maureen Harris, PhD, Dir.
**Activities/Fields:** Distribution and determinants of Type 1 diabetes and its complications in populations, including community-based groups and large patient populations.

**★ 9070 ★ U.S. Department of Health and Human Services**
**National Institutes of Health**
**National Institute of Diabetes and Digestive and Kidney Diseases**
**Division of Digestive Diseases and Nutrition**
**(Epidemiology and Data Systems Program)**
MSC 5450
6707 Democracy Blvd., Rm. 673
Bethesda, MD 20892-5450
**Phone:** (301)594-8878 **Fax:** (301)480-8300
**Email:** everhartj@extra.niddk.nih.gov
**Website:** http://www.niddk.nih.gov/fund/program/A-Elist.htmDDNE
James Everhart, MD, Ch.
**Activities/Fields:** Collection, analysis, and dissemination of data on digestive diseases and their complications.

**★ 9071 ★ U.S. Department of Health and Human Services**
**National Institutes of Health**
**National Institute of Diabetes and Digestive and Kidney Diseases**
**Renal Diseases Epidemiology**
Natcher Bldg.
45 Center Dr.
Bethesda, MD 20892
**Email:** jonesc@extra.niddk.nih.gov
**Website:** http://www.niddk.nih.gov/fund/program/M-Rlist.htmRDEP
Camille A. Jones, MD, Dir.
**Activities/Fields:** Descriptive and analytic research, including development and analysis of surveillance databases, cross-sectional surveys, prospective observational studies, and case-control studies (for evaluating rare diseases). Key areas include disease prevention; developing early markers of injury; defining risk factors for morbidity and mortality; increasing evaluation of kidney disease measurements and outcomes in ongoing observational studies.

**★ 9072 ★ U.S. Department of Health and Human Services**
**National Institutes of Health**
**National Institute of Diabetes and Digestive and Kidney Diseases**
**Urologic Diseases Epidemiology Program**
2 Democracy Pl., Rm. 615
Bethesda, MD 20892
**Phone:** (301)594-8305
**Email:** eggersp@extra.niddk.nih.gov
**Website:** http://www.niddk.nih.gov/fund/program/S-Zlist.htmUDEP
Paul Eggers, PhD, Dir.
**Activities/Fields:** Dedicated to preventing disease, developing early markers of injury, defining risk factors for morbidity and mortality, and increasing evaluation of urologic disease measurements and outcomes in ongoing observational studies. Dedicated to increasing availability of epidemiologic data through new databases and full utilization of existing federal, state, and private sources of data.

**★ 9073 ★ U.S. Department of Health and Human Services**
**National Institutes of Health**
**National Institute of Environmental Health Sciences**
**Division of Extramural Research and Training**
**(Chemical Exposures and Molecular Biology Branch)**
PO Box 12233
Research Triangle Park, NC 27709
**Phone:** (919)541-4943　　　**Fax:** (919)316-4606
**Email:** dearry@niehs.nih.gov
**Website:** http://www.niehs.nih.gov/dert/dertcemb/cembb.htm
Dr. Allen Dearry, Ch.
**Activities/Fields:** Environmental chemical exposures, environmental and molecular epidemiology.


**★ 9074 ★ U.S. Department of Health and Human Services**
**National Institutes of Health**
**National Institute of Environmental Health Sciences**
**Epidemiology Branch**
M/D A3-05
PO Box 12233
Research Triangle Park, NC 27709
**Phone:** (919)541-4660　　　**Fax:** (919)541-2511
**Email:** wilcox@niehs.nih.gov
**Website:** http://dir.niehs.nih.gov/direb/
Allen J. Wilcox, Ch.
**Activities/Fields:** Reproductive epidemiology and environmental and molecular epidemiology.


**★ 9075 ★ University of Cincinnati**
**Division of Epidemiology and Biostatistics**
PO Box 670183
Cincinnati, OH 45267-0183
**Phone:** (513)558-1410　　　**Fax:** (513)558-4838
**Email:** charles.buncher@uc.edu
**Website:** http://www.uc.edu
Dr. C.R. Buncher, Hd.
**Activities/Fields:** Epidemiologic and biostatistical research, especially in environmental, occupational, and medical fields.


**★ 9076 ★ University of Connecticut Health Center**
**Center for Microbial Pathogenesis**
263 Farmington Ave.
Farmington, CT 06030
**Phone:** (860)679-8129　　　**Fax:** (860)679-8130
**Email:** swikel@up.uchc.edu
**Website:** http://cmp.uchc.edu/
Stephen Wikel, PhD, Dir.
**Activities/Fields:** Parasitic strategies which enable microbial pathogens to cause disease.


**University of Iowa**
**Center for Health Effects of Environmental Contamination (CHEEC)**
*See:* Entry 8983


**★ 9077 ★ University of Michigan**
**Michigan Bone Health Study**
Department of Epidemiology
School of Public Health
Ann Arbor, MI 48109-2029
**Phone:** (734)936-3892　　　**Fax:** (734)763-4552
**Email:** peter_weyer@uiowa.edu
**Website:** http://www.cheec.uiowa.edu
Mary Fran Sowers, PhD, Chm.
**Activities/Fields:** Epidemiology of health and disease, including investigation of origins, nature, and interrelations of major chronic disorders, particularly cardiovascular diseases, diabetes, arthritis, chronic respiratory diseases, and cancer. Also studies biological, social, and physical variables of chronic disease, including environmental factors and stresses as observed in families, households, and other subgroups of the population. Focuses on interactions between constitutional/genetic factors and environmental influences. The Tecumseh Community Health Study, a continuing multidisciplinary, multifaceted investigation, has been underway since 1957 in a total community of 10,000 inhabitants, with the aim of identifying disease precursors and indices of susceptibility as early in life as possible, with a view to prevention. **Frmly:** Tecumseh Community Health Study.


**★ 9078 ★ University of Pennsylvania**
**Center for Clinical Epidemiology and Biostatistics**
824 Blockley Hall
Sch. of Medicine
423 Guardian Dr.
Philadelphia, PA 19104-6021
**Phone:** (215)898-2368　　　**Fax:** (215)573-5315
**Email:** bstrom@cceb.med.upenn.edu
**Website:** http://cceb.med.upenn.edu
Dr. Brian L. Strom, Dir.
**Activities/Fields:** Epidemiology of disease and risk factors of clinical importance, especially pharamacoepidemiology, molecular epidemiology, cancer, cardiovascular disease, renal disease, women's health, reproductive epidemiology, emergency medicine, injury, and aging. **Frmly:** Clinical Epidemiology Unit.


**★ 9079 ★ University of Pittsburgh**
**Nutrition Biochemistry Laboratory**
503 Parran Hall
Department of Epidemiology
Graduate Sch. of Public Health
Pittsburgh, PA 15261
**Phone:** (412)624-2020　　　**Fax:** (412)624-3120
Dr. Rhobert Evans, Dir.
**Activities/Fields:** Etiology and treatment of chronic diseases, including study of lipids, lipoproteins, osteoporsis, diabetes, hypertension, cancer, and aging.


**★ 9080 ★ University of Quebec**
**National Institute for Scientific Research-Armand-Frappier Institute**
**Epidemiology and Biostatistics Unit**
531 Blvd. des Prairies
Laval, QC, Canada H7V 1B7
**Phone:** (450)687-5010　　　**Fax:** (450)686-5501
**Email:** Jack_Siemiatycki@iaf.uquebec.ca
Dr. Jack Siemiatycki, Dir.
**Activities/Fields:** Epidemiological studies on cancer and other chronic diseases. Research focuses on occupational and environmental risk factors for cancer and juvenile onset diabetes mellitus II, water quality and gastrointestinal illness, air pollution and human health, and data collection and methodological issues in statistical analysis. **Frmly:** Epidemiology and Preventive Medicine Research Centre.


**★ 9081 ★ University of Southern California**
**International Twin Study**
1441 Eastlake Ave.
Los Angeles, CA 90033
**Phone:** (323)865-0445　　　**Fax:** (323)865-0141
**Email:** tmack@usc.edu
Dr. Thomas Mack, Dir.
**Activities/Fields:** Epidemiologic investigation of the etiology of various chronic diseases in twins, including cancers (breast, gastrointestinal tract, and melanoma), multiple sclerosis, diabetes, and other chronic diseases.


**University of Texas—Houston Health Science Center**
**Human Genetics Center**
*See:* Entry 9519


**★ 9082 ★ University of Toronto**
**Centre for Health Promotion**
**Ontario Tobacco Research Unit**
33 Russell St.
Toronto, ON, Canada M5S 2S1
**Phone:** (416)595-6888　　　**Fax:** (416)595-6068
**Email:** otru@camh.net
**Website:** http://www.camh.net/otru
Roberta Ferrence, Dir.
**Activities/Fields:** Tobacco control, including epidemiology of tobacco use and cessation, tobacco and youth, gender issues in tobacco use, ethnicity and tobacco use, economic factors in tobacco use, tobacco policy attitudes, policy and program evaluation, community interventions, and enviromental tobacco smoke. **Pub:** *Current Abstracts on Tobacco.* • *Directory, literature reviews, special reports, annotated bibliographies, information updates.* • *Working papers.*


**★ 9083 ★ Utah State University**
**Institute for Antiviral Research**
5600 Old Main Hill
Logan, UT 84322-5600
**Phone:** (435)797-1902　　　**Fax:** (435)797-3959
**Email:** rsidwell@cc.usu.edu
**Website:** http://www.usu.edu/iar/index.html
Dr. Robert W. Sidwell, Dir.
**Activities/Fields:** Control of viral diseases. **Pub:** *Reports.*


**★ 9084 ★ Virginia Health and Human Resources Secretariat**
**Health Department**
**Epidemiology Office**
1500 E Main St.
PO Box 2448
Richmond, VA 23219
**Phone:** (434)786-6029　　　**Fax:** (434)786-1076
**Email:** rstroube@vdh.state.va.us
Dr. Robert Stroube, Dir.
**Activities/Fields:** Epidemiology.

## Federal Government Agencies

**U.S. Department of Health and Human Services**
**National Institutes of Health (NIH)**
**National Institute of Diabetes, Digestive and Kidney Diseases (NIDDK)**
*See:* Entry 8657

## Foundations & Other Funding Organizations

### Other Funding Organizations

★ **9085** ★ **American Gastroenterological Association (AGA)**
7910 Woodmont Ave., 7th Fl.
Bethesda, MD 20814
**Phone:** (301)654-2055     **Fax:** (301)652-3890
**Email:** webinfo@gastro.org
**Website:** http://www.gastro.org
D. Montgomery Bissell, MD, Vice Chair
**Desc:** Physicians of internal medicine certified in gastroenterology; radiologists, pathologists, surgeons, and physiologists with special interest and competency in gastroenterology. Studies normal and abnormal conditions of the digestive organs and problems connected with their metabolism; conducts scientific research; offers placement services. **Awards:** Advanced Research Training Award (annual) for advanced fellow, usually in second full research year; Elsevier Research Initiative Award for junior faculty, senior faculty, or established investigator; Fiterman Clinical Research Award (annual) for senior faculty or established investigator; Funderberg Scholar Award for junior faculty, senior faculty, or established investigator; Industry Research Scholar Award (annual) for junior faculty; International Travel Award for junior faculty, senior faculty, or established investigator; Sponsored Symposia (biennial) for senior faculty or established investigator; Student Abstract Prize for high school, undergraduate, medical, and graduate students; Student Research Fellowship Award (annual) for high school undergraduate, medical, and graduate students.

★ **9086** ★ **American Lithotripsy Society (ALS)**
305 Second Ave., Ste. 200
Waltham, MA 02451
**Phone:** (781)895-9098     **Fax:** (781)895-9088
**Email:** als@lithotripsy.org
**Website:** http://www.lithotripsy.org
Wesley E. Harrington, CAE, Contact
**Desc:** Promotes trade and public awareness of Lithotripsy. (Lithotripsy is a non-invasive procedure to treat kidney stones and gall stones.) Disseminates information; conducts educational programs, quality improvement and certification programs. **Awards:** Distinguished Guest Lecturer (annual).

★ **9087** ★ **Crohn's and Colitis Foundation of America (CCFA)**
386 Park Ave. S, 17th Fl.
New York, NY 10016-8804
**Phone:** (212)685-3440     **Free:** 800-932-2423
**Fax:** (212)779-4098
**Email:** info@ccfa.org
**Website:** http://www.ccfa.org
Rodger L. DeRose, CEO
**Desc:** Supports research to find the cause and cure of Crohn's Disease (ileitis) and ulcerative colitis. Provides educational programs for patients, physicians, and the public, support groups, chapter newsletters, a national magazine, informational brochures and books, professional medical forums, and research publications, and a website. **Awards:** Research Fellowship (semiannual) for training; Research Grant (semiannual) for research.

## National & International Organizations

★ **9088** ★ **Alagille Syndrome Alliance (ASA)**
c/o Cindy L. Hahn
10630 SW Garden Park Pl.
Tigard, OR 97223
**Phone:** (503)639-6217
**Email:** alagille@earthlink.net
**Website:** http://www.alagille.org
Cindy L. Hahn, Pres.
**Fnded:** 1993. **Desc:** Works to provide a support network for family, friends and healthcare providers as well as children and adults with Alagille Syndrome, a liver disorder affecting the bile ducts and/or the pulmonary arteries, heart and lungs, spinal column, eyes, facial features and less frequently, the pancreas, renal system and arteries in the brain. **Pub:** *Fact Sheet.* • *LiverLink*, bimonthly. Newsletter. Back issues are available. • Brochure.Available for schools.

★ **9089** ★ **American Association for the Study of Liver Diseases (AASLD)**
1729 King St.
Alexandria, VA 22314
**Phone:** (703)299-9766     **Fax:** (703)299-9622
**Email:** lclaassen@aasld.org
**Website:** http://www.aasld.org
Sherrie H. Cathcart, Exec. Dir.
**Fnded:** 1950. **Mem:** 2,300. **Nat'l Groups:** 1. **Desc:** The leading organization focused solely on the science and practice of hepatology, promoting liver wellness and high-quality, cost-effective, compassionate care of patients with hepatobiliary diseases. **Pub:** *Hepatology*, monthly. Journal. • *Liver Transplantation and Surgery*, monthly. Journal. • Newsletter, bimonthly.

**American Board of Colon and Rectal Surgery (ABCRS)**
*See:* Entry 19475

**American Broncho-Esophagological Associat ion (ABEA)**
*See:* Entry 18729

★ **9090** ★ **American Celiac Society/ Dietary Support Coalition (ACS/DSC)**
59 Crystal Ave.
West Orange, NJ 07052-3570
**Phone:** (973)325-8837     **Fax:** (973)669-8808
**Email:** amerceliacsoc@netscape.net
**Website:** http://www.abea.net/
Annette Bentley, Exec. Officer
**Fnded:** 1970. **Mem:** 7,000. **Nat'l Groups:** 4. **Reg. Groups:** 76. **Local Groups:** 57. **Desc:** Individuals interested in a gluten-free diet; physicians who diagnose and care for individuals with gluten-sensitive intestinal disease, dietitians, nutritionists, and agencies that serve or have an interest in individuals with gluten-sensitive enteropathy, also known as celiac sprue. Provides information on how to follow a gluten-free diet; assists members in locating specialty foods that are gluten-free; encourages retailers to make gluten-free products available. Coordinates activities with other international celiac societies. Maintains speakers' bureau for patients and health care professionals. **Pub:** *Whoo's Report*, 3/year. Newsletter. **Frmly:** (1990) America Celiac Society.

★ **9091** ★ **American College of Gastroenterology (ACG)**
4900B S 31st St.
Arlington, VA 22206-1656
**Phone:** (703)820-7400     **Fax:** (703)931-4520
**Website:** http://www.acg.gi.org
Thomas F. Fise, Dir.
**Fnded:** 1932. **Mem:** 7,000. **Desc:** Professional society of physicians and surgeons specializing in diseases and disorders of the gastrointestinal tract and accessory organs of digestion, including disorders due to nutrition. **Pub:** *American Journal of Gastroenterology*, monthly. Journal. **Frmly:** (1934) Society for the Advancement of Gastroenterology; (1954) National Gastroenterological Association.

★ **9092** ★ **American Gastroenterological Association (AGA)**
7910 Woodmont Ave., 7th Fl.
Bethesda, MD 20814
**Phone:** (301)654-2055     **Fax:** (301)652-3890
**Email:** webinfo@gastro.org
**Website:** http://www.gastro.org
D. Montgomery Bissell, MD, Vice Chair
**Fnded:** 1897. **Mem:** 8,600. **Desc:** Physicians of internal medicine certified in gastroenterology; radiolo-

gists, pathologists, surgeons, and physiologists with special interest and competency in gastroenterology. Studies normal and abnormal conditions of the digestive organs and problems connected with their metabolism; conducts scientific research; offers placement services. **Pub:** *AGA News*, monthly. *Price:* Included in membership dues. • *Directory of Researchers in Gastroenterology*, annual. Directory. • *Gastroenterology*, monthly. *Price:* $135 for individuals; $212 for institutions.

### ★ 9093 ★ American Liver Foundation (ALF)
75 Maiden Ln., Ste. 603
New York, NY 10038
**Phone:** (212)668-1000　　　　**Free:** 800-223-0179
**Fax:** (212)483-8179
**Email:** webmail@liverfoundation.org
**Website:** http://www.liverfoundation.org
Alan P. Brownstein, Pres.

**Fnded:** 1976. **Mem:** 24,000. **Desc:** Health agency working to fund research, promote the understanding and prevention of hepatitis and other liver diseases, and find cures for hepatitis and other liver diseases. Disseminates public and patient information on liver diseases, liver functions, and preventive measures. Provides information about support groups for liver disease patients and their families. Offers physician referral service. Sponsors seminars on disease diagnosis and management for physicians and other health professionals. Sponsors programs, which enables liver disease patients and concerned individuals to meet specialists and learn of recently developed information on treatment and research. Operates continuing organ donor awareness campaign in order to increase the number of organs available for transplant; monitors legislation (nationally and regionally) in areas affecting liver patients. Serves as trustee of funds raised to cover costs related to liver transplant surgery. Sponsors Corporate Wellness Program to provide information on liver disease for use in employee publications. **Pub:** *American Liver Foundation–Annual Report. Price:* Free. • *American Liver Foundation–Progress*, 3/year. Newsletter. Covers foundation programs; reports on research, news of liver diseases. *Price:* Included in membership dues. • *Liver Update: Function and Disease*, semiannual. Newsletter. *Price:* Included in membership dues. • Also publishes brochures, leaflets, and information sheets.

### ★ 9094 ★ American Motility Society (AMS)
230 E Ohio St., Ste. 400
Chicago, IL 60611-3265
**Phone:** (312)644-0828　　　　**Fax:** (312)644-8557
**Email:** ams@bostrom.com
James Ryan, PhD, Treas.

**Fnded:** 1980. **Mem:** 220. **Desc:** Professionals interested in the study of gastrointestinal (GI) motility. Promotes basic science and clinical research on the neural, humoral, and paracrine control of GI tract motility in health and disease.

### American Society of Abdominal Surgeons (ASAS)
*See:* Entry 19488

### ★ 9095 ★ American Society for Gastrointestinal Endoscopy (ASGE)
13 Elm St.
Manchester, MA 01944-1314
**Phone:** (978)526-8330　　　　**Fax:** (978)526-4018
**Email:** asge@shore.net
**Website:** http://www.asge.org
William T. Maloney, Exec. Dir.

**Fnded:** 1941. **Mem:** 7,300. **Desc:** Gastroenterologists, internists, and surgeons who perform gastroscopic, esophagoscopic, coloscopic, and peritoneoscopic examinations. Works to further the knowledge of digestive disease by endoscopic methods (visual inspection of the intestinal tract). **Pub:** *Gastrointestinal*

*Endoscopy*, bimonthly. Journal. Includes index, book reviews, case reports, and new materials and methods. *Price:* Included in membership dues. **Frmly:** American Gastroscopic Club; American Gastroscopic Society.

### ★ 9096 ★ Argentine Society of Gastroenterology (Sociedad Argentina de Gastroenterologia)
Santa Fe 1171
1059 Buenos Aires, Argentina
**Phone:** 54 1 411633
**Fnded:** 1927.

### ★ 9097 ★ Asian Federation of Coloproctology (AFC)
Mackay Memorial Hospital, Apt. 92 - Section II
Chung-San N Rd.
Taipei, Taiwan
**Phone:** 886 2 543355　　　　**Fax:** 886 2 5433642
**Lang(s):** Chinese, English. **Desc:** Coloproctologists. Seeks to advance the study, teaching, and practice of coloproctology; encourages continuing professional development of members. Formulates and enforces standards of coloproctological practice; sponsors training courses.

### ★ 9098 ★ Asian Ostomy Association (AOA)
11. Rd. 12, Minden Heights
Gelugor
11700 Penang, Malaysia
**Phone:** 60 4 6572717　　　　**Fax:** 60 4 2618691
**Lang(s):** English, Malay. **Desc:** Physicians and other health care personnel with an interest in ostomy and the care of ostomy patients. Seeks to improve the quality of life of ostomy patients; promotes advancement in the practice of ostomy medicine. Serves as a clearinghouse on ostomy; sponsors research and continuing professional development programs.

### ★ 9099 ★ Asian Pacific Association for the Study of the Liver (APASL)
c/o Academy of Medicine
College of Medicine Bldg.
16 College Rd., Ste. 01-01
Singapore 169854, Singapore
**Phone:** 65 2238968　　　　**Fax:** 65 2255155
**Lang(s):** Chinese, English. **Desc:** Physicians, hepatologists, and other health care professionals and scientists with an interest in the liver and its functions. Seeks to advance the hepatological scholarship. Facilitates exchange of information among members; conducts research and educational programs.

### Asian Pan-Pacific Society for Paediatric Gastroenterology and Nutrition
*See:* Entry 5619

### Asian Society for Hepato-Biliary-Pancreatic Surgery (ASHBPS)
*See:* Entry 19510

### ★ 9100 ★ Association of European Coeliac Societies (AECS)
Ave. Louis Bertrand 100, Boite A20
B-1030 Brussels, Belgium
**Phone:** 32 2 2168347　　　　**Fax:** 32 2 2168347
**Email:** hbp2001@cuhk.edu.hk

**Lang(s):** English, French. **Desc:** Health care professionals with an interest in coeliac disease and related disorders; individuals with coeliac disease and their families. Promotes improved diagnosis and treatment of coeliac disease; seeks to improve the quality of life of people with coeliac disease. Facilitates exchange of information among health researchers and practition-

ers working with coeliac disease; provides support and services to people with coeliac disease.

### ★ 9101 ★ Association of Gastrointestinal Motility Disorders (AGMD)
11 North St.
Lexington, MA 02420
**Phone:** (781)861-3874
**Email:** AGMDInc@aol.com
**Website:** http://www.digestivemotility.org
Mary-Angela DeGrazia-DiTucci, Pres. -CEO

**Fnded:** 1991. **Mem:** 550. **Desc:** Non-profit international organization which serves as an integral educational resource concerning digestive motility disorders. Also functions as an important information base for members of the medical community. **Pub:** *AGMD Beacon*, quarterly. Newsletter. Updates members about organization and medical alerts. *Price:* included in membership dues. • *AGMD Search and Research*, quarterly. Newsletter. Poses questions from members and provides responses. • Bulletin, quarterly. Updates professional members about organization and medical alerts. • Also publishes educational materials concerning digestive motility disorders and diseases. **Frmly:** (2000) American Society of Adults with Pseudo-Obstruction.

### ★ 9102 ★ Association of National, European and Mediterranean Societies of Gastroenterology (Association des Societes Nationales, Europeennes et Mediterraneennes de Gastroenterologie — ASNEMGE)
c/o Margariet van Dijk-Meijer
Wolkendek 5
NL-3454 TG De Meern, Netherlands
**Phone:** 31 30 6667400　　　　**Fax:** 31 30 6622808
**Email:** info@asnemge.org
**Website:** http://www.ashemge.org

**Fnded:** 1947. **Mem:** 37. **Reg. Groups:** 1. **Lang(s):** English, French, German. **Desc:** A branch of the World Organization of Gastroenterology. National societies for gastroenterology in 37 European and Mediterranean countries. Promotes the exchange of scientific information in the field of gastroenterology and co-organizer of yearly United European Gastroenterology week. **Pub:** Proceedings, quadrennial.

### ★ 9103 ★ Bockus International Society of Gastroenterology (BISG)
300 Community Dr.
Manhasset, NY 11030
**Phone:** (516)562-4281　　　　**Fax:** (516)663-4617
**Email:** bernste@nshs.edu
Dr. David Bernstein, Sec. Gen.

**Fnded:** 1958. **Mem:** 440. **Nat'l Groups:** 1. **Desc:** Physicians in 22 countries specializing in gastroenterology (the study of the anatomy, physiology, and pathology of the stomach and intestines). Furthers scientific advances in gastroenterology worldwide. (The society is named for noted gastroenterologist H.L. Bockus of Philadelphia, PA.) **Pub:** Proceedings, biennial.

### ★ 9104 ★ British Colostomy Association
15 Station Rd.
Reading RG1 1LG, United Kingdom
**Phone:** 44 118 9391537　　　　**Fax:** 44 118 9569095
**Email:** sue@bcass.org.uk
**Website:** http://www.bcass.org.uk

**Fnded:** 1967. **Mem:** 13,500. **Reg. Groups:** 26. **Lang(s):** English. **Desc:** Anyone who has a colostomy and/or their carer. Exists to offer help and encouragement to anyone who has had or is about to have a colostomy. Home and hospital visits by arrangement. **Pub:** *Living With a Colostomy.* Booklet. • *Tidings*, semiannual. Newsletter.

**★ 9105 ★ British Society of Gastroenterology**
3 St Andrews Pl.
London NW1 4LB, United Kingdom
**Phone:** 44 171 3873534 **Fax:** 44 171 4873734
**Email:** bsg@mailbox.ulcc.ac.uk
**Website:** http://www.bsg.org.uk
**Fnded:** 1937. **Mem:** 2,400. **Reg. Groups:** 16. **Desc:** Physicians and surgeons with a special interest in gastroenterology. Associate nurse/clinical members. Concerned with the advancement of gastroenterology and the promotion of friendship amongst those who have a special interest in the subject. **Pub:** *Gut*, monthly.

**★ 9106 ★ Canadian Association of Gastroenterology (CAG) (Association Canadienne de Gastroenterologie — ACG)**
2902 S Sheridan Way
Oakville, ON, Canada L6J 7L6
**Phone:** (905)829-2504 **Fax:** (905)829-0242
**Email:** cagoffice@cag-acg.org
**Website:** http://www.cag-acg.org
**Lang(s):** English, French. **Desc:** Gastroenterologists and other health care professionals with an interest in gastroenterology. Seeks to advance gastroenterological practice. Conducts continuing professional education programs.

**Canadian Association of Nephrology Nurses and Technologists (CANNT)**
*See:* Entry 15679

**★ 9107 ★ Canadian Celiac Association (CCA) (L'Association Canadienne de la Maladie Coeliaque — ACMC)**
5170 Dixie Rd., Ste. 204
Mississauga, ON, Canada L4W 1E3
**Phone:** (905)507-6208 **Free:** 800-363-7296
**Fax:** (905)507-4673
**Email:** celiac@look.ca
**Website:** http://www.celiac.ca
**Fnded:** 1926. **Mem:** 6,000. **Nat'l Groups:** 1. **Reg. Groups:** 25. **Lang(s):** English, French. **Desc:** Individuals with celiac sprue; health care professionals with an interest in gastrointestinal diseases. Seeks to improve the quality of life of people with celiac sprue and related disorders; promotes advancement in the diagnosis and treatment of gastrointestinal maladies. Provides support and assistance to people with celiac sprue and related disorders; conducts research and educational programs. **Pub:** *Celiac News*, 3/year. Newsletter.

**Canadian Society of Gastroenterology Nurses and Associates (CSGNA)**
*See:* Entry 15697

**★ 9108 ★ Celiac Disease Foundation (CDF)**
13251 Ventura Blvd., Ste. 1
Studio City, CA 91604-1838
**Phone:** (818)990-2354 **Fax:** (818)990-2379
**Email:** cdf@celiac.org
**Website:** http://www.celiac.org
Elaine Monarch, Exec. Dir.
**Fnded:** 1990. **Desc:** Provides services and support for persons with Celiac Disease/Dermatitis Herpetiformis (CD/DH) through programs of education advocacy, and research; telephone information and referral services; medical advisory board; and special educational seminars and general meetings. (CD is a digestive disorder found in genetically susceptible individuals, in which the surface of the small intestine is damaged by the ingestion of food products containing proteins commonly known as gluten. Toxic glutens are found in all forms of wheat, rye, barley, and possibly oats.) **Pub:** *Celiac Disease Foundation Newsletter*, quarterly.

Newsletter. Includes information about the disease, treatment, nutrition, food and drug updates, support articles, and recipes. *Price:* Included in membership dues.

**★ 9109 ★ Celiac Sprue Association/ United States of America (CSA/USA)**
PO Box 31700
Omaha, NE 68131-0700
**Phone:** (402)558-0600 **Fax:** (402)558-1347
**Email:** celiacs@csaceliacs.org
**Website:** http://www.csaceliacs.org
Mary Schluckebier, Exec. Dir.
**Fnded:** 1986. **Mem:** 9,143. **Nat'l Groups:** 1. **Reg. Groups:** 6. **State Groups:** 6. **Local Groups:** 90. **Desc:** Individuals with the conditions of celiac sprue and dermatitis herpetiformis; parents of celiac children. (Celiac sprue is a genetic disorder resulting in digestive malabsorption of the protein portion of wheat, rye, and other cereal grains, causing symptoms such as intestinal lesions, diarrhea, vomiting, weight loss, and abdominal discomfort; dermatitis herpetiformis is a gluten-related skin disorder. Successful treatment usually calls for removing all gluten-containing cereal grains and their derivatives from the diet.) Serves as a vehicle for the provision of mutual support groups and facilitates interaction with other organizations involved in digestive disorders. Encourages and supports research on celiac disease. Disseminates educational materials on gluten-free foods and research on results; exchanges information on maintaining a gluten-free diet. **Pub:** *Cookbooks for Diets Free of Cereal Grains*. Books. • *Lifeline*, quarterly. Newsletter. • *On the Celiac Condition: A Handbook for Celiacs and Their Families, 2nd Ed.*. Handbook. • Brochures. • Pamphlets. **Frmly:** (1979) Midwestern Celiac Sprue Association.

**★ 9110 ★ Chron's and Colitits Foundation of America (CCFA)**
386 Park Ave. South, 17th Fl.
New York, NY 10016-8840
**Phone:** (212)685-3440 **Free:** 800-932-2423
**Fax:** (212)779-4098
**Email:** info@ccfa.org
**Website:** http://www.ccfa.org/
**Fnded:** 1967. **Nat'l Groups:** 55. **Desc:** Lay and physician volunteers. Dedicated to improving the quality of life for persons with Crohn's disease or ulcerative colitis, collectively known as inflammatory bowel diseases (IBD). **Pub:** *Foundation Focus*. Magazine. Contains in-depth features about research and coping issues.

**★ 9111 ★ Coeliac Society of the United Kingdom (CSUK)**
Box 220
High Wycombe HP11 2HY, United Kingdom
**Phone:** 44 1494 437278 **Fax:** 44 1494 474349
**Email:** admin@coeliac.co.uk
**Website:** http://www.coeliac.co.uk
**Mem:** 30,000. **Local Groups:** 55. **Desc:** National support organisation for people with intolerance to Gluten. **Pub:** *List of Gluten-Free Manufactured Products*, annual. Directory. Directory of manufacturers and suppliers.

**★ 9112 ★ Crohn's and Colitis Foundation of America (CCFA)**
386 Park Ave. S, 17th Fl.
New York, NY 10016-8804
**Phone:** (212)685-3440 **Free:** 800-932-2423
**Fax:** (212)779-4098
**Email:** info@ccfa.org
**Website:** http://www.ccfa.org
Rodger L. DeRose, CEO
**Fnded:** 1967. **Mem:** 60,000. **State Groups:** 55. **Local Groups:** 300. **Desc:** Supports research to find the cause and cure of Crohn's Disease (ileitis) and ulcerative colitis. Provides educational programs for patients, physicians, and the public, support groups, chapter newsletters, a national magazine, information-

al brochures and books, professional medical forums, and research publications, and a website. **Pub:** *Foundation Focus*, 3/year. Magazine. Contains personal accounts of persons living with colitis and ileitis. *Price:* Included in membership dues. • *Inflammatory Bowel Disease: A Guide for Patients and Their Families*. Book. • *Inflammatory Bowel Diseases*, quarterly. Journal. • *Managing Your Child's Crohn's Disease or Ulcerative Colitis*. Book. • *The New People Not Patients: A Source Book for Living with IBD*. Book. **Frmly:** (1969) Foundation for Ileitis and Colitis; (1992) National Foundation for Ileitis and Colitis.

**Cystic Fibrosis Foundation (CFF)**
*See:* Entry 9316

**★ 9113 ★ Danish Society of Gastroenterology (Dansk Gastroenterologisk Selskab — DGS)**
Kohenhavns Amts Sygehus Herlev
DK-2730 Herlev, Denmark
**Email:** info@cff.org
**Website:** http://www.cff.org
**Fnded:** 1970.

**★ 9114 ★ Digestive Disease National Coalition (DDNC)**
507 Capital Court NE, Ste. 200
Washington, DC 20002
**Phone:** (202)544-7497 **Fax:** (202)546-7105
**Website:** http://www.ddnc.org
Dale P. Dirks, Washington Rep.
**Fnded:** 1979. **Mem:** 30. **Desc:** Lay and professional medical organizations concerned with digestive diseases. Objectives are to: inform the public and the health care community about digestive diseases and related nutrition; seek federal funding for research, education, and training. Represents members' interests regarding federal and state legislation that affects digestive diseases research, health care, and education. **Frmly:** (1986) Coalition of Digestive Disease Organizations.

**★ 9115 ★ Digestive Disorders Foundation**
PO Box 251
Edgware
Middlesex HA8 6HG, United Kingdom
**Phone:** 44 20 74860341 **Fax:** 44 20 72242012
**Email:** ddf@digestivedisorders.org.uk
**Website:** http://www.digestivedisorders.org.uk
**Fnded:** 1971. **Reg. Groups:** 3. **Desc:** Aims to raise money for research into disorders of the gastrointestinal tract, liver and pancreas. Patient information leaflets are available on receipt of a stamped self-addressed envelope. These cover the most common digestive disorders. **Pub:** *Annual Review*, annual.

**★ 9116 ★ European Association for the Study of the Liver (EASL)**
149, rue de Sevres
F- 75747 Paris, France
**Phone:** 33 1 44495126 **Fax:** 33 1 44495165
**Email:** isabelle.porteret@nck.ap-hop-paris.fr
**Fnded:** 1966.

**★ 9117 ★ European Gastro Club**
c/o Prof. Wolfram Domschke, MD
Department of Medicine
University of Munster
Albert-Schweitzer-Str. 33
D-48129 Munster, Germany
**Phone:** 49 251 8347661 **Fax:** 49 251 8347570
**Email:** domschke@uni-muenster.de
**Fnded:** 1968. **Mem:** 52. **Nat'l Groups:** 20. **Desc:** Promotes exchange of scientific information regarding the stomach and its diseases from various points of view, including: epidemiology, morphology, physiology, biochemistry, immunology, cell and molecular

biology, and clinics. Fosters exchange of information among members.

## ★ 9118 ★ European Hernia Society (Groupe de recherche europeen sur la paroi abdominale — GREPA)

74, rue Marcel Cachin
F-93017 Bobigny, France
**Phone:** 33 1 48369722 **Fax:** 33 1 48369731
**Email:** chevrel@compuserve.com
**Fnded:** 1978. **Desc:** Promotes research on all anatomic, physiologic and pathologic problems relating to the abdominal wall.

## ★ 9119 ★ European Ostomy Association

c/o Deutsche ILCO
PO Box 1265
D-85112 Freising, Germany
**Phone:** 49 81 61934301 **Fax:** 49 81 61934304
**Email:** info@ilco.de
**Website:** http://www.ilco.de
**Desc:** Umbrella ostomy Association that provides "member Associations information and management guidelines, helps to inform new ostomy Associations, and advocates on all related matters and policies."

## ★ 9120 ★ European Society of Comparative Gastroenterology (ESCG)

50, rue Jeanne d'Arc
F-69003 Lyon, France

## ★ 9121 ★ European Society of Neurogastroenterology and Gastrointestinal Motility

Herestr 49
3000 Leuven, Belgium
**Fax:** 32 1 6345757
**Email:** theo.peeters@med.kuleuven.ac.be
**Website:** http://www.neurogastro.org/
**Fnded:** 1981. **Desc:** Promotes research in the field of gastrointestinal motility; forum for presentation or discussion.

## ★ 9122 ★ European Society of Paediatric Gastroenterology, Hepatology and Nutrition (ESPGHAN)

c/o Prof. Dr. M.J. Lentze
Children's Hospital Medical Center of the University of Bonn
Bonn, Germany
**Phone:** 49 228 2873213 **Fax:** 49 228 2873314
**Email:** lentze@mailer.meb.uni-bonn.de
**Fnded:** 1968. **Mem:** 300. **Desc:** Works to establish uniform nutrition standards for children in Europe. Fosters the improved treatment of gastrointestinal diseases of children. Promotes scientific exchange among research groups in Europe. Offers training programs and workshops for physicians.

## ★ 9123 ★ European Society for Primary Care Gastroenterology

c/o Christine van der Laan
Department of General Practice
PO Box 80045
3508 BA Utrecht, Netherlands
**Phone:** 31 30 2538195 **Fax:** 31 30 2539028
**Email:** webmaster@espcg.org
**Website:** http://www.espcg.org
**Desc:** Promotes high standards in the management of gastrointestinal problems in primary care throughout Europe.

## ★ 9124 ★ Foundation for Digestive Health and Nutrition (FDHN)

7910 Woodmont Ave., Ste. 610
Bethesda, MD 20814-3015
**Phone:** (301)222-4002 **Fax:** (301)222-4010
**Email:** info@fdhn.org
**Website:** http://www.fdhn.org
David Lee, Dir. Operations
**Fnded:** 2001. **Desc:** FDHN is the foundation of the American Gastroenterological Association. The goal of the FDHN is to be the largest source of funds for research and public education in digestive diseases. **Frmly:** (2001) American Digestive Health Foundation.

## ★ 9125 ★ Gastro-Intestinal Research Foundation (GIRF)

c/o Joseph B. Kirsner, M.D.
70 E Lake St., Ste. 1015
Chicago, IL 60601-5907
**Phone:** (312)332-1350
**Email:** girf@girf.org
**Website:** http://www.girf.org
Joseph B. Kirsner, MD, Contact
**Fnded:** 1967. **Desc:** Physician-clinicians and physician-scientists. Committed to the goal of solving the problems of digestive diseases.

## ★ 9126 ★ Gluten Intolerance Group of North America (GIGNA)

15110 10th Ave., SW
Ste. A
Seattle, WA 98116-1820
**Phone:** (206)246-6652 **Fax:** (206)246-6531
**Email:** info@gluten.net
**Website:** http://www.gluten.net
Cynthia Kupper, CRD, CDE, Exec. Dir.
**Fnded:** 1974. **Mem:** 2,000. **Local Groups:** 2. **Desc:** Persons with gluten-sensitive enteropathy (celiac sprue) or dermatitis herpetiformis, family members, physicians, dietitians, and celiac sprue societies. (Gluten is a protein found in wheat, rye, oats, and barley. Gluten-sensitive enteropathy is an inherited disorder characterized by gluten-related destruction of the small intestine. Symptoms include diarrhea, weight loss, fatigue, and anemia.) Works to educate patients, health care personnel, and the public; to offer psychological support to celiac sprue patients and their families in dealing with the adjustment and nutritional limitations of the disease; to conduct research into the causes. Promotes practical application in specific food research, such as recipe development and information on gluten content of products. Offers children's services and group and individual counseling. **Pub:** *GIG Cookbook*. Book. Contains instructions for a gluten-free diet. *Price:* $22.50. • *GIG Newsletter*, quarterly. Newsletter. Provides book reviews, product information, recipes, and research reports to help in monitoring diets for persons with celiac sprue and dermatitis. *Price:* $30/year in U.S. • Videos. • Also publishes cookbook and fact sheets. **Frmly:** (1985) Gluten Intolerance Group.

## ★ 9127 ★ Hepatitis Foundation International

c/o Martha Young
504 Elick Dr.
Silver Spring, MD 20904
**Phone:** (973)239-1035 **Free:** 800-891-0707
**Fax:** (973)857-5044
**Email:** mail@hepfi.org
**Website:** http://www.hepfi.org
Thelma King Thiel, Chm. and C. E. O.
**Fnded:** 1994. **Mem:** 50,000. **Local Groups:** 425. **Desc:** Individuals concerned about those with hepatitis. Provides education and information for distribution to the general public, patients, educators, and medical professionals about the diagnosis, treatment, and prevention of viral hepatitis. Maintains database of hepatitis support groups and website information. Conducts train-the-trainer programs for those interested in the topic. **Pub:** *Hepatitis Alers*, quarterly. Newsletter. Contains current articles about the latest research and developments in combating viral hepatitis.

## ★ 9128 ★ Hong Kong Society of Gastroenterology (HKSG)

Room 1203, Bank of America Tower
12 Harcourt Rd. Central
Hong Kong, People's Republic of China
**Phone:** 852 28695933 **Fax:** 852 28699533
**Email:** gastro@netvigator.com
**Website:** http://www.fmshk.com.hk/hksg
**Fnded:** 1981. **Mem:** 155. **Lang(s):** Chinese, English.
**Desc:** Gastroenterologists and other individuals with an interest in gastroenterology. Seeks to advance gastroenterological research, teaching, and practice; promotes continuing professional development among members. Serves as a clearinghouse on gastroenterology; sponsors research and educational programs.

## ★ 9129 ★ Hong Kong Stoma Association

14-15 Lung Fook House, G/F
Lower Wong Tai Sin Estate
Wong Tai Sin
Hong Kong, People's Republic of China
**Phone:** 852 28346096 **Fax:** 852 28383873
**Email:** hkstoma@netvigator.com
**Fnded:** 1979. **Mem:** 1,500. **Lang(s):** Cantonese, English. **Desc:** Individuals with stoma (small surgical openings in their gastrointestinal systems allowing for the elimination of urine and feces when the body's normal excretory functions are impaired) are members. Seeks to improve the quality of life of people with stoma. Provides support, information, and counseling for people planning on undergoing stoma surgery; conducts educational and support group meetings for members. **Pub:** Newsletter, bimonthly.

## ★ 9130 ★ Ileostomy and Internal Pouch Support Group

PO Box 132
Scunthorpe DN15 9YW, United Kingdom
**Fax:** 44 1724 721601
**Email:** ia@ileostomypouch.demon.co.uk
**Website:** http://www.ileostomypouch.demon.co.uk
**Fnded:** 1956. **Mem:** 9,636. **Desc:** To help people who have had or are about to have their colon removed, to return to a fully active and normal life as soon as possible. The activities of IA include hospital and home visiting, members' meetings, equipment exhibitions, medical research, stoma-care clinics, advisory services, lectures and demonstrations. **Pub:** *IA Journal*, quarterly. Journal.

## ★ 9131 ★ Inter American Society of Digestive Endoscopy (Sociedad Interamericana de Endoscopia Digestiva — SIED)

Calle 11, no 1129 1e A
1900 La Plata, Argentina
**Phone:** 54 21241991 **Fax:** 54 1225111

## ★ 9132 ★ International Association Colon Hydro Therapy (I-ACT)

PO Box 461285
San Antonio, TX 78246-1285
**Phone:** (210)366-2888 **Fax:** (210)366-2999
**Email:** iact@healthy.net
**Website:** http://www.i-act.org
A.R. Hoenninger, PhD, Exec. Dir.
**Fnded:** 1988. **Mem:** 1,000. **Reg. Groups:** 15. **Desc:** Designed to heighten the awareness of the colon hydrotherapy profession, ensure continuing and progressive education in the field of colon hydrotherapy and implement professionalism beyond reproach. **Pub:** *I-ACT Quarterly*, quarterly. Newsletter. *Price:* Free for members.

## ★ 9133 ★ International Association of Colon Therapy (I-ACT)

c/o A.R. Hoenninger III, N.D.
PO Box 461285
San Antonio, TX 78246-1285
**Phone:** (210)366-2888 **Fax:** (210)366-2999
**Email:** iact@healthy.net

**Website:** http://www.iact.org
A.R: Hoenninger, PhD, Exec. Dir.
**Fnded:** 1988. **Mem:** 25,000. **Desc:** Professional colon hydrotherapists and other health care practitioners. Works to unite the community of colon hydrotherapy professionals and increase visibility and recognition in the health care industry. Promotes the establishment of uniform guidelines and standards of practice and the establishment of accredited colon hydrotherapy schools. Conducts research and educational programs; plans to operate referral service. Maintains library. **Pub:** *I-ACT Newsletter*, quarterly. Newsletter. Provides organization updates, convention schedule, and continuing education course schedule. *Price:* Included in membership dues. **Frmly:** (1993) American Colon Therapy Association.

★ 9134 ★ **International Association for Gastrointestinal Motility in Children (GIMIC)**
Av de la Cote de Nacre
F-14033 Caen, France
**Fnded:** 1989. **Desc:** Promotes Research on gastrointestinal motility in children and its disturbances.

★ 9135 ★ **International Association for the Study of the Liver (IASL) (Association Internationale pour l'Etude du Foie)**
c/o Jenny Heathcote
Toronto Western Hospital
399 Bathhurst St., 6BF, Rm. 170
Toronto, ON, Canada M5T 2S8
**Phone:** (416)603-5914 **Fax:** (416)603-7175
**Email:** elise_iasl@hotmail.com
**Website:** http://www.iaslonline.org
**Fnded:** 1958. **Mem:** 879. **Lang(s):** English. **Desc:** Members of regional societies for the study of the liver representing 67 countries. Supports the training of experts in hepatology; encourages basic and clinical research on the liver and its diseases; acts to facilitate prevention, recognition, and treatment of diseases of the liver. **Pub:** Newsletter, biennial.

**International Bronchoesophagological Society (IBES)**
*See:* Entry 18747

★ 9136 ★ **International Continence Society (ICS)**
c/o Victoria Rees, Admin.
Southmead Hospital
Bristol BS10 5NB, United Kingdom
**Phone:** 44 117 9503510 **Fax:** 44 117 9503469
**Email:** vicky@icsoffice.org
**Website:** http://www.icsoffice.org
**Fnded:** 1971. **Mem:** 1,400. **Lang(s):** English. **Desc:** Physicians, surgeons, nurses, physicists, physiotherapists, bio-engineers, and scientists. Promotes the study of the storage and voiding function of the lower urinary tract, its diagnosis, and the management of lower urinary tract dysfunction. Encourages research into pathophysiology, diagnostic techniques, and treatment. **Pub:** *Neurourology and Urodynamics*, bimonthly. Journal.

★ 9137 ★ **International Foundation for Functional Gastrointestinal Disorders (IFFGD)**
PO Box 178064
Milwaukee, WI 53217-8076
**Phone:** (414)964-1799 **Free:** 888-964-2001
**Fax:** (414)964-7176
**Email:** iffgd@iffgd.org
**Website:** http://www.iffgd.org
**Desc:** Promotes gastrointestinal disorders research and provides a voice for patients. **Pub:** *Participate*, quarterly. Offers state-of-the-art information about functional GI disorders.

★ 9138 ★ **International Hepato-Pancreato-Biliary Association (IHPBA)**
c/o Vanderbilt Transplant Center
Oxford House, Ste. 801
Nashville, TN 37232
**Phone:** (615)343-2735 **Fax:** (615)343-5365
**Email:** hannah.wilson@vanderbilt.edu
**Website:** http://www.ahpba.org
Henry A. Pitt, Pres.
**Fnded:** 1978. **Mem:** 2,000. **Desc:** Endoscopists, hepatologists, radiologists, and surgeons in 25 countries. Provides a forum for the presentation of papers concerning diagnostic and treatment modalities of lymphatic, pancreatic, and biliary disorders. Promotes exchange of ideas, reviews current standards of practice, and seeks to establish prospective controlled protocols in the field. Initiates research regarding factors involved in biliary, pancreatic, and liver diseases. **Frmly:** International Hepato-Biliary Pancreatic Association; (1988) International Biliary Association.

★ 9139 ★ **International Organization for Specialized Studies on Diseases of the Esophagus (OESO) (Organisation Internationale d'Etudes Specialisees pour les Maladies de l'Oesophage — OESO)**
c/o Robert Giuli, M.D.
Hopital Beaujon
2 blvd. Pershing
F-75017 Paris, France
**Phone:** 33 1 55379015 **Fax:** 33 1 55379040
**Email:** robert.giuli@oeso.org
**Fnded:** 1979. **Lang:** English, French. **Desc:** Thoracic and digestive surgeons, ear, nose, and throat specialists, intensive care specialists, pathologists, nutritionists, endoscopists, radio- and chemotherapists, and others who diagnose and treat patients suffering from cancer and other diseases of the esophagus. Acts as a forum for specialists to meet, study, and discuss the epidemiology, histological classification, and treatments of esophageal diseases. Conducts research programs. **Pub:** *Program of the International Polydisciplinary Congress*, periodic. **Frmly:** (2001) International Organization for Statistical Studies on Diseases of the Esophagus.

★ 9140 ★ **International Ostomy Association (IOA)**
43 Raananstreet
34385 Haifa, Israel
**Phone:** 972 48388080 **Fax:** 972 48388080
**Email:** eoawolff@inter.net.il
**Website:** http://www.ostomyinternational.org
**Desc:** Aims to provide information and management guides lines to its Member Associations. Helps to form new Ostomy Associations. Represents worldwide the interests of all ostomoates and those with related surgeries by advocating on all Ostomy-related matters and policies.

**International Society for Digestive Surgery**
*See:* Entry 19571

★ 9141 ★ **International Society for Diseases of the Esophagus (ISDE) (Kokusai Shokudo Shikkan Kaigi)**
Institute of Gastroentrology
Tokyo Women's Medical College
8-1, Kawada-cho
Shinjuku-ku
Tokyo 162, Japan
**Phone:** 81 3 33581435 **Fax:** 81 3 33581424
**Email:** isde@home.email.ne.jp
**Fnded:** 1979. **Mem:** 800. **Lang(s):** English. **Desc:** Physicians, researchers, and academicians in 44 countries. Purpose is to broaden scientific and medical understanding of diseases of the esophagus through the sharing of research information. Conducts scholastic meetings and symposia. **Pub:** *Disease of the Esophagus*, quarterly. Journal. • *ISDE News*, semiannual. Newsletter.

★ 9142 ★ **Intestinal Disease Foundation**
Landmarks Bldg.
1 Station Sq., Ste. 525
Pittsburgh, PA 15219-1138
**Phone:** (412)261-5888 **Free:** 877-587-9606
**Fax:** (412)471-2722
**Email:** intdis@stargate.net
**Website:** http://www.intestinalfoundation.org
Linda E. Schorr, Exec. Dir.
**Fnded:** 1986. **Mem:** 1,200. **Local Groups:** 1. **Desc:** Provides information, guidance and emotional support to persons with chronic intestinal illness and their families. Offers volunteer phone network, quarterly newsletter and "readerfriendly" educational materials. **Pub:** *Intestinal Fortitude*, quarterly. Newsletter. *Price:* Free. For members only.

★ 9143 ★ **Latin American Society for Pediatric Gastroenterology and Nutrition (Sociedad Latinoamericana de Gastroenterologia Pediatrica y Nutricion — SLAGPN)**
Rua Pedro de Toledo 441
04039-031 Sao Paulo, Brazil
**Phone:** 55 11 5705834 **Fax:** 55 11 5705834
**Email:** slagpn@mandic.com.br
**Fnded:** 1974. **Desc:** Supports research of the functions of gastrointestinal tract, liver and nutrition in normal and abnormal conditions in children.

★ 9144 ★ **National Association of Colitis and Crohn's Disease (NACC)**
4 Beaumont House
Sutton Rd.
Saint Albans AL1 5HH, United Kingdom
**Phone:** 44 1727 830038 **Fax:** 44 1727 862550
**Email:** nacc@nacc.org.uk
**Website:** http://www.nacc.org.uk
**Fnded:** 1979. **Mem:** 30,000. **Reg. Groups:** 70. **Lang(s):** English. **Desc:** Patients, relatives, health professionals, and anyone interested in colitis and Crohn's disease. Provides support and information for patients and families living with these conditions. **Pub:** Newsletter, quarterly.

★ 9145 ★ **National Digestive Diseases Information Clearinghouse (NDDIC)**
2 Information Way
Bethesda, MD 20892-3570
**Phone:** (301)654-3810 **Free:** 800-891-5389
**Fax:** (301)907-8906
**Email:** nddic@info.niddk.nih.gov
**Website:** http://www.niddk.nih.gov
Kathy Kranzfelder, Dir.
**Fnded:** 1980. **Desc:** An information and referral service of the National Institute of Diabetes and Digestive and Kidney Diseases. Serves as a central information resource on the prevention and management of digestive diseases. Responds to written inquiries, develops and distributes publications about digestive diseases, and provides referrals to digestive disease organizations, including support groups. Maintains a database of patient and professional education materials, from which literature searches are generated. Provides bulk orders of publications to health and information professionals planning patient health education programs. **Pub:** *Age Page: Constipation.* • *Cirrhosis of the Liver.* • *Constipation.* • *Crohn's Disease.* • *Digestive Diseases Statistics.* • *Diverticulosis and Diverticulitis.* • *Facts and Fallacies About Digestive Diseases.* • *Gallstones.* • *Gas in the Digestive Tract.* • *Gastroesophageal Reflux Disease (Hiatal Hernia and Heartburn).* • *Harmful Effects of Medicines on the Adult Digestive System.* • *Hemorrhoids.* • *Irritable Bowel Syndrome.* • *Lactose Intolerance.* • *Pancreatitis.* • *Smoking and Your Digestive System.* • *Stomach and Duodenal Ulcers.* • *Ulcerative Colitis.* • *Your Digestive System and How it Works.* **AKA:**

Digestive Diseases Clearinghouse. **Frmly:** (1985) National Digestive Diseases Education and Information Clearinghouse.


★ **9146** ★ **National Hepatitis C Coalition**

PO Box 5058
Hemet, CA 92544
**Phone:** (909)658-4414
**Email:** support@nationalhepatitis-c.org
**Website:** http://nationalhepatitis-c.org/

**Desc:** Hepatitis C patients and families. Dedicated to providing education and support through online communications. Promotes research for treatments and promotes awareness.


★ **9147** ★ **National Pressure Ulcer Advisory Panel (NPUAP)**

11250 Roger Bacon Dr., Ste. 8
Reston, VA 20190-5202
**Phone:** (703)464-4849          **Fax:** (703)435-4390
**Email:** rguggolz@drohanmgmt.com
**Website:** http://www.npuap.org
Rick Guggolz, Exec. Dir.

**Fnded:** 1987. **Desc:** Dedicated to the prevention and management of pressure ulcers. Acts as information resource for health care professionals, government, public and health care agencies. Promotes research and legislative action. **Pub:** Newsletter, quarterly.


**North American Society for Pediatric Gastroenterology, Hepatology and Nutrition (NASPGHAN)**
*See:* Entry 5737


**Norwegian Cystic Fibrosis Association (NCFA)**
**(Norsk Forening for Cystisk Fibrose — NFCF)**
*See:* Entry 9355


★ **9148** ★ **Norwegian Ostomy Association (Norsk Forening for Stomi-og Reservoaropererte)**

Postboks 5327
Majorstua
N-0304 Oslo, Norway
**Phone:** 47 22593000          **Fax:** 47 22853696
**Email:** norilco@kreft.no
**Website:** http://www.cfnorge.no

**Fnded:** 1971. **Mem:** 6,000. **Local Groups:** 22. **Lang(s):** English, Norwegian. **Desc:** Individuals representing the interests of ostomy patients. Promotes information exchange among members. Works to improve quality of health care before and after surgery. **Pub:** *NORILCO-NYTT*, bimonthly. Magazine.


**Pediatric Digestion and Motility Disorders Society (PEDS)**
*See:* Entry 5742


★ **9149** ★ **Rainbow Celebration of Hope Network**

16507 Parkridge Ct.
Houston, TX 77053
**Phone:** (713)326-8571
**Email:** rainchope@aol.com
**Website:** http://www.wecaretoo.com/Organizations/TX/rainbowcelebration.html
Shelia Robey-Bailey, Contact

**Fnded:** 1999. **Mem:** 10. **Desc:** Provides spiritual and educational resources for individuals on dialysis; also provides means of support. **Pub:** Newsletter, annual. Covers past and future events and organizations.


**Reach Out for Youth with Ileitis and Colitis**
*See:* Entry 5749


★ **9150** ★ **Scandinavian Association for Gastrointestinal Motility**

c/o Einar Bjornsson
Department of Medicine II
Sahlgren's Hospital
S-413 45 Goteborg, Sweden
**Email:** einar.bjornsson@medicine.gu.sef
**Website:** http://www.reachoutforyouth.org

**Fnded:** 1987. **Desc:** Seeks to increase scientific knowledge of gastrointestinal motility and neurogastroenterology. Works to improve diagnosis and treatment of motility disturbances. **Pub:** Newsletter, periodic.


★ **9151** ★ **Scientific Society of Forensic Meidlogy and Gastrointestinal Endoscopy**

5th City Clinical Hospital
Clinic of Internal Medicine
Stoletov 67-A
BG-1233 Sofia, Bulgaria
**Phone:** 359 2 9268105          **Fax:** 359 2 325141
**Email:** mechkov@techno-link.com

**Fnded:** 1973. **Mem:** 200. **Nat'l Groups:** 2. **Reg. Groups:** 1. **Lang(s):** English, French. **Desc:** Fosters research in hepatology, gastroenterology and gastrointestinal endoscopy. **Pub:** *Bulgarian Journal of Hepatogastroenterology*, quarterly. **Frmly:** Bulgarian Gastro-Surgical Club; Bulgarian Association of Surgeons and Gastroenterologists.


★ **9152** ★ **Sociedad Chilena de Gastroenterologia**

Casilla 166, Correo 55
Santiago, Chile
**Phone:** 56 2 6343106          **Fax:** 56 2 3413836
**Fnded:** 1938.


★ **9153** ★ **Society of American Gastrointestinal Endoscopic Surgeons (SAGES)**

2716 Ocean Park Blvd., Ste. 3000
Santa Monica, CA 90405
**Phone:** (310)314-2404          **Fax:** (310)314-2585
**Email:** sagesmail@aol.com
**Website:** http://www.sages.org
Sallie Matthews, Exec. Dir.

**Fnded:** 1980. **Mem:** 3,900. **Desc:** Surgeons who perform gastrointestinal endoscopy and laparascopy. Promotes the concepts of gastrointestinal endoscopy as an integral part of surgery and encourages academic, clinical, and research achievements in the field. Establishes standards of training and practice and guidelines for privileging. Provides a forum for the exchange of ideas on gastrointestinal endoscopy and related sciences. Conducts scientific studies. Offers Corporate Council membership that facilitates communication between the corporate sector and surgeons. **Pub:** *Surgical Endoscopy*, monthly. Journal. Contains information on Surgical Endoscopy. *Price:* $135/year. • Also publishes numerous guidelines on Gastrointestinal Endoscopic Surgery, privileging and standards of practice.


★ **9154** ★ **Society of Gastroenterology Nurses and Associates (SGNA)**

401 N Michigan Ave.
Chicago, IL 60611-4267
**Phone:** (312)321-5165          **Free:** 800-245-7462
**Fax:** (312)527-6658
**Email:** sgna@sba.com
**Website:** http://www.sgna.org
Mary Beth Hepp, Exec. Dir.

**Fnded:** 1974. **Mem:** 6,000. **Reg. Groups:** 60. **Desc:** To unite personnel engaged in the field of gastroenterology/endoscopy in order to promote the highest professional standards for gastroenterology nurses and associates. Conducts national and regional educational courses and research programs. Cooperates with other professional associations, hospitals, universities, industries, technical societies, research organizations, and governmental agencies. **Pub:** *Gastroenterology Nursing*, bimonthly. Includes subject and author indexes, book reviews, new product information. *Price:* $52/year for individuals; $80/year for institutions; $25/year for students; $15/copy. • *Gastroenterology Nursing - A Core Curriculum.* • *Job Description Handbook.* • *Manual of Gastrointestinal Procedures.* • *Pediatric Supplement.* • *Pulmonary Supplement.* • *SGNA News*, bimonthly. Newsletter. Contains regional directory, regional news, and articles on research and finance. *Price:* Free to members. **Frmly:** (1989) Society of Gastrointestinal Assistants.


★ **9155** ★ **Society of Gastrointestinal Radiologists (SGR)**

c/o International Meeting Managers, Inc.
4550 Post Oak Place, Ste. 342
Houston, TX 77027
**Phone:** (713)965-0566          **Fax:** (713)960-0488
**Email:** administration@sgr.org
**Website:** http://www.sgr.org/sgr_main.htm
Eric vanSonnenberg, MD, Pres.

**Fnded:** 1971. **Desc:** Strive to furnish leadership and foster advances in diagnostic, interventional, gastrointestinal and abdominal radiology; work to exchange knowledge pertaining to research practice and education in gastrointestinal and abdominal radiology. Annual lecture in memory of Walter B. Cannon, the pioneer physiologist who initiated gastrointestinal radiology and an annual postgraduate course in gastrointestinal radiology.


★ **9156** ★ **United European Gastroenterology Federation (UEGF)**

c/o Prof. Juan R. Malagelada
Hospital General Vall d'Hebron
Pg. Val d'Hebron, 119-129
E-08035 Barcelona, Spain
**Phone:** 34 3 4281883          **Fax:** 34 3 2096205
**Email:** arthom@email.msn.com

**Fnded:** 1988. **Desc:** Promotes exchange of information in the field of gastroenterology.


★ **9157** ★ **United Ostomy Association (UOA)**

19772 MacArthur Blvd., Ste. 200
Irvine, CA 92612-2405
**Free:** 800-826-0826
**Email:** director@uoa.org
**Website:** http://www.uoa.org
Nancy Italia, Exec. Dir.

**Fnded:** 1962. **Mem:** 34,000. **Reg. Groups:** 12. **Local Groups:** 500. **Desc:** Individuals who have lost the normal function of their bowel or bladder necessitating colostomy, ileostomy, ileal conduit, or ureterostomy surgery, known as ostomy. Aids in rehabilitation of these persons through mutual aid, moral support, and exchange of practical information in managing the stoma and its necessary prosthetic appliances; sponsors visiting program allowing patients to ask nonmedical questions of individuals who have experienced a similar condition. Works to educate the public as to the nature of ostomy, with a view to ending job and insurance discrimination. Encourages research on management of ostomy and prosthetic equipment and appliances; also encourages study of the costs for rehabilitating ostomy patients. Prepares exhibits for medical conventions. Maintains speakers' bureau; compiles statistics. **Pub:** *Ostomy Quarterly*. Magazine. Contains information on ostomy management, human interest stories, organizational news, nutrition tips, and ostomy and alternate procedures. • *Services of the United Ostomy Association*. Brochure. • Annual Report, quarterly.


★ **9158** ★ **World Council of Coloproctology (WCCP)**

Prince of Wales Private Hopsital
Barker St.
Randwick, NSW 2031, Australia
**Phone:** 61 2 96504954          **Fax:** 61 2 96504898
**Fnded:** 1990.

**★ 9159 ★ World Organization of Gastroenterology (OMGE) (Organisation Mondiale de Gastroenterologie — OMGE)**
Brunnsteinstrabe 10
D-81541 Munich, Germany
**Phone:** 49 89 41419240    **Fax:** 49 89 41419245
**Email:** omge@omge.org
**Website:** http://www.omge.org
**Fnded:** 1958. **Mem:** 75. **Reg. Groups:** 3. **Lang(s):** English, French, Spanish. **Desc:** National gastroenterology societies. Promotes research in the field of gastroenterology (the study of the diseases and pathology of the stomach and intestines). Fosters exchange of information among members. Compiles statistics. **Pub:** *Directory*, quadrennial. Directory. • *Nomenclature of Digestive Diseases.* • *OMGE Bulletin*, quadrennial. Bulletin. • *OMGE Newsletter*, annual. Newsletter. • *OMGE Statutes*, quadrennial.

## Research Centers

**★ 9160 ★ Albert Einstein College of Medicine**
**Marion Bessin Liver Research Center**
Ullman Bldg., Rm. 625
1300 Morris Park Ave.
Bronx, NY 10461
**Phone:** (718)430-2098    **Fax:** (718)430-8975
**Email:** shafritz@aecom.yu.edu
**Website:** http://www.aecom.yu.edu/liver
Dr. David A. Shafritz, Dir.
**Activities/Fields:** Mechanisms of liver cell injury and repair, gene regulation, membrane structure/function, cirrhosis, genetic diseases, heavy metal toxicity, cellular growth control, liver progenitor cells, livery cell transplanation, somatic gene therapy, hepatitis virus infection, chronic liver diseases, and hepatic carcinogenesis.

**★ 9161 ★ American Association for the Study of Liver Diseases**
1729 King St., Ste. 100
Alexandria, VA 22314-2720
**Phone:** (703)299-9766    **Fax:** (703)299-9622
**Email:** scathcart@aasld.org
**Website:** http://www.aasld.org
Sherrie Cathcart, Contact
**Activities/Fields:** Liver disease and hepatic research.

**Case Western Reserve University**
**Cystic Fibrosis and Pediatric Pulmonary Center**
*See:* Entry 9378

**★ 9162 ★ Center for Basic Research in Digestive Diseases**
Guggenheim 17
Mayo Clinic
Rochester, MN 55905
**Phone:** (507)284-1006    **Fax:** (507)284-0762
**Email:** larusso.nicholas@mayo.edu
Dr. N.F. LaRusso, Dir.
**Activities/Fields:** Cell biology, focusing on molecular and biochemical mechanisms of secretion in digestive tissues.

**★ 9163 ★ Center for Human Nutrition, Inc.**
502 S 44th St., Rm. 3007
Omaha, NE 68105
**Phone:** (402)559-5500    **Fax:** (402)559-7302
**Email:** chn_icsn@unmc.edu
Dr. Ann Grandjean, Exec. Dir.
**Activities/Fields:** Basic and clinical nutrition studies, clinical trials, intervention studies, and post marketing studies.

**Emory University**
**Cystic Fibrosis Care, Teaching and Research Center**
*See:* Entry 9394

**★ 9164 ★ McMaster University**
**Intestinal Disease Research Program (IDRP)**
Health Sciences Centre, Rm. 3N5C
1200 Main St. W
Hamilton, ON, Canada L8N 3Z5
**Phone:** (905)525-9140    **Fax:** (905)522-3454
**Email:** idrp@mcmaster.ca
**Website:** http://www.fhs.mcmaster.ca/idrp/
Dr. Mary Perdue, Dir.
**Activities/Fields:** Intestinal diseases, especially within the following themes: immunophysiology, enteric infection, mucosal immunology, gut-brain interactions, physiology, pharmacology.

**Medical College of Wisconsin**
**Cystic Fibrosis Research Center**
*See:* Entry 9414

**★ 9165 ★ Stanford University**
**Liver Transplant Program**
750 Welch Rd., Ste. 210
Palo Alto, CA 94304-1509
**Phone:** (650)725-3360    **Fax:** (650)498-5692
**Email:** ggarcia@leeland.stanford.edu
Dr. Gabriel Garcia, Contact
**Activities/Fields:** Gastroenterology, focusing on treatment of viral hepatitis. **Frmly:** Gastroenterology Clinic.

**★ 9166 ★ Temple University**
**Motility Laboratory/Gastroenterology**
Parkinson Bldg.
School of Medicine
3401 N Broad St.
Philadelphia, PA 19140
**Phone:** (215)707-3428    **Fax:** (215)707-2684
**Email:** hparkman@nimbus.temple.edu
Dr. Robert Fisher, Dir.
**Activities/Fields:** Neurohumoral control of gastrointestinal motility, including mechanical properties and neuropeptide receptor characteristics of gastrointestinal tract smooth muscle and neurohormonal interactions in gastrointestinal motility; applied clinical research. **Frmly:** Institute of Gastroenterology.

**U.S. Department of Health and Human Services**
**National Institute of Diabetes and Digestive and Kidney Diseases**
**Division of Diabetes, Endocrinology, and Metabolic Diseases**
**Cystic Fibrosis Research Program**
*See:* Entry 9441

**★ 9167 ★ U.S. Department of Health and Human Services**
**National Institute of Diabetes and Digestive and Kidney Diseases (NIDDK)**
**Division of Digestive Diseases and Nutrition (DDDN)**
31 Center Dr., Ste. 9A27
Bethesda, MD 20892-2560
**Phone:** (301)496-1333    **Fax:** (301)480-7926
**Email:** hoofnaglej@extra.niddk.nih.gov
**Website:** http://www.niddk.nih.gov/fund/program/a-elist.htmcystic
Dr. Jay H. Hoofnagle, Dir.
**Activities/Fields:** Fundamental and clinical studies of the normal functions of the digestive tract (esophagus, stomach, intestines) and changes associated with diseases of the liver, gallbladder, biliary tract, and exocrine pancreas; and basic nutrition, nutritional requirements, trace minerals, dietary fiber, obesity, and clinical nutrition. Principal Division components include the Digestive Diseases Branch, Nutritional Sciences Branch, and Special Programs Branch.

**★ 9168 ★ U.S. Department of Health and Human Services**
**National Institute of Diabetes and Digestive and Kidney Diseases**
**Division of Digestive Diseases and Nutrition**
**Digestive Diseases Programs Branch (GI Transport and Absorption Program)**
Two Democracy Plaza Room 663
6707 Democracy Blvd. MSC 5450
Bethesda, MD 20892-5450
**Phone:** (301)594-8884    **Fax:** (301)480-8300
**Email:** mm102i.@nih.gov
Dr. Michael Kenneth May, Prog. Dir.
**Activities/Fields:** Process of food digestion in the gastrointestinal tract (GIT). Other areas of research focus on the regulation of gene expression in the developing GIT; the structure and function of the gut mucosa; the cytoskeletal structure and contractility in brush border; the growth and differentiation of gastrointestinal cells in normal and disease states; intestinal transplantation, storage, and preservation; and gastrointestinal tissue injury, repair, and regeneration. Also supported are studies on gastrointestinal diseases such as maldigestion and malabsorption syndromes, celiac sprue, diarrhea, inflammatory bowel disease, gastric and duodenal ulcers, diseases of the salivary glands (excluding cystic fibrosis), and the effects of prostaglandins and other treatment modalities on the gastrointestinal tract and their possible role in the pathogenesis and treatment of digestive diseases.

**★ 9169 ★ U.S. Department of Health and Human Services**
**National Institute of Diabetes and Digestive and Kidney Diseases**
**Division of Digestive Diseases and Nutrition**
**Digestive Diseases Programs Branch (Liver and Biliary Tract Diseases Program)**
6700 Rockledge Dr., Rm. 5229
Bethesda, MD 20892
**Phone:** (301)435-3762    **Fax:** (301)402-3171
**Email:** tk13v@nih.gov
Thomas F. Kresina, PhD, Dir.
**Activities/Fields:** Office coordinates research to investigate opportunistic infections related to liver and enteric diseases, in particular, hepatitis C in the context of HIV infection, as well as, International Research related to HIV, liver disease, and substance abuse. Research focus also targets minority, and special populations with emphasis on specific issues related to HIV infection, and liver disease; safer behavior and health services; and impacr of HIV exposure in lives of the minority community. Both adults and children of all underrepresented racial, and ethnic populations are emphasized in this research focus. Biomedical research investigations support minority- related aspects of alcohol metabolism, organ damage to the liver and pancreas by alcohol and enhanced progression of AIDS-defining opportunistic infections, such as tuberculosis and hepatitis C by addiction to alcohol.

## ★ 9170 ★ U.S. Department of Health and Human Services
National Institute of Diabetes and Digestive and Kidney Diseases
Division of Digestive Diseases and Nutrition
**Epidemiology and Clinical Trials Branch (Clinical Trials Program)**
2 Democracy Plaza
6707 Democracy Blvd., MSC 5450
Bethesda, MD 20892-5450
**Phone:** (301)594-8879 **Fax:** (301)480-8300
**Email:** pr132q@nih.gov
Patricia R. Robuck, PhD, Dir.

**Activities/Fields:** Administers multi- and single center clinical trials in digestive and nutritional diseases and disorders. **Frmly:** Digestive Diseases Centers Branch.

U.S. Department of Health and Human Services
National Institute of Diabetes and Digestive and Kidney Diseases
Division of Extramural Activities
*See:* Entry 8781

## ★ 9171 ★ U.S. Department of Health and Human Services
National Institute of Diabetes and Digestive and Kidney Diseases
Division of Intramural Research
**Digestive Diseases Branch**
NIH Bldg. 10, Rm. 9C-103
10 Center Dr. MSC 1804
Bethesda, MD 20892-1804
**Phone:** (301)496-4201 **Fax:** (301)402-0600
**Email:** hammond2@extra.niddk.nih.gov
**Website:** http://www.niddk.nih.gov/funds/divisions/dea/deaintro.htm
Dr. Robert T. Jensen, Chf.

**Activities/Fields:** Diseases and disorders of the digestive tract, including the physiology, biochemistry, and etiology of diseases of the gastrointestinal tract and the liver, enzymes and metabolic pathways, disturbances in gastrointestinal tract function, and the effect of various treatments and therapies. Activities are carried out in sections for gastroenterology and liver diseases.

## ★ 9172 ★ U.S. Department of Health and Human Services
National Institutes of Health
National Institute of Diabetes and Digestive and Kidney Diseases
**Diabetic Nephropathy Program**
2 Democracy Blvd., Rm. 639
Bethesda, MD 20892
**Phone:** (301)594-7713
**Email:** kimmelp@extra.niddk.nih.gov
**Website:** http://www.niddk.nih.gov/fund/program/A-Elist.htmdianep
Paul L. Kimmel, MD, Dir.

**Activities/Fields:** Pathophysiology and pathogenesis of diabetic nephropathy, natural history studies, and clinical trials through R01 mechanism, including molecular pathogenesis of extracellular matrix expansion and glomerulosclerosis, the role of the renin-angiotension system and growth factors, and the identification of treatments to prevent renal scarring.

U.S. Department of Health and Human Services
National Institutes of Health
National Institute of Diabetes and Digestive and Kidney Diseases
Division of Diabetes, Endocrinology, and Metabolic Diseases
**(Acquired Immunodeficiency Syndrome (AIDS) and Human Immunodeficiency Virus (HIV) Program)**
*See:* Entry 11934

## ★ 9173 ★ U.S. Department of Health and Human Services
National Institutes of Health
National Institute of Diabetes and Digestive and Kidney Diseases
Division of Diabetes, Endocrinology, and Metabolic Diseases
**(Adipocyte Biology Research Program)**
DEM 2/605
Bethesda, MD 20892
**Phone:** (301)594-7689 **Fax:** (301)435-6047
**Email:** naftc@extra.niddk.nih.gov
**Website:** http://www.niddk.nih.gov/fund/program/A-Elist.htmadipocyte
Carol Haft, PhD, Dir.

**Activities/Fields:** Development and physiology of the adipocyte cell, including studies on the properties of transcription factors that regulate adipocyte differentiation; consequences of insulin action on adipocyte physiology; and use of animal and tissue culture models to understand adipocyte biology.

## ★ 9174 ★ U.S. Department of Health and Human Services
National Institutes of Health
National Institute of Diabetes and Digestive and Kidney Diseases
Division of Digestive Diseases and Nutrition
**(Gastrointestinal Transport and Absorption Program)**
MSC 5450
6707 Democracy Blvd., Rm. 663
Bethesda, MD 20892-5450
**Phone:** (301)594-8884 **Fax:** (301)480-8300
**Email:** maym@extra.niddk.nih.gov
**Website:** http://www.niddk.nih.gov/fund/program/F-Llist.htmGTAP
Michael Ken May, PhD, Dir.

**Activities/Fields:** Process of food digestion, and absorption and transport in the gastrointestinal tract, including the synthesis and assembly of digestive enzymes; the transport of water, ions, sugars, amino acids, peptides, lipids, vitamins, and macromolecules; and the formation, structure, and function of chylomicrons. Other areas of research focus on the regulation of gene expression in the gastrointestinal tract; structure and function of the gut mucosa; cytoskeletal structure and contractility in brush borders; the growth and differentiation of gastrointestinal cells in normal and disease states; intestinal transplantation, storage, and preservation; and gastrointestinal tissue injury, repair, and regeneration. Also supported are studies on gastrointestinal diseases such as maldigestion and malabsorption syndromes.

## ★ 9175 ★ U.S. Department of Health and Human Services
National Institutes of Health
National Institute of Diabetes and Digestive and Kidney Diseases
Division of Digestive Diseases and Nutrition
**(Gastrointestinal Neuroendocrinology Research Program)**
MSC 5450
6707 Democracy Blvd., Rm. 663
Bethesda, MD 20892-5450
**Phone:** (301)594-8884 **Fax:** (301)480-8300
**Email:** maym@extra.niddk.nih.gov
**Website:** http://www.niddk.nih.gov/fund/program/F-Llist.htmGNP
Michael Ken May, PhD, Dir.

**Activities/Fields:** Basic and clinical studies on normal and abnormal function of both the enteric nervous system and the elements within the central nervous system that control the enteric nervous system, including histochemical and neurochemical analyses of the enteric nervous system, electrical properties of enteric ganglia, chemical neurotransmission, neural control of effector function, and extrinsic nervous input. Emphasis is on gastrointestinal hormones and peptides, including their structure, biological actions, structure-activity relationships, receptors, distribution, quantitation, metabolism, release, correlation with physiological events, deficiency, and the role of time variation in the data collected in the above studies. In addition, the program supports studies on disease conditions associated with excessive or inadequate secretion of neuropeptides.

## ★ 9176 ★ U.S. Department of Health and Human Services
National Institutes of Health
National Institute of Diabetes and Digestive and Kidney Diseases
Division of Digestive Diseases and Nutrition
**(Clinical Trials in Digestive Diseases)**
2 Democracy Pl., Rm. 659
Bethesda, MD 20892
**Phone:** (301)594-8879 **Fax:** (301)480-8300
**Email:** robuckp@extra.niddk.nih.gov
**Website:** http://www.niddk.nih.gov/fund/program/A-Elist.htmDDCT
Patrick R. Robuck, PhD, Dir.

**Activities/Fields:** Evaluation of experimental interventions in comparison with a standard treatment and/or placebo control in digestive diseases.

## ★ 9177 ★ U.S. Department of Health and Human Services
National Institutes of Health
National Institute of Diabetes and Digestive and Kidney Diseases
**End-Stage Renal Disease Program**
6707 Democracy Blvd.
Bethesda, MD 20892
**Phone:** (301)496-4000
**Email:** agodoal@extra.niddk.nih.gov
**Website:** http://www.niddk.nih.gov/fund/program/A-Elist.htmend
Lawrence Y. Agodoa, MD, Dir.

**Activities/Fields:** Strives to reduce morbidity and mortality from bone, blood, nervous system, metabolic, gastrointestinal, cardiovascular, and endocrine abnormalities in end-stage kidney failure; aims to improve the effectiveness of dialysis and transplantation. Special areas of interest include hemodialysis membrane reuse and alternative dialyzer sterilization methods; biocompatible membranes; high-flux hemodialysis; criteria for adequacy of dialysis.

## ★ 9178 ★ U.S. Department of Health and Human Services
National Institutes of Health
National Institute of Diabetes and Digestive and Kidney Diseases
**Kidney, Urology, and Hematology Centers Program**
MSC 5458
2 Democracu Blvd., Rm. 621
Bethesda, MD 20892-5458
**Phone:** (301)594-7717 **Fax:** (301)480-3510
**Email:** badmand@extra.niddk.nih.gov
**Website:** http://www.niddk.nih.gov/fund/program/F-Llist.htm
David Badman, PhD, Dir.

**Activities/Fields:** Strives to reduce adult and pediatric mortality and morbidity from kidney, urologic, and hematologic diseases.

**★ 9179 ★ U.S. Department of Health and Human Services**
**National Institutes of Health**
**National Institute of Diabetes and Digestive and Kidney Diseases**
**Pediatric Nephrology Programs**
630-2 Democracy Plz.
Bethesda, MD 20892-5458
**Phone:** (301)594-7717          **Fax:** (301)480-3510
**Email:** gladys_hirschman@nih.gov
**Website:** http://www.niddk.nih.gov/fund/program/M-Rlist.htmpednep
Gladys H. Hirschman, MD, Dir.
**Activities/Fields:** Aims to characterize the scope, nature, and impact of kidney diseases of children, including the causes, treatment, and prevention of these disorders.

**★ 9180 ★ U.S. Department of Health and Human Services**
**National Institutes of Health**
**National Institute of Diabetes and Digestive and Kidney Diseases**
**Urology Program**
2 Democracy Blvd.
Bldg. 45, Rm. 6AS-136
Bethesda, MD 20892
**Phone:** (301)594-7717          **Fax:** (301)480-3510
**Email:** nybergl@ep.niddk.nih.gov
**Website:** http://www.niddk.nih.gov/fund/program/S-Zlist.htmuroprog
Leroy M. Nyberg, Jr.,MD, Dir.
**Activities/Fields:** Normal and abnormal development, structure, and function of the genitourinary tract and studies on the genitourinary effects of diabetes mellitus, spinal cord injury, and multiple sclerosis. Research includes etiology, diagnosis, pathophysiology, therapy, and prevention of major adult urological disease and disorders, including shock-wave and laser lithotripsy, urolithiasis inhibitors, bladder substitution procedures and devices, and prostate growth inhibitor and reduction therapies.

**★ 9181 ★ University of Alabama at Birmingham**
**Liver Center**
MCLM Bldg., 2nd Fl.
1900 University Blvd.
Birmingham, AL 35294-0005
**Phone:** (205)975-9698          **Fax:** (205)975-9777
**Email:** jbloomer@uab.edu
**Website:** http://info.dom.uab.edu/gastro/livercenter/LC.html
Joseph R. Bloomer, MD, Dir.
**Activities/Fields:** Diagnosis and treatment of liver disease and related disorders.

**★ 9182 ★ University of Calgary**
**Gastrointestinal Research Group**
Health Science Centre
3330 Hospital Dr. NW
Calgary, AB, Canada T2N 4N1
**Phone:** (403)220-7611          **Fax:** (403)220-0995
**Email:** swain@ucalgary.ca
**Website:** http://www.ucalgary.ca/~girg/
Mark G. Swain, Ch.
**Activities/Fields:** Neuroendocrine control of gastrointestinal (GI) function, secretory functions in the GI tract, motility of the biliary tract and intestine, intestinal absorption, membrane physiology, immunology of the GI tract, intestinal inflammation, inflammatory bowel disease, developmental physiology, hepatobiliary disease, hepatic receptors, malnutrition, satiety and appetite control, intestinal adaptation, gut hormone, and splanchnic blood flow.

**★ 9183 ★ University of California, Davis**
**Gastroenterology and Nutrition Center**
Pediatric GI
UCD Medical Center
2516 Stockton Blvd.
Sacramento, CA 95817
**Phone:** (916)734-3750          **Fax:** (916)734-4098
**Email:** michael.haight@ucdmc.ucdavis.edu
**Website:** http://www.ucdmc.ucdavis.edu
Dr. Michael Haight, Ch., Pediatric Gastroenterology
**Activities/Fields:** Pediatric nutritional support, and feeding problems in children, Pediatric Short Bowel Syndrome, outcomes and lactation. **Pub:** *Educational booklets, videos.*

**★ 9184 ★ University of California, Los Angeles**
**CURE: Digestive Diseases Research Center**
Bldg. 115, Rm. 115
VAGLAHS
Los Angeles, CA 90073-1792
**Phone:** (310)312-9284          **Fax:** (310)268-4963
**Email:** ytache@ucla.edu
**Website:** http://www.cure.med.ucla.edu
Yvette Tache, PhD, Dir.
**Activities/Fields:** Peptic ulcer disease, relationship of Helicobacter pylori infection to ulcers. Etiology and treatment of functional bowel disease, cell proliferation, gastrointestinal neoplasm, and nutritional intestinal absorption. **Frmly:** Center for Ulcer Research and Education.

**★ 9185 ★ University of California, Los Angeles**
**Harbor-UCLA Medical Center**
**Center for the Study of Inflammatory Bowel Disease**
1124 W Carson St., Bldg. N-21
Torrance, CA 90502
**Phone:** (310)222-2475          **Fax:** (310)212-7837
**Email:** Veysselein@rei.edu
Viktor E. Eysselein, MD, Ch.
**Activities/Fields:** Inflammatory bowel disease, particularly the origin, causes, and treatment of ulcerative colitis and Crohn's disease. Conducts related studies in molecular biology, cell biology, and immunology. Performs clinical trials of new drugs.

**★ 9186 ★ University of Chicago**
**Inflammatory Bowel Disease Research Center**
Department of Medicine, MC 6084
5841 S Maryland Ave.
Chicago, IL 60637-6084
**Phone:** (773)702-6458          **Fax:** (773)702-2281
**Email:** echang@medicine.bsd.uchicago.edu
Dr. Eugene B. Chang, Dir.
**Activities/Fields:** Pathophysiology and treatment of inflammatory bowel diseases, including molecular and cellular immunology, epithelial cell biology, human genetics, inflammation, therapeutic clinical trials, and clinical epidemiology. **Pub:** *IBD Center Newsletter*, quarterly. Newsletter.

**★ 9187 ★ University of Chicago**
**Joseph B. Kirsner Center for the Study of Digestive Diseases**
5841 S Maryland Ave.
Chicago, IL 60637
**Phone:** (773)702-9790          **Fax:** (773)702-2182
**Email:** bhunt@medicine.bsd.uchicago.edu
Dr. Stephen Hanauer, Dir.
**Activities/Fields:** Gastroenterology, including colon cancer, inflammatory bowel disease, irritable bowel syndrome, disorders of the esophagus, and pancreatic cancer.

**★ 9188 ★ University of Chicago**
**Liver Study Unit**
MC 4076
5841 S Maryland Ave.
Chicago, IL 60637-4076
**Phone:** (773)702-6145          **Fax:** (773)834-1288
Dr. Alfred L. Baker, Dir.
**Activities/Fields:** Role of nutrition in avoiding or managing liver diseases and new therapeutic approaches for treatment of specific liver diseases. Provides comprehensive care for patients with liver diseases, including assessment of severity using noninvasion methods and management of chronic hepatitis patients.

**★ 9189 ★ University of Iowa**
**James A. Clifton Center for Digestive Diseases**
Internal Medicine, 4500 JCP
Iowa City, IA 52242
**Phone:** (319)356-3127
**Email:** joel-weinstock@uiowa.edu
**Website:** http://www.uiowa.edu/~vpr/research/organize/clifton.htm
Joel V. Weinstock, Dir.
**Activities/Fields:** Diseases and conditions of the digestive system, including nutrition, inflammatory bowel disease, abdominal pain, and liver disease. Other basic medical research areas emphasized are motility, absorption, organ-regeneration, and transplantion.

**★ 9190 ★ University of Miami**
**Center for Liver Diseases**
Division of Hepatology
School of Medicine
1500 NW 12th Ave., No. 1101
Miami, FL 33136
**Phone:** (305)243-5787
**Website:** http://www.med.miami.edu/hepatology/index.html
Dr. Eugene R. Schiff, Dir.
**Activities/Fields:** Diseases of the liver and biliary tract.

**University of Miami**
**Cystic Fibrosis Research Center**
*See:* Entry 9506

**★ 9191 ★ University of Michigan**
**Michigan Gastrointestinal Peptide Research Center**
6520 MSRB I
1150 W Medical Dr.
Ann Arbor, MI 48109-0682
**Phone:** (734)647-2942          **Fax:** (734)763-2535
**Email:** jcole@umich.edu
**Website:** http://www.med.umich.edu/mgpc
Chung Owyang, MD, Dir.
**Activities/Fields:** Gastroenterology, including chemistry and biology of gut hormones as they relate to the physiology and pathology of the digestive tract, liver cell differentiation, effect of nutrients on pancreatic endocrine and exocrine secretions, and neuroendocrine modulation of smooth muscle cell function and gut motility. **Frmly:** Gastroenterology Research Laboratory.

**University of Minnesota**
**Cystic Fibrosis Center**
*See:* Entry 9508

**University of Missouri—Columbia**
**Cystic Fibrosis Research Center**
*See:* Entry 9510

**University of Nebraska at Omaha**
**Pediatric Pulmonary and Cystic Fibrosis**
**Research Center**
*See:* Entry 9513

### ★ 9192 ★ University of North Carolina at Chapel Hill
**Center for Gastrointestinal Biology and Diseases (CGIBD)**
CB 7555
Mason Farm Rd., Unit 49
Chapel Hill, NC 27599-7555
**Phone:** (919)966-1757     **Fax:** (919)966-7592
**Email:** cgibd@med.unc.edu
**Website:** http://www.niddk.nih.gov/
Robert Sandler, MD, Co-Dir.

**Activities/Fields:** Mechanisms of inflammation and fibrosis in the liver and intestine as they relate to inflammatory bowel disease.

### ★ 9193 ★ University of Southern California
**Liver Office**
7601 E Imperial Hwy.
Downey, CA 90242
**Phone:** (562)401-8961     **Fax:** (562)401-7615
Dr. Bruce A. Runyon, Prog. Ch.

**Activities/Fields:** Liver diseases, including both clinical and basic biochemical and virologic studies of cirrhosis and viral hepatitis.

**University of Utah**
**Intermountain Cystic Fibrosis Center**
*See:* Entry 9523

### ★ 9194 ★ University of Virginia
**Digestive Health Center of Excellence**
Division of GI/Hepatology
PO Box 800708
Charlottesville, VA 22908
**Phone:** (434)924-2959
**Email:** barbara.chatfield@hsc.utah.edu
**Website:** http://www.hsc.virginia.edu/internal/digestive-health/home.html
Fabio Cominelli, MD, Dir.

**Activities/Fields:** Underlying causes of many gastrointestinal diseases. The research program is centered around five themes: mucosal immunology and gut inflammation, gastrointestinal cancer, bacterial/viral-host interactions, epithelial cell and hepatocyte transport, clinical epidemiology and outcomes research.

### ★ 9195 ★ University of Washington
**Children's Hospital and Medical Center**
**Exstrophy Center of Excellence**
4800 Sand Point Way NE
PO Box 5371/CH-78
Seattle, WA 98105
**Phone:** (206)526-2509     **Fax:** (206)526-2131
**Email:** mmitch@chmc.org
Michael Mitchell, MD, Dir.

**Activities/Fields:** Cloacal or bladder exstrophy in children. **Pub:** *Meeting Reports.*

### ★ 9196 ★ Virginia Commonwealth University
**Hepatology Section and Liver Transplant Program**
PO Box 980341
Richmond, VA 23298-0711
**Phone:** (434)828-4060     **Fax:** (434)828-4945
**Email:** mshiffma@hsc.vcu.edu
Dr. Shiffman, Dir.

**Activities/Fields:** Anti-viral therapy for chronic viral hepatitis B and C; new treatments for chronic liver disease; complications of chronic liver disease including ascites, variceal hemorrhage, and hepatic enceph-

alopathy; liver transplantation including the development of new immunosupressive therapies.

**Washington University in St. Louis**
**Cystic Fibrosis Center**
*See:* Entry 9528

### ★ 9197 ★ Yale University
**Yale Liver Center**
Department of Medicine
PO Box 208019
New Haven, CT 06520-8019
**Phone:** (203)785-5279     **Fax:** (203)785-7273
**Email:** James.boyer@yale.edu
**Website:** http://livercenter.yale.edu
James L. Boyer, MD, Dir.

**Activities/Fields:** Studies of liver structure, function, and disease. **Pub:** *Newsletter*, semiannually.

---

# State & Regional Organizations

## Crohn's & Colitis

*State chapters of the Crohn's and Colitis Foundation of America are listed below. The national office is located at 386 Park Ave. S, 17th Fl., New York, NY 10016-8804. Additional information can be obtained by calling the national office at (800) 932-2423, or by consulting their web site at http://www.ccfa.org/.*

### Alabama

### ★ 9198 ★ Crohn's and Colitis Foundation of America
**Alabama/Northwest Florida Chapter**
244 Goodwin Crest Dr., Ste.. 120
Birmingham, AL 35209
**Phone:** (205)941-9900     **Free:** 800-249-1993
**Fax:** (205)941-1411
**Email:** alabama@ccfa.org
**Website:** http://www.ccfa.org/chapters/alabama/
Pat Talty, Exec Director

### Arizona

### ★ 9199 ★ Crohn's and Colitis Foundation of America
**Arizona Chapter**
1815 W Missouri Ave., Ste. 103
Phoenix, AZ 85015
**Phone:** (602)589-7233     **Free:** 800-582-7460
**Fax:** (602)589-0087
**Website:** http://www.ccfa.org/chapters/arizona/

### California

### ★ 9200 ★ Crohn's and Colitis Foundation of America
**Greater Los Angeles Chapter**
3701 Wilshire Blvd., Ste. 1120
Los Angeles, CA 90010
**Phone:** (213)380-3800     **Fax:** (213)380-5593
**Email:** losangeles@ccfa.org
**Website:** http://www.ccfa.org/chapters/losangeles/
Hank Borenstein, Exec Director
**Remarks:** Also serves Hawaii.

### ★ 9201 ★ Crohn's and Colitis Foundation of America
**Greater San Diego and Desert Area Chapter**
2180 Garnet Ave., Ste. 3L
San Diego, CA 92109
**Phone:** (858)274-8898     **Fax:** (858)274-8896

**Email:** sandiego@ccfa.org
**Website:** http://www.ccfa.org/chapters/sandiego/
Pamela Meistrell, Exec Director

### ★ 9202 ★ Crohn's and Colitis Foundation of America
**Long Beach Affiliate**
Long Beach Memorial Medical Center
2801 Atlantic Ave., 5th Fl.
Long Beach, CA 90801-1428
**Phone:** (562)424-9000

### ★ 9203 ★ Crohn's and Colitis Foundation of America
**Northern California Chapter**
1730 S Amphlett Blvd., Ste. 230
San Mateo, CA 94402
**Phone:** (650)578-6590     **Free:** 800-241-0758
**Fax:** (650)578-6599
**Email:** ccfagba@pacbell.net
**Website:** http://www.ccfa.org/chapters/greaterbay/
Carol Gerstein, Exec Director
**Frmly:** Greater Bay Area Chapter.

### ★ 9204 ★ Crohn's and Colitis Foundation of America
**Orange County Chapter**
2030 E 4th St., Ste. 104
Santa Ana, CA 92705
**Phone:** (714)547-8500     **Fax:** (714)547-8585
**Email:** orangecounty@ccfa.org
**Website:** http://www.ccfa.org/chapters/orangecounty/
Kathy Castaneda, Exec Director

### Colorado

### ★ 9205 ★ Crohn's and Colitis Foundation of America
**Rocky Mountain Chapter**
1777 S Bellaire St., Ste. 120
Denver, CO 80222
**Phone:** (303)639-9163     **Free:** (866)768-2232
**Fax:** (303)639-9166
**Email:** RockyMountain@ccfa.org
**Website:** http://www.ccfa.org/chapters/rockymountain/

**Remarks:** Serves Colorado, Nebraska, Utah, and Wyoming.

### Connecticut

### ★ 9206 ★ Crohn's and Colitis Foundation of America
**Central Connecticut Chapter**
PO Box 185431
Hamden, CT 06518
**Phone:** (203)876-1693     **Fax:** (203)876-1693
**Email:** ctccfa@aol.com
**Website:** http://www.ccfa.org/chapters/centralct/

### ★ 9207 ★ Crohn's and Colitis Foundation of America
**Northern Connecticut Affiliate**
PO Box 370614
West Hartford, CT 06137-0614
**Email:** ccfanorthct@aol.com

### Florida

### ★ 9208 ★ Crohn's and Colitis Foundation of America
**Gold Coast/South Florida Chapter**
8177 W Glades Rd., Ste. 216
Boca Raton, FL 33434
**Phone:** (561)218-2929     **Free:** 877-664-2929
**Fax:** (561)218-2240
**Email:** goldcoast@ccfa.org
**Website:** http://www.ccfa.org/chapters/goldcoast/

**★ 9209 ★ Crohn's and Colitis Foundation of America**
**South Florida Chapter**
1380 NE Miami Gardens Dr., Ste. 250
North Miami Beach, FL 33179
**Phone:** (305)354-2788        **Fax:** (305)354-7244
**Email:** southflorida@ccfa.org
**Website:** http://www.ccfa.org

## Georgia

**★ 9210 ★ Crohn's and Colitis Foundation of America**
**Georgia/Tennessee Chapter**
2250 N Druid Hills Rd., Ste. 250
Atlanta, GA 30329
**Phone:** (404)982-0616        **Free:** 800-472-6795
**Fax:** (404)982-0656
**Website:** http://www.ccfa.org/chapters/georgia/
Marcia Greenburg, Exec Director

## Illinois

**★ 9211 ★ Crohn's and Colitis Foundation of America**
**Illinois/Carol Fisher Chapter**
2250 E Devon Ave., Ste. 244
Des Plaines, IL 60018
**Phone:** (847)827-0404        **Free:** 800-886-6664
**Fax:** (847)827-6593
**Website:** http://www.ccfa.org/chapters/illinois/

## Indiana

**★ 9212 ★ Crohn's and Colitis Foundation of America**
**Indiana Chapter**
931 E 86th St., Ste. 102
Indianapolis, IN 46240
**Phone:** (317)259-8071        **Free:** 800-332-6029
**Fax:** (317)259-8091
**Website:** http://www.ccfa.org/chapters/indiana/
Jan Koontz, Exec Director

## Iowa

**★ 9213 ★ Crohn's and Colitis Foundation of America**
**Eastern Iowa Affiliate**
712 26th St. SE
Cedar Rapids, IA 52403-2917
**Phone:** (319)393-7876
**Email:** easterniowa@ccfa.org
**Website:** http://www.ccfa.org/chapters/easterniowa/
Allison Allen, Contact

**★ 9214 ★ Crohn's and Colitis Foundation of America**
**Iowa State Chapter**
PO Box 57562
Des Moines, IA 50322
**Phone:** (515)252-6179        **Fax:** (515)266-1512
**Email:** iowa@ccfa.org
**Website:** http://www.ccfa.org/chapters/iowa/

## Kentucky

**★ 9215 ★ Crohn's and Colitis Foundation of America**
**Kentucky Chapter**
4801 Sherburn Ln., Ste. 201
Louisville, KY 40207
**Phone:** (502)893-3535        **Fax:** (502)893-3553
**Email:** kyccfai@aol.com
**Website:** http://www.ccfa.org/chapters/kentucky/
**Remarks:** Serves Kentucky and southern Indiana.

## Louisiana

**★ 9216 ★ Crohn's and Colitis Foundation of America**
**Louisiana Chapter**
4141 Veterans Blvd., Ste. 336
Metairie, LA 70002
**Phone:** (504)888-1135        **Free:** 800-799-0157
**Fax:** (504)888-1132
**Email:** louisiana@ccfa.org
**Website:** http://www.ccfa.org/chapters/louisiana/
Dr. Robert Hammer, President

## Maryland

**★ 9217 ★ Crohn's and Colitis Foundation of America**
**Maryland/South Delaware Chapter**
1107 Kenilworth Dr., Ste. 320
Baltimore, MD 21204
**Phone:** (410)825-5199        **Free:** 800-618-5583
**Fax:** (410)825-5431
**Website:** http://www.ccfa.org/chapters/md-southde/

## Massachusetts

**★ 9218 ★ Crohn's and Colitis Foundation of America**
**New England Chapter**
280 Hillside Ave.
Needham, MA 02494
**Phone:** (781)449-0324        **Fax:** (781)449-0325
**Email:** ne@ccfa.org
**Website:** http://www.ccfa.org/chapters/ne/

## Michigan

**★ 9219 ★ Crohn's and Colitis Foundation of America**
**Michigan Chapter**
31313 Northwestern Hwy., Ste. 209
Farmington Hills, MI 48334
**Phone:** (248)737-0900        **Fax:** (248)737-0904
**Email:** Miccfa@aol.com
**Website:** http://www.ccfa.org/chapters/michigan/
Bernie Riker, Exec Director

**★ 9220 ★ Crohn's and Colitis Foundation of America**
**Western Michigan Office**
125 Ottawa Ave. NW, Ste. 350
Grand Rapids, MI 49503
**Phone:** (616)774-0805        **Fax:** (616)774-4096
**Email:** westernmichigan@ccfa.org
**Website:** http://www.ccfa.org/chapters/westmich/
Pam Seymour, Contact

## Minnesota

**★ 9221 ★ Crohn's and Colitis Foundation of America**
**Minnesota/Dakotas Chapter**
1885 University Ave. W, Ste. 355
Saint Paul, MN 55104
**Phone:** (651)917-2424        **Free:** 888-422-3266
**Fax:** (651)917-2425
**Website:** http://www.ccfa.org/chapters/minnesota/

## Mississippi

**★ 9222 ★ Crohn's and Colitis Foundation of America**
**Mississippi Affiliate**
PO Box 631
Ridgeland, MS 39158
**Phone:** (601)605-1849
**Email:** mississippi@ccfa.org
**Website:** http://www.ccfa.org/chapters/mississippi/

## Missouri

**★ 9223 ★ Crohn's and Colitis Foundation of America**
**Gateway Chapter**
8420 Delmar Ave., Ste. 500A
Saint Louis, MO 63124
**Phone:** (314)991-0220        **Free:** 800-783-8006
**Fax:** (314)991-8756
**Website:** http://www.ccfa.org/chapters/gateway/
**Remarks:** Serves Missouri, Kansas, southern Illinois, and northeast Arkansas.

## New Jersey

**★ 9224 ★ Crohn's and Colitis Foundation of America**
**New Jersey Chapter**
45 Wilson Ave.
Manalapan, NJ 07726
**Phone:** (732)786-9960        **Fax:** (732)786-9964
**Email:** newjersey@ccfa.org
**Website:** http://www.ccfa.org/chapters/newjersey/
Rosemarie Golombos, Exec Director

## New York

**★ 9225 ★ Crohn's and Colitis Foundation of America**
**Central NY Affiliate**
PO Box 47
Syracuse, NY 13206-0047
**Free:** 877-352-3621
**Email:** centralny@ccfa.org
**Website:** http://www.ccfa.org/chapters/centralny

**★ 9226 ★ Crohn's and Colitis Foundation of America**
**Fairfield/Westchester Chapter**
200 Bloomingdale Rd., 2nd Fl.
White Plains, NY 10605
**Phone:** (914)328-2874        **Fax:** (914)328-2946
**Email:** westfield@ccfa.org
**Website:** http://www.ccfa.org/chapters/westfield/
Renee Krutoff, Exec Director
**Remarks:** Serves Fairfield County, Connecticut, as well as Westchester, Putnam, Rockland, and Orange counties, New York.

**★ 9227 ★ Crohn's and Colitis Foundation of America**
**Greater New York Chapter**
386 Park Ave. S, 14th Fl.
New York, NY 10016-8804
**Phone:** (212)679-1570        **Fax:** (212)679-3567
**Website:** http://www.ccfa.org/chapters/newyork/

**★ 9228 ★ Crohn's and Colitis Foundation of America**
**Long Island Chapter**
585 Stewart Ave., Ste. 414
Garden City, NY 11530
**Phone:** (516)222-5530        **Fax:** (516)222-5535
**Email:** longisland@ccfa.org
**Website:** http://www.ccfa.org/chapters/longisland/

**★ 9229 ★ Crohn's and Colitis Foundation of America**
**Rochester Chapter**
1279 Chili Ave.
Rochester, NY 14624
**Phone:** (716)349-4144

**★ 9230 ★ Crohn's and Colitis Foundation of America**
**Upstate/Northeastern New York Chapter**
4 Normanskill Blvd.
Delmar, NY 12054

**Phone:** (518)439-0252
**Email:** capitalny@ccfa.org
**Website:** http://www.ccfa.org/chapters/capitalny/
Linda Winston, President

**★ 9231 ★ Crohn's and Colitis Foundation of America**
**Western New York Chapter**
PO Box 224
Williamsville, NY 14231-0224
**Phone:** (716)833-2870
**Email:** westernny@ccfa.org
**Website:** http://www.ccfa.org/chapters/westernny/

## North Carolina

**★ 9232 ★ Crohn's and Colitis Foundation of America**
**Carolinas Chapter**
**Charlotte Office**
442 S Main St., Ste. 1
Davidson, NC 28036
**Phone:** (704)894-9751          **Free:** 888-455-3338
**Fax:** (704)894-9752
**Email:** northcarolina@ccfa.org
**Website:** http://www.ccfa.org

**★ 9233 ★ Crohn's and Colitis Foundation of America**
**Carolinas Chapter**
**Columbia Office**
134 McSwain Dr.
West Columbia, NC 29169
**Phone:** 888-455-3338          **Fax:** (704)894-9752
**Email:** carolinas@ccfa.org
**Website:** http://www.ccfa.org/chapters/scarolina/

**★ 9234 ★ Crohn's and Colitis Foundation of America**
**Carolinas Chapter**
**Raleigh Office**
8408 Glenwood Ave., Ste. H
Raleigh, NC 27612
**Phone:** (919)786-9852          **Free:** 800-360-1433
**Fax:** (919)786-9854
**Email:** raleigh@ccfa.org
**Website:** http://www.ccfa.org/chapters/northcarolina/

## Ohio

**★ 9235 ★ Crohn's and Colitis Foundation of America**
**Central Ohio Chapter**
2021 E Dublin Granville Rd., Ste. 125
Columbus, OH 43229
**Phone:** (614)781-9970          **Free:** 800-625-5977
**Fax:** (614)781-9972
**Email:** centralohio@ccfa.org
**Website:** http://www.ccfa.org/chapters/centralohio/

**★ 9236 ★ Crohn's and Colitis Foundation of America**
**Greater Cincinnati Chapter**
2139 Auburn Ave.
Cincinnati, OH 45219
**Phone:** (513)585-1775          **Free:** 877-283-7513
**Fax:** (513)585-3071
**Email:** cincinnati@ccfa.org
**Website:** http://www.ccfa.org/chapters/cincinnati/
Andrea Sothfelder, Contact
**Remarks:** Also serves the greater Dayton area and northern Kentucky.

**★ 9237 ★ Crohn's and Colitis Foundation of America**
**Northeast Ohio Chapter**
23366 Commerce Park Rd., Ste. 210
Beachwood, OH 44122
**Phone:** (216)831-2692          **Fax:** (216)831-2792

**Email:** neohio@ccfa.org
**Website:** http://www.ccfa.org/chapters/neohio/

## Oklahoma

**★ 9238 ★ Crohn's and Colitis Foundation of America**
**Oklahoma Chapter**
4504 E 67th St., Ste. 125
Tulsa, OK 74136
**Phone:** (918)523-8540          **Free:** 800-658-1533
**Fax:** (918)523-8560
**Website:** http://www.ccfa.org/chapters/oklahoma/

## Pennsylvania

**★ 9239 ★ Crohn's and Colitis Foundation of America**
**Philadelphia/Delaware Valley Chapter**
367 E St. Rd.
Trevose, PA 19053
**Phone:** (215)396-9100          **Free:** 888-340-4744
**Fax:** (215)396-1170
**Email:** philadelphia@ccfa.org
**Website:** http://www.ccfa.org/chapters/philadelphia/

**★ 9240 ★ Crohn's and Colitis Foundation of America**
**Western Pennsylvania/West Virginia Chapter**
580 S Aiken Ave., Ste. 202
Pittsburgh, PA 15232
**Phone:** (412)687-9775          **Free:** 800-627-6467
**Fax:** (412)687-8544
**Email:** wpawv@ccfa.org
**Website:** http://www.ccfa.org/chapters/wpawv/

## Puerto Rico

**★ 9241 ★ Crohn's and Colitis Foundation of America**
**Puerto Rico Affiliate**
56 Marbella St.
San Juan, PR 00907
**Phone:** (787)727-4481          **Fax:** (787)727-4481
**Email:** puertorico@ccfa.org
**Website:** http://www.ccfa.org/chapters/puertorico/

## Texas

**★ 9242 ★ Crohn's and Colitis Foundation of America**
**Houston Gulf Coast/South Texas Chapter**
5120 Woodway, Ste. 8008
Houston, TX 77056
**Phone:** (713)572-2232          **Free:** 800-785-2232
**Fax:** (713)572-2433
**Email:** houston@ccfa.org
**Website:** http://www.ccfa.org/chapters/houston/
Monique Bossett, Exec Director

**★ 9243 ★ Crohn's and Colitis Foundation of America**
**North Texas Chapter**
9601 White Rock Trail, Ste. 102
Dallas, TX 75238
**Phone:** (972)243-8959          **Fax:** (972)243-8954
**Email:** grankin@coserv.net
**Website:** http://www.ccfa.org/chapters/ntexas/
Greg Rankin, Director

## Virginia

**★ 9244 ★ Crohn's and Colitis Foundation of America**
**Greater Washington DC/Virginia Chapter**
901 King St., Ste 101
Alexandria, VA 22314
**Phone:** (703)739-2548          **Free:** 877-807-5271
**Fax:** (703)739-9657

**Email:** washingtondc@ccfa.org
**Website:** http://www.ccfa.org/chapters/washingtondc/

## Washington

**★ 9245 ★ Crohn's and Colitis Foundation of America**
**Northwest Chapter**
320 Andover Park E, Ste. 270
Seattle, WA 98188
**Phone:** (206)574-0698          **Free:** 877-703-6900
**Fax:** (206)574-0869
**Email:** northwest@ccfa.org
**Website:** http://www.ccfa.org/chapters/northwest/
**Remarks:** Serves Alaska, Idaho, Montana, Oregon, and Washington.

## Wisconsin

**★ 9246 ★ Crohn's and Colitis Foundation of America**
**Wisconsin Chapter**
2401 N Mayfair Rd., Ste. 19
Wauwatosa, WI 53226
**Phone:** (414)475-5520          **Free:** 877-586-5588
**Fax:** (414)475-5502
**Email:** wisconsin@ccfa.org
**Website:** http://www.ccfa.org/chapters/wisconsin/

# Liver Diseases

*State chapters of the American Liver Foundation are listed below. The national office is located at 75 Maiden Lane, Ste. 603, New York, NY 10038. Additional information can be obtained by calling the national office at (800) GO-LIVER, or by consulting their web site at http://www.liverfoundation.org/.*

## Alabama

**★ 9247 ★ American Liver Foundation**
**Alabama Chapter**
617 Lorna Sq.
Birmingham, AL 35216
**Phone:** (205)822-1126          **Fax:** (205)824-2009
**Email:** paalliver@aol.com
Pamela Gallagher, Director

## Arizona

**★ 9248 ★ American Liver Foundation**
**Arizona Chapter**
4545 E Shea Blvd., Ste. 164
Phoenix, AZ 85028
**Phone:** (602)953-1800          **Fax:** (602)953-1806
**Email:** alfofaz@qwest.net
Leanne Marco, Director

## California

**★ 9249 ★ American Liver Foundation**
**Greater Los Angeles Chapter**
5777 Century Blvd., Ste. 865
Los Angeles, CA 90045
**Phone:** (310)670-4624          **Fax:** (310)670-4672
**Email:** dgracon@liver411.com
**Website:** http://www.liver411.com
Donna Gracon, Director

**★ 9250 ★ American Liver Foundation**
**Northern California Chapter**
870 Market St., Ste. 1046
San Francisco, CA 94102
**Phone:** (415)248-1060          **Free:** 800-292-9099
**Fax:** (415)248-1066
**Email:** info@liverlifeline.com
**Website:** http://www.liverlifeline.com
Linden Young, Director

**★ 9251 ★ American Liver Foundation**
**San Diego Chapter**
4452 Park Blvd., Ste. 102
San Diego, CA 92116
**Phone:** (619)291-5483     **Fax:** (619)295-7181
**Email:** alfsandiego@aol.com
Kristina Furrow, Director

## Colorado

**★ 9252 ★ American Liver Foundation**
**Rocky Mountain Chapter**
3593 S Teller St., Ste. 403
Lakewood, CO 80235-2030
**Phone:** (303)988-4388     **Fax:** (303)988-4398
**Email:** rockymtnliver@qwest.com
Katherine Kinch, Director

## Connecticut

**★ 9253 ★ American Liver Foundation**
**Connecticut Chapter**
110 Washington Ave, 3rd Fl.
North Haven, CT 06473
**Phone:** (203)234-6304     **Fax:** (203)234-6327
**Email:** info@ctalf.org
**Website:** http://www.ctalf.org
JoAnn Thompson, Director

## District of Columbia

**★ 9254 ★ American Liver Foundation**
**Greater Washington DC Chapter**
1875 Eye St. NW, Ste. 1200
Washington, DC 20006
**Phone:** (202)872-6600     **Fax:** (202)872-6603
**Email:** alfdc@starpower.net
**Website:** http://www.liverdc.org
Yao P. Tyus, Director

## Florida

**★ 9255 ★ American Liver Foundation**
**Gulf Coast Chapter**
101 American Center Place, Ste. 201
Tampa, FL 33619-4400
**Phone:** (813)740-0045     **Fax:** (813)740-2524
**Email:** alfgcc@aol.com
Maria Eddy, Director

## Georgia

**★ 9256 ★ American Liver Foundation**
**Georgia Chapter**
1201 Clairmont Rd., Ste. 120
Decatur, GA 30030
**Phone:** (404)633-9169     **Free:** (866)-GA-LIVER
**Fax:** (404)633-8709
**Email:** alfga@mindspring.com
Charlotte Thompson, Director

## Illinois

**★ 9257 ★ American Liver Foundation**
**Illinois Chapter**
27 E Monroe St., Ste. 700A
Chicago, IL 60603
**Phone:** (312)377-9030     **Fax:** (312)377-9035
**Email:** jackie@illinois-liver.org
**Website:** http://www.illinois-liver.org
Paul Ladniak, Contact

## Massachusetts

**★ 9258 ★ American Liver Foundation**
**New England Chapter**
88 Winchester St.
Newton, MA 02461
**Phone:** (617)527-5600     **Free:** 800-298-6766
**Fax:** (617)527-5636
**Email:** info@liverfoundation-ne.org
**Website:** http://www.liverfoundation-ne.org
Judi Kaplan Elkin, Contact

## Michigan

**★ 9259 ★ American Liver Foundation**
**Michigan Chapter**
31700 W 12 Mile Rd, Ste. 201
Farmington Hills, MI 48334
**Phone:** (248)489-5400     **Fax:** (248)489-0376
**Email:** miliver@coast.com
Ryan Ambrozaitis, Director

## Minnesota

**★ 9260 ★ American Liver Foundation**
**Minnesota Chapter**
1500 McAndrews Rd. W, Ste. 214
Burnsville, MN 55337
**Phone:** (952)892-8441     **Fax:** (952)892-8442
**Email:** amlivermn@yahoo.com
**Website:** http://www.angelfire.com/mn2/amlivermn
Scott A. Suckow, Director
**Remarks:** Serves Minnesota and eastern North Dakota and South Dakota.

## Missouri

**★ 9261 ★ American Liver Foundation**
**Missouri Chapter**
16 Hampton Village Plaza, Ste. 215
Saint Louis, MO 63109
**Phone:** (314)352-7377     **Free:** (866)455-4837
**Fax:** (314)352-7875
**Email:** alfmo@mcleodusa.net
Katherine Auble, Director
**Remarks:** Serves Missouri and southern Illinois.

## New York

**★ 9262 ★ American Liver Foundation**
**Greater New York Chapter**
80 Wall St., Ste. 509
New York, NY 10005
**Phone:** (212)943-1059     **Free:** 877-307-7507
**Fax:** (212)943-1314
**Email:** nyliverfoundation@yahoo.com
**Website:** http://www.nyliverfoundation.com
Scott Suckow, Exec Director
**Remarks:** Also serves northeastern New Jersey.

**★ 9263 ★ American Liver Foundation**
**Western New York Chapter**
25 Canterbury Rd., Ste. 316
New York, NY 10025
**Phone:** (716)271-2859     **Fax:** (716)271-8642
**Email:** livrlady@aol.com
Nancy Koris, Director

## North Carolina

**★ 9264 ★ American Liver Foundation**
**North Carolina Triangle Chapter**
PO Box 268
Morrisville, NC 27560
**Phone:** (919)481-3024     **Fax:** (919)481-9571
**Email:** ncalf@worldnet.att.net
**Website:** http://www.ntwrks.com/~tbordeaux/ncalf.htm
Larry Bordeaux, Director

## Ohio

**★ 9265 ★ American Liver Foundation**
**Northern Ohio Chapter**
5755 Granger Rd., Ste. 335
Independence, OH 44131-1455
**Phone:** (216)635-2780     **Free:** (866)-OHIO-ALF
**Fax:** (216)635-2781
**Email:** morganalf@usalogin.net
Terri L. Manns, Director

## Pennsylvania

**★ 9266 ★ American Liver Foundation**
**Delaware Valley Chapter**
111 Presidential Blvd., Ste. 214
Bala Cynwyd, PA 19004
**Phone:** (610)668-0152     **Fax:** (610)668-0155
**Email:** alfdelval@aol.com
**Website:** http://www.netaxs.com/~emagroup/alfdel-va.htm
Peggy Gilbey McMackin, Director
**Remarks:** Serves Pennsylvania, Delaware, and souther New Jersey.

## Tennessee

**★ 9267 ★ American Liver Foundation**
**Mid-South Chapter**
5583 Murray Rd., Ste. 205
Memphis, TN 38119
**Phone:** (901)766-7668     **Fax:** (901)766-2061
**Email:** midsouthalf@yahoo.com
Laura Jackson, Director

## Texas

**★ 9268 ★ American Liver Foundation**
**South Texas Chapter**
2425 W Loop S, Ste. 660
Houston, TX 77027
**Phone:** (713)622-1318     **Fax:** (713)622-1376
**Email:** LiverSTX@aol.com
Patti Wittlif, Director

## Washington

**★ 9269 ★ American Liver Foundation**
**Pacific Northwest Chapter**
2033 6th Ave., Ste. 260
Seattle, WA 98121
**Phone:** (206)443-3805     **Fax:** (206)443-1511
**Email:** pnwliver@uswest.net
Barbara Hernandez, Director

## Wisconsin

**★ 9270 ★ American Liver Foundation**
**Wisconsin Chapter**
4929 N Lyndell Ave.
Glendale, WI 53217
**Phone:** (414)961-4936     **Fax:** (414)961-7288
**Email:** alfwisc@aol.com
Dee Eberle, Director

## Federal Government Agencies

**★ 9271 ★ U.S. Department of Health and Human Services**
National Institutes of Health
National Human Genome Research Institute
9000 Rockville Rd.
Bethesda, MD 20892
**Phone:** (301)496-0844
**Website:** http://www.nhgri.nih.gov/
Francis S. Collins, MD, Director
**Desc:** The Center formulates research goals and long-range plans to accomplish the mission of the human genome project, including the study of ethical, legal, and social implications of human genome research. It supports and administers research and research training programs in human genome research including chromosome mapping, DNA sequencing, database development, and technology development for genome research; provides coordination of genome research and with industry and academia; and conducts research on human genetic disease.

## Foundations & Other Funding Organizations

### Other Funding Organizations

**★ 9272 ★ A-T Medical Research Foundation**
c/o Pam Smith
5241 Round Meadow Rd.
Hidden Hills, CA 91302
**Phone:** (818)704-8146          **Fax:** (818)704-8310
**Website:** http://www.gspartners.com/at
George Smith, Pres.
**Desc:** Works to fund medical research to find a cure for Ataxia-Telangiectasia (A-T), a degenerative genetic disease of the nervous system. Sponsors pioneering research as well as advanced work. **Awards:** Grant to support research.

**★ 9273 ★ American Porphyria Foundation (APF)**
PO Box 22712
Houston, TX 77227
**Phone:** (713)266-9617          **Fax:** (713)871-1788
**Email:** porphyrus@juno.com
**Website:** http://www.enterprise.net/apf
Desiree H. Lyon, Exec. Dir.
**Desc:** Persons interested in advancing awareness and treatment of the porphyrias; affected patients. Porphyria is a class of seven rare (and usually inherited) metabolic disorders of varying severity affecting the nervous system or the skin. It is character-

ized by a deficiency of an enzyme used in making heme (a ring-shaped molecule called a porphyrin), which in turn is used in making hemoglobin. One of porphyria's recurrent though not requisite symptoms is purple-red urine. The foundation's purposes are to: provide financial support for researchers in porphyria; improve the diagnosis and treatment of porphyria through educational programs; locate porphyria patients. Maintains a lending library of videotapes, papers, and pamphlets. **Awards:** Research Grant (annual).

**★ 9274 ★ Association for Glycogen Storage Disease (AGSD)**
PO Box 896
Durant, IA 52747
**Phone:** (563)785-6038          **Fax:** (563)785-6038
**Website:** http://www.agsdus.org
Hollie Swain, Pres.
**Desc:** Individuals afflicted with glycogen storage disease; families of GSD sufferers; health care professionals. (GSD is a hereditary condition characterized by a lack of or deficiency in any of the enzymes used by the body to break down glycogen, resulting in hypoglycemia and related disorders, and requiring diet modifications and frequent or continual feeding, and in extreme cases resulting in death.) Acts as a forum for the discussion of GSD, its treatment, and the problems faced by parents raising children with GSD. Disseminates medical information; fosters communication between the families of GSD patients and health care professionals. Conducts fundraising drive. Aids members in obtaining equipment necessary for home care of GSD patients; provides referral services for individuals seeking GSD treatment facilities. **Awards:** AGSD Grant (annual) for work with GSD.

**Children's PKU Network (CPN)**
*See:* Entry 5594

**★ 9275 ★ Cystic Fibrosis Foundation (CFF)**
6931 Arlington Rd.
Bethesda, MD 20814
**Phone:** (301)951-4422          **Free:** 800-344-4823
**Fax:** (301)951-6378
**Email:** info@cff.org
**Website:** http://www.cff.org
Robert J. Beall, PhD, Pres. & CEO
**Desc:** Supports medical research, professional education, and care centers to benefit patients with cystic fibrosis (CF), an inherited fatal disease among children and adults. With this disease a thick mucus clogs the lungs, creating breathing difficulties and high susceptibility to infection; the digestive system and other organs are also affected. More than 113 care centers affiliated with the foundation provide patient services. Medical programs provide support for a national network of multidisciplinary basic and clinical research grants. **Awards:** Fellowship for clinical or research training, professional education, accreditation, and development of treatment centers; grant for the study and treatment of CF.

**★ 9276 ★ Cystinosis Foundation (CF)**
2516 Stockbridge Dr.
Oakland, CA 94611
**Free:** 800-392-8458          **Fax:** (209)222-7997
**Email:** jd2hotz@qnis.net
**Website:** http://www.cystinosisfoundation.org
Jean Hotz, Pres.
**Desc:** Parents, relatives, and friends of cystinotic children; interested members of the medical community and the public. (Cystinosis is a genetic metabolic disease in which abnormal amounts of the amino acid cystine collect in the cells, leading to kidney failure.) Purposes are to increase public awareness about cystinosis; to act as a support group to parents of children with the disease; to raise funds for research. Maintains speakers' bureau. **Awards:** Grant for research; Volunteer of the Year Award.

**★ 9277 ★ Dysautonomia Foundation**
633 3rd Ave., 12th Fl.
New York, NY 10017
**Phone:** (212)949-6644          **Fax:** (212)682-7625
**Email:** dys212@aol.com
**Website:** http://www.familialdysautonomia.org/
Lenore F. Roseman, Exec. Dir.
**Desc:** Parents, relatives, friends, and benefactors of children afflicted with Familial dysautonomia, a Jewish genetic disease of the autonomic nervous system. Now that the FD Gene has been located and there is a carrier available, we must now fund research into discovering the function the gene plays within the body. **Awards:** Research Grants (annual) for post doctoral research into FD.

**★ 9278 ★ Dystrophic Epidermolysis Bullosa Research Association of America (DEBRA)**
5 W 36th St., No. 404
New York, NY 10018
**Phone:** (212)868-1573          **Fax:** (212)863-9296
**Email:** mrivera@debra.org
**Website:** http://www.debra.org
Martin Hassner, Exec. Dir.
**Desc:** People with Epidermolysis Bullosa and their families; other interested individuals. (Epidermolysis Bullosa represents a group of inherited disorders of the skin characterized by formation of blisters resulting from the most minimal trauma.) To raise funds to promote and support research into the cause, nature, and treatment of EB in all its forms; to relieve the physical and mental distress of victims by providing practical advice, guidance, support, and other assistance. Distributes educational material to the public and medical professionals. Works for federal funding for biomedical research of EB and related disorders. Offers children's services; conducts educational programs. conducts educational programs. **Awards:** Debra Research Grants (annual) scientific research in EB.

**Facioscapulohumeral (FSH) Society**
*See:* Entry 13523

### ★ 9279 ★ Fanconi Anemia Research Fund (FARF)

1801 Willamette St., Ste. 200
Eugene, OR 97401-4030
**Phone:** (541)687-4658          **Free:** 800-828-4891
**Fax:** (541)687-0548
**Email:** info@fanconi.org
**Website:** http://www.fanconi.org
Mary Ellen Eiler, Exec. Dir.

**Desc:** Families with children afflicted with Fanconi anemia, a genetic disorder. Seeks to offer support to families, help them network, and keep them apprised of research relating to Fanconi anemia; assists research on this disorder. Operates support group. Conducts fundraising for research through public awareness programs and special projects. Funds research projects. **Awards:** Grant.

### ★ 9280 ★ Hereditary Disease Foundation (HDF)

1303 Pico Blvd.
Santa Monica, CA 90405-1553
**Phone:** (310)450-9913          **Fax:** (310)450-9532
**Email:** cures@hdfoundation.org
**Website:** http://www.hdfoundation.org
Milton Wexler, Chair

**Desc:** To fund basic biomedical research on the causes, prevention, diagnosis, treatment, and cure of genetic disorders and in particular Huntington's Disease, an inherited neurological disorder. Maintains grant programs to support scientific projects in major medical and basic science laboratories throughout the U.S. Offers grants and postdoctoral fellowships. Sponsors a series of interdisciplinary workshops to stimulate new ideas and approaches to understanding hereditary problems. Helps maintain two tissue banks for research purposes. Disseminates information to organizations and individuals. **Awards:** John J. Wasmuth Award postdoctoral fellowships; Lieberman Award (annual) innovative research for treatment or cure of huntington's disease; Milton Wexler Award postdoctoral fellowships.

### ★ 9281 ★ International Rett Syndrome Association (IRSA)

9121 Piscataway Rd.
Clinton, MD 20735
**Phone:** (301)856-3334          **Free:** 800-818-RETT
**Fax:** (301)856-3336
**Email:** irsa@rettsyndrome.org
**Website:** http://www.rettsyndrome.org
Kathy Hunter, Pres.

**Desc:** Parents of children with Rett Syndrome; interested professionals and supporters. (A child afflicted with Rett Syndrome, which strikes only females, seems normal until 7 to 18 months of age, when autistic-like withdrawal sets in; though this symptom eases in time, higher brain functions continue to deteriorate, leading to severe retardation. The child also loses purposeful use of her hands, wringing them in a constant "hand-washing" movement in front of the face or chest. The syndrome is named for Dr. Andreas Rett, of Vienna, Austria, who described it in 1966. The cause of Rett Syndrome has been traced to a defective gene, called the MeCP2 on the X chromosome.) Provides support to parents; encourages research; collects and disseminates information. Assists in identifying syndrome victims; conducts activities aimed at the prevention, treatment, and eventual eradication of Rett Syndrome. **Awards:** Research Grant (annual) for individuals approved by a Professional Advisory board.

### ★ 9282 ★ Iron Overload Diseases Association (IOD)

433 Westwind Dr.
North Palm Beach, FL 33408-5123
**Phone:** (561)840-8512          **Fax:** (561)842-9881
**Email:** iod@ironoverload.org
**Website:** http://www.ironoverload.org
Roberta Crawford, Pres.

**Desc:** Physicians and patients. Purposes are to: serve hemochromatosis patients and families; encourage

research and public information; press for earlier diagnosis and more effective treatment. (Hemochromatosis is a genetic condition of iron overload in which excess iron damages organs and tissues, producing varying late-stage symptoms including liver cirrhosis, diabetes, heart failure, arthritis, and skin pigmentation, leading to death unless diagnosed early and treated adequately.) Specific plans are: to organize chapters and to develop a public relations plan, television interviews, and press releases; to sponsor screening programs and patient referral service; prepare diagnosis sheets for doctors and medical schools. Current emphasis is on alerting the public to the dangers of excess iron, since the disease is more prevalent than previously believed, and most susceptible individuals are unaware of the hazard. Authorities believe that five in 1000 carry both genes and that one in eight carries a single gene. Acts as a clearinghouse for doctors to call on for research materials and plans to establish a toll-free number for the public. Sponsors fundraising program. Is also in the process of setting up an index of laboratory research in progress. Conducts programs; compiles statistics; maintains speakers' bureau; conducts research programs. **Awards:** Grant for research.

### ★ 9283 ★ Lowe Syndrome Association (LSA)

222 Lincoln St.
West Lafayette, IN 47906
**Phone:** (765)743-3634
**Email:** info@lowesyndrome.org
**Website:** http://www.lowesyndrome.org
Kaye McSpadden, Dir. of Public & Scientific Affairs

**Desc:** Parents, friends, and relatives of individuals with Lowe syndrome; medical, educational, and social service professionals and agencies. Fosters communication among families; provides medical and educational information; promotes a better understanding of Lowe syndrome; supports and encourages medical research. **Awards:** Medical Research Grant (annual) potential to further the understanding of Lowe syndrome or lead to better treatments.

### ★ 9284 ★ National Ataxia Foundation (NAF)

2600 Fernbrook Ln. N, No. 119
Minneapolis, MN 55447
**Phone:** (763)553-0020          **Fax:** (763)553-0167
**Email:** naf@mail.ataxia.org
**Website:** http://www.ataxia.org
Donna Gruetzmacher, Exec. Dir.

**Desc:** Membership is open to any individual who wishes to contribute to the eradication of ataxia (a genetic disease characterized by the degeneration of the nerves of the spinal cord and the cerebellum, causing a loss of coordination and disturbance in gait and related conditions such as peroneal muscular atrophy, hereditary spastic paraplegia, and hereditary tremor. Ataxia may be inherited as a recessive or dominant trait and may strike persons from a very early age up to and even beyond 50 years of age. Ataxia is very similar to multiple sclerosis; however, multiple sclerosis is not inherited and has a different origin.) Objectives are: to make an early diagnosis of ataxia by locating all potential victims and encouraging them to have an examination; to educate the public and the helping professions about ataxia; to initiate basic research and coordinate efforts of worldwide research centers. Emphasis is on locating and understanding the genes responsible. Provides services and information to ataxia victims and their families. **Awards:** Ataxia Research Grant (annual).

### ★ 9285 ★ National Foundation for Jewish Genetic Diseases (NFJGD)

250 Park Ave., Ste. 1000
New York, NY 10177
**Phone:** (212)371-1030          **Fax:** (212)319-5808
**Website:** http://www.nfjgd.org
George Crohn, Pres.

**Desc:** Individuals concerned with the eradication of the seven known genetic diseases that affect children

of predominantly Ashkenazi Jewish heritage. (These diseases include Gaucher's disease, Dystonia, Dysautonomia, Tay-Sachs, Bloom's Syndrome, Niemann-Pick, and Mucolipidosis IV.) Seeks to accomplish its goal by establishing carrier identification tests, providing genetic counseling which includes prenatal testing procedures, and conducting a nationwide education campaign to inform the public that these diseases exist and attack without warning. Supports basic medical research in the prevention and cure of these diseases. Acts as referral agency. Has sponsored symposia on chromosome breakage and neoplasia, Gaucher's disease, and cellular molecular biology of neuronal development. **Awards:** Scholarship.

### National Marfan Foundation (NMF)

*See:* Entry 13528

### ★ 9286 ★ National Neurofibromatosis Foundation (NNFF)

95 Pine St., 16th Fl.
New York, NY 10005
**Phone:** (212)344-6633          **Free:** 800-323-7938
**Fax:** (212)747-0004
**Email:** nnff@nf.org
**Website:** http://www.nf.org/
Michelle Messinger, Dir. of Public Education

**Desc:** The leading resource on neurofibromatosis, a genetic disorder that causes tumors to grow along nerves throughout the body. Provides direct services to children and adults with NF, as well as information and resources to the public and medical professionals via a toll-free number and a website. **Awards:** Basic Grant (annual) for research in neurofibromatosis; Young Investigator Grant (annual) for research in neurofibromatosis.

### ★ 9287 ★ National Society of Genetic Counselors (NSGC)

c/o Bea Leopold
233 Canterbury Dr.
Wallingford, PA 19086-6617
**Phone:** (610)872-7608          **Fax:** (610)872-1192
**Email:** fyi@nsgc.org
**Website:** http://www.nsgc.org
Bea Leopold, Exec. Dir.

**Desc:** The leaing voice, authority and advocate for the genetic counseling profession. **Awards:** Jane Engelberg Memorial Fellowship (annual); Natalie Weissberger Paul National Achievement Award (annual); Special Project Fund (annual).

### ★ 9288 ★ Neurofibromatosis (NF)

8855 Annapolis Rd., Ste. 110
Lanham, MD 20706-2924
**Phone:** (301)918-4600          **Free:** 800-942-6825
**Fax:** (301)918-0009
**Email:** nfinc1@aol.com
**Website:** http://www.nfinc.org
John C. Vickerman, CMP, Exec. Dir.

**Desc:** Organizations providing support for individuals with neurofibromatosis (NF) and their families, physicians, and other health care providers. (NF is a genetic neurological disorder that can cause tumors to form on nerves and is linked to learning disabilities, hearing loss, vision impairment, epilepsy, and cancer.) Increases public awareness of NF through information dissemination; informs federal, state, and local legislators of the needs of NF families. Promotes, supports, and funds medical, clinical, educational, and sociological research that addresses the need to diagnose, treat, cure, and prevent NF. Identifies local NF support and peer counseling groups; offers referrals to medical resources and scientifically-evaluated research. Participates in networking of voluntary health organizations. **Awards:** NF Inc. Scholar (annual) for contribution to the NF cause.

**★ 9289 ★ Osteogenesis Imperfecta Foundation (OIF)**
804 W Diamond Ave., Ste. 210
Gaithersburg, MD 20878
**Phone:** (301)947-0083     **Free:** 800-981-2663
**Fax:** (301)947-0456
**Email:** bonelink@oif.org
**Website:** http://www.oif.org
Ms. Mary Beth Huber, Information & Resource Dir.
**Desc:** Osteogenesis Imperfecta Foundation, Inc. is a voluntary national health organization dedicated to helping people cope with osteogenesis imperfecta. The mission of the OI Foundation is to improve the quality of life for individuals affected by OI through education, awareness, mutual support and research into the treatment and potential cure of the disorder. Information is provided to individuals who have OI and their families, medical professionals and other members of the community. Resources and programs include a quarterly newsletter, a physician information service, written literature, informative videos, national conferences and local support groups. Compiles statistics. **Awards:** Michael Geisman Memorial Fellowship and Seed Awards (annual) for research contribution; monetary for OI research projects.

**★ 9290 ★ Prader-Willi Foundation**
267 Oxford St.
Rochester, NY 14607
**Phone:** (716)442-1655     **Free:** 800-442-1655
**Fax:** (716)271-2782
**Email:** alliance@proder-willi.org
**Website:** http://www.prader-willi.org
Sheldon L. Tarakan, Pres.
**Desc:** Devoted to serving individuals with Prader-Willi Syndrome. Provides information on subjects related to Prader-Willi Syndrome. Finances related projects such as residential development, family support, behavorial research, and awareness. Works with other Prader-Willi organizations. **Awards:** Grant for other Prader-Willi organizations for development and publication.

**PXE International**
*See:* Entry 13532

**★ 9291 ★ Tuberous Sclerosis Alliance (TS Allianc)**
c/o Beth Michaels
801 Roeder Rd., Ste. 750
Silver Spring, MD 20910
**Phone:** (301)562-9890     **Free:** 800-225-6872
**Fax:** (301)562-9870
**Email:** beth.michaels@tsalliance.org
**Website:** http://www.tsalliance.org
Beth Michaels, Dir. /Comm.
**Desc:** Encourages and provides grants for research into the diagnosis, cause, management, and cure of tuberous sclerosis. (Tuberous sclerosis is a genetic disease characterized by one or more of the following: epileptic seizures, mental retardation, behavioral problems, non-malignant tumors, or skin lesions.) Provides support to families affected by the disease through a nationwide network of volunteer area representatives and the distribution of informational packets. Conducts educational programs for medical and allied professionals. **Awards:** Grant; NTSA Awards (annual).

**★ 9292 ★ VHL Family Alliance (VHLFA)**
171 Clinton Rd.
Brookline, MA 02445
**Phone:** (617)277-5667     **Free:** 800-767-4VHL
**Fax:** (617)734-8233
**Email:** info@vhl.org
**Website:** http://www.vhl.org
Joyce Graff, Chair
**Desc:** Patients affected by Von Hippel-Lindau Disease; their families; medical professionals; interested others. Von Hippel-Lindau Disease is a genetic disorder involving abnormal growth forming "knots" of blood vessels in the retina, brain, or spinal cord areas. These knots are hemangiomas, a kind of tumor. Promotes education of the medical community, pa-

tients, and the general public about the disease. Provides an international support network to families affected by VHL. Conducts research and educational programs; maintains speakers' bureau. **Awards:** Minster Volunteer Award (annual); Research Award (annual) for a proposal approved by research board.

---

# National & International Organizations

**★ 9293 ★ A-T Medical Research Foundation**
c/o Pam Smith
5241 Round Meadow Rd.
Hidden Hills, CA 91302
**Phone:** (818)704-8146     **Fax:** (818)704-8310
**Website:** http://www.gspartners.com/at
George Smith, Pres.
**Fnded:** 1989. **Desc:** Works to fund medical research to find a cure for Ataxia-Telangiectasia (A-T), a degenerative genetic disease of the nervous system. Sponsors pioneering research as well as advanced work. **Pub:** Newsletter, annual.

**★ 9294 ★ Acid Maltase Deficiency Association (AMDA)**
PO Box 700248
San Antonio, TX 78270-0248
**Phone:** (210)494-6144     **Fax:** (210)497-3810
**Email:** tianrama@aol.com
**Website:** http://www.amda-pompe.org/
**Desc:** Promotes awareness of Acid Maltase Deficiency, also known as Pompe's Disease; assists in funding research.

**★ 9295 ★ Aicardi Syndrome Newsletter**
c/o Denise Parsons
1510 Polo Fields Ct.
Louisville, KY 40245
**Phone:** (502)244-9152     **Fax:** (502)244-9152
**Email:** AICNews@aol.com
**Website:** http://www.aicardi.com
Denise Parsons, Trustee
**Fnded:** 1983. **Mem:** 200. **Desc:** Families with daughters affected by Aicardi Syndrome (Aicardi Syndrom is a rare genetic disorder affecting females only; and characterized by absence of the corpus callosum, and retinal lesions, seizures, and mental retardation). Provides information, research opportunities, networking, and communication. Acts as a reference and resource contact for medical, educational, and professional organizations. Conducts research programs. **Pub:** *Aicardi Syndrome Newsletter*, 2-3/year. Newsletter. • *ASN Brief*, bimonthly. Newsletter. • Brochure. • Directory.

**★ 9296 ★ Alpha One Foundation**
2937 SW 27th Ave., Ste. 302
Miami, FL 33133
**Phone:** (305)567-9888     **Free:** 877-228-7321
**Fax:** (305)567-1317
**Website:** http://www.alphaone.org
John W. Walsh, Pres.
**Fnded:** 1995. **Desc:** Strives to provide leadership and resources that will result in increased research, improved health, worldwide detection and a cure for Alpha1-Antitrypsin Deficiency (Alpha-1). Devoted solely to research and a cure through grant award programs, research registry, DNA and tissue bank and various programs.

**★ 9297 ★ Alstrom Syndrome International**
14 Whitney Farm Rd.
Mount Desert, ME 04660
**Phone:** (207)288-6385     **Free:** 800-371-3628
**Fax:** (207)288-6078
**Email:** jdm@jax.org

**Website:** http://www.jax.org/alstrom
Jan D. Marshall, Ch.
**Fnded:** 1995. **Nat'l Groups:** 3. **Desc:** Individuals with Alstrom's syndrome (a genetic disorder resulting in multiple organ failures) and their families; health care professionals with an interest in the syndrome and its diagnosis and treatment. Seeks to improve the quality of life of people with Alstrom's syndrome. Serves as a clearinghouse on the syndrome and its treatment; functions as a support group for people with Alstrom's syndrome and their families. Encourages and fosters genetic and clinical research on Alstion Syndrome. **Pub:** *The Alstrom Syndrome Handbook*. Book. • *The Alstrom Syndrome Newsletter*, 3/year. Newsletter. **Frmly:** (2002) International Society for Alstrom Syndrome Families.

**★ 9298 ★ American Board of Genetic Counseling (ABGC)**
9650 Rockville Pike
Bethesda, MD 20814-3998
**Phone:** (301)571-1825     **Fax:** (301)571-1895
**Email:** tvogel@genetics.faseb.org
**Website:** http://www.abgc.net
Sharon Robinson, Admin.
**Fnded:** 1993. **Mem:** 1,400. **Desc:** Individuals who have passed the board's examination. Certifies individuals for the delivery of genetic counseling services; accredits genetic counseling master's degree granting programs. **Pub:** *American Board of Genetic Counseling–Membership Directory*, biennial. Membership Directory. Includes the ABGC, Genetics Society of America, American Society of Human Genetics, American College of Medical Genetics, and the American Board of Medical Genetics. *Price:* Included in membership dues; $50/copy for nonmembers.

**★ 9299 ★ American College of Medical Genetics (ACMG)**
9650 Rockville Pike
Bethesda, MD 20814
**Phone:** (301)530-7127     **Fax:** (301)571-0677
**Email:** acmg@faseb.org
**Website:** http://www.asmg.net
Edward R. B. McCabe, MD,PhD, Pres.
**Fnded:** 1991. **Mem:** 1,100. **Desc:** Physicians and others with an interest in genetics and the delivery of medical genetics services to the public. Works to insure the availability of genetic services without regard to considerations of race, gender, sexual orientation, disability, or ability to pay. Promotes and supports genetics research. Establishes and maintains scientific and professional standards for medical genetics education, research, and practice. Lobbies for effective and fair health policies and legislation; provides information and technical assistance to government agencies engaged in health care regulation or policy formation. Makes available continuing professional education programs; represents members' interests. Conducts advocacy campaigns for people with genetic problems; sponsors public education programs. **Pub:** *Genetics in Medicine; Standards and Guidelines*, bimonthly. Journal. *Price:* $215/yr. US individual; $435/yr. US in training; $85/yr. Outside US.

**Association for Glycogen Storage Disease (AGSD)**
*See:* Entry 8677

**Ataxia - UK**
*See:* Entry 13949

**Behavior Genetics Association (BGA)**
*See:* Entry 12417

**★ 9300 ★ Brazilian Genetics Society (Sociedade Brasileira de Genetica)**
Departamento de Genetica
Faculdade de Medicina, USP
14049 Ribeirao Preto, Brazil

**Phone:** 55 16 6331610
**Email:** office@ataxia.org.uk
**Website:** http://www.bga.org
**Fnded:** 1955.


**Brazilian Muscular Dystrophy Association (Associacao Brasileira de Distrofia Muscular)**
*See:* Entry 13959


★ **9301** ★ **Canadian College of Medical Geneticists (CCMG) (College Canadien de Geneticiens Medicaux — CCGM)**
c/o Royal College of Physicians and Surgeons of Canada
774 Echo Dr.
Ottawa, ON, Canada K1S 5N8
**Phone:** (613)730-6250          **Fax:** (613)730-1116
**Email:** ccmg@rcpsc.edu
**Website:** http://ccmg.medical.org
**Fnded:** 1975. **Mem:** 180. **Lang(s):** English, French. **Desc:** Physicians and other health care professionals with an interest in genetics. Promotes professional development of members; seeks to advance medical genetic research and practice. Facilitates exchange of information among members; conducts research and educational programs.


★ **9302** ★ **Canadian Cystic Fibrosis Foundation (CCFF) (Fondation Canadienne de la Fibrose Kystique — FCFK)**
2221 Yonge St., Ste. 601
Toronto, ON, Canada M4S 2B4
**Phone:** (416)485-9149          **Free:** 800-378-2233
**Fax:** (416)485-0960
**Email:** info@cysticfibrosis.ca
**Website:** http://www.cysticfibrosis.ca
**Fnded:** 1960. **Lang(s):** English, French. **Desc:** Individuals with cystic fibrosis and their families, health care and other professionals working with people with cystic fibrosis. Promotes CF research in Canadian universities and hospitals by funding research grants and major research development programs and gives special grants for training and research to students, fellows, scholars and visiting scientists skilled in such areas as respiratory, pediatrics and behavioral sciences. Promotes the regular exchange of information among researchers, scholars and clinical personnel and offers incentive grants to Canadian cystic fibrosis clinics. Provides support and services to people with cystic fibrosis and their families; sponsors research and educational programs. **Pub:** *Candid Facts*, quarterly. Newsletter.


★ **9303** ★ **Canadian Down Syndrome Society (CDSS)**
811 14th St. NW
Calgary, AB, Canada T2N 2A4
**Phone:** (403)270-8500          **Free:** 800-883-5608
**Fax:** (403)270-8291
**Email:** dsinfo@cdss.ca
**Website:** http://www.cdss.ca
**Fnded:** 1987. **Mem:** 2,000. **Local Groups:** 50. **Lang(s):** English, French. **Pub:** *Babies with Down syndrome.* • *CDSS Quarterly*, quarterly. Newsletter.


★ **9304** ★ **Canadian Genetic Diseases Network**
2125 East Mall, Rm. 349
Vancouver, BC, Canada V6T 1Z4
**Phone:** (604)822-7217          **Fax:** (604)822-7945
**Email:** c.smith@cgdn.ubc.ca
**Website:** http://www.cgdn.generes.ca/
**Fnded:** 1990. **Mem:** 37. **Reg. Groups:** 13. **Lang(s):** English, French. **Desc:** Canadian scientists and health care professionals engaged in medical genetic research. Works to develop and commercialize basic research in genetically related diseases including

cancer, cystic fibrosis, myotonic dystrophy, and huntington's disease. Forms partnerships with industry to develop basic research technologies; trains students in genetic research, with particular focus on the graduate and post-doctoral levels. **Pub:** *The Scanner*, semiannual. Newsletter. Relates advances in genetically related disease research for members, related industries and government agencies.


**Canadian Hemochromatosis Society (CHS)**
*See:* Entry 8686


★ **9305** ★ **Canadian Marfan Association (CMA)**
Central Plaza Postal Outlet
128 Queen St. S
PO Box 42257
Mississauga, ON, Canada L5M 4Z0
**Phone:** (905)826-3223          **Fax:** (905)826-2125
**Email:** info@marfan.ca
**Website:** http://www.marfan.ca
**Fnded:** 1986. **Mem:** 600. **Reg. Groups:** 4. **Lang(s):** English, French. **Desc:** People with Marfan Syndrome (a genetic disorder of the connective tissue), their families, and health care providers and other individuals with an interest in the disorder. Promotes an improved quality of life for people with Marfan Syndrome; seeks to prove diagnostic techniques and treatments of Marfan. Serves as a clearinghouse on Marfan Syndrome; provides support and services to people with Marfan and their families; conducts educational campaigns to raise public awareness of the disorder. Maintains network of local Marfan support groups. **Pub:** *Newslinks*, 3/year. Newsletter.


**Celiac Sprue Association/United States of America (CSA/USA)**
*See:* Entry 9109


**Charcot-Marie-Tooth Association (CMTA)**
*See:* Entry 13974


★ **9306** ★ **CHERUBS - Association of Congenital Diaphragmatic Hernia Research (CDH)**
c/o Dawn M. Torrence
PO Box 1150
Creedmoor, NC 27522
**Phone:** (919)693-8158          **Free:** 877-403-1944
**Fax:** (919)924-1114
**Email:** cmtassoc@aol.com
**Website:** http://www.cherubs-cdh.org/
Dawn M. Torrence, Pres.
**Mem:** 650. **Nat'l Groups:** 27. **State Groups:** 50. **Desc:** Parents, grandparents, foster parents, pediatric surgeons, genetic counselors, pediatricians, nurses, ECMO directors, respiratory therapists, and epidemiologists. Dedicated to helping families of children born with Congenital Diaphragmatic Hernia (CDH); promotes research into possible causes and better treatments.


★ **9307** ★ **Children's PKU Network (CPN)**
3790 Via De La Valle, Ste. 120
Del Mar, CA 92014-4248
**Phone:** (858)509-0767          **Free:** 800-377-6677
**Fax:** (858)509-0768
**Email:** pkunetwork@aol.com
**Website:** http://www.pkunetwork.org
Cindy Neptune, Exec. Dir.
**Fnded:** 1991. **Mem:** 8. **Nat'l Groups:** 1. **Desc:** Works to address the special needs of all people involved in the treatment of Phenylketonuria (PKU), a genetic metabolic disease whereby the body is unable to process the amino acid phenylalanine. Networks families and individuals with each other; provides discount dietary aids; offers financial assistance and support groups; provides crisis intervention; advocates mandatory guidelines for insurance carriers to cover

expenses of medical food treatment of PKU individuals; conducts fundraisers; endows research benefiting PKU and other metabolic disorders. **Pub:** *UPDATE*, semiannual. Newsletter.


★ **9308** ★ **Chromosome Deletion Outreach (CDO)**
c/o Linda Sorg
PO Box 724
Boca Raton, FL 33429-0724
**Free:** 888-236-6880          **Fax:** (561)395-4252
**Email:** cdo@att.net
**Website:** http://www.chromodisorder.org
Linda Sorg, Contact
**Fnded:** 1992. **Mem:** 1,600. **Desc:** Promotes research and understanding of chromosome disorders, including partial duplications (trisomies), inversions, translocations, rings and sex chromosome disorders; provides support to families of children born with these rare disorders; gathers and disseminates information; promotes research and a positive community understanding of these disorders. **Pub:** *Chromosome Deletion Outreach*, quarterly. Newsletter. Contains articles submitted by members and a column offering advice from doctors.


★ **9309** ★ **Chromosome 18 Registry and Research Society**
c/o Jannine D. Cody
6302 Fox Head
San Antonio, TX 78247
**Phone:** (210)657-4968          **Fax:** (210)657-4968
**Email:** office@chromosome18.org
**Website:** http://www.chromosome18.org
Jannine Cody, PhD, Pres.
**Fnded:** 1990. **Mem:** 500. **Reg. Groups:** 12. **Desc:** Individuals with the chromosome 18 disorder, their families, and physicians. (Chromosome 18 anomalies cover a wide range of disorders, including: Trisomy 18, 18q-, 18p-, and Ring 18.) Purposes are: to locate persons with chromosome 18 anomalies; to educate the families, as well as the public about the prognoses and treatments of these disorders; to encourage, conduct, and publish research into areas that impact these families; and to link affected families and physicians to the research community. Offers educational programs. **Pub:** *Chromosome 18 Communique*, quarterly. Newsletter. • Brochure.


★ **9310** ★ **Chromosone 9P Network (9P)**
393 N Grass Valley Rd.
Pine Valley, UT 84781
**Phone:** (435)574-1121          **Fax:** (435)574-2000
**Email:** beverly.udell@9pminus.org
**Website:** http://www.9pminus.org
Jon Storr, Exec. Dir.
**Fnded:** 1984. **Mem:** 200. **Desc:** Parents and caregivers of children that have Monosomy 9P. Offers support to families. (Monosomy 9P is a rare chromosome disorder in which a piece of the 9th chromosome pair is broken off. It results in mental retardation, physical deformity, and triganocephaly of the forehead.) Acts as a clearinghouse for information on the disorder. Maintains a roster of families having a child with Monosomy 9P. Partakes in research, and holds an annual conference. **Pub:** Brochures. **Frmly:** (1999) Support Groups for Monosomy 9P.


★ **9311** ★ **Coalition For Heritable Disorders Of Connective Tissue**
23 Mountain Rd.
Sharon, MA 02067
**Phone:** (781)784-6672
**Email:** info@chdct.org
**Website:** http://www.chdct.org
Sharon Terry, Pres.
**Fnded:** 1989. **Desc:** Strives to bring about greater awareness of heritable disorders of connective tissue in the medical professions and in the public; encourages teaching about these conditions in medical schools; encourages the training of health practition-

ers to identify, diagnose and treat various heritable connective tissue disorders; fosters research.

---

**★ 9312 ★ Coffin-Lowry Syndrome Foundation**
3045 255th Ave. SE
Sammamish, WA 98075
**Phone:** (425)427-0939
**Email:** clsfoundation@yahoo.com
**Website:** http://clsfoundation.tripod.com
Mary Hoffman, Chair

**Fnded:** 1991. **Desc:** Serves as a clearinghouse for information on Coffin-Lowry Syndrome. (CLS is an inherited syndrome causing retardation, developmental delay, dysmorphic features, and skeletal anomolies.) Offers support services for families dealing with CLS. **Pub:** *CLSF News*, monthly. Newsletter. *Price:* Free.

---

**Cooley's Anemia Foundation (CAF)**
*See:* Entry 10154

---

**★ 9313 ★ Corp. for Menke's Disease (CMD)**
5720 Buckfield Ct.
Fort Wayne, IN 46804
**Phone:** (219)436-0137     **Fax:** (219)436-0137
**Email:** bjswiss@aol.com
**Website:** http://www.thalassemia.org
Jane Swiss, Pres.

**Mem:** 86. **Desc:** Families with children born with Menke's disease; medical professionals. (Menke's disease is a terminal genetic disorder, primarily found in males, in which the body is unable to process copper.) Supports research; promotes experimental treatments. **Pub:** Newsletter, annual.

---

**★ 9314 ★ Cri du Chat Syndrome Mutual Help Group**
c/o R. Clarke, Ph.D.
10640 SW 129th Ct.
Miami, FL 33186
R. Clarke, PhD, Contact

**Fnded:** 1997. **Mem:** 5. **Nat'l Groups:** 1. **State Groups:** 1. **Local Groups:** 1. **Desc:** Family members of people with Cri du Chat Syndrome, a genetic disorder usually resulting in profound mental retardation. Promotes understanding of the syndrome and its manifestations. Facilitates communication and mutual support among members; conducts educational programs; makes available children's services. **Pub:** *Cri du Chat Newsletter*, periodic. Newsletter. *Price:* With membership. • *Just Getting Started.*

---

**★ 9315 ★ Cystic Fibrosis Association of Ireland (CFAI)**
CF House
24 Lower Rathmines Rd.
Dublin 6, Ireland
**Phone:** 353 1 4962433     **Fax:** 353 1 4962201
**Email:** cfhouse@internet-ireland.ie
**Website:** http://cfireland.ie

**Fnded:** 1963. **Mem:** 900. **Reg. Groups:** 8. **Lang(s):** English, Irish. **Desc:** People with cystic fibrosis and their families; individuals and organizations providing support and services to people with cystic fibrosis. Seeks to improve the quality of life of people with cystic fibrosis. Provides backup services for young people with cystic fibrosis. **Pub:** Magazine, annual.

---

**★ 9316 ★ Cystic Fibrosis Foundation (CFF)**
6931 Arlington Rd.
Bethesda, MD 20814
**Phone:** (301)951-4422     **Free:** 800-344-4823
**Fax:** (301)951-6378
**Email:** info@cff.org
**Website:** http://www.cff.org
Robert J. Beall, PhD, Pres. & CEO

**Fnded:** 1955. **Local Groups:** 85. **Desc:** Supports medical research, professional education, and care centers to benefit patients with cystic fibrosis (CF), an inherited fatal disease among children and adults. With this disease a thick mucus clogs the lungs, creating breathing difficulties and high susceptibility to infection; the digestive system and other organs are also affected. More than 113 care centers affiliated with the foundation provide patient services. Medical programs provide support for a national network of multidisciplinary basic and clinical research grants. **Pub:** *Commitment*, quarterly. Newsletter. Features updates on research news and fund-raising news. *Price:* Free. • Annual Report, annual. • Also publishes consumer fact sheets.

---

**★ 9317 ★ Cystic Fibrosis Trust**
11 London Rd.
Bromley BR1 1BY, United Kingdom
**Phone:** 44 208 4647211     **Fax:** 44 208 3130472
**Email:** enquires@cftrust.org.uk
**Website:** http://www.cftrust.org.uk

**Fnded:** 1964. **Mem:** 62,500. **Desc:** Individuals affected by Cystic Fibrosis. **Pub:** *CF News*, quarterly. Newsletter. Contains medical and clinical articles, experiences of people involved with cystic fibrosis, welfare issues. Publishes booklets, leaflets, and fact sheets.

---

**★ 9318 ★ Cystinosis Foundation (CF)**
2516 Stockbridge Dr.
Oakland, CA 94611
**Free:** 800-392-8458     **Fax:** (209)222-7997
**Email:** jd2hotz@qnis.net
**Website:** http://www.cystinosisfoundation.org
Jean Hotz, Pres.

**Fnded:** 1983. **Mem:** 150. **Reg. Groups:** 20. **Desc:** Parents, relatives, and friends of cystinotic children; interested members of the medical community and the public. (Cystinosis is a genetic metabolic disease in which abnormal amounts of the amino acid cystine collect in the cells, leading to kidney failure.) Purposes are to increase public awareness about cystinosis; to act as a support group to parents of children with the disease; to raise funds for research. Maintains speakers' bureau. **Pub:** *Cystinosis Foundation Newsletter*, quarterly. Newsletter. • *Facts About Cystinosis*. Brochure. • *National Directory of Information*, periodic. Directory. For physicians engaged in cystinosis research. • Directory, periodic. For parents of children with cysinosis. **Frmly:** Alliance of Genetic Support Groups; (1986) Cystinosia Foundation of California.

---

**DEBRA Ireland**
*See:* Entry 6809

---

**★ 9319 ★ Disorders of Chromosome 16 Foundation (DOC16)**
c/o Karen Lange
331 Haddon Cir.
Vernon Hills, IL 60061
**Phone:** (847)816-0627     **Fax:** (847)367-4031
**Email:** wlango@aol.com
**Website:** http://members.aol.com/wlango
Karen Lange, Pres.

**Desc:** Promotes research into Disorders of Chromosome 16 and provides information on abnormalities; offers information, education and support to families of children living with the disorder and to expectant parents confronting a similar diagnosis; serves as a resource aiding families, friends, caregivers, and medical professionals in their supportive roles. Provides referrals and a database of registered families. **Pub:** Newsletter, quarterly.

---

**★ 9320 ★ Down Syndrome Ireland (DSI)**
30 Mary St.
Dublin 1, Ireland
**Phone:** 353 1 8730999     **Fax:** 353 1 8731064
**Email:** dsi@tinet.ie
**Website:** http://www.downsyndrome.ie

**Fnded:** 1972. **Mem:** 2,200. **Reg. Groups:** 23. **Lang(s):** English, Irish. **Desc:** People with Down syndrome and their families; health care and service providers working with people with Down syndrome. Seeks to improve the quality of life of people with Down syndrome. Provides support and services to people with Down syndrome and their families; conducts educational programs. **Pub:** Magazine, quarterly. • Newsletter, 5/year.

---

**Ehlers Danlos National Foundation (EDNF)**
*See:* Entry 13584

---

**★ 9321 ★ European Alliance Genetic Support Groups**
31 Vredehofstraat
NL-3761 HA Soestdijk, Netherlands
**Phone:** 31 356028155     **Fax:** 31 356027440
**Email:** i.roelofsz@vsop.nl
**Website:** http://www.ednf.org

**Fnded:** 1992. **Mem:** 30. **State Groups:** 15. **Desc:** Individuals with genetic disorders and their families. Promote services which meet the needs of those with genetic disorders and their families. Hold conferences, participate in patient organizations.

---

**★ 9322 ★ European Down's Syndrome Association (EDSA)**
c/o Richard Bonjean
rue V. Close, 41
B-4800 Polleur-Verviers, Belgium
**Phone:** 32 87 223355     **Fax:** 32 87 220716

**Desc:** Professionals and family members of those with Down's syndrome. Promotes the right's and welfare of persons with Down's syndrome to receive health care and educational services; implements a network of local groups of parents and professionals; dedicated to the principles of normalization for those with Down's syndrome; strives to advance health programs for persons with Down's syndrome.

---

**★ 9323 ★ European Federation of Hereditary Ataxias (Euro-ATAXI)**
Haagwindelaan 19
3090 Overijse, Belgium
**Phone:** 32 2 6576176     **Fax:** 32 2 6571510
**Email:** dk.euro-ataxia@skynet.be
**Website:** http://home.wanadoo.nl/euro-ataxia/
**Fnded:** 1989.

---

**European Federation for Immunogenetics (EFI)**
*See:* Entry 3210

---

**European Neurofibromatosis**
*See:* Entry 13998

---

**★ 9324 ★ European Society of Gene Therapy (ESGT)**
c/o Prof. Meral Ozguc
Hacettepe University
Medical Biology Faculty of Medicine Sihhiye
TR-06100 Ankara, Turkey
**Phone:** 90 312 3052483     **Fax:** 90 312 3110777
**Email:** mozguc@gen.hun.edu.tr
**Website:** http://www.esgt2001.org

**Desc:** Promotes clinical research in gene therapy. Fosters communication among members related to gene transfer and therapy. Liaises with regulatory bodies in Europe.

---

**★ 9325 ★ European Society for Phenylketonuria and Allied Disorders (ESPKU)**
Woestijne 16
9880 Aalter, Belgium
**Phone:** 32 5 3630657     **Fax:** 32 5 3622708

**Desc:** Promotes medical and scientific research in phenylketonuria; obliges the postnatal screening to detect the illness.

**European Study Group on Lysosomal Diseases (ESGLD)**
*See:* Entry 8699

**Facioscapulohumeral (FSH) Society**
*See:* Entry 13591

★ **9326** ★ **Fanconi Anemia Research Fund (FARF)**
1801 Willamette St., Ste. 200
Eugene, OR 97401-4030
**Phone:** (541)687-4658     **Free:** 800-828-4891
**Fax:** (541)687-0548
**Email:** info@fanconi.org
**Website:** http://www.fanconi.org
Mary Ellen Eiler, Exec. Dir.
**Fnded:** 1989. **Mem:** 2,000. **Nat'l Groups:** 13. **Desc:** Families with children afflicted with Fanconi anemia, a genetic disorder. Seeks to offer support to families, help them network, and keep them apprised of research relating to Fanconi anemia; assists research on this disorder. Operates support group. Conducts fundraising for research through public awareness programs and special projects. Funds research projects. **Pub:** *FA Family Directory*, annual. Directory. *Price:* $5 in US; $7 all other countries. • *FA Family Newsletter*, semiannual. Newsletter. • *Fanconi Anemia: A Handbook for Families and Their Physicians*. Handbook. **Frmly:** (1989) Fanconi's Anemia Support Group.

**Foundation for Ichthyosis and Related Skin Types (FIRST)**
*See:* Entry 6817

★ **9327** ★ **Fragile X Society**
c/o Mrs. Lesley Walker
53 Winchelsea Lane
Hastings TN35 4LG, United Kingdom
**Phone:** 44 142 4813147
**Email:** lesleywalker@fragile.k-web.co.uk
**Website:** http://www.fragilex.org.uk
**Fnded:** 1990. **Mem:** 1,200. **Desc:** Aims to provide support and comprehensive information to families whose children and adult relatives have fragile X syndrome, to raise awareness of fragile X and to encourage research.

★ **9328** ★ **French Society of Genetics (SFG)**
3b, rue de la Ferollerie
F-45071 Orleans, France
**Phone:** 33 2 38515438
**Fnded:** 1987.

**Gaucher's Association (GA)**
*See:* Entry 8703

★ **9329** ★ **Genetic Alliance (GA)**
4301 Connecticut Ave. NW, Ste. 404
Washington, DC 20008
**Phone:** (202)966-5557     **Free:** 800-336-4363
**Fax:** (202)966-8553
**Email:** info@geneticalliance.org
**Website:** http://www.geneticalliance.org
Mary E. Davisdon, MSW, Exec. Dir.
**Fnded:** 1986. **Mem:** 884. **Desc:** Voluntary genetic organizations; professionals and other interested individuals. Promotes the health and well-being of individuals and families affected by genetic disorders. Provides a forum for the discussion of cross-disability similarities and the identification of available resources. Fosters a partnership among consumers and professionals to enhance education and service for and represent the needs of individuals affected by genetic disorders. Supports networking efforts of members with government agencies, professional groups, service providers, and organizations. Provides technical assistance to genetic support groups. Disseminates information to the public on available resources and referrals. Makes available traveling educational exhibit for member organizations. **Pub:** *Alliance Alert*, monthly. Newsletter. Includes announcements, calendar of events, and membership information. *Price:* For members only. • *Alliance Health Insurance Resource Guide*. • *Informed Consent: Participation in Genetic Research Studies*. • *International Directory of Genetic Advocacy Organizations and Related Resources*. Directory. • *Media Reporting in the Genetic Age*. • Brochures. **Frmly:** (2001) Alliance of Genetic Support Groups.

★ **9330** ★ **Genetic and Inherited Disorders Organization (GIDO)**
Carmichael House
N Brunswick St.
Dublin 7, Ireland
**Phone:** 353 1 8721501
**Email:** inherited.disorders@ireland.com
**Fnded:** 1989. **Lang(s):** English, Irish. **Desc:** An umbrella organization for voluntary organizations in Ireland involved with genetic disorders.

★ **9331** ★ **Genetics Society of China**
917 Datun Rd., Andingmenwai
Beijing 100101, People's Republic of China
**Phone:** 852 10 64919944     **Fax:** 852 10 64914896

**Gluten Intolerance Group of North America (GIGNA)**
*See:* Entry 9126

**Hemochromatosis Foundation (HF)**
*See:* Entry 8706

★ **9332** ★ **Hereditary Disease Foundation (HDF)**
1303 Pico Blvd.
Santa Monica, CA 90405-1553
**Phone:** (310)450-9913     **Fax:** (310)450-9532
**Email:** cures@hdfoundation.org
**Website:** http://www.hdfoundation.org
Milton Wexler, Chair
**Fnded:** 1968. **Desc:** To fund basic biomedical research on the causes, prevention, diagnosis, treatment, and cure of genetic disorders and in particular Huntington's Disease, an inherited neurological disorder. Maintains grant programs to support scientific projects in major medical and basic science laboratories throughout the U.S. Offers grants and postdoctoral fellowships. Sponsors a series of interdisciplinary workshops to stimulate new ideas and approaches to understanding hereditary problems. Helps maintain two tissue banks for research purposes. Disseminates information to organizations and individuals. **Pub:** *Hereditary Disease Foundation*, 4/yr.Newsletter. *Price:* Free.

**HHT Foundation International**
*See:* Entry 5014

★ **9333** ★ **Hong Kong Society of Medical Genetics (HKSMG)**
c/o Clinical Genetic Service
2 Kwong Lee Rd., 3/F
Sham Shui Po Kowloon
Hong Kong, People's Republic of China
**Phone:** 852 23605479     **Fax:** 852 27291440
**Email:** hhtinfor@hht.com
**Website:** http://www.fmshk.com.hk/hksmg
**Fnded:** 1986. **Lang(s):** Chinese, English. **Desc:** Geneticists and health care personnel working in the field of genetics. Seeks to advance the study and practice of medical genetics. Facilitates exchange of information among members; conducts research and educational programs; maintains speakers' bureau.

**Huntington Society of Canada (HSC)**
*See:* Entry 14018

**Huntington's Disease Association (HDA)**
*See:* Entry 14019

**Huntington's Disease Association of Ireland (HDAI)**
*See:* Entry 14020

**Huntington's Disease Society of America (HDSA)**
*See:* Entry 14021

**Indian Muscular Dystrophy Association (IMDA)**
*See:* Entry 14024

★ **9334** ★ **International Association for Research on Epstein Barr Virus**
080
F-94800 Villejuif, France
**Email:** hdsainfo@hdsa.org
**Website:** http://www.hdsa.org

★ **9335** ★ **International Behavioural and Neural Genetics Society (IBANGS)**
c/o Fred van Leuven
Experimental Genetics Group - EGG
Department of Human Genetics - CME
K.U. Leuven - Campus Gasthuisberg O&N 06
B-3000 Leuven, Belgium
**Email:** fredvl@med.kuleuven.ac.be
**Website:** http://www.ibngs.org/
**Fnded:** 1996. **Mem:** 500. **Desc:** Scientists and students in the field of behavioural neurogenetics. Promotes excellence in the field of neurobehavioural genetics. **Pub:** *Genes, Brain and Behavior*.

★ **9336** ★ **International Fibrodysplasia Ossificans Progressiva Association (IFOPA)**
PO Box 196217
Winter Springs, FL 32719-6217
**Phone:** (407)365-4194     **Fax:** (407)365-3213
**Email:** together@ifopa.org
**Website:** http://www.ifopa.org
Jeannie L. Peeper, Pres.
**Fnded:** 1988. **Mem:** 250. **Desc:** Individuals affected by FOP, their families and friends, and health care professionals. (FOP, also known as fibrodysplasia ossificans progressiva, is a rare genetic disorder in which normal bone is produced in abnormal locations, causing joints to become rigid and immobile. Onset usually occurs during childhood and may eventuate in the complete immobilization of nearly every joint in the body. The cause is currently unknown.) Provides support services to those affected by FOP, including medical resources. Encourages and funds medical research into causes of FOP and other bone-related disorders; promotes public education regarding the disorder and its effects. Facilitates communication among those affected by FOP. **Pub:** *FOP Connection*, quarterly. Newsletter. Including articles on daily coping skills new members, research updates. *Price:* Included in membership dues. **AKA:** International FOP Association.

**International Huntington Association (IHA)**
*See:* Entry 14031

**International Joseph Disease Foundation (IJDF)**
*See:* Entry 14032

**Iron Overload Diseases Association (IOD)**
*See:* Entry 8710

**★ 9337 ★ Joubert Syndrome Foundation**
12348 Summer Meadow Rd.
Rock, MI 49880-9552
**Phone:** (906)359-4707     **Fax:** (906)359-4205
**Email:** joubert@up.net
**Website:** http://www.joubertfoundation.com
Mary Van Damme, Co-Founder & Family Resource Coordinator

**Fnded:** 1992. **Mem:** 320. **Nat'l Groups:** 1. **Reg. Groups:** 7. **Desc:** Support and information exchange group for families of people afflicted with Joubert's Syndrome, a genetically transmitted syndrome in which the cerebellar vermis, a section of the brain controlling balance and coordination, is partially or completely missing. Brain stem abnormality causes problems with breathing and eye movements. Physical manifestations of JS include disturbances in breathing patterns, ataxia (unsteadiness), abnormal eye movements, hypotonia, and possible mental retardation. Promotes continuing education for medical professionals. **Pub:** *Rainbow*, quarterly. Newsletter. • *Registry of Families.* **Frmly:** (1999) Joubert Syndrome Parents in Touch Network.

**★ 9338 ★ Klinefelter Syndrome and Associates (KSA)**
PO Box 119
Roseville, CA 95678-0119
**Phone:** (916)773-2999     **Free:** 800-999-9428
**Fax:** (916)773-1449
**Email:** ksinfo@genetic.org
**Website:** http://www.genetic.org/ks
Melissa Aylstock, Exec. Officer

**Fnded:** 1989. **Mem:** 2,000. **Reg. Groups:** 3. **Desc:** Individuals affected by Klinefelter Syndrome and their families. (Klinefelter syndrome is a genetic alteration, occurring only in males, identified by the presence of an extra "X" chromosome on the chromosome chain that determines gender.) Provides support services; facilitates networking and exchange of information. Conducts educational programs. **Pub:** *The Even Exchange*, periodic. Newsletter. • Brochure.Contains information Klinefelter Syndrome. **AKA:** KS and Associates.

**Klippel-Trenaunay Support Group (KTSG)**
*See:* Entry 13608

**★ 9339 ★ Late-Onset Tay-Sachs Foundation (LOTSF)**
1303 Paper Mill Rd.
Erdenheim, PA 19038
**Phone:** (215)836-9426     **Free:** 800-672-2022
**Email:** contactkt@hotmail.com
**Website:** http://www.lotsf.org/

**Desc:** Devoted to research and treatment of Late-onset Tay-Sachs disease, including clinical symptoms, molecular basis of the disease, and pattern of inheritance. **Pub:** *Horizon.* Newsletter.

**★ 9340 ★ Latin American Association for Genetics**
**(Asociacion Latinoamericana de Genetica — ALAG)**
University de Chile
Facultad de Medicine
Santiago, Chile

**★ 9341 ★ Laurence-Moon-Bardet-Biedl Syndrome Network (LMBBSN)**
306 Mirfield Ln.
Lexington Park, MD 20653
**Phone:** (301)863-5658
**Email:** josiahsmom@hotmail.com
**Website:** http://www.geocities.com/hotsprings/spa/1761/
Barbara Mielcarek, Contact

**Fnded:** 1984. **Desc:** Provides a network for individuals with Laurence-Moon-Bardet-Biedl syndrome, a genetic disorder. (Persons with LMBBS suffer from general developmental delay and exhibit symptoms of retinitis pigmentosa, a degenerative eye disease; hypogenitalism; polydactyly; obesity.) **Pub:** *LMBBS Network News*, periodic. Newsletter. Includes list of member families. **AKA:** Laurence-Moon-Biedl Syndrome Network; LMBS Network.

**★ 9342 ★ LMBS Network**
c/o Sonya Coster
124 Lincoln Ave.
Purchase, NY 10577
**Phone:** (914)251-1163
**Email:** josiahsmum@hotmail.com
**Website:** http://www.blindness.org
Sonya Coster, Contact

**Fnded:** 1980. **Mem:** 50. **Nat'l Groups:** 1. **Desc:** Individuals with LMBS and family members. Offers support to individuals and family members. **Pub:** *Network*, semiannual. Newsletter. Profiles and information. *Price:* Free. • Brochure, annual. Contains general information on disease, profile of cases, addresses of contacts.

**★ 9343 ★ Lowe Syndrome Association (LSA)**
222 Lincoln St.
West Lafayette, IN 47906
**Phone:** (765)743-3634
**Email:** info@lowesyndrome.org
**Website:** http://www.lowesyndrome.org
Kaye McSpadden, Dir. of Public & Scientific Affairs

**Fnded:** 1983. **Mem:** 400. **Desc:** Parents, friends, and relatives of individuals with Lowe syndrome; medical, educational, and social service professionals and agencies. Fosters communication among families; provides medical and educational information; promotes a better understanding of Lowe syndrome; supports and encourages medical research. **Pub:** *Living with Lowe Syndrome.* • *On the Beam*, 3/year. Membership newsletter for families affected by Lowe syndrome. *Price:* Included in membership dues.

**★ 9344 ★ Malignant Hyperthermia Association of the United States (MHAUS)**
PO Box 1069
39 E State St.
Sherburne, NY 13460-1069
**Phone:** (607)674-7901     **Fax:** (607)674-7910
**Email:** info@mhaus.org
**Website:** http://www.mhaus.org
Janice L. Bays, Exec. Dir.

**Fnded:** 1981. **Mem:** 2,500. **Desc:** Malignant Hyperthermia (MH) patients and health care providers. MH is a genetically transmitted, often fatal, muscular disorder triggered in susceptible individuals by certain general anesthetic agents. Objectives are to: save lives by making information about MH available; discuss problems that confront families affected by MH; fund research on the causes, detection, and management of MH; disseminate research information. **Pub:** *The Communicator*, quarterly. Newsletter. Contains MH updates for MHS patients and medical professionals. *Price:* $35 per year. • *Emergency Treatment for MH.* • *Malignant Hyperthermia, Four Cases (for medcial professionals).* Video. • *Malignant Hyperthermia, Knowing Your Role (for medical professionals).* Video. • *Managing MH - Clinical Updates.* Pamphlet. • *Preventing MH - An Anesthesia Protocol.* Pamphlet. • *Testing for Susceptibility to MH.* Pamphlet. • *Understanding MH.* Booklet.

**★ 9345 ★ MedPed**
University of Utah
410 Chipeta Way, Rm. 161
Salt Lake City, UT 84108
**Free:** 888-244-2465     **Fax:** (801)581-5402
**Email:** slarri@ucvg.med.utah.edu

**Website:** http://www.medped.org
Stacey Larrinaga-Shum, Prog. Mgr.

**Fnded:** 1989. **Desc:** Promotes early diagnosis, proper treatment, and prevention of premature deaths for people with inherited cholesterol disorders, specifically Familial Hypercholesterolemia (FH).

**★ 9346 ★ Michael Fund (International Foundation for Genetic Research) (MF-IFGR)**
500A Garden City Dr.
Monroeville, PA 15146-1128
**Phone:** (412)823-6380     **Fax:** (412)373-7713
**Email:** randy@michaelfund.org
**Website:** http://www.michaelfund.org
Randy Engel, Exec. Dir.

**Fnded:** 1978. **Desc:** Intertwines the funding of scientific research on Down's Syndrome and related genetic disorders with a pro-life philosophy. Supports research on prevention, cure, or reduction of the effects of Down's Syndrome; enlists support from professionals; and advocates working in this field. Opposes intrauterine detection and abortion of the affected unborn as well as deliberate euthanasia of children and adults with birth defects. Aims to make research findings available to others conducting similar research and to advocate and encourage efforts to improve the care, treatment, education, evaluation and habilitation of children and adults with mental and physical handicaps, to the benefit of their families and communities. **Pub:** *Friends of the Michael Fund Newsletter*, semiannual. Newsletter. Contains topics on eugenics, genetics, prenatal diagnosis. *Price:* Donation.

**★ 9347 ★ MUMS National Parent-to-Parent Network (MUMS)**
c/o Julie Gordon
150 Custer Ct.
Green Bay, WI 54301-1243
**Phone:** (920)336-5333     **Free:** 877-336-5333
**Fax:** (920)339-0995
**Email:** mums@netnet.net
**Website:** http://www.netnet.net/mums/
Julie Gordon, Pres.

**Fnded:** 1979. **Mem:** 18,000. **Nat'l Groups:** 1. **Reg. Groups:** 61. **State Groups:** 32. **Local Groups:** 28. **Desc:** Parents or care providers of a child with any disability, rare disorder, chromosomal abnormality or health condition. Seeks to provide support to parents in the form of a networking system that matches parents with other parents whose children have the same or similar condition, including rare disorders. Informs and updates families and professionals about services available. Refers parents to support groups & assists in forming new groups. **Pub:** *MUMS National Parent to Parent Network Matchmaker*, quarterly. Newsletter. **Frmly:** Mothrs United for Moral Support.

**National Ataxia Foundation (NAF)**
*See:* Entry 14070

**National Center for the Study of Wilson's Disease (NCSWD)**
*See:* Entry 8718

**★ 9348 ★ National Down's Syndrome Association (NDSA)**
NDSA Inst. of Genetics
Hospital for Genetic Diseases
O.U. Begumpet
Hyderabad 500 016, Andhra Pradesh, India
**Phone:** 91 44 3313681
**Email:** info@msgiinteractive.com
**Website:** http://www.ataxia.org

**Fnded:** 1987. **Mem:** 250. **Lang(s):** English. **Desc:** Interested individuals promoting the spread of knowledge about Down's Syndrome (a congenital condition resulting in moderate to severe mental deficiency). Stresses importance of improvement in quality of life for persons with Down's Syndrome. Furnishes the latest research available on the medical, psychosocial, and educational/vocational aspects of the disease; assists in the formation of selfhelp groups; provides training programs for children with the disease; works toward the establishment of special schools for Down's Syndrome children in India. Holds lectures and seminars. **Pub:** *Bulletin on Down's Syndrome*, semi-annual. Bulletin. Also publishes public education material in Telugu, the local language of Andhra Pradesh, India.

### ★ 9349 ★ National Foundation for Ectodermal Dysplasias (NFED)

410 E Main
Box 114
Mascoutah, IL 62258
**Phone:** (618)566-2020          **Fax:** (618)566-4718
**Email:** nfed1@aol.com
**Website:** http://www.nfed.org
Mary Kaye Richter, Exec. Dir.

**Fnded:** 1981. **Mem:** 3,000. **Desc:** Families of ectodermal dysplasia patients and the medical community. (Ectodermal dysplasia is a genetic birth defect usually resulting in an abnormal development of the outer layer of cells in the embryo. The disorder may be characterized by absent or poorly functioning sweat glands, sparse hair follicles, abnormal hair texture, absence of hair and skin oils, disfigured finger and toe nails, hearing or sight deficiencies, abnormalities of the limbs and cleft palate. With proper medical care, ED patients can live fairly normal lives.) Locates patients and provides them with support and information. Assists the medical community in acquiring the necessary information for treating an ED patient, locates treatment facilities and provides referral services. Makes funds available to qualified applicants for dental and other necessary care. Conducts educational meetings and assists with research projects. Provides children's services; compiles statistics. Supports researchers financially and through access to patients when approved. **Pub:** *A Multi-Syndrome Guide to ED.* • *A Skin Guide to Ectodermal Dysplasia.* • *Dental Guide to the Ectodermal Dysplasia.* • *The EDucator*, bimonthly. Newsletter. **Price:** $25/year. • *Evan's New Teeth.* Booklet. Booklet for children. • *Eye, Ear, Nose and Throat Guide to the Ectodermal Dysplasias.* • *Family Guide to the Ectodermal Dysplasias.*

### ★ 9350 ★ National Foundation for Jewish Genetic Diseases (NFJGD)

250 Park Ave., Ste. 1000
New York, NY 10177
**Phone:** (212)371-1030          **Fax:** (212)319-5808
**Website:** http://www.nfjgd.org
George Crohn, Pres.

**Fnded:** 1974. **Desc:** Individuals concerned with the eradication of the seven known genetic diseases that affect children of predominantly Ashkenazi Jewish heritage. (These diseases include Gaucher's disease, Dystonia, Dysautonomia, Tay-Sachs, Bloom's Syndrome, Niemann-Pick, and Mucolipidosis IV.) Seeks to accomplish its goal by establishing carrier identification tests, providing genetic counseling which includes prenatal testing procedures, and conducting a nationwide education campaign to inform the public that these diseases exist and attack without warning. Supports basic medical research in the prevention and cure of these diseases. Acts as referral agency. Has sponsored symposia on chromosome breakage and neoplasia, Gaucher's disease, and cellular molecular biology of neuronal development. **Pub:** Books. • Brochures.

### ★ 9351 ★ National Fragile X Foundation (NFXF)

PO Box 190488
San Francisco, CA 94119
**Phone:** (925)938-9300          **Free:** 800-688-8765
**Fax:** (925)938-9315
**Email:** natlfx@fragilex.org
**Website:** http://www.fragilex.org
Robert Miller, Exec. Dir.

**Fnded:** 1984. **Mem:** 1,000. **State Groups:** 80. **Desc:** Fragile X patients and their families; other individuals

and institutions interested in the syndrome including health care professionals, special education teachers, genetics centers, hospitals, and libraries. (Fragile X syndrome is an X-linked genetic condition which causes varying degrees of mental retardation in affected males, and can cause mental retardation or psychological disorders in carrying females. FXS can be diagnosed by a DNA analysis test.) Seeks to increase awareness of the characteristics and treatment of FXS among members and the public. Works to stimulate research into the causes and treatment of the syndrome. Supports and provides assistance and advice to parents of children with FXS. Conducts research and educational programs. **Pub:** *Boys with Fragile X Syndrome.* Book. • *Children With Fragile X Syndrome: A Parents Guide.* Book. • *Fragile X Syndrome and Hand Book For Parents and Professionals.* Booklets. • *Fragile X Syndrome The Basics.* Brochure. • *Issues and Strategies for Educating Children With FXS*, bimonthly. Videos. • *National Fragile X Foundation Newsletter*, bimonthly. Newsletter. • Also publishes family and professional information packets.

### National Gaucher Foundation (NGF)
*See:* Entry 8719

### National Hemophilia Foundation (NHF)
*See:* Entry 10233

### National Marfan Foundation (NMF)
*See:* Entry 13636

### National MPS Society
*See:* Entry 8723

### National Niemann Pick Disease Foundation (NPD)
*See:* Entry 8724

### National Organization for Albinism and Hypopigmentation (NOAH)
*See:* Entry 8725

### ★ 9352 ★ National Society of Genetic Counselors (NSGC)

c/o Bea Leopold
233 Canterbury Dr.
Wallingford, PA 19086-6617
**Phone:** (610)872-7608          **Fax:** (610)872-1192
**Email:** fyi@nsgc.org
**Website:** http://www.nsgc.org
Bea Leopold, Exec. Dir.

**Fnded:** 1979. **Mem:** 2,000. **Reg. Groups:** 6. **Desc:** The leaing voice, authority and advocate for the genetic counseling profession. **Pub:** *Journal of Genetic Counseling*, bimonthly. Journal. • *Perspectives in Genetic Counseling*, quarterly. Newsletter. • Also publishes high school and college level career packets.

### National Tay-Sachs and Allied Diseases Association (NTSAD)
*See:* Entry 8726

### Neurofibromatosis (NF)
*See:* Entry 14087

### ★ 9353 ★ Norwegian Association for People with Restricted Growth (NIK) (Norsk Interesseforening for Kortvokste — NIK)

Postboks 4568
0404 OSLO Torshov, Norway
**Phone:** 47 88001584
**Email:** nfinc1@aol.com
**Website:** http://www.nfinc.org

**Fnded:** 1983. **Mem:** 150. **Nat'l Groups:** 1. **Lang(s):** English, Norwegian. **Desc:** Represents the interests of small people. **Pub:** *NIK-Posten*, quarterly. Newsletter.

### ★ 9354 ★ Norwegian Bardet-Biedl Syndrome Association (NLMBBSA) (Interesseforeningen fur LMBB i Norge)

PO Box 4568
Torshov
N-0404 Oslo, Norway
**Phone:** 47 62578219
**Email:** btrodahl@frisurf.no

**Fnded:** 1984. **Mem:** 70. **Lang(s):** English, German. **Desc:** Persons with Laurence-Moon-Bardet-Biedl syndrome and their families. (LMBB is a genetic disorder; symptoms include retinitis pigmentosa, hypogenitalism, polydactyly, and obesity.) Offers assistance to children with LMBB and their parents as well as adults with LMBB, especially those newly diagnosed. **Frmly:** (1998) Norwegian LMBB's Syndrome Association.

### ★ 9355 ★ Norwegian Cystic Fibrosis Association (NCFA) (Norsk Forening for Cystisk Fibrose — NFCF)

Postboks 4568
Torshov
N-0404 Oslo, Norway
**Phone:** 47 88004108          **Fax:** 47 22799199
**Email:** cfblad@folio.no
**Website:** http://www.cfnorge.no

**Fnded:** 1976. **Mem:** 700. **Nat'l Groups:** 1. **Reg. Groups:** 4. **Lang(s):** English, Norwegian. **Desc:** Persons with cystic fibrosis and interested individuals. Promotes improvements in the methods of care for persons with cystic fibrosis. Disseminates information; coordinates clinical research. **Pub:** *Nordic Cystic Fibrosis Magazine*, quarterly. Magazine.

### ★ 9356 ★ Norwegian Osteogenesis Imperfecta Foundation (NFOI) (Norsk Forening for Osteogenesis Imperfecta)

Postboks 4568
Nyaalen
N-0404 Oslo, Norway
**Phone:** 47 22799100          **Fax:** 47 22799198
**Email:** nfei@c2i.net
**Website:** http://home.c2i.net/nfoi/

**Fnded:** 1979. **Mem:** 460. **Reg. Groups:** 2. **Lang(s):** English. **Desc:** Persons with OI and others interested in OI. (OI is a hereditary disease that causes various symptoms such as brittle bones, loose joints, short stature, poor teeth, and bad hearing.) NFOI is connected to a competence center: Trenings-OG Radgivningj Senteret (TRS) at Sunnaas Hospital. The center provides advice on different issues concerning OI. NFOI is also member of OI-NORDEN (Scandinavian Organization) and OIFE (European Foundation). **Pub:** *OI-NYTT*, quarterly. Journal. • *OI-permen*, periodic. Includes medical and technical information. Also publishes brochures and pamphlets.

### Organic Acidemia Association (OAA)
*See:* Entry 8729

### Organization of Teratology Information Services
*See:* Entry 4890

### ★ 9357 ★ Osteogenesis Imperfecta Foundation (OIF)

804 W Diamond Ave., Ste. 210
Gaithersburg, MD 20878
**Phone:** (301)947-0083          **Free:** 800-981-2663
**Fax:** (301)947-0456
**Email:** bonelink@oif.org
**Website:** http://www.oif.org
Ms. Mary Beth Huber, Information & Resource Dir.

**Fnded:** 1970. **Mem:** 4,500. **State Groups:** 43. **Desc:** Osteogenesis Imperfecta Foundation, Inc. is a voluntary national health organization dedicated to helping people cope with osteogenesis imperfecta. The mission of the OI Foundation is to improve the quality of life for individuals affected by OI through education, awareness, mutual support and research into the treatment and potential cure of the disorder. Information is provided to individuals who have OI and their families, medical professionals and other members of the community. Resources and programs include a quarterly newsletter, a physician information service, written literature, informative videos, national conferences and local support groups. Compiles statistics. **Pub:** *Growing Up With OI: A Guide for Children*. Book. • *Growing Up With OI: A Guide for Families & Caregivers*. Book. • *Managing Osteogenesis Imperfecta: A Medical Manual*. Book. *Price:* $28.50. • *Osteogenesis Imperfecta Foundation–Breakthrough*, quarterly. Newsletter. Contains medical reports, foundation news, and activities. *Price:* Free to members; $12/year for nonmembers. • *You Are Not Alone.* Videos. *Price:* $7.50. • Also publishes other medical and general literature.

**★ 9358 ★ Prader-Willi Foundation**
267 Oxford St.
Rochester, NY 14607
**Phone:** (716)442-1655　　　**Free:** 800-442-1655
**Fax:** (716)271-2782
**Email:** alliance@proder-willi.org
**Website:** http://www.prader-willi.org
Sheldon L. Tarakan, Pres.

**Fnded:** 1994. **Desc:** Devoted to serving individuals with Prader-Willi Syndrome. Provides information on subjects related to Prader-Willi Syndrome. Finances related projects such as residential development, family support, behavorial research, and awareness. Works with other Prader-Willi organizations. **Pub:** *Moris A. Angulo, MD Prader-Willi Syndrom: A Guide for Families & Others.* • *News & Notes*, quarterly. Newsletter. *Price:* Free.

**PXE International**
*See:* Entry 13655

**★ 9359 ★ Share and Care Cockayne Syndrome Network**
c/o Shirley Rodriguez
PO Box 570618
Dallas, TX 75357
**Phone:** (972)613-4590　　　**Free:** (866)COCKAYNE
**Fax:** (972)613-4590
**Email:** j93082@aol.com
**Website:** http://www.cockayne-syndrome.org
Shirley Rodriguez, contact

**Fnded:** 1993. **Mem:** 1,500. **Desc:** Professionals and families. Works to provide information on Cockayne Syndrome, a rare form of dwarfism, to help parents and doctors to make informed decisions in the care of these children. Provides support for families; encourages research. **Pub:** *Newsletter*, quarterly. Brochure. Research updates and articles on individual children.

**★ 9360 ★ Sociedad de Genetica de Chile**
Casilla 70061, Correo 7
Santiago, Chile
**Phone:** 56 2 776560
**Fnded:** 1964.

**Society for Mucopolysaccharide Diseases (MPS)**
*See:* Entry 8736

**Society for the Study of Inborn Errors of Metabolism (SSIEM)**
*See:* Entry 8737

**★ 9361 ★ Sotos Syndrome Support Association (SSSA)**
Three Danada Sq. E, No. 235
Wheaton, IL 60187
**Phone:** (402)556-2445
**Email:** sssa@well.com
**Website:** http://www.well.com/user/sssa
Eilene Thomas, Pres.

**Fnded:** 1984. **Mem:** 125. **Desc:** Health care professionals and families of children with Sotos Syndrome. (Sotos Syndrome, also known as Cerebral Giantism, is a genetic disorder resulting in exceptional and rapid growth in the first five years, mental retardation, and speech and coordination impairments.) Purposes are to disseminate information to families of children diagnosed with Sotos Syndrome, form support groups, and provide referral and networking services. **Pub:** *SSSA Notes*, quarterly. Newsletter. Includes question and answer section, doctor's column, news updates, and comments from parents. *Price:* Included in membership dues. • Brochure. • Also publishes guidebook.

**Sudden Arrythmia Death Syndromes Foundation (SADS)**
*See:* Entry 5074

**★ 9362 ★ Support Organization for Trisomy 18/13 (SOFT 18/13)**
c/o Barb VanHerreweghe
2982 S Union St.
Rochester, NY 14624
**Phone:** (716)594-4621　　　**Free:** 800-716-SOFT
**Fax:** (716)594-1957
**Email:** barbsoft@aol.com
**Website:** http://www.trisomy.org
Barb VanHerreweghe, Contact

**Fnded:** 1979. **Mem:** 2,100. **Nat'l Groups:** 1. **State Groups:** 50. **Local Groups:** 1. **Desc:** Families, friends, and professionals involved with children born with Trisomy 18 or Trisomy 13. (Trisomy 18 and 13 are genetic disorders in which there are three no. 18 or no. 13 chromosomes rather than the usual two. The disorders are characterized by mental retardation, neurological problems, and respiratory and circulatory deficiencies, and occur in approximately 1000 births per year in the U.S.) Offers support, understanding, and encouragement to families of affected individuals. Provides the public with information on these conditions and birth defects in general. Makes available to families and professionals a file of medical information. Representatives participate in workshops, seminars, lectures, and group studies at universities and hospitals. Conducts surveys and compiles statistics about medical treatment and problems. Maintains speakers' bureau and placement service. **Pub:** *Care of Infant & Child with T18 & T13*. *Price:* $10.95. • *Soft Notes*, bimonthly. • *The SOFT Touch*, 6/yr. Newsletter. Includes reader's forum and chapter news. *Price:* $25. • *Trisomy 18 - A Book for Families*. *Price:* $10.95. • *Trisomy 13 - A Guidebook for Families*. *Price:* $10.95. • Brochures.

**★ 9363 ★ Treacher Collins Foundation (TCF)**
PO Box 683
Norwich, VT 05055-0683
**Phone:** (802)649-3050　　　**Free:** 800-823-2055
**Email:** geomrf@hotmail.com
**Website:** http://www.treachercollinsfnd.org
Hope Charkins, M.S.W., Exec. Dir.

**Fnded:** 1988. **Desc:** Families, individuals, and professionals interested in developing and sharing knowledge about Treacher Collins Syndrome and related conditions. (Treacher Collins Syndrome, also known as Franceschetti-Klein Syndrome, is a rare genetic condition involving underdevelopment of the structures of the head and face.) Promotes research to improve the quality of life of individuals with Treacher Collins Syndrome. Provides networking and support. Operates referral and resource listing service. **Pub:** *Adults with Treacher Collins Syndrome Talk About Their Lives*. Video. • *American Resource List*. • *First Things First: Early Issues for Children with Treacher*

*Collins Syndrome*. Video. • *Genetic Update: Treacher Collins Syndrome*. Offers information about the discovery of the gene which causes Treacher Collins; diagnostic and pre-natal testing; and TCF position on the discovery. • *The Genetics of Treacher Collins Syndrome*. Video. • *Parents Talk About Treacher Collins Syndrome*. Video. • *The Psycho/Social Implications of Treacher Collins Syndrome*. Video. • *Rare Should Not Mean Alone*. Video. Covers Treacher Collins syndrome and the services of the foundation. • *The Surgical Creation of an Ear*. Video. • *Terminology List*. • *Treacher Collins Syndrome - An Overview*. Booklet. • *Treacher Collins Syndrome: Nutrition, Feeding, and Eating*. Booklet. • Newsletter, annual. *Price:* Donations accepted. • Pamphlet. • Also publishes a networking list. **Frmly:** Treacher Collins Family Network.

**★ 9364 ★ Tuberous Sclerosis Alliance (TSAlliance)**
c/o Beth Michaels
801 Roeder Rd., Ste. 750
Silver Spring, MD 20910
**Phone:** (301)562-9890　　　**Free:** 800-225-6872
**Fax:** (301)562-9870
**Email:** beth.michaels@tsalliance.org
**Website:** http://www.tsalliance.org
Beth Michaels, Dir. /Comm.

**Fnded:** 1974. **Mem:** 4,000. **Nat'l Groups:** 1. **Desc:** Encourages and provides grants for research into the diagnosis, cause, management, and cure of tuberous sclerosis. (Tuberous sclerosis is a genetic disease characterized by one or more of the following: epileptic seizures, mental retardation, behavioral problems, non-malignant tumors, or skin lesions.) Provides support to families affected by the disease through a nationwide network of volunteer area representatives and the distribution of informational packets. Conducts educational programs for medical and allied professionals. **Pub:** *Perspective*, quarterly. Newsletter. Contains research articles, resources for patients and parents, legislative news. *Price:* Available to members. • Also publishes brochures, fact sheets. **Frmly:** (2001) National Tuberous Sclerosis Association.

**★ 9365 ★ Turner Syndrome Society of the U.S. (TSSUS)**
14450 T. C. Jester, Ste. 260
Houston, TX 77014
**Phone:** (832)249-9988　　　**Free:** 800-365-9944
**Fax:** (832)249-9987
**Email:** manager@turner-syndrome-us.org
**Website:** http://www.turner-syndrome-us.org
Merriott Terry, National Exec. Dir.

**Fnded:** 1987. **Mem:** 2,000. **Local Groups:** 36. **Desc:** Provides assistance, support and education to girls and women with Turners Syndrome, their families, physicians and the interested public. Mission is to enable innovations in health for Turner syndrome women by: working with health care professionals to expand knowledge about the condition, its diagnosis, treatment and prevention through research; promoting the successful rearing, affirmation and support of individuals affected by the condition, and to enable innovations in learning for Turner syndrome women by: providing a public forum for communication of state-of-the-art information, exchange of ideas and social support, and increasing public awareness of Turner syndrome, its effects and its possibilities. **Pub:** Videos. • Newsletter, quarterly.

**★ 9366 ★ Turner's Syndrome Society (TSS)**
814 Glencairn Ave.
Toronto, ON, Canada M6B 2A3
**Phone:** (416)781-2086　　　**Free:** 800-465-6744
**Fax:** (416)781-7245
**Email:** tssincan@web.net
**Website:** http://www.turnersyndrome.ca
**Fnded:** 1983. **Mem:** 500. **Lang(s):** English, French. **Desc:** Individuals with Turner's Syndrome (a chromosomal disorder affecting women), their families, and health care professionals and organizations with an

interest in the disorder. Promotes an improved quality of life for people with Turner's Syndrome; seeks to advance research into living with Turner's Syndrome. **Pub:** *Turner's Syndrome News*, quarterly. Newsletter.


**Velo-Cardio-Facial Syndrome (VCFS)**
*See:* Entry 5080


★ **9367** ★ **VHL Family Alliance (VHLFA)**
171 Clinton Rd.
Brookline, MA 02445
**Phone:** (617)277-5667          **Free:** 800-767-4VHL
**Fax:** (617)734-8233
**Email:** info@vhl.org
**Website:** http://www.vhl.org
Joyce Graff, Chair
**Fnded:** 1993. **Mem:** 10,000. **Nat'l Groups:** 9. **State Groups:** 29. **Desc:** Patients affected by Von Hippel-Lindau Disease; their families; medical professionals; interested others. Von Hippel-Lindau Disease is a genetic disorder involving abnormal growth forming "knots" of blood vessels in the retina, brain, or spinal cord areas. These knots are hemangiomas, a kind of tumor. Promotes education of the medical community, patients, and the general public about the disease. Provides an international support network to families affected by VHL. Conducts research and educational programs; maintains speakers' bureau. **Pub:** *VHL Family Forum*, quarterly. Newsletter. Contains the latest information on VHL, research into the disease, and support network information. *Price:* Included in membership. • *VHL Patient Handbook*. Booklet. • *What is VHL?*. Brochures. *Price:* $2 for 25. • *Your Family Health Tree*. Booklet. **AKA:** Von Hippel-Lindau Family Alliance.


**Wilson's Disease Association (WDA)**
*See:* Entry 8739


**World Federation of Hemophilia (WFH)
(Federation Mondiale de l'Hemophilie —
 FMH)**
*See:* Entry 10261

---

## Research Centers


★ **9368** ★ **Albany Medical College
Pediatric Pulmonary and Cystic Fibrosis
 Care, Research and Teaching Center**
47 New Scotland Ave., Mail Code A112
Albany, NY 12208
**Phone:** (518)262-6880          **Fax:** (518)262-6884
**Email:** kaslovr@mail.amc.edu
**Website:** http://wfh.org
Robert Kaslovsky, MD, Dir.
**Activities/Fields:** Cystic fibrosis, asthma clinical studies of patients. **Frmly:** Cystic Fibrosis Care Research and Teaching Center.


★ **9369** ★ **Alberta Children's Hospital
 Research Centre
Medical Genetics Group**
1820 Richmond Rd. SW
Calgary, AB, Canada T2T 5C7
**Phone:** (403)229-7373          **Fax:** (403)543-9100
**Email:** snyder@ucalgary.ca
**Website:** http://www.ucalgary.ca/UofC/faculties/medicine/medgenetics/index.htm
Dr. Floyd Snyder, Hd.
**Activities/Fields:** Genetics, including mammalian developmental genetics, genetic control of meiosis, gene mapping and linkage, population genetics, genetic susceptibility to multifactorial inherited disorders such as insulin-dependent diabetes mellitus, use of recombinant DNA methods in clinical medicine, syndrome identification, congenital anomaly surveillance and epidemiology, chromosomal abnormalities in human

sperm and eggs, asymmetry, metacarpophalangeal pattern profile studies, regulatory and genetic aspects of nucleotide metabolism, molecular characterization of inherited enzyme abnormalities, and MSAFP - Down Syndrome screen. **Pub:** *Bulletin of the Hereditary Diseases Program of Alberta*, quarterly.


★ **9370** ★ **American Type Culture
Collection
National Stem Cell Resource**
10801 University Blvd.
Manassas, VA 20110-2209
**Phone:** (703)365-2802          **Fax:** (703)365-2790
**Email:** dbarnes@atcc.org
David W. Barnes, PhD, Prin. Investigator
**Activities/Fields:** Characterization of nonhuman embryonal stem cells, and lineage- or tissue-specific neonatally derived stem cells from a variety of species with regard to germline chimerism, marker expression, differentiative potential, transfectability, selective agent sensitivity and vector suitability.


★ **9371** ★ **Baylor College of Medicine
Baylor DNA Diagnostic Laboratory**
Department of Molecular & Human Genetics
1 Baylor Plz., Rm. 210D
Houston, TX 77030
**Phone:** (713)798-6536          **Fax:** (713)798-6584
**Email:** dnalb@bcm.tmc.edu
**Website:** http://www.bcmgeneticlabs.org/dnadiagnostic.htm
Dr. Benjamin Roa, Dir.
**Activities/Fields:** DNA-based testing for diagnosis, including carrier detection, prenatal diagnosis of more than 35 genetic diseases, densitometric detection of deletion and duplication mutations, estimations of carrier risk for cystic fibrosis, and rapid diagnosis of Duchenne muscular dystrophy with the multiplex amplication assay.


**Baylor College of Medicine
Biochemical Genetics Laboratory**
*See:* Entry 8743


★ **9372** ★ **Baylor College of Medicine
Center for Cell and Gene Therapy**
Methodist Hospital, Ste. 1100
Houston, TX 77030-2399
**Phone:** (832)824-4663          **Fax:** (832)825-4668
**Email:** mbrenner@bcm.tmc.edu
**Website:**      http://www.bcm.tmc.edu/catalog/center_for_cell_and_gene_thera.html
Malcolm K. Brenner, MD, Dir.
**Activities/Fields:** Correction of hereditary and acquired disorders in humans by delivery of therapeutic genes or cells in patients. Five major areas of research in gene therapy have been targeted: genetic disorders, heart disease, infectious diseases, cancer, and neurological disorders.


★ **9373** ★ **Baylor College of Medicine
Department of Molecular and Human
 Genetics**
1 Baylor Plz., Rm. T619
Houston, TX 77030
**Phone:** (713)798-6522          **Fax:** (713)798-7773
**Email:** abeaudet@bcm.tmc.edu
**Website:** http://www.imgen.bcm.tmc.edu/molgen/
Dr. Arthur L. Beaudet, Chm.
**Activities/Fields:** Genetics including human genome sequencing, mouse genome sequencing, gene replacement therapy, gene expression, structure of human chromosome, gene mapping, cell protein synthesis, recombinant DNA techniques, teratology, dysmorphology, clinical cytogenetics, somatic gene transfer, human lipid storage diseases, molecular biology of immune development and human immunodeficiencies, DNA repair and replication, molecular genetics of heritable eye diseases, prenatal diagnosis of congenital malformations and characterization of families of transgenic mice that show mutant phenotypes. Also

coordinates research and patient services in the field of molecular genetics. **Frmly:** Institute for Molecular Genetics.


★ **9374** ★ **Baylor College of Medicine
Kleberg Cytogenetics Laboratory**
1 Baylor Plz., Rm. 15E
Houston, TX 77030
**Phone:** (713)798-4984          **Fax:** (713)798-3157
**Email:** kcl@bcm.tmc.edu
**Website:** http://www.bcmgeneticlabs.org/klebergcytogenetics.htm
Lisa Shaffer, PhD, Dir.
**Activities/Fields:** High-resolution chromosome analysis and development of molecular diagnostic methods for cytogenetic disorders and chromosomal studies.


★ **9375** ★ **Boston University
Center for Human Genetics**
715 Albany St.
Boston, MA 02118-2394
**Phone:** (617)638-7083          **Fax:** (617)638-7092
**Email:** amilunsk@bu.edu
**Website:** http://www.bumc.bu.edu/Departments/HomeMain.asp?DepartmentID=118
Aubrey Milunsky, MD, Dir.
**Activities/Fields:** Routine and specialized chromosome studies, prenatal diagnosis of genetic disorders, molecular genetic (DNA) analysis for diagnosis and carrier detection, maternal serum quadruple screening, biochemical genetic studies, cancer cytogenetics, paternity testing with DNA analysis, and genetic counseling and birth defects evaluation.


**Boys Town National Research Hospital
Center for Hereditary Communication
 Disorders**
*See:* Entry 6134


★ **9376** ★ **Canadian Genetic Diseases
 Network**
NCE Bldg.
2125 East Mall, Rm. 349
Vancouver, BC, Canada V6T 1Z4
**Phone:** (604)822-7217          **Fax:** (604)822-7945
**Email:** csmith.cgdn@ubc.ca
**Website:** http://www.cgdn.generes.ca/welnav.html
Dr. Ron Woznow, Dir.
**Activities/Fields:** Genetic causes of diseases, including myotonic dystrophy, Huntington's disease, and Wilson's disease; genetic predisposition to cancer, including colerectal cancer, tuberculosis, and diabetes; carrier screening and mutation and distribution in populations, including cystic fibrosis, cleft palate, thalassemia, and ricketts; cost effective diagnostic testing, including retinoblastoma and alkaline phosphatase deficiency; biochemical genetics and models of disease, including Huntington's disease, Tay Sachs, lipoprotein lipase deficiency, retinal myopathies, and metabolic diseases; and new therapy trials, including muscular dystrophy and DNA modification strategies.


★ **9377** ★ **Case Western Reserve
 University
Center for Human Genetics**
University Hospitals of Cleveland
11100 Euclid Ave., Lakeside Bldg. 1500
Cleveland, OH 44106-9959
**Phone:** (216)844-3936          **Fax:** (216)844-7497
**Website:** http://genetics.cwru.edu/cfhg.html
Huntington F. Willard, PhD, Dir.
**Activities/Fields:** Human genetics, clinical genetics, molecular genetics, and cytogenetics. **Frmly:** Genetics Center.


**Case Western Reserve University
Center for Inherited Disorders of Energy
 Metabolism (CIDEM)**
*See:* Entry 8744

**★ 9378 ★ Case Western Reserve University**
**Cystic Fibrosis and Pediatric Pulmonary Center**
Rainbow Babies & Childrens Hospital, Rm. 3001
11100 Euclid Ave.
Cleveland, OH 44106
**Phone:** (216)844-3267 **Fax:** (216)844-5916
**Email:** mwk3@po.cwru.edu
**Website:** http://www.cwru.edu/med/CIDEM/cidem.htm
Michael W. Konstan, Dir.

**Activities/Fields:** Cystic fibrosis and pulmonary physiology in children, including basic and clinical studies on evolution and pathology of pulmonary lesion in cystic fibrosis, abnormal mucous secretions of patients with cystic fibrosis, developmental biology of the lung, pulmonary physiology, treatment of chronic obstructive pulmonary disease, intracellular signalling, electrolyte transport and membrane permeability of intestinal, sweat, and respiratory epithelial and individual cells and membrane biopotentials, gene therapy of pulmonary diseases, and inflammation in the cystic fibrosis lung. Asthma studies include basic cell biology of airways and studies of therapeutic regimens for safety and efficacy. Seeks to develop a comprehensive therapeutic regimen for cystic fibrosis.

**★ 9379 ★ Center for Human Genetics**
PO Box 770
Bar Harbor, ME 04609-0770
**Phone:** (207)288-5815
Melba Wilson, Dir.

**Activities/Fields:** Epidemiological and laboratory studies in human genetics, including studies on retinitis pigmentosa, hemochromatosis, hemophilia, Down's syndrome, and cystic fibrosis. **Pub:** *Newsletter*, 3/ year. **Frmly:** Genetic Counseling Center.

**★ 9380 ★ Center for the Improvement of Human Functioning International, Inc.**
3100 N Hillside Ave.
Wichita, KS 67219
**Phone:** (316)682-3100 **Fax:** (316)682-5054
**Email:** staff@brightspot.org
**Website:** http://www.brightspot.org
Hugh Riordan, MD, Dir.

**Activities/Fields:** Human genetic variability and its effects on body chemistry, health and disease, and diagnosis and treatment, especially cancer. Also investigates the measurement of naturally occurring low-energy emission from the human body and effects of extracorporeal subtle energies. **Frmly:** Olive W. Garvey Center for the Improvement of Human Functioning Inc.

**★ 9381 ★ Children's Hospital**
**Cystic Fibrosis Research Center**
3705 5th Ave.
Pittsburgh, PA 15213
**Phone:** (412)692-5630 **Fax:** (412)692-6645
**Email:** davido@pitt.edu
David M. Orenstein, MD, Dir.

**Activities/Fields:** Cystic fibrosis and related diseases, including pediatric pulmonary and pediatric gastrointestinal diseases. Also studies pediatric exercise physiology, and lung cellular immunology.

**★ 9382 ★ Children's Hospital**
**Molecular Diagnostics Lab**
Pathology Department, B120
1056 E 19th Ave.
Denver, CO 80218
**Phone:** (303)837-2725 **Fax:** (303)831-4112
**Email:** wei.qi@tchden.org
Qi Wei, PhD, Supvr.

**Activities/Fields:** Research and testing for genetic diseases, focusing on cancer. DNA diagno stics testing services include both major and minor breakpoint cluster region (BCR) rearrangments; pre-B cell ALL t(1;19) PCR analysis; Y DNA PCR and probe analysis; retinoblastoma gene deletion and linkage analysis; Wilms' tumor gene deletion analysis; and DNA and RNA isolation for special studies. Research efforts, both basic and applied, are focused on mechanisms of carcinogenesis, emphasizing the development of sensitive methods and techniques for the early (pre-clinical) detection of cancer; measuring biological (genetic) damage induced by human exposure to toxic agents; and determining genetic markers of diagnostic and prognostic value in the clinical care of cancer patients.

**★ 9383 ★ Children's Hospital and Medical Center**
**Cystic Fibrosis Research Center**
Mail Stop CH18
4800 Sand Point Way NE
PO Box C5371
Seattle, WA 98105
**Phone:** (206)526-2024 **Fax:** (206)528-2639
**Email:** bramsey@u.washington.edu
Bonnie W. Ramsey, Dir.

**Activities/Fields:** Cystic fibrosis, particularly cardiopulmonary and infectious disease-related pathophysiology, gene therapy, and evaluation of treatment of patients with cystic fibrosis and cardiorespiratory diseases, including clinically oriented research on lung mechanics, and sputum microbiology.

**★ 9384 ★ Children's Memorial Hospital**
**Cystic Fibrosis Research Center**
2300 Children's Plz., Box 43
Northwestern University
Chicago, IL 60614
**Phone:** (773)880-4382 **Fax:** (773)880-6300
**Email:** smccolley@northwestern.edu
Dr. Susanna McColley, Dir.

**Activities/Fields:** Cystic fibrosis, particularly airways inflammation, exercise, psychosocial issues, fat absorption, outcomes research, nutrition, and epidemiology. **Pub:** *Cystic Fibrosis Center News*, quarterly.

**★ 9385 ★ Child's Health Hospital**
**Research Centre**
1820 Richmond Rd. SW
Calgary, AB, Canada T2T 5C7
**Phone:** (403)229-7241 **Fax:** (403)543-9111
Dr. R. Brent Scott, Dir.

**Activities/Fields:** Centre houses two research groups: the Medical Genetics Research Group which conducts research on genetic epidemiology, genetic linkage, molecular genetics, human sperm chromosome analysis, experimental mammalian teratology, developmental genetics, cytogenetics, and birth defects; and the Behavioural Research Group with programs in childhood conditions such as hyperactivity, diet and behavior, learning disorders, and stress-related disorders. Research and development of diagnostic services in biochemical genetics, cytogenetic and molecular genetics are supported through the Alberta Hereditary Diseases Program and are integrated in the Centre. Also sponsors pediatric research in respirology, gastroenterology, vision research, infectious diseases, neonatology, and other allied health disciplines. **Pub:** *Alberta Children's Hospital Research Centre Annual Reports.* • *Bulletin of the Alberta Hereditary Diseases Program*, quarterly. **Frmly:** Kinsmen Pediatric Research Centre.

**★ 9386 ★ Colorado State University**
**Macromolecular Resources**
Department of Biochemistry, 355 MRB
Fort Collins, CO 80523
**Phone:** 800-491-0424 **Free:** 800-4DN-AFAX
**Email:** cfiol@mmr.bmb.colostate.edu
**Website:** http://mmr.bmb.colostate.edu/
Carol J. Fiol, PhD, Dir.

**Activities/Fields:** Produces custom oligonucleotides for DNA researchers and custom peptides. Also offers mass spectrophotometry, protein sequencing and DNA sequencing services.

**★ 9387 ★ Columbia-Presbyterian Medical Center**
**Columbia Genome Center**
630 W 168th St.
New York, NY 10032-3784
**Phone:** (212)305-3440 **Fax:** (212)305-1191
**Email:** ise1@columbia.edu
I.S. Edelman, MD, Dir.

**Activities/Fields:** DNA and human disease conditions in chromosome 13. The center contains six laboratory sections: Molecular Genetics, Physical mapping, DNA sequencing, Cancer Genetics, Genomic Informatics, and Molecular Bioinformatics.

**★ 9388 ★ Columbia University**
**Center for Reproductive Sciences**
630 W 168th St.
New York, NY 10032
**Phone:** (212)305-2304 **Fax:** (212)305-3869
**Email:** nm274@columbia.edu
**Website:** http://cpmcnet.columbia.edu/dept/obgyn/patient-care-services/contact-us.htmlsciences
Dr. Rogerio A. Lobo, MD, Dir.

**Activities/Fields:** Biology of reproduction, including neuroendocrinology, male and female gametogenesis, reproductive endocrinology, genetics, perinatology, angiogenesis, and reproductive oncology.

**★ 9389 ★ Columbia University**
**Molecular Genetics Laboratory**
1051 Riverside Dr.
New York, NY 10032
**Phone:** (212)543-5868 **Fax:** (212)543-6211
Dr. James Knowles, Dir.

**Activities/Fields:** Human molecular genetics, including genetic and physical mapping of human chromosomes, and the mapping and characterization of human disease genes.

**★ 9390 ★ Cystic Fibrosis Center (Portland, OR)**
Pediatric Pulmonary Division, CDRCP
707 SW Gaines Rd.
Portland, OR 97201
**Phone:** (503)494-8023 **Fax:** (503)494-8898
**Email:** powersm@ohsu.edu
Michael R. Powers, MD, Res. Dir.

**Activities/Fields:** Cystic fibrosis, including laboratory and clinical studies of molecular abnormalities in cystic fibrosis and lyses of pulmonary mucus.

**★ 9391 ★ Cystic Fibrosis Foundation**
6931 Arlington Rd., Ste. 200
Bethesda, MD 20814
**Phone:** (301)951-4422 **Free:** 800-344-4823
**Fax:** (301)951-6378
**Email:** info@cff.org
**Website:** http://www.cff.org
Robert Beall, PhD, Pres. /CEO

**Activities/Fields:** Causes and treatment of cystic fibrosis. The Research Development Program involves a network of research centers supported by the Foundation; also supports many care centers throughout the United States. **Pub:** *Annual Report.* • *Commitment*, quarterly.

**Dalhousie University**
**Atlantic Research Centre**
*See:* Entry 4637

**★ 9392 ★ Duke University**
**Center for Human Genetics (CHG)**
DUMC Box 3445
Durham, NC 27710
**Free:** 800-283-4316 **Fax:** (919)684-2275
**Email:** center@chg.mc.duke.edu
**Website:** http://www.chg.duke.edu/
Margaret A. Pericak-Vance, PhD, Dir.

**Activities/Fields:** Genetic and epidemiologic basis of human disease, both rare and common.

**★ 9393 ★ Duke University**
**Cystic Fibrosis Research Center**
PO Box 2994
Durham, NC 27710
**Phone:** (919)684-3364     **Fax:** (919)684-2292
**Email:** eates004@mc.duke.edu
Maria D. Martinez, MD, Dir.
**Activities/Fields:** Cystic fibrosis and related respiratory diseases of children.

**Eleanor Roosevelt Institute**
*See:* Entry 4640

**★ 9394 ★ Emory University**
**Cystic Fibrosis Care, Teaching and**
**Research Center**
1547 Clifton Rd. NE
Atlanta, GA 30322
**Phone:** (404)727-5728     **Fax:** (404)727-4828
**Email:** dcaplan@emory.edu
**Website:** http://www.eri.uchsc.edu
Dr. Daniel B. Caplan, Dir.
**Activities/Fields:** Cystic fibrosis and respiratory and gastrointestinal diseases of children.

**★ 9395 ★ Genome Sequencing Center**
CB 8501
Washington University in St. Louis
4444 Forest Park Blvd.
Saint Louis, MO 63108
**Phone:** (314)286-1800     **Fax:** (314)286-1810
**Website:** http://genome.wustl.edu/gsc/
Robert H. Waterston, MD, Dir.
**Activities/Fields:** Genome mapping and sequencing, technology development, and informatics.

**★ 9396 ★ Houston Advanced Research**
**Center**
**DNA Technology Laboratory**
4800 Research Forest Dr.
The Woodlands, TX 77381
**Phone:** (281)363-7947     **Fax:** (281)363-7946
**Email:** dao@harc.edu
**Website:** http://www.harc.edu/dna/
Dr. Dat D. Dao, Dir.
**Activities/Fields:** Development and application of DNA technologies, especially applications of genosensor technology, which are miniaturized DNA chips that can quickly analyze genetic alterations.

**★ 9397 ★ Indiana University Bloomington**
**Howard Hughes Medical Institute**
**Research Laboratory**
Jordan Hall, Rm. A507
Bloomington, IN 47405
**Phone:** (812)855-3033     **Fax:** (812)855-2577
**Email:** kaufman@bio.indiana.edu
Thomas C. Kaufman, Dir.
**Activities/Fields:** Understanding the genetic basis of the developmental program of higher organisms. Efforts focus on the homeotic genes that play a crucial role in the development of the fruit fly Drosphilia melanogaster.

**★ 9398 ★ Indiana University-Purdue**
**University at Indianapolis**
**Cystic Fibrosis and Pediatric Pulmonary**
**Clinic**
702 Barnhill Dr., Rm. 2750
Indianapolis, IN 46202-5225
**Phone:** (317)274-5652     **Fax:** (317)278-0927
**Email:** heigen@iupui.edu
Howard Eigen, MD, Dir.
**Activities/Fields:** Cystic fibrosis and chronic lung diseases, including clinical studies of pediatric pulmo-

nary, gastrointestinal, genetic problems, and lung inflammation.

**★ 9399 ★ The Institute for Genomic**
**Research (TIGR)**
9712 Medical Center Dr.
Rockville, MD 20850
**Phone:** (301)838-0200     **Fax:** (301)838-0208
**Email:** cmfraser@tigr.org
**Website:** http://www.tigr.org
Claire M. Fraser, PhD, Pres.
**Activities/Fields:** Structural, functional and comparative analysis of genomes and gene products from a wide variety of organisms including viruses, eubacteria (both pathogens and non-pathogens), archaea (the so-called third domain of life), and eukaryotes (plants, animals, fungi and protists such as the malarial parasite).

**★ 9400 ★ Institute for Systems Biology**
**(ISB)**
1441 N 34th St.
Seattle, WA 98103-8904
**Phone:** (206)732-1200     **Fax:** (206)732-1299
**Email:** lhood@systemsbiology.org
**Website:** http://www.systemsbiology.org/
Dr. Leroy Hood, Dir.
**Activities/Fields:** Study of genes and proteins, especially how genomic DNA, mRNA, proteins, functional proteins, informational pathways and informational networks work together. The goal is to predict and prevent disease.

**★ 9401 ★ International Center for**
**Skeletal Dysplasia**
St. Joseph Medical Center
7601 Osler Dr.
Towson, MD 21204
**Phone:** (410)337-1250     **Fax:** (410)337-1042
Dr. Steven Kopits, Dir.
**Activities/Fields:** Skeletal dysplasia, particularly dwarfism. Studies include metatropic dysplasia, a rare form of dwarfism identified in 1966.

**★ 9402 ★ Jackson Laboratory**
600 Main St.
Bar Harbor, ME 04609-1500
**Phone:** (207)288-6000     **Free:** 800-422-6423
**Fax:** (207)288-6150
**Email:** pubinfo@jax.org
**Website:** http://www.jax.org
Kenneth Paigen, PhD, Dir.
**Activities/Fields:** Formal genetics, molecular genetics, developmental genetics, physiological genetics, immunology, cell biology, and biochemistry as related to cancer, diabetes, anemias, other human diseases, as well as normal growth and development. Annually produces 2,000,000 genetically standardized mutant and inbred mice strains for its own research staff and research workers throughout the world. Five major areas of research include, Cancers, development and aging-related, immune system and blood disorders, neurological and sensory disorders, and metabolic diseases. **Pub:** *Animal Health & Genetic Quality Control Report*, quarterly. • *Annual Report.* • *Handbook of Genetically Standardized JAX Mice.* • *Inside the Jackson Laboratory*, 3/year. • *Scientific Report.*

**★ 9403 ★ Jackson Laboratory**
**Induced Mutant Resource**
600 Main St.
Bar Harbor, ME 04609
**Phone:** (207)288-6223     **Fax:** (207)288-6149
**Email:** mtd@jax.org
**Website:** http://www.jax.org
Muriel T. Davisson, PhD, Contact
**Activities/Fields:** Imports, establishes on defined genetic background and phenotypically characterizes transgenic, targeted mutation and induced (eg, ENU mutagenesis) mutation mice; develops sperm cryopreservation methodology, assisted reproduction tech-

nology, high throughput genotyping and speed congeic methodology.

**★ 9404 ★ Jeanette Kennelly Kroch**
**Center for Twin Studies**
Prentice Pavilion
Northwestern Memorial Hospital
333 E Superior St., Rm. 410
Chicago, IL 60611
**Phone:** (312)926-7519     **Fax:** (312)926-0367
**Email:** apeacema@nmh.org
Alan M. Peaceman, MD, Dir.
**Activities/Fields:** Multiple births. Conducts ultrasound and genetic research for the early detection of identical or fraternal twins; longitudinal ultrasound studies to determine normal growth patterns in multiple-birth pregnancies; clinical studies of methods to prevent premature labor and delivery, which result in low-birthweight twins; and studies related to specific aspects of twin development, such as speech patterns.

**★ 9405 ★ Johns Hopkins University**
**Adolescent Idiopathic Scoliosis**
**Laboratory (AIS)**
Ross Bldg., Rm. 232
720 Rutland Ave.
Baltimore, MD 21205
**Phone:** (410)614-3717     **Fax:** (410)502-6414
**Email:** bmarosy@jhmi.edu
**Website:** http://www.med.jhu.edu/ais/
Dr. Nancy H. Miller, Contact
**Activities/Fields:** Genetics of adolescent idiopathic scoliosis, a condition characterized by a lateral curvature of the spine.

**★ 9406 ★ Johns Hopkins University**
**Bipolar Pedigree Collection**
Affective Disorders Section
Department of Psychiatry & Behavioral Sciences
600 N Wolfe St., Meyer 3-181
Baltimore, MD 21287-7381
**Phone:** (410)955-5212     **Fax:** (410)955-0152
Dr. J. Raymond DePaulo, Jr., Prin. Investigator
**Activities/Fields:** Genetics of bipolar disorder (manic-depressive illness), involving families in which someone is suffering from this condition.

**Johns Hopkins University**
**Center for Hereditary Eye Diseases**
*See:* Entry 21116

**★ 9407 ★ Johns Hopkins University**
**Center for Inherited Disease Research**
Triad Technology Center
333 Cassell Dr., Ste. 2000
Baltimore, MD 21224
**Email:** jhched@jhmi.edu
**Website:** http://www.cidr.jhmi.edu/main.html
Dr. David Valle, Prin. Investigator
**Activities/Fields:** Provides genotyping and statistical genetics services for investigators seeking to identify genes that contribute to human disease, primarily on multifactorial hereditary disease.

**★ 9408 ★ Johns Hopkins University**
**Cystic Fibrosis Research Center**
202 Physiology
725 N Wolfe St.
Baltimore, MD 21205
**Phone:** (410)955-7166     **Fax:** (410)955-0461
**Email:** wguggino@jhmi.edu
**Website:** http://www.johnshopkinscfresearch.org/researchlab.htm
Dr. William B. Guggino, Dir.
**Activities/Fields:** Cystic fibrosis and related fields, including epithelial cell transport, molecular genetics, respiratory cell biology, and biochemistry.

**La Jolla Institute for Molecular Medicine**
*See:* Entry 10361


**★ 9409 ★ Laval University**
**Medical Research Centre**
**Human Genetics Unit**
2705 Blvd. Laurier
Sainte Foy, QC, Canada G1V 4G2
**Phone:** (418)654-2244      **Fax:** (418)654-2714
**Email:** sec.drs@crchul.hlaval.ca
**Website:** http://www.crchul.ulaval.ca/crchul/en/cen-tre/default_pres.htm
Jack Puymirat, MD, Dir.

**Activities/Fields:** Molecular mechanisms controlling genetic expression; thyroid hormones and central nervous system development; molecular genetics of myotonic dystrophy; implication of cytoskeletal and nucleoskeletal proteins in morphonogenetic and differentiation processes; molecular genetics of Charcot-Marie-Tooth disease; control of cell cycle; gene therapy; myoblasts transplantation for Duchenne's disease, Myotonia congenita, and genetic testing.


**★ 9410 ★ Laval University**
**Molecular Microbiology and Protein**
**    Engineering Group**
Departemente de Biologie Medicale
4142 Pavillon Charles-Eugene-Marchand
Faculte de Medecine
Sainte Foy, QC, Canada G1K 7P4
**Phone:** (418)656-2131      **Fax:** (418)656-7176
**Email:** rclevesq@rsvs.ulaval.ca
Roger C. Levesque, Dir.

**Activities/Fields:** Structure-function analysis of B-lactamases, dihydrofolate reductase and superoxide dismutase in pathogenic microorganisms. Studies also include molecular genetics, phylogeny, and evolution of multiresistant transposons, and sequencing pseudomonas genome.


**Laval University**
**Saint-Francois-d'Assise Hospital Research**
**    Centre**
*See:* Entry 18400


**★ 9411 ★ Lawrence Berkeley National**
**    Laboratory**
**Life Sciences Division**
Mail Stop 83-101
1 Cyclotron Rd.
Berkeley, CA 94720
**Phone:** (510)486-4365      **Fax:** (510)486-5586
**Email:** mjbissell@lbl.gov
**Website:** http://www.lbl.gov/lifesciences/
Mina J. Bissell, PhD, Div. Dir.

**Activities/Fields:** Human Genome Project; mutagenesis and carcinogenesis, emphasizing DNA repair and recombination; mechanisms of tissue-specific gene expression, focusing on mammary gland cells and hemopoiesis; structural biology, concentrating on the three-dimensional structure of integral membrane proteins; and radiobiology, stressing molecular and cellular mechanisms and the risks associated with radiation as an environmental hazard.


**★ 9412 ★ Louisiana State University in**
**    Shreveport**
**Genetics Section of Pediatrics**
Medical Center
1501 Kings Hwy.
Shreveport, LA 71130
**Phone:** (318)675-6083      **Fax:** (318)675-6089
**Email:** tthurm@lsumc.edu
T.F. Thurmon, MD, Dir.

**Activities/Fields:** Clinical applications of genetics, biochemical genetics, and cytogenetics. Studies include chromatographic diagnostic techniques, heredity of dysmorphic syndromes, and chromosome aberrations in cancer. **Frmly:** Birth Defects Center.


**★ 9413 ★ McMaster University**
**Centre for Gene Therapeutics**
Health Science Centre
1200 Main St. W
Hamilton, ON, Canada L8N 3Z5
**Phone:** (905)521-2100      **Fax:** (905)577-0198
**Email:** gauldie@mcmaster.ca
**Website:** http://www.fhs.mcmaster.ca/cgt/main.html
Jack Gauldie, Dir.

**Activities/Fields:** Delivery of genes as therapeutic agents in the treatment of human and animal disease. This entails basic investigations to target gene product involvement, creation of vector systems for appropriate delivery of therapeutic genes and rapid translation of promising medicines to the clinical setting. The center is focused on developing cures for cancer, inflammatory diseases and infectious diseases.


**★ 9414 ★ Medical College of Wisconsin**
**Cystic Fibrosis Research Center**
Specialty Clinic
Milwaukee Children's Hospital of Wisconsin
9000 W Wisconsin Ave., Ste. 211
Milwaukee, WI 53201
**Phone:** (414)266-6731      **Fax:** (414)266-6742
**Email:** splain@mcw.edu
Dr. M.L. Splaingard, Dir.

**Activities/Fields:** Cystic fibrosis, chest impedance measurements, and newborn screening studies. Provides patient care as a service to referring physicians and instruction for small groups of medical students from the College.


**★ 9415 ★ Medical College of Wisconsin**
**Human and Molecular Genetic Center**
8701 Watertown Plank Rd.
Milwaukee, WI 53226
**Phone:** (414)456-4887      **Fax:** (414)456-6516
**Email:** jacob@mcw.edu
**Website:** http://brc.mcw.edu/lgr
Dr. Howard J. Jacob, Dir.

**Activities/Fields:** Identification of the genes involved in multifactorial diseases, such as cancer, cardiovascular disease, obesity, insulin dependent diabetes mellitus, and non-insulin dependent diabetes. **Frmly:** Laboratory for Genetics Research.


**Metro Health Medical Center**
**Department of Epidemiology and**
**    Biostatistics**
**Human Genetic Analysis Resource**
*See:* Entry 9054


**Miami Children's Hospital Research**
**    Institute**
*See:* Entry 5804


**★ 9416 ★ Michael Fund/International**
**    Foundation for Genetic Research**
500 A Garden City Dr.
Monroeville, PA 15146
**Phone:** (412)823-6380      **Fax:** (412)373-7713
**Email:** tengel@bellatlantic.net
**Website:** http://www.michaelfund.org
Randy Engel, Contact

**Activities/Fields:** Down's Syndrome and related genetic disorders with a pro-life philosophy, focusing on funding, prevention, cure or reducing the effects of Down's Syndrome. Also opposes abortion of the unborn, including deliberate euthanasia of children and adults with birth defects. **Pub:** *Friends of the Michael Fund Newsletter.*


**★ 9417 ★ Molecular Genetics Laboratory**
Davis, 2069
Cedars-Sinai Medical Center
110 George Burns Rd.
Los Angeles, CA 90048
**Phone:** (310)423-7627      **Fax:** (310)423-0302
**Email:** julie.korenberg@cshs.org


**Website:** http://www.csmc.edu/genetics/korenberg/korenberg.html
Dr. Julie Korenberg, Contact

**Activities/Fields:** Human genome analysis and novel applications; primate evolutionary mechanisms; molecular basis of cognition; genetic origins of congenital heart disease; Down Syndrome; Wiliams Syndrome; DNA isolation and diagnostics, including Southern blotting, libraryscreening, subcloning, probe growth, and preparation. **Frmly:** Molecular Diagnostics Laboratory.


**National Science Foundation**
**Directorate for Biological Sciences**
**Division of Molecular and Cellular**
**    Biosciences**
**Microbial Genetics Program**
*See:* Entry 4664


**★ 9418 ★ North York General Hospital**
**North York Regional Genetics Centre**
4001 Leslie St.
Toronto, ON, Canada M2K 1E1
**Phone:** (416)756-6345      **Fax:** (416)756-6727
**Email:** pwyatt@nygh.on.ca
**Website:** http://www.nsf.gov/bio/mcb/mcbgenetics.htmmg
Dr. Philip Wyatt, Dir.

**Activities/Fields:** Clinical genetics, prenatal biology, and chromosomal and metabolic diseases.


**★ 9419 ★ Oklahoma Medical Research**
**    Foundation**
**Functional Proteomics Laboratory**
825 NE 13th St.
Oklahoma City, OK 73104
**Phone:** (405)271-6673      **Fax:** (405)271-3980
**Email:** xin-li-lin@omrf.ouhsc.edu
**Website:** http://www.omrf.org/OMRF/Research/16/Program.asp
Xinli Lin, Prog. Hd.

**Activities/Fields:** Structural genomics and functional proteomics.


**★ 9420 ★ Oregon Health and Science**
**    University**
**Biochemical Genetics Laboratory**
Department of Molecular & Medical Genetics
3181 SW Sam Jackson Pk. Rd., BH-2029
Portland, OR 97201
**Phone:** (503)494-5400      **Fax:** (503)494-7645
**Email:** gibsonm@ohsu.edu
K. Michael Gibson, PhD, Dir.

**Activities/Fields:** Inborn errors of metabolism and mitochondrial myopathies.


**★ 9421 ★ Oregon Health and Science**
**    University**
**Portland Alcohol Research Center (PARC)**
VA Medical Center, R&D 12
Portland, OR 97201
**Phone:** (503)220-8262      **Fax:** (503)721-1029
**Email:** rutledgm@ohsu.edu
**Website:** http://www.ohsu.edu/som-BehNeuro/PARC/Center.html
Mark Rutledge-Gorman, Admin.

**Activities/Fields:** Genetics of neuroadaptation to ethanol, specifically how the brain adapts to alcohol, and mapping the genes underlying alcoholism risk.


**Pope Paul VI Institute for the Study of**
**    Human Reproduction, Inc.**
*See:* Entry 18404

**★ 9422 ★ Queen's University at Kingston**
**Cytogenetics and DNA Research**
**Laboratory**
Ongwanada
191 Portsmouth Ave.
Kingston, ON, Canada K7M 8A6
**Phone:** (613)548-4417 **Fax:** (613)548-8135
**Email:** cytodna@post.queensu.ca
**Website:** http://www.ongwanada.com/research.html
Jeanette J.A. Holden, PhD, Dir.

**Activities/Fields:** Cytogenetics, DNA markers, linkage studies, fragile-X syndrome, X-linked mental retardation, x-linked hydrocephalus, Down's syndrome, autism, affective disorders, schizophrenia, melanoma, and chromosome instability.

**★ 9423 ★ Rockefeller University**
**Laboratory of Biochemical Genetics and**
**Metabolism**
1230 York Ave.
PO Box 179
New York, NY 10021
**Phone:** (212)327-7700 **Fax:** (212)327-7165
**Email:** breslow@rockefeller.edu
Prof. Jan L. Breslow, MD, Contact

**Activities/Fields:** Human genetic susceptibility to atherosclerosis, especially the molecular genetics and clincial significance of the apolipoproteins, a group of proteins that coat the lipoprotein particles and determine their metabolism.

**★ 9424 ★ Rockefeller University**
**Laboratory of Human Genetics and**
**Hematology**
1230 York Ave.
New York, NY 10021
**Phone:** (212)327-8000 **Fax:** (212)327-8862
**Email:** auerbac@mail.rockefeller.edu
**Website:** http://www.rockefeller.edu/labheads/auerbach/auerbach.html
Arleen D. Auerbach, Dir.

**Activities/Fields:** Fanconi anemia (FA), an autosomal recessive disorder characterized clinically by progressive pancytopenia, variable skeletal and other congenital abnormalities, predisposition to malignancy, particularly acute myelogenous leukemia (AML), prenatal diagnosis of FA, and identification of genes that cause FA.

**★ 9425 ★ Rockefeller University**
**Starr Center for Human Genetics**
1230 York Ave.
New York, NY 10021
**Phone:** (212)327-8000 **Free:** 888-920-9100
**Fax:** (212)327-7373
**Website:** http://www.rockefeller.edu/graduate/cen-starr.htm
Dr. Jeffrey M. Friedman, Dir.

**Activities/Fields:** Genetic analysis of human disease and biology, including heart disease, obesity, diabetes, schizophrenia, hearing loss, obsessive-compluvsive disorder, and addictive disorders.

**★ 9426 ★ Saginaw Valley State**
**University**
**Genetic Research Laboratory**
7400 Bay Rd.
University Center, MI 48710
**Phone:** (517)790-4358 **Fax:** (517)790-2717
**Email:** cfp@svsu.edu
**Website:** http://www.svsu.edu/biology/
Dr. Charles F. Pelzer, Hd.

**Activities/Fields:** Molecular genetics, emphasizing electrophoresis and Southern Blots of human DNA, isoelectric focusing of blood proteins in health and disease such as breast cancer, and biochemical genetics of red cell isozymes in the mouse. Performs restriction fragment length polymorphism (RFLP) analysis to help map human chromosone number 10 and Southern blotting to identify tumor suppressor genes.

**★ 9427 ★ St. Christopher's Hospital for**
**Children**
**Cystic Fibrosis Center**
Erie Ave. at Front St.
Philadelphia, PA 19134
**Phone:** (215)427-5183 **Fax:** (215)427-4621
**Email:** daniel.schidlow@drexel.edu
Daniel Schidlow, MD, Dir.

**Activities/Fields:** Cystic fibrosis and other chronic respiratory diseases, including cystic fibrosis of the pancreas in children, epidemiology of lung infections, airway injury in children, lung mechanics in infants, developmental respiratory physiology, and clinical trials for new therapies against cystic fibrosis.

**Sidney Kimmel Cancer Center (SKCC)**
*See:* Entry 10414

**★ 9428 ★ Southern Louisiana Cystic**
**Fibrosis Clinical Care and Research**
**Center/Pediatric Pulmonary Center**
Tulane University
1430 Tulane Ave.
New Orleans, LA 70112
**Phone:** (504)588-5601 **Fax:** (504)588-5490
**Email:** rbecker@tmcpop.tmc.tulane.edu
**Website:** http://www.skcc.org/
Dr. Robert C. Beckerman, Dir.

**Activities/Fields:** Cystic fibrosis, childhood asthma, apnea, sleep disorders and sleep disordered breathing, SIDS, control of breathing in immature mammal models.

**★ 9429 ★ Southwest Foundation for**
**Biomedical Research**
**Genetics Core Laboratory**
Department of Genetics
PO Box 760549
San Antonio, TX 78245-0147
**Phone:** (210)258-9688 **Fax:** (210)670-3344
**Email:** scole@darwin.sfbr.org
**Website:** http://www.sfbr.org
Dr. Shelley Cole, Dir.

**Activities/Fields:** Molecular genetics of chronic diseases in humans and nonhuman primates. **Frmly:** Molecular Genetics Laboratory.

**★ 9430 ★ Stanford University**
**Beckman Center for Molecular and**
**Genetic Medicine**
Sch. of Medicine
Stanford, CA 94305
**Phone:** (650)725-7657 **Fax:** (650)725-7739
**Email:** shapiro@cmgm.stanford.edu
Dr. Lucy Shapiro, Dir.

**Activities/Fields:** Molecular understanding of critical biological functions and how these are affected by disease, including study of genes related to human disease, development of new diagnostic tests for known and newly recognized diseases, and development of therapies based on gene or cell replacement models.

**★ 9431 ★ Stanford University**
**Interdepartmental Medical Genetics**
**Program**
Howard Hughes Medical Institute
Beckman Center
Stanford, CA 94305-5323
**Phone:** (650)725-8089 **Fax:** (650)725-8112
**Email:** francke@cmgm.stanford.edu
Dr. Uta Francke, Trng. Prog. Dir.

**Activities/Fields:** Molecular basis of heritable disorders, including polygenic and multi-factorial diseases, chromosome structure and function, and genome and gene mapping. Develops methods to manipulate and study large fragments of DNA and animal models and new treatment modalities of human genetic disease by homologous recombination.

**★ 9432 ★ Stanford University**
**Stanford Human Genome Center**
975 California
Palo Alto, CA 94306
**Phone:** (650)320-5800 **Fax:** (650)320-5801
**Email:** myers@shgc.stanford.edu
**Website:** http://shgc.stanford.edu/
Richard Myers, Dir.

**Activities/Fields:** Construction of high resolution Radiation Hybrid maps of the human genome and the sequencing of large, contiguous genomic relations.

**★ 9433 ★ State University of New York**
**Upstate Medical University at Syracuse**
**Robert C. Schwartz Cystic Fibrosis**
**Center and Pediatric Pulmonary Center**
750 E Adams, 5th Fl., Pediatrics
Syracuse, NY 13210
**Phone:** (315)464-6323 **Fax:** (315)464-6322
**Email:** anbarr@mail.upstate.edu
Dr. Ran D. Anbar, Dir.

**Activities/Fields:** Cystic fibrosis, asthma, and hypnosis, including clinical studies.

**★ 9434 ★ Stowers Institute for Medical**
**Research**
1000 E 50th St.
Kansas City, MO 64110
**Phone:** (816)926-4000 **Fax:** (816)444-8644
**Email:** info@stowers-institute.org
**Website:** http://www.stowers-institute.org/Splash.asp
Robert E. Krumlauf, PhD, Sci. Dir.

**Activities/Fields:** Complex genetic systems to unlock the mysteries of disease and find the keys to their causes, treatment and prevention. **Pub:** *The Stowers Report*, quarterly.

**Temple University**
**Center for Neurovirology and Cancer**
**Biology**
**Laboratory of Immunobiology**
*See:* Entry 14284

**★ 9435 ★ Texas A&M University**
**Alkek Institute of Biosciences and**
**Technology**
**Center for Genome Research**
2121 W Holcombe Blvd.
Houston, TX 77030-3303
**Phone:** (713)677-7651 **Fax:** (713)677-7689
**Email:** rwells@ibt.tamu.edu
Dr. Robert D. Wells, Dir.

**Activities/Fields:** Structure and biology of DNA in living cells and viruses and its role in the developmental expression of genetic information. Specific research areas include cancer and other human genetic diseases, maintenance and stability of chromosome ends, and the processing of information from DNA into functional messenger ribonucleic acid (RNA) for expression into proteins.

**★ 9436 ★ Trinity University**
**Genetics Laboratory for Typing**
**Nonhuman Primates**
Department of Biology
715 Stadium Dr.
San Antonio, TX 78212-7200
**Phone:** (210)999-8347 **Fax:** (210)999-7229
**Email:** wstone@trinity.edu
**Website:** http://www.trinity.edu/
William H. Stone, PhD, Dir.

**Activities/Fields:** Genetic typing of nonhuman primates of various species. The aim is to define as many genetic markers as possible in nonhuman primates. Research in DNA typing focuses population genetics; identification of markers for other traits, such as major genes in polymorphic systems; control of genetic variation; and monitoring of breeding, control of inbreeding, and development of breeding programs. Resources and diagnostic services include: genetic profiling of several different genetic systems, plus DNA, which together can define an almost unlimited number of different phenotypes; STR typings; performs DNA typing of rhesus monkeys, chimpanzees and other great apes; genotyping and quantification of genetic variability using short tandem repeat DNA markers and PCR, restriction site RFLPs. Genetic advice for research strategy. Works toward the development of the nonhuman primate as an animal model for human disease.

**★ 9437 ★ Tulane University**
**Gene Therapy Center**
1430 Tulane Ave., S-99
New Orleans, LA 70112
**Phone:** (504)988-7711    **Fax:** (504)988-7710
**Email:** d.procko@tulane.edu
**Website:** http://www.som.tulane.edu/gene_therapy/
Dr. Darwin J. Prockop, Dir.
**Activities/Fields:** Gene therapy of bone and cartilage diseases, Parkinson's Disease and brain tumors. **Pub:** *Peer reviewed research reports.*

**★ 9438 ★ United Cerebral Palsy**
**Research and Educational Foundation**
1660 L St. NW, Ste. 700
Washington, DC 20036
**Phone:** (202)776-0406    **Free:** 800-872-5827
**Fax:** (202)776-0414
**Email:** lsmithslade@ucp.org
**Website:** http://ucp.org
Murray Goldstein, DO, Contact
**Activities/Fields:** Cerebral palsy, focusing on improving the treatment, management, and functioning of persons with cerebral palsy.

**★ 9439 ★ U.S. Department of Energy**
**Department of Energy Program Offices—**
**Environment, Safety and Health**
**Office of Biological and Environmental**
**Research**
**((Medical Sciences Division)**
**Genome Instrumentation Research**
**Program)**
19901 Germantown Rd., SC-73
Germantown, MD 20874-1290
**Phone:** (301)903-9009
**Email:** roland.hirsch@science.doe.gov
**Website:** http://www.sc.doe.gov/production/ober/ msd_genome_instrum.html
Roland F. Hirsch, PhD, Prog. Mgr.
**Activities/Fields:** Advanced sequencing technologies to enable sequencing rates up to one million bases per day; automation stages of chromosomes mapping and sequencing for efficiency and cost effectiveness. New sequencing technology includes development of advanced, highly multiplexed capillary gel electrophoresis systems, electrophoresis separations in liquid media without gels and applications of mass spectrometry and flow cytometry to analysis of sequencing fragments.

**U.S. Department of Health and Human**
**Services**
**Food and Drug Administration**
**Center for Bilogics Evaluation and**
**Research**
**Division of Cellular and Gene Therapies**
*See:* Entry 4695

**U.S. Department of Health and Human**
**Services**
**Food and Drug Administration**
**Center for Bilogics Evaluation and**
**Research**
**Laboratory Cellular Immunology**
**(Division of Cellular and Gene Therapies)**
*See:* Entry 4696

**U.S. Department of Health and Human**
**Services**
**Food and Drug Administration**
**Center for Biologics Evaluation and**
**Research**
**Molecular Medical Genetics Staff**
*See:* Entry 4722

**U.S. Department of Health and Human**
**Services**
**Food and Drug Administration**
**National Center for Toxicological**
**Research**
**Genetic Toxicology Division**
*See:* Entry 17380

**U.S. Department of Health and Human**
**Services**
**National Cancer Institute**
**Division of Cancer Control and**
**Population Sciences**
**Extramural Epidemiology and Genetics**
**Program**
*See:* Entry 10440

**U.S. Department of Health and Human**
**Services**
**National Cancer Institute**
**Laboratory of Genetics**
*See:* Entry 10485

**★ 9440 ★ U.S. Department of Health and**
**Human Services**
**National Center for Research Resources**
**Biological Models and Materials Resource**
**Program**
**Caenorhabditis Genetics Center**
Univ. of Minnesota
250 Biological Sciences Center
1445 Gortner Ave.
Saint Paul, MN 55108-1095
**Phone:** (612)625-2265    **Fax:** (612)625-5754
**Email:** stier@biosci.cbs.umn.edu
**Website:** http://biosci.cbs.umb/cgc
Bob Herman, Dir.
**Activities/Fields:** Provides genetic stocks of Caenorhabditis elegans and other Caenorhabditis species for use by investigators initiating or continuing research on this nematode. The Center also acquires new strains described in current literature and evaluates methods for permanent storage of genetic stocks. Current research includes: resolution of conflicting genetic data received from research laboratories, improving the resolution of the genetic map, and alignment of the genetic and physical maps. **Pub:** *Worm Breeders Gazette.* Newsletter.

**U.S. Department of Health and Human**
**Services**
**National Heart, Lung, and Blood Institute**
**Molecular Hematology Branch**
*See:* Entry 10504

**U.S. Department of Health and Human**
**Services**
**National Institute of Allergy and**
**Infectious Diseases (NIAID)**
**Division of Allergy, Immunology, and**
**Transplantation**
**Genetics and Transplantation Branch**
*See:* Entry 3276

**U.S. Department of Health and Human**
**Services**
**National Institute of Allergy and**
**Infectious Diseases**
**Laboratory of Immunogenetics**
*See:* Entry 3283

**★ 9441 ★ U.S. Department of Health and**
**Human Services**
**National Institute of Diabetes and**
**Digestive and Kidney Diseases**
**Division of Diabetes, Endocrinology, and**
**Metabolic Diseases**
**Cystic Fibrosis Research Program**
Natcher Bldg.
6707 Democracy Blvd.
Rm. 6103, MSC 5460
Bethesda, MD 20892-5460
**Phone:** (301)594-8810    **Fax:** (301)480-3503
**Email:** McKeonC@extra.niddk.nih.gov
**Website:** http://www.niddk.nih.gov/fund/program/a-el-ist.htmcystic
Dr. Catherine McKeon, Contact
**Activities/Fields:** Supports investigator-initiated research projects related to the etiology, pathogenesis, diagnosis, and treatment of cystic fibrosis (CF). In addition, the Program supports a cystic fibrosis research centers and small Business Innovation Research Grants.

**★ 9442 ★ U.S. Department of Health and**
**Human Services**
**National Institute of Diabetes and**
**Digestive and Kidney Diseases**
**Division of Intramural Research**
**Genetics and Biochemistry Branch**
NIH Bldg. 10, Rm. 9D08
10 Center Dr. MSC 1810
Bethesda, MD 20892-1810
**Phone:** (301)496-2710    **Fax:** (301)496-9878
Dr. R. Daniel Camerini-Otero, Chf.
**Activities/Fields:** Clinical, biochemical, developmental, and molecular genetics. The range of current projects covers a wide field, from the very basic (e.g., mechanisms of genetic recombination and gene conversion in mammalian cells, DNA-mediated gene transfer, the regulation of gene expression, the molecular biology of early development in *Xenopus laevis*, biosynthesis and transport of lysosomal proteins, the molecular mechanisms of endocytosis, and the biochemical and molecular bases of human genetic disorders) to the more applied (i.e., development of new diagnostic tests and carrier detection for a number of human genetic diseases and the development of new techniques for gene purification and transfer).

**U.S. Department of Health and Human**
**Services**
**National Institute of Diabetes and**
**Digestive and Kidney Diseases**
**Laboratory of Chemical Biology**
*See:* Entry 4730

**U.S. Department of Health and Human**
**Services**
**National Institute of Environmental Health**
**Sciences**
**Division of Environmental Carcinogenesis**
**Experimental Carcinogenesis and**
**Mutagenesis Laboratory**
*See:* Entry 8964

**★ 9443 ★ U.S. Department of Health and Human Services**
**National Institute of General Medical Sciences**
**Division of Genetics and Developmental Biology**
Bldg. 45, Rm. 2AS-25
45 Center Dr., MSC 6200
Bethesda, MD 20892-6200
**Phone:** (301)594-0943     **Fax:** (301)480-2228
**Email:** greenbej@nigms.nih.gov
**Website:** http://www.nih.gov/nigms
Judith H. Greenberg, PhD, Dir.
**Activities/Fields:** Genetics research and developmental biology to better understand the fundamental processes and mechanisms of inheritance. An objective of the program is the eventual prevention and improved treatment of genetic ills in man, including multifactoral diseases with a strong hereditary component, such as diabetes, atherosclerosis, hypertension, and schizophrenia. Research training support provided by the Division includes: institutional predoctoral programs, which sponsor research training in the broad field of genetic principles and mechanisms; individual postdoctoral awards, which support training for research that will lead to further understanding of genetics and development; and institutional postdoctoral programs (with emphasis on medical genetics), which provide advanced and special research training in genetics. Research is concerned with basic genetic and developmental studies. Research topics include the replication, repair, and recombination of DNA; regulation of gene expression; population genetics and evolution; cell cycle control; developmental genetics; chromosomal organization and mechanics; and neurogenetics.

**U.S. Department of Health and Human Services**
**National Institute of Mental Health**
**Intramural Research Programs Division (Clinical Research)**
**Clinical Neurogenetics Branch**
*See:* Entry 12736

**U.S. Department of Health and Human Services**
**National Institute of Neurological Disorders and Stroke**
**Division of Intramural Research (Basic Neurosciences Program)**
**Laboratory of Developmental Neurogenetics**
*See:* Entry 14301

**U.S. Department of Health and Human Services**
**National Institute of Neurological Disorders and Stroke**
**Division of Intramural Research (Clinical Neurosciences Program)**
**Developmental and Metabolic Neurology Branch**
*See:* Entry 14310

**★ 9444 ★ U.S. Department of Health and Human Services**
**National Institutes of Health**
**Baylor College of Medicine**
**Human Genome Sequencing Center**
One Baylor Plaza
MSC-226
Houston, TX 77030
**Phone:** (713)798-6539     **Fax:** (713)798-5741
**Email:** hgsc-help@bcm.tmc.edu
**Website:** http://www.hgsc.bcm.tmc.edu/
Richard Gibbs, Dir.

**Activities/Fields:** Human Genome Project, Dictyostelium sequencing, Drosophila sequencing, Mouse sequencing, and cDNA sequencing.

**U.S. Department of Health and Human Services**
**National Institutes of Health (NIH)**
**National Cancer Institute (NCI)**
**Division of Basic Sciences**
**((Laboratory of Biosystems and Cancer)**
**Structure and Function of Mammalian Centromere Section)**
*See:* Entry 10510

**U.S. Department of Health and Human Services**
**National Institutes of Health**
**National Cancer Institute**
**Division of Basic Sciences**
**(Laboratory of Biosystems and Cancer)**
*See:* Entry 10512

**U.S. Department of Health and Human Services**
**National Institutes of Health**
**National Cancer Institute**
**Division of Basic Sciences**
**((Laboratory of Experimental Immunology)**
**Cellular and Molecular Immunology Section)**
*See:* Entry 10514

**U.S. Department of Health and Human Services**
**National Institutes of Health**
**National Cancer Institute**
**Division of Basic Sciences**
**(Laboratory of Genomic Diversity — LGD)**
*See:* Entry 10516

**U.S. Department of Health and Human Services**
**National Institutes of Health**
**National Cancer Institute**
**Division of Basic Sciences**
**((Experimental Immunology Branch)**
**Dinah Singer Laboratory)**
*See:* Entry 10523

**U.S. Department of Health and Human Services**
**National Institutes of Health**
**National Cancer Institute**
**Division of Basic Sciences**
**((Experimental Immunology Branch)**
**Andre Nussenzweig Laboratory)**
*See:* Entry 10525

**U.S. Department of Health and Human Services**
**National Institutes of Health**
**National Cancer Institute**
**Division of Cancer Control and Population Sciences (DCCPS)**
**((Epidemiology and Genetics Research Program)**
**Analytic Epidemiology Research Branch — AERB)**
*See:* Entry 10540

**U.S. Department of Health and Human Services**
**National Institutes of Health**
**National Cancer Institute**
**Division of Cancer Control and Population Sciences (DCCPS)**
**((Epidemiology and Genetics Research Program)**
**Clinical and Genetic Epidemiology Research Branch — CGERB)**
*See:* Entry 10542

**U.S. Department of Health and Human Services**
**National Institutes of Health**
**National Cancer Institute**
**Division of Cancer Epidemiology and Genetics**
**(Laboratory of Population Genetics)**
*See:* Entry 10548

**U.S. Department of Health and Human Services**
**National Institutes of Health**
**National Cancer Institute**
**Division of Cancer Epidemiology and Genetics**
**(Human Genetics Program)**
*See:* Entry 10549

**U.S. Department of Health and Human Services**
**National Institutes of Health**
**National Cancer Institute**
**Division of Cancer Epidemiology and Genetics**
**(Viral Epidemiology Branch)**
*See:* Entry 10550

**U.S. Department of Health and Human Services**
**National Institutes of Health**
**National Cancer Institute**
**Division of Cancer Epidemiology and Genetics**
**(Occupational Epidemiology Branch)**
*See:* Entry 10551

**U.S. Department of Health and Human Services**
**National Institutes of Health**
**National Cancer Institute**
**Division of Cancer Epidemiology and Genetics**
**(Radiation Epidemiology Branch)**
*See:* Entry 10552

**U.S. Department of Health and Human Services**
**National Institutes of Health**
**National Cancer Institute**
**Division of Cancer Epidemiology and Genetics**
**(Environmental Epidemiology Branch)**
*See:* Entry 10553

**U.S. Department of Health and Human Services**
**National Institutes of Health**
**National Cancer Institute**
**Division of Cancer Epidemiology and Genetics**
**(Nutritional Epidemiology Branch)**
*See:* Entry 10554

**U.S. Department of Health and Human Services**
**National Institutes of Health**
**National Cancer Institute**
**Division of Clinical Sciences**
**(Urologic Oncology Branch)**
*See:* Entry 10560

**U.S. Department of Health and Human Services**
**National Institutes of Health**
**National Cancer Institute**
**Division of Clinical Sciences**
**(Laboratory of Pathology)**
*See:* Entry 10561

**U.S. Department of Health and Human Services**
**National Institutes of Health**
**National Cancer Institute**
**Laboratory of Molecular Technology**
*See:* Entry 10563

**★ 9445 ★ U.S. Department of Health and Human Services**
**National Institutes of Health**
**National Eye Institute**
**Intramural Research**
**(Ophthalmic Genetics and Visual Function Branch)**
Bldg. 10, Rm. 10N226
10 Center Dr., MSC 1860
Bethesda, MD 20892-1860
**Phone:** (301)496-3577          **Fax:** (301)402-1214
**Email:** kaiserm@box-k.nih.gov
**Website:**          http://www.nei.nih.gov/intramural/ogcsb.htmocg
Muriel I. Kaiser, Ch.

**Activities/Fields:** Gene expression and molecular interactions important to the eye to prevent, diagnose, and treat diseases of the eye and visual system, including corneal disease, cataract, retinal disease, and abnormalities of visual pathways.

**U.S. Department of Health and Human Services**
**National Institutes of Health (NIH)**
**National Eye Institute (NEI)**
**Intramural Research**
**((Laboratory of Mechanisms of Ocular Diseases)**
**Molecular Therapeutics)**
*See:* Entry 21160

**★ 9446 ★ U.S. Department of Health and Human Services**
**National Institutes of Health**
**National Human Genome Research Institute (NHGRI)**
31 Ctr. Dr., Rm. 4B09
Bethesda, MD 20892
**Phone:** (301)496-0844          **Fax:** (301)402-0837
**Email:** fc23a@nih.gov
**Website:** http://www.nhgri.nih.gov
Francis S. Collins, Dir.

**Activities/Fields:** The Institute's mission is to head the Human Genome Project for the National Institutes of Health.

**★ 9447 ★ U.S. Department of Health and Human Services**
**National Institutes of Health**
**National Human Genome Research Institute (NHGRI)**
**Division of Extramural Research**
**(Ethical Legal and Social Implications Research Program — ELSI)**
Bldg. 31, Rm. B2B07
31 Center Dr., MSC 2033
Bethesda, MD 20892-6050
**Phone:** (301)402-4997          **Fax:** (301)402-1950
**Email:** et22s@nih.gov
**Website:**          http://www.nhgri.nih.gov/About_NHGRI/Der/Elsi/
Elizabeth Thomson, MS, Prog. Dir.

**Activities/Fields:** The program supports research that identifies and analyzes the ethical, legal, and social issues surrounding human genetics research.

**★ 9448 ★ U.S. Department of Health and Human Services**
**National Institutes of Health**
**National Human Genome Research Institute (NHGRI)**
**Division of Extramural Research**
**(Genome Informatics Program)**
Bldg. 31, Rm. B2B07
31 Ctr. Dr., MSC 2033
Bethesda, MD 20892
**Phone:** (301)496-7531          **Fax:** (301)480-2770
**Email:** lisa_brooks@nih.gov
**Website:**          http://www.nhgri.nih.gov/About_NHGRI/Der/ginform.htm
Lisa D. Brooks, PhD, Prog. Dir.

**Activities/Fields:** Fund grants on genomic data analysis, including sequence analysis, gene mapping, complex trait mapping and genetic variation; the development of database tools; and the development and maintenance of databases and genetic data.

**★ 9449 ★ U.S. Department of Health and Human Services**
**National Institutes of Health**
**National Human Genome Research Institute (NHGRI)**
**Division of Extramural Research**
**(Genetic Variation Program)**
Bldg. 31, Room B2B07
31 Center Dr., MSC 2033
National Institutes of Health
Bethesda, MD 20892-2033
**Phone:** (301)496-7531          **Fax:** (301)480-2770
**Email:** lisa_brooks@nih.gov
**Website:**          http://www.nhgri.nih.gov/About_NHGRI/Der/variat.htm
Lisa D. Brooks, PhD, Prog. Dir.

**Activities/Fields:** Funds research on the discovery Discovering and scoring of single nucleotide polymorphisms and other types of sequence variation, and the developmenting of high-resolution maps of genetic variation, and the developmenting of methods for the large-scale analysis of genetic variation, relating to phenotype and the analysis of complex traits.

**★ 9450 ★ U.S. Department of Health and Human Services**
**National Institutes of Health**
**National Human Genome Research Institute (NHGRI)**
**Division of Extramural Research**
**(Model Organisms Program)**
Bldg. 31, Rm. B2B07
31 Center Dr., MSC 2033
Bethesda, MD 20892-6050
**Phone:** (301)496-7531          **Fax:** (301)480-2770
**Email:** jp22d@nih.gov
**Website:**          http://www.nhgri.nih.gov/About_NHGRI/Der/model.htm
Jane Peterson, PhD, Prog. Dir.

**Activities/Fields:** Mapping and sequencing of the genomes of model organisms, including E. coli, S. cerevisiae, C. elegans, D. melanogaster and the laboratory mouse.

**★ 9451 ★ U.S. Department of Health and Human Services**
**National Institutes of Health**
**National Human Genome Research Institute (NHGRI)**
**Division of Extramural Research**
**(Large Scale Sequencing Program)**
Bldg. 31, Rm. B2B07
31 Center Dr., MSC 2033
Bethesda, MD 20892-2033
**Phone:** (301)496-7531          **Fax:** (301)480-2770
**Email:** jp22d@nih.gov
**Website:**          http://www.nhgri.nih.gov/about.nhgri/der/bigseq.htm
Jane Peterson, PhD, Prog. Dir.

**Activities/Fields:** Construction of physical maps and sequencing entire genomes, focusing on the human, mouse and Drosophila genomes.

**★ 9452 ★ U.S. Department of Health and Human Services**
**National Institutes of Health**
**National Human Genome Research Institute (NHGRI)**
**Division of Extramural Research**
**(Functional Analysis of the Genome Program)**
Bldg. 31, Rm. B2B07
31 Center Dr.
Bethesda, MD 20892
**Phone:** (301)496-7531          **Fax:** (301)480-2770
**Email:** ef5j@nih.gov
**Website:**          http://www.nhgri.nih.gov/About_NHGRI/Der/function.htm
Elise Feingold, PhD, Prog. Dir.

**Activities/Fields:** Development of improved techniques and strategies for efficient identification and functional analysis of genes, coding regions, and other functional elements of the genome on a high throughput, genome-wide basis.

**★ 9453 ★ U.S. Department of Health and Human Services**
**National Institutes of Health**
**National Human Genome Research Institute (NHGRI)**
**Division of Extramural Research**
**(Sequencing Technology Program)**
Bldg. 31, Rm. B2-B07
Bethesda, MD 20892-2033
**Phone:** (301)496-7531          **Fax:** (301)480-2770
**Email:** js173g@nih.gov
**Website:**          http://www.nhgri.nih.gov/About_NHGRI/Der/seqtech.htm
Jeffery Schloss, PhD, Prog. Dir.

**Activities/Fields:** Development of new methods, technologies, and instruments for rapid, low-cost determination of DNA sequence.

**★ 9454 ★ U.S. Department of Health and Human Services**
**National Institutes of Health**
**National Human Genome Research Institute (NHGRI)**
**Division of Intramural Research**
**(Clinical Gene Therapy Branch)**
10 Center Dr., Bldg. 10, Rm. 10C103
Bethesda, MD 20892
**Phone:** (301)435-2944          **Fax:** (301)496-7194
**Email:** fabio@nhgri.nih.gov
**Website:**          http://www.nhgri.nih.gov/Intramural_research/Clinical_therapy/
Fabio Candotti, MD, Branch Hd.

**Activities/Fields:** Basic and applied science important to gene therapy and its application to the treatment of human diseases.

**★ 9455 ★ U.S. Department of Health and Human Services**
**National Institutes of Health**
**National Human Genome Research Institute (NHGRI)**
**Division of Intramural Research (Cancer Genetics Branch)**
49 Convent Dr., Bldg. 49, Rm. 4A22
Bethesda, MD 20892
**Phone:** (301)402-2023 **Fax:** (301)402-2040
**Email:** jtrent@nhgri.nih.gov
**Website:** http://www.nhgri.nih.gov/Intramural_research/Lab_cancer/
Jeffrey M. Trent, PhD, Chf.

**Activities/Fields:** The Branch's focus it to define the genetic changes that lead to the initiation and progression of cancer.

**★ 9456 ★ U.S. Department of Health and Human Services**
**National Institutes of Health**
**National Human Genome Research Institute (NHGRI)**
**Division of Intramural Research (Inherited Disease Research Branch)**
49 Convent Dr., Bldg. 49, Rm. 4A72
Bethesda, MD 20892
**Phone:** (301)402-2039 **Fax:** (301)402-2170
**Email:** rlnuss@nhgri.nih.gov
**Website:** http://www.nhgri.nih.gov/Intramural_research/IDRB/
Robert L. Nussbaum, MD, Chf.

**Activities/Fields:** The Branch's focus it to develop and apply tools in statistics, genetics and computer science to locate genes that contribute to multifactorial genetic disease.

**★ 9457 ★ U.S. Department of Health and Human Services**
**National Institutes of Health**
**National Human Genome Research Institute (NHGRI)**
**Division of Intramural Research (Genetic Disease Research Branch)**
49 Convent Dr., Bldg. 49, Rm. 4A72
Bethesda, MD 20892
**Phone:** (301)402-2039 **Fax:** (301)402-2170
**Email:** rlnuss@nhgri.nih.gov
**Website:** http://www.nhgri.nih.gov/DIR/LGDR
Robert L. Nussbaum, MD, Chf.

**Activities/Fields:** The Branch's focus is to identify the genetic abnormalities responsible for human disease and elucidate the mechanisms by which they cause abnormalities in structure and function.

**★ 9458 ★ U.S. Department of Health and Human Services**
**National Institutes of Health**
**National Human Genome Research Institute**
**Division of Intramural Research (Medical Genetics Branch)**
Gerontology Research Center
PO Box 4
5600 Nathan Shock Dr.
Baltimore, MD 21224-6825
**Phone:** (410)558-8201 **Fax:** (410)558-8087
**Email:** francomanocl@grc.nih.gov
**Website:** http://www.grc.nia.nih.gov/branches/lg/hgims/hgims.htm
Clair A. Francomano, MD, Chf.

**Activities/Fields:** The laboratory examines patients and families affected by inherited disorders to identify and characterize novel disorders of human development.

**★ 9459 ★ U.S. Department of Health and Human Services**
**National Institutes of Health**
**National Human Genome Research Institute (NHGRI)**
**Division of Intramural Research (Genetics and Molecular Biology Branch)**
49 Convent Dr., Bldg. 49, Rm. 3A14
Bethesda, MD 20892-4442
**Phone:** (301)402-2194 **Fax:** (301)402-4929
**Email:** jp82a@nih.gov
**Website:** http://www.nhgri.nih.gov/Intramural_research/Lab_transfer
Jennifer M. Puck, MD, Br. Chf.

**Activities/Fields:** The Branch uses molecular genes involved in the normal development and function of many tissues, including blood and epithelial cells, the immune system and the nervous system.

**★ 9460 ★ U.S. Department of Health and Human Services**
**National Institutes of Health**
**National Human Genome Research Institute (NHGRI)**
**Division of Intramural Research (Genome Technology Branch)**
50 S Dr., Bldg. 50, Rm.5523
Bethesda, MD 20892
**Phone:** (301)402-0201 **Fax:** (301)402-4735
**Email:** egreen@nhgri.nih.gov
**Website:** http://www.nhgri.nih.gov/DIR/GTB/
Eric D. Green, MD, Chf.

**Activities/Fields:** The Branch's focus is contemporary technologies for performing genome analysis.

**★ 9461 ★ U.S. Department of Health and Human Services**
**National Institutes of Health**
**National Human Genome Research Institute**
**Human Genome Project**
Bldg. 31, Rm. 4B09
Bethesda, MD 20892
**Phone:** (301)496-0844 **Fax:** (301)402-8037
**Email:** francisc@exchange.nih.gov
**Website:** http://www.nhgri.nih.gov/index.html
Francis Collins, MD, Dir.

**Activities/Fields:** Constructs detailed genetic and physical maps of human genome to determine complete nucleotide sequence of human DNA in order to localize the estimated 50,000-100,000 genes within the human genome; performs analyses of genomes in several organisms.

**★ 9462 ★ U.S. Department of Health and Human Services**
**National Institutes of Health (NIH)**
**National Institute on Aging**
**Intramural Research Programs (Laboratory of Genetics)**
Gerontology Research Center
5600 Nathan Shock Dr.
Baltimore, MD 21224
**Phone:** (410)558-8337
**Email:** schlessingerd@grc.nia.nih.gov
**Website:** http://www.grc.nia.nih.gov/branches/lg/lg.htm
David Schlessinger, PhD, Ch.

**Activities/Fields:** Studies of genetic determinants as an integrated part of human development.

**U.S. Department of Health and Human Services**
**National Institutes of Health (NIH)**
**National Institute on Aging**
**Intramural Research Programs (Cancer Molecular Genetics Unit)**
*See:* Entry 10565

**★ 9463 ★ U.S. Department of Health and Human Services**
**National Institutes of Health (NIH)**
**National Institute on Aging**
**Intramural Research Programs (Cell Cycle Control Unit)**
Gateway
7201 Wisconsin Ave., Ste. 3C309
Bethesda, MD 20892-9205
**Email:** gorospem@grc.nia.nih.gov
**Website:** http://www.grc.nia.nih.gov/branches/lbc/cccu.htm
Myriam Gorospe, PhD, Hd.

**Activities/Fields:** Cellular response to stress and gene expression; post-transcriptional control of cell cycle regulatory genes; functional analysis of the von Hippel-Lindau (VHL) tumor suppressor gene.

**★ 9464 ★ U.S. Department of Health and Human Services**
**National Institutes of Health**
**National Institute of Child Health and Human Development**
**Division of Intramural Research (Laboratory of Mammalian Genes and Development)**
Bldg.6B, Rm. 413
Bethesda, MD 20892
**Phone:** (301)496-1855
**Email:** hw@helix.nih.gov
**Website:** http://dir2.nichd.nih.gov/labs/lab.php3?13
Heinrich J. Westphal, Hd.

**Activities/Fields:** Advanced gene targeting and transgenic technologies to study genes that control specific stages of mouse development, particularly development of central and peripheral nervous systems, pituitary and thymus development and mechanisms of genomic imprinting.

**★ 9465 ★ U.S. Department of Health and Human Services**
**National Institutes of Health**
**National Institute of Child Health and Human Development**
**Division of Intramural Research (Laboratory of Gene Regulation and Development)**
Bldg. 1st, Rm. 106
Bethesda, MD 20892-2425
**Phone:** (301)496-8391
**Email:** alanh@box-a.nih.gov
**Website:** http://dir2.nichd.nih.gov/labs/lab.php3?10
Alan Hinnebusch, Ch.

**Activities/Fields:** Regulation of gene expression in two model eukaryotic systems, the yeasts saccharomyces cerevisiae and Schizosaccharomyces pombe.

**★ 9466 ★ U.S. Department of Health and Human Services**
**National Institutes of Health**
**National Institute of Child Health and Human Development**
**Division of Intramural Research (Laboratories of the Scientific Director)**
Bldg. 31, Rm. 2A50
31 Center Dr.
Bethesda, MD 20892
**Phone:** (301)496-2133
**Website:** http://dir2.nichd.nih.gov/labs/lab.php3?17
Igor Dawid, Ch.

**Activities/Fields:** Molecular events that influence fidelity of the genome, facilitating both evolution and species stability.

**★ 9467 ★ U.S. Department of Health and Human Services**
**National Institutes of Health**
**National Institute of Child Health and Human Development**
**Division of Intramural Research**
**(Perinatology Research Branch)**
Bldg. 31, Rm. 2A32
31 Center Dr., MSC 2425
Bethesda, MD 20892-2425
**Phone:** (301)993-2700
**Email:** romeror@mail.nih.gov
**Website:** http://dir2.nichd.nih.gov/labs/lab.php3?18
Roberto Romero, Hd.

**Activities/Fields:** Conditions responsible for perinatal morbidity and mortality, especially the study of human parturition (premature labor), intrauterine growth retardation, congenital anomalies, and pre-eclampsia.


**★ 9468 ★ U.S. Department of Health and Human Services**
**National Institutes of Health**
**National Institute of Child Health and Human Development**
**Division of Intramural Research**
**(Heritable Disorders Branch)**
Bldg. 10, Rm. 9S241
10 Center Dr.
Bethesda, MD 20892
**Phone:** (301)496-6683
**Email:** marinij@mail.nih.gov
**Website:** http://dir2.nichd.nih.gov/labs/lab.php3?4
Joan C. Marini, Head

**Activities/Fields:** Etiology, diagnosis therapy of human genetic disorders, particularly clinically, inborn errors of metabolism and connective tissue disorders.


**★ 9469 ★ U.S. Department of Health and Human Services**
**National Institutes of Health**
**National Institute of Dental and Craniofacial Research**
**Division of Intramural Research**
**(Matrix Metalloproteinase Section)**
Bldg. 30, Rm. 132
30 Convent Dr., MSC 4326
Bethesda, MD 20892-4326
**Phone:** (301)496-1483          **Fax:** (301)402-1512
**Email:** henning.birkedal-hansen@nih.gov
**Website:** http://wwwdir.nidcr.nih.gov/dirweb/cores/mms/mms.asp
Dr. Henning Birkedal-Hansen, Actg. Ch.

**Activities/Fields:** Factors controlling synthesis, genetic regulation and function of matrix metalloproteinases in homeostasis and disease; defines role of metalloproteinases in cellular regulation and collagen degradation; characterizes biological function of matrix metalloproteinase inhibitors, TIMPs, and regulation of TIMP synthesis.


**★ 9470 ★ U.S. Department of Health and Human Services**
**National Institutes of Health**
**National Institute of Dental and Craniofacial Research**
**Division of Intramural Research**
**(Functional Genomics Unit)**
Bldg. 30, Rm. 529
30 Convent Dr., MSC 4326
Bethesda, MD 20892-4326
**Phone:** (301)435-2887          **Fax:** (301)435-2888
**Email:** ashok.kulkarni@nih.gov
**Website:** http://wwwdir.nidcr.nih.gov/dirweb/cores/fgu/fgu.asp
Dr. Ashok Kulkarni, Dir.

**Activities/Fields:** Seeks to delineate precise in vivo functions of specific genes involved in molecular processes underlying disease conditions involving degenerative processes, metabolic defects and immune disorders.


**U.S. Department of Health and Human Services**
**National Institutes of Health**
**National Institute of Dental and Craniofacial Research**
**Division of Intramural Research**
**(Molecular and Genetic Epidemiology Section)**
*See:* Entry 9066


**U.S. Department of Health and Human Services**
**National Institutes of Health**
**National Institute of Dental and Craniofacial Research**
**Division of Intramural Research**
**(Craniofacial Epidemiology and Genetics Branch)**
*See:* Entry 9067


**U.S. Department of Health and Human Services**
**National Institutes of Health**
**National Institute of Dental and Craniofacial Research**
**Division of Intramural Research**
*See:* Entry 6629


**U.S. Department of Health and Human Services**
**National Institutes of Health**
**National Institute of Diabetes and Digestive and Kidney Diseases**
**Division of Diabetes, Endocrinology, and Metabolic Diseases**
**(Steroid Metabolism Program)**
*See:* Entry 8792


**★ 9471 ★ U.S. Department of Health and Human Services**
**National Institutes of Health**
**National Institute of Diabetes and Digestive and Kidney Diseases**
**Division of Diabetes, Endocrinology, and Metabolic Diseases**
**(Genetics of Complications Program)**
2 Democracy Pl., Rm. 699
Bethesda, MD 20892
**Phone:** (301)594-0021
**Email:** linderb@extra.niddk.nih.gov
**Website:** http://www.niddk.nih.gov/fund/program/F-Llist.htm
Barbara Linder, MD, Dir.

**Activities/Fields:** Discovery of genes that increase an individual's susceptibility to complications of diabetes. Basic mechanisms involved organs including kidneys, nervous system, eye, and vasculature.


**★ 9472 ★ U.S. Department of Health and Human Services**
**National Institutes of Health**
**National Institute of Diabetes and Digestive and Kidney Diseases**
**Division of Diabetes, Endocrinology, and Metabolic Diseases**
**(Genetics of Diabetes Program)**
6707 Democracy Blvd., Rm. 6103
Bethesda, MD 20892-5460
**Phone:** (301)594-8810          **Fax:** (301)480-3503
**Email:** mckeonc@extra.niddk.nih.gov
**Website:** http://www.niddk.nih.gov/fund/program/F-Llist.htm
Catherine McKeon, PhD, Sr. Adv.

**Activities/Fields:** Identification of genes that contribute to type 1 and 2 diabetes mellitus.


**★ 9473 ★ U.S. Department of Health and Human Services**
**National Institutes of Health**
**National Institute of Diabetes and Digestive and Kidney Diseases**
**Division of Diabetes, Endocrinology, and Metabolic Diseases**
**(Gene Therapy and Cystic Fibrosis Centers Program)**
MSC-5460
6707 Democracy Blvd., Rm. 6103
Bethesda, MD 20892-5460
**Phone:** (301)594-8810          **Fax:** (301)480-3503
**Email:** mckeonc@extra.niddk.nih.gov
**Website:** http://www.niddk.nih.gov/fund/program/F-Llist.htm
Catherine McKeon, PhD, Sr. Adv.

**Activities/Fields:** Development of gene therapy techniques; fosters multidisciplinary collaboration in the development of clinical trials for the treatment of cystic fibrosis and other genetic metabolic diseases.


**★ 9474 ★ U.S. Department of Health and Human Services**
**National Institutes of Health**
**National Institute of Diabetes and Digestive and Kidney Diseases**
**Division of Diabetes, Endocrinology, and Metabolic Diseases**
**(Gene Therapy Program)**
MSC-5460
6707 Democracy Blvd., Rm. 6103
Bethesda, MD 20892-5460
**Phone:** (301)594-8810          **Fax:** (301)480-3503
**Email:** mckeonc@extra.niddk.nih.gov
**Website:** http://www.niddk.nih.gov/fund/program/F-Llist.htm
Catherine McKeon, PhD, Sr. Adv.

**Activities/Fields:** Development of basic and applied gene therapy for genetic metabolic diseases, particularly pilot and feasibility studies to improve gene delivery systems; basic science of AAV, adenovirus, retrovirus, and lentivirus vectors; nonviral methods of gene transfer such as liposomes or DNA conjugates; studies targeting gene delivery to specific cell types; gene therapy of stem cells to treat genetic metabolic disease.


**U.S. Department of Health and Human Services**
**National Institutes of Health**
**National Institute of Environmental Health Sciences**
**Environmental Genome Project**
*See:* Entry 8971


**★ 9475 ★ U.S. Department of Health and Human Services**
**National Institutes of Health**
**National Institute of Environmental Health Sciences**
**Environmental Genomic SNP Database Platform**
PO Box 12233
Research Triangle Park, NC 27709
**Phone:** (919)541-2548          **Fax:** (919)541-5002
**Email:** selkirk@niehs.nih.gov
**Website:** http://manuel.niehs.nih.gov/egsnp/home.htm
Dr. James Selkirk, Dir.

**Activities/Fields:** Identification of functionally important polymorphisms in environmental response genes that may determine differences in disease risks to environmental exposures.

**U.S. Department of Health and Human Services**
**National Institutes of Health**
**National Institute of Environmental Health Sciences**
**Laboratory of Molecular Carcinogenesis (Molecular and Genetic Epidemiology)**
*See:* Entry 10573

**U.S. Department of Health and Human Services**
**National Institutes of Health**
**National Institute of Environmental Health Sciences**
**Laboratory of Molecular Carcinogenesis (Gene Regulation Group)**
*See:* Entry 10577

**★ 9476 ★ U.S. Department of Health and Human Services**
**National Institutes of Health**
**National Institute of Environmental Health Sciences**
**Laboratory of Molecular Carcinogenesis (Cell Adhesion and Migration)**
M/D A2-01
PO Box 12233
Research Triangle Park, NC 27709
**Phone:** (919)541-7797
**Email:** akiyama@niehs.nih.gov
**Website:** http://dir.niehs.nih.gov/dirlmc/home.htm
Steven K. Akiyama, PhD, Prin. Investigator
**Activities/Fields:** Contributes to normal processes such as cellular differentiation, embryonic development, and would healing as well as to the progression of diseases and pathological conditions such as cancer, inflammatory responses, and developmental abnormalities that can arise from acute or chronic exposure to environmental toxicants.

**★ 9477 ★ U.S. Department of Health and Human Services**
**National Institutes of Health**
**National Institute of Environmental Health Sciences**
**Laboratory of Molecular Carcinogenesis**
M/D A2-01
PO Box 12233
Research Triangle Park, NC 27709
**Phone:** (919)541-7797
**Email:** letvinc1@niehs.nih.gov
**Website:** http://dir.niehs.nih.gov/dirlmc/
Donna Letvinchik, Sec.
**Activities/Fields:** Critical target genes in carcinogenesis to understand how chemicals act upon these genes to influence cancer development, including cancer prevention, diagnosis, and treatment.

**★ 9478 ★ U.S. Department of Health and Human Services**
**National Institutes of Health**
**National Institute of Environmental Health Sciences**
**Laboratory of Structural Biology (Mass Spectrometry Group)**
PO Box 12233
Research Triangle Park, NC 27709
**Phone:** (919)541-1966 **Fax:** (919)541-0022
**Email:** tomer@niehs.nih.gov
**Website:** http://dir.niehs.nih.gov/dirlsb/msshome.htm
Kenneth B. Tomer, PhD, Prin. Investigator
**Activities/Fields:** Mass spectrometry to identify unknown proteins and components of protein complexes and to study the macromolecular interactions within the complexes, including spermiation, protein-protein and protein-DNA interactions during mammalian base excision repair; investigates non-covalent complexes between CD4 and HIV gp120.

**★ 9479 ★ U.S. Department of Health and Human Services**
**National Institutes of Health**
**National Institute of Environmental Health Sciences**
**Laboratory of Structural Biology (DNA Repair and Nucleic Acid Enzymology Group)**
PO Box 12233
Research Triangle Park, NC 27709
**Phone:** (919)541-3267 **Fax:** (919)541-3592
**Email:** wilsons@niehs.nih.gov
**Website:** http://dir.niehs.nih.gov/dirlsb/naehome.htm
Dr. Samuel H. Wilson, Prin. Investigator
**Activities/Fields:** Physical, biochemical, cell and molecular biology studies of mammalian base excision repair enzymes and DNA polymerases, in particular studies gap-filling DNA synthesis and other gap repair reactions during Mammalian DNA repair.

**★ 9480 ★ U.S. Department of Health and Human Services**
**National Institutes of Health**
**National Institute of Environmental Health Sciences**
**Laboratory of Structural Biology (DNA Replication Fidelity Group)**
PO Box 12233
Research Triangle Park, NC 27709
**Phone:** (919)541-2644 **Fax:** (919)541-7613
**Email:** kunkel@niehs.nih.gov
**Website:** http://dir.niehs.nih.gov/dirlsb/drfhome.htm
Thomas A. Kunkel, PhD, Prin. Investigator
**Activities/Fields:** Understanding the fidelity of normal DNA replication and repair processes that control spontaneous and induced mutation rates in organisms from viruses to humans, and understanding how these processes are perturbed by polymorphisms or mutations in critical genes or by DNA damage resulting from intracellular metabolism or exposure to the external environment.

**U.S. Department of Health and Human Services**
**National Institutes of Health**
**National Institute of Environmental Health Sciences**
**Laboratory of Structural Biology**
*See:* Entry 8972

**★ 9481 ★ U.S. Department of Health and Human Services**
**National Institutes of Health**
**National Institute of Environmental Health Sciences**
**Microarray Center**
111 Alexander Dr., Bldg. 101, Rm. D228
M/D F1-09
PO Box 12233
Research Triangle Park, NC 27709
**Phone:** (919)541-1310 **Fax:** (919)541-1506
**Email:** afshari@niehs.nih.gov
**Website:** http://dir.niehs.nih.gov/microarray/
Dr. Cindy Afshari, Co-Dir.
**Activities/Fields:** Identification of toxicants on the basis of tissue-specific patterns of gene expression (molecular signature); mechanisms of action of environmental agents through identification of gene expression networks; uses toxicant-induced gene expression as a biomarker to assess human exposure; effects of toxicants from one species to another; interactions of mixtures of chemicals; effects of low dose exposures versus high dose exposures; development of public database of expression profiles.

**★ 9482 ★ U.S. Department of Health and Human Services**
**National Institutes of Health**
**National Institute of Environmental Health Sciences**
**National Center for Toxicogenomics**
PO Box 12233
Research Triangle Park, NC 27709
**Phone:** (919)541-4141 **Fax:** (919)541-1460
**Email:** tennant@niehs.nih.gov
**Website:** http://www.niehs.nih.gov/nct/home.htm
Dr. Raymond W. Tennant, Dir.
**Activities/Fields:** Genomics science to improve understanding of basic biological responses to environmental stressors/toxicants; aims to catalyze the application of toxicogenomics to improve human health.

**★ 9483 ★ U.S. Department of Health and Human Services**
**National Institutes of Health**
**National Institute of Mental Health**
**Experimental Therapeutics Branch (Section on Developmental Genetic Epidemiology)**
MSC 1381
Bldg. 10, Rm. 4n222
Bethesda, MD 20892-1381
**Phone:** (301)496-4183 **Fax:** (301)480-8348
**Email:** nimhinfo@nih.gov
**Website:** http://intramural.nimh.nih.gov/research/etpb/
Kathleen R. Merikankangas, PhD, Ch.
**Activities/Fields:** Identification of risk factors for mood and anxiety disorders, their association with other psychiatric and medical disorders, including epidemiology, clinical psychology, developmental psychology, genetic epidemiology, psychiatry, and biostatistics.

**U.S. Department of Health and Human Services**
**National Institutes of Health**
**National Institute of Mental Health**
**Experimental Therapeutics Branch (Section on Behavioral Neuropharmacology)**
*See:* Entry 14346

**U.S. Department of Health and Human Services**
**National Institutes of Health**
**National Institute of Mental Health**
**Experimental Therapeutics Branch (Section on Clinical and Experimental Neurospychology)**
*See:* Entry 14332

**U.S. Department of Health and Human Services**
**National Institutes of Health**
**National Institute of Mental Health**
**Laboratory of Biochemical Genetics**
*See:* Entry 14347

**★ 9484 ★ U.S. Department of Health and Human Services**
**National Institutes of Health**
**National Institute of Mental Health**
**Laboratory of Cellular and Molecular Regulation (Unit on Temporal Gene Expression)**
Bldg. 36, Rm. 2A09
36 Convent Dr.
Bethesda, MD 20892
**Phone:** (301)496-7522 **Fax:** (301)402-1748
**Email:** abri@codon.nih.gov
**Website:** http://intramural.nimh.nih.gov/lcmr/
Rubin Baler, PhD, Contact

**Activities/Fields:** Understanding the molecular underpinnings of transcriptional specificity in circadian transcriptional loops, focusing on the DNA determinants of circadian regulated genes and the identification of circadian accessory proteins with role sin the fine tuning of key temporal parameters.

**U.S. Department of Health and Human Services**
**National Institutes of Health**
**National Institute of Mental Health**
**Laboratory of Cellular and Molecular Regulation**
**(Section on Neural Gene Expression)**
*See:* Entry 14349

**★ 9485 ★ U.S. Department of Health and Human Services**
**National Institutes of Health**
**National Institute of Mental Health**
**Laboratory of Genetics**
**(Gene Discovery Unit)**
Bldg. 36, Rm. 3A31
9000 Rockville Pike
Bethesda, MD 20892
**Phone:** (301)496-5351
**Email:** nimhinfo@nih.gov
**Website:** http://intramural.nimh.nih.gov/research/log/
Tom Bonner, PhD, Ch.

**Activities/Fields:** Identification of candidate genes in restricted regions of the genome identified by linkage studies of complex genetic diseases, i.e. those that are not expected to show perfect cosegregation with any single locus.

**★ 9486 ★ U.S. Department of Health and Human Services**
**National Institutes of Health**
**National Institute of Mental Health**
**Laboratory of Genetics**
Bldg. 36, Rm. 3A31
9000 Rockville Pike
Bethesda, MD 20892
**Phone:** (301)496-5351
**Email:** nimhinfo@nih.gov
**Website:** http://intramural.nimh.nih.gov/research/log/
Michael Brownstein, PhD, Ch.

**Activities/Fields:** Complex genetic traits in humans and rodents, including whole genome genetic scans to the physiology of neuronal systems and protein structure activity relationships when appropriate.

**★ 9487 ★ U.S. Department of Health and Human Services**
**National Institutes of Health**
**National Institute of Mental Health**
**Laboratory of Molecular Biology**
**(Section on Molecular Neurobiology)**
Bldg. 36, Rm. 1B08
9000 Rockville Pike
Bethesda, MD 20892
**Phone:** (301)496-4864          **Fax:** (301)402-0245
**Email:** nimhinfo@nih.gov
**Website:** http://intramural.nimh.nih.gov/research/lmb/
Barry B. Kaplan, PhD, Ch.

**Activities/Fields:** Strives to define the function and origins of the mRNA population, and establish the existence of new inter- and/or intra-cellular macromolecular communication pathways in the nervous system.

**★ 9488 ★ U.S. Department of Health and Human Services**
**National Institutes of Health**
**National Institute of Mental Health**
**Laboratory of Molecular Biology**
Bldg. 36, Rm. 1B08
9000 Rockville Pike
Bethesda, MD 20892

**Phone:** (301)496-4864          **Fax:** (301)402-0245
**Email:** nimhinfo@nih.gov
**Website:** http://intramural.nimh.nih.gov/research/lmb/
Howard Nash, MD, Ch.

**Activities/Fields:** Mechanistic aspects of diverse biological processes, including biochemistry coupled with genetics and cell and molecular biology.

**★ 9489 ★ U.S. Department of Health and Human Services**
**National Institutes of Health**
**National Institute of Mental Health**
**Laboratory of Molecular Biology**
**(Section on Molecular Genetics)**
Bldg. 36, Rm. 1B08
9000 Rockville Pike
Bethesda, MD 20892
**Phone:** (301)496-4864          **Fax:** (301)402-0245
**Email:** nimhinfo@nih.gov
**Website:** http://intramural.nimh.nih.gov/research/lmb/
Howard Nash, MD, Ch.

**Activities/Fields:** Identification of conserved genes that encode or control the physiological targets of an important class of pharmacological agents using molecular genetic and biochemical experiments.

**★ 9490 ★ U.S. Department of Health and Human Services**
**National Institutes of Health**
**National Institute of Mental Health**
**Laboratory of Molecular Pathophysiology**
Bldg. 1, Rm. 3B310
1 Center Dr.
Bethesda, MD 20892-0135
**Phone:** (301)594-1089          **Fax:** (301)480-3610
**Email:** alzonae@intra.nimh.nih.gov
**Website:** http://intramural.nimh.nih.gov/research/lmp/
Husseini Manji, MD, Ch.

**Activities/Fields:** Investigation of disease- and treatment-induced changes in gene and protein expression profiles that regulate neuroplasticity and cellular resilience in mood disorders.

**U.S. Department of Health and Human Services**
**National Institutes of Health**
**National Institute of Mental Health**
**Laboratory of Neurotoxicology**
**(Unit on Neuroimmunology)**
*See:* Entry 14359

**U.S. Department of Health and Human Services**
**National Institutes of Health**
**National Institute of Mental Health**
**Molecular Neuropsychiatry Section**
*See:* Entry 12749

**★ 9491 ★ U.S. Department of Health and Human Services**
**National Institutes of Health**
**National Institute of Neurological Disorders and Stroke**
**Division of Extramural Research**
**(Neurogenetics Program)**
NSC/2136
6001 Executive Blvd.
Bethesda, MD 20892
**Phone:** (301)496-5745          **Fax:** (301)402-1501
**Email:** rf45c@nih.gov
**Website:** http://www.ninds.nih.gov/about_ninds/clusters/neurogenetics.htm
Robert Finkelstein, PhD, Dir.

**Activities/Fields:** Identification of neurological disease genes; mechanisms by which genetic mutations cause neurological disease; aims to develop gene-based therapeutics for neurological disorders.

**★ 9492 ★ U.S. Department of Health and Human Services**
**National Institutes of Health (NIH)**
**National Institute of Neurological Disorders and Stroke**
**Division of Intramural Research**
**(Clinical Stroke Research Unit)**
Bldg. 36, Rm. 4A03
36 Convent Dr., MSC 4128
Bethesda, MD 20892-4128
**Phone:** (301)295-1755          **Fax:** (301)295-0863
**Email:** degrabat@ninds.nih.gov
**Website:** http://www.ninds.nih.gov/about_ninds/labs/92.htm
Thomas J. DeGraba, MD, Investigator

**Activities/Fields:** Atherosclerosis, focused on the study of association of gene polymorphisms in the regulators of inflammation, T-lymphocyte profile, and altered gene expression in symptomatic versus asymptomatic patients.

**★ 9493 ★ U.S. Department of Health and Human Services**
**National Institutes of Health**
**Office of Recombinant DNA Activities**
6000 Executive Blvd. Ste. 302
Bethesda, MD 20892-7010
**Phone:** (301)496-9838          **Fax:** (301)496-9839
**Website:** http://www.nih.gov/
Debra Knorr, Actg. Dir.

**Activities/Fields:** Administers the recombinant DNA research activities supported and monitored by the National Institutes of Health. (Recombinant DNA is prepared through laboratory transplantation or splicing of genes from one organism to another.) ORDA reviews all special requests submitted to NIH involving recombinant DNA technology and implements NIH policies and procedures for conducting this research.
**Pub:** *NIH Guidelines for Research Involving Recombinant DNA Molecules.*

**★ 9494 ★ University of Alabama at Birmingham**
**Gregory Fleming James Cystic Fibrosis Research Center**
790 McCallum Bldg.
Birmingham, AL 35294-0005
**Phone:** (205)934-7210          **Fax:** (205)934-7593
**Email:** sorscher@uab.edu
Dr. Eric J. Sorscher, Dir.

**Activities/Fields:** Cystic fibrosis, including electrolyte transport and metabolism, mucin secretion and biochemistry, genetics, regulation of immune mechanisms, membrane traffic regulation, gene therapy, and pharmacologic therapy.

**★ 9495 ★ University of Arkansas at Little Rock**
**Arkansas Children's Hospital Cystic Fibrosis Center**
800 Marshall
Little Rock, AR 72202-3591
**Phone:** (501)320-1018          **Fax:** (501)320-3930
Dr. John L. Caroll, Dir.

**Activities/Fields:** Cystic fibrosis and related respiratory diseases of children, including aerosol deposition and pulmonary function testing in children.

**★ 9496 ★ University of British Columbia**
**Centre for Molecular Medicine and Therapeutics (CMMT)**
950 W 28th Ave.
Vancouver, BC, Canada V5Z 4H4
**Phone:** (604)875-3535          **Fax:** (604)875-3819
**Email:** info@cmmt.ubc.ca
**Website:** http://www.cmmt.ubc.ca/about.htm
Michael Hayden, Dir.

**Activities/Fields:** Determination and control of genetic susceptibility to disease.

**★ 9497 ★ University of California, Davis**
**Division of Agriculture and Natural Resources**
**Genetic Resources Conservation Program**
1 Shields Ave.
Davis, CA 95616-8602
**Phone:** (530)754-8501          **Fax:** (530)754-8505
**Email:** grcp@ucdavis.edu
**Website:** http://www.grcp.ucdavis.edu
Dr. Calvin O. Qualset, Dir.

**Activities/Fields:** Facilitates the collection and maintenance of animal, plant, and microbial genetic resources; identifies animal, plant, and microbial genetic resources critical to California and supports their conservation; and develops improved methods and strategies for procuring and maintaining genetic resources.

**★ 9498 ★ University of California, Davis**
**Genetics Typing Laboratory**
Department of Anthropology
209 Young Hall
Davis, CA 95616
**Phone:** (530)752-6343          **Fax:** (530)752-8885
**Email:** dgsmith@ucdavis.edu
David Glenn Smith, PhD, Prin. Investigator

**Activities/Fields:** Identification and characterization of previously unknown polymorphisms; the effectiveness of alternative genetic management strategies and the effect of demographic factors on the population/genetic structure of captive groups of primates; identification of marker loci for genes that influence susceptibility to retroviral, B-virus, and other infections; and employment of both ancient and contemporary mitochondrial DNA and microsatellite DNA loci for studies of ancestor-descendant relationships.

**★ 9499 ★ University of California, San Diego**
**Ludwig Institute for Cancer Research**
**Laboratory of Cancer Biology**
9500 Gilman Dr.
La Jolla, CA 92093
**Phone:** (619)534-7802
**Email:** rkolodner@ucsd.edu
**Website:** http://ludwig.ucsd.edu/
Dr. Richard Kolodner, Hd.

**Activities/Fields:** Genetic and biochemical dissection of the processes of DNA recombination and repair.

**★ 9500 ★ University of California, San Diego**
**Ludwig Institute for Cancer Research**
**Laboratory of Cell Biology**
9500 Gilman Dr.
La Jolla, CA 92093
**Phone:** (619)534-7802
**Email:** dcleveland@ucsd.edu
**Website:** http://ludwig.ucsd.edu/
Don W. Cleveland, Hd.

**Activities/Fields:** How chromosomes are faithfully moved into each daughter cell just prior to division, how neurofilaments structure the cytoplasm of neurons, and the use of transgenic mice to investigate mechanisms of motor neuron disease.

**★ 9501 ★ University of California, San Diego**
**Ludwig Institute for Cancer Research**
**Laboratory of Tumor Biology**
9500 Gilman Dr.
La Jolla, CA 92093
**Phone:** (619)534-7802
**Email:** wcavenee@ucsd.edu
**Website:** http://ludwig.ucsd.edu/
W.K. Cavenee, Dir.

**Activities/Fields:** Genetic dissection of human cancer.

**University of Colorado**
**B.F. Stolinsky Research Laboratories**
*See:* Entry 6906

**★ 9502 ★ University of Colorado at Boulder**
**Institute for Behavioral Genetics**
CB 447
Boulder, CO 80309
**Phone:** (303)492-2342
**Email:** Toni.Smolen@colorado.edu
Dr. Toni N. Smolen, Asst. Dir.

**Activities/Fields:** Application of behavioral genetics to pharmacogenetics, learning disabilities, cognitive development, and vulnerability to drug abuse. Specific interests include genetics of aging, reading disability, genetic and neurobiological correlates of animal behavior, human alcohol studies, and genetic factors in personality and cognitive development of twins and adopted children.

**★ 9503 ★ University of Florida**
**Center for Mammalian Genetics**
1600 Archer Rd.
PO Box 100245
Gainesville, FL 32611
**Phone:** (352)392-3054          **Fax:** (352)392-9053
**Email:** jennyj@ufl.edu
**Website:** http://cmg.health.ufl.edu/
Thomas P. Yang, PhD, Dir.

**Activities/Fields:** Genetic and physical mapping of human disease genes, mutation analysis of human disease genes, gene therapy, somatic genome stability, cytogenetics, clinical genetics and dysmorphology, viral genetics, immunogenetics, neurogenetics, population and evolutionary genetics, and regulation of eukaryotic gene expression.

**University of Iowa**
**Birth Defects and Genetic Disorders Unit**
*See:* Entry 4900

**★ 9504 ★ University of Iowa**
**Cystic Fibrosis Research Center**
Internal Medicine, 500 EMRB
Iowa City, IA 52242
**Phone:** (319)335-7619
**Email:** michael-welsh@uiowa.edu
Michael J. Welsh, Dir.

**Activities/Fields:** Cystic fibrosis. Because cystic fibrosis is caused by gene mutations, the center is especially interested in the development of gene therapy for this disease.

**★ 9505 ★ University of Louisville**
**Louisville Twin Study**
Medical-Dental Research Bldg.
Health Science Center
Louisville, KY 40292
**Phone:** (502)852-1090          **Fax:** (502)852-1093
Dr. Kay Phillip, Actg. Dir.

**Activities/Fields:** Human behavior genetics, including a longitudinal study of twins and siblings from birth to early adulthood, assessment of temperament and mental development, biomedical studies of twins, and multivariate analyses of their cognitive, perceptual, and motor skills.

**University of Maryland at Baltimore**
**Center for Celiac Research (CFCR)**
*See:* Entry 3305

**★ 9506 ★ University of Miami**
**Cystic Fibrosis Research Center**
PO Box 016820
Miami, FL 33101-6820
**Phone:** (305)243-6641          **Fax:** (305)243-6708
**Email:** gpiedimo@med.miami.edu

**Website:** http://www.celiaccenter.org/
Dr. Giovanni Piedimonte, Dir.

**Activities/Fields:** Cystic fibrosis, asthma, pulmonary manifestations of pediatric AIDS, and respiratory diseases of children. Also studies pediatric exercise physiology and sleep and apnea disorders.

**University of Miami**
**Mailman Center for Child Development**
*See:* Entry 5826

**★ 9507 ★ University of Minnesota**
**Caenorhabditis Genetics Center**
250 Biological Science Center
1445 Gortner Ave.
Saint Paul, MN 55108-1095
**Phone:** (612)625-2265          **Fax:** (612)625-5754
**Email:** stier@biosci.cbs.umn.edu
**Website:** http://pediatrics.med.miami.edu
Dr. Robert K. Herman, Dir.

**Activities/Fields:** Acquisition, banking, distribution, and coordination of genetic nomenclature of Caenorhabditis elegans strains maintained for distribution to researchers. **Pub:** *Celegans Genetic Map.* • *Worm Breeder's Gazette.*

**★ 9508 ★ University of Minnesota**
**Cystic Fibrosis Center**
University of Minnesota Hospital
420 Delaware St. SE
Minneapolis, MN 55455
**Phone:** (612)626-4440          **Fax:** (612)624-0696
**Email:** milla005@tc.umn.edu
Dr. Carlos E. Milla, Dir.

**Activities/Fields:** Cystic fibrosis, pediatric pulmonary diseases, pulmonary physiology, infant pulmonary function, biochemistry of cystic fibrosis, nutrition, liver disease, inflamation, psychosocial intervention, home monitoring, heart-lung and lung transplantation, sweat test, bioengineering, biophysics, and physical therapy. Activities include development of high frequency compression therapy. **Pub:** *CF Guidebook.*

**★ 9509 ★ University of Minnesota**
**Institute of Human Genetics**
Box 206
Mayo Memorial Bldg.
420 Delaware St. SE
Minneapolis, MN 55455-0374
**Phone:** (612)624-3110          **Fax:** (612)626-7031
**Email:** faras@gene.med.umn.edu
**Website:** http://www.ihg.med.umn.edu/index.html
Dr. Anthony J. Faras, Dir.

**Activities/Fields:** Human genetics and developmental biology, including biochemical, molecular, and clinical genetics, cytogenetics, metabolism, and genetic counseling. Current research involves tumor viruses; gene transfer; eukaryotic gene regulation; rearrangement and regulation of immunoglobulin genes; molecular genetics of the major histocompatibility complex; genetic defects of human pigment genes; and bone marrow transplantation. **Pub:** *MicroChem News.*

**★ 9510 ★ University of Missouri—Columbia**
**Cystic Fibrosis Research Center**
Health Science Center
Department of Child Health
Columbia, MO 65212
**Phone:** (573)882-6978          **Fax:** (573)882-2742
**Email:** konigp@missouri.edu
Peter Konig, MD, Dir.

**Activities/Fields:** Intracellular control mechanisms of secretion as they relate to cystic fibrosis, secretory mechanisms for water and electroytes in exocrine glands, structure and function of pulmonary glycoproteins in cystic fibrosis and other chronic pulmonary diseases, and therapies for pulmonary disease in cystic fibrosis.

**★ 9511 ★ University of Nebraska Medical Center**
**Hattie B. Munroe Center for Human Genetics**
985440 Nebraska Medical Center
Omaha, NE 68198-5440
**Phone:** (402)559-5070    **Fax:** (402)559-9463
**Email:** wgsanger@unmc.edu
**Website:** http://www.unmc.edu/services/geneticslab
Warren G. Sanger, PhD, Dir.

**Activities/Fields:** Research and treatment concentrating in cancer cytogenetics and prenatal diagnosis, including lymphoma, leukemia, and solid tumor research, chromosome changes in response to treatment, diagnostics of chromosome abnormalities, and treatment of prenatal genetic conditions associated with mental retardation and disability.

**★ 9512 ★ University of Nebraska Medical Center**
**Signal Transduction Laboratory**
983255 Nebraska Medical Center
Omaha, NE 68198-3255
**Website:** http://www.unmc.edu/Olson/research/lab-sig.htm
John S. Davis, PhD, Dir.

**Activities/Fields:** Cellular and molecular mechanisms that are responsible for relaying the actions of gonadotropins, growth factors, and cytokines in ovarian cells. The laboratory examines novel intracellular signal transduction pathways that govern cell survival and death, cell proliferation, cellular differentiation, gene expression, and steroidogenesis.

**★ 9513 ★ University of Nebraska at Omaha**
**Pediatric Pulmonary and Cystic Fibrosis Research Center**
985190 NE Medical Center
Omaha, NE 68198-5190
**Phone:** (402)559-6275    **Fax:** (402)559-7062
**Email:** jcolombo@unmc.edu
Dr. John L. Colombo, Dir.

**Activities/Fields:** Cystic fibrosis, including optimal use of antibiotics and respiratory therapy modalities; optimal use of aerosolized drug therapy; pancreatic function; effects of chronic aspiration, particularly on airway hyperactivity and inflammation; and bronchoalveolar lavage cytology in acute and chronic pediatric diseases.

**★ 9514 ★ University of Oklahoma**
**Pulmonary and Cystic Fibrosis Center**
Children's Hospital of Oklahoma, Rm. 3316B
940 NE 13th St.
Oklahoma City, OK 73104
**Phone:** (405)271-6390    **Fax:** (405)271-5055
**Email:** james-royall@ouhsc.edu
James Royall, Dir.

**Activities/Fields:** Cystic fibrosis and other respiratory diseases of children.

**University of Oklahoma Health Sciences Center**
**Center for American Indian Health Research**
*See:* Entry 2710

**★ 9515 ★ University of Pennsylvania**
**Institute for Human Gene Therapy (IHGT)**
Wistar Institute, Rm. 204
University of Pennsylvania School of Medicine
3601 Spruce St.
Philadelphia, PA 19104
**Phone:** (215)898-3000    **Fax:** (215)898-6588
**Email:** wilsonjm@mail.med.upenn.edu
**Website:** http://www.uphs.upenn.edu/ihgt/
Jim Wilson, Dir.

**Activities/Fields:** Human gene therapy as a means of treating disease.

**University of Pennsylvania**
**Referral Center for Animal Models of Human Genetic Disease**
*See:* Entry 20690

**University of Quebec**
**National Institute for Scientific Research-Armand-Frappier Institute**
**Human Health Research Centre**
*See:* Entry 3308

**★ 9516 ★ University of Rochester**
**Aab Institute of Biomedical Sciences**
**Center for Human Genetics and Molecular Pediatric Disease (CHGMPD)**
School of Medicine & Dentistry
601 Elmwood Ave., Box 703
Rochester, NY 14642
**Phone:** (716)273-2428    **Fax:** (716)271-7512
**Email:** richard_insel@urmc.rochester.edu
**Website:** http://www.urmc.rochester.edu/Aab/geneped/
Richard A. Insel, MD, Dir.

**Activities/Fields:** Identifying, characterizing, and understanding gene-disease relationships and environmental contributions, defining the molecular basis and pathogenesis of human disease, identifying pathways of gene expression, and elucidating targets and interventions for the prevention and therapy of human disease.

**★ 9517 ★ University of Sherbrooke**
**Molecular Biology Research Centre**
**RNA Group**
Departement de Microbiologie et Infectiologie
Faculte de Medecine
3001 12e Ave. Nord
Sherbrooke, QC, Canada J1H 5N4
**Phone:** (819)564-5321    **Fax:** (819)564-5392
Benoit Chabot, Contact

**Activities/Fields:** Gene expression in vitro and in vivo, including the recombination of viral and cellular genes, alternative splicing of RNA, expression and function of transformation genes, replication of telomeres and clinical applications of PCR.

**★ 9518 ★ University of Texas—Houston Health Science Center**
**Genetic Marker Laboratory**
School of Public Health
1200 Hermann Pressler, Ste. E-453
Houston, TX 77030
**Phone:** (713)500-9816    **Fax:** (713)500-0900
**Email:** eric.boerwinkle@uth.tmc.edu
Dr. Eric Boerwinkle, Dir.

**Activities/Fields:** Investigates DNA polymorphisms to find genetic bases for diseases, with special emphasis on common chronic diseases such as diabetes and heart disease. Approaches include linkage and pedigree analysis, DNA automated typing, and sequencing.

**★ 9519 ★ University of Texas—Houston Health Science Center**
**Human Genetics Center**
School of Public Health
1200 Hermann Pressler, Ste. E-453
Houston, TX 77030
**Phone:** (713)500-9816    **Fax:** (713)500-0900
**Email:** eric.boerwinkle@uth.tmc.edu
Dr. Eric Boerwinkle, Dir.

**Activities/Fields:** Genetic analysis of the common chronic diseases to identify and characterize the genes contributing to morbidity and mortality in most westernized populations. Research involves genetic linkage studies to localize and characterize genes contributing to disease susceptibility. Such information provides the opportunity to better predict the occurrence of disease onset and better understand mechanisms of disease etiology and pathophysiology. The

research activities in the Center emphasize the evolutionary origin of disease susceptibility mutations, the genetic analysis of cardiovascular disease risk factors, and chronic disease among the Mexican-American population in South Texas. **Pub:** *Center for Demographic and Population Genetics Reports.*

**★ 9520 ★ University of Texas**
**Southwestern Medical Center at Dallas**
**Eugene McDermott Center for Human Growth and Development**
6000 Harry Hines Blvd., 10th Fl., Rm. 10.204
Dallas, TX 75390-8591
**Phone:** (214)648-1600    **Fax:** (214)648-1666
**Email:** helen.hobbs@utsouthwestern.edu
**Website:** http://mcdermott.swmed.edu
Dr. Helen H. Hobbs, Dir.

**Activities/Fields:** Genetic factors that contribute to human health and disease. The center promotes research in diverse areas including lipid metabolism, atherosclerosis, energy metabolism, chromosomal rearrangements, DNA repair, human growth and development, reproduction, cancer genetics, and biotechnology.

**★ 9521 ★ University of Toronto**
**Centre for Cardiovascular Research**
**Cardiac Gene Unit**
Department of Laboratory Medicine and Pathobiology
100 College St., Rm. 418A
Toronto, ON, Canada M5G 1L5
**Phone:** (416)978-8758    **Fax:** (416)978-5650
**Email:** liewcc@tcgu.med.utoronto.ca
**Website:** http://www.tcgu.med.utoronto.ca
C.C. Liew, PhD, Dir.

**Activities/Fields:** Genes that may be associated with cardiovascular disease. **Pub:** *Monographs, papers, and abstracts.*

**University of Utah**
**Cardiovascular Genetic Research Clinic**
*See:* Entry 5200

**★ 9522 ★ University of Utah**
**DNA Diagnostic Laboratory**
Center for Advanced Medical Technologies, Rm. 150
729 S Arapeen Dr.
Salt Lake City, UT 84108
**Phone:** (801)581-8334    **Free:** 888-DNA-MAPS
**Fax:** (801)585-3876
**Email:** ken.ward@hsc.utahh.edu
**Website:** http://www-medlib.med.utah.edu/dnadx/index.html
Kenneth Ward, MD, Dir.

**Activities/Fields:** Gene mapping, genetic diagnosis, preimplantation testing, pregnancy loss, birth defect genes, and preeclampsia genes.

**★ 9523 ★ University of Utah**
**Intermountain Cystic Fibrosis Center**
School of Medicine
50 N Medical Dr., Rm. 2C454
Salt Lake City, UT 84132
**Phone:** (801)581-2410    **Fax:** (801)587-9620
**Email:** barbara.chatfield@hsc.utah.edu
**Website:** http://www.med.utah.edu/pulm/cf.htm
Barbara Chatfield, Pediatrics Dir.

**Activities/Fields:** Cystic fibrosis and pulmonary disease, including studies electrolyte metabolism in the lung, lung mechanics, clinical studies of new therapies, and antibiotic pharmacology. **Pub:** *CF Informer Newletter*, quarterly.

**University of Washington**
**Alzheimer's Disease Research Center**
*See:* Entry 14471

## ★ 9524 ★ University of Washington
## Comprehensive Biology-Exploiting the
## Yeast Genome
Box 357360
Departments of Genetics, Molecular Biotechnology,
& Biochemi
Seattle, WA 98195-7360
**Phone:** (206)543-5345 **Fax:** (206)685-1792
**Email:** tdavis@u.washington.edu
**Website:** http://depts.washington.edu/~yeastrc/
Trisha Davis, PhD, Prin. Investigator

**Activities/Fields:** Complete genome sequence of the
yeast Saccharomyces cerevisiae using the methods of
mass spectrometry, the two-hybrid system, and microscopy.

## ★ 9525 ★ University of Washington
## Genome Center
Fluke Hall, Box 352145
Mason Rd.
Seattle, WA 98195
**Phone:** (206)685-7366 **Fax:** (206)685-7344
**Email:** uwgchelp@u.washington.edu
**Website:** http://www.genome.washington.edu/
UWGC/
Maynard Olson, Dir.

**Activities/Fields:** Mapping of human genomic DNA.

## ★ 9526 ★ University of Wisconsin—
## Madison
## Pediatric Pulmonary Center
Clinical Science Center
University Hospitals
600 Highland Ave.
Madison, WI 53792-4108
**Phone:** (608)263-8555 **Fax:** (608)263-0510
**Email:** cggreen@facstaff.wisc.edu
**Website:** http://www2.medsch.wisc.edu/children-
shosp/ppc/ppchome.html
Dr. Christopher G. Green, Dir.

**Activities/Fields:** Cystic fibrosis and other respiratory
diseases of children; home care of technology-depen-
dent children.

## ★ 9527 ★ Vanderbilt University
## Vanderbilt Addiction Center (VAC)
Psychiatric Hospital at Vanderbilt
1601 23rd Ave. S
Nashville, TN 37212-8645
**Phone:** (615)322-3527 **Free:** 800-365-2270
**Email:** vac.webmail@mcmail.vanderbilt.edu
**Website:** http://www.mc.vanderbilt.edu/addiction/
Peter R. Martin, MD, Dir.

**Activities/Fields:** Drug and alcohol dependence, especially genetic-environmental interactions.

## ★ 9528 ★ Washington University in St.
## Louis
## Cystic Fibrosis Center
1 Children's Pl.
Saint Louis, MO 63110
**Phone:** (314)454-2694 **Fax:** (314)454-2515
**Email:** ferkol_t@kids.wustl.eduu
Dr. Thomas Ferkol, Dir.

**Activities/Fields:** Cystic fibrosis and pulmonary diseases, plus nutrition and malabsorption in relation to
cystic fibrosis and liver diseases and effects of mechanisms of inflammatory response in cyctic fibrosis-relat-
ed diseases. Conducts research on lung transplantation and nutrition in cystic fibrosis, as well as basic
studies of immune mechanisms. Provides clinical
material to departments of the University engaged in
related research and offers educational programs for
patients, parents, and professionals.

## ★ 9529 ★ Wayne State University
## Center for Molecular Medicine and
## Genetics
Scott Hall, Rm. 3216
540 E Canfield
Detroit, MI 48201
**Phone:** (313)577-5323 **Fax:** (313)577-8083
**Email:** info@genetics.wayne.edu
**Website:** http://cmmg.biosci.wayne.edu
Dr. Mark Hughes, PhD, Dir.

**Activities/Fields:** Development and differentiation,
including studies into meiotic differentiation, cell type-
specific gene regulation, protein structure and function, and genome organization and stability; cancer
and metastasis, including mapping of cancer genes,
induction of carcinogenesis, gene regulation in cancer,
and mechanisms of metastasis; human genetics and
disease, comprising the genetic cause of Huntington's
disease, arthritis and tissue remodeling, and diabetes
and insulin action; viral disease, including papilloma
viruses in cervical cancer; and gene therapeutics,
including fetal gene therapy, and gene therapy for
lymphoma and leukemia.

## ★ 9530 ★ Wayne State University
## Cystic Fibrosis Care, Teaching and
## Resource Center
Children's Hospital of Michigan
3901 Beaubien
Detroit, MI 48201
**Phone:** (313)745-5541 **Fax:** (313)993-2948
**Email:** dtoder@med.wayne.edu
Debbie Toder, MD, Dir.

**Activities/Fields:** Cystic fibrosis and pediatric pulmonary diseases. Also participates in multi-centered
clinical trials.

## ★ 9531 ★ Wayne State University
## Pre-Natal/Cancer-Cytogenetics Laboratory
Hutzel Professional Bldg., Ste. 401-412
Department of Pathology
4727 St. Antoine
Detroit, MI 48201
**Phone:** (313)966-0680 **Fax:** (313)966-0687
**Email:** sebrahim@med.wayne.edu
Dr. Salah Ebrahim, Dir.

**Activities/Fields:** Cytogenetics, including studies in
the areas of neonatal development and endocrinology.
Performs tests on amniotic fluids, CVS, bloods, bone
marrows, and solid tissues.

## ★ 9532 ★ Wayne State University
## Sickle Cell Center
Children's Hospital of Michigan
3901 Beaubien
Detroit, MI 48201
**Phone:** (313)745-5613 **Fax:** (313)745-5237
**Email:** ssarnaik@wayne.med.edu
Dr. S. Sarnaik, Dir.

**Activities/Fields:** Sickle cell diseases, including clinical trials of new drugs, psychosocial research, and
newborn screening and follow-up of infants with sickle
cell diseases.

## ★ 9533 ★ Yale University
## Pediatric Cystic Fibrosis Research Center
Sch. of Medicine
333 Cedar St.
PO Box 208064
New Haven, CT 06520-8064
**Phone:** (203)785-2480 **Fax:** (203)785-6337
**Email:** regina.palazoo@yale.edu
Dr. Regina M. Palazzo, Dir.

**Activities/Fields:** Cystic fibrosis and related respiratory diseases of children, with special emphasis on
control of respiration.

# State & Regional Organizations

## Cystic Fibrosis

*Listed below are chapters of the Cystic Fibrosis
Foundation, 6931 Arlington Rd., Bethesda, MD
20814, (800)FIGHT-CF, http://www.cff.org/.*

### Alabama

## ★ 9534 ★ Cystic Fibrosis Foundation
## Alabama Chapter
502 Montgomery Hwy., Ste. 101
Birmingham, AL 35216
**Phone:** (205)870-8565 **Free:** 800-523-2357
**Email:** alabama@cff.org
**Website:** http://www.cff.org
Kathleen Ash, Director

### Arizona

## ★ 9535 ★ Cystic Fibrosis Foundation
## Arizona Chapter
3800 N Central Ave. Ste 700
Phoenix, AZ 85012
**Phone:** (602)224-0068 **Fax:** (602)224-0432
**Email:** arizona@cff.org
**Website:** http://www.cff.org
Jan Lee Sproat, Director

### Arkansas

## ★ 9536 ★ Cystic Fibrosis Foundation
## Arkansas Chapter
1604 Merrill Dr. Ste. D
Little Rock, AR 72211
**Phone:** (501)224-5888 **Free:** 800-264-0030
**Fax:** (501)663-6711
**Email:** arkansas@cff.org
**Website:** http://www.cff.org
Gloria Redman, Director

### California

## ★ 9537 ★ Cystic Fibrosis Foundation
## Northern California Chapter
1939 Harrison St. Ste. 207
Oakland, CA 94612
**Phone:** (415)677-0155 **Fax:** (415)267-9695
**Email:** no-calif@cff.org
**Website:** http://www.cff.org

## ★ 9538 ★ Cystic Fibrosis Foundation
## Southern California Chapter
9820 Willow Creek Rd., Ste. 245
San Diego, CA 92123
**Phone:** (858)578-2945 **Fax:** (858)578-2865
**Email:** san-diego@cff.org
**Website:** http://www.cff.org
Michele Mason, Director

## ★ 9539 ★ Cystic Fibrosis Foundation
## Southern California Chapter—Los Angeles
## Office
1950 Santelle Blvd., Ste. 328
Los Angeles, CA 90025
**Phone:** (310)479-8585 **Fax:** (310)473-7307
**Email:** so-calif-la@cff.org
**Website:** http://www.cff.org
Katherine Caulfield, Director

## ★ 9540 ★ Cystic Fibrosis Foundation
## Southern California / Utah Office
2150 Town Center Pl., Ste. 120
Anaheim, CA 92806
**Phone:** (714)938-1393 **Free:** 800-232-8731
**Fax:** (714)938-1462

**Website:** http://www.cff.org
Helen Johnson, Director

## Colorado

**★ 9541 ★ Cystic Fibrosis Foundation**
**Colorado Chapter**
1755 Blake St.
Denver, CO 80202
**Phone:** (303)296-6610
**Email:** colorado@cff.org
**Website:** http://www.cff.org
Penny Barnow, Director

**★ 9542 ★ Cystic Fibrosis Foundation**
**Colorado Chapter**
**Pikes Peak Office**
118 N Tejon St., Ste. 200
Colorado Springs, CO 80903
**Phone:** (719)444-8966    **Fax:** (719)444-0926
**Email:** pikes-peak@cff.org
**Website:** http://www.cff.org
Barbara Furr-Cassidy, Director

## Connecticut

**★ 9543 ★ Cystic Fibrosis Foundation**
**Connecticut Chapter**
185 Filas Dean Hwy.
Wethersfield, CT 06109
**Phone:** (860)257-6907    **Free:** 800-841-2828
**Fax:** (860)257-6903
**Email:** conn@cff.org
**Website:** http://www.cff.org
Rosemary Hoffmann, Director

## Florida

**★ 9544 ★ Cystic Fibrosis Foundation**
**Florida Chapter**
2 Prospect Park Business Center
3443 NW 55th St., Bldg. 7
Fort Lauderdale, FL 33309
**Phone:** (954)739-5006    **Fax:** (954)739-2890
**Email:** florida@cff.org
**Website:** http://www.cff.org
Christina Landshut, Director

**★ 9545 ★ Cystic Fibrosis Foundation**
**Florida Chapter**
**Tampa Regional Office**
1315 S Howard Ave., Ste 102
Tampa, FL 33606
**Phone:** (813)258-0266    **Fax:** (813)258-3380
**Email:** tampa-fl@cff.org
**Website:** http://www.cff.org
Susan Baty, Director

**★ 9546 ★ Cystic Fibrosis Foundation**
**Jacksonville Regional Office**
2121 A Corporate Sq. Blvd, Ste. 170
Jacksonville, FL 32216
**Phone:** (904)724-0064    **Free:** 800-344-4823
**Fax:** (904)724-0280
**Email:** jax-fl@cff.org
**Website:** http://www.cff.org/jacksonville.htm
Claudia Werner, Director

**★ 9547 ★ Cystic Fibrosis Foundation**
**Orlando Regional Office**
1080 Woodcock Rd., Ste. 245
Orlando, FL 32803
**Phone:** (407)896-1113
**Email:** orlando-fl@cff.org
**Website:** http://www.cff.org
Suzanne Beranek, Director

**★ 9548 ★ Cystic Fibrosis Foundation**
**Palm Beach Regional Office**
2200 N Florida Mango Rd., Ste. 304
West Palm Beach, FL 33409
**Phone:** (561)683-9965
**Email:** palm-beach-fl@cff.org
**Website:** http://www.cff.org
Marie Cook, Director

## Georgia

**★ 9549 ★ Cystic Fibrosis Foundation**
**Georgia Chapter**
2250 N Druid Hills Rd., Ste. 275
Atlanta, GA 30329
**Phone:** (404)325-6973    **Free:** 800-476-4483
**Fax:** (404)325-7921
**Email:** georgia@cff.org
**Website:** http://www.cff.org
Maureen A. Fraser, Director

## Illinois

**★ 9550 ★ Cystic Fibrosis Foundation**
**Greater Illinois Chapter**
150 N Michigan Ave., Ste. 400
Chicago, IL 60601
**Phone:** (312)236-4491    **Free:** 800-824-5064
**Fax:** (312)236-2797
**Email:** illinois@cff.org
**Website:** http://www.cff.org
Ashton Chase, Director

## Indiana

**★ 9551 ★ Cystic Fibrosis Foundation**
**Indiana Chapter**
1261 W 86th St., Ste. E2
Indianapolis, IN 46260
**Phone:** (317)202-9210    **Free:** 800-622-4826
**Fax:** (317)202-9215
**Email:** indiana@cff.org
**Website:** http://www.cff.org
Linda Moritz, Director

## Iowa

**★ 9552 ★ Cystic Fibrosis Foundation**
**Iowa Chapter**
2600 72nd St., Ste. M
Des Moines, IA 50322
**Phone:** (515)252-1530    **Free:** 800-798-5151
**Fax:** (515)252-7684
**Email:** iowa@cff.org
**Website:** http://www.cff.org
Lisa Werner, Director

## Kentucky

**★ 9553 ★ Cystic Fibrosis Foundation**
**Kentucky / West Virginia Chapter**
1941 Bishop Ln., Ste. 507
Louisville, KY 40218
**Phone:** (502)452-6353    **Free:** 800-526-8126
**Fax:** (502)456-2936
**Email:** kent-wv@cff.org
**Website:** http://www.cff.org
Mary Lee Stevens, Director
**Program(s):** Medical Education and Training Therapeutics Development Program.

## Louisiana

**★ 9554 ★ Cystic Fibrosis Foundation**
**Louisiana Chapter**
4621 W Napoleon Ave., Ste. 207
Metairie, LA 70001
**Phone:** (504)455-5194    **Free:** 800-257-4166
**Fax:** (504)889-2592
**Email:** louisiana@cff.org
**Website:** http://www.cff.org
Renee Ganucheau, Director

**★ 9555 ★ Cystic Fibrosis Foundation**
**Louisiana Chapter**
**Baton Rouge Regional Office**
7354 Alberta Dr. Ste E
Baton Rouge, LA 70808
**Phone:** (225)769-9994    **Free:** 877-753-9990
**Email:** baton-rouge@cff.org
**Website:** http://www.cff.org
Nancy Wertz, Director

## Maryland

**★ 9556 ★ Cystic Fibrosis Foundation**
**Maryland Chapter**
10616 Beaver Dam Rd., Ste. 6
Hunt Valley, MD 21030
**Phone:** (410)771-9000    **Free:** 800-731-2873
**Email:** maryland@cff.org
**Website:** http://www.cff.org
Josephine Schaeffer, Director

## Massachusetts

**★ 9557 ★ Cystic Fibrosis Foundation**
**Massachusetts/Rhode Island Chapter**
220 N Main, Ste. 104
Natick, MA 01760
**Phone:** (508)655-6000    **Free:** 800-966-0444
**Email:** mass-ri@cff.org
**Website:** http://www.cff.org
Pamela Spitzer, Director

**★ 9558 ★ Cystic Fibrosis Foundation**
**Rhode Island Chapter**
220 N Main St., Ste. 104
Natick, MA 01760
**Phone:** (508)655-6000    **Free:** 800-966-0444
**Email:** mass-ri@cff.org
**Website:** http://www.cff.org
Pamela Spitzer, Director

## Michigan

**★ 9559 ★ Cystic Fibrosis Foundation**
**Ann Arbor Office**
1100 N Main St.
Ann Arbor, MI 48104
**Phone:** (734)998-1234
**Email:** ann-arbor-mi@cff.org
**Website:** http://www.cff.org

**★ 9560 ★ Cystic Fibrosis Foundation**
**Genesee Valley Regional Office**
10775 S Saginaw, Ste. J
Grand Blanc, MI 48439
**Phone:** (810)603-3271    **Fax:** (810)603-3274
**Email:** geneseevalleyregional@cff.org
**Website:** http://www.cff.org
Kaygie Goggins, Director

**★ 9561 ★ Cystic Fibrosis Foundation**
**Greater Michigan Chapter-Eastern Region**
3064 Boardwalk
Saginaw, MI 48603
**Phone:** (989)790-2233    **Free:** 800-968-7169
**Fax:** (989)790-1050
**Email:** saginaw-mi@cff.org
**Website:** http://www.cff.org

**★ 9562 ★ Cystic Fibrosis Foundation**
**Greater Michigan Chapter—Western Region**
3835 28th St. SE, Ste. 105
Grand Rapids, MI 49512
**Phone:** (616)285-8140    **Free:** 800-968-1050
**Fax:** (616)285-4530
**Email:** grapids-mi@cff.org
**Website:** http://www.cff.org
Beth Heyboer, Director

**★ 9563 ★ Cystic Fibrosis Foundation**
**Metro Detroit Chapter**
2265 Livernois, Ste. 410
Troy, MI 48083
**Phone:** (248)269-8759　　　　**Fax:** (248)362-2608
**Email:** detroit@cff.org
**Website:** http://www.cff.org
Patricia Lee, Director

## Minnesota

**★ 9564 ★ Cystic Fibrosis Foundation**
**Minnesota Chapter**
1611 W County Rd. B, Ste. 221
Saint Paul, MN 55113
**Phone:** (651)631-3290　　　　**Fax:** (651)631-3296
**Email:** minn@cff.org
**Website:** http://www.cff.org
Nancy L. Viking, Director
**Remarks:** Foundation raises money for research to find a cure for cystic fibrosis and to improve the quality of life for persons with the disease. **Program(s):** Gene Therapy; Clinical Research; Research and Development Program Centers; CFF-NIH Gene Therapy Centers; CF Care Centers.

## Missouri

**★ 9565 ★ Cystic Fibrosis Foundation**
**Gateway Chapter**
200 S Hanley, Ste. 620
Saint Louis, MO 63105
**Phone:** (314)721-2490　　　　**Free:** 800-727-1464
**Fax:** (314)721-2809
**Email:** gateway@cff.org
**Website:** http://www.cff.org/gateway.htm
Bert Merrell, Director

## Nebraska

**★ 9566 ★ Cystic Fibrosis Foundation**
**Nebraska Chapter**
10838 Old Mill Rd., Ste. 6
Omaha, NE 68154
**Phone:** (402)330-6164
**Email:** nebraska@cff.org
**Website:** http://www.cff.org
Penny Biever, Director

## New Hampshire

**★ 9567 ★ Cystic Fibrosis Foundation**
**Northern New England Chapter**
114 Perimeter Rd., Unit E
Nashua, NH 03063
**Phone:** (603)598-8191　　　　**Free:** 800-757-0203
**Fax:** (603)598-8167
**Email:** no-new-eng@cff.org
**Website:** http://www.cff.org
Christopher Hendry, Director

## New Mexico

**★ 9568 ★ Cystic Fibrosis Foundation**
**New Mexico Chapter**
4004 Carlisle NE, Ste. B
Albuquerque, NM 87107
**Phone:** (505)883-1455　　　　**Fax:** (505)883-3998
**Email:** new-mexico@cff.org
**Website:** http://www.cff.org
Carolyn Jackson, Director

## New York

**★ 9569 ★ Cystic Fibrosis Foundation**
**Central New York Chapter**
6700 Old Collamer Rd.
East Syracuse, NY 13057
**Phone:** (315)463-7965　　　　**Free:** 800-962-6578
**Fax:** (315)463-8221
**Email:** central-ny@cff.org

**Website:** http://www.cff.org
Jennifer Janes, Director

**★ 9570 ★ Cystic Fibrosis Foundation**
**Greater New York Chapter**
60 E 42nd St., Ste. 1563
New York, NY 10165
**Phone:** (212)986-8783　　　　**Fax:** (212)697-4282
**Email:** greater-ny@cff.org
**Website:** http://www.cff.org
Doris F. Tulcin, Exec Director

**★ 9571 ★ Cystic Fibrosis Foundation**
**Greater New York Chapter**
**Long Island Office**
420 Jericho Tpk., Ste. 320
Jericho, NY 11753
**Phone:** (516)827-1290　　　　**Fax:** (516)827-1295
**Email:** long-island@cff.org
**Website:** http://www.cff.org
Yolan J. Wolf, Director

**★ 9572 ★ Cystic Fibrosis Foundation**
**Northeastern New York Chapter**
12 Avis Dr.
Latham, NY 12110
**Phone:** (518)783-7361　　　　**Fax:** (518)783-7394
**Email:** ne-ny@cff.org
**Website:** http://www.cff.org
Linda Traylor, Director

**★ 9573 ★ Cystic Fibrosis Foundation**
**Rochester Chapter**
301 Exchange Blvd., Ste. 206
Rochester, NY 14608
**Phone:** (585)546-5890　　　　**Fax:** (585)546-3903
**Email:** rochester-ny@cff.org
**Website:** http://www.cff.org
Kelly Hallenbeck, Director

## North Carolina

**★ 9574 ★ Cystic Fibrosis Foundation**
**Carolinas Chapter**
1005 Bullard Ct., Ste. 105
Raleigh, NC 27615
**Phone:** (919)878-5040　　　　**Free:** 800-822-9941
**Fax:** (919)878-5049
**Email:** carolinas@cff.org
**Website:** http://www.cff.org
Nancy Mallory, Director

**★ 9575 ★ Cystic Fibrosis Foundation**
**Charlotte Office**
1428 Orchard Lake Dr., No. B
Charlotte, NC 28270
**Phone:** (704)321-7852　　　　**Free:** 800-336-0329
**Fax:** (704)321-7856
**Email:** charlotte-nc@cff.org
**Website:** http://www.cff.org
Janice Dumsha, Director

## Ohio

**★ 9576 ★ Cystic Fibrosis Foundation**
**Central Ohio Chapter**
960 Kingsmill Pkwy., Ste. 101
Columbus, OH 43229
**Phone:** (614)846-2440　　　　**Fax:** (614)846-2472
**Email:** central-oh@cff.org
**Website:** http://www.cff.org
Alyce Elbert, Director

**★ 9577 ★ Cystic Fibrosis Foundation**
**Rainbow Chapter**
2000 E 9th St., Ste. 420
Cleveland, OH 44115
**Phone:** (216)902-8140　　　　**Free:** 800-368-2150
**Email:** rainbow@cff.org

**Website:** http://www.cff.org
Jennifer Basel, Director

## Oklahoma

**★ 9578 ★ Cystic Fibrosis Foundation**
**Sooner Chapter**
2642 E 21st St., Ste. 100
Tulsa, OK 74114
**Phone:** (918)744-6354　　　　**Free:** 800-814-5766
**Email:** sooner@cff.org
**Website:** http://www.cff.org
JoAnn Winn, Director

## Oregon

**★ 9579 ★ Cystic Fibrosis Foundation**
**Oregon / Idaho / Montana Chapter**
5331 SW Macadam, Ste. 340
Portland, OR 97239
**Phone:** (503)226-3435　　　　**Free:** 800-448-8404
**Fax:** (503)226-4165
**Email:** oregon@cff.org
**Website:** http://www.cff.org
Charlotte Governale, Director

## Pennsylvania

**★ 9580 ★ Cystic Fibrosis Foundation**
**Central Pennsylvania Chapter**
55 S Progress Ave.
Harrisburg, PA 17109
**Phone:** (717)671-4000　　　　**Free:** 800-671-2262
**Fax:** (717)671-4007
**Email:** central-pa@cff.org
**Website:** http://www.cff.org
Lisa Schlager, Director

**★ 9581 ★ Cystic Fibrosis Foundation**
**Delaware Valley Chapter**
2004 Sproul Rd., Ste. 208
Broomall, PA 19008
**Phone:** (610)325-6001　　　　**Free:** 800-378-8423
**Fax:** (610)325-6588
**Email:** del-valley@cff.org
**Website:** http://www.cff.org
Susan Yannessa, Director

**★ 9582 ★ Cystic Fibrosis Foundation**
**Northeastern Pennsylvania Chapter**
1541 Alta Dr., Ste. 102
Whitehall, PA 18052
**Phone:** (610)820-0206　　　　**Free:** 800-552-2199
**Fax:** (610)820-9367
**Email:** ne-pa@cff.org
**Website:** http://www.cff.org
Cynthia Phillips, Director
**Program(s):** Gene Therapy Studies.

**★ 9583 ★ Cystic Fibrosis Foundation**
**Western Pennsylvania Chapter**
810 River Ave., Ste. 100
Pittsburgh, PA 15212
**Phone:** (412)321-4422　　　　**Free:** 800-562-5395
**Fax:** (412)321-9305
**Email:** west-pa@cff.org
**Website:** http://www.cff.org
Mary Pat Root Joseph, Director

## Tennessee

**★ 9584 ★ Cystic Fibrosis Foundation**
**Tennessee Chapter**
209 10th Ave S, Ste. 426
Nashville, TN 37203
**Phone:** (615)255-1167
**Email:** tenn@cff.org
**Website:** http://www.cff.org
Belinda Dinwiddie, Contact

**★ 9585 ★ Cystic Fibrosis Foundation
Tennessee Chapter
Memphis Office**
1028 Crest Haven, Ste. 203
Memphis, TN 38119
**Phone:** (901)818-9090
**Email:** memphis@cff.org
**Website:** http://www.cff.org
JoAnne Knox, Director

## Texas

**★ 9586 ★ Cystic Fibrosis Foundation
Lone Star Chapter**
8620 N New Braunsels, Ste. 110
San Antonio, TX 78217
**Phone:** (210)829-7267　　　**Fax:** (210)829-4204
**Website:** http://www.cff.org/
Beth Morgan, Director

**★ 9587 ★ Cystic Fibrosis Foundation
Northeast Texas Chapter**
2929 Carlisle, Ste. 230
Dallas, TX 75204
**Phone:** (214)871-2222　　　**Fax:** (214)969-7439
**Email:** ne-texas@cff.org
**Website:** http://www.cff.org
Sila N. Foote, Contact

**★ 9588 ★ Cystic Fibrosis Foundation
Texas Gulf Coast Chapter**
50 Briah Hollow Ln., Ste. 495 E
Houston, TX 77027
**Phone:** (713)621-0006　　　**Fax:** (713)621-2542
**Email:** texas-gulf@cff.org
**Website:** http://www.cff.org
Sissy Boyd, Director

## Washington

**★ 9589 ★ Cystic Fibrosis Foundation
Washington/Alaska Chapter**
100 W Harrison N Towers, Ste. 510
Seattle, WA 98119
**Phone:** (206)282-4770　　　**Free:** 800-647-7774
**Email:** washington@cff.org
**Website:** http://www.cff.org
Dottie Moore, Director

**★ 9590 ★ Cystic Fibrosis Foundation
Washington/Alaska Chapter**
100 W Harrison N Towers, Ste. 510
Seattle, WA 98119
**Phone:** (206)282-4770　　　**Free:** 800-647-7774
**Fax:** (206)283-8359
**Email:** washington@cff.org
**Website:** http://www.cffwa.org/
Dottie Moore, Director

## Wisconsin

**★ 9591 ★ Cystic Fibrosis Foundation
Wisconsin Chapter**
2421 Mayfair Rd., Ste. 320
Milwaukee, WI 53226
**Phone:** (414)778-4820　　　**Free:** 800-472-7720
**Fax:** (414)778-4824
**Email:** wisconsin@cff.org
**Website:** http://www.cff.org
Lisa Weisman, Director

# Chapter 28
# Health Care Administration

## Federal Government Agencies

**★ 9592 ★ U.S. Department of Health and Human Services (HRSA)**
**Health Resources and Services Administration**
5600 Fishers Ln.
Rockville, MD 20857
**Phone:** (301)443-2086
**Website:** http://www.hrsa.gov
**Desc:** HRSA is the principle primary health care service agency of the federal government. Its mission is to make essential primary care services accessible to the poor, uninsured, and geographically isolated–populations severely underserved by the private health care system.

## Foundations & Other Funding Organizations

### Other Funding Organizations

**★ 9593 ★ American Society for Healthcare Risk Management (ASHRM)**
One N Franklin
Chicago, IL 60606
**Phone:** (312)422-3989      **Fax:** (312)422-4580
**Email:** esummy@aha.org
**Website:** http://www.ashrm.org
Elizabeth Summy, Exec. Dir.
**Desc:** Employees actively involved in the risk management functions of hospitals or other health care providers, and others involved in insurance, brokerage, and consulting. Purposes are to: promote professional development of hospital risk managers; provide educational resources and programs on healthcare risk management; address risk management issues affecting the health care industry. **Awards:** Innovation and Research Awards (annual).

**★ 9594 ★ American Society of Ophthalmic Administrators (ASOA)**
4000 Legato Rd., No. 850
Fairfax, VA 22033
**Phone:** (703)591-2220      **Free:** 800-451-1339
**Fax:** (703)591-0614
**Email:** asoa@asoa.org
**Website:** http://www.asoa.org
Lucy Santiago, Exec. Dir.
**Desc:** A division of the American Society of Cataract and Refractive Surgery . Persons involved with the administration of an ophthalmic office or clinic. Facilitates the exchange of ideas and information in order to improve management practices and working conditions. Offers placement services. **Awards:** William A. Rose Pinnacle Award (annual) to ophthalmology prac-

tices demonstrating exemplary effort to eliminate potential abusive billing practices and maintain compliance with government regulations.

**★ 9595 ★ Foundation of American College of Health Care Administrators (FACHCA)**
300 N Lee St., No. 301
Alexandria, VA 22314-2807
**Phone:** (703)739-7900      **Free:** 888-88A-CHCA
**Fax:** (703)739-7901
**Email:** mtn@achca.org
**Website:** http://www.achca.org
Mary Tellis-Nayak, Pres. /CEO
**Desc:** Individuals dedicated to the improvement of the administration of long-term care facilities. Conducts professional training programs and research in administration. **Awards:** Administrator in Training Scholarship (annual) for an administrator-in-training in a long-term care facility; Director of Nursing Award (annual); Research Award (annual) for research pertaining to long-term care.

**★ 9596 ★ National Association of Directors of Nursing Administration in Long Term Care (NADONA/LTC)**
10101 Alliance Rd., No. 140
Cincinnati, OH 45242
**Phone:** (513)791-3679      **Free:** 800-222-0539
**Fax:** (513)791-3699
**Email:** info@nadona.org
**Website:** http://www.nadona.org
Joan C. Warden-Saunders, R.N., Exec. Dir.
**Desc:** Directors, assistant directors, and former directors of nursing in long term care. Goals are: to create and establish an acceptable ethical standard for practices in long term care nursing administration and to promote and encourage research in the profession; to develop and provide a consistent program of education and certification for the positions of director, associate director, and assistant director; to promote a positive image of the long term health care industry. Encourages members to share concerns and experiences; sponsors research programs. Advocates legislation pertaining to the practice of professional nursing. Maintains speakers' bureau. nursing. Maintains speakers' bureau. **Awards:** Above and Beyond (annual) upon request; Caring (annual) members conference; Upward Bound (annual).

**★ 9597 ★ National Association of Health Services Executives (NAHSE)**
8630 Fenton St., No. 126
Silver Spring, MD 20910
**Phone:** (301)588-2255      **Fax:** (301)588-0011
**Email:** nahse_hq@compuserve.com
**Website:** http://www.nahse.org/
Dr. Hilda Richards, Pres.
**Desc:** Black health care executive managers, planners, educators, advocates, providers, organizers, researchers, and consumers participating in academic ventures, educational forums, seminars, workshops, systems design, legislation, and other activities. Con-

ducts National Work-Study Program and sponsors educational programs. **Awards:** Haynes Rice Scholarship (annual) for students majoring in healthcare; Humanitarian Award (annual) for outstanding service in the field of human services; NAHSE Scholarship (annual).

## Medical & Allied Health Schools

### Health Services Administration

*The following health services administration programs are accredited by the Accrediting Commission on Education for Health Services Administration. For further information on these programs, and for listings of undergraduate programs, contact the Association of University Programs in Health Administration, 730 11th St. NW, 4th Floor, Washington, DC 20001-4510, (202) 638-1448, http://www.aupha.org/.*

### Alabama

**★ 9598 ★ University of Alabama, Birmingham**
**Department of Health Services Administration**
**Master of Science in Health Administration Program**
506 Webb Bldg.
1530 3rd Ave. S
Birmingham, AL 35294-3361
**Phone:** (205)934-1735      **Fax:** (205)975-6608
**Email:** msha@uab.edu
**Website:** http://www.hsa.uab.edu
Stephen J. O'Conner, PhD, Director
**Fnded:** 1965.

### Alberta

**★ 9599 ★ University of Alberta**
**Department of Public Health Sciences**
**Graduate Program in Health Services Administration**
13-103 Clinical Sciences Bldg.
University of Alberta
Edmonton, AB, Canada T6G 2G3
**Phone:** (780)492-8608      **Fax:** (780)492-0364
**Email:** kent.rondeau@alberta.ca
**Website:** http://www.med.ualberta.ca/PHS/
Kent V. Rondeau, PhD, Director

## Arizona

**★ 9600 ★ Arizona State University**
**College of Business**
**School of Health Administration and Policy**
**Graduate Program in Health Services Administration**
Box 874506
Tempe, AZ 85287-4506
**Phone:** (602)965-7778          **Fax:** (602)965-6654
**Email:** asuhap@asu.edu
**Website:** http://www.cob.asu.edu/hap/index.html
Eugene S. Schneller, Director

**★ 9601 ★ Arizona State University**
**School of Health Administration and Policy**
**Graduate Program in Health Services and Policy**
College of Business
Box 874506
Tempe, AZ 85287-4506
**Email:** asuhap@atsasu.edu
**Website:** http://www.cob.asu.edu/hap/index/html

## Arkansas

**★ 9602 ★ University of Arkansas, Little Rock**
**College of Professional Professional Studies**
**Graduate Program in Health Services Administration**
2801 S University Ave.
Little Rock, AR 72204-1099
**Phone:** (501)569-3293          **Fax:** (501)569-8365
**Email:** jbwayne@ualr.edu
**Website:** http://www.ualr.edu/~hsadmin/index.htm
John B. Wayne, PhD, Director

## California

**★ 9603 ★ San Diego State University**
**Graduate School of Public Health**
**Division of Health Services Administration**
San Diego, CA 92182-4162
**Phone:** (619)594-4443          **Fax:** (619)594-6112
**Email:** swilliam@mail.sdsu.edu
**Website:** http://www.sdsu.edu
Stephen J. Williams, Director

**★ 9604 ★ University of California, Berkeley**
**Haas School of Business**
**Graduate Program in Health Services Management**
Haas School of Business, mail code 1900
Berkeley, CA 94720
**Phone:** (510)643-1399          **Fax:** (510)642-4700
**Email:** raube@haas.berkeley.edu
**Website:** http://www.haas.berkeley.edu/advantage/health.htm
Kristiana Raube, PhD, Exec Director

**★ 9605 ★ University of California, Los Angeles**
**School of Public Health**
**Department of Health Services**
**Health Policy and Management Program**
PO Box 951772
10833 Le Conte Ave.
Los Angeles, CA 90095-1772
**Phone:** (310)825-7863          **Fax:** (310)825-3317
**Email:** almer@ph.ucla.edu
**Website:** http://www.ph.ucla.edu/hs
Diana W. Hilberman, Dr.PH, Director
**Fnded:** 1960.

**★ 9606 ★ University of Southern California**
**School of Policy, Planning and Development**
**Health Services Administration Program**
Los Angeles, CA 90089-0626
**Phone:** (213)740-4280          **Fax:** (213)740-1801
**Email:** myrtle@usc.edu
**Website:** http://www.usc.edu/dept/sppd
LaVonna Lewis, PhD, Director

## Colorado

**★ 9607 ★ University of Colorado, Denver**
**Graduate School of Business Administration**
**Programs in Health Services Administration**
Campus Box 165
PO Box 173364
Denver, CO 80217-3364
**Phone:** (303)556-5845          **Fax:** (303)556-5899
**Email:** elbiggs@aol.com
**Website:** http://www.business.cudenver.edu
Errol L. Biggs, PhD, Director

**★ 9608 ★ University of Colorado, Denver**
**Network for Healthcare Management**
**Executive Master of Business Administration in Health Administration**
PO Box 480006
Denver, CO 80248-0006
**Phone:** (303)623-1888          **Fax:** (303)623-6228
**Email:** peter_taffe@cao.cudenver.edu
**Website:** http://www.execed.colorado.edu
Errol L. Biggs, PhD, Director

## Connecticut

**★ 9609 ★ University of Connecticut**
**School of Business**
**Center for Health Systems Management**
368 Fairfield Rd., U-41
Storrs, CT 06269-2041
**Phone:** (860)486-4122          **Fax:** (860)486-4230
**Email:** jkramer@sba.uconn.edu
**Website:** http://www.sba.uconn.edu/HealthSystems/
Jeffrey A. Kramer, PhD, Director

**★ 9610 ★ Yale University**
**School of Medicine**
**Department of Epidemiology and Public Health**
**Division of Health Policy and Administration**
60 College St.
PO Box 208034
New Haven, CT 06520-8034
**Phone:** (203)785-2854          **Fax:** (203)785-6287
**Website:** http://www.yale.edu/yaleinfo/gradprof.html
Mark Schlesinger, PhD, Director
**Fnded:** 1947.

## District of Columbia

**★ 9611 ★ The George Washington University**
**Department of Health Services Management and Policy**
2175 K St. NW, Ste. 700
Washington, DC 20037
**Phone:** (202)467-2288          **Fax:** (202)416-0075
**Website:** http://www.gwumc.edu/sphhs/heaser.htm
Brian Biles, MD, Director
**Fnded:** 1959.

## Florida

**★ 9612 ★ Florida International University**
**Program in Health Services Administration**
N Miami Campus
3000 NE 151st St.
North Miami, FL 33181-3600
**Phone:** (305)919-5890          **Fax:** (305)919-5848
**Email:** spm@fiu.edu
**Website:** http://www.fiu.edu/~cupa/hsa-grad.html
Gloria J. Deckard, PhD, Director

**★ 9613 ★ University of Central Florida**
**College of Health and Public Affairs**
**Health Services Administration Program**
13-103 Clinical Sciences Bldg.
University of Alberta
Orlando, FL 32816
**Phone:** (407)823-6318          **Fax:** (407)823-6318
**Email:** hsainfo@mail.ucf.edu
**Website:** http://www.cohpa.ucf.edu/health.pro/hsa/graduate/
Myron Fottler, PhD, Exec Director

**★ 9614 ★ University of Florida**
**Colleges of Health Professions**
**Graduate Program in Health Administration**
PO Box 100195
Gainesville, FL 32610-0195
**Phone:** (352)392-7590          **Fax:** (352)392-7109
**Email:** hsa-info@hp.ufl.edu
**Website:** http://www.hp.ufl/hsa
Niccie L. McKay, PhD, Director

**★ 9615 ★ University of Miami**
**Academic Programs in Health Administration and Policy**
PO Box 248505
Coral Gables, FL 33124-6524
**Phone:** (305)284-5926          **Fax:** (305)284-5905
**Email:** mfrench@miami.edu
**Website:** http://www.bus.miami.edu/gbp/ealth/index.html
Michael T. French, PhD, Director

**★ 9616 ★ University of South Florida**
**College of Public Health**
**Department of Health Policy and Management**
13201 Bruce B. Downs Blvd.
MDC 56
Tampa, FL 33612-3805
**Free:** 888-873-2674          **Fax:** (813)974-6741
**Email:** advisor@hsc.usf.edu
**Website:** http://www.hsc.usf.edu/PUBHEALTH/hpm
Barbara Langland Orban, PhD, Director
**Fnded:** 1988.

## Georgia

**★ 9617 ★ Georgia State University**
**Graduate Program in Health Administration**
**Institute of Health Administration**
University Plaza
Atlanta, GA 30303
**Phone:** (404)651-2637          **Fax:** (404)651-1230
**Email:** asumner@gsu.edu
**Website:** http://www.gsu.edu/~wwwiha/
Andrew T. Sumner, Director
**Fnded:** 1965.

## Illinois

### ★ 9618 ★ Governors State University
**College of Health Professions**
**Health Administration Program**
University Park, IL 60466
**Phone:** (708)534-4032     **Fax:** (708)534-8041
**Email:** c-crawford@atsgovst.edu
**Website:** http://www.govst.edu
Catherine M. Crawford, PhD, Director

### ★ 9619 ★ Northwestern University
**Kellogg Graduate School of Management**
**Program in Health Industry Management**
Nathaniel Leverone Hall
2001 Sheridan Rd.
Evanston, IL 60208
**Phone:** (847)491-5540     **Fax:** (847)491-2683
**Email:** myrogers@nwu.edu
**Website:** http://www.kellogg.nwu.edu
Joel I. Shalowitz, MD, Director

### ★ 9620 ★ Rush University
**Health Systems Management**
Rush-Presbyterian /St. Luke's Medical Center
1653 W Congress Pkwy.
Chicago, IL 60612-3833
**Phone:** (312)942-5402     **Fax:** (312)942-4957
**Email:** rushhsm@rushu.rush.edu
**Website:** http://www.rushu.rush.edu/hsm
Denise M. Oleske, PhD, Director

### ★ 9621 ★ University of Chicago
**Graduate Program in Health**
**Administration and Policy**
969 E 60th St.
Box 6011
Chicago, IL 60637
**Phone:** (773)702-1324     **Fax:** (773)702-7222
**Email:** lawlor@atschas.uchicago.edu
**Website:** http://www.uchicago.edu
Edward F. Lawlor, PhD, Director
**Fnded:** 1934.

## Indiana

### ★ 9622 ★ Indiana University
**School of Public and Environmental**
**Affairs**
**Graduate Program in Health**
**Administration**
1110 W Michigan St.
Rm. LO 227
Indianapolis, IN 46202-5152
**Phone:** (317)278-4898     **Free:** 877-292-9321
**Fax:** (317)274-4444
**Email:** MHASPEA@iupui.edu
**Website:** http://www.mha.iupui.edu/
Stephen L. Walston, PhD, Director

## Iowa

### ★ 9623 ★ Des Moines University
**Health Care Administration Program**
3200 Grand Ave.
Des Moines, IA 50312
**Phone:** (515)271-1364     **Free:** 800-240-2767
**Fax:** (515)271-1614
**Email:** HM.Admit@dmu.edu
**Website:** http://www.dmu.edu/cohs/dhm/hca/index.htm
Mary Pat Wohlford-Wessels, Director

### ★ 9624 ★ University of Iowa
**College of Medicine and Graduate**
**College**
**A Division of Health Management and**
**Policy**
2700 Steindler Bldg.
Iowa City, IA 52242
**Phone:** (319)335-9814     **Fax:** (319)335-9772
**Email:** student-affairs-administrator@mail.pmeh.uiowa.edu
**Website:** http://www.pmeh.uiowa.edu/hmp/MHAdegree.html
Douglas S. Wakefield, PhD, Director

## Kansas

### ★ 9625 ★ University of Kansas
**School of Medicine**
**Department of Health Policy and**
**Management**
Student Services Office
Edwards Campus
12600 Quivira Rd.
Overland Park, KS 66213
**Phone:** (913)897-8585     **Fax:** (913)897-8681
**Email:** ks_hsa@kumc.edu
**Website:** http://www.kumc.edu/som/hpm
Cynthia Carter Haddock, PhD, Director

## Kentucky

### ★ 9626 ★ University of Kentucky
**Martin School of Public Policy &**
**Administration**
**Master of Health Administration Program**
419 Patterson Office Tower
Lexington, KY 40506-0027
**Phone:** (859)252-5594     **Fax:** (859)323-1937
**Email:** rcr@pop.uky.edu
**Website:** http://www.uky.edu/RGS/Martin School
Robert C. Rodgers, PhD, Director
**Alt. Contact:** For Program information: 413 Patterson Office Tower, Lexington, KY 40506-0027; email: (Sarah Lee) solee@pop.uky.edu.

## Louisiana

### ★ 9627 ★ Tulane University
**School of Public Health and Tropical**
**Medicine**
**Tulane University Health Sciences Center**
**Department of Health Systems**
**Management**
1440 Canal St., Ste. 1900
New Orleans, LA 70112
**Phone:** (504)988-7700     **Fax:** (504)988-7701
**Email:** hsm@hsm.tulane.edu
**Website:** http://www.tulane.hsm.edu
Judith W. Overall, Director

## Maryland

### ★ 9628 ★ The Johns Hopkins University
**School of Hygiene and Public Health**
**Department of Health Policy and**
**Management**
**Masters of Health Science in Health**
**Finance and Management**
624 N Broadway, Rm. 406
Baltimore, MD 21205-1995
**Phone:** (410)955-5317     **Fax:** (410)955-6959
**Email:** dshiloh@jhsph.edu
**Website:** http://www.jhsph.edu/Departments/HPM/mhs/htm
William J. Ward, Jr., Director
**Fnded:** 1972.

## Massachusetts

### ★ 9629 ★ Boston University
**School of Management**
**Health Care Management Program**
595 Commonwealth Ave., Rm. 106
Boston, MA 02215
**Phone:** (617)353-2730     **Fax:** (617)353-9498
**Email:** smghcmp@bu.edu
**Website:** http://management.bu.edu
Alan B. Cohen, ScD, Director

### ★ 9630 ★ Clark University
**Graduate School of Management**
**Health Administration Program**
Carlson Hall
950 Main St.
Worcester, MA 01610-1477
**Phone:** (508)793-7670     **Fax:** (508)793-8822
**Email:** eottensmeyer@atsclark.edu
**Website:** http://www.mba.clark.edu
Edward Ottensmeyer, PhD, Director

### ★ 9631 ★ Simmons College
**Graduate Program in Health Care**
**Administration**
300 The Fenway
S309
Boston, MA 02115
**Phone:** (617)521-2377     **Fax:** (617)521-3406
**Email:** gshsadm@simmons.edu
**Website:** http://www.simmons.edu/programs/gshs/gphca.html
Linda Roemer, PhD, Director

## Michigan

### ★ 9632 ★ University of Michigan
**School of Public Health**
**Department of Health Management and**
**Policy**
University of Michigan
School of Public Health
Ann Arbor, MI 48109-2029
**Phone:** (734)763-9900     **Fax:** (734)764-4338
**Email:** sph.hmp.inquiries@umich.edu
**Website:** http://www.sph.umich.edu
William G. Weissert, PhD, Director

## Minnesota

### ★ 9633 ★ University of Minnesota
**Program in Healthcare Administration**
Carlson School of Management, Rm. 3-140
321 19th Ave. S
Minneapolis, MN 55455-9940
**Phone:** (612)624-8818     **Free:** 877-MHA-UOFM
**Fax:** (612)624-8804
**Email:** mha@carlsonschool.umn.edu
**Website:** http://www.carlsonschool.umn.edu/mha
James W. Begun, PhD, Director
**Fnded:** 1946.

## Missouri

### ★ 9634 ★ Saint Louis University
**School of Public Health**
**Department of Health Administration**
3663 Lindell Blvd.
Saint Louis, MO 63108
**Phone:** (314)977-8112     **Free:** 800-782-6769
**Fax:** (314)977-8150
**Email:** laxm@slu.edu
**Website:** http://www.slu.edu/colleges/sph/
Claudia R. Campbell, PhD, Director
**Fnded:** 1947.

**★ 9635 ★ University of Missouri,
Columbia
Health Services Management**
324 Clark Hall
Columbia, MO 65211
**Phone:** (573)882-1849          **Free:** 800-877-4764
**Fax:** (573)882-6158
**Email:** mha@health.missouri.edu
**Website:** http://www.hmi.missouri.edu
Gordon D. Brown, PhD, Director

**★ 9636 ★ Washington University
School of Medicine
Health Administration Program**
4547 Clayton Ave.
Saint Louis, MO 63110-1501
**Phone:** (314)362-4277          **Fax:** (314)362-3265
**Email:** marilyn@medicine.wustl.edu
**Website:** http://www.medicine.wustl.edu/~hap
Stuart B. Boxerman, Director
**Fnded:** 1946.

## Nebraska

**★ 9637 ★ Creighton University
Master of Health Services Administration**
2500 California Plaza
Omaha, NE 68178
**Phone:** (402)280-3268          **Fax:** (402)280-3332
**Email:** mclean@creighton.edu
**Website:** http://hsa.creighton.edu
Robert A. McLean, Director

## New Hampshire

**★ 9638 ★ University of New Hampshire
School of Health and Human Services
Department of Health Management and
Policy
Master of Health Administration Program**
Hewitt Hall
4 Library Way
Durham, NH 03824
**Phone:** (603)862-2733          **Fax:** (603)862-3461
**Email:** mha.info@unh.edu
**Website:** http://www.unh.edu.hmp/
James B. Lewis, Director

## New Jersey

**★ 9639 ★ Seton Hall University
Graduate Department of Public and
Health Administration**
Seton Hall University
South Orange, NJ 07079
**Phone:** (973)761-9510          **Fax:** (973)275-2463
**Email:** wishnaom@shu.edu
**Website:** http://www.setonworldwide.com
Naomi Wish, PhD, Contact

## New York

**★ 9640 ★ City University of New York
Baruch College
Mount Sinai School of Medicine
Graduate Program in Health Care
Administration**
17 Lexington Ave., Box F1215
New York, NY 10010
**Phone:** (212)802-6706          **Fax:** (212)802-6705
**Email:** Ted_Joyce@Baruch.cuny.edu
**Website:** http://www.baruch.cuny.edu
Ted Joyce, PhD, Director

**★ 9641 ★ Cornell University
College of Human Ecology
Department of Policy Analysis and
Management
Sloan Program in Health Services
Administration**
N231 Martha Van Rensselaer Hall
Ithaca, NY 14853-4401
**Phone:** (607)255-2594          **Fax:** (607)255-4071
**Email:** dsk@cornell.edu
**Website:** http://www.human.cornell.edu/pam/sloan
Donald S. Kenkel, PhD, Director

**★ 9642 ★ New York University
Robert F. Wagner Graduate School of
Public Service
Program in Health Policy and
Management**
40 W 4th St.
Tisch Hall, Rm. 600
New York, NY 10012-1118
**Phone:** (212)998-7440          **Fax:** (212)995-4162
**Email:** wagner.admissions@nyu.edu
**Website:** http://www.nyu.edu/wagner
Anthony Kovner, PhD, Director

**★ 9643 ★ Union College
Graduate Management Institute
Program in Health Systems
Administration**
807 Union Ave.
Lamont House Graduate Center
Schenectady, NY 12308
**Phone:** (518)388-6238          **Fax:** (518)388-6754
**Email:** mba@union.edu
**Website:** http://www.mba.union.edu
Martin A. Strosberg, PhD, Director

## North Carolina

**★ 9644 ★ Duke University
The Fuqua School of Businesss
Health Sector Management Program**
PO Box 90120
Durham, NC 27708-0120
**Phone:** (919)660-7989          **Fax:** (919)660-7843
**Email:** hsm@fuqua.duke.edu
**Website:** http://www.fuqua.duke.edu/programs/hsm
Kevin A. Schulman, MD, Director

**★ 9645 ★ University of North Carolina,
Chapel Hill
School of Public Health
Department of Health Policy and
Administration**
CB 7400, McGavran-Greenburg Hall
Chapel Hill, NC 27599-7400
**Phone:** (919)966-7350          **Fax:** (919)966-6961
**Email:** kkilpatr@sph.unc.edu
**Website:** http://www.sph.unc.edu/hpaa/
Kerry E. Kilpatrick, PhD, Director

**★ 9646 ★ University of North Carolina,
Charlotte
Health Administration**
9201 University City Boulevard
Macy 103
Charlotte, NC 28223
**Phone:** (704)687-4522          **Fax:** (704)687-4347
**Email:** WFPilkin@email.uncc.edu
**Website:**          http://www.uncc.edu/gradmiss/hltad-
mas.htm
William F. Pilkington, Director

## Nova Scotia

**★ 9647 ★ Dalhousie University
Faculty of Health Professions
School of Health Services Administration**
5599 Fenwick St.
Halifax, NS, Canada B3H 1R2
**Phone:** (902)494-7097          **Fax:** (902)494-6849
**Email:** health.services.administration@dal.ca
**Website:** http://www.dal.ca/shsa
Thomas A. Rathwell, PhD, Director

## Ohio

**★ 9648 ★ Cleveland State University
College of Business Administration
Graduate Study in Health Care
Administration**
College of Business Administration Bldg. 434
Cleveland, OH 44112
**Phone:** (216)687-4711          **Fax:** (216)687-9354
**Email:** b.marshall@csuohio.edu
**Website:** http://www.csuohio.edu/hca/
Brenda Stevenson Marshall, PhD, Director

**★ 9649 ★ Ohio State University
Graduate Program in Health Services
Management and Policy**
1583 Perry St., Rm. 246
Columbus, OH 43210-1234
**Phone:** (614)292-9708          **Fax:** (614)292-3572
**Email:** hsmp@sosu.edu
**Website:** http://www.med.ohio-state.edu/hsmp/
Stephen F. Loebs, PhD, Director

**★ 9650 ★ Xavier University
Graduate Program in Health Services
Administration**
3800 Victory Pkwy.
Cincinnati, OH 45207-7331
**Phone:** (513)745-3392          **Fax:** (513)745-4301
**Email:** schicki@admin.xu.edu
**Website:** http://www.xu.edu/dpets/mhsa
Ida Critelli Schick, PhD, Director
**Fnded:** 1958.

## Oklahoma

**★ 9651 ★ University of Oklahoma
Health Sciences Center
College of Public Health
Department of Health Administration and
Policy**
PO Box 26901
Oklahoma City, OK 73190
**Phone:** (405)271-2114          **Fax:** (405)271-1868
**Email:** edward-brandt@ouhsc.edu
**Website:** http://w3.uokhsc.edu/hap
Edward N. Brandt, Jr,PhD, Director

## Ontario

**★ 9652 ★ University of Ottawa
Master's Program in Health
Administration**
136 Jean-Jacques Lussier Private
Vanier Bldg.
Faculty of Administration
Ottawa, ON, Canada K1N 6N5
**Phone:** (613)562-5884          **Fax:** (613)562-5912
**Email:** mha@admin.uottowa.ca
**Website:** http://www.admin.uottowa.ca.mha
Douglas E. Angus, Director

**★ 9653 ★ University of Toronto
Health Administration Program**
2nd Fl., McMurrich Bldg.
12 Queen's Park Crescent W
Toronto, ON, Canada M5S 1A8
**Phone:** (416)946-3023          **Fax:** (416)978-7350

**Email:** tina.smith@utoronto.ca
**Website:** http://www.utoronto.ca/hltadmin/
Tina Smith, Director

## Oregon

### ★ 9654 ★ Oregon State University
**Department of Public Health**
**Health Care Administration Program**
Waldo Hall 256
Corvallis, OR 97331-6406
**Phone:** (541)737-2686  **Fax:** (541)737-4001
**Email:** leonard.friedman@atsorst.edu
**Website:** http://www.osu.orst.edu
Leonard H. Friedman, PhD, Director

## Pennsylvania

### ★ 9655 ★ King's College
**McGowan School of Business**
**Master of Science Health Care**
**Administration**
133 N River St.
Wilkes-Barre, PA 18711
**Phone:** (570)208-6083  **Fax:** (570)208-5989
**Email:** bjhealey@kings.edu
**Website:** http://www.kings.edu/hca
Bernard J. Healey, PhD, Director

### ★ 9656 ★ Penn State Great Valley
**The Pennsylvania State University**
**Great Valley School of Graduate**
**Professional Studies**
**Health Care Master of Business**
**Administration Program**
30 E Swedesford Rd.
Malvern, PA 19355
**Phone:** (610)648-3269  **Fax:** (610)889-1334
**Email:** jld13@psu.edu
**Website:** http://www.gv.psu.edu
Janice L. Dreachslin, Director

### ★ 9657 ★ Pennsylvania State University
**Department of Health Policy and**
**Administration**
**Concurrent Master Business**
**Administration/Master Health**
**Administration Program**
116 Henderson Bldg.
University Park, PA 16802
**Phone:** (814)863-2859  **Fax:** (814)865-2905
**Email:** bgf2@psu.edu
**Website:** http://www.hhdev.psu.edu/hpa/hpa.htm
S. Diane Brannon, PhD, Director

### ★ 9658 ★ Temple University
**School of Business and Management**
**Department of Risk, Insurance, and**
**Healthcare Management**
**Graduate Program in Health Management**
Ritter Annex (004-00)
Philadelphia, PA 19122
**Phone:** (215)204-8468  **Fax:** (215)204-3851
**Email:** zinn@vm.temple.edu
**Website:** http://www.sbm.temple.edu
Jacqueline Zinn, PhD, Director

### ★ 9659 ★ University of Pennsylvania
**The Wharton School**
**Graduate Program in Health Care**
**Management**
Colonial Penn Center
3641 Locust Walk
Philadelphia, PA 19104-6218
**Phone:** (215)898-6861  **Fax:** (215)573-2157
**Email:** pauly@wharton.upenn.edu
**Website:** http://www.wharton.upenn.edu
Mark V. Pauly, PhD, Director

### ★ 9660 ★ University of Pittsburgh
**Health Administration Program**
A-646 Crabtree Hall
130 DeSoto St.
Pittsburgh, PA 15261
**Phone:** (412)624-3123  **Fax:** (412)624-3146
**Email:** lave@pitt.edu
**Website:** http://www.edc.gsph.pitt.edu/hsa/
Judith R. Lave, PhD, Director

### ★ 9661 ★ University of Scranton
**Panuska College of Professional Studies**
**Graduate Program in Health**
**Administration**
417 McGurrin Hall
Scranton, PA 18510-4597
**Phone:** (570)941-4242  **Fax:** (570)941-5882
**Email:** oldenp1@uofs.edu
**Website:** http://www.academic.uofs.edu/department/
HAHR/mha_program.htm
Peter C. Olden, PhD, Director

### ★ 9662 ★ Widener University
**Graduate Program in Health and Medical**
**Services Administration**
One University Place
Chester, PA 19013
**Phone:** (610)499-4384  **Fax:** (610)499-4615
**Email:** health.administration@widener.edu
**Website:** http://www.sba.widener.edu/hmsahome/
html
Caryl E. Carpenter, PhD, Director

## Puerto Rico

### ★ 9663 ★ University of Puerto Rico
**Graduate School of Public Health**
**Master in Health Services Administration**
Medical Sciences Campus Bldg.
GPO Box 5067
San Juan, PR 00936-5067
**Phone:** (787)758-2525  **Fax:** (787)758-2783
**Email:** roramirez@rcm.upr.edu
**Website:** http://www.rcm.upr.edu
Roberto Ramirez, PhD, Director

## South Carolina

### ★ 9664 ★ Medical University of South Carolina
**Department of Health Administration and**
**Policy**
**Master of Health Administration Program**
19 Hagwood Ave., Ste. 408
PO Box 250807
Charleston, SC 29425
**Phone:** (843)792-2118  **Fax:** (843)792-3327
**Email:** dhapinfo@musc.edu
**Website:** http://www.musc.edu/hap/
Andrea W. White, PhD, Director

### ★ 9665 ★ University of South Carolina
**School of Public Health**
**Graduate Program in Health Services**
**Administration**
**Department of Health Administration**
Columbia, SC 29208
**Phone:** (803)777-6096  **Fax:** (803)777-1836
**Email:** dcdodson@sph.sc.edu
**Website:** http://www.hadm.sc.edu
Don C. Dodson, PhD, Director

## Tennessee

### ★ 9666 ★ Meharry Medical College
**Health Services Administration Program**
1005 D.B. Todd Blvd.
Box 53-A
Nashville, TN 37208-9989
**Phone:** (615)327-6069  **Fax:** (615)327-6717

**Email:** elbrown@mail.mmc.edu
**Website:** http://www.mmc.edu
Herman M. Ellis, MD, Director

### ★ 9667 ★ University of Memphis
McCord Hall, Rm. 119
Memphis, TN 38152
**Phone:** (901)678-1465  **Fax:** (901)678-2981
**Email:** peftzgrl@memphis.edu
**Website:** http://www.people.memphis.edu/~gaheal-
thadmin
Paul E. Fitzgerald, Jr,PhD, Director

## Texas

### ★ 9668 ★ Houston Baptist University
**Center For Health Studies**
**Graduate Programs in Health**
**Administration**
7502 Fondren Rd.
Houston, TX 77074-3298
**Phone:** (281)649-3419  **Fax:** (281)649-3340
**Email:** hgriffin@hbu.edu
**Website:** http://www.hbu.edu/Pages/acad/
H3Fmsha.html
Harold Ray Griffin, PhD, Director

### ★ 9669 ★ Midwestern State University
**College of Health and Human Services**
**Health and Public Administration**
3410 Taft Blvd.
Wichita Falls, TX 76308
**Phone:** (940)397-4752  **Fax:** (940)397-4845
**Email:** russell.porter@nexus.mwsu.edu
**Website:** http://www.mwsu.edu/~hsa/hsaintro.html
Russel D. Porter, PhD, Director

### ★ 9670 ★ Southwest Texas State University
**Graduate Program in Health Care**
**Administration**
601 University Dr.
San Marcos, TX 78666-4616
**Phone:** (512)245-3556  **Fax:** (512)245-8712
**Email:** ws06@swt.edu
**Website:** http://www.health.swt.edu
Wayne B. Sorensen, PhD, Director
**Fnded:** 1973.

### ★ 9671 ★ Texas Tech University
**College of Business Administration**
**The MBA & MD/MBA Program in Health**
**Organization Management**
Lubbock, TX 79409-2101
**Phone:** (806)742-1236  **Fax:** (806)742-2308
**Email:** hom@ba.ttu.edu
**Website:** http://www.ba.ttu.edu
Timothy W. Nix, PhD, Director

### ★ 9672 ★ Texas Woman's University, Houston
**Program in Health Care Administration**
1130 MD Anderson Blvd.
Houston, TX 77030
**Phone:** (713)794-2061  **Fax:** (713)794-2350
**Email:** kmoseley@twu.edu
**Website:** http://www.twu.edu/houston/
S. Kelley Moseley, PhD, Director

### ★ 9673 ★ Trinity University
**On-Campus Graduate Program in Health**
**Care Administration**
715 Stadium Dr., No. 58
Chapman Graduate Center-N400
San Antonio, TX 78212-7200
**Phone:** (210)999-8107  **Fax:** (210)999-8108
**Email:** hca@trinity.edu

**Website:** http://www.trinity.edu/departments/health-care
Stephen L. Tucker, Contact
**Fnded:** 1965.

**★ 9674 ★ U.S. Army/Baylor University Center for Healthcare Education and Studies**
**Academy of Health Sciences**
**Graduate Program in Health Care Administration**
3151 Scott Rd. (MCCS-HRA)
Fort Sam Houston, TX 78234-6135
**Phone:** (210)221-6345  **Fax:** (210)221-6051
**Email:** charles.wainright@cen.amedd.army.mil
**Website:** http://www.cs.amedd.army.mil/baylorhca
LTC Charles F. Wainright, III, PhD, Director

**★ 9675 ★ University of Houston, Clear Lake**
**School of Business and Public Administration**
**Healthcare Administration Program**
2700 Bay Area Blvd.
Mail Code 73
Houston, TX 77058-1098
**Phone:** (281)283-3130  **Fax:** (281)283-3136
**Email:** hadm@cl.uh.edu
**Website:** http://www.cl.uh.edu/bpa/hadm
Phillip J. Decker, Director

**★ 9676 ★ University of Mary Hardin-Baylor**
**Graduate Program in Health Services Management**
900 College St.
UMHB Station Box 8405
Belton, TX 76513-2599
**Phone:** (254)295-4558  **Free:** 800-727-UNMB
**Fax:** (254)295-5300
**Email:** mhsm@umhb.edu
**Website:** http://www.umhb.edu/programs/Graduate/MHSM.htm
Dr. Mary Anne Franklin, Contact

### Virginia

**★ 9677 ★ Virginia Commonwealth University**
**Medical College of Virginia**
**School of Allied Health Professions**
**Department of Health Administration**
Box 980203
Richmond, VA 23298-0203
**Phone:** (804)828-0719  **Fax:** (804)828-1894
**Email:** shavasy@hsc.vcu.edu
**Website:** http://www.had.vcu.edu
Jan Clement, PhD, Director

### Washington

**★ 9678 ★ University of Washington, Seattle**
**Graduate Program in Health Services Administration**
Box 357660
Seattle, WA 98195-7660
**Phone:** (206)543-8778  **Fax:** (206)543-3964
**Email:** alinew@u.washington.edu
**Website:** http://depts.washington.edu/mhap
Dr. William E. Welton, PhD, Director

**★ 9679 ★ Washington State University**
**Graduate Program in Health Policy and Administration**
668 N Riverpoint Blvd., Box B
Spokane, WA 99202-1162
**Phone:** (509)358-7980  **Fax:** (509)358-7900
**Email:** venzon@wsu.edu

**Website:** http://www.hpa.spokane.wsu.edu
Winsor C. Schmidt, Contact

### Wisconsin

**★ 9680 ★ University of Wisconsin, Madison**
**Administrative Medicine Program**
734 WARF Bldg.
610 N Walnut St.
Madison, WI 53705-2397
**Phone:** (608)263-4889  **Fax:** (608)262-6404
**Email:** hwilde@facstaff.wisc.edu
**Website:** http://www.medsch.wisc.edu/adminmed/
David Kindig, MD,PhD, Director
Mark Covaleski, PhD, Director

# National & International Organizations

**★ 9681 ★ Accrediting Commission on Education for Health Services Administration (ACEHSA)**
730 11th St. NW, No. 400
Washington, DC 20001
**Phone:** (202)638-5131  **Fax:** (202)638-3429
**Email:** acehsa@aupha.org
**Website:** http://www.acehsa.org
Jeptha W. Dalton, PhD, Pres. & CEO
**Fnded:** 1968. **Mem:** 67. **Desc:** Accredits graduate degree programs in health services administration, health planning, and health policy. Goal is the improvement of professional education. **Pub:** *Official List of Accredited Programs*, semiannual. *Price:* Free. **Frmly:** (1976) Accrediting Commission on Graduate Education for Hospital Administration.

**★ 9682 ★ American Academy of Ambulatory Care Nursing (AAACN)**
East Holly Ave., Box 56
Pitman, NJ 08071-0056
**Phone:** (856)256-2350  **Free:** 800-262-6877
**Fax:** (856)589-7463
**Email:** aaacn@ajj.com
**Website:** http://www.aaacn.org
Cynthia R. Nowicki, EdD,RN, Contact
**Fnded:** 1978. **Mem:** 1,900. **Local Groups:** 17. **Desc:** AAACN is the association of professional nurses who identify ambulatory care nursing as essential to the continuum of high quality, cost-effective patient care. The mission of the Academy is to advance the art and science of ambulatory care nursing. The goals of the Academy are to be the voice of ambulatory care nursing, promote professional practices, stimulate innovative thinking, build collaborating relationships, and strengthen the AAACN resource base. **Pub:** *Ambulatory Care Nursing Administration and Practice Standards*, periodic. Manual. Reference manual. *Price:* $15 for members; $25 for nonmembers. • *American Academy of Ambulatory Care Nursing Administration Membership Directory*, annual. Directory. Arranged alphabetically and geographically. *Price:* Included in membership dues. • *Dermatology Nursing.* Journal. • *MedSurg Nursing.* Journal. • *Nursing Economics*, bimonthly. Journal. • *Pediatric Nursing.* Journal. • *Viewpoint*, bimonthly. Newsletter. Includes legislative updates and synopses of articles in current journals. *Price:* Included in membership dues; $80 institutional. **Frmly:** American Academy of Ambulatory Nursing Administration.

**★ 9683 ★ American Academy of Medical Administrators (AAMA)**
701 Lee St., Ste. 600
Des Plaines, IL 60016
**Phone:** (847)759-8601  **Fax:** (847)759-8602
**Email:** info@aameda.org
**Website:** http://www.aameda.org
Renee S. Schleicher, CAE, Pres. /CEO

**Fnded:** 1957. **Mem:** 2,800. **Reg. Groups:** 8. **State Groups:** 50. **Desc:** Individuals involved in healthcare management at all levels. Promotes healthcare administration through educational courses and research. **Pub:** *American Academy of Medical Administrators–Executive*, quarterly. Newsletter. Covers membership activities. Includes triennial membership directory;also contains calendar of events, book reviews, and lists of new members. *Price:* Included in membership dues; $60/year for nonmembers. • *Journal of Cardiovascular Management*, bimonthly. Journal. • *Journal of Oncology Management*, bimonthly. Journal.

**★ 9684 ★ American Academy of Medical Administrators Research and Educational Foundation (AAMA)**
701 Lee St., Ste. 600
Des Plaines, IL 60016
**Phone:** (847)759-8601  **Fax:** (847)759-8602
**Email:** info@aameda.org
**Website:** http://www.aameda.org/AboutAAMA/about-foundation.html
Renee S. Schleicher, CAE, Pres.
**Fnded:** 1957. **Mem:** 3,800. **Reg. Groups:** 7. **State Groups:** 50. **Desc:** Individuals with health care backgrounds. Conducts research in the health care field and seminars geared toward professional development. Maintains placement services. **Pub:** *AAMA Executive*, bimonthly. Newsletter. Covers management topics, industry trends, current developments in health care administration, and association news. Includes book reviews. *Price:* Included in membership dues; $110/year for nonmembers.

**★ 9685 ★ American Academy of Podiatric Practice Management**
707 Turnpike St.
North Andover, MA 01845
**Phone:** (978)686-6185  **Fax:** (978)685-9410
**Email:** aappmexecdir@aol.com
**Website:** http://www.aappm.com
Harvey Lederman, D.P.M., Pres.
**Fnded:** 1961. **Mem:** 200. **Desc:** Doctors of podiatric medicine interested in practice administration. Works to standardize office management procedures to create more efficient podiatry practices; conducts research on the administration and function of podiatry offices; develops formalized procedures for obtaining and training podiatry office assistants. Disseminates pedal information and material on practice management. Investigates methods of delivering improved podiatric care to an increasing number of patients; seeks effective participation in the public health team. Maintains collection of newsletters and position papers; sponsors seminars and workshops. Compiles statistics. **Pub:** *AAPA Newsletter*, quarterly. Newsletter. • *Directory of Membership*, annual. Directory. **Frmly:** (1969) American Academy of Practice Management in Podiatry; (1970) American Academy of Podiatric Management; (1993) American Academy Podiatric Administration.

**★ 9686 ★ American Academy of Professional Coders (AAPC)**
309 West 700 South
Salt Lake City, UT 84101-2608
**Free:** 800-626-2633  **Fax:** (801)236-2258
**Email:** info@aapc.com
**Website:** http://www.aapc.org
Lan C. England, Exec. Dir.
**Fnded:** 1988. **Mem:** 24,000. **State Groups:** 50. **Local Groups:** 250. **Desc:** Certified professional coders. Promotes high standards of physician and outpatient facility coding through education and cerification. **Pub:** *AAPC Coding Edge*, monthly. Newsletter. **Frmly:** (2001) American Academy of Procedural Coders.

**★ 9687 ★ American Association for Continuity of Care (AACC)**
PO Box 532
Dunedin, FL 34697-0532
**Phone:** (727)738-1030  **Fax:** (727)738-8099

**Email:** phudsonsommers@ij.net
Pat Hudson-Sommers, Pres.

**Fnded:** 1982. **Mem:** 500. **Reg. Groups:** 6. **Desc:** Health care professionals involved in discharge planning, social work, hospital administration, home care, long-term care, home health agencies, and continuity of care. Studies and researches issues; proposes and supports legislation concerning Medicare changes and home health care. Maintains speakers' bureau. **Pub:** *ACCESS*, bimonthly. Newsletter. Includes calendar of events, regional reports, member notes, and committee reports. *Price:* Included in membership dues. • *American Association for Continuity of Care–Membership Directory*, annual. Membership Directory. *Price:* Included in membership dues.

---

**★ 9688 ★ American Association of Healthcare Administrative Management (AAHAM)**
11240 Waples Mill Rd., Ste. 400
Fairfax, VA 22030
**Phone:** (703)281-4043　　　**Fax:** (703)359-7562
**Email:** debra@statmarketing.com
**Website:** http://www.aaham.org
Sharon Rosenblatt Galler, Exec. Dir.

**Fnded:** 1968. **Mem:** 2,000. **State Groups:** 39. **Desc:** Business offices, credit and collection managers, and admitting officers for hospitals, clinics, and other health care organizations. To educate members, exchange information and techniques, and keep members abreast of new regulations relating to their field. Seeks proper recognition for the financial aspect of hospital and clinic management. Offers certification program. Administers examinations in April and October for qualification as Certified Patient Account Manager (CPAM) and Certified Clinic Account Manager (CCAM). Maintains placement services; sponsors seminars and workshops on a local, regional, and national level. Operates speakers' bureau. **Pub:** *Journal of Healthcare Administrative Management*, quarterly. Journal. Lists employment opportunities; includes industry news. *Price:* Included in membership dues; $30/year for nonmembers. **Frmly:** (1981) American Guild of Patient Account Managers; (1999) American Guild of Patient Account Management.

---

**★ 9689 ★ American Association of Integrated Healthcare Delivery Systems**
4435 Waterfront Dr., Ste. 101
PO Box 4913
Glen Allen, VA 23058-4913
**Phone:** (804)747-5823　　　**Fax:** (804)747-5316
**Email:** bwilliams@aaihds.org
**Website:** http://www.aaihds.org
Douglas L. Chaet, Chm.

**Fnded:** 1993. **Mem:** 900. **Desc:** Physicians, hospital executives and board members, health plan executives, and other key entities and professionals employed by all forms of IDDSs including PHOS, IPA POSOS, AND MSOS. Seeks to provide advocacy for issues related to integrated healthcare through research, education, and communication. Conducts educational and research programs; maintains speakers' bureau and information clearinghouse. **Pub:** *Integrated Healthcare Delivery System*, quarterly. Newsletter. **Frmly:** (1998) American Association of Physician-Hospital Organizations.

---

**★ 9690 ★ American Association of Psychiatric Administrators (AAPA)**
c/o Dr. Dave Davis
1938 Peachtree Rd. NW, Ste. 505
Atlanta, GA 30309
**Phone:** (404)355-2914　　　**Fax:** (404)355-2917
**Email:** drdavis@whstarmail.com
**Website:** http://www.psychiatricadministrators.org/
Dr. Dave Davis, Contact

**Fnded:** 1960. **Mem:** 300. **Reg. Groups:** 3. **State Groups:** 6. **Desc:** Psychiatrists who occupy the position of chief administrative or clinical officer of a public or private neuropsychiatric hospital or clinic. Provides for the efficient consolidation and dissemination of information concerning the treatment, care, and rehabilitation of the mentally ill or handicapped; the effective application of training and research; and the development of the highest standards and qualifications for administrators of public neuropsychiatric hospitals. Conducts educational programs. Acts as a forum through which the common voice of the membership may be expressed and publicized. **Pub:** *Journal of American Association of Psychiatric Administrators*, periodic. Journal. • *List of Members*, biennial. Membership Directory. • Newsletter, quarterly. **Frmly:** (1975) Association of Medical Superintendents of Mental Hospitals.

---

**★ 9691 ★ American College of Addiction Treatment Administrators (ACATA)**
c/o Ronald J. Hunsicker, D.Min.
313 W Liberty St., Ste. 129
Lancaster, PA 17603
**Phone:** (717)392-8480　　　**Fax:** (717)392-8481
**Email:** rhunsicker@naatp.org
Ronald Hunsicker, Pres. /CEO

**Fnded:** 1984. **Mem:** 250. **Desc:** Administrators of addiction treatment facilities. Promotes educational and professional standards in the field of addiction treatment administration. Encourages continuing education and training of members. Recognizes individuals who have provided outstanding service in the field. Seeks to educate members and the public on issues surrounding the administration of treatment programs. Sponsors workshops. **Pub:** *Visions*, monthly. Newsletter.

---

**★ 9692 ★ American College of Cardiovascular Administrators (ACCA)**
701 Lee St., Ste. 600
Des Plaines, IL 60016
**Phone:** (847)759-8601　　　**Fax:** (847)759-8602
**Email:** info@aameda.org
**Website:** http://www.aameda.org
Renee S. Schleicher, Contact

**Fnded:** 1986. **Mem:** 900. **Reg. Groups:** 7. **State Groups:** 50. **Desc:** A specialty college of the American Academy of Medical Administrators. Upperand middle-level managers of health care professionals in the cardiovascular health care field; associate members are junior supervisors, salespersons, and individuals. Represents members within the medical industry; provides credentialing of cardiology administrators. Serves as a forum for the exchange of information. Conducts educational programs. **Pub:** *Journal of Cardiovacular Management*, bimonthly. Journal. *Price:* included in membership dues.

---

**★ 9693 ★ American College of Health Care Administrators (ACHCA)**
300 N Lee St., No. 301
Alexandria, VA 22314
**Phone:** (703)739-7900　　　**Free:** 888-88-ACHCA
**Fax:** (703)739-7901
**Email:** mtn@achca.org
**Website:** http://www.achca.org
Mary Tellis-Nayak, Pres. & CEO

**Fnded:** 1962. **Mem:** 6,360. **Reg. Groups:** 11. **State Groups:** 48. **Desc:** Persons actively engaged in the administration of long-term care facilities, such as nursing homes, retirement communities, assisted living facilities, and subacute care programs. ACHCA administers professional certification programs for assisted living, subacute and nursing home administrators. Works to elevate the standards in the field and to develop and promote a code of ethics and standards of education and training. Seeks to inform allied professions and the public that good administration of long-term care facilities calls for special formal academic training and experience. Encourages research in all aspects of geriatrics, the chronically ill, and administration. Maintains placement service. Holds special education programs; facilitates networking among administrators. **Pub:** *Balance*, bimonthly. Journal. Contains original research and practical applications, commentaries, and book reviews. • *E-Compass*, bimonthly. Newsletter. Contains information on initiatives and industry updates. • Also publishes educa-

tional materials. **Frmly:** American College of Nursing Home Administrators.

---

**★ 9694 ★ American College of Healthcare Executives (ACHE)**
1 N Franklin, Ste. 1700
Chicago, IL 60606-3491
**Phone:** (312)424-2800　　　**Fax:** (312)424-0023
**Email:** ache@ache.org
**Website:** http://www.ache.org
Thomas C. Dolan, PhD., FACHE, CAE, Pres. and CEO

**Fnded:** 1933. **Mem:** 30,000. **Local Groups:** 110. **Desc:** Healthcare executives. Conducts credentialing and educational programs and an annual Congress on Healthcare Management. Conducts ground-breaking research and career development and public policy programs. Publishing division, Health Administration Press, publishes books and journals on health services management and textbooks for use in college and university courses. Works toward goal of improving the health status of society by advancing healthcare leadership management excellence. Works toward goal of improving the health status of society by advancing healthcare management excellence. by advancing healthcare management excellence. **Pub:** *Frontiers of Health Services Management*, quarterly. Journal. Contains articles debating current healthcare topics and commentaries from outstanding scholars and practitioners in the field. *Price:* $75/year; in U.S. • *Healthcare Executive*, bimonthly. Magazine. Provides in-depth analysis of emerging trends in healthcare management and includes strategies for confronting healthcare management issues. *Price:* $118/year outside U.S. institution; $75/year outside U.S.; $65/year in U.S. • *Journal of Healthcare Management*, bimonthly. Journal. Provides healthcare management research and articles on topics such as leadership and managed care. *Price:* $85/year outside U.S.; $75/year (U.S.). • *Member Directory*. Directory. Available online, free of charge to members. • Also publishes case studies, books, journals, manuals, and newsletters; offers cassette tapes. **Frmly:** (1985) American College of Hospital Administrators.

---

**American College of Home Health Administrators (ACHHA)**
*See:* Entry 1891

---

**★ 9695 ★ American College of Managed Care Administrators (ACMCA)**
701 Lee St., No. 600
Des Plaines, IL 60016-4516
**Phone:** (224)540-4310　　　**Fax:** (224)645-0590
**Email:** info@aamed.org
**Website:** http://www.aameda.org
Scott Robillard, Contact

**Fnded:** 1994. **Mem:** 600. **Reg. Groups:** 7. **State Groups:** 50. **Desc:** Specialty college of the American Academy of Medical Administrators. Managers of professionals who are directly or indirectly providing managed healthcare. Works to promote the advancement of members' professional standing, education, and personal achievement and develop innovative concepts in managed care administration. Conducts an employment referral and educational programs. **Pub:** *Executive*, bimonthly. Journal.

---

**★ 9696 ★ American College of Managed Care Medicine (ACMCM)**
4435 Waterfront Dr., Ste. 101
PO Box 4765
Glen Allen, VA 23060
**Phone:** (804)527-1906　　　**Fax:** (804)747-5316
**Email:** info@acmcm.org
**Website:** http://www.acmcm.org
Dr. William Tindall, Contact

**Fnded:** 1995. **Mem:** 2,000. **Desc:** Physicians and other health care providers working for managed care organizations. Seeks to advance the effectiveness of managed care health services. Conducts continuing professional development courses for health care providers and prepares members for a managed care certificate examination; facilitates exchange of information among members; sponsors research; maintains speakers' bureau. **Pub:** *American Journal of Integrated Health Care*, quarterly. Journal.

### ★ 9697 ★ American College of Medical Practice Executives (ACMPE)

104 Inverness Ter. E
Englewood, CO 80112-5306
**Free:** 877-275-6462          **Fax:** (303)643-4439
**Email:** acmpe@mgma.com
**Website:** http://www.mgma.com/acmpe
Andrea M. Rossiter, Sr. VP

**Fnded:** 1956. **Mem:** 3,000. **Desc:** Professional credentialing organization. Membership is drawn from Medical Group Management Association and beyond. Works to encourage medical group practice administrators to improve and maintain their proficiency and to provide appropriate recognition; to establish a program with uniform standards of admission, advancement, certification and fellowship in order to achieve the highest possible standards in the profession of medical group practice administration; to participate in the development of educational and research programs for the advancement of the profession; to inform the medical profession and the public of the value of trained and experienced men and women in the management of the administrative affairs of all forms of group practice; to instill in its membership a constant awareness of the high ideals and traditions of the medical profession and medical group administration so that its members will conduct themselves in such a manner as to augment those ideals and traditions. Conducts educational programs such as Management Education Programs and Group Practice Governance Leadership Institute. **Pub:** *College Review*, semiannual. Professional manuscripts submitted to the College for advancement to fellow status; arranged by subject and author. *Price:* $10/copy to members; $16/copy to affiliates; $22/copy to nonmembers. • *Your Pathway to Excellence*. Brochure. Provides general information regarding ACMPE membership application. **Frmly:** (1976) American College of Clinic Managers; (1993) American College of Medical Group Administrators.

### ★ 9698 ★ American College of Medical Practice Management

6855 Jimmy Carter Blvd., Ste. 2100
Norcross, GA 30071
**Phone:** (770)734-9904          **Fax:** (770)734-9709
**Email:** webmaster@practicemanagement.com
Roger G. Bonds, Exec. Dir.

**Fnded:** 1990. **Mem:** 400. **Desc:** Health care administrators with an interest in continuing professional development; continuing medical education programs. Seeks to increase the quality and availability of continuing medical education courses. Serves as a clearinghouse on continuing medical education; formulates model practice management and recruitment and physician employment contracts; sponsors fellowship and certification programs for continuing medical educators. **Pub:** *Medical Staff Development Professional*, periodic. Journal. **Frmly:** (2000) American College of Medical Staff Development.

### ★ 9699 ★ American College of Mental Health Administration (ACMHA)

324 Freeport Rd.
Pittsburgh, PA 15238-3422
**Phone:** (412)820-0670          **Fax:** (412)820-0669
**Email:** lawhel@aol.com
**Website:** http://www.acmha.org
Dr. Lawrence A. Heller, PhD, Exec. Dir.

**Fnded:** 1980. **Mem:** 200. **Desc:** Mental health clinician administrators. **Pub:** *ACMHA Newsletter*, quarterly. Newsletter. Includes organization news and critical essays. *Price:* $12/year.

## American College of Oncology Administrators (ACOA)

*See:* Entry 10101

### ★ 9700 ★ American College of Physician Executives (ACPE)

4890 W Kennedy Blvd., Ste. 200
Tampa, FL 33609
**Phone:** (813)287-2000          **Free:** 800-562-8088
**Fax:** (813)287-8993
**Email:** acpe@acpe.org
**Website:** http://www.acpe.org
Roger S. Schenke, Exec. VP

**Fnded:** 1974. **Mem:** 14,000. **Desc:** Physicians whose primary professional responsibility is the management of health care organizations. Provides for continuing education and certification of the physician executive and the advancement and recognition of the physician executive and the profession. Offers specialized career planning, counseling, recruitment and placement services, and research and information data on physician managers. **Pub:** *American College of Physician Executives–Membership Directory*, annual. Membership Directory. *Price:* Included in membership dues. • *Fundamentals of Medical Management: A Guide for the Physician Executive*. Book. Includes discussion of organizational theory, effective communication, negotiating skills, conflict management, and organizational politics. *Price:* $40 for members; $50 for nonmembers. • *International Health Care: A Bibliography*. Bibliography. Contains material on international health care systems such as up-to-date lists of citations from the literature. *Price:* $20 for members; $40 for nonmembers. • *Managing in an Academic Health Care Environment*. Book. Provides an overview of managing in this unique environment. *Price:* $40 for members; $50 for nonmembers. • *Medical Directors: What, Why, How*. Monograph. Covers the possible responsibilities for the position of Medical Director. *Price:* $15 for members; $20 for nonmembers. • *New Leadership in Health Care Management–The Physician Executive*. Book. Outlines the knowledge base physician executives must master in order to effectively compete and succeed. *Price:* $35 for members; $49 for nonmembers. • *New Leadership in Healthcare Management, 2nd Edition*. Monograph. Outlines a step-by-step strategy to planning a successful job pursuit, with advice on structuring your resume and setting up personal networking. *Price:* $15 for members; $25 for nonmembers. • *The Physician Executive Journal of Management*, bimonthly. Newsletter. *Price:* Included in membership dues. • *Physician Executive: Journal of Management*, monthly. Journal. Includes recurring columns on health economics and health law. *Price:* Included in membership dues; $48/year for nonmembers. • *Roads to Medical Management: Physician Executives' Career Decisions*. Monograph. Tracks the career moves of 15 physician executives into medical management. *Price:* $19.95 for members.

### ★ 9701 ★ American Healthcare Radiology Administrators (AHRA)

PO Box 334
Sudbury, MA 01776
**Phone:** (978)443-7591          **Free:** 800-334-2472
**Fax:** (978)443-8046
**Email:** info@ahraonline.org
**Website:** http://www.ahraonline.org
Mary S. Reitter, Exec. Dir.

**Fnded:** 1973. **Mem:** 3,300. **Desc:** Radiology and healthcare managers. Works to improve management of radiology departments in hospitals, physician practices, and other health care facilities; to provide a forum for publication of educational, scientific, and professional materials. Has established code of ethics for the profession. Provides liaison between related organizations such as radiology, health care and management groups, and government agencies. Compiles statistics; conducts specialized education programs. Energize! **Pub:** *Link*, monthly. Newsletter. *Price:* for members. • *Membership Directory*, annual. Membership Directory. • *Radiology Management*, bimonthly. **Frmly:** (1986) American Hospital Radiology Administrators.

### ★ 9702 ★ American Health Planning Association (AHPA)

7245 Arlington Blvd., Ste. 300
Falls Church, VA 22042
**Phone:** (703)573-3103          **Fax:** (703)573-1276
**Email:** tpiper@mail.state.mo.us
**Website:** http://www.ahpanet.org/
Dean Montgomery, Contact

**Fnded:** 1970. **Desc:** State and local health planning agencies and affiliated organizations and individuals. Conducts research; disseminates information; serves as clearinghouse for health planning activities and concepts; sponsors programs of technical assistance; provides continuing education. **Pub:** *National Directory of Health Planning, Policy, and Regulatory Agencies*, annual. Directory. *Price:* $125. • *TODAY in Health Planning*, quarterly. **Frmly:** (1977) American Association for Comprehensive Health Planning.

### ★ 9703 ★ American Organization of Nurse Executives (AONE)

325 Seventh St. NW
Washington, DC 20004
**Phone:** (202)626-2240          **Fax:** (202)638-5499
**Email:** aone@aha.org
**Website:** http://www.aone.org
Pamela Thompson, RN, Exec. Dir.

**Fnded:** 1967. **Mem:** 4,000. **State Groups:** 69. **Desc:** Provides leadership, professional development, advocacy, and research to advance nursing practice and patient care, promote nursing leadership and excellence, and shape healthcare public policy. Supports and enhances the management, leadership, educational, and professional development of nursing leaders. Offers placement service through Career Development and Referral Center. **Pub:** *AONE Updates*, 3/weeks. Newsletter. Bulleted update of information related to nursing administration. • Books. • Membership Directory, annual. *Price:* Included in membership dues. • Monographs. • Videos. **Frmly:** (1977) American Society for Hospital Nursing Service Administrators; (1984) American Society for Nursing Service Administrators.

### ★ 9704 ★ American Society for Healthcare Food Service Administrators (ASHFSA)

One N Franklin
Chicago, IL 60606
**Phone:** (312)422-3870          **Fax:** (312)422-4581
**Email:** pburton@aha.org
**Website:** http://www.ashfsa.org
Patricia Burton, Exec. Dir.

**Fnded:** 1967. **Mem:** 1,200. **Local Groups:** 50. **Desc:** Serves individuals with healthcare food service management responsibilities, educators, suppliers and consultants to the profession, is the driving force in the healthcare food service industry and provides healthcare professionals with the resources to compete and succeed. **Pub:** *Healthcare Food Service TRENDS*, quarterly. Magazine. • Also publishes food service reference works on administration, budgeting, cafeteria and financial management, and hospital food service system planning. **Frmly:** American Society for Hospital Food Service Administrators.

### ★ 9705 ★ American Society for Healthcare Human Resources Administration (ASHHRA)

c/o American Hospital Association
One N Franklin, 31st Fl.
Chicago, IL 60606
**Phone:** (312)422-3720          **Fax:** (312)422-4577
**Email:** ashhra@aha.org
**Website:** http://www.ashhra.org
Brandon Melton, Pres.

**Fnded:** 1964. **Mem:** 2,400. **Desc:** Purposes are: to provide effective and continuous leadership in the field of health care human resources administration; to promote cooperation with hospitals and allied associations in matters pertaining to hospital human resources administration; to further the professional and educational development of members; to encourage and promote research; to encourage and assist local groups in chapter formation through regular programs and institutes on health care human resources issues. Offers placement service. **Pub:** *Directory of Health Care Human Resources Consultants*, annual. Directory. • *Hospitals*, bimonthly. • *The Pulse*, quarterly. Journal. Reports on professional ethics and legislative activity. Includes calendar of events and chapter and member news. *Price:* Included in membership dues. • *Roster of Membership*, annual. Membership Directory.

### ★ 9706 ★ American Society for Healthcare Risk Management (ASHRM)
One N Franklin
Chicago, IL 60606
**Phone:** (312)422-3989　　　**Fax:** (312)422-4580
**Email:** esummy@aha.org
**Website:** http://www.ashrm.org
Elizabeth Summy, Exec. Dir.

**Fnded:** 1980. **Mem:** 4,300. **State Groups:** 47. **Desc:** Employees actively involved in the risk management functions of hospitals or other health care providers, and others involved in insurance, brokerage, and consulting. Purposes are to: promote professional development of hospital risk managers; provide educational resources and programs on healthcare risk management; address risk management issues affecting the health care industry. **Pub:** *Journal of Healthcare Risk Management*, quarterly. Journal. Covers research, trends, and new developments in the field of healthcare risk management. Includes educational program calendar and legal update. *Price:* Included in membership dues.

### ★ 9707 ★ American Society of Ophthalmic Administrators (ASOA)
4000 Legato Rd., No. 850
Fairfax, VA 22033
**Phone:** (703)591-2220　　　**Free:** 800-451-1339
**Fax:** (703)591-0614
**Email:** asoa@asoa.org
**Website:** http://www.asoa.org
Lucy Santiago, Exec. Dir.

**Fnded:** 1986. **Mem:** 2,000. **Desc:** A division of the American Society of Cataract and Refractive Surgery . Persons involved with the administration of an ophthalmic office or clinic. Facilitates the exchange of ideas and information in order to improve management practices and working conditions. Offers placement services. **Pub:** *A Manager's Survival Guide to Employee Rights.* • *Administrative Eyecare*, quarterly. Magazine. • *Effective Interviews for Every Situation.* • *Federal Employment Law. Price:* $95 for members; $125 for nonmembers. • *Guidebook to Medical Practice Finances Reporting.* • *Managed Care and Contracting.* Manual. *Price:* $150 for members; $225 for nonmembers. • *Marketing Ophthalmology.* • *Ophthalmic Practice Management I & II.* • *Ophthalmic Regulatory Manual.* Handbook. *Price:* $100 for members; $150 for nonmembers. • *Ophthalmic Reimbursement Manual.* Manual. *Price:* $90 for members; $145 for nonmembers. • *Performance Appraisals: The Latest Legal Nightmare.*

### ★ 9708 ★ Associated Medical Services (AMS)
14 Prince Arthur Ave., Ste. 101
Toronto, ON, Canada M5R 1A9
**Phone:** (416)924-3368　　　**Fax:** (416)323-3338
**Email:** ams@ams-inc.on.ca
**Website:** http://www.ams-inc.on.ca

**Fnded:** 1937. **Lang(s):** English, French. **Desc:** Health services. Promotes increased availability of quality health care. Facilitates communication and cooperation among members; represents members' interests before government agencies, professional medical organizations, and the public. **Pub:** *Corporate Report*, biennial. Report. • Newsletter, 3/year.

### ★ 9709 ★ Association of Behavioral Healthcare Management (ABHM)
12300 Twinbrook Pkwy, Ste. 320
Rockville, MD 20852
**Phone:** (301)984-6200　　　**Fax:** (301)881-7159
**Email:** davids@nccbh.org
**Website:** http://www.nccbh.org/abhm/index.htm
Alan Mabry, PhD, Chair

**Fnded:** 1959. **Mem:** 900. **Desc:** Administrators of services for the emotionally disturbed, mentally ill, mentally retarded, developmentally disabled, and those with problems of alcohol and substance abuse. Objectives are to: further the education of administrators; develop criteria for and certify the competence of administrators; promote adherence to a code of ethics. Aids in developing professional administrative skills and administration of services. Sponsors educational workshops. **Pub:** *AMHA Leader*, bimonthly. Newsletter. Current news and information on mental health administration issues. *Price:* $90/year. • *Journal of Mental Health Administration*, quarterly. Journal. Covers management practice, research, and policy issues in the mental health field. **Frmly:** (1969) American Society of Mental Health Business Administrators; (1997) Association of Mental Heath Administrators.

### ★ 9710 ★ Association of Family Practice Residency Directors (AFPRD)
PO Box 11210
Shawnee Mission, KS 66207-1210
**Phone:** (913)906-6000　　　**Free:** 800-274-2237
**Fax:** (913)906-6105
**Email:** afprd@aafp.org
**Website:** http://www.afprd.org
Stacy Singleton, Mgr.

**Fnded:** 1990. **Mem:** 406. **Desc:** Promotes excellence in family practice graduate education. Provides representation for residency directors at a national level and provides a political voice for them in appropriate arenas. Promotes cooperation and communication between residency programs and different branches of the family practice specialty. Dedicated to improving of education of family physicians. Provides a network for mutual assistance among FP. residency directors. **Pub:** *Highlights*, quarterly. Newsletter. *Price:* Free for members.

### ★ 9711 ★ Association of Healthcare Internal Auditors (AHIA)
PO Box 449
Onsted, MI 49265-0449
**Phone:** (517)467-7729　　　**Free:** 888-275-2442
**Fax:** (517)467-6104
**Email:** pbogusz@ahia.org
**Website:** http://www.ahia.org
Pat Bogusz, Exec. Dir.

**Fnded:** 1981. **Mem:** 1,000. **Desc:** Health care internal auditors and other interested individuals. Promotes cost containment and increased productivity in health care institutions through internal auditing. Serves as a forum for the exchange of experience, ideas, and information among members; provides continuing professional education courses and informs members of developments in health care internal auditing. Offers employment clearinghouse services. **Pub:** *New Perspectives on Healthcare Auditing*, quarterly. Journal. Contains book reviews, audit findings, and local and regional group news. **Frmly:** (1989) Healthcare Internal Audit Group.

### ★ 9712 ★ Association of Health Facility Survey Agencies (AHFSA)
Missouri Department of Health
Bureau of Health Facility Regulation
912 Wildwood Dr.
PO Box 570
Jefferson City, MO 65102
**Phone:** (573)751-6302　　　**Fax:** (573)526-3621
Shanna E. Schopp, Interim Admin.

**Fnded:** 1968. **Mem:** 51. **Desc:** Directors of state or territorial health facility licensure and certification programs; staff members of a state or territorial health facility licensure and certification agency; employees of the federal Health Care Financing Administration; interested individuals. (The term health facilities refers to health/medical institutions including hospitals, nursing homes, rehabilitation centers, reproductive health centers, independent clinical laboratories, hospices, and ambulatory surgical centers.) Purposes are to exchange information among members and between members and the Association of State and Territorial Health Officials; constitute a "reservoir of expertise" to aid in the guidance of ASTHO; improve the quality of health facility licensure and certification programs; provide a forum for state and territorial issues at the national level. Has a representative on an ASTHO standing committee and liaises with the federal Department of Health and Human Services and the HCFA. Has developed new training programs with the HHS and testified before the U.S. Senate Special Committee on Aging on survey and certification procedures. Bestows annual Surveyor of the Year Award. **Pub:** *AHFSA Directory*, annual. Directory. • *Association of Health Facility Survey Agencies Newsletter*, semiannual. Newsletter. Reports on the quality of health facility licensure and certification programs and related issues. Includes calendar of events. *Price:* Included in membership dues. • Papers. **Frmly:** (1991) Association of Health Facility Licensure and Certification Directors.

### ★ 9713 ★ Association of Operating Department Practitioners (AODP)
Lewes Enterprise Centre
112 Malling St.
Lewes BN7 2RJ, United Kingdom
**Phone:** 44 870 7460984　　　**Fax:** 44 870 7460985
**Email:** office@aodp.org
**Website:** http://www.aodp.org

**Fnded:** 1945. **Mem:** 4,000. **Desc:** Seeks to maintain quality standards among operating department practitioners. **Pub:** *Technic*, monthly. Journal.

### ★ 9714 ★ Association for Quality in Healthcare
Regents Park House
Regent St.
Leeds LS2 7QJ, United Kingdom
**Phone:** 44 113 2237296　　　**Fax:** 44 113 2237298
**Email:** aqh@virgin.net

**Fnded:** 1986. **Mem:** 600. **Reg. Groups:** 9. **Lang(s):** English. **Desc:** Anyone interested in promoting measurable and continuous improvement in the quality of healthcare for the benefit of the public. Dedicated solely to all aspects of the subject of measuring and improving the quality of healthcare services. **Pub:** *Journal for the Association for Quality Healthcare*, quarterly. Journal. • *Quality Times*, quarterly. Newsletter.

### ★ 9715 ★ Association of State and Territorial Dental Directors (ASTDD)
322 Cannondale Rd.
Jefferson City, MO 65109
**Phone:** (573)636-0453
**Email:** astdd@socket.net
**Website:** http://www.hs.state.az.us/cfhs/ooh/
M. Dean Perkins, DDS, Exec. Dir.

**Mem:** 53. **Desc:** Directors of state and territorial dental programs. Provides a forum for consideration of dental health administrative problems and policies on the state and territorial level; promotes constructive plans for better administrative procedures.

### ★ 9716 ★ Association of State and Territorial Health Officials (ASTHO)
1275 K St., NW, Ste. 800
Washington, DC 20005-4006
**Phone:** (202)371-9090　　　**Fax:** (202)371-9797
**Email:** ghardy@astho.org
**Website:** http://www.astho.org
George E. Hardy, Jr., Exec. Dir.

**Fnded:** 1942. **Mem:** 57. **Desc:** Represents the executive officer of the department of public health of each of the U.S. states, territories and possessions and is engaged in a wide range of legislative, educational, scientific and programmatic issues and activities on behalf of public health. Seeks to"formulate and influence sound national public health policy and to assist state health officials in the development and implementation of programs and policies to promote health and prevent disease, injury and disability." Serves as a primary information resource to state health agencies on a wide range of issues, including HIV/AIDS, immunizations, tobacco-use control, primary care, maternal and child health, school health and the environment. Its sixteen affiliate organizations represent state public health specialty associations for chronic disease programs, dental health, emergency medical services, epidemiology, health facility survey agencies, HIV/AIDS, local health liaisons, maternal and child health programs, nursing services, nutrition services, public health laboratories, public health promotion and education, public health statistics and information systems, social work and vector control services. **Pub:** *ASTHO Annual Report*, annual. Annual Report. *Price:* Free. • *Conference Proceedings*, annual. Proceedings. • *State Public Health Agencies*, biennial. Directory. Lists state health departments. *Price:* $150. • Membership Directory, biennial. • Newsletter, periodic. **Frmly:** (1975) Association of State and Territorial Health Officers.

★ 9717 ★ **Association of University Programs in Health Administration (AUPHA)**
730 11th St. NW, Fl. 4
Washington, DC 20001-4510
**Phone:** (202)638-1448          **Fax:** (202)638-3429
**Email:** aupha@aupha.org
**Website:** http://www.aupha.org
Jeptha W. Dalston, Ph.D., FACHE, Pres. /CEO
**Fnded:** 1948. **Mem:** 1,200. **Desc:** Universities offering graduate and undergraduate study in health services and hospital administration. To improve the quality of education in health services administration. Undertakes research and educational programs, such as studies of the criteria used for selection of students and curriculum patterns adopted by various universities. Conducts faculty institutes on topics relating to health administration. Compiles statistics. **Pub:** *AUPHA Exchange*, bimonthly. Newsletter. • *Health Services Administration Education*, biennial. Directory. • *Journal of Health Administration Education*, quarterly. Journal. **Frmly:** (1973) Association of University Programs in Hospital Administration.

★ 9718 ★ **Australian Association of Practice Managers (AAPM)**
PO Box 1108
Carlton, VIC 3058, Australia
**Fax:** 61 3 96631960
**Email:** vic@aapm.org.au
**Website:** http://www.aapm.org.au
**Fnded:** 1979. **Lang(s):** English. **Desc:** Practice managers in the healthcare industry. Promotes professional excellence in healthcare practice management.

★ 9719 ★ **Australian College of Health Service Executives (ACHSE)**
PO Box 341
North Ryde, NSW 1670, Australia
**Phone:** 61 2 98050431          **Fax:** 61 2 98782272
**Email:** achse@achse.org.au
**Website:** http://www.achse.org.au
**Fnded:** 1945. **Mem:** 3,000. **Lang(s):** English. **Desc:** Aims to develop and foster excellence in Health Service Management through education and ongoing professional development of existing and potential health service managers.

★ 9720 ★ **Biotech Medical Management Association (BMMA)**
10592 Perry Hwy., No. 300
Wexford, PA 15090
**Free:** 888-990-2662          **Fax:** (724)934-8449
**Email:** contactus@bioastec.com

**Website:** http://www.bmma.org
Mark G. Fuller, MD, Contact
**Fnded:** 1993. **Desc:** Physicians and pharmacists involved in managed care insurance programs; insurance companies, pharmaceutical manufacturers, and other firms with an interest in managed care medicine; academic institutions, medical and insurance consultants, and health care representatives. Promotes establishment of national standards regulating medical and drug policies and the administration of medical and pharmacy benefits. Represents members before government agencies, industrial organizations, and the public; facilitates communication between biotechnology manufacturers and health care payers and providers; supports pharmaceutical research; conducts educational programs. **Pub:** *Journal of the Biotech Medical Management Association*, quarterly. Journal. Dedicated to new developments in biotechnology. *Price:* $120/yr.

★ 9721 ★ **British Association of Medical Managers**
Petersgate House, 3rd Fl.
St. Petersgate
Stockport SK1 1HE, United Kingdom
**Phone:** 44 161 4741141          **Fax:** 44 161 4747167
**Email:** bamm@bamm.co.uk
**Website:** http://www.bamm.co.uk
**Fnded:** 1991. **Mem:** 1,800. **Desc:** Doctors from all specialties and at all levels of interest in management are invited to apply for membership. Junior doctors are warmly welcomed and non medical managers are welcome to apply for associate membership. Concerned with the promotion of quality healthcare by improving and supporting the contribution of doctors in management. Unites doctors with an interest in healthcare management. Members are keen to learn from, and work with each other to ensure a meaningful and effective contribution to the management of organisations. **Pub:** *Clinician in Management*, bimonthly. • Newsletter.

★ 9722 ★ **British Dental Practice Managers Association**
Norman House
16 Asfordby Rd.
Melton Mowbray LE13 0HR, United Kingdom
**Phone:** 44 870 8400341          **Fax:** 44 870 8400342
**Email:** info@bdpma.org.uk
**Website:** http://www.bdpma.org.uk
**Fnded:** 1992. **Mem:** 400. **Reg. Groups:** 10. **Desc:** Promote co-operation and provide a way to communicate and support those actively involved in Dental Practice Management. **Pub:** *Networking*, quarterly. Newsletter.

★ 9723 ★ **Canadian College of Health Service Executives**
350 Sparks St., Ste. 402
Ottawa, ON, Canada K1R 7S8
**Phone:** (613)235-7218          **Fax:** (613)235-5451
**Email:** cchse@cchse.org
**Website:** http://www.cchse.org
**Fnded:** 1970. **Mem:** 3,000. **Reg. Groups:** 20. **Desc:** Health service executives in Canada. **Pub:** *Healthcare Management Forum*, quarterly, always March, June, September, and December. Journal. Contains articles on innovations in health services.

★ 9724 ★ **Canadian Council on Health Services Accreditation (CCHSA)**
1730 St. Laurent Blvd., Ste. 100
Ottawa, ON, Canada K1G 5L1
**Phone:** (613)738-3800          **Fax:** (613)738-1244
**Email:** huto@cchsa.ca
**Website:** http://www.cchsa.ca
**Fnded:** 1958. **Mem:** 1,541. **Lang(s):** English, French. **Desc:** Agencies and organizations accrediting health care services including mental health care, cancer treatment centers, home health care, and community health. Seeks to ensure high standards of ethics, practice, and equipment and facilities among Canadi-

an health services. Formulates and enforces standards; conducts research and educational programs. **Pub:** *The Accreditation Standard*, quarterly. Newsletter. • *Standards*. Manual. • Annual Report. • Reports. **Frmly:** (1995) Canadian Council on Health Facilities Accreditation.

★ 9725 ★ **Canadian Health Care Material Management Association (CHCMMA)**
c/o Lions Gate Hospital
231 E 15th St.
North Vancouver, BC, Canada V7L 2L7
**Phone:** (604)984-5800          **Fax:** (604)984-5838
**Email:** bharber@nshr.hnet.bc.ca
**Lang(s):** English, French. **Desc:** Materials management professionals employed by health care facilities. Promotes excellence in the field of health care materials management. Facilitates communication and cooperation among members; sponsors continuing professional development courses.

★ 9726 ★ **Canadian Health Coalition (CHC) (Coalition Canadienne de la Sante — CCS)**
2841 Riverside Dr.
Ottawa, ON, Canada K1V 8X7
**Phone:** (613)521-3400          **Fax:** (613)521-9638
**Email:** info@healthcoalition.ca
**Website:** http://www.healthcoalition.ca
**Lang(s):** English, French. **Desc:** Individuals and organizations with an interest in health care. Promotes increased availability and quality of health services. Monitors the performance of health care facilities and services and makes recommendations for their improvement.

★ 9727 ★ **Canadian Health Record Association (CHRA) (College des Archivists Medicale du Canada — CAMC)**
1090 Don Mills Rd., Ste. 501
Don Mills, ON, Canada M3C 3R6
**Phone:** (416)447-4900          **Fax:** (416)447-4598
**Email:** info@chra.ca
**Website:** http://www.chra.ca
**Fnded:** 1949. **Mem:** 3,000. **Lang(s):** English, French. **Desc:** Librarians, archivists, and other individuals engaged in the maintenance of medical records. Promotes excellence in the practice of medical records management. Facilitates communication and cooperation among members; sponsors continuing professional development courses for medical records managers.

★ 9728 ★ **Canadian Healthcare Engineering Society (CHES) (Societe Canadienne d'Ingenierie des Services de Sante — SCIH)**
The Woolen Mill
4 Cataraqui St., Ste. 310
Kingston, ON, Canada K7K 1Z7
**Phone:** (613)531-2661          **Fax:** (613)531-0626
**Email:** info@ches.org
**Website:** http://www.ches.org
**Lang(s):** English, French. **Desc:** Hospital maintenance engineers and other individuals responsible for the physical plant of health care facilities. Promotes excellence in hospital engineering. Serves as a forum for the exchange of information among members; sponsors educational and training programs. **Frmly:** (2000) Canadian Hospital Engineering Society.

★ 9729 ★ **Canadian Institute of Health Care and Business (CIHCB)**
No. 7 Hayden St., Ste. 303
Toronto, ON, Canada M4Y 2P2
**Phone:** (416)925-4417
**Email:** can_inst@istar.ca
**Website:** http://home.istar.ca/~can_inst

**Lang(s):** English, French. **Desc:** Business professionals working in the field of health care. Promotes effective application of business principles within the health care industries. Sponsors continuing professional education courses for members.

**★ 9730 ★ Canadian Register of Health Service Providers in Psychology (CRHSPP)**
**(Repertoire Canadien des Psychologues Offrant des Services de Sante — RCPOSS)**
368 Dalhousie St., Ste. 300
Ottawa, ON, Canada K1N 5P4
**Phone:** (613)562-0900     **Fax:** (613)562-0902
**Email:** info@crhspp.ca
**Website:** http://www.crhspp.ca
**Fnded:** 1985. **Mem:** 3,000. **Lang(s):** English, French. **Desc:** Provides psychologists' credentials. Promotes increased availability of psychological services. Serves as a clearinghouse on psychological and related services; sponsors research and educational programs.

**★ 9731 ★ Case Management Society of America (CMSA)**
8201 Cantrell Rd., Ste. 230
Little Rock, AR 72227-2448
**Phone:** (501)225-2229     **Fax:** (501)221-9068
**Email:** cmsa@cmsa.org
**Website:** http://www.cmsa.org
Jeanne Boling, Exec. Dir.
**Fnded:** 1990. **Mem:** 7,500. **State Groups:** 1. **Local Groups:** 72. **Desc:** Case management and allied healthcare professionals. Offers members a voice in the future through opportunities for professional leadership and networking opportunities, case management legislative impact and visibility, publications, educational workshops, seminars, conferences, recognition and fellowship opportunities. **Pub:** *The Case Manager*, bimonthly. Journal. • *Case Report*, bimonthly. Newsletter. Published in The Case Manager, CMSA's official journal. • *Standards of Practice.* • Brochure, annual. • Membership Directory, annual.

**★ 9732 ★ Center for Research in Ambulatory Health Care Administration (CRAHCA)**
104 Inverness Ter. E
Englewood, CO 80112-5306
**Phone:** (303)397-7897     **Fax:** (303)397-1827
**Email:** gtn@mgma.com
**Website:** http://www.mgma.com
Glenn T. Hammons, MD, VP
**Fnded:** 1973. **Desc:** Seeks to advance the art and science of medical group practice management to improve the health of our communtities. Vision is to be the source of excellence and innovation as the leading association in providing quality and timely services and resources for medical practice management and leadership. Develops and advances research-based knowledge in the field of ambulatory health care by improving education, management technology, publications, and database services. Research is directed toward health care economics, policy development and analysis, alternative organizational models for health care delivery, evaluation methodologies, models of provider team leadership, and the social aspects of health services organizations and the communities in which they serve. Research interests include provider reimbursement and the analysis of ambulatory health care and medical practice costs. The evolution and impact of integrated and managed care systems and the role of access and quality in the production and management of ambulatory care services will be examined. The impact of these areas on health system reform will be studied. **Pub:** *Actuarial Issues in the Fee-for-Service/Prepaid Medical Group.* Book. *Price:* $32/copy. • *Case Management in Primary Care.* Manual. *Price:* $24/copy. • *Geriatric Collaborative Care Model.* Book. *Price:* $17/copy. • *Getting Started in Geriatrics.* Handbook. *Price:* $29/copy. • *Health Information Management Medical Record Processes*

*in Group Practice.* Book. *Price:* $39/copy. • *Integrated Health Care.* Book. *Price:* $44/copy. • *Making Integrated Care Work.* Book. *Price:* $49/copy. • *Medical Group Practice Chart of Accounts.* Book. *Price:* $49/copy. • *Performance Efficiency Evaluation*, annual. Report. *Price:* $695/year. • *Prepare for Eldercare.* Handbook. *Price:* $14/copy. • *Quality Improvement.* Book. *Price:* $39/copy. **AKA:** CRAHCA.

**★ 9733 ★ CPRI-HOST**
4915 St. Elmo Ave., Ste. 401
Bethesda, MD 20814-6052
**Phone:** (301)657-5918     **Fax:** (301)657-1296
**Email:** administration@cpri-host.org
**Website:** http://www.cpri-host.org/
Patricia Wise, MA,MSN, Exec. Dir.
**Fnded:** 1992. **Desc:** Working to provide vision and leadership to promote the universal and effective use of electronic health care information systems to improve health and the delivery of health care. **Frmly:** (2002) Computer-based Patient Record Institute and Healthcare Open Systems and Trials.

**★ 9734 ★ European Health Management Association (EHMA)**
Vergemount Hall
Clonskeagh
Dublin 6, Ireland
**Phone:** 353 1 2839299     **Fax:** 353 1 2838653
**Email:** rdooley@ehma.org
**Website:** http://www.ehma.org
**Fnded:** 1966. **Mem:** 200. **Lang(s):** English, French. **Desc:** Policy makers, senior managers, personnel directors, academic institutions, and research organizations in the healthcare sector. Seeks to improve healthcare in Europe by raising standards of managerial performance in the health sector. Fosters cooperation between health service organizations and institutions in the field of healthcare management education and training. Promotes the continuing education and development of healthcare managers. Offers advice and support to national governments in Europe; evaluates members' management development programs. **Pub:** *Conference Proceedings*, annual. Journal. • *Health Services Administration Education and Research*, annual. Directory. • *Management Development for Health Care: An International Perspective.* • *Management Education and Training in the Health Sector: A Perspective for Italy.* • Newsletter, bimonthly. **Frmly:** (1987) European Association of Programmes in Health Services Studies.

**Federation of American Hospitals (FAHS)**
*See:* Entry 11491

**★ 9735 ★ Foundation of American College of Health Care Administrators (FACHCA)**
300 N Lee St., No. 301
Alexandria, VA 22314-2807
**Phone:** (703)739-7900     **Free:** 888-88A-CHCA
**Fax:** (703)739-7901
**Email:** mtn@achca.org
**Website:** http://www.achca.org
Mary Tellis-Nayak, Pres. /CEO
**Fnded:** 1971. **Mem:** 2,000. **Desc:** Individuals dedicated to the improvement of the administration of long-term care facilities. Conducts professional training programs and research in administration. **Pub:** *Foundation Focus in Long-term Care Administration*, quarterly. Newsletter. Includes research updates. *Price:* Included in membership dues. • *The Journal of Long-Term Care Administration*, quarterly. *Price:* $70/year. **Frmly:** (1983) Foundation of American College of Nursing Home Administrators.

**★ 9736 ★ Health Science Center (HSC)**
10180 Committee Medical College
Hanoi, Vietnam
**Phone:** 84 4 63514     **Fax:** 84 4 63514

**Lang(s):** English, French, Vietnamese. **Desc:** Health care providers. Seeks to increase access to quality health services among previously underserved populations. Makes available primary medical care; sponsors research and educational programs.

**★ 9737 ★ Health Systems Trust - South Africa (HNSA)**
PO Box 808
Durban 4000, Republic of South Africa
**Phone:** 27 31 3072954     **Fax:** 27 31 3040775
**Email:** webmaster@hst.org.za
**Website:** http://www.hst.org.za
**Lang(s):** Afrikaans, English. **Desc:** Hospitals, clinics, and other health care facilities; telecommunications and satellite communications networks. Promotes improved communication and cooperation among health care facilities. Serves as a clearinghouse on medicine and telecommunications; maintains electronic network linking members; conducts educational and training programs for health care and telecommunications professionals.

**★ 9738 ★ Healthcare Information and Management Systems Society (HIMSS)**
230 E Ohio St., Ste. 500
Chicago, IL 60611-3269
**Phone:** (312)664-4467     **Fax:** (312)664-6143
**Email:** membership@himss.org
**Website:** http://www.himss.org
Stephen Lieber, CAE, Pres. /CEO
**Fnded:** 1961. **Mem:** 12,000. **Reg. Groups:** 37. **Local Groups:** 35. **Desc:** Healthcare professionals. Provides leadership in healthcare for management of technology, information, and change through educational opportunities and services; supports professionals developing key innovations in healthcare delivery and administration, including telemedicine, computer-based patient records, community health information networks, and portable/wireless healthcare computing. **Pub:** *HIMSS News*, monthly. Newsletter. Contains society news. • *Journal of Healthcare Information Management*, quarterly. Journal. Features the latest research and opinions in the industry.

**★ 9739 ★ Healthcare Leadership Council (HLC)**
900 17th St. NW, Ste. 600
Washington, DC 20006
**Phone:** (202)452-8700     **Fax:** (202)296-9561
**Email:** dwiermanski@hlc.org
**Website:** http://hlc.org
Mary Grealey, Pres.
**Fnded:** 1988. **Desc:** Health care industry executives. Promotes the advancement of a market-based health care system that values innovation and provides affordable, high-quality health care; presents its system idea to Congress, administration, media, the research community and the public.

**★ 9740 ★ HealthNet Zimbabwe (HZ)**
Computer Science Department
University of Zimbabwe
Harare, Zimbabwe
**Phone:** 263 4 303211     **Fax:** 263 4 333407
**Email:** borland@healthnet.zw
**Lang(s):** English. **Desc:** Health care professionals. Promotes increased use of electronic communications to advance the practice of health care. Serves as a clearinghouse on medicine.

**★ 9741 ★ Hong Kong Society of Health Services Executives**
PO Box 70875
Kowloon Central Post Office
Hong Kong, People's Republic of China
**Email:** fng@ouhk.edu.hk
**Website:** http://www.medicine.org.hk/hkshse/
**Mem:** 200. **Desc:** Promotes the professional advancement of health service management. Seeks to achieve excellence in health care service in Hong Kong

through the advancement of professional and ethical standards in service management. Organizes educational activities.

★ **9742** ★ **Institute of Healthcare Management**
46 Grosvenor Gardens
London SW1, United Kingdom
**Phone:** 44 207 8819235    **Fax:** 44 207 8819236
**Email:** enquires@ihm.org.uk
**Website:** http://www.ihm.org.uk/home.cfm
**Fnded:** 1902. **Mem:** 8,000. **Reg. Groups:** 8. **State Groups:** 3. **Desc:** Those involved in the management and administration of health care. To promote excellence in health services management and the development of good managers, to affect health services policy and its implementation and to create and sustain a professional community of health services managers. It is a forum, network and management development association for individuals both inside and outside the NHS. **Pub:** *Health Management*, monthly. Magazine. Contains in-house journal for IHSM members. • *The IHSM Health and Social Services Yearbook*, annual. Book. **Frmly:** (2000) Institute of Health Services Management.

★ **9743** ★ **Intergovernmental Health Policy Project (IHPP)**
444 N Capital St. Ste 515
Washington, DC 20001
**Phone:** (202)624-8698    **Fax:** (202)737-1069
**Email:** dick.merritt@ncsl.org
Richard E. Merritt, Dir.
**Fnded:** 1979. **Desc:** Health policy researchers. Provides information on state health legislation and programs to state executive officials, legislators, legislative staff, and others. Serves as information clearinghouse; responds to specific information requests on state programs. Compiles statistics. Offers a customized legislative tracking service to customers. **Pub:** *State Health Notes*, semimonthly. Newsletter. *Price:* $297. • Newsletter, bimonthly. • Newsletter, 10/year. • Monograph, annual. Summarizes state legislation relating to health care.

**International Association of Healthcare Central Service Materiel Management (IAHCSMM)**
*See:* Entry 11496

★ **9744** ★ **International Federation of Health Records Organizations (IFHRO)**
c/o Philip Roxborough
2/365 Richardson Rd.
Mount Roskill
Auckland, New Zealand
**Phone:** 64 9 6267975    **Fax:** 64 9 6267975
**Email:** philipr@ahsl.co.az
**Website:** http://www.iahcsmm.com
**Fnded:** 1968. **Mem:** 200. **Nat'l Groups:** 2. **Lang(s):** English. **Desc:** Organizations in 21 countries working in the health records field; persons involved in the field of health records in countries where no national organizations exist are associate members; individuals who have made significant contributions to the federation are honorary members. Objectives are to: improve health records standards in hospitals, dispensaries, and various health and medical institutions; promote efficient methods of health records in patient care, statistics, research, and teaching; provide a worldwide forum for individuals working in the health records field; encourage the international exchange of education requirements and training programs in the field of health records. Works closely with the World Health Organization and jointly sponsors workshops and research and educational projects in the health records field. **Pub:** *International Health Records*, quarterly. Newsletter.

★ **9745** ★ **Laboratory Animal Management Association (LAMA)**
7300 Metro Blvd., Ste. 585
Edina, MN 55439
**Phone:** (952)250-6201    **Fax:** (952)835-4774
**Email:** imartinez@rcm.upr.edu
**Website:** http://www.lama-online.org
Ivette Martinez-Palma, Pres.
**Fnded:** 1984. **Mem:** 435. **Reg. Groups:** 3. **Desc:** Laboratory animal facility managers. Seeks to evaluate and update basic and advanced management techniques and to educate laboratory animal facility managers. Makes available resource material; coordinates exchange programs for management personnel. Offers consulting on management techniques. **Pub:** *LAMA Lines*, bimonthly. Includes branch news and a listing for employment opportunities. *Price:* Included in membership dues. • *Lama Review*, quarterly. Journal. • Membership Directory, annual. **Frmly:** Laboratory Animal Managers Association.

★ **9746** ★ **Management Society for Healthcare Professionals**
88 Lockhart Rd., 8/F
Hong Kong, People's Republic of China
**Fnded:** 1984. **Lang(s):** Chinese, English. **Desc:** Managerial and adminstrative staff of health care services; medical, paramedical, and nursing professionals. Promotes effective delivery of health care and patient care and management services. Seeks to facilitate the professional development of members. Represents members' interests; collaborates with government agencies in establishment of public health policies and programs; facilitates exchange of information among members. Conducts educational programs; sponsors social activities.

★ **9747** ★ **Medical Group Management Association (MGMA)**
104 Inverness Terr. E
Englewood, CO 80112-5306
**Phone:** (303)799-1111    **Free:** 877-275-6462
**Fax:** (303)643-4439
**Email:** infocenter@mgma.com
**Website:** http://www.mgma.com
William F. Jessee, MD, CEO
**Fnded:** 1926. **Mem:** 18,000. **Nat'l Groups:** 1. **Reg. Groups:** 4. **Desc:** For professionals involved in the business management of groups in medical practice. Products and services include education, benchmarking, surveys, national advocacy and networking opportunities for members. **Pub:** *Academic Practice Faculty Compensation and Production Survey Report*, annual. Report. A census of academic clinical science Departments designed to assist Department admins. in evaluating the scope of compensation and production of med. school fac. *Price:* $225/copy for members; $275/copy for affiliates; $375/copy for nonmembers. • *Academic Practice Management Compensation Survey Report*, annual. Report. A census of academic clinical science Departments and practice plans designed to provide comparative Information to academic medical practices and others. *Price:* $90/copy for members; $120/copy for affiliates; $150/copy for nonmembers. • *Ambulatory Surgery Center Performance Survey Report*, annual. Report. Provides comparative measures to assess annual ambulatory surgery center (ASC) financial and operational results. *Price:* $90/copy for members; $120/copy for affiliates; $150/copy for nonmembers. • *Cost Survey Report*, annual. Report. Covers every facet of medical group operating costs, bring over- and under-spending into sharp relief, enabling readers to right-size their practice. *Price:* $240/copy for members; $290/copy for affiliates; $450/copy for nonmembers. • *Management Services Organization Performance Survey Report*, annual. Report. Provides comparative measures useful in benchmarking annual MSO corporate financial and operational results. *Price:* $240/copy for members; $290/copy for affiliates; $450/copy for nonmembers. • *Physician Compensation and Production Survey*, annual. Report. **Frmly:** (1946) Association of Clinic Managers; (1963) National Association of Clinical Managers.

**National Alliance of State and Territorial AIDS Directors**
*See:* Entry 11810

**National Association of Boards of Examiners of Long Term Care Administrators (NABE)**
*See:* Entry 15919

★ **9748** ★ **National Association of County Health Facility Administrators (NACHFA)**
c/o National Association of Counties
440 First St., NW
Washington, DC 20001
**Phone:** (202)393-6226    **Fax:** (202)393-2630
**Email:** nab@bostromdc.com
**Website:** http://www.naco.org
Frank Colb, Staff Liaison
**Fnded:** 1977. **Mem:** 250. **Desc:** Administrators of freestanding and hospital-based long-term care facilities owned and operated by county governments or city-county consolidations; elected local officials. Promotes interests of county long-term care facilities; offers guidance in relevant legislative and regulatory areas. Provides technical assistance; conducts training workshops. Compiles statistics on public policy changes, such as changes in the Medicaid program, which affect long-term care facilities.

★ **9749** ★ **National Association of Directors of Nursing Administration in Long Term Care (NADONA/LTC)**
10101 Alliance Rd., No. 140
Cincinnati, OH 45242
**Phone:** (513)791-3679    **Free:** 800-222-0539
**Fax:** (513)791-3699
**Email:** info@nadona.org
**Website:** http://www.nadona.org
Joan C. Warden-Saunders, R.N., Exec. Dir.
**Fnded:** 1986. **Mem:** 4,600. **Reg. Groups:** 5. **State Groups:** 35. **Desc:** Directors, assistant directors, and former directors of nursing in long term care. Goals are: to create and establish an acceptable ethical standard for practices in long term care nursing administration and to promote and encourage research in the profession; to develop and provide a consistent program of education and certification for the positions of director, associate director, and assistant director; to promote a positive image of the long term health care industry. Encourages members to share concerns and experiences; sponsors research programs. Advocates legislation pertaining to the practice of professional nursing. Maintains speakers' bureau. nursing. Maintains speakers' bureau. **Pub:** *The Director*, quarterly. Journal. Includes research, clinical papers and news items. *Price:* Included in membership dues.

★ **9750** ★ **National Association of Health Services Executives (NAHSE)**
8630 Fenton St., No. 126
Silver Spring, MD 20910
**Phone:** (301)588-2255    **Fax:** (301)588-0011
**Email:** nahse_hq@compuserve.com
**Website:** http://www.nahse.org/
Dr. Hilda Richards, Pres.
**Fnded:** 1968. **Mem:** 500. **Reg. Groups:** 16. **Local Groups:** 7. **Desc:** Black health care executive managers, planners, educators, advocates, providers, organizers, researchers, and consumers participating in academic ventures, educational forums, seminars, workshops, systems design, legislation, and other activities. Conducts National Work-Study Program and sponsors educational programs. **Pub:** *NAHSE Notes*, quarterly. Newsletter. *Price:* Free.

★ **9751** ★ **National Association Medical Staff Services (NAMSS)**
PO Box 140647
Austin, TX 78714-0647

**Phone:** (512)454-7928      **Fax:** (512)454-3036
**Email:** namss@namss.org
**Website:** http://www.namss.org
Sandra Young-Mattson, CMSC, CPCS, Pres.

**Fnded:** 1971. **Mem:** 4,000. **Reg. Groups:** 5. **State Groups:** 48. **Local Groups:** 32. **Desc:** Individuals involved in the management and administration of healthcare provider services. Seeks to: enhance the knowledge and experience of medical staff services professionals; promote the certification of those involved in the profession. **Pub:** *Credentialing and Medical Staff Law.* • *Guidebook: Developing a Policy and Procedure Manual.* Manual. • *Medical Staff Leadership Orientation Manual.* • *NAMSS Membership Roster*, annual. Membership Directory. • *Synergy*, bimonthly. Magazine. *Price:* Included in membership dues; $65/year for nonmembers.

**National Association of Professional Geriatric Care Managers (PGCM)**
*See:* Entry 3004

★ **9752** ★ **National Association of State Alcohol and Drug Abuse Directors (NASADAD)**
808 17th St. NW, Ste. 410
Washington, DC 20006
**Phone:** (202)293-0090      **Fax:** (202)293-1250
**Email:** dcoffice@nasadad.org
**Website:** http://www.nasadad.org
Lewis E. Gallant, PhD, Exec. Dir.

**Fnded:** 1971. **Mem:** 56. **Desc:** Purposes are: to represent the interests of state alcohol and drug abuse directors and their agencies before Congress and federal agencies; to foster development of comprehensive alcohol and drug abuse programs on state resources/services, alcohol and drug issues related to AIDS, drunk driving, and criminal justice activities in each state. Operates Project for Addiction Counselor Training, AIDS Policy Project, Criminal Justice Programs, Methadone Treatment Quality Assurance System project, and the National Prevention Network (NPN). Serves as an information clearinghouse. Conducts seminars on current and emerging alcohol and drug abuse issues. **Pub:** *Directory of State Alcohol and Drug Abuse Directors*, monthly. Directory. • *Special Report. Price:* $80/year. • *State Alcohol and Drug Abuse Profile*, annual. Report. Provides data on state fiscal resources, services to clients, drug trends, model products, and special needs. *Price:* $45. • *State Resource and Services Related to Alcohol and Drug Problems*, annual. • *State Substance Abuse Quarterly*, quarterly. Newsletter. Covers significant national and state development. *Price:* $80. • *Treatment Works.* **Frmly:** (1978) National Association of State Drug Abuse Program Coordinators.

★ **9753** ★ **National Association of State EMS Directors (NASEMSD)**
111 Park Pl.
Falls Church, VA 22046-4513
**Phone:** (703)538-1799      **Fax:** (703)241-5603
**Email:** info@nasemsd.org
**Website:** http://www.nasemsd.org
Elizabeth B. Armstrong, CAE, Exec. Dir.

**Fnded:** 1981. **Mem:** 56. **Reg. Groups:** 4. **Desc:** Provides vision and leadership in the development and improvement of EMS systems and national EMS policy. **Pub:** *EMS Office, Structure, and Functioning. Price:* $35. • *EMT Certification, Licensing, and Reciprocity Requirements. Price:* $25. • *NASEMSD Scanner*, quarterly. Newsletter. Includes information on state EMS programs. • *Training and Certification of EMS Personnel. Price:* $50. • *Trauma Center Designation Survey*. Survey. *Price:* $28.

★ **9754** ★ **National Association of State Medicaid Directors (NASMD)**
810 1st St. NE, Ste. 500
Washington, DC 20002
**Phone:** (202)682-0100      **Fax:** (202)682-3706
Lee Partridge, Dir.

**Fnded:** 1979. **Desc:** Representatives of state Medicaid agencies. Promotes effective and efficient management of federal and state health care programs. Facilitates communication and cooperation between state and federal Medicaid authorities; serves as a clearinghouse on Medicaid benefits.

★ **9755** ★ **National Association of State Mental Health Program Directors (NASMHPD)**
66 Canal Center Plz., Ste. 302
Alexandria, VA 22314
**Phone:** (703)739-9333      **Fax:** (703)548-9517
**Email:** bob.glover@nasmhpd.org
**Website:** http://www.nasmhpd.org
Dr. Robert W. Glover, Exec. Dir.

**Fnded:** 1963. **Mem:** 55. **Desc:** State commissioners in charge of the state mental disability programs; associate members are assistant commissioners for children and youth, aged, legal services, forensic services, and adult services. Promotes cooperation of state government agencies in delivery of services to mentally disabled persons; fosters the exchange of scientific and programmatic information in the administration of public mental health programs including mental illness treatment programs, community and hospital care of persons who are mentally ill, mentally retarded, alcoholic, and drug addiction. Monitors state and federal and congressional activities; gathers and analyzes information on organization, structure, funding, and programming of state government mental health programs. A cooperating agency of the National Governors' Association and the Council of State Governments.

★ **9756** ★ **National Association of Supervisors and Administrators of Health Occupations Education (NASAHOE)**
c/o Jo Ann Wakelyn
Virginia Department of Education
PO Box 2120
Richmond, VA 23218-2060
**Phone:** (804)225-2842      **Fax:** (804)371-2456
**Email:** jwakelyn@pen.k12.va.us
Jo Ann Wakelyn, Pres.

**Mem:** 35. **Desc:** State administrators and local supervisors of health occupations education. Acts as resource sharing group, particularly in the area of curriculum development. Seeks to develop shared resources for recruitment. **Pub:** *NASAHOE News*, quarterly. Newsletter. **Frmly:** (1988) National Association for State Administrators of Health Occupations Education.

★ **9757** ★ **National Council of State Pharmacy Association Executives (NCSPAE)**
c/o Rebecca Snead
Virginia Pharmacists Association
5501 Patterson Ave., No. 200
Richmond, VA 23226
**Phone:** (804)285-4145      **Fax:** (804)285-4227
**Email:** rrsnead@erols.com
**Website:** http://www.ncspae.org
Jo An Condie, Pres.

**Fnded:** 1927. **Mem:** 52. **State Groups:** 52. **Desc:** Professional society of the executive officers of state pharmacy associations. **Frmly:** (1964) National Conference of State Pharmaceutical Association Secretaries; (1992) National Council of State Pharmaceutical Association.

★ **9758** ★ **National Minority Health Association (NMHA)**
PO Box 11876
Harrisburg, PA 17108
**Free:** (866)347-9959      **Fax:** (717)232-9733
Dr. David Dalton, Chm.

**Fnded:** 1987. **Mem:** 53,000. **Reg. Groups:** 5. **State Groups:** 1. **Local Groups:** 50. **Desc:** Health care providers and associations, consumers, executives and administrators, educators, pharmaceutical and health insurance companies, and other corporations with an interest in health care. Seeks to identify and focus attention on the health needs of minorities. Promotes: more effective research in minority health issues; better training of health care practitioners; development of programs that encourage minorities to pursue careers in the health care industry and educate minority communities on the importance of good health. Initiates discussions with professional health organizations, academic institutions, state and federal governments, and health departments to develop strategies to improve the quality and availability of health care, health delivery systems, and health professionals to minority communities. Maintains speakers' bureau, conducts research and educational programs; sponsors children's programs; complies statistics. **Pub:** *The National Minority Health Association News*, quarterly.

★ **9759** ★ **National Renal Administrators Association (NRAA)**
1904 Naomi Pl.
Prescott, AZ 86303-5061
**Phone:** (928)717-2772      **Fax:** (928)441-3857
**Email:** nraa@nraa.org
**Website:** http://www.nraa.org
Michael Paget, Exec. Dir.

**Fnded:** 1977. **Mem:** 475. **Desc:** Administrative personnel involved with dialysis programs for patients suffering from kidney failure. Provides a vehicle for the development of educational and informational services for members. Maintains contact with health care facilities and government agencies. Operates placement service; compiles statistics; conducts political action committee. **Pub:** *NRAA Journal*, annual. Journal. Serves as an educational and informational resource for administrative personnel involved in the End Stage Renal Disease Program. *Price:* Free; $50 for nonmembers. • *Presidents Letter*, monthly. *Price:* Free to members; $10 nonmembers.

★ **9760** ★ **Professional Association of Health Care Office Management (PAHCOM)**
461 E Ten Mile Rd.
Pensacola, FL 32534
**Phone:** (850)474-9460      **Free:** 800-451-9311
**Fax:** (850)474-6352
**Email:** pahcom@pahcom.com
**Website:** http://www.pahcom.com
Rose Chambers, Contact

**Fnded:** 1988. **Mem:** 3,200. **Nat'l Groups:** 1. **Local Groups:** 40. **Desc:** Office managers of small group and solo medical practices. Operates certification program for health care office managers. **Pub:** *Compliance Program Guide.* Manual. • *Medical Law & Ethics.* Manual. • *Medical Office Management*, bimonthly. Newsletter. Provides current event information. *Price:* Free. For members only. • *Personnel Management.* Manual. • *Practice Enhancement.* Manual. • *Revenue Management.* Manual. **Frmly:** (2001) Professional Association of Health Care Office Managers.

★ **9761** ★ **PSRC of America**
200 Madison Ave., Ste. 2108
New York, NY 10016
**Phone:** (212)686-9147      **Fax:** (212)779-9307
**Email:** cwielk@psrc-of-america.org
**Website:** http://www.psrc-of-america.org
Carol A. Wielk, Exec. Dir.

**Fnded:** 1977. **Desc:** Physicians, nurses, health care administrators, and consumers. Monitors the quality, appropriateness, and cost of health care given to patients in hospitals, ambulatory clinics, nursing facilities, and physicians' offices. Carries out work on behalf of managed care companies, health care institutions and facilities, insurance carriers and governmental entities. **Pub:** *Informational Health Care Bulletin*, periodic. **Frmly:** (1999) Professional Standards Review Council of America.

## ★ 9762 ★ Radiology Business Management Association (RBMA)

65 Enterprise
Aliso Viejo, CA 92656
**Phone:** 888-224-RBMA                  **Fax:** (949)376-3456
**Email:** info@rbma.org
**Website:** http://www.rbma.org
Sharon Urch, Exec. Dir.

**Fnded:** 1968. **Mem:** 1,600. **Reg. Groups:** 4. **State Groups:** 50. **Local Groups:** 10. **Desc:** Business managers for private radiology groups; corporate members include: vendors of equipment, services, or supplies. Purposes are to improve business administration of radiologists' practices to better serve patients and the medical profession; and to provide opportunities for professional development and recognition. Offers extensive educational and networking opportunities and informal placement service. Maintains information services emphasizing those aspects unique to the business of radiology. **Pub:** *Radiology Business Management Association–Bulletin*, bimonthly. Newsletter. Covers organizational topics, industry trends, and legislative developments affecting the private practice of radiology; includes annual index. *Price:* Included in membership dues; $100/year for nonmembers. • *Radiology Business Management Association–HIPAA Bulletin*, monthly. Bulletin. A radiology resource for education, implementation and compliance. • *Radiology Business Management Association–Membership Directory*, annual. Membership Directory. **Frmly:** (1990) Radiologists Business Managers Association.

## ★ 9763 ★ Society of Medical Administrators (SMA)

c/o Dr. Ronald P. Kaufman
Montefiore Medical Center
111 E 210th St.
Bronx, NY 10467
**Phone:** (718)920-2001                  **Fax:** (718)652-2161
Dr. Spencer Foreman, Pres.

**Fnded:** 1920. **Mem:** 50. **Desc:** Medical doctors in hospital or health care administration. Discusses issues concerning health care administration. **Pub:** Directory, annual. • Also publishes minutes of the Annual Meeting. **Frmly:** (1951) Medical Superintendents Club.

## Society of Medical-Dental Management Consultants (SMD)

*See:* Entry 9995

## Society of Nursery Nursing (SNN)

*See:* Entry 5757

## ★ 9764 ★ Society for Radiation Oncology Administrators (SROA)

PO Box 51687
Albuquerque, NM 87181-1687
**Phone:** (505)571-9065                  **Free:** (866)458-7762
**Fax:** (505)298-5063
**Email:** sroa@asrt.org
**Website:** http://www.sroa.org/
Robyn Blatter, Sec.

**Fnded:** 1984. **Mem:** 500. **Desc:** Individuals with managerial responsibilities in radiation oncology at the executive, divisional, or departmental level, and whose functions include personnel, budget, and development of operational procedures and guidelines for therapeutic radiology departments. Strives to improve the administration of the business and nonmedical management aspects of therapeutic radiology, to promote the field of therapeutic radiology administration, to provide a forum for communication among members, and to disseminate information among members. Maintains speakers' bureau; offers placement service. **Pub:** *SROA Membership Directory*, annual. Membership Directory. *Price:* Included in membership dues. • *SROA Newsletter*, quarterly. Newsletter. Includes calendar of events and employment listings. *Price:* Included in membership dues; $50 for non-members in

U.S.; $60 for non-members outside U.S. **Frmly:** (1985) Radiation Oncology Administrators.

## ★ 9765 ★ Women in Managed Care (WMC)

4435 Waterfront Dr., Ste. 101
PO Box 6026
Glen Allen, VA 23058-6026
**Phone:** (804)527-1905                  **Fax:** (804)747-5316
**Email:** info@wimc.org
**Website:** http://www.wimc.org
Laura Bousquet, Exec. Dir.

**Fnded:** 1996. **Mem:** 1,000. **Desc:** Women working for managed care health services providers. Promotes professional advancement of members. Conducts research and educational programs. **Pub:** *Women in Managed Care*, monthly. Newsletter.

---

# Research Centers

## ★ 9766 ★ Academy for Health Services Research and Health Policy

1801 K St. NW, Ste. 701
Washington, DC 20006
**Phone:** (202)292-6700                  **Fax:** (202)292-6800
**Email:** info@ahsrhp.org
**Website:** http://www.academyhealth.org
David Helms, Pres. /CEO

**Activities/Fields:** Healthcare services and policy, focusing on education, improvements, cooperation, funding, and development and implementation of national and state legislative and administrative policies. **Pub:** *Academy reports.* • *Connection: A Newsletter Linking the Users and Producers of Drug Abuse Services Research.* • *Forum: Translating Research into Quality Health Care for Veterans.* • *Frontlines: Linking Alcohol Services Research and Practice.* • *HCFO Findings Briefs.* • *HCFO News & Progress.* • *Issue briefs.* • *National Health Care Purchasing Institute Newsletters, briefs.* • *State Coverage Initiatives Newsletter.*

## ★ 9767 ★ American Academy of Pediatrics
### Division of Health Policy Research

141 NW Point Blvd.
Elk Grove Village, IL 60009-0927
**Phone:** (847)434-7627                  **Fax:** (847)228-9651
**Email:** hlthpoly@aap.org
**Website:** http://www.aap.org
Beth K. Yudkowsky, Dir.

**Activities/Fields:** Organization, financing, and delivery of child health care, including studies on third-party payment programs, health care for low-income and high-risk children, office practices, the distribution of pediatricians, evaluations of pediatric programs, health workforce, and practice parameters/guidelines development. **Pub:** *Newsletter.* **Frmly:** Department of Research.

## ★ 9768 ★ American Medical Association Center for Health Policy Research

515 N State St.
Chicago, IL 60610
**Phone:** (312)464-5387                  **Fax:** (312)464-5849
**Email:** david_emmons@ama-assn.org
**Website:** http://www.ama-assn.org
David W. Emmons, PhD, Dir.

**Activities/Fields:** Physician practice arrangements, medical practice costs and revenues, physician workforce, competitiveness of insurance markets, health system reform, and access to care. **Pub:** *Physician Marketplace Statistics*, annually. • *Socioeconomic Characteristics of Medical Practice*, annually.

## ★ 9769 ★ Baylor College of Medicine Center for Medical Ethics and Health Policy

1 Baylor Plz.
Houston, TX 77030
**Phone:** (713)798-6290                  **Fax:** (713)798-5678
**Email:** bbrody@bcm.tmc.edu
Dr. Baruch Brody, Dir.

**Activities/Fields:** Priorities for health care services, methods of funding health care services, and social controls on health care service, including studies on ethics in clinical decision making and value issues in controlling the cost of medicine. **Pub:** *News Bulletin*, semimonthly.

## ★ 9770 ★ Brandeis University Schneider Institute for Health Policy

Mail Stop 035
Heller School for Social Policy and Management
PO Box 549110
Waltham, MA 02454-9110
**Phone:** (781)736-3900                  **Fax:** (781)736-3928
**Email:** wallack2@brandeis.edu
**Website:** http://www.heller.brandeis.edu/sihp.asp
Stanley S. Wallack, PhD, Exec. Dir.

**Activities/Fields:** Health services research and policy analysis, focusing on the design, development, implementation, and evaluation of innovative financing and delivery systems. Specific areas of research include establishing and implementing national health care expenditure limits, all-payer payment systems, an Alcohol and Drug Services Survey, the changing trends of substance abuse, financing and reimbursement of drug abuse treatment programs, and long-term care for the elderly, including home care services for the disabled elderly and cost effective models and standards for assisted living. Operates the Center for Health Policy Analysis and Research; Health Policy Center; Bigel Institute for Health Policy.

## ★ 9771 ★ Center for Research on Services for Severe Mental Illness

Hampton House
624 N Broadway, No. 482
Baltimore, MD 21205-1996
**Phone:** (410)955-3625                  **Fax:** (410)614-9152
**Email:** dsteinwa@jhsph.edu
**Website:** http://www.jhsph.edu/~c-smi
Dr. Donald M. Steinwachs, Dir.

**Activities/Fields:** Issues of organization and finance of services for persons with severe mental illnesses (SMI) and their impact on utilization, quality of care, patient outcomes, and costs. The goals of the Center are to develop further, refine and validate methods (including quality of care criteria) to assure the appropriate match between patient needs and services that can lead to the best outcomes for persons with SMI, and to develop guidelines for the financing and organization of care that meet cost and effectiveness criteria and that take into account variations in patient needs, available resources, and community, social support, and family characteristics. The specific aims of the center are directed at four policy relevant areas; (1) to assess the impact of the course of severe mental illnesses, and their associated problems, on service needs and patterns of treatment; (2) to assess the effectiveness and costs of alternative treatment approaches for persons with SMI which are based on treatment models with established efficacy or accepted practice, and develop and test quality of care criteria for matching treatment needs to services for patients with severe mental illnesses; (3) to examine the role of financing mechanisms as a means to encourage efficiency, assure access to appropriate care for the SMI, and provide incentives for enhancing patient outcomes, including dimensions of mental status, physical status, adequacy of living arrangements, and quality of life; and (4) to examine alternative organizational and system approaches for managing resources, coordinating services to persons with SMI, and evaluating their impact on utilization, housing, general medical care, and resources including income support and payment for treatment and related services. **Frmly:** Center on the Organization and Financing of Care for the Severely Mentally Ill.

★ **9772** ★ **Columbia University**
**Center for the Study of Society and**
**Medicine**
College of Physicians & Surgeons
630 W 168th St.
New York, NY 10032
**Phone:** (212)305-4184          **Fax:** (212)305-6416
**Email:** jc1466@columbia.edu
**Website:** http://www.societyandmedicine.org
Dr. David J. Rothman, Dir.

**Activities/Fields:** Issues that arise in clinical and research settings, including studies in bioethics and health policy, bioethics and medical decision-making, social policy, analyses of the social history of patient-hood.

★ **9773** ★ **Connecticut Hospital**
**Association**
110 Barnes Rd.
PO Box 90
Wallingford, CT 06492-0090
**Phone:** (203)265-7611          **Fax:** (203)284-9318
**Website:** http://www.chime.org
Jennifer Jackson, Pres.

**Activities/Fields:** Hospital industry, including hospital administration, manpower development and training, quality of care, shared services and facilities, financial reimbursement, ancillary service utilization, and mental health planning.

★ **9774** ★ **Dartmouth College**
**Center for Evaluative Clinical Sciences**
Dartmouth Medical Sch.
7251 Strasenburgh
Hanover, NH 03755-3863
**Phone:** (603)650-1684          **Fax:** (603)650-1225
**Website:** http://www.dartmouth.edu/dms/cecs/
John E. Wennberg, Dir.

**Activities/Fields:** Evaluative clinical science and health care delivery, including medical care epidemiology, health policy, health behavior, efficacy of medical procedures, quality of medical and surgical care, distribution of health care resources, medical interventions and consequences for patients, care at the end of life, distribution of health care resources across hospital market areas, geriatric health, and sociology of medical organizations.

★ **9775** ★ **Harvard University**
**Center for Quality of Care Research and**
**Education (QCARE)**
677 Huntington Ave.
Boston, MA 02115
**Phone:** (617)432-2027          **Fax:** (617)432-3199
**Email:** qcare@hsph.harvard.edu
**Website:** http://www.hsph.harvard.edu/qcare
Dr. R. Heather Palmer, Dir.

**Activities/Fields:** Clinical performance measures for application in a wide range of health care delivery settings.

★ **9776** ★ **Harvard University**
**Division of Health Policy Research and**
**Education**
180 Longwood Ave.
Boston, MA 02115
**Phone:** (617)432-1325          **Fax:** (617)432-0173
**Email:** newhouse@hcp.med.harvard.edu
Dr. Joseph Newhouse, Dir.

**Activities/Fields:** Coordinates health policy resources throughout the University, including suggestion of new research initiatives, stimulation of educational activities, coordination of research and educational efforts, promotion of multidisciplinary analysis of complex health policy issues, and dissemination of health policy findings. **Pub:** *Annual Report.*

★ **9777** ★ **The Institute for Rehabilitation**
**and Research**
**Independent Living Research Utilization**
**(ILRU)**
2323 S Shepherd, Ste. 1000
Houston, TX 77019
**Phone:** (713)520-0232          **Fax:** (713)520-5785
**Email:** ilru@ilru.org
**Website:** http://www.ilru.org/ilru-projects_2.html
Lex Frieden, PhD, Dir.

**Activities/Fields:** Strategies for developing and implementing techniques for providing high quality consumer-directed services; addressing the independent living needs of persons who may be unserved or under-served because of barriers related to culture, language, disability type, geographic locale, or other distinguishing factors; and preparing individuals to work in independent living service and advocacy settings. **Pub:** *Monographs.* ● *Newsletter*, bimonthly. ● *Technical report series.*

★ **9778** ★ **Johns Hopkins University**
**Health Services Research and**
**Development Center**
624 N Broadway, Rm. 482
Baltimore, MD 21205-1996
**Phone:** (410)955-3625          **Fax:** (410)955-0470
**Email:** dsteinwa@jhsph.edu
Dr. Donald M. Steinwachs, Dir.

**Activities/Fields:** Conducts health services research, including studies on the following: determinants of health outcomes; the impacts of alternative health care systems on cost and quality; effective strategies for health promotion and disease prevention; and methods of meeting the needs of high risk populations such as the poor, elderly, mentally ill, disabled, and children. Research is conducted using experimental (randomized controlled trials) or nonexperimental methods, and relies to varying degrees on primary data sources obtained through interviews and observation and secondary data sources obtained from management information systems, financial reports, and existing regional and national data sources and surveys.

★ **9779** ★ **McMaster University**
**Centre for Health Economics and Policy**
**Analysis (CHEPA)**
Facility of Health Sciences
1200 Main St. W
Hamilton, ON, Canada L8N 3Z5
**Phone:** (905)525-9140          **Fax:** (905)546-5211
**Email:** chepa@fhs.mcmaster.ca
Brian Hutchison, Actg. Dir.

**Activities/Fields:** Health economics and health policy analysis, including organization, funding, and delivery of health care; the evaluation of health care programs and technologies; the measurement of health at the individual and population level; the determinants of population health; and the processes of health policy making. **Pub:** *CHSPA Working Papers Series*, quarterly.

★ **9780** ★ **Medical College of Wisconsin**
**Health Policy Institute (HPI)**
8701 Watertown Plank Rd.
Milwaukee, WI 53226
**Phone:** (414)456-8762          **Fax:** (414)456-6529
**Website:** http://www.mcw.edu/html/body_ov_-hpi.html
Dr. Richard A. Cooper, Dir.

**Activities/Fields:** Health care policies and issues, including bioethics, health services, epidemiology, and biostatistics.

★ **9781** ★ **MGMA Center for Research**
104 Inverness Ter. E
Englewood, CO 80112-5306
**Phone:** (303)397-7879          **Fax:** (303)397-1827
**Email:** npiland@mgma.com
**Website:** http://www.mgma.com/research
Dr. Neill F. Piland, Res. Dir.

**Activities/Fields:** Health services, health economics, patient safety, new management technologies, tools for effective and efficient administration of healthcare organizations, and outcomes research. **Pub:** *Medical Group Management Journal*, bimonthly. **Frmly:** Center for Research in Ambulatory Health Care Administration.

★ **9782** ★ **Northwestern University**
**Institute for Health Services Research**
**and Policy Studies**
629 Noyes St.
Evanston, IL 60208-4170
**Phone:** (847)491-5643          **Fax:** (847)491-2202
**Email:** ihsrps@northwestern.edu
**Website:** http://www.northwestern.edu/ihsrps
Dr. Peter P. Budetti, Dir.

**Activities/Fields:** Health services research and policy analysis focusing on the relationship between health care delivery systems and health outcomes, health economics, organization behavior in health, competition in the delivery of health services, physician and institutional incentives. **Pub:** *Working paper series.*

★ **9783** ★ **Pacific Institute for Research**
**and Evaluation**
**Decision Sciences Institute**
120 Wayland Ave., Ste. 7
Providence, RI 02906
**Phone:** (401)751-1314          **Fax:** (401)751-1592
**Email:** dwight@pire.org
**Website:** http://www.pire.org/centers/DSI.htm
Pamela Dwight, Contact

**Activities/Fields:** Decision-making in areas such as long-term cost-effectiveness of alcohol treatment, impact of addictions and mental health treatment on general medical care, and managed care.

★ **9784** ★ **Rockburn Institute**
6581 Belmont Woods Rd.
Elkridge, MD 21075
**Phone:** (410)796-4554          **Fax:** (410)796-3173
Dale N. Schumacher, MD, Pres.

**Activities/Fields:** Health care services and effective and efficient management of health care institutions.

★ **9785** ★ **Rush University**
**Center for Health Management Studies**
Rush-Presbyterian-St. Luke's Medical Center
1653 W Congress Pky.
Chicago, IL 60612-3833
**Phone:** (312)942-5402          **Fax:** (312)942-4957
**Email:** gglandon@rushu.rush.edu
**Website:** http://www.rushu.rush.edu
Gerald Glandon, Dir.

**Activities/Fields:** Health care organizations, including studies in organization and administration, organizational behavior, research design and statistics, cost containment, health economics, health care financial management, quantitative methods and epidemiology, long-term care, and information systems. **Pub:** *Annual Report.* ● *Working Paper Series*, semiannually.

★ **9786** ★ **Tulane University**
**Center for International Resource**
**Development**
Sch. of Public Health & Tropical Medicine
1440 Canal St., Ste. 2200
New Orleans, LA 70112
**Phone:** (504)584-3655          **Fax:** (504)584-3653
**Email:** mock@mailhost.tcs.tulane.edu
**Website:** http://www.tulane.edu/~inhl/inhl.htm
Dr. Nancy Mock, Dir.

**Activities/Fields:** Research and evaluation of international health and development. Center conducts family planning and reproductive health projects in Africa and South and Central America, nutritional epidemiology, family planning impact evaluations worldwide, and health and human resources analysis for Africa.

**★ 9787 ★ University of Alabama at Birmingham**
**Lister Hill Center for Health Policy**
330 Ryals Public Health Bldg.
1665 University Blvd.
Birmingham, AL 35294-0022
**Phone:** (205)975-8966      **Fax:** (205)934-3347
**Email:** morrisey@uab.edu
**Website:** http://www.healthpolicy.uab.edu
Michael A. Morrisey, PhD, Dir.

**Activities/Fields:** Health policy research, focusing on health care markets and managed care, maternal and child health, management in public health organizations, aging policy, and outcomes research. **Pub:** *Health Policy Abstract*, 10/year.

**★ 9788 ★ University of California, San Francisco**
**Institute for Health Policy Studies**
3333 California St., Ste. 265
San Francisco, CA 94143-0936
**Phone:** (415)476-4921      **Fax:** (415)476-0705
**Email:** hluft@itsa.ucsf.edu
**Website:** http://ihps.ucsf.edu
Harold S. Luft, Dir.

**Activities/Fields:** Health policy and health services.

**★ 9789 ★ University of Cincinnati**
**Institute for Health Policy and Health Services Research (IHPHSR)**
Mail Location 0840
University of Cincinnati Medical Center
French Bldg. East, Ste. 275
Cincinnati, OH 45267-0840
**Phone:** (513)558-2756      **Fax:** (513)558-2744
**Email:** alfred.tuchfarber@uc.edu
**Website:** http://www.ihphsr.uc.edu
Dr. Alfred Tuchfarber, Dir.

**Activities/Fields:** Health policy and health services, especially cost effectiveness and outcomes.

**★ 9790 ★ University of Cincinnati**
**Institute for Health Policy and Health Services Research**
**Center for Clinical Effectiveness**
University of Cincinnati Medical Center
202 Goodman Dr., Ste. 275
Cincinnati, OH 45267-0840
**Phone:** (513)558-2756      **Fax:** (513)558-2744
**Email:** alfred.tuchfarber@uc.edu
Dr. Alfred Tuchfarber, Dir.

**Activities/Fields:** Health-related quality of life, cost effectiveness of diagnostic and treatment strategies, pharmacoeconomics, outcomes, and severity of illness.

**★ 9791 ★ University of Colorado—Denver**
**Center for Human Investment Policy**
1445 Market St., Ste. 350
Denver, CO 80202
**Phone:** (303)820-5631      **Fax:** (303)820-5656
**Email:** jbasso@carbon.cudenver.edu
Donna Garnett, Proj. Dir.

**Activities/Fields:** Ethical and policy issues in health care, including health care for the medically indigent, cost of care, rural health care, medical malpractice costs, prenatal care, public health, euthanasia, and the role of public opinion in policy formation. **Pub:** *Front-Lines*.

**★ 9792 ★ University of Florida**
**Institute for Health Policy Research**
Health Science Center
JHMHC PO Box 100177
Gainesville, FL 32610-0177
**Phone:** (352)265-8035      **Fax:** (352)265-8047
**Email:** admin@hpe.ufl.edu
**Website:** http://www.hpe.ufl.edu
Prof. Michael K. Miller, Dir.

**Activities/Fields:** Policy research and evaluations of long-term care and aging, hospital cost controls, regulatory and administrative methods in the health sector, health economics and financing, maternal and child health, HIV/AIDS, community epidemiology, outcomes research.

**★ 9793 ★ University of Iowa**
**Public Policy Center**
**Health Policy Research Program**
212 South Quadrangle
Iowa City, IA 52242-1192
**Phone:** (319)335-6813      **Fax:** (319)335-6801
**Email:** peter-damiano@uiowa.edu
**Website:** http://www.uiowa.edu/~ppc/hlth.html
Peter C. Damiano, Dir.

**Activities/Fields:** Effects of policy initiatives and government activities on the cost, access, and quality of health care.

**★ 9794 ★ University of Kentucky**
**Center for Excellence in Rural Health**
100 Airport Gardens Rd., Ste. 10
Hazard, KY 41701-9500
**Phone:** (606)439-3557      **Fax:** (606)436-8833
**Email:** ltkepfe@pop.uky.edu
**Website:** http://www.mc.uky.edu/ruralhealth
Loyd Kepferle, Dir.

**Activities/Fields:** Rural health in Kentucky, focusing on health manpower needs, health care delivery, health care policy, and health problems unique to rural populations. Specific areas of study include assessments of new health policy, legislation, and regulation and their impact on rural health delivery, health problems among rural low-income persons and rural population needs in the areas of mental health, substance abuse and prevention. Policy oriented studies include surveys of local attitudes and perceptions of health care, rural and small hospitals, longitudinal study on the impact of rural-based health professions education, and health professionals distribution; and a survey of small businesses in Kentucky and their experiences with health insurance; a survey of physicians and midwives to determine the nature, scope, and future of obstetrical practice; and a household health survey of health needs, perceptions of health status and the health care system, and functional status of the elderly. Participatory action research being conducted in 16 countries which revolves around stimulating rural economics by increasing local health services utilization. **Pub:** *Rural Health Initiative*. Newsletter.

**★ 9795 ★ University of Memphis**
**Center for Health Services Research**
119 Mccord Hall
Division of Health Administration
Memphis, TN 38152
**Phone:** (901)678-2794      **Fax:** (901)678-2981
**Email:** peftzgrl@memphis.edu
Dr. Paul Fitzgerald, Dir.

**Activities/Fields:** Health services research, including health administration, health utilization and access, health finance, health policy and law, guardianship, medical malpractice, mental health policy and law, health ethics, research methodology in health services research, and health decision making.

**★ 9796 ★ University of Minnesota**
**Division of Health Services Research and Policy**
Box 729
Mayo Memorial Bldg.
Minneapolis, MN 55455
**Phone:** (612)624-6151      **Fax:** (612)624-2196
**Email:** foote003@tc.umn.edu
Susan Bartlett Foote, Div. Hd.

**Activities/Fields:** Long-term care, health insurance, managed health care, patient care outcomes, rural health services, and health policy analysis. **Pub:** *Institute News*, 3/year. • *Research brief*, monthly. **Frmly:** Institute for Health Services Research.

**★ 9797 ★ University of Pennsylvania**
**Center for Health Outcomes and Policy Research**
School of Nursing
Nursing Education Bldg.
420 Guardian Dr., Fl. 3R
Philadelphia, PA 19104-6096
**Phone:** (215)898-5673      **Fax:** (215)573-2062
**Email:** laiken@nursing.upenn.edu
**Website:** http://www.nursing.upenn.edu/chopr/
Linda H. Aiken, Dir.

**Activities/Fields:** Health care and workforce organization, financing, and outcomes; and public policies that influence nursing and health care delivery nationally and internationally.

**★ 9798 ★ University of Texas—Houston**
**Health Science Center**
**Center for Health Policy Studies (CHAMPS)**
1200 Herman Pressler, Ste. E-735
Houston, TX 77025
**Phone:** (713)500-9390      **Fax:** (713)500-9359
**Website:** http://www.sph.uth.tmc.edu:8052/champs/champs.html
Frank I. Moore, PhD, Dir.

**Activities/Fields:** Health policy options and program effects, including community health needs assessments in metropolitan counties and underserved regions of Texas; studies concerned with health expenditures and with supply and distribution of the health professions workforce in Texas; program evaluations of teen pregnancy prevention, managed care and community-oriented primary care programs; public health internships in the Lower Rio Grande Valley; and health workforce development in third world countries.

**★ 9799 ★ University of Texas—Houston**
**Health Science Center**
**Health Policy Institute**
1200 Hermann Pressler, Ste. 901
PO Box 20186
Houston, TX 77225
**Phone:** (713)500-9485      **Fax:** (713)500-9493
**Email:** david.low@uth.tmc.edu
Dr. M. David Low, Dir.

**Activities/Fields:** Health policy issues at the local, state, national, and international level, including cost, access, quality of health care, and the social ecology of health. **Pub:** *Discussion Papers*, occasionally.

**★ 9800 ★ University of Washington**
**Western Network for Education in Health Administration**
**Center for Health Management Research**
Seattle, WA 98105

**Activities/Fields:** New ways to organize and manage patient care, physical-organization relations, and implementation of new approaches to managing quality.

**★ 9801 ★ University of Waterloo**
**Centre for Applied Health Research**
Faculty of Applied Health Science
Burt Matthews Hall
Waterloo, ON, Canada N2L 3G1
**Phone:** (519)888-4567      **Fax:** (519)746-6776
**Email:** deanahs@healthy.uwaterloo.ca
**Website:** http://www.ahs.uwaterloo.ca
Dr. Michael Sharratt, Dean

**Activities/Fields:** Research conducted through several centers: Murray Alzheimer Research and Education Program; Health Behaviour Research Group; Functional Independence for Seniors; Program Training and Consultation Centre; and Ergonomics and Safety Consulting Services. **Pub:** *CAHR News*.

**★ 9802 ★ University of Wisconsin— Madison**
**Center for Health Systems Research and Analysis**
WARF Bldg., Rm. 1163
610 Walnut St.
Madison, WI 53705-2397
**Phone:** (608)263-5722   **Fax:** (608)263-4523
**Email:** david_zimmerman@chsra.wic.edu
**Website:** http://www.chsra.wisc.edu
Dr. David R. Zimmerman, Dir.
**Activities/Fields:** Five major research areas: quality assessment and improvement, long term care, public health policy and program evaluation, consumer decision making, and patient education and support.

**★ 9803 ★ West Virginia University**
**Office of Health Services Research**
Health Science Center
PO Box 9190
Morgantown, WV 26506-9190
**Phone:** (304)293-2601   **Fax:** (304)293-6685
**Email:** cpollard@hsc.wvu.edu
Cecil Pollard, Dir.
**Activities/Fields:** Health services research, manpower studies, resource allocation, demography, and computer technology support. **Pub:** *Newsletter*, quarterly.

# State Government Agencies

## Health Planning & Development

**★ 9804 ★ Alabama Health Planning and Development Agency**
100 N Union St, Ste. 870
PO Box 303025
Montgomery, AL 36130-3025
**Phone:** (334)242-4103   **Fax:** (334)242-4113
**Email:** info@shpda.state.al.us
**Website:** http://shpda.state.al.us/

**★ 9805 ★ Arizona Department of Health Services**
**Planning Office**
1740 W Adams St.
Phoenix, AZ 85007
**Phone:** (602)542-1000   **Fax:** (602)542-1062
**Website:** http://www.hs.state.az.us/

**★ 9806 ★ Arkansas Department of Health**
**Planning Bureau**
4815 W Markham
Little Rock, AR 72205
**Phone:** (501)661-2238   **Fax:** (501)661-2414
**Website:** http://health.state.ar.us

**★ 9807 ★ California Health and Welfare Agency**
**Statewide Health Planning and Development Office**
1600 9th St., Ste. 435
Sacramento, CA 95814
**Phone:** (916)654-1499   **Fax:** (916)653-2854
**Website:** http://www.oshpd.cahwnet.gov/

**★ 9808 ★ Colorado Department of Human Services**
**Health Care Policy and Financing Division**
**Health Plans Operations**
1575 Sherman St.
Denver, CO 80203-1714
**Phone:** (303)866-2993   **Fax:** (303)866-4411
**Email:** diane.rodriguez@state.co.us
**Website:** http://www.chcpf.state.co.us/index.html
Karen Reinertson, Contact

**★ 9809 ★ Connecticut Department of Public Health**
**Policy, Planning, and Evaluation Office**
**Health Information Systems**
410 Capitol Ave.
PO Box 340308
Hartford, CT 06134-0308
**Phone:** (860)509-7163   **Fax:** (860)509-7160
**Email:** webmaster.dph@po.state.ct.us
**Website:** http://www.state.ct.us/dph/OPPE/hphis.htm
Daniel J. Saviano, Director

**★ 9810 ★ Delaware Department of Health and Social Services**
**Management Services Division**
1901 N DuPont Hwy.
New Castle, DE 19720
**Phone:** (302)577-4515   **Fax:** (302)577-4539
**Email:** dhssinfo@state.de.us
**Website:**   http://www.state.de.us/dhss/dms/dmshome.htm
Valencia L. Beaty, Director

**★ 9811 ★ Florida Agency Health Care Administration**
Fort Knox Executive Center, Bldg. 3
2727 Mahan Dr.
Tallahassee, FL 32308-5407
**Free:** 888-419-3456
**Email:** ahca@fdhc.state.fl.us
**Website:** http://www.fdhc.state.fl.us/

**★ 9812 ★ Georgia Department of Community Health**
**Division of Health Planning**
2 Peachtree St. NW
Atlanta, GA 30303
**Phone:** (404)656-0655   **Fax:** (404)656-0654
**Website:** http://www.communityhealth.state.ga.us/
Valerie Hepburn, Contact

**★ 9813 ★ Hawaii Department of Health**
**Hawaii State Health Planning and Development Agency**
1177 Alakea St. Rm.402
Honolulu, HI 96813
**Phone:** (808)587-0788   **Fax:** (808)587-0783
**Email:** shpda@health.state.hi.us
**Website:** http://www.state.hi.us/health/shpda/

**★ 9814 ★ Idaho Department of Health and Welfare**
**Bureau of Vital Records and Health Statistics**
450 W State St.
PO Box 83720
Boise, ID 83720-0036
**Phone:** (208)334-5976   **Free:** 800-926-2588
**Fax:** (208)334-6558
**Website:** http://www2.state.id.us/dhw/index.htm
Jane Smith, Contact

**★ 9815 ★ Illinois Department of Public Health**
**Epidemiology and Health Systems Development Office**
525 W Jefferson St., 2nd Fl.
Springfield, IL 62761
**Phone:** (217)785-2040   **Fax:** (217)785-4308
**Email:** mrichard@idph.state.il.us
**Website:**   http://www.idph.state.il.us/about/epistudies.htm
Margaret Richards, PhD, Contact

**★ 9816 ★ Indiana Department of Health**
**Health and Planning Division**
2 N Meridian St.
Indianapolis, IN 46204
**Phone:** (317)233-1325
**Website:** http://www.state.in.us/isdh/

**★ 9817 ★ Iowa Department of Public Health**
**Division of Administration and Regulatory Affairs**
Lucas State Office Bldg.
321 E 12th St.
Des Moines, IA 50319-0075
**Phone:** (515)281-5787
**Email:** webmaster@idph.state.ia.us
**Website:** http://www.idph.state.ia.us/ar.htm
David Fries, Contact

**★ 9818 ★ Kansas Department of Health and Environment**
**Health Division**
Charles Curtis State Office Bldg.
1000 SW Jackson, suite 300
Topeka, KS 66612-1365
**Phone:** (785)296-1343   **Fax:** (785)296-1562
**Email:** info@kdhe.state.ks.us
**Website:** http://www.kdhe.state.ks.us/health/
J. Michael Moser, MD, Director

**★ 9819 ★ Kentucky Families and Children Cabinet**
**Health Planning and Certification Office**
275 E Main St.
Frankfort, KY 40621
**Phone:** (502)564-7130   **Fax:** (502)564-3866
**Email:** dean.crawford@mail.state.ky.us
**Website:** http://cfc.state.ky.us/

**★ 9820 ★ Louisiana Department of Health and Hospitals**
**Division of Community Health**
**Health Resources Management Bureau**
1201 Capitol Access Rd.
PO Box 629
Baton Rouge, LA 70821-0629
**Phone:** (504)342-9513   **Fax:** (504)342-8098
**Email:** ophweb@.dhh.state.la.us
**Website:** http://www.dhh.state.la.us/OPH/resmgt.htm

**★ 9821 ★ Maryland Department of Health and Mental Hygiene**
**Health Care Commission**
4201 Patterson Ave., 5th Fl.
Baltimore, MD 21215
**Phone:** (410)764-3460   **Free:** 877-245-1762
**Fax:** (410)358-1236
**Email:** webmaster@mhcc.state.md.us
**Website:** http://www.mhcc.state.md.us/
Barbara McLean, Director

**★ 9822 ★ Massachusetts Executive Office of Health and Human Services**
**Public Health Department**
**Policy and Planning Office**
250 Washington St.
Boston, MA 02108-4619
**Phone:** (617)624-6000
**Email:** dph.info@state.ma.us
**Website:** http://www.state.ma.us/dph/dphhome.htm

**★ 9823 ★ Michigan Community Health Department**
**Policy and Legal Affairs**
**Health Legislation and Policy Development**
Lewis Cass Bldg., 6th Fl.
320 S Walnut St.
Lansing, MI 48913
**Phone:** (517)373-3500
**Email:** arias@.mi.gov
**Website:** http://www.mdch.state.mi.us/
Carol Isaacs, Contact

**★ 9824 ★ Mississippi Department of Health**
**Health Regulation Office**
**Health Planning and Resource Development Division**
PO Box 1700
570 Woodrow Wilson Blvd.
Jackson, MS 39215-1700
**Phone:** (601)576-7874          **Fax:** (601)576-7530
**Email:** harmstrong@msdh.state.ms.us
**Website:** http://www.msdh.state.ms.us/planning/index.htm

**★ 9825 ★ Missouri Department of Health and Senior Services**
**Director's Office**
920 Wildwood Dr.
PO Box 570
Jefferson City, MO 65102
**Phone:** (573)751-6001          **Fax:** (573)751-6041
**Email:** info@mail.health.state.mo.us
**Website:** http://www.health.state.mo.us/AbouttheDepartment/DS3.html

**★ 9826 ★ Montana Department of Public Health and Human Services**
**Health Policy and Services Division**
1400 Broadway
PO Box 202951
Helena, MT 59620
**Phone:** (406)444-4540          **Fax:** (406)444-1861
**Email:** dphhstech@state.mt.gov
**Website:** http://www.dphhs.state.mt.us/divisions/hps/hps_phone.htm
Maggie Bullock, Contact

**★ 9827 ★ Nebraska Department of Health and Human Services**
**Health Policy and Service Planning**
PO Box 95007
301 Centennial Mall S
Lincoln, NE 68509
**Phone:** (402)471-9433          **Free:** 800-254-4202
**Fax:** (402)471-9449
**Email:** hhsinfo@www.hhs.state.ne.us
**Website:** http://www.hhs.state.ne.us/poc/pocindex.htm
Chris Peterson, Contact

**★ 9828 ★ Nevada Department of Human Resources**
**Health Division**
**Health Planning Bureau**
505 E King St., Rm. 102
Carson City, NV 89701
**Phone:** (775)684-4218          **Fax:** (775)684-4156
**Email:** oitsupport@nvhd.state.nv.us
**Website:** http://www.state.nv.us/health/

**★ 9829 ★ New Hampshire Department of Health and Human Services**
**Public Health Services Division**
**Health Services Planning and Review Bureau**
129 Pleasant St.
Concord, NH 03301

**Phone:** (603)271-4606          **Fax:** (603)271-4141
**Website:** http://www.dhhs.state.nh.us

**★ 9830 ★ New Jersey Department of Health**
**Health Care Systems Analysis Division**
John Fitch Plaza
PO Box 360
Trenton, NJ 08625-0360
**Phone:** (609)984-3939
**Website:** www.state.nj.us/health/hcsa/hcsadmin.htm
Marilyn Dahl, Contact

**★ 9831 ★ New Mexico Health Policy Commission**
2055 S Pacheco St., Ste. 200
Santa Fe, NM 87505
**Phone:** (505)424-3200
**Email:** hpcwebteam@hpc.state.nm.us
**Website:** http://hpc.state.nm.us/

**★ 9832 ★ North Carolina Department of Health and Human Services**
**Facility Services Division**
**State Medical Facilities Planning Section**
701 Barbour Dr.
2714 Mail Service Ctr.
Raleigh, NC 27699-2714
**Phone:** (919)855-3865          **Fax:** (919)715-4413
**Website:** http://facility-services.state.nc.us/planpage.htm

**★ 9833 ★ North Dakota Department of Health**
**Administrative Services Section**
**Health Information Systems Division**
600 E Boulevard Ave.
Bismarck, ND 58505-0200
**Phone:** (701)328-2392          **Fax:** (701)328-4727
**Website:** http://www.health.state.nd.us/ndhd/admin/index.htm
Arvy Smith, Contact

**★ 9834 ★ The Office for Oregon Health Plan Policy and Research**
255 Capitol St. NE, 5th Fl.
Salem, OR 97310
**Phone:** (503)378-2422          **Free:** 800-359-9517
**Fax:** (503)378-5511
**Email:** dhr.info@state.or.us
**Website:** http://www.ohppr.state.or.us
John Santa, MD, Director

**★ 9835 ★ Oklahoma Department of Health**
**Health Promotion and Policy Analysis Office**
**Health Planning**
1000 NE 10th St., Rm. 1106
Oklahoma City, OK 73117
**Phone:** (405)271-1685
**Email:** philiph@health.state.ok.us
**Website:** http://www.health.state.ok.us/PROGRAM/planning/index.html

**★ 9836 ★ Pennsylvania Department of Health**
**Quality Assurance**
**Health Care Financing Bureau**
PO Box 90
Health and Welfare Bldg.
Harrisburg, PA 17108
**Phone:** (717)787-5193          **Free:** 888-466-2787
**Fax:** (717)705-0947
**Email:** webmaster@health.state.pa.us
**Website:** http://www.health.state.pa.us/QA/HMO/default.htm

**★ 9837 ★ South Carolina Environmental Control**
**State Health Plan**
2600 Bull St.
Columbia, SC 29201
**Phone:** (803)898-3432
**Email:** WhitesAN@Columb54.dhec.state.sc.us
**Website:** http://www.scdhec.net/Health_Reg/hrshp.htm

**★ 9838 ★ South Dakota Department of Health**
**Policy and External Affairs Office**
600 E Capitol
Pierre, SD 57501-2536
**Phone:** (605)773-3361          **Free:** 800-738-2301
**Email:** DOH.INFO@state.sd.us
**Website:** http://www.state.sd.us/doh/
Doneen Hollingsworth, Contact

**★ 9839 ★ State Health Planning and Development Agency**
825 N Capitol St. NE
Washington, DC 20002
**Phone:** (202)442-5875
**Website:** http://www.dchealth.com/shpda

**★ 9840 ★ Tennessee Department of Health**
**TennCare**
729 Church St.
Nashville, TN 37243
**Phone:** (615)532-7542          **Free:** 800-669-1851
**Fax:** (615)741-0213
**Email:** ssharpe@mail.state.tn.us
**Website:** http://www.state.tn.us/tenncare
Mark Reynolds, Director

**★ 9841 ★ Texas Department of Health**
**Health Data and Policy Analysis Bureau**
1100 W 49th St.
Austin, TX 78756-3199
**Phone:** (512)458-7111          **Free:** 888-963-7111
**Website:** http://www.tdh.state.tx.us/data.htm

**★ 9842 ★ Vermont Agency of Human Services**
**Social and Rehabilitation Services Department**
**Planning and Evaluation Division**
103 S Main St.
State Complex
Waterbury, VT 05671-2401
**Phone:** (802)241-2100          **Fax:** (802)241-2980
**Email:** webmaster@srs.state.vt.us
**Website:** http://www.state.vt.us/srs

**★ 9843 ★ Virginia Office of Health and Human Resources**
**Medical Assistance Services Department**
**Policy and Budget Division**
600 E Broad St., Ste. 1300
Richmond, VA 23219
**Phone:** (804)371-7561          **Fax:** (804)786-0729
**Email:** jsmith@dmas.state.va.us
**Website:** http://www.cns.state.va.us/dmas/

**★ 9844 ★ Washington State Health Care Authority**
676 Woodland Sq. Loop SE
PO Box 42682
Olympia, WA 98504-2682
**Phone:** (360)923-2600
**Email:** adminwww@hca.wa.gov
**Website:** http://www.wa.gov/hca/

**★ 9845 ★ Wisconsin Department of
  Health and Family Services**
**Health Division**
**Management and Policy Office**

PO Box 7850
Madison, WI 53707-7850
**Phone:** (608)266-6954

**Website:** http://www.dhfs.state.wi.us/aboutdhfs/dmt/
dmt.htm
Sue Reinardy, Contact

## Federal Government Agencies

**★ 9846 ★ Railroad Retirement Board**
844 N Rush St.
Chicago, IL 60611-2092
**Phone:** (312)751-4776
**Website:** http://www.rrb.gov/
Cherryl T. Thomas, Chairman of the Board
**Desc:** The Railroad Retirement Board administers comprehensive retirement-survivor and unemployment-sickness benefit programs for the nation's railroad workers and their families.

**★ 9847 ★ U.S. Department of Health and Human Services**
**Health Care Financing Administration (HCFA)**
200 Independence Ave. SW
Washington, DC 20201
**Phone:** (202)690-6726    **Fax:** (202)690-6262
**Website:** http://www.hcfa.gov/
Thomas Scully, Dir of Admin
**Desc:** The Health Care Financing Administration oversees the Medicare program, a federal health insurance program for persons over 65 years of age and certain disabled persons; the Medicaid program, which supplies grants to states to provide medical services to the needy; and related federal medical care quality control staffs.

**★ 9848 ★ U.S. Social Security Administration (SSA)**
6401 Security Blvd.
Baltimore, MD 21235
**Phone:** (410)965-1234    **Fax:** (410)966-1463
**Website:** http://www.ssa.gov/
William A. Halter, Contact
**Desc:** The Social Security Administration manages the Nation's social insurance program, consisting of retirement, survivors, and disability insurance programs. It also administer the Supplemental Security Income program for the aged, blind and disabled. The Administration is responsible for studying the problems of poverty and economic insecurity among Americans and making recommendations on effective methods of solving these problems through social insurance. The Administration also assigns Social Security numbers to U.S citizens and maintains earnings records for workers under their Social Security numbers.

## Foundations & Other Funding Organizations

### Private Foundations

**★ 9849 ★ Claude R. Lambe Charitable Foundation**
1450 G. St. Northwest, Ste. 445
Washington, DC 20005
**Phone:** (202)393-2354    **Fax:** (202)842-4667
Kelly Young, Vice President
**Fnded:** 1982. **Philosophy:** The foundation favors research and study organizations, primarily those concerned with economics and public policy issues. **Priorities:** *Arts & Humanities:* About 36%. *Civic & Public Affairs:* 58%. Economic policy, free enterprise, and law and justice. *Education:* 39%. Primarily targeting colleges, universities and institutes that focus on social sciences. *Note:* Total contributions made in 1998. **Typ. Recipients:** Health Policy/Cost Containment.

**★ 9850 ★ John A. Hartford Foundation**
55 East 59th St.
New York, NY 10022-1178
**Phone:** (212)832-7788    **Fax:** (212)593-4913
**Email:** mail@jhartfound.org
**Website:** http://www.jhartfound.org
James O'Sullivan, Grants Manager
**Fnded:** 1929. **Philosophy:** The John A. Hartford Foundation's primary program emphasis is its Aging and Health Program, which seeks to strengthen the capacity of the American health care system to meet the needs of an aging population. Giving is focused on increasing the capacities of academic geriatricians and health professionals and on integrating and improving services for the elderly. Examples of ongoing grant programs include: The Centers of Excellence program, in which selected academic medical centers use Foundation grants to strengthen recruitment to academic geriatric careers and provide training and research opportunities for faculty geriatricians, and, The Beeson Scholars career development awards, administered by the American Federation for Aging Research, to develop a new cadre of physician-scientists to be leaders in geriatric research and care. The program,"Improving Depression Care for Elders, seeks to assist the office-based primary care physician be developing, implementing and evaluating a disease management model for the care of depressed elders. The Social Work Initiative is broadly designed to improve social work practice with older adults through the development of better education and training programs, which builds on the Foundation's Geriatric Interdisciplinary Team Training and General Physician programs." The Social Work Initiative also parallels the Foundation's Academic Geriatrics and Nursing Institute. 1998 Annual Report. **Priorities:** *International:* 99%. Supports geriatric health. *Note:* Total contributions made in 1999. **Typ. Recipients:** Arthritis, Cancer, Clinics/Medical Centers, Geriatric Health, Health Funds, Health Organizations, Health Policy/

Cost Containment, Health-General, Home-Care Services, Hospitals, Long-Term Care, Medical Education, Medical Rehabilitation, Medical Research, Medical Training, Mental Health, People with Disabilities, Public Health, Research/Studies Institutes. **Geo. Dist:** nationally.

**John M. Olin Foundation**
*See:* Entry 421

**John Randolph and Dora Haynes Foundation**
*See:* Entry 426

**Joyce Foundation**
*See:* Entry 8542

**Philip M. McKenna Foundation**
*See:* Entry 591

**★ 9851 ★ Rosenberg Foundation**
47 Kearny St., Ste. 804
San Francisco, CA 94108
**Phone:** (415)421-6105    **Fax:** (415)421-0141
**Email:** rosenfdn@rosenbergfdn.org
**Website:** http://www.rosenbergfdn.org
Kirke Wilson, President, Secretary
**Fnded:** 1935. **Philosophy:** The Rosenberg Foundation currently has three program priorities: children and their families in poverty in rural and urban areas in California, the changing population of California, and child support reform. Regarding the first priority, the foundation supports programs that reduce dependency, promote self-help, create access to the economic mainstream, or address the causes of poverty among children and families. Programs under the second priority receiving prime consideration will be those that promote the full social, economic, and cultural integration of immigrants and minorities into a pluralistic society. The Rosenberg Foundation is seeking projects which test new ideas and which show significant and permanent improvement in public social policy. Regarding the third priority, the foundation supports projects that are working to improve the child support system through advocacy and public education in the areas of paternity establishment, collection and distribution of support orders, and development of the national child support assurance program. **Priorities:** *Civic & Public Affairs:* 69%. Funds legal centers and child support system reform. *Education:* 1%. *Environment:* 29%. Supports programs that help to improve the situations of children and their families in poverty. *Note:* Total contributions made in 1998. **Typ. Recipients:** Health Policy/Cost Containment. **Geo. Dist:** CA, grantss are made outside California to operate productions in California and to national organisation benefiting Californians.

**Russell Sage Foundation**
*See:* Entry 648

## Corporate Foundations

**Guardian Life Insurance Co. of America**
*See:* Entry 1103

**Waste Management Inc.**
*See:* Entry 1493

**Xerox Foundation**
*See:* Entry 5476

# National & International Organizations

**★ 9852 ★ American Academy of Insurance Medicine (AAIM)**
c/o Robert W. Watson, MD
Allianz Life Insurance Co. of North America
5701 Golden Hills Dr.
Minneapolis, MN 55416-1297
**Phone:** (763)765-6533          **Fax:** (763)765-6520
**Email:** robert-watson@allianzlife.com
**Website:** http://www.aaimedicine.org
Richard E. Brown, Pres.
**Fnded:** 1889. **Mem:** 600. **Desc:** Professional society of medical directors of life insurance companies. **Pub:** *Journal of Insurance Medicine*, quarterly. Journal. *Price:* Included in membership dues; $65/year for nonmembers. **Frmly:** (1992) Association of Life Insurance Medical Directors of America.

**★ 9853 ★ American Association of Health Plans (AAHP)**
1129 20th St. NW, Ste. 600
Washington, DC 20036-3421
**Phone:** (202)778-3200          **Fax:** (202)331-7487
**Email:** aahp@aahp.org
**Website:** http://www.aahp.org
Karen Ignagni, Pres.
**Fnded:** 1959. **Mem:** 1,000. **Desc:** Supports the managed health care industry. Lobbies; conducts research programs and workshops; Maintains placement service. **Pub:** *healthplan*, bimonthly. Magazine. *Price:* $75/year.

**American Association of Managed Care Nurses (AAMCN)**
*See:* Entry 15639

**★ 9854 ★ American Association of Preferred Provider Organizations**
PO Box 429
Jeffersonville, IN 47131-0429
**Phone:** (812)246-4376          **Free:** 800-642-2515
**Fax:** (812)246-4630
**Email:** kgreenrose@aappo.org
**Website:** http://www.aappo.org
Karen Greenrose, Pres.
**Fnded:** 1983. **Mem:** 1,100. **Reg. Groups:** 4. **State Groups:** 9. **Desc:** Seeks to advance the development, growth and success of network-based managed health care organizations(PPOs PSOs IPAs, etc.). Provides its members with a variety of educational and networking opportunities. Advocates the needs and interests of its members before local, state and federal legislators and regulators. Promotes network-based managed health care to payors, employers and the general public through a variety of media outlets. **Pub:** *AAPPO Legislative Bulletin*, periodic. Newsletter. Provides information on legislation and regulations affecting the PPO industry. *Price:* Free to members; $75/year for nonmembers. • *Directory of Operational PPOs*, annual. Directory. Contains information on approximately 1000 PPO organizations and products. *Price:* Free to organizational members; $225 for individual members; $425 for nonmembers. • *Health Care Innovations*, bimonthly. Magazine. Contains in-

formation on product innovations, systems, trends, and individuals in the managed care field. *Price:* Included in membership dues; $50/year for nonmembers. • *PPO Market Report*, annual. Provides summary data and charts on the PPO industry. *Price:* Free to organizational members; $62.50 for individual members; $125 for nonmembers. **Frmly:** (1999) Association of Managed Healthcare Organizations.

**★ 9855 ★ Association of Health Insurance Advisors**
2901 Telestar Ct.
Falls Church, VA 22042
**Phone:** (703)770-8200          **Fax:** (703)770-8201
**Email:** ahia@naifa.org
**Website:** http://www.ahia.net
Michael L. Kerley, Exec. VP
**Fnded:** 1990. **Mem:** 5,000. **Desc:** Insurance agents and advisors specializing in health, disability, long term care insurance and/or employee benefits.

**★ 9856 ★ Blue Cross and Blue Shield Association (BCBSA)**
225 N Michigan Ave.
Chicago, IL 60611
**Phone:** (312)297-6000          **Fax:** (312)297-6609
**Website:** http://www.bluecares.com
Patrick G. Hays, Pres. and CEO
**Fnded:** 1982. **Desc:** Local Blue Cross and Blue Shield Plans in the U.S., and other licensees in Europe, Japan, and Jamaica. To promote the betterment of public health and security; to secure the widest public acceptance of voluntary nonprofit, prepayment of health services; to provide services to Blue Cross and Blue Shield Plans and licensees. Contracts with federal government as administrative agency for federal health progams; sponsors and conducts programs on health care and prepayment issues. Also publishes reports and pamphlets.

**★ 9857 ★ Canadian Association of Blue Cross Plans (CABCP) (Association Canadienne des Croix Bleue)**
185 The West Mall, Ste. 600
Etobicoke, ON, Canada M9C 5P1
**Phone:** (416)626-1688          **Fax:** (416)626-6445
**Email:** gerry.devlin@ont.bluecross.ca
**Website:** http://www.bluecross.ca
**Fnded:** 1955. **Mem:** 6. **Lang(s):** English, French. **Desc:** Independent Blue Cross health plans. Seeks to promote, enhance and protect association trademarks and trade names across Canada; facilitates communication and cooperation among members in support of regional and national growth and development.

**★ 9858 ★ Canadian Health Economics Research Association (CHERA) (Association Canadienne pour la Recerche en Economie de la Sante — ACRES)**
Abramsky Hall, 3rd Fl.
Queen's University
Kingston, ON, Canada K7L 3N6
**Phone:** (613)533-6675          **Fax:** (613)533-6353
**Email:** swanb@post.queensu.ca
**Fnded:** 1983. **Mem:** 330. **Desc:** Economists, administrators, political scientists, sociologists, social workers, policymakers, and other individuals with an interest in the economics of health care. Facilitates communication and exchange of information among members. Gathers and disseminates health economics information. Promotes quality research in health economics and related fields. Maintains registry of health economics researchers and research projects in Canada. Maintains Internet server. **Pub:** *CHERAction*, quarterly. Newsletter. • *Membership Registry*, annual. Directory.

**★ 9859 ★ Council for Affordable Health Insurance (CAHI)**
112 S West St., Ste. 400
Alexandria, VA 22314
**Phone:** (703)836-6200          **Fax:** (703)836-6550
**Email:** mail@cahi.org
**Website:** http://www.cahi.org
**Fnded:** 1992. **Mem:** 200. **Desc:** Companies and individuals with an interest in the health care financing system in the United States. Promotes health care reform that "enact positive, market-based reforms that preserve freedom of choice for individuals and encourage a competitive health care market." Devises model health care reform plans; conducts lobbying and advocacy campaigns; sponsors educational programs.

**Delta Dental Plans Association (DDPA)**
*See:* Entry 6505

**★ 9860 ★ Health Benefits Coalition for Affordable Choice and Quality**
1201 F St. NW, Ste. 200
Washington, DC 20004
**Email:** cs@ddpa.org
**Website:** http://www.hbcweb.com/
**Mem:** 3000,000. **Desc:** Employers providing health care coverage. Promotes affordable, quality health care, through broader coverage, choice and competition in the marketplace, rather than government mandates.

**★ 9861 ★ Healthcare Financial Management Association (HFMA)**
2 Westbrook Corporate Financial Center, Ste. 700
Westchester, IL 60154-5700
**Phone:** (708)531-9600          **Free:** 800-252-HFMA
**Fax:** (708)531-0032
**Email:** tarya@hfma.org
**Website:** http://www.hfma.org
Richard L. Clarke, Pres. & CEO
**Fnded:** 1946. **Mem:** 34,000. **State Groups:** 70. **Desc:** Financial management professionals employed by hospitals and long-term care facilities, public accounting and consulting firms, insurance companies, medical groups, managed care organizations, government agencies, and other organizations. Conducts conferences, including annual conference in late June, audio teleconferences. Publishes books on healthcare financial issues. A Fellowship in Healthcare Financial Management (FHFMA) as well as the Certified Healthcare Professional (CHFP) in Fianace and Accounting, Financial Management of Physician Practices, Managed Care, and Patient Financial Services are offered. **Pub:** *Healthcare Financial Management*, monthly. Magazine. Includes industry news, articles on financial management in all types of facilities across the healthcare continuum. *Price:* $82 /year for nonmembers. • *Notes from National*, monthly. Newsletter. *Price:* Included in membership dues. • *Patient Accounts*, monthly. Newsletter. Covers the financial operations of business office and patient accounting functions, including preadmission information gathering. *Price:* $60/year for members; $108/year for nonmembers. • Books. • Videos. **Frmly:** (1968) American Association of Hospital Accountants; (1982) Hospital Financial Management Association.

**★ 9862 ★ Healthcare Financing Study Group (HFSG)**
1666 K St. NW, Ste. 500
Washington, DC 20006
**Fax:** (202)466-3215
**Fnded:** 1973. **Mem:** 40. **Desc:** Investment banking, law, consulting, and accounting firms involved in providing capital financing for health care institutions. Analyzes legislative and regulatory proposals from the standpoint of the health care financial community. Provides forum for exchange of information concerning health care financing. **Pub:** Bulletin, periodic. • Newsletter, monthly. **Frmly:** (1981) Hospital Financing Study Group.

**★ 9863 ★ Health Industry Group Purchasing Association (HIGPA)**
1444 Eye St., NW, Ste. 410
Washington, DC 20005
**Phone:** (202)393-7306     **Fax:** (202)628-2310
**Email:** info@higpa.org
**Website:** http://www.higpa.org
**Fnded:** 1990. **Desc:** For-profit and not-for-profit corporations, purchasing groups, associations, multi hospital systems and health care provider alliances. **Pub:** *CapitoLine.* Newsletter.

**★ 9864 ★ Healthcare Billing and Management Association**
1540 S Coast Hwy., No. 203
Laguna Beach, CA 92651
**Phone:** 877-640-4262     **Fax:** (949)376-3456
**Email:** info@hbma.com
**Website:** http://www.hbma.com
Sanford J. Hill, Pres.
**Desc:** Companies who provide third paty medical billing services.

**★ 9865 ★ Healthcare Financial Management Association (HFMA)**
1301 Connecticut Ave., NW, Ste. 300
Washington, DC 20036-3417
**Phone:** (202)296-2920     **Free:** 800-252-HFMA
**Fax:** (202)223-9771
**Email:** webmaster@hfma.org
**Website:** http://www.hfma.org
Terry Arya, Contact
**Mem:** 33,000. **Desc:** Healthcare management associates. Strives to help its members excel in their jobs and careers. Hosts seminars and conferences. **Pub:** *Healthcare Financial Management*, monthly. Magazine. Contains information related to the healthcare industry. • *HFMA Express News*, weekly. Newsletter. E-mailed to members. • *HFMA Wants You to Know*, biweekly. Newsletter. Available via e-mail to members and public. *Price:* Free. • *Patient Accounts*, monthly. Newsletter. Contains information related to patient financial services.

**★ 9866 ★ International Committee for Life Disability and Health Assurance Medicine**
c/o Hannover RE
7, rue montauvet
F-75008 Paris, France
**Phone:** 33 1 42668778     **Fax:** 33 1 42668798
**Fnded:** 1899. **Mem:** 81. **Lang(s):** English. **Desc:** Medical doctors working in life insurance and reinsurance companies in 41 countries. Promotes fraternal benefit life insurance; facilitates contact and cooperation among members. Establishes societies of life assurance medicine in countries where they do not exist. **Pub:** *Annals of Life Assurance Medicine*, triennial.

**★ 9867 ★ Long Term Care Campaign (LTCC)**
PO Box 27394
Washington, DC 20038
**Phone:** (202)434-3744     **Fax:** (202)434-6403
**Email:** info@ltccampaign.org
**Website:** http://www.ltccampaign.org
Kevin Donnellan, Chair
**Fnded:** 1987. **Mem:** 143. **Nat'l Groups:** 143. **Desc:** Consumer, provider, business, labor, ciuk, older adult, and disability groups. Works to make long term health care accessible and affordable for all families. **Pub:** *The Campaigner*, quarterly. Newsletter. Long Term Care issues and legislative updates. • *The Time Is Now*. Videos.

**★ 9868 ★ National Association of Managed Care Physicians (NAMCP)**
4435 Waterfront Dr., Ste. 101
PO Box 4765
Glen Allen, VA 23060
**Phone:** (804)527-1905     **Free:** 800-722-0376
**Fax:** (804)747-5316
**Email:** info@namcp.com
**Website:** http://www.namcp.com
Dr. W.C. Williams, MD, Sr. VP
**Fnded:** 1991. **Mem:** 12,000. **Reg. Groups:** 2. **State Groups:** 5. **Desc:** Licensed physicians and allied health professionals working in managed health care programs; medical residents and students interested in managed health care; corporations or agencies providing services or goods to the industry; interested others. Enhances the ability of practicing physicians to proactively participate within the managed health care arena through research, communication, and education. Provides a forum for members to communicate their concerns about the changing health care environment, integrate into managed health care delivery systems, and assure continuous improvement in the quality of health care services provided. Develops practice criteria, quality assurance measures, and appropriate utilization management criteria. Offers educational programs; maintains speakers' bureau and placement services; conducts research programs; developing informational clearinghouse. **Pub:** *Managed Care Medicine*, bimonthly. Journal. *Price:* $95. • *NAMCP Guide to Managed Care*. Monograph.

**★ 9869 ★ National Association of Medicaid Directors (NASMD)**
810 1st St. NE, Ste. 500
Washington, DC 20002-4267
**Phone:** (202)682-0100     **Fax:** (202)289-6555
**Email:** lpartridge@aphsa.org
**Website:** http://www.aphsa.org
Lee Partridge, Dir. Health Policy
**Mem:** 54. **Desc:** Directors and senior staff of state and territorial medical assistance programs. Promotes effective Medicaid policy and program administration; works with the federal government on issues through technical advisory groups. Conducts forums on policy and technical issues. **Pub:** *MMI Bulletin*, monthly. Newsletter. Summary of legal decisions, legislation, regulations, waivers relating to Medicaid program. *Price:* $90/year. **Frmly:** (1995) State Medicaid Directors Association.

**★ 9870 ★ National Association of Primary Care**
Lettsom House
11 Chandos St.
Cavendish Sq.
London W1M 9DE, United Kingdom
**Phone:** 44 207 6361677     **Fax:** 44 171 6361601
**Email:** napc@primarycare.co.uk
**Website:** http://www.primarycare.co.uk
**Fnded:** 1991. **Mem:** 1,000. **Desc:** GP fundholding practices in England, Scotland, Wales & N Ireland. Aims to: promote good communication amongst fundholding practices; develop and extend the scope of services to patients offered by fundholding practices; encourage education research for and within fundholding practices; maintain the highest ethical standards on the part of practitioners in fundholding practices; encourage the creation of new fundholding practices. **Frmly:** (2000) National Association of Fundholding Practices.

**★ 9871 ★ National Coalition on Health Care**
1200 G St., NW, Ste. 750
Washington, DC 20005
**Phone:** (202)638-7151
**Email:** info@nchc.org
**Website:** http://www.nchc.org
**Fnded:** 1990. **Mem:** 100000,000. **Reg. Groups:** 96. **Desc:** Large and small businesses, labor unions, consumer groups, religious groups, and primary care providers. United to achieve better, more affordable healthcare for all Americans.

**★ 9872 ★ National Committee for Quality Assurance (NCQA)**
2000 L St., NW, Ste. 500
Washington, DC 20036
**Phone:** (202)955-3500     **Free:** 888-275-7585
**Fax:** (202)955-3599
**Website:** http://www.ncqa.org
Margaret E. O'Kane, Pres.
**Fnded:** 1979. **Desc:** Board of Directors representing employers, consumer and labor representatives, health plans, quality experts, regulators and representatives from organized medicine. mission: To improve the quality of health care delivered everywhere. Accredits quality assurance programs in prepaid managed health care organizations. Develops and coordinates programs for assessing the quality of care and service in the managed health care industry. Conducts research; holds training and educational seminars; operates speakers' bureau. **Pub:** *Health Plan Employer Data and Information Set*, annual. Handbook. • *Quality Matters*, 3/year. Newsletter. Discusses quality-related activities in the managed care industry and at NCQA. *Price:* $90/year.

**★ 9873 ★ National Council of Health Facilities Finance Authorities (NCHFFA)**
PO Box 61482
Denver, CO 80206
**Website:** http://www.nchffa.org
**Fnded:** 1990. **Desc:** Serves the common interests and improves effectiveness of member authorities through communication, education, and advocacy, with emphasis on issues which directly influence the availability of or access to tax-exempt financing for healthcare facilities. **Pub:** Newsletter.

**National CPA Health Care Advisors Association (HCAA)**
*See:* Entry 9989

**★ 9874 ★ National Health Care Anti-Fraud Association (NHCAA)**
1255 23rd St. NW
Washington, DC 20037
**Phone:** (202)659-5955     **Fax:** (202)785-6764
**Email:** fraud@nhcaa.org
**Website:** http://www.nhcaa.org
William Mahon, Exec. Dir.
**Fnded:** 1985. **Mem:** 900. **Desc:** Network of private insurance companies and public and private agencies that work against health insurance fraud. **Pub:** *NHCAA Network*, quarterly. Newsletter. • Also plans to make available educational materials.

**★ 9875 ★ National Organization of Life and Health Insurance Guaranty Associations (NOLHGA)**
13873 Park Center Rd., Ste. 329
Herndon, VA 20171
**Website:** http://www.nolhga.com
**Mem:** 52. **Desc:** Promotes the life and health insurance guaranty industry.

**★ 9876 ★ Office of Health Economics**
12 Whitehall
London SW1A 2DY, United Kingdom
**Phone:** 44 207 9309203     **Fax:** 44 207 7471419
**Email:** laulsford@ohe.org
**Website:** http://www.ohe.org
**Fnded:** 1962. **Desc:** Undertakes research on the economic aspects of medical care, with particular reference to the pharmaceutical industry. **Pub:** Papers.

## ★ 9877 ★ Physician Insurers Association of America (PIAA)
2275 Research Blvd., Ste. 250
Rockville, MD 20850
**Phone:** (301)947-9000          **Fax:** (301)947-9090
**Email:** dshearin@thepiaa.org
**Website:** http://www.thepiaa.org
Lawrence E. Smarr, Pres.
**Fnded:** 1977. **Mem:** 60. **Desc:** Physician liability insurance companies, including domestic physician and dental liability insurers, international affiliates, and reinsurers. Seeks to further the best interests of member companies in areas related to physician liability insurance. Focuses on the availability and affordability of professional liability insurance and the effective delivery of quality healthcare. Conducts research and educational programs; monitors and advocates for legislation. **Pub:** *The Physician Insurer*, quarterly. Magazine. *Price:* $45/year. • *PIAA Membership Directory*, annual. Membership Directory. • Also publishes studies of major liability concerns in the insurance industry, including issues related to treatment of breast, lung, and colon cancer; medication errors; and laparoscopy procedures.

# Research Centers

**Academy for Health Services Research and Health Policy**
*See:* Entry 9766

## ★ 9878 ★ Center for Health Economics Research
411 Waverley Oaks Rd., Ste. 330
Waltham, MA 02452-8414
**Phone:** (781)788-8100          **Fax:** (781)788-8101
**Email:** inso@her-cher.org
**Website:** http://www.her-cher.org
Dr. Janet B. Mitchell, Pres.
**Activities/Fields:** Health economics, including alternative ways of reimbursing capital under the Medicare prospective payment system, access to care, physician payment, hospital costs, black-white treatment differences, and cost-effectiveness of technology.

## ★ 9879 ★ Cornell University
**Health Benefits Research Unit**
225 E 64th St., Ste. 202
New York, NY 10021-6660
**Phone:** (212)746-1240          **Fax:** (212)888-5663
Dr. Eugene G. McCarthy, Dir.
**Activities/Fields:** Health benefits, including a study on whether physicians offering a second opinion concurred with the original recommendation for elective surgery and a program to identify and direct patients to ambulatory surgical facilities. Arranges appointments between patients and approximately 28,000 board certified surgeons throughout the U.S.

## ★ 9880 ★ Council for Affordable Health Insurance (CAHI)
112 S West St., Ste. 400
Alexandria, VA 22314
**Phone:** (703)836-6200          **Fax:** (703)836-6550
**Email:** mail@cahi.org
**Website:** http://www.cahi.org/About/whatwedo.htm
Nona B. Wegner, Pres. /Exec. Dir.
**Activities/Fields:** Free market solutions to America's health care challenges. **Pub:** *Reports*.

**Johns Hopkins University**
**Primary Care Policy Center for Underserved Populations (PCPC)**
*See:* Entry 10009

## ★ 9881 ★ Olive View-UCLA Medical Center Foundation
14445 Olive View Dr., North Annex
Sylmar, CA 91342-1495
**Phone:** (818)364-3686          **Fax:** (818)364-4584
**Email:** ovinfo@earthlink.net
**Website:** http://www.oliveviewfoundation.org
Beverly Froelich, Dir.
**Activities/Fields:** Community based needs assessments.

**State University of New York at Stony Brook**
**Center for Health Policy and Management**
*See:* Entry 10016

## ★ 9882 ★ U.S. Department of Health and Human Services
**Health Care Financing Administration**
**Office of Research and Demonstrations**
7500 Security Blvd., Rm. C3-20-11
Baltimore, MD 21244-1850
**Phone:** (410)786-6503          **Fax:** (410)786-6511
**Email:** ospinquiry@hcfa.gov
**Website:** http://www.hcfa.gov
Thomas M. Kickham, PhD, Actg. Dir.
**Activities/Fields:** Develops and manages long-term strategic planning processes for the Health Care Financing Administration. Provides analytic support and information to Administration programs. Identifies and evaluates emerging trends in health care delivery and financing. Coordinates demonstration activities; participates in experimental health care delivery projects; develops research and educational materials. **Pub:** *Active Projects Report*, annually. • *Health Care Financing Review*, quarterly. **Frmly:** Office of Research and Demonstrations.

## ★ 9883 ★ U.S. Department of Health and Human Services
**Office of Research and Demonstrations**
**Beneficiary Studies Division**
**Research and Evaluation Group**
C3-19-07
7500 Security Blvd.
Baltimore, MD 21244
**Phone:** (410)786-6507          **Fax:** (410)786-5515
Renee Mentnech, PhD, Dir.
**Activities/Fields:** Designs and conducts research and evaluations to study the impacts of CHFA and other health care programs, focusing particularly on beneficiary issues. Designs and conducts general studies related to beneficiaries. Evaluates demonstration projects, pilot projects and other innovations in HCFA programs. Designs demonstration projects. Develops data bases and evaluation methods/tools to evaluate the impact of HCFA programs on beneficiary issues. Provides technical research and evaluation related support to HCFA, HHS and others related to beneficiary issues. **Pub:** *Health Care Financing Annual Review.* **Frmly:** Office of Research and Demonstrations; Beneficiary Studies Division.

## ★ 9884 ★ U.S. Department of Health and Human Services
**Office of Research and Demonstrations**
**Office of Demonstrations and Evaluations**
**Long-Term Care Experimentation Division**
**(Division of Health Systems Research)**
C3-20-17
7500 Security Blvd.
Baltimore, MD 21244
**Phone:** (410)786-6640          **Fax:** (410)786-6511
Brigid Goody, Dir.
**Activities/Fields:** Designs and conducts research and evaluations to study the impacts of HCFA and other health care programs; Designs and conducts general studies related to health care systems; Evaluates demonstration projects, pilot projects and other innovations in HCFA programs; Designs demonstration projects, particularly related to innovative delivery systems, models for long term care and dually-eligible beneficiaries; Develops databases and evaluation methods/tools to evaluate the impact of HCFA programs; Provides technical research and evaluation related support to HCFA, HHS, and others. **Frmly:** Office of Demonstrations and Evaluations; Long Term Care Experimentation Division.

## ★ 9885 ★ U.S. Department of Health and Human Services
**Office of Research and Demonstrations**
**Office of Demonstrations and Evaluations**
**Research and Evaluation Group**
C3-21-28
7500 Security Blvd.
Baltimore, MD 21244
**Phone:** (410)786-6500          **Fax:** (410)786-5515
Al Esposito, Dir.
**Activities/Fields:** Research and Evaluation Group provides leadership and executive direction within HCFA for a wide range of health care financing research and demonstration activities. Designs and conducts research and evaluation of the health care delivery system including HCFA and other health care programs. Develops data bases and conducts analyses of the health care market. **Pub:** *Health Care Financing Review*, quarterly. • *Supplement*, annually.

## ★ 9886 ★ University of California at Berkeley
**Center for Mental Health Services Research (CMHSR)**
2020 Milvia St., Ste. 405
Berkeley, CA 94720-5610
**Phone:** (510)643-3555          **Fax:** (510)643-3522
**Email:** snowden@uclink4.berkeley.edu
**Website:** http://socrates.berkeley.edu/~cmhsr
Dr. Lonnie Snowden, Ch.
**Activities/Fields:** Organization and financing of care for severely mentally ill persons, including financing and economics, organization of services and systems, and methods and measurement.

## ★ 9887 ★ University of California, Los Angeles
**Center for Health Policy Research**
10911 Weyburn Ave., Ste. 300
Los Angeles, CA 90024
**Phone:** (310)794-0909          **Fax:** (310)794-2686
**Email:** chpr@ucla.edu
**Website:** http://www.healthpolicy.ucla.edu
E. Richard Brown, PhD, Dir.
**Activities/Fields:** Cost-effectiveness of health programs and services and their effects on health of communities and consumers; policy analysis and develops policy tools that address issues of health promotion and disease prevention.

**University of Cincinnati**
**Institute for Health Policy and Health Services Research (IHPHSR)**
*See:* Entry 9789

**University of Cincinnati**
**Institute for Health Policy and Health Services Research**
**Center for Clinical Effectiveness**
*See:* Entry 9790

## ★ 9888 ★ University of Colorado
**Center for Health Services Research**
1355 S Colorado Blvd., Ste. 306
Denver, CO 80222
**Phone:** (303)756-8350          **Fax:** (303)759-8196
**Email:** pete.shaughnessy@uchsc.edu
**Website:** http://www.ihphsr.uc.edu
Peter W. Shaughnessy, PhD, Dir.

**Activities/Fields:** Health services research and health policy research for federal and state governments, foundations, and related organizations, emphasizing general health policy topics and issues in long-term care quality, access, cost and cost effectiveness. Studies emphasize Medicare and Medicaid quality assurance and reimbursement for long-term care providers, including home health agencies, subacute care facilities, swing-bed hospitals, and traditional nursing homes. Studies focus on the collection and analysis of extensive primary and secondary cross-sectional and longitudinal data at the patient and facility levels. Contributes to federal and state policy deliberations on regulatory and reimbursement issues in long-term care, and to clinical practice and decision making (especially in quality assurance.).

**University of Iowa**
**National Maternal and Child Health**
**Resource Center**
*See:* Entry 5823

**University of Maryland, Baltimore County**
**Center for Health Program Development**
**and Management (CHPDM)**
*See:* Entry 10024

**University of Memphis**
**Center for Health Services Research**
*See:* Entry 9795

**★ 9889 ★ University of Pennsylvania**
**Health Services Research Unit (HSRU)**
Blockley Hall, Rm. 1211
Division of General Internal Medicine
423 Guardian Dr.
Philadelphia, PA 19104-6021
**Phone:** (215)898-6868      **Fax:** (215)898-0611
**Email:** hlthsvrs@mail.med.upenn.edu
**Website:** http://www.uphs.upenn.edu/dgimhsr/
Dr. Henry Glick, Dir.

**Activities/Fields:** Allocation and appropriate use of health care resources, including cost-effectiveness of new pharmaceuticals, managed care and the physician workforce, and methodology of cost analysis.

**★ 9890 ★ University of Washington**
**Center for Cost and Outcomes Research**
**(CCOR)**
Box 358853
Seattle, WA 98195
**Phone:** (206)543-4943
**Email:** deyo@u.washington.edu
**Website:** http://depts.washington.edu/ccor/
Richard A. Deyo, MD, Co-Dir.

**Activities/Fields:** Cost-effective approaches to improving the health of patients and populations and identification of ways to put these improvements into practice. **Pub:** *Annual report.*

**University of Washington**
**Child Health Institute (CHI)**
*See:* Entry 5835

**University of West Florida**
**Behavioral Medicine Laboratory**
*See:* Entry 12781

# State Government Agencies

## Medicaid

**★ 9891 ★ Alabama Medicaid Agency**
501 Dexter Ave.
PO Box 5624
Montgomery, AL 36103-5624
**Phone:** (334)242-5000      **Fax:** (334)242-5097
**Email:** webmaster@www.medicaid.state.al.us
**Website:** http://www.medicaid.state.al.us

**★ 9892 ★ Alaska Department of Health**
**and Social Services**
**Public Health Division**
**Division of Medical Assistance**
PO Box 110660
Juneau, AK 99811-0610
**Phone:** (907)465-3355      **Fax:** (907)465-2204
**Email:** bob_labbe@health.state.ak.us
**Website:** http://www.hss.state.ak.us/dma/table.htm
Bob Labbe, Director

**★ 9893 ★ Arizona Health Care Cost**
**Containment System**
**Medicaid Program**
801 E Jefferson St.
Phoenix, AZ 85034
**Phone:** (602)417-4000
**Email:** flopez@ahcccs.state.az.us
**Website:** http://www.ahcccs.state.az.us/

**★ 9894 ★ Arkansas Department of**
**Human Services**
**Medical Services Division**
Donaghey Plaza S
PO Box 1437, Slot 1100
Little Rock, AR 72203-1437
**Phone:** (501)682-8292      **Fax:** (501)682-1197
**Website:** http://www.medicaid.state.ar.us/
Ray Hanley, Contact

**★ 9895 ★ Colorado Department of**
**Human Services**
**Health Care Policy and Financing**
**Division**
**Medicaid Management Information System**
1575 Sherman St.
Denver, CO 80203-1714
**Email:** comments@www.state.co.us
**Website:** http://www.chcpf.state.co.us/index.html

**★ 9896 ★ Connecticut Department of**
**Social Services**
**Medical Assistance**
**Medicaid Program**
25 Sigourney St.
Hartford, CT 06105-5033
**Phone:** (860)424-5126      **Free:** 800-842-1508
**Fax:** (860)951-9544
**Email:** pgr.dss@po.state.ct.us
**Website:** http://www.dss.state.ct.us/svcs/medical.htm

**★ 9897 ★ Delaware Department of Health**
**and Social Services**
**Social Services Division**
**Medicaid Unit**
Lewis Bldg.
1901 N DuPont Hwy.
New Castle, DE 19720
**Free:** 800-372-2022      **Fax:** (302)255-9500
**Email:** dhssinfo@state.de.us
**Website:** http://www.state.de.us/dhss/dss/dsshome.htm, Sr.

**★ 9898 ★ Florida Agency for Health Care**
**Administration**
**Medicaid Office**
2727 Mahan Dr., Mail Stop 8
Tallahassee, FL 32308
**Phone:** (850)488-3560      **Free:** 888-419-3456
**Fax:** (850)488-2520
**Website:** http://www.fdhc.state.fl.us/Medicaid/index.shtml
Bob Sharpe, Contact

**★ 9899 ★ Georgia Department of**
**Community Health**
**Division of Medical Assistance**
2 Peachtree St. NW
Atlanta, GA 30303
**Phone:** (404)651-8681
**Website:** http://www.communityhealth.state.ga.us/
Mark Trail, Contact

**★ 9900 ★ Idaho Department of Health**
**and Welfare**
**Medicaid Division**
450 W State St., 5th Floor
PO Box 83720
Boise, ID 83720-0036
**Phone:** (208)334-5747      **Fax:** (208)334-6558
**Website:** http://www2.state.id.us/dhw/medicaid/index.htm
Joe Brunson, Director

**★ 9901 ★ Illinois Department of Public**
**Aid**
**Medical Programs Division**
201 S Grand Ave. E
Springfield, IL 62763-0001
**Phone:** (217)782-2570      **Fax:** (217)782-5672
**Email:** aidd2372@mail.idpa.state.il.us
**Website:** http://WWW.STATE.il.us/dpa/html/medical_news.htm

**★ 9902 ★ Indiana Family and Social**
**Services Administration**
**Medicaid Policy and Planning Office**
402 W Washington St.
PO Box 7083
Indianapolis, IN 46207-7083
**Phone:** (317)233-4455      **Free:** 800-457-4584
**Fax:** (317)233-4693
**Website:** http://www.in.gov/fssa/
Melanie Bella, Contact

**★ 9903 ★ Iowa Department of Human**
**Services**
**Medical Services Division**
**Medicaid Program**
Hoover State Office Bldg.
1305 E Walnut
Des Moines, IA 50319
**Phone:** (515)281-8621      **Free:** 800-972-2017
**Email:** fdhs@dhs.state.ia.us
**Website:** http://www.dhs.state.ia.us/dhsphone.asp

**★ 9904 ★ Kansas Department of Social**
**and Rehabilitation Services**
**Adult Medical Services Commission**
Docking State Office Bldg.
915 SW Harrison St., Rm 603N
Topeka, KS 66612
**Phone:** (785)296-3959
**Email:** libby@srsexec.wpo.state.ks.us
**Website:** http://www.srskansas.org/srsadult-comm.html
Ann Koci, Contact

**★ 9905 ★ Kentucky Health Services Cabinet**
**Medicaid Services Department**
275 E Main St, 6th Floor
Frankfort, KY 40621
**Phone:** (502)564-4321     **Fax:** (502)564-0509
**Email:** chs.dmsweb@mail.state.ky.us
**Website:** http://chs.state.ky.us/dms/

**★ 9906 ★ Louisiana Department of Health and Hospitals**
**Health Services Financing Bureau**
1201 Capitol Access Rd.
PO Box 91030
Baton Rouge, LA 70821-9030
**Phone:** (225)342-5774     **Fax:** (225)342-3893
**Email:** medweb@dhhmail.dhh.state.la.us
**Website:** http://www.dhh.state.la.us/medicaid/index.htm

**★ 9907 ★ Maine Department of Human Services**
**Medical Services Bureau**
**Policy and Provider Services Division**
**Medicaid Program**
442 Civic Center Dr.
11 State House Station
Augusta, ME 04333-0011
**Phone:** (207)287-3094     **Free:** 800-321-5557
**Email:** Sandy.Goldman@state.me.us
**Website:** http://www.state.me.us/bms/bmshome.htm
Sandy Goldman, Director

**★ 9908 ★ Massachusetts Executive Office of Health and Human Services**
**Medical Assistance Division**
1 Ashburton Place, rm 1109
Boston, MA 02108
**Phone:** (617)727-7600     **Fax:** (617)727-5134
**Email:** contactdma@nt.dma.state.ma.us
**Website:** http://www.state.ma.us/dma/

**★ 9909 ★ Michigan Community Health Department**
**Health Programs Administration**
**Medicaid Operations Bureau**
320 South Walnut St.
Lewis Cass Bldg., 6th Floor
Lansing, MI 48913
**Phone:** (517)373-3500
**Email:** barriep@.michigan.gov
**Website:** http://www.michigan.gov/mdch

**★ 9910 ★ Minnesota Department of Human Services**
**Health and Continuing Care Strategies Division**
**Medicaid Program**
444 Lafayette Rd. N
Saint Paul, MN 55155
**Phone:** (651)296-8517     **Free:** 800-657-3659
**Fax:** (651)297-3230
**Email:** dhs.webmaster@state.mn.us
**Website:** http://www.dhs.state.mn.us/hlthcare/asstprog/mmap.htm

**★ 9911 ★ Mississippi Office of the Governor**
**Medicaid Division**
239 N Lamar St.
801 Robert E Lee Bldg.
Jackson, MS 39201-1399
**Phone:** (601)359-6050     **Free:** 800-421-2408
**Fax:** (601)359-6048
**Email:** webmaster@medicaid.state.ms.us
**Website:** http://www.dom.state.ms.us/
Rica Lewis-Payton, Director

**★ 9912 ★ Missouri Department of Social Services**
**Medical Services Division**
615 Howerton Ct.
PO Box 6500
Jefferson City, MO 65102-6500
**Phone:** (573)751-3425     **Fax:** (573)751-6564
**Email:** webmaster@mail.medicaid.state.mo.us
**Website:** http://www.dss.state.mo.us/dms/index.htm

**★ 9913 ★ Nebraska Department of Health and Human Services**
**Medicaid Division**
301 Centennial Mall S
PO Box 95026
Lincoln, NE 68509-5026
**Phone:** (402)471-9567     **Fax:** (402)471-9449
**Email:** hhs_system_information@hhs.state.ne.us
**Website:** http://www.hhs.state.ne.us/med/medindex.htm
Bob Seiffert, Director

**★ 9914 ★ Nevada Department of Human Resources**
**Welfare Division**
**Medicaid Program**
1470 E College Parkway
Carson City, NV 89706
**Phone:** (775)684-0500
**Email:** sallsip@welfare.state.nv.us
**Website:** http://welfare.state.nv.us/

**★ 9915 ★ New Hampshire Department of Health and Human Services**
**Office of Health Planning and Medicaid**
**Medical Services Bureau**
129 Pleasant St.
Concord, NH 03301
**Phone:** (603)271-5254     **Free:** 800-852-3345
**Fax:** (603)271-8431
**Website:** http://www.dhhs.state.nh.us/DHHS/ContactDirectory/default.htm

**★ 9916 ★ New Jersey Department of Human Services**
**Medical Assistance and Health Services Division**
Quakerbridge Plaza
PO Box 712
Trenton, NJ 08625-0712
**Phone:** (609)588-2600     **Free:** 800-356-1561
**Fax:** (609)588-3583
**Email:** webmaster@dhs.state.nj.us
**Website:** http://www.state.nj.us/humanservices/dmahs/index.html

**★ 9917 ★ New Mexico Department of Human Services**
**Medical Assistance Division**
PO Box 2348
Santa Fe, NM 87504-2348
**Phone:** (505)827-3100     **Free:** 888-997-2583
**Fax:** (505)827-3185
**Website:** http://www.state.nm.us/hsd/mad/Index.html

**★ 9918 ★ New York State Department of Health**
**Office of Continuing Care**
**New York State Partnership for Long-Term Care**
1 Commerce Plaza
Room 726
99 Washington Ave.
Albany, NY 12260
**Phone:** (518)473-8083     **Free:** 888-697-7582
**Email:** pltc@health.state.ny.us
**Website:** http://www.nyspltc.org/about/index.html

**★ 9919 ★ North Carolina Department of Health and Human Services**
**Medical Assistance Division**
1985 Umstead Dr.
2501 Mail Service Ctr.
Raleigh, NC 27699-2501
**Phone:** (919)857-4011     **Fax:** (919)733-6608
**Website:** http://www.dhhs.state.nc.us/docs/division.htm
Nina Yeager, Director

**★ 9920 ★ North Dakota Department of Human Services**
**Medical Services Division**
600 E Boulevard Ave.
Department 325
Bismarck, ND 58505-0250
**Phone:** (701)328-2321     **Free:** 800-755-2604
**Fax:** (701)328-1544
**Email:** dhsmed@.state.nd.us
**Website:** http://lnotes.state.nd.us/dhs/dhsweb.nsf/ServicePages/MedicalServices

**★ 9921 ★ Ohio Department of Job and Family Services**
**Medicaid Bureau**
30 E Broad St., 31st Fl.
Columbus, OH 43215
**Phone:** (614)644-0140
**Website:** http://www.state.oh.us/odjfs/ohp/index.stm
**Frmly:** Ohio Department of Human Services.

**★ 9922 ★ Oklahoma Health Care Authority**
4545 N Lincoln Blvd., Ste. 124
Oklahoma City, OK 73105
**Phone:** (405)522-7300
**Website:** http://www.ohca.state.ok.us/

**★ 9923 ★ Oregon Department of Human Resources**
**Medical Assistance Program Office**
500 Summer St. NE E37
Salem, OR 97301-1079
**Phone:** (503)945-5772     **Free:** 800-527-5772
**Email:** dhr.info@state.or.us
**Website:** http://www.omap.hr.state.or.us/

**★ 9924 ★ Pennsylvania Department of Public Welfare**
**Medical Assistance Office**
PO Box 2675
Health & Welfare Bldg., Rm. 515
Harrisburg, PA 17105-2675
**Phone:** (717)787-1870
**Website:** http://www.dpw.state.pa.us/omap/dpwomap.asp

**★ 9925 ★ Rhode Island Department of Human Services**
**Medical Services Division**
600 New London Ave.
Cranston, RI 02920
**Phone:** (401)462-6500     **Fax:** (401)464-6504
**Website:** http://www.dhs.state.ri.us/

**★ 9926 ★ South Carolina Health and Human Services Department**
**Health Services Bureau**
**Medicaid Program**
1801 Main St.
PO Box 8206
Columbia, SC 29202-8206
**Phone:** (803)898-2640     **Fax:** (803)898-4515
**Email:** Adams@dhhs.state.sc.us
**Website:** http://www.state.sc.us/dhhs/

**★ 9927 ★ South Dakota Department of Social Services**
**Program Management Division**
**Medical Services Office**
700 Governors Dr.
Pierre, SD 57501
**Phone:** (605)773-3495　　　**Fax:** (605)773-5246
**Email:** Medicaid@dss.state.sd.us
**Website:** http://www.state.sd.us/social/medicaid/index.htm

**★ 9928 ★ Tennessee Department of Health**
**Tenncare Division**
729 Church St.
Nashville, TN 37243
**Phone:** (615)532-7542　　　**Free:** 800-669-1851
**Fax:** (615)741-0882
**Email:** you@yours.gov
**Website:** http://www.state.tn.us/tenncare/
Lola Potter, Contact

**★ 9929 ★ Texas Department of Health**
**Health Care Financing Division**
**Medicaid Managed Care Bureau**
1100 W 49th St.
Austin, TX 78756-3199
**Phone:** (512)338-6508　　　**Free:** 888-963-7111
**Email:** susan.milam@tdh.state.tx.us
**Website:** http://www.tdh.state.tx.us/hcf/mcstart.htm
Susan Milan, PhD, Director

**★ 9930 ★ Utah Department of Health**
**Health Care Financing Division**
**Medicaid Policy and Planning Bureau**
288 N 1460 W
PO Box 143106
Salt Lake City, UT 84114-3106

**Phone:** (801)538-6406　　　**Free:** 800-662-9651
**Fax:** (801)538-6412
**Email:** gsix@utah.gov
**Website:** http://www.health.state.ut.us/medicaid/index.html
Michael Deily, Director

**★ 9931 ★ Vermont Agency of Human Services**
**Prevention, Assistance, Transition and Health Access Department**
**Health Access Office**
103 S Main St.
Waterbury, VT 05671
**Phone:** (802)241-2880　　　**Free:** 800-529-4060
**Fax:** (802)241-2897
**Email:** WebMaster@wpath.state.vt.us
**Website:** http://www.dpath.state.vt.us/

**★ 9932 ★ Virginia Office of Health and Human Resources**
**Medical Assistance Services Department**
600 E Broad St., Ste. 1300
Richmond, VA 23219
**Phone:** (804)786-4231
**Email:** webmaster@dmas.state.va.us
**Website:** http://165.176.249.159/

**★ 9933 ★ Washington Department of Social and Health Services**
**Medical Assistance Administration**
617 8th Ave SE
PO Box 45100
Olympia, WA 98504-5100
**Free:** 800-562-3022
**Website:** http://fortress.wa.gov/dshs/maa/

**★ 9934 ★ West Virginia Department of Health and Human Resources**
**Medical Services Bureau**
350 Capitol St., Rm. 251
Charleston, WV 25301-3706
**Phone:** (304)926-1703　　　**Fax:** (304)558-1451
**Email:** medcomm@wvdhhr.org
**Website:** http://www.wvdhhr.org/bms/
Nancy Atkins, Director

**★ 9935 ★ Wisconsin Department of Health and Family Services**
**Health Division**
**Health Care Financing Bureau**
PO Box 309
Madison, WI 53701-0309
**Phone:** (608)266-2522
**Email:** webmaster@dhfs.state.wi.us
**Website:** http://www.dhfs.state.wi.us/aboutdhfs/DHCF/dhcf.htm
Peggy Handrich, Contact

**★ 9936 ★ Wyoming Department of Health**
**Health Care Financing Division**
**Minimum Medical Program**
Hathaway Bldg., 4th Fl.
6101 Yellowstone Rd.
Cheyenne, WY 82002
**Phone:** (307)777-6004　　　**Fax:** (307)777-3617
**Email:** molson@state.wy.us
**Website:** http://wdhfs.state.wy.us/dcfh/
Mary Olson, Contact

# Chapter 30
# Health Care Industry

## Federal Government Agencies

**★ 9937 ★ Federal Trade Commission (FTC)**
600 Pennsylvania Ave. NW
Washington, DC 20580
**Phone:** (202)326-2222        **Fax:** (202)326-3676
**Website:** http://www.ftc.gov/
Timothy J. Muris, Chairman of the Board
**Desc:** The objective of the FTC is to maintain competitive enterprise as the keystone of the American economic system, and to prevent the free enterprise system from being fettered by monopoly or restraints on trade or corrupted by unfair or deceptive trade practices. The Commission is charged with keeping competition both free and fair.

**★ 9938 ★ U.S. Department of Health and Human Services**
**Agency for Healthcare Research and Quality**
2101 E Jefferson St.
Rockville, MD 20852
**Phone:** (301)594-6662
**Email:** info@ahrq.gov
**Website:** http://www.ahrq.gov/
John M. Eisenberg, Director
**Desc:** The Agency for Healthcare Research and Quality supports research aimed at reducing healthcare costs, medical errors, and patient safety concerns, as well as improving the quality and availability of care.

**U.S. Department of Health and Human Services**
**Food and Drug Administration**
**Center for Biologics Evaluation and Research**
*See:* Entry 17862

**U.S. Department of Health and Human Services**
**Food and Drug Administration**
**Center for Devices and Radiological Health**
*See:* Entry 18088

**U.S. Department of Health and Human Services**
**Food and Drug Administration**
**Center for Drug Evaluation and Research**
*See:* Entry 17863

## Foundations & Other Funding Organizations

### Private Foundations

**Joyce Foundation**
*See:* Entry 8542

**Rosenberg Foundation**
*See:* Entry 9851

### Other Funding Organizations

**★ 9939 ★ American Association of Medical Assistants (AAMA)**
20 N Wacker Dr., Ste. 1575
Chicago, IL 60606-2963
**Phone:** (312)899-1500        **Free:** 800-228-2262
**Fax:** (312)899-1259
**Email:** rosenfdn@rosenbergfdn.org
**Website:** http://www.aama-ntl.org
Donald A. Balasa, Exec. Dir.
**Desc:** Medical assistants are allied health professionals who work primarily in anbilatory (out patient) settings and perform clinical and administrative procedures. Activities include a certification program consisting of study and an examination, passage of which entitles the individual to become credentialed as a Certified Medical Assistant. Conducts accreditation of one- and two-year programs in medical assisting in conjunction with the commission on Accreditation of Allied Health Education Programs. Provides assistance and information to institutions of higher learning desirous of initiating courses for medical assistants. Awards continuing education units for selected educational programs. **Awards:** Maxine Williams Scholarship.

**★ 9940 ★ American Health Care Association (AHCA)**
1201 L St. NW
Washington, DC 20005
**Phone:** (202)842-4444        **Fax:** (202)842-3860
**Website:** http://www.ahca.org
Dr. Charles H. Roadman, II, CEO
**Desc:** Federation of state associations of long-term health care facilities. Promotes standards for professionals in long-term health care delivery and quality care for patients and residents in a safe environment. Focuses on issues of availability, quality, affordability, and fair payment. Operates as liaison with governmental agencies, Congress, and professional associations. Compiles statistics. **Awards:** James Durante Nurse Scholarship (annual) for nursing student working in a long term care facility.

**★ 9941 ★ American Society for Healthcare Food Service Administrators (ASHFSA)**
One N Franklin
Chicago, IL 60606
**Phone:** (312)422-3870        **Fax:** (312)422-4581
**Email:** pburton@aha.org
**Website:** http://www.ashfsa.org
Patricia Burton, Exec. Dir.
**Desc:** Serves individuals with healthcare food service management responsibilities, educators, suppliers and consultants to the profession, is the driving force in the healthcare food service industry and provides healthcare professionals with the resources to compete and succeed. **Awards:** Dorothy Killian Scholarship hotel, restaurant, food management or dietetics programs.

**★ 9942 ★ National Association for Healthcare Quality (NAHQ)**
4700 W Lake Ave.
Glenview, IL 60025-1485
**Phone:** (847)375-4720        **Free:** 800-966-9392
**Fax:** 877-218-7939
**Email:** dsimmons@nahq.com
**Website:** http://www.nahq.org
Diane K. Simmons, Exec. Dir.
**Desc:** Healthcare professionals in quality assessment and improvement, utilization and risk management, case management, infection control, managed care, nursing, and medical records. Objectives are: to encourage, develop, and provide continuing education for all persons involved in health care quality; to give the patient primary consideration in all actions affecting his or her health and welfare; to promote the sharing of knowledge and encourage a high degree of professional ethics in health care quality. Offers accredited certification in the field of healthcare quality, utilization, and risk management. Facilitates communication and cooperation among members, medical staff, and health care government agencies. Conducts educational seminars and conferences. **Awards:** Award for Association Excellence (annual); Clare Glover Distinguished Member Award (annual); Stumph Award for Excellence in Publication (annual).

## National & International Organizations

**★ 9943 ★ Academy Health Sciences**
2578 Broadway, Ste. 112
New York, NY 10025
**Phone:** (212)932-2381
**Email:** naturaltherapy@verizon.net
**Website:** http://www.naturaltherapy.com
Dr. Shoshana Margolin, Coord.
**Fnded:** 1996. **Mem:** 120. **Desc:** Arranges conferences where researchers and practitioners share innovative ideas on upgrading the skills of healthcare professionals. Conducts research and educational programs.

**★ 9944 ★ Accrediting Bureau of Health Education Schools (ABHES)**
803 W Broad St., Ste. 730
Falls Church, VA 22046
**Phone:** (703)533-2082          **Fax:** (703)998-2550
**Email:** info@abhes.org
**Website:** http://www.abhes.org
Carol A. Moneymaker, Exec. Dir.

**Fnded:** 1964. **Mem:** 180. **Desc:** Serves as a nationally recognized accrediting agency of health education institutions and schools conducting medical laboratory technician and medical assistant education programs. Establishes criteria and standards for the administration and operation of health education institutions. Seeks to enhance the profession through the improvement of schools, courses, and the competence of graduates. Schools must apply voluntarily for accreditation; once accredited, they must report to the bureau annually and be reexamined at least every 6 years. Has accredited 15 programs for medical laboratory technicians, 124 medical assistants, and 80 institutions of allied health. **Pub:** *Accrediting Bureau of Health Education Schools–Directory of Accredited Schools and Programs*, annual. Directory. Lists education institutions and programs accredited by the com missioners of the ABHES. • *Advantage*, quarterly. Newsletter. Includes calendar of events, news, lists personnel and comissioners. **Frmly:** Accrediting Bureau of Medical Laboratory Schools.

**★ 9945 ★ Advocate Health Care (AHC)**
2025 Windsor Dr.
Oak Brook, IL 60523
**Phone:** (630)572-9393          **Free:** 800-323-8622
**Fax:** (630)572-9139
**Website:** http://www.advocatehealth.com/
Richard Risk, Pres.

**Fnded:** 1995. **Mem:** 10. **Desc:** Health care corporations. Promotes the philosophy that good health care involves an understanding of human ecology and must meet the emotional and spiritual as well as the physical needs of patients. (Human ecology is the "understanding and care of human beings as whole persons in light of their relationships to God, themselves, their families, and the society in which they live.") Supports the concept of holistic health care. Sponsors teaching programs at hospitals; maintains support groups. Sponsors the Park Ridge Center, an institute for the study of health, faith, and ethics; and Parkside Alcoholic Research Foundation, which studies the cause and course of alcoholism and substance abuse. Maintains speakers' bureau. **Pub:** *Human Ecology Booklet*, semiannual. Booklet. • *Ounce of Prevention*, quarterly. • *Second Opinion: Health, Faith, and Ethics*, 3/year. Journal. *Price:* $35/year. • Annual Report. • Bulletin, bimonthly.

**★ 9946 ★ African Medical and Research Foundation - Tanzania (AMREF)**
PO Box 2773
Upanga Rd.
Dar es Salaam, United Republic of Tanzania
**Phone:** 255 51 116610          **Fax:** 255 51 115823
**Email:** amreftz@africaonline.co.tz
**Website:** http://www.amref.org

**Fnded:** 1957. **Desc:** Works to develop health programs among communities in Africa. Conducts research; compiles and disseminates information on health issues. Networks with other organizatins with similar objectives, providing a forum for information exchange and cooperation in projects and research.

**★ 9947 ★ Alliance of Community Health Plans (ACHP)**
2000 M St., NW, Ste. 201
Washington, DC 20036-3307
**Phone:** (202)785-2247          **Fax:** (202)785-4060
**Email:** jebeler@achp.org
**Website:** http://www.achp.org
Jack C. Ebeler, Pres.

**Fnded:** 1984. **Desc:** Members are twenty-two not-for-profit and provider-based health plans, non-investor owned and provider-based, that serve more than 12 million Americans in 18 states and the District of Columbia. These plans have distinguished themselves through the National Committee for Quality Assurance accreditation, and with superior scores in both the Health Plan Data and Information Set and the Consumer Assessment of Health Plan Survey. The Alliance provides aid to contributing plans to enhance the wellbeing of their members and their communities and promotes the improvement in health care services of member plans by supporting activities which focus on the achievement of the highest standards of health care delivery. **Frmly:** The HMO Group.

**★ 9948 ★ Alliance for Health Reform (AHR)**
1900 L St. NW, Ste. 512
Washington, DC 20036
**Phone:** (202)466-5626          **Fax:** (202)466-6525
**Email:** edhoward@allhealth.org
**Website:** http://www.allhealth.org
Edward F. Howard, Exec. V. Pres.

**Fnded:** 1991. **Desc:** Individuals and organizations with an interest in health care. Promotes increased public awareness of health care issues and proposals for health care reform in the United States. Serves as a clearinghouse on health care reform.

**★ 9949 ★ American Accreditation Healthcare Commission (URAC)**
1275 K St. NW, Ste. 1100
Washington, DC 20005
**Phone:** (202)216-9010          **Fax:** (202)216-9006
**Email:** gcarneal@urac.org
**Website:** http://www.urac.org
Garry Carneal, Pres. /CEO

**Fnded:** 1990. **Mem:** 300. **Desc:** Accreditation body for the managed health care industry. Seeks to establish and enforce standards for the managed care industry. Examines managed health care providers and bestows accreditation upon qualifying case management, health utilization management, health network, health plan, practitioner credentialling, credentials verification, workers' compensation utilization management, workers' compensation network, and health call center programs. **Pub:** *Directory of Accredited Organizations*, annual. Directory. *Price:* $39/copy. • *Models of Care: Case Studies of Healthcare Delivery Innovation.* Book. *Price:* $195/copy.

**★ 9950 ★ American Association of Healthcare Consultants (AAHC)**
1926 Waukegan Rd., Ste. 1
Glenview, IL 60025-1770
**Phone:** (847)657-6964          **Free:** 800-362-4674
**Fax:** (847)657-6819
**Email:** info@aahc.net
**Website:** http://www.aahc.net
David L. Stumph, Exec. Dir.

**Fnded:** 1949. **Mem:** 200. **Desc:** Professional association of individuals (185) and firms (50) exclusively devoted to health care consultation. Serves as a resource for health care providers; offers continuing education to members. Provides information concerning the role of health consulting. **Pub:** Membership Directory, annual. **Frmly:** (1984) American Association of Hospital Consultants.

**★ 9951 ★ American Health Care Advisory Association (AHCAA)**
PO Box 11369
Robinson
Waco, TX 76716
Nick Keeling, Pres.

**Fnded:** 1982. **Mem:** 25,000. **Desc:** Acts as an advisory organization promoting improved health care and reduction in medical costs. Gathers information concerning medical and insurance costs. **Pub:** *Vitality Health Gram*, quarterly.

**★ 9952 ★ American Health Decisions (AHD)**
1445 Market St., Ste. 380
Denver, CO 80202
**Email:** garlandm@ohsu.edu
**Website:** http://www.ahd.org/
Michael J. Garland, Chm.

**Fnded:** 1989. **Mem:** 21. **Desc:** Confederation of state health programs. Assists in establishing public education programs about health care and policy; works to increase availability of quality medical care. Promotes personal autonomy on ethical issues, such as patients making the decision to refuse or accept treatment. Addresses problems arising from ethical conflicts over new medical technologies and disease prevention. Maintains research and educational programs; disseminates information.

**★ 9953 ★ American Medical Network**
15429 N Florida Ave.
Tampa, FL 33613
**Free:** (866)346-2354          **Fax:** (813)264-0647
**Email:** benefits@americanmednetwork.com
**Website:** http://www.americanmednetwork.com

**Fnded:** 1996. **Desc:** Practicing physicians. Represents doctors' concerns for their patients; establishes a national quality database for use in negotiating managed care contracts; educates laymen and policy makers on quality of care issues; and influences health care policy.

**★ 9954 ★ American Medical Resources Foundation (AMRF)**
56 Oak Hill Way
PO Box 3609
Brockton, MA 02304
**Phone:** (508)580-3301          **Fax:** (508)580-3306
**Email:** amrf@amrf.com
**Website:** http://www.amrf.com
Kay H. Barney, Chm.

**Fnded:** 1988. **Desc:** Donates used, but fully functional, medical equipment to hospitals and clinics serving the poor in Third World and developing nations. The equipment is donated to AMRF by over 300 hospitals and industries in the U.S. and by private physicians and dentists. Donated equipment includes beds and patient transports; through monitors; x-rays; infant warmers; infant transformers; patient handling equipment; pulmonary, cardiac or ultrasonic diagnostic equipment; and diverse equipment for general and specialized use in prenatal, natal, pediatric and adult departments. Coordinates volunteer procedures and assists in the setting up and calibration of all equipment at the recipient hospitals. Provides training for the hospital biomedical technicians. **Pub:** *AMRF News*, quarterly. Newsletter.

**American Society Bioethics and Humanities**
*See:* Entry 1924

**★ 9955 ★ American Society for Healthcare Food Service Administrators (ASHFSA)**
1 N Franklin
Chicago, IL 60606
**Phone:** (312)422-3870          **Fax:** (312)422-4581
**Email:** ashfsa@aha.org
**Website:** http://www.ashfsa.org
Eliana Schultz, Pres.

**Fnded:** 1967. **Desc:** Individuals with healthcare food service management responsibilities, educators, suppliers and consultants to the profession. Seeks to advance the practice of healthcare food service management in a broad range of healthcare settings. **Pub:** Video.Cassette recordings of ASHFSA Internet-based conferences.

**Argentina Association of Medical Advisers (AAMA)**
**(Association Agentes de Propaganda Medica de la Republica Argentina — AAPMRA)**
*See:* Entry 1939

**★ 9956 ★ Association for Education in Healthcare Information Technology**
4500 Hugh Howell Rd., Ste. 340
Tucker, GA 30084
**Phone:** (770)270-9611 **Fax:** (770)270-0632
**Email:** insight@pami.org
**Website:** http://64.239.40.35/
**Desc:** Employees, consultants in healthcare industry. Works to provide its members with information on the healthcare industry and related information technology issues.

**★ 9957 ★ Association of the European Self-Medication Industry (AESGP)**
**(Europaischer Fachverband der Arzneimittel-Hersteller)**
7, ave. de Tervuren
B-1040 Brussels, Belgium
**Phone:** 32 2 7355130 **Fax:** 32 2 7355222
**Email:** info@aesgp.be
**Website:** http://www.aesgp.be
**Fnded:** 1964. **Mem:** 25. **Lang(s):** English. **Desc:** National European proprietary medicines associations. (Proprietary medicines are packaged, over-the-counter drugs.) Advocates self-medication, defined as the therapeutic use of drugs that are safe, effective, and available without prescription. Objectives are to: encourage the involvement of the pharmaceutical industry in European national health care systems; promote and maintain high standards of production, distribution, and advertising of proprietary drugs; ensure that the interests of the proprietary drug industry are recognized by institutions responsible for health legislation; enhance cooperation and the exchange of information among members, and with international professional, industrial, and governmental organizations; represent member associations in World Self-Medication Industry (WSMI). Compiles statistics. **Pub:** *Annual Meeting Proceedings.* • *Developing Self-Medication in Central and Eastern Europe.* • *Self-Medication and the Pharmacist,* periodic. • *Summary of Product Characteristics for Non-Prescription Medicines in the EC.*

**★ 9958 ★ Association of German Dental Manufacturers**
**(Verband der Deutschen Dental-Industrie — VDDI)**
Postfach 40 06 63
D-50836 Cologne, Germany
**Phone:** 49 221 9486280 **Fax:** 49 221 483428
**Email:** h.russegger@vddi.de
**Website:** http://www.vddi.de
**Fnded:** 1917. **Mem:** 190. **Lang(s):** German. **Desc:** Companies manufacturing dental equipment and supplies. Establishes international standards and technical harmonization for dental equipment. Represents members' interests before government bodies, international agencies, and the public. Maintains liaison with organizations representing dentists, dental technicians, and dental supply dealers and distributors. Compiles statistics. **Pub:** *The German Dental Industry,* biennial. Brochure.

**★ 9959 ★ Association for Healthcare Resource and Materials Management (AHRMM)**
c/o American Hospital Association
1 N Franlkin
Chicago, IL 60606
**Phone:** (312)422-3840 **Fax:** (312)422-4573
**Email:** ahrmm@aha.org
**Website:** http://www.ahrmm.org
Deborah Sprindzunas, Exec. Dir.

**Fnded:** 1962. **Mem:** 2,700. **Local Groups:** 45. **Desc:** Individuals active in the field of purchasing, inventory and distribution, and materials management as performed in hospitals, related patient care institutions, or government and voluntary health organizations, and who are employed by an organization eligible for institutional membership in the American Hospital Association; associate members are individuals active in the areas of health care supply manufacturing, distributing, and consulting. Purposes are to: assist members with their responsibilities; provide access to the latest ideas, methods, developments, information, and techniques in the field of hospital purchasing and materials management; establish associations with others in the profession; provide recognition in the profession through participation in policy-making; provide a link with the AHA. Conducts certification program in health care management. **Pub:** *Association for Healthcare Resource & Materials Management–Conference Proceedings,* annual. Proceedings. Presents case studies. *Price:* $45/year for members; $65/year for nonmembers. • *Association for Healthcare Resource & Materials Management–Membership Roster,* annual. Membership Directory. *Price:* Included in membership dues. • *Healthcare Resource & Materials Management News,* bimonthly. Newsletter. Contains reviews of educational programs, current legal and legislative problems, new resources and materials management techniques, and assoc. news. *Price:* Included in membership dues. • *Resource Catalog,* annual. **Frmly:** (1976) American Society for Hospital Purchasing Agents; (1983) American Society for Hospital Purchasing and Materials Management; (1994) American Society for Hospital Materials Management; (1998) American Society for Healthcare Materials Management.

**Berufsverband der Pharmaberater (BP)**
*See:* Entry 2008

**Berufsverband der Pharmarefenten Osterreichs (BPO)**
*See:* Entry 2009

**★ 9960 ★ Better Sleep Council (BSC)**
501 Wythe St.
Alexandria, VA 22314
**Phone:** (703)683-8371 **Fax:** (703)683-4503
**Email:** bsc@sleepproducts.org
**Website:** http://www.bettersleep.org
Andrea Herman, Dir.
**Fnded:** 1978. **Desc:** Bedding manufacturers and suppliers organized to increase public awareness of the importance of sleep to good health, quality of life, and the role of the sleep system in pursuit of a good night's sleep. **Pub:** *Better Sleep Guide.* Brochure. A consumer guide to sleep and mattresses. • Also publishes press kits. **Frmly:** (1987) Better Sleep Council (of the National Association of Bedding Manufacturers); (1993) Better Sleep Council (of the International Sleep Products Association).

**★ 9961 ★ Britain - Nepal Medical Trust (BNMT)**
c/o Export House
130 Yale Rd.
Tonbridge TN9 1SP, United Kingdom
**Phone:** 44 1732 360284 **Fax:** 44 1732 363876
**Fnded:** 1968. **Lang(s):** English. **Desc:** Health care professionals and health organizations. Seeks to improve the health of the people of Nepal. Works with Nepalese government agencies to increase delivery of health services in underserved areas. Evaluates health programs and makes recommendations for their improvement; distributes medical equipment, medications, and other supplies.

**★ 9962 ★ British Dental Trade Association (BDTA)**
Mineral Ln.
Chesham HP5 1NL, United Kingdom
**Phone:** 44 1494 782873 **Fax:** 44 1494 786659

**Email:** admin@bdta.org.uk
**Website:** http://www.bdta.org.uk
**Fnded:** 1923. **Mem:** 116. **Lang(s):** English. **Desc:** Companies manufacturing dental equipment and supplies. Establishes international standards and technical harmonization for dental equipment. Represents members' interests before government bodies, international agencies, and the public. Maintains liaison with organizations representing dentists, dental technicians, and dental supply dealers and distributors. Compiles statistics. **Pub:** *Dental Trader,* quarterly. Journal.

**Business Alliance for Commerce in Hemp (IASPA)**
**(Associazione Italiana Informatori Scientifici del Farmaco — AIISF)**
*See:* Entry 2017

**Canadian Health Coalition (CHC)**
**(Coalition Canadienne de la Sante — CCS)**
*See:* Entry 9726

**Center for the Well Being of Health Professionals**
*See:* Entry 16771

**Coalition for Nonprofit Health Care Research and Development (CNHCRD)**
*See:* Entry 2065

**CPRI-HOST**
*See:* Entry 9733

**Cyprus Medical Representatives Association (CMRA)**
*See:* Entry 2077

**★ 9963 ★ Danish Dental Manufacturers**
Borsen
DK-1217 Copenhagen K, Denmark
**Phone:** 45 33950500 **Fax:** 45 33325216
**Email:** administration@cpri-host.org
**Website:** http://www.cpri-host.org/
**Lang(s):** Danish, English. **Desc:** Companies manufacturing dental equipment and supplies. Establishes international standards and technical harmonization for dental equipment. Represents members' interests before government bodies, international agencies, and the public. Maintains liaison with organizations representing dentists, dental technicians, and dental supply dealers and distributors. Compiles statistics.

**★ 9964 ★ DENIP**
c/o Unamec
Leuvenstraat 29
B-1800 Vivoorde, Belgium
**Phone:** 32 2 2570590 **Fax:** 32 2 2524398
**Email:** n.vanlent@unamec.be
**Lang(s):** Dutch, French, German. **Desc:** Companies manufacturing dental equipment and supplies. Establishes international standards and technical harmonization for dental equipment. Represents members' interests before government bodies, international agencies, and the public. Maintains liaison with organizations representing dentists, dental technicians, and dental supply dealers and distributors.

**★ 9965 ★ ECRI**
c/o Laurie D. Menyo, Communications Dept.
5200 Butler Pke.
Plymouth Meeting, PA 19462
**Phone:** (610)825-6000 **Fax:** (610)834-1275
**Email:** info@ecri.org
**Website:** http://www.healthcare.org
Jeffrey C. Lerner, PhD, Pres. /CEO

**Fnded:** 1955. **Mem:** 5,000. **Desc:** Improves the safety, performance, reliability, and cost effectiveness of health care technology through research testing, and publication of results. Provides technical consulting and accident investigation and educational programs. Functions as a worldwide information clearinghouse for health care technology assessment and hazards and deficiencies in medical devices; sponsors seminars. Provides information and technical assistance for planning, procurement and management of medical equipment. Conducts research; compiles statistics and operates speakers' bureau. **Pub:** *Health Devices*, weekly. • *Health Devices Alerts*, weekly. • *Health Devices Sourcebook*, annual. Directory. • *Health Technology Trends*, monthly. Newsletter. • *Healthcare Environmental Management*, monthly. • *Healthcare Product Comparison System*, monthly. • *Healthcare Risk Control*, monthly. • *Healthcare Technology Assessment Reports: Executive Briefings*, monthly. • *Hospital Hazardous Materials Management*, monthly. Newsletter. • *Operating Room Risk Management*, bimonthly. • *Technology for Anesthesia*, periodic. Includes information on medical equipment and research updates. *Price:* $125/year. • *Technology for Cardiology*, monthly. Newsletter. Reports on ECRI comparative product evaluations; offers hazard reports on medical devices and device operation data. Includes research updates. *Price:* $125/year. • *Technology for Respiratory Therapy*, monthly. Newsletter. Evaluates medical devices and summarizes reported problems, hazards, and recalls. Includes research updates and health care technology abstracts. *Price:* $125/year. **Frmly:** (1968) Graduate Pain Research Foundation; (1979) Emergency Care Research Institute.

★ **9966** ★ **Families U.S.A. Foundation**
1334 G St. NW
Washington, DC 20005
**Phone:** (202)628-3030     **Fax:** (202)347-2417
**Email:** info@familiesusa.org
**Website:** http://www.familiesusa.org
Ronald F. Pollack, Exec. Dir.

**Fnded:** 1981. **Desc:** Issues reports and other materials on health care and long term care for use by consumer organizations, policymakers, the media, and state-based coalitions working on health care and long term care reform. **Pub:** *Crossing to Mexico: Priced Out of American Health Care.* Survey. Surveys Mexican doctors and American consumers about the reasons Americans go to Mexico for routine medical care. *Price:* $5. • *The Crunch: The Health Insurance Crisis Comes to America's Charities.* Covers the problems of the small business market for health insurance by examining the experiences of 500 non-profit groups surveyed. *Price:* $5. • *Half of Us: Families Priced Out of Health Protection.* Provides an analysis of government survey data. *Price:* $10. • *The Health Cost Squeeze on Older Americans.* Provides an analysis of elderly out-of-pocket health care costs; compares current costs to those prior to the enactment of Medicare. *Price:* $5. • *The Heavy Burden of Home Care.* Provides an analysis of home care expenditures and the high out-of-pocket costs consumers pay to provide home care. *Price:* $5. • *Making Them Wait For Social Security Disability Benefits.* Provides an analysis of the waiting times and backlogs for people applying for Social Security and SSI Disability benefits. *Price:* $5. • *The Medicare Buy-in: A Promise Unfulfilled.* Describes the Medicare buy-in benefits, the Qualified Medicare Beneficiary and Specified Low-income Medicare Beneficiary. *Price:* $5. • *No Sale: The Failure of Barebones Insurance.* Examines state barebones policies and their ability to provide affordable coverage and to expand insurance to the uninsured population. *Price:* $15. • *Nursing Home Insurance: Who Can Afford It?.* Provides an analysis of the affordability of providing nursing home insurance policies for today's elderly population. *Price:* $5. • *Prescription Costs: America's Other Drug Crisis.* Provides an analysis (for years 1985-1991) of the prices of America's 20 top selling drugs and the pharmaceutical companies' profits. *Price:* $5. • *They Make That Much.* Survey. Contains salaries of medical specialists, CEOs of dru. **Frmly:** (1989) Villers Foundation.

★ **9967** ★ **Federation of the European Dental Industry**
**(Federation de l'Industrie Dentaire en Europe — FIDE)**
Kirchweg 2
D-50858 Cologne, Germany
**Phone:** 49 221 9486280     **Fax:** 49 221 483428
**Fnded:** 1957. **Mem:** 10. **Lang(s):** English. **Desc:** National associations of companies engaged in the manufacture of dental instruments and supplies. Functions as a platform for coordination of development and works to harmonize international standards within the industry; represents members' interests before government and European Community agencies. Promotes environmental protection, bar coding (HIBC), market statistics (project). **Pub:** *FIDE - European Dental Industry*, biennial. Brochure. Membership brochure. • *FIDE News*, 1-2/year. Newsletter.

★ **9968** ★ **Federation of the Trade Unions in Health Care**
Maria Luiza 45
BG-1202 Sofia, Bulgaria
**Phone:** 359 2 882097     **Fax:** 359 2 831814
**Fnded:** 1990. **Mem:** 33,953. **Reg. Groups:** 28. **Local Groups:** 448. **Lang(s):** English, French, Russian. **Desc:** Defends and represents members' interests.

★ **9969** ★ **Forum for Health Care Planning (Forum)**
314 Vistade Valle
Mill Valley, CA 94941-4107
**Phone:** (415)381-1846     **Fax:** (415)381-1104
Cornelia Hinz, Contact
**Fnded:** 1950. **Mem:** 500. **Reg. Groups:** 5. **Desc:** Is dedicated to the promotion of quality health care. Provides opportunities for advocacy and continuing education programs for persons committed to planning quality health care services and facilities. Disseminates and exchanges information on hospital and health care planning. **Pub:** Membership Directory, annual. • Newsletter, quarterly. **Frmly:** (1986) American Association for Hospital Planning.

★ **9970** ★ **Health Care Compliance Association (HCCA)**
1211 Locust St.
Philadelphia, PA 19107
**Phone:** (215)545-3334     **Free:** 888-580-8373
**Fax:** (215)545-8107
**Email:** info@hcca-info.org
**Website:** http://www.hcca-info.org
Bill Ward, Contact
**Fnded:** 1997. **Mem:** 3,200. **Nat'l Groups:** 1. **Reg. Groups:** 10. **Desc:** Healthcare professionals involved in compliance in the health care industry. Promotes quality compliance programs in health care. Offers educational programs, professional network and discussion groups. **Pub:** *Compliance Today*, monthly. Magazine.

★ **9971** ★ **Health Care Liability Alliance (HCLA)**
PO Box 19008
Washington, DC 20036-9008
**Phone:** (202)293-4255     **Fax:** (202)296-7689
**Website:** http://www.hcla.org/
**Desc:** Medical organizations. Dedicated to improving America's health care system through reform.

★ **9972** ★ **Health Care Supplies Association**
32 Etron Close
Chester House
Datchet
Slough SL3 9BE, United Kingdom
**Phone:** 44 1753 580176     **Fax:** 44 1753 580176
**Fnded:** 1960. **Mem:** 490. **Desc:** To promote maintain and seek continuously to improve professional standards and training relating to supplies and associated services within the healthcare sector. To establish and maintain a professional link with appropriate statutory bodies. To liaise with professional and other organizations. Activities include two annual training schools for junior grades in the supplies discipline and an annual conference. **Pub:** *Official Procurement Guide*, annual. Book.

★ **9973** ★ **Health Industry Business Communications Council (HIBCC)**
2525 E Arizona Biltmore Clr., Ste. 127
Phoenix, AZ 85016-2129
**Phone:** (602)381-1091     **Fax:** (602)381-1093
**Email:** info@hibcc.org
**Website:** http://www.hibcc.org/
Robert A. Hankin, PhD, Pres.
**Fnded:** 1984. **Mem:** 1,000. **Desc:** Individuals and companies in the health care industry. To improve the quality and economic efficiency of health care by instituting and overseeing a uniform system of computer bar coding (for identification of health care equipment) and by promoting the use of this and other automated technologies in the health care industry. **Pub:** *Health Industry Lines*, quarterly. Newsletter. *Price:* Included in membership dues. • *Standards*, periodic. **Frmly:** (1987) Health Industry Bar Code Council.

★ **9974** ★ **Health Services Union of Australia (HSUA)**
171 Drummond St.
Carlton, VIC 3053, Australia
**Phone:** 61 3 96507466     **Fax:** 61 3 96542386
**Email:** hsua@hsua.asn.au
**Website:** http://www.hsua.asn.au
**Mem:** 90,000. **Lang(s):** English. **Desc:** Workers in the health care industries. Seeks to advance the economic well-being and improve the conditions of employment of members. Represents members in negotiations with employers.

★ **9975** ★ **HealthCare Compliance Packaging Council (HCPC)**
252 N Washington St., Ste. A
Falls Church, VA 22046
**Phone:** (703)538-4030     **Fax:** (703)538-6305
**Email:** pgmayberry@aol.com
**Website:** http://www.unitdose.org
Peter G. Mayberry, Exec. Dir.
**Fnded:** 1990. **Mem:** 80. **Desc:** Promotes the use of "unit-dose blister packaging" for pharmaceutical as a means of insuring better patient compliance with drug regimens. Sponsors research and provides educational programs. **Pub:** *Compliance News and Views*, quarterly. Newsletter. • *Unit Dose Alert*, bimonthly. Newsletter.

★ **9976** ★ **Healthcare Forum**
180 Montgomery St., Ste. 1520
San Francisco, CA 94104-4230
Kathryn E. Johnson, CEO & Pres.
**Fnded:** 1927. **Mem:** 1,100. **Desc:** Healthcare leaders and executives. Promotes visionary leadership and motivation in healthcare. Conducts leadership development education programs; produces computer based educational materials. Sponsors research activities. **Pub:** *Healthcare Forum Journal*, bimonthly. Journal. *Price:* $55.

★ **9977** ★ **INDENT, Dutch Dental Association**
Postbus 190
NL-2700 AD Zoetermeer, Netherlands
**Phone:** 31 79 3531269     **Fax:** 31 79 3531365
**Email:** indent@fme.nl
**Fnded:** 1978. **Mem:** 22. **Lang(s):** Dutch. **Desc:** Companies manufacturing dental equipment and supplies. Establishes international standards and technical harmonization for dental equipment. Represents members' interests before government bodies, international agencies, and the public. Maintains liaison

with organizations representing dentists, dental technicians, and dental supply dealers and distributors. Compiles statistics. **Pub:** *INDENT Export Group, the Netherlands.* Brochure. Contains information regarding products and activities of members of the INDENT export group. **Frmly:** (1993) VNFTP.

**★ 9978 ★ Institute of Certified Healthcare Business Consultants (ICHBC)**
307 N Michigan Ave., Ste. 800
Chicago, IL 60601-5309
**Phone:** (312)360-0384       **Free:** 800-447-1684
**Fax:** (312)360-0388
**Email:** info@ichbc.org
**Website:** http://www.ichbc.org
Barbara Boden, Exec. Dir.

**Fnded:** 1975. **Mem:** 295. **Desc:** Individuals providing business advisory services to physicians and dentists. Maintains code of ethics, rules of professional conduct, and certification program; administers examination and conducts review course. Membership by successful completion of certification examination only. **Pub:** *Institute of Certified Healthcare Business Consultants–Certified News*, quarterly. Newsletter. *Price:* available to members only. • *Institute of Certified Healthcare Business Consultants–Membership Directory*, annual. Membership Directory. **Frmly:** (1999) Institute of Certified Professional Business Consultants.

**★ 9979 ★ Intercare**
900 Wilshire Blve., Ste. 500
Los Angeles, CA 90017
**Phone:** (213)627-8878       **Fax:** (213)627-9183
**Email:** info@intercare.com
**Website:** http://www.intercare.com/
Theodore Carcich, Jr., Pres.

**Fnded:** 1976. **Mem:** 600. **Desc:** Individuals involved or interested in the long-term health care of the chronically ill. Works to improve long-term health care; to encourage high standards of professional care and administration; to interact with professional groups, academic institutions, and governmental agencies; to provide opportunities for individual research; to discover solutions to the problems of the aged, chronically ill, and disabled; to establish a clearinghouse of research findings and resources. Maintains speakers' bureau. Provides semi-quarterly educational program in various countries. **Pub:** *Intercare, International Directory*, annual. Directory. • Journal, quarterly.

**★ 9980 ★ International Association of Medical Equipment Remarketers (IAMER)**
183 Lucy Ln.
Wylie, TX 75098-7244
**Free:** 877-304-2637       **Fax:** (480)575-0891
**Email:** radlady@att.net
**Website:** http://www.iamers.org/
Tom Norman, Pres.

**Fnded:** 1994. **Mem:** 150. **Desc:** Dealers, lessors, refurbishers, and services of medical equipment. Promotes ethical business practices and delivers high quality previously owned medical equipment. Offers educational and research programs and maintains a speakers bureau. **Pub:** Newsletter. • Directory. • Brochure.

**★ 9981 ★ International Health Evaluation Association (IHEA)**
846 S Hotel St., Ste. 303
Honolulu, HI 96813-2583
**Phone:** (808)524-4411       **Fax:** (808)524-5559
**Website:** http://www.ihea.net
William Rakowski, Chair

**Fnded:** 1971. **Mem:** 300. **Reg. Groups:** 3. **Desc:** Users, suppliers, and manufacturers of computer-based health evaluation systems including clinics, hospitals, physicians, medical students, and research institutions. Is dedicated to the improvement of health care through: the advancement of computer-based health testing and evaluation techniques; the refine-

ment of associated data-processing systems and biomedical devices; the development of a low-cost, high-quality health programs. Believes the technique of computer-based health evaluation can be used in the areas of testing industrial workers and others exposed to environmental hazards, mandatory tests conducted by governmental agencies, and pre-admission hospital testing. Sponsors seminars on clinical preventive medicine for the discussion of medical results, operational techniques, new applications, and cost-effectiveness data. Conducts research; compiles statistics; maintains library; operates speakers' bureau. **Pub:** *Proceedings of Annual Symposia*, quarterly. Proceedings. *Price:* Free. • *Regional Newsletter*, periodic. Newsletter. • Newsletter, quarterly.

**International Union of Medical Advisers Associations (IUMAA) (Union Internationale des Associations de Delegues Medicaux — UIADM)**
*See:* Entry 2225

**★ 9982 ★ Kaiser Family Foundation**
2400 Sand Hill Rd.
Menlo Park, CA 94025
**Phone:** (650)854-9400       **Fax:** (650)854-4800
**Website:** http://www.kff.org
Drew Altman, Pres.

**Desc:** Works to research and promote health care issues. Focuses on health policy, media and public education, and health and development in South Africa.

**★ 9983 ★ Medical Information Bureau (MIB)**
PO Box 105, Essex Station
Boston, MA 02112
**Phone:** (781)329-4500       **Fax:** (781)329-3379
**Email:** infoline@mib.com
**Website:** http://www.mib.com
James F. Cook, Pres.

**Fnded:** 1902. **Mem:** 750. **Desc:** Life, health, and disability insurance companies. Seeks to reduce insurance fraud by providing member companies with information previous claims.

**★ 9984 ★ National Association for Healthcare Recruitment (NAHCR)**
307 Park Lake Cir.
Orlando, FL 32803
**Phone:** (407)843-6981       **Fax:** (407)423-4648
**Email:** ruthw@fha.org
**Website:** http://www.nahcr.com
Ruth Welke, Project Manager

**Fnded:** 1975. **Mem:** 1,000. **Reg. Groups:** 57. **Local Groups:** 50. **Desc:** Individuals employed directly by hospitals and other health care organizations which are involved in the practice of professional health care recruitment. Promotes sound principles of professional health care recruitment. Provides financial assistance to aid members in planning and implementing regional educational programs. Offers technical assistance and consultation services. Compiles statistics. **Pub:** *Annual Recruitment Survey*, annual. Survey. • *NAHCR Directions*, bimonthly. *Price:* $200/year. • *Recruiter Handbook*. Handbook. • *Who's Who in Recruitment and Resources*, annual. **Frmly:** National Association of Nurse Recruiters; (1987) National Association of Healthcare Recruiters.

**★ 9985 ★ National Association of Healthcare Consultants**
1255 23rd St. NW
Washington, DC 20037-1174
**Phone:** (202)452-8282       **Free:** 800-313-6242
**Fax:** (202)833-3636
**Email:** consultants@healthcon.org
**Website:** http://www.healthcon.org
Melissa Forburger, Exec. Dir.

**Fnded:** 1994. **Mem:** 350. **Nat'l Groups:** 1. **Desc:** Consultants who "provide ethical, confidential, and

professional advice to the healthcare industry." Promotes professional development of members; works to improve the standard of health care consulting services. Facilitates exchange of information among members; conducts educational and training programs; encourages members to attain Certified Healthcare Business Consultant (CHBC) status. Compiles statistics; makes available legal and marketing advice; provides group purchasing discount programs to members; maintains speakers' bureau. **Pub:** *Update*, periodic. Newsletter. *Price:* Not for sale. • Newsletter, periodic.

**National Association of Medical Advisers of Morocco (NAMAA) (Association Nationale des Delegues Medicaux du Maroc — ANDMM)**
*See:* Entry 2279

**★ 9986 ★ National Association of Physician Recruiters (NAPR)**
PO Box 150127
Altamonte Springs, FL 32715-0127
**Phone:** (407)774-7880       **Free:** 800-726-5613
**Fax:** (407)774-6440
**Email:** kmg-assn@worldnet.att.net
**Website:** http://www.napr.com
Bill Kautter, CAE, Exec. VP

**Fnded:** 1983. **Mem:** 300. **Desc:** Physician search firms (companies that recruit resident physicians or practicing physicians to fill positions nationwide). Promotes a positive public image of physician recruiting services. Seeks to establish accreditation standards for the field. Provides marketing services to the physician recruiting industry. Maintains speakers' bureau. Sponsors educational programs and seminars. Compiles statistics. **Pub:** *NAPA Business Report (Newsletter)*, annual, Client Brochure. Brochures. *Price:* $.75. • *NAPR Business Report*, quarterly. Newsletter.

**National Business Coalition on Health**
*See:* Entry 2284

**★ 9987 ★ National Coalition of Mental Health Professionals and Consumers**
PO Box 438
Commack, NY 11725
**Phone:** (631)424-5232       **Free:** 888-729-6662
**Fax:** (516)549-3942
**Email:** ncmhpc@aol.com
**Website:** http://www.nomanagedcare.org/
Deborah Peel, MD, Pres.

**Desc:** Mental health professionals, consumers and consumer advocates. Works to address the negative impact of managed care on patients and professionals in mental health care; promotes pro-patient, pro-quality alternatives that preserve a patient's right to choice, privacy, and control over treatment, expose abuses in managed care, and bring about regulation of the managed care industry. **Pub:** *Consumer Protection Manual.* Manual. • Newsletter.

**★ 9988 ★ National Committee for Quality Health Care (NCQHC)**
1800 Massachusetts Ave. NW, Ste. 545
Washington, DC 20036
**Phone:** (202)331-7535       **Fax:** (202)331-7532
**Email:** ncqhc@erols.com
**Website:** http://www.ncqhc.org/
Catherine E. McDermott, Pres.

**Fnded:** 1978. **Mem:** 151. **Desc:** Coalition of health care professionals and organizations principally involved in the health care industry; includes hospitals, physicians, health maintenance organizations, nursing homes, manufacturers of health care equipment, investment bankers, architects, contractors, and accountants. Works to maintain and strengthen quality health care in the U.S. **Pub:** *An American Health Strategy: Ensuring the Availability of Quality Health Care.* • *Critical Condition: America's Health Care in*

*Jeopardy.* • *Quality Bulletin*, bimonthly. Bulletin. • *Quality Outlook*, bimonthly. • Pamphlets. • Papers. **Frmly:** National Committee on Hospital Capital Expenditures.

## ★ 9989 ★ National CPA Health Care Advisors Association (HCAA)

111 E Wacker Dr., Ste. 990
Chicago, IL 60601
**Free:** 800-869-0491                    **Fax:** (312)729-9800
**Email:** info@hcaa.com
**Website:** http://www.hcaa.com
Lisa Bruno, Exec. Dir.
**Fnded:** 1992. **Mem:** 47. **Desc:** Certified public accountant (CPA) firms providing financial and consulting services to health care professionals. Seeks to enhance members' ability to serve the health care industry. Facilitates resource sharing and the establishment of joint ventures among members; provides marketing services to members; conducts industry surveys; sponsors continuing professional development and training courses. **Pub:** *Practice Management Advisor*, quarterly. Newsletter. A customizable newsletter for clients of members.

## ★ 9990 ★ National Emergency Equipment Dealers Association (NEEDA)

c/o Kenton H. Pattie
8421 Frost Way
Annandale, VA 22003
**Phone:** (703)280-4622              **Fax:** (703)280-0942
**Email:** kentonp1@aol.com
**Website:** http://www.needa.org
Pattie H. Kenton, Exec. Dir.
**Fnded:** 1996. **Mem:** 88. **Desc:** Dealers and services of fire, rescue, and emergency medical service vehicles, supplies and equipment. Preserves and strengthens the free market systems for dealers through advocacy, information and training. **Pub:** *NEEDA Newsletter*, monthly. Newsletter. Appears daily on Web site. *Price:* $100 per year.

## National Union of Medical Advisers Associations (NUMAA) (Syndicat National Professionel Autonome des Deleges Visiteurs Medicaux — SNPADVM)

*See:* Entry 2314

## ★ 9991 ★ Pakistan Voluntary Health and Nutrition Association (PVHNA)

9C, 18th Commercial St.
Karachi 29, Pakistan
**Phone:** 92 21 446709              **Fax:** 92 21 437653
**Fnded:** 1979. **Mem:** 30. **Lang(s):** English, Urdu. **Desc:** Seeks to improve public health in Pakistan. Promotes education in nutrition and family planning. Provides family planning organizations with training manuals. Conducts training programs in: water sanitation, child care, health care, and vocational education. Offers immunization services.

## Partnership for Patient Safety (P4PS)

*See:* Entry 2344

## Professional Association of Medical Advisers (PAMA) (Association Professionelle des Deleges Medicaux — APDM)

*See:* Entry 2362

## Professional Union of French-Speaking Medical Advisers (PUFSMA) (Union Professionelle des Deleges Medicaux Francophones — UPDMF)

*See:* Entry 2363

## ★ 9992 ★ Qualified Private Medical Practitioners and Hospitals' Association (QPMPA)

Ashoka Bhavan
Kayamkulam 690 502, India
**Phone:** 91 479 445532              **Fax:** 91 479 474911
**Email:** kumarkishore@satyam.net.in
**Website:** http://www.qpmpa.com
**Desc:** Promotes the private medical practitioners profession and hospitals industry.

## ★ 9993 ★ Regulatory Affairs Professionals Society (RAPS)

11300 Rockville Pike, Ste. 1000
Rockville, MD 20852
**Phone:** (301)770-2920              **Fax:** (301)770-2924
**Email:** raps@raps.org
**Website:** http://www.raps.org
Sherry Keramidas, PhD, CAE
**Fnded:** 1976. **Mem:** 8,200. **Desc:** Represents the regulatory affairs profession and the individuals who are part of this dynamic field. RAPS members are the health regulatory leaders of today and tomorrow in areas such as medical devices, pharmaceuticals, biologics, biotechnology, and in vitro diagnostics. **Pub:** *Regulatory Affairs Focus*, monthly. Magazine. *Price:* $120 for nonmembers.

## ★ 9994 ★ Society for Clinical Data Management (SCDM)

203 Towne Centre Dr.
Hillsborough, NJ 08844-4693
**Phone:** (908)359-0623              **Fax:** (908)359-7619
**Email:** info@scdm.org
**Website:** http://www.scdm.org
**Desc:** Promotes the discipline of clinical data management as a profession in the pharmaceutical and health care industries; supports educational opportunities; provides information and experience exchange to members; promotes standards of good practice. **Pub:** *Data Basics*, quarterly. Newsletter. • Papers.

## Society for Health and Human Values (SHHV)

*See:* Entry 2401

## ★ 9995 ★ Society of Medical-Dental Management Consultants (SMD)

3646 E Ray Rd., B16-45
Phoenix, AZ 85044
**Free:** 800-826-2264              **Fax:** (602)759-3530
**Email:** chuck@smdmc.org
**Website:** http://www.smdmc.org
Charles R. Wold, CPA, Exec. Sec.
**Fnded:** 1968. **Mem:** 60. **State Groups:** 50. **Desc:** Professional medical and/or dental management consultants associated for educational and information sharing purposes. Objectives are to: advance the profession; share management techniques; improve individual skills; provide clients with competent and capable business management. Provides information on insurance and income tax. Conducts surveys; compiles statistics. **Pub:** *Membership Roster*, annual. Membership Directory. • *SMD Statistics*. • *Society of Medical-Dental Management Consultants–Newsletter*, monthly. Newsletter. *Price:* Included in membership dues. • Bulletin.

## Spanish Confederation of Medical and Technical Advisers Associations (SCMTAA) (Confederacion Espanola de Asociaciones de Informadores Tecnicos Sanitarios — CEATIMEF)

*See:* Entry 2412

## ★ 9996 ★ Stratis Health

2901 Metro Dr., Ste. 400
Bloomington, MN 55425
**Phone:** (612)854-3306              **Fax:** (612)853-8503
**Email:** info@stratishealth.org
**Website:** http://www.stratishealth.org
Patsy Riley, CEO
**Fnded:** 1971. **Mem:** 3,500. **Desc:** Physicians interested in ensuring the availabilty of quality health care at reasonable costs. Evaluates health care services at hospitals, retirement homes, and other facilities. Develops health care standards for hospitals and offers consultation services to operators of health care facilities to improve efficiency in services. Conducts research and development on latest treatments and medical technologies. Tests new medical technologies.

## ★ 9997 ★ Swedish Dental Trade Association (Foreningen Svensk Dentalhandel — FSD)

Box 1416
S-111 84 Stockholm, Sweden
**Phone:** 46 8 50893800              **Fax:** 46 8 50893801
**Email:** fsd@branschkansliet.se
**Website:** http://www.dentalhandel.se
**Fnded:** 1989. **Mem:** 60. **Lang(s):** English, Swedish. **Desc:** Companies manufacturing dental equipment and supplies. Establishes international standards and technical harmonization for dental equipment. Represents members' interests before government bodies, international agencies, and the public. Maintains liaison with organizations representing dentists, dental technicians, and dental supply dealers and distributors. Compiles statistics.

## Swiss Association of Medical Advisers (SWMA) (Association Suisse Deleges Medicaux — ASDM)

*See:* Entry 2418

## Syllogos Iatrikon Episkepton Elladas (SIEE)

*See:* Entry 2420

## ★ 9998 ★ VHA

220 E Las Colinas Blvd.
Irving, TX 75039-5500
**Free:** 877-847-1450              **Fax:** (972)830-0332
**Email:** feedback@vha.com
**Website:** http://www.vhahealthfoundation.org
C. Thomas Smith, Pres. & CEO
**Fnded:** 1977. **Mem:** 2,150. **Reg. Groups:** 22. **Desc:** Health care alliance that represents 1,600 healthcare organizations nationwide, offering its members programs and services to help them improve their operational and clinical efficiency as well as community health. **Pub:** *Alliance*, monthly. Newsletter. Publication about VHA programs, And services and member activities. *Price:* available to members only. • Annual Report, annual. **Frmly:** (1995) Voluntary Hospitals of America.

## ★ 9999 ★ Workgroup for Electronic Data Interchange (WEDI)

12020 Sunrise Valley Dr., Ste 100
Reston, VA 20191
**Phone:** (703)391-2716              **Fax:** (703)391-2759
**Email:** webmaster@wedi.org
**Website:** http://www.wedi.org
James A. Schuping, Contact
**Desc:** Promotes Electronic Commerce in the Health Care Industry.

## World Research Foundation (WRF)

*See:* Entry 8932

**★ 10000 ★ Zero to Three: National Center for Infants, Toddlers and Families**
2000 M St. NW, Ste. 2000
Washington, DC 20036
**Phone:** (202)638-1144 **Free:** 800-899-4301
**Fax:** (202)638-0851
**Email:** info@wrf.org
**Website:** http://www.zerotothree.org
Matthew E. Melmed, Exec. Dir.
**Fnded:** 1977. **Desc:** Professionals and researchers in the health care industry, policymakers, and parents working to improve the healthy physical, cognitive and social development of infants, toddlers, and their families. Members share their expertise about infants, toddlers, and their families. Sponsors training and technical assistance activities. **Pub:** *Zero to Three*, 6/year. Bulletin. Includes research and practice reports, book and video reviews, calendar of events, funding source information, and lists of training opportunities. *Price:* $60/year; $102/2 years; $144/3 years; Order in bulk for discounts. **Frmly:** (1992) National Center for Clinical Infant Programs; (2001) National Center for Infants, Toddlers and Families.

# Research Centers

**★ 10001 ★ Center for Health Care Strategies**
1009 Lenox Dr., Ste. 204
Lawrenceville, NJ 08648
**Phone:** (609)895-8101 **Fax:** (609)895-9648
**Email:** sas@chcs.org
**Website:** http://www.chcs.org
Stephen A. Somers, Pres.
**Activities/Fields:** Development and implementation of effective health and social policy for all Americans.

**Center for Human Services**
*See:* Entry 11849

**★ 10002 ★ Columbia University Center for Molecular Therapeutics (CMT)**
Department of Pharmacology
630 W 168th St.
New York, NY 10032
**Phone:** (212)305-8754 **Fax:** (212)305-8351
**Email:** mrr1@columbia.edu
**Website:** http://cpmcnet.columbia.edu/dept/cmt/
Michael Rosen, MD, Contact
**Activities/Fields:** Strategies, drugs, and devices for delivery of health care.

**★ 10003 ★ Cross Cultural Health Care Program (CCHCP)**
1200 12th Ave. S
Seattle, WA 98144
**Phone:** (206)326-4161 **Fax:** (206)326-2471
**Email:** xculture@pacmed.org
**Website:** http://www.xculture.org/
Tom Lonner, PhD, Mgr.
**Activities/Fields:** Cultural competency in health and human services, focusing on organizational practices. Research focuses on services provided to non-mainstream, limited English-speaking populations in the Seattle area.

**Dalhousie University Atlantic Health Promotion Research Centre (AHPRC)**
*See:* Entry 2480

**Dalhousie University Population Health Research Unit (PHRU)**
*See:* Entry 2481

**★ 10004 ★ Health Research and Educational Trust of New Jersey**
760 Alexander Rd.
Princeton, NJ 08543-0001
**Phone:** (609)275-4145 **Fax:** (609)275-4228
**Email:** fvali@njha.com
**Website:** http://www.njha.com
Valerie Sellers, Sr. VP, Health Plan. & Res.
**Activities/Fields:** Health services, particularly access to primary healthcare in New Jersey; geographic variations of hospitalizations for ambulatory care sensitive conditions; domestic violence, medical and social management of care for the victims covering Kids New Jersey; Health Access Initiative for Low-Income Uninsured Children; Breast Cancer Awareness project; newborn screening; quality improvement analysis; race and ethnicity coding; electronic birth certificate data analysis. **Pub:** *Bring Your Baby Back.* • *Building Healthier Communities: A Profile of the Community's Health.* • *Comparative Clinical Outcomes Report.* • *Directory of New Jersey FamilyCare Outreach and Application Assistance Sites.* • *A Networking Guide to Hospital Educational Programs for Children and Adolescents.* • *New Jersey FamilyCare Educational/Awareness Video.* • *New Jersey Family-Care Outreach Worker Training Manual.* • *Outreach Toolkit for Faith-Based Organizations.* • *Outreach Toolkit for Hospitals.* • *Parenting Guide.* • *Shaping Healthier Tomorrows.* • *A Women's Resource Guide to Breast Cancer Services in New Jersey.*

**★ 10005 ★ Institute for Clinical Evaluative Sciences (ICES)**
2075 Bayview Ave., Rm. G106
Toronto, ON, Canada M4N 3M5
**Phone:** (416)480-4055 **Fax:** (416)480-6048
**Email:** info@ices.on.ca
**Website:** http://www.ices.on.ca/
Dr. Andreas Laupacis, Pres. /CEO
**Activities/Fields:** Effectiveness, quality, equity and efficiency of health care in Ontario. **Pub:** *ICES Practice Atlas series.* • *Newsletters.* • *Technical papers.*

**★ 10006 ★ Institute of Health Economics**
10405 Jasper Ave., No. 1200
Edmonton, AB, Canada T5J 3N4
**Phone:** (780)448-4881 **Fax:** (780)448-0018
**Email:** webmaster@ihe.ab.ca
**Website:** http://www.ihe.ca
Donna Angus, Dir. Commun. & Res. Transfer
**Activities/Fields:** Health and pharmaceutical economic, outcome and policy research. **Pub:** *IHE News.*

**★ 10007 ★ Institute for Urban Family Health**
16 E 16th St.
New York, NY 10003
**Phone:** (212)633-0800 **Fax:** (212)691-4610
**Website:** http://www.institute2000.org/
Neil Calman, MD, Pres.
**Activities/Fields:** Primary health care delivery and primary care education.

**★ 10008 ★ Johns Hopkins School of Public Health**
**Risk Sciences and Public Policy Institute**
615 N Wolfe St., Rm. W6033
Baltimore, MD 21205-2179
**Phone:** (410)614-4962 **Fax:** (410)955-0863
**Email:** mschwab@jhsph.edu
**Website:** http://www.jhsph.edu/Research/Centers/rsppi
Dr. Margo Schwab, Asst. Dir.
**Activities/Fields:** Interpretation, synthesis, and organization of scientific information for analysis risk; evaluation of the implications of risk assessments for alternative management decisions; and evaluation of risk management outcomes for public health. **Pub:** *Newsletter.*

**Johns Hopkins University Center for Epidemiology and Policy**
*See:* Entry 9050

**★ 10009 ★ Johns Hopkins University Primary Care Policy Center for Underserved Populations (PCPC)**
452 Hampton House
Department of Health Policy and Management
624 N Broadway
Baltimore, MD 21205
**Phone:** (410)955-9725 **Fax:** (410)614-9046
**Email:** bstarfie@jhsph.edu
**Website:** http://www.jhsph.edu/hao/pcpc/
Dr. Barbara Starfield, Dir.
**Activities/Fields:** Organization, financing, and mode of delivery for primary care to underserved and vulnerable populations. **Pub:** *White papers.*

**★ 10010 ★ Johns Hopkins University Women's and Children's Health Policy Center (WCHPC)**
615 N Wolfe St.
Baltimore, MD 21205
**Phone:** (410)502-5443 **Fax:** (410)955-2303
**Website:** http://www.med.jhu.edu/wchpc/overview.htm
Holly Grason, Contact
**Activities/Fields:** Health system reforms impacting the health of women, children, and adolescents. **Pub:** *Research and technical resource briefs.*

**★ 10011 ★ Laval University Health Services Research Group**
Pavillon des Sciences de l'administration
Cite universitaire
Sainte Foy, QC, Canada G1K 7P4
**Phone:** (418)656-3503 **Fax:** (418)656-2624
Prof. Clermont Begin, Contact
**Activities/Fields:** Health care organizations, including planning, financing, decision making, information systems, evaluation of health policies, socio-political aspects of organization and evaluation of health services.

**★ 10012 ★ Medical Research Modernization Committee**
3200 Morley Rd.
Shaker Heights, OH 44122
**Phone:** (216)283-6702 **Fax:** (216)283-6702
**Email:** stkaufman@mindspring.com
**Website:** http://www.mrmcmed.org/
Stephen R. Kaufman, MD, Contact
**Activities/Fields:** Research modalities, focusing on their medical and scientific merits in order to identify outdated research methods and promote reliable and efficient methods. **Pub:** *Perspectives on Medical Research*, occasionally. Monograph.

**★ 10013 ★ New Jersey Health and Senior Services Department**
**Health Planning and Regulation**
**Health Care Systems Analysis**
**Research and Development**
225 East State St., 8th Fl.
PO Box 360
Trenton, NJ 08625-0360
**Phone:** (609)292-9354 **Fax:** (609)292-6523
**Email:** enoggoh@doh.state.nj.us
Emmanuel Noggoh, Dir.
**Activities/Fields:** Health care.

**★ 10014 ★ Oregon Health and Science University**
**Center on Self-Determination**
3608 SE Powell Blvd.
Portland, OR 97202
**Phone:** (503)232-9154 **Fax:** (503)232-6423
**Email:** powersl@ohsu.edu

**Website:** http://cdrc.ohsu.edu/selfdetermination/
Laurie Powers, PhD, Co-Dir.
**Activities/Fields:** Identification, development, validation on and communication of policies and practices that promote the self-determination of people with and without disabilities. **Pub:** *Educational materials.*


**Southern Illinois University at Carbondale
Center for Rural Health and Social
    Service Development (CRHSSD)**
*See:* Entry 2591


**★ 10015 ★ Stanford University
Stanford Medical Informatics (SMI)**
MSOB X-215
251 Campus Dr.
Stanford, CA 94305-5479
**Phone:** (650)723-6979        **Fax:** (650)725-7944
**Email:** musen@smi.stanford.edu
**Website:** http://www-camis.stanford.edu/main.html
Prof. Mark A. Musen, MD, Hd.
**Activities/Fields:** Methods for acquiring, representing, processing, and managing knowledge and data within health care and the biomedical sciences.


**★ 10016 ★ State University of New York
    at Stony Brook
Center for Health Policy and Management**
Stony Brook, NY 11794-8402
**Phone:** (631)444-3198        **Fax:** (631)444-6266
Nancy Rice, Dir.
**Activities/Fields:** Social policy regarding health care, access to care, cost efficiency of care, effectiveness of health care, health education and manpower planning and the assessment and testing of treatment protocols in New York. Same specific projects include a quality and standards analysis of information available to consumers of healthcare information in New York, including assessment of complementary and alternative medicine utilization; efficiency analyses of hospitals and nursing homes operating in New York as well as the University Hospital Department of Medicine. **Pub:** *Monographs.*


**U.S. Department of Health and Human
    Services
National Institute of Neurological
    Disorders and Stroke
Small Business Innovation Research
    Program**
*See:* Entry 14318


**★ 10017 ★ U.S. Department of Health
    and Human Services
Public Health Service
Agency for Health Care Policy and
    Research
Center for Organization and Delivery
    Studies**
2101 E Jefferson St., Ste. 605
Rockville, MD 20852
**Phone:** (301)594-1410        **Fax:** (301)594-2314
**Email:** info@ahrq.gov
**Website:** http://www.ahcpr.gov/about/cods/
Irene Fraser, Dir.
**Activities/Fields:** Health care markets, health care delivery systems, and health care organizations. **Pub:** *Monographs.* • *Reports.*


**U.S. Department of Veterans Affairs
Veterans Health Administration
Office of Research and Development
Health Services Research and
    Development Service
(Service Directed Research Program)**
*See:* Entry 13499


**U.S. Department of Veterans Affairs
Veterans Health Administration
Office of Research and Development
Health Services Research and
    Development Service
(Investigator Initiated Research Program)**
*See:* Entry 13500


**U.S. Department of Veterans Affairs
Veterans Health Administration
Office of Research and Development
Health Services Research and
    Development Service
(Management Decision and Research
    Center)**
*See:* Entry 13501


**U.S. Department of Veterans Affairs
Veterans Health Administration
Office of Research and Development
Health Services Research and
    Development Service
(Center for the Study of Healthcare
    Provider Behavior)**
*See:* Entry 13502


**U.S. Department of Veterans Affairs
Veterans Health Administration
Office of Research and Development
Health Services Research and
    Development Service
(Northwest Center for Outcomes
    Research in Older Adults)**
*See:* Entry 13503


**U.S. Department of Veterans Affairs
Veterans Health Administration
Office of Research and Development
Health Services Research and
    Development Service
(Center for Chronic Disease Outcomes
    Research)**
*See:* Entry 13504


**U.S. Department of Veterans Affairs
Veterans Health Administration
Office of Research and Development
Health Services Research and
    Development Service
(Center for Mental Healthcare and
    Outcomes Research)**
*See:* Entry 13505


**U.S. Department of Veterans Affairs
Veterans Health Administration
Office of Research and Development
Health Services Research and
    Development Service
(Center for Health Services Research in
    Primary Care)**
*See:* Entry 13506


**★ 10018 ★ University of Alabama at
    Birmingham
Center for Outcomes and Effectiveness
    Research and Education (COERE)**
MT 412
1530 3rd Ave. S
Birmingham, AL 35294-4410
**Phone:** (205)934-6838        **Fax:** (205)934-4888
**Email:** coere@uab.edu
**Website:** http://www.dopm.uab.edu/coere
Catarina I. Kiefe, PhD,MD, Co-Dir.


**Activities/Fields:** Analysis of the outcomes and effectiveness of health services that takes patients' experiences, preferences, and values into account.


**University of Alaska Anchorage
Institute for Circumpolar Health Studies
    (ICHS)**
*See:* Entry 2650


**★ 10019 ★ University of Alberta
John Dossetor Health Ethics Centre**
5-16 University Extension Centre
Edmonton, AB, Canada T6G 2T4
**Phone:** (780)492-6676        **Fax:** (780)492-0673
**Email:** dossetor.centre@ualberta.ca
**Website:** http://www.ualberta.ca/BIOETHICS/
Vangie Bergum, PhD, Dir.
**Activities/Fields:** Ethical and moral issues in the provision of healthcare.


**★ 10020 ★ University of Arkansas for
    Medical Sciences
Centers for Mental Healthcare Research
Center for Outcomes Research and
    Effectiveness (CORE)**
Department of Psychiatry
5800 W 10th St., Ste. 712
Little Rock, AR 72204
**Phone:** (501)660-7550        **Fax:** (501)660-7543
**Email:** coreinfo@exchange.uams.edu
**Website:** http://www.uams.edu/CORE/home.htm
Dr. G. Richard Smith, Jr., Dir.
**Activities/Fields:** Impact of treatment on the outcomes of health care, particularly while adjusting for prognostic characteristics in a diagnostically similar patient population. **Pub:** *Annual report.*


**University of California, Los Angeles
Center for Health Policy Research**
*See:* Entry 9887


**★ 10021 ★ University of Connecticut
    Health Center
Health Policy and Primary Care Research
    Center**
263 Farmington Ave., Ste. 260
Farmington, CT 06030-6325
**Phone:** (860)679-5487
**Email:** chpr@uchc.edu
**Website:** http://www.hlth-pol-ctr.uchc.edu/
Dr. Howard Bailit, Dir.
**Activities/Fields:** Health care, especially community delivery systems, alcohol and addiction services, mental health, dental health.


**★ 10022 ★ University of Houston
Institute for Health Care Marketing**
Department of Marketing
College of Business Administration
Houston, TX 77204-6283
**Phone:** (713)743-4558        **Fax:** (713)743-4572
**Email:** gelb@uh.edu
**Website:** http://marketing.cba.uh.edu/gelb/health_
care_marketing/intro.htm
Prof. Betsy D. Gelb, Dir.
**Activities/Fields:** Health care marketing and health promotion.


**★ 10023 ★ University of Kentucky
Center for Health Services Management
    and Research**
College of Applied Health Professions Bldg., Rms.
102 & 109
121 Washington Ave.
Lexington, KY 40536-0003
**Phone:** (859)257-6504        **Fax:** (859)257-2454
**Email:** scutch@pop.uky.edu

**Website:** http://www.mc.uky.edu/CHSMR
F. Douglas Scutchfield, MD, Dir.

**Activities/Fields:** Improvement of access to, and the use, quality, accessibility, delivery, organization, financing, and outcomes of health care services and an increase in knowledge and understanding of the structure, processes, and effects of health services for individuals and populations. **Pub:** *Newsletter.* • *White papers.*

### ★ 10024 ★ University of Maryland, Baltimore County
**Center for Health Program Development and Management (CHPDM)**
1000 Hilltop Cir.
Baltimore, MD 21250
**Phone:** (410)455-6854          **Fax:** (410)455-6850
**Email:** jkaelin@chpdm.umbc.edu
**Website:** http://www.umbc.edu/chpdm/
John Kaelin, Exec. Dir.

**Activities/Fields:** Healthcare programs and policies, focusing on improving overall quality and purchaser value.

### ★ 10025 ★ University of Massachusetts Lowell
**Center for Public Health Research and Health Promotion**
3 Solomont Way, Ste. 3
Lowell, MA 01854
**Phone:** (978)934-4461          **Fax:** (978)934-3006
**Email:** Barbara_Mawn@uml.edu
**Website:** http://www.uml.edu/res/misc/health.html
Dr. Barbara Mawn, Co. -Dir.

**Activities/Fields:** Health professions. **Frmly:** Center for Health Promotion; Center for Health Sciences, Health Promotion, and Public Health.

**University of Montreal
Interdisciplinary Health Research Group**
*See:* Entry 18016

### ★ 10026 ★ University of Nebraska Medical Center
**Nebraska Center for Rural Health Research**
984350 Nebraska Medical Center
Omaha, NE 68198-4350
**Phone:** (402)559-5260          **Fax:** (402)559-7259
**Email:** kmueller@unmc.edu
**Website:** http://www.unmc.edu/rural/page2.htm
Keith J. Mueller, PhD, Dir.

**Activities/Fields:** Improvement of health care delivery in rural areas.

### ★ 10027 ★ University of Nebraska Medical Center
**Nebraska Center for Rural Health Research**
984350 Nebraska Medical Center
Omaha, NE 68198-4350
**Phone:** (402)559-5260          **Fax:** (402)559-7259
**Email:** kmueller@unmc.edu
**Website:** http://www.unmc.edu/rural/page2.htm
Keith J. Mueller, PhD, Dir.

**Activities/Fields:** Improvement of health care delivery in rural areas. The center focuses on special populations among rural residents, including the elderly, children, minorities, mentally ill, under and uninsured, and new immigrants whose needs for assistance are unique.

### ★ 10028 ★ University of Pittsburgh
**Center for Research on Health Care (CRHC)**
UPMC Montefiore, Ste. E820
Pittsburgh, PA 15213
**Phone:** (412)692-4853          **Fax:** (412)692-4838
**Email:** ctrrhc@pitt.edu
**Website:** http://www.pitt.edu/~ctrrhc/
Wishwa N. Kapoor, MD, Dir.

**Activities/Fields:** Health services.

**University of Toronto
Centre for Health Promotion
Quality of Life Research Unit**
*See:* Entry 2735

### ★ 10029 ★ University of Toronto
**Home and Community Care Evaluation and Research Centre**
50 St. George St.
Toronto, ON, Canada M5S 3H4
**Phone:** (416)978-8369          **Fax:** (416)978-8222
**Email:** peter.coyte@utoronto.ca
**Website:** http://www.hcerc.utoronto.ca
Dr. Peter Coyte, Co-Dir.

**Activities/Fields:** People, technologies, and health care settings. **Pub:** *Annual report.* • *Children and Youth Home Care Newsletter.* • *Newsletter.* • *Working Papers Series.* **Frmly:** Home Care Evaluation and Research Centre.

### ★ 10030 ★ University of Virginia
**Center for Improving Minority Health (CIMH)**
Ste. 800729 UVa Health System
Charlottesville, VA 22908
**Phone:** (434)924-1165          **Fax:** (434)243-2916
**Website:** http://www.med.virginia.edu/cimh/
Dr. M. Norman Oliver, Dir.

**Activities/Fields:** Health care delivery, access, and outcomes among minority populations, especially disparities in health care and outcomes.

### ★ 10031 ★ University of Washington
**End of Life Care Research Program**
Harborview Medical Center, Box 359762
325 9th Ave.
Seattle, WA 98104
**Phone:** (206)731-2106          **Fax:** (206)731-8584
**Email:** jrc@u.washington.edu
**Website:** http://depts.washington.edu/eolcare/
J. Randall Curtis, Co-Dir.

**Activities/Fields:** Improvement of end-of-life care, including quality of care and communication about end-of-life care.

### ★ 10032 ★ Veterans Health Administration
**Office of Research and Development
Center for Health Care Evaluation (CHCE)**
795 Willow Rd. (152-MPD)
Menlo Park, CA 94025
**Phone:** (650)493-5000
**Email:** christine.timko@med.va.gov
**Website:** http://www.chce.research.med.va.gov/chce/content/main.htm
Christine Timko, PhD, Actg. Dir.

**Activities/Fields:** Improvement in the organization and delivery of health care services; improvement in diagnostic assessment, screening procedures, and clinical decision making; improvement in treatment for substance use and psychiatric disorders; and improvement in health services research methods.

### ★ 10033 ★ Veterans Health Administration
**Office of Research and Development
Center for Health Equity Research and Promotion (CHERP)**
VA Pittsburgh Healthcare System
University Dr. C, 11E130-B (130-U)
Pittsburgh, PA 15213
**Phone:** (412)688-6000          **Fax:** (412)688-6916
**Email:** mary.walsh3@med.va.gov
**Website:** http://www.upenn.edu/ldi/healthdisparities.html
Michael J. Fine, MD, Dir.

**Activities/Fields:** Health and health care disparities among vulnerable groups of veterans.

### ★ 10034 ★ Virginia Commonwealth University
**Outcomes Research Institute**
Virginia Biotechnology Research Park, Biotech One
800 E Leigh St., Ste 115B
PO Box 980219
Richmond, VA 23298-0219
**Phone:** (434)225-3450          **Fax:** (434)827-0087
**Email:** rwenzel@hsc.vcu.edu
**Website:** http://www.trials-outcomes.clt.vcu.edu/outcomes/mission.html
Richard P. Wenzel, MD, Exec. Dir.

**Activities/Fields:** Delivery of the best medical care with the best possible outcome to patients in a health care system.

### ★ 10035 ★ Wayne State University
**Center for Healthcare Effectiveness Research (CHER)**
121 Shiffman Medical Library
4325 Brush
Detroit, MI 48201
**Phone:** (313)577-5189          **Fax:** (313)577-1773
**Email:** mmassana@med.wayne.edu
**Website:** http://www.med.wayne.edu/cher/opener.htm
Dr. Mike Massanari, Contact

**Activities/Fields:** Health care services and their effectiveness.

### ★ 10036 ★ York University
**Centre for Health Studies (YCHS)**
Rm. 214 York Lanes
4700 Keele St.
Toronto, ON, Canada M3J 1P3
**Phone:** (416)736-5941          **Fax:** (416)736-5986
**Email:** ychs@yorku.ca
**Website:** http://www.yorku.ca/ychs/
Georgina Feldberg, PhD, Dir.

**Activities/Fields:** Political economy of health; health policy, institutions and professions; women and health; culture, ethnicity and health; mental and physical fitness; and health and the environment. **Pub:** *Newsletter.*

# Chapter 31
# Hematology & Oncology

## Federal Government Agencies

**U.S. Department of Health and Human Services**
**National Institutes of Health (NIH)**
**National Heart, Lung, and Blood Institute (NHLBI)**
*See:* Entry 4916

★ **10037** ★ **U.S. Department of Health and Human Services**
**National Institutes of Health (NIH)**
**National Institute of Cancer (NIC)**
9000 Rockville Pike
Bethesda, MD 20892
**Phone:** (301)435-3848        **Free:** 800-422-6237
**Website:** http://www.cancer.gov
Richard Klausner, MD, Director

**Desc:** NIC has developed a national cancer program to expand existing scientific knowledge on cancer cause and prevention, as well as on the diagnosis, treatment, and rehabilitation of cancer patients. Research activities cover a broad spectrum encompassing basic biological, clinical, prevention, and behavioral research.

## Foundations & Other Funding Organizations

### Private Foundations

★ **10038** ★ **Alexander and Margaret Stewart Trust**
Brawner Bldg., Ste. 210
888 17th St. Northwest
Washington, DC 20006-3939
**Phone:** (202)785-9892        **Fax:** (202)785-0918
Doris Lustine, Executive Secretary

**Fnded:** 1951. **Philosophy:** "The Alexander and Margaret Stewart Trust makes grants to organizations, primarily in Washington, D.C., that provide care or treatment for those suffering from cancer or childhood afflictions." "Cancer: Under the will of Mary E. Stewart, the Trustees entertain grant applications for care and treatment of people afflicted with cancer. The Trust occasionally may fund the purchase of equipment used in cancer diagnosis and treatment. It rarely funds the education of students or doctors engaged in cancer research. The Trust is supporting research of emerging cancer therapies, but does not accept proposals for such research, working instead with experts to fund research at selected institutions." "Child Health: Under the will of Helen S. Devore, grants are made for the care of children who are physically or mentally ill or handicapped, and for research, education, or prevention of diseases common to early childhood. This includes societal behavioral patterns that have a negative impact on the welfare of children." "The Trustees welcome evidence that a requested program has ongoing community support and acceptance before funding is considered and will consider funding start-up costs (not 'planning' projects) for a new program with the intention that the donee organization will continue the program using alternate sources of funding. Programs aiding the economically deprived are favored." 1997 Application Guidelines **Priorities:** *International:* 100%. Supports trust solicited cancer research, cancer care, and hospices. **Typ. Recipients:** Cancer, Child Abuse, Children's Health/Hospitals, Clinics/Medical Centers, Eyes/Blindness, Family Planning, Health Organizations, Health-General, Hospices, Hospitals, Long-Term Care, Medical Education, Mental Health, Nursing Services, People with Disabilities, Prenatal Health Issues, Single-Disease Health Associations. **Geo. Dist:** Washington, DC, metropolitan area.

★ **10039** ★ **Allegheny Foundation**
One Oxford Center
301 Grant St., Ste. 3900
Pittsburgh, PA 15219-6401
**Phone:** (412)392-2900
**Website:** http://www.scaife.com
Joanne Beyer, President

**Fnded:** 1953. **Philosophy:** The foundation reports that it "confines most of its grant awards to programs for historic preservation, civic development, education, youth development, and animal welfare." Although the foundation makes grants to local chapters of national organizations for programs which benefit the local economy, preference is shown for locally based and operated organizations and programs. **Priorities:** *Arts & Humanities:* 25%. Museums, theater, and historical societies. *Civic & Public Affairs:* 27%. Public policy, economic development, and community services. *Education:* 27%. Supports educational funds and associations. *Environment:* 16%. Youth organizations and animal welfare. *Note:* Total contributions made in 1999. **Typ. Recipients:** Cancer, Medical Education, People with Disabilities. **Geo. Dist:** PA, including western Pennsylvania.

**Assisi Foundation of Memphis**
*See:* Entry 11687

**Beneficia Foundation**
*See:* Entry 73

★ **10040** ★ **Bingham Trust**
PO Box 2004
New York, NY 10109
**Phone:** (212)852-1000
**Email:** hm6085@pitcairn.com
Patricia Davidson, Trustee

**Fnded:** 1934. **Philosophy:** Every five years, the trust shifts its primary focus to entirely new fields of interest. Funds available in the grant cycle beginning January 1, 1996, and ending December 31, 2000, have been entirely committed to four institutions providing transitional housing for certain psychiatric patients, four public middle schools to improve the schools' coordination with families and social services, two organizations developing and distributing contraceptives in underdeveloped countries, a program for the application of DNA technology in the fields of anthropology and archaeology, and a small number of minor grants selected by the trustees. The trust's fields of interest in the cycle starting January 1, 2001, will not be determined until the year 2000. **Priorities:** *Civic & Public Affairs:* 9%. Giving includes foundations, clubs and housing. *Education:* 22%. Funding to middle schools, universities, school for the deaf and other school programs. *Environment:* 22%. Supports United Way, shelters, child welfare, homes and human development services. *International:* 15%. Supports children's health, hospitals, health centers, and arthritis. *Note:* Totl contributions made in 2000. **Typ. Recipients:** Arthritis, Cancer, Children's Health/Hospitals, Clinics/Medical Centers, Eyes/Blindness, Health-General, Home-Care Services, Hospitals, Mental Health. **Geo. Dist:** nationwide.

★ **10041** ★ **Bruce McMillan, Jr. Foundation**
PO Box 9
Overton, TX 75684
**Phone:** (903)834-3148        **Fax:** (903)834-3947
Ralph Ward, Jr., President

**Fnded:** 1951. **Philosophy:** The Bruce McMillan, Jr., Foundation supports the areas of education, religion, scientific, literary and charitable. Educational funding favors colleges and universities and agricultural programs. Scholarships are generally restricted to students from eight high schools in the Overton, TX, area. Health care support goes to cancer research, blood centers, and treatment centers. Religious support favors individual churches in the Overton, TX, area, and social services support includes youth organizations. **Priorities:** *Arts & Humanities:* 4%. For a museum. *Civic & Public Affairs:* 1%. *Education:* 62%. Supports educational endowments for secondary schools and colleges. *Environment:* 5%. Youth and family services programs. *International:* 8%. Health centers. *Note:* Total contributions made in fiscal 1999. **Typ. Recipients:** Cancer, Child Abuse, Children's Health/Hospitals, Domestic Violence, Emergency/Ambulance Services, Family Planning, Health Organizations, Heart, Heart, Prenatal Health Issues, Public Health, Sexual Abuse, Single-Disease Health Associations, Substance Abuse, Transplant Networks/Donor Banks. **Geo. Dist:** TX, emphasis on the Overton area.

**Carl J. Herzog Foundation**
*See:* Entry 105

**Chisholm Foundation**
*See:* Entry 125

**Clara Blackford Smith and W. Aubrey Smith Charitable Foundation**
*See:* Entry 128

## ★ 10042 ★ D and DF Foundation

1 Maritime Plz., Ste. 1400
San Francisco, CA 94111
**Phone:** (415)288-0540
Donald Fisher, Trustee

**Fnded:** 1986. **Priorities:** *Arts & Humanities:* 4%. Funds museums, dance, and music. *Civic & Public Affairs:* 69%. Supports parks, community foundations, and clubs. *Education:* 19%. Supports pre-college education and universities. *Environment:* 6%. Supports United Way, social services agencies, children's organizations, and volunteer services. *International:* 2%. Supports medical research and women's health. *Note:* Total contributionss in fiscal 1999. **Typ. Recipients:** AIDS/HIV, Cancer, Clinics/Medical Centers, Health Funds, Health Organizations, Health-General, Hospitals, Medical Education, Medical Research, People with Disabilities. **Geo. Dist:** CA.


## E. L. Wiegand Foundation

*See:* Entry 188


## ★ 10043 ★ Elizabeth Morse Genius Charitable Trust

231 S Lasalle St.
Chicago, IL 60697-0246
**Phone:** (312)828-8028     **Fax:** (312)987-0806
Charles Slamar, Jr., Trust Officer

**Fnded:** 1992. **Priorities:** *Arts & Humanities:* 36%. Supports performing arts, public broadcasting and local orchestras. *Civic & Public Affairs:* 17%. Supports community development and legal advocacy. *Education:* 12%. Supports educational insitutions. *Environment:* 12%. Supports social services, youth concerns and the homeless shelters. *International:* 19%. Supports hospitals and medical/wellness centers. *Religion:* 4%. Supports museums of natural history and science and industry. *Note:* Contributions were made in fiscal 1999. **Typ. Recipients:** Cancer, Children's Health/Hospitals, Clinics/Medical Centers, Domestic Violence, Emergency/Ambulance Services, Hospitals, Long-Term Care, Public Health. **Geo. Dist:** Chicago, IL.


## Elmer and Mamdouha Bobst Foundation

*See:* Entry 219


## ★ 10044 ★ Elsa U. Pardee Foundation

Box 2767
Midland, MI 48641-2767
**Phone:** (517)832-3691
**Email:** info@pardeefoundation.org
**Website:** www.pardeefoundation.org
Lucille Dougherty, Staff Assistant

**Fnded:** 1944. **Philosophy:** The purpose of the foundation is "to support research in the field of cancer, and to provide for others those advantages of knowledge and techniques still undiscovered in the treatment of cancer." Current foundation policy allocates one-third to cancer treatment, one-third to cancer research projects and one-third to established cancer-research institutes. Grants support hospitals, universities, and research institutes for projects to study control of, and cures for, cancer. Assistance with the cost of cancer treatment to families was also an area of interest to the founder, and her niece, Elsa G. Allen. Besides increasing its commitment to cancer research, the foundation also continues to fund high quality endeavors that have proven their significance. Each year the foundation devotes about one-third of funding to proposals recommended by its Medical Committee as innovative new projects. **Priorities:** *Education:* 5%. *International:* 95%. Cancer research. Approximately one-third goes to new research; one-third to ongoing programs; and about one-third for treatment costs for cancer victims. *Note:* Total contributions made in 2000. **Typ. Recipients:** Cancer, Clinics/Medical Centers, Hospitals, Medical Research, Transplant Networks/Donor Banks. **Geo. Dist:** nationally.


## Fannie E. Rippel Foundation

*See:* Entry 2889


## Ford Family Foundation

*See:* Entry 246


## ★ 10045 ★ Jane Coffin Childs Memorial Fund for Medical Research

c/o Yale University School of Medicine
333 Cedar St.
Rm. LW 300
New Haven, CT 06510
**Phone:** (203)785-4612     **Fax:** (203)785-3301
**Email:** jccfund@yale.edu
**Website:** http://www.jccfund.org
Elizabeth Ford, Administrative Director

**Fnded:** 1937. **Philosophy:** The fund traditionally has supported basic cancer research, rather than the investigation of the clinical aspects of the disease. Current funding is limited to post-doctoral fellowships for physicians and scientists. **Priorities:** *Education:* 66%. Supports scientific education, medical education, colleges, and universities. *International:* 32%. Majority of supports is for cancer research. *Religion:* 2%. Supports Scripps Research Institute Department of Chemistry. *Note:* Total contributions made in fiscal 2000. **Typ. Recipients:** Cancer, Children's Health/Hospitals, Clinics/Medical Centers, Medical Education, Medical Research, Medical Training, Research/Studies Institutes. **Geo. Dist:** national and international.


## ★ 10046 ★ John Templeton Foundation

5 Radnor Corporate Center, Ste. 100
100 Matsonford Rd.
PO Box 8322
Radnor, PA 19087-8322
**Phone:** (610)687-8942     **Fax:** (610)687-8961
**Email:** info@templeton.org
**Website:** http://www.templeton.org

**Fnded:** 1988. **Philosophy:** The John Templeton Foundation was established in 1987 by renowned international investor, Sir John Templeton, to encourage a fresh appreciation of the critical importance, for all peoples and cultures, of the moral and spiritual dimensions of life. Through it's programs, the Foundations seeks to encourage the world to catch the vision of the tremendous possibilities for spiritual progress in an open and humble approach to life; encourage institutions of learning to incorporate training towards excellence in character in their efforts to prepare the next generation for service; to encourage growth in appreciating the potential of free societies; and to promote the understanding of the significant responsibilities associated with freedom in its several aspects, moral, spiritual, political and economic. "Website." **Typ. Recipients:** Cancer, Health Organizations, Health-General, Medical Research, Mental Health.


## Joseph Alexander Foundation

*See:* Entry 435


## ★ 10047 ★ Life Sciences Research Foundation

Princeton University
Washington Rd.
Princeton, NJ 08544
**Phone:** (609)258-3551
**Email:** sdirenzo@molbio.princeton.edu
**Website:** http://lsrf.molbio.princeton.edu
Susan DiRenzo, Assistant Director

**Fnded:** 1984. **Priorities:** *Education:* 100%. Awards postdoctoral research fellowships to graduates of graduate schools in the biological sciences for basic research in life sciences. The purpose of the grants is to train and support high quality young scientists in the very best research environments. *Note:* Total contributions made in 1999. **Typ. Recipients:** Cancer, Children's Health/Hospitals, Hospitals (University Affiliated), Medical Education, Medical Research.


## ★ 10048 ★ Louis and Sandra Berkman Foundation

PO Box 820
Steubenville, OH 43952
**Phone:** (614)283-3722
John Koren, Secretary

**Fnded:** 1952. **Philosophy:** The foundation primarily supports higher education. Minimal funding goes to health organizations and religious welfare causes. **Priorities:** *Education:* 97%. Colleges and universities, with major grants to Bethany College and Franciscan University. *International:* 1%. Medical centers, cancer research, and public health. *Note:* Total contributions made in 1998. **Typ. Recipients:** Cancer, Children's Health/Hospitals, Clinics/Medical Centers, Emergency/Ambulance Services, Eyes/Blindness, Family Planning, Health Organizations, Heart, Hospices, Hospitals, Medical Research, Prenatal Health Issues, Public Health, Single-Disease Health Associations, Transplant Networks/Donor Banks. **Geo. Dist:** MA; OH; PA.


## ★ 10049 ★ Loyola Foundation, Inc.

308 C St., Northeast
Washington, DC 20002
**Phone:** (202)546-9400
Albert McCarthy, III, Executive Director, Secretary

**Fnded:** 1957. **Philosophy:** The Loyola Foundation was established "to assist overseas Catholic mission activities. In the beginning we hoped to assist, in a very small and limited way, a vast area of the world." Over the last thirty years, the foundation has broadened its interests, but primarily supports four areas: vehicles; construction, renovation, and repairs; equipment and furnishings; and agricultural and water projects. The foundation funds basic, durable vehicles to missions that apply. It will not fund buses to be used by the local population or trucks for hauling equipment. Construction, renovation, and repair projects include schools, churches, and community centers. Grants for equipment have primarily been to church-run trade schools, health centers, religious educational projects, and self-help centers. Grants for furnishings include churches, rectories, convents, classrooms, and schools. Water projects include some well digging and storage tank construction. The foundation has supported missions around the world and often visits the locations it funds. The areas include Africa, the Middle East, Asia, the Caribbean, and Central and South America. **Priorities:** *Civic & Public Affairs:* 9%. Supports community and neighborhood development. *Education:* 11%. Religious schools and universities. *Environment:* 5%. Funds family and social services. *Note:* Total contributions made in fiscal 1999. **Typ. Recipients:** Cancer, Public Health, Substance Abuse. **Geo. Dist:** internationally.


## ★ 10050 ★ Mary Moody Northen Foundation

PO Box 1300
Galveston, TX 77553
**Phone:** (409)765-9770     **Fax:** (409)762-7055
Betty Massey, Executive Administrator & Treasurer

**Fnded:** 1964. **Philosophy:** While the foundation supports charitable activities in Texas and Virginia, it primarily concentrates its charitable activities to two foundation-administered programs, including the restoration of the W. L. Moody, Jr., residence in Galveston, TX. The foundation will develop the residence as a "house museum" and research center dedicated to the Moody family and its role in the history of Galveston. The foundation also supports Mountain Lake Properties, which is comprised of 2,600 acres of mountain timberland, meadows, and a volcanic lake. The foundation will preserve and operate this property for the benefit of the public in the same manner as national and state forest properties. **Priorities:** *Arts & Humanities:* About 76%. Support for Museums. *Environment:* 1%. Funds the Galveston Partnership for better living. *Note:* Total contributions made in fiscal 1999. **Typ. Recipients:** Cancer. **Geo. Dist:** TX; VA.


## Mary Stuart Rogers Foundation

*See:* Entry 5560

**Monterey Fund**
*See:* Entry 5561


**Oberkotter Foundation**
*See:* Entry 13857


**★ 10051 ★  Oliver S. and Jennie R. Donaldson Charitable Trust**
114 West 47th St.
New York, NY 10036
**Phone:** (212)852-1000        **Fax:** (212)852-3377
**Email:** George_Nofer@SHSL.com
Linda Franciscovich, Senior Vice President

**Fnded:** 1969. **Philosophy:** The foundation makes grants across the major categories of support. Most of the grants are made in the areas of education, health, civic affairs, and social services. Educational funding favors colleges and universities. Funding for health care goes to support cancer treatment and research at a number of facilities, hospitals, and health organizations. In civic affairs, interests primarily include conservation and preservation organizations. Social service funding supports community centers, homes, and animal protection organizations. **Priorities:** *Arts & Humanities:* 1%. Supports public libraries, theater, and a radio club. *Civic & Public Affairs:* 6%. Supports civic and community affairs. *Education:* 4%. Supports colleges, universities, and educational programs. *Environment:* 53%. Supports volunteer consulting and youth services. *International:* 31%. Supports hospitals, children's health, and cancer research. *Note:* Contributions were made in 1998. **Typ. Recipients:** Cancer, Children's Health/Hospitals, Clinics/Medical Centers, Emergency/Ambulance Services, Health Organizations, Hospitals, Medical Research, Mental Health, Nursing Services, People with Disabilities, Preventive Medicine/Wellness Organizations, Research/Studies Institutes, Single-Disease Health Associations. **Geo. Dist:** northeastern United States.


**★ 10052 ★  Park Foundation**
PO Box 550
Ithaca, NY 14851
**Phone:** (607)272-9124        **Fax:** (607)272-6057
Joanne Florino, Executive Director

**Fnded:** 1966. **Priorities:** *Arts & Humanities:* 21%. Provides major support to public broadcasting; also funds libraries and arts organizations. *Education:* 78%. Supports colleges and universities, with particular focus on funding projects and fellowships. *Note:* Total contributions made in 2000. **Typ. Recipients:** Cancer, Diabetes, Eyes/Blindness, Heart, Hospices, Hospitals, Medical Rehabilitation, Prenatal Health Issues. **Geo. Dist:** NY, Central New York.


**Randolph Foundation**
*See:* Entry 11691


**★ 10053 ★  Sabbah Family Foundation**
PO Box 19608
Greensboro, NC 27419-9608
**Phone:** (336)294-4494        **Fax:** (336)547-0840
**Email:** lw@hrhroffice.org
Maurice Sabbah, President, Treasurer & Director

**Fnded:** 1987. **Priorities:** *Arts & Humanities:* Less than 1%. Funds art foundation. *Civic & Public Affairs:* 86%. Funds civic foundations. Major grant to Oklahoma Community Foundation ($18,000,000). *Education:* Less than 1%. Funds secondary and higher education. *Environment:* Less than 1%. Funds Young Men's Christian Association. *Note:* Total contributions made in fiscal 2000. **Typ. Recipients:** Cancer, Children's Health/Hospitals. **Geo. Dist:** Oklahoma City, OK.


**★ 10054 ★  Samuel Freeman Charitable Trust**
114 West 47th St.
New York, NY 10036-1532
**Phone:** (212)852-3683        **Fax:** (212)852-3377
Carolyn Larke, Contact

**Fnded:** 1981. **Philosophy:** The Samuel Freeman Charitable Trust makes grants across the major categories of support. Major interests include municipalities, colleges, cancer research, museums, and social services. **Priorities:** *Arts & Humanities:* 19%. Supports museum, public broadcasting, ballet and historic preservation. *Civic & Public Affairs:* 6%. Supports community safety. *Education:* 60%. Supports colleges, universities, and schools *Environment:* 5%. Supports YMCA and the Scouts. *International:* 5%. Supports single-disease health associations and health organizations. *Note:* Total contributions made in 1998. **Typ. Recipients:** AIDS/HIV, Cancer, Clinics/Medical Centers, Diabetes, Eyes/Blindness, Family Planning, Health-General, Hospitals, Medical Education, Medical Research, Multiple Sclerosis, People with Disabilities, Single-Disease Health Associations, Substance Abuse. **Geo. Dist:** mid-Atlantic region.


**Sarita Kenedy East Foundation**
*See:* Entry 663


**Sidney J. Weinberg, Jr. Foundation**
*See:* Entry 11413


**Skillman Foundation**
*See:* Entry 683


**Skirball Foundation**
*See:* Entry 11414


**★ 10055 ★  T. J. Brown and C. A. Lupton Foundation**
PO Box 1629
Fort Worth, TX 76101-1629
**Phone:** (817)332-1541
**Email:** kschlachtenhaufen@skillman.org
**Website:** http://www.skillman.org
Sam Woodson, III, President

**Fnded:** 1942. **Philosophy:** The T. J. Brown and C. A. Lupton Foundation primarily supports education, particularly the Texas Christian University. Other educational support goes to legal training. Other interests include civic affairs, mainly zoos, and the arts. **Priorities:** *Arts & Humanities:* 29%. Supports the performing arts, the Fort Worth Symphony, and museums and opera. *Civic & Public Affairs:* 11%. The Fort Worth Zoological Society, philanthropic organizations and law & justice. *Education:* 50%. Major support is given to Texas Christian University, as well as schools and learning centers. *Environment:* 1%. Funds the Young Men's Christian Association, food banks, children's welfare, and shelters. *International:* 4%. Supports cancer, diabetes, and a health foundation. *Religion:* 5%. Supports a science museum. *Note:* Total contributions made in 2000. **Typ. Recipients:** Cancer, Diabetes, People with Disabilities, Public Health, Substance Abuse. **Geo. Dist:** Ft. Worth, TX.


**★ 10056 ★  Vollmer Foundation**
PO Box 704
Butler, NJ 07405
**Phone:** (973)492-2309        **Fax:** (973)492-2309
Albert Ennist, Assistant Secretary

**Fnded:** 1965. **Philosophy:** The purpose of the Vollmer Foundation is "to make charitable distributions that will in some way benefit the people of Venezuela." The main areas of interest to the foundation are education, community foundations and scientific investigation. **Priorities:** *Civic & Public Affairs:* 11%. Funds Hispanic American Center for Economic Research. *Note:* Total contributions made in 1998. **Typ. Recipients:** Cancer.


**★ 10057 ★  Walton Family Foundation**
PO Box 2030
Bentonville, AR 72712
**Phone:** (479)464-1570        **Fax:** (501)464-1580
**Website:** http://www.wffhome.com
Buddy Philpot, Director

**Fnded:** 1987. **Philosophy:** The Foundation's main focus is systemic reform in education, with special emphasis on primary and secondary education. The Foundation also supports several university level programs that involve K-12 education and that address issues directly relating to children. The Foundation also currently funds three scholarship programs: Walton Scholarship–awarded to the children of Wal-Mart associates who are high school seniors and have exhibited superior standards academically and have been active in positions of leadership and responsibility. International Scholarship Program–recruits students from Belize, Costa Rica, El Salvador, Guatemala, Honduras, Mexico, Nicaragua, and Panama to attend college in the United States. Walton Delta Scholarship Program–awards grants to students from the Arkansas Delta region who are high school seniors interested in pursuing a career in teaching. The Foundation also has particular interest in the Mississippi River's delta region of Arkansas and Mississippi, concentrating on economic development in the area and on enhancing the educational opportunities for students and adults. **Priorities:** *Arts & Humanities:* Supports museums, performing arts, and art centers. *Civic & Public Affairs:* 19%. Focus on free enterprise, community affairs, and philanthropic organizations. *Education:* 61%. Supports private precollege education, colleges and universities, and education reform. *Environment:* 10%. Supports scouting, familu services, family planning, and YMCA. *International:* 2%. *Religion:* 2%. *Note:* Total contributions made in 1998. **Typ. Recipients:** Cancer, Health Organizations, Long-Term Care, Mental Health, Research/Studies Institutes, Substance Abuse. **Geo. Dist:** AR.


**★ 10058 ★  William and Mary Greve Foundation**
630 Fifth Ave., Ste. 1750
New York, NY 10111
**Phone:** (212)307-7850        **Fax:** (212)262-8340
**Email:** williamary@msn.com
Anthony Kiser, President & Director

**Fnded:** 1964. **Philosophy:** The foundation's primary interests are the performing and visual arts, with a focus on off-Broadway theater. Another priority is basic education programs aimed at improving the quality of secondary education. Public policy groups dealing with East-West relations also receive support. **Priorities:** *Arts & Humanities:* 37%. Supports symphony orchestra, performing arts, music schools, and public libraries. *Civic & Public Affairs:* 9%. Supports community development and services. *Education:* 34%. Supports colleges, universities, educational institutions and programs. *Environment:* 2%. Supports children and youth services, employment, and social services. *Note:* Contributions were made in 1998. **Typ. Recipients:** Cancer, Eyes/Blindness, People with Disabilities. **Geo. Dist:** nationally; NY.


## Corporate Foundations

**AMR/American Airlines Foundation**
*See:* Entry 836


**Avon Products Foundation, Inc.**
*See:* Entry 857


**Bandai Foundation**
*See:* Entry 11694


**Barclays Capital**
*See:* Entry 871


**Bassett Furniture Industries Foundation**
*See:* Entry 875


**★ 10059 ★  Bechtel Foundation**
PO Box 193965
San Francisco, CA 94119-3965
**Phone:** (415)768-5974        **Fax:** (415)768-0263

**Email:** lmlang@bechtel.com
**Website:** http://www.bechtel.com/bechfoun.html
Leeanne Lang, Assistant Secretary

**Priorities:** *Civic & Public Affairs:* 8%. Supports a public garden, municipalities, ethnic organizations, and other civic organizations. *Education:* 68%. Focus on math, science, and engineering education. Support is given for educational enrichment programs such as local science fairs, special educational activities, or regional museum programs in math or science for young people around the world; and engineering and business schools at selected colleges and universities around the world (divided between unrestricted support and support for scholarship programs). *Environment:* 18%. Primarily supports the United Way or similar campaigns in the communities where Bechtel offices or major projects. *Note:* Total contributions made in 1999. **Typ. Recipients:** Adolescent Health Issues, AIDS/HIV, Cancer, Children's Health/Hospitals, Emergency/Ambulance Services, Hospitals, Medical Education, Prenatal Health Issues, Research/Studies Institutes, Substance Abuse. **Geo. Dist:** internationally, in major operating locations.

★ 10060 ★ **Ben & Jerry's Foundation**
30 Community Dr.
South Burlington, VT 05403-6828
**Phone:** (802)846-1500          **Fax:** (802)846-1610
**Website:** http://www.benjerry.com/foundation
Rebecca Golden, Executive Director

**Fnded:** 1977. **Priorities:** *Civic & Public Affairs:* 62%. Focus is on public policy, justice issues, minority issues, and human rights. *Education:* 1%. *Environment:* 4%. Funds family and youth services. *Note:* Total foundation contributions made in 2000. **Typ. Recipients:** AIDS/HIV, Cancer, Mental Health, People with Disabilities. **Geo. Dist:** U.S.-based organizations; VT, focusing on Community Action Teams.

**Benjamin Jacobson & Sons Foundation**
*See:* Entry 884

★ 10061 ★ **Boler Co. Foundation**
500 Park Blvd., Ste. 1010
Itasca, IL 60143-1285
**Phone:** (630)773-9111          **Fax:** (630)773-9121
John Boler, Chairman, President & Chief Executive
  Of

**Fnded:** 1987. **Priorities:** *Education:* 99%. Primary support for a religions high school; also funds universities. *Note:* Total contributions in 2000. **Typ. Recipients:** Cancer, Children's Health/Hospitals, Hospices, Hospitals, Long-Term Care. **Geo. Dist:** IL; IN; OH.

**Boswell Foundation, Inc.**
*See:* Entry 897

★ 10062 ★ **Central Newspapers
Foundation**
care of Gannett Co., Inc.
1100 Wilson Boulevard
Arlington, VA 22234
**Phone:** (703)633-1299          **Fax:** (703)656-1435
Sandy Harless, Executive Director

**Fnded:** 1935. **Priorities:** *Education:* 100%. The majority of the foundation's support goes to grants and scholarship programs in journalism education at major colleges and universities in Indiana and Arizona. Also provides higher education scholarships to children of employees and paper carriers. *Note:* Total foundation contributions made in fiscal 2001. **Typ. Recipients:** Cancer, Eyes/Blindness, People with Disabilities, Preventive Medicine/Wellness Organizations. **Geo. Dist:** AZ; IN.

**Collins & Aikman Foundation**
*See:* Entry 953

**Copolymer Foundation**
*See:* Entry 13520

★ 10063 ★ **CSR America Companies
Foundation**
1501 Belvedere Rd.
West Palm Beach, FL 33406
**Phone:** (561)833-5555          **Fax:** (561)820-8359
**Email:** flaplaca@wpbcentral.csra.com
Frank LaPlaca, Administrator

**Fnded:** 1957. **Priorities:** *Arts & Humanities:* 2%. Supports the Raymond F. Kravis Center. *Civic & Public Affairs:* 5%. Supports community foundations and other civic organizations. *Education:* 59%. Funds universities and colleges. *Environment:* 27%. Supports United Way, scouts, and substance abuse initiatives. **Typ. Recipients:** Cancer, Children's Health/Hospitals, Substance Abuse. **Geo. Dist:** FL, Dade County; FL, Palm Beach County.

★ 10064 ★ **Domino's Pizza Inc.**
PO Box 997
Ann Arbor, MI 48106
**Phone:** (734)930-3674          **Fax:** (734)668-1946
**Email:** ryanh@dominos.com
**Website:** http://www.dominos.com
Holly Ryan, Public Affairs Director

**Typ. Recipients:** Cancer, Children's Health/Hospitals, People with Disabilities. **Geo. Dist:** nationally for religion-oriented grants; MI, including southeast Michigan.

**E.L. Craig Foundation**
*See:* Entry 1012

**Ecolab Foundation**
*See:* Entry 8548

**F.K. Bemis Family Foundation**
*See:* Entry 1036

**FBW Foundation**
*See:* Entry 7878

**FINA Foundation**
*See:* Entry 1046

**GenAmerican Foundation**
*See:* Entry 1077

★ 10065 ★ **Genesis Foundation**
2600 Kettering Tower
Dayton, OH 45423
**Phone:** (937)910-9300
**Email:** cendicott@genam.com
**Website:** http://www.genamerica.com
Robert Reithman, Treasurer

**Fnded:** 1952. **Priorities:** *Arts & Humanities:* 31%. Supports music, dance, libraries, public television, and art institutes. *Civic & Public Affairs:* 7%. Supports minority business, parks, and community foundations. *Education:* 27%. Supports schools, community colleges, and scholarship funds. *Environment:* 16%. Supports YMCA, Boy Scouts of America, United Way, and Big Brothers/Big Sisters. *International:* 15%. Supports hospitals and health funds. *Religion:* 1%. Supports science Olympiad. *Note:* Total foundation contributions made in 2000. **Typ. Recipients:** Cancer, Children's Health/Hospitals, Clinics/Medical Centers, Clinics/Medical Centers, Emergency/Ambulance Services, Hospices, Hospitals, Long-Term Care, People with Disabilities, Transplant Networks/Donor Banks. **Geo. Dist:** NY; OH.

**Halliburton Foundation, Inc.**
*See:* Entry 1109

**IFF Foundation Inc.**
*See:* Entry 1144

**J.D. Edwards Foundation**
*See:* Entry 1154

**J.T. Tai and Co. Foundation, Inc.**
*See:* Entry 1159

**Kupferberg Foundation**
*See:* Entry 5577

**Leviton Foundation New York**
*See:* Entry 1202

**Milacron Foundation**
*See:* Entry 1241

★ 10066 ★ **Monroe Auto Equipment Co.
Foundation**
PO Box 75000
MC 3462
Detroit, MI 48275-3462
**Phone:** (313)222-5067
**Email:** hleviton@leviton.com
**Website:** http://www.halliburton.com/corp/about.asp

**Priorities:** *Arts & Humanities:* 11%. Funds museums. *Civic & Public Affairs:* 9%. Funds housing and civic foundations. *Education:* 31%. Funds schools, colleges, and universities. *Environment:* 48%. Funds United Way and recreation. *Note:* Total contributions made in 2000. **Typ. Recipients:** Cancer, Emergency/Ambulance Services, Health Organizations, Home-Care Services, Hospices, Hospitals, Substance Abuse. **Geo. Dist:** nationally, including any U.S. possessions.

**OMC Foundation**
*See:* Entry 11458

★ 10067 ★ **Oshkosh Truck Foundation**
2307 Oregon St.
PO Box 2566
Oshkosh, WI 54903-2566
**Phone:** (920)235-9151
Robert Bohn, Jr., President

**Fnded:** 1960. **Priorities:** *Arts & Humanities:* 5%. Supports art centers, music, and historic preservation. *Education:* 18%. Supports schools, and educational foundations. *Environment:* 76%. Supports YMCA, United Way, substance abuse programs, and youth organizations. *International:* 1%. Primarily supports health organizations. *Note:* Total contributions made in fiscal 2000. **Typ. Recipients:** Cancer, Clinics/Medical Centers, Domestic Violence, Heart, Public Health, Sexual Abuse, Substance Abuse. **Geo. Dist:** Brandenton, FL; Oshkosh, WI.

**Publix Supermarkets Charities**
*See:* Entry 11462

★ 10068 ★ **Regis Foundation**
7201 Metro Boulevard
Minneapolis, MN 55439
**Phone:** (612)947-7777          **Fax:** (612)947-7900
**Website:**      http://www.publix.com/comm_involvement.htm
Mr. Myron Kunin, President

**Fnded:** 1981. **Priorities:** *Arts & Humanities:* 14%. Supports art museums and a theater. *Civic & Public Affairs:* 1%. Supports housing initiatives and other civic causes. *Education:* 32%. Funds universities and scholarship funds. *Environment:* 1%. Supports United Way. *Note:* Total contributions in 1998. **Typ. Recipients:** Cancer, People with Disabilities. **Geo. Dist:** Minneapolis, MN.

**Robbins and Myers Foundation**
*See:* Entry 8554

**Saint Paul Companies Inc.**
*See:* Entry 1368

**Sentry Insurance Foundation Inc.**
*See:* Entry 1382

**Spang & Co. Charitable Trust**
*See:* Entry 5588

**★ 10069 ★ Sprint Foundation**
2330 Shawnee Mission Parkway
Westwood, KS 66205
**Phone:** (913)624-3343      **Fax:** (913)624-3490
**Website:** http://www.sprint.com/sprint/overview/commun.html
David Thomas, Executive Director
**Priorities:** *Arts & Humanities:* 17%. Supports major visual and performig arts organizations, museums and other cultural organizations, and activities which have effective outreach programs that broaden the cultural experience of the general public and bring cultural opportunity to the economically disadvantaged. *Civic & Public Affairs:* 23%. Supports economic development, legal and women's issues, and civic organizations. Special project grants targeted to encourage resource-sharing efforts among not-for-profit agencies are also considered. *Education:* 30%. Supports activities that will prepare people for the challenges of the workplace and enable them to be productive participants in the economy by addressing educational needs and initiatives covering the childhood through early adult years. Targets public school renewal and reform, programs that enhance educational opportunities for minorities and/or the disadvantaged, excellence in teaching and retention of quality educators, encourages employee and public support of education, and the use of new communications technology in education. Also sponsors matching gifts program. *Environment:* 29%. Supports youth organizations with drug and alcohol education, minority youth endeavors, community youth activities, and United Way. *International:* 2%. Supports medical centers. *Note:* Total contributions in 1998. **Typ. Recipients:** Cancer, Children's Health/Hospitals, Heart, Public Health. **Geo. Dist:** principally near operating locations and to national organizations; also to areas where the company's subsidiaries have major concentrations of employees.

**SunTrust Banks Foundation**
*See:* Entry 1420

**Sverdrup Corp. Charitable Trust**
*See:* Entry 1422

**Synetic Foundation**
*See:* Entry 5589

**★ 10070 ★ Toro Foundation**
8111 Lyndale Ave. South
Bloomington, MN 55420-1196
**Phone:** (612)887-8960
Donald St. Dennis, Community Relations
**Fnded:** 1989. **Priorities:** *Arts & Humanities:* 5%. Supports music, museums, and theaters. *Civic & Public Affairs:* 7%. Supports economic development, municipalities, and foundation councils. *Education:* 18%. Supports higher education and schools. *Environment:* 49%. Primary support for the United Way; also supports food banks. *International:* 2%. Primarily supports hospitals and cancer institutions. *Note:* Total fnd contributions made in 2000. **Typ. Recipients:** AIDS/HIV, Cancer, Diabetes, Emergency/Ambulance Services, Heart, People with Disabilities, Public Health, Public Health, Substance Abuse. **Geo. Dist:** headquarters and operating communities.

**Tribune New York Foundation**
*See:* Entry 1446

**Truland Foundation**
*See:* Entry 5590

**United Co. Charitable Foundation**
*See:* Entry 1455

**Universal Studios Foundation**
*See:* Entry 1463

**USAA Foundation, A Charitable Trust**
*See:* Entry 1468

## Other Funding Organizations

**★ 10071 ★ American Association for Cancer Research (AACR)**
Public Ledger Bldg., Ste. 826
150 S Independence Mall W
Philadelphia, PA 19106-3483
**Phone:** (215)440-9300      **Fax:** (215)440-9313
**Email:** membership@aacr.org
**Website:** http://www.aacr.org
Margaret Foti, Ph.D, Exec. Dir.
**Desc:** Works to facilitate communication and dissemination of information among scientists and others dedicated to cancer research; seeks to advance understanding of cancer etiology, prevention, diagnosis and treatment throughout the world. Fosters research on cancer, public and science education and training. **Awards:** American Cancer Society Award (annual); Bruce F. Cain Memorial Award (annual); C.P. Rhoads Memorial Award (annual); G.H.A. Clowes Memorial Award (annual); Gertrude Elion Cancer Research Award (annual); Travel Award-Annual Meeting (annual) for medical or graduate students.

**★ 10072 ★ American College of Phlebology (ACP)**
100 Webster St., Ste. 101
Oakland, CA 94607-3724
**Phone:** (510)834-6500      **Fax:** (510)832-7300
**Email:** acp@amsinc.org
**Website:** http://www.phlebology.org
Craig Feied, MD, Pres.
**Desc:** Physicians and medical students with an interest in the evaluation and management of patients with varicose veins, thrombophlebitis, thrombosis, and venous leg ulcers. Seeks to advance the study, teaching, and practice of phlebology; promotes continuing professional development of members. Serves as a network facilitating cooperation and exchange of information among medical professionals with an interest in phlebology; conducts educational programs; functions as a clearinghouse on medical techniques and technologies applicable to the practice of phlebology. **Awards:** BSN-JOBST Research Grant (annual); Walter DeGroot Fellowship Award (annual).

**★ 10073 ★ American Institute for Cancer Research (AICR)**
1759 R St., NW
Washington, DC 20009
**Phone:** (202)328-7744      **Free:** 800-843-8114
**Fax:** (202)328-7226
**Email:** aicrweb@aicr.org
**Website:** http://www.aicr.org
**Desc:** Fosters research and provides information related to diet, nutrition and cancer. **Awards:** AICR Research Grants.

**★ 10074 ★ American Society of Cytopathology (ASC)**
400 W 9th St., Ste. 201
Wilmington, DE 19801
**Phone:** (302)429-8802      **Fax:** (302)429-8807
**Email:** asc@cytopathology.org
**Website:** http://www.cytopathology.org
Elizabeth A. Jenkins, Exec. Admin.
**Desc:** Physicians, Cytotechnologists and scientists dedicated to the cytologic method of diagnostic pathology. **Awards:** Papanicoluau Award (annual) for a cytopathologist selected by committee.

**★ 10075 ★ Aplastic Anemia and MDS International Foundation (AAFA)**
PO Box 613
Annapolis, MD 21404-0613
**Phone:** 800-747-2820      **Fax:** (410)867-0240
**Email:** help@aamds.org
**Website:** http://www.aplastic.org
Marilyn Baker, Exec. Dir.
**Desc:** Serves as an information source for persons with aplastic anemia and myelodysplastic syndromes. (Aplastic anemia is an often fatal disease in which the bone marrow fails to produce new blood cells.) Provides free educational materials and medical information. Financially supports research. Hosts annual International Patient Conferences presenting the latest in medical research findings and networking opportunities for patients and their families. **Awards:** New Research Award (annual).

**★ 10076 ★ Cancer Federation (CFI)**
PO Box 1298
Banning, CA 92220-0009
**Phone:** (909)849-4325      **Free:** 800-207-2873
**Fax:** (909)849-0156
**Email:** cancerfederation@yahoo.com
**Website:** http://www.cancerfed.com
Karen Alene, Admin.
**Desc:** Physicians, scientists, nurses, and laymen (both cancer patients and nonpatients). Promotes research and education in the field of cancer immunology. Seeks to discover appropriate cancer therapies using natural biological modifiers. Funds research at major centers throughout the U.S., including the University of California (Riverside and Santa Barbara), University of Hawaii, and University of Pittsburgh, on biological modifiers, such as lymphokines; killer cells; Interleukin I and II; diet; and psychological aspects of cancer. Compiles statistics; conducts research and education in cancer therapy, including vaccines, and in psychological programming for patients. Offers counseling program for cancer patients and their families. Sponsors public medical conferences and in-service courses for nurses on the psychology of cancer, and research projects at many universities and hospitals in the field of immunology. Sponsors charitable program. **Awards:** Scholarship (annual) for high school and college seniors in the field of microbiology; Science, Communication, and Service Awards (annual).

**★ 10077 ★ Cancer Research Foundation of America**
1600 Duke St., Ste. 110
Alexandria, VA 22314
**Phone:** (703)836-4412      **Free:** 800-227-2732
**Fax:** (703)836-4413
**Website:** http://www.preventcancer.org
**Desc:** Foundations, individuals and companies. Aims to prevent cancer through research and education. Sponsors grants and fellowships, publishes educational materials. **Awards:** Fellowship; grant.

**★ 10078 ★ Children's Leukemia Research Association (NLA)**
585 Stewart Ave., Ste. LL18
Garden City, NY 11530
**Phone:** (516)222-1944      **Fax:** (516)222-0457
**Email:** clra@erols.com
**Website:** http://www.childrensleukemia.org/
Allan D. Weinberg, Exec. Dir.
**Desc:** Promotes leukemia research and public awareness of the disease. Provides financial aid to leukemia patients and their families, based on need. **Awards:** Grant (annual) for research; recognition.

### ★ 10079 ★ Cooley's Anemia Foundation (CAF)

129-09 26th Ave., No. 203
Flushing, NY 11354
**Phone:** (718)321-2873          **Free:** 800-522-7222
**Fax:** (718)321-3340
**Email:** info@cooleysanemia.org
**Website:** http://www.thalassemia.org
Jayne Restivo, Exec. Dir.

**Desc:** Parents of children afflicted with Cooley's anemia; doctors, technicians, nurses, and others interested in the treatment and eventual cure of the disease. (Cooley's anemia is an incurable blood disease requiring frequent blood transfusions to keep its victims alive; it is named after Dr. Thomas B. Cooley, a Detroit, MI, physician who first described it in 1925.) Distributes therapy materials including infusion pumps and batteries, at no charge, to victims of the disease. Presents awards for scientific and humanitarian achievement. Sponsors medical symposia to educate physicians and scientists about new drugs or therapies for Cooley's anemia or other thalassemias. Sponsors Thalassemia Action Group, a networking task force of young adult victims of thalassemia. Operates speakers' bureau. Conducts blood drives. **Awards:** Fellowship Grant (annual) for fellowships and innovative and promising research projects; Humanitarian Achievement; Patient Scholarship (annual); recognition for scientific and humanitarian achievement.

### ★ 10080 ★ Diabetes Exercise and Sports Association (DESA)

PO Box 1935
Litchfield Park, AZ 85340
**Phone:** (623)535-4593          **Free:** 800-898-4322
**Fax:** (623)535-4741
**Email:** desa@diabetes-exercise.org
**Website:** http://www.diabetes-exercise.org
Paula Harper, RN, CDE, Pres.

**Desc:** Individuals with diabetes and healthcare professionals. Promotes the participation of individuals with diabetes in sports activities. Provides a network and support group for athletes with diabetes. Conducts educational programs to increase self care skills for individuals with diabetes and counseling skills for healthcare professionals. Offers blood sugar screenings; sponsors volunteer services and speakers' bureau. Conducts children's services. **Awards:** Lifescan Prize for Athletic Achievement (annual) athletic achievements, potential for further success in endeavors potential for grant to assist in goal, how prize will be used to promote value of exercise for people w/ diabetes.

### ★ 10081 ★ Hepatitis Foundation International

c/o Martha Young
504 Elick Dr.
Silver Spring, MD 20904
**Phone:** (973)239-1035          **Free:** 800-891-0707
**Fax:** (973)857-5044
**Email:** mail@hepfi.org
**Website:** http://www.hepfi.org
Thelma King Thiel, Chm. and C. E. O.

**Desc:** Individuals concerned about those with hepatitis. Provides education and information for distribution to the general public, patients, educators, and medical professionals about the diagnosis, treatment, and prevention of viral hepatitis. Maintains database of hepatitis support groups and website information. Conducts train-the-trainer programs for those interested in the topic. **Awards:** Career Development Award (annual) for epidemiology and outcomes research of viral hepatitis.

### ★ 10082 ★ Histiocytosis Association of America

302 N Broadway
Pitman, NJ 08071
**Phone:** (856)589-6606          **Free:** 800-548-2758
**Fax:** (856)589-6614
**Email:** president@histio.org

**Website:** http://www.histio.org/us
Jeffrey M. Toughill, Pres.

**Desc:** Patients, families, and friends of those suffering from histiocytic disorders; physicians, oncologists, and hematologists working in the field of histiocytosis research. (Histiocytosis is a rare disease that causes histiocytes, a type of white blood cell, to multiply and attack organs, body systems, or bones.) Works to provide support for patients and their families and friends. Funds research on the cause and treatment of histiocytosis. Acts as a referral service. Maintains speakers' bureau. **Awards:** Medical Research (annual).

### ★ 10083 ★ International Atherosclerosis Society (IAS)

6550 Fannin, Ste. 1211
Houston, TX 77030-2704
**Phone:** (713)797-0401          **Fax:** (713)797-8853
**Email:** info@athero.org
**Website:** http://www.athero.org
Ann S. Jackson, Exec. Dir.

**Desc:** Scientists and other professionals involved in research in the field of atherosclerosis; corporations and firms supporting aims of the IAS. Promotes the advancement of science, research, and teaching in the field of atherosclerosis throughout the world. (Atherosclerosis is a form of arteriosclerosis characterized by the deposition of fatty substances in and fibrosis of the inner layer of the arteries.) Advocates an interdisciplinary approach to the study of atherosclerosis and related diseases. Facilitates international communication and exchange of knowledge among scientists in the field. Assists in the organization of exchange visits among scientists at various research centers. Fosters and encourages young researchers by arranging contacts, and offering travel support to world gatherings in the field. Coordinates activities in atherosclerosis research. **Awards:** Scholarship; Visiting Fellowship Award (semiannual).

### ★ 10084 ★ International Myeloma Foundation

12650 Riverside Dr., Ste. 206
North Hollywood, CA 91607
**Phone:** (818)487-7455          **Free:** 800-452-CURE
**Fax:** (818)487-7454
**Email:** TheIMF@myeloma.org
**Website:** http://www.myeloma.org
Stephanie Colman, Director of Community Relations

**Desc:** The International Myeloma Foundation is a nonprofit organization dedicated to the eduction, treatment and research of multiple myeloma, a little-known cancer of the bone marrow. We provide a variety of patient and physician education and support programs and services. **Awards:** Brian D. Novis Research Grant (annual) for a doctor or researcher actively working on multiple myeloma.

### ★ 10085 ★ International Society for Experimental Hematology (ISEH)

2025 M St. NW, Ste. 800
Washington, DC 20036
**Phone:** (202)367-1183          **Fax:** (202)367-2183
**Email:** iseh@dc.sba.com
**Website:** http://www.iseh.org
Thomas Reiser, Exec. Dir.

**Desc:** Scientists and health care professionals in the field of experimental hematology. Seeks to advance the science and practice of hematology; promotes professional development of members. Serves as a forum for the exchange of information on experimental hematology and related topics; sponsors research and educational programs. **Awards:** Young Investigators Awards (annual) for depth of research in abstracts.

### ★ 10086 ★ Leukemia and Lymphoma Society

1311 Mamaroneck Ave.
White Plains, NY 10605
**Phone:** (914)949-5213          **Free:** 800-955-4572
**Fax:** (914)949-6691

**Email:** irc_lls@hotmail.com
**Website:** http://www.leukemia.org
Dwayne Howell, PhD, Pres. /CEO

**Desc:** Raises funds to combat leukemia, lymphoma, Hodgkin's Disease and myeloma through research, patient service, and public and professional education and advocacy. Sponsors medical symposia; conducts research; provides financial aid for patients and free information; sponsors support groups. Free information available through 1-800-955-4LSA or website: www.leukemia.org. **Awards:** Fellowship; recognition; scholarship.

### ★ 10087 ★ Lymphatic Research Foundation (LRF)

39 Pool Dr.
Roslyn, NY 11576-2038
**Phone:** (516)625-9862          **Fax:** (516)625-9410
**Email:** lrf@lymphaticresearch.org
**Website:** http://www.lymphaticresearch.org
Wendy Chaite, Esq., Pres.

**Desc:** Health care professionals, scientists, and researchers with an interest in lymphatic diseases and related disorders. Seeks to advance the prevention, diagnosis, and treatment of lymphatic diseases. Serves as a clearinghouse on lymphatic research; facilitates exchange of information among members; advocates the creation of a nationally supported lymphatic research program; functions as a liaison linking public and private-sector lymphatic research institutions and programs. **Awards:** Andrew Moisoff Young Investigator Award (periodic) for lymphatic research.

### ★ 10088 ★ National Alliance of Breast Cancer Organizations (NABCO)

9 E 37th St., 10th Fl.
New York, NY 10016
**Phone:** (212)889-0606          **Free:** 888-80-NABCO
**Fax:** (212)689-1213
**Email:** NABCOinfo@aol.com
**Website:** http://www.nabco.org
Amy Langer, Exec. Dir.

**Desc:** The National Alliance of Breast Cancer Organization (NABCO) is the leading non-profit information and education resource on breast cancer and a network of over 400 member organizations nationwide. NABCO provides information to medical professionals and their organizations and to patients and their families, and advocates for beneficial regulatory change and legislation. With public and corporate partners, NABCO has collaborated on educational and medical programs thast have reached a national audience, heightening public awareness and connecting women with needed services. centers, and hospital programs. Services are free of charge. **Awards:** Within Our Reach (a NABCO program) (annual) for community programs serving poor and medically underserved women.

### ★ 10089 ★ National Blood Foundation (NBF)

8101 Glenbrook Rd.
Bethesda, MD 20814-2749
**Phone:** (301)215-6552          **Fax:** (301)907-6895
**Email:** nbf@aabb.org
**Website:** http://www.aabb.org

**Desc:** Promotes the safety and adequacy of America's blood supply by supporting research and education for blood banking and transfusion medicine. **Awards:** Scientific Research Grants Program (annual) one or two year grants to prepare or support new investigators in the fields of blood banking, transfusion medicine, and tissue transplantation.

### ★ 10090 ★ National Ovarian Cancer Coalition (NOCC)

500 NE Spanish River Blvd., Ste. 14
Boca Raton, FL 33431
**Phone:** (561)393-0005          **Free:** 888-OVA-RIAN
**Fax:** (561)393-7275
**Email:** nocc@ovarian.org

**Website:** http://www.ovarian.org
Gail Hayward, Pres.

**Desc:** Individuals with ovarian cancer and their families; health care professionals treating people with ovarian cancer. Seeks to advance the prevention, diagnosis, and treatment of ovarian cancer. Serves as a clearinghouse on ovarian cancer; provides support and services to members; conducts educational programs. **Awards:** Research Fund (annual).

### ★ 10091 ★ Skin Cancer Foundation (SCF)

245 5th Ave., Ste. 1403
New York, NY 10016
**Phone:** (212)725-5176    **Free:** 800-SKIN-490
**Fax:** (212)725-5751
**Email:** info@skincancer.org
**Website:** http://www.skincancer.org
Perry Robins, MD, Pres.

**Desc:** Sponsors medical symposia and public education programs on the prevention and early recognition of skin cancer. Grants its Seal of Recommendation to sunscreen products that meet the criteria and standards established by the SCF as effective aids in the prevention of sun-induced damage to the skin. **Awards:** The Frederic E. Mohs Award (annual) bestowed to qualified researchers and institutions; The Henry W. Menn Memorial Award (annual); The Henry W. Shotmeyer Award (annual).

### ★ 10092 ★ Society of Surgical Oncology (SSO)

c/o Rick Slawny
85 W Algonquin Rd., Ste. 550
Arlington Heights, IL 60005
**Phone:** (847)427-1400    **Fax:** (847)427-1294
**Website:** http://www.surgonc.org/
Rick Slawny, Exec. Dir.

**Desc:** Physicians and scientists working in the field of cancer. **Awards:** Monetary for outstanding cancer basic scientist; monetary for outstanding clinical scientist; monetary for outstanding clinical layman; recognition (annual) for medical resident who is performing an original research project.

### ★ 10093 ★ Society of Vascular Technology (SVT)

4601 Presidents Dr., Ste. 260
Lanham, MD 20706-4831
**Phone:** (301)459-7550    **Fax:** (301)459-5651
**Email:** info@svtnet.org
**Website:** http://www.svtnet.org
Suzanne Stone, Exec. Dir.

**Desc:** Vascular technologists and others in the field of noninvasive vascular technology. (Noninvasive vascular technology is a highly technical and specialized method of monitoring the blood flow in arms and legs and veins and arteries away from the heart in order to better diagnose disease and blood clots.) Seeks to establish an information clearinghouse providing reference and assistance in matters relating to noninvasive vascular technology; facilitate cooperation among noninvasive vascular facilities and other health professions; provide continuing education for individuals in the field. **Awards:** Pioneer Award (annual).

### ★ 10094 ★ Susan G. Komen Breast Cancer Foundation (SGKF)

5005 LBJ, Ste. 250
Dallas, TX 75244
**Phone:** (972)855-1600    **Free:** 800-IM-AWARE
**Fax:** (972)855-1605
**Website:** http://www.breastcancerinfo.com
Susan Braun, CEO/Pres.

**Desc:** Breast cancer patients, health care professionals, and other interested individuals. Works to: increase the recovery and survival rates of breast cancer patients; heighten public awareness of the risks of breast cancer and the need for early detection. Establishes breast screening and training in self-examination procedures; provides funding through grants for research and screening programs. Spon-

sors educational programs. Bestows awards; sponsors competitions; maintains speakers' bureau. **Awards:** Fellowship (annual); grant (annual).

# National & International Organizations

### ★ 10095 ★ Action Cancer

1 Marlborough Park
Belfast BT9 6XS, United Kingdom
**Phone:** 44 2890 803344    **Fax:** 44 2890 803356
**Email:** info@actioncancer.org
**Website:** http://www.actioncancer.org
**Fnded:** 1973. **Local Groups:** 40. **Desc:** Works to heighten awareness of the importance of early cancer detection. Offers breast and cervical cancer screening services for women, and testicular and prostatic screening services for men. Provides counselling for cancer patients, families, and friends. Maintains research lab. Disseminates information. **Pub:** *Action Cancer News*, quarterly. Magazine. • Annual Report. Selection of Cancer informatioin leaflets.

### ★ 10096 ★ African American Breast Cancer Alliance (AABCA)

PO Box 8981
Minneapolis, MN 55408-0981
**Phone:** (612)825-3675    **Fax:** (612)825-3675
**Email:** aabcainc@yahoo.com
**Website:** http://www.geocities.com/aabcainc/
**Fnded:** 1990. **Desc:** Committed to helping Black women, people of color, families and communities cope with breast cancer. Sponsors a breast cancer support group for patients and survivors at various stages of their experiences; addresses the specific needs of Black women diagnosed with breast cancer; also sponsors celebrations and health events for survivors, families, friends and communities. **Pub:** *Being There*. Brochure. Contains advice to empower women to take charge of their health and care of their lives by becoming more informed about breast cancer.

### ★ 10097 ★ American Association for Cancer Research (AACR)

Public Ledger Bldg., Ste. 826
150 S Independence Mall W
Philadelphia, PA 19106-3483
**Phone:** (215)440-9300    **Fax:** (215)440-9313
**Email:** membership@aacr.org
**Website:** http://www.aacr.org
Margaret Foti, Ph.D, Exec. Dir.

**Fnded:** 1907. **Mem:** 16,000. **Local Groups:** 3. **Desc:** Works to facilitate communication and dissemination of information among scientists and others dedicated to cancer research; seeks to advance understanding of cancer etiology, prevention, diagnosis and treatment throughout the world. Fosters research on cancer, public and science education and training. **Pub:** *Cancer Epidemiology, Biomarkers & Prevention*, 8/year. Journal. Contains original research on causes and prevention of cancer. *Price:* $155/year for individual nonmembers. • *Cancer Research*, semimonthly. Journal. Contains reports in subfields of cancer research: biochemistry, biophysics, carcinogenesis, endocrinology, immunology, and molecular biology. *Price:* Included in membership; $610/year for individual nonmembers. • *Cell Growth and Differentiation*, monthly. Journal. Contains in vitro and in vivo studies of mechanisms underlying normal and abnormal cell behavior and cell growth control. *Price:* Included in membership dues; $140/year for nonmembers. • *Clinical Cancer Research*, monthly. Journal. Features articles on clinical and translational cancer research. *Price:* $215/year for individual nonmembers. • *Supplement to Journal*, periodic. Journal. • Directory, annual. • Proceedings, annual.

### ★ 10098 ★ American Board of Chelation Therapy (ABCT)

1407-1/2 N Wells St.
Chicago, IL 60610-1305
**Free:** 800-356-2228    **Fax:** (312)266-3685
**Email:** jackhank@mindspring.com
**Website:** http://www.abct.info
Jack Hank, Exec. Dir.

**Fnded:** 1982. **Mem:** 220. **Desc:** Works to define and establish qualifications required of licensed physicians and surgeons for certification in the field of chelation therapy. (Chelation therapy is used in cases of blood poisoning and involves the use of metal binding and bio-inorganic agents intravenously infused into the bloodstream to "pick up" and remove calcium, lead, or other toxic heavy metals and restore cellular homeostasis. Because of lack of controlled studies for conditions other than calcinosis, digitalis toxicity, and excessive body storage of heavy metals, chelation therapy is not considered standard medical procedure.) Stresses that proper use of chelation therapy requires knowledge of nutrition and exercise and expertise in assisting patients in implementing lifestyle changes. Refers candidate physicians to sponsor ingorganizations for teaching workshops, audio and video learning aids, and reading and study materials. Has created series of testing procedures designed to be comprehensive and unbiased. Administers oral and written examinations and conducts reviews of candidates' background experience and patient records. Maintains standards through process of recertification and reexamination. Sponsored by the American Holistic Medical Association, American College for Advancement in Medicine, Great Lakes Association of Clinical Medicine, and the International Oxidative Medical Association.

### ★ 10099 ★ American Cancer Society (ACS)

2200 Century Pky., Ste. 950
Atlanta, GA 30345
**Phone:** (404)816-4994    **Free:** 800-ACS-2345
**Fax:** (404)315-9348
**Website:** http://www.cancer.org
John R. Seffrin, PhD, CEO

**Fnded:** 1913. **Reg. Groups:** 17. **Local Groups:** 3400. **Desc:** The American Cancer Society is the nationwide, community-based, voluntary health organization dedicated to eliminating cancer as a major health problem by preventing cancer, saving lives and diminishing suffering from cancer, through research, education, advocacy, and service. **Pub:** *American Cancer Society*. Annual Report. *Price:* Free. • *CA-A Cancer Journal for Clinicians*, bimonthly. Covers cancer treatment, prevention, and diagnosis. *Price:* Free for health professionals. • *Cancer*, semimonthly. Medical journal covering cancer prevention, research, diagnosis, and treatment. Includes proceedings supplements covering ACS conferences. *Price:* $219/year for individuals; $437/year for institutions. • *Cancer Facts and Figures*, annual. Report providing statistical information on the major sites of cancer including incidence, mortality and survival rates, and risk factors. *Price:* Free. **Frmly:** (1944) American Society for the Control Cancer.

### ★ 10100 ★ American College of MOHS Micrographic Surgery and Cutaneous Oncology (ACMMSCO)

930 E Woodfield Rd.
Schaumburg, IL 60173-4927
**Phone:** (847)330-9830    **Free:** 800-500-7224
**Fax:** (847)330-1135
**Email:** bpaez@aad.org
**Website:** http://www.mohscollege.org
Kimberly A. Hoarle, Exec. Dir.

**Fnded:** 1967. **Mem:** 600. **Desc:** Physicians, dermatologists, surgeons, plastic surgeons, and other specialists who have had a minimum of one year of training in Mohs surgery at an approved institution. (Mohs surgery is used for the microscopically controlled excision of skin cancer.) Provides a means for accreditation of physicians who have become proficient in the method; to facilitate education and the exchange of ideas. **Frmly:** (1987) American College of Chemosurgery.

## ★ 10101 ★ American College of Oncology Administrators (ACOA)
701 Lee St., Ste. 600
Des Plaines, IL 60016
**Phone:** (847)759-8601          **Fax:** (847)759-8602
**Email:** info@aameda.org
**Website:** http://www.aameda.org
Scott Robillard, Contact

**Fnded:** 1991. **Mem:** 500. **Reg. Groups:** 7. **State Groups:** 50. **Desc:** Specialty College of the American Academy of Medical Administrators. Oncology administrators, managers and consultants. Brings together all components of oncology management to develop creative strategies, quality programs, and sound evaluation mechanisms. Promotes advancement of members through continuing education and research in oncology management. Conducts educational programs. **Pub:** *Journal of Oncology Management*, bimonthly. Journal. Contains information and ideas for professionals involved in managing cancer programs.

## ★ 10102 ★ American College of Phlebology (ACP)
100 Webster St., Ste. 101
Oakland, CA 94607-3724
**Phone:** (510)834-6500          **Fax:** (510)832-7300
**Email:** acp@amsinc.org
**Website:** http://www.phlebology.org
Craig Feied, MD, Pres.

**Fnded:** 1985. **Mem:** 915. **Desc:** Physicians and medical students with an interest in the evaluation and management of patients with varicose veins, thrombophlebitis, thrombosis, and venous leg ulcers. Seeks to advance the study, teaching, and practice of phlebology; promotes continuing professional development of members. Serves as a network facilitating cooperation and exchange of information among medical professionals with an interest in phlebology; conducts educational programs; functions as a clearinghouse on medical techniques and technologies applicable to the practice of phelbology. **Pub:** *Journal of Dermatologic Surgery*, monthly. Journal. • *Vein Line*, quarterly. Newsletter. **Frmly:** (1997) North American Society of Phlebology.

## ★ 10103 ★ American Head and Neck Society (AHNS)
601 N Caroline, Rm. 6254
Baltimore, MD 21287
**Phone:** (410)647-2227          **Fax:** (410)647-8944
**Email:** rwagner@pitt.edu
**Website:** http://www.headandneckcancer.org
Keith S. Heller, MD, Pres.

**Fnded:** 1959. **Mem:** 1,635. **Desc:** Otolaryngologists and other physicians with board certification whose primary interest is head and neck oncology. Associate membership is for other other practioners who treat head and neck cancer. Seeks to advance knowledge relevant to treatment of diseases of the head and neck, including reconstruction and rehabilitation. Promotes development of programs of training in head and neck oncology. **Pub:** *Head and Neck Cancer Practice Guidelines*. Practice Guidelines for Head and Neck Oncology. *Price:* $5 members; $10 non-members. **Frmly:** (1998) Society of Head and Neck Surgeons; (1999) American Society for Head and Neck Surgery; (2000) American Society of Head and Neck Surgeons.

## ★ 10104 ★ American Institute for Cancer Research (AICR)
1759 R St., NW
Washington, DC 20009
**Phone:** (202)328-7744          **Free:** 800-843-8114
**Fax:** (202)328-7226
**Email:** aicrweb@aicr.org
**Website:** http://www.aicr.org

**Fnded:** 1983. **Desc:** Fosters research and provides information related to diet, nutrition and cancer. **Pub:** Newsletter, quarterly.

## ★ 10105 ★ American Joint Committee on Cancer (AJCC)
633 North St. Clair St.
Chicago, IL 60611
**Phone:** (312)202-5313          **Fax:** (312)202-5009
**Email:** sburkhardt@facs.org
**Website:** http://www.cancerstaging.org
Susan Burkhardt, AJCC Administrator

**Fnded:** 1959. **Mem:** 40. **Desc:** Surgeons, physicians, radiologists, pathologists, American Cancer Society representatives, and National Cancer Institute representatives. Formulates and publishes systems of classification for cancer staging and end results reporting for the purpose of selecting the most effective treatment, determining prognosis, and continuing evaluation of cancer control measures. Promotes the use of developed systems of classification of cancer and evaluates systems of recording and reporting data. **Pub:** *AJCC Manual for Staging of Cancer, 5th ed.*, quadrennial. Manual. Includes classification for cancer staging & end results reporting for selecting treatment, determining prognosis and evaluating cancer. *Price:* $49. **Frmly:** (1981) American Joint Committee for Cancer Staging and End Results Reporting.

## ★ 10106 ★ American Radium Society (ARS)
820 Jorie Blvd.
Oak Brook, IL 60523-2251
**Phone:** (630)590-7713          **Fax:** (630)571-7837
**Email:** ars@rsna.org
**Website:** http://www.americanradiumsociety.org
Jay S. Cooper, MD, Pres.

**Fnded:** 1916. **Mem:** 774. **Desc:** Professional society promoting the study of cancer in all its aspects, including the scientific study of the treatment of cancer patients. Encourages liaison among medical specialists and allied scientists concerned with cancer treatment. **Pub:** *American Radium Society–Membership Directory*, annual. Directory. *Price:* Included in membership dues.

## ★ 10107 ★ American Sickle Cell Anemia Association
10300 Carnegie Ave.
Cleveland Clinic/East Office Bldg. (EEb18)
Cleveland, OH 44106
**Phone:** (216)229-8600          **Fax:** (216)229-4500
**Email:** irabragg@ascaa.org
**Website:** http://ascaa.org
Ira Bragg-Grant, Exec. Dir.

**Fnded:** 1971. **Desc:** Ensures the availability and accessibility of quality, comprehensive sickle cell services. Provides quality and quantity counseling, education, testing services, and promotes public professional awareness about sickle cell anemia and its hemoglobin diseases and trait variants. **Frmly:** (2001) American Sickle Cell Society; (2002) American Sickle Cell Anemia Society.

## ★ 10108 ★ American Society for Blood and Marrow Transplantation (ASBMT)
85 W Algonquin Rd., Ste. 550
Arlington Heights, IL 60005
**Phone:** (847)427-0224          **Fax:** (847)427-9656
**Email:** mail@asbmt.org
**Website:** http://www.asbmt.org
Alan K. Leahigh, Exec. Dir.

**Fnded:** 1993. **Mem:** 1,000. **Desc:** Individuals, organizations, and corporations with an interest in blood and marrow transplantation. Seeks to advance blood and marrow transplantation techniques; promotes professional advancement of physicians and support personnel engaged in blood and marrow transplantations. Facilitates exchange of information among members; serves as a clearinghouse on blood and marrow transplantation; sponsors educational programs. **Pub:** *ASBMT News*, quarterly. Newsletter. • *Biology of Blood and Marrow Transplantation*, monthly. Journal. • *Blood and Marrow Transplantation Reviews*, quarterly. Bulletin.

## ★ 10109 ★ American Society of Clinical Oncology (ASCO)
1900 Duke St., Ste. 200
Alexandria, VA 22314
**Phone:** (703)299-0150          **Fax:** (703)299-1044
**Email:** asco@asco.org
**Website:** http://www.asco.org
Charles M. Balch, Exec. VP/CEO

**Fnded:** 1964. **Mem:** 15,400. **Desc:** Physicians who treat people with cancer. Sets the standard for patient care worldwide, and leads the fight for more effective cancer treatments, increased funding for clinical and translational research. **Pub:** *ASCO News*, quarterly. Newsletter. • *Journal of Clinical Oncology*, monthly. Journal. • Directory, annual. • Proceedings, annual.

## ★ 10110 ★ American Society of Hematology (ASH)
1900 M St., NW, Ste. 200
Washington, DC 20036
**Phone:** (202)776-0544          **Fax:** (202)776-0545
**Email:** ash@hematology.org
**Website:** http://www.hematology.org
Martha Liggett, Exec. Dir.

**Fnded:** 1958. **Mem:** 9,500. **Desc:** Hematologists (specialists in the study of blood) and other persons holding doctorate degrees with an interest in the field. Promotes exchange of information and ideas related to blood and blood-forming tissues and investigation of hematologic problems. Offers educational programs. **Pub:** *ASH News*, 3/year. Newsletter. • *Blood*, bimonthly. Journal. • *Meeting Program*, annual.

## American Society of Pediatric Hematology/Oncology (ASPHO)
*See:* Entry 5614

## American Society of Preventive Oncology (ASPO)
*See:* Entry 17795

## American Society for Therapeutic Radiology and Oncology (ASTRO)
*See:* Entry 18119

## ★ 10111 ★ Aplastic Anemia and MDS International Foundation (AAFA)
PO Box 613
Annapolis, MD 21404-0613
**Phone:** 800-747-2820          **Fax:** (410)867-0240
**Email:** help@aamds.org
**Website:** http://www.aplastic.org
Marilyn Baker, Exec. Dir.

**Fnded:** 1983. **Mem:** 15,000. **Desc:** Serves as an information source for persons with aplastic anemia and myelodysplastic syndromes. (Aplastic anemia is an often fatal disease in which the bone marrow fails to produce new blood cells.) Provides free educational materials and medical information. Financially supports research. Hosts annual International Patient Conferences presenting the latest in medical research findings and networking opportunities for patients and their families. **Pub:** *Aplastic Anemia and MDS International Foundation*, quarterly. Newsletter. Provides information on aplastic and other bone marrow failure dise s. *Price:* Free. • *Aplastic Anemia: MDS Basic Explanations*, periodic. Describes the course of the disease and current treatment options. Includes glossary of medical terms. *Price:* Free. • *Communicating Patient and Family Needs to the Medical Care Team.* • *Families Coping with Hospital Life*, periodic. • Booklets. • Brochures. • Newsletter, quarterly. **Frmly:** (1999) Aplastic Anemia Foundation of America.

## ★ 10112 ★ Aplastic Anemia and Myeldysphasia Association of Canada (AAAC)
22 Aikenhead Rd.
Etobicoke, ON, Canada M9R 2Z3
**Phone:** (416)235-0468          **Fax:** (416)235-1756

**Website:** http://www.aplastic.ualberta.ca
**Fnded:** 1987. **Mem:** 600. **Reg. Groups:** 4. **State Groups:** 3. **Lang(s):** English, French. **Desc:** Individuals with aplastic anemia or myelodysplasia; health care professionals, family members of people with aplastic anemia or myelodysplasia, and others with an interest in this condition. Promotes research into the cause, treatment, and cure of aplastic anemia and myelodysplasia. Conducts charitable and educational programs. **Pub:** Newsletter, periodic. **Frmly:** (1999) Aplastic Anemia of Canada.

★ **10113** ★ **Argentine Society of Hematology (SAH) (Sociedad Argentina de Hematologia)**
Av Angel Gallardo 899
1405 Buenos Aires, Argentina
**Fnded:** 1948.

★ **10114** ★ **The Arlin J. Brown Information Center (TAJBIC)**
PO Box 191
Stafford, VA 22555-0191
**Phone:** (540)752-9511        **Fax:** (540)752-4324
Arlin J. Brown, Dir. & Pres.
**Fnded:** 1963. **Mem:** 215. **Desc:** Cancer patients, holistic health practitioners, and other interested individuals. Works to educate the public about nontoxic, holistic therapies for cancer and other diseases via advertising and printed material. Offers phone consultation. **Pub:** *Comprehensive Cancer Therapy.* Monograph. • *Health Victory Bulletin*, monthly. Bulletin. Includes updates on alternative cancer treatments and other holistic health information. *Price:* $25. • *March of Truth on Cancer.*

★ **10115** ★ **Asian Clinical Oncology Society (ACOS)**
Churchill Communications Japan
Churchill Bldg.
2-8-16 Yutenji
Meguro-ku
Tokyo 153, Japan
**Phone:** 81 3 57210632        **Fax:** 81 3 57210415
**Lang(s):** English, Japanese. **Desc:** Oncologists and other health care professionals with an interest in clinical oncology. Seeks to advance the study, teaching, and practice of clinical oncology. Serves as a forum for the exchange of information among members; sponsors research and educational programs.

★ **10116** ★ **Asian and Pacific Federation of Organizations for Cancer Research and Control (APFOCRC)**
Seoul National University Hospital
28 Yunkun-dong
Conggno-ku
Seoul 110-744, Republic of Korea
**Phone:** 82 2 7602314        **Fax:** 82 2 7448307
**Lang(s):** English, Korean. **Desc:** Cancer researchers and research institutions; organizations providing care to people with cancer. Seeks to discover more effective methods for the treatment and eventual cure of cancer; works to improve the quality of life of people with cancer. Serves as a clearinghouse on cancer and cancer research; facilitates exchange of information among cancer researchers; provides support and services to people with cancer.

★ **10117** ★ **Asociacion Nacional Contra el Cancer (ANCEC)**
Apdo 7358, Zona 5
Ciudad de Panama
Panama City, Panama
**Phone:** 507 2252512        **Fax:** 507 2255366
**Website:** http://www.panamatravel.com/ancec.htm
**Fnded:** 1970. **Mem:** 150. **Nat'l Groups:** 1. **Reg. Groups:** 21. **State Groups:** 9. **Lang(s):** Spanish. **Desc:** Works to educate Panamanian people on prevention and detection of cancer. Informs women on prevention, self-testing, and importance of regular gynecological examinations. Maintains clinics offering mammograms, Pap smears, and prostate examinations. **Pub:** *Revista ANCEC*, biennial. Magazine. Contains articles on cancer, ongoing activities, and projects.

★ **10118** ★ **Association of American Cancer Institutes (AACI)**
c/o Dr. Edwin A. Mirand
200 Lathrop St.
Iroquois Bldg., No. 305
Pittsburgh, PA 15213
**Phone:** (412)647-2076        **Fax:** (412)647-3659
**Website:** http://www.roswellpark.org
Barbara Duffy Stewart, Exec. Dir.
**Fnded:** 1959. **Mem:** 85. **Desc:** Directors of cancer centers. Informs members of important legislative and program developments in the field. Promotes discussion among cancer center leadership throughout the world; fosters collaboration between members on research, education, and service programs; works to further educational and training opportunities in related biomedical sciences; advises federal, state, and local governments, and private and civic organizations concerning cancer research and related health topics. **Pub:** *AACI Newsletter*, periodic. Newsletter. *Price:* Free. **Frmly:** (1968) Association of Cancer Institute Directors.

★ **10119** ★ **Association of Community Cancer Centers (ACCC)**
11600 Nebel St., Ste. 201
Rockville, MD 20852
**Phone:** (301)984-9496        **Fax:** (301)770-1949
**Website:** http://www.accc-cancer.org
Edward L. Braud, MD, Pres.
**Fnded:** 1974. **Mem:** 6,000. **State Groups:** 17. **Desc:** Institutions (650) and 17 state oncology societies involved in the provision of community cancer care. Fosters communication among providers of community cancer care; seeks to improve the quality of care available to cancer patients in community settings; encourages clinical research utilizing the community as a setting. **Pub:** *Community Cancer Programs in the U.S.*, annual. Reference guide to freestanding and hospital-based cancer programs. *Price:* $50 non-profit organizations; $150 others. • *Compendia-Based Drug Bulletin*, quarterly. Bulletin. • *Critical Pathways*, periodic. • *Oncology Issues*, bimonthly. Journal. Provides information on community cancer programs for association members, who are physicians, nurses, social workers, and other health professionals. *Price:* $40/year. • *Standards for Cancer Programs*, periodic.

★ **10120** ★ **Association of European Cancer Leagues (AECL)**
c/o Cancer Society of Finland
Liisankatu 21B
SF-00170 Helsinki, Finland
**Phone:** 358 9 13533238        **Fax:** 358 9 1351093
**Email:** mervi.perkinen@cancer.fi
**Website:** http://ecl.uicc.org/
**Lang(s):** English, Irish Gaelic. **Desc:** National cancer societies. Promotes advancement in the prevention, diagnosis, and treatment of cancer; seeks to improve the quality of life of people with cancer and their families. Facilitates communication and cooperation among members; sponsors research and educational programs; provides support and services to people with cancer.

**Association of Freestanding Radiation Oncology Centers (AFROC)**
*See:* Entry 18124

★ **10121** ★ **Association for International Cancer Research (AICR)**
Madras House
South St.
North Haugh
Saint Andrews KY16 9EH, United Kingdom
**Phone:** 44 1334 477910        **Fax:** 44 1334 478667
**Email:** info@AFROC.org
**Website:** http://www.aicr.org.uk/
**Fnded:** 1979. **Mem:** 14. **Desc:** Funds cancer research. Disseminates research results. **Pub:** *Progress*, 3/year.

★ **10122** ★ **Association of Nordic Cancer Registries (ANCR)**
c/o Norwegian Cancer Registry
Montebello
N-0310 Oslo, Norway
**Phone:** 47 22451300        **Fax:** 47 22451370
**Lang(s):** English, Norwegian. **Desc:** National cancer registries. Promotes availability of data on cancer patients; seeks to advance the prevention, diagnosis, and treatment of cancer. Serves as a clearinghouse on cancer and its treatment; sponsors health screenings and other services; conducts research.

**Association of Pediatric Oncology Nurses (APON)**
*See:* Entry 5628

**Association of Pediatric Oncology Social Workers (APOSW)**
*See:* Entry 19077

**Association for Research of Childhood Cancer (AROCC)**
*See:* Entry 5630

**Association of Residents in Radiation Oncology (ARRO)**
*See:* Entry 18126

★ **10123** ★ **Australasian Lymphology Association**
Reul-Hirche
Physiotherapist Department
Royal Brisbane Hospital
Herston, QLD 4029, Australia
**Email:** arro@astro.org
**Website:** http://www.arro.org/

★ **10124** ★ **Australian Cancer Society**
500 George St
Sydney, NSW 2000, Australia
**Fnded:** 1999.

★ **10125** ★ **Barbados Cancer Society (BCS)**
Lefferts Pl.
River Rd.
Saint Michael, Barbados
**Phone:** (246)436-8888        **Fax:** (246)429-3227
**Email:** info@barbacan.com
**Fnded:** 1980. **Mem:** 2,500. **Local Groups:** 1. **Lang(s):** English. **Desc:** Doctors, nurses, social workers, and other concerned individuals. Researches cancer prevention methods and treatment strategies for cancer patients. Assists in coordinating efforts to reduce Barbadian mortality from cancer. Provides occupational therapy, transportation, and early detection services. Encourages efforts to educate the public in the problems, symptoms, and treatment of cancer; disseminates information. Aids in establishing and furthering cancer research activities. Sponsors researchers to attend international conferences and training sessions. Visits schools and distributes literature; offers financial assistance to children who have lost a parent to cancer. Maintains speakers' bureau. Works in cooperation with the American Cancer Society. **Pub:** *Newsletter*, 3/year. Newsletter.

### ★ 10126 ★ Brain Tumor Foundation of Canada (BTFC)
**(La Fondation Canadienne des tumeurs cerebrales)**
650 Waterloo St., Ste. 100
London, ON, Canada N6B 2R4
**Phone:** (519)642-7755     **Free:** 800-265-5106
**Fax:** (519)642-7192
**Email:** btfc@btfc.org
**Website:** http://www.btfc.org/

**Fnded:** 1982. **Desc:** Provides support services to those affected by brain tumors; promotes public awareness, education and funding. **Pub:** Handbooks.

### The Brain Tumor Society (TBTS)
*See:* Entry 13957

### ★ 10127 ★ Breast Cancer Action (BCA)
55 New Montgomery St., Ste. 323
San Francisco, CA 94105
**Phone:** (415)243-9301     **Free:** 877-278-6722
**Fax:** (415)243-3996
**Email:** info@bcaction.org
**Website:** http://www.ccac-art.edu
Barbara Brenner, Exec. Dir.

**Fnded:** 1990. **Mem:** 8,500. **Nat'l Groups:** 1. **Reg. Groups:** 1. **Desc:** Women living with breast cancer. Seeks to carry "the voices of people affected by breast cancer to inspire and compel the changes necessary to end the breast cancer epidemic." Monitors and publicizes developments in breast cancer detection and treatment; sponsors lobbying programs; advocates for increased access to breast cancer screening and treatment services; facilitates environmental protection initiatives; works to ensure accurate reporting of breast cancer issues in public media. **Pub:** *Breast Cancer Action Newsletter*, bimonthly. Newsletter. Information on developments in treatment, research, detection and politics of breast-cancer. *Price:* $35 per year.

### ★ 10128 ★ Breast Cancer Care
Kiln House
210 New Kings Rd.
London SW6 4NZ, United Kingdom
**Phone:** 44 207 3842984     **Fax:** 44 207 3843387
**Email:** bcc@breastcancercare.org.uk
**Website:** http://www.breastcancercare.org.uk

**Fnded:** 1973. **Reg. Groups:** 2. **Lang(s):** English. **Desc:** Provides information and support to those affected by breast cancer. Operates advice line, one-to-one volunteer support, and aftercare services, including prosthesis fitting. **Pub:** Books. • Newsletter, quarterly. • Pamphlets. Contains information on breast cancer awareness and breast cancer treatments. **Frmly:** (1993) Breast Care and Masectomy Association.

### ★ 10129 ★ Breast Cancer Society
401 St. Clair St.
Point Edward, ON, Canada N7V 1P2
**Free:** 800-567-8767
**Email:** bcsc@bcsc.ca
**Website:** http://www.bcsc.ca/

**Fnded:** 1991. **Desc:** Private charity dedicated to funding breast cancer research to improve the detection, prevention, and treatment, and ultimately a cure for the disease. Sponsors golf tournaments, fashions shows, and other fundraising events, as well as the sale of pins to show support.

### ★ 10130 ★ Breast Cancer Support Service - Northern Ireland
c/o Ulster Cancer Foundation
40 Eglantine Ave.
Belfast BT9 6DX, United Kingdom
**Phone:** 44 2890 663281     **Fax:** 44 2890 660081
**Email:** ulstercancer@btconnect.com
**Website:** http://www.ulstercancer.co.uk

**Fnded:** 1974. **Reg. Groups:** 13. **Local Groups:** 18. **Desc:** Promotes awareness of breast care and early

detection of breast cancer. Supports the rehabilitation of women who have breast cancer and breast surgery. **Pub:** *Coping with Breast Cancer*. Booklet. **Frmly:** Breast Care and Mastectomy Support Service.

### ★ 10131 ★ British Association for Cancer Research (BACR)
Institute of Cancer Research
15 Cotswold Rd.
Sutton SM2 5NG, United Kingdom
**Phone:** 44 208 7224208     **Fax:** 44 208 7701395
**Email:** bacr@icr.ac.uk
**Website:** http://www.icr.ac.uk/bacr/Home.htm

**Fnded:** 1960. **Mem:** 1,300. **Lang(s):** English. **Desc:** Laboratory and clinical cancer research workers. Conducts and promotes research into the prevention, causes, treatment, and cure of cancer. **Pub:** *British Journal of Cancer*, monthly. Journal.

### ★ 10132 ★ British Society for Haematology
2 Carlton House Terr.
London SW1Y 5AF, United Kingdom
**Phone:** 44 208 6437305     **Fax:** 44 208 7700933
**Email:** janice@bshhya.demon.co.uk
**Website:** http://www.blackwell-science.com/uk/society/bsh/default.htm

**Fnded:** 1960. **Mem:** 1,079. **Lang(s):** English. **Desc:** Medical practitioners specialising in haematology; scientific graduates who are active in haematology research; MLSOs grade 3 and above who have worked in the specialty for at least 3 years and have shown evidence of research. To advance the practice and study of haematology, promote good haematological practice and facilitate contact between persons interested in haematology. **Pub:** *British Journal of Haematology*, 16/year. Journal. • *BSH Bulletins*, quarterly. Bulletins.

### Canadian Association of Pharmacy in Oncology (CAPhO)
*See:* Entry 17523

### ★ 10133 ★ Canadian Association of Psychological Oncology
**(Association Canadienne d'Oncologie Psychosociale)**
c/o St. Boniface Hospital
409 Tache Ave.
Winnipeg, MB, Canada R2H 2A6
**Phone:** (204)235-3141     **Fax:** (204)237-6048
**Email:** viola.giesbrecht@cancercare.mb.ca
**Website:** http://capho.ca

**Lang(s):** English, French. **Desc:** Oncologists and psychologists with an interest in oncology. Promotes improved care of oncology patients through interdisciplinary use of oncological and psychological treatment strategies. Sponsors research and educational programs.

### ★ 10134 ★ Canadian Association of Radiation Oncologists (CARO)
600 W 10th Ave.
Vancouver, BC, Canada V5Z 4E6
**Phone:** (604)877-6193     **Fax:** (604)877-0505
**Email:** sbroadbe@caro-acro.ca
**Website:** http://www.caro-acro.ca

**Fnded:** 1986. **Mem:** 300. **Lang(s):** English, French. **Desc:** Radiation oncologists and oncology residents and fellows. Promotes advancement of the science and practice of radiation oncology. Seeks to facilitate professional advancement of members. Conducts continuing professional education programs.

### ★ 10135 ★ Canadian Breast Cancer Foundation
790 Bay St., Ste. 1000
Toronto, ON, Canada M5G 1N8
**Phone:** (416)596-6773     **Free:** 800-387-9816
**Fax:** (416)596-7857

**Email:** cseidman@cbcf.org
**Website:** http://www.cbcf.org

**Fnded:** 1986. **Reg. Groups:** 4. **Lang(s):** English. **Desc:** Health care professionals, women with breast cancer, their families, and others interested in breast cancer issues. Promotes the advancement of breast cancer research, education, diagnosis and treatment through various programs and fundraising events.

### ★ 10136 ★ Canadian Cancer Society (CCS)
10 Alcorn Ave., Ste. 200
Toronto, ON, Canada M4V 3B1
**Phone:** (416)961-7223     **Fax:** (416)961-4189
**Email:** ccs@cancer.ca
**Website:** http://www.cancer.ca

**Fnded:** 1938. **Lang(s):** English, French. **Desc:** Community-based volunteers. Promotes research into the causes, detection, and cure of cancer; seeks to improve the quality of life of people with cancer. Conducts fundraising activities benefitting cancer research; sponsors volunteer training programs; makes available educational courses. **Pub:** *Progress Against Cancer*, 3/year. Magazine.

### ★ 10137 ★ Canadian Hematology Society (CHS)
**(Societe Canadienne d'Hematologie — SCH)**
199-435 St. Laurent Blvd.
Ottawa, ON, Canada K1K 2Z8
**Phone:** (613)748-9613     **Fax:** (613)748-6392
**Email:** cag@magi.com

**Lang(s):** English, French. **Desc:** Hematologists and other scientists and health care professionals with an interest in hematology. Seeks to advance the study, teaching, and practice of hematology. Serves as a forum for the exchange of information among members; conducts continuing professional education courses. **Pub:** *Canadian Hematology Society*, 3/year. Newsletter.

### ★ 10138 ★ Canadian Hemophilia Society (CHS)
**(Societe Canadienne de l'Hemophilie — SCH)**
625 President Kennedy Ave., Ste. 1210
Montreal, QC, Canada H3A 1K2
**Phone:** (514)848-0503     **Free:** 800-668-2686
**Fax:** (514)848-9661
**Email:** chs@hemophilia.ca
**Website:** http://www.hemophilia.ca

**Fnded:** 1953. **Mem:** 2,500. **Nat'l Groups:** 1. **Reg. Groups:** 5. **State Groups:** 10. **Lang(s):** English, French. **Desc:** People with hemophilia and their families; health care professionals with an interest in hematological disorders. Seeks to advance the diagnosis and treatment of hemophilia; promotes improvement in the quality of life of people with hemophilia. Provides support and services to people with hemophilia and their families; conducts educational programs. **Pub:** *Hemophilia Today*, quarterly. Newsletter.

### ★ 10139 ★ Canadian Oncology Society (COS)
**(Societe d'Oncologie du Canada — SOC)**
82-84 Barrie St.
Kingston, ON, Canada K7L 3N6
**Phone:** (613)533-6000     **Fax:** (613)533-2941
**Email:** bvandersluis@ctg.queensu.ca
**Website:** http://www.cos.ca

**Lang(s):** English, French. **Desc:** Oncologists and other health care professionals with an interest in oncology. Seeks to advance the study and practice of oncology. Serves as a clearinghouse on oncology; sponsors research and educational programs.

★ 10140 ★ **Canadian Sickle Cell Society (CSCS)**
**(La Societe de l'Anemie Falciforme du Canada — SAFC)**
6999 Cote-Des-Neiges Rd., Ste. 33
Montreal, QC, Canada H3S 2B8
**Phone:** (514)735-5109          **Fax:** (514)735-5100
**Email:** cslaf@total.net
**Lang(s):** English, French. **Desc:** People with sickle cell anemia and their families; health care professionals with an interest in sickle cell anemia. Seeks to improve the quality of life of people with sickle cell anemia; promotes advancement in the prevention and treatment of the disease. Provides support and assistance to people with sickle cell anemia and their families; sponsors research and educational programs.

★ 10141 ★ **Cancer Biotherapy Research Group**
PO Box 680757
Franklin, TN 37068-0757
**Phone:** (615)791-6393          **Fax:** (615)791-4719
**Email:** cbrg_cancer@compuserve.com
Carol DePriest, Exec. Dir.
**Fnded:** 1987. **Mem:** 100. **Desc:** Practicing oncologists, cancer management professionals, hospitals, and biopharmaceutical companies interested in using biologicals alone and with other agents in the treatment of all types of cancer. Promotes and sponsors research into biotherapy and other innovative cell biology technologies such as tumor-infiltrating lymphocytes, autologous vaccines and activated lymphocytes, pulsed LAK cells, and peripheral and bone marrow stem cells. Conducts cancer trials, and studies; provides networking opportunities. Publishes research results. **Frmly:** (1997) National Biotherapy Study Group.

★ 10142 ★ **Cancer Care (CC)**
275 7th Ave.
New York, NY 10001-6708
**Phone:** (212)712-8400          **Free:** 800-813-4673
**Fax:** (212)719-0263
**Email:** info@cancercare.org
**Website:** http://www.cancercare.org/
Diane Blum, Exec. Dir.
**Fnded:** 1944. **Mem:** 80,000. **Local Groups:** 38. **Desc:** The oldest and largest national non-profit agency dedicated to providing emotional support, information and practical help to people with cancer, and their loved ones. Has assisted over two million people nationwide through telephone counseling, referral services, teleconference programs, office-based services, and via the internet. All services are provided free of charge and are available to people of all ages, with all types of cancer, at any stage of the disease. All services, including cancer awareness initiatives, extend also to family members, caregivers and professionals. **Pub:** *Cancer Care*. Annual Report. *Price:* Free. • *Currents*, quarterly. Newsletter. • Also publishes symposia proceedings, social research studies, professional papers, and brochures; distributes films and videotapes. **Frmly:** (1986) National Cancer Foundation; (1991) National Cancer Care Foundation.

★ 10143 ★ **Cancer Control Society (CCS)**
2043 N Berendo St.
Los Angeles, CA 90027
**Phone:** (323)663-7801
**Website:** http://www.cancercontrolsociety.com
Norman Fritz, Pres.
**Fnded:** 1973. **Mem:** 5,500. **Desc:** Cancer patients, doctors, and interested individuals. Educates the public on the prevention and control of cancer and other diseases through nutrition, tests, and nontoxic alternative therapies, such as Laetrile, Gerson, Hoxsey, Koch, Enzymes, Wheat Grass, Immunology, Mega-Vitamins and Minerals, Detoxification and Nutrition, and DMSO and Chelation Therapy. Provides information through a 12-hour telephone hot line, direct mail, doctor and patient lists, speakers, films, cancer clinic tours, and Cancer Book House. **Pub:** *Cancer Book House List*, biennial. • *Cancer Control Journal*, periodic. Journal. Reports on one specific cancer-related topic in each issue. *Price:* Included in membership dues. • *Doctor and Clinic Directory*, 6/year. Directory. • *Patient Directory*, 6/year. Directory.

★ 10144 ★ **Cancer Federation (CFI)**
PO Box 1298
Banning, CA 92220-0009
**Phone:** (909)849-4325          **Free:** 800-207-2873
**Fax:** (909)849-0156
**Email:** cancerfederation@yahoo.com
**Website:** http://www.cancerfed.com
Karen Alene, Admin.
**Fnded:** 1977. **Mem:** 1,500. **Desc:** Physicians, scientists, nurses, and laymen (both cancer patients and nonpatients). Promotes research and education in the field of cancer immunology. Seeks to discover appropriate cancer therapies using natural biological modifiers. Funds research at major centers throughout the U.S., including the University of California (Riverside and Santa Barbara), University of Hawaii, and University of Pittsburgh, on biological modifiers, such as lymphokines; killer cells; Interleukin I and II; diet; and psychological aspects of cancer. Compiles statistics; conducts research and education in cancer therapy, including vaccines, and in psychological programming for patients. Offers counseling program for cancer patients and their families. Sponsors public medical conferences and in-service courses for nurses on the psychology of cancer, and research projects at many universities and hospitals in the field of immunology. Sponsors charitable program. **Pub:** *Challenge of the Cancer Federation*, quarterly. Newsletter. Provides general information on cancer research and treatments. Contains information on federation activities and book reviews. *Price:* Included in membership dues. • Audiotapes. • Booklets. • Books. • Monographs. • Videos.

★ 10145 ★ **Cancer Information Service (CIS)**
NCI/NIH, Bldg. 31, 10A03
31 Center Dr., MSC2580
Bethesda, MD 20892-2580
**Free:** 800-4-CANCER          **Fax:** (301)402-0555
**Website:** http://cis.nci.nih.gov/
Chris Thomsen, Chief
**Fnded:** 1975. **Reg. Groups:** 19. **Desc:** Funded by the National Cancer Institute. Trained counselors provide information about cancer causes, prevention, detection, diagnosis, rehabilitation, and research. Provides technical assistance to state and regional organizations conducting cancer education activities.

★ 10146 ★ **Cancer Registry of Norway**
Montebello
N-0310 Oslo, Norway
**Phone:** 47 22451300          **Fax:** 47 22451370
**Email:** kreftregisteret@kreftreg.no
**Website:** http://www.kreftregisteret.no
**Lang(s):** English, Norwegian. **Desc:** National cancer registries. Promotes availability of data on cancer patients; seeks to advance the prevention, diagnosis, and treatment of cancer. Serves as a clearinghouse on cancer and its treatment; sponsors health screenings and other services; conducts research. **Frmly:** (1999) Norweigan Cancer Registry.

★ 10147 ★ **Cancer Research Foundation of America**
1600 Duke St., Ste. 110
Alexandria, VA 22314
**Phone:** (703)836-4412          **Free:** 800-227-2732
**Fax:** (703)836-4413
**Website:** http://www.preventcancer.org
**Fnded:** 1985. **Desc:** Foundations, individuals and companies. Aims to prevent cancer through research and education. Sponsors grants and fellowships, publishes educational materials.

**Cancer Research Society (CRS)**
**(Societe de Recherche sur le Cancer — SRC)**
*See:* Entry 12078

**Candlelighters Childhood Cancer Foundation (CCCF)**
*See:* Entry 5648

★ 10148 ★ **Childhood Cancer Foundation - Candlelighters Canada**
55 Eglinton Ave. E, Ste. 401
Toronto, ON, Canada M4P 1G8
**Phone:** (416)489-6440          **Fax:** (416)489-9812
**Email:** staff@candlelighters.ca
**Website:** http://www.candlelighters.ca
**Fnded:** 1987. **Local Groups:** 50. **Lang(s):** English, French. **Desc:** Volunteers. Seeks to improve the quality of life of children with cancer and their families. Provides assistance to children with cancer and their families; maintains support groups; sponsors educational and recreational programs. **Pub:** *Contact*, every 6 months. Newsletter.

**Children's Blood Foundation (CBF)**
*See:* Entry 5656

★ 10149 ★ **Children's Brain Tumor Foundation (CBTF)**
274 Madison Ave., No. 1301
New York, NY 10016
**Phone:** (212)448-9494          **Free:** (866)CBT-HOPE
**Fax:** (212)448-1022
**Email:** info@cbtf.org
**Website:** http://www.cbtf.org
Judy Hurley, Exec. Dir.
**Fnded:** 1988. **Desc:** Works to improve the outlook for children with brain and spinal cord tumors. Raises funds for research; provides counseling, education and support services for families and survivors. **Pub:** *A Resource Guide for Parents of Children with Brain and Spinal Cord Tumors.* Booklet. Contains technical and practical information for parents. *Price:* Free. • *The Challenge.* Newsletter.

★ 10150 ★ **Children's Leukemia Research Association (NLA)**
585 Stewart Ave., Ste. LL18
Garden City, NY 11530
**Phone:** (516)222-1944          **Fax:** (516)222-0457
**Email:** clra@erols.com
**Website:** http://www.childrensleukemia.org/
Allan D. Weinberg, Exec. Dir.
**Fnded:** 1965. **Desc:** Promotes leukemia research and public awareness of the disease. Provides financial aid to leukemia patients and their families, based on need. **Frmly:** (1994) National Leukemia Association.

★ 10151 ★ **China Anticancer Association (CACA)**
52 Fucheng Rd.
Beijing 100036, People's Republic of China
**Phone:** 86 22 3359958          **Fax:** 86 22 23526512
**Email:** xuzhigang@caca.or.cn
**Website:** http://www.caca.org.cn
**Fnded:** 1985. **Mem:** 20,000. **Nat'l Groups:** 1. **Reg. Groups:** 3. **State Groups:** 26. **Local Groups:** 33. **Lang(s):** Chinese, English. **Desc:** Physicians, researchers, and interested individuals in the People's Republic of China. Conducts research programs concentrating on the prevention of cancer. Sponsors research exchange with cancer experts in other countries. Maintains 23 academic commissions. Offers educational programs; disseminates information to the public about cancer prevention. Organizes academic conferences and symposia. **Pub:** *Cancer Research on Prevention and Treatment*, quarterly. Journal. • *Chinese Journal for Cancer Research*, quarterly. Journal. • *Chinese Journal of Clinical Oncology*, monthly. Journal. Includes English abstracts.

## ★ 10152 ★ Colombian Institute of Pediatric Oncology
**(Instituto Colombiano de Oncologia Pediatrica)**
Calle 120, No 8-23
Santa Fe de Bogota, Colombia
**Phone:** 57 1 2133067
**Fnded:** 1982.

## ★ 10153 ★ Cooleycare
Centro Trasfusionale e di Immunologia dei Trapianti
Ospedale Policlinico
Via Francesco Sforza 35
I-20122 Milan, Italy
**Phone:** 39 2 55034012      **Fax:** 39 2 5458129
**Email:** info@ctit.org
**Website:** http://www.ctit.org
**Fnded:** 1984. **Mem:** 36. **Lang(s):** English. **Desc:** Hematologists and specialists dealing with thalassemia-related problems. (Thalassemia, also known as Cooley's Anemia, is a dysfunction of the red blood cells that occurs in individuals of Mediterranean descent.) Promotes regular studies on thalassemia; provides children's services. Offers professional training. **Pub:** *Meeting Proceedings*, biennial. Proceedings. • *Thalassemia Today*, periodic. Journal.

## ★ 10154 ★ Cooley's Anemia Foundation (CAF)
129-09 26th Ave., No. 203
Flushing, NY 11354
**Phone:** (718)321-2873      **Free:** 800-522-7222
**Fax:** (718)321-3340
**Email:** info@cooleysanemia.org
**Website:** http://www.thalassemia.org
Jayne Restivo, Exec. Dir.
**Fnded:** 1954. **Mem:** 8,000. **Nat'l Groups:** 16. **State Groups:** 4. **Local Groups:** 6. **Desc:** Parents of children afflicted with Cooley's anemia; doctors, technicians, nurses, and others interested in the treatment and eventual cure of the disease. (Cooley's anemia is an incurable blood disease requiring frequent blood transfusions to keep its victims alive; it is named after Dr. Thomas B. Cooley, a Detroit, MI, physician who first described it in 1925.) Distributes therapy materials including infusion pumps and batteries, at no charge, to victims of the disease. Presents awards for scientific and humanitarian achievement. Sponsors medical symposia to educate physicians and scientists about new drugs or therapies for Cooley's anemia or other thalassemias. Sponsors Thalassemia Action Group, a networking task force of young adult victims of thalassemia. Operates speakers' bureau. Conducts blood drives. **Pub:** *Lifeline*, quarterly. Newsletter. • Also publishes 'What It Means to be a Carrier' and 'What Is Cooley's Anemia. **Frmly:** (1977) Cooley's Anemia Blood and Research Foundation for Children.

## ★ 10155 ★ Cord Blood Donor Foundation (CBDF)
1200 Bayhill Dr., Ste. 301
San Bruno, CA 94066
**Phone:** (650)635-1452      **Fax:** (650)635-1428
**Email:** information@cordblooddonor.org
**Website:** http://www.cordblooddonor.org
**Desc:** Promotes education awareness and further research in the use of cord blood stem cells. Cord blood is blood that remains in the umbilical cord and placenta following birth. Cord blood stem cells are used to treat life-threatening diseases including leukemia, other cancers and blood and immune disorders.

## ★ 10156 ★ Corporate Angel Network (CAN)
Westchester County Airport
One Loop Rd.
White Plains, NY 10604
**Phone:** (914)328-1313      **Fax:** (914)328-4201
**Email:** info@corpangelnetwork.org
**Website:** http://www.CorpAngelNetwork.org
Thomas J. Robertazzi, Exec. Dir.
**Fnded:** 1981. **Mem:** 500. **Desc:** Arranges free air transportation for cancer patients traveling to and from recognized cancer treatment centers, using empty seats on corporate aircraft. All ambulatory cancer patients and bone marrow donors not needing on-board care are eligible. **Pub:** *FlightLines*, quarterly. Newsletter.

## ★ 10157 ★ Damon Runyon Cancer Research Foundation
675 3rd Ave., 25 Fl.
New York, NY 10017
**Phone:** (212)697-9100      **Free:** 800-445-2494
**Fax:** (212)697-4050
**Email:** crfinfo@drcrf.org
**Website:** http://www.drcrf.org
Lorraine W. Egan, Exec. Dir.
**Fnded:** 1946. **Desc:** Nonprofit organization dedicated to advancing cancer research through the funding of initial postdoctoral fellowships and junior faculty awards nationwide. Monies are raised through the Fund's Broadway Tickets theater service and the solicitation of individuals, foundations and corporations. **Pub:** Annual Report, annual. • Brochures. • Newsletter, 3/year. **Frmly:** Damon Runyon Foundation for Cancer Research; (1973) Damon Runyon Memorial Fund for Cancer Research; (1988) Damon Runyon - Walter Winchell Cancer Fund; (1993) Damon Runyon - Walter Winchell Cancer Research Fund.

## ★ 10158 ★ Dana-Farber Cancer Institute
44 Binney St.
Boston, MA 02115
**Phone:** (617)632-3000
**Email:** dana-farbercontact-us@dfci.harvard.edu
**Website:** http://www.dfci.harvard.edu
**Fnded:** 1947. **Desc:** Physicians and scientists. Disseminates innovative patient therapies and scientific discoveries worldwide to aid the fight against cancer and AIDS. Committed to providing compassionate care and support to both children and adults with cancer, AIDS, and related diseases.

## ★ 10159 ★ Danish Cancer Society
Strandboulevarden 49
DK-2100 Copenhagen, Denmark
**Phone:** 45 35257500      **Fax:** 45 35257701
**Email:** info@cancer.dk
**Website:** http://www.cancer.dk
**Fnded:** 1928. **Mem:** 250,000. **Local Groups:** 260. **Lang(s):** Danish, English. **Desc:** Health care professionals and medical researchers and organizations with an interest in cancer; people with cancer and their families. Seeks to: prevent the development of cancer; improve the recovery rate of people with cancer; and limit the "physical, psychological, and social side-effects of cancer." Establishes "new, vital initiatives in the areas of prevention, research and patient support;" works to persuade public sector agencies to take over operation of these initiatives. Monitors existing treatment systems and makes recommendations for their improvement; provides support and services to people with cancer and their families. Maintains cancer registry.

## ★ 10160 ★ European Association for Cancer Research (EACR)
c/o Paul Sanders, Sec.
University of Nottingham
Cancer Research Laboratories
Nottingham NG7 2RD, United Kingdom
**Phone:** 44 115 9515114    **Fax:** 44 115 9515115
**Email:** paul.saunders@nottingham.ac.uk
**Website:** http://www.eacr.org/
**Fnded:** 1968. **Mem:** 1,500. **Lang(s):** English. **Desc:** Persons who have worked actively in cancer research for at least 2 years and who have an academic degree or the equivalent; membership in 40 countries. Seeks to advance cancer research by facilitating communication among research workers, particularly by organizing meetings. Sponsors: EACR Italian Fellowship Program, providing financial support for researchers to spend from 3 months to 1 year in Italian research institutions; EACR Travel Fellowship Program, awarding travel expenses for member researchers to and from host institutions. **Pub:** *Directory of the EACR*, biennial. Directory. • *EACR Newsletter*, semiannual. Newsletter. • *European Journal of Cancer and Clinical Oncology*, monthly. Journal.

## ★ 10161 ★ European Association for NeuroOncology (EANO)
c/o B. Mueller
Klinik Bavaria
An der Wodlfsschlucht 1-2
D-01731 Kreischa, Germany
**Fax:** 49 35 20662954
**Email:** mueler@eano.de
**Website:** http://www.eano.de
**Fnded:** 1990. **Mem:** 350. **Desc:** Physicians, epidemiologists, biostatisticians, scientists and health professionals worldwide with an interest in any field of neurooncology. Fosters international cooperation in neurooncologic research and clinical training. **Pub:** *Journal of Neuro-Oncology*. Journal. • Newsletter, periodic.

## ★ 10162 ★ European Cancer Prevention Organization (ECP)
c/o M.C. Gueur
rue Martin v, 40 (Bte 5)
B-1200 Brussels, Belgium
**Phone:** 32 2 7790668      **Fax:** 32 2 7790668
**Website:** http://www3.uicc.org/others/ecp/ecp.html
**Fnded:** 1983. **Mem:** 120. **Lang(s):** English. **Desc:** Scientists interested in cancer prevention research. Seeks to coordinate studies in cancer prevention and to inform the scientific community as well as the public. Conducts workshops. **Pub:** *ECP News*, quarterly. • *ECP Symposium Proceedings*, annual. • *European Journal of Cancer Prevention*, bimonthly. Journal.

## European Oncology Nursing Society (EONS)
*See:* Entry 15710

## ★ 10163 ★ European Organization for Research and Treatment of Cancer (EORTC)
**(Organisation Europeenne pour la Recherche et le Traitement du Cancer)**
83, ave. Mounier, bte. 11
B-1200 Brussels, Belgium
**Phone:** 32 2 7741641      **Fax:** 32 2 7723545
**Email:** eortc@eortc.be
**Website:** http://www.eortc.be
**Fnded:** 1962. **Mem:** 2,500. **Reg. Groups:** 36. **Lang(s):** English. **Desc:** Doctors, pharmacologists, clinicians, statisticians, computer analysts, and others in 25 countries involved in the development of anticancer therapies. Aims to develop cancer research in Europe through the coordination of joint research projects by hospitals and laboratories. Maintains screening program of potential anticancer agents and clinical research groups formed to carry out trials with new therapeutic agents. Maintains EORTC New Drug Development Program to coordinate the development of new anticancer medications; operates EORTC Central Office and Data Center to coordinate and conduct cancer clinical trials performed by a network of 2000 doctors in over 300 hospitals in Europe; conducts educational and research programs as well as health, economics, and quality of life studies. Compiles statistics. **Pub:** *EORTC Organisation, Activities and Current Research*, annual. Directory. • *European Journal of Cancer*, monthly. **Frmly:** (1968) Groupe Europeen de Chimiotherapie Anticancereuse.

## European Research Organization of Genital Infection and Neoplasia (EUROGIN)
*See:* Entry 18892

**European Society of Gynaecological Oncology (ESGO)**
*See:* Entry 16673

**★ 10164 ★ European Society for Hyperthermic Oncology (ESHO)**
University Hospital Rotterdam-Daniel
Groene Hilledijk 301
NL-3075 EA Rotterdam, Netherlands
**Phone:** 31 10 4391806      **Fax:** 31 10 4391022
**Email:** rhoon@hyph.azr.nl

**Fnded:** 1987. **Mem:** 150. **Lang(s):** English. **Desc:** Oncologists and medical researchers with an interest in hyperthermic oncology. Promotes advancement in the techniques and technology of hyperthermic oncology. Facilitates "integration and exchange of information between different disciplines in the study of the biological effects of heat in the treatment of cancer." **Pub:** Newsletter, periodic.

**★ 10165 ★ European Society for Medical Oncology (ESMO)**
Annals of Oncology
Via la Santa 7
CH-6962 Lugano Cedex, Switzerland
**Phone:** 33 45 35454090      **Fax:** 33 45 31356906
**Email:** mbjsekfc@rh.dk
**Website:** http://www.esmo.org/

**Fnded:** 1975. **Mem:** 520. **Lang(s):** English. **Desc:** Medical oncologists; associate members are biologists, surgeons, radiotherapists, and other specialists. Sponsors and contributes to education in oncology. **Pub:** *Proceedings of Meeting*, annual. Journal.

**★ 10166 ★ European Society of Surgical Oncology (ESSO)**
Institut Jules Bordet
rue Heger-Bordet 1
B-1000 Brussels, Belgium
**Phone:** 32 2 5373106      **Fax:** 32 2 5390374
**Email:** eursso@skynet.be
**Website:** http://www.esso-surgeonline.be

**Fnded:** 1981. **Mem:** 1,020. **Desc:** Surgical oncologists. Sponsors educational programs. Fosters multidisciplinary collaboration in the clinical management of cancer patients. **Pub:** *European Journal of Surgical Oncology*, monthly. Journal.

**★ 10167 ★ European Society for Therapeutic Radiology and Oncology (ESTRO)**
Av. E Mounier 83
B-1200 Brussels, Belgium
**Phone:** 32 2 7759347      **Fax:** 32 2 7795494
**Email:** info@estro.be
**Website:** http://www.estro.be

**Fnded:** 1980. **Mem:** 5,000. **Lang(s):** English. **Desc:** Individuals from 84 countries involved in the fields of radiotherapy and oncology. Works to improve standards of cancer treatment by fostering the exchange with other specialties involved in the treatment of cancer. Develops educational and training guidelines; makes available basic and continuing medical education courses. **Pub:** *ESTRO Newsletter*, periodic. Newsletter. Society's life. • *Journal of Radiotherapy and Oncology*, monthly. Journal.

**★ 10168 ★ European Working Group for Psychosomatic Cancer Research**
c/o Intern Psychooncology Project
Bergstrasse 10
D-26122 Oldenburg, Germany
**Phone:** 49 441 12147      **Fax:** 49 441 884462
**Fnded:** 1962. **Mem:** 50. **Desc:** Encourages research, cooperation and exchange among scientists by regular symposia.

**★ 10169 ★ Federation of European Cancer Societies (FECS)**
Ave. E Mounier 83
B-1200 Brussels, Belgium
**Phone:** 32 2 7750202      **Fax:** 32 2 7750200
**Email:** info@fecs.be
**Website:** http://www.fecs.be

**Fnded:** 1981. **Lang(s):** English, French. **Desc:** European societies active in the fields of clinical and experimental oncology and oncology nursing. Promotes collaboration among members; seeks to advance the prevention, diagnosis, and treatment of cancer. Encourages international cooperation in oncology research; represents members' interests at the European level. **Pub:** *European Journal of Cancer*, periodic.

**Foundation for Advancement in Cancer Therapy (FACT)**
*See:* Entry 4258

**★ 10170 ★ Foundation for the Children's Oncology Group (NCCF)**
440 E Huntington Dr., Ste. 402
PO Box 60012
Arcadia, CA 91066-6012
**Phone:** (626)447-1674      **Free:** 800-458-6223
**Fax:** (626)447-6359
**Email:** info@conquerkidscancer.org
**Website:** http://www.conquerkidscancer.org

**Desc:** Physician-scientists. Supports a network of childhood cancer treatment and research institutions caring for infants, children, teens and young adults. **Frmly:** (2002) National Childhood Cancer Foundation.

**★ 10171 ★ Friends of the Jose Carreras International Leukemia Foundation**
1100 Fairview Ave. N, D5-100
PO Box 19024
Seattle, WA 98109-1024
**Phone:** (206)667-7108      **Fax:** (206)667-6498
**Email:** friendsjc@carrerasfoundation.org
**Website:** http://www.carrerasfoundation.org
Karen Carbonneau, Admin.

**Fnded:** 1990. **Desc:** Raises funds for fellowship awards focused on research into the treatment and cure of leukemia and related blood disorders. **Pub:** *Friends to Friends*, 3/year. Newsletter. Current news about the Foundation.

**★ 10172 ★ Friends of St. Luke's Hospital**
c/o St. Luke's Hospital
Highfield Rd.
Rathgar
Dublin 6, Ireland
**Phone:** 353 1 4065102      **Fax:** 353 1 4976237
**Email:** foslh@iol.ie
**Website:** http://www.friendsofstlukes.ie

**Fnded:** 1981. **Mem:** 15. **Desc:** Seeks to enhance the care, comfort and management of cancer patients at Dublin's St. Luke's Hospital. Works to ensure that patients benefit to the fullest extent from the advances in techniques and equipment.

**★ 10173 ★ Gilda Radner Familial Ovarian Cancer Registry**
c/o Cathy Fahey
Roswell Park Cancer Institute
Elm & Carlton Sts.
Buffalo, NY 14263-0001
**Phone:** (716)845-4503      **Free:** 800-682-7426
**Fax:** (716)845-8266
**Email:** gradner@roswellpark.org
**Website:** http://www.ovariancancer.com/grwp.html
Cathy Fahey, Mgr.

**Fnded:** 1990. **Desc:** Committed to the identification of new genes associated with familial ovarian cancer, thereby improving genetic and psychosocial counseling for individuals and families. Characterizes lifestyle choices (i.e., oral contraceptive use, hormone replacement therapy, number of pregnancies) that reduce ovarian cancer risk in women who may be susceptible to the disease. Strives for better methods for detecting ovarian cancer, for reliable predictive testing for cancer predisposition and prevention.

**★ 10174 ★ Gilda's Club**
322 Eighth Ave.
New York, NY 10001
**Phone:** (212)686-9898      **Fax:** (212)686-9290
**Email:** info@gildasclub.org
**Website:** http://www.gildasclub.org

**Fnded:** 1995. **Desc:** Provides places where people with cancer and their families and friends join with others to build social and emotional support as a supplement to medical care. The free program consists of The Basic III: I. Support and Networking groups; II. Lectures and Workshops; and III. Social Activities.

**★ 10175 ★ Gynecologic Oncology Group (GOG)**
PO Box 60167
Philadelphia, PA 19102-0167
**Phone:** (215)854-0770      **Fax:** (215)854-0716
**Email:** cgaloppo@acog.org
**Website:** http://www.gog.org
Dr. Robert C. Parks, Chm.

**Fnded:** 1970. **Mem:** 65. **Desc:** Institutions and teaching hospitals conducting research in gynecological oncology. Sponsored by the American College of Obstetricians and Gynecologists.

**★ 10176 ★ Haitian Association Against Cancer (HAAAC)**
c/o Jacques-Albert Calixte
1001 NE 125 St.
North Miami, FL 33161
**Phone:** (305)899-9922      **Fax:** (305)895-2767
**Website:** http://www.haaac.org/
Jacques-Albert Calixte, Founder

**Fnded:** 1997. **Desc:** Provides information on detection services of cancer to the public, particularly Haitians and Haitian-Americans who are uninsured and/or not being served. Serves as a support center for cancer survivors, particularly Haitians and Haitian-Americans, who are suffering from the emotional stress of cancer. Offers counseling, community outreach, and support groups. **Pub:** Pamphlets.Provides alternative information in the fight against cancer. • Videos.Provides alternatives in the crusade against cancer.

**★ 10177 ★ Histiocytosis Association of America**
302 N Broadway
Pitman, NJ 08071
**Phone:** (856)589-6606      **Free:** 800-548-2758
**Fax:** (856)589-6614
**Email:** president@histio.org
**Website:** http://www.histio.org/us
Jeffrey M. Toughill, Pres.

**Fnded:** 1985. **Mem:** 5,200. **Desc:** Patients, families, and friends of those suffering from histiocytic disorders; physicians, oncologists, and hematologists working in the field of histiocytosis research. (Histiocytosis is a rare disease that causes histiocytes, a type of white blood cell, to multiply and attack organs, body systems, or bones.) Works to provide support for patients and their families and friends. Funds research on the cause and treatment of histiocytosis. Acts as a referral service. Maintains speakers' bureau. **Pub:** *The Facts About HLH/FHL*. Brochure. *Price:* Free. • *The Facts about Langerhans Cell Histiocytosis*. Brochure. *Price:* Free. • *The Facts about Langerhans Cell Histiocytosis and Diabetes Insipidus*. Brochure. • *Patient Directory*, periodic. Directory. • Newsletter, quarterly. Reports on histiocytosis patients, their families, physicians, researchers, and other interested parties. *Price:* Free. **Frmly:** (1987) Histiocytosis-X Association of America.

## ★ 10178 ★ Hong Kong Anti-Cancer SOC (HKACS)

8/F, Comprehensive Services Block
Nam Long Hospital
30 Nam Long Shan Rd.
Hong Kong, People's Republic of China
**Phone:** 852 28140950     **Fax:** 852 28731405
**Email:** hkacs@netvigator.com
**Website:** http://www.ha.org.hk/org/hkacs
**Fnded:** 1964. **Mem:** 126. **Lang(s):** Chinese, English. **Desc:** Coordinates and promotes activities against cancer. Seeks to identify the causes of cancer and educate the public regarding cancer prevention. Sponsors cancer research and organizes educational programs.

## ★ 10179 ★ Hong Kong Association of Blood Transfusion and Haematology

15 King's Park Rise
Hong Kong, People's Republic of China
**Phone:** 852 27101383     **Fax:** 852 27804277
**Email:** channk@ha.org.hk
**Website:** http://www.fmshk.com.hk/hkabth
**Fnded:** 1992. **Mem:** 140. **Lang(s):** Chinese, English. **Desc:** Health care professionals operating in the fields of hematology and blood transfusion; corporations and organizations with an interest in hematology. Seeks to advance the practice of hematology and transfusion. Establishes and enforces standards of practice and professional conduct for members; serves as a forum for discussion of developments in hematology and transfusion; facilitates formation of contacts between members and their counterparts worldwide. **Pub:** Newsletter, 3/year.

## ★ 10180 ★ Hong Kong Cancer Chemotherapy Society

c/o Dr. Anthony Chan
810 Melbourne Plz.
33 Queens Rd.
Central, Central
Hong Kong, People's Republic of China
**Phone:** 852 25861726     **Fax:** 852 25960802
**Email:** anthonytcchan@cuhk.edu.hk
**Website:** http://www.fmshk.com.hk/hkccs
**Fnded:** 1990. **Mem:** 81. **Lang(s):** Chinese, English. **Desc:** Physicians practicing cancer chemotherapy. Seeks to advance the study and practice of chemotherapy; promotes continuing professional development of members. Facilitates exchange of knowledge, skill, and experience among members.

## ★ 10181 ★ Hong Kong Cancer Institute

Faculty of Medicine
Prince Wales Hospital
Hong Kong, People's Republic of China
**Phone:** 852 26322119     **Fax:** 852 26497426
**Email:** pjjohnson@cuhk.edu.hk
**Fnded:** 1989. **Desc:** Coordinates cancer research efforts. Disseminates information.

## ★ 10182 ★ Hong Kong Paediatric Haematology and Oncology Study Group (HKPHOSG)

c/o Dr. Chi Wai Anselm Lee
Department of Pediatrics
Tuen Mun Hospital
Tuen Mun
Hong Kong, People's Republic of China
**Phone:** 852 24685111     **Fax:** 852 24569111
**Email:** aclee@netvigator.com
**Website:** http://www.fmshk.com.hk/hkphosg
**Fnded:** 1993. **Mem:** 43. **Lang(s):** Chinese, English. **Desc:** Physicians with an interest in pediatric hematology and oncology. Seeks to advance methods of diagnosis and treatment of pediatric hematological and oncological problems. Conducts educational and continuing professional development courses for members. Compiles statistics. **Pub:** Newsletter, monthly.

## ★ 10183 ★ Indian Association of Surgical Oncology (IASO)

c/o Dr. Ravi Kent
Department of Surgery
Maulana Azad Medical College
New Delhi 110 002, Delhi, India
**Phone:** 91 11 4353320     **Fax:** 91 11 3230316
**Email:** ravibina@hotmail.com
**Fnded:** 1977. **Desc:** Cancer surgeons, radiologists, pathologists, and biochemists. Promotes advancement and practice of surgical oncology. **Pub:** Annual Report. • Journal, periodic.

## ★ 10184 ★ Indian Cancer Society

74 Jerbai Wadia Rd.
Parel, Bhoiwada
Bombay 400 012, Maharashtra, India
**Phone:** 91 22 4125238
**Fnded:** 1951. **Local Groups:** 30. **Desc:** Provides educational, diagnostic, therapeutic, and related services relating to cancer. Promotes cancer detection, treatment, and prevention through mobile cancer detection service. Offers rehabilitation services. Sponsors public and professional educational programs.

## ★ 10185 ★ Inter-American Society for Chemotherapy (IASC)

Azcuenaga 769, Piso 2, Apt 7
1029 Buenos Aires, Argentina
**Phone:** 54 11 49542365     **Fax:** 54 1 49528255
**Fnded:** 1983. **Desc:** Promotes acquisition and dissemination of knowledge in chemotherapy and related areas.

## ★ 10186 ★ International Agency for Research on Cancer (IARC) (Centre International de Recherche sur le Cancer — CIRC)

150, cours Albert Thomas
F-69372 Lyon, France
**Phone:** 33 4 72738485     **Fax:** 33 4 72738575
**Email:** lastname@iarc.fr
**Website:** http://www.iarc.fr
**Fnded:** 1965. **Mem:** 16. **Lang(s):** English, French. **Desc:** Cancer research arm of the World Health Organization. Representatives of nations involved in international collaboration in cancer research. Generates and disseminates information on the causes and prevention of cancer; conducts research in the field of cancer epidemiology, biostatistics, and environmental carcinogenesis. Evaluates and examines populations with unusually high or low frequencies of cancer and identifies the role of environmental factors including cultural and dietary habits and chemicals. Assists governments in cancer control programs. Maintains laboratories and collaborates with scientists working in national laboratories. Organizes training courses; compiles statistics. **Pub:** *Directory of On-Going Research in Cancer Epidemiology*, biennial. • *Technical Report Series*, periodic.

## International Association of Cancer Registries (IACR) (Association Internationale des Registres du Cancer)

*See:* Entry 12088

## ★ 10187 ★ International Association of Cancer Victors and Friends (IACVF)

5336 Harwood Rd.
San Jose, CA 95124-5711
**Phone:** (408)448-4094     **Free:** 888-613-6733
**Fax:** (408)264-9659
**Email:** cmckenna@best.com
**Website:** http://www.cancervictors.org
C. McKenna, Coord.
**Fnded:** 1963. **Mem:** 4,000. **Nat'l Groups:** 10. **Reg. Groups:** 13. **State Groups:** 2. **Desc:** Encourages independent research on cancer therapies and disseminates information on "nontoxic" chemotherapies.

Works directly with cancer patients providing one-on-one services. Offers educational programs on topics including carcinogens in air, food, and water and nutrition in relation to cancer. **Pub:** *Cancer Victors Journal*, quarterly. Journal. Provides news on nontoxic cancer treatments and breakthroughs in cancer research; includes studies on carcinogenic conditions. *Price:* Included in membership dues. • Audiotapes. • Books. • Pamphlets. • Reprints. **Frmly:** (1985) International Association of Cancer Victims and Friends.

## ★ 10188 ★ International Association for Comparative Research on Leukemia and Related Diseases (IACRLRD)

c/o The de Burlo Group
50 Federal St.
Boston, MA 02110
**Phone:** (617)483-0275     **Fax:** (617)338-6077
**Email:** deBurlo@erols.com
C. Russell de Burlo, PhD, Treas.
**Fnded:** 1963. **Mem:** 500. **Desc:** Promotes cooperation and coordination of basic and clinical research on leukemia and related diseases. Emphasizes comparative aspects of different disciplines in order to develop new hypotheses and introduce comparable working methods. Sponsors educational programs. **Pub:** *Symposium Proceedings*, biennial. Proceedings. *Price:* Free for members only; $35/issue for nonmembers.

## ★ 10189 ★ International Association for the Study of Lung Cancer

9 Blegdamsvej
DK-2100 Copenhagen, Denmark
**Phone:** 45 35453445     **Fax:** 45 35356909
**Email:** hansenhh@iaslc.org
**Website:** http://www.iaslc.org/
**Fnded:** 1974. **Desc:** Promotes the study of prevention, diagnosis, treatment, and all aspects of lung cancer.

## International Bone Marrow Transplant Registry (IBMTR)

*See:* Entry 20332

## ★ 10190 ★ International Cytokine Societies (ICS)

c/o Dr. Sherwood M. Reichard
1021 15th St., Ste. 9
Augusta, GA 30910
**Phone:** (706)722-7511     **Fax:** (706)722-7515
**Email:** maps@csranet.com
**Website:** http://www.ibmtr.org
Dr. Sherwood M. Reichard, Exec. Dir.
**Fnded:** 1975. **Mem:** 3,000. **Desc:** Reticuloendothelial and related research societies concerned with the body's defenses against disease and cancer. Works to advance research and understanding of the reticuloendothelial system. (RES is a diffuse system of cells arising from mesenchyme and comprising all phagocytic cells of the body excluding circulating leukocytes.) Fosters and maintains scientific cooperation and communication among individual scientists and regional and national societies worldwide. Maintains liaison with the International Council of Scientific Unions, World Health Organization, and similar organizations to facilitate the appropriate representation of RES research. Sponsors international scientific conferences, seminars, workshops, and training courses. **Pub:** *Proceedings of International Meetings*, biennial. **Frmly:** (1998) International Union of Retoculoendothelial Societies.

## ★ 10191 ★ International Federation of Blood Donor Organizations (IFBDO) (Federazione Internazionale delle Organizzazioni dei Donatori di Sangue)

c/o Ms. Nicole Patterson
34 place Raoul-Dautry
F-75748 Paris Cedex 15, France
**Phone:** 33 1 45387193

**Fnded:** 1955. **Mem:** 43. **Lang(s):** English, French, Spanish. **Desc:** National voluntary blood donor associations united to promote voluntary blood giving. Considers problems of common interest such as voluntary donations from which all political and religious considerations are excluded, and medical progress of blood transfusions. Seeks laws related to voluntary blood giving and governmental action prohibiting blood commerce. Exchanges information; acts as liaison with the European Council, League of Red Cross and Red Crescent Societies, United Nations Educational, Scientific and Cultural Organization, and World Health Organization. Provides specialized education. **Pub:** *FIODS Revue*, quarterly.

### ★ 10192 ★ International Myeloma Foundation
12650 Riverside Dr., Ste. 206
North Hollywood, CA 91607
**Phone:** (818)487-7455          **Free:** 800-452-CURE
**Fax:** (818)487-7454
**Email:** TheIMF@myeloma.org
**Website:** http://www.myeloma.org
Stephanie Colman, Director of Community Relations
**Fnded:** 1990. **Mem:** 75,000. **Desc:** The International Myeloma Foundation is a non-profit organization dedicated to the eduction, treatment and research of multiple myeloma, a little-known cancer of the bone marrow. We provide a variety of patient and physician education and support programs and services. **Pub:** *A Concise Review of the Disease and Treatment Options*. Book. • *Myeloma Today*, bimonthly. Newsletter. *Price:* $25 6/year for U.S. subscribers; $35 6/year for international subscribers. • *Patient Hankbook*. Book. • *"So You're Considering..."*. Brochure.

### ★ 10193 ★ International Network for Cancer Treatment and Research (INCTR)
c/o Dr. Philip Schein
15200 Shady Grove Rd., Ste. 350
Rockville, MD 20850
**Phone:** (301)296-4541          **Fax:** (301)330-0740
**Website:** http://www.inctr.org/
Dr. Philip Schein, Pres.
**Fnded:** 1998. **Desc:** Seeks to build capacities for cancer treatment and research in countries where such capacities are currently limited. **Pub:** Newsletter, quarterly.

### International Psycho-Oncology Society (IPOS)
*See:* Entry 12521

### ★ 10194 ★ International Society of Blood Purification
c/o Prof. Thomas A. Golper
S-3301 MCN
Vanderbilt University Medical Center
Nashville, TN 37232
**Phone:** (615)343-2220          **Fax:** (615)343-2675
**Email:** info@ipos-aspboa.org
**Website:** http://www.ipos-aspboa.org
Dr. Michael J. Lysaght, Contact
**Fnded:** 1982. **Mem:** 140. **Desc:** Blood purification professionals.

### ★ 10195 ★ International Society for Cutaneous Lymphomas (ISCL)
c/o Dr. Nicola Pimpinelli
Department Dermatological Sciences
University of Florence Medical School
Via degli Alfani 37
I-50121 Florence, Italy
**Phone:** 39 55 2344422          **Fax:** 39 55 2758303
**Email:** pimpi@ngi.it
**Website:** http://www.cutaneouslymphoma.org
**Fnded:** 1992. **Mem:** 215. **Lang(s):** English. **Desc:** Fosters communication and cooperation among individuals and groups interested in the diagnosis, treat-

ment, and investigation of primary cutaneous lymphomas.

### ★ 10196 ★ International Society for Experimental Hematology (ISEH)
2025 M St. NW, Ste. 800
Washington, DC 20036
**Phone:** (202)367-1183          **Fax:** (202)367-2183
**Email:** iseh@dc.sba.com
**Website:** http://www.iseh.org
Thomas Reiser, Exec. Dir.
**Fnded:** 1972. **Mem:** 1,400. **Desc:** Scientists and health care professionals in the field of experimental hematology. Seeks to advance the science and practice of hematology; promotes professional development of members. Serves as a forum for the exchange of information on experimental hematology and related topics; sponsors research and educational programs. **Pub:** *Experimental Hematology*, monthly. Journal. *Price:* included in membership dues. • *Membership Directory*, periodic. Directory.

### ★ 10197 ★ International Society of Hematology (ISH) (Societe Internationale d'Hematologie)
Diaz Ordaz 808, Anzures
72530 Puebla, Puebla, Mexico
**Phone:** 52 22 438100          **Fax:** 52 22 438428
**Fnded:** 1946. **Mem:** 3,000. **Reg. Groups:** 3. **Lang(s):** English. **Desc:** Doctors of medicine and persons holding Ph.D. degrees who have completed at least 5 years in the practice or research of hematology (branch of medical science dealing with the blood, its formation, functions, and diseases). Works to promote hematology research and the advancement and recognition of hematology as a biological science. **Pub:** *Membership List*, biennial. • Newsletter, semiannual.

### ★ 10198 ★ International Society of Hematology - European African Division
Hematology Laboratory Department
Hospital Clinic I Provincial
Calle Villarroel, 170
E-08036 Barcelona, Spain
**Phone:** 34 3 4548229          **Fax:** 34 3 4548229
**Fnded:** 1946. **Mem:** 1,300. **Lang(s):** English. **Desc:** Scientists and physicians in 85 countries with at least 5 years experience in the field of hematology. Promotes the exchange of ideas and information relating to blood and blood forming tissues; provides an international forum for the dissemination of new information concerning hematological problems. Aims to standardize hematological methods and nomenclature on an international scale and to heighten awareness of clinical hematological problems among scientific investigators while recognizing hematology as a legitimate branch of the biological sciences. Sponsors educational programs. **Pub:** *ISH*, biennial. Newsletter. • *ISH Newsletter*, semiannual. Newsletter.

### ★ 10199 ★ International Society of Lymphology (ISL)
c/o Dr. Marlys H. Witte
University of Arizona
College of Medicine/Surgery
1501 N Campbell Ave., No. 4406
Tucson, AZ 85724-5063
**Phone:** (520)626-6118          **Fax:** (520)626-0822
**Email:** lymph@u.arizona.edu
**Website:** http://www.u.arizona.edu/~witte/ISL.htm
Marlys H. Witte, MD, Sec. Gen.
**Fnded:** 1966. **Mem:** 385. **Nat'l Groups:** 9. **Desc:** Professionals active in the medical, biological, and technical sciences. Promotes the study of lymphology and seeks to advance and disseminate knowledge in the field. Activities include: stimulating and strengthening experimentation and clinical investigation in lymphology; establishing relations between researchers and clinicians in the different fields of lymphology; encouraging contact and exchange of ideas among members and national and international organizations.

Organizes postgraduate courses. **Pub:** *Lymphology*, quarterly. Journal. *Price:* $75 with 10% discount for vendors. • *Progress in Lymphology*, biennial. Proceedings.

### International Society of Pediatric Oncology (SIOP) (Societe Internationale d'Oncologie Pediatrique — SIOP)
*See:* Entry 5703

### International Society for Peritoneal Dialysis (ISPD)
*See:* Entry 20386

### ★ 10200 ★ International Society for Preventive Oncology (ISPO)
c/o Mr.Nieburgs
55 Lake Ave. North, Box 20
Worcester, MA 01655
**Phone:** (508)856-1822          **Fax:** (508)856-1824
**Email:** editor@cancerprev.org
**Website:** http://www.cancerprev.org
Herbert E. Nieburgs, MD, Ed.
**Fnded:** 1980. **Mem:** 400. **Desc:** Physicians and other professionals at the doctoral level; individuals with professional equivalence who are actively engaged in preventive oncology. Promotes the prevention of cancer through the identification and control of cancer causing factors; fosters secondary prevention through detection and treatment of cancer in its earliest, most curable stages. Sponsors basic research on cancer prevention and early detection and provides a forum for information exchange between scientists engaged in research and those working on preventive and clinical oncology. Conducts workshops. **Pub:** *Cancer Detection and Prevention*, 6/year. • *Proceedings of International Symposium on Immunobiology of Cancer and Allied Immune Dysfunctions*, biennial. • *Proceedings of the International Conference on Human Tumor Markers*, biennial. • *Proceedings of the International Symposium on Prevention and Detection of Cancer*, biennial.

### ★ 10201 ★ International Society for Radiation Oncology (ISRO)
Av E Mounier 83-4
1200 Brussels, Belgium
**Phone:** 32 2 7795494          **Fax:** 32 2 7759342
**Email:** frederique.artus@isro.be
**Website:** http://www.isro.be
**Fnded:** 1981. **Desc:** Fosters the fields of radiotherapy and oncology, by promoting studies and research.

### ★ 10202 ★ International Society of Radiolabelled Blood Elements (ISORBE)
c/o Dr. Margarida Rodrigues
ISOTOPIX
Hariannengasse 30
A-1090 Vienna, Austria
**Phone:** 43 1 4020902          **Fax:** 43 1 4029292
**Email:** rodrigues@hotmail.com
**Website:** http://www.isorbe.org
**Fnded:** 1990. **Mem:** 201. **State Groups:** 28. **Lang(s):** English. **Desc:** Scientists working in the field of labeled blood cells. Seeks to promote the study of radiolabeled blood elements. Protects archives and promotes standardization.

### ★ 10203 ★ International Society on Thrombosis and Haemostasis (ISTH)
CB 7035
UNC Medical School
Chapel Hill, NC 27599-7035
**Phone:** (919)929-3807          **Fax:** (919)929-3935
**Email:** headquarters@isth.org
**Website:** http://www.isth.org
Uri Seligsohn, Chm.
**Fnded:** 1969. **Mem:** 2,000. **Desc:** Biomedical scientists in over 50 countries interested in thrombosis (the

presence of a clot in a blood vessel) and hemostasis (the arrest of bleeding). Engages in research and education concerning thrombosis, hemostasis, blood clotting, and vascular biology. **Pub:** *Thrombosis and Haemostasis*, monthly. Journal. • Abstracts of congressional proceedings and lectures published as special issues of journal, and annual reports of SSC Scientific subcommittees. **Frmly:** (2002) International Society on Thrombosis and Hemostasis.

★ **10204** ★ **International Union Against Cancer (UICC)**
**(Union Internationale Contre le Cancer)**
3, rue du Conseil General
CH-1205 Geneva, Switzerland
**Phone:** 41 22 8091811     **Fax:** 41 22 8091810
**Email:** info@uicc.org
**Website:** http://www.uicc.ch/
**Fnded:** 1933. **Mem:** 286. **Lang(s):** English. **Desc:** Voluntary cancer leagues and societies, national organizations, private or public cancer research institutions, and ministries of health in 86 countries. Promotes a comprehensive international campaign against cancer. Directs activities in fields of prevention, research, and treatment; sponsors special projects in fields including cervical cancer, head and neck cancer, and exchange of information on unproven methods in cancer treatment. Facilitates training courses for researchers and health professionals; makes available advisory visits by cancer experts. **Pub:** *International Calendar of Meetings on Cancer*, semiannual. • *International Journal of Cancer and Predictive Oncology*, 30/year. Journal. • *UICC International Directory of Cancer Institutes and Organizations*, quadrennial. Directory. • *UICC News*, quarterly. Also publishes monographs, reports, publication lists, and new book announcements; produces cancer education packs and workshop guidelines.

★ **10205** ★ **International Union of Angiology (IUA)**
1, av J Poulhes
F-31403 Toulouse, France
**Phone:** 33 5 61552637     **Fax:** 33 5 61322634
**Email:** angio@wanadoo.fr
**Website:** http://www.i.u.angiology.org/
**Fnded:** 1958. **Desc:** Stimulates scientific knowledge in the whole field of angiology and diseases of blood vessels.

★ **10206** ★ **Irish Cancer Society (ICS)**
5 Northumberland Rd.
Dublin 4, Ireland
**Phone:** 353 1 2310500     **Fax:** 353 1 668759
**Email:** reception@irishcancer.ie
**Website:** http://www.irishcancer.ie
**Lang(s):** English, Irish Gaelic. **Desc:** National cancer societies. Promotes advancement in the prevention, diagnosis, and treatment of cancer; seeks to improve the quality of life of people with cancer and their families. Facilitates communication and cooperation among members; sponsors research and educational programs; provides support and services to people with cancer.

★ **10207** ★ **Irish Haemophilia Society (IHS)**
Iceland House
Arran Ct.
Arran Quay
Dublin 7, Ireland
**Phone:** 353 1 8724466     **Fax:** 353 1 8724494
**Email:** haemophiliasociety@eircom.net
**Website:** http://www.haemophilia-society.ie
**Fnded:** 1968. **Mem:** 300. **Nat'l Groups:** 1. **Lang(s):** English, Irish. **Desc:** Individuals and organizations. Seeks to improve the quality of life of people with hemophilia and their families. Makes available support and services; conducts educational and advocacy campaigns; supports hematological research. **Pub:** Newsletter, annual, 3 monthly.

★ **10208** ★ **Israel Cancer Association (ICA)**
**(Haagudah Lemilchama Besartan Beyisrael)**
7 Revivim St.
PO Box 437
IL-53104 Givatayim, Israel
**Phone:** 972 3 5721616     **Fax:** 972 3 5719578
**Email:** info@cancer.org.il
**Website:** http://www.cancer.org.il
**Fnded:** 1952. **Local Groups:** 52. **Lang(s):** Arabic, English, Hebrew, Russian. **Desc:** Encourages and facilitates research on cancer prevention and early diagnosis. Supports cancer medical treatment services, and finances rehabilitation and social welfare programs for cancer patients. Provides educational programs. **Pub:** *Adcan*, semiannual. • *Bama*, periodic. Journal. Includes information on medical, psychosocial, and welfare aspects of cancer.

★ **10209** ★ **Jamaica Cancer Society (JCS)**
16 Lady Musgrave Rd.
Kingston 5, Jamaica
**Phone:** (876)927-4933     **Fax:** (876)978-1918
**Email:** jcs@ns.com.jm
**Website:** http://www.jamaicacancersociety.org
**Fnded:** 1955. **Mem:** 1,200. **Nat'l Groups:** 1. **Reg. Groups:** 1. **Local Groups:** 1. **Desc:** Health care professionals, people with cancer and their families, and other interested individuals. Promotes and encourages research into the causes and cure of cancer, and improved treatments for people with cancer. Conducts public education programs on cancer detection and treatment; offers specialized training for cancer doctors and nurses. Operates cancer screening clinics. **Pub:** *Can Survive*, biennial. Newsletter. • Brochure.

★ **10210** ★ **Kidney Cancer Association**
1234 Sherman Ave., Ste. 203
Evanston, IL 60202-1375
**Phone:** (847)332-1051     **Free:** 800-850-9132
**Fax:** (847)332-2978
**Email:** office@kidneycancerassociation.org
**Website:** http://www.kidneycancerassociation.org
**Fnded:** 1990. **Desc:** Provides a broad range of services related to kidney cancer, including patient meetings, annual convention for patients and doctors, sponsors research and advocates for changes.

★ **10211** ★ **Leukemia and Lymphoma Society**
1311 Mamaroneck Ave.
White Plains, NY 10605
**Phone:** (914)949-5213     **Free:** 800-955-4572
**Fax:** (914)949-6691
**Email:** irc_lls@hotmail.com
**Website:** http://www.leukemia.org
Dwayne Howell, PhD, Pres. /CEO
**Fnded:** 1949. **Local Groups:** 57. **Desc:** Raises funds to combat leukemia, lymphoma, Hodgkin's Disease and myeloma through research, patient service, and public and professional education and advocacy. Sponsors medical symposia; conducts research; provides financial aid for patients and free information; sponsors support groups. Free information available through 1-800-955-4LSA or website: www.leukemia.org. **Pub:** *Educational Literature*. Brochures. *Price:* Free. • *Leukemia Society of America–Newsline*, quarterly. Newsletter. Provides information on advances in the research into leukemia, lymphoma, Hodgkin's Disease and Myeloma. Includes research updates. *Price:* Free. **Frmly:** (1955) Robert Roesler de Villiers Foundation; (2000) Leukemia Society of America.

★ **10212** ★ **Lymphatic Research Foundation (LRF)**
39 Pool Dr.
Roslyn, NY 11576-2038
**Phone:** (516)625-9862     **Fax:** (516)625-9410
**Email:** lrf@lymphaticresearch.org
**Website:** http://www.lymphaticresearch.org
Wendy Chaite, Esq., Pres.
**Fnded:** 1998. **Desc:** Health care professionals, scientists, and researchers with an interest in lymphatic diseases and related disorders. Seeks to advance the prevention, diagnosis, and treatment of lymphatic diseases. Serves as a clearinghouse on lymphatic research; facilitates exchange of information among members; advocates the creation of a nationally supported lymphatic research program; functions as a liaison linking public and private-sector lymphatic research institutions and programs. **Pub:** *Lymphatic Research & Biology*, quarterly. Journal.

★ **10213** ★ **Lymphoma Association**
PO Box 386
Aylesbury HP20 2GA, United Kingdom
**Phone:** 44 1296619400     **Fax:** 44 1296619414
**Email:** support@lymphoma.org.uk
**Website:** http://www.lymphoma.org.uk
**Fnded:** 1986. **Mem:** 2,000. **Desc:** Provides information and emotional support for anyone affected by lymphoma. Provides a Help line; telephone links to helpers with similar experience of lymphoma; a network of regional support groups and a quarterly newsletter for members. **Pub:** *Fundraising News*, quarterly. • *Lymphoma News*, quarterly. Newsletter.

★ **10214** ★ **Lymphoma Research Foundation (LRF)**
c/o Donna Shu
8800 Venice Blvd., Ste. 207
Los Angeles, CA 90034
**Phone:** (310)204-7040     **Free:** 800-500-9976
**Fax:** (310)204-7043
**Email:** helpline@lymphoma.org
**Website:** http://www.lymphoma.org
Suzanne Bliss, Exec. Dir.
**Fnded:** 2001. **Desc:** Provides support and information for lymphoma patients and their families regarding diagnosis, treatments, clinical trials, support services, literature, and physician referrals. Serves patients with a buddy support program. Supports lymphoma specific education for both patients and healthcare professionals. Promotes advocacy. **Pub:** *Lymphoma Update*, quarterly. Newsletter. Provides information about lymphoma and the Foundation, as well as current events.

★ **10215** ★ **Make Today Count (MTC)**
1235 E Cherokee St.
Springfield, MO 65804-2203
**Phone:** (417)885-2588     **Fax:** (417)888-8761
Connie Zimmerman, Exec. Dir.
**Fnded:** 1974. **Mem:** 5,000. **Local Groups:** 200. **Desc:** Cancer patients and others with life-threatening illnesses, and their immediate families. Works to bring members and their neighbors together to discuss openly the false implications and the realities of life-threatening diseases. Takes a positive approach to the problems of serious illness in order to lessen the emotional trauma for all concerned. Assists professionals in communicating with and meeting the needs of seriously ill patients. Maintains speakers' bureau and referral service; plans educational programs, films, and tapes. **Pub:** *Chapter Directory*, annual. Directory. • *Make Today Count Newsletter*, bimonthly. Newsletter. Offers emotional support to people with cancer or other life-threatening illnesses, and to their family members, friends, and professionals. *Price:* $10/year. • *Make Today Count - Until Tomorrow Comes*.

★ **10216** ★ **Marie Curie Cancer Care (MCCC)**
89 Albert Embankment
London SE1 7TP, United Kingdom
**Phone:** 44 207 5997729     **Fax:** 44 207 5997708
**Email:** info@mariecurie.org.uk
**Website:** http://www.mariecurie.org.uk
**Fnded:** 1948. **Lang(s):** English. **Desc:** Health care professionals working with people who have cancer.

Seeks to improve the quality of life of people with cancer; promotes increased availability and effectiveness of cancer care. Operates nationwide network of Marie Curie Nurses in the community and operates ten hospices across England, Scotland, Wales, and Northern Ireland; provides specialist care for people with cancer; conducts cancer research. Conducts educational programs. **Pub:** *Marie Curie News*, quarterly. Newsletter. • Pamphlets.

**★ 10217 ★ Mautner Project for Lesbians with Cancer**
1707 L St. NW, Ste. 500
Washington, DC 20036
**Phone:** (202)332-5536 **Fax:** (202)332-0662
**Email:** mautner@mautnerproject.org
**Website:** http://www.mautnerproject.org/

**Fnded:** 1990. **Desc:** Dedicated to lesbians with cancer, their partners and caregivers; provides education and information to the lesbian community regarding cancer; promotes understanding to the health care community about special concerns of lesbians with cancer and their families; advocates for lesbian health issues in national arenas.

**★ 10218 ★ Men Against Breast Cancer (MABC)**
2379 Lewis Ave.
Rockville, MD 20851-2335
**Free:** (866)547-6222 **Fax:** (301)770-5697
**Email:** info@menagainstbreastcancer.org
**Website:** http://www.menagainstbreastcancer.org/
Marc Heyison, Pres. /Co-Founder

**Desc:** Strives to eradicate breast cancer as a life-threatening disease by mobilizing and supporting men as active participants in the fight against the disease.

**★ 10219 ★ Mothers Supporting Daughters with Breast Cancer (MSDBC)**
c/o Charmayne Dierker
21710 Bayshore Rd.
Chestertown, MD 21620
**Phone:** (410)778-1982 **Fax:** (410)778-1411
**Email:** msdbc@dmv.com
**Website:** http://www.mothersdaughters.org
Charmayne Dierker, Pres.

**Fnded:** 1995. **Desc:** Assists mothers of daughters with breast cancer. Provides basic medical information about breast cancer as a disease and the various treatments that patients may receive. Also offers a local, regional, and national communication network for mothers and daughters. Our main goal is to offer emotional support to mothers of daughters newly-diagnosed with breast cancer. **Pub:** *Daughter's Brochure.* Brochure. Provides information about the difficulties a mother may be experiencing and how to help. *Price:* Free. • *Mother's Handbook.* Handbook. Prepared for mothers who have had a daughter diagnosed with breast cancer. Provides a list of free resources.

**★ 10220 ★ National Alliance of Breast Cancer Organizations (NABCO)**
9 E 37th St., 10th Fl.
New York, NY 10016
**Phone:** (212)889-0606 **Free:** 888-80-NABCO
**Fax:** (212)689-1213
**Email:** NABCOinfo@aol.com
**Website:** http://www.nabco.org
Amy Langer, Exec. Dir.

**Fnded:** 1986. **Mem:** 400. **Desc:** The National Alliance of Breast Cancer Organization (NABCO) is the leading non-profit information and education resource on breast cancer and a network of over 400 member organizations nationwide. NABCO provides information to medical professionals and their organizations and to patients and their families, and advocates for beneficial regulatory change and legislation. With public and corporate partners, NABCO has collaborated on educational and medical programs thast have reached a national audience, heightening public awareness and connecting women with needed ser-

vices. centers, and hospital programs. Services are free of charge. **Pub:** *NABCO News*, quarterly. Newsletter. Monitors developments relating to breast cancer. *Price:* Included in membership dues. • *NABCO's Resource List*, annual. Contains information on materials and organizations that provide information about breast cancer. *Price:* Included in membership dues; $5/copy.

**★ 10221 ★ National Association for Proton Therapy**
7910 Woodmont Ave., Ste. 1303
Bethesda, MD 20814
**Phone:** (301)913-9360 **Fax:** (301)913-0372
**Email:** lenarzt@compuserve.com
**Website:** http://proton-therapy.org
Leonard Arzt, Contact

**Fnded:** 1989. **Mem:** 3. **Desc:** Oncologists and other health care professionals with an interest in the treatment of cancer. Promotes use of proton therapy to treat cancer patients. Conducts research and educational programs; gathers and disseminates information. **Pub:** *Proton News*, periodic. Newsletter.

**★ 10222 ★ National Blood Foundation (NBF)**
8101 Glenbrook Rd.
Bethesda, MD 20814-2749
**Phone:** (301)215-6552 **Fax:** (301)907-6895
**Email:** nbf@aabb.org
**Website:** http://www.aabb.org

**Fnded:** 1983. **Desc:** Promotes the safety and adequacy of America's blood supply by supporting research and education for blood banking and transfusion medicine.

**★ 10223 ★ National Brain Tumor Foundation (NBTF)**
414 13th St., No. 700
Oakland, CA 94612-2603
**Phone:** (510)839-9777 **Free:** 800-934-CURE
**Fax:** (510)839-9779
**Email:** nbtf@braintumor.org
**Website:** http://www.braintumor.org
Janis Brewer, Exec. Dir.

**Fnded:** 1981. **Desc:** Medical researchers, doctors, brain tumor patients, and relatives working together to improve the quality of life for brain tumor patients and their families and find a cure through research. Raises funds for brain tumor research; offers patient services such as educational materials, a toll-free brain tumor information line, a quarterly newsletter, information about support groups and patient networks, and national and regional conferences. **Pub:** *Brain Tumors: A Guide.* Booklet. Contains information on brain tumors. *Price:* 1st copy free; $6 each additional copy. • *SEARCH*, quarterly. Newsletter. Informs readers of advances in treatment and psychosocial support. • Pamphlets. **Frmly:** (1989) Friends of Brain Tumor Research.

**★ 10224 ★ National Breast Cancer Coalition (NBCC)**
1707 L St. NW, Ste. 1060
Washington, DC 20036
**Phone:** (202)296-7477 **Free:** 800-622-2838
**Fax:** (202)265-6854
**Email:** info@natlbcc.org
**Website:** http://www.stopbreastcancer.org
Fran Visco, Pres.

**Fnded:** 1991. **Mem:** 60,000. **Desc:** Promotes research into the cause of, optimal treatments and cure for breast cancer, aims to improve coordination and distribution of research funds and recruitment and training of scientists; strives to improve access to breast cancer screening, diagnosis, treatment and care for all women, particularly the underserved and uninsured, through legislation and change in regulation and delivery of breast health care; dedicated to increasing involvement and influence of those living with breast cancer in the areas of legislation, regulatory processes and all aspects of clinical trial design,

including access to clinical trials. advocacy activities; formulated national action plan on breast cancer, to which the Clinton Administration committed in 1993. Operates: Aspen Project, which brings together industrial, scientific, governmental, and consumer representatives to develop innovative approaches to the prevention and treatment of breast cancer; Project LEAD, which trains grass roots advocates to influence public policies affecting people with breast cancer; Clinical Trials Project, which trains NBCC members to collaborate with scientific and industrial organizations to expedite clinical trials of breast cancer drugs and treatments. Sponsors The Face of Breast Cancer, a travelling **Pub:** *End the Breast Cancer Epidemic*, quarterly. Newsletter.

**★ 10225 ★ National Cancer Center (NCC)**
88 Sunnyside Blvd., Ste. 307
Plainview, NY 11803
**Phone:** (516)349-0610 **Fax:** (516)349-1755
**Email:** info@nationalcancercenter.org
Regina English, Exec. Dir.

**Fnded:** 1953. **Desc:** Supports cancer research and educational programs. Concentrates on cytology, immunology, detection, and prevention of cancer, and on invention and perfection of new methods and instruments for early diagnosis of cancer. **Frmly:** (1954) Eugene L. Garey Cancer Foundation; (1965) Cancer Cytology Foundation of America; (1986) National Cancer Cytology Center.

**★ 10226 ★ National Cancer Institute (NCI)**
NCI Public Inquiries Office
Ste. 3036A
6116 Executive Blvd., MSC 8322
Bethesda, MD 20892-8322
**Phone:** (301)435-3848
**Email:** webmaster@cancer.gov
**Website:** http://www.nci.nih.gov

**Fnded:** 1937. **Desc:** Dedicated to defeat cancer through research in cancer biology, causation, prevention, detection, treatment, and survivorship.

**★ 10227 ★ National Cancer Institute of Canada (NCIC) (Institut National du Cancer du Canada — INCC)**
10 Alcorn Ave., Ste. 200
Toronto, ON, Canada M4V 3B1
**Phone:** (416)961-7223 **Fax:** (416)961-7327
**Email:** ncic@cancer.ca
**Website:** http://www.ncic.cancer.ca

**Fnded:** 1947. **Mem:** 48. **Lang(s):** English, French. **Desc:** Coordinates and correlates the efforts of individuals and organized bodies with the goal of reducing the morbidity and mortality of cancer. This role is fulfilled through the support of clinical and laboratory-based research activities and research personnel. **Pub:** *Breast Cance Bulletin*, semiannual. Newsletter. • *Canadian Cancer Statistics*, annual. • *Scientific Report*, annual. • *UPDATE*, quarterly. Newsletter. • Annual Report, annual.

**★ 10228 ★ National Cancer Registrars Association (NCRA)**
1310 Braddock Place, Ste. 102
Alexandria, VA 22314
**Phone:** (703)299-6640 **Fax:** (703)299-6620
**Email:** info@ncra-usa.org
**Website:** http://www.ncra-usa.org
Linda G. Mulvihill, RHIT, Pres.

**Fnded:** 1974. **Mem:** 2,500. **Desc:** Persons involved in central, state, regional, and hospital-based tumor registries including physicians, hospital administrators, and health care planners who maintain ongoing records of the cancer patient's history, diagnosis, therapy, and outcome. Purposes are to: promote research and education in tumor registry administration and practice; improve service to cancer patients; establish standards of education and provide a standardized course of study for tumor registrars; raise the level of knowledge and performance of tumor registrars through continuing education; disseminate information regarding current activities, research, and trends in the cancer field; initiate and/or participate in programs to improve and standardize the compiling of tumor - related information; interact with professional and governmental organizations that use data derived from tumor registries. Has conducted national educational programs including: coding and tumor registry workshops; symposia on head and neck tumors, lymphatic and hematopoietic neoplasms, and non-Hodgkin's lymphoma; tumor registry training program and seminars. Sponsors registry management training program at the University of Pittsburgh School of Health Related Professions to instruct tumor registrars. Offers certification examinations for tumor registrars; provides continuing education program to help members maintain certification; offers educational assistance for new registrars. **Pub:** *Connection,* quarterly. Newsletter. • *National Cancer Registrars Association–Membership Roster,* annual. *Price:* Included in membership dues. • *National Cancer Registrars Association–Proceedings/Annual Report,* annual. *Price:* Included in membership dues. • *National Cancer Registrars Association–The Journal of Registry Management.* Journal. Includes book reviews, peer reviewed scientific articles and lists of employment opportunities. *Price:* Included in membership dues; $40/year for nonmembers; $55/year for international subscriptions. • Surveys.Contains information on compensation. • Also publishes educational materials. **Frmly:** National Tumor Registrars Association.

★ **10229** ★ **National Coalition for Cancer Research (NCCR)**
426 C St. NE
Washington, DC 20002
**Phone:** (202)544-1880          **Fax:** (202)543-2565
**Email:** md@capitolassociates.com
**Website:** http://www.cancercoalition.org/
Marguerite Donoghue Baxtor, Exec. Dir.

**Fnded:** 1986. **Mem:** 19. **Desc:** Lay and professional organizations committed to the eradication of cancer. Dedicated to strengthening the National Cancer Program through public education and communication about the value of cancer research, treatment, and prevention.

★ **10230** ★ **National Coalition for Cancer Survivorship (NCCS)**
1010 Wayne Ave., Ste. 770
Silver Spring, MD 20910-5600
**Phone:** (301)650-9127          **Free:** 877-622-7937
**Fax:** (301)565-9670
**Email:** info@cansearch.org
**Website:** http://www.cansearch.org
Ellen Stovall, Pres. /CEO

**Fnded:** 1986. **Mem:** 2,500. **Reg. Groups:** 7. **Desc:** Ensures quality of cancer care for all Americans. Provides leadership and education, supports research, promotes responsible advocacy. helping survivors deal with life after cancer is diagnosed. Operates speakers' bureau. **Pub:** *Charting the Journey: An Almanac of Resources for Cancer Survivors.* Book. • *NCCS Networker,* quarterly. Newsletter. News and articles on cancer survivorship, interviews, and reviews. • *Survivors.* Book. • *Teamwork: The Cancer Patient's Guide to Talking With Your Doctor.* Booklet. • *What Cancer Survivors Need to Know About Health Insurance.* Booklet. • Also publishes many booklets on cancer-related topics.

★ **10231** ★ **National Comprehensive Cancer Network (NCCN)**
50 Huntington Pike, Ste. 200
Rockledge, PA 19046
**Phone:** (215)728-4788          **Free:** 888-909-6226
**Fax:** (215)728-3877
**Email:** information@nccn.org
**Website:** http://www.nccn.org
Tricia Wilson, Contact

**Fnded:** 1995. **Mem:** 19. **Desc:** Established to provide cancer care to the greatest number of patients in need;

to advance cancer prevention, screening, diagnosis and treatment through excellence in basic and clinical research; to enhance the effectiveness and efficiency of cancer care delivery through the ongoing collection, synthesis and analysis of outcomes data. **Pub:** *The Complete Library of Practice Guidelines in Oncology.*

★ **10232** ★ **National Foundation for Cancer Research (NFCR)**
4600 W West Hwy., Ste. 525
Bethesda, MD 20814
**Phone:** (301)654-1250          **Free:** 800-321-2873
**Fax:** (301)654-5824
**Email:** fcsjr@nfcr.org
**Website:** http://www.researchforacure.com/site/PageServer
Franklin C. Salisbury, Jr., Pres.

**Fnded:** 1974. **Desc:** Purpose is to conduct basic scientific research and scientific investigation of the structure and function of normal and abnormal cells. This research is based on the belief that cancer is a disturbance of normal cellular function at the submolecular level. Funds 40 laboratories in the U.S. and 7 other countries. **Pub:** *National Cancer Bulletin,* periodic. Newsletter. *Price:* Free to donors. • Also publishes booklets and papers. **Frmly:** (1975) Bethesda National Foundation of Massachusetts.

★ **10233** ★ **National Hemophilia Foundation (NHF)**
116 West 32nd St., 11th floor
New York, NY 10001
**Phone:** (212)328-3700          **Free:** 800-42-HANDI
**Fax:** (212)328-3777
**Email:** info@hemophilia.org
**Website:** http://www.hemophilia.org
Mark Skinner, Pres.

**Fnded:** 1948. **Mem:** 1,500. **Local Groups:** 48. **Desc:** Voluntary health organization consisting of individuals with hemophilia, their families, medical and paramedical professionals, and other interested persons. (Hemophilia is a hereditary disease in which blood clotting is abnormally delayed.) Supports research through postgraduate fellowship program; disseminates literature for the public and medical and paramedical personnel. Conducts educational programs. Operates information center to provide research assistance, referrals, and comprehensive resources on hemophilia, HIV/AIDS, and related topics. Chapters help in blood recruitment drives and referral services for patients and sponsor summer camps for young people with hemophilia. Maintains library. **Pub:** *Directory of Hemophilia Treatment Centers,* periodic. Directory. **Frmly:** (1956) Hemophilia Foundation.

★ **10234** ★ **National Immunotherapy Cancer Research Foundation**
PO Box 1027
Flemington, NJ 08822
**Phone:** (908)806-4300          **Fax:** (908)806-3548
Dale A. Facchina, Pres. & CEO

**Fnded:** 1990. **Desc:** Promotes the use of immune system stimulation including vaccines, biological response modifiers, and other immuno-augmentative treatments as a cure for cancer. Raises funds for immunotherapy and immunology research in the prevention and treatment of cancer.

**National Marrow Donor Program (NMDP)**
*See:* Entry 20341

★ **10235** ★ **National Ovarian Cancer Coalition (NOCC)**
500 NE Spanish River Blvd., Ste. 14
Boca Raton, FL 33431
**Phone:** (561)393-0005          **Free:** 888-OVA-RIAN
**Fax:** (561)393-7275
**Email:** nocc@ovarian.org
**Website:** http://www.ovarian.org
Gail Hayward, Pres.

**Fnded:** 1996. **Mem:** 16,000. **State Groups:** 25. **Desc:** Individuals with ovarian cancer and their families; health care professionals treating people with ovarian cancer. Seeks to advance the prevention, diagnosis, and treatment of ovarian cancer. Serves as a clearinghouse on ovarian cancer; provides support and services to members; conducts educational programs.

★ **10236** ★ **Native American Cancer Research (NACR)**
c/o Linda Burhansstipanov
3022 S Nova Rd
Pine, CO 80470-7830
**Phone:** (303)838-9359          **Fax:** (303)838-7629
**Website:** http://members.aol.com/natamcan/
Linda Burhansstipanov, Pres. /Exec. Dir.

**Fnded:** 1999. **Desc:** Strives to reduce Native American cancer incidence and mortality, and to increase survival from cancer among Native Americans; implements cancer primary prevention, secondary prevention, risk reduction, screening (early detection), education, training, research, diagnoses, control, treatment, support, quality of life, and/or studies of cancer among Native Americans. **Pub:** *Native American Cancer Research Program Newsletter,* 3/year. Newsletter. Informs native and non-natives of Native American cancer prevention and control.

**Oncology Nursing Society (ONS)**
*See:* Entry 15765

★ **10237** ★ **Ovarian Cancer National Alliance**
910 17th St. NW, Ste. 413
Washington, DC 20006
**Phone:** (202)331-1332          **Fax:** (202)292-2292
**Email:** ovarian@aol.com
**Website:** http://www.ovariancancer.org/
Ann Kolker, Contact

**Fnded:** 1997. **Desc:** Works to promote knowledge about breast cancer and works toward a cure.

★ **10238** ★ **Panamerican Society of Phlebology and Lymphology (Sociedad Panamericana de Flebologia y Linfologia)**
Avellaneda 198
1642 San Isidro, Argentina
**Phone:** 54 11 47472373          **Fax:** 54 11 47472373
**Email:** cesanchez@intramed.net.ar
**Fnded:** 1978. **Desc:** Promotes exchange of scientific knowledge through congresses, meetings and workshops.

★ **10239** ★ **Patient Advocates for Advanced Cancer Treatment (PAACT)**
1143 Parmelee NW
Grand Rapids, MI 49504-3844
**Phone:** (616)453-1477          **Fax:** (616)453-1846
**Email:** rhprofit@aol.com
**Website:** http://www.paactusa.org
Janet Ney, Sr., Exec. Officer

**Fnded:** 1984. **Mem:** 36,000. **Desc:** Prostate cancer patients and physicians. Engages in advocacy activities. Provides educational materials to those with prostate cancer. Conducts protocol studies and research. **Pub:** *Cancer Communication,* quarterly. Newsletter. • *Prostate Cancer Report.* Report.

★ **10240** ★ **People Against Cancer (PAC)**
604 East St.
PO Box 10
Otho, IA 50569-0010
**Phone:** (515)972-4444          **Fax:** (515)972-4415
**Email:** info@peopleagainstcancer.com
**Website:** http://www.peopleagainstcancer.com
Frank D. Wiewel, Contact

**Fnded:** 1985. **Mem:** 2,000. **Desc:** Promotes research into alternative cancer therapy and prevention. Conducts educational, charitable, and research programs.

**Pub:** *Options*, quarterly. Newsletter. • Bulletin. • Directory.

**★ 10241 ★ Pituitary Network Association (PNA)**
PO Box 1958
Thousand Oaks, CA 91358
**Phone:** (805)499-9973   **Fax:** (805)499-1523
**Email:** ptna@pituitary.org
**Website:** http://www.pituitary.org
Robert Knutzen, Contact
**Fnded:** 1993. **Mem:** 5,000. **Nat'l Groups:** 4. **Reg. Groups:** 8. **State Groups:** 4. **Desc:** Patients supplying information to other patients, families and health care professionals. Publishes books and news magazines on pituitary issues. **Pub:** *Pituitary Patient Resource Guide*, biennial. Book. Reference guide for pituitary patients, their families, physicians, and all health care providers. *Price:* $39.95 for members; $49.95 for nonmembers. • *PNA Newsletter*, bimonthly. Newsletter. **Frmly:** (1993) PTNA; (2002) Pituitary Tumor Network Association.

**★ 10242 ★ Plasma Protein Therapeutics Association (PPTA)**
1350 I St., NW, Ste. 830
Washington, DC 20005
**Phone:** (202)789-3100   **Fax:** (202)789-4197
Yan Bult, Pres.
**Fnded:** 1992. **Desc:** Works for consensus development of industry-wide initiatives and primary advocate for the world's leading producers of plasma-based and recombinant biological therapeutics.

**★ 10243 ★ R. A. Bloch Cancer Foundation**
4400 Main St., Ste. 500
Kansas City, MO 64111
**Phone:** (816)932-8453   **Free:** 800-433-0464
**Fax:** (816)931-7486
**Email:** hotline@hrbloch.com
**Website:** http://www.blochcancer.org
Donna O'Connor, Contact
**Fnded:** 1980. **Desc:** Sponsors the Cancer Hot Line, a support group that matches cancer patients with volunteers who are survivors of the same type of cancer. Also offers resource information and provides the book "Fighting Cancer" free of charge to anyone dealing with cancer. **Pub:** *Cancer. . .There's Hope*. Book. • *Cancer Hot Line News*, quarterly. • *Fighting Cancer*. Book. • *Guide for Cancer Supporters*. Book. **Frmly:** (1989) Cancer Connection.

**★ 10244 ★ Radiation Therapy Oncology Group (RTOG)**
1101 Market St., 14th Fl.
Philadelphia, PA 19107
**Phone:** (215)574-3189   **Free:** 800-277-5463
**Fax:** (215)923-1737
**Email:** tmckeough@phila.acr.org
**Website:** http://www.rtog.org
Tim McKeough, Admin.
**Fnded:** 1971. **Mem:** 290. **Desc:** Clinical radiation therapy investigative centers united to conduct cooperative clinical trials and studies to improve the care of patients with cancer. Maintains 50 committees. **Pub:** *RTOG Report*. Reprint.

**★ 10245 ★ Reach to Recovery**
c/o American Cancer Society
1599 Clifton Rd.
Atlanta, GA 30329
**Free:** 800-ACS-2345   **Fax:** (404)982-3691
**Website:** http://www.cancer.org/eprise/main/docroot/shr/content/shr_2.1_x_reach_to_r    ecovery?sitearea=shr
Ena Wanless, Mgr. Breast Cancer Programs
**Fnded:** 1952. **Desc:** A peer support program for people with a personal concern about breast cancer; sponsored by the American Cancer Society. Trained volunteers provide support and information for people

and help them meet the physical, emotional and cosmetic needs related to their disease and its treatment. Patient and volunteer may meet face to face or by telephone. Volunteers are able to provide support and up-to-date information, including literature for spouses, partners, children, other loved ones, and friends. **Pub:** *Reach to Recovery Program*. Brochure.

**★ 10246 ★ Rose Kushner Breast Cancer Advisory Center (RKBCAC)**
PO Box 757
Palos Verdes Estates, CA 90274
**Phone:** (310)897-3445   **Fax:** (310)897-3444
**Email:** lkkushner@yahoo.com
**Website:** http://www.rkbcac.org/
Harvey D. Kushner, Ed.
**Fnded:** 1975. **Desc:** Information service for people, mostly women concerned about or with breast cancer. Provides information to public, patients and physicians concerning current knowledge about breast cancer detection, diagnosis, treatment and follow-up. **Pub:** *If You've Thought About Breast Cancer by Rose Kushner*, biennial. Booklet. *Price:* Free. **Frmly:** Breast Cancer Advisory Center; (1991) Women's Breast Cancer Advisory Center; (1991) Women's Breast Cancer Advisory Center.

**Sargent Cancer Care for Children (SCCC)**
*See:* Entry 5751

**★ 10247 ★ Sickle Cell Disease Association of America (SCDAA)**
200 Corporate Pointe, Ste. 495
Culver City, CA 90230-8727
**Phone:** (310)216-6363   **Free:** 800-421-8453
**Fax:** (310)215-3722
**Email:** scdaa@sicklecelldisease.org
Lynda King Anderson, Pres. /COO
**Fnded:** 1971. **Mem:** 65. **Local Groups:** 86. **Desc:** Community groups involved in sickle cell anemia programs throughout the U.S. (Sickle cell anemia is an inherited blood disease that primarily affects black people and is a major health problem within the black community.) Purposes are to: provide leadership on a national level in order to create awareness in all circles of the negative impact of sickle cell anemia on the health and economic, social, and educational well-being of the individual and his/her family and to create awareness of the requirements for resolution; prepare and distribute substantive educational materials; develop and promote implementation of service program standards that will be in the best interest of the affected population; provide ongoing technical assistance to interested groups; encourage adequate support for research. Resources include: counselor training; workshops and seminars; blood banks; screening and testing; tutorial services; camps for children with sickle cell disease; vocational rehabilitation; scholarships. Operates Charles F. Whitten Sickle Cell Summer Research Apprenticeships, Roland J. Nyman Research Fund, and Rick Berry Fund. **Pub:** *Comprehensive Guide to Sickle Cell Disease & SCDAA Services*. • *HELP, A Guide to Sickle Cell Disease Programs and Services*, periodic. • *SCD Parent/Teacher Guide*. • *Sickle Cell Disease Association of America Newsletter*, quarterly. Newsletter. *Price:* Free. • *Sickle Cell Disease Association of America Viewpoint*, periodic. • *Sickle Cell Disease Fact Brochures*. • Brochures. • Pamphlets. **Frmly:** National Association for Sickle Cell Disease.

**★ 10248 ★ Sisters Network**
8787 Broadway Dr., Ste. 4206
Houston, TX 77063
**Phone:** (713)781-0255   **Fax:** (713)780-8998
**Email:** sisnet4@aol.com
**Website:** http://sistersnetworkinc.org
Karen E. Jackson, Contact
**Fnded:** 1994. **Mem:** 800. **Nat'l Groups:** 1. **Reg. Groups:** 6. **State Groups:** 13. **Local Groups:** 25. **Desc:** African-American women who have survived breast cancer. Promotes improved breast health

among African-American women; seeks to reduced the incidence of breast cancer. Gathers and disseminates information on breast cancer prevention and self detection; provides emotional and psychological support to AfricanAmerican women with breast cancer; supports breast cancer research initiatives and advocacy training. **Pub:** Newsletter, periodic.

**★ 10249 ★ Skin Cancer Foundation (SCF)**
245 5th Ave., Ste. 1403
New York, NY 10016
**Phone:** (212)725-5176   **Free:** 800-SKIN-490
**Fax:** (212)725-5751
**Email:** info@skincancer.org
**Website:** http://www.skincancer.org
Perry Robins, MD, Pres.
**Fnded:** 1977. **Desc:** Sponsors medical symposia and public education programs on the prevention and early recognition of skin cancer. Grants its Seal of Recommendation to sunscreen products that meet the criteria and standards established by the SCF as effective aids in the prevention of sun-induced damage to the skin. **Pub:** *Flash!*. Newsletter. *Price:* $5.00. • *Melanoma Letter*, quarterly. Newsletter. Contains articles and commentary on advances in the prevention and treatment of skin cancer. *Price:* $25/year (minimum donation). • *Play it Safe in the Sun*. Book. *Price:* $9.95. • *Skin Cancer Foundation Journal*, annual. Journal. Contains short articles on the prevention, early detection, and treatment of skin cancer. Includes publications list. *Price:* $8/copy. • *Sun and Skin News*, quarterly. Newsletter. Provides practical advice on the prevention, treatment, and early detection of skin cancer. Includes research updates. *Price:* $25/year (minimum donation). • *Sun Sense: A Complete Guide*. Book. *Price:* $14.95. • *Understanding Melanoma, What you need to know*. Book. *Price:* $14.95. • *Worldwide Melanoma Update*. Newsletter. *Price:* $6. Also publishes posters, charts, sun protection guidelines, slide sets, audiovisuals, CD-rom manuals and brochures. **Frmly:** (1978) National Skin Cancer Foundation.

**★ 10250 ★ Sociedad Chilena de Hematologia**
Casilla 166, Correo 55
Santiago, Chile
**Phone:** 56 2 3413113   **Fax:** 56 2 2693394
**Fnded:** 1943.

**★ 10251 ★ Society of Gynecologic Oncologists (SGO)**
401 N Michigan Ave.
Chicago, IL 60611
**Phone:** (312)644-6610   **Fax:** (312)527-6640
**Email:** sgo@sba.com
**Website:** http://www.sgo.org
M. Eileen Widner, Exec. Dir.
**Fnded:** 1969. **Mem:** 772. **Desc:** Purposes are to: improve the care of patients with gynecological cancer; encourage research in gynecologic oncology; advance knowledge in the field; upgrade standards of practice. Evaluates and seeks to address the trends in gynecologic oncology; assesses the future of the field.

**★ 10252 ★ Society for Hematopathology (SH)**
1 Cloister Ct.
Box 101
Bethesda, MD 20814
**Phone:** (301)402-0174   **Fax:** (301)402-0174
**Email:** shollis@mail.nih.gov
**Website:**    http://www.dartmouth.edu/~nlevy/wwwx.html
Stephanie Hollis, Coord.
**Fnded:** 1981. **Mem:** 500. **Desc:** Physicians; doctors of science, osteopathy, veterinary medicine, and dental surgery. Promotes exchange of information and encourages clinical, morphologic, and functional investigation of the hematopoietic (pertaining to the formation of blood cells) and lymphoreticular (regarding reticu-

loendothelial cells of the lymph glands) systems. **Pub:** Newsletter.

## Society for Radiation Oncology Administrators (SROA)
*See:* Entry 9764

## ★ 10253 ★ Society of Surgical Oncology (SSO)
c/o Rick Slawny
85 W Algonquin Rd., Ste. 550
Arlington Heights, IL 60005
**Phone:** (847)427-1400          **Fax:** (847)427-1294
**Email:** sroa@asrt.org
**Website:** http://www.surgonc.org/
Rick Slawny, Exec. Dir.

**Fnded:** 1940. **Mem:** 1,700. **Desc:** Physicians and scientists working in the field of cancer. **Pub:** *Annals of Surgical Oncology*, 10/year. Journal. Includes proceedings of the society's annual scientific sessions. **Frmly:** (1974) James Ewing Society.

## ★ 10254 ★ Susan G. Komen Breast Cancer Foundation (SGKF)
5005 LBJ, Ste. 250
Dallas, TX 75244
**Phone:** (972)855-1600          **Free:** 800-IM-AWARE
**Fax:** (972)855-1605
**Website:** http://www.breastcancerinfo.com
Susan Braun, CEO/Pres.

**Fnded:** 1982. **Mem:** 45,000. **Nat'l Groups:** 114. **Desc:** Breast cancer patients, health care professionals, and other interested individuals. Works to: increase the recovery and survival rates of breast cancer patients; heighten public awareness of the risks of breast cancer and the need for early detection. Establishes breast screening and training in self-examination procedures; provides funding through grants for research and screening programs. Sponsors educational programs. Bestows awards; sponsors competitions; maintains speakers' bureau. **Pub:** *Frontline*, quarterly. Newsletter. Highlights current breast cancer issues and Komen events. *Price:* Free. **Frmly:** (1989) Susan G. Komen Foundation.

## ★ 10255 ★ Swedish Hemophilia Society (FBIS)
Box 55507
S-102 04 Stockholm, Sweden
**Phone:** 46 8 54640510          **Fax:** 46 8 54640514
**Email:** info@tbis.se
**Website:** http://www.tbis.se

**Fnded:** 1964. **Mem:** 1,325. **Nat'l Groups:** 1. **Reg. Groups:** 8. **Lang(s):** English, Swedish. **Desc:** Individuals with hemophilia and their families; health care professionals and other individuals providing support to people with hemophilia. Seeks to improve the quality of life of people with hemophilia; works to advance the treatment of hemophilia and related disorders. Facilitates communication and cooperation among members; sponsors educational programs.

## ★ 10256 ★ Terry Fox Foundation (TFF)
789 Don Mills Rd., Ste. 802
Toronto, ON, Canada M3C 1T5
**Phone:** (416)962-7866          **Fax:** (416)962-5677
**Email:** national@terryfoxrun.org
**Website:** http://www.terryfoxrun.org

**Fnded:** 1981. **Lang(s):** English, French. **Desc:** Individuals and organizations. Seeks to "maintain the vision and principles of Terry Fox;" promotes and supports research into the causes and treatment of cancer. Conducts fundraising activities benefitting cancer research. **Pub:** Newsletter, periodic. • Brochure.

## ★ 10257 ★ Ulster Cancer Foundation (UCF)
40-42 Eglantine Ave.
Belfast BT9 6DX, United Kingdom

**Phone:** 44 1232 663281          **Fax:** 44 1232 660081
**Email:** ucf1@unite.net
**Website:** http://www.ulstercancer.org

**Fnded:** 1970. **Local Groups:** 60. **Lang(s):** English. **Desc:** Encourages and facilitates research on cancer and its prevention and early diagnosis. Seeks to help patients and their families cope with cancer. Works for new and better treatments for cancer, helps people reduce their risk of developing the disease. Conducts educational programs including clinics and training sessions for health care professionals; makes available children's services; sponsors competitions and bestows awards. Compiles statistics. **Pub:** *Cancer Control in Practice*. Book. A training and resource park for practice nurses. • *Cancer Education and Care in the Workplace*. Book. • *Environmental Health Perspectives on Cancer*. • *Focus on Cancer in Schools*. • *Smoking Matters for Young People*.

## Veterinary Cancer Society (VCS)
*See:* Entry 20656

## ★ 10258 ★ Woman To Woman
c/o Dr. Lucie A. DiMaggio
1807 Elmwood Ave., Ste. 165
Buffalo, NY 14207-2434
**Email:** info@womantowomanvideos.org
**Website:** http://www.vetcancersociety.org
Dr. Lucie A. DiMaggio, Founder

**Desc:** Provides videos and resource guides for newly diagnosed breast-cancer patients. Offers education, support and comfort. **Pub:** *NWL*. • Videos.

## ★ 10259 ★ Women's Cancer Network (WCN)
401 N Michigan Ave.
Chicago, IL 60611
**Phone:** (312)644-6610
**Email:** gcp@sba.com
**Website:** http://www.wcn.org

**Desc:** Disseminates information about various types of gynecologic cancer. Educates women on the prevention and treatment of cancer.

## ★ 10260 ★ Women's Healthcare Educational Network (WHEN)
9 Jackson St.
Tiffin, OH 44883
**Free:** 800-991-8877          **Fax:** (419)443-0785
**Email:** info@whenusa.org
**Website:** http://www.whenusa.org
Georgette O-Brien, Pres.

**Fnded:** 1990. **Mem:** 75. **Desc:** An organization of businesses providing services to women who have undergone cancer surgery. Seeks to "increase awareness of the post breast cancer women, the medical communities, managed care providers, and support groups to the importance of proper external breast form fitting procedures." Assists corporations in the development of breast prostheses and clothing for women who have undergone breast cancer surgery; conducts educational programs for busines owners. **Pub:** *One Voice*, quarterly. Newsletter. Contains information on breast cancer and women's health issues. *Price:* $10/yr to non-members; Included in membership.

## ★ 10261 ★ World Federation of Hemophilia (WFH) (Federation Mondiale de l'Hemophilie — FMH)
1425 Rene-Levesque West
Ste. 1010
Montreal, QC, Canada H3G 1T7
**Phone:** (514)875-7944          **Fax:** (514)875-8916
**Email:** wfh@wfh.org
**Website:** http://wfh.org

**Fnded:** 1963. **Mem:** 1,000. **Nat'l Groups:** 88. **Reg. Groups:** 3. **Lang(s):** French, Spanish. **Desc:** Representatives of national hemophilia committees or societies. Assists individuals with hemophilia and persons

with related disorders. Aims to stimulate interest in the development and improvement of diagnosis, treatment, rehabilitation, education, and research in hemophilia. Serves as a coordinating body to develop the collection, distribution and exchange of useful information and to make relevant investigations throughout the world. Encourages the establishment and development of other hemophilia organizations. Compiles statistics. **Pub:** *Hemophilia World*, quarterly. Newsletter. • *Information Update*, periodic. Bulletin.

## ★ 10262 ★ Y-ME National Breast Cancer Organization (Y-ME)
212 W Van Buren, 5th Fl.
Chicago, IL 60607
**Phone:** (312)986-8338          **Free:** 800-221-2141
**Fax:** (312)294-8597
**Email:** ymeone@aol.com
**Website:** http://www.y-me.org
Susan N. Nathanson, Ph.D, Exec. Dir.

**Fnded:** 1978. **Mem:** 15,000. **Nat'l Groups:** 25. **State Groups:** 23. **Local Groups:** 23. **Desc:** Purpose is to provide peer support, education and information to women who have or suspect they have breast cancer. Activities include presurgical counseling inservice programs for health professionals, hot line volunteer training, and technical assistance. Administers the Deborah David Dewar Fund, the Billie Klein Memorial Fund, Shellie Broutman Memorial, Eve & Susan Feldman Memorial and Mimi Kaplan Memorial. Provides a Latino program, teen breast health program, and adult workshops regarding mammography screening and breast self-exam. **Pub:** *A Women's Guide to Breast Cancer*. Brochure. • *Every Women's Guide to Breast Cancer*. Price: One copy is free. • *I Still Buy Green Bananas: Living with Hope...Breast Cancer*. Brochure. • *Just For Teens*. Brochure. • *When the Woman You Love Has Breast Cancer*. • *Y-ME Hotline*, bimonthly. Newsletter. • Breast Cancer Just for Teens!; A Woman's Guide to Breast Care. All brochures available in English and Spanish. **Frmly:** (1989) Y-Me Breast Cancer Support; (1994) Y-Me National Organization for Breast Cancer Information and Support.

# Research Centers

## ★ 10263 ★ Abbott Northwestern Hospital David F. Hickok Memorial Cancer Research Laboratory
800 E 28th St.
Minneapolis, MN 55407
**Phone:** (612)863-4339
**Email:** editor@epress.com
**Website:** http://www.msi.umn.edu/Projects/mg90601/anwhome.html
Lester F. Harris, PhD, Sci. Dir.

**Activities/Fields:** Breast cancer.

## ★ 10264 ★ Albany Medical College Center for Cancer and Blood Disorders
47 New Scotland Ave., Mail Code 52
Albany, NY 12208
**Phone:** (518)262-5297          **Fax:** (518)262-5975
**Email:** lymang@mail.amc.edu
Dr. Gary Lyman, Hd.

**Activities/Fields:** Cancer and blood disorders, focusing on medical oncology, hematology, radiotherapy, pathology, surgery, and bone marrow transplantation.

## ★ 10265 ★ Albert Einstein College of Medicine Albert Einstein Clinical Cancer Center
Chanin Bldg., Rm. 209
1300 Morris Park Ave.
Bronx, NY 10461
**Phone:** (718)430-2302          **Fax:** (718)430-8550
**Email:** igoldman@aecom.yu.edu

**Website:** http://www.aecom.yu.edu/cancer
I. David Goldman, MD, Dir.

**Activities/Fields:** Cancer, including studies on carcinogenesis and chemotherapeutic agents, regulation of growth and function in normal and cancer cells, cell structure and metabolism in normal and cancer cells, immuno-oncology, viral oncology, genetics, membrane synthesis, nucleic acid synthesis, gene expression in malignant cells, and cell function and regulation. Conducts clinical cancer studies. **Frmly:** Montefiore Medical Center; Cancer Research Center.

**★ 10266 ★ AMC Cancer Research Center and Foundation**
1600 Pierce St.
Denver, CO 80214
**Phone:** (303)233-6501       **Free:** 800-321-1557
**Fax:** (303)239-3400
**Email:** slagat@amc.org
**Website:** http://www.amc.org
Thomas J. Slaga, PhD, Pres. /CEO

**Activities/Fields:** Cancer prevention and control, focusing on early diagnosis, nutrition, chemoprevention, metabolic epidemiology, and intervention trials in human populations, particularly women and underserved populations. Promotes the application of knowledge to reduce cancer incidence and mortality rates.

**★ 10267 ★ American Association for Cancer Research**
Public Ledger Bldg., Ste. 826
150 S Independence Mall W
Philadelphia, PA 19106-3483
**Phone:** (215)440-9300       **Fax:** (215)440-9313
**Email:** foti@aacr.org
**Website:** http://www.aacr.org
Margaret Foti, Contact

**Activities/Fields:** Cancer, focusing on observation, problems, and new significant research.

**★ 10268 ★ American Health Foundation**
1 Dana Rd.
Valhalla, NY 10595
**Phone:** (914)789-7158
**Website:** http://www.ahf.org
Daniel W. Nixon, MD, Pres.

**Activities/Fields:** Improves methods of prevention of cancer and other diseases, trains health professionals, and teaches the public how to reduce risk factors of disease. Conducts collaborative laboratory studies with hospitals in cellular and molecular biology, chemical and environmental carcinogenesis, cell genetics, and the nutritional aspects of disease. **Pub:** *Preventive Medicine*, monthly.

**★ 10269 ★ American Institute for Cancer Research (AICR)**
1759 R St. NW
Washington, DC 20009
**Phone:** (202)328-7744       **Free:** 800-843-8114
**Fax:** (202)328-7226
**Email:** aicrweb@aicr.org
**Website:** http://www.aicr.org
Glen Weldon, Contact

**Activities/Fields:** Provides grants to universities and nonprofit institutions on the role of diet and nutrition in the prevention and adjuvant treatment of cancer. **Pub:** *AICR Newsletter*, quarterly. • *Cancer Resource for cancer patients*. • *Children's newsletter*. • *Meal Planning Reference Book for Dietians*.

**★ 10270 ★ American Italian Cancer Foundation**
112 E 71st St., Ste. 2b
New York, NY 10021-4121
**Phone:** (212)628-9090       **Fax:** (212)517-6089
**Email:** aicf@aicfonline.com
**Website:** http://www.aicfonline.org
Daniele Bodini, Chairman

**Activities/Fields:** Cancer prevention and treatment.

**★ 10271 ★ Arizona State University Cancer Research Institute**
Tempe, AZ 85287-2404
**Phone:** (480)965-0186       **Fax:** (480)965-8558
**Email:** BPettit@asu.edu
**Website:** http://www.asu.edu/clas/cancer_research/
Dr. George R. Pettit, Dir.

**Activities/Fields:** Discovery of new cancer chemotherapeutic drugs for human treatment employing organic chemistry, biochemistry, and biology, including a unique program concerned with isolation, structural identification, and syntheses of naturally occurring anticancer agents from marine animals, plants, and microorganisms.

**★ 10272 ★ Association of American Cancer Institutes**
Iroquois Bldg., Ste. 305
200 Lothrop St.
Pittsburgh, PA 15213
**Phone:** (412)647-2076       **Fax:** (412)647-3659
**Email:** stewartbd@msx.upmc.edu
**Website:** http://www.aaci-cancer.org
Barbara Duffy Stewart, Exec. Dir.

**Activities/Fields:** Causes, nature, prevention, treatment, and rehabilitation of cancer.

**★ 10273 ★ Association for Research of Childhood Cancer**
PO Box 251
Buffalo, NY 14225-0251
**Phone:** (716)681-4433
**Website:** http://www.arocc.org
Ann O'Donnell, Pres.

**Activities/Fields:** Pediatric cancer, focusing on funding, expanding, and continuing of research centers. Also provides seed money for pilot projects in cancer research.

**★ 10274 ★ Barbara Ann Karmanos Cancer Institute**
4100 John R
Detroit, MI 48201
**Phone:** (313)966-7170       **Free:** 800-527-6266
**Fax:** (313)966-7173
**Email:** vaitkevi@karmanos.org
**Website:** http://www.karmanos.org
Dr. Vainutis Vaitkevicius, Dir.

**Activities/Fields:** Treatment, diagnosis, and prevention of cancer. **Pub:** *Karmanos*, weekly. **Frmly:** Detroit Institute for Cancer Research, Michigan Cancer Foundation.

**★ 10275 ★ Bastyr University Bastyr University Cancer Research Center (BUCRC)**
14500 Juanita Dr. NE
Kenmore, WA 98028
**Phone:** (425)823-1300       **Fax:** (425)823-6222
**Email:** buri@bastyr.edu
**Website:** http://www.bastyr.edu/research/bucrc/
Leanna J. Standish, PhD, Res. Dir.

**Activities/Fields:** Natural medical therapies for treatment and prevention of cancer.

**★ 10276 ★ Baton Rouge Regional Tumor Registry**
4950 Essen Ln.
Baton Rouge, LA 70809
**Phone:** (225)767-0430       **Fax:** (225)215-1356
**Email:** gayd@marybird.com
Gay Duke, Dir.

**Activities/Fields:** Provides a base of statistical information of cancer incidence in the Baton Rouge area and serves as a useful tool for physicians investigating the success rates of various forms of cancer treatment. Conducts specialized studies in conjunction with the American Cancer Society, National Cancer Institute, and the American College of Surgeons. **Pub:** *Annual Report*. • *Louisiana Tumor Registry*.

**★ 10277 ★ Bay Area Tumor Institute**
400 30th St., Ste. 301
Oakland, CA 94609-3305
**Phone:** (510)465-8570       **Fax:** (510)465-8588
**Email:** bsiegel@bati.org
**Website:** http://www.bati.org
Barry B. Siegel, Pres.

**Activities/Fields:** Phase 2 and phase 3 clinical drug trials for cancer therapy.

**Baylor College of Medicine Center for Cell and Gene Therapy**
*See:* Entry 9372

**Baylor University Medical Center Blood and Bone Marrow Transplant Program**
*See:* Entry 20348

**★ 10278 ★ The Blood Center**
PO Box 2178
Milwaukee, WI 53201-2178
**Phone:** (414)933-5000       **Fax:** (414)937-6284
**Email:** rlgnerlich@bcsew.edu
**Website:** http://www.bloodctrwise.org
John W. Adamson, MD, Exec. VP/Res.

**Activities/Fields:** Blood-related research in the areas of platelets, hemostasis/thrombosis, immunogenetics, vascular biology, stem cell biology, and transfusion medicine. Major activities include the collection and distribution of blood and blood products, basic research, clinical laboratory testing, and bone marrow donor recruitment. **Pub:** *Annual Report*.

**Blood and Marrow Transplant Laboratory**
*See:* Entry 20349

**★ 10279 ★ Boston Comprehensive Sickle Cell Center**
FGH Bldg., 2nd Fl.
Boston Medical Center
820 Harrison Ave.
Boston, MA 02118
**Phone:** (617)414-5727       **Fax:** (617)414-5739
**Email:** lillian.mcmahon@bmc.org
Dr. Lillian E.C. McMahon, Nurse/Mgr.

**Activities/Fields:** Sickle cell trait and sickle cell anemia/disease, including molecular, cellular, tissue, and organ studies. Investigates glucose 6-phosphate dehydrogenase deficiency, coagulation and carbomylation of hemoglobin S, anti-sickling compounds, red cell membrane alterations, fetal jeopardy, fetal hemoglobin synthesis, cardiac manifestations, lung function, and infection. Conducts ultrastructural and clinical studies and seeks to translate basic and clinical research to improved health care at the community level. **Pub:** *Educational Booklets*.

**★ 10280 ★ Boston University Cancer Research Center (CRC)**
715 Albany St., K-703
Boston, MA 02118
**Phone:** (617)638-8265       **Fax:** (617)638-6518
**Email:** sfenness@bu.edu
**Website:** http://www.bumc.bu.edu/Departments/HomeMain.asp?DepartmentID=109
Salli Fennessey, Contact

**Activities/Fields:** Cancer, including cellular and molecular biology, receptors, carcinogenesis, immunology, toxicology, molecular genetics, nucleic acid damage and repair, mechanism of action of chemotherapeutic agents, and new approaches to cancer treatment. Affiliated hospitals provide a wide variety of specialized approaches to clinical management of cancer, including surgery, radiation therapy, chemotherapy, and immunotherapy. Patients entered on local, regional, and national treatment protocols. **Frmly:** Hubert H. Humphrey Cancer Research Center.

## ★ 10281 ★ Brigham Young University Cancer Research Center
S125 Eyring Science Center
PO Box 24629
Provo, UT 84602-4629
**Phone:** (801)378-3913      **Fax:** (801)378-5474
**Email:** cancer_research@byu.edu
**Website:** http://cancerresearch.byu.edu
Daniel L. Simmons, PhD, Dir.
**Activities/Fields:** Chemistry and biochemistry of nucleic acids and their derivatives as potential medicinal agents, including synthesis of antiviral and antitumor agents, detection of carcinogenic materials in the environment, isolation and study of antitumor agents from natural products, and study of the biochemical mechanism of action of various antitumor agents. **Pub:** *The Cancer Chronicle*, bimonthly.

## ★ 10282 ★ British Columbia Cancer Agency
**British Columbia Cancer Research Centre**
601 W 10th Ave.
Vancouver, BC, Canada V5Z 1L3
**Phone:** (604)877-6152      **Fax:** (604)877-6010
**Email:** vling@bccancer.bc.ca
**Website:** http://www.bccancer.bc.ca/research
Dr. Victor Ling, VP, Res.
**Activities/Fields:** Maintains eight departments for cancer research: Advanced Therapeutics - developing and testing new and more effective treatments for cancer. Cancer Control Research - working to understand the risk factors of cancer and developing cancer prevention strategies. Cancer Endocrinology - finding new treatments for endocrine-related cancers, such as prostate cancer. Cancer Genetics and developmental Biology (Centre for Intergrated Genomics) - a specialty lab for identifying genomic changes and the signalling and metabolic pathways associated with tumour development. Cancer Imaging - Focusing on developing new technology for early detection and localization of cancer and pre-cancerous lesions. Genome Sequence Centre- A high-throughput genomic science centre dedicated to cancer research. Medical Biophysics - Making inroads into understanding cancer biology and the practical aspects of radiotherapy and related treatments. Terry Fox Lab - Developing new technology for diagnosis and treatment of cancers of the blood and lymphatic system, and new understanding of the control of cell growth and differentiation, aging and gene regulation. **Pub:** *Annual Report*.

## ★ 10283 ★ British Columbia Cancer Agency
**British Columbia Cancer Research Centre**
**Department of Cancer Endocrinology**
600 W 10th Ave.
Vancouver, BC, Canada V5Z 4E6
**Phone:** (604)877-6015      **Fax:** (604)877-6011
**Email:** schou@bccancer.bc.ca
**Website:** http://www.bccancer.bc.ca
**Activities/Fields:** Molecular basis of early progression of prostate cancer to androgen independence, and early detection of primary and metastatic disease. New therapies under development include Intermittent Androgen Suppression (IAS) and peptide memetics to prevent lygand independent activation of the androgen receptor. The experimental Nb2 node lymphoma is also maintained for studies on the mitogenic properties of prolactin and growth hormone.

## ★ 10284 ★ British Columbia Cancer Agency
**British Columbia Cancer Research Centre**
**Medical Biophysics Department**
601 W 10th Ave.
Vancouver, BC, Canada V5Z 4E6
**Phone:** (604)877-6010      **Fax:** (604)877-6002
**Email:** rdurand@bccancer.bc.ca
**Website:** http://http://www.bccrc.ca/mb/
Dr. R.E. Durand, Hd.
**Activities/Fields:** Laboratory and clinical studies on control of cancer, particularly radiation therapy and adjuncts to radiation therapy, including radiosensitizers and chemotherapy. Also conducts basic studies of tumor growth, angiogenesis mutagenesis and radiation damage mechanisms.

## ★ 10285 ★ British Columbia Cancer Agency
**British Columbia Cancer Research Centre**
**Terry Fox Laboratory for Hematology/ Oncology**
601 W 10th Ave.
Vancouver, BC, Canada V5Z 1L3
**Phone:** (604)877-6070      **Fax:** (604)877-0712
**Email:** allen@terryfox.ubc.ca
**Website:** http://www.bccrc.ca/tfl/index.html
Dr. Allen C. Eaves, Dir.
**Activities/Fields:** Hematology and oncology, particularly the regulation of growth and differentiation in normal and malignant hemopoiesis and lymphopoiesis. Research activities focus on studies of hemopoietic progenitors, bone marrow transplantation, gene therapy, aging, cell adhesion, metastasis, growth factors and receptors, and signal transduction mechanisms.

## ★ 10286 ★ British Columbia Cancer Agency
**British Columbia Cancer Research Centre**
**Vancouver Cancer Centre**
601 W 10th Ave.
Vancouver, BC, Canada V5Z 1L3
**Phone:** (604)877-6000      **Free:** 800-663-3333
**Fax:** (604)877-0585
Dr. Susan O'Reilly, Hd.
**Activities/Fields:** Development of new therapeutic and diagnostic procedures for cancer patients, use of biological agents such as interferon and IL-2, new methods of delivery of anticancer drugs, including use of liposomes, mechanisms of mutations to resistance within tumors, and development of genetically engineered tumor cell vaccines.

## ★ 10287 ★ British Columbia Children's Hospital
**Children's and Women's Health Centre of British Columbia**
980 W 28th Ave.
CMMT Bldg., Rm. 2092
Vancouver, BC, Canada V5Z 4H4
**Phone:** (604)875-3602      **Fax:** (604)875-3601
**Email:** dkalousek@cw.bc.ca
Prof. Dagmar K. Kalousek, Dir.
**Activities/Fields:** Chromosomal mosaicism and its effect on human intrauterine development, specifically the correlation between chromosomal complement of placenta and intrauterine development of the fetus.

## ★ 10288 ★ Burnham Institute
10901 N Torrey Pines Rd.
La Jolla, CA 92037
**Phone:** (858)646-3100      **Fax:** (858)646-3199
**Email:** ruoslahti@burnham.org
**Website:** http://www.burnham.org/
Erkki Ruoslahti, MD, Pres. /CEO
**Activities/Fields:** Cell adhesion and extracellular matrix, neurobiology, glycobiology, gene regulation, oncogene and tumor suppressor gene, apoptosis and cell death, degenerative disease research and aging, and bioinformatics and biological complexity. **Pub:** *Annual Report*.

## ★ 10289 ★ Burzynski Research Institute
9432 Old Katy Rd., Ste. 200
Houston, TX 77055
**Phone:** (713)335-5697      **Fax:** (713)335-5699
**Email:** info@burzynskiclinic.com
**Website:** http://www.cancermed.com
Dr. Stanislaw R. Burzynski, Founder
**Activities/Fields:** Antineoplastons A 10 and AS21 in the treatment of cancer. Antineoplastons are peptides and amino acid derivatives that are apoptosis inducers, working at the level of p53 tumor suppressor genes and ras oncogenes.

## ★ 10290 ★ Cancer Biotherapy Research Group (CBRG)
PO Box 680757
Franklin, TN 37068-0757
**Phone:** (615)791-6393      **Fax:** (615)791-4719
**Email:** cbrg_cancer@compuserve.com
**Website:** http://www.cbrg.org
Rosalie A. Crispin, Exec. Dir.
**Activities/Fields:** Clinical cancer research, focusing on the treatment of solid cancer tumors in adults and the use of biologicals and biological response modifiers alone or in combination with other treatment modalities. **Pub:** *NBSG Newsletter*, biennially. **Frmly:** National Biotherapy Study Group.

## ★ 10291 ★ Cancer Care Ontario
620 University Ave.
Toronto, ON, Canada M5G 2L7
**Phone:** (416)971-5100      **Fax:** (416)971-6888
**Email:** Kristin.Jenkins@cancercare.on.ca
**Website:** http://www.cancercare.on.ca
Dr. Alan Hudson, Pres. /CEO
**Activities/Fields:** Cancer prevention, early detection, diagnosis, treatment, and supportive care. Supports basic and clinical scientists at eight Regional Cancer Centers throughout Ontario and in the Division of Preventive Oncology. **Pub:** *Cancer Care.* ● *Publications on cancer incidence and mortality.* **Frmly:** Ontario Cancer Treatment and Research Foundation.

## ★ 10292 ★ Cancer Care Ontario
**London Regional Cancer Centre**
790 Commissioners Rd. E
London, ON, Canada N6A 4L6
**Phone:** (519)685-8600      **Fax:** (519)685-8614
**Email:** research@lrcc.on.ca
**Website:** http://www.lrcc.on.ca/
Dr. James Koropatnick, Dir.
**Activities/Fields:** Molecular biology of cancer, with emphasis on tumor metastasis and progression and on drug resistance studies; molecular endocrinology, with emphasis on intracellular transportation of steroid hormones; and steroid receptors in breast cancer. Studies include physics and radiation oncology, including 3-D imaging, brachytherapy, portal imaging, and clinical trials. Medical oncology research program focuses on bone marrow transplantation, biological response modifiers, and dose intensity.

## ★ 10293 ★ Cancer and Leukemia Group B
208 S LaSalle St., Ste. 2000
Chicago, IL 60604-1104
**Phone:** (773)702-9171      **Fax:** (773)345-0117
**Email:** ksartell@midway.uchicago.edu
**Website:** http://www.calgb.org/
Richard L. Schilsky, MD, Gp. Chm.
**Activities/Fields:** Cooperative group conducting therapeutic multi-modal, multi-institutional, randomized cancer clinical trials primarily in seven disease areas: leukemia, lymphoma, breast, gastrointestinal, genitourinary, respiratory and melanoma. Aims to increase the number of cases brought under complete remission from cancer by increasing knowledge of the disease process and appropriate treatments. Affiliated with several pathology, immunology, and cytogenetic laboratories.

## ★ 10294 ★ Cancer Research Center
3501 Berrywood Dr.
Columbia, MO 65201
**Phone:** (573)875-2255      **Fax:** (573)443-1202
**Email:** eisenstarkA@missouri.edu
**Website:** http://www.cancerresearchcenter.org
Dr. Abraham Eisenstark, Scientific Dir.
**Activities/Fields:** Basic oncology and studies in immunology, microbiology, protein biochemistry, bioengi-

neering, carcinogenesis, and cancer detection. Specific studies include biochemical markers for early detection of cancer cells, environmental carcinogenesis, and oxidative cellular damage. **Pub:** *The Mirror*, quarterly.

**★ 10295 ★ Cancer Research Foundation**
PO Box 0493
Chicago, IL 60690-0493
**Phone:** (312)630-0055          **Fax:** (312)630-0075
**Email:** crf@cancerresearchfdn.org
**Website:** http://www.cancerresearchfdn.org
Merle Goldblatt Cohen, Pres.
**Activities/Fields:** Funds laboratory and clinical cancer research at Chicago universities and medical schools. **Pub:** *Annual Report.* • *Newsletters.*

**★ 10296 ★ Cancer Research Institute, Inc.**
681 5th Ave.
New York, NY 10022
**Phone:** (212)688-7515          **Free:** 800-992-2623
**Fax:** (212)832-9376
**Email:** info@cancerresearch.org
**Website:** http://www.cancerresearch.org
Carlos A. Ferrer, Chm.
**Activities/Fields:** Supports research projects in fundamental immunology and cancer immunology that seek to develop cancer therapies based on the immune system. **Pub:** *Annual Report.* • *Cancer and the Immune System: The Vital Connection.* • *The Cancer Research Institute Help Book: What to Do If Cancer Strikes.* • *Prostate cancer and melanoma brochures.*

**★ 10297 ★ Cancer Research Laboratory**
Children's Hospital of Orange County
455 S Main St.
Orange, CA 92868
**Phone:** (714)532-8548          **Fax:** (714)516-4277
**Email:** vslone@choc.org
Dr. Leonard Sender, Dir.
**Activities/Fields:** Experimental hematopoiesis, tumor vaccines. **Frmly:** Pediatric Cancer Research Laboratory.

**★ 10298 ★ Cancer Resource Center**
4600 Valley Rd., Ste. 336
Lincoln, NE 68510
**Phone:** (402)483-2827          **Free:** 800-487-8786
**Fax:** (402)483-2882
**Email:** dseuss@lmef.org
**Website:** http://www.lmef.org
Barb Morton, Dir.
**Activities/Fields:** Oncology, especially pathology and radiotherapy, and drug studies for pharmaceutical companies. **Frmly:** Lincoln Cancer Center.

**★ 10299 ★ CancerCare Manitoba**
675 McDermot Ave.
Winnipeg, MB, Canada R3E 0V9
**Phone:** (204)787-2241          **Fax:** (204)787-1184
**Email:** brent.schacter@cancercare.mb.ca
**Website:** http://www.cancercare.mb.ca
Dr. Brent A. Schacter, Pres. /CEO
**Activities/Fields:** Cancer treatment and research, including radiation oncology, psychosocial oncology, surgical oncology, hematology, medical oncology, pediatric oncology, gynecologic oncology, medical physics, epidemiology, biostatistics, molecular biology, biochemical pharmacology, and immunology. Clinical trial research in association with NSABP, NCIC, CCSG. **Pub:** *Annual Report.*

**★ 10300 ★ Carcinoid Cancer Foundation, Inc.**
1751 York Ave.
New York, NY 10128
**Phone:** (212)722-3132          **Free:** 888-722-3132
**Fax:** (212)831-3031
**Email:** mwarner@carcinoid.org
**Website:** http://www.carcinoid.org
Monica Warner, Res. Coord.
**Activities/Fields:** Carcinoid tumors, carcinoid syndrome, and other related neuroendocrine tumors.

**★ 10301 ★ Carson-Newman College Cancer Research Project**
Jefferson City, TN 37760
**Phone:** (865)475-9061          **Fax:** (865)471-3578
**Activities/Fields:** Provides compounds for testing against tumors in animals and the AIDS virus; and tuberculosis; and drug delivery targeting.

**★ 10302 ★ Center for Blood Research**
800 Huntington Ave.
Boston, MA 02115
**Phone:** (617)731-6470          **Fax:** (617)731-5676
**Email:** lanner@cbr.med.harvard.edu
Michael Lanner, Exec. VP
**Activities/Fields:** Human blood, including multidisciplinary studies on heart disease, diabetes, cancer, AIDS, hemophilia, sickle cell anemia, mental illness, hepatitis, Rh factor in pregnancy, serum proteins, blood collection methods, preservation of formed elements, methods of plasma fractionation, and characterization of plasma components.

**Center for Molecular Medicine and Immunology**
*See:* Entry 3242

**★ 10303 ★ Center for Radiation Therapy**
MC 9006
5758 S Maryland Ave.
Chicago, IL 60637
**Phone:** (773)702-0817          **Fax:** (773)834-7233
**Email:** rrw@radonc.uchospitals.edu
Ralph Weichselbaum, MD, Ch.
**Activities/Fields:** Cancer and treatment, including studies in radiation oncology, radiation biology, chemotherapy, and oncology information systems.

**★ 10304 ★ Center for Research in Thrombolysis**
Brigham & Women's Hospital
75 Francis St.
Boston, MA 02115
**Phone:** (617)732-5537          **Fax:** (617)732-5343
**Email:** jotten@bics.bwh.harvard.edu
Jeff Otten, Pres.
**Activities/Fields:** Biochemistry and molecular biology of the mammalian fibrinolytic system. Projects include isolating and cloning membrane receptors and constructing and characterizing mutant forms of fibrinolytic inhibitors.

**★ 10305 ★ Centre for Integrated Genomics (CIG)**
Biotechnology Laboratory
University of British Columbia
6174 University Blvd., No. 237
Vancouver, BC, Canada V6T 1Z3
**Phone:** (604)822-4838          **Fax:** (604)822-2114
**Email:** biotech@interchange.ubc.ca
**Website:** http://www.biotech.ubc.ca
Dr. Doug Kilburn, Co-Dir.
**Activities/Fields:** Structural and functional genomics as they relate to cancer and the identification of genes involved in, or responsible for, oncogenesis and tumor progression. Although cancer research is the main focus of the center, applying genome science to problems in the basic life sciences and biotechnology is also a consideration.

**★ 10306 ★ Charity Hospital of New Orleans**
**Oncology Treatment Unit**
Medical Center of Louisiana
1532 Tulane Ave.
New Orleans, LA 70112
**Phone:** (504)568-3214          **Fax:** (504)568-3653
Walter Smith, Dir.
**Activities/Fields:** Cancer, including clinical studies in chemotherapy, immunotherapy, surgery, and hyperthermia.

**★ 10307 ★ Chicago Medical School**
**H.M. Bligh Cancer Research Laboratories**
3333 Green Bay Rd.
North Chicago, IL 60064
**Phone:** (847)578-3230          **Fax:** (847)578-3349
**Email:** kimy@finchcms.edu
Prof. Yoon Burn Kim, MD, Actg. Dir.
**Activities/Fields:** Human cancer research, especially breast and lung cancer. Research activities include early immuno-detection of carcinomas, and active use of T/Tn antigen vaccine to prevent recurrence of advanced breast carcinoma.

**★ 10308 ★ Children's Center for Cancer and Blood Disorders**
Richland Memorial Hospital
University of South Carolina School of Medicine
7 Richland Medical Pk., Ste. 203
Columbia, SC 29203
**Phone:** (803)434-3533          **Fax:** (803)434-3094
**Email:** ronnie.neuberg@palmettohealth.edu
Dr. Ronnie W. Neuberg, Dir.
**Activities/Fields:** Causes, treatments, and prevention of childhood cancer.

**★ 10309 ★ Children's Leukemia Research Association**
585 Stewart Ave., Ste. 18
Garden City, NY 11530
**Phone:** (516)222-1944          **Fax:** (516)222-0457
**Email:** clra@erols.com
**Website:** http://www.childrensleukemia.org
Allan D. Weinberg, Exec. Dir.
**Activities/Fields:** Leukemia research and public awareness of the disease.

**★ 10310 ★ Children's Oncology Group Research Data Center**
104 N Main St., Ste. 600
Gainesville, FL 32601
**Phone:** (352)392-5633          **Fax:** (352)392-8162
**Website:** http://www.childrensoncologygroup.org
Dr. Stephen Hunger, Contact
**Activities/Fields:** Pathobiology of childhood cancers, focusing on control measures and improving treatment outcomes.

**★ 10311 ★ Colorado Cancer Research Program**
2253 S Oneida, 3rd Fl, Ste. B
Denver, CO 80224-2522
**Phone:** (303)777-2663          **Free:** 888-785-6789
**Fax:** (303)777-2642
**Email:** ccrp@co-cancerresearch.org
**Website:** http://www.co-cancerresearch.org
Peter C. Raich, MD, Prin. Investigator
**Activities/Fields:** Cancer and clinical oncology.

**★ 10312 ★ Colorado Neurological Institute**
**CNI Brain Tumor Program**
701 E Hampden Ave., Ste. 160
Englewood, CO 80110
**Phone:** (303)806-7420
**Email:** jbriles@thecni.org
**Website:** http://thecni.org/braintumor/
Edward B. Arenson, MD, Co-Dir.

**Activities/Fields:** Photodynamic therapy for the treatment of brain tumors.

### ★ 10313 ★ Columbia University
**Herbert Irving Comprehensive Cancer Center**
622 W 168th St., PH 18-200
New York, NY 10032
**Phone:** (212)305-9327     **Fax:** (212)305-7846
**Email:** kha4@columbia.edu
**Website:** http://www.ccc.columbia.edu/
Karen Antman, MD, Dir.

**Activities/Fields:** Molecular tumor virology, oncogenes, molecular and clinical genetics, biophysics, cell biology, basic mechanisms of carcinogenesis, molecular epidemiology, biochemistry, endocrinology, developmental biology, cancer epidemiology, sociomedical sciences, occupational health, and biostatistics and data management. **Frmly:** Columbia Presbyterian Cancer Center.

### ★ 10314 ★ Comprehensive Sickle Cell Center (Cincinnati, OH)
Children's Hospital Medical Center
3333 Burnet Ave.
Cincinnati, OH 45229
**Phone:** (513)636-4541     **Free:** 800-344-2462
**Fax:** (513)636-5562
**Email:** clint.joiner@CHMCC.org
Dr. Clinton Joiner, Dir.

**Activities/Fields:** Sickle cell disease, including molecular, cellular, tissue, and organ studies. Conducts clinical trials and seeks to translate research to improved health care.

### ★ 10315 ★ Creighton University
**Hereditary Cancer Prevention Clinic**
School of Medicine
2500 California Plz.
Omaha, NE 68178-0403
**Phone:** (402)280-1796     **Fax:** (402)280-1734
**Email:** tinley@creighton.edu
**Website:** http://medicine.creighton.edu/medschool/prevmed/hc.html
Prof. Henry T. Lynch, MD, Dir.

**Activities/Fields:** Hereditary cancer, including studies of its incidence and patterns. Disseminates current genetic, diagnostic, and therapeutic information to patients. **Pub:** *Newsletter*. **Frmly:** Institute for Familial Cancer Management and Control Inc.

### ★ 10316 ★ Cross Cancer Institute
11560 University Ave.
Edmonton, AB, Canada T6G 1Z2
**Phone:** (780)432-8320     **Fax:** (780)432-8425
**Email:** carolcas@cancerboard.ab.ca
**Website:** http://www.ualberta.ca/.–oncology
Dr. Carol E. Cass, Assoc. Dir.

**Activities/Fields:** Molecular oncology, medical physics and biophysics, radiation and solid tumor biology, tumor immunobiology, and experimental radiotherapy and chemotherapy.

### ★ 10317 ★ CTRC Research Foundation
14960 Omicron Dr.
San Antonio, TX 78245
**Phone:** (210)677-3800     **Fax:** (210)677-0058
**Email:** jcole@saci.org
**Website:** http://www.ctrc.saci.org
John F. Cole, PhD, COO

**Activities/Fields:** Causes and treatment of cancer, emphasizing the development of new anticancer agents. Maintains the Cancer Therapy and Research Center.

### ★ 10318 ★ Dana-Farber Cancer Institute
44 Binney St.
Boston, MA 02115
**Phone:** (617)632-4266     **Fax:** (617)632-2161
**Email:** edward_benz@dfci.harvard.edu

**Website:** http://www.dana-farber.net
Dr. Edward J. Benz, Jr., Pres.

**Activities/Fields:** Medical oncology, cancer pharmacology, pediatric oncology, cell growth and regulation, cancer genetics, human retrovirology, tumor immunology and virology, immunogenetics, lymphocyte biology, biostatistics and epidemiology, molecular carcinogenesis, biochemical pharmacology, neoplastic disease mechanisms, structural molecular biology, membrane immunochemistry, cancer control, tumor virus genetics, immunopathology, gene regulation, eukaryotic transcription, molecular biology, molecular genetics, molecular immunology, molecular immunobiology, medicine, gynecologic oncology, oncodiagnostic radiology and nuclear medicine, radiotherapy, and surgical oncology. **Pub:** *Scientific Report*, biennially. **Frmly:** Children's Cancer Research Foundation; Sidney Farber Cancer Institute.

### ★ 10319 ★ Dana-Farber Cancer Institute
**Department of Biostatistical Science**
44 Binney St.
Boston, MA 02115
**Phone:** (617)632-3012     **Fax:** (617)632-2444
**Email:** dph@jimmy.harvard.edu
**Website:** http://www.biowww.dfci.harvard.edu
Dr. David P. Harrington, Ch.

**Activities/Fields:** Organized into the laboratories of biostatistics and computing, which carry on a multifaceted program combining independent research, collaboration, and consulting in quantitative methods as they apply to cancer research. Project areas include methodological research in statistics, mathematical models in chronic disease epidemiology, bioinformatics, statistical computing, and applied probability and database research. Conducts multi-institutional cancer clinical trials.

### ★ 10320 ★ Drew/Meharry/Morehouse Consortium Cancer Center
1005 D.B. Todd Blvd.
Nashville, TN 37208
**Phone:** (615)327-6927     **Fax:** (615)327-5844
**Email:** mhargreaves@mmc.edu
Margaret Hargreaves, MD, Dir.

**Activities/Fields:** Cancer prevention and control, including epidemiological and behavioral research planning and implementation, and therapeutic clinical cancer trials.

### ★ 10321 ★ Duke University
**Comprehensive Sickle Cell Center**
Medical Center
Box 3939
Durham, NC 27710
**Phone:** (919)684-6464     **Fax:** (919)681-6174
**Email:** telen002@mc.duke.edu
Marilyn J. Telen, MD, Dir.

**Activities/Fields:** Sickle cell disease, including molecular, cellular, tissue, and organ studies. Conducts clinical trials. Seeks to translate basic and clinical research to improved health care at the community level.

**Duke University**
**Division of Pediatric Hematology Oncology**
*See:* Entry 5790

### ★ 10322 ★ Duke University
**Duke Comprehensive Cancer Center**
Medical Center
PO Box 3843
Durham, NC 27710
**Phone:** (919)684-3377     **Fax:** (919)684-5653
**Email:** rosof001@mc.duke.edu
**Website:** http://www.canctr.mc.duke.edu
Dr. O. Michael Colvin, Dir.

**Activities/Fields:** Prevention, detection, diagnosis, and treatment of cancer, including multidisciplinary studies in cellular and molecular biology, chemical and

environmental carcinogenesis, ultrastructure, cell genetics, virology, tumor immunology, epidemiology, and biostatistics. Conducts clinical investigations. **Pub:** *Annual Progress Report*. • *Cancer Patient Support Program*. • *Duke Cancer Center Notes*, quarterly. • *Melanoma*. • *Newsletters on Pediatric Brain Tumors*. • *Recreation Therapy*.

### ★ 10323 ★ Eastern Cooperative Oncology Group (ECOG)
303 Boylston St.
Brookline, MA 02445
**Phone:** (617)632-3610     **Fax:** (617)632-2990
Dr. Robert Comis, Chm.

**Activities/Fields:** Multidisciplinary cancer trials, including treatment, biologic and basic research, and cancer control and prevention. **Pub:** *Newsletter*, semi-annually.

### ★ 10324 ★ Emory University
**Georgia Center for Cancer Statistics**
Rollins School of Public Health
1518 Clifton Rd.
Atlanta, GA 30322
**Phone:** (404)727-3069     **Fax:** (404)727-7261
**Email:** jandr04@sph.emory.edu
**Website:** http://www.sph.emory.edu/GCCS/
Judy Andrews, Proj. Coord.

**Activities/Fields:** Serves as a cancer registry for five counties of metropolitan Atlanta and ten rural counties in central Georgia. Seeks to monitor the incidence of cancer in a geographically defined population, identify groups with unusual risks of cancer, monitor oncologic practices within the community, assess the survival experience of cancer patients, and provide a resource for epidemiological and biostatistical studies and training. Studies racial differences in cancer survival, cancers especially prevalent among blacks, passive exposure to cigarette smoke and risk of lung cancer, exposure to agent orange and risk of lymphoma and soft tissue sarcoma, risk factors for selected uterine malignancies, barriers to the early detection of cervical cancer, and viral infection and T-cell leukemias. **Frmly:** Atlanta Cancer Surveillance Center.

### ★ 10325 ★ Emory University
**Winship Cancer Institute**
1365 Clifton Rd. NE, Bldg. B, Ste. 4100
Atlanta, GA 30322
**Phone:** (404)778-5180     **Fax:** (404)778-5048
**Email:** jonathan_simons@emory.edu
**Website:** http://www.emory.edu/WHSC/WCI
Dr. Jonathan W. Simons, Dir.

**Activities/Fields:** A university-based cancer center coordinating multidisciplinary basic and clinical cancer research, improving methods of treatment, diagnosis, and prevention, training health professionals, and transferring cancer knowledge to surrounding communities.

### ★ 10326 ★ Fitzpatrick Oncology Center
Champlain Valley Physicians Hospital
75 Beekman St.
Plattsburgh, NY 12901
**Phone:** (518)562-7100     **Fax:** (518)562-7531
Janice Hess, Dir.

**Activities/Fields:** Oncological clinical research.

### ★ 10327 ★ Florida Hospital Cancer Institute
**Clinical and Research Laboratories**
2501 N Orange Ave., Ste. 786
Orlando, FL 32804
**Phone:** (407)303-2440     **Fax:** (407)303-2441
**Email:** john.francis@flhosp.org
John L. Francis, PhD, Dir.

**Activities/Fields:** Cell biology, cancer metastasis, anticoagulants, hemostasis and thrombosis. **Frmly:** Walt Disney Memorial Cancer Institute; Hemostasis and Thrombosis Research Unit.

**★ 10328 ★ Foundation for Advanced Cancer Studies, Inc.**
333 Briarwood Ave. SE
Grand Rapids, MI 49506-1739
**Website:** http://www.facsi.org
Dr. G. Vande Woude, Pres.

**Activities/Fields:** Basic cancer research, focusing on the rapid dissemination of new research information to scientists, clinicians, and the public.


**★ 10329 ★ Foundation for Blood Research**
69 US Rte. 1
PO Box 190
Scarborough, ME 04070-0190
**Phone:** (207)883-4131 **Free:** 800-639-8605
**Fax:** (207)883-1527
**Email:** ritchie@fbr.org
**Website:** http://www.fbr.org
Robert F. Ritchie, MD, Pres.

**Activities/Fields:** Health science education, epidemiology, genetics, immunology, oncology, perinatalogy, rheumatology, prenatal diagnosis, and cancer. Immunochemical analysis of human blood and other body fluids is performed and coupled with epidemiological data both for research on and for use in computer applications in disease diagnosis. Also performs clinical testing. **Pub:** *AFP Office Update Newsletter*, quarterly. • *Clinical Genetics Newsletter*, quarterly. • *Genetics Digest Newsletter*, 5/year. • *Proceedings of Scarborough Meetings*, periodically. • *RDL Newsletter*, quarterly.


**★ 10330 ★ Foundation for Research and Treatment of Cancer**
4800 Fillmore Ave., No. 1359
Alexandria, VA 22311
**Phone:** (703)575-8987
Dr. Nour Safi, Dir.

**Activities/Fields:** Studies in mice of monoclonal antibodies as a diagnostic tool and treatment for cancer.


**★ 10331 ★ Fox Chase Cancer Center**
7701 Burholme Ave.
Philadelphia, PA 19111
**Phone:** (215)728-6900 **Free:** 888-369-2427
**Fax:** (215)728-2594
**Email:** rc_young@fccc.edu
**Website:** http://www.fccc.edu
Robert C. Young, MD, Pres.

**Activities/Fields:** Cancer, including biomolecular structure and function, cellular and developmental biology, immunobiology, molecular oncology, virology, medical oncology, nursing research, imaging and spectroscopy, pathology, pharmacology, therapeutic radiology, surgical oncology, behavioral research, epidemiology and biostatistics. **Pub:** *President's Report*. • *Scientific Report*, annually.


**★ 10332 ★ Fred Hutchinson Cancer Research Center**
1100 Fairview Ave. N
PO Box 19024
Seattle, WA 98109-1024
**Phone:** (206)667-5000 **Free:** 800-4-CANCER
**Fax:** (206)667-5268
**Email:** lhartwel@fhcrc.org
**Website:** http://www.fhcrc.org
Dr. Leland Hartwell, Dir.

**Activities/Fields:** Cancer, including basic, clinical, and public health sciences. Research programs include basic science, human biology, human immunogenetics, marrow transplantation, organ systems, pain and toxicity, pediatric oncology, transplantation biology, biostatistics, cancer biology, cancer prevention research, and epidemiology.


**★ 10333 ★ Garden State Cancer Center John P. Caufield Technology Extension Center for Investigational Cancer Treatment**
520 Belleville Ave.
Belleville, NJ 07109
**Phone:** (973)844-7000 **Fax:** (973)844-7020
**Email:** gscancer@att.net
Dr. David M. Goldenberg, Dir.

**Activities/Fields:** Develops and provides new and more effective technologies for the early detection, diagnosis, and treatment of cancer; facilitates the transfer of investigational, diagnostic and treatment methods to New Jersey practitioners and hospitals; provides minority populations with access to state-of-the-art cancer protocols and treatment within their own community.


**★ 10334 ★ Georgetown University Vincent T. Lombardi Cancer Center**
Main Campus
3800 Reservoir Rd. NW
Washington, DC 20007
**Phone:** (202)687-2223 **Fax:** (202)687-6402
**Website:** http://lombardi.georgetown.edu
Marc Lippman, MD, Dir.

**Activities/Fields:** Prevention, detection, diagnosis, and treatment of cancer, including clinical and basic science activities in all oncologic specialties (surgery, medicine, gynecology, pediatrics, radiology, pathology, urology, and immunology) and basic science studies in pharmacology, biochemistry, radiation biology, virology, molecular genetics, analytic chemistry, flow cytometry, and electron microscopy.


**★ 10335 ★ Geraldine Brush Cancer Research Institute**
California Pacific Medical Center
Sterm Bldg.
2330 Clay St.
San Francisco, CA 94115
**Phone:** (415)561-1728 **Fax:** (415)561-1390
**Email:** nml@cooper.cpmc.org
Dr. Nancy M. Lee, Assoc. Dir.

**Activities/Fields:** Advanced molecular and cellular biology studies of human cancer. Special emphasis on breast cancer.


**★ 10336 ★ H.L. Snyder Memorial Research Foundation**
1407 Wheat Rd.
Winfield, KS 67156
**Phone:** (316)221-4080 **Fax:** (316)221-2684
**Email:** lsmith@snyderrf.com
**Website:** http://www.snyderrf.org
Larry D. Smith, Dir.

**Activities/Fields:** Biochemical and molecular biological studies of diseases, especially cancer. Develops clinical assays for early cancer detection.


**★ 10337 ★ H. Lee Moffitt Cancer Center and Research Institute**
12902 Magnolia Dr.
Tampa, FL 33612
**Phone:** (813)972-4673 **Fax:** (813)972-3919
**Email:** ruckdeschel@moffitt.usf.edu
**Website:** http://www.moffitt.usf.edu
John C. Ruckdeschel, MD, Dir. /CEO

**Activities/Fields:** Basic, clinical, and cancer control programs in immunology, molecular oncology, experimental therapeutics, genetic immunotherapy, behavioral oncology, cancer prevention, tobacco intervention, digital medical imaging. Conducts clinical programs in all disease sites, including breast; thoracic oncology, cutaneous, and bone marrow transplantation, etc. **Pub:** *Cancer Control*, quarterly. • *Lifetime Choices*, 3/year. • *Today's Tomorrows*, quarterly.


**★ 10338 ★ Hamilton Regional Cancer Center**
699 Concession St.
Hamilton, ON, Canada L8V 5C2
**Phone:** (905)387-9495 **Fax:** (905)575-6326
**Email:** george.browman@hrcc.on.ca
Dr. George Browman, CEO

**Activities/Fields:** Basic research focusing on tumor cell signalling and experimental therapeutics and clinical trials and supportive care research in cancer. Translational research focusing on new therapeutics from basic to clinical is highly encouraged.


**★ 10339 ★ Harvard University Harvard Center for Cancer Prevention**
Harvard School of Public Health
665 Huntington Ave., Bldg. 2, Rm. 105
Boston, MA 02115
**Phone:** (617)432-0038 **Fax:** (617)432-1722
**Email:** hccp@hsph.harvard.edu
**Website:** http://www.hsph.harvard.edu/cancer/index.html
David J. Hunter, MD, Dir.

**Activities/Fields:** Cancer prevention. **Pub:** *Newsletter*, bimonthly.


**★ 10340 ★ Harvard University Harvard Cyclotron Laboratory**
44 Oxford St.
Cambridge, MA 02138
**Phone:** (617)495-2885 **Fax:** (617)495-8054
**Email:** jsisterton@partners.org
**Website:** http://neurosurgery.mgh.harvard.edu/hcl/
Dr. Janet Sisterton, Contact

**Activities/Fields:** Proton beam technology for medical applications in both experimental and routine treatment of benign and cancerous tumors, including associated technical developments and clinical trials of proton radiation therapy and radiobiology. Other interests include proton activation analysis and other uses of proton beams, accelerator design study, and occasional radiation damage studies for commercial uses from aerospace and similar industries.


**Harvard University Laboratory for Cell and Molecular Biology**
*See:* Entry 4644


**★ 10341 ★ Head and Neck Center**
2157 Main St.
Buffalo, NY 14214
**Phone:** (716)862-1900 **Fax:** (716)862-1899
**Website:** http://www.sisters-buffalo.org/home/cancer/headneck/
Dr. John M. Lore, Jr., Hd.

**Activities/Fields:** Basic and clinical studies on head and neck cancer, especially in the areas of wound healing, bone regeneration, and biomaterials. **Frmly:** Center of Excellence in Otolaryncology.


**Health Research, Inc.**
*See:* Entry 17983


**★ 10342 ★ Hipple Cancer Research Center**
4100 S Kettering Blvd.
Dayton, OH 45439
**Phone:** (937)293-8508 **Free:** (866)447-7538
**Fax:** (937)293-7652
**Email:** hipple@hipple.org
**Website:** http://www.hipple.org/mission.htm
Hans J. Berkel, MD, Pres. /CEO

**Activities/Fields:** Cancer prevention and control. **Pub:** *Newsletter*.

**★ 10343 ★ Howard University**
**Cancer Center**
2041 Georgia Ave. NW
Washington, DC 20060
**Phone:** (202)806-7697      **Fax:** (202)667-1686
**Email:** adams-campbell@howard.edu
Dr. Lucille Adams-Campbell, Dir.

**Activities/Fields:** Multidisciplinary genomic research of African-Americans. Basic research includes molecular biology of cancer, mechanisms of metastases, tumor immunology, pharmacology of antineoplastic drugs, clinical chemotherapeutic research, pilot studies for the treatment of various neoplasms, and radiotherapeutic research, including intraoperative radiation therapy, hyperthermia, and combined modality therapy. Epidemiological research includes nutrition, cancer treatment effectiveness and various studies on the medically underserved targeted participants. Purpose is to better understand the biomedical significance of genomic variability underlying susceptability and/or resistance to common, chronic debilitating diseases and disorders using breast cancer as a prototype.

**★ 10344 ★ Howard University**
**Center for Sickle Cell Disease**
2121 Georgia Ave. NW
Washington, DC 20059
**Phone:** (202)806-7930      **Fax:** (202)806-4517
Dr. Oswaldo Castro, Dir.

**Activities/Fields:** Sickle cell disease, including basic and clinical investigations of its nature, causes, effects, and potential control. Develops and implements high quality total care for victims of the disease. Develops and evaluates methods of prevention through screening for sickle and other abnormal hemoglobins and participates in the Mid-Atlantic Regional Genetic Counseling Program. **Pub:** *Annual Report.*

**★ 10345 ★ Huntsman Cancer Institute**
**(HCI)**
2000 Circle of Hope
Salt Lake City, UT 84112
**Phone:** (801)585-0303      **Free:** 877-585-0303
**Email:** public.affairs@hci.utah.edu
**Website:** http://www.hci.utah.edu/
Stephen M. Prescott, MD, Exec. Dir.

**Activities/Fields:** Genetic basis of cancer.

**★ 10346 ★ Illinois Oncology Research**
**Association**
900 Main St., Ste. 780
Peoria, IL 61602
**Phone:** (309)671-5180      **Fax:** (309)672-4138
**Email:** info@ohaci.com
**Website:**      http://www.ohaci.com/research/research.htm

**Activities/Fields:** Cancer treatment and control, including chemotherapy, immunotherapy, hormonal therapy, and radiation therapy.

**★ 10347 ★ Indiana University**
**Herman B. Wells Center for Pediatric**
**Research**
Sch. of Medicine
702 Barnhill Dr., Rm. 2600
Indianapolis, IN 46202
**Phone:** (317)274-8900      **Fax:** (317)274-9906
**Email:** tnoonan@iupui.edu
**Website:** http://www.iupui.edu/~wellsctr/
Dr. Mary Dinauer, Dir.

**Activities/Fields:** Hematology and oncology, cell biology of polarized cells (including the blood-brain barrier), protein sorting in eukaryotic cells, bone marrow transplantation, clinical oncology research, pediatric oncology, DNA repair, gene therapy, developmental biology of neuroblastoma, gene transfer into stem cells, tumor immunology, clinical aspects of childhood acute myelogenous leukemia, the role of protein phosphorylation in control of cell proliferation and differentiation, clinical aspects and molecular biology of neutrophil disorders, neurooncology, late effects of CNS therapy, clinical aspects of supportive care of oncology patients, therapy for neuroblastoma, clinical use of hemotopoietic growth factors, secondary leukemias, clinical aspects of hemostasis, molecular biology of myeloid-specific gene expression, cancer biogenesis using neuroblastoma as a model, and molecular biology of nuclear retinoic acid receptors in myeloid leukemia, neuroblastoma cells, endocrinology, neonatology, pulmonary, cardiovascular development.

**★ 10348 ★ Indiana University-Purdue**
**University at Indianapolis**
**Laboratory for Experimental Oncology**
Sch. of Medicine
699 West Dr.
Indianapolis, IN 46202-5119
**Phone:** (317)274-7921      **Fax:** (317)274-3939
**Email:** gw1@iupui.edu
Prof. George Weber, MD, Dir.

**Activities/Fields:** Biochemical pharmacology and chemotherapy of experimental and clinical cancer. **Pub:** *Advances in Enzyme Regulation.*

**★ 10349 ★ Institute for Cancer and**
**Blood Diseases**
MS412
Hahnemann University
Broad & Vine Sts.
Philadelphia, PA 19102
**Phone:** (215)762-7026      **Fax:** (215)762-8857
**Email:** hbw22@drexel.edu
Dr. Isadore Brodsky, Dir.

**Activities/Fields:** Basic research program with possible clinical trials in the following areas: interferon, oncogenesis, differentiation, molecular biology, viral oncogenesis, immunology, cell biology, and cytogenesis, autoimmune diseases. **Frmly:** Herbert L. Orlowitz Institute for Cancer and Blood Diseases.

**★ 10350 ★ Institute for Cancer and**
**Blood Research**
150 N Robertson Blvd., Ste. 316
Beverly Hills, CA 90211
**Phone:** (310)657-4706      **Fax:** (310)657-2185
Dr. Howard R. Bierman, Sci. Dir.

**Activities/Fields:** Biochemical regulation of cell growth and control of leukocyte maturation in leukemias, including clinical studies to isolate and purify substances that stimulate cell division and maintain normal maturation of neoplastic cells; ultrastructural immunolocalization of novel protein products in myeloid leukemias; prediagnostic detection of cancer, oncogenes, and products for antioncogenes; detailed computer analysis of predictive-oriented data acquired from healthy subjects and patients with neoplastic disease; investigation of tumor diathesis, including preclinical diagnosis of multiple primary neoplasms and studies of families to define increased susceptibility to develop neoplasms; and continuing studies of dermatoglyphics, predictive profiles, and other genetic markers as they relate to neoplasia.

**★ 10351 ★ Institute for Cancer Research**
Fox Chase Cancer Center
7701 Burholme Ave.
Philadelphia, PA 19111
**Phone:** (215)728-2490      **Fax:** (215)728-2778
**Email:** am_skalka@fccc.edu
**Website:** http://www.fccc.edu
Dr. Anna Marie Skalka, Dir.

**Activities/Fields:** Causes, nature, diagnosis, and treatment of cancer, including studies in cellular, molecular, and developmental biology, immunology, molecular oncology, structural biology, and virology. **Pub:** *Scientific Report,* annually.

**Institute for Clinical Research, Inc.**
*See:* Entry 5109

**★ 10352 ★ Iowa Oncology Research**
**Association**
1223 Center St., Ste. 19
Des Moines, IA 50309-1014
**Phone:** (515)244-7586      **Free:** 888-244-6061
**Fax:** (515)244-3037
**Email:** sherrijr@iora.org
**Website:** http://www.iora.org
Sherri Rickabaugh, Admin.

**Activities/Fields:** Clinical cancer studies, including new chemotherapy agents and radiation therapy techniques.

**★ 10353 ★ Jerome H. Holland Laboratory**
American Red Cross
15601 Crabbs Branch Way
Rockville, MD 20855
**Phone:** (301)738-0600      **Fax:** (301)738-0553
Leon W. Hoyer, MD, Dir.

**Activities/Fields:** Blood cells, blood proteins, cytokines, receptors, blood services technology, tissue biology, epidemiology of transfusion-transmitted diseases, plasma derivatives, adhesion factors, angiogenesis, inflammation. Conducts basic and applied research and development for the Biomedical Services Division of the American Red Cross. **Pub:** *R&D Annual Report.* Annual report. **Frmly:** American Red Cross National Headquarters Lab.

**Johns Hopkins University**
**Center for Cancer Complementary**
**Medicine**
*See:* Entry 4330

**★ 10354 ★ Johns Hopkins University**
**Johns Hopkins Thyroid Tumor Center**
Johns Hopkins Hospital
1830 E Monument St., Ste. 333
Baltimore, MD 21287-0003
**Phone:** (410)955-3663      **Fax:** (410)955-8172
**Email:** ladenson@welchlink.welch.jhu.edu
**Website:** http://www.med.jhu.edu/thyroid
Paul W. Ladenson, MD, Dir.

**Activities/Fields:** Causes and treatment of thyroid cancer.

**★ 10355 ★ Johns Hopkins University**
**Physiological Mechanics and Transport**
**Laboratory**
Department of Biomedical Engineering
School of Medicine
720 Rutland Ave.
611 Traylor Research Bldg.
Baltimore, MD 21205
**Phone:** (410)955-6419      **Fax:** (410)614-8796
**Email:** apopel@jhu.edu
**Website:** http://www.bme.jhu.edu/~apopel/PMTL.html
Prof. Aleksander S. Popel, PhD, Contact

**Activities/Fields:** Mechanics and regulation of blood flow, oxygen transport to tissue, blood flow and molecular transport in the cerebral circulation, and the mechanics and electromotility of the cochlear outer hair cell.

**★ 10356 ★ Johns Hopkins University**
**Sidney Kimmel Comprehensive Cancer**
**Center**
The Harry and Jeanette Weinberg Bldg.
401 N Broadway, Ste. 1100
Baltimore, MD 21231
**Phone:** (410)955-8822      **Fax:** (410)955-6787
**Email:** abeloma@jhmi.edu
**Website:** http://www.hopkinscancercenter.org
Martin D. Abeloff, MD, Dir.

**Activities/Fields:** Cancer and related disorders, with bone marrow transplantation, cancer biology, medical oncology, pediatric oncology, pharmacology and experimental therapeutics, and radiological sciences. Activities emphasize the application of new knowledge to management of patients with cancer and prevention of neoplastic diseases and their complications, with major aim of the several complementary research programs of the Center being an increased understanding of human neoplasia and more effective clinical management. **Pub:** *Promise and Progress Magazine*, annually. • *Scientific Report*, biennially. **Frmly:** Oncology Center.

★ **10357** ★ **Kansas City Clinical Oncology Program**
6601 Rockhill Rd.
Kansas City, MO 64131-9000
**Phone:** (816)823-0555 **Fax:** (816)823-0563
**Email:** kccop@kccop.org
**Website:** http://www.kccop.org
Leslie Herst, Exec. Dir.
**Activities/Fields:** Oncological clinical trials.

★ **10358** ★ **Kansas State University Center for Basic Cancer Research**
1500 Hayes Dr., Ste. B
Manhattan, KS 66502-5014
**Phone:** (785)532-6705 **Fax:** (785)532-6707
**Email:** terryj@ksu.edu
**Website:** http://www.ksu.edu/cancer.center
Dr. Terry C. Johnson, Dir.
**Activities/Fields:** Cancer autonomy and metastasis; tumor initiation, promotion, and progression; chemotherapeutic compounds; growth regulation, the immune system, and other cellular interactions; and oncogene expression. **Pub:** *Accepting a Challenge Magazine*. • *A Day with Dr. Waddle (children's workbook on cancer).*

★ **10359** ★ **Kellogg Cancer Care Center (KCCC)**
Evanston Northwestern Health Care
2650 Ridge Ave.
Evanston, IL 60201
**Phone:** (847)570-2110 **Fax:** (847)570-2918
**Email:** J.Kmandeicar@nwu.edu
**Website:** http://www.enh.org
Dr. J.D. Khandekar, Dir.
**Activities/Fields:** Treatment and diagnosis of cancer, including phase 1 and 2 studies, evaluation of new drug protocols, and brain tumor studies. Basic and clinical research also includes studies of breast, head and neck, lung, bladder, and pancreatic cancers, blood clotting and fibrinolytic mechanisms in tumor patients, thromboembolic problems in cancer patients, pituitary tumor surgery, immunology/virology, microbiology, hematology, clinical biochemistry, pharmacology, diagnosis by fine needle aspiration techniques, oncogens, medical oncology, and psychiatry. Also conducts studies in flow cytometry and magnetic resonance imaging and spectroscopy. **Frmly:** Evanston Cancer Care Center.

★ **10360** ★ **Kentucky Cancer Program**
2365 Harrodsburg Rd., Ste. A230
Lexington, KY 40504-3381
**Phone:** (859)219-0772 **Fax:** (859)219-0548
**Email:** dka@kcp.uky.edu
**Website:** http://www.kcr.uky.edu/kcp/
Debra Armstrong, Dir.
**Activities/Fields:** Cancer control. Collects and disseminates information leading to improved prevention, diagnosis, and treatment of cancer. Serves communities throughout the Commonwealth through identified intermediaries, working through District Cancer Councils and community cancer coalitions. The Cancer Control Program developed the computerized Kentucky Cancer Registry (KCR), and has recently been designated a SEER site to which Kentucky hospitals are legislatively mandated to report cancer incidence. Supports a community-based research component to evaluate cancer control efforts of joint interventions and information dissemination. **Pub:** *CHOICES*. • *For Your Peace of Mind Video*. • *KCR Cancer Incidence Report*. • *Literacy Curriculum for Breast and Cervical Cancer*. • *Pathfinder*. • *Research Findings*. • *Woman Talk*, a video about cervical health.

★ **10361** ★ **La Jolla Institute for Molecular Medicine**
4570 Executive Dr., Ste. 100
San Diego, CA 92121
**Phone:** (858)587-8788 **Fax:** (858)587-6742
**Email:** moubre@ljimm.org
**Website:** http://www.ljimm.org/
Dr. Mario A. Bourdon, Sci. Dir.
**Activities/Fields:** Cause and cures of cancer, immune diseases and genetic disorders.

★ **10362** ★ **Laboratory of Signal Transduction**
Memorial Sloan-Kettering Cancer Center
1275 York Ave., Box 254
New York, NY 10021
**Phone:** (212)639-8573 **Fax:** (212)794-4342
**Email:** rkolesnick@ski.mskcc.org
Dr. Richard Kolesnick, Prin. Investigator
**Activities/Fields:** Signal transduction for cytokines and hormones, including tumor necrosis factor-alpha, interleukin-1, and activin.

★ **10363** ★ **Laboratory of Tumor Antigen Immunochemistry**
Memorial Sloan-Kettering Cancer Center
1275 York Ave.
New York, NY 10021
**Phone:** (212)639-2257 **Fax:** (212)717-3379
**Email:** k-lloyd@ski.mskcc.org
Dr. Kenneth O. Lloyd, Contact
**Activities/Fields:** Monoclonal antibodies and carbohydrate antigens. **Frmly:** Laboratory of Human Cancer Immunology.

★ **10364** ★ **Laval University Cancer Research Centre**
Hotel-Dieu de Quebec
9 McMahon
Quebec, QC, Canada G1R 2J6
**Phone:** (418)691-5281 **Fax:** (418)691-5439
**Email:** Luc.Belanger@crhdq.ulaval.ca
Dr. Luc Belanger, Sci. Dir.
**Activities/Fields:** Cellular and molecular mechanisms relating differentiation and cancer, including genomic organization and molecular regulation of fetoprotein, histones, metallothionein, oncogenes, cytochromes P-450 and developmental tyrosine kinase genes, developmental genes in embryonic stem cell mice, structure of active versus inactive chromatin, nature of neoplastic liver cell progenitors, role of growth factor-cell interactions in tissue growth, differentiation and neoplasia, cell surface markers of bladder cancer, hormone receptors, mechanisms of ribosomal transcription, action of DNA intercalating drugs, carcinogen activation, and mutagenesis. Also conducts research and development activities in clinical oncology, cancer epidemiology and psycho-oncology. Serves as a reference center for flow cytometry, hormone receptor measurements, confocal microscopy, and genetic probes in cancer.

**Laval University Medical Research Centre Oncology and Molecular Endocrinology Research Center**
*See:* Entry 8756

★ **10365** ★ **Loma Linda University Cancer Institute**
11360 Mountain View Ave., Ste. E
PO Box 2000
Loma Linda, CA 92354
**Phone:** (909)588-6003 **Fax:** (909)558-6020
**Email:** fernand.labrie@crchul.ulaval.ca
**Website:** http://www.llu.edu/llu/ci/
James M. Slater, MD, Dir.
**Activities/Fields:** Cancer prevention and treatment, specifically molecular genetics, neurosciences, and cancer cell and molecular biology and their relation-

ships to cancer; and translating basic science findings into clinical applications.

★ **10366** ★ **Mary Bird Perkins Cancer Center**
4950 Essen Ln.
Baton Rouge, LA 70809
**Phone:** (225)767-0847 **Fax:** (225)766-0218
**Email:** infor@marybird.com
**Website:** http://www.marybird.org
Todd D. Stevens, Pres. /CEO
**Activities/Fields:** Radiation treatment, including participation in national clinical trials of the Radiation Therapy Oncology Group and the Southwest Oncology Group, as well as pharmaceutical and in-house studies.

★ **10367** ★ **Massachusetts General Hospital East Cancer Center**
13th St., Bldg. 149
Charlestown, MA 02129
**Phone:** (617)726-5610 **Fax:** (617)726-5637
**Email:** isselbacher@helix.mgh.harvard.edu
Kurt Isselbacher, MD, Dir.
**Activities/Fields:** Cell cycle regulation and cancer genetics, including breast, colon, and melanoma, and metastasis.

★ **10368** ★ **Massachusetts Institute of Technology Center for Cancer Research**
77 Massachusetts Ave., E17-110
Cambridge, MA 02139
**Phone:** (617)253-6403 **Fax:** (617)252-1891
**Email:** crays@mit.edu
**Website:** http://web.mit.edu/ccrhq/www/
Dr. Richard Hynes, Dir.
**Activities/Fields:** Cancer biology, emphasizing molecular biology, genetics, cell biology, developmental biology, and immunology. Specific areas of research include split genes and RNA splicing, cloning oncogenes and tumor suppressor genes from human tumors, T-cell receptors, integrin receptors and cell adhesion, mechanisms, used by tumor cells to evade chemotherapy, gene identification for myotonic dystrophy, Huntington's disease, and Wilm's tumor, the generation of various strains of mutant mice, biochemical mechanisms controlling RNA transcription and splicing, HIV gene studies, cytotoxic and helper T lymphocytes, lymphocyte antigen-specific receptors, molecular mechanisms of antigen presentation, cell surface proteins and cellular adhesion and migration, and cytoskeletal proteins and cell motility and shape.

★ **10369** ★ **Mayo Clinic Cancer Center**
200 1st St. SW
Rochester, MN 55905
**Phone:** (507)284-9589 **Fax:** (507)284-9349
**Email:** prendergast@mayo.edu
**Website:** http://www.mayo.edu/research/cnacerc
Dr. Franklyn G. Prendergast, PhD, Dir.
**Activities/Fields:** Broad-based cancer research program ranging from basic and clinical science to clinical studies on prevention, detection, diagnosis, and treatment of cancer. Participates as a comprehensive cancer center for conducting research, improving methods of treatment, diagnosis, and prevention, training health professionals, and transferring cancer knowledge to surrounding communities in National Cancer Institute's nationwide coordination program, established under National Cancer Act of 1971.

★ **10370** ★ **McGill University McGill Cancer Centre**
McIntyre Medical Sciences Bldg.
3655 Promenade Sir-William Osler
Montreal, QC, Canada H3G 1Y6
**Phone:** (514)398-3535 **Fax:** (514)398-6769
**Email:** tremblay@med.mcgill.ca

**Website:** http://www.medserv.mcgill.ca/cancer
Dr. Michel L. Tremblay, Dir.

**Activities/Fields:** Cancer, including molecular biology of human and murine carcinoembryonic antigen, family nature and regulation of mammalian origins of DNA replication, molecular biology of dominant and recessive oncogenes, cancer related cellular surface sugar-containing molecules, and molecular basis of spatial differentiation in mice and its aberration in tumors.

★ 10371 ★ **McGill University**
**McGill Centre for Translational Research in Cancer**
**Clinical Research Unit**
3755 Cote Ste. Catherine Rd.
Montreal, QC, Canada H3T 1E2
**Phone:** (514)340-8222
**Email:** wmiller@ldi.jgh.mcgill.ca
**Website:** http://www.mctrc.org/en/Default.htm
Wilson Miller, MD, Dir.

**Activities/Fields:** Novel cancer therapeutics, including pharmacokinetics/dynamics.

★ 10372 ★ **McGill University**
**Montreal Neurological Institute**
**Brain Tumour Research Centre**
Neuro Development Office
3801 University St.
Montreal, QC, Canada H3A 2B4
**Phone:** (514)398-1958 **Fax:** (514)398-8072
**Website:** http://www.mni.mcgill.ca/brain.htm
Dr. David Kaplan, Res. Dir.

**Activities/Fields:** Causes and treatment of brain tumors.

★ 10373 ★ **Medical College of Georgia**
**Sickle Cell Center**
AC 1004
Augusta, GA 30912-3128
**Phone:** (706)721-9640 **Fax:** (706)721-9637
**Email:** akutlar@mail.mcg.edu
Dr. Abdullah Kutlar, Dir.

**Activities/Fields:** Hemoglobinopathy detection, identification, and characterization, including studies of factors determining severity of sickle cell anemia in adults and the young child, cardiac evaluation of children with sickle cell anemia, thalassemia in association with sickle cell syndromes, biochemical studies in sickle cell anemia and related disorders with special emphasis on heterogeneity of Hb F, immunological identification, DNA gene mapping of hemoglobin variants, nucleotide sequence, and thalassemia genes, and characterization of hemoglobin variants. **Pub:** *Hemoglobin: International Journal for Hemoglobin Research*, bimonthly. • *SPHERE*, bimonthly.

★ 10374 ★ **Medical College of Ohio**
**Cancer Research Division**
Department of Pathology, HE 202
3055 Arlington Ave.
Toledo, OH 43614-5806
**Phone:** (419)383-4918 **Fax:** (419)383-3089
**Email:** hschut@mco.edu
Dr. Herman A.J. Schut, Contact

**Activities/Fields:** Cancer, including chemical carcinogenesis, chemoprevention, molecular biology, toxicology, and tissue culture. Specific research includes oncogene activation and suppressor gene inactivation in cancer, inhibition of cancer by dietary components, and regulation of tumor promotion.

★ 10375 ★ **Medical College of Wisconsin**
**Cancer Center**
8701 Watertown Plank Rd.
Milwaukee, WI 53226
**Phone:** (414)805-5583
**Email:** bcampbell@mcw.edu
Bruce H. Campbell, MD, Interim Dir.

**Activities/Fields:** Experimental Therapy program focuses on developing new agents and strategies for the treatment of cancer, including photodynamic therapy; understanding cell resistance, focusing on glutathione, iron metabolism and nitric oxide; and limiting the toxicity and side effects of cancer treatment, focusing on gastrointestinal effects and chronic renal damage caused by radiation therapy; Cancer Biologyand Molecular Genetics Program studies regulatory mechanisms at the structural, cellular and molecular levels in the following areas: regulation of cell growth and orcogenesis, development, virology and viral transformation, and molecular diagnostics; Cancer Prevention and Control Program conducts several multi-year studies in behavioral interventions are on-going in the areas of environmental hazards (pesticides and cancer risk), smoking cessation interventions, skin cancer prevention education, early screening education and nutrition education; research interest in quality of life issues in the areas of pediatric, breast and head/neck cancers; and studies in chemotherapeutic agents in cancer prevention; Bone Marrow Transplantation/Immunology Program conducts ongoing studies in T-cell depletion, cytokines, graft-vs-host disease; autologous, allogenic, and unrelated donor therapies; lymphocyte infusion; International Bone Marrow Transplant Registry.

★ 10376 ★ **Memorial Sloan-Kettering**
**Cancer Center**
1275 York Ave.
New York, NY 10021
**Phone:** (212)639-2000 **Fax:** (212)639-5850
**Email:** varmus@mskcc.org
**Website:** http://www.mskcc.org
Dr. Harold Varmus, Pres.

**Activities/Fields:** Molecular biology, cell biology and genetics, cellular biochemistry and biophysics, immunology, and molecular pharmacology and therapeutics. Aims to advance the understanding of the nature and fundamental causes of cancer and improve the means available for its prevention, diagnosis, and treatment. **Pub:** *Annual Report.* • *Center Newsletter.* • *Memorial Sloan-Kettering Cancer Center Research and Educational Programs.*

★ 10377 ★ **Michigan State University**
**Carcinogenesis Laboratory**
**College of Osteopathic Medicine**
341 Food Safety & Toxicology Bldg.
East Lansing, MI 48824
**Phone:** (517)353-7785 **Fax:** (517)353-9004
**Email:** maher@msu.edu
**Website:** http://www.com.msu.edu/carcino/
Prof. Veronica M. Maher, PhD, Co-Dir.

**Activities/Fields:** Carcinogenesis, including research in cellular and molecular biology, mutagenesis, mammalian cell DNA repair, and homologous recombination. **Pub:** *Monographs.* • *Newsletter,* occasionally. • *Papers.*

★ 10378 ★ **Montreal Cancer Institute**
1560 Sherbrooke St. E
Montreal, QC, Canada H2L 4M1
**Phone:** (514)890-8213 **Fax:** (514)412-7591
**Email:** info@icm.qc.ca
**Website:** http://www.icm.qc.ca
Ms. Maral Tersakian, Dir.

**Activities/Fields:** Viral carcinogenesis, molecular biology, genetic engineering, biochemical changes associated with neoplastic transformation, epidemiology of cancer, and clinical pharmacology.

★ 10379 ★ **Mountain States Tumor**
**Institute, Inc.**
100 E Idaho
Boise, ID 83712-6241
**Phone:** (208)381-3132 **Fax:** (208)381-3124
**Email:** frelless@slrmc.org
Sharon Frelleson, RN, Clin. Res. Coord.

**Activities/Fields:** Adult and pediatric oncology clinical trials.

★ 10380 ★ **National Black Leadership**
**Initiative on Cancer II (NBLIC)**
720 Westview Dr., SW
Atlanta, GA 30310
**Phone:** (404)756-5205
**Email:** hamilts@msm.edu
**Website:** http://www.nblic.org
Joyce Q. Sheets, Prog. Dir.

**Activities/Fields:** Cancer prevention and mortality in the black community.

★ 10381 ★ **National Cancer Institute of**
**Canada**
**Clinical Trials Group (CTG)**
Queen's University
10 Alcorn Ave., Ste. 200
Toronto, ON, Canada M4V 3B1
**Phone:** (613)533-6430 **Fax:** (613)533-2941
**Email:** jpater@ctg.queensu.ca
**Website:** http://www.ncic.cancer.ca/progs/ctge.htm
Dr. J.L. Pater, Dir.

**Activities/Fields:** Cancer, cancer therapy, and supportive care.

★ 10382 ★ **National Foundation for**
**Cancer Research (NFCR)**
4600 East West Hwy., Ste. 525
Bethesda, MD 20814
**Phone:** (301)654-1250 **Free:** 800-321-2873
**Fax:** (301)654-5824
**Email:** fcsjr@nfcr.org
**Website:** http://www.researchforacure.com
Franklin Salisbury, Jr., Pres.

**Activities/Fields:** Contracts with major universities for basic science cancer research in the fields of biophysics, theoretical physics and chemistry, biochemistry, chemistry, and biological sciences. **Pub:** *Annual Scientific Report.* • *NFCR Annual Report.*

★ 10383 ★ **National Surgical Adjuvant**
**Breast and Bowel Project (NSABP)**
East Commons Professional Bldg.
4 Allegheny Center, 5th Fl.
Pittsburgh, PA 15212-5234
**Phone:** (412)330-4600 **Fax:** (412)330-4660
**Email:** normanwolmark@nsabp.org
**Website:** http://www.nsabp.pitt.edu
Dr. Norman Wolmark, Chm.

**Activities/Fields:** Breast and bowel cancer treatments and breast cancer prevention. Operates in cooperation with over 300 member institutions throughout the U.S., Canada, Puerto Rico, and Australia. **Pub:** *Progress Reports,* semiannually.

★ 10384 ★ **New England Medical Center**
**Hospitals, Inc.**
**Gynecologic Oncology Group (GOG)**
Box 232
750 Washington St.
Boston, MA 02111
**Phone:** (617)636-6058 **Fax:** (617)636-3258
**Website:** http://www.nemc.org
Cornelius O. Granai, MD, Dir.

**Activities/Fields:** Treatment of gynecologic cancer. Evaluates surgical techniques, radiation therapy, and new chemotherapeutic agents. Emphasizes trophoblastic disease and cancers of the uterus, cervix, vulva, and ovaries.

★ 10385 ★ **New York Medical College**
**Institute of Breast Diseases**
Munger Pavillion, Rm. G-13
Valhalla, NY 10595
**Phone:** (914)493-8770 **Fax:** (914)493-1651
**Email:** zachrau@nymc.edu
Reinhard E. Zachrau, MD, Contact

**Activities/Fields:** Breast diseases, including skin window reactivity and second primary breast cancer.

**★ 10386 ★ New York University**
**Kaplan Comprehensive Cancer Center**
School of Medicine
550 1st Ave.
New York, NY 10016
**Phone:** (212)263-6485          **Fax:** (212)263-8210
**Website:** http://kccc-www.med.nyu.edu/
Dr. Steven J. Burakoff, Dir.

**Activities/Fields:** Cancer research is carried out in designated program units of cancer epidemiology and prevention, cell interactions, clinical oncology, environmental carcinogenesis, genetic and molecular toxicology, growth regulation, molecular and tumor immunology, and molecular and viral oncology. **Pub:** *Kaplan Center Newsletter*, semiannually.

**★ 10387 ★ Norris Cotton Cancer Center**
**(NCCC)**
Dartmouth-Hitchcock Medical Center
Lebanon, NH 03756
**Phone:** (603)650-6300          **Free:** 800-639-6918
**Fax:** (603)650-6333
**Email:** norris.cotton.cancer.center@dartmouth.edu
**Website:** http://www.dartmouth.edu/dms/nccc
Mark A. Israel, MD, Contact

**Activities/Fields:** Clinical treatment trials, including bone marrow transplantation, chemotherapy trials, intraoperative radiation therapy, and monoclonal antibody treatment. Studies are conducted in the areas of tumor immunology, radiobiology, chemical carcinogenesis, cancer epidemiology, cancer control, cytogenetics, tumor endocrinology, molecular genetics, cancer risk, and palliative care. Participates as one of a group of regional clinical and nonclinical centers conducting multidisciplinary cancer research, improving methods of treatment, diagnosis, and prevention, training health professionals, and transferring cancer knowledge to surrounding communities.

**★ 10388 ★ North Central Cancer**
**Treatment Group**
Operations Office
Plummer Bldg.
200 1st St. SW
Rochester, MN 55905
**Phone:** (507)284-2511          **Fax:** (507)284-1902
**Email:** kuhlmann.marilyn@mayo.edu
**Website:** http://ncctg.mayo.edu
Dr. Michael J. O'Connell, Chm.

**Activities/Fields:** Cancer research and therapy, including surgery, medical oncology, therapeutic radiology, pathology, and cancer control. Seeks to transfer nationwide cancer research and therapy to patients at the community level. Group maintains a patient base of 7,000 and operates 112 separate research protocols.

**★ 10389 ★ Northern California Cancer**
**Center**
32960 Alvarado-Niles Rd., Ste. 600
Union City, CA 94587
**Phone:** (510)429-2500          **Fax:** (510)429-2550
**Email:** dwest@nccc.org
**Website:** http://www.nccc.org
Dee W. West, PhD, Exec. Dir.

**Activities/Fields:** Conducts multidisciplinary studies in epidemiology and related fields. Also conducts cancer research and demonstration activities (detection, psychosocial, prevention, nutrition) with communities in the Center's service area, focusing on the minority populations and the underserved. **Pub:** *Cancer Calendar*, quarterly. • *Estate Planning Brochure.* • *Highlights.* • *Registry Newsletters.*

**★ 10390 ★ Northwestern University**
**John I. Brewer Trophoblastic Disease**
**Center**
Prentice Women's Hospital
333 E Superior, Ste. 420
Chicago, IL 60611
**Phone:** (312)926-7365          **Fax:** (312)926-2188

**Email:** jlurain@nmh.org
John R. Lurain, MD, Dir.

**Activities/Fields:** Pathology, epidemiology, and experimental chemotherapy in patients with trophoblastic diseases; experimental protocols and new chemotherapeutic agents and combinations of agents; pathologic studies of choriocarcinoma and hydatidiform mole; and the effect of oral contraceptive use on the development of gestational trophoblastic diseases.

**★ 10391 ★ Northwestern University**
**Robert H. Lurie Comprehensive Cancer**
**Center of Northwestern University**
Olson Pavillion, Ste. 8250
303 E Chicago Ave.
Chicago, IL 60611-3008
**Phone:** (312)908-5250          **Fax:** (312)908-1372
**Email:** s-rosen@northwestern.edu
**Website:** http://www.cancer.northwestern.edu
Steven T. Rosen, MD, Dir.

**Activities/Fields:** The Center has ten established research programs. Basic science programs include Viral Oncogenesis, Tumor Invasion, Metastasis and Angiogenesis; Hormone Action and Signal Transduction in Cancer; and Cancer Genes and Molecular Regulation. Clinical science research is conducted in the areas of Breast Cancer, Prostate Cancer, Hematologic Malignancies, Pediatric Oncology, Cancer Prevention and Control. Coordinates multidisciplinary, basic, and clinical cancer research; seeks improved methods of cancer treatment, diagnosis and prevention; trains health care professionals; and transfers cancer knowledge to surrounding communities. **Pub:** *Community Newsletter.* • *Journal of the Robert H. Lurie Cancer Center of Northwestern University*, semiannually. • *Lurie Cancer Center News and Calendar*, bimonthly.

**★ 10392 ★ Ohio Cancer Research**
**Associates**
50 W Broad St., Ste. 1132
Columbus, OH 43215-3388
**Phone:** (614)224-1127          **Fax:** (614)224-0654
**Email:** ocra@ohiocancer.org
**Website:** http://www.ohiocancer.org
Dennis Zack, Exec. Dir.

**Activities/Fields:** Cancer "seed money" research projects.

**★ 10393 ★ Ohio State University**
**Caligiuri Laboratory**
A458 Starling-Loving Hall
320 W 10th Ave.
Columbus, OH 43210
**Phone:** (614)293-7521          **Fax:** (614)293-7522
**Email:** caligiuri-1@medctr.osu.edu
**Website:** http://www.jamesline.com/caligiuri
Michael Caligiuri, MD, Dir.

**Activities/Fields:** Research, patient service, and training through a fellowship program on various aspects of hematology and oncology, including cancer immunology, human cancer genetics, lymphocyte signaling, importance of complement in host defense against malignancy, the role of oxygen radicals in mononuclear effector cells and tumor cell targets, and clinical research in the development, implementation, and assessment of protocols in the treatment of leukemia, lymphoma, bone marrow transplantation, and solid tumors. The training program is designed to provide postdoctoral fellowship experience in the development and performance of clinical and laboratory research projects related to hematology and medical oncology.

**★ 10394 ★ Ohio State University**
**Comprehensive Cancer Center**
300 W 10th Ave., Ste. 519
Columbus, OH 43210
**Phone:** (614)293-7518          **Free:** 800-293-5066
**Fax:** (614)293-3305
**Email:** jones-8@medctr.osu.edu

**Website:** http://www.jamesline.com/output/content/cccsite/ccc/ccsite.html
Clara D. Bloomfield, MD, Dir.

**Activities/Fields:** Carcinogenesis, cancer chemoprevention, cancer control, immunology, developmental therapeutics, hormones and cancer, molecular biology, RNA oncogenic virus, neuro-oncology, head and neck oncology, urologic oncology, and pediatric oncology. Investigations also cover bone marrow transplantation, biochemistry and genetics, breast cancer, clinical trials, and pharmacology and toxicology. **Pub:** *Scientific Report*, biennially.

**★ 10395 ★ Oklahoma Medical Research**
**Foundation**
**Immunobiology and Cancer Research**
**Program**
825 NE 13th St.
Oklahoma City, OK 73104
**Phone:** (405)271-6673          **Fax:** (405)271-3980
**Email:** paul-kincade@omrf.ouhsc.edu
**Website:** http://www.omrf.ouhsc.edu/omrf/research/14
Paul W. Kincade, PhD, Hd.

**Activities/Fields:** Mechanisms for regulation of B lymphocyte production in lymphopoietic tissues, including cytokines, hormones, and cell adhesion molecules.

**★ 10396 ★ Ontario Cancer Institute/**
**Princess Margaret Hospital**
610 University Ave.
Toronto, ON, Canada M5G 2M9
**Phone:** (416)946-2000          **Fax:** (416)340-2967
**Website:** http://www.ocipmh.org
Dr. Alan Hudson, CEO

**Activities/Fields:** Cancer research, including studies on mechanisms regulating cellular growth and differentiation (with emphasis on the hemopoietic system), cellular and molecular immunology (particularly mechanisms involved in immune-recognition), molecular structure (including physical and molecular biological approaches to macromolecular structure and interactions), experimental therapy (including radiobiology and chemotherapy), clinical physics and epidemiology (including research in preventative oncology, quality of life, and clinical trials methodology). Participates in local, national, and international trials, including studies of all sites and types of malignancies, imaging techniques, and therapeutic trials. **Pub:** *Annual Report.*

**★ 10397 ★ Oregon Health and Science**
**University**
**Oregon Cancer Institute (OCI)**
CR 145
3181 SW Sam Jackson Park Rd.
Portland, OR 97201-3098
**Phone:** (503)494-1617
**Email:** cancer@ohsu.edu
**Website:** http://www.ohsu.edu/oci/
Dr. Grover C. Bagby, Jr., Dir.

**Activities/Fields:** Prevention, treatment, diagnosis and control of cancer by identifying the specific pathophysiologically significant molecular defects in cancer cells.

**Palo Alto Institute of Molecular Medicine**
*See:* Entry 4673

**★ 10398 ★ Parker Hughes Cancer Center**
2699 Patton Rd.
Roseville, MN 55113
**Phone:** (651)796-5400          **Free:** 800-815-7505
**Email:** info@parkerhughes.org
**Website:** http://www.ih.org/
Fatih M. Uckun, MD, Med. Dir.

**Activities/Fields:** Cancer treatments, especially the development of new, effective anti-cancer drugs.

## ★ 10399 ★ Pediatric Oncology Group

Operations Office
645 N Michigan Ave., Ste. 910
Chicago, IL 60611
**Phone:** (312)482-9944     **Fax:** (312)482-9460
**Website:** http://www.pog.ufl.edu
Dr. Sharon B. Murphy, Hd.

**Activities/Fields:** Investigations of childhood cancers. Provides a national cooperative mechanism to promote new treatment methods through comparison of patients who receive different treatments.

## ★ 10400 ★ Purdue University Cancer Center

Life Science Research Bldg.
1524 Hansen
West Lafayette, IN 47907-1524
**Phone:** (765)494-9129     **Fax:** (765)494-9193
**Website:** http://www.cancer.purdue.edu
Richard F. Borch, MD, Dir.

**Activities/Fields:** Experimental therapeutics and diagnostics, structural biology, cell growth and differentiation. **Pub:** *Annual report.*

## ★ 10401 ★ Queen's University Cancer Research Laboratories (QCRL)

Botterell Hall, 3rd Fl.
Kingston, ON, Canada K7L 3N6
**Phone:** (613)533-2778     **Fax:** (613)533-6830
**Email:** deeleyr@post.queensu.ca
**Website:** http://meds-ss10.meds.queensu.ca/medicine/crl/
Roger G. Deeley, PhD, Dir.

**Activities/Fields:** Cancer biology, including drug resistance and metabolism; tumor progression; and the regulation of cell growth, proliferation and differentiation.

## Radiation Oncology Research and Development Center

*See:* Entry 18171

## Revici Foundation for Lipid Research

*See:* Entry 20202

## Rockefeller University Laboratory of Human Genetics and Hematology

*See:* Entry 9424

## ★ 10402 ★ Roger Williams Hospital Roger Williams Cancer Center

Roger Williams Medical Center
825 Chalkstone Ave.
Providence, RI 02908
**Phone:** (401)456-6565     **Fax:** (401)456-6793
**Email:** auerbac@mail.rockefeller.edu
**Website:** http://www.rockefeller.edu/labheads/auerbach/auerbach.html
Sharon Harpel, Contact

**Activities/Fields:** Cellular immunotherapy of tumors, stem cell plasticity, molecular biology of breast and prostate cancer, molecular regulation of myelopoiesis, clinical stem cell transplantation, and cancer prevention and early detection.

## ★ 10403 ★ Roswell Park Cancer Institute

Elm & Carlton Sts.
Buffalo, NY 14263
**Phone:** (716)845-2300     **Free:** 800-685-6825
**Fax:** (716)845-8261
**Email:** askrpci@roswellpark.org
**Website:** http://www.roswellpark.org

**Activities/Fields:** Genetics, biophysical therapies, immunology, experimental therapeutics,and epidemiology of cancer, including the clinical application of recent findings in cancer research and the effectiveness of surgery, chemotherapy, and radiation in cancer therapy. Research program includes work in drug develop-

ment, pharmacokinetics, crystallography, photodynamic therapy, and biological response modifiers.
**Pub:** *Annual Scientific Report.* • *Cancer Report.* • *Monday Morning Oncology Update.* • *Roswellness.*

## ★ 10404 ★ Roswell Park Cancer Institute Laboratory of Flow Cytometry

Elm & Carlton Sts.
Buffalo, NY 14263
**Phone:** (716)845-8471     **Fax:** (716)845-8806
**Email:** flow@attglobal.net
**Website:** http://rpciflowcytometry.com
Dr. Carleton Stewart, Dir.

**Activities/Fields:** Licensed reference laboratory for the classification by immunophenotyping of leukemias and lymphomas, monitoring of transplant patients, and evaluation of DNA in solid tumors. Also uses multiparameter flow cytometry to study normal myeloid cell differentiation and the development of molecular phenotyping. Provides clinical research support for protocols that require specific immunophenotyping follow-up to monitor the progress of therapy and develops new tests to improve cancer management.

## ★ 10405 ★ Roswell Park Cancer Institute Transgenic Facility

Elm & Carlton Sts.
Buffalo, NY 14263
**Phone:** (716)845-5843     **Fax:** (716)845-5908
**Email:** paul.soloway@roswellpark.org
Paul Soloway, PhD, Dir.

**Activities/Fields:** Transgenics, including genome modification.

## ★ 10406 ★ Rumbaugh-Goodwin Institute for Cancer Research Inc.

1850 NW 69th Ave., Ste. 5
Plantation, FL 33313
**Phone:** (954)587-9020     **Fax:** (954)321-5311
**Email:** mgicr@mindspring.com
**Website:** http://www.gicr.com
Michael J. Dauphinee, PhD, Dir.

**Activities/Fields:** Biological sciences using specific pathogen-free animals to develop human tumor xenograft models to improve cancer therapy by drug synergism, immunotherapy and improved delivery of treatment modalities. Studies cover hybridoma technology and application, tumor therapy, immunohistochemistry, hemopoietic and tumor stem cell growth (promotion and inhibition), and tumor behavior in immunosuppressed animals. Research services include preclinical trials for anticancer agents, monoclonal antibody production in mouse ascites or in vitro and downstream processing. Maintains laboratories in biochemistry, immunology, immunohistochemistry, flow cytometry, molecular biology, and cell culture.
**Frmly:** Germfree Life Research Center; Goodwin Institute for Cancer Research.

## ★ 10407 ★ Rush University Bone Marrow Transplant Center

Rush-Presbyterian-St. Luke's Medical Center
1653 W Congress Pky.
Chicago, IL 60612
**Phone:** (312)942-6173     **Fax:** (312)733-1590
**Email:** hklingem@rush.edu
**Website:** http://www.rush.edu/bmt
Dr. Hans Klingemann, Dir.

**Activities/Fields:** Bone marrow transplantation in the treatment of leukemia, malignant lymphoma, myeloma, breast cancer, and graft-versus host disease in allogenic bone marrow transplantation.

## ★ 10408 ★ Rush University Rush Cancer Institute

Professional Bldg. I, Ste. 809
Rush-Presbyterian-St. Luke's Medical Center
1725 W Harrison St.
Chicago, IL 60612
**Phone:** (312)563-2190     **Free:** 800-224-7874
**Fax:** (312)455-9635

**Email:** hpreisle@rush.edu
Harvey D. Preisler, MD, Dir.

**Activities/Fields:** Cancer, including biochemistry, immunology surveillance, virology, lymphomal leukemia, and psychosocial studies. Participates in the National Cancer Institute's nationwide program for coordinating multidisciplinary basic and clincial cancer research, improving methods of treatment, diagnosis, and prevention, training health professionals, and transferring cancer knowledge to surrounding communities. **Pub:** *Rush Center Institute Newsletter.*

## ★ 10409 ★ Rutgers University Laboratory for Cancer Research

Department of Chemical Biology
College of Pharmacy
164 Frelinghuysen Rd.
Piscataway, NJ 08854-8020
**Phone:** (732)445-3400     **Fax:** (732)445-0687
**Email:** aconney@rci.rutgers.edu
**Website:** http://eohsi.rutgers.edu/lcr/
Prof. Allan H. Conney, Dir.

**Activities/Fields:** Mechanisms of chemical carcinogenesis and mutagenesis; mechanisms of inhibition of carcinogenesis; factors influencing the metabolism and action of drugs, carcinogens, environmental chemicals and steroid hormones; regulation and biological significance of multiple cytochromes P-450; drug interactions; induced synthesis of microsomal enzymes.

## ★ 10410 ★ St. Francis Hospital (Tulsa, OK) Natalie Warren Bryant Cancer Center

Warren Cancer Research Foundation
6151 S Yale, Ste. B103
Tulsa, OK 74136
**Phone:** (918)491-5878     **Fax:** (918)494-1527
Dr. Kenneth Manning, Contact

**Activities/Fields:** Bone marrow transplants, medical oncology, radiotherapy, pathology, and surgery. Conducts clinical trials.

## St. Louis University Institute for Molecular Virology

*See:* Entry 4682

## ★ 10411 ★ Salk Institute for Biological Studies Cancer Center

PO Box 85800
San Diego, CA 92186-5800
**Phone:** (858)453-4100     **Fax:** (858)457-4765
**Email:** eckhart@salk.edu
**Website:** http://www.salk.edu
Dr. Walter Eckhart, Dir.

**Activities/Fields:** Participates as one of a group of selected nonclinical cancer centers in National Cancer Institute's nationwide program for coordinating multidisciplinary basic and clinical cancer research, improving methods of treatment, diagnosis, and prevention, training health professionals, and transferring cancer knowledge to surrounding communities, established under National Cancer Act of 1971. Areas of research include molecular biology, virology, cell biology, and developmental biology. Conducts basic research into mechanisms of cell regulation and growth control.
**Frmly:** Armand Hammer Center for Cancer Biology.

## ★ 10412 ★ Saskatchewan Cancer Agency Cancer Research Unit

20 Campus Dr.
Saskatoon, SK, Canada S7N 4H4
**Phone:** (306)655-2778     **Fax:** (306)655-2639
**Email:** scarlsen@scf.sk.ca
Dr. S.A. Carlsen, Dir.

**Activities/Fields:** Basic cancer research, including elucidation of the properties of signal transduction, oncogene expression, tumor metastasis, drug sensitivity, and genetic engineering of novel biological reagents for tumor diagnosis and therapy.

**★ 10413 ★ Sickle Cell Association of the Texas Gulf Coast**
2626 S Loop W, Ste. 245
Houston, TX 77054
**Phone:** (713)666-0300 **Fax:** (713)666-0217
**Email:** scatgc@sicklecell-texas.org
Kenneth G. Beatty, Exec. Dir.
**Activities/Fields:** Performs laboratory tests to identify persons with sickle cell disease. **Pub:** *Consumer Chronicles*, bimonthly. • *Sickle Cell Anemia Fast Facts*. • *Sickle Scope Newsletter*, quarterly. **Frmly:** Sickle Cell Disease Research Foundation of Texas Inc.

**★ 10414 ★ Sidney Kimmel Cancer Center (SKCC)**
10835 Altman Row
San Diego, CA 92121
**Phone:** (858)450-5990 **Fax:** (858)450-3251
**Website:** http://www.skcc.org/
Albert B. Deisseroth, MD, Pres. /CEO
**Activities/Fields:** Cancer diagnosis, treatment and prevention, based on understanding the genetic components of cancer which may lead to gene therapy, vaccine therapy and immunotherapy. **Pub:** *SKCC News*.

**★ 10415 ★ Society for the Study of Blood**
VA Medical
800 Poly Pl.
Brooklyn, NY 11209
**Phone:** (718)836-6600 **Fax:** (718)630-2822
**Email:** luhrs.carol@new-york.va.gov
Dr. Carol Luhrs, Contact
**Activities/Fields:** Hematology, blood groupings, transfusion, physiology, and pathology of blood.

**★ 10416 ★ Stehlin Foundation for Cancer Research**
1315 St. Joseph Pky., Ste. 1818
Houston, TX 77002
**Phone:** (713)659-1336 **Fax:** (713)659-1503
**Website:** http://www.stehlin.org
Robert Anderson, Exec. Dir.
**Activities/Fields:** Tissue culture of human cancers, transplantation of human cancers into athymic mice, experimental chemotherapy of human cancers growing in tissue culture or nude mice, investigation and development of new anticancer drugs, immunology of human cancers, effects of heat on human cancers, development and treatment of breast cancer, relationships between virus and human cancer, rapid screening of anticancer drugs and clinical trials for potential anti-cancer drugs.

**★ 10417 ★ Strang Cancer Prevention Center**
428 E 72nd St.
New York, NY 10021
**Phone:** (212)794-4900 **Fax:** (212)396-1244
**Email:** mosborne@strang.org
**Website:** http://www.strang.org
Dr. Michael P. Osborne, Pres. /CEO
**Activities/Fields:** Molecular genetics; hormonal carcinogenics; evaluation of new preventive agents for colon, breast and prostate cancer. **Pub:** *Progressions Newsletter*. Newsletter. • *Strang Cancer Genetics Newsletter*. Newsletter.

**★ 10418 ★ Susan Love MD Breast Cancer Foundation**
427 E Carrillo St.
Santa Barbara, CA 93101
**Phone:** (805)963-2877 **Fax:** (805)963-6877
**Email:** slovebcf@aol.com

**Website:** http://www.susanlovemdfoundation.org
Elizabeth Thompson, Exec. Dir.
**Activities/Fields:** Breast cancer, including methods of detection and treatment, with special emphasis on the intraductal approach. **Frmly:** Santa Barbara Breast Cancer Institute.

**★ 10419 ★ Swedish Tumor Institute**
1221-1225 Madison St.
Seattle, WA 98104
**Phone:** (206)386-2323 **Fax:** (206)386-2393
Donald W. Tesh, MD, Dir.
**Activities/Fields:** Cancer, including research, treatment, prevention, pain management, early detection, genetics, and related psychosocial issues. Center also conducts on Phase I-III clinical trials in treatment, prevention, control, and epidemiology of cancer, and investigates methods of instruction in cancer pain management. **Pub:** *Cancer Institute Annual Report*.

**★ 10420 ★ Syracuse Cancer Research Institute**
600 E Genesee St.
Syracuse, NY 13202-3111
**Phone:** (315)472-6616 **Fax:** (315)476-5722
**Website:** http://www.ngen.com/hs-cancer
Joseph Gold, MD, Dir.
**Activities/Fields:** Cachexia, or weight loss and debilitation as a result of cancer. Specifically studies the drug hydrazine sulfate, a chemical that acts to block the body's chemical machinery which converts lactic acid, amino acids, and other carbon 2-5 molecules to glucose and thus depletes the normal body energy pools; and experimental combinations of chemotherapy with hydrazine sulfate and cytotoxic chemotherapeutic agents, hormones, and recombinant DNA products.

**Temple University**
**Center for Neurovirology and Cancer Biology**
**Laboratory of AIDS Pathogenesis and Molecular Therapeutics**
*See:* Entry 14283

**★ 10421 ★ Temple University**
**Center for Neurovirology and Cancer Biology**
**Laboratory of Cancer Biology and Intervention**
BioLife Sciences Bldg.
College of Science & Technology
1900 N 12th St.
Philadelphia, PA 19122
**Phone:** (215)204-0620 **Fax:** (215)204-0679
**Email:** jayrapp@astro.temple.edu
**Website:** http://www.temple.edu/cnvcb
Dr. Krzysztof Reiss, MD, Prin. Investigator
**Activities/Fields:** Molecular pathways involved in the development of cancer, especially brain cancer.

**★ 10422 ★ Temple University**
**Fels Institute for Cancer Research and Molecular Biology**
Sch. of Med.
3307 N Broad St., Rm. 150
Philadelphia, PA 19140
**Phone:** (215)707-4300 **Fax:** (215)707-4588
**Email:** reddy@unix.temple.edu
**Website:** http://www.temple.edu/fels/
E. Premkumar Reddy, Dir.
**Activities/Fields:** Basic sciences, with emphasis on biochemical, molecular, and genetic aspects of cancer, including molecular biology, cell biology, and biochemistry. **Pub:** *Annual Report*.

**★ 10423 ★ Texas Cancer Data Center**
1515 Holcombe Blvd.-573
Houston, TX 77030

**Phone:** (713)792-2277 **Fax:** (713)794-1951
**Email:** tcdc@txcancer.org
**Website:** http://www.txcancer.org
Lewis E. Foxhill, MD, Contact
**Activities/Fields:** Reduction of human suffering and economic impact of cancer on Texans by the collection of computerized information on cancer resources, services, and statistics.

**★ 10424 ★ Thomas Jefferson University Cardeza Foundation for Hematologic Research**
1015 Walnut St.
Philadelphia, PA 19107
**Phone:** (215)955-7786 **Fax:** (215)955-2366
**Email:** steven.mckenzie@mail.tju.edu
Steven E. McKenzie, MD, Dir.
**Activities/Fields:** Hematology, especially vascular biology.

**★ 10425 ★ Thomas Jefferson University Kimmel Cancer Center**
1050 Bluemle Life Sciences Bldg.
233 S 10th St.
Philadelphia, PA 19107-6799
**Phone:** (215)503-4645 **Fax:** (215)923-3528
**Email:** carlo.croce@mail.tju.edu
**Website:** http://www.kcc.tju.edu/default.htm
Carlo M. Croce, MD, Dir.
**Activities/Fields:** Genetics, including molecular genetic analysis of the normal human genome, cytogenetics of aneuploidy syndromes, genetics of the immune system, genetics of collagen and extracellular matrix genes, and molecular genetics of human hematopoietic neoplasias and solid tumors; immunology, including antigen presentation, autoimmunity, B-cell development, cancer immunology, cell growth regulation and differentiation, cellular immunology, cell activation and signal transduction, cytokines, developmental immunology, and immunochemistry; and microbiology and molecular virology, including chemical and antigenic structure of virus particles, viral replication, antiviral agents, regulation of viral gene expression, viral oncogenes, virus-cell interactions, latent virus infections, neurovirology, microbial immunology, microbial pathogenesis, antiparasite vaccine development, cell biology of malaria, and immunobiology of river blindness. **Frmly:** Jefferson Cancer Institute.

**★ 10426 ★ Thompson Cancer Survival Center**
1915 White Ave.
Knoxville, TN 37916
**Phone:** (865)541-1678 **Fax:** (865)541-2823
**Website:** http://www.thompsoncancer.com
**Activities/Fields:** Oncology, including phase I, II, and III trials of drug, radiation, or biology therapies and laser treatments. Center comprises the following research departments: Clinical Trials; Laser Photodynamic Therapy; and Bone Marrow Transplant Laboratory.

**★ 10427 ★ Tom Baker Cancer Centre**
1331 29th St. NW
Calgary, AB, Canada T2N 4N2
**Phone:** (403)670-1711 **Fax:** (403)283-1651
**Email:** gavinst@cancerboard.ab.ca
Dr. Gavin C.E. Stuart, Dir.
**Activities/Fields:** Cancer, concentrating on interleukins, cell and molecular biology, metastasis, oncogenes, immunology of melanoma, and neuroblastoma and small cell lung cancer. Clinical trials focus on cancer therapy, biotherapy, epidemiology, and prevention. **Frmly:** Southern Alberta Cancer Centre.

**★ 10428 ★ Tulane University Cancer Center**
1430 Tulane Ave., Box SL-68
New Orleans, LA 70112-2699
**Phone:** (504)585-6060 **Fax:** (504)585-6077
**Email:** rweiner@tulane.edu

**Website:** http://www.som.tulane.edu/cancer
Dr. Roy S. Weiner, Dir.

**Activities/Fields:** Cancer, including AIDS-related cancers, biochemistry, bone marrow transplant, breast cnacer, chemotherapy, diet and nutrition, endocrine, environmental carcinogens, epidemiology, eye, ear, nose, and throat, gastro-intestinal cancer, general cancer research, genetics, genito-urinary, gynecological and obstetric, head and neck cancer, hepatocellular cancer, Hodgkin's disease, Kidney cancer, leukemia, lung and esophageal cancer, lymphoma, melanoma, myeloma, occupational carcinogens, opthamology, otolaryngology, ovarian and cervical cancers, pain and anesthesia, pediatric oncology, prevention of cancer, prostate cancer, psych-oncology, racial and ethnic factors, radiation and radiotherapy, skin cancer, surgical oncology, and Wilms' tumor. **Pub:** *Inside the Tulane Cancer Center*, 3/year.


**★ 10429 ★ U.S. Department of Energy**
**Department of Energy Program Offices—Environment, Safety and Health**
**Office of Biological and Environmental Research**
**((Medical Sciences Division)**
**Boron Neutron Capture Therapy)**
19901 Germantown Rd., SC-73
Germantown, MD 20874-1290
**Phone:** (301)903-9106
**Email:** peter.kirchner@science.doe.gov
**Website:** http://www.sc.doe.gov/production/ober/msd_bnct.html
Peter Kirchner, MD, Prog. Mgr.

**Activities/Fields:** Experimental approach to cancer treatment based on a dual step technique utilizing two linked treatment components. **Pub:** *Reports*.


**★ 10430 ★ U.S. Department of Health and Human Services**
**Centers for Disease Control and Prevention**
**National Institute for Occupational Safety and Health**
**National Occupational Research Agenda**
**(Cancer Research Methods)**
NIOSH 4676
Columbia Pkwy. (C-14)
Cincinnati, OH 45226
**Phone:** (513)533-8481          **Free:** 800-356-4676
**Fax:** (513)533-8588
**Email:** pas4@cdc.gov
**Website:** http://www.cdc.gov/niosh/nrcanc.html
Paul A. Schulte, PhD, Team Ldr.

**Activities/Fields:** Prevention of occupational cancer by identifying exposures that have carcinogenic potential and eliminate or reduce their presence in the workplace.


**U.S. Department of Health and Human Services**
**Food and Drug Administration**
**Center for Bilogics Evaluation and Research**
**Laboratory of Hemostasis**
*See:* Entry 4697


**U.S. Department of Health and Human Services**
**Food and Drug Administration**
**Center for Biologics Evaluation and Research**
**Bone Marrow Growth Factors Staff**
*See:* Entry 4699

**U.S. Department of Health and Human Services**
**Food and Drug Administration**
**Center for Biologics Evaluation and Research**
**Division of Hematology**
**(Laboratory of Plasma Derivatives)**
*See:* Entry 4702


**U.S. Department of Health and Human Services**
**Food and Drug Administration**
**Center for Biologics Evaluation and Research**
**Division of Hematology**
*See:* Entry 4703


**U.S. Department of Health and Human Services**
**Food and Drug Administration**
**Center for Biologics Evaluation and Research**
**Laboratory of Cellular Hematology**
*See:* Entry 4708


**U.S. Department of Health and Human Services**
**Food and Drug Administration**
**Center for Biologics Evaluation and Research**
**Molecular Tumor Biology Staff**
*See:* Entry 4723


**★ 10431 ★ U.S. Department of Health and Human Services**
**National Cancer Institute**
Cancer Information Products & Systems
6116 Executive Blvd., Ste. 300
Rockville, MD 20852
**Phone:** (301)496-9096          **Fax:** (301)480-8105
**Email:** cancernetstaff@mail.nih.gov
Gisele Sarosy, PhD, Actg. Assoc. Dir.

**Activities/Fields:** Develops, maintains, and refines information on cancer treatment, screening, prevention, genetics, and supportive care for patients, health professionals, and the public, using editorial boards and scientific review processes. CIPS manages the production of this evidence-based information and its dissemination utilizing a variety of technologies (e.g., NCI Web sites such as CancerNet, facsimile, e-mail, etc.) and through partnerships with organizations that license NCI information. Also investigates new technologies and their applicability to gather, organize, and disseminate cancer information. ncer-related research and demonstration encompassing basic research, diagnosis, treatment, rehabilitation, and public and patient education. These centers also educate and train professionals in various clinical and research specialties. Research activities conducted at NCI's laboratories or supported through grants and contracts include many investigative approaches to cancer, including research in chemistry, biochemistry, biology, molecular biology, immunology, radiation physics, experimental chemotherapy, epidemiology, biometry, radiotherapy, and pharmacology. Major components of NCI include: Cancer Biology, Diagnosis and Centers Division; Cancer Etiology Division;.


**★ 10432 ★ U.S. Department of Health and Human Services**
**National Cancer Institute**
**Basic Sciences Division**
**Basic Research Laboratory**
NCI-Frederick
Bldg. 469, Rm. 101
Frederick, MD 21702
**Phone:** (301)846-1318          **Fax:** (301)846-6164
**Email:** kcannon@mail.ncifcrf.gov
Karen Cannon, Sec.

**Activities/Fields:** Plans and conducts research on the cellular, molecular, genetic, biochemical and immunological mechanism affecting the progression, diagnosis and treatment of cancer; and collaborates with scientists from other research programs within the National Cancer Institute and the National Institutes of Health. **Pub:** *Proceedings.* • *Research Reports*. **Frmly:** (1996) Laboratory of Molecular Oncology.


**★ 10433 ★ U.S. Department of Health and Human Services**
**National Cancer Institute**
**Division of Basic Sciences**
**Intramural Research Program**
NIH Bldg. 31, Ste. 3A11
9000 Rockville Pike
Bethesda, MD 20892
**Phone:** (301)496-4345          **Fax:** (301)496-0775
Dr. J. Carl Barrett, Dir.

**Activities/Fields:** Program comprises branches for Immunology and laboratories for studies in biochemistry, cell biology, cellular oncology, genetics, immunobiology, mathematical biology, molecular biology, tumor immunology and biology.


**★ 10434 ★ U.S. Department of Health and Human Services**
**National Cancer Institute**
**Division of Cancer Biology**
Executive Pl. N, Ste. 5000
6130 Executive Blvd.
EPN Bldg., Ste. 500
Bethesda, MD 20892
**Phone:** (301)496-7028          **Fax:** (301)496-1037
**Email:** bs62d@nih.gov
**Website:** http://www3.cancer.gov/dcb/dcbhom.htm
Barbara Spalholz, PhD, Dir.

**Activities/Fields:** Extramural and basic and applied research on cancer cell biology and immunology, including the biological and health effects of exposures to ionizing and non-ionizing radiation, and the role of chemical, physical and biological agents, acting separately or together, in the development of cancer. Principal components include the Cancer Biology Branch, Cancer Immunology Branch, Cancer Genetics Branch Biological Carcinogenesis Branch, Chemical and Physical Carcinogenesis Branch, and Radiation Effects Branch. **Pub:** *Annual Report*.


**★ 10435 ★ U.S. Department of Health and Human Services**
**National Cancer Institute**
**Division of Cancer Biology**
**Cancer Biology Branch**
6130 Executive Blvd., Ste. 5000
Bethesda, MD 20892
**Phone:** (301)496-7028          **Fax:** (301)402-1037
**Email:** cf33a@nih.gov
**Website:** http://www3.cancer.gov/dcb/cbbhom.htm
Colette S. Freeman, PhD, Chf.

**Activities/Fields:** Facilitates and supports basic biological research aimed at defin ing elements of the phenotype of the malignant cell through interdisciplinary approaches. Areas of emphasis include both positive and negative regulation of cell growth and differentiation, mechanisms involved in the process of metastasis and of angiogenesis, the influence of the extracellular environment on the tumor cell, GENE EXPRESSION, PATHWAYS OF SIGNAL TRANSDUCTION, MODELS FOR CANCER BIOLOGY and the molecular biology of cancer cells.


**★ 10436 ★ U.S. Department of Health and Human Services**
**National Cancer Institute**
**Division of Cancer Biology**
**Cancer Genetics Branch**
6130 Executive Blvd., EPN 700
Bethesda, MD 20892
**Phone:** (301)496-1591          **Fax:** (301)402-7819
Dr. Sheila E. Taube, Chf.

**Activities/Fields:** Early detection, diagnosis (including staging, grading, and prognosis), and monitoring of changes during therapy or progression of disease. Projects in these areas are frequently concerned with improvement of existing techniques as well as the development of new tests and procedures. Supports research in the areas of immunodiagnosis, pathology/cytology, and biochemistry and genetics.

**★ 10437 ★  U.S. Department of Health**
**    and Human Services**
**National Cancer Institute**
**Division of Cancer Biology**
**Cancer Immunology Branch**
Executive Plaza N, Rm. 501
6130 Executive Blvd.
Bethesda, MD 20892-7381
**Phone:** (301)496-7815          **Fax:** (301)480-2844
**Email:** am214t@nih.gov
**Website:** http://www.nci.nih.gov/dcb/cibhom.htm
Robert A. Mufson, PhD, Chf.

**Activities/Fields:** Molecular immunology and cellular immunology, with special emphasis on understanding the role of the immune system in the development, growth, and spread of tumors as it relates to the problems of cause, prevention, treatment, and diagnosis of malignant diseases.

**★ 10438 ★  U.S. Department of Health**
**    and Human Services**
**National Cancer Institute**
**Division of Cancer Biology**
**Chemical and Physical Carcinogenesis**
**    Program**
6130 Executive Blvd., Ste. 5000
MSC 7386
Bethesda, MD 20892-7055
**Phone:** (301)496-5471          **Fax:** (301)496-1040
**Email:** dl58s@nih.gov
**Website:** http://www.nci.nih.gov/DCB/DCBhom.htm
Dr. David Longfellow, Branch Chf.

**Activities/Fields:** Occurrence of cancer caused or promoted by chemical or physical agents, acting separately or together, or in combination with biological agents; and provides a broad spectrum of information, advice, and consultation to individual scientists and institutional science management officials relative to NIH and NCI funding and scientific review policies and procedures, preparation of grant applications, and choice of funding instruments. The Branch also: provides NCI management with recommendations as to funding needs, priorities, and strategies for the support of relevant research areas consistent with the current state of development of individual research activities and the promise of new initiatives; plans, develops, and manages research resources necessary for the conduct of the coordinated research program; and plans, organizes, and conducts meetings and workshops to further program objectives and maintains contact with the relevant scientific community to identify and evaluate new research trends relating to its program responsibilities. **Pub:** *National Cancer Institute's Annual Report.*

**★ 10439 ★  U.S. Department of Health**
**    and Human Services**
**National Cancer Institute**
**Division of Cancer Biology**
**Radiation Effects Branch**
6130 Executive Blvd.
Rockville, MD 20852-7391
**Phone:** (301)496-9326          **Fax:** (301)496-1224
**Website:** http://www.nih.gov
Bruce Wachholz, Chf.

**Activities/Fields:** Mechanisms of radiation-induced mutagenesis and carcinogenesis including supportive studies in radiation chemistry, radiation physics, molecular biology, cytogenetics and cell transformation; studies of cancer among selected populations exposed to radionuclides intentionally or accidentally released into the environment.

**★ 10440 ★  U.S. Department of Health**
**    and Human Services**
**National Cancer Institute**
**Division of Cancer Control and**
**    Population Sciences**
**Extramural Epidemiology and Genetics**
**    Program**
6130 Executive Blvd., Rm. 5114
MSC 7395
Bethesda, MD 20892-7395
**Phone:** (301)594-9499          **Fax:** (301)435-5477
**Email:** winnde@mail.nih.gov
**Website:** http://epi.grants.cancer.gov/index.html
Dr. Deborah Winn, PhD, Actg. Assoc. Dir.

**Activities/Fields:** Plans, develops, directs and manages a national extramural program of basic and applied research in biometry, epidemiology, and related multidisciplinary activities; establishes program priorities and evaluates program effectiveness; provides a broad spectrum of information, advice, and consultation to individual scientists and institutional sciences management officials concerning National Institutes of Health and National Cancer Institute (NCI) funding and scientific review policies and procedures, preparation of grant applications, and choice of funding instruments; provides (NCI) management with recommendations as to funding needs, priorities and strategies for the support of relevant research areas consistent with the current state of development of individual research activities and the promise of new initiatives; plans, develops, and manages research resources necessary for the conduct of the coordinated research program; and plans, organizes, and conducts meetings and workshops to further program objectives.

**★ 10441 ★  U.S. Department of Health**
**    and Human Services**
**National Cancer Institute**
**Division of Cancer Epidemiology and**
**    Genetics**
6120 Executive Blvd., Rm. 8070
Bethesda, MD 20892
**Phone:** (301)496-1611          **Fax:** (301)402-3256
Dr. Joseph F. Fraumeni, Jr., Contact

**Activities/Fields:** The Division of Cancer Epidemiology and Genetics (DCEG) is the primary focus within the National Cancer Institute for population-based research on environmental and genetic determinants of cancer. Intramural and collaborative interdisciplinary studies are conducted on the distribution, causes and natural history of cancer, and the means for its prevention. Research areas of special interest include genetic predisposition, lifestyle factors, environmental contaminants, occupational exposures, medications, radiation and infectious agents, as well as statistics and methods development.

**★ 10442 ★  U.S. Department of Health**
**    and Human Services**
**National Cancer Institute**
**Division of Cancer Epidemiology and**
**    Genetics**
**Epidemiology and Biostatistics Program**
EPS - 7018
Bethesda, MD 20892-7236
**Phone:** (301)496-5785          **Fax:** (301)402-4489
Dr. Peggy Tucker, Chf.

**Activities/Fields:** Activities of the Clinical Epidemiology Branch include: status and future prospects for research in specific areas of clinical observations of cancer patients and from clinical studies of families epistimology. and occupational groups and correlation of these results with laboratory findings; studies of the late effects of childhood cancer and the therapy of childhood cancer; operation of a clinic dealing with the genetics of human cancer to evaluate factors affecting risks of specific types of cancer such as neurofibromatosis; and preparation of analytical reviews to define current status and future prospects for research in specific areas of clinical epidemiology.

**★ 10443 ★  U.S. Department of Health**
**    and Human Services**
**National Cancer Institute**
**Division of Cancer Prevention and**
**    Control**
**Cancer Control Research Program**
**(Public Health Applications Branch)**
6130 Executive Blvd., Rm. 241
Bethesda, MD 20892
**Phone:** (301)496-8585          **Fax:** (301)496-8675
Mark Manley, Chf.

**Activities/Fields:** Responsible for the development, implementation, and evaluation of an extramural research program aimed at reducing risk factors for cancer and increasing early detection of cancer. **Pub:** *Monographs.* • *Professional journals.* **Frmly:** Health Promotion Science Branch.

**★ 10444 ★  U.S. Department of Health**
**    and Human Services**
**National Cancer Institute**
**Division of Cancer Prevention and**
**    Control**
**Cancer Control Research Program**
6130 Executive Blvd, Rm. 232
Rockville, MD 20852
**Phone:** (301)496-8594          **Fax:** (301)480-6637
Thomas J. Glynn, PhD, Chf.

**Activities/Fields:** Widespread use of proven health promotion and other cancer prevention and management techniques by health professionals, patients and their families, populations at elevated risk, and the general public; monitor basic and clinical research activities in order to identify new interventions that will reduce cancer rates in populations and to facilitate research on their application; provide training opportunities for research and/or application of cancer prevention and management interventions; establish program priorities, allocate resources, and integrate the projects of the various participating branches; and provide programmatic and consultative support to other divisional, institute, governmental, and private sector organizations that facilitate the application of proven cancer control interventions in populations. Program comprises branches for Cancer Control Applications, Health Promotion Science, and Special Population Studies. (A fourth unit, the Cancer Training Branch, no longer exists.).

**★ 10445 ★  U.S. Department of Health**
**    and Human Services**
**National Cancer Institute**
**Division of Cancer Prevention and**
**    Control**
**Cancer Prevention Program**
**(Chemoprevention Branch)**
Executive Plaza N, Rm. 2118 M
6130 Executive Blvd.
M.S 7322
Bethesda, MD 20892
**Phone:** (301)496-8563          **Fax:** (301)402-0553
Dir. James Crowell, MD, Chf.

**Activities/Fields:** Chemoprevention involves the study and development of selected micronutrients or other small molecular weight substances for the purposes of reducing cancer incidence. Research has focused on identifying or demonstrating (in animal models, epidemiological studies, and human clinical trials) natural or synthetic agents that can lower cancer incidence. Activities include 68 ongoing clinical trials nationally and internationally with 200,000 subjects. Also develops drugs.

**★ 10446 ★  U.S. Department of Health**
**    and Human Services**
**National Cancer Institute**
**Division of Cancer Prevention and**
**    Control**
**Cancer Prevention Program**
9000 Rockville Pike
Bethesda, MD 20892

**Phone:** (301)496-8567          **Fax:** (301)402-0553
Dr. Winfred Malone, Actg. Assoc. Dir.

**Activities/Fields:** Cancer detection to determine which technique s for early detection of cancer can reduce morbidity and mortality from cancer; chemo-prevention research to determine whether selected micronutrients or synthetic compounds can be shown in human trials to reduce cancer incidence; and diet and cancer research to determine whether changes in the diet can be shown to reduce cancer incidence in human trials. Principal components are the Prevention Program.


★ **10447** ★ **U.S. Department of Health and Human Services**
**National Cancer Institute**
**Division of Cancer Prevention and Control**
**Early Detection and Community Oncology Program**
c/o Barnett S Kramer
Office of Medical Applications of Research
31 Center Dr., Rm. 1B01
Bethesda, MD 20892
**Phone:** (301)496-9569          **Fax:** (301)496-9931
Dr. Barnett S. Kramer, Dep. Dir., DCPC

**Activities/Fields:** Cancer centers and scientific investigations to improve cancer treatment, rehabilitation, and continuing care. EDCOP encourages collaboration and transfer of technology and information among cancer centers, community hospitals, physicians, and other health professionals; seeks ways to enhance the efforts of centers and community resources to advance cancer control; and stimulates integrated research, both basic and clinical, for specific cancers (breast, large bowel, pancreas, prostate, and urinary bladder). Support of community programs generating basic and clinical data about cancer and accelerates transfer of knowledge to health professionals and to the general public. In the areas of treatment, continuing care, and rehabi litation, EDCOP supports comparative and demonstration research on effective techniques, procedures, and protocols that have specific applicability to physical, cosmetic, functional, social, and psychological problems related to cancer. Program comprises the Cancer Centers Branch, Centers and Community Oncology Program.


★ **10448** ★ **U.S. Department of Health and Human Services**
**National Cancer Institute**
**Division of Cancer Prevention and Population Sciences**
**Cancer Surveillance Research Program**
6116 Executive Blvd., MSC 8315
Bethesda, MD 20892-8315
**Phone:** (301)496-8506          **Fax:** (301)480-4077
Dr. Brenda K. Edwards, Assoc. Dir.

**Activities/Fields:** Impact of cancer and monitor the effects of cancer prevention and control activities in research, prevention, screening, treatment, and rehabilitation. Program also provides application research support for a broad range of activities in the Cancer Prevention and Control Division. Principal areas of interest are incidence, survival, and mortality of cancer in the United States as monitored through the Surveillance, Epidemiology, and End Results (SEER) Program; health behavior and chemical practice patterns; economics of cancer; and cancer control resource allocations. Program comprises branches for Computer Systems, Cancer Statistics, and Applied Research.
**Pub:** *Annual Cancer Statistics Review.*


★ **10449** ★ **U.S. Department of Health and Human Services**
**National Cancer Institute**
**Division of Cancer Treatment and Diagnosis**
**Developmental Therapeutics Program (Natural Products Branch)**
NCI-Frederick
Fairview Center, Ste. 206
PO Box B 2-1201
Frederick, MD 21702-1201
**Phone:** (301)846-5387          **Fax:** (301)846-6178
**Email:** cragg@dtpax2.ncifcrf.gov
**Website:**        http://dtp.nci.nih.gov/branches/npb/index.html
Dr. Gordon Cragg, Chf.

**Activities/Fields:** Acquisition of novel natural products for testing for anticancer anti-HIV activity via fermentation programs; and plant and marine organism collection and extraction projects.


★ **10450** ★ **U.S. Department of Health and Human Services**
**National Cancer Institute (NCI)**
**Division of Cancer Treatment and Diagnosis (DCTD)**
**Developmental Therapeutics Program (DTP)**
**(Toxicology and Pharmacology Branch — T&PB)**
Executive Plaza N, Ste. 8034
6130 Executive Blvd.
Bethesda, MD 20892-7451
**Phone:** (301)496-8777          **Fax:** (301)480-4836
**Email:** tomaszej@mail.nih.gov
**Website:**        http://epsws1.ncifcrf.gov:2345/dis3d/dtp.html
Dr. Joseph E. Tomaszewski, Chf.

**Activities/Fields:** Provides the safety and toxicity information required for the scientific evaluation of new antitumor and anti-HIV drugs and vaccines by the Cancer Treatment Division's Drug Development Group or through the RAID Program for Phase I clinical trials. It is responsible for the acquisition of toxicology data on both new and established agents. The data accumulated are evaluated, and, for new drugs, provide the database for deriving the initial clinical dose and the toxicological base required for an Investigational New Drug Application to the Food and Drug Administration. The Branch also plans and guides developmental research for organ-specific toxicity assays such as bone marrow and heart, provides assistance for the development of new toxicology assays, tests new radiosensitizers and radioprotectors and assists the Pharmaceutical Resources Branch in the evaluation of experimental drug formulations.


★ **10451** ★ **U.S. Department of Health and Human Services**
**National Cancer Institute**
**Division of Cancer Treatment and Diagnosis**
**Developmental Therapeutics Program (Grants and Contracts Operations Branch)**
Executive Plaza N, Rm. 8153
9000 Rockville Pike
Bethesda, MD 20892-7456
**Phone:** (301)496-8783          **Fax:** (301)402-5200
**Email:** wolpertm@exchange.nih.gov
**Website:** http://dtp.nci.nih.gov
Dr. Mary Wolpert, Chf.

**Activities/Fields:** Preclinical anticancer drug discovery and development.


★ **10452** ★ **U.S. Department of Health and Human Services**
**National Cancer Institute**
**Division of Cancer Treatment, Diagnosis, and Centers**
NIH Bldg. 31, 3A44
31 Center Dr., MSC 2440
Bethesda, MD 20892-2440
**Phone:** (301)496-4291          **Fax:** (301)496-0826
**Email:** ef30d@nih.gov
**Website:** http://www3.cancer.gov/dctd/index.html
Dr. Ellen Feigal, Actg. Dir.

**Activities/Fields:** Cancer treatment activities with the objective of curing or controlling cancer in man by utilizing combination modalities (including chemical, surgical, radiological, and certain immunological techniques); administers a total drug development program; and serves as the national focal point for information and data on cancer treatment studies. Division components are: Cancer Therapy Evaluation Program; Developmental Therapeutics Program; Radiation Research Program; Biomedical Imaging Program; Cancer Diagnosis Program.


★ **10453** ★ **U.S. Department of Health and Human Services**
**National Cancer Institute**
**Division of Cancer Treatment, Diagnosis, and Centers**
**Biological Response Modifiers Program (Biological Resources Branch)**
Frederick Cancer Research and Development Center
Bldg. 1052, Rm. 253
PO Box B
Frederick, MD 21701
**Phone:** (301)846-1098          **Fax:** (301)846-5429
Dr. Stephen Creckmore, Chf.

**Activities/Fields:** Preclinical and clinical biological response modifiers re search in the biomedical community. The Branch monitors Phase I and early Phase II clinical studies that assess biological effects of biological response modifiers in cancer patients and correlate changes in the biological modifications with antitumor activity. In addition, Branch has established a preclinical screening program for the selection and preclinical assessment of the efficacy of biological response modifiers. A resource distribution system involving information acquisition and assessment as well as agent acquisition and testing has also been established.


★ **10454** ★ **U.S. Department of Health and Human Services**
**National Cancer Institute**
**Division of Cancer Treatment, Diagnosis, and Centers**
**Cancer Centers Branch**
6116 Executive Blvd., Ste. 700
MSC8345
Bethesda, MD 20892-8345
**Phone:** (301)496-8531          **Fax:** (301)402-0181
**Email:** lw187q@nih.gov
**Website:** http://www3.cancer.gov/cancercenters/
Linda K. Weiss, PhD, Chf.

**Activities/Fields:** Multidisciplinary cancer research efforts in the areas of basic, clinical and cancer prevention, control and population sciences. The Cancer Center Support Grant (CCSG) is intended to provide infrastructure for academic and research institutions for establishing and sustaining an interdisciplinary research focus on cancer. **Pub:** *Proceedings.* • *Research Reports.*

**★ 10455 ★ U.S. Department of Health and Human Services**
**National Cancer Institute**
**Division of Cancer Treatment, Diagnosis, and Centers**
**Clinical Oncology Program**
**(Radiation Oncology Branch)**
NIH Bldg. 10, Rm. B3B69
9000 Rockville Pike
Bethesda, MD 20892
**Phone:** (301)496-5457　　**Fax:** (301)480-5439
Dr. C. Norm Coleman, Dir.

**Activities/Fields:** Clinical investigation of cancer treatment using X-ray technology; and laboratory investigation of radiobiology of human tumor cell lines, mechanisms of action of various compounds and their effects on radiosensitization/radioprotection, and phototherapy and radioimmunoglobulin for prescriptions. Emphasis is on radiation sensitizing compounds, radioprotecting compounds, intraoperative irradiation, and atypical fractionation schemes. Areas of investigation include primary breast cancer, carcinoma of the bladder, small cell carcinoma of the lung, lymphoma, Hodgkin's disease, gliomas, mycosis fungoides, soft tissue sarcomas, and pediatric neoplasms. **Pub:** *Proceedings.*

**★ 10456 ★ U.S. Department of Health and Human Services**
**National Cancer Institute**
**Division of Cancer Treatment, Diagnosis, and Centers**
**Clinical Oncology Program**
**(NCI-Navy Medical Oncology Branch)**
NCI-NNMC
8901 Wisconsin
Bethesda, MD 20889-5105
**Phone:** (301)496-0901　　**Fax:** (301)496-0047
Dr. Barry Gause, Chf.

**Activities/Fields:** New modes of detection, staging, and treatment of human cancers by integrat ing clinical and laboratory research with an emphasis on understanding the fundamental biology of human tumor cells and applying these lessons to the clinic. By combining the most recent techniques of cellular and molecular biology with innovative clinical treatment studies, entering patients into other NCI protocols, and providing clinical care to Department of Defense patients for the Naval Hospital, the Branch represents a unique resource to both the National Cancer Institute and the Naval Hospital. The Branch is concerned with the primary care and clinical investigation of patients with a variety of solid tumors and hematologic malignancies. A major effort involves the staging and treatment of carcinomas of the breast, lung, and gastrointestinal tract. Performs chemotherapeutic protocols.

**★ 10457 ★ U.S. Department of Health and Human Services**
**National Cancer Institute**
**Division of Cancer Treatment, Diagnosis, and Centers**
**Developmental Therapeutics Program**
Executive Plaza N, Rm. 8000
6130 Executive Blvd.
Bethesda, MD 20892-7458
**Phone:** (301)496-8720　　**Fax:** (301)402-0831
**Email:** eslb@nih.gov
**Website:** http://dtp.nci.nih.gov/
Dr. Edward A. Sausville, Assoc. Dir.

**Activities/Fields:** Preclinical discovery and development of anticancer and anti-HIV agents for the Division of Cancer Treatment and Diagnosis, focusing on chemotherapy and comprising both extramural and intramural elements. The extramural component includes nine branches: Biological Resources Branch; Biological Testing Branch; Drug Synthesis and Chemistry Branch; Grants and Contracts Operations Branch; Information Technology Branch; Natural Products Branch; Pharmaceutical Resources Branch; Pharmacology and Toxicology Branch; Screening Technologies Branch. The intramural program includes the Laboratory of Drug Discovery Research and Development. Program is responsible for all preclinical phases of development, including acquisition and synthesis of materials, screening, production of diverse products, pharmaceutical development, toxicology, and pharmacology.

**★ 10458 ★ U.S. Department of Health and Human Services**
**National Cancer Institute**
**Division of Cancer Treatment, Diagnosis, and Centers**
**Developmental Therapeutics Program**
**(Information Technology Branch)**
Executive Plaza N, Rm. 811
6130 Executive Blvd.
Rockville, MD 20852
**Phone:** (301)496-8747　　**Fax:** (301)480-4808
**Email:** zaharevitz@dtpax2.ncifcrf.gov
**Website:** http://dtp.nci.nih.gov
Kenneth Paull, Chf.

**Activities/Fields:** All data associated with the Developmental Therapeutics Program. This includes data pertaining to the acquisition of chemicals and their structure and estimated properties as well as data derived from biological screening and from toxicology measurements. A developmental effort within the Branch is directed at improved methodologies of large file searching, new techniques for chemical structure manipulation, and studies of the relationships between chemical structure and physical and biological properties of molecules. **Pub:** *Proceedings.* • *Research Reports.*

**★ 10459 ★ U.S. Department of Health and Human Services**
**National Cancer Institute**
**Division of Cancer Treatment, Diagnosis, and Centers**
**Developmental Therapeutics Program**
**(Drug Synthesis and Chemistry Branch)**
Executive Plaza N, Ste. 8028
6130 Executive Blvd.
Bethesda, MD 20892-7448
**Phone:** (301)496-8795　　**Fax:** (301)480-4817
Dr. Ven Narayanan, Chf.

**Activities/Fields:** Acquiring and managing the flow of unique synthetic compounds for evaluation as potential anticancer agents.

**★ 10460 ★ U.S. Department of Health and Human Services**
**National Cancer Institute (NCI)**
**Division of Cancer Treatment, Diagnosis, and Centers**
**Diagnostic Imaging Program**
Executive Plaza N, Rm. 6000
6130 Executive Blvd.
Bethesda, MD 20892
**Phone:** (301)496-9531　　**Fax:** (301)480-5785
**Email:** sullivand@dtpepn.nci.nih.gov
**Website:** http://cancer.gov/bip
Dr. Daniel C. Sullivan, Assoc. Dir.

**Activities/Fields:** Responsible for both the stimulation of research in need-determined areas and the administration of grants, contracts, and cooperative agreements in support of development and evaluation of radiologic diagnostic imaging systems and related technology, including instrumentation and methodology to improve diagnosis of cancer and other diseases. This includes rapidly developing nonionizing modalities such as magnetic resonance imaging (MRI), diaphanography, and ultrasound as well as improvements in X-ray computed tomography (CT), digital radiography, positron emission tomography (PET), single photon emission computed tomography (SPECT), and other research in nuclear medicine and nuclide imaging such as the diagnostic applications of radio-labeled monoclonal antibodies.

**★ 10461 ★ U.S. Department of Health and Human Services**
**National Cancer Institute**
**Division of Cancer Treatment, Diagnosis, and Centers**
**Radiation Research Program**
**(Radiotherapy Development Branch)**
Executive Plaza N, 6015-A
6130 Executive Blvd.
Bethesda, MD 20892-7440
**Phone:** (301)496-9360　　**Fax:** (301)480-5785
**Email:** fmahoney@mail.nih.gov
Francis J. Mahoney, PhD, Actg. Chf.

**Activities/Fields:** Cancer treatment. The scientific disciplines represented are radiation oncology, radiobiology, radiation chemistry, and radiation physics. Major areas of research in terms of funding are particle radiotherapy (photons, electrons, and particles), hyperthermia, radiation modifiers, radioimmunotherapy, radiobiology, expert systems, and radiation physics.

**★ 10462 ★ U.S. Department of Health and Human Services**
**National Cancer Institute**
**Division of Cancer Treatment, Diagnosis, and Centers**
**Radiation Research Program**
Executive Plaza N 6015-A
6130 Executive Blvd., MSC 7440
Bethesda, MD 20892-7440
**Phone:** (301)496-6111　　**Fax:** (301)480-5785
**Email:** ccoleman@mail.nih.gov
Dr. C. Norman Coleman, Dir.

**Activities/Fields:** Diagnosis, staging, treatment, and post-treatmen t evaluation for the cancer patient for whom radiation and related forms of energy are used. It is an extramural radiation research program which establishes program priorities, allocates resources, maintains project integration, evaluates program effectiveness, and represents the program area in the management and scientific decision-making processes of the National Cancer Institute. This requires the coordination of research program activities with related programs elsewhere at NCI and NIH, with other federal agencies, and with national and international research organizations. The Program's branches are Diagnostic Imaging Research and Radiotherapy Development.

**★ 10463 ★ U.S. Department of Health and Human Services**
**National Cancer Institute**
**Division of Clinical Sciences**
NIH Bldg. 10, Rm. 12N214
10 Center Dr. MSC 1904
Bethesda, MD 20892-1904
**Phone:** (301)496-4251　　**Fax:** (301)496-9962
**Email:** gc45e@nih.gov
Dr. Gregory A. Curt, Clin. Dir.

**Activities/Fields:** Intramural treatment-research arm of the e National Cancer Institute. It comprises branches for: Clinical Pharmacology, Medicine, NCI-Navy Medical Oncology, Pediatrics, Radiation Oncology, and Surgery.

**★ 10464 ★ U.S. Department of Health and Human Services**
**National Cancer Institute**
**Division of Clinical Sciences**
**Cancer Prevention Studies Branch**
Executive Plaza N, Rm. 211, MS 7326
6060 Executive Blvd.
Bethesda, MD 20892-7326
**Phone:** (301)496-8559　　**Fax:** (301)435-8644
**Email:** pt1@nih.gov
**Website:** http://www-dcs.nci.nih.gov/branches/cpsb
Philip R. Taylor, MD, Chf.

**Activities/Fields:** Cancer control. It conducts intramural research in the areas of die t, nutrition, and cancer; genetics and cancer; cancer chemoprevention; and other cancer prevention strategies aimed at lowering human cancer risk. Current focus is on nutrition, primarily through development of prevention trials. Research includes studies in cancer epidemiology, clinical nutrition, and genetic epidemiology; and development of cancer prevention trials and epidemiologic methods.


**★ 10465 ★ U.S. Department of Health and Human Services**
**National Cancer Institute**
**Division of Clinical Sciences**
**Cancer Therapy Evaluation Program**
**(Biometric Research Branch)**
Executive Plaza N, Rm. 739
Bethesda, MD 20892
**Phone:** (301)496-4836     **Fax:** (301)402-0560
**Website:** http://ctep.info.nih.gov/BRB
Dr. Richard Simon, Chf.

**Activities/Fields:** Integral unit of Cancer Treatment and Diagnosis Division. It develops and evaluates clinical and biological data relating to cancer treatment.


**★ 10466 ★ U.S. Department of Health and Human Services**
**National Cancer Institute**
**Division of Clinical Sciences**
**Cancer Therapy Evaluation Program**
6130 Executive Blvd.
Ste. 7018
Bethesda, MD 20892
**Phone:** (301)496-6138     **Fax:** (301)402-0084
Dr. Michele Christian, Dir.

**Activities/Fields:** Responsible for the administration and coordination of the majority of the extramural clinical trials supported by the Cancer Treatment Division. These programs include the activities of the clinical cooperative groups, the Phase I and Phase II drug development contractors, and the holders of investigator-initiated grants relating to cancer treatment. (Certain programs in developmental radiotherapy, such as high LET radiation, are administered in the Radiation Research Program; and the Phase I development of biologic response modifiers is handled by the Biological Response Modifiers Program.) Principal components of CTEP are: the Biometric Research Branch, Clinical Investigations Branch, Investigational Drug Branch, and the Regulatory Affairs Branch.


**★ 10467 ★ U.S. Department of Health and Human Services**
**National Cancer Institute**
**Division of Clinical Sciences**
**Hypoxia and Tumorigenesis Unit**
Bldg. 37, Rm. 2C08
37 Convent Dr.
Bethesda, MD 20892-4255
**Phone:** (301)496-7279     **Fax:** (301)496-0497
**Email:** huange@mail.nih.gov
**Website:** http://www.nci.nih.gov/intra/LHC/hypoxia.htm
Eric Huang, Prin. Investigator

**Activities/Fields:** Mechanisms by which hypoxia contributes to tumorigenesis. Research focuses on hypoxia-inducible factor 1 (HIF1), and its role in tumor formation, progression, and metastasis.


**★ 10468 ★ U.S. Department of Health and Human Services**
**National Cancer Institute**
**Division of Clinical Sciences**
**Intramural Research Program**
**(Metabolism Branch)**
NIH Bldg. 10, Rm. 4N115
10 Center Dr. MSC1374
Bethesda, MD 20892-1374
**Phone:** (301)496-6653     **Fax:** (301)496-9956
**Email:** tawald@helix.nih.gov
Dr. Thomas A. Waldmann, Chf.

**Activities/Fields:** Clinical and laboratory investigations focusing on performing molecular analyses of lymphocyte development and function, including purification of transactivating factors and the genes that encode them; functional genomics involving cDNA microarray analysis of human leukemia/lymphoma; developing antigen processing and the presentation to T lymphocytes with applications to vaccine design for AIDS and cancer; characterizing the multisubunit IL-2 and IL-15 receptors and developing their use as a target for immunotherapy using humanized monoclonal antibodies armed with toxins and alpha and beta emitting radionuclides; studying the arrangement of immunoglobulin and T-cell antigen receptor genes in normal and neoplastic cells; and evaluating biochemical events that accompany cell growth and the hormonal control of this growth as they relate to the study of malignancies.


**★ 10469 ★ U.S. Department of Health and Human Services**
**National Cancer Institute**
**Division of Clinical Sciences**
**Laboratory of Human Carcinogenesis**
37 Convent Dr.
Bldg. 37, Rm. 2COS
Bethesda, MD 20892-4255
**Phone:** (301)496-2048     **Fax:** (301)496-0497
**Email:** curtis_harris@nih.gov
**Website:**     http://www.nci.nih.gov/intra/LHC/LHCPAGE.htm
Curtis C. Harris, MD, Ch.

**Activities/Fields:** Molecular mechanisms of human carcinogenesis; experimental approaches in biological systems for the extrapolation of carcinogenesis data and mechanisms from experimental animals to human situation; and host factors that determine differences in carcinogenesis susceptibility among individuals.
**Pub:** *Bibliography*, annually.


**★ 10470 ★ U.S. Department of Health and Human Services**
**National Cancer Institute**
**Division of Clinical Sciences**
**Medicine Branch**
NIH Bldg. 10, Rm. 12N226
9000 Rockville Pike
Bethesda, MD 20892
**Phone:** (301)496-4916     **Fax:** (301)402-0172
Dr. Carmen Allegra, Actg. Ch.

**Activities/Fields:** Adult medical oncology unit with clinical programs emphasizing the broad area of internal medicine as related to cancer. Clinical emphasis is given to the diagnosis, staging, and treatment of Hodgkin's disease, malignant lymphomas, breast cancer, ovarian carcinoma, sarcomas, melanoma, AIDS/Kaposi's Sarcoma, chronic leukemias, and testicular carcinoma. The research program focuses on the general areas of drug resistance and cytogenetics of neoplastic and hemopoietic cells, tumor immunology, and the biochemical pharmacology of antineoplastic agents. A collaborative effort with the Clinical Pharmacology Branch and other groups concerned with pharmacokinetics is maintained. In addition, an active research program is in progress in the fields of hormone receptors and the molecular biology of hormone action.


**★ 10471 ★ U.S. Department of Health and Human Services**
**National Cancer Institute**
**Division of Clinical Sciences**
**Surgery Branch**
NIH Bldg. 10, Rm. 2B42
10 Center Dr.
Bethesda, MD 20892
**Phone:** (301)496-4164     **Fax:** (301)402-1738
Dr. Steven Rosenberg, Chf.

**Activities/Fields:** Treatment of solid tumors and a broad program of laboratory research in c ancer. A wide variety of malignancies are studied, including melanomas, sarcomas, rectal cancer, breast carcinoma, pancreatic cancers, and head and neck cancers. The Branch investigates the use of adjuvant chemotherapy and immunotherapy and develops surgical techniques. Laboratory efforts of the Surgery Branch are closely related to its clinical activities and include programs in tumor immunology and surgical metabolism. Branch staff also serve as general surgeons to the entire National Institutes of Health and provide a variety of general surgical consultations not necessarily related to the field of cancer medicine.


**★ 10472 ★ U.S. Department of Health and Human Services**
**National Cancer Institute**
**Division of Extramural Activities**
6116 Executive Blvd., Ste. 8000
Mail Stop 8327
Bethesda, MD 20892
**Phone:** (301)496-5147     **Fax:** (301)402-0956
**Email:** mk74s@nih.gov
**Website:** http://www.nci.nih.gov
Marvin R. Kalt, PhD, Dir.

**Activities/Fields:** Administers and directs the National Cancer Institute's grant and contract review and processing activities; provides initial technical and scientific merit review of grants and contracts for the Institute; represents NCI on overall NIH extramural and collaborative program policy committees, coordinates such policy within NCI, and develops and recommends NCI policies and procedures as related to the review of grants and contracts; coordinates the Institute's review of research grant and training programs with the National Cancer Advisory Board; coordinates the implementation of committee management policies within NCI and provides the Institute's staff support for the National Cancer Advisory Board; coordinates program planning and evaluation in the extramural area; and provides scientific reports and analyses to the Institute's grant and contract programs. Principal components are the Grants Review Branch, Special Review and Resources Branch, Program Coordination and Referral Branch, Applied Information Systems Branch, and the Research Analysis and Evaluation Branch, which analyzes and indexes the scientific content of all grants awarded by NCI as well as NCI contracts and extramural programs.


**★ 10473 ★ U.S. Department of Health and Human Services**
**National Cancer Institute**
**Division of Extramural Activities**
**Special Review and Resources**
6130 Executive Blvd. EPN Rm. 605
Bethesda, MD 20892
**Phone:** (301)496-7903     **Fax:** (301)402-0742
Wilna A. Woods, Ch.

**Activities/Fields:** Branch reviews the technical merit of all research and development, scientific resource, and scientific support contract proposals submitted to NCI in response to Requests for Proposals (RFPs).


**★ 10474 ★ U.S. Department of Health and Human Services**
**National Cancer Institute**
**Frederick Cancer Research and Development Center**
Bldg. 427, Rm. 1
PO Box B
Frederick, MD 21702-1201
**Phone:** (301)846-1113     **Fax:** (301)846-6628
**Email:** rd5lm@nih.gov
**Website:** http://web.neifcrf.gov
Dr. Ronald H. DeFelice, Chf.

**Activities/Fields:** Genetic and biochemical events related to the development and expression for the malignant phenotype; and develops strategies for therapeutic intervention in the malignant process based on these findings.

**★ 10475 ★ U.S. Department of Health and Human Services**
**National Cancer Institute**
**International Cancer Information Center**
6116 Executive Blvd.
Ste. 300-A
Rockville, MD 20852
**Phone:** (301)496-9096     **Fax:** (301)480-8105
Gisele Sarosy, MD, Actg. Assoc. Dir.
**Activities/Fields:** Purpose of ICRDB is to collect, analyze, and disseminate all data useful in prevention, diagnosis, treatment and supportive care of cancer and, as feasible, to disseminate results of cancer research undertaken in any country for the use of anyone conducting cancer research in any country. **Pub:** *Overviews.* • *Recent Reviews.*

**★ 10476 ★ U.S. Department of Health and Human Services**
**National Cancer Institute**
**Laboratory of Biochemistry**
NIH Bldg. 37, Rm. 6106C, MSC 4255
9000 Rockville Pike
Bethesda, MD 20892-4255
**Phone:** (301)496-5957     **Fax:** (301)402-3095
**Email:** ckl@helix.nih.gov
Dr. Claude Klee, MD, Chf., Lab. of Biochem.
**Activities/Fields:** Relationship between structure and function in biological systems and on the regulation of cellular processes. The research involves prokaryotes and a range of eukaryote systems selected because of their potential for yielding important information on cellular structure, function, regulation, development, and differentiation. The study of regulation encompasses regulation of gene expression, regulation by interaction of macromolecules, and regulation of cells by hormones and ions. Work is carried out on both the molecular and cellular level. Techniques include those of biochemistry, physical chemistry, cell biology, and molecular genetics. **Pub:** *Proceedings.*

**★ 10477 ★ U.S. Department of Health and Human Services**
**National Cancer Institute**
**Laboratory of Biological Chemistry**
NIH Bldg. 37
9000 Rockville Pike
Bethesda, MD 20892
**Phone:** (301)496-4116     **Fax:** (301)496-5839
Dr. Richard Cysyk, Chf.
**Activities/Fields:** Cellular reactions that are critical to the control of tumor cell proliferation or differentiation. Recent advances in cell biology are evaluated for possible targets, and agents are designed to interact with these targets and are evaluated for biochemical and antitumor effectiveness. An important aspect of this mission is to develop appropriate in vivo systems to evaluate the chemotherapeutic effectiveness of agents shown to be active in simpler in vitro model systems. Accordingly, the Laboratory is involved in identifying endogenous factors present in vivo that modify drug action and influence differential toxicity with the aim of manipulating these factors to enhance antitumor activity.

**★ 10478 ★ U.S. Department of Health and Human Services**
**National Cancer Institute**
**Laboratory of Cell Biology**
NIH Bldg. 37, Rm. 1A09
Convent Dr., MSC 4254
Bethesda, MD 20892-4255
**Phone:** (301)496-1530     **Fax:** (301)402-0450
**Email:** mgottesman@nih.gov
Dr. Michael M. Gottesman, MD, Chf., Lab. of Cel Biology
**Activities/Fields:** Basic cell biology in relation to cancer immunology. Major emphasis is on characterization of tumor antigens biochemically and immunologically and the immune responses they evoke. Studies include antigens isolated from sarcomas, leukemias, and melanomas. As a corollary to this study, the biologic properties of alien histocompatibility antigens and variant antigens in neoplasms are also under study.

**★ 10479 ★ U.S. Department of Health and Human Services**
**National Cancer Institute**
**Laboratory of Cellular Carcinogenesis and Tumor Promotion**
National Cancer Institute Bldg. 37 Rm. 3B25
37 Convent Dr. MSC 4255
Bethesda, MD 20892-4255
**Phone:** (301)496-2162     **Fax:** (301)496-8709
**Email:** yuspas@mail.nih.gov
Dr. Stuart Yuspa, Chf.
**Activities/Fields:** Molecular and biological changes that occur at the cellular and tissue level during the process of carcinogenesis. Objectives are to: define normal regulatory mechanisms for cellular growth and differentiation; determine the mechanism by which carcinogens alter normal regulation and the biological nature of these alterations; investigate the mechanism by which tumor promoters enhance the expression of carcinogen-induced alterations; identify cellular determinants for enhanced susceptibility or resistance to carcinogens and tumor promoters; and elucidate the mechanism by which certain pharmacologic agents inhibit carcinogenesis.

**★ 10480 ★ U.S. Department of Health and Human Services**
**National Cancer Institute**
**Laboratory of Chemoprevention**
NIH Bldg. 41, Rm. C629
4 Library Dr., MSC 5055
Bethesda, MD 20892
**Phone:** (301)496-6108     **Fax:** (301)496-8395
**Email:** Robertsa@dce41.nci.nih.gov
**Website:** http://rex.nci.nih.gov/RESEARCH/basic/lc/lcpage.htm
Dr. Anita Roberts, PhD, Chf.
**Activities/Fields:** Cell regulation by transfering growth factor-B; carcinogenesis. **Frmly:** (1998) Laboratory of Chemoprevention.

**★ 10481 ★ U.S. Department of Health and Human Services**
**National Cancer Institute**
**Laboratory of Comparative Carcinogenesis**
NCI At Frederick
Bldg. 538
Frederick, MD 21702-1201
**Phone:** (301)846-1241     **Fax:** (301)846-5946
**Email:** keefer@mail.ncifcrf.gov
Dr. Larry Keefer, PhD, Chf.
**Activities/Fields:** Effects of chemical carcinogens in rodents and nonhuman primates in order to identify differences between species that are important for interspecies extrapolations of the effects of chemical agents, including extrapolations to man, and that afford experimental approaches to the elucidation of mechanisms in chemical carcinogenesis. Research is oriented toward identification of susceptibility and resistance to chemical carcinogenesis and toward identification, description, and investigation of mechanisms for interspecies differences and for cell and organ specificity in chemical carcinogenesis. The Laboratory investigates the roles of perinatal age period and pregnancy in modifying susceptibility to chemical carcinogens; studies mechanisms of action of the carcinogenic metals, cadmium, and nickel; and utilizes synthetic nitric oxide carrier compounds (NO-NOates) to investigate the biologic effects of this multifunctional bioregulatory compound.

**★ 10482 ★ U.S. Department of Health and Human Services**
**National Cancer Institute**
**Laboratory of Experimental Carcinogenesis**
NIH Bldg. 37, Rm. 3C28
37 Convent Dr.
Bethesda, MD 20892
**Phone:** (301)496-1935     **Fax:** (301)496-0734
**Email:** fran_williams@nih.gov
**Website:** http://neoplasia.nci.nih.gov
Dr. Snorri S. Thorgeirsson, Chf.
**Activities/Fields:** Elucidate mechanisms of malignant transformation in human and animal cells by chemical carcinogens; determine critical cellular and genetic factors involved in initiation, promotion, and progression of transformed cells; and apply the knowledge obtained from studying animal models toward effective prevention of cancer in man. Principal areas of research interest are the use of transgenic mouse models in cancer research, molecular and cellular aspects of hepatic stem cells; multidrug resistant gene family; chemical carcinogenesis and mutagenesis; molecular biology; and protein chemistry.

**★ 10483 ★ U.S. Department of Health and Human Services**
**National Cancer Institute**
**Laboratory of Experimental Immunology**
NCI-CCR
Bldg. 560, Rm. 3193 NCI
Frederick, MD 21702-1201
**Phone:** (301)846-1323     **Fax:** (301)846-1673
Dr. John Ortaldo, Chf.
**Activities/Fields:** Cellular and humoral components of the immune response that may be involved in resistance to tumor growth; studies growth factors and other biological response modifiers (BRMs) that may be involved in the regulation of tumor growth; studies the mechanism of action of various biologicals at the cellular and molecular level; develops new biologicals and BRMs and investigates the effects of selected BRMs on the host and on tumor growth; and develops protocols for optimal biological response modification and evaluates the therapeutic efficacy of these substances in experimental animal tumor systems and cancer patients.

**★ 10484 ★ U.S. Department of Health and Human Services**
**National Cancer Institute**
**Laboratory of Experimental Pathology**
Federal Bldg., Rm. 618D
7500 Wisconsin
Bethesda, MD 20892-9123
**Phone:** (301)496-2818     **Fax:** (301)402-1829
Dr. Umberto Saffiotti, Chf.
**Activities/Fields:** Neoplastic transformation and its underlying mechanisms, with particular emphasis on epithelial target cells. It plans, develops, and implements research on the experimental pathology of carcinogenesis, and is especially concerned with the induction of neoplasia by chemical and physical factors in epithelial tissues. Activities include: development, characterization, and evaluation of experimental pathology models of human cancer, such as cancers of the respiratory tract, by in vivo and in vitro carcinogenesis methods; development and characterization of tissue culture systems for quantitative study of the effects of carcinogens alone or in combination; and research on mechanisms of carcinogenesis correlating different levels of biological organization, from human and animal whole organisms, organs, and tissue, to the cellular, subcellular, and molecular levels. **Pub:** *Proceedings.*

## ★ 10485 ★ U.S. Department of Health and Human Services
**National Cancer Institute**
**Laboratory of Genetics**
NIH Bldg. 37, Rm. 2B04
37 Convent Dr.
Bethesda, MD 20892-4256
**Phone:** (301)496-1734      **Fax:** (301)402-1031
Dr. Michael Potter, Chf.

**Activities/Fields:** Role of genes that determine susceptibility and resistance to neoplastic development and special genes and their products that are associated with the neoplastic state (oncogenes, retroviral gene products, tumor associated antigens). Past activities have involved studies of the plasma cell tumor system in mice, and research continues on the organization of immunoglobulin genes and gene families and structure-function correlations with monoclonal antibodies. Areas of current research interest include: amino acid and DNA sequences, recombinant DNA technology, tissue culture, and hybridoma-monoclonal and antibody production.

## ★ 10486 ★ U.S. Department of Health and Human Services
**National Cancer Institute**
**Laboratory of Human Carcinogenesis**
NIH Bldg. 37, Rm. 2C05
37 Convent Dr.
Bethesda, MD 20892-4255
**Phone:** (301)496-2048      **Fax:** (301)496-0497
Curtis Harris, Chf.

**Activities/Fields:** Mechanisms of carcinogenesis in epithelial cells from humans and experimental animals; experimental approaches in biological systems for the extrapolation of carcinogenesis data and mechanisms from experimental animals to the human situation; and host factors that determine differences in carcinogenic susceptibility among individuals. Research is carried out in three areas: molecular and biochemical epidemiology; carcinogen macromolecular interaction; and in vitro carcinogenesis.

## ★ 10487 ★ U.S. Department of Health and Human Services
**National Cancer Institute**
**Laboratory of Immunobiology**
Frederick Cancer Research and Development
 Center
Ft. Detrick
Immunobiology Bldg. 560, Rm. 12-71
Frederick, MD 21702-1201
**Phone:** (301)846-1557      **Fax:** (301)846-6145
Dr. Berton Zbar, Chf.

**Activities/Fields:** Mechanisms of the effector arm of the immune system and cancer genetics. Its program comprises three interacting areas: the Office of the Chief, the Immunopathology Section, and the Cellular Immunity Section. Areas of research interest have included studies on cellular effectors of the immune system; the chemotaxis of leukocytes; the mechanisms of activation of macrophages to kill tumor cells; identification of genetic changes; human solid tumors; cloning of recessive oncogenes; and the suppression of malignant phenotype by gene replacement.

## ★ 10488 ★ U.S. Department of Health and Human Services
**National Cancer Institute**
**Laboratory of Mathematical Biology**
Frederick Cancer Research and Development
 Center
Bldg. 469, Rm. 151
Frederick, MD 21702-1201
**Phone:** (301)846-5532      **Fax:** (301)846-5598
**Email:** jmaizel@ncifcrf.gov
**Website:** http://www-lecb.ncifcrf.gov
Dr. Jacob V. Maizel, Chf.

**Activities/Fields:** Studies nucleic acid sequences, protein sequences, and macromolecular structure (including prediction of molecular structure) using methods of computation; kinetics of metabolic systems using computational and modeling methodology; applications of image analysis to micrographs and two-dimensional gels; theoretical immunology; and membrane biophysics and structure.

## ★ 10489 ★ U.S. Department of Health and Human Services
**National Cancer Institute**
**Laboratory of Medicinal Chemistry**
NIH Bldg. 37, Rm. 5CO2
37 Convent Dr. MSC 4255
Bethesda, MD 20892-4255
**Phone:** (301)496-8065      **Fax:** (301)402-2275
Victor E. Marquez, Chf.

**Activities/Fields:** Rational discovery of antitumor agents; implements basic research on the mechanisms of antitumor drug action and drug toxicity; incorporates knowledge of biochemical/molecular mechanisms into a drug synthesis program aimed at optimizing drug efficacy through enhancement of antitumor activity/selectivity and/or minimization of toxicity; and develops strategies for improving the clinical utility of new or existing anticancer drugs by overcoming tumor resistance and/or by protection of normal tissues against toxicity. Compounds with potential antitumor activity are synthesized and effects of such agents are assessed in experimental tumor systems in vitro and in vivo and on a variety of potential subcellular target sites (e.g., nucleic acids, nuclear proteins, microtubular protein, and enzyme systems). Analytical methodology for in vivo studies with new agents is developed, and, where warranted, biological studies with these agents are extended to the preclinical and Phase I stages. A wide range of methodologies is currently in use.

## ★ 10490 ★ U.S. Department of Health and Human Services
**National Cancer Institute**
**Laboratory of Molecular Biology**
NIH Bldg. 37, Rm. 5106
37 Convent Dr. MSC-4255
Bethesda, MD 20892-4255
**Phone:** (301)496-4797      **Fax:** (301)402-1344
**Email:** pasta@helix.nih.gov
Dr. Ira H. Pastan, Chf.

**Activities/Fields:** Immunotoxins for treatment of human cancer. To accomplish this, Pseudomonas exotoxin is coupled to monoclonal antibodies that react with specific human cancers. The activity of these conjugates is assessed in cell culture and animal models. Toxicity studies are conducted with monkeys, and the first promising immunotoxins are being prepared for clinical testing. The mechanisms by which immunotoxins enter and kill cells is studied by biochemical, genetic, and cell biological approaches in order to devise ways to improve the therapeutic efficiency of these agents. **Pub:** *Proceedings.*

## ★ 10491 ★ U.S. Department of Health and Human Services
**National Cancer Institute**
**Laboratory of Molecular Carcinogenesis**
NIH Bldg. 37, Rm. 3E24
9000 Rockville Pike
Bethesda, MD 20892
**Phone:** (301)496-6849      **Fax:** (301)496-8419
Harry V. Gelboin, PhD, Chf.

**Activities/Fields:** Cellular and biochemical events and mechanisms involved in carcinogenesis. Activities include: examination of the unusual properties of cells from patients who may be predisposed to cancer because of hereditary disease and investigation of various mechanisms of DNA repair using DNA transfection and sequencing to define the genomic changes observed; investigation of the genetics, multiplicity, and structure of the drug and carcinogen metabolizing enzyme systems; studies using monoclonal antibodies to gain an understanding of individual differences and their relationship to drug and carcinogen sensitivity; investigation of the mutation, recombination, and repair caused by carcinogen treatment using shuttle vectors that replicate in mammalian and bacterial cells; and studies of the relationship between the structure and function in chromatin (using biochemical and immunological methods), including evaluation of the regulatory properties of the non-histone proteins.

## ★ 10492 ★ U.S. Department of Health and Human Services
**National Cancer Institute**
**Laboratory of Molecular Immunoregulation**
Frederick Cancer Research and Development
 Center
Bldg. 560 Rm. 21-89A
Frederick, MD 21702-1201
**Phone:** (301)846-1551      **Fax:** (301)846-7042
**Email:** oppenhei@ncifcrf.gov
**Website:** http://rex.nci.nih.gov/RESEARCH/basic/lmi/lmipage.htm
Dr. Joost Oppenheim, Chf.

**Activities/Fields:** Biochemical and molecular effects of biological response modifiers on host resistance to cancer. It investigates at a molecular level the inter- and intracellular processes that regulate host defense mechanisms, including isolation of proteins, RNA, and DNA that regulate production and activities of lymphokines, cytokines, and their receptors. It utilizes in vitro and in vivo models to study the modulation by lymphokines/cytokines of cellular functions that participate in host defense. In addition, Laboratory devises new tests for diagnosis of cancer and for better definition of the immune status and more critical evaluation of biological response modifiers (BRMs). It evaluates the effects of BRMs on immunoregulatory pathways and host defense mechanisms; and generates BRMs that modify host defense mechanisms.

## ★ 10493 ★ U.S. Department of Health and Human Services
**National Cancer Institute**
**Laboratory of Molecular Pharmacology**
NIH Bldg. 37, Rm. 5D02
37 Convent Dr. MSC 4255
Bethesda, MD 20892-4255
**Phone:** (301)496-5944      **Fax:** (301)402-0752
Dr. Yves Sommier, Chf.

**Activities/Fields:** Mechanisms of action of anticancer agents are studied in culture and subcellular systems, with particular attention to effects involving DNA and nuclear proteins. Investigations focus on the relation between drug-induced macromolecular damage (and its repair) and cell survival. Drugs are also used as probes of the structure and function of DNA and chromatin. Experimental approaches include cell culture, DNA macromolecular damage measurements, DNA sequence analysis, and nuclear protein fractionation techniques. Major areas of current interest are the effects of anticancer drugs on topoisomerase enzymes and on cell cycle regulation. **Pub:** *Proceedings.* • *Research Reports.*

## ★ 10494 ★ U.S. Department of Health and Human Services
**National Cancer Institute**
**Laboratory of Molecular Virology**
NIH Bldg. 41, Rm. B602
41 Library Dr., MSC 5055
Bethesda, MD 20892
**Phone:** (301)496-9867      **Fax:** (301)496-4951
**Email:** hagerg@exchange.nih.gov
**Website:** http://rex.nci.nih.gov/RESEARCH/basic/lrbge/lrbge.htm
Dr. Gordon Hager, Ch.

**Activities/Fields:** Normal and abnormal regulation of gene expression. Studies employ methods from molecular biology, immunology, virology, and cell biology in an attempt to determine in specific cases what signals regulate gene expression. Current efforts involve both viral and eukaryotic genetic units. Research focuses on genes which are regulated at the level of transcription and which, in some cases, are responsive to induction by hormones or transacting proteins. Studies involve oncogenes and the mutations which are responsible for activation of these genes in neoplasia; and histocompatibility antigens and the roles of these genes in immune surveillance and tumor immunity. **Frmly:** (1996) Laboratory of Molecular Virology.

**★ 10495 ★ U.S. Department of Health and Human Services**
**National Cancer Institute**
**Laboratory of Pathology**
NIH Bldg. 10, Rm. 2A33
10 Center Dr. MSC 1500
Bethesda, MD 20892-1500
**Phone:** (301)496-3185　　**Fax:** (301)402-0043
Dr. Lance Liotta, Chf.

**Activities/Fields:** Surgical pathology and autopsy services at the Clinical Center of the NIH. Offers diagnostic electron microscopy studies and cytopathologic services, including exfoliative and fine needle aspiration; provides all types of histological services and staining procedures for National Cancer Institute scientists; and conducts research programs in various areas of experimental cancer research. It also provides a fully accredited residency program in anatomic pathology. Component sections of the Laboratory are: Biochemical Pathology Section, Cytopathology Section, Gene Regulation Section, Hematopathology Section, Surgical Pathology Section, Postmortem Section, Tumor Invasion and Metastases Section, Ultrastructural Pathology Section, Molecular Pathology Section, Extracellular Matrix Pathology Section, Molecular Immune Activation Secion, and Women's Cancers Section. **Pub:** *Proceedings.* • *Research Reports.*

**★ 10496 ★ U.S. Department of Health and Human Services**
**National Cancer Institute**
**Laboratory of Tumor Cell Biology**
NIH Bldg. 37, Rm. 6A11
9000 Rockville Pike
Bethesda, MD 20892
**Phone:** (301)496-6007　　**Fax:** (301)496-8394
Dr. Genoveffa Franchini, Chf.

**Activities/Fields:** Cellular proliferation, cell differentiation, and biochemical growth characteristics of normal and malignant mammalian cells both in vivo and in vitro, which will permit the optimal use of antitumor agents in the treatment of cancer and AIDS. Particular attention is given to human leukemias and lymphomas, acquired immunodeficiency syndrome (AIDS), Kaposi's sarcoma, antiviral agents, and vaccine development.

**★ 10497 ★ U.S. Department of Health and Human Services**
**National Cancer Institute**
**Laboratory of Tumor Immunology and Biology**
**Laboratory of Tumor Immunology and Biology**
NIH Bldg. 10, Rm. 8B07
10 Center Dr., MSC 1750
Bethesda, MD 20892
**Phone:** (301)496-4343　　**Fax:** (301)496-2756
**Email:** js141c@nih.gov
**Website:** http://rex.nci.nih.gov/RESEARCH/basic/ltib/ltibpage.htm
Jeffrey Schlom, PhD, Chf.

**Activities/Fields:** Immunologic markers specific for or associated with various human neoplasms, with the ultimate aim of applying these toward the diagnosis, prognosis, and treatment of human cancer. Activities focus on: the generation and characterization of monoclonal antibodies to tumor-associated determinants, with particular emphasis on the study of human carcinomas; conjugation of monoclonal antibodies to isotopes or toxins to aid in the diagnosis, localization, and potential elimination of tumor cells; studies on the association between specific murine and human genetic elements and tumorigenesis using techniques of gene cloning and molecular hybridization; and devel-

opment of immunoassays to aid in the characterization of human tumor cell populations and in the diagnosis or prognosis of certain human cancers.

**★ 10498 ★ U.S. Department of Health and Human Services**
**National Cancer Institute**
**Laboratory of Viral Carcinogenesis**
Frederick Cancer Research and Development Center
Bldg. 560, Rm. 21-105
Frederick, MD 21702-1201
**Phone:** (301)846-1296　　**Fax:** (301)846-1686
Dr. Stephen O'Brien, PhD, Chf.

**Activities/Fields:** Genetic and cellular mechanism of neoplastic transformation in man and mammalian model systems. Studies are conducted on the specific cellular genes that participate in transformation from several distinct approaches. Interests include studies on: endogenous mammalian retroviruses and their role in gene regulation and neoplasia; the expression of transforming viruses, their included oncogenes, and their ancestral cellular homologs during development and carcinogenesis using recombinant DNA technologies and systems; molecular processes of chemical carcinogenesis using gene cloning, cell transfection, and cell biology procedures; somatic cell genetic approaches to neoplastic transformation and the cytogenetic consequences of transformation; and activities of hormone-like growth factors and tumor promoters to determine their regulation of transformation sensitivity genes and transforming genes and of the progressive stages of transformation of cells in vitro and in vivo.

**★ 10499 ★ U.S. Department of Health and Human Services**
**National Cancer Institute**
**Memorial Sloan-Kettering Cancer Center**
**Institute for Cancer Research**
**(Clinical Nutrition Research Unit)**
1250 1st Ave.
New York, NY 10021
**Phone:** (212)639-8352　　**Fax:** (212)639-5115
Dr. Richard S. Rivlin, Prog. Dir.

**Activities/Fields:** Nutrition and cancer prevention; bone and mineral metabolism; energy intake expenditure; immunology and infection; lipid metabolism; cellular growth; vitamins and trace elements; DNA repair and gene expression; hormonal regulation.

**★ 10500 ★ U.S. Department of Health and Human Services**
**National Cancer Institute**
**Office of the Deputy Directory for Extramural Sciences**
**Comprehensive Minority Biomedical Section**
6116 Executive Blvd.
Ste. 7028
M.SC. 8350
Bethesda, MD 20892
**Phone:** (301)496-7344　　**Fax:** (301)402-4551
Dr. Sanya A. Springfield, PhD, Dir.

**Activities/Fields:** Program reflects a broad-based approach to every aspect of the minority cancer problem, with particular focus on the cancer incidence mortality disparity between the black community and the general population. Emphasis is on increased funding for research by minority scientists, concerted enrollment of minority physicians and patients in clinical trials programs, cancer prevention and awareness heightening, and training and manpower development.

**★ 10501 ★ U.S. Department of Health and Human Services**
**National Cancer Institute**
**Office of International Affairs**
6130 Executive Blvd. Ste 100
Bethesda, MD 20892-7301
**Phone:** (301)496-4761　　**Fax:** (301)496-3954

**Email:** nc6@cu.nih.gov
**Website:** http://www.icic.nci.nih.gov/oia/master.html
Dr. Federico Welsch, Assoc. Dir.

**Activities/Fields:** Promotes cooperative research through exchange programs with institutes in foreign countries; provides cancer research information worldwide, directly and through other institutions; and maintains liaison with international organizations and agencies involved in cancer research.

**★ 10502 ★ U.S. Department of Health and Human Services**
**National Cancer Institute**
**Office of Technology Development**
Executive Plaza South, Rm. 450
6120 Executive Blvd.
Rockville, MD 20852
**Phone:** (301)496-0477　　**Fax:** (301)402-2117
**Website:** http://www.otd.nci.nih.gov
Dr. Kathleen Sybert, Dir.

**Activities/Fields:** Responsible for administering cooperative research and development agreements with industry and universities; and providing patent management and licensing support.

**U.S. Department of Health and Human Services**
**National Heart, Lung, and Blood Institute**
*See:* Entry 5146

**U.S. Department of Health and Human Services**
**National Heart, Lung, and Blood Institute**
**Division of Epidemiology and Clinical Applications**
*See:* Entry 5147

**U.S. Department of Health and Human Services**
**National Heart, Lung, and Blood Institute**
**Division of Epidemiology and Clinical Applications**
**Clinical Applications and Prevention Program**
*See:* Entry 5148

**U.S. Department of Health and Human Services**
**National Heart, Lung, and Blood Institute**
**Division of Extramural Affairs**
*See:* Entry 5149

**★ 10503 ★ U.S. Department of Health and Human Services**
**National Heart, Lung, and Blood Institute**
**Division of Intramural Research**
**Hematology Branch**
NIH Bldg. 10, Rm. 7C103
10 Center Dr. MSC 1652
Bethesda, MD 20892-1652
**Phone:** (301)496-5093　　**Fax:** (301)496-8396
**Email:** youngn@nih.gov
**Website:** http://www.nhlbi.nih.gov/
Dr. Neal S. Young, Chf.

**Activities/Fields:** Normal and abnormal hematopoiesis. Clinical research is conducted on patients with bone marrow failure syndromes, especially aplastic anemia, Fancon's anemia, and myelodysplasia; inherited anemias, including sickle cell anemia and thalassemia; and hematologic malignancies, including chronic myelogenous leukemia and multiple myeloma. The major areas of laboratory investigation are: immune suppression of hematopoiesis; viral interactions with bone marrow cells, especially of the human parvovirus; gene transduction into hematopoietic stem cells; and modulation of graft-versus-leukemia and graft-versus-host disease in allogeneic bone marrow transplantation. Techniques from cell biology, immunology, virology, and molecular biology are all employed in these efforts.

**U.S. Department of Health and Human Services**
**National Heart, Lung, and Blood Institute**
**Division of Intramural Research**
**Molecular Disease Branch**
**(Experimental Atherosclerosis Section)**
*See:* Entry 5158

**U.S. Department of Health and Human Services**
**National Heart, Lung, and Blood Institute**
**Laboratory of Biochemical Genetics**
*See:* Entry 5160

**U.S. Department of Health and Human Services**
**National Heart, Lung, and Blood Institute**
**Laboratory of Biophysical Chemistry**
*See:* Entry 5161

**U.S. Department of Health and Human Services**
**National Heart, Lung, and Blood Institute**
**(NHLBI)**
**Laboratory of Cell Biology (LCB)**
*See:* Entry 5163

**U.S. Department of Health and Human Services**
**National Heart, Lung, and Blood Institute**
**Laboratory of Cell Signaling**
*See:* Entry 5164

**★ 10504 ★ U.S. Department of Health and Human Services**
**National Heart, Lung, and Blood Institute**
**Molecular Hematology Branch**
NIH Bldg. 10, Rm. 7D18
9000 Rockville Pike
Bethesda, MD 20892
**Phone:** (301)496-5844        **Fax:** (301)496-9985
**Email:** besafer@helix.nih.gov
Brian Safer, Actg. Chf.

**Activities/Fields:** Mechanism and regulation of mammalian gene expression to develop the understanding and technology necessary to carry out human gene therapy. The types of diseases being targeted are genetic cancer, viral, and cardiovascular. Major areas of research include gene cloning and adeno-associated virus (AAV) gene transfer, AAV vector development and isolation and characterization of genes, and expression of trans-acting factors involved in the regulation of gene expression, both at the transcriptional and translational level. **Pub:** *Proceedings.* • *Research Reports.*

**★ 10505 ★ U.S. Department of Health and Human Services**
**National Heart, Lung, and Blood Institute**
**Sickle Cell Disease Scientific Research Group**
2 Rockledge Centre
6701 Rockledge Dr. MSC 7950
Bethesda, MD 20892-7950
**Phone:** (301)435-0055        **Fax:** (301)480-0868
**Activities/Fields:** Provides a bridge for rapid translation and transfer of basic and clinical research on sickle cell disease to health care at the community level. The centers combine fundamental and clinical research, clinical trials, training and community service in an approach designed to concentrate resources, facilities, and personnel in a focused approach to the problems posed by sickle cell disease. Specific research projects include: molecular, cellular, tissue,

and organ studies in sickle cell disease, clinical trials, training, and education.

**U.S. Department of Health and Human Services**
**National Institute of Diabetes and Digestive and Kidney Diseases**
**Division of Kidney, Urologic, and Hematologic Diseases**
*See:* Entry 20403

**★ 10506 ★ U.S. Department of Health and Human Services**
**National Institute of Diabetes and Digestive and Kidney Diseases**
**Division of Kidney, Urologic, and Hematologic Diseases**
**Hematology Program**
6707 Democracy Blvd., Rm. 621
MSC 5458
Bethesda, MD 20892-5458
**Phone:** (301)594-7717        **Fax:** (301)480-3510
**Email:** badmand@extra.niddk.nih.gov
**Website:** http://www.niddk.nih.gov/fund/programs/f-list.htmbasic
David G. Badman, PhD, Prog. Dir.

**Activities/Fields:** Blood, including: hemoglobin structure and genetics; anemias of chronic diseases such as chronic renal failure; molecular and cellular role of erythropoietin; iron metabolism, transport, and storage; iron overload and deficiency; white blood cell metabolism and function; development of new iron chelating compounds for clinical use and testing the toxicity of these compounds; and hematologic aspects of AIDS, including bone marrow suppression; hematopoiesis, including stem cell biology; and gene therapy research.

**★ 10507 ★ U.S. Department of Health and Human Services**
**National Institutes of Health**
**Frederick Cancer Research and Development Center**
PO Box B
Frederick, MD 21702-1201
**Phone:** (301)846-1108        **Fax:** (301)846-1494
**Activities/Fields:** Cancer causes, biology, diagnosis, and treatment, and AIDS studies. The basic research program (operated by the biomedical research firm Advanced BioScience Laboratories, Inc.) and the NCI intramural research programs involve studies in macromolecular structure and function; mechanisms for inducing cancer using carcinogens; activation and expression of oncogenes; mechanisms, evolution, and control of transformation; in vitro and in vivo screening for cancer and AIDS therapeutic agents; regulation of host defense mechanisms; therapeutic use of immune effector mechanisms; phase I and II clinical trials of biological and chemotherapeutic agents; identification and regulation of AIDS virus genes and proteins; and genetics of cell differentiation and development. Support services are provided by the other four FCRDC contractors (see above). In addition, FCRDC provides research opportunities for researchers, pre- and postdoctoral fellows, professors on sabbatical from universities, clinicians, individuals sponsored by outside grants or fellowships, collaborative workers, student interns, and others in the scientific community to participate in research at the Center. **Pub:** *Research Reports.*

**★ 10508 ★ U.S. Department of Health and Human Services**
**National Institutes of Health**
**National Cancer Institute**
PO Box B
Frederick, MD 21702-1201
**Phone:** (301)846-1108        **Fax:** (301)846-1494
**Email:** strobel@ncifcrf.gov
**Website:** http://web.ncifcrf.gov/
Marjorie C. Strobel, Sci. Oper. Mgr.

**Activities/Fields:** Causes of cancer, AIDS, and related diseases.

**★ 10509 ★ U.S. Department of Health and Human Services**
**National Institutes of Health**
**National Cancer Institute**
**Analytical Chemistry Laboratory**
PO Box B
Frederick, MD 21702-1201
**Phone:** (301)846-7286        **Fax:** (301)846-6037
**Email:** venstra@ncifcrf.gov
**Website:** http://web.ncifcrf.gov/rtp/labs/ACL/ACL.asp
Dr. Timothy D. Veenstra, Lab. Hd.

**Activities/Fields:** Techniques and methods for separating, analyzing, characterizing, and identifying compounds ranging from small molecules to complex biological samples such as proteins and polynucleotides.

**★ 10510 ★ U.S. Department of Health and Human Services**
**National Institutes of Health (NIH)**
**National Cancer Institute (NCI)**
**Division of Basic Sciences**
**((Laboratory of Biosystems and Cancer) Structure and Function of Mammalian Centromere Section)**
Bldg. 49, Rm. 4A56
Bethesda, MD 20892
**Phone:** (301)496-0541        **Fax:** (301)480-2772
**Email:** vl19x@nih.gov
**Website:**        http://ccr.cancergov/staff/staff.asp?staffid=310
Vladimir Larionov, PhD, Actg. Hd.

**Activities/Fields:** Centromeric regions of human chromosomes; determines minimal structural requirements for functional centromere and to generate portable human artificial chromosome (HAC) for gene delivery; isolation and characterization of human disease genes.

**★ 10511 ★ U.S. Department of Health and Human Services**
**National Institutes of Health (NIH)**
**National Cancer Institute (NCI)**
**Division of Basic Sciences**
**((Laboratory of Biosystems and Cancer) Cancer and Aging Section)**
Bldg. 40, Rm. 2609
Bethesda, MD 20892
**Phone:** (301)594-8516
**Email:** barrett@mail.nih.gov
**Website:**        http://rex.nci.nih.gov/RESEARCH/basic/LBCCASBarrett.html
J. Carl Barrett, PhD, Ch.

**Activities/Fields:** Environmental causes of cancer as well as endogenous causes of cancer, including spontaneous mutations, aging, and hormones.

**★ 10512 ★ U.S. Department of Health and Human Services**
**National Institutes of Health**
**National Cancer Institute**
**Division of Basic Sciences**
**(Laboratory of Biosystems and Cancer)**
Bldg. 37, Rm. 5032
37 Convent Dr., MSC-4264
Bethesda, MD 20892
**Phone:** (301)594-8516
**Email:** barrett@mail.nih.gov
**Website:**        http://rex.nci.nih.gov/RESEARCH/basic/LBCBarrettsLab.html
J. Carl Barrett, PhD, Ch.

**Activities/Fields:** Molecular and environmental causes of cancer; identification of new cancer genes; understanding mechanisms of action of specific genes in cell signaling cell proliferation, and cell death.

**★ 10513 ★ U.S. Department of Health and Human Services**
**National Institutes of Health**
**National Cancer Institute**
**Division of Basic Sciences**
**((Laboratory of Experimental Immunology) Leokocyte Cell Biology Section)**
NCI-FCRDC
Bldg. 560, Rm. 31-93
Frederick, MD 21702-1201
**Phone:** (301)846-1323　　　**Fax:** (301)846-1673
**Email:** ORTALDO@NCIFCRF.GOV
**Website:** http://www3.cancer.gov/intra/lei/lcbs1.htm
John R. Ortaldo, PhD, Actg. Sect. Hd.

**Activities/Fields:** Differentiation and activation of human and murine leukocytes and the role of the cellular immune system in mediation antitumor immune responses.


**★ 10514 ★ U.S. Department of Health and Human Services**
**National Institutes of Health**
**National Cancer Institute**
**Division of Basic Sciences**
**((Laboratory of Experimental Immunology) Cellular and Molecular Immunology Section)**
NCI at Frederick
Bldg. 560, Rm. 31-23
Frederick, MD 21702-1201
**Phone:** (301)846-5700　　　**Fax:** (301)846-1673
**Website:** http://www3.cancer.gov/intra/lei/cm1s1.htm
Howard A. Young, PhD, Sect. Hd.

**Activities/Fields:** Molecular regulation of gene expression.


**★ 10515 ★ U.S. Department of Health and Human Services**
**National Institutes of Health**
**National Cancer Institute**
**Division of Basic Sciences**
**((Laboratory of Experimental Immunology) Experimental Therapeutics Section)**
NCI-FCRDC
Bldg. 560, Rm. 31-93
Frederick, MD 21702-1201
**Phone:** (301)846-1258　　　**Fax:** (301)846-1673
**Email:** wiltroutr@mail.ncifcrf.gov
**Website:** http://www3.cancer.gov/intra/eei/e7s1.htm
Robert H. Wiltrout, PhD, Sect. Hd.

**Activities/Fields:** Models that parallel the growth and dissemination observed clinically in human tumors; treatment of primary tumors and/or metastases; immunological and cell biological mechanisms by which biological response modifiers mediate antitumor/antimetastatic effects; regulation and mobilization of committed hematopoietic progenitor and pluripotent stem cells.


**★ 10516 ★ U.S. Department of Health and Human Services**
**National Institutes of Health**
**National Cancer Institute**
**Division of Basic Sciences**
**(Laboratory of Genomic Diversity — LGD)**
Frederick Cancer Res. and Dev. Ctr.
Bldg. 560, Rm. 11-82
Frederick, MD 21702-1201
**Phone:** (301)846-1296　　　**Fax:** (301)846-1686
**Email:** obrien@.ncifcrf.gov
**Website:** http://home.ncifcrf.gov/ccr/lgd/
Stephen J. O'Brien, PhD, Chf.

**Activities/Fields:** Virus-host relationships in viral-induced cancers; the interaction of viral and cellular genes; host immune mechanisms related to the control of virus-induced cancers; and molecular processes in viral carcinogenesis.


**★ 10517 ★ U.S. Department of Health and Human Services**
**National Institutes of Health**
**National Cancer Institute**
**Division of Basic Sciences**
**(Laboratory of Leukocyte Biology)**
Frederick Cancer Res. and Dev. Ctr.
Frederick, MD 21702-1201
**Phone:** (301)846-1504　　　**Fax:** (301)846-7034
**Email:** ruscettif@mail.ncifcrf.gov
**Website:** http://rex.nci.nih.gov/RESEARCH/basic/llb/llbpage.htm
Francis W. Ruscetti, PhD, Chf.

**Activities/Fields:** Regulation of the biological response of hematopoietic and stem cells to humoral factors, the signal transduction pathways which control these stem cells, the cellular and viral aspects of pathogenesis caused by infection of these cells by human retroviruses and the application of these studies to the development of new therapies for cancer and AIDS.


**★ 10518 ★ U.S. Department of Health and Human Services**
**National Institutes of Health**
**National Cancer Institute (NCI)**
**Division of Basic Sciences**
**(HIV Drug Resistance Program — DRP)**
NCI-Frederick
PO Box B
Frederick, MD 21702
**Phone:** (301)846-5943　　　**Fax:** (301)846-6013
**Email:** jcoffin@ncifcrf.gov
**Website:** http://www.ncifcrf.gov/hivdrp/index.html
John Coffin, PhD, Prog. Dir.

**Activities/Fields:** Effective antiviral therapy is the only hope for survival for the nearly one million Americans and 35 million individuals worldwide infected with HIV. Recognizing that evolution of resistant virus is the principal obstacle to such therapy, the HIV Drug Resistance Program is applying basic, translational, and clinical research to problems central to understanding the mechanism and evolution of antiviral drug resistance. Current research activities include: structural and biochemical analysis of reverse transcriptase variants; mechanism of genetic variation during virus replication; virion structure and assembly; virus-host interaction; development of model systems for the study of HIV in vivo; identification of novel replication inhibitors; clinical studies on the genetic structure and dynamics of HIV populations in vivo. Conducts in vitro drug resistance selection assays, genotypic and phenotypic analyses, and a range of other techniques, such as Polymerase Chain Reaction (PCR), site mutagenesis, viral load monitoring, and viral enzyme analysis for the HIV drug resistance program.


**★ 10519 ★ U.S. Department of Health and Human Services**
**National Institutes of Health**
**National Cancer Institute**
**Division of Basic Sciences**
**(Laboratory of Molecular Cell Biology — LMCB)**
Bethesda, MD 20892
**Phone:** (301)496-3029
**Email:** cw1m@nih.gov
**Website:** http://rex.nci.nih.gov/RESEARCH/basic/lmcb/lmcbpage.htm
Carl Wu, PhD, Chf.

**Activities/Fields:** The laboratory investigates basic cellular processes of homeostasis, growth, division, and differentiation, with an emphasis on the molecular biology of chromosomes and the cell nucleus.


**★ 10520 ★ U.S. Department of Health and Human Services**
**National Institutes of Health**
**National Cancer Institute**
**Division of Basic Sciences**
**(Laboratory of Metabolism)**
Bldg. 37, Rm. 3E24
Bethesda, MD 20892
**Phone:** (301)496-9067　　　**Fax:** (301)496-8419
**Email:** fjgonz@helix.nih.gov
**Website:** http://rex.nci.nih.gov/RESEARCH/basic/lm/lmpage.htm
Frank J. Gonzalez, PhD, Lab Chf.

**Activities/Fields:** Research for the National Cancer Institute on metabolism.


**★ 10521 ★ U.S. Department of Health and Human Services**
**National Institutes of Health**
**National Cancer Institute**
**Division of Basic Sciences**
**(Laboratory of Immune Cell Biology — LICB)**
NIH Bldg. 10, Rm. 1B40
Bethesda, MD 20892-1152
**Phone:** (301)496-4931
**Email:** jda@box-j.nih.gov
**Website:** http://www3.cancer.gov/intra/licb/licbpage.htm
Jonathan D. Ashwell, MD, Chf.

**Activities/Fields:** Biology of the immune system at the molecular and cellular levels, including the mechanisms and consequences of apoptosis (regulated cell death) and T cell receptor engagement.


**★ 10522 ★ U.S. Department of Health and Human Services**
**National Institutes of Health**
**National Cancer Institute**
**Division of Basic Sciences**
**(Laboratory of Cell Regulation and Carcinogenesis)**
NIH/NCI/LCRC, Bldg. 41, Rm. C629
41 Library Dr.
MSC 5055
Bethesda, MD 20892-5055
**Phone:** (301)496-5391　　　**Fax:** (301)496-8395
**Email:** robertsa@dce41.nci.nih.gov
**Website:** http://rex.nci.nih.gov/RESEARCH/basic/lc/lcpage.htm
Anita Roberts, PhD, Chf.

**Activities/Fields:** The laboratory focuses on mechanisms of carcinogenesis and on the role of the peptide growth factor, transforming growth factor-beta (TGF-beta), in homeostasis and pathophysiologic processes.


**★ 10523 ★ U.S. Department of Health and Human Services**
**National Institutes of Health**
**National Cancer Institute**
**Division of Basic Sciences**
**((Experimental Immunology Branch) Dinah Singer Laboratory)**
Bldg.10, Rm. 4B36, NIH
Bethesda, MD 20892-1360
**Phone:** (301)496-9097　　　**Fax:** (301)480-8499
**Email:** ds13j@nih.gov
**Website:** http://rex.nci.nih.gov/RESEARCH/basic/eib/singerd.htm
Dinah Singer, PhD, Chf., Molecular Regulation Sect.

**Activities/Fields:** Research interest is the molecular mechanisms regulating MHC gene expression.

**★ 10524 ★ U.S. Department of Health and Human Services**
**National Institutes of Health**
**National Cancer Institute**
**Division of Basic Sciences**
**((Experimental Immunology Branch)**
**Alfred Singer Laboratory)**
Bldg.10, Rm. 4B17, NIH
Bethesda, MD 20892-1360
**Phone:** (301)496-5461          **Fax:** (301)496-0887
**Email:** as38y@nih.gov
**Website:** http://rex.nci.nih.gov/RESEARCH/basic/eib/
singera.htm
Alfred Singer, MD, Chf., Experimental Immunology Br.
**Activities/Fields:** Research interests include T cell development, T cell receptor structure and function and intrathymic signaling.

**★ 10525 ★ U.S. Department of Health and Human Services**
**National Institutes of Health**
**National Cancer Institute**
**Division of Basic Sciences**
**((Experimental Immunology Branch)**
**Andre Nussenzweig Laboratory)**
Bldg.10, Rm. 4B36, NIH
Bethesda, MD 20892-1360
**Phone:** (301)402-1894          **Fax:** (301)496-0887
**Email:** an62h@nih.gov
**Website:** http://rex.nci.nih.gov/RESEARCH/basic/eib/
nusenzwg.htm
Andre Nussenzweig, PhD, Investigator
**Activities/Fields:** Research interests include the function of DNA repair during lymphocyte development and aging.

**★ 10526 ★ U.S. Department of Health and Human Services**
**National Institutes of Health**
**National Cancer Institute**
**Division of Basic Sciences**
**((Experimental Immunology Branch)**
**Richard Hodes Laboratory)**
Bldg.10, Rm. 4B17, NIH
Bethesda, MD 20892-1360
**Phone:** (301)496-3129          **Fax:** (301)496-0887
**Email:** rh32z@nih.gov
**Website:** http://rex.nci.nih.gov/RESEARCH/basic/eib/
hodes.htm
Richard Hodes, MD, Chf., Immune Regulation Sect.
**Activities/Fields:** Research interests include cellular and molecular regulation of T cell and B cell activation.

**★ 10527 ★ U.S. Department of Health and Human Services**
**National Institutes of Health**
**National Cancer Institute**
**Division of Basic Sciences**
**((Experimental Immunology Branch)**
**Pierre Henkart Laboratory)**
Bldg.10, Rm. 4B36, NIH
Bethesda, MD 20892-1360
**Phone:** (301)496-1554          **Fax:** (301)496-0887
**Email:** ph8j@nih.gov
**Website:** http://rex.nci.nih.gov/RESEARCH/basic/eib/
henkart.htm
Pierre A. Henkart, PhD, Investigator
**Activities/Fields:** Research interests include molecular mechanisms of lymphocyte-mediated cytoxicity and molecular mechanisms of T lymphocyte apoptosis.

**★ 10528 ★ U.S. Department of Health and Human Services**
**National Institutes of Health**
**National Cancer Institute**
**Division of Basic Sciences**
**((Experimental Immunology Branch)**
**Michael Kuehn Laboratory)**
Bldg.10, Rm. 4B17, NIH
10 Center Dr.
Bethesda, MD 20892-1360
**Phone:** (301)496-9341          **Fax:** (301)496-0887
**Email:** mk16m@nih.gov
**Website:** http://rex.nci.nih.gov/RESEARCH/basic/eib/
kuehn.htm
Michael Kuehn, PhD, Investigator
**Activities/Fields:** Research interest is genetic control of vertebrate embryonic development.

**★ 10529 ★ U.S. Department of Health and Human Services**
**National Institutes of Health**
**National Cancer Institute**
**Division of Basic Sciences**
**((Experimental Immunology Branch)**
**Paul Roche Laboratory)**
Bldg.10, Rm. 4B36, NIH
9000 Rockville Pke.
Bethesda, MD 20892-1360
**Phone:** (301)496-7177          **Fax:** (301)496-0887
**Email:** pr17m@nih.gov
**Website:** http://rex.nci.nih.gov/RESEARCH/basic/eib/
roche.htm
Paul A. Roche, PhD, Prin. Investg.
**Activities/Fields:** Research area is protein trafficking in lymphocytes.

**★ 10530 ★ U.S. Department of Health and Human Services**
**National Institutes of Health**
**National Cancer Institute**
**Division of Basic Sciences**
**((Experimental Immunology Branch)**
**Gene Shearer Laboratory)**
Bldg.10, Rm. 4B17, NIH
Bethesda, MD 20892-1360
**Phone:** (301)402-3246          **Fax:** (301)496-0887
**Email:** gs22y@nih.gov
**Website:** http://rex.nci.nih.gov/RESEARCH/basic/eib/
shearer.htm
Gene Shearer, PhD, Prin. Investg. /Sect. Chf.
**Activities/Fields:** Research areas include immune regulation and immune responses and AIDS immunology and tumor immunology.

**★ 10531 ★ U.S. Department of Health and Human Services**
**National Institutes of Health**
**National Cancer Institute**
**Division of Basic Sciences**
**((Experimental Immunology Branch)**
**Stephen Shaw Laboratory)**
Bldg.10, Rm. 4B36, NIH
Bethesda, MD 20892-1360
**Phone:** (301)496-3626          **Fax:** (301)496-0887
**Email:** sshaw@nih.gov
**Website:** http://rex.nci.nih.gov/RESEARCH/basic/eib/
shaw.htm
Stephen Shaw, MD, Sec. Chf.
**Activities/Fields:** Research areas include genetics of the human histocompatability locus (HLA) and T cell differentiation, T cell adhesion, and their regulation.

**★ 10532 ★ U.S. Department of Health and Human Services**
**National Institutes of Health**
**National Cancer Institute**
**Division of Basic Sciences**
**((Experimental Immunology Branch)**
**David Segal Laboratory)**
Bldg.10, Rm. 4B36, NIH
9000 Rockville Pke.
Bethesda, MD 20892-1360
**Phone:** (301)496-4746          **Fax:** (301)496-0887
**Email:** dave_segal@nih.gov
**Website:** http://rex.nci.nih.gov/RESEARCH/basic/eib/
segal.htm
David M. Segal, PhD, Prin. Investg. /Sect. Chf.
**Activities/Fields:** Research area is innate immunity.

**★ 10533 ★ U.S. Department of Health and Human Services**
**National Institutes of Health**
**National Cancer Institute**
**Division of Basic Sciences**
**((Experimental Epidemiology Branch)**
**Flow Cytometry Laboratory)**
Bldg.10, Rm. 4B17, NIH
Bethesda, MD 20892-1360
**Phone:** (301)496-2776          **Fax:** (301)496-0887
**Email:** ss71k@nih.gov
**Website:** http://rex.nci.nih.gov/RESEARCH/basic/eib/
sharrow.htm
Susan Sharrow, Sr. Investg. & Fac. Mgr.
**Activities/Fields:** Research area is Flow Cytometry in Immunology.

**★ 10534 ★ U.S. Department of Health and Human Services**
**National Institutes of Health**
**National Cancer Institute**
**Division of Cancer Control and Population Sciences (DCCPS)**
**(Applied Research Program — ARP)**
313 EPN
6130 Executive Blvd., MSC 7344
Bethesda, MD 20892
**Phone:** (301)496-8500          **Fax:** (301)435-3710
**Email:** barbashr@mail.nih.gov
**Website:** http://appliedresearch.cancer.gov
Rachel Ballard-Barbash, Assc. Dir.
**Activities/Fields:** Patterns and trends in cancer related risk factors, health behaviors, economics, outcomes, and health services and influences of those factors, including databases for cancer related surveillance research.

**★ 10535 ★ U.S. Department of Health and Human Services**
**National Institutes of Health**
**National Cancer Institute**
**Division of Cancer Control and Population Sciences (DCCPS)**
**(Surveillance, Epidemiology and End Results Program — SEER)**
6116 Executive Blvd., Ste.504
Rockville, MD 20852
**Phone:** (301)496-5288          **Fax:** (301)496-9949
**Email:** bh43a@.nih.gov
**Website:** http://seer.cancer.gov
Benjamin F. Hankey, ScD, Br. Chf.
**Activities/Fields:** The program collects and publishes incidence and survival data from 11 population-based cancer registries and three supplemental registries covering approximately 14 percent of the U.S. population. **Pub:** *The Cancer Statistics Review 1973-1996.*

**★ 10536 ★ U.S. Department of Health and Human Services**
National Institutes of Health
National Cancer Institute
Division of Cancer Control and
　Population Sciences (DCCPS)
Office of the Director
6130 Executive Blvd.
Executive Plaza N, Rm. 6134
Rockville, MD 20852
**Phone:** (301)594-6776　**Fax:** (301)594-6787
**Email:** barbara.rimer@.nih.gov
**Website:** http://dccps.nci.nih.gov/index.html
Dr. Barbara Rimer, Dir.

**Activities/Fields:** Cancer genetic, epidemiologic, behavioral, social and surveillance research to reduce the risk, incidence and deaths from cancer.


**★ 10537 ★ U.S. Department of Health and Human Services**
National Institutes of Health
National Cancer Institute
Division of Cancer Control and
　Population Sciences (DCCPS)
((Behavioral Research Program)
Helath Promotion Research Branch —
　HPRB)
6130 Executive Blvd., EPN 4078
Bethesda, MD 20892-7335
**Phone:** (301)435-2841　**Fax:** (301)480-2087
**Website:** http://dccps.nci.nih.gov/HPRB/default.html
Linda Nebeling, Br. Chf.

**Activities/Fields:** Non-tobacco behavioral prevention of cancer, including the areas of diet, physical activity, energy balance, virus exposure and sun exposure.


**★ 10538 ★ U.S. Department of Health and Human Services**
National Institutes of Health
National Cancer Institute
Division of Cancer Control and
　Population Sciences (DCCPS)
((Behavioral Research Program)
Basic Biobehavioral Research Branch —
　BBRB)
6130 Executive Blvd./EPN 4066
Bethesda, MD 20892
**Phone:** (301)496-8776　**Fax:** (301)435-7547
**Email:** ms496r@nih.gov
**Website:** http://dccps.nci.nih.gov/BBRB/default.html
Michael Stefanek, Br. Chf.

**Activities/Fields:** Preintervention research, including genetic testing for cancer, psychophysiological and genetic processes, genetic determinants of individual differences in the reinforcing effects of smoking, eating and/or physical activity and stress, immunity and cancer etiology and/or progression.


**★ 10539 ★ U.S. Department of Health and Human Services**
National Institutes of Health
National Cancer Institute
Division of Cancer Control and
　Population Sciences (DCCPS)
((Behavioral Research Program)
Tobacco Control Research Branch —
　TCRB)
Executive Pl. N, Rm. 4039B
6130 Executive Blvd.
Bethesda, MD 20892
**Phone:** (301)435-8638
**Email:** cb270r@nih.gov
**Website:** http://dccps.nci.nih.gov/TCRB/default.html
Cathy Backinger, Br. Chf.

**Activities/Fields:** Tobacco use, with the aim of reversing the epidemic of tobacco-related cancers.


**★ 10540 ★ U.S. Department of Health and Human Services**
National Institutes of Health
National Cancer Institute
Division of Cancer Control and
　Population Sciences (DCCPS)
((Epidemiology and Genetics Research
　Program)
Analytic Epidemiology Research Branch
　— AERB)
6130 Executive Blvd.
Rm. 5100
Bethesda, MD 20892
**Phone:** (301)435-4914　**Fax:** (301)402-4279
**Email:** sm33k@nih.gov
**Website:** http://epi.grants.cancer.gov/aerb
Sandra Melnick, Br. Chf.

**Activities/Fields:** Cancer etiology and modifying factors, in areas ranging from nutritional epidemiology, infectious disease epidemiology, hormonal studies, molecular epidemiology, metabolic/enzymatic pathways, physical and chemical agents, environmental epidemiology, to spatial studies.


**★ 10541 ★ U.S. Department of Health and Human Services**
National Institutes of Health
National Cancer Institute
Division of Cancer Control and
　Population Sciences (DCCPS)
((Surveillance Epidemiology and End
　Results Program — SRP)
Statistical Research and Applications
　Branch — SRAB)
Executive Plaza N, Ste. 4103
6116 Executive Blvd., MSC 8317
Bethesda, MD 20892
**Phone:** (301)480-2047　**Fax:** (301)435-3710
**Email:** srab@nih.gov
**Website:** http://srab.cancer.gov
Eric Feuer, PhD, Br. Chf.

**Activities/Fields:** The branch plans, conducts, and supports statistical research, modeling, collaboration and consultation related to the cancer surveillance and the cancer control missions of the National Cancer Institute.


**★ 10542 ★ U.S. Department of Health and Human Services**
National Institutes of Health
National Cancer Institute
Division of Cancer Control and
　Population Sciences (DCCPS)
((Epidemiology and Genetics Research
　Program)
Clinical and Genetic Epidemiology
　Research Branch — CGERB)
6130 Executive Blvd., Rm. 5114, MSC 7395
Bethesda, MD 20892
**Phone:** (301)594-9499　**Fax:** (301)435-5477
**Website:** http://epi.grants.cancer.gov/cgerb
Deborah M. Winn, Act. Chf.

**Activities/Fields:** Clinical and genetic epidemiology, ranging from elucidating determinants or progression and prognosis, pre-malignant conditions, clinical diagnostic strategies, clinical population genetics, clinical bioethics, genetic epidemiology, gene-gene and gene-modifier interactions, characterization of cancer susceptibility genes, and clinical and genetic networks and family registries.


**★ 10543 ★ U.S. Department of Health and Human Services**
National Institutes of Health
National Cancer Institute
Division of Cancer Control and
　Population Sciences (DCCPS)
((Applied Research Program)
Risk Factor Monitoring and Methods
　Branch)
6130 Executive Blvd.- MSC 7344
Bethesda, MD 20892
**Phone:** (301)496-4766　**Fax:** (301)435-3710
**Email:** SK52r@nih.gov
**Website:** http://riskfactor.cancer.gov
Sue Krebs-Smith, Branch. Chf.

**Activities/Fields:** The branch supports surveys designed to assess the prevalence of individual and societal risk factors in cancer prevention and research methods to improve their assessment.


**★ 10544 ★ U.S. Department of Health and Human Services**
National Institutes of Health
National Cancer Institute
Division of Cancer Control and
　Population Sciences (DCCPS)
((Applied Research Program)
Outcomes Research Branch — ORB)
6310 Executive Blvd.
Bethesda, MD 20892
**Phone:** (301)496-8500　**Fax:** (301)435-3710
**Email:** lipscomj@mail.nih.gov
**Website:** http://healthservices.cancer.gov/outcomes.html
Joseph Liscomb, Branch Chf.

**Activities/Fields:** Cancer outcomes measurement and analysis.


**★ 10545 ★ U.S. Department of Health and Human Services**
National Institutes of Health
National Cancer Institute
Division of Cancer Control and
　Population Sciences (DCCPS)
((Applied Research Program)
Health Services and Economics Branch)
6310 Executive Blvd.
Bethesda, MD 20892
**Phone:** (301)496-8500　**Fax:** (301)435-3710
**Email:** mbrown@mail.nih.gov
**Website:** http://healthservices.cancer.gov/economics/econdesc.html
Martin Brown, Branch Chf.

**Activities/Fields:** The study of cancer related health services for cancer sites which contribute most to cancer burden.


**★ 10546 ★ U.S. Department of Health and Human Services**
National Institutes of Health
National Cancer Institute
Division of Cancer Control and
　Population Sciences (DCCPS)
(Epidemiology and Genetics Research
　Program — EGRP)
6130 Executive Blvd., Rm. 5114, MSC 7395
Bethesda, MD 20892
**Phone:** (301)496-9600　**Fax:** (301)435-5477
**Email:** winnde@mail.nih.gov
**Website:** http://epi.grants.cancer.gov
Deborah M. Winn, Ph.D, Act. Assoc. Dir.

**Activities/Fields:** The program plans, develops and manages a program of grant-supported, population-bases research on the etiology and prevention of cancer.

**★ 10547 ★ U.S. Department of Health and Human Services**
**National Institutes of Health**
**National Cancer Institute**
**Division of Cancer Control and Population Sciences (DCCPS)**
**(Behavioral Research Program)**
6130 Executive Blvd., MSC 7326
Bethesda, MD 20892-7326
**Phone:** (301)435-6816    **Fax:** (301)435-7547
**Email:** bc136e@.nih.gov
**Website:** http://dccps.nci.nih.gov/BRP
Robert T. Croyle, Assoc. Dir.

**Activities/Fields:** Behavioral research in areas such as tobacco use, screening, dietary behavior, health communication, and sun protection to increase cancer prevention.

**★ 10548 ★ U.S. Department of Health and Human Services**
**National Institutes of Health**
**National Cancer Institute**
**Division of Cancer Epidemiology and Genetics**
**(Laboratory of Population Genetics)**
Bldg. 41/D702
41 Library Dr.
Bethesda, MD 20892-5055
**Phone:** (301)435-8953    **Fax:** (301)435-8963
**Email:** kb52s@nih.gov
**Website:** http://dceg.cancer.gov/hgp/chg/index.html
Dr. Kenneth H. Buetow, Chf.

**Activities/Fields:** The Laboratory investigates genetic determinants of cancer in human populations.

**★ 10549 ★ U.S. Department of Health and Human Services**
**National Institutes of Health**
**National Cancer Institute**
**Division of Cancer Epidemiology and Genetics**
**(Human Genetics Program)**
6120 Executive Blvd.
MSC 7236
Bethesda, MD 20892-7335
**Phone:** (301)496-4375
**Email:** fraumenj@mail.nih.gov
**Website:** http://dceg.cancer.gov/hgp/address.html
Dr. Joseph F. Fraumeni, Jr.M.D, Actg. Dir.

**Activities/Fields:** The program plans, directs, manages and evaluates a diverse program of population-based research in genetic susceptibility to cancer, including clinical genetics, genetic epidemiology and population genetics.

**★ 10550 ★ U.S. Department of Health and Human Services**
**National Institutes of Health**
**National Cancer Institute**
**Division of Cancer Epidemiology and Genetics**
**(Viral Epidemiology Branch)**
6120 Executive Blvd.
MSC 7248
EPS Rm. 8012
Bethesda, MD 20892-7335
**Phone:** (301)496-8115    **Fax:** (301)402-0817
**Email:** goedertj@mail.nih.gov
**Website:** http://dceg.cancer.gov/ebp/veb/index.html
Dr. James J. Goedert, Chf.

**Activities/Fields:** The Branch conducts studies aimed at identifying the role of RNA and DNA viruses and other infectious agents in the etiology of human cancer.

**★ 10551 ★ U.S. Department of Health and Human Services**
**National Institutes of Health**
**National Cancer Institute**
**Division of Cancer Epidemiology and Genetics**
**(Occupational Epidemiology Branch)**
6120 Executive Blvd.
MSC 7240
EPS Rm. 8118
Bethesda, MD 20892-7335
**Phone:** (301)496-9093    **Fax:** (301)402-1819
**Email:** blaira@mail.nih.gov
**Website:** http://dceg.cancer.gov/ebp/oeb/index.html
Dr. Aaron Blair, Chf.

**Activities/Fields:** The Branch conducts studies to identify occupational groups at high risk of cancer.

**★ 10552 ★ U.S. Department of Health and Human Services**
**National Institutes of Health**
**National Cancer Institute**
**Division of Cancer Epidemiology and Genetics**
**(Radiation Epidemiology Branch)**
6120 Executive Blvd.
MSC 7238
Bethesda, MD 20892
**Phone:** (301)496-6600
**Email:** eron@mail.nih.gov
**Website:** http://dceg.cancer.gov/ebp/reb/address.html
Dr. Elaine Ron, Chf.

**Activities/Fields:** The Branch conducts research to identify and quantify the risk of cancer in populations exposed to ionizing and non-ionizing radiation.

**★ 10553 ★ U.S. Department of Health and Human Services**
**National Institutes of Health**
**National Cancer Institute**
**Division of Cancer Epidemiology and Genetics**
**(Environmental Epidemiology Branch)**
6120 Executive Blvd.
MSC 7234
Bethesda, MD 20892-7335
**Phone:** (301)402-0916
**Email:** brintonl@mail.nih.gov
**Website:** http://dceg.cancer.gov/ebp/eeb/address.html
Dr. Louise A. Brinton, Chf.

**Activities/Fields:** The Branch conducts population-base studies to detect lifestyle, hormonal and other environmental and genetic determinants of cancer and coordinates studies to identify mechanisms of human carcinogenesis.

**★ 10554 ★ U.S. Department of Health and Human Services**
**National Institutes of Health**
**National Cancer Institute**
**Division of Cancer Epidemiology and Genetics**
**(Nutritional Epidemiology Branch)**
6120 Executive Blvd.
EPS Rm. 7040
Bethesda, MD 20892-7335
**Phone:** (301)594-2931    **Fax:** (301)496-6829
**Email:** schatzka@mail.nih.gov
**Website:** http://dceg.cancer.gov/ebp/neb/index.html
Dr. Arthur Schatzkin, Chf.

**Activities/Fields:** The Branch conducts population-base studies to assess etiologic hypotheses on the relationship of cancer risk to diet and nutrition; tests for associations between dietary factors, hormones, and risk at specific cancer; develops methods for nutritional epidemiology.

**★ 10555 ★ U.S. Department of Health and Human Services**
**National Institutes of Health**
**National Cancer Institute (NCI)**
**Division of Cancer Treatment and Diagnosis (DCTD)**
**((Cancer Diagnosis Program — CDP) Technology Development Branch — TDB)**
Executive Plaza N, Rm. 6035A
6130 Executive Blvd.
Bethesda, MD 20892
**Phone:** (301)402-4185    **Fax:** (301)402-7819
**Email:** jj37d@nih.gov
**Website:** http://www-cdp.ims.nci.nih.gov/tdb.html
Dr. James Jacobson, Chf.

**Activities/Fields:** The Branch supports the development of novel technologies and devices that will result in better tools to aid in the clinical management of cancer patients.

**★ 10556 ★ U.S. Department of Health and Human Services**
**National Institutes of Health**
**National Cancer Institute**
**Division of Cancer Treatment and Diagnosis**
**((Cancer Diagnosis Program — CDP) Resources Development Branch — RDB)**
Executive Plaza N, Rm. 700
6130 Executive Blvd.
Bethesda, MD 20892
**Fax:** (301)402-7819
**Email:** ra32u@nih.gov
**Website:** http://www.cdp.ims.nci.nih.gov/rdb.html
Dr. Roger Aamodt, Branch Chf.

**Activities/Fields:** The Branch stimulates, develops and supports human tissue resources to ensure availability of the tissue specimens needed to facilitate basic and translational cancer research.

**★ 10557 ★ U.S. Department of Health and Human Services**
**National Institutes of Health**
**National Cancer Institute**
**Division of Cancer Treatment and Diagnosis**
**((Cancer Diagnosis Program — CDP) Diagnostics Research Branch)**
Executive Plaza N, Rm. 6035A
6130 Executive Blvd.
Bethesda, MD 20892
**Phone:** (301)496-1591    **Fax:** (301)402-7819
**Email:** TL82S@nih.gov
**Website:** http://www-cdp.ims.nci.nih.gov/drb.html
Tracy G. Lugo, PhD, Prog. Dir.

**Activities/Fields:** Supports research into new tools for cancer diagnosis, covering the entire process from the identification of potentially useful tumor cell characteristics to assuring that promising approaches to diagnosis and prognosis are moved from the laboratory to clinical practice in a timely way.

**★ 10558 ★ U.S. Department of Health and Human Services**
**National Institutes of Health**
**National Cancer Institute**
**Division of Cancer Treatment and Diagnosis**
**(Cancer Diagnosis Program — CDP)**
9000 Rockville Pike
Bethesda, MD 20892
**Phone:** (301)496-8639
**Email:** st29f@nih.gov
**Website:** http://www.cdp.ims.nci.nih.gov
Sheila E. Taube, PhD, Assoc. Dir.

**Activities/Fields:** Stimulates and supports research aimed at the development of better tools to aid in the clinical management of cancer patients.

★ 10559 ★ **U.S. Department of Health and Human Services**
**National Institutes of Health**
**National Cancer Institute**
**Division of Clinical Sciences**
**(HIV and AIDS Malignancy Branch — HAMB)**
Bldg. 10, Rm. 12N226
Bethesda, MD 20892
**Phone:** (301)496-0328     **Fax:** (301)402-3645
**Email:** yarchoan@helix.nih.gov
**Website:** http://www-dcs.nci.nih.gov/branches/aidstrials/index.html
Robert Yarchoan, MD, Chf.

**Activities/Fields:** HIV infection and AIDS-related malignancies in children and adults.

★ 10560 ★ **U.S. Department of Health and Human Services**
**National Institutes of Health**
**National Cancer Institute**
**Division of Clinical Sciences**
**(Urologic Oncology Branch)**
10 Center Dr., MSC 1501
Bldg. 10, Rm. 2B47
Bethesda, MD 20892-1501
**Phone:** (301)496-6353     **Fax:** (301)402-0922
**Email:** linehanm@mail.nih.gov
**Website:** http://www-dcs.nci.nih.gov/branches/urology/
W. Marston Linehan, MD, Chf.

**Activities/Fields:** Cancer genes and molecular aspects of hereditary as well as sporadic forms of kidney, prostrate and bladder cancer.

★ 10561 ★ **U.S. Department of Health and Human Services**
**National Institutes of Health**
**National Cancer Institute**
**Division of Clinical Sciences**
**(Laboratory of Pathology)**
National Institutes of Health
Bldg. 10, Rm. 2A33
9000 Rockville Pike
Bethesda, MD 20892
**Phone:** (301)496-3185     **Fax:** (301)480-0853
**Email:** lance@helix.nih.gov
**Website:** http://home.ccr.cancer.gov/lop/clinical
Dr. Lance A. Liotta, Chf.

**Activities/Fields:** Genetic mechanisms of human tumor progression, gene regulation, molecular immunology, invasion and metastasis, and cellular interaction with the extracellular matrix.

★ 10562 ★ **U.S. Department of Health and Human Services**
**National Institutes of Health**
**National Cancer Institute**
**Division of Clinical Sciences**
**((HIV and AIDS Malignancy Branch — HAMB)**
**Pediatric HIV Working Group — PHWG)**
Bldg. 10, Rm. 10s255
Bethesda, MD 20892
**Phone:** (301)402-1391     **Fax:** (301)480-1562
**Email:** yarchoan@helix.nih.gov
**Website:** http://www-dcs.nci.nih.gov/aidstrials/pdshm.html
Robert Yarchoan, MD, Ch.

**Activities/Fields:** The group conducts clinical trials and provides family-centered care for HIV-infected children and families who participate in those trials.

★ 10563 ★ **U.S. Department of Health and Human Services**
**National Institutes of Health**
**National Cancer Institute**
**Laboratory of Molecular Technology**
PO Box B
Frederick, MD 21702-1201
**Phone:** (301)846-5676     **Fax:** (301)846-6100
**Email:** mtlseq@ncifcrf.gov
**Website:** http://web.ncifcrf.gov/rtp/lmt.asp
Dr. David J. Munroe, Hd.

**Activities/Fields:** Gene discovery and analysis capabilities, including advanced sequencing, genetics, genomics, and proteomics technologies.

★ 10564 ★ **U.S. Department of Health and Human Services**
**National Institutes of Health**
**National Cancer Institute**
**Protein Chemistry Laboratory**
PO Box B
Frederick, MD 21702-1000
**Phone:** (301)846-5154     **Fax:** (301)846-6065
**Email:** fisher@ncifcrf.gov
**Website:** http://web.ncifcrf.gov/rtp/PCL.asp
Dr. Robert J. Fisher, Hd.

**Activities/Fields:** N-terminal amino acid sequencing from PVDF-blotted proteins; GMP amino acid sequencing; protein digestion and separation resultant peptides by HPLC, MALDI-TOF mass spectrometry; and the study of macromolecular interactions using surface plasmon resonance spectroscopy (BIAcore analysis).

**U.S. Department of Health and Human Services**
**National Institutes of Health**
**National Human Genome Research Institute (NHGRI)**
**Division of Intramural Research**
**(Cancer Genetics Branch)**
*See:* Entry 9455

**U.S. Department of Health and Human Services**
**National Institutes of Health (NIH)**
**National Institute on Aging**
**Intramural Research Programs**
**(Laboratory of Molecular Gerontology)**
*See:* Entry 3089

★ 10565 ★ **U.S. Department of Health and Human Services**
**National Institutes of Health (NIH)**
**National Institute on Aging**
**Intramural Research Programs**
**(Cancer Molecular Genetics Unit)**
Gerontology Research Center
5600 Nathan Shock Dr.
Baltimore, MD 21224-6825
**Phone:** (410)558-8506     **Fax:** (410)558-8386
**Email:** morinp@grc.nia.nih.gov
**Website:** http://www.grc.nia.nih.gov/branches/lbc/cmgu.htm
Patrice Jean-Luc Morin, PhD, Hd.

**Activities/Fields:** Ovarian cancer and the Wnt pathway in human cancer.

★ 10566 ★ **U.S. Department of Health and Human Services**
**National Institutes of Health**
**National Institute of Dental and Craniofacial Research**
**Division of Extramural Research**
**(Neoplastic Diseases Branch)**
Bldg. 45, Rm. 4AN-24A
45 Center Dr., MSC 6402
Bethesda, MD 20892-6402

**Phone:** (301)594-2419     **Fax:** (301)480-8318
**Email:** ann.sandberg@nih.gov
**Website:** http://www.nidcr.nih.gov/research/extramural/neoplast.asp
Ann L. Sandberg, PhD, Ch.

**Activities/Fields:** Basic, translational, clinical, and epidemiological research on cancers of the oral cavity, including etiology and early detection of oral cancers; progression of oral cancers; invasion and metastasis of oral cancer cells; therapy or oral cancers.

★ 10567 ★ **U.S. Department of Health and Human Services**
**National Institutes of Health**
**National Institute of Dental and Craniofacial Research**
**Division of Intramural Research**
**(Proteases and Tissue Remodeling Unit)**
Bldg. 30, Rm. 211
30 Convent Dr., MSC 4340
Bethesda, MD 20892-4340
**Phone:** (301)435-1840     **Fax:** (301)402-0823
**Email:** thomas.bugge@nih.gov
**Website:** http://wwwdir.nidcr.nih.gov/dirweb/opcb/ptru.asp
Dr. Thomas Bugge, Ch.

**Activities/Fields:** Understanding the function of matrix degrading proteolytic enzymes in physiological and pathological tissue remodeling processes, including cancer invasion and metastasis.

★ 10568 ★ **U.S. Department of Health and Human Services**
**National Institutes of Health**
**National Institute of Dental and Craniofacial Research**
**Division of Intramural Research**
**(Molecular Therapeutics Unit)**
Bldg. 30, Rm. 211
30 Convent Dr., MSC 4340
Bethesda, MD 20892-4340
**Phone:** (301)594-5270     **Fax:** (301)402-0823
**Email:** adrian.senderowicz@nih.gov
**Website:** http://wwwdir.nidcr.nih.gov/dirweb/opcb/mtu.htm
Dr. Adrian Senderowicz, Ch.

**Activities/Fields:** Mechanism-based therapeutic approaches for head and neck cancer, especially the study of antiproliferative mechanisms of novel small molecules, including the identification of pathways necessary for induction of apoptosis, differentiation, and cell cycle arrest.

**U.S. Department of Health and Human Services**
**National Institutes of Health**
**National Institute of Dental and Craniofacial Research**
**Division of Intramural Research**
**(Peptide and Immunochemistry Unit)**
*See:* Entry 3293

★ 10569 ★ **U.S. Department of Health and Human Services**
**National Institutes of Health**
**National Institute of Dental and Craniofacial Research**
**Division of Intramural Research**
**(Molecular and Cellular Biochemistry Unit)**
Bldg. 30, Rm. 211
30 Convent Dr., MSC 4340
Bethesda, MD 20892-4340
**Phone:** (301)496-4069     **Fax:** (301)402-0823
**Email:** frank.robey@nih.gov
**Website:** http://wwwdir.nidcr.nih.gov/dirweb/opcb/mcbu.asp
Dr. Myung Hee Park, Dir.

**Activities/Fields:** Understanding normal control mechanisms underlying regulation of proliferation, differentiation and apoptosis of human oral keratinocytes and the multistep genotypic and phenotypic changes associated with oral carcinogenesis.

**★ 10570 ★ U.S. Department of Health and Human Services**
**National Institutes of Health**
**National Institute of Dental and Craniofacial Research**
**Division of Intramural Research (Cell Growth Regulation Section)**
Bldg. 30, Rm. Rm. 211
30 Convent Dr., MSC 4340
Bethesda, MD 20892-4340
**Phone:** (301)496-6259      **Fax:** (301)402-0823
**Email:** silvio.gutkind@nih.gov
**Website:** http://wwwdir.nidcr.nih.gov/dirweb/opcb/cgr.asp
Dr. J. Silvio Gutkind, Ch.
**Activities/Fields:** Oral and pharyngeal cancer, including molecular mechanisms controlling normal and aberrant cell growth.

**★ 10571 ★ U.S. Department of Health and Human Services**
**National Institutes of Health**
**National Institute of Dental and Craniofacial Research**
**Division of Intramural Research (Molecular Carcinogenesis Unit)**
Bldg. 30, Rm. 211
30 Convent Dr., MSC 4340
Bethesda, MD 20892-4340
**Phone:** (301)496-6259      **Fax:** (301)402-0823
**Email:** silvio.gutkind@nih.gov
**Website:** http://wwwdir.nidcr.nih.gov/dirweb/opcb/mcs.asp
Dr. J. Silvio Gutkind, Ch.
**Activities/Fields:** Oral and pharyngeal cancer, including molecular mechanisms involved in squamous cell carcinogenesis.

**★ 10572 ★ U.S. Department of Health and Human Services**
**National Institutes of Health**
**National Institute of Dental and Craniofacial Research**
**Division of Intramural Research (Oral and Pharyngeal Cancer Branch)**
Bldg. 30, Rm. 211
30 Convent Dr., MSC 4340
Bethesda, MD 20892-4340
**Phone:** (301)496-6259      **Fax:** (301)402-0823
**Email:** silvio.gutkind@nih.gov
**Website:** http://wwwdir.nidcr.nih.gov/dirweb/opcb/opcbhome.asp
J. Silvio Gutkind, PhD, Ch.
**Activities/Fields:** Normal and aberrant functions of tissues, cells, and molecules as they relate to oral disease states, with emphasis on etiology, diagnosis, treatment, and prevention of oral tumors.

**★ 10573 ★ U.S. Department of Health and Human Services**
**National Institutes of Health**
**National Institute of Environmental Health Sciences**
**Laboratory of Molecular Carcinogenesis (Molecular and Genetic Epidemiology)**
M/D A2-01
PO Box 12233
Research Triangle Park, NC 27709
**Phone:** (919)541-7797
**Email:** taylor@niehs.nih.gov
**Website:** http://dir.niehs.nih.gov/dirlmc/
Jack A. Taylor, PhD, Prin. Investigator

**Activities/Fields:** Interaction between genes and environmental exposures in human carcinogenesis, focus on understanding human genetic variation in susceptibility to DNA damage, and frequency and pattern of DNA mutation from environmental exposure.

**★ 10574 ★ U.S. Department of Health and Human Services**
**National Institutes of Health**
**National Institute of Environmental Health Sciences**
**Laboratory of Molecular Carcinogenesis (Regulatory Protein Section)**
M/D2 - 04
PO Box 12233
Research Triangle Park, NC 27709
**Phone:** (919)541-1531      **Fax:** (919)541-4704
**Email:** merrick@niehs.nih.gov
**Website:** http://dir.niehs.nih.gov/dirlmc/
B. Alex Merrick, PhD, Prin. Investigator
**Activities/Fields:** Relates specific phosphorylation sites on p53 and p21-waf1 proteins with cell growth, DNA damage and apoptosis in normal and tumor cells.
**Frmly:** Laboratory of Molecular Cardinogenesis; Regulatory Protein Section.

**★ 10575 ★ U.S. Department of Health and Human Services**
**National Institutes of Health**
**National Institute of Environmental Health Sciences**
**Laboratory of Molecular Carcinogenesis (Molecular Toxicology Group)**
M/D A2-01
PO Box 12233
Research Triangle Park, NC 27709
**Phone:** (919)541-7797
**Email:** devereux@niehs.nih.gov
**Website:** http://dir.niehs.nih.gov/dirlmc/home.htm
Theodora Devereux, Prin. Investigator
**Activities/Fields:** Mechanisms of environmental carcinogenesis with emphasis on detection and identification of activated protooncogenes and inactivated tumor suppressor genes in human and rodent tumors.

**★ 10576 ★ U.S. Department of Health and Human Services**
**National Institutes of Health**
**National Institute of Environmental Health Sciences**
**Laboratory of Molecular Carcinogenesis (Eicosanoid Biochemistry Section)**
M/D A2-01
PO Box 12233
Research Triangle Park, NC 27709
**Phone:** (919)541-7797
**Email:** eling@niehs.nih.gov
**Website:** http://dir.niehs.nih.gov/dirlmc/home.htm
Thomas Eling, PhD, Prin. Investigator
**Activities/Fields:** Enzymes (prostaglandin H synthase or Cox and lipoxygenases or Lox) which metabolize the cis-unsaturated fatty acids, arachidonic acid and linoleic acid to prostaglandins and other related metabolites.

**★ 10577 ★ U.S. Department of Health and Human Services**
**National Institutes of Health**
**National Institute of Environmental Health Sciences**
**Laboratory of Molecular Carcinogenesis (Gene Regulation Group)**
M/D A2-01
PO Box 12233
Research Triangle Park, NC 27709
**Phone:** (919)541-7797
**Email:** afshari@niehs.nih.gov
**Website:** http://dir.niehs.nih.gov/dirlmc/home.htm
Cynthia A. Afshari, PhD, Prin. Investigator

**Activities/Fields:** Molecular events involved in the loss of negative growth controls and the evolution of cancer, including the discovery and cloning of novel tumor suppressor genes, function of thee genes from a cell biology and transduction approach.

**★ 10578 ★ U.S. Department of Health and Human Services**
**National Institutes of Health**
**National Institute of Environmental Health Sciences**
**Laboratory of Molecular Carcinogenesis (Hormones and Cancer Section)**
M/D A2-01
PO Box 12233
Research Triangle Park, NC 27709
**Phone:** (919)541-7797
**Email:** diaugus2@niehs.nih.gov
**Website:** http://dir.niehs.nih.gov/dirlmc/home.htm
Dr. Richard DiAugustine, Prin. Investigator
**Activities/Fields:** Ovarian steroids and how they regulate growth and contribute to oncogenesis in target organs such as the uterus and mammary gland.

**★ 10579 ★ U.S. Department of Health and Human Services**
**National Institutes of Health**
**National Institute of Environmental Health Sciences**
**Laboratory of Molecular Carcinogenesis (Metastasis Section)**
M/D A2-01
PO Box 12233
Research Triangle Park, NC 27709
**Phone:** (919)541-7797
**Email:** olden@niehs.nih.gov
**Website:** http://dir.niehs.nih.gov/dirlmc/
Ken Olden, PhD, Contact
**Activities/Fields:** Characteristics of metastatic tumor cells, such as the ability to adhere to and migrate on extracellular matrix molecules; activation of integrins in the adhesion of human breast carcinoma cells to basement membrane proteins (1,2).

**U.S. Department of Health and Human Services**
**National Institutes of Health**
**National Institute of Environmental Health Sciences**
**Laboratory of Molecular Carcinogenesis**
*See:* Entry 9477

**★ 10580 ★ U.S. Department of Health and Human Services**
**National Institutes of Health**
**National Institute of Mental Health**
**Laboratory of Molecular Biology (Section on Biophysical Chemistry)**
Bldg. 36, Rm. 1B08
9000 Rockville Pike
Bethesda, MD 20892
**Phone:** (301)496-4864      **Fax:** (301)402-0245
**Email:** nimhinfo@nih.gov
**Website:** http://intramural.nimh.nih.gov/research/lmb/
David M. Neville, Jr., MD
**Activities/Fields:** Development of anti T-cell immunotoxins that deplete blood and lymph node T-cells by 2-3 logs in vivo; engineering these immunotoxins as both single fusion and coupled proteins for use in preclinical and clinical trials.

**★ 10581 ★ University of Alabama at Birmingham**
**Comprehensive Cancer Center**
1824 6th Ave. S, Rm. 237
Birmingham, AL 35294-3300
**Phone:** (205)934-5077      **Free:** 800-822-0933
**Fax:** (205)975-7428
**Email:** al.lobuglio@ccc.uab.edu

**Website:** http://www.ccc.uab.edu/
Dr. Albert F. LoBuglio, Dir.

**Activities/Fields:** Oncology, involving medicine, dentistry, surgery, bone marrow transplantation, basic science, pathology, radiation oncology, obstetrics and gynecology, virology, biophysics, molecular biology, epidemiology, and pediatrics. Programs concentrate on the molecular biology and molecular genetics of malignant tranformation, (including oncogene and retroviral mechanisms), nature of the transformed membrane, structure of its antigens and their biologic function, and role and interaction of T and B cells in protection against cancer. Also concerned with models for assessment of effect of surgery, immunotherapy and chemotherapy in intact animals, possessing models for myeloma and osteogenic sarcoma, and crystalline and solution biochem istry of anticancer agents. Conducts clinical activities, including investigations into biology and usefulness of certain tumor scanning agents, including monoclonal antibodies, magnetic resonance imaging, and use of new agents for treatment of a wide variety of human tumors. **Pub:** *Cancer Center Magazine*, quarterly. • *Communications Newsletter*, 8/year.

**University of Alberta**
**Faculty of Pharmacy and Pharmaceutical Sciences**
**Noujaim Institute for Pharmaceutical Oncology Research**
*See:* Entry 17571

**★ 10582 ★ University of Arizona**
**Arizona Cancer Center**
1515 N Campbell Ave.
PO Box 245024
Tucson, AZ 85724
**Phone:** (520)626-7925        **Fax:** (520)626-6898
**Email:** dvonhoff@azcc.arizona.edu
**Website:** http://www.arizonacancercenter.org
Dr. Daniel D. Von Hoff, MD, Dir.

**Activities/Fields:** Clinical and laboratory cancer studies, including microarray technology, tumor cell kinetics, clinical pharmacology and pharmacokinetics, new targeted drug development, drug resistance mechanisms, human tumor cloning, markers of cellular activity in malignant tumors, cell and molecular biology, immunology, carcinogenesis, medical imaging, cancer prevention and control, cytogenetics, pain management, stereotactic radiosurgery, bone marrow transplantation, gene therapy, epidemiology, and biostatistics. Clinical studies focus on histological tumor types, staging of disease, tumor kinetics, measurement of tumor burden, and new approaches to chemotherapy. New approaches to biological therapy include developing interleukins, interferons, colony stimulating factors, and tumor vaccines. Ongoing projects focus on developing new cytotoxic derivatives of anticancer drugs and pharmacokinetics in tumor systems. Conducts reversal of clinical drug resistance studies, clinical pharmacology of anticancer drugs research, and drug interaction evaluations. Performs clinical cancer research on patients with all types of tumors, with special competence in treating breast, colon, ovarian, pancreatic, lung, and prostate cancers; melanoma; sarcoma; Hodgkin's disease; lymphoma, including mycosis fungoids; head and neck cancers; and brain tumors. **Pub:** *Annual Report.* • *Newsletter.* • *Scientific Report.* • *Special Interest Periodicals.*

**★ 10583 ★ University of Arkansas for Medical Sciences**
**Arkansas Cancer Research Center**
4301 W Markham, Slot 623
Little Rock, AR 72205
**Phone:** (501)686-8300        **Fax:** (501)686-8165
**Website:** http://www.acrc.uams.edu
James Suen, MD, Dir.

**Activities/Fields:** Molecular, cellular, and genetic mechanisms of cancer therapies, including studies in immunology, mechanisms of metastases, radiation enteropathy, cell surface proteases, growth factors and cytokines, angiogenesis, cell genesis and differ-

entiation. Clinical research projects concentrate on hematologic malignancies and solid tumors, including their etiology, epidemiology, and the role of diet; mechanisms of growth; improved methods of diagnosis; responses to new therapies; and patient outreach, education, outcomes, and quality of life.

**★ 10584 ★ University of Arkansas for Medical Sciences**
**Myeloma and Transplantation Research Center (MTRC)**
4301 W Markham, Slot 776
Little Rock, AR 72205
**Phone:** (501)686-8250        **Fax:** (501)686-6442
**Email:** mtrc@exchange.uams.edu
**Website:** http://myeloma.uams.edu
Guido Tricot, MD, Dir.

**Activities/Fields:** Treatment of multiple myeloma as well as other hematological malignancies.

**★ 10585 ★ University of Calgary**
**Cancer Biology Research Group**
Health Science Centre
3330 Hospital Dr. NW
Calgary, AB, Canada T2N 4N1
**Phone:** (403)220-8695        **Fax:** (403)270-0834
**Email:** karl@ucalgary.ca
**Website:**        http://www.acs.ucalgary.ca/~resoff/index.html
Dr. Karl Riabowol, Chm.

**Activities/Fields:** Cell and molecular biology and their importance in the development and treatment of human cancers, including growth regulation, cell adhesion and metastasis, tumor differentiation, gene expression, cell surface markers, experimental cancer therapy, and relationship of cancer and aging. **Pub:** *Annual Report.*

**★ 10586 ★ University of California at Berkeley**
**Cancer Research Laboratory**
447 Life Science Addition
Berkeley, CA 94720-2751
**Phone:** (510)642-4711        **Fax:** (510)642-5741
**Email:** jallison@uclink4.berkeley.edu
Dr. James P. Allison, Dir.

**Activities/Fields:** Biology of epithelial neoplasia, with special emphasis on mammary and hepatic cancers; molecular pathogenesis of leukemia; factors involved in transformation of normal cells to neoplastic cells; and mechanism of neoplasia. Also studies production of monoclonal antibodies to cell surface structures altered during neoplastic transformation.

**University of California at Berkeley**
**Center for Family and Community Health**
*See:* Entry 2658

**★ 10587 ★ University of California, Irvine**
**Cancer Research Institute**
Biology Science II, Rm. 3221
Irvine, CA 92697-3905
**Phone:** (949)824-5886        **Fax:** (949)824-4023
**Email:** hyfan@uci.edu
**Website:** http://socrates.berkeley.edu/~sph/CFCH
Dr. Hung Fan, Dir.

**Activities/Fields:** Focuses on immunology, virology, and growth factors, emphasizing basic research in various aspects of cancer. Also conducts studies in other areas central to understanding regulation in eukaryotic cells.

**★ 10588 ★ University of California, Irvine**
**Chao Family Comprehensive Cancer Center**
101 The City Dr., Bldg. 23
Rte. 81
Orange, CA 92868

**Phone:** (714)456-8200
**Email:** ssmaxwell@uci.edu
**Website:** http://ucihs.uci.edu/cancer/
Dr. Frank L. Meyskens, Jr., Dir.

**Activities/Fields:** Cancer treatment.

**University of California, Los Angeles**
**Marrow and Stem Cell Transplantation Program**
*See:* Entry 20357

**★ 10589 ★ University of California, Los Angeles**
**UCLA Jonsson Comprehensive Cancer Center**
8-684 Factor Bldg.
PO Box 951781
Los Angeles, CA 90095-1781
**Phone:** (310)825-5268        **Fax:** (310)206-5553
**Email:** kirwin@mednet.ucla.edu
**Website:** http://www.cancer.mednet.ucla.edu
Dr. Judith C. Gasson, Dir.

**Activities/Fields:** Cancer, including both basic science research in molecular, cellular, and developmental biology, signal transduction, tumor immunology, and viral and chemical carcinogenesis and clinical/translational research in breast and women's reproductive cancers, hematopoietic malignancies and bone marrow transplantation, prostate oncology, and solid tumor oncology in the following fields: central nervous system, thoracic, gastrointestinal, musculoskeletal, melanoma, and head and neck. Also conducts cancer prevention and control demonstration and research projects under the headings of patients and survivors, and healthy and at-risk populations. Sponsors support groups for cancer patients. **Pub:** *Discoveries*, annually.

**★ 10590 ★ University of California, San Diego**
**Cancer Center**
9500 Gilman Dr., MC 0658
La Jolla, CA 92093-0658
**Phone:** (858)822-1222        **Fax:** (858)534-7628
**Email:** dedavis@ucsd.edu
**Website:** http://cancer.ucsd.edu
Dr. David Tarin, Dir.

**Activities/Fields:** Cancer, including clinical trials, outreach (education, prevention and treatment), and basic/clinical/prevention studies, including cancer biology, cancer genetics, cancer pharmacology, cancer prevention and control, cancer symptom control, translational oncology, and viral malignancy.

**University of California, San Diego**
**Ludwig Institute for Cancer Research**
**Laboratory of Cancer Biology**
*See:* Entry 9499

**University of California, San Diego**
**Ludwig Institute for Cancer Research**
**Laboratory of Tumor Biology**
*See:* Entry 9501

**University of California, San Francisco**
**Brain Tumor Research Center**
*See:* Entry 14402

**★ 10591 ★ University of California, San Francisco**
**Comprehensive Cancer Center**
Box 0128
San Francisco, CA 94143-0128
**Phone:** (415)476-2201        **Fax:** (415)502-3179
**Email:** cceditor@cc.ucsf.edu
**Website:** http://cc.ucsf.edu/
Frank McCormick, PhD, Dir.

**Activities/Fields:** Cancer and hematology, endocrinology, fundamental properties of cell membranes, role of interferon and cell-cell interactions in immune response to cancer, surface markers on leukemic cells, role of viruses in cancer, management of breast cancer, factors involved in control of cell proliferation and differentiation, use of liposomes to deliver drug and macromolecules into cells, mechanism of membrane fusion, molecular pharmacology of antineoplastic drugs, and interaction between the coagulation and fibrinolytic systems and cancer cells.

★ 10592 ★ **University of California, San Francisco**
**Northern California Comprehensive Sickle Cell Center**
San Francisco General Hospital
1001 Potrero Ave., Rm. 331, Bldg. 100
San Francisco, CA 94110
**Phone:** (415)206-5169          **Fax:** (415)206-3071
**Email:** wmentzer@sfghpeds.ucsf.edu
William C. Mentzer, MD, Dir.

**Activities/Fields:** Sickle cell disease, including molecular, cellular, tissue, and organ studies. Conducts clinical trials. Seeks to translate research on sickle cell disease to improved health care at the community level.

**University of California, San Francisco Radiation Oncology Research Laboratory**
*See:* Entry 18183

★ 10593 ★ **University of Chicago**
**Ben May Institute for Cancer Research**
MC 6027
5841 S Maryland Ave.
Chicago, IL 60637-6027
**Phone:** (773)702-0380          **Fax:** (773)702-4634
**Email:** admin@ben-may.bsd.uchicago.edu
**Website:** http://ben-may.bsd.uchicago.edu
Dr. Marsha Rosner, Dir.

**Activities/Fields:** Cancer and hormone-dependent tumors, including cancer of breast and prostate through studies in immunobiology, biochemistry, clinical medicine, experimental pathology, organic chemistry, and physiology on morphology and function of cells.

★ 10594 ★ **University of Chicago**
**Cancer Research Center**
5841 S Maryland Ave., MC 1140
Chicago, IL 60637-1470
**Phone:** (773)702-6180          **Fax:** (773)702-9311
**Email:** mscofiel@medicine.bsd.uchicago.edu
**Website:** http://www-uccrc.bsd.uchicago.edu
Nicholas J. Vogelzang, MD, Dir.

**Activities/Fields:** Cause, prevention, and treatment of cancer, including investigations of gynecologic cancers, lung cancer, head and neck cancer, pediatric cancers, gastro-intestinal cancers, breast cancer, lymphoma, leukemia, autologous bone marrow transplantation. Conducts research in cancer biology, molecular genetics, tumor immunology, developmental therapeutics, clinical research, diagnostics using radiology and radionuclide imaging, radiotherapy, radiation physics, radiation biology, developmental biology, and biochemistry. Major program areas include: molecular biology of cell growth and differentiation, chromosomes and cancer, immunology and cancer, developmental therapeutics, clinical investigations, cancer prevention and control, and advanced medical imaging. Developing programs include cancer prevention, breast cancer and prostate cancer. **Pub:** *Annual scientific report.* • *UCCRC Update.*

★ 10595 ★ **University of Cincinnati**
**Barrett Cancer Center**
234 Goodman St.
Cincinnati, OH 45267-4281
**Phone:** (513)558-3300          **Fax:** (513)558-5680

**Website:** http://www.med.uc.edu/medcente/barrett/BARRETT.htm
John C. Winkelmann, MD, Assoc. Dir., Clin. Svcs.

**Activities/Fields:** Cancer, in conjunction with the National Surgical Adjuvant Breast Project, Southwest Oncology Group, Gynecologic Oncology Group, and Radiation Therapy Oncology Group. Also studies gynecologic oncology, surgical oncology, neurologic oncology, and radiation therapy and radiation oncology. **Pub:** *Annual Reports.* Annual report.

★ 10596 ★ **University of Colorado**
**Cancer Center**
4200 E 9th Ave., B188
Denver, CO 80262
**Phone:** (303)315-3007          **Fax:** (303)315-3304
**Email:** paul.bunn@uchsc.edu
**Website:** http://uch.uchsc.edu/uccc
Dr. Paul A. Bunn, Jr., Dir.

**Activities/Fields:** Prevention, early detection, and treatment of cancer.

★ 10597 ★ **University of Florida**
**Computational Neuroengineering Laboratory (CNEL)**
Center Dr., Bldg. 33, Rm. NEB486
PO Box 116130
Gainesville, FL 32611
**Phone:** (352)392-2682          **Fax:** (352)392-0044
**Email:** principe@cnel.ufl.edu
**Website:** http://www.cnel.ufl.edu/leftframe1.php
Dr. Jose C. Principe, Dir.

**Activities/Fields:** Adaptive information processing systems, particularly nonlinear adaptive signal processing, pattern recognition, neuromorphic computation and neurobiologically inspired models and devices. **Pub:** *Papers.* • *Dissertations.* • *Theses.* • *Reports.*

★ 10598 ★ **University of Florida**
**Division of Hematology and Medical Oncology**
Department of Medicine
College of Medicine
PO Box 100277
Gainesville, FL 32610
**Phone:** (352)392-3000          **Fax:** (352)392-8530
**Website:** http://www.medicine.ufl.edu/hemaonc/index.shtml
Dr. William Stratford-May, Div. Ch.

**Activities/Fields:** Oncology, including medicine, radiotherapy, pathology, and surgery. Focuses on growth regulation of normal and malignant cells.

**University of Florida**
**Radiation Oncology Clinic**
*See:* Entry 18184

**University of Georgia**
**Drug Discovery Group**
*See:* Entry 11945

★ 10599 ★ **University of Hawaii**
**Cancer Research Center of Hawaii**
1236 Lauhala St.
Honolulu, HI 96813
**Phone:** (808)586-3013          **Fax:** (808)586-3052
**Email:** dchu@rx.uga.edu
**Website:** http://www.crch.org
Carl-Wilhelm Vogel, MD, Dir.

**Activities/Fields:** Cancer, with major emphasis in cancer epidemiology, focused on multidisciplinary cancer etiology studies that utilize Hawaii's unique ethnic population distribution for basic and demographic research; basic science, including environmental carcinogenesis, experimental therapeutics, and cell transformation and differentiation; and prevention and control; research, including clinical treatment trials, chemoprevention and other cancer control interven-

tions. **Pub:** *Annual reports.* • *Newsletters.* • *Scientific Report,* triennially.

**University of Illinois at Chicago**
**Surgical Oncology**
*See:* Entry 19624

★ 10600 ★ **University of Iowa**
**Holden Comprehensive Cancer Center**
University of Iowa Hospitals and Clinics
200 Hawkins Dr.
Iowa City, IA 52242-1002
**Phone:** (319)353-8620          **Free:** 800-237-1225
**Fax:** (319)353-8988
**Email:** george-weiner@uiowa.edu
**Website:** http://www.ccihealthcare.com/cancer
George J. Weiner, MD, Dir.

**Activities/Fields:** The Holden is organized into seven research programs including: Cancer Epidemiology; Cellular Activation in Cancer; Experimental Therapeutics; Free Radicals and Membranes; Molecular and Tumor Virology; Molecular Mechanisms of Metastasis, and prostate. **Pub:** *Newsletter.* **Frmly:** Cancer Center.

★ 10601 ★ **University of Kansas**
**Kansas Cancer Institute**
University of Kansas Medical Center
3901 Rainbow Blvd.
Kansas City, KS 66160-7312
**Phone:** (913)588-4700          **Fax:** (913)588-4701
**Email:** agaier@kumc.edu
**Website:** http://www2.kumc.edu/kci/
Amy E. Gaier, Proj. Dir.

**Activities/Fields:** Cancer, including interdisciplinary studies on its prevention, detection, and diagnosis. Programs focus on hormonally regulated cancers, chemotherapy, radiation therapy, immunotherapy, surgical therapy, psychosocial rehabilitation of pediatric patients and families, drug development, cellular and molecular biology, chemical and environmental carcinogenesis, tumor immunology, epidemiology, and biostatistics. Also conducts clinical trial investigations.

★ 10602 ★ **University of Kentucky**
**Children's Cancer Study Group**
College of Medicine
Lexington, KY 40536
**Phone:** (859)323-5694          **Fax:** (859)257-6048
**Email:** mfgree0@pop.uky.edu
M.F. Greenwood, MD, Dir.

**Activities/Fields:** Pediatric oncology, including clinical trials and bone marrow transplantation.

★ 10603 ★ **University of Kentucky**
**Lucille Parker Markey Cancer Center**
800 Rose St.
Lexington, KY 40536-0093
**Phone:** (859)257-4500          **Fax:** (859)323-2074
**Email:** acohen@pop.uky.edu
**Website:** http://www.mc.uky.edu/markey
Dr. Alfred M. Cohen, MD, Dir. /CEO

**Activities/Fields:** Cancer research, including tumor immunology, molecular genetics, signal transduction, mechanisms of carcinogenesis, experimental therapeutics, and clinical trials. Core facilities include macromolecular structure, flow cytometry, tissue procurement, clinical research office, NMR spectroscopy, and transgenic cell construction. **Pub:** *Annual Report.* • *Quarterly Newsletter.*

**University of Kentucky**
**Radiation Therapy Oncology Center**
*See:* Entry 18186

★ 10604 ★ **University of Louisville**
**Henry Vogt Cancer Research Institute**
James Graham Brown Cancer Center
529 S Jackson St., Rm. 430
Louisville, KY 40202-3256

Phone: (502)562-4369          Fax: (502)562-4368
Email: caw@bcc.louisville.edu
Website: http://www.bcc.louisville.edu/vogt/
Stephen C. Peiper, MD, Dir.

**Activities/Fields:** Molecular hematology/oncology, marrow transplantation, horomone receptors, anticancer drug development, molecular carcinogenesis, methods of drug delivery, laser therapy, growth factors, and drug disposition (clinical pharmacy).

### ★ 10605 ★ University of Maryland at Baltimore
**Greenbaum Cancer Center**
22 S Greene St., Rm. N9E17
Baltimore, MD 21201
Phone: (410)328-5506          Fax: (410)328-8667
Website: http://www.umm.edu/cancer
Sanford Stass, MD, Dir.

**Activities/Fields:** Pharmacology, clinical pharmacology, infectious diseases, molecular biology, pathology, cytogenetics, immunology, electron microscopy, and drug and blood and marrow transplantation and combined modality treatment of cancer patients, with emphasis on acute leukemia, breast cancer, sarcomas, lymphomas, lung cancer, prostate cancer, breast and neck cancers and other solid tumors. Maintains programs in the following areas: the chemotherapeutic approach to cancer therapy and the development of experimental protocols; infectious disease relationship to cancer; cell component therapy and cellular replacement; critical care of cancer patients; angiogenesis; signal transduction; molecular and structure biology; hormonal therapy; biomarkers, viral carcinogenesis; pharmacology and the use of cancer chemotherapeutic agents; anti-cancer drug development; combined modalities treatments, biological treatment; cellular and molecular biology of cancer; supportive care; and pharmacokinetics and pharmacodynamics of antineoplastic agents.

### ★ 10606 ★ University of Medicine and Dentistry of New Jersey
**The Cancer Institute of New Jersey**
195 Little Albany St.
New Brunswick, NJ 08901
Phone: (732)235-2465          Fax: (732)235-6949
Website: http://www.cinj.umdnj.edu
William N. Hait, MD, Dir.

**Activities/Fields:** Basic, clinical, population and translational cancer.

### ★ 10607 ★ University of Miami
**Sylvester Comprehensive Cancer Center**
School of Medicine
1475 NW 12 Ave.
Miami, FL 33136
Phone: (305)243-4918          Fax: (305)243-4901
Email: wgoodwin@miami.edu
Dr. Goodwin, Dir.

**Activities/Fields:** Cancer, including clinical investigation related to treatment of cancer, especially solid tumors and malignancies adults; molecular and cell biology as related to causation and pathogenesis of cancer; epidemiological research as related to environmental etiology of cancer in Florida and its prevention; and cellular differentation, cell population kinetics, epidemiology of cancer, viral oncology, and immunology.

### ★ 10608 ★ University of Michigan
**Comprehensive Cancer Center**
Cancer Research Committee
6303 Cancer Center
Ann Arbor, MI 48109
Phone: (734)763-2532          Fax: (734)647-9271
Email: efearon@mmg.im.med.umich.edu
Website: http://www.cancer.med.umich.edu/
Dr. Eric Fearon, Assoc. Dir.

**Activities/Fields:** Responsible for stimulating interest in cancer and clinical research in cell biology among

faculty and students of the University and procurement of funds for support of their research. Funds dispensed on basis of formal applications submitted to the Committee.

### ★ 10609 ★ University of Minnesota
**Hematology, Oncology and Transplantation Division**
420 Delaware St. SE, Box 480
Minneapolis, MN 55455
Phone: (612)625-2654          Free: 800-888-8642
Fax: (612)625-6919
Paul Sommers, Contact

**Activities/Fields:** Pediatric, surgical, medical, and radiation oncology in the areas of breast cancer, acute leukemia, lung cancer, lymphomas, testicular cancer, ovarian cancer, melanoma, and autologous marrow transplantation. Participates in cooperative group research, investigates local protocol, performs clinical analyses of malignancies. Conducts laboratory studies in signal transduction, gene regulation, biologic markers, cell differentiation, monoclonal antibodies, pharmacokinetics, cytogenetics, and molecular biology of normal and malignant cells. **Pub:** *Masonic Cancer Center News*, quarterly. **Frmly:** Masonic Cancer Center.

**University of Missouri—Columbia**
**Radiation Oncology Program**
*See:* Entry 18189

### ★ 10610 ★ University of Nebraska
**Medical Center**
**Eppley Institute for Research in Cancer and Allied Diseases**
986805 Nebraska Medical Center
Omaha, NE 68198-6805
Phone: (402)559-4090          Fax: (402)559-4651
Email: vcerino@unmc.edu
Website: http://www.unmc.edu/Eppley/default.htm
Dr. Kenneth H. Cowan, Dir.

**Activities/Fields:** Mechanisms, causes, prevention, early diagnosis, and treatment of cancer, including programs in molecular, cellular and structural biology, and developmental therapeutics. **Pub:** *Annual Report.* • *Cancer Update Newsletter.* • *Eppley Facts.* • *Graduate Brochure.* • *Scientific Report.*

### ★ 10611 ★ University of Nevada, Reno
**Allie M. Lee Cancer Research Laboratory**
Department of Biochemistry, Mail Stop 330
Reno, NV 89557
Phone: (775)784-4107          Fax: (775)784-1419
Email: ronp@cabnr.unr.edu
Dr. Ronald S. Pardini, Dir.

**Activities/Fields:** Nutritional intervention in the treatment of cancer with omega-3 fatty acids. Role of dietary fat in regulating tumor growth by altering expression of tumor suppressor genes and oncogenes, pharmacological investigations of natural products for the treatment of cancer.

**University of Nevada, Reno**
**Natural Products Lab**
*See:* Entry 4769

### ★ 10612 ★ University of New Mexico
**Cancer Research and Treatment Center**
900 Camino de Salud NE
Albuquerque, NM 87131-5636
Phone: (505)272-2151          Fax: (505)272-2841
Email: lkvols@salud.unm.edu
Dr. Larry K. Kvols, Dir. & CEO

**Activities/Fields:** Clinical investigations in growth-factor-supplemented high dose chemotherapy, hyperthermia, and various national cooperative group trials; tumor immunology; non-invasive diagnostic technology and development of magnetic resonance imaging; cell surface marker studies in hematopoetic and solid tumors; HPV/cervical cancer; hepatitis virus replica-

tion; HTLV-I and II; and cancer in Hispanics and Native Americans. Studies also include biology of natural killer cells and molecular mechanisms of immunosuppression, gene expression, signal transduction, oncogenes, and immune regulation.

### ★ 10613 ★ University of New Mexico
**Cancer Research and Treatment Center**
**New Mexico Tumor Registry**
2325 Camino de Salud NE
Albuquerque, NM 87131-5306
Phone: (505)272-5541          Fax: (505)272-8572
Email: ckey@nmtr.unm.edu
Dr. Charles R. Key, Co-Dir.

**Activities/Fields:** Cancer epidemiology, with emphasis on Hispanics and American Indians. Participates in the NCI's SEER (Surveillance Epidemiology and End Results) Program. **Pub:** *New Mexico Tumor Registry Newsletter*, quarterly.

**University of New Mexico**
**Clinical and Magnetic Resonance Research Center**
*See:* Entry 18190

### ★ 10614 ★ University of North Carolina at Chapel Hill
**Center for Thrombosis and Hemostasis**
CB 7015
Burnett-Womack Bldg.
School of Medicine
Manning Dr.
Chapel Hill, NC 27599-7015
Phone: (919)966-3704          Fax: (919)966-6012
Email: margo-price@med.unc.edu
Website: http://www.med.unc.edu/thromb/
Gilbert C. White, II, MD, Dir.

**Activities/Fields:** Thrombosis and hemostasis; the genetics and molecular biology of blood coagulation, including recombinant factors VIII and VIIA and the rationale for treatment or prophylaxis of thrombosis and hemorrhage, including research on peptide growth factors, platelets, lipoprotein metabolism, von Willebrand factor, factor VIII, fibrinogen and fibrin assembly, fibronectin, protease inhibitors, heparin and antithrombins, endothelial cell culture, thrombin and prothrombin, and factor IX and its variants, factor X, acute phase reactants, actin filament system, and gene replacement therapy.

### ★ 10615 ★ University of North Carolina at Chapel Hill
**UNC Lineberger Comprehensive Cancer Center**
CB 7295, Lineberger
School of Medicine
Chapel Hill, NC 27599-7295
Phone: (919)966-3036          Fax: (919)966-3015
Email: dgs@med.unc.edu
Website: http://cancer.med.unc.edu
Dr. Dianne Shaw, Contact

**Activities/Fields:** Cancer cell biology, immunology, molecular carcinogenesis, molecular therapeutics, virology, cancer genetics clinical research, breast cancer, radiobiology and imaging, cancer epidemiology, and cancer prevention and control. **Pub:** *Newsletter.*

### ★ 10616 ★ University of Notre Dame
**W.M. Keck Center for Transgene Research (CTR)**
229 Nieuwland Science Hall
College of Science
Notre Dame, IN 46556
Phone: (219)631-6375
Website: http://www.nd.edu/~transgen/
Dr. Francis J. Castellino, Dir.

**Activities/Fields:** Pathophysiological roles of the genes of the blood coagulation, anticoagulation, and fibrinolytic pathways in hemostasis, with associated relevance to embryonic development, vessel wall development, cancer, pulmonary fibrosis, and arteriosclerosis.

**★ 10617 ★ University of Oklahoma
Thrombosis and Coagulation Laboratory**
Oklahoma University Hospital, Rm. EB 400
PO Box 26307
Oklahoma City, OK 73126
**Phone:** (405)271-6161 **Fax:** (405)271-3620
**Email:** bill-kern@ouhsc.edu
William Kern, MD, Dir., Clinical Hematopathology

**Activities/Fields:** Thrombosis, fibrinolysis, and anticoagulation. Develops clinical assays for protein C and protein S.

**★ 10618 ★ University of Pennsylvania
Cancer Center**
16 Penn Tower
3400 Spruce St.
Philadelphia, PA 19104-4283
**Phone:** (215)662-6065 **Fax:** (215)349-5325
**Email:** glickjh@mail.med.upenn.edu
**Website:** http://oncolink.upenn.edu
John H. Glick, MD, Dir.

**Activities/Fields:** Cancer biology, diagnosis, cause, prevention, treatment, control, and rehabilitation, including programs in immunobiology, cell biology, virology, clinical investigations, pediatric oncology, cancer epidemiology, melanoma, stem cell biology and therapeutic breast cancer prevention, neuro-oncology, behavioral sciences and health sciences.

**★ 10619 ★ University of Pennsylvania
Comparative Leukemia Unit**
New Bolton Center
382 W St. Rd.
Kennett Square, PA 19348
**Phone:** (610)444-2284 **Fax:** (610)925-8123
**Email:** jfferrer@vet.upenn.edu
Jorge Ferrer, MD, Dir.

**Activities/Fields:** Cancer research focusing primarily on the etiology and pathogenesis of bovine leukemia for the development of a new relevant animal model system for studies on the etiology, pathogenesis, and immunoprophylaxis of viral-induced leukemia in humans. Studies include bovine leukemia virus (BLV) and its relationship to other retroviruses, particularly human T-cell lymphotropic virus type one (HTLV-I) and acquired immune deficiency syndrome (AIDS) virus. Also studies vaccine development.

**University of Pennsylvania
Specialized Center for Research in
Hyperbaric Oxygen Therapy**
*See:* Entry 4344

**★ 10620 ★ University of Pittsburgh
Cancer Institute**
Iroquois Bldg., Ste. 206
3600 Forbes Ave.
Pittsburgh, PA 15213
**Free:** 800-237-4724 **Fax:** (412)624-1936
**Email:** pci-info@msx.upmc.edu
**Website:** http://www.upci.upmc.edu
Ronald B. Herberman, MD, Dir.

**Activities/Fields:** Cancer's causes, course and cure.

**★ 10621 ★ University of Puerto Rico
Puerto Rico Cancer Center**
PO Box 365067
San Juan, PR 00936-5067
**Phone:** (787)763-2443 **Fax:** (787)751-6242
**Email:** n_figueroa@rcmaca.upr.clu.edu
Dr. Nayda Figueroa, Asst. Dir.

**Activities/Fields:** Cancer biology and carcinogenesis, solid-state carcinogenesis, bioactivation of precarcinogens, asbestos carcinogenesis, synthesis of antineoplastic agents, synthesis of radiosensitizers, tumor immunology, dietary factors in carcinogenesis, and radiation. Seeks cancer control through the Center's

Cancer Tumor Registry, Detection Program, and public education. Cancer control research involves epidemiology, biostatistics, health management, and economics. **Pub:** *Cancer in Puerto Rico*, annually.

**University of Quebec
National Institute for Scientific Research-
Armand-Frappier Institute
Human Health Research Centre**
*See:* Entry 3308

**★ 10622 ★ University of Rhode Island
Cancer Prevention Research Center
(CPRC)**
2 Chafee Rd.
Kingston, RI 02881
**Phone:** (401)874-2830
**Email:** cprc@etal.uri.edu
**Website:** http://www.uri.edu/research/cprc/
Prof. James O. Prochaska, PhD, Dir.

**Activities/Fields:** Prevention of cancer, other chronic diseases, and premature death by developing better solutions to the most common killers and cripplers today, namely life-style factors like smoking, substance abuse, high-risk sex, unhealthy diets, and sedentary life styles.

**★ 10623 ★ University of Rochester
James P. Wilmot Cancer Center**
601 Elmwood Ave.
PO Box 704
Rochester, NY 14642
**Phone:** (716)275-9484 **Fax:** (716)273-1042
**Email:** richard.fisher@urmc.rochester.edu
**Website:** http://www.urmc.rochester.edu/cancercenter/index.html
Richard I. Fisher, MD, Dir.

**Activities/Fields:** Diagnosis and therapy of cancer, with particular emphasis on experimental therapeutics. Conducts laboratory research in biochemical genetics, radiation biology, immunology, endocrine biochemistry, and cancer pharmacology, utilizing animal tumor research, biomathematics/statistics, cell culture, nucleic acid sequencing, and ultrastructure facilities. Participant in five national cooperative groups.

**★ 10624 ★ University of Southern
California
Comprehensive Sickle Cell Center**
2025 Zonal Ave., Rm. 304
Los Angeles, CA 90033
**Phone:** (323)442-1259 **Fax:** (323)442-1255
**Email:** cagejohn@hsc.usc.edu
Dr. Cage S. Johnson, Dir.

**Activities/Fields:** Sickle cell disease, including studies on molecular biology of red cells, fetal hemoglobin identification, and renal, cardiovascular, and endocrine functions.

**★ 10625 ★ University of Southern
California
Hematology, Hematologic Malignancy and
Retrovial Research Program**
Division of Hematology
1441 Eastlake Ave., Rm. 3468
Los Angeles, CA 90033
**Phone:** (323)865-3913 **Fax:** (323)865-0060
**Email:** hornor@hsc.usc.edu
**Website:** http://www.uscnorris.com
Alexandra Levine, MD, Hd.

**Activities/Fields:** Hematologic malignancies, including non-Hodgkin's lymphoma, Hodgkin's disease, leukemia and multiple myeloma; bone marrow transplantation program, including state-of-the-art gene therapy and marking program; HIV, and AIDS-related cancers, including lymphoma, Kaposi's sarcoma, and cervical cancer; and immune-based therapy for malignant disease. Other areas include hemostasis, including studies on blood coagulation, platelets, etiology of thrombosis, chemical separation and characterization

of blood clotting factors and antibody to blood clotting factors; sickle cell disease and other hemoglobinopathies. **Frmly:** Hematology Research Laboratory.

**★ 10626 ★ University of Southern
California
Hematopathology Unit**
1200 N State St., Rm. 2422
Los Angeles, CA 90033
**Phone:** (323)226-7064 **Fax:** (323)226-7119
**Email:** nathwani@hsc.usc.edu
Dr. Bharat N. Nathwani, Ch.

**Activities/Fields:** Investigates neoplasms of hematopoietic system, molecular biology, and polymerase chain reactions.

**★ 10627 ★ University of Southern
California
Medical Oncology Research Program**
1441 Eastlake Ave.
Los Angeles, CA 90033
**Phone:** (323)865-3963 **Fax:** (323)865-0061
**Email:** dmoody@hsc.usc.edu
Derek Raghavan, MD, Dir.

**Activities/Fields:** Medical oncology, chemotherapy, and immunotherapy of cancer. Conducts laboratory and clinical investigations into the biology and treatment of cancer, including studies on innovative treatments, new drugs and biological agents, locoregional therapy such as hyperthermia, and preclinical and clinical pharmacology. Major studies are also conducted in autologous bone marrow transplantation for solid tumors and in biological response modifiers, including interleukin-2 interferons, monoclonal antibodies, and melanoma vaccines.

**★ 10628 ★ University of Southern
California
Norris Comprehensive Cancer Center**
1441 Eastlake Ave.
Los Angeles, CA 90081-9181
**Phone:** (323)865-0816 **Fax:** (323)865-0102
**Email:** jones_p@ccnt.hsc.usc.edu
**Website:** http://ccnt.hsc.usc.edu/
Peter A. Jones, PhD, Dir.

**Activities/Fields:** Multidisciplinary basic, clinical, epidemiological and translational studies in the following program areas: molecular genetics, regulatory biology, developmental therapeutics and clinical trials, cancer epidemeology, cancer control research, gemitourinary cancer, gastrointestinal cancer, breast cancer, and hematologic malignancies/retroviral disease. **Pub:** *Cancer Center Report*, 3/year.

**★ 10629 ★ University of Tennessee
Memphis Cancer Center**
910 Madison Ave., Ste. 917
Memphis, TN 38163
**Phone:** (901)448-5150 **Fax:** (901)448-5033
**Email:** hniel@utmem.edu
Harvey B. Niell, MD, Dir.

**Activities/Fields:** Detection, evaluation, and treatment of cancer, specifically, clinical therapeutic research, cancer drug development, cell growth and regulation, and gene regulation and expression. **Pub:** *Cancer Education Bulletin*, monthly.

**★ 10630 ★ University of Tennessee,
Knoxville
Experimental Oncology Laboratory**
College of Veterinary Medicine
2407 River Dr.
Knoxville, TN 37996
**Phone:** (865)974-8217 **Fax:** (865)974-5616
**Email:** hmsch@utk.edu
Dr. Hildegard M. Schuller, Dir.

**Activities/Fields:** Oncology research, focusing on role of receptor mediated signal transduction pathways and their role in chemical carcinogenesis mechanisms.

**★ 10631 ★ University of Tennessee, Knoxville**
**Human Immunology and Cancer Program (HICP)**
1924 Alcoa Hwy.
Knoxville, TN 37920-6999
**Phone:** (865)544-9165          **Fax:** (865)544-6865
**Email:** asolomon@mc.utmck.edu
**Website:** http://www.utmck.edu/hicp/default.asp
Alan Solomon, MD, Dir.

**Activities/Fields:** Multiple myeloma, AL amyloidosis, and monoclonal B cell-related neoplasms. Conducts basic and clinical investigations related to the pathogenesis, diagnosis, and treatment of patients with B cell immunoproliferative diseases. **Pub:** *Scientific journals.*


**★ 10632 ★ University of Texas**
**M.D. Anderson Cancer Center**
Texas Medical Center
1515 Holcombe Blvd.
Houston, TX 77030
**Phone:** (713)792-6161          **Free:** 800-392-1611
**Website:** http://www.mdanderson.org
John Mendelsohn, MD, Pres.

**Activities/Fields:** Research includes basic science programs in biochemistry and molecular biology, biomathematics, carcinogenesis, cancer biology, metastasis and angiogenesis; immunology and molecular genetics; clinical research programs in brain tumor, breast cancer, gastrointestinal oncology, gynecological and ovarian cancer, head and neck oncology, leukemia/lymphoma and hematologic malignancies, lung cancer, pediatric oncology, prostate and genitourinary cancer, sarcoma and skin cancer; thematic research programs in bone marrow transplantation, cancer bioimmunotherapy, diagnostic oncology including laboratory medicine, pathology, and nuclear medicine, cancer drug development, gene therapy and molecular therapeutics, radiation oncology and biology, cancer supportive care, and veterinary medicine and surgery; and population-based research programs in behavioral science, clinical cancer prevention and epidemiology. Extensive translational research projects anchor the continuum from basic research to clinical application to improve early detection, diagnostic techniques, multidisciplinary therapy, rehabilitation, and cancer prevention. **Pub:** *OncoLog*, quarterly. • *Reports*, biennially.


**★ 10633 ★ University of Texas**
**M.D. Anderson Cancer Center**
**Levit Radiologic-Pathologic Institute**
Mail Stop 208
1515 Holcombe Blvd.
Houston, TX 77030
**Phone:** (713)792-6214          **Fax:** (713)792-0812
**Email:** shildebr@mdanderson.org
**Website:** http://www.manderson.org/departments/levitrpi
Stan Hildebrand, Dir.

**Activities/Fields:** Treatment of cancer patients and the diagnosis and prevention of cancer. Also involved in imaging support for multi-disciplinary treatment conferences, electronic publishing, and simplified communication of patient records between referring consulting physicians.


**★ 10634 ★ University of Texas Medical Branch at Galveston**
**Sealy Center for Cancer Cell Biology**
301 University Blvd.
Galveston, TX 77550-1048
**Phone:** (409)747-1935          **Fax:** (409)747-1938
**Email:** afields@utmb.edu
**Website:** http://www2.utmb.edu/scccb/
Alan P. Fields, PhD, Dir.

**Activities/Fields:** Cancer cell biology to reduce incidence, morbidity, and mortality of cancer. **Frmly:** Educational Cancer Research Center; Sealy Center for Oncology and Hematology/Educational Cancer Center.


**★ 10635 ★ University of Texas**
**Southwestern Medical Center at Dallas**
**Cancer Immunobiology Center (CIC)**
5323 Harry Hines Blvd.
Dallas, TX 75390-8576
**Phone:** (214)648-1200          **Fax:** (214)649-1252
**Email:** ellen.vitetta@utsouthwestern.edu
**Website:** http://www2.utsouthwestern.edu/cic/
Dr. Ellen Vitetta, Dir.

**Activities/Fields:** Immunologically-based strategies for the diagnosis and therapy of cancer and AIDS.


**University of Texas Southwestern Medical Center at Dallas**
**Center for Biomedical Inventions (CBI)**
*See:* Entry 4782


**University of Texas Southwestern Medical Center at Dallas**
**Hamon Center for Basic Research in Cancer**
*See:* Entry 2733


**★ 10636 ★ University of Texas**
**Southwestern Medical Center at Dallas**
**Hamon Center for Therapeutic Oncology Research**
6000 Harry Hines Blvd., NB8.206
Dallas, TX 75390-8593
**Phone:** (214)648-4900          **Fax:** (214)648-4940
**Email:** brenda.zielke@utsouthwestern.edu
**Website:** http://www.utsouthwestern.edu/cancer/
Brenda Zielke, Contact

**Activities/Fields:** Prevention, early detection, diagnosis, prognostic assessment, and treatment of human cancer.


**★ 10637 ★ University of Texas**
**Southwestern Medical Center at Dallas**
**Sickle Cell Case Management Program**
5323 Harry Hines Blvd.
Dallas, TX 75390-9063
**Phone:** (214)648-8594          **Fax:** (214)648-3122
**Email:** gbuch2@mednet.swmed.edu
Dr. George Buchanan, Dir.

**Activities/Fields:** Researches morbidity and mortality of pediatric sickle cell patients.


**★ 10638 ★ University of Vermont**
**Vermont Cancer Center**
Health Science Research Facility
149 Beaumont Ave.
Burlington, VT 05405-0075
**Phone:** (802)656-4414          **Fax:** (802)656-8788
**Email:** vcc@uvm.edu
**Website:** http://www.vermontcancer.org/
Dr. David W. Yandell, Dir.

**Activities/Fields:** Cancer, including multidisciplinary programs in terminal cancer, clinical research, cancer prevention and control research, genome stability and cell signaling and control. Conducts clinical studies in cancer chemotherapy, surgical oncology, radiotherapy and pediatric hematology-oncology. Trains health professionals and transfers cancer knowledge to surrounding communities as part of NCI's nationwide coordinated program to reduce incidence, morbidity, and mortality of cancer established under National Cancer Act of 1971. **Pub:** *Innovations Newsletter*, quarterly.


**★ 10639 ★ University of Virginia**
**Cancer Center**
Box 800334
Charlottesville, VA 22908-0334
**Phone:** (434)924-9333          **Free:** 800-251-3627
**Fax:** (434)982-0049
**Email:** ba4n@virginia.edu
**Website:** http://www.med.virginia.edu/medcntr/cancer/home.html
Barry Anderson, Jr., Admin.

**Activities/Fields:** Cancer.


**★ 10640 ★ University of Wisconsin—Madison**
**Comprehensive Cancer Center**
600 Highland Ave.
Madison, WI 53792-6164
**Phone:** (608)263-8600          **Free:** 800-622-8922
**Fax:** (608)263-8613
**Website:** http://www.cancer.wisc.edu/
John E. Niederhuber, MD, Dir.

**Activities/Fields:** Biology of cancer, focused on human-oriented problems in cause, prevention, tumor localization, and treatment. Organized into eight collaborative research programs: Cancer Control and Population Sciences; Cancer Genetics; Cell Signaling and Growth Control; Etiology and Chemoprevention; Experimental Therapeutics; Human Cancer Virology; Imaging and Radiation Sciences; Immunology and Immunotherapy. Four of these programs have clinical trial activity and all eight interact closely with fourteen Disease Oriented Multidisciplinary Working Groups. **Pub:** *Annual Report.* • *Newsletter.*


**★ 10641 ★ University of Wisconsin—Madison**
**Hematology Research Laboratory**
Medical Science Center, Rm. 4459
1300 University Ave.
Madison, WI 53706
**Phone:** (608)262-1576          **Fax:** (608)263-4969
**Email:** dfmosher@facstaff.wisc.edu
Dr. Deane Mosher, Dir.

**Activities/Fields:** Biology and biochemistry. Conducts studies on cell cultures, particularly the plasma proteins, fibronectin, vitronectin, and the platelet protein thrombospondin. Characterizes proteins for biomedical applications.


**★ 10642 ★ University of Wisconsin—Madison**
**McArdle Laboratory for Cancer Research**
Department of Oncology
1400 University Ave.
Madison, WI 53706-1599
**Phone:** (608)262-2177          **Fax:** (608)262-2824
**Email:** drinkwater@oncology.wisc.edu
**Website:** http://www.mcardle.wisc.edu
Dr. Norman R. Drinkwater, Dir.

**Activities/Fields:** Cellular, developmental, molecular, animal cell, and viral biology; and genetics, biochemistry, and immunology. Emphasizes mechanisms and controls of transcription, translation, and replication in cells and viruses; mechanisms of environmental, chemical, and viral carcinogenesis; and chemistry and metabolism of nucleic acids and proteins.


**Van Andel Research Institute (VARI)**
*See:* Entry 2752


**★ 10643 ★ Vanderbilt University**
**Vanderbilt-Ingram Cancer Center (VICC)**
649 Preston Bldg.
Nashville, TN 37232-6838
**Phone:** (615)936-1782          **Fax:** (615)936-1790
**Email:** george.vandewoude@vai.org
**Website:** http://www.mc.vanderbilt.edu/vumc/centers/cancer/
Harold L. Moses, MD, Dir.

**Activities/Fields:** Cancer treatment, diagnosis, and prevention.

**★ 10644 ★ Virginia Commonwealth University**
**Massey Cancer Center**
401 College St.
Richmond, VA 23298-0037
**Phone:** (434)828-0450          **Fax:** (434)828-8453
**Email:** ginder@vcu.edu
**Website:** http://www.vcu.edu/mcc/
Dr. Gordon D. Ginder, Dir.
**Activities/Fields:** Molecular biology, immunobiology, developmental therapeutics, neurooncology, carcinogenesis, genetics, hematopoiesis, bone marrow transplantation, cancer prevention, and structural biology. Clinical studies include translational research and participation in national cooperative groups. Focuses on decision analysis methodologies for evaluation of cancer treatment outcomes and costs through a Health Sciences Research Program. **Pub:** *Advance*, semiannually. • *In-Advance*, monthly.

**★ 10645 ★ Wake Forest University Comprehensive Cancer Center**
Medical Center Blvd.
Winston Salem, NC 27157
**Phone:** (336)716-7971          **Fax:** (336)716-0293
**Email:** ftorti@wfubmc.edu
**Website:** http://www.wfubmc.edu/cancer/
Dr. Frank M. Torti, Dir.
**Activities/Fields:** Cause and therapy of cancer, in a multidisciplinary effort to determine cause of cancer and to develop more effective means of treating malignant disease. **Frmly:** Oncology Research Center.

**★ 10646 ★ Walt Disney Memorial Cancer Institute**
**Cancer Research Division**
12722 Research Pky.
Orlando, FL 32826-3227
**Phone:** (407)380-9977          **Fax:** (407)380-9978
**Email:** barry@sneezy.fhis.net
Barry Schweitzer, PhD, Contact
**Activities/Fields:** Cancer, including cell biology and cell regulation, molecular biology, structural biology and drug design, and hemostasis and thrombosis.

**★ 10647 ★ Walther Cancer Institute, Inc.**
3202 N Meridian St.
Indianapolis, IN 46208
**Phone:** (317)921-2040          **Fax:** (317)924-4688
**Email:** fhaslam@walther.org
**Website:** http://www.walther.org
Joseph E. Walther, MD, Pres. /CEO
**Activities/Fields:** Treatment, prevention, and cure of cancer and studies on the care of cancer patients and families. **Pub:** *Annual Report.* • *Newsletter*, quarterly. **Frmly:** Walther Medical Research Institute.

**★ 10648 ★ Walther Cancer Institute, Inc.**
**Mary Margaret Walther Program for Cancer Care Research**
School of Nursing
Indiana University
1111 Middle Dr., Rm. 340
Indianapolis, IN 46202
**Phone:** (317)274-9970          **Fax:** (317)278-2021
**Email:** vchampio@iupui.edu
Dr. Victoria L. Champion, Dir.
**Activities/Fields:** Cancer prevention/control, survivorship, and cancer care delivery, focusing on developing an interdisciplinary effort to conduct behavioral research improving the quality of life for cancer patients and their families. Research addresses the psychological, economic, sociological and spiritual needs of those going through the cancer experience; increasing early detection of cancer and decreasing the occurrence of cancer through individual, family, and community behaviors; and improving the delivery of cost-effective cancer care by health professionals to cancer patients and their families. **Pub:** *Brochures*, annually.

**★ 10649 ★ Walther Cancer Institute, Inc.**
**Walther Oncology Center**
Indiana University School of Medicine
1044 W Walnut St., Rm. 302
Indianapolis, IN 46202-5254
**Phone:** (317)274-7510          **Fax:** (317)274-7592
**Email:** hbroxmey@iupui.edu
**Website:** http://www.iupui.edu/~woc/
Hal E. Broxmeyer, PhD, Sci. Dir.
**Activities/Fields:** Blood cell and solid tumor studies, including regulation of the production of normal and cancer cells and umbilical cord blood transplantation, growth factors, suppressor molecules, receptors, gene regulation, oncogenes, differentiation, signal transduction, phosphorylation, cell division cycle genes, and protein tyrosine phosphatases.

**★ 10650 ★ Washington University in St. Louis**
**Siteman Cancer Center**
Box 8100
660 S Euclid
Saint Louis, MO 63110-1093
**Phone:** (314)747-7222          **Free:** 800-600-3606
**Website:** http://www.siteman.wustl.edu/
Timothy J. Eberlein, MD, Dir.
**Activities/Fields:** Cancer prevention and treatment. Areas of interest include cancer genetics, cellular proliferation, oncologic imaging, stem cell biology, tumor immunology.

**Wayne State University**
**Center for Molecular Medicine and Genetics**
*See:* Entry 9529

**Wayne State University**
**Laura S. Nye Surgical Research Fund for Desmoid Tumors**
*See:* Entry 14484

**★ 10651 ★ West Virginia University**
**Mary Babb Randolph Cancer Center**
Health Science Center
PO Box 9300
Morgantown, WV 26506
**Phone:** (304)293-3528          **Fax:** (304)293-4667
**Email:** dfsurg@aol.com
**Website:** http://www.hsc.wvu.edu/mbrcc/
Eddie Reed, Dir.
**Activities/Fields:** Cancer, especially among residents of West Virginia.

**★ 10652 ★ Wood Hudson Cancer Research Laboratory**
931 Isabella St.
Newport, KY 41071-4701
**Phone:** (859)581-7249          **Fax:** (859)581-2392
**Email:** woodhdsn@iac.net
**Website:** http://woodhudson.org
Julia Carter, Pres.
**Activities/Fields:** Cancer, particularly the study of clinical cases and animal models to learn new methods for diagnosing and treating cancer and the study of environmental causes of cancer. **Pub:** *Abstracts, articles.* • *Newsletter.*

**★ 10653 ★ Yale University**
**Boyer Center for Molecular Medicine**
School of Medicine
295 Congress Ave., Rm. 109
New Haven, CT 06536-0812
**Phone:** (203)737-2266          **Fax:** (203)737-2267
**Email:** vincent.machesi@yale.edu
**Website:** http://www.info.med.yale.edu/bcmm/
Dr. Vincent Machesi, Dir.
**Activities/Fields:** Molecular oncology and medicine, focusing on multicellular oncology and organisms.

**★ 10654 ★ Yale University**
**Yale Cancer Center**
333 Cedar St.
PO Box 208028
New Haven, CT 06520-4095
**Phone:** (203)785-4371          **Fax:** (203)785-4116
**Email:** vincent.devita@yale.edu
**Website:** http://www.med.yale.edu/ycc
Dr. Vincent T. DeVita, Jr., Dir.
**Activities/Fields:** Cell biology, developmental therapeutics, immunology, molecular oncology and development, molecular virology, as well as cancer prevention and control, and cancer genetics. Clinical research programs include therapeutic radiology, ovarian cancer, stem cell biology and transplantation, genetic therapy, medical oncology, breast cancer, and lymphoma. Therapeutic clinical trials are conducted in various disease specific areas. **Pub:** *Cancer Connections.* • *Cancer Genetic Counseling Newsletter.* • *Caring Newsletter*, semiannually. • *Protocols.* • *Yale Cancer Center Referring Physicians Directory.*

# State & Regional Organizations

## Cancer

*Divisions of the American Cancer Society are listed below. The national office is located at 1599 Clifton Rd. NE, Atlanta, GA 30329, (800)ACS-2345, http://www.cancer.org/.*

### Alabama

**★ 10655 ★ American Cancer Society**
**Baldwin County Office**
26148 Capital Dr., Ste. F
Daphne, AL 36526
**Phone:** (251)621-7996          **Fax:** (251)447-0271

**★ 10656 ★ American Cancer Society**
**Birmingham Branch**
1100 Ireland Way, Ste. 201
Birmingham, AL 35205
**Phone:** (205)879-2242          **Fax:** (205)930-8895
**Website:** http://www2.cancer.org/state/al/index.html

**★ 10657 ★ American Cancer Society**
**Dothan Office**
2346 W Main St., Ste. 3
Dothan, AL 36303
**Phone:** (334)793-1012          **Fax:** (334)792-7278

**★ 10658 ★ American Cancer Society**
**Florence Office**
130 S Poplar St.
Florence, AL 35630
**Phone:** (256)767-0823          **Fax:** (256)767-0894

**★ 10659 ★ American Cancer Society**
**Huntsville Office**
2515-B Memorial Pkwy. SW
Huntsville, AL 35801
**Phone:** (256)536-1855          **Fax:** (256)534-0843

**★ 10660 ★ American Cancer Society**
**Mobile Office**
900 Western America Cir., Ste. 101
Mobile, AL 36609
**Phone:** (251)344-9856          **Fax:** (251)344-9882

**★ 10661 ★ American Cancer Society**
**Montgomery Office**
3054-C McGehee Rd.
Montgomery, AL 36111

**Phone:** (334)288-3432    **Fax:** (334)612-8181

★ 10662 ★ **American Cancer Society**
**Tuscaloosa Office**
2132 McFarland Blvd. E, Ste. C
Tuscaloosa, AL 35404
**Phone:** (205)758-0700    **Fax:** (205)758-0116

## Alaska

★ 10663 ★ **American Cancer Society**
**Anchorage Branch**
1057 W Fireweed Ln., Ste. 204
Anchorage, AK 99503
**Phone:** (907)277-8696    **Free:** 800-478-9355
**Fax:** (907)263-2073
**Email:** cindy.emery@cancer.org
**Website:** http://www.cancer.org

## Arizona

★ 10664 ★ **American Cancer Society**
**Central Arizona Division**
2929 E Thomas Rd.
Phoenix, AZ 85016-8034
**Phone:** (602)553-7129    **Fax:** (602)381-3096
**Website:** http://www2.cancer.org/state/az/index.html

★ 10665 ★ **American Cancer Society**
**Northern Arizona Region**
2724 E Lakin, Ste. 9
Flagstaff, AZ 86004
**Phone:** (928)526-3800    **Fax:** (928)526-5870

★ 10666 ★ **American Cancer Society**
**Northwest Valley Office**
12211 W Bell Rd., No. 102
Surprise, AZ 85374
**Phone:** (623)583-2828    **Fax:** (623)583-1163

★ 10667 ★ **American Cancer Society**
**Rural Communities Region**
2929 E Thomas Rd.
Phoenix, AZ 85016
**Phone:** (602)224-0524    **Fax:** (602)381-3096
**Remarks:** Serves Arizona, Nevada, and New Mexico.

★ 10668 ★ **American Cancer Society**
**Southeastern Arizona Region**
1636 N Swan, Ste. 151
Tucson, AZ 85712
**Phone:** (520)321-7989    **Fax:** (520)321-7988

★ 10669 ★ **American Cancer Society**
**Western Yavapai and Mingus Verde**
**Office**
917 E Gurley St., Ste. 1B
Prescott, AZ 86301
**Phone:** (928)541-9270

## Arkansas

★ 10670 ★ **American Cancer Society**
**Arkansas Division**
901 N University Ave.
Little Rock, AR 72207
**Phone:** (501)664-3480    **Fax:** (501)666-0068
**Website:** http://www2.cancer.org/state/ar/index.html

## California

★ 10671 ★ **American Cancer Society**
**Amador County Office**
1765 Challenge Way, Ste. 115
Sacramento, CA 95815
**Phone:** (916)446-7933    **Fax:** (916)325-2351

★ 10672 ★ **American Cancer Society**
**Antelope Valley-Eastern Sierra Unit**
1043 W Ave. 4, Ste. B
Palmdale, CA 93551
**Phone:** (661)945-7585    **Fax:** (661)945-9039

★ 10673 ★ **American Cancer Society**
**Auburn Unit**
333 Sunrise Ave., Ste. 344
Roseville, CA 95661
**Phone:** (916)783-4181    **Fax:** (916)783-4175

★ 10674 ★ **American Cancer Society**
**Bakersfield Unit**
1523 California Ave.
Bakersfield, CA 93304
**Phone:** (661)327-2424    **Fax:** (661)327-2921

★ 10675 ★ **American Cancer Society**
**Bishop Unit**
c/o Antelope Valley-Eastern Sierra Unit
1043 W Ave. 4, Ste. B
Palmdale, CA 93551
**Phone:** (661)945-7585    **Fax:** (661)945-9039

★ 10676 ★ **American Cancer Society**
**Border Regional Office**
2655 Camino del Rio N, Ste. 100
San Diego, CA 92108
**Phone:** (619)299-4200    **Free:** 800-ACS-2345
**Fax:** (619)296-0928

★ 10677 ★ **American Cancer Society**
**Brawley Regional Unit**
Pioneers Memorial Hospital
207 W Legion Rd.
Brawley, CA 92227
**Phone:** (760)344-4195    **Fax:** (760)352-0316

★ 10678 ★ **American Cancer Society**
**Central Alameda County Unit**
1900 Mowry Ave., Ste. 405
Fremont, CA 94538
**Phone:** (510)742-8346    **Fax:** (510)742-8417

★ 10679 ★ **American Cancer Society**
**Central Coast Counties Unit**
1184 Monroe St., Stes. 1 & 2
Salinas, CA 93906
**Phone:** (831)442-2992    **Fax:** (831)442-2710

★ 10680 ★ **American Cancer Society**
**Central Contra Costa County Unit**
1885 Oak Park Blvd.
Pleasant Hill, CA
**Phone:** (925)934-7640    **Fax:** (925)934-5372

★ 10681 ★ **American Cancer Society**
**Central Los Angeles Unit**
3333 Wilshire Blvd., Ste. 900
Los Angeles, CA 90010
**Phone:** (213)386-6102    **Fax:** (213)480-0806

★ 10682 ★ **American Cancer Society**
**Central Valley Regional Office**
2222 W Shaw Ave., Ste. 201
Fresno, CA 93711
**Phone:** (559)451-0722    **Fax:** (559)451-0744
**Email:** mary.johnson@cancer.org
**Website:** http://www.cancer.org

★ 10683 ★ **American Cancer Society**
**Central Ventura County Unit**
250 W Citrus Grove, Ste. 200
Oxnard, CA 93030
**Phone:** (805)983-8864    **Fax:** (805)983-3751

★ 10684 ★ **American Cancer Society**
**Corona/Norco Unit**
1240 Palmyrita Ave., Ste. A
Riverside, CA 92507
**Phone:** (909)683-6415    **Fax:** (909)682-6804

★ 10685 ★ **American Cancer Society**
**Desert Palms Unit**
74-140 El Paseo, Ste. 1
Palm Desert, CA 92260
**Phone:** (760)568-2691    **Fax:** (760)341-8783

★ 10686 ★ **American Cancer Society**
**Desert Sierra Regional Office**
1240 Palmyrita Ave., Unit A
Riverside, CA 92507
**Phone:** (909)320-7142    **Free:** 800-ACS-2345
**Fax:** (909)682-6804

★ 10687 ★ **American Cancer Society**
**Downey/Rio Hondo Unit**
9901 Paramount Blvd., Ste. 245
Downey, CA 90240
**Phone:** (562)776-0201    **Fax:** (562)776-0373

★ 10688 ★ **American Cancer Society**
**East Bay Regional Office**
1700 Webster St.
Oakland, CA 94612
**Phone:** (510)452-5229    **Free:** 800-ACS-2345
**Fax:** (510)763-8826

★ 10689 ★ **American Cancer Society**
**East Contra Costa County Unit**
1885 Oak Park Blvd.
Pleasant Hill, CA 94523
**Phone:** (925)934-7640    **Fax:** (925)934-5372

★ 10690 ★ **American Cancer Society**
**East Inland Valley Unit**
8560 Vineyard Ave., Ste. 108
Rancho Cucamonga, CA 91730
**Phone:** (909)949-6115    **Fax:** (909)949-6813

★ 10691 ★ **American Cancer Society**
**East San Gabriel Valley Unit**
339 E Rowland St.
Covina, CA 91723
**Phone:** (626)966-9994    **Fax:** (626)966-8664

★ 10692 ★ **American Cancer Society**
**El Dorado/Alpine Unit**
333 Sunrise Ave., Ste. 344
Roseville, CA 95661
**Phone:** (916)783-4181    **Fax:** (916)783-4175

★ 10693 ★ **American Cancer Society**
**Elk Grove/Laguna Unit**
1765 Challenge Way, Ste. 115
Sacramento, CA 95815
**Phone:** (916)446-7933    **Fax:** (916)325-2351

★ 10694 ★ **American Cancer Society**
**Fontana Unit**
8560 Vineyard Ave., Ste. 108
Rancho Cucamonga, CA 91730
**Phone:** (909)949-6115    **Fax:** (909)949-6813

★ 10695 ★ **American Cancer Society**
**Fresno County Unit**
2222 W Shaw Ave., Ste. 201
Fresno, CA 93711
**Phone:** (559)451-0722    **Fax:** (559)451-0744

**★ 10696 ★ American Cancer Society**
**Gold Coast Regional Office**
426 E Barcellus, Ste. 304
Santa Maria, CA 93454
**Phone:** (805)925-8190　　　**Fax:** (805)925-1424

**★ 10697 ★ American Cancer Society**
**Greater Conejo Valley Unit**
50 W Hillcrest Dr., Ste. 208
Thousand Oaks, CA 91360
**Phone:** (805)497-0114　　　**Fax:** (805)497-9800

**★ 10698 ★ American Cancer Society**
**Greater North Unit**
Alton Deere Plaza
1940 E Deere Ave., Ste. 100
Santa Ana, CA 92705
**Phone:** (949)261-9446　　　**Fax:** (949)261-9419

**★ 10699 ★ American Cancer Society**
**Greater Petaluma Area**
400 N McDowell Blvd.
Petaluma, CA 94954
**Phone:** (707)766-8066　　　**Fax:** (707)545-3179

**★ 10700 ★ American Cancer Society**
**Greater San Bernardino Area**
1240 Palmyrita Ave., Ste. A
Riverside, CA 92507
**Phone:** (909)683-6415　　　**Fax:** (909)682-6804

**★ 10701 ★ American Cancer Society**
**Greater Ventura Unit**
3737 Telegraph Rd., Ste. D
Ventura, CA 93003
**Phone:** (805)644-6656　　　**Fax:** (805)644-6626

**★ 10702 ★ American Cancer Society**
**High Desert Unit**
14815 7th St.
Victorville, CA 92392
**Phone:** (760)245-2443

**★ 10703 ★ American Cancer Society**
**Humboldt-Del Norte Counties Unit**
2942 "F" St.
Eureka, CA 95501
**Phone:** (707)442-1436　　　**Fax:** (707)442-6427

**★ 10704 ★ American Cancer Society**
**Imperial Central Unit**
400 S 8th St.
El Centro, CA 92243
**Phone:** (760)352-6656　　　**Fax:** (760)352-0316

**★ 10705 ★ American Cancer Society**
**Indian Wells Valley Unit**
129 E Ridgecrest Blvd.
Ridgecrest, CA 93556
**Phone:** (760)371-1312　　　**Fax:** (760)371-2333

**★ 10706 ★ American Cancer Society**
**Inland Mendocino Unit**
497 Leslie St.
Ukiah, CA 95482
**Phone:** (707)462-7642　　　**Fax:** (707)462-0281

**★ 10707 ★ American Cancer Society**
**Irvine Unit**
Alton Deere Plaza
1940 E Deere Ave., Ste. 100
Santa Ana, CA 92705
**Phone:** (949)261-9446　　　**Fax:** (949)261-9419

**★ 10708 ★ American Cancer Society**
**Kings County Unit**
823 W Lacey Blvd.
Hanford, CA
**Phone:** (559)584-6691　　　**Fax:** (559)584-2815

**★ 10709 ★ American Cancer Society**
**Lakeport Unit**
1031 Jefferson St.
Napa, CA 94559
**Phone:** (707)255-5911　　　**Fax:** (707)255-3823

**★ 10710 ★ American Cancer Society**
**Lodi Unit**
207 E Alpine Ave.
Stockton, CA 95204
**Phone:** (209)941-2676　　　**Fax:** (209)941-2824

**★ 10711 ★ American Cancer Society**
**Lompoc Valley Unit**
604 E Ocean Ave.
Lompoc, CA 93436
**Phone:** (805)736-2610　　　**Fax:** (805)736-9413

**★ 10712 ★ American Cancer Society**
**Long Beach-Harbor-Southeast Unit**
936 Pine Ave.
Long Beach, CA 90813
**Phone:** (562)437-0791　　　**Fax:** (562)495-1782

**★ 10713 ★ American Cancer Society**
**Los Angeles Coastal Cities, South Bay Branch**
514 N Prospect Ave., Ste. 150
Redondo Beach, CA 90277
**Phone:** (310)937-2605　　　**Fax:** (310)937-2717

**★ 10714 ★ American Cancer Society**
**Los Angeles Coastal Cities Unit**
5731 W Slauson Ave., Ste. 200
Culver City, CA 90230
**Phone:** (310)348-0356　　　**Fax:** (310)645-1428

**★ 10715 ★ American Cancer Society**
**Los Angeles Region**
3333 Wilshire Blvd., Ste. 900
Los Angeles, CA 90010
**Phone:** (213)386-7660　　　**Fax:** (213)380-6286

**★ 10716 ★ American Cancer Society**
**Los Banos Unit**
PO Box 462
Los Banos, CA 93635
**Phone:** (209)827-4340　　　**Fax:** (209)722-6628

**★ 10717 ★ American Cancer Society**
**Madera County Unit**
425 N Gateway, Ste. C
Madera, CA 93637
**Phone:** (559)673-9425　　　**Fax:** (559)673-9432

**★ 10718 ★ American Cancer Society**
**Marin County Unit**
25 Bellam Blvd., Ste. 150
San Rafael, CA 94901
**Phone:** (415)454-8464　　　**Fax:** (415)456-1477

**★ 10719 ★ American Cancer Society**
**Mendocino Coast Area**
497 Leslie St.
Ukiah, CA 95482
**Phone:** (707)462-7642　　　**Fax:** (707)462-0281

**★ 10720 ★ American Cancer Society**
**Merced/Mariposa County Unit**
301 W 18th St., Ste. 101
Merced, CA 95340
**Phone:** (209)722-3341　　　**Fax:** (209)722-6628

**★ 10721 ★ American Cancer Society**
**Mission Oaks Unit**
274 Heather Ct.
Templeton, CA 93465
**Phone:** (805)238-9657　　　**Fax:** (805)434-3947

**★ 10722 ★ American Cancer Society**
**Modoc County Unit**
3290 Bechelli Ln.
Redding, CA 96002
**Phone:** (530)222-1058　　　**Fax:** (530)222-1409

**★ 10723 ★ American Cancer Society**
**Mojave Valley Unit**
1240 Palmyrita Ave., Ste. A
Riverside, CA 92507
**Phone:** (909)683-6415　　　**Fax:** (909)682-6804

**★ 10724 ★ American Cancer Society**
**Morongo Basin Unit**
56351 Twentynine Palms, Ste. B
Yucca Valley, CA 92284
**Phone:** (760)365-9828　　　**Fax:** (760)365-8317

**★ 10725 ★ American Cancer Society**
**Mountain Valley Unit**
2889 Cohasset Rd., Ste. 6
Chico, CA 95973
**Phone:** (530)342-4567　　　**Fax:** (530)345-5871

**★ 10726 ★ American Cancer Society**
**Multi-Cities Unit**
1240 Palmyrita Ave., Ste. A
Riverside, CA 92507
**Phone:** (909)683-6415　　　**Fax:** (909)682-6804

**★ 10727 ★ American Cancer Society**
**Napa County Unit**
1031 Jefferson St.
Napa, CA 94559
**Phone:** (707)255-5911　　　**Fax:** (707)255-3823

**★ 10728 ★ American Cancer Society**
**Nevada City/Grass Valley Unit**
618 5th St.
Marysville, CA 95901
**Phone:** (530)741-1366　　　**Fax:** (530)741-1383

**★ 10729 ★ American Cancer Society**
**Newport-Mesa Unit**
Alton Deere Plaza
1940 E Deere Ave., Ste. 100
Santa Ana, CA 92705
**Phone:** (949)261-9446　　　**Fax:** (949)261-9419

**★ 10730 ★ American Cancer Society**
**North Coast Border Unit**
1301 Northcrest Dr.
Crescent City, CA
**Phone:** (707)464-8277　　　**Fax:** (707)465-6710

**★ 10731 ★ American Cancer Society**
**North State Unit**
3290 Bechelli Ln.
Redding, CA 96002
**Phone:** (530)222-1058　　　**Fax:** (530)222-1409

★ 10732 ★ **American Cancer Society**
**North Valley Region**
1765 Challenge Way, Ste. 115
Sacramento, CA 95815
**Phone:** (916)446-7933  **Fax:** (916)325-4955

★ 10733 ★ **American Cancer Society**
**Northern California Chinese Unit**
39277 Liberty St., Ste. D-14
Fremont, CA 94538
**Phone:** (510)797-0600  **Fax:** (510)797-0698

★ 10734 ★ **American Cancer Society**
**Orange County Regional Office**
Alton Deere Plaza
1940 E Deere Ave., Ste. 100
Santa Ana, CA 92705
**Phone:** (949)261-9446  **Free:** 800-ACS-2345
**Fax:** (949)261-9419

★ 10735 ★ **American Cancer Society**
**Palo Verde Valley Unit**
74-140 El Paseo, Ste. 1
Palm Desert, CA 92260
**Phone:** (760)568-2691  **Fax:** (760)341-8783

★ 10736 ★ **American Cancer Society**
**Perris Valley Unit**
1240 Palmyrita Ave., Ste. A
Riverside, CA 92507
**Phone:** (909)683-6415  **Fax:** (909)682-6804

★ 10737 ★ **American Cancer Society**
**Redlands/Yucaipa Unit**
1240 Palmyrita Ave., Ste. A
Riverside, CA 92507
**Phone:** (909)683-6415  **Fax:** (909)682-6804

★ 10738 ★ **American Cancer Society**
**Redwood Empire Region**
c/o East Bay Region
1700 Webster St.
Oakland, CA 94612
**Phone:** (510)452-5229  **Fax:** (510)763-8826

★ 10739 ★ **American Cancer Society**
**Riverside Unit**
1240 Palmyrita Ave., Ste. A
Riverside, CA 92507
**Phone:** (909)683-6415  **Fax:** (909)682-6804

★ 10740 ★ **American Cancer Society**
**Sacramento Unit**
1765 Challenge Way, Ste. 115
Sacramento, CA 95815
**Phone:** (916)446-7933  **Fax:** (916)325-2351

★ 10741 ★ **American Cancer Society**
**Saddleback Valley Unit**
Alton Deere Plaza
1940 E Deere Ave., Ste. 100
Santa Ana, CA 92705
**Phone:** (949)261-9446  **Fax:** (949)261-9419

★ 10742 ★ **American Cancer Society**
**San Diego County Unit**
2655 Camino Del Rio N, Ste. 100
San Diego, CA 92108
**Phone:** (619)299-4200  **Fax:** (619)296-0928

★ 10743 ★ **American Cancer Society**
**San Fernando Valley Unit**
4940 Van Nuys Blvd., Ste. 301
Sherman Oaks, CA 91403
**Phone:** (818)905-7766  **Fax:** (818)905-9058

★ 10744 ★ **American Cancer Society**
**San Francisco County Unit**
235 Montgomery St., Ste. 320
San Francisco, CA 94104
**Phone:** (415)394-7100  **Free:** 800-ACS-2345
**Fax:** (415)394-7101

★ 10745 ★ **American Cancer Society**
**San Gabriel Valley Unit**
50 N Hill Ave., Ste. 200
Pasadena, CA 91106
**Phone:** (626)795-7774  **Fax:** (626)568-2888

★ 10746 ★ **American Cancer Society**
**San Joaquin/Calaveras Unit**
207 E Alpine Ave.
Stockton, CA 95204
**Phone:** (209)941-2676  **Fax:** (209)941-2824

★ 10747 ★ **American Cancer Society**
**San Luis Obispo Unit**
1428 Phillips Ln., Ste. 201
San Luis Obispo, CA 93401
**Phone:** (805)543-1481  **Fax:** (805)543-1515

★ 10748 ★ **American Cancer Society**
**San Mateo County Unit**
1650 S Amphlett Blvd., Ste. 110
San Mateo, CA 94402
**Phone:** (650)578-9902  **Fax:** (650)578-9940

★ 10749 ★ **American Cancer Society**
**Santa Barbara Unit**
1432 Chapala St.
Santa Barbara, CA 93101
**Phone:** (805)963-1576  **Fax:** (805)963-6093

★ 10750 ★ **American Cancer Society**
**Santa Clara County Unit**
1715 S Bascom Ave., Ste. 100
Campbell, CA 95008
**Phone:** (408)879-1032  **Fax:** (408)879-1031

★ 10751 ★ **American Cancer Society**
**Santa Clarita Valley Unit**
20655 Soledad Canyon Rd., Ste. 17
Santa Clarita, CA 91351
**Phone:** (661)298-0886  **Fax:** (661)298-0885

★ 10752 ★ **American Cancer Society**
**Santa Cruz County Unit**
Dominican Hospital Education Ctr.
1555 Soquel Dr.
Santa Cruz, CA 95065
**Phone:** (831)477-9523  **Fax:** (831)477-9506

★ 10753 ★ **American Cancer Society**
**Santa Maria Valley Unit**
220 S Palisade Dr., Ste. 103
Santa Maria, CA 93454
**Phone:** (805)922-2354  **Fax:** (805)928-6054

★ 10754 ★ **American Cancer Society**
**Santa Rosa Unit**
1451 Guerneville Rd., Ste. 220
Santa Rosa, CA 95403
**Phone:** (707)545-6720  **Fax:** (707)545-3179

★ 10755 ★ **American Cancer Society**
**Sierra View Unit**
456 W Putnam
Porterville, CA 93257
**Phone:** (559)782-7666

★ 10756 ★ **American Cancer Society**
**Silicon Valley/Central Coast Regional**
**Office**
1715 S Bascom Ave., Ste. 100
Campbell, CA 95008
**Phone:** (408)879-1032  **Fax:** (408)879-1030

★ 10757 ★ **American Cancer Society**
**Simi Valley Unit**
1445 E Los Angeles Ave., Ste. 207
Simi Valley, CA 93065
**Phone:** (805)527-5360  **Fax:** (805)527-3357

★ 10758 ★ **American Cancer Society**
**Siskiyou County Unit**
3290 Bechelli Ln.
Redding, CA 96002
**Phone:** (530)222-1058  **Fax:** (530)222-1409

★ 10759 ★ **American Cancer Society**
**Solano County Unit**
1652 W Texas St., Ste. 110
Fairfield, CA 94533
**Phone:** (707)425-5006  **Fax:** (707)425-5639

★ 10760 ★ **American Cancer Society**
**Sonoma Valley Area Office**
400 N McDowell Blvd.
Petaluma, CA 94954
**Phone:** (707)766-8066  **Fax:** (707)545-3179

★ 10761 ★ **American Cancer Society**
**South Central Los Angeles Unit**
641 E El Segundo Blvd.
Los Angeles, CA 90059
**Phone:** (323)757-9992  **Fax:** (323)757-9995

★ 10762 ★ **American Cancer Society**
**South Contra Costa County Unit**
1885 Oak Park Blvd.
Pleasant Hill, CA 94523
**Phone:** (925)934-7640  **Fax:** (925)934-5372

★ 10763 ★ **American Cancer Society**
**South Placer Unit**
333 Sunrise Ave., Ste. 344
Roseville, CA 95661
**Phone:** (916)783-4181  **Fax:** (916)783-4175

★ 10764 ★ **American Cancer Society**
**Stanislaus Unit**
1604 Ford Ave., Ste. 8
Modesto, CA 95350
**Phone:** (209)524-7242  **Fax:** (209)524-7454

★ 10765 ★ **American Cancer Society**
**Tehama County Unit**
3290 Bechelli Ln.
Redding, CA 96002
**Phone:** (530)222-1058  **Fax:** (530)222-1409

★ 10766 ★ **American Cancer Society**
**Temecula/Murrieta Unit**
1240 Palmyrita Ave., Ste. A
Riverside, CA 92507
**Phone:** (909)683-6415  **Fax:** (909)682-6804

★ 10767 ★ **American Cancer Society**
**Tri-Cities Unit**
1900 Mowry Ave., Ste. 405
Fremont, CA 94538
**Phone:** (510)742-8346  **Fax:** (510)742-8417

**★ 10768 ★ American Cancer Society**
**Tri-Valley Unit**
7000 Village Pkwy., Ste. E
Dublin, CA 94568
**Phone:** (925)833-2784          **Fax:** (925)833-9137

**★ 10769 ★ American Cancer Society**
**Tulare County Unit**
211 N Encina
Visalia, CA
**Phone:** (559)734-1391          **Fax:** (559)734-0429

**★ 10770 ★ American Cancer Society**
**Tuolumne County Unit**
1604 Ford Ave., Ste. 8
Modesto, CA 95350
**Phone:** (209)524-7242          **Fax:** (209)524-7454

**★ 10771 ★ American Cancer Society**
**Upper Napa Valley/Lake County Area**
**Office**
1031 Jefferson St.
Napa, CA 94559
**Phone:** (707)255-5911          **Fax:** (707)255-3823

**★ 10772 ★ American Cancer Society**
**West Bay Regional Office**
235 Montgomery St., Ste. 320
San Francisco, CA 94104
**Phone:** (415)394-7100          **Fax:** (415)394-7101

**★ 10773 ★ American Cancer Society**
**West Contra Costa County Unit**
2023 Vale Rd., Ste. 4
San Pablo, CA 94806
**Phone:** (510)236-6905          **Fax:** (510)236-6970

**★ 10774 ★ American Cancer Society**
**West Inland Valley Unit**
8560 Vineyard Ave., Ste. 108
Rancho Cucamonga, CA 91730
**Phone:** (909)949-6115          **Fax:** (909)949-6813

**★ 10775 ★ American Cancer Society**
**West Unit**
Alton Deere Plaza
1940 E Deere Ave., Ste. 100
Santa Ana, CA 92705
**Phone:** (949)261-9446          **Fax:** (949)261-9419

**★ 10776 ★ American Cancer Society**
**Yolo County Unit**
1765 Challenge Way, Ste. 115
Sacramento, CA 95815
**Phone:** (530)662-3464          **Fax:** (916)325-2351

**★ 10777 ★ American Cancer Society**
**Yuba Sutter Colusa Unit**
618 5th St.
Marysville, CA 95901
**Phone:** (530)741-1366          **Fax:** (530)741-1383

### Colorado

**★ 10778 ★ American Cancer Society**
**Boulder County Office**
2130 Mountain View Ave., Ste. A
Longmont, CO 80501
**Phone:** (303)776-2689          **Fax:** (303)776-2875

**★ 10779 ★ American Cancer Society**
**Colorado Springs Office**
1445 N Union, Ste. B-100
Colorado Springs, CO 80909
**Phone:** (719)636-5101          **Fax:** (719)636-1480

**★ 10780 ★ American Cancer Society**
**Grand Junction Office**
2754 Compass Dr., Ste. 328
Grand Junction, CO 81506
**Phone:** (970)242-9593          **Fax:** (970)242-2283

**★ 10781 ★ American Cancer Society**
**Larimer County Office**
344 E Foothills Pkwy., Ste. 2E
Fort Collins, CO 80525
**Phone:** (970)226-0148          **Fax:** (970)223-6214

**★ 10782 ★ American Cancer Society**
**Mile High Office**
2253 S Oneida St.
Denver, CO 80224
**Phone:** (303)758-2030          **Free:** 800-882-9455
**Fax:** (303)759-1615

**★ 10783 ★ American Cancer Society**
**Pueblo Office**
720 N Main St., Ste. 418
Pueblo, CO 81003
**Phone:** (719)543-2824          **Fax:** (719)543-2877

**★ 10784 ★ American Cancer Society**
**Southwest Colorado Office**
3801 N Main Ave.
Durango, CO 81301
**Phone:** (970)247-0278          **Fax:** (970)247-4200

**★ 10785 ★ American Cancer Society**
**Weld County Office**
1020 9th Ave.
Greeley, CO 80631
**Phone:** (970)356-9727

### Connecticut

**★ 10786 ★ American Cancer Society**
**Rhode Island & Eastern Connecticut**
**Division**
**Norwich Office**
238 W Town St.
Norwich, CT 06360
**Phone:** (860)887-2547          **Fax:** (860)885-0820

**★ 10787 ★ American Cancer Society**
**Southern New England Regional Office**
Meriden Executive Pk.
538 Preston Ave.
Meriden, CT 06450
**Phone:** (203)379-4700          **Fax:** (203)379-5060

**★ 10788 ★ American Cancer Society**
**Southwest New England Regional Office**
372 Danbury Rd.
Wilton, CT 06897
**Phone:** (203)563-0740          **Fax:** (203)563-0738

### Delaware

**★ 10789 ★ American Cancer Society**
**New Castle Office**
92 Read's Way, Ste. 205
New Castle, DE 19720
**Phone:** (302)324-4227          **Free:** 800-ACS-2345
**Fax:** (302)324-4233

### District of Columbia

**★ 10790 ★ American Cancer Society**
**District of Columbia Division**
1875 Connecticut Ave. NW, Ste. 730
Washington, DC 20009
**Phone:** (202)483-2600          **Fax:** (202)483-1174

### Florida

**★ 10791 ★ American Cancer Society**
**Alachua Unit**
2119 SW 16th St.
Gainesville, FL 32608
**Phone:** (352)376-6866          **Fax:** (352)336-3861

**★ 10792 ★ American Cancer Society**
**Baker Office**
1732 Kingsley Ave., Ste. 3
Orange Park, FL 32067
**Phone:** (904)264-6039          **Fax:** (904)264-6272

**★ 10793 ★ American Cancer Society**
**Bartow Office**
809 S Florida Ave.
Lakeland, FL 33801
**Phone:** (863)688-2326          **Fax:** (863)687-6939

**★ 10794 ★ American Cancer Society**
**Bay Area Office**
2012-A Lisenby Ave.
Panama City, FL 32405
**Phone:** (850)785-9205          **Fax:** (850)872-9431

**★ 10795 ★ American Cancer Society**
**Big Bend Committee Office**
241 John Knox Rd., Ste. 100
Tallahassee, FL 32308
**Phone:** (850)297-0588          **Fax:** (850)297-0592

**★ 10796 ★ American Cancer Society**
**Brevard Area Office**
4356-B Fortune Pl.
Melbourne, FL 32904
**Phone:** (321)723-7737          **Fax:** (321)723-3344

**★ 10797 ★ American Cancer Society**
**Broward Office**
3407 NW 9th Ave., Ste. 100
Fort Lauderdale, FL 33309
**Phone:** (954)564-0880          **Fax:** (954)561-8072

**★ 10798 ★ American Cancer Society**
**Calhoun Office**
2012-A Lisenby Ave.
Panama City, FL 32405
**Phone:** (850)785-9205          **Fax:** (850)872-9431

**★ 10799 ★ American Cancer Society**
**Capital Area Office**
241 John Knox Rd., Ste. 100
Tallahassee, FL 32308
**Phone:** (850)297-0588          **Fax:** (850)297-0592

**★ 10800 ★ American Cancer Society**
**Charlotte Office**
22107 Elmira Blvd.
Port Charlotte, FL 33952
**Phone:** (941)627-3000          **Fax:** (941)627-5229

**★ 10801 ★ American Cancer Society**
**Citrus Unit**
140 N Sportsman Pt.
Inverness, FL 34453
**Phone:** (352)637-5577          **Fax:** (352)637-2590

**★ 10802 ★ American Cancer Society**
**Clay Unit**
1732 Kingsley Ave., Ste. 3
Orange Park, FL 32073
**Phone:** (904)264-6039          **Fax:** (904)264-6272

**★ 10803 ★ American Cancer Society**
**Collier Office**
990 1st Ave. S, Ste. 200
Naples, FL 34102
**Phone:** (239)261-0337 **Fax:** (239)649-5571

**★ 10804 ★ American Cancer Society**
**Dade Office**
3901 NW 79th Ave., Ste. 224
Miami, FL 33166
**Phone:** (305)594-4363 **Fax:** (305)592-5140

**★ 10805 ★ American Cancer Society**
**DeSoto Office**
2100 S Tamiami Tr., Ste. A
Venice, FL 34293
**Phone:** (941)497-4309 **Fax:** (941)497-4752

**★ 10806 ★ American Cancer Society**
**Duval Office**
4030 Boulevard Center Dr.
Jacksonville, FL 32207
**Phone:** (904)398-0537 **Fax:** (904)396-0240

**★ 10807 ★ American Cancer Society**
**East Polk Unit**
192 Ave. D NW
Winter Haven, FL 33880
**Phone:** (863)294-0661 **Fax:** (863)293-3906

**★ 10808 ★ American Cancer Society**
**East/Southeast Volusia Office**
146 Orange Ave.
Daytona Beach, FL 32114
**Phone:** (386)253-1633 **Fax:** (386)253-1636

**★ 10809 ★ American Cancer Society**
**Escambia Unit**
701 E Cervantes St.
Pensacola, FL 32501
**Phone:** (850)438-4491 **Fax:** (850)433-5003

**★ 10810 ★ American Cancer Society**
**First Coast Area Office**
4030 Boulevard Center Dr.
Jacksonville, FL 32207
**Phone:** (904)398-0537 **Fax:** (904)396-0240

**★ 10811 ★ American Cancer Society**
**Flagler Office**
146 Orange Ave.
Daytona Beach, FL 32114
**Phone:** (386)439-3507 **Fax:** (386)253-1633

**★ 10812 ★ American Cancer Society**
**Franklin Office**
2012-A Lisenby Ave.
Panama City, FL 32405
**Phone:** (850)785-9205 **Fax:** (850)872-9431

**★ 10813 ★ American Cancer Society**
**Gadsden/Chattahoochee Office**
241 John Knox Rd., Ste. 100
Tallahassee, FL 32308
**Phone:** (850)297-0588 **Fax:** (850)297-0592

**★ 10814 ★ American Cancer Society**
**Greater Tampa Office**
1001 S MacDill Ave.
Tampa, FL 33629
**Phone:** (813)254-3630 **Free:** 800-ACS-2345
**Fax:** (813)349-4431
**Website:** http://www2.cancer.org/state/fl/index.htm

**★ 10815 ★ American Cancer Society**
**Gulf Coast Area Office**
701 E Cervantes St.
Pensacola, FL 32501
**Phone:** (850)438-4491 **Fax:** (850)438-9871

**★ 10816 ★ American Cancer Society**
**Gulf Office**
2012-A Lisenby Ave.
Panama City, FL 32405
**Phone:** (850)785-9205 **Fax:** (850)872-9431

**★ 10817 ★ American Cancer Society**
**Hardee/Manatee/Highlands Unit**
600 U.S. 301 Blvd. W, Ste. 136
Bradenton, FL 34205
**Phone:** (863)773-0333 **Fax:** (941)745-1760

**★ 10818 ★ American Cancer Society**
**Hernando Office**
8159 State Rd. 52
Hudson, FL 34667
**Phone:** (727)863-1019 **Fax:** (727)869-7228

**★ 10819 ★ American Cancer Society**
**High-Five Unit**
2119 SW 16th St.
Gainesville, FL 32608
**Phone:** (352)376-6866 **Fax:** (352)336-3861

**★ 10820 ★ American Cancer Society**
**Holmes/Emerald Coast Office**
4 Jackson St. NE
Fort Walton Beach, FL 32548
**Phone:** (850)244-3813 **Fax:** (850)664-5366

**★ 10821 ★ American Cancer Society**
**Indian River Office**
3375 20th St., Ste. 100
Vero Beach, FL 32960
**Phone:** (561)562-2272 **Fax:** (561)562-2666

**★ 10822 ★ American Cancer Society**
**Jackson Office**
2012-A Lisenby Ave.
Panama City, FL 32405
**Phone:** (850)785-9205 **Fax:** (850)872-9431

**★ 10823 ★ American Cancer Society**
**Jacksonville Beaches/Ponte Vedra Office**
2850 Isabella Blvd., Ste. 20
Jacksonville Beach, FL 32250
**Phone:** (904)249-0022 **Fax:** (904)270-0976

**★ 10824 ★ American Cancer Society**
**Lake/Sumter Office**
1411 E Main St., Ste. 3
Leesburg, FL 34748
**Phone:** (352)326-9599 **Fax:** (352)326-3855

**★ 10825 ★ American Cancer Society**
**Lee/Cape Coral Office**
4575 Via Royale, Ste. 110
Fort Myers, FL 33919
**Phone:** (239)936-1113 **Fax:** (239)936-3763

**★ 10826 ★ American Cancer Society**
**Leon Office**
241 John Knox Rd., Ste. 100
Tallahassee, FL 32308
**Phone:** (850)297-0588 **Fax:** (850)297-0592

**★ 10827 ★ American Cancer Society**
**Liberty Office**
2012-A Lisenby Ave.
Panama City, FL 32405
**Phone:** (850)785-9205 **Fax:** (850)872-9431

**★ 10828 ★ American Cancer Society**
**Marco Island Office**
917 N Collier Blvd.
Marco Island, FL 34145
**Phone:** (941)642-8800 **Fax:** (941)642-0027

**★ 10829 ★ American Cancer Society**
**Marion Unit**
2100 SE 17th St., Ste. 110
Ocala, FL 34471
**Phone:** (352)629-4727 **Fax:** (352)629-5107

**★ 10830 ★ American Cancer Society**
**Martin Office**
865 SE Monterey Commons Blvd.
Stuart, FL 34996
**Phone:** (772)287-7467 **Fax:** (772)287-7925

**★ 10831 ★ American Cancer Society**
**Miami Beach/North Dade Office**
3901 NW 79 Ave., Ste. 224
Miami, FL 33166
**Phone:** (305)594-4363 **Fax:** (305)947-8737

**★ 10832 ★ American Cancer Society**
**Monroe/Keys Office**
2502-B Roosevelt Blvd.
Key West, FL 33040
**Phone:** (305)292-2333 **Fax:** (305)294-3964

**★ 10833 ★ American Cancer Society**
**Nassau Office**
2850 Isabella Blvd., Ste. 20
Jacksonville Beach, FL 32250
**Phone:** (904)249-0022 **Fax:** (904)270-0976

**★ 10834 ★ American Cancer Society**
**North Central Area Office**
2119 SW 16th St.
Gainesville, FL 32608
**Phone:** (352)376-6866 **Fax:** (352)336-3861

**★ 10835 ★ American Cancer Society**
**North Okaloosa Office**
4 Jackson St. NE
Fort Walton Beach, FL 32548
**Phone:** (850)244-3813 **Fax:** (850)664-5366

**★ 10836 ★ American Cancer Society**
**Okeechobee Office**
3375 20th St., Ste. 100
Vero Beach, FL 32960
**Phone:** (561)562-2272 **Fax:** (561)562-2666

**★ 10837 ★ American Cancer Society**
**Orlando Metro Office**
1601 W Colonial Dr.
Orlando, FL 32804
**Phone:** (407)843-8680 **Fax:** (407)649-6502

**★ 10838 ★ American Cancer Society**
**Osceola Unit**
1601 W Colonial Dr.
Orlando, FL 32804
**Phone:** (407)843-8680 **Fax:** (407)423-2383

**★ 10839 ★ American Cancer Society**
**Palm Beach Benefit Office**
235 S County Rd., No. 20
Palm Beach, FL 33480
**Phone:** (561)655-3449     **Fax:** (561)655-3686

**★ 10840 ★ American Cancer Society**
**Pasco Office**
8159 State Rd. 52
Hudson, FL 34667
**Phone:** (727)863-1019     **Fax:** (727)869-7228

**★ 10841 ★ American Cancer Society**
**Pinellas Office**
4801 86th Ave. N
Pinellas Park, FL 33782
**Phone:** (727)546-9822     **Fax:** (727)545-3753

**★ 10842 ★ American Cancer Society**
**Putnam Office**
600 Zeigler Dr.
Palatka, FL 32177
**Phone:** (386)328-6224     **Fax:** (904)325-8086

**★ 10843 ★ American Cancer Society**
**Saint Johns Office**
2850 Isabella Blvd., Ste. 20
Jacksonville Beach, FL 32250
**Phone:** (904)249-0022     **Fax:** (904)270-0976

**★ 10844 ★ American Cancer Society**
**Saint Lucie Office**
3375 20th St., Ste. 100
Vero Beach, FL 32960
**Phone:** (561)562-2272     **Fax:** (561)562-2666

**★ 10845 ★ American Cancer Society**
**Santa Rosa Unit**
701 E Cervantes St.
Pensacola, FL 32501
**Phone:** (850)438-4491     **Fax:** (850)438-5003

**★ 10846 ★ American Cancer Society**
**Sarasota Office**
1750 17th St., Ste. A
Sarasota, FL 34234
**Phone:** (941)365-2858     **Fax:** (941)365-3256

**★ 10847 ★ American Cancer Society**
**Seminole Unit**
1601 W Colonial Dr.
Orlando, FL 32804
**Phone:** (407)843-8680     **Fax:** (407)649-6502

**★ 10848 ★ American Cancer Society**
**South Palm Beach Office**
3350 NW Boca Raton Blvd., Ste. A-34
Boca Raton, FL 33431
**Phone:** (561)394-7751     **Fax:** (561)394-7909

**★ 10849 ★ American Cancer Society**
**South Sarasota Office**
2100 S Tamiami Tr., Ste. A
Venice, FL 34293
**Phone:** (941)497-4309     **Fax:** (941)497-4752

**★ 10850 ★ American Cancer Society**
**Suburban Hillsborough Unit**
1462 Oakfield Dr.
Brandon, FL 33511
**Phone:** (813)685-0670     **Fax:** (813)689-1320

**★ 10851 ★ American Cancer Society**
**Tri-City Office**
22107 Elmira Blvd.
Port Charlotte, FL 33952
**Phone:** (941)627-3000     **Fax:** (941)627-5229

**★ 10852 ★ American Cancer Society**
**Tri-County Office**
2119 SW 16th St.
Gainesville, FL 32608
**Phone:** (352)376-6866     **Fax:** (352)336-3861

**★ 10853 ★ American Cancer Society**
**Washington Office**
2012-A Lisenby Ave.
Panama City, FL 32405
**Phone:** (850)785-9205     **Fax:** (850)872-9431

**★ 10854 ★ American Cancer Society**
**West Palm Beach Office**
5 Harvard Cir., Ste. 110
West Palm Beach, FL 33409
**Phone:** (561)616-9370     **Fax:** (561)616-9371

**★ 10855 ★ American Cancer Society**
**West Polk Unit**
809 S Florida Ave.
Lakeland, FL 33801
**Phone:** (863)688-2326     **Fax:** (863)687-6939

**★ 10856 ★ American Cancer Society**
**West Volusia Office**
218-A E New York Ave.
DeLand, FL 32724
**Phone:** (386)734-7836     **Fax:** (386)738-2215

## Georgia

**★ 10857 ★ American Cancer Society**
**Albany Office**
323 Pine Ave.
Albany, GA 31701
**Phone:** 800-282-4914     **Fax:** (229)446-7709

**★ 10858 ★ American Cancer Society**
**Athens Office**
1060 Gaines School Rd., Ste. B-2
Athens, GA 30605
**Phone:** 800-282-4914     **Fax:** (706)549-2314

**★ 10859 ★ American Cancer Society**
**Atlanta Office**
2200 Century Pkwy., Ste. 950
Atlanta, GA 30345
**Phone:** (404)816-4994     **Fax:** (404)315-9348
**Website:** http://www2.cancer.org/state/ga/index.html

**★ 10860 ★ American Cancer Society**
**Augusta Office**
2623 Washington Rd., Bldg F, Ste. 104
Augusta, GA 30904
**Phone:** 800-282-4914     **Fax:** (706)731-0979

**★ 10861 ★ American Cancer Society**
**Brunswick Office**
2311 Heron St.
Brunswick, GA 31520
**Phone:** 800-282-4914     **Fax:** (912)262-0773

**★ 10862 ★ American Cancer Society**
**Columbus Office**
1233 12th St.
Columbus, GA 31902
**Phone:** 800-282-4914     **Fax:** (706)324-4749

**★ 10863 ★ American Cancer Society**
**Dalton Office**
300 W Emery St., Ste. 106
Dalton, GA 30720
**Phone:** 800-282-4914     **Fax:** (706)226-7531

**★ 10864 ★ American Cancer Society**
**Fayetteville Office**
135 Bradford Sq., Ste. B
Fayetteville, GA 30215
**Phone:** (404)816-4994     **Fax:** (770)460-1641

**★ 10865 ★ American Cancer Society**
**Gainesville Office**
2565 Thompson Bridge Rd, Ste. 114
Gainesville, GA 30501
**Phone:** (404)816-4994     **Fax:** (770)297-7418

**★ 10866 ★ American Cancer Society**
**Gwinnett Office**
6500 Sugarloaf Pkwy., Ste. 260
Duluth, GA 30097
**Phone:** (404)816-4994     **Fax:** (770)814-9517

**★ 10867 ★ American Cancer Society**
**Macon Office**
804 Cherry St., Ste. A
Macon, GA 31201
**Phone:** 800-282-4914     **Fax:** (478)741-5905

**★ 10868 ★ American Cancer Society**
**Marietta Office**
1825 Barrett Lakes Blvd., Ste. 280
Kennesaw, GA 30144
**Phone:** (404)816-4994     **Fax:** (770)429-9824

**★ 10869 ★ American Cancer Society**
**Savannah Office**
5102 Paulsen St., Bldg. 4
Savannah, GA 31405
**Phone:** 800-282-4914     **Fax:** (912)355-0955

**★ 10870 ★ American Cancer Society**
**Statesboro Office**
515 Denmark St., Ste. 500
Statesboro, GA 30458
**Phone:** 800-282-4914     **Fax:** (912)764-3089

**★ 10871 ★ American Cancer Society**
**Waycross Office**
406 Tebeau St.
Waycross, GA 31501
**Phone:** 800-282-4914     **Fax:** (912)283-9694

## Guam

**★ 10872 ★ American Cancer Society**
**Guam Unit**
140 Aspinall St., Ste. 102
Agana, GU 96910
**Phone:** (671)477-9451     **Fax:** (671)477-9450

## Hawaii

**★ 10873 ★ American Cancer Society**
**Central/Leeward Unit**
98-029 Hekaha St., Bldg 5, Ste. 6
Aiea, HI 96701
**Phone:** (808)486-8420     **Fax:** (808)935-9780

**★ 10874 ★ American Cancer Society**
**East Hawaii Unit**
614 Kilauea Ave., Ste. 2
Hilo, HI 96720
**Phone:** (808)935-9763     **Fax:** (808)935-9780

★ 10875 ★ **American Cancer Society**
**Honolulu Office**
2370 Nuuanu Ave.
Honolulu, HI 96817
**Phone:** (808)595-7544　　**Free:** 800-ACS-2345
**Fax:** (808)595-7545
**Website:** http://www.hi-cancer.org


★ 10876 ★ **American Cancer Society**
**Kauai Unit**
3535 Kuhio Hwy.
Lihue, HI 96766
**Phone:** (808)245-2942　　**Fax:** (808)245-2302


★ 10877 ★ **American Cancer Society**
**Maui-Molokai-Lanai Unit**
Cameron Ctr.
95 Mahalani St.
Wailuku, HI 96793
**Phone:** (808)244-5553　　**Fax:** (808)244-6195


★ 10878 ★ **American Cancer Society**
**Molokai Branch**
PO Box 1618
Kaunakakai, HI 96748
**Phone:** (808)553-5154


★ 10879 ★ **American Cancer Society**
**West Hawaii Unit**
74-5588 R Pawai Pl.
Kailua Kona, HI 96740
**Phone:** (808)334-0442　　**Fax:** (808)334-0443


★ 10880 ★ **American Cancer Society**
**Windward Unit**
130 Kailua Rd., Ste. 102B
Kailua, HI 96734
**Phone:** (808)262-5124　　**Fax:** (808)262-4212

### Idaho

★ 10881 ★ **American Cancer Society**
**Eastern Idaho Office**
900 E Harmony
Blackfoot, ID 83221
**Phone:** (208)785-2516　　**Fax:** (208)785-6457


★ 10882 ★ **American Cancer Society**
**Magic Valley Office**
149 W 50 S
Rupert, ID 83350
**Phone:** (208)436-5238　　**Fax:** (208)436-5267


★ 10883 ★ **American Cancer Society**
**Northern Idaho Office**
1602 Sherman Ave., Ste. 104
Coeur d'Alene, ID 83814
**Phone:** (208)667-9749　　**Fax:** (208)765-5733


★ 10884 ★ **American Cancer Society**
**Treasure Valley Office**
2676 Vista Ave.
Boise, ID 83705
**Phone:** (208)343-4609　　**Free:** 800-632-5934
**Fax:** (208)343-9922
**Website:** http://www2.cancer.org/state/id/index.html

### Illinois

★ 10885 ★ **American Cancer Society**
**Chicago Regional Office**
77 E Monroe St., 12th Fl.
Chicago, IL 60603
**Phone:** (312)372-0471　　**Free:** 800-227-2345
**Fax:** (312)372-0910
**Website:** http://www.il.cancer.org


★ 10886 ★ **American Cancer Society**
**DuPage County Regional Office**
999 Main St.
Glen Ellyn, IL 60137
**Phone:** (630)469-3011　　**Free:** 800-ACS-2345
**Fax:** (630)469-3065
**Email:** shammes@cancer.org
**Website:** http://www.il.cancer.org/


★ 10887 ★ **American Cancer Society**
**Eastern Illinois Office**
2509 S Neil St.
Champaign, IL 61820
**Phone:** (217)356-9076　　**Free:** 800-ACS-2345
**Fax:** (217)356-7721
**Website:** http://www.il.cancer.org/


★ 10888 ★ **American Cancer Society**
**Fox Valley Regional Office**
11 E Wilson St.
Batavia, IL 60510
**Phone:** (630)879-9009　　**Free:** 800-ACS-2345
**Fax:** (630)879-9047
**Website:** http://www.il.cancer.org/


★ 10889 ★ **American Cancer Society**
**Lake County Regional Office**
777 Central Ave.
Highland Park, IL 60035
**Phone:** (847)432-0577　　**Fax:** (847)432-0599


★ 10890 ★ **American Cancer Society**
**Metro East Regional Office**
118 S Seminary St.
Collinsville, IL 62234
**Phone:** (618)345-7911　　**Fax:** (618)345-8320


★ 10891 ★ **American Cancer Society**
**North Shore Illinois Office**
820 Davis St., Ste. 340
Evanston, IL 60201
**Phone:** (847)328-5147　　**Free:** 800-ACS-2345
**Fax:** (847)570-6043
**Website:** http://www.il.cancer.org


★ 10892 ★ **American Cancer Society**
**Northern Illinois Regional Office**
4312 E State St.
Rockford, IL 61108
**Phone:** (815)229-1287　　**Free:** 800-ACS-2345
**Fax:** (815)229-1363
**Website:** http://il.cancer.org/


★ 10893 ★ **American Cancer Society**
**Northwest Illinois Regional Office**
3727 Blackhawk Rd.
Rock Island, IL 61201
**Phone:** (309)794-0601　　**Free:** 800-ACS-2345
**Fax:** (309)793-3251
**Website:** http://www.il.cancer.org/


★ 10894 ★ **American Cancer Society**
**Northwest Suburban Regional Office**
100 W Palatine Rd., Ste. 150
Palatine, IL 60067
**Phone:** (847)358-3965　　**Free:** 800-ACS-2345
**Fax:** (847)358-9218
**Website:** http://www.il.cancer.org/


★ 10895 ★ **American Cancer Society**
**Prairie Land Regional Office**
17060 Oak Park Ave.
Tinley Park, IL 60477
**Phone:** (708)633-7770　　**Free:** 800-ACS-2345
**Fax:** (708)633-7773
**Website:** http://www.il.cancer.org/


★ 10896 ★ **American Cancer Society**
**Riverside Regional Office**
7234 W Ogden Ave., Ste. 3 S
Riverside, IL 60546
**Phone:** (708)484-8541　　**Fax:** (708)484-3179


★ 10897 ★ **American Cancer Society**
**Southern Regional Office**
805 W DeYoung St., Ste. B
Marion, IL 62959
**Phone:** (618)998-9898　　**Fax:** (618)997-8456


★ 10898 ★ **American Cancer Society**
**West Central Regional Office**
4234 N Knoxville Ave., Ste. B
Peoria, IL 61614
**Phone:** (309)688-3488　　**Free:** 800-ACS-2345
**Fax:** (309)688-9493
**Website:** http://www.il.cancer.org/


★ 10899 ★ **American Cancer Society**
**Western Illinois Regional Office**
1305 Wabash
Springfield, IL 62704
**Phone:** (217)546-7586　　**Free:** 800-ACS-2345
**Fax:** (217)546-7631
**Website:** http://www.il.cancer.org/

### Indiana

★ 10900 ★ **American Cancer Society**
**Central Indiana Area Service Center**
6030 W 62nd St.
Indianapolis, IN 46278
**Phone:** (317)347-6670　　**Free:** 800-233-6303
**Fax:** (317)347-6679
Denice Kallmyer, Exec Director


★ 10901 ★ **American Cancer Society**
**Evansville Branch**
1510 W Franklin St.
Evansville, IN 47710
**Phone:** (812)424-8281　　**Free:** 800-227-2345
**Fax:** (812)424-1059
Gene Watson, Exec Director


★ 10902 ★ **American Cancer Society**
**Indianapolis Office**
6030 W 62nd St.
Indianapolis, IN 46278
**Phone:** (317)347-6670　　**Fax:** (317)347-6679


★ 10903 ★ **American Cancer Society**
**Lower Eastern Indiana Area Service Center**
923 4th St.
PO Box 689
Columbus, IN 47201
**Phone:** (812)376-6781　　**Fax:** (812)376-8031
Amy Eden, Exec Director


★ 10904 ★ **American Cancer Society**
**Lower Eastern Indiana Area Service Center**
Jenkins Hall
1401 Chester Blvd.
Richmond, IN 47374
**Phone:** (765)962-4180　　**Fax:** (765)966-8023


★ 10905 ★ **American Cancer Society**
**Mid-Indiana Area Service Center**
2831 N Oakwood
Muncie, IN 47304-2254
**Phone:** (765)284-1696　　**Fax:** (765)289-3254

**★ 10906 ★ American Cancer Society**
**Mid-Indiana Area Service Center**
707 W Historic 8th St.
Anderson, IN 46016
**Phone:** (765)642-6603      **Fax:** (765)642-6711
Gloria Collins, Contact


**★ 10907 ★ American Cancer Society**
**Mid-Indiana Area Service Center**
**Kokomo Office**
1150 S Dixon Rd.
Kokomo, IN 46902
**Phone:** (765)457-9173      **Fax:** (765)457-0595
Jim Seidel, Exec Director


**★ 10908 ★ American Cancer Society**
**Mid-Indiana Area Service Center**
**Lafayette Office**
401 S Earl St., Ste. 2C
Lafayette, IN 47904
**Phone:** (765)449-4799      **Fax:** (765)449-4065


**★ 10909 ★ American Cancer Society**
**Mid-Indiana Area Service Center**
**Marion Office**
1315 Gillespie St.
Marion, IN 46952
**Phone:** (765)668-7188      **Fax:** (265)668-7188


**★ 10910 ★ American Cancer Society**
**Mid-Southwestern Area Service Center**
318 Main St.
Vincennes, IN 47591
**Phone:** (812)886-9007      **Fax:** (812)886-9008


**★ 10911 ★ American Cancer Society**
**Mid-Southwestern Indiana Area Service**
  **Center**
1500 Meridian Rd.
Jasper, IN 47546
**Phone:** (812)482-7545      **Fax:** (812)482-6962
Christine Hopson, Exec Director


**★ 10912 ★ American Cancer Society**
**North Central Indiana Area Service**
  **Center**
535 W Edison, Unit 6
Mishawaka, IN 46545
**Phone:** (574)257-9789      **Fax:** (574)257-9790


**★ 10913 ★ American Cancer Society**
**Northeast Indiana Area Service Center**
2420 N Coliseum Blvd., Ste. 200
Fort Wayne, IN 46805
**Phone:** (219)471-3911      **Fax:** (219)483-5344
Peter Rinn, Exec Director


**★ 10914 ★ American Cancer Society**
**Northwest Indiana Area Service Center**
107 W 78th Pl.
Merrillville, IN 46410
**Phone:** (219)793-1030      **Fax:** (219)793-1033
Bill Lieber, Exec Director


**★ 10915 ★ American Cancer Society**
**Northwest Indiana Area Service Center**
410 E Lincolnway
Valparaiso, IN 46383
**Phone:** (219)464-2895      **Fax:** (219)465-1044
**Email:** Judy.Rooney-Davis@cancer.org
**Website:** http://www.cancer.org
Judy Rooney-Davis, Exec Director


**★ 10916 ★ American Cancer Society**
**South Central Indiana Area Service**
  **Center**
710 N Walnut St.
Bloomington, IN 47404
**Phone:** (812)336-8423      **Fax:** (812)339-9213
**Email:** jbretz@cancer.org
**Website:** http://www.cancer.org
Jim Bretz, Exec Director


**★ 10917 ★ American Cancer Society**
**Southeast Indiana Area Service Center**
230 Montgomery St., Ste. 105
Clarksville, IN 47129
**Phone:** (812)282-4266      **Free:** 800-227-2345
**Fax:** (812)282-5334
David Dougherty, Director


**★ 10918 ★ American Cancer Society**
**Southwestern Indiana Area Service**
  **Center**
1510 W Franklin St.
Evansville, IN 47710
**Phone:** (812)424-8281      **Fax:** (812)424-1059


**★ 10919 ★ American Cancer Society**
**Wabash Valley Indiana Area Service**
  **Center**
705 Putnam St.
Terre Haute, IN 47802
**Phone:** (812)232-2679      **Fax:** (812)232-2741
Julie Hansen, Exec Director


## Iowa

**★ 10920 ★ American Cancer Society**
**Burlington Office**
1223 S Gear, Ste. 009
West Burlington, IA 52655
**Phone:** (319)752-4008      **Fax:** (319)752-6750


**★ 10921 ★ American Cancer Society**
**Carroll Office**
628 N Main St., Ste. 101
Carroll, IA 51401
**Phone:** (712)794-0100      **Fax:** (712)794-0101


**★ 10922 ★ American Cancer Society**
**Cedar Rapids Office**
4080 1st Ave. NE
Cedar Rapids, IA 52402
**Phone:** (319)365-5241      **Fax:** (319)365-1739


**★ 10923 ★ American Cancer Society**
**Council Bluffs Office**
2705 E Kanesville Blvd.
Council Bluffs, IA 51503
**Phone:** (712)323-6611      **Fax:** (712)323-7250


**★ 10924 ★ American Cancer Society**
**Davenport Office**
1351 W Central Park Ave., Ste. 1100
Davenport, IA 52804
**Phone:** (563)421-4227      **Fax:** (563)421-4229


**★ 10925 ★ American Cancer Society**
**Des Moines Office**
8364 Hickman, Ste. D
Des Moines, IA 50325
**Phone:** (515)253-0147      **Fax:** (515)253-0806


**★ 10926 ★ American Cancer Society**
**Dubuque Office**
367 Cedar Cross Rd.
Dubuque, IA 52003
**Phone:** (563)583-8249      **Fax:** (563)583-8240


**★ 10927 ★ American Cancer Society**
**Fort Dodge Office**
900 Central Ave., Ste. 21
Fort Dodge, IA 50501
**Phone:** (515)576-7078      **Fax:** (515)576-8353


**★ 10928 ★ American Cancer Society**
**Iowa City Office**
301 S Clinton St., 2nd Fl.
Iowa City, IA 52240
**Phone:** (319)337-8958      **Fax:** (319)337-8978


**★ 10929 ★ American Cancer Society**
**Mason City Office**
130 4th St. SW
Mason City, IA 50401
**Phone:** (641)422-9055      **Fax:** (641)422-9091


**★ 10930 ★ American Cancer Society**
**Sioux City Office**
Terra Ctr.
600 4th St., Ste. 229
Sioux City, IA 51101
**Phone:** (712)233-1148      **Fax:** (712)233-1507


**★ 10931 ★ American Cancer Society**
**Storm Lake Office**
541 Cayuga St.
Storm Lake, IA 50588
**Phone:** (712)732-9022      **Fax:** (712)732-9026


**★ 10932 ★ American Cancer Society**
**Waterloo Office**
200 E Ridgeway, Ste. 300
Waterloo, IA 50702
**Phone:** (319)272-2880      **Fax:** (319)272-2881


## Kansas

**★ 10933 ★ American Cancer Society**
**Kansas City Metro Office**
6700 Antioch Rd., Ste. 100
Merriam, KS 66204-1200
**Phone:** (913)432-3277      **Free:** 800-ACS-2345
**Fax:** (913)432-1732
**Website:** http://www.cancer.org/state/heartland/


**★ 10934 ★ American Cancer Society**
**Manhattan Office**
3100 Heritage Ct., Ste. 80
Manhattan, KS 66503
**Phone:** (785)539-1547      **Free:** 800-359-1025
**Fax:** (785)539-1547
**Website:** http://www.cancer.org/state/heartland/in-
dex.html


**★ 10935 ★ American Cancer Society**
**Southwest Kansas/Northwest Oklahoma**
  **Office**
1712 32nd St.
Great Bend, KS 67530
**Phone:** (620)792-4994


**★ 10936 ★ American Cancer Society**
**Topeka Office**
1315 SW Arrowhead Rd.
Topeka, KS 66604
**Phone:** (785)273-4422      **Free:** 800-359-1025
**Fax:** (785)273-1503
**Website:** http://www.cancer.org/state/heartland/


**★ 10937 ★ American Cancer Society**
**Wichita Office**
435 S Broadway, Ste. 100
Wichita, KS 67202
**Phone:** (316)265-3400      **Free:** 800-478-4788
**Fax:** (316)265-3490

## Kentucky

**★ 10938 ★ American Cancer Society**
**Ashland Office**
4338 13th St.
Ashland, KY 41102
**Phone:** (606)324-1819     **Fax:** (606)327-1744
Website: http://www2.cancer.org/state/ky/index.html

**★ 10939 ★ American Cancer Society**
**Bowling Green Office**
Greenwood Courtyard
2425 Scottsville Rd., Ste. 123
Bowling Green, KY 42104-4457
**Phone:** (270)782-3654     **Fax:** (270)846-0202
Website: http://www2.cancer.org/state/ky/

**★ 10940 ★ American Cancer Society**
**Lexington Office**
160 Moore Dr., Ste. 201
Lexington, KY 40503
**Phone:** (859)276-3223     **Fax:** (859)276-3056
Website: http://www2.cancer.org/state/ky/

**★ 10941 ★ American Cancer Society**
**Louisville Area**
**Clark, Floyd Counties**
701 W Muhammad Ali Blvd.
Louisville, KY 40203
**Phone:** (502)584-6782     **Free:** 800-ACS-2345
**Fax:** (502)584-8946

**★ 10942 ★ American Cancer Society**
**Louisville Office**
701 W Muhammad Ali Blvd.
Louisville, KY 40203
**Phone:** (502)584-6782     **Fax:** (502)584-6767
Website: http://www2.cancer.org/state/ky/index.html

**★ 10943 ★ American Cancer Society**
**Northern Kentucky Office**
Nicholas Center, Ste. A2
6612 Dixie Hwy.
Florence, KY 41042
**Phone:** (859)647-2200     **Fax:** (859)647-2246
Website: http://www2.cancer.org/state/ky/

**★ 10944 ★ American Cancer Society**
**Owensboro Office**
319 W 10th St.
Owensboro, KY 42301
**Phone:** (270)683-0425     **Fax:** (270)683-1471
Website: http://www2.cancer.org/state/ky/index.html

**★ 10945 ★ American Cancer Society**
**Paducah Office**
3140 Parisa Dr.
Paducah, KY 42003
**Phone:** (270)444-0375     **Free:** 800-ACS-2345
**Fax:** (270)444-0380

**★ 10946 ★ American Cancer Society**
**Purchase District**
3140 Parisa Dr.
Paducah, KY 42003
**Phone:** (502)444-0375     **Fax:** (502)444-0380
Website: http://www2.cancer.org/state/ky/index.html

**★ 10947 ★ American Cancer Society**
**Somerset Kentucky Office**
402 Coomer St.
Somerset, KY 42503
**Phone:** (606)679-6143     **Free:** 800-ACS-2345
**Fax:** (606)677-1943

## Louisiana

**★ 10948 ★ American Cancer Society**
**Alexandria Office**
605C Medical Center Dr.
Alexandria, LA 71301
**Phone:** (318)445-4190     **Fax:** (318)445-5008

**★ 10949 ★ American Cancer Society**
**Baton Rouge Office**
4919 Jamestown Ave., Ste. 104
Baton Rouge, LA 70808
**Phone:** (225)927-0782     **Fax:** (225)927-0785

**★ 10950 ★ American Cancer Society**
**Houma Office**
614 Barrow St.
Houma, LA 70360
**Phone:** (985)851-7776     **Fax:** (985)851-5939

**★ 10951 ★ American Cancer Society**
**Kenner Office**
2200 Veterans Memorial Blvd., Ste. 214
Kenner, LA 70062
**Phone:** (504)469-0021     **Fax:** (504)469-0033
Website: http://www2.cancer.org/state/la/index.html

**★ 10952 ★ American Cancer Society**
**Lafayette Office**
1604 W Pinhook Rd., Ste. 182
Lafayette, LA 70508
**Phone:** (337)237-3736     **Fax:** (337)237-6907

**★ 10953 ★ American Cancer Society**
**Lake Charles Office**
1 Lakeshore Dr., Ste. 1585
Lake Charles, LA 70629
**Phone:** (337)433-5131     **Fax:** (337)439-9620

**★ 10954 ★ American Cancer Society**
**Monroe Office**
1761 N 19th St.
Monroe, LA 71201
**Phone:** (318)398-7248     **Fax:** (318)361-0718

**★ 10955 ★ American Cancer Society**
**Shreveport Office**
920 Pierremont Rd., Ste. 300
Shreveport, LA 71106
**Phone:** (318)227-8901     **Fax:** (318)865-4831

## Maine

**★ 10956 ★ American Cancer Society**
**Northeast New England Region**
**Topsham Office**
1 Main St., Ste. 300
Topsham, ME 04086-1240
**Phone:** (207)373-3700     **Free:** 800-464-3102
**Fax:** (207)725-6680

## Maryland

**★ 10957 ★ American Cancer Society**
**Cumberland Office**
111 S George St.
Cumberland, MD 21502
**Phone:** (301)722-2145     **Fax:** (301)724-6179

**★ 10958 ★ American Cancer Society**
**Eldersburg Office**
1393 Progress Way, Ste. 908
Eldersburg, MD 21784
**Phone:** (410)781-4316     **Fax:** (410)781-4317

**★ 10959 ★ American Cancer Society**
**Gambrills Office**
1041 Rte. 3 N, Bldg. A
Gambrills, MD 21054
**Phone:** (410)721-4304     **Fax:** (410)721-4307

**★ 10960 ★ American Cancer Society**
**Hagerstown Office**
1037 Haven Rd.
Hagerstown, MD 21742
**Phone:** (301)733-8272     **Fax:** (301)733-0285

**★ 10961 ★ American Cancer Society**
**Salisbury Office**
1138 Parsons Rd.
Salisbury, MD 21803
**Phone:** (410)749-1624     **Fax:** (410)860-0832

**★ 10962 ★ American Cancer Society**
**Silver Spring Office**
11331 Amherst Ave.
Silver Spring, MD 20902
**Phone:** (301)933-9350     **Fax:** (301)929-8243

**★ 10963 ★ American Cancer Society**
**White Marsh Office**
8219 Town Center Dr.
Baltimore, MD 21236
**Phone:** (410)931-6850     **Free:** 888-640-0427
**Fax:** (410)931-6875
Website:   http://www.inet.net/imc/acsworking/md/index.shtml?md&total

## Massachusetts

**★ 10964 ★ American Cancer Society**
**Central New England Regional Office**
Natick Business Park
6 Strathmore Rd.
Natick, MA 01760
**Phone:** (508)652-4300     **Fax:** (508)655-4907

**★ 10965 ★ American Cancer Society**
**Massachusetts Bay Regional Office**
25 Stuart St., 4th Fl.
Boston, MA 02116
**Phone:** (617)556-7400     **Fax:** (617)426-0383

**★ 10966 ★ American Cancer Society**
**Midcoastal New England Region**
**Byfield Office**
12 Kent Way, Ste. 209
Byfield, MA 01922
**Phone:** (978)462-0571     **Free:** 800-227-2345
**Fax:** (978)462-1566

**★ 10967 ★ American Cancer Society**
**New England Division**
30 Speen St.
Framingham, MA 01701
**Free:** 800-ACS-2345

**★ 10968 ★ American Cancer Society**
**Southeast New England Regional Division**
**Brockton Office**
1115 W Chestnut St., Ste. 301
Brockton, MA 02301
**Phone:** (508)584-9600     **Fax:** (508)584-9699

**★ 10969 ★ American Cancer Society**
**Southeast New England Regional Office**
1115 W Chestnut St.
Brockton, MA 02301
**Phone:** (508)584-9600     **Fax:** (508)584-9699

**★ 10970 ★ American Cancer Society**
**Western New England Region**
**Pittsfield Office**
39 Wahconah St., 2nd Fl.
Pittsfield, MA 01201
**Phone:** (413)734-6000　　　**Fax:** (413)445-0007

**★ 10971 ★ American Cancer Society**
**Western New England Region**
**West Springfield Office**
31 Capital Dr.
West Springfield, MA 01089
**Phone:** (413)734-6000　　　**Free:** 800-227-2345
**Fax:** (413)746-4099

## Michigan

**★ 10972 ★ American Cancer Society**
**Barry County Office**
PO Box 509
Hastings, MI 49058
**Phone:** (616)945-4107

**★ 10973 ★ American Cancer Society**
**Bay Area Service Center**
1480 W Center Rd., Ste. 1
Essexville, MI 48732
**Phone:** (989)895-1730　　　**Free:** 800-728-2323
**Fax:** (989)895-1745
**Website:** http://www.gl.cancer.org
Linda Johnson, Exec Director

**★ 10974 ★ American Cancer Society**
**Capital Area Service Center**
1755 Abbey Rd.
East Lansing, MI 48823
**Phone:** (517)332-3300　　　**Fax:** (517)887-8152

**★ 10975 ★ American Cancer Society**
**East Michigan Area Service Center**
2353 S Linden Rd., Ste. B
Flint, MI 48532
**Phone:** (810)733-3702　　　**Fax:** (810)733-1480
**Website:** http://www.gl.cancer.org/
Becky Langtry, Exec Director

**★ 10976 ★ American Cancer Society**
**Gladwin County Office**
110 Ross St.
Beaverton, MI 48612
**Phone:** (989)895-1730　　　**Fax:** (989)435-8011

**★ 10977 ★ American Cancer Society**
**Huron Valley Area Service Center**
2010 Hogsback Rd., Ste. 6
Ann Arbor, MI 48105
**Phone:** (734)971-4300　　　**Fax:** (734)971-2818
**Website:** http://www.gl.cancer.org/
Amy Thompson-Boyk, Exec Director

**★ 10978 ★ American Cancer Society**
**Ionia County Office**
PO Box 45
Ionia, MI 48846
**Phone:** (866)364-6284

**★ 10979 ★ American Cancer Society**
**Lakeshore Area Service Center**
854 S Washington Ave., Ste. 410
Holland, MI 49423
**Phone:** (616)396-5576　　　**Fax:** (616)396-2673
**Website:** http://www.gl.cancer.org/
Jeff Compagner, Exec Director

**★ 10980 ★ American Cancer Society**
**Livingston County Office**
7208 W Grand River
Brighton, MI 48114
**Phone:** (810)225-8590　　　**Free:** (734)971-2818
**Website:** http://www.gl.cancer.org
Amy Thompson-Boyk, Exec Director

**★ 10981 ★ American Cancer Society**
**Macomb Office**
39425 Garfield, Ste. 24
Clinton Township, MI 48038
**Phone:** (586)263-8000　　　**Fax:** (586)263-5650
**Website:** http://www.gl.cancer.org/
Megan White, Exec Director

**★ 10982 ★ American Cancer Society**
**Metro Detroit Area Service Center**
18505 W 12 Mile Rd.
Southfield, MI 48076
**Phone:** (248)557-5353　　　**Free:** 800-227-2345
**Fax:** (248)557-6128
Megan White, Exec Director

**★ 10983 ★ American Cancer Society**
**Montcalm County Office**
PO Box 701
Greenville, MI 48838
**Phone:** (866)364-6284

**★ 10984 ★ American Cancer Society**
**Muskegon Office**
1383 E Laketon Ave.
Muskegon, MI 49442
**Phone:** (231)722-7407　　　**Fax:** (231)722-6267
Jeff Compagner, Director

**★ 10985 ★ American Cancer Society**
**Northern Michigan Area Service Center**
525 W 14th St., Ste. 5
Traverse City, MI 49684
**Phone:** (231)947-0860　　　**Free:** 800-723-0370
**Fax:** (231)947-0830
**Website:** http://www.gl.cancer.org/
Bob Burian, Exec Director

**★ 10986 ★ American Cancer Society**
**South Central Michigan Service Center**
715 W Michigan Ave.
Jackson, MI 49201
**Phone:** (517)787-0382　　　**Fax:** (517)787-1613
**Email:** sandysummerfelt@cancer.org
**Website:** http://www.gl.cancer.org/
Kathey Maitland, Exec Director

**★ 10987 ★ American Cancer Society**
**Southwest Michigan Area Service Center**
5110 Sprinkle Rd.
Portage, MI 49002
**Phone:** (616)349-8719　　　**Fax:** (616)349-0846

**★ 10988 ★ American Cancer Society**
**Upper Peninsula Area Office**
1400 S Carpenter Ave.
Iron Mountain, MI 49801
**Phone:** (906)776-2150　　　**Fax:** (906)776-2155

**★ 10989 ★ American Cancer Society**
**West Michigan Area Service Center**
400 Ann St. NW, Ste. 202
Grand Rapids, MI 49504
**Phone:** (616)364-6121　　　**Fax:** (616)364-6451
**Website:** http://www.gl.cancer.org/
Deb Sprague, Exec Director

## Minnesota

**★ 10990 ★ American Cancer Society**
**Bemidji Office**
750 Paul Bunyan Dr. NW, Ste. 7
Bemidji, MN 56601
**Phone:** (218)444-2810　　　**Fax:** (218)444-2811

**★ 10991 ★ American Cancer Society**
**Brainerd Office**
17 Washington St., Ste. 2
Brainerd, MN 56401
**Phone:** (218)829-6212　　　**Fax:** (218)829-6258

**★ 10992 ★ American Cancer Society**
**Duluth Office**
130 W Superior St., LL2, Ste. 200
Duluth, MN 55802
**Phone:** (218)727-7439　　　**Free:** 800-582-5152
**Fax:** (218)727-8069
**Website:** http://www2.cancer.org/state/mw/

**★ 10993 ★ American Cancer Society**
**Grand Rapids Office**
Grand Rapids Community Cancer Center
2101 S Hwy. 169, Ste. 2
Grand Rapids, MN 55744
**Phone:** (218)326-4235　　　**Fax:** (218)326-5420

**★ 10994 ★ American Cancer Society**
**Mankato Office**
227 E Main, Ste. 110
Mankato, MN 56001
**Phone:** (507)345-1451　　　**Fax:** (507)345-3093

**★ 10995 ★ American Cancer Society**
**Marshall Office**
348 W Main St.
Marshall, MN 56258
**Phone:** (507)929-5000　　　**Fax:** (507)929-5005

**★ 10996 ★ American Cancer Society**
**Minneapolis Office**
3316 W 66th St.
Edina, MN 55435
**Phone:** (952)925-2772　　　**Free:** 800-582-5152
**Fax:** (952)925-6333
**Website:** http://www2.cancer.org/state/mn/

**★ 10997 ★ American Cancer Society**
**Moorhead Office**
1001 Center Ave., Ste. K
Moorhead, MN 56560
**Phone:** (218)233-6114　　　**Free:** 800-225-0289
**Fax:** (218)236-6307
**Website:** http://www2.cancer.org/state/mw/

**★ 10998 ★ American Cancer Society**
**Rochester Office**
882 7th St. NW
Rochester, MN 55901
**Phone:** (507)287-2044　　　**Free:** 800-582-5152
**Fax:** (507)287-2178
**Website:** http://www2.cancer.org/state/mw/

**★ 10999 ★ American Cancer Society**
**Saint Cloud Office**
3721 23rd St. S, Ste. 102
Saint Cloud, MN 56301
**Phone:** (320)255-0220　　　**Free:** 800-293-7028
**Fax:** (320)255-5517
**Website:** http://www2.cancer.org/state/mw/

★ 11000 ★ American Cancer Society
**St. Paul Office**
1096 Raymond Ave.
Saint Paul, MN 55108
**Phone:** (651)644-1224          **Free:** 800-349-0087
**Fax:** (651)644-2819

★ 11001 ★ American Cancer Society
**Willmar Office**
333 Litchfield Ave. SW
Willmar, MN 56201
**Phone:** (320)235-7237          **Fax:** (320)235-0796

### Mississippi

★ 11002 ★ American Cancer Society
**Gulfport Office**
417 Security Sq.
Gulfport, MS 39507
**Phone:** (228)896-7024          **Fax:** (228)896-8620

★ 11003 ★ American Cancer Society
**Hattiesburg Office**
204 W Front St.
Hattiesburg, MS 39401
**Phone:** (601)545-7770          **Fax:** (601)545-7774

★ 11004 ★ American Cancer Society
**Jackson Office**
1380 Livingston Ln.
Jackson, MS 39213
**Phone:** (601)362-8874          **Free:** 800-227-2345
**Fax:** (601)362-8876
**Website:** http://www.cancer.org/ms.html

★ 11005 ★ American Cancer Society
**Meridian Office**
4825-A Poplar Springs Dr.
Meridian, MS 39305
**Phone:** (601)481-1712          **Fax:** (601)482-0258

### Missouri

★ 11006 ★ American Cancer Society
**Cape Girardeau Office**
937 Broadway, Ste. 302
Cape Girardeau, MO 63701
**Phone:** (573)334-9197          **Fax:** (573)334-5115
**Website:**      http://www.cancer.org/state/heartland/index.html

★ 11007 ★ American Cancer Society
**Columbia Office**
33 E Broadway, Ste. 100
Columbia, MO 65203
**Phone:** (573)443-1496          **Free:** 800-429-7753
**Fax:** (573)442-9955

★ 11008 ★ American Cancer Society
**Hannibal Office**
714 Broadway, Ste. 2
Hannibal, MO 63401
**Phone:** (573)221-4660          **Free:** 800-684-2733
**Fax:** (573)221-3326

★ 11009 ★ American Cancer Society
**Heartland Division**
1100 Pennsylvania Ave.
Kansas City, MO 64105
**Free:** 800-227-2345

★ 11010 ★ American Cancer Society
**Jefferson City Office**
2413 Hyde Park Rd.
Jefferson City, MO 65109
**Phone:** (573)635-4821          **Free:** 800-635-9194
**Fax:** (573)635-7821

★ 11011 ★ American Cancer Society
**Joplin Office**
2700 McClelland Blvd., Bldg. A, Ste. 110
Joplin, MO 64804
**Phone:** (417)624-6808          **Free:** 800-ACS-2345
**Fax:** (417)782-2348

★ 11012 ★ American Cancer Society
**O'Fallon Office**
105 W Pitman
O'Fallon, MO 63366
**Phone:** (636)379-8971          **Fax:** (636)379-8975

★ 11013 ★ American Cancer Society
**Osage Beach Office**
5740 Hwy. 54, Ste. 1002
Osage Beach, MO 65065
**Phone:** (573)302-7895          **Fax:** (573)317-1523

★ 11014 ★ American Cancer Society
**St. Joseph Office**
3931 Sherman Ave.
Saint Joseph, MO 64506
**Phone:** (816)233-2558          **Free:** 800-356-3161
**Fax:** (816)233-6952

★ 11015 ★ American Cancer Society
**St. Louis Office**
4207 Lindell Blvd.
Saint Louis, MO 63108
**Phone:** (314)286-8100          **Fax:** (314)286-8160
**Email:** june.shinners@cancer.org
**Website:** http://www.cancer.org

★ 11016 ★ American Cancer Society
**Sikeston Office**
201 N New Madrid St.
Sikeston, MO 63801
**Phone:** (573)471-1823          **Free:** 800-ACS-2345
**Fax:** (573)471-1372

★ 11017 ★ American Cancer Society
**Springfield Office**
3322 S Campbell, Ste. R
Springfield, MO 65807
**Phone:** (417)881-4668          **Fax:** (417)881-7955

★ 11018 ★ American Cancer Society
**Trenton Office**
406 E 9th St.
Trenton, MO 64683
**Phone:** (660)359-4484          **Fax:** (660)359-2115

### Montana

★ 11019 ★ American Cancer Society
**Billings Office**
550 N 31st St., Ste. 103
Billings, MT 59101
**Phone:** (406)256-7150          **Free:** 800-252-5470
**Fax:** (406)256-7170

★ 11020 ★ American Cancer Society
**Missoula Office**
3550 Mullan Rd., Ste. 105
Missoula, MT 59808
**Phone:** (406)542-2191          **Fax:** (406)327-0146

### Nebraska

★ 11021 ★ American Cancer Society
**Kearney Office**
3710 Central Ave.
Kearney, NE 68847
**Phone:** (308)237-7481          **Fax:** (308)236-2016

★ 11022 ★ American Cancer Society
**Lincoln Office**
5733 S 34th St., Ste. 500
Lincoln, NE 68516
**Phone:** (402)423-4888          **Free:** 877-232-4787
**Fax:** (402)423-4915

★ 11023 ★ American Cancer Society
**Omaha Office**
9850 Nicholas St., Ste. 200
Omaha, NE 68114
**Phone:** (402)393-5800          **Fax:** (402)393-7790

### Nevada

★ 11024 ★ American Cancer Society
**Greater Las Vegas Regional Office**
1325 E Harmon Ave.
Las Vegas, NV 89119
**Phone:** (702)798-6877          **Free:** 800-ACS-2345
**Fax:** (702)798-0530

★ 11025 ★ American Cancer Society
**Northern Nevada Regional Office**
6490 S McCarran Blvd., Ste. 40
Reno, NV 89509
**Phone:** (775)329-0609          **Fax:** (775)329-8592

### New Hampshire

★ 11026 ★ American Cancer Society
**Midcoastal New England Regional Office**
**Bedford Office**
Gail Singer Memorial Bldg.
360 State Rte. 101, Unit 8
Bedford, NH 03110
**Phone:** (603)472-8899          **Free:** 800-640-7101
**Fax:** (603)472-7093
**Website:** http://www.ne-cancer.org

### New Jersey

★ 11027 ★ American Cancer Society
**Central New Jersey Region**
**Fords Office**
846 Main St.
Fords, NJ 08863
**Phone:** (732)738-6800          **Fax:** (732)738-8984

★ 11028 ★ American Cancer Society
**Central New Jersey Region**
**Lawrenceville Office**
3076 Princeton Pike
Lawrenceville, NJ 08648
**Phone:** (609)895-0101          **Fax:** (609)895-0944

★ 11029 ★ American Cancer Society
**Jersey Shore Region**
**Shrewsbury Office**
801 Broad St.
Shrewsbury, NJ 07702
**Phone:** (732)758-8220          **Fax:** (732)758-8225

★ 11030 ★ American Cancer Society
**Jersey Shore Region**
**Toms River Office**
1035 Hooper Ave.
Toms River, NJ 08753
**Phone:** (732)914-1000          **Fax:** (732)914-1004

★ 11031 ★ American Cancer Society
**Metro New Jersey Region**
**Elizabeth Office**
507 Westminster Ave.
Elizabeth, NJ 07208
**Phone:** (908)354-7373          **Fax:** (908)354-0284

★ 11032 ★ **American Cancer Society**
**Metro New Jersey Region**
**Secaucus Office**
150 Meadowlands Pkwy.
Secaucus, NJ 07094
**Phone:** (201)866-1020 **Fax:** (201)866-2401

★ 11033 ★ **American Cancer Society**
**Metro New Jersey Region**
**West Orange Office**
767 Northfield Ave.
West Orange, NJ 07052
**Phone:** (973)736-7770 **Fax:** (973)669-5817

★ 11034 ★ **American Cancer Society**
**New Jersey Chinese Unit**
**Fords Office**
846 Main St.
Fords, NJ 08863
**Phone:** (732)225-8588 **Fax:** (732)225-8589

★ 11035 ★ **American Cancer Society**
**New Jersey Chinese Unit**
**Parsippany Office**
669 Littleton Rd.
Parsippany, NJ 07054
**Phone:** (973)334-2249 **Fax:** (973)331-5944

★ 11036 ★ **American Cancer Society**
**New Jersey Chinese Unit**
**Shrewsbury Office**
801 Broad St.
Shrewsbury, NJ 07702
**Phone:** (732)224-8868 **Fax:** (732)224-8821

★ 11037 ★ **American Cancer Society**
**Northern New Jersey Region**
**Hackensack Office**
20 Mercer St.
Hackensack, NJ 07601
**Phone:** (201)343-2222 **Fax:** (201)343-1839

★ 11038 ★ **American Cancer Society**
**Northern New Jersey Region**
**Wayne Office**
468 Parish Dr., No. 6
Wayne, NJ 07470
**Phone:** (973)696-1885 **Fax:** (973)696-1916

★ 11039 ★ **American Cancer Society**
**Northwest New Jersey Region**
**Flemington Office**
84 Park Ave.
Flemington, NJ 08822
**Phone:** (908)782-6112 **Fax:** (908)782-3995

★ 11040 ★ **American Cancer Society**
**Northwest New Jersey Region**
**Oxford Office**
4 Opdyke's Ln.
Oxford, NJ 07863
**Phone:** (908)453-2103 **Fax:** (908)453-3724

★ 11041 ★ **American Cancer Society**
**Northwest New Jersey Region**
**Parsippany Office**
669 Littleton Rd.
Parsippany, NJ 07054
**Phone:** (973)331-9300 **Fax:** (973)331-9444

★ 11042 ★ **American Cancer Society**
**Northwest New Jersey Region**
**Raritan Office**
600 1st Ave.
Raritan, NJ 08869
**Phone:** (908)725-4664 **Fax:** (908)707-1858

★ 11043 ★ **American Cancer Society**
**South Jersey Region**
**Absecon Office**
626 N Shore Rd.
Absecon, NJ 08201
**Phone:** (609)645-7272 **Fax:** (609)641-9469

★ 11044 ★ **American Cancer Society**
**South Jersey Region**
**Cape May Court House Office**
Burdette Tomlin Memorial Hospital
2 Stone Harbor Blvd.
Cape May Court House, NJ 08210
**Phone:** (609)465-9587

★ 11045 ★ **American Cancer Society**
**South Jersey Region**
**Cherry Hill Office**
1851 Old Cuthbert Rd.
Cherry Hill, NJ 08034
**Phone:** (856)616-1650 **Fax:** (856)616-8449

★ 11046 ★ **American Cancer Society**
**South Jersey Region**
**Vineland Office**
1400 W Landis Ave.
Vineland, NJ 08360
**Phone:** (856)692-1364 **Fax:** (856)691-9130

## New Mexico

★ 11047 ★ **American Cancer Society**
**Albuquerque Regional Office**
5800 Lomas Blvd. NE
Albuquerque, NM 87110-6539
**Phone:** (505)260-2105 **Free:** 800-ACS-2345
**Fax:** (505)266-9513
**Website:** http://www2.cancer.org/state/nm/index.html

★ 11048 ★ **American Cancer Society**
**Clovis Office**
PO Box 1856
Clovis, NM 88101
**Phone:** (505)762-5112 **Fax:** (505)742-1710

★ 11049 ★ **American Cancer Society**
**Northern New Mexico Regional Office**
531 Harkle Rd., Ste. B
Santa Fe, NM 87505
**Phone:** (505)988-5548 **Fax:** (505)986-1940

## New York

★ 11050 ★ **American Cancer Society**
**Brooklyn Regional Office**
148 Pierrepont St.
Brooklyn, NY 11201
**Phone:** (718)237-7850 **Fax:** (718)852-9422

★ 11051 ★ **American Cancer Society**
**Capital New York Region**
**Loudonville Office**
260 Osborne Rd.
Loudonville, NY 12211
**Phone:** (518)438-7841 **Fax:** (518)438-9608

★ 11052 ★ **American Cancer Society**
**Capital New York Region**
**Queensbury Office**
Mt. Royal Plaza
959 State Rte. 9
Queensbury, NY 12804
**Phone:** (518)792-5358 **Fax:** (518)792-9204

★ 11053 ★ **American Cancer Society**
**Central New York Region**
**East Syracuse Office**
6725 Lyons St.
PO Box 7
East Syracuse, NY 13057
**Phone:** (315)437-7025 **Fax:** (315)437-8233
**Website:** http://www2.cancer.org/states/index.cfm?id=35

★ 11054 ★ **American Cancer Society**
**Central New York Region**
**Malone Office**
94 E Main St.
Malone, NY 12953
**Phone:** (518)483-3636 **Fax:** (518)483-3906

★ 11055 ★ **American Cancer Society**
**Central New York Region**
**Utica Office**
430 Court St., Ste. 205
Utica, NY 13502
**Phone:** (315)724-8125 **Fax:** (315)738-0517

★ 11056 ★ **American Cancer Society**
**Hudson Valley Region**
**Kingston Office**
95 Schwenk Dr.
Kingston, NY 12401
**Phone:** (845)331-8300 **Fax:** (845)331-4109

★ 11057 ★ **American Cancer Society**
**Hudson Valley Region**
**Middletown Office**
Wisner Professional Bldg.
419 E Main St.
Middletown, NY 10940
**Phone:** (845)343-5612 **Fax:** (845)343-8023

★ 11058 ★ **American Cancer Society**
**Hudson Valley Region**
**Poughkeepsie Office**
Vassar Brother's Hospital
45 Reade Pl.
Poughkeepsie, NY 12601
**Phone:** (845)452-2635 **Fax:** (845)452-8067

★ 11059 ★ **American Cancer Society**
**Hudson Valley Region**
**Suffern Office**
1 Executive Blvd., No. 206
Suffern, NY 10901
**Phone:** (845)368-1251 **Fax:** (845)368-1255

★ 11060 ★ **American Cancer Society**
**Lakes Region Office**
1400 Winton Rd. N
Rochester, NY 14609
**Phone:** (585)288-1950 **Fax:** (585)288-6467

★ 11061 ★ **American Cancer Society**
**Manhattan/Bronx Regional Office**
271 W 125th St., Ste. 210
New York, NY 10027
**Phone:** (212)663-8800 **Fax:** (212)663-8835

★ 11062 ★ **American Cancer Society**
**Manhattan/Bronx Regional Office**
19 W 56th St.
New York, NY 10019
**Phone:** (212)586-8700 **Fax:** (212)237-3855

★ 11063 ★ **American Cancer Society**
**Nassau Regional Office**
839 Stewart Ave.
Garden City, NY 11530

**Phone:** (516)229-4100        **Fax:** (516)229-4110

**★ 11064 ★ American Cancer Society**
**New York Chinese Unit**
**Flushing Office**
41-60 Main St., No. 206
Flushing, NY 11355
**Phone:** (718)886-8890        **Fax:** (718)886-8981

**★ 11065 ★ American Cancer Society**
**Queens Regional Office**
97-77 Queens Blvd., Ste. 1110
Rego Park, NY 11374
**Phone:** (718)263-2224        **Fax:** (718)261-0758

**★ 11066 ★ American Cancer Society**
**Southern New York Region**
**Elmira Office**
627 W Church St.
Elmira, NY 14905
**Phone:** (607)734-1552        **Fax:** (607)734-2435

**★ 11067 ★ American Cancer Society**
**Southern New York Region**
**Endicott Office**
31 Adams Ave.
Endicott, NY 13760
**Phone:** (607)786-7736        **Fax:** (607)785-6087

**★ 11068 ★ American Cancer Society**
**Southern New York Region**
**Sidney Office**
5 Oak Ave.
Sidney, NY 13838
**Phone:** (607)563-8462        **Fax:** (607)563-9044

**★ 11069 ★ American Cancer Society**
**Staten Island Regional Office**
58 New Dorp Plaza
Staten Island, NY 10306
**Phone:** (718)987-8871        **Fax:** (718)351-0361

**★ 11070 ★ American Cancer Society**
**Suffolk Regional Office**
20 Hampton Rd.
Southampton, NY 11968
**Phone:** (631)287-6277

**★ 11071 ★ American Cancer Society**
**Suffolk Regional Office**
75 Davids Dr.
Hauppauge, NY 11788
**Phone:** (631)436-7070        **Free:** 800-ACS-2345
**Fax:** (631)436-5380

**★ 11072 ★ American Cancer Society**
**Westchester Regional Office**
2 Lyon Pl.
White Plains, NY 10601
**Phone:** (914)949-4800        **Fax:** (914)949-8851

**★ 11073 ★ American Cancer Society**
**Western New York Region**
**Amherst Office**
101 John James Audubon Pkwy.
Amherst, NY 14228
**Phone:** (716)689-6981        **Fax:** (716)689-4923

**★ 11074 ★ American Cancer Society**
**Western New York Region**
**Buffalo Office**
1490 Jefferson Ave.
Buffalo, NY 14208
**Phone:** (716)882-6428        **Fax:** (716)885-4956

**★ 11075 ★ American Cancer Society**
**Western New York Region**
**Jamestown Office**
113 E 2nd St.
Jamestown, NY 14701
**Phone:** (716)487-1129        **Fax:** (716)661-3381

### North Carolina

**★ 11076 ★ American Cancer Society**
**Asheville Administrative Resource Center**
120 Executive Park, Bldg. 1
Asheville, NC 28801
**Phone:** 800-282-4914        **Fax:** (828)252-8890

**★ 11077 ★ American Cancer Society**
**Greenville Administrative Resource**
**Center**
930-B Wellness Dr.
Greenville, NC 27834
**Phone:** 800-282-4914        **Fax:** (252)695-0671

**★ 11078 ★ American Cancer Society**
**Hope Lodge Office**
930-A Wellness Dr.
Greenville, NC 27834
**Phone:** (252)816-4994        **Fax:** (252)695-6557

**★ 11079 ★ American Cancer Society**
**Metrolina Administrative Resource Center**
500 E Morehead St., Ste. 211
Charlotte, NC 28202
**Phone:** 800-282-4914        **Fax:** (704)376-0516

**★ 11080 ★ American Cancer Society**
**Raleigh Administrative Resource Center**
11 S Boylan Ave., Ste. 221
Raleigh, NC 27603
**Phone:** (919)834-8463        **Free:** 800-282-4914
**Fax:** (919)839-0551

**★ 11081 ★ American Cancer Society**
**Triad Administrative Resource Center**
4-A Oak Branch Dr.
Greensboro, NC 27407
**Phone:** 800-282-4914        **Fax:** (336)834-8777

**★ 11082 ★ American Cancer Society**
**Wilmington Administrative Resource**
**Center**
3131 Wrightsville Ave.
Wilmington, NC 28403
**Phone:** 800-282-4914        **Fax:** (910)763-1936

### North Dakota

**★ 11083 ★ American Cancer Society**
**Bismarck Office**
1102 S Washington St., Ste. 105
Bismarck, ND 58504
**Phone:** (701)224-9954        **Fax:** (701)250-9145

**★ 11084 ★ American Cancer Society**
**Fargo Office**
121 Roberts St.
Fargo, ND 58102
**Phone:** (701)232-1385        **Free:** 800-342-4535
**Fax:** (701)232-1109
**Website:** http://www.cancer.org/nd.html

**★ 11085 ★ American Cancer Society**
**Grand Forks Office**
1832 S Washington St.
Grand Forks, ND 58201
**Phone:** (701)792-3333        **Fax:** (701)792-3334

**★ 11086 ★ American Cancer Society**
**Minot Office**
600 22nd Ave. NW
Minot, ND 58701
**Phone:** (701)838-5550        **Fax:** (701)838-4710

### Ohio

**★ 11087 ★ American Cancer Society**
**Allen Area Office**
616 S Collett St.
Lima, OH 45805
**Phone:** (419)225-8860        **Free:** 888-227-6446
**Fax:** (419)225-8862
**Website:** http://www.oh.cancer.org

**★ 11088 ★ American Cancer Society**
**Clark/Miami Area Office**
1130 Vester Ave.
Springfield, OH 45503
**Phone:** (937)399-0809        **Free:** 888-227-6446
**Fax:** (937)399-2060
**Website:** http://www.oh.cancer.org

**★ 11089 ★ American Cancer Society**
**Cuyahoga County Office**
10501 Euclid Ave.
Cleveland, OH 44106
**Phone:** (216)241-1177        **Free:** 888-227-6446
**Fax:** (216)241-0334
**Website:** http://www.oh.cancer.org

**★ 11090 ★ American Cancer Society**
**Defiance Area Office**
419 5th St., Ste. 2030
Defiance, OH 43512
**Phone:** (419)782-6866        **Free:** 888-227-6446
**Fax:** (419)782-4372
**Website:** http://www.oh.cancer.org

**★ 11091 ★ American Cancer Society**
**Fairfield Area Office**
151 Lake St.
Lancaster, OH 43130
**Phone:** (740)653-5632        **Free:** 888-227-6446
**Fax:** (740)653-5677
**Website:** http://www.oh.cancer.org

**★ 11092 ★ American Cancer Society**
**Franklin County Office**
870 Michigan Ave.
Columbus, OH 43215
**Phone:** (614)228-8466        **Free:** 888-227-6446
**Fax:** (614)228-4456
**Website:** http://www.oh.cancer.org

**★ 11093 ★ American Cancer Society**
**Geauga Area Office**
7861 Crile Rd.
Concord, OH 44077
**Phone:** (440)358-0864        **Free:** 888-227-6446
**Fax:** (440)358-9073
**Website:** http://www.oh.cancer.org

**★ 11094 ★ American Cancer Society**
**Hamilton County Office**
11117 Kenwood Rd.
Cincinnati, OH 45242
**Phone:** (513)891-1600        **Free:** 888-227-6446
**Fax:** (513)891-5583
**Website:** http://www.oh.cancer.org

**★ 11095 ★ American Cancer Society**
**Hancock Office**
110 S Main St.
Findlay, OH 45840
**Phone:** (419)423-0456        **Free:** 888-227-6446
**Fax:** (419)423-1120

Website: http://www.oh.cancer.org


**★ 11096 ★ American Cancer Society**
**Lorain Area Office**
43099 N Ridge Rd.
Elyria, OH 44035
Phone: (440)324-2211　　　Free: 888-227-6446
Fax: (440)324-4217
Website: http://www.oh.cancer.org


**★ 11097 ★ American Cancer Society**
**Lucas County Office**
135 Chesterfield Dr., No. 100
Maumee, OH 43537
Phone: (419)891-9200　　　Free: 888-227-6446
Fax: (419)891-9223
Website: http://www.oh.cancer.org


**★ 11098 ★ American Cancer Society**
**Mahoning County Office**
525 N Broad St.
Canfield, OH 44406
Phone: (330)533-0546　　　Free: 888-227-6446
Fax: (330)533-1678
Website: http://www.oh.cancer.org


**★ 11099 ★ American Cancer Society**
**Marion Area Office**
253 E Church St.
Marion, OH 43302
Phone: (740)387-3202　　　Free: 888-227-6446
Fax: (740)383-2988
Website: http://www.oh.cancer.org


**★ 11100 ★ American Cancer Society**
**Mercer Area Office**
105 S Walnut St.
Celina, OH 45822
Phone: 888-227-6446　　　Fax: (419)486-3490


**★ 11101 ★ American Cancer Society**
**Montgomery Area Office**
40 S Perry St., Ste. 120
Dayton, OH 45402
Phone: 888-227-6446　　　Fax: (937)223-5435


**★ 11102 ★ American Cancer Society**
**Montgomery Area Office**
40 S Perry St., Ste. 120
Dayton, OH 45402
Phone: (937)223-8521　　　Free: 888-227-6446
Fax: (937)223-5435
Website: http://www.oh.cancer.org


**★ 11103 ★ American Cancer Society**
**Muskingum Area Office**
3612 Maple Ave.
Zanesville, OH 43702
Phone: (740)454-2589　　　Free: 888-227-6446
Fax: (740)374-5168
Website: http://www.oh.cancer.org


**★ 11104 ★ American Cancer Society**
**Pickaway Area Office**
469 E Ohio St.
PO Box 67
Circleville, OH 43113
Phone: 888-227-6446　　　Fax: (740)474-6078


**★ 11105 ★ American Cancer Society**
**Ross Area Office**
138 Marietta Rd., Ste. D
Chillicothe, OH 45601
Phone: (740)702-1160　　　Free: 888-227-6446
Fax: (740)702-1163
Website: http://www.oh.cancer.org


**★ 11106 ★ American Cancer Society**
**Southwest Ohio Area Office**
5378-A Cox Smith Rd.
Mason, OH 45040
Phone: 888-227-6446　　　Fax: (513)229-4994


**★ 11107 ★ American Cancer Society**
**Stark Area Office**
925 S Main St.
North Canton, OH 44720
Phone: (330)497-7100　　　Free: 888-227-6446
Fax: (330)966-0436
Website: http://www.oh.cancer.org


**★ 11108 ★ American Cancer Society**
**Summit Area Office**
1900 W Market St.
Akron, OH 44313
Phone: (330)865-1200　　　Free: 888-227-6446
Fax: (330)865-1205
Website: http://www.cancer.org
Kathy Singer, Exec Director


**★ 11109 ★ American Cancer Society**
**Trumbull Area Office**
525 N Broad, Rte. 46
Canfield, OH 44406
Phone: 888-227-6446　　　Fax: (330)533-1678


**★ 11110 ★ American Cancer Society**
**Tuscarawas Area Office**
201A W Ohio Ave.
Dover, OH 44622
Phone: 888-227-6446　　　Fax: (330)602-5062


**★ 11111 ★ American Cancer Society**
**Washington Area Office**
215 Marion St.
Marietta, OH 45750
Phone: (740)374-5464　　　Free: 888-227-6446
Fax: (740)374-5464
Website: http://www.oh.cancer.org


**★ 11112 ★ American Cancer Society**
**Wood Area Office**
1045 N Main St., Ste. 8
Bowling Green, OH 43402
Phone: (419)353-5645　　　Free: 888-227-6446
Fax: (419)352-8041
Website: http://www.oh.cancer.org


## Oklahoma


**★ 11113 ★ American Cancer Society**
**Lawton Office**
1305 W Gore Blvd., Ste. A
Lawton, OK 73501
Phone: (580)353-8145　　　Fax: (580)353-8146
Website: http://www.cancer.org/state/heartland/


**★ 11114 ★ American Cancer Society**
**Norman Office**
2420 Springer Dr., Ste. 205
Norman, OK 73069
Phone: (405)329-1332　　　Free: 888-320-3757
Fax: (405)329-1334
Email: amcgrew@cancer.org
Website: http://www.cancer.org/state/heartland/


**★ 11115 ★ American Cancer Society**
**Oklahoma City Office**
8400 Silver Crossing, Ste. H
Oklahoma City, OK 73132
Phone: (405)843-9888　　　Free: 800-733-9888
Fax: (405)848-0795
Website: http://www.cancer.org/state/heartland/


**★ 11116 ★ American Cancer Society**
**Tulsa Office**
5110 S Yale, Ste. 101
Tulsa, OK 74135
Phone: (918)743-6767　　　Free: 888-376-1725
Fax: (918)743-9655
Website: http://www.cancer.org/state/heartland


## Oregon


**★ 11117 ★ American Cancer Society**
**Eugene Office**
2350 Oakmont Way, Ste. 200
Eugene, OR 97401
Phone: (541)484-2211　　　Fax: (541)687-9624


**★ 11118 ★ American Cancer Society**
**Medford Office**
31 W 6th
Medford, OR 97501
Phone: (541)779-6091　　　Fax: (541)779-1470


**★ 11119 ★ American Cancer Society,**
**Northwest Division**
**Portland Office**
0330 SW Curry St.
Portland, OR 97201
Phone: (503)295-6422　　　Free: 800-577-6552
Fax: (503)228-1062


## Pennsylvania


**★ 11120 ★ American Cancer Society**
**Adams Office**
424 E Middle St.
Gettysburg, PA 17325
Phone: (717)334-5352　　　Fax: (717)334-3974


**★ 11121 ★ American Cancer Society**
**Bedford Office**
322 S Juliana St., Ste. 8
Bedford, PA 15522
Phone: (814)623-8819　　　Fax: (814)623-6518


**★ 11122 ★ American Cancer Society**
**Berks Office**
498 Bellevue Ave.
Reading, PA 19605
Phone: (610)921-2328　　　Fax: (610)921-9521


**★ 11123 ★ American Cancer Society**
**Blair Office**
1004 N Juniata St.
Hollidaysburg, PA 16648
Phone: (814)695-9511　　　Fax: (814)695-8986


**★ 11124 ★ American Cancer Society**
**Bux-Mont Office**
High Point Professional Bldg.
700 Horizon Cir., Ste. 201
Chalfont, PA 18914
Phone: (215)712-3290　　　Fax: (215)712-3298


**★ 11125 ★ American Cancer Society**
**Cambria Office**
351 Budfield St.
Johnstown, PA 15904
Phone: (814)266-8744　　　Fax: (814)266-7754


**★ 11126 ★ American Cancer Society**
**Cameron Office**
135 W 4th St.
Emporium, PA 15834
Phone: (814)486-0911　　　Fax: (814)486-0825

★ 11127 ★ **American Cancer Society**
**Capital Regional Office**
3211 N Front St., Ste. 100
Harrisburg, PA 17110
**Phone:** (717)231-5780        **Fax:** (717)231-5784

★ 11128 ★ **American Cancer Society**
**Carbon-Tamaqua Office**
33 W Ridge St.
Lansford, PA 18232
**Phone:** (610)921-2328        **Fax:** (570)645-8845

★ 11129 ★ **American Cancer Society**
**Centre Office**
123 S Sparks St.
State College, PA 16801
**Phone:** (814)238-8908        **Fax:** (814)238-3236

★ 11130 ★ **American Cancer Society**
**Chester County Office**
428 Exton Commons
Exton, PA 19341
**Phone:** (610)363-6720

★ 11131 ★ **American Cancer Society**
**Clarion Office**
133B W Main St.
PO Box 408
Clarion, PA 16214
**Phone:** (814)226-7261        **Fax:** (814)226-8352

★ 11132 ★ **American Cancer Society**
**Clearfield Office**
119 E Market St.
Clearfield, PA 16830
**Phone:** (814)765-6988        **Fax:** (814)765-6744

★ 11133 ★ **American Cancer Society**
**Corry Area Office**
2 S Center St.
PO Box 103
Corry, PA 16407
**Phone:** (814)665-1691        **Fax:** (814)664-3851

★ 11134 ★ **American Cancer Society**
**Crawford Office**
464 Pine St.
Meadville, PA 16335
**Phone:** (814)337-8300        **Fax:** (814)337-8303

★ 11135 ★ **American Cancer Society**
**Delaware County Office**
600 N Jackson St., 2nd Fl.
Media, PA 19063
**Phone:** (610)565-1009        **Fax:** (610)892-9438

★ 11136 ★ **American Cancer Society**
**DuBois Gateway Area Office**
993 Beaver Dr.
Du Bois, PA 15801
**Phone:** (814)375-3548        **Fax:** (814)375-4430

★ 11137 ★ **American Cancer Society**
**Elk Office**
117 N Michael St.
Saint Marys, PA 15857
**Phone:** (814)834-9796        **Fax:** (814)834-7149

★ 11138 ★ **American Cancer Society**
**Erie Office**
2115 W 38th St.
Erie, PA 16508
**Phone:** (814)866-5077        **Fax:** (814)866-3890

★ 11139 ★ **American Cancer Society**
**Franklin Office**
452 E King St.
Chambersburg, PA 17201
**Phone:** (717)264-4412        **Fax:** (717)264-0765

★ 11140 ★ **American Cancer Society**
**Fulton Office**
452 E King St.
Chambersburg, PA 17201
**Phone:** (717)264-4412        **Fax:** (717)264-0765

★ 11141 ★ **American Cancer Society**
**Hanover Office**
1 Center Sq., Ste. 4
Hanover, PA 17331
**Phone:** (717)632-4918

★ 11142 ★ **American Cancer Society**
**Huntingdon Office**
RD 1, Box 33D
Huntingdon, PA 16652
**Phone:** (814)627-0083        **Fax:** (814)627-0089

★ 11143 ★ **American Cancer Society**
**Jefferson Office**
103 N Gilpin St.
Punxsutawney, PA 15767
**Phone:** (814)938-6460        **Fax:** (814)938-9437

★ 11144 ★ **American Cancer Society**
**Lancaster Office**
314 Good Dr.
Lancaster, PA 17603
**Phone:** (717)397-3744        **Fax:** (717)397-1526

★ 11145 ★ **American Cancer Society**
**Lebanon Office**
701 Cumberland St.
Lebanon, PA 17042
**Phone:** (717)273-4582        **Fax:** (717)273-3891

★ 11146 ★ **American Cancer Society**
**Lehigh Valley Office**
2121 City Line Rd.
Bethlehem, PA 18017
**Phone:** (610)921-2328        **Fax:** (610)882-5861

★ 11147 ★ **American Cancer Society**
**McKean Office**
121 Main St.
Bradford, PA 16701
**Phone:** (814)368-6183        **Fax:** (814)368-1174

★ 11148 ★ **American Cancer Society**
**Mercer Office**
19 Jefferson Ave.
Sharon, PA 16146
**Phone:** (724)346-3529        **Fax:** (724)346-1896

★ 11149 ★ **American Cancer Society**
**Mifflin-Juniata Office**
26 N Brown St.
Lewistown, PA 17044
**Phone:** (717)248-1421        **Fax:** (717)248-8015

★ 11150 ★ **American Cancer Society**
**North Central Regional Office**
1948 E 3rd St.
Williamsport, PA 17701
**Phone:** (570)326-4149        **Fax:** (570)326-7767

★ 11151 ★ **American Cancer Society**
**Northeast Region**
**Greater Hazleton Unit**
St. Gabriel House
132 S Wyoming St.
Hazleton, PA 18201
**Phone:** (570)459-1212        **Fax:** (570)454-2544

★ 11152 ★ **American Cancer Society**
**Northeast Region**
**Monroe Unit**
Business 209
RR 2, Box 2138
Stroudsburg, PA 18360
**Phone:** (570)421-7010        **Fax:** (570)421-8891

★ 11153 ★ **American Cancer Society**
**Northeast Region**
**Susquehanna/Wyoming Unit**
PO Box 4
Montrose, PA 18801
**Phone:** (570)278-1694        **Fax:** (570)278-2021

★ 11154 ★ **American Cancer Society**
**Northeast Region**
**Wayne Unit**
627 Main St., Lower Level
Honesdale, PA 18431
**Phone:** (570)253-3350        **Fax:** (570)253-9426

★ 11155 ★ **American Cancer Society**
**Northeast Region**
**Wyoming Valley Unit**
71 N Franklin St., Rm. 110
Wilkes Barre, PA 18701
**Phone:** (570)825-7763        **Fax:** (570)822-8673

★ 11156 ★ **American Cancer Society**
**Northeast Region Office**
**Lackawanna Office**
1101 Hill St.
Jessup, PA 18434
**Phone:** (570)383-4700        **Fax:** (570)383-4707

★ 11157 ★ **American Cancer Society**
**Northeast Regional Office**
**Jessup Unit**
1101 Hill St.
Jessup, PA 18434
**Phone:** (570)383-4700        **Fax:** (570)383-4707

★ 11158 ★ **American Cancer Society**
**Northeast Regional Office**
**Pike Unit**
110 W Harford St.
Milford, PA 18337
**Phone:** (570)296-7676

★ 11159 ★ **American Cancer Society**
**Potter Office**
538 E 2nd St., Rm. 1
Coudersport, PA 16915
**Phone:** (814)274-8330        **Fax:** (814)274-7724

★ 11160 ★ **American Cancer Society**
**Schuylkill Office**
512 N Centre St., Ste. 1-B
Pottsville, PA 17901
**Phone:** (610)921-2328        **Fax:** (570)622-8549

★ 11161 ★ **American Cancer Society**
**Somerset Office**
168 W Union St.
Somerset, PA 15501
**Phone:** (814)445-2584        **Fax:** (814)443-9585

**★ 11162 ★ American Cancer Society**
**Southeast Philadelphia Regional Office**
1626 Locust St.
Philadelphia, PA 19103
**Phone:** (215)985-5400          **Free:** 800-ACS-2345
**Fax:** (215)985-5406

**★ 11163 ★ American Cancer Society**
**Southwest Region**
**Beaver Unit**
320 Bilmar Dr.
Pittsburgh, PA 15205
**Phone:** (412)919-1100          **Free:** 888-227-5445
**Fax:** (412)919-1101

**★ 11164 ★ American Cancer Society**
**Southwest Regional Office**
320 Bilmar Dr.
Pittsburgh, PA 15205
**Phone:** (412)919-1100          **Fax:** (412)919-1101

**★ 11165 ★ American Cancer Society**
**Venango-Forest Office**
10 W Front St.
Oil City, PA 16301
**Phone:** (814)677-3077          **Fax:** (814)676-1995

**★ 11166 ★ American Cancer Society**
**Warren Office**
2 S State St.
North Warren, PA 16365
**Phone:** (814)723-5780          **Fax:** (814)723-0135

**★ 11167 ★ American Cancer Society**
**York Office**
924 N Colonial Ave.
York, PA 17403
**Phone:** (717)848-1841          **Fax:** (717)852-0919

### Puerto Rico

**★ 11168 ★ American Cancer Society**
**Puerto Rico Division**
**Arecibo Office**
**(Sociedad Americana del Cancer de**
**Puerto Rico, Inc.)**
URB Radioville
Calle No. 2, Casa No. 4
Arecibo, PR 00612
**Phone:** (787)879-0656          **Free:** 800-ACS-2345
**Fax:** (787)879-0656
**Email:** diananunzpr/acs/us@cancer.org
**Website:** http://www.cancer.org

**★ 11169 ★ American Cancer Society**
**Puerto Rico Division**
**Caguas Office**
**(Sociedad Americana del Cancer de**
**Puerto Rico, Inc.)**
San Juan Bautista Medical Ctr.
Primer Piso Carr. 172
Caguas, PR 00725
**Phone:** (787)743-4040          **Fax:** (787)744-4336
**Website:** http://www@cancer.org

**★ 11170 ★ American Cancer Society**
**Puerto Rico Division**
**Mayaguez Office**
**(Sociedad Americana del Cancer de**
**Puerto Rico, Inc.)**
Calle Prolongacion Vadi 203
Mayaguez, PR 00680
**Phone:** (787)833-3320          **Fax:** (787)833-3320

**★ 11171 ★ American Cancer Society**
**Puerto Rico Division**
**Ponce Office**
**(Sociedad Americana del Cancer de**
**Puerto Rico, Inc.)**
716 Calle Ferrocarril
Ponce, PR 00717
**Phone:** (787)844-1037          **Fax:** (787)844-1037

### Rhode Island

**★ 11172 ★ American Cancer Society**
**Rhode Island Division**
**East Bay Unit**
400 Main St.
Pawtucket, RI 02860-2996
**Phone:** (401)722-8480          **Free:** 800-364-5520
**Fax:** (401)727-9449
**Website:** http://www.ne-cancer.org

**★ 11173 ★ American Cancer Society**
**Rhode Island & Eastern Connecticut**
**Division**
**Providence Office**
222 Richmond St., Ste. 200
Providence, RI 02903
**Phone:** (401)722-8480          **Fax:** (401)421-0535

### South Carolina

**★ 11174 ★ American Cancer Society**
**Aiken Office**
115 Greenville St.
Aiken, SC 29801
**Phone:** 800-282-4914          **Fax:** (803)648-5094

**★ 11175 ★ American Cancer Society**
**Central Midlands Office**
Westpark Plaza
128 Stonemark Ln.
Columbia, SC 29210
**Phone:** (803)750-1693          **Free:** 800-282-4914
**Fax:** (803)750-4000
**Website:** http://www.cancer.org/state/sc/

**★ 11176 ★ American Cancer Society**
**Charleston Office**
5900 Core St., Ste. 504
North Charleston, SC 29406
**Phone:** 800-282-4914          **Fax:** (843)747-2761

**★ 11177 ★ American Cancer Society**
**Greenville Office**
154 Milestone Way
Greenville, SC 29615
**Phone:** 800-282-4914          **Fax:** (864)458-8454

**★ 11178 ★ American Cancer Society**
**Greenwood Office**
Hampton & Merriman
3 Village Square
Greenwood, SC 29648
**Phone:** 800-282-4914          **Fax:** (864)229-7653

**★ 11179 ★ American Cancer Society**
**Hilton Head Office**
15 Palmetto Business Park
Palmetto Bay Rd.
Hilton Head Island, SC 29928
**Phone:** 800-282-4914          **Fax:** (843)842-9898

**★ 11180 ★ American Cancer Society**
**Myrtle Beach Office**
950-48th Ave. N
Myrtle Beach, SC 29577
**Phone:** 800-282-4914          **Fax:** (843)213-0055

### South Dakota

**★ 11181 ★ American Cancer Society**
**Aberdeen Office**
310 NW 8th Ave., Ste. 407
Aberdeen, SD 57401
**Phone:** (605)229-5906          **Fax:** (605)229-1019

**★ 11182 ★ American Cancer Society**
**Mitchell Office**
209 E 4th
Mitchell, SD 57301
**Phone:** (605)996-0121          **Fax:** (605)996-0204

**★ 11183 ★ American Cancer Society**
**Pierre Office**
221 S Central Ave.
Pierre, SD 57501
**Phone:** (605)224-7836          **Fax:** (605)224-7847

**★ 11184 ★ American Cancer Society**
**Rapid City Office**
2465 W Chicago St.
Rapid City, SD 57702
**Phone:** (605)342-7740          **Fax:** (605)399-2062

**★ 11185 ★ American Cancer Society**
**Sioux Falls Office**
4101 S Carnegie Pl.
Sioux Falls, SD 57106
**Phone:** (605)361-8277          **Free:** 800-660-7703
**Fax:** (605)361-8537
**Website:** http://www2.cancer.org/state/mw/

**★ 11186 ★ American Cancer Society**
**Watertown Office**
525 5th St. SE, Ste. 4
Watertown, SD 57201
**Phone:** (605)882-2957          **Fax:** (605)882-1701

### Tennessee

**★ 11187 ★ American Cancer Society**
**Chattanooga Office**
850 Fort Wood St.
Chattanooga, TN 37403
**Phone:** (423)267-8613          **Fax:** (423)266-8494
**Website:** http://www2.cancer.org/state/tn/

**★ 11188 ★ American Cancer Society**
**Jackson Office**
2935 U.S. Hwy. 45 Bypass
Jackson, TN 38305
**Phone:** (731)664-4663          **Fax:** (731)664-7858

**★ 11189 ★ American Cancer Society**
**Johnson City Office**
508 Princeton Rd., Ste. 102
Johnson City, TN 37601
**Phone:** (423)926-2921          **Free:** 800-ACS-2345
**Fax:** (423)283-7112
**Email:** strivett@cancer.org
**Website:** http://www2.cancer.org/state/tn/

**★ 11190 ★ American Cancer Society**
**Knoxville Office**
871 Weisgarber Rd.
Knoxville, TN 37909
**Phone:** (865)584-1668          **Fax:** (865)584-1673
**Website:** http://www2.cancer.org/state/tn/

**★ 11191 ★ American Cancer Society**
**Memphis Office**
1378 Union Ave.
Memphis, TN 38104
**Phone:** (901)278-2000          **Free:** 800-227-2345
**Fax:** (901)278-2020

**★ 11192 ★ American Cancer Society**
**Nashville Office**
2000 Charlotte Ave.
Nashville, TN 37203
**Phone:** (615)327-0991        **Fax:** (615)327-4038
**Website:** http://www2.cancer.org/state/tn/

### Texas

**★ 11193 ★ American Cancer Society**
**Abilene Office**
209 S Danville, Bldg. B, Ste. 107
Abilene, TX 79605
**Phone:** (915)692-6446        **Fax:** (915)691-9920
**Website:** http://www.acs-tx.org/Texas.nsf

**★ 11194 ★ American Cancer Society**
**Amarillo Office**
3915 Bell St.
Amarillo, TX 79109
**Phone:** (806)353-4306        **Fax:** (806)354-0668
**Website:** http://www.acs-tx.org/Texas.nsf

**★ 11195 ★ American Cancer Society**
**Austin Office**
2433 Ridgepoint Dr. B
Austin, TX 78754
**Phone:** (512)919-1870        **Fax:** (512)919-1846
**Website:** http://www.acs-tx.org/Texas.nsf

**★ 11196 ★ American Cancer Society**
**Beaumont Office**
755 S 11th St., Ste. 212
Beaumont, TX 77701-3723
**Phone:** (409)835-2138

**★ 11197 ★ American Cancer Society**
**Bryan Office**
3207 Briarcrest Dr.
Bryan, TX 77802
**Phone:** (979)776-1463        **Fax:** (979)774-0865

**★ 11198 ★ American Cancer Society**
**Corpus Christi Office**
4101 S Alameda
Corpus Christi, TX 78411
**Phone:** (361)857-0134        **Fax:** (361)854-3260

**★ 11199 ★ American Cancer Society**
**Dallas Office**
8900 Carpenter Fwy.
Dallas, TX 75247
**Phone:** (214)819-1200        **Fax:** (214)631-3869

**★ 11200 ★ American Cancer Society**
**El Paso Office**
909 E San Antonio
El Paso, TX 79901
**Phone:** (915)544-4425        **Fax:** (915)532-3748

**★ 11201 ★ American Cancer Society**
**Fort Worth Office**
3301 W Freeway
Fort Worth, TX 76107
**Phone:** (817)737-9990        **Fax:** (817)737-9977

**★ 11202 ★ American Cancer Society**
**Houston Office**
6301 Richmond
Houston, TX 77057
**Phone:** (713)266-2877        **Fax:** (713)266-4159

**★ 11203 ★ American Cancer Society**
**Laredo Office**
Plaza 3, Ste. 1
2329 E Saunders
Laredo, TX 78043
**Phone:** (956)723-7933        **Fax:** (956)723-6303

**★ 11204 ★ American Cancer Society**
**Lubbock Office**
3411 73rd St.
Lubbock, TX 79423
**Phone:** (806)792-7126        **Fax:** (806)793-0148

**★ 11205 ★ American Cancer Society**
**Lufkin Office**
4000 S Medford Dr., Ste. 17E
Lufkin, TX 75901
**Phone:** (936)634-2883        **Free:** 800-277-2345
**Fax:** (936)634-2792
**Email:** l.tullas@cancer.org
**Website:** http://www.cancer.org

**★ 11206 ★ American Cancer Society**
**Midland Office**
2304 W Wadley
Midland, TX 79705
**Phone:** (915)683-6374        **Fax:** (915)687-5360
**Email:** vhavins@cancer.org
**Website:** http://www.cancer.org

**★ 11207 ★ American Cancer Society**
**Odessa Office**
811 Central
Odessa, TX 79761
**Phone:** (915)334-6121        **Fax:** (915)334-7830

**★ 11208 ★ American Cancer Society**
**Rio Grande Valley Office**
5413 S McColl Rd.
Edinburg, TX 78539
**Phone:** (956)682-8320        **Free:** 800-227-2345
**Fax:** (956)682-8410

**★ 11209 ★ American Cancer Society**
**San Angelo Office**
3228 College Hills Blvd.
San Angelo, TX 76904
**Phone:** (915)944-2509        **Fax:** (915)949-4398

**★ 11210 ★ American Cancer Society**
**San Antonio Office**
8115 Datapoint Dr.
San Antonio, TX 78229
**Phone:** (210)614-4211        **Fax:** (210)615-7724

**★ 11211 ★ American Cancer Society**
**Texarkana Office**
5501 Plaza Dr.
Texarkana, TX 75503
**Phone:** (903)831-5422        **Fax:** (903)831-6521

**★ 11212 ★ American Cancer Society**
**Texas City Office**
9002 FM 1764
Texas City, TX 77591
**Phone:** (409)938-0672        **Fax:** (409)938-0007

**★ 11213 ★ American Cancer Society**
**Tyler Office**
1301 S Broadway
Tyler, TX 75701
**Phone:** (903)597-1348        **Free:** 800-ACS-2345
**Fax:** (903)531-2350

**★ 11214 ★ American Cancer Society**
**Upper Valley Office**
5413 S McColl Rd.
Edinburg, TX 78539
**Phone:** (956)682-8320        **Fax:** (956)682-8410

**★ 11215 ★ American Cancer Society**
**Victoria Office**
4401 Lilac
Victoria, TX 77901
**Phone:** (361)578-2849        **Free:** 800-ACS-2345
**Fax:** (361)578-8071
**Website:** http://www.acstx.org

**★ 11216 ★ American Cancer Society**
**Waco Office**
1311 New Rd.
Waco, TX 76710
**Phone:** (254)753-0806        **Free:** 800-227-2345
**Fax:** (254)753-0544
**Email:** jmadden@cancer.org
**Website:** http://www.cancer.org

**★ 11217 ★ American Cancer Society**
**Wichita Falls Office**
2304 Midwestern Pkwy., Ste. 206
Wichita Falls, TX 76308
**Phone:** (940)691-7201        **Free:** 800-227-2345
**Fax:** (940)696-0656
**Email:** mwaggone@cancer.org
**Website:** http://www.cancer.org

### Utah

**★ 11218 ★ American Cancer Society**
**Central Utah Office**
819 Palisade Rd.
Sterling, UT 84665
**Phone:** (435)835-6351        **Fax:** (435)835-6350

**★ 11219 ★ American Cancer Society**
**Greater Salt Lake Office**
941 East 3300 South
Salt Lake City, UT 84106
**Phone:** (801)483-1500        **Fax:** (801)483-1558
**Website:** http://www2.cancer.org/state/ut/

**★ 11220 ★ American Cancer Society**
**Ogden Office**
2404 Washington Blvd., Ste. 218
Ogden, UT 84401
**Phone:** (801)393-8657        **Fax:** (801)393-2260

**★ 11221 ★ American Cancer Society**
**Provo Office**
286 South 600 East, Ste. A
Provo, UT 84606
**Phone:** (801)373-5886        **Fax:** (801)373-8220

**★ 11222 ★ American Cancer Society**
**Southern Utah Office**
592 N Mall Dr.
Saint George, UT 84790
**Phone:** (435)674-9707

### Vermont

**★ 11223 ★ American Cancer Society**
**Northwest New England Region**
**Montpelier Office**
11 Loomis St.
Montpelier, VT 05602
**Phone:** (802)223-2348        **Fax:** (802)223-4818
**Website:** http://www.ne-cancer.org/

**★ 11224 ★ American Cancer Society**
**Northwest New England Region**
**Rutland Office**
734-9 US Rte. 4 E
Box H
Rutland, VT 05701
**Phone:** (802)775-0514　　**Fax:** (802)773-8359

**★ 11225 ★ American Cancer Society**
**Northwest New England Region**
**South Burlington Office**
150 Kennedy Dr., Ste. 4
South Burlington, VT 05403
**Phone:** (802)658-0626

### Virgin Islands

**★ 11226 ★ American Cancer Society**
**Saint Croix Office**
PO Box 6987
Saint Croix, VI 00823
**Phone:** (340)778-2882　　**Fax:** (340)778-2116

**★ 11227 ★ American Cancer Society**
**Saint Thomas/Saint John Office**
PO Box 10427
Saint Thomas, VI 00801
**Phone:** (340)775-5373　　**Fax:** (340)775-5373

### Virginia

**★ 11228 ★ American Cancer Society**
**Abingdon Office**
205 W Main St., Ste. 23
Abingdon, VA 24210
**Phone:** (276)739-7780　　**Fax:** (276)739-7781

**★ 11229 ★ American Cancer Society**
**Charlottesville Office**
3042-D Berkmar Dr.
Charlottesville, VA 22901
**Phone:** (434)978-7423　　**Fax:** (434)978-1258

**★ 11230 ★ American Cancer Society**
**Glen Allen Office**
4240 Park Pl. Ct.
Glen Allen, VA 23060
**Phone:** (804)527-3700　　**Fax:** (804)527-3700
**Website:** http://www.inet.net/imc/acsworking/va/

**★ 11231 ★ American Cancer Society**
**Harrisonburg Office**
1920 H Medical Ave.
Harrisonburg, VA 22801
**Phone:** (540)434-3360　　**Fax:** (540)432-1621

**★ 11232 ★ American Cancer Society**
**Lynchburg Office**
2316 Atherholt Rd., Ste. 108
Lynchburg, VA 24501
**Phone:** (434)845-0973　　**Fax:** (434)845-8719

**★ 11233 ★ American Cancer Society**
**Martinsville Office**
1079 Spruce St.
Martinsville, VA 24115
**Phone:** (276)638-8944　　**Fax:** (276)638-3778

**★ 11234 ★ American Cancer Society**
**Norfolk Office**
2730 Ellsmere Ave.
Norfolk, VA 23513
**Phone:** (757)853-6638　　**Fax:** (757)853-7006

**★ 11235 ★ American Cancer Society**
**Peninsula Office**
895 Middleground Blvd., Ste. 154
Newport News, VA 23606
**Phone:** (757)591-8330　　**Fax:** (757)591-8328

**★ 11236 ★ American Cancer Society**
**Roanoke Office**
9 E Church Ave.
Roanoke, VA 24011
**Phone:** (540)344-8699　　**Fax:** (540)345-2361

**★ 11237 ★ American Cancer Society**
**Vienna Office**
124 Park St. SE
Vienna, VA 22180
**Phone:** (703)938-5550　　**Fax:** (703)938-6779

**★ 11238 ★ American Cancer Society**
**Winchester Office**
2654 Valley Ave., Ste. B
Winchester, VA 22601
**Phone:** (540)667-2315　　**Fax:** (540)667-7798

### Washington

**★ 11239 ★ American Cancer Society**
**Everett Office**
728 134th St. SW, Ste. 101
Everett, WA 98204
**Phone:** (425)741-8949　　**Free:** 800-729-5588
**Fax:** (425)741-9638
**Website:** http://www2.cancer.org/states/index.cfm?id=50

**★ 11240 ★ American Cancer Society**
**Kennewick Office**
7325 W Deschutes Ave., Ste. A
Kennewick, WA 99336
**Phone:** (509)783-5108　　**Fax:** (509)737-9702
**Website:** http://www2.cancer.org/states/index.cfm?id=50

**★ 11241 ★ American Cancer Society**
**Spokane Office**
1403 W Third
Spokane, WA 99204
**Phone:** (509)455-3440　　**Free:** 800-227-2345
**Fax:** (509)455-3990

**★ 11242 ★ American Cancer Society**
**Tacoma Office**
1551 Broadway, Ste. 200
Tacoma, WA 98402
**Phone:** (253)272-5767　　**Free:** 800-729-3880
**Fax:** (253)272-4485
**Website:** http://www2.cancer.org/states/index.cfm?id=50

### West Virginia

**★ 11243 ★ American Cancer Society**
**Bluefield Office**
1808 Jefferson St.
Bluefield, WV 24701
**Phone:** (304)327-8770　　**Fax:** (304)323-3161

**★ 11244 ★ American Cancer Society**
**Charleston Office**
301 RHL Blvd., Stes. 6 and 7
Charleston, WV 25309
**Phone:** (304)746-9950　　**Free:** 800-288-3618
**Fax:** (304)746-9962

**★ 11245 ★ American Cancer Society**
**Huntington Office**
1336 Hal Greer Blvd.
Huntington, WV 25701
**Phone:** (304)523-7989　　**Fax:** (304)523-7996

**★ 11246 ★ American Cancer Society**
**Morgantown Office**
300A Scott Ave.
Morgantown, WV 26505
**Phone:** (304)296-8155　　**Fax:** (304)296-6172

**★ 11247 ★ American Cancer Society**
**Parkersburg Office**
3901 Briscoe Rd.
PO Box 4451
Parkersburg, WV 26104
**Phone:** (304)422-1472　　**Fax:** (304)422-9569

### Wisconsin

**★ 11248 ★ American Cancer Society**
**Appleton Office**
14 Tri Park Way, Bldg. 2
Appleton, WI 54914
**Phone:** (920)739-1201　　**Fax:** (920)739-2442

**★ 11249 ★ American Cancer Society**
**Eau Claire Office**
2427 N Hillcrest Pkwy., Ste. 7
Altoona, WI 54720
**Phone:** (715)832-0181　　**Fax:** (715)832-8570

**★ 11250 ★ American Cancer Society**
**Franklin Office**
9809 S Franklin Dr., Ste. 102
Franklin, WI 53132
**Phone:** (414)423-8570　　**Fax:** (414)423-8538

**★ 11251 ★ American Cancer Society**
**Green Bay Office**
3311 S Packerland Dr.
De Pere, WI 54115
**Phone:** (920)338-1541　　**Fax:** (920)338-1545

**★ 11252 ★ American Cancer Society**
**La Crosse Office**
1285 Rudy St., Ste. 103
Onalaska, WI 54650
**Phone:** (608)783-5000　　**Fax:** (608)783-5005

**★ 11253 ★ American Cancer Society**
**Madison Office**
8317 Elderberry Rd.
Madison, WI 53717
**Phone:** (608)833-4555　　**Fax:** (608)833-1195

**★ 11254 ★ American Cancer Society**
**Pewaukee Office**
N19 W24350 Riverwood Dr.
Waukesha, WI 53188
**Phone:** (262)523-5500　　**Fax:** (262)523-9433
**Website:** http://www2.cancer.org/state/mw/

**★ 11255 ★ American Cancer Society**
**Rhinelander Office**
3716 Country Dr., Ste. 4
Rhinelander, WI 54501
**Phone:** (715)362-2400　　**Fax:** (715)362-2433

**★ 11256 ★ American Cancer Society**
**Sheboygan Office**
515 Superior Ave.
Sheboygan, WI 53081
**Phone:** (920)457-5661　　**Fax:** (920)457-8760

★ 11257 ★ **American Cancer Society**
**Wausau Office**
903 S 17th Ave., Ste. B
Wausau, WI 54401
**Phone:** (715)848-2881     **Fax:** (715)848-3797

★ 11258 ★ **American Cancer Society**
**West Bend Office**
237 N Main St.
West Bend, WI 53095
**Phone:** (262)338-4060     **Fax:** (262)338-3850

## Wyoming

★ 11259 ★ **American Cancer Society**
**Casper Office**
152 N Durbin St., Ste. 312
Casper, WY 82601
**Phone:** (307)577-4892     **Fax:** (307)577-4892

★ 11260 ★ **American Cancer Society**
**Cheyenne Office**
4202 Ridge Rd.
Cheyenne, WY 82001
**Phone:** (307)638-3331     **Fax:** (307)638-1199
**Website:** http://www.cancer.org/state/wy/

★ 11261 ★ **American Cancer Society**
**Green River Office**
560 Uinta Dr., Ste. 3
Green River, WY 82935
**Phone:** (307)875-5020     **Fax:** (307)875-5024

★ 11262 ★ **American Cancer Society**
**Northwest Wyoming Office**
1411 E Fremont St.
Riverton, WY 82501
**Phone:** (307)857-3265     **Fax:** (307)857-3267

## Hemophilia

*The following are state affiliates of the National Hemophilia Foundation, 116 W 32nd St., 11th Fl., New York, NY 10001, (800)42-HANDI, http://www.hemophilia.org/.*

### Arizona

★ 11263 ★ **Hemophilia Association, Inc.**
4001 N 24th St.
Phoenix, AZ 85016
**Phone:** (602)955-3947     **Fax:** (602)955-1962
**Email:** mike@hemophiliaz.org
**Website:** http://www.hemophiliaz.org
Michael Rosenthal, Exec Director

### Arkansas

★ 11264 ★ **Hemophilia Foundation of Arkansas, Inc.**
PO Box 1135
Greenbrier, AR 72058
**Phone:** (501)679-7300     **Free:** 800-484-9064
Laveane Lovelady, President
John Little, Vice President

### California

★ 11265 ★ **Central California Hemophilia Foundation**
PO Box 163689
Sacramento, CA 95816
**Phone:** (916)448-0370     **Fax:** (916)489-1569
**Email:** hubbert@pacbell.net
**Website:** http://www.cchfsac.org
Sean Hubbert, President

★ 11266 ★ **Hemophilia Association of San Diego**
3570 Camino Del Rio N, Ste. 108
San Diego, CA 92108
**Phone:** (619)325-3570     **Fax:** (619)325-4350
**Email:** hemoofsd@aol.com
**Website:** http://www.hemophiliasd.org
Jessica Swann, Exec Director
Antonio Pascucci, President

★ 11267 ★ **Hemophilia Foundation of Northern California**
7700 Edgewater Dr., Ste. 710
Oakland, CA 94621
**Phone:** (510)568-6243     **Fax:** (510)568-6111
**Email:** consultvb@aol.com
**Website:** http://www.hfnconline.org
Val Bias, President

★ 11268 ★ **Hemophilia Foundation of Southern California**
33 S Catalina Ave., Ste. 102
Pasadena, CA 91106
**Phone:** (626)793-6192     **Free:** 800-371-4123
**Fax:** (626)796-5605
**Email:** hfsc@earthlink.net
**Website:** http://www.hemosocal.org
Rosemary Hutton, President

### Colorado

★ 11269 ★ **Hemophilia Society of Colorado**
10020 E Girard Ave., Ste. 100
Denver, CO 80231
**Phone:** (303)750-6990     **Free:** 888-687-CLOT
**Fax:** (303)750-7035
**Email:** irarhojani@worldnett.att.net
**Website:** http://www.cohemo.org
Sherri Rhojani, President
Donna Reiner, President

### Florida

★ 11270 ★ **Hemophilia Foundation of Greater Florida**
1350 N Orange Ave., Ste. 227
Winter Park, FL 32789
**Phone:** (407)629-0000     **Free:** 800-293-6527
**Fax:** (407)629-9600
**Email:** Hemofoundation@earthlink.net
**Website:** http://www.hemophiliaflorida.org
Fran Haynes, Exec Director
Barbara Burgeson, President

★ 11271 ★ **National Hemophilia Foundation**
**Florida Chapter**
17810 Littlewood Dr.
Spring Hill, FL 34610-7357
**Phone:** (727)856-7057     **Fax:** (727)856-2257
**Email:** dphilipsen@aol.com
**Website:** http://www.geocities.com/hotsprings/1809
Natalie Philipsen, Exec Director
Aleida Wiggins, President

### Georgia

★ 11272 ★ **Hemophilia of Georgia, Inc.**
8800 Roswell Rd., Ste. 170
Atlanta, GA 30350
**Phone:** (770)518-8272     **Fax:** (770)518-3310
**Email:** mail@hog.org
**Website:** http://www.hog.org
Patricia Dominic, Exec Director
Hiram Allen, President

### Hawaii

★ 11273 ★ **Hemophilia Foundation of Hawaii**
Kapiolani Medical Center
1164 Bishop St., Ste. 1501
Honolulu, HI 96813
**Phone:** (808)521-5483     **Fax:** (808)528-7430
**Email:** hemofdhi@pixi.com
Stanley Yates, President

### Illinois

★ 11274 ★ **Hemophilia Foundation of Illinois**
332 S Michigan Ave., Ste. 1135
Chicago, IL 60604
**Phone:** (312)427-1495     **Fax:** (312)427-1602
**Email:** info@hemophiliaillinois.org
**Website:** http://www.hemophiliaillinois.org
Thomas Gauthier, Exec Director
Robert Robinson, President

### Indiana

★ 11275 ★ **Hemophilia of Indiana, Inc.**
2216 E 44th St.
Indianapolis, IN 46205
**Phone:** (317)543-1299     **Fax:** (317)543-1291
Stephen Bassett, Exec Director
Othor Aldridge, President

### Kentucky

★ 11276 ★ **Kentucky Hemophilia Foundation, Inc.**
Kosair Charities Center
982 Eastern Parkway
Louisville, KY 40217-1566
**Phone:** (502)634-8161     **Fax:** (502)634-9995
**Email:** kyhemo@bellsouth.net
**Website:** http://www.kyhemo.org
Ursela M. Lacer, Exec Director

### Louisiana

★ 11277 ★ **Louisiana Hemophilia Foundation**
3636 S Sherwood Forest Blvd., Ste. 450
Baton Rouge, LA 70816-2285
**Phone:** (225)291-1675     **Fax:** (225)291-1679
**Email:** lahemophilia@etigers.net
**Website:** http://www.louisianahemophilia.org
Lori Keels, Exec Director
Howard Young, President

### Massachusetts

★ 11278 ★ **New England Hemophilia Association**
180 Rustcraft Rd., Ste. 101
Dedham, MA 02026-4596
**Phone:** (781)326-7645     **Fax:** (781)329-5122
**Email:** neha@world.std.com
Catherine Cornell, Exec Director
Steve Jelinek, President

### Michigan

★ 11279 ★ **Hemophilia Foundation of Michigan**
905 W Eisenhower Circle, Ste. 107
Ann Arbor, MI 48103
**Phone:** (734)332-4226     **Fax:** (734)332-4204
**Email:** harner@hfmich.org
**Website:** http://www.hfmich.org
Ivan C. Harner, Exec Director
Andrew Voegtle, President

## Minnesota

**★ 11280 ★ Hemophilia Foundation of Minnesota & the Dakotas**
750 S Plaza Dr., Ste. 207
Mendota Heights, MN 55120
**Phone:** (651)406-8655   **Free:** 800-994-4363
**Fax:** (651)406-8656
**Email:** hfmd1@aol.com
Richard Baker, Exec Director
Shirley Wilson, Exec Director

## Nebraska

**★ 11281 ★ National Hemophilia Foundation**
**Nebraska Chapter**
3610 Dodge St., No. 110-W
Omaha, NE 68131
**Phone:** (402)342-3329   **Fax:** (402)342-4329
**Email:** Mrye@hemophiliaone.com
**Website:** http://www.nebraskanhf.org
Matt Rye, President

## Nevada

**★ 11282 ★ Hemophilia Foundation of Nevada**
PO Box 90158
Henderson, NV 89009
**Phone:** (702)564-4368   **Fax:** (702)564-2299
**Email:** hfnv@earthlink.net
**Website:** http://www.hemophilianevada.org
Brad Rassuchine, President
Renee Paper, Exec Director

## New Mexico

**★ 11283 ★ Sange de Oro, Inc.**
**Hemophilia Foundation of New Mexico**
PO Box 7188
Albuquerque, NM 87194-7188
**Phone:** (505)341-9321
**Email:** Bjor@aol.com
Elisabeth Ortega Rangel, Exec Director

## New York

**★ 11284 ★ Bleeding Disorders Association of Northeastern New York**
PO Box 3703
Albany, NY 12203
**Phone:** (518)782-9787   **Fax:** (518)782-9787
**Email:** hemovw@hotmail.com
**Website:** http://www.geocities.com/hotsprings/oasis/9190
Tom Brownell, President

**★ 11285 ★ Hemophilia Center of Western New York, Inc.**
462 Grider St.
Buffalo, NY 14215
**Phone:** (716)896-2470   **Fax:** (716)898-5537
**Email:** hemoctr@pce.net
**Website:** http://www.wnyhemophilia.com
Rosemary Holmberg, Exec Director
Thomas Long, President

**★ 11286 ★ Mary M. Gooley Hemophilia Center, Inc.**
1415 Portland Ave., Ste. 425
Rochester, NY 14621
**Phone:** (716)922-5700   **Fax:** (716)922-5775
**Email:** robert.fox@viahealth.org
**Website:** http://www.hemocenter.org
Robert Fox, Exec Director

## North Carolina

**★ 11287 ★ Hemophilia of North Carolina**
2 Centerview Dr., Ste. 51
Greensboro, NC 27407
**Free:** 800-990-5557   **Fax:** (704)587-0815
**Email:** srfarr@worldnet.att.net
Jody Throckmorton, President

## Ohio

**★ 11288 ★ National Hemophilia Foundation**
**Central Ohio Chapter**
670 Suntree Dr.
Worthington Highlands
Westerville, OH 43081-5013
**Phone:** (614)847-5634
Mike Capsel, President

**★ 11289 ★ National Hemophilia Foundation**
**Greater Cincinnati/Northern Kentucky Chapter**
1008 Marshall Ave., Ste. 3
Cincinnati, OH 45225
**Phone:** (513)961-4366   **Fax:** (513)871-6803
**Email:** ly113@aol.com
Linda Young, Exec Director

**★ 11290 ★ Northern Ohio Hemophilia Foundation, Inc.**
Independence Tower
5755 Granger Rd., Ste. 790
Cleveland, OH 44131
**Phone:** (216)739-1755   **Free:** 800-554-HEMO
**Fax:** (216)739-1758
**Email:** hemo@earthlink.net
**Website:** http://www.bleedingdisordersnorohio.org
Randi Paltrow, Exec Director

**★ 11291 ★ Northwest Ohio Hemophilia Foundation**
1 Stranahan Sq., Ste. 540
Toledo, OH 43604
**Phone:** (419)242-9587   **Fax:** (419)242-6316
**Email:** stephanieb@uhs-toledo.org
**Website:** http://www.uhs-toledo.org
Stephanie Branco, Director

**★ 11292 ★ Southwestern Ohio Hemophilia Foundation**
82 Elva Ct., Ste. B
Vandalia, OH 45377
**Phone:** (937)415-0644   **Fax:** (937)415-0604
**Email:** jlswohf@aol.com
Rita Falkenback, President

## Oklahoma

**★ 11293 ★ Oklahoma Hemophilia Foundation**
1501 N Classen Blvd., Ste. B
Oklahoma City, OK 73106
**Phone:** (405)524-7069   **Free:** 800-735-3855
**Fax:** (405)524-7916
**Email:** mmorseohf@aol.com
Mike Morse, Exec Director

## Pennsylvania

**★ 11294 ★ National Hemophilia Foundation**
**Delaware Valley Chapter**
222 S Easton Rd., Ste. 107
Glenside, PA 19038
**Phone:** (215)885-6500   **Fax:** (215)885-6074
**Email:** hemophilia@navpoint.com
**Website:** http://www.hemophiliasupport.org
Clifford Cohn, President

**★ 11295 ★ National Hemophilia Foundation**
**Western Pennsylvania Chapter**
532 S Aiken Ave., Ste. 102
Pittsburgh, PA 15232
**Phone:** (412)683-2231   **Fax:** (412)683-2568
**Email:** wpcnhf@pgh.net
Patricia Enright, Exec Director

## Rhode Island

**★ 11296 ★ Rhode Island Hemophilia Foundation**
160 Plainfield St.
Providence, RI 02909
**Phone:** (401)944-6950   **Fax:** (401)944-4161
Emili Vaziri, President

## South Carolina

**★ 11297 ★ Hemophilia of South Carolina**
PO Box 2386
Irmo, SC 29063
**Free:** 888-829-4849   **Fax:** 888-829-4849
**Email:** Factoreight@aol.com
Brandy Stewart, President

## Tennessee

**★ 11298 ★ Tennessee Hemophilia & Bleeding Disorders Foundation**
7003 Chadwick Dr., Ste. 269
Brentwood, TN 37027
**Phone:** (615)373-0351   **Fax:** (615)373-4394
**Email:** thbdf@worldnet.att.net
**Website:** http://www.home.att.net/~thbdf
Sandy Jones, Contact

## Texas

**★ 11299 ★ National Hemophilia Foundation**
**Lone Star Chapter**
16910 Shady Square Ct.
Houston, TX 77095
**Phone:** (281)861-6644   **Fax:** (281)861-6644
Debbie de la Riva, Exec Director

## Utah

**★ 11300 ★ Utah Hemophilia Foundation**
880 E 3375 S
Salt Lake City, UT 84106
**Phone:** (801)484-0325   **Fax:** (801)484-4177
**Email:** soleil@hemophiliautah.org
**Website:** http://www.hemophiliautah.org
Susan Soleil, Exec Director

## Virginia

**★ 11301 ★ Hemophilia Association of the Capital Area**
3251 Old Lee Hwy., Ste. 3
Fairfax, VA 22030-1504
**Phone:** (703)352-7641   **Fax:** (703)352-2145
**Email:** info@hacacares.org
**Website:** http://www.hacacares.org
Sandi Qualley, Exec Director

**★ 11302 ★ National Hemophilia Foundation**
**United Virginia Chapter**
9801 Husting Terrace
Chesterfield, VA 23832
**Phone:** (804)748-7896   **Fax:** (804)796-9043
**Email:** pader55@cs.com
Patricia DeRatto, Exec Director

## Wisconsin

### ★ 11303 ★ Great Lakes Hemophilia Foundation
PO Box 704
Milwaukee, WI 53210-0704
**Phone:** (414)257-0200 **Free:** 888-797-4543
**Fax:** (414)257-1225
**Email:** Kmarquardt@glhf.org
**Website:** http://www.glhf.org
Kathleen M. Marquardt, Exec Director

## Leukemia

*State chapters of The Leukemia and Lymphoma Society are listed below. The national office is located at 1311 Mamaroneck Ave., White Plains, NY 10605. Additional information can be obtained by calling the national office at (800) 955-4LSA, or by consulting their web site at http://www.leukemia.org/.*

## Alabama

### ★ 11304 ★ The Leukemia and Lymphoma Society
**Alabama Chapter**
100 Chase Park S, Ste. 220
Birmingham, AL 35244
**Phone:** (205)989-0098 **Fax:** (205)989-0099
Valerie Hunton, Exec Director

## Arizona

### ★ 11305 ★ The Leukemia and Lymphoma Society
**Desert Mountain States Chapter**
2990 E Northern Ave., Ste. E-100
Phoenix, AZ 85028
**Phone:** (602)788-8622 **Free:** 800-568-1372
**Fax:** (602)788-3455
Tim Metzer, Exec Director
**Remarks:** Serves Arizona, Utah, and western Texas.

## California

### ★ 11306 ★ The Leukemia and Lymphoma Society
**Greater Los Angeles Chapter**
6033 W Century Blvd., Ste. 300
Los Angeles, CA 90045
**Phone:** (310)216-7600 **Fax:** (310)216-1500
Barbara Howell, Exec Director

### ★ 11307 ★ The Leukemia and Lymphoma Society
**Greater Sacramento Area Chapter**
3105 Fite Circle, Ste. 101
Sacramento, CA 95827
**Phone:** (916)369-7581 **Fax:** (916)369-0812
Tracy Newman, Exec Director
**Remarks:** Also serves much of Nevada.

### ★ 11308 ★ The Leukemia and Lymphoma Society
**Northern California Chapter**
1390 Market St., Ste. 1200
San Francisco, CA 94102
**Phone:** (415)625-1100 **Fax:** (415)625-1155

### ★ 11309 ★ The Leukemia and Lymphoma Society
**San Diego/Hawaii Chapter**
8575 Gibbs Dr., Ste. 262
San Diego, CA 92123
**Phone:** (858)277-1800 **Free:** 800-215-1098
**Fax:** (858)277-1748
Keith Turner, Exec Director
**Alt. Contact:** Hawaii Number: (808) 534-1222.

### ★ 11310 ★ The Leukemia and Lymphoma Society
**Tri-County Chapter**
2333 N Broadway, Ste. 320
Santa Ana, CA 92706
**Phone:** (714)881-0610 **Free:** 888-535-9300
**Fax:** (714)881-0616
**Email:** quinteroj@ca-tri.leukemia.org
**Website:** http://www.ca-tri.leukemia.org
Sam Thomas, Exec Director
**Remarks:** Also serves the Las Vegas, Nevada, area.

## Colorado

### ★ 11311 ★ The Leukemia and Lymphoma Society
**Rocky Mountain Chapter**
5353 W Dartmouth Ave.
Denver, CO 80227
**Phone:** (303)984-2110 **Fax:** (303)984-2352
**Remarks:** Serves Colorado, Idaho, Montana, and Wyoming.

## Connecticut

### ★ 11312 ★ The Leukemia and Lymphoma Society
**Connecticut Chapter**
300 Research Pkwy., Ste. 310
Meriden, CT 06450
**Phone:** (203)379-0445 **Free:** 888-282-9465
**Fax:** (203)379-0451
Elizabeth Garrigan, Exec Director

### ★ 11313 ★ The Leukemia and Lymphoma Society
**Fairfield County Chapter**
25 3rd St., 4th Fl.
Stamford, CT 06905
**Phone:** (203)967-8326 **Fax:** (203)325-8559
**Email:** fairfieldinfo@yahoo.com
Michael Angarola, Exec Director

## Delaware

### ★ 11314 ★ The Leukemia and Lymphoma Society
**Delaware Chapter**
100 W 10 St., Ste. 209
Wilmington, DE 19801
**Phone:** (302)661-7300 **Free:** 800-220-1617
**Fax:** (302)661-0363

## Florida

### ★ 11315 ★ The Leukemia and Lymphoma Society
**Central Florida Chapter**
3319 Maguire St., Ste. 101
Orlando, FL 32803
**Phone:** (407)898-0733 **Fax:** (407)896-8645
Tracy Tucker, Exec Director

### ★ 11316 ★ The Leukemia and Lymphoma Society
**Northern Florida Chapter**
9143 Phillips Hwy., Ste. 130
Jacksonville, FL 32256
**Phone:** (904)538-0721 **Free:** 800-868-0072
**Fax:** (904)538-9245
Eden Carr, Exec Director

### ★ 11317 ★ The Leukemia and Lymphoma Society
**Palm Beach Area Chapter**
4360 Northlake Blvd., Ste. 109
Palm Beach Gardens, FL 33410
**Phone:** (561)775-9954 **Free:** 888-478-8550
**Fax:** (561)775-0930
**Email:** McDonaldP@FL-wpb.leukemia.org
**Website:** http://www.FL-wpb.leukemia.org
Patricia McDonald, Exec Director

### ★ 11318 ★ The Leukemia and Lymphoma Society
**Southern Florida Chapter**
3325 Hollywood Blvd., Ste. 400
Hollywood, FL 33021
**Phone:** (954)961-3234 **Fax:** (954)961-7376
**Email:** silvermanb@fl-so.leukemia-lymphoma.org
**Website:** http://www.fl-so.leukemia-lymphoma.org
Barbara Silverman, Exec Director

### ★ 11319 ★ The Leukemia and Lymphoma Society
**Suncoast Chapter**
13907 N Dale Mabry Hwy., Ste. 101
Tampa, FL 33618
**Phone:** (813)963-6461 **Fax:** (813)963-1306
Anna Maria Gentile, Exec Director

## Georgia

### ★ 11320 ★ The Leukemia and Lymphoma Society
**Georgia Chapter**
2625 Cumberland Pkwy, Ste. 205
Atlanta, GA 30339
**Phone:** (770)438-6006 **Free:** 800-399-7312
**Fax:** (770)438-6563
Laurie Papelian, Exec Director

## Illinois

### ★ 11321 ★ The Leukemia and Lymphoma Society
**Illinois Chapter**
100 W Monroe Ave., Ste. 1610
Chicago, IL 60603
**Phone:** (312)726-0003 **Fax:** (312)726-4769
Lee J. Brown, Exec Director

## Indiana

### ★ 11322 ★ The Leukemia and Lymphoma Society
**Indiana Chapter**
921 E 86th St., Ste. 205
Indianapolis, IN 46240
**Phone:** (317)726-2270 **Fax:** (317)726-2280
Dennis Norris, Exec Director

## Iowa

### ★ 11323 ★ The Leukemia and Lymphoma Society
**Iowa Chapter**
8033 University Blvd., Ste. A
Des Moines, IA 50325
**Phone:** (515)270-6169 **Free:** 800-347-1074
**Fax:** (515)270-5392
**Email:** janna@crn.org
**Website:** http://www.crn.org
Janna LaCock, Exec Director

## Kansas

### ★ 11324 ★ The Leukemia and Lymphoma Society
**Kansas Chapter**
555 N Woodlawn, Bldg. 1, Ste. 113
Wichita, KS 67208
**Phone:** (316)687-2222 **Free:** 800-779-2417
**Fax:** (316)687-1122
**Email:** kansas@ks.leukemia-lymphoma.org
**Website:** http://www.ks.leukemia-lymphoma.org

**★ 11325 ★ The Leukemia and Lymphoma Society**
**Mid-America Chapter**
Cloverleaf Bldg. 1, Ste. 202
6811 W 63rd St.
Shawnee Mission, KS 66202
**Phone:** (913)262-1515　　**Free:** 800-256-1075
**Fax:** (913)262-2167
**Email:** janna@crn.org
**Website:** http://www.crn.org
Janna LaCock, Contact
**Remarks:** Serves western Missouri and eastern Kansas.

## Kentucky

**★ 11326 ★ The Leukemia and Lymphoma Society**
**Kentucky Chapter**
710 W Main St., Ste. 201
Louisville, KY 40202
**Phone:** (502)584-8490　　**Free:** 800-955-2566
**Fax:** (502)589-5316
Janelle Sumner, Exec Director

## Louisiana

**★ 11327 ★ The Leukemia and Lymphoma Society**
**Louisiana Chapter**
3636 S I-10 Service Rd., Ste. 304
Metairie, LA 70001
**Phone:** (504)837-0945　　**Free:** 888-290-0945
**Fax:** (504)837-9193
Susan Krilov, Exec Director

## Maryland

**★ 11328 ★ The Leukemia and Lymphoma Society**
**Maryland Chapter**
Chester Bldg., Ste. 314
8600 La Salle Rd.
Baltimore, MD 21286
**Phone:** (410)825-2500　　**Fax:** (410)825-2515
**Website:** http://www.mdleukemia.org
Sharon Yateman, Exec Director

## Massachusetts

**★ 11329 ★ The Leukemia and Lymphoma Society**
**Massachusetts Chapter**
495 Old Connecticut Path, Ste. 220
Framingham, MA 01701
**Phone:** (508)879-5083　　**Free:** 800-688-6572
**Fax:** (508)879-8163
Iris Gleason, Exec Director
**Remarks:** Serves Massachusetts, Maine, and New Hampshire.

## Michigan

**★ 11330 ★ The Leukemia and Lymphoma Society**
**Michigan Chapter**
1421 E 12 Mile Rd., Bldg. A
Madison Heights, MI 48071
**Phone:** (248)582-2900　　**Free:** 800-456-5413
**Fax:** (248)582-2925
**Email:** bizzisj@mi.leukemia-lymphoma.org
**Website:** http://www.mi.leukemia-lymphoma.org
Julia K. Bizzis, Exec Director

## Minnesota

**★ 11331 ★ The Leukemia and Lymphoma Society**
**Minnesota Chapter**
5217 Wayzata Blvd., Ste. 221
Saint Louis Park, MN 55416
**Phone:** (952)545-3309　　**Fax:** (952)545-5926
Murray Schmidt, Exec Director
**Remarks:** Serves Minnesota, North Dakota, and South Dakota.

## Mississippi

**★ 11332 ★ The Leukemia and Lymphoma Society**
**Mississippi Chapter**
405 Fontaine Pl., Ste. 103
Ridgeland, MS 39157
**Phone:** (601)956-7447　　**Free:** 877-538-5364
**Fax:** (601)956-6957
Julie Levanway, Exec Director

## Missouri

**★ 11333 ★ The Leukemia and Lymphoma Society**
**Gateway Chapter**
77 W Port Plaza, Ste. 101
Saint Louis, MO 63146
**Phone:** (314)878-0780　　**Free:** 800-264-2873
**Fax:** (314)878-4050
Judith Swiecicki, Exec Director
**Remarks:** Serves eastern Missouri and southern Illinois.

## Nebraska

**★ 11334 ★ The Leukemia and Lymphoma Society**
**Nebraska Chapter**
2665 Farnam St.
Omaha, NE 68131
**Phone:** (402)344-2242　　**Free:** 888-847-4974
**Fax:** (402)344-2422
**Email:** opbroekr@ne.leukemia.org
**Website:** http://www.ne.leukemia.org
Rosemary Opbroek, Exec Director

## New Jersey

**★ 11335 ★ The Leukemia and Lymphoma Society**
**Northern New Jersey Chapter**
45 Springfield Ave.
Springfield, NJ 07081
**Phone:** (973)376-9559　　**Fax:** (973)376-7072
Lorraine Seidel, Exec Director

**★ 11336 ★ The Leukemia and Lymphoma Society**
**Southern New Jersey Chapter**
216 Haddon Ave., Ste. 328
Westmont, NJ 08108
**Phone:** (856)869-0200　　**Free:** 888-920-8557
**Fax:** (856)869-7383
Nanette Forte, Exec Director

## New Mexico

**★ 11337 ★ The Leukemia and Lymphoma Society**
**New Mexico Chapter**
3150 Carlisle NE, Ste. 35
Albuquerque, NM 87110
**Phone:** (505)830-6040　　**Free:** 888-286-7846
**Fax:** (505)830-6041
Cindi Ankiewicz, Exec Director
**Remarks:** Serves New Mexico and the Greater El Paso, Texas, area.

## New York

**★ 11338 ★ The Leukemia and Lymphoma Society**
**Central New York Chapter**
Learbury Centre
401 N Salina St.
Syracuse, NY 13203
**Phone:** (315)471-1050　　**Free:** 800-690-8944
**Fax:** (315)471-6434
Toni E. Bennett, Exec Director

**★ 11339 ★ The Leukemia and Lymphoma Society**
**Long Island Chapter**
555 Broad Hollow Rd., Ste. 403
Melville, NY 11747
**Phone:** (631)752-8500　　**Fax:** (631)752-9066
Kerri Kaplan, Exec Director

**★ 11340 ★ The Leukemia and Lymphoma Society**
**New York City Chapter**
475 Park Ave. S, 21st Fl.
New York, NY 10016
**Phone:** (212)448-9206　　**Fax:** (212)448-9214
Mary Kozik, Exec Director

**★ 11341 ★ The Leukemia and Lymphoma Society**
**Westchester/Hudson Valley Chapter**
1311 Mamaroneck Ave., Ste. 330
White Plains, NY 10605
**Phone:** (914)949-0084　　**Fax:** (914)949-0391
Jean Montano, Exec Director

**★ 11342 ★ The Leukemia and Lymphoma Society**
**Western New York/Finger Lakes Chapter**
4053 Maple Rd., Ste. 110
Amherst, NY 14226
**Phone:** (716)635-9111　　**Fax:** (716)837-0335
Nancy Hails, Exec Director

## North Carolina

**★ 11343 ★ The Leukemia and Lymphoma Society**
**North Carolina Chapter**
5950 Fairview Rd., Ste. 250
Charlotte, NC 28210
**Phone:** (704)998-5012　　**Free:** 800-888-9934
**Fax:** (704)998-5010
Selena Rogers, Exec Director

## Ohio

**★ 11344 ★ The Leukemia and Lymphoma Society**
**Central Ohio Chapter**
2225 City Gate Dr., Ste. E
Columbus, OH 43219
**Phone:** (614)476-7194　　**Free:** 800-686-2873
William Carnes, Exec Director

**★ 11345 ★ The Leukemia and Lymphoma Society**
**Northern Ohio Chapter**
902 Westpoint Pkwy., Ste. 300
Cleveland, OH 44145
**Phone:** (440)617-2873　　**Fax:** (440)617-2879
Nathaniel A. Cross, Exec Director

★ **11346** ★ **The Leukemia and Lymphoma Society**
**Southern Ohio Chapter**
Fourth and Race Towers
105 W 4th St.
Cincinnati, OH 45202
**Phone:** (513)361-2100          **Fax:** (513)361-2109
Nancy Brinker, Exec Director

### Oklahoma

★ **11347** ★ **The Leukemia and Lymphoma Society**
**Oklahoma Chapter**
3613 NW 56th St., Ste. 230
Oklahoma City, OK 73112
**Phone:** (405)943-8888          **Fax:** (405)945-8355
**Email:** odonnells@ok.leukemia-lymphoma.org
**Website:** http://www.ok.leukemia-lymphoma.org
Suzanne O'Donnell, Exec Director

### Oregon

★ **11348** ★ **The Leukemia and Lymphoma Society**
**Oregon Chapter**
6501 SW Macadam Ave.
Portland, OR 97201
**Phone:** (503)245-9866          **Fax:** (503)245-9865
Gregory Knox, Exec Director

### Pennsylvania

★ **11349** ★ **The Leukemia and Lymphoma Society**
**Central Pennsylvania Chapter**
800 Corporate Cir., Ste. 100
Harrisburg, PA 17110
**Phone:** (717)652-6520          **Free:** 800-822-2873
**Fax:** (717)652-8614

★ **11350** ★ **The Leukemia and Lymphoma Society**
**Eastern Pennsylvania Chapter**
2 International Plaza, Ste. 245
Philadelphia, PA 19113
**Phone:** (610)521-8274          **Fax:** (610)521-6132
Joanne Spink, Exec Director

★ **11351** ★ **The Leukemia and Lymphoma Society**
**Western Pennsylvania and West Virginia Chapter**
2 Gateway Ctr.
13 North
Pittsburgh, PA 15222

**Phone:** (412)395-2873          **Free:** 800-726-2873
**Fax:** (412)395-2888
George Omiros, Exec Director

### Rhode Island

★ **11352** ★ **The Leukemia and Lymphoma Society**
**Rhode Island Chapter**
75 Sockanosset Crossroad, Ste. 206
Box 8099
Cranston, RI 02920
**Phone:** (401)943-8888          **Fax:** (401)943-1377
Lynn Aaronson, Exec Director

### South Carolina

★ **11353** ★ **The Leukemia and Lymphoma Society**
**South Carolina Chapter**
1247 Lake Murray Blvd.
Irmo, SC 29063
**Phone:** (803)749-4299          **Fax:** (803)749-4088
**Email:** canningf@sc.leukemia-lymphoma.org
**Website:** http://www.sc.leukemia-lymphoma.org
Frank Canning, Exec Director

### Tennessee

★ **11354** ★ **The Leukemia and Lymphoma Society**
**Tennessee Chapter**
446 Metroplex Dr., Ste. A-200
Nashville, TN 37211
**Phone:** (615)331-2980          **Free:** 800-332-2980
**Fax:** (615)331-2941
**Email:** llstennchap@netscape.net
Karen Rudzinski, Exec Director

### Texas

★ **11355** ★ **The Leukemia and Lymphoma Society**
**North Texas Chapter**
12850 Spurling Dr., Ste. 220
Dallas, TX 75230
**Phone:** (972)239-0959          **Fax:** (972)239-0892
Richard Reader, Exec Director

★ **11356** ★ **The Leukemia and Lymphoma Society**
**South/West Texas Chapter**
950 Isom Rd., Ste. 104
San Antonio, TX 78216
**Phone:** (210)377-1775          **Free:** 800-683-2458
**Fax:** (210)344-3717
Cindy Atmar, Exec Director

★ **11357** ★ **The Leukemia and Lymphoma Society**
**Texas Gulf Coast Chapter**
5005 Mitchelldale, Ste. 115
Houston, TX 77092
**Phone:** (713)680-8088          **Fax:** (713)683-9504
Joan Jarrett, Exec Director

### Virginia

★ **11358** ★ **The Leukemia and Lymphoma Society**
**National Capital Area Chapter**
5845 Richmond Hwy., Ste. 630
Alexandria, VA 22303
**Phone:** (703)960-1100          **Fax:** (703)960-0920
**Email:** samuelsc@dc-cap.leukemia-lymphoma.org
**Website:** http://www.tntdc.org
Darcy Valentine, Director
**Remarks:** Serves Washington DC, west-central Maryland, and northeastern Virginia.

★ **11359** ★ **The Leukemia and Lymphoma Society**
**Virginia Chapter**
2101 Executive Dr.
Tower Box 21
Hampton, VA 23666
**Phone:** (757)838-9351          **Free:** 800-866-4483
**Fax:** (757)827-7337
Diane Hagemann, Exec Director

### Washington

★ **11360** ★ **The Leukemia and Lymphoma Society**
**Washington and Alaska Chapter**
530 Dexter Ave. N, Ste. 300
Seattle, WA 98109
**Phone:** (206)628-0777          **Free:** 888-345-4572
**Fax:** (206)292-9791
**Email:** WAChapter@wa.leukemia-lymphoma.org
**Website:** http://www.wa.leukemia-lymphoma.org
Kathryn Bennett, Exec Director

### Wisconsin

★ **11361** ★ **The Leukemia and Lymphoma Society**
**Wisconsin Chapter**
1126 S 70th St., Ste. N405-A
Milwaukee, WI 53214
**Phone:** (414)256-4020          **Free:** 800-261-7399
**Fax:** (414)256-4025
Bede Barth, Exec Director

## Foundations & Other Funding Organizations

### Private Foundations

**★ 11362 ★ Abney Foundation**
100 Vine St.
Anderson, SC 29621
**Phone:** (864)964-9201 **Fax:** (864)964-9209
**Email:** info@abneyfoundation.org
**Website:** http://www.abneyfoundation.org
Carl Edwards, Executive Director
**Fnded:** 1957. **Philosophy:** The Abney Foundation primarily supports higher education in South Carolina. Interests include colleges, technical schools, and universities. The foundation also supports hospitals, hospices, homes, food distribution, youth organizations, and churches. **Priorities:** *Arts & Humanities:* 2%. Supports theater, music, arts funds. *Civic & Public Affairs:* 1%. Supports community affairs. *Education:* 78%. Supports colleges, universities and scholarship. *Environment:* 3%. Supports youth services, special olympics, meals on wheels, and the elderly Young Men's Christian Association. *International:* 8%. Supports hospices, health clinics, diabetes and medical research. *Note:* Total contributions made in 1998. **Typ. Recipients:** Cancer, Clinics/Medical Centers, Diabetes, Home-Care Services, Hospices, Hospitals, Medical Education, Medical Research. **Geo. Dist:** SC.

**Alex Hillman Family Foundation**
*See:* Entry 33

**★ 11363 ★ Amelia Peabody Charitable Fund**
10 Post Office Square North, Ste. 995
Boston, MA 02109
**Phone:** (617)451-6178
JoAnne Borek, Executive Director
**Fnded:** 1942. **Philosophy:** The purpose of the Amelia Peabody Charitable Fund is to assist local charitable and educational organizations, with emphasis on hospitals, cultural programs, education institutions, and conservation groups. **Priorities:** *Arts & Humanities:* 14%. Primary support for museums and art centers. *Civic & Public Affairs:* 14%. Community affairs. *Education:* 16%. Supports colleges and universities and special education. *Environment:* 21%. Emphasis on youth organizations. *International:* 30%. Focus on hospitals, single-disease health associations, pediatric health, and medical research. *Religion:* 2%. Funds laboratories. *Note:* Total contributions made in 1999. **Typ. Recipients:** Alzheimers Disease, Arthritis, Cancer, Children's Health/Hospitals, Clinics/Medical Centers, Diabetes, Emergency/Ambulance Services, Eyes/Blindness, Family Planning, Geriatric Health, Health Organizations, Health-General, Heart, Home-Care Services, Hospitals, Long-Term Care, Medical Education, Medical Research, Medical Training, Nursing Services, People with Disabilities, Prenatal Health Issues, Public Health, Single-Disease Health Associations, Speech & Hearing, Substance Abuse. **Geo. Dist:** New England; Boston, MA, metropolitan area.

**Amelia Peabody Foundation**
*See:* Entry 41

**★ 11364 ★ American Foundation Corp.**
629 Euclid Ave., Ste. 720
Cleveland, OH 44114
**Phone:** (216)241-6664 **Fax:** (216)241-6693
**Website:** http://www.ameliapeabody.org
Maria Muth, Treasurer
**Fnded:** 1974. **Philosophy:** The American Foundation Corporation makes most of its grants in the areas of civic affairs, education, the arts, and social services. In civic affairs, interests include an arboretum, conservation and environmental affairs, and wildlife resources. Educational funding favors private academies, colleges and universities, and technical education. Support for the arts goes to art associations and institutes, the performing arts, and museums. Social service funding includes child welfare, youth organizations, and animal protection. The foundation also supports other recipient areas. **Priorities:** *Arts & Humanities:* 5%. Supports museums. *Civic & Public Affairs:* 33%. Supports parks, gardens, municipalities, fire departments, and a zoo. *Education:* 17%. Supports secondary schools and education organizations. *Environment:* 24%. Funds animal protection, women's organizations, and family planning services. *International:* 12%. Supports hospitals. *Religion:* 1%. Supports scientific research. *Note:* Total contributions made in 1998. **Typ. Recipients:** Cancer, Children's Health/Hospitals, Clinics/Medical Centers, Emergency/Ambulance Services, Family Planning, Heart, Hospices, Hospitals, Hospitals (University Affiliated), Long-Term Care, Medical Education, Medical Rehabilitation, Mental Health, Nursing Services, People with Disabilities. **Geo. Dist:** nationally; OH.

**Andersen Foundation**
*See:* Entry 43

**Arie and Ida Crown Memorial**
*See:* Entry 50

**Assisi Foundation of Memphis**
*See:* Entry 11687

**★ 11365 ★ B. B. Owen Trust**
PO Box 830068
Richardson, TX 75083
**Phone:** (972)783-7170 **Fax:** (972)783-7175
**Email:** aicm@crown-chicago.com
Monty Jackson, Trustee
**Fnded:** 1974. **Philosophy:** The B. B. Owen Charitable Trust primarily contributes most of its grants to health care, specifically medical centers in Texas. Other areas of interest include food and clothing distribution, community centers, homes, religion, and civic affairs. **Priorities:** *Arts & Humanities:* 10%. Funds ballet. *Civic & Public Affairs:* 28%. City of McKinney parks, and local Texas government. *Education:* 6%. Supports the University of Dallas and Junior Achievement. *Environment:* 19%. Boys & Girls Clubs, YMCA, YWCA, childrens charities. *International:* About 16%. Supports pediatric health, hospitals, and health funds. *Note:* Total contributions made in fiscal 1999. **Typ. Recipients:** Children's Health/Hospitals, Clinics/Medical Centers, Eyes/Blindness, Family Planning, Hospitals, Hospitals (University Affiliated), Kidney, Medical Research, Nursing Services, People with Disabilities, Preventive Medicine/Wellness Organizations. **Geo. Dist:** TX, Dallas.

**★ 11366 ★ Bat Hanadiv Foundation No. 3**
c/o Carter Leoyard & Milburn
2 Wall St., 13th Floor
New York, NY 10005
**Fax:** (212)732-3232
Jerome Caufield, Attorney
**Fnded:** 1981. **Philosophy:** The Bat Hanadiv Foundation No. 3 gives primarily to Jewish causes in Israel. The foundation's three main interests include educational institutions, civic groups, and the arts. In the area of education, grants fund universities and scientific education. **Priorities:** *Arts & Humanities:* 1%. Funds the Jerusalem Music Center. *Civic & Public Affairs:* 32%. Supports the Ramat Hanadiv Memorial Gardens. *Education:* 50%. Supports science education, Jewish studies, and special education. *Religion:* 12%. Funding the Weizmann Institute of Science. *Note:* Total contributions made in 1997. **Typ. Recipients:** Hospices, Hospitals, Substance Abuse.

**Beatrice P. Delany Charitable Trust**
*See:* Entry 67

**Benjamin and Mary Siddons Measey Foundation**
*See:* Entry 74

**★ 11367 ★ Benjamin and Roberta Russell Educational Foundation**
PO Box 369
Alexander City, AL 35011-0272
**Phone:** (256)329-1320 **Fax:** (256)329-5346
James Nabors, Secretary & Treasurer
**Fnded:** 1944. **Philosophy:** The foundation's primary interest is education, with a focus on higher education. Support often goes to universities, community colleges, and private academies. The foundation also will contribute to hospitals, health relief agencies, single-disease associations, and children's welfare organizations. **Priorities:** *Arts & Humanities:* 6%. Libraries and the performing arts. *Civic & Public Affairs:* 1%. Supports municipal projects. *Education:* 56%. Scholarships, colleges, universities, and secondary schools. *Environment:* 26%. Scouting and youth organizations, and humane societies. *International:* 11%. Single-disease health organizations, hospitals, health funds, and

hospices. *Note:* Total contributions made in 1998. **Typ. Recipients:** Alzheimers Disease, Children's Health/Hospitals, Diabetes, Emergency/Ambulance Services, Hospices, Hospitals, Kidney, Multiple Sclerosis, Single-Disease Health Associations. **Geo. Dist:** Southeastern USA; AL.


### ★ 11368 ★ Benson and Edith Ford Fund
100 Renaissance Ctr., 34th Fl.
Detroit, MI 48243
**Phone:** (313)259-7777　　**Fax:** (313)393-7579
David Hempstead, Secretary & Trustee
**Fnded:** 1943. **Philosophy:** The foundation makes grants in the areas of youth organizations and child welfare, hospitals, civic affairs, the arts, and education. A wide variety of grants are given in each of these areas. **Priorities:** *Arts & Humanities:* 45%. Funds support the fine arts, historical societies, the performing arts, and music; a major grant went to the Henry Ford Museum and Greenfield Village. *Civic & Public Affairs:* 6%. Supports the Detroit Zoological Society, a neighborhood club, and parks. *Education:* 5%. Supports private pre-college education, colleges and universities, and college funds. *Environment:* 13%. Gives to scouts, food banks, youth programs, homes, United Way, and animal protection. *International:* 8%. Supports hospitals, health centers, and single-disease health associations. *Religion:* 22%. Supports the Edison Institute and Woods Hole Oceanographic Institute. *Note:* Total contributions made in 2000. **Typ. Recipients:** Alzheimers Disease, Cancer, Children's Health/Hospitals, Clinics/Medical Centers, Emergency/Ambulance Services, Eyes/Blindness, Family Planning, Health Organizations, Hospitals, Long-Term Care, People with Disabilities, Preventive Medicine/Wellness Organizations, Public Health, Substance Abuse. **Geo. Dist:** MI, especially Detroit.


### Booth-Bricker Fund
*See:* Entry 85


### Broyhill Family Foundation
*See:* Entry 91


### ★ 11369 ★ Caleb C. and Julia W. Dula Educational and Charitable Foundation
112 South Hanley Rd., 2nd Floor
Saint Louis, MO 63105-3418
**Phone:** (314)726-2800　　**Fax:** (314)863-3821
James Mauze, General Counsel
**Fnded:** 1939. **Philosophy:** The foundation primarily supports the arts and civic affairs. Art funding favors libraries, symphonies, and historic preservation. Civic affairs support goes to foundations, zoos and botanical gardens, and environmental affairs. The foundation also makes contributions to education, hospitals and nursing services, and social services. **Priorities:** *Arts & Humanities:* 23%. Supports theaters, music, dance, and historical societies. *Civic & Public Affairs:* 20%. Botanical gardens, zoos, and foundations were funded. *Education:* 27%. Secondary schools and universities received grants. *Environment:* 14%. Supports people with disabilities, youth organizations, family services, and animal welfare. *International:* 12%. Funding went to hospitals and single-disease health associations. *Note:* Total contributions made in 1998. **Typ. Recipients:** Alzheimers Disease, Cancer, Children's Health/Hospitals, Clinics/Medical Centers, Diabetes, Emergency/Ambulance Services, Family Planning, Health Organizations, Hospitals, Medical Education, Nursing Services, People with Disabilities, Preventive Medicine/Wellness Organizations, Single-Disease Health Associations. **Geo. Dist:** MO; NY.


### California Wellness Foundation
*See:* Entry 5547


### ★ 11370 ★ Camp Younts Foundation
PO Box 813
Franklin, VA 23851
**Phone:** (757)562-3439　　**Fax:** (757)569-7839

**Website:** http://www.tcwf.org
Bobby Worrell, Executive Director
**Fnded:** 1955. **Philosophy:** The foundation typically supports small colleges, private academies, and military institutes. Another priority is civic affairs, specifically, Southampton County, VA, and through the Elms Foundation. Other areas of support include churches, homes, and child welfare organizations. **Priorities:** *Arts & Humanities:* 11%. Funds museums and historical organisation. *Civic & Public Affairs:* 20%. Funds philanthropic organizations, botanical gardens and local histori cal society. *Education:* 57%. Higher education and seminars. *Environment:* 2%. People with disabilities and recreation and athletics. *International:* 3%. Primarily supports the Southampton Memorial Hospital in addition to single dise ase associations. *Religion:* 1%. *Note:* Contributions were made in 1998. **Typ. Recipients:** Cancer, Hospitals, Medical Education, Nursing Services, People with Disabilities, Single-Disease Health Associations. **Geo. Dist:** southeastern states; VA.


### Cannon Foundation
*See:* Entry 8538


### ★ 11371 ★ The Cannon Foundation, Inc.
PO Box 548
Concord, NC 28026-0548
**Phone:** (704)786-8216　　　**Fax:** (704)785-2052
Frank Davis, Executive Director
**Fnded:** 1943. **Philosophy:** The foundation is dedicated to carrying out the donor's "commitment to the people of Cabarrus County and the state of North Carolina through his philanthropy in health, education, and religion." **Priorities:** *Arts & Humanities:* 10%. Gives to museums and historic preservation. *Civic & Public Affairs:* 25%. Primary support for family services and youth organizations. *Education:* 23%. Funds colleges, universities, and elementary education. *International:* 36%. Supports hospitals, hospices, clinics, and health services. *Note:* Total contributions made in fiscal 1999. Percentages were provided by foundation and are approximate. **Typ. Recipients:** Adolescent Health Issues, AIDS/HIV, Children's Health/Hospitals, Clinics/Medical Centers, Domestic Violence, Emergency/Ambulance Services, Family Planning, Geriatric Health, Health Organizations, Health-General, Home-Care Services, Hospices, Hospitals, Nutrition, People with Disabilities, People with Disabilities, Prenatal Health Issues, Public Health, Research/Studies Institutes, Substance Abuse, Transplant Networks/Donor Banks. **Geo. Dist:** NC.


### ★ 11372 ★ Carl B. and Florence E. King Foundation
5956 Sherry Lane, Ste. 620
Dallas, TX 75225
**Phone:** (214)750-1884　　**Fax:** (214)750-1651
Carl Yeckel, President
**Fnded:** 1966. **Philosophy:** "The Foundation contributes to a variety of concerns and organizations, including Goodwill Industries, the YMCA and YWCA, the Boy Scouts of America, and a wide range of Texas youth groups. Even before the value and popularity of academic scholarships became evident, the King Foundation was providing a number of deserving college students with financial assistance. That focus continues today." "The King Foundation also provides funds for the construction of schools, hospitals, and homes for the aged, handicapped, and indigent. Selected grants assist medical research organizations and other charitable or scientific associations. The Foundation makes contributions to educational institutions as well." The Carl B. and Florence E. King Foundation 1997 brochure and guidelines **Priorities:** *Arts & Humanities:* 14%. Public broadcasting, symphonies, and theater programs for young audiences. *Education:* About 76%. Focus on Texas universities, scholarships, 4-H programs, prep schools, and religious education. *International:* About 10%. Supports health organizations. *Note:* Total contributions made in 1998. **Typ. Recipients:** Cancer, Children's Health/Hospitals, Clinics/Medical Centers, Diabetes, Emer-

gency/Ambulance Services, Eyes/Blindness, Family Planning, Health Funds, Health Organizations, Hospitals, Medical Education, Medical Rehabilitation, Medical Research, Nursing Services, People with Disabilities, Prenatal Health Issues, Substance Abuse. **Geo. Dist:** Dallas, TX, including metropolitan area.


### Carrie Estelle Doheny Foundation
*See:* Entry 108


### ★ 11373 ★ Charles M. Bair Memorial Trust
c/o U.S. Bank & Trust National Association of Montana
PO Box 30678
Billings, MT 59115
**Phone:** (406)657-8004　　　**Fax:** (406)657-8034
**Email:** doheny@dohenyfoundation.org
**Website:** http://www.dohenyfoundation.org
Helen Hancock, Contact
**Fnded:** 1978. **Philosophy:** The trust's priorities include hospitals and medical centers in Montana that were named in the original trust document, Christian Science churches, and scholarships to graduates of Harlowton and White Sulphur Springs high schools. High school graduates in Meagher and Wheatland counties also are supported. **Priorities:** *International:* 97%. Emphasis on hospitals and medical centers. **Typ. Recipients:** Clinics/Medical Centers, Hospitals. **Geo. Dist:** MT, Meagher County; MT, Wheatland County.


### ★ 11374 ★ Christ is Our Salvation Foundation (CIOS)
PO Box 20815
Waco, TX 76702-0815
**Phone:** (254)752-5551　　　**Fax:** (254)752-4711
Paul Piper, Sr., Trustee
**Fnded:** 1952. **Philosophy:** The foundation primarily is interested in supporting Christian religious organizations. Churches, missions, conventions, and bible classes all are given support. Religious education is a secondary interest, along with support for civic affairs, social services, and the arts. **Priorities:** *Civic & Public Affairs:* 1%. Supports community foundations. *Education:* 5%. Supports colleges and universities. *Environment:* 1%. Supports community service organizations. *International:* 35%. Primarily supports hospitals. *Note:* Total contributions made in fiscal 1999. **Typ. Recipients:** Cancer, Children's Health/Hospitals, Clinics/Medical Centers, Health Organizations, Hospitals, People with Disabilities, Public Health, Substance Abuse. **Geo. Dist:** midwestern states; TX.


### ★ 11375 ★ Clark Foundation (NY)
One Rockefeller Plaza, 31st Floor
New York, NY 10020-2102
**Phone:** (212)977-6900　　　**Fax:** (212)977-3424
Charles Hamilton, Executive Director
**Fnded:** 1931. **Philosophy:** The foundation continues to support the hospitals and the museums in Cooperstown, NY. Funding is also given for educational, youth, employment, and social service organizations. An important area of foundation activity is the scholarship program for students from the Cooperstown area. Students may attend any college of their choice. Funds are earmarked for each particular student and administered through the college. **Priorities:** *Arts & Humanities:* 5%. Funds opera, museums, and historical associations. *Civic & Public Affairs:* 16%. Supports community development, women's issues, housing, business issues, and employment services. *Education:* 16%. Supports scholarships, precollege and college education, and outward bound programs. *Environment:* 33%. Supports united funds, children's organizations, and family services. *International:* 2%. *Note:* Total contributions made in fiscal 2000. **Typ. Recipients:** AIDS/HIV, Cancer, Clinics/Medical Centers, Emergency/Ambulance Services, Family Planning, Health Funds, Health Organizations, Hospitals, Kidney, Medical Education, Medical Training, Mental Health, Outpatient Health Care, People with Disabili-

ties, Substance Abuse. **Geo. Dist:** nationally; Cooperstown, NY; New York, NY.


**Coleman Foundation (IL)**
*See:* Entry 137


★ **11376 ★ Constantin Foundation**
4809 Cole Ave., LB-127
Dallas, TX 75205-3578
**Phone:** (214)522-9300     **Fax:** (214)521-7025
**Email:** Coleman@colemanfoundation.org
**Website:** http://www.colemanfoundation.org
Betty Hillin, Executive Director
**Fnded:** 1947. **Philosophy:** Traditionally, most grants have been awarded to private colleges, universities, and secondary schools. The remainder of funds have supported hospitals and medical centers, and social service organizations. **Priorities:** *Arts & Humanities:* 2%. Supports performing arts for youth. *Education:* 53%. Private schools and the University of Dallas. *Environment:* 41%. Supports shelters, volunteer centers and youth organizations. *International:* 4%. Supports the Arthritis Foundation. *Note:* Total contributions made in 1998. **Typ. Recipients:** Arthritis, Cancer, Child Abuse, Children's Health/Hospitals, Clinics/Medical Centers, Family Planning, Health Organizations, Hospitals, Hospitals (University Affiliated), Medical Research, Mental Health, People with Disabilities, Single-Disease Health Associations, Substance Abuse. **Geo. Dist:** TX, Dallas County; Dallas, TX, including metropolitan area.


★ **11377 ★ CTW Foundation, Inc.**
PO Box 2205
Wilmington, DE 19899-0911
**Phone:** (302)425-2501     **Fax:** (908)719-6725
Robert Tucker, President
**Fnded:** 1954. **Priorities:** *Arts & Humanities:* 16%. Supports art foundations, performing arts, and museums. *Education:* 22%. Supports universities, colleges, and schools. *Environment:* 55%. Supports domestic violence services and people with disabilities. *International:* 4%. Supports medical centers and single-disease health associations. *Note:* Total contributions made in 2000. **Typ. Recipients:** Cancer, Children's Health/Hospitals, Clinics/Medical Centers, Domestic Violence, Health Funds, Health Organizations, Hospitals, Medical Education, Medical Rehabilitation, Medical Research, Medical Training, People with Disabilities, Preventive Medicine/Wellness Organizations, Public Health. **Geo. Dist:** nationally.


**Dale J. Bellamah Foundation**
*See:* Entry 155


**Dan Murphy Foundation**
*See:* Entry 156


**Davenport-Hatch Foundation**
*See:* Entry 160


★ **11378 ★ David, Helen, and Marian Woodward Fund-Atlanta**
PO Box 4148
GA31221
Atlanta, GA 30302
**Phone:** (404)332-6677     **Fax:** (404)332-1389
Beverly Blake, Principal Manager
**Fnded:** 1975. **Philosophy:** The fund focuses its giving in the Atlanta, GA, area. Contributions reflect an emphasis on health care and education; social services, religious organizations, civic groups, and the arts also receive support from the fund. **Priorities:** *Arts & Humanities:* 17%. Supports historic preservation; music, and general architects. *Civic & Public Affairs:* 28%. Supports community foundations, clubs, parks, and ethnic organizations. *Education:* 36%. Primarily funding private precollege education. Also supports religious education. *Environment:* 9%. Supports scouting, young men's christian association and

camps. *International:* 6% Supports medicine centers, alzheimers, and health organizations. *Note:* Total contributions made in fiscal 1999. **Typ. Recipients:** Child Abuse, Children's Health/Hospitals, Clinics/Medical Centers, Health Organizations, Health Policy/Cost Containment, Hospitals, Long-Term Care, People with Disabilities, Public Health, Single-Disease Health Associations, Substance Abuse. **Geo. Dist:** GA, emphasis on Atlanta and neighboring states.


★ **11379 ★ de Kay Foundation**
1211 Ave. of America
New York, NY 10036
**Phone:** (646)366-0852
Adreanne Gorman, Contact
**Fnded:** 1967. **Philosophy:** The de Kay Foundation makes grants to a few organizations. One-third of contributions goes to St. Barnabas Hospital in New York. Another one-third of funds was split between the Federation for Protestant Welfare Agencies and the Community Service Society of New York. The remaining one-third funds the groups which enable elderly individuals (over age 65) in the Tri-State region to remain in their homes. Applications must be submitted through social service agencies. Individuals applying directly will be rejected. **Priorities:** *Environment:* 25%. Supports the Community Service Society of New York and the Federation of Protestant Welfare agencies. *International:* 50%. Supports St. Barnabas Hospital. *Note:* Total contributions made in fiscal 1999. **Typ. Recipients:** Hospitals. **Geo. Dist:** New York, NY.


**Dellora A. and Lester J. Norris Foundation**
*See:* Entry 165


★ **11380 ★ DeRoy Testamentary Foundation**
4000 Southfield Town Center, Ste. 1450
Southfield, MI 48075
**Phone:** (248)827-0920     **Fax:** (248)827-0922
**Email:** DeRoyFdtn@aol.com
Julie Holly, Vice President
**Fnded:** 1979. **Philosophy:** The foundation makes most of its grants in the areas of education, social services, the arts, and health care. Educational funding favors university English departments, arts and business education, scholarship funds, and drop-out programs. Funding for social service organizations favors animal protection, family services, homes for the aged, and community centers. The foundation also funds health foundations and hospitals. **Priorities:** *Arts & Humanities:* 11%. Historical societies, music, museums, and libraries. *Civic & Public Affairs:* 6%. Funds women's affairs, justice issues, and a zoo. *Education:* 31%. Supports colleges, univesities, and local schools. *Environment:* 21%. Funds a humane society, family services, child welfare, and united funds. *International:* 18%. Funds hospitals, home care, and hospices. *Note:* Total contributions made in 1999. **Typ. Recipients:** Cancer, Children's Health/Hospitals, Clinics/Medical Centers, Domestic Violence, Emergency/Ambulance Services, Eyes/Blindness, Family Planning, Health Organizations, Hospices, Hospitals, Long-Term Care, Medical Education, Medical Rehabilitation, Medical Research, Mental Health, Nursing Services, People with Disabilities, Prenatal Health Issues, Public Health, Trauma Treatment. **Geo. Dist:** Metropolitan Detroit, MI.


**DeWitt Wallace-Reader's Digest Fund**
*See:* Entry 166


★ **11381 ★ Dr. C. C. and Mabel L. Criss Memorial Foundation**
1700 Farnam St.
Omaha, NE 68102
**Phone:** (402)348-6364     **Fax:** (402)348-6666
**Email:** dwrd@wallacefunds.org
**Website:** http://www.wallacefunds.org
James Strasheim, Trustee

**Fnded:** 1978. **Philosophy:** The foundation primarily supports organizations and institutions in Omaha, NE. Colleges and universities receive major contributions. Private secondary education is also a priority. Large grants usually support the construction and expansion of schools. Health care, research, and hospitals are supported. Local cultural associations and historical preservation organizations are of interest to the foundation. Community services also receive funding. **Priorities:** *Arts & Humanities:* 23%. Supports performing arts, university of Nebraska library, and museums. *Education:* 71%. Supports leadership training colleges and universities and religious education in Nebraska. *Environment:* 4%. Supports family services, the United Way, people with disabilities, scouts, and substance abuse and treatment. *International:* 1%. Funds Hospice programs. *Note:* Contributions were made in fiscal 1999. **Typ. Recipients:** Children's Health/Hospitals, Heart, Hospices, Hospitals, Prenatal Health Issues. **Geo. Dist:** Omaha, NE.


**Dora Roberts Foundation**
*See:* Entry 177


**Dover Foundation**
*See:* Entry 181


**Duke Endowment**
*See:* Entry 183


★ **11382 ★ E. J. Grassmann Trust**
PO Box 4470
Warren, NJ 07059
**Phone:** (908)753-2440     **Fax:** (908)753-9384
**Email:** droberson@tde.org
**Website:** http://www.dukeendowment.org
William Engel, Executive Director & Trustee
**Fnded:** 1979. **Philosophy:** The trust attempts to fund the types of organizations that Mr. Grassmann supported during his lifetime. Preferred organizations include local hospitals and health organizations; organizations engaged in ecological endeavors; educational institutions; and organizations that help the needy, particularly children. "Preference will be given to organizations with low administration expenses, that show efforts to encourage individuals to help themselves, and that make efforts to achieve a broad base of funding sources." **Priorities:** *Arts & Humanities:* 9%. Historical societies, performing arts, museums and theatres. *Civic & Public Affairs:* 6%. Community support, urban nature concerns, and housing. *Education:* 25% Supports colleges, academies and secondary schools. *Environment:* 10%. Children's and outreach services, Young Men's Christian Association, camps, and family planning services. *International:* 21% Associations, hospitals and cancer. *Note:* Total contributions made in 1998. **Typ. Recipients:** AIDS/HIV, Cancer, Children's Health/Hospitals, Clinics/Medical Centers, Emergency/Ambulance Services, Family Planning, Health Organizations, Hospices, Hospitals, Medical Education, Medical Rehabilitation, Nursing Services, People with Disabilities, Public Health, Trauma Treatment. **Geo. Dist:** GA; NJ, Union County and surounding area.


★ **11383 ★ Eleanor and Edsel Ford Fund**
100 Renaissance Ctr., Ste. 3400
Detroit, MI 48243
**Phone:** (313)259-7777     **Fax:** (313)393-7579
David Hempstead, Secretary & Trustee
**Fnded:** 1944. **Philosophy:** Contributions are "committed pursuant to testamentary direction left by Eleanor Clay Ford." The purpose of the fund is to provide financial support to corporations, trusts, community chests, funds, or foundations, organized and operated solely for religious, charitable, scientific, literary or educational purposes, or for the prevention of cruelty to children or animals. **Priorities:** *Arts & Humanities:* 24%. Supports music and Arts Founders Society. *Education:* 43%. Supports arts/humanities education and schools. *International:* 21%. Funds support the Henry Ford Health System. *Religion:* 11%.

Supports the Edison Institute. *Note:* Total contributions made in 2000. **Typ. Recipients:** Health Organizations, Hospitals, Public Health. **Geo. Dist:** Detroit, MI, including metropolitan area.


**Elizabeth Morse Genius Foundation**
*See:* Entry 213


**Ellen Browning Scripps Foundation**
*See:* Entry 216


**★ 11384 ★ English-Bonter-Mitchell Foundation**
110 West Berry, 10th Floor
Fort Wayne, IN 46802
**Phone:** (219)426-0555          **Fax:** (219)461-6198
**Website:** http://www.scrippsfoundation.org
Teresa Tracey, Trust Officer

**Fnded:** 1972. **Philosophy:** The foundation's giving focuses on culture and youth programs. Support also is directed toward higher education, hospitals, churches and religious organizations, social services, and community development. **Priorities:** *Arts & Humanities:* 27%. Supports public broadcasting, arts funds, historical preservation, orchestra, music, and theater. *Civic & Public Affairs:* 6%. Supports parks and zoos. *Education:* 34%. Supports Junior Achievement, education associations, colleges, and universities. *Environment:* 28%. Supports Big Brothers/Big Sisters, scouting, the disabled, YMCA, and United Way. *International:* 4%. Supports hospital foundations, medical centers, and hospice. *Note:* Total contributions made in 2000. **Typ. Recipients:** Children's Health/Hospitals, Clinics/Medical Centers, Emergency/Ambulance Services, Health Funds, Health Organizations, Hospices, Hospitals, Medical Education, Medical Rehabilitation, Mental Health, People with Disabilities, Public Health, Single-Disease Health Associations, Substance Abuse. **Geo. Dist:** IN, primarily Fort Wayne.


**★ 11385 ★ Evan and Marion Helfaer Foundation**
735 North Water St.
Milwaukee, WI 53202-4188
**Phone:** (414)276-3600          **Fax:** (414)276-0172
Thomas Smallwood, Co-Trustee & Administrator

**Fnded:** 1971. **Philosophy:** The foundation makes grants across the major categories of support. Educational funding favors universities, colleges, medical and engineering schools, and private high schools. Health service support goes to hospitals and cancer and blood centers. Funding for the arts includes performing arts, museums, and historic preservation. Social service interests include youth organizations, united funds, and community centers. The foundation will make grants to other recipient areas as well. **Priorities:** *Arts & Humanities:* 10%. Focus on museums, libraries, arts funds, theater, and music. *Civic & Public Affairs:* 55%. Funds stadiums and community projects. *Education:* 17%. Primary and secondary schools and colleges and universities are funded. *Environment:* 12%. Grants are made to youth organizations, united funds, child welfare, services. *International:* 1%. Support goes to a health education center and hospitals. *Note:* Total contributions made in fiscal 1999. **Typ. Recipients:** Child Abuse, Children's Health/Hospitals, Clinics/Medical Centers, Geriatric Health, Heart, Hospitals, Medical Education, Medical Research, Mental Health, Nursing Services, People with Disabilities, Public Health, Single-Disease Health Associations, Substance Abuse. **Geo. Dist:** Milwaukee, WI.


**Fannie E. Rippel Foundation**
*See:* Entry 2889


**Fletcher Jones Foundation**
*See:* Entry 240


**Fondren Foundation**
*See:* Entry 245


**Forest Lawn Foundation**
*See:* Entry 249


**Forrest C. Lattner Foundation**
*See:* Entry 250


**★ 11386 ★ Fritz B. Burns Foundation**
4001 West Alemeda Ave., Ste. 203
Burbank, CA 91505
**Phone:** (818)840-8802          **Fax:** (818)849-0468
**Email:** fletcherjones2@1wilshire.com
**Website:** http://www.forestlawnfoundation.org
Joseph Rawlinson, President

**Fnded:** 1955. **Philosophy:** The foundation emphasizes areas of funding established by the donor during his lifetime. The foundation offers "educational contributions with an emphasis on buildings, equipment, endowments, student scholarship and loan funds, and faculty fellowships." Hospitals, hospital equipment, and medical research also are supported. **Priorities:** *Arts & Humanities:* 1%. *Civic & Public Affairs:* 2%. *Education:* About 62%. Supports colleges, universities, and precollege educational institutions. *Environment:* 3%. *International:* About 20%. Primarily hospitals and medical centers. *Note:* Total contributions made in fiscal 1995. **Typ. Recipients:** Children's Health/Hospitals, Clinics/Medical Centers, Emergency/Ambulance Services, Family Planning, Health Organizations, Hospitals, Medical Research, Nursing Services, Nutrition, People with Disabilities, Prenatal Health Issues, Research/Studies Institutes, Single-Disease Health Associations. **Geo. Dist:** Los Angeles, CA, metropolitan area.


**Fullerton Foundation**
*See:* Entry 268


**Gebbie Foundation**
*See:* Entry 274


**★ 11387 ★ Generoso Pope Foundation**
211 West 56th St., 5th Fl.
New York, NY 10019
**Phone:** (212)765-4156          **Fax:** (212)765-4157
**Email:** cjbonner@fullertonfoundation.org
Mr. Anthony Pope, President & Secretary

**Fnded:** 1947. **Philosophy:** The foundation reflects the personal philanthropic interests of the Pope family, especially their interest in Roman Catholic institutions and in organizations that study and record the experience of Italian immigrants in America. Many recipients are given funds annually. Other foundation interests include welfare funds, higher and secondary education, and hospitals. **Priorities:** *Arts & Humanities:* 7% supports museums, public radio, performing arts, journalism, and art. *Civic & Public Affairs:* 12% supports police benevolence and community services. *Education:* 18% supports colleges, universities, educational programs. *Environment:* 9%. Supports March of Dimes, Meals on Wheels, and battered women's services. *International:* 45%. Supports hospitals, medical centers, pediatric medicine, rehabilitation, disease and disorder concerns. *Note:* Contributions were made in 1998. **Typ. Recipients:** Children's Health/Hospitals, Clinics/Medical Centers, Diabetes, Domestic Violence, Eyes/Blindness, Geriatric Health, Health Funds, Health Organizations, Hospitals, Long-Term Care, Medical Education, Medical Rehabilitation, Medical Research, Mental Health, People with Disabilities, Prenatal Health Issues, Public Health, Single-Disease Health Associations. **Geo. Dist:** New York, NY, metropolitan area; limited support elsewhere. **Frmly:** Pope Foundation.


**George F. Baker Trust**
*See:* Entry 276


**★ 11388 ★ Gladys Brooks Foundation**
P O Box 7689
Garden City, NY 11530
**Phone:** (516)746-6103
**Website:** http://www.gladysbrooksfoundation.org
Jessica Rutledge, Administrative Assistant

**Fnded:** 1981. **Philosophy:** The foundation was created "to provide for the intellectual, moral, and physical welfare of the people of this country by establishing and supporting non-profit libraries, educational institutions, hospitals, and clinics. The foundation will consider grant applications in the fields of libraries, education, hospitals, and clinics." Library grant applications will be considered for endowments, construction, and equipment. In education, grant applications will be considered generally for educational endowments to fund scholarships based solely on leadership and academic ability of the student; endowments to support salaries of educators who confine their activities primarily to classroom instruction in the liberal arts, mathematics, and the sciences during the academic year; and erection or endowment of buildings, wings, or additions thereto of buildings for educational purposes. Grant applications from hospitals and clinics will be considered generally where the proposal demonstrates one or more of the following: (a) a new health need; (b) an improvement in the quality of health care; or (c) reduced health costs with better patient outcomes. "No grant will be considered that is to support a laboratory research project." **Priorities:** *Arts & Humanities:* 8%. Supports museums, libraries and historic preservation. *Civic & Public Affairs:* 6%. Cathedral Community Cares. *Education:* 42%. Supports Colleges and universities, education foundations, tutoring programs, and schools. *Environment:* 11%. *International:* 28%. Supports hospitals and cancer research. *Note:* Total contributions made in 2000. **Typ. Recipients:** Cancer, Children's Health/Hospitals, Clinics/Medical Centers, Emergency/Ambulance Services, Hospitals, Medical Education, Medical Research, Nursing Services, People with Disabilities, Research/Studies Institutes, Single-Disease Health Associations. **Geo. Dist:** CT; DE; DC; IN; ME; MD; MA; NH; NJ; NY; NC; OH; PA; RI; SC; VT; VA; WA; WV.


**Gladys and Roland Harriman Foundation**
*See:* Entry 291


**The Grainger Foundation**
*See:* Entry 300


**H. A. and Mary K. Chapman Charitable Trust**
*See:* Entry 309


**Hagedorn Fund**
*See:* Entry 312


**Harden Foundation**
*See:* Entry 315


**★ 11389 ★ Harkness Foundation for Dance**
145 East 48th St., Ste. 26C
New York, NY 10017-0025
**Phone:** (212)755-5540          **Fax:** (212)755-5542
**Website:** http://www.grainger.com
Theodore Bartwink, Treasurer

**Fnded:** 1986. **Philosophy:** The Harkness Foundation for Dance focuses on funding for the performing arts, dance venues, and dance scholarships. Limited funding is also available for non-performing arts organizations, with some funding going to health and social service causes. **Priorities:** *Arts & Humanities:* 56%. Supports dance ballet, theater, arts, institutes, arts councils, libraries, history, and opera. *Civic & Public Affairs:* 2%. Supports festival and women's affairs. *Education:* 17%. Supports arts/humanities education, colleges, and universities. *Environment:* 15%. Supports youth organizations and YM & YWHA. *Interna-*

tional: 8%. Supports hospital. *Note:* Total contributions made in 1998. **Typ. Recipients:** AIDS/HIV, Cancer, Hospitals. **Geo. Dist:** New York, NY.


**Harold K. L. Castle Foundation**
*See:* Entry 317


**Harriet Ford Dickenson Foundation**
*See:* Entry 18209


**Harriett Ames Charitable Trust**
*See:* Entry 319


**Hartford Courant Foundation**
*See:* Entry 11689


**★ 11390 ★ Harvey and Bernice Jones Charitable Trust**
PO Box 2035
Springdale, AR 72765
**Phone:** (501)756-0611          **Fax:** (501)750-7444
**Email:** hcfoundation@courant.com
**Website:** http://www.jonesnet.org
Joel Carver, Trustee
**Fnded:** 1989. **Philosophy:** The trust concentrates its grant program on education, medical services, and religious organizations in Arkansas. The primary emphasis is on assisting organizations near Springdale, AR, where Bernice Jones lives. The trust concentrates on helping a few select organizations with ongoing support. **Priorities:** *Education:* 5%. Supports colleges. *Environment:* 95%. Major support in this area goes to the Harvey and Bernice Jones Center for Families. *Note:* Contributions were made in fiscal 1998. **Typ. Recipients:** Children's Health/Hospitals, Clinics/Medical Centers, Eyes/Blindness, Health-General, Hospitals, Long-Term Care. **Geo. Dist:** AR, Northwest Arkansas.


**Hawn Foundation**
*See:* Entry 331


**Helen Brach Foundation**
*See:* Entry 333


**★ 11391 ★ Helen Clay Frick Foundation**
3 Mellon Bank Center, 40th Floor
Pittsburgh, PA 15259
**Phone:** (412)234-5784          **Fax:** (412)234-1073
**Email:** robinson.bk@mellon.com
Barbara Robinson, Trust Administrator
**Fnded:** 1947. **Philosophy:** The major focus of the Frick Foundation has been on the fine arts, which stems from its founder's interest in art and the collection acquired by her father. Much of the annual funds go to the Frick Collection in New York City. Other areas of interest are the environment and education. **Priorities:** *Arts & Humanities:* 36%. Supports arts museums, historic preservation, and the performing arts. *Civic & Public Affairs:* 12%. Supports botanical gardens, clubs. *Education:* 8%. Funds medical education, religious education, and universities. *Environment:* 2%. Supports community service organizations, animal protection, and child welfare. *Religion:* 13%. Supports science museums, general-science, and science centers. *Note:* Total contributions made in 1998. **Typ. Recipients:** Hospitals, Medical Education. **Geo. Dist:** New York, NY; Pittsburgh, PA.


**Henry and Lucy Moses Fund**
*See:* Entry 340


**★ 11392 ★ The Hoover Foundation**
101 East Maple St.
North Canton, OH 44720
**Phone:** (216)499-9200          **Fax:** (216)497-5857
Lawrence Hoover, Chairman

**Fnded:** 1945. **Philosophy:** The Hoover Foundation makes most of its grants in the areas of education, civic affairs, social services, and the arts. Educational funding favors educational enhancement programs, colleges, private high schools, and technical education. Funding for civic affairs goes to municipalities, the environment, and consumer affairs. Social service support includes united funds, community centers, and animal protection. In the arts, interests include libraries, art institutes, historical preservation, and the performing arts. **Priorities:** *Arts & Humanities:* 35%. Supports libraries, museums, music, and the performing arts. *Civic & Public Affairs:* 6%. Supports employment/job training and a community foundation. *Education:* 17%. Supports religious education, education reform, colleges and public schools. *Environment:* 40%. Supports domestic violence/child abuse services, community centers, YMCA, United Way, and family planning services. *International:* 1%. Supports single-disease health associations, medical centers, and medical research. *Note:* Total contributions made in 2000. **Typ. Recipients:** Children's Health/Hospitals, Domestic Violence, Emergency/Ambulance Services, Eyes/Blindness, Family Planning, Health Funds, Health Organizations, Heart, Hospitals, Medical Research, Multiple Sclerosis, People with Disabilities, Respiratory, Substance Abuse, Transplant Networks/Donor Banks. **Geo. Dist:** OH, Stark County.


**★ 11393 ★ Hudson-Webber Foundation**
333 West Fort St., Ste. 1310
Detroit, MI 48226
**Phone:** (313)963-7777          **Fax:** (313)963-2818
David Egner, President
**Fnded:** 1943. **Philosophy:** The Hudson-Webber Foundation's objective is "to improve the vitality and quality of life of the metropolitan Detroit community." The foundation has a particular interest in the revitalization of downtown Detroit and institutions and programs that directly benefit its citizens. The foundation concentrates its efforts and resources in five program areas: the Detroit Medical Center, economic development of southeastern Michigan (with emphasis on the creation of employment opportunities), Detroit physical revitalization, the arts, and crime abatement in Detroit. **Priorities:** *Arts & Humanities:* 14%. Supports historical preservation, art institutes, orchestra and opera. *Civic & Public Affairs:* 25%. Supports community foundations and job training. *Education:* 10%. Supports universities. *Environment:* 12%. Supports United Way, family services and youth programs. *International:* 30%. Supports hospital research and medical centers. *Religion:* 8%. Supports science center. *Note:* Total contributions made in 1998. **Typ. Recipients:** Cancer, Child Abuse, Children's Health/Hospitals, Clinics/Medical Centers, Domestic Violence, Family Planning, Health Organizations, Hospitals, Prenatal Health Issues, Public Health, Substance Abuse, Transplant Networks/Donor Banks. **Geo. Dist:** MI, Oakland County; MI, Southeastern Michigan; MI, Wayne County; Detroit, MI.


**★ 11394 ★ Hugoton Foundation**
900 Park Ave.
New York, NY 10021
**Phone:** (212)734-5447          **Fax:** (212)734-5448
Joan Stout, President
**Fnded:** 1981. **Philosophy:** The Hugoton Foundation makes most of its grants in the areas of health care and education. Funding for health care favors hospitals. Education support goes primarily to medical and nursing schools, colleges, and secondary education. The foundation also supports other recipient areas on a limited basis. **Priorities:** *Arts & Humanities:* 3%. Supports libraries and museums. *Education:* 28%. Supports universities, science, education, religious education, and nursing soos. *Environment:* 2%. Supports recreation/athletics, emergency relief, child welfare, and animal protection. *International:* 51%. Supports hospital, medical centers, hospices, heart research, nursing services, and cancer research. *Religion:* 5%. Supports a natural history museum. *Note:* Total contributions made in 1999. **Typ. Recipients:** Alzheimers Disease, Cancer, Children's Health/Hospitals, Clinics/Medical Centers, Emergency/Ambulance

Services, Eyes/Blindness, Geriatric Health, Health Organizations, Heart, Hospitals, Medical Education, Medical Rehabilitation, Medical Research, Mental Health, Nursing Services, Nursing Services, People with Disabilities, Research/Studies Institutes, Respiratory, Single-Disease Health Associations, Transplant Networks/Donor Banks. **Geo. Dist:** New York, NY.


**★ 11395 ★ J. Aron Charitable Foundation**
126 East 56th St., Ste. 2300
New York, NY 10022
**Phone:** (212)832-8352
Mr. Peter Aron, President & Executive Director
**Fnded:** 1934. **Philosophy:** The foundation generally supports arts and cultural programs, educational institutions, hospitals and health organizations, and social service agencies. **Priorities:** *Arts & Humanities:* 75%. Supports museums, with major funding to the South Street Seaport Museum. *Civic & Public Affairs:* 3%. Emphasis on Community foundations. *Education:* 6%. Colleges and universities, and secondary education received grants. *Environment:* 6%. Emphasis on the Phoenix House Development Fund and shelters. *International:* 9%. Gives to hospitals, medical centers, and medical research. *Note:* Total contributions made in 1998. **Typ. Recipients:** Clinics/Medical Centers, Emergency/Ambulance Services, Eyes/Blindness, Family Planning, Geriatric Health, Hospitals, Hospitals (University Affiliated), Medical Education, Medical Research, Mental Health, People with Disabilities, Research/Studies Institutes, Respiratory, Single-Disease Health Associations, Single-Disease Health Associations, Substance Abuse. **Geo. Dist:** New Orleans, LA, including metropolitan area; New York, NY.


**★ 11396 ★ J. E. and L. E. Mabee Foundation, Inc.**
3000 Mid-Continent Tower
401 South Boston Ave., 30th Floor
Tulsa, OK 74103-4017
**Phone:** (918)584-4286
John Conway, Jr., Vice Chairman, Secretary, Treasurer & Tr
**Fnded:** 1948. **Philosophy:** The general objectives of the foundation are to assist religious, charitable, and educational organizations. The foundation generally makes its largest grants in the area of education, specifically to construct and renovate facilities. Such capital grants are given to institutions of higher learning. Youth issues are also an important foundation focus. Grants in this area generally fund building programs. In the health field, the foundation funds capital projects for hospitals, health agencies, and institutions engaged in the discovery, treatment, and care of diseases. **Priorities:** *Arts & Humanities:* 2%. Funding for renovations at museums and other cultural institutes. *Education:* 34%. Emphasis on college and university building funds. *Environment:* 45%. Primarily for youth organizations. *International:* 14%. Focus on capital campaigns at hospitals. *Note:* Total contributions made in fiscal 2000. **Typ. Recipients:** Cancer, Children's Health/Hospitals, Clinics/Medical Centers, Diabetes, Domestic Violence, Health Funds, Health Organizations, Health-General, Heart, Hospices, Hospitals, Long-Term Care, Medical Education, Medical Rehabilitation, Medical Research, Mental Health, Nursing Services, People with Disabilities, Public Health, Research/Studies Institutes, Single-Disease Health Associations, Substance Abuse. **Geo. Dist:** AR; KS; MO; NM; OK; TX.


**Jackson Hole Preserve**
*See:* Entry 392


**Jay and Betty Van Andel Foundation**
*See:* Entry 402


**★ 11397 ★ The John L. Weinberg Foundation**
375 Park Ave., Ste. 1002
New York, NY 10152-1099

**Phone:** (212)902-8555          **Fax:** (212)888-7559
John Weinberg, Contact

**Fnded:** 1959. **Philosophy:** The John L. Weinberg Foundation primarily supports hospitals and university-level education. Other areas of interest include civic affairs, the arts, and social services. **Priorities:** *Arts & Humanities:* 56%. Supports libraries, museums, public broadcasting, and historic preservation. *Civic & Public Affairs:* 3%. Supports historic homes and parks. *Education:* 20%. Colleges and universities, minority education, private precollege education, arts and humanities education, and scholarship funds. *Environment:* 1%. Supports animal protection, food distribution programs, Young Men's Christian Association, United Way, and scouting. *International:* 17%. Supports hospital, medical centers, single disease health associations, and mental health. *Note:* Total contributions made in fiscal 2000. **Typ. Recipients:** AIDS/HIV, Cancer, Children's Health/Hospitals, Clinics/Medical Centers, Diabetes, Emergency/Ambulance Services, Geriatric Health, Health Funds, Hospitals, Medical Research, People with Disabilities, Single-Disease Health Associations, Substance Abuse. **Geo. Dist:** nationally; Greenwich, CT; New York, NY.


★ **11398** ★ **John M. Hopwood Charitable Trust**
PNC Bank
2 PNC Plaza, 25th Floor
620 Liberty Ave.
Pittsburgh, PA 15222-2705
**Phone:** (412)762-3502          **Fax:** (412)705-1043
**Email:** bruce.bickel@pncbank.com
Bruce Bickel, Senior Vice President and Manager

**Fnded:** 1948. **Philosophy:** Though the trust makes grants across the major categories of support, medical organizations its primary interest. In health services, interests include hospital foundations, health programs, and hospitals. Arts support favors museums, libraries, festivals, theater, and other performing arts. Support for education includes giving to colleges, universities, and private schools. Social service support goes to united funds, community centers, and community activities. The trust also places emphasis on environmental concerns. **Priorities:** *Arts & Humanities:* 4%. Supports performing arts, museums, art centers, and public broadcasting. *Civic & Public Affairs:* 12%. Gives to civic leagues, economic development, and housing. *Education:* 33%. Contributes to colleges, universities, private schools, education funds, scholarships, and literacy. *Environment:* 14%. Funds youth groups, Young Men's Christian Association, Big Brothers/Big Sisters, scouts, drug awareness and United Way. *International:* 27%. Supports hospitals and hospital associated foundations, mental health and single disease health associations. *Note:* Total contributions made in 2000. **Typ. Recipients:** Cancer, Children's Health/Hospitals, Clinics/Medical Centers, Domestic Violence, Emergency/Ambulance Services, Health Organizations, Hospices, Hospitals, Kidney, Long-Term Care, Medical Education, Medical Rehabilitation, Mental Health, Multiple Sclerosis, Nursing Services, People with Disabilities, Public Health, Single-Disease Health Associations, Speech & Hearing, Substance Abuse. **Geo. Dist:** PA, Western part of state.


★ **11399** ★ **John McShain Charities**
300 East Lancaster Ave., Ste. 200
Wynnewood, PA 19096-2105
**Fax:** (215)564-2343
Mary McShain, President

**Fnded:** 1949. **Philosophy:** The foundation's purpose is to make donations primarily to education, as well as to benefit Roman Catholic churches, religious organizations, and welfare funds. The foundation has also supported music, community organizations, and hospitals. **Priorities:** *Arts & Humanities:* 1%. Supports museums, libraries and a fine arts committee. *Civic & Public Affairs:* 2%. Supports community foundations. *Education:* 72%. Emphasis on secondary and preparatory schools, colleges, and universities. *Environment:* 1%. Funds human services. *International:* 1%. Supports hospitals. *Note:* Total contributions made in

fiscal 1999. **Typ. Recipients:** AIDS/HIV, Clinics/Medical Centers, Health Organizations, Hospitals, Long-Term Care, People with Disabilities. **Geo. Dist:** some grants nationally; Philadelphia, PA, some national grants.


**John P. Murphy Foundation**
*See:* Entry 424


★ **11400** ★ **John R. McCune Charitable Trust**
PO Box 1749
Pittsburgh, PA 15230
**Phone:** (412)644-7796          **Fax:** (412)644-8059
James Edwards, Executive Director

**Fnded:** 1972. **Philosophy:** The trust primarily provides grants to health-care institutions, institutions of secondary and higher education, and social service agencies. The trust does not make pledges beyond one year. The majority of the trust's grants are awarded to institutions or agencies located in western Pennsylvania. **Priorities:** *Arts & Humanities:* 1%. Supports arts councils. *Civic & Public Affairs:* 6%. Primarily for community foundations and development, and training centers. *Education:* 34%. Supports colleges, universities, and pre-college education. and scholarships. *Environment:* 25%. Funds children's centers, YMCAs, youth groups, animal protection senior concerns,and food banks. *International:* 20%. Gives to hospitals, health care centers, medical research, and Alzheimers. *Note:* Total contributions made in fiscal 1999. **Typ. Recipients:** Alzheimers Disease, Child Abuse, Children's Health/Hospitals, Children's Health/Hospitals, Clinics/Medical Centers, Diabetes, Health Funds, Health Organizations, Hospitals, Medical Research, Mental Health, Multiple Sclerosis, People with Disabilities, Prenatal Health Issues, Public Health, Research/Studies Institutes, Single-Disease Health Associations, Substance Abuse, Transplant Networks/Donor Banks. **Geo. Dist:** Pittsburgh, PA, including western Pennsylvania.


★ **11401** ★ **John Stauffer Charitable Trust**
301 North Lake Ave., 10th Floor
Pasadena, CA 91101-4108
**Phone:** (626)793-9400          **Fax:** (626)793-5900
Mr. H. Senecal, Trustee

**Fnded:** 1974. **Philosophy:** The trust is limited to supporting colleges, universities, and hospitals. Giving to colleges and universities emphasizes efforts to acquire and erect buildings and other facilities; obtain equipment, instruments, books, and furnishings; and provide scholarships, fellowships, and professorships that specifically target science and chemistry. Support to hospitals is more limited and goes toward acquiring land, erecting buildings and other facilities, and obtaining equipment, instruments, and furnishings. The trust prefers to give grants to institutions that maintain balanced operating budgets and avoid deficit financing. The trustees encourage the use of plaques to memorialize the name of John Stauffer. **Priorities:** *Education:* 37%. Primarily supports colleges and universities. *International:* 63%. Supports hospitals. *Note:* Total contributions made in fiscal 1999. **Typ. Recipients:** Cancer, Children's Health/Hospitals, Clinics/Medical Centers, Emergency/Ambulance Services, Family Planning, Health Organizations, Heart, Hospitals, Medical Rehabilitation, Medical Research, Mental Health, Outpatient Health Care, People with Disabilities, Public Health, Substance Abuse. **Geo. Dist:** CA.


**Joseph Alexander Foundation**
*See:* Entry 435


★ **11402** ★ **Joseph Meyerhoff Fund**
25 S Charles St.
Ste. 2100
Baltimore, MD 21201
**Phone:** (410)727-3200          **Fax:** (410)727-3207
**Email:** tmr@magnajm.com
Ms. Terry Rubenstein, Executive Director

**Fnded:** 1953. **Philosophy:** The fund supports a wide variety of charitable organizations. Jewish religious organizations are favored along with the Baltimore Symphony Orchestra and Jewish historical preservation societies. Peace initiatives and interests in Israel also are major interests. A range of educational support is also given by the fund. **Priorities:** *Arts & Humanities:* 16%. Funds the symphony orchestra, public broadcasting, libraries, performing arts and the B&O Railroad Museum. *Civic & Public Affairs:* 3%. Funds parks, civic and community affairs. *Education:* 4%. Funds colleges, universities, and educational programs. *Environment:* 1%. Funds community services. *International:* 4%. Funds the Sinai Hospital Department for Development. *Religion:* 5%. *Note:* Contributions were made in 1998. **Typ. Recipients:** Hospitals, Speech & Hearing. **Geo. Dist:** Baltimore, MD; New York, NY.


**Josiah W. and Bessie H. Kline Foundation**
*See:* Entry 440


**Joyce Mertz-Gilmore Foundation**
*See:* Entry 11690


**Julius Frankel Foundation**
*See:* Entry 443


**June Rockwell Levy Foundation**
*See:* Entry 444


**Kresge Foundation**
*See:* Entry 459


★ **11403** ★ **L. G. Balfour Foundation**
c/o Fleet National Bank
75 State St., 7th Floor
Mail Code: MABOFO7B
Boston, MA 02109
**Phone:** (617)346-2484          **Fax:** (617)346-2495
**Email:** rebecca.mcdade@harrisbank.com
**Website:** http://www.kresge.org
Kerry Sullivan, Director, Grants

**Fnded:** 1973. **Philosophy:** L. G. Balfour built his fortune through his long association with educational institutions. His foundation reflects this by giving primarily to programs designed to improve access to education for all potentially qualified students. The foundation funds various scholarship programs and is particularly interested in supporting programs designed to eliminate barriers to education for capable but financially needy students, especially minorities. The foundation concentrates on programs carried out by qualified charitable institutions in Massachusetts and the New England area. The foundation will consider proposals for any charitable purpose in Attleboro, MA, or the surrounding area. Primary consideration, however, will be given to the educational and medical needs of the community. In addition to the competitive grant programs described above, the foundation funds a scholarship program for L. G. Balfour Company employees and provides grants to specific educational, fraternal, and medical institutions named by L. G. Balfour before his death. **Priorities:** *Education:* 100%. Supports various programs for students in New England, especially minorities or youth with a financial need. **Typ. Recipients:** Hospitals. **Geo. Dist:** New England area; MA.


**Lannan Foundation**
*See:* Entry 5467


★ **11404** ★ **Laura Moore Cunningham Foundation**
510 Main St.
Boise, ID 83702
**Phone:** (208)365-2512
**Email:** jo@lannan.org

**Website:** http://www.lannan.org
Harry Bettis, Contact

**Fnded:** 1964. **Philosophy:** The Laura Moore Cunningham Foundation is primarily interested in providing business scholarships through educational institutions located in Idaho. The foundation also contributes to several Idaho hospitals. In addition, the foundation awards various smaller grants to support social services, civic organizations, and the arts. **Priorities:** *Arts & Humanities:* 13%. Public broadcasting, museums, music, and arts festivals. *Civic & Public Affairs:* 5%. Supports fire department. *Education:* 47%. Primarily to colleges and universities for scholarship funding. *Environment:* 20%. Supports homes, family planning, and programs for seniors. *International:* 6%. Supports medical centers and emergency services. *Note:* Total contributions made in fiscal 1999. **Typ. Recipients:** Child Abuse, Children's Health/Hospitals, Clinics/Medical Centers, Emergency/Ambulance Services, Family Planning, Health Organizations, Health-General, Heart, Hospices, Hospitals, Hospitals (University Affiliated), Long-Term Care, Medical Education, Nursing Services, People with Disabilities, Prenatal Health Issues, Single-Disease Health Associations. **Geo. Dist:** ID.


**Longwood Foundation**
*See:* Entry 476


**★ 11405 ★ Louis and Harold Price Foundation**
450 Park Ave., Ste. 1102
New York, NY 10022-2605
**Phone:** (212)753-0240          **Fax:** (212)752-9338
**Email:** grantinquiry@pricefoundation.org
**Website:** http://www.pricefoundation.org
Timothy Jones, President

**Fnded:** 1951. **Philosophy:** The foundation supports a business institute, Jewish welfare funds, hospitals, community funds, and higher education, including scholarship funds. Grants also are given to youth agencies, camps for children, temple support, medical research, the arts, and services for the blind and other disabled persons. The foundation responds more favorably to proposals from organizations in California, Colorado and New York. **Priorities:** *Arts & Humanities:* 6%. *Civic & Public Affairs:* 13%. *Education:* 32%. Includes a large grant to the Price Institute for Entrepreneurial Studies. *Environment:* 11%. Supports community services, child welfare, and programs for the disabled. *International:* 35%. Funds hospitals, medical research, mental health, and single-disease health organizations. *Note:* Total contributions made in 2000. **Typ. Recipients:** AIDS/HIV, Alzheimers Disease, Arthritis, Cancer, Children's Health/Hospitals, Clinics/Medical Centers, Emergency/Ambulance Services, Eyes/Blindness, Health Funds, Health Organizations, Health-General, Heart, Hospitals, Kidney, Long-Term Care, Medical Rehabilitation, Medical Research, Mental Health, Multiple Sclerosis, Outpatient Health Care, People with Disabilities, Research/Studies Institutes, Single-Disease Health Associations. **Geo. Dist:** Los Angeles, CA, including the metropolitan area; New York, NY, including the metropolitan area.


**Louise H. and David S. Ingalls Foundation**
*See:* Entry 482


**Lucius N. Littauer Foundation**
*See:* Entry 485


**Lutheran Brotherhood Foundation**
*See:* Entry 487


**Marion I. and Henry J. Knott Foundation**
*See:* Entry 504


**Marion O. and Maximilian E. Hoffman Foundation**
*See:* Entry 505


**★ 11406 ★ Marmot Foundation**
100 West 10TH St., Ste. 1109
Wilmington, DE 19801-1694
**Phone:** (302)998-5195
**Email:** knott@knottfoundation.org
**Website:** http://www.knottfoundation.org
Charles Gummey, Contact

**Fnded:** 1968. **Philosophy:** The foundation's primary focus is social service organizations, including united funds and community center support. Youth organizations are also a major priority. The trustees are also interested in education, from day schools to high schools to the university level. Health services are considered a secondary interest, with most support going directly to hospitals. **Priorities:** *Arts & Humanities:* 12%. Supports Bear Library and Winterthur Museum. *Civic & Public Affairs:* 12%. Supports civic and community affairs. *Education:* 19%. Supports educational insitutions and programs. *Environment:* 21%. Supports United Way, children and family services, planned parenthood, and senior citizen services. *International:* 29%. Supports hospitals, hospice, medical centers, disease and disorder concerns. *Religion:* 1%. Supports the South Florida Science Museum. *Note:* Contributions were made in 1998. **Typ. Recipients:** Arthritis, Cancer, Children's Health/Hospitals, Clinics/Medical Centers, Diabetes, Emergency/Ambulance Services, Eyes/Blindness, Family Planning, Health Funds, Health Organizations, Heart, Hospices, Hospitals, Hospitals (University Affiliated), Medical Education, Mental Health, Outpatient Health Care, People with Disabilities, Preventive Medicine/Wellness Organizations, Public Health, Research/Studies Institutes, Substance Abuse, Trauma Treatment. **Geo. Dist:** DE; FL.


**Marshall L. and Perrine D. McCune Charitable Foundation**
*See:* Entry 5558


**★ 11407 ★ Mary J. Hutchins Foundation**
45 John St.
New York, NY 10038
**Phone:** (212)964-3859
**Email:** fsowers@swcp.com
**Website:** http://www.nmmccune.org
Richard Mirabella, Vice President

**Fnded:** 1935. **Philosophy:** The Mary J. Hutchins Foundation primarily supports health care and social service organizations. Health support goes to general and specialty hospitals. Nursing also is supported. Social service support favors homes and shelters, charity and welfare organizations, and youth clubs. Civic affairs agencies are supported on a limited basis. The foundation also endeavors to provide aid to poor and needy adults regardless of age, race, and creed. **Priorities:** *Arts & Humanities:* 2%. Supports visual arts. *Civic & Public Affairs:* 5%. Suppports foundations and philanthropic organizations. *Education:* 2%. The Summit Speech School received support. *Environment:* 36%. Youth clubs, homes, scouting, family planning services, and United Way. *International:* 38%. Hospitals and medical centers, hospice, visiting nurses, and Multiple Sclerosis. *Note:* Total contributions made in 1999. **Typ. Recipients:** Clinics/Medical Centers, Emergency/Ambulance Services, Eyes/Blindness, Family Planning, Hospices, Hospitals, Hospitals (University Affiliated), Medical Rehabilitation, Medical Research, Mental Health, Multiple Sclerosis, Nursing Services, People with Disabilities, Sexual Abuse, Single-Disease Health Associations. **Geo. Dist:** New York, NY.


**Massey Foundation**
*See:* Entry 518


**★ 11408 ★ Millbrook Tribute Garden**
PO Box AC
Millbrook, NY 12545
**Phone:** (845)677-3434
Kathy Shanks, Trustee

**Fnded:** 1943. **Philosophy:** The Millbrook Tribute Garden makes grants across the major categories of support. Educational support favors Millbrook's private schools. Religious support goes to individual churches and religious welfare. Health care interests include hospitals. **Priorities:** *Arts & Humanities:* 8%. Supports a library and the performing arts. *Civic & Public Affairs:* 3%. Supports community development, botanical gardens and a horticultural society. *Education:* 30%. Supports secondary and preparatory schools, colleges, and universities. *Environment:* 22%. Supports youth services, senior citizens services, volunteer services, and planned parenthood. *International:* 10%. Supports hospitals and centers for women with AIDS. *Note:* Total contributions made in fiscal 1998. **Typ. Recipients:** AIDS/HIV, Family Planning, Hospices, Hospitals, Medical Rehabilitation. **Geo. Dist:** Millbrook, NY, and vicinity.


**Monterey Fund**
*See:* Entry 5561


**Nicholas H. Noyes, Jr. Memorial Foundation**
*See:* Entry 14913


**★ 11409 ★ O'Donnell Foundation**
100 Crescent Court, Ste. 1660
Dallas, TX 75201
**Phone:** (214)871-5800          **Fax:** (214)855-8988
**Email:** admin@noyesfoundation.org
**Website:** http://www.noyesfoundation.org
Carolyn Bacon, Executive Director

**Fnded:** 1957. **Philosophy:** The foundation's primary focus is on education, especially science and engineering. It also funds civic and public affairs organizations, medical centers, and the arts. **Priorities:** *Arts & Humanities:* 1%. Funds art museums. *Civic & Public Affairs:* 1%. Supports other foundations. *Education:* 96%. Supports public primary and secondary schools in Texas. Major building grant to University of Texas at Austin. *Environment:* 1%. Supports Life Sciences Research Foundation. *Religion:* 1%. Supports science research. *Note:* Total contributions made in fiscal 1999. **Typ. Recipients:** Clinics/Medical Centers, Hospitals (University Affiliated), Medical Education, Respiratory. **Geo. Dist:** TX.


**★ 11410 ★ Offield Family Foundation**
400 North Michigan Ave., Room 407
Chicago, IL 60611
**Phone:** (312)467-5480          **Fax:** (312)467-0473
Marie Larson, Secretary

**Fnded:** 1940. **Philosophy:** The foundation supports a wide variety of charitable organizations. Most of the support goes to civic affairs, including conservation issues and women's affairs. Health is also a major priority, mainly supporting hospitals. Public broadcasting and family planning are consistently supported, while public education remains a minor interest. **Priorities:** *Arts & Humanities:* 19%. Cultural parks, arts centers, and public broadcasting. *Civic & Public Affairs:* 10%. Women's resources, clubs, and community foundations. *Education:* 8%. Public precollege education, colleges, and universities. *Environment:* 15%. Planned Parenthood, youth clubs, and food banks. *International:* 14%. Medical centers, burn centers, and hospitals. *Note:* Contributions made in fiscal 1998. **Typ. Recipients:** Cancer, Children's Health/Hospitals, Clinics/Medical Centers, Emergency/Ambulance Services, Family Planning, Health Funds, Health Organizations, Hospices, Hospitals, Hospitals (University Affiliated), Medical Education, Medical Research, People with Disabilities, Public Health, Substance Abuse, Transplant Networks/Donor Banks, Trauma Treatment. **Geo. Dist:** nationally.

**Overbrook Foundation**
*See:* Entry 573

**Park Foundation**
*See:* Entry 10052

**Pauline Allen Gill Foundation**
*See:* Entry 579

**Philip L. Van Every Foundation**
*See:* Entry 590

**Philip M. McKenna Foundation**
*See:* Entry 591

**Prospect Hill Foundation**
*See:* Entry 598

**Raymond John Wean Foundation**
*See:* Entry 609

**★ 11411 ★ Reeves Foundation (OH)**
PO Box 441
Dover, OH 44622-0441
**Phone:** (330)364-4660
**Email:** RJWeanFdn@aol.com
**Website:** http://www.fdncenter.org/grantmaker/prospecthill
Don Ulrich, Executive Director
**Fnded:** 1966. **Philosophy:** Foundation interests include hospitals, historic preservation, municipalities, and educational projects. The foundation will also fund other recipient areas. **Priorities:** *Arts & Humanities:* 27%. Supports libraries, public broadcasting, and historic preservation. *Civic & Public Affairs:* 18%. Supports towns/municipalities, parks/gardens, safety, and community foundations. *Education:* 17%. Supports scholarships, educational funds, religious education, and schools. *Environment:* 4%. Supports counseling, family services, Young Men's Christian Association, and emergency relief. *International:* 25%. Supports hospital, cancer research, and health organizations. *Note:* Total contributions made in 1998. **Typ. Recipients:** Alzheimers Disease, Cancer, Children's Health/Hospitals, Clinics/Medical Centers, Emergency/Ambulance Services, Hospices, Hospitals, Hospitals, People with Disabilities, Public Health. **Geo. Dist:** OH, Tuscarawas County.

**Robert R. Young Foundation**
*See:* Entry 629

**Robert Russell Memorial Foundation**
*See:* Entry 630

**Rosamond Gifford Charitable Corp.**
*See:* Entry 640

**★ 11412 ★ Rowland Foundation**
PO Box 13
Cambridge, MA 02238
**Phone:** (617)497-4634          **Fax:** (617)497-4627
**Email:** christmas@rowland.org
**Website:** http://www.giffordfd.org
Dr. Philip DuBois, President
**Fnded:** 1960. **Philosophy:** The foundation primarily funds "academic institutions, social welfare, hospitals, museums, conservation, historical associations, medical research, and the arts." **Priorities:** *Civic & Public Affairs:* 5%. Funds community foundations. *Education:* 5%. Supports universities. *Religion:* 90%. Major support is awarded to the Rowland Institute for science. *Note:* Total contributions made in 1998. **Typ. Recipients:** Cancer, Children's Health/Hospitals, Eyes/Blindness, Family Planning, Health Funds, Health Organizations, Heart, Hospitals, Medical Education, Medical Rehabilitation, Medical Research, People with

Disabilities, Single-Disease Health Associations. **Geo. Dist:** primarily New England.

**Samuel Rubin Foundation**
*See:* Entry 657

**Sapirstein-Stone-Weiss Foundation**
*See:* Entry 660

**Seymour H. Knox Foundation**
*See:* Entry 675

**Shubert Foundation**
*See:* Entry 678

**★ 11413 ★ Sidney J. Weinberg, Jr. Foundation**
Tax Department, 30th Fl.
85 Broad St.
New York, NY 10004
**Phone:** (212)902-1000
**Email:** kbojw@aol.com
**Website:** http://www.samuelrubinfoundation.org
Sydney Weinberg, Jr., Trustee
**Fnded:** 1979. **Philosophy:** The foundation makes most of its grants in the areas of health care, education, and civic affairs. Health care funding favors hospitals, cancer research, pediatrics, and single disease associations. Funding in education emphasizes colleges, universities, and business education. Support for civic affairs goes to the Carnegie Institute in Washington, DC, and economic development. The foundation also will fund the arts, religion, and social services. **Priorities:** *Arts & Humanities:* 8%. *Civic & Public Affairs:* 3%. *Education:* 57%. Precollege private education, colleges and universities, and business education. *Environment:* About 1%. *International:* 3%. Hospitals, Cystic Fibrosis research, aging research, and medical centers. *Religion:* 23%. Carnegie Institution and oceanography. *Note:* Total contributions made in fiscal 1999. **Typ. Recipients:** Cancer, Children's Health/Hospitals, Clinics/Medical Centers, Emergency/Ambulance Services, Family Planning, Geriatric Health, Health Funds, Health Organizations, Health-General, Heart, Hospices, Hospitals, Hospitals (University Affiliated), Medical Education, Medical Research, Mental Health, Nursing Services, People with Disabilities, Preventive Medicine/Wellness Organizations, Single-Disease Health Associations, Substance Abuse. **Geo. Dist:** nationally; New York, NY.

**★ 11414 ★ Skirball Foundation**
767 Fifth Ave., 50th Floor
New York, NY 10153
**Phone:** (212)832-8500          **Fax:** (212)593-6241
Martin Blackman, President & Trustee
**Fnded:** 1950. **Philosophy:** The Skirball Foundation has had close ties with Hebrew Union College and the University of Southern California. The Skirballs helped fund the Hubbard Chair in British History, in honor of USC president emeritus John Hubbard. Mr. Skirball, a member and vice chairman of the board of governors at Hebrew Union College, was actively involved in the college's decision to accept then USC president Norman Topping's invitation to the college to locate its Los Angeles campus adjacent to the University The Skirball Cancer Pharmacology Laboratory is part of a major addition to the Kenneth Norris Jr. Cancer Hospital and Research Institute that opened in late 1991 on USC's Health Sciences Campus. The foundation is also a supporter of the arts and created the Skirball Museum at Hebrew Union College, one of the world's finest museums of Jewish culture. The Skirball Center serves biblical scholars, archaeologists, and students of biblical and ancient Near Eastern history, and preserves and exhibits the findings of excavations. The fund will also make possible a research and fellowships award program for study in the archaeology of the ancient Near East. **Priorities:** *Education:* 30%. Supports colleges and universities and religious education. *International:* 17%. Focus on medical re-

search, and single-disease health associations. *Note:* Total contributions made in 1998. **Typ. Recipients:** Arthritis, Cancer, Children's Health/Hospitals, Clinics/Medical Centers, Eyes/Blindness, Geriatric Health, Health Organizations, Health-General, Heart, Hospitals, Long-Term Care, Medical Education, Medical Education, Medical Research, People with Disabilities, Research/Studies Institutes, Single-Disease Health Associations, Speech & Hearing, Substance Abuse. **Geo. Dist:** Los Angeles, CA; New York, NY; Cincinnati, OH.

**South Texas Charitable Foundation**
*See:* Entry 690

**Starr Foundation**
*See:* Entry 697

**★ 11415 ★ Statler Foundation**
107 Delaware Ave., Ste. 680
Buffalo, NY 14202
**Phone:** (716)852-1104          **Fax:** (716)852-3968
**Email:** grants@starrfoundation.org
**Website:** http://fdncenter.org/grantmaker/starr/
Carlo Perfetto, Chairman, Scholarship Committee
**Fnded:** 1934. **Philosophy:** Following the interests of Mr. Statler, the foundation supports education, training, and research in the hotel and food industry. It contributes to educational institutions that teach hotel and food management, and food preparation. Its main emphasis is on scholarships. **Priorities:** *Civic & Public Affairs:* 2%. *Education:* 89%. Includes universities and scholarships. *Environment:* 3%. Supports construction, training and renovations. *Note:* Total contributions made in 1998. **Typ. Recipients:** Children's Health/Hospitals, Hospitals. **Geo. Dist:** internationally; nationally; NY.

**Steele-Reese Foundation**
*See:* Entry 699

**★ 11416 ★ Sunderland Foundation**
PO Box 25900
Overland Park, KS 66225
**Phone:** (913)451-8900          **Fax:** (913)319-6191
**Email:** sunderlandfoundation@ashgrove.com
**Website:** http://www.sunderlandfoundation.org
James Sunderland, President
**Fnded:** 1945. **Philosophy:** The foundation primarily supports education, with emphasis on colleges and universities in the Midwest. Secondary interests include the arts, civic affairs, social services, religion, and hospitals. **Priorities:** *Arts & Humanities:* 20%. Museums, music, historical preservation, and art programs for youth. *Civic & Public Affairs:* 6%. Community and foundation grants, mostly in the Kansas City, Missouri area. *Education:* 36%. Colleges and universities, mainly in Missouri, Kansas, and Nebraska. *Environment:* 22%. Scouting, 4-H programs, children's homes, and YMCAs. *International:* 9%. Children's health and hospitals, the American Red Cross, and arthritis research. *Note:* Total contributions made in 1999. **Typ. Recipients:** Cancer, Children's Health/Hospitals, Clinics/Medical Centers, Domestic Violence, Eyes/Blindness, Family Planning, Health Organizations, Hospitals, Mental Health, People with Disabilities, Research/Studies Institutes. **Geo. Dist:** AR; KS; MO; NE.

**Teagle Foundation**
*See:* Entry 716

**Thelma Doelger Charitable Trust**
*See:* Entry 719

**Theodore H. Barth Foundation**
*See:* Entry 720

**★ 11417 ★ Theresa and Edward O'Toole Foundation**
1290 Ave. of the Americas, 5th Fl.
New York, NY 10104
**Phone:** (212)635-1520
Peter McDermott, Contact
**Fnded:** 1971. **Philosophy:** The foundation is primarily interested in supporting Catholic churches and organizations. Some educational support goes to Catholic unions, universities, and schools. **Priorities:** *Education:* 46%. Primarily supports religious secondary schools and colleges. *Environment:* 1%. Shelters, food distribution. *International:* 12%. Supports hospitals, medical centers and programs. *Note:* Total contributions made in fiscal 1999. **Typ. Recipients:** Cancer, Clinics/Medical Centers, Health Organizations, Hospitals, Long-Term Care. **Geo. Dist:** nationally; NJ; NY.

**Thomas and Agnes Carvel Foundation**
*See:* Entry 722

**Thomas Anthony Pappas Charitable Foundation**
*See:* Entry 723

**Thomas J. Emery Memorial**
*See:* Entry 726

**★ 11418 ★ Timken Foundation of Canton**
200 Market Ave, North, Ste. 210
Canton, OH 44702-1437
**Phone:** (330)452-1144          **Fax:** (330)452-2306
**Email:** dickesd@timkenfoundation.org
Don Dickes, Secretary & Treasurer
**Fnded:** 1934. **Philosophy:** The foundation allocates major support for charitable organizations that will benefit the citizens in local areas, in the United States, Australia, Canada, France, Italy, Poland, Romania, South Africa, England, Germany, and Brazil where the Timken Company has manufacturing facilities. **Priorities:** *Arts & Humanities:* 7%. Makes donations to museums, art centers, and public libraries. *Education:* 45%. Funds colleges and universities and precollege education. *Environment:* 13%. Supports YMCAs, youth groups, and women's concerns. *International:* 11%. *Note:* Total contributions made in fiscal 1999. **Typ. Recipients:** Cancer, Clinics/Medical Centers, Domestic Violence, Emergency/Ambulance Services, Geriatric Health, Heart, Hospitals, Medical Education, Substance Abuse. **Geo. Dist:** internationally; national; operating locations; OH.

**Tozer Foundation**
*See:* Entry 730

**★ 11419 ★ Weezie Foundation**
345 Park Ave.
New York, NY 10019
**Phone:** (212)464-2744
Irina Shea, Contact
**Fnded:** 1961. **Philosophy:** The Weezie Foundation makes most of its grants in the areas of social services and education. Social service funding favors employment and job training and youth organizations. Funding for education goes to private schools and specialty colleges. The foundation also supports hospitals as a secondary interest. Other support areas are funded on a limited basis. **Priorities:** *Civic & Public Affairs:* 17%. Support community associations, Pittsburgh Zoo, libraries and MA Horticultural Society. *Education:* 50%. Provides supports to Massachusetts elementary schools and academies. *Environment:* 11%. Funds youth and family services. *International:* 13%. Supports local hospital and physical therapy program. *Religion:* 8%. Provides funding for the Cold Spring Harbor Laboratory. *Note:* Total contributions made in 1998. **Typ. Recipients:** Clinics/Medical Centers, Eyes/Blindness, Hospitals, Hospitals (University Affiliated), Medical Education, Medical Rehabilitation, Mental Health, People with Disabilities, Substance Abuse. **Geo. Dist:** Northeastern USA.

**Whitehall Foundation**
*See:* Entry 756

**★ 11420 ★ Wilbur May Foundation**
2716 Ocean Park Blvd, Ste. 2011
Santa Monica, CA 90405
**Phone:** (310)314-2400          **Fax:** (310)314-2401
**Email:** Email@Whitehall.org
**Website:** http://www.whitehall.org
Mary Turner, Section
**Fnded:** 1948. **Philosophy:** The foundation focuses its giving on programs for the young and hospitals. **Priorities:** *Arts & Humanities:* 2%. Supports libraries, music, and film & video. *Civic & Public Affairs:* 3%. Supports community foundations and clubs. *Education:* About 41%. Supports colleges and universities, scholarships, and education associations. *Environment:* 26%. Emphasis on parks and recreation, child welfare, youth organizations, scouts, Young Men's Christian Association, United Way, and camps. *International:* About 28%. Focus on an eye institute, single-disease health associations, and hospitals. *Note:* Total contributions made in fiscal 1997. **Typ. Recipients:** AIDS/HIV, Cancer, Child Abuse, Children's Health/Hospitals, Children's Health/Hospitals, Clinics/Medical Centers, Diabetes, Eyes/Blindness, Health Organizations, Heart, Hospitals, Medical Education, Medical Rehabilitation, Medical Research, People with Disabilities, Prenatal Health Issues, Public Health, Research/Studies Institutes, Respiratory, Single-Disease Health Associations, Substance Abuse. **Geo. Dist:** CA, Southern California; Los Angeles, CA; Reno, NV.

**William K. Warren Foundation**
*See:* Entry 772

**William T. Kemper Charitable Trust**
*See:* Entry 778

**William T. Morris Foundation**
*See:* Entry 780

**Woods Fund of Chicago**
*See:* Entry 784

**Zemurray Foundation**
*See:* Entry 792

## Corporate Foundations

**A.O. Smith Foundation, Inc.**
*See:* Entry 793

**Advanced Micro Devices, Inc.**
*See:* Entry 799

**AEGON U.S.A. Charitable Foundation**
*See:* Entry 800

**Agrilink Foods/Pro-Fac Foundation**
*See:* Entry 804

**Allianz Life Insurance Co. of North America**
*See:* Entry 817

**America West Airlines Foundation**
*See:* Entry 822

**Ameritech Michigan**
*See:* Entry 2893

**AMP Foundation**
*See:* Entry 835

**Amsted Industries Foundation**
*See:* Entry 837

**AOL Time Warner Foundation**
*See:* Entry 5569

**Baltimore Gas & Electric Foundation**
*See:* Entry 862

**Bank of Hawaii Charitable Foundation**
*See:* Entry 866

**Bank of New York Co., Inc.**
*See:* Entry 868

**Bank One, Texas-Houston Office**
*See:* Entry 869

**BD**
*See:* Entry 879

**★ 11421 ★ Belk Foundation**
2801 West Tyvola Rd.
Charlotte, NC 28217-4500
**Phone:** (704)357-1000          **Fax:** (704)357-1883
**Email:** Malinda.B.Small@constellation.com
**Website:** http://www.bd.com/responsibility/
Paul Wyche, Jr., Trustee
**Fnded:** 1988. **Priorities:** *Arts & Humanities:* 8%. Interests include museums and the performing arts. *Civic & Public Affairs:* 3%. Supports community-oriented organizations. *Education:* 63%. More than three-fourths generally supports colleges and universities in North Carolina, South Carolina, and Georgia. Other interests include child care, education funds, economic education, and precollege public education. *Environment:* 12%. More than one-fourth supports united funds. Remaining funds support recreation, youth organizations, and family planning. *International:* 8%. Grants support building funds at North Carolina hospitals. *Note:* Total contributions in fiscal 1999. **Typ. Recipients:** Arthritis, Cancer, Children's Health/Hospitals, Emergency/Ambulance Services, Family Planning, Health Funds, Health Organizations, Heart, Hospitals, Hospitals (University Affiliated), Medical Education, Medical Rehabilitation, Substance Abuse. **Geo. Dist:** GA; NC; SC.

**Belo Foundation**
*See:* Entry 882

**Berwind Group**
*See:* Entry 885

**Boise Cascade Corp.**
*See:* Entry 8547

**Boler Co. Foundation**
*See:* Entry 10061

**Bourns Foundation**
*See:* Entry 898

**Bowater Inc.**
*See:* Entry 899

**★ 11422 ★ Brown Shoe Co. Charitable Trust**
c/o Suntrust Bank, Atlanta
PO Box 4655
Atlanta, GA 30302
**Phone:** (314)854-4000
**Email:** tmalecek@brownshoe.com

**Website:** http://www.bowater.com
Thomas G. Malecek, Secretary, Board of Control

**Priorities:** *Arts & Humanities:* 18%. Funds symphony and opera societies in the St. Louis, MO, area. Other interests include public broadcasting, historic preservation, art museums, and theater. Matches employee gifts to cultural organizations. *Civic & Public Affairs:* 12%. Interests include botanical gardens, housing, zoos, the environment, and economic development. *Education:* 10%. Primarily supports private colleges and universities with degree programs. Recipients also include minority college funds and seminaries. Matches employee gifts to private colleges and universities. *Environment:* 55%. Primarily supports united funds and youth organizations. Also supports recreation and athletics and community service organizations. *Note:* Total foundation contributions made in 2000. **Typ. Recipients:** Alzheimers Disease, Children's Health/Hospitals, Domestic Violence, Emergency/Ambulance Services, Eyes/Blindness, Hospitals, Medical Research, Multiple Sclerosis, People with Disabilities, Prenatal Health Issues, Preventive Medicine/Wellness Organizations. **Geo. Dist:** principally near operating locations and to national organizations; St. Louis, MO.


**Bucyrus-Erie Foundation**
*See:* Entry 907


★ 11423 ★ **Burlington Industries Foundation**
PO Box 21207
Greensboro, NC 27420-1207
**Phone:** (336)379-2303          **Fax:** (336)379-4504
**Email:** windham.dick@burlington.com
C. Windham, Executive Director

**Priorities:** *Arts & Humanities:* 4%. Contributions primarily channeled through local arts councils. Interests include museums, libraries, music, and public broadcasting. *Civic & Public Affairs:* 2%. Supports programs that benefit employees and the community, with interests in environmental concerns; civil rights; law and justice; economic development; safety; and business and free enterprise. *Education:* 53%. Primarily supports colleges and universities located in areas where there is a high concentration of employees and from which the company recruits. Interests include textiles-related education, and technological, engineering, and business education. Education associations and funds, public secondary education, university libraries, economic, arts, fashion design, and math education all receive funding. Grants in this field, awarded in the Southeast and nationally, generally range between $1,000 and $10,000. *Environment:* 29%. Primarily supports united funds and youth organizations. Interests also include crime and delinquency prevention, employment, and community service organizations. Also supports organizations where employees volunteer. *International:* 5%. Supports local hospitals, generally preferring capital projects rather than operating expenses. Also supports local health care facilities in operating locations. Generally does not support other health-related organizations. *Voluntarism:* Company does not have a formal employee volunteer program, but it provides meeting space on the premises or time off to individual employees who volunteer for Junior Achievement. Company also sponsors two Red Cross Blood Drives annually. *Note:* Total contributions in fiscal 1999. **Typ. Recipients:** AIDS/HIV, Children's Health/Hospitals, Clinics/Medical Centers, Emergency/Ambulance Services, Health Organizations, Hospices, Hospitals, Multiple Sclerosis, Outpatient Health Care, People with Disabilities, Preventive Medicine/Wellness Organizations, Respiratory, Single-Disease Health Associations, Substance Abuse. **Geo. Dist:** principally near operating locations and to national organizations; NC; SC; VA.


★ 11424 ★ **Burlington Resources Foundation**
5051 Westheimer, Ste. 1400
Houston, TX 77056-5604
**Phone:** (817)347-2000
Gavin Smith, President

**Priorities:** *Arts & Humanities:* 6%. Interests include theater, performing arts, visual arts, and other related activities. *Civic & Public Affairs:* 1%. Supports affordable housing, zoos, municipalities, and crime prevention. *Education:* 63%. Gives to colleges and universities, with priority given to technical colleges and educational programs and mining education. Grants of an exceptional nature may be made to vocational and noncollege schools. Also matches employee gifts to institutions of higher learning. *Environment:* 11%. Primarily supports child welfare, youth camps and organizations, services for the disabled, community service organizations, and athletics/recreation programs. *International:* 9%. Supports hospitals, cancer and heart centers, hospices, pregnancy centers, and single-disease health associations. *Religion:* 2%. Gives to the Houston Museum of Natural Science. *Note:* Total foundation contributions made in 2000. **Typ. Recipients:** Alzheimers Disease, Child Abuse, Children's Health/Hospitals, Emergency/Ambulance Services, Heart, Hospices, Medical Research, Nursing Services, People with Disabilities, Prenatal Health Issues, Preventive Medicine/Wellness Organizations, Public Health, Single-Disease Health Associations.


**Carrier Corp.**
*See:* Entry 918


**CCB Foundation**
*See:* Entry 923


★ 11425 ★ **Century 21 Associates Foundation**
22 Cortlandt St.
New York, NY 10007
**Website:** http://www.utc.com/commun
Abraham Gindi, Trustee

**Fnded:** 1982. **Priorities:** *Education:* 2%. *Environment:* 1%. *International:* 12%. Funds medical centers, cancer research, hospitals, and other medical research. *Note:* Total contributions made in 1999. **Typ. Recipients:** Cancer, Diabetes, Hospitals, Hospitals (University Affiliated), Long-Term Care, People with Disabilities. **Geo. Dist:** NJ; NY.


★ 11426 ★ **Citigroup Foundation**
850 Third Ave., 13th Floor
New York, NY 10022
**Phone:** (212)559-9163          **Fax:** (212)793-5944
**Website:** http://www.citigroup.com
Paul Ostergard, Vice President, Director, Corporate Cont

**Priorities:** *Arts & Humanities:* 7%. Museums and performing arts groups receive significant support. Special interest in groups that encourage new talent and outreach programs that bring the arts to broad audiences, including public schools and the disadvantaged. Cultural support also includes historical preservation, libraries, public broadcasting, arts councils, zoos, botanical gardens, and arts education. Matches employee contributions to cultural groups. *Civic & Public Affairs:* 37%. Funds neighborhood development, including groups concerned with economic development and affordable housing. Increasing emphasis is on community development financial institutions. Also supports employment training, civic groups, nonprofit technical assistance, and groups concerned with urban issues. *Education:* 34%. Supports efforts to improve education at all levels. Increasing efforts on K-12 programs within inner-city schools; early childhood and public education; and programs that focus on equal access to quality education for minorities and women. Also interested in programs to prepare young people for employment. Supports organizations conducting research on free enterprise, economics, and public policy; graduate schools of business; and other institutions from which employees are recruited. Matches employees' gifts to education. *Environment:* 7%. Support goes largely to the United Way of the Tri-State Area. Other united funds in major operating locations also receive support. *International:* 10%. Focuses on education to prevent health problems and health care cost containment. *Voluntarism:* The corpo-

ration's volunteer incentive program provides up to $500 for organizations to which employees volunteer. *Note:* Contributions analysis based on Headquarters Program Grants for 1999. **Typ. Recipients:** Children's Health/Hospitals, Emergency/Ambulance Services, Health Organizations, Health Policy/Cost Containment, Hospices, Hospitals, Hospitals (University Affiliated), Medical Research, People with Disabilities, Single-Disease Health Associations, Substance Abuse, Transplant Networks/Donor Banks. **Geo. Dist:** headquarters and operating communities; New York, NY.


**Citizens Charitable Foundation**
*See:* Entry 946


**CLARCOR Foundation**
*See:* Entry 947


**CNA Foundation**
*See:* Entry 950


**Comerica Charitable Foundation**
*See:* Entry 957


**Commonwealth Edison Co.**
*See:* Entry 960


★ 11427 ★ **Corning Inc. Foundation**
MP-LB-02
Corning, NY 14831
**Phone:** (607)974-8746          **Fax:** (607)974-4756
**Email:** leslie.jackson@exeloncorp.com
**Website:** http://www.corning.com/inside_corning/foundation.asp
Kristin Swain, President

**Priorities:** *Arts & Humanities:* 39%. Emphasis is on cultural programs that support art preservation, art museums, performing arts, opera, and art workshops. Usually supports large cultural organizations. Support to cultural organizations includes art education, arts organizations, libraries, museums, and public broadcasting. *Civic & Public Affairs:* 11%. Community and civic issues funding includes youth organizations including scouts and Boys & Girls Clubs, community foundations, public policy research, natural disaster relief, emergency relief, and international organizations that directly benefit the US. Supports U.S.-based organizations with an international focus. Interests include community development in the Third World and foreign policy and international relations. *Education:* 41%. Recipients include colleges and universities, private elementary and secondary schools and public schools. Program supports the engineering grants-in-aid project, which provides assistance to women and other minority students enrolled at selected colleges of engineering. Also supports engineering education and career development projects, predoctoral science fellowships and special projects, with emphasis on the physical sciences. *Environment:* 9%. Supports the United Way. *Note:* Total contributions made in 2000. **Typ. Recipients:** Clinics/Medical Centers, Emergency/Ambulance Services, Family Planning, Hospices, Hospitals (University Affiliated), Medical Rehabilitation. **Geo. Dist:** headquarters and operating communities and nationally; internationally to U.S.-based organizations.


★ 11428 ★ **CP&L Foundation**
PO Box 1551
Raleigh, NC 27602
**Phone:** (919)546-4112          **Fax:** (919)546-4338
Tammy Brown, Manager, Corporate Community Relations

**Priorities:** *Arts & Humanities:* 27%. Supports local arts groups, including museums and art centers. *Civic & Public Affairs:* 22%. Funds business and free enterprise. *Education:* 47%. Supports engineering, minority, liberal arts, science, and math education. *Environment:* 4%. *Note:* Total foundation contributions in 1998. **Typ. Recipients:** Child Abuse, Emergency/Ambulance Services, Health Organizations, Hospitals, Single-Disease Health Associations. **Geo. Dist:** principally near operating locations and to national organizations.

**Cranston Foundation**
*See:* Entry 976

**Crestar Foundation**
*See:* Entry 978

**Crown Books Foundation**
*See:* Entry 5571

**CSR America Companies Foundation**
*See:* Entry 10063

**Demoulas Foundation**
*See:* Entry 994

**★ 11429 ★ Dow Jones Foundation**
PO Box 300
Princeton, NJ 08543
**Phone:** (609)520-5143     **Fax:** (609)520-5180
**Email:** len.doherty@dowjones.com
Leonard Doherty, Administrative Officer
**Priorities:** *Arts & Humanities:* Less than 5%. Museums, libraries, and musical organizations receive limited support. *Civic & Public Affairs:* 40% to 50%. Majority of giving supports the Dow Jones Newspaper Fund in a single grant. Professional and trade associations, primarily in journalism, also receive significant support. Other interests include organizations concerned with First Amendment issues and civil rights. *Education:* 30% to 35%. Donations to colleges and universities receive highest priority. Journalism education is also of significant interest. Other support goes to minority education and independent college funds. *Environment:* 20% to 30%. Primarily supports united funds. Child welfare also receives a substantial portion of social services funds. Other interests include youth groups and community service organizations. **Typ. Recipients:** Clinics/Medical Centers, Hospitals, People with Disabilities. **Geo. Dist:** principally near operating locations and to national organizations.

**Duchossois Foundation**
*See:* Entry 1006

**E.L. Craig Foundation**
*See:* Entry 1012

**Eaton Charitable Fund**
*See:* Entry 1016

**Equitable Resources, Inc.**
*See:* Entry 1030

**Ethyl Corp.**
*See:* Entry 1032

**Fidelity Investments Charitable Gift Fund Foundation, Inc.**
*See:* Entry 1044

**FINA Foundation**
*See:* Entry 1046

**★ 11430 ★ First American Foundation**
First American Center
315 Deaderick St., 11th Floor
Nashville, TN 37237
**Phone:** (615)736-6679

**Website:** http://www.fidelityfoundation.org
Ashley Webster, Contact
**Fnded:** 1993. **Priorities:** *Arts & Humanities:* 13% Supppots museums, opera, dance, and the performing arts. *Civic & Public Affairs:* 12%. Public policy, zoos, parks, historical sites, and community foundations are supported. *Education:* 8%. Focus is on colleges and universities. *Environment:* 60%. Supports United Way, YMCA, and youth organizations. *International:* 7%. Supports Ronald McDonald House, hospice and health care systems. *Religion:* Less than 1%. Funds a science center. *Note:* Total foundation contributions made in 1999. **Typ. Recipients:** Children's Health/Hospitals, Children's Health/Hospitals, Clinics/Medical Centers, Health Organizations, Hospices, Hospitals, Hospitals (University Affiliated), Medical Education, Public Health. **Geo. Dist:** headquarters and operating communities.

**First Evergreen Foundation**
*See:* Entry 1048

**★ 11431 ★ FMC Foundation**
200 E Randolph Dr.
Chicago, IL 60601
**Phone:** (312)861-6105     **Fax:** (312)861-6141
**Email:** fmcfoundation@fmc.com
Ms. Catherine Swigon, Executive Director
**Priorities:** *Arts & Humanities:* 12%. Museums, libraries, and performing arts supported. *Civic & Public Affairs:* 14%. Supports civic organizations that address recreational needs and environmental, urban, and governmental issues. *Education:* 12%. Generally, almost half of foundation's education contributions are made through employee matching gifts program. In addition, supports student associations at colleges and universities across the country that graduate a significant number of future employees. Grants are made to minority programs in fields relevant to company. Also supports free enterprise and economic education through colleges, universities, and other organizations for younger students. *Environment:* 50%. United Way, Salvation Army, and youth organizations are supported. *International:* 4%. Primarily funds single-disease associations. *Religion:* 4%. Supports research and science museums. *Voluntarism:* Encourages employee volunteerism by matching a portion of their contributions to United Way and by giving special consideration to organizations in which employees have been actively involved. *Note:* Total contributions made in fiscal 2000. **Typ. Recipients:** Children's Health/Hospitals, Emergency/Ambulance Services, Health Funds, Health Organizations, Health Policy/Cost Containment, Heart, Hospitals, Medical Education, Medical Rehabilitation, Public Health. **Geo. Dist:** nationally; operating locations.

**★ 11432 ★ Forest City Enterprises Charitable Foundation, Inc.**
50 Public Square, Ste. 1100
Cleveland, OH 44113-2203
**Phone:** (216)621-6060     **Fax:** (216)263-6208
Allan Krulak, Vice President
**Fnded:** 1976. **Priorities:** *Arts & Humanities:* 17%. Supports orchestras, theater, art museums, and historical societies. *Civic & Public Affairs:* 2%. Funds organizations concerned with economic development, civil rights, youth, urban affairs, crime prevention, and employment. *Education:* 23%. Majority supports scholarships. High priorities include science and technology education and religious education. *International: (Health and Welfare)* 58%. Welfare funding supports the United Way and a variety of other social service groups, including religious welfare organizations. Majority of health support focuses on hospitals. Interests also include medical research and single-disease health associations. *Note:* Total contributions made in fiscal 2000. **Typ. Recipients:** AIDS/HIV, Alzheimers Disease, Cancer, Children's Health/Hospitals, Clinics/Medical Centers, Diabetes, Emergency/Ambulance Services, Health Organizations, Hospices, Hospitals, Multiple Sclerosis, Prenatal Health Issues, Public Health, Sexual Abuse, Single-Disease Health Associ-

ations, Substance Abuse. **Geo. Dist:** operating locations; New York, NY, including metropolitan area; OH; Cleveland, OH, including metropolitan area.

**Franklin Electric, Edward J. Schaefer, and T. W. KehoeCharitable and Educational Foundation**
*See:* Entry 5572

**Gallo Foundation**
*See:* Entry 1072

**GEICO Philanthropic Foundation**
*See:* Entry 1076

**General Mills Foundation**
*See:* Entry 1081

**Genesis Foundation**
*See:* Entry 10065

**Gillette Co.**
*See:* Entry 1090

**Goldman Sachs Foundation**
*See:* Entry 8550

**★ 11433 ★ GPU Foundation**
2800 Pottsville Pike
Reading, PA 19640-0001
**Phone:** (610)929-3601     **Fax:** (610)921-6571
**Email:** cathy_chizauskas@gillette.com
**Website:** http://www.gillette.com/community/corpcontributions.asp
Cynthia Wandishin, Contact
**Fnded:** 1999. **Priorities:** *Arts & Humanities:* 12%. Funds cultural centers, performing arts, public broadcasting, and theater. *Civic & Public Affairs:* 16%. Supports parks, women's centers, and community development. *Education:* 6%. Supports colleges and universities. *Environment:* 50%. Funds youth organizations and children's welfare groups, YMCA, and human service organizations. *International:* 10%. Funds the American Red Cross. *Note:* Total foundation contributions made in 2000. **Typ. Recipients:** Emergency/Ambulance Services, Hospitals, People with Disabilities, Substance Abuse. **Geo. Dist:** headquarters and operating communities.

**★ 11434 ★ Habig Foundation**
1600 Royal St.
Jasper, IN 47549
**Phone:** (812)482-1600     **Fax:** (812)482-8166
Douglas Habig, Chairman & Chief Executive Officer
**Fnded:** 1951. **Priorities:** *Arts & Humanities:* 2%. Supports arts programs. *Civic & Public Affairs:* 10%. Supports festivals, free enterprise, safety, women's affairs public policy, and community foundations. *Education:* 55%. Supports colleges, elementary and secondary schools, and organizations promoting education. *Environment:* 10%. Supports athletics, child welfare, counseling, Girl Scouts, and youth organizations. *International:* 1%. Funds hospitals and health organizations. *Note:* Total contributions made in fiscal 1999. **Typ. Recipients:** Home-Care Services, Hospices, Hospitals, Medical Education, Mental Health. **Geo. Dist:** headquarters and operating communities.

**Halliburton Foundation, Inc.**
*See:* Entry 1109

**Harsco Corp. Fund**
*See:* Entry 1118

## ★ 11435 ★ Hasbro Children's Foundation

32 West 23rd St.
New York, NY 10010
**Phone:** (212)645-2400　　　**Fax:** (917)606-6264
**Email:** pat.george@halliburton.com
**Website:** http://www.hasbro.org
Jane Englebardt, Executive Director

**Typ. Recipients:** Hospitals, Mental Health, Nutrition, People with Disabilities. **Geo. Dist:** nationally.

## ★ 11436 ★ Herman O. West Foundation

101 Gordon Dr.
Exton, PA 19341-0645
**Phone:** (610)594-2945　　　**Fax:** (610)594-3011
**Email:** maureen_goebel@westpharma.com
Maureen Goebel, Administrator

**Priorities:** *Arts & Humanities:* 2%. Recipients include theaters, museums, orchestras, and arts councils. *Civic & Public Affairs:* 10%. Supports community service agencies, economic development, minority and women's groups, and zoos. *Education:* 29%. Support goes to colleges and universities, minority education, and community education programs. Also provides scholarships. *Environment:* 40%. Primarily supports United Way. Also funds youth organizations and human services. *International:* 14%. Focus on hospitals and health organizations. *Note:* Total contributions made in 2000. **Typ. Recipients:** Cancer, Children's Health/Hospitals, Emergency/Ambulance Services, Family Planning, Health Organizations, Hospitals, Medical Education, Medical Rehabilitation, Medical Research, Nursing Services, People with Disabilities, Prenatal Health Issues, Public Health, Substance Abuse, Trauma Treatment. **Geo. Dist:** headquarters and operating communities; FL; NE; NJ; NC; PA.

## ★ 11437 ★ Hershey Foods Corp.

100 Crystal A Dr.
Hershey, PA 17033-0810
**Phone:** (717)534-7880　　　**Fax:** (717)534-7015
**Website:** http://www.hersheys.com
Jennifer Goss, Corporate Communications

**Priorities:** *Arts & Humanities:* 10%. Supports museums, public broadcasting, symphonies, and art education and associations. *Civic & Public Affairs:* About 15%. Emphasis is on economic development, safety organizations, research programs, and organizations that promote economic freedom and the protection of private and individual enterprise. *Education:* About 40%. Approximately one-third of educational giving represents matched employee gifts. Supports education funds, with emphasis on nutrition, economic, science and business administration programs, and programs that promote a better understanding of the competitive economic system. *International:* 15% to 20%. Emphasis is on local United Way campaigns and food bank donations. Also supports youth groups, community service centers, and organizations serving minority and disadvantaged groups. **Typ. Recipients:** Clinics/Medical Centers, Hospitals, Nutrition, People with Disabilities, Substance Abuse. **Geo. Dist:** principally near operating locations and to national organizations.

## Hewlett-Packard Co. Foundation

*See:* Entry 1127

## ★ 11438 ★ Hickory Tech Corp. Foundation

221 E Hickory St.
PO Box 3248
Mankato, MN 56002-3248
**Phone:** (507)387-1866　　　**Fax:** (507)625-9191
**Email:** janerush@hickorytech.com
**Website:** http://www.hp.com/go/grants
Jane Rush, Administrator

**Fnded:** 1963. **Priorities:** *Arts & Humanities:* About 9%. Supports local music and theater groups. *Civic & Public Affairs:* Less than 2%. Supports the chamber of commerce and community-school partnerships. *Education:* 65%. Supports public and private colleges and universities in company's headquarters area. The foundation also provides scholarships for children of employees, accounting for approximately one-third of education support, and has established scholarship programs at local universities. *Environment:* 21%. Primarily supports the United Way. Also supports youth organizations, shelters, clothes distribution and food distribution. *International:* 3%. *Note:* Contributions made in fiscal 1999. **Typ. Recipients:** Cancer, Children's Health/Hospitals, Emergency/Ambulance Services, Health-General, Heart, Hospitals, Medical Rehabilitation, Multiple Sclerosis, Prenatal Health Issues, Trauma Treatment. **Geo. Dist:** Mankato, MN.

## ★ 11439 ★ Hoffer Foundation

500 Collins St.
South Elgin, IL 60177
**Phone:** (847)741-5841
**Email:** hofferpl@inil.com
Robert Hoffer, Chairman, President & Chief Executive Of

**Fnded:** 1966. **Priorities:** *Arts & Humanities:* 21%. *Civic & Public Affairs:* 1%. *Education:* 49%. *Environment:* 18%. *International:* 5%. *Note:* Total contributions made in 1998. **Typ. Recipients:** Children's Health/Hospitals, Hospitals. **Geo. Dist:** IL.

## ★ 11440 ★ HON Industries Charitable Foundation

414 East Third St.
Muscatine, IA 52761-0071
**Phone:** (319)264-7400　　　**Fax:** (319)264-7217
**Website:** http://www.honi.com/CorporateResponsibility.htm
Susan Cradick, Secretary-Treasurer

**Fnded:** 1985. **Priorities:** *Arts & Humanities:* 5%. Gives to libraries and museums. *Civic & Public Affairs:* 11%. Donations are given mainly to organizations that benefit the business community. Emphasis on the city of Muscatine, IA. *Education:* 48%. Interests include colleges and universities, Junior Achievement, and secondary schools. *Environment:* 27%. Supports local United Ways, day care, youth groups, youth sports, and domestic abuse prevention. *International:* 5%. Funds health centers, community health initiatives, American Red Cross, and the March of Dimes. *Note:* Total foundation contributions made in fiscal 2000. **Typ. Recipients:** Cancer, Children's Health/Hospitals, Domestic Violence, Emergency/Ambulance Services, Health Organizations, Hospitals, Preventive Medicine/Wellness Organizations, Public Health, Speech & Hearing. **Geo. Dist:** headquarters and operating communities; Muscatine, IA.

## Hubbard Foundation

*See:* Entry 1136

## Hunt Corp.

*See:* Entry 11696

## ★ 11441 ★ IBP Foundation

PO Box 515
Dakota City, NE 68731
**Phone:** (402)235-2061
**Email:** cheryl_walmsley@Hunt-Corp.com
**Website:** http://www.hunt-corp.com
Gene Leman, Chairman

**Fnded:** 1979. **Priorities:** *Arts & Humanities:* Less than 1%. Supports a library. *Civic & Public Affairs:* 27%. Supports foundations, community groups, and public safety (including fire, rescue, and police departments). *Education:* 8%. Funds colleges, Junior Achievement, pre-college schools, and Head Start. *Environment:* 65%. The majority of social services funding supports the Red Cross and United Ways in various communities. Also funds child welfare and community centers. *International:* Less than 1%. Funds a health service for pregnant women. *Note:* Total contributions made in 1999. **Typ. Recipients:** Children's Health/Hospitals, Clinics/Medical Centers, Emergency/Ambulance Services, Hospitals, Prenatal Health Issues. **Geo. Dist:** Boise, ID; Joslin, IL; Logansport, IN; Columbus Junction, IA; Denison, IA; Perry, IA; Sioux City, IA; Storm Lake, IA; Waterloo, IA; Emporia, KS; Garden City, KS; Dakota City, NE; Lexington, NE; Madison, NE; South Sioux City, NE; West Point, NE; Amarillo, TX; Pasco, WA.

## IFF Foundation Inc.

*See:* Entry 1144

## ★ 11442 ★ James M. Cox Foundation

PO Box 105720
Atlanta, GA 30348
**Phone:** (404)843-5000　　　**Fax:** (404)843-5599
**Email:** LeighAnn.Launius@cox.com
Leigh Launius, Assistant Secretary

**Priorities:** *Arts & Humanities:* 21%. Recipients include museums, arts centers and institutes, and musical groups such as orchestras. *Civic & Public Affairs:* 21%. Supports public policy, housing, parks and zoos, and community services. *Education:* 17%. Supports educational programs, schools, universities and colleges. *Environment:* 10%. Funds youth foundations, recreational groups, councils for victims, and shelters. *International:* 7%. Funds hospitals, medical treatment centers. *Note:* Total foundation contributions made in 2000. **Typ. Recipients:** Cancer, Child Abuse, Children's Health/Hospitals, Emergency/Ambulance Services, Health Policy/Cost Containment, Health-General, Hospices, Hospitals, Medical Education, Medical Rehabilitation, Multiple Sclerosis, Preventive Medicine/Wellness Organizations, Public Health, Single-Disease Health Associations. **Geo. Dist:** headquarters and operating communities; Atlanta, GA.

## James S. Copley Foundation

*See:* Entry 1164

## Kerr-McGee Foundation

*See:* Entry 1183

## ★ 11443 ★ Key Foundation

127 Public Square
Cleveland, OH 44114
**Phone:** (216)689-7598　　　**Fax:** (216)689-3865
**Email:** bruce_akers@keybank.com
Bruce Akers, Senior Vice President, Public Affairs

**Priorities:** *Voluntarism:* Company employees volunteer at Neighbors Make The Difference Day, a program where key closes its office for one afternoon and send its employees to perform volunteer services. **Typ. Recipients:** Hospitals. **Geo. Dist:** primarily service area.

## ★ 11444 ★ KeySpan Foundation

175 East Old Country Rd.
Hicksville, NY 11801
**Phone:** (516)545-6100　　　**Fax:** (516)545-6094
**Email:** foundation@keyspanenergy.com
**Website:** http://www.keyspanenergy.com/foundation
David Okorn, Executive Director

**Fnded:** 1998. **Priorities:** *Arts & Humanities:* 15%. Supports musical performance, libraries, art museums, public broadcasting, and other cultural organizations. *Civic & Public Affairs:* 10%. Funds community development, legal aid, and botanical gardens. *Education:* 13%. Supports colleges and universities, business and arts education, public schools, and literacy initiatives. *Environment:* 42%. Supports the United Way, food distribution, boy and girl scouts, and the Salvation Army. *International:* 8%. Gives to organizations that address cancer, heart, and birth defect issues. *Note:* Total contributions made in 2000. **Typ. Recipients:** Cancer, Health Organizations, Heart, Hospices, Hospitals, Kidney, Mental Health, People with Disabilities, Prenatal Health Issues, Single-Disease Health Associations.

## Kupferberg Foundation

*See:* Entry 5577

## ★ 11445 ★ L.L. Bean, Inc.
15 Casco St.
Freeport, ME 04033
**Phone:** (207)865-4761      **Fax:** (207)552-6821
**Website:** http://www.llbean.com
Janet Wyper, Manager, Community Relations

**Priorities:** *Arts & Humanities:* Limited funding is available for local Maine cultural and arts organizations, such as the Portland Museum of Art and the Maine State Music Theater. *Education:* Educational reform in local public schools (K-12) in Maine is the second priority. Focus is on curriculum development and restructuring efforts to improve the quality of education and life choices of children of employees and their neighbors. Organizations that have been supported include Junior Achievement and the Maine Career Advantage Program. *Environment:* Support is also given to health and human services in the local area, primarily through gifts to the United Way. **Typ. Recipients:** Hospitals. **Geo. Dist:** nationally; Brunswick, ME; Freeport, ME; Lewiston, ME; Portland, ME.

## Laclede Gas Charitable Trust
*See:* Entry 5578

## ★ 11446 ★ Ladish Co. Foundation
5481 South Packard Ave.
Cudahy, WI 53110
**Phone:** (414)747-2863      **Fax:** (414)747-2915
**Email:** wlarson@ladishco.com
Jim Miller, Trustee

**Priorities:** *Arts & Humanities:* 3%. *Civic & Public Affairs:* 2%. *Education:* 50%. Majority of funding supports the Wisconsin Foundation of Independent Colleges and the Michigan Tech Fund. The remainder funds colleges, universities, and secondary schools in Wisconsin. *Environment:* 24%. Primarily supports the United Way of Milwaukee, WI. Also supports youth organizations, food distribution, child welfare, the disabled, and community service organizations. *International:* 17%. Hospitals and health-care foundations in Milwaukee, WI, and organizations for blindness and disease prevention. *Note:* Total contributions made in fiscal 1999. **Typ. Recipients:** Alzheimers Disease, Arthritis, Cancer, Children's Health/Hospitals, Clinics/Medical Centers, Emergency/Ambulance Services, Eyes/Blindness, Health Organizations, Heart, Hospitals, Medical Research, Multiple Sclerosis, Nursing Services, People with Disabilities, Prenatal Health Issues, Respiratory, Single-Disease Health Associations, Speech & Hearing, Transplant Networks/Donor Banks. **Geo. Dist:** Cudahy, WI; Milwaukee, WI.

## Landmark Communications Foundation
*See:* Entry 1196

## Leviton Foundation New York
*See:* Entry 1202

## LG&E Energy Foundation
*See:* Entry 8551

## ★ 11447 ★ Lincoln Electric Foundation
22801 St. Clair Ave.
Cleveland, OH 44117
**Phone:** (216)481-8100      **Fax:** (216)486-6476
**Email:** hleviton@leviton.com
Paul Beddia, Vice President, Government & Community A

**Priorities:** *Arts & Humanities:* 8%. Supports the Cleveland Orchestra, ballet, opera, theater, and fine arts museums. *Civic & Public Affairs:* About 8%. Interests include environmental affairs, law enforcement, Cleveland civic associations, international organizations, and philanthropic organizations. *Education:* 21%. Most funds support local colleges and universities. Education funds and Junior Achievement also receive support. *Environment:* 40%. Majority of funds support the United Way. Remaining funds typically benefit youth organizations, recreation, and religious welfare. *International:* 19%. Primarily assists area

hospitals. Support also goes to single-disease health organizations. *Religion:* 4%. Funds the Great Lakes Museum. *Note:* Total contributions in 1999. **Typ. Recipients:** Cancer, Children's Health/Hospitals, Clinics/Medical Centers, Diabetes, Emergency/Ambulance Services, Family Planning, Health Organizations, Hospitals, Long-Term Care, Medical Rehabilitation, Mental Health, Multiple Sclerosis, Nursing Services, People with Disabilities, Preventive Medicine/Wellness Organizations, Public Health, Respiratory, Single-Disease Health Associations, Substance Abuse. **Geo. Dist:** Cleveland, OH, including metropolitan area.

## ★ 11448 ★ Louisiana-Pacific Foundation
111 Southwest Fifth Ave.
Portland, OR 97204
**Phone:** (503)221-0800      **Fax:** (503)821-5322
**Email:** kim.miller@lpcorp.com
Kim Miller, Contact

**Priorities:** *Civic & Public Affairs:* About 20%. Environmental affairs, economic development, and community affairs organizations and Habitat for Humanity. *Education:* About 80%. Virtually all funding supports a foundation-sponsored scholarship program for dependents of company employees. Limited support to public education and junior colleges, as well as to the Horatio Alger Association, a youth education and scholarship program. **Typ. Recipients:** Cancer, Children's Health/Hospitals, Emergency/Ambulance Services, Health Organizations, Heart, Hospices, Hospitals, Medical Research, People with Disabilities, Prenatal Health Issues, Public Health, Single-Disease Health Associations, Substance Abuse. **Geo. Dist:** primarily headquarters and operating communities.

## Lowe's Charitable and Educational Foundation
*See:* Entry 1212

## ★ 11449 ★ Mallinckrodt Inc.
675 McDonnel Blvd.
PO Box 5840
Saint Louis, MO 63134
**Phone:** (314)654-2000      **Fax:** (314)654-5381
**Website:** http://www.mallinckrodt.com
June Fowler, Corporate Communications Coordinator

**Typ. Recipients:** Hospitals, People with Disabilities, Substance Abuse. **Geo. Dist:** headquarters and operating communities.

## Mamiye Foundation
*See:* Entry 1216

## M&T Charitable Foundation
*See:* Entry 5580

## Marshall & Ilsley Foundation, Inc.
*See:* Entry 1221

## ★ 11450 ★ The May Department Stores Co. Foundation
611 Olive St.
Saint Louis, MO 63101
**Phone:** (314)342-6299      **Fax:** (314)342-4461
Joni Baker, Manager, Corporate Communications

**Fnded:** 1945. **Priorities:** *Arts & Humanities:* 15%. Supports major museums, music groups, dance, and dramatic arts organizations. *Civic & Public Affairs:* 11%. Support includes improving downtowns and neighborhoods, local festivals, and civil rights. *Education:* 25%. Contributes to higher education. Company is also the national sponsor for OASIS, the national health and wellness program for adults over 55. Members meet in paticipating May Department Stores and are involved in volunteer programs, including the OASIS Intergenerational Tutoring program to help grade school children in reading. Supports literacy efforts, scholarships, and internship programs. *Environment:* 30%. Priorities include United Way, Big

Brothers/Big Sisters, Boys and Girls Clubs, youth centers, family services, and YMCA. *International:* 19%. Supports hospitals, single-disease health associations, and federated organizations. Supports hunger relief, services for the homeless and victims of domestic abuse, AIDS and cancer efforts. *Note:* Except for civic grants, employee matching gifts are included in all areas of giving. Contributions made in 1999. **Typ. Recipients:** AIDS/HIV, Cancer, Children's Health/Hospitals, Clinics/Medical Centers, Emergency/Ambulance Services, Health Funds, Health Organizations, Heart, Hospitals, Medical Education, Multiple Sclerosis, People with Disabilities, Respiratory, Substance Abuse. **Geo. Dist:** operating locations.

## ★ 11451 ★ McDermott International Inc.
1450 Poydras St.
New Orleans, LA 70112-6058
**Phone:** (504)587-4411      **Fax:** (504)587-5677
Don Washington, Director, Corporate Communications

**Typ. Recipients:** Hospitals. **Geo. Dist:** national organizations; operating locations.

## MGIC Investment Corp.
*See:* Entry 1240

## Monroe Auto Equipment Co. Foundation
*See:* Entry 10066

## ★ 11452 ★ Morgan Stanley Dean Witter Foundation
1221 Ave. of the Americas, 27th Floor
New York, NY 10020
**Phone:** (212)762-6484      **Fax:** (212)762-7790
**Email:** whatadifference@morganstanley.com
**Website:** http://www.morganstanley.com/about/inside/community.html

**Fnded:** 1961. **Priorities:** *Arts & Humanities:* 12%. Museums, libraries, and performing arts centers and public broadcasting in New York City receive support. *Civic & Public Affairs:* 11%. Supports organizations that promote diversity and programs that provide job preparation and business/financial services education for minorities, women, and the disabled. Also funds libraries, parks, and community foundations. *Education:* 18%. Interests include economic education, graduate schools of business, college counseling, public and private school drop-out prevention initiatives, and arts-in-education programs. Also includes matching gifts. *Environment:* (Health and Human Services) 51%. Funds are distributed across a broad spectrum of interests, including counseling, youth, employment, recreational, and community service organizations, food distribution, and housing initiatives. Supports hospitals and pediatric health-related services. *Voluntarism:* Morgan Stanley employees are associated with several organizations addressing critical human service needs. Programs include employment training for the homeless, shelters for homeless women, scholarships for students from Chicago's housing projects, shelters in San Francisco, summer vacations for NYC youngsters, mental illness services, camps for youngsters, employment programs for runaways, and educational services to Chicago public schools. The company sponsors a Volunteer Incentive Program (VIP) which provides grants to health and human service charities where employees are active and ongoing volunteers. Grants through VIP typically range from $500 to $5,000. *Note:* Total contributions made in 2000. **Typ. Recipients:** AIDS/HIV, Cancer, Children's Health/Hospitals, Family Planning, Home-Care Services, Hospitals, Hospitals (University Affiliated), Medical Rehabilitation, Mental Health, Multiple Sclerosis, Prenatal Health Issues, Substance Abuse. **Geo. Dist:** Los Angeles, CA, branch locations; San Francisco, CA, branch locations; Chicago, IL, branch locations; New York, NY, branch locations.

## ★ 11453 ★ Murphy Oil Corp.
200 Peach St.
El Dorado, AR 71730

**Phone:** (870)864-6222          **Fax:** (870)864-6480
**Email:** Betty_LeBrescu@murphyoilcorp.com
**Website:** http://www.murphyoilcorp.com
Betty LeBrescu, Manager, Community & Public Relations

**Typ. Recipients:** Hospitals. **Geo. Dist:** headquarters and operating communities.

**Nabisco Foundation Trust**
*See:* Entry 1252

**National City Bank of Ohio**
*See:* Entry 1254

★ 11454 ★ **National Fuel Gas Co.**
10 Lafayette Square
Buffalo, NY 14203
**Phone:** (716)857-7000          **Fax:** (716)857-7413
**Website:** http://www.nationalcity.com
Ms. P. Watkins, Supervisor, Corporate Communications

**Priorities:** *Arts & Humanities:* Arts associations and centers, historic preservation, museums, music, public broadcasting, and theater. *Civic & Public Affairs:* Interests include better government, civil rights, consumer affairs, the environment, housing, safety, and zoos. *Education:* Supports colleges and universities; education associations; engineering, elementary, minority, and health education; and literacy. *Environment:* Supports programs for the aged, animal protection, community centers, drug and alcohol programs, employment and job training, the disabled, youth organizations, and united funds. *International:* Funds geriatric health, cost containment, hospitals and hospices, mental health, and single-disease associations. *Voluntarism:* The company reports that it participates in volunteer programs in conjunction with the United Way, and sponsors a mentoring program at specific schools. **Typ. Recipients:** Hospices, Hospitals, Mental Health, People with Disabilities, Substance Abuse. **Geo. Dist:** headquarters and operating communities.

**National Starch & Chemical Foundation**
*See:* Entry 1260

**Nationwide Foundation**
*See:* Entry 1261

★ 11455 ★ **New York Stock Exchange Foundation, Inc.**
11 Wall St., 6th Floor
New York, NY 10005
**Phone:** (212)656-5290          **Fax:** (212)656-5629
**Website:**     http://www.nationwide.com/about_us/involve/fndatn.htm
James Buck, Secretary

**Priorities:** *Arts & Humanities:* 21%. Mainly supports public broadcasting, the performing arts, libraries, and museums in New York City. *Civic & Public Affairs:* 19%. Activities supported include public policy, community affairs, and economic development. *Education:* 26%. Supports Junior Achievement and other national educational programs and organizations. *Environment:* 28%. Major support is awarded to the United Way. Other organizations supported include camps, youth organizations, and recreation programs. *International:* 6%. Primarily supports hospitals and single-disease centers. *Note:* Total contributions made in 1999. **Typ. Recipients:** Adolescent Health Issues, Cancer, Hospitals, Medical Education, People with Disabilities. **Geo. Dist:** New York, NY.

★ 11456 ★ **North American Royalties Foundation**
200 E 8th St.
Chattanooga, TN 37402
**Phone:** (423)265-3181
Lorie Mallchok, Vice President, Corporate Affairs

**Priorities:** *Arts & Humanities:* 22%. Funds public broadcasting and museums. *Civic & Public Affairs:* 5%. Supports community development and a community coalition. *Education:* 35%. Supports arts education, funds an elementary school, and provides scholarships. *Environment:* 33%. Supports the United Way and youth organizations and social services for boys. *International:* Less than 1%. Supports hospitals and medical research organizations. *Note:* Total contributions made in 2000. **Typ. Recipients:** Cancer, Clinics/Medical Centers, People with Disabilities. **Geo. Dist:** Chattanooga, TN.

**Northern Indiana Public Service Co.**
*See:* Entry 1276

★ 11457 ★ **Olin Corp. Charitable Trust**
501 Merritt 7
PO Box 4500
Norwalk, CT 06856-4500
**Phone:** (203)750-3301          **Fax:** (203)750-3065
**Email:** cpiacentini@corp.olin.com
**Website:** http://www.olin.com/about/charitable.asp
Carmella Piacentini, Administrator

**Priorities:** *Arts & Humanities:* 7%. Major support for the Buffalo Bill Memorial Association. Also supports theaters, the performing arts, museums, libraries, ballet, and art centers. Predominant means of arts support is matching gifts program. *Civic & Public Affairs:* 13%. Recipients include local community affairs associations; minority and urban affairs groups; economics, business, free enterprise, and public policy organizations; municipal beautification projects; and an aquarium. *Education:* 39%. Primary support to higher education institutions, with emphasis on engineering, science, and technology. Private secondary schools are supported through matching gifts. Minority and pre-college programs also supported. The remainder supports educational associations, including scholarship programs. Sponsors matching gifts program for higher and secondary educational institutions. *Environment:* 23%. Primarily supports the United Way. Also funds youth groups and children's charities. *International:* 12%. Primary interests are hospitals and medical centers. Also supports single-disease health associations and ambulatory services. *Religion:* 1%. Funds a science museum. *Voluntarism:* Supports programs which include employee volunteers. Also awards Volunteer Recognition grants; organizations where employees volunteer receive grants of $500 to $3,000. *Note:* Total foundation contributions made in 2000. **Typ. Recipients:** Cancer, Children's Health/Hospitals, Clinics/Medical Centers, Emergency/Ambulance Services, Geriatric Health, Health Organizations, Hospices, Hospitals, Medical Education, Medical Rehabilitation, Mental Health, Nursing Services, Public Health, Single-Disease Health Associations, Substance Abuse. **Geo. Dist:** communities where employees work and live; some support for national organizations.

★ 11458 ★ **OMC Foundation**
100 Sea Horse Dr.
Waukegan, IL 60085
**Phone:** (847)689-7165          **Fax:** (847)689-5555
Lauren Baker, Director, Public Affairs

**Fnded:** 1945. **Typ. Recipients:** Cancer, Clinics/Medical Centers, Diabetes, Health-General, Heart, Hospitals, Respiratory, Single-Disease Health Associations, Substance Abuse. **Geo. Dist:** headquarters and operating communities.

**OSG Foundation**
*See:* Entry 1293

**Peoples Energy Corp.**
*See:* Entry 1309

**Philips Electronics North America Corp.**
*See:* Entry 1314

★ 11459 ★ **Phillips Petroleum Co.**
Phillips Bldg., 16th Floor
Bartlesville, OK 74004
**Phone:** (918)661-6171          **Fax:** (918)662-1347
**Email:** cgbradl@ppco.com
Clara Bradley, Administrator

**Priorities:** *Arts & Humanities:* 5% to 10%. Arts associations, including almost one-third to educational television. Other interests include art centers, theater, and historical societies. Programs which introduce K-12 students to the arts and humanities are favored. *Civic & Public Affairs:* 5% to 10%. Organizations involved with energy industry-related issues, tourism in operating communities, and international relations and trade. Special emphasis on theheadquarters community, Bartlesville, OK. *Education:* 50% to 58%. Primarily reflects the interests of the company, such as engineering and geoscience. Fellowship and research grants account for about one-tenth of this support and encompass agronomy and graduate education and research in chemistry, engineering, geophysics, geology, combustion, and polymer science. Significant support also goes to colleges and universities for miscellaneous purposes including scholarships; programs in chemistry, science, and technology; and unrestricted operating support. Educational contributions are limited to schools or organizations whose location, facilities, or curricula are beneficial to the communities from whichthe company recruits. Company also sponsors a matching gifts program and a scholarship program for employees' children. Also funds educational film series to promote interest in mathematics and science careers. Phillips is the national sponsor of the U.S. Swimming and Mathcounts. *Environment:* 5% to 10%. Youth organizations, including child welfare programs, boys' and girls' clubs, Junior Achievement, and boy and girl scouts in locations where company operates. *International:* About 10%. United funds, community services, substance abuse prevention, and health agencies. Emphasis on Oklahoma and Texas. **Typ. Recipients:** Clinics/Medical Centers, Domestic Violence, Geriatric Health, Health Organizations, Hospitals, Medical Education, Medical Rehabilitation, Medical Research, Mental Health, Nutrition, People with Disabilities, Public Health, Substance Abuse. **Geo. Dist:** headquarters and operating communities.

**Pioneer Investments Management USA Inc.**
*See:* Entry 1318

★ 11460 ★ **Pitney Bowes Inc.**
1 Elmcroft Rd.
Stamford, CT 06926-0700
**Phone:** (203)351-6669          **Fax:** (203)351-6303
**Email:** obrienpo@pb.com
**Website:** http://www.pb.com
Polly O'Brien, Director, Community Affairs

**Priorities:** *Arts & Humanities:* Less than 5%. Supports various arts activities near corporate operating locations. *Civic & Public Affairs:* About 15%. Supports urban affairs, civil rights, and community development. *Education:* About 20%. Interests include Head Start and similar programs; school-wide and grade-wide tutorial programs; parenting skills and guidance programs; and before- and after-school programs that provide activities and enrichment. Other interests include high school mathematics and science programs. *International:* About 45%. Supports United Way and human service organizations involved in developing affordable housing via building or renovation, as well as those that provide temporary shelter. *Voluntarism:* Employee volunteerism is encourage through the company's National Week of Caring and PB People: Building Stronger Communities programs. **Typ. Recipients:** Hospitals. **Geo. Dist:** headquarters and operating communities.

**PNC Foundation**
*See:* Entry 1321

## ★ 11461 ★ Potlatch Foundation II
601 West Riverside Ave., Ste. 1100
Spokane, WA 99201
**Phone:** (509)835-1518          **Fax:** (509)835-1559
**Email:** foundation@potlatchcorp.com
**Website:** http://www.potlatchcorp.com/company/foundations/html
Hugh Travaille, Foundation President

**Priorities:** *Arts & Humanities:* 3%. Performing arts centers and museums. *Civic & Public Affairs:* 15%. Local economic development and environmental efforts. *Education:* 55%. Supports the Potlatch Foundation for Higher Education, which provides for scholarships; colleges and universities; and pre-college education. *Environment:* 16%. Funds United Way, athletics, and youth organizations. *International:* 1%. Supports community hospitals. *Note:* Total foundation contributions made in 2000. **Typ. Recipients:** Hospitals. **Geo. Dist:** AR; San Francisco, CA; ID; MN.

## Providence Journal Charitable Foundation
*See:* Entry 1332

## Public Service Electric & Gas Foundation
*See:* Entry 8553

## ★ 11462 ★ Publix Supermarkets Charities
PO Box 407
Lakeland, FL 33802
**Phone:** (863)686-8754
**Email:** mary_ellen_ahern@projo.com
**Website:** http://www.publix.com/comm_involvement.htm
Carol Barnett, Chairperson

**Fnded:** 1967. **Priorities:** *Arts & Humanities:* 2%. Funds art festivals, and children, youth and art museums. *Civic & Public Affairs:* 1%. Supports Florida Olympic campaign, public affairs, the Florida aquarium, and civic organizations. *Education:* 12%. Supports colleges, universities, public schools and educational programs in Florida. *Environment:* 80%. Majority of social service funding is donated to the United Way; also supports youth services, YMCA, the homeless, family services, and the handicapped. *International:* 1%. Funds clinics, hospitals, and single-disease health associations. *Note:* Contributions were made in 2000. **Typ. Recipients:** Cancer, Clinics/Medical Centers, Emergency/Ambulance Services, Family Planning, Geriatric Health, Hospices, Hospitals, People with Disabilities, Single-Disease Health Associations, Substance Abuse, Transplant Networks/Donor Banks. **Geo. Dist:** AL; FL; GA; SC.

## Questar Corp.
*See:* Entry 1340

## R.R. Donnelley & Sons Co.
*See:* Entry 5474

## Reliant Energy Foundation
*See:* Entry 5587

## Revlon Foundation Inc.
*See:* Entry 1350

## Riggs Bank NA
*See:* Entry 1355

## Robert I. Wishnick Foundation
*See:* Entry 1356

## Ryder System Charitable Foundation
*See:* Entry 1364

## Saint Paul Companies Inc.
*See:* Entry 1368

## Salomon Smith Barney
*See:* Entry 18224

## Sentry Insurance Foundation Inc.
*See:* Entry 1382

## Solo Cup Foundation
*See:* Entry 1397

## ★ 11463 ★ Southern New England Telephone Co.
310 Orange St.
New Haven, CT 06510
**Phone:** (203)771-3114          **Fax:** (203)865-5198
**Email:** marybeth-jones@riggsbank.com
**Website:** http://www.smithbarney.com/abt_sb/community/index.html
Kathleen Buccy, Manager, Contributions

**Priorities:** *Education:* Focus is on technical edcuation. Company grant programs include "Narrowing the Digital Divide," to improve computer literacy in adults through grants to colleges, universities, and technical schools; a grant to the University of Connecticut for research in information technology; small grants supporting high school band and music programs; and free Internet access and websites for Connecticut schools and libraries. The companies also funds Amistad America, SeniorNet Learning Centers, the Sporting Geography education program, the Celebration of Excellence Program (recognizing outstanding teachers), and educational conferences. SNET is a business partner with Katherine Brennan School. **Typ. Recipients:** Hospitals, People with Disabilities, Substance Abuse. **Geo. Dist:** New Haven, CT.

## Springs Industries, Inc.
*See:* Entry 1402

## Sprint/United Telephone
*See:* Entry 1403

## ★ 11464 ★ State Farm Companies Foundation
One State Farm Plz., SC3
Bloomington, IL 61710-0001
**Phone:** (309)766-2161          **Fax:** (309)766-2314
**Email:** jill.jones.A3RI@statefarm.com
**Website:** http://www.statefarm.com/foundati/foundati.htm
Jill Jones, Assistant Secretary

**Fnded:** 1963. **Priorities:** *Arts & Humanities:* 3%. Supports arts and culture organizations with an emphasis on history museums and societies. *Civic & Public Affairs:* 1%. Funds leadership foundations, law organizations and women's organizations. *Education:* 66%. Supports colleges and universities, insurance education, fellowships, and doctoral awards. *Environment:* 27%. Supports the United Way, youth activities, and a wide variety of health and human service organizations. *International:* 3%. Funds medical programs. *Voluntarism:* Company-sponsored volunteer programs include loaned executives for United Way campaigns, Junior Achievement advisors, and Red Cross Blood drives. Interested employees complete a questionnaire, then receive a newsletter of volunteer activities. Employees participate in activities on their own initiative. *Note:* Total contributions made in 1998. **Typ. Recipients:** Cancer, Children's Health/Hospitals, Clinics/Medical Centers, Hospitals, Medical Education, Medical Rehabilitation, Public Health, Substance Abuse. **Geo. Dist:** near major offices.

## Stonecutter Foundation
*See:* Entry 1413

## ★ 11465 ★ Sunoco Inc.
Ten Penn Center
1801 Market St.
Philadelphia, PA 19103
**Phone:** (215)977-3924          **Fax:** (215)246-8562
**Website:** http://www.suncoinc.com
Edward Hazzouri, Manager Contributions

**Priorities:** *Arts & Humanities:* 10% to 15%. Museums, theaters, dance companies, and visual and performing arts programs. *Civic & Public Affairs:* 15% to 20%. Organizations that promote economic development and employment opportunities. (Public Policy) About 15%. Non-partisan organizations engaged in public policy issues and economic research important to company interests; groups promoting government efficiency; and organizations concerned with the allocation of public funds. *Education:* About 25%. Major support to higher education. Other recipients include minority education and education associations. *International:* 30% to 35%. Primarily supports the United Way. Also supports hospitals, community service organizations, and youth organizations. **Typ. Recipients:** Hospitals, People with Disabilities, Public Health, Substance Abuse. **Geo. Dist:** operating locations; Philadelphia, PA.

## Susquehanna-Pfaltzgraff Foundation
*See:* Entry 1421

## Sverdrup Corp. Charitable Trust
*See:* Entry 1422

## Tektronix Foundation
*See:* Entry 8557

## Telcordia Technologies
*See:* Entry 8558

## Textron Charitable Trust
*See:* Entry 1434

## Thomasville Furniture Industries Foundation
*See:* Entry 1435

## Torchmark Corp.
*See:* Entry 1443

## Tribune New York Foundation
*See:* Entry 1446

## TRW Foundation
*See:* Entry 1449

## Union Pacific Foundation
*See:* Entry 1454

## ★ 11466 ★ United Airlines Foundation
PO Box 66100
Chicago, IL 60666
**Phone:** (847)700-5714          **Fax:** (847)700-7345
**Email:** uafoundation@UAL.com
**Website:** http://www.up.com/found/index.htm
Eileen Younglove, Manager-Contributions

**Priorities:** *Arts & Humanities:* 18%. Keen interest in projects designed to introduce young people to museums, music, dance, and other creative areas. Also supports museums and libraries. *Civic & Public Affairs:* 5%. Programs that directly improve life in the community. Funds Habitat for Humanity projects around the world and supports their mission of decent, affordable housing for all. *Education:* 16%. Tutoring and mentoring systems, Adopt-a-School projects, and School To Work initiatives. *Environment:* 42%. Majority of funds go to United Way chapters across the United States and Canada. *International:* 4%. Programs that help individuals with disabilities and disease through grants, airline tickets for medical transport, and employee volunteerism. *Religion:* 15%. Funds science centers and museums. *Voluntarism:* Co. sponsors employee volunteer programs such as: Believers

Program-an educational mentoring and tutoring program; Habitat for Humanity; Take Your Community to Work Day; and AIDS walks. Through its United We Care Program, co. also awards grants to organizations where employees volunteer. *Note:* Total contributions made in 1999. **Typ. Recipients:** Alzheimers Disease, Cancer, Children's Health/Hospitals, Heart, Hospitals, Medical Research, Single-Disease Health Associations. **Geo. Dist:** internationally; focusing on major cities served by the company.

★ **11467** ★ **Universal Foods Foundation**
777 East Wisconsin Ave.
Milwaukee, WI 53202-5304
**Phone:** (414)271-6755
Stephen Rolfs, Secretary & Treasurer
**Priorities:** *Arts & Humanities:* (Culture & Art) 21%. Supports historic preservation, art museums, public broadcasting, libraries, and performing arts. *Civic & Public Affairs:* (Civic Activity) 21%. Recipients include chambers of commerce, job training, law enforcement and fire departments, economic development programs, community festivals and activities, women's affairs, zoos, and community foundations. *Education:* 24%. Major support goes to colleges and universities, with some emphasis on medical and education. Other recipients include literacy groups and education funds. *Environment:* (Health and Welfare) 34%. Supports the United Way and youth organizations. Primarily supports hospitals, but funding also goes to medical research and United Way agencies. *Note:* Total contributions made in fiscal 2000. **Typ. Recipients:** Cancer, Children's Health/Hospitals, Clinics/Medical Centers, Emergency/Ambulance Services, Heart, Hospitals, Medical Education, Medical Research, Multiple Sclerosis, People with Disabilities, Single-Disease Health Associations, Transplant Networks/Donor Banks. **Geo. Dist:** headquarters and operating communities.

**USX Foundation, Inc.**
*See:* Entry 1472

**Valspar Foundation**
*See:* Entry 1474

★ **11468** ★ **Verizon Foundation**
1095 Ave. of the Americas
New York, NY 10036
**Phone:** 800-360-7955           **Fax:** (212)398-0951
**Email:** Fresa.Kooi@verizon.com
**Website:** http://foundation.verizon.com
Fresa Kooi, Executive Assistant to the President
**Fnded:** 2000. **Priorities:** *Arts & Humanities:* 10%. Supports libraries, performing arts, monuments, museums, and preservation. *Civic & Public Affairs:* 16%. Funds minority and women's affairs, nonprofit management, public safety, urban affairs, and public policy. *Education:* 37%. Supports literacy initiatives, colleges and universities, primary and secondary education, and education assistance for the disadvantaged. *Environment:* 31%. Provides major support to the United Way. Also funds youth organizations, human services, disaster relief, and other social service organizations. funds for nonprofit organizations across the country through organized pledge-a-thons, such as walk-a-thons or bike-a-thons. Under the program, the foundation matches funds collected by each team up to $25,000 per team to qualified nonprofit organizations. *International:* 2%. Funds national single-disease health organizations and hospitals and medical centers. *Religion:* 4%. Supports science centers and museums. *Voluntarism:* The Verizon Incentive Program recognizes employees' contribution of time and talent to nonprofit organizations where they live and work. Under the program, employees apply for a grant for the qualified organization where they volunteered at least 50 hours in a 12 month period. The foundation rewards them with a $500 check for presentation to the designated organization. Employees may request VIP grants on behalf of two separate organizations in a 12 month period for a total of $1,000. The Verizon Team Incentive Program rewards teams of ten or more eligible employees

to collectively raise funds for nonprofit organizations across the country through organized pledge-a-thons, such as walk-a-thons or bike-a-thons. Under the program, the foundation matches funds collected by each team up to $25,000 per team to qualified nonprofit organizations. *Note:* Total contributions made in 2000. **Typ. Recipients:** Domestic Violence, Emergency/Ambulance Services, Geriatric Health, Health Policy/Cost Containment, Hospitals, People with Disabilities, Substance Abuse. **Geo. Dist:** operating locations.

★ **11469** ★ **Vesper Foundation**
8223 Brecksville Rd., Ste. 100
Brecksville, OH 44141
**Phone:** (440)838-4700        **Fax:** (440)838-4702
John Curci, Vice President & Treasurer
**Priorities:** *Arts & Humanities:* 10%. Supports libraries, museums, and historic preservation. *Civic & Public Affairs:* 43%. Supports zoos and parks. Major grant to New York Botanical Garden. *Education:* 31%. Supports colleges and universities and art education. *Environment:* 4%. Primarily supports United Way, youth organizations, and animal shelters. *International:* 1%. *Religion:* 1%. Supports Woods Hole Oceanographic Institute. *Note:* Total contributions made in 1999. **Typ. Recipients:** Cancer, Hospitals, Hospitals (University Affiliated), Single-Disease Health Associations. **Geo. Dist:** nationally, focusing on the Northeast USA.

★ **11470** ★ **Warren Alpert Foundation**
27 Warren Way, PO Box 72743
Providence, RI 02907
**Phone:** (401)781-9900
John Dziedzic, Treasurer
**Fnded:** 1988. **Priorities:** *Education:* 54%. Foundation makes awards to individuals, selected after consultation with a panel of medical experts in concert with the faculty of Harvard Medical School. Also funds medical research. *International:* 22%. Supports medical centers and hospitals. *Religion:* 2%. *Note:* Total foundation contributions made in 2000. **Typ. Recipients:** Eyes/Blindness, Heart, Hospitals, Long-Term Care, Medical Education.

**Waste Management Inc.**
*See:* Entry 1493

★ **11471** ★ **Wausau Paper Mills Foundation**
1244 Kronenwetter Dr.
Mosinee, WI 54455-9099
**Phone:** (715)693-4470
**Website:** http://www.wm.com
Thomas Howatt, Foundation Officer
**Priorities:** *Arts & Humanities:* 9%. Aids an art museum, and an historical museum, and performing arts. *Civic & Public Affairs:* 20%. Funds community involvement, junior achievement, fire departments, and community foundations. *Education:* 5%. Supports an indiana college foundation. *Environment:* 62%. Supports scouting, the United Way, and the YMCA. *Religion:* 4%. Funds paper science at University of Wisconsin. *Note:* Total contributions made in 1999. **Typ. Recipients:** Health Organizations, Hospitals, Public Health, Respiratory. **Geo. Dist:** WI.

★ **11472** ★ **Weldon F. Osborne Foundation**
Krystal Bldg.
1 Union Square, Ste. 210
Chattanooga, TN 37402-2501
**Phone:** (423)267-0931        **Fax:** (423)267-0931
Harold Wilson, Executive Director
**Priorities:** *Arts & Humanities:* 2%. Funds an urban art institute. *Civic & Public Affairs:* 30%. Priorities include: community revitalization, the police force, foundations, community centers, and self monitoring neighborhood programs. *Education:* 17%. Supports colleges and schools. *Environment:* 33%. Funds the Salvation Army

United Way, YMCA, and youth programs. *International:* 6%. Funding supports the Chattanooga Heart Institute. *Note:* Contributions made in 2001. **Typ. Recipients:** Children's Health/Hospitals, Hospitals. **Geo. Dist:** TN; Chattanooga, TN.

**Westvaco Foundation Trust**
*See:* Entry 1499

**Wisconsin Energy Corp. Foundation, Inc.**
*See:* Entry 1508

**Wolfe Associates, Inc.**
*See:* Entry 5591

**Wolverine World Wide Foundation**
*See:* Entry 1512

★ **11473** ★ **Woodward Governor Co. Charitable Trust**
61111 North Second St.
Rockford, IL 61125
**Phone:** (815)877-7441        **Fax:** (815)639-6033
**Email:** comrel@dispatch.com
**Website:** http://www.dispatch.com
Thomas Winking, Contributions Committee Chairman
**Priorities:** *Arts & Humanities:* 4%. The arts, including symphonies and various museums. *Civic & Public Affairs:* 9%. Housing, crime prevention, legal aid, and safety are also priorities. *Education:* 16%. Educational programs including schools and literacy councils. *Environment:* 64%. Food distribution centers, community services, minority groups, youth organizations, United Way, and various programs for child welfare. *International:* 4%. Most recipients are single-disease health organizations. Funds also support the handicapped, mental health groups, and some clinics and hospitals. *Religion:* 2%. Funds science museums, natural history museums and the discovery center. *Note:* Total contributions made in 1998. **Typ. Recipients:** Alzheimers Disease, Cancer, Children's Health/Hospitals, Clinics/Medical Centers, Emergency/Ambulance Services, Geriatric Health, Health Organizations, Hospices, Hospitals, Medical Rehabilitation, Medical Research, Mental Health, People with Disabilities, Public Health, Research/Studies Institutes, Single-Disease Health Associations, Speech & Hearing, Substance Abuse, Transplant Networks/Donor Banks. **Geo. Dist:** headquarters and operating communities.

★ **11474** ★ **Zenith Electronics Corp.**
2000 Milbrook Dr.
Lincolnshire, IL 60069
**Phone:** (847)941-8184        **Fax:** (847)941-8177
John Taylor, Vice President, Public Affairs & Communi
**Priorities:** *Arts & Humanities:* Less than 5%. Preference to public radio and television stations. *Civic & Public Affairs:* (United Funds & United Way) Around 40% of budget. Supports United Ways and other federated campaigns in Chicago and other plant communities. Between 10% and 15%. Preference given to organizations that serve and involve minorities, the handicapped, and youth. *Education:* Between 20% and 25%. Contributes to institutions where company recruits employees or with which there are significant corporate relationships, such as joint research projects, board leadership by Zenith executives, and employee involvement or benefits. Generally does not support precollegiate educational institutions. *International:* Between 15% and 20%. Priority given to hospitals serving Zenith plant communities or significant numbers of employees and their families. **Typ. Recipients:** Hospitals, People with Disabilities. **Geo. Dist:** nationally; preference is given to organizations located near corporate operating locations.

★ **11475** ★ **Zilkha Foundation, Inc.**
767 5th Ave., Ste. 4605
New York, NY 10153

**Phone:** (212)758-7750          **Fax:** (212)758-7803
Ezra Zilkha, President
**Fnded:** 1948. **Priorities:** *Arts & Humanities:* 70%. Support includes operas, libraries, museums, ballet, and historic preservation. *Civic & Public Affairs:* 9%. Funds public policy organizations. *Education:* 6%. Major support includes the Waterford Institute and universities. *Environment:* 2%. Support goes to the disabled, youth groups, and housing. *International:* 1%. Supports hospitals, medical centers, and research. *Note:* Total contributions made in fiscal 1999. **Typ. Recipients:** AIDS/HIV, Alzheimers Disease, Cancer, Clinics/Medical Centers, Emergency/Ambulance Services, Eyes/Blindness, Geriatric Health, Hospitals, Hospitals (University Affiliated), Medical Education, Medical Research, People with Disabilities, People with Disabilities, Public Health, Research/Studies Institutes, Substance Abuse, Transplant Networks/Donor Banks. **Geo. Dist:** New York, NY.

# National & International Organizations

## ★ 11476 ★ American Association of Eye and Ear Hospitals (AAEEH)
1444 Eye St., NW, Ste. 410
Washington, DC 20005
**Phone:** (202)347-1993          **Fax:** (202)628-2310
**Email:** rbetz@aaeeh.org
**Website:** http://www.aaeeh.org
Robert Betz, Ph.D, Exec. Dir.
**Fnded:** 1983. **Mem:** 18. **Desc:** Chief executive officers and administrators of eye and ear specialty hospitals. Seeks to advance, at the federal level, fair economic treatment for eye and ear specialty hospitals; to share business functions such as purchasing, planning, and information and data collection. Compiles statistics. **Pub:** *Washington Eyeline*, monthly. Newsletter.

## American Association of Hospital Podiatrists (AAHP)
*See:* Entry 17700

## American Association of Integrated Healthcare Delivery Systems
*See:* Entry 9689

## ★ 11477 ★ American Hospital Association (AHA)
1 N Franklin
Chicago, IL 60606-3421
**Phone:** (312)422-3000          **Fax:** (312)422-4796
**Email:** hromero@aha.org
**Website:** http://www.aha.org
Richard J. Davidson, PhD, Pres.
**Fnded:** 1898. **Mem:** 54,500. **Desc:** Health care provider organizations. Seeks to advance the health of individuals and communities. Leads, represents, and serves health care provider organizations that are accountable to the community and committed to health improvement. **Pub:** *AHANews*, weekly. • *Guide to the Health Care Field*, annual. • *Hospital Statistics*, annual. • *Hospitals and Health Networks*, biweekly. **Frmly:** (1906) Association of Hospital Superintendents of U.S. and Canada.

## ★ 11478 ★ American Osteopathic Healthcare Association (AOHA)
5550 Friendship Blvd., Ste., 300
Chevy Chase, MD 20815
**Phone:** (301)968-2642          **Fax:** (301)968-4195
**Email:** aoha@osteohdq.org
David Kushner, Pres. & CEO
**Fnded:** 1934. **Mem:** 160. **Reg. Groups:** 6. **Desc:** AOHA's mission is to serve its members by promoting the health and welfare of the American public through effective leadership; serving as the unified voice in areas of common interest for the advancement of osteopathic health care; and providing advocacy and eduation to ensure members' success. **Pub:** *Osteopathic Membership Directory*, annual. Membership Directory. Lists osteopathic hospitals; contains statistical data. *Price:* Included in membership dues; $125 for non-members. • *Osteopathic Progress*, monthly. Newsletter. *Price:* Included in membership dues. **Frmly:** (1993) American Osteopathic Hospital Association.

## ★ 11479 ★ American Society for Healthcare Engineering of the American Hospital Association (ASHE)
c/o American Hospital Association
One N Franklin, 27th Fl.
Chicago, IL 60606
**Phone:** (312)422-3800          **Fax:** (312)422-4571
**Email:** ashe@aha.org
**Website:** http://www.ashe.org
Albert J. Sunseri, PhD, Exec. Dir.
**Fnded:** 1962. **Mem:** 5,500. **Local Groups:** 75. **Desc:** Hospital engineers, facilities managers, directors of buildings and grounds, assistant administrators, directors of maintenance, directors of clinical engineering, design and construction professionals, and safety officers. Works to: promote better patient care by encouraging and assisting members to develop their knowledge and increase their competence in the field of facilities management; cooperate with hospitals and allied associations in matters pertaining to facilities management; bring about closer cooperation among members; provide a medium for interchange of material relative to facilities management. Maintains library; conducts educational programs. Offers Actions for Professional Excellence Recognition Program (APEx). **Pub:** *American Society for Healthcare Engineering–Management and Compliance Series*, semiannual. Provides comprehensive coverage of a specific facilities management topic. *Price:* $75/volume for members; $98/volume for nonmembers. • *American Society for Healthcare Engineering–Technical Document Series*, monthly. Report. Covers a specific topic in clinical/biomedical engineering, facilities management engineering, or design and construction. • *American Society for Hospital Engineering–Yearbook.* Membership Directory. Arranged alphabetically by name, hospital, and city and state; includes vendor directory. • *Health Facilities Management Magazine*, monthly. Journal. • *Publications Catalog*, semiannual. Lists books, films, tapes, documents, and publications available from the society. *Price:* Free. • Also publishes books. **Frmly:** American Society for Hospital Engineering.

## ★ 11480 ★ American Society for Healthcare Environmental Services of the American Hospital Association (ASHES)
1 N Franklin St.
Chicago, IL 60606
**Phone:** (312)422-3860          **Fax:** (312)422-4572
**Email:** ashes@aha.org
**Website:** http://www.ashes.org
Patti Costello, Exec. Dir.
**Fnded:** 1986. **Mem:** 1,600. **Nat'l Groups:** 1. **Reg. Groups:** 16. **Desc:** Managers and directors of hospital environmental services, laundry and linen services, housekeeping departments and waste management (non-hazardous and hazardous). Provides a forum for discussion among members of common challenges, Professional development, and career advancement. Maintains liaison between members and governmental and standards setting bodies. Bestows Accolades Awards, Phoenix Award, Years of Service Award. Certified Healthcare Environmental Services Professional (CHESP) available through education and Examination. **Pub:** *ASHES Newsletter*, quarterly. Newsletter. • *Professional Development Series*, quarterly. • Multiple publications related to env. svc. and technical issues.

## American Society for Healthcare Food Service Administrators (ASHFSA)
*See:* Entry 9704

## American Society for Healthcare Risk Management (ASHRM)
*See:* Entry 9706

## American Society of Health System Pharmacists (ASHP)
*See:* Entry 17512

## ★ 11481 ★ American Women's Hospitals Service Committee of AMWA (AWHS/AMWA)
801 N Fairfax St., Ste. 400
Alexandria, VA 22314
**Phone:** (703)838-0500          **Fax:** (703)549-3864
**Email:** info@amwa-doc.org
**Website:** http://www.amwa-doc.org
Omega L. Logan Silva, Pres.
**Fnded:** 1917. **Desc:** A project of the American Medical Women's Association Foundation. International philanthropic medical relief service that supports medical and hospital services conducted by women doctors and nurses for the care of the indigent sick and prevention of disease. Current activities, carried on in Haiti, and the U.S., fostering health education through demonstrations, home visits, and giving financial aid to hospitals and clinics. **Frmly:** (1959) American Women's Hospitals; (1982) American Women's Hospitals Service.

## Association of Air Medical Services (AAMS)
*See:* Entry 8571

## ★ 11482 ★ Association of Canadian Academic Health Care Organizations (Association Canadienne des Institutions de Sante Universtaires)
4500 Oak St., Rm. E405
Vancouver, BC, Canada V6H 3N1
**Phone:** (604)875-3468          **Fax:** (604)872-3290
**Email:** secretariat@acaho.org
**Website:** http://www.acaho.org
**Fnded:** 1973. **Mem:** 16. **Lang(s):** English, French. **Desc:** Teaching hospitals. Promotes advancement of medical education and residency. Represents the interests of medical residents and teaching hospitals; sponsors research and conducts educational programs. **Frmly:** (2000) Association of Canadian Teaching Hospitals.

## ★ 11483 ★ Association for Healthcare Philanthropy (AHP)
313 Park Ave., Ste. 400
Falls Church, VA 22046
**Phone:** (703)532-6243          **Fax:** (703)532-7170
**Email:** bill@go-ahp.org
**Website:** http://www.go-ahp.org
Dr. William C. McGinly, Pres.,CEO
**Fnded:** 1967. **Mem:** 2,800. **Reg. Groups:** 7. **Desc:** Persons employed by healthcare organizations in the field of healthcare resource development and fundraising; hospital administrators and trustees; hospitals; interested individuals. Purposes are to create a cohesive body of healthcare development executives to advance the interests and knowledge of healthcare fund development; to encourage and stimulate better understanding of healthcare needs; to accomplish common goals through an exchange of ideas and information. Conducts educational programs. Holds regional seminars. Compiles statistics. Conducts research; sponsors competitions. Maintains library. **Pub:** *AHP Connect*, 8/year. Newsletter. • *Association for Healthcare Philanthropy–Directory*, annual. Directory. Lists members and allied firms. Includes calendar of events. *Price:* Included in membership dues. • *Association for Healthcare Philanthropy–Journal*, semiannu-

al. Journal. *Price:* Included in membership dues; $38/year for nonmembers. • *Report on Giving.* • *Salary and Benefits.* **Frmly:** (1967) Developpartners; (1991) National Association for Hospital Development.

★ **11484** ★ **Association for Hospital Medical Education (AHME)**
419 Beulah Rd.
Pittsburgh, PA 15235
**Phone:** (412)244-9302          **Free:** (866)617-4780
**Fax:** (412)243-4692
**Email:** AHMEinPGH@aol.com
**Website:** http://ahme.med.edu
Margie Kleppick, Exec. Dir.

**Fnded:** 1956. **Mem:** 683. **Desc:** Dedicated to the comprehensive support of medical education professionals; supports continuum if medical education. **Pub:** *AHME Membership Directory*, annual. Membership Directory. Online version only. • *AHME News*, semiannual. Newsletter. • *Guide to Graduate Medical Education (Guide I and II).* • *Resource and Reference Center.* • *Transitional Year Program Directory (Purple Book)*, annual. **Frmly:** (1968) Association of Hospital Directors of Medical Education.

★ **11485** ★ **Association for Responsible Medicine (AARM)**
c/o Ray McEachern
PO Box 270986
Tampa, FL 33688
**Phone:** (813)909-0776          **Fax:** (813)933-6236
**Email:** armxd@sprynet.com
Ray McEachern, Exec. Dir.

**Fnded:** 1994. **Mem:** 1,200. **Desc:** Individuals requiring the services of acute care hospitals; individuals the group feels are victims of medical malpractice. Seeks to "reduce the incidence of medical mistakes that cause injury to patients." Gathers and disseminates information on malpractice suits and publishes on website. **Pub:** *Patient Advocate*, quarterly. Newsletter. • Brochure.

★ **11486** ★ **Australian Private Hospitals Association (APHA)**
Level 1
25 Napier Close
Deakin, ACT 2600, Australia
**Phone:** 61 2 62852716          **Fax:** 61 2 62852243
**Email:** michael.roff@apha.org.au
**Website:** http://www.apha.org.au

**Lang(s):** English. **Desc:** Represents private hospitals in Australia.

★ **11487** ★ **Canadian Friends of the Bene Berak Hospital (CRBBH)**
579 Old Orchard Grove
Toronto, ON, Canada M5M 2H2
**Phone:** (416)783-5773          **Fax:** (416)537-0437
**Fnded:** 1979. **Lang(s):** English, French. **Desc:** Individuals and organizations. Promotes continuation and expansion of the activities of the Bene Berak Hospital. Conducts fundraising activities; sponsors charitable programs. **Pub:** Brochure, periodic.

★ **11488** ★ **Canadian Healthcare Association**
17 York St., Ste. 100
Ottawa, ON, Canada K1N 9J6
**Phone:** (613)241-8005          **Fax:** (613)241-5055
**Email:** info@canadian-healthcare.org
**Website:** http://www.canadian-healthcare.org

**Fnded:** 1931. **Mem:** 13. **State Groups:** 13. **Lang(s):** French. **Desc:** Promotes a humane, effective, efficient health system of the highest quality. **Pub:** *Guide to Canadian Healthcare Facilities*, annual. Directory. Lists health care facilities in Canada.

**Canadian Society of Hospital Pharmacists (CSHP)**
**(Societe Canadienne des pharmaciens d'Hopitaux — SCPH)**
*See:* Entry 17530

★ **11489** ★ **Community Hospitals Association**
Meadow Brow
Broadway Rd.
Ilminster TA19 9RG, United Kingdom
**Phone:** 44 1460 55951          **Fax:** 44 1460 53207
**Email:** irh@rural-health.ac.uk
**Website:** http://www.rural-health.ac.uk/cha.htm

**Fnded:** 1969. **Mem:** 409. **Desc:** Community hospitals within and outside the NHS. Works towards developing the range and continuing improvement of services provided by community hospitals. Gathers and disseminates information on all aspects of work carried out in community hospitals; gives help and advice to members in furthering the interests of community hospitals. **Pub:** *Community Hospital Association Newletter*, quarterly.

★ **11490** ★ **Council of Teaching Hospitals (COTH)**
2450 N St. NW
Washington, DC 20037-1127
**Phone:** (202)828-0400          **Fax:** (202)828-1125
**Email:** amcas@aamc.org
**Website:** http://www.wamc.com
Robert M. Dickler, VP

**Fnded:** 1965. **Mem:** 400. **Desc:** Teaching hospitals. Provides activities and programs relating to specific problems and opportunities in medical school-affiliated or university-owned teaching hospitals. Distributes communications analyzing congressional activities, Executive Branch actions, court decisions affecting teaching hospitals, and teaching hospital reimbursement regulations; disseminates special interest bibliographies, surveys of housestaff policies, comparative hospital financial data, and other materials. Appoints study groups and ad hoc advisory task forces. **Pub:** *COTH Report*, 8-10/year. Newsletter. Reviews current federal and state legislation and general activities of the association and its affiliates. *Price:* $30/year. • *Survey of House Staff Stipends, Benefits, and Funding*, annual.

★ **11491** ★ **Federation of American Hospitals (FAHS)**
801 Pennsylvania Ave. NW, Ste. 245
Washington, DC 20004-2604
**Phone:** (202)624-1500          **Fax:** (202)737-6462
**Email:** info@americashospitals.com
**Website:** http://www.fahs.com
Charles N. Kahn, III, Pres.

**Fnded:** 1966. **Mem:** 1,700. **Desc:** Privately- or investor-owned (for-profit) hospitals. **Pub:** *Hospital Outlook*, monthly. Newsletter. Monitors health legislation, regulatory and reimbursement matters and developments in the health care industry. *Price:* Included in membership dues; $150/year for nonmembers. • Annual Report. **Frmly:** (2001) Federation of American Health Systems.

★ **11492** ★ **Floating Hospital (FH)**
Pier 11 Wall at South St.
New York, NY 10005
**Phone:** (212)514-7440          **Fax:** (212)785-0290
Ken Berger, Exec. VP & COO

**Fnded:** 1866. **Desc:** Provides medical, dental and health education services. Programs occur within a 4-deck ship, docked in the East River at Wall Street. Provides health services to homeless children and their families, children in kinship foster care and their kinship families, and adolescents who engage in high risk behaviors. Programs take place dockside and while sailing around New York harbor. The ship is open during day and evening hours, six days each week. All programs integrate health education and nutrition, the keys of disease prevention, with compre-

hensive and continuous primary care. **Frmly:** (1980) St. John's Guild - The Floating Hospital.

★ **11493** ★ **German Hospital Federation (GHF)**
**(Deutsche Krankenhausgesellschaft — DKG)**
Munsterstr. 169
D-40476 Dusseldorf, Germany
**Phone:** 49 211 454730          **Fax:** 49 211 4547361
**Email:** dkg.mail@dkgev.de
**Website:** http://www.dkgev.de

**Fnded:** 1949. **Mem:** 28. **Nat'l Groups:** 12. **Reg. Groups:** 16. **State Groups:** 12. **Lang(s):** English, French. **Desc:** Federal state hospital associations and welfare federations in Germany. Publicizes members' accomplishments in public health. Works to maintain and improve the performance of hospitals; fosters exchange of information among members. Serves as liaison between members and government and other organizations; makes recommendations to legislative bodies. **Pub:** *das Krankenhaus*, monthly. Magazine. **Frmly:** (1998) German Hospital Association.

**Healthcare Information and Management Systems Society (HIMSS)**
*See:* Entry 12083

**Hospital Organization of Pedagogues in Europe (HOPE)**
*See:* Entry 5686

★ **11494** ★ **Hungarian Hospital Association (HHA)**
**(Magyar Korhazszovetseg — MKSZ)**
Fogaskereku u.4-6
H-1125 Budapest, Hungary
**Phone:** 36 1 2145159          **Fax:** 36 1 2149715
**Email:** cogels@pedi.ucl.ac.be
**Website:** http://www.connect-to-hope.org

**Fnded:** 1931. **Mem:** 155. **Local Groups:** 14. **Desc:** Doctors, nurses, and technical and administrative hospital personnel in Hungary. Disseminates research results and information based on the operation of hospitals and other health institutions. Fosters utilization of national and foreign medical achievements. Bestows awards. **Pub:** *A Korhaz*, quarterly. • Directory, quinquennial. Includes Dutch and English supplements.

★ **11495** ★ **Institute for Health Care Management**
Postbus 9697
NL-3506 GR Utrecht, Netherlands
**Phone:** 31 30 2739700          **Fax:** 31 30 2739560
**Email:** nzi@nzi.nl

**Fnded:** 1968. **Local Groups:** 7. **Lang(s):** Dutch, English, French, German. **Desc:** Seeks to develop a "sound, humane, and financially feasible health service" in the Netherlands. Conducts scientific research; offers advisory services; maintains educational programs. Disseminates information to health institutions and health care services. **Pub:** *NZI Notities*, bimonthly. Magazine. **Frmly:** (1999) Institute for Health Management.

★ **11496** ★ **International Association of Healthcare Central Service Materiel Management (IAHCSMM)**
213 W Institute Pl., Ste. 307
Chicago, IL 60610
**Phone:** (312)440-0078          **Free:** 800-962-8274
**Fax:** (312)440-9474
**Email:** mailbox@iahcsmm.com
**Website:** http://www.iahcsmm.com
Betty Hanna, Exec. Dir.

**Fnded:** 1958. **Mem:** 9,000. **State Groups:** 35. **Desc:** Professional personnel responsible for management and distribution of supplies from central service materiel management departments of a hospital. Works to improve the quality of central service materiel management departments in hospitals; share information and ideas; research hospital central service materiel management methods and practices; conduct and promote continuing education programs. Sponsors management correspondence courses, technician training and materials management courses through Purdue University in Indiana. Has established a certification program to recognize exceptional achievement. Maintains technician registry and placement service. Surveys salaries. Conducts research programs; compiles statistics. Maintains 23 committees. **Pub:** *Communique*, bimonthly. • Also publishes technical management and training manuals. **Frmly:** (1969) National Association of Hospital Central Service Personnel; (1989) International Association of Hospital Central Service Management.

**★ 11497 ★ International Association for Healthcare Security and Safety (IAHSS)**
PO Box 637
Lombard, IL 60148
**Phone:** (630)871-9936        **Free:** 888-353-0990
**Fax:** (630)871-9938
**Email:** nancy@iahss.org
**Website:** http://www.iahss.org
Bradley W. Williams, Pres.

**Fnded:** 1968. **Mem:** 1,700. **Reg. Groups:** 17. **Local Groups:** 53. **Desc:** Administrative and supervisory personnel in the field of hospital security and safety. To develop, promote, and coordinate better security/safety programs in medical care facilities. Offers placement services; conducts specialized education programs. **Pub:** *Healthcare Protection Management*, semiannual. Journal. • Membership Directory, annual. • Newsletter, quarterly. **Frmly:** (1990) International Association for Hospital Security.

**★ 11498 ★ International Hospital Federation (IHF) (Federacion Internacional de Hospitales)**
c/o Christa Obenaus, Events Coor.
46 Grosvenor Gardens
London SW1W 0EB, United Kingdom
**Phone:** 44 20 78819222    **Fax:** 44 20 78819223
**Email:** christao@ihf.co.uk
**Website:** http://www.hospitalmanagement.net

**Fnded:** 1929. **Mem:** 1,694. **Reg. Groups:** 1. **Lang(s):** English, French, Spanish. **Desc:** Individuals (1117); organizations (388); professional firms (114); government representatives (75). Promotes improvement in the planning and management of hospitals and health services through study tours, information services, and research and development projects. Serves as an advocate for hospitals and related health service organizations in world health affairs. Sponsors regional conferences and courses for senior hospital and health services managers from developing countries. Compiles statistics. **Pub:** *Health Service International*, quarterly. Newsletter. • *Hospitals International*, quarterly. Newsletter. • *World Hospitals*, 3/year. Journal. Includes summaries in French and Spanish.

**National Association of Children's Hospitals and Related Institutions (NACHRI)**
*See:* Entry 5716

**★ 11499 ★ National Association of Healthcare Access Management (NAHAM)**
2025 M St. NW, Ste. 800
Washington, DC 20036
**Phone:** (202)367-1125        **Fax:** (202)367-2125
**Email:** info@naham.org
**Website:** http://www.naham.org
Rita Borowski, Pres.

**Fnded:** 1974. **Mem:** 850. **Reg. Groups:** 6. **Desc:** Healthcare access managers united to improve patient care and community relations. Promotes professional recognition and provides educational resources for the

healthcare patient access field. Serves as a central source of technical information on changes and trends in healthcare that affect patient access services. Advocates progressive changes in healthcare practices; provides information on admissions and registration procedures. **Pub:** *Connections*, bimonthly. Newsletter. Contains list of employment opportunities. *Price:* Included in membership dues; $75/year for nonmembers. • *The NAHAM Management Journal*, quarterly. Journal. Contains reports on trends affecting admissions, patient registration, and patient access; includes descriptions of techniques, systems, and services. *Price:* Included in membership dues; $90/year for nonmembers. • *National Association of Healthcare Access Management–Membership Directory*, annual. Membership Directory. **Frmly:** (1990) National Association of Hospital Admitting Managers.

**★ 11500 ★ National Association of Health Unit Coordinators (NAHUC)**
1947 Madron Rd.
Rockford, IL 61107-1716
**Phone:** (815)633-4351        **Free:** 888-22-NAHUC
**Fax:** (815)633-4438
**Email:** office@nahuc.org
**Website:** http://www.nahuc.org
Faylua Core, Pres.

**Fnded:** 1980. **Mem:** 1,700. **Reg. Groups:** 9. **Local Groups:** 30. **Desc:** Coordinators of nonclinical nursing unit activities; educators, supervisors, students, and graduates in the field. Promotes the professional practice of unit coordinating. Has established standards of practice defining the role and responsibilities of health unit coordinators in the nonclinical area of health care and ensuring delivery of quality patient care. Works to establish certification guidelines for individual practitioners with a goal of national certification. Seeks recognition of the change in job title from clerk to that of coordinator, which the group believes better describes the nature of the position. Promotes continuing education and research; endeavors to develop accreditation of educational programs and standards of education for job entry. Provides vocational information to prospective students in the field; recruits students into the profession. Represents members' interests before allied health professionals, educational institutions, governmental bodies, and the community. Sponsors regional workshops, seminars, and other educational programs; compiles statistics. Maintains certification board and speakers' bureau; offers annual national certification exam and annual educational conference. **Pub:** *Information Booklet*, annual. Booklet. *Price:* Free. • *National Association of Health Unit Coordinators–Coordinator*, quarterly. Newsletter. *Price:* Included in membership dues; $15/year for nonmembers. • *National Association of Health Unit Coordinators - Education Program Procure Guide.* Booklet. Provides information to assist in the development or evaluation of a formal educational program. *Price:* $30 for members; $50 for nonmembers. • *National Association of Health Unit Coordinators–Membership Directory*, annual. Membership Directory. *Price:* Included in membership dues. • *Question & Answer Brochures.* Brochures. **Frmly:** (1990) National Association of Health Unit Clerks-Coordinators.

**★ 11501 ★ National Association of Hospital Hospitality Houses (NAHHH)**
PO Box 18087
Asheville, NC 28814-0087
**Phone:** (828)253-1188        **Free:** 800-542-9730
**Fax:** (828)253-8082
**Email:** helpinghomes@nahhh.org
**Website:** http://www.nahhh.org
Celena E. Grey, Exec. Dir.

**Fnded:** 1986. **Mem:** 175. **Reg. Groups:** 10. **Desc:** Hospitals, hospital hospitality houses (HHH), charitable foundations, and interested individuals. (Hospital hospitality houses are temporary residential facilities for patients and their families.) Provides assistance to members and offers information and guidance to those who wish to establish an HHH. Conducts educational programs; operates resource center and speakers'

bureau; compiles statistics. **Pub:** *Inside Hospitality*, quarterly. Newsletter. *Price:* Free. • *National Association of Hospitality Houses: Home Away From Home.* Brochure. Sent to members, hospitals, and healthcare agencies.

**★ 11502 ★ National Association of Psychiatric Health Systems (NAPHS)**
325 7th St., NW, Ste. 625
Washington, DC 20004-2802
**Phone:** (202)393-6700        **Fax:** (202)783-6041
**Email:** naphs@naphs.org
**Website:** http://www.naphs.org
Mark Covall, Exec. Dir.

**Fnded:** 1933. **Mem:** 292. **Desc:** Advocates for behavioral health. Represents provider systems that are committed to the delivery of responsive, accountable, and clinically effective preventing treatment, and care for children, adolescents, and adults with mental and substance use disorders. **Frmly:** (1993) National Association of Private Psychiatric Hospitals.

**★ 11503 ★ National Association of Public Hospitals and Health Systems (NAPH)**
1301 Pennsylvania Ave., NW, Ste. 950
Washington, DC 20004
**Phone:** (202)585-0100        **Fax:** (202)585-0101
**Email:** naph@naph.org
**Website:** http://www.naph.org
Christine Capito Burch, Exec. Dir.

**Fnded:** 1980. **Mem:** 70. **Desc:** Urban public hospitals. Promotes the development of federal, state, and local legislative and policy agendas for members. **Pub:** *Safety Net*, quarterly. • Newsletter, periodic. **Frmly:** (1998) National Association of Public Hospitals.

**★ 11504 ★ National Perinatal Information Center**
144 Wayland Ave., Ste. 300
Providence, RI 02906
**Phone:** (401)274-0650        **Fax:** (401)455-0377
**Email:** npic@npic.org
**Website:** http://www.npic.org
David E. Gagnon, Exec. Dir.

**Fnded:** 1985. **Mem:** 2,000. **Desc:** Gathers extensive patient data on hospital stays. Serves as perinatal research center for Maternal and Child Health Clearinghouse. Provides educational and research programs. Maintains speakers' bureau Performs children's services. **Pub:** *NPIC Newsletter*, quarterly. Contains articles on NPIC research. *Price:* included in membership dues. • Brochure, annual. • Directory.

**★ 11505 ★ New Zealand Private Hospitals Association (NZPHA)**
PO Box 12 481
Wellington 6015, New Zealand
**Phone:** 64 4 4733159        **Fax:** 64 4 4733554
**Email:** lesley@nzpha.org.nz
**Website:** http://www.nzpha.org.nz

**Fnded:** 1946. **Lang(s):** English. **Desc:** Private hospitals in New Zealand. Represents, protects, and advocates the interests of its members and their associated services.

**★ 11506 ★ Premier Advocacy**
444 N Capitol St. NW, Ste. 625
Washington, DC 20001-1511
**Phone:** (202)393-0860        **Fax:** (202)393-0864
**Website:** http://my.premierinc.com/frames/index.jsp?pagelocation=/all/advocacy/
Herb Kuhn, Corporate VP

**Fnded:** 1984. **Mem:** 40. **Desc:** Nonprofit multi-hospital systems. Sponsors educational programs for corporate officers and trustees of multi-hospital systems. Monitors, investigates, and develops policy positions on developments in the health care field. **Frmly:** Association AMHS Institute; (1988) American Healthcare Institute; (1998) AMHS Institute; (1999) Premier.

### ★ 11507 ★ Section for Metropolitan Hospitals (SMH)

c/o American Hospital Association
1 N Franklin, Ste. 27
Chicago, IL 60606
**Phone:** (312)422-3000          **Fax:** (312)422-4583
**Email:** jsupplitt@aha.org
**Website:** http://www.aha.org/MemberRelations/metroh.asp
John T. Supplitt, Dir.

**Fnded:** 1984. **Mem:** 1,365. **Desc:** Institutional members of the American Hospital Association that are located within a metropolitan statistical area and/or provide a significant proportion of Medicare, Medicaid, and uncompensated care; participate in undergraduate and/or graduate medical education programs and research; provide high volumes of ambulatory care; offer specialized services; and are involved in professional and paraprofessional education and training programs. Represents views of members to the AHA and assists in the development and implementation of policies and programs to promote recognition, support, and growth for its members within the health care field. Serves as clearinghouse for metropolitan hospital delivery, finance, governanc e, management, and organizational issues. Compiles statistics; maintains databases; conducts forums.

### ★ 11508 ★ Section for Psychiatric and Substance Abuse Services (SPSPAS)

c/o American Hospital Association
One N Franklin
Chicago, IL 60606
**Phone:** (312)422-3000          **Free:** 800-242-4890
**Fax:** (312)422-4796
**Email:** hromero@aha.org
**Website:** http://www.aha.org/memberrelations/psas.org
Gary A. Mecklenburg, Pres.

**Fnded:** 1969. **Mem:** 3,000. **Desc:** Institutional members, both general hospitals and freestanding specialty hospitals, of the American Hospital Association who provide psychiatric, substance abuse, clinical psychology, and other behavioral health services. Assists the AHA in development and implementation of policies and programs to promote improvement of and advocacy for the nation's behavioral health care providers. Active in formulating and commenting on federal legislation and regulations relating to psychiatric and substance abuse services. Develops and maintains liaison relationships with key organizations important to behavioral health providers. **Frmly:** (1972) Psychiatric Hospital Section; (1984) Psychiatric Services Section; (1991) Special Constituency Section for Mental Health and Psychiatric Services; (1997) Special Constituency Section for Psychiatric and Substance Abuse Services.

### ★ 11509 ★ Shriners Hospitals for Children

2900 Rocky Point Dr.
Tampa, FL 33607-1460
**Phone:** (813)281-0300          **Free:** 800-237-5055
**Website:** http://www.shrinershq.org/Hospitals/
Lewis K. Molnar, Exec. VP

**Fnded:** 1922. **Mem:** 22. **Desc:** SHC operated orthopedic hospitals (19) and burn hospitals (4) founded by and affiliated with the Imperial Council of the Ancient Arabic Order of the Nobles of the Mystic Shrine for North America. Provides no-cost orthopedic and burn care to children under 18 years of age. Maintains the Shriners Hospitals for Children Endowment Fund. Conducts research; compiles statistics. **Pub:** *Between Us*, 3/year. Magazine. *Price:* Free. • *Imperial Council of the Ancient Arabic Order of the Nobles of the Mystic Shrine for North America.* • Booklet. • Brochures. • Pamphlets. • Also publishes fact sheets.

### Society for Healthcare Epidemiology of America

*See:* Entry 9043

### ★ 11510 ★ Society for Healthcare Strategy and Market Development of the American Hospital Association

1 N Franklin
Chicago, IL 60606
**Phone:** (312)422-3888          **Fax:** (312)422-4579
**Email:** stratsoc@aha.org
**Website:** http://www.stratsociety.org
Nancy Wilson, Pres.

**Fnded:** 1996. **Mem:** 4,000. **Local Groups:** 57. **Desc:** Persons in hospitals, health systems and networks, managed care plans, ambulatory care and physician groups who are engaged in strategic planning, business development, marketing, or public relations activities. **Pub:** *Directory of Health Care Strategic Management and Communications Consultants*, annual. Directory. *Price:* Free to members; $40/copy for nonmembers. • *Membership Directory Society for Healthcare Strategy and Market Development*, annual. Membership Directory. *Price:* Included in membership dues. • *Spectrum*, bimonthly. Tabloid; includes calendar of events. *Price:* Included in membership dues. **Frmly:** (1984) American Society for Hospital Public Relations; (1990) American Society for Hospital Marketing and Public Relations; (1998) American Society for Healthcare Marketing and Public Relations.

### ★ 11511 ★ Standing Committee of the Hospitals of the European Union (HOPE)

35 Kapucijnenvoer
B-3000 Leuven, Belgium
**Phone:** 32 16 336902          **Fax:** 32 16 336906
**Email:** sg@hope.be
**Website:** http://www.hope.be
**Fnded:** 1966. **Mem:** 22. **Lang(s):** English, French, German. **Desc:** Works to develop the range and continuing improvement of services provided by hospitals. Gathers and disseminates information. **Pub:** *Hospital Healthcare Europe*, annual. Book. Official HOPE reference book.

### ★ 11512 ★ Swiss Hospital Association (SHA)
### (H Die Spitaler der Schweiz)

Lorrainestrasse 4A
CH-3013 Bern, Switzerland
**Phone:** 41 31 3351111          **Fax:** 41 31 3351170
**Email:** geschaeftsstelle@hplus.ch
**Fnded:** 1930. **Mem:** 729. **Lang(s):** English, French, German. **Desc:** Safeguards, promotes, and represents the political, economic, and legal interests of public and private hospitals, clinics, and nursing homes. Serves as a liaison between health care authorities, health insurers and facilities. Plays an active role in defining medical, economic, social, and educations politics within the Swiss system of public health. Develops guidelines for compiling medical and administrative statistics, quality management, performance assessment, and controlling. Operates a publishing house and two education centers. **Pub:** *List of Members*, periodic. • *Medizinische Gesamtstatistik der Schweizer Spitaler.* • *Schweizer Spital*, monthly.

### ★ 11513 ★ Trinity Medical Center

2701 17th St.
Rock Island, IL 61201-5393
**Phone:** (309)779-5000          **Fax:** (309)779-2303
**Website:** http://www.trinityqc.com
William Leaver, Pres.

**Mem:** 110. **Desc:** Hospitals sponsored by a Lutheran church or bearing the title Lutheran. Offers periodic grants for the advancement of health care chaplaincy programs. **Pub:** *Lutheran Health Resources Directory*, periodic. Directory. • Newsletter, quarterly.

### ★ 11514 ★ Volunteer Trustees of Not-for-Profit Hospitals

818 18th St. NW, Ste. 900
Washington, DC 20006
**Phone:** (202)659-0338          **Fax:** (202)659-0116
**Email:** vt@sprintmail.com
**Website:** http://www.volunteertrustees.org
Linda B. Miller, Pres.

**Fnded:** 1980. **Mem:** 150. **State Groups:** 45. **Desc:** Representatives of 155 not-for-profit hospitals and their voluntary governing boards. Objectives are to: provide a trustee voice in policy-making and legislative activities; develop a communications network among trustees in order to provide the highest quality medical care at the lowest possible price; provide educational services to hospital governing boards; facilitate accurate portrayal of not-for-profit hospitals in the media and Congress. Areas of concern include: Medicare; controlling hospital costs; strategic planning for the not-for-profit hospital community. Compiles information on governing boards. Conducts roundtables.

## Research Centers

**U.S. Department of Health and Human Services**
**National Center for Infectious Diseases**
**Hospital Infections Program**
*See:* Entry 11901

## State Government Agencies

### Hospital Licensure

### ★ 11515 ★ Alaska Department of Health and Social Services
**Medical Assistance Division**
**Health Facilities Licensing and Certification Office**
4730 Business Park Blvd., Ste. 18
Anchorage, AK 99503
**Phone:** (907)334-2483          **Fax:** (907)561-3011
**Email:** shelby_larsen@health.state.ak.us
**Website:** http://www.hss.state.ak.us/dma/HFLC.HTM
Shelby Larsen, Contact

### ★ 11516 ★ Arizona Department of Health Services
**Health Care Licensure Office**
1647 E Morten Ave., Ste. 240
Phoenix, AZ 85020
**Phone:** (602)674-4340          **Fax:** (602)861-0463
**Email:** jhaaske@hs.state.az.us
**Website:** http://www.hs.state.az.us/als/index.html

### ★ 11517 ★ Arkansas Department of Health
**Health Resources Bureau**
**Health Facility Services and Systems Division**
5800 W Tenth St. Ste. 400
Little Rock, AR 72204
**Phone:** (501)661-2201
**Website:** http://health.state.ar.us

### ★ 11518 ★ California Health and Welfare Agency
**Health Services Department**
**Licensing and Certification Division**
7801 Folsom Blvd., Ste. 200
PO Box 942732
Sacramento, CA 95826
**Phone:** (916)229-3400          **Free:** 800-554-0354
**Fax:** (916)229-3465
**Website:** http://www.dhs.ca.gov/lnc/index.htm

**★ 11519 ★ Colorado Public Health and Environment Department**
**Health Office**
**Health Facilities Division**
4300 Cherry Creek Dr. S
Denver, CO 80246-1530
**Phone:** (303)692-2800
**Email:** health.facilities@state.co.us
**Website:** http://www.cdphe.state.co.us/hf/

**★ 11520 ★ Connecticut Department of Public Health**
**Regulatory Services Bureau**
**Health Systems Regulation Division**
410 Capitol Ave.
PO Box 340308
Hartford, CT 06134-0308
**Phone:** (860)509-7406        **Fax:** (860)509-7539
**Email:** webmaster.dph@po.state.ct.us
**Website:** http://www.state.ct.us/dph/DPH_Main/About_DPH/brs/brs.htm
Cynthia Denne, Contact

**★ 11521 ★ District of Columbia Department of Consumer and Regulatory Affairs**
**Service Facility Regulations Administration**
**Health Facility Division**
941 N Capital St. NE, Rm. 1100
Washington, DC 20002
**Phone:** (202)442-4400
**Website:** http://dcra.dc.gov/main.shtm

**★ 11522 ★ Florida Department of Health**
**Licensure and Certification Office**
4052 Bald Cypress Way, Bin A00
Tallahassee, FL 32399
**Phone:** (850)245-4443
**Email:** health@doh.state.fl.us
**Website:** http://www.doh.state.fl.us/

**★ 11523 ★ Georgia Department of Human Resources**
**Regulatory Services Office**
**Health Care Section**
2 Peachtree St. NW,
Atlanta, GA 30303
**Phone:** (404)657-5550        **Fax:** (404)657-8934
**Email:** mapalli@dhr.state.ga.us
**Website:** http://www2.state.ga.us/departments/dhr/ors/orshcs.htm

**★ 11524 ★ Hawaii Department of Health**
**Office of Health Care Assurance**
601 Kamokila Blvd.
Rm. 395
Kapolei, HI 96707
**Phone:** (808)586-4080        **Fax:** (808)586-4444
**Email:** webmail@health.hi.us
**Website:** http://www.state.hi.us/health/about/dohphn01.htm
Helen Yoshimi, Contact

**★ 11525 ★ Idaho Department of Health and Welfare**
**Medicaid Division**
**Facility Standards Bureau**
450 West State St.
Boise, ID 83720-0036
**Phone:** (208)334-6626
**Website:** http://www2.state.id.us/dhw/FacilStandards/bfs_index.htm
Debra Ransom, Director

**★ 11526 ★ Illinois Department of Public Health**
**Health Care Regulation Office**
**Health Care Facilities and Programs Division**
**Hospital Licensing Section**
525 W Jefferson St., 5th Fl.
Springfield, IL 62761
**Phone:** (217)782-2913        **Fax:** (217)524-6292
**Email:** bbell@idph.state.il.us
**Website:** http://www.idph.state.il.us/about/ohcr.htm

**★ 11527 ★ Indiana Department of Health**
**Acute Care Division**
2 N Meridian St.
Indianapolis, IN 46204
**Phone:** (317)233-1325
**Website:** http://www.state.in.us/isdh/regsvcs/acc/acute.htm

**★ 11528 ★ Iowa Department of Inspections and Appeals**
**Health Facilities Division**
Lucas State Office Bldg.
321 E 12th St.
Des Moines, IA 50319-0001
**Phone:** (515)281-4115
**Email:** mtooman@dia.state.ia.us
**Website:** http://www.dia-hfd.state.ia.us/
Marvin L. Tooman, Director

**★ 11529 ★ Kansas Department of Health and Environment**
**Health Division**
**Adult and Child Care Facilities Bureau**
**Hospital Program**
1000 SW Jackson St., Ste. 330
Topeka, KS 66612
**Phone:** (785)296-1240        **Fax:** (785)296-1266
**Email:** healthfacilities@kdhe.state.ks.us
**Website:** http://www.kdhe.state.ks.us/bhfr/

**★ 11530 ★ Kentucky Health Services Cabinet**
**Inspector General Office**
**Community Health Services Division**
275 E Main St, 5E-A
Frankfort, KY 40621
**Phone:** (502)564-2800        **Fax:** (502)564-6546
**Website:** http://chs.state.ky.us/oig/community/
Floyd B. Parrish, Director

**★ 11531 ★ Louisiana Department of Health and Hospitals**
**Health Standards Section**
**Licensing and Certification Division**
PO Box 3767
Baton Rouge, LA 70821-3767
**Phone:** (225)342-0415        **Fax:** (225)342-5292
**Email:** ldeaton@dhh.state.la.us
**Website:** http://www.dhh.state.la.us/boards.htm
Lisa M. Deaton, Contact

**★ 11532 ★ Maine Department of Human Services**
**Medical Services Bureau**
**Licensing and Certification Division**
11 State House Station
35 Anthony Ave
Augusta, ME 04333-0011
**Phone:** (207)624-5443        **Fax:** (207)624-5378
**Email:** lou.dorogi@state.me.us
**Website:** http://www.state.me.us/bms/
Lou Dorogi, Director

**★ 11533 ★ Maryland Department of Health and Mental Hygiene**
**Office of Health Care Quality**
Spring Grove Hospital Center
Bland Bryant Bldg.
55 Wade Ave.
Catonsville, MD 21228
**Phone:** (410)402-8000
**Email:** ohcqweb@dhmh.state.md.us
**Website:** http://www.dhmh.state.md.us/ohcq/

**★ 11534 ★ Massachusetts Executive Office of Health and Human Services**
**Public Health Department**
**Health Care Quality Division**
10 W St, 5th Fl.
Boston, MA 02111
**Phone:** (617)753-8000        **Fax:** (617)753-8125
**Email:** paul.l.dreyer@state.ma.us
**Website:** http://www.state.ma.us/dph/hcqskel.htm
Paul Dreyer, Director

**★ 11535 ★ Michigan Department of Consumer and Industry Services**
**Commercial Services Bureau**
**Licensing Division**
PO Box 30018
Lansing, MI 48909
**Phone:** (517)241-9223        **Fax:** (517)241-9280
**Email:** bcsinfo@cis.state.mi.us
**Website:** http://www.cis.state.mi.us/bcs/licdiv.htm
Jean Boven, Director

**★ 11536 ★ Minnesota Department of Health**
**Health Systems and Special Populations Bureau**
**Facility and Provider Compliance Division**
PO Box 64975
Saint Paul, MN 55164-0975
**Phone:** (651)215-5800
**Email:** fpcmail@mdh-fpc.health.state.mn.us
**Website:** http://www.health.state.mn.us/divs/fpc/fpc.html

**★ 11537 ★ Mississippi Department of Health**
**Health Regulation Office**
**Licensure Division**
570 Woodrow Wilson Blvd. Ste. 200
PO Box 1700
Jackson, MS 39216
**Phone:** (601)576-7300        **Fax:** (601)576-7225
**Email:** vphipps@msdh.state.ms.us
**Website:** http://www.msdh.state.ms.us/licensure/index.htm

**★ 11538 ★ Missouri Department of Health**
**Health Standards and Licensure Division**
**Hospital Licensing and Certification Bureau**
930 Wildwood
PO Box 570
Jefferson City, MO 65102
**Phone:** (573)751-6271        **Fax:** (573)526-3621
**Email:** info@mail.health.state.mo.us
**Website:** http://www.health.state.mo.us/AbouttheDepartment/DS6.html

**★ 11539 ★ Montana Department of Public Health and Human Services**
**Health Facilities Division**
2401 Colonial Dr.
PO Box 202953
Helena, MT 59620-2953
**Phone:** (406)444-2037        **Fax:** (406)444-1742
**Email:** ddavis@state.mt.gov

**Website:** http://www.dphhs.state.mt.us/divisions/qad/qad_phone.htm
Mary Dalton, Director

**★ 11540 ★ Nebraska Department of Health and Human Services**
**Environmental Health**
**Health Facilities Licensure Division**
301 Centennial Mall S
PO Box 95007
Lincoln, NE 68509-5044
**Phone:** (402)471-0179        **Fax:** (402)471-0555
**Email:** hmeeks@doh.state.ne.us
**Website:** http://www.hhs.state.ne.us/enh/enh-index.htm
Helen Meeks, Contact

**★ 11541 ★ Nevada Department of Human Resources**
**Health Division**
**Licensure and Certification Bureau**
1550 E College Parkway, St.158
Carson City, NV 89706
**Phone:** (775)687-4475        **Fax:** (775)687-6588
**Website:** http://www.state.nv.us/health/
Luana Ritch, Contact

**★ 11542 ★ New Hampshire Department of Health and Human Services**
**Public Health Services Division**
**Health Facilities Administration Bureau**
129 Pleasant St.
Concord, NH 03301-3857
**Phone:** (603)271-4592        **Fax:** (603)271-4968
**Website:** http://www.dhhs.state.nh.us

**★ 11543 ★ New Jersey Department of Health**
**Health Facilities Evaluation and Licensing Division**
**Licensing, Certification, and Standards Office**
120 S Stockton St.
PO Box 367
Trenton, NJ 08625-0367
**Phone:** (609)633-9051        **Free:** 800-792-9770
**Fax:** (609)633-9087
**Email:** ltc@doh.state.nj.us
**Website:** http://www.state.nj.us/health/ltc/

**★ 11544 ★ New Mexico Department of Health**
**Public Health Division**
**Licensing and Certification Bureau**
2040 S Pacheco St. 2nd Flr., Rm 413
Santa Fe, NM 87505
**Phone:** (505)476-9025        **Fax:** (505)476-9053
**Website:**        http://www.health.state.nm.us/dhi/HFLC.htm

**★ 11545 ★ North Carolina Department of Health and Human Services**
**Facility Services Division**
2706 Mail Service Ctr.
2701 Mail Service Ctr.
Raleigh, NC 27699-2701
**Phone:** (919)733-2342        **Free:** 800-624-3004
**Fax:** (919)733-2757
**Email:** Michelle.Penny@ncmail.net
**Website:** http://facility-services.state.nc.us/
Lynda McDaniel, Director

**★ 11546 ★ North Dakota Department of Health**
**Health Resources Section**
**Health Facilities Division**
600 E Boulevard, Department 301
Bismarck, ND 58505-0200

**Phone:** (701)328-2352        **Fax:** (701)328-1890
**Email:** ajohnson@state.nd.us
**Website:**        http://www.health.state.nd.us/ndhd/resource/facilities/about/
Allen Johnson, Director

**★ 11547 ★ Ohio Department of Health**
**Quality Assurance Division**
**Regulatory Compliance Bureau**
246 N High St.
PO Box 118
Columbus, OH 43216-0118
**Phone:** (614)644-6220        **Fax:** (614)752-4157
**Email:** BRC@gw.odh.state.oh.us
**Website:** http://www.odh.state.oh.us/
Alan Curtis, Director

**★ 11548 ★ Oklahoma Department of Health**
**Special Health Services**
**Medical and Facilities Services**
1000 NE 10th St.
Rm. 1114
Oklahoma City, OK 73117-1299
**Phone:** (405)271-6576        **Fax:** (405)271-1308
**Email:** Medicalfacilities@health.state.ok.us
**Website:** http://www.health.state.ok.us/PROGRAM/medfac/index.html

**★ 11549 ★ Oregon Department of Human Resources**
**Health Division**
**Health Care Licensure and Certification Section**
Portland State Office Bldg.
800 NE Oregon St.
Portland, OR 97232
**Phone:** (503)731-4013        **Fax:** (503)731-3184
**Website:**        http://www.ohd.hr.state.or.us/hclc/welcome.htm
Kathleen Smail, Contact

**★ 11550 ★ Pennsylvania Department of Health**
**Quality Assurance Bureau**
PO Box 90
Health and Welfare Bldg.
Harrisburg, PA 17108
**Free:** 877-724-3258
**Email:** webmaster@health.state.pa.us
**Website:** http://www.health.state.pa.us/qa/
Richard Lee, Contact

**★ 11551 ★ Rhode Island Department of Health**
**Health Services Regulations Office**
**Facilities Regulations Division**
3 Capitol Hill, Rm. 306
Providence, RI 02908
**Phone:** (401)222-2566        **Free:** 800-745-5555
**Website:**        http://www.health.state.ri.us/hsr/facreg/facreg.htm

**★ 11552 ★ South Carolina Department of Health and Environmental Control**
**Health Services Office**
**Health Facilities Regulation Bureau**
2600 Bull St.
PO Box 101106
Columbia, SC 29211-1708
**Phone:** (803)545-4663        **Fax:** (803)545-4212
**Website:** http://www.scdhec.net/hr

**★ 11553 ★ South Dakota Department of Health**
**Licensure and Certification Program**
615 E 4th St.
Pierre, SD 57501

**Phone:** (605)773-3356        **Fax:** (605)773-6667
**Email:** DOH.INFO@doh.state.sd.us
**Website:**        http://www.state.sd.us/doh/Facility/index.htm

**★ 11554 ★ Tennessee Department of Health**
**Manpower and Facilities Bureau**
**Health Care Facilities Division**
Cordell Hull Bldg., 1st Fl.
425 5th Ave., N
Nashville, TN 37247-0508
**Phone:** (615)741-7221
**Email:** Diane.Denton@state.tn.us
**Website:** http://www2.state.tn.us/health/HCF/

**★ 11555 ★ Texas Department of Health**
**Bureau of Licensing and Compliance**
**Health Facility Licensing and Compliance Division**
1100 W 49th St.
Austin, TX 78756
**Phone:** (512)834-6650        **Fax:** (512)834-6653
**Email:** infohflc@tdh.state.tx.us
**Website:** http://www.tdh.state.tx.us/hfc/hfc-web.htm
Nance Stearman, Director

**★ 11556 ★ Utah Department of Health**
**Health Systems Improvement Division**
**Health Facilities and Child Care Licensing Bureau**
288 N 1460 W
PO Box 142003
Salt Lake City, UT 84114-2003
**Phone:** (801)538-6152        **Free:** 888-287-3704
**Fax:** (801)538-6325
**Email:** mbentley@doh.state.ut.us
**Website:** http://www.health.state.ut.us/hsi/hfl/
Debra Wynkoop, Contact

**★ 11557 ★ Vermont Agency of Human Services**
**Health Department**
**Medical Care Regulation Division**
108 Cherry St.
PO Box 70
Burlington, VT 05402-0070
**Phone:** (802)863-7200        **Fax:** (802)865-7754
**Email:** Webkeeper@vdh.state.vt.us
**Website:** http://www.healthyvermonters.info/

**★ 11558 ★ Virginia Office of Health and Human Resources**
**Health Department**
**Center for Quality Health Care Services and Consumer Protection**
3600 W Broad St., St. 216
Richmond, VA 23230
**Phone:** (804)367-2106        **Free:** 800-955-1819
**Fax:** (804)367-2804
**Website:**        http://www.vdh.state.va.us/quality/default.htm

**★ 11559 ★ Washington Department of Health**
**Facility and Services Licensing Division**
PO Box 47852
Olympia, WA 98504-7852
**Phone:** (360)705-6652        **Fax:** (360)705-6654
**Website:** http://www.doh.wa.gov/hsqa/fsl/default.htm

**★ 11560 ★ West Virginia Department of Health and Human Resources**
**Public Health Bureau**
**Health Facility Licensure and Certification Office**
350 Capitol St.
Room 206
Charleston, WV 25301
**Phone:** (304)558-0050
**Email:** RobWest@wvdhhr.org
**Website:** http://www.wvdhhr.org/ohflac/default.htm
John Wilkinson, Director

**★ 11561 ★ Wisconsin Department of Health and Family Services**
**Health Division**
**Quality Compliance Bureau**
PO Box 7851
Madison, WI 53707-7851
**Phone:** (608)266-0554
**Email:** webmaster@dhfs.state.wi.us
**Website:** http://www.dhfs.state.wi.us/aboutdhfs/DSL/dsl.htm
Sinikka McCabe, Contact

# State & Regional Organizations

## Hospitals

*Listed below are state hospital associations that are allied with the American Hospital Association, 1 N Franklin, Chicago, IL 60606, (312)422-3000, http://www.aha.org/.*

### Alabama

**★ 11562 ★ Alabama Hospital Association**
500 N East Blvd.
Montgomery, AL 36117
**Phone:** (334)272-8781 **Fax:** (334)270-9527
J. Michael Horsley, CEO & Pres

### Alaska

**★ 11563 ★ Alaska State Hospital and Nursing Home Association**
426 Main St.
Juneau, AK 99801
**Phone:** (907)586-1790 **Fax:** (907)463-3573
Laraine Derr, CEO & Pres

### Alberta

**★ 11564 ★ Provincial Health Authorities of Alberta**
44 Capital Blvd.
200/10044-108 St. NW
Edmonton, AB, Canada T5J 3S7
**Phone:** (780)426-8503 **Fax:** (780)424-4309
E. Michael Higgins, Exec Director

### Arizona

**★ 11565 ★ Arizona Hospital and Healthcare Association**
2901 N Central Ave.
Phoenix, AZ 85012-2729
**Phone:** (602)445-4300 **Fax:** (602)445-4299
John R. Rivers, CEO & Pres

### Arkansas

**★ 11566 ★ Arkansas Hospital Association**
419 Natural Resources Dr.
Little Rock, AR 72205-1539

**Phone:** (501)224-7878 **Fax:** (501)224-0519
James R. Teeter, CEO & Pres

### California

**★ 11567 ★ California Healthcare Association**
1201 K St., Ste. 800
Sacramento, CA 95814
**Phone:** (916)552-7547 **Fax:** (916)552-7618
C. Duane Dauner, President
**Alt. Contact:** PO Box 1100, Sacramento, CA 95814.
**Frmly:** California Association of Hospitals and Health Systems.

**★ 11568 ★ Healthcare Association of San Diego and Imperial Counties**
402 W Broadway, 22nd Flr.
San Diego, CA 92101-3542
**Phone:** (619)544-0777 **Fax:** (619)544-0888
Stephen A. Escoboza, CEO & Pres

**★ 11569 ★ Healthcare Association of Southern California**
515 S Figueroa St., Ste. 1300
Los Angeles, CA 90071-3322
**Phone:** (213)538-0700 **Fax:** (213)629-4272
James D. Barber, CEO & Pres

**★ 11570 ★ Hospital Council of Northern and Central California**
1215 K. St., Ste. 730
Sacramento, CA 95814
**Phone:** (916)552-7608 **Fax:** (916)552-2618
Gregg Schnepple, CEO & Pres

### Colorado

**★ 11571 ★ Colorado Health and Hospital Association**
7335 E Orchard Rd., Ste. 100
Englewood, CO 80111
**Phone:** (720)489-1630 **Fax:** (720)489-9400
Larry Wall, President

### Connecticut

**★ 11572 ★ Connecticut Hospital Association**
110 Barnes Rd.
PO Box 90
Wallingford, CT 06492-0090
**Phone:** (203)294-7200 **Fax:** (203)269-7713
Jennifer Jackson, President

### Delaware

**★ 11573 ★ Delaware Healthcare Association**
1280 S Governors Ave.
Dover, DE 19904-4802
**Phone:** (302)674-2853 **Fax:** (302)734-2731
Joseph M. Letnaunchyn, President

### District of Columbia

**★ 11574 ★ District of Columbia Hospital Association**
1250 Eye St. NW, Ste. 700
Washington, DC 20005-3930
**Phone:** (202)682-1581 **Fax:** (202)371-8151
Robert A. Malson, President

### Florida

**★ 11575 ★ Florida Hospital Association**
307 Park Lake Cir.
PO Box 531107
Orlando, FL 32803-1107

**Phone:** (407)841-6230 **Fax:** (407)422-5948
Charles F. Pierce, Jr., President

**★ 11576 ★ South Florida Hospital and Healthcare Association, Inc.**
6363 Taft St., Ste. 200
Hollywood, FL 33024
**Phone:** (954)964-1660 **Fax:** (954)962-1260
Linda S. Quick, President

### Georgia

**★ 11577 ★ Georgia Hospital Association**
**An Association of Hospitals and Health Systems**
1675 Terrell Mill Rd.
Marietta, GA 30067
**Phone:** (770)955-0324 **Fax:** (770)955-5801
Joseph A. Parker, President

### Hawaii

**★ 11578 ★ Healthcare Association of Hawaii**
932 Ward Ave., Ste. 430
Honolulu, HI 96814-2126
**Phone:** (808)521-8961 **Fax:** (808)599-2879
Richard E. Meiers, CEO & Pres

### Idaho

**★ 11579 ★ Idaho Hospital Association**
615 N 7th St.
Boise, ID 83701-1278
**Phone:** (208)338-5100 **Fax:** (208)338-7800
Steven A. Millard, President

### Illinois

**★ 11580 ★ Illinois Hospital and HealthSystems Association**
1151 E Warrenville Rd.
PO Box 3015
Naperville, IL 60566-7015
**Phone:** (630)505-7777 **Fax:** (630)505-9457
Kenneth C. Robbins, President

**★ 11581 ★ Metropolitan Chicago Healthcare Council**
222 S Riverside Plaza, 19th Flr.
Chicago, IL 60606
**Phone:** (312)906-6000 **Fax:** (312)993-0779
Earl C. Bird, President

### Indiana

**★ 11582 ★ Indiana Hospital and Health Association**
1 American Sq.
PO Box 82063
Indianapolis, IN 46282
**Phone:** (317)633-4870 **Fax:** (317)633-4875
Kenneth G. Stella, President
**Frmly:** Indiana Hospital Association.

### Iowa

**★ 11583 ★ Iowa Hospital Association**
100 E Grand Ave., Ste. 100
Des Moines, IA 50309
**Phone:** (515)288-1955 **Fax:** (515)283-9366
Stephen F. Brenton, President
**Frmly:** Iowa Hospitals Association.

**★ 11584 ★ Iowa Hospital Association**
100 E Grand Ave., Ste. 100
Des Moines, IA 50309
**Phone:** (515)288-1955 **Fax:** (515)283-9366
Stephen F. Brenton, President

## Kansas

★ **11585** ★ **Kansas Hospital Association**
215 SE 8th St.
Topeka, KS 66603
**Phone:** (785)233-7436     **Fax:** (785)233-6955
Donald A. Wilson, President
**Alt. Contact:** PO Box 2308, Topeka, KS 66601-2308.

## Kentucky

★ **11586** ★ **Kentucky Hospital Association**
**An Association of Kentucky Hospitals and Health Systems**
2501 Nelson Miller Pky.
PO Box 436629
Louisville, KY 40253-6629
**Phone:** (502)426-6220     **Fax:** (502)426-6226
Michael T. Rust, President

## Louisiana

★ **11587** ★ **Louisiana Hospital Association**
9521 Brookline Ave.
Baton Rouge, LA 70809-1431
**Phone:** (225)928-0026     **Fax:** (225)923-1004
Lynn B. Nicholas, CEO & Pres
**Alt. Contact:** PO Box 80720, Baton Rouge, LA 70898-0720.

★ **11588** ★ **Metropolitan Hospital Council of New Orleans**
2450 Severn Ave., Ste. 210
Metairie, LA 70001
**Phone:** (504)837-1171     **Fax:** (504)837-1174
John J. Finn, PhD, President

## Maine

★ **11589** ★ **Maine Hospital Association**
150 Capitol St.
Augusta, ME 04330
**Phone:** (207)622-4794     **Fax:** (207)622-3073
Steven R. Michaud, President

## Maryland

★ **11590** ★ **Healthcare Council of the National Capital Area**
8201 Corporate Dr., Ste. 410
Landover, MD 20785-2229
**Phone:** (301)731-4700     **Fax:** (301)731-8286
Joseph P. Burns, CEO & Pres

★ **11591** ★ **Maryland Hospital Association**
**The Association of Maryland Hospitals & Health Systems**
6820 Deerpath Rd.
Elkridge, MD 21075-6234
**Phone:** (410)379-6200     **Fax:** (410)379-8239
Calvin M. Pierson, President

## Massachusetts

★ **11592** ★ **Massachusetts Hospital Association**
5 New England Executive Park
Burlington, MA 01803
**Phone:** (781)272-8000     **Fax:** (781)272-0466
Ronald M. Hollander, President

## Michigan

★ **11593** ★ **Healthcare Council of MidMichigan**
3927 Beecher Rd.
Flint, MI 48532-3803

**Phone:** (810)766-8898     **Fax:** (810)762-4108
Marlene Soderstrom, President

★ **11594** ★ **Hospital Council of East Central Michigan**
141 Harrow Ln., Ste. 11
Saginaw, MI 48603
**Phone:** (517)792-1725     **Fax:** (517)792-3099
Elizabeth S. Schnettler, President

★ **11595** ★ **Michigan Health and Hospital Association**
6215 W St. Joseph Hwy.
Lansing, MI 48917
**Phone:** (517)323-3443     **Fax:** (517)323-0946
Spencer C. Johnson, President

★ **11596** ★ **North Central Council of the Michigan Hospital Association**
616 Petoskey St., Ste. 202
Petoskey, MI 49770
**Phone:** (231)439-9812     **Fax:** (231)439-9813
Elizabeth Gertz, Exec Director

★ **11597** ★ **Southeast Michigan Health and Hospital Council**
24725 W Twelve Mile Rd., Ste. 104A
Southfield, MI 48034
**Phone:** (248)358-2950     **Fax:** (248)358-1098
Donald P. Potter, President

★ **11598** ★ **Southwestern Michigan Hospital Council**
6215 W St. Joseph Hwy.
Lansing, MI 48917
**Phone:** (517)323-3443     **Fax:** (517)323-0946
Clark R. Ballard, President

## Minnesota

★ **11599** ★ **Minnesota Hospital and Healthcare Partnership**
2550 University Ave. W, Ste. 350S
Saint Paul, MN 55114-1900
**Phone:** (651)641-1121     **Fax:** (651)659-1477
Bruce J. Rueben, President
**Frmly:** Minnesota Hospital Association.

## Mississippi

★ **11600** ★ **Mississippi Hospital Association**
6425 Lakeover Rd.
PO Box 16444
Jackson, MS 39236-6444
**Free:** 800-289-8884     **Fax:** (601)368-3200
Sam W. Cameron, CEO & Pres

## Missouri

★ **11601** ★ **The Health Alliance of MidAmerica**
10401 Holmes Rd., Ste. 280
Kansas City, MO 64131-3368
**Phone:** (816)941-3800     **Fax:** (816)941-0818
Michael R. Dunaway, Senior VP

★ **11602** ★ **Missouri Hospital Association**
PO Box 60
Jefferson City, MO 65102-0060
**Phone:** (573)893-3700     **Fax:** (573)893-2809
Marc D. Smith, President

## Montana

★ **11603** ★ **Montana Hospital Association**
**An Association of Montana Health Care Providers**
1720 9th Ave.
PO Box 5119
Helena, MT 59604
**Phone:** (406)442-1911     **Fax:** (406)443-3894
James F. Ahrens, President

## Nebraska

★ **11604** ★ **Nebraska Association of Hospitals and Health Systems**
1640 L St., Ste. D
Lincoln, NE 68508
**Phone:** (402)458-4900     **Fax:** (402)475-4091
Laura J. Redoutey, CHE, President

## Nevada

★ **11605** ★ **Nevada Hospital Association**
4600 Kietzke Ln., Ste. I-206
Reno, NV 89502
**Phone:** (775)827-0184     **Fax:** (775)827-0190
Bill M. Welch, CEO & Pres
**Frmly:** Nevada Hospital Association.

## New Brunswick

★ **11606** ★ **New Brunswick Healthcare Association**
861 Woodstock Rd.
Fredericton, NB, Canada E3B 7R7
**Phone:** (506)451-0750     **Fax:** (506)451-0760
Michel J. Poirier, Exec Director

## New Hampshire

★ **11607** ★ **New Hampshire Hospital Association**
**Foundation for Healthy Communities**
125 Airport Rd.
Concord, NH 03301-7300
**Phone:** (603)225-0900     **Fax:** (603)225-4346
Michael J. Hill, President

## New Jersey

★ **11608** ★ **New Jersey Hospital Association**
PO Box 1
760 Alexander Rd., CN1
Princeton, NJ 08543-0001
**Phone:** (609)275-4000     **Fax:** (609)452-8097
Gary S. Carter, FACHE, CEO & Pres

## New Mexico

★ **11609** ★ **New Mexico Hospitals and Health Systems Association**
2121 Osuna Rd. NE
Albuquerque, NM 87113
**Phone:** (505)343-0010     **Fax:** (505)343-0012
Maureen L. Boshier, CEO & Pres

## New York

★ **11610** ★ **Greater New York Hospital Association, Subsidiaries, and Affiliates**
555 W 57th St., 15th Flr.
New York, NY 10019
**Phone:** (212)246-7100     **Fax:** (212)262-6350
Kenneth E. Raske, President

★ **11611** ★ **Healthcare Association of New York State**
1 Empire Dr.
Rensselaer, NY 12144

**Phone:** (518)431-7600          **Fax:** (518)431-7915
Daniel Sisto, President

★ **11612** ★ **Iroquois Healthcare Alliance**
17 Halfmoon Executive Park Dr.
Clifton Park, NY 12065
**Phone:** (518)383-5060          **Fax:** (518)383-2616
Gary J. Fitzgerald, President
**Alt. Contact:** 5740 Commons Pk., E Syracuse, NY 13057; ph: 315445-1851, fax: 315445-2293.

★ **11613** ★ **Nassau—Suffolk Hospital Council, Inc.**
3001 Expressway Dr. N, Ste. 300
Islandia, NY 11749-5308
**Phone:** (631)435-3000          **Fax:** (631)435-2343
Peter M. Sullivan, CEO & Pres

★ **11614** ★ **Northern Metropolitan Hospital Association**
400 Stony Brook Ct.
Newburgh, NY 12550
**Phone:** (845)562-7520          **Fax:** (845)562-0187
Arthur E. Weintraub, President

★ **11615** ★ **Rochester Regional Healthcare Association**
3445 Winton Pl.
Rochester, NY 14623
**Phone:** (716)273-8180          **Fax:** (716)273-8189
Robert M. Swinnerton, CEO & Pres

★ **11616** ★ **Western New York Healthcare Association**
1876 Niagara Falls Blvd.
Tonawanda, NY 14150-6439
**Phone:** (716)695-0843          **Fax:** (716)695-0073
William D. Pike, President

### Newfoundland

★ **11617** ★ **Newfoundland & Labrador Health Boards Association**
PO Box 8234
Saint John's, NF, Canada A1B 3N4
**Phone:** (709)364-7701          **Fax:** (709)364-6460
John F. Peddle, Exec Director

### North Carolina

★ **11618** ★ **North Carolina Hospital Association**
**An Association of Hospitals and Health Networks**
PO Box 4449
Cary, NC 27519-4449
**Phone:** (919)677-2400          **Fax:** (919)677-4200
William A. Pully, President

### North Dakota

★ **11619** ★ **North Dakota Healthcare Association**
1121 N 13th St., Ste. 1
Bismarck, ND 58501
**Phone:** (701)224-9732          **Fax:** (701)224-9529
Arnold R. Thomas, President
**Frmly:** North Dakota Hospital Association.

### Northwest Territories

★ **11620** ★ **Northwest Territories Health Care Association**
PO Box 1709
Yellowknife, NT, Canada X1A 2P3
**Phone:** (867)873-9253          **Fax:** (867)873-9254
Sharon Ehaloak, Exec Director

### Nova Scotia

★ **11621** ★ **Nova Scotia Association of Health Organizations**
Bedford Professional Centre
2 Dartmouth Rd.
Bedford, NS, Canada B4A 2K7
**Phone:** (902)832-8500          **Fax:** (902)832-8505
Robert A. Cook, CEO & Pres

### Ohio

★ **11622** ★ **Akron Regional Hospital Association**
190 Montrose W Ave., Ste. 201
Akron, OH 44321-2786
**Phone:** (330)668-6180          **Fax:** (330)668-2013
Marianne G. Lorini, President

★ **11623** ★ **Center for Health Affairs**
1226 Huron Rd. E
Cleveland, OH 44115
**Phone:** (216)696-6900          **Fax:** (216)696-1837
C. Wayne Rice, PhD, CEO & Pres

★ **11624** ★ **Greater Cincinnati Health Council**
2100 Sherman Ave., Ste. 100
Cincinnati, OH 45212-2775
**Phone:** (513)531-0200          **Fax:** (513)531-0278
Lynn R. Olman, President

★ **11625** ★ **Greater Dayton Area Hospital Association**
32 N Main St., Ste. 1441
Dayton, OH 45402
**Phone:** (937)228-1000          **Fax:** (937)228-1035
Joseph M. Krella, President

★ **11626** ★ **Hospital Council of Northwest Ohio**
3231 Central Park W Dr., Ste. 200
Toledo, OH 43614
**Phone:** (419)842-0800          **Fax:** (419)843-8889
W. Scott Fry, CEO & Pres

★ **11627** ★ **Ohio Hospital Association**
**The Association for Hospitals and Health Systems**
155 E Broad St.
Columbus, OH 43215
**Phone:** (614)221-7614          **Fax:** (614)221-4771
James R. Castle, CEO & Pres

### Oklahoma

★ **11628** ★ **Greater Oklahoma City Hospital Council**
4000 Lincoln Blvd.
Oklahoma City, OK 73105
**Phone:** (405)359-5530          **Fax:** (405)359-5500
Jerry Maier, Chairman of the Board

★ **11629** ★ **Oklahoma Hospital Association**
4000 Lincoln Blvd.
Oklahoma City, OK 73105
**Phone:** (405)427-9537          **Fax:** (405)424-4507
Craig W. Jones, President

### Ontario

★ **11630** ★ **Catholic Health Association of Canada**
1247 Kilborn Pl.
Ottawa, ON, Canada K1H 6K9
**Phone:** (613)731-7148          **Fax:** (613)731-7797
Richard Haughian, D.Th., President

★ **11631** ★ **Ontario Hospital Association**
200 Front St. W, Ste. 2800
Toronto, ON, Canada M5V 3L1
**Phone:** (416)205-1300          **Fax:** (416)205-1310
David MacKinnon, President

### Oregon

★ **11632** ★ **Oregon Association of Hospitals and Health Systems**
4000 Kruse Way Pl.
Bldg. 2, Ste. 100
Lake Oswego, OR 97035-2543
**Phone:** (503)636-2204          **Fax:** (503)636-8310
Kenneth M. Rutledge, President

### Pennsylvania

★ **11633** ★ **Delaware Valley Healthcare Council of HAP**
121 S Broad St., 20th Fl.
Philadelphia, PA 19107
**Phone:** (215)735-9695          **Fax:** (215)790-1267
Andrew B. Wigglesworth, President

★ **11634** ★ **Hospital Council of Western Pennsylvania**
500 Commonwealth Dr.
Warrendale, PA 15086
**Phone:** (724)776-6400          **Fax:** (724)776-6969
Ian G. Rawson, PhD, President

★ **11635** ★ **Hospital and Healthsystem Association of Pennsylvania**
4750 Lindle Rd.
PO Box 8600
Harrisburg, PA 17105-8600
**Phone:** (717)564-9200          **Fax:** (717)561-5334
Carolyn F. Scanlan, CEO & Pres
**Frmly:** Hospital Association of Pennsylvania.

### Prince Edward Island

★ **11636** ★ **Health Association of Prince Edward Island, Inc.**
10 Pownal St.
Charlottetown, PE, Canada C1A 3V6
**Phone:** (902)368-3901          **Fax:** (902)368-3231
Ken Ezeard, President

### Puerto Rico

★ **11637** ★ **Puerto Rico Hospital Association**
Villa Nevarez Professional Center, Officina 101-103
Centro Commercial Villa Nevarez
San Juan, PR 00927
**Phone:** (787)764-0290          **Fax:** (787)753-9748
Juan Rivera, Exec VP

### Quebec

★ **11638** ★ **Quebec Hospital Association**
505 blvd. de Maisonneuve W, Ste. 400
Montreal, QC, Canada H3A 3C2
**Phone:** (514)842-4861          **Fax:** (514)282-4271
Daniel Adam, Exec VP

### Rhode Island

★ **11639** ★ **Hospital Association of Rhode Island**
880 Butler Dr., Ste. 1
Providence, RI 02906
**Phone:** (401)274-4274          **Fax:** (401)274-1838
Edward Quinlan, President

## Saskatchewan

★ **11640** ★ **Saskatchewan Association of Health Organizations**
1445 Park St.
Regina, SK, Canada S4N 4C5
**Phone:** (306)347-5500          **Fax:** (306)347-5500
Louise Simard, CEO & Pres

## South Carolina

★ **11641** ★ **South Carolina Hospital Association**
101 Medical Circle
PO Box 6009
West Columbia, SC 29171-6009
**Phone:** (803)796-3080          **Fax:** (803)796-2938
Ken A. Shull, FACHE, President

## South Dakota

★ **11642** ★ **South Dakota Association of Healthcare Organizations**
3708 Brooks Pl.
Sioux Falls, SD 57106
**Phone:** (605)361-2281          **Fax:** (605)361-5175
David R. Hewett, CEO & Pres
**Frmly:** South Dakota Hospital Association.

## Tennessee

★ **11643** ★ **Tennessee Hospital Association**
500 Interstate Blvd. S
Nashville, TN 37210
**Phone:** (615)256-8240          **Fax:** (615)242-4803
Craig A. Becker, President

## Texas

★ **11644** ★ **Dallas—Fort Worth Hospital Council**
250 Decker Dr.
Irving, TX 75062
**Phone:** (972)719-4900          **Fax:** (972)719-4009
John C. Gavras, President

★ **11645** ★ **Greater San Antonio Hospital Council**
8620 N New Braunfels, Ste. 420
San Antonio, TX 78217
**Phone:** (210)820-3500          **Fax:** (210)820-3888
William Dean Rasco, CEO & Pres

★ **11646** ★ **Texas Hospital Association**
6225 US Hwy. 290 E
PO Box 15587
Austin, TX 78761-5587
**Phone:** (512)465-1000          **Fax:** (512)465-1090
Richard Betts, FACHE, CEO & Pres

## Utah

★ **11647** ★ **Utah Health Association**
**Utah Hospital and Health Systems Association**
2180 S 1300 E, Ste. 440
Salt Lake City, UT 84106-2843
**Phone:** (801)486-9915          **Fax:** (801)486-0882
Richard B. Kinnersley, President

## Vermont

★ **11648** ★ **Vermont Association of Hospitals and Health Systems**
148 Main St.
Montpelier, VT 05602
**Phone:** (802)223-3461          **Fax:** (802)223-0364
Norman E. Wright, President
**Frmly:** Vermont Hospital Association.

## Virginia

★ **11649** ★ **Virginia Hospital and Healthcare Association**
4200 Innslake Dr.
PO Box 31394
Richmond, VA 23294
**Phone:** (804)747-8600          **Fax:** (804)965-0475
Laurens Sartoris, President
**Frmly:** Virginia Hospital Association.

## Washington

★ **11650** ★ **Washington State Hospital Association**
300 Elliott Ave. W, Ste. 300
Seattle, WA 98119-4118
**Phone:** (206)281-7211          **Fax:** (206)283-6122
Leo F. Greenawalt, CEO & Pres

## West Virginia

★ **11651** ★ **West Virginia Hospital Association**
100 Association Dr.
Charleston, WV 25311-1571
**Phone:** (304)344-9744          **Fax:** (304)344-9745
Steven J. Summer, President

## Wisconsin

★ **11652** ★ **Wisconsin Health and Hospital Association**
5721 Odana Rd.
Madison, WI 53719-1289
**Phone:** (608)274-1820          **Fax:** (608)274-8554
Mark Knight, CEO & Pres
**Frmly:** Wisconsin Hospital Association.

## Wyoming

★ **11653** ★ **Wyoming Hospital Association**
PO Box 249
Cheyenne, WY 82003
**Phone:** (307)632-9344          **Fax:** (307)632-9347
Robert C. Kidd, II, President

# Foundations & Other Funding Organizations

## Other Funding Organizations

**★ 11654 ★ American Society of Clinical Hypnosis - Education and Research Foundation (ASCH-ERF)**
130 E Elm Ct., No. 201
Roselle, IL 60172-2000
**Phone:** (630)980-4740 **Fax:** (630)351-8490
**Email:** info@asch.net
**Website:** http://www.asch.net
Philip R. Appell, PhD, Pres.

**Desc:** Teaching and research arm of the American Society of Clinical Hypnosis. Physicians, dentists, and psychologists. Underwrites workshops in the U.S. and Canada to train professionals in hypnosis and broaden their knowledge of psychotherapy. Basic section is designed to familiarize physicians, psychologists, and dentists with hypnosis and its applications to problems of the psychologically normal patient including preparation for childbirth, comfort in the dental chair, and other problems and complaints complicated by emotional conflicts, such as smoking and obesity. Advanced section deals with techniques that can be used in addition to hypnotherapy in treating patients. **Awards:** Mutter Fund for ASCH Regional Workshops for financial hardship students.

# National & International Organizations

**★ 11655 ★ Academy of Scientific Hypnotherapy (ASH)**
PO Box 12041
San Diego, CA 92112
**Phone:** (619)427-6225 **Fax:** (619)427-5650
**Email:** docbill@e-machines.net
**Website:** http://www.health.gov/nhic/NHICScripts/Entry.cfm?HRCode=HR0670
William E. Kemery, PhD, Pres.

**Fnded:** 1977. **Mem:** 250. **Desc:** Professionals in the healing arts who have been properly trained in hypnosis, and who are known to the academy to be ethical and of good professional reputation. The academy plans to fill the need for training programs, continuing education, and certification throughout the U.S. Maintains placement and referral service; compiles statistics. **Pub:** *Hypnotherapy in Review*, periodic. Newsletter. Reports on medical and psychological research in hypnotherapy. Includes book reviews. *Price:* Included in membership dues. • Bulletin, periodic. • Monograph, periodic. *Price:* Included in membership dues.

**★ 11656 ★ American Academy of Medical Hypnoanalysts (AAMH)**
5628 Murray Rd., Ste. 4
Memphis, TN 38119-3876
**Phone:** 888-454-9766 **Free:** 888-454-9766
**Fax:** (901)683-1224
**Website:** http://www.aamh.com
John Scott, Jr., Admin.

**Fnded:** 1974. **Mem:** 125. **Reg. Groups:** 8. **Desc:** Medical doctors, doctors of osteopathy, psychologists, social workers, and professional counselors. Provides training in and promotes the use of medical hypnoanalysis. (Medical hypnoanalysis employs an analytic approach to resolving emotional disorders that is applied while the subject is hypnotized.) Conducts 3-month residency training programs. **Pub:** *Medical Hypnoanalysis Journal*, quarterly. Journal. *Price:* $40/year; $10 single copy. • Membership Directory, annual.

**★ 11657 ★ American Association of Professional Hypnotherapists (AAPH)**
4149A El Camino Way
Palo Alto, CA 94306-4036
**Phone:** (650)323-3224
**Email:** josie@deepideas.com
**Website:** http://www.aaph.org
Josie Hadley, Exec. Dir.

**Fnded:** 1980. **Mem:** 1,525. **Desc:** Hypnotherapists, marriage and family therapists, psychologists, clinical social workers, physicians, pastoral counselors, and others trained and experienced in hypnosis therapy. Promotes public awareness of hypnosis as applied to personal motivation and improvement, habit control, and assisting the healing process. Acts as forum for the exchange of ideas and techniques; encourages a high level of professional ethics; promotes positive image of hypnotherapy. **Pub:** *Hypnotherapy Today*, quarterly. Newsletter. Covers techniques, new theories and innovations, case descriptions, and new uses of hypnotherapy. *Price:* Included in membership dues. • *National Register of Professional Hypnotherapists*, annual. Arranged by state and country. *Price:* Included in membership dues.

**★ 11658 ★ American Board of Psychological Hypnosis (ABPH)**
c/o Samuel M. Migdole, Ed.D., ABPH
North Shore Counseling Center
23 Broadway
Beverly, MA 01915
**Phone:** (978)922-2280 **Fax:** (978)927-1758
**Email:** pres.abph@prodigy.net
Samuel M. Migdole, Ed.D., Pres.

**Fnded:** 1959. **Desc:** Awards specialty diplomas to qualified licensed doctoral level psychologists in experimental and clinical hypnosis. Purpose is to raise the standards of individuals conducting research in hypnosis and those using it in clinical practice by requiring specialized training and experience in the field as evidenced by advanced educational credentials in psychology, published research, written and oral examinations, and recommendations of colleagues. **Frmly:** American Board of Examiners in Psychological Hypnosis; American Board of Professional Psychology in Hypnosis.

**★ 11659 ★ American Council of Hypnotist Examiners (ACHE)**
700 S Central Ave.
Glendale, CA 91204
**Phone:** (818)242-1159 **Fax:** (818)247-9379
**Email:** hypnotismla@earthlink.net
Gil Boyne, Exec. Dir.

**Fnded:** 1980. **Mem:** 8,200. **Nat'l Groups:** 4. **Reg. Groups:** 8. **State Groups:** 1. **Local Groups:** 1. **Desc:** Educates, examines, and awards certification in the field of hypnotherapy. Maintains speakers' bureau. Sponsors educational programs. **Pub:** *American Hypnotherapy Report*, annual. Report. Contains news and information on the hypnotherapy profession. *Price:* Included in membership dues. • *Directory of Certified Members*, periodic. Membership Directory. • *International Hypnotherapy Report*, quarterly. Magazine. *Price:* Free to members. • Newsletter, periodic. *Price:* Free to members. **AKA:** Hypnotists Examining Council.

**★ 11660 ★ American Guild of Hypnotherapists (AGH)**
2200 Veterans Blvd., No. 108
Kenner, LA 70062-4005
**Phone:** (504)468-3223 **Fax:** (504)468-3213
**Email:** southwest@southwest.edu
Reg Sheldrick, PhD, Pres.

**Fnded:** 1975. **Mem:** 877. **Desc:** Hypnotherapists and professional hypnotists; mental health, medical, dental, and chiropractic professionals who use hypnosis in their practices. Offers home study course in hypnosis/hypnotherapy. Is approved by many state licensing boards as a provider of continuing education credit. **Pub:** *Journal of Hypnotherapy*, quarterly. Journal. • Newsletter, periodic.

**★ 11661 ★ American Hypnosis Association (AHA)**
18607 Ventura Blvd., Ste. 310
Tarzana, CA 91356
**Fax:** (818)344-2262
**Email:** info@hypnosismotivation.com
**Website:** http://www.hypnosismotivation.com
George Kappas, Pres.

**Fnded:** 1972. **Mem:** 1,000. **State Groups:** 2. **Desc:** Professionals and paraprofessionals in hypnotherapy. Acts as a resource center for members. **Pub:** *American Hypnotherapist*, quarterly. Newsletter.

**★ 11662 ★ American Society of Clinical Hypnosis (ASCH)**
130 E Elm Ct., Ste. 201
Roselle, IL 60172-2000
**Phone:** (630)980-4740 **Fax:** (630)351-8490
**Email:** asch@asch.net
**Website:** http://www.asch.net
John E. Kasper, PhD, Exec. VP

**Fnded:** 1957. **Mem:** 3,000. **Reg. Groups:** 36. **State Groups:** 17. **Local Groups:** 19. **Desc:** Physicians, dentists, psychologists with doctoral or masters degrees, and clinical social workers and counselors, and nurses with master's degrees. Brings together professional people in medical, dental, and psychological fields using hypnosis; sets up standards of training; conducts teaching sessions and workshops at basic and advanced levels. Offers instruction on clinical hypnosis and various simple forms of psychotherapy and psychodynamics. Cooperates with all scientific disciplines with regard to use of hypnosis. Maintains speakers' bureau. **Pub:** *American Journal of Clinical Hypnosis*, quarterly. Journal. *Price:* $88. • *American Society of Clinical Hypnosis–Newsletter*, quarterly. Promotes the acceptance of hypnosis as a tool in clinical medicine and scientific research. Includes member news and calendar of events. *Price:* Included in membership dues. • Directory, annual.

★ **11663** ★ **American Society of Clinical Hypnosis - Education and Research Foundation (ASCH-ERF)**
130 E Elm Ct., No. 201
Roselle, IL 60172-2000
**Phone:** (630)980-4740      **Fax:** (630)351-8490
**Email:** info@asch.net
**Website:** http://www.asch.net
Philip R. Appell, PhD, Pres.
**Fnded:** 1957. **Mem:** 2,400. **Reg. Groups:** 37. **Desc:** Teaching and research arm of the American Society of Clinical Hypnosis. Physicians, dentists, and psychologists. Underwrites workshops in the U.S. and Canada to train professionals in hypnosis and broaden their knowledge of psychotherapy. Basic section is designed to familiarize physicians, psychologists, and dentists with hypnosis and its applications to problems of the psychologically normal patient including preparation for childbirth, comfort in the dental chair, and other problems and complaints complicated by emotional conflicts, such as smoking and obesity. Advanced section deals with techniques that can be used in addition to hypnotherapy in treating patients. **Pub:** *American Journal of Clinical Hypnosis*, quarterly. Journal. Contains research and clinical articles on hypnosis. *Price:* $70 in U.S., individual; $125 for institutions. • *Newsletter of American Society of Clinical Hypnosis*, quarterly. Newsletter. **Frmly:** (1962) Seminars on Hypnosis Foundation.

★ **11664** ★ **Association of Qualified Curative Hypnotherapists**
10 Balaclava Rd.
Kings Heath
Birmingham B14 7SG, United Kingdom
**Phone:** 44 121 4411775
**Email:** info@aqch.org
**Website:** http://www.aqch.org
**Fnded:** 1985. **Mem:** 60. **Nat'l Groups:** 1. **Local Groups:** 5. **Desc:** Curative hypnotherapists. Maintains and advances the standards of hypnotherapy. Promotes professional development and training programs. Registered charity. **Pub:** *Hypnotherapy Journal*, semiannual. Journal. Continuing professional development.

★ **11665** ★ **Australian Society of Clinical Hypnotherapists**
PO Box 471
Eastwood, NSW 2122, Australia
**Phone:** 61 2 98742776      **Fax:** 61 2 98742776
**Email:** referrals@asch.com.au
**Website:** http://www.asch.com.au/
**Fnded:** 1974. **Mem:** 390. **Nat'l Groups:** 1. **State Groups:** 3. **Lang(s):** English. **Desc:** Clinical hypnotherapists. Seeks to maintain high ethical and professional standards in the practice of clinical hypnotherapy. Promotes advancement of hypnotherapeutic techniques. Informs members about developments in clinical hypnotherapy; conducts continuing professional education programs; operates referral service. **Pub:** *The Australian Journal of Clinical Hypnotherapy and Hypnosis*, semiannual. Journal.

★ **11666** ★ **British Society of Experimental and Clinical Hypnosis**
c/o Phyllis A. Alden, Hon.Sec.
Psychology Consultancy
District General Hospital
Scartho Rd.
Grimsby DN33 2BA, United Kingdom
**Phone:** 44 1472 873423      **Fax:** 44 1472 879238
**Email:** honsec@bsech.demon.co.uk
**Website:** http://www.alden-residence.demon.co.uk
**Fnded:** 1977. **Mem:** 300. **Lang(s):** English. **Desc:** Medical doctors, dentists, psychologists, other health service personnel. A learned society for doctors, dentists, psychologists and other health care professionals interested in theory, research and therapeutic applications of hypnosis. It organizes meetings, training events and an annual conference. **Pub:** *Contemporary Hypnosis*, quarterly. Journal.

★ **11667** ★ **British Society of Hypnotherapists**
37 Orbain Rd.
London SW6 7JZ, United Kingdom
**Phone:** 44 207 73851166      **Fax:** 44 207 73851166
**Email:** sy@bsh1950.fsnet.co.uk
**Website:** http://www.bsh1950.fsnet.co.uk
**Fnded:** 1950. **Mem:** 20. **Desc:** Specialising in the treatment of nervous disorders and addictions. Provides information service for public; conducts research on behalf of members and distributes information to them.

★ **11668** ★ **British Society of Medical and Dental Hypnosis**
4 Kirkwood Ave.
Cookridge
Leeds LS16 7JU, United Kingdom
**Phone:** 44 7000 560309      **Fax:** 44 1709 554558
**Email:** secretary@bsmdh.org
**Website:** http://www.bsmdh.org
**Fnded:** 1952. **Mem:** 398. **Desc:** Qualified doctors, dentists and other registered health professionals Promotes the study and training in the principles and practice of hypnosis. It encourages research and publication of work relating to hypnosis. **Pub:** Journal, annual. • Newsletter, 3/year. **Frmly:** British Society of Dental Hypnosis; The Dental and Medical Society for the Study of Hypnosis.

★ **11669** ★ **Canadian Institute of Hypnotism (CIH)**
110 rue Greystone
Pointe Claire, QC, Canada H9R 5T6
**Phone:** (514)426-1010      **Fax:** (514)426-4680
**Email:** mmker@qc.aibn.com
**Fnded:** 1953. **Mem:** 486. **Lang(s):** English, French. **Desc:** Health care professionals making use of hypnosis in their practices. Promotes improved training in and application of hypnosis as a medical care technique. Conducts research and educational programs; makes available children's services; maintains speakers' bureau. **Pub:** *Newsletter of CIH*, quarterly. Newsletter. Classical Format. • Bulletin, periodic. • Brochure.

★ **11670** ★ **Hypnotherapy Association**
14 Crown St.
Chorley
Lancashire PR7 7QX, United Kingdom
**Phone:** 44 207 7234443
**Website:** http://www.zednet.co.uk/bhahypnotherapy/
**Fnded:** 1958. **Mem:** 483. **Lang(s):** Spanish. **Desc:** Practitioners with at least 4 years post graduate of training in psychotherapy and hypnotherapy who comply with the Association's code of competence and ethics. Concerned with professional standards in the treatment of nervous disorders by trained psychotherapists who use hypnosis when appropriate to facilitate recall by the patient, as well as using other methods proven by research into long-term results. Referrals, research, lectures, broadcasts, talks, papers, articles, books and seminars arranged.

★ **11671** ★ **Institute for Research in Hypnosis and Psychotherapy (IRHP)**
1991 Broadway, Apt. 18B
New York, NY 10023
**Phone:** (212)874-5290      **Fax:** (914)764-1445
Dr. Milton V. Kline, Dir.
**Fnded:** 1954. **Desc:** Psychologists, psychiatrists, physicians, and social workers trained in clinical hypnosis, hypnotherapy, and hypnoanalysis. Sponsors research in clinical and experimental hypnosis; offers postgraduate training in hypnosis and its applications; develops standards and procedures for advanced education in clinical and experimental hypnosis. Operates Morton Prince Centers, low-cost treatment centers for outpatients who cannot afford hypnotherapy or hypnoanalysis in private practice. Conducts consulting and educational training services. Compiles statistics; maintains databases and speakers' bureau. **Frmly:** (1982) Institute for Research in Hypnosis.

★ **11672** ★ **International Center of Medical and Psychological Hypnosis (ICMPH)**
**(Centro Internazionale di Ipnosi Medica e Psicologica)**
Istituto di Indagini Psicologiche
Corso XXII Marzo 57
I-20129 Milan, Italy
**Phone:** 39 2 7388427      **Fax:** 39 2 7491051
**Email:** uimpsico@tin.it
**Website:** http://www.uim-psico.org
**Fnded:** 1969. **Mem:** 340. **Reg. Groups:** 15. **Desc:** Physicians, psychologists, and teachers of psychology and psychiatry at universities. Seeks to advance the knowledge of hypnosis and its applications. Organizes courses in psychosomatic medicine and medical and psychological hypnosis for physicians and psychologists. Conducts research on hypnosis, hypnoanesthesia, hypnotherapy, hypnotic eugenics, childbirth, and hypnotic contraception. Holds seminars and workshops. Also handles courses in psychology of handwriting, expert analysis for handwriting or forensic issues, autogenous training, and naturopathy. **Pub:** *Literature*, semiannual. Also publishes *Dictionary of Hypnopsychology and Handwriting Psychology*.

★ **11673** ★ **International Medical and Dental Hypnotherapy Association (IMDHA)**
4110 Edgeland, Ste. 800
Royal Oak, MI 48073-2285
**Phone:** (248)549-5594      **Free:** 800-257-5467
**Fax:** (248)549-5421
**Email:** aspencer@infinityinst.com
**Website:** http://www.infinityinst.com
Anne H. Spencer, PhD, Exec. Dir.
**Fnded:** 1987. **Mem:** 1,500. **State Groups:** 18. **Local Groups:** 2. **Desc:** Certified hypnotherapists; associate members are non-certified hypnotherapists and individuals interested in hypnosis. Hypnotherapists help to mentally prepare patients to deal with the stress and pain involved with medical and dental procedures. Offers certification courses. Maintains an International Referral Directory which lists certified members. Maintains speakers' bureau and library on hypnosis and mind development. Offers educational programs. Has affiliate Hypnosis training schools. Has free Email Hypnosis and Holistic Living Journal written monthly. Offers Specialty Certifications to certified members at annual Educational Conference. **Pub:** *Hypnosis and Holistic Health*. Journal. • *Subconsciously Speaking: You Can Change Your Life Through the Powers of Your Mind*, bimonthly. Newsletter. Contains articles of interest including hypnosis, imagery, holistic health, and consciousness. *Price:* Included in membership dues; $12/year to nonmembers in U.S. • Articles.

★ **11674** ★ **International Society of Hypnosis**
c/o Behavioural Medicine Unit
Austin and Repatriation Medical Centre
Repat Campus

Locked Bag 1
Heidelberg West, VIC 3081, Australia
**Phone:** 61 3 94964105          **Fax:** 61 3 94964107
**Email:** ish-central.office@medicine.unimelb.edu.au
**Lang(s):** English. **Desc:** Hypnotists and medical professionals. Promotes increased use of hypnosis in the treatment of diseases and as an adjunct to traditional medical therapies. Fosters interdisciplinary research into the medical benefits of hypnosis; facilitates exchange of information among members; sponsors training and continuing professional development programs.

★ **11675** ★ **International Society for Medical and Psychological Hypnosis (ISMPH)**

**(Centro Internazionale di Ipnosi Medica e Psicologica — CIIMP)**
c/o Dr. Aurora Zavertanik, Sec.
Corso XXII Marzo 57
I-20129 Milan, Italy
**Phone:** 39 2 70126489          **Fax:** 39 2 7491051
**Email:** uimpsico@tin.it
**Website:** http://www.uim-psico.org
**Fnded:** 1985. **Mem:** 172. **Reg. Groups:** 18. **Local Groups:** 15. **Lang(s):** English, Italian. **Desc:** Professional medical doctors and psychologists. Promotes the study and use of hypnotherapeutic treatments. Conducts annual courses for members.

★ **11676** ★ **International Society for Medical and Psychological Hypnosis, U.S.A. Office (ISMPH)**
1991 Broadway, Apt. 18B
New York, NY 10023
**Phone:** (212)874-5290          **Fax:** (914)764-1445
Dr. Milton V. Kline, Dir.
**Fnded:** 1982. **Mem:** 4,000. **Desc:** Health care professionals involved with medical and psychological hypnosis. Supports clinical research in hyponosis and research in psychotherapy strategies and tactics; offers advanced training and certification for hypnotherapists. Maintains speakers' bureau; compiles statistics. **Pub:** *Conference Proceedings*, annual. Proceedings. • *Morton Price Mental Health Center*, quarterly. Newsletter. Contains original research, membership news, book reviews, and conference reports.

★ **11677** ★ **Milton H. Erickson Foundation (MHEF)**
3606 N 24th St.
Phoenix, AZ 85016
**Phone:** (602)956-6196          **Fax:** (602)956-0519
**Email:** office@erickson-foundation.org
**Website:** http://www.erickson-foundation.org
Jeffrey K. Zeig, Dir.
**Fnded:** 1979. **Desc:** Seeks to promote and advance the contributions made to health sciences by Milton H. Erickson, M.D. (1901-1980), regarded as an authority on hypnotherapy and brief strategic therapy. Dedicated to the training of health and restricted to mental health professionals. **Pub:** *A Teaching Seminar with Milton H. Erickson, M.D.*. Book. Transcript with com-

mentary of a one-week teaching seminar. • *Ericksonian Methods: The Essence of the Story*. Book. • *Ericksonian Monographs*, up to 3/year. Monographs. Contains selected articles on Ericksonian hypnosis and psychotherapy, including technique, theory, and research topics. • *M.H. Erickson Foundation Newsletter*, 3/year. Newsletter. Contains articles and notices relating to Ericksonian approaches to psychotherapy and hypnosis. *Price:* Optional donation, available to professionals. • *The Process of Hypnotic Induction: A Training Videotape Featuring Inductions Conducted by Milton H. Erickson in 1964*. Video. Discusses the process and describes the microdynamics of Erickson's techniques. • *Symbolic Hypnotherapy*. Video. Presents information regarding the use of symbols in psychotherapy and hypnosis. • *What Is Psychotherapy?: Contemporary Perspectives*. Book. Contains edited commentaries of eminent clinicians.

★ **11678** ★ **National College of Hypnosis and Psychotherapy**
12 Cross St.
Nelson BB9 7EN, United Kingdom
**Phone:** 44 1282 699378          **Fax:** 44 1282 698633
**Email:** hypnosis_nchp@compuserve.com
**Website:** http://www.hypnotherapyuk.net
**Fnded:** 1977. **Mem:** 200. **Desc:** Mature students seeking a reputable, externally accredited (by the British Accreditation Council) training with a view to running their own practices, for interest or to augment their existing professional skills. Concerned with training in hypnotherapy/psychotherapy/counselling on part-time basis to appropriate, suitably motivated, mature students in London, Liverpool, Glasgow, and Northern Ireland. Courses are held at regular intervals throughout the year. Member of United Kingdom Council for Psychotherapy and European Association for Hypnopsychotherapy. Higher Education. Courses are held at regular intervals throughout the year. Member of United Kingdom Council for Psychotherapy.

★ **11679** ★ **National Guild of Hypnotists (NGH)**
PO Box 308
Merrimack, NH 03054-0308
**Phone:** (603)429-9438          **Fax:** (603)424-8066
**Email:** ngh@ngh.net
**Website:** http://www.ngh.net
Dr. Dwight F. Damon, Pres.
**Fnded:** 1951. **Mem:** 7,000. **State Groups:** 65. **Desc:** Certified and registered hypnotherapists, demonstrational (stage) hypnotists, and interested individuals. Objective is to unite all persons sharing a professional interest in hypnotism. Seeks to: establish standards for professional conduct; increase members' knowledge in there respective areas of specialization; improve members' professional skills to enhance the quality of services provided to clients; register individuals as hypnotherapists; encourage educational programs to further the knowledge and understanding of hypnosis; promote the acceptance of hypnosis; stimulate scientific research in the field and dissemination of results; cooperate with other professional societies that share mutual goals, ethics, and interests; provide members

with group benefits; improve members' individual skills in the marketing of their services and management of their practices. Offers ongoing educational seminars and workshops, and certification program. Compiles statistics; conducts research programs. Operates speakers' bureau. Maintains hall of fame. Publishes Journal of Hypnotism and Hypno-Gram-quarterlies for members. Hypnosis Today-A hypnosis magazine for the general public. **Pub:** *Hypno-Gram*, quarterly. Newsletter. • *Hypnosis Today*, annual. Magazine. *Price:* $3.95. • *The Journal of Hypnotism*, quarterly. Magazine. *Price:* Included in membership dues. • *NGH Video Rental Library*. Videos. *Price:* for members. • Audiotapes. • Books.

★ **11680** ★ **National Register of Hypnotherapists and Psychotherapists**
12 Cross St.
Nelson BB9 7EN, United Kingdom
**Phone:** 44 1282 716839          **Fax:** 44 1282 698633
**Email:** nrhp@btconnect.com
**Website:** http://www.nrhp.co.uk
**Fnded:** 1985. **Mem:** 390. **Desc:** Therapists who have graduated from the National College of Hypnosis and Psychotherapy or equivalent trainings. Promotes and protects the professional status, standards, ethics and interest of its members and also promotes the interests of those members of the public who seek professional help, and for whom it provides a nationwide referral service. Member of the United Kingdom Council for Psychotherapy. **Pub:** *Directory of Practitioners*, annual. Directory. Contains a listing of qualified hypno-psychotherapists in UK. • *Information Leaflet*. • *Reports and Statistical Analyses of Membership*. Report.

★ **11681** ★ **Society for Clinical and Experimental Hypnosis (SCEH)**
PO Box 642114
Pullman, WA 99164-2114
**Phone:** (509)332-7555          **Fax:** (509)335-2097
**Email:** sceh@pullman.com
**Website:** http://sunsite.utk.edu/IJCEH/scehframe.htm
Cindy Scott, Exec. Dir.
**Fnded:** 1949. **Mem:** 950. **Desc:** United States constituent society of the International Society of Hypnosis. Professional society of physicians, dentists, doctoral level psychologists, and certain psychiatric social workers interested in research in hypnosis and its boundary areas as well as the therapeutic use of hypnosis in clinical practice. Encourages cooperation among professional and scientific disciplines in use of hypnosis; promotes educational standards; conducts introductory and advanced workshops and continuing education seminars in therapeutic hypnosis. Offers continuing education seminars in New York City and San Francisco, CA. **Pub:** *Focus*, quarterly. Newsletter. Contains research and clinical notes, society news, book reviews, and obituaries. *Price:* $11/year. • *International Journal of Clinical and Experimental Hypnosis*, quarterly. Journal. Contains book reviews, statistics, and research and clinical reports. *Price:* Included in membership dues; $49/year for nonmembers. • Membership Directory, annual.

# Chapter 34
# Infectious Diseases

## Federal Government Agencies

★ 11682 ★ **Executive Office of the President**
**Office of Policy Development**
**Domestic Policy Council**
**Director of National AIDS Policy**
Eisenhower Executive Office Bldg., Rm. 216
Washington, DC 20502
**Phone:** (202)456-2216
Sandra Thurman, Director

★ 11683 ★ **U.S. Department of Health and Human Services**
**Centers for Disease Control and Prevention**
**National Center for HIV, STD, and TB Prevention**
1600 Clifton Rd. NE
Atlanta, GA 30333
**Phone:** (404)639-3311
**Website:** http://www.cdc.gov/nchstp/od/nchstp.html

★ 11684 ★ **U.S. Department of Health and Human Services**
**Centers for Disease Control and Prevention**
**National Center for Infectious Diseases**
1600 Clifton Rd. NE
Atlanta, GA 30333
**Phone:** (404)639-3311　　**Fax:** (404)639-3039
**Website:** http://www.cdc.gov/ncidod/
**Desc:** The Center for Infectious Diseases coordinates a national program to improve the identification, investigation, diagnosis, prevention, and control of infectious diseases. It maintains programs dealing with AIDS, hospital infections, sexually transmitted diseases, bacterial diseases, host factors, mycotic diseases, parasitic diseases, viral diseases, and vector-borne viral diseases.

★ 11685 ★ **U.S. Department of Health and Human Services**
**Health Resources and Services Administration**
**HIV/AIDS Bureau**
5600 Fishers Lane
Rockville, MD 20857
**Phone:** (301)443-3376
**Website:** http://hab.hrsa.gov/
**Desc:** The Bureau administers the Ryan White Comprehensive AIDS Resources Emergency (CARE) Act and conducts a wide range of programs which provide primary care and support services to low-income, uninsured, and underinsured individuals and families affected by HIV/AIDS. It also provides HIV emergency relief grants to eligible metropolitan areas, and HIV care grants to States and U.S Territories; funds the AIDS Drug Assistance Program for all States and eligible territories; and supports projects examining economic changes and managed care effects of the Nation's network of HIV/AIDS care delivery.

**U.S. Department of Health and Human Services**
**National Institutes of Health (NIH)**
**National Institute of Allergy and Infectious Diseases (NIAID)**
*See:* Entry 3173

## Foundations & Other Funding Organizations

### Private Foundations

★ 11686 ★ **The Andy Warhol Foundation for the Visual Arts**
65 Bleecker St., 7th Fl.
New York, NY 10012
**Phone:** (212)387-7555　　**Fax:** (212)387-7560
**Website:** http://www.warholfoundation.org
Pamela Clapp, Program Director
**Fnded:** 1987. **Philosophy:** The foundation's mission is the "advancement of the visual arts." According to the foundation's statement of purpose, the visual arts include painting, sculpture, printmaking, photography, film, video, decorative arts, and art publishing. The foundation's objective is to "foster innovative expression and the creative process by encouraging and supporting cultural organizations that in turn, directly or indirectly, support artists and their work... The foundation is focused primarily on supporting work of a challenging and often experimental nature, while noting that the interpretation of those terms may vary from place to place and culture to culture." The foundation will only consider proposals from performing arts groups (dance, theater, and music groups) for specific aspects of their activity that incorporate the visual arts in their performances. Grants are awarded to curatorial programs at museums, artists' organizations, and other cultural organizations in the United States and abroad to assist in the innovative presentation of the visual arts with an emphasis on projects that cultivate new, expanded, and diverse audiences. Projects may include exhibitions, catalogs, audience development, and other organizational activities directly related to these areas. This category also supports the work of choreographers and performing artists where the visual arts are an inherent element of the production. The historic preservation program awards grants to organizations seeking to preserve and enhance historic buildings, districts, and landscapes, and to organizations seeking to increase public participation in the urban planning process. In addition to its grant making, the foundation has worked with the DIA Center for the Arts and the Carnegie Institute to establish the Andy Warhol Museum in Pittsburgh, PA–the artist's hometown. The foundation has provided the museum with art work and archival material for its permanent collection. The foundation has also supported the museum with grants. The foundation does not fund exhibitions or other activities relating to Andy Warhol's work. **Priorities:** *Arts & Humanities:* 100%. Supports visual arts, curatorial programs, and historic preservation and historic restoration. *Note:* Total contributions made in fiscal 2000. **Typ. Recipients:** AIDS/HIV. **Geo. Dist:** nationally.

★ 11687 ★ **Assisi Foundation of Memphis**
PO Box 381437
Memphis, TN 38183
**Phone:** (901)684-1564
Barry Flynn, Executive Director
**Fnded:** 1994. **Priorities:** *Arts & Humanities:* 8%. Gives to libraries, museums, and public broadcasting. *Education:* 30%. Provides major support to the University of Tennessee; also funds public pre-college schools, literacy programs, colleges, and charter/private schools. *International:* 31%. Supports clinics, hospitals, pediatric health, medical research institutes, medical foundations, single-disease health associations, and hospice. *Note:* Total contributions made in 2000. **Typ. Recipients:** AIDS/HIV, Cancer, Children's Health/Hospitals, Clinics/Medical Centers, Health Organizations, Hospitals, Medical Research. **Geo. Dist:** TN.

★ 11688 ★ **Columbia Foundation**
One Lombard St., Ste. 305
San Francisco, CA 94111
**Phone:** (415)986-5179　　**Fax:** (415)986-1732
**Website:** http://www.columbia.org
Susan Clark, Executive Director
**Fnded:** 1940. **Philosophy:** "While the foundation's broad philanthropic purpose has given it flexibility to respond to changing social conditions, it has nevertheless maintained its long-standing interest in world peace, human rights, the environment, cross-cultural and international understanding, the quality of urban life, and the arts." "Arts and Culture: institutional advancement of San Francisco's major arts organizations and the creation of art by individual artists or groups of artists engaged in a new collaboration or in community service through their art." "Environment: enhanced understanding and application of principles of sustainability according to which the future capacity of the earth to support life is preserved with a focus on non-polluting agriculture and the preservation and restoration of biological diversity and wild ecosystems including ancient forest, wetlands, and other endangered wilderness areas." "Human rights: work to stop the use of capital punishment, to advocate for the right to die with dignity, to normalize attitudes toward homosexuality and eradicate homophobia, the right to express convictions, to be free from discrimination, and the right of every person to physical and mental integrity." "Urban community: Promote the viability and quality of life over time without using up the natural processes and products on which life itself depends. In the context of sustainable urban commu-

nity development, an integral part of this goal is community planning which fosters a healthy, mutually-reinforcing balance between ecological, economic, and social concerns." 1996 & 1997 Application, 1999 guidelines. "Priority is given to the following types of projects: those that promote social change rather than providing an ongoing service; venture funding for new ideas or for efforts to address controversial issues; programs in the early stages of development when the potential is high out funding is scarce; programs that promote the renewal or advancement of major community institutions of long-term interest to the foundation; and programs that educate and train community leaders in sustainability as a new governing principle for all community and economic development." **Priorities:** *Arts & Humanities:* About 17%. Opera, orchestras, art exhibits. *Civic & Public Affairs:* 31%. Gay/Lesbian rights, violence prevention, urban community development. *Education:* 13%. University and bilingual programs. *Environment:* 1%. *International:* 6%. Supports single-disease health associations. *Note:* Total contributions made in fiscal 1999. **Typ. Recipients:** AIDS/HIV, Domestic Violence, Emergency/Ambulance Services, Health Funds, Health Policy/Cost Containment, Hospices, Long-Term Care, Medical Research, Nutrition, Preventive Medicine/Wellness Organizations, Public Health. **Geo. Dist:** CA, especially northern California; San Francisco, CA, including metropolitan area; London.


**Edna McConnell Clark Foundation**
*See:* Entry 196


**Edward W. Hazen Foundation**
*See:* Entry 204


**F. B. Heron Foundation**
*See:* Entry 5466


**Frances and Benjamin Benenson Foundation**
*See:* Entry 253


★ 11689 ★ **Hartford Courant Foundation**
285 Broad St.
Hartford, CT 06115
**Phone:** (860)241-6472          **Fax:** (860)520-6988
**Email:** hcfoundation@courant.com
**Website:** http://www.hartfordcourantfoundation.org
Kate Miller, Executive Director
**Fnded:** 1950. **Priorities:** *Arts & Humanities:* 19%. Supports public television, the theater, museums, orchestras, and historic preservation. *Civic & Public Affairs:* 23%. Funds community development, parks, cultural centers, and foundations. *Education:* 10%. Supports literacy, private education (precollege), public education (precollege), colleges/universities. *Environment:* 18%. Funds programs for children and for families in need. *International:* 3%. Supports health-related programs and health centers. *Religion:* 22%. Provides major donation to the Science Center of Connecticut. *Note:* Total contributions made in 1999. **Typ. Recipients:** AIDS/HIV, Child Abuse, Children's Health/Hospitals, Clinics/Medical Centers, Domestic Violence, Family Planning, Hospitals, Hospitals (University Affiliated), Medical Rehabilitation, Medical Research, Mental Health, Nursing Services, People with Disabilities, Prenatal Health Issues, Public Health, Substance Abuse. **Geo. Dist:** CT, Central Connecticut.


**Ittleson Foundation**
*See:* Entry 12273


**Joseph Alexander Foundation**
*See:* Entry 435


★ 11690 ★ **Joyce Mertz-Gilmore Foundation**
218 East 18th St.
New York, NY 10003-3694
**Phone:** (212)475-1137          **Fax:** (212)777-5226
**Email:** jmgf@jmgf.org
**Website:** http://www.jmgf.org
Robert Crane, President
**Fnded:** 1959. **Philosophy:** "The Joyce Mertz-Gilmore Foundation has environment, human rights, peace and security, and New York City grantmaking programs. The Foundation prefers to make general support grants to organizations whose work closely parallels its interests. The Foundation also supports specific programs or projects when appropriate." Environment: "The Foundation supports organizations promoting increased energy efficiency and the development and use of renewable energy sources for the future. Key areas of interest include: promoting efficiency and renewables through revision of state and local utility regulations and sound national policies; increasing public awareness and interest in energy efficiency; and promoting renewable energy in developing countries." Human Rights: "The Foundation supports organizations which investigate and publicize human rights abuses, advocate non-political applications of international human rights law, encourage the free flow of information within and between countries or work to build the capacity of non-governmental human rights groups in developing countries, Central Europe and former Soviet republics. The Foundation supports policy efforts, advocacy and information dissemination related to the fair and humane treatment of the growing, worldwide refugee population. The Foundation also promotes development approaches which draws upon resources and knowledge of the refugees themselves, and empowers refugees to press for their own needs and rights. The Foundation supports national or regional efforts to protect and extend the rights of immigrants and refugees, and lesbian and gay men. The Foundation makes grants to groups which undertake advocacy and policy work, citizen awareness activities and/or litigation to establish clear precedents for protecting the civil rights of these groups. The Foundation supports voluntary sector capacity- and infrastructure-building in Central Europe and the former Soviet republics." New York City Human and Built Environment: "The Foundation supports HIV/AIDS public education and policy work with and emphasis on the involvement of underserved communities in the policy making process. The Foundation supports efforts to ensure that all New Yorkers have access to public parks, open space, waterfronts and green spaces in their neighborhoods, emphasizing the relationship between public spaces and community development and stabilization. The Foundation supports technical assistance providers working with community-based organizations. The Foundation supports organizations making small grants and/or providing technical assistance and training programs for local community leadership and resource development in underserved neighborhoods." 1995-1996 Annual Report **Priorities:** *Arts & Humanities:* 41%. Dance, theater, arts associations, and museums. *Civic & Public Affairs:* 16%. Supports the New York City Human and Built Environment program. *Note:* Total contributions made in 1998. **Typ. Recipients:** AIDS/HIV, Hospitals (University Affiliated). **Geo. Dist:** internationally; nationally; New York, NY.


**Marshall L. and Perrine D. McCune Charitable Foundation**
*See:* Entry 5558


**Norcross Wildlife Foundation**
*See:* Entry 562


★ 11691 ★ **Randolph Foundation**
255 East 49th St., Ste. 23D
New York, NY 10017
**Phone:** (212)752-7148          **Fax:** (212)752-7316
**Email:** lw@hrhroffice.org
**Website:** http://www.norcrossws.org
Heather Higgins, Trustee

**Fnded:** 1990. **Philosophy:** "The Randolph Foundation will continue to focus on public policy issues, but from a slightly different perspective: we are particularly concerned with fostering those underlying values and attitudes that enable free-market and democratic systems to function and flourish. We believe those values are reflected in individual character, and are central to the institutional foundations of a free society; morality and public life, family and community, and competitive educational structures affecting the preservation and continuing development of American Civilization." "The Randolph Foundation has defined this program area under the broad heading of 'Cultural Values, Civic Virtues'. This would include reemphasizing such concepts as: obligations as well as rights; self-control as well as self-expression; personal ethics over legal obligations; responsibility as opposed to dependency; individual merit in contrast to group entitlement; reliance on the private sphere before government; and values that are superior, not relative." "Within this area, the Randolph Foundation is also interested in investing its limited resources to encourage new and worthwhile ideas, individuals, projects, and organizations. Solicitations for support which do not meet these criteria, however worthwhile, will almost certainly be declined." 1997 **Priorities:** *Arts & Humanities:* 8%. Supports the visual arts. *Civic & Public Affairs:* 76%. Primary support for public policy groups. *Education:* 14%. Focus on colleges, universities, and education associations. *International:* 2%. *Note:* Total contributions made in fiscal 1998. **Typ. Recipients:** AIDS/HIV, Cancer, Medical Research, Outpatient Health Care. **Geo. Dist:** nationally.


★ 11692 ★ **Trust for Mutual Understanding**
30 Rockefeller Plaza, Rm. 5600
New York, NY 10112
**Phone:** (212)632-3405          **Fax:** (212)632-3409
**Email:** tmu@tmuny.org
**Website:** http://www.tmuny.org
Richard Lanier, Director
**Fnded:** 1984. **Philosophy:** The Trust for Mutual Understanding primarily is interested in supporting professional exchanges between the United States, the former Soviet Union, and East Central Europe in the areas of environmental conservation and the arts. "As a result of the Trust's primary commitment to encouraging the exchange of individuals, usually by providing assistance for travel and related expenses of project participants, priority consideration is given to those requests in which professional interaction plays a major role and in which there is a significant degree of collaborative effort." **Priorities:** *Arts & Humanities:* 43%. Includes the visual and the performing arts, and exchanges eligible for consideration include exhibitions, performaces given in conjunction with lecture/demonstrations, creative collaborations, curatorial research projects, art conservation and historic preservation initiatives, arts management programs, and cultural documentation activities. *Civic & Public Affairs:* 8%. Funds business/nonprofit management and public policy. *Education:* 18%. Supports colleges and universities. *Religion:* 5%. Supports biological science/research. *Note:* Total contributions made in 1999. **Typ. Recipients:** AIDS/HIV, Health-General, Medical Education. **Geo. Dist:** nationally.


★ 11693 ★ **Wenner-Gren Foundation for Anthropological Research**
220 Fifth Ave., 16th Fl.
New York, NY 10001-7708
**Phone:** (212)683-5000          **Fax:** (212)683-9151
**Email:** info@wennergren.org
**Website:** http://www.wennergren.org
Dr. Richard Fox, President
**Fnded:** 1951. **Philosophy:** The foundation's interest is the support of basic research in all branches of anthropology, including social/cultural anthropology, ethnology, biological/physical anthropology, archaeology, and anthropological linguistics, and in closely related disciplines concerned with human origins, development, and variation. The foundation particularly invites projects employing comparative perspectives

or integrating two or more subfields of anthropology. The foundation supports small grants of up to $20,000 for general anthropological research; predoctoral grants to aid doctoral dissertation or thesis research; Richard Carley Hunt Memorial Postdoctoral Fellowships of up to $15,000 for scholars within five years of receipt of the doctorate; Developing Countries Training Fellowships of up to $12,500 per year, for periods from six months to three years, for scholars from developing countries seeking additional training in anthropology; and conference support in the form of grants to conference organizers and the foundation's own sponsored conferences. The foundation runs an International Collaborative Research Grants Program. This program awards up to $25,000 to assist anthropological research projects undertaken by two or more investigators from different countries. The foundation also has Historical Archives grants program to assist individuals holding significant records and personal papers with the expenses of preparing and transferring them for archival deposit and to assist individuals conducting oral history interviews. This program awards up to $15,000. **Priorities:** *Education:* 99%. Supports research and promotion of anthropological issues through fellowships and scholarships. *Note:* Total contributions made in 2000. **Typ. Recipients:** AIDS/HIV, Children's Health/Hospitals, Prenatal Health Issues. **Geo. Dist:** nationally.


**Winthrop Rockefeller Foundation**
*See:* Entry 7874


## Corporate Foundations

**★ 11694 ★ Bandai Foundation**
c/o The Carmen Group
1299 Penn. Ave. NW, Eigth Fl.
Washington, DC 20004
**Phone:** (301)836-7777          **Fax:** (301)558-0627
**Website:** http://www.wrockefellerfoundation.org
Alison Miller, Contact

**Fnded:** 1994. **Priorities:** *Arts & Humanities:* 2%. Supports preservation of archived films. *Civic & Public Affairs:* 7% Funds civic and community groups. *Education:* 18%. Supports higher education and children's after school educational activities. *Environment:* 46% Funds primarily children's social services. *International:* 27%. Supports primarily children's health care and research. *Note:* Total contributions made for 1999. **Typ. Recipients:** AIDS/HIV, Arthritis, Cancer, Children's Health/Hospitals, Hospitals (University Affiliated), Medical Education, Medical Research, Single-Disease Health Associations. **Geo. Dist:** nationally.


**Ecolab Foundation**
*See:* Entry 8548


**★ 11695 ★ Gap Foundation/Gap Inc. Community Relations**
1 Harrison St.
San Francisco, CA 94105
**Phone:** (415)427-2757          **Fax:** (415)427-2504
**Website:** http://www.gapinc.com/community/community.htm
Dotti Hatcher, Senior DRC

**Fnded:** 1969. **Priorities:** *Note:* Gap divisional programs will initiate community activities by individual Gap, Inc. brands, with an emphasis on the metropolitan areas of Chicago, Los Angeles, New York, and San Francisco. Gap's Sourcing pilot program will focus giving on garment workers and the communities in which they live, especially overseas. **Typ. Recipients:** AIDS/HIV, Cancer, Clinics/Medical Centers, Domestic Violence, Emergency/Ambulance Services, Health Funds, Health Organizations, Hospices, Hospitals, Medical Research, Prenatal Health Issues, Preventive Medicine/Wellness Organizations, Public Health, Research/Studies Institutes, Single-Disease Health Associations, Transplant Networks/Donor Banks, Trauma Treatment. **Geo. Dist:** headquarters and operating locations; Los Angeles, CA; San Francisco, CA; Chicago, IL; New York, NY.


**GenAmerican Foundation**
*See:* Entry 1077


**Gerber Foundation**
*See:* Entry 5573


**★ 11696 ★ Hunt Corp.**
1 Commerce Sq.
2005 Market St.
Philadelphia, PA 19103-7085
**Phone:** (215)841-2398          **Fax:** (215)656-3714
**Email:** cheryl_walmsley@Hunt-Corp.com
**Website:** http://www.hunt-corp.com
Cheryl Walmsley, Grant Administrator

**Priorities:** *Arts & Humanities:* 25%. Supports programs which enable young people in low-income neighborhoods t participate in creative activities in their respective neighbothoods so far as such opportunities are either inadequate or non-existent. *Civic & Public Affairs:* 50%. Supports selected civic organizations which provide leadership on issues of importance to Philadelphians. Also contributes to programs where significant Hunt employee involvement has been demonstrated. Unusual approaches to problems outside of the above priority areas such as research projects or public policy forums are also considered. *Education:* 25%. Foundation places special emphasis on educational inititatives which provide art-related educational programs to lower-income and/or educationally disadvantaged populations at the elementary and secondary levels, promote literacy, or contribute to curriculum development, specific skills training and/or educational innovation. *Note:* Total contributions made in 1998. **Typ. Recipients:** AIDS/HIV, Child Abuse, Children's Health/Hospitals, Domestic Violence. **Geo. Dist:** headquarters.


**John Wiley & Sons, Inc.**
*See:* Entry 1171


**★ 11697 ★ Navcom Charities Foundation**
9815 Godwin Dr.
Manassas, VA 20110-4156
**Phone:** (703)361-0884
**Website:** http://www.wiley.com
Liz Johnson, Administrative Assistant to the Presiden

**Fnded:** 1992. **Typ. Recipients:** AIDS/HIV. **Geo. Dist:** headquarters area only.


**Principal Financial Group Foundation, Inc.**
*See:* Entry 1329


**Saint Paul Companies Inc.**
*See:* Entry 1368


**Synetic Foundation**
*See:* Entry 5589


**Target Foundation**
*See:* Entry 1425


**UPS Foundation**
*See:* Entry 1466


**★ 11698 ★ WPWR-TV Channel 50 Foundation**
2151 N Elston Ave.
Chicago, IL 60614-3999
**Phone:** (773)292-5016          **Fax:** (773)276-6477
**Email:** mail@wpwr50fund.org
**Website:** http://www.community.ups.com
Laura Sampson, Program Officer

**Fnded:** 1992. **Priorities:** *Arts & Humanities:* 57%. Supports museums, ballet, theater, arts councils, and public broadcasting. *Civic & Public Affairs:* 16%. Funds law and justice issues, advocacy, and parks.


*Education:* 14%. Funds colleges and universities and arts education. *Environment:* 6%. Funds United Way, youth organizations, and services for immigrants and the disadvantaged. *International:* 6%. Supports AIDS research. *Note:* Total foundation contributions made in fiscal 2000. **Typ. Recipients:** AIDS/HIV, Health Policy/Cost Containment. **Geo. Dist:** Chicago, IL, including metropolitan area; IN, Northwest part of the state.


## Other Funding Organizations

**★ 11699 ★ American Lyme Disease Foundation (ALDF)**
Mill Pond Offices
293 Rte. 100
Somers, NY 10589
**Phone:** (914)277-6970          **Free:** 800-876-LYME
**Fax:** (914)277-6974
**Email:** inquire@aldf.com
**Website:** http://www.aldf.com
David L. Weld, Contact

**Desc:** Health care professionals and other individuals with an interest in Lyme Disease, a disorder transmitted to humans by the deer tick. Works to control the spread of Lyme Disease, and to improve treatments for the disorder. Maintains physician referral service; produces educational materials and conducts public and professional education programs; supports Lyme Disease research. **Awards:** Research Fund (annual) for prevention and control of tick-borne diseases.


**★ 11700 ★ Elton John AIDS Foundation (EJAIDSF)**
PO Box 17139
Beverly Hills, CA 90209-3139
**Phone:** (310)535-1775
**Email:** AmgejAIDSF@ejaf.org
**Website:** http://ejaf.org
Alexandra Crane, Contact

**Desc:** Individuals and organizations. Promotes increased access to, and improved quality of, patient care services for people with AIDS. Provides financial assistance to AIDS care programs and prevention projects; conducts fundraising activities. **Awards:** Service and Prevention Grants (quarterly).


**★ 11701 ★ Herpes Resource Center - American Social Health Association (HRC)**
PO Box 13827
Research Triangle Park, NC 27709
**Phone:** (919)361-8488          **Fax:** (919)361-8425
**Email:** phidra@ashastd.org
**Website:** http://www.ashastd.org/hrc

**Desc:** Individuals with recurrent genital herpes infections; individuals interested in the dissemination of information about genital herpes. (Herpes is a sexually transmitted disease which is as yet incurable.) Works to give emotional support to individuals, and to provide current information about herpes. Maintains the National Herpes Hotline. Offers referrals to local support groups (HELP) throughout the U.S. and Canada for people living with herpes; HELP groups provide a safe, confidential environment in which to obtain accurate information about HSV and share experiences with other people concerned about herpes. Compiles statistics. **Awards:** Fellowship; grant.


**★ 11702 ★ National AIDS Fund**
1030 15th St. NW, Ste. 860
Washington, DC 20005-2208
**Phone:** (202)408-4848          **Fax:** (202)408-1818
**Email:** info@aidsfund.org
**Website:** http://www.aidsfund.org
Mary Wilson-Byrom, CEO

**Desc:** Promotes leadership and generates resources for effective community responses to HIV/AIDS. **Awards:** Scholarship activists to participate in conference/training.

## ★ 11703 ★ National Catholic AIDS Network (NCAN)

PO Box 960
Occidental, CA 95465
**Phone:** (707)874-3031          **Fax:** (707)874-1433
**Email:** info@ncan.org
**Website:** http://www.ncan.org
Fr. Rodney DeMartini, Exec. Dir.

**Desc:** Provides support and exchange of information among Roman Catholic HIV/AIDS service workers and pastoral ministers. Disseminates educational materials on HIV/AIDS. **Awards:** Lumina Award (annual) for creative and effective pastoral leadership in HIV/AIDS ministry; monetary (annual) for an individual with HIV from an economically impoverished area or service providers who qualify to attend annual ministry conference.

## ★ 11704 ★ National Foundation for Infectious Diseases (NFID)

4733 Bethesda Ave., Ste. 750
Bethesda, MD 20814
**Phone:** (301)656-0003          **Fax:** (301)907-0878
**Email:** info@nfid.org
**Website:** http://www.nfid.org
Susan J. Rehm, MD, Pres.

**Desc:** Supports research into the causes and cures of infectious diseases; assists in the education of both professionals and the public in infectious diseases. Conducts programs in prevention of infectious diseases. **Awards:** Jimmy & Rosalynn Carter Award for Humanitarian Contributions (annual) for humanitarian contributions to the health of humankind; Maxwell Finland Award for Scientific Achievement (annual) for scientific achievements which contribute to improving medical research; New Investigator Matching Grants (annual); NFID Postdoctoral Fellowships (annual) for physicians specializing in infectious diseases.

## ★ 11705 ★ National Minority AIDS Council (NMAC)

1931 13th St. NW
Washington, DC 20009-4432
**Phone:** (202)483-6622          **Free:** 800-544-0586
**Fax:** (202)483-1135
**Email:** info@nmac.org
**Website:** http://www.nmac.org
Paul A. Kawata, Exec. Dir.

**Desc:** Public health departments and AIDS service organizations. Serves as a clearinghouse of information on AIDS as it affects minority communities in the U.S. Facilitates discussion among national minority organizations about AIDS. Maintains Project Health, Education, and AIDS Leadership, which provides computer usage, strategic planning, financial management, and volunteer program development assistance to AIDS service organizations, and Project Volunteer Information, Technical Assistance, and Leadership, which provides technical assistance in volunteer program development and maintenance. Conducts training conferences. Offers educational and research programs; compiles statistics. Maintains speakers' bureau. **Awards:** Recognition; scholarship.

## ★ 11706 ★ Pediatric AIDS Foundation

2950 31st St., Ste. 125
Santa Monica, CA 90405-3037
**Phone:** (310)314-1459          **Fax:** (310)314-1469
**Email:** info@pedAIDS.org
**Website:** http://www.pedaids.org
Kate Carr, CEO

**Desc:** Confronts medical problems unique to children infected with HIV/AIDS, and focuses on finding medical answers that will bring hope. Identifies and funds critically needed pediatric AIDS research worldwide. Provides funds to hospitals around the country which serve children with HIV/AIDS through an Emergency Assistance Program. Encourages students to enter the field of pediatric AIDS through a Student Intern Award Program. Develops and distributes national Parent Education Program for parents of elementary and pre-school age children. **Awards:** Research Grant; Student Internship.

## ★ 11707 ★ Society of Infectious Diseases Pharmacists (SIDP)

1717 W 6th, Ste. 214
Austin, TX 78703
**Phone:** (512)708-0611          **Fax:** (512)708-0627
**Email:** sidp@aams-texas.com
**Website:** http://www.sidp.org/

**Desc:** Pharmacists with a primary interest and practice in infectious diseases pharmacotherapy, and who have spent at least two years performing pharmacotherpeutic research are active members; pharmacists and other individuals not meeting the requirements for active membership, but who share an interest in infectious diseases pharmacotherapy, are associate members. Seesk to advance the study and practice of infectious diseases pharmacotherapy, and to enhance the professional status of members. Serves as a forum for discussion and exchange of information among members. Encourages pharmacotherapeutic research. **Awards:** SIDP/Abbott Award for Outcomes Research (annual) for established researcher making a significant contribution to the field of infectious diseases pharmacotherapy; SIDP/Ortho McNeil Scientist Preceptorship Award (annual) for research groups wishing to visit their collaborators; SIDP Young Investigator's Award (annual) for outstanding young pharmacotherapeutic researcher.

# National & International Organizations

## ★ 11708 ★ ACT UP

332 Bleecker St., No. G5
New York, NY 10014-2980
**Phone:** (212)966-4873          **Fax:** (212)966-4873
**Email:** actupny@panix.com
**Website:** http://www.actupny.org

**Fnded:** 1987. **Desc:** Individuals "united in anger and committed to direct action to end the AIDS crisis." Seeks to increase public awareness and government involvement in the fight against AIDS. Conducts rallies and demonstrations aimed at public figures or institutions that the group feels should be doing more to combat AIDS. Lobbies for quicker availabiltiy of experimental AIDS drugs. **Pub:** *Act Up Americans*. Catalog. • *ACT UP Reports*, quarterly. Newsletter. • *AIDS, Act Up and Activism*. Handbook. • *Merchandise Catalog. Price:* Free upon request. • *Women and AIDS Handbook*. Handbook. **AKA:** AIDS Coalition to Unleash Power.

## ★ 11709 ★ AFAPAC Foundation

Daalwijk 29
NL-1102 AA Amsterdam, Netherlands
**Phone:** 31 20 6003454          **Fax:** 31 20 6006269
**Email:** 1.afapac@wxs.nl

**Fnded:** 1993. **Desc:** Seeks to prevent the spread of the AIDS virus. Provides counseling services.

## ★ 11710 ★ African Council of AIDS Service Organizations

c/o ENDA Tiers Monde
54 rue Cannot
Boite Postale 3370
Dakar, Senegal
**Phone:** 221 8231935          **Fax:** 221 8236615
**Email:** icaso@endadak.gn.apc.org
**Website:** http://www.africaso.org

**Lang(s):** English, French. **Desc:** Organizations providing services to people with AIDS. Seeks to improve the quality of life of people with aids; promotes increased availability of AIDS services; works to stop the spread of AIDS. Serves as a forum for communication among members; coordinates members' activities; functions as a clearinghouse on AIDS and AIDS services.

## ★ 11711 ★ African Network on HIV/AIDS - Europe

Focus Consultancy
32B Warwick Sq.
London SW1 V2AQ, United Kingdom
**Phone:** 44 171 9320072     **Fax:** 44 171 9320074
**Email:** london@fcwsq.demon.co.uk

**Lang(s):** English. **Desc:** National European AIDS organizations with an interest in the AIDS epidemic in Africa. Seeks to slow the spread of AIDS and increase the availability of AIDS treatment services in African countries. Makes available educational and consulting services.

## ★ 11712 ★ Africans in Partnership Against AIDS

517 College St., Ste. 338
Toronto, ON, Canada M8G 4A2
**Phone:** (416)924-5256          **Fax:** (416)924-6575
**Email:** apaa@on.aibn.com

**Fnded:** 1993. **Mem:** 150. **Lang(s):** English, French. **Desc:** Individuals of African descent. Seeks to slow the spread of AIDS and HIV among Africans. Conducts educational programs on AIDS prevention. Provides a supportive environment for those infected or affected by HIV/AIDS, their partners, friends, and families. **Pub:** *Childminding*, semiannual. Newsletter.

## ★ 11713 ★ Africans United to Control AIDS

c/o African Community Health Services
219-339 Bloor St. W
Toronto, ON, Canada M5S 1W7
**Phone:** (416)519-7600          **Fax:** (416)519-7317
**Email:** aches@globalserve.net

**Lang(s):** English, French. **Desc:** Individuals of African descent. Seeks to stop the spread of AIDS and HIV among Africans. Conducts educational programs on AIDS prevention.

## ★ 11714 ★ Aggressive Aids Prevention

Federal PO Box 26227
San Francisco, CA 94126-6227
**Phone:** (415)255-6022
**Email:** bod@aggressive.org
**Website:** http://www.aggressive.org
Devin Kordt-Thomas, Media

**Fnded:** 1998. **Desc:** Promotes HIV/AIDS awareness. Provides information, materials and education.

## ★ 11715 ★ AIDS Action

1906 Sunderland Place NW
Washington, DC 20036
**Phone:** (202)530-8030          **Fax:** (202)530-8031
**Email:** aidsaction@aidsaction.org
**Website:** http://www.aidsaction.org

**Fnded:** 1984. **Mem:** 3,200. **Desc:** National AIDS service organizations. Dedicated to responsible federal policy for improved HIV/AIDS care and services, vigorous medical research and effective prevention. Operates the Pedro Zamora Center national AIDS youth advocacy program.

## ★ 11716 ★ AIDS Action Now! (AAN) (Le groupe d'action sida)

517 College St. S, Ste. 420
Toronto, ON, Canada M6G 4A2
**Phone:** (416)928-2206          **Fax:** (416)928-2185
**Email:** info@catie.ca
**Website:**          http://www.gaycanada.com/aan/aan-frame.htm

**Lang(s):** English, French. **Desc:** Individuals and organization. Seeks to prevent the spread of AIDS and HIV; promotes research into a cure for AIDS. Makes available support and services to people with HIV and AIDS; conducts educational programs to increase awareness of AIDS and HIV prevention techniques. **Pub:** *VESS Newsletter*, quarterly. Newsletter.

**★ 11717 ★ AIDS Care Education and Training (ACET)**
PO Box 3693
London SW15 2BS, United Kingdom
**Phone:** 44 20 87800400    **Fax:** 44 20 87800400
**Email:** acet@acetuk.org
**Website:** http://www.acetuk.org
**Fnded:** 1988. **Nat'l Groups:** 7. **Reg. Groups:** 6.
**Lang(s):** English. **Desc:** Promotes effective and un-
conditional care for people with HIV and AIDS world-
wide. Conducts educational and training programs for
AIDS care providers; works with national and interna-
tional AIDS care organizations to improve the quality
and availability of AIDS care. **Pub:** *ACET Newsletter*,
3/year. Newsletter. • *HIV - Facts for Life*. Booklet.

**★ 11718 ★ AIDS Education and Research Trust (AVERT)**
4 Brighton Rd.
Horsham RH13 5BA, United Kingdom
**Phone:** 44 1403 210202    **Fax:** 44 1403 211001
**Email:** info@avert.org
**Website:** http://www.avert.org
**Fnded:** 1986. **Lang(s):** English. **Desc:** Sponsors
AIDS control programs in England. Seeks to improve
the quality of life for persons with AIDS. Conducts
research and educational programs. Provides free
information on AIDS, both within the U.K. and over-
seas. **Pub:** *AIDS: Working with Young People*. Book.
Active learning resource for those working with young
people. • *Condoms, Pills & Other Useful Things: A
Young Person's Guide to Contraception and STDs*.
Booklet. • *Not Under My Roof: Families Talking about
Sex & AIDS*. Book. • *Prisons, HIV and AIDS: Risks
and Experiences in Custodial Care*. Book. • *Sexual
Feelings & Relationships*. Booklet. • Pamphlets. •
Reports.

**★ 11719 ★ AIDS Evaluation**
Swiss Federal Office of Public Health
Evaluation Computer Centre
CH-3003 Bern, Switzerland
**Phone:** 41 31 3238023    **Fax:** 41 31 3238805
**Lang(s):** English, French, German, Italian. **Frmly:**
Bureau Central pour le SIDA.

**★ 11720 ★ AIDS Foundation of Canada**
885 Dunsmuir St., Ste. 1000
Vancouver, BC, Canada V6C 1N5
**Phone:** (604)688-7294    **Fax:** (604)689-4888
**Email:** ganapath@axionet.com
**Fnded:** 1986. **Mem:** 6. **Lang(s):** English, French.
**Desc:** Individuals and corporations with an interest in
the prevention and treatment of AIDS and HIV.
Promotes an improved quality of life for people with
HIV and AIDS; seeks to advance AIDS and HIV
treatment and prevention techniques. Conducts public
awareness programs to slow the spread of AIDS;
provdies financial and other assistance to innovative
programs assisting people with HIV and AIDS. Sponsors charitable programs.

**★ 11721 ★ AIDS Helpline**
c/o The Centre at the Warehouse
7 James St. S
Belfast BT2 8DN, United Kingdom
**Phone:** 44 28 90249268    **Fax:** 44 28 90329845
**Email:** thecentre@dnet.co.uk
**Website:** http://www.aidshelpline.org.uk
**Fnded:** 1985. **Mem:** 48. **Desc:** Makes available
counselors to offer advice to those affected by AIDS.
Offers home support. Conducts preventative educa-
tion and a outreach programs. Promotes fundraising.
Provides a range of complementary therapies free-
phone helpline, health enquiries, advice line.

**★ 11722 ★ AIDS Prevention League (APPLE)**
199 King Ct.
Akron, OH 44303-2322
Saiom Lehman, Exec. Officer
**Fnded:** 1987. **Desc:** Coalition promoting non-dairy
vegetarianism as a deterrent to AIDS. Works to
educate the public about the alleged correlation between animal products and AIDS. Believes that ingest-
ing animal products weakens the immune system,
making it vulnerable to the AIDS virus. (Group believes that out of all AIDS patients, not a single one is
vegetarian.) Promotes the use of intravenous vitamin
C and a raw fruit diet as a possible cure for or means
of causing remission of AIDS. **Pub:** *AIDS News*,
periodic.

**★ 11723 ★ AIDS Resource Foundation for Children (ARFC)**
St. Clare's Home for Children
182 Roseville Ave.
Newark, NJ 07107
**Phone:** (973)483-4250    **Fax:** (973)483-1998
**Website:** http://www.aidsresource.org/default.asp
Terrence P. Zealand, Exec. Dir.
**Fnded:** 1985. **Desc:** Operates homes for children
ages birth thru 12 years of age with HIV, AIDS, or
AIDS-Related Complex (ARC) medically fragile (ie:
cerebral palsy, menigitis, mentally retarded, etc.) who
are well enough to be released from the hospital but
are in need of foster care placement or respite care;
provides support services to families coping with AIDS
or related diseases. Operates foster parent recruitment, training, and support programs; collects and
distributes toys and clothing. Sponsors summer camp
for families. Conducts HIV training workshops, community outreach programs, and agency networking;
maintains speakers' bureau. Provides referrals, bereavement counseling, and emergency assistance.
Acts as a model program for transitional foster homes
nationwide; although all homes are currently operating
in the New Jersey area, any child with AIDS or a
related disease is eligible for assistance. **Pub:** Newsletter, periodic. **AKA:** St. Clare's Home for Children;
St. Clare's Home Health; St. Clare's Home Properties.

**★ 11724 ★ AIDS School Education Resource Centre**
c/o Programme of Education for the Prevention of
AIDS
UNESCO
Section de l'Education Preventive
Division de la Renovation de l'Enseignement
   Secondaire et Pr
7 Place de Fontenoy
F-75352 Paris, France
**Phone:** 33 1 45681622    **Fax:** 33 1 45685621
**Email:** s.bahri@unesco.org
**Lang(s):** English, French. **Desc:** AIDS education
programs and institutions. Seeks to slow the spread of
AIDS through increasing public awareness of the
disease. Sponsors educational programs and pro-
duces and distributes curricular materials.

**★ 11725 ★ AIDS Secreatariat - Antigua-Barbuda**
Ministry of Health and Civil Service Affairs
AIDS Secretariat
AFLAK Bldg.
Friar's Hill Rd.
Saint Johns, Antigua-Barbuda
**Phone:** (268)462-5039    **Fax:** (268)462-5039
**Email:** aidssec@candw.ag
**Fnded:** 1989. **Lang(s):** English. **Desc:** Individuals in
Antigua-Barbuda interested in fighting the spread of
HIV/AIDS. Conducts public awareness and health
programs.

**★ 11726 ★ AIDS Society for Asia and the Pacific**
c/o Wednesday Friends Club
Edmund Blacket Bldg., 1st Fl. S Wing
Prince of Wales Hospital
Randwick, NSW 2031, Australia
**Phone:** 61 2 93822775    **Fax:** 61 2 93822787
**Email:** j.dwyer@unsw.edu.au
**Fnded:** 1990. **Mem:** 3,600. **Nat'l Groups:** 3. **Lang(s):**
English. **Desc:** AIDS organizations and agencies.
Seeks to prevent the spread of AIDS through in-
creased public awareness of the disease and its
prevention; promotes improved treatment of AIDS and
HIV. Sponsors educational programs; conducts re-
search.

**★ 11727 ★ All Africa Leprosy, Tuberculosis and Rehabilitation Training Centre (ALERT)**
PO Box 165
Addis Ababa, Ethiopia
**Phone:** 251 1 711110    **Fax:** 251 1 711199
**Email:** leprosytb@telecom.net.et
**Website:** http://www.telecom.net.et/~tdalert
**Fnded:** 1965. **Lang(s):** English. **Desc:** Health care
services working with people with leprosy. Seeks to
advance the diagnosis, prevention, and treatment of
leprosy. Makes available medical services; conducts
training programs for health care personnel. Main
emphasis is on international training related to leprosy
and tuberculosis.

**★ 11728 ★ Alliance for South Asian AIDS Prevention (ASAAP)**
20 Carlton St., Ste. 126, Fl. M
Toronto, ON, Canada M5B 2H5
**Phone:** (416)599-2727    **Fax:** (416)599-6011
**Email:** asaap@asaap.ca
**Website:** http://www.asaap.ca
**Fnded:** 1989. **Mem:** 120. **Lang(s):** Bengali, English,
Gujarati, Hindi, Punjabi, Tamil, Urdu. **Desc:** Seeks to
stop the spread of HIV and AIDS in Toronto's South
Asian communities. Provides support and services to
South Asian individuals affected by HIV/AIDS. Con-
ducts AIDS and HIV advocacy, networking, preven-
tion, and education programs. **Pub:** *WASPNews*,
periodic. Newsletter.

**★ 11729 ★ American Academy of Tropical Medicine (AATM)**
16126 E Warren
PO Box 24224
Detroit, MI 48224
**Phone:** (313)882-0641    **Fax:** (313)882-5110
Ben Allie, MD, Pres.
**Fnded:** 1984. **Mem:** 2,600. **Nat'l Groups:** 10. **Reg.
Groups:** 10. **Desc:** Physicians and allied health
professionals interested in tropical medicine. Provides
postgraduate continuing medical education; confers
certificates and diplomas. Maintains speakers' bureau;
provides placement service. Conducts research and
compiles statistics. Conducts educational programs;
offers children's services. **Pub:** *Journal of the American Academy of Tropical Medicine*, semiannual. Journal. Includes book reviews, employment opportunities,
and information on new diagnostic equipment. *Price:*
$125/year. • Monographs. • Newsletter, periodic. •
Also publishes case studies and plans to publish
directory of physicians and hospitals in tropical countries.

**★ 11730 ★ American Board of Tropical Medicine (ABTM)**
PO Box 24224
Detroit, MI 48224
**Phone:** (313)882-0641    **Fax:** (313)882-5110
Dr. Ben Alli, Assoc. Dir.
**Fnded:** 1980. **Mem:** 2,100. **State Groups:** 2. **Desc:**
Physicians including pediatricians, dermatologists,
surgeons, professionals of public health and preventive medicine, and pathologists interested in tropical
medicine. United to preserve the quality of care in
tropical medicine. Investigates qualifications and determines the competency of candidates applying for
membership and provides continuing medical education programs to specialists in tropical medicine.
Issues certificate as evidence of meeting continuing
medical education requirements. Compiles statistics.
**Pub:** Newsletter, annual. *Price:* $100. • Publishes

*Directory of Specialists in Tropical Medicine.* **AKA:** American College of Tropical Medicine.

★ **11731** ★ **American Foundation for AIDS Research (amfAR)**
120 Wall St., 13th floor
New York, NY 10005-3902
**Phone:** (212)806-1600       **Free:** 800-39-AMFAR
**Fax:** (212)806-1601
**Email:** teresa.coffey@amfar.org
**Website:** http://www.amfar.org
William F. Zabel, Secretary
**Fnded:** 1985. **Reg. Groups:** 2. **Desc:** Dedicated to the support of AIDS research and prevention, treatment education, and advocacy of AIDS-related public policy. **Pub:** *amfAR Treatment Insider*, bimonthly. Reprint. • *HIV/AIDS Treatment Directory*, semiannual. Directory. *Price:* Most distributed free. • Bulletin, periodic.

★ **11732** ★ **American Foundation for the Prevention of Venereal Disease (AFPVD)**
799 Broadway, Ste. 638
New York, NY 10003
**Phone:** (212)253-9778
Mary O'Connell, Sec.
**Fnded:** 1967. **Desc:** Provides educational material to the public on the prevention of sexually transmitted diseases. Encourages every individual to assume responsibility for his or her own health; stresses the importance of proper personal hygiene. Seeks to eliminate the feelings of guilt and shame that are associated with sexually transmitted diseases. **Pub:** *Sexually Transmitted Disease Prevention for Everyone*, periodic. Brochure. **Frmly:** (1967) New York Alliance for the Eradication of Venereal Disease, Inc.

★ **11733** ★ **American Institute for Teen AIDS Prevention**
PO Box 395
Oberlin, OH 44074-0395
**Phone:** (440)774-5411       **Fax:** (440)233-6455
**Email:** TeenAIDS@msn.com
Duane Crumb, Pres.
**Fnded:** 1987. **Desc:** Provides HIV/STD education programs to schools and churches. Maintains speakers' bureau. Develops and distributes HIV/STD education materials. **Pub:** *Developing Your Church AIDS Policy.* Book. Leads church leaders through the process of researching, drafting, and implementing an AIDS policy. *Price:* $8. • *Don't Let AIDS Catch You!* Brochure. HIV/AIDS education for teens. • *Guide to Positive HIV/AIDS Education.* Book. • *It's Your Choice.* Video. • *Making Love without Doing It.* Brochure. • *Staying Current*, bimonthly. *Price:* Free. **Frmly:** AIDS Information Ministries; American Institute for Teen Aids Prevention.

★ **11734** ★ **American Leprosy Missions (ALM)**
1 ALM Way
Greenville, SC 29601
**Phone:** (864)271-7040       **Free:** 800-543-3135
**Fax:** (864)271-7062
**Email:** amlep@leprosy.org
**Website:** http://www.leprosy.org
David Galvin, Org. /Donor Svcs. Mgr.
**Fnded:** 1906. **Desc:** Provides medical, rehabilitative, and social care for people with leprosy, also known as Hansen's disease, in over 20 countries. Conducts specialized training for medical workers; supports medical and social rehabilitation; provides special literature on leprosy to medical personnel abroad. Sponsors research in the U.S., Brazil, India, and Ethiopia. Assists the national leprosy control programs of Brazil, Angola, Burma, Mexico, and The Philippines. Provides management assistance for the *International Journal of Leprosy*. Maintains hall of fame, museum of leprosy, and speakers' bureau. Maintains hall of fame, museum of leprosy, and speakers' bureau. **Pub:** *Word*

*and Deed*, quarterly. Newsletter. Includes ALM news. *Price:* Free.

★ **11735** ★ **American Social Health Association (ASHA)**
PO Box 13827
Research Triangle Park, NC 27709
**Phone:** (919)361-8400       **Fax:** (919)361-8425
**Email:** phidra@ashastd.org
**Website:** http://www.ashastd.org
William C. Parra, CEO
**Fnded:** 1914. **Desc:** A national voluntary health agency dedicated to stopping sexually transmitted diseases and their harmful consequences to individuals, families and communities. Works to expand biomedical research, provide information and education programs, upgrade clinical care, and improve public policy. Provides leadership in public policy issues. Supplies public health agencies with patient education materials. Engages directly in biomedical research through its ASHA Research Fund. Operates Herpes Resource Center, a national program for those infected with the genital herpes virus, and HPV Support Program, a national program for those infected with the human papilloma virus. **Pub:** *Helper*, quarterly. Newsletter. Reports on the latest research on the herpes simplex virus; includes information on strategies for coping with the virus and on treatments. *Price:* $25/yr. • *HPV News*, quarterly. Includes latest research on HPV/genital warts and information on coping strategies. *Price:* $25/yr. • *Managing Herpes*. *Price:* $19.75 includes shipping and handling. • Brochures. • Pamphlets. **Frmly:** (1959) American Social Hygiene Association.

★ **11736** ★ **American Society of Tropical Medicine and Hygiene (ASTMH)**
60 Revere Dr., Ste. 500
Northbrook, IL 60062
**Phone:** (847)480-9592       **Fax:** (847)480-9282
**Email:** astmh@astmh.org
**Website:** http://www.astmh.org
Kevin Hacke, Exec. Dir.
**Fnded:** 1951. **Mem:** 3,000. **Desc:** Professional society of physicians and scientists interested in tropical medicine and hygiene, including the areas of arbovirology, entomology, medicine, nursing, parasitology, immunology, infectious disease, and travelers' health. **Pub:** *American Journal of Tropical Medicine and Hygiene*, monthly. Journal. *Price:* $400/yr North America; $450/yr outside North America. • *Health Hints for the Tropics.* • *Tropical Medicine and Hygiene News*, bimonthly.

★ **11737** ★ **Anti-Tuberculosis Association Afghanistan Programme (ATA)**
35/E Canal Rd.
University Town
Peshawar, Afghanistan
**Phone:** 92 91 840126
**Fnded:** 1990. **Desc:** Works to control the spread of tuberculosis in Afghanistan. Operates tuberculosis clinics. Makes available medications.

★ **11738** ★ **Asia-Pacific Council of AIDS Services Organizations (APCASO)**
Yayasan Citra Usadha Indonesia
Jalan Belimbing Gang Y No. 4
80231 Denpasar, Indonesia
**Phone:** 62 361 246757       **Fax:** 62 361 246757
**Email:** doetomo@indo.net.id
**Lang(s):** English, Indonesian. **Desc:** Organizations providing services to people with AIDS and their families. Promotes increased availability of AIDS services in Asia and the Pacific. Facilitates communication and cooperation among members; coordinates provision of AIDS services by multiple agencies.

★ **11739** ★ **Asia-Pacific Network of People With HIV/AIDS**
c/o Paul Tohh
Race Course Rd.
Singapore 218568, Singapore
**Phone:** 65 2951153       **Fax:** 65 2955567
**Email:** paultoh@pacific.net.sg
**Website:** http://www.xs4all.nl/~gnp/asap.html
**Fnded:** 1994. **Lang(s):** Chinese, English. **Desc:** People with AIDS and HIV and their families; organizations providing services to people with AIDS and HIV. Seeks to improve the quality of life of people with AIDS and HIV; promotes increased availability of social and medical services for people with AIDS and HIV. Coordinates members' programs; sponsors research on AIDS services.

★ **11740** ★ **Association of French-Language Leprologists (AFLL) (Association des Leprologues de Lange Francaise — ALLF)**
4 rue Jean Jacques Bel
F-33000 Bordeaux, France
**Phone:** 33 5 56523214       **Fax:** 33 5 56523214
**Email:** pibobin@fr.packardbell.org
**Fnded:** 1984. **Mem:** 500. **Lang(s):** English, French. **Desc:** Health care professionals with an interest in leprosy and Buruli Ulcer. Promotes advancement in the prevention, diagnosis, and treatment of leprosy; seeks to improve the quality of life of people with leprosy. Facilitates communication and cooperation among members; serves as a clearinghouse on leprosy and its treatment; sponsors research; makes available services to people with leprosy. **Pub:** *Bulletin de l'ALLF*, semiannual. Journal. Information and continuous training about Leprosy and Buruli Ulcer.

**Association of Nurses in AIDS Care (ANAC)**
*See:* Entry 15666

★ **11741** ★ **Association for Professionals in Infection Control and Epidemiology (APIC)**
1275 K St. NW, Ste. 1000
Washington, DC 20005
**Phone:** (202)789-1890       **Fax:** (202)789-1899
**Email:** apicinfo@apic.org
**Website:** http://www.apic.org
Christopher E. Laxton, Exec. Dir.
**Fnded:** 1972. **Mem:** 11,800. **Nat'l Groups:** 1. **State Groups:** 50. **Local Groups:** 112. **Desc:** Physicians, microbiologists, nurses, epidemiologists, medical technicians, sanitarians, and pharmacists. Purpose is to improve patient care by improving the profession of infection control through the development of educational programs and standards. Promotes quality research and standardization of practices and procedures. Develops communications among members, and assesses and influences legislation related to the field. Conducts seminars at local level. **Pub:** *American Journal of Infection Control*, bimonthly. Journal. Academic Peer Reviewed Journal. *Price:* Free. For members only. • *APIC News*, bimonthly. Newsletter. **Frmly:** (1997) Association for Practitioners in Infection Control.

★ **11742** ★ **Australasian Society for HIV Medicine (ASHM)**
LMB 5057
Surry Hills, NSW 1300, Australia
**Phone:** 61 2 93682700       **Fax:** 61 2 93809528
**Email:** ashm@ashm.org.au
**Website:** http://www.ashm.org.au
**Fnded:** 1989. **Lang(s):** English. **Desc:** Physicians, medical scientists, health care professionals, and other individuals involved in the field of HIV/AIDS medicine. Seeks to advance the study, teaching, and practice of HIV/AIDS medicine; works to stop the spread of AIDS. Serves as a clearinghouse on HIV/AIDS medicine; maintains journal club; conducts lob-

bying campaigns; sponsors national HIV Education Program for Australasian Doctors; develops and distributes educational materials. Facilitates establishment of international HIV/AIDS medical networks. Advises government agencies responsible for public health and other policies relating to HIV/AIDS. **Pub:** *Directory of Australasian HIV Medical Services*, annual. Directory. • *HN Journal Club*, monthly. Newsletter. • *Noah's Arc*, quarterly. Newsletter.

### ★ 11743 ★ Australian National Council on AIDS and Related Diseases (ANCARD)

GPO Box 9848
Mail Drop 13
Department of Health and Family Services
Canberra, ACT 2601, Australia
**Phone:** 61 2 62897029     **Fax:** 61 2 62898098
**Website:** http://www.ancahrd.org

**Fnded:** 1988. **Mem:** 27. **Lang(s):** English. **Desc:** Provides independent and expert advice to the Minister of Health on the implementation of the National HIV/AIDS Strategy. Identifies national objectives and priorities. Disseminates information to increase community understanding. **Pub:** Bulletin, periodic. **Frmly:** (1998) Australian National Council on AIDS.

### ★ 11744 ★ Black Coalition for AIDS Prevention (BCAP)

790 Bay St., Ste 940
Toronto, ON, Canada M5G 1N8
**Phone:** (416)977-9955     **Fax:** (416)977-2325
**Email:** blackcap@black-cap.com

**Lang(s):** English, French. **Desc:** Individuals concerned about the spread of HIV and AIDS in African Canadian communities. Promotes increased awareness of AIDS prevention techniques. Conducts educational programs; serves as a clearinghouse on AIDS prevention.

### ★ 11745 ★ Body Positive

19 Fulton St., Ste. 308B
New York, NY 10038
**Phone:** (212)566-7333     **Free:** 800-566-6599
**Fax:** (212)566-4539
**Email:** bodypositive@bodypos.org
**Website:** http://www.thebody.com/
Michael Dentato, Exec. Dir.

**Fnded:** 1987. **Mem:** 15,000. **Desc:** Provides support services for people who are HIV-infected or have AIDS, and their families and friends. Organizes seminars on treatment issues and socials. Provides outreach programs and recreational services. **Pub:** *Body Positive*, monthly. Newsletter. *Price:* $35 invidual. • *Positive Options*. Book. Book for people living with HIV/AIDS. • *Resource Directory*, 2/year. • *SIDA*, 6/year.

### ★ 11746 ★ Brazilian Interdisciplinary AIDS Association (ABIA) (Associacao Brasileiar Interdisciplinar de AIDS)

Rua da Candelaria 79, Andar 10
20050-000 Rio de Janeiro, RJ, Brazil
**Phone:** 55 21 2231040     **Fax:** 55 21 22538495
**Email:** abia@ax.apc.org
**Website:** http://www.alternex.com.br/~abia/

**Fnded:** 1986. **Mem:** 17. **Lang(s):** English, Portuguese, Spanish. **Desc:** Advocates a multidisciplinary approach to issues raised by AIDS. Assesses AIDS-related government initiatives and works to develop adequate prevention, education, and information policies. Studies the social impact of AIDS in Brazil; compiles and disseminates updated information on HIV-infection prevention and control; critiques available information and works to lessen the spread of misinformation; provides consultancy and advisory services. Serves as a clearing house and resource center; maintains database in cooperation with the Brazilian Institute of Social and Economic Analyses. Conducts seminars on ethical, moral, and social aspects of the disease and educational and research

programs. **Pub:** *ABIA Bulletin*, quarterly. Newsletter. • *Acao Anti AIDS*, bimonthly. Magazine. • *AIDS in Brazil*. Book. • Books.

### ★ 11747 ★ British Infection Society

Nuffield Department of Medicine, Level 7
John Radcliffe Hospital
Oxford 0X3 9DU, United Kingdom
**Phone:** 44 1865 220154     **Fax:** 44 1865 222962
**Website:**     http://www.britishinfectionsociety.org/society2.html

**Fnded:** 1997. **Mem:** 900. **Desc:** Members of the medical profession and others working in related spheres which are relevant to the society's objectives. Established to relieve sickness by the study of all aspects of infection and to promote the wide dissemination of relevant knowledge. **Pub:** *The Journal of Infection*, bimonthly. Journal. **Frmly:** (1997) British Society for the Study of Infection.

### ★ 11748 ★ Canadian AIDS Society (CAS)

309 Cooper St., 4th Fl.
Ottawa, ON, Canada K2P 0G5
**Phone:** (613)230-3580     **Fax:** (613)563-4998
**Email:** casinfo@cdnaids.ca
**Website:** http://www.cdnaids.ca

**Fnded:** 1986. **Mem:** 103. **Nat'l Groups:** 62. **Reg. Groups:** 98. **Local Groups:** 36. **Lang(s):** English, French. **Desc:** National coalition of over one hundred community-based AIDS organizations across Canada. **Pub:** *Quarterly Update*, quarterly. Newsletter.

### ★ 11749 ★ Canadian AIDS Treatment Information Exchange (CATIE)

555 Richmond St. W, Ste. 505
Box 1104
Toronto, ON, Canada M5V 3B1
**Phone:** (416)203-7122     **Free:** 800-263-1638
**Fax:** (416)203-8284
**Email:** info@catie.ca
**Website:** http://www.catie.ca

**Fnded:** 1991. **Mem:** 700. **Lang(s):** English, French. **Desc:** Seeks to assist people with AIDS and health care providers in making informed treatment decisions. Gathers and disseminates information on AIDS treatments. Facilitates access by health care professionals to the latest information on advances in AIDS care. Conducts educational programs. **Pub:** *Factsheet*, periodic. Pamphlet. • *HIV+ Peers as Treatment Information Counselors*. Handbook. • *HIV-Related Clinical Trials in Ontario*, periodic. Directory. • *Hooking Up to Social Services*. Report. • *Managing Your Health*. Book. • *TreatmentUpdate*, 10/year. Journal. • Newsletter, quarterly.

### Canadian Association for Clinical Microbiology and Infectious Diseases (CACMID) (Association Canadienne de Microbiologie Clinique et des Maladies — ACMCM)

See: Entry 4597

### ★ 11750 ★ Canadian Association of Medical Microbiologists (CAMM) (Association Canadienne des Medecins Microbiologistes — ACMM)

London, ON, Canada N6A 5A5
**Email:** camm@megma.ca
**Website:** http://www.cacmid.ca

**Lang(s):** English, French. **Desc:** Medical microbiologists. Seeks to advance the science of medical microbiology; promotes professional advancement of members. Facilitates communication and cooperation among members; conducts research and educational programs.

### Canadian Association of Nurses in AIDS Care (Association Canadienne des Infirmieres et Infirmiers en Sidologie)

See: Entry 15681

### ★ 11751 ★ Canadian Foundation for AIDS Research (CANFAR) (Fondation canadienne de recherche sur le SIDA — FCRS)

165 University Ave., Ste. 901
Toronto, ON, Canada M5H 3B8
**Phone:** (416)361-6281     **Free:** 800-563-2873
**Fax:** (416)361-5736
**Email:** cure@canfar.com
**Website:** http://www.canfar.com

**Fnded:** 1988. **Mem:** 75. **Lang(s):** English, French. **Desc:** Seeks to advance AIDS and HIV research and services. Provides support and assistance to Canadian AIDS and HIV research projects; conducts educational programs to raise public awareness of AIDS and HIV. **Pub:** *Catalyst*, semiannual. Newsletter.

### Canadian HIV/AIDS Legal Network (Reseau Juridique Canadien VIH/SIDA)

See: Entry 12233

### ★ 11752 ★ Canadian Infectious Disease Society (CIDS) (Societe Canadienne de Maladies Infectieuses — SCMI)

2197 promenade Riverside Dr.
Ste./piece 504
Ottawa, ON, Canada K1H 7X3
**Phone:** (613)260-3233     **Fax:** (613)260-3235
**Email:** cids@magma.ca
**Website:** http://www.cids.medical.org

**Lang(s):** English, French. **Desc:** Promotes excellence in the prevention, diagnosis, and management of human infectious diseases. **Pub:** *The Canadian Journal of Infectious Diseases*, bimonthly. Journal.

### ★ 11753 ★ CAVDA-Citizens AIDS Project (CAP)

Ste. 128
800 W Central Rd.
Mount Prospect, IL 60056
**Phone:** (847)398-3378     **Fax:** (847)398-7309
**Email:** cavdarx@earthlink.net
Howard A. Mirsky, Dir.

**Fnded:** 1986. **Mem:** 125. **Desc:** A project of the Citizens Alliance for VD Awareness. Physicians, pharmacists, nurses, health professionals, and interested others. Seeks to provide information and educational programs to professionals and the public in order to dispel myths associated with sexually transmitted diseases and Acquired Immune Deficiency Syndrome. Conducts research programs and disseminates information and surveys through media and group presentations. Compiles statistics; maintains speakers' bureau. **Pub:** *STD Spotlight*, quarterly. Newsletter. *Price:* $30/year. • Pamphlets.

### ★ 11754 ★ CDC National Prevention Information Network (NPIN)

PO Box 6003
Rockville, MD 20849-6003
**Phone:** (800)458-5231     **Free:** 800-243-7012
**Fax:** (301)562-1050
**Email:** info@cdcpin.org
**Website:** http://www.cdcnpin.org
Jesse Milan, Jr., Project Dir.

**Fnded:** 1987. **Desc:** A service of the Centers for Disease Control and Prevention. Collects, analyzes, and disseminates information on HIV/AIDS, STDs, and TB primarily for healthcare professionals, educators, social service workers, attorneys, employers and human resource professionals, state HIV/AIDS programs, community organizations, and service associations. Responds to the information needs of health professionals. Offers referral service, and Business and Labor Resource Service (BLRS). **Pub:** *List of Materials*, quarterly. Booklet. • Brochures. **Frmly:** (1991) National AIDS Information Clearinghouse; (1992) National AIDS Clearinghouse.


★ **11755** ★ **CFIDS Association of America**
PO Box 220398
Charlotte, NC 28222-0398
**Free:** 800-442-3437          **Fax:** (704)365-9755
**Email:** info@cfids.org
**Website:** http://www.cfids.org
Kim Kenney, Exec. Officer

**Fnded:** 1986. **Mem:** 23,000. **Desc:** Individuals with chronic fatigue and immune dysfunction syndrome (chronic viral illness associated with dysfunction of the immune system; formerly called chronic Epstein-Barr virus); doctors, nurses, and government officials. Advocates continued research into the cause and cure of the syndrome. Funds pilot medical research projects. **Pub:** *The CFIDS Chronicle and Research Review*, 4/year. Journal. Contains research and medical articles, advocacy efforts reports, practical tips on living with CFIDS and book and media reviews. *Price:* Included in membership dues. • Also publishes patient guide and other educational materials. **Frmly:** (1994) CFIDS Association.


★ **11756** ★ **Children's AIDS Fund**
PO Box 16433
Washington, DC 20041
**Phone:** (703)433-1560          **Free:** (866)829-1560
**Fax:** (703)433-1561
**Email:** info@childrensaidsfund.org
**Website:** http://www.childrensaidsfund.org
Anita M. Smith, Pres.

**Fnded:** 1987. **Desc:** Serves children and families who are HIV impacted through direct assistance referrals, counseling, and resource materials. Advisory board of doctors, public health professionals, legislators, educators, and clergy assisting in the formulation of a sound public policy on HIV/AIDS that will be understood and promoted by the public. Encourages the public to react compassionately toward persons affected, infected, or ill with HIV or AIDS. Advocates early diagnosis; promotes reducing transmission of the epidemic through public health intervention strategies such as confidential and voluntary partner notification. Supports development of treatments, diagnostics, vaccines, and an eventual cure for the disease. Promotes health care access for individuals infected with HIV and AIDS. Testifies before national, state, and local government agencies. Operates speakers' bureau. **Pub:** *AIDS/HIV News*, bimonthly. *Price:* $25/year. • *The Church's Response to the Challenge of AIDS/HIV*. Compiled in conjunction with MAP International. • *Guide to Federal Funding of HIV Disease*, periodic. • Audiotapes. • Brochures. • Videos. • Also issues literature, conference transcripts, and testimonies. **Frmly:** (1993) Americans for a Sound AIDS Policy; (1998) Americans for a Sound AIDS/HIV Policy.


★ **11757** ★ **China AIDS Network (CAN)**
5 Dong Dan San Tiao
Peking Union Medical College
Beijing 100005, People's Republic of China
**Phone:** 86 10 65288167     **Fax:** 86 10 65288170
**Email:** klzhang@bj.col.com.cn

**Desc:** Works to minimize the incidence of AIDS through education. Develops and distributes materials on AIDS and its transmission.


★ **11758** ★ **China Leprosy Association**
126 Gulou Xidajie
Xicheng District
Beijing 100009, People's Republic of China
**Phone:** 86 10 64033787     **Fax:** 86 10 64033787
**Email:** cla2000@163.com
**Website:** http://skinstd.com

**Fnded:** 1985. **Mem:** 9,192. **State Groups:** 23. **Lang(s):** English. **Desc:** Individuals (9192) and orga-

nizations (23) in the People's Republic of China. Seeks to prevent leprosy; works to develop advanced treatment methods. Fosters exchange and cooperation with leprosy organizations in other countries. Conducts research and educational programs. **Pub:** *China Leprosy and Skin Diseases Journal*, quarterly. Journal. Contains scientific reports and papers on operational activities related to leprosy skin diseases and STD control in China. • *Selected Papers of Foreign Leprosy Journals*. Translated in Chinese. • Films.


★ **11759** ★ **Chinese Anti-Tuberculosis Society**
42 Dung-si-xi-da St.
Beijing, People's Republic of China
**Phone:** 852 10 553685


★ **11760** ★ **Citizens Alliance for VD Awareness (CAVDA)**
Ste. 128
800 W Central Rd.
Mount Prospect, IL 60056
**Phone:** (847)398-3378          **Fax:** (847)398-7909
**Email:** cavdarx@earthlink.net
Howard A. Mirsky, Pres.

**Fnded:** 1972. **Mem:** 125. **Desc:** Businessmen, corporations, social service agencies, public health agencies, physicians, nurses, and pharmacists. Provides information to the public, especially to high incidence groups, about symptoms, treatment, and prevention of sexually transmitted diseases, including AIDS (acquired immune deficiency syndrome). Seeks to increase commitment of health professionals and the public to venereal disease and AIDS control. Conducts demonstrations, public service messages, and surveys. **Pub:** *STD Spotlight: Dedicated to Thought and Activity in STD Information-Education Programs*, quarterly. Newsletter. *Price:* $30/year. • Pamphlets. • Also publishes fact sheets.


★ **11761** ★ **Comissao Nacional de Luta Contra a SIDA (CNLCS)**
Palacio Bensaude
Estrada da Luz 153
P-1600-153 Lisbon, Portugal
**Phone:** 351 21 7220820     **Fax:** 351 21 7220822
**Email:** cnlcs@cnlcs.min-saude.pt

**Fnded:** 1985. **Reg. Groups:** 20. **Lang(s):** English, French, Portuguese, Spanish. **Desc:** Works to prevent the spread of HIV and AIDS. Advises governmental and nongovernmental agencies. Conducts educational programs, compiles and disseminates information. Coordinates health care and social support activities, screening, and viral load testing. Offers financial support to NGO's. **Pub:** *Contra Sida*, quarterly. Bulletin. Contains epidemiological data on AIDS in Portugal and Europe. • Pamphlets.


★ **11762** ★ **Community and Hospital Infection Control Association - Canada (CHICA)**
PO Box 46125
RPO Westdale
Winnipeg, MB, Canada R3R 3S3
**Phone:** (204)897-5990          **Fax:** (204)895-9595
**Email:** chicacda@mb.sympatico.ca
**Website:** http://www.chica.org

**Fnded:** 1971. **Mem:** 800. **Lang(s):** English, French. **Desc:** Health care professionals engaged in the prevention and control of infections. Seeks to improve the health of Canadians by promoting excellence in the practice of infection prevention and control. Serves as a clearinghouse on infection control standards and practices; facilitates communication and exchange of information among members; conducts continuing professional education programs for members. Collaborates with government agencies responsible for public health in the formulation and enforcement of certification standards and in the development of public policies. Provides advice and assistance to organizations and agencies concerned with specific

diseases, including AIDS. Maintains speakers' bureau. **Pub:** *Canadian Journal of Infection Control*, quarterly. Journal.


★ **11763** ★ **Corporacion Chilena de Prevencion del SIDA (CChPS)**
Casilla 49, Correo 22
General Jofre 179
Santiago, Chile
**Phone:** 56 2 2225255          **Fax:** 56 2 2228356
**Email:** chilaids@cchps.mic.cl

**Fnded:** 1987. **Mem:** 125. **Lang(s):** English, Spanish. **Desc:** Promotes AIDS awareness, operating safe-sex educational programs and distributing information on the facts of AIDS. Conducts HIV testing and research programs. Offers counseling and referral to medical and social services. Maintains speakers' bureau. Organizes HIV-positive persons to advocate for improved services. **Pub:** *Rapport Annuel*, annual. Report. De Amores y Sombras: Poblaciones y Culturas Homo y Bisexuales de Hombres en Santiago **Frmly:** Corporacion Chilena contra el SIDA; Comite Nationale de Lutte contre le SIDA.


★ **11764** ★ **Dale and Keith Foundation**
12 Rossner
Brunswick, ME 04011
**Phone:** (207)729-5823
Keith Brooks, Pres.

**Fnded:** 1994. **Desc:** Strives to help stop the spread of AIDS through Southeast Asia by "curbing the sex industry in Thailand" through education and job training. Also works to help abandoned children of American servicemen, and to provide homes for children and families of individuals with the HIV virus in the U.S.


★ **11765** ★ **Damien Dutton Society for Leprosy Aid (DDSLA)**
616 Bedford Ave.
Bellmore, NY 11710
**Phone:** (516)221-5829          **Fax:** (516)221-5909
Howard E. Crouch, Pres.

**Fnded:** 1944. **Mem:** 8,000. **Nat'l Groups:** 1. **Desc:** Religious leaders and laypeople interested in aiding victims of Hansen's disease (leprosy). Provides relief, research, and recreation to victims of leprosy all over the world regardless of race, color, or creed. **Pub:** *After Damien: Dutton*. Book. • *Brother Dutton of Molokai*. Book. • *Damien-Dutton Call*, quarterly. Newsletter. *Price:* available to members only. • *Once Over and Lightly*. Book. • *This One Is For Gussie*. Book. • *Two Hearts - One Fire*. Book. • *Two Josephs on Molokai*. Book. **Frmly:** (1972) Damien-Dutton Society.


★ **11766** ★ **Damien Foundation - Belgium (DFB) (Fondation Damien)**
263, Leopold II Laan
B-1081 Brussels, Belgium
**Phone:** 32 2 4225911          **Fax:** 32 2 4225900
**Email:** secret@damien-foundation.be
**Website:** http://www.damienactie.be

**Fnded:** 1964. **Mem:** 3,000. **Lang(s):** Dutch, English, French. **Desc:** Volunteers working to eradicate leprosy and tuberculosis. Promotes control of the disease through detection, treatment, training, and research. Supports field training as well as formal training in specialized institutions; maintains charitable programs. **Pub:** *Perspectives*, quarterly.


**Dana-Farber Cancer Institute**
*See:* Entry 10158


★ **11767** ★ **DEBRA International**
13 Wellington Business Pk.
Duke's Ride
Crowthorne RG45 6LS, United Kingdom
**Phone:** 44 1344 771961          **Fax:** 44 1344 762661
**Email:** admin@debra.org.uk

**Website:** http://www.debra-international.org
**Fnded:** 1997. **Mem:** 29. **Desc:** Seeks to promote the well being of people with EB and to promote research in the area.

### ★ 11768 ★ Design Industries Foundation Fighting AIDS (DIFFA)
101 W 23rd St.
PMB 2261
New York, NY 10011
**Phone:** (212)727-3100     **Fax:** (212)727-2574
**Email:** info@diffa.org
**Website:** http://www.diffa.org
David Sheppard, Exec. Dir.
**Fnded:** 1984. **Local Groups:** 15. **Desc:** Serves as a foundation bestowing grants to AIDS organizations and programs providing direct patient care and services; preventive, post-diagnostic, and community education; housing, meals, emergency assistance, and legal advocacy; treatment and community-based research. **Pub:** *Good Magazine*, quarterly. Magazine. Contains information on managing care and commerce. *Price:* $35. **Frmly:** Design Industries Foundation for AIDS.

### ★ 11769 ★ Disinfected Mail Study Circle (DMSC)
25 Sinclair Grove
London NW11 9JH, United Kingdom
**Phone:** 44 208 4559190
**Fnded:** 1974. **Mem:** 170. **Lang(s):** English. **Desc:** Postal historians, doctors, researchers, libraries, and research foundations in 25 countries. Studies the historic treatment of mail so as to prevent the spread of contagious diseases. The study circle is continuing the research work of the late Dr. K. F. Meyer and his associates, many of whom are members. The study has been extended to include health certificates and passports, anti-vaccination postal propaganda, and related subjects. Maintains speakers' bureau; conducts research programs. **Pub:** *Cumulative Indexes.* • *Pratique*, 3/year. Magazine. Contains research articles and notices of meetings.

### ★ 11770 ★ Elton John AIDS Foundation (EJAIDSF)
PO Box 17139
Beverly Hills, CA 90209-3139
**Phone:** (310)535-1775
**Email:** AmgejAIDSF@ejaf.org
**Website:** http://ejaf.org
Alexandra Crane, Contact
**Fnded:** 1992. **Nat'l Groups:** 1. **Desc:** Individuals and organizations. Promotes increased access to, and improved quality of, patient care services for people with AIDS. Provides financial assistance to AIDS care programs and prevention projects; conducts fundraising activities.

### ★ 11771 ★ European Society of Clinical Microbiology and Infectious Diseases (ESCMID)
PO Box 11 31
D-82018 Taufkirchen, Germany
**Phone:** 41 61 6867799     **Fax:** 41 61 6867798
**Email:** info@escmid.org
**Website:** http://www.escmid.org
**Fnded:** 1983. **Mem:** 2,700. **Desc:** Professionals working in the fields of clinical microbiology and/or infectious diseases.

### ★ 11772 ★ European Society for Clinical Virology (ESCV)
Regional Public Health Laboratory
Department of Virology
van Ketwich Verschuurlaan 92
NL-9721 SW Groningen, Netherlands
**Phone:** 31 50 5215160     **Fax:** 31 50 5271488
**Email:** schirmjslg@compuserve.com
**Website:** http://www.escv.org

**Fnded:** 1997. **Mem:** 600. **Lang(s):** English, French. **Desc:** Virologists and other health care professionals; researchers and scientists with an interest in viruses. Seeks to advance the practice of virology and rapid viral diagnosis. Sponsors continuing professional education programs for virologists; conducts research. **Frmly:** (2000) European Group for Rapid Viral Diagnosis.

### European Society for Infectious Diseases in Obstetrics and Gynaecology (ESIDOG)
*See:* Entry 16675

### Every Child by Two
*See:* Entry 5681

### ★ 11773 ★ Exotic Pathology Society (EPS) (Societe de Pathologie Exotique)
Institut Pasteur
25, rue du Docteur-Roux
F-75724 Paris Cedex 15, France
**Phone:** 33 1 45668869     **Fax:** 33 1 45664485
**Email:** socpatex@pasteur.fr
**Website:** http://www.pasteur.fr/sante/socpatex/pages
**Fnded:** 1908. **Mem:** 850. **Lang(s):** French. **Desc:** Doctors, bacteriologists, biologists, entomologists, epidemiologists, parapsychologists, pharmacists, veterinarians, and virologists. Promotes the study of tropical diseases. Provides a forum for the presentation and discussion of research findings in the field. **Pub:** *Annuaire*, quadrennial. Yearbook. • *Bulletin de la Societe de Pathologie Exotique*, quarterly. Newsletter.

### ★ 11774 ★ Gay Men's Health Crisis (GMHC)
119 W 24th St.
The Tisch Bldg.
New York, NY 10011-1913
**Phone:** (212)807-6655     **Free:** 800-243-7692
**Fax:** (212)367-1236
**Email:** hotline@gmhc.org
**Website:** http://www.gmhc.org
Ana Oliveira, Exec. Dir.
**Fnded:** 1982. **Desc:** GMHC is "the world's most experienced and comprehensive not-for-profit AIDS service organization." Provides direct social services to people coping with HIV/AIDS, educates the public about HIV, and advocates at all levels of government for sound AIDS policies. **Pub:** *GMHC News*, quarterly. Newsletter. • *Medical Answers About AIDS.* Booklet. • *Program Service News*, monthly. Newsletter. • *Treatment Issues*, monthly. Newsletter. *Price:* Free. • *The Volunteer*, bimonthly. Newsletter. Updates medical, clinical, political, and referral information on AIDS. Includes calendar of events. *Price:* Free. • *When A Friend has AIDS.* Booklet. • Catalog.Contains marketed education materials. • Pamphlets.Prevention of AIDS materials.

### ★ 11775 ★ Global Human Research Foundation (GHR)
14-4-14 Satyakrishna Nivas
Kolagatlavari St.
Vizianagaram 535 002, Andhra Pradesh, India
**Phone:** 91 892227283     **Fax:** 91 892227283
**Lang(s):** English, Hindi. **Desc:** Seeks to curtail the spread of infectious diseases, with particular emphasis on slowing the AIDS epidemic. Conducts preventive health education programs; serves as a clearinghouse for development organizations interested in public health issues. Makes available health care services.

### Group B Strep Association
*See:* Entry 16679

### ★ 11776 ★ Haitian Coalition on AIDS (HCA)
50 Court St., Ste. 1010
Brooklyn, NY 11201
**Phone:** (718)855-7275     **Fax:** (718)852-5377
**Email:** info@haitiancentercouncil.org
**Website:** http://www.haitiancentercouncil.org/programs.htm
Henry Frank, Exec. Dir.
**Fnded:** 1983. **Mem:** 70. **Reg. Groups:** 8. **State Groups:** 7. **Local Groups:** 6. **Desc:** Community centers; professional groups of doctors, journalists, lawyers, nurses, social workers, and civil rights and media representatives. Purpose is to educate the public concerning what the coalition feels is the discriminatory classification of Haitians as an ethnonational group that runs a high risk of contracting AIDS. Seeks to heighten AIDS awareness within the Haitian community. Offers social services and placement for persons with AIDS; provides counseling to their families. Sponsors conferences and seminars at churches and universities. Compiles statistics; maintains speakers' bureau.

### ★ 11777 ★ Herpes Resource Center - American Social Health Association (HRC)
PO Box 13827
Research Triangle Park, NC 27709
**Phone:** (919)361-8488     **Fax:** (919)361-8425
**Email:** phidra@ashastd.org
**Website:** http://www.ashastd.org/hrc
**Fnded:** 1979. **Local Groups:** 98. **Desc:** Individuals with recurrent genital herpes infections; individuals interested in the dissemination of information about genital herpes. (Herpes is a sexually transmitted disease which is as yet incurable.) Works to give emotional support to individuals, and to provide current information about herpes. Maintains the National Herpes Hotline. Offers referrals to local support groups (HELP) throughout the U.S. and Canada for people living with herpes; HELP groups provide a safe, confidential environment in which to obtain accurate information about HSV and share experiences with other people concerned about herpes. Compiles statistics. **Pub:** *The Helper*, quarterly. Journal. *Price:* $25/yr. • *Herpes: Questions & Answers.* Pamphlet. *Price:* Free. • *Managing Herpes: How to Live and Love with a Chronic STD.* Book. *Price:* $24.95. • *Telling Your Partner About Herpes.* Pamphlet. • *Understanding Herpes.* Booklet. *Price:* $6. • *When Your Partner Has Herpes.* Pamphlet.

### ★ 11778 ★ Herpes Viruses Association
41 North Rd.
London N7 9DP, United Kingdom
**Website:** http://www.herpes.org.uk
**Fnded:** 1985. **Mem:** 1,300. **Local Groups:** 7. **Lang(s):** English, French, Spanish. **Desc:** Provides accurate information on herpes simplex virus (to counteract the "herpes hype"), to the media, health professionals and the public. **Pub:** *Sphere*, quarterly. Journal.

### ★ 11779 ★ HIV/AIDS Program
c/o United States Conference of Mayors
1620 Eye St. NW
Washington, DC 20006
**Phone:** (202)293-7330     **Fax:** (202)293-2352
**Email:** info@usmayors.org
**Website:** http://www.usmayors.org
Richard C. Johnson, Contact
**Fnded:** 1983. **Desc:** AIDS prevention program of the United States Conference of Mayors. Acts as a forum for information exchange among members; provides policy information to the media. Operates speakers' bureau and conducts educational programs. **Pub:** *AIDS Information Exchange*, bimonthly. Newsletter. • *Local AIDS Policy.* • *Local AIDS Services: A National Directory*, periodic. Directory.

## ★ 11780 ★ HIV/AIDS Treatment Information Service (ATIS)

PO Box 6303
Rockville, MD 20849-6303
**Phone:** (301)519-0459     **Free:** 800-448-0440
**Fax:** (301)519-6616
**Email:** atis@hivatis.org
**Website:** http://hivatis.org/
**Desc:** Provides bilingual health information regarding HIV/AIDS treatment options.

## ★ 11781 ★ Hong Kong Society for Infectious Diseases

c/o Dept. of Pediatrics
Princess Margaret Hospital
Lai Chi Kok
Hong Kong, People's Republic of China
**Phone:** 852 29903402     **Fax:** 852 29903481
**Email:** ccwleung@netvigator.com
**Website:** http://www.fmshk.com.hk/hksid/home.htm
**Fnded:** 1995. **Mem:** 90. **Lang(s):** Chinese, English. **Desc:** Health care professionals, researchers, scientists, medical practitioners and other persons who are interested in infectious diseases. The objectives are to promote the study of infectious diseases. Conducts public education programs and continuing professional development courses; sponsors research projects. **Pub:** *Bulletin of the Hong Kong Society for Infectious Diseases*, quarterly. Bulletin. Includes Scientific articles and calendar of local and international meetings on infectious diseases. • *Bulletin of the Hong Kong Society for Infectious Diseases*, quarterly. Newsletter.

## ★ 11782 ★ HPV Support Program - American Social Health Association

PO Box 13827
Research Triangle Park, NC 27709
**Phone:** (919)361-8400     **Fax:** (919)361-8425
**Email:** bonrei@ashastd.org
**Website:** http://www.ashastd.org
**Fnded:** 1991. **Local Groups:** 15. **Desc:** Disseminates information and educational materials about human papillomavirus (HPV). Offers assistance to local support groups and/or people living with HPV. **Pub:** *HPV News*, quarterly. Journal. Covers medical and psychosocial information about HPV and genital warts. *Price:* $25/yr. • *HPV Questions and Answers*. Pamphlet.

## Ibero-Latin American College of Dermatology (ILACD)

## (Colegio Ibero-Latino-Americano de Dermatologia — CILAD)

*See:* Entry 6822

## ★ 11783 ★ Immunization Action Coalition (IAC)

1573 Selby Ave., Ste. 234
Saint Paul, MN 55104
**Phone:** (651)647-9009     **Fax:** (651)647-9131
**Email:** admin@immunize.org
**Website:** http://www.immunize.org
Deborah L. Wexler, MD, Exec. Dir.
**Fnded:** 1990. **Mem:** 6,000. **Desc:** Works to boost immunization rates. Promotes awareness of and responsibility for immunization of all people against all vaccine-preventable diseases. Conducts educational and outreach programs; develops print and audiovisual educational materials. **Pub:** *IAC Express*. Newsletter. • *Needle Tips and the Hepatitis B Coalition News*, semiannual. Newsletter. Discuss all vaccine-preventable diseases and hepatitis B. *Price:* Free. • *Vaccinate Adults!*, semiannual. Newsletter. *Price:* Free.

## Infection Control Nurses' Association

*See:* Entry 15718

## ★ 11784 ★ Infectious Diseases Society of Southern Africa (IDSSA) (Aansteeklike Siektesvereniging van Suider Afrika — ASVSA)

Department of Medical Microbiology
SAIMR
Johannesburg, Republic of South Africa
**Phone:** 27 11 4899183     **Fax:** 27 11 4899184
**Email:** lucilleb@mail.saimr.wits.ac.za
**Website:** http://home.global.co.za/~tropids/id-news.html
**Fnded:** 1983. **Mem:** 150. **Lang(s):** English. **Desc:** Health care professionals including doctors, medical researchers and technologists, and trade representatives in 4 countries. Stimulates interest among doctors in infectious disease; seeks to alleviate the current shortage of infectious disease specialists in southern Africa. Compiles statistics. **Pub:** *Infectious Diseases Update*, 3/month. • *Southern African Journal of Epidemiology and Infection*, quarterly.

## ★ 11785 ★ Infoshare International (II)

584 Castro St., Ste. 671
San Francisco, CA 94114
**Phone:** (415)437-1873     **Fax:** (415)843-4066
**Email:** infoshare1@aol.com
**Website:** http://www.spiral.com/infoshare/welcome.html
Julie Stachowiak, Exec. Dir.
**Fnded:** 1993. **Desc:** AIDS organizations in Russia and the United States. Promotes increased public awareness of AIDS and HIV and their prevention and treatment. Serves as a clearinghouse on AIDS and HIV; provides clothing, food, and support services to people with HIV and their families; makes available technical and administrative assistance to grass roots AIDS organizations; conducts educational programs.

## ★ 11786 ★ Interagency Coalition on AIDS and Development

1 Nicholas St., Ste. 726
Ottawa, ON, Canada K2P 1B7
**Phone:** (613)233-7440     **Fax:** (613)233-8361
**Email:** info@icad-cisd.com
**Website:** http://www.icad-cisd.com
**Fnded:** 1990. **Mem:** 117. **Lang(s):** French. **Desc:** Seeks to lessen the impact of HIV/AIDS in resource-poor communities and countries. We are a coalition of Canadian international development organizations, AIDS service organizations and other interested organizations and individuals. **Pub:** *ICAD Member News*, quarterly. Newsletter. Contains articles, Internet sites, and upcoming events.

## ★ 11787 ★ International AIDS Society (IAS)

PO Box 4249
Folkungagatan 49
SE-102 65 Stockholm, Sweden
**Phone:** 46 8 55697050     **Fax:** 46 8 55697059
**Email:** secretariat@ias.se
**Website:** http://www.ias.se/
**Fnded:** 1988. **Mem:** 5,700. **Desc:** Promotes the study of AIDS internationally. **Pub:** *IAS Membership Directory*. Newsletter. • *IAS Newsletter*, 3/year.

## ★ 11788 ★ International AIDS Vaccine Initiative (IAVI)

110 William St.
New York, NY 10038-3901
**Phone:** (212)847-1111     **Fax:** (212)847-1112
**Email:** info@iavi.org
**Website:** http://www.iavi.org
**Fnded:** 1996. **Desc:** Works to speed the development and distribution of preventative AIDS vaccines.

## ★ 11789 ★ International Association of Physicians in AIDS Care (IAPAC)

33 N LA Salle St. Ste. 1700
Chicago, IL 60602-2601
**Phone:** (312)795-4930     **Fax:** (312)795-4938
**Email:** iapac@iapac.org
**Website:** http://www.iapac.org
Gordon Nary, Pres.
**Fnded:** 1995. **Mem:** 7,500. **Desc:** Provides educational programs to caregivers, physicians and patients. Promotes public policy reform and research. **Pub:** *Journal of the International Association of Physicians In AIDS Care*, monthly. Journal. Clinical and Social Articles-peer reviewed. *Price:* $60/year. • Also publishes Themis–Public policy and AIDS law.

## ★ 11790 ★ International Christian Leprosy Mission (ICLM)

PO Box 596
Forest Grove, OR 97116
**Phone:** (503)285-9098     **Fax:** (503)285-6535
**Email:** HealingHands8414@aol.com
Dr. Daniel Pulliam, Pres.
**Fnded:** 1943. **Mem:** 12. **Reg. Groups:** 3. **Desc:** Carries on evangelical missionary work and assists in physical treatment of people with leprosy and their children. **Pub:** *Global Missions*, quarterly. Newsletter. *Price:* Free. • *KLM Healing Hands*, monthly. Newsletter. *Price:* Free.

## ★ 11791 ★ International Federation of Anti-Leprosy Associations (ILEP) (Federation Internationale des Associations Contre la Lepre — ILEP)

234 Blythe Rd.
London W14 0HJ, United Kingdom
**Phone:** 44 20 76026925     **Fax:** 44 20 73711621
**Email:** ilep@ilep.org.uk
**Website:** http://www.ilep.org.uk
**Fnded:** 1966. **Mem:** 17. **Lang(s):** English, French, German. **Desc:** International federation of autonomous non-governmental anti-leprosy organizations, most of which generate their income by raising funds from private donors to support more than a thousand projects in 97 countries. Members support medical, scientific, social, and humanitarian activities throughout the world to cure and rehabilitate people affected by leprosy and to prevent and eventually eradicate the disease. **Pub:** *ILEP Connection*, quarterly. Newsletter.

## ★ 11792 ★ International Leprosy Association (Societe Internationale Contre la Lepre)

Royal Tropical Institute
135 Wibautstraat
NL-1097 DN Amsterdam, Netherlands
**Phone:** 31 20 6939297     **Fax:** 31 20 6680823
**Lang(s):** Dutch, English. **Desc:** Health care professionals and medical researchers. Seeks to lessen the incidence of leprosy worldwide; promotes development of more effective leprosy treatments. Serves as a clearinghouse on leprosy and its prevention, diagnosis, and treatment. Sponsors research; conducts educational programs.

## International Organization Against Trachoma (IOAT) (Organisation Internationale pour la Lutte Contre le Trachome)

*See:* Entry 20993

## ★ 11793 ★ International Polio Network (IPN)

4207 Lindell Blvd., No. 110
Saint Louis, MO 63108
**Phone:** (314)534-0475     **Fax:** (314)534-5070
**Email:** gini_intl@msn.com
**Website:** http://www.post-polio.org
Joan L. Headley, Dir.
**Fnded:** 1985. **Mem:** 6,500. **Desc:** Individuals who have had polio; rehabilitation health professionals. Promotes networking and the exchange of information among the post-polio community; encourages research into the long-term effects of polio. **Pub:** *Hand-*

book on the Late Effects of Poliomyelitis for Physicians and Survivors (Revised Edition). Handbook. *Price:* $12. • *Polio Network News*, quarterly. Newsletter. *Price:* $22. • *Post-Polio Directory*, annual. Directory. Contains directory of clinics, health professionals, and support groups. *Price:* $8. • *Rehabilitation Gazette, Int'l Ventilator Users Network (IVUN) News*.

★ 11794 ★ **International Scientific Council for Trypansomiasis Research and Control (Conseil Scientifique International de Recherches sur les Trypanosomiases et leur Controle)**
Secretariat OAU/STRC
Ports Authority Bldg.
26/28 Marina
Private Mail Bag 2359
Lagos, Lagos, Nigeria
**Phone:** 234 1 2633430          **Fax:** 234 1 2636093
**Lang(s):** English. **Desc:** Medical and public health professionals with an interest in tryposomiasis and related disorders. (Tryposomiasis, also known as sleeping sickness, is one of a group of diseases caused by the parasitic family of paramecia, trypanosomatidae.) Seeks to advance the prevention, diagnosis, and treatment of tryposomiasis and related disorders. Serves as a clearinghouse on trypanosomatidae and the diseases they cause; facilitates exchange among experts on tryposomiasis and related disorders; conducts research and educational programs.

**International Society of Neurovirology**
*See:* Entry 14039

★ 11795 ★ **International Union Against Sexually Transmitted Infections, Regional Office for North America**
c/o Jonathon Zenilman
Johns Hopkins Hospital - Division of ID
1159 Ross Research Bldg.
720 Rutland Ave.
Baltimore, MD 21205
**Phone:** (410)955-7635          **Fax:** (410)614-9775
**Email:** jzenil@jhmi.edu
**Website:** http://www.iusti.org
Julius Schachter, Pres.
**Fnded:** 1923. **Desc:** U.S. office of the International Union Against Sexually Transmitted Diseases. Governmental and nongovernmental agencies and individuals working in the field of venereal disease control. Encourages campaigns, both medical and social, against venereal diseases and treponematoses. **Pub:** Proceedings, biennial. **Frmly:** (1998) International Union Against the Veneral Diseases and the Treponematoses, Regional Office for North America.

★ 11796 ★ **International Union Against Sexually Transmitted Infections - United Kingdom (IUSTI)**
c/o Dr. James Bingham
Department of Genito-Urinary Medicine
Thomas Guy House, 2nd floor
St. Thomas' St.
London 5000, United Kingdom
**Phone:** 44 171 9555000          **Fax:** 44 171 4036459
**Email:** james.bingham@gstt.stjames.nhs.uk
**Website:** http://www.iusti.org
**Fnded:** 1923. **Lang(s):** English, French, Spanish. **Desc:** Promotes international cooperation in the control of sexually transmitted diseases, including HIV infection, with an emphasis on the medical, social, and epidemiological aspects.

**International Union against Sexually Transmitted Infections - Australia**
*See:* Entry 18901

★ 11797 ★ **Japanese Association for Infectious Diseases**
Sankei 8 Bldg., 6F
1-8-7 Ebisu
Shibuya-ku
Tokyo 150-0013, Japan
**Email:** info@kansensho.or.jp
**Desc:** Healthcare professionals, researchers, and scientists working to advance the study and treatment of infectious diseases. **Pub:** Journal, periodic.

★ 11798 ★ **Leonard Wood Memorial (American Leprosy Foundation) (LWM)**
11600 Nebel St., Ste. 210
Rockville, MD 20852
**Phone:** (301)984-1336          **Fax:** (301)770-0580
**Email:** lwm-alf@erols.com
**Website:** http://www.ilep.org.uk/ilep_member_lwm.htm
Douglas S. Walsh, MD, Acting Scientific Dir.
**Fnded:** 1928. **Desc:** Health and research foundation concerned with microbiological research of Hansen's Disease (leprosy), and other related diseases. Conducts research programs in the U.S. and the Philippines. Supports clinical and basic laboratory research and epidemiological surveys. Sponsors exchange programs. Conducts collaborative studies with the Philippine Leprosy Mission, Culion Foundation, Colorado State University, Rockefeller University, the Delta Primate Center, American Leprosy Missions, International Sasakawa Memorial Health Foundation, Damien-Dutton Society, World Health Organization, UCLA School of Medicine, Ethiopia, India, Korea. **Pub:** Annual Report, annual. *Price:* Free. **AKA:** American Leprosy Foundation. **Frmly:** (1978) Leonard Wood Memorial for the Eradication of Leprosy.

★ 11799 ★ **LEPRA - England**
Fairfax House
Causton Rd.
Colchester CO1 1PU, United Kingdom
**Phone:** 44 1206 562286          **Fax:** 44 1206 762151
**Email:** lepra@lepra.org.uk
**Website:** http://www.lepra.org.uk
**Fnded:** 1924. **Mem:** 50. **Local Groups:** 2. **Lang(s):** English, French, Portuguese, Spanish. **Desc:** Objective is to eradicate leprosy throughout the world. Operates training programs for medical personnel. Supports research for the development of leprosy drugs and vaccines, and research projects of the World Health Organization. Concentrates efforts in Africa, Asia, and Brazil. Maintains special children's, eye, and hand remobilization funds. Investigates potential for treatment of leprosy in conjunction with that of other diseases. Sponsors competitions; bestows awards. **Pub:** *Leprosy Review*, quarterly. Journal.

**Lyme Disease Foundation (LDF)**
*See:* Entry 13616

★ 11800 ★ **Malawi Against Physical Disabilities (MAP)**
PO Box 256
Blantyre, Malawi
**Phone:** 265 674634          **Fax:** 265 674604
**Email:** map@malawi.net
**Website:** http://www.lyme.org
**Fnded:** 1980. **Mem:** 130. **Local Groups:** 300. **Lang(s):** English. **Desc:** Rehabilitation of people with physical disabilities caused by polio, burns, tuberculous of the spine, amputations, congenital deformities, cerebral palsy, strokes etc. **Pub:** *Annual Report*, annual. • *Financial Report.* • *MAP Feedback.* • *MAP Newsletter.* Newsletter. • Journal, semiannual.

★ 11801 ★ **Medical Mycological Society of the Americas (MMSA)**
c/o Dr. James Harris
2501 Timberline Dr.
Austin, TX 78746
**Phone:** (512)458-7566          **Fax:** (512)458-7697
**Email:** jim.harris@tdh.state.tx.us
Dr. James L. Harris, Sec. Treas.
**Fnded:** 1966. **Mem:** 300. **Desc:** Medical professionals interested in fungi and fungal diseases. Seeks to exchange professional information; promotes continuing education in medical mycology in association with American Society for Microbiology. **Pub:** Bulletin, quarterly. • Directory, periodic.

★ 11802 ★ **Mobilization Against AIDS (MAA)**
584 Castro St., No. 416
San Francisco, CA 94114-1465
**Phone:** (415)863-4676          **Fax:** (415)863-4740
Phillip Machingura, Prog. Asst.
**Fnded:** 1984. **Mem:** 1,000. **Local Groups:** 1. **Desc:** Individuals supporting increased government expenditure on AIDS research, treatment, and social services. Purposes are to: lobby Congress, the Food and Drug Administration, and the National Institutes of Health to provide support and funding to AIDS organizations; mobilize people into public expressions of support for persons with AIDS; oppose civil rights attacks on persons with AIDS. Organizes annual International AIDS candlelight vigil, marches, and the Just Sign IT postcard campaign. Provides speakers on the civil rights ramifications of the AIDS crisis. **Pub:** *Action Alert*, quarterly. Newsletter. *Price:* Included in membership. • *International AIDS Candlelight Memorial and Mobilization.* Booklet. **Frmly:** (1987) Mobilization Against AIDS; (1992) National Mobilization Against AIDS.

★ 11803 ★ **Mothers' Voices**
165 W 46th St., Ste. 701
New York, NY 10036
**Phone:** (212)730-2777          **Fax:** (212)730-4378
**Email:** mvoices@mvoices.org
**Website:** http://www.mvoices.org
Trish Maylan Turruella, Exec. Dir.
**Fnded:** 1992. **Reg. Groups:** 5. **Desc:** Only national, grassroots, non-profit organizations mobilizing mothers as AIDS and sexual health educators and advocates. Provides resources for mothers to educate their children regarding sexuality and drug use, and how better understanding can help prevent HIV infection. **Pub:** *Speaking from the Heart*, quarterly. Newsletter.

★ 11804 ★ **Names Project Foundation (NPF)**
PO Box 5552
Atlanta, GA 31107
**Phone:** (404)688-5500          **Fax:** (404)688-5552
**Email:** bac@aidsquilt.net
**Website:** http://www.aidsquilt.org
Andy Ilves, Exec. Dir.
**Fnded:** 1987. **Nat'l Groups:** 38. **Local Groups:** 53. **Desc:** Promotes creation of AIDS Memorial Quilt as an "appropriate, compassionate response" to the AIDS epidemic. Goals of the project are to provide a creative means of remembrance and healing; to illustrate the enormity of the AIDS epidemic; to increase public awareness of AIDS; to assist with HIV prevention education; and to raise funds for community-based AIDS service organizations. The 25 acre quilt currently contains 43,000 panels from each of the 50 states and 39 foreign countries bearing the names of persons who have died as a result of AIDS. Among materials sewn into the panels are stuffed animals, merit badges, records, feather boas, and a baseball jersey. jersey. jersey. **Pub:** *A Promise To Remember*. Book. • *Always Remember*. Book. • *"On Display"*, quarterly. Newsletter. *Price:* Donation. • *The Quilt: Stories From the NAMES Project*. Book. • Also publishes fact sheets, flyers, and press releases. **Frmly:** Names Project.

★ 11805 ★ **National AIDS Committee - Germany (Nationaler AIDS-Beirat — NAB)**
Federal Ministry for Health
D-53108 Bonn, Germany

**Phone:** 49 1888 4413210  **Fax:** 49 1888 4414932 **Email:** miesala@bmg.bund.de
**Fnded:** 1987. **Mem:** 27. **Lang(s):** German. Does not correspond in English. **Desc:** Organizations and individual experts interested in preventing the spread of HIV/AIDS. Counsels German government on AIDS related matters. **Pub:** *Voten des Nationalen AIDS-Beirates - 1987-1997.* Brochure.

★ **11806** ★ **National AIDS Committee - Mexico (CONASIDA)**
**(Centro Nacional para la Prevencion y Control del VIH/SIDA)**
Calz. de Tlalfan 4585, 20. piso
Col. Toriello Guerra
14050 Mexico City, DF, Mexico
**Phone:** 52 5 55284848          **Fax:** 52 5 5284220
**Email:** conasida@prodigy.net.mx
**Website:** http://www.ssa.gob.mx/conasida
**Fnded:** 1986. **Mem:** 143. **State Groups:** 31. **Lang(s):** English, Spanish. **Desc:** Individual interested in preventing the spread of HIV/AIDS in Mexico. Offers public education programs on the transmission and effects of the disease. Campaigns to raise awareness and fund research. **Pub:** *Guia de Atencion Domiciliaria,* periodic. Booklet. Information for patients, consultants and hospitals on HIV/AIDS. • *Guia de Atencion Psicologica.* • *Guia para la Atencion Medica de Pacientes con Infeccion por VIH/SIDA en Consulta Externa y Hospitales.* • *Guias para Enfermeras.*

★ **11807** ★ **National AIDS Committee - Seychelles**
Ministry of Health
PO Box 52
Victoria, Seychelles
**Phone:** 248 388000          **Fax:** 248 224792
**Fnded:** 1987. **Mem:** 7. **Desc:** Promotes the study of AIDS.

★ **11808** ★ **National AIDS Fund**
1030 15th St. NW, Ste. 860
Washington, DC 20005-2208
**Phone:** (202)408-4848          **Fax:** (202)408-1818
**Email:** info@aidsfund.org
**Website:** http://www.aidsfund.org
Mary Wilson-Byrom, CEO
**Fnded:** 1988. **Mem:** 200. **State Groups:** 27. **Desc:** Promotes leadership and generates resources for effective community responses to HIV/AIDS. **Pub:** *News from the National AIDS Fund,* quarterly. Newsletter. • AIDS-in the workplace publications list available. **Frmly:** (1996) Rational Community AIDS Partnership.

★ **11809** ★ **National AIDS Trust**
New City Cloisters
188/196 Old St.
London EC1V 9FR, United Kingdom
**Phone:** 44 207 8146767     **Fax:** 44 207 2160111
**Email:** info@nat.org.uk
**Website:** http://www.nat.org.uk
**Fnded:** 1987. **Nat'l Groups:** 2. **Lang(s):** English. **Desc:** Individuals and organizations in the United Kingdom interested in preventing the spread of HIV/AIDS. Conducts educational programs, fundraising, policy work, employers initiatives, research, lobbying, and parliamentary liaison. **Pub:** *Impact,* 10/year. Magazine. Research reports.

★ **11810** ★ **National Alliance of State and Territorial AIDS Directors**
444 N Capitol St. NW, Ste. 339
Washington, DC 20001
**Phone:** (202)434-8090          **Fax:** (202)434-8092
**Email:** jscofield@nastad.org
**Website:** http://www.nastad.org
Julie M. Scofield, Exec. Dir.
**Fnded:** 1992. **Mem:** 59. **State Groups:** 59. **Desc:** State and territorial directors of public state health HIV/

AIDS programs and services. Dedicated to reducing the incidence of HIV infection in the U.S. and territories, providing comprehensive, compassionate, and quality care to all persons living with HIV/AIDS, and the development of responsible and compassionate public policies. **Pub:** *HIV Prevention Bulletin,* monthly. Newsletter.

★ **11811** ★ **National Association of People With AIDS (NAPWA)**
1413 K St. NW
Washington, DC 20005-3442
**Phone:** (202)898-0414          **Fax:** (202)898-0435
**Email:** napwa@napwa.org
**Website:** http://www.napwa.org
Terje Anderson, Exec. Dir.
**Fnded:** 1987. **Desc:** Serves as the collective voice and national consumer health education and advocacy resource for all people living with HIV disease in the United States, and those who care for us NAPWA advocates on behalf of all people living with HIV and AIDS in order to end the epidemic and the human suffering caused by HIV/AIDS. **Pub:** *Active Voice,* quarterly. Provides information about healthcare and advocacy issues. *Price:* Free. • *An Ounce of Prevention.* Informs family members and caregivers about the prevention of further HIV infection. • *Facts About AIDS.* Provides an introduction of HIV and related issues. • *Living with HIV.* Provides information on resources for treatment and offers prevention against further infection. • *Medical Alert,* quarterly. Identifies new approaches to treating HIV/AIDS, explains what new drugs are being tested and how they work, and provides treatment strategies. *Price:* Free.

★ **11812** ★ **National Catholic AIDS Network (NCAN)**
PO Box 960
Occidental, CA 95465
**Phone:** (707)874-3031          **Fax:** (707)874-1433
**Email:** info@ncan.org
**Website:** http://www.ncan.org
Fr. Rodney DeMartini, Exec. Dir.
**Fnded:** 1989. **Mem:** 4,500. **Reg. Groups:** 5. **Desc:** Provides support and exchange of information among Roman Catholic HIV/AIDS service workers and pastoral ministers. Disseminates educational materials on HIV/AIDS. **Pub:** *Connections,* quarterly. Newsletter. *Price:* Membership benefit.

★ **11813** ★ **National Chronic Fatigue Syndrome and Fibromyalgia Association (NCFSFA)**
PO Box 18426
Kansas City, MO 64133
**Phone:** (816)313-2000          **Fax:** (816)524-6782
**Email:** information@ncfsfa.org
**Website:** http://www.ncfsfa.org
Orvalene Prewitt, Pres.
**Fnded:** 1985. **Mem:** 2,000. **Reg. Groups:** 2. **State Groups:** 14. **Local Groups:** 400. **Desc:** Individuals suffering from chronic fatigue syndrome and Fibromyalgia health care professionals. Chronic fatigue syndrome, also known as Chronic Epstein-Barr Virus syndrome, is characterized by persistent, recurring feelings of general weakness; other symptoms include sore throat, unexplained muscle pain, new headaches, devastating fatigue, impaired memory or concentration, tender lymph nodes, unrefreshing sleep and post-exertion malaise. Fibromyalgia is characterized as pain, generally felt all over, and can be compounded by fatigue, sleep disturbances, changes in mood, headaches and gastro-intestinal problems. Sponsors educational programs. Maintains speakers' bureau. **Pub:** *A Guide for Physicians When Considering a Diagnosis of Chronic Fatigue Syndrom in Children.* Brochure. • *A School's Guide for Students with CFS.* • *CFS: Addressing the Realities of a Chronic Illness.* Video. Includes educational information. • *CFS and School Success.* Brochure. • *CFS in the Workplace.* Brochure. • *CFS: Thief of Vitality.* Brochure. • *Chronic Fatigue Syndrome.* Bibliography. • *Coping Skills.* Brochure. • *Heart of America News,* quarterly. News-

letter. *Price:* Free for members. • *How to be a Phone Contact Packet.* • *How to Start a Support Group Packet.* • *Neuro-Psychological Rehabilitation Techniques.* Brochure. • *Patient Information Packet.* • *Physician Information Packet.* • *Social Security Disability Benefits.* Brochure. • *Understanding the Emotions Surrounding CFS.* Brochure. **Frmly:** (1985) National Chronic Epstein-Barr Virus Association; (1993) National Chronic Fatigue Syndrome Association.

★ **11814** ★ **National Episcopal AIDS Coalition (NEAC)**
520 Clinton Ave.
Brooklyn, NY 11238
**Phone:** (718)857-9445          **Free:** 800-588-6628
**Fax:** (718)638-3039
**Email:** neac@neac.org
**Website:** http://www.neac.org
Richard F. Brewer, Admin.
**Fnded:** 1988. **Mem:** 1,400. **Desc:** Works to educate all Episcopalians about HIV/AIDS issues. Advocates for the physical, emotional and spiritual health of and the pastoral care for HIV/AIDS infected people. Develops support networks and communities. **Pub:** *Neaction,* quarterly. Newsletter.

★ **11815** ★ **National Foundation for Infectious Diseases (NFID)**
4733 Bethesda Ave., Ste. 750
Bethesda, MD 20814
**Phone:** (301)656-0003          **Fax:** (301)907-0878
**Email:** info@nfid.org
**Website:** http://www.nfid.org
Susan J. Rehm, MD, Pres.
**Fnded:** 1973. **Desc:** Supports research into the causes and cures of infectious diseases; assists in the education of both professionals and the public in infectious diseases. Conducts programs in prevention of infectious diseases. **Pub:** *Coccidiomycosis and Host-Fungus Interplay.* Proceedings. • *Double Helix,* quarterly. Newsletter. Reports on public welfare and support of research, education, and prevention of infectious disease. Monitors legislation. *Price:* Free. • *National Foundation for Infectious Diseases–Annual Report.* Annual Report. • *Recognition and Management of Nursing Home Infections.*

★ **11816** ★ **National Minority AIDS Council (NMAC)**
1931 13th St. NW
Washington, DC 20009-4432
**Phone:** (202)483-6622          **Free:** 800-544-0586
**Fax:** (202)483-1135
**Email:** info@nmac.org
**Website:** http://www.nmac.org
Paul A. Kawata, Exec. Dir.
**Fnded:** 1986. **Mem:** 480. **Reg. Groups:** 2. **State Groups:** 20. **Local Groups:** 160. **Desc:** Public health departments and AIDS service organizations. Serves as a clearinghouse of information on AIDS as it affects minority communities in the U.S. Facilitates discussion among national minority organizations about AIDS. Maintains Project Health, Education, and AIDS Leadership, which provides computer usage, strategic planning, financial management, and volunteer program development assistance to AIDS service organizations, and Project Volunteer Information, Technical Assistance, and Leadership, which provides technical assistance in volunteer program development and maintenance. Conducts training conferences. Offers educational and research programs; compiles statistics. Maintains speakers' bureau. **Pub:** *Computer Technical Assistance Manual.* • *Leadership Reprint Series,* quarterly. Includes information on strategies for addressing HIV/AIDS and scientific updates. • *Legislative Update,* bimonthly. • *NMAC HEALer,* bimonthly. Includes updates on projects, community needs, and statistics. • *NMAC Update,* bimonthly. Newsletter. Includes association information and coverage of HIV/AIDS issues. • *Technical Assistance Manual for Volunteer Program Development.* • *Technical Assistance Newsletter,* bimonthly. Newsletter.

**★ 11817 ★ National Native American AIDS Prevention Center**
436-14th St., Ste. 1020
Oakland, CA 94612
**Phone:** (510)444-2051 **Fax:** (510)444-1593
**Email:** information@nnaapc.org
**Website:** http://www.nnaapc.org
Ron Rowell, Exec. Dir.

**Fnded:** 1987. **Desc:** Network of concerned Native people. Works to stop the spread of HIV and related diseases, including sexually transmitted disease and tuberculosis, among American Indians, Alaska Natives, and Native Hawaiians by improving their health status through empowerment and self determination. Serves as a resource to Native communities and to support community efforts by providing education and information services, thereby ehancing the physical, spiritual, and economic health of Native people. Sponsors educational programs. Maintains speakers' bureau. Compiles statistics. **Pub:** *Season*, annual. Journal. **Frmly:** (1998) National Indian AIDS Hotline.

**★ 11818 ★ National Tuberculosis Controllers Association**
2951 Flowers Rd. S, Ste. 102
Atlanta, GA 30341-4000
**Phone:** (770)455-0801 **Free:** 888-455-0801
**Fax:** (770)455-4221
**Email:** ntca@ntca-tb.org
**Website:** http://www.ntca-tb.org
Walter Q. Page, Exec. Dir.

**Fnded:** 1995. **Mem:** 459. **Desc:** Seeks to provide a collective voice for TB controllers to advance and advocate for tuberculosis control and elimination activities in the U.S. Advocates for policies and laws to advance tuberculosis control and elimination at the sate, local, and territorial levels. **Pub:** *The Red Snapper Review*, quarterly. Newsletter. Contains organizational and scientific news.

**★ 11819 ★ Organization for Coordination and Cooperation in the Struggle Against Endemic Diseases - Burkina Faso (OCCSED)**
**(Organisation de Coordination et de Cooperation pour la Lutte Contre les Grandes Endemies — OCCGE)**
01 Boite Postale 153
Bobo-Dioulasso 01, Burkina Faso
**Phone:** 226 970101 **Fax:** 226 970099
**Email:** occgoas@fasonet.bf

**Fnded:** 1960. **Mem:** 7. **Lang(s):** English, French. **Desc:** Health care professionals, researchers, and services. Seeks to eradicate selected contagious diseases. Conducts medical research; delivers medical services to populations prone to endemic diseases.

**Pediatric AIDS Foundation**
*See:* Entry 5741

**★ 11820 ★ Philippine National AIDS Council**
3F, Bldg. 12, Department of Health
Sta. Cruz
Manila, Philippines
**Phone:** 63 2 7430512
**Email:** naspcp@doh.gov.ph
**Website:** http://www.doh.gov.ph/aids/

**Fnded:** 1988. **Reg. Groups:** 16. **Lang(s):** English. **Desc:** Provides AIDS information and education; offers AIDS counseling training. Implements programs for the management and care of HIV-infected individuals and persons with AIDS. Conducts research; compiles statistics. Maintains speakers' bureau; serves as a clearinghouse on AIDS and other sexually transmitted diseases; provides laboratory services. **Pub:** *Monthly Update*, quarterly. Newsletter. **Frmly:** (1998) National AIDS/STD Prevention and Control Program.

**★ 11821 ★ Polio Society (PS)**
4200 Wisconsin Ave. NW, PMB 106-273
Washington, DC 20016
**Phone:** (301)897-8180 **Fax:** (202)466-1911
Becky Evans, Contact

**Fnded:** 1984. **Mem:** 3,500. **Local Groups:** 3. **Desc:** Polio survivors and health care professionals interested in the long-term health of patients who have had the disease. Gathers and disseminates information on post-polio syndrome. (PPS is a condition in which polio survivors suffer unaccustomed fatigue, joint and muscle pain, weakening or loss of muscle function, and respiratory problems.) Acts as liaison between members and medical facilities; maintains outreach program and referral service; sponsors support groups. Advocates on issues of disability and benefits. **Pub:** *Options*, quarterly. Newsletter. • Brochures.Informational brochures. • Also publishes information packets. **Frmly:** Post-Polio League for Information and Outreach.

**★ 11822 ★ Positively Women**
347-349 City Rd.
London EC1V 1LR, United Kingdom
**Phone:** 44 171 7130444 **Fax:** 44 171 7131020

**Fnded:** 1987. **Lang(s):** English, French, Luganda, Swahili. **Desc:** Offers peer support and self-help services to women with HIV and/or AIDs and their children. Provides information; maintains a resource facility. **Pub:** *Positively Women Newsletter*, bimonthly. Newsletter.

**★ 11823 ★ Project Inform (PI)**
205 13th St., No. 2001
San Francisco, CA 94103
**Phone:** (415)558-8669 **Free:** 800-822-7422
**Fax:** (415)558-0684
**Email:** web@projectinform.org
**Website:** http://www.projectinform.org
Avi Rose, Exec. Dir.

**Fnded:** 1985. **Mem:** 70,000. **Desc:** Information clearinghouse and hot line providing updated information on drug treatments for persons with AIDS or the Human Immunodeficiency Virus. Also provides information on organizations through which the drug treatments can be obtained. Works to speed up research process and focus on promising new treatments. **Pub:** *PI Perspective*, quarterly. Journal. Contains treatment information and focuses on advocacy issues. *Price:* Free. • Also publishes information packet and fact sheets on treatments and standards of care.

**★ 11824 ★ Remedios AIDS Foundation**
1066 Remedios St.
Malate
Manila 1004, Philippines
**Phone:** 63 2 5240924 **Fax:** 63 2 5223431
**Email:** raf@phil.gn.apc.org

**Fnded:** 1991. **Mem:** 100. **Reg. Groups:** 4. **Lang(s):** English, Tagalog. **Desc:** Provides quality reproductive health information and services to targetted communities. Programs include counseling, resource center, Information Education Communicates materials, the Youth Zone, Clinica Remedios, support services, networking and advocacy. **Pub:** *Remedios Newsletter*, quarterly. Newsletter. • *Sourcebook on HIV/AIDS-STD Counseling*. Book.

**★ 11825 ★ Royal Society of Tropical Medicine and Hygiene (RSTMH)**
Manson House
26 Portland Pl.
London W1B 1EY, United Kingdom
**Phone:** 44 207 5802127 **Fax:** 44 207 4361389
**Email:** mail@rstmh.org
**Website:** http://www.rstmh.org/

**Fnded:** 1907. **Mem:** 3,000. **Lang(s):** English. **Desc:** Medical and veterinary practititioners, scientists, and interested others representing 88 countries. Promotes health and seeks to advance the study, control, and prevention of tropical diseases in humans and animals. Encourages information exchange and facilitates discussion. **Pub:** *Bulletin of Tropical Medicine & International Health.* • *Transactions of the Royal Society of Tropical Medicine and Hygiene*, bimonthly. Journal. • *Yearbook of the Royal Society of Tropical Medicine and Hygiene.*

**★ 11826 ★ San Francisco AIDS Foundation (SFAF)**
995 Market St. Ste. 200
San Francisco, CA 94103
**Phone:** (415)487-3000 **Free:** 800-367-AIDS
**Fax:** (415)487-3009
**Email:** feedback@staf.org
**Website:** http://www.sfaf.org
Pat Christen, Exec. Dir.

**Fnded:** 1982. **Desc:** Regional organization whose goals are to educate the public on the prevention of AIDS and to make various social service programs accessible to people with AIDS. Provides community forums; develops and distributes educational materials. Provides assistance to people with AIDS in obtaining emergency housing, social security and veterans' benefits, medical and insurance benefits, and legal referral services. Works with legislators, corporations, public health coalitions, activists, and the media to advance public health policy and improve media coverage. Maintains speakers' bureau. **Pub:** *Bulletin of Experimental Treatments for AIDS*, quarterly. Bulletin. Covers AIDS-related diseases, research, care, treatment, and clinical trials. *Price:* Free for individuals; Free for institutions. • Booklets. • Brochures. • Videos. • Also distributes AIDS educational materials. **Frmly:** AIDS/Kaposi's Sarcoma Research and Education Foundation.

**★ 11827 ★ Scientific Society of Mycology**
National Center of Infectious Diseases
26, Yanko Sakazov Blvd.
BG-1504 Sofia, Bulgaria
**Phone:** 359 2 465520 **Fax:** 359 2 655878

**Fnded:** 1992. **Mem:** 39. **Lang(s):** English. **Desc:** Fosters research in mycology.

**★ 11828 ★ Sequella Global Tuberculosis Foundation**
c/o Carol A. Nacy
9610 Medical Center Dr., Ste. 220
Rockville, MD 20850
**Phone:** (301)762-3100 **Fax:** (301)762-2122
**Email:** information@sequellafoundation.org
**Website:** http://www.sequellafoundation.org
Carol A. Nacy, PhD, Pres.

**Fnded:** 1977. **Desc:** Researchers. Established as a resource for the Tuberculosis Research Community to help identify and develop concepts and tools for controlling the global epidemic.

**★ 11829 ★ Sexually Transmitted Infections Prevention Committee (STIPC)**
37/39 rue D'Argens
Msida MSD 05, Malta
**Phone:** 356 322306 **Fax:** 356 319243
**Email:** lilian.a.debono@magnet.mt

**Fnded:** 1986. **Mem:** 5. **Lang(s):** English. **Desc:** Makes recommendations for national AIDS and other sexually transmitted diseases policy formulation; advises Director General of Health, Malta. **Frmly:** (1999) National Committee for AIDS Prevention and Control.

**★ 11830 ★ Society of Infectious Diseases Pharmacists (SIDP)**
1717 W 6th, Ste. 214
Austin, TX 78703
**Phone:** (512)708-0611 **Fax:** (512)708-0627
**Email:** sidp@aams-texas.com
**Website:** http://www.sidp.org/

**Desc:** Pharmacists with a primary interest and practice in infectious diseases pharmacotherapy, and who have spent at least two years performing pharmacotherpeutic research are active members; pharmacists and other individuals not meeting the requirements for active membership, but who share an interest in infectious diseases pharmacotherapy, are associate members. Seesk to advance the study and practice of infectious diseases pharmacotherapy, and to enhance the professional status of members. Serves as a forum for discussion and exchange of information among members. Encourages pharmacotherapeutic research. **Pub:** *News Update*, monthly. Newsletter. • *SIDP*, 3/year. Newsletter.

**Society for Prevention of Infertility (SPI)**
*See:* Entry 18377

### ★ 11831 ★ Southern Africa AIDS Information Dissemation Service

Morkel House
17 Beveridge Rd.
Avondale
Harare, Zimbabwe
**Phone:** 263 4 336193          **Fax:** 263 4 336195
**Email:** info@safaids.org.zw
**Website:** http://www.safaids.org.zw
**Fnded:** 1994. **Lang(s):** English. **Desc:** Social welfare and health care organizations. Promotes increased awareness of AIDS and HIV and their prevention; seeks to improve the quality of life of people with AIDS and their families. Serves as a clearinghouse on AIDS and HIV. **Frmly:** (2000) Southern Africa Federation for AIDS.

### ★ 11832 ★ Southern African Network of AIDS Service Organizations

PO Box 6690
Harare, Zimbabwe
**Phone:** 263 4 745748
**Email:** sanaso@mango.zw
**Fnded:** 1991. **Mem:** 900. **Nat'l Groups:** 145. **Reg. Groups:** 1. **State Groups:** 10. **Local Groups:** 44. **Lang(s):** English, Portuguese. **Desc:** Social service organizations working with NGO's and community based organizations working on HIV/AIDS in Southern Africa and with people living with HIV/AIDS in Southern Africa. Promotes increased access to information among people with AIDS; encourages coordination of members' activities. Serves as a clearinghouse on HIV and AIDS and their prevention; conducts advocacy lobbying programs to promote adequate resources and create supportive environments for an appropriate and effective response to HIV/AIDS. **Pub:** *SANASO Newsletter*, quarterly. Newsletter.

### ★ 11833 ★ Swaziland Network of AIDS Service Organizations

c/o TASC
PO Box 1279
Manzini, Swaziland
**Phone:** 268 5054790          **Fax:** 268 5054752
**Fnded:** 1989. **Lang(s):** English. **Desc:** Organizations providing service to people with AIDS. Seeks to improve the quality of life of people with AIDS; promotes advancement of AIDS services; works for the full integration of people with AIDS and HIV into society. Facilitates communication and cooperation among members; sponsors research and educational programs; provides support and services to people with AIDS. **Pub:** *AIDS Awareness*, annual. Newsletter. Booklets, pamphlets, and reports.

### ★ 11834 ★ Teens Teaching AIDS Prevention (TEENS TAP)

3030 Walnut
Kansas City, MO 64108
**Phone:** (816)561-8784          **Free:** 800-234-8336
**Fax:** (816)531-7199
Elizabeth Spaur, Youth Outreach Coor.
**Fnded:** 1987. **Mem:** 300. **Desc:** Sponsored by the Good Samaritan Project. Provides teenagers with information on AIDS through peer counseling. Also provides information to interested adults. Maintains

speakers' bureau for schools and youth groups. Provides companions for children and teens with AIDS and their families. Makes available training and technical guidance to groups interested in organizing teen peer education programs. **Pub:** Brochures. • Manuals.

### ★ 11835 ★ Treatment Action Group (TAG)

611 Broadway, Ste. 612
New York, NY 10012
**Phone:** (212)253-7922          **Fax:** (212)253-7923
**Email:** tag-nyc@msn.com
**Website:** http://www.treatmentactiongroup.org
Regina Gillis, Admin. Dir.
**Fnded:** 1992. **Mem:** 50. **Desc:** Individuals who are HIV positive and individuals interested in AIDS treatment research. Promotes AIDS research; advocates for research and treatment. Conducts educational programs. **Pub:** *Tagline*, monthly. Newsletter. Features AIDS research and policy. *Price:* $30/year. • Also publishes various reports on AIDS research and treatments.

### ★ 11836 ★ UNAIDS

20, avenue Appia
CH-1211 Geneva 27, Switzerland
**Phone:** 41 22 7913666          **Fax:** 41 22 7914187
**Email:** unaids@unaids.org
**Website:** http://www.unaids.org
**Fnded:** 1995. **Lang(s):** English, French, German, Italian. **Desc:** Health care personnel and other individuals and organizations interested in stopping the global AIDS epidemic. Seeks to reduce the suffering of people with HIV and AIDS; works to "counter the impact of the pandemic on individuals, communities, and societies." Conducts educational programs in areas including AIDS prevention and treatment; makes available health and social services to people with HIV and AIDS.

### ★ 11837 ★ Women Organized to Respond to Life-Threatening Diseases (WORLD)

414 13th St., 2nd Fl.
Oakland, CA 94612-2603
**Phone:** (510)986-0340          **Fax:** (510)986-0341
**Website:** http://www.womenhiv.org/
Deborah McSmith, Exec. Dir.
**Fnded:** 1991. **Mem:** 12,000. **Desc:** An empowerment organization by and for women infected or affected by the HIV virus. Offers support and information to women who have AIDS and HIV. Offers retreats and educational classes. Maintains speakers bureau. **Pub:** *WORLD*, monthly. Newsletter. Personal testimonies of infected women; medical and political information. Easy-to-understand women specific HIV/AIDS treatment. **AKA:** WORLD.

### ★ 11838 ★ World Association on Sarcoidosis and Other Granulomatous Disorders (WASOG)

149 Harley St.
London W1N 1HG, United Kingdom
**Phone:** 44 171 9354444
**Email:** rizzatog@tin.it
**Website:** http://pinali.unipd.it/sarcoid
**Fnded:** 1958. **Mem:** 300. **Lang(s):** English. **Desc:** Physicians in 40 countries. Promotes and sponsors research and clinical activities on sarcoidosis concerning damage to the brain, eyes, heart, lungs, and skin. (Sarcoidosis is characterized by inflammation of the lungs, eyes, skin, and other tissue and results in immunological upset; its cause is unknown.) Maintains speakers' bureau and hall of fame. **Pub:** *Sarcoidosis*, semiannual. • *Transactions of the World Congress on Sarcoidosis*, biennial. **Frmly:** (1987) International Committee of Sarcoidosis.

**World Association of Veterinary Microbiologists, Immunologists, and Specialists in Infectious Diseases (WAVMI)**
**(Association Mondiale des Veterinaires Microbiologistes, Immunologistes et Specialistes des Maladies Infectieuses — AMVMI)**
*See:* Entry 20665

### ★ 11839 ★ Zambia National AIDS Network

c/o FHT
Private Bag 243
Lusaka, Zambia
**Phone:** 260 1 222834          **Fax:** 260 1 222834
**Lang(s):** English. **Desc:** Individuals and organizations working with people with AIDS. Promotes increased public awareness of AIDS and HIV and their prevention; seeks to improve the quality of life of people with AIDS. Coordinates members' activities; serves as a clearinghouse on AIDS and HIV; sponsors research and educational programs.

### ★ 11840 ★ Zimbabwe AIDS Network

PO Box CY 3006
Causeway
Harare, Zimbabwe
**Phone:** 263 4 700924          **Fax:** 263 4 700330
**Email:** zansec@zol.co.zw
**Fnded:** 1991. **Mem:** 150. **Nat'l Groups:** 150. **Lang(s):** English. **Desc:** Individuals and organizations working with people with HIV and AIDS. Seeks to increase public awareness of AIDS and its prevention; works to improve the quality of life of people with HIV and their families. Serves as a clearinghouse on AIDS and HIV; provides support and services to people with AIDS. **Pub:** *The Web*, quarterly. Newsletter. Features national and regional news on HIV/AIDS.

## Research Centers

### ★ 11841 ★ Aaron Diamond AIDS Research Center

455 1st Ave., 7th Fl.
New York, NY 10016
**Phone:** (212)448-5000          **Fax:** (212)725-1126
**Website:** http://www.adarc.org
David D. Ho, MD, Dir.
**Activities/Fields:** Pathogenesis of HIV-1 in vivo, maternal-fetal transmission of HIV-1, antibody responses to HIV and vaccine development, mechanism of HIV entry into CD4+ and CD4- cells, anti-HIV therapeutics and viral resistance, search for the causative agent of HIV-negative cases of immunodeficiency, cellular immune responses to HIV-1 in the pathogenesis of AIDS, cellular immune responses to HIV-1 in vaccine development, development of the scid mouse model for HIV studies, receptors for human retroviruses (HIV and HTLV), assembly of HIV virion, function of accessory genes of HIV, interaction of HIV envelope with the cellular receptor, mechanism of viral entry, and mapping of the functional determinants of HIV envelope glycoprotein.

### ★ 11842 ★ African Medical and Research Foundation, U.S.A.

19 W 44th St., Ste. 710
New York, NY 10036
**Phone:** (212)768-2440          **Fax:** (212)768-4230
**Email:** amrefusa@amrefusa.org
**Website:** http://www.amref.org/usa.html
Dr. Jane Carter, Contact
**Activities/Fields:** The spread and prevention of AIDS, malaria, and hydatid disease. Also creates health care & training models used by developing countries worldwide.

**★ 11843 ★ AIDS Research Consortium of Atlanta, Inc.**
131 Ponce de Leon Ave. NE, Ste. 130
Atlanta, GA 30308-1962
**Phone:** (404)876-2317 **Fax:** (404)872-1701
**Email:** arca@aidsresearchatlanta.org
**Website:** http://www.aidsresearchatlanta.org
Melanie Thompson, MD, Prin. Investigator
**Activities/Fields:** HIV clinical trials and epidemiology.

**★ 11844 ★ American Academy of Tropical Medicine and Surgery**
16126 E Warren
PO Box 24224
Detroit, MI 48224-0224
**Phone:** (313)882-0641 **Fax:** (313)882-0979
Dr. Ben Allie, Chm.
**Activities/Fields:** Tropical diseases, including diarrhea and ankle edema, and evaluation of disease spectrum. **Pub:** *Journal of the American Academy of Tropical Medicine and Surgery.*

**Arizona Health Services Department**
**Public Health Services**
**Bureau of Epidemiology and Disease Control**
**Office of Infectious Disease Services Office**
*See:* Entry 9046

**★ 11845 ★ Bastyr University**
**Bastyr University AIDS Research Center (BUARC)**
Bastyr University Research Institute
14500 Juanita Dr. NE
Kenmore, WA 98028
**Phone:** (425)602-3165 **Fax:** (425)602-3079
**Email:** buri@bastyr.edu
**Website:** http://www.bastyr.edu/research/buarc/
Leanna J. Standish, PhD, Dir.
**Activities/Fields:** Alternative medical treatments for HIV/AIDS.

**★ 11846 ★ Biomedical Research Institute**
12111 Parklawn Dr.
Rockville, MD 20852
**Phone:** (301)881-3300 **Fax:** (301)881-7640
**Email:** biomed@afbr-bri.com
**Website:** http://www.afbr-bri.com
Dr. James L. Leef, Dir.
**Activities/Fields:** Conducts research on malaria and schistosomiasis, manages a low temperature repository, and performs large scale freeze-drying.

**Brigham and Women's Hospital**
**Channing Laboratory**
*See:* Entry 9049

**★ 11847 ★ Canadian Bacterial Diseases Network**
Heritage Medical Research Bldg., Rm. 282
3300 Hospital Dr. NW
Calgary, AB, Canada T2N 4N1
**Phone:** (403)220-2564 **Fax:** (403)283-5241
**Email:** woods@acs.uca/gary.ca
**Website:** http://www.cbdn.ca
Dr. Donald E. Woods, Sci. Dir.
**Activities/Fields:** Bacterial diseases of humans, animals, fish, and plants. Eight program areas include: antibiotics, including structure/activity relationships at the molecular level, mechanisms of antibiotic resistance, and outer membrane permeability; intracellular bacteria, adherence, and macrophages; live attenuated and subcellular vaccines, including novel attenuated strains as vaccine carriers, outer membrane proteins as carriers for peptide epitopes, and vaccine projects on human and fish pathogens; diagnostics, including analysis of DNA sequences, monoclonal antibodies, and other methods for use as diagnostic agents for Chlamydia, Pseudomonas, Salmonella, Campylobacter, Anaerobes, toxins, beta-lactamases, Neisseria, Yersinia, Bordetella, and major fish, animal, and plant pathogens; fish vaccines and diagnostics; toxins, including toxic shock syndrome, pertussis toxin, and Pasteurella haemolytica toxin; helicobacter, including mechanisms of ineffectivenss of antibiotics, molecular biology and genetics, and surface molecule studies; and sexually transmitted diseases, including molecular biology of surface antigens and molecular typing methods.

**★ 11848 ★ Center for Complex Infectious Diseases (CCID)**
3328 Stevens Ave., 2nd Fl.
Rosemead, CA 91770
**Phone:** (626)572-7288 **Fax:** (626)572-9288
**Website:** http://www.ccid.org/
Dr. John Martin, Contact
**Activities/Fields:** Nature, origin, disease associations, modes of transmission, methods of diagnosis and responses to therapy of complex infectious diseases. **Pub:** *Articles.* • *Lab reports.*

**★ 11849 ★ Center for Human Services**
7200 Wisconsin Ave., Ste. 600
Bethesda, MD 20814-4811
**Phone:** (301)654-8338 **Fax:** (301)941-8427
**Email:** dnicholas@urc-chs.com
**Website:** http://www.urc-chs.com
Dr. David Nicholas, Dir.
**Activities/Fields:** Applies quality assurance methods in health care settings around the world and conducts comparative studies of quality assessment, quality assurance costs, and quality relationship. **Pub:** *QA Brief.*

**★ 11850 ★ City of Hope**
**National Medical Center and Beckman Research Institute**
**Strategic Program for Innovative Research in AIDS Therapy**
Virology & Infectious Diseases/Department of Pediatrics
1500 E Duarte Rd.
Duarte, CA 91010
**Phone:** (626)359-2495 **Fax:** (626)301-8458
**Email:** jzaia@cityofhope.org
Dr. John A. Zaia, Prin. Investigator
**Activities/Fields:** Developmental gene therapy in the treatment of AIDS, including development and delivery of antiviral DNA and RNA; and pathogenesis and treatment of cytomegalovirus infection; and development of CMV vaccine.

**★ 11851 ★ Dana-Farber Cancer Institute**
**Department of Cancer Immunology and AIDS**
44 Binney St.
Boston, MA 02115
**Phone:** (617)632-3348 **Fax:** (617)632-4630
**Email:** harvey_cantor@dfci.harvard.edu
Harvey Cantor, Ch.
**Activities/Fields:** T-cell development and function.

**Duke University**
**Pediatric Rheumatoid Clinic**
*See:* Entry 5792

**Emory University**
**Emory Vaccine Research Center**
*See:* Entry 3245

**Family Health International (FHI)**
*See:* Entry 18395

**★ 11852 ★ Foundation for Research in Infectious Diseases**
PO Box 2734
Saratoga, CA 95070
**Email:** brobinson@fhi.org
**Website:** http://www.fhi.org
Ruth Walzer, Pres.
**Activities/Fields:** Infectious diseases, particularly invasive mycoses. **Pub:** *Minutes.* • *Scholarly papers.*

**★ 11853 ★ George Washington University Center for Virology, Immunology and Infectious Disease Research**
Children's National Medical Center
111 Michigan Ave. NW
Washington, DC 20010
**Phone:** (202)884-3981 **Fax:** (202)884-3985
**Email:** chhollan@cnmc.org
Dr. Christie A. Holland, Dir.
**Activities/Fields:** Virologic and immunologic problems relating to infectious diseases and vaccine development, hospital acquired nosocomial infections.

**★ 11854 ★ Georgia State University Herpes B-Virus Diagnosis: National Resource Laboratory**
Viral Immunology Center
Department of Biology
50 Decatur St.
Atlanta, GA 30302-4118
**Phone:** (404)651-0808 **Fax:** (404)651-0814
**Email:** biojkh@panther.gsu.edu
**Website:** http://www.gsu.edu/bvirus
Julia K. Hilliard, PhD, Prin. Investigator
**Activities/Fields:** Identification of B-virus infections in humans and macaques and the basic pathogenesis mechanisms of this and other neurotropic herpesviruses; development of control and prevention strategies for B-virus infections in both humans and macaques.

**Georgia State University**
**Viral Immunology Center**
**National B Virus Resource Laboratory**
*See:* Entry 4643

**★ 11855 ★ Great Lakes Regional Center for AIDS Research**
North Bldg.
3220 School of Information
University of Michigan
1075 Beal Ave.
Ann Arbor, MI 48109-2112
**Phone:** (734)764-6132 **Fax:** (734)647-8045
**Email:** steasley@umich.edu
**Website:** http://www.greatlakescfar.org/index.html
Stephanie Teasley, PhD, Collaboratory Dir.
**Activities/Fields:** Acquired immune deficiency syndrome in adults, molecular virology of human immunodeficiency virus (HIV), and experimental therapy of HIV. **Frmly:** Northwestern University; Comprehensive AIDS Center.

**HIV Center for Clinical and Behavioral Studies**
*See:* Entry 12691

**★ 11856 ★ Independent Agencies**
**U.S. International Development Cooperation Agency**
**U.S. Agency for International Development**
**Bureau for Global Programs, Field Support and Research**
**((Center for Population, Health and Nutrition)**
**HIV/AIDS Division — HIV-AIDS)**
USAID/G/PHN/HN/HIV-AIDS
Ronald Reagan Bldg.
Washington, DC 20523-1000
**Phone:** (202)712-4810       **Fax:** (202)216-3524
**Email:** ehrharda@child.cpmc.columbia.edu
**Website:** http://www.usaid.gov/pop_health/aids/
**Activities/Fields:** Reducing "high risk" sexual behavior; treatment and control of sexually transmitted infections and disearse; and development of surveillance systems to more clearly understand the dynamics of transmission, the impact of the epidemics and the effect of the interventions designed to curtail them.

**★ 11857 ★ Indiana University**
**Mid-America Adolescent Sexually Transmitted Disease Cooperative Research Center**
1120 South Dr.
Indianapolis, IN 46202
**Phone:** (317)274-1427       **Free:** 800-274-4862
**Email:** dporr@iupui.edu
Donald Orr, MD, Dir.
**Activities/Fields:** Chlamydia trachomatous, papilloma virus, gonorrhea and HIV, as well as opportunistic diseases such as pneumocystis pneumonia; genital ulcers, including herpes; and drug-resistant strains of gonorrhea.

**★ 11858 ★ Indiana University-Purdue University at Indianapolis**
**Indiana AIDS Clinical Trials Unit**
550 N University Blvd., No. 5550
Indianapolis, IN 46202
**Phone:** (317)274-8456       **Free:** 800-421-3316
**Fax:** (317)274-1876
**Email:** actg.indiana@fstrf.org
**Website:** http://www.iupui.edu/it/indyactu/index.html
Joseph Wheat, Princ. Investigator
**Activities/Fields:** AIDS treatment, including an antiretroviral approach; treatment and prevention of AIDS complications, including pneumocystis, pneumonia, cryptococcal meningitis, histoplasmosis, cytomegalovirus infection, Kaposi's sarcoma, and dementia.

**Institute for Clinical Research, Inc.**
*See:* Entry 5109

**★ 11859 ★ Irvington Institute for Immunological Research**
245 5th Ave., Rm. 2101
New York, NY 10016-8728
**Phone:** (212)576-1005       **Fax:** (212)576-1006
**Email:** irving1@ix.netcom.com
**Website:** http://www.irvingtoninstitute.org
Kerry W. Walsh, Exec. Dir.
**Activities/Fields:** Diseases and dysfunctions involving the immune system, including AIDS, cancer, diabetes, rheumatoid arthritis, allergies, organ rejection, and systemic lupus erythematosus. **Pub:** *Irvington Institute Newsletter*, quarterly. Newsletter.

**★ 11860 ★ Johns Hopkins University**
**STD Research Group**
Ross Bldg., Rm. 1159
School of Medicine
720 Rutland Ave.
Baltimore, MD 21205
**Phone:** (410)955-7636       **Fax:** (410)955-7889
**Email:** jzenilma@welchlink.welch.jhu.edu

**Website:** http://www.med.jhu.edu/jhustd/
Jonathan M. Zenilman, MD, Dir.
**Activities/Fields:** Edidemiology, prevention and behavioral aspects of sexually transmitted diseases (STDs), and establishing rapid and reliable testing and diagnoses of STDs.

**★ 11861 ★ Kansas City AIDS Research Consortium**
4050 Pennsylvania, Ste. 230
Kansas City, MO 64111
**Fax:** (816)756-5121
**Email:** jmeier@kcarc.org
Jan Meier, Clinical Dir.
**Activities/Fields:** HIV and AIDS clinical trials, opportunistic infections, anti-retrovirals, and HIV wasting treatment. **Pub:** *KCARC Research Report*, bimonthly.

**Kuzell Institute for Arthritis and Infectious Diseases**
*See:* Entry 13693

**★ 11862 ★ Laval University**
**Infectious Disease Research Centre**
2705, blvd. Laurier
Sainte Foy, QC, Canada G1V 4G2
**Phone:** (418)654-2705       **Fax:** (418)654-2715
**Email:** michel.g.bergeron@crchul.ulaval.ca
Michel G. Bergeron, Dir.
**Activities/Fields:** Molecular basis of action of antimicrobial agents and the mechanisms involved in microbial resistance against these agents. Develops new transportation vehicles of antimicrobials in bacteria, parasites, and viruses; works on metabolic particularities of parasites; develops new diagnostic kits for quick detection of bacterial and viral infections; and works on new vaccines. Studies AIDS, treatments for HIV-infected patients, and the immunological, pharmacodynamic, and psychosocial factors controlling HIV infections.

**★ 11863 ★ Legislative, Judicial, and Executive Offices**
**National Science and Technology Council**
**Committee on International Science, Engineering, and Technology**
**Task Force on Emerging Infectious Diseases**
Executive Secretariat
CISET Task Force on Emerging Infectious Diseases
2201 C St. NW
Washington, DC 20520
**Website:** http://www.state.gov/www/global/oes/health/task_force/index.html
**Activities/Fields:** Supports researchers and regional and international resources to focus on diagnostic reagents for low incidence diseases and identification of rare and unusual diseases. Provides research and training assistance to WHO and other organizations for establishment of guidelines for proper use of antimicrobial drugs and for development of new chemotherapeutic agents; promotes collaborations among U.S. agencies.

**★ 11864 ★ McGill University**
**Centre for the Study of Host Resistance**
Montreal General Hospital
1650 Cedar Ave., Rm. A6.149
Montreal, QC, Canada H3G 1A4
**Phone:** (514)934-8038       **Fax:** (514)933-7146
**Email:** md88@musica.mcgill.ca
Dr. Emil Skamene, Dir.
**Activities/Fields:** Genetic regulation of host susceptibility and resistance in diseases of adulthood, including cancer, tuberculosis, malaria, and other infectious diseases.

**★ 11865 ★ McGill University**
**McGill Centre for Tropical Diseases**
Montreal General Hospital, Rm. D7-153
1650 Cedar Ave.
Montreal, QC, Canada H3G 1A4
**Phone:** (514)934-8049       **Fax:** (514)933-9385
**Email:** md10@musica.mcgill.ca
Dr. J. Dick MacLean, Dir.
**Activities/Fields:** Tropical medicine and clinical parasitology, including studies of giardiases, malaria, cryptospridum, micronutrients, toxoplasma, ciguatera, trichinosis, and the epidemiology of medical problems in refugees and travelers. Maintains surveillance of Canadians traveling to, living in, or emigrating from the tropics.

**★ 11866 ★ Medical College of Wisconsin**
**Center for AIDS Intervention Research (CAIR)**
2071 North Summit Ave.
Milwaukee, WI 53202
**Phone:** (414)456-7700       **Fax:** (414)287-4206
**Website:** http://www.cair.mcw.edu/
Dr. Jeffrey Kelly, Contact
**Activities/Fields:** New intervention strategies to prevent HIV infection in populations vulnerable to the disease, including inner-city women, homeless men and women, gay men, youth at risk, and chronic mentally ill adults.

**★ 11867 ★ Meharry Medical College**
**Center on Tropical Diseases**
Division of Sponsored Research
1005 D.B. Todd Blvd.
Nashville, TN 37208
**Phone:** (615)327-6193       **Fax:** (615)327-5621
**Email:** gchill@mmc.edu
Dr. George C. Hill, Contact
**Activities/Fields:** Molecular, biochemical, and immunological aspects of tropical disease. Specific research includes studies on African trypanosomiasis, Chagas' disease, schistosomiasis, malaria, and leprosy. **Pub:** *Tropical Diseases Newsletter*. Newsletter.

**★ 11868 ★ National Center for Infectious Diseases**
**Division of Vector-Borne Infectious Diseases**
**Arbovirus Diseases Branch**
PO Box 2087
Fort Collins, CO 80522-2087
**Phone:** (970)221-6442       **Fax:** (970)266-3544
Dr. John T. Roehrig, Br. Ch.
**Activities/Fields:** Epidemiology of mosquito and tick-borne viral diseases. Provides consultation and on-site investigations for local, state, national, and international health agencies during arthropod-borne viral disease outbreaks. Conducts a national surveillance of arboviral diseases. **Pub:** *Research Reports.*

**★ 11869 ★ National Center for Infectious Diseases**
**Division of Vector-Borne Infectious Diseases**
**Bacterial Zoonosis Branch**
**Plague Section**
PO Box 2087
Fort Collins, CO 80522
**Phone:** (970)221-6400       **Fax:** (970)221-6476
**Email:** dvdid@cdc.gov
**Website:** http://www.cdc.gov/ncidod/dvbid/plague/index.htm
**Activities/Fields:** Diagnosis, therapy, epidemiology, and control of bubonic plague; maintains a surveillance system in collaboration with state and federal health agencies to detect fluctuations of infection in animal populations; and serves as a WHO Reference Center for plague diagnosis and control. **Pub:** *CDC Surveillance Reports.* • *Reference and Research*, biennially.

**★ 11870 ★ Northwestern University**
**Samuel Sackett Research Laboratory**
680 N Lakeshore Dr., Ste. 1106
Chicago, IL 60611
**Phone:** (312)908-9137　　　**Fax:** (312)908-5820
Dr. Steven M. Wolinsky, Dir.
**Activities/Fields:** HIV/AIDS cellular and humoral resistance to infection, viral central nervous system infections, pharmacology of antimicrobial agents, investigation of infectious diarrhea, and natural history of infectious diseases.


**★ 11871 ★ Ohio State University**
**Center for Retrovirus Research**
1925 Coffey Rd.
Columbus, OH 43210-1093
**Phone:** (614)292-7317　　　**Fax:** (614)292-6473
**Email:** mathes.2@osu.edu
Dr. Lawrence Mathes, Dir.
**Activities/Fields:** Animal and human retroviruses, including HIV in humans, feline immunodeficiency virus, equine infectious anemia, and leukemia virus of cats. **Pub:** *Newsletter*, quarterly.


**★ 11872 ★ Ohio State University**
**Division of Infectious Diseases**
410 W 10th Ave.
Columbus, OH 43210
**Phone:** (614)293-8732　　　**Fax:** (614)293-5240
Dr. Robert J. Fass, Dir.
**Activities/Fields:** Pathogenesis, prophylaxis, therapy, pathology, serology of infectious diseases (including Legionnaire's disease, herpes infections, acquired immune deficiency syndrome, and other opportunistic infections), and extensive in vitro and clinical evaluations of antimicrobial agents.


**Revici Foundation for Lipid Research**
*See:* Entry 20202


**Rockefeller University**
**Laboratory of Bacteriology, Pathogenesis**
**and Immunology**
*See:* Entry 3260


**★ 11873 ★ Rural Center for AIDS/STD**
**Prevention (RCAP)**
801 E 7th St.
Bloomington, IN 47405-3085
**Phone:** (812)855-1718　　　**Free:** 800-566-8644
**Fax:** (812)855-3717
**Email:** aids@indiana.edu
**Website:** http://www.indiana.edu/~aids/
William L. Yarber, Dir.
**Activities/Fields:** AIDS, HIV, and STD prevention in rural areas.


**★ 11874 ★ Rutgers University**
**AIDS Research Group**
Institute for Health
30 College Ave.
New Brunswick, NJ 08901-1293
**Phone:** (732)932-8579　　　**Fax:** (732)932-6872
**Email:** scrystal@rci.rutgers.edu
**Website:** http://www.ihhcpar.rutgers.edu
Stephen Crystal, PhD, Dir.
**Activities/Fields:** Social and behavioral research on AIDS, focusing on policy issues and applying social science methodology to the planning and evaluation of programs and policies designed to meet public health objectives. Specific areas of research include HIV health services, long-term care, social networks, mental health programs, the social context of health-related behavior in Hispanic and black subcultures, health cognition and health belief systems, legal aspects of serving endangered and high-risk populations, and cost of care and services utilization studies.


**★ 11875 ★ St. Clare's Hospital and**
**Health Center**
**Spellman Center for HIV-Related Disease**
415 W 51st St.
New York, NY 10019
**Phone:** (212)459-8130　　　**Fax:** (212)459-8353
**Email:** vlrobles@netscape.net
Victoria Robles, Dir.
**Activities/Fields:** Clinical drug trials, including immune modulators, anti-retrovirals, prophylactic therapies for infections, DDI, and granulocyte-macrophage colony-stimulating activity factors.


**St. Louis University**
**Institute for Molecular Virology**
*See:* Entry 4682


**★ 11876 ★ Stanford University**
**AIDS Clinical Trials Unit**
Division of Infectious Diseases, Rm. S-156
Stanford, CA 94305-5107
**Phone:** (650)723-6231　　　**Fax:** (650)725-2395
**Email:** merigan@stanford.edu
**Website:** http://www-leland.stanford.edu/group/aids/
index.html
Dr. Thomas C. Merigan, Dir.
**Activities/Fields:** Antiviral drug studies, including inhibitors of HIV, HBV, and herpes replication using in vitro and in vivo antiviral models.


**★ 11877 ★ State University of New York**
**at Buffalo**
**Infectious and Chronic Disease Center**
**(ICDC)**
Sch. of Dental Medicine
Department of Oral Biology
115 Foster Hall
3435 Main St.
Buffalo, NY 14214
**Phone:** (716)829-2844　　　**Fax:** (716)829-2387
**Email:** rjgenco@acsu.buffalo.edu
**Website:** http://research.sdm.buffalo.edu/
Dr. Robert J. Genco, Prin. Investigator
**Activities/Fields:** Interactions of infections, such as periodontal disease, with chronic diseases including heart disease, respiratory disease, and osteoporosis.


**★ 11878 ★ State University of New York**
**at Buffalo**
**Witebsky Center for Microbial**
**Pathogenesis and Immunology**
243 Biomedical Research Bldg.
Buffalo, NY 14260
**Phone:** (716)829-2848　　　**Fax:** (716)829-3534
**Website:** http://www.smbs.buffalo.edu/wcmpi/
Noreen Williams, PhD, Dir.
**Activities/Fields:** Molecular mechanisms of infectious diseases.


**★ 11879 ★ State University of New York**
**at Stony Brook**
**Stony Brook HIV Treatment Development**
**Center**
State University of New York Health Science
Center, HSC T-15
Stony Brook, NY 11794-8153
**Phone:** (631)444-1658　　　**Fax:** (631)444-7518
**Email:** rsteigb@mail.som.sunysb.edu
**Website:** http://www.informatics.sunysb.edu/internalmed/AidsHIV/HIVhome.html
Roy T. Steigbigel, MD, Dir.
**Activities/Fields:** Treatment of HIV infection.


**★ 11880 ★ Temple University**
**Center for Neurovirology and Cancer**
**Biology**
**Laboratory of NeuroAIDS and Gene**
**Therapy**
BioLife Sciences Bldg.
College of Science & Technology
1900 N 12th St.
Philadelphia, PA 19122
**Phone:** (215)204-0604　　　**Fax:** (215)204-0679
**Email:** s.amini@astro.temple.edu
Dr. Shohreh Amini, Prin. Investigator
**Activities/Fields:** Human immunodeficiency virus (HIV) bacterial antigens.


**★ 11881 ★ Terry Beirn Community**
**Programs for Clinical Research on**
**AIDS (CPCRA)**
8757 Georgia Ave., 12th Fl.
Silver Spring, MD 20910-3714
**Phone:** (301)230-9670　　　**Fax:** (301)230-7190
**Email:** mdiggins@s-3.com
**Website:** http://www.cpcra.org/
Meg Diggins, Clinical Sec. Corrd.
**Activities/Fields:** Day-to-day medical management of HIV disease; treatment and therapies for AIDS.


**★ 11882 ★ Tulane University**
**Center for Infectious Diseases (CID)**
J. Bennett Johnston Bldg., 5th Fl.
Tulane University Medical Center
1430 Tulane Ave., SL-71
New Orleans, LA 70112-2699
**Phone:** (504)584-3552　　　**Fax:** (504)988-6686
**Email:** center.infecdis@tulane.edu
**Website:** http://www.tulane.edu/~cid/
Dr. Donald J. Krogstad, Dir.
**Activities/Fields:** Emerging and re-emerging infectious diseases, both in the United States and abroad.


**U.S. Department of Defense**
**Army Medical Research and Materiel**
**Command**
**Army Medical Research Institute of**
**Infectious Diseases**
*See:* Entry 13473


**U.S. Department of Defense**
**Army Medical Research and Materiel**
**Command**
**Walter Reed Army Institute of Research**
**Communicable Diseases and Immunology**
**Division**
*See:* Entry 3267


**U.S. Department of Health and Human**
**Services**
**Centers for Disease Control and**
**Prevention**
**National Institute for Occupational Safety**
**and Health**
**National Occupational Research Agenda**
**(Infectious Diseases)**
*See:* Entry 16812


**U.S. Department of Health and Human**
**Services**
**Centers for Disease Control and**
**Prevention**
**National Institute for Occupational Safety**
**and Health**
**National Occupational Research Agenda**
**(Indoor Environment)**
*See:* Entry 16813

**U.S. Department of Health and Human Services**
**Food and Drug Administration**
**Center for Bilogics Evaluation and Research**
**Division of Bacterial Products**
*See:* Entry 4694

**U.S. Department of Health and Human Services**
**Food and Drug Administration**
**Center for Biologics Evaluation and Research**
**Laboratory of Hepatitis Viruses**
*See:* Entry 4713

**U.S. Department of Health and Human Services**
**Food and Drug Administration**
**Center for Biologics Evauluation and Research**
**Laboratory of Enteric and Sexually Transmitted Diseases**
*See:* Entry 4725

**★ 11883 ★ U.S. Department of Health and Human Services**
**Health Resources and Services Administration**
**Gillis W. Long Hansen's Disease Center**
1770 Physician Park Dr.
Baton Rouge, LA 70816
**Phone:** (225)756-3700 **Fax:** (225)756-3806
**Email:** kopecko@cber.fda.gov
**Website:** http://www.bthc.hrsa.gov/nhdp
Charles Stanley, Dir.
**Activities/Fields:** Care and rehabilitation of patients with Hansen's disease (leprosy) and for basic and applied research related to all aspects of the disease. In addition, Center provides a training facility for professionals and paraprofessionals involved with the diagnosis and treatment of Hansen's disease, both within the United States and abroad. Areas of research interest include studies of the causative organism of leprosy and its effect on the body as well as research in methods of clinical treatment and rehabilitation; mycobacterioses including tuberculosis. Accomplishments have included the infection of armadillos with the leprosy organism, the first experimental animal to be found naturally susceptible to the disseminated form of this disease, and earlier, the discovery of sulfone therapy, the first effective treatment for the disease. Tuberculosis studies include comprehensive evaluation of 50,000 candidate anti-TB drugs. **Pub:** *International Journal of Leprosy*, quarterly. • *The Star*, quarterly. **Frmly:** (2000) Gillis W. Long Hansen's Disease Center.

**★ 11884 ★ U.S. Department of Health and Human Services**
**National Center for Infectious Diseases**
1600 Clifton Rd. NE, MSC-C12
Atlanta, GA 30333
**Phone:** (404)371-5329 **Fax:** (404)371-5449
**Email:** jem3@cdc.gov
**Website:** http://www.cdc.gov/ncidod/
Joseph E. McDade, Dep. Dir.
**Activities/Fields:** Coordinates a national program to improve the identification, investigation, diagnosis, prevention, and control of infectious diseases. Principal Center components include: Arctic Investigations Program; Bacterial and Mycotic Diseases Division; Hospital Infections Program; Division of AIDS, STD, DTB Lab Research; Division of Parisitic Diseases; Vector-Borne Infectious Diseases Division; and Division of Viral and Rickettsial Diseases; Division of Quarantine; and Scientific Resources Program.

**★ 11885 ★ U.S. Department of Health and Human Services**
**National Center for Infectious Diseases**
**Arctic Investigations Program**
4055 Tudor Centre Dr.
Anchorage, AK 99508
**Phone:** (907)729-3400 **Fax:** (907)729-3429
**Email:** jcb3@cdc.gov
**Website:** http://www.cdc.gov/ncidod/aip/aip.htm
Dr. Jay C. Butler, Dir.
**Activities/Fields:** Mission is to prevent infectious diseases and improve the quality of life of people living in the arctic and subarctic through: investigation of the causes of infectious diseases; evaluation of methods for disease prevention and control; dissemination of information; provision of epidemiologic, statistical, and laboratory consultation and technical assistance; and assistance in training of personnel to perform studies of conditions that impact health. Activities focus on studies of conditions that occur at high incidence, are unique to, or may be of potential benefit to populations in (and outside of) the arctic and subarctic. Emphasis is on acute infectious diseases, but investigations are also conducted on select chronic diseases that are sequelae of infectious diseases and/or in which an infectious disease is suspected to play a role. Specific disease areas of interest include: Hepatitis B, Streptococcus pneumoniae, Haemophilus influenzae b, Helicobacter pylori, respiratory syncytial virus. **Pub:** *Proceedings.* • *Research Reports.*

**★ 11886 ★ U.S. Department of Health and Human Services**
**National Center for Infectious Diseases**
**Division of AIDS, STD, and Tuberculosis Laboratory Research**
**Tuberculosis/Mycobacteriology Branch**
1600 Clifton Rd. NE
Bldg. 7, Rm. SSB5
MS G35
Atlanta, GA 30333
**Phone:** (404)639-1280 **Fax:** (404)639-1287
**Email:** tms1@cdc.gov
Dr. Tim Shinnick, Ch.
**Activities/Fields:** Tuberculosis and other mycobacterial diseases, emphasizing etiologic agents of tuberculosis, leprosy, and other mycobacterioses; surveillance of the incidence of these diseases; and diagnostic procedures for rapid identification and drug resistance patterns. Principal research interest are moleucular biology, rapid diagnostic procedures, subtyping mechanisms, immunology, genetics, drug development, virulence factors, and taxonomy. **Pub:** *Proceedings.* **Frmly:** Division of Bacterial and Mycotic Diseases; Emerging Bacterial and Mycotic Diseases Branch; Tuberculosis and Other Mycobacteriosis Laboratory Section.

**★ 11887 ★ U.S. Department of Health and Human Services**
**National Center for Infectious Diseases**
**Division of AIDS, STDS, Tuberculosis Laboratories**
**Immunology Branch**
1600 Clifton Rd., NE, Bldg. 17 Rm. 3016 (MSA-25)
Atlanta, GA 30333
**Phone:** (404)639-3434 **Fax:** (404)639-2108
**Email:** jsm3@cdc.gov
Dr. J. Steven McDougal, Chf.
**Activities/Fields:** Immunology and Acquired Immunodeficiency Syndrome (AIDS). **Frmly:** Division of Host Factors.

**★ 11888 ★ U.S. Department of Health and Human Services**
**National Center for Infectious Diseases**
**Division of AIDS, STDS, and Tuberculosis Laboratories**
**Retrovirus Diseases Branch**
1600 Clifton Rd. NE, G19
Atlanta, GA 30333
**Phone:** (404)639-1024 **Fax:** (404)639-1174
Dr. Thomas M. Folks, PhD, Chf.
**Activities/Fields:** Retrovirus diseases and retroviral etiologies of chronic diseases.

**★ 11889 ★ U.S. Department of Health and Human Services**
**National Center for Infectious Diseases**
**Division of Bacterial and Mycotic Diseases**
**Childhood and Respirtory Diseases Branch**
Mail Stop C23
1600 Clifton Rd., NE
Atlanta, GA 30333
**Phone:** (404)639-2215 **Fax:** (404)639-3970
Tiffany Neal, Contact
**Activities/Fields:** Laboratory and epidemiologic investigations of organisms except enteric and sexually transmitted diseases. Principal subjects of study are influenzae, type b; meningitidis; Group A streptococcus; Group B streptococcus; Brazilian purpuric fever; sipneumoniae, legionella infections, chlamydia and mycoplasma infections, and otitis media.

**★ 11890 ★ U.S. Department of Health and Human Services**
**National Center for Infectious Diseases**
**Division of HIV / AIDS**
1600 Clifton Rd., NE
Mail Stop E-49
Atlanta, GA 30333
**Phone:** (404)639-0900 **Fax:** (404)639-2007
**Email:** rxj1@cdc.gov
**Website:** http://www.cdc.gov/hiv/dhap.htm
Robert Janssen, Dir.
**Activities/Fields:** Epidemiologic and laboratory investigations, surveillance, and studies to determine risk factors, transmission patterns, prevalence/incidence of HIV/AIDS, and case reporting for acquired immunodeficiency syndrome. Program also develops and evaluates laboratory methods and procedures for the isolation and characterization of human immunodeficiency virus (HIV) and serodiagnosis and understanding of viral pathogenesis. Principal component units are: Office of the Director, Epidemiology Branch, Laboratory Investigations Branch, Statistics and Data Management Branch, HIV Seroepidemiology Branch, Field Services Branch, Technical Information Activity, International Activity, Surveillance Branch, Hematologic Diseases Branch, and Immunology Branch.

**★ 11891 ★ U.S. Department of Health and Human Services**
**National Center for Infectious Diseases**
**Division of Parasitic Diseases**
4770 Buford Hwy., MS F22
Chamblee, GA 30341-3724
**Phone:** (770)488-7750 **Fax:** (770)488-7794
**Email:** kelz1@cdr.gov
**Website:** http://www.cdc.gov/ncidod/dpd/
Kay Lawton, RN, MN, Deputy Dir.
**Activities/Fields:** Parasitic diseases to define disease etiology, mode of transmission, and populations at risk; works to develop effective methods for diagnosis, prevention, and control; participates in clinical, field, and laboratory research to develop, evaluate, and improve laboratory methodologies and materials and therapeutic practices used for rapid and accurate diagnosis and treatment of parasitic diseases; and sponsors laboratory studies of selected parasitic infections, with emphasis on animal in vitro model systems for parasitic relationships, chemotherapy, and immu-

nology, in order to develop effective methods for diagnosis, prevention, and control.

**★ 11892 ★ U.S. Department of Health and Human Services**
**National Center for Infectious Diseases**
**Division of Parasitic Diseases**
**Entomology Branch**
**(Vector Biology and Toxicology Section)**
4770 Buford Hwy., MS F22
Chamblee, GA 30341-3724
**Phone:** (770)488-4240     **Fax:** (770)488-4258
**Email:** bew5@cdc.gov
**Website:** http://www.cdc.gov/ncidod/dpd/aboutdpd/default.htmorg.structure
Robert A. Wirtz, Chf. Entomology Branch

**Activities/Fields:** Vector control strategies and disseminates the results; conducts research on vector biology and the molecular and biochemical mechanisms for insecticide resistance; develops biochemical and bioassay field tests to assess vector insecticide susceptibility; develops and validates chemical tests for the detection of parasitic disease drugs and their metabolites in body fluids and tissues, and determines the pharmacologic response to such drugs; develops chemical procedures to detect new and existing pesticides in various formulations.

**★ 11893 ★ U.S. Department of Health and Human Services**
**National Center for Infectious Diseases**
**Division of Parasitic Diseases**
**Epidemiology Branch**
**(Parasitic Diseases Section)**
4770 Buford Hwy., MS F22
Atlanta, GA 30341-3724
**Phone:** (770)488-7760     **Fax:** (770)488-7794
Mark Eberhardt, Actg. Dir.

**Activities/Fields:** Surveillance and epidemiologic investigations of parasitic diseases, other than malaria, in the U.S. and abroad. Monitors the efficacy and safety of antiparasitic drugs. Monitors and investigates water source disease outbreaks. **Frmly:** (2000) Epidemiology Branch; Parasitic Diseases Section.

**★ 11894 ★ U.S. Department of Health and Human Services**
**National Center for Infectious Diseases**
**Division of Parasitic Diseases**
**Epidemiology Branch**
**(Malaria Section)**
4770 Buford Hwy., MS F22
Atlanta, GA 30341-3724
**Phone:** (770)488-7789     **Fax:** (770)488-7761
Rick Steketer, Chf.

**Activities/Fields:** Malaria in the U.S. and among U.S. citizens abroad; monitors the efficacy and safety of antimalarial drugs for chemoprophylaxis and chemotherapy; and provides clinical advice and epidemiologic assistance on the treatment, control, and prevention of malaria in the U.S. and abroad.

**★ 11895 ★ U.S. Department of Health and Human Services**
**National Center for Infectious Diseases**
**Division of Parasitic Diseases**
**Epidemiology Branch**
4770 Buford Hwy., MS F22
Atlanta, GA 30341-3724
**Phone:** (770)488-7760     **Fax:** (770)488-7761
James Maguire, Chf.

**Activities/Fields:** Parasitic diseases in the U.S. and abroad; monitors the efficacy and safety of antiparasitic drugs; provides clinical advice and epidemiologic assistance to state and local health departments, other federal agencies, and national and international health organizations, on the diagnosis, treatment, control, and prevention of parasitic diseases.

**★ 11896 ★ U.S. Department of Health and Human Services**
**National Center for Infectious Diseases**
**Division of Vector-Borne Infectious Diseases**
**Dengue Branch**
1324 Calle Canada
San Juan, PR 00920-3860
**Phone:** (787)706-2399     **Fax:** (787)706-2496
**Email:** ggc1@cdc.gov
Gary G. Clark, Chf.

**Activities/Fields:** Study of dengue, a viral disease spread by mosquitoes. Research includes investigation of vectors, reservoirs of disease, viruses that cause disease, and methods for surveillance prevention and control. **Pub:** *Dengue Surveillance Summary.*
• *Research Reports.*

**★ 11897 ★ U.S. Department of Health and Human Services**
**National Center for Infectious Diseases**
**Division of Viral and Rickettsial Diseases**
1600 Clifton Rd. NE (MS A-30)
Atlanta, GA 30333
**Phone:** (404)639-3574     **Fax:** (404)639-3163
**Website:** http://www.cdc.gov/ncidod/dvrd/index.htm
James W. LeDuc, Actg. Dir.

**Activities/Fields:** Viral and rickettsial diseases of national and international importance. The Division addresses significant disease problems by the integrated application of modern virologic and epidemiologic methodologies–from molecular biologic methodologies (including nucleic acid and protein biochemistry) to immunologic and pathophysiologic methodologies to epidemiologic and statistical methodologies. Division comprises the Biometrics Activity, Infectious Disease Pathology Activity, Influenza Branch, Respiratory and Enteric Virus Branch, Special Pathogens Branch, Viral Exanthems and Herpesvirus Branch, and Viral and Rickettsial Zoonoses Branch. Branch. **Pub:** *Proceedings.* • *Research Reports.* **Frmly:** Viral Diseases Division.

**★ 11898 ★ U.S. Department of Health and Human Services**
**National Center for Infectious Diseases**
**Division of Viral and Rickettsial Diseases**
**Hepatitis Branch**
1600 Clifton Rd., NE, MS A33
MS G37
Atlanta, GA 30333
**Phone:** (404)371-5900     **Fax:** (404)371-5221
**Email:** hsm1@cdc.gov
**Website:** http://www.cdc.gov/ncidod/diseases/hepatitis/index.htm
Richard Conlon, MD, Actg. Dep. Dir.

**Activities/Fields:** Hepatitis A, B, C, D, and E. Works to implement hepatitis B and hepatitis A immunization programs nationally and internationally. **Pub:** *Hepatitis Surveillance Report*, annually.

**★ 11899 ★ U.S. Department of Health and Human Services**
**National Center for Infectious Diseases**
**Division of Viral and Rickettsial Diseases**
**Influenza Branch**
1600 Clifton Rd., NE
G-16
Atlanta, GA 30333
**Phone:** (404)639-3591     **Fax:** (404)639-2334
**Email:** NJC1@CDC.GOV
Nancy Cox, Chf.

**Activities/Fields:** Focal point within CDC for studies pertaining to influenza viruses, their variation and occurrence in populations, and their control.

**U.S. Department of Health and Human Services**
**National Center for Infectious Diseases**
**Division of Viral and Rickettsial Diseases**
**Respiratory and Enteric Virus Branch**
*See:* Entry 18764

**★ 11900 ★ U.S. Department of Health and Human Services**
**National Center for Infectious Diseases**
**Division of Viral and Rickettsial Diseases**
**Viral and Rickettsial Zoonoses Branch**
Epidemiology Section
1600 Clifton Rd., NE
Atlanta, GA 30333
**Phone:** (404)639-1087     **Fax:** (404)639-4436
**Email:** jfc5@cdc.gov
**Website:** http://www.cdc.gov/ncidod/dvrd/branch/vrzb.htm
Dr. James Childs, Consult.

**Activities/Fields:** Rickettsial agents (such as those of Rocky Mountain spotted fever and Q fever).

**★ 11901 ★ U.S. Department of Health and Human Services**
**National Center for Infectious Diseases**
**Hospital Infections Program**
1600 Clifton Rd. NE
Mail Stop E-69
Atlanta, GA 30333
**Phone:** (404)639-6400     **Fax:** (404)639-6459
**Email:** wrj1c@cdc.gov
**Website:** http://www.cdc.gov/ncidod/hip/hip.htm
Dr. William Jarvis, Chf.

**Activities/Fields:** Hospital-associated infections. The Program serves as the focal point within the National Center for Infectious Diseases for the issuance of recommendations and guidelines on prevention and control of hospital infections. The Program involves research on methods for preventing and controlling hospital infections and for rapid diagnosis of disease and identification of unusual sources of infection; and research to identify methods for antimicrobial susceptibility testing of groups of microorganisms and to determine the role of drug-resistant microorganisms in hospital infections. Program also provides epidemic aid and epidemiological consultation, upon request from state health departments, to institutions and public health organizations regarding the identification and control of nosocomial infections, provides basic diagnostic services in support of field investigations and cooperates with other components of CID for more definitive diagnosis of nosocomial infections and identification of etiologic agents, provides antimicrobial susceptibility consultation and services to other components of CID, provides intramural and extramural technical expertise and assistance in professional training activities; and serves as designated national and international reference centers for certain nosocomial infections. Components of the Hospital Infections Program are: Anti-Hospital Environmental Laboratory Branch, Nosocomial Pathogens Laboratory Branch, Investigation and Prevention Branch, and HIV Infectious Branch. **Pub:** *Guidelines for the Prevention and Control of Nosocomial Infections.* • *National Nosocomial Infections Surveillance System Reports.*

**★ 11902 ★ U.S. Department of Health and Human Services**
**National Center for Infectious Diseases**
**Scientific Resources Program**
1600 Clifton Rd., NE
Atlanta, GA 30333
**Phone:** (404)639-3466     **Fax:** (404)639-3199
**Email:** bzm9@cdc.gov
**Website:** http://www.cdc.gov/ncidod/about.htm
Carolyn Black, Dir.

**Activities/Fields:** Procures, manages, and distributes the resources required by CDC investigators for research and service activities; conducts protocol reviews for research and diagnostic activities involving laboratory animals, and produces cell cultures, cell culture media, and microbiologic media, using modern methods and exhaustive quality assurance testing; maintains an active applied research program in cell biology, and conducts research leading to the development of new cell culture systems and cell lines; procures, prepares, and distributes sterile glassware and plasticware, and provides packing, shipping, and receiving services for etiologic agents, diagnostic specimens, and reagents from the CDC catalog; and provides services for maintaining and developing laboratory equipment; provides to the NCID research environments the instrumentation and expertise required to develop, refine, and apply modern technologies pertinent to the prevention and control of infectious, autoimmune, neoplastic, and hemotolgic diseases.

**U.S. Department of Health and Human Services**
**National Institute of Allergy and Infectious Diseases**
**Division of Acquired Immuniodeficiency Syndrome (AIDS)**
**Basic Science Program**
**(Epidemiology Branch)**
*See:* Entry 9064

**★ 11903 ★ U.S. Department of Health and Human Services**
**National Institute of Allergy and Infectious Diseases**
**Division of Acquired Immunodeficiency Syndrome (AIDS)**
6007 Rockledge Dr.
Bldg. 6700 B, Rm. 4142
Bethesda, MD 20892
**Phone:** (301)496-0545          **Fax:** (301)402-1505
**Email:** et89f@nih.gov
**Website:** http://www.niaid.nih.gov/daids/default.htm
Dr. Edmond C. Tramont, MD, Dir.

**Activities/Fields:** Basic knowledge of the pathogenesis, natural history, and transmission of HIV. Promotes progress in the detection, treatment, and prevention of HIV.

**★ 11904 ★ U.S. Department of Health and Human Services**
**National Institute of Allergy and Infectious Diseases**
**Division of Acquired Immunodeficiency Syndrome (AIDS)**
**Basic Science Program**
**(Pathogenesis and Basic Research Branch)**
Room 2140; Mail Stop 7610
6700B Rockledge Dr.
Bethesda, MD 20892-7610
**Phone:** (301)496-8666          **Fax:** (301)402-0369
**Email:** gm16s@nib.gov
**Website:** http://www.niaid.nih.gov
Gregory Milman, PhD, Dir.

**Activities/Fields:** Bioterrorism-related research, electronic research administration, small business opportunities, distance learning, and Internet training.

**★ 11905 ★ U.S. Department of Health and Human Services**
**National Institute of Allergy and Infectious Diseases**
**Division of Acquired Immunodeficiency Syndrome (AIDS)**
**Basic Science Program**
**(Targeted Interventions Branch)**
6700 B Rockledge Dr.
Room 4254
Bethesda, MD 20892
**Phone:** (301)496-8197          **Fax:** (301)402-3211
**Email:** te35m@nih.gov
Dr. Sandra Bridges, Chf.

**Activities/Fields:** Discovery of effective vaccines and therapies for the prevention and treatment of HIV infection and disease.

**★ 11906 ★ U.S. Department of Health and Human Services**
**National Institute of Allergy and Infectious Diseases**
**Division of Acquired Immunodeficiency Syndrome (AIDS)**
**Basic Science Program**
6700 B Rockledge Dr. MSC 7626
Bethesda, MD 20892-7626
**Phone:** (301)496-0637          **Fax:** (301)402-3211
Dr. Carl Dieffenbach, PhD, Assoc. Dir.

**Activities/Fields:** Pathogenesis, basic virology, immunobiology, pathobiology, the discovery of novel therapeutic approaches, and epidemiology.

**★ 11907 ★ U.S. Department of Health and Human Services**
**National Institute of Allergy and Infectious Diseases**
**Division of Acquired Immunodeficiency Syndrome (AIDS)**
**Biostatistics Research Branch**
6700-B Rockledge Dr.
Bethesda, MD 20892
**Phone:** (301)496-0694          **Fax:** (301)480-5703
Dennis Dixon, Chf.

**Activities/Fields:** Methodologic and biostatistical oversight and assistance.

**★ 11908 ★ U.S. Department of Health and Human Services**
**National Institute of Allergy and Infectious Diseases**
**Division of Acquired Immunodeficiency Syndrome (AIDS)**
**Epidemiology Project Team**
6700-B Rockledge Dr., Rm. 4131
Bethesda, MD 20892
**Phone:** (301)402-0135          **Fax:** (301)402-3211
Carlie Williams, MD, Actg. Chf.

**Activities/Fields:** Epidemiology of HIV.

**★ 11909 ★ U.S. Department of Health and Human Services**
**National Institute of Allergy and Infectious Diseases**
**Division of Acquired Immunodeficiency Syndrome (AIDS)**
**Office of Program Operations and Scientific Information**
6007 Rockledge Dr., Rm. 4143
Bethesda, MD 20892
**Phone:** (301)496-0545          **Fax:** (301)402-1505
**Email:** tlasalvia@niaid.nih.gov
**Website:** http://www.niaid.nih.gov/daids/org/daidsorg.htm
Thomas Lasalvia, RN, Contact

**Activities/Fields:** Collects and maintains scientific data and composes reports for the Division of Acquired Immunodeficiency Syndrome.

**★ 11910 ★ U.S. Department of Health and Human Services**
**National Institute of Allergy and Infectious Diseases**
**Division of Acquired Immunodeficiency Syndrome (AIDS)**
**Pediatric Project Team**
6700-B Rockledge Dr. Rm. 5225
Bethesda, MD 20892
**Phone:** (301)402-2300          **Fax:** (301)402-3171
J. McNamara, MD, Chf.

**Activities/Fields:** HIV disease in relation to infants, children, and adolescents.

**★ 11911 ★ U.S. Department of Health and Human Services**
**National Institute of Allergy and Infectious Diseases**
**Division of Acquired Immunodeficiency Syndrome (AIDS)**
**Pharmaceutical and Regulatory Affairs Branch**
6700-B Rockledge Dr.
Bethesda, MD 20892
**Phone:** (301)496-8213          **Fax:** (301)402-1506
Anna Martinez, PhD, Chf.

**Activities/Fields:** Assures that all clinical trials sponsored by DAIDS are conducted in accordance with FDA and Federal regulations.

**★ 11912 ★ U.S. Department of Health and Human Services**
**National Institute of Allergy and Infectious Diseases**
**Division of Acquired Immunodeficiency Syndrome (AIDS)**
**Scientific Assessment and Resource Branch**
6003 Executive Blvd.
North Bethesda, MD 20852
**Phone:** (301)402-0755          **Fax:** (301)480-5703
P. Sager, PhD, Chf.

**Activities/Fields:** Conducts reviews to ensure that the Division's activities effectively address the stated scientific goals and priorities.

**★ 11913 ★ U.S. Department of Health and Human Services**
**National Institute of Allergy and Infectious Diseases**
**Division of Acquired Immunodeficiency Syndrome (AIDS)**
**Therapeutics Research Program**
**(Pediatric Medicine Branch)**
Bldg. 31, Rm. 7A50
31 Center Dr.
Bethesda, MD 20892-2520
**Phone:** (301)402-2300          **Fax:** (301)402-0120
Dr. James G. McNamara, Dir.

**Activities/Fields:** Therapeutic strategies directed at: the clinical conditions associated with HIV infection in children and adolescents; and intervention to reduce the risk of transmission of HIV from infected mothers to the infant or fetus.

**★ 11914 ★ U.S. Department of Health and Human Services**
**National Institute of Allergy and Infectious Diseases**
**Division of Acquired Immunodeficiency Syndrome (AIDS)**
**Therapeutics Research Program**
**(Opportunistic Infections Research Branch)**
6700-B Rockledge Dr., Rm. 5108
MSC 7624
Bethesda, MD 20892
**Phone:** (301)402-2304          **Fax:** (301)402-3171
**Email:** bl17u@nih.gov
**Website:** http://www.niaid.nih.gov/daids/org/daidstrp.htm
B. Laughon, PhD, Chf.

**Activities/Fields:** Improved therapies for the treatment and prophylaxis of OIs tuberculosis associated with HIV disease.

**★ 11915 ★ U.S. Department of Health and Human Services**
**National Institute of Allergy and Infectious Diseases**
**Division of Acquired Immunodeficiency Syndrome (AIDS)**
**Therapeutics Research Program (Coordinating Centers Branch)**
Solar Bldg., Rm. 3A-06
6003 Executive Blvd.
Bethesda, MD 20892-7630
**Phone:** (301)496-7728 **Fax:** (301)402-2508
D.M. Dixon, PhD, Chf.

**Activities/Fields:** Oversees the technical and administrative management of a program of research grants and contracts that provide coordinating support for the clinical trials organization supported by the TRP. This includes data management, biostatistical analysis, information processing, laboratory specimen tracking, coordinating, monitoring, and operations support. Oversight of the Division of AIDS Treatment Research Initiative (DATRI) is coordinated by this branch.

**★ 11916 ★ U.S. Department of Health and Human Services**
**National Institute of Allergy and Infectious Diseases**
**Division of Acquired Immunodeficiency Syndrome (AIDS)**
**Therapeutics Research Program (HIV Research Branch)**
6700-B Rockledge Dr., Rm. 5102
Bethesda, MD 20892
**Phone:** (301)496-0700 **Fax:** (301)480-4582
**Email:** cp22n@nih.gov
Carla Pettinelli, MD, Chf.

**Activities/Fields:** Preclinical and clinical research on: therapeutic strategies directed at the treatment of adult primary HIV infection; the augmentation of specific HIV immune responses and general host immunity in HIV-infected individuals; and the neurological complications of HIV infection.

**★ 11917 ★ U.S. Department of Health and Human Services**
**National Institute of Allergy and Infectious Diseases**
**Division of Acquired Immunodeficiency Syndrome (AIDS)**
**Therapeutics Research Program (Clinical Site Management Branch)**
6700-B Rockledge Dr., Rm. 5157
Bethesda, MD 20892
**Phone:** (301)402-0143 **Fax:** (301)480-4582
**Email:** mm154j@nih.gov
Margaret Matula, Actg. Chf.

**Activities/Fields:** Oversees the technical and administrative management of a program of research grants and contracts supporting clinical research sites carrying out DAIDS-supported clinical trials. These programs include: the Adult and Pediatric AIDS Clinical Trials Group (ACTG); the Terry Beirn Community Programs for Clinical Research on AIDS (CPCRA); the National Hemophilia Foundation (NHF); and the Acute Infection and Early Disease Research Program (AIEDRP).

**★ 11918 ★ U.S. Department of Health and Human Services**
**National Institute of Allergy and Infectious Diseases**
**Division of Acquired Immunodeficiency Syndrome (AIDS)**
**Therapeutics Research Program**
6700-B Rockledge Dr., Rm. 5102
Bethesda, MD 20892
**Phone:** (301)496-8210 **Fax:** (301)480-4582
**Email:** fbl0C@nih.gov
Frederick Batzold, Actg. Dir.

**Activities/Fields:** Therapies against HIV disease, including associated opportunistic infections (OIs) and cancer in adults, infants, children, and adolescents.

**★ 11919 ★ U.S. Department of Health and Human Services**
**National Institute of Allergy and Infectious Diseases**
**Division of Acquired Immunodeficiency Syndrome (AIDS)**
**Vaccine and Prevention Research Program (Preclinical Research Branch)**
6700-B Rockledge Dr., Rm. 4102
Bethesda, MD 20892
**Phone:** (301)402-0121 **Fax:** (301)402-3684
**Email:** jbradac@niaid.nih.gov
**Website:** http://www.niaid.nih.gov/daids/vaccine
James Bradac, PhD, Chf.

**Activities/Fields:** Preclinical development and evaluation of safe and effective AIDS vaccines and adjuvants for the prevention of AIDS. **Frmly:** (2000) Preclinical Research Branch.

**★ 11920 ★ U.S. Department of Health and Human Services**
**National Institute of Allergy and Infectious Diseases**
**Division of Acquired Immunodeficiency Syndrome (AIDS)**
**Vaccine and Prevention Research Program (Efficacy Trials Branch)**
Solar Bldg., Rm. 2A-12
6003 Executive Blvd.
Bethesda, MD 20892
**Phone:** (301)496-6177 **Fax:** (301)402-3684
R. Hoff, Chf.

**Activities/Fields:** Large-scale and domestic and international clinical trials of HIV vaccines and other biomedical and behavioral interventions.

**U.S. Department of Health and Human Services**
**National Institute of Allergy and Infectious Diseases**
**Division of Extramural Activities**
*See:* Entry 3277

**U.S. Department of Health and Human Services**
**National Institute of Allergy and Infectious Diseases**
**Division of Extramural Activities**
**Contract Management Branch**
*See:* Entry 3278

**U.S. Department of Health and Human Services**
**National Institute of Allergy and Infectious Diseases**
**Division of Extramural Activities**
**Grants Management Branch**
*See:* Entry 3279

**U.S. Department of Health and Human Services**
**National Institute of Allergy and Infectious Diseases**
**Division of Intramural Research**
*See:* Entry 3280

**★ 11921 ★ U.S. Department of Health and Human Services**
**National Institute of Allergy and Infectious Diseases**
**Division of Microbiology and Infectious Diseases**
**Bacteriology and Mycology Branch**
6700 B. Rockledge Dr., MSC-7630
Bethesda, MD 20892-7630
**Phone:** (301)496-7728 **Fax:** (301)402-2508
**Email:** tk9c@nih.gov
**Website:** http://www.niaid.nih.gov/dir/default.htm
Dr. Dennis M. Dixon, Chf.

**Activities/Fields:** Diseases of man caused by bacteria and fungi, including: investigations on the biology and physiology of bacteria and fungi, their morphology, antigenic structure and composition, and toxins and endotoxins; and studies on pathogenesis, immunopathology, host defense mechanisms, diagnostic procedures, therapeutic measures, animal models, and the epidemiology of disease. Specific disease program areas include: medical mycology, turberculosis, and leprosy; hospital-associated infections; and streptococcal diseases and sequelae; and vector-borne bacterial diseases including Lyme disease. Other diseases and problem areas, such as Legionnaires' disease, listeriosis, mycoplasma infections, brucell osis, and anaerobic infections, are also investigated.

**★ 11922 ★ U.S. Department of Health and Human Services**
**National Institute of Allergy and Infectious Diseases**
**Division of Microbiology and Infectious Diseases**
**Enteric Diseases Branch**
6700 B Rockledge Dr.
Room 3109
MSC 7630
Bethesda, MD 20892
**Phone:** (301)496-7051 **Fax:** (301)402-1456
Dr. Leslye Johnson, Chf.

**Activities/Fields:** Bacterial and viral enteric diseases, viral hepatitis, hepatitis antiviral drug development, hepatitis C, helicobacter pylori, and mucosal immunity.

**★ 11923 ★ U.S. Department of Health and Human Services**
**National Institute of Allergy and Infectious Diseases**
**Division of Microbiology and Infectious Diseases**
**Parasitology and International Programs Branch**
Solar Bldg., Rm. 3A10
Bethesda, MD 20892
**Phone:** (301)496-2544 **Fax:** (301)402-0659
**Email:** sj13y@nih.gov
**Website:** http://www.niaid.nih.gov/dmid/dmidover.htm
Dr. Stephanie James, Chf.

**Activities/Fields:** Host/parasite and vector relationships, with the ultimate goal of controlling parasitic diseases through such procedures as chemoprophylaxis, immunoprophylaxis, chemotherapy, and vector control. Research projects involve parasitology and medical entomology and use a broad spectrum of multidisciplinary approaches, including immunology, molecular biology, and biochemistry. Emphasis is directed toward studies on the infectious diseases of developing countries, through special programs on tropical disease research. As a means of stimulating research on schistosomiasis and filariasis, NIAID also supports two contracts to provide investigators with animals and vectors infected with various species of both these parasites.

★ 11924 ★ **U.S. Department of Health and Human Services**
**National Institute of Allergy and Infectious Diseases**
**Division of Microbiology and Infectious Diseases**
**Respiratory Diseases Branch**
6700B Rockledge Dr.
Room 3143
Bethesda, MD 20892
**Phone:** (301)496-1884     **Fax:** (301)480-4528
**Email:** pm23v@nih.gov
Dr. Pamela McInnes, Deputy Director

**Activities/Fields:** Acute respiratory disease. Maintains programs in influenza, bacterial and viral respiratory disease, bacterial and viral vaccines, tuberculosis, pertussis, and pneumonia.

★ 11925 ★ **U.S. Department of Health and Human Services**
**National Institute of Allergy and Infectious Diseases**
**Division of Mirobiology and Infectious Diseases**
**Virology Branch**
7600-B Rockledge Dr.
Bethesda
Bethesda, MD 20892
**Phone:** (301)496-7453     **Fax:** (301)480-1594
**Email:** cl28r@nih.gov
Dr. Catherine Laughlin, Chf.

**Activities/Fields:** SUPs grant and contract research on viral infections other than HIV and on prevention and treatment of these infections.

**U.S. Department of Health and Human Services**
**National Institute of Allergy and Infectious Diseases**
**Laboratory of Clinical Investigation**
*See:* Entry 3282

★ 11926 ★ **U.S. Department of Health and Human Services**
**National Institute of Allergy and Infectious Diseases**
**Laboratory of Infectious Diseases**
NIH 50 Room 6134
9000 Rockville Pike
Bethesda, MD 20892
**Phone:** (301)496-2024     **Fax:** (301)496-8312
Robert M. Chanock, MD, Sr. Investigator

**Activities/Fields:** Defines the cause and epidemiology of medically important viral diseases and develops means for their control. Activities range from identification and antigenic characterization of viruses that cause acute disease of the respiratory and gastrointestinal tracts and liver to basic molecular studies of viral structure, function, and genome organization. Molecular biologic techniques are used to elucidate pathogenesis of disease as well as to develop purified subunit antigens and attenuated viral mutants for use in prevention of respiratory, gastrointestinal, and hepatic viral diseases.

★ 11927 ★ **U.S. Department of Health and Human Services**
**National Institute of Allergy and Infectious Diseases**
**Laboratory of Microbial Structure and Function**
Rocky Mountain Laboratories
903 S 4th St.
Hamilton, MT 59840
**Phone:** (406)363-3211     **Fax:** (406)363-9394
**Email:** jmusser@niaid.nih.gov
**Website:** http://www.niaid.nih.gov
Dr. James Musser, Chf.

**Activities/Fields:** Structural and functional elements of pathogenic bacterial surface components involved in pathogenesis and/or virulence of selected organisms or in genesis of host immunological responses to infections by these agents. Studies involve *Neissera gonorrhoeae*, *Borellia burgdorferi*, and others; both protein and nonprotein components of these gram-negative organism outer membrane are prime study candidates as mediators of interactions between bacterium and host and as likely vaccine components. Chemical characteristics, immunochemical properties, and genetic control of selected surface proponents are investigated to delineate their relationship to infectious disease phenomena of these bacteria. **Pub:** *Proceedings.* • *Research Reports*.

★ 11928 ★ **U.S. Department of Health and Human Services**
**National Institute of Allergy and Infectious Diseases**
**Laboratory of Molecular Microbiology**
NIH Bldg. 4, Rm. 315
4 Center Dr., MSC 0460
Bethesda, MD 20892-0460
**Phone:** (301)496-4012     **Fax:** (301)402-0226
Dr. Malcolm A. Martin, Chf.

**Activities/Fields:** Microorganisms and their capacity to produce disease in vertebrate hosts. Of prime importance in this effort is the biochemical characterization of viral genomes and the detailed analyses of gene products regulating expression or giving rise to mature structural proteins. A principal area of investigation has been the human immunodeficiency virus (HIV), with classical virological procedures used for the detection, quantitation, and biological characterization of HIV isolates of diverse origin. Biochemical and molecular biological techniques such as nucleic acid hybridization, gene cloning, DNA sequencing, in vitro mutagenesis, and transfection are used in combination with procedures such as immunoprecipitation or protein purification to study individual viral genes or potentially infectious proviral DNAs in order to assess structure/function relationships. Programs involving murine retroviruses concentrate on those portions of the viral genome that encode proteins that initiate and/or maintain the transformed state. The roles of host cellular determinants that augment or diminish disease/oncogenesis are also investigated.

**U.S. Department of Health and Human Services**
**National Institute of Allergy and Infectious Diseases (NIAID)**
**Laboratory of Molecular Structure**
*See:* Entry 3287

★ 11929 ★ **U.S. Department of Health and Human Services**
**National Institute of Allergy and Infectious Diseases**
**Laboratory of Persistent Viral Diseases**
Rocky Mountain Laboratories
903 S 4th St.
Hamilton, MT 59840
**Phone:** (406)363-9354     **Fax:** (406)363-9286
**Email:** bchesebro@nih.gov
Bruce Chesebro, MD, Chf.

**Activities/Fields:** Virus-host interaction, with the primary aim of elucidating mechanisms involved in establishment, maintenance, and elimination of persistent viral infections. Particular emphasis is placed on persistent viral infections involving cells of the hemopoietic and lymphoid systems and the central nervous system. The role of persistent infection in the development of autoimmune or immune complex disease is also studied. Models examined include human AIDS retrovirus and murine retroviruses, rabies virus, Aleutian disease virus of mink, and the agent of scrapie and other transmissable spongiform encephalopathies of humans and animals.

★ 11930 ★ **U.S. Department of Health and Human Services**
**National Institute of Allergy and Infectious Diseases**
**Laboratory of Viral Diseases**
NIH Bldg. 4, Rm. 229A
4 Center Dr., MSC0445
Bethesda, MD 20892-0445
**Phone:** (301)496-9869     **Fax:** (301)480-1147
**Email:** bmoss@nih.gov
**Website:** http://www.niaid.nih.gov/dir/labs/lvd.htm
Dr. Bernard Moss, Chf.

**Activities/Fields:** Genetic organization, expression, replication, assembly, and pathogenicity of viruses. Live recombinant viruses are genetically engineered for use as immunological tools and as vaccines against a variety of infectious agents. Current research topics include: regulation of gene expression in vitro and in vivo; mechanisms of DNA replication in vitro and in vivo; structure and function of RNA and DNA polymerases; genetic engineering of recombinant viruses as live vaccines; antiviral agents; determinants of virus virulence; host resistance genes; viral growth factors; and targets of humoral and cell-mediated immunity.

**U.S. Department of Health and Human Services**
**National Institute of Allergy and Infectious Diseases**
**Office of Administrative Management**
**Extramural Administrative Management Branch**
*See:* Entry 3288

**U.S. Department of Health and Human Services**
**National Institute of Allergy and Infectious Diseases**
**Office of Communications**
*See:* Entry 3289

**U.S. Department of Health and Human Services**
**National Institute of Allergy and Infectious Diseases**
**Office of Policy Analysis**
*See:* Entry 3290

**U.S. Department of Health and Human Services**
**National Institute of Allergy and Infectious Diseases**
**Rocky Mountain Laboratories**
**Administrative and Facilities Management Section**
*See:* Entry 3291

**U.S. Department of Health and Human Services**
**National Institute of Dental Research**
**Division of Extramural Research**
**Oral Soft Tissue Diseases and AIDS Program**
*See:* Entry 6620

**U.S. Department of Health and Human Services**
**National Institutes of Health**
**Frederick Cancer Research and Development Center**
*See:* Entry 10507

**U.S. Department of Health and Human Services**
**National Institutes of Health**
**National Cancer Institute**
*See:* Entry 10508

**U.S. Department of Health and Human Services**
**National Institutes of Health**
**National Cancer Institute**
**Division of Basic Sciences**
**(Laboratory of Leukocyte Biology)**
*See:* Entry 10517

**U.S. Department of Health and Human Services**
**National Institutes of Health**
**National Cancer Institute (NCI)**
**Division of Basic Sciences**
**(HIV Drug Resistance Program — DRP)**
*See:* Entry 10518

**U.S. Department of Health and Human Services**
**National Institutes of Health**
**National Cancer Institute**
**Division of Clinical Sciences**
**(HIV and AIDS Malignancy Branch — HAMB)**
*See:* Entry 10559

**U.S. Department of Health and Human Services**
**National Institutes of Health**
**National Cancer Institute**
**Division of Clinical Sciences**
**((HIV and AIDS Malignancy Branch — HAMB)**
**Pediatric HIV Working Group — PHWG)**
*See:* Entry 10562

**★ 11931 ★ U.S. Department of Health and Human Services**
**National Institutes of Health**
**National Institute of Allergy and Infectious Diseases**
**Division of Intramural Research**
**(Laboratory of Host Defenses)**
Bldg. 10, Rm. 11N113
10 Center Dr.
MSC 1886
Bethesda, MD 20892-1886
**Phone:** (301)496-1343　　**Fax:** (301)402-4369
**Email:** jg21z@nih.gov
**Website:** http://www.niaid.nih.gov/dir/labs/lhd.htm
John I. Gallin, MD, Ch.

**Activities/Fields:** Mechanisms of host defense against bacterial and fungal infections, particularly the biochemistry, function and structure of phagocytic cells, including peripheral blood polymorphonuclear leukocytes (neutrophils), eosinophils, and monocytes, and fixed-tissue macrophages.

**★ 11932 ★ U.S. Department of Health and Human Services**
**National Institutes of Health**
**National Institute of Allergy and Infectious Diseases**
**Division of Intramural Research**
**(Laboratory of Intracellular Parasites)**
Rocky Mountain Laboratories
903 S 4th St.
Hamilton, MT 59840
**Phone:** (406)363-9233　　**Fax:** (406)363-9355
**Email:** harlan_caldwell@nih.gov
**Website:** http://www.niaid.nih.gov/dir/labs/licp.htm
Harlan D. Caldwell, PhD, Ch.

**Activities/Fields:** Immunologic and pathologic aspects of infections caused by intracellular prokaryotes, including chlamydia, mycobacteria, and chlamydia trachomatis.

**★ 11933 ★ U.S. Department of Health and Human Services**
**National Institutes of Health**
**National Institute of Dental and Craniofacial Research**
**Division of Intramural Research**
**(Oral Infection and Immunity Branch)**
Bldg. 30, Rm. 332
30 Convent Dr., MSC 4352
Bethesda, MD 20892-4352
**Phone:** (301)496-9218　　**Fax:** (301)402-1064
**Email:** sharon.wahl@nih.gov
**Website:** http://wwwdir.nidcr.nih.gov/dirweb/oiib/oiib.asp
Dr. Sharon M. Wahl, Dir.

**Activities/Fields:** Infectious pathogens, their unique attributes and virulence factors to provide insight into mechanisms of disarming them, especially the mucosal immune system.

**U.S. Department of Health and Human Services**
**National Institutes of Health**
**National Institute of Dental and Craniofacial Research**
**Division of Intramural Research**
**(Peptide and Immunochemistry Unit)**
*See:* Entry 3293

**★ 11934 ★ U.S. Department of Health and Human Services**
**National Institutes of Health**
**National Institute of Diabetes and Digestive and Kidney Diseases**
**Division of Diabetes, Endocrinology, and Metabolic Diseases**
**(Acquired Immunodeficiency Syndrome (AIDS) and Human Immunodeficiency Virus (HIV) Program)**
2 Democracy Plz., Rm. 669
Bethesda, MD 20892
**Phone:** (301)594-8877
**Email:** hamiltonf@ep.niddk.nih.gov
**Website:** http://www.niddk.nih.gov/program/A-El-ist.htmauto
Frank Hamilton, MD, Dir.

**Activities/Fields:** Characterization of intestinal injury, mechanisms of maldigestion, and intestinal mucosal functions, as well as hepatic and biliary dysfunction in patients with AIDS or in appropriate animal models.

**★ 11935 ★ U.S. Department of Health and Human Services**
**National Institutes of Health**
**National Institute of Mental Health**
**Laboratory of Cellular and Molecular Regulation**
**(Section on Molecular Virology)**
Bldg. 10, Rm. 3A05
9000 Rockville Pike
Bethesda, MD 20892
**Phone:** (301)402-1641
**Email:** m_eiden@codon.nih.gov
**Website:** http://intramural.nimh.nih.gov/research/lcmr
Maribeth Eiden, PhD, Ch.

**Activities/Fields:** Use of retroviruses such as gibbon ape leukemia virus (GALV) to study the process of viral entry. Aims to identify new intracellular protein actors as well as development of efficient viral vectors.

**★ 11936 ★ U.S. Department of Health and Human Services**
**National Institutes of Health**
**National Institute of Mental Health**
**Laboratory of Molecular Biology**
**(Unit on Lymphocyte Function)**
Bldg. 36, Rm. 1B08
9000 Rockville Pike
Bethesda, MD 20892
**Phone:** (301)496-4864　　**Fax:** (301)402-0245
**Email:** nimhinfo@nih.gov
**Website:** http://intramural.nimh.nih.gov/research/lmb/
Jon W. Marsh, PhD, Ch.

**Activities/Fields:** Immunological and central nervous system (CNS) dysfunction. Studies the cellular biochemical alterations generated by the expression of HIV accessory proteins, in particular, the HIV virulence factor NEF, the way this protein associated with an active serine kinase, Pak, and affects activation pathways critical to normal function of both the immunological and nervous systems, and the role these proteins play in pathogenesis.

**★ 11937 ★ U.S. Department of Health and Human Services**
**National Institutes of Health**
**Office of AIDS Research**
Bldg. 2 Room 4E 14
Two Center Dr. MSC 0250
Bethesda, MD 20892
**Phone:** (301)496-0357　　**Fax:** (301)496-2119
Dr. Jack Whitescarvre, Act. Dir.

**Activities/Fields:** Advises the Director, NIH, and senior staff on the development of NIH-wide policy related to AIDS research, and coordinates NIH intramural and extramural AIDS research activities; Represents the Director, NIH, on all outside AIDS-related committees requiring NIH participation; Provides staff support to the NIH AIDS Advisory Committee; Recommends Intramural/Extramural AIDS research priorities to the Director, NIH; Develops an NIH annual plan and budget for AIDS research; Develops and maintains an information database on Intramural/Extramural AIDS activities and prepares special or recurring reports as needed; Develops information strategies to assure the public is informed of NIH AIDS research activities; Recommends solutions to ethical/legal issues arising from AIDS research; Facilitates cooperation in AIDS research between government, industry, and universities; and Fosters and develops plans for NIH involvement in international AIDS research activities.

**U.S. Department of Veterans Affairs**
**Veterans Health Administration**
**Office of Research and Development**
**Medical Research Service**
**(AIDS Research Center )**
*See:* Entry 13509

**U.S. Department of Veterans Affairs**
**Veterans Health Administration**
**Office of Research and Development**
**Medical Research Service**
**(AIDS Research Center )**
*See:* Entry 13510

**University of Alabama at Birmingham**
**Ob/Gyn Infectious Disease Research Laboratory**
*See:* Entry 16740

**★ 11938 ★ University of California, Davis**
**AIDS Virus Diagnostic Laboratory**
1 Shields Ave.
Davis, CA 95616-8542
**Phone:** (530)752-8242　　**Fax:** (530)752-4816
**Email:** jcarlson@clb.ucdmc.ucdavis.edu
James R. Carlson, PhD, Dir.

**Activities/Fields:** Human immunodeficiency virus (HIV) serology, HIV production and purification, bioassays of HIV inactivation, comparative retrovirology, and vaccine development.

**★ 11939 ★ University of California, Davis**
**Center for Comparative Medicine (CCM)**
1 Shields Ave.
Davis, CA 95616
**Phone:** (530)752-7913　　　　**Fax:** (530)752-7914
**Website:** http://ccm.ucdavis.edu
Stephen Barthold, PhD, Dir.

**Activities/Fields:** Persistent infectious diseases common to humans and animals, especially host-agent interactions and intervention strategies.

**★ 11940 ★ University of California, San Diego**
**Center for AIDS Research (CFAR)**
9500 Gilman Dr., MC 0616
La Jolla, CA 92093-0616
**Phone:** (858)534-5545　　　　**Fax:** (858)822-1934
**Email:** csussman@ucsd.edu
**Website:** http://www.ari.ucsd.edu/cfar/cfar.html
Douglas Richman, MD, Dir.

**Activities/Fields:** Development of improved vaccines and therapies for HIV infection and associated diseases through the study of molecular pathogenesis and immunopathogenesis of HIV infection and clinical trials of therapies and vaccines. **Pub:** *Newsletter.*

**★ 11941 ★ University of California, San Francisco**
**AIDS Research Institute (ARI)**
CB 0886
74 New Montgomery, Ste. 600
San Francisco, CA 94105
**Phone:** (415)597-9203　　　　**Fax:** (415)597-9213
**Email:** ari@psg.ucsf.edu
**Website:** http://hivinsite.ucsf.edu/ari
Thomas J. Coates, PhD, Dir.

**Activities/Fields:** AIDS vaccine, new therapies, transmission dynamics and prevention, AIDS policy and ethics. **Pub:** *ARI Newsletter.*

**★ 11942 ★ University of California, San Francisco**
**California AIDS Research Center (C-ARC)**
Department of Stomatology, Rm. S-612
PO Box 0422
San Francisco, CA 94143-0422
**Phone:** (415)476-5415　　　　**Fax:** (415)476-4204
**Email:** greenspanj@dentistry.ucsf.edu
Dr. John S. Greenspan, Dir.

**Activities/Fields:** Understanding the mechanisms by which HIV infection is avoided or slowed and translational studies to understand how to make these findings clinically relevant. The center is organized around 4 research themes: natural immunity resistance to infection, role of CXCR4 signaling in CD8+ T-cell apoptosis during HIV infection, dissecting the molecular basis for virologic but not immunologic failure in HIV-infected patients receiving protease inhibitor therapy, and transmission of drug-resistant HIV-1.

**University of California, San Francisco**
**Center for AIDS Prevention Studies (CAPS)**
*See:* Entry 17838

**★ 11943 ★ University of California, San Francisco**
**George Williams Hooper Foundation**
513 Parnassus Ave., HSW1501
San Francisco, CA 94143-0552
**Phone:** (415)476-5157　　　　**Fax:** (415)476-6185
**Email:** gracest@itsa.ucsf.edu

**Website:** http://www.caps.ucsf.edu/capsweb
Dr. J. Michael Bishop, Dir.

**Activities/Fields:** Cancer biology; genetics and physiology of mammalian cells and organisms; animal models resembling human cancers; and cell biology, immunology and the pathogenesis of infectious diseases.

**★ 11944 ★ University of California, San Francisco**
**Oral AIDS Center (OAC)**
513 Parnassus Ave.
San Francisco, CA 94143-0422
**Phone:** (415)476-5415　　　　**Fax:** (415)476-4204
**Email:** greenspanj@dentistry.ucsf.edu
**Website:** http://itsa.ucsf.edu/~ucstoma/Oac.htm
Dr. John S. Greenspan, Dir.

**Activities/Fields:** Oral manifestations of HIV infection.

**★ 11945 ★ University of Georgia**
**Drug Discovery Group**
College of Pharmacy
Athens, GA 30602-2352
**Phone:** (706)542-5379　　　　**Fax:** (706)542-5381
**Email:** dchu@rx.uga.edu
**Website:** http://www.rx.uga.edu/main/home/chug-roup/
Prof. David C.K. Chu, Contact

**Activities/Fields:** Design and discovery of compounds for the treatment of various emerging infectious diseases. The main area of research includes the structure-based drug design and synthesis of novel agents against human immunodeficiency virus (HIV), hepatitis B virus (HBV), hepatitis C virus (HCV), and drug resistant bacteria as well as agents against cancer.

**★ 11946 ★ University of Hawaii**
**Hawaii AIDS Clinical Research Program**
Leahi Hospital
Young Bldg., 6th Fl.
3675 Kilauea Ave.
Honolulu, HI 96816
**Phone:** (808)737-2751　　　　**Fax:** (808)735-7047
**Email:** shikuma@hawaii.edu
Cecilia M. Shikuma, MD, Dir.

**Activities/Fields:** AIDS, HIV, and complications of HIV.

**★ 11947 ★ University of Maryland**
**Division of Infectious Diseases**
Medical Sch. Teaching Facility
10 S Pine St., Rm. 900
Baltimore, MD 21201
**Phone:** (410)706-7560　　　　**Fax:** (410)706-8700
Michael Bonnenberg, Hd.

**Activities/Fields:** Infections in the elderly, including infection from urinary catheterization, epidemiology of nursing home patients, tests of antimicrobial agents, and pharmacokinetics and microbiology using animal models and clinical techniques.

**★ 11948 ★ University of Maryland**
**Medical Biotechnology Center**
**Institute of Human Virology**
725 W Lombard St.
Baltimore, MD 21201
**Phone:** (410)706-8614　　　　**Fax:** (410)706-1952
Robert C. Gallo, MD, Dir.

**Activities/Fields:** Chronic viral diseases and virally-linked cancers, specifically HIV/AIDS. **Pub:** *Discovery,* quarterly. • *Journal of Human Virology,* bimonthly.

**★ 11949 ★ University of Maryland at Baltimore**
**Center for Vaccine Development (CVD)**
685 W Baltimore St., Rm. 480
Baltimore, MD 21201-1509

**Phone:** (410)706-5328　　　　**Fax:** (410)706-6205
**Email:** cvd@medicine.umaryland.edu
**Website:** http://medschool.umaryland.edu/CVD/
Myron M. Levine, MD, Dir.

**Activities/Fields:** Bacterial diseases, parasitic diseases, viral diseases, novel delivery systems, combination vaccines and public health and policy.

**University of Medicine and Dentistry of New Jersey**
**Lyme Disease Center**
*See:* Entry 13728

**★ 11950 ★ University of Miami**
**Center for Tropical and Parasitic Diseases**
Medical School
1600 NW 10th Ave.
Miami, FL 33136
**Phone:** (305)243-3116　　　　**Fax:** (305)243-3888
**Email:** aager@med.miami.edu
Dr. Arba Ager, Dir.

**Activities/Fields:** All aspects of malaria, including malaria drug testing in rodents. Also conducts nutritional and chemotherapy research.

**★ 11951 ★ University of North Carolina at Chapel Hill**
**Center for AIDS Research (CFAR)**
Lineberger Comprehensive Cancer Center, CB 7295
Chapel Hill, NC 27599
**Phone:** (919)966-8645
**Email:** mohr4me@med.unc.edu
**Website:** http://www.cfar.unc.edu/
Ronald I. Swanstrom, PhD, Dir.

**Activities/Fields:** Prevention, detection, and treatment of HIV infection.

**University of Oklahoma Health Sciences Center**
**Center for American Indian Health Research**
*See:* Entry 2710

**★ 11952 ★ University of Quebec**
**National Institute for Scientific Research-Armand-Frappier Institute**
**Virology Research Centre**
531 Blvd. des Prairies
PO Box 100
Laval, QC, Canada H7N 4Z3
**Phone:** (450)686-5515　　　　**Fax:** (450)686-5626
**Email:** chris-mcglory@ouhsc.edu
**Website:** http://w3.ouhsc.edu/coph/CophSub/CAIHRtxt.htm
Dr. Max Arella, Dir.

**Activities/Fields:** Molecular virology, ecovirology, and biotechnology, including studies on the mechanisms of viral transmission, interactions between viruses-hosts and environment, new viral vaccines, applications of monoclonal antibodies and DNA probes to viral diagnostics, use of insect viruses as expression vectors and biological control agents. **Pub:** *Annual Report.* • *Triennial Plan.*

**★ 11953 ★ University of Rochester**
**Aab Institute of Biomedical Sciences**
**Center for Vaccine Biology and Immunology**
601 Elmwood Ave., Box 609
Rochester, NY 14642
**Phone:** (716)275-9120　　　　**Fax:** (716)273-2452
**Email:** tim_mosmann@urmc.rochester.edu
**Website:** http://www.urmc.rochester.edu/Aab/vacc-bio/
Tim Mosmann, PhD, Dir.

**Activities/Fields:** Vaccines for difficult infectious diseases such as tuberculosis, malaria and AIDS, and creation of new types of vaccines for treating cancer, allergy and autoimmunity.

**★ 11954 ★ University of South Florida**
**Center for HIV Education and Research**
13301 Bruce B. Downs Blvd.
Tampa, FL 33612-3899
**Phone:** (813)974-4430  **Fax:** (813)974-8451
**Email:** knox@fmhi.usf.edu
**Website:** http://www.fmhi.usf.edu/hiv
Prof. Michael D. Knox, Dir.
**Activities/Fields:** Treatment of persons infected with HIV, study of HIV risk factors, and AIDS prevention. Provides current AIDS and HIV information to physicians, psychologists, dentists, nurses, and other health care providers.

**★ 11955 ★ University of Southern**
**California**
**Infectious Disease Research Laboratories**
General Research Laboratory, Rm. 2G4
LAC-USC Med. Center
1801 E Marengo
Los Angeles, CA 90033
**Phone:** (323)226-3825  **Fax:** (323)226-3827
**Email:** holtom@hsc.usc.edu
Dr. Paul Holtom, Dir.
**Activities/Fields:** Infectious diseases, bacteriology, and miscellaneous antibiotic trials.

**University of Texas Southwestern Medical**
**Center at Dallas**
**Cancer Immunobiology Center (CIC)**
*See:* Entry 10635

**★ 11956 ★ University of Virginia**
**Myles Thaler Center for AIDS and Human**
**Retrovirus Research**
PO Box 800743
Charlottesville, VA 22908
**Phone:** (434)982-1597  **Fax:** (434)982-1590
**Email:** thalercenter@virginia.edu
**Website:** http://www.med.virginia.edu/medcntr/centers/thaler/home.html
Prof. David Rekosh, PhD, Dir.
**Activities/Fields:** Human retrovirus life cycle, viral regulatory genes, viral assembly and viral entry.

**Wayne State University**
**Center for Molecular Medicine and**
**Genetics**
*See:* Entry 9529

## State Government Agencies

### AIDS

**★ 11957 ★ Alabama Department of**
**Public Health**
**HIV / AIDS Division**
RSA Tower
201 Monroe St., Ste. 1450
PO Box 303017
Montgomery, AL 36130-3017
**Phone:** (334)206-5364  **Fax:** (334)206-2092
**Email:** info@genetics.wayne.edu
**Website:** http://www.adph.org/aids/
Jane B. Cheeks, JD, Director

**★ 11958 ★ Alaska Department of Health**
**and Social Services**
**Public Health Division**
**Epidemiology Section**
3601 C St., Ste. 540
PO Box 240249
Anchorage, AK 99524-0249
**Phone:** (907)269-8000  **Free:** 800-478-0084
**Fax:** (907)562-7802
**Email:** epiweb@epi.hss.state.ak.us
**Website:** http://www.epi.hss.state.ak.us/

**★ 11959 ★ Arizona Department of Health**
**Services**
**Office of Infectious Diseases**
**Offices of HIV / STD Services**
3815 N Black Canyon Hwy.
Phoenix, AZ 85015
**Phone:** (602)230-5932  **Fax:** (602)263-4943
**Email:** webmaster@hs.state.az.us
**Website:** http://www.hs.state.az.us/edc/hivpage.html
Christopher Brown, MBA, Director

**★ 11960 ★ California Health and Welfare**
**Agency**
**Health Services Department**
**Office of AIDS**
611 N 7th St., Ste. A
Sacramento, CA 95814-0208
**Phone:** (916)445-0553  **Fax:** (916)323-4642
**Email:** adarr@dhs.ca.gov
**Website:** http://www.dhs.cahwnet.gov/org/ps/ooa/ooaindex.htm

**★ 11961 ★ Connecticut Department of**
**Public Health**
**Bureau of Community Health**
**AIDS Division**
410 Capitol Ave.
PO Box 340308
Hartford, CT 06134-0308
**Phone:** (860)509-7801  **Free:** 800-509-7900
**Fax:** (860)509-7853
**Email:** webmaster.dph@po.state.ct.us
**Website:** http://www.dph.state.ct.us/BCH/AIDS/HPAIDS.html
Rosa M. Biaggi, MPH, Director

**★ 11962 ★ Delaware Department of**
**Health and Social Services**
**Division of Public Health**
**Disease Prevention and Control**
**HIV / AIDS Epidemiology Program**
Jesse Cooper Bldg.
Federal & Water St.
PO Box 637
Dover, DE 19903
**Phone:** (302)739-2354  **Fax:** (302)739-6659
**Email:** dhsinfo@state.de.us
**Website:** http://www.delaware-epi.org/aids1.htm

**★ 11963 ★ Florida Department of Health**
**Health & Human Services**
**Bureau of HIV / AIDS**
4052 Bald Cypress Way, Bin A09
Tallahassee, FL 32399-1715
**Phone:** (850)245-4444
**Email:** health@doh.state.fl.us
**Website:** http://www9.myflorida.com/aids/index.html
Tom Liberti, Director

**★ 11964 ★ Georgia Department of**
**Human Resources**
**Public Health Division**
**Epidemiology Branch**
**HIV/STD Epidemiology Unit**
2 Peachtree St. NW
Atlanta, GA 30303-3186
**Phone:** (404)657-2588

**Email:** gaepinfo@dhr.state.ga.us
**Website:** http://www.ph.dhr.state.ga.us/epi/aidsunit.shtml
John F. Beltrami, MD, Director

**★ 11965 ★ Hawaii Department of Health**
**Health Resources Adminstration**
**STD / AIDS Prevention Branch**
3627 Kilauea Ave., Room 306
Honolulu, HI 96816
**Phone:** (808)733-9010  **Fax:** (808)733-9015
**Website:** http://www.state.hi.us/health/resource/comm_dis/std_aids/index.html
Peter M. Whiticar, Director

**★ 11966 ★ Illinois Department of Public**
**Health**
**Office of Health Protection**
**AIDS Activities Section**
525 W Jefferson St., 2nd Fl.
Springfield, IL 62761-0001
**Phone:** (217)782-3984  **Fax:** (217)524-0802
**Email:** thughes@idph.state.il.us
**Website:** http://www.idph.state.il.us/about/ohp.htm
Tom Hughes, Director

**★ 11967 ★ Iowa Department of Public**
**Health**
**Bureau of Disease Prevention**
**HIV / AIDS Program**
Lucas State Office Bldg.
321 E 12th St.
Des Moines, IA 50319-0075
**Phone:** (515)242-5838  **Fax:** (515)281-4958
**Email:** pyoung@idph.state.ia.us
**Website:** http://www.idph.state.ia.us/fch/inf_dis/hiv-aids.htm
Patricia Young, Director

**★ 11968 ★ Kansas Department of Health**
**and Environment**
**Division of Health**
**HIV - STD Section**
1000 SW Jackson, Ste. 210
Topeka, KS 66612-1274
**Phone:** (785)296-6173  **Fax:** (785)296-4197
**Email:** kmilhon@kdhe.state.ks.us
**Website:** http://www.kdhe.state.ks.us/hiv-std/index.html
Karl Milhon, Director

**★ 11969 ★ Louisiana Department of**
**Health and Hospitals**
**Office of Public Health**
**HIV / AIDS Services**
234 Loyola Ave., 5th Floor
New Orleans, LA 70112
**Phone:** (504)568-7474  **Fax:** (504)568-7044
**Email:** hivweb@dhh.state.la.us
**Website:** http://www.dhh.state.la.us/OPH/hivstd/Default.htm
Beth Scalco, Director

**★ 11970 ★ Maine Department of Human**
**Services**
**Health Bureau**
**Disease Control Division**
11 State House Station
Augusta, ME 04333
**Phone:** (207)287-6448  **Fax:** (207)287-3498
**Email:** sallylou.patterson@state.me.us
**Website:** http://www.state.me.us/dhs/boh/ddc/HIV_STD.htm
Sally-Lou Patterson, Director

**★ 11971 ★ Massachusetts Executive Office of Health and Human Services**
**Public Health Department**
**HIV / AIDS Bureau**
250 Washington St., 3d Fl.
Boston, MA 02108
**Phone:** (617)624-5300　　**Fax:** (617)624-5399
**Email:** dph.info@state.ma.us
**Website:** http://www.state.ma.us/dph/aids/hivaids.htm
Jean Flatley McGuire, PhD, Director

**★ 11972 ★ Michigan Department of Community Health**
**HIV / AIDS - STD Division**
Ste. 300
2479 Woodlake Circle
Okemos, MI 48864
**Phone:** (517)241-5900　　**Fax:** (517)241-5911
**Email:** arias@state.mi.us
**Website:** http://www.mdch.state.mi.us/dch/hiv_aids.htm
James K. Haveman, Jr., Director

**★ 11973 ★ Minnesota Department of Health**
**STD and HIV Section**
717 Delaware St. SE
PO Box 64975
Saint Paul, MN 55164-0975
**Phone:** (651)215-5800　　**Fax:** (651)623-5743
**Email:** jan.wiehle@health.state.mn.us
**Website:** http://www.health.state.mn.us/divs/dpc/aids-std/aids-std.htm
Jan Wiehle, Contact

**★ 11974 ★ Missouri Department of Health & Senior Services**
**Section of STD / HIV**
930 Wildwood Dr.
PO Box 570
Jefferson City, MO 65102-0570
**Phone:** (573)751-6439　　**Free:** 800-392-0272
**Fax:** (573)751-6447
**Email:** info@dhss.state.mo.us
**Website:** http://www.health.state.mo.us/sshapcs/SSHAPCS.html

**★ 11975 ★ Montana Department of Public Health and Human Services**
**Health Policy and Services Division**
**Disease Prevention & Control**
**STD / AIDS Program**
1400 Broadway
PO Box 202951
Helena, MT 59620-2951
**Phone:** (406)444-9028　　**Fax:** (406)444-6842
**Email:** bdeitle@state.mt.us
**Website:** http://www.dphhs.state.mt.us/hpsd/pubheal/disease/stdhiv/index.htm
Bruce Deitle, Director

**★ 11976 ★ Nebraska Department of Health and Human Services**
**Health Promotion and Disease Prevention**
**Communicable Disease Section**
**HIV Prevention Program**
301 Centennial Mall S
PO Box 94817
Lincoln, NE 68509-4817
**Phone:** (402)471-9098　　**Free:** 800-782-2437
**Fax:** (402)471-0382
**Email:** charles.housman@hhss.state.ne.us
**Website:** http://www.hhs.state.ne.us/dpc/HIV.htm
Dan Cillessen, Director

**★ 11977 ★ New Hampshire Department of Health and Human Services**
**Office of Community & Public Health**
**HIV Prevention Program**
6 Hazen Dr.
Concord, NH 03301
**Phone:** (603)271-4502　　**Free:** 800-852-3345
**Fax:** (603)271-4934
**Website:** http://www.dhhs.state.nh.us/DHHS/HIVPREVENTION/default.htm/

**★ 11978 ★ North Carolina Department of Health and Human Services**
**HIV / STD Prevention & Care Branch**
1902 Mail Service Ctr.
Raleigh, NC 27699-1902
**Phone:** (919)733-7301　　**Fax:** (919)733-1020
**Email:** betsy.school@ncmail.net
**Website:** http://www.schs.state.nc.us/epi/hiv/

**★ 11979 ★ North Dakota Department of Health**
**Disease Control Division**
**HIV / AIDS Section**
**AIDS Program**
600 E Boulevard, 2nd Fl.
Bismarck, ND 58505-0200
**Phone:** (701)328-2378　　**Free:** 800-472-2180
**Fax:** (701)328-2499
**Email:** kmongeon@state.nd.us
**Website:** http://www.health.state.nd.us/ndhd/prevent/disease/hiv
Karin Mongeon, Director

**★ 11980 ★ Ohio Department of Health**
**Prevention Division**
**AIDS Client Resources Section**
246 N High St.
PO Box 118
Columbus, OH 43216-0118
**Phone:** (614)466-6374　　**Fax:** (614)564-2432
**Email:** BCHSSD@gw.odh.state.oh.us
**Website:** http://www.odh.state.oh.us/ODHPrograms/AIDS/aids1.htm

**★ 11981 ★ Oklahoma Department of Health**
**Personal Health Services**
**HIV / STD Services**
1000 NE 10th St.
Oklahoma City, OK 73117
**Phone:** (405)271-4636　　**Free:** 800-535-2437
**Fax:** (405)271-3431
**Email:** michelgg@health.state.ok.us
**Website:** http://www.health.state.ok.us/PROGRAM/hivstd/index.html
Michelle Green-Gilbert, Contact

**★ 11982 ★ Oregon Department of Human Resources**
**Public Health Services**
**Sexually Transmitted Diseases Program**
800 NE Oregon St.
Portland, OR 97232
**Phone:** (503)731-4026　　**Fax:** (503)731-4608
**Email:** janet.j.karius@state.or.us
**Website:** http://www.ohd.hr.state.or.us/std/welcome.htm
Jan Karius, Director

**★ 11983 ★ Pennsylvania Department of Health**
**Public Health Programs**
**HIV and AIDS Programs**
Health and Welfare Bldg.
PO Box 90
Harrisburg, PA 17108
**Phone:** (717)783-0479　　**Free:** 877-724-3258
**Fax:** (717)772-6959

**Email:** webmaster@health.state.pa.us
**Website:** http://www.health.state.pa.us/php/HIV/default.htm

**★ 11984 ★ South Carolina Department of Health and Environmental Control**
**Bureau of Disease Control**
**STD HIV Program**
Mills/Jarrett Comples
PO Box 101106
Columbia, SC 29211-0106
**Phone:** (803)898-0749　　**Free:** 800-277-0873
**Email:** Kettinld@Columb60.dhec.state.sc.us
**Website:** http://www.scdhec.net/hs/diseasecont/disease.htm
Lynda Kettinger, Director

**★ 11985 ★ South Dakota Department of Health**
**Disease Prevention**
**HIV / AIDS Program**
615 E 4th St.
Pierre, SD 57501
**Phone:** (605)773-3737　　**Free:** 800-592-1861
**Fax:** (605)773-5509
**Email:** DOH.INFO@state.sd.us
**Website:** http://www.state.sd.us/doh/Disease/index.htm

**★ 11986 ★ Tennessee Department of Health**
**AIDS Program**
Cordell Hull Bldg.
435 5th Ave. N
Nashville, TN 37247-5281
**Phone:** (615)741-3111　　**Free:** 800-525-2437
**Fax:** (615)741-2491
**Email:** DDenton@mail.state.tn.us
**Website:** http://www.state.tn.us/health/

**★ 11987 ★ Texas Department of Health**
**HIV / STD Prevention Bureau**
1100 W 49th St.
Austin, TX 78756-3199
**Phone:** (512)490-2505　　**Free:** 888-963-7111
**Fax:** (512)458-9368
**Email:** hivstd.infoline@tdh.state.tx.us
**Website:** http://www.tdh.state.tx.us/hivstd/default.htm

**★ 11988 ★ Utah Department of Health**
**Bureau of Communicable Disease Control**
**HIV and AIDS Bureau**
288 N 1460 W
PO Box 142105
Salt Lake City, UT 84114-2105
**Phone:** (801)538-6096　　**Fax:** (801)538-9913
**Email:** tgarrett@doh.state.ut.us
**Website:** http://www.health.state.ut.us/els/hivaids/index.html

**★ 11989 ★ Vermont Department of Health**
**HIV / AIDS Program**
108 Cherry St.
PO Box 70
Burlington, VT 05402-0070
**Phone:** (802)863-7245　　**Free:** 800-244-7639
**Fax:** (802)863-7314
**Email:** webkeeper@vdh.state.vt.us
**Website:** http://www.state.vt.us/health/_hs/aids/aids.htm

**★ 11990 ★ Virginia Department of Health**
**Division of HIV / STD**
1500 E Main St., Rm.112
PO Box 2448
Richmond, VA 23218
**Phone:** (804)786-6267　　**Free:** 800-533-4148
**Fax:** (804)225-3517

**Email:** lbranch@vdh.state.va.us
**Website:** http://www.vdh.state.va.us/std/index.htm
Casey Riley, Director

**★ 11991 ★ Washington Department of Health**
**Community and Family Health Services Division**
**HIV Client Services**
PO Box 47841
Olympia, WA 98504-7841
**Phone:** (360)236-3426     **Free:** 800-272-2437
**Fax:** (360)664-2616
**Email:** Darren.Layman@doh.wa.gov
**Website:** http://www.doh.wa.gov/cfh/HIV_AIDS/Client_Svcs/default.htm
Darren Layman, Contact

**★ 11992 ★ West Virginia Department of Health and Human Resources**
**Bureau for Public Health**
**Division of Surveillance and Disease Control**
**AIDS Program**
350 Capitol St., Rm. 125
Charleston, WV 25301-3715
**Phone:** (304)558-2950     **Free:** 800-642-8244
**Fax:** (304)558-6335
**Email:** lorettahaddy@wvdhhr.org
**Website:** http://www.wvdhhr.org/bph/oehp/sdc/aids.htm
Loretta Haddy, Contact

**★ 11993 ★ Wisconsin Department of Health and Family Services**
**Public Health**
**Communicable Disease Program**
**AIDS / HIV Program**
1 W Wilson St
Madison, WI 53702
**Phone:** (608)266-1865     **Fax:** (608)264-6078
**Email:** webmaildph@dhfs.state.wi.us
**Website:** http://www.dhfs.state.wi.us/aids-hiv/index.htm

**★ 11994 ★ Wyoming Department of Health**
**HIV / AIDS / Hepatitis Program**
Hathaway Bldg., 4th Fl.
Cheyenne, WY 82002
**Phone:** (307)777-5932     **Fax:** (307)777-7382
**Email:** srente@state.wy.us
**Website:** http://wdhfs.state.wy.us/AIDS/
Sharon G. Renter, MS, Director

# Chapter 35
# Information & Communications

## Federal Government Agencies

**★ 11995 ★ U.S. Department of Health and Human Services**
**Centers for Disease Control and Prevention (CDCP)**
**National Center for Health Statistics (NCHS)**
1600 Clifton Rd. NE
Atlanta, GA 30333
**Phone:** (404)639-3311
**Website:** http://www.cdc.gov/nchs/

**Desc:** The NCHS mission is to collect, analyze, and disseminate national health statistics; conduct research in survey and statistical methodology; provide specialized training programs and technical assistance; and coordinate cooperative programs with state, national, and international organizations. NCHS maintains data systems that produce data in the following areas: extent of illness and disability in the population; distribution and normative standards for physiological and nutritional measurements; national vital statistics, including births, deaths, marriages, and divorces; hospital, nursing home, and ambulatory care utilization; health expenditures; family formation, growth, and dissolution; and other major health topics.

**★ 11996 ★ U.S. Department of Health and Human Services (NIH)**
**National Institutes of Health (CSR)**
**Center for Scientific Review**
9000 Rockville Pike
Bethesda, MD 20892
**Phone:** (301)435-1111
**Website:** http://www.csr.nih.gov

**Desc:** The Center receives and assigns applications for peer reviews to scientific review groups whose members hold advanced degrees and are established investigators in the extramural community. After review, applications are referred to funding components for potential award. The Center develops and implements innovative, flexible ways to conduct referral and review for all aspects of science.

**★ 11997 ★ U.S. Department of Health and Human Services**
**National Institutes of Health (NIH)**
**National Library of Medicine (NLM)**
9000 Rockville Pike
Bethesda, MD 20892
**Phone:** (301)496-6308
**Website:** http://www.nlm.nih.gov/
Donald A.B. Lindberg, MD, Director

**Desc:** The National Library of Medicine is the Nation's primary medical information source and is authorized to provide medical library services and online bibliographic search capabilities to public and private agencies, organizations, institutions, and individuals. It sponsors and conducts research and development in biomedical communications, in such areas as telemedicine, expert systems, and advanced medical imaging projects.

**★ 11998 ★ U.S. Library of Congress**
**National Library Service for the Blind and Physically Handicapped**
1291 Taylor St. NW
Washington, DC 20542-4960
**Phone:** (202)707-5100

**Desc:** Talking and braille books and magazines are distributed through 142 regional and subregional libraries to blind and physically handicapped residents of the U.S. and its territories.

## Foundations & Other Funding Organizations

### Other Funding Organizations

**★ 11999 ★ American Academy of Professional Coders (AAPC)**
309 West 700 South
Salt Lake City, UT 84101-2608
**Free:** 800-626-2633          **Fax:** (801)236-2258
**Email:** info@aapc.com
**Website:** http://www.aapc.org
Lan C. England, Exec. Dir.

**Desc:** Certified professional coders. Promotes high standards of physician and outpatient facility coding through education and cerification. **Awards:** Coder of the Year (annual) for excellence in medical coding; Networker of the Year (annual) for connecting coders together for discussion leading to correct solutions of reimbursement problems.

**★ 12000 ★ Association of Medical Illustrators (AMI)**
2965 Flowers Rd. S Ste. 105
Atlanta, GA 30341-5520
**Phone:** (770)454-7933          **Fax:** (770)351-3348
**Email:** assnhq@mindspring.com
**Website:** http://www.medical-illustrators.org/
William H. Just, CAECMP, Exec. Dir.

**Desc:** Medical illustrators and individuals engaged in related pursuits. Promotes the study and encourages the advancement of medical illustration and allied fields of visual education. Works to advance medical education and to promote understanding and cooperation with medical and related professions. Offers placement services. Maintains speakers' bureau; accredits six postgraduate medical illustration programs. Offers continuing education program; provides professional certification; conducts research; compiles statistics. **Awards:** Recognition; scholarship.

**★ 12001 ★ Chinese American Medical Society (CAMS)**
c/o Dr. H.H. Wang
281 Edgewood Ave.
Teaneck, NJ 07666
**Phone:** (201)833-1506          **Fax:** (201)833-8252
**Email:** hw5@columbia.edu
**Website:** http://www.camsociety.org
Dr. Daisy Saw, MD, Pres.

**Desc:** Physicians of Chinese origin residing in the U.S. and Canada. Seeks to advance medical knowledge, scientific research, and interchange of information among members and to promote the health status of Chinese Americans. Conducts educational meetings; supports research. Maintains placement service. Sponsors limited charitable program. **Awards:** Scholarship (annual); Scientific Award (annual) for member with highest scholastic achievements.

**★ 12002 ★ Drug Information Association (DIA)**
501 Office Center Dr., Ste. 450
Fort Washington, PA 19034-3211
**Phone:** (215)628-2288          **Fax:** (215)641-1229
**Email:** dia@diahome.org
**Website:** http://www.diahome.org
Joseph R. Assenzo, PhD, Exec. Dir.

**Desc:** Provides neutral, global forum promoting exchange of information critical to professional performance and achievement in the discovery, development, regulation, surveillance, or marketing of pharmaceuticals or related products. **Awards:** Research Award Grant (annual).

**★ 12003 ★ Gazette International Networking Institute (GINI)**
4207 Lindell Blvd., No. 110
Saint Louis, MO 63108-2915
**Phone:** (314)534-0475          **Fax:** (314)534-5070
**Email:** gini_intl@msn.com
**Website:** http://www.post-polio.org
Joan L. Headley, Dir.

**Desc:** Polio survivors, ventilator users, other individuals with neuromuscular diseases, health care personnel, insurance agencies, government agencies, independent living centers, and interested others. Works to inform, encourage, dignify, and sustain people with disabilities. Seeks to create a communications network to provide information on issues related to disabilities. Serves as clearinghouse for information on polio, ventilators, neuromuscular diseases, and independent living. Sponsors seminars. Coordinates International Polio Network and International Ventilator Users Network. **Awards:** Research Awards (periodic).

**★ 12004 ★ Healthcare Information and Management Systems Society (HIMSS)**
230 E Ohio St., Ste. 500
Chicago, IL 60611-3269
**Phone:** (312)664-4467          **Fax:** (312)664-6143
**Email:** himss@himss.org
**Website:** http://www.himss.org/
H. Stephen Lieber, CAE, Pres.

**Desc:** Persons who, by education and/or appropriate experience, are professionally qualified to engage in the analysis, design, and operation of health care information systems, management engineering, telecommunications, and clinical systems professions. Provides leadership in health care for the management of systems, information, and change, while striving for high quality, efficient and effective patient care through analysis and technology implementation. Maintains speakers' bureau. Offers placement service. **Awards:** Richard P. Covert Scholarship (annual) for student member in field of study consistent with HIMSS service areas.

★ **12005** ★ **National Organization for Rare Disorders (NORD)**
PO Box 8923
New Fairfield, CT 06812-8923
**Phone:** (203)746-6518 **Free:** 800-999-6673
**Fax:** (203)746-6481
**Email:** orphan@rarediseases.org
**Website:** http://www.rarediseases.org
Susan Olivo, Admin. Assistant
**Desc:** Doctors, professionals, academics, voluntary health organizations, and individuals interested in rare disorders. Serves as a clearinghouse for information concerning rare disorders. Objectives are: to monitor the Orphan Drug Act; to link individuals with rare disorders together for mutual support; to stimulate research on rare diseases; to foster communication among voluntary agencies, health-related industries, and government bodies. (Orphan drugs are used in the treatment of rare disorders. Since their use is not widespread, most drug companies cannot expect to profit from the development and manufacture of these drugs. The Orphan Drug Act gives financial assistance and tax incentives to drug companies that develop these drugs.) Provides information on rare disorders and referrals to organizations. **Awards:** NORD Research Grant (biennial) bestowed to scientists for clinical research on new treatments for rare diseases; recognition (annual) bestowed to individuals and corporations for outstanding service in health or orphan drug development.

# Medical & Allied Health Schools

## Health Information Administration

*The following baccalaureate, post-baccalaureate, and master's degree programs in health information (medical record) administration have been accredited by the Commission on Accreditation of Allied Health Education Programs (35 E Wacker Dr., Ste. 1970, Chicago, IL 60601-2208, (312)553-9355, http://www.caahep.org/) in collaboration with the Council on Accreditation of the American Health Information Management Association, 233 N Michigan Ave., Ste. 2150, Chicago, IL 60601-5519, (312)233-1100, http://www.ahima.org/. Contact either of these organizations for a listing of accredited academic programs for health information (medical record) technicians.*

### Alabama

★ **12006** ★ **Alabama State University**
**Health Information Administrator Program**
PO Box 271
Montgomery, AL 36101-0271
**Phone:** (334)229-5058 **Fax:** (334)229-4964
**Email:** sholt@asunet.alasu.edu
Sandria K. Holt, Director

★ **12007** ★ **University of Alabama, Birmingham**
**Health Information Administrator Program**
University Station
Birmingham, AL 35294-3361
**Phone:** (205)934-1678 **Fax:** (205)934-5980
**Email:** sgrostic@uab.edu
**Website:** http://www.uab.edu
Sara S. Grostick, Director

### Arkansas

★ **12008** ★ **Arkansas Tech University**
**Health Information Administrator Program**
105 Wilson Hall
Russellville, AR 72801
**Phone:** (501)968-0441 **Fax:** (501)964-0504
**Email:** melinda.wilkins@mail.atu.edu
**Website:** http://pls.atu.edu/biosci/him/him.htm
Melinda Wilkins, Director

### California

★ **12009** ★ **Loma Linda University**
**Health Information Administrator Program**
1905 Nichol Hall
Loma Linda, CA 92350
**Phone:** (909)558-4976 **Fax:** (909)558-0404
**Email:** marilyn-davidian@sahp.llu.edu
**Website:** http://www.llu.edu/llu/sahp/
Marilyn R. Davidian, Director

### Colorado

★ **12010** ★ **Regis University**
**Health Information Administrator Program**
3333 Regis Blvd.
Denver, CO 80221-1099
**Phone:** (303)458-4157 **Fax:** (303)964-5533
**Email:** scarlon@regis.edu
**Website:** http://www.regis.edu/shcp/hsam.htm
Sheila A. Carlon, PhD, Director

### Florida

★ **12011** ★ **Florida A&M University**
**Health Information Administrator Program**
Tallahassee, FL 32307
**Phone:** (904)599-3822 **Fax:** (904)561-2457
**Website:** http://www.famu.edu/ahs/him.html
Barbara W. Mosley, PhD, Director

★ **12012** ★ **Florida International University**
**Health Information Administrator Program**
N Campus
3000 NE 151 St.
ACI, Rm. 394C
Miami, FL 33181-3000
**Phone:** (305)919-5631 **Fax:** (305)919-4864
**Email:** martinez@fiu.edu
**Website:** http://www.fiu.edu/~cohealth/
Odalys Martinez, Director

★ **12013** ★ **Lake-Sumter Community College**
**Health Information Administrator Program**
9501 US Hwy. 441
Leesburg, FL 34788-8751
**Phone:** (352)365-3581 **Fax:** (352)365-3501
**Email:** ziesemerb@lscc.cc.fl.us
Brandy G. Ziesemer, Director

★ **12014** ★ **University of Central Florida**
**Health Information Administrator Program**
PO Box 162205
Orlando, FL 32816-2205
**Phone:** (407)823-2353 **Fax:** (407)823-6138
**Email:** barr@pegasus.cc.ucf.edu
**Website:** http://www.cohpa.ucf.edu/health.pro/
Carol J. Barr, Director

### Georgia

★ **12015** ★ **Clark Atlanta University**
**Health Information Administrator Program**
James P. Brawley Dr. at Fair St. SW
Atlanta, GA 30314
**Phone:** (404)880-8115 **Fax:** (404)880-6165
**Website:** http://www.cau.edu/
Barbara Brice, PhD, Director

★ **12016** ★ **Macon State College**
**Health Information Administrator Program**
100 College Station Dr.
Macon, GA 31206-5144
**Phone:** (912)471-2788 **Fax:** (912)417-2787
**Email:** nsayle@mail.maconstate.edu
Nanette Sayles, Director

★ **12017** ★ **Medical College of Georgia**
**Health Information Administrator Program**
AL-130
Augusta, GA 30912-0400
**Phone:** (706)721-3436 **Fax:** (706)721-6067
**Email:** cacampbe@mail.mcg.edu
**Website:** http://www.mcg.edu/sah/him
Carol A. Campbell, Director

### Illinois

★ **12018** ★ **Chicago State University**
**Health Information Administrator Program**
9501 S King Dr.
BHS 610
Chicago, IL 60628-1598
**Phone:** (773)995-2593 **Fax:** (773)995-4484
**Email:** L_thomas@email.com
**Website:** http://www.csu.edu/CollegeOfHealthSciences/HealthInformationAdministration/
Leona M. Thomas, Director

★ **12019** ★ **Illinois State University**
**Health Information Administrator Program**
Felmley Hall 305
Normal, IL 61790-5220
**Phone:** (309)438-8329 **Fax:** (309)438-2450
**Email:** fwaterst@ilstu.edu
**Website:** http://www.cast.ilstu.edu/hsc/courses/under/hsc-u.htm
Francis L. Waterstraat, Jr., Director

★ **12020** ★ **University of Illinois, Chicago**
**College of Health and Human Development Sciences**
**Health Information Administrator Program**
1919 W Taylor, Rm. 811
M/C520
Chicago, IL 60612
**Phone:** (312)996-3530 **Fax:** (312)413-0205
**Email:** patena@uic.edu
**Website:** http://www.sbhis.uic.edu/GradBk98-99/him_main.htm
Karen Patena, Director

### Indiana

★ **12021** ★ **Indiana University, Northwest**
**Health Information Technician Program**
3400 Broadway
Gary, IN 46408
**Phone:** (219)980-6654 **Fax:** (219)980-6649
**Email:** mskurk@iunhaw1.iun.indiana.edu
**Website:** http://www.iun.edu/~ahealth/
Margaret A. Skurka, Director

## Kansas

**★ 12022 ★ University of Kansas Medical Center**
**Health Information Administrator Program**
3901 Rainbow Blvd.
Kansas City, KS 66160-7607
**Phone:** (913)588-2422          **Fax:** (913)588-2428
**Email:** dkellogg@kumc.edu
**Website:** http://www.kumc.edu/SAH/HIM/
Don Kellogg, Director

## Kentucky

**★ 12023 ★ Eastern Kentucky University**
**Health Information Administrator Program**
521 Lancaster Ave.
Richmond, KY 40475-3102
**Phone:** (859)622-1915          **Fax:** (859)622-2013
**Email:** hrshinds@acs.eku.edu
**Website:** http://www.healthinfo.eku.edu
Frances A. Hindsman, Director

## Louisiana

**★ 12024 ★ Louisiana Tech University**
**Health Information Administrator Program**
PO Box 3171
Ruston, LA 71272
**Phone:** (318)257-2854          **Fax:** (318)257-4896
**Email:** davison@him.latech.edu
**Website:** http://www.ans.latech.edu/him-index.html
Lou H. Davison, Director

**★ 12025 ★ University of Louisiana, Lafayette**
**College of Sciences**
**Health Information Administrator Program**
PO Box 41007
Lafayette, LA 70504
**Phone:** (337)482-6629          **Fax:** (337)482-5902
**Email:** venable@louisiana.edu
**Website:** http://www.usl.edu/departments/HealthInfoMgmt/
Carol A. Venable, Director

## Massachusetts

**★ 12026 ★ Northeastern University**
**Health Information Administrator Program**
266 Ryder Hall
Boston, MA 02115
**Phone:** (617)373-2525          **Fax:** (617)373-2325
**Email:** a.collins@nunet.neu.edu
**Website:** http://www.neu.edu/uc/
Annalee Collins, Director

## Michigan

**★ 12027 ★ Baker College of Flint**
**Health Information Administrator Program**
1050 W Bristol Rd.
Flint, MI 48507
**Phone:** (810)766-4147          **Fax:** (810)766-4049
**Email:** savag_am@acadfl.baker.edu
**Website:** http://www.baker.edu/
Amy Savage, Director

**★ 12028 ★ Ferris State University**
**College of Allied Health Sciences**
**Health Information Administrator Program**
200 Ferris Dr.
VFS 402
Big Rapids, MI 49307-2740
**Phone:** (231)591-2313          **Fax:** (231)591-3788
**Email:** ellen_j_haneline@ferris.edu
**Website:** http://www.ferris.edu/htmls/colleges/allied-he/hinfoman.htm
Ellen J. Haneline, Director

## Minnesota

**★ 12029 ★ College of Saint Scholastica**
**Health Information Administrator Program**
1200 Kenwood Ave.
Duluth, MN 55811
**Phone:** (218)723-6011          **Fax:** (218)733-2239
**Email:** klatour@css.edu
**Website:** http://www.ccs.edu
Kathleen M. LaTour, Director

## Mississippi

**★ 12030 ★ University of Mississippi Medical Center**
**Health Information Administrator Program**
2500 N State St.
Jackson, MS 39216
**Phone:** (601)984-6305          **Fax:** (601)984-6344
**Email:** byates@shrp.umsmed.edu
**Website:** http://shrp3.unsmed.edu/him/index.html
Rebecca J. Yates, Director

## Missouri

**★ 12031 ★ Saint Louis University Health Sciences Center**
**Department of Health Information Management**
**Health Information Administrator Program**
3437 Caroline St.
Saint Louis, MO 63104
**Phone:** (314)577-8516          **Fax:** (314)577-8503
**Email:** smithjk@slu.edu
**Website:** http://www.slu.edu/colleges/AH/Departments/him.html
Karen Jody Smith, Director

**★ 12032 ★ Stephens College**
**Health Information Administrator Program**
Campus Box 2083
1200 E Broadway
Columbia, MO 65215
**Phone:** (573)876-7283          **Fax:** (573)876-7248
**Email:** joanr@wc.stephens.edu
**Website:** http://www.stephens.edu/www/PR/GradConEd/GCE_HIM.html
Joan T. Rines, PhD, Director

## Nebraska

**★ 12033 ★ College of Saint Mary**
**Health Information Administrator Program**
1901 S 72nd St.
Omaha, NE 68124
**Phone:** (402)399-2611          **Fax:** (402)399-2657
**Email:** ejacobs@csm.edu
**Website:** http://www.csm.edu
Ellen B. Jacobs, Director

## New Jersey

**★ 12034 ★ Kean University**
**Health Information Administrator Program**
Morris Ave.
Union, NJ 07083
**Phone:** (908)527-3010
**Website:** http://www.Kean.edu/%7Emedrec/him.html
Natalie Sartori, Director

## New York

**★ 12035 ★ Long Island University**
**Health Information Administrator Program**
CW Post Campus
Northern Blvd.
Greenvale, NY 11548
**Phone:** (516)299-2485          **Fax:** (516)299-2527
**Email:** healprof@cwpost.liu.edu
**Website:** http://www.cwpost.liunet.edu/cwis/cwp/hscience/healinfo/healinfo.html
Joann Johansmeyer, Director

**★ 12036 ★ State University of New York Health Science Center, Brooklyn (SUNY)**
**Health Information Administrator Program**
450 Clarkson Ave.
PO Box 105
Brooklyn, NY 11203
**Phone:** (718)270-7770          **Fax:** (718)270-7739
**Email:** itopor@netmail.hscbklyn.edu
**Website:** http://www.hscbklyn.edu/CHRP/him.html
Isaac Topor, EdD, Director

**★ 12037 ★ State University of New York Institute of Technology, Utica/Rome**
**Health Information Administrator Program**
PO Box 3050
Utica, NY 13504-3050
**Phone:** (315)792-7391          **Fax:** (315)792-7138
**Email:** fdls1@sunyit.edu
**Website:** http://www.sunyit.edu/pubm/academic/undrgrad/hlthinfo/degrees.htm
Donna L. Silsbee, Director

## North Carolina

**★ 12038 ★ East Carolina University**
**School of Allied Health Sciences**
**Health Information Administrator Program**
Greenville, NC 27858
**Phone:** (252)328-4426          **Fax:** (252)328-4470
**Email:** laymane@mail.ecu.edu
**Website:** http://www.news.ecu.edu/experts/healthinfo_manage.html
Elizabeth Layman, PhD, Director

**★ 12039 ★ Western Carolina University**
**Health Information Administrator Program**
Moore Hall
Cullowhee, NC 28723
**Phone:** (828)227-3513          **Fax:** (828)227-7071
**Email:** floreani@wcu.edu
**Website:** http://www.wcu.edu/aps/healths/him-home.html
Walter R. Floreani, Director

## Ohio

**★ 12040 ★ Ohio State University**
**Health Information Administrator Program**
1583 Perry St.
Columbus, OH 43210
**Phone:** (614)292-0567          **Fax:** (614)292-0210
**Email:** brodnik.2@osu.edu
**Website:** http://www.amp.ohio-state.edu/!sampweb/hi-1.htm
Melanie Brodnik, PhD, Director

## Oklahoma

**★ 12041 ★ East Central University**
**Health Information Administrator Program**
Ada, OK 74820
**Phone:** (580)332-8000          **Fax:** (580)332-4616
**Email:** sdixon@mailclerk.ecok.edu
**Website:** http://www.ecok.edu/acaddept/him/
Sandra A. Dixon, Director

**★ 12042 ★ Southwestern Oklahoma State University**
**Health Information Administrator Program**
100 Campus Dr.
Weatherford, OK 73096
**Phone:** (580)774-3287          **Fax:** (580)774-3795
**Email:** pricham@swosu.edu
**Website:** http://164.58.39.105/academic/arts_sci.htm
Marion Prichard, Director

## Pennsylvania

**★ 12043 ★ Duquesne University**
**Department of Health Management**
**  Systems**
**Health Information Administrator Program**
429 Fisher Hall
Pittsburgh, PA 15282-0001
**Phone:** (412)396-4772        **Fax:** (412)396-5554
**Website:** http://www.duq.edu/index.html
Joan M. Kiel, PhD, Director

**★ 12044 ★ Gwynedd-Mercy College**
**Health Information Administrator Program**
Gwynedd Valley, PA 19437
**Phone:** (215)646-7300        **Fax:** (215)641-5559
**Email:** hornung.j@gmc.edu
**Website:** http://www.gmc.edu/academic/schools/al-
liedhealth/himgmt.htm
Jennifer Hornung, Director

**★ 12045 ★ Temple University**
**College of Allied Health Professions**
**Health Information Administrator Program**
3307 N Broad St.
Philadelphia, PA 19140
**Phone:** (215)707-4823        **Fax:** (215)707-5852
**Email:** lharman@vm.temple.edu
**Website:** http://www.temple.edu/HIM/
Laurinda Harman, PhD, Director

**★ 12046 ★ University of Pittsburgh**
**Health Information Administrator Program**
6051 Forbes Tower
Pittsburgh, PA 15260
**Phone:** (412)647-1190        **Fax:** (412)647-1199
**Email:** madelhak@pitt.edu
**Website:** http://www.him.upmc.edu
Mervat Abdelhak, PhD, Director

**★ 12047 ★ York College of Pennsylvania**
**Health Information Administrator Program**
Country Club Rd.
York, PA 17405-7199
**Phone:** (717)849-1616        **Fax:** (717)849-1619
**Email:** jfultz@ycp.edu
**Website:** http://goose.ycp.edu/department/biology/in-
dex.html
Jean A. Fultz, Director

## Puerto Rico

**★ 12048 ★ University of Puerto Rico**
**Health Information Administrator Program**
GPO Box 5067
San Juan, PR 00936-5067
**Phone:** (787)764-3609        **Fax:** (787)764-3609
**Email:** anaorabona@cprs.rcm.upr.edu
**Website:** http://cprsweb.rcm.upr.edu/HealthInfoAd-
ministration.htm
Anna Orabona-Ocasio, Director

## South Dakota

**★ 12049 ★ Dakota State University**
**Health Information Administrator Program**
East Hall
Madison, SD 57042-1799
**Phone:** (605)256-5137        **Fax:** (605)256-5060
**Email:** bennettd@pluto.dsu.edu
**Website:** http://www.dsu.edu
Dorine Bennett, Director

## Tennessee

**★ 12050 ★ Tennessee State University**
**Health Information Administrator Program**
3500 John A. Merritt Blvd.
Nashville, TN 37209-1561
**Phone:** (615)963-7441        **Fax:** (615)963-7498

**Email:** kunnu@harpo.tnstate.edu
**Website:** http://www.tnstate.edu/alhp/
Elizabeth Kunnu, Director

**★ 12051 ★ University of Tennessee,**
**  Memphis**
**Department of Health Information**
**  Management**
**Health Information Administrator Program**
822 Beale St., Rm. 300
Memphis, TN 38163
**Phone:** (901)448-6486        **Fax:** (901)448-7545
**Email:** mmcain@utmem.edu
**Website:** http://www.utmen.edu/him/homepage.htm
Mary C. McCain, Director

## Texas

**★ 12052 ★ Southwest Texas State**
**  University**
**Health Information Administrator Program**
San Marcos, TX 78666
**Phone:** (512)245-8242        **Fax:** (512)245-8258
**Email:** sbo2@swt.edu
**Website:** http://www.health.swt.edu/catalog/himma-
jor.html
Sue E. Biedermann, Director

**★ 12053 ★ Texas Southern University**
**Health Information Administrator Program**
3100 Cleburne St.
Houston, TX 77004
**Phone:** (713)327-7265        **Fax:** (713)313-1094
**Email:** fannyhawkins@hotmail.com
**Website:** http://www.tsu.edu/pharmacy/index.htm
Fanny Hawkins, EdD, Director

**★ 12054 ★ University of Texas Medical**
**  Branch, Galveston**
**Health Information Administrator Program**
301 University Blvd.
Galveston, TX 77555-1028
**Phone:** (409)772-3051        **Fax:** (409)772-9574
**Email:** dglemire@utmb.edu
**Website:** http://www.sahs.utmb.edu
Diane Lemire, Director

## Utah

**★ 12055 ★ Weber State University**
**Health Information Administrator Program**
3911 University Circle
Ogden, UT 84408-3911
**Phone:** (801)626-7298        **Fax:** (801)626-7683
**Email:** celliott@weber.edu
**Website:** http://weber.edu/has/Default.html
Chris Elliott, Director

## Washington

**★ 12056 ★ University of Washington**
**Health Information Administrator Program**
1107 NE 45th, Ste. 400
Mail Stop JD-02
Seattle, WA 98105
**Phone:** (206)543-8810        **Fax:** (206)543-9345
**Email:** gcmurphy@u.washington.edu
**Website:** http://www.edoutreach.washington.edu/ex-
tinfo/certprog/hia/default.htm
Gretchen Murphy, Director

## Wisconsin

**★ 12057 ★ University of Wisconsin,**
**  Milwaukee**
**Health Information Administrator Program**
PO Box 413
Milwaukee, WI 53201
**Phone:** (414)229-3862        **Fax:** (414)906-3962
**Email:** madsen@uwm.edu

**Website:** http://www.uwm.edu/sahp/ugp/hia/hiamen-
u.html
Mary K. Madsen, PhD, Director

## <u>Medical Illustration</u>

*Schools listed below offer degree programs that are
accredited by the Association of Medical Illustrators
(2965 Flowers Rd. S, Ste. 105 Atlanta, GA 30341,
(770) 454-7933, http://www.medical-illustrators.org/)
in conjunction with the Commission on Accreditation of
Allied Health Education Programs (35 E Wacker Dr.,
Ste. 1970, Chicago, IL 60601-2208, (312)553-9355,
http://www.caahep.org/).*

### Georgia

**★ 12058 ★ Medical College of Georgia**
**Allied Health and Graduate Studies**
**Graduate Program in Medical Illustration**
1120 15th St.
Augusta, GA 30912-0300
**Phone:** (706)721-3266        **Fax:** (706)721-7855
**Email:** medart@mail.mcg.edu
**Website:** http://www.mcg.edu/SAH/MedIll/index.html
Steven J. Harrison, Director

### Illinois

**★ 12059 ★ University of Illinois, Chicago**
**College of Health and Human**
**  Development Sciences**
**Department of Biomedical Visualization**
**Program in Medical Illustration**
MC-527
Chicago, IL 60612
**Phone:** (312)996-8344        **Fax:** (312)996-8342
**Email:** sbarrows@uic.edu
**Website:** http://www.sbhis.uic.edu/GradBk98-99/bvis/
main.htm
Scott Barrows, PhD, Director

### Maryland

**★ 12060 ★ Johns Hopkins School of**
**  Medicine**
**Department of Art as Applied to Medicine**
**Program in Medical Illustration**
1830 E Monument St., Ste. 7000
Baltimore, MD 21205
**Phone:** (410)955-3213        **Fax:** (410)955-1085
**Email:** glees@medart.jhu.edu
**Website:** http://www.med.jhu.edu/medart
Gary P. Lees, Director

### Michigan

**★ 12061 ★ University of Michigan**
**  Medical Center**
**School of Medical and Biological**
**  Illustration**
**Program in Medical Illustration**
2000 Bonisteel Blvd., Rm. 1075
1327 Jones Dr.
Ann Arbor, MI 48109
**Phone:** (734)647-3504        **Fax:** (734)647-0469
**Email:** brdsmith@umich.edu
**Website:** http://www.umich.edu/~medill/index.html
Bradley R. Smith, PhD, Director

### Texas

**★ 12062 ★ University of Texas**
**  Southwestern Medical Center, Dallas**
**Department of Biomedical**
**  Communications—Exchange Park**
**Program in Medical Illustration/Graduate**
**  Program in Medical Illustration**
5323 Harry Hines Blvd.
Dallas, TX 75235-8881
**Phone:** (214)648-4699        **Fax:** (214)648-5353

**Email:** lewis.calver@email.swmed.edu
**Website:** http://www.swmed.edu/medillus
Lewis E. Calver, Director

# National & International Organizations

**Accrediting Bureau of Health Education Schools (ABHES)**
*See:* Entry 9944

## ★ 12063 ★ American Association for Medical Transcription (AAMT)
100 Sycamore Ave.
Modesto, CA 95354-0550
**Phone:** (209)527-9620          **Free:** 800-982-2182
**Fax:** (209)527-9633
**Email:** aamt@aamt.org
**Website:** http://www.aamt.org
Kimberly Andosca, CEO

**Fnded:** 1978. **Mem:** 7,500. **State Groups:** 26. **Local Groups:** 120. **Desc:** Medical transcriptionists, their supervisors, teachers and students of medical transcription, owners and managers of medical transcription services, and other interested health personnel. Purpose is to provide information about the profession of medical transcription and to provide continuing education for medical transcriptionists. (Medical transcriptionists translate patients' records of medical care and treatment from oral dictation to printed form.) Advocates professional recognition of medical transcriptionists in county, state, and national medical societies and in health care facilities nationwide. Sponsors voluntary certification/credentialing program. Offers updates on developments in medicine and curricula, and on new transcription methods and equipment; sponsors and encourages research in the field. Establishes guidelines for education of medical transcriptionists. Fosters positive relations among medical transcriptionists, the public, members of allied health services, and the legislature. **Pub:** *The AAMT Book of Style for Medical Transcription, 2nd Ed..* Book. • *Cert Alert*, quarterly. Newsletter. • *Journal of the American Association for Medical Transcription*, bi-monthly. Journal. Offers guidance in quality assurance for medical transcription, medican and nonmedical educational articles, word lists, and technology updates. *Price:* Included in membership dues; $150/year for nonmembers; $30/issue. • *The Leading Edge*, monthly. Newsletter. • Also publishes medical transcription modules and medical transcription video programs.

## ★ 12064 ★ American College of Medical Administrators (ACMA)
701 Lee St., Ste. 600
Des Plaines, IL 60016
**Phone:** (847)759-8601          **Fax:** (847)759-8602
**Email:** info@aameda.org
**Website:** http://www.aameda.org
Nancy Anderson, Contact

**Fnded:** 1991. **Mem:** 225. **Reg. Groups:** 7. **State Groups:** 50. **Desc:** Specialty College of the American Academy of Medical Administrators. Healthcare information leaders serving in management positions. Works to promote the advancement of members' knowledge, professional standing, credentialing, and personal achievements in information technology, management, and strategic planning. Conducts educational programs. **Pub:** *Executive*, bimonthly. Journal.

## ★ 12065 ★ American Health Information Management Association (AMRA)
233 N Michigan Ave., Ste. 2150
Chicago, IL 60601-5519
**Phone:** (312)233-1100          **Fax:** (312)233-1500
**Email:** info@ahima.org

**Website:** http://www.ahima.org
Barbara P. Fuller, JD, Pres.

**Fnded:** 1928. **Mem:** 40,000. **State Groups:** 52. **Desc:** Registered record administrators; accredited record technicians with expertise in health information management, biostatistics, classification systems, and systems analysis. Sponsors Independent Study Programs in Medical Record Technology and coding. Conducts annual qualification examinations to credential medical record personnel as Registered Record Administrators (RRA), Accredited Record Technicians (ART) and Certified Coding Specialists (CCS). Maintains Foundation of Research and Education Library, Scholarships and loans. **Pub:** *From the Couch: Official Newsletter of the Mental Health Record Section of the American Medical Record Association*, quarterly. Newsletter. *Price:* Included in membership dues. • *Journal of AHIMA*, 10/year. Journal. Contains articles on the theory, practice, and current issues in health information management. Includes book reviews and calendar of events. *Price:* $72. • *Leader: AHIMA Volunteer*, quarterly. Newsletter. *Price:* Included in membership dues. • *QA Section Connection*, bimonthly. Newsletter. Provides educational information on the management and methodology of health care quality assurance programs. Includes annual subject index. *Price:* Included in membership dues. • *Spectrum*, quarterly. Newsletter. *Price:* Included in membership dues. • Also publishes guides, workbooks, and other materials on medical record management and related subjects. **Frmly:** (1928) American Association of Medical Record Librarians; (1938) Association of Record Librarians of North America; (1991) American Medical Records Association.

## ★ 12066 ★ American Medical Informatics Association (AMIA)
4915 St. Elmo Ave., Ste. 401
Bethesda, MD 20814
**Phone:** (301)657-1291          **Fax:** (301)657-1296
**Email:** dennis@mail.amia.org
**Website:** http://www.amia.org
Dennis Reynolds, Exec. Dir.

**Fnded:** 1990. **Mem:** 3,200. **Nat'l Groups:** 1. **Desc:** Medical personnel, physicians, physical scientists, engineers, data processors, researchers, educators, hospital administrators, nurses, medical record administrators, and computer professionals. Objectives are: to apply advanced systems and information technologies to scientific, literary, and educational activities; to promote excellence in health care; to promote patient care, teaching, research, and health administration. **Pub:** *Abstract Book*, annual. Book. Contains abstracts of sessions of the association's Spring Congress. *Price:* $50 plus shipping and handling. • *Journal of the American Medical Informatics Association*, bimonthly. Journal. • *Proceedings of Symposium on Computer Applications in Medical Care*. Proceedings.

**American Nursing Informatics Association (ANIA)**
*See:* Entry 15653

## ★ 12067 ★ American Podiatric Medical Writers Association (APMWA)
PO Box 750129
Forest Hills, NY 11375
**Phone:** (718)897-9700          **Fax:** (718)896-5747
**Email:** bblock@prodigy.net
**Website:** http://www.ania.org
Dr. Barry H. Block, Exec. Dir.

**Fnded:** 1985. **Mem:** 100. **Desc:** Podiatric medical writers. Promotes the improvement of writing on podiatric topics. **Pub:** *American Podiatric Medical Writers Association–Membership Directory*, annual. Membership Directory. *Price:* Free. • *American Podiatric Medical Writers Association–Newsletter*, quarterly. Newsletter. Lists new members. *Price:* Free with self-addressed stamped envelope.

## ★ 12068 ★ American Printing House for the Blind (APH)
PO Box 6085
1839 Frankfort Ave.
Louisville, KY 40206-0085
**Phone:** (502)895-2405          **Free:** 800-223-1839
**Fax:** (502)899-2274
**Email:** cs@aph.org
**Website:** http://www.aph.org
Dr. Tuck Tinsley, III, Pres.

**Fnded:** 1858. **Desc:** Produces literature in all media (braille, large type, recorded, computer disc) for the blind. Manufactures special products for use by visually impaired students and adults, such as preschool and vocational materials and talking software. Conducts ongoing educational research program. Conducts art contest, tours of the plant and of the APH Museum of artifacts from the education of the blind field. **Pub:** *APH Slate*, quarterly. Newsletter. Provides information on new products for the visually impaired; also includes organization news and activities. *Price:* Free. • *APH Technology Update: Technology for People Who Are Visually Impaired*, annual. Newsletter. Covers computer and other high-tech products designed for blind persons. *Price:* Free. • Makes available Newsweek, Readers Digest, and Weekly Reader in braille, tape, or large type.

## ★ 12069 ★ Asian Pacific Association for Medical Informatics (APAMI)
National University Hospital
Department of Community, Occupational and Family Medicine
Lower Kent Ridge Rd.
Singapore 0511, Singapore
**Phone:** 65 7724296          **Fax:** 65 7791489
**Email:** lunkc@nusvm.bitnet
**Website:** http://www.apami.org

**Lang(s):** Chinese, English. **Desc:** Medical information and information management organizations. Seeks to advance the practice of medical information management; promotes development and implementation of new medical informatics technologies. Serves as a clearinghouse on medical information management; sponsors research and educational programs.

## ★ 12070 ★ Association of Biomedical Communication Directors (ABCD)
c/o Beverly E. Hill Ed. D
Medical Educational Resources Program
Indiana University School of Medicine
1226 W Michigan St., BR 156
Indianapolis, IN 46202-5178
**Fax:** (317)274-4638
Beverly E. Hill, Ed.D.. Sec.

**Fnded:** 1972. **Mem:** 87. **Desc:** Individuals with common managerial concerns in health science communications, such as persons with direct administrative responsibility for operations of a biomedical communications facility in a school or academic health science center. Provides a forum for the sharing and dissemination of information, materials, and ideas. Promotes research and education in administrative practices with regard to health sciences communications. Works to develop information materials such as surveys and profiles helpful in the management of biomedical communications. **Pub:** *Exchange*, quarterly. Journal. • *Membership Roster*, annual. Journal. • *Report of Annual Survey of The Directors of Biomedical Communications*.

## ★ 12071 ★ Association of Medical Illustrators (AMI)
2965 Flowers Rd. S Ste. 105
Atlanta, GA 30341-5520
**Phone:** (770)454-7933          **Fax:** (770)351-3348
**Email:** assnhq@mindspring.com
**Website:** http://www.medical-illustrators.org/
William H. Just, CAECMP, Exec. Dir.

**Fnded:** 1945. **Mem:** 1,000. **Desc:** Medical illustrators and individuals engaged in related pursuits. Promotes the study and encourages the advancement of medical illustration and allied fields of visual education.

Works to advance medical education and to promote understanding and cooperation with medical and related professions. Offers placement services. Maintains speakers' bureau; accredits six postgraduate medical illustration programs. Offers continuing education program; provides professional certification; conducts research; compiles statistics. **Pub:** *Journal of Biocommunication*, quarterly. Journal. • *Medical Illustration Sourcebook*, annual. • Directory, annual. • Newsletter, bimonthly.


★ **12072** ★ **Association for Public Health Statistics and Information Systems**
c/o Tiffany Mandis Emami
1220 19th St. NW, Ste. 802
Washington, DC 20036
**Phone:** (202)463-8851          **Fax:** (202)463-4870
**Email:** hq@naphsis.org
**Website:** http://www.naphsis.org
Alfrod G. Zangri, Pres.

**Fnded:** 1933. **Mem:** 300. **Desc:** Officials of state and local health agencies responsible for registration, tabulation, and analysis of births, deaths, fetal deaths, marriages, divorces, and other health statistics. **Pub:** Journal, bimonthly. **Frmly:** (1958) American Association of Registration Executives; (1980) American Association for Vital Records and Public Health Statistics; (1997) Association for Vital Records and Health Statistics.


★ **12073** ★ **Benjamin Franklin Literary and Medical Society (BFLMS)**
1100 Waterway Blvd.
Indianapolis, IN 46202
**Phone:** (317)636-8881          **Fax:** (317)639-0126
**Email:** satevepst@aol.com
**Website:** http://www.health.gov/nhic/NHICScripts/Entry.cfm?HRCode=HR1637
Dr. Cory SerVaas, Pres. /CEO

**Fnded:** 1976. **Mem:** 2300,000. **Desc:** Individuals, industries, and businesses united to support research and promote sciences, literature, and the arts in order to achieve greater public understanding of science and the humanities. Major emphasis is on the dissemination of health, preventive medicine, and nutrition information to the health community and the public. Advocates a preventive approach to health care including proper nutrition, daily exercise, and good health habits. Offers training in cardiopulmonary resuscitation and other life-saving skills; conducts health education programs. Sponsors the Children's Better Health Institute, which publishes material designed to educate children of preschool through elementary school levels on health, nutrition, safety, and exercise, and provides parents with medical information concerning infants and children. Operates Medical Education and Research Foundation, which disseminates medical information in lay terms, covering concepts and developments in preventive medicine, safety procedures and techniques, health dangers, proper dietary habits, and reports on new and developing treatments and medications for cancer patients and techniques used for early detection of cancer. Sponsors the Saturday Evening Post Society which conducts national health surveys; publicizes advances in science, medicine, nutrition, and preventive medicine; funds research projects; and encourages commercial manufacturers to produce innovative health equipment. Is named for Benjamin Franklin (1706-90), who founded the Pennsylvania Gazette in 1728, which eventually became the Saturday Evening Post. (The society purchased this magazine from the Curtis Publishing Company in 1982.) Franklin was also a strong supporter of the arts and sciences. **Pub:** *Child Life*, 8/year. Magazine. Promotes reading and good health habits in children between the ages of seven and nine. Includes "Ask the Doctor" column, poems, and short stories. *Price:* $14.95/year. • *Children's Digest*, 8/year. Magazine. Promotes reading and good health habits in children between the ages of eight and ten. Includes book reviews. *Price:* $14.95/year. • *Children's Playmate Magazine*, 8/year. Magazine. Promotes reading and good health habits for children between the ages of five and seven. Includes book

reviews. *Price:* $14.95/year. • *Humpty Dumpty*, 8/year. Magazine. Promotes reading and good health habits for children between the ages of four and six. *Price:* $14.95/year. • *Jack and Jill*, 8/year. Magazine. Promotes reading and good health habits for children between the ages of six and eight. *Price:* $14.95/year. • *Mecidal Update Newsletter*, monthly. Newsletter. Includes foundation news and research updates. *Price:* $12/year. • *Saturday Evening Post*, bimonthly. • *Turtle Magazine for Preschool Kids*, 8/year. Magazine. Promotes reading and good health, safety, and nutrition habits for children between the ages of two and five. Includes book reviews. *Price:* $14.95/year.


★ **12074** ★ **BioCommunications Association (BCA)**
115 Stoneridge Dr.
Chapel Hill, NC 27514-9737
**Phone:** (919)967-8246          **Fax:** (919)967-8246
**Email:** bcaoffice@aol.com
**Website:** http://bca.org
Nancy Hurtgen, Central Office Admin.

**Fnded:** 1931. **Mem:** 450. **Local Groups:** 29. **Desc:** Photographers, technicians, doctors, scientists, educators, and others concerned with photography in the health sciences and related fields. Seeks to advance the techniques of biophotography and biomedical communications through meetings, seminars, and workshops. Has established Board of Registry to offer qualifying examinations for Registered Biological Photographer. **Pub:** *Journal of Biocommunication*. Journal. Published jointly with two other associations. **Frmly:** (2001) Biological Photographic Association.


★ **12075** ★ **Canada's Health Informatics Association**
2 Carlton St., Ste. 1304
Toronto, ON, Canada M5B 1J3
**Phone:** (416)979-5551          **Fax:** (416)979-1144
**Email:** info@coachorg.com
**Website:** http://www.coachorg.com/

**Fnded:** 1975. **Mem:** 850. **Lang(s):** English. **Desc:** Health care and information systems professionals. Promotes education and the exchange of ideas in the field of medical information systems. **Pub:** *Guidelines for the Protection of Health Information*. Book. Contains a framework for developing and implementing security and privacy programs. **Frmly:** (1999) Canadian Organization for Advancement of Computers in Health.


★ **12076** ★ **Canadian Institute for Health Information (CIHI)**
377 Dalhousie St., Ste. 200
Ottawa, ON, Canada K1N 9N8
**Phone:** (613)241-7860          **Fax:** (613)241-8120
**Email:** lpoirier@cihi.ca

**Fnded:** 1994. **Lang(s):** English, French. **Desc:** Working to improve the health of Canadians and the health care system, provides quality health information, committed to safeguarding the privacy and confidentiality of personal health information. Seeks to coordinate the development and maintenance of a common approach to health information for Canada, provides accurate and timely information that needed to establish sound health policies, manages the Canadian health system effectively and creates public awareness of factors affecting good health.


★ **12077** ★ **Canadian Medicalert Foundation (CMAF)**
**(La Fondation Canadienne MedicAlert — FCMA)**
2005 Sheppard Ave. E, Ste. 800
Toronto, ON, Canada M2J 5B4
**Phone:** (416)696-0267          **Free:** 800-668-1507
**Fax:** 800-392-8422
**Email:** medinfo@medicalert.ca
**Website:** http://www.medicalert.ca

**Fnded:** 1961. **Mem:** 1000,000. **Lang(s):** English, French. **Desc:** Provides life-long access to personal and medical information in order to protect and save

member's lives; offers immediate access to medical information in emergencies, unlimited record updates, a MedicAlert bracelet or necklet (engraved with ID number, 24-hour emergency hotline number and specific medical conditions) and a wallet card with additional medical data. A complete record is available to emergency responders and medical professionals worldwide in 140 languages on the 24-hour hotline, in order to assist in making accurate diagnosis and to administer proper treatment. **Pub:** *MedicAlert Connects*, semiannual. Newsletter. Provides information to members and donors regarding CMAF activities, accomplishments, etc.


★ **12078** ★ **Cancer Research Society (CRS)**
**(Societe de Recherche sur le Cancer — SRC)**
402 - 625 Ave Du President-Kennedy
Montreal, QC, Canada H3A 3S5
**Phone:** (514)861-9227          **Fax:** (514)861-9220
**Email:** info@cancer-research-society.ca
**Website:** http://www.cancer-research-society.ca

**Fnded:** 1946. **Lang(s):** English, French. **Desc:** Health care professionals and research scientists with an interest in cancer. Seeks to advance cancer research. Serves as a forum for the exchange of information among members; sponsors research and educational programs; provides financial support to cancer research and treatment institutions.


**Coalition of National Health Education Organizations (CNHEO)**
*See:* Entry 2064


★ **12079** ★ **Council on Health Information and Education (CHIE)**
2272 Colorado Blvd., No. 1228
Los Angeles, CA 90041
**Fax:** (818)637-7809
**Email:** ecapwell@otterbein.edu
**Website:** http://hsc.usf.edu/CFH/cnheo/
D. Andre, Dir.

**Fnded:** 1978. **Desc:** Promotes health and fitness of Americans through the dissemination of information on health care, nutrition, and exercise. Warns against fads in health and nutrition; conducts research on health and exercise products; reviews books on health, fitness, nutrition, sexuality, and sports. **Pub:** Pamphlets.


**Council for Sex Information and Education (CSIE)**
*See:* Entry 18890


★ **12080** ★ **Drug Information Association (DIA)**
501 Office Center Dr., Ste. 450
Fort Washington, PA 19034-3211
**Phone:** (215)628-2288          **Fax:** (215)641-1229
**Email:** dia@diahome.org
**Website:** http://www.diahome.org
Joseph R. Assenzo, PhD, Exec. Dir.

**Fnded:** 1965. **Mem:** 27,000. **Desc:** Provides neutral, global forum promoting exchange of information critical to professional performance and achievement in the discovery, development, regulation, surveillance, or marketing of pharmaceuticals or related products. **Pub:** *DIA Forum*, 3/year. Magazine. • *DIA Today*, quarterly. Newsletter. • *Drug Information Association–Membership Directory*, annual. Directory. *Price:* Included in membership dues; $100/copy for nonmembers. • *Drug Information Journal*, quarterly. Journal. *Price:* Included in membership dues.


★ **12081** ★ **Friends of the National Library of Medicine**
1555 Connecticut Ave., NW
Ste. 200
Washington, DC 20036

**Phone:** (202)462-0992          **Fax:** (202)462-9043
**Email:** info@fnlm.org
**Website:** http://www.fnlm.org
Beverly R. Hoffmann, CAE, Exec. Dir.

**Fnded:** 1986. **Mem:** 500. **Desc:** Seeks to improve health by increasing the use of the latest, most effective medical and scientific information by health care professionals, scientists, and the general public. Strives to educate the health, corporate, and public communities about the National Library of Medicine by building a coalition of financial and others supporters.

**Gazette International Networking Institute (GINI)**
*See:* Entry 7989

**★ 12082 ★ Health Academy (HA)**
c/o Public Relations Society of America
33 Irving Pl.
New York, NY 10003-2376
**Phone:** (212)995-2230          **Fax:** (212)995-0757
**Email:** hq@prsa.org
**Website:** http://www.healthacademy.prsa.org/
Ricky DeGenaro, Dir.

**Fnded:** 1989. **Mem:** 600. **Nat'l Groups:** 1. **Desc:** A professional section of the Public Relations Society of America. Senior public relations professionals working in hospitals, multi-hospital systems, medical and dental organizations, insurance companies and Health Maintenance Organizations, foundations, rehabilitation facilities, pharmaceutical firms, government health care units, or health education and research organizations; public relations consultants working in the health care industry. Seeks to enhance the quality and stature of health care public relations. Conducts professional development seminars. **Pub:** *By-laws and Membership Directory*, annual. Directory. • *Health Academy News*, bimonthly. • Monographs.

**★ 12083 ★ Healthcare Information and Management Systems Society (HIMSS)**
230 E Ohio St., Ste. 500
Chicago, IL 60611-3269
**Phone:** (312)664-4467          **Fax:** (312)664-6143
**Email:** himss@himss.org
**Website:** http://www.himss.org/
H. Stephen Lieber, CAE, Pres.

**Fnded:** 1961. **Mem:** 12,000. **Reg. Groups:** 40. **Desc:** Persons who, by education and/or appropriate experience, are professionally qualified to engage in the analysis, design, and operation of health care information systems, management engineering, telecommunications, and clinical systems professions. Provides leadership in health care for the management of systems, information, and change, while striving for high quality, efficient and effective patient care through analysis and technology implementation. Maintains speakers' bureau. Offers placement service. **Pub:** *Annual Conference*, annual. Proceedings. • *HIMSS News*, monthly. Newsletter. *Price:* Included in membership dues. • *Journal of Healthcare Information Management*, quarterly. Journal. Technical peer reviewed journal. *Price:* Included in membership dues. • Monographs, periodic. • Books, periodic. • Handbooks, periodic. **Frmly:** (1987) Hospital Management Systems Society.

**★ 12084 ★ Health Education Resource Organization (HERO)**
101 W Read St., Ste. 825
Baltimore, MD 21201
**Phone:** (410)685-1180          **Fax:** (410)752-3353
**Email:** heroprogrg@aol.com

**Fnded:** 1983. **Desc:** Provides client care services and preventive education regarding AIDS to Maryland residents; disseminates information on AIDS prevention and treatment to interested individuals nationwide. Provides social service and mental health counseling, support groups, legal aid, emergency funding, referrals, and case management. **Pub:** *Hero News*, monthly. Newsletter. • Also produces a wide range of

educational materials on AIDS prevention. **AKA:** HERO.

**Health Information Resource Center (HIRC)**
*See:* Entry 2141

**★ 12085 ★ Health Sciences Communications Association (HESCA)**
39 Wedgewood Dr., Ste. A
Jewett City, CT 06351
**Phone:** (860)376-5915          **Fax:** (860)376-6621
**Email:** hesca@hesca.org
**Website:** http://www.hesca.org/
Ronald Sokolowski, Exec. Dir.

**Fnded:** 1959. **Mem:** 400. **Reg. Groups:** 9. **Desc:** Media managers, graphic artists, biomedical librarians, producers, faculty members of health science and veterinary medicine schools, health professional organizations, and industry representatives. Acts as a clearinghouse for information used by professionals engaged in health science communications. Coordinates Media Festivals Program which recognizes outstanding media productions in the health sciences. Offers placement service. **Pub:** *Feedback*, 5/year. Provides members with information on the field of biocommunications and on work of colleagues. Includes employment listings and regional news. *Price:* Included in membership dues; $30/year for nonmembers. • *Health Sciences Communications Association–Who's Who*, annual. Membership Directory. *Price:* Included in membership dues. • *HESCA Learning Resources Center Catalog*, annual. Catalog. • *Journal of Biocommunication*, quarterly. Journal. Includes abstracts of biocommunication literature, gallery of medical art, and video and other media reviews. *Price:* Included in membership dues; $25 for nonmembers; $28 for institutions; $20 for students. • *Patient Education Sourcebook*. • Brochures. • Monographs. • Also publishes indexes; distributes audiovisual materials. **Frmly:** (1972) Council on Medical Television.

**★ 12086 ★ HEATH Resource Center (GWHRC)**
George Washington University
2121 K St. NW, Ste. 220
Washington, DC 20037
**Phone:** (202)973-0905          **Free:** 800-544-3284
**Fax:** (202)973-0908
**Email:** askheath@heath.gwu.edu
**Website:** http://www.heath.gwu.edu
Pamela Ekpone, Dir.

**Fnded:** 1977. **Desc:** National information Clearinghouse. Works to aid in the postsecondary education of people who are disabled. Provides information on educational support services, procedures, policies, adaptations, campus opportunities, vocational technical schools, adult education programs, and independent living centers. **Pub:** *Fact Sheet*, quarterly. Newsletter. • *Information*, 3/year. Directory. • *Resource Directory*, semiannual. Directory. • Also publishes topical informational materials.

**★ 12087 ★ Hong Kong Society of Medical Informatics (HKSMI)**
c/o Dr. C.P. Wong
Ruttonjee Hospital
266 Queen's Rd. E
Hong Kong, People's Republic of China
**Phone:** 852 22911345          **Fax:** 852 22911335
**Email:** cpwong@iohk.com

**Fnded:** 1986. **Mem:** 800. **Lang(s):** Chinese, English. **Desc:** Medical practitioners. Promotes the use of medical informatics in health care. Sponsors research and educational programs.

**★ 12088 ★ International Association of Cancer Registries (IACR) (Association Internationale des Registres du Cancer)**
c/o International Agency for Research on Cancer
150, cours Albert Thomas
F-69372 Lyon Cedex 08, France
**Phone:** 33 4 72738485          **Fax:** 33 4 72738575
**Email:** whelan@iarc.fr
**Website:** http://www-dep.iarc.fr/iacr.htm

**Fnded:** 1966. **Mem:** 410. **Lang(s):** English. **Desc:** Population-based cancer registries in 100 countries. Encourages the development and application of cancer registration and morbidity techniques to studies of defined populations. Endeavors to increase global awareness of the importance of producing accurate and comparable morbidity and mortality data which can be used to generate etiological hypotheses for cancer and as a basis for epidemiological studies, health planning, and other aspects of cancer control. **Pub:** *Cancer Incidence in Five Continents*, 5/year. Book. • *International Association of Cancer Registries' Newsletter*, biennial. Newsletter.

**★ 12089 ★ International Medical Informatics Association (IMIA)**
5782 172th St.
Edmonton, AB, Canada T6M 134
**Phone:** (780)489-4531          **Fax:** (780)489-3290
**Email:** imia@v-wave.com
**Website:** http://www.imia.org

**Fnded:** 1978. **Mem:** 72. **Reg. Groups:** 4. **Lang(s):** English. **Desc:** National organizations in the field of medical and health informatics. Objective is the international exchange of knowledge concerning health care and biomedical research through medical informatics. Sponsors conferences. **Pub:** *IMIA Medical Informatics Newsletter*. Newsletter.

**Intersociety Committee on Pathology Information (ICPI)**
*See:* Entry 17145

**★ 12090 ★ Japanese Association of Healthcare Information Systems Industry (JAHIS)**
c/o Tranomon TBL Building
1-19-9, Toranomon
Minato-ku
Tokyo 105-0001, Japan
**Phone:** 81 3 35068010          **Fax:** 81 3 35068070
**Email:** icpi@pathol.faseb.org
**Website:** http://www.jahis.gr.jp

**Lang(s):** English, Japanese. **Desc:** Corporations and organizations involved in the healthcare information system industry. Promotes the sound development of the healthcare information system industry and contributes to people's health, medical care, and welfare by improving technology and promoting the standardization of healthcare information systems. **Pub:** *JAHIS News*. Annual Report.

**★ 12091 ★ Media Access Group at WGBH (NCAM)**
PO Box 200
Boston, MA 02134
**Phone:** (617)300-5400          **Fax:** (617)300-1035
**Email:** access@wgbh.org
**Website:** http://www.wgbh.org/access

**Desc:** Dedicated to information equity to make media accessible to underserved populations such as disabled persons, minority-language users, and people with low literacy skills. **Pub:** *Media Access*, annual. Newsletter. **Frmly:** (2001) CPB/WGBH National CTR for Accessible Media

### ★ 12092 ★ Medical Records Institute (MRI)

567 Walnut St.
PO Box 600770
Newton, MA 02460
**Phone:** (617)964-3923          **Fax:** (617)964-3926
**Email:** cust_service@medrecinst.com
**Website:** http://www.medrecinst.com
C. Peter Waegemann, Exec. Dir.

**Fnded:** 1979. **Desc:** Conducts research and education in the fields of medical documentation and computerization of patient information. Maintains committees and network groups. Compiles statistics. **Pub:** *Handbook of Optical Memory Systems*. Handbook. Monthly updates available. *Price:* $100.50. • *Toward An Electronic Patient Record*, 10/year. *Price:* $145. • Proceedings. **Frmly:** (1988) Institute for Medical Record Economics.

### ★ 12093 ★ National Association of Health Data Organizations (NAHDO)

375 Chipeta Way, Ste. A
Salt Lake City, UT 84108
**Phone:** (801)587-9104          **Fax:** (801)587-9125
**Email:** info@nahdo.org
**Website:** http://www.nahdo.org
Denise Love, Exec. Dir.

**Fnded:** 1986. **Mem:** 112. **Desc:** Members include state, federal, nonprofit and private health data organizations, employee benefits consultants, professional review organizations, data analysis firms, software vendors, and health services consultants, health care researchers, third-party payers, hospital associations, managed care organizations. Seeks to improve health care through the collection, dissemination, and application of health care data. Promotes public availability of and access to health data; supports use of health care data to guide formulation of health policy, purchasing, and establishment of needed health services. Sponsors educational programs, workshops, & seminars. Conducts surveys and comparative studies; maintains speakers' bureau. **Pub:** *Inventory of Statewide Hospital Discharge Data Activities*. Manual. *Price:* $225. • *NAHDO Annual Report*, annual. Annual Report. *Price:* Free.

### National Association for Public Health Statistics and Information Systems (NAPHSIS)

*See:* Entry 17955

### National Cancer Registrars Association (NCRA)

*See:* Entry 10228

### National Council on Patient Information and Education (NCPIE)

*See:* Entry 17545

### National Families in Action (NFIA)

*See:* Entry 19325

### National Institute of Electromedical Information (NIEI)

*See:* Entry 4517

### ★ 12094 ★ NEA Health Information Network (NEA HIN)

1201 16th St., NW, Ste. 521
Washington, DC 20036
**Phone:** (202)822-7570          **Free:** 800-718-8387
**Fax:** (202)822-7775
**Email:** info@neahin.org
**Website:** http://www.neahin.org

**Fnded:** 1987. **Desc:** Dedicated to improve health, safety, and student achievement by providing school employees with vital, effective and timely health information. **Frmly:** (2001) Health Information Network.

### R. A. Bloch Cancer Foundation

*See:* Entry 10243

### Recording for the Blind and Dyslexic (RFB)

*See:* Entry 21060

### ★ 12095 ★ Tel-Med

24769 Redlands Blvd., Ste. L
Loma Linda, CA 92354
**Phone:** (909)478-0330          **Fax:** (909)478-3312
**Email:** telmed@ix.netcom.com
**Website:** http://www.tel-med.com
Michael Carpenter, CFO

**Fnded:** 1971. **Mem:** 200. **Desc:** Hospitals, medical societies, universities, medical centers, public libraries, and other organizations offering the Tel-Med program. Tel-Med is a library of three to five minute recorded health related messages created to be played over the telephone for public use, free of charge. Provides messages to communities; local libraries are established where individuals from the community can call to listen to messages. Operates as an information service intended to educate and assist in recognizing early signs of illness and is not designed to diagnose or treat medical problems. Scripts are written by medical professionals and examined by a team of physicians; messages are reviewed at least annually. Offers services and information on a wide range of medical subjects including alcoholism, arthritis, bee stings, cancer, diabetes, drug abuse, influenza, medical costs, mental health, nutrition, parenting, sex education, smoking, vasectomies, and vaginitis. **Pub:** *Tel-Med Newsletter*, quarterly. Newsletter. • Annual Report, annual. • Brochures. • Also publishes tape listings and literature on implementation of the Tel-Med program.

## Research Centers

### ★ 12096 ★ George Washington University Biostatistics Center

6110 Executive Blvd., Ste. 750
Rockville, MD 20852
**Phone:** (301)881-9260          **Fax:** (301)881-3742
**Website:** http://biostat.bsc.gwu.edu
Sarah Fowler, Dir.

**Activities/Fields:** Biostatistics, focusing on data management and analysis for medical research projects.

### ★ 12097 ★ Georgetown University Imaging Science and Information Systems Research Center

Medical Center, Department of Radiology
Georgetown University Medical Center
2115 Wisconsin Ave. NW, Ste. 603
Washington, DC 20007
**Phone:** (202)687-5990          **Fax:** (202)784-3479
**Email:** cleary@isis.imac.georgetown.edu
**Website:** http://www.isis.georgetown.edu
Kevin R. Cleary, PhD, Dir.

**Activities/Fields:** Health care improvement through innovations in computers, communication, imaging and information technologies.

### ★ 12098 ★ Harvard University Center for Biostatistics in AIDS Research

FXB Bldg.
Harvard Sch. of Public Health
651 Huntington Ave.
Boston, MA 02115
**Phone:** (617)432-2829          **Fax:** (617)432-3163
**Email:** lagakos@sdac.harvard.edu
Stephen W. Lagakos, Dir.

**Activities/Fields:** Treatments for persons infected with HIV. **Frmly:** Statistical Data and Analysis Center.

### Johns Hopkins University Center for Clinical Trials

*See:* Entry 2514

### ★ 12099 ★ Johns Hopkins University Center for Communication Programs

111 Market Pl., Ste. 310
Baltimore, MD 21202-4024
**Phone:** (410)659-6300          **Fax:** (410)659-6266
**Email:** jbertran@jhuccp.org
**Website:** http://www.jhuccp.org
June Bertrand, PhD, Dir.

**Activities/Fields:** Behavior change communication in the areas of family health, reproductive health, maternal and child health, and AIDS/STD prevention. Develops communication programs using mass media, interpersonal communication/counseling, advocacy, and community mobilization. Uses behavioral, attitudinal, and other social science research techniques to enhance and document the impact of communication on family planning and related health behavior. **Pub:** *Communication Impact*. Newsletter. • *Field Reports*. • *Population Reports*, quarterly. • *Working Papers*.

### ★ 12100 ★ Maryland Medical Research Institute

600 Wyndhurst Ave.
Baltimore, MD 21210-2425
**Phone:** (410)435-4200          **Fax:** (410)323-8622
**Email:** mterrin@mmri.org
**Website:** http://www.mmri.org
Dr. Michael Terrin, Pres.

**Activities/Fields:** Data gathering, analysis, and design for large-scale clinical trials and epidemiological studies in medical areas such as heart disease, cancer, blood disease, septicemia, AIDS, surgical treatment and laser therapy, and in retinal diseases, and the effects of diet on health status. **Pub:** *Controlled Clinical Trials*, quarterly.

### ★ 12101 ★ Massachusetts Health Data Consortium

460 Totten Pond Rd., Ste. 385
Waltham, MA 02451
**Phone:** (781)890-6040          **Fax:** (781)768-2510
**Email:** estone@mahealthdata.org
**Website:** http://www.mahealthdata.org
Elliot M. Stone, Exec. Dir. /CEO

**Activities/Fields:** Health services research, including studies of hospitals, patient and physician databases, and discharged patients since 1978. **Pub:** *Datagram*. • *Health Data News*, quarterly. • *Public Meeting Report*, annually. • *Webmasters Digest*.

### ★ 12102 ★ McGill University Lady Davis Institute for Medical Research McGill AIDS Centre

3755 Chemin de la Cote-Sainte-Catherine, Rm 318
Montreal, QC, Canada H3T 1E2
**Phone:** (514)340-8260          **Fax:** (514)340-7502
**Email:** wainberg@ldi.jgh.mcgill.ca
Mark A. Wainberg, MD, Dir.

**Activities/Fields:** Promotes research on all aspects of HIV/AIDS, the development of new drugs, treatments, and vaccines for HIV/AIDS, as well as the development of comprehensive cost-effective models of care and treatment for HIV infection and AIDS. Sponsors basic, clinical, epidemiological, preventive, and psychosocial studies of HIV/AIDS. Topics include residential drug abuse treatment models for AIDS prevention, immune response in AIDS, regulation of interferon gene expression, HIV-1 resistance to AZT and other drugs, Canadian women and HIV, HIV prevention through peer intervention among youth, assessment of social support for patients with HIV/AIDS, knowledge of HIV/AIDS among daycare workers and parents, and personal strivings and levels of self-determination in predicting adjustments in AIDS. **Pub:** *Newsletter*, quarterly.

**National Disease Research Interchange**
*See:* Entry 9055

**Texas Cancer Data Center**
*See:* Entry 10423

**U.S. Department of Defense**
**Army Medical Research and Materiel Command**
**Walter Reed Army Institute of Research**
**Medical Audio-Visual Services Division**
*See:* Entry 13482

**★ 12103 ★ U.S. Department of Health and Human Services**
**Food and Drug Administration**
**Center for Drug Evaluation and Research**
**Office of Drug Standards**
**(Marketing Practices and Communications Branch)**
Mail Code HFD-040
5600 Fishers Ln.
Rockville, MD 20857
**Phone:** (301)827-2828      **Fax:** (301)594-6759
**Email:** abramst@cder.fda.gov
**Website:** http://www.fda.gov/cder/ddmac/index.htm
Thomas Abrams, Dir.
**Activities/Fields:** Industry-wide marketing practices of the pharmaceutical industry and improvement of drug communications between FDA, health professionals, and the public. Specific research areas include prescription drugs, marketing practices, and health communications. **Frmly:** Drug Labeling Education and Research Branch.

**★ 12104 ★ U.S. Department of Health and Human Services**
**Health Care Financing Administration**
**Bureau of Data Management and Strategy**
**Office of Health Care Information Systems**
7500 Security Blvd.
N-3-13-15
Baltimore, MD 21244-1850
**Phone:** (410)786-1951      **Fax:** (410)786-1783
**Website:** http://www.hcfa.gov
Joe Broseker, Dir.
**Activities/Fields:** Development and implementation of pl ans and policies for the classification, standardization, identification, development, and security of data, procedures, and standards to meet the Health Care Financing Administration's information requirements and to provide health care data for research purposes. **Pub:** *ICD-9-CM Errata Addenda*, annually. • *Research reports*.

**★ 12105 ★ U.S. Department of Health and Human Services**
**Health Resources and Services Administration**
**Bureau of Health Professions**
**Office of Policy and Research**
**(Information Resource Management Branch)**
5600 Fishers Ln., Rm. 8808
Park Lawn Bldg.
Rockville, MD 20857
**Phone:** (301)443-1355      **Fax:** (301)443-4414
Art Smith, Chf.
**Activities/Fields:** Provides health and health-related data available at the county level; compatible and consistent health-related data in a variety of forms in order to be of use to the broadest possible range of users; and flexible analytical capabilities for analysis of health and health-related data. **Frmly:** Information Systems Branch of the Office of Data Analysis and Management.

**★ 12106 ★ U.S. Department of Health and Human Services**
**Indian Health Service**
**Office of Planning, Evaluation, and Legislation**
**Division of Program Statistics**
Twinbrook Metro Plaza
12300 Twinbrook Pkwy., Ste. 450
Rockville, MD 20852
**Phone:** (301)443-1180      **Fax:** (301)443-1522
**Email:** epaisano@hqe.ihs.gov
**Website:** http://www.ihs.gov/nonmedicalprograms/ihs_stats/index.sp
Edna Paisano, Supv. Stat.
**Activities/Fields:** Main function is to satisfy the American Indian and Alaska Native health statistics information needs of its clients. The Division manages a number of information systems that provide data for measuring the health status of the American Indian and Alaska Native population and appraising IHS program activities. Division's primary duty is to serve IHS management, but it also has numerous dealings with other government agencies, government contractors, academia, researchers, the media, and the general public. Division is responsible for: vital events statistics, patient care statistics, and population statistics. In addition to providing statistical data, Division also provides statistical advice on analyzing the data. **Pub:** *Indian health status reports*, occasionally. • *Regional Differences in Indian Health*, annually. • *Trends in Indian Health*, annually.

**U.S. Department of Health and Human Services**
**National Cancer Institute**
**Division of Cancer Treatment, Diagnosis, and Centers**
**Developmental Therapeutics Program**
**(Information Technology Branch)**
*See:* Entry 10458

**U.S. Department of Health and Human Services**
**National Cancer Institute**
**International Cancer Information Center**
*See:* Entry 10475

**★ 12107 ★ U.S. Department of Health and Human Services**
**National Center for Health Statistics**
6525 Belcrest Rd.
Hyattsville, MD 20782
**Phone:** (301)458-4500      **Fax:** (301)929-2802
**Email:** efs2@cdc.gov
**Website:** http://www.cdc.gov/nchs/
Edward Sondik, Dir.
**Activities/Fields:** National health statistics; conduct research in survey and statistical methodology; provide specialized training programs and technical assistance; and coordinate cooperative programs with state, national, and international organizations. Principal components include the Office of Analysis and Epidemiology, Office of Research and Methodology, and Office of Vital and Health Statistics Systems (Health Care Statistics Division, Health Examination Statistics Division, Health Interview Statistics Division, and Vital Statistics Division). Data Base NCHS maintains data systems that produce data in the following areas: extent of illness and disability in the population; distribution and normative standards for physiological and nutritional measurement; national vital statistics, including births, deaths, marriages, and divorces; hospital, nursing home, and ambulatory care utilization; health expenditures; family formation, growth, and dissolution; and other major health topics. **Pub:** *Advance Data*. • *Health U S*, annually. • *National Vital Statistics Report*. • *Vital and Health Statistics Series*. • *Vital Statistics of the U S*, annually.

**U.S. Department of Health and Human Services**
**National Institute on Alcohol Abuse and Alcoholism**
**Biometry and Epidemiology Division**
*See:* Entry 19368

**U.S. Department of Health and Human Services**
**National Institute of Allergy and Infectious Diseases**
**Office of Communications**
*See:* Entry 3289

**★ 12108 ★ U.S. Department of Health and Human Services**
**National Institute of Diabetes and Digestive and Kidney Diseases**
**Division of Intramural Research**
**Mathematical Research Branch**
BSA Bldg., Ste. 350
9190 Rockville Pike
Bethesda, MD 20892-2690
**Phone:** (301)496-4325      **Fax:** (301)402-0535
**Email:** asherman@nih.gov
**Website:** http://mrb.niddk.nih.gov
Dr. Arthur S. Sherman, Ch.
**Activities/Fields:** Mathematical and theoretical aspects of biological problems and the development of analytical and numerical methodology underlying such an approach. The research programs are designed to provide a formal basis and theoretical apparatus for the rational analysis and quantitative interpretation of biological phenomena. Research is organized around biological subject-matter areas rather than around subdisciplines of mathematics. Primary areas of research include neuroscience, physiology, cell biology, and endocrimology.

**U.S. Department of Health and Human Services**
**National Institute of Mental Health**
**Division of State and Community Systems Development**
**Survey and Analysis Branch**
*See:* Entry 12721

**U.S. Department of Health and Human Services**
**National Institute of Mental Health**
**Office of Scientific Information**
*See:* Entry 12747

**U.S. Department of Health and Human Services**
**National Institute of Neurological Disorders and Stroke**
**Division of Demyelinating, Atrophic, and Dementing Disorders**
**Huntington's Disease Research Roster**
*See:* Entry 14296

**U.S. Department of Health and Human Services**
**National Institute for Occupational Safety and Health**
**Education and Information Division**
**Information Resources Branch**
*See:* Entry 16826

**U.S. Department of Health and Human Services**
**National Institutes of Health**
**Office of Medical Applications of Research**
*See:* Entry 18004

**★ 12109 ★ U.S. Department of Health and Human Services**
**National Library of Medicine**
Bldg. 38, 2S15
8600 Rockville Pike
Bethesda, MD 20894
**Phone:** (301)496-6308 **Fax:** (301)496-4450
**Email:** publicinfo@nlm.nih.gov
**Website:** http://www.nlm.nih.gov
Dr. Donald A.B. Lindberg, Dir.

**Activities/Fields:** World's largest research library in a single scientific and professional field. The Library collects materials in all major areas of the health sciences and, to a lesser degree, in chemistry, physics, botany, and zoology. The Library's extensive collections and information services may be used by health professionals and health-science students. In addition, NLM serves as a national resource for all U.S. health science libraries through its National Network of Libraries of Medicine. This network, which offers lending and other services, includes 4000 basic unit libraries (mostly at hospitals), 125 Resource Libraries (at medical schools), and eight Regional Medical Libraries (covering all geographic areas of the United States), and the NLM itself. **Pub:** *Index Medicus*, monthly.


**★ 12110 ★ U.S. Department of Health and Human Services**
**National Library of Medicine**
**Extramural Programs Division**
6705 Rockledge Dr., Ste. 301
Bethesda, MD 20894
**Phone:** (301)496-4621 **Fax:** (301)402-2952
**Email:** cornm@mail.nlm.nih.gov
**Website:** http://www.nlm.nih.gov/ep/extramural.html
Dr. Milton Corn, Dir.

**Activities/Fields:** Administers the National Library of Medicine's program of grants fo r support of fundamental and applied work in the organization, representation, utilization, and dissemination of health knowledge, with special interest in medical informatics and biotechnology information. Grants are generally awarded in three main categories: Research, Development, and Demonstration awards are investigator-initiated projects that address problems of health information access, retrieval, and utilization. Projects may investigate fundamental research problems, may undertake development of theoretical findings into practical applications, or may demonstrate the value of new technologies in operating situations. First Independent Research Support and Transition (FIRST) Awards are small project awards to young investigators. Eligibility is limited to those who have received the doctorate within five years but have not yet served as principal investigator on a research grant or contract. Research Career Development Awards are available to young scientists with three or more years of postdoctoral experience. These awards enable the scientist to devote full time to research.


**★ 12111 ★ U.S. Department of Health and Human Services**
**National Library of Medicine**
**Office of Computer and Communications Systems**
**Special Assistant for Research and Development**
Bldg. 38A, Rm. 9F904
8600 Rockville Pike
Bethesda, MD 20894
**Phone:** (301)496-9300 **Fax:** (301)496-0673
Dr. Tamas E. Doszkocs, Computer Sci.

**Activities/Fields:** Information processing, including information retrieval, ergonomics, natural language processing, artificial intelligence, and database management.


**★ 12112 ★ University of Alberta**
**Telehealth Technology Research Institute (TTRI)**
508
Butterworth Way
Edmonton, AB, Canada T6R 2G8
**Phone:** (780)436-7221 **Fax:** (780)988-5660
**Email:** masako.miyazaki@ualberta.ca
**Website:** http://www.e-ttri.com
Masako Miyazaki, Pres.

**Activities/Fields:** Research and development of e-health technology at consumer level. Technology supported community base healthcare.


**University of Cincinnati**
**Division of Epidemiology and Biostatistics**
*See:* Entry 9075


**★ 12113 ★ University of Minnesota**
**Coordinating Centers for Biometric Research**
Division of Biostatistics
2221 University Ave. SE, Ste. 200
Minneapolis, MN 55414-3080
**Phone:** (612)626-8887 **Fax:** (612)626-9054
**Email:** biostat@ccbr.umn.edu
**Website:** http://www.biostat.umn.edu
John Connett, Div. Hd.

**Activities/Fields:** Cancer, AIDS, chronic obstructive pulmonary disease, coronary heart disease, otitis media (ear infection), and hypertension. Research activities include developing new statistical methodology; collaborating on applied projects that influence clinical, public health, and public policy; and applied and methodological research.


**★ 12114 ★ University of Vermont**
**Medical Biostatistics/Biometry Facility**
27 Hills Science Bldg.
Burlington, VT 05405
**Phone:** (802)656-2526 **Fax:** (802)656-0632
**Email:** tashikag@zoo.uvm.edu
Taka Ashikaga, PhD, Dir.

**Activities/Fields:** Survey research of health behaviors; epidemiologic surveys for respiratory disease, cancer, and lower back pain; clinical trials; and evaluative research in the areas of public education, school health education, patient education, and health professional education. Also performs psychiatric patient follow-up studies, cancer mortality studies, studies on genetic-based disease factors, and studies of impact of acid rain on forest ecosystems. Conducts surveys of public opinion, mass media patterns, marketing practices, and health status.


# State Government Agencies

## Vital Statistics

**★ 12115 ★ Alabama Department of Public Health**
**Health Statistics Center**
**Quality Assurance Division**
PO Box 5618
Montgomery, AL 36103-5618
**Phone:** (334)206-5418 **Fax:** (334)206-2733
**Website:** http://www.alapubhealth.org/


**★ 12116 ★ Alaska Department of Health and Social Services**
**Public Health Division**
**Vital Statistics Section**
PO Box 110675
Juneau, AK 99811-0675
**Phone:** (907)465-3392 **Fax:** (907)465-3618

**Website:** http://www.hss.state.ak.us/dph/bvs/
Al Zangri, Director


**★ 12117 ★ Arizona Department of Health Services**
**Vital Records Office**
1740 West Adams St.
Phoenix, AZ 85007
**Phone:** (602)542-1216 **Fax:** (602)542-2940
**Email:** webmaster@hs.state.az.us
**Website:** http://www.hs.state.az.us/plan/ohpes.htm


**★ 12118 ★ Arkansas Department of Health**
**Health Resources Bureau**
**Vital Records Division**
4815 W Markham, Slot 44
Little Rock, AR 72205-3867
**Phone:** (501)661-2371
**Website:** http://www.healthyarkansas.com/services/services_ts2_all.htmlVital
Sharon Leinbach, Contact


**★ 12119 ★ California Health and Welfare Agency**
**Health Services Department**
**Vital Records Branch**
304 S St.
PO Box 730241
Sacramento, CA 94244-0241
**Phone:** (916)445-2684
**Website:** http://www.dhs.cahwnet.gov/org/hisp/chs/chsindex.htm


**★ 12120 ★ Colorado Public Health and Environment Department**
**Administration and Support Office**
**Health Statistics and Vital Records Division**
4300 Cherry Creek Dr. S
Denver, CO 80246-1530
**Phone:** (303)692-2160 **Fax:** (303)691-7704
**Email:** health.statistics@state.co.us
**Website:** http://www.cdphe.state.co.us/hs/hsshom.asp


**★ 12121 ★ Connecticut Department of Public Health**
**Policy, Planning, and Evaluation Office**
**Vital Records Division**
410 Capitol Ave.
PO Box 340308
MS 11VRS
Hartford, CT 06134-0308
**Phone:** (860)509-7163 **Fax:** (860)509-7160
**Email:** angela.kasek@po.state.ct.us
**Website:** http://www.state.ct.us/dph/OPPE/hpvital.htm
Daniel J. Savino, Director


**★ 12122 ★ Delaware Department of Health and Social Services**
**Public Health Division**
**Office of Vital Statistics**
PO Box 637
Dover, DE 19903
**Phone:** (302)739-4721 **Fax:** (302)736-1862
**Email:** dhssinfo@state.de.us
**Website:** http://www.state.de.us/dhss/dph/vs.htm


**★ 12123 ★ District of Columbia Department of Human Services**
**State Center for Health Statistics**
**Vital Records Branch**
825 N Capitol St. NE
First Floor
Washington, DC 20002
**Phone:** (202)442-9009 **Fax:** (202)442-4833

**Website:** http://www.dchealth.com/vitalrecords.htm

**★ 12124 ★ Florida Department of Health and Rehabilitative Services**
**Vital Records & Statistics Office**
PO Box 210
Jacksonville, FL 32231-0042
**Phone:** (904)359-6900     **Fax:** (904)359-6931
**Email:** vitalstats@doh.state.fl.us
**Website:** http://www9.myflorida.com/planning_eval/phstats/index.html
Ken T. Jones, Contact


**★ 12125 ★ Georgia Department of Human Resources**
**Public Health Division**
**Vital Records Office**
2600 Skyland Dr. NE
Atlanta, GA 30319-3640
**Phone:** (404)679-4701
**Email:** gdphinfo@dhr.state.ga.us
**Website:** http://www.ph.dhr.state.ga.us/programs/vitalrecords/index.shtml


**★ 12126 ★ Hawaii Department of Health**
**Health Status Monitoring Office**
**Vital Records Section**
1250 Punchbowl St., Rm. 103
PO Box 3378
Honolulu, HI 96801
**Phone:** (808)586-4400     **Fax:** (808)586-4444
**Email:** vr-info@mail.health.state.hi.us
**Website:** http://www.state.hi.us/health/records/index.html


**★ 12127 ★ Idaho Department of Health and Welfare**
**Health Division**
**Vital Records and Health Statistics Bureau**
Pete T. Cenarrusa Bldg. 1st Fl.
450 W State St.
PO Box 83720
Boise, ID 83720-0036
**Phone:** (208)334-5500     **Fax:** (208)334-6558
**Email:** dhwinfo@idhw.state.id.us
**Website:** http://www2.state.id.us/dhw/hwgd_www/contentlist.htmlVitalStats
Davalee Leavitt, Contact


**★ 12128 ★ Illinois Department of Public Health**
**Finance and Administration Office**
**Vital Records Division**
605 W Jefferson St.
Springfield, IL 62702-5097
**Phone:** (217)782-6554     **Fax:** (217)523-2648
**Email:** mailus@idph.state.il.us
**Website:** http://www.idph.state.il.us/vital/vitalhome.htm


**★ 12129 ★ Indiana Department of Health**
**Public Health Statistics Division**
2 N Meridian St.
Indianapolis, IN 46204
**Phone:** (317)233-2700     **Fax:** (317)233-7210
**Website:** http://www.state.in.us/isdh/bdcertifs/birth_and_death_certificates.htm


**★ 12130 ★ Iowa Department of Public Health**
**Planning and Administration Division**
**Vital Records Bureau**
Lucas State Office Bldg.
321 E 12th St.
Des Moines, IA 50319-0075
**Phone:** (515)281-4944
**Email:** webmaster@idph.state.ia.us
**Website:** http://idph.state.ia.us/pa/vr.htm


**★ 12131 ★ Kansas Department of Health and Environment**
**Health and Environment Statistics Division**
**Vital Statistics Office**
1000 SW Jackson, Ste. 120
Topeka, KS 66612-2221
**Phone:** (785)296-1400     **Fax:** (785)296-8075
**Email:** Vital.Records@kdhe.state.ks.us
**Website:** http://www.kdhe.state.ks.us/vital/
Gabriel Faimon, Director


**★ 12132 ★ Kentucky Health Services Cabinet**
**Department for Public Health**
**Vital Statistics Division**
275 E Main St, 1E-A
Frankfort, KY 40621
**Phone:** (502)564-4212     **Fax:** (502)227-0032
**Website:** http://publichealth.state.ky.us/vital.htm


**★ 12133 ★ Louisiana Department of Health and Hospitals**
**Health Information Division**
**Vital Records Registry**
PO Box 60630
New Orleans, LA 70160
**Phone:** (504)568-8353     **Fax:** (504)568-6909
**Email:** vitalweb@ddhh.state.la.us
**Website:** http://oph.dhh.state.la.us/recordsstatistics/vitalrecords/


**★ 12134 ★ Maine Department of Human Services**
**Research and Vital Statistics Division**
11 State House Station
221 State St
Augusta, ME 04333-0011
**Phone:** (207)287-3181
**Email:** lorraine.wilson@state.me.us
**Website:** http://janus.state.me.us/dhs/welcome.htm


**★ 12135 ★ Maryland Department of Health and Mental Hygiene**
**Health Services Analysis and Evaluation Administration**
201 W Preston St., 5th Fl.
Baltimore, MD 21201
**Phone:** (410)767-5806     **Fax:** (410)767-6489
**Email:** corddrym@dhmh.state.md.us
**Website:** http://www.dhmh.state.md.us/hsaea/


**★ 12136 ★ Massachusetts Executive Office of Health and Human Services**
**Public Health Department**
**Vital Records and Statistics Division**
150 Mt. Vernon St., 1st Fl.
Dorchester, MA 02125-3105
**Phone:** (617)740-2600
**Email:** jean.lorusso@state.ma.us
**Website:** http://www.state.ma.us/dph/rvr.htm


**★ 12137 ★ Michigan Community Health Department**
**State Registrar and Health Statistics Center**
3423 N Martin Luther King Blvd.
PO Box 30691
Lansing, MI 48909
**Phone:** (517)335-8677     **Fax:** (517)335-9513
**Email:** Humphrysk@state.mi.us
**Website:** http://www.mdch.state.mi.us/PHA/OSR/index.htm


**★ 12138 ★ Minnesota Department of Health**
**Center for Health Statistics**
**Vital Records Section**
717 Delaware St. SE
PO Box 9441
Minneapolis, MN 55440-9441
**Phone:** (612)676-5120
**Email:** chs1@health.state.mn.us
**Website:** http://www.health.state.mn.us/divs/chs/data/bd_1.htm


**★ 12139 ★ Mississippi Department of Health**
**Community Health Services Office**
**Vital Statistics Division**
571 Stadium Dr.
PO Box 1700
Jackson, MS 39215-1700
**Phone:** (601)576-7960     **Fax:** (601)576-7505
**Email:** vrinfo@msdh.state.ms.us
**Website:** http://www.msdh.state.ms.us/phs/index.htm


**★ 12140 ★ Missouri Department of Health**
**Health Information Management and Epidemiology Center**
**Vital Records Bureau**
930 Wildwood Dr.
PO Box 570
Jefferson City, MO 65102
**Phone:** (573)751-6381
**Email:** info@mail.health.state.mo.us
**Website:** http://www.health.state.mo.us/BirthAndDeathRecords/BirthAndDeathRecords.html


**★ 12141 ★ Montana Department of Public Health and Human Services**
**Vital Records and Statistics Bureau**
PO Box 4210
111 N Sanders
Helena, MT 59604-4210
**Phone:** (406)444-1756     **Fax:** (406)444-1803
**Email:** kferlicka@state.mt.us
**Website:** http://www.dphhs.state.mt.us/divisions/otd/vital_stats.htm
Bruce Schwartz, Contact


**★ 12142 ★ Nebraska Department of Health and Human Services**
**Vital Records Office**
Nebraska Department of HHS Finance and Support
Vital Records
PO Box 95065
Lincoln, NE 68509-5065
**Phone:** (402)471-2871     **Fax:** (402)471-0383
**Email:** Vitalrecords@hhss.state.ne.us
**Website:** http://www.hhs.state.ne.us/ced/cedindex.htm


**★ 12143 ★ Nevada Department of Human Resources**
**Health Division**
**Vital Records Bureau**
505 E King St.
Rm. 102
Carson City, NV 89701
**Phone:** (775)684-4242     **Fax:** (775)684-4156
**Website:** http://www.state.nv.us/health/


**★ 12144 ★ New Hampshire Department of Health and Human Services**
**Public Health Services Division**
**Vital Records and Health Statistics Bureau**
6 Hazen Dr.
Concord, NH 03301

**Phone:** (603)271-4650  **Free:** 800-852-3345
**Fax:** (603)271-3447
**Email:** vitalrecords@dhhs.state.nh.us
**Website:** http://www.dhhs.state.nh.us/

**★ 12145 ★ New Jersey Department of Health**
**Health Care Systems Analysis Division**
**Center for Health Statistics**
PO Box 360
Trenton, NJ 08625-0360
**Phone:** (609)984-6702  **Fax:** (609)984-7633
**Email:** chs@doh.state.nj.us
**Website:** http://www.state.nj.us/health/chs/
Katherine Hempstead, Director

**★ 12146 ★ New Mexico Department of Health**
**Public Health Division**
**Vital Statistics Section**
1105 St. Francis Dr.
1190 St. Francis Dr.
Santa Fe, NM 87505
**Phone:** (505)827-0121
**Website:** http://dohewbs2.health.state.nm.us/Vital-Rec/

**★ 12147 ★ North Carolina Department of Health and Human Services**
**North Carolina Center for Health Statistics**
**Vital Records Section**
1903 Mail Service Ctr.
Raleigh, NC 27699-1903
**Phone:** (919)733-3526
**Email:** SCHS.Info@ncmail.net
**Website:** http://www.schs.state.nc.us/SCHS/about/branches/vital.html

**★ 12148 ★ North Dakota Department of Health**
**Administrative Services Section**
**Vital Records Division**
600 E Boulevard Ave.
Bismarck, ND 58505-0200
**Phone:** (701)328-2360  **Fax:** (701)328-1850
**Email:** vitalrec@state.nd.us
**Website:** http://www.health.state.nd.us/ndhd/admin/vital/
Beverly Wittmann, Director

**★ 12149 ★ Oklahoma Department of Health**
**Administrative Services**
**Vital Records Division**
1000 NE 10th St.
Rm. 111
Oklahoma City, OK 73117
**Phone:** (405)271-4040
**Website:** http://www.health.state.ok.us/PROGRAM/vital/index.html

**★ 12150 ★ Oregon Department of Human Resources**
**Health Division**
**Vital Statistics Section**
Portland State Office Bldg.
800 NE Oregon St., Ste. 215
PO Box 14050
Portland, OR 97293-0050
**Phone:** (503)731-4109
**Website:** http://www.ohd.hr.state.or.us/chs/welcome.htm
Jennifer Woodward, Contact

**★ 12151 ★ Pennsylvania Department of Health**
**Public Health Assessment**
**Vital Records Division**
101 S Mercer St.
PO Box 1528
New Castle, PA 16103-1528
**Phone:** (717)783-2548  **Fax:** (724)772-3258
**Email:** webmaster@health.state.pa.us
**Website:** http://www.health.state.pa.us/hpa/Stats/vital/

**★ 12152 ★ Rhode Island Department of Health**
**Management Services**
**Vital Record Division**
3 Capitol Hill, Rm. 101
Providence, RI 02908
**Phone:** (401)222-2811
**Email:** library@health.state.ri.us
**Website:** http://www.health.state.ri.us/yhd05.htm

**★ 12153 ★ South Carolina Department of Health and Environmental Control**
**Vital Records and Public Health Statistics Office**
2600 Bull St.
Columbia, SC 29201
**Phone:** (803)898-3630  **Fax:** (803)799-0301
**Email:** goodinj@columb20.dhec.state.sc.us
**Website:** http://www.scdhec.net/vr/index.htm

**★ 12154 ★ South Dakota Department of Health**
**Vital Records Program**
600 E Capitol
Pierre, SD 57501-2536
**Phone:** (605)773-4961
**Email:** DOH.INFO@state.sd.us
**Website:** http://www.state.sd.us/doh/VitalRec/index.htm

**★ 12155 ★ Tennessee Department of Health**
**Administrative Services Bureau**
**Health Statistics Division**
**Vital Records Section**
Central Services Bldg.
421 5th Ave. N, 1st Fl.
Nashville, TN 37247-0460
**Phone:** (615)741-1763  **Fax:** (615)741-9860
**Email:** DDenton@mail.state.tn.us
**Website:** http://www2.state.tn.us/health/vr/

**★ 12156 ★ Texas Department of Health**
**Vital Statistics Bureau**
1100 W 49th St.
PO Box 12040
Austin, TX 78711-2040
**Phone:** (512)458-7111  **Free:** 888-963-7111
**Fax:** (512)458-7233
**Email:** register@tdh.state.tx.us
**Website:** http://www.tdh.state.tx.us/bvs/default.htm

**★ 12157 ★ Utah Department of Health**
**Health Statistics and Vital Records Bureau**
288 N 1460 W
PO Box 141012
Salt Lake City, UT 84114-1012
**Phone:** (801)538-6105
**Email:** vrequest@doh.state.ut.us
**Website:** http://www.health.state.ut.us/bvr/

**★ 12158 ★ Vermont Agency of Human Services**
**Health Department**
**Public Health, Analysis and Policy Division**
**Vital Records Unit**
108 Cherry St.
PO Box 70
Burlington, VT 05402-0070
**Phone:** (802)863-7275  **Free:** 800-439-5008
**Fax:** (802)828-3710
**Website:** http://www.state.vt.us/health/_hs/vitals/records/vitalrecords.htm

**★ 12159 ★ Virginia Office of Health and Human Resources**
**Health Department**
**Vital Records Office**
PO Box 1000
Richmond, VA 23218-1000
**Phone:** (804)662-6200
**Email:** lwhitaker@vdh.state.va.us
**Website:** http://www.vdh.state.va.us/vitalrec/f_08.htm
Deborah Little-Bowser, Director

**★ 12160 ★ Washington Department of Health**
**Health Statistics Center**
1112 SE Quince St.
PO Box 47890
Olympia, WA 98504-7890
**Phone:** (360)236-4300
**Email:** glenda.moore@doh.wa.gov
**Website:** http://www.doh.wa.gov/EHSPHL/CHS/cert.htm

**★ 12161 ★ West Virginia Department of Health and Human Resources**
**Public Health Bureau**
**Epidemiology and Health Promotion Office**
**Health Statistics Division**
350 Capitol St., Rm. 165
Charleston, WV 25301-3715
**Phone:** (304)558-9100
**Email:** danchristy@wvdhhr.org
**Website:** http://www.wvdhhr.org/bph/oehp/hsc/hschome.htm

**★ 12162 ★ Wisconsin Department of Health and Family Services**
**Health Division**
**Vital Statistics Office**
PO Box 309
Madison, WI 53701-0309
**Phone:** (608)266-1371  **Fax:** (608)261-4971
**Email:** VitalRecords@dhfs.state.wi.us
**Website:** http://www.dhfs.state.wi.us/VitalRecords/index.htm

**★ 12163 ★ Wyoming Department of Health**
**Preventive Health and Safety Division**
**Vital Records Section**
Hathaway Bldg., 4th Fl.
Cheyenne, WY 82002
**Phone:** (307)777-7591
**Email:** cmccaf@missc.state.wy.us
**Website:** http://wdhfs.state.wy.us/vital_records/index.htm
Lucinda McCaffrey, Director

# Foundations & Other Funding Organizations

## Other Funding Organizations

**★ 12164 ★ American Society for Clinical Laboratory Science (ASCLS)**
7910 Woodmont Ave., Ste. 530
Bethesda, MD 20814
**Phone:** (301)657-2768          **Fax:** (301)657-2909
**Email:** ascls@ascls.org
**Website:** http://www.ascls.org
Elissa Passiment, EdM, Exec. VP

**Desc:** Primarily clinical laboratory personnel who have an associate or baccalaureate degree and clinical training and specialists who hold at least a master's degree in one of the major fields of clinical laboratory science such as bacteriology, mycology, or biochemistry; also includes technicians, specialists, and educators with limited certificates and students enrolled in approved programs of clinical laboratory studies and military medical technology schools. Promotes and maintains high standards in clinical laboratory methods and research and advances standards of education and training of personnel. Conducts educational program of seminars and workshops. Sponsors award competition to encourage the writing of scientific papers. Approves programs of continuing education and maintains records on participation in continuing education programs for members. **Awards:** Scholarship for training in clinical laboratory science.

**★ 12165 ★ Clinical Laboratory Management Association (CLMA)**
989 Old Eagle School Rd., Ste. 815
Wayne, PA 19087
**Phone:** (610)995-9580          **Fax:** (610)995-9568
**Email:** rneri@lcma.org
**Website:** http://www.clma.org
Robert A. Neri, Exec. VP

**Desc:** Individuals holding managerial or supervisory positions with clinical laboratories; persons engaged in education of such individuals; manufacturers or distributors of equipment or services to clinical laboratories. Objectives are: to enhance management skills and promote more efficient and productive department operations; to further exchange of professional knowledge, new technology, and colleague experience; to encourage cooperation among those engaged in management or supervisory functions. Activities include: workshops, seminars, and expositions; dissemination of information about legislation and other topics. **Awards:** Chapter of the Year (annual); Educational Scholarship (annual); Industry Awards (annual); Sterling Service (annual).

**★ 12166 ★ Clinical Ligand Assay Society (CLAS)**
3139 S Wayne Rd.
Wayne, MI 48184
**Phone:** (734)722-6290          **Fax:** (734)722-7006

**Email:** clas@clas.org
**Website:** http://www.clas.org
Daisy S. McCann, PhD, Exec. Dir.

**Desc:** Seeks to establish and promote high standards in the science and application of ligand assay technology by encouraging research, education practitioners, and fostering communication and cooperation among individuals in laboratories in medicine, academia, and industry. Sponsors job placement service. Sponsors job placement service. **Awards:** CLAS Distinguished Scientist Award (annual) distinguished record in ligand assay technology.

**★ 12167 ★ National Society for Histotechnology (NSH)**
4201 Northview Dr., Ste. 502
Bowie, MD 20716-2604
**Phone:** (301)262-6221          **Fax:** (301)262-9188
**Email:** histo@nsh.org
**Website:** http://www.nsh.org
Roberta Mosedale, Exec. Dir.

**Desc:** Histology laboratory technicians, pathologists, laboratory equipment manufacturers' representatives, and interested individuals. Encourages the professional growth and advancement of histoprofessionals and promotes the exchange of ideas and knowledge significant to histotechnology. Assists in the establishment and mutual understanding of related societies. Provides continuing education training courses. Investigates health hazards in the laboratory; ensures the safety of the laboratory; and participates in formulating federal laboratory regulations. **Awards:** Histotechnologist of the Year Award (annual); J.B. McCormick Award (annual); Newsletter of the Year Award (annual); scholarship.

# Medical & Allied Health Schools

## Blood Bank Technology

*Facilities listed below offer Specialist in Blood Bank (SBB) education programs accredited by the American Association of Blood Banks (8101 Glenbrook Rd., Bethesda, MD 20814-2749, (301)907-6977, http://www.aabb.org) in collaboration with the Commission on Accreditation of Allied Health Education Programs (35 E Wacker Dr., Ste. 1970, Chicago, IL 60601-2208, (312)553-9355, http://www.caahep.org/).*

## Alabama

**★ 12168 ★ University of Alabama, Birmingham**
**American Red Cross Blood Services, Birmingham Region**
**Specialist in Blood Bank Technology Program**
SHRP Bldg., Rm. 381
1714 Ninth Ave. S
Birmingham, AL 35294-1270
**Phone:** (205)934-5987          **Fax:** (205)975-7302
**Email:** fritsman@uab.edu
**Website:** http://www.ua.edu
Margaret G. Fritsman, Director
Shu T. Huang, MD, Contact

## California

**★ 12169 ★ Sacramento Medical Foundation Education Program**
**Specialist in Blood Bank Technology Program**
1625 Stockton Blvd.
Sacramento, CA 95816
**Phone:** (916)453-3661          **Fax:** (916)452-1664
**Email:** sacblood@concentric.net
Sally Morgan-Gannon, DIR
Paul V. Holland, MD, CNT

## District of Columbia

**★ 12170 ★ Walter Reed Army Medical Center**
**Department of Pathology**
**U.S. Army Blood Bank Fellowship Program**
**Specialist in Blood Bank Technology Program**
6900 Georgia Ave.
Washington, DC 20307-5001
**Phone:** (202)782-6210          **Fax:** (202)782-4502
**Email:** william.turcan@na.amedo.army.mil
**Website:** http://www.wramc.amedd.army.mil/
William Turcan, Director
Maj. D. Joe Chaffin, MD, Contact

## Florida

**★ 12171 ★ Florida Blood Services**
**Transfusion Medicine Academic Center**
**Specialist in Blood Bank Technology Program**
10100 Ninth St. N
Saint Petersburg, FL 33713
**Phone:** (727)568-5433          **Fax:** (727)568-2177
**Website:** http://www.fbsblood.org/academic.asp
Alice Cox Putman, Director
German Felix LeParc, MD, Contact

## Illinois

★ **12172** ★ **University of Illinois, Chicago**
**Specialist in Blood Bank Technology**
**Program**
808 S Wood St.
Rm. 690 M/C 518
Chicago, IL 60612-7305
**Phone:** (312)996-6721 **Fax:** (312)996-9296
**Email:** sbb_program@uic.edu
**Website:** http://www.sbhis.uic.edu
Veronica N. Lewis, DIR
Sanobar Kahn, MD, CNT

## Louisiana

★ **12173** ★ **Medical Center of Louisiana**
**Charity Hospital**
**Specialist in Blood Bank Technology**
**Program**
1532 Tulane Ave.
New Orleans, LA 70112-2860
**Phone:** (504)568-3502 **Fax:** (504)568-2635
**Email:** kkirkl@lsumc.edu
Karen C. Kirkley, DIR
Yuan S Kao, MD, CNT

## Maryland

★ **12174** ★ **Johns Hopkins Hospital**
**Specialist in Blood Bank Technology**
**Program**
Carnegie Bldg., No. 667
600 N Wolfe St.
Baltimore, MD 21287-6667
**Phone:** (410)955-6580 **Fax:** (410)955-0618
**Email:** deirdre@welchlink.welch.jhu.edu
Deirdre Parsons, DIR
Paul Ness, MD, CNT

★ **12175** ★ **U.S. Department of Health**
**and Human Services**
**National Institutes of Health (NIH)**
**Clinical Center Blood Bank**
**Specialist in Blood Bank Technology**
**Program**
NIH/CC/DTM Bldg. 10, Rm. 1C 711
10 Center Dr., MSC 1184
Bethesda, MD 20892
**Phone:** (301)496-8335 **Fax:** (301)402-1360
**Email:** kcipolone@dtm.cc.nih.gov
**Website:** http://www.nih.gov
Karen Cipolone, DIR
David F. Stroncek, MD, CNT

## Ohio

★ **12176** ★ **Ohio State University Medical**
**Center Blood Bank**
**American Red Cross Blood Services,**
**Central Ohio Region**
**Specialist in Blood Bank Technology**
**Program**
995 E Broad St.
Columbus, OH 43205
**Phone:** (614)253-2740 **Fax:** (614)253-2487
Joanne Kosanke, DIR
Mary Wissel, MD, CNT

★ **12177** ★ **University of Cincinnati**
**Medical Center**
**Hoxworth Blood Center**
**Specialist in Blood Bank Technology**
**Program**
3130 Highland Ave.
PO Box 670055
Cincinnati, OH 45267-0055
**Phone:** (513)558-1259 **Fax:** (513)588-1279
**Email:** nefftp@email.uc.edu
**Website:** http://www2.hoxworth.org/hoxworth/ed-uopp.htm
Terri P. Neff, DIR
Thomas Zuck, MD, CNT

## Texas

★ **12178** ★ **Gulf Coast Regional Blood**
**Center**
**School of Blood Bank Technology**
**Specialist in Blood Bank Technology**
**Program**
1400 La Concha Lane
Houston, TX 77054-1802
**Phone:** (713)791-6201 **Fax:** (713)791-6610
**Email:** cwong@giveblood.org
**Website:** http://www.giveblood.org
Clare Wong, Director
Arthur Bracey, MD, Contact

★ **12179** ★ **University of Texas Health**
**Science Center**
**University Health System**
**Specialist in Blood Bank Technology**
**Program**
4502 Medical Dr., MS 29
San Antonio, TX 78229-4493
**Phone:** (210)358-2807 **Fax:** (210)358-4762
**Email:** smithla@uthscsa.edu
**Website:** http://www.uthscsa.edu
Bonnie M. Fodermaier, DIR
Chantal Harrison, MD, CNT

★ **12180** ★ **University of Texas Medical**
**Branch, Galveston**
**Specialist in Blood Bank Technology**
**Program**
301 University Blvd.
Galveston, TX 77555-0717
**Phone:** (409)772-4866 **Fax:** (409)772-3193
**Email:** jvincent@utmb.edu
**Website:** http://www.utmb.edu
Janet Vincent, DIR
Alexander Indrikovs, MD, CNT

★ **12181** ★ **University of Texas**
**Southwestern Medical Center, Dallas**
**Specialist in Blood Bank Technology**
**Program**
5323 Harry Hines Blvd.
Dallas, TX 75390-8878
**Phone:** (214)648-1785 **Fax:** (214)648-1029
**Email:** barbara.fryer@email.swmed.edu
**Website:** http://www.swmed.edu/education/allied/
Lynn M. Little, PhD, Director
Harold Kaplan, MD, Contact

## Wisconsin

★ **12182** ★ **Blood Center of Southeast**
**Wisconsin**
**Specialist in Blood Bank Technology**
**Program**
638 N 18th St.
Milwaukee, WI 53233
**Phone:** (414)937-6274 **Fax:** (414)937-6461
**Email:** stjohnson@bcsew.edu
**Website:** http://www.bloodctrwise.org
Susan T. Johnson, DIR
Janice G. McFarland, MD, CNT

# National & International Organizations

★ **12183** ★ **Academy of Clinical**
**Laboratory Physicians and Scientists**
**(ACLPS)**
c/o William L. Roberts
500 Chipeta Way
Salt Lake City, UT 84108
**Phone:** (801)583-2787 **Fax:** (801)584-5207
**Email:** william.roberts@aruplab.com
**Website:** http://www.aclps.org
William L. Roberts, MD, Ph, Sec. -Treas.

**Fnded:** 1966. **Mem:** 500. **Desc:** Physicians, Scientists, and Educators. Encourages and promotes the highest standards of education, service and research in clinical pathology at universities and medical schools. Sponsors journal. **Pub:** *ACLPS Newsletter*, periodic. Newsletter. *Price:* Included with membership. • *The American Journal of Clinical Pathology*. Journal. Publication sponsored by ACLPS and the American Society for clinical pathology.

★ **12184** ★ **American Association of**
**Bioanalysts (AAB)**
917 Locust St., Ste. 1100
Saint Louis, MO 63101-1419
**Phone:** (314)241-1445 **Fax:** (314)241-1449
**Email:** aab@aab.org
**Website:** http://www.aab.org
Mark S. Birenbaum, PhD, Admin.

**Fnded:** 1956. **Mem:** 1,000. **Desc:** Professional organization of directors, owners, managers, supervisors, technologists and technicians of bioanalytical clinical laboratories devoting their efforts to clinical laboratory procedure and testing. Sponsors Proficiency Testing Service open to individuals engaged in the clinical laboratory field. Provides specialized education and representation before federal and state legislatures and regulatory agencies. **Pub:** *AAB Bulletin*, bimonthly. Bulletin. • *AAB Update*, periodic.

★ **12185** ★ **American Association of**
**Bioanalysts Board of Registry**
917 Locust St., Ste. 1100
Saint Louis, MO 63101-1419
**Phone:** (314)241-1445 **Fax:** (314)241-1449
**Email:** aab@aab.org
**Website:** http://www.aab.org
Mark S. Birenbaum, PhD, Admin.

**Fnded:** 1962. **Desc:** Autonomous certifying agency for medical technologists, laboratory technicians, and physician office laboratory technicians. Maintains Continuing Education for Professional Advancement (CEPA) program to approve and record continuing education unit credits. **Frmly:** Accrediting Commission; (2000) Credentialing Commission.

★ **12186** ★ **American Association of**
**Blood Banks (AABB)**
8101 Glenbrook Rd.
Bethesda, MD 20814-2749
**Phone:** (301)907-6977 **Fax:** (301)907-6895
**Email:** aabb@aabb.org
**Website:** http://www.aabb.org
Sara Foer, Contact

**Fnded:** 1947. **Mem:** 11,500. **Desc:** Community and hospital blood centers and transfusion and transplantation services, physicians, nurses, technologists, administrators, blood donor recruiters, scientists, and individuals involved in related activities. Encourages the voluntary donation of blood and other tissues and organs through education, public information, and research. Operates the National Blood Exchange; inspects and accredits blood banks and parentage testing laboratories; sponsors the National Blood Foundation; maintains a rare donor file and reference laboratory system. Maintains over 40 scientific, technical, and administrative committees and three councils. **Pub:** *AABB News Briefs*, 11/year. Newsletter. Includes calendar of events, employment listings, and government affairs update. *Price:* Included in membership dues. • *American Association of Blood Banks–Membership Directory*, biennial. Directory. Lists institutional and individual members in alphabetical and geographic order. *Price:* Included in membership dues; $50 for nonmembers. • *Blood Bank Week*. Newsletter. Covers scientific, legislative, and regulatory events affecting blood banking and transfusion medicine. *Price:* $98/year for members; $128/year for nonmembers. • *Directory of Community Blood Centers*, biennial. Directory. *Price:* $25 for participating members; $50 for nonmembers. • *Standards for Blood Banks and Transfusion Services*, every 18 months. *Price:* $20 for members; $35 for nonmembers. • *Technical Manual*, triennial. Manual. *Price:* $48 for members; $60 for nonmembers; $45 for students. • *Transfusion*, monthly. Journal. Presents scientific, technical, and administrative papers relating to the field of blood banking. Includes advertisers index and convention abstract. *Price:* Included in membership dues; $135/year for nonmember individuals; $195/year for institutions. • Books. • Monographs.

### ★ 12187 ★ American Association for Clinical Chemistry (AACC)
2101 L St. NW, Ste. 202
Washington, DC 20037-1558
**Phone:** (202)857-0717          **Free:** 800-892-1400
**Fax:** (202)887-5093
**Email:** info@aacc.org
**Website:** http://www.aacc.org
Richard Flaherty, Exec. VP

**Fnded:** 1948. **Mem:** 11,000. **Local Groups:** 22. **Desc:** Clinical laboratory scientists and others engaged in the practice of clinical chemistry in independent laboratories, hospitals, and allied institutions. Maintains Endowment Fund for Research in Clinical Chemistry. Maintains employment service. Sponsors: therapeutic drug monitoring and endocrinology programs; continuing education programs; quality control programs. Compiles statistics; sponsors speakers' bureau. **Pub:** *Clinical Chemistry Journal*, monthly. Journal. • *Clinical Laboratory News*, monthly. • *Clinical Laboratory Strategies*, monthly. • Annual Report, annual. • Books. • Membership Directory, annual. **Frmly:** (1976) American Association of Clinical Chemists.

### ★ 12188 ★ American Clinical Laboratory Association (ACLA)
1250 H St. NW, Ste. 880
Washington, DC 20005
**Phone:** (202)637-9466          **Fax:** (202)637-2050
**Email:** chawk@clinical-labs.org
**Website:** http://www.clinical-labs.org
David N. Sundwall, MD, Pres.

**Fnded:** 1971. **Desc:** Corporations, partnerships, or individuals owning or controlling one or more independent clinical laboratory facilities operating for a profit and licensed under the Clinical Laboratories Improvement Act of 1967 or the Clinical Laboratories Improvement Amendment of 1988, or accredited by the Medicare program. Promotes the development of uniformly high quality laboratory testing; eliminates the present inequalities in the standards applied to different segments of the clinical laboratory market; discourages the enactment of restrictive legislative or regulatory policies that may impede the free flow of commerce or operate to the detriment of the public. Examines federal and state health care and laboratory regulatory and legislative proposals and submi ts comments and opinions to the appropriate agencies or legislative bodies.

### ★ 12189 ★ American Federation for Medical Research
227 Massachusetts Ave., NE, Ste. 303
Washington, DC 20002
**Phone:** (202)543-7032          **Fax:** (202)543-7062
**Email:** admin@afmr.org
**Website:** http://www.afmr.org
Kevin D. O'Brien, Pres.

**Fnded:** 1940. **Mem:** 6,000. **Reg. Groups:** 4. **Local Groups:** 19. **Desc:** Provides a forum for young clinical scientists (under 43); promotes and encourages original research in clinical and laboratory medicine. Offers specialized education program; maintains information services on membership status, files, and National Abstracting Processing. Annual scientific program presents sections on: Cardiovascular; Dermatology; Endocrinology; Gastroenterology; Genetics; Hematology; Immunology and Connective Tissue; Infectious Disease; Metabolism; Neoplastic Disease; Patient Care; Pulmonary; Renal and Electrolytes. **Pub:** *Journal of Investigative Medicine*, bimonthly. Journal. **Frmly:** (1998) American Federation for Clinical Research.

### ★ 12190 ★ American Medical Technologists (AMT)
710 Higgins Rd.
Park Ridge, IL 60068-5765
**Phone:** (847)823-5169          **Free:** 800-275-1268
**Fax:** (847)823-0458
**Email:** mail@amt1.com
**Website:** http://www.amt1.com
Christopher A. Damon, J.D., Exec. Dir.

**Fnded:** 1939. **Mem:** 25,000. **State Groups:** 38. **Desc:** National professional association and certifying body for medical laboratory technologists, technicians, medical assistants, dental assistants, and phlebotomists. Maintains job information service. Sponsors AMT Institute for Education, evaluates and recommends continuing education programs. **Pub:** *AMT Events and Continuing Education Supplement*, 6/yr. Journal. Includes book reviews and legislative updates. *Price:* Included in membership dues; $35/year for nonmembers in the U.S.; $45/year for foreign nonmembers.

### ★ 12191 ★ American Society for Apheresis (ASFA)
3900 E Timrod
Tucson, AZ 85711
**Phone:** (520)327-8584          **Fax:** (520)322-6778
**Email:** asfa@azstarnet.com
**Website:** http://www.apheresis.org
Phillip Gutt, Contact

**Fnded:** 1981. **Mem:** 800. **Desc:** Physicians, nurses, technologists, scientists, and other allied health professionals active in the field of apheresis, the separation and removal of components from blood. Aims to: promote training and research in apheresis therapy for patients; improve the care and management of apheresis donors; encourage the use of apheresis technology; assist in forming standards and regulations in the field of apheresis. Provides opportunity for the exchange of experiences and opinions through discussions, presentations, and publications; offers consulting on problems in the practice of apheresis. Conducts studies and courses. Plans to establish a central registry of apheresis information. **Pub:** *ASFA Newsletter*, periodic. Newsletter. • *Journal of Clinical Apheresis*, quarterly. Journal. *Price:* $124/year.

### ★ 12192 ★ American Society for Clinical Laboratory Science (ASCLS)
7910 Woodmont Ave., Ste. 530
Bethesda, MD 20814
**Phone:** (301)657-2768          **Fax:** (301)657-2909
**Email:** ascls@ascls.org
**Website:** http://www.ascls.org
Elissa Passiment, EdM, Exec. VP

**Fnded:** 1932. **Mem:** 13,000. **Reg. Groups:** 10. **State Groups:** 50. **Desc:** Primarily clinical laboratory personnel who have an associate or baccalaureate degree and clinical training and specialists who hold at least a master's degree in one of the major fields of clinical laboratory science such as bacteriology, mycology, or biochemistry; also includes technicians, specialists, and educators with limited certificates and students enrolled in approved programs of clinical laboratory studies and military medical technology schools. Promotes and maintains high standards in clinical laboratory methods and research and advances standards of education and training of person-

nel. Conducts educational program of seminars and workshops. Sponsors award competition to encourage the writing of scientific papers. Approves programs of continuing education and maintains records on participation in continuing education programs for members. **Pub:** *ASCLS Today*, monthly. Newsletter. *Price:* Included in membership dues. • *Clinical Laboratory Science*, quarterly. Journal. *Price:* Included in membership dues; $40 for individuals; $60 for corporations. • Books. • Brochures. • Manuals. • Videos. **Frmly:** American Society of Medical Technologists; (1936) American Society of Clinical Laboratory Technicians; (1993) American Society for Medical Technology.

### ★ 12193 ★ American Society for Clinical Pathology (ASCP)
2100 W Harrison
Chicago, IL 60612
**Phone:** (312)738-1336          **Free:** 800-621-4142
**Fax:** (312)738-1619
**Email:** info@ascp.org
**Website:** http://www.ascp.org
Nadine M. Filipiak, Dir. /Comm. & Membership

**Fnded:** 1922. **Mem:** 150,C00. **Desc:** Works to promote public health and safety by the appropriate application of pathology and laboratory medicine. Provides educational, scientific, and charitable services. **Pub:** *American Journal of Clinical Pathology*, monthly. Journal. • *ASCP Member News*, monthly. Newsletter. • *Laboratory Medicine*, monthly. Journal. • *Pathology Patterns*, semiannual. • Membership Directory, triennial. **Frmly:** (2002) American Society of Clinical Pathologists.

### ★ 12194 ★ American Society of Cytopathology (ASC)
400 W 9th St., Ste. 201
Wilmington, DE 19801
**Phone:** (302)429-8802          **Fax:** (302)429-8807
**Email:** asc@cytopathology.org
**Website:** http://www.cytopathology.org
Elizabeth A. Jenkins, Exec. Admin.

**Fnded:** 1951. **Mem:** 3,500. **Desc:** Physicians, Cytotechnologists and scientists dedicated to the cytologic method of diagnostic patholcgy. **Pub:** *Acta Cytologica*, bimonthly. Journal. • *The ASC Bulletin*, 8/year. Bulletin. • *Consider a Career in Cytotechnology*. Brochure. • *Cytopathology Review Course Syllabus*. **Frmly:** Inter-Society Cytology Council; American Society of Cytology.

### ★ 12195 ★ American Society for Cytotechnology (ASCT)
1500 Sunday Dr., Ste. 102
Raleigh, NC 27607
**Phone:** (919)787-5181          **Free:** 800-948-3947
**Fax:** (919)787-4916
**Email:** info@asct.com
**Website:** http://www.asct.com
Kathleen Norris, Exec. Dir.

**Fnded:** 1979. **Mem:** 1,500. **Reg. Groups:** 10. **Desc:** Cytotechnologists (technologists trained in the identification of cells and cellular abnormalities such as cancer), students of cytotechnology, and medical doctors in the field of cytopathology. Seeks to: enhance the role of the cytotechnologist in the health care system; stimulate communication and cooperation among cytotechnologists and other health professionals; inform members of current legislative and legal issues pertaining to the profession of cytotechnology and other related professions; support and promote educational opportunities. Urges participation in educational programs ava lable through the American Society of Cytopathology. **Pub:** *ASCT News*, 8/year. Newsletter. Covers educational, legislative, and other developments affecting the profession. Includes book reviews, calendar of events and employment listings. *Price:* available to members only.

### ★ 12196 ★ America's Blood Centers
725 15th St. NW, Ste. 700
Washington, DC 20005

**Phone:** (202)393-5725          **Free:** 888-USB-LOOD
**Fax:** (202)393-1282
**Email:** bthaler@americasblood.org
**Website:** http://www.americasblood.org
Brooke Thaler, Contact

**Fnded:** 1962. **Mem:** 75. **Desc:** Independent, nonprofit, federally licensed blood centers serving defined geographic areas that collectively provide about half of the nation's volunteer donor blood supply. Purpose is to ensure an optimal supply of blood, blood components, and blood derivatives and the development of a comprehensive range of the highest quality blood services to meet the needs of the American people. Compiles data and statistics; conducts research concerning organizational, administrative, fiscal, and operational phases of blood banking; establishes liaison and conducts cooperative activities of all kinds with national, regional, and local associations, groups, and organizations having a relationship of any kind to the drawing, processing, storing, or distribution of blood. **Pub:** *CCBC Newsletter*, weekly. Newsletter. Includes calendar of events and list of employment opportunities. *Price:* Free to members; $216/year for nonmembers (U.S. and Canada); $240/year for nonmembers (outside the U.S. and Canada). • Membership Directory, semiannual. **Frmly:** (1971) Community Blood Bank Council; (1998) Council of Community Blood Centers.


★ **12197** ★ **Association of Clinical
   Scientists**
PO Box 1287
Middlebury, VT 05753
**Phone:** (802)462-2507          **Fax:** (802)462-2673
**Email:** clinsci@sover.net
**Website:** http://www.clinicalscience.org
Robert E. Brown, MD, Pres.

**Fnded:** 1949. **Mem:** 500. **Desc:** Professional society of physicians and scientists working in various fields of laboratory medicine. Seeks to promote education and research in clinical science by practical methods; maintain and improve the accuracy of measurements in clinical laboratories and promote uniformity in clinical laboratory procedures; encourage cooperation between physicians and nonphysicians concerned with the application of scientific methods to medical practice. **Pub:** *Annals of Clinical and Laboratory Science*, quarterly. Journal. Scientific peer-reviewed journal. *Price:* Included in membership dues; $120 / year for nonmembers. • *Clinical Science Trumpet*, bimonthly. Newsletter. • Membership Directory, annual. **Frmly:** (1956) Clinical Science Club.


**Canadian Association of Medical
   Microbiologists (CAMM)
(Association Canadienne des Medecins
   Microbiologistes — ACMM)**
*See:* Entry 11750


★ **12198** ★ **Canadian Society for Medical
   Laboratory Science**
PO Box 2830 LCD 1
Hamilton, ON, Canada L8N 3N8
**Phone:** (905)528-8642          **Fax:** (905)528-4968
**Email:** toupitch@csmls.org
**Website:** http://www.csmls.org

**Fnded:** 1937. **Mem:** 14,000. **Lang(s):** English, French. **Desc:** Laboratory technologists in 20 countries. Seeks to maintain high standards of medical laboratory technology to insure effective and economical laboratory services. Promotes the interests of medical laboratory technologists. Emphasizes the importance of continuing education; sponsors courses. Communicates with government authorities concerning issues affecting members. Offers insurance program to members. Organizes national medical laboratory week annually. Bestows awards. **Pub:** *Annual Roster*. • *Canadian Journal of Medical Laboratory Science*, bimonthly. Journal. • *Catalogs of Continuing Education*. • *Guidelines for Laboratory Safety*. Manual.


★ **12199** ★ **Clinical Laboratory
   Management Association (CLMA)**
989 Old Eagle School Rd., Ste. 815
Wayne, PA 19087
**Phone:** (610)995-9580          **Fax:** (610)995-9568
**Email:** rneri@lcma.org
**Website:** http://www.clma.org
Robert A. Neri, Exec. VP

**Fnded:** 1976. **Mem:** 6,500. **Nat'l Groups:** 90. **Local Groups:** 103. **Desc:** Individuals holding managerial or supervisory positions with clinical laboratories; persons engaged in education of such individuals; manufacturers or distributors of equipment or services to clinical laboratories. Objectives are: to enhance management skills and promote more efficient and productive department operations; to further exchange of professional knowledge, new technology, and colleague experience; to encourage cooperation among those engaged in management or supervisory functions. Activities include: workshops, seminars, and expositions; dissemination of information about legislation and other topics. **Pub:** *Clinical Laboratory Management Association–Membership Directory*, annual. Directory. Arranged alphabetically and geographically. *Price:* Included in membership dues, online for members. • *Clinical Laboratory Management Review*, bimonthly. Journal. Covers concepts and techniques of management and issues and trends in health care that affect the clinical laboratory. *Price:* Included in membership dues; $130/year for nonmembers; $176/year for U.S. institutions. • *CLMA Vantage Point*, monthly. Newsletter. Contains articles on time management, employee performance appraisals, selecting a laboratory, information system and communication skills. *Price:* Included in membership dues. **Frmly:** (1976) American Association of Clinical Laboratory Supervisors and Administrators.


★ **12200** ★ **Clinical Ligand Assay Society
   (CLAS)**
3139 S Wayne Rd.
Wayne, MI 48184
**Phone:** (734)722-6290          **Fax:** (734)722-7006
**Email:** clas@clas.org
**Website:** http://www.clas.org
Daisy S. McCann, PhD, Exec. Dir.

**Fnded:** 1976. **Mem:** 5,000. **Reg. Groups:** 12. **Desc:** Seeks to establish and promote high standards in the science and application of ligand assay technology by encouraging research, education practitioners, and fostering communication and cooperation among individuals in laboratories in medicine, academia, and industry. Sponsors job placement service. Sponsors job placement service. **Pub:** *Journal of Clinical Ligand Assay*, quarterly. Journal. Contains reviews and articles on clinical ligand assay techniques. Includes bibliography of recent articles and manufacturers' directory. *Price:* Included in membership dues. • Directory, biennial. • Also publishes syllabi for annual meeting, and a newsletter. **Frmly:** (1981) Clinical Radioassay Society.


★ **12201** ★ **College of American
   Pathologists (CAP)**
325 Waukegan Rd.
Northfield, IL 60093-2750
**Phone:** (847)832-7000          **Free:** 800-323-4040
**Fax:** (847)832-8000
**Email:** acoeminfo@acoem.org
**Website:** http://www.cap.org
Lee VanBremen, PhD., Exec. VP

**Fnded:** 1947. **Mem:** 15,116. **Desc:** Physicians practicing the specialty of pathology (diagnosis, treatment, observation, and understanding of the progress of disease or medical condition) obtained by morphologic, microscopic, chemical, microbiologic, serologic, or any other type of laboratory examination made on the patient. Fosters improvement of education, research, and medical laboratory service to physicians, hospitals, and the public. Provides job placement information for members. Conducts laboratory accreditation program and laboratory proficiency testing surveys. Maintains spokepersons network; provides free health information to the public; compiles statistics; sponsors

educational programs. **Pub:** *Archives of Pathology and Laboratory Medicine*, monthly. Journal. *Price:* Free to members; $135 US and Canada; $185 other countries. • *CAP TODAY*, monthly. Newspaper. Includes scientific abstracts. *Price:* Included in membership dues; $40 US; $60 US possessions and the rest of North America; $95 other Countries. • *College of American Pathologists–Directory*, annual. Directory. *Price:* Included in membership dues. • *College of American Pathologists–Job Placement Bulletin*, bimonthly. Bulletin. Updating service providing job listings. *Price:* Included in membership dues. • Also publishes other materials of interest to pathologists and the public.


★ **12202** ★ **European Association for
   Professions in Biomedical Science
   (EPBS)**
c/o Ms Kristina Malm Janson
Box 3260
S-103 65 Stockholm, Sweden
**Phone:** 46 8 147700          **Fax:** 46 8 204096
**Email:** kristina.malm.janson@vardforbundet.se
**Website:** http://www.european-epbs.org

**Fnded:** 1998. **Lang(s):** English. **Desc:** Professional organizations representing medical laboratory technologists in the European Community. Offers advice to the European Commission in matters concerning medical laboratory technological profession. For those who work in the frontline of biomedical science in healthcare. EPBS is the organization to develop and promote cooperation in key areas such as education, continuing professional education, competencies and accreditation.


★ **12203** ★ **European Bank of Frozen
   Blood of Rare Groups (EBFBRG)
   (Banque Europeenne de Sange Congele
   de Groupes Rares)**
Sanquib Blood Supply Foundation
Plesmanlaan 125
NL-1066 CX Amsterdam, Netherlands
**Phone:** 31 20 5123373          **Fax:** 31 20 5123685
**Email:** m_overbeeke@clb.nl
**Website:** http://www.clb.nl

**Fnded:** 1969. **Mem:** 54. **Lang(s):** English, French, German. **Desc:** Individuals representing national blood banks and research centers.


★ **12204** ★ **International Association of
   Medical Laboratory Technologists
   (IAMLT)
(Association Internationale des
   Technologistes de Laboratoire Medical)**
Adolf Fredriks Kyrkogata 11
S-111 37 Stockholm, Sweden
**Phone:** 46 8 103031          **Fax:** 46 8 109061
**Email:** office@iamlt.org
**Website:** http://www.iamlt.org

**Fnded:** 1954. **Mem:** 39. **Reg. Groups:** 1. **State Groups:** 39. **Lang(s):** English, French, German. **Desc:** Member of the World Health Organization. National societies united to provide a means of communication among medical laboratory technologists in 39 countries. Promotes the continued education of health laboratory workers; plans curriculum for courses in health laboratory technology and management. Advises governments and governmental agencies on these matters and on validation of examinations leading to qualifications in medical laboratory. Maintains science development fund. **Pub:** *Curriculum for a Course in Health Safety*. Journal. • *International Directory of Medical Laboratory Science Education*, periodic. Directory. Details medical lab education worldwide. • *MedTec International*, semiannual. Journal. Covers information for medical laboratory technologists.

★ 12205 ★ **International Society of Blood Transfusion (ISBT)**
**(Societe Internationale de Transfusion Sanguine — SITS)**
PO Box 111
Royal Lancaster Infirmary
Ashton Rd.
Lancaster LA1 4GT, United Kingdom
**Phone:** 44 1524 306273    **Fax:** 44 1524 306273
**Website:**    http://www.iccbba.com/oldwebsite/internationalsocietyofbloodtransfusionshort.htm
**Fnded:** 1937. **Mem:** 1,300. **Nat'l Groups:** 105. **Lang(s):** English, French. **Desc:** Members of national blood bank societies in 105 countries. Works toward solving the scientific, technical, social, and ethical problems related to the transfusion of blood. Encourages closer relations among individuals dealing with such problems; standardizes methods and equipment. Facilitates the exchange of information among members. **Pub:** *Transfusion Today*, quarterly. • *Vox Sanguinis*, quarterly. Also publishes congress proceedings and technical guides.

★ 12206 ★ **National Accrediting Agency for Clinical Laboratory Sciences (NAACLS)**
8410 W Bryn Mawr Ave., Ste. 670
Chicago, IL 60631
**Phone:** (773)714-8880    **Fax:** (773)714-8886
**Email:** info@naacls.org
**Website:** http://www.naacls.org
Olive Kimball, CEO
**Fnded:** 1973. **Mem:** 695. **Desc:** Independently accredits academic programs in hospitals, colleges, and universities for the following health professional classifications: Clinical Laboratory Scientist/Medical Technologist, Clinical Laboratory Technician/Medical laboratory Technician, Histologic Technician, Histotechnologist, Pathologists' Assistant. Independently approves academic programs in hospitals and colleges for the following: Cytogenetic Technologist, Phlebotomist, Clinical Assistant. Establishes standards for quality educational programs; determines if hospitals and colleges are maintaining standards through self-study and on-site visits. Provides workshops for program officials on self-study and accreditation. **Pub:** *Guide to Accreditation*. • *NAACLS News*, quarterly. Newsletter. Includes news related to allied health professions and listing of position vacancies. *Price:* Free to members and accredited program officials; $15/year for nonmembers. • *NAACLS Program Approval Guide*. • *National Accrediting Agency for Clinical Laboratory Sciences–Annual Report*. Annual Report. • *National Accrediting Agency for Clinical Laboratory Sciences–Essentials*. **Frmly:** (1973) Board of Schools of the ASCP.

★ 12207 ★ **National Blood Transfusion Service**
PO Box A101
Avondale
Harare, Zimbabwe
**Phone:** 263 4 707801    **Fax:** 263 4 707820
**Email:** lloyd@healthnet.zw
**Website:** http://www.epicnewmedia.net/nbts
**Fnded:** 1986. **Desc:** Promotes the availability of blood supplies for tranfusions in Zimbabwe. Disseminates information. **Pub:** *Annual Report*. • Booklet. AIDS awareness and giving blood.

★ 12208 ★ **National Credentialing Agency for Laboratory Personnel (NCA)**
PO Box 15945-289
Lenexa, KS 66285
**Phone:** (913)438-5110    **Fax:** (913)541-0156
**Email:** nca-info@goamp.com
**Website:** http://www.nca-info.org
Kathryn Sudduth, Sec. -Treas.
**Fnded:** 1977. **Mem:** 65,000. **Desc:** Persons who direct, educate, supervise, or practice in clinical laboratory science. To assure the public and employers of the competence of clinical laboratory personnel; to

provide a mechanism for individuals demonstrating competency in the field to achieve career mobility. Develops and administers competency-based examinations for certification of clinical laboratory personnel; provides for periodic recertification by examination or through documentation of continuing education. Compiles statistics. **Frmly:** (2001) National Certification Agency for Medical Lab Personnel.

★ 12209 ★ **National Phlebotomy Association (NPA)**
1901 Brightseat Rd.
Landover, MD 20785
**Phone:** (301)386-4200    **Fax:** (301)386-4203
**Email:** naltphle@aol.com
Diane Crawford, CEO
**Fnded:** 1978. **Mem:** 12,000. **Desc:** Offers educational programs for phlebotomists; to accredit phlebotomy programs; to give national certification examinations in phlebotomy at the request of approved program. (Phlebotomy is the collection of a blood specimen for analysis in the treatment of disease.) Conducts regional workshops and educational programs. Compiles statistics. **Pub:** *National Phlebotomy Association Certified Phlebotomists Registry*, periodic. • *Self Study Modules in Phlebotomy*. • *The Tourniquet*, annual. Newsletter. Includes list of employment opportunities, research reports, and profiles of members. *Price:* Free.

★ 12210 ★ **National Rare Blood Club (NRBC)**
Associated Health Foundation
99 Madison Ave.
New York, NY 10016
**Phone:** (212)889-8245    **Free:** 800-772-8668
**Fax:** (212)448-1811
Edward Birnbaum, Pres.
**Fnded:** 1978. **Mem:** 16,000. **Desc:** Persons ages 18-65 with rare blood types who are physically able to donate blood. Operates as a voluntary community service with no fees or dues involved.

★ 12211 ★ **National Registry of Certified Chemists (NRCC)**
815 15th St. NW, Ste. 508
Washington, DC 20005
**Phone:** (202)393-7140    **Fax:** (202)393-4059
**Email:** nrcc6@aol.com
**Website:** http://www.nrcc6.org
Gilbert E. Smith, PhD, Exec. Dir.
**Fnded:** 1967. **Mem:** 700. **Desc:** Certification programs for chemical hygiene officers, clinical chemists, clinical chemistry technologists, environmental analytical chemists, environmental analytical technicians, and toxicological chemists based on education, experience, and examination. **Pub:** Directory, annual. **Frmly:** (2001) National Registry in Clinical Chemistry.

★ 12212 ★ **National Society for Histotechnology (NSH)**
4201 Northview Dr., Ste. 502
Bowie, MD 20716-2604
**Phone:** (301)262-6221    **Fax:** (301)262-9188
**Email:** histo@nsh.org
**Website:** http://www.nsh.org
Roberta Mosedale, Exec. Dir.
**Fnded:** 1973. **Mem:** 4,800. **Reg. Groups:** 9. **State Groups:** 42. **Desc:** Histology laboratory technicians, pathologists, laboratory equipment manufacturers' representatives, and interested individuals. Encourages the professional growth and advancement of histoprofessionals and promotes the exchange of ideas and knowledge significant to histotechnology. Assists in the establishment and mutual understanding of related societies. Provides continuing education training courses. Investigates health hazards in the laboratory; ensures the safety of the laboratory; and participates in formulating federal laboratory regulations. **Pub:** *Journal of Histotechnology*, quarterly. Journal. Topics include anatomy, pathology, enzyme histochemistry, special stains, immunohistochemistry,

cytology, and electron microscopy. *Price:* Included in membership dues; $70/year for nonmembers; $100/year for nonmembers outside U.S. • *NSH In Action*, quarterly. Annual Report. *Price:* for members. • *NSH in Action*, quarterly. Newsletter. • Booklets.Pertains to careers. • Also publishes training aids.

★ 12213 ★ **NCCLS**
940 W Valley Rd., Ste. 1400
Wayne, PA 19087-1898
**Phone:** (610)688-0100    **Fax:** (610)688-0700
**Email:** info@nccls.org
**Website:** http://www.nccls.org
John V. Bergen, PhD, Exec. Dir.
**Fnded:** 1968. **Mem:** 2,100. **Desc:** Government agencies, professional societies, clinical laboratories, and industrial firms with interests in medical testing. Purposes are to promote the development of national and international standards for medical testing and to provide a consensus mechanism for defining and resolving problems that influence the quality and cost of healthcare work performed. **Pub:** *Member/Volunteer Directory*. Directory. Information on NCCLS programs, projects, committees, members, volunteers, and staff. *Price:* Included in membership dues. • *NCCLS Update*, monthly. Newsletter. Includes new member information and meeting calendar. *Price:* Free. • Reports. • Videos. • Also publishes standards and guidelines and documents. **Frmly:** (1994) National Committee for Clinical Laboratory Standards; (1997) NCCLS: The Clinical Laboratory Standards Organization; (2000) National Committee for Clinical Laboratory Standards.

★ 12214 ★ **Pan American Federation for Voluntary Bloodgiving**
**(Federacion Panamericana pro Donacion Voluntaria de Sangre)**
Apartado Postal 5830
Caracas, Venezuela
**Desc:** Promotes voluntary bloodgiving throughout the Americas. Collects and diffuses blood for hospitals and clinics throughout the region.

★ 12215 ★ **Scottish National Blood Transfusion Association (SNBTA)**
2 Otterburn Park
Edinburgh EH14 1JX, United Kingdom
**Phone:** 44 131 4437636
**Fnded:** 1940. **Mem:** 250,000. **Lang(s):** English. **Desc:** Blood donors. Promotes donation of blood; seeks to insure a reliable and safe supply of blood and plasma for use in medical transfusions. Represents the interests of blood and bone marrow donors before medical organizations and government agencies; provides support and assistance to the Scottish National Blood Transfusion Service; consults with medical organizations to improve blood donation and transfusion techniques. Maintains speakers' bureau. **Pub:** *Annual Report and Statement of Accounts*, annual. Annual Report.

★ 12216 ★ **Society of Medical Laboratory Technologists of South Africa (SMLTSA)**
**(Vereniging van Geneeskundige Laboratorium Tegnoloe van Suid-Afrika — VGLTSA)**
PO Box 6014
Roggebaai
Cape Town 8012, Republic of South Africa
**Phone:** 27 21 4194857    **Fax:** 27 21 4212566
**Email:** smltsa@smltsa.org.za
**Website:** http://www.smltsa.org.za
**Fnded:** 1951. **Mem:** 1,700. **Local Groups:** 15. **Lang(s):** Afrikaans, English. **Desc:** Medical technologists, students, and interested persons organized to promote the medical technology profession. Works to: establish standards of practice; influence public policy; provide a forum for the exchange of ideas. Acts as an advisory and consulting body. Represents the profes-

sion before certifying, educational, employment, and registering authorities. Sponsors activities that advance scientific knowledge and encourage original work. **Pub:** *Constitution of the Society of Medical Laboratory Technologists of South Africa.* Book. • *Medical Technology*, semiannual. Journal. • *Medical Technology News*, periodic. Newspaper. • Newsletter.

★ **12217** ★ **Zimbabwe Institute of Medical Laboratory Scientists**
PO Box 8220
Causeway
Harare, Zimbabwe
**Phone:** 263 705639          **Fax:** 263 792588
**Mem:** 250. **Nat'l Groups:** 1. **Reg. Groups:** 2. **Lang(s):** English. **Desc:** Medical laboratory scientists. Seeks to maintain high standards in the practice of medical laboratory science, and to insure effective and economical laboratory services. Promotes continuing professional education of members. **Pub:** *Journal of the Zimbabwe Institute of Med. Lab. Scientists*, annual. Journal. **Frmly:** (1990) Association of Medical Laboratory Technologists of Zimbabwe.

## Research Centers

★ **12218** ★ **International Institute for the Advancement of Medicine (IIAM)**
1232 Mid-Valley Dr.
Jessup, PA 18434-1823
**Phone:** (570)496-3400          **Fax:** (570)343-6993
**Email:** gina_smith@.prtb.org
**Website:** http://www.iiam.org
Gina Dunne Smith, PhD, Dir.
**Activities/Fields:** Placement of non-transplantable human organs and tissues for research; serological testing for infectious diseases in donors; and fresh and frozen tissue slices, cells, and subcellular fractions.

**Johns Hopkins University**
**Medical Imaging Laboratory**
*See:* Entry 2520

★ **12219** ★ **Medical University of South Carolina**
**Molecular Morphology and Imaging Core**
644 Basil Science Bldg.
Department of Cell Biology & Anatomy
173 Ashley Ave.
Charleston, SC 29425-2204
**Phone:** (843)792-3779          **Fax:** (843)792-0664
**Email:** litkell@musc.edu
**Website:** http://www.musc.edu/mmi/
Dr. Larry L. Litke, Dir.
**Activities/Fields:** Cell biology and cellular and molecular influences on cardiovascular development.

**San Francisco State University**
**Center for Biomedical Laboratory Science**
*See:* Entry 4684

★ **12220** ★ **South Carolina Health and Environmental Control Department**
**Health Services Division**
**Bureau of Laboratories**
8231 Parklane Rd.
Columbia, SC 29223
**Phone:** (803)896-0800          **Fax:** (803)896-0983
**Email:** dowdahe@columb68.dhec.state.sc.us
**Website:** http://www.scdhec.net/hs/lab/lab.htm
Harold Dowda, PhD, Ch.
**Activities/Fields:** Health issues. **Pub:** *Bureau of Laboratories Annual Report.*

★ **12221** ★ **South Carolina Health and Environmental Control Department**
**Health Services Division**
**Bureau of Laboratories**
**Diagnostic Microbiology Division**
8231 Parklane Rd.
Columbia, SC 29223

**Phone:** (803)896-0965          **Fax:** (803)896-0657
**Email:** wozniaka@columb68.dhec.state.sc.us
Dr. Arthur Wozniak, Dir.
**Activities/Fields:** Arboviruses, emerging diseases.
**Frmly:** Virology/Serology Division.

★ **12222** ★ **South Carolina Health and Environmental Control Department**
**Health Services Division**
**Bureau of Laboratories**
**Division of Clinical Cytology**
8231 Parklane Rd.
Columbia, SC 29223
**Phone:** (803)896-0892          **Fax:** (803)896-0983
Marc S. Busnardo, MD, Dir.
**Activities/Fields:** Nature of diseases and the changes caused by them.

**U.S. Department of Health and Human Services**
**National Cancer Institute**
**Laboratory of Pathology**
*See:* Entry 10495

★ **12223** ★ **U.S. Department of Health and Human Services**
**National Institute of General Medical Sciences**
**Diagnostic Laboratory**
1230 York Ave.
Box 2
New York, NY 10021
**Phone:** (212)327-8522          **Fax:** (212)327-8536
Michael D. Hayre, DVM, Dir.
**Activities/Fields:** Provides diagnostic services and prospective and retrospective clinical studies in conjunction with disease screening and laboratory animal diagnostics at Rockefeller University. Research includes: transgenic animal technology; PCR; macrophage biology; and clinical case reviews. Provides a complete laboratory animal diagnostic program.

# Chapter 37
# Law & Medicine

## Foundations & Other Funding Organizations

### Private Foundations

**Greenwall Foundation**
*See:* Entry 304

### Other Funding Organizations

**★ 12224 ★ American College of Legal Medicine (ACLM)**
1111 N Plaza Dr., Ste. 550
Schaumburg, IL 60173
**Phone:** (847)969-0283   **Free:** 800-433-9137
**Fax:** (847)517-7229
**Email:** aclm@wjweiser.com
**Website:** http://www.aclm.org
Miles Zaremski, Pres.
**Desc:** Persons who hold degrees in medicine, dentistry, law and nursing. Promotes and advances the field of legal medicine or medical jurisprudence; arranges for meetings with medical, legal, and professional groups and legislative, judicial, and enforcement bodies interested in any province where law and medicine are contiguous; fosters and encourages centers for study and research in the field of legal medicine and publishes materials pertaining to legal medicine. **Awards:** Hirsh Award (annual) bestowed to a dentistry, podiatry, nursing, pharmacy, health science or health care administration student for outstanding original paper on legal medicine; Letourneau Award (annual) bestowed to a law student for outstanding original paper on legal medicine; Schwartz Award (annual) bestowed to a medical student for outstanding original paper on legal medicine.

## National & International Organizations

**★ 12225 ★ African Commission of Health and Human Rights Promoters (ACHHRP)**
Rabito Clinic
PO Box 7286
North
Accra, Ghana
**Phone:** 233 21 774526   **Fax:** 233 21 777465
**Lang(s):** English. **Desc:** Health and human rights organizations. Promotes respect for the rights of the individual and the rule of law; seeks to increase availability of health care services among previously underserved populations. Publicizes human rights abuses; makes available health care programs.

**★ 12226 ★ American Association of Legal Nurse Consultants (AALNC)**
4700 W Lake Ave.
Glenview, IL 60025-1485
**Phone:** (847)375-4713   **Free:** 877-402-2562
**Fax:** 877-734-8668
**Email:** info@aalnc.org
**Website:** http://www.aalnc.org/
Rosie Oldham, Pres.
**Fnded:** 1989. **Mem:** 4,000. **State Groups:** 48. **Desc:** Promotes the professional advancement of registered nurses consulting with the legal arena by providing a forum for education and exchange of information. Conducts annual educational program. **Pub:** *The Journal of Legal Nurse Consulting*, quarterly. Journal. Includes legal and legislative updates, and networking information. *Price:* Free to members. • *Legal Nurse Consulting: Principles and Practice.* *Price:* $70 for members; $80 non-members.

**★ 12227 ★ American Association of Nurse Attorneys (TAANA)**
7794 Grow Dr.
Pensacola, FL 32514
**Phone:** (850)474-3646   **Free:** 877-532-2262
**Fax:** (850)484-8762
**Email:** taana@puetzamc.com
**Website:** http://www.taana.org
Belinda E. Puetz, Ph.D, RN, Exec. Dir.
**Fnded:** 1982. **Mem:** 400. **Local Groups:** 24. **Desc:** Nurse attorneys, nurses in law school, and attorneys in nursing school. Aims to better nurse attorneys and inform the public on matters of nursing, health care, and law. Goals are to facilitate communication and information sharing between professional groups; to establish an employment network; to assist new and potential nurse attorneys; to develop the profession; to promote the image of nurse attorneys as experts and consultants in nursing and law. Maintains educational foundation. **Pub:** *Demonstrating Financial Responsibility in Nursing Practice.* Brochure. Contains information for nurses considering the purchase of professional liability insurance. *Price:* $2. • *Guidelines for the Selection of Counsel for the State Nurses Association.* • *Inside TAANA*, 3/year. Newsletter. Contains reports from committees and chapters, legislative information, and member notes. *Price:* Included in membership dues. • *Journal of Nursing Law*, quarterly. Journal. • *Making the Transition: From Nursing to the Law.* • *Model Curriculum for Legal Content in Nursing Education.* • *On Becoming A Nurse Attorney.* • *TAANA Membership Resource Directory*, annual. Membership Directory.

**★ 12228 ★ American Board of Forensic Anthropology (ABFA)**
c/o Dr. Frank P. Saul
Lucas County Coroner's Office
2595 Arlington Ave.
Toledo, OH 43614-2674
**Phone:** (419)213-3908
**Email:** fsaul@mco.edu
**Website:** http://www.csuchico.edu/anth/ABFA
Dr. Frank P. Saul, Contact
**Fnded:** 1977. **Mem:** 50. **Desc:** Board for certification of physical anthropologists who wish to become forensic anthropologists. (Forensic anthropology refers to application of the science of physical anthropology in assistance of law enforcement agencies; forensic anthropologists identify and glean information from human remains.) Promotes improvement in the practice of forensic anthropology and encourages adherence to high standards in the field. Conducts written and practical examinations for prospective forensic anthropologists; awards certificates of qualification. Compiles statistics. **Pub:** *Diplomates, American Board of Forensic Anthropology Directory*, annual. Directory. Contains listings of current diplomates in forensic anthropology.

**★ 12229 ★ American College of Legal Medicine (ACLM)**
1111 N Plaza Dr., Ste. 550
Schaumburg, IL 60173
**Phone:** (847)969-0283   **Free:** 800-433-9137
**Fax:** (847)517-7229
**Email:** aclm@wjweiser.com
**Website:** http://www.aclm.org
Miles Zaremski, Pres.
**Fnded:** 1960. **Mem:** 1,450. **Desc:** Persons who hold degrees in medicine, dentistry, law and nursing. Promotes and advances the field of legal medicine or medical jurisprudence; arranges for meetings with medical, legal, and professional groups and legislative, judicial, and enforcement bodies interested in any province where law and medicine are contiguous; fosters and encourages centers for study and research in the field of legal medicine and publishes materials pertaining to legal medicine. **Pub:** *American College of Legal Medicine–Newsletter*, quarterly. Newsletter. Contains basic news and information of the College. *Price:* Included in membership dues. • *College of Legal Medicine Membership Directory*, annual. Membership Directory. *Price:* Included in membership dues; $50/copy for nonmembers. • *Journal of Legal Medicine*, periodic. Journal. Offers discussion of topics of interest in legal medicine, health law, food and drug law, and medicolegal research and education. *Price:* Included in membership dues; $134/year for nonmembers. • *Legal Medicine Perspectives*, bimonthly. • *Medical Legal Lessons*, bimonthly. Includes summaries of prominent cases and discussions of recent statutes.

**★ 12230 ★ American Society of Law, Medicine and Ethics (ASLME)**
765 Commonwealth Ave., Ste. 1634
Boston, MA 02215
**Phone:** (617)262-4990   **Fax:** (617)437-7596
**Email:** info@aslme.org
**Website:** http://www.aslme.org
Benjamin W. Moulton, Exec. Dir.
**Fnded:** 1972. **Mem:** 4,500. **Desc:** Physicians, attorneys, health care management executives, nurses, insurance company personnel, members of the judiciary, and others interested in medicolegal relations, health law, and ethics. Purpose is to provide opportunities for continuing education through publications,

conferences, and information clearinghouse. Maintains speakers' bureau. **Pub:** *American Journal of Law & Medicine*, quarterly. Journal. Health care law review containing annotations of recent court decisions, book releases, and student case and note section. *Price:* $90 /year for individuals; $170 /year for institutions. • *Journal of Law, Medicine & Ethics*, quarterly. Journal. Reports on medically related legal and social issues such as managed care, genetics, pain management, physician-assisted suicide. Peer reviewed. *Price:* $90 /year for individuals; $170 /year for institutions. **Frmly:** (1911) Massachusetts Society of Examing Physicians; (1973) Massachusetts Society of Law and Medicine; (1993) American Society of Law and Medicine.


★ **12231** ★ **American Society for Pharmacy Law (ASPL)**
1224 Centre W, Ste. 200B
Springfield, IL 62704
**Phone:** (217)391-0219          **Fax:** (217)793-0041
**Email:** bobplye@assn-srvs.com
**Website:** http://www.aspl.org
Robert E. Pyle, Exec. Dir.

**Fnded:** 1974. **Mem:** 1,000. **Desc:** Pharmacists, lawyers, and students. Purposes are to: further legal knowledge; communicate accurate legal information to pharmacists; foster knowledge and education pertaining to the rights and duties of pharmacists; distribute information of interest to members; provide a forum for exchange of information pertaining to pharmacy law. **Pub:** *Pharmacy Law Annual*, annual. Membership Directory. Contains legal pharmacy law articles. • *RX Ipsa Loquitur*, monthly.


**Arab Disabled Confederation (ADC)**
*See:* Entry 7919


★ **12232** ★ **Association of Police Surgeons**
Clarke House
18A Mount Parade
Harrogate HG1 1BX, United Kingdom
**Phone:** 44 1423 509727
**Email:** chris@forensic-science-society.org.uk
**Website:** http://www.apsweb.org.uk

**Fnded:** 1951. **Mem:** 1,050. **Desc:** Members are medical practitioners who regularly assist or advise the police in medical or forensic cases. To promote the best interests of police surgeons; advancement of medico legal knowledge in all its aspects; liaison between appointed police surgeons and other medical practitioners; practical and theoretical study of the subject by lectures, discussions, correspondence and any other means.


★ **12233** ★ **Canadian HIV/AIDS Legal Network**
**(Reseau Juridique Canadien VIH/SIDA)**
417 Saint-Pierre St., Ste. 408
Montreal, QC, Canada H2Y 2M4
**Phone:** (514)397-6828          **Fax:** (514)397-8570
**Email:** info@aidslaw.ca
**Website:** http://www.aidslaw.ca

**Fnded:** 1992. **Mem:** 300. **Lang(s):** English, French. **Desc:** Legal professionals and other individuals with an interest in the legal rights and status of people with HIV and AIDS. Promotes increased respect for the civil and human rights of people with HIV and AIDS. Conducts research and educational programs.


★ **12234** ★ **Canadian Medical Malpractice Prevention Association (CMMPA)**
2900 Warden Ave. No. 92093
Scarborough, ON, Canada M1W 3Y8
**Phone:** (416)969-1587

**Fnded:** 1987. **Lang(s):** English, French. **Desc:** Individuals with an interest in medical malpractice and related issues. Promotes effective medical treatment and reform of legal medical malpractice procedures. Maintains speakers' bureau.


★ **12235** ★ **Child Care Law Center (CCLC)**
221 Pine St., 3rd Fl.
San Francisco, CA 94104
**Phone:** (415)394-7144          **Fax:** (415)495-6734
**Email:** info@childcarelaw.org
**Website:** http://www.childcarelaw.org
Nancy Strohl, Exec. Dir.

**Fnded:** 1978. **Desc:** Provides legal services, technical assistance, and training programs to attorneys and others working to improve child care for low-income families. Develops legislative and regulatory policies; monitors legislative issues. **Pub:** *The ADA and Child Care: Information for Parents of Children with Disabilities.* • *Caring for Children with HIV or AIDS in Child Care.* • *Caring for Children with Special Needs: The ADA and Child Care.* • *Child Care Contracts: Information for Parents.* • *Child Care Contracts: Information for Providers.* • *The Child Care Tax Credit: A Booklet for Parents.* Booklet. • *Employing People with Disabilities: The ADA and Child Care.* • *Family Day Care Zoning Advocacy Guide.* • *Legal Update*, quarterly. Newsletter. • *Liability Insurance: Insuring Your Program.* • *Working For Change*, quarterly. • Offers various additional publications.


**Children's Healthcare Is a Legal Duty (CHILD)**
*See:* Entry 5657


★ **12236** ★ **European Association of Centres of Medical Ethics (EACME)**
Kapucijnenvoer 35
B-3000 Louvain, Belgium
**Phone:** 32 16 336951          **Fax:** 32 16 336952
**Email:** paul.schotsmans@med.kuleuven.ac.be
**Website:** http://www.childrenshealthcare.org

**Fnded:** 1985. **Mem:** 59. **Lang(s):** English, French. **Desc:** Medical ethics centers. Promotes critical public and professional concern regarding ethical issues encountered in the practice of medicine. Gathers and disseminates information; conducts research and makes research tools available to members; coordinates collaborative research efforts among members. Encourages continuing ethical education for health care professionals. **Pub:** *EACME News*, periodic. Bulletin.


★ **12237** ★ **European Council of Legal Medicine**
**(ECLM)**
Institute of Legal Medicine
190 Winterthurstrasse
CH-8057 Zurich, Switzerland
**Fax:** 41 1 6356815
**Website:** http://www.irm.unizh.ch/eclm

**Fnded:** 1992. **Mem:** 51. **Nat'l Groups:** 20. **Lang(s):** English, French, German, Italian. **Desc:** Representatives of member states of the European Free Trade Agreement in which legal medicine is recognized as a professional discipline. (Legal medicine refers to the medical examination of unexpected or unnatural deaths within the framework of the legal system.) Seeks to advance the study and practice of legal medicine. Represents the profession at the European level; serves as a clearinghouse on scientific, educational, and professional matters pertaining to legal medicine.


★ **12238** ★ **International Association of Coroners and Medical Examiners (IACME)**
PO Box 899
Mansfield, LA 71052
**Phone:** (318)872-0516          **Fax:** (318)872-4495
Jack Grindle, MD, Contact

**Fnded:** 1938. **Mem:** 335. **Desc:** Educational seminar involving all aspects of death investigation such as pathology, autopsy, crime scene investigation, mass disasters and anthropology. Offers continuing medical

education credit. **Pub:** *RECAP*, quarterly. Newsletter. *Price:* Included in membership dues.


**International Lawyers in Alcoholics Anonymous (ILAA)**
*See:* Entry 19299


**International Organization for Forensic Odonto-Stomatology (IOFOS)**
*See:* Entry 6557


★ **12239** ★ **Japanese Society of Legal Medicine (JSLM)**
c/o Department of Forensic Medicine
Graduate School of Medicine
University of Tokyo
7-3-1 Hongo, Bunkyo-ku
Tokyo 113-0033, Japan
**Phone:** 81 3 58005416
**Email:** grahamr@co.clark.nv.us
**Website:** http://www.ilaa.org

**Desc:** Pathologists, toxicologists, lawyers, police criminalists, and professors of legal medicine in Japan. Conducts educational programs. **Pub:** Journal, periodic.


★ **12240** ★ **Legal Action for Women (LAW)**
PO Box 11061
Pensacola, FL 32524
**Phone:** (334)962-3554          **Free:** 888-9-WOMENS
**Email:** law@gulftel.com
**Website:** http://www.legalactionforwomen.org
Vicky Conroy, Contact

**Fnded:** 1985. **Desc:** Provides legal referral for women injured by abortions. Conducts research on medical malpractice; promotes action on abortion safety.


★ **12241** ★ **Medical Protection Society (MPS)**
33 Cavendish Sq.
London W16 0PS, United Kingdom
**Phone:** 44 207 3991301          **Fax:** 44 207 3991300
**Email:** info@mps.org.uk
**Website:** http://www.mps.org.uk/

**Lang(s):** English. **Desc:** Physicians, dentists, and other health care professionals. Seeks to assist members in protecting themselves from customer complaints and litigation. Provides technical and customer service assistance to members in matters involving disputes with clients and litigation arising from patient care. Represents members before health boards, hospital inquiries, and other professional misconduct or incompetence proceedings. Makes available legal and ethical advice to members.


★ **12242** ★ **National Association of Disability Evaluating Professionals (NADEP)**
PO Box 35407
Richmond, VA 23235-0407
**Phone:** (804)378-8809          **Fax:** (804)272-9257
**Email:** mayrehab@aol.com
**Website:** http://www.nadep.com
Virgil Robert May, III, Dir.

**Fnded:** 1984. **Mem:** 1,000. **Nat'l Groups:** 1. **Desc:** Lawyers, doctors, psychologists, employers, and others interested or involved in disability claims process, evaluation, and case management. Provides a forum for the exchange of information. Serves as a training center which prepares health professionals to qualify for the Certified Disability Examiner credential offered by the Commission on Disability Examiner Certification. **Pub:** *Disability Evaluation and Rehabilitation Review*, quarterly. Newsletter. *Price:* Included in membership. • *NADEP Guide to Functional Capacity Evaluation with Department Rating Applications Textbook.* Book. *Price:* $140 for nonmembers; $120 for members. **Frmly:** (1991) International Health Consultants.

★ 12243 ★ **National Association of**
**Medical Examiners (NAME)**
1402 S Grand Blvd.
Saint Louis, MO 63104
**Phone:** (314)577-8298     **Fax:** (314)268-5971
**Email:** name@slu.edu
**Website:** http://www.thename.org
Denise Settlemoir, Exec. Dir.

**Fnded:** 1966. **Mem:** 950. **Desc:** Medical examiners, pathologists, and other licensed physicians who have responsibilities in connection with the official investigation of sudden, suspicious, and violent deaths. Attempts to establish greater understanding and support for the medical examiner system among the public, government officials, and the medical and legal professions. Has established standards for inspection and accreditation of a modern medico-legal investigative system. **Pub:** *American Journal of Forensic Medicine and Pathology*, quarterly. Journal.

★ 12244 ★ **National Committee for**
**Medical Research Ethics (NEM)**
**(Den Nasjonale Forskningsetiske Komite**
**for Medisin — NEM)**
Prinsensgate 18
PB 522 Sentrum
N-0105 Oslo, Norway
**Phone:** 47 23318300     **Fax:** 47 23318301
**Email:** knut.ruyter@etikkom.no
**Website:** http://www.etikkom.no

**Fnded:** 1990. **Mem:** 12. **Reg. Groups:** 5. **Lang(s):** English, Norwegian. **Desc:** Health care professionals, attorneys, ethicists, and others with an interest in ethical aspects of medical research. Promotes increased awareness of ethical issues within the medical research industry; conducts continuing professional education and public education programs.

★ 12245 ★ **Scandinavian Society of**
**Forensic Medicine (SSFM)**
**(Nordisk Rattsmedicinsk Forening)**
University of Iceland
Faculty of Medicine
Armula 30
IS-108 Reykjavik, Iceland
**Phone:** 354 1 5602480     **Fax:** 354 1 56019047
**Email:** ggeiss@rhi.hi.is

**Fnded:** 1961. **Lang(s):** Danish, English, Norwegian, Swedish. **Desc:** Experts on forensic medicine from 7 northern European countries. Promotes cooperation among members; mediates exchange of scientific and practical experiences. **Pub:** *Conference Proceedings*, triennial.

★ 12246 ★ **Society of Medical**
**Jurisprudence (SMJ)**
PO Box 1304
New York, NY 10008-1304
**Phone:** (212)473-0523

**Fnded:** 1883. **Mem:** 150. **Desc:** Lawyers, physicians, surgeons, health professionals, chemists, and law and medical school professors. Promotes the investigation, study, and advancement of medical jurisprudence and high standards of medical expert testimony. Sponsors individual lectures and serial presentations of medicolegal interest. **Pub:** *Ligature*, 9/year. Newsletter. Contains legislative and regulatory information. • Directory. • Also plans to publish essays on current issues of medico-legal interest. **Frmly:** (1883) Medico-Legal Society; (1891) Society of Medical Jurisprudence and State Medicine.

★ 12247 ★ **World Medical Law**
**Association**
UZ-1K3, De Pintelaan 185
9000 Gent, Belgium
**Phone:** 32 9 2403859     **Fax:** 32 9 2404380
**Fnded:** 1967.

# Research Centers

**Bureau of Legal Dentistry (BLD)**
*See:* Entry 6600

★ 12248 ★ **Case Western Reserve**
**University**
**Center for Biomedical Ethics**
Sch. of Medicine
10900 Euclid Ave.
Cleveland, OH 44106-4976
**Phone:** (216)368-6196     **Free:** 800-773-2633
**Fax:** (216)368-8713
**Email:** sxy2@po.cwru.edu
**Website:** http://www.cwru.edu/med/bioethics/bioethics/htm
Stuart J. Youngner, MD, Dir.

**Activities/Fields:** Bioethics, including human genetics, decisions to end life, aging, and reproductive alternatives. **Pub:** *CenterViews Newsletter*, 3/year.

★ 12249 ★ **Georgetown University**
**Kennedy Institute of Ethics**
Box 571212
Washington, DC 20057-1212
**Phone:** (202)687-8099     **Fax:** (202)687-8089
**Email:** kicourse@georgetown.edu
**Website:** http://www.georgetown.edu/research/kie/
Dr. Madison Powers, Dir.

**Activities/Fields:** Social and ethical issues in biomedical sciences, such as resource allocation in health care, human experimentation, genetic engineering, euthanasia, death and dying, reproductive technologies, physician-patient relations, in vitro fertilization, abortion, and organ transplantation. Also researches other fields of applied ethics–international relations, government, law, journalism, business, and technology policy. **Pub:** *Bibliography of Bioethics*, annually. • *Bioethics Thesaurus*, annually. • *Encyclopedia of Bioethics*. • *International Directory of Bioethics Organizations*. • *Kennedy Institute of Ethics Journal*. • *New Titles in Bioethics*, quarterly. • *Scope Notes*. • *Searching BIOETHICSLINE*. **Frmly:** Joseph and Rose Kennedy Institute for the Study of Human Reproduction and Bioethics.

★ 12250 ★ **Harvard University**
**Francois-Xavier Bagnoud Center for**
**Health and Human Services (FXB)**
School of Public Health
651 Huntington Ave., 7th Fl.
Boston, MA 02115
**Phone:** (617)432-0656     **Fax:** (617)432-4310
**Email:** fxbcenter@igc.org
**Website:** http://www.hsph.harvard.edu/fxbcenter/
Stephen P. Marks, Dir.

**Activities/Fields:** Health and human rights. **Pub:** *Reports*. • *Health and Human Rights: An International Journal*. • *Working papers*.

★ 12251 ★ **Institute for Jewish Medical**
**Ethics**
645 14th Ave.
San Francisco, CA 94118
**Phone:** (415)752-7333     **Fax:** (415)752-5851
**Email:** ijmeaa@flash.net
**Website:** http://www.ijme.org
Miriam Real, Contact

**Activities/Fields:** Jewish principles of medical ethics, including Jewish law and human and animal experimentation, physician compassion for the patient, artificial insemination, in-vitro fertilization, surrogate motherhood and abortion, allocation of health care resources, organ transplantation (with emphasis on kidney and developments in Israel), and the right to die.

★ 12252 ★ **Laval University**
**Medical and Environmental Research**
**Group**
Philosophy Department
Pavillon Felix Antoine Savard
Quebec, QC, Canada G1K 7P4
**Phone:** (418)656-2244     **Fax:** (418)656-7267
Marie-Helene Parizeau, Dir.

**Activities/Fields:** Bioethics, human experimentation, ethical committees, education in ehtics for health professionals.

★ 12253 ★ **McGill University**
**Centre for Medicine, Ethics, and Law**
3690 Peel St.
Montreal, QC, Canada H3A 1W9
**Phone:** (514)398-7400     **Fax:** (514)398-4668
**Email:** somerville@falaw.lan.mcgill.ca
M.A. Somerville, Dir.

**Activities/Fields:** Social and policy issues which have medical, ethical, and legal dimensions, including medical research, reproductive technology, aging, population, AIDS, euthanasia, genetics, and biotechnology.

★ 12254 ★ **McGill University**
**Clinical Trials Research Group (CTRG)**
Biomedical Ethics Unit
3690 Peel St.
Montreal, QC, Canada H3A 1W9
**Phone:** (514)398-6945
**Email:** glass@falaw.lan.mcgill.ca
**Website:** http://www.mcgill.ca/ctrg/
Prof. Kathleen Cranley Glass, Contact

**Activities/Fields:** Ethical and legal issues in the design, review, and implementation of clinical trials.

★ 12255 ★ **Milton Helpern Institute of**
**Forensic Medicine**
520 1st Ave.
New York, NY 10016
**Phone:** (212)447-2030     **Fax:** (212)447-2716
Dr. Charles S. Hirsch, Dir.

**Activities/Fields:** Promotes medical-legal research, particularly the problems arising out of the official investigation of sudden, suspicious, violent, and unusual deaths, including those occuring in legal custody. Serves as a repository for material and a reference source in legal medicine, including medical-legal books, journals, and films. **Pub:** *International Microform Journal of Legal Medicine and Forensic Sciences*, quarterly.

★ 12256 ★ **Oregon Health and Science**
**University**
**Center for Ethics in Health Care**
3181 SW Sam Jackson Park Rd., UHN-86
Portland, OR 97201-3098
**Phone:** (503)494-1260
**Email:** ehtics@ohsu.edu
**Website:** http://www.ohsu.edu/ethics
Dr. Susan W. Tolle, Dir.

**Activities/Fields:** Ethics in contemporary health care, including end-of-life care.

★ 12257 ★ **St. Louis University**
**Center for Health Care Ethics**
Health Science Center
3545 Lafayette Ave.
Saint Louis, MO 63104
**Phone:** (314)577-8195     **Fax:** (314)268-5150
**Email:** magill@slu.edu
**Website:** http://www.slu.edu/centers/chce
Prof. Gerrard Magill, PhD, Dir.

**Activities/Fields:** Issues in health care ethics, including human genomics, stem cell research, organ transplants, end of life concerns, organizational ethics in health care, empirical research in health ethics. **Pub:** *Health Care Ethics USA Newsletter*, quarterly.

**★ 12258 ★ Serological Research Institute (SERI)**
3053 Research Dr.
Richmond, CA 94806-5206
**Phone:** (510)223-7374 **Fax:** (510)222-8887
**Email:** bwraxall@serological.com
**Website:** http://www.serological.com/
Brian Wraxall, Exec. Dir.

**Activities/Fields:** Analyzing blood and other body fluids encountered as evidence in criminal and civil matters, including genetic marker typing in blood and other bodily fluid stains and new or improved methods of analysis of serological evidence.

**★ 12259 ★ Stanford University Center for Biomedical Ethics**
701A Welch Rd., Ste. 1105
Palo Alto, CA 94304
**Phone:** (650)723-5760 **Fax:** (650)725-6131
**Email:** BKoenig@stanford.edu
**Website:** http://scbe.stanford.edu
Dr. Barbara Koenig, Exec. Dir.

**Activities/Fields:** Scientific and biomedical ethics, focusing on applying ethical reasoning to actual moral problems in the practice of medicine and science; contributing to the national and international discussion of biomedical and scientific issues through research, with a focus on empirical bioethics studies; convening scholars, professionals, and policymakers to debate and propose policy solutions regarding biomedical and scientific ethical issues; and serving as a scholarly resource for the University and the community.

**★ 12260 ★ U.S. Department of Health and Human Services**
**Office of Assistant Secretary for Health**
**Office Of Research Integrity**
Rockwall Bldg. 2
5515 Security Ln., Ste. 700
Rockville, MD 20852
**Phone:** (301)443-3400 **Fax:** (301)443-5351
**Email:** cpascal@osophs.dhhs.gov
**Website:** http://ori.dhhs.gov
Chris Pascal, Dir.

**Activities/Fields:** Responds to any allegations of scientific misconduct occurring in research supported by the Public Health Service.

**★ 12261 ★ U.S. Department of Health and Human Services**
**Office of Assistant Secretary for Health**
**Office of Research Integrity**
**Research Investigations Division**
Rockwall Bldg. 2
5515 Security Ln., Ste. 700
Rockville, MD 20852
**Phone:** (301)443-5330 **Fax:** (301)594-0043
**Website:** http://ori.dhhs.gov/html/programs/rapidresponse.asp
Alan R. Price, Dir.

**Activities/Fields:** Responds to allegations of scientific misconduct occurring in research supported by the Public Health Service.

**★ 12262 ★ University of Chicago Center for Clinical Medical Ethics**
MC 6098
Department of Medicine
5841 S Maryland Ave.
Chicago, IL 60637-6098
**Phone:** (773)702-1453 **Fax:** (773)702-0090
**Email:** msiegler@medicine.bsd.uchicago.edu
Mark Siegler, MD, Dir.

**Activities/Fields:** Clinical medical ethics, bioethics, technology assessment, and medical outcomes research.

**★ 12263 ★ University of North Texas Health Science Center at Fort Worth**
**Institute of Forensic Medicine**
3500 Camp Bowie Blvd.
Fort Worth, TX 76107-2699
**Phone:** (817)735-2429 **Fax:** (817)735-2424
**Email:** lnancy@hsc.unt.edu
Stephen L. Putthoff, DO, Chm.

**Activities/Fields:** Sudden death due to cardiovascular disease, sudden infant death syndrome, gunshot wounds, blunt and sharp force injuries, and forensic aspects of mass disasters.

**University of Pennsylvania**
**Social Work Mental Health Research Center (SWMHRC)**
*See:* Entry 12770

**★ 12264 ★ University of Pittsburgh Center for Bioethics and Health Law**
Medical Arts Bldg., Ste. 300
3708 5th Ave.
Pittsburgh, PA 15213
**Phone:** (412)647-5700 **Fax:** (412)647-5877
**Email:** bioethic@pitt.edu
**Website:** http://www.law.pitt.edu/~bioethic/faculty.htm
Dr. Alan Meisel, Dir.

**Activities/Fields:** Theoretical and clinical analysis of the complex ethical issues surrounding the health care process from a multidisciplinary perspective. Research areas include ethical issues surrounding the recruitment of patients to cancer chemotherapy clinical trials, effectiveness of required request laws and policies for organ and tissue donation, quality of nursing care provided to patients with AIDS, doctor-patient communication regarding advance directives, doctor-family communication in an intensive care unit, coercion in management of psychiatric patients, and comparison of ethical issues in engineering with medical ethics issues. **Frmly:** Center for Medical Ethics.

**★ 12265 ★ University of Virginia Center for Biomedical Ethics**
PO Box 800758
Charlottesville, VA 22908
**Phone:** (434)924-5974 **Fax:** (434)982-3971
**Email:** jdm8n@virginia.edu
**Website:** http://www.med.virginia.edu/bioethics
Jonathan D. Moreno, Dir.

**Activities/Fields:** Identification, analysis, and resolution of ethical problems in health care.

**★ 12266 ★ West Virginia University Center for Health Ethics and Law**
1195 Health Sciences N
Robert C. Byrd Health Sciences Center
PO Box 9022
Morgantown, WV 26506-9022
**Phone:** (304)293-7618 **Fax:** (304)293-7442
**Email:** amoss@hsc.wvu.edu
**Website:** http://www.hsc.wvu.edu/chel/
Alvin H. Moss, MD, Dir.

**Activities/Fields:** Health ethics and law.

## Federal Government Agencies

**★ 12267 ★ U.S. Department of Health and Human Services**
**National Institutes of Health (NIH)**
**National Institute of Mental Health (HIMH)**
9000 Rockville Pike
Bethesda, MD 20892
**Phone:** (301)443-3673     **Fax:** (301)443-0008
**Website:** http://www.nimh.nih.gov/
Steven E. Hyman, MD, Director

**Desc:** The Institute supports and conducts fundamental research in neuroscience, genetics, molecular biology, and behavior as the foundation of an extensive clinical research portfolio which seeks to expand and refine treatments available for illnesses such as schizophrenia; depressive disorders; severe anxiety; childhood mental disorders; and other mental disorders. It supports research on treatment outcomes in actual practice settings, including primary care settings and seeks to establish a sound scientific basis for the prevention of mental illness.

**★ 12268 ★ U.S. Department of Health and Human Services**
**Substance Abuse and Mental Health Services Administration**
**Center for Mental Health Services**
5600 Fishers Lane
Rockville, MD 20857
**Phone:** (301)443-0001
**Website:** http://www.samhsa.gov/centers/cmhs/cmhs.html
Gail P. Hutchings, Director

**Desc:** The Center provides national leadership to promote the improved state of mental health and the rehabilitation of people with mental disorders and others affected. The Center administers grants, contracts, and cooperative agreements which support the development and application of new knowledge in the health care field; supports activities to improve management of mental health care; collects data on the various forms of mental illness; cooperates with other Federal components to coordinate disaster assistance, community response, and other mental health emergency services as a consequence of national disasters; and collaborates with the alcohol, drug abuse, and mental health institutes on services research issues.

## Foundations & Other Funding Organizations

### Private Foundations

**Annie E. Casey Foundation**
*See:* Entry 5545

**Arcana Foundation**
*See:* Entry 49

**Bingham Trust**
*See:* Entry 10040

**★ 12269 ★ Blowitz-Ridgeway Foundation**
One Northfield Plaza
570 Frontage Rd., Ste. 528
Northfield, IL 60093-1213
**Phone:** (847)446-1010
**Website:** http://www.aecf.org
Tina Erickson, Administrator

**Fnded:** 1984. **Philosophy:** One of the primary funding areas of the foundation is "the support of non-profit agencies which provide health care to economically disadvantaged children and adolescents." Additional interests include child welfare, family services, and youth organizations. In 1998, the foundation reported funding medical research in targeted subject areas: Parkinson's Disease, prostate cancer, and childhood asthma, as well as applied research in orphan diseases, Hepatitis C, and breast cancer. **Priorities:** *Education:* 6%. Supports a high schools, arts education, and educational foundations. *Environment:* 32%. Supports homeless shelters, food distribution, family services, services for victims of violence, youth organizations, and early childhood development initiatives. *International:* 62%. Funds healthcare services and medical research. *Note:* Total contributions for fiscal 2000. **Typ. Recipients:** AIDS/HIV, Alzheimers Disease, Arthritis, Cancer, Child Abuse, Children's Health/Hospitals, Clinics/Medical Centers, Domestic Violence, Emergency/Ambulance Services, Eyes/Blindness, Family Planning, Health Organizations, Health-General, Home-Care Services, Hospices, Hospitals, Hospitals (University Affiliated), Long-Term Care, Medical Rehabilitation, Medical Research, Mental Health, Nursing Services, Outpatient Health Care, People with Disabilities, Prenatal Health Issues, Public Health, Respiratory, Sexual Abuse, Single-Disease Health Associations, Speech & Hearing. **Geo. Dist:** IL.

**Blumenthal Foundation**
*See:* Entry 82

**Cannon Foundation**
*See:* Entry 8538

**★ 12270 ★ Christopher Reynolds Foundation**
267 5th Ave.
New York, NY 10021
**Phone:** (212)532-1606     **Fax:** (212)532-1403
**Email:** crfny@aol.com
**Website:** http://www.blumenthalfoundation.org
Andrea Panaritis, Executive Director & Secretary

**Fnded:** 1952. **Philosophy:** The Christopher Reynolds Foundation makes most of its grants in the areas of international development, policy, and social science. Civic affairs contributions are a major priority, with interests in international policy and national security. Educational funding supports large universities with international studies programs. **Priorities:** *Arts & Humanities:* 2%. Supports museums, and historic preservation. *Civic & Public Affairs:* 26%. Supports environmental and economic justice programs, and democracy. *Education:* 7%. Education funds, science research, and universities. *Environment:* 4%. Supports youth organizations, and community service foundations. *International:* 2%. Primarily supports health institutes. *Religion:* 4%. Supports scientific organizations. *Note:* Total contributions made in fiscal 1999. **Typ. Recipients:** Medical Education, Mental Health, Public Health, Speech & Hearing. **Geo. Dist:** U.S. organizations working in Indochina; MI; NY; OH.

**Dale J. Bellamah Foundation**
*See:* Entry 155

**Davenport-Hatch Foundation**
*See:* Entry 160

**Edward W. Hazen Foundation**
*See:* Entry 204

**★ 12271 ★ Essel Foundation**
2500 Westchester Ave.
Purchase, NY 10577
**Phone:** (914)698-7133
**Website:** http://www.hazenfoundation.org
Constance Lieber, President

**Fnded:** 1966. **Philosophy:** The Essel Foundation is primarily interested in supporting mental illness research. Regular contributions are made to support depression and schizophrenia treatment and research. Higher education is an additional area of interest. **Priorities:** *Education:* 2%. Colleges and universities. *International:* 92%. Major support to the National Alliance for Research on Schizophrenia and Depression. *Note:* Total contributons made in fiscal 1999. **Typ. Recipients:** Cancer, Clinics/Medical Centers, Geriatric Health, Medical Research, Mental Health, Single-Disease Health Associations. **Geo. Dist:** New York, NY.

**Eugene B. Casey Foundation**
*See:* Entry 224

**Forrest C. Lattner Foundation**
*See:* Entry 250

---

**★ 12272 ★ Freed Foundation**
3050 K St. Northwest, Ste. 220
Washington, DC 20007
**Phone:** (202)337-5487
Elizabeth Freed, President
**Fnded:** 1954. **Philosophy:** The Freed Foundation is "interested in non-traditional learning environments, especially those which benefit children. Whether related to socio-economic issues, traumatic childhood experiences, absense of positive role models, or other influences, many children cannot be reached through mainstream educational settings and do not have access to appropriate alternatives. We hope to focus on educational grants in the areas on environmental awareness, artistic creativity, and/or cultural enrichment. We feel connected and interested in learning. Programs focused on enriching children's lives by improving self-esteem, mental health and overall wellbeing are top priorities. We sincerely hope to make a difference by investing our resources in this manner." President's Message, 1996 Annual Report **Priorities:** *Arts & Humanities:* 25%. Supports history, theater, and the performing arts. *Civic & Public Affairs:* 2%. Supports botanical gardens. *Education:* 18%. Supports minority education, afterschool/enrichment programs, and literacy. *Environment:* 6%. Supports camps, youth programs, family services, and crime prevention. *International:* 12%. Supports prenatal health issues, eyes/blindness, and AIDS. *Note:* Total contributions made in 1999. **Typ. Recipients:** AIDS/HIV, Alzheimers Disease, Cancer, Child Abuse, Children's Health/Hospitals, Clinics/Medical Centers, Domestic Violence, Emergency/Ambulance Services, Eyes/Blindness, Family Planning, Hospices, Hospitals, Medical Education, Medical Rehabilitation, Mental Health, Nutrition, People with Disabilities, Public Health, Research/Studies Institutes, Sexual Abuse, Single-Disease Health Associations, Substance Abuse. **Geo. Dist:** Washington, DC, including metropolitan area.

---

**Hugh Kaul Foundation Trust**
*See:* Entry 366

---

**Irving I. Moskowitz Foundation**
*See:* Entry 379

---

**★ 12273 ★ Ittleson Foundation**
15 East 67th St.
New York, NY 10021
**Phone:** (212)794-2008          **Fax:** (212)794-0351
**Website:** http://www.ittlesonfoundation.org
Anthony Wood, Executive Director
**Fnded:** 1932. **Philosophy:** The foundation currently is interested in programs which address issues associated with AIDS, mental health, and the environment. The foundation's literature states, "While our strategies change from year to year, our interest is in a sense constant. We want the United States to be a stronger and healthier country tomorrow than it is today. Our fields of interest by their very nature express benchmarks toward that goal. A democracy is only worthy of that name when it both forcefully and compassionately addresses the needs of the most sick (and) the most disturbed..." The foundation focuses on projects that address the consequences of AIDS on the mental health of people with the disease, their families, and caregivers. The foundation is also supportive of innovative prevention efforts, especially those that address the needs of youth. In environment, the foundation is interested in the education of a new generation of environmentalists, urban environmental issues, and efforts at resource protection. The foundation supports programs that provide new opportunities to recruit young people into the environmental studies field, and it seeks pilot projects that will test new approaches to solving environmental problems, and bring about changes through policy research or applied research, such as tests of innovative technology; analyses of regulations and laws; innovative recycling projects; and similar efforts. The foundation encour-

ages projects that link formal professional competence with community-based efforts. The foundation promotes the well-being of mankind through support of mental health, psychiatric research, and behavioral science research. Since 1932, mental health has been the primary focus and will continue to be a strong interest. The foundation is especially interested in innovative projects that address underserved populations, such as the elderly, poor, and minorities. The foundation encourages projects that link formal professional competence to informal networks of support in order to make services available. The foundation is interested in providing seed money for the start-up of innovative programs that improve the social welfare of citizens. Preference is given to pilot projects, test and demonstration projects, and applied research of public policy. Projects should be of nationally in scope or significance beyond the local area of implementation and should result in a product or outcome of some consequence in the real world. **Priorities:** *Civic & Public Affairs:* 10%. Supports aquariums, public policy, womens affairs, civil rights, housing, and legal aid. *Education:* Supports universities, schools, and religious education. *Environment:* 13%. Supports food distribution, homes, shelter/homeless. *International:* 47%. Major supportis for AIDS/HIV. Also supports nursing services, and mental health. *Note:* Total contributions made in 1998. **Typ. Recipients:** AIDS/HIV, Cancer, Child Abuse, Children's Health/Hospitals, Emergency/Ambulance Services, Geriatric Health, Health Organizations, Hospitals, Medical Education, Medical Research, Mental Health, Nutrition, People with Disabilities, Prenatal Health Issues, Preventive Medicine/Wellness Organizations, Public Health, Research/Studies Institutes, Single-Disease Health Associations, Substance Abuse. **Geo. Dist:** nationally.

---

**★ 12274 ★ John D. and Catherine T. MacArthur Foundation**
140 South Dearborn St., Ste. 1100
Chicago, IL 60603-5285
**Phone:** (312)726-8000          **Fax:** (312)920-6258
**Email:** 4answers@macfdn.org
**Website:** http://www.macfound.org
Richard Kaplan, Director, Grants Management
**Fnded:** 1970. **Philosophy:** "The Foundation is dedicated to helping groups and individuals foster lasting improvements in the human condition. The foundation seeks the development of healthy individuals and effective communities; peace within and among nations; responsible choices about human reproduction; and a global ecosystem capable of supporting healthy human societies. The Foundation pursues this mission by supporting research, policy development, dissemination, education and training, and practice." The Foundation makes grants through two major integrated programs. The Program on Human and Community Development supports work in community development, the arts, economic opportunity, youth development, education, mental health, research and other areas. The Program on Global Security and Sustainability focuses upon issues of peace, population and the environment. The Foundation's special programs are the General Program, through which a number of special initiatives that promote excellence and diversity in the media, and the MacArthur Fellows Program. **Priorities:** *Arts & Humanities:* 3%. Through the general program, support goes to media projects that increase the diversity of viewpoints on film, television, and radio, especially documentary works. *Civic & Public Affairs:* 21%. Focus on economic opportunity, building community capacity, cross-cutting initiatives, and land grants/donations to Florida. *Education:* 9%. Supports fellowships, colleges, and universities. *Environment:* 14%. Child and youth development, and population issues. *International:* 3%. Mental health policy and research. *Note:* Total contributions made in 1998. **Typ. Recipients:** Clinics/Medical Centers, Family Planning, Geriatric Health, Health Organizations, Health Policy/Cost Containment, Medical Education, Medical Research, Mental Health, Preventive Medicine/Wellness Organizations, Public Health, Research/Studies Institutes. **Geo. Dist:** internationally; nationally; FL, Palm Beach County: human and community development grants; Chicago, IL, education

reform grants; Chicago, IL, human and community development grants; global security and sustainability grants; global security and sustainability grants; global security and sustainability grants; global security and sustainability grants.

---

**John Templeton Foundation**
*See:* Entry 10046

---

**Lyndhurst Foundation**
*See:* Entry 5468

---

**Marion I. and Henry J. Knott Foundation**
*See:* Entry 504

---

**Ordean Foundation**
*See:* Entry 570

---

**Powell Foundation**
*See:* Entry 5469

---

**★ 12275 ★ R. J. Maclellan Charitable Trust**
Provident Bldg., Ste. 501
Chattanooga, TN 37402
**Phone:** (423)755-8142          **Fax:** (423)755-1640
**Email:** hugh@maclellan.net
**Website:** http://www.maclellanfdn.org
Hugh Maclellan, Jr., Trustee
**Fnded:** 1954. **Philosophy:** Its indenture states that the trust gives to institutions "organized and operated exclusively for religious, charitable, scientific, literary or educational purposes." However, the trust makes grants primarily for religious purposes and education. Religious funding favors Christian leadership development, saturation church planting, theological institutions, ministries, Bible institutes, and international missions. Educational support goes to religious education and preselected private schools. The foundation also supports other recipient areas. **Priorities:** *Environment:* 2%. Includes family services. *Note:* Total contributions made in 1998. **Typ. Recipients:** Mental Health, Sexual Abuse. **Geo. Dist:** nationally; Atlanta, GA; Chattonooga, TN, and surrounding area.

---

**Russell Sage Foundation**
*See:* Entry 648

---

**Schumann Fund for New Jersey**
*See:* Entry 666

---

**★ 12276 ★ Spencer Foundation**
875 North Michigan Ave., Ste. 3930
Chicago, IL 60611-1803
**Phone:** (312)337-7000          **Fax:** (312)337-0282
**Email:** vicepres@spencer.org
**Website:** http://www.spencer.org
Paul Goren, Vice President
**Fnded:** 1962. **Philosophy:** "The Foundation has as its primary mission, by the intent of its founder, 'to investigate ways in which education can be improved, around the world.' To achieve this goal, the Foundation is committed to supporting high quality investigation of education through its research programs and to strengthening and renewing the educational research community through fellowship programs and related activities. The Foundation defines education broadly to include all the situations and institutions in which education proceeds, across the entire life span. An important expectation of the Foundation is that the activities it supports, taken together over the years, will contribute significantly to the enhancement of educational opportunity for all people." "The Foundation's programs are organized within three divisions: Research, Fellowships, and Training. In addition, a handful of programs are also operated out of the Office of the Vice President. Programs in the Research Division support work that shows promise of contribut-

ing new knowledge, understanding, and improvement of educational thought and practice. Programs in the Fellowship Division support educational researchers at different stages of their professional careers, providing resources to both beginning and senior researchers to pursue concentrated intellectual activity. Programs in the Training Division are aimed at improving the work and performance of agencies and institutions, mainly universities and graduate schools of education at universities, which hold a mission of training and apprenticing educational researchers. Funding programs within the Vice President's Office are experimental or developmental, spanning and augmenting the other divisions' programmatic objectives." 2000 Application and Review Information **Priorities:** *Education:* 98%. Includes colleges and universities, foreign schools, and research institutes. Within education, the foundation supports a broad range of disciplinary and interdisciplinary categories. *Note:* Total contributions made in fiscal 2000. **Typ. Recipients:** Children's Health/Hospitals, Mental Health. **Geo. Dist:** internationally; nationally.

★ 12277 ★ **Staunton Farm Foundation**
Center City Tower, Ste. 210
650 Smithfield St.
Pittsburgh, PA 15222
**Phone:** (412)281-8020          **Fax:** (412)232-3115
**Website:** http://www.stauntonfarm.org
Joni Schwager, Program Officer, Foundation Manager
**Fnded:** 1937. **Philosophy:** The foundation continues to adhere to Mrs. McCready's philosophy of helping "the sick and unfortunate." The foundation focuses on programs designed to address the needs of those suffering from mental illness. A primary interest is taken in projects which represent new and different approaches for organizations which provide patient care. The foundation supports work in the fields of mental health and social services. All organizations that are funded by Staunton Farm deal with mental health problems and the welfare of the emotionally handicapped, and are located in Southwestern Pennsylvania. The foundation emphasizes organizations addressing the needs of children with mental illness, or agencies collaborating in providing those services. **Priorities:** *Civic & Public Affairs:* 1%. *Education:* 12%. Mental health education programs. *Environment:* 58%. Counseling services, youth programs, and therapy. *International:* 23%. Mental health, AIDS, and therapeutic services. *Note:* Total contributions made in 2000. **Typ. Recipients:** AIDS/HIV, Children's Health/Hospitals, Clinics/Medical Centers, Domestic Violence, Eyes/Blindness, Family Planning, Health Funds, Health Organizations, Health-General, Hospices, Hospitals, Medical Education, Medical Rehabilitation, Mental Health, People with Disabilities, Public Health, Sexual Abuse, Single-Disease Health Associations, Substance Abuse. **Geo. Dist:** PA, Southwestern Pennsylvania.

**Swalm Foundation**
*See:* Entry 713

★ 12278 ★ **van Ameringen Foundation, Inc.**
509 Madison Ave.
New York, NY 10022-5501
**Phone:** (212)758-6221          **Fax:** (212)688-2105
**Website:** http://www.vanamfound.org
Henry Van Ameringen, President
**Fnded:** 1950. **Philosophy:** The foundation's primary interest is furthering "prevention, education, and direct care in the mental health field with an emphasis on those individuals and populations having a disadvantaged background and deprived opportunities." Priority interest areas include preventive and early-intervention strategies, particularly those which work in tandem with educational programs; programs to link existing resources for clients, particularly the mixing of public and private efforts; programs which increase the accessibility of the poor to mental health services; and programs which include a self-help model. Recently supported projects include programs dealing with parental stress, programs for abused children and

their parents, crisis centers for runaways, services for the elderly, and education for minorities. Some funding is directed to arts projects related to mental health issues. **Priorities:** *Arts & Humanities:* 1%. Supports Lichtenstein Creative Media. *Civic & Public Affairs:* 3%. Community affairs and housing. *Education:* About 1%. Supports colleges and universities. *Environment:* 4%. Veterans services, child welfare, and counseling. *International:* 89%. Mental health, university-affiliated hospitals, and children's health. *Note:* Total contributions made in 1998. **Typ. Recipients:** AIDS/HIV, Cancer, Children's Health/Hospitals, Clinics/Medical Centers, Domestic Violence, Emergency/Ambulance Services, Geriatric Health, Health Organizations, Health-General, Hospitals, Hospitals (University Affiliated), Long-Term Care, Medical Education, Medical Rehabilitation, Medical Research, Mental Health, People with Disabilities, Prenatal Health Issues, Preventive Medicine/Wellness Organizations, Single-Disease Health Associations, Substance Abuse. **Geo. Dist:** Northeastern USA.

**Walton Family Foundation**
*See:* Entry 10057

★ 12279 ★ **Wasie Foundation**
4999 France Ave. South, Ste. 250
601 Second Ave. South
Minneapolis, MN 55410
**Phone:** (612)332-3883          **Fax:** (612)455-6888
**Email:** rachel@wasie.org
**Website:** http://www.wffhome.com
Rachel Pearson, Program Associate
**Fnded:** 1966. **Philosophy:** The Wasie Foundation strives to fulfill the interest of its donors by funding organizations whose goals and missions reflect the interests of the late Stanley and Marie Wasie: greater opportunity for young people of Polish descent through education; hope and recovery for people with schizophrenia; a higher quality of life for people with arthritis; a brighter future for children with medical problems and improved treatment and care for people with cancer. **Priorities:** *Civic & Public Affairs:* 1%. Supports associations of small foundations. *Education:* 26%. Funds colleges, universities, scholarships, and medical education. *Environment:* 22%. Supports camps. community organizations and services primarily for those with arthritis and for children. *International:* 51%. Provides funding for organizations supporting cancer research, services for the mentally ill, cerebral palsy research and children's health. *Note:* Total contributions made in 1999. **Typ. Recipients:** Arthritis, Cancer, Children's Health/Hospitals, Clinics/Medical Centers, Health-General, Hospices, Long-Term Care, Medical Education, Medical Research, Mental Health, Research/Studies Institutes, Single-Disease Health Associations, Speech & Hearing. **Geo. Dist:** MN.

**William T. Grant Foundation**
*See:* Entry 5567

## Corporate Foundations

**AGL Resources Inc.**
*See:* Entry 803

**Alabama Power Foundation**
*See:* Entry 808

**Ben & Jerry's Foundation**
*See:* Entry 10060

**The Boeing Co. Charitable Trust**
*See:* Entry 5472

**Carrier Corp.**
*See:* Entry 918

★ 12280 ★ **Central Vermont Public Service Corp.**
77 Grove St.
Rutland, VT 05701
**Phone:** (802)747-5672          **Fax:** (802)747-2188
**Email:** sbush@aglresources.com
**Website:** http://www.cvps.com
Andrea Bove, Exec. Asst.
**Typ. Recipients:** Mental Health. **Geo. Dist:** VT.

**Comerica Charitable Foundation**
*See:* Entry 957

**Eli Lilly Foundation**
*See:* Entry 1022

**First Evergreen Foundation**
*See:* Entry 1048

★ 12281 ★ **Gannett Foundation**
7950 Jones Branch Dr.
Mc Lean, VA 22107
**Phone:** (703)854-6069
**Email:** isimpson@gci1.gannett.com
**Website:** http://www.gannettfoundation.org/apply.htm
Irma Simpson, Manager
**Priorities:** *Arts & Humanities:* 16% Supports arts and culture organizations (11%) and media (5%). *Civic & Public Affairs:* 12%. *Education:* 15%. *Environment:* 16%. *International:* 9%. *Note:* Total contributions made in 2000. **Typ. Recipients:** Mental Health, People with Disabilities. **Geo. Dist:** operating locations.

**GenCorp Foundation**
*See:* Entry 1078

**Habig Foundation**
*See:* Entry 11434

**H&R Block Foundation**
*See:* Entry 1111

**Hasbro Children's Foundation**
*See:* Entry 11435

★ 12282 ★ **Heller Financial, Inc.**
500 West Monroe St.
Chicago, IL 60661
**Phone:** (312)441-6748          **Fax:** (312)441-6728
**Email:** jkorba@hellerfin.com
**Website:** http://www.hellerfinancial.com
Judy Korba, Contributions Manager
**Priorities:** *Voluntarism:* The company has a volunteer committee, an incentive program, and has adopted a public school. **Typ. Recipients:** Mental Health. **Geo. Dist:** headquarters and operating communities.

**Household International Inc.**
*See:* Entry 1132

**Laclede Gas Charitable Trust**
*See:* Entry 5578

**Lotus Development Philanthropy Program**
*See:* Entry 1210

**National Fuel Gas Co.**
*See:* Entry 11454

**National Life Group**
*See:* Entry 1257

**Nationwide Foundation**
*See:* Entry 1261

**R.R. Donnelley & Sons Co.**
*See:* Entry 5474

**Truland Foundation**
*See:* Entry 5590

**Varian Medical Systems, Inc.**
*See:* Entry 1477

**Vulcan Materials Co. Foundation**
*See:* Entry 1482

**Waste Management Inc.**
*See:* Entry 1493

**Wells Fargo Bank Nebraska, N.A.**
*See:* Entry 1496

**Woodward Governor Co. Charitable Trust**
*See:* Entry 11473

## Other Funding Organizations

**★ 12283 ★ American Association for Marriage and Family Therapy (AAMFT)**
112 S Alfred St.
Alexandria, VA 22314
**Phone:** (703)838-9808          **Fax:** (703)838-9805
**Email:** exec@aamft.org
**Website:** http://www.aamft.org
James Morris, Pres.

**Desc:** Professional society of marriage and family therapists. Assumes a major role in developing & maintaining the highest standards of excellence in this field. Has 76 accredited training programs throughout the U.S. Sponsors educational and research programs. **Awards:** Cumulative Contribution to Family Therapy Research Award (annual); Distinguished Leadership Award (annual); Distinguished Professional Contribution to Family Therapy Award (annual); Divisional Contribution Award (annual); Ethnic Minority Fellowships Awards; Ethnic Minority Honorable Mention Awards; Graduate Student Research Grant Award (annual); Organizational Contribution Award (annual); Outstanding Scholarly Publication in Family Therapy Research Award (annual); Significant Contribution to the Field of Marriage and Family Therapy Award (annual).

**★ 12284 ★ American Foundation for Suicide Prevention**
120 Wall St., Fl. 22
New York, NY 10005-4001
**Phone:** (212)363-3500          **Free:** 888-333-AFSP
**Fax:** (212)363-6237
**Email:** inquiry@afsp.org
**Website:** http://www.afsp.org
Robert Gebbia, Exec. Dir.

**Desc:** Medical professionals, community leaders, and suicide survivors. Provides funding for research on the causes and prevention of suicide. Trains professionals in the treatment of suicidal individuals; offers support programs for suicide survivors. **Awards:** AFSP Institutional Grants (annual) for research centers exploring innovative ideas in the prevention of suicide; Established Researcher Award (annual) for senior researchers in suicidology investigating new aspects of the field; Post-Doctoral Research Fellowship (annual) for full-time research by an investigator who has received a Ph.D. degree within the previous 5 years but has not had 3 years of fellowship support.

**★ 12285 ★ American Nouthetic Psychology Association (ANPA)**
c/o Dr. David M. Carnrike
PO Box 801
Hardwick, GA 31034
**Phone:** (334)660-7675          **Fax:** (334)666-8003
**Website:** http://www.alltel.net/~biblepsy
Dr. David M. Carnrike, Pres.

**Desc:** Psychologists and other individuals with an interest in nouthetic psychology. Promotes high standards of training, ethics, and practice in the field. Conducts research and educational programs. **Awards:** Alice M. Camp Award (annual) for first year college psychology students.

**★ 12286 ★ American Psychological Society (APS)**
1010 Vermont Ave. NW, Ste. 1100
Washington, DC 20005-4907
**Phone:** (202)783-2077          **Fax:** (202)783-2083
**Email:** aps@aps.washington.dc.us
**Website:** http://www.psychologicalscience.org
Alan G. Kraut, Contact

**Desc:** Scientists and academics. Works for the advancement of the discipline of psychology and the promotion of human welfare through research and application. Conducts research programs; educates policy makers on the role human behavior plays in societal problems; offers liability insurance plans. **Awards:** William James Fellow (annual).

**★ 12287 ★ American Psychopathological Association (APPA)**
Department of Psychiatry
Washington University School of Medicine
4940 Children's Pl.
Saint Louis, MO 63110
**Email:** zorumskc@psychiatry.wustl.edu
**Website:** http://www.appassn.org
Chuck Zorumski, MD, Pres.

**Desc:** Physicians and scientists interested in the field of psychopathology. To investigate scientific problems of abnormal psychology including: study of phenomena arising from abnormal mental processes; study of organic pathological conditions directly connected with abnormal mental processes; study of means which may remove or modify social or individual factors operating in the production of mental disease; study of relationship between psychopathological and social or cultural problems. **Awards:** Paul Moch Award (annual) for academy distinction; Samuel Hamilton Award (annual); Zubin Award (annual).

**★ 12288 ★ Association for Advancement of Behavior Therapy (AABT)**
305 7th Ave., Ste. 16A
New York, NY 10001-6008
**Phone:** (212)647-1890          **Free:** 800-685-AABT
**Fax:** (212)647-1865
**Email:** mjeimer@aabt.org
**Website:** http://www.aabt.org/
Mary Jane Eimer, CAE, Exec. Dir.

**Desc:** Psychologists primarily, but also psychiatrists, social workers, counselors, physicians, dentists, nurses, students, and other professionals interested in the issues, problems, and development of the field of behavior therapy and cognitive behavior therapy, with specific emphasis on research and clinical applications. Sponsors training programs and lectures for professionals; maintains speakers' bureau; handles referrals for the public to locate behavior therapists in their area; facilitates communication between behavior therapists interested in specific problems or information. AABT local affiliates hold training meetings, workshops, seminars, case demonstrations, and discussion groups. discussion groups. **Awards:** Career/Lifetime Achievement (annual); Distinguished Friend to Behavior Therapy (annual); Distinguished/Outstanding Contribution by an Individual for Education/Training (triennial); Elsie Ramos Awards (annual) for the best student poster submitted at annual convention; Outstanding Training Program (annual); Presi-

dent's New Researcher Award (annual); Student Dissertation Award (annual).

**★ 12289 ★ Association for Child Psychoanalysis (ACP)**
PO Box 253
Ramsey, NJ 07446
**Phone:** (201)825-3138          **Fax:** (201)825-3138
**Email:** childanalysis@compuserve.com
**Website:** http://www.westnet.com/acp/
Erna Furman, Pres.

**Desc:** Child psychoanalysts united to provide a forum for discussion and dissemination of information in their field. Conducts national and international scientific meetings. **Awards:** Monetary (annual).

**★ 12290 ★ Association for Women in Psychology (AWP)**
423 N Albany St.
Ithaca, NY 14850
**Phone:** (607)735-1907
**Email:** support@awpsych.org
**Website:** http://www.awpsych.org
Diane Maluso, Contact

**Desc:** Seeks to: end the role that the association feels psychology has had in perpetuating unscientific and unquestioned assumptions about the "natures" of women and men; encourage unbiased psychological research on sex and gender in order to establish facts and expose myths; encourage research and theory directed toward alternative sex-role socialization, child rearing practices, life-styles, and language use; educate and sensitize the science and psychology professions as well as the public to the psychological, social, political, and economic rights of women; combat the oppression of women of color; encourage research on issues of concern to women of color; achieve equality of opportunity for women and men within the profession and science of psychology. Conducts business and professional sessions at meetings of regional psychology associations. Maintains Hall of Fame and speakers' bureau. Monitors sexism in the American Psychological Association. **Awards:** Distinguished Publication Award (annual) selection by committee; Jewish Women's Caucus Award for Scholarship (annual) for projects and papers published, also unpublished documents; Lesbian Psychologies Unpublished Manuscript Award (annual); Student Research Prize (annual) for research on women and gender; Women of Color Psychologies Award (annual).

**★ 12291 ★ Depression and Related Affective Disorders Association (DRADA)**
Johns Hopkins Hospital Meyer 3-181
600 N Wolfe St.
Baltimore, MD 21287-7381
**Phone:** (410)955-4647          **Fax:** (410)614-3241
**Email:** drada@jhmi.edu
**Website:** http://www.drada.org
Cathy Pollock, Dir.

**Desc:** Individuals with affective disorders, their families and friends, and mental health professionals. (Affective disorders include depressive illnesses and manic-depression.) Provides support services including referrals, educational programs, networking, and consultation. Encourages and facilitates the formation of local support groups for those with affective disorders; provides training for support group leaders. Cosponsors with Johns Hopkins annual mood disorders symposium. Maintains speakers' bureau. **Awards:** Scholarship (annual) bestowed to a research student.

**★ 12292 ★ Family Therapy Network (FTN)**
7705 13th St. NW
Washington, DC 20012
**Phone:** (202)829-2452          **Fax:** (202)726-7983
**Email:** info@psychnetworker.org
Richard Simon, Dir.

**Desc:** Promotes the exchange of ideas and information among psychotherapists. **Awards:** Innovations in Training (annual) for those who demonstrate history of preparing therapists to work with underserved populations, increasing cultural diversity of skilled practitioners and developing more effective training and supervision programs.

**International Society of Psychiatric
Mental Health Nurses (ISPN)**
*See:* Entry 14925

**★ 12293 ★ International Transactional
Analysis Association (ITAA)**
436 14th St. Ste. 1301
Oakland, CA 94612-2710
**Phone:** (510)625-7720      **Fax:** (510)625-7725
**Email:** itaa@itaa-net.org
**Website:** http://www.itaa-net.org
Gordon B. Hewitt, PhD, Pres.
**Desc:** Educational corporation of persons in medical and behavioral sciences, including psychiatrists, psychologists, social workers, nurses, educators, marriage and family counselors, clergy, and organizational consultants. Maintains standards of practice and teaching of transactional analysis, which involves group therapy, social dynamics, and personality theory based on analysis of the "transactions" or interactions between persons. (The book, *Games People Play*, covers basic transactional analysis theory; its author, Dr. Eric Berne, was ITAA founder.) **Awards:** Eric Berne Memorial Award (annual) scientific research in transactional analysis; Eric Berne Research Grant.

**★ 12294 ★ Milton H. Erickson
Foundation (MHEF)**
3606 N 24th St.
Phoenix, AZ 85016
**Phone:** (602)956-6196      **Fax:** (602)956-0519
**Email:** office@erickson-foundation.org
**Website:** http://www.erickson-foundation.org
Jeffrey K. Zeig, Dir.
**Desc:** Seeks to promote and advance the contributions made to health sciences by Milton H. Erickson, M.D. (1901-1980), regarded as an authority on hypnotherapy and brief strategic therapy. Dedicated to the training of health and restricted to mental health professionals. **Awards:** Lifetime Achievement Award (periodic); scholarship (periodic).

**NADD - An Association for Persons with
Developmental Disabilities and Mental
Health Needs**
*See:* Entry 6864

**★ 12295 ★ National Alliance for
Research on Schizophrenia and
Depression (NARSAD)**
60 Cutter Mill Rd., Ste. 404
Great Neck, NY 11021
**Phone:** (516)829-0091      **Free:** 800-829-8289
**Fax:** (516)487-6930
**Email:** info@narsad.org
**Website:** http://www.mhsource.com/narsad.html
Constance Lieber, Pres.
**Desc:** Raises funds for research on schizophrenia, depression, and other mental illnesses. **Awards:** Lieber Prize (annual) for established scientific investigator; Young Investigators (annual) for scientific research.

**★ 12296 ★ Psi Beta**
1027 Westbridge Ln.
PO Box 4838
Chattanooga, TN 37405
**Phone:** (423)265-6555      **Free:** 888-PSI-BETA
**Fax:** (423)265-0033
**Email:** psibeta@psibeta.org
**Website:** http://www.psibeta.org
Carol Tracy, Exec. Dir.

**Desc:** Honor society - community, and junior college psychology students. Participates in psychology conventions. Provides means for contact with professors in students' areas of interest. Conducts educational programs and sponsors national awards. Promotes excellence in scholarship, leadership, research and community service. **Awards:** Allyn & Bacon Research Paper Award (annual) for 3 original emperical research papers written in APA style; Ann G. Robinson College Life (annual) for a unique promotion of the quality of 2-year college life that advances psychology and Psi Beta's mission; Carol Tracy Community Service Award (annual) for outstanding community service project; Harcourt College Publishers National Chapter Award (annual) active chapter that demonstrates outstanding programming; Virginia Sexton Faculty Advisor Award (annual) for outstanding service as faculty advisor.

**★ 12297 ★ Psychohistory Forum (PF)**
627 Dakota Trail
Franklin Lakes, NJ 07417
**Phone:** (201)891-7486      **Fax:** (201)891-6866
**Email:** pelovitz@aol.com
Paul H. Elovitz, PhD, Dir.
**Desc:** Psychologists, psychiatrists, Psychotherapists, social workers, historians, psychohistorians, and laypeople having a scholarly interest in the integration of depth psychology and history. (Psychohistory is the study of psychobiography, group process, the mechanisms of defense, the history of childhood, creativity, dreams, and the difference between stated intention and actual behavior). Seeks to further psychohistory through the exchange of information. Conducts bimonthly workshops on topics related to psychohistory and training seminars on dream analysis, innovation, teaching, and methodology. Aids individuals in psychohistorical research. Holds lecture series. lecture series. **Awards:** Halpern Award for the Best Psychohistorical Idea (annual); Halpren Graduate Student Award (annual) for the best psychohistorical idea; Student Award year's membership.

**★ 12298 ★ Psychometric Society (PS)**
c/o Dr. Terry Ackerman
UNCG
207 Curry Bldg.
Greensboro, NC 27402-6171
**Phone:** (336)334-3474      **Fax:** (336)334-4120
**Email:** taackerm@uncg.edu
**Website:** http://www.psychometricsociety.org/
Dr. Terry Ackerman, Sec.
**Desc:** Persons interested in development of quantitative models for psychological phenomena and quantitative methodology in the social and behavioral sciences. **Awards:** Psychometric Society Dissertation Award (annual) review of dissertation by a committee of three past presidents.

**★ 12299 ★ Society for the Psychological
Study of Social Issues (SPSSI)**
1901 Pennsylvania Ave. NW, No. 901
Washington, DC 20006-3405
**Phone:** (202)223-5100      **Fax:** (202)223-5555
**Email:** spssi@spssi.org
**Website:** http://www.spssi.org
Jennifer Crocker, Pres.
**Desc:** Psychologists, sociologists, anthropologists, psychiatrists, political scientists, and social workers. Works to: obtain and disseminate to the public scientific knowledge about social change and other social processes; promote psychological research on significant theoretical and practical questions of social issues; encourage application of findings to problems of society. **Awards:** Award for Best Paper (annual); Internship research grant (annual); Research Grants (annual).

**★ 12300 ★ Society for a Science of
Clinical Psychology**
c/o Raymond P. Lorion
University of Pennsylvania

Graduate School of Education
Psychology in Education Division
3700 Walnut St.
Philadelphia, PA 19104-6216
**Phone:** (215)898-7367      **Fax:** (215)573-2115
**Email:** lorion@gse.upenn.edu
**Website:** http://pantheon.yale.edu/~tat22/
Thomas D. Borkovec, PhD, Pres.
**Desc:** Promotes the integration of the scientist and the practitioner in training, research and applied undertakings in the field of clinical psychology. **Awards:** Dissertation Grant Awards; Distinguished Scientist Award; Outstanding Dissertation Award.

**★ 12301 ★ World Organization and
Public Education Corp. of the National
Association for the Advancement of
Psychoanalysis**
80 8th Ave., Ste. 1501
New York, NY 10011-5126
**Phone:** (212)741-0515      **Fax:** (212)366-4347
**Email:** naap72@aol.com
**Website:** http://www.naap.org
Margery Quackenbush, Admin.
**Desc:** Works for public education for the National Association for the Advancement of Psychoanalysis. **Awards:** Gradiva Awards (annual) for work that advances psychoanalysis; Vision Awards (annual) for work that advances psychoanalysis.

# Medical & Allied Health Schools

## Psychoanalysis

*The psychoanalytic training institutes listed below are accredited by the National Association for the Advancement of Psychoanalysis, 80 8th Ave., Ste. 1501, New York, NY 10011, (212)741-0515, http://www.naap.org.*

### Colorado

**★ 12302 ★ Colorado Center for Modern
Psychoanalytic Studies**
2240 Linden Ave.
Boulder, CO 80304-1617
**Phone:** (303)447-1159      **Fax:** (303)473-1963
**Email:** lbloom2240@aol.com
Miriam K. Bloom, PhD, Director

### New Jersey

**★ 12303 ★ New Jersey Center for
Modern Psychoanalysis**
14-25 Plaza Rd. Ste. 215
Fair Lawn, NJ 07410
**Phone:** (201)794-1222      **Fax:** (201)796-3432
Stanley Hayden, PhD, Director

**★ 12304 ★ Psychoanalytic Center of
Northern New Jersey**
769 Northfield Ave., No LL2
West Orange, NJ 07052
**Phone:** (973)736-7600      **Fax:** (973)736-6519
**Email:** SPEUD@aol.com
Vicki Semel, PsyD, Director

**★ 12305 ★ Psychoanalytic Training
Institute of New Jersey**
800 Catalpa Ave.
Teaneck, NJ 07666
**Phone:** (201)836-1065      **Fax:** (201)836-3902
**Email:** njinstitut@aol.com
Neil Wilson, PhD, Director

## New York

### ★ 12306 ★ Blanton-Peale Graduate Institute
3 West 29 St.
New York, NY 10001
**Phone:** (212)725-7850     **Fax:** (212)689-3212
Dr. Holly Harrison Johnson, Director

### ★ 12307 ★ C.G. Jung Institute of New York
28 E 39th St.
New York, NY 10016-2587
**Phone:** (212)986-5458     **Fax:** (212)867-0920
**Email:** cgjungnyc@worldnet.att.net
**Website:** http://www.cgjungpage.com
Soren Ekstrom, PhD, President

### ★ 12308 ★ Institute for Expressive Analysis
240 East 93 St., Ste. 12
New York, NY 10024
**Phone:** (212)362-2167     **Fax:** (212)595-6053
**Email:** SMRSTN@aol.com
**Website:** http://iea-ny.org/
Joel M. Gavriele-Gold, PhD, Director

### ★ 12309 ★ International University for Graduate Studies
239 Central Park West, Ste. 1AS
New York, NY 10019
**Free:** 888-660-0686     **Fax:** 888-660-0686
**Email:** CarolynWest@compuserve.com
Norma Ross, Director

### ★ 12310 ★ Mid-Manhattan Institute for Psychoanalysis
239 Central Park West, Ste. 1AS
New York, NY 10024
**Phone:** (212)799-8558     **Fax:** (212)799-8135
**Email:** mmi@mmi.edu
Deborah Bershatsky, PhD, Director

### ★ 12311 ★ National Psychological Association for Psychoanalysis Training Institute
150 W 13th St.
New York, NY 10011
**Phone:** (212)924-7440     **Fax:** (212)989-7543
**Email:** info@npap.org
**Website:** http://www.npap.org
Gary Ahlskog, PhD, President

### ★ 12312 ★ New York Center for Jungian Studies
41 Park Ave., Ste. 1D
New York, NY 10016
**Phone:** (212)689-8238     **Fax:** (212)889-7634
**Email:** aryeh@hvi.com
Aryeh Maidenbaum, PhD, Director

### ★ 12313 ★ Psychoanalytic Psychotherapy Study Center
80 Fifth Ave., Ste. 903
New York, NY 10011
**Phone:** (212)254-4422     **Fax:** (212)675-4386
**Email:** ppsc@worldnet.att.net
**Website:** http://www.nonprofitpages.com/ppsc/
Judy Levitz, PhD, Director

### ★ 12314 ★ Training and Research Institute for Self Psychology
15 W 96 St.Ste. 2
New York, NY 10025
**Phone:** (212)663-3508
**Email:** TrispNYC@msn.com
**Website:** http://www.selfpsychology.org/trisp/
R.B. Ulman, PhD, Director

### ★ 12315 ★ Washington Square Institute
41 E 11th St.
New York, NY 10003
**Phone:** (212)477-2600     **Fax:** (212)477-2600
**Email:** info@WSI.org
**Website:** http://www.wsi.org/
Gerd H. Fenchel, PhD, Director

### ★ 12316 ★ Westchester Institute for Training in Psychoanalysis and Psychotherapy
105 S Bedford Rd., Ste. 302
PO Box 89
Mount Kisco, NY 10549
**Phone:** (914)666-0163     **Fax:** (914)666-0390
Donald E. Kalsched, PhD, Director

## Pennsylvania

### ★ 12317 ★ Institute for Psychoanalytic Psychotherapies
26 Summit Grove Ave., Ste. 217
Bryn Mawr, PA 19010
**Phone:** (215)635-5368     **Fax:** (215)635-5601
**Email:** HHCOVITZ@aol.com
Howard H. Covitz, PhD, Director

### ★ 12318 ★ Philadelphia School of Psychoanalysis
313 S 16 St.
Philadelphia, PA 19102
**Phone:** (215)732-8244     **Fax:** (215)732-8454
**Email:** psp@libertynet.org
**Website:** http://www.libertynet.org/psp/
Stephen Day Ellis, PhD, Contact

---

# National & International Organizations

### ★ 12319 ★ AboutFace International (AF)
123 Edward St., Ste. 1003
Toronto, ON, Canada M5G 1E2
**Phone:** (416)597-2229     **Free:** 800-665-3223
**Fax:** (416)597-8494
**Email:** info@aboutfaceinternational.org
**Website:** http://www.aboutfaceinternational.org
**Fnded:** 1985. **Mem:** 6,000. **Lang(s):** Portuguese, Spanish. **Desc:** Individuals with facial difference resulting from birth conditions, surgery, or accidents; family members and health care providers. Serves as a network for mutual support and information exchange on coping skills and resources for recovery. Offers continuing education program to medical, nursing, and allied health professionals concerned with facial difference. Provides phone consultation services. Booklets of information/resources on specific conditions, a quarterly newsletter; hospital visits, school programs and local chapter across North America. **Pub:** *The About Face Newsletter.* Newsletter. ● *Apert, Crouzon, and Other Craniosynostosis Syndromes.* Booklet. ● *Unwrapping the Package: Dispelling Myths About Unusual Appearances.* ● *You, Your Child and the Craniofacial Team: My Newborn Has a Facial Difference,* periodic. Brochures. ● Video.

### ★ 12320 ★ Academy of Counseling Psychology (ACoP)
514 E Capitol Ave.
Jefferson City, MO 65101
**Phone:** (573)634-7157     **Fax:** (573)634-7157
**Website:** http://academyofabpps.org/
W. James Cosse, PhD, Pres.
**Fnded:** 1992. **Desc:** Counseling psychologists. Promotes standards of professional practice and conduct within the specialization of Counseling Psychology; seeks to protect the well-being of the public, the profession, and the Academy. Provides education and training. **Pub:** *ACoP.* Newsletter.

### ★ 12321 ★ Academy for Eating Disorders (AED)
6728 Old McLean Village Dr.
Mc Lean, VA 22101
**Phone:** (703)556-9222     **Fax:** (703)556-8729
**Email:** aed@degnon.org
**Website:** http://www.aedweb.org/
**Fnded:** 1993. **Desc:** Eating disorders research and treatment, particularly anorexia nervosa, bulimia nervosa, binge eating disorder, and related disorders; promotes effective treatment and care to patients; develops and advances primary and secondary preventions; disseminates information; advocates on behalf of patients, the public and eating disorder professionals; assists in developing guidelines for training, practice and professionals within the field. **Pub:** Newsletter.

### ★ 12322 ★ Academy of Organizational and Occupational Psychiatry (AOOP)
717 Princess St.
Alexandria, VA 22314
**Free:** 877-789-2667     **Fax:** 877-789-6050
**Email:** staff@aoop.com
**Website:** http://www.aoop.org
Carol Deck, Contact
**Fnded:** 1990. **Mem:** 160. **Desc:** Strives to provide a forum for exchanging ideas between psychiatry and the world of work. The association is dedicated to the advancement of psychiatric solutions to the problems of organizations, workers, and leaders. **Pub:** *The Bulletin of Organizational and Occupational Psychiatry,* biennial. Bulletin. Contains scholarly articles regarding occupational and organizational psychiatry for publication. ● Membership Directory.

### ★ 12323 ★ Academy of Psychosomatic Medicine (APM)
5824 N Magnolia
Chicago, IL 60660
**Phone:** (773)784-2025     **Fax:** (773)784-1304
**Email:** apsychmed@aol.com
**Website:** http://www.apm.org
Evelyne A. Hallberg, Exec. Dir.
**Fnded:** 1954. **Mem:** 1,000. **Desc:** Interdisciplinary organization of health care professionals dedicated to the concept of total health care of the physical and emotional needs of the patient. Objectives are: to advance scientific knowledge and the practice of medicine relating to the interaction of mind, body, and environment through study and research; to cooperate with other workers in these and related disciplines; to provide a forum for the presentation and discussion of these problems; to publish the results of research; to facilitate total and comprehensive care. **Pub:** *Academy of Psychosomatic Medicine–Directory,* annual. Directory. ● *Psychosomatics,* bimonthly. Journal. Includes book reviews and calendar of events. *Price:* Included in membership dues; $99/year for nonmembers.

### ★ 12324 ★ African Regional Council of the World Federation for Mental Health (ARCWFMH)
PO Box 50209
Lusaka, Zambia
**Phone:** 260 1 2822880     **Fax:** 260 5 224585
**Email:** arcofwfmh@zamnet.zm
**Lang(s):** English. **Desc:** Mental health professionals and organizations. Seeks to advance the diagnosis and treatment of mental illness. Facilitates exchange of information among members; provides assistance and consulting services to mental health care programs.

**★ 12325 ★ Agoraphobic Foundation of Canada (AFC)**
**(Fondation Canadienne pour les Agoraphobes — FCA)**
PO Box 132
Station Chomedey
Laval, QC, Canada H7W 4K2
**Phone:** (514)628-5215

**Lang(s):** English, French. **Desc:** People with agoraphobia (fear of leaving home or being in public places) and their families; mental health professionals with an interest in agoraphobia. Seeks to improve the quality of life of people with agoraphobia. Serves as a clearinghouse on agoraphobia and its treatment; makes available support and services to members. **Pub:** *Animal Concern News*, quarterly. Newsletter.

**★ 12326 ★ Albert Ellis Institute**
45 E 65th St.
New York, NY 10021
**Phone:** (212)535-0822          **Free:** 800-323-4738
**Fax:** (212)249-3582
**Email:** info@rebt.org
**Website:** http://www.rebt.org
Dominic J. DiMattia, Ed.D, Exec. Dir.

**Fnded:** 1968. **Desc:** Provides professional training; moderate-cost treatment services, including individual and group psychotherapy, marriage and family counseling, and crisis intervention; consultative services for mental health professionals, corporations, and community agencies; research programs in applied psychology. Operates speakers' bureau. Rational emotive behavior therapy, the institute's chief treatment approach, is a psychological theory and technique devised in 1955 based on the assumption that human beings become disturbed through acquiring irrational thoughts, beliefs, philosophies, or attitudes. REBT asserts that people can be taught to change their negative and disturbed feelings and behaviors by consciously correcting the false beliefs and inaccurate perceptions that underlie and accompany these feelings. **Frmly:** (1978) Institute for Advanced Study in Rational Psychotherapy; (1996) Institute for Rational-Emotive Therapy.

**★ 12327 ★ Alfred Adler Institute (AAI)**
24 E 21st St., Fl. 8
New York, NY 10010-7200
**Phone:** (212)254-1048          **Fax:** (212)254-8271
**Website:** http://www.alfredadler-ny.org/
Robert Ellenbogen, PhD, Exec. Dir.

**Fnded:** 1948. **Mem:** 220. **Desc:** Offers training in psychotherapy, analytic psychotherapy, and analysis to psychiatrists, psychologists, social workers, teachers, clergymen, lawyers, counselors and other related professional persons. Conducts part-time, evening three-year-plus program to provide an understanding of the dynamics of personality and interpersonal relationships and to teach therapeutic methods and techniques. Presents the theory of Individual Psychology as formulated by the Austrian psychiatrist Alfred Adler (1870-1937). Maintains the Alfred Adler Consultation Center. **Pub:** *Journal of Individual Psychology*, quarterly. Journal. • Bulletin, annual. • Newsletter, quarterly. **Frmly:** Alfred Adler Institute for Individual Psychology.

**★ 12328 ★ Alliance for the Mentally Ill**
Colonial Place Three, 2107 Wilson Blvd., Ste. 300
Arlington, VA 22201-3042
**Phone:** (703)524-7600          **Fax:** (703)524-9094
**Email:** nnv2info@nami.org
**Website:** http://www.nami.org
Rick Birkel, Exec. Dir.

**Fnded:** 1979. **Mem:** 160,000. **Nat'l Groups:** 1. **State Groups:** 50. **Local Groups:** 1300. **Desc:** Mentally ill persons and their families. Works to inform the public about mental illness and enhance the lives of people who are mentally ill. Conducts research and educational programs. **Pub:** *The Advocate*, bimonthly. Newsletter. • *Decade of the Brain Research*, quarterly.

**★ 12329 ★ Alzheimer's Association Japan**
Kyoto Social Welfare Hall
Horikawa-Marutamachi
Kamigyo
Kyoto 602-8143, Japan
**Phone:** 81 75 8118195          **Fax:** 81 75 8118188
**Email:** afcdejpn@mbox.kyoto-inet.or.jp
**Website:** http://www.alzheimer.or.jp

**Fnded:** 1980. **Mem:** 7,000. **Reg. Groups:** 39. **Lang(s):** English, Japanese. **Desc:** Family caregivers, medical professionals, and volunteers involved with and concerned for people affected with dementia, including Alzheimer's disease. Seeks to raise awareness of Alzheimer's Disease and other forms of dementia in Japan, and to help dementia patients and their families. Provides public education and professional training; appeals to the Ministry of Health and Welfare and local governments. **Pub:** *Caring for the Elderly*, monthly. Newsletter.

**★ 12330 ★ Alzheimer's Disease Foundation Malaysia (ADFM)**
14, Lorong Utara A
46200 Petaling Jaya, Malaysia
**Phone:** 60 3 79581522          **Fax:** 60 3 79581507
**Email:** alzheimers@pd.jaring.my
**Website:** http://www.adfm.org.my

**Fnded:** 1997. **Mem:** 18. **State Groups:** 3. **Lang(s):** English. **Desc:** Seeks to raise awareness of Alzheimer's Disease and other forms of dementia in Malaysia, and to help dementia patients and their families. **Pub:** *Sharing*, quarterly. Newsletter. Includes information on past and future activities, caregiver stories, and tips.

**★ 12331 ★ Alzheimer's and Related Disorders Society of India (ARDSI)**
PO Box 53
Kunnamkulam 680 503, Kerala, India
**Phone:** 91 488 522939          **Fax:** 91 488 523801
**Email:** alzheimr@md2.vsnl.net.in
**Website:** http://www.alzheimerindia.org

**Fnded:** 1984. **Lang(s):** English. **Desc:** Seeks to raise awareness of Alzheimer's Disease and other forms of dementia in India, and to help dementia patients and their families.

**American Academy of Addiction Psychiatry (AAAP)**
*See:* Entry 19248

**American Academy of Child and Adolescent Psychiatry (AACAP)**
*See:* Entry 5604

**★ 12332 ★ American Academy of Clinical Psychiatrists (AACP)**
PO Box 458
Glastonbury, CT 06033
**Phone:** (860)633-5045          **Fax:** (860)633-6023
**Email:** info@aacp.com
**Website:** http://www.aacp.com
Gregory Teas, MD, Pres.

**Fnded:** 1975. **Mem:** 600. **Desc:** Practicing board-eligible or board-certified psychiatrists. Promotes the scientific practice of psychiatric medicine. Conducts educational and teaching research. **Pub:** *Annals of Clinical Psychiatry*, quarterly. Journal. *Price:* Included in membership dues.

**★ 12333 ★ American Academy of Health Care Providers**
314 W Superior St., Ste. 702
Duluth, MN 55802
**Phone:** (218)727-3940          **Fax:** (218)722-0347
**Email:** info@americanacademy.org
**Website:** http://www.americanacademy.org
Richard E. Rogers, Exec. Dir.

**Fnded:** 1989. **Desc:** Nurses, doctors, psychologists, psychiatrists, social workers, and counselors. Establishes and maintains Certified Addiction Specialist (CAS) credentials. Strives to create a national unity of standards.

**★ 12334 ★ American Academy on Mental Retardation (AAMR)**
c/o Dr. Marsha Seltzer
Waisman Center
University of Wisconsin-Madison
1500 Highland Ave.
Madison, WI 53705
**Email:** mseltzer@waisman.wisc.edu
**Website:** http://www.academyonmr.org/
Dr. Marsha Malick Seltzer, Contact

**Fnded:** 1960. **Mem:** 250. **Desc:** Scientists actively engaged in research in any discipline relating to mental retardation; active membership is limited to scientists possessing a doctorate degree. Encourages and promotes investigative work in the clinical and experimental field of mental retardation; provides a forum for research workers in this field. Facilitates relations between various disciplines and stimulates cooperative research. Cooperates with national and international organizations and cosponsors colloquia, symposia, and other meetings. **Pub:** Newsletter, semiannual.

**★ 12335 ★ American Academy of Psychoanalysis (AAP)**
PO Box 30
1 Regency Dr.
Bloomfield, CT 06002-0030
**Phone:** (860)243-0437          **Free:** 888-691-8281
**Fax:** (860)286-0787
**Email:** aap@ssmgt.com
**Website:** http://aapsa.org
Jacquelyn Coleman, Exec. Dir.

**Fnded:** 1956. **Mem:** 750. **Desc:** Psychoanalysts are fellows of the academy; psychiatric members are psychiatrists who meet specific requirements; associates are psychiatrists, scientists, or educators; candidates. Seeks to develop communication among psychoanalysts and persons in other disciplines in science and the humanities; provides a forum for inquiry into the phenomena of individual motivation and social behavior; encourages and supports research in psychoanalysis; fosters acceptance of psychoanalysis. Sponsors seminars and symposia. **Pub:** *Academy Forum*, biennial. Magazine. Contains articles on psychoanalysis and related topics and book reviews. *Price:* $20. • *Academy News*. Newsletter. • *Journal of the American Academy of Psychoanalysis*, quarterly. Journal. *Price:* $35. **Frmly:** (1966) Academy of Psychoanalysis; (2001) American Foundation for Psychoanalysis and Psychoanalysis in Groups.

**★ 12336 ★ American Academy of Psychotherapists (AAP)**
PO Box 1611
New Bern, NC 28563
**Phone:** (252)634-3066          **Fax:** (252)634-3067
**Email:** aapoffice@coastalnet.com
**Website:** http://www.coe.iup.edu/aap/main.html
Nancy R. Hunt, Dir.

**Fnded:** 1955. **Mem:** 725. **Reg. Groups:** 4. **Desc:** Professional society of psychologists, psychiatrists, clergy, and social workers engaged in the practice of psychotherapy. Provides meeting ground for psychotherapists of differing backgrounds and orientations. Facilitates cross-discipline thinking, planning, and research in psychotherapy. Sponsors workshops. **Pub:** *AAP Newsletter*, monthly. Newsletter. • *VOICES*, quarterly. Journal. *Price:* $30/year. • Directory, biennial.

**★ 12337 ★ American Art Therapy Association (AATA)**
1202 Allanson Rd.
Mundelein, IL 60060-3808

**Phone:** (847)949-6064　　　　**Free:** 888-290-0878
**Fax:** (847)566-4580
**Email:** info@arttherapy.org
**Website:** http://www.arttherapy.org
Shaun McNiff, Pres.

**Fnded:** 1969. **Mem:** 4,300. **Local Groups:** 30. **Desc:** Art therapists, students, and individuals in related fields. Supports the progressive development of therapeutic uses of art, the advancement of research, and improvements in the standards of practice. Has established specific professional criteria for training art therapists. Facilitates the exchange of information and experience. Compiles statistics. **Pub:** *American Art Therapy Association–Newsletter*, quarterly. Newsletter. Provides information on related organizations and available resources; includes calendar of events, legislative news, and member news. *Price:* Included in membership dues; $16/year for nonmembers. • *Art Therapy*, quarterly. Journal. Includes referred articles and illustrations, news and summaries of national conferences, books reviews, media, and commentaries. *Price:* Included in membership dues; $40/year for nonmembers; $57/year for institutions; $64/year for nonmembers outside the U.S. • *Proceedings of Annual Conference*. Proceedings.

### ★ 12338 ★ American Association of Chairs of Departments of Psychiatry (AACDP)

AACDP
UCHC-Dept Psychiatry, MC 1935
263 Farmington Ave.
Farmington, CT 06030-1935
**Phone:** (860)679-8113　　　**Fax:** (860)679-1246
**Email:** info@aacdp.org
**Website:** http://www.aacdp.org
Daniel K. Winstead, MD, Pres.

**Fnded:** 1967. **Mem:** 136. **Desc:** Chairmen of departments of psychiatry in colleges of medicine. Purposes are: to promote medical education, research, and patient care, particularly as these concern psychiatry; to promote the growth and continuing development of psychiatry; to provide a forum for discussion and exchange of ideas among the chairmen of departments of psychiatry in medical schools; to provide appropriate liaison between chairmen and individuals and organizations whose activities bear on the objectives of the association. Membership list.

### ★ 12339 ★ American Association of Community Psychiatrists (AACP)

PO Box 282189
Dallas, TX 75228-0218
**Phone:** (972)686-5227　　　**Fax:** (972)613-5532
**Email:** frda1@airmail.net
**Website:** http://www.communitypsychiatry.org/
Francis M. Roton, Admin. Dir.

**Fnded:** 1984. **Mem:** 350. **Reg. Groups:** 7. **Desc:** Psychiatrists and psychiatry residents practicing in community mental health centers (CMHCs) or similar programs that provide care to populations of the mentally ill regardless of their ability to pay. Works to address issues faced by psychiatrists who practice within CMHCs, with the goal of ensuring quality patient care. Purposes are to: increase the number of psychiatrists who choose careers in community mental health; clarify and solve mutual problems regarding community mental health psychiatric practice; inform and educate the public about the community psychiatrist's role in treating the mentally ill; encourage research and training in psychiatry in the community mental health setting; establish liaison with similar professional associations and foster local and regional groups interested in public community psychiatry. Works to deal with issues such as professional burnout, the function of the psychiatrist within CMHCs, assuring relevant continuing medical education, and improving care in CMHCs. Proposes and promotes standards and guidelines of psychiatric practice and staffing in CMHCs; fosters a multidisciplinary approach to CMHC psychiatric care employing nurses, psychiatrists, psychologists, and social workers. Operates work groups in areas such as residency and fellowship training, standards of care, psychiatric

leadership in community settings, and CMHCs and the homeless. Disseminates information on legislative activities, local and regional programs, treatment methods, and other matters relating to community psychiatry. **Pub:** *AACP Membership Directory*, annual. Membership Directory. • *Community Psychiatrist*, quarterly. Newsletter.

### ★ 12340 ★ American Association of Directors of Psychiatric Residency Training (AADPRT)

Executive Office
University of Connecticut Health Center
Department of Psychiatry
263 Farmington Ave., LG066
Farmington, CT 06030-1935
**Phone:** (860)679-8112　　　**Fax:** (860)679-1246
**Email:** aadprt@psychiatry.uchc.edu
**Website:** http://www.aadprt.org
David Goldberg, MD, Exec. Dir.

**Fnded:** 1973. **Mem:** 428. **Desc:** Creates, Reviews and maintains standards for Psychiatric residency training programs **Pub:** *Academic Psychiatry*, quarterly. • Newsletter, quarterly.

### American Association for Geriatric Psychiatry (AAGP)

*See:* Entry. 2918

### ★ 12341 ★ American Association for Marriage and Family Therapy (AAMFT)

112 S Alfred St.
Alexandria, VA 22314
**Phone:** (703)838-9808　　　**Fax:** (703)838-9805
**Email:** exec@aamft.org
**Website:** http://www.aamft.org
James Morris, Pres.

**Fnded:** 1942. **Mem:** 23,000. **Reg. Groups:** 53. **Desc:** Professional society of marriage and family therapists. Assumes a major role in developing & maintaining the highest standards of excellence in this field. Has 76 accredited training programs throughout the U.S. Sponsors educational and research programs. **Pub:** *Family Therapy Glossary*. Includes an overview of family therapy terms aimed at new MFTs. *Price:* $8.95. • *Family Therapy News*, bimonthly. Includes research news, interviews, reports on legislative and organization acivities, and activities calendar. *Price:* Included in membership dues; $25/year for nonmembers; $40/year for institutions. • *Journal of Marital and Family Therapy*, quarterly. Journal. Also includes articles on clinical practice, research, theory, and training. Includes book reviews. *Price:* Included in membership dues; $45/year for nonmembers; $75/year for institutions. • Also publishes other brochures and books; produces series of professional training videos. **Frmly:** (1970) American Association of Marriage Counselors; (1978) American Association of Marriage and Family Counselors.

### ★ 12342 ★ American Association of Mental Health Professionals in Corrections (AAMHPC)

PO Box 160208
Sacramento, CA 95816-0208
**Email:** corrmentalhealth@aol.com
J.S. Zil, MD, JD, National Pres.

**Fnded:** 1940. **Mem:** 2,000. **Nat'l Groups:** 1. **Desc:** Psychiatrists, psychologists, social workers, nurses, and other mental health professionals; individuals working in correctional settings. Fosters the progress of behavioral sciences related to corrections. Goals are: to improve the treatment, rehabilitation, and care of the mentally ill, mentally retarded, and emotionally disturbed; to promote research and professional education in psychiatry and allied fields in corrections; to advance standards of correctional services and facilities; to foster cooperation between individuals concerned with the medical, psychological, social, and legal aspects of corrections; to share knowledge with other medical practitioners, scientists, and the public. Conducts scientific meetings to contribute to the

advancement of the therapeutic community in all its institutional settings, including correctional institutions, hospitals, churches, schools, industry, and the family. **Pub:** *Corrective and Social Psychiatry*, quarterly. Journal. Includes book reviews, calendar of events, and research reports. *Price:* Included in membership dues; $35/year for nonmembers. • Papers. **Frmly:** (1978) Medical Correctional Society of the American Correctional Association.

### American Association of Psychiatric Administrators (AAPA)

*See:* Entry 9690

### ★ 12343 ★ American Association of Psychiatric Technicians (AAPT)

2000 "O" St., Ste. 250
Sacramento, CA 95814-5286
**Phone:** (916)443-1701　　　**Free:** 800-391-7589
**Fax:** (916)329-9145
**Email:** appt@psych-health.com
**Website:** http://www.psychiatricadministrators.org/
Keith Hearn, Exec. Dir.

**Fnded:** 1991. **Mem:** 2,500. **Desc:** Administers the Nationally Certified Psychiatric Technician examination to non-licensed direct-care workers in the fields of mental illness, developmental disabilities and substance abuse. September as "Mental Health Workers Week." Conducts educational programs; offers placement information; compiles statistics.

### ★ 12344 ★ American Association of Spinal Cord Injury Psychologists and Social Workers (AASCIPSW)

75-20 Astoria Blvd.
Jackson Heights, NY 11372
**Phone:** (718)803-3782　　　**Fax:** (718)803-0414
**Email:** aascipsw@epva.org
**Website:** http://www.aascipsw.org
Vivian Beyda, PhD, Assoc. Exec. Dir.

**Fnded:** 1986. **Mem:** 430. **Desc:** Psychologists and social workers who treat patients with spinal cord impairment; others interested in the spinal injury field. Promotes improved psychsocial care of spinal cord injury patients; develops and enhances related education and research programs. Focuses on topics such as sexuality and spinal cord injury, alcohol and drug dependent spinal cord injury patients, adjusting to spinal cord injuries, and planning for care in the community. Sponsors research grant program. **Pub:** *SCI Psychosocial Process*, quarterly. Journal. *Price:* Included in membership dues. • Also publishes suggested reading list and practice guidelines.

### ★ 12345 ★ American Association of Suicidology (AAS)

4201 Connecticut Ave. NW, Ste. 408
Washington, DC 20008
**Phone:** (202)237-2280　　　**Fax:** (202)237-2282
**Email:** info@suicidology.org
**Website:** http://www.suicidology.org
Dr. Alan Berman, Exec. Dir.

**Fnded:** 1968. **Mem:** 1,100. **Reg. Groups:** 5. **Desc:** Psychologists, psychiatrists, social workers, nurses, health educators, physicians, directors of suicide prevention centers, clergy, and others from various disciplines and fields of experience who share a common interest in the advancement of studies of suicide prevention and life-threatening behavior. Seeks to recognize and encourage suicidology (the study of suicide, suicide prevention, and related phenomena of self-destruction). Advances education, disseminates information through programs and publications, and cooperates with other organizations in suicidology. **Pub:** *AAS Membership Roster*, periodic. Arranged by state and region. *Price:* $10/copy. • *American Association of Suicidology–Newslink*, quarterly. Newsletter. Includes association news and calendar of events. *Price:* Included in membership dues. • *Crisis Center Directory*, periodic. Directory. Lists approximately 600 suicide prevention and crisis intervention agencies in the United States. *Price:* $20/

copy. • *Directory of Survivors of Suicide Support Groups*, periodic. Directory. *Price:* $10. • *Proceedings of Annual Meeting. Price:* $30. • *Suicide and Life-Threatening Behavior*, quarterly. Journal. *Price:* available to members only. • *Surviving Suicide*, quarterly. Newsletter. *Price:* $20/year.

**★ 12346 ★ American Board of Examiners of Psychodrama, Sociometry, and Group Psychotherapy (ABEPSGP)**
PO Box 15572
Washington, DC 20003
**Phone:** (202)483-0514
Dale Richard Buchanan, Exec. Dir.
**Fnded:** 1975. **Mem:** 389. **Desc:** Certifying body for professionals in the fields of group psychotherapy, psychodrama, and sociometry. (Psychodrama was developed by Dr. Jacob L. Moreno, 1889-1974, and is used to afford catharsis and social relearning. Sociometry studies interpersonal relationships in groups of people.) Works to establish and maintain national professional standards. Administers annual exam which includes on-site observation. Compiles statistics. **Pub:** *Board News*, semiannual. *Price:* available to members only. • Directory, annual. *Price:* Free. • Also publishes standards for psychodramatists.

**American Board of Professional Neuropsychology**
*See:* Entry 13906

**★ 12347 ★ American Board of Professional Psychology (ABPP)**
514 E Capitol Ave.
Jefferson City, MO 65101-3008
**Phone:** (573)634-5607          **Free:** 800-255-7792
**Fax:** (573)634-7157
**Email:** office@abpp.org
**Website:** http://www.abpp.org
Ted Packard, PhD, Pres.
**Fnded:** 1947. **Mem:** 3,950. **Nat'l Groups:** 11. **Desc:** Certification board which conducts oral examinations and awards diplomas to advanced specialists in 11 professional specialties: psychoamalysis, rehabilitation psychology, behavioral psychology, clinical psychology, industrial and organizational psychology, forensic psychology, counseling psychology, clinical neuropsychology, family psychology, health psychology, and school psychology. Candidates must have three years of qualifying experience in psychological practice. **Pub:** *American Board of Professional Psychology–Diplomat*, semiannual. Newsletter. *Price:* Included in membership dues. • *Directory of Diplomats*, biennial. Directory. • *Manual for Oral Examinations*, annual. • *Policies and Procedures*, annual. **Frmly:** (1968) American Board of Examiners in Professional Psychology.

**★ 12348 ★ American Board of Psychiatry and Neurology (ABPN)**
500 Lake Cook Rd., Ste. 335
Deerfield, IL 60015-5249
**Phone:** (847)945-7900          **Fax:** (847)945-1146
**Email:** webmaster@abpn.com
**Website:** http://www.abpn.com
Pedro Ruiz, MD, Pres.
**Fnded:** 1934. **Desc:** Physicians with specialized training in psychiatry, neurology, child neurology, child adolescent psychiatry, clinical neurophysiology, and geriatric psychiatry. Determines eligibility requirements, administers examinations, and certifies physicians.

**American College of Mental Health Administration (ACMHA)**
*See:* Entry 9699

**American College of Neuropsychiatrists (ACN)**
*See:* Entry 16988

**American College of Neuropsychopharmacology (ACNP)**
*See:* Entry 17324

**★ 12349 ★ American College of Psychiatrists (ACP)**
732 Addison St., Ste. B
Berkeley, CA 94710
**Phone:** (510)704-8020          **Fax:** (510)704-0113
**Email:** aliceacp@aol.com
**Website:** http://www.acpsych.org
Jack W. Bonne, III, Pres.
**Fnded:** 1963. **Mem:** 1,000. **Desc:** Established to honor men and women who have made a significant contribution to psychiatry. Members, in turn, invite into membership younger psychiatrists whose scholarly work and demonstrated clinical excellence indicate that they show promise of becoming leaders in the field. **Pub:** *ACP News*, quarterly. Newsletter. • Handbook. • Membership Directory, annual.

**★ 12350 ★ American College of Psychoanalysts (ACPA)**
520 Breck Ct.
Benicia, CA 94510-1372
**Phone:** (707)745-2070          **Fax:** (707)746-7677
**Email:** amercolpsa@aol.com
Angela Clark, Exec. Sec.
**Fnded:** 1969. **Mem:** 240. **Desc:** Physician psychoanalysts. Honorary, scientific, and professional organization. Goal is to contribute to the development of psychoanalysis. Provides professional leadership and supports high standards in the practice of psychoanalysis. Offers a scientific forum for theoretical points of view and encourages the understanding, acceptance, and constructive utilization of sound analytic concepts by an informed public. Offers specialized education program. **Pub:** Bulletin, biennial.

**★ 12351 ★ American Dance Therapy Association (ADTA)**
2000 Century Plz., Ste. 108
Columbia, MD 21044
**Phone:** (410)997-4040          **Fax:** (410)997-4048
**Email:** info@adta.org
**Website:** http://www.adta.org
Dianne Dulicai, PhD, ADTR, Pres.
**Fnded:** 1966. **Mem:** 1,200. **Desc:** Individuals professionally practicing dance therapy, students interested in becoming dance therapists, university departments with dance therapy programs, and individuals in related therapeutic fields. Purpose is to establish and maintain high standards of professional education and competence in dance therapy. Acts as information center; develops guidelines for educational programs and for approval of programs; maintains registry of qualified dance therapists. Maintains Marian Chace Memorial Fund to be used for educational, literary, or scientific projects related to dance in the field of mental health. **Pub:** *American Journal of Dance Therapy*, semiannual. Journal. • *Conference Proceedings*. Proceedings. • *Dance Therapy Bibliography*. Bibliography. • Membership Directory, annual. • Monographs. • Newsletter, quarterly.

**★ 12352 ★ American Group Psychotherapy Association (AGPA)**
25 E 21st St., 6th Fl.
New York, NY 10010
**Phone:** (212)477-2677          **Free:** 877-668-2472
**Fax:** (212)979-6627
**Email:** info@agpa.org
**Website:** http://www.agpa.org
Marsha S. Block, CEO
**Fnded:** 1942. **Mem:** 4,500. **Reg. Groups:** 40. **Desc:** Psychiatrists, psychologists, social workers, psychiatric nurses, and other mental health professionals who meet specific educational and professional requirements. Sponsors educational and research programs. **Pub:** *The Group Circle*, bimonthly. Newsletter. • *Group Works!*, quarterly. Brochure. Information about group psychotherapy. *Price:* Included in membership dues. • *Guidelines for Training of Group Psychotherapists*, quarterly. Journal. Includes calendar of events and research updates. *Price:* Included in membership dues. • *International Journal of Group Psychotherapy*, quarterly. Journal. • Membership Directory, biennial.

**★ 12353 ★ American Institute of Stress (AIS)**
124 Park Ave.
Yonkers, NY 10703
**Phone:** (914)963-1200          **Fax:** (914)965-6267
**Email:** stress124@earthlink.net
**Website:** http://www.stress.org
Paul J. Rosch, MD, Pres. & Chm.
**Fnded:** 1979. **Mem:** 2,000. **Desc:** Physicians, health professionals, scholars, and others from varied disciplines constitute board of trustees. Explores the personal and social consequences of stress. Compiles research data on topics such as: relationships between emotional factors and cardiovascular disease; stress and the immune system with specific emphasis on cancer; stress reduction programs for industry; occupational stress (for example, that of law enforcement officers or air traffic controllers); executive stress ("burn out"); and pharmacological and holistic methods of stress reduction. Seeks a definition of health that recognizes the need for harmony between the individual and the physical and social environments as well as the effects of positive emotions such as creativity, faith, and humor on health. Evaluates ongoing research efforts and stress management programs in the U.S. and abroad. Disseminates information to individuals, institutions, and organizations. Serves as a network for rapid communication among individuals in different disciplines. Sponsors consulting services. **Pub:** *Health and Stress: The Newsletter of the American Institute of Stress*, monthly. Newsletter. *Price:* $35 in U.S.; $45 outside U.S. • *Readings in Oncology*. Book. • Also publishes papers and speeches and issues reprints on stress.

**★ 12354 ★ American Managed Behavioral Healthcare Association (AMBHA)**
c/o Pamela Greenberg, Director
1101 PA Ave., NW, 6th Fl.
Washington, DC 20004
**Phone:** (202)756-7308          **Fax:** (202)434-4564
**Website:** http://www.ambha.org
Pamela Greenberg, MPP, Exec. Dir.
**Fnded:** 1994. **Mem:** 10. **Desc:** Managed behavioral healthcare organizations. Works to advance the value of managed behavioral healthcare and promotes the inclusion of mental illnesses and addiction disorders in benefit coverage. **Pub:** *Catalog of Special Reports*. Catalog.

**★ 12355 ★ American Mental Health Counselors Association (AMHCA)**
801 N Fairfax, Ste. 304
Alexandria, VA 22314
**Phone:** (703)548-6002          **Free:** 800-326-2642
**Fax:** (703)548-5233
**Email:** vmoore@amhca.org
**Website:** http://www.amhca.org
W. Mark Hamilton, Ph.d.D., Exec. Dir.
**Fnded:** 1976. **Mem:** 7,000. **State Groups:** 50. **Desc:** Professional counselors employed in mental health services; students. Aims to: deliver quality mental health services to children, youth, adults, families, and organizations; improve the availability and quality of counseling services through licensure and certification, training standards, and consumer advocacy. Supports specialty and special interest networks. Fosters communication among members. A division of the American Counseling Association. **Pub:** *Advocate*, 6/year. Newsletter. Contains current information on the mental health profession. *Price:* Included in membership dues; $25 nonmembers. • *Journal of Mental Health Counseling*, quarterly. Journal. • *Mental Health Brights*. Brochures. Contains information on divorce, eating disorders, child abuse, parenting young children, handling conflict, caring for aging parents.

### ★ 12356 ★ American Music Therapy Association (AMTA)

8455 Colesville Rd., Ste. 1000
Silver Spring, MD 20910
**Phone:** (301)589-3300          **Fax:** (301)589-5175
**Email:** info@musictherapy.org
**Website:** http://www.musictherapy.org
Dr. Andrea Farbman, Exec. Dir.

**Fnded:** 1950. **Mem:** 4,000. **Reg. Groups:** 8. **Desc:** Supports the therapeutic use of music in hospital, rehabilitation, educational and community settings. Monitors the clinical practice of music therapy to insure the services provided to persons with disabilities are the highest quality possible. Serves as the national voice advocating for the development and expansion of music therapy services and programs. **Pub:** *AMTA Membership Sourcebook*, annual. Membership Directory. Contains statistical information and association documents. *Price:* Included in membership dues; $30/year for nonmembers. • *Journal of Music Therapy*, quarterly. Journal. *Price:* Included in membership dues. • *Music Therapy Clinical Training Facilities Handbook*. Handbook. Lists approved facilities and programs offering music therapy internships, available on Website. • *Music Therapy Matters*, quarterly. Newsletter. *Price:* Included in membership dues. • *Music Therapy Perspectives*, semiannual. *Price:* Included in membership dues. **Frmly:** (1998) National Association for Music Therapy; (2001) American Association for Music Therapy.

### ★ 12357 ★ American Neuropsychiatric Association (ANPA)

c/o Thomas McAllister, M.D.
Department of Psychiatry
Dartmonth-Hitchcock, Med. Ctr.
One Memorial Center Dr.
Lebanon, NH 03756
**Email:** anpa@osu.edu
**Website:** http://www.neuropsychiatry.com/ANPA
Pat Arnold, Account Exec.

**Fnded:** 1987. **Mem:** 425. **Desc:** Conducts educational and research programs. **Pub:** *Journal of Neuropsychiatry and Clinical Neurosciences*. Journal.

### ★ 12358 ★ American Nouthetic Psychology Association (ANPA)

c/o Dr. David M. Carnrike
PO Box 801
Hardwick, GA 31034
**Phone:** (334)660-7675          **Fax:** (334)666-8003
**Website:** http://www.alltel.net/~biblepsy
Dr. David M. Carnrike, Pres.

**Fnded:** 1986. **Mem:** 800. **Reg. Groups:** 7. **State Groups:** 50. **Desc:** Psychologists and other individuals with an interest in nouthetic psychology. Promotes high standards of training, ethics, and practice in the field. Conducts research and educational programs.

### ★ 12359 ★ American Orthopsychiatric Association (ORTHO)

330 7th Ave., 18th Fl.
New York, NY 10001-3010
**Phone:** (212)564-5930          **Fax:** (212)564-6180
**Email:** amerortho@aol.com
**Website:** http://www.amerortho.org
Kathy Purtill, Admin.

**Fnded:** 1924. **Mem:** 4,500. **Desc:** Psychiatrists, psychologists, social workers, and educators; psychiatric nurses and lawyers; others in related fields, including anthropology, sociology, and economics. Seeks to unite and provide a common meeting ground for those engaged in the study and treatment of problems of human behavior. Fosters research and disseminates information concerning scientific work in the field of mental health. **Pub:** *American Journal of Orthopsychiatry*, quarterly. Journal. Covers therapeutic work with children and adults, community mental health, studies in interpersonal relations, and other related topics. *Price:* Included in membership dues; $60/year for nonmember individuals; $85/year for institutions. • *Readings: A Journal of Reviews and Commentary in Mental Health*, quarterly. Journal. *Price:* Included in

membership dues; $25/year for nonmember individuals; $35/year for institutions. • Books. • Catalog. • Monographs.

### ★ 12360 ★ American Psychiatric Association (APA)

1400 K St. NW
Washington, DC 20005
**Phone:** (202)682-6000          **Free:** 888-357-7924
**Fax:** (202)682-6850
**Email:** apa@psych.org
**Website:** http://www.psych.org
Richard K. Harding, Pres.

**Fnded:** 1844. **Mem:** 40,000. **Reg. Groups:** 77. **Desc:** Psychiatrists. Seeks to further the study of the nature, treatment, and prevention of mental disorders. Assists in formulating programs to meet mental health needs; compiles and disseminates facts and figures about psychiatry; furthers psychiatric education and research. **Pub:** *American Journal of Psychiatry*, monthly. Journal. Includes book reviews. *Price:* Included in membership dues; $60/year for nonmembers; $30/year for students; $90/year for institutions. • *Psychiatric News*, semimonthly. • *Psychiatric Services*, monthly. Journal. Covers the delivery of mental health services in organized settings. Includes book reviews and research reports. *Price:* $40/year for members; $20/year for students; $60/year for institutions. • Books. • Membership Directory, biennial. • Pamphlets. **Frmly:** (1892) Association of Medical Superintendents of American Institutions for Insane; (1921) American Medico Psychological Association.

**American Psychiatric Nurses Association (APNA)**
*See:* Entry 15654

### ★ 12361 ★ American Psychoanalytic Association (APsaA)

309 E 49th St.
New York, NY 10017
**Phone:** (212)752-0450          **Fax:** (212)593-0571
**Email:** central.office@apsa.org
**Website:** http://www.apsa.org/
Ellen B. Fertig, Admin. Dir.

**Fnded:** 1911. **Mem:** 3,500. **Local Groups:** 43. **Desc:** Psychoanalysts who have graduated from or are currently attending an accredited institute. Seeks to establish and maintain standards for the training of psychoanalysts and for the practice of psychoanalysis; fosters the integration of psychoanalysis with other branches of medicine; encourages research. Conducts educational programs. **Pub:** *The American Psychoanalyst*, quarterly. Newsletter. • *Journal of the American Psychoanalytic Association*, quarterly. Journal. • *Roster*, biennial. • *Title Key Word and Author Index to Psychoanalytic Journals*. • Also publishes material on psychoanalytic education and research.

### ★ 12362 ★ American Psychological Association (APA)

750 First St. NE
Washington, DC 20002-4242
**Phone:** (202)336-5500          **Free:** 800-374-2721
**Fax:** (202)336-6069
**Email:** mhonaker@apa.org
**Website:** http://www.apa.org/
L. Michael Honaker, PhD, CEO

**Fnded:** 1892. **Mem:** 154,000. **Reg. Groups:** 7. **State Groups:** 58. **Desc:** Scientific and professional society of psychologists. Students participate as affiliates. Works to advance psychology as a science, a profession, and as a means of promoting human welfare. **Pub:** *American Psychologist*, monthly. Journal. Publishes articles on current issues in psychology as well as empirical, theoretical, and practical articles on broad aspects of psychology. *Price:* Included in membership dues; $180/year for nonmembers in the U.S.; $220/year for nonmembers outside the U.S.; $332/year for institutions in the U.S. • *APA Monitor*, monthly. Newspaper. Reports on the science, profession, and social responsibility of psychology, plus legislative

developments affecting mental health and education. *Price:* Included in membership dues; $30/year for nonmembers in the U.S.; $48/year for institutions in the U.S.; $35/year for nonmembers outside the U.S. • *Behavioral Neuroscience*, bimonthly. Journal. Publishes original research papers in the broad field of the biological bases of behavior. Includes reviews and theoretical articles. *Price:* $83/year for members; $166/year for nonmembers in the U.S.; $186/year for nonmembers outside the U.S.; $332/year for institutions in the U.S. • *Clinician's Research Digest*, monthly. Newsletter. Contains selections and summaries of articles from clinical research journals. *Price:* $46/year for U.S. members; $83/year for U.S. nonmembers; $123/year for nonmembers outside of the U.S.; $110/year for U.S. institutions. • *Contemporary Psychology*, monthly. Journal. Contains critical reviews of books, films, tapes, and other media relevant to psychology. *Price:* $73/year for members; $145/year for nonmembers in the U.S.; $185/year for nonmembers outside the U.S.; $291/year for institutions in the U.S. • *Developmental Psychology*, bimonthly. Journal. Publishes articles that advance knowledge and theory about human development across the life span. *Price:* $72/year for members; $144/year for nonmembers in the U.S.; $164/year for nonmembers outside the U.S.; $284/year for institutions in the U.S. • *Directory of the American Psychological Association*, quinquennial. Me.

### ★ 12363 ★ American Psychological Association Division of Independent Practice (APADIP)

919 W Marshall
Phoenix, AZ 85013
**Phone:** (602)246-6768          **Fax:** (602)246-6577
**Email:** div42apa@primenet.com
**Website:** http://www.apa.org/about/division/div42.html
Jeannie Beeaff, Administrator

**Fnded:** 1982. **Mem:** 8,600. **Desc:** Members of the American Psychological Association (APA) engaged in independent practice. Works to insure that the needs and concerns of independent psychology practitioners are considered by the APA. Gathers and disseminates information on legislation affecting the practice of psychology, managed care and other developments in the health care industries, office management, malpractice risk and insurance, hospital management. Offers continuing professional education programs. **Pub:** *Independent Practitioner*, quarterly. Bulletin.

### ★ 12364 ★ American Psychological Association - Division of Psychotherapy

6557 E Riverdale St.
Mesa, AZ 85215
**Phone:** (602)363-9211          **Fax:** (480)854-8966
**Website:** http://www.apa.org/about/division/div29.html

**Fnded:** 1964. **Mem:** 6,500. **Desc:** A division of the American Psychological Association. Psychologists and psychotherapists interested in exchanging scientific and technical information about psychotherapy. Conducts continuing education workshops. **Pub:** *Psychotherapy Bulletin*, quarterly. Bulletin. • *Psychotherapy Journal*, quarterly. Journal.

### ★ 12365 ★ American Psychological Society (APS)

1010 Vermont Ave. NW, Ste. 1100
Washington, DC 20005-4907
**Phone:** (202)783-2077          **Fax:** (202)783-2083
**Email:** aps@aps.washington.dc.us
**Website:** http://www.psychologicalscience.org
Alan G. Kraut, Contact

**Fnded:** 1988. **Mem:** 15,000. **Desc:** Scientists and academics. Works for the advancement of the discipline of psychology and the promotion of human welfare through research and application. Conducts research programs; educates policy makers on the role human behavior plays in societal problems; offers liability insurance plans. **Pub:** *APS Observer*, monthly. Newsletter. Features current society activities and world events affecting noteworthy research. • *Current Directions in Psychological Science*, bimonthly. Journal. Provides informative reviews on important trends and controversies in psychological research. • *Psychological Science*, bimonthly. Journal. • *Psychological Science in the Public Interest*. Monographs.

**★ 12366 ★ American Psychopathological Association (APPA)**
Department of Psychiatry
Washington University School of Medicine
4940 Children's Pl.
Saint Louis, MO 63110
**Email:** zorumskc@psychiatry.wustl.edu
**Website:** http://www.appassn.org
Chuck Zorumski, MD, Pres.

**Fnded:** 1912. **Mem:** 500. **Desc:** Physicians and scientists interested in the field of psychopathology. To investigate scientific problems of abnormal psychology including: study of phenomena arising from abnormal mental processes; study of organic pathological conditions directly connected with abnormal mental processes; study of means which may remove or modify social or individual factors operating in the production of mental disease; study of relationship between psychopathological and social or cultural problems. **Pub:** *Comprehensive Psychiatry*, quarterly. Journal. General psychiatry journal. • *Proceedings of Annual Meeting*.

**★ 12367 ★ American Psychosomatic Society (APS)**
6728 Old McLean Village Dr.
Mc Lean, VA 22101
**Phone:** (703)556-9222     **Fax:** (703)556-8729
**Email:** info@psychosomatic.org
**Website:** http://www.psychosomatic.org
Laura Degnon, Assoc. Exec. Dir.

**Fnded:** 1943. **Mem:** 950. **Desc:** Promotes scientific understanding of interrelationships among biological, psychological, social and behavioral factors in human health and disease, and the integration of the fields of science that separately examine them, fosters this understanding in education and improved health care. **Pub:** *APS Newsletter*, semiannual. Newsletter. • *Psychosomatic Medicine*, 6/year. Journal. **Frmly:** (1948) American Society for Research in Psychosomatic Problems.

**★ 12368 ★ American Psychotherapy Association (APA)**
2750 E Sunshine
Springfield, MO 65804
**Phone:** (417)823-0173     **Free:** 800-205-9165
**Fax:** (417)823-9959
**Email:** member@americanpsychotherapy.com
**Website:** http://www.americanpsychotherapy.com
Daphne Greenlee, Chief Association Officer

**Fnded:** 1997. **Mem:** 5,000. **Desc:** Counselors, social workers, psychologists, psychiatrists, marriage and family therapists, nurse psychotherapists, and pastoral counselors. Seeks to enhance public perception of psychotherapy. Serves as a forum for the discussion, development, and dissemination of ethical and professional standards for psychotherapists. but rather function as a completely separate and distinct discipline exte nd cooperation to associations with similar goals and objectives. Recent activities include: challenging the misuse of psychotherapy in institutional settings; organizing therapists under nondiscipline lines; combatting economic, sexual, class, and racial exploitation. Operates library and biographical archives. Compiles statistics; sponsors competitions. Maintains Board of Examiners in Psychotherapy to evaluate training, experience, and professional excellence of individuals. **Pub:** *Annals of American Psychotherapy Association*, bimonthly. Newsletter. Covers developments in psychotherapeutic practice; includes book reviews and calendar of events. *Price:* $125.

**American Society for Adolescent Psychiatry (ASAP)**
*See:* Entry 5613

**★ 12369 ★ American Society of Group Psychotherapy and Psychodrama (ASGPP)**
301 N Harrison St., Ste. 508
Princeton, NJ 08540
**Phone:** (609)452-1339     **Fax:** (609)936-1659
**Email:** asgpp@asgpp.org
**Website:** http://www.asgpp.org
Eduardo Garcia, Exec. Dir.

**Fnded:** 1942. **Mem:** 650. **Nat'l Groups:** 4. **State Groups:** 8. **Local Groups:** 6. **Desc:** Social workers, psychologists, psychiatrists, clergy members, nurses, and others interested in group psychotherapy, psychodrama, and sociometry. Conducts educational programs; compiles statistics. **Pub:** *The International Journal of Action Methods, Psychodrama Skill Training and Role Playing*, quarterly. Journal. Application of Action methods to the fields of psycotherapy, counseling, education & organizational development. • *Psychodrama Network News*, quarterly. Newsletter.

**★ 12370 ★ American Society for Philosophy Counseling and Psychotherapy (ASPCP)**
c/o Dr. Kenneth F.T. Cust
Central Missouri State University
Center for Applied & Professional Ethics
Warrensburg, MO 64093
**Phone:** (660)543-4268     **Fax:** (660)543-8544
**Email:** kencust@philosophical-services.com
**Website:** http://www.aspcp.org/Documents/documents.html
Dr. Kenneth F.T. Cust, Interim Exec. Dir.

**Desc:** Promotes both the professional and academic sides of philosophical counseling and philosophy as a private practice profession. **Pub:** Newsletter.

**★ 12371 ★ American Society of Psychoanalytic Physicians (ASPP)**
4804 Jasmine Dr.
Rockville, MD 20853
**Phone:** (301)929-1470     **Fax:** (301)929-1491
**Email:** cheesick@casbah.acns.nwu.edu
**Website:** http://pubweb.northwestern.edu/~chessick/aspp.htm
Janice S. Wright, Exec. Dir.

**Fnded:** 1985. **Mem:** 275. **Desc:** Physicians, psychiatrists, and psychoanalysts united to: foster a wider understanding and utilization of psychoanalytic concepts; provide an opportunity to study psychoanalytic theory from all schools of thought; encourage clinical and didactic research; promote social and professional fraternalism among members in the field and maintain good relationships with other professional groups. Offers lectures on therapy that combines psychoanalytic orientation with other disciplines. **Pub:** *The Bulletin*, semiannual. Bulletin. *Price:* Included in membership dues.

**★ 12372 ★ American Society of Psychopathology of Expression (ASPE)**
c/o Dr. Irene Jakab
74 Lawton St.
Brookline, MA 02446
**Phone:** (617)738-9821     **Fax:** (617)975-0411
Dr. Irene Jakab, Pres.

**Fnded:** 1964. **Mem:** 137. **Desc:** Psychiatrists, psychologists, art therapists, sociologists, art critics, artists, social workers, linguists, educators, criminologists, writers, and historians. At least two-thirds of the members are physicians. Fosters collaboration among specialists in the United States who are interested in the problems of expression and in the artistic activities connected with psychiatric, sociological, and psychological research. Disseminates information about research and clinical applications in the field of psychopathology of expression. Sponsors

consultations, seminars, and lectures on art therapy. **Pub:** *American Society of Psychopathology of Expression–Newsletter*, semiannual. Newsletter. Includes obituaries and book reviews. *Price:* Included in membership dues. • *Art Media as a Vehicle of Communication*. *Price:* $33. • *The Personality of the Therapist*. • *The Role of the Imagination in the Healing Process*. • *Stress Management Through Art*. *Price:* $18. • Proceedings, annual.

**★ 12373 ★ Anorexia Bulimia Nervosa Association (ABNA)**
Woodwards House, 1st Fl.
47-49 Waymouth St.
Adelaide, SA 5000, Australia
**Phone:** 61 8 82121644     **Fax:** 61 8 82127991
**Email:** mail@abnasa.asn.au

**Fnded:** 1983. **Desc:** Individuals with eating disorders, their families, and friends. Promotes prevention and effective treatment of eating disorders

**★ 12374 ★ Anorexia Nervosa and Related Eating Disorders (ANRED)**
PO Box 5102
Eugene, OR 97405
**Phone:** (541)344-1144
**Email:** jarinor@rio.com
**Website:** http://www.anred.com
Dr. J. Bradley Rubel, Pres.

**Fnded:** 1979. **Mem:** 20,000. **Desc:** Provides comprehensive information about anorexia nervosa, bulimia, binge eating disorder, and other lesser known eating disorders. eating, and compulsive exercising. eating, and compulsive exercising. **Pub:** Pamphlets. • Also publishes resource material and fact sheets.

**★ 12375 ★ Argentine Society of Psychology (Sociedad Argentina de Psicologia)**
Callao 435
1022 Buenos Aires, Argentina
**Phone:** 54 1 4323760
**Fnded:** 1930.

**★ 12376 ★ ASEAN Federation for Psychiatric and Mental Health**
Panpreecha AFPMH
Somdet Chaopraya Hospital
Klongsan
Bangkok 10600, Thailand
**Phone:** 66 2 4371298     **Fax:** 66 2 4375456
**Lang(s):** English, Thai. **Desc:** Psychiatrists and other mental health professionals; mental health care facilities. Promotes increased access to mental health care; seeks to advance the study, teaching, and practice of psychiatry. Facilitates exchange of information among members; provides support and assistance to mental health care institutions.

**★ 12377 ★ Asia-Pacific Association of Psychotherapists (APAP)**
4/4 Charles St.
Petersham 2049, Australia
**Lang(s):** English. **Desc:** Psychotherapists. Seeks to advance the study and practice of psychotherapy; promotes adherence to high standards of ethics and practice by members. Serves as a forum for the exchange of information among members; sponsors research and educational programs.

**★ 12378 ★ Asian Association of Social Psychology (AASP)**
Department of Psychology
The University of Melbourne
Melbourne, VIC 3010, Australia
**Phone:** 61 3 83446312     **Fax:** 61 3 93476618
**Email:** y.kashima@psych.unimelb.edu.au
**Website:** http://www.sites.psych.unimelb.edu.au/aasp

**Lang(s):** English. **Desc:** Psychologists and other individuals with an interest in social psychology. Seeks to advance the study, teaching, and practice of social psychology. Serves as a forum for the exchange of information among members; sponsors research and educational programs. **Pub:** *Asian Journal of Social Psychology*, 3/year.


**Asian-South Pacific Association for Sport Psychology (ASPASP)**
*See:* Entry 19144


★ **12379** ★ **Asperger Syndrome Coalition of the United States (ASC-US)**
PO Box 49267
Jacksonville, FL 32240-9267
**Free:** (866)4AS-PRGR
**Email:** info@asc-us.org
**Website:** http://www.asperger.org/

**Desc:** Individuals, families, professionals such as doctors, psychologists, educators, therapists. Promotes understanding of Asperger Syndrome and related conditions, including pervasive developmental disorder, not otherwise specified; high functioning autism; nonverbal learning disability; semantic-pragmatic disorder, hyperlexia. Seeks to develop a nationwide support group assistance program, provide leadership training, and produce products, services and educational materials.


★ **12380** ★ **Association for Advanced Training in the Behavioral Sciences (AATBS)**
5126 Ralston St.
Ventura, CA 93003
**Free:** 800-472-1931          **Fax:** (805)676-3033
**Website:** http://www.aatbs.com/

**Desc:** Aims to produce study materials in order to provide education and training for psychologists, marriage and family therapists, social workers, mental health counselors and alcohol/drug counselors to pass professional exams.


★ **12381** ★ **Association for Advancement of Behavior Therapy (AABT)**
305 7th Ave., Ste. 16A
New York, NY 10001-6008
**Phone:** (212)647-1890        **Free:** 800-685-AABT
**Fax:** (212)647-1865
**Email:** mjeimer@aabt.org
**Website:** http://www.aabt.org/
Mary Jane Eimer, CAE, Exec. Dir.

**Fnded:** 1966. **Mem:** 4,500. **Desc:** Psychologists primarily, but also psychiatrists, social workers, counselors, physicians, dentists, nurses, students, and other professionals interested in the issues, problems, and development of the field of behavior therapy and cognitive behavior therapy, with specific emphasis on research and clinical applications. Sponsors training programs and lectures for professionals; maintains speakers' bureau; handles referrals for the public to locate behavior therapists in their area; facilitates communication between behavior therapists interested in specific problems or information. AABT local affiliates hold training meetings, workshops, seminars, case demonstrations, and discussion groups. **Pub:** *Association for Advancement of Behavior Therapy–Membership Directory*, semiannual. Membership Directory. Contains alphabetical, and geographic listings; includes degree, license, specialties, diplomates, and boards. *Price:* Included in membership dues; $50 for nonmembers. ● *The Behavior Therapist*, 10/year. Newsletter. Reports the latest research and includes book reviews, association news, professionals and legislative issues reports, training updates, job listings. *Price:* Included in membership dues; $60/year for nonmembers. ● *Behavior Therapy*, quarterly. Journal. An international journal devoted to the application of behavioral and cognitive sciences to clinical problems. *Price:* $75/year for nonmembers; $145/year for institutions. ● *Cognitive and Behavioral Practice*, quarterly. Journal. Integrates

behavior therapy principles and research with clinical practice techniques. *Price:* $75/for nonmembers; $145/for institutions. ● *Directory of Graduate Training in Behavior Therapy and Experimental-Clinical Psychology*, biennial. Lists over 300 psychology, special education, and counseling programs that offer training in behavior therapy. *Price:* $20 for members; $25 for non-members. ● *Directory of Psychology Internships: Programs Offering Behavioral Training*, periodic. Contains information on admission requirements, application deadlines, and program structure; statistics. *Price:* $20 for members; $25 for nonmembers. ● Also publishes a series of Fact Sheets to educate lay audiences about a variety of psychological disorders, including panic attacks, obsessive-compulsive disorder, post-traumatic stress syndrome, depression, eating disorders, and more. Call for a complete list of available titles. **Frmly:** (1968) Association for Advancement of the Behavioral Therapies.


★ **12382** ★ **Association for the Advancement of Gestalt Therapy (AAGT)**
c/o Carol Brockman
7861 Spring Ave.
Elkins Park, PA 19027
**Phone:** (215)782-1484        **Fax:** (215)635-2391
**Email:** info@aagt.org
**Website:** http://www.azagt.org
Carol Brockmon, Pres.

**Desc:** Psychiatrists, psychologists, social workers, teachers, academics, writers, artists, performers, organizational consultants and political and social analysts, activists, and students. Seeks to advance theory, philosophy, practice and research in Gestalt Therapy and its various applications, including but not limited to, personal growth, mental health, education, organization and systems development, political and social development and change, and the fine and performing arts.


★ **12383** ★ **Association for Advancement of Psychoanalysis (of the Karen Horney Psychoanalytic Institute and Center) (AAP)**
329 E 62nd St.
New York, NY 10021
**Phone:** (212)838-4333        **Fax:** (212)838-7158
**Email:** karenhorneyclnic@aol.com
**Website:** http://www.karenhorneycenter.org
Judith Fox-Fliesser, MD, Contact

**Fnded:** 1941. **Mem:** 80. **Desc:** Certified psychoanalysts interested in encouraging training in psychoanalysis and disseminating psychoanalytic principles to the medical-psychiatric profession and the general community. Conducts scientific meetings. Maintains a consultation and referral service, placement service, and speakers' bureau. Supports research programs; sponsors public educational lectures; maintains library of 4000 volumes. **Pub:** *The American Journal of Psychoanalysis*, quarterly. Journal. Includes book reviews. *Price:* $24 for individuals; $50 for libraries and institutions. ● Newsletter, semiannual.


★ **12384** ★ **Association for the Advancement of Psychological Understanding of Human Nature (VPM)**
Postfach 2161
CH-8033 Zurich, Switzerland
**Phone:** 41 1 2610031        **Fax:** 41 1 2610561
**Email:** vpm@compuserve.com
**Website:** http://www.vpm.ch

**Fnded:** 1986. **Mem:** 700. **Lang(s):** English, French, German, Italian. **Desc:** Psychologists and other scientists with an interest in human behavior. Seeks to advance scholarship on the psychological components of human behavior. Facilitates exchange of information among members; sponsors research and educational programs.

★ **12385** ★ **Association for Advancement of Psychology (AAP)**
PO Box 38129
Colorado Springs, CO 80937
**Phone:** (719)520-0688        **Free:** 800-869-6595
**Fax:** (719)520-0375
**Email:** smpfeiffer@aapnet.org
**Website:** http://www.aapnet.org/
Stephen M. Pfeiffer, PhD, Exec. Dir.

**Fnded:** 1974. **Mem:** 6,000. **Desc:** Members of the American Psychological Association or other national psychological associations, students of psychology, and organizations with a primarily psychological focus. Purposes are to advance psychology and represent the interests of all psychologists (professional, social, and scientific) in the public policy arena. Maintains Psychologists For Legislative Action Now, a political action and education committee. **Pub:** *Association for Advancement of Psychology–Advance*, quarterly. Newsletter. Includes calendar of events and research updates. *Price:* Included in membership dues.


★ **12386** ★ **Association for the Advancement of Psychotherapy (AAP)**
c/o T. Byram Karasu, M.D.
Albert Einstein College of Medicine
Belfer Education Center, Rm. 405
1300 Morris Park Ave.
Bronx, NY 10461-1602
**Phone:** (718)430-3503        **Fax:** (718)430-8907
**Email:** info@ajp.org
**Website:** http://www.ajp.org
T. Byram Karasu, MD, Editor-in-Chief

**Fnded:** 1939. **Mem:** 400. **Desc:** Works to create a forum where all concepts of psychotherapeutic thought can be aired for the advancement of psychotherapy in practice, research, and training. **Pub:** *American Journal of Psychotherapy*, quarterly. Journal. Includes book reviews and software reviews. *Price:* $64 for individuals; $91 for institutions; $70 for individuals in Canada; $98 for institutions in Canada.


★ **12387** ★ **Association for Ambulatory Behavioral Healthcare**
2301 Mount Vernon Ave., Ste. 100
Alexandria, VA 22301
**Phone:** (703)836-2274        **Fax:** (703)836-0083
**Email:** aabh@aabh.org
**Website:** http://www.aabh.org
James K. Finley, Exec. Off.

**Fnded:** 1965. **Mem:** 1,100. **Reg. Groups:** 26. **Desc:** Individuals interested in the development and improvement of the continuum of psychiatric treatment. To support, encourage, and stimulate the expansion of ambulatory behavioral health services. Sponsors educational discussions on partial hospitalization, intensive outpatient and rehabilitative services including clinical research and administrative issues. Provides consultation services to stimulate and support the study, evaluation, and implementation of ambulatory behavioral health services. Collaborates with other groups in establishing standards of operation and performance in the field. Monitors local and national legislative activity directly related to behavioral healthcare. **Pub:** *AAPH Membership Directory*, annual. Membership Directory. ● *Bibliography*, triennial. ● *Bibliography of Child and Adolescent Partial Hospitalization*. ● *Continuum: Developments in Ambulatory Mental Health Care*, quarterly. Journal. ● *Inside AAPH*, bimonthly. Newsletter. ● *Insurance and Partial Hospitalization*. ● *Standards and Guidelines for Child and Adolescent Partial Hospitalization*. ● *Standards and Guidelines for Partial Hospitalization*. **Frmly:** (1975) Partial Hospitalization Study Group; (1979) Federation of Partial Hospitalization Study Groups; (1996) American Association for Partial Hospitalization.


★ **12388** ★ **Association for Analytic and Bodymind Therapy and Training**
Princes House
8 Princes Ave.
Muswell Hill
London N10 3LR, United Kingdom

**Phone:** 44 181 8835418

**Fnded:** 1974. **Mem:** 4. **Desc:** Qualified and experienced psychotherapists. To extend psychotherapy from quiet, controlled talking therapy to vocal and bodily awareness and participation. To promote experiential therapy.

**★ 12389 ★ Association for Applied Poetry (AAP)**
60 N Main St.
Johnstown, OH 43031-1015
**Phone:** (740)967-6060
**Email:** pudding@johnstown.net
**Website:** http://www.puddinghouse.com
Jennifer Bosveld, pres.

**Fnded:** 1984. **Desc:** Poets, teachers, therapists, social workers, creative artists, librarians, and interested individuals. Promotes the application of poetry and creative writing to human services, healing, and self-awareness and self-actualization. Conducts support groups and tutorials. Operates Pudding House Bed and Breakfast retreat at Puddings House Writiers Resource Center. Maintains speakers'bureau. Conducts educational programs. **Pub:** *Pudding Magazine: The International Journal of Applied Poetry*, periodic. Journal. Contains poetry essays and reviews applicable to education and human services and art. *Price:* Included with membership. • *Topics for Getting in Touch: A Poetry Therapy Sourcebook.* • Also publishes articles, chapbooks, and educational materials.

**Association of Behavioral Healthcare Management (ABHM)**
*See:* Entry 9709

**★ 12390 ★ Association for Birth Psychology (ABP)**
444 E 82nd St.
New York, NY 10028
**Phone:** (212)988-6617
**Email:** davids@nccbh.org
**Website:** http://birthpsychology.org
Leslie Feher, PhD, Exec. Dir.

**Fnded:** 1978. **Mem:** 352. **Desc:** Obstetricians, pediatricians, midwives, nurses, psychotherapists, psychologists, counselors, social workers, sociologists, and others interested in birth psychology, a developing discipline concerned with the experience of birth and the correlation between the birth process and personality development. Seeks to promote communication among professionals in the field; encourage commentary, research, and theory from different points of view; establish birth psychology as an autonomous science of human behavior; develop guidelines and give direction to the field. **Pub:** *Birth Psychology Bulletin*, semiannual. Journal. Covers conception to the first year of life. Includes book reviews, research reports, calendar of events, and case reports. *Price:* Included in membership dues; $20/year for nonmembers. • Books.

**★ 12391 ★ Association of Black Psychologists (ABPsi)**
PO Box 55999
Washington, DC 20040-5999
**Phone:** (202)722-0808          **Fax:** (202)722-5941
**Email:** admin@abpsi.org
**Website:** http://www.abpsi.org
Ann E. Pharr, PhD, Exec. Dir.

**Fnded:** 1968. **Mem:** 1,400. **Reg. Groups:** 4. **State Groups:** 29. **Local Groups:** 35. **Desc:** Professional psychologists and others in associated disciplines. Aims to: enhance the psychological well-being of black people in America; define mental health in consonance with newly established psychological concepts and standards; develop policies for local, state, and national decision-making that have impact on the mental health of the black community; support established black sister organizations and aid in the development of new, independent black institutions to enhance the psychological, educational, cultural, and economic situation. Offers training and information on

AIDS. Conducts seminars, workshops, and research. **Pub:** *Association of Black Psychologists Publications Manual.* Manual. • *Journal of Black Psychology*, quarterly. Journal. Provides research results. Includes book reviews. *Price:* $30/year for individuals; $50/year for institutions. • *Monographs From the Journal of Black Psychology*, biennial. Monographs. • *Proceedings of Annual Convention.* Proceedings. • *Psych Discourse*, monthly. Journal. Includes calendar of events and research updates. *Price:* Included in membership dues; $95/year for nonmembers. • *Resource Manual for Black Psychology Students.* Manual. • *Sourcebook on the Teaching of Black Psychology.* • Also publishes brochures, bulletins, and research projects; distributes videotapes on issues in black psychology.

**Association for Child Psychoanalysis (ACP)**
*See:* Entry 5620

**Association for Child Psychology and Psychiatry (ACPP)**
*See:* Entry 5621

**Association of Child Psychotherapists (ACP)**
*See:* Entry 5622

**★ 12392 ★ Association for Clinical Psychosocial Research (ACPR)**
685 W Baltimore St.
Baltimore, MD 21209-1549
**Phone:** (215)842-4550          **Fax:** (215)843-3441
**Email:** ldixon@umaryland.edu
**Website:** http://www.wpic.pitt.edu/acpr
Katherine Shear, MD, Pres.

**Desc:** Professionals active in psychosocial research who show promise as independent investigators. Seeks to improve research and enhance prevention, treatment and rehabilitation. Conducts annual meetings and seminars.

**★ 12393 ★ Association for Comprehensive Energy Psychology (ACEP)**
c/o Dr. Dorothea Hover-Kramer
12307 Oak Knoll Rd.
Poway, CA 92064
**Phone:** (858)748-5963          **Fax:** (858)748-3119
**Email:** acep@energypsych.org
**Website:** http://www.energypsych.org/
Dr. Dorothea Hover-Kramer, Contact

**Fnded:** 1999. **Mem:** 550. **Reg. Groups:** 11. **Desc:** Professionals in psychotherapeutic practice, allied health professionals, researchers, organizations, students, and interested laypersons. Promotes understanding of energy psychology in order to establish the field's credibility among health professionals, particularly psychotherapists; creates collegial atmosphere for collaboration in order to produce treatments for the public. **Pub:** Newsletter.

**★ 12394 ★ Association of European Psychiatrists (AEP)**
Clinique Psychiatrique
CHU
Place de l'Hopital
F-67091 Strasbourg, France
**Phone:** 33 3 88115406          **Fax:** 33 3 88116189
**Email:** aep.strasbourg@wanadoo.fr
**Website:** http://www.aep.lu
**Fnded:** 1983. **Mem:** 1,200. **Lang(s):** English, French. **Desc:** Psychiatrists. Seeks to advance psychiatric scholarship and practice. Facilitates communication and cooperation among members; sponsors research and continuing professional development programs.

**★ 12395 ★ Association for Humanistic Psychology (AHP)**
1516 Oak St., No. 320A
Alameda, CA 94501-2947
**Phone:** (510)769-6495          **Fax:** (510)769-6433
**Email:** ahpoffice@aol.com
**Website:** http://www.ahpweb.org
Leland Baggett, Pres.

**Fnded:** 1962. **Mem:** 2,000. **Nat'l Groups:** 2. **State Groups:** 1. **Local Groups:** 2. **Desc:** Psychologists, social workers, clergy, educators, psychiatrists, and others engaged in humanistic practice. Functions as an international community of people who are dedicated to the exploration, healing, and expansion of the human mind, body and soul, and to building a society that advances our ability to choose, to grow, and to create. Aims to realize a vision of the possible for humanity. **Pub:** *AHP Perspective*, bimonthly. Newsletter. Covers growth therapies, holistic education, interdisciplinary humanistic practices, and social concerns. Includes calendar of events. *Price:* Included in membership dues. • *Journal of Humanistic Psychology*, quarterly. Journal. **Frmly:** American Association for Humanistic Psychology.

**★ 12396 ★ Association of Humanistic Psychology Practitioners (AHPP)**
BCM AHPP
London WC1N 3XX, United Kingdom
**Phone:** 44 8457 660326
**Fnded:** 1980. **Mem:** 250. **Lang(s):** English, French, German, Italian, Swedish. **Desc:** Provides accreditation of humanistic psychotherapists as member organization of the U.K. Council for Psychotherapy and for other therapists and counsellors; makes available referral services; conducts training and professional development programs. Disseminates information to members.

**★ 12397 ★ Association Internationale de Psychologie du Travail de Langue Francaise (AIPTLF)**
Universite Lille 3
Pr Claude Lemoine, AIPTLF
UFR Psychologie
BP 149
F-59653 Villeneuve D'Ascq cedex, France
**Phone:** 33 3 20416315          **Fax:** 33 3 20416324
**Email:** lemoine@univ-lille3.fr
**Website:** http://www.psp.ucl.ac.be/aiptlf2002
**Fnded:** 1980. **Mem:** 1,000. **Nat'l Groups:** 1. **Lang(s):** French. Does not correspond in English. **Desc:** Doctors, personnel directors, industrial psychologists, and sociologists in 30 countries. Promotes the French language within the field of industrial psychology. Seeks to keep members informed and to aid in the perfection of their work. Facilitates the exchange of current research and information among members. **Pub:** *Actes de Congres*, biennial. Journal. • *Psychologie du Travail et des Organisations*, quarterly. Journal. **Frmly:** French-Language Association of Work Psychology.

**★ 12398 ★ Association for Psychoanalytic Medicine (APM)**
4560 Delafield Ave.
Bronx, NY 10471-3905
**Phone:** (718)548-6088          **Fax:** (718)548-8302
**Email:** gsagi@aol.com
**Website:** http://theapm.org
Dr. George Sagi, Treas.

**Fnded:** 1945. **Mem:** 241. **Desc:** Organization of physicians who are psychoanalysts. Provides forum on psychoanalytic developments for membership and community. Conducts postgraduate seminars. Sponsors speakers for community or medical groups. Is conducting research on psychoanalytic involvement in social issues. **Pub:** *Between Analyst and Patient.* Book. • *The Psychology of Men.* Book. • *Roster*, biennial. • Bulletin, every 9 months. **Frmly:** (1946) Association for Psychoanalytic and Psychosomatic Medicine.

### ★ 12399 ★ Association for Psychological Type (APT)

4700 W Lake Ave.
Glenview, IL 60025
**Phone:** (847)375-4717　　　**Fax:** (847)375-4777
**Email:** staff@aptcentral.org
**Website:** http://www.aptcentral.org
Marvin Rytting, Pres.

**Fnded:** 1979. **Mem:** 5,000. **Reg. Groups:** 7. **Local Groups:** 60. **Desc:** Individuals involved in organizational development, religion, management, education, and counseling, and who are interested in psychological type, the Myers-Briggs Type Indicator, and the works of Carl G. Jung (1875-1961). Purpose is to bring together and share ideas related to the uses of MBTI and the application of psychological type theory in any area; promotes research, development, and education in the field. Sponsors seminars conferences and training sessions on the use of psychological type. **Pub:** *Association for Psychological Type–Membership Directory*, biennial. Membership Directory. Arranged by name, ZIP code, and psychological-type interest. *Price:* Included in membership dues. • *Bulletin of Psychological Type*, quarterly. Bulletin. Covers interest area issues, upcoming events, and book reviews. *Price:* Included in membership dues. • *Journal of Psychological Type*, quarterly. Journal. Discusses type theory and research. *Price:* Included in membership dues.

### ★ 12400 ★ Association of Psychology Postdoctoral and Internship Centers (APPIC)

10 G St., Ste. 750
Washington, DC 20002
**Phone:** (202)589-0600　　　**Fax:** (202)589-0603
**Email:** appic@aol.com
**Website:** http://www.appic.org
Connie Hercey, Exec. Officer

**Fnded:** 1968. **Mem:** 550. **Desc:** Veterans Administration hospitals, medical centers, state hospitals, university counseling centers, and other facilities that provide internship and postdoctoral programs in professional psychology. Promotes activities that assist in the development of professional psychology training programs. Serves as a clearinghouse to provide Ph.D. candidates with internship placement assistance at member facilities. Conducts workshops and seminars on training procedures in clinical psychology at the Ph.D. level. **Pub:** *APPIC Newsletter*, semiannual. Newsletter. *Price:* $10 free for members. • *Internship and Postdoctoral Programs in Professional Psychology*, annual. Directory. **Frmly:** (1991) Association of Psychology Internship Centers.

### ★ 12401 ★ Association for Research in Nervous and Mental Disease (ARNMD)

630 West 168th St.
Box 23
New York, NY 10032
**Phone:** (212)740-7608　　　**Fax:** (212)305-4548
**Email:** arnmd@arnmd.org
**Website:** http://www.arnmd.org/arnmd/
James E. Goldman, MD, Sec. Treas.

**Fnded:** 1920. **Mem:** 950. **Desc:** Individuals engaged in the practice or research of neurology, neurosurgery, or psychiatry who are members of neurologic or psychiatric societies. **Pub:** *Proceedings*, annual. **Frmly:** (1922) Neuropsychiatric Research Society.

### ★ 12402 ★ Association of State and Provincial Psychology Boards

c/o Randolph P. Reaves
PO Box 241245
7177 Halcyon Summit Dr.
Montgomery, AL 36124
**Phone:** (334)832-4580　　　**Free:** 800-448-4069
**Fax:** (334)269-6379
**Email:** asappb@asppb.org
**Website:** http://www.asppb.org
Randolph P. Reaves, J.D., Exec. Off.

**Fnded:** 1961. **Mem:** 62. **Desc:** State boards of psychology from across the U.S. and Canada. Pro-

motes the development and administration of the national EPPP examination for certification for the practice of psychology. Provides legal counsel to the member boards as well as keeping them abreast of changes in the field of psychology. Provides Certificate of Professional Qualification in Psychology (CPQ) to qualified psychologists for licensure in multiple jurisdictions. **Pub:** *ASPPB*, quarterly. Newsletter. *Price:* $8/year. **Frmly:** American Association of State Psychology Boards.

### ★ 12403 ★ Association of Stress Consultants

BSY Group
Stanhope Sq.
Holsworthy EX22 6DF, United Kingdom
**Phone:** 44 1409 259214　　　**Free:** 800-731-9271
**Fax:** 44 1409 259215
**Email:** info@bsygroup.co.uk
**Fnded:** 1946. **Desc:** Stress consultants.

### ★ 12404 ★ Association of Stress Therapists

8 Greenriggs
Wigmore
Luton LU29TQ, United Kingdom
**Phone:** 44 1582 452964
**Fnded:** 1991. **Mem:** 30. **Local Groups:** 1. **Desc:** Promotes stress therapy as a complementary therapy used to alleviate the physical and mental symptoms caused by stress.

### ★ 12405 ★ Association for the Study of Dreams (ASD)

PO Box 1592
Merced, CA 95341-1592
**Phone:** (209)724-0889　　　**Fax:** (209)724-9319
**Email:** asdreams@aol.com
**Website:** http://www.asdreams.org
Sue Moreno, Contact

**Fnded:** 1984. **Mem:** 900. **Desc:** Medical professionals, sociologists, counselors, educators, researchers, students, and others whose disciplines are involved in the study of dreams and dreaming. Provides an international interdisciplinary forum for the promotion and public dissemination of information regarding research into the physiological and therapeutic aspects of dreams and their interpretation. **Pub:** *Dream Time*, quarterly. Magazine. Contains research reports, clinical reports, interviews, case studies, and book reviews. *Price:* Included in membership dues. • *Dreaming*, quarterly. Journal. Contains scholarly articles on every aspect of dreams and dreaming. Includes book reviews. • Audiotapes.Contains conference lectures.

### ★ 12406 ★ Association for the Teaching of Psychology

c/o British Psychological Society
48 Princess Rd., E
St. Andrew's House
Leicester LE1 7DR, United Kingdom
**Phone:** 44 116 2549568
**Website:** http://www.a-t-p.org.uk
**Mem:** 1,000. **Desc:** Teachers of psychology in Secondary Schools, Further Education Colleges and Colleges of Higher Education. Supports teachers of psychology at pre-degree level. Provides help and advice. Organizes an annual updating conference for members and distributes resources produced by teachers for teachers. **Pub:** *Psychology Teaching Journal*, annual. Journal.

### ★ 12407 ★ Association of Therapeutic Communities (ATC)

c/o Pine St. Day Centre
13-15 Pine St.
London EC1R 0JG, United Kingdom
**Phone:** 44 20 89509557　　　**Fax:** 44 20 89509557
**Email:** post@therapeuticcommunities.org
**Website:** http://www.therapeuticcommunities.org

**Desc:** Nurses, social workers, researchers, psychologists, creative therapists, managers, residential care staff, teachers, psychotherapists, psychiatrists, and academics. Conducts training and education programs. **Pub:** *Therapeutic Communities Journal*, periodic. Journal.

### ★ 12408 ★ Association for Therapeutic Philosophy (ATP)

33 Marlborough Rd.
Swindon SN3 1PH, United Kingdom
**Phone:** 44 1793 538586　　　**Fax:** 44 1793 538586
**Email:** psycountrg@aol.com
**Website:** http://members.aol.com/psycountrg
**Fnded:** 1983. **Mem:** 450. **Desc:** Seeks to develop therapeutic philosophy concepts and treatment type. **Frmly:** (2001) Association of Psychological Counselling and Training.

### ★ 12409 ★ Association for Women in Psychology (AWP)

423 N Albany St.
Ithaca, NY 14850
**Phone:** (607)735-1907
**Email:** support@awpsych.org
**Website:** http://www.awpsych.org
Diane Maluso, Contact

**Fnded:** 1969. **Mem:** 2,400. **Desc:** Seeks to: end the role that the association feels psychology has had in perpetuating unscientific and unquestioned assumptions about the "natures" of women and men; encourage unbiased psychological research on sex and gender in order to establish facts and expose myths; encourage research and theory directed toward alternative sex-role socialization, child rearing practices, life-styles, and language use; educate and sensitize the science and psychology professions as well as the public to the psychological, social, political, and economic rights of women; combat the oppression of women of color; encourage research on issues of concern to women of color; achieve equality of opportunity for women and men within the profession and science of psychology. Conducts business and professional sessions at meetings of regional psychology associations. Maintains Hall of Fame and speakers' bureau. Monitors sexism in the American Psychological Association. **Pub:** *AWP Membership Directory*, annual. Membership Directory. *Price:* Free with membership. • *AWP Newsletter*, quarterly. Newsletter. **Frmly:** (1970) Association for Women Psychologists.

### ★ 12410 ★ Association of Workers for Children with Emotional and Behavioural Difficulties

Charlton Ct.
East Sutton
Maidstone ME17 3DQ, United Kingdom
**Phone:** 44 1622 843104　　　**Fax:** 44 1622 844220
**Email:** awcebd@mistral.co.uk
**Website:** http://www.awcebd.co.uk
**Fnded:** 1953. **Mem:** 1,000. **Reg. Groups:** 6. **Desc:** All professions involved in work with children and young people with emotional and behavioural difficulties and those who are involved in training. Promotes meeting the needs of children and young people with emotional and/or behavioural difficulties, in a variety of settings including education. **Pub:** *Emotional and Behavioral Difficulties*, 3/year. Journal. Multidisciplinary practitioners journal. • Newsletter, semiannual.

### ★ 12411 ★ Australasian Society for Traumatic Stress Studies (ASTSS)

288 Walsh St.
South Yarra, VIC 3141, Australia
**Phone:** 61 3 96504205
**Email:** valentp@msn.com.au
**Website:** http://www.astss.org.au
**Fnded:** 1990. **Lang(s):** English. **Desc:** Scientists and health care professionals with an interest in traumatic stress. Promotes "advancement of knowledge about the nature, consequences, treatment and prevention of highly stressful experiences." Gathers and dissemi-

nates information on traumatic stress and its diagnosis and treatment; sponsors research and educational programs.

**★ 12412 ★ Australian Psychological Society**
PO Box 38
Flinders Ln. PO
Melbourne, VIC 8009, Australia
**Phone:** 61 3 86623300 **Fax:** 61 3 96636177
**Email:** natoff@psychsociety.com.au
**Website:** http://www.psychsociety.com.au/
**Fnded:** 1966. **Mem:** 13,000. **Lang(s):** English. **Desc:** Psychologists. Seeks to "represent, promote and advance psychology and psychologists within the context of improving community well-being and scientific knowledge." Develops and maintains standards of training and practice; lobbies government agencies on matters of social welfare, justice, education, and health; conducts educational programs for members and the public. **Pub:** *In Psych*, bimonthly. Magazine.

**★ 12413 ★ Autism Network International (ANI)**
PO Box 35448
Syracuse, NY 13235-5448
**Phone:** (315)476-2462 **Fax:** (315)425-1978
**Email:** ani@caltcentral.com
**Website:** http://www.ani.ac
Jim Sinclair, Coord.
**Fnded:** 1992. **Mem:** 400. **Desc:** Autistic-run self-help and advocacy organization for autistic individuals. Seeks to provide a forum for autistic people to share information and tips for coping and problem-solving; advocates for appropriate services and civil rights for all autistic people at all levels of functioning. Provides information and referrals for parents and teachers of autistic people; sponsors group lobbying and educational campaigns. Serves as a support group. **Pub:** *Our Voice*, quarterly. **Price:** Included in membership dues. • *Pen Pal List*. Directory. Lists people interested in correspondence. **Price:** available to members only.

**★ 12414 ★ Autism Services Center (NAH)**
605 9th St.
PO Box 507
Huntington, WV 25710-0507
**Phone:** (304)525-8014 **Fax:** (304)525-8026
Dr. Ruth C. Sullivan, PhD, Exec. Dir.
**Fnded:** 1979. **Desc:** Service agency for individuals with autism and other developmental disabilities, and their families. (Autism is a disorder of communication and behavior which often manifests itself in social isolation, severe language deficiency, and compulsive insistence on routine and ritual in daily activities.) Assists families and agencies attempting to meet the unique needs of individuals with autism and other developmental disabilities; makes available technical assistance in designing programs. Provides supervised apartments, group homes, respite services, independent living services, and job-coached employment. Conducts workshops and consulting in autismD-isseminates information regarding autism and its treatment. **Frmly:** (1993) National Autism Hotline.

**★ 12415 ★ Autism Society of America (ASA)**
7910 Woodmont Ave., Ste. 300
Bethesda, MD 20814-3067
**Phone:** (301)657-0881 **Free:** 800-3AU-TISM
**Fax:** (301)657-0869
**Email:** info@autism-society.org
**Website:** http://www.autism-society.org/
Audrey Horne, Pres.
**Fnded:** 1965. **Mem:** 23,000. **Local Groups:** 230. **Desc:** Parents, teachers, psychologists, speech therapists, pediatricians, neurologists, and others interested in the welfare of children with severe disorders of communication and behavior. Informs the public of the symptoms and problems of children and adults with autism; promotes better understanding of the condition in general; aids physicians in making earlier and more

accurate diagnoses. Committed to the alleviation of this disorder through support of research, public and professional education, and development of habilitative services. Sponsors two mail-order book stores with over 100 titles on autism. **Pub:** *Advocate*, bimonthly. Newsletter. Promotes better understanding of autism by informing the public of the symptoms and problems of children and adults with autism. **Price:** Included in membership dues. • Audiotapes.Covers conference. • Booklets. • Handbooks. • Pamphlets. • Proceedings, annual. • Reprints. **Frmly:** (1981) National Society for Autistic Children; (1987) NSAC, The National Society for Children and Adults with Autism.

**★ 12416 ★ Befrienders International (BI)**
26-27 Market Pl.
Kingston Upon Thames KT1 1JH, United Kingdom
**Phone:** 44 208 5414949 **Fax:** 44 208 5411544
**Email:** admin@befrienders.org
**Website:** http://www.befrienders.org
**Fnded:** 1974. **Mem:** 30,000. **Nat'l Groups:** 34. **Reg. Groups:** 7. **Local Groups:** 318. **Lang(s):** English. **Desc:** Mission is to build effective suicide prevention services resourced by volunteers throughout the world. **Pub:** *Befriending Worldwide*, quarterly. Newsletter. **Frmly:** (1991) Befrienders International Samaritans Worldwide.

**★ 12417 ★ Behavior Genetics Association (BGA)**
c/o Hermine Maes, Ph.D.
Virginia Commonwealth University
PO Box 98003
Richmond, VA 23298-0003
**Website:** http://www.bga.org
Matt McGue, Pres.
**Fnded:** 1971. **Mem:** 400. **Desc:** Individuals engaged in teaching or research in some area of behavior genetics. Purposes are: to promote the scientific study of the interrelationship of genetic mechanisms and human and animal behavior through sponsorship of scientific meetings, publications, and communications among and by members; to encourage and aid the education and training of research workers in the field of behavior genetics; to aid in public dissemination and interpretation of information concerning the interrelationship of genetics and behavior and its implications for health, human development, and education. **Pub:** *Behavior Genetics*, bimonthly. Journal. Includes research reports. **Price:** Included in membership dues; $240/year for nonmembers in the U.S.; $267/year for nonmembers outside the U.S.

**★ 12418 ★ Belgian Federation of Psychologists**
Grasmarkt 105/18
B-1000 Brussels, Belgium
**Phone:** 32 2 5147509 **Fax:** 32 2 5147510
**Email:** bfp@skynet.be
**Website:** http://www.bfp-fbp.be
**Desc:** Umbrella organization for psychological societies in Belgium.

**★ 12419 ★ Black Mental Health Alliance (BMHA)**
2901 Druid Park Dr., Ste. A110
Business Ctr. at Park Circle
Baltimore, MD 21215
**Phone:** (410)837-2642 **Fax:** (410)837-2646
**Email:** bhealthall@aol.com
**Website:** http://bmhaec.org
Tracee E. Bryant, Exec. Dir.
**Fnded:** 1984. **Mem:** 250. **Reg. Groups:** 1. **State Groups:** 1. **Local Groups:** 1. **Desc:** Seeks to increase clinicians, clergy, educators, and social service professionals awareness of African-Americans mental health needs and concerns on issues including stress, violence, racism, susbstance abuse, and parenting. Provides consultation, public information, and resource referrals. Conducts a public awareness campaign; educates the community about available resources; develops programs that benefit African-

American children and families. Offers training to human service workers, teachers, police officers, and other service providers who work with culturally diverse populations. Maintains speakers' bureau. The support group provides emotional support, education and interaction for family members experiencing the stresses of caring for and/or living with a mentally ill relative. Provides a resource referral service; maintains an extensive list of African American mental health professionals who are sensitive to and appreciate cultural differences. Offers programs that invest in the needs of African American adult and adolescent females who are at risk of, or have, HIV or AIDS. Offers the "Free Yourself Stop Smoking and Prevention" program. **Pub:** *Visions*, quarterly. Newsletter. Contains updates, information, employment opportunities, community service information, and calendar. **Price:** Included in membership dues.

**★ 12420 ★ BODYWHYS: Help, Support, Understanding for Anorexia and Bulimia Nervosa**
PO Box 105
Blackrock, Dublin, Ireland
**Phone:** 353 1 2834963 **Fax:** 353 1 2834963
**Email:** info@bodywhys.ie
**Website:** http://www.bodywhys.ie
**Fnded:** 1995. **Local Groups:** 5. **Desc:** Offers support to people with/affected by eating disorders. Disseminates information to promote a better understanding of eating disorders. Runs self-help and support groups. **Frmly:** (2000) BODYWHYS, Organization for Anorexia and Bulimia Nervosa.

**★ 12421 ★ British Association for Behavioural and Cognitive Psychotherapies**
BABCP General Office
PO Box 9
Accrington BB5 2GD, United Kingdom
**Phone:** 44 1254 875277 **Fax:** 44 1254 239114
**Email:** babcp@babcp.com
**Website:** http://www.babcp.org.uk
**Fnded:** 1972. **Mem:** 2,000. **Lang(s):** English. **Desc:** Health, Social Service, education staff and therapists in private practice; individuals interested in psychotherapies and accredited/registered psychotherapists. Promotion of behavioural and cognitive therapy approaches in health, educational and social problem areas. **Pub:** *BABCP Newsletter*, 3/year. Newsletter. • *Behavioural & Cognitive Psychotherapy Journal*, quarterly. Journal.

**★ 12422 ★ British Association for Counselling and Psychotherapy (BACP)**
1 Regent Pl.
Rugby CV21 2PJ, United Kingdom
**Phone:** 44 870 4 435252 **Fax:** 44 870 4 435160
**Email:** bacp@bacp.co.uk
**Website:** http://www.counselling.co.uk
**Fnded:** 1977. **Mem:** 17,000. **Desc:** Individual or organisational membership for those working as counsellors or those using counselling skills as part of their role. Aims to promote awareness of counselling internationally and raise standards of training and practice through its Ethical Framework for Good Practice in Counselling and Psychotherapy. It provides support for members including an information service for members and the public, divisions for special interest groups and local affiliated groups. **Pub:** *Training in Counselling & Psychotherapy*, annual. • *United Kingdom Counseling & Psychotherapy Directory 2000*, annual. Directory. The most comprehensive & widely used way to find a counselor in the UK. **Frmly:** (2001) British Association for Counselling.

**★ 12423 ★ British Association for Dramatherapists**
41 Broomhouse Ln.
Hurlingham Park
London SW6 3DP, United Kingdom
**Phone:** 44 207 17310160 **Fax:** 44 207 17310160

**Email:** gllian@badth.demon.co.uk
**Fnded:** 1976. **Mem:** 630. **Desc:** Aims to: educate the public about dramatherapy, support dramatherapists wherever they work and increase the availability of properly-trained and supervised dramatherapists. Also aims to ensure that high standards are maintained and to implement Equal Opportunities policies. It responds to increasing demands for information and represents dramatherapy at a national and international level. **Pub:** *Dramatherapy*, quarterly. Newsletter. • *The Journal of Dramatherapy*, 3/year. Journal. Also publishes an information pack.

**British Association for Psychopharmacology (BAP)**
*See:* Entry 17331

★ 12424 ★ **British Association of Psychotherapists (BAP)**
37 Mapesbury Rd.
London NW2 4HJ, United Kingdom
**Phone:** 44 20 84529823     **Fax:** 44 20 84525182
**Email:** mail@bap-psychotherapy.org
**Website:** http://www.bap-psychotherapy.org
**Fnded:** 1951. **Mem:** 500. **Desc:** Full, Associate and Student Members, trained and qualified by BAP in either adult or child psychotherapy. Aims to promote the knowledge and application of psychotherapy and the training of both Adult and Child Psychotherapists. External courses were begun in 1989 for the benefit of interested members of the helping professions. A clinical service is also operated to help people find a qualified psychotherapist. An Msc. Training is also available. **Pub:** Journal, semiannual.

★ 12425 ★ **British False Memory Society**
Bradford-on-Avon BA15 1NF, United Kingdom
**Phone:** 44 1225 868682     **Fax:** 44 1225 862251
**Email:** bfms@compuserve.com
**Website:** http://www.bfms.org.uk
**Fnded:** 1993. **Mem:** 1,200. **Desc:** Seeks to raise awareness of the dangers of recovered memory therapy. Collaborates with associated organizations. Offers telephone support to family members falsely accused of childhood sexual abuse. Fosters research. **Pub:** *BFMS Newsletter*, 2-3 times a year. Newsletter.

★ 12426 ★ **British Psycho-Analytical Society (BP-AS)**
Byron House
112A-114 Shirland Rd.
London W9 2EQ, United Kingdom
**Phone:** 44 20 7563 5000   **Fax:** 44 20 7563 5001
**Email:** editors@psychoanalysis.org.uk
**Website:** http://www.ijpa.org
**Fnded:** 1913. **Mem:** 500. **Lang(s):** English. **Desc:** Psychoanalysts in the United Kingdom. Offers instructional programs. Promotes members' interests. **Pub:** *International Journal of Psycho-Analysis*, bimonthly. • Newsletter. Also publishes calendar of events.

★ 12427 ★ **British Psychodrama Association**
Heather Cottage
The Clachan
Helensburgh G84 0RF, United Kingdom
**Phone:** 44 143 6831838
**Website:** http://www.psychodrama.org.uk
**Fnded:** 1984. **Mem:** 250. **Desc:** Promotes the use of psychodrama and sociodrama as a creative and effective approach to working with a wide range of people in a variety of different settings. Psychodrama, sociometry, and group psychotherapy developed from the work of Jacob Levy Moreno (1889-1974). **Pub:** Journal, semiannual. • Bulletin, quarterly.

★ 12428 ★ **British Psychological Society (BPS)**
St. Andrews House
48 Princess Rd. E
Leicester LE1 7DR, United Kingdom
**Phone:** 44 116 2549568     **Fax:** 44 116 2470787
**Email:** mail@bps.org.uk
**Website:** http://www.bps.org.uk
**Fnded:** 1901. **Mem:** 33,000. **Nat'l Groups:** 24. **Local Groups:** 7. **Lang(s):** English. **Desc:** Academic, research, and all branches of applieed psychology. Promotes the advancement of psychological study and works to ensure high standards of professional education and conduct. Offers courses. **Pub:** *British Journal of Clinical Psychology*, quarterly, in February, May, September, and November. Journal. • *British Journal of Developmental Psychology*, quarterly, in March, June, September, and November. Journal. • *British Journal of Health Psychology*, quarterly, in February, May, September, and November. Journal. • *British Journal of Mathematical and Statistical Psychology*, semiannual, in May and November. Journal. • *British Journal of Medical Psychology*, quarterly, in March, June, September, and December. Journal. • *British Journal of Psychology*, quarterly, in February, May, August, and November. Journal. • *British Journal of Social Psychology*, quarterly, in March, June, September, and December. Journal. • *Journal of Occupational and Organizational Psychology*, quarterly, in March, June, September, and December. Journal.

★ 12429 ★ **Bulimia Anorexia Nervosa Association (BANA)**
300 Cabana Rd. E
Windsor, ON, Canada N9G 1A3
**Phone:** (519)969-2112       **Fax:** (519)969-0227
**Email:** info@bana.ca
**Website:** http://www.bana.ca
**Fnded:** 1982. **Mem:** 200. **Lang(s):** English, French. **Desc:** Individuals with eating disorders; health care professionals and others with an interest in the treatment of people with eating disorders; interested others. Promotes prevention and effective treatment of eating disorders. Conducts therapy groups for people with eating disorders; sponsors research and educational programs; makes available children's services; maintains speakers' bureau. **Pub:** *Positive Direction*, quarterly. Directory.

★ 12430 ★ **C. G. Jung Foundation for Analytical Psychology**
28 E 39th St.
New York, NY 10016
**Phone:** (212)697-6430       **Fax:** (212)953-3989
**Email:** cgjungny@aol.com
**Website:** http://www.cgjungpage.org/nyfound.html
Janet M. Careswell, Exec. Dir.
**Fnded:** 1963. **Mem:** 1,000. **Desc:** Analysts who follow the precepts of Carl G. Jung (1875-1961), Swiss psychologist; persons interested in analytical psychology. Provides information on analytical psychology. Sponsors public lectures, films, continuing education courses and professional seminars. Operates book service which provides publications on analytical psychology and related topics, and lectures on audiocassettes. **Pub:** *Quadrant*, semiannual. • Annual Report.

★ 12431 ★ **Canadian Alliance of Physiotherapy Regulators**
1243 Islington Ave., Ste. 501
Etobicoke, ON, Canada M8X 1Y9
**Phone:** (416)234-8800       **Fax:** (416)234-8820
**Website:** http://www.alliancept.org/
**Desc:** Advocates on national regulatory issues for physiotherapy regulators; seeks to develop a national consistency of registration requirements, national consistency of standards, and to have the Physiotherapy National Exam used throughout Canada. **Pub:** Annual Report. • Bulletin.

★ 12432 ★ **Canadian Association for Music Therapy (CAMT) (Association de Musicotherapie du Canada — AMC)**
Wilfrid Laurier University
Waterloo, ON, Canada N2L 3C5
**Phone:** (519)884-1970       **Free:** 800-996-CAMT
**Fax:** (519)884-8853
**Email:** camt@musictherapy.ca
**Website:** http://www.musictherapy.ca
**Fnded:** 1974. **Mem:** 400. **Reg. Groups:** 6. **Local Groups:** 1. **Lang(s):** English, French. **Desc:** Promotes the use and development of music for health and well-being in prevention and treatment with all age groups. Establishes, maintains, and improves standards of treatment and service in music therapy; encourages and develops research. Acts as a forum for the exchange of ideas, advice, guidance, and professional experience. Represents the interests of music therapists in matters relating to governmental legislation, jobs, and salary scales. Offers professional accreditation to music therapists. **Pub:** *CAMT Newsletter*, 3/year. Newsletter. News on professional issues concerning music therapists. • *Canadian Journal of Music Therapy*, annual. Journal. • *Conference Proceedings*, published from 1979-1992. • *Membership Directory*, annual.

**Canadian Association of Psychological Oncology (Association Canadienne d'Oncologie Psychosociale)**
*See:* Entry 10133

★ 12433 ★ **Canadian Association for Suicide Prevention (CASP) (Association Canadienne pour la Prevention du Suicide — ACPS)**
11456 Jasper Ave., Ste. 301
Edmonton, AB, Canada T5K 0M1
**Phone:** (780)482-0198       **Fax:** (780)488-1495
**Email:** casp@suicideprevention.ca
**Website:** http://www.suicideprevention.ca
**Fnded:** 1985. **Mem:** 300. **Lang(s):** English, French. **Desc:** Individuals and organizations. Seeks to reduce the incidence of suicide through advocacy, support, and advising. **Pub:** *CASP News*, 3/year. Newsletter.

★ 12434 ★ **Canadian Centre for Stress and Well-Being**
1 Yonge St., Ste. 1801
Toronto, ON, Canada M5E 1W7
**Phone:** (416)363-6204       **Fax:** (416)369-0515
**Lang(s):** English, French. **Desc:** Individuals suffering from stress; health care professionals and organizations with an interest in stress. Seeks to advance the diagnosis and treatment of stress and related disorders; works to improve the quality of life of people suffering from stress. Provides support and assistance to victims of stress and their families; sponsors research and educational programs.

★ 12435 ★ **Canadian Counselling Association (CCA)**
116 Albert St., Ste. 702
Ottawa, ON, Canada K1P 5G3
**Phone:** (613)237-1099       **Free:** 877-765-5565
**Fax:** (613)237-9786
**Email:** info@ccacc.ca
**Website:** http://www.ccacc.ca
**Fnded:** 1965. **Mem:** 1,900. **Lang(s):** English, French. **Desc:** Professionally trained counselors in the fields of education, employment and career development, social work, business, industry, mental health, public service agencies, government, and private practice. Promotes the counseling profession in Canada.

**Canadian Federation of Mental Health Nurses (CFMHN)**
*See:* Entry 15686

**★ 12436 ★ Canadian Mental Health Association**
**(Association Canadienne pour la Sante Mentale)**
2160 Yonge St., 3rd Fl.
Toronto, ON, Canada M4S 2Z3
**Phone:** (416)484-7750        **Fax:** (416)484-4617
**Email:** national@cmha.ca
**Website:** http://www.cmha.ca
**Fnded:** 1918. **Local Groups:** 135. **Lang(s):** English, French. **Desc:** Mental health professionals and other individuals with an interest in community mental health. Works to enable individuals, groups, and communities to increase control over and enhance their mental health. Serves as a social advocate to encourage public action to strengthen community mental health services; conducts lobbying activities. Promotes mental health research; organizes and operates grass roots programs to help people whose mental health is at risk make use of the services available to them. Sponsors educational programs. **Pub:** Newsletter, quarterly. • Pamphlets.

**★ 12437 ★ Canadian Psychiatric Association (CPA)**
**(Association des Psychiatres du Canada — APC)**
260-441 MacLaren St.
Ottawa, ON, Canada K2P 2H3
**Phone:** (613)234-2815        **Fax:** (613)234-9857
**Email:** cpa@cpa-apc.org
**Website:** http://www.cpa-apc.org
**Fnded:** 1951. **Mem:** 2,700. **State Groups:** 10. **Lang(s):** English, French. **Desc:** Works to improve mental health and psychiatric care delivery systems in Canada. Fosters high standards among Canadian psychiatrists; promotes continuing education of members; encourages and participates in educational programs for patient care providers; promotes research into psychiatric disorders; represents members before government bodies and licensing bureaus, universities, and related organizations. **Pub:** Canadian Journal of Psychiatry, 10/year. Journal. • CPA Bulletin, bimonthly. • CPA News Bulletin, quarterly.

**★ 12438 ★ Canadian Psychoanalytic Society (CPS)**
**(Societe et Institut Canadiens de Psychanalyse — SICP)**
7000 Cote Des Neiges
Montreal, QC, Canada H3S 2C1
**Phone:** (514)342-7444        **Fax:** (514)342-1062
**Email:** psyanal@aei.ca
**Website:**                http://www.psychoanalysis.ca/main.asp?P=287A5CPS5B
**Lang(s):** English, French. **Desc:** Psychoanalysts and other mental health professionals with an interest in psychoanalysis. Seeks to advance the study, teaching, and practice of psychoanalysis. Serves as a forum for the exchange of information among members; conducts educational and continuing professional development courses; sponsors research.

**★ 12439 ★ Canadian Psychological Association (CPA)**
**(Societe Canadienne de Psychologie — SCP)**
151 Slater St., Ste. 205
Ottawa, ON, Canada K1P 5H3
**Phone:** (613)237-2144        **Fax:** (613)237-1674
**Email:** cpa@cpa.ca
**Website:** http://www.cpa.ca
**Fnded:** 1939. **Mem:** 5,000. **Lang(s):** English, French. **Desc:** Psychologists and other individuals with an interest in psychology. Seeks to advance the study, teaching, and practice of psychology; promotes ongoing professional development of members. Facilitates exchange of information among members. **Pub:** Canadian Psychology, periodic. Journal. • Psynopsis, periodic. Newsletter.

**Canadian Register of Health Service Providers in Psychology (CRHSPP)**
**(Repertoire Canadien des Psychologues Offrant des Services de Sante — RCPOSS)**
See: Entry 9730

**★ 12440 ★ Canadian Schizophrenia Foundation (CSF)**
16 Florence Ave.
Toronto, ON, Canada M2N 1E9
**Phone:** (416)733-2117        **Fax:** (416)733-2352
**Email:** centre@orthomed.org
**Website:** http://www.orthomed.org/csf/csf.htm
**Fnded:** 1969. **Lang(s):** English. **Desc:** People with schizophrenia and their families, mental health professionals, and others with an interest in schizophrenia and related conditions. Promotes an improved quality of life for people with schizophrenia; seeks to identify more effective treatments for the disorder. Faciltates communication among mental health professionals studying schizophrenia; sponsors research. **Pub:** Nutrition and Mental Health, quarterly. Newsletter.

**★ 12441 ★ Canadian Society for Psychomotor Learning and Sport Psychology**
**(Societe Canadienne d'Apprentissage Psychomoteur et de Psychologie du Sport)**
School of Human Kinetics
University of British Columbia
6081 University Blvd., Ste. 210
Vancouver, BC, Canada V6T 1Z1
**Phone:** (604)492-2187        **Fax:** (604)492-2364
**Email:** webmaster@scapps.org
**Website:** http://www.scapps.org
**Lang(s):** English, French. **Desc:** Health care professionals and other individuals with an interest in psychomotor learning and sports psychology. Seeks to advance the study and practice of sports psychology. Gathers and disseminates information; sponsors research and educational programs.

**★ 12442 ★ Center for Applications of Psychological Type (CAPT)**
2815 NW 13th St., Ste. 401
Gainesville, FL 32609
**Phone:** (352)375-0160        **Free:** 800-777-2278
**Fax:** (352)378-0503
**Email:** info@capt.org
**Website:** http://www.capt.org
Mary H. McCaulley, PhD, Pres.
**Fnded:** 1975. **Desc:** Works to disseminate information on Isabel Briggs Myers' works and encourage practical applications of Carl G. Jung's (1875-1961) theory of psychological types; seeks to foster understanding and constructive use of personality differences. Primary focus is on the theory of psychological types utilizing the Myers-Briggs Type Indicator (for young people and adults, created by Myers and her mother, Katharine Briggs) and the Murphy-Meisgeier Type Indicator For Children to identify Jungian types. (Jung's theory states that seemingly random variations in behavior are actually consistent and orderly if one understands differences in the ways people process information and make decisions.) Conducts introductory and advanced training through workshops, consultation, and other training sessions for psychologists in the areas of counseling, education, religion, organizations, and research; offers continuing education courses. Sponsors research and offers research consultation; provides computer scoring of MBTI forms to professionally qualified users. Provides consultation on the applications of the MBTI and on-site development of MBTI skills of qualified personnel. Operates the Isabel Briggs Myers Memorial Library containing MBTI- and Jungian-related material. Distributes teaching aids, question booklets, answer sheets, scoring keys, and computer software for MBTI analyses. Sponsors exhibits on professional conferences. Works closely with Association for Psychological Type. **Pub:**

Atlas of Type Tables. • Bibliography of the MBTI, semiannual. Bibliography. • Books. • Reports. • Also publishes papers, training exercises, and other materials.

**★ 12443 ★ Center for Professional Well-Being (CWBHP)**
21 W Colony Pl., Ste. 150
Durham, NC 27705
**Phone:** (919)489-9167        **Fax:** (919)419-0011
**Email:** cpwb@mindspring.com
**Website:** http://www.cpwb.org
Margaret Seeman, Program Dir./Office Mgr.
**Fnded:** 1979. **Mem:** 800. **Nat'l Groups:** 1. **Reg. Groups:** 1. **Desc:** Society serving health and other professional associations. Promotes the well-being of health professionals and their families through: preventive education on manifestations of disabilities; increased awareness about the stresses inherent in the system of providing health services; efforts to improve and maintain effectiveness. Conducts research and supports efforts to study the incidence and causes of professional impairment, with prevention as a goal. Maintains speakers' bureau; provides individual consulting and counseling. Offers workshops on The Joy of Medicine, Physician Burnout, and Preventive Malpractice Strategies; sponsors retreats, seminars, and lectures. **Pub:** Being Well: Bulletin of the Society for Professional Well-Being, quarterly. Bulletin. **Price:** Included in membership dues; $55. • Booklets. • Monographs. • Videos. **Frmly:** (1993) Center for the Well-Being of Health Professionals.

**★ 12444 ★ Center for the Study of Psychiatry and Psychology**
4628 Chestnut St.
Bethesda, MD 20814
**Phone:** (301)652-5580        **Fax:** (301)652-5924
**Website:** http://www.icspp.org
Peter R. Breggin, MD, Dir.
**Fnded:** 1971. **Desc:** Fosters prevention and treatment of mental and emotional disorders. Promotes alternatives to administering psychiatric drugs to children. Biannual convention/meeting. **Pub:** Ethical Human Sciences and Services (EHSS), quarterly. Journal. **Frmly:** (1995) Center for the Study of Psychiatry.

**★ 12445 ★ Chinese Association for Mental Health**
c/o Cai Zhuo Ji, Pres.
5 An Kang Hutong
De Wai
Beijing 100088, People's Republic of China
**Phone:** 86 10 82085385        **Fax:** 86 10 62359838
**Fnded:** 1985. **Mem:** 20,000. **Local Groups:** 26. **Lang(s):** Chinese. **Desc:** Physicians, psychologists, sociologists. Seeks to increase people's psychological health, to elevate their social adaptation ability, and to prevent psychological disorders.

**★ 12446 ★ Chinese Psychological Society**
Institute of Psychology
Chinese Academy of Sciences
Beijing 100101, People's Republic of China
**Phone:** 852 10 64888946  **Fax:** 852 10 64872070
**Email:** icp2004@atspsych.ac.cn
**Website:** http://www.icp2004.psych.ac.cn
**Desc:** Promotes academic communication through congresses, conferences, meetings, organizing research projects, publishing books, providing counseling services and suggestions to related institutions and departments.

**★ 12447 ★ Christian Association for Psychological Studies (CAPS)**
c/o Dr. Randolph K. Sanders
PO Box 310400
New Braunfels, TX 78131-0400
**Phone:** (830)629-2277        **Fax:** (830)629-2342
**Email:** capsintl@compuvision.net

**Website:** http://www.caps.net
Dr. Randolph K. Sanders, PhD, Exec. Dir.
**Fnded:** 1956. **Mem:** 2,100. **Reg. Groups:** 7. **Local Groups:** 65. **Desc:** Psychologists, marriage and family therapists, social workers, educators, physicians, nurses, ministers, researchers, pastoral counselors, and rehabilitation workers and others professionally engaged in the fields of psychology, counseling, psychiatry, pastoring, and related areas. Association is based upon a genuine commitment to superior clinical, pastoral, and scientific enterprise in the theoretical and applied social sciences and theology, assuming persons in helping professions will be guided to professional and personal growth and a greater contribution to others in this way. Aims to help members cooperatively as Christians to explore the fields of psychology, pastoring, and psychotherapy for a better insight into perso nality and interpersonal relations and to articulate and promote the lordship of Christ in these scientific disciplines. **Pub:** *CAPS Report*, quarterly. Newsletter. Includes information on membership activities and schedule of events. *Price:* Free. • *Christian Monograph Series*, periodic. Monograph. • *International Directory of the Christian Association for Psychological Studies*, annual. Membership Directory. Arranged geographically, with separate listings for libraries. *Price:* $10. • *Journal of Psychology and Christianity*, quarterly. Journal. Contains articles on clinical and theoretical topics. Includes book reviews and professional employment opportunities. *Price:* Included in membership dues; $40/year for nonmembers; $50/year for libraries.

**Collegium Internationale Neuro-Psychopharmacologicum (CINP)**
*See:* Entry 13978

★ **12448** ★ **Colombian Association of Psychiatry**
**(Asociacion Colombiana de Psiquiatria)**
Apdo 52053
Santa Fe de Bogota, Colombia
**Phone:** 57 1 2561148
**Email:** asocopsi@col1.telecom.com.co
**Website:** http://www.psiquiatria.org.co/
**Fnded:** 1961.

★ **12449** ★ **Committee for Truth in Psychiatry (CTIP)**
PO Box 1214
New York, NY 10003
**Phone:** (212)665-6587
**Website:** http://dspace.dial.pipex.com/comcare/cftip.html
Linda Andre, Dir.
**Fnded:** 1984. **Mem:** 500. **Desc:** Former psychiatric patients who have had electroconvulsive therapy (ECT), working to bring about truthfully informed consent to shock treatment. Works to retain ECT's current FDA classification as a high-risk procedure. Has submitted a proposal to the Food and Drug Administration regarding a statement of information about ECT that would be given to patients before they give consent for treatment. Seeks endorsements for the CTIP statement. Also has petitioned the FDA for an animal and human CAT scan study of ECT. Provides counseling for individuals/families facing a decision about ECT, or recovering from ECT. **Pub:** *A Synopsis of the Conflict Over ECT at the FDA*. Pamphlet. *Price:* Free. • *FDA's Regulatory Proceedings Concerning ECT*. Pamphlet. *Price:* Free. • *Shockwaves*, quarterly. Newsletter. *Price:* $10/year for survivors and supporters; $5/year for low-income subscribers; $25/year for professionals, agencies, institutions. • *What You Need to Know about ECT*. *Price:* Free.

★ **12450** ★ **Community Dreamsharing Network (CDN)**
PO Box 8032
Hicksville, NY 11802-8032
**Phone:** (516)735-1969       **Fax:** (516)796-9455
**Email:** comdream@aol.com

**Website:** http://yalenewhavenhealth.org/Library/HealthGuide/SelfHelp/Topic.asp?hwid=shc63dre
Harold Roger Ellis, PhD, Dir.
**Fnded:** 1982. **Mem:** 600. **Nat'l Groups:** 150. **Reg. Groups:** 7. **State Groups:** 5. **Local Groups:** 10. **Desc:** Social groups of individuals interested in discussing and understanding their dreams. Works to organize local dreamsharing groups which meet weekly and encourages networking between these groups. Refers qualified dreamsharing activity helpers to schools and groups. Trains elementary and high school teachers in using the dreams of students. Sponsors training sessions in dream understanding methods; conducts research. Maintains speakers' bureau and placement service. Maintains a database of dreamsharing groups. **Pub:** *Dream Switchboard*, quarterly. Newsletter. Includes networking notices. *Price:* $15 /year for individuals. **Frmly:** (1970) Center for Dream Drama; (1982) New York/New Jersey DreamSharing Network; (1988) Dreamsharing Grassroots Network.

★ **12451** ★ **Community Guidance Service (CGS)**
133 E 73rd St.
New York, NY 10021
**Phone:** (212)724-1091       **Fax:** (212)724-1091
Alphrodite Clamar, PhD, Dir.
**Fnded:** 1953. **Desc:** Service agency providing low-cost psychotherapy services at private offices throughout the New York City area. Staff includes psychiatrists, psychologists, and social workers. **Frmly:** Group for Community Guidance Centers.

★ **12452** ★ **Congres Des Psychoanalyses De Langue Francaise (CPLF)**
187, rue St-Jacques
F-75005 Paris, France
**Phone:** 33 1 43296670       **Fax:** 33 1 44070744
**Mem:** 500. **Lang(s):** French. **Desc:** Psychoanalysts and students of the International Psycho-Analytical Association. Sponsors research work groups, plenary sessions, and meetings. **Frmly:** Congress of Romance Language Psychoanalysts.

★ **12453** ★ **Council for the National Register of Health Service Providers in Psychology (CNRHSPP)**
1120 G St. NW, Ste. 330
Washington, DC 20005
**Phone:** (202)783-7663       **Fax:** (202)347-0550
**Email:** judy@nationalregister.org
**Website:** http://www.nationalregister.org
Judy E. Hall, PhD, Contact
**Fnded:** 1974. **Mem:** 14,000. **Desc:** Psychologists who are licensed or certified by a state/provincial/territorial board of examiners of psychology and who have met council criteria as health service providers in psychology. **Pub:** *Designated Doctoral Programs in Psychology*. • *National Register of Health Service Providers in Psychology*, annual. • *The Register Report*, semiannual. Magazine. Includes current issues in practice.

★ **12454** ★ **Czech-Moravian Psychological Society**
**(Ceskomoravska psychologicka spolecnost)**
Kladenska 48
CZ-160 00 Prague 6, Czech Republic
**Phone:** 42 2 35360477
**Email:** cmps@ecn.cz
**Website:** http://www.ecn.cz/cmps/
**Lang(s):** Czech, English. **Desc:** Psychologists in the Czech Republic. Promotes psychology as a field of knowledge and as a profession. Comments on psychological publications; promotes ethical practices and principles; provides information and counseling service. **Pub:** Bulletin, quarterly.

★ **12455** ★ **Danish Psychologists' Association**
**(Dansk Psykolog Forening — DP)**
Stockholmsgade 27
DK-2100 Copenhagen, Denmark
**Phone:** 45 35269955       **Fax:** 45 35269755
**Email:** dp@dp.dk
**Website:** http://www.dp.dk
**Fnded:** 1947.

★ **12456** ★ **Danubian Psychiatric Association**
c/o pro mente Oberosterreich
Figulystrasse 32
A-4020 Linz, Austria
**Phone:** 43 732 656103       **Fax:** 43 732 651321
**Email:** donausymposion@promenteooe.at
**Fnded:** 1964. **Mem:** 61. **State Groups:** 16. **Lang(s):** English. **Desc:** Provides international scientific contracts with psychiatrists. Organizes a biannual symposium of psychiatry in different countries.

**Deaf-REACH**
*See:* Entry 6029

★ **12457** ★ **Depression Alliance**
35 Westminster Bridge Rd.
London SE1 7JB, United Kingdom
**Phone:** 44 20 76330557       **Fax:** 44 20 76330559
**Email:** information@depressionalliance.org
**Website:** http://www.depressionalliance.org
**Fnded:** 1979. **Mem:** 3,000. **Desc:** Provides information and support to anyone affected by depression. Services include a self-help groups, correspondence schemes and a unique range of literature. **Pub:** Newsletter, quarterly.

★ **12458** ★ **Depression and Related Affective Disorders Association (DRADA)**
Johns Hopkins Hospital Meyer 3-181
600 N Wolfe St.
Baltimore, MD 21287-7381
**Phone:** (410)955-4647       **Fax:** (410)614-3241
**Email:** drada@jhmi.edu
**Website:** http://www.drada.org
Cathy Pollock, Dir.
**Fnded:** 1986. **Mem:** 1,300. **Desc:** Individuals with affective disorders, their families and friends, and mental health professionals. (Affective disorders include depressive illnesses and manic-depression.) Provides support services including referrals, educational programs, networking, and consultation. Encourages and facilitates the formation of local support groups for those with affective disorders; provides training for support group leaders. Cosponsors with Johns Hopkins annual mood disorders symposium. Maintains speakers' bureau. **Pub:** *A Patients Perspective: Dick Cavett*. Video. • *A Patients Perspective: Mike Wallace*. Video. • *Day for Night: Recognizing Teenage Depression*. Video. • *Depressive Illness: What You Need to Know*. Video. • *Downtime: A Workplace Guide to Understanding Clinical Depression*. Video. • *DRADA Update*, bimonthly. Brochure. • *Manual for Affective Disorder Support Groups*. Manual. • *Smooth Sailing*, quarterly. Newsletter. *Price:* Included in membership dues.

★ **12459** ★ **Depressives Anonymous: Recovery From Depression (DARFD)**
4625 Douglas Ave.
Bronx, NY 10471
Dr. Helen DeRosis, Founder
**Fnded:** 1977. **Mem:** 3,000. **Desc:** Individuals suffering from depression or anxiety. A selfhelp organization which helps people deal with their anxiety or depression through weekly meeting and sharing of experiences. Conducts research; offers classes. Disseminates information. Interested people may send a SASE or ask for a collect call at the above number.

**Pub:** Newsletter, 3-4/year. • Also publishes brochures and pamphlets.

★ **12460** ★ **Division of Family Psychology**
c/o American Psychological Association
750 First St. NE
Washington, DC 20002-4242
**Phone:** (202)336-6013 **Fax:** (202)218-3599
**Email:** brhamp@aol.com
**Website:** http://www.apa.org/divisions/div43
Terrence Patterson, EdD, ABPP, Pres.
**Fnded:** 1984. **Mem:** 2,000. **Desc:** A division of the American Psychological Association. Psychologists interested in research, teaching, prevention, treatment, evaluation, and public interest initiatives in family psychology. seeks to promote human welfare through the development, dissemination, and application of knowledge about the dynamics, structure, and functioning of the family. Conducts research and specialized education programs. Maintains speakers' bureau. **Pub:** *The Family Psychologist*, quarterly. Bulletin.

**Dual Disorders Anonymous**
*See:* Entry 19276

★ **12461** ★ **Eating Disorders Association (EDA)**
Wensum House, 1st Fl.
103 Prince of Wales Rd.
Norwich NR1 1DW, United Kingdom
**Phone:** 44 1603 619090 **Fax:** 44 1603 664915
**Email:** info@edauk.com
**Website:** http://www.edauk.com
**Fnded:** 1989. **Mem:** 3,500. **Local Groups:** 54. **Lang(s):** English. **Desc:** Individuals affected by anorexia, bulimia nervosa, and related eating disorders, their families, and friends. Offers information, help, and support. Seeks to enhance awareness and understanding of these illnesses. Communicates with related organizations and individuals in the medical and counseling professions. Disseminates information. Organizes regional support days. Offers training for professionals. **Pub:** *European Eating Disorders Review*, 5/year. Journal. • *Signpost*, quarterly. Magazine.

★ **12462** ★ **Eating Disorders Northern Ireland**
78 Glengoland Pk.
Belfast BT17 0JB, United Kingdom
**Phone:** 44 2890 621627
**Fnded:** 1992. **Mem:** 20. **Reg. Groups:** 2. **Local Groups:** 3. **Desc:** Support group for carers and sufferers of anorexia and other eating disorders. Disseminates information.

★ **12463** ★ **Emotions Anonymous International Service Center (EA)**
PO Box 4245
2233 University Ave. W, Ste. 402
Saint Paul, MN 55104-0245
**Phone:** (651)647-9712 **Fax:** (651)647-1593
**Email:** eaisc@mtn.org
**Website:** http://www.emotionsanonymous.org
Karen Mead, Exec. Dir.
**Fnded:** 1971. **Mem:** 5,000. **Nat'l Groups:** 1175. **State Groups:** 35. **Local Groups:** 20. **Desc:** "Fellowship of men and women who share their experience, strength, and hope with each other, that they may solve their common problem and help each other recover from emotional illness." Uses the Twelve Steps of Alcoholics Anonymous World Services, adapted to emotional problems. Disseminates literature and information; provides telephone referrals to worldwide chapters. **Pub:** *Emotions Anonymous*. Book. Available in both soft and hard cover editions. *Price:* $15. • *The New Message*, quarterly. Magazine. Provides stories from EA members and their recovery through EA. • *Today*. Book.

★ **12464** ★ **European Association of Experimental Social Psychology (EAESP)**
c/o Sibylle Classen
PO Box 420 143
D-48068 Muenster, Germany
**Fax:** 49 2533 281144
**Email:** sibylle@eaesp.org
**Website:** http://www.eaesp.org/
**Fnded:** 1964. **Mem:** 800. **Lang(s):** English. **Desc:** Individuals in 28 countries working in the field of experimental and theoretical social psychology. Promotes theoretical and experimental social psychology and arranges for the exchange of information among members and related associations worldwide. Conducts summer schools for young researchers. **Pub:** *European Bulletin of Social Psychology*, 3/year. Newsletter. • *European Journal of Social Psychology*, bimonthly. Journal. • *European Monographs*, periodic.

★ **12465** ★ **European Association of Multidisciplinary Practice in Child, Adolescent and Family Mental Health (Association Europeene de Pratiques Multidisciplinaires en Sante Mentale de l'Enfant, l'Adolescent et de la Familie)**
c/o CMPP
4 rue Ed Branly
Case Postale 1484
F-77000 Melun, France
**Phone:** 33 1 60689990 **Fax:** 33 1 64377024
**Lang(s):** English, French. **Desc:** Mental health practitioners. Promotes a multidisciplinary approach in the provision of child, adolescent, and family mental health services. Encourages cooperation among members and arranges joint mental health programs; conducts research and continuing professional training programs.

★ **12466** ★ **European Association of Personality Psychology (EAPP)**
Henri Dunantlaan 2
B-9000 Gent, Belgium
**Phone:** 32 9 2646499 **Fax:** 32 9 2646473
**Email:** flip.defruyt@rug.ac.be
**Website:** http://allserv.rug.ac.be/~fdefruyt/eapp.html
**Fnded:** 1984. **Desc:** Develops empirical and theoretical personality psychology by exchange of information.

★ **12467** ★ **European Association of Psychological Assessment (EAPA)**
c/o Prof. M. Forns-Santacana
Universidad de Barcelona
Dep. Personalidad, Evaluacion y Tratamiento Psicologico
Paseo Vall d'Hebron 171
E-08035 Barcelona, Spain
**Fnded:** 1990. **Desc:** Works to increase scientific interest in psychological assessment in Europe. Fosters communication and scientific exchange. **Pub:** *European Journal of Psychological Assessment*. Journal. • Newsletter, annual.

★ **12468** ★ **European Association for Psychotherapy**
Krieglergasse 11/5
A-1030 Vienna, Austria
**Phone:** 43 1 7144243 **Fax:** 43 1 7159963
**Email:** eap.headoffice@magnet.at
**Website:** http://www.psychother.com/eap
**Fnded:** 1991. **Mem:** 650. **Desc:** Psychotherapists from 28 European countries. Fosters the free and independent practice of psychotherapy. Develops ethical guidelines for the protection of patients Promotes high training standards. **Pub:** *International Journal of Psychotherapy*. Journal.

★ **12469** ★ **European Council on Eating Disorders (ECED)**
Department of Psychiatry
St. George's Hospital Medical School
London SW17 0RE, United Kingdom
**Phone:** 44 208 7253463 **Fax:** 44 208 7253350
**Email:** eced@sghms.ac.uk
**Fnded:** 1989. **Mem:** 500. **Lang(s):** English. **Desc:** European medical clinicians and researchers with an interest in eating disorders. Seeks to advance the diagnosis and medical treatment of eating disorders. Facilitates exchange of information and clinical skills among members. **Pub:** Newsletter, periodic.

★ **12470** ★ **European Federation of Family Associations of People with Mental Illness (EUFAMI)**
151 Groeneweg
B-3001 Heverlee, Belgium
**Phone:** 32 16 232382 **Fax:** 32 16 238818
**Email:** admin@eumafi.org
**Website:** http://www.eufami.org
**Fnded:** 1992. **Nat'l Groups:** 26. **Lang(s):** Danish, English, French, German. **Desc:** Promotes the interests of people with mental illness and their careers. Works to remove the stigma surrounding mental illness by promoting a positive image to counteract misinformation. Lobbies for improved equality of legislation throughout Europe which benefits both the health and social care of people with mental illness and those who care for them. Sponsors research into the causes and treatments of mental illness. **Pub:** *Silent Partners*. Research document into careers' needs. • *Working Together*, 3/year. Newsletter. **Frmly:** (2001) European Federation of Associations of Families of Mentally Ill People.

★ **12471** ★ **European Federation for Pscyhoanalytic Psychotherapy**
5 Windsor Rd.
Finchley
London, United Kingdom
**Phone:** 44 20 84399873 **Fax:** 44 20 83433197
**Email:** joycepiper@compuserve.com
**Desc:** Umbrella organization that links together national networks of adult, child, and adolescent and group psychoanalytic psychotherapists, and psychoanalysts involved in public sector services.

★ **12472** ★ **European Psycho-Analytical Federation (EPF) (Federation Europeenne de Psychanalyse — FEP)**
37 Wooddsome Rd.
London NW5 15A, United Kingdom
**Phone:** 44 207 4857269 **Fax:** 44 207 2099963
**Email:** d.tuckett@ucl.ac.uk
**Website:** http://www.epf-ev.org
**Fnded:** 1969. **Reg. Groups:** 26. **Lang(s):** English, French, German. **Desc:** Psychoanalysts from 19 countries belonging to European psychoanalytical societies. Seeks to further psychoanalysis as a comprehensive theory of personality and therapeutic method based on the teachings of Sigmund Freud (1856-1939), Austrian neurologist and founder of psychoanalysis. Works to maintain and improve standards of education and scientific inquiry and to foster theoretical research. Disseminates information on theoretical and practical aspects of psychoanalysis. Stimulates communication among psychoanalysts; provides a forum for discussion of psychoanalytic and related topics. Encourages the integration of psychoanalysis and other disciplines. Organizes seminars and symposia. **Pub:** *Bulletin*, semiannual. • *Psychoanalytic Training in Europe: 10 Years of Discussion*. • *Pulsion de Mort*.

## European Society of Child and Adolescent Psychiatry (ESCAP) (Societe Europeene de Psychiatrie de l'Enfant et de l'Adolescent — SEPEA)
*See:* Entry 5676

### ★ 12473 ★ European Society for Cognitive Psychology (ESCP)
c/o Andre Vandierendonck
Department of Experimental Psychology
University of Ghent
Henri Dunantlaan 2
B-9000 Gent, Belgium
**Email:** andre.vandierundonck@rug.ac.be
**Website:** http://www.ulb.ac.be/assoc/escop
**Fnded:** 1985. **Mem:** 512. **Desc:** Stimulates research within the field of Cognitive Psychology and related subjects, particularly with respect to collaboration and exchange of information between researchers in different European countries. **Pub:** *European Journal of Cognitive Psychology*, quarterly. Journal.

### ★ 12474 ★ European Society for Communicative Psychotherapy
c/o The School of Psychotherapy and Counselling
Regent's College
Inner Cir.
Regent's Park
London, United Kingdom
**Phone:** 44 20 78477584     **Fax:** 44 20 78477446
**Email:** info@escp.org
**Desc:** Psychiatrists and psychotherapists in Europe.

### ★ 12475 ★ European Society of Handwriting Psychology (ESHP) (Europaische Gesellschaft fur Schriftpsychologie und Schriftexpertise — EGS)
Klebestrasse 6
Postfach 2077
CH-8041 Zurich, Switzerland
**Phone:** 41 1 4816218     **Fax:** 41 1 4816288
**Email:** egs_sekretariat@web.ch
**Website:** http://www.graphology-europe.com
**Fnded:** 1972. **Mem:** 468. **Nat'l Groups:** 10. **Lang(s):** English, French, German. **Desc:** Psychologists, psychiatrists, physicians, personnel consultants, criminal investigators, and university professors. **Pub:** *EGS-ESHP Bulletin*, annual. Newsletter.

### ★ 12476 ★ Families of Adults Afflicted with Asperger's Syndrome (FAAAS)
PO Box 514
Centerville, MA 02632-0514
**Phone:** (508)790-1930     **Fax:** (508)790-1930
**Email:** faaas@faaas.org
**Website:** http://www.faaas.org/
Karen E. Rodman, Pres. /Founder
**Fnded:** 1997. **Desc:** Provides support to family members of adult individuals afflicted with the neurological disorder, Asperger's Syndrome. Promotes public awareness to families and medical communities.

### ★ 12477 ★ Family Therapy Section of the National Council on Family Relations (FTSNCFR)
3989 Central Ave. NE, No. 550
Minneapolis, MN 55421
**Phone:** (763)781-9331     **Free:** 888-781-9331
**Fax:** (763)781-9348
**Email:** nikki@ncfr.org
**Website:** http://www.oakland.edu/~blume/ncfr/
**Fnded:** 1955. **Desc:** A section of the National Council on Family Relations. Practicing family therapists and family therapy supervisors, educators, and researchers. Seeks to improve the practice of family therapy through the development of theory, research, and training. Promotes communication between family therapy researchers and clinicians; functions as a network for family therapy research projects; conducts educational programs. **Frmly:** (1991) National Council on Family Relations Family Therapy Section.

### Federation of Families for Children's Mental Health (FFCMH)
*See:* Entry 5682

### ★ 12478 ★ Finnish Association for Mental Health (FAMH) (Suomen Mielenterveysseura)
Maistraatinportti 4 A
FIN-00240 Helsinki, Finland
**Phone:** 358 9 615516     **Fax:** 358 9 61551770
**Email:** ffcmh@ffcmh.org
**Website:** http://www.mielenterveysseura.fi
**Fnded:** 1897. **Mem:** 90. **Lang(s):** English, Finnish, German, Swedish. **Desc:** Voluntary organization for professional and lay people. Promotes mental health through programs of prevention. Introduces new procedures in voluntary and statutory mental health work. Provides support and crisis services; offers vocational training programs. Maintains 15 crisis centers. **Pub:** *Mielenterveys*, bimonthly. Includes mental health information. • *Perheterapia*, quarterly. Provides family therapy information. • Books. • Journals. • Newsletter, annual.

### ★ 12479 ★ First Steps to Freedom
7 Avon Ct.
School Lane
Kenilworth CV8 2GX, United Kingdom
**Phone:** 44 1926 864473     **Fax:** 44 870 1640567
**Email:** info@firststeps.demon.co.uk
**Website:** http://www.firststeps.demon.co.uk
**Fnded:** 1991. **Mem:** 1,500. **Desc:** People who suffer from phobias, panic attacks, general anxiety, obsessive compulsive disorders, and tranquilizer withdrawal. Makes available telephone help line, support groups, relaxation audio tapes. Conducts educational programs. **Pub:** *NWL*, quarterly.

### ★ 12480 ★ French-Language Association of Scientific Psychology (Association de Psychologie Scuentifique de Langue Francaise — APSLF)
29, av R Schumann
F-13621 Aix-en-Provence, France
**Fax:** 33 4 542590312
**Fnded:** 1950. **Desc:** Stimulates contacts between psychologists using the French language.

### ★ 12481 ★ French-Language Society of Medical Psychology
95, bd Pinel
F-69677 Bron, France
**Phone:** 33 4 72358694     **Fax:** 33 4 72358593
**Fnded:** 1960.

### French-Speaking Neuropsychological Society (Societe de Neuropsychologie de Langue Francaise)
*See:* Entry 14009

### ★ 12482 ★ General Hypnotherapy Registry
Hazelwood Broadmead
Sway Lymington
Lymington S041 6DH, United Kingdom
**Phone:** 44 1590 683770     **Fax:** 44 1590 683770
**Email:** admin@general-hypnotherapy-register.com
**Website:** http://www.general-hypnotherapy-register.com
**Fnded:** 1971. **Mem:** 750. **Desc:** Counselors and therapists, mainly offering short-term treatment in private practice. Most members offer hypnotherapy as their main method of treatment. To represent and protect the interests of independent therapists and hypnotherapists. To provide referrals lists of practitioners in which the public may have full confidence by maintaining high standards of practice and conduct among members. Provides register of practitioners. **Pub:** Bulletin, bimonthly. **Frmly:** (1997) National Council of Psychotherapists and Hypnotherapy Register; (2000) National Council of Psychotherapists.

### ★ 12483 ★ German Academy for Psychoanalysis (GAP) (Deutsche Akademie fur Psychoanalyse — DAP)
c/o Maria Ammon
Goethestrasse 54
D-80336 Munich, Germany
**Phone:** 49 89 539674     **Fax:** 49 89 5328837
**Fnded:** 1969. **Mem:** 90. **Lang(s):** English, German. **Desc:** Psychoanalysts, psychiatrists, and psychotherapists in Germany. Promotes training and research in psychoanalysis and psychotherapy within the framework of "dynamic psychiatry" as developed by the group's former president, Gunter Ammon. **Pub:** *Dynamic Psychiatry*, bimonthly. Journal. • *Handbook of Dynamic Psychiatry*. Handbook.

### German Association of Sport Psychology
*See:* Entry 19157

### ★ 12484 ★ German Group Psychotherapeutic Society (GGPS) (Deutsche Gruppenpsychotherapeutische Gesellschaft — DGG)
c/o Dr. Dorothy Doldinger
Kantstrabe 120-121
D-10625 Berlin, Germany
**Phone:** 49 30 3132698     **Fax:** 49 30 3136959
**Email:** dgg@dynpsych.de
**Website:** http://www.uni-leipzig.de/~asp/english
**Fnded:** 1968. **Mem:** 150. **Lang(s):** German. **Desc:** Group psychotherapists and experts in group dynamics. Practices in the field of prevention based on the concept of psychoanalytical group dynamics of the Berlin School founded by Dr. G. Ammon. Conducts research and therapy sessions; provides training to individuals interested in group dynamics. Holds group dynamic weekends. **Pub:** *Dynamic Psychiatry*, bimonthly.

### ★ 12485 ★ German Society for Humanistic Psychology (Deutsche Gesellschaft fur Humanistische Psychologie)
Schubbendenweg 4
D-52249 Eschweiler, Germany
**Phone:** 49 2403 4726     **Fax:** 49 2403 20447
**Fnded:** 1972. **Mem:** 60. **Desc:** Psychologists and laypeople. Serves as a network for the development of human sciences in ways that recognize distinctive human qualities and work toward fulfilling the innate capacities of people, both as individuals and in society. Works to link individuals holding a humanistic vision of the person, and to encourage others to share this view. **Pub:** *Humanistiche Psychologie Halbjehrbuch*, semiannual. Journal.

### ★ 12486 ★ Group for the Advancement of Psychiatry (GAP)
PO Box 28218
Dallas, TX 75228
**Phone:** (972)613-3044     **Fax:** (972)613-5532
**Website:** http://www.groupadpsych.org/
Frances Roton, Contact
**Fnded:** 1946. **Mem:** 300. **Desc:** Independent group of psychiatrists organized in working committees interested in applying the principles of psychiatry toward the study of human relations. Works closely with specialists in many other disciplines. Investigates such subjects as school desegregation, use of nuclear energy, religion, psychiatry in the armed forces, mental retardation, cross-cultural communication, medical

uses of hypnosis, and the college experience. Maintains 25 committees. **Pub:** Reports.

★ **12487** ★ **Group-Analytic Society**
258 Belize Rd.
London NW6 4BT, United Kingdom
**Phone:** 44 207 3161824    **Fax:** 44 207 3161880
**Email:** info@groupanalyticsociety.org
**Fnded:** 1952. **Mem:** 600. **Desc:** Group-analysts, doctors, psychiatrists, professors, educationalists, caring professions. Receives and administers funds to be used for the promotion and development of group analysis as a treatment, prophylaxis and science; its advancement through study, research and teaching, and the provision of advisory services, lectures and publications. **Pub:** *Journal - Group Analysis*, quarterly. Journal.

★ **12488** ★ **Guild of Psychotherapists**
47 Nelson Sq.
London SE1 0QA, United Kingdom
**Phone:** 44 181 5404454    **Fax:** 44 181 5405483
**Email:** guild@psycho.org.uk
**Website:** http://www.psycho.org.uk
**Fnded:** 1974. **Mem:** 170. **Lang(s):** French, German, Greek, Hebrew, Spanish. **Desc:** Qualified and registered psychoanalytic psychotherapists practising in London and all parts of the country. Aims to train psychoanalytic psychotherapists and to offer a clinical referral service with qualified psychotherapists in all areas of the country. Reduced fees available.

★ **12489** ★ **Hellenic Psychological Society (HPS)**
Psychological Laboratory
Aristotle University of Thessaloniki
GR-540 06 Thessaloniki, Greece
**Phone:** 30 310 997374    **Fax:** 30 310 997384
**Email:** efklides@psy.auth.gr
**Desc:** Psychologists in Greece. Promotes the advancement of psychological study.

★ **12490** ★ **Hong Kong Alzheimer's Disease and Brain Failure Association**
c/o GF Wang Lai House
Wang Tau Hom Estate
Kowloon
Hong Kong, People's Republic of China
**Phone:** 852 27943010    **Fax:** 852 23384820
**Fnded:** 1995. **Lang(s):** English. **Desc:** Advocates improvement in services and resources for patients affected by dementia and their families. Works to increase public awareness; assists and provides sponsorship for local research.

★ **12491** ★ **Hungarian Psychological Association**
PO Box 220
H-1536 Budapest, Hungary
**Phone:** 36 1 3500555138   **Fax:** 36 1 3500555138
**Email:** vakata@izabell.elte.hu
**Website:** http://www.mpt.hu
**Desc:** Fosters increased knowledge regarding psychology through educational programs and conferences.

★ **12492** ★ **Indian Psychological Association**
J.L. Nehru Marg
New Delhi 110 002, India
**Phone:** 91 11 6447189
**Email:** satsang@mailcity.com

★ **12493** ★ **Indonesian Psychologist Association (Himpsi)**
Kebayoran Centre A16
12240 Jakarta, Indonesia
**Phone:** 62 21 7254040    **Fax:** 62 21 7254040
**Email:** pusat@himpsi.org

**Website:** http://www.himpsi.org
**Fnded:** 1959. **Mem:** 6,500. **Reg. Groups:** 10. **Lang(s):** English, Indonesian. **Desc:** Professors, researchers, and graduate students in psychology as well as psychologists in the Republic of Indonesia. Promotes the development of psychological sciences and professions in Indonesia.

★ **12494** ★ **The Information Exchange (TIE)**
120 N Main St.
New City, NY 10956
**Phone:** (845)634-0050    **Fax:** (845)634-1690
**Email:** bertpepper@aol.com
Bert Pepper, MD, Exec. Dir.
**Fnded:** 1983. **Desc:** Information dissemination for individuals with serious ongoing mental/emotional disorders. The psychiatric disorder may be a major mental illness or personality disorder, or a mixture of emotional problems with substance abuse or other disabilities. Goals are to gather information and effective program initiatives; to disseminate information to professionals and the public; to create an awareness of the needs of this population. Provides consultation and teaching about the patients and on effective ways of meeting their needs. Conducts presentations for professional and community groups. meeting their needs. Conducts presentations for professional and community groups. **Pub:** Bulletin, quarterly. **Frmly:** (1994) The Information Exchange on Young Adult Chronic Patients.

★ **12495** ★ **Institute for the Advancement of Human Behavior (IAHB)**
4370 Alpine Rd., Ste. 209
Portola Valley, CA 94028
**Phone:** (650)851-8411    **Free:** 800-258-8411
**Fax:** (650)851-0406
**Website:** http://www.ibh.com
G. W. Piaget, Pres.
**Fnded:** 1977. **Desc:** Continuing educational organization for health care professionals. Provides training opportunities in behavioral topics such as: the psychology of health care; human sexuality; brief therapy, PTSD, couples therapy, maintaining long-term health behaviors, and the role of imagery in health care. **Pub:** Audiotapes, periodic. **AKA:** Institute for Behavioral Healthcare.

★ **12496** ★ **Institute for Applied Psychology (IAP)**
Av de Stalingrad 23
1000 Brussels, Belgium
**Phone:** 32 2 5112411    **Fax:** 32 2 5117181
**Email:** kvonvietinghoff@skynet.be
**Fnded:** 1993.

★ **12497** ★ **Institute of Athletic Motivation (IAM)**
2308 Crystal Ct.
Antioch, CA 94509
**Phone:** (925)754-2828    **Free:** 800-288-2992
**Fax:** (925)978-1503
**Email:** winslowwri@aol.com
William J. Winslow, Pres.
**Fnded:** 1962. **Desc:** Originated by sports psychologists to: enhance the performance of athletes in competitive and recreational sports; enable coaches to better understand and coach athletes; provide athletes with self-knowledge for self-improvement and development. Prepares reports on athletic attitudes of athletes based on results of Athletic Motivation Inventory and Athletic Success Profile, written questionnaires prepared specifically for sports to measure 11 traits related to success: agressiveness, drive, determination, responsibility, leadership, self-confidence, emotional control, mental toughness, coachability, conscientiousness, and trust. Markets programs to high schools, colleges, amateur athletes, professional teams, and recreational athletes. Maintains software licensing program for sports organizations and consultants. Operates speakers' bureau. **AKA:** (2001) Athlet-

ic Success Institute. **Frmly:** (1971) Institute for Study of Athletic Motivation; (1998) Institute for Study of Athletic Motivation and Institute of Athletic Motivation.

★ **12498** ★ **Institute for the Development of Emotional and Life Skills/ National Institute of Relationship Enahancement (IDEALS)**
4400 East- West Hwy., Ste. 28
Bethesda, MD 20814
**Phone:** (301)986-1479    **Free:** 800-THE-NIRE
**Fax:** (301)680-3756
**Email:** niremd@nire.org
**Website:** http://www.nire.org
Dr. William Nordling, Exec. Dir.
**Fnded:** 1972. **Mem:** 12. **Desc:** Strives to develop and research effective programs for improving emotional and interpersonal skills and providing high-quality training and supervision for mental health professionals, managers, workers, and the public. Conducts training programs for professionals in the areas of mental health, health care, human services, education, and business; sponsors training programs for laypeople in the areas of improving interpersonal relations, problem solving, and effective functioning in family and in business settings. Offers programs for workers and managers in communication, goal planning, motivation, negotiation, stress and time management, personnel management, and supervision. **Pub:** *A Scriptural Guide to a Fulfilling Marriage.* • *Parenting: A Skills Training Manual.* • *Relationship Skills Manual.* • Bibliography.Contains training programs, research articles, books and films. **Frmly:** (2000) Institute for the Development of Emotional and Life Skills.

★ **12499** ★ **Institute for Expressive Analysis (IEA)**
205 W 89th
New York, NY 10024
**Phone:** (212)362-2167
Joel Gavriele Gold, Exec. Dir.
**Fnded:** 1976. **Mem:** 64. **Local Groups:** 1. **Desc:** Practicing art, dance, and music therapists, social workers, art teachers, and psychotherapists trained in expressive analysis (a psychotherapy that strives to develop the left and right brain activities to achieve body-mind integration and the mobilization of creative energies). Sponsors lectures and workshops for the public and professionals. Provides advanced courses leading to certification as associate, fellow, or full member of the institute. Maintains educational and counseling center. **Pub:** Journal, annual. **Frmly:** Center for Expressive Analysis; Center for Expressive Psychotherapy.

★ **12500** ★ **Institute of Group Analysis**
1 Daleham Gardens
London NW3 5BY, United Kingdom
**Phone:** 44 171 4312693    **Fax:** 44 171 4317246
**Email:** iga@igalondon.org.uk
**Website:** http://www.igalondon.org.uk
**Fnded:** 1971. **Mem:** 300. **Desc:** Counsellors, social workers, psychologists, psychiatrists, caring professionals, probation officers. Responsible for the establishment of a widely recognised professional qualification in group-analytic psychotherapy. The principal aim is to promote and forward the selection, education and training of persons in order to qualify them for the conduct and study of group analysis and related forms of psychotherapy. **Pub:** *Dialogue*, 4 times a month. Newsletter.

**Institute for Labor and Mental Health (ILMH)**
*See:* Entry 16776

★ **12501** ★ **Institute for Mental Health Initiatives (IMHI)**
2175 K St., NW, Ste. 700
Washington, DC 20037

**Phone:** (202)467-2285 **Fax:** (202)467-2289
**Email:** imhi-info@gwumc.edu
**Website:** http://www.gwumc.edu/sphhs/imhi/
Suzanne Stutman, Pres.

**Fnded:** 1982. **Desc:** Uses a public health approach to promote mental health and prevent emotional disorders. Seeks to transform complex mental health concepts into positive models of human interaction. Gathers knowledge derived from clinical and research findings on good mental health, which it then adapts for use by the media, educators, health and mental health professionals, community leaders, and parents. Conducts meetings and workshops; consults with media professionals; creates training videos, discussion guides, and public service announcements. Works to influence perceptions and attitudes through the power of commercial mass media. **Pub:** *Dialogue*, quarterly. Newsletter. Provides information on human emotions for media professionals. *Price:* $30. • *Exploring First Feelings.* Video. • *Intiatives*, quarterly. Newsletter. Reports on current issues and new developments in mental health. • *The Rethink Workout for Teens: Learning to Manage Anger.* Video. • *Take Another Look: Learning to Rethink Anger.* Video. • *The Violence Framework: Guidelines for Understanding, Reporting, and Portraying Violence.* Handbook. • *What Do You Tell the Children? How to Help Children Deal with Disasters.* Handbook.

**★ 12502 ★ Institute of Mental Health Research and Postgraduate Training**
35 Poplar Rd.
Parkville, VIC 3052, Australia
**Fnded:** 1955.

**★ 12503 ★ Institute on Psychiatric Services/American Psychiatric Association**
1400 K St. NW
Washington, DC 20005
**Phone:** (202)682-6314 **Free:** 888-357-7924
**Fax:** (202)682-6850
**Email:** apa@psych.org
**Website:** http://www.psych.org
Jill L. Gruber, Coord.

**Fnded:** 1949. **Desc:** Annual meeting sponsored by the American Psychiatric Association. Open to employees of all psychiatric and related health and educational facilities. Includes lectures by experts in the field and workshops and accredited courses on problems, programs, and trends. Offers on-site Job Bank, which lists opportunities for mental health professionals. Organized scientific exhibits. **Pub:** *Psychiatric Services*, monthly. Journal. *Price:* $45/individuals; $75/institutions; $22.50/students. **Frmly:** (1995) Institute on Hospital and Community Psychiatry.

**★ 12504 ★ Institute of Psychiatry**
c/o University of London
De Crespigny Park
Denmark Hill
London SE5 8AF, United Kingdom
**Phone:** 44 171 7035411

**Fnded:** 1948. **Desc:** To promote excellence in the research, development and teaching of psychiatry and its allied subjects and to apply and disseminate this knowledge through the development of treatment for the relief of suffering. **Pub:** Annual Report, annual.

**★ 12505 ★ Institute of Psychosexual Medicine**
12 Chandos St.
Cavendish Sq.
London W1G 9DR, United Kingdom
**Phone:** 44 207 5800631 **Fax:** 44 207 5800631
**Email:** ipm@telinco.co.uk
**Website:** http://www.ipm.org.uk

**Fnded:** 1974. **Mem:** 450. **Desc:** Medical practitioners only. Seeks to promote the study and practice of psychosexual medicine through seminar training and research. **Pub:** *Journal of the Institute of Psychosocial Medicine*, 3/year. Journal.

**★ 12506 ★ Institute of Social Psychiatry**
c/o Sutton Manor Clinic
London Rd.
Stapleford Tawney
Romford RM4 1SR, United Kingdom
**Phone:** 44 1992 814661 **Fax:** 44 1708 688583

**Fnded:** 1947. **Desc:** Aims to further and finance, if feasible, research into psychiatry. Runs a nursing home for elderly mentally handicapped. The Institute of Social Psychiatry is a Registered Charity.

**★ 12507 ★ Institute of Transactional Analysis**
6 Princes St.
Oxford OX4 1DD, United Kingdom
**Phone:** 44 186 5728012 **Fax:** 44 186 5728012
**Email:** admin@ita.org.uk
**Website:** http://www.ita.org.uk

**Fnded:** 1973. **Mem:** 900. **Desc:** Professional members, qualified to teach and supervise the practice of TA. Certified TA analysts and trainee TA analysts. Also those interested in TA. Promotes and maintains the practice of TA, sets and maintains standards of professional practice and training. **Pub:** *ITA News*, quarterly.

**★ 12508 ★ International Academy of Behavioral Medicine, Counseling and Psychotherapy (IABMCP)**
12830 Hillcrest Rd., Ste. 111
Dallas, TX 75230-1517
**Phone:** (972)437-3370 **Fax:** (972)437-1190
**Website:** http://www.iabmcp.org
George Mount, Exec. Sec.

**Fnded:** 1988. **Mem:** 1,100. **Desc:** Psychologists, psychiatrists, physicians, social workers, health care specialists, educators, and others in the field of behavioral medicine. Provides liaison between members and other health professionals and disciplines; educates the public and health professionals about the benefits of behavioral medicine; assists in developmental training guidelines for behavioral medicine practice; develops guidelines for implementation of behavioral medicine for the American Psychological Association and other organizations. Disseminates behavioral/biomedical information; sponsors continuing education program. **Pub:** *American Academy of Behavioral Medicine–Newsletter*, quarterly. Newsletter. *Price:* Included in membership dues. • *Membership Roster*, annual. • Journal, 1-3/year.

**International Association for Child and Adolescent Psychiatry and Allied Professions (IACAPAP)**
*See: Entry 5691*

**★ 12509 ★ International Association of Counselors and Therapists (IACT)**
10915 Bonita Beach Rd., Ste. 1101
Bonita Springs, FL 34135-9049
**Phone:** (941)498-9710 **Fax:** (941)498-1215
**Email:** iactnow@aol.com
**Website:** http://www.iact.org
Jillian R. LaVelle, Pres.

**Fnded:** 1990. **Mem:** 7,000. **Desc:** Mental health professionals, medical professionals, social workers, clergy, educators, hypnotherapists, counselors, and individuals interested in the helping professions. Promotes enhanced professional image and prestige for complementary therapy. Provides a forum for exchange of information and ideas among practitioners of traditional and nontraditional therapies and methodologies; fosters unity among "grassroots" practitioners and those with advanced academic credentials. Facilitates the development of new therapy programs. Conducts educational, research, and charitable programs. Awards credits for continuing education. Maintains speakers' bureau and library; operates referral and placement services; compiles statistics. Assists in the development of local chapters. **Pub:** *Unlimited Human!*, quarterly. Magazine. Includes health and wellness articles. *Price:* Included in membership dues.

**★ 12510 ★ International Association for Cross-Cultural Psychology (IACCP)**
c/o Klaus Boehnke, Sec.Gen.
Chemnitz University of Technology
2000-2004
Department of Sociology
D-09107 Chemnitz, Germany
**Phone:** 49 371 5313925 **Fax:** 49 371 5314450
**Email:** klaus.boehnke@phil.tu-chemnitz.de
**Website:** http://www.iaccp.org

**Fnded:** 1972. **Mem:** 700. **Reg. Groups:** 6. **Lang(s):** English. **Desc:** Serves as a forum for exchanges among psychologists and other researchers who are interested in comparative research into human behavior and experience. Pursues the universal validity of psychological theories in all branches of psychology and related disciplines. **Pub:** *Cross-Cultural Psychology Bulletin*, quarterly. Bulletin. Contains news of IACCP, brief reports, and other items of interest. • *Cross-Cultural Psychology Monographs*, semiannual. Monograph. • *Journal of Cross-Cultural Psychology*, bimonthly. Journal. • Proceedings, biennial.

**★ 12511 ★ International Association of Eating Disorders Professionals (IAEDP)**
PO Box 196459
Winter Springs, FL 32719
**Phone:** (407)831-7099 **Free:** 800-800-8126
**Fax:** (407)831-2661
**Email:** info@iaedp.com
**Website:** http://www.iaedp.com
Dr. Marie Shafe, Exec. Dir.

**Fnded:** 1985. **Mem:** 800. **Desc:** Eating disorders counselors, specialists, and associates. Establishes and develops curricula; operates and implements a system for certifying eating disorders specialists and associates; provides public education and information on eating disorders. Offers professional consulting and assistance to the medical community, hospitals, courts, law enforcement agencies, schools, churches, and social welfare agencies. Facilitates networking among members; makes available employment opportunity information. Sponsors workshops; maintains speakers' bureau and annual symposia. **Pub:** *Clinical Quorum. Price:* Included in membership dues. • Bulletin, monthly. Contains association news and activities and certification update. *Price:* included in membership dues. • Also publishes certification manual and curriculum for higher education.

**★ 12512 ★ International Association of French-Language Labor Psychology (Association Internationale de Psychologie du Travail de Langue Francais — AIPTLF)**
Pr. Claude Lemoine-Aiptlf
Universite Lille 3, VFR Psychologie
BP 149
F-76821 Villeneuve d'Ascq Cedex, France
**Phone:** 33 3 20116315 **Fax:** 33 3 20116324
**Email:** lemoine@univ-lille3.fr

**Fnded:** 1980. **Lang(s):** English, French. **Desc:** French-speaking psychologists specializing in labor psychology. Seeks to advance scholarship and practice in the field of labor psychology. Facilitates exchange of information among members; sponsors research and training programs. **Pub:** *Psychologie du Travail et des Organisations*, quarterly. Journal. • *Top-Actualite.* Newsletter.

**★ 12513 ★ International Association of Group Psychotherapy (IAGP)**
c/o D. Mattke
Auf Der Steige 5
D-53129 Bonn, Germany
**Phone:** 49 228 232897 **Fax:** 49 228 232897
**Email:** djmattke@aol.com
**Website:** http://www.psych.mcgill.ca/labs/iagp/IAGP.html

**Fnded:** 1954. **Mem:** 800. **Desc:** Physicians, psychologists, social workers, nurses, and mental health workers in 32 countries interested in group psychotherapy.

Seeks to further communication and education between professionals in the practice and study of group psychotherapy. **Pub:** *Forum*, quarterly. Articles and member information. • Directory, triennial.

**★ 12514 ★ International Association for the History of Psychoanalysis (IAHP)**
8, rue du Commandant Mouchotte
F-75014 Paris, France
**Phone:** 33 1 40478933    **Fax:** 33 1 40470449
**Email:** aihp@magic.fr
**Website:** http://www.aihp-iahp.com/
**Fnded:** 1985. **Desc:** Promotes a thorough knowledge of the history of psychoanalysis and of its founder; bridges differences among national approaches to psychoanalysis and overcomes them through exposure.

**★ 12515 ★ International Association of Individual Psychology (IAIP)**
c/o Horst Groner
Marut Str. 12
D-99867 Gotha, Germany
**Phone:** 49 3621 401060    **Fax:** 49 3621 401060
**Email:** horst.groener@t-online.de
**Website:** http://www.iaiponline.org
**Fnded:** 1954. **Mem:** 26. **Lang(s):** English, French, German, Italian. **Desc:** Societies, associations, and institutes of Adlerian or Individual Psychology. Seeks to expand and deepen the scientific and practical aspects of Alfred Adler's (1870-1937) theory of Individual Psychology. Fosters cooperation and information exchange among members. **Pub:** *Directory and Constitution*, triennial. Directory.

**★ 12516 ★ International Association of Psychosocial Rehabilitation Services (IAPSRS)**
601 N Hammonds Ferry Rd., Ste. A
Linthicum, MD 21090
**Phone:** (410)789-7054    **Fax:** (410)789-7675
**Email:** general@iapsrs.org
**Website:** http://www.iapsrs.org
Ruth A. Hughes, PhD, CEO
**Fnded:** 1976. **Mem:** 1,900. **Nat'l Groups:** 2. **Reg. Groups:** 2. **State Groups:** 32. **Local Groups:** 32. **Desc:** Individuals (1200) and organizations (700) serving adults with a psychiatric disability. Promotes the advancement of the role, scope, and quality of service designed to facilitate the readjustment into the community of the adults with psychiatric disabilities. Provides a forum for the exchange of ideas, experiences, and contributions to the field. Offers technical assistance to organizational members; sponsors regional training conferences. **Pub:** *PSR Connection*, quarterly. Newsletter. *Price:* Included in membership dues. • *Psychosocial Rehabilitation Journal*, quarterly. Journal. Includes calendar of events and research reports. *Price:* Included in membership dues. • *Weekly Email Report: What's New in Psyciatric Rehabilitation*. Newsletter. • Also publishes legislative bulletins, documents, and professional information.

**International Association of Spiritual Psychiatry (IASP)**
*See:* Entry 4276

**★ 12517 ★ International Balint Federation (IBF) (Federation Internationale Balint)**
c/o Dr. John Salinsky
32 Wentworh Hill
Wembley HA9 9SG, United Kingdom
**Phone:** 44 181 9042844
**Email:** info@essence-euro.org
**Website:** essence-euro.org
**Fnded:** 1975. **Lang(s):** English, French. **Desc:** Groups and corresponding members in 34 countries. Promotes group training and practice according to the principles of Michael Balint (1896-1970), psychiatrist and author. Studies the patient-physician relationship

on a psychosocial level and encourages improved psychological training and research in practice.

**★ 12518 ★ International Committee Against Mental Illness (ICAMI)**
PO Box 1921, Grand Central Sta.
New York, NY 10163-1921
**Phone:** (212)263-6214    **Fax:** (212)263-8135
**Email:** rc31@nyu.edu
Dr. Robert Cancro, Pres.
**Fnded:** 1958. **Desc:** Fosters psychosocial rehabilitation and mental health research, services, and information systems. Provides technical assistance to professional rehabilitation organizations in expanding or installing computer information systems in psychiatry and in planning workshops, symposia, and conferences. Organizes international consortium of voluntary agencies and rehabilitation groups. Conducts research; operates speakers' bureau. Has worked on projects in Colombia, Indonesia, Iran, Israel, Kuwait, Liberia, Nepal, Pakistan, and Yugoslavia. The committee is a direct outgrowth of a pioneering psychiatric treatment project in Haiti that is now operated by the Haitian government.

**★ 12519 ★ International Federation of Psychoanalytic Societies (IFPS)**
c/o Dr. Sonia Gojman
Callejon del Horno No. 6
04000 Villa Coyoacan, Mexico
**Phone:** 525 5546383    **Fax:** 525 5540925
**Email:** sgojman@yahoo.com
**Website:** http://www.ifp-s.org
**Fnded:** 1962. **Mem:** 22. **Lang(s):** English, German, Spanish. **Desc:** Psychoanalytic societies in 13 countries. Promotes interest in psychoanalytic theory; encourages information exchange and discussion; fosters practice of psychoanalytic theory. **Pub:** *International Federation of Psychoanalytic Societies–Membership Directory*, periodic. Directory. • *International Forum of Psychoanalysis*, quarterly. Journal. • *Papers*, periodic.

**★ 12520 ★ International Organization of Psychophysiology (IOP) (Organisation Internationale de Psychophysiologie — IOP)**
Douglas Hospital, McGill University
6875 LaSalle Blvd.
Montreal, QC, Canada H4H 1R3
**Phone:** (514)761-6131    **Fax:** (514)762-3031
**Email:** iop@iop-world.org
**Website:** http://www.iop-world.org
**Fnded:** 1982. **Nat'l Groups:** 45. **Lang(s):** English, French. **Desc:** Scientists who hold a Ph.D., M.D., or equivalent degree and who specialize in psychophysiology or one of the neurosciences. (Psychophysiology is the study of the physiology of the psychic functions through the brain-body-behavior interrelationships of the living organism in conjunction with the environment.) Undertakes and promote psychophysiological research, teaching, and applications worldwide. Seeks to develop guidelines for the improvement of the human psychophysiological condition throughout the world. Disseminates information on subjects including aggression and defense, evolution and development of behavior, information processing, interhemispneric relations, learning and memory, motivation and emotion, and psychophysiological disorders. Collaborates with the United Nations and its specialized agencies with the aim of reinforcing international scientific cooperation in psychophysiology and related fields for the good of the human race. Maintains International Centre of Psychophysiology, providing research, practice, and training opportunities for qualified graduates; assists participants in becoming contemporary psychophysiologists. **Pub:** *International Journal of Psychophysiology*, monthly. Journal. • *IOP Newsletter*, quarterly. Newsletter.

**★ 12521 ★ International Psycho-Oncology Society (IPOS)**
1242 Second Ave.
New York, NY 10021
**Phone:** (212)639-3919    **Fax:** (212)717-3763
**Email:** info@ipos-aspboa.org
**Website:** http://www.ipos-aspboa.org
Uwe Koch, MD,PhD, Contact
**Desc:** Addresses the two major psychological dimensions of cancer: the psychological response of patients to cancer and the behavioral and social factors that influence risk, detection and survival.

**★ 12522 ★ International Psychoanalytical Association (IPA) (Association Psychanalytique Internationale)**
Broomhills
Woodside Ln.
London N12 8UD, United Kingdom
**Phone:** 44 208 4468324    **Fax:** 44 208 4454729
**Email:** ipa@ipa.org.uk
**Website:** http://www.ipa.org.uk
**Fnded:** 1910. **Mem:** 10,100. **Nat'l Groups:** 62. **Reg. Groups:** 1. **Lang(s):** English, French, German, Spanish. **Desc:** Organizations in 30 countries involved in psychoanalysis. Encourages communication among members and promotes high educational standards. Organizes training programs, conferences, and gives research grants. **Pub:** *Bulletin*, annual. Bulletin. • *Information Booklet*, periodic. Booklet. • *Newsletter*, semiannual. Newsletter. • *Roster*, annual. • Monographs, annual.

**International Psychogeriatric Association (IPA)**
*See:* Entry 2980

**★ 12523 ★ International REST Investigators Society (IRIS)**
c/o Thomas H. Fine
Medical College of Ohio
Department of Psychiatry
Toledo, OH 43614
**Phone:** (419)383-5695    **Fax:** (419)383-3031
**Email:** tfine@mco.edu
**Website:** http://www.ipa-online.org
Thomas H. Fine, Pres.
**Fnded:** 1983. **Desc:** Scientists and individuals interested in exploring the psychophysiological effects of floating. Serves as an information exchange for researchers, therapists, and individuals interested in restricted environmental stimulation techniques (REST). (Restricted environmental stimulation techniques include methods of producing a relaxed environment to create changes in consciousness and behavior such as floatation or isolation tanks.) Clinically, REST is being used in conjunction with relaxation training, biofeedback, psychotherapy, and a variety of stress-related disorders. Organizes meetings where members and other interested individuals can communicate current interests, exchange ideas and suggestions, and form collaborative research groups. **Pub:** *REST and Self-Regulation Conference Proceedings*, periodic. • Bulletin, 3/year. • Also publishes bibliography.

**★ 12524 ★ International Rorschach Society (IRS) (Societe Rorschach Internationale)**
c/o Ms. Trudi Finger, Treas.
c/o Hans Huber Publishers
Langgass-Strasse 76
CH-3000 Bern 9, Switzerland
**Phone:** 41 31 3004500    **Fax:** 41 31 3004590
**Email:** webmaster@rorschach.com
**Website:** http://www.rorschach.com
**Fnded:** 1948. **Mem:** 1,700. **Lang(s):** English, French, Italian, Spanish. **Desc:** Societies (12) and individuals (76). Develops international contacts between Rorschach specialists and other interested individuals;

promotes theoretical and practical knowledge of Rorschach and other projective techniques. (Rorschach test, named after Hermann Rorschach, a Swiss psychiatrist, is a test in which personality characteristics are made accessible to analysis by the subject's interpretation of the nature and meaning of a series of standard inkblot patterns.) Organizes regional and international meetings. Conducts research. **Pub:** *Bulletin of the International Rorschach Society*, annual. Bulletin. • *Rorschachiana*, triennial. Yearbook. Includes congress proceedings.

★ **12525** ★ **International School Psychology Association**
Hans Knudsens Plads 1A, 1st Floor
DK-2100 Copenhagen, Denmark
**Phone:** 45 44982106          **Fax:** 45 39293700
**Email:** ispa-denmark@web4you.dk
**Website:** http://www.ispaweb.org/
**Fnded:** 1974. **Desc:** Promotes communication between professionals committed to improvement of mental health of children.

★ **12526** ★ **International Society of Analytical Trilogy (ISAT)**
**(Sociedade Internacional de Trilogia Analitica)**
Avenida Reboucas 3819
05401-450 Sao Paulo, SP, Brazil
**Phone:** 55 11 2103616
**Website:** http://www.trilogiaanalitica.com.br
**Fnded:** 1970. **Mem:** 762. **Nat'l Groups:** 9. **Reg. Groups:** 6. **Lang(s):** English, French, German, Portuguese, Spanish. **Desc:** Accredited psychoanalysts having scientific training in Brazil, England, Finland, Portugal, and Sweden; individuals with a medical, human, or social science degree who are currently studying analytical trilogy; students working with accredited analysts. Promotes analytical trilogy, a form of psychoanalysis that uses dialogue to cure mental as well as physical illness through a technique called interiorization. (Also known as integral psychoanalysis, analytical trilogy was founded by Prof. Norberto R. Keppe as a continuation of the psychoanalytical discoveries of Sigmund Freud and his colleagues.) Conducts research and therapy for treatment of emotional and psychosomatic problems and encourages study of humanistic culture in all its forms including social, philosophical, religious, educational, and artistic. Promotes scientific investigation of psychoanalysis, philosophy, and theology. Fosters training in the integral psychoanalytical and trilogical fields. Activities include: group and individual analysis for treating neurosis, psychosis, and organic illness without drugs; children's services; radio and television programs; introductory courses for the public. Operates publishing company, bookshop, and cultural center. Is currently organizing a collection of case studies including written declarations, X-rays, medical examination data, and documented results obtained through the use of analytical trilogy. **Pub:** *Integral Psychoanalysis Magazine*, semiannual. Magazine. • *Trilogy*, quarterly. • Bulletin, monthly. Also publishes booklets and books. **Frmly:** (1982) Society of Integral Psychoanalysis.

★ **12527** ★ **International Society of Art and Psychopathology**
**(Societe Internationale de Psychopathologie de l'Expression — SIPE)**
27, rue du Marechal Joffre
F-64000 Pau, France
**Phone:** 33 5 9276974          **Fax:** 33 5 9276974
**Fnded:** 1959.

★ **12528** ★ **International Society of Behavioral Medicine**
Blegdamsvej 3
DK-2200 Copenhagen, Denmark
**Phone:** 45 35327965
**Email:** p.due@socmed.ku.dk

**Website:** http://www.isbm.miami.edu/

★ **12529** ★ **International Society for Comparative Psychology (ISCP)**
PO Box 1897
Lawrence, KS 66044-8897
**Phone:** (913)843-1235          **Fax:** (913)843-1274
**Email:** rmmurphey@ucdavis.edu
**Website:** http://www.er.uquam.ca/nobel/iscp
Robert M. Murphey, Sec.
**Fnded:** 1983. **Mem:** 80. **Desc:** Psychologists, biologists, anthropologists, and neuroscientists who work in or are interested in comparative psychology. Aims: to promote the international development of comparative psychology; establish worldwide communication among comparative psychologists; encourage the study of the development and evolution of behavior. **Pub:** *Advances in Comparative Psychology*, semiannual. *Price:* $35. • *International Journal of Comparative Psychology*, quarterly. Journal. *Price:* Free to members; $95. • *ISCP Newsletter*, bimonthly. Newsletter.

★ **12530** ★ **International Society for Developmental Psychobiology (ISDP)**
c/o Dr. Robert Lickliter
Virginia Tech
Blacksburg, VA 24061-0436
**Phone:** (540)231-5346          **Fax:** (540)231-3652
**Email:** rsullivan@ou.edu
**Website:** http://www.isdp.org
Regina Sullivan, Sec.
**Fnded:** 1967. **Mem:** 335. **Desc:** Research scientists in the field of developmental psychobiology; biology and psychology students. Promotes research in the field of developmental psychobiology, the study of the brain and behavior throughout the life span and in relation to other biological processes. Stimulates communication and interaction among scientists in the field. Provides the editorship for the journal, *Development Psychobiology*. Compiles statistics. **Pub:** *Developmental Psychobiology*, bimonthly. Journal. Addresses the anatomical, physiological, biochemical, hormonal, pharmacological, genetic, and evolutionary aspects of behavioral development. *Price:* Included in membership dues. • Membership Directory, every 1-2 years. • Newsletter, 2-3/year.

★ **12531** ★ **International Society for Ecological Psychology (ISEP)**
c/o William M. Mace
Department of Psychology
300 Summit St.
Hartford, CT 06106-3100
**Phone:** (860)297-2343          **Fax:** (860)297-2538
**Email:** william.mace@mail.trincoll.edu
William M. Mace, Contact
**Fnded:** 1981. **Mem:** 330. **Nat'l Groups:** 7. **Desc:** Promotes ecological psychology. **Pub:** *Ecological Psychology: The Journal*, quarterly. Journal. • *Resources for Ecological Psychology*.

★ **12532** ★ **International Society for Music in Medicine (ISMM)**
**(Internationale Gesellschaft fur Musik in der Medizin)**
Paulmannshoher Str. 17
D-58515 Ludenscheid, Germany
**Phone:** 49 2351 9452260          **Fax:** 49 2351 94517
**Fnded:** 1982. **Mem:** 80. **Reg. Groups:** 1. **Lang(s):** English. **Desc:** Medical doctors, scientists, and music therapists. Initiates and coordinates interdisciplinary research into the psychological and physiological basis for and applications of music in medicine. **Pub:** *International Journal of Arts Medicine*, quarterly. Journal. • *Music Medicine, Vol. I, 1993*. Book. • *Music Medicine, Vol. 2, 1996*. Book. • *Music Medicine Vol 3, 1998*. Book.

★ **12533** ★ **International Society for Oneiric Mental Imagery Techniques (ISMIT)**
**(Societa Internazionale per le Techniche d'Imagerie Mentale Onirique)**
c/o Chez Mme Odile Dorkel, Pres.
56 rue Sedaive
F-75011 Paris, France
**Phone:** 33 1 01484681
**Email:** odile.dorkel@wanadoo.fr
**Website:** http://www.arbrevert.org
**Fnded:** 1966. **Mem:** 80. **Desc:** Fosters inquiry and interaction among researchers and practitioners of mental imagery techniques in psychotherapy. Conducts research on mental imagery psychotherapy; disseminates research results. Organizes seminars on psychotherapeutic practice. **Pub:** *Decentration*, periodic. • *Mental Imagery*. • *Vocabulary of Psychotherapies*. Additional publications available on request.

★ **12534** ★ **International Society of Political Psychology (ISPP)**
c/o Dana Ward, Exec. Dir.
ISPP Central Office
Pitzer College
1050 N Mills Ave.
Claremont, CA 91711
**Phone:** (909)621-8442          **Fax:** (928)395-2224
**Email:** ispp@pitzer.edu
**Website:** http://ispp.org/ispp/centraloffice.html
Dana Ward, Exec. Dir.
**Fnded:** 1978. **Mem:** 1,400. **Nat'l Groups:** 3. **Reg. Groups:** 8. **Desc:** Psychologists, psychiatrists, psychoanalysts, political scientists, historians, sociologists, economists, anthropologists, media representatives, and government officials. Promotes understanding and scientific interest in the relationship between psychological, political, social, and economic processes. Seeks to facilitate communication among members and to increase the quality and application of work in political psychology. Examines relationships between psychological and political events. Areas of interest include: political violence and terrorism; socialization and the media; human rights conflict resolution; bureaucracy negotiation and mediation; totalitarianism. Sponsors the Summer Institute in Political Psychology in conjunction with Ohio State University. Conducts panel discussions. **Pub:** *ISPPNews*, semiannual. Newsletter. Contains information on activities and news of the organization; includes availability of fellowships, grants, and visiting scholar programs. *Price:* Free for members. • *Political Psychology*, quarterly. Journal. Covers classics in political psychology, interdisciplinary foundations of political psychology, and issues in professional development.

**International Society of Psychiatric Mental Health Nurses (ISPN)**
*See:* Entry 5704

★ **12535** ★ **International Society of Psychology of Handwriting (ISPH)**
**(Societa Internazionale di Psicologia della Scrittura — SIPS)**
Istituto di Indagini Psicologiche
Corso XXII Marzo 57
I-20129 Milan, Italy
**Phone:** 39 2 70126489          **Fax:** 39 2 7491051
**Email:** uimpsico@tin.it
**Website:** http://www.uim-psico.org
**Fnded:** 1961. **Mem:** 192. **Reg. Groups:** 12. **Lang(s):** English, German, Spanish. **Desc:** Physicians, psychologists, psychiatrists, teachers, and others. Promotes study and research in the psychology of handwriting. Has prepared documentaries on the subject for classroom and public instruction. Offers children's services. **Pub:** *Albo dei Docenti e Specialisti dell'UIM*, semiannual. Newsletter. Contains information on activities, research, schedule of courses, and professional updates. • *Catalog of Publications*. Catalog. • Directory.

**★ 12536 ★ International Society for Psychophysics (ISP)**
c/o Prof. Ana Garriga-Trillo
Psychology Faculty
UNED
Ciudad Universitaria
E-28040 Madrid, Spain
**Website:** http://www.psy.ulaval.ca/~ispp/
**Fnded:** 1985. **Mem:** 114. **Lang(s):** English. **Desc:** Promotes research in psychophysics. **Pub:** *Fechner Day*, annual, same year as meeting. Book. Contains all contributions to the yearly meetings.

**International Society of Sports Psychology (ISSP)**
*See:* Entry 19160

**★ 12537 ★ International Society for the Study of Dissociation (ISSD)**
60 Revere Dr., Ste. 500
Northbrook, IL 60062
**Phone:** (847)480-0899    **Fax:** (847)480-9282
**Email:** issd@issd.org
**Website:** http://www.issd.org
Richard Koepke, Exec. Dir.
**Fnded:** 1982. **Mem:** 1,200. **Desc:** Promotes research and training in the identification and treatment of dissociative disorders. Supports international communications and cooperation among professional clinicians and investigators working in the field of dissociation. **Pub:** *ISSD Membership Directory*, periodic. Membership Directory. Ongoing electronic directory. • *ISSD News*, bimonthly. Newsletter. • *The Journal of Trauma and Dissociation*, quarterly. Journal. • *Standards of Practice Guidelines for treating Dissociative Identity Disorder in Adults. Price:* Included in membership dues; $5/additional copy for members; $10 for nonmembers. **Frmly:** International Society for the Study of Multiple Personalities and Dissociation.

**★ 12538 ★ International Society for the Study of Individual Differences (ISSID)**
c/o Dr. Alois Angleitner, Sec.Treas.
Department of Psychology
University of Bielefeld
Postfach 10 01 31
D-33501 Bielefeld, Germany
**Phone:** 49 521 1064540    **Fax:** 49 521 1066422
**Email:** matthegd@email.uc.edu
**Fnded:** 1983. **Mem:** 255. **Lang(s):** English. **Desc:** People with a university degree (or equivalent) who are contributing to the development of empirical and/or theoretical psychology of individual differences. Fosters research and the worldwide interchange of information relating to the individual differences in personality, temperament, intelligence, attitudes, abilities, moods, and psychopathology. **Pub:** *Personality and Individual Differences*. Journal.

**★ 12539 ★ International Society for Traumatic Stress Studies (ISTSS)**
60 Revere Dr., Ste. 500
Northbrook, IL 60062
**Phone:** (847)480-9028    **Fax:** (847)480-9282
**Email:** istss@istss.org
**Website:** http://www.istss.org
Rick Koepke, Exec. Dir.
**Fnded:** 1985. **Mem:** 2,500. **Desc:** Professionals who treat individuals suffering from traumatic stress. (Traumatic stress is a medical term applied to persons who experience severe mental or emotional reactions to extraordinary stressful situations such as war, crime, natural disasters, and high-stress occupations.) Conducts research in the treatment of these cases; disseminates information. Holds seminars. Bestows awards. **Pub:** *ISTSS Membership Directory*, annual. Membership Directory. *Price:* Not for sale, for members only. • *Journal of Traumatic Stress*, bimonthly. Journal. Reports on the latest findings and innovations in the study and treatment of those affected by traumatic stress. *Price:* $275 $275/year for nonmembers; $320/year for nonmembers (outside U.S.); $52/

year for personal subscription. • *Membership List*, periodic. *Price:* $61/year for personal subscription (outside U.S.); $500. • *Traumatic Stress Points*, quarterly. Newsletter. Contains book reviews, topical articles, and association news. *Price:* Included in membership dues; Included in membership dues. **Frmly:** Society for Traumatic Stress Studies.

**★ 12540 ★ International Transactional Analysis Association (ITAA)**
436 14th St. Ste. 1301
Oakland, CA 94612-2710
**Phone:** (510)625-7720    **Fax:** (510)625-7725
**Email:** itaa@itaa-net.org
**Website:** http://www.itaa-net.org
Gordon B. Hewitt, PhD, Pres.
**Fnded:** 1958. **Mem:** 2,500. **Desc:** Educational corporation of persons in medical and behavioral sciences, including psychiatrists, psychologists, social workers, nurses, educators, marriage and family counselors, clergy, and organizational consultants. Maintains standards of practice and teaching of transactional analysis, which involves group therapy, social dynamics, and personality theory based on analysis of the "transactions" or interactions between persons. (The book, *Games People Play*, covers basic transactional analysis theory; its author, Dr. Eric Berne, was ITAA founder.) **Pub:** *International Transactional Analysis Membership Directory*, annual. Contains alphabetical and geographical listing of members. *Price:* $10. • *ITAA Membership Directory*, annual. Membership Directory. • *Script*, 9/year. Newsletter. • *Transactional Analysis Journal*, quarterly. Journal. **Frmly:** (1961) San Francisco Social Psychiatry Seminar.

**★ 12541 ★ International Union of Psychological Science (IUPsyS)**
School of Psychology
University of Ottawa
145 Jean-Jacques Lussier
C.P. 450, Sta. A
Ottawa, ON, Canada K1N 6N5
**Phone:** (613)562-5800    **Fax:** (613)562-5169
**Email:** pritchie@uottawa.ca
**Website:** http://www.iupsys.org
**Fnded:** 1951. **Mem:** 66. **Lang(s):** English, French. **Desc:** National psychological societies and committees united for: the development of psychological science through exchange of ideas and scientific information; the exchange of scholars and students; the organization of international congresses of psychology; publication and documentation; cooperation with related scientific groups interested in the development of psychology as a discipline and a profession. Conducts educational programs and international research network project. **Pub:** *International Directory of Psychologists*, quinquennial. Directory. • *International Journal of Psychology*, bimonthly. Journal. Peer reviewed scholarly journal including International Platform.

**★ 12542 ★ Irish Psycho-Analytical Association**
89 Grosvenor Sq.
Rathmines
Dublin 6, Ireland
**Phone:** 353 1 4967288    **Fax:** 353 1 4978766
**Fnded:** 1942. **Mem:** 21. **Lang(s):** English. **Desc:** Practicing psychoanalysts and psychoanalytic psychotherapists. Represents members in dealings with government agencies, both Irish and within the European Union, and maintains standards of psychoanalytic practice in Ireland in conjunction with sister organizations.

**★ 12543 ★ Irish Society for Autism (ISA)**
Unity Bldg.
16/17 Lower O'Connell St.
Dublin 1, Ireland
**Phone:** 353 1 8744684    **Fax:** 353 1 8744224
**Email:** autism@isa.iol.ie

**Website:** http://www.iol.ie/~isal
**Fnded:** 1963. **Lang(s):** English, Irish. **Desc:** Individuals and organizations. Seeks to improve the quality of life of people with autism and their families. Makes available support and services; conducts educational and advocacy campaigns. **Pub:** Newsletter, bimonthly.

**★ 12544 ★ Israel Psychological Association (IPA)**
PO Box 11497
IL-61114 Tel Aviv, Israel
**Phone:** 972 3 5239393    **Fax:** 972 3 5230763
**Email:** psycho@zahav.net.il
**Website:** http://psychology.org.il
**Fnded:** 1958. **Mem:** 2,900. **Lang(s):** Hebrew. **Desc:** Psychologists in Israel. Promotes high ethical standards in patient treatment. Represents members' interests; disseminates information. **Pub:** *Psychologia*, semiannual. Journal. Contains local articles and publications.

**★ 12545 ★ Japanese Society of Adlerian Psychology (JSAP)**
c/o Adler Guild
Futaba Bldg. 3F
5-12-15 Nishi-Nakajima, Yodogawa
Osaka 532-0011, Japan
**Phone:** 81 6 63064699    **Fax:** 81 6 63060160
**Fnded:** 1984. **Mem:** 1,200. **Desc:** Individuals interesting in studying and developing the psychology of Alfred Adler.

**★ 12546 ★ Jean Piaget Society: Society for the Study of Knowledge and Development (JPSSSKD)**
Human Development
Larsen Hall 702
Harvard GS Education
Cambridge, MA 02138
**Phone:** (617)495-3614    **Fax:** (617)495-3626
**Email:** Kurt_Fischer@harvard.edu
**Website:** http://www.piaget.org
Kurt Fischer, Contact
**Fnded:** 1970. **Mem:** 500. **Desc:** Scholars, teachers, and researchers interested in exploring the nature of the developmental construction of human knowledge. Purpose is to further research on knowledge and development, especially in relation to the work of Jean Piaget (1896-1980), a Swiss developmentalist noted for his work in child psychology, the study of human development, and the origin and growth of human knowledge. Conducts small meetings and programs. **Pub:** *Genetic Epistemologist*, quarterly. Newsletter. Covers the nature of human knowledge. *Price:* Included in membership dues. • *Jean Piaget Symposium Series*, annual. *Price:* Included in membership dues; $80 for nonmembers. **Frmly:** (1989) Jean Piaget Society.

**★ 12547 ★ Karen Horney Clinic (KHC)**
329 E 62nd St.
New York, NY 10021
**Phone:** (212)838-4333    **Fax:** (212)838-7158
**Website:** http://www.karenhorneycenter.org
Dr. Giselle Galdi, Dir.
**Fnded:** 1955. **Desc:** Promotes psychoanalytic and psychotherapeutic treatment of individuals and groups focusing on the special problems of children, adolescents, victims of violent crimes, adult survivors of childhood sexual abuse, and persons with psychoneurotic and emotional problems. Named for Karen Horney (1885-1952), German/American psychoanalyst and author of several books on neurosis, psychoanalysis, and related topics. Conducts children's services. **Pub:** *American Journal of Psychoanalysis*, quarterly. Journal. • *Association for the Advancement of Psychoanalysis*, periodic. **Frmly:** (1979) Karen Horney Psychoanalytic Clinic.

**Klingenstein Third Generation Foundation**
*See:* Entry 5710

★ **12548** ★ **Korean Academy of Psychotherapists (KAP)**
c/o Dr. Rhee Dongshick
178-23 Song-buk dong
Song-buk-ku
Seoul 136-020, Republic of Korea
**Phone:** 82 2 7620273          **Fax:** 82 2 7659776
**Email:** sally@ktgf.org
**Website:** http://kap.kams.or.kr
**Fnded:** 1974. **Mem:** 150. **Local Groups:** 1. **Lang(s):** English, Korean. **Desc:** Psychiatrists and psychologists united to study and integrate the principles of psychoanalysis and psychotherapy with those of Eastern Tao. (Eastern Tao is based on Taoist, Confucian, and Buddhist philosophies.) Operates training program. Conducts research; maintains speakers' bureau; compiles statistics. **Pub:** *Eastern Tao and Western Psychotherapy.* • *KAP Membership Directory,* annual. Directory. • *KAP Newsletter,* monthly. Newsletter. • *Psychotherapy,* semiannual. Includes abstract in English. • *Psychotherapy Protocol,* monthly. Plans to publish case books.

★ **12549** ★ **Leadership Council for Mental Health, Justice and the Media**
191 Presidential Blvd., Ste. C-132
Bala Cynwyd, PA 19004
**Phone:** (610)664-5007          **Fax:** (610)664-5279
**Website:** http://www.leadershipcouncil.org
**Desc:** Scientists, clinicians, educators, legal scholars, journalists and public policy analysts. Promote psychological science and provide current materials and information for mental health issues.

★ **12550** ★ **Lithuanian Psychological Association**
Didlaukio Str. 47
2057 Vilnius, Lithuania
**Phone:** 370 2 761890          **Fax:** 370 2 761890
**Email:** irue.pociute@fsf.vu.lt
**Website:** http://www.psd.fsf.vu.it/lps/index.html
**Desc:** Psychologists in Lithuania. Promotes the advancement of psychological study.

★ **12551** ★ **London Association of Primal Psychotherapists**
West Hill House
6 Swains Ln.
London N6 6QS, United Kingdom
**Phone:** 44 207 2679616          **Fax:** 44 207 4820858
**Email:** info@lapp.org
**Website:** http://www.lapp.org
**Fnded:** 1986. **Mem:** 55. **Lang(s):** Croatian, French, German, Spanish. **Desc:** Student membership open to trainees; associate membership open to people with an interest in the field of psychotherapy; full membership open to those qualified to work as primal psychotherapists. Aims to refine and develop primal psychotherapy. To this end a four year training programme is run that is recognized by the United Kingdom Council for Psychotherapy. Also has a trust fund devoted to working with people facing life threatening illness.

★ **12552** ★ **Malta Union of Professional Psychologists**
PO Box 341
Valletta, Malta
**Email:** vcasl@educ.um.edu.mt
**Desc:** Psychologists in Malta. Promotes the advancement of psychological study.

★ **12553** ★ **Mental After Care Association (MACA)**
25 Bedford Sq.
London WC1B 3HW, United Kingdom
**Phone:** 44 207 4366194          **Fax:** 44 207 6371980
**Email:** maca-bs@maca.org.uk
**Website:** http://www.maca.org.uk
**Fnded:** 1879. **Mem:** 100. **Reg. Groups:** 3. **Lang(s):** English. **Desc:** MACA is a leading mental health charity providing high quality services in the community, hospitals and prisons. With up to 80 services throughout the country, we support more than 1,500 people with severe and enduring mental health needs and their carers. We work in partnership with health authorities, local authorities, housing associations and other voluntary agencies. **Pub:** *Annual Report.* • Pamphlets, periodic.

★ **12554** ★ **Mental Health Association of Ireland (MHAI)**
Mensana House
6 Adelaide St.
Dun Laoghaire, Dublin, Ireland
**Phone:** 353 1 2841166          **Fax:** 353 1 2841736
**Email:** info@mensana.org
**Website:** http://mhai.healthyirish.com
**Local Groups:** 90. **Lang(s):** English. **Desc:** Seeks to help those who are mentally ill and to promote positive mental health in Ireland. Works to provide various types of accommodation outside the hospital, to set-up workshops, to visit and befriend those affected, and to arrange social events.

★ **12555** ★ **Mental Health Corp.s of America (MHCA)**
1876-A Elder Ct.
Tallahassee, FL 32308
**Phone:** (850)942-4900
**Email:** twilliams@mhca.com
**Website:** http://www.mhca.com/2WhatIsMHCA.htm
**Desc:** Behavioral healthcare organizations. Strives to enhance the business performance of members, while preserving its social mission.

★ **12556** ★ **Mental Health Foundation**
20/21 Cornwall Terrace
London NW1 4QL, United Kingdom
**Phone:** 44 207 5357400          **Fax:** 44 207 5357474
**Email:** mhf@mhf.org.uk
**Website:** http://www.mentalhealth.org.uk
**Fnded:** 1949. **Desc:** Plays a vital role in pioneering new approaches to prevention, treatment and care. Allocates grants for research and community projects, contributes to public debate and strives to reduce the stigma attached to mental illness and learning disabilities.

★ **12557** ★ **Mental Health Media**
356 Holloway Rd.
London N7 6PA, United Kingdom
**Phone:** 44 20 77008171          **Fax:** 44 20 76860959
**Email:** info@mhmedia.com
**Website:** http://www.mhmedia.com
**Fnded:** 1965. **Lang(s):** German. **Desc:** Specializes in the use of the full range of communications media to promote understanding of mental health or learning difficulties issues from a user perspective in order to reduce discrimination and prejudice. Recently established a media bureau, which supports mental health service users in working with journalists, writers, and broadcasters to improve their coverage of mental health issues. Also acts as a production house for a full range of information publications, including videos and CDs, about mental health and learning difficulties issues from the user perspective. **Frmly:** Mental Health Film Council; (1996) Mental Health Media Council.

★ **12558** ★ **Mental Research Institute (MRI)**
555 Middlefield Rd.
Palo Alto, CA 94301
**Phone:** (650)321-3055          **Fax:** (650)321-3785
**Email:** mri@mri.org
**Website:** http://www.mri.org
Wendel Ray, Dir.
**Fnded:** 1959. **Desc:** Psychiatrists, psychologists, and licensed therapists skilled in the disciplines related to the behavioral sciences. Conducts research, training, and service programs in the field of human behavior, with special emphasis on the family as a social unit. Research programs are primarily funded by foundation grants and private donations. Offers year-long courses, short-term residency programs, and short- and long-term workshops on family therapy, brief therapy, narrative therapy, communication, and related subjects. Operates family-oriented and brief therapy-oriented sliding scale fee clinic, which also serves as a training and research base. Maintains speakers' bureau. Current research programs focus on longitudinal study of families of alcoholics, youth, violence, bullying, and pain management.

★ **12559** ★ **Midwestern Psychological Association (MPA)**
c/o Ralph Erber
DePaul University
Department of Psychology
2219 N Kenmore
Chicago, IL 60614
**Website:** http://www.ssc.msu.edu/~mpa/
**Mem:** 3,000. **Desc:** Psychological association, with interests in the physiology of vision to social stereotyping, from political psychology to medical psychology, from organizational behavior to children's language development, from memory to depression, from sex roles to drug addiction.

★ **12560** ★ **MIND - Mental Health Charity**
Granta House
15-19 Broadway
London E15 4BQ, United Kingdom
**Phone:** 44 20 85192122          **Fax:** 44 20 85221725
**Email:** contact@mind.org.uk
**Website:** http://www.mind.org.uk
**Fnded:** 1948. **Mem:** 1,700. **Reg. Groups:** 7. **Local Groups:** 208. **Lang(s):** English. **Desc:** Promotes mental health and encourages a better understanding of mental health problems. Seeks to eliminate the stigma associated with mental illness. Conducts research; disseminates information. Offers legal referral services. Sponsors charitable program. Maintains information service. Conducts training and educational courses and seminars. **Pub:** *Annual Report.* • *OpenMIND,* bimonthly. Magazine. • *Publications from MIND,* periodic. Catalog.

★ **12561** ★ **Mothers Against Munchausen Syndrome by Proxy Allegations (MAMA)**
1407 Ranch Dr.
Senatobia, MS 38668
**Fax:** (662)562-6669
**Website:** http://www.msbp.com/
**Desc:** Dedicated to ending accusations against parents from Munchausen Syndrome by Proxy (MSBP) allegations.

★ **12562** ★ **Multidisciplinary Association for Psychedelic Studies (MAPS)**
2105 Robinson Ave.
Sarasota, FL 34232
**Phone:** (941)924-6277          **Free:** 888-868-6277
**Fax:** (941)924-6265
**Email:** info@maps.org
**Website:** http://www.maps.org
Dr. Rick Doblin, Pres.
**Fnded:** 1986. **Mem:** 1,800. **Desc:** Promotes the development of beneficial, socially sanctioned uses of psychedelic drugs and marijuana. Helps researchers design, obtain government approval for, fund, conduct and report on psychedelic research in human volunteers; funds MDMA psychotherapy studies; facilitates research and FDA approval for marijuana to be prescribed for medical uses. **Pub:** *Maps Bulletin,* quarterly. Magazine. Contains reports on MAPS activities, current research and feature articles. *Price:* $10/ sample issue. • The Secret Chief: Conversations with a Pioneer of the Underground Psychedelic Therapy Movement.

**NADD - An Association for Persons with Developmental Disabilities and Mental Health Needs**
*See:* Entry 6887


**National Academy of Neuropsychology (NAN)**
*See:* Entry 14069


**★ 12563 ★ National Alliance for the Mentally III (NAMI)**
Colonial Place Three
2107 Wilson Blvd., Ste. 300
Arlington, VA 22201-3042
**Phone:** (703)524-7600          **Free:** 800-950-NAMI
**Fax:** (703)516-7238
**Email:** bobc@nami.org
**Website:** http://www.nami.org
Jerry Radke, Exec. Dir.
**Fnded:** 1979. **Mem:** 220,000. **State Groups:** 50. **Local Groups:** 1200. **Desc:** Nations leading organization dedicated to improving the lives of children and adults with severe mental illness through support, education, research, and advocacy. Focus includes schizophrenia, bipolar disorder, major depression, and anxiety disorder. **Pub:** *NAMI Advocate*, quarterly. Newsletter. *Price:* Included in membership dues. • Brochures. • Handbooks. • Newsletters.


**★ 12564 ★ National Alliance for Research on Schizophrenia and Depression (NARSAD)**
60 Cutter Mill Rd., Ste. 404
Great Neck, NY 11021
**Phone:** (516)829-0091          **Free:** 800-829-8289
**Fax:** (516)487-6930
**Email:** info@narsad.org
**Website:** http://www.mhsource.com/narsad.html
Constance Lieber, Pres.
**Fnded:** 1986. **Desc:** Raises funds for research on schizophrenia, depression, and other mental illnesses. **Pub:** *NARSAD Research*, quarterly. Newsletter. Highlights current scientific research. *Price:* Contribution.


**★ 12565 ★ National Association for the Advancement of Psychoanalysis (NAAP)**
80 8th Ave., Ste. 1501
New York, NY 10011-1501
**Phone:** (212)741-0515          **Fax:** (212)366-4347
**Email:** naap72@aol.com
**Website:** http://www.naap.org
Margery Quackenbush, Admin.
**Fnded:** 1972. **Mem:** 1,700. **Desc:** Psychoanalytic organizations and individual psychoanalysts from a variety of schools of psychoanalytic thought united for the advancement of psychoanalysis as a profession. Establishes standards for psychoanalytic training and works to improve its quality. Sets standards for certification of individual psychoanalysts; registers those who have met its training standards. **Pub:** *NAAP News*, quarterly. Covers institute, committee, and membership activities. Includes legislative news, calendar of events, and obituaries. *Price:* Included in membership dues; $12/year for nonmembers. • *Registry of Psychoanalysts*, annual. Directory. Lists qualified psychoanalysts and candidates-in-training. Includes list of member organizations and geographic index. *Price:* $15/copy. **Frmly:** (2000) National Association for the Advancement of Psychoanalysis and the American Accreditation in Psychoanalysis.


**★ 12566 ★ National Association of Anorexia Nervosa and Associated Disorders (ANAD)**
Box 7
Highland Park, IL 60035
**Phone:** (847)831-3438          **Fax:** (847)433-4632
**Email:** anad20@aol.com

**Website:** http://www.anad.org
Vivian Hanson Meehan, RN, Pres. /Founder
**Fnded:** 1976. **Desc:** Anorexics and bulimics, their families, health professionals, and others interested in the problems of anorexia nervosa and bulimia. Maintains chapters in 45 states, Canada, South Africa, Ghana, France, Italy, Puerto Rico, Argentina, England, Slovenia, Ireland, Switzerland, Colombia, Spain and Germany. Aims to: seek a better understanding of, prevent, and cure anorexia nervosa and associated eating disorders; educate the public and health professionals on illnesses relating to eating disorders and methods of treatment. Encourages and promotes research on the cause of eating disorders, methods of prevention, types of treatment and their effectiveness, and basic facts about victims. Acts as a resource center, compiling and providing information about eating disorders. Serves as an advocacy agency for those concerned with eating disorders. Works to end insurance discrimination against sufferers of eating disorders. Fights against the production, marketing, and distribution of dangerous diet aids and the use of misleading advertisements. Encourages and cosponsors local and regional meetings. Maintains speakers' bureau; provides children's services; compiles statistics. Conducts referral service, surveys, education, and early detection programs. Organizes selfhelp groups. **Pub:** *Working Together*, quarterly. Newsletter. *Price:* Included in membership dues. **Frmly:** (1980) Anorexia Nervosa and Associated Disorders.


**★ 12567 ★ National Association of Cognitive-Behavioral Therapists (NACBT)**
PO Box 2195
Weirton, WV 26062
**Phone:** (304)723-3982          **Free:** 800-853-1135
**Fax:** (304)723-3982
**Email:** nacbt@nacbt.org
**Website:** http://www.nacbt.org/
Aldo R. Pucci, Pres.
**Fnded:** 1995. **Desc:** Promotes and supports the teaching and practice of cognitive-behavior psychotherapy and to support those professionals and students seeking to practice it; sets standards for credentialing.


**★ 12568 ★ National Association of Counsellors, Hypnotherapists and Psychotherapists**
PO Box 719
Cambridge CB5 0NX, United Kingdom
**Phone:** 44 163 8741363          **Fax:** 44 163 8744190
**Email:** mail@nachp.org
**Website:** http://www.nachp.org
**Desc:** Aims to maintain a register of qualified therapists which is available to members of the public seeking treatment.


**★ 12569 ★ National Association of County Behavioral Health Directors (NACBHD)**
1555 Connecticut Ave. NW, Ste. 200
Washington, DC 20036
**Phone:** (202)234-7543          **Fax:** (202)462-9043
**Email:** lauren@nacbhd.org
**Website:** http://www.nacbhd.org
Lauren Wolfe, MS, Dep. Exec. Dir.
**Fnded:** 1996. **Mem:** 300. **Desc:** County/local behavioral health authorities responsible for the planning and delivery of mental health, developmental disabilities and substance abuse services and the state associations representing their interests. Promotes excellence in the delivery of county/local behavioral health services. **Pub:** *Consumer Viewpoints: Mental Health in America Update.* • *Mental Health in America: County Behavioral Health Authorities Speak Out.* • *NACBHD Bulletin*, bimonthly. Newsletter. Contains policy information, articles of interest on local programs, association announcements, and job bank. *Price:* for members.

**★ 12570 ★ National Association for Drama Therapy (NADT)**
733 15th St. NW, Ste. 330
Washington, DC 20005
**Phone:** (202)966-7409          **Fax:** (202)638-7895
**Email:** nadt@dmg-dc.com
**Website:** http://www.nadt.org
Rod Daniel, Contact
**Fnded:** 1979. **Mem:** 425. **Reg. Groups:** 2. **Desc:** Drama therapists (those trained in the therapeutic applications of creative drama and theatre) and others interested in the field of drama therapy, including those in the psychotherapy, rehabilitation, and education professions. (The association defines drama therapy as the intentional use of drama and theatrical processes to achieve the therapeutic goals of symptom relief, emotional and physical integration, and personal growth. It is used with individuals, groups, and families to maintain health and to treat emotional disorders, learning difficulties, geriatric problems, and social maladjustments.) Purposes are to: develop criteria and standards of training for drama therapists; maintain a system of registration and peer review; encourage research and development of professional training opportunities in drama therapy; represent the interests of members to legislative and regulatory agencies regarding the inclusion of drama therapy in mental health and education bills, state job lines, and insurance policies. Sponsors educational events; maintains speakers' bureau. **Pub:** *Dramascope*, semi-annual. Newsletter. Includes book reviews, calendar of events, employment listings, descriptions of treatment programs and methods, and commentaries and reports. *Price:* Included in membership dues. • *Membership List/Registry*, annual. • *Proceedings of Annual Conference*, annual. Proceedings. • Bibliography. • Monographs. • Survey. • Also publishes information on workshops and courses in drama therapy.


**★ 12571 ★ National Association for Poetry Therapy (NAPT)**
733 15th St. NW, Ste. 330
Washington, DC 20005
**Phone:** (202)966-2536          **Fax:** (202)638-7895
**Email:** napt@dmg-dc.com
**Website:** http://www.poetrytherapy.org
Nancy Scherlong, Pres.
**Fnded:** 1981. **Mem:** 380. **Reg. Groups:** 16. **Desc:** Psychiatrists, psychologists, social workers, teachers, nurses, librarians, occupational therapists, paraprofessionals, ministers, counselors, recreation and rehabilitation specialists, and poets and professors of English and psychology. Objective is to promulgate the principles and techniques of poetry therapy for healing and personal growth. (Poetry therapy is used with patients in a variety of mental states ranging from "normal neurosis" to acute psychosis, as well as the physically handicapped and the learning disabled. Methods of using poetry for therapy vary and include reading poems and encouraging clients to write their own poetry. The general purpose is to lead the person into talking or writing about himself or herself and bringing out emotions not previously shown or discussed). Sponsors two degrees in the field of poetry therapy: Certified Poetry Therapist (CPT) and Registered Poetry Therapist (RPT). **Pub:** *Journal of Poetry Therapy*, quarterly. Magazine. *Price:* Included in membership dues. • *NAPT Museletter*, 3/year. Includes training and conference information. *Price:* $15/year for nonmembers. • *Trainee's and Trainer's Guide. Price:* $20. **Frmly:** World Poetry Therapy Association; (1981) Association for Poetry Therapy.


**National Association of Postpartum Care Services**
*See:* Entry 18342


**National Association of Psychiatric Health Systems (NAPHS)**
*See:* Entry 11502

**National Association of Psychiatric Treatment Centers for Children (NAPTCC)**
*See:* Entry 5717

**★ 12572 ★ National Association for Rural Mental Health (NARMH)**
3700 W Division St., Ste. 105
Saint Cloud, MN 56301
**Phone:** (320)202-1820          **Free:** 800-809-5879
**Fax:** (320)202-1833
**Email:** narmh@facts.ksu.edu
**Website:** http://www.narmh.org
Donald Sawyer, Pres.
**Fnded:** 1977. **Mem:** 500. **Desc:** Mental health practitioners and administrators and others dedicated to improving mental health services in rural areas. Promotes effective rural mental health services. Promotes the use of services by rural community dwellers. **Pub:** *Rural Mental Health*, quarterly. Newsletter.

**★ 12573 ★ National Association of School Psychologists (NASP)**
4340 East West Hwy., Ste. 402
Bethesda, MD 20814
**Phone:** (301)657-0270          **Fax:** (301)657-0275
**Website:** http://www.nasponline.org
Charlie Deupree, Pres.
**Fnded:** 1969. **Mem:** 23,000. **Reg. Groups:** 5. **State Groups:** 51. **Desc:** School psychologists. Serves the mental health and educational needs of all children and youth. Encourages and provides opportunities for professional growth of individual members. Informs the public on the services and practice of school psychology, and advances the standards of the profession. Operates national school psychologist certification system. Sponsors children's services. **Pub:** *Communique Newspaper*, 8/year. Newspaper. • *School Psychology Review*, quarterly. Journal. • Catalog.Lists publications. • Monographs. • Reports.

**★ 12574 ★ National Association for Self Esteem**
2000 N Linden, N-234
Normal, IL 61761
**Free:** 800-488-NASE
**Email:** betty@selfesteem.org
**Website:** http://www.self-esteem-nase.org
**Desc:** Strives to integrate self-esteem within families, schools, and the workplace. **Pub:** *Self Esteem Today*. Magazine.

**★ 12575 ★ National Center for American Indian and Alaska Native Mental Health Research (NCAIANMHR)**
UCHSC Psychiatry Department
4455 E 12th Ave., Box. A011-13
Denver, CO 80220
**Phone:** (303)315-9232          **Free:** 800-820-9299
**Fax:** (303)315-9579
**Email:** billie.greene@uchsc.edu
**Website:** http://www.uchsc.edu/ai/ncaianmhr/
Billie K. Green, Journal Mgr.
**Fnded:** 1987. **Desc:** Faculty, staff, and research associates in the mental health field. Conducts and supports research on management, prevention, and investigation of mental illness among Native Americans and Alaska Natives. Assists organizations in conducting and implementing mental health research. Disseminates information and statistics to public. **Pub:** *Behavioral Health Issues Among American Indians and Alaska Natives: Explorations on the Frontiers of the Biobehavioral Sciences*. Monograph. *Price:* $20. • *Calling From the Rim: Suicidal Behavior Among American Indian and Alaska Native Adolescents*. Monograph. *Price:* $20. • *Journal of the National Center for American Indian and Alaska Native Mental Health Research*, 3/year. Journal. Includes empirical research, case studies, unpublished dissertations, and articles on behavioral and social health sciences. *Price:* Free on-line. • *Mental Health Programs for*

*American Indians: Their Logic, Structure and Function*. Monograph. *Price:* $20. • *New Directions in Prevention Among American Indian and Alaska Native Communities*. Monograph. *Price:* $14.95. • *The People Who Give More: Health and Mental Health Among the Contemporary Puyallup Indian Tribal Community*. Monograph. *Price:* $20.

**★ 12576 ★ National Coalition of Creative Arts Therapy Associations (NCCATA)**
c/o AMTA
8455 Colesville Rd., Ste. 1000
Silver Spring, MD 20910
**Phone:** (714)751-0103
**Email:** mb33@nyu.edu
**Website:** http://www.ncata.com
Miriam Roskin Berger, Chair
**Fnded:** 1979. **Mem:** 8,000. **Nat'l Groups:** 6. **Desc:** Creative arts therapists. Promotes therapeutic and rehabilitative uses of the arts in medicine, mental health, special education, and forensic and social services; coordinates member associations' activities and efforts in meeting common objectives while supporting and advancing each group's discipline. Works to: represent members' interests in legislative activities; define joint positions on public policy issues; facilitate communication among members; initiate educational and research programs. Compiles statistics. **Frmly:** (2002) National Coalition of Arts Therapy Associations.

**★ 12577 ★ National Coalition of Psychiatrists Against Motorcoach Therapy (NCPAMT)**
c/o Dr. Anne Rose
4909 Briarwood Ave., No. 7
Royal Oak, MI 48073-1318
Jonathon Steele, PhD, Exec. Dir.
**Fnded:** 1985. **Mem:** 430. **Desc:** Psychiatrists, psychotherapists, psychologists, social workers, counselors, and mental health officials. Objective is to stop the practice of "Motorcoach Therapy," described by the coalition as the "escalating and unethical practice of procuring one-way bus fares for habitual and undesirable mental health patients" upon their release from local mental health facilities. Provides for information exchange; has launched an awareness campaign targeted primarily at mental health officials.

**National College of Hypnosis and Psychotherapy**
*See:* Entry 11678

**★ 12578 ★ National Council for Community Behavioral Healthcare**
12300 Twinbrook Pkwy., No. 320
Rockville, MD 20852
**Phone:** (301)984-6200          **Fax:** (301)881-7159
**Email:** davids@nccbh.org
**Website:** http://www.nccbh.org
Charles Ray, Contact
**Fnded:** 1969. **Mem:** 900. **State Groups:** 38. **Desc:** Conducts educational programs. Maintains speakers' bureau **Pub:** *National Council News*, monthly. Newsletter. **Frmly:** (1997) National Council on Community Mental Health Centers; (1999) National Community Mental Healthcare Council.

**★ 12579 ★ National Depressive and Manic Depressive Association (NDMDA)**
730 N Franklin, Ste. 501
Chicago, IL 60610-7204
**Phone:** (312)642-0049          **Free:** 800-826-3632
**Fax:** (312)642-7243
**Email:** nbunch@ndmda.org
**Website:** http://www.ndmda.org
Lydia Lewis, Exec. Dir.
**Fnded:** 1986. **Mem:** 65,000. **Reg. Groups:** 6. **Local Groups:** 275. **Desc:** Seeks to educate patients, families, professionals, and the public concerning the nature of depressive and manic-depressive illnesses

as treatable medical diseases; to foster self-help for patients and families; to eliminate discrimination and stigma; to improve access to care; and to advocate for research toward the elimination of these illnesses. **Pub:** *A Guide to Depressive and Manic Depressive Illness: Diagnosis, Treatment and Support*. Pamphlet. Contains patient information on depression and bipolar illnesses. • *Dark Glasses and Kaleidoscopes: Living with Manic Depression*. Video. • *Outreach*, quarterly. Newsletter. Includes book reviews, calendar of events, articles on research and treatment, consumer awareness, and advocacy. **Frmly:** (1978) Manic Depressive and Depressive Association.

**★ 12580 ★ National Eating Disorder Information Centre (NEDIC)**
College Wing, 1-211
200 Elizabeth St.
Toronto, ON, Canada M5G 2C4
**Phone:** (416)340-4156          **Fax:** (416)340-3430
**Email:** nedic@uhn.on.ca
**Website:** http://www.nedic.ca
**Fnded:** 1985. **Lang(s):** English. **Desc:** Provides information and resources on causes, symptoms of, and therapeutic and health care treatments for eating disorders and the preoccupation with food and weight. Aims to raise awareness on eating disorders through conducting lectures and workshops. Sponsors Eating Disorder Awareness Week in Canada and publishes bulletins. **Pub:** Bulletin, 5/year. Provides information and resources on range of topics related to food and weight preoccupation.

**★ 12581 ★ National Eating Disorders Association**
603 Stewart St., Ste. 803
Seattle, WA 98101
**Phone:** (206)382-3587          **Fax:** (206)829-8501
**Email:** info@edap.org
**Website:** http://www.nationaleatingdisorders.org
**Fnded:** 2001. **Desc:** Formed to provide educational programming, prevention efforts, research, advocacy, treatment and outreach for those suffering from eating disorders such an anorexia and bulimia. Sponsors National Eating Disorders Awareness Week, in its 14th year, celebrated in fifty states. Distributes educational brochures, sponsors a Prevention Puppet Project designed to teach elementary school children about health self-esteem and body image. Created the GO GIRLS! program, designed to help high school girls learn more about body image and the role that the media plays in the way the feel about themselves and their bodies. Runs a national media advocacy campaign. **Pub:** *A Guide to the Primary Prevention of Eating Disorders*. Brochure. *Price:* $20 per 100. **Frmly:** (1980) Anorexia Nervosa Aid Society; (1983) American Anorexia Nervosa Association.

**★ 12582 ★ National Federation for Biblio/ Poetry Therapy (NFBPT)**
c/o Sherry Reiter
1904 E 1st St.
Brooklyn, NY 11223
**Phone:** (718)998-4572
**Email:** sreiter@erols.com
Sherry Reiter, Exec. Dir.
**Fnded:** 1983. **Mem:** 10. **Desc:** Establishes standards for individuals, organizations, and institutions engaged in the training of biblio/poetry therapists or the practice of biblio/poetry therapy as a profession. (Biblio/poetry therapy uses literature or poetry to help patients "respond to an emotional impact which can then be integrated in self-awareness and self-understanding.") A credentialing committee grants certification and the most advanced level, registration as a poetry therapist.

**★ 12583 ★ National Foundation for Depressive Illness (NAFDI)**
PO Box 2257
New York, NY 10116
**Phone:** (212)268-4260          **Free:** 800-239-1265
**Fax:** (212)268-4434

**Website:** http://www.depression.org
Amy Russell, Administrator

**Fnded:** 1983. **Desc:** Provides public and professional education and information on recent medical advances in affective mood disorders. Conducts seminars on affective disorders, pharmaceutical development, and disease-related loss of productivity. Maintains speakers' bureau. Provides support group and referral services to appropriate doctors. **Pub:** *NAFDI News*, quarterly. Newsletter. • *Now We Can Treat the Illness Called Depression.* • Brochures.

### ★ 12584 ★ National Institute for Clinical Application of Behavioral Medicine (NICABM)

PO Box 523
Mansfield Center, CT 06250
**Phone:** (860)456-1153     **Free:** 800-743-2226
**Fax:** (860)423-4512
**Email:** info@nicabm.com
**Website:** http://www.nicabm.com
Ruth M. Buczynski, PhD, Pres.

**Fnded:** 1988. **Desc:** Works to provide information to behavioral health professionals. Conducts educational programs. **Pub:** Newsletter, quarterly.

### ★ 12585 ★ National Institute of Mental Health (NIMH)

6001 Executive Blvd., Rm. 8184
MSC 9663
Bethesda, MD 20892-9663
**Phone:** (301)443-4513     **Free:** 800-421-4211
**Fax:** (301)443-4279
**Email:** nimhinfo@nih.gov
**Website:** http://www.nimh.nih.gov

**Desc:** Strives to achieve better understanding, treatment, and eventually prevention of mental illness.

### ★ 12586 ★ National Mental Health Association (NMHA)

1021 Prince St.
Alexandria, VA 22314-2971
**Phone:** (703)684-7722     **Free:** 800-969-NMHA
**Fax:** (703)684-5968
**Email:** infoctr@nmha.org
**Website:** http://www.nmha.org
Michael Faenza, CEO/Pres.

**Fnded:** 1909. **Mem:** 416,000. **Reg. Groups:** 340. **Desc:** Addresses all aspects of mental health and mental illness and is dedicated to improving mental health, preventing mental disorders, and achieving victory over mental illnesses. NMHA, in partnership with more than 340 affiliates across the country, accomplishes its mission through advocacy, public education, research, and service. **Pub:** *The ADA and People with Mental Illness: An Employer's Manual.* Book. A guide to accommodations for people w/mental & emotional disorders. *Price:* $40. • *Aiding People in Conflict: A Guide for Law Enforcement.* • *The Bell,* 12/year. Newsletter includes association news, calendar of events, legislative news, mental health/health trends and research news. **Frmly:** National Association for Mental Health; (1980) Mental Health Association.

### ★ 12587 ★ National Mental Health Consumers' Self-Help Clearinghouse (NMHCSHC)

1211 Chestnut St., Ste. 1207
Philadelphia, PA 19107
**Phone:** (215)751-1810     **Free:** 800-553-4539
**Fax:** (215)636-6312
**Email:** info@mhselfhelp.org
**Website:** http://www.mhselfhelp.org
Joseph Rogers, Exec. Dir.

**Fnded:** 1985. **Desc:** Serves mental health consumers/ex-patients and consumer/ex-patients, self-help groups, and consumer-run services. Provides technical assistance in the development of self-help projects, including advocacy groups, support groups, consumer-run services and self-advocacy efforts. Offers infor-

mational referrals, written material, and consulting services. **Pub:** *Advocacy and Recovery Using the Internet.* • *Art and Science of Writing Proposals That Win.* • *Consumer-Run Businesses and Services.* • *Consumer-Run Drop-In Centers.* • *Fighting Stigma.* • *History of the Consumer Movement.* • *Organizing and Operating a Speakers Bureau.* • *Raising Money for a Self-Help/Advocacy Group.* • *Self-Advocacy.* • *Serving on Boards and Committees.* • *Starting a Self-Help/ Advocacy Group.* • *Systems Advocacy.*

### ★ 12588 ★ National Phobics Society

Zion Centre
339 Stratford Rd.
Hulme
Manchester M15 4ZY, United Kingdom
**Phone:** 44 161 7700456     **Fax:** 44 161 2279862
**Email:** natphob.soc@good.co.uk
**Website:** http://www.phobics-society.org.uk

**Fnded:** 1970. **Mem:** 6,000. **Desc:** Provides information, support, and advice to anyone affected by anxiety disorders, including panic attacks, OCD, BDD, agoraphobia, social phobia, and PTSD.

### ★ 12589 ★ National Psychological Association for Psychoanalysis (NPAP)

150 W 13th St.
New York, NY 10011
**Phone:** (212)924-7440     **Fax:** (212)989-7543
**Email:** info@npap.org
**Website:** http://www.npap.org
Harvey Kaplan, Pres.

**Fnded:** 1948. **Mem:** 365. **Desc:** Professional society for practicing psychoanalysts. Conducts training program leading to certification in psychoanalysis. Offers information and private referral service for the public. Operates speakers' bureau. **Pub:** *National Psychological Association for Psychoanalysis–Bulletin,* biennial. Bulletin. *Price:* Free. • *National Psychological Association for Psychoanalysis–News and Reviews,* semiannual. *Price:* Included in membership dues. • *Psychoanalytic Review,* bimonthly. Journal. Includes book reviews.

### ★ 12590 ★ National Register of Health Service Providers in Psychology

1120 G St., NW, Ste. 330
Washington, DC 20005
**Phone:** (202)783-7663
**Email:** judy@nationalregister.com
**Website:** http://www.nationalregister.com
Judy E. Hall, PhD, Exec. Officer

**Fnded:** 1974. **Mem:** 14,000. **Desc:** Licensed psychologists. Goal is to contribute to the continuous improvement of health services to the public by developing, reviewing and disseminating standards for evaluating credentials, disseminating information, conducting ethics programs, and evaluating education programs. Developed the subsidiary, HSP Verified, to develop electronic solutions for providing credentialing services. **Pub:** *The Register Report,* 3/year. Magazine.

### National Register of Hypnotherapists and Psychotherapists
*See:* Entry 11680

### ★ 12591 ★ National Remotivation Therapy Organization (NRTO)

PO Box 440
York Harbor, ME 03911
**Phone:** (207)363-7577     **Fax:** (207)351-1915
**Email:** nrhp@btconnect.com
**Website:** http://www.remotivation.fws1.com
Michael L. Stotts, Exec. Dir.

**Fnded:** 1971. **Mem:** 412. **State Groups:** 5. **Desc:** Certified remotivation therapists organized to provide a forum for the discussion of ideas and information related to the field. Remotivation therapy involves the use of small group sessions to stimulate and revitalize individuals who have experienced a decline in interest in their surroundings, themselves, and other people.

Conducts discussions of methods that allow patients an opportunity for verbal expression, renewal of listening skills, and resocialization. **Pub:** *NRTO Newsletter,* quarterly. Newsletter. *Price:* $20/year. • *Remotivation Therapy Information.* Brochure. • *Remotivator,* quarterly. Newsletter. **AKA:** National Remotivation Technique Organization.

### ★ 12592 ★ National Runaway Switchboard (NRS)

3080 N Lincoln Ave.
Chicago, IL 60657
**Phone:** 800-621-4000     **Fax:** (773)929-5150
**Email:** info@nrscrisisline.org
**Website:** http://www.nrscrisisline.org
Lora Thomas, Exec. Dir.

**Fnded:** 1974. **Desc:** A 24-hour, toll-free national switchboard for runaways, families of runaways, and other troubled youth. Provides names and phone numbers of centers for shelter and other social services across the country, including counseling centers, referral lines, drug treatment facilities, and family planning services. Offers to relay messages between young people and their families if desired; can also set up conferences calls between youths and parents or agencies. The caller's confidentiality is maintained. Maintains speakers' bureau. Funded in part by the Family and Youth Services Bureau of the U.S. Department of Health and Human Services. Also provides free Bus ride home for qualified runaways. Access to AT&T Language Line. **Pub:** *FrontLine,* quarterly. Newsletter. Contains statistical data and reports on activities.

### ★ 12593 ★ National Schizophrenia Fellowship (NSF)

30 Tabernacle St.
London EC2A 4DD, United Kingdom
**Phone:** 44 20 73309100     **Fax:** 44 20 73309102
**Email:** info@london.nsf.org.uk
**Website:** http://www.at-ease.nsf.org.uk

**Fnded:** 1972. **Mem:** 7,102. **Reg. Groups:** 8. **Local Groups:** 150. **Desc:** Exists to improve the lives of everyone affected by schizophrenia and other severe mental illnesses by providing quality support, services, and information and by influencing local, regional, and national policies. **Pub:** *A Meeting Of Minds - A Positive Response To Mental Disorder.* Video. Features the perspectives of schizophrenia sufferers, their careers, CPNs, social workers, and police officers. • *Cognitive Therapy.* Report. Covers a complimentary form of treatment. • *Does Severe Mental Illness Run In Families?.* • *Finding The Right Medication.* Handbook. A guide to drugs available to treat schizophrenia. • *500 Million More - Where and Why it is Needed.* Report. Highlights the underfunding of community care for people with a severe mental illness. • *Is Cost A Factor.* Survey. • *One in Ten.* Report. Covers suicide and other unnatural deaths involving people with schizophrenia. • *Schizophrenia.* Pamphlet. Covers the causes and symptoms of schizophrenia, including treatment. • *Schizophrenia And Research - UK.* Report. • *Schizophrenia - Notes for Relatives and Friends.* Pamphlet. • *The Silent Partners - The Needs and Experiences of People Who Care For People With A Severe Mental Illness.* Reprint. • *What is Schizophrenia?.*

### ★ 12594 ★ Network Against Coercive Psychiatry (NACP)

172 W 79th St., No. 2E
New York, NY 10024
**Phone:** (212)560-7288     **Fax:** (212)799-9026
**Email:** seth17279@aol.com
Dr. Seth Farber, PhD, Contact

**Fnded:** 1989. **Desc:** Comprised of psychotherapists including psychiatrists, survivors of psychiatric incarceration, scholars and other concerned citizens. Promotes the idea of mental illness as a misleading and degrading metaphor. Works towards the possible development of a social movement against the mental health system.

## ★ 12595 ★ New Zealand Psychological Society (NZPsS)

PO Box 4092
Wellington, New Zealand
**Phone:** 64 4 8015414          **Fax:** 64 4 8015366
**Email:** office@psychology.org.nz
**Website:** http://www.psychology.org.nz

**Fnded:** 1967. **Mem:** 700. **Local Groups:** 8. **Lang(s):** English. **Desc:** Professional association for psychologists and interested individuals. Promotes psychology as a science. Represents interests of professional psychologists; provides services to members. Publishes "New Zealand Journal of Psychology." **Pub:** *AGM Agenda*, annual. • *Connections*, monthly. Newsletter. • *New Zealand Journal of Psychology*, semiannual. Journal. Two issues per volume. • *NZPSS Bulletin*, quarterly. Bulletin. • *Practice Issues for Clinical and Applied Psychologists in New Zealand*. Book. • *The Practice of Psychology & the Law: A Handbook*. Handbook.

## ★ 12596 ★ Nordic Association for Psychiatric Epidemiology (NAPE)

c/o Kristinn Tomasson
Bildshofoa 16
IS-110 Reykjavik, Iceland
**Phone:** 354 5504650

**Fnded:** 1997. **Desc:** Professionals within psychiatric epidemiology research. Promotes research within psychiatric epidemiology; recruits and supervises young researchers; aims to expand collaboration between Nordic and global countries; disseminates research results.

## ★ 12597 ★ North American Society of Adlerian Psychology (NASAP)

65 E Wacker Pl., No. 1710
Chicago, IL 60601
**Phone:** (312)629-8801          **Fax:** (312)629-8859
**Email:** nasap@msn.com
**Website:** http://www.alfredadler.org/
Jerianne Garber, Admin.

**Fnded:** 1951. **Mem:** 1,200. **Local Groups:** 34. **Desc:** Psychiatrists, psychologists, educators, social workers, clergy, and others interested in promoting the knowledge, training, and teaching of individual psychology, developed by the Austrian psychiatrist Alfred Adler (1870-1937). Encourages development of professional workers and groups in individual psychology; establishes standards for professional activities of members. Conducts research in child behavior and psychology, counseling, psychotherapy, group therapy, and treatment of the mentally ill. Sponsors training institutes and summer school program. Promotes establishment of family education associations and parent study groups. **Pub:** *Alfred Adler: As We Remember Him*. Book. • *An Adlerian Resource Book*. • *Individual Psychology: Journal of Adlerian Theory, Research and Practice*, quarterly. Journal. • *Membership List*, biennial. • *North American Society of Adlerian Psychology–Newsletter*, bimonthly. Newsletter. Includes calendar of events. *Price:* Included in membership dues; $20/year for nonmembers. **Frmly:** (1977) American Society of Alderian Psychology.

## ★ 12598 ★ Northern Ireland Association for Mental Health

80 University St.
Beacon House
Belfast BT7 1HE, United Kingdom
**Phone:** 44 28 90328474     **Fax:** 44 28 90232940
**Fnded:** 1959. **Mem:** 280. **Local Groups:** 32. **Desc:** Promotes dignity, choice, integration and participation for those with mental health needs living in the community. Aims to offer services of the highest standard to people with mental health needs; inform and educate the public about mental health; and press for high standards in the provision of mental health services. **Pub:** *Mental Health Matters*, quarterly.

## ★ 12599 ★ Northern Ireland Chest Heart and Stroke Association

21 Dublin Rd.
Belfast BT2 7HB, United Kingdom
**Phone:** 44 28 90320184     **Fax:** 44 28 90333487
**Website:** http://www.nichsa.com

**Fnded:** 1946. **Reg. Groups:** 16. **Lang(s):** English. **Desc:** Promotes the prevention of, and alleviate the suffering resulting from chest, heart, and stroke illnesses in Northern Ireland. Supports rehabilitation facilities; offers subsidized vacations for families affected by these diseases; provides nebulizers for asthmatic children and adults; provides help and advice; provides grants for people with low incomes; funds research.

## ★ 12600 ★ Norwegian Psychological Association

PO Box 8733
Youngstorget
N-0028 Oslo, Norway
**Phone:** 47 23103130          **Fax:** 47 22424292
**Email:** npfpsot@psykol.no
**Website:** http://www.psykol.no

**Desc:** Psychologists in Norway. Promotes the advancement of psychological study.

## ★ 12601 ★ Obsessive-Compulsive Anonymous (OCA)

PO Box 215
New Hyde Park, NY 11040
**Phone:** (516)739-0662          **Fax:** (212)768-4679
Roy C., Contact

**Fnded:** 1988. **Mem:** 1,000. **Nat'l Groups:** 70. **Reg. Groups:** 70. **Desc:** Individuals suffering from obsessive-compulsive disorders. (OCD is characterized by recurrent unpleasant thoughts and/or repetitive, irrational mannerisms the sufferer feels compelled to perform.) Follows the 12-step method originated by Alcoholics Anonymous World Services to assist members in their recovery. **Pub:** *Obsessive Compulsive Anonymous Second Edition - 1999*. Book. *Price:* $19.00. • *Obsessive Compulsive Disorder: A Survival Guide for Family and Friends*. *Price:* $9.95.

## ★ 12602 ★ Obsessive-Compulsive Foundation (OCF)

337 Notch Hill Rd.
North Branford, CT 06471
**Phone:** (203)315-2190          **Fax:** (203)315-2196
**Email:** info@ocfoundation.org
**Website:** http://www.ocfoundation.org
Patty Perkins Doyle, Exec. Dir.

**Fnded:** 1986. **Mem:** 11,000. **State Groups:** 9. **Desc:** Individuals with obsessive-compulsive disorders and their families and friends; professionals involved in the treatment of OCD. (OCD is often chronic and characterized by recurrent unpleasant thoughts and/or repetitive behaviors that the person feels driven to perform. Individuals with OCD realize their obsessions and compulsions are irrational or excessive, yet find they have no control over them. Individuals with OCD often become demoralized, depressed, and anxious.) Seeks to control and find a cure for OCD while improving the welfare of its individuals with OCD. Disseminates information on OCD and possible new therapies. Offers educational programs for professionals and the public. Assists with fundraising and forming local support groups; fosters communication between members. Funds research into causes and treatments. **Pub:** *Kidscope*, semiannual. Newsletter. For children and teens with OCD. • *OCD*. Brochure. • *OCD Newsletter*, bimonthly. Newsletter. • Also produces educational materials. **Frmly:** (1988) Obsessive Compulsive Disorder Foundation.

## ★ 12603 ★ Option Institute and Fellowship (OIF)

2080 S Undermountain Rd.
Sheffield, MA 01257
**Phone:** (413)229-2100          **Free:** 800-714-2779
**Fax:** (413)229-8931
**Email:** happiness@option.org
**Website:** http://www.option.org
Lauren Astor, Pub. Rel. Mgr.

**Fnded:** 1983. **Desc:** Provides individuals, couples, families, businesses and groups empowering personal growth programs and seminars using life-changing, experiential learning techniques that can greatly improve relationships, career, health and quality of life. Option Process counseling sessions with Certified Option Process Mentors/Counselors are offered. **Pub:** *A Miracle to Believe In*. Book. • *A Sacred Dying*. Book. • *Giant Steps*. Book. • *Happiness Is a Choice*. Book. • *Out-Smarting Your Karma*. Book. • *Power Dialogues*. Book. • *Son-Rise: The Miracle Continues*. Book. • *To Love Is To Be Happy With*. Book.

## Orthodox Christian Association of Medicine, Psychology and Religion (OCAMPR)

*See:* Entry 2333

## ★ 12604 ★ Postgraduate Center for Mental Health (PCMH)

c/o Vocational Services Department
344 W 36th St.
New York, NY 10018
**Phone:** (212)560-6720          **Fax:** (212)563-1291
**Email:** pcmhvoc@bigfoot.com
**Website:** http://www.webstrats.com/pcmhvoc.htm
Dr. Jacob Barak, Pres. & CEO

**Fnded:** 1945. **Desc:** Provides: therapy for individuals, groups, couples, and families; training; psychiatric day and evening care program; community services and public educational programs. Conducts research. Maintains: social rehabilitation clinic; child/adolescent and family clinic; adult clinic; employee support service; group residence for the mentally ill preparing for independent living. Training opportunities include: Adult Fellowship, Advanced Training for Social Workers, Child and Adolescent Counseling, Family Therapy, Group Therapy, Pastoral Counseling, Psychology Internship, and Social Work Internship. Offers mental health and organizational consultation to industry and government agencies. Maintains six residential facilities (supported housing) for homeless mentally ill. Oversees distribution of funds for programs providing housing and supportive services to people with HIV/AIDS. **Pub:** *Psychoanalysis and Psychotherapy*, semiannual. Journal. Includes professional book reviews and author and title indexes. *Price:* $37.50/year. **Frmly:** Institute for Research in Psychotherapy; (1962) Postgraduate Center for Psychotherapy.

## ★ 12605 ★ Psi Beta

1027 Westbridge Ln.
PO Box 4838
Chattanooga, TN 37405
**Phone:** (423)265-6555          **Free:** 888-PSI-BETA
**Fax:** (423)265-0033
**Email:** psibeta@psibeta.org
**Website:** http://www.psibeta.org
Carol Tracy, Exec. Dir.

**Fnded:** 1981. **Mem:** 17,000. **Nat'l Groups:** 1. **Reg. Groups:** 5. **Local Groups:** 160. **Desc:** Honor society - community, and junior college psychology students. Participates in psychology conventions. Provides means for contact with professors in students' areas of interest. Conducts educational programs and sponsors national awards. Promotes excellence in scholarship, leadership, research and community service. **Pub:** *Psi Beta Chapter Handbook*, annual. Handbook. *Price:* $16/copy. • *Psi Beta Newsletter*, 3/year. Newsletter. *Price:* Included in membership fee; $7.50/year for nonmembers.

## ★ 12606 ★ Psi Chi, National Honor Society in Psychology

PO Box 709
825 Vine St.
Chattanooga, TN 37401-0709
**Phone:** (423)774-2443          **Fax:** (423)265-1529
**Email:** psichi@psichi.org

**Website:** http://www.psichi.org
Kay Wilson, Exec. Officer

**Fnded:** 1929. **Mem:** 380,000. **Reg. Groups:** 7. **Local Groups:** 985. **Desc:** Honor society - men and women, psychology. **Pub:** *Chapter Handbook*, annual. Manual. • *Eye on Psi Chi*, quarterly. Magazine. *Price:* Included in membership dues. • *Psi Chi Journal of Undergraduate Research*, quarterly. Journal.


**Psychiatric Nurses Association of Ireland**
*See:* Entry 15769


★ 12607 ★ **Psychiatric Rehabilitation Services (PRS)**
500 W Annandale Rd.
Falls Church, VA 22046
**Phone:** (703)536-9000        **Fax:** (703)533-9858
**Email:** pstilton@prsinc.org
**Website:** http://www.prsinc.org

**Fnded:** 1963. **Desc:** Working to help people with serious mental illness develop the skills and resources to recover and live satisfying and more self-sufficient lives in the community.


★ 12608 ★ **Psychoanalytic Research Society**
c/o Joseph Turkel
6 W 77th St., Ste. 1B
New York, NY 10024
**Phone:** (212)787-4092
**Email:** joeturkel@aol.com
**Website:** http://www.columbia.edu/~hc137/prs/
Harold Cook, Pres.

**Desc:** Promotes psychoanalytic research of an empirical, theoretical and clinical nature, including the planning and conducting of psychoanalytic research and dissemination of findings. **Pub:** *Bulletin of the Psychoanalytic Research Society*. Bulletin.


★ 12609 ★ **Psychohistory Forum (PF)**
627 Dakota Trail
Franklin Lakes, NJ 07417
**Phone:** (201)891-7486        **Fax:** (201)891-6866
**Email:** pelovitz@aol.com
Paul H. Elovitz, PhD, Dir.

**Fnded:** 1983. **Mem:** 100. **Desc:** Psychologists, psychiatrists, Psychotherapists, social workers, historians, psychohistorians, and laypeople having a scholarly interest in the integration of depth psychology and history. (Psychohistory is the study of psychobiography, group process, the mechanisms of defense, the history of childhood, creativity, dreams, and the difference between stated intention and actual behavior.) Seeks to further psychohistory through the exchange of information. Conducts bimonthly workshops on topics related to psychohistory and training seminars on dream analysis, innovation, teaching, and methodology. Aids individuals in psychohistorical research. Holds lecture series. lecture series. **Pub:** *Clio's Psyche: Understanding the Why of Culture Current Events, History and Society*, quarterly. Journal. *Price:* $25 for nonmembers in U.S.; $29 for nonmembers outside U.S.; $45 for nonmembers in U.S. for 2 years. • *Immigrant Experience: Personal Narrative and Psychological Analysis*. Monograph.


★ 12610 ★ **Psychological Society Ireland**
CX House
2A Corn Exchange Pl.
Poolbeg St.
Dublin 2, Ireland
**Phone:** 353 1 6717122        **Fax:** 353 1 6717048
**Email:** psihq@eircom.net

**Fnded:** 1970. **Mem:** 1,600. **Desc:** Strives to advance psychology as a pure and applied science. Maintains a code of ethics and standards of conduct. Provides professional diploma schemes.


★ 12611 ★ **Psychology of Religion**
c/o Nancy S. Thurston
Department of Psychology
George Fox University
414 N Meridian St.
Newberg, OR 97132-2697
**Fax:** (503)538-8383
Dr. Nancy Thurston, Sec.

**Fnded:** 1948. **Mem:** 1,350. **Desc:** A division of the American Psychological Association. Seeks to encourage and accelerate research, theory, and practice in the psychology of religion and related areas. Facilitates the dissemination of data on religious and allied issues and on the integration of these data with current psychological research, theory, and practice. **Pub:** *Psychology of Religion–Newsletter*, quarterly. Newsletter. Contains articles, interviews, book reviews, and announcements focusing on psychology and religion. *Price:* Free to members; $5/year to nonmembers. **Frmly:** (1971) American Catholic Psychological Association; (1993) Psychologists Interested in Religious Issues.


★ 12612 ★ **Psychology Society (PS)**
100 Beekman St.
New York, NY 10038-1810
**Phone:** (212)285-1872
Dr. Pierre C. Haber, Exec. Dir.

**Fnded:** 1960. **Mem:** 4,600. **Nat'l Groups:** 5. **Reg. Groups:** 5. **Local Groups:** 5. **Desc:** Professional membership is limited to psychologists who have a doctorate and are certified/licensed as such in the state where they practice. Associate membership is intended for teachers and researchers as well as persons who will attain professional status shortly. Seeks to further the use of psychology in therapy, family and social problems, behavior modification, and treatment of drug abusers and prisoners. Encourages the use of psychology in the solution of social and political conflicts. Operates an information bureau to answer inquiries of authors and media. Sponsors biennial overseas trip to enable members and their spouses to observe other programs and institutions. Collaborates with other associations. Evaluates programs in the use of psychology. Recommends legislation; appears in court cases where issues of mental health occur as expert and impartial witness. **Pub:** *PS Newsletter*, monthly. Newsletter. Includes book reviews, calendar of events, and research updates. *Price:* Included in membership dues. • *PS Quarterly*. Journal. *Price:* Included in membership dues. • *Psychology Society–Membership List*, biennial. Membership Directory.


★ 12613 ★ **Psychometric Society (PS)**
c/o Dr. Terry Ackerman
UNCG
207 Curry Bldg.
Greensboro, NC 27402-6171
**Phone:** (336)334-3474        **Fax:** (336)334-4120
**Email:** taackerm@uncg.edu
**Website:** http://www.psychometricsociety.org/
Dr. Terry Ackerman, Sec.

**Fnded:** 1935. **Mem:** 2,200. **Desc:** Persons interested in development of quantitative models for psychological phenomena and quantitative methodology in the social and behavioral sciences. **Pub:** *Psychometrika*, quarterly. Journal. Covers statistical models of psychological phenomena. Includes book and software reviews. *Price:* $100 for organizations and nonmembers.


★ 12614 ★ **Psychonomic Society (PS)**
1710 Fortview Rd.
Austin, TX 78704
**Phone:** (512)462-2442        **Fax:** (512)462-1101
**Email:** cinnamon@psychonomic.org
**Website:** http://www.psychonomic.org
Robert F. Lorch, Jr., Sec. -Treas.

**Fnded:** 1959. **Mem:** 2,500. **Desc:** Persons qualified to conduct and supervise scientific research in psychology or allied sciences; members must hold a Ph.D. degree or its equivalent and must have published significant research other than the doctoral dissertation. Promotes the communication of scientific research in psychology and allied sciences. **Pub:** *Animal Learning and Behavior*, quarterly. Journal. Covers animal learning, motivation, emotion, and behavior, including classical and operant conditioning, sensory effects, and imprinting. *Price:* $36/year for individuals; $78/year for institutions. • *Behavior Research Methods, Instruments, and Computers*, quarterly. Journal. Contains articles in the areas of methods, techniques, and instrumentation of research in experimental psychology. *Price:* $46/year for individuals; $99/year for institutions. • *Cognitive, Affective, & Behavioral Neuroscience*, quarterly. Journal. • *Memory and Cognition*, bimonthly. Journal. Covers human memory and learning, conceptual processes, thinking, decision making, and skilled performance. *Price:* $50/year for individuals; $107/year for institutions. • *Perception and Psychophysics*, monthly. Journal. Provides articles on sensory processes, perception, and psychophysics, including reports of experimental investigations. *Price:* $68/year for individuals; $149/year for institutions. • *Program of the Annual Meeting of the Psychonomic Society*. Schedule and abstracts. *Price:* Included in membership dues; $7/copy to nonmembers in North America; $8.50/copy to nonmembers outside North America. • *Psychobiology*, quarterly. Journal. Encompasses all of the allied fields of the neurosciences relating directly to behavior; includes experimental, review, and theoretical papers. *Price:* $36/year for individuals; $73/year for institutions. • *Psychonomic Bulletin and Review*, quarterly. Journal. Contains short reports and full length review articles covering all areas of experimental psychology. *Price:* $42/year for individuals; $89/year for institutions.


★ 12615 ★ **Rabbinic Center for Research and Counseling (RCRC)**
128 E Dudley Ave.
Westfield, NJ 07090
**Phone:** (908)233-0419        **Fax:** (908)233-6459
**Email:** ihf@rcrconline.org
**Website:** http://www.rcrconline.org
Rabbi Irwin H. Fishbein, Dir.

**Fnded:** 1970. **Desc:** Individuals interested in the marriage relationship and marriage counseling with special emphasis on interfaith marriage. Purpose is to provide courses, workshops and counseling for intermarried couples, and to establish and operate outpatient clinics for treatment of emotional and mental disabilities by the application of both psychotherapeutic knowledge and religious guidance. Conducts research; maintains list of rabbis who officiate at interfaith marriages; distributes literature.


★ 12616 ★ **Radical Caucus in Psychiatry (RCP)**
c/o Carl Cohen, M.D.
SUNY Downstate Med. Center
Box 1203
450 Clarkson Ave.
Brooklyn, NY 11203
**Phone:** (718)270-2907        **Fax:** (718)287-0337
**Email:** cohen_c@hscbklyn.edu
Carl Cohen, MD, Coord.

**Fnded:** 1969. **Mem:** 75. **Desc:** Members of the American Psychiatric Association and individuals interested in mental health issues who take a politically progressive stand in psychiatry. Objective is to examine the socioeconomic and sociopolitical aspects of mental health issues from a left-oriented perspective. Areas of study have included a critical analysis of biological psychiatry, patient rights, and psychiatric treatment of mental patients in Latin America. Presents research findings to professionals and laypersons. Maintains speakers' bureau. **Pub:** Newsletter, annual.


★ 12617 ★ **Radix Institute (RI)**
3212 Monte Vista, NE
Albuquerque, NM 87106-2120
**Free:** 888-777-2349
**Email:** information@radix.org

**Website:** http://www.radix.org
Dale Cummings, Dir.

**Fnded:** 1963. **Mem:** 60. **Desc:** Educational and scientific organization dedicated to studying the creative process in nature as described by Wilhelm Reich. Reich, a psychoanalyst who began his work with Sigmund Freud, discovered and described the existence of the "muscular armor," or how blocked emotion is held in the chronic patterns of tension in the body. The Radix flow is experienced as feeling or emotion and is expressed in spontaneous movements of the body. Offers classes, workshops, and individual sessions in "Education in Feeling." Conducts teacher training and programs for professionals and research on the nature of the Radix. training and programs for professionals and research on the nature of the Radix. **Pub:** *List of Radix Teachers Worldwide*, annual. *Price:* Free. • *The Radix Journal*, biennial. Journal. *Price:* $26/year. • *Radix Newsletter*, 3/year. Newsletter. • Also publishes books and a newsletter. **Frmly:** Interscience Research Institute.


★ 12618 ★ **Reclamation Inc.**
2502 Waterford Dr.
San Antonio, TX 78217
**Phone:** (210)822-3569
Don H. Culwell, Dir.

**Fnded:** 1974. **Mem:** 20. **Local Groups:** 1. **Desc:** Former mental patients; interested others. Seeks to eliminate the stigma of mental illness and reclaim members' "human dignity." Serves as a voice for mental health patients in consumer, social, and political affairs. Helps members to live outside a hospital setting by providing assistance in the areas of resocialization, employment, and housing. Monitors media coverage; encourages "positive" presentations of mental health patients and increased coverage of mental health community service projects and events. **Pub:** *Positive Visibility*, quarterly. Newsletter. *Price:* included in membership dues.


★ 12619 ★ **Recovery**
802 N Dearborn St.
Chicago, IL 60610
**Phone:** (312)337-5661          **Fax:** (312)337-5756
**Email:** inquiries@recovery-inc.com
**Website:** http://www.recovery-inc.com
Shirley Sachs, Exec. Dir.

**Fnded:** 1937. **Mem:** 10,000. **Local Groups:** 800. **Desc:** Community mental health organization offering a self-help method developed by the neuropsychiatrist Dr. Abraham A. Low at the Psychiatric Institute of the University of Illinois Medical School. (The Recovery method is a system of techniques for controlling temperamental behavior and changing attitudes toward nervous symptoms and fears.) **Pub:** *Recovery Reporter*, bimonthly. Newsletter. *Price:* Included in membership dues. • *Recovery, Inc. Reports*. Newsletter. For professionals. • *Recovery, The Association of Nervous and Former Mental Patients–Directory*, annual. Directory. Lists the location and time of group meetings in the United States, Canada, and abroad. *Price:* $3 available to members only. **AKA:** Recovery, Inc., The Association of Nervous and Former Mental Patients.


★ 12620 ★ **Richmond Fellowship of Austria (RFA)**
Society for Mental Health
Hoffmanngasse 12
A-9020 Klagenfurt, Austria
**Phone:** 43 46355112          **Fax:** 43 463501256
**Email:** kuna.pmk@carinthia.com
**Fnded:** 1979. **Mem:** 400. **Nat'l Groups:** 2. **Lang(s):** English, Slovene. **Desc:** Community mental health services. Seeks to insure ethical and efficient administration of community mental health care programs and institutions. Conducts training programs for community mental health personnel; participates in charitable activities. **Pub:** *Pro Mente Kaouten*, quarterly. Newsletter.


★ 12621 ★ **Richmond Fellowship International (RFI)**
16 Europoint
5-11 Lavington St.
London SE1 0NZ, United Kingdom
**Phone:** 44 20 79456187          **Fax:** 44 20 79456190
**Email:** rfi.uk@virgin.net
**Website:** http://freespace.virgin.net/rfi.uk
**Fnded:** 1981. **Mem:** 18. **Nat'l Groups:** 26. **Reg. Groups:** 1. **State Groups:** 6. **Lang(s):** English, French, Spanish. **Desc:** Promotes the establishment and operation of halfway houses and day centers for abused children, former psychiatric patients and recovering drug addicts. Organizes mental health training programs for social workers, psychologists, psychotherapists, and psychiatric nurses. Supports development of community based psychosocial rehabilitation services and service user advocacy. **Pub:** *Annual Report*. • Newsletter, periodic.


★ 12622 ★ **Romanian Alzheimer Society**
Bd. Mihail Kogalniceanu 95A
Sc. A. Et. 1, Ap. 8, Sector 5
Bucharest, Romania
**Phone:** 40 1 6863470          **Fax:** 40 1 3113471
**Email:** alzsocro@fx.ro
**Website:** http://www.alz.co.uk/help/associations.html
**Fnded:** 1992. **Mem:** 250. **Lang(s):** English. **Desc:** Family caregivers, medical professionals, and volunteers involved with and concerned for people affected with dementia, including Alzheimer's disease. Works to support the elderly affected with mental disorders, particularly Alzheimer patients and their families.


★ 12623 ★ **Royal Australian and New-Zealand College of Psychiatrists (RANZCP)**
Maudsley House
390 La Trobe St.
Melbourne, VIC 3000, Australia
**Phone:** 61 3 96400646          **Fax:** 61 3 96425652
**Fnded:** 1963.


★ 12624 ★ **Royal College of Psychiatrists**
17 Belgrave Sq.
London SW1X 8PG, United Kingdom
**Phone:** 44 20 72352351          **Fax:** 44 20 72451231
**Email:** rcpsych@rcpsych.ac.uk
**Website:** http://www.rcpsych.ac.uk
**Fnded:** 1971. **Mem:** 10,000. **Desc:** Psychiatrists. **Pub:** *British Journal of Psychiatry, Psychiatric Bulletin*, monthly. Journal.


★ 12625 ★ **SAFE - Self Abuse Finally Ends**
c/o Karen Conterio
7115 W North Ave., PMB 319
Oak Park, IL 60302
**Phone:** (708)783-0171          **Free:** 800-DONT-CUT
**Website:** http://www.safe-alternatives.com
Karen Conterio, Contact
**Fnded:** 1984. **Local Groups:** 1. **Desc:** Professional group assisting self-injurious individuals in the treatment of their addictive behavior patterns. Maintains speakers' bureau; compiles statistics. **Pub:** *Bodily Harm*. Book. *Price:* $14.95. **Frmly:** (1987) Self-Mutilators Support Group.


★ 12626 ★ **Samaritans - England**
10 The Grove
Slough SL1 1QP, United Kingdom
**Phone:** 44 1753 216500          **Fax:** 44 1753 775787
**Email:** admin@samaritans.org.uk
**Website:** http://www.samaritans.org.uk
**Fnded:** 1953. **Mem:** 19,500. **Local Groups:** 203. **Desc:** A nationwide charity providing confidential, emotional support to anyone in crisis, 24 hours a day, 365 days a year. Not a religious or political organization. **Pub:** *Educational Materials*, periodic. • *Samaritan News*, quarterly. • Books, periodic. • Videos, periodic.


★ 12627 ★ **Schizophrenia Association of Great Britain**
International Schizophrenia Centre
Bryn Hyfryd, The Crescent
Bangor LL57 2AG, United Kingdom
**Phone:** 44 124 8354048
**Email:** info@sagb.co.uk
**Website:** http://www.sagb.co.uk
**Fnded:** 1970. **Mem:** 3,000. **Desc:** Provides information about schizophrenia for patients and families to increase understanding of the illness. **Pub:** Newsletter, semiannual. Contains articles on recent findings in Schizophrenia including nutritional aspects.


★ 12628 ★ **Schizophrenia Ireland (SI)**
38 Blessington St.
Dublin 7, Ireland
**Phone:** 353 1 8601620          **Fax:** 353 1 8601602
**Email:** schizi@iol.ie
**Website:** http://www.iol.ie/lucia
**Lang(s):** English, Irish. **Desc:** Individuals and organizations. Seeks to improve the quality of life of people with schizophrenia and their families. Makes available support and services; conducts educational and advocacy campaigns.


★ 12629 ★ **Schizophrenia Society of Canada (Societe canadienne de schizophrenie)**
75 The Donway W, Ste. 814
Don Mills, ON, Canada M3C 2E9
**Phone:** (416)445-8204          **Free:** 888-772-4673
**Email:** info@schizophrenia.ca
**Website:** http://www.schizophrenia.ca/
**Fnded:** 1979. **Reg. Groups:** 100. **Local Groups:** 10. **Desc:** Support group providing understanding of schizophrenia; disseminates information concerning the latest developments in schizophrenia research and treatment and society activities; advocates for legislation and improvements in services. Provides public awareness and education programs, family support, fundraising, or administration at various levels. **Pub:** *SSC Bulletin*. Bulletin. • Annual Report.


★ 12630 ★ **Schizophrenics Anonymous (SA)**
1209 California Rd.
Eastchester, NY 10709
**Phone:** (914)337-2252
**Website:** http://www.schizophrenia.com
Elizabeth A. Plante, Dir.
**Fnded:** 1967. **Mem:** 100. **Desc:** Self-help organization. Groups are comprised of diagnosed schizophrenics who meet to share experiences, strengths, and hopes in an effort to help each other cope with common problems and recover from the disease; rehabilitation program follows the 12 principles of Alcoholics Anonymous World Services. Discussion topics include: symptoms and how to deal with them; the need to be responsible even though one is ill; overcoming guilt related to the illness. Each of the local groups attempts to recruit a volunteer mental health consultant from the area. The volunteer aids in program development and group discussion. **Pub:** Newsletter, semiannual. Provides health information. *Price:* $20. • Also distributes guidelines for establishing SA groups.


★ 12631 ★ **Scientific Society of Psychiatry**
Psihiatrichna Klinika
Sv.G.Sofiiski 1
BG-1431 Sofia, Bulgaria
**Phone:** 359 2 523503          **Fax:** 359 2 594094
**Desc:** Fosters research in psychiatry.


★ 12632 ★ **Scientific Society of Psychosomatic Medicine**
State University Hospital of Neurology and Psychiatry

Tzarigradsko chaussee IVth km
BG-1113 Sofia, Bulgaria
**Phone:** 359 2 520333      **Fax:** 359 2 594094
**Fnded:** 1990. **Mem:** 103. **Reg. Groups:** 4. **Local Groups:** 16. **Lang(s):** English, French, Russian. **Desc:** Fosters research in the relationship between the mind and the body. Develops new therapeutical strategies in psychosomatic disorders in different ethnic groups. **Pub:** *Psychosomatic Medicine*, quarterly. Journal.

★ 12633 ★ **Scottish Association for Mental Health**
Cumbrae House
15 Carlton Ct.
Glasgow G5 9JP, United Kingdom
**Phone:** 44 141 5687000      **Fax:** 44 141 5687001
**Email:** enquire@samh.org.uk
**Website:** http://www.samh.org.uk
**Fnded:** 1923. **Mem:** 239. **Local Groups:** 23. **Desc:** Health Boards, Regional Councils, District Councils, Psychiatric Hospitals, local and regional voluntary organisations, Trade Unions, Professional Bodies Universities, individuals, local associations for mental health. Campaigns for better hospital and community services; seeks to increase understanding of mental distress; provides direct services to people who have suffered from mental health problems, namely supported accommodation and training for employment on projects all over Scotland. Information, training and a development consultancy are also offered to local groups, professionals and affiliated local mental health associations. **Pub:** *Mental Health Matters*, quarterly. Newsletter.

**Section for Psychiatric and Substance Abuse Services (SPSPAS)**
*See:* Entry 11508

★ 12634 ★ **Sidran Traumatic Stress Foundation**
200 E Joppa Rd., Ste. 207
Baltimore, MD 21286
**Phone:** (410)825-8888      **Free:** 888-825-8249
**Fax:** (410)337-0747
**Email:** sidran@sidran.org
**Website:** http://www.sidran.org
Esther Giller, Exec. Dir.
**Fnded:** 1986. **Desc:** Supports people with trauma-generated psychological disorders. Educates trauma survivors, their support people and caregivers through the development of programs, projects, and publications. Provides advocacy services; maintains speakers' bureau; information clearinghouse; professional training. **Pub:** *Sidran Bookshelf on Trauma and Dissociation*, annual. Catalog. • *Training Materials*. • *Workbooks*. • Books.Books for professional and lay audiences about the mental health effects of extremely traumatic experiences. **Frmly:** (2000) Sidran Foundation and Press.

★ 12635 ★ **Sigmund Freud Archives (SFA)**
c/o Harold P. Blum, M.D.
23 The Hemlocks
Roslyn, NY 11576
**Phone:** (516)621-6850      **Fax:** (516)621-3014
**Email:** haroldpblum@cs.com
Harold P. Blum, MD, Exec. Dir.
**Fnded:** 1951. **Mem:** 18. **Desc:** Psychoanalysts interested in the preservation and collection of scientific and personal writings of Sigmund Freud (1856-1939), Austrian neurologist and founder of psychoanalysis. Assists in research on Freud's life and work and the evolution of psychoanalytic thought; collects and classifies all documents, papers, publications, personal correspondence, and historical data written by, to, and on Freud.

★ 12636 ★ **Singapore Association for Counselling (SAC)**
c/o Singapore Professional Centre
People's Association
Youth Block, Rm. 4
9 Stadium Link
Singapore 397750, Singapore
**Phone:** 65 3482586      **Fax:** 65 4409450
**Desc:** Counselors, social workers, psychologists, and others active in the profession of counseling. Encourages high standards of professional ethics, competence, conduct, educational qualifications, and achievement. Promotes research in counseling.

★ 12637 ★ **Singapore Association for Mental Health (SAMH)**
Block 69 Lorong 4
Toa Payho, Ste. 01-365
Singapore 310069, Singapore
**Phone:** 65 2553222      **Fax:** 652526834
**Desc:** Promotes services for the social and mental well-being of people in Singapore. Works to improve the care and rehabilitation of the mentally ill and emotionally disturbed.

★ 12638 ★ **Singapore Psychiatric Association (SPA)**
PO Box 177
Hougang Central Post Office
Singapore 915306, Singapore
**Desc:** Psychiatrists in Singapore. Fosters high standards. Promotes continuing education of members.

★ 12639 ★ **Singapore Psychological Society (SPS)**
PO Box 192
Newton Post Office
Singapore 912207, Singapore
**Website:** http://www.angelfire.com/sc2/sps/
**Fnded:** 1979. **Lang(s):** English. **Desc:** Psychologists, professors, and students. Promotes the advancement of psychology as a science and as a profession in Singapore.

★ 12640 ★ **Social Psychiatry Research Institute (SPRI)**
150 E 69th St., Ste. 2H
New York, NY 10021
**Phone:** (212)628-4800      **Fax:** (212)249-8546
Ari Kiev, MD, JD, Pres.
**Fnded:** 1970. **Desc:** Promotes, supports, and conducts, in and outside the U.S., research in the fields of mental health and psychiatry; to assemble data and findings for mental health and psychiatry. Is presently conducting double-blind psychopharmacological studies of antidepressant and antianxiety medications with volunteers. Has supported several suicide prevention and drug abuse projects. Has developed a 15-week home-study program on panic and agoraphobia.

★ 12641 ★ **Social/Vocational Rehabilitation Clinic (SVRC)**
c/o Post-Graduate Center West
344 W 36th St.
New York, NY 10018
**Phone:** (212)971-3200      **Fax:** (212)244-2034
Michelle Sternchos, Contact
**Fnded:** 1959. **Desc:** Clinic employing a comprehensive therapeutic clinical program for psychiatric outpatients. Aims at reducing hospital admissions and creating a therapeutic and social experience resulting in independent living, improved interpersonal relationships, and productivity in the work field. Offers a program of "therapeutic groups of creative, recreational, experiential, and work activities." Provides individual counseling, activity and therapy, and medication therapy; offers placement service; operates case management services. Sponsors vocational activities, family therapy, internship program, and community outreach activities. Functions as a psychotherapeutic

service of the Postgraduate Center for Mental Health. **Frmly:** The Living Room; (1975) Social Rehabilitation Clinic; (1977) Psychiatric Day and Evening Clinic; (1988) Social Rehabilitation Clinic.

★ 12642 ★ **Society of Behavioral Medicine (SBM)**
7600 Terrace Ave., Ste. 203
Middleton, WI 53562
**Phone:** (608)827-7267      **Fax:** (608)831-5485
**Email:** sbm@tmahq.com
**Website:** http://www.sbmweb.org
David B. Abrams, PhD, Pres.
**Fnded:** 1978. **Mem:** 2,300. **Desc:** Behavioral and biomedical researchers and clinicians studying health promotion and disease prevention, with primary focus on the interactions between health and behavior. Seeks to function as a forum for the exchange of ideas and information between health care providers and basic scientists and medical researchers. Gathers and disseminates information to members and the public; conducts educational programs for health care professionals; works to integrate behavioral and biomedical research. **Pub:** *Annals of Behavioral Medicine*, quarterly. Journal. Features comprehensive area reviews of topics affecting biobehavioral research and practice; also contains abstracts of recent articles in the field. *Price:* $145 in US; $175 foreign. • *Annual Meeting Proceedings*. Proceedings. Supplement to *Annals of Behavioral Medicine*. • *Education and Training Directory*. Directory. *Price:* Directory is available on website. • *SBM Outlook*, quarterly. Newsletter. • *Membership Directory*, biennial. Directory is available only on website.

★ 12643 ★ **Society of Biological Psychiatry (SBP)**
Mayo Clinic of Jacksonville, Research-Birdsall 310
4500 San Pablo Rd.
Jacksonville, FL 32224
**Phone:** (904)953-2842      **Fax:** (904)953-7117
**Email:** peterson.maggie@mayo.edu
**Website:** http://www.sobp.org
Maggie Peterson, Mgr.
**Fnded:** 1945. **Mem:** 950. **Desc:** International professional society of psychiatrists, neurologists, neurosurgeons, pharmacologists, neuropharmacologists, physiologists, psychologists, and physicians in related biological studies. Studies the neuronal basis of human behavior and the biological basis of psychiatry. Compiles statistics. **Pub:** *Biological Psychiatry*, bimonthly. • *Membership Roster*, annual. Membership Directory.

★ 12644 ★ **Society for Chaos Theory in Psychology and Life Sciences**
Arizona State University, Dept. of Industrial Engineering
PO Box 875906
Tempe, AZ 85287-5906
**Email:** kevin.dooley@asu.edu
**Website:** http://www.societyforchaostheory.org
Kevin Dooley, Pres.
**Fnded:** 1991. **Mem:** 300. **Desc:** Researchers, theoriticians, and practitioners. Examines the application of "dynamical systems theory, far-from-equilibrium thermodynamics, self-organization, neural nets, evolutionary computation, fractals, cellular automata, related forms of chaos, catastrophes, bifurcations, nonlinear dynamics, and complexity theories to psychology and the life sciences." **Pub:** Newsletter. • Books. • Journal.

**Society for Developmental and Behavioral Pediatrics (SDBP)**
*See:* Entry 5756

★ 12645 ★ **Society for the Exploration of Psychotherapy Integration (SEPI)**
134 Wooleys Ln.
Great Neck, NY 11023
**Phone:** (516)877-4803      **Fax:** (516)877-4805

**Email:** stricker@adelphi.edu
**Website:** http://www.cyberpsych.org/sepi/
Dr. George Stricker, Treas.

**Fnded:** 1984. **Mem:** 750. **Reg. Groups:** 15. **Desc:** Mental health professionals interested in the integration of theories and methods of psychotherapy. Encourages communication among members. Promotes collaborative work among psychotherapists who adhere to different theories and methods. **Pub:** *Journal of Psychotherapy Integration*, quarterly. Journal. Contains professional articles and book reviews. • *SEPI Newsletter*, quarterly. Newsletter.

★ **12646** ★ **Society for Industrial and Organizational Psychology (SIOP)**
PO Box 87
Bowling Green, OH 43402-0087
**Phone:** (419)353-0032　　　　**Fax:** (419)352-2645
**Email:** lhakel@siop.bgsu.edu
**Website:** http://www.siop.org
Ann Marie Ryan, Pres.

**Fnded:** 1982. **Mem:** 6,000. **Nat'l Groups:** 1. **Desc:** Dedicated to promoting human welfare through various applications of psychology to all types of organizations providing goods and services. **Pub:** *The Industrial-Organizational Psychologist (TIP)*, quarterly. Newsletter. Contains information about Society activities and articles of interest to those in the field. *Price:* included in membership dues, or for a small charge to others.

★ **12647** ★ **Society for Life History Research (SLHR)**
c/o Joan McCord
Temple University
Philadelphia, PA 19122
**Fax:** (610)667-0568
Joan McCord, Exec. Off.

**Fnded:** 1970. **Mem:** 700. **Desc:** Members are drawn from a wide range of disciplines, including behavior genetics, medicine, statistics, psychology, psychiatry, and sociology. Research programs are carried out by individual members; the society reports and publishes research results. **Pub:** *Human Functioning in Longitudinal Perspective.* • *Life History Research in Psychopathology.* • *Origins and Course of Psychopathology.* • *Origins of Psychopathology.* • *Proceedings,* every 18 months. • *Research and Public Policy.* • *Straight and Devious Pathways from Childhood to Adulthood.* **Frmly:** (1984) Society for Life History Research in Psychopathology.

★ **12648** ★ **Society of Multivariate Experimental Psychology (SMEP)**
PO Box 400400
Charlottesville, VA 22904-4400
**Phone:** (804)924-3374
**Email:** mfaccallum.l@osu.edu
**Website:** http://www.smep.org/
Joe Rodgers, Sec. -Treas.

**Fnded:** 1960. **Mem:** 65. **Desc:** Psychologists interested in the branch of experimental psychology that centers on multivariate designs and associated special forms of analysis. Promotes substantive research and scientific discovery to develop mathematical/statistical models leading to their evaluation and integration into the development of psychological theory. **Pub:** *Multivariate Behavioral Research*, quarterly.

★ **12649** ★ **Society for Pediatric Psychology (SPP)**
c/o Center for Alcoholism and Addiction Studies
Brown University
Box GBH
Providence, RI 02912
**Phone:** (401)444-1833　　　　**Fax:** (401)444-1888
**Email:** anthony_spirito@brown.edu
**Website:** http://www.neuropsychiatry.com/DPHB
Anthony Spirito, PhD, Pres.

**Fnded:** 1968. **Mem:** 995. **Desc:** A section of the American Psychological Association. Psychologists working in children's hospitals, developmental clinics,

and pediatric and medical group practices. Fosters the development of theory, research, training, and professional practice in pediatric psychology and the application of psychology to medical and psychological problems of children, youths, and their families. Supports legislation benefiting children's health and welfare. Sponsors colloquia and symposia; provides speakers. **Pub:** *Journal of Pediatric Psychology*, quarterly. Journal. Includes research reports, literature and book reviews, case studies, graphs, tables, charts, and society meeting minutes. *Price:* Included in membership dues; $50 for nonmembers. • *Progress Notes, Newsletter of the Society for Pediatric Psychology*, 3/year. Newsletter. Contains research articles on pediatric psychology. Includes abstracts of published literature, society news, and lists of employment opportunities. *Price:* Included in membership dues.

★ **12650** ★ **Society for Personality Assessment (SPA)**
6109 H Arlington Blvd.
Falls Church, VA 22044
**Phone:** (703)534-4772　　　　**Fax:** (703)534-6905
**Email:** klecksen@aol.com
**Website:** http://www.personality.org
Dr. Stephen Finn, Pres.

**Fnded:** 1938. **Mem:** 3,000. **Desc:** Psychologists, behavioral scientists, anthropologists, and psychiatrists. Promotes the study, research, development, and application of personality assessment. **Pub:** *Journal of Personality Assessment*, 6/year. Journal. Includes book reviews, case reports, and annual directory. *Price:* Included in membership dues; $70/year for nonmembers; $270/year for institutions. • *SPA Exchange*, semiannual. Newsletter. **Frmly:** (1938) Rorschach Research Exchange; (1958) Society for Projective Techniques and Rorschach Institute; (1970) Society for Projective Techniques and Personality Assessment.

★ **12651** ★ **Society for Personality and Social Psychology (SPSP)**
c/o Gina Reisinger
University of Rochester
Department of Psychology
Rochester, NY 14627
**Phone:** (716)275-8724
**Email:** spsp@scp.rochester.edu
**Website:** http://www.spsp.org/
Claude Steele, Pres.

**Fnded:** 1974. **Mem:** 3,000. **Desc:** Social and personality psychologists. Conducts and disseminates research on social and personality psychology. Sponsors SPSP Diversity Programs. **Pub:** *Personality and Social Psychology Review*, quarterly. Journal. Contains original theoretical papers and conceptual review articles in personality and social psychology. *Price:* $50 for individuals, $170 for institutions. • *Personalty and Social Psychology Bulletin*, monthly. Journal. Contains original empirical papers in all areas of personality and social psychology. *Price:* $575 for regular institution; $50 for single issues, regular institution; $102 /year for nonmembers; $11 for single issues, for nonmembers.

★ **12652** ★ **Society for Police and Criminal Psychology**
c/o A. Steven Dietz
City of Austin
8409 Ganttcrest Dr.
Austin, TX 78749
**Phone:** (512)530-8211
**Email:** steven.dietz@ci.austin.tx.us
**Website:** http://cep.jmu.edu/spcp/
A. Steven Dietz, Pres.

**Desc:** Promotes the scientific study of the criminal justice system, focusing on law enforcement, the judicial, and the corrections elements in criminal justice. Research includes the full range of human behaviors, motivations, and actions within the criminal justice system, along with causation of crime, victimization, and organizational influences. **Pub:** *Journal of Police and Criminal Psychology*, semiannual, spring

and fall. Journal. Contains information on issues relevant to practitioners and academicians in the field of criminal justice.

★ **12653** ★ **Society of Professors of Child and Adolescent Psychiatry (SPCAP)**
3615 Wisconsin Ave. NW
Washington, DC 20016-3007
**Phone:** (202)966-7300　　　　**Fax:** (202)966-2891
**Email:** mgomez@aacap.org
Matthew Gomez, Admin. Mgr.

**Fnded:** 1969. **Mem:** 150. **Desc:** Division directors from university psychiatric departments who meet annually to discuss issues in child and adolescent psychiatry. **Pub:** *SPCAP Membership Directory*, annual. Directory. **Frmly:** (1987) Society of Professors of Child Psychiatry.

**Society for the Psychological Study of Lesbian, Gay and Bisexual Issues (SPSLGBI)**
*See:* Entry 18912

★ **12654** ★ **Society for the Psychological Study of Social Issues (SPSSI)**
1901 Pennsylvania Ave. NW, No. 901
Washington, DC 20006-3405
**Phone:** (202)223-5100　　　　**Fax:** (202)223-5555
**Email:** spssi@spssi.org
**Website:** http://www.spssi.org
Jennifer Crocker, Pres.

**Fnded:** 1936. **Mem:** 2,600. **Desc:** Psychologists, sociologists, anthropologists, psychiatrists, political scientists, and social workers. Works to: obtain and disseminate to the public scientific knowledge about social change and other social processes; promote psychological research on significant theoretical and practical questions of social issues; encourage application of findings to problems of society. **Pub:** *Journal of Social Issues*, quarterly. Journal. *Price:* $55 for nonmembers. • *Social Psychological Applications to Social Issues.* Books. • *SPSSI Newsletter*, 3/year. Newsletter. **AKA:** American Psychological Association, Division 9.

★ **12655** ★ **Society for Psychophysiological Research (SPR)**
c/o Connie Duncan
1010 Vermont Ave., Ste. 1100
Washington, DC 20005
**Phone:** (202)393-4810　　　　**Fax:** (202)783-2083
**Email:** spr@aps.washington.dc.us
**Website:** http://www.wlu.edu/~spr

**Fnded:** 1960. **Mem:** 906. **Desc:** Research group comprising representatives from psychology, psychiatry, physiology, medicine, and biomedical engineering concerned with the interrelationship between behavioral and biological processes. Conducts research including the evaluation of biofeedback in the treatment of disease states. Maintains historical archives. Conducts workshops. **Pub:** *Psychophysiology*, bimonthly.

★ **12656** ★ **Society for Psychotherapy Research (SPR)**
308 Moore Bldg.
University Park, PA 16802
**Website:** http://www.psychotherapyresearch.org/
Louis G. Castonguay, PhD, Pres.

**Mem:** 1,000. **Reg. Groups:** 4. **Desc:** Committed to the scientific study of psychotherapy. **Pub:** Newsletter.

★ **12657** ★ **Society for a Science of Clinical Psychology**
c/o Raymond P. Lorion
University of Pennsylvania
Graduate School of Education
Psychology in Education Division

3700 Walnut St.
Philadelphia, PA 19104-6216
**Phone:** (215)898-7367          **Fax:** (215)573-2115
**Email:** lorion@gse.upenn.edu
**Website:** http://pantheon.yale.edu/~tat22/
Thomas D. Borkovec, PhD, Pres.

**Fnded:** 1966. **Desc:** Promotes the integration of the scientist and the practitioner in training, research and applied undertakings in the field of clinical psychology.

**Sozialverband Vdk Deutschland**
*See:* Entry 3037

**★ 12658 ★ Spiritual Emergence Network (SEN)**
1453 Mission St.
San Francisco, CA 94103
**Phone:** (415)648-2610
**Email:** info@ciis.edu
**Website:** http://www.ciis.edu/comserv/sen.html
Craig Turek, Dir.

**Fnded:** 1980. **Mem:** 10,000. **Desc:** Seeks to develop an expanded model of mental health care to help people in crisis by using scientific and spiritual assistance. Operates an information and referral service. Offers educational programs. Maintains speakers' bureau. **Pub:** *Spiritual Emergence Network Newsletter*, 2-3/year. Newsletter. • *Spiritual Emergency*. Book. • Brochure.

**★ 12659 ★ Stress and Anxiety Research Society (STAR)**
c/o Dr. Dennis Hocevar
WPH-600
School of Education
University of Southern California
Los Angeles, CA 90089-0031
**Fax:** (213)740-2367
**Email:** hocevar@usc.edu
**Website:** http://www.star-society.org/
Dr. Volker Hodapp, Sec.

**Fnded:** 1980. **Desc:** Researchers sharing an interest in problems of stress, coping, and anxiety. Promotes international and multidisciplinary analysis of stress and related topics. Serves as a forum for exchange of scientific information regarding stress; gathers and disseminates stress research results; facilitates cooperative research among members. **Pub:** *Anxiety, Stress and Coping*, annual. Journal. Contains reprints of research reports, theoretical papers, and interpretive literature reviews; includes case studies and other correspondence. • *STAR Newsletter*, semiannual. Newsletter.

**★ 12660 ★ Sufi Psychology Association (SPA)**
PO Box 2221
Davis, CA 95617-2221
**Website:** http://sufi-psychology.org/

**Fnded:** NNfo. **Mem:** unding ,pro. **Desc:** Psychologists, psychotherapists, psychiatrists and researchers. Promotes Sufi Psychology. **Pub:** *SPA Journal*, semiannual. Journal.

**★ 12661 ★ Swedish Psychological Association (SPA) (Sveriges Psykologforbund — SPF)**
Vasagatan 48
Box 3287
S-103 65 Stockholm, Sweden
**Phone:** 46 8 56706400          **Fax:** 46 8 56706499
**Fnded:** 1955. **Mem:** 7,500. **Desc:** Union of psychologists in Sweden.

**★ 12662 ★ THEO BC**
1910 Quebec St.
Vancouver, BC, Canada V5T 4K1
**Phone:** (604)872-0770          **Fax:** (604)873-1758
**Email:** tcostello@theobc.org
**Website:** http://www.theobc.org

**Fnded:** 1976. **Mem:** 36. **Lang(s):** English, French. **Desc:** Individuals working with people with psychiatric, emotional, and social disabilities. Seeks to improve the quality of life of people with emotional and psychiatric disabilities. Conducts vocational and educational programs to enable people with emotional and psychiatric disabilities to join the mainstream of society; sponsors charitable activities. **Pub:** Newsletter, periodic. • Bulletin, periodic. • Brochure. **Frmly:** (2000) Arbutus Vocational Society.

**★ 12663 ★ Turkish Psychological Association (TPA)**
Mesrutiyet Cad. 22/12
TR-06640 Ankara, Turkey
**Phone:** 90 312 4256765          **Fax:** 90 312 4174059
**Email:** bilgi@psikolog.org.tr
**Website:** http://www.psikolog.org.tr

**Fnded:** 1976. **Mem:** 1,600. **Reg. Groups:** 3. **Lang(s):** English, Turkish. **Desc:** Psychologists and psychology faculty. Represents the science and the profession of psychology in Turkey. **Pub:** *Turk Psikoloji Dergisi (Turkish Journal of Psychology)*. Journal. Includes empirical articles, review papers, and articles concerning national policies for psychologists.

**★ 12664 ★ Uganda Association for the Mentally Handicapped (UAMH)**
5 Kms. Bombo Rd. Off 200 m. Kawaala Rd.
PO Box 9177
Kampala, Uganda
**Phone:** 256 41 566404          **Fax:** 256 41 566404
**Fnded:** 1983. **Mem:** 548. **Nat'l Groups:** 1. **Reg. Groups:** 4. **Local Groups:** 18. **Lang(s):** English, Luganda, Swahili. **Desc:** Provides for the education and care of mentally handicapped individuals in Uganda. Seeks to increase public awareness of the needs of the mentally handicapped. Offers programs to increase self-help, leisure, and communication skills. Conducts research and periodic courses, seminars, and workshops; offers children's services. Organizes competitions including the Special Olympics and Very Special Arts. Operates placement service. Maintains vocational training and respite care programs. **Pub:** *Information to Africa Network - FEPAPHAM*, quarterly. • *Parent-to-Parent Help: Contact Service*, annual. **Frmly:** (1999) Inclusion Uganda.

**★ 12665 ★ United Kingdom Council for Psychotherapy**
167-169 Great Portland St.
London W1N 5FB, United Kingdom
**Phone:** 44 20 74363002          **Fax:** 44 20 74363013
**Email:** ukcp@psychotherapy.org.uk
**Website:** http://www.psychotherapy.org.uk

**Fnded:** 1989. **Mem:** 79. **Desc:** Psychotherapy organisations. The protection of the public by the promotion of appropriate standards for training, research, education and the practice of psychotherapy and by the dissemination of information. The publication of a register of psychotherapists. Liaison with Government and the European Commission as necessary. **Pub:** *Directory of Member Organisations*, annual. Directory. • *National Register of Psychotherapists*, annual.

**★ 12666 ★ Well Spouse Foundation (WSF)**
PO Box 30093
Elkins Park, PA 19027
**Free:** 800-838-0879
**Email:** info@wellspouse.org
**Website:** http://www.wellspouse.org
Marty Beilin, Pres.

**Fnded:** 1988. **Mem:** 3,000. **Nat'l Groups:** 50. **Desc:** Husbands, wives, and partners of chronically ill patients. An emotional support network functioning to raise public consciousness about and advocate for the caregivers and families of the chronically ill. Establishes local support groups and supplies information and materials. Compiles statistics; conducts educational programs. **Pub:** *Mainstay*, quarterly. Newsletter. Contains membership news and information, advoca-

cy issues, and helpful hints. *Price:* Included in membership dues. **Frmly:** National Well Spouse Foundation.

**★ 12667 ★ William Glasser Institute**
22024 Lassen St., No. 118
Chatsworth, CA 91311
**Phone:** (818)700-8000          **Free:** 800-899-0688
**Fax:** (818)700-0555
**Email:** wginst@earthlink.net
William Glasser, MD, Pres.

**Fnded:** 1967. **Reg. Groups:** 9. **Desc:** Teaches Reality Therapy, Choice Theory, and Lead Management concepts to those who wish to use the knowledge in various working environments. **Pub:** *Journal of Reality Therapy*, semiannual. Journal. • Newsletter, 3/year. **Frmly:** Institute for Reality Therapy; (1998) Institute for Control Therapy, Reality Therapy, and Quality Management.

**★ 12668 ★ World Association for Dynamic Psychiatry (WADP)**
c/o Maria Ammon
Dynamic-Psychiatric Clinic
Geiselgasteigstrasse 203
Menterschwaige
D-81545 Munich, Germany
**Phone:** 49 89 6427230          **Fax:** 49 89 64272395
**Website:** http://www.dynpsych.de

**Fnded:** 1980. **Mem:** 500. **Nat'l Groups:** 22. **Lang(s):** English, German. **Desc:** Disseminates the theory and practice of dynamic psychiatry developed at Gunter Ammon's Berlin School of Dynamic Psychiatry. Fosters and creates opportunities for dynamic psychiatry study in universities and other institutions. Promotes continuous advanced training in dynamic psychiatry for better patient care and improvement of public health. Conducts research into disease prevention, therapeutic method efficiency, and education standards; disseminates results. **Pub:** *Dynamische Psychiatrie/Dynamic Psychiatry*, bimonthly. • *WADP*, semiannual. Newsletter.

**World Association for Infant Mental Health (WAIMH)**
*See:* Entry 5771

**★ 12669 ★ World Association of Psychoanalysis (Association Mondiale de Psychanalyse — AMP)**
5 rue de Lille
F-75007 Paris, France
**Phone:** 33 1 45485672          **Fax:** 33 1 45487938
**Email:** wapol@wapol.org
**Website:** http://www.wapol.org/

**Fnded:** 1992. **Mem:** 1,800. **Lang(s):** English, French. **Desc:** Mental health care professionals. Promotes advancement in psychoanalytical scholarship and practice. Serves as a clearinghouse on psychoanalysis and its applications; conducts research and educational programs.

**★ 12670 ★ World Association for Psychosocial Rehabilitation - U.S. Branch (WAPR)**
c/o Martin Gittelman
Manhattan Psychiatric Center
Wards Island
New York, NY 10035
**Phone:** (212)369-0500          **Fax:** (212)369-0935
**Email:** gittem01@popmail.med.nyu.edu
Dr. Zebulon Taintor, Pres.

**Fnded:** 1987. **Mem:** 500. **Desc:** Professionals in the mental health field concerned with research, study, and training in psychosocial rehabilitation. (Psychosocial rehabilitation assists individuals whose primary problems or pathologies are related to psychiatric dysfunctions that limit their social, personal, or occupational functioning.) Conducts research and educational programs; maintains speakers' bureau and placement services. **Pub:** *Bulletin WAPR*, periodic. Bulletin. *Price:* Free. For members only. • *International Journal of Mental Health*, quarterly. Journal. *Price:* $50 to members. • Newsletter, periodic.


**★ 12671 ★ World Association for Social Psychiatry (WASP)**
656 Romero Canyon Rd.
Santa Barbara, CA 93108
**Phone:** (805)969-1376          **Fax:** (805)969-1376
John L. Carleton, MD, Honorary Pres.
**Fnded:** 1964. **Mem:** 3,000. **Reg. Groups:** 26. **Desc:** Professionals, contributors, and interested individuals active in allied fields of social psychiatry including anthropology, social work, nursing, or occupational therapy. Objectives are to: study the nature of man and his surrounding culture; research methods to prevent and treat internal changes and behavioral disorders; advance the physical, social, and philosophic well-being of mankind. Fosters collaboration among members and distributes theoretical and practical information. Conducts workshops and demonstrations of rehabilitation centers. **Pub:** *French Journal of Social Psychiatry*, quarterly. Journal. • *International Journal of Social Psychiatry*, quarterly. Journal. • *World Journal of Social Psychiatry*, quarterly. Journal. **Frmly:** (1978) International Association for Social Psychiatry.


**★ 12672 ★ World Federation for Mental Health (WFMH)**
1021 Prince St.
Alexandria, VA 22314-2971
**Phone:** (703)838-7543          **Fax:** (703)519-7648
**Email:** wfmh@erols.com
**Website:** http://www.wfmh.org
Richard Hunter, Dep. Sec. Gen.
**Fnded:** 1948. **Mem:** 3,500. **Reg. Groups:** 9. **Desc:** Associations and individuals dedicated to achieving the highest level of public mental health. Objectives include charitable, scientific, literary, and educational activities in the field of mental health. Organizes training programs. Sponsors World Mental Health Day. **Pub:** Newsletter, quarterly. *Price:* Free to members. **Frmly:** (1948) International Committee for Mental Hygiene.


**★ 12673 ★ World Forensic Psychiatry and Psychology Association (WFPPA)**
Rue Franklin 140
1000 Brussels, Belgium
**Fax:** 32 2 7365176


**★ 12674 ★ World Organization and Public Education Corp. of the National Association for the Advancement of Psychoanalysis**
80 8th Ave., Ste. 1501
New York, NY 10011-5126
**Phone:** (212)741-0515          **Fax:** (212)366-4347
**Email:** naap72@aol.com
**Website:** http://www.naap.org
Margery Quackenbush, Admin.
**Fnded:** 1995. **Desc:** Works for public education for the National Association for the Advancement of Psychoanalysis. **Pub:** Brochure. **Frmly:** (2000) Public Education Corp. of the National Association for the Advancement of Psychoanalysis.


**★ 12675 ★ World Psychiatric Association (WPA)**
c/o Mt. Sinai School of Medicine-CUNY
University of NY
Fifth Ave. & 100th St.
Box 1093
New York, NY 10029-6574
**Phone:** (718)334-5094          **Fax:** (718)334-5096
**Email:** wpa@dti.net
**Website:** http://www.wpanet.org
Prof. Juan E. Mezzich, Jr., Sec. Gen.

**Fnded:** 1950. **Mem:** 116. **Nat'l Groups:** 114. **Reg. Groups:** 18. **Desc:** Psychiatric societies and individuals in 90 countries. Objectives are: to promote international cooperation in the field of psychiatry; to advance inquiry into the etiology, pathology, and treatment of mental illness; to strengthen relations among psychiatrists working in various fields. Encourages the exchange of information concerning the medical problems of mental diseases; sponsors educational and research programs. Comprises 40 sections representing different specialties in psychiatry. **Pub:** *WPA News*, quarterly. Newsletter. *Price:* for members.


**★ 12676 ★ Zimbabwe National Association for Mental Health**
PO Box A 196
Avondale
Harare, Zimbabwe
**Phone:** 263 4 731272          **Fax:** 263 4 792946
**Email:** zimnamh@africaonline.co.zw
**Fnded:** 1981. **Mem:** 1,700. **Nat'l Groups:** 6. **Local Groups:** 250. **Desc:** Works to educate and rehabilitate the mentally ill. Informs the public about mental health issues. Promotes mental health for all throughout Zimbabwe. Contributes to increased awareness on the negative impact of child sexual abuse on children and to facilitate action to prevent and protect the child from all forms of sexual exploitation and sexual abuse. Promotes mental health for all through lobbying and advocacy and networks with other relevant stakeholders. **Pub:** *Zimnamh Newsletter*, quarterly. Newsletter. Containing information about mental health. • Pamphlets. Containing information about mental health. • Video.


# Research Centers

**★ 12677 ★ Ackerman Institute for the Family**
149 E 78th St.
New York, NY 10021
**Phone:** (212)879-4900          **Fax:** (212)744-0206
**Email:** psteinglass@ackerman.org
**Website:** http://www.ackerman.org
Peter Steinglass, MD, Exec. Dir.
**Activities/Fields:** Cancer and other chronic illnesses, catastrophic illness, AIDS/AIDS-Related Complex (ARC), school problems, women's issues, family violence, stressful life events, family life cycle issues, family factors in psychiatric disorders, alcoholism, and drug abuse.


**★ 12678 ★ Allan Memorial Institute**
1025 Pine Ave. W
Montreal, QC, Canada H3A 1A1
**Phone:** (514)842-1231          **Fax:** (514)843-1644
Paul Beaudry, MD, Dir.
**Activities/Fields:** Clinical and field investigation in the areas of clinical psychopharmacology, mood disorders, child and adolescent psychiatry, family studies (including family therapy), consultation-liaison psychiatry and cognitive therapy.


**Association for Research in Nervous and Mental Disease**
*See:* Entry 14140


**★ 12679 ★ Aurora Mental Health Research Institute**
14301 E Hampden Ave.
Aurora, CO 80014
**Phone:** (303)617-2300          **Fax:** (303)617-2397
**Email:** arnmd@arnmd.org
Dr. Randy C. Stith, Ch. Admin.
**Activities/Fields:** Community-based mental health services and the support systems they require. Provides technical assistance to private and public agen-

cies with special emphasis on person-machine issues relating to microcomputer and mainframe computers.


**★ 12680 ★ Autism Research Institute**
4182 Adams Ave.
San Diego, CA 92116
**Phone:** (619)281-7165          **Fax:** (619)563-6840
**Website:** http://www.autismresearchinstitute.com
Dr. Bernard Rimland, Dir.
**Activities/Fields:** Causes and treatment of severe behavior disorders in children, particularly autism. Conducts computerized analyses of its diagnostic reports on individual children with severe behavior disorders, and studies the relationship between nutrition and learning and behavior disorders. Serves as an international clearinghouse of information on autism, disseminating information to parents, researchers, hospitals, schools, and professional practitioners. **Pub:** *Autism Research Review International*, quarterly. **Frmly:** Institute for Child Behavior Research.


**Blanchette Rockefeller Neurosciences Institute**
*See:* Entry 14148


**★ 12681 ★ Boston University Center for Anxiety and Related Disorders (CARD)**
Kenmore Sq.
648 Beacon St., 6th Fl.
Boston, MA 02215
**Phone:** (617)353-9610          **Fax:** (617)353-9609
**Email:** dhbarlow@bu.edu
**Website:** http://www.bu.edu/anxiety/adult.html
David H. Barlow, PhD, Dir.
**Activities/Fields:** Anxiety disorders in adults and children, including generalized anxiety disorder, panic disorder, agoraphobia, obsessive-compulsive disorder, social phobia, depression, and various sexual-function disorders.


**Boston University Laboratory of Neuropsychology**
*See:* Entry 14150


**Center for Research on Services for Severe Mental Illness**
*See:* Entry 9771


**★ 12682 ★ Center for the Research and Treatment of Anorexia Nervosa**
10921 Wilshire Blvd., Ste. 702
Los Angeles, CA 90024
**Phone:** (213)824-5881
**Email:** dsteinwa@jhsph.edu
**Website:** http://www.jhsph.edu/~c-smi
Dr. Burt Crausman, PhD, Dir.
**Activities/Fields:** Anorexia nervosa and other eating disorders, including research into their causes, detection, and treatment.


**★ 12683 ★ Centre for Addiction and Mental Health Clarke Division**
33 Russell St.
Toronto, ON, Canada M5T 2S1
**Phone:** (416)535-8501
**Email:** public_affairs@camh.net
**Website:** http://www.camh.net
Dr. Paul Garfinkel, Pres. /CEO
**Activities/Fields:** Addiction and mental health. Studies include use and effects of alcohol, tobacco, and other drugs, with concentration in preovention and health promotion, drug and alcoholism treatment; socio-behavioral, medical, bio-behavioral, and biochemical research; and program evaluation. Develops and evaluates effectiveness of different treatment methods. Epidemiological studies of alcohol and drug use among general population and sub-groups. Effec-

tive strategies for prevention and early intervention, as well as behavioral, psychological, physical, and social/environmental factors that contribute to abuse. Problem gambling. Mental health research and treatment, such as group therapy, crisis management, stress managment, nutritional counselling, case management, living skills, training, therapeutic recreation and relapse prevention. Gender identity, anger managment, mood disorders, neurological impairment, concurrent disorders, developmental handicaps, and psychosocial intervention. **Frmly:** Addiction and Mental Health Services Corp.; Clarke Institute of Psychiatry Division.

**Child's Health Hospital Research Centre**
*See:* Entry 9385

**★ 12684 ★ Concordia University**
**(Montreal, QC, Canada)**
**Centre for Research in Human**
**Development (CRHD)**
7141 Sherbrooke St W
Montreal, QC, Canada H4B 1R6
**Phone:** (514)848-2240 **Fax:** (514)848-2815
**Email:** lserbin@vax2.concordia.ca
**Website:** http://www-psychology.concordia.ca/department/graduate/res-cen.html
Dr. Lisa Serbin, Dir.

**Activities/Fields:** Psychological development across the human life-span, focusing on normal social and cognitive development; atypical developmental patterns; and the study of competence in elderly populations. Specific fields of study include developmental, clinical, cognitive and social psychology; education; applied statistics; medicine; pediatrics; and gerontology. **Pub:** *Research Bulletins*, monthly.

**★ 12685 ★ Dave Garroway Laboratory for**
**the Study of Depression**
Pennsylvania Hospital, Mezzanine Fl.
210 W Washington Sq.
Philadelphia, PA 19106
**Phone:** (215)829-7314 **Fax:** (215)829-7315
Howard S. Sudak, MD, Dir.

**Activities/Fields:** Longitudinal studies of depression, including recurring depression, anxiety, and personality disorders in individuals with major depression. Examines predictors of recurrence, objective and subjective measures of symptom severity, and patient vulnerability. Applies multiperspective approach, including biological, behavioral, social, interpersonal, psychoanalytical, and cognitive aspects of depression. **Pub:** *American Journal of Psychiatry.* • *Archives of General Psychiatry.* • *Psychiatry Research.*

**★ 12686 ★ Douglas Hospital Research**
**Centre**
6875 La Salle Blvd.
Verdun, QC, Canada H4H 1R3
**Phone:** (514)761-6131 **Fax:** (514)762-3033
**Email:** quirem@douglas.mcgill.ca
**Website:** http://www.mcgill.ca/douglas
Dr. Rémi Quirion, Sci. Dir.

**Activities/Fields:** Mental health, including aging, psychoneuroendocrinology, cognitive measurements, and behavior; Alzheimer's disease, incorporating animal models, neurochemistry, and trials of nootropic drugs; depression and its biological markers, with clinical trials of new antidepressants; schizophrenia and alcoholism, including neurochemical studies and new treatment methods; violence neurobiological studies and new treatment methods; social psychiatry and epidemiology; and eating disorders.

**★ 12687 ★ Duke University**
**Anxiety and Traumatic Stress Program**
Medical Center
PO Box 3812
Durham, NC 27710
**Phone:** (919)684-2880 **Fax:** (919)684-8866

**Email:** jonathan.davidson@duke.edu
Dr. Jonathan Davidson, Prog. Dir.

**Activities/Fields:** Activities focus on diagnosis and treatment of anxiety disorders, including panic disorder, agoraphobia, social phobias, Post-Traumatic Stress Disorder (PTSD), obsessive-compulsive disorder (OCD), and generalized anxiety, as well as complementary and alteractive medicine.

**★ 12688 ★ Duke University**
**Behavioral Medicine Research Center**
Duke Medical Center
PO Box 3926
Durham, NC 27710
**Phone:** (919)684-3863 **Fax:** (919)681-8960
**Email:** rbw@bmrc.mc.duke.edu
Dr. Redford Williams, Dir.

**Activities/Fields:** Behavior, including emotional stress and personality factors as they affect physical diseases with emphasis on coronary disease and cancer. Uses epidemiological and experimental approaches.

**Duke University**
**Occupational Mental Health Programs**
*See:* Entry 16787

**★ 12689 ★ Emory University**
**Emory Alzheimer's Disease Center (ADC)**
Wesley Woods Health Center, 2nd Fl.
1841 Clifton Rd.
Atlanta, GA 30329
**Phone:** (404)728-6950
**Email:** emoryadc@emory.edu
**Website:** http://www.emory.edu/WHSC/MED/ADC/
Allan Levey, MD, Dir.

**Activities/Fields:** Alzheimer's disease.

**★ 12690 ★ Fountain House, Inc.**
**Van Ameringen Center for Research**
425 W 47th St.
New York, NY 10036
**Phone:** (212)582-0340 **Fax:** (212)265-5482
**Email:** rodiau@compuserve.com
**Website:** http://www.fountainhouse.org/research.html
Kenneth J. Dudek, Exec. Dir.

**Activities/Fields:** Rehabilitation, symptomatology, and stigma of serious mental illness with a focus on member self-determination in recovery. Evaluates the effectiveness of clubhouse model programs of psychiatric rehabilitation in facilitating post-hospital community adjustment and evaluates the effectiveness of transitional employment and other employment models. **Pub:** *Fountain House Annual.*

**★ 12691 ★ HIV Center for Clinical and**
**Behavioral Studies**
New York State Psychiatric Institute
1051 Riverside Dr., Unit 15
New York, NY 10032
**Phone:** (212)543-5969 **Fax:** (212)543-6003
**Email:** ehrharda@child.cpmc.columbia.edu
**Website:** http://www.hivcenternyc.org
Anke A. Ehrhardt, PhD, Dir. & Prin. Investigator

**Activities/Fields:** Investigates high risk sexual behaviors leading to HIV infection among heterosexual adults (especially women), adolescents, and gay men. Studies include prevention among depressed adolescent girls and gay and lesbian adolescents, development of interventions aimed at heterosexual women and men, serodiscordant male couples, and homeless mentally ill men and women. Methods development and quality assurance proceed in the domains of psychosocial and qualitative assessment, psychosexual assessment, biostatistics, data management, and epidemiology. Conducts programs in community liaison, media-based interventions and education, and ethical, legal, and policy issues. **Pub:** *Bibliography.*

**Indiana University-Purdue University at**
**Indianapolis**
**Riley Child and Adolescent Psychiatry**
**Clinic**
*See:* Entry 5796

**★ 12692 ★ Institute for Psychoanalysis**
122 S Michigan, Ste. 1300
Chicago, IL 60603-6107
**Phone:** (312)922-7474 **Fax:** (312)922-5656
**Email:** cmcdougl@iupui.edu
**Website:** http://www.chicagoanalysis.org
Dr. Jerome Winer, Dir.

**Activities/Fields:** Psychoanalysis, psychosomatic medicine, psychiatry, and related behavioral sciences. Topics of interest include parent loss, mourning, and stuttering. **Pub:** *Annual of Pychoanalysis.* • *Classics in Psychoanalysis.* • *Emotions and Behavior Monographs.*

**Johns Hopkins University**
**Bipolar Pedigree Collection**
*See:* Entry 9406

**★ 12693 ★ Laval University**
**Robert Giffard Research Centre**
2601, Chemin de la Canardiere
Beauport, QC, Canada G1J 2G3
**Phone:** (418)663-5741 **Fax:** (418)663-9540
**Email:** michel.maziade@psa.ulaval.ca
Michel Maziade, Dir.

**Activities/Fields:** Mental disorders, including Alzheimer's disease, bipolar disorders, and autism. Center searches for diagnostics and treatments for neurological and psychiatric disorders, and works to identify susceptible genes by identifying and characterizing a linkage marker. Specific program includes the mapping and characterization of major genes that result in schizophrenia and mental depression.

**★ 12694 ★ Margaret S. Mahler**
**Psychiatric Research Foundation**
254 Kent Rd.
Wynnewood, PA 19096
**Phone:** (610)645-5524 **Fax:** (610)645-5524
**Email:** wsingletarymd@aol.com
Dr. William M. Singletary, Pres.

**Activities/Fields:** Issues related to child development, education for parenting, and prevention and early intervention.

**★ 12695 ★ Matrix Research Institute**
**Research Employment, Training and**
**Rehabilitation Services for People with**
**Mental Illness**
Robert Morris Bldg., 10th Fl.
100 N 17th St.
Philadelphia, PA 19103
**Phone:** (215)569-2240 **Fax:** (215)569-2806
**Email:** pkpmri@aol.com
**Website:** http://www.matrixresearch.org
Daniel Raudenbush, PhD, Dir.

**Activities/Fields:** Employment needs of persons with serious psychiatric disabilities, specifically improving access to the Social Security Work Incentives; evaluating alternatives to rehabilitation systems; improving access to employment services; women and work; a multicultural perspective on rehabilitation; the nature of the employer/employee relationship; long-term career paths of persons with serious mental illness; costs of employment services; and the impact of managed care on employment services. **Pub:** *Training manuals and educational materials.*

**★ 12696 ★ MCP Hahnemann University**
**of the Health Sciences**
**Eastern Pennsylvania Psychiatric Institute**
3200 Henry Ave.
Philadelphia, PA 19129

**Phone:** (215)842-4100          **Fax:** (215)843-9672
**Email:** tp26@drexel.edu
Trevor Price, MD, Ch., Dept. of Psychiatry

**Activities/Fields:** Neurosciences, mental health, and pharmacology, including basic, clinical, and applied studies on etiology and treatment modalities in mental disability, mental health of normal children, and prevention of mental disorders. Provides residency training programs and training for psychologists, social service workers, student nurses, and occupational therapists at both undergraduate and graduate levels.

★ **12697** ★ **Menninger Clinic**
**Department of Research**
PO Box 829
Topeka, KS 66601-0829
**Phone:** (785)350-5357          **Fax:** (785)350-5392
**Email:** sargenj@menninger.edu
**Website:** http://www.menninger.edu
John Sargent, MD, Res. Dir.

**Activities/Fields:** Mental health and illness from an interdisciplinary perspective, presently focused on three major content areas: developmental psychopathology, clinical applications of attachment theory, and treatment outcome research. **Pub:** *Bulletin of the Menninger Clinic*, bimonthly. • *Monographs.*

★ **12698** ★ **Michael Reese Hospital and Medical Center**
Singer Pavillion
2959 S Cottage Grove
Chicago, IL 60616
**Phone:** (312)791-3800          **Fax:** (312)791-8060
Dr. Bruce Gober, Ch. of Svcs.

**Activities/Fields:** Mental health and mental illness, its etiology, treatment, and prevention, including psychiatry, psychophysiology, clinical psychology, and neurophysiology. Studies ego functions, schizophrenia, the modal adolescent, normal and disturbed adolescents, family dynamics, and comparison of scales of manifest anxiety. Conducts biological and clinical investigations of affective disorder in children and adolescents; patterns of self-image in normal, delinquent, and disturbed adolescents; and the psychosomatic aspects of juvenile diabetes.

★ **12699** ★ **Mid-Missouri Mental Health Center**
3 Hospital Dr.
Columbia, MO 65201
**Phone:** (573)884-1300          **Fax:** (573)884-1010
**Website:** http://www.modmh.state.mo.us/mid_mo/index.htm
Dennis R. Canote, CEO

**Activities/Fields:** Mental health issues among children and adolscents, including epidemiology of psychiatric disorders, family violence, violence among adolescents, and outcome studies.

★ **12700** ★ **Nathan S. Kline Institute for Psychiatric Research**
140 Old Orangeburg Rd.
Orangeburg, NY 10962
**Phone:** (845)398-5500          **Fax:** (845)398-5510
**Website:** http://www.rfmh.org/nki/
Robert Cancro, MD, Dir.

**Activities/Fields:** Mental illness, including multidisciplinary studies on its etiology, epidemiology, treatment, and control; computer sciences, emphasizing clinical and administrative services; and biochemical, genetic, physiological, neurochemical, and psychopharmacological research. Collaborates in research with investigators from other institutions and many countries. Consists of nine divisions: information sciences, statistical sciences and epidemiology, molecular biology, clinical research, analytical psychopharmacology, neurochemistry, neurophysiology, geriatric physchiatry, MICA, and research support.

★ **12701** ★ **National Alliance for Research on Schizophrenia and Depression (NARSAD)**
60 Cutter Mill Rd., Ste. 404
Great Neck, NY 11021
**Phone:** (516)829-5576          **Free:** 800-829-8289
**Fax:** (516)487-6930
**Email:** amoran@narsad.org
**Website:** http://www.narsad.org
Audra L. Moran, Dir., Res. Grants Prog.

**Activities/Fields:** Causes, cure, treatments, and prevention of severe mental illnesses, primarily schizophrenia and depression. Emphasizes biomedical studies of brain diseases. Awards research grants and supports university-based research centers. **Pub:** *NARSAD Research Newsletter.*

★ **12702** ★ **National Association of State Mental Health Program Directors Research Institute, Inc.**
66 Canal Center Plz., Ste. 302
Alexandria, VA 22314-1591
**Phone:** (703)739-9333          **Fax:** (703)548-9517
**Email:** noel.mazade@nasmhpd.org
**Website:** http://www.rdmc.org/nri
Dr. Noel A. Mazade, Exec. Dir.

**Activities/Fields:** Mental health services and management of state mental health programs. Also compiles data and conducts research activities on various aspects of state mental health agencies financing, staffing, clinical services, and mental health service systems. **Pub:** *Outlook*, periodically.

★ **12703** ★ **New Hampshire-Dartmouth Psychiatric Research Center**
105 Pleasant St.
Concord, NH 03301
**Phone:** (603)271-5747          **Fax:** (603)271-5265
**Website:** http://www.dartmouth.edu/dms/psychrc
Robert E. Drake, MD, Dir.

**Activities/Fields:** Development of effective services for people with dual psychiatric disorders. Research focuses on cost-effective rehabilitation services; relationships between substance abuse, trauma, and victimization, and HIV risk behaviors; alternative service models for older adults; and models for shared decision making between clients and treatment providers.

★ **12704** ★ **New York Institute for Medical Research, Inc.**
PO Box 832
Nyack, NY 10960
**Phone:** (845)359-7160          **Fax:** (845)359-3801
**Email:** nyinstitut@aol.com
Esin Cig, Exec. Admin.

**Activities/Fields:** Behavioral, psychophysiological, and psychopharmacological research. Topics of interest include depression in young and elderly patients, dementia, anxiety neurosis, behavior and sleep disorders, and phase I studies on healthy volunteers. The Institute provides evaluation and treatment of selected psychiatric outpatients, such as psychiatric assessments, experimental psychological testing, physical and neurological examinations, clinical and diagnostic EEG, computer analyzed resting and sleep EEG, ECG, and clinical chemistry, including hormonal evaluations. **Pub:** *Newsletter*, occasionally.

★ **12705** ★ **New York State Psychiatric Institute**
1051 Riverside Dr.
New York, NY 10032
**Phone:** (212)543-5000          **Fax:** (212)543-6012
**Email:** jmo2@clumbia.edu
**Website:** http://www.nyspi.org/
Dr. John Oldham, Dir.

**Activities/Fields:** Psychiatry and neurosciences, including basic and clinical studies in biochemistry, psychoneuropharmacology, neuroendocrinology, neurotoxicology, psychosocial sciences, research and

clinical psychology, genetics, nosology, psychophysiology, developmental psychobiology, sociology, epidemiology, communication sciences and psychoanalysis. **Pub:** *Annual report*.

**New York University Medical Center**
**William and Sylvia Silberstein Aging and Dementia Research Center (ADRC)**
*See:* Entry 3059

★ **12706** ★ **Northwestern University Asher Center for the Study and Treatment of Depressive Disorders**
Ward Bldg., 9th Fl.
303 E Chicago
Chicago, IL 60611
**Phone:** (312)908-9380          **Fax:** (312)503-0466
**Email:** b-mckinney@nwu.edu
**Website:** http://www.ashercenter.nwu.edu/
Dr. William McKinney, Dir.

**Activities/Fields:** Depressive disorders, especially the neurobiological processes and mechanisms that underlie their development. Three central themes have been emphasized, including animal models of depression, neurobiological substrates of depressive disorders, and developmental perspectives.

★ **12707** ★ **Ohio State University Laboratory of Psychobiology**
Townsend Hall, Rm. 48
1885 Neil Ave.
Columbus, OH 43210
**Phone:** (614)292-1749          **Fax:** (614)292-4537
**Email:** berntson.2@osu.edu
Dr. Gary G. Berntson, Contact

**Activities/Fields:** Psychobiology and comparative psychology, including studies on recovery of function after brain damage, psychopharmacology, psychophysiology, developmental processes, and animal cognition. **Frmly.** Laboratory of Comparative and Physiological Psychology.

★ **12708** ★ **Psychiatric Research Institute**
1100 N St. Francis, Ste. 200
Wichita, KS 67214-2878
**Phone:** (316)291-4774
**Email:** kendra_frey@via-christi.org
**Website:** http://www.pri-research.org
Dr. W. Dale Horst, Admin. Dir.

**Activities/Fields:** Clinical drug testing for depression in adults and children, Alzheimer's disease, schizophrenia (inpatient and outpatient), centralized anxiety disorder, panic disorder, antiobesity, and pharmacokinetic drug testing.

★ **12709** ★ **Research Center on Managed Care for Psychiatric Disorders**
10920 Wilshire Blvd., Ste. 300
Los Angeles, CA 90024-6505
**Phone:** (310)794-3725          **Fax:** (310)794-3724
**Email:** punzalan@ucla.edu
**Website:** http://www.npi.ucla.edu/centers/hsrc/
Kenneth Wells, MD, Dir.

**Activities/Fields:** Managed care for vulnerable populations with psychiatric disorders. **Pub:** *Working papers series.*

**Rockefeller University**
**Laboratory of Human Behavior and Metabolism**
*See:* Entry 8763

**★ 12710 ★ Royal Ottawa Health Care Group**
**Institute of Mental Health Research (IMHR)**
Royal Ottawa Hospital, LG 2044
1145 Carling Ave.
Ottawa, ON, Canada K1Z 7K4
**Phone:** (613)722-6521 **Fax:** (613)722-5871
**Email:** imhr@rohcg.on.ca
Arun Ravindran, Actg. Dir. Gen.

**Activities/Fields:** Biopsychosocial research into the major psychiatric disorders, including schizophrenia, affective disorders, and anxiety disorders. Other areas of interest are geriatrics, forensics, addictions, and children's mental health.


**★ 12711 ★ Rush University**
**Center for Suicide Research and Prevention**
Rush-Presbyterian-St. Luke's Medical Center
600 S Paulina, Ste. 529
Chicago, IL 60612
**Phone:** (312)942-3351 **Fax:** (312)942-6876
**Email:** dclark@rush.edu
David C. Clark, PhD, Dir.

**Activities/Fields:** Suicidal behavior, including epidemiological and prevention research.


**★ 12712 ★ Rush University**
**Rush Institute for Mental Well-Being**
1720 W Polk St.
Chicago, IL 60612
**Phone:** (312)942-5372 **Fax:** (312)942-3113
Dr. Jan Fawcett, MD, Dir.

**Activities/Fields:** Clinical treatment of depression and related disorders, including alcoholism, anxiety disorders, and psychoses; treatment for damages caused by such disorders, including social and work impairment, recurrent episodes, and suicides; methods for prevention of depression and related disorders; and stress management techniques.


**★ 12713 ★ Rutgers University**
**Center for Research on the Organization and Financing of Care for the Severely Mentally Ill**
30 College Ave.
New Brunswick, NJ 08901-1293
**Phone:** (732)932-8415 **Fax:** (732)932-6872
**Email:** mechanic@rci.rutgers.edu
**Website:** http://www.ihhcpar.rutgers.edu/
Dr. David Mechanic, Dir.

**Activities/Fields:** Mental health services and policy in the state and nationally. Research agenda includes health and mental health policy; barriers to successful patient outcomes following hospitalization; economic consequences of mental illness; facilitating appropriate housing for the severely mentally ill; insurance coverage for young mentally ill adults; improving general medical care for the severely mentally ill; impact of mental health services under managed care; mental health aspects of the AIDS epidemic; psychiatric care in general hospitals; relationships between the general medical and the specialty psychiatric sectors; relationships between minority families and the public mental health system; service elements and the quality of functioning among the chronically mentally ill; study of post-World War II mental health policy; trends in children's mental health services; depression among the elderly; post treatment distress on breast cancer patients; using managed care to improve mental health services; improving compliance to antipsychotic medications; the impact of the deinstitutionalization on communities; diversion programs for individuals with a mental illness who are in the criminal justice system; and cultural issues in mental health treatment.


**★ 12714 ★ Social Psychiatry Research Institute**
150 E 69th St.
New York, NY 10021
**Phone:** (212)628-4800 **Fax:** (212)249-8546
Dr. Ari Kiev, Pres.

**Activities/Fields:** Mental health and psychiatry, including psychopharmacological studies of antidepressant, anti-anxiety, and Alzheimer's medications. Conducts clinical drug trials. Assembles data for the mental health and psychiatric professions.


**State University of New York Health Science Center at Brooklyn**
**Child Psychiatry Research Program**
*See:* Entry 5811


**State University of New York Health Science Center at Brooklyn**
**Infant and Child Behavior Laboratory**
*See:* Entry 5812


**State University of New York Health Science Center at Brooklyn**
**Neurodynamic Laboratory**
*See:* Entry 14278


**★ 12715 ★ State University of New York Health Science Center at Stony Brook**
**Institute for Mental Health Research**
Department of Psychiatry & Behavioral Science
Stony Brook, NY 11794-8101
**Phone:** (631)444-2990 **Fax:** (631)444-7534
**Email:** hb@cns.hscbklyn.edu
**Website:** http://www.uhmc.sunysb.edu:80/psychiatry/
Mark J. Sedler, MD, Actg. Chm.

**Activities/Fields:** Seeks to determine neurobiological factors in mental illnesses that can be used to aid in the development of improved treatments. Conducts basic neurobiological research and applied clinical studies. Areas of interest include psychopharmacology, molecular neurobiology, child psychopathology, behavioral biology, and behavioral medicine. **Frmly:** Long Island Research Institute.


**U.S. Department of Health and Human Services**
**National Institute on Aging**
**Laboratory of Personality and Cognition**
*See:* Entry 3084


**U.S. Department of Health and Human Services**
**National Institute on Alcohol Abuse and Alcoholism**
**Prevention Research Center**
*See:* Entry 19373


**★ 12716 ★ U.S. Department of Health and Human Services**
**National Institute of Mental Health (NIMH)**
6001 Executive Blvd., Rm. 8235
Bethesda, MD 20892-9669
**Phone:** (301)443-3673 **Fax:** (301)443-2578
**Email:** rn3p@nih.gov
**Website:** http://www.nimh.nih.gov
Richard K. Nakamura, PhD, Actg. Dir.

**Activities/Fields:** Brain, mental illness, and mental health, particularly the causes, prevention, diagnosis, and treatment of mental illnesses. Principal components are: the Divisions of Neuroscience and Behavioral Science, Clinical and Treatment Research, Epidemiology and Services Research, Extramural Activities, and Intramural Research Programs; Offices of Prevention, Equal Employment Opportunity, Rural Mental Health Research, Legislative Analysis and Coordination, Scientific Information, Resource Management, and Science Policy and Program Planning;

Office for Special Populations; and Office on AIDS. Operates the Neuropsychiatric Research Hospital on the St. Elizabeth's Hospital campus in Washington, D.C.


**★ 12717 ★ U.S. Department of Health and Human Services**
**National Institute of Mental Health**
**Division of Clinical and Treatment Research**
5600 Fishers Ln., Rm. 17C-20
Rockville, MD 20857
**Phone:** (301)443-3683 **Fax:** (301)443-7264
David Shore, MD, Actg. Dir.

**Activities/Fields:** Service delivery and health economics at the clinical, institutional, and systems levels; the understanding, treatment, and prevention of antisocial and violent behavior and their effects, including law and mental health interaction; and the prevention, control, and treatment of rape, other sexual assault, and their effects. The Division consists of: the Child and Family Support Branch, Services Research Branch, Statistical Research Branch, and Systems Development and Community Support Branch. **Frmly:** (1990) Biometry and Applied Sciences Division; Applied and Services Research Division.


**★ 12718 ★ U.S. Department of Health and Human Services**
**National Institute of Mental Health**
**Division of Clinical and Treatment Research**
**Child and Adolescent Disorders Research Branch**
6001 Executive Loop, Rm. 6200
MSC 9617
Bethesda, MD 20892-9617
**Phone:** (301)443-5944 **Fax:** (301)480-4415
**Email:** dkoretz@mail.nih.gov
Doreen Koretz, PhD, Chf.

**Activities/Fields:** Child and adolescent disorders, including attention deficit disorder, depression, conduct disorders, and autism. Also investigates suicide among children and adolescents. Focuses on classification, assessment, etiology, genetics, clinical course, outcome, and pharmacologic, somatic, and psychosocial treatment and rehabilitation of disorders affecting children and adolescents. **Frmly:** (1997) Division of Clinical and Treatment Research; Child and Adolescent Disorders Research Branch; (2000) Developmental Psychopathology Disorders Research Branch.


**★ 12719 ★ U.S. Department of Health and Human Services**
**National Institute of Mental Health**
**Division of Clinical and Treatment Research**
**Mental Disorders of the Aging Research Branch**
5600 Fishers Ln., Rm. 10-75
Rockville, MD 20857
**Phone:** (301)443-1185 **Fax:** (301)594-6784
Dr. Barry Lebowitz, Chf.

**Activities/Fields:** Mental health and illness implications of the aging process and old age. This includes studies on: causes, treatment, and prevention of Alzheimer's disease, senile dementia, and related disorders, with emphasis on differential diagnosis, test of memory-enhancing agents, and issues of coexisting illness and excess ability; causes, treatment, and prevention of depression in older persons (including investigations of the relationship of depression to dementing disorders, suicide, alcoholism, medical disease, and other behavioral disorders); causes, treatment, and prevention of behavioral disturbance and dysfunction, with special reference to agitation, assaultive/aggressive behavior, confusion, disorientation, and other behavioral problems; development and refinement of pharmacologic and psychosocial treatments, with special attention to efficacy, safety, side-effects, mechanisms of action, and drug/drug interaction; behavioral medicine and the interface of physical illness and mental disorders in later life; chronically mentally ill elderly, with special attention to treatment and management of schizophrenia and to psychosocial and behavioral approaches to quality of life; design and refinement of methods for treatment intervention, clinical trials, and service delivery models for the elderly; mental illness in nursing homes; effects of families, support systems, and self-help groups on the care of older persons with significant mental disorders; family stress and the care of Alzheimer's disease victims; and prevention of pathology among elderly at risk for mental illness. Support is provided through a wide range of mechanisms, including the Geriatric Mental Health Academic Award; Scientist Development Awards; and National Research Service Awards, including individual fellowships and institutional awards at pre-doctoral or postdoctoral levels. In addition, the Clinical Research Centers on Psychopathology of the Elderly Program provides support to a limited number of centers situated in clinical treatment settings with demonstrable interest in the study of mental health and aging.

★ **12720** ★ **U.S. Department of Health and Human Services**
**National Institute of Mental Health**
**Division of Extramural Activities**
6001 Executive Blvd., Rm. 6154
MSC 9609
Bethesda, MD 20892-9609
**Phone:** (301)443-3367          **Fax:** (301)443-4720
**Email:** jsteinbe@nih.gov
**Website:** http://www.nimh.nih.gov/dea/index.htm
Jane Steinberg, PhD, Dir.

**Activities/Fields:** Provides leadership and advice in developing, implementing, and coordinating extramural programs and policies; represents the Institute on extramural program and policy issues within the Department and with outside organizations; provides scientific and technical review of applications for grants, cooperative agreements, and contracts; and oversees National Advisory Mental Health Council activities. The Division consists of the Office of the Director and the following branches: Clinical, Epidemiological, and Services Review Branch; Neuroscience and Behavioral Science Review Branch; Research Development and Special Projects Review Branch; and Extramural Policy Branch. Division does not provide direct grant support. Copies of all current grant announcements may be obtained from this office, but consultation with regard to the development of grant applications should be obtained directly from the research support divisions of the National Institute of Mental Health.

★ **12721** ★ **U.S. Department of Health and Human Services**
**National Institute of Mental Health**
**Division of State and Community Systems Development**
**Survey and Analysis Branch**
5600 Fishers Ln.
Parklawn, Rm. 15C-04
Rockville, MD 20857
**Phone:** (301)443-3343          **Fax:** (301)443-7926
**Email:** rmanders@samhsa.gov
**Website:** http://www.mentalhealth.org
Ronald W. Manderscheid, Chf.

**Activities/Fields:** Statistics on the major characteristics of the nation's mental health service systems, their resources, staffing, utilization patterns, costs, and financing; develops methodology for statistical data collection and demography; and conducts ecological and demographic studies on the need and demand for mental health services. In addition, Branch provides consultation to state and local mental health agencies on statistical methodology, mental health information systems, and the use of data. **Pub:** *Information Systems Series.* • *Mental Health National Statistics Series.* **Frmly:** (1992) Statistical Research Branch.

★ **12722** ★ **U.S. Department of Health and Human Services**
**National Institute of Mental Health**
**Epidemiology and Services Research Division**
6001 Executive Blvd.
Bethesda, MD 20892-9629
**Phone:** (301)443-3648          **Fax:** (301)443-4045
**Email:** gnorquis@nih.gov
**Website:** http://www.nimh.nih.gov
Dr. Grayson Norquist, Dir.

**Activities/Fields:** Clinical epidemiology, classification, assessment, etiology, clinical course, outcome, treatment, and prevention of mental disorders and servcies research. **Frmly:** Clinical Research Division; Epidemiology and Services Research Division.

★ **12723** ★ **U.S. Department of Health and Human Services**
**National Institute of Mental Health**
**Epidemiology and Services Research Division**
**Epidemiology and Psychopathology Research Branch**
60001 Executive Blvd., Rm. 7219
MSC-9649
Bethesda, MD 20892-9649
**Phone:** (301)443-3774          **Fax:** (301)443-7895
Charles T. Kaelber, MD, Actg. Chf.

**Activities/Fields:** Assessing mental health/mental illness status of populations in terms of incidence and prevalence; describing the natural history of disorders and identifying illness syndromes in the community as well as in clinical patient populations; developing new epidemiologic, statistical, demographic, and other quantitatively oriented methodologies for assessing the mental illness/health of a population; conducting epidemiologic studies to identify etiologic factors of mental health/mental disorder in different groups in terms of inheritance, experience, behavior, biologic factors, and environment in community or patient populations; conducting case-control studies to test the efficacy of some positive action of intervention; and conducting clinical research in the classification, assessment, etiology, genetics, clinical course, outcome, and treatment of general psychopathology and other mental outcome and treatment of general psychopathology and other mental disorders. Support is provided through research grants, conference grants, small grants, specifically announced cooperative agreements, and institutional research training grants, as well as Research Scientist Development, Research Scientist, Clinical Scientist, and Physician Scientist Awards, and pre- and postdoctoral individual fellowships. Branch comprises the Development and Application of Epidemiology Methods Section, Development and Testing of Epidemiology Hypotheses Section, Experimental Epidemiology and Evaluation Section, and General Psychopathology Section.

★ **12724** ★ **U.S. Department of Health and Human Services**
**National Institute of Mental Health**
**Epidemiology and Services Research Division**
**Prevention Research Branch**
5600 Fishers Ln., Rm. 10C09
Rockville, MD 20857
**Phone:** (301)443-4283          **Fax:** (301)443-4045
Eve K. Moscicki, Chf.

**Activities/Fields:** Prevention of mental disorders and behavioral dysfunctions and the promotion of mental health, including preventing socio-emotional problems among infants and young children at risk; preventing conduct and other behavioral disorders in school-aged children; preventing anxiety and depressive disorders in children and adults; promoting mental health through the enhancement of protective factors, including coping mechanisms; preventing suicide and suicidality in preclinical populations; and preventing affective and anxiety disorders in HIV-infected individuals, people at high-risk for infection, their families, caretak-

ers, and loved ones. **Pub:** *Proceedings.* • *Research Reports.*

★ **12725** ★ **U.S. Department of Health and Human Services**
**National Institute of Mental Health**
**Epidemiology and Services Research Division**
**Violence and Traumatic Stress Research Branch**
5600 Fishers Ln., Parklawn, 18C-14
Rockville, MD 20857
**Phone:** (301)443-1636          **Fax:** (301)443-4611
Koretz Doreen, PhD, Contact

**Activities/Fields:** Support research and research training concerned with the development and prevention of adult psychopathology and mental disorders. Included within the Branch are studies aimed at the major brain disorders (e.g., schizophrenia, bipolar disorder, major depression), antisocial and other personality disorders, and co-morbid physical and mental disorders, as well as cross cutting epidemiological studies and studies that examine traumatic stress and victimization as a risk factor for psychopathology. priority areas but are relevant to NIMH and Branch missions. The Branch does not support research that is not clearly relevant to mental health concerns or research that more appropriately falls within the mission of other federal programs. **Frmly:** Antisocial and Violent Behavior Branch.

★ **12726** ★ **U.S. Department of Health and Human Services**
**National Institute of Mental Health**
**Intramural Research Programs Division**
Bldg. 10, Rm. 4N222
MSC 2108
10 Central Dr.
Bethesda, MD 20892
**Phone:** (301)496-3501          **Fax:** (301)480-8348
**Email:** rd31o@nih.gov
**Website:** http://intramural.nimh.nih.gov
Robert Desimone, PhD, Dir.

**Activities/Fields:** Clinical and behavioral, biological, and special research dealing with the causes, diagnosis, treatment, and prevention of mental disorders and the biological and psychosocial factors that determine human behavior and development; provides a focus for national attention in the area of mental health research; and provides technical support through development and maintenance of electronic and mechanical instrumentation and equipment. **Pub:** *ADAMHA News*, biweekly. • *NIH Record*, biweekly.

★ **12727** ★ **U.S. Department of Health and Human Services**
**National Institute of Mental Health**
**Intramural Research Programs Division**
**Experimental Therapeutic Branch**
NIH Bldg. 10, Rm. 4F-229A
10 Center Dr., MSC 1380
Bethesda, MD 20892-1380
**Phone:** (301)496-4303          **Fax:** (301)480-5135
David Pickar, MD, Chf. of Expmt. Therapeutics

**Activities/Fields:** Basic and clinical neuroscience and attempts to integrate data on the biochemistry and pharmacology of the central nervous system with an understanding of the pathogenesis and treatment of major psychiatric diseases. Branch comprises the Clinical and Pharmacology Section, Clinical Studies Section, Molecular Neurogenetics Section, and Molecular Pharmacology Section. **Frmly:** Clinical Neuroscience Branch.

**★ 12728 ★ U.S. Department of Health
and Human Services**
**National Institute of Mental Health**
**Intramural Research Programs Division**
**Socio-Environmental Studies Laboratory**
Federal Bldg., Rm. B1A-14
7550 Wisconsin Ave.
Bethesda, MD 20892-9005
**Phone:** (301)496-3383          **Fax:** (301)402-0621
**Email:** carmi.schooler@nih.gov
Carmi Schooler, PhD, Sect. Ch.

**Activities/Fields:** Social structure and personality, and cognition, including studies on basic cognitive and interpersonal processes in normal and schizophrenic individuals throughout the life span.


**★ 12729 ★ U.S. Department of Health
and Human Services**
**National Institute of Mental Health**
**Intramural Research Programs Division
(Basic Research)**
**Cell Biology Laboratory**
NIH Bldg. 36, Rm. 2A-11
9000 Rockville Pike
Bethesda, MD 20892
**Phone:** (301)496-9444          **Fax:** (301)402-1748
Michael J. Brownstein, Chf.

**Activities/Fields:** Light and electron microscope-level neuroanatomy, chronobiology, developmental neurobiology, biosynthesis of biologically active molecules, isolation of novel peptide hormones, and regulation of intracellular processes by chemical messenger. Laboratory has a section on biochemical pharmacology.


**★ 12730 ★ U.S. Department of Health
and Human Services**
**National Institute of Mental Health**
**Intramural Research Programs Division
(Basic Research)**
**Cerebral Metabolism Laboratory**
NIH Bldg. 36, Rm. 1A-05
9000 Rockville Pike
Bethesda, MD 20892
**Phone:** (301)496-1371          **Fax:** (301)480-1668
**Website:** http://www.shiloh.nimh.nih.gov
Louis Sokoloff, MD, Chf.

**Activities/Fields:** Neurochemistry and neurophysiology using biochemical methods for measuring local cerebral glucose utilization, local cerebral blood flow, and local cerebral protein synthesis in vivo. Laboratory comprises sections on clinical brain imaging and developmental neurochemistry.


**★ 12731 ★ U.S. Department of Health
and Human Services**
**National Institute of Mental Health**
**Intramural Research Programs Division
(Basic Research)**
**General and Comparative Biochemistry
Laboratory**
NIH Bldg. 36, Rm. 3D28
36 Convent Dr., MSC 4094
Bethesda, MD 20892-4094
**Phone:** (301)496-3241          **Fax:** (301)402-4747
Giulio L. Cantoni, MD, Sci. Emeritus

**Activities/Fields:** Mechanisms and pathways of biological methylation, alkaloid biosynthesis, peptides, cellular differentiation, and gene expression in eukaryotes. Focus is on the enzymatic mechanisms in methyl transfer reactions, mechanism of drug addiction, muscle differentiation in cell culture, and genetic engineering. **Pub:** *Annual Report.*


**★ 12732 ★ U.S. Department of Health
and Human Services**
**National Institute of Mental Health**
**Intramural Research Programs Division
(Basic Research)**
**Molecular Biology Laboratory**
NIH Bldg. 36, Rm. 1B-08
9000 Rockville Pike
Bethesda, MD 20892
**Phone:** (301)496-6945          **Fax:** (301)402-0245
**Email:** davidn@helix.nih.gov
David Neville, MD, Chf.

**Activities/Fields:** Comprises sections on biophysical chemistry, molecular genetics, and regulatory proteins.


**★ 12733 ★ U.S. Department of Health
and Human Services**
**National Institute of Mental Health**
**Intramural Research Programs Division
(Clinical Research)**
**Biological Psychiatry Branch**
NIH Bldg. 10, Rm. 3S-239
10 Center Dr.
Bethesda, MD 20892-1272
**Phone:** (301)496-4805          **Fax:** (301)402-0052
Dr. Robert Post, Chf.

**Activities/Fields:** Clinical psychiatric problems, including manic-depressive and schizo-affective illness, recurrent depression, and panic-anxiety disorders. The Branch's goal is to develop programs to investigate psychologic, biochemical, and neuroanatomic contributions to the study of manic-depressive illness, anxiety disorders, and related symptoms. Focus is on psychobiology, involving studies in psychiatry, psychology, neurology, genetics, pharmacology, and biochemistry. Specific research interests are the biochemistry of neurotransmission and the action of mood stabilizers, brain imaging of affective illness, and the models of sensitization and kindling. Branch comprises Anxiety and Affective Disorders Unit, Behavioral Biology Unit, Psychobiology Section, Molecular Neurobiology Section, and Behavioral Pharmacology Unit.


**★ 12734 ★ U.S. Department of Health
and Human Services**
**National Institute of Mental Health**
**Intramural Research Programs Division
(Clinical Research)**
**Child Psychiatry Branch**
NIH Bldg. 10, Rm. 3N-202
10 Center Dr., MSC 1600
Bethesda, MD 20892-1600
**Phone:** (301)496-6080          **Fax:** (301)402-0296
**Email:** rapoport@helix.nih.gov
**Website:** http://intramural.nimh.nih.gov/research/chp/index2.html
Judith L. Rapoport, MD, Chf.

**Activities/Fields:** Biological aspects of child psychiatry, including childhood schizophrenia, obsessive compulsive disorder, and hyperactivity. Areas of interest include pediatric psychopharmacology and brain imaging in child psychiatry. **Pub:** *Annual Report.*


**★ 12735 ★ U.S. Department of Health
and Human Services**
**National Institute of Mental Health**
**Intramural Research Programs Division
(Clinical Research)**
**Clinical Neuroendocrinology Branch**
NIH Bldg. 10, Rm. 2D-46
10 Center Dr.
Bethesda, MD 20892-1284
**Phone:** (301)496-6884          **Fax:** (301)402-1561
Philip W. Gold, MD, Chf.

**Activities/Fields:** Physiological organization of neuroendocrine systems and on the relevance of alterations in neuroendocrine function to the pathophysiology and etiology of major psychiatric disorders.


**★ 12736 ★ U.S. Department of Health
and Human Services**
**National Institute of Mental Health**
**Intramural Research Programs Division
(Clinical Research)**
**Clinical Neurogenetics Branch**
NIH Bldg. 10, Rm. 2D46
9000 Rockville Pike
Bethesda, MD 20892
**Phone:** (301)496-0373          **Fax:** (301)402-0859
**Website:** http://intramural.nimh.nih.gov/research/nsb/index.htm
Ellen Sidransky, MD, Sect. Ch.

**Activities/Fields:** Clinical and basic biologic and pharmacologic studies relating to the genetics of manic-depressive illness and schizophrenia. **Pub:** *Conference proceedings.*


**★ 12737 ★ U.S. Department of Health
and Human Services**
**National Institute of Mental Health**
**Intramural Research Programs Division
(Clinical Research)**
**Clinical Psychobiology Branch**
NIH Bldg. 10, Rm. 4S-239
10 Center Dr., MSC 1390
Bethesda, MD 20892-1390
**Phone:** (301)496-2141          **Fax:** (301)496-5439
Thomas A. Wehr, MD, Chf.

**Activities/Fields:** Clinical psychiatric and psychobiological research. Research interest includes sleep physiology and biological rythmns, seasonal affective disorder, (SAD) and light treatment. **Pub:** *Proceedings.*


**★ 12738 ★ U.S. Department of Health
and Human Services**
**National Institute of Mental Health**
**Intramural Research Programs Division
(Clinical Research)**
**Laboratory of Clinical Science**
NIH Bldg. 10, Rm. 3D41
10 Center Dr., MSC 1264
Bethesda, MD 20892-1264
**Phone:** (301)496-2757          **Fax:** (301)402-0188
**Email:** murphy.dl@helix.nih.gov
Dr. Dennis L. Murphy, MD, Chf.

**Activities/Fields:** Medical research related to mental health. Principal components include the Analytical Biochemistry Section, Pharmacology Section, Geriatric Psychiatry Section, Histopharmacology Section, and Clinical Neuropharmacology Section. **Pub:** *Proceedings of national and international conferences.*


**★ 12739 ★ U.S. Department of Health
and Human Services**
**National Institute of Mental Health**
**Intramural Research Programs Division
(Clinical Research)**
**Neurophsiology Laboratory**
NIHAC Bldg. 110, Rm. 119
Poolesville, MD 20837
**Phone:** (301)496-1201          **Fax:** (301)402-0236
Charles Gerfen, Actg. Chf.

**Activities/Fields:** Neurophysiology.


**★ 12740 ★ U.S. Department of Health
and Human Services**
**National Institute of Mental Health**
**Intramural Research Programs Division
(Clinical Research)**
**Neuropsychology Laboratory**
NIH Bldg. 49, Rm. 1B80
49 Convent Dr., MSC 4415
Bethesda, MD 20892-4415
**Phone:** (301)496-5625          **Fax:** (301)402-0046
Dr. Robert Desimore, Dir.

**Activities/Fields:** Relationships between neural structures and behavior in nonhuman primates using a multidisciplinary approach to study cognitive functions such as perception, attention, memory, and emotion in Old World monkeys.

**★ 12741 ★ U.S. Department of Health and Human Services**
**National Institute of Mental Health**
**Intramural Research Programs Division (Clinical Research)**
**Psychology and Psychopathology Laboratory**
NIH Bldg. 15K, Rm. 101A
15 North Dr.
Bethesda, MD 20892-2668
**Phone:** (301)496-2551          **Fax:** (301)402-1218
Allan F. Mirsky, PhD, Section Chf.

**Activities/Fields:** Genetic and neurobehavioral factors in psychopathology, and on normal cognition, emphasizing the pathology of attention.

**★ 12742 ★ U.S. Department of Health and Human Services**
**National Institute of Mental Health**
**Intramural Research Programs Division (Neuropsychiatric Research at Saint Elizabeth's Hospital)**
**Biochemical Genetics Laboratory**
Bldg. 10, Rm. 2D-54
9000 Rockville Pike
Bethesda, MD 20892
**Phone:** (301)435-3583          **Fax:** (301)480-9862
**Email:** merrilc@helix.nih.gov
Dr. Carl R. Merril, MD, Chf.

**Activities/Fields:** Affects of aging on the central nervous system. Primarily concerned with studies of protein variations in the brain, focusing on proteins and protein detection in normal and disease states. Exploring new approaches to increase the sensitivity of protein detection methods. Also, exploring the use of bacterial viruses, or bacteriophage, that display specific ligands or antibodies that can bind to proteins to provide a detection amplification system with a sensitivity to permit identification and characterization of proteins from single cells, or for the examination of trace proteins from tissues. Investigating the use of bacteriophage to treat infectious diseases caused by bacterial infections, as well as bacteriophage evolution, genomics, and molecular biology. The emergence of antibiotic-resistant bacterial strains requires the exploration of alternate antibacterial therapies, which led to study of the ability of bacterial viruses (bacteriophage, or phage) to rescue mice bacteremic from VRE. **Frmly:** Preclinical Pharmacology Laboratory.

**★ 12743 ★ U.S. Department of Health and Human Services**
**National Institute of Mental Health**
**Intramural Research Programs Division (Neuropsychiatric Research at Saint Elizabeth's Hospital)**
**Clinical and Services Branch**
Clinical Brain Disorders Branch
Bldg. 10 Center Dr., Rm. 4S-241
MSC1377
Bethesda, MD 20814-9692
**Phone:** (301)435-8966          **Fax:** (301)480-7795
**Email:** eganm@intra.nimh.nih.gov
Michael Egan, MD, Actg. Dir.

**Activities/Fields:** Schizophrenia, focusing on molecular genetic and epidemiological studies of the new physiological alternatives associated with schizophrenia using patients and their families.

**★ 12744 ★ U.S. Department of Health and Human Services**
**National Institute of Mental Health**
**Neuroscience and Behavioral Science Division**
5600 Fishers Ln., Rm. 11-103
Rockville, MD 20857
**Phone:** (301)443-3563          **Fax:** (301)443-1731
**Website:** http://www.nimh.nih.gov
Stephen L. Foote, PhD, Actg. Dir.

**Activities/Fields:** Programs of research, research training, and resource development in basic and clinical neuroscience; reviews and assesses the performance of such programs; collaborates with other federal agencies and with outside organizations. The Division consists of the Behavioral and Integrative Neuroscience Research Branch, Molecular and Cellular Neuroscience Research Branch, Genetics Research Branch, Preclinical and Clinical Therapeutics Research Branch, the Research Training and Research Development Program, and the Translational Research and Scientific Technology Program. **Pub:** Conference proceedings. **Frmly:** Basic Sciences Division; (1993) Basic Brain and Behavioral Sciences Division.

**★ 12745 ★ U.S. Department of Health and Human Services**
**National Institute of Mental Health**
**Neuroscience and Behavioral Science Division**
**Behavioral, Cognitive, and Social Science Research Branch**
6001 Exec. Blvd., Rm. 7215
Bethesda, MD 20892-9651
**Phone:** (301)443-3942          **Fax:** (301)443-9876
**Email:** moliveri@nih.gov
Dr. Mary Ellen Oliveri, Chf.

**Activities/Fields:** Programs of research, research training, and resource development in the behavioral sciences to increase understanding of psychological, psychosocial, emotional, and cognitive factors influencing behavior. **Frmly:** Behavioral Sciences Research Branch.

**★ 12746 ★ U.S. Department of Health and Human Services**
**National Institute of Mental Health**
**Neuroscience and Behavioral Sciences Division**
**Molecular and Cellular Neuroscience Research Branch**
Neuroscience Ctr. Bldg.
6001 Executive Blvd.
Rockville, MD 20857
**Phone:** (301)443-1504          **Fax:** (301)443-4822
Dr. Stephen Zalcman, Chf.

**Activities/Fields:** Behavior and brain function in order to develop knowledge of basic biological/molecular mechanisms underlying mental disorders and to understand the basic processes involved in the action of psychoactive drugs. Activities involve biobehavioral research, neurobiological research, and psychopharmacological research, which includes support for clinical and preclinical studies on the physiological sites and mechanisms of actions of psychoactive drugs. Branch comprises the Neuroimaging and Applied Neuroscience Research Branch.

**★ 12747 ★ U.S. Department of Health and Human Services**
**National Institute of Mental Health**
**Office of Scientific Information**
6001 Executive Blvd., Rm. 8184, MSC 9663
Bethesda, MD 20892-9663
**Phone:** (301)443-4513          **Free:** 800-421-4211
**Fax:** (301)443-4279
**Email:** nimhpubs@nih.gov
**Website:** http://www.nimh.nih.gov/ocpl/index.htm
Clarissa Wittenberg, Dir.

**Activities/Fields:** Administers the Institute's public communication, scientific information dissemination, and media relations activities. Prepares materials for professionals and the general public based on current research developments. Is responsible for a national program to educate the public, primary care providers, and mental health specialists about mental disorders, including anxiety disorders and depressive illnesses. Office is comprised of two branches, the Public Affairs and Science Reports Branch and the Information Resources and Inquiries Branch.

**U.S. Department of Health and Human Services**
**National Institute of Nursing Research**
**Intramural Research Division**
**Laboratory for the Study of Human Responses to Health and Illness**
*See:* Entry 15787

**U.S. Department of Health and Human Services**
**National Institute for Occupational Safety and Health**
**Biomedical and Behavioral Science Division**
**Applied Psychology and Ergonomics Branch**
*See:* Entry 16823

**U.S. Department of Health and Human Services**
**National Institutes of Health**
**National Institute of Mental Health**
**Experimental Therapeutics Branch (Section on Cognitive Neuropsychology)**
*See:* Entry 14331

**U.S. Department of Health and Human Services**
**National Institutes of Health**
**National Institute of Mental Health**
**Experimental Therapeutics Branch (Geriatric Psychiatry Branch)**
*See:* Entry 3095

**U.S. Department of Health and Human Services**
**National Institutes of Health**
**National Institute of Mental Health**
**Experimental Therapeutics Branch (Clinical Neuroendocrinology Branch)**
*See:* Entry 14341

**U.S. Department of Health and Human Services**
**National Institutes of Health**
**National Institute of Mental Health**
**Experimental Therapeutics Branch (Section on Clinical Studies)**
*See:* Entry 14342

**★ 12748 ★ U.S. Department of Health and Human Services**
**National Institutes of Health**
**National Institute of Mental Health**
**Experimental Therapeutics Branch (Section on Neuropathology)**
Bldg. 10, Rm. 3n212
9000 Rockville Pike
Bethesda, MD 20892
**Phone:** (301)496-4805          **Fax:** (301)402-0052
**Email:** nimhinfo@nih.gov
**Website:** http://intramural.nimh.nih.gov/research/cbdb/
Joel Kleinman, MD, Ch.

**Activities/Fields:** Postmortem studies of schizophrenia, suicide, alcohol, other drug addictions, movement disorders, and dementias.

**U.S. Department of Health and Human Services**
**National Institutes of Health**
**National Institute of Mental Health**
**Experimental Therapeutics Branch**
**(Section on Developmental Genetic Epidemiology)**
*See:* Entry 9483

**★ 12749 ★ U.S. Department of Health and Human Services**
**National Institutes of Health**
**National Institute of Mental Health**
**Molecular Neuropsychiatry Section**
6001 Executive Blvd., Rm. 5213
MSC 2668
Bethesda, MD 20892-9561
**Phone:** (410)550-2953          **Fax:** (410)550-1477
**Email:** jcadet@intra.nida.nih.gov
**Website:** http://www.nida.nih.gov/DIR/molec-neuro.html
Jean Lud Cadet, MD, Ch.

**Activities/Fields:** Investigates biochemical, cellular and genetic abnormalities in neurobehavioral disorders; assesses effects of drugs at the cellular and molecular level; development of RNA isolation and gene cloning techniques to study disorders at the genomic level.

**★ 12750 ★ U.S. Department of Health and Human Services**
**National Institutes of Health**
**National Institute of Mental Health**
**Pediatrics and Developmental Neuropsychiatry Branch**
Bldg. 10, Rm. 4N208
9000 Rockville Pike
Bethesda, MD 20892
**Phone:** (301)496-5323          **Fax:** (301)402-8497
**Email:** swedos@irp.nimh.nih.gov
**Website:** http://intramural.nimh.nih.gov/research/pdn/
Susan Swedo, MD, Ch.

**Activities/Fields:** Identification of factors influencing the onset and expression of psychiatric symptomatology; development of treatment and prevention strategies for pediatric psychopathology.

**★ 12751 ★ U.S. Department of Health and Human Services**
**National Institutes of Health**
**National Institute of Mental Health**
**Section on Biological Rhythms**
Bldg. 10, Rm. 3S231
9000 Rockville Pike
Bethesda, MD 20892
**Phone:** (301)496-2141          **Fax:** (301)496-5439
**Email:** tawehr@box-t.nih.gov
**Website:** http://intramural.nimh.nih.gov/research/sbr/
Thomas A. Wehr, MD, Ch.

**Activities/Fields:** Human circadian and seasonal rhythms and their role in the pathogenesis of mood and sleep disorders; investigates how light regulates the timing of these rhythms and how it can be used for treatment.

**U.S. Department of Health and Human Services**
**National Institutes of Health**
**National Institute of Mental Health**
**Section on Pharmacology**
*See:* Entry 8812

**★ 12752 ★ U.S. Department of Health and Human Services**
**National Institutes of Health**
**National Institute of Mental Health**
**Section on Socio-Environmental Studies**
Bldg. 10, Rm. 4N222
9000 Rockville Pike
Bethesda, MD 20892
**Phone:** (301)496-3383
**Email:** schoolec@irp.nimh.nih.gov
**Website:** http://intramural.nimh.nih.gov/research/ses
Carmi Schooler, PhD, Ch.

**Activities/Fields:** Determinants of normal and abnormal psychological functioning during the life span, including cognitive processing and self-direction or autonomy.

**U.S. Department of Veterans Affairs**
**National Center for Post-Traumatic Stress Disorder**
**Behavioral Science Division**
*See:* Entry 13488

**U.S. Department of Veterans Affairs**
**National Center for Post-Traumatic Stress Disorder**
**Clinical Neurosciences Division**
*See:* Entry 13489

**U.S. Department of Veterans Affairs**
**National Center for Post-Traumatic Stress Disorder**
**Education Division**
*See:* Entry 13490

**U.S. Department of Veterans Affairs**
**National Center for Post-Traumatic Stress Disorder**
**Executive Division**
*See:* Entry 13491

**U.S. Department of Veterans Affairs**
**National Center for Post-Traumatic Stress Disorder**
**Northeast Program Evaluation Center**
*See:* Entry 13492

**U.S. Department of Veterans Affairs**
**National Center for Post-Traumatic Stress Disorder**
**Pacific Islands Division**
*See:* Entry 13493

**U.S. Department of Veterans Affairs**
**National Center for Post-Traumatic Stress Disorder**
**Women's Health Sciences Division**
*See:* Entry 13494

**U.S. Department of Veterans Affairs**
**Veterans Health Administration**
**Office of Research and Development**
**Medical Research Service**
**(Schizophrenia Research Center)**
*See:* Entry 13511

**U.S. Department of Veterans Affairs**
**Veterans Health Administration**
**Office of Research and Development**
**Medical Research Service**
**(Schizophrenia Research Center)**
*See:* Entry 13512

**University of California at Berkeley**
**Center for Mental Health Services Research (CMHSR)**
*See:* Entry 9886

**★ 12753 ★ University of California, Los Angeles**
**Harbor-UCLA Medical Center**
**Research and Education Institute**
1124 W Carson St.
Torrance, CA 90502-2006
**Phone:** (310)222-4266          **Fax:** (310)222-4264
**Email:** snowden@uclink4.berkeley.edu
**Website:** http://www.rei.edu
Gail V. Anderson, MD, Dir.

**Activities/Fields:** Role of ethnicity (including culture) and biological variables in the mental health of ethnic minority populations. Conducts studies using pharmacokinetic, pharmacodynamic, and pharmacogenetic research techniques to examine ethnic and individual differences in responses to psychotropic drugs.

**★ 12754 ★ University of California, Los Angeles**
**Neuropsychiatric Institute**
760 Westwood Plz.
Los Angeles, CA 90024
**Phone:** (310)206-1233          **Fax:** (310)825-3942
**Website:** http://www.npi.ucla.edu
Dr. Peter C. Whybrow, Dir.

**Activities/Fields:** Genetics, pharmacology, mental retardation; developmental neurobiology; behavioral sciences, including anthropology; biochemistry, neurophysiology, cognitive neuroscience, brain imaging, health services and social policy.

**★ 12755 ★ University of California, Los Angeles**
**Program on Psychosocial Adaptation and the Future**
Neuropsychiatric Institute
760 Westwood Plz.
Los Angeles, CA 90024-1759
**Phone:** (310)825-0463          **Fax:** (310)825-3002
**Email:** preadapt@ucla.edu
Roderic Gorney, PhD, Dir.

**Activities/Fields:** Studies psychosocial and cultural determinants of behavior, including impact of television on adults and the clinical role of the sense of the future in mental illness.

**★ 12756 ★ University of California, San Francisco**
**Langley Porter Psychiatric Institute**
401 Parnassus Ave.
San Francisco, CA 94143
**Phone:** (415)476-7000          **Free:** 800-723-7140
**Fax:** (415)476-7320
**Email:** cvd@lppi.ucsf.edu
**Website:** http://www.ucsf.edu/psych/home.htm
Craig Van Dyke, MD, Dir.

**Activities/Fields:** Clinical studies of psychiatric disorders and psychotherapy and basic research studies in psychopharmacology, neurobiology, cellular and molecular biology, behavioral biology, and social sciences.

**★ 12757 ★ University of Colorado**
**National Center for American Indian and Alaska Native Mental Health Research**
University North Pavilion
Department of Psychiatry
4455 E 12th Ave., A011-13
Denver, CO 80220
**Phone:** (303)315-9232          **Fax:** (303)315-9579
**Email:** jan.beals@uchsc.edu
**Website:** http://www.uchsc.edu/sm/ai/ncaianmhr
Dr. Jan Beals, PhD, Dir.

**Activities/Fields:** Determination and improvement of the performance characteristics of self-report measures of serious psychological dysfunction and diagnostic interviews for assessing alcohol, drug, and mental (ADM) disorders; establishment of the prevalence and incidence of ADM disorders and related risk factors through descriptive and experimental epidemiological investigations; development and evaluation of methods for detecting and managing ADM disorders presented in human service settings; and examination of the effectiveness of interventions for preventing ADM disorders and promoting well-being. Ongoing studies include the Services Utilization and Psychiatric Epidemiology Project, which seeks to obtain prevalence rates of the major ADM disorders among American Indians; the Choices Project, which is designed to develop reliable and valid measures of pregnancy intentionality by more fully and carefully elucidating the cultural, familial, and individual contexts of this phenomenon; the Healthy Ways Project, which studies the behavioral and biomedical epidemiology of HIV/AIDS and STDs in two American Indian tribes and uses this information to design individual and community level preventive interventions; the American Indian Pathways to Abstinence Project, which investigates how problem drinking and abstinence are meaningfully construed and experienced by American Indian men and women; and the Early Head Start Project which seeks to understand normative infant and toddler development and parenting practices within a Northern Plains culture. **Pub:** *American Indian and Alaska Native Mental Health Research Journal*, 3/year. • *Annual Monograph*.


**University of Florida**
**Center for Ambulatory Studies**
*See:* Entry 4560


★ **12758** ★ **University of Illinois at**
**Chicago**
**National Research and Training Center**
**on Psychiatric Disability**
104 S Michigan Ave., Ste. 900
Chicago, IL 60603
**Phone:** (312)422-8180          **Fax:** (312)422-0740
**Email:** jcook@ripco.com
**Website:** http://www.psych.uic.edu/uicnrtc
Judith A. Cook, PhD, Dir.
**Activities/Fields:** Psychiatric disabilities. Activities focus on five core areas that emphasize self-determination for people with psychiatric disabilities, including choice in treatment decision-making, economic self-sufficiency, consumer advocacy under managed care, career development through real jobs and real wages, and strengthening self-determination skills and self-advocacy.


**University of Illinois at Chicago**
**Psychiatric Institute**
*See:* Entry 5821


**University of Illinois at Chicago**
**Rehabilitation Research and Training**
**Center on Aging with Developmental**
**Disabilities (RRTCADD)**
*See:* Entry 3105


★ **12759** ★ **University of Kansas**
**Alzheimer's Disease Center (ADC)**
G043 Delp Pavilion
3901 Rainbow Blvd.
Kansas City, KS 66160
**Phone:** (913)588-6981          **Fax:** (913)588-6965
**Email:** glopez@kumc.edu
**Website:** http://adc.kumc.edu/
Grisel Lopez, MD, Dir.
**Activities/Fields:** Causes and treatments for Alzheimer's disease and other dementing illnesses.


**University of Kansas**
**Child and Family Research Center**
*See:* Entry 5824


**University of Louisville**
**Louisville Twin Study**
*See:* Entry 9505


★ **12760** ★ **University of Maryland**
**Maryland Psychiatric Research Center**
PO Box 21247
Baltimore, MD 21228-0747
**Phone:** (410)402-7666          **Fax:** (410)402-7198
**Email:** wcarpent@mprc.umaryland.edu
**Website:** http://www.mprc.umaryland.edu
Dr. William T. Carpenter, Jr., Dir.
**Activities/Fields:** Etiology and treatment of chronic schizophrenia and including assessment of therapeutic efficacy of treatment, design of safer approaches to antipsychotic and other drug treatments, definition of subgroups of patients to permit clinicians to match patients and treatments, design and implementation of experimental treatments. Neuroscience program studies brain mechanisms involved in the causes, manifestations, and treatment of mental illness. Provides clinical and diagnostic services and education for families and patients.


★ **12761** ★ **University of Massachusetts**
**Eunice Kennedy Shriver Center for**
**Mental Retardation, Inc.**
Medical School
200 Trapelo Rd.
Waltham, MA 02452-6319
**Phone:** (781)642-0001          **Fax:** (781)893-5340
**Email:** william.mcilvane@umassmed.edu
**Website:** http://www.umassmed.edu/shriver
Dr. William McIlvane, Dir.
**Activities/Fields:** Interdisciplinary studies in mental retardation and developmental disabilities, conducted through two research departments: Biomedical Sciences and Psychological Sciences. **Pub:** *Newsletter*, quarterly.


★ **12762** ★ **University of Michigan**
**Mental Health Research Institute**
205 Zina Pitcher Pl.
Ann Arbor, MI 48109-0720
**Phone:** (734)764-4235          **Fax:** (734)647-4130
**Email:** rpfreed@umich.edu
**Website:** http://www.med.umich.edu/mhri
Ruth P. Freedman, Admin.
**Activities/Fields:** Biological and behavioral studies relevant to normal and pathological human behavior and treatment of mental illness. Conducts studies on basic biological mechanisms relevant to normal and pathological behavior. Emphasis on neuroscience and biological psychiatry. **Pub:** *MHRI Annual Report*, biennially.


★ **12763** ★ **University of Missouri—**
**Columbia**
**Missouri Institute of Mental Health**
5400 Arsenal St.
Saint Louis, MO 63139-1494
**Phone:** (314)644-8851          **Fax:** (314)644-8834
**Email:** mimhdw@showme.missouri.edu
**Website:** http://www.mimh.edu
Danny Wedding, PhD, Dir.
**Activities/Fields:** Mental health policy and ethics, mental health information systems, computer applications for the assessment and treatment of the mentally retarded and mentally ill, outcomes assessments, and mental health program evaluation research. **Frmly:** Missouri Institute of Psychiatry.


★ **12764** ★ **University of Missouri—St.**
**Louis**
**Center for Trauma Recovery**
Weinman Bldg.
Department of Psychology
8001 Natural Bridge Rd.
Saint Louis, MO 63121
**Phone:** (314)516-5391          **Fax:** (314)516-5392
**Email:** resick@umsl.edu
**Website:** http://www.umsl.edu/divisions/artsscience/psychology/CVRPResearch.html
Patricia A. Resick, PhD, Dir.
**Activities/Fields:** Posttraumatic stress disorder (PTSD), its causes and treatments.


★ **12765** ★ **University of Montreal**
**Riviere-des-Prairies Hospital Research**
**Centre**
7070 Blvd. Perras
Montreal, QC, Canada H1E 1A4
**Phone:** (514)323-7260          **Fax:** (514)323-4163
**Email:** jj.breton.hrdp@ssss.gouv.qc.ca
Dr. Jean-Jacques Breton, Dir.
**Activities/Fields:** Epidemiology of mental disorders, screening, suicide, autism, sleep disorders. **Pub:** *Journal Articles*.


**University of North Carolina at Chapel**
**Hill**
**Clinical Research Unit**
*See:* Entry 2706


★ **12766** ★ **University of Pennsylvania**
**Center for Cognitive Therapy**
Department of Psychiatry
School of Medicine
3600 Market St., 8th Fl.
Philadelphia, PA 19104-2649
**Phone:** (215)898-4100          **Fax:** (215)898-1865
**Email:** psycct@mail.med.upenn.edu
**Website:** http://www.med.upenn.edu/psycct
Cory F. Newman, PhD, Dir.
**Activities/Fields:** Psychiatric outpatient clinic, engaged in developing different assessment instruments to measure constructs of cognitive theory, extending the cognitive approach to anxiety and other psychiatric disorders, assessing and predicting suicidal risks, studying outpatient populations, and assessing different training models for cognitive therapists. **Pub:** *Center for Cognitive Therapy Newsletter*.


★ **12767** ★ **University of Pennsylvania**
**Center for Mental Health Policy and**
**Services Research**
3600 Market St., 7th Fl.
Philadelphia, PA 19104-2648
**Phone:** (215)662-2886          **Fax:** (215)349-8715
**Email:** trevor@cmhpsr.upenn.edu
**Website:** http://www.uphs.upenn.edu/~cmhpsr/
Trevor Hadley, PhD, Dir.
**Activities/Fields:** Mental health policy and services.


★ **12768** ★ **University of Pennsylvania**
**Depression Research Unit**
University City Science Center
3600 Market St., 8th Fl.
Philadelphia, PA 19104-2649
**Phone:** (215)662-3462          **Fax:** (215)662-6443
**Email:** jamsterd@mail.med.upenn.edu
Jay D. Amsterdam, MD, Dir.
**Activities/Fields:** Affective disorders. Research areas include psychopharmacology, particularly development of new antidepressant drugs; clinical neuroendocrinology; and the biochemical causes of major depression.

**★ 12769 ★ University of Pennsylvania**
**Mood and Anxiety Disorders Section**
3535 Market St., Ste. 670
Philadelphia, PA 19104-3309
**Phone:** (215)898-4301 **Fax:** (215)898-0509
**Email:** krickels@mail.med.upenn.edu
Dr. Karl Rickels, Dir.

**Activities/Fields:** Psychopharmacology, including short- and long-term clinical trials on the effects of antidepressive and antianxiety medications. **Frmly:** Psychopharmacology Research Unit.

**★ 12770 ★ University of Pennsylvania**
**Social Work Mental Health Research**
 **Center (SWMHRC)**
School of Social Work
3701 Locust Walk
Philadelphia, PA 19104-6214
**Phone:** (215)573-9688
**Email:** solomonp@ssw.upenn.edu
**Website:** http://www.ssw.upenn.edu/SWMHRC/index.htm
Phyllis L. Solomon, PhD, Co-Dir.

**Activities/Fields:** Mental health services and the social welfare of persons with severe mental illnesses. The center focuses on three areas of intervention: legal, mental health managed care, and mental health and supportive services.

**★ 12771 ★ University of Pennsylvania**
**Weight and Eating Disorders Program**
Department of Psychiatry
3535 Market St., Ste. 3108
Philadelphia, PA 19104
**Phone:** (215)898-7314 **Fax:** (215)898-2878
**Email:** wadden@mail.med.upenn.edu
**Website:** http://www.uphs.upenn.edu/~weight
Dr. Thomas A. Wadden, Dir.

**Activities/Fields:** Obesity, binge eating disorder, bulimia (including behavioral treatments for all). body image, metabolic rate and body fat measures, and predictors of adiposity in infancy.

**★ 12772 ★ University of Pittsburgh**
**Center for Mental Health Services**
 **Research (CMHSR)**
Cathedral of Learning, Rm. 2217
Pittsburgh, PA 15260
**Phone:** (412)624-6572 **Fax:** (412)624-1159
**Email:** cmhsr@pitt.edu
**Website:** http://server.socialwork.pitt.edu/~cmhsr/
Carol M. Anderson, PhD, Dir.

**Activities/Fields:** Understanding of individual, community and mental health service systems factors that facilitate or discourage the use of treatment resources; identification of barriers and modification of pathways to mental health care; and adaptation, design, and testing interventions for low income, minority, and other community populations.

**★ 12773 ★ University of Pittsburgh**
 **Medical Center**
**Western Psychiatric Institute and Clinic**
3811 O'Hara St.
Pittsburgh, PA 15213
**Phone:** (412)624-2100 **Fax:** (412)624-8015
**Email:** bourdl@msx.upmc.edu
**Website:** http://www.wpic.pitt.edu
Donna L. Bour, Contact

**Activities/Fields:** Advancement of basic and clinical knowledge in psychological, biological, environmental, and social interactions related to mental health and psychiatric care. Conducts research on psychiatric disorders, including depression, manic-depression, schizophrenia, anorexia nervosa, Alzheimer's disease, autism, anxiety, obsessive-compulsive disorders, and borderline disorders. Clinical services are organized around comprehensive treatment modules in the following areas: adolescent and young adult disorders, adult affective disorders, geriatrics, schizophrenia, chemical dependency, and children's services. Clinical

laboratory investigations include studies in clinical pharmacology, neuroendocrinology, psychophysiology, neuropharmacology, neurophysics, molecular neurobiology and genetics, and EEG sleep. Also researches health habits and precursors of medical disease states such as hypertension, diabetes, obesity, effects of drug abuse, and epidemiology of psychiatric disorders.

**★ 12774 ★ University of South Florida**
**Louis de la Parte Florida Mental Health**
 **Institute**
13301 Bruce B. Downs Blvd.
Tampa, FL 33612-3807
**Phone:** (813)974-4602 **Fax:** (813)974-4699
**Email:** leone@fmhi.usf.edu
**Website:** http://www.fmhi.usf.edu
Dr. David Shern, Dean

**Activities/Fields:** Mental health care, including aging and mental health, child and family studies, community mental health, and mental health law and policy. **Pub:** *Journal of Behavioral Health Services and Research*, quarterly. • *Journal of Mental Health and Aging*, quarterly. • *Mental Health Reviews.* **Frmly:** Florida Mental Health Institute.

**University of South Florida**
**Research and Training Center for**
 **Children's Mental Health**
*See:* Entry 5831

**University of South Florida**
**Roskamp Institute for Research into**
 **Neurodegenerative Diseases**
*See:* Entry 14458

**★ 12775 ★ University of Tennessee**
**Children's Mental Health Services**
 **Research Center**
128 Henson Hall
Knoxville, TN 37996-3332
**Phone:** (865)974-1707 **Fax:** (865)974-1662
**Email:** roskamp@hsc.usf.edu
**Website:** http://utcmhsrc.csw.utk.edu
Dr. Charles A. Glisson, Dir.

**Activities/Fields:** Children's mental health, especially children who are at risk, the factors which place them at risk, the quality of the services being provided to them, and the long-term outcomes.

**★ 12776 ★ University of Tennessee,**
 **Knoxville**
**Children's Mental Health Services**
 **Research Center**
128 Henson Hall
Knoxville, TN 37996-3332
**Phone:** (865)974-1707 **Fax:** (865)974-1662
**Email:** cglisson@utk.edu
**Website:** http://utcmhsrc.csw.utk.edu/
Dr. Charles Glisson, Dir.

**Activities/Fields:** Children who are at risk for mental illness, the factors which place them at risk, the quality of the services being provided to them, and the long-term outcomes.

**★ 12777 ★ University of Texas—Houston**
 **Health Science Center**
**Mental Sciences Institute**
1300 Moursund Ave.
Houston, TX 77030
**Phone:** (713)500-2500 **Fax:** (713)500-2553
**Email:** robert.w.guynn@uth.tmc.edu
**Website:** http://www.msi.uth.tmc.edu
Dr. Robert Guynn, Dir.

**Activities/Fields:** Biochemical and behavioral aspects of psychiatric diseases, particularly psychopathology and pharmacology of alcohol and drug addiction, and affective and anxiety disorders. Performs basic and clinical studies in neuroendocrinology, me-

tabolism, behavioral science, disorders, mental retardation, neurochemistry, psychophysiology, biochemistry, crime and delinquency, and gerontology. **Frmly:** Houston State Psychiatric Institute; Texas Research Institute of Mental Science.

**University of Vermont**
**Clinical Neuroscience Research Unit**
 **(CNRU)**
*See:* Entry 14468

**★ 12778 ★ University of Virginia**
**Center for the Study of Mind and Human**
 **Interaction (CSMHI)**
PO Box 800657
Charlottesville, VA 22908-0657
**Phone:** (434)982-1045 **Fax:** (434)982-2524
**Email:** mind@virginia.edu
**Website:** http://hsc.virginia.edu/csmhi/
Dr. Vamik D. Volkan, Dir.

**Activities/Fields:** Large-group dynamics, including ethnic tension, racism, national identity, terrorism, societal trauma, leader-follower relationships, and other aspects of national and international conflict. **Pub:** *Mind and Human Interaction.*

**★ 12779 ★ University of Virginia**
**Southeastern Rural Mental Health**
 **Research Center**
Health Science Center, Box 800782
Charlottesville, VA 22908-0782
**Phone:** (434)982-3273 **Fax:** (434)982-3275
**Email:** srmhrc@virginia.edu
**Website:** http://www.virginia.edu/~srmhrc
Elizabeth Merwin, Dir.

**Activities/Fields:** Rural mental health, focusing African-Americans and impoverished mentally ill individuals and their families. Specific area of study include the incidence and prevalence of mental disorders and co-occurring physical health problems, informal and formal care networks and interventions accessed and utilized by rural high risk populations in need of mental health and health service, and the cost and effectiveness of outreach and alternative models linking mental health, social service, and health care providers in the delivery of services to seriously mentally ill adults, the elderly, women, and children.

**★ 12780 ★ University of Washington**
**Alcohol and Drug Abuse Institute**
1107 NE 45th St., Ste. 120
PO Box 354805
Seattle, WA 98105-4631
**Phone:** (206)543-0937 **Fax:** (206)543-5473
**Email:** ddonovan@u.washington.edu
**Website:** http://depts.washington.edu/adai
Dennis M. Donovan, PhD, Dir.

**Activities/Fields:** Social, clinical, and psychological aspects of alcohol and drug abuse. **Pub:** *ADAI Technical Reports.*

**★ 12781 ★ University of West Florida**
**Behavioral Medicine Laboratory**
Department of Psychology
11000 University Pky.
Pensacola, FL 32514
**Phone:** (850)474-2041 **Fax:** (850)474-2042
**Email:** fandrasi@uwf.edu
**Website:** http://uwf.edu/psych/b_med.html
Dr. Frank Andrasik, Dir.

**Activities/Fields:** Interface between the biomedical and behavioral sciences; treatments for medical disorders and the most cost-effective delivery mechanisms for these treatments.

**★ 12782 ★ University of Wisconsin—Madison**
**HealthEmotions Research Institute**
6001 Research Pk. Blvd.
Madison, WI 53719-1176
**Phone:** (608)263-6685    **Fax:** (608)263-9340
**Email:** kalin@healthemotions.org
**Website:** http://www.healthemotions.org
Ned H. Kalin, MD, Dir.
**Activities/Fields:** Relationships between positive emotions, physiological systems, and health.

**University of Wisconsin—Madison**
**Neuropsychology Laboratory**
*See:* Entry 14473

**★ 12783 ★ Vanderbilt University**
**Center for Mental Health Policy**
1207 18th Ave. S
Nashville, TN 37212
**Phone:** (615)322-8435    **Fax:** (615)322-7049
**Email:** bickman@attglobal.net
**Website:** http://www.vanderbilt.edu/VIPPS/CMHP/cmhphome.html
Dr. Leonard Bickman, Dir.
**Activities/Fields:** Evaluation of homeless family programs, effects of family empowerment on children's mental health, patterns of psychiatric hospitalization of children, and evaluation of school mental health services.

**★ 12784 ★ Washington Institute for**
**Mental Illness Research and Training**
Eastern Branch
PO Box A
Medical Lake, WA 99022-0045
**Phone:** (509)299-4501    **Fax:** (509)299-4664
**Email:** dyck@wsu.edu
**Website:** http://www.spokane.wsu.edu/research&service/wimirt/wimirthome.html
Dennis G. Dyck, PhD, Dir.
**Activities/Fields:** Mental health clinical and services research for persons with severe and persistent mental illness; family and patient psychoeducation and support; and immune function and mental illness.

**★ 12785 ★ Washington University in St. Louis**
**Center for Mental Health Services**
**Research (CMHSR)**
CB 1093
Saint Louis, MO 63130-4899
**Phone:** (314)935-5687    **Fax:** (314)935-7508
**Email:** cmhsr@gwbmail.wustl.edu
**Website:** http://gwbweb.wustl.edu/Users/cmhsr/
Enola K. Proctor, PhD, Dir.
**Activities/Fields:** Mental health services from a variety of care providers, ranging from mental health specialists to family members.

**★ 12786 ★ Yale University**
**Ribicoff Research Facilities of the**
**Connecticut Mental Health Center**
34 Park St.
New Haven, CT 06508
**Phone:** (203)974-7726    **Fax:** (203)974-7724
**Email:** ronald.duman@yale.edu
Dr. Ronald S. Duman, Dir.
**Activities/Fields:** Preclinical and clinical studies of the neurobiological basis of severe mental disorders, including depression, anxiety, schizophrenia, and drug addiction. Conducts basic research programs in molecular, biochemical, neurophysiological, neuropharmacological, and behavioral fields. **Pub:** *Yale Psychiatry*.

**★ 12787 ★ Yeshiva University**
**Sound View-Throgs Neck Community**
**Mental Health Center**
2527 Glebe Ave.
Bronx, NY 10461
**Phone:** (718)904-4400    **Fax:** (718)931-7307
Dr. Thomas Betzler, Exec. Dir.
**Activities/Fields:** Mental health, mental illness, and recovery from mental illness.

# State Government Agencies

## Mental Health

**★ 12788 ★ Alabama Department of**
**Mental Health and Mental Retardation**
RSA Union
100 N Union St., Ste. 518
Montgomery, AL 36130-1410
**Phone:** (334)242-3107    **Fax:** (334)242-0684
**Website:** http://www.mh.state.al.us/
Kathy Sawyer, Director

**★ 12789 ★ Alaska Department of Health**
**and Social Services**
**Mental Health and Developmental**
**Disabilities Division**
350 Main St., Rm. 217
PO Box 110620
Juneau, AK 99811-0620
**Phone:** (907)465-3370    **Free:** 800-465-4828
**Fax:** (907)465-2668
**Email:** dmhdd_webmaster@health.state.ak.us
**Website:** http://www.hss.state.ak.us/dmhdd/
Leonard Abel, Contact

**★ 12790 ★ Arizona Department of Health**
**Services**
**Behavioral Health Services Division**
2122 E Highland
Phoenix, AZ 85016
**Phone:** (602)381-8999    **Fax:** (602)553-9140
**Email:** csmallw@hs.state.az.us
**Website:** http://www.hs.state.az.us/bhs/home.htm

**★ 12791 ★ Arkansas Department of**
**Human Services**
**Mental Health Services Division**
4313 W Markham
Little Rock, AR 72205
**Phone:** (501)686-9164    **Fax:** (501)686-9182
**Email:** sheila.duncan@mail.state.ar.us
**Website:** http://www.state.ar.us/dhs/dmhs/
Sheila Duncan, Contact

**★ 12792 ★ California Health and Welfare**
**Agency**
**Mental Health Department**
1600 9th St., Rm. 151
Sacramento, CA 95814
**Phone:** (916)654-2309    **Free:** 800-896-2512
**Fax:** (916)654-3198
**Email:** webmastr@dmhhq.state.ca.us
**Website:** http://www.dmh.cahwnet.gov/

**★ 12793 ★ Colorado Department of**
**Human Services**
**Mental Health Division**
3824 W Princeton Cir.
Denver, CO 80236
**Phone:** (303)866-7400    **Fax:** (303)866-7428
**Email:** debbie.kupfer@state.co.us
**Website:** http://www.cdhs.state.co.us/ohr/mhs/index.html

**★ 12794 ★ Connecticut Department of**
**Mental Health and Addiction Services**
**Mental Health Services**
410 Capitol Ave., 4th Fl.
PO Box 341431
Hartford, CT 06134
**Phone:** (860)418-7000    **Free:** 800-446-7348
**Website:** http://www.dmhas.state.ct.us/

**★ 12795 ★ Delaware Department of**
**Health and Social Services**
**Alcoholism, Drug Abuse, and Mental**
**Health Division**
1901 N Dupont Hwy.
New Castle, DE 19720
**Phone:** (302)255-9399    **Fax:** (302)577-4486
**Email:** dhssinfo@state.de.us
**Website:** http://www.state.de.us/dhss/dadamh/dmhhome.htm
Renata J. Henry, Director

**★ 12796 ★ District of Columbia**
**Department of Human Services**
**Mental Health Commission**
2700 Martin Luther King Ave., SE
Washington, DC 20032
**Phone:** (202)673-7440    **Free:** 800-793-4357
**Website:** http://dc.gov/contact/index.htm

**★ 12797 ★ Florida Department of**
**Children and Families**
**Alcohol, Drug Abuse and Mental Health**
**Office**
1317 Winewood Blvd.
Tallahassee, FL 32399-0700
**Phone:** (850)487-2920
**Website:** http://www.state.fl.us/cf_web/adm/

**★ 12798 ★ Georgia Department of**
**Human Resources**
**Mental Health, Mental Retardation and**
**Substance Abuse Division**
2 Peachtree St. NW
Atlanta, GA 30303-3142
**Phone:** (404)657-2272    **Fax:** (404)657-2256
**Email:** irmcilvaine@dhr.state.ga.us
**Website:** http://www2.state.ga.us/departments/dhr/mhmrsa/index.html

**★ 12799 ★ Hawaii Department of Health**
**Behavioral Health Administration**
1250 Punchbowl St.
Honolulu, HI 96813
**Phone:** (808)586-4400    **Fax:** (808)586-4444
**Website:** http://www.state.hi.us/health/about/behavior.html
Anita Swanson, Director

**★ 12800 ★ Idaho Department of Health**
**and Welfare**
**Family and Community Services Division**
**Mental Health Bureau**
1720 Westgate Dr. Ste.s A-D
PO Box 83720
Boise, ID 83720-0026
**Phone:** (208)334-0800    **Free:** 800-600-6474
**Fax:** (208)334-0828
**Email:** connorc@idhw.state.id.us
**Website:** http://www2.state.id.us/dhw/mentalhealth/index.htm
Kathy Tidwell, Contact

**★ 12801 ★ Illinois Department of Human**
**Services**
**Office of Developmental Disabilities**
100 S Grand Ave.
Springfield, IL 62762-0002
**Phone:** (217)524-0260    **Free:** 800-843-6154

**Email:** nsanchez@dhs.state.il.us
**Website:** http://www.state.il.us/agency/dhs/ddnp.html

**★ 12802 ★ Indiana Family and Social Services Administration**
**Mental Health Division**
**Office of Communications**
402 W Washington St.
PO Box 7083
Indianapolis, IN 46207-7083
**Phone:** (317)232-7800    **Free:** 800-901-1133
**Fax:** (317)233-4693
**Website:** http://www.ai.org/fssa/dmh/index.html
Janet Corson, Director

**★ 12803 ★ Iowa Department of Human Services**
**Mental Health, Mental Retardation and Developmental Disabilities Division**
Hoover State Office Bldg.
1305 E Walnut
Des Moines, IA 50319-0114
**Phone:** (515)281-8472    **Free:** 800-972-2017
**Fax:** (515)281-8512
**Email:** jchesni@dhs.state.ia.us
**Website:** http://www.dhs.state.ia.us/HomePages/DHS/MIandDD.htm
Jim Chesnik, Contact

**★ 12804 ★ Kansas Department of Social and Rehabilitation Services**
**Mental Health and Development Disabilities Division**
915 SW Harrison
Topeka, KS 66612
**Phone:** (785)296-3959    **Free:** 888-582-3759
**Fax:** (785)296-2173
**Website:** http://www.srskansas.org/hcp/mhsatr/mhsatr.htm

**★ 12805 ★ Kentucky Health Services Cabinet**
**Mental Health and Mental Retardation Department**
100 Fair Oaks Ln.
Frankfort, KY 40621
**Phone:** (502)564-4448    **Fax:** (502)564-3844
**Email:** BruceW.Scott@mail.state.ky.us
**Website:** http://dmhmrs.chr.state.ky.us/MH/
Bruce W. Scott, Director

**★ 12806 ★ Louisiana Department of Health and Hospitals**
**Mental Health Office**
Louisiana Office of Mental Health
PO Box 4049, Bin 12
Baton Rouge, LA 70821
**Phone:** (225)342-2540    **Fax:** (225)342-5066
**Email:** vroyal@dhh.state.la.us
**Website:** http://www.dhh.state.la.us/OMH/index.htm

**★ 12807 ★ Maine Department of Mental Health and Mental Retardation**
**Mental Health Division**
40 State House Station
Augusta, ME 04333-0040
**Phone:** (207)287-4200    **Fax:** (207)287-4268
**Email:** Lynn.F.Duby@state.me.us
**Website:** http://www.state.me.us/dmhmrsa/mhservices/MHservices.htm
Lynn F. Duby, Director

**★ 12808 ★ Maryland Department of Health and Mental Hygiene**
**Mental Hygiene Administration**
Spring Grove Hospital Center
55 Wave Ave.
Dix Bldg.
Catonsville, MD 21228
**Phone:** (410)402-8300    **Free:** 800-888-1965
**Fax:** (410)402-8301
**Website:** http://www.dhmh.state.md.us/mha/

**★ 12809 ★ Massachusetts Executive Office of Health and Human Services**
**Mental Health Department**
25 Staniford St.
Boston, MA 02114
**Phone:** (617)727-5600    **Free:** 800-221-0053
**Fax:** (617)727-4350
**Email:** richard.copp@state.ma.us
**Website:** http://www.state.ma.us/eohhs/agencies/dmh.htm
Marylou Sudders, Contact

**★ 12810 ★ Michigan Department of Community Health**
Lewis Cass Bldg., 6th Fl.
320 S Walnut
Lansing, MI 48913
**Phone:** (517)373-3500    **Fax:** (517)335-3090
**Email:** arias@state.mi.us
**Website:** http://www.mdch.state.mi.us/
James K. Haveman, Contact

**★ 12811 ★ Minnesota Department of Human Services**
**Health and Continuing Care Strategies**
**Mental Health Services Division**
444 Lafayette Rd. N
Saint Paul, MN 55155
**Phone:** (651)297-3933
**Email:** dhs.webmaster@state.mn.us
**Website:** http://www.dhs.state.mn.us/contcare/mhhome.htm

**★ 12812 ★ Mississippi Department of Mental Health**
1101 Robert E Lee Bldg.
239 N Lamar St.
Jackson, MS 39201
**Phone:** (601)359-1288    **Free:** 877-210-8513
**Fax:** (601)359-6295
**Website:** http://www.dmh.state.ms.us/
Albert R. Hendrix, PhD, Director

**★ 12813 ★ Missouri Department of Mental Health**
**Mental Health Administration Office**
1706 E Elm St.
PO Box 687
Jefferson City, MO 65102
**Phone:** (573)751-4122    **Free:** 800-364-9687
**Fax:** (573)751-8224
**Email:** dmhmail@mail.dmh.state.mo.us
**Website:** http://www.modmh.state.mo.us/cps/cps.html

**★ 12814 ★ Montana Department of Public Health and Human Services**
**Mental Health Division**
1400 Broadway
PO Box 202951
Helena, MT 59620
**Phone:** (406)444-2706    **Fax:** (406)444-4435
**Email:** rpoulsen@state.mt.gov
**Website:** http://www.dphhs.state.mt.us/hot/mhap.htm
Randy Poulsen, Contact

**★ 12815 ★ Nebraska Department of Health and Human Services**
**Community Mental Health Division**
PO Box 95044
Lincoln, NE 68509
**Phone:** (402)471-2306
**Website:** http://www.hhs.state.ne.us/beh/mh/mh.htm

**★ 12816 ★ Nevada Department of Human Resources**
**Mental Health and Developmental Services Division**
505 E King St., Rm. 602
Carson City, NV 89701-3790
**Phone:** (775)684-5943    **Fax:** (775)684-5966
**Email:** mhds@govmail.state.nv.us
**Website:** http://mhds.state.nv.us/
Carlos Brandenburg, PhD, Contact

**★ 12817 ★ New Hampshire Department of Health and Human Services**
**Office of Family Services**
**Community Mental Health Division**
6 Hazen Dr.
Concord, NH 03301-5404
**Phone:** (603)271-4638    **Fax:** (603)271-8705
**Website:** http://www.dhhs.state.nh.us/

**★ 12818 ★ New Jersey Department of Human Services**
**Mental Health Services Division**
50 E State St.
PO Box 727
3535 Quackerbridge Rd.
Trenton, NJ 08625-0727
**Phone:** (609)777-0702    **Free:** 800-382-6717
**Fax:** (609)777-0835
**Email:** dmhsmail@dhs.state.nj.us
**Website:** http://www.state.nj.us/humanservices/DMHS/index.html
Alan Kaufman, Director

**★ 12819 ★ New Mexico Department of Health**
**Mental Health Division**
Harold Runnels Bldg.
1190 St. Francis Dr.
Suite North 3200
Santa Fe, NM 87503
**Phone:** (505)827-2601    **Free:** 800-962-8963
**Website:** http://www.health.state.nm.us/bhsd/bhsdonline

**★ 12820 ★ New York State Office of Mental Health**
44 Holland Ave.
Albany, NY 12229
**Phone:** (518)474-4403    **Free:** 800-597-8481
**Fax:** (518)474-2149
**Email:** webadmin@omh.state.ny.us
**Website:** http://www.omh.state.ny.us/

**★ 12821 ★ North Carolina Department of Health and Human Services**
**Mental Health, Developmental Disabilities and Substance Abuse Services Division**
3014 Mail Service Center
325 N Salisbury
Raleigh, NC 27699-3014
**Phone:** (919)571-4980    **Fax:** (919)571-4984
**Email:** susan.m.kelley@ncmail.net
**Website:** http://www.dhhs.state.nc.us/mhddsas/
Don Willis, Contact

**★ 12822 ★ North Dakota Department of Human Services**
**Mental Health and Substance Abuse Services**
**Mental Health Issues**
600 S Second St., Ste 1D
Bismarck, ND 58504
**Phone:** (701)328-8940    **Free:** 800-755-2719
**Fax:** (701)328-8969
**Email:** solunj@state.nd.us

**Website:** http://lnotes.state.nd.us/dhs/dhsweb.nsf/ServicePages/MentalHealthandSubstanceAbuseServices

**★ 12823 ★ Ohio Department of Mental Health**
30 E Broad St., 8th Fl.
Columbus, OH 43266-0414
**Phone:** (614)466-2596
**Email:** swankd@mhmail.mh.state.oh.us
**Website:** http://www.mh.state.oh.us

**★ 12824 ★ Oklahoma Department of Mental Health**
1200 NE 13th St.
PO Box 53277
Oklahoma City, OK 73152
**Phone:** (405)522-3908
**Website:** http://www.odmhsas.org/

**★ 12825 ★ Oregon Department of Human Resources**
**Mental Health and Developmental Disabilities Services Division**
**Mental Health Services Office**
2575 Bittern St. NE
PO Box 14250
Salem, OR 97309-0740
**Phone:** (503)945-9700  **Fax:** (503)373-7327
**Email:** karen.wickizer@mail.mhd.hr.state.or.us
**Website:** http://omhs.mhd.hr.state.or.us/

**★ 12826 ★ Pennsylvania Department of Public Welfare**
**Mental Health Office**
PO Box 2675
333 Health & Welfare Bldg., Rm. 502
Harrisburg, PA 17105
**Phone:** (717)787-6443  **Fax:** (717)787-5394
**Website:** http://www.dpw.state.pa.us/omhsas/dpwmh.asp

**★ 12827 ★ Rhode Island Department of Mental Health, Retardation and Hospitals**
**Integrated Mental Health Services**
14 Harrington Rd.
Cranston, RI 02920
**Phone:** (401)462-3201  **Fax:** (401)462-3204
**Website:** http://www.mhrh.state.ri.us/Mental%20Health.htm

**★ 12828 ★ South Carolina Department of Mental Health**
2414 Bull St.
Columbia, SC 29202
**Phone:** (803)898-8581
**Email:** webmaster@dmh.state.sc.us
**Website:** http://www.state.sc.us/dmh/

**★ 12829 ★ South Dakota Department of Human Services**
**Mental Health Division**
Hillsview Plaza, E Hwy 34
500 E Capitol
Pierre, SD 57501-5070
**Phone:** (605)773-5991  **Fax:** (605)773-7076
**Email:** infoMH@dhs.state.sd.us
**Website:** http://www.state.sd.us/dhs/dmh/index.htm

**★ 12830 ★ Tennessee Department of Mental Health and Mental Retardation**
**Mental Health Services Division**
425 Fifth Ave. N
Cordell Hull Bldg. 3rd Fl.
Nashville, TN 37243
**Phone:** (615)532-6767
**Email:** mrobinson2@mail.state.tn.us

**Website:** http://www.state.tn.us/mental/mhs.html

**★ 12831 ★ Texas Department of Mental Health and Mental Retardation**
**Mental Health Division**
909 W 45th St.
PO Box 12668
Austin, TX 78711-2668
**Phone:** (512)454-3761
**Email:** ellen.hurst@mhmr.state.tx.us
**Website:** http://www.mhmr.state.tx.us/
Karen F. Hale, Director

**★ 12832 ★ Utah Department of Human Services**
**Mental Health Division**
120 N 200 W, Ste. 415
PO Box 142200
Salt Lake City, UT 84144-2200
**Phone:** (801)538-4270  **Fax:** (801)538-9892
**Email:** jchilton@hs.state.ut.us
**Website:** http://www.hsmh.state.ut.us/

**★ 12833 ★ Vermont Agency of Human Services**
**Developmental and Mental Health Services Department**
**Mental Health Division**
Weeks Bldg.
103 S Main St.
Waterbury, VT 05671-1601
**Phone:** (802)241-2610  **Fax:** (802)241-1129
**Email:** webmaster@ddmhs.state.vt.us
**Website:** http://www.state.vt.us/dmh

**★ 12834 ★ Virginia Office of Health and Human Resources**
**Mental Health, Retardation and Substance Abuse Services Department**
**Mental Health Services Division**
109 Governor St.
Richmond, VA 23219
**Phone:** (804)786-4837  **Free:** 800-451-5544
**Fax:** (804)786-9621
**Email:** bbrenzovich@dmhmrsas.state.va.us
**Website:** http://www.dmhmrsas.state.va.us/

**★ 12835 ★ Washington Department of Social and Health Services**
**Health and Rehabilitative Services Office**
**Mental Health Division**
PO Box 45130
Olympia, WA 98504-5130
**Phone:** (360)902-8070  **Free:** 888-713-6010
**Fax:** (360)902-0809
**Website:** http://www.wa.gov/dshs/hrsa/hrsa3ov.htmlMHD

**★ 12836 ★ West Virginia Department of Health and Human Resources**
**Community Support Bureau**
**Office of Behavioral Health Services Division**
350 Capitol St., Rm. 350
Charleston, WV 25301-3702
**Phone:** (304)558-0627  **Fax:** (304)558-1008
**Email:** obhs@wvdhhr.org
**Website:** http://www.wvdhhr.org/obhs/mhcr.htm

**★ 12837 ★ Wisconsin Department of Health and Family Services**
**Supportive Living Division**
**Community Mental Health Bureau**
1 W Wilson St., Rm 433
PO Box 7851
Madison, WI 53707-7851
**Phone:** (608)267-7792  **Fax:** (608)267-7793
**Email:** webmaster@dhfs.state.wi.us

**Website:** http://www.dhfs.state.wi.us/MH_BCMH/index.htm

# State & Regional Organizations

## Autism

*State chapters of the Autism Society of America are listed below. The national office is located at 7910 Woodmont Ave., Ste. 300, Bethesda, MD 20814-3015. Additional information can be obtained by calling the national office at (800) 3-AUTISM, or by consulting their web site at http://www.autism-society.org/.*

### Alabama

**★ 12838 ★ Autism Society of Alabama**
771 2nd St.
Helena, AL 35080
**Phone:** (205)621-0548  **Free:** 877-428-8476
**Fax:** (205)681-1514
**Email:** director@autism-alabama.org
**Website:** http://www.autism-alabama.org

### Arizona

**★ 12839 ★ Autism Society of America Greater Phoenix Chapter**
PO Box 10543
Phoenix, AZ 85064-0543
**Phone:** (480)940-1093
**Website:** http://aztec.asu.edu/phxautism/index.html

### California

**★ 12840 ★ Autism Society of America Inland Empire Chapter**
PO Box 8932
Moreno Valley, CA 92552
**Phone:** (909)242-4413  **Free:** 800-328-8476
**Fax:** (909)242-4413
**Email:** dar4mar@aol.com
**Website:** http://www.inlandempireasa.org
Debbie Rosenbrook, President

**★ 12841 ★ Autism Society of America San Diego County Chapter**
PO Box 420908
San Diego, CA 92124
**Phone:** (619)298-1981  **Fax:** (619)587-9788
**Email:** sdasa@icestorm.net
**Website:** http://www.sd-autism.org/home/index.htm
Kay Freeman, President

**★ 12842 ★ Autism Society of Los Angeles**
**United Autism Alliance**
1612 W Olive Ave., Ste. 201
Burbank, CA 91506
**Phone:** (818)953-3855  **Fax:** (818)953-3850
**Email:** info@unitedautismalliance.org
**Website:** http://www.unitedautismalliance.org

### Connecticut

**★ 12843 ★ Autism Society of Connecticut**
125 Harrington St.
Meriden, CT 06451
**Phone:** (203)235-7629
**Email:** ideasb@cshore.com
**Website:** http://www.autismsocietyofct.org

## Delaware

**★ 12844 ★ Autism Society of Delaware**
PO Box 7336
Wilmington, DE 19803-0336
**Phone:** (302)777-7273
**Email:** DelAutism@aol.com
**Website:** http://www.wserv.com/delautism/
Artie Kempner, President

## Florida

**★ 12845 ★ Manasota Autism Society**
PO Box 18934
Sarasota, FL 34276-1934
**Phone:** (941)328-0121          **Fax:** (941)328-0121
**Email:** mas@saraweb.com
**Website:** http://www.saraweb.com/MAS/

## Kentucky

**★ 12846 ★ Autism Society of Western Kentucky**
PO Box 1647
Henderson, KY 42419-1647
**Phone:** (270)826-0510
**Email:** tawanda@dynasty.net
**Website:** http://www.kentucky-autism.org
Nancy Boyett, Contact

## Michigan

**★ 12847 ★ Autism Society of Michigan**
6035 Executive Dr., Ste. 109
Lansing, MI 48911
**Phone:** (517)882-2800          **Free:** 800-223-6722
**Fax:** (517)882-2816
**Email:** miautism@aol.com
**Website:** http://www.autism-mi.org/
Chris Swartwout, President

## Minnesota

**★ 12848 ★ Twin Cities Autism Society**
970 Raymond Ave., Ste. 101
Saint Paul, MN 55114-1146
**Phone:** (651)647-1083          **Fax:** (651)642-1230
**Email:** mpowell@goldengate.net
**Website:** http://www.tcas.org/

## North Carolina

**★ 12849 ★ Autism Society of North Carolina, Inc.**
505 Oberlin Rd., Ste. 230
Raleigh, NC 27605-1345
**Phone:** (919)743-0204          **Free:** 800-442-2762
**Fax:** (919)743-0208
**Email:** jlawson@autismsociety-nc.org
**Website:** http://www.autismsociety-nc.org/

## Ohio

**★ 12850 ★ Autism Society of Greater Cincinnati**
CCDD Bldg. E
3333 Burnet Ave., Rm. 4-32
Cincinnati, OH 45229
**Phone:** (513)636-7203          **Fax:** (513)636-2224
**Email:** asgc@fuse.net
**Website:** http://www.autismcincy.org/

## Oregon

**★ 12851 ★ Autism Society of Oregon**
PO Box 13884
Salem, OR 97309
**Phone:** (503)234-5729          **Free:** 888-AUTISM-1
**Fax:** (503)363-9110
**Email:** aso@teleport.com
**Website:** http://www.autismoregon.com

## Tennessee

**★ 12852 ★ Autism Society of Middle Tennessee**
480 Craighead St., Ste. 200
Nashville, TN 37204
**Phone:** (615)385-2077          **Fax:** (615)383-1176
**Email:** asmt@bellsouth.net
**Website:** http://www.autismmidtenn.org

## Washington

**★ 12853 ★ Autism Society of Washington**
PO Box 310
East Olympia, WA 98540
**Phone:** (360)943-2205          **Fax:** (360)330-2240
**Email:** autismsociety@hotmail.com
**Website:** http://www.autismsocietyofwa.org
Kitsie Morris, Exec Director

## Wisconsin

**★ 12854 ★ Autism Society of Wisconsin**
103 W College Ave., Ste. 601
Appleton, WI 54911-5744
**Phone:** (920)993-0279          **Free:** 888-4-AUTISM
**Fax:** (920)993-0279
**Email:** asw@asw4autism.org
**Website:** http://www.asw4autism.org/

## Depression

*State chapters of the National Depressive and Manic-Depressive Association are listed below. The national office is located at 730 N Franklin St., Ste. 501, Chicago, Illinois 60610-7204. Additional information can be obtained by calling the national office at (800) 826-3632, or by consulting their web site at http://www.ndmda.org/.*

## Alabama

**★ 12855 ★ National Depressive and Manic-Depressive Association Huntsville Chapter**
PO Box 2933
Huntsville, AL 35804-2933
**Phone:** (256)536-3471
**Email:** dmda_huntsville@yahoo.com
**Website:** http://www.geocities.com/dmda_huntsville
Elayne Fountain, Contact

**★ 12856 ★ National Depressive and Manic-Depressive Association Huntsville MDSG Chapter**
660 Gallatin St.
Huntsville, AL 35801
**Phone:** (256)533-1970          **Fax:** (256)532-4112
Bernice Maze, Contact

**★ 12857 ★ National Depressive and Manic-Depressive Association Morgan County Chapter**
PO Box 1502
Decatur, AL 35602
**Phone:** (256)353-1160          **Fax:** (256)353-1163
**Email:** cvance1530@aol.com
Sue Brantley, Contact

**★ 12858 ★ National Depressive and Manic-Depressive Association SOMI Bipolar Group**
Mobile, AL
**Phone:** (251)340-6189
Eddy Jones, Contact

**★ 12859 ★ National Depressive and Manic-Depressive Association Southeast Alabama Chapter**
Dothan, AL
**Phone:** (334)794-7008
Robin Saliba, Contact

**★ 12860 ★ National Depressive and Manic-Depressive Association Tuscaloosa Chapter**
PO Box 1731
Tuscaloosa, AL 35403
**Phone:** (205)349-8791
**Email:** harley-1929@yahoo.com
Harley Sullivan, Contact

## Arizona

**★ 12861 ★ National Depressive and Manic-Depressive Association Bipolar Bears of Phoenix Chapter**
936 W Impala Center
Mesa, AZ 85210
**Phone:** (480)838-3716          **Fax:** (480)994-4744
**Email:** psawyer@wd4fak.org
**Website:** http://www.wd4fak.org
Phil Sawyer, Contact

**★ 12862 ★ National Depressive and Manic-Depressive Association Maricopa County Chapter**
6411 E Thomas
Scottsdale, AZ 85251
**Phone:** (480)994-4407          **Fax:** (480)994-4744
**Email:** mhaaz@uswest.net
**Website:** http://www.mhaaz.com
Sue Armstrong, Contact

## Arkansas

**★ 12863 ★ National Depressive and Manic-Depressive Association Arkansas Chapter**
PO Box 94339
North Little Rock, AR 72190
**Phone:** (501)753-4767          **Fax:** (501)771-1226
**Email:** jerjun@juno.com
Jerry Quick, Contact

## California

**★ 12864 ★ National Depressive and Manic-Depressive Association Coachella Valley Chapter**
100 S Sunrise Way, Box 357
Palm Springs, CA 92262-6737
**Phone:** (760)343-2781          **Fax:** (760)323-2404
**Email:** mwslas@juno.com
Merrill Seroy, Contact

**★ 12865 ★ National Depressive and Manic-Depressive Association Depression Support/Visalia Chapter**
11002 Ave. 352
Visalia, CA 93291
**Phone:** (559)733-7362          **Fax:** (559)733-7362
**Email:** rillmitch@thegrid.net
Rill Mitchell, Contact

**★ 12866 ★ National Depressive and Manic-Depressive Association Escondido Chapter**
1540 E Valley Pkwy.
Escondido, CA 92027
**Phone:** (760)739-2971          **Free:** 800-336-2000
**Fax:** (760)735-9067
**Email:** kls5@pphs.org
**Website:** http://www.pphs.org
Bryan Heath, Contact

**★ 12867 ★ National Depressive and Manic-Depressive Association**
**Fontana/Upland Chapter**
Fontana, CA
**Phone:** (909)947-1307     **Fax:** (909)947-4081
Samantha Johns, Contact

**★ 12868 ★ National Depressive and Manic-Depressive Association**
**Foundations Support Group**
c/o MDDA of Riverside
16280 Whispering Spur
Riverside, CA 92504
**Phone:** (909)658-5013
**Email:** mddaofriv@aol.com
**Website:** http://www.geocities.com/mddariv
Patricia Wilson, Contact

**★ 12869 ★ National Depressive and Manic-Depressive Association**
**Glendale Chapter**
Glendale, CA
**Phone:** (323)662-5564
**Email:** getout@earthlink.net

**★ 12870 ★ National Depressive and Manic-Depressive Association**
**Greater Long Beach Chapter**
4634 Ostrom Ave.
Lakewood, CA 90713
**Phone:** (714)960-7922
**Email:** celtic1100@yahoo.com
Neil Young, Contact

**★ 12871 ★ National Depressive and Manic-Depressive Association**
**High Desert Chapter**
20318 Thunderbird Rd., No. 2
Apple Valley, CA 92307
**Phone:** (760)946-0308
**Email:** galucla@aol.com
Gerri Logan, Contact

**★ 12872 ★ National Depressive and Manic-Depressive Association**
**Humboldt County**
PO Box 7118
Eureka, CA 95502-7118
**Phone:** (707)839-4353
**Email:** les58paul@cs.com
**Website:** http://http://www.chargette.com/client/dmda/dmda.html
James Selle, Contact

**★ 12873 ★ National Depressive and Manic-Depressive Association**
**Indian Wells Valley Chapter**
China Lake, CA
**Phone:** (760)377-3223
**Email:** ramer@ridgenet.net
Robert Millsop, Contact

**★ 12874 ★ National Depressive and Manic-Depressive Association**
**La Jolla Chapter**
8950 Villa La Jolla Dr., No. 2142
La Jolla, CA 92037
**Phone:** (858)535-4783     **Free:** 888-274-3637
**Fax:** (858)457-8527
**Email:** pmcgrath@ucsd.edu

**★ 12875 ★ National Depressive and Manic-Depressive Association**
**Los Angeles Chapter**
PO Box 341201
Los Angeles, CA 90034-1201
**Phone:** (818)893-7363
Doreen Scott, Contact

**★ 12876 ★ National Depressive and Manic-Depressive Association**
**Monterey Chapter**
Monterey, CA
**Phone:** (831)646-8800     **Fax:** (831)637-9369
**Email:** mdmda@msn.com
Rod Guthrie, Contact

**★ 12877 ★ National Depressive and Manic-Depressive Association**
**Mt. Shasta Chapter**
PO Box 557
Mount Shasta, CA 96067
**Phone:** (530)918-7233     **Fax:** (530)926-2668
Kareen Thomas, Contact

**★ 12878 ★ National Depressive and Manic-Depressive Association**
**Oceanside Chapter**
Oceanside, CA
**Phone:** (760)597-9754
**Email:** dmdaca@aol.com
Robert Jr., Jones, Jr., Contact

**★ 12879 ★ National Depressive and Manic-Depressive Association**
**Orange County Chapter**
PO Box 223
Tustin, CA 92781-0223
**Phone:** (714)744-8718
**Email:** gdierking@aol.com
**Website:** http://www.angelfire.com/ca/dmdaoc/index.html
Gloria Dierking, Contact

**★ 12880 ★ National Depressive and Manic-Depressive Association**
**Pasadena Chapter**
Pasadena, CA
**Phone:** (626)446-0458
Jill Hall, Contact

**★ 12881 ★ National Depressive and Manic-Depressive Association**
**Riverside Chapter**
Riverside, CA
**Phone:** (909)780-3366     **Fax:** (909)780-5758
**Email:** cdmda@aol.com
Jo Ann Martin, Contact

**★ 12882 ★ National Depressive and Manic-Depressive Association**
**Riverside Chapter**
16280 Whispering Spur
Riverside, CA 92504
**Phone:** (909)780-3366     **Fax:** (909)780-5758
**Email:** mddaofriv@ad.com
**Website:** http://www.geocities.com/mddariv/index.html

**★ 12883 ★ National Depressive and Manic-Depressive Association**
**Sacramento Chapter**
2521 Key West Way
Sacramento, CA 95826
**Phone:** (916)684-1358     **Fax:** (916)363-3184
Marilyn Hillerman, Contact

**★ 12884 ★ National Depressive and Manic-Depressive Association**
**San Diego County Chapter**
11878 Ave. of Industry
San Diego, CA 92128
**Phone:** (619)487-3200     **Fax:** (619)485-5418
Kent Layton, Contact

**★ 12885 ★ National Depressive and Manic-Depressive Association**
**San Francisco Chapter**
900 Hyde St., 3rd Fl.
San Francisco, CA 94109
**Phone:** (415)995-4792     **Fax:** (510)436-3144
**Email:** info@sfdmda.org
**Website:** http://www.sfdmda.org
Ted Goto, Contact

**★ 12886 ★ National Depressive and Manic-Depressive Association**
**San Joaquin Chapter**
PO Box 403
Lodi, CA 95241
**Phone:** (209)334-4642
**Email:** dmda_sanjoaquin@yahoo.com
**Website:** http://www.geocities.com/dmda_sanjoaquin
Glenda Lee, Contact

**★ 12887 ★ National Depressive and Manic-Depressive Association**
**Stanford Young Persons' Support Group**
Stanford, CA
**Phone:** (650)245-1048
**Email:** dianaphrodite@yahoo.com
Diana Galbraith, Contact

**★ 12888 ★ National Depressive and Manic-Depressive Association**
**Stanislaus County Chapter**
Modesto, CA
**Phone:** (209)544-8473     **Fax:** (209)869-1758
**Email:** dmda55@hotmail.com
Scott Hill, Contact

**★ 12889 ★ National Depressive and Manic-Depressive Association**
**Temecula Chapter**
Temecula, CA
**Phone:** (909)926-8393
**Email:** threez@pe.net
**Website:** http://www.geocities.com/tdmda

**★ 12890 ★ National Depressive and Manic-Depressive Association**
**UCLA/West Los Angeles Chapter**
300 Medical Plaza, 2nd Fl., Conf. Rm. 1
Los Angeles, CA 90095-8346
**Phone:** (310)836-2275
Rob Barrett, Contact

**★ 12891 ★ National Depressive and Manic-Depressive Association**
**Uplifters/Riverside Chapter**
19880 Kirkpatrick Rd.
Perris, CA 92570
**Phone:** (909)780-0379     **Fax:** (909)780-5758
**Email:** arleekirk@juno.com
Arlie Kirkpatrick, Contact

**★ 12892 ★ National Depressive and Manic-Depressive Association**
**Visalia/Hanford Chapter**
118 W Myrtle St.
Hanford, CA 93230
**Phone:** (559)585-1227
**Email:** mettee@lemoorenet.com
Irene Spindler, Contact

## Colorado

**★ 12893 ★ National Depressive and Manic-Depressive Association**
**Aurora Chapter**
8000 E 12th Ave., No. 4B1
Denver, CO 80220
**Phone:** (303)329-9894

**Email:** cstowell@softhome.net
Carol Stowell, Contact

**★ 12894 ★ National Depressive and
Manic-Depressive Association
Boulder Chapter**
PO Box 1343
Boulder, CO 80306-1343
**Phone:** (303)449-3529
**Email:** tani.pierce@colorado.edu
Laurie Domeron, Contact

**★ 12895 ★ National Depressive and
Manic-Depressive Association
Colorado Springs/Initiatives Chapter**
PO Box 366
Colorado Springs, CO 80901-0366
**Phone:** (719)477-1515      **Fax:** (719)477-1515
**Email:** dmdacolospgs@pcisys.net
Jason Cellan, Contact

**★ 12896 ★ National Depressive and
Manic-Depressive Association
North Star Chapter**
Westminster, CO
**Phone:** (303)584-1957      **Fax:** (303)404-9264
Sharron Thomas, Contact

**★ 12897 ★ National Depressive and
Manic-Depressive Association
Pueblo Chapter**
1600 Grand Ave., No. 125
Pueblo, CO 81003
**Phone:** (719)583-9798      **Free:** 800-976-5929
**Fax:** (719)544-5708
**Email:** jackselway@puebloadvocacy.com
**Website:** http://www.puebloadvocacy.com/dmda
Jack Selway, Contact

**★ 12898 ★ National Depressive and
Manic-Depressive Association
Southwest Chapter**
455 S Lee St.
Lakewood, CO 80226
**Phone:** (303)331-2599      **Fax:** (303)830-8918
Joe Petrovich, Contact

### Connecticut

**★ 12899 ★ National Depressive and
Manic-Depressive Association
Greenwich Chapter**
c/o Greenwich Hospital
5 Perryridge Rd.
Greenwich, CT 06830
**Phone:** (203)975-2451      **Fax:** (203)863-4445
**Email:** fbtworld@aol.com
**Website:** http://www.greenhosp.org
Peter Flierl, Contact

**★ 12900 ★ National Depressive and
Manic-Depressive Association
Northwest Connecticut Chapter**
Torrington, CT
**Phone:** (860)567-8928
Doyle Finan, Contact

### Delaware

**★ 12901 ★ National Depressive and
Manic-Depressive Association
New Directions/Delaware Chapter**
6 Hilton Rd.
Wilmington, DE 19810
**Phone:** (302)286-1161      **Fax:** (302)475-1574
**Email:** newdirectionsdelaware@yahoo.com
**Website:** http://www.newdirectionsdelaware.org
Dolores Grimes, Contact

### District of Columbia

**★ 12902 ★ National Depressive and
Manic-Depressive Association
Capital Area Chapter**
Washington, DC
**Phone:** (703)566-1699
**Email:** cadma_99@yahoo.com
Alvin Martin, Contact

**★ 12903 ★ National Depressive and
Manic-Depressive Association
Washington DC Chapter**
4228 Wisconsin Ave. NW
Washington, DC 20016
**Phone:** (202)885-5653
Lois Morris, Contact

### Florida

**★ 12904 ★ National Depressive and
Manic-Depressive Association
Broward County Chapter**
7425 N University Dr.
Tamarac, FL 33321-2901
**Phone:** (954)969-0291
**Email:** glennk@bellsouth.net
**Website:** http://www.bcdmda.org
Glenn Krate, Contact
**Crisis Phone(s):** 24-hour line, (954) 463-0911.

**★ 12905 ★ National Depressive and
Manic-Depressive Association
Central Brevard Chapter**
1407 N Lakemont Dr.
Cocoa, FL 32922
**Phone:** (321)632-9164
**Email:** cocoalocal@aol.com
Carolyn C. Hubbard, Contact

**★ 12906 ★ National Depressive and
Manic-Depressive Association
Collier County Chapter**
1055 Rordon Ave.
Naples, FL 34103
**Phone:** (941)649-6241
Charis Nelson, Contact

**★ 12907 ★ National Depressive and
Manic-Depressive Association
Fellowship Chapter**
919 SE 14th St.
Ocala, FL 34471-3917
**Phone:** (352)732-0879
Bob Rile, Contact

**★ 12908 ★ National Depressive and
Manic-Depressive Association
Fort Meyers Chapter**
1846 Braman Ave.
Fort Myers, FL 33901
**Phone:** (941)931-9170
Anna Montoro, Contact

**★ 12909 ★ National Depressive and
Manic-Depressive Association
Gainesville Chapter**
PO Box 140604
Gainesville, FL 32614-0604
**Phone:** (352)335-0081
Sandy Wentworth, Contact

**★ 12910 ★ National Depressive and
Manic-Depressive Association
Gold Coast Chapter**
3501 Johnson St.
Hollywood, FL 33021

**Phone:** (954)565-3585      **Fax:** (954)985-6183
**Email:** pamelaames@attbi.com
Pamela Ames, Contact

**★ 12911 ★ National Depressive and
Manic-Depressive Association
Greater Jacksonville Chapter**
6271-24 St. Augustine Rd., No. 3126
Jacksonville, FL 32217
**Phone:** (904)751-9121      **Fax:** (904)448-8965
**Email:** juliuan@aol.com
Julie Livesay, Contact

**★ 12912 ★ National Depressive and
Manic-Depressive Association
Hillsborough Chapter**
Brandon, FL
**Phone:** (813)685-4818
**Email:** revrev@prodigy.net
Andrew Newelski, Contact

**★ 12913 ★ National Depressive and
Manic-Depressive Association
Inverness Chapter**
Inverness, FL
**Phone:** (352)341-5688
**Email:** korestis@tampabay.rr.net
Kelsey Orestis, Contact

**★ 12914 ★ National Depressive and
Manic-Depressive Association
Jacksonville Beach Chapter**
Jacksonville Beach, FL
**Phone:** (904)399-5468
Susan Seimer, Contact

**★ 12915 ★ National Depressive and
Manic-Depressive Association
The Manic Blues Chapter**
8638 Knotty Pine Ln.
Orlando, FL 32825
**Phone:** (407)277-7976      **Fax:** (407)468-6803
**Email:** themanicblues@flashmail.com
Marian Becker, Contact

**★ 12916 ★ National Depressive and
Manic-Depressive Association
Mental Health Association of Volusia
County, Inc.**
Daytona Beach, FL
**Email:** dbfla@bellsouth.net
Jack Paulden, Contact

**★ 12917 ★ National Depressive and
Manic-Depressive Association
North Palm Beach County Chapter**
18601 Misty Lake Dr.
Jupiter, FL 33458
**Phone:** (561)575-9787      **Fax:** (561)575-9787
**Email:** wsdgbp@aol.com
Joan Angle, Contact

**★ 12918 ★ National Depressive and
Manic-Depressive Association
Palm Beaches Chapter**
6347 Lacosta Dr., No. F
Boca Raton, FL 33433
**Phone:** (561)391-3401
**Email:** pbdmda@webtv.net
Harlan Friedman, Contact

**★ 12919 ★ National Depressive and
Manic-Depressive Association
Pensacola Chapter**
PO Box 2041
Pensacola, FL 32513-2041
**Phone:** (850)291-9753      **Fax:** (850)474-8775

**Email:** dmdapensacola@aol.com
Jack White, Contact

**★ 12920 ★ National Depressive and
Manic-Depressive Association
Sarasota Chapter**
5220 Ventura Ave.
Sarasota, FL 34235
**Phone:** (941)745-3518     **Fax:** (941)374-6235
Pat Schmidt, Contact

**★ 12921 ★ National Depressive and
Manic-Depressive Association
South Brevard Chapter**
Melbourne, FL 32901
**Phone:** (407)729-0888
Margaret Lee, Contact

**★ 12922 ★ National Depressive and
Manic-Depressive Association
Suncoast Center Chapter**
4024 Central Ave.
Saint Petersburg, FL 33711
**Phone:** (727)327-7656     **Fax:** (727)323-8978
Kristi Yatchak, Contact

**★ 12923 ★ National Depressive and
Manic-Depressive Association
Tallahassee Chapter**
4825 Six Oaks Dr.
Tallahassee, FL 32303
**Phone:** (850)514-1900     **Fax:** (850)541-1941
**Email:** bendahuston@aol.com
Barbara Benda, Contact

**★ 12924 ★ National Depressive and
Manic-Depressive Association
Tampa Bay Chapter**
PO Box 340572
Tampa, FL 33694
**Phone:** (813)878-2906
**Email:** tbdmda@tbdmda.org
**Website:** http://www.tbdmda.org
Susan Shaw, Contact

**★ 12925 ★ National Depressive and
Manic-Depressive Association
West Pasco Chapter**
15012 Dennis Dr.
Hudson, FL 34669
**Phone:** (727)819-9427     **Fax:** (727)819-9427
Bob Thompson, Contact

### Georgia

**★ 12926 ★ National Depressive and
Manic-Depressive Association
Greater Augusta Chapter**
PO Box 1927
Augusta, GA 30903
**Phone:** (706)722-0010     **Fax:** (706)722-8819
Dan Cook, Contact

**★ 12927 ★ National Depressive and
Manic-Depressive Association
Greater Savannah Chapter**
455 Mall Blvd., No. 49
Savannah, GA 31406
**Phone:** (912)927-2064
John Ralston, Contact

**★ 12928 ★ National Depressive and
Manic-Depressive Association
Jesup Chapter**
1950 S Hwy. 301, No. 704
Jesup, GA 31546

**Phone:** (912)427-9281
Nina Howerton, Contact

**★ 12929 ★ National Depressive and
Manic-Depressive Association
Metropolitan Atlanta Chapter**
8198 Brookwood Valley Cir.
Atlanta, GA 30309
**Phone:** (404)355-8815
**Email:** info@atlantamoodsupport.com
**Website:** http://www.atlantamoodsupport.com
Stephen Propst, Contact

**★ 12930 ★ National Depressive and
Manic-Depressive Association
Thomasville Chapter**
PO Box 1378
Thomasville, GA 31799-1378
**Phone:** (229)227-9851
**Email:** ahansard@rose.net
Renee Hansard, Contact

### Hawaii

**★ 12931 ★ National Depressive and
Manic-Depressive Association
United Self Help Chapter**
Honolulu, HI
**Phone:** (808)926-0466
Bud Bowles, Contact

### Idaho

**★ 12932 ★ National Depressive and
Manic-Depressive Association
New Beginnings Chapter**
Idaho Falls, ID
**Phone:** (208)238-7073
**Email:** drmaddox670@aol.com
Debra Maddox, Contact

**★ 12933 ★ National Depressive and
Manic-Depressive Association
North Idaho Chapter**
Coeur d'Alene, ID
**Phone:** (208)666-3740     **Fax:** (208)666-2977
Rosemarie Olsen, Contact

**★ 12934 ★ National Depressive and
Manic-Depressive Association
Saint Alphonsus Chapter**
7470 Holbrook Ln., No. 112
Boise, ID 83704-5806
**Phone:** (208)658-9126
Fred Freeman, Contact

### Illinois

**★ 12935 ★ National Depressive and
Manic-Depressive Association
Aurora Chapter**
1N286 Woods Ave.
Wheaton, IL 60188
**Phone:** (630)653-3560
**Email:** sneezercat@aol.com
Thomas E. Johnson, Contact

**★ 12936 ★ National Depressive and
Manic-Depressive Association
Belleville Chapter
St. Elizabeth's Hospital**
211 S 3rd St.
Belleville, IL 62222
**Phone:** (618)234-2120     **Fax:** (618)222-4761
Richard Avdoian, Contact

**★ 12937 ★ National Depressive and
Manic-Depressive Association
Berwyn Chapter**
Berwyn, IL
**Phone:** (708)524-1794
**Email:** dmda_berwyn@yahoo.com
Pamela Strening, Contact

**★ 12938 ★ National Depressive and
Manic-Depressive Association
Bloomington/Normal Chapter**
710 E Front St.
Bloomington, IL 61701-5414
**Phone:** (309)821-1448
**Email:** seventenfronthouse@netscape.com
Kathy Brown, Contact

**★ 12939 ★ National Depressive and
Manic-Depressive Association
CAMDA Chapter**
4109 E Oaks Rd.
Urbana, IL 61802
**Phone:** (217)344-7901
**Email:** camda@compuserve.com
Sten Johansen, Contact

**★ 12940 ★ National Depressive and
Manic-Depressive Association
Fox Valley Chapter**
2365 Coach and Surrey Lane
Aurora, IL 60506
**Phone:** (630)859-8035
**Email:** bmj923@aol.com
**Website:** http://www.geocities.com/foxvalleydmda
Blanche Jones, Contact

**★ 12941 ★ National Depressive and
Manic-Depressive Association
Gurnee Chapter**
c/o Village Church of Gurnee
1319 N Hunt Club Rd.
Gurnee, IL 60031
**Phone:** (847)263-7079     **Fax:** (847)244-0413
**Email:** deniseanderson2@yahoo.com
**Website:** http://www.dmdagurnee.org
Denise Anderson, Contact

**★ 12942 ★ National Depressive and
Manic-Depressive Association
Hinsdale Chapter**
244 E Ogden, No. 114
Hinsdale, IL 60521
**Phone:** (708)788-3858
Kate Moran, Contact

**★ 12943 ★ National Depressive and
Manic-Depressive Association
Illinois Valley Chapter**
207 15th St.
Mendota, IL 61342-1311
**Phone:** (815)539-6432
**Email:** doris22737@yahoo.com
Doris J. Meyer, Contact
**Frmly:** Depressive and Manic-Depressive Association, Northern Illinois.

**★ 12944 ★ National Depressive and
Manic-Depressive Association
Joliet Chapter**
Joliet, IL
**Phone:** (815)773-7000
Stacey Stone, Contact

★ **12945** ★ **National Depressive and Manic-Depressive Association**
**Libertyville Chapter**
PO Box 8911
Waukegan, IL 60079-8911
**Phone:** (847)336-8346  **Fax:** (847)360-4296
John Philipp, Contact

★ **12946** ★ **National Depressive and Manic-Depressive Association**
**Metropolitan Chicago Chapter**
4725 N Western Ave., No. 220
Chicago, IL 60625
**Phone:** (773)465-3280  **Fax:** (773)465-3385
**Email:** dmdamc@ameritech.net
**Website:** http://members.tripod.com/dmda-mc/index.htm
Chet Taranowski, Contact

★ **12947** ★ **National Depressive and Manic-Depressive Association**
**Mood Challenge Chapter**
PO Box 6074
Peoria, IL 61601-6074
**Phone:** (309)686-4382
James B. Staley, Contact

★ **12948** ★ **National Depressive and Manic-Depressive Association**
**Mood Tides Chapter**
Decatur, IL
**Phone:** (217)429-2132
**Email:** devore@family-net.net
Carolyn DeVore, Contact

★ **12949** ★ **National Depressive and Manic-Depressive Association**
**New Hope Elmhurst Chapter**
PO Box 1332
Elmhurst, IL 60126
**Phone:** (630)415-3266
Pam Wagner, Contact

★ **12950** ★ **National Depressive and Manic-Depressive Association**
**North Shore Chapter**
Kenilworth Union Church
211 Kenilworth Ave.
Kenilworth, IL 60043
**Phone:** (847)251-4272  **Fax:** (847)251-4289
Elizabeth Cobb, Contact

★ **12951** ★ **National Depressive and Manic-Depressive Association**
**Northwestern Medical Campus Chapter**
675 N St. Clair, No. 20-250
Chicago, IL 60611
**Phone:** (312)695-3511
**Email:** vbrooks@nmff.org
Verna Brooks, Contact

### Indiana

★ **12952** ★ **National Depressive and Manic-Depressive Association**
**BehaviorCorp**
Carmel, IN
**Phone:** (317)587-0500  **Fax:** (317)574-1234
**Email:** lburch@behaviorcorp.org
**Website:** http://www.behaviorcorp.org
Larry L. Burch, Contact

★ **12953** ★ **National Depressive and Manic-Depressive Association**
**Central Indiana Chapter**
Indianapolis, IN
**Phone:** (317)290-9686  **Fax:** (317)290-9685
**Email:** info@dmdacentralindiana.org
**Website:** http://www.dmdacentralindiana.org
Marchell K. Hunt, Contact

★ **12954** ★ **National Depressive and Manic-Depressive Association**
**Elkhart County Chapter**
54470 Saddlebrook Crossing
Elkhart, IN 46514
**Phone:** (219)264-4053
Mary Kay Froschauer, Contact

★ **12955** ★ **National Depressive and Manic-Depressive Association**
**Four County Counseling Center**
Logansport, IN
**Phone:** (219)722-5151  **Fax:** (219)722-9523
**Email:** ulrich@fourcounty.org
**Website:** http://www.fourcounty.org
Lawrence R. Ulrich, Contact

★ **12956** ★ **National Depressive and Manic-Depressive Association**
**Fulton County Chapter**
321 E 8th St.
Rochester, IN 46975
**Phone:** (219)223-6870  **Fax:** (219)224-6870
**Email:** gsmokermhafc@rtcol.com
Ginelle Smoker, Contact

★ **12957** ★ **National Depressive and Manic-Depressive Association**
**Hamilton County Chapter**
942 N 10th St.
Noblesville, IN 46060
**Phone:** (317)776-3455  **Fax:** (317)776-1155
**Email:** mhahc@juno.com
Kelli Spence, Contact

★ **12958** ★ **National Depressive and Manic-Depressive Association**
**Indiana Chapter**
55 Monument Circle, No. 700
Indianapolis, IN 46204-2918
**Phone:** (317)686-0588  **Fax:** (317)638-3540
**Email:** mha@mentalhealthassociation.com
**Website:** http://www.mentalhealthassociation.com
Kevin Kilty, Contact

★ **12959** ★ **National Depressive and Manic-Depressive Association**
**Indianapolis Chapter**
2506 Willowbrook Pkwy., No. 100
Indianapolis, IN 46205
**Phone:** (317)251-0005  **Fax:** (317)254-2800
**Email:** jspray@mcmha.org
Lynn Carson, Contact

★ **12960** ★ **National Depressive and Manic-Depressive Association**
**North West Indiana Chapter**
1083 N 475 E
Chesterton, IN 46304
**Phone:** (219)926-3424
**Email:** rkowal@netnitco.net
Ron Kowalski, Contact

★ **12961** ★ **National Depressive and Manic-Depressive Association**
**Northeastern Center, Inc.**
220 S Main St.
PO Box 817
Kendallville, IN 46755
**Phone:** (219)347-2453  **Fax:** (219)347-2456
**Email:** necinfo@northeasterncenter.org
**Website:** http://www.northeasterncenter.org
Corey Walker, Contact

★ **12962** ★ **National Depressive and Manic-Depressive Association**
**South West Indiana Chapter**
123 NW 4th St., No. 614
Evansville, IN 47708
**Phone:** (812)426-2640  **Fax:** (812)426-7207
**Email:** vcmha@juno.com
Donna Carr, Contact

### Iowa

★ **12963** ★ **National Depressive and Manic-Depressive Association**
**Des Moines Chapter**
1120 E 6th St., No. 7
Des Moines, IA 50316
**Phone:** (515)244-9411
**Email:** suplu@aol.com
Ellie Philips, Contact

★ **12964** ★ **National Depressive and Manic-Depressive Association**
**Dubuque Mental Health Support Group**
4950 Angel View Dr.
Dubuque, IA 52002
**Phone:** (563)556-2873
**Email:** pagronen1@mchsi.com
Penny Gronen, Contact

★ **12965** ★ **National Depressive and Manic-Depressive Association**
**Quad Cities Chapter**
2720 Middle Rd.
Davenport, IA 52803
**Phone:** (319)355-3977  **Fax:** (319)359-2779
**Email:** dirko@netexpress.net
Kathy Kuhl, Contact

★ **12966** ★ **National Depressive and Manic-Depressive Association**
**Siouxland Chapter**
PO Box 1917
Sioux City, IA 51102
**Phone:** (712)252-4489  **Fax:** (712)252-3871
Katherine Potter, Contact
**Remarks:** Serves Iowa and South Dakota.

★ **12967** ★ **National Depressive and Manic-Depressive Association**
**Tri-State Consumers Group Chapter**
4501 West St.
Sioux City, IA 51108
**Phone:** (712)277-4687
Denny Wilshire, Contact
**Remarks:** Serves Iowa and South Dakota.

### Kansas

★ **12968** ★ **National Depressive and Manic-Depressive Association**
**El Dorado Chapter**
El Dorado, KS
**Phone:** (316)541-2935
Esther Fitzgerald, Contact

★ **12969** ★ **National Depressive and Manic-Depressive Association**
**Flint Hills Chapter**
2919 Northwood Dr.
Milford, KS 66514
**Phone:** (785)776-1332  **Fax:** (785)239-2251
**Email:** flinthillsdmda@hotmail.com
Jim Walker, Contact

**★ 12970 ★ National Depressive and Manic-Depressive Association**
**Kansas City Southside Chapter**
2226 S 29th St.
Kansas City, KS 66106-5512
**Phone:** (913)384-0782
**Email:** babble@kc.rr.com
**Website:** http://www.depressionsupport.org
Janet Northcott, Contact

**★ 12971 ★ National Depressive and Manic-Depressive Association**
**Topeka Chapter**
PO Box 4335
Topeka, KS 66604-0335
**Phone:** (785)272-1360          **Fax:** (785)272-1360
**Email:** ksbryce@aol.com
Bryce Miller, Contact

**★ 12972 ★ National Depressive and Manic-Depressive Association**
**Wichita Chapter**
1451 N Woodlawn
Wichita, KS 67208
**Phone:** (316)269-2534          **Fax:** (316)269-1409
**Email:** director30@hotmail.com
Barbara Andres, Contact

### Kentucky

**★ 12973 ★ National Depressive and Manic-Depressive Association**
**Bluegrass Chapter**
Frankfort, KY
**Phone:** (502)564-7510
**Email:** don.thurber@mail.state.ky.us
Don Thurber, Contact

**★ 12974 ★ National Depressive and Manic-Depressive Association**
**Louisville Chapter**
Louisville, KY
**Phone:** (502)595-8309          **Fax:** (502)587-8212
**Email:** leo@leoweekly.com
Carl Brown, Contact

**★ 12975 ★ National Depressive and Manic-Depressive Association**
**Western Kentucky Chapter**
2544 Bittle Rd.
Owensboro, KY 42301
**Phone:** (270)683-3893
Clara Heintz, Contact

### Louisiana

**★ 12976 ★ National Depressive and Manic-Depressive Association**
**New Orleans Chapter**
1212 Melody Dr.
Metairie, LA 70002
**Phone:** (504)835-2413
**Email:** mzaeringer@aol.com
Marilyn Zaeringer, Contact

### Maine

**★ 12977 ★ National Depressive and Manic-Depressive Association**
**Portland Chapter**
Portland, ME
**Phone:** (207)878-8317
**Email:** khess1@maine.rr.com
Ken Hess, Contact

**★ 12978 ★ National Depressive and Manic-Depressive Association**
**York County Chapter**
2 Lyman Ave., No. 11
Saco, ME 04072-1954
**Phone:** (207)283-9375
**Email:** marensta@maine.rr.com
Dr. Michael Arenstam, Contact

### Manitoba

**★ 12979 ★ Mood Disorders Association of Manitoba, Inc.**
4-1000 Notre Dame Ave.
Winnipeg, MB, Canada R3E 0N3
**Phone:** (204)786-0987          **Fax:** (204)786-1906
**Email:** sdmdm@depression.mb.ca
**Website:** http://www.depression.mb.ca

### Maryland

**★ 12980 ★ National Depressive and Manic-Depressive Association**
**Maryland Chapter**
DRADA Meyer 3-181
600 N Wolfe St.
Baltimore, MD 21287-7381
**Phone:** (410)955-4647          **Fax:** (410)614-3241
**Email:** drada@jhmi.edu
**Website:** http://www.med.jhu.edu/drada
Wendy Resnick, Contact

### Massachusetts

**★ 12981 ★ National Depressive and Manic-Depressive Association**
**Attleboro Chapter**
140 Park St.
Attleboro, MA 02703
**Phone:** (508)222-7525
**Email:** info@mddaboston.org
**Website:** http://www.mddaboston.org
Chantal Polsonetti, Contact

**★ 12982 ★ National Depressive and Manic-Depressive Association**
**Boston Chapter**
PO Box 102
Belmont, MA 02478
**Phone:** (617)855-2795          **Fax:** (617)855-3666
**Email:** info@mddaboston.org
**Website:** http://www.mddaboston.org
Everett Page, Contact

**★ 12983 ★ National Depressive and Manic-Depressive Association**
**Northeast Chapter**
PO Box 2624
Worcester, MA 01653
**Phone:** (508)791-0060
**Email:** jeebee1952@msn.com
Jo-Ellen Stone, Contact

**★ 12984 ★ National Depressive and Manic-Depressive Association**
**Northern Worcester County Chapter**
Leominster, MA
**Phone:** (978)874-2713
Eric Hawkins, Contact

**★ 12985 ★ National Depressive and Manic-Depressive Association**
**Westwood Lodge Hospital Chapter**
45 Clapboardtree St.
Westwood, MA 02090
**Phone:** (781)431-9704
**Email:** jacqueline.swerling@cgey.com
Jacquie Swerling, Contact

### Michigan

**★ 12986 ★ National Depressive and Manic-Depressive Association**
**Cadillac Area Chapter**
Cadillac, MI
**Phone:** (231)839-5670          **Fax:** (231)775-6454
**Email:** jamesfitz@netonecom.net
Theresa Surs, Contact

**★ 12987 ★ National Depressive and Manic-Depressive Association**
**Grand Rapids Chapter**
858 Reynard St. SE
Grand Rapids, MI 49507
**Phone:** (616)246-0280
Tim Griffin, Contact

**★ 12988 ★ National Depressive and Manic-Depressive Association**
**Greater Flint Area/Rising Above Chapter**
Lot 62 Merry Lane
Mount Morris, MI 48458-2426
**Phone:** (810)789-3609          **Fax:** (810)789-3609
**Email:** mvallet@gfn.org
Ellie M. Vallet, Contact

**★ 12989 ★ National Depressive and Manic-Depressive Association**
**Hillsdale & Jackson Counties Chapter**
1200 N West Ave.
Jackson, MI 49202
**Phone:** (517)780-3384          **Fax:** (517)789-9981
**Email:** lesia.pikaart@lifewaysmco.com

**★ 12990 ★ National Depressive and Manic-Depressive Association**
**Metropolitan Detroit Chapter**
PO Box 132
Dearborn, MI 48121
**Phone:** (313)532-4217
**Email:** lifeinbalance@mdda-metro-detroit.org
**Website:** http://www.mdda-metro-detroit.org
Gary Wyatt, Contact

**★ 12991 ★ National Depressive and Manic-Depressive Association**
**Northeast Michigan Chapter**
PO Box 715
Alpena, MI 49707
**Phone:** (517)354-4470
**Email:** nemdmda@netscape.net
Bruce Fowler, Contact

**★ 12992 ★ National Depressive and Manic-Depressive Association**
**Traverse Bay Area/Suttons Bay Chapter**
701 S Elmwood, No. 19
Traverse City, MI 49684
**Phone:** (231)342-3076
Jim Brubaker, Contact

**★ 12993 ★ National Depressive and Manic-Depressive Association**
**Tri-Cities Michigan Chapter**
609 N Trumbull
Bay City, MI 48708
**Phone:** (989)662-7897
**Email:** richpe55@yahoo.com
Richard M. Philipp, Contact

### Minnesota

**★ 12994 ★ National Depressive and Manic-Depressive Association**
**Help, Hope & Healing Chapter**
Columbia Heights, MN

**Phone:** (763)571-6070
Joe Kunza, Contact

★ **12995** ★ **National Depressive and Manic-Depressive Association**
**Minnesota Chapter**
2021 E Hennepin Ave., No. 412
Minneapolis, MN 55413
**Phone:** (612)379-7933        **Fax:** (612)331-1630
**Email:** dmdaminnesota@juno.com
Nikita Godette, Contact

### Mississippi

★ **12996** ★ **National Depressive and Manic-Depressive Association**
**Gulf Coast Chapter**
4803 Harrison Cir.
Gulfport, MS 39507
**Phone:** (228)864-4579        **Free:** 800-584-6274
J. B. Morgan, Contact

### Missouri

★ **12997** ★ **National Depressive and Manic-Depressive Association**
**Greater Saint Louis Chapter**
1905 S Grand Blvd.
Saint Louis, MO 63104
**Phone:** (314)776-3969        **Fax:** (314)776-7071
**Email:** dmdastl@aol.com
Helen Minth, Contact

★ **12998** ★ **National Depressive and Manic-Depressive Association**
**Kansas City Fairway Chapter**
901 Tamoshanter
Kansas City, MO 64145
**Phone:** (816)942-5802        **Fax:** (913)281-3977
**Email:** tterwelp@worldnet.att.net
Tony Terwelp, Contact

★ **12999** ★ **National Depressive and Manic-Depressive Association**
**Southeast Missouri Chapter**
PO Box 658
Cape Girardeau, MO 63702-0658
**Phone:** (573)332-0650        **Fax:** (573)334-4416
Kathryn Myers, Contact

### Montana

★ **13000** ★ **National Depressive and Manic-Depressive Association**
**Cascade County Outreach Chapter**
PO Box 3305
Great Falls, MT 59403
**Phone:** (406)453-7767        **Fax:** (406)453-7767
Rebecca L. Hewitt, Contact

### Nebraska

★ **13001** ★ **National Depressive and Manic-Depressive Association**
**Greater Omaha Chapter**
5157 Jackson St.
Omaha, NE 68106
**Phone:** (402)551-3275
**Email:** dmda@home.com
**Website:** http://www.discoveromaha.com/community/groups/dmda
Kate Ryan, Contact

### New Hampshire

★ **13002** ★ **National Depressive and Manic-Depressive Association**
**Nashua Chapter**
PO Box 3761
Nashua, NH 03061
**Phone:** (603)930-5920
**Email:** winw@dmdanashua.org
**Website:** http://www.dmdanashua.org
W. E. Warren, Contact

### New Jersey

★ **13003** ★ **National Depressive and Manic-Depressive Association**
**Bergen County Recovery Group**
PO Box 1296
Paramus, NJ 07653
**Phone:** (973)423-4394        **Fax:** (201)525-0844
**Email:** bergendmda@aol.com
**Website:** http://community.nj.cm/cc/dmda

★ **13004** ★ **National Depressive and Manic-Depressive Association**
**Colts Neck Chapter**
Colts Neck, NJ
**Phone:** (732)919-7739
**Email:** rcallen@monmouth.com
Rick Allen, Contact

★ **13005** ★ **National Depressive and Manic-Depressive Association**
**Essex County Chapter**
187 Bellevue Ave.
Montclair, NJ 07043
**Phone:** (973)744-5230
**Email:** margoatwell@msn.com
**Website:** http://community.nj.com/cc/dmda.essexcounty
Margo Atwell, Contact

★ **13006** ★ **National Depressive and Manic-Depressive Association**
**First New Jersey/Morristown Chapter**
1 Stony Hill Pl.
Livingston, NJ 07039
**Phone:** (973)994-1143        **Free:** 800-367-6274
**Email:** LSB1@panix.com
**Website:** http://community.nj.com/cc/1stnjdmdsg
Linda Boginsky, Contact

★ **13007** ★ **National Depressive and Manic-Depressive Association**
**Middlesex County Chapter**
61 Glenn Oaks Ct.
Old Bridge, NJ 08857
**Phone:** (732)910-8614        **Fax:** (732)679-6346
**Email:** mcdmda@hotmail.com
**Website:** http://community.nj.com/cc/mcdmda
Sekhar Subramani, Contact

★ **13008** ★ **National Depressive and Manic-Depressive Association**
**Sussex County Chapter**
2 Smith St.
Newton, NJ 07860
**Phone:** (973)383-3808
Jean Bodner, Contact

★ **13009** ★ **National Depressive and Manic-Depressive Association**
**Union County Chapter**
99 Beauvoir Ave.
Summit, NJ 07901
**Phone:** (908)233-7074
**Email:** margoatwell@msn.com
**Website:** http://www.community.nj.com/cc/dmda.wes
Theldora Hawkins, Contact

### New Mexico

★ **13010** ★ **National Depressive and Manic-Depressive Association**
**Albuquerque Chapter**
PO Box 27619
Albuquerque, NM 87125-7619
**Phone:** (505)857-3778
**Email:** dmda4albq@yahoo.com
Victoria Cain, Contact

★ **13011** ★ **National Depressive and Manic-Depressive Association**
**Valencia County Chapter**
Los Lunas, NM
**Phone:** 888-547-9475
Rick Swift, Contact

### New York

★ **13012** ★ **National Depressive and Manic-Depressive Association**
**Albany Chapter**
Albany, NY
**Phone:** (518)346-6800
**Email:** consumer@capital.net
Barbara Schumaker, Contact

★ **13013** ★ **National Depressive and Manic-Depressive Association**
**Binghamton Chapter**
PO Box 1236
Binghamton, NY 13901
**Phone:** (607)778-2532
Jude Trepa, Contact

★ **13014** ★ **National Depressive and Manic-Depressive Association**
**Capitol District Mood Disorder Support Group**
Albany, NY
**Phone:** (518)465-9413
Peter Berkery, Contact

★ **13015** ★ **National Depressive and Manic-Depressive Association**
**Dutchess County Chapter**
510 Haight Ave.
Poughkeepsie, NY 12603
**Phone:** (914)473-2500        **Fax:** (914)473-4870
**Email:** mhadc@frontiernet.com
**Website:** http://www.mhadc.com

★ **13016** ★ **National Depressive and Manic-Depressive Association**
**Finger Lakes Chapter**
375-377 W Church St.
Elmira, NY 14901
**Phone:** (607)734-4789        **Fax:** (607)737-6274
**Email:** info@dmdaotfl.com
**Website:** http://www.dmdaotfl.com
George A. Griffith, Contact

★ **13017** ★ **National Depressive and Manic-Depressive Association**
**Ithaca Bipolar Explorers Club Chapter**
1013 N Tioga St.
Ithaca, NY 14850
**Phone:** (607)255-7053        **Fax:** (607)255-5684
**Email:** cs19@cornell.edu
Carole Stone, Contact
**Frmly:** Depressive and Manic-Depressive Association, Ithaca Bipolar.

**★ 13018 ★ National Depressive and Manic-Depressive Association**
**Long Island Chapter**
110 Grove St.
Merrick, NY 11566-2246
**Phone:** (516)379-1238

**★ 13019 ★ National Depressive and Manic-Depressive Association**
**MDSG New York Chapter**
PO Box 30377
New York, NY 10011
**Phone:** (212)533-6374          **Fax:** (212)675-0218
**Email:** info@mdsg.org
**Website:** http://www.mdsg.org
Tory Masters, Contact

**★ 13020 ★ National Depressive and Manic-Depressive Association**
**Rochester Chapter**
120 Holyoke St., No. 7
Rochester, NY 14615
**Phone:** (585)594-5988
**Email:** rochdmda@aol.com
**Website:** http://www.geocities.com/rocdmda
Sue Harkins, Contact

**★ 13021 ★ National Depressive and Manic-Depressive Association**
**Westchester Chapter**
White Plains Hospital Center
Davis Ave. at E Post Rd.
White Plains, NY 10601
**Phone:** (914)476-4720
**Email:** wcdmda@aol.com
**Website:**          http://hometown.aol.com/wcdmda/index.html

### North Carolina

**★ 13022 ★ National Depressive and Manic-Depressive Association**
**North Carolina Chapter**
1046 Washington St.
Raleigh, NC 27605-1258
**Phone:** (919)821-4343          **Fax:** (919)821-4043
**Email:** ncdmda01@aol.com
Charles Hinton, Contact

### North Dakota

**★ 13023 ★ National Depressive and Manic-Depressive Association**
**Fargo Chapter**
124 8th St. N
Fargo, ND 58102
**Phone:** (701)237-5871          **Fax:** (701)237-0562
**Email:** mharrv@juno.com
Susan Helgeland, Contact

### Ohio

**★ 13024 ★ National Depressive and Manic-Depressive Association**
**Above the Moods Chapter**
9299 State Rte. 66 N
Delphos, OH 45833
**Phone:** (419)692-2785
Irene Blockberger, Contact

**★ 13025 ★ National Depressive and Manic-Depressive Association**
**Athens Chapter**
PO Box 225
Athens, OH 45701
**Phone:** (740)594-0022
**Email:** dmdaathens@earthlink.net
Linda Bauer, Contact

**★ 13026 ★ National Depressive and Manic-Depressive Association**
**Cleveland Chapter**
11501 Mayfield Rd., No. 100
Cleveland, OH 44106
**Phone:** (216)229-4841
J. Thomas Kalka, Contact

**★ 13027 ★ National Depressive and Manic-Depressive Association**
**Consumers Union of Lucas County**
Toledo, OH
**Phone:** (419)242-1801
**Email:** dmdatol@amplex.net
Sandy Chambers, Contact

**★ 13028 ★ National Depressive and Manic-Depressive Association**
**Findlay Chapter**
2330 S Main St.
Findlay, OH 45840
**Phone:** (419)427-2502
Karen McClellan, Contact

**★ 13029 ★ National Depressive and Manic-Depressive Association**
**Four County ADAM Board Chapter**
115 Deerfield Circle
Bryan, OH 43506
**Phone:** (419)636-2076          **Fax:** (419)267-3353
**Email:** lougoblu@bnnorth.net
Caroline Gretick, Contact

**★ 13030 ★ National Depressive and Manic-Depressive Association**
**Greater Toledo Chapter**
961 S Reynolds Rd., No. 37
Toledo, OH 43615
**Phone:** (419)255-1459          **Fax:** (419)255-4823
**Email:** dmdatol@amplex.net
Dorene Sherman, Contact

**★ 13031 ★ National Depressive and Manic-Depressive Association**
**Medina Chapter**
Human Services Bldg.
246 Northland Dr.
Medina, OH
**Phone:** (330)769-4884
**Email:** dmdamedina@hotmail.com
**Website:** http://dmdamedina.tripod.com
Sally Williamson, Contact

**★ 13032 ★ National Depressive and Manic-Depressive Association**
**Northwest Columbus Chapter**
360 Meadow View Dr.
Powell, OH 43065
**Phone:** (740)548-6487
**Email:** dmdacolumbus@insight.rr.com
Barbara Ryan, Contact

**★ 13033 ★ National Depressive and Manic-Depressive Association**
**Tri-County and Akron Chapter**
Akron General Medical Center
400 Wabash Ave.
Akron, OH 44307
**Phone:** (330)384-6475          **Fax:** (330)996-5802
**Email:** ccihlar@agmc.org
**Website:** http://www.agmc.org
Claudia Cihlar, RN, Contact

**★ 13034 ★ National Depressive and Manic-Depressive Association**
**Wayne County Chapter**
Wooster, OH
**Phone:** (330)264-1590

**Email:** whudson54@aol.com
Walter Hudson, Contact

### Oklahoma

**★ 13035 ★ National Depressive and Manic-Depressive Association**
**Edmond Chapter**
Edmond, OK
**Phone:** (405)844-7967
Gerri Hames, Contact

**★ 13036 ★ National Depressive and Manic-Depressive Association**
**El Reno Chapter**
El Reno, OK
**Phone:** (405)262-3909
Larry Bolain, Contact

**★ 13037 ★ National Depressive and Manic-Depressive Association**
**Midwest City Chapter**
Midwest City, OK
**Phone:** (405)737-1923
Jackie Skaggs, Contact

**★ 13038 ★ National Depressive and Manic-Depressive Association**
**Norman Chapter**
Norman, OK
**Phone:** (405)447-5819
Sharon Willis, Contact

**★ 13039 ★ National Depressive and Manic-Depressive Association**
**Northside Oklahoma City Chapter**
14832 NW Expy.
Piedmont, OK 73078
**Phone:** (405)840-0607
Mary McCormick, Contact

**★ 13040 ★ National Depressive and Manic-Depressive Association**
**Oklahoma Chapter**
5313 S May Ave.
Oklahoma City, OK 73119
**Phone:** (405)681-8073
**Email:** bth@aol.com
W. D. Thomas, Contact

**★ 13041 ★ National Depressive and Manic-Depressive Association**
**Southside Oklahoma City Chapter**
1821 Classen Blvd., No. 223
Oklahoma City, OK 73106
**Phone:** (405)521-1911          **Fax:** (405)373-2275
Jess Allen, Contact

**★ 13042 ★ National Depressive and Manic-Depressive Association**
**Southwest Oklahoma Chapter**
2328 NW 47th St.
Lawton, OK 73505
**Phone:** (405)692-2644
Monica Scott, Contact

**★ 13043 ★ National Depressive and Manic-Depressive Association**
**Yukon Chapter**
Yukon, OK
**Phone:** (405)373-0059
Iva Cook, Contact

## Ontario

**★ 13044 ★ Mood Disorders Association of Ontario**
40 Orchard View Blvd., Ste. 222
Toronto, ON, Canada M4R 1B9
**Phone:** (416)486-8046     **Free:** 888-486-8236
**Fax:** (416)486-8127
**Email:** info@mooddisorders.on.ca
**Website:** http://www.mooddisorders.on.ca
Leona Chase, Contact

## Oregon

**★ 13045 ★ National Depressive and Manic-Depressive Association**
**Clackamas County Chapter**
Oregon City, OR
**Phone:** (503)722-6500
**Email:** dmda_clackamas_county@hotmail.com
Casadi Marino, Contact

**★ 13046 ★ National Depressive and Manic-Depressive Association**
**Hillsboro Depression Support Group**
Portland, OR
**Phone:** (503)357-6331
Gen Horlacher, Contact

**★ 13047 ★ National Depressive and Manic-Depressive Association**
**Lane County Chapter**
557 Fenster St.
Eugene, OR 97401
**Phone:** (541)484-6090
**Email:** tazlady@uswest.net
Sheila Denney, Contact

## Pennsylvania

**★ 13048 ★ National Depressive and Manic-Depressive Association**
**Allegheny County Chapter**
1945 5th Ave.
Pittsburgh, PA 15219
**Phone:** (412)391-3820     **Fax:** (412)391-3825
**Email:** mhaac@sgi.net
Delores Burgess, Contact

**★ 13049 ★ National Depressive and Manic-Depressive Association**
**Beaver County Chapter**
219 3rd St.
Beaver, PA 15009
**Phone:** (724)775-9152     **Fax:** (724)775-9153
**Email:** svs2u@hotmail.com
Suzanne Vogel-Scibilia, MD, Contact

**★ 13050 ★ National Depressive and Manic-Depressive Association**
**Bipolar/Pottstown Chapter**
Pottstown Memorial Medical Center
1600 E High St.
Pottstown, PA 19464
**Phone:** (610)327-7633     **Fax:** (610)327-7641
Linda W. Thompson, Contact

**★ 13051 ★ National Depressive and Manic-Depressive Association**
**Delaware County Chapter**
Upper Darby, PA
**Phone:** 877-687-9552     **Fax:** 877-687-9552
**Email:** dmda562@msn.com
Joseph T. Bunting, Contact

**★ 13052 ★ National Depressive and Manic-Depressive Association**
**Delaware Valley Chapter**
PO Box 911
Bala Cynwyd, PA 19004-0901
**Phone:** (215)581-5438
**Email:** dmda562@msn.com
Ronald Berman, Contact

**★ 13053 ★ National Depressive and Manic-Depressive Association**
**Depressive & Manic Depressive Illness Support Group/WPIC**
3811 O'Hara St.
Pittsburgh, PA 15213
**Phone:** (412)624-2211     **Fax:** (412)642-5734
Joan Buttenfield, RN, Contact

**★ 13054 ★ National Depressive and Manic-Depressive Association**
**Erie Chapter**
1101 Peach St.
Erie, PA 16501
**Phone:** (814)452-4462     **Fax:** (814)456-6593
**Email:** shirleyf@surferie.net
Shirley Ruth French, Contact

**★ 13055 ★ National Depressive and Manic-Depressive Association**
**Friends for Friends Chapter**
4641 Roosevelt Blvd.
Philadelphia, PA 19124-2399
**Phone:** (215)831-7809
Michael Solomon, Contact

**★ 13056 ★ National Depressive and Manic-Depressive Association**
**HUP Chapter**
9639 James St.
Philadelphia, PA 19114
**Phone:** (215)552-8737
**Email:** hupdmda2dhazam@aol.com
Denis Hazam, Contact

**★ 13057 ★ National Depressive and Manic-Depressive Association**
**Lehigh Valley Chapter**
2552 W South St.
Allentown, PA 18104
**Phone:** (610)252-2395
**Email:** info@dmda-lv.org
**Website:** http://www.dmda-lv.org
Regina Weppel, Contact

**★ 13058 ★ National Depressive and Manic-Depressive Association**
**New Directions/Abington Chapter**
PO Box 181
Hatboro, PA 19040
**Phone:** (215)887-4059
**Email:** boris@home.com
Amy Russell, Contact

**★ 13059 ★ National Depressive and Manic-Depressive Association**
**Pocono Mountain Chapter**
19 Crystal St.
East Stroudsburg, PA 18301
**Phone:** (570)420-8070     **Fax:** (570)424-6487
Lisa Butz, Contact

**★ 13060 ★ National Depressive and Manic-Depressive Association**
**Reach Out Foundation**
229 Plaza Blvd., No. 101
Morrisville, PA 19067
**Phone:** (215)428-0404
**Email:** rofbucks@aol.com

## Quebec

**★ 13061 ★ Alliance for the Mentally Ill Quebec, Inc.**
**(Alliance pour les Malades Mentaux Inc.)**
5253 Decarie, Ste. 150
Montreal, QC, Canada H3W 3C3
**Phone:** (514)486-1448     **Fax:** (514)486-6157
**Email:** amique@dsuper.net
**Website:** http://www.dsuper.net/~amique
Ella Amir, Contact

## Rhode Island

**★ 13062 ★ National Depressive and Manic-Depressive Association**
**Rhode Island Chapter**
Providence, RI
**Phone:** (401)254-2573     **Fax:** (401)254-0609
**Email:** jmcnulty@nami.org
Jim McNulty, Contact

## South Carolina

**★ 13063 ★ National Depressive and Manic-Depressive Association**
**Charleston Chapter**
Charleston, SC
**Phone:** (843)723-2618
**Email:** manicgh@bellsouth.net
Melinda G. Harmon, Contact

**★ 13064 ★ National Depressive and Manic-Depressive Association**
**Greenwood County/Winding Paths Chapter**
Greenwood, SC
**Phone:** (864)229-3570
**Email:** tjdorsey@emeraldis.com
Janet W. Dorsey, Contact

**★ 13065 ★ National Depressive and Manic-Depressive Association**
**South Carolina Chapter, Inc.**
Myrtle Beach, SC
**Phone:** (843)347-3035     **Fax:** (843)347-9375
**Email:** nscrauder@sc.rr.com
George Wright, Contact

**★ 13066 ★ National Depressive and Manic-Depressive Association**
**Ups & Downs**
Greenville, SC
**Phone:** (864)455-3798     **Fax:** (864)455-4540
Robert Parker, Contact

## Tennessee

**★ 13067 ★ National Depressive and Manic-Depressive Association**
**Madison Chapter**
Madison, TN
**Phone:** (615)356-1622
**Email:** TeenaR@AOL.com
Teena Rodgers, Contact

**★ 13068 ★ National Depressive and Manic-Depressive Association**
**Memphis Chapter**
Memphis, TN
**Phone:** (901)377-4763
**Email:** dmda-memphis@hotmail.com
Leah Ann Kelley, Contact

**★ 13069 ★ National Depressive and Manic-Depressive Association**
**Nashville Centennial Chapter**
Nashville, TN
**Phone:** (615)228-4810
**Email:** LizBeth782@aol.com
Elizabeth Reed, Contact

**★ 13070 ★ National Depressive and Manic-Depressive Association**
**Pendulum of Chattanooga**
Chattanooga, TN
**Phone:** (423)698-2384          **Fax:** (423)698-6617
**Email:** coatsfh@aol.com
Marilou Coats, Contact

**★ 13071 ★ National Depressive and Manic-Depressive Association**
**Pendulum of Knoxville**
Knoxville, TN
**Phone:** (865)545-7863          **Fax:** (865)545-3049
Laura Menefee Green, Contact

**★ 13072 ★ National Depressive and Manic-Depressive Association**
**Two Rivers Chapter**
Nashville, TN
**Phone:** (615)884-2160
Becky Barrett, Contact

### Texas

**★ 13073 ★ National Depressive and Manic-Depressive Association**
**Austin Chapter**
Austin, TX
**Phone:** (512)326-9396
**Email:** austindmda@yahoo.com
**Website:** http://www.main.org/dmda/index.html
L. J. Smith, Contact

**★ 13074 ★ National Depressive and Manic-Depressive Association**
**Bay Area Chapter**
Friendswood, TX
**Phone:** (281)335-1000
**Email:** brew1@houston.rr.com
Paul Koll, Contact

**★ 13075 ★ National Depressive and Manic-Depressive Association**
**Brazos Valley Area Chapter**
Bryan, TX
**Phone:** (979)779-7336
**Email:** o.firstfixer@gte.net
Suzanne Helland, Contact

**★ 13076 ★ National Depressive and Manic-Depressive Association**
**Dallas Chapter**
Dallas, TX
**Phone:** (817)654-7100
Bill Drissel, Contact

**★ 13077 ★ National Depressive and Manic-Depressive Association**
**El Paso Chapter**
El Paso, TX
**Phone:** (915)541-1400          **Fax:** (915)544-5992
**Email:** epdmda@aol.com
**Website:** http://www.epdmda.org
William E. Myers, Contact

**★ 13078 ★ National Depressive and Manic-Depressive Association**
**Ft. Worth and Tarrant Counties Chapter**
Fort Worth, TX
**Phone:** (817)654-7100

**★ 13079 ★ National Depressive and Manic-Depressive Association**
**Georgetown Chapter**
Georgetown, TX
**Phone:** (512)863-5560
Anita Smith, Contact

**★ 13080 ★ National Depressive and Manic-Depressive Association**
**Greater Austin Chapter**
Austin, TX
**Phone:** (512)331-6866
**Email:** kjazz68-1999@yahoo.com
Karen Brown, Contact

**★ 13081 ★ National Depressive and Manic-Depressive Association**
**Houston and Harris County Chapter**
Houston, TX
**Phone:** (713)528-1546          **Fax:** (281)514-2570
**Email:** jim.yeomans@compaq.com
**Website:** http://www.dmdahouston.org

**★ 13082 ★ National Depressive and Manic-Depressive Association**
**San Antonio Chapter**
San Antonio, TX
**Phone:** (210)661-2693
**Email:** sadmda2002@yahoo.com
Charlotte Dallas, Contact

**★ 13083 ★ National Depressive and Manic-Depressive Association**
**Texas Chapter**
Austin, TX
**Phone:** 888-716-2807          **Fax:** (512)478-5223
Paul Koll, Contact

**★ 13084 ★ National Depressive and Manic-Depressive Association**
**Tyler Chapter**
Tyler, TX
**Phone:** (903)566-8401
Mary Mathison, Contact

### Utah

**★ 13085 ★ National Depressive and Manic-Depressive Association**
**Uplift Chapter**
444 W Stonehedge Dr., No. 8L
Salt Lake City, UT 84107
**Phone:** (801)264-8193
John Kreipl, Contact

### Virginia

**★ 13086 ★ National Depressive and Manic-Depressive Association**
**Lynchburg Depressive Disorders Chapter**
PO Box 216
Lynchburg, VA 24505
**Phone:** (804)237-5768          **Fax:** (804)237-6140
**Email:** phil@dmdav.org
**Website:** http://www.dmdav.org
Linda Theisen, Contact

**★ 13087 ★ National Depressive and Manic-Depressive Association**
**Norfolk Chapter**
6157 Westwood Terrace
Norfolk, VA 23508
**Phone:** (757)483-1003
**Email:** rpcline@exis.net
Linda Matthews, Contact

**★ 13088 ★ National Depressive and Manic-Depressive Association**
**Richmond Chapter**
12189 Stokesley Ct.
Richmond, VA 23233
**Phone:** (804)360-4305          **Fax:** (804)360-8020
Allan Lassiter, Contact

**★ 13089 ★ National Depressive and Manic-Depressive Association**
**Roanoke Anxiety & Depressive Disorders Chapter**
2944 Lockridge Rd. SW
Roanoke, VA 24014
**Phone:** (540)344-0723          **Fax:** (540)344-1610
Susan Whately, Contact

### Washington

**★ 13090 ★ National Depressive and Manic-Depressive Association**
**Clark County Chapter**
Vancouver, WA
**Phone:** (360)686-3496
Susan Plummer, Contact

**★ 13091 ★ National Depressive and Manic-Depressive Association**
**Greater Seattle Chapter**
PO Box 22344
Seattle, WA 98122
**Phone:** (206)748-1577
**Website:** http://www.behavenet.com/seattledmda
Ken Clark, Contact

**★ 13092 ★ National Depressive and Manic-Depressive Association**
**Skagit Valley Chapter**
Mount Vernon, WA
**Phone:** (360)424-8224
**Email:** oroboros@gte.net
Diana Dodds, Contact

**★ 13093 ★ National Depressive and Manic-Depressive Association**
**Tacoma Chapter**
**Hope for Depression and Bipolar Support Group**
Tacoma, WA
**Email:** laurie@tacid.org
**Website:** http://www.tacid.org

**★ 13094 ★ National Depressive and Manic-Depressive Association**
**Tri-City Bi-Polar Support Group**
35202 N Flagstone Dr.
Benton City, WA 99320
**Phone:** (509)946-9230
**Email:** cider_house_rules@yahoo.com

**★ 13095 ★ National Depressive and Manic-Depressive Association**
**Whatcom County Chapter**
PO Box 4124
Bellingham, WA 98227
**Phone:** (360)733-1627          **Fax:** (360)676-4697
Jean Danielson, Contact

### West Virginia

**★ 13096 ★ National Depressive and Manic-Depressive Association**
**Wheeling Chapter**
Wheeling, WV
**Phone:** (304)242-0154
Penny Stenger, Contact

## Wisconsin

**★ 13097 ★ National Depressive and
Manic-Depressive Association
La Crosse Area Chapter**
1515 State St.
La Crosse, WI 54601
**Phone:** (608)786-2360     **Fax:** (608)783-4996
**Email:** rpavenue@aol.com
Ray Pauloski, Contact

**★ 13098 ★ National Depressive and
Manic-Depressive Association
Menomonee Falls Chapter**
W167 N 8633 Jacobson Dr.
Menomonee Falls, WI 53051
**Phone:** (262)251-2697
Tom Malone, Contact

**★ 13099 ★ National Depressive and
Manic-Depressive Association
Mood Disorders of Green Bay Chapter**
N 8272 State Hwy. 55
Seymour, WI 54165
**Phone:** (920)833-6324
Deloris Clausen, Contact

**★ 13100 ★ National Depressive and
Manic-Depressive Association
Ozaukee County Chapter**
2141 N Briar Dr.
West Bend, WI 53095
**Phone:** (262)338-1614
**Email:** kkatty2@yahoo.com
Jane Kleinowski, Contact

**★ 13101 ★ National Depressive and
Manic-Depressive Association
Southeastern Wisconsin Chapter**
PO Box 510214
Milwaukee, WI 53202-0041
**Phone:** (414)964-2586
**Email:** dmdasewmilw@hotmail.com
Roseanne Schmidt, Contact

## Mental Health

*Associations listed below are state affiliates of the
National Mental Health Association, 1021 Prince St.,
Alexandria, VA 22314-2971, (800)969-NMHA, http://
www.nmha.org/. Contact the national association for
information on states not listed here.*

## Alabama

**★ 13102 ★ National Mental Health
Association in Etowah County**
901 Goodyear Ave.
Gadsden, AL 35903
**Phone:** (256)492-3381     **Fax:** (256)494-5536
**Email:** mhaofet@internetpro.net
Cathy Spivey, Director

**★ 13103 ★ National Mental Health
Association in Madison County**
701 Andrew Jackson Way
Huntsville, AL 35801
**Phone:** (256)536-9441     **Fax:** (256)534-7533
**Email:** director@mentalhealthalabama.org
**Website:** http://www.mentalhealthalabama.org
Sandra Moon, Director

**★ 13104 ★ National Mental Health
Association in Montgomery**
1116 S Hull St.
Montgomery, AL 36104
**Phone:** (334)262-5500     **Fax:** (334)262-1576

**Email:** mhamontg@hiwaay.net
Darold Dunlavy, Exec Director

**★ 13105 ★ National Mental Health
Association in Morgan County**
PO Box 1502
Decatur, AL 35602
**Phone:** (256)353-1160     **Fax:** (256)353-1163
**Email:** sue@mhainmc.org
**Website:** http://www.mhainmc.org
Sue Brantley, Director

**★ 13106 ★ National Mental Health
Association in Southwestern Alabama**
PO Box 282
Montrose, AL 36559-0282
**Phone:** (334)626-9585
**Email:** mhaswa@msn.com

**★ 13107 ★ National Mental Health
Association in Tuscaloosa County**
2123 9th St.
Tuscaloosa, AL 35401
**Phone:** (205)752-2689     **Fax:** (205)758-5773
Joan Brown, Director

## Alaska

**★ 13108 ★ National Mental Health
Association in Alaska**
4050 Lake Otis Pkwy., Ste. 204-A
Anchorage, AK 99508
**Phone:** (907)563-0880     **Fax:** (907)563-0881
**Email:** mhaa@alaska.net
**Website:** http://www.alaska.net/~mhaa/
Jan McGillivary, Director

## Arizona

**★ 13109 ★ National Mental Health
Association of Arizona, Scottsdale**
6411 E Thomas Rd.
Scottsdale, AZ 85251
**Phone:** (480)994-4407     **Fax:** (480)994-4744
**Email:** mhaaz@qwest.net
**Website:** http://www.mhaaz.com

**★ 13110 ★ National Mental Health
Association of Southern Arizona**
1905 E 7th St., Bldg. 4
Tucson, AZ 85719
**Phone:** (520)882-4806     **Fax:** (520)882-0124
**Email:** mhatucson1@aol.com
**Website:** http://www.mhaaz.com
Cheryl Collier Becker, Director

## Arkansas

**★ 13111 ★ National Mental Health
Association in Northwest Arkansas**
PO Box 1993
Fayetteville, AR 72702-1993

## California

**★ 13112 ★ National Mental Health
Association of Alameda County**
1801 Adeline St., Rm. 203
Oakland, CA 94607
**Phone:** (510)835-5010     **Fax:** (510)835-9232
**Email:** mhaac@wenet.net
**Website:** http://www.mhaac.org

**★ 13113 ★ National Mental Health
Association of California**
1127 11th St., Ste. 830
Sacramento, CA 95814
**Phone:** (916)557-1167     **Fax:** (916)447-2350
**Email:** rselix@mhac.org

**Website:** http://www.mhac.org
Rusty Selix, Director

**★ 13114 ★ National Mental Health
Association Los Angeles County**
1336 Wilshire Blvd., 2nd Fl.
Los Angeles, CA 90017-1705
**Phone:** (213)413-1130     **Fax:** (213)413-1114
**Email:** rvanhorn@mhala.org
**Website:** http://www.mhala.org

**★ 13115 ★ National Mental Health
Association in Los Angeles County**
1336 Wilshire Blvd., 2nd Fl.
Los Angeles, CA 90017
**Phone:** (213)413-1130
**Email:** mailbox@mhala.org     **Fax:** (213)413-1114
**Website:** http://www.mhala.org

**★ 13116 ★ National Mental Health
Association in Sacramento**
9719 Lincoln Village Dr., St. 407
Sacramento, CA 95827
**Phone:** (916)366-4600     **Fax:** (916)855-5448
**Email:** information@mhasc.org
**Website:** http://www.mhasc.org

**★ 13117 ★ National Mental Health
Association in Sacramento**
9719 Lincoln Village Dr., Ste. 407
Sacramento, CA 95827
**Phone:** (916)366-4600     **Fax:** (916)855-5448
**Email:** information@mhasc.org
**Website:** http://www.mhasc.org/open.htm

**★ 13118 ★ National Mental Health
Association in San Diego County**
2047 El Cajun Blvd.
San Diego, CA 92104-1091
**Phone:** (619)543-0412     **Fax:** (619)543-0748
**Email:** mhasd@flash.net
**Website:** http://www.mhasd.org

**★ 13119 ★ National Mental Health
Association in San Diego County**
2047 El Cajon Blvd.
San Diego, CA 92104
**Phone:** (619)543-0412     **Fax:** (619)543-0748
**Email:** mhasd@flash.net

**★ 13120 ★ National Mental Health
Association of San Francisco**
1095 Market St., Ste. 408
San Francisco, CA 94103
**Phone:** (415)241-2926     **Fax:** (415)241-2928
**Email:** mhaofsf@aol.com

**★ 13121 ★ National Mental Health
Association of Santa Barbara**
2017 Chapala St.
Santa Barbara, CA 93105
**Phone:** (805)569-1607     **Fax:** (805)682-0906
**Email:** sbmha@aol.com

**★ 13122 ★ National Mental Health
Association in Santa Barbara**
2017 Chapala St.
Santa Barbara, CA 93105
**Phone:** (805)569-1607     **Fax:** (805)682-0906
**Email:** sbmha@aol.com
Annmarie Cameron, Exec Director

**★ 13123 ★ Riverside Mental Health
Advocacy Program**
3634 Elizabeth St.
Riverside, CA 92506
**Phone:** (909)686-3706     **Fax:** (909)686-7267

**Website:** http://www.familyserviceriv.ca.com
Aggie Jenkins, President

## Colorado

**★ 13124 ★ National Mental Health
Association of Colorado**
6795 E Tennessee Ave., No. 425
Denver, CO 80224
**Phone:** (303)377-3040 **Free:** 800-456-3249
**Fax:** (303)377-4920
**Email:** jmrohner@mhacolorado.org
**Website:** http://www.mhacolorado.org
Victoria Simonsen, Director

**★ 13125 ★ National Mental Health
Association of El Paso County**
12 N Meade Ave.
Colorado Springs, CO 80909
**Phone:** (719)633-4601 **Fax:** (719)633-0845
**Email:** mha@pppartnership.org
**Website:** http://www.pppartnership.org

**★ 13126 ★ National Mental Health
Association of the Midwest**
PO Box 1468
Paonia, CO 81428
**Phone:** (970)527-4388 **Fax:** (970)527-6761
**Email:** rt.rt@juno.com

**★ 13127 ★ National Mental Health
Association of the Midwest**
PO Box 1468
Paonia, CO 81428
**Phone:** (970)527-4388 **Fax:** (970)527-6761

**★ 13128 ★ National Mental Health
Association of Pueblo**
PO Box 4623
Pueblo, CO 81003
**Phone:** (719)583-9798 **Fax:** (719)544-5708
**Email:** jackselway@puebloadvocacy.com
**Website:** http://www.puebloadvocacy.com

## Connecticut

**★ 13129 ★ National Mental Health
Association of Connecticut**
20-30 Beaver Rd.
Wethersfield, CT 06109
**Phone:** (860)529-1970 **Fax:** (860)529-6833
**Email:** webmaster@mhact.org
**Website:** http://www.mhact.org

## Delaware

**★ 13130 ★ National Mental Health
Association in Delaware**
812-D Philadelphia Pike
Wilmington, DE 19809
**Phone:** (302)765-9740 **Fax:** (302)765-9745
**Email:** dtreacy@dca.net
**Website:** http://www.mhainde.org

## District of Columbia

**★ 13131 ★ National Mental Health
Association of Washington DC**
1628 16th St. NW
Washington, DC 20009
**Phone:** (202)265-6363 **Fax:** (202)265-3265
**Email:** info@mhadc.org
**Website:** http://www.mhadc.org

## Florida

**★ 13132 ★ National Mental Health
Association of Bay County**
PO Box 2245
Panama City, FL 32402
**Phone:** (850)769-5441 **Fax:** (850)769-5528
**Email:** mhabay@knology.net

**★ 13133 ★ National Mental Health
Association of Broward County**
7145 W Oakland Park Blvd.
Lauderhill, FL 33313
**Phone:** (954)746-2055 **Fax:** (954)746-6373
**Email:** mhaceo@aol.org
**Website:** http://www.mhabroward.org

**★ 13134 ★ National Mental Health
Association of Central Florida**
608 Mariposa St.
Orlando, FL 32801
**Phone:** (407)843-1563 **Fax:** (407)843-4245
**Email:** mhacf@aol.com
**Website:** http://www.mhacf.com
Juanita Hernandez-Black, CEO & Pres

**★ 13135 ★ National Mental Health
Association of Collier County**
2335 9th St. N, Ste. 404
Naples, FL 34103
**Phone:** (941)261-5405 **Fax:** (941)261-2931
**Email:** ccmha@mindspring.com
**Website:** http://www.ccmha.org

**★ 13136 ★ National Mental Health
Association of Greater Tampa Bay, Inc.**
20505 U.S. Hwy. 19 N, Ste. 19
Clearwater, FL 33764
**Phone:** (727)669-1385 **Fax:** (727)669-1394
**Email:** mha@mha-tampabay.com
**Website:** http://www.mha-tampabay.com
Kelly Stuart Williams, CEO & Pres

**★ 13137 ★ National Mental Health
Association of Indian River County**
2001 9th Ave., Ste. 301
Vero Beach, FL 32960
**Phone:** (561)569-9788 **Fax:** (561)569-2088

**★ 13138 ★ National Mental Health
Association in Northeast Florida, Inc.**
4615 Phillips Hwy.
Jacksonville, FL 32207-2363
**Phone:** (904)399-5468 **Fax:** (904)399-3908
**Email:** mentalhealth@fcol.com
**Website:** http://www.mhajax.org
Claud Myers, CEO & Pres

**★ 13139 ★ National Mental Health
Association of Okaloosa and Walton
Counties**
PO Box 505
Fort Walton Beach, FL 32549
**Phone:** (850)244-1040 **Fax:** (850)244-2573
**Email:** mhaowfl@gnt.net
**Website:** http://www.mhaow.org
**Program(s):** Mental Health Education; 'Kids Link'
Children's Mental Health Information and Referral
Program; Mental Health Career Counseling; Domestic
Violence Awareness.

**★ 13140 ★ National Mental Health
Association of Palm Beach County,
Inc.**
909 Fern St.
West Palm Beach, FL 33401
**Phone:** (561)832-3755 **Fax:** (561)832-3900
**Email:** info@mentalhealthpbc.com

**Website:** http://www.mentalhealthpbc.com

**★ 13141 ★ National Mental Health
Association of Palm Beach County,
Inc.**
909 Fern St.
West Palm Beach, FL 33401
**Phone:** (561)832-3755 **Fax:** (561)832-3990
**Email:** info@mentalhealthpbc.com
**Website:** http://www.mentalhealthpbc.com

**★ 13142 ★ National Mental Health
Association of Volusia and Flagler
Counties**
531 S Ridgewood Ave.
Daytona Beach, FL 32114-2554
**Phone:** (386)252-5785 **Fax:** (386)255-7560
**Email:** mhadbfl@bellsouth.net
**Website:** http://www.mhavolusia.org

**★ 13143 ★ National Mental Health
Association of West Florida, Inc.**
840 W Lakeview Ave.
Pensacola, FL 32501
**Phone:** (850)438-9879 **Free:** 888-723-6544
**Fax:** (850)438-5901
**Email:** kgarber@mhawfl.org
**Website:** http://www.mhawfl.org
Karen Garber, CEO & Pres

## Georgia

**★ 13144 ★ National Mental Health
Association of Clayton County**
PO Box 524
Morrow, GA 30260-9998
**Phone:** (770)991-8509 **Fax:** (770)991-8507
**Email:** deborah_hanks@msn.com

**★ 13145 ★ National Mental Health
Association of Georgia**
100 Edgewood Ave. NE, Ste. 502
Atlanta, GA 30303-3068
**Phone:** (404)527-7175 **Fax:** (404)527-7187
**Email:** executiveoffice@nmhag.org
**Website:** http://www.nmhag.org

**★ 13146 ★ National Mental Health
Association of Greater Augusta, Inc.**
1720 Central Ave.
Augusta, GA 30904
**Phone:** (706)736-4339 **Fax:** (706)738-3548
**Email:** friendshipcenter@hotmail.com

**★ 13147 ★ National Mental Health
Association of Middle Flint**
PO Box 1063
Oglethorpe, GA 31068
**Phone:** (478)472-4738

**★ 13148 ★ National Mental Health
Association of Newton County**
PO Box 206
Covington, GA 30015-0206
**Phone:** (770)786-0807
**Email:** nccp@bellsouth.net

**★ 13149 ★ National Mental Health
Association of North Georgia
Mountains**
Stephens County Police Department
PO Box 579
Toccoa, GA 30577
**Phone:** (706)886-8655 **Fax:** (706)282-3316
**Email:** toccoagapd@alltel.net
Curtis Scott, President

★ 13150 ★ National Mental Health
Association of Northeast Georgia
PO Box 6384
Athens, GA 30604
**Phone:** (706)549-7888          **Fax:** (706)549-1651
**Email:** mhanega@bellsouth.net

★ 13151 ★ National Mental Health
Association of South Coastal Georgia
PO Box 189
Brunswick, GA 31521-0189
**Phone:** (912)638-2320          **Fax:** (912)638-1446
**Email:** mhaone@adelphia.org

★ 13152 ★ National Mental Health
Association of Wayne County
PO Box 935
Jesup, GA 31598
**Phone:** (912)579-2205

### Hawaii

★ 13153 ★ National Mental Health
Association in Hawaii
200 N Vineyard Blvd., No. 300
Honolulu, HI 96817
**Phone:** (808)521-1846          **Fax:** (808)533-6995
**Email:** mha@i-one.com
**Website:** http://www.mhahawaii.org/

★ 13154 ★ National Mental Health
Association in Hawaii County
HCR 1, Box 5822
Keaau, HI 96749
**Phone:** (808)965-6601          **Fax:** (808)966-9825
**Email:** grogan@ilhawaii.net
**Website:** http://mhahawaii.org

★ 13155 ★ National Mental Health
Association in Kauai County
200 N Vineyard Blvd., No. 300
Honolulu, HI 96817
**Phone:** (808)521-1846
**Website:** http://www.mhahawaii.org

★ 13156 ★ National Mental Health
Association in Maui County
95 Mahalani St.
Wailuku, HI 96793
**Phone:** (808)242-6461          **Fax:** (808)242-1857
**Website:** http://www.mhahawaii.org

### Idaho

★ 13157 ★ National Mental Health
Association of Idaho
PO Box 4725
Boise, ID 83711-4725
**Phone:** (208)893-9983          **Fax:** (208)327-0510
**Email:** kalek@juno.com

### Illinois

★ 13158 ★ National Mental Health
Association of DuPage County
188 W Randolph St., Ste. 2225
Chicago, IL 60601
**Phone:** (312)368-9070          **Fax:** (312)368-0283

★ 13159 ★ National Mental Health
Association of Fayette County
2120 Lincoln St.
Evanston, IL 60201
**Phone:** (847)328-6198          **Fax:** (847)869-4701
**Email:** madel513653@aol.com

★ 13160 ★ National Mental Health
Association in Illinois
188 W Randolph St., Ste. 2225
Chicago, IL 60601
**Phone:** (312)368-9070          **Fax:** (312)368-0283
**Email:** mhai@mhai.org
**Website:** http://www.mhai.org
Jan Holcomb, Director

★ 13161 ★ National Mental Health
Association of Illinois Valley, Inc.
5407 N University
Peoria, IL 61614
**Phone:** (309)692-1766          **Fax:** (309)692-2966
**Email:** mhaiv@mhaiv.org
**Website:** http://www.mhaiv.org

★ 13162 ★ National Mental Health
Association of Macon County, Inc.
1314 N Main
Decatur, IL 62526
**Phone:** (217)422-2988          **Fax:** (217)422-1108
**Email:** smartinmha@aol.com
**Website:** http://www.dps61.org

★ 13163 ★ National Mental Health
Association in McLean County
PO Box 795
Bloomington, IL 61702-0795
**Phone:** (309)862-4408          **Fax:** (309)862-1542
**Email:** bisbeejk@aol.com

★ 13164 ★ National Mental Health
Association of the North Shore
2120 Lincoln St.
Evanston, IL 60201-2282
**Phone:** (847)328-6198          **Fax:** (847)869-4701
**Email:** mhans@megsinet.net

★ 13165 ★ National Mental Health
Association of the Rock River Valley
PO Box 4061
Rockford, IL 61110
**Phone:** (815)395-1839          **Fax:** (815)395-9117

★ 13166 ★ National Mental Health
Association of Southwestern Illinois
PO Box 285
Edwardsville, IL 62025
**Phone:** (618)650-7216          **Fax:** (618)650-7216
**Email:** info@mhaswil.org

### Indiana

★ 13167 ★ National Mental Health
Association in Allen County
227 E Washington Blvd.
Fort Wayne, IN 46802
**Phone:** (219)422-6441          **Fax:** (219)423-3400

★ 13168 ★ National Mental Health
Association in Blackford County
814 N Richmond
Hartford City, IN 47348
**Phone:** (765)348-7040          **Fax:** (765)348-7046
**Email:** dmitchell@towfin.com

★ 13169 ★ National Mental Health
Association in Boone County
127 W Main St., Ste. 314
Lebanon, IN 46052
**Phone:** (765)482-3020          **Fax:** (765)482-9001
**Email:** mhabc@in-motion.net

★ 13170 ★ National Mental Health
Association in Cass County
421 12th St.
Logansport, IN 46947
**Phone:** (219)722-3984

★ 13171 ★ National Mental Health
Association in Clark County
6815 Hwy. 311
Sellersburg, IN 47172
**Phone:** (812)256-6291

★ 13172 ★ National Mental Health
Association in Clay County
1211 E National Ave.
Brazil, IN 47834
**Phone:** (812)448-8801
Pat Heffner, Exec Director

★ 13173 ★ National Mental Health
Association in Clinton County
51 W Clinton St., Ste. 101
Frankfort, IN 46041-1931
**Phone:** (765)659-3825

★ 13174 ★ National Mental Health
Association in Daviess County
PO Box 183
Washington, IN 47501
**Phone:** (812)254-2423

★ 13175 ★ National Mental Health
Association in Dearborn County
PO Box 354
Lawrenceburg, IN 47025
**Phone:** (812)577-5440

★ 13176 ★ National Mental Health
Association in Dekalb County
902 Deer Ridge Crossing
Auburn, IN 46706
**Phone:** (219)925-2963          **Fax:** (219)925-1733
Cheryl Taylor, Exec Director

★ 13177 ★ National Mental Health
Association in Delaware County
413 S Liberty St.
Muncie, IN 47305
**Phone:** (765)288-1924          **Fax:** (765)288-1956
**Email:** kwalkmhadc@aol.com
Vickie Strahan, Exec Director

★ 13178 ★ National Mental Health
Association in Dubois County
PO Box 566
Jasper, IN 47547-0566
**Phone:** (812)482-3020
Leah Hayworth, President

★ 13179 ★ National Mental Health
Association in Elkhart County
421 S 2nd St., Ste. 340
Elkhart, IN 46516
**Phone:** (219)295-8935          **Fax:** (219)295-1460
**Email:** mhaec@peoplepc.com

★ 13180 ★ National Mental Health
Association in Floyd County
PO Box 63
New Albany, IN 47151
**Phone:** (812)941-0308

**★ 13181 ★ National Mental Health Association in Franklin County**
1216 N Main St.
PO Box 94
Brookville, IN 47012
**Phone:** (513)524-5371
Lisa Stiener, Exec Director

**★ 13182 ★ National Mental Health Association in Fulton County**
401 E 8th St., Ste. C
Rochester, IN 46975
**Phone:** (574)223-6870    **Fax:** (574)224-6870
**Email:** gsmokermhafc@rtcol.com
Genelle Smoker, Exec Director

**★ 13183 ★ National Mental Health Association in Gibson**
RR 3, Box 67
Owensville, IN 47665
**Phone:** (812)724-2141
Ruth Braselton, President

**★ 13184 ★ National Mental Health Association in Greene County**
RR 2, Box 132
Solsberry, IN 47459
**Phone:** (812)825-7108
Norman Sullivan, President

**★ 13185 ★ National Mental Health Association in Hamilton County**
942 N 10th St.
Noblesville, IN 46060
**Phone:** (317)776-3455    **Fax:** (317)776-3456

**★ 13186 ★ National Mental Health Association in Hancock County**
98 E North St.
Greenfield, IN 46140
**Phone:** (317)462-2877    **Fax:** (317)462-2877
**Email:** HCMHA98@aol.com
Ann Osborne, Exec Director

**★ 13187 ★ National Mental Health Association in Hendricks County**
6845 E U.S. 36, Ste. 880
Avon, IN 46123
**Phone:** (317)272-0027    **Fax:** (317)272-1176

**★ 13188 ★ National Mental Health Association in Henry County**
PO Box 449
New Castle, IN 47362
**Phone:** (765)529-4403    **Fax:** (765)593-2510

**★ 13189 ★ National Mental Health Association in Howard County**
507 N Webster St.
Kokomo, IN 46904-2221
**Phone:** (765)459-0309    **Fax:** (765)459-0300
**Email:** mhahowardco@aol.com
Jennifer Trobaugh, Exec Director

**★ 13190 ★ National Mental Health Association in Indiana**
55 Monument Cir., Ste. 455
Indianapolis, IN 46204
**Phone:** (317)638-3501    **Fax:** (317)638-3540
**Email:** MHAI@mentalhealthassociation.com
**Website:** http://www.mentalhealthassociation.com
Steve McCaffrey, President

**★ 13191 ★ National Mental Health Association in Jackson County**
PO Box 51
Seymour, IN 47274

**Phone:** (812)522-3480

**★ 13192 ★ National Mental Health Association in Jay County**
964 S Meridian St.
Portland, IN 47371
**Phone:** (219)726-8614
Sheron McClung, Exec Director

**★ 13193 ★ National Mental Health Association in Johnson County**
PO Box 748
Franklin, IN 46131
**Phone:** (317)535-6960

**★ 13194 ★ National Mental Health Association in Knox County**
PO Box 859
Vincennes, IN 47591
**Phone:** (812)895-1007    **Fax:** (812)885-2723

**★ 13195 ★ National Mental Health Association in Kosciusko County**
920 Fisher
PO Box 822
Warsaw, IN 46581
**Phone:** (219)269-2102    **Fax:** (219)269-3554
**Email:** mha@kconline.com
Sandra Frush, Exec Director

**★ 13196 ★ National Mental Health Association in Lake County**
9722 Parkway Dr.
Highland, IN 46322
**Phone:** (219)922-3822    **Fax:** (219)922-3825
**Email:** mhainlakecounty@yahoo.com

**★ 13197 ★ National Mental Health Association in Lawrence County**
RR 11, Box 23
Bedford, IN 47421
**Phone:** (812)275-3028

**★ 13198 ★ National Mental Health Association in Marion County**
2506 Willowbrook Pkwy., No. 100
Indianapolis, IN 46205-1542
**Phone:** (317)251-0005    **Fax:** (317)254-2800
**Email:** mtowell@mcmha.org
Marge Towell, Exec Director

**★ 13199 ★ National Mental Health Association in Marshall County**
401 W Jefferson St.
Plymouth, IN 46563
**Phone:** (219)935-5314

**★ 13200 ★ National Mental Health Association in Monroe County**
441 S College Ave.
Bloomington, IN 47403
**Phone:** (812)323-9720    **Fax:** (812)323-9132
**Email:** mha@bloomington.in.us
Elaine Moore, Exec Director

**★ 13201 ★ National Mental Health Association in Morgan County**
118 E Morgan St.
Martinsville, IN 46151
**Phone:** (765)342-1515
**Email:** mhamorg@scican.net

**★ 13202 ★ National Mental Health Association in Parke County**
RR 4, PO Box 250
Rockville, IN 47872

**Phone:** (765)245-2719

**★ 13203 ★ National Mental Health Association in Perry County**
PO Box 366
Tell City, IN 47586-0366
**Phone:** (812)547-7905    **Fax:** (812)547-5146
**Email:** wcwagner@psci.net

**★ 13204 ★ National Mental Health Association in Porter County, Inc.**
402 E Indiana Ave.
Valparaiso, IN 46383
**Phone:** (219)462-6267    **Fax:** (219)464-7483
**Email:** mha@netnitco.net
Margaret Stevens, Exec Director

**★ 13205 ★ National Mental Health Association in Putnam County**
10 ½ N Jackson St.
Greencastle, IN 46135
**Phone:** (765)653-3310    **Fax:** (765)653-2565
**Email:** mhapc2@ccrtc.com

**★ 13206 ★ National Mental Health Association in Randolph County**
430 S Meridian St.
Winchester, IN 47394
**Phone:** (765)932-2004

**★ 13207 ★ National Mental Health Association in Rush County**
Rush County Courthouse, 3rd Fl.
201 E 2nd St.
Rushville, IN 46173
**Phone:** (765)932-2004

**★ 13208 ★ National Mental Health Association in St. Joseph County**
211 W Madison St.
South Bend, IN 46601
**Phone:** (219)234-1049    **Fax:** (219)234-1040
**Email:** rjtraz@mindspring.com
Ryan J. Trzaskowski, Exec Director

**★ 13209 ★ National Mental Health Association in Spencer County**
HCR 68, Box 575
Saint Meinrad, IN 47577
**Phone:** (812)547-9630
**Email:** sschaefer@psci.net
Mary Posner, President

**★ 13210 ★ National Mental Health Association in Steuben County**
PO Box 372
Angola, IN 46703
**Phone:** (219)665-5981
Betty Bemesderfer, Exec Director

**★ 13211 ★ National Mental Health Association in Tippecanoe County**
915 Columbia St., Ste. 1
Lafayette, IN 47901-1476
**Phone:** (765)742-1800    **Fax:** (765)742-2085
**Email:** edir@dcwi.com
**Website:** http://dcwi.com/~mha/welcome.htm

**★ 13212 ★ National Mental Health Association in Vanderburgh County**
123 NW 4th St., Ste. 707
Evansville, IN 47708-1715
**Phone:** (812)426-2640    **Fax:** (812)426-7207
**Email:** vcmha@juno.com
Donna Carr, Exec Director

**★ 13213 ★ National Mental Health Association in Vigo County**
620 8th Ave.
Terre Haute, IN 47804
**Phone:** (812)232-5681 **Fax:** (812)234-2863
**Email:** mhavc@indy.net
Kathy Alexander, Exec Director

**★ 13214 ★ National Mental Health Association in Wabash County**
Box 310
North Manchester, IN 46962
**Phone:** (219)982-7766 **Fax:** (219)774-3432
**Email:** mamast@kconline.com
Mary Ann Mast, Exec Director

**★ 13215 ★ National Mental Health Association in Wayne County**
750 NW 13th St.
Richmond, IN 47374
**Phone:** (765)966-0221 **Fax:** (765)966-5915
**Email:** mha@infocom.com

**★ 13216 ★ National Mental Health Association in Wells County**
223 W Washington St.
Bluffton, IN 46714-2050
**Phone:** (219)824-1514

**★ 13217 ★ National Mental Health Association in White County**
Monticello Health Care
1120 N Main St.
Monticello, IN 47960
**Phone:** (219)583-9221
Pam Ashton, President

## Iowa

**★ 13218 ★ National Mental Health Association in Dubuque County**
PO Box 283
Dubuque, IA 52004-0283
**Phone:** (563)582-2233 **Fax:** (319)584-0730
**Email:** dbqiamha@aol.com
Betty Allen, Secretary

**★ 13219 ★ National Mental Health Association of Hamilton County**
PO Box 334
Hamilton, IA 50116
**Phone:** (515)832-9620 **Fax:** (515)832-9591
Darren Helton, President

## Kansas

**★ 13220 ★ National Mental Health Association of the Heartland**
739 Minnesota Ave.
Kansas City, KS 64101
**Phone:** (913)281-2221 **Fax:** (913)281-3977
**Email:** evans@mhah.org
**Website:** http://www.mhah.org
**Frmly:** Mental Health Association of the Heartland (Kansas).

**★ 13221 ★ National Mental Health Association of Kansas**
3745 SW Wanamaker Rd.
Topeka, KS 66610-1369
**Phone:** (785)252-8038 **Fax:** (985)233-5440
**Email:** asknbeg@terraworld.net
Gary W. Long, II, Director

**★ 13222 ★ National Mental Health Association in Reno County**
1520 N Plum
PO Box 2021
Hutchinson, KS 67504-2021
**Phone:** (316)663-7772 **Fax:** (316)665-4497
**Email:** mha_candace@yahoo.com

**★ 13223 ★ National Mental Health Association of South Central Kansas**
555 N Woodlawn, Ste. 3105
Wichita, KS 67208-4385
**Phone:** (316)685-1821 **Fax:** (316)685-0768
**Email:** rosemary@mhasck.org
**Website:** http://www.mhasck.org

## Kentucky

**★ 13224 ★ National Mental Health Association of Kentucky**
120 Sears Ave., Ste. 213
Louisville, KY 40207
**Phone:** (502)893-0460 **Free:** 888-702-0463
**Fax:** (502)896-1306
**Email:** mhaky@kih.net
**Website:** http://www.mhaky.org
Sheriall Cunningham, Director

**★ 13225 ★ National Mental Health Association of Northern Kentucky**
605 Madison Ave.
Covington, KY 41011
**Phone:** (859)292-2487 **Fax:** (859)292-2485
**Email:** mhnky@aol.com
**Website:** http://members.aol.com/mhnky/mhnky.html

## Louisiana

**★ 13226 ★ National Mental Health Association in Caddo-Bossier**
3825 Gilbert St., Ste. 209
Shreveport, LA 71104
**Phone:** (318)861-5971 **Fax:** (318)861-5972
**Email:** mhaincb@aol.com

**★ 13227 ★ National Mental Health Association in Caldwell Parish**
PO Box 136
Columbia, LA 71418
**Phone:** (318)649-5066
**Email:** hefnerp@aol.com

**★ 13228 ★ National Mental Health Association in Catahoula Parish**
403 Willow St.
Jonesville, LA 71343
**Phone:** (318)339-8562
Robbie M. Wilson, President

**★ 13229 ★ National Mental Health Association in Franklin Parish**
PO Box 128
Winnsboro, LA 71295
**Phone:** (318)435-3334
Drew Dunn, President

**★ 13230 ★ National Mental Health Association in Louisiana**
200 Lafayette St., Ste. 709
Baton Rouge, LA 70801
**Phone:** (225)343-1921 **Free:** 800-241-6425
**Fax:** (225)343-1983
**Email:** mhal15@aol.com

**★ 13231 ★ National Mental Health Association in Metropolitan New Orleans**
PO Box 850407
New Orleans, LA 70185
**Phone:** (504)897-1140 **Fax:** (504)897-2368
**Email:** mhamno@bellsouth.net

**★ 13232 ★ National Mental Health Association in Red River County**
Rte. 1, Box 274
Coushatta, LA 71019-7505
**Phone:** (318)932-5494
Betty Sullivan, President

**★ 13233 ★ National Mental Health Association in Southwest Louisiana**
PO Box 805
Lake Charles, LA 70602-0805
**Phone:** (337)582-1430 **Fax:** (337)582-1430
**Email:** melliott61@juno.com

**★ 13234 ★ Tri Parish National Mental Health Association**
PO Box 166
Jonesville, LA 71343
**Phone:** (318)339-8562

## Maryland

**★ 13235 ★ National Mental Health Association of Howard County**
11702 Lightfall Ct.
Columbia, MD 21044
**Phone:** (410)995-3323 **Fax:** (410)997-4227
Donna Rawlings, Contact

**★ 13236 ★ National Mental Health Association of the Lower Shore**
PO Box 269
Snow Hill, MD 21863
**Phone:** (410)543-2057 **Fax:** (410)632-3224
**Email:** foxtrot@shore.intercom.net

**★ 13237 ★ National Mental Health Association of Maryland**
711 W 40th St., Ste. 460
Baltimore, MD 21211
**Phone:** (410)235-1178 **Fax:** (410)235-1180
**Email:** info@mhamd.org
**Website:** http://www.mhamd.org
Linda Raines, Director

**★ 13238 ★ National Mental Health Association of Metropolitan Baltimore**
711 W 40th St., Ste. 460
Baltimore, MD 21211
**Phone:** (410)235-1178 **Fax:** (410)235-1180
**Email:** mhaofmd@aol.com
Diane Cabot, Exec Director

**★ 13239 ★ National Mental Health Association of Montgomery County**
1000 Twinbrook Pkwy.
Rockville, MD 20851
**Phone:** (301)424-0656 **Fax:** (301)738-1030
**Email:** info@mhamc.org
**Website:** http://www.mhamc.org

**★ 13240 ★ National Mental Health Association of Prince George's County**
PO Box 89
Hyattsville, MD 20781
**Phone:** (301)699-2737 **Fax:** (301)699-2746
**Website:** http://www.mhapgc.freeservers.com

**★ 13241 ★ National Mental Health Association of Southern Maryland**
1170 Overlook Dr.
Accokeek, MD 20607-3516
**Phone:** (301)283-2410
Vivian Mills, President

**★ 13242 ★ National Mental Health Association in Talbot County**
108 Maryland Ave., Ste. 103
Easton, MD 21601
**Phone:** (410)822-0444       **Fax:** (410)820-7283
**Email:** bjadams@mhamdes.org
**Website:** http://www.mhamdes.org

**★ 13243 ★ National Mental Health Association of Washington County**
8162 Arcadia Ln.
Boonsboro, MD 21713
**Phone:** (301)739-4138
Sue Farrell, President

## Michigan

**★ 13244 ★ National Mental Health Association of Michigan**
15920 W 12 Mile Rd.
Southfield, MI 48076
**Phone:** (248)557-6777       **Fax:** (248)557-5995
**Email:** mhamich@aol.com
**Website:** http://www.geocities.com/CapitolHill/Lobby/468

## Mississippi

**★ 13245 ★ National Mental Health Association of the Capitol Area**
409 Briarwood Dr., Ste. 310
Jackson, MS 39206
**Phone:** (601)956-2800       **Fax:** (601)956-6380
**Email:** mhajxn@aol.com

**★ 13246 ★ National Mental Health Association of Mississippi**
PO Box 7329
Gulfport, MS 39506
**Phone:** (228)864-6274       **Fax:** (228)864-1310
**Email:** Keenminds@aol.com

## Missouri

**★ 13247 ★ National Mental Health Association of Greater Saint Louis**
1905 S Grand Blvd.
Saint Louis, MO 63104
**Phone:** (314)773-1399       **Fax:** (314)773-5930
**Email:** mhagstl@aol.com
James House, II, CEO & Pres

**★ 13248 ★ National Mental Health Association of the Heartland**
739 Minnesota Ave.
Kansas City, MO 66101
**Phone:** (913)281-2221       **Fax:** (913)281-3977
**Email:** mevans@mhah.org
**Website:** http://www.mhah.org

## Montana

**★ 13249 ★ National Mental Health Association of Billings**
3308 2nd Ave. N
PO Box 20891
Billings, MT 59104
**Phone:** (406)245-0697       **Fax:** (406)259-0624
**Email:** mhabillings@imt.net
Leanne Swanson, Exec Director

**★ 13250 ★ National Mental Health Association of Daniels County**
Box 746
Scobey, MT 59263
**Phone:** (406)487-2671
Esther Kramer, President

**★ 13251 ★ National Mental Health Association of Great Falls**
PO Box 2774
Great Falls, MT 59403
**Phone:** (406)268-6254

**★ 13252 ★ National Mental Health Association of Montana**
25 S Ewing, Ste. 200
Helena, MT 59601
**Phone:** (406)442-4276       **Fax:** (406)442-4986
**Email:** mham@in-tch.com
**Website:** http://www.mhamontana.org
Andrea Merrill, Director

**★ 13253 ★ National Mental Health Association of Sheridan County**
736 Shippe Canyon
Plentywood, MT 59254
**Phone:** (406)286-5625

**★ 13254 ★ National Mental Health Association of Sweet Grass County**
Box 372
Big Timber, MT 59011
**Phone:** (406)932-5594
Nora Hansen, President

## Nebraska

**★ 13255 ★ National Mental Health Association of Nebraska**
PO Box 23001
Lincoln, NE 68504
**Phone:** (402)474-3183       **Fax:** (402)474-3274
**Email:** info@mha-ne.org
**Website:** http://www.mha-ne.org

## New Jersey

**★ 13256 ★ National Mental Health Association in Atlantic County**
1147 N New Rd.
Absecon, NJ 08201
**Phone:** (609)272-1700       **Fax:** (609)484-0123
**Email:** mhaac@aol.com
**Website:** http://mhanj.org

**★ 13257 ★ National Mental Health Association of Essex County**
33 S Fullerton Ave.
Montclair, NJ 07042
**Phone:** (973)509-9777       **Fax:** (973)509-9888
**Email:** mhaecdavison@aol.com

**★ 13258 ★ National Mental Health Association of Hudson County**
3000 Kennedy Blvd., Ste. 305
Jersey City, NJ 07306
**Phone:** (201)653-4700       **Fax:** (201)653-4100
**Email:** mhahc@aol.com

**★ 13259 ★ National Mental Health Association of Monmouth County**
59 Broad St.
Eatontown, NJ 07724
**Phone:** (732)542-6422       **Fax:** (732)389-3163
**Email:** mhamonmouth@monmouth.com
**Website:** http://www.mentalhealthmonmouth.org

**★ 13260 ★ National Mental Health Association of Morris County**
28 Walnut St., Box 9
Madison, NJ 07940
**Phone:** (973)377-9280       **Fax:** (973)377-8608
**Email:** mhamc@aol.com

**★ 13261 ★ National Mental Health Association of Morris County**
28 Walnut St.
Box 9
Madison, NJ 07940
**Phone:** (973)377-9280       **Fax:** (973)377-8608
**Email:** mhamc@aol.com

**★ 13262 ★ National Mental Health Association in New Jersey**
88 Pompton Ave.
Verona, NJ 07044
**Phone:** (973)571-4100       **Free:** 800-367-8850
**Fax:** (973)857-1777
**Email:** info@mhanj.org
**Website:** http://www.mhanj.org

**★ 13263 ★ National Mental Health Association of Ocean County**
681 River Ave., Ste. 2J
Lakewood, NJ 08701
**Phone:** (732)905-1132       **Fax:** (732)905-0906
**Email:** mhaoc@aol.com

**★ 13264 ★ National Mental Health Association in Passaic County**
404 Clifton Ave.
Clifton, NJ 07011
**Phone:** (973)478-4444       **Fax:** (973)478-0941
**Email:** mhapc@aol.com
Joanne Green, Exec Director

**★ 13265 ★ National Mental Health Association in Southwestern New Jersey**
505 Cooper St.
Camden, NJ 08102
**Phone:** (856)966-6767       **Fax:** (856)541-3986
**Email:** mhaswnj2@aol.com

**★ 13266 ★ National Mental Health Association of Union County**
23 North Ave. E
Cranford, NJ 07016
**Phone:** (908)272-0300       **Fax:** (908)272-5696
Edmund Murphy, Exec Director

**★ 13267 ★ Trenton Advocacy Association**
121 Broad St., 2nd Fl.
Trenton, NJ 08628
**Phone:** (609)656-0110       **Fax:** (609)656-8078
**Email:** mhanjtrenton@aol.com

## New Mexico

**★ 13268 ★ National Mental Health Association in New Mexico**
PO Box 1417
506 N Prince Dr.
Espanola, NM 87532
**Phone:** (505)753-4131       **Fax:** (505)382-4778
**Email:** mhanm@cybermesa.com

**★ 13269 ★ National Mental Health Association in New Mexico**
506 N Prince Dr.
PO Box 1417
Espanola, NM 87532
**Phone:** (505)753-4131       **Fax:** (801)382-4778

Email: mhanm@cybermesa.com
Deborah Fickling, Director

## New York

★ 13270 ★ National Mental Health
Association in Albany County
500 Central Ave.
Albany, NY 12206
Phone: (518)435-9931     Fax: (518)435-9937
Email: kimballm@crisny.org
Website: http://www.crisny.org
Michel Kimball, Exec Director

★ 13271 ★ National Mental Health
Association in Allegany County
45 N Broad St.
Wellsville, NY 14895
Phone: (716)593-1991     Fax: (716)593-7104

★ 13272 ★ National Mental Health
Association in Cattaraugus County, Inc.
129 N Union St.
PO Box 833
Olean, NY 14760
Phone: (716)372-0208     Fax: (716)372-0222

★ 13273 ★ National Mental Health
Association in Cayuga County
PO Box 184
Cayuga, NY 13034
Phone: (315)258-9531     Fax: (315)258-3185
Email: arleenie@yahoo.com
Arleen Egry, President

★ 13274 ★ National Mental Health
Association in Chautauqua County
413 Main St.
Jamestown, NY 14701
Phone: (716)487-0616     Fax: (716)483-3524
Email: chautmha@hotmail.com

★ 13275 ★ National Mental Health
Association in Clinton County
159 Margaret St., Ste. 201
Plattsburgh, NY 12901
Phone: (518)563-8206     Fax: (518)563-9958
Email: hcook@bhsn.org
Website: http://www.bhsn.org

★ 13276 ★ National Mental Health
Association of Columbia/Green
Counties
713 Union St.
Hudson, NY 12534
Phone: (518)828-4619     Fax: (518)828-1196
Jeffrey Rovitz, Exec Director

★ 13277 ★ National Mental Health
Association of Cortland County, Inc.
25 Clinton Ave.
PO Box 282
Cortland, NY 13045
Phone: (607)758-3107     Fax: (607)758-3107

★ 13278 ★ National Mental Health
Association in Dutchess County
510 Haight Ave.
Poughkeepsie, NY 12603
Phone: (845)473-2500     Fax: (845)473-4870
Email: mhadc@hvc.rr.com
Website: http://www.mhadc.com

★ 13279 ★ National Mental Health
Association of Erie County, Inc.
999 Delaware Ave.
Buffalo, NY 14209

Phone: (716)886-1242     Fax: (716)881-6428
Email: mhaec@localnet.com
Website: http://members.localnet.com/~mhaec

★ 13280 ★ National Mental Health
Association in Essex County
RD 1, Box 1012
Westport, NY 12993-9702
Phone: (518)962-2077     Free: 800-440-8074
Fax: (518)962-8233
Email: mha@mhainessex.org

★ 13281 ★ National Mental Health
Association in Franklin County
52 Broadway, Ste. 2B
Saranac Lake, NY 12983
Phone: (518)891-0504     Free: 800-776-9992
Fax: (518)891-6423
Email: mhafc@northnet.org

★ 13282 ★ National Mental Health
Association in Fulton/Montgomery
Counties
73 N Main St., Ste. 106
Gloversville, NY 12078
Phone: (518)725-2790     Free: 800-734-5864
Fax: (518)775-1076
Email: jcharney@mybizz.net
Website: http://www.mentalhealthassociation.org

★ 13283 ★ National Mental Health
Association in Genessee County
25 Liberty St.
Batavia, NY 14020
Phone: (585)344-2611     Fax: (585)345-1418
Email: gencomha@2ki.net

★ 13284 ★ National Mental Health
Association in Jefferson County
212 William St.
Watertown, NY 13601-2602
Phone: (315)788-0970     Fax: (315)788-8092
Email: mhajc@northnet.org
Roberta Hagerty, Contact

★ 13285 ★ National Mental Health
Association of Nassau County, Inc.
186 Clinton St.
Hempstead, NY 11550
Phone: (516)489-2322     Fax: (516)489-2784
Email: mhanc@mhanc.org
Website: http://www.mhanc.org

★ 13286 ★ National Mental Health
Association in New York City, Inc.
666 Broadway, Rm. 200
New York, NY 10012
Phone: (212)254-0333     Fax: (212)529-1959
Email: mhaofnyc@aol.com

★ 13287 ★ National Mental Health
Association in New York State, Inc.
194 Washington Ave., Ste. 415
Albany, NY 12210
Phone: (518)434-0439     Free: 800-766-6177
Fax: (518)427-8676
Email: mhanys@mhanys.org
Website: http://www.mhanys.org/

★ 13288 ★ National Mental Health
Association in Niagara County, Inc.
36 Pine St.
Lockport, NY 14094
Phone: (716)433-3780     Fax: (716)433-3847
Email: mhancny@aol.com
Website: http://www.mhanc.com

★ 13289 ★ National Mental Health
Association of Onondaga County
3049 E Genesse St.
Syracuse, NY 13224
Phone: (315)445-5606     Fax: (315)445-1828
Email: fuscoaa@clrc.org
Website: http://www.mha-oc.org

★ 13290 ★ National Mental Health
Association in Orange County
20 Walker St.
Goshen, NY 10924
Phone: (914)294-7411     Free: 800-832-1200
Fax: (914)294-7348
Email: mha@mhaorangeny.com
Website: http://www.mhaorangeny.com

★ 13291 ★ National Mental Health
Association in Orleans County
113 E State St.
PO Box 269
Albion, NY 14411
Phone: (716)589-1158     Fax: (716)589-1158
Email: ritbo@aol.com

★ 13292 ★ National Mental Health
Association of Oswego County
70 Bunner St.
Oswego, NY 13126-3703
Phone: (315)349-3533     Fax: (315)349-3533
Email: mhaosw@scsinter.net

★ 13293 ★ National Mental Health
Association in Putnam County, Inc.
Brewster Town Ctr.
1620 Rte. 22
Brewster, NY 10509
Phone: (914)278-7600     Fax: (914)278-0600
Email: mhaputnm@bestweb.net
Website: http://www.bestweb.net/~mhaputnm/

★ 13294 ★ National Mental Health
Association in Rochester/Monroe
Counties, Inc.
339 East Ave., Ste. 201
Rochester, NY 14604
Phone: (585)325-3145     Fax: (585)325-3188
Email: pwoods@mharochester.org
Website: http://www.mharochester.org

★ 13295 ★ National Mental Health
Association of Rockland County, Inc.
20 Squadron Blvd.
New City, NY 10956
Phone: (845)639-7400     Fax: (845)639-7419
Email: mharc@aol.com
Website: http://www.mharockland.org/

★ 13296 ★ National Mental Health
Association in Schuyler County
106 Shannon St.
PO Box 141
Watkins Glen, NY 14891
Phone: (607)535-7426     Fax: (607)535-8284

★ 13297 ★ National Mental Health
Association of the Southern Tier, Inc.
82 Oak St.
Binghamton, NY 13905
Phone: (607)771-8888     Fax: (607)771-8892
Email: mhaofst@tier.net
Website: http://www.tier.net/mhaofst
Casemiro Epe, Exec Director

★ 13298 ★ National Mental Health
Association in Steuben County
115 Liberty
Bath, NY 14810

**Phone:** (607)776-6577          **Fax:** (607)776-7895

**★ 13299 ★ National Mental Health Association in Suffolk County**
199 N Wellwood Ave., Ste. 2
Lindenhurst, NY 11757
**Phone:** (631)226-3900          **Fax:** (631)225-1708
**Email:** louischerry@earthlink.net
**Website:** http://www.mhasuffolk.org

**★ 13300 ★ National Mental Health Association in Tompkins County**
518 W State St.
Ithaca, NY 14850
**Phone:** (607)273-9250          **Fax:** (607)272-5343
**Email:** info@mhaedu.org
**Website:** http://info.mhaedu.org

**★ 13301 ★ National Mental Health Association in Ulster County**
PO Box 2304
Kingston, NY 12402
**Phone:** (914)336-4747          **Fax:** (845)336-0192
**Email:** ependegar@mhainulster.com
**Website:** http://mhainulster.com

**★ 13302 ★ National Mental Health Association in Warren/Washington**
York Plaza
3043 State Route 4
Hudson Falls, NY 12839
**Phone:** (518)747-2284          **Fax:** (518)747-2253
**Email:** peter@wwamh.org
**Website:** http://www.wwamh.org

**★ 13303 ★ National Mental Health Association of Westchester County, Inc.**
2269 Saw Mill River Rd., Bldg. 1A
Elmsford, NY 10523
**Phone:** (914)345-5900          **Fax:** (914)347-8859
**Email:** help@mhawestchester.org
**Website:** http://www.mhawestchester.org

## North Carolina

**★ 13304 ★ National Mental Health Association in Beaufort County**
4814 River Rd., Ste. 10
Washington, NC 27889
**Phone:** (252)946-9538
**Email:** nakreisher@aol.com

**★ 13305 ★ National Mental Health Association in Burke County**
PO Drawer 1266
Morganton, NC 28680
**Phone:** (828)439-4421          **Fax:** (828)439-4444

**★ 13306 ★ National Mental Health Association in Caldwell County**
247 Commercial St.
Lenoir, NC 28645
**Phone:** (828)757-5710          **Fax:** (828)757-5718
**Email:** weschester1@angelfire.com

**★ 13307 ★ National Mental Health Association in Carteret County**
PO Box 425
Swansboro, NC 28584
**Phone:** (252)393-2426          **Fax:** (252)745-2080
**Email:** patp@coastalnet.com

**★ 13308 ★ National Mental Health Association in Cleveland County**
201 W Marion St., Rm. 306
Shelby, NC 28150

**Phone:** (704)481-8637          **Fax:** (704)481-1960
**Email:** mha@cetlink.net

**★ 13309 ★ National Mental Health Association in Columbus County**
PO Box 534
Whiteville, NC 28472
**Phone:** (910)642-5168          **Fax:** (910)640-1010
Colene B. Stanley, President

**★ 13310 ★ National Mental Health Association in Craven County**
474 State Hwy. 306 S
Vanceboro, NC 28586
**Phone:** (252)745-4352

**★ 13311 ★ National Mental Health Association in Cumberland County**
310 Green St., Ste. 201-A
Fayetteville, NC 28302
**Phone:** (336)323-1954
**Email:** rmhacc@aol.com
Dana Covington, Contact

**★ 13312 ★ National Mental Health Association in Davidson County**
PO Box 1642
Lexington, NC 27293
**Phone:** (336)956-2952          **Fax:** (336)956-1647
**Email:** kaysaintsing@lexcominc.net

**★ 13313 ★ National Mental Health Association in Forsyth County, Inc.**
1 Brownsboro Plaza, Ste. 100
4265 Brownsboro Rd.
Winston-Salem, NC 27106
**Phone:** (336)759-9370          **Fax:** (336)759-3248
**Email:** andy@mha-fc.org
**Website:** http://www.mha-fc.org

**★ 13314 ★ National Mental Health Association in Greensboro**
1004 N Elm St.
Greensboro, NC 27401
**Phone:** (336)373-1402          **Fax:** (336)286-9642
**Email:** swalker@mhag.org
**Website:** http://www.greensboro.com/mha

**★ 13315 ★ National Mental Health Association in High Point**
910 Mill Ave.
PO Box 5693
High Point, NC 27260
**Phone:** (336)883-7480          **Fax:** (336)883-4013
**Email:** inncom@greensboro.com

**★ 13316 ★ National Mental Health Association in Johnston County**
26 Noble St.
Smithfield, NC 27577
**Phone:** (919)934-0311          **Fax:** (919)934-0311
**Email:** angelsamongus42@aol.com
**Website:** http://www.ncneighbors.com/1352/

**★ 13317 ★ National Mental Health Association in McDowell**
25 Academy St.
Marion, NC 28752
**Phone:** (828)652-3001          **Fax:** (828)652-1884
**Email:** tclontz@mcdowell.main.nc.us

**★ 13318 ★ National Mental Health Association in Mecklenburg/Cabarrus Counties**
3701 Latrobe Dr., Ste. 140
Charlotte, NC 28211
**Phone:** (704)365-3454          **Fax:** (704)365-9973

**Email:** mhameck@aol.com
**Website:** http://groups.gocarolinas.com/mhameck

**★ 13319 ★ National Mental Health Association in Nash-Rocky Mount**
PO Box 8773
Rocky Mount, NC 27804
**Phone:** (252)937-8820          **Fax:** (252)937-6702
**Email:** mhanrm@hotmail.com
Susan Smith, Director

**★ 13320 ★ National Mental Health Association in New Hanover**
301 N Front St., Ste. 4
PMD 265
Wilmington, NC 28401
**Phone:** (910)251-9005          **Fax:** (910)762-2265
**Email:** LauraWillisMHANC@aol.com

**★ 13321 ★ National Mental Health Association in North Carolina**
3820 Bland Rd.
Raleigh, NC 27609
**Phone:** (919)981-0740          **Fax:** (919)954-7238
**Email:** sgoff@mha-nc.org
**Website:** http://www.mha-nc.org

**★ 13322 ★ National Mental Health Association in Onslow County**
PO Box 425
Swansboro, NC 28584
**Phone:** (252)393-2426
**Email:** patp@coastalnet.com

**★ 13323 ★ National Mental Health Association in Orange County**
302 W Weaver St., Ste. F
PO Box 2253
Chapel Hill, NC 27515-2253
**Phone:** (919)942-8083          **Fax:** (919)688-4887
**Email:** mhaoc@intrex.net
**Website:** http://www.mhaoc.org
Megan L. Risley, Exec Director

**★ 13324 ★ National Mental Health Association in Pamlico County**
PO Box 425
Swansboro, NC 28584
**Phone:** (252)393-2426
**Email:** patp@coastalnet.com

**★ 13325 ★ National Mental Health Association in Pitt County**
101 W 14th St., Ste. 3
Greenville, NC 27835
**Phone:** (252)752-7448          **Fax:** (252)752-2729
**Email:** faeriename@aol.com

**★ 13326 ★ National Mental Health Association in Randolph, Inc.**
513-D White Oak St.
PO Box 4397
Asheboro, NC 27204-4397
**Phone:** (336)625-5551          **Fax:** (336)625-2331
**Email:** mharc@atomic.net

**★ 13327 ★ National Mental Health Association of Rowan County**
650 Statesville Blvd., Ste. 1
Salisbury, NC 28144
**Phone:** (704)636-9912          **Fax:** (704)639-0695
**Website:** http://www.dantana.com/mha

**★ 13328 ★ National Mental Health Association in Rutherford County**
286 Burch Hutchins Rd.
Forest City, NC 28043

Phone: (828)286-8884          Fax: (828)286-8330
Carolyn Osbourne, Exec Director


★ 13329 ★ National Mental Health
Association in Stanly County
124 S 1st St.
PO Box 237
Albemarle, NC 28002
Phone: (704)982-7516          Fax: (704)982-7516
Email: lahnorwood@vnet.net
Linda Hoy, Exec Director


★ 13330 ★ National Mental Health
Association of Stokes County
3868 Piney Mountain Rd.
Walnut Cove, NC 27052


★ 13331 ★ National Mental Health
Association in Vance County
1221 Alpha St.
Henderson, NC 27536
Phone: (919)438-3412
Ralph Glover, President


★ 13332 ★ National Mental Health
Association in Wake County
3820 Bland Rd.
Raleigh, NC 27609
Phone: (910)425-5971          Fax: (910)323-1954
Romaine Dougherty, Contact


★ 13333 ★ National Mental Health
Association in Wayne County
719 E Ash St.
PO Box 1476
Goldsboro, NC 27534
Phone: (919)734-3530          Fax: (919)731-1186
Email: mhawc@esn.net
Website: http://www.ww2.esn.net/mhawc


★ 13334 ★ National Mental Health
Association in Wilson County
509 W Nash St.
PO Box 652
Wilson, NC 27894
Phone: (252)242-2773          Fax: (252)237-6118
Email: mha_wc@bbnp.com
Rebecca R. Boyette, Exec Director


★ 13335 ★ National Mental Health
Association in Yancey
PO Box 284
Burnsville, NC 28714
Phone: (828)682-7498


★ 13336 ★ Outreach and Prevention
Services of Alamance, Inc.
711 Hermitage Rd.
Burlington, NC 27216
Phone: (336)438-2050          Fax: (336)438-2059
Email: hudsonjanA2@netscape.net


### North Dakota


★ 13337 ★ Missouri Valley Mental Health
Association
2817 Hawkens St., No. 4
Bismarck, ND 58503
Phone: (701)258-5169
Email: kipknaup@hotmail.com


★ 13338 ★ National Mental Health
Association of the Lake Region
4746 76th Ave. NE
Devils Lake, ND 58301-9232
Phone: (701)662-8482
Grace Sharbono, President


★ 13339 ★ National Mental Health
Association in North Dakota
1459 Interstate Loop
PO Box 4106
Bismarck, ND 58502-4106
Phone: (701)255-3692          Free: 800-472-2911
Fax: (701)255-2411
Email: director@mha-nd.org
Website: http://www.btigate.com/mhand


★ 13340 ★ National Mental Health
Association of North Valley
136 Rolling Hills Circle
Grand Forks, ND 58201
Phone: (701)772-8792          Fax: (701)775-8645
Email: joschristy@juno.com
Website: http://www.btigate.com/~mhand
Jo Christenson, President


★ 13341 ★ National Mental Health
Association in Souris Valley
1459 Interstate Loop
PO Box 160
Minot, ND 58702-0160
Phone: (701)255-3692          Fax: (701)255-2411
Email: mchand@btigate.com
Jennifer Bartsch, President


★ 13342 ★ National Mental Health
Association of the South Central
Region
2605 Circle Dr.
Jamestown, ND 58401-3924
Phone: (701)253-3842          Fax: (701)253-3204
Email: giedtd@state.nd.us
Nancy Schultz, President


★ 13343 ★ National Mental Health
Association of South Valley
124 8th St. N
Fargo, ND 58102-4915
Phone: (701)237-5871          Free: 800-472-2911
Fax: (701)237-0562
Email: mharry@juno.com
Susan Helgeland, Exec Director


★ 13344 ★ National Mental Health
Association of the Southwest
117 1st St. E
Dickinson, ND 58601
Phone: (701)227-7611          Fax: (701)227-7618
Email: 88buck@state.nd.us
Karen McConnell, President


★ 13345 ★ National Mental Health
Association in the Tri-County Region
1402 9th Ave. W
Williston, ND 58801
Phone: (701)572-2651
Email: rhickok@dia.net
Rick Hickock, President


### Ohio


★ 13346 ★ Mental Health Associations of
Ohio
538 E Town St., Ste. D
Columbus, OH 43215
Phone: (614)221-1441          Fax: (614)221-1491
Email: mhafcoh@aol.com
Laura Moskow Sigal, Director


★ 13347 ★ National Mental Health
Association of the Cincinnati Area, Inc.
2400 Reading Rd., Ste. 412
Cincinnati, OH 45202
Phone: (513)721-2910          Fax: (513)287-8544
Email: mhacincinnati@fuse.net
Website: http://www.mentalhealthassn.org


★ 13348 ★ National Mental Health
Association of Franklin County
538 E Town St., Ste. D
Columbus, OH 43215
Phone: (614)221-1441          Fax: (614)221-1491
Email: mhafcoh@aol.com
Website: http://www.mhafc.org


★ 13349 ★ National Mental Health
Association in Knox County
11 W Gambier St.
Mount Vernon, OH 43050-3301
Phone: (740)397-3088
Email: fladen4@yahoo.com


★ 13350 ★ National Mental Health
Association in Licking County
65 Messimer Dr.
Newark, OH 43055
Phone: (740)522-1341          Fax: (740)522-4464
Email: mhalc@alink.com
Website: http://www.mhalc.org


★ 13351 ★ National Mental Health
Association in Lucas County
1 Stranahan Sq., Ste. 540
Toledo, OH 43604-1900
Phone: (419)242-9587          Fax: (419)242-6316
Email: judyr@uhs-toledo.org
Website: http://www.uhs-toledo.org


★ 13352 ★ National Mental Health
Association of Miami County
1100 Wayne St., Ste. 4002
Troy, OH 45373
Phone: (937)332-9293          Fax: (937)332-9293
Email: mhamc@mail2.wesnet.com
Website: http://www.mhamc.com


★ 13353 ★ National Mental Health
Association of Ottawa County
1 Stranahan Sq., Ste. 540
Toledo, OH 43604-1900
Phone: (419)242-9587          Fax: (419)242-6316
Email: uhs@uhs-toledo.org
Website: http://www.uhs-toledo.org


★ 13354 ★ National Mental Health
Association of Summit County
405 Tallmadge Rd.
Cuyahoga Falls, OH 44221
Phone: (330)923-0688          Free: 800-991-1311
Fax: (330)923-7573
Email: rlibertini@mhasc.net
Website:                                     http://
www.mentalhealthassociationofsummitcounty.org


★ 13355 ★ National Mental Health
Association in Union County
131 N Main St.
Marysville, OH 43040
Phone: (937)642-0935          Fax: (937)644-9543
Email: paulus@netexp.net


### Oklahoma


★ 13356 ★ National Mental Health
Association in Tulsa
1870 S Boulder
Tulsa, OK 74119-5234
Phone: (918)585-1213          Fax: (918)585-1263
Email: mbrose@mhat.org
Website: http://www.mhat.org
Michael W. Brose, Exec Director

★ **13357 ★ National Mental Health Association in Tulsa**
1870 S Boulder
Tulsa, OK 74119-5234
**Phone:** (918)585-1213          **Fax:** (918)585-1263
**Email:** mbrose@mhat.org
**Website:** http://www.mhat.org
Mike Brose, Exec Director

## Oregon

★ **13358 ★ National Mental Health Association of Oregon**
812 SW Washington St., Ste. 640
Portland, OR 97204
**Phone:** (503)227-8496          **Fax:** (503)227-8496
**Email:** beckie@quik.com

## Pennsylvania

★ **13359 ★ The Advocacy Alliance, A National Mental Health Association**
846 Jefferson Ave.
PO Box 1368
Scranton, PA 18501
**Phone:** (570)342-7762          **Fax:** (570)207-9194
**Email:** teo@theadvocacyalliance.org
**Website:** http://www.theadvocacyalliance.org

★ **13360 ★ National Mental Health Association of Adams County, Inc.**
223 Baltimore St.
Gettysburg, PA 17325
**Phone:** (717)334-3139          **Fax:** (717)633-7104
**Email:** cmentzer@netrax.net

★ **13361 ★ National Mental Health Association of Allegheny County**
1945 5th Ave.
Pittsburgh, PA 15219-5543
**Phone:** (412)391-3820          **Fax:** (412)391-3825
**Email:** mha@mhaac.net
**Website:** http://www.mhaac.net

★ **13362 ★ National Mental Health Association of the Capital Region**
3 Crossgates Dr., Ste. 120
Mechanicsburg, PA 17055-2459
**Phone:** (717)796-0601          **Fax:** (717)796-0603
**Email:** astritemhacdp@paonline.com
**Website:** http://www.mentalhealthassoc.org

★ **13363 ★ National Mental Health Association of the Central Susquehanna Valley**
37 Main St., Ste. 206
Bloomsburg, PA 17815
**Phone:** (570)784-9583          **Free:** 800-874-3220
**Fax:** (570)784-3220
**Email:** mhacsv@jlink.net

★ **13364 ★ National Mental Health Association in Cumberland, Dauphin & Perry**
3 Crossgates Dr., Ste. 120
Mechanicsburg, PA 17055-2459
**Phone:** (717)796-0601          **Fax:** (717)796-0603
**Email:** johnc@mentalhealthassoc.org
**Website:** http://www.mentalhealthassoc.org/

★ **13365 ★ National Mental Health Association in Franklin/Fulton Counties**
154 S 2nd St.
Chambersburg, PA 17201
**Phone:** (717)264-4301          **Fax:** (717)264-3591
Lisa Boice, Exec Director

★ **13366 ★ National Mental Health Association in Lancaster County**
630 Janet Ave.
Lancaster, PA 17601
**Phone:** (717)397-7461          **Fax:** (717)397-2530
**Email:** mhalc@redrose.net
Mary Steffy, Director

★ **13367 ★ National Mental Health Association in Lebanon County**
136 N 9th St.
Lebanon, PA 17046-4903
**Phone:** (717)273-5781          **Fax:** (717)273-6908
**Email:** mhaleb@lmf.net
Judith Feather, Director

★ **13368 ★ National Mental Health Association of Mercer County**
19 N Water Ave.
Sharon, PA 16146-1343
**Phone:** (724)347-1303          **Fax:** (724)347-3199
Dr. James D. Robb, Director

★ **13369 ★ National Mental Health Association of Northwest Pennsylvania**
1101 Peach St.
Erie, PA 16501-1812
**Phone:** (814)452-4462          **Fax:** (814)456-6593
**Email:** eccmhc@nc.inter.net

★ **13370 ★ National Mental Health Association in Pennsylvania**
1414 N Cameron, Ste. C
Harrisburg, PA 17103
**Phone:** (717)236-8110          **Fax:** (717)236-0192
**Email:** swalther@paonline.com

★ **13371 ★ National Mental Health Association of Reading and Berks County**
122 W Lancaster Ave., Ste. 207
Shillington, PA 19607-1348
**Phone:** (610)775-3000          **Fax:** (610)775-4000
**Email:** mharbc@ptd.net
**Frmly:** Berks County Mental Health Association.

★ **13372 ★ National Mental Health Association of Southeastern Pennsylvania**
1211 Chestnut St., 11th Fl.
Philadelphia, PA 19107
**Phone:** (215)751-1800          **Fax:** (215)636-6300
**Email:** mha@mhasp.org
**Website:** http://www.mhasp.org

★ **13373 ★ National Mental Health Association in Westmoreland County**
409 Coulter Ave., Ste. 4
Greensburg, PA 15601
**Phone:** (724)834-6351          **Fax:** (724)834-6352
**Email:** mhawc@westol.com
**Website:** http://www.westol.com/mhawc
Laura Hawkins, Director

★ **13374 ★ National Mental Health Association of York County**
303 E Market St.
York, PA 17403-5614
**Phone:** (717)843-6973          **Fax:** (717)843-0185
**Email:** mentalhealth@mhay.org
**Website:** http://www.mhay.org
Kristin Keech, Director

## Rhode Island

★ **13375 ★ National Mental Health Association of Rhode Island**
Independence Sq.
500 Prospect St.
Pawtucket, RI 02860
**Phone:** (401)726-2285          **Fax:** (401)365-6170
**Email:** mmhari@mhari.org
**Website:** http://www.mhari.org

## South Carolina

★ **13376 ★ National Mental Health Association in Abbeville County**
761 Mt. Lebanon Rd.
Donalds, SC 29638
**Phone:** (864)379-2479

★ **13377 ★ National Mental Health Association in Aiken County**
104 Florence St. SW
PO Box 1074
Aiken, SC 29801
**Phone:** (803)641-4164          **Fax:** (803)641-4166
**Email:** mhaac@duesouth.net
**Website:** http://www.mha-aikensc.org

★ **13378 ★ National Mental Health Association in Anderson County**
PO Box 663
Anderson, SC 29622
**Phone:** (864)260-2221
Claudia Robinson, Contact

★ **13379 ★ National Mental Health Association in Bamberg County**
PO Box 276
Denmark, SC 29042
**Phone:** (803)793-5786

★ **13380 ★ National Mental Health Association in Barnwell County**
302 N Lartigue St.
Blackville, SC 29817
**Phone:** (803)284-3229

★ **13381 ★ National Mental Health Association in Beaufort/Jasper Counties**
7 Office Park Dr., Ste. 228
PO Box 22538
Hilton Head Island, SC 29925
**Phone:** (843)842-5855          **Fax:** (843)842-5865

★ **13382 ★ National Mental Health Association in Calhoun County**
Rte. 3, Box 504
Saint Matthews, SC 29135
**Phone:** (803)823-2612

★ **13383 ★ National Mental Health Association in Cherokee County**
714 S Limestone St.
Gaffney, SC 29340
**Phone:** (803)489-8191
Shirley Tisdale, Contact

★ **13384 ★ National Mental Health Association in Chester County**
PO Box 392
Chester, SC 29706
**Phone:** (803)385-2191

**★ 13385 ★ National Mental Health Association in Claredon County**
PO Box 278
Summerton, SC 29148
**Phone:** (803)485-2510

**★ 13386 ★ National Mental Health Association in Colleton County**
119 Charles St.
PO Box 1547
Walterboro, SC 29488
**Phone:** (843)549-1732 **Fax:** (843)549-2359

**★ 13387 ★ National Mental Health Association in Darlington County**
PO Box 131
Hartsville, SC 29551
**Phone:** (843)332-1481

**★ 13388 ★ National Mental Health Association in Florence County**
514-B S Dargen St.
Florence, SC 29506
**Phone:** (843)661-5407 **Fax:** (843)661-3859
**Email:** susanisrael@aol.com

**★ 13389 ★ National Mental Health Association in Georgetown County**
226 Queen St.
Georgetown, SC 29442
**Phone:** (843)527-6919 **Fax:** (843)527-2325
**Email:** jfenhagen@earthlink.net

**★ 13390 ★ National Mental Health Association in Greenville County**
301 University Ridge, Ste. 5600
Greenville, SC 29601-3675
**Phone:** (864)467-3344 **Fax:** (864)467-3547

**★ 13391 ★ National Mental Health Association in Horey County**
First Union Bank
2110 Oak St.
Myrtle Beach, SC 29577
**Phone:** (803)448-2688
Nick Sherfesee, President

**★ 13392 ★ National Mental Health Association in Kershaw County**
PO Box 586
Camden, SC 29020-2335
**Phone:** (803)432-7955 **Fax:** (803)425-0030
**Email:** whspence4@worldnet.att.net

**★ 13393 ★ National Mental Health Association in Lancaster County**
1769 Charles Ave.
Lancaster, SC 29720
**Phone:** (803)285-7471
**Email:** pbarry@gwm.sc.edu
Dr. Peter Barry, Contact

**★ 13394 ★ National Mental Health Association in Laurens County**
PO Box 81
Laurens, SC 29360
**Phone:** (864)984-1809

**★ 13395 ★ National Mental Health Association in Lee County**
261 Luckey Rd.
Bishopville, SC 29010
**Phone:** (803)428-5738

**★ 13396 ★ National Mental Health Association in Marion County**
3914 Elm Ct.
Mullins, SC 29574
**Phone:** (803)464-0630

**★ 13397 ★ National Mental Health Association in Marlboro County**
707 Crestview Dr.
Bennettsville, SC 29512
**Phone:** (803)479-4016
Beulah C. Black, President

**★ 13398 ★ National Mental Health Association in McCormick County**
PO Box 227
McCormick, SC 29835
**Phone:** (803)391-2131

**★ 13399 ★ National Mental Health Association in Mid-Carolina**
PO Box 1657
Columbia, SC 29202-1657
**Phone:** (803)733-5425 **Fax:** (803)733-5427

**★ 13400 ★ National Mental Health Association in Oconee County**
PO Box 915
Walhalla, SC 29691
**Phone:** (864)638-3058

**★ 13401 ★ National Mental Health Association in Orangeburg County**
801 Shillings Bridge Rd.
Orangeburg, SC 29116
**Phone:** (803)533-0018 **Fax:** (803)516-0242
Brannon Underwood, Contact

**★ 13402 ★ National Mental Health Association in Pickens County**
3600 Pumkintown Hwy.
Pickens, SC 29671
**Phone:** (864)878-3974

**★ 13403 ★ National Mental Health Association of the Piedmont**
153 N Spring St.
Spartanburg, SC 29306
**Phone:** (864)582-3104 **Fax:** (864)582-3322

**★ 13404 ★ National Mental Health Association in Saluda County**
PO Box 191
Saluda, SC 29138
**Phone:** (803)356-9398

**★ 13405 ★ National Mental Health Association in South Carolina**
1823 Gadsden St.
Columbia, SC 29201
**Phone:** (803)779-5363 **Fax:** (803)779-0017
**Email:** mha@mha-sc.org
**Website:** http://www.mha-sc.org

**★ 13406 ★ National Mental Health Association in Sumter County**
c/o Sumter National Bank
PO Box 1629
Sumter, SC 29151
**Phone:** (803)755-7701
Lucy Thomas, President

**★ 13407 ★ National Mental Health Association in York County**
2778 Woodbridge Dr.
Fort Mill, SC 29715

**Phone:** (803)548-0952

### Tennessee

**★ 13408 ★ National Mental Health Association of Greater Knoxville**
PO Box 52405
Knoxville, TN 37950-2405
**Phone:** (865)584-9125 **Fax:** (865)584-9125
**Email:** mhagk@lock-net.com
**Website:** http://www.korrnet.org/mha
Ben Harrington, Director

**★ 13409 ★ National Mental Health Association of the Mid-South**
200 Jefferson Ave., Ste. 1107
Memphis, TN 38103-2328
**Phone:** (901)323-0633 **Fax:** (901)323-0858
**Email:** mha@netten.net

**★ 13410 ★ National Mental Health Association of Middle Tennessee**
2416 21st Ave. S, Ste. 201
Nashville, TN 37212
**Phone:** (615)269-5355 **Fax:** (615)269-5413
**Email:** forinfo@mhamt.org
**Website:** http://www.ichope.com
Elizabeth Lentchner, Director

**★ 13411 ★ National Mental Health Association of Tennessee**
2416 21st Ave., Ste. 20
Nashville, TN 37212-5318
**Phone:** (615)242-7122 **Fax:** (615)242-9637
**Email:** anitab@mhatn.org
**Website:** http://www.mhatn.org

### Texas

**★ 13412 ★ National Mental Health Association in Abilene**
PO Box 7282
Abilene, TX 79608
**Phone:** (915)673-2300 **Fax:** (915)673-2671
**Email:** mhaa@bitstreet.com
**Website:** http://www.abilenementalhealth.org

**★ 13413 ★ National Mental Health Association in Beaumont/Jefferson Counties**
670 N 7th St.
Beaumont, TX 77702-1741
**Phone:** (409)833-9657 **Fax:** (409)833-3522
**Website:** http://www.mentalhealthbeaumont.org
Pat Hays, President

**★ 13414 ★ National Mental Health Association in Fort Bend County**
10435 Greenbough Dr., Bldg. II, Ste. 200
Stafford, TX 77477
**Phone:** (281)261-1876 **Fax:** (281)261-1833
**Email:** mhafbc@wt.net
**Website:** http://www.mhafbc.org

**★ 13415 ★ National Mental Health Association of Greater Dallas**
624 N Good-Latimer Expy., Ste. 200
Dallas, TX 75204
**Phone:** (214)871-2420 **Fax:** (214)954-0611
**Email:** tsimmons@mhadallas.org
**Website:** http://www.mhadallas.org

**★ 13416 ★ National Mental Health Association of Greater Houston**
2211 Norfolk, Ste. 810
Houston, TX 77098
**Phone:** (713)523-8963 **Fax:** (713)522-0698
**Email:** bschwartz@mhahouston.org

**Website:** http://www.mhahouston.org
**Program(s):** Information and Referral Services, Advocacy, Self-Help Resource Center.

**★ 13417 ★ National Mental Health Association in Greater San Antonio**
8431 Fredricksburg Rd., Ste. 110
San Antonio, TX 78229
**Phone:** (210)614-7566          **Fax:** (210)614-7589
**Email:** mhasatx@axs4u.net

**★ 13418 ★ National Mental Health Association in Tarrant County**
3136 W 4th St.
Fort Worth, TX 76107-2113
**Phone:** (817)335-5405          **Fax:** (817)334-0025
**Email:** mhatc@mhatc.org
Lauralee Harris, President

**★ 13419 ★ National Mental Health Association in Texas**
8401 Shoal Creek Blvd.
Austin, TX 78757-7597
**Phone:** (512)454-3706          **Fax:** (512)454-3725
**Email:** mhainfo@mhatexas.org
**Website:** http://www.mhatexas.org
Clare Hudspeth, Exec Director

**★ 13420 ★ National Mental Health Association in Texas**
8401 Shoal Creek Blvd.
Austin, TX 78757-7597
**Phone:** (512)454-3706          **Fax:** (512)454-3725
**Email:** whatinfo@mhatexas.org
**Website:** http://www.mhatexas.org
Stella Mullins, President

**★ 13421 ★ National Mental Health Association in Tyler**
113 E Houston
Tyler, TX 75702
**Phone:** (903)592-0582          **Fax:** (903)592-7318
Tim King, President

### Utah

**★ 13422 ★ National Mental Health Association in Utah**
1800 SW Temple, Ste. 503
Salt Lake City, UT 84115-3040
**Phone:** (801)596-3705          **Fax:** (801)596-3658
**Email:** mhaut@xmission.com
**Website:** http://www.xmission.com/~mhaut/index.htm

### Vermont

**★ 13423 ★ National Mental Health Association in Vermont**
PO Box 165
Montpelier, VT 05601
**Phone:** (802)223-6263          **Fax:** (802)828-5252
**Email:** vamh1@aol.com
**Website:** http://www.vamh.org
Ken Libertoff, Director

### Virginia

**★ 13424 ★ National Mental Health Association of Augusta**
Professional Bldg., Rm. 206
Staunton, VA 24401
**Phone:** (540)886-7181          **Fax:** (540)885-0640

**★ 13425 ★ National Mental Health Association of Central Virginia**
1010 Miller Park Sq.
Lynchburg, VA 24501
**Phone:** (804)847-9055          **Fax:** (804)847-3600
**Email:** mhacvexdir@aol.com

**★ 13426 ★ National Mental Health Association of Charlottesville/Albemarle, Inc.**
513 Stewart St., Ste. J
Charlottesville, VA 22902
**Phone:** (434)977-4673
**Email:** mha@avenue.org
**Website:** http://www.monticelloavenue.org

**★ 13427 ★ National Mental Health Association in Chesterfield**
PO Box 2188
Chesterfield, VA 23832
**Phone:** (804)748-7938
**Email:** kmorrow52@hotmail.com
Kenneth Marrow, President

**★ 13428 ★ National Mental Health Association in Danville/Pittsylvania County**
1225 W Main St.
PO Box 1106
Danville, VA 24543
**Phone:** (434)792-3700          **Fax:** (434)791-3187
**Email:** mha@gamewood.net
**Website:** http://pws.gamewood.net/~mha/

**★ 13429 ★ National Mental Health Association of Fauquier County**
PO Box 3549
Warrenton, VA 20188
**Phone:** (540)341-8732          **Fax:** 800-349-9057
**Email:** mhafc@mindspring.com
**Website:** http://www.fauquier-mha.org

**★ 13430 ★ National Mental Health Association in Fredericksburg**
2217 Princess Anne St., Ste. 219-1
Fredericksburg, VA 22401
**Phone:** (540)371-2704          **Free:** 800-684-6423
**Fax:** (540)372-3709
**Email:** mhaf@infi.net
**Website:** http://www.fls.infi.net/~mhaf

**★ 13431 ★ National Mental Health Association in Halifax County**
PO Box 329
South Boston, VA 24592
**Phone:** (804)572-3992          **Fax:** (804)572-8959
Irene Gravitt, Exec Director

**★ 13432 ★ National Mental Health Association in Hanover**
203 S Taylor St.
Ashland, VA 23005
**Phone:** (804)798-5902          **Fax:** (804)752-8373
**Email:** sunrisehse@aol.com
**Website:** http://www.hanovermentalhealth.org

**★ 13433 ★ National Mental Health Association in Martinsville/Henry Counties**
117 Broad St.
PO Box 582
Martinsville, VA 24114
**Phone:** (276)638-7801          **Fax:** (276)638-7960
**Email:** mha638@intelos.net
**Website:** http://intelos.net/mha638

**★ 13434 ★ National Mental Health Association of New River Valley**
303 Church St.
Blacksburg, VA 24060
**Phone:** (540)951-4990          **Fax:** (540)951-5015
**Email:** mhanry@bellatlantic.net
**Website:** http://donthide.org
Amy Forsyth-Stephens, Exec Director

**★ 13435 ★ National Mental Health Association of Roanoke Valley**
PO Box 592
Roanoke, VA 24004
**Phone:** (540)344-0931          **Fax:** (540)344-0932
**Email:** mharv@roanoke.infi.net

**★ 13436 ★ National Mental Health Association of Rockbridge County**
PO Box 1088
Lexington, VA 24450
**Phone:** (540)463-2911
Linda Munsey, Exec Director

**★ 13437 ★ National Mental Health Association in South Hampton Roads**
1513 E Sewells Point Rd.
Norfolk, VA 23502
**Phone:** (757)853-2606          **Fax:** (757)566-2013
**Email:** lhowards@aol.com

**★ 13438 ★ National Mental Health Association of Virginia**
503 E Main St., Ste. 707
Richmond, VA 23219
**Phone:** (804)225-5591          **Fax:** (804)225-5593
**Email:** vmfisher@hsc.vcu.edu
**Website:** http://www.mhav.org

**★ 13439 ★ National Mental Health Association of Warren County**
PO Box 358
Front Royal, VA 22630
**Phone:** (276)635-6223

**★ 13440 ★ Peninsula Mental Health Association**
2501 Washington Ave., 5th Fl.
Newport News, VA 23607
**Phone:** (757)245-0217          **Fax:** (757)245-5126
Bonnie Kelly, President

### Washington

**★ 13441 ★ National Mental Health Association of Washington Washington Advocates for the Mentally Ill**
802 NW 70th St.
Seattle, WA 98117
**Phone:** (206)789-7722          **Free:** 800-782-9264
**Fax:** (206)784-0957
**Email:** wami@wolfenet.com
**Website:** http://www.nami-wami.com
Eleanor Owen, Exec Director

### West Virginia

**★ 13442 ★ National Mental Health Association in the Greater Kanawha Valley, Inc.**
1 United Way Sq.
Charleston, WV 25301-1098
**Phone:** (304)340-3512          **Fax:** (304)340-3508
**Email:** mha@wvinter.net
Ellen Ward, Director

**★ 13443 ★ National Mental Health Association in Monongalia County**
PO Box 1533
Morgantown, WV 26507
**Phone:** (304)292-0525
Penny Fletcher, Director

## Wisconsin

★ 13444 ★ **National Mental Health Association in Brown County**
612 Skyline Blvd.
PO Box 1016
Green Bay, WI 54305
**Phone:** (920)468-6720
Barbara Bauer, President

★ 13445 ★ **National Mental Health Association in Calumet County**
W2643 St. Charles
Chilton, WI 53014
**Phone:** (920)849-1450     **Fax:** (920)894-2506
**Email:** wayne@tcei.com
Diane Kuckenbecker, President

★ 13446 ★ **National Mental Health Association in Milwaukee County**
734 N 4th St., No. 325
Milwaukee, WI 53203-2102
**Phone:** (414)276-3122     **Fax:** (414)276-3124
**Email:** mha@mhamilw.org
**Website:** http://www.mhamilw.org
Karen Robison, CEO & Pres

★ 13447 ★ **National Mental Health Association in Sheboygan County**
2020 Erie Ave.
Sheboygan, WI 53081
**Phone:** (920)458-3951     **Fax:** (920)458-3441
**Email:** mhasheb@bytehead.com
Beverly Randall, Director

## Federal Government Agencies

**★ 13448 ★ U.S. Department of Defense**
**Department of the Air Force**
**Air Staff**
**Surgeon General of the Air Force**
1670 Air Force Pentagon
Washington, DC 20330-1670
**Phone:** (703)697-6061
**Website:** www.af.mil
Paul K. Carlton, Jr., Surgeon General of the Air Force
**Desc:** The Surgeon General is part of the Air Staff, independent of the basic staff structure, providing advisory and support services to both the Chief of Staff and the Air Staff. Operating components are: (1) Assistant Surgeon General for Dental Services, (2) Biomedical Sciences Corps, (3) Congressional and Public Affairs, (4) Health Care Studies and Evaluations, (5) Medical Programs and Resources, (6) Medical Support, and (7) Nursing Services.

**★ 13449 ★ U.S. Department of Defense**
**Department of the Army**
**Army Medical Command (MEDCOM)**
Washington, DC 20310
**Phone:** (703)681-3000
**Website:** http://www.armymedicine.army.mil/
Lt.Gen. James B. Peake, Director
**Desc:** The U.S. Army Medical Command provides direction and planning for the Army Medical Department in conjunction with the Office of the Surgeon General. It develops and integrates doctrine, training, leader development, organization, and material for Army health services. MEDCOM also allocates resources and evaluates delivery of services.

**★ 13450 ★ U.S. Department of Defense**
**Department of the Army**
**Army Staff**
**Office of the Army Surgeon General**
c/o Department of the Army
The Pentagon
Washington, DC 20310
**Phone:** (703)695-2442
**Website:** http://www.army.mil/
Lt.Gen. James B. Peake, Surgeon General of the Army
**Desc:** The office of the Surgeon General manages health services for the Army and, as directed, for other services, agencies, and organizations. Other responsibilities include health standards for Army personnel; health professional education and training; career management for missioned and warrant officer personnel of the Army Medical Department; medical research, material development and test and evaluation; policies concerning health aspects of Army environmental programs and prevention of diseases; and planning, programming, and budgeting for Army-wide health services. Major components of the Office

of the Surgeon General include: (1) Dental Services/Dental Corps; (2) Veterinary Services/Veterinary Corps; (3) Army Medical Specialist Corps; (4) Army Nurse Corps; and (5) the Health Facility Planning Agency.

**★ 13451 ★ U.S. Department of Defense**
**Department of the Navy**
**Bureau of Medicine and Surgery**
c/o Department of the Navy
23rd and E Sts. NW
Washington, DC 20372-5120
**Phone:** (202)762-3701          **Fax:** (202)762-3211
**Website:** http://www.navy.mil
R.A. Nelson, Chief, Bureau of Medicine and Surgery
**Desc:** The Bureau directs the provision of medical and dental services for Navy and Marine Corps personnel and their dependants; administers the execution and implementation of contingency support plans and programs to provide effective medical and dental readiness capability; provides professional and technical medical and dental services to the fleet, fleet marine force, and shore activities of the Navy; and ensures cooperation with civil authorities in matters pertaining to public health disasters and other emergencies.

**★ 13452 ★ U.S. Department of Defense**
**Department of the Navy**
**United States Marine Corps**
**Office of Health Services**
2 Navy Annex
Washington, DC 20380-1775
**Phone:** (703)614-1034
**Website:** http://www.usmc.mil/

**★ 13453 ★ U.S. Department of Defense**
**Office of Assistant Secretary of Defense**
**for Health Affairs**
The Pentagon
Washington, DC 20301-1155
**Phone:** (703)545-6700          **Fax:** (703)614-3537
**Website:** http://www.defenselink.mil/
**Desc:** Office is responsible for Department of Defense health matters, including preventive medicine; medical readiness; health care delivery; drug and alcohol abuse prevention; and procurement, development, and retention of medical personnel.

**★ 13454 ★ U.S. Department of Defense**
**Office of Assistant Secretary of Defense**
**for Health Affairs**
**TRICARE Management Activity (TMA)**
c/o The Pentagon
Skyline 5, Ste. 810
5111 Leesburg Pike
Falls Church, VA 22041-3206
**Phone:** (703)681-1730          **Fax:** (703)681-3665
**Website:** http://www.tricare.osd.mil
**Desc:** TRICARE was formed from the consolidation of the TRICARE Support Office, the Defense Medical

Programs Activity, and the integration of health management program functions formerly located in the Office of the Assistant Secretary of Defense for Health Affairs. The TMA mission is to manage TRICARE; administer and manage the Defense Health Program appropriation; provide operational direction and support to the Uniformed Services in the management and administration of the TRICARE program; and administer CHAMPUS. medical/dental services provided to active duty service members by civilian medical personnel.

**★ 13455 ★ U.S. Department of Defense**
**Uniformed Services University of the**
**   Health Sciences (USUHS)**
4301 Jones Bridge Rd.
Bethesda, MD 20814-4799
**Phone:** (301)295-3030          **Fax:** (301)295-1960
**Website:** http://www.usuhs.mil
James A. Zimble, MD, President
**Desc:** The Uniformed Services University of the Health Sciences was established to educate career-oriented medical officers for the Military Departments and the Public Health Service. The University currently incorporates the F. Edward Hebert School of Medicine and the Graduate School of Nursing.

**★ 13456 ★ U.S. Department of Veterans**
**   Affairs**
**Veterans Health Administration**
810 Vermont Ave. NW
Washington, DC 20420
**Phone:** (202)273-4800
**Website:** http://www.va.gov/
**Desc:** The Veterans Health Administration (formerly Health Services and Research Administration) provides hospital, nursing home and domiciliary care, and outpatient medical and dental care to eligible veterans of military service in the Armed Forces. It operates medical centers, domiciliaries, clinics, and nursing home units in the U.S., the Commonwealth of Puerto Rico, and the Republic of the Philippines, and provides for similar care under VA auspices in non-VA hospitals and community nursing homes, and for visits by veterans to non-VA physicians and dentists for outpatient treatment. Under the Civilian Health and Medical Program, dependents of certain veterans are provided with medical care supplied by non-VA institutions and physicians. The Administration conducts both individual medical and health-care delivery research projects and multi-hospital research programs. It assists in the education of physicians and dentists, and with training of many other health care professionals through affiliations with educational institutions and organizations.

# National & International Organizations

## ★ 13457 ★ Army Nurse Corps Association (ANCA)
PO Box 39235, Serna Sta.
San Antonio, TX 78218-1235
**Phone:** (210)650-3534          **Fax:** (210)650-3534
**Email:** ranca@juno.com
**Fnded:** 1977. **Mem:** 2,100. **Desc:** Army Nurse Corps officers from active, or retiree status or those serving honorably for shorter periods, or reserve duty. Provides educational and social opportunities for members; disseminates information to the public. Seeks to preserve history of the U.S. Army Nurse Corps. **Pub:** *Connection*, quarterly. Newsletter. **Frmly:** (2001) Retired Army Nurse Corps Association.

## ★ 13458 ★ Association of Military Surgeons of the U.S. (AMSUS)
9320 Old Georgetown Rd.
Bethesda, MD 20814
**Phone:** (301)897-8800          **Free:** 800-761-9320
**Fax:** (301)530-5446
**Email:** amsus@amsus.org
**Website:** http://www.amsus.org
RADM Frederic G. Sanford, MC USN, Ret. Contact
**Fnded:** 1891. **Mem:** 11,000. **Nat'l Groups:** 1. **Local Groups:** 10. **Desc:** Physicians, dentists, veterinarians, nurses, pharmacists, dietitians, therapists, and others of commissioned rank (or grades E5 through E9) or equivalent in the Army, Navy, Air Force, Public Health Service, and Veterans Administration; Reserve and National Guard officers are also eligible for membership. Advances all phases of federal medicine and allied sciences related to federal health services. Provides group insurance. **Pub:** *AMSUS Newsletter*, quarterly. Newsletter. • *Military Medicine*, monthly.

## ★ 13459 ★ Hospitalized Veterans Writing Project (HVWP)
5920 Nall, Rm. 105
Mission, KS 66202
**Phone:** (913)432-1214
Barbara Sauvan, Pres.
**Fnded:** 1946. **Desc:** Individuals and organizations united to encourage hospitalized U.S. veterans to write for pleasure and rehabilitation during their hospital stay. Maintains speakers' bureau and slide program with commentary. Conducts writing sessions in hospitals. **Pub:** *Veterans' Voices*, 3/year. Magazine. Contains prose, poetry, artwork, and cartoons submitted by hospitalized veterans. *Price:* $8/year for hospitalized veterans and outpatients; $15/year for others.

## ★ 13460 ★ Indian Military Historical Society
33 High St., Tilbrook
Huntington PE18 0JP, United Kingdom
**Phone:** 44 20 85744425
**Fnded:** 1983. **Mem:** 201. **Desc:** Conducts research into the military history of the Indian sub-continent.

## ★ 13461 ★ International Committee of Military Medicine (ICMM) (Comite International de Medecine Militaire — CIMM)
Queen Astrid Military Hospital
B-1120 Brussels, Belgium
**Phone:** 32 2 2644348          **Fax:** 32 2 22644367
**Email:** cimm.icmm@smd.be
**Fnded:** 1921. **Mem:** 89. **Lang(s):** English, French. **Desc:** Medical representatives of the military forces of nations worldwide. Works to encourage and maintain professional cooperation among those in various countries whose mission is to care for the sick and wounded of the armed forces. Aims to improve such care by standardization of related disciplines and techniques, complete documentation and dissemination of military-medical information, and development of an international medical law. Conducts courses. **Pub:** *International Review of the Armed Forces Medical Services*, quarterly. Journal. **Frmly:** (1990) International Committee of Military Medicine and Pharmacy.

## ★ 13462 ★ National Association of VA Physicians and Dentists (NAVAPD)
11 Canal Centre Plz., Ste. 110
Alexandria, VA 22314-1595
**Phone:** (703)548-0280          **Fax:** (703)683-7939
**Email:** navapd@dgsys.com
**Website:** http://www.navapd.org
Robert M. Conroy, Pres.
**Fnded:** 1975. **Mem:** 2,000. **Desc:** Physicians and dentists at Department of Veterans Affairs Medical Centers. Purpose is to strengthen and improve the quality of care and conditions at VA health care facilities. Works to assure that veterans receive quality care. **Pub:** *NAVAPD News*, bimonthly. Newsletter. *Price:* Included in membership. • *NAVAPD Notes*, bimonthly.

## ★ 13463 ★ Navy Anesthesia Society (NAS)
c/o LCDR David G. Elkins
Department of Anesthesiology
Naval Medical Center
San Diego, CA 92134-5000
**Phone:** (619)532-8943          **Fax:** (619)532-8945
**Email:** elkinsdave@aol.com
**Website:** http://www.geocities.com/Vienna/2209/nas.html
LCDR David G. Elkins, Sec.
**Fnded:** 1988. **Mem:** 400. **Desc:** Military physicians and nurse anesthetists. Committed to the delivery of anesthesia and critical care services, trauma care and combat casualty transport in a military environment, including natural or man-made disasters and in underdeveloped countries. **Pub:** *NAS Newsletter*. Newsletter.

## Nurses Organization of Veterans Affairs (NOVA)
*See:* Entry 15763

## ★ 13464 ★ Society of Air Force Physicians (SAFP)
HQ AFMOA/SGOC
Bolling Air Force Base
110 Luke Ave., Ste. 400
Washington, DC 20332-7050
**Phone:** (202)767-4073          **Fax:** (202)404-7366
**Email:** nova@vanurse.org
**Website:** http://www.vanurse.org
Jim Cox, Contact
**Fnded:** 1958. **Mem:** 300. **Desc:** Air Force internists, family practitioners, and specialists in emergency medicine, dermatology, allergy/immunology, and neurology. Objectives are to foster advancement of the art and science of medicine in the Air Force; encourage clinical and laboratory investigation; disseminate information.

## ★ 13465 ★ Society of Army Physician Assistants (SAPA)
6762 Candlewood Dr.
Fort Myers, FL 33919
**Phone:** (941)482-2162          **Fax:** (941)482-2162
**Email:** sapamed@aol.com
**Website:** http://www.sapa.org/
**Fnded:** 1976. **Desc:** Represents and supports the U.S. Army Physician Assistant, including, former, active, retired, reserve and National Guard PA's. Aims to provide a forum for discussion, representation with the AAPA; provides low cost continuing medical education (CME) to members and the PA profession. **Pub:** Newsletter, bimonthly. • Membership Directory.

## ★ 13466 ★ Society of Medical Consultants to the Armed Forces (SMCAF)
4301 Jones Bridge Rd., A1050
Bethesda, MD 20814
**Phone:** (301)295-9822          **Fax:** (301)295-3627
**Email:** jhutton@usuhs.mil
**Website:** http://www.smcaf.org
John E. Hutton, MD, Pres.
**Fnded:** 1945. **Mem:** 1,000. **Desc:** Professional society of physicians and surgeons who have been in active military service and who have acted as consultants to the Surgeons General of the Army, Navy, or Air Force. To preserve and encourage the association of civilian consultants and military medical personnel and to assist in the development and maintenance of the highest standards of medical practice in the Armed Forces. **Pub:** *Roster*, every 2-3 years. • Newsletter, 3/year. **Frmly:** Society of U.S. Medical Consultants in World War II.

## ★ 13467 ★ Society of Military Otolaryngologists - Head and Neck Surgeons (SMO-HNS)
c/o Sue Pearce
9231 Shawdow Lawn Circle
Converse, TX 78109
**Phone:** (210)945-9006          **Fax:** (210)945-9024
**Email:** spearce@worldnet.att.net
Sue Pearce, Admn. Sec.
**Fnded:** 1952. **Mem:** 320. **Nat'l Groups:** 1. **Desc:** Otolaryngologists, head and neck surgeons and residents in training of the U.S. Army, Air Force, Navy, and former active duty members. Purposes are to further the social and professional contacts of military otolaryngologists and to advance the science and art of the field. **Frmly:** (1952) Society of Military Otolaryngologists.

## Sozialverband Vdk Deutschland
*See:* Entry 3037

# Research Centers

## ★ 13468 ★ Henry M. Jackson Foundation for the Advancement of Military Medicine
1401 Rockville Pke., Ste. 600
Rockville, MD 20852
**Phone:** (301)424-0800          **Fax:** (301)424-5771
**Email:** commdept@hjf.org
**Website:** http://www.hjf.org
John W. Lowe, Pres.
**Activities/Fields:** Infectious diseases, HIV research, immunology, wound healing, sepsis, shock and traumatic injury, telemedicine, prostate cancer, cardiovascular disease, addiction medicine, pediatrics and preventive medicine, emergency medical training, diagnostic radiology, head injury, and occupational health. Coordinates clinical trials sponsored by private industry. **Pub:** *Annual Report*. Annual report.

## ★ 13469 ★ Johns Hopkins University Center for Civilian Biodefense Studies
Candler Bldg., Ste. 850
111 Market Pl.
Baltimore, MD 21202
**Phone:** (410)223-1667          **Fax:** (410)223-1665
**Website:** http://www.hopkins-biodefense.org
D.A. Henderson, MD, Dir.
**Activities/Fields:** Medical and public health threats posed by biological weapons, their expected clinical manifestations, available treatment strategies, epidemiology, and potential methods of prophylaxis.

## ★ 13470 ★ U.S. Department of Defense Army Medical Research and Materiel Command

Ft. Detrick, Bldg. 660
Frederick, MD 21702-5012
**Phone:** (301)619-7613 **Fax:** (301)619-2982
Brig.Gen. Russell Zajtchuk, Comdr.

**Activities/Fields:** Solving medical problems of military importance. The program, which is designed to maintain or restore the health of the individual soldier, involves: assessment, prevention, diagnosis, and treatment of infectious diseases that would hamper military operations; disease vector surveillance; combat casualty care and rapid return to duty of injured soldiers; management of maxillofacial injury; assessment and prevention of oral diseases; research in dental materials; studies on health hazards of military materiel; studies on factors limiting soldier effectiveness; medical countermeasures to chemical warfare agents, including pretreatment and antidote drugs, skin decontamination compounds and medical management of chemical casualties. Command has nine major research and development laboratories including Letterman Army Institute of Research; Aeromedical Research Laboratory; Biomedical Research and Development Laboratory; Institute of Dental Research; Institute of Surgical Research; Medical Research Institute of Chemical Defense; Medical Research Institute of Infectious Diseases; Medical Research Institute of Environmental Medicine; and Walter Reed Army Institute of Research. **Pub:** *Technical reports.*

## ★ 13471 ★ U.S. Department of Defense Army Medical Research and Materiel Command

**Army Institute of Surgical Research**

Ft. Sam Houston, Bldg. 3611
3400 Rawley E Chambers Ave.
San Antonio, TX 78234-6315
**Phone:** (210)916-2720 **Fax:** (210)227-8502
Col. Cleon W. Goodwin, Comdr. & Dir.

**Activities/Fields:** Investigation of problems of mechanical and thermal injuries; care of patients with such injuries; education and training of physicians and ancillary medical personnel in the principles of management of injured patients; and investigative studies at both the basic and clinical levels. Principal subject of research (basic and applied) is burn and trauma care, including studies in fluid resuscitation, host resistance, metabolic response, nutrition, leukocyte dysfunction, thyroid hormone kinetics, wound care, surgical infection, inhalation injury, surgical critical care, skin substitutes, and mechanical trauma. **Pub:** *USAISR Anniversary Symposia.* • *USAISR Annual Research Reports.*

## ★ 13472 ★ U.S. Department of Defense Army Medical Research and Materiel Command

**Army Medical Research Institute of Chemical Defense**

Attn: MCMR-UV-RC
3100 Ricketts Point Rd.
Aberdeen Proving Ground, MD 21010-5400
**Phone:** (410)436-3628 **Fax:** (410)436-1960
**Website:** http://chemdef.apgea.army.mil/
Col. James A. Romano, Comdr.

**Activities/Fields:** Medical defense of chemical warfare (CW). This includes basic research on mechanisms of action of CW agents and antidotes to establish a database from which to devise improved methods for the prevention, resuscitation, treatment, and management of chemical casualties; and assistance in the integration of products into the logistical system, doctrine development, and training of medical and nonmedical personnel in the management and prevention of chemical casualties. Basic research is conducted on neuronal, physiologic, and pharmacologic mechanisms of chemical warfare agents and pretreatment and treatment compounds. Applied research is directed toward the development of biomedical models; standardization of methods and procedures; pretreatment and treatment drug screening; biomedical data acquisition; analysis, prediction, and information transfer; toxicological and behavioral effects of sublethal doses of CW agents; tolerance to chronic CW agent exposure; toxicological effects of chemotherapeutics; safety and efficacy of pretreatment compounds; sensory effects of CW agents; vesicant treatment technology; soldier and patient decontamination technology; skin protection technology; skin toxicology; and management and treatment of mass chemical casualties. Research efforts are supplemented by a complementary research and development contract program and by collaboration with USAMRMC sister institutes, other government laboratories, universities, and research efforts with allied countries. **Pub:** *Bioscience review proceedings.* • *Historical Report,* annually. • *Proceedings.* • *Research Reports.*

## ★ 13473 ★ U.S. Department of Defense Army Medical Research and Materiel Command

**Army Medical Research Institute of Infectious Diseases**

Ft. Detrick
1425 Porter St.
Frederick, MD 21702-5011
**Phone:** (301)619-2833 **Fax:** (301)619-4625
**Email:** usamriidweb@amedd.army.mil
**Website:** http://www.usamriid.army.mil
Col. Gerald W. Parker, Comdr.

**Activities/Fields:** USAMRIID develops vaccines, drugs and diagnostics to protect U.S. forces from biological warfare threats and endemic infectious diseases requiring special containment. The Institute also develops and conducts educational programs on medical management of builogical casualties, and maintains a world-class reference laboratory capability for identification of biological threat agents. While USAMRIID's primary focus in on protecting the military, its research has civilian applications as well. **Pub:** *Conference Proceedings.* • *Research Reports.*

## ★ 13474 ★ U.S. Department of Defense Army Medical Research and Materiel Command

**Army Research Institute of Environmental Medicine**

Bldg. 42, Kansas St.
Natick, MA 01760-5007
**Phone:** (508)233-4811 **Fax:** (508)233-5298
**Website:** http://www.usariem.army.mil
Col. Marie Stephens, Contact

**Activities/Fields:** Effects of temperature, altitude, work, chemical defense, and military nutrition on the soldier's life processes, performance, and health; defining the complex interaction of environmental stress, the body's defenses, and the techniques, equipment, and procedures best calculated to protect the soldier and make the soldier operationally effective; assessing decrements to soldier performance caused by the synergy of environmental extremes and protective measures against chemical agents; and conducting research in the physiology and health effects of Army physical fitness training. In coordination with the U.S. Army Natick Research, Development, and Engineering Center, Institute conducts nutrition research for the Department of Defense Food and Nutrition Research, Development, Testing, and Engineering Program to develop feeding strategies for operational rations and supplements to minimize decrements in the soldier's performance under sustained combat conditions. USARIEM also assists the Natick center in the development of personal clothing and equipment by assessing the physiological impact of these items under all climatic conditions. In addition, Institute acts as a liaison with other federal agencies to develop the research technology base to discharge the Army Surgeon General's responsibilities as DoD executive agent for nutrition. USARIEM also provides technical advice and consultant services to Army commanders, installations, and activities in support of the Army Preventive Medicine Program and, on request, to other federal agencies.

## ★ 13475 ★ U.S. Department of Defense Army Medical Research and Materiel Command

**Army Research Institute of Environmental Medicine**

**Military Nutrition and Biochemistry Division**

Natick, MA 01760-5007
**Phone:** (508)233-4194 **Fax:** (508)233-4869
**Email:** rfrancesconi@natick-ccmail.army.mil
**Website:** http://www.usariem.army.mil/nbd/milnut.htm
Ralph P. Francesconi, PhD, Chf.

**Activities/Fields:** Nutrition research, development, testing, evaluation, and engineering support to the Department of Defense Food and Nutrition Research, Development, Test, and Evaluation and Engineering Program; and provides technical assistance to the Surgeon General of the Army on biomedical aspects of nutrition and performance. **Pub:** *Proceedings.* • *Research Reports.*

## ★ 13476 ★ U.S. Department of Defense Army Medical Research and Materiel Command

**Army Research Institute of Environmental Medicine**

**Occupational Health and Performance Directorate**

Bldg. 42
Natick, MA 01760-5007
**Phone:** (508)233-4800 **Fax:** (508)233-4195
**Email:** richard.johnson@na.amedd.army.mil
Dr. Richard F. Johnson, Dir.

**Activities/Fields:** Interactive effects of environment, nutrition, and the physiologic and psychologic demands of military operations on soldier health and performance. Objectives focus on the identification and quantification of military operational stressors, characterization of dose-response or energy-injury manifestation, development of attenuation or prevention measures, and development of predictive health and performance models. Research activities include: a program on epidemiologic field survey methods and models of environmental operational factors affecting soldier health and performance, designed to identify and relate environmental/operational stressors to soldier health and performance and develop predictive epidemiologic models for field validation; studies on the impact of the environment and sustained operations on military performance, which use military tasks involving specified psychomotor and cognitive skills in laboratory/field experiments to determine task components most influenced by environmental stressors; and assessment of the interactive effects of chemical defense factors and environmental stressors with animal/human performance models in order to evaluate independent and synergistic effects of environmental stressors and chemical defense factors (e.g., agents, antidotes, pretreatments) on performance parameters, determine dose-response relationships, develop attenuation/preventive measures of performance decrements, and develop and validate predictive models. **Frmly:** Occupational Health and Performance Division.

## ★ 13477 ★ U.S. Department of Defense Army Medical Research and Materiel Command

**Army Research Institute of Environmental Medicine**

**Thermal and Mountain Medicine Division**

Kansas St. Bldg. 42
Natick, MA 01760-5007
**Phone:** (508)233-4832 **Fax:** (508)233-5298
**Email:** michael.sawka@na.amedd.army.mil
Michael Sawka, Dir.

**Activities/Fields:** Illnesses, injuries, and physiological performance effects associated with exposure to the environmental extremes of heat, cold, and high altitude.

**★ 13478 ★ U.S. Department of Defense Army Medical Research and Materiel Command**
**Walter Reed Army Institute of Research**
Washington, DC 20307-5100
**Phone:** (202)782-3551    **Fax:** (202)782-3114
Col. E.T. Takafuji, Commander

**Activities/Fields:** Biologically-active substances such as bacteria, viruses, biological and chemical threat agents, and toxic environmental contaminants; trauma and high-energy (wound infections, traumatic organ failure, blood substitutes, laser injury, and high-power microwaves); and stress and performance (combat psychiatric casualties, and sustained operations). Maintains permanent subordinate laboratories in Thailand, Brazil, Kenya, and Germany. Maintains subordinate detachments collocated with Navy or Air Force at Brooks Air Force Base, TX; Wright Patterson Air Force Base, Dayton, OH; and Bethesda Naval Center, MD.

**★ 13479 ★ U.S. Department of Defense Army Medical Research and Materiel Command**
**Walter Reed Army Institute of Research Biochemistry Division**
Steven Sitter Ave.
Washington, DC 20307-5100
**Phone:** (202)782-3001    **Fax:** (202)782-6304
**Website:** http://wrair-www.army.mil/divisions.htm
Bhupendra P. Doctor, Dir.

**Activities/Fields:** Divisional components include the Departments of Biological Chemistry, Applied Biochemistry and Membrane Biochemistry. The Department of Biological Chemistry investigates the use of biological products, such as exogenous cholinesterases, and pharmaceutical products, such as huperzine, as pretreatment drugs for organophosphate exposure. Work also includes studies designed to elucidate the three-dimensional structure of the cholinesterases, the mechannisms of inhibition by reversible nonreversible inhibitors, and the reactivation of cholinesterases by oximes. The Department of Membrane Biochemistry develops liposomes and liposome-adjuvant formulatins, evaluating the immunogenicity of various liposome-adjuvant vaccine formulations, developing method for the manufacture of liposomal vaccines according to current Good Manufacturing Pratices (cGMP) of the U.S. Food and Drug Administration, and using the cGMP methods developed to manufacture liposomal vaccines for use in clinical trials.

**★ 13480 ★ U.S. Department of Defense Army Medical Research and Materiel Command**
**Walter Reed Army Institute of Research Biometrics Division**
Washington, DC 20307-5100
**Phone:** (202)782-3151    **Fax:** (202)782-6950
Lt.Col. John P. Litrio, Dir.

**Activities/Fields:** Provides automation, biomedical engineering, and biostatistics services and support to all elements of the Institute; manages the WRAIR automation program; and advises and provides consultative services on experimental design, data analysis, data processing, systems engineering, and data communications.

**★ 13481 ★ U.S. Department of Defense Army Medical Research and Materiel Command**
**Walter Reed Army Institute of Research Department of Applied Biochemistry**
Washington, DC 20307-5100
**Phone:** (202)782-6361    **Fax:** (202)782-7651
Peter Chiang, Chf.

**Activities/Fields:** Develops novel drugs to treat military diseases or threats and to elucidate the attendant biochemical pharmacology. Focus areas include pharmacology of Anatoxin-A; medical countermeasures for Botulinum Toxin; nerve agent countermeasures advanced anticonvulsants; prevention of military HIV infection; medical countermeasures for physiologically active compounds; and medical countermeasures for Ricin.

**★ 13482 ★ U.S. Department of Defense Army Medical Research and Materiel Command**
**Walter Reed Army Institute of Research Medical Audio-Visual Services Division**
Washington, DC 20307-5100
**Phone:** (202)782-7106    **Fax:** (202)782-2136
Imre L. Toth, Dir.

**Activities/Fields:** Provides medical scientific illustration, medical research photography, motion picture production, and classroom/auditorium support meetings (held at WRAIR) for WRAIR research activities; serves as production agency for medical training films involving medical and/or paramedical subjects.

**★ 13483 ★ U.S. Department of Defense Army Medical Research and Materiel Command**
**Walter Reed Army Institute of Research Medicine Division**
Washington, DC 20307-5100
**Phone:** (202)782-7300    **Fax:** (202)782-0703
Col. Charles E. McQueen, Dir.

**Activities/Fields:** Resolving military medical problems that fall within the general domain of the disciplines of internal medicine through study, laboratory experiments, and consultation. Divisional components include departments of Clinical Physiology, Gastroenterology, Hematology, Medical Research Fellowship, Nephrology, and Respiratory Research. **Pub:** *Proceedings.* • *Research Reports.*

**★ 13484 ★ U.S. Department of Defense Army Medical Research and Materiel Command**
**Walter Reed Army Institute of Research (WRAIR)**
**Preventive Medicine Division**
503 Robert Grant Rd.
Silver Spring, MD 20910
**Phone:** (301)319-9600    **Fax:** (301)319-9104
Col. Patrick W. Kelley, Dir.

**Activities/Fields:** Plans, conducts, and coordinates graduate education programs in the field of military preventive medicine; assists in the production of technical information concerned with this specialty; and designs and conducts epidemiologic studies. Division also provides epidemiologic consultation services. Components of this Division are departments of Advanced Preventive Medicine Studies, Epidemiology, and Field Studies, the Accession Medical Standards Analysis and Research Activity, and the Department of Defense Global Emerging Infections System.

**★ 13485 ★ U.S. Department of Veterans Affairs**
**GI Research Laboratory**
4150 Clement St., 151-M2
San Francisco, CA 94121
**Phone:** (415)750-2095    **Fax:** (415)750-2196
**Email:** youngk@itsa.ucsf.edu
Dr. Young S. Kim, Dir.

**Activities/Fields:** Molecular biology and cell biology, including studies on DNA cloning and sequencing, PCR, vector construction, site-directed mutagenesis, eukaryotic gene transfection, and oncogene and tumor suppressor gene molecular biology.

**★ 13486 ★ U.S. Department of Veterans Affairs**
**Hines Veterans Administration Hospital**
**Midwest Center for Health Services and Policy Research**
151H
PO Box 5000
Hines, IL 60141
**Phone:** (708)202-2414    **Fax:** (708)202-2316
**Email:** weiss@research.hines.med.va.gov
**Website:** http://research.hines.med.va.gov
Kevin Weiss, MD, Dir.

**Activities/Fields:** Conduct relevant, high quality health services research; stimulate health services research and provide technical assistance in its development. Research objectives focus on accountability of the health care delivery system; examination of patient and health system outcomes including utilization, cost, mortality and morbidity, quality; evaluation of continuum of care for veterans with chronic conditions; assessing the effect of VA health care programs and policies on patient outcomes. **Pub:** *Newsletter*, monthly. • *Newsbrief*, quarterly. Newsletter.

**★ 13487 ★ U.S. Department of Veterans Affairs**
**National Center for Post Traumatic Stress Disorder**
Veterans Affairs Medical & Regional Office Center
215 N Main St.
White River Junction, VT 05009-0001
**Phone:** (802)296-5132    **Fax:** (802)296-5135
**Email:** ncptsd@ncptsd.org
**Website:** http://www.ncptsd.org
Matt Friedman, Dir.

**Activities/Fields:** Post Traumatic Stress Disorder, caused by the traumatic stress of war; dangerous peacekeeping operations; interpersonal violence, such as assault, rape, and child abuse; disaster; and severe accidental and violent trauma in the civilian arena.

**★ 13488 ★ U.S. Department of Veterans Affairs**
**National Center for Post-Traumatic Stress Disorder**
**Behavioral Science Division**
VA Medical Center (116B-2)
150 S Huntington Ave.
Boston, MA 02130
**Phone:** (617)232-9500    **Fax:** (617)278-4501
**Email:** andrea.carney@med.va.gov
**Website:** http://www.ncptsd.org
Andrea Carney, Contact

**Activities/Fields:** Develops scientifically validated measures of post-traumatic stress disorder (PTSD), including psychological and psychophysiological procedures, identifies basic mechanisms of PTSD as related to neuroscience, psychological, and behavioral processes, and health-related aspects of stress and trauma.

**★ 13489 ★ U.S. Department of Veterans Affairs**
**National Center for Post-Traumatic Stress Disorder**
**Clinical Neurosciences Division**
VA Medical Center
Psychiatry Service (116A)
950 Campbell Ave.
West Haven, CT 06516
**Phone:** (203)932-5711    **Fax:** (203)937-3481
**Email:** charney.dennis@west-haven.va.gov
**Website:** http://www.ncpsd.org/about/divisions/west_haven/index.html
Dennis Charney, MD, Dir.

**Activities/Fields:** Research on post-traumatic stress syndrome, including the effects of severe stress on brain function and new treatments for trauma victims.

**★ 13490 ★ U.S. Department of Veterans Affairs**
**National Center for Post-Traumatic Stress Disorder**
**Education Division**
VA Palo Alto Health Care System
3801 Miranda Ave.
Palo Alto, CA 94304
**Phone:** (650)493-5000        **Fax:** (650)617-2869
**Email:** fdg@icon.palo-alto.med.va.gov
**Website:** http://www.ncptsd.org/about/divisions/education/index.html
Fred W. Gusman, MSW, Dir.

**Activities/Fields:** Research on post-traumatic stress disorder, including inpatient research protocols, sleep studies, and cross-cultural investigations.


**★ 13491 ★ U.S. Department of Veterans Affairs**
**National Center for Post-Traumatic Stress Disorder**
**Executive Division**
VA Medical Center (116D)
White River Junction, VT 05009
**Phone:** (802)296-5132        **Fax:** (802)296-5135
**Email:** ptsd@dartmouth.edu
**Website:** http://www.ncptsd.org/about/divisions/executive/index.html
Matthew J. Friedman, MD, Exec. Dir.

**Activities/Fields:** Directs the research operations of the Center and its divisions. **Pub:** *PTSD Research Quarterly*, quarterly.


**★ 13492 ★ U.S. Department of Veterans Affairs**
**National Center for Post-Traumatic Stress Disorder**
**Northeast Program Evaluation Center**
VA Connecticut Health Care System (182)
950 Campbell Ave.
West Haven, CT 06516
**Phone:** (203)937-3851        **Fax:** (203)937-3433
**Email:** robert.rosenheck@yale.edu
**Website:** http://www.ncptsd.org/about/divisions/nepec/index.html
Linda Scelfo-Appio, Contact

**Activities/Fields:** Performs evaluation and monitoring of all VA hospital-based posttraumatic stress disorder programs throughout the nation.


**★ 13493 ★ U.S. Department of Veterans Affairs**
**National Center for Post-Traumatic Stress Disorder**
**Pacific Islands Division**
1132 Bishop St., Ste. 307
Honolulu, HI 96813
**Phone:** (808)566-1546        **Fax:** (808)566-1885
**Email:** kay.winona@honolulu.va.gov
**Website:** http://www.ncptsd.org/about/divisions/pacific/index.html
Winona Kay, Contact

**Activities/Fields:** Research on cross-cultural factors affecting the expression, assessment, and treatment of PTSD among ethnic minorities, particularly Pacific Islander and Asian Americans.


**★ 13494 ★ U.S. Department of Veterans Affairs**
**National Center for Post-Traumatic Stress Disorder**
**Women's Health Sciences Division**
VA Boston Health Care System
150 S Huntington St.
Boston, MA 02130
**Phone:** (617)232-9500        **Fax:** (617)278-4515
**Email:** dorsey.cheryl@boston.va.gov
**Website:** http://www.ncptsd.org/about/divisions/womens/index.html
Peggy Shea, Prog. Asst.

**Activities/Fields:** Research on the psychological impact of military service on women veterans, including the effect of post-traumatic stress disorder on women's health and medical problems.


**★ 13495 ★ U.S. Department of Veterans Affairs**
**Rehabilitation Research and Development Center**
VA Medical Center (153)
3801 Miranda Ave.
Palo Alto, CA 94304
**Phone:** (650)493-5000        **Fax:** (650)852-3474
**Email:** zajac@roses.stanford.edu
**Website:** http://www.palo-alto.med.va.gov/programs.htm
James Golf, Dir.

**Activities/Fields:** State-of-the-art technological aids and treatments for disabled veterans to improve their independence and quality of life, especially in their mobility. Specific research areas include orthopedic biomechanics, neuromuscular systems, human-machine integration, fracture healing and implant design, skeletal biology and physical activity, coordination of human movement, surgery simulation, neuromuscular diagnosis and repair, robotics, patient-handling, functional assessment, and technology transfer. **Pub:** *Conference proceedings.* • *Progress Report.*


**★ 13496 ★ U.S. Department of Veterans Affairs**
**Rehabilitation Research and Development Center**
**Design Development**
**Laboratory of Neuromuscular Biomechanics**
VA Medical Center
3801 Miranda Ave.
Palo Alto, CA 94304-1530
**Phone:** (650)493-5000        **Fax:** (650)493-4919
Christopher Jacobs, Dir.

**Activities/Fields:** Supports research on coordination of human lower extremity muscles during functional activities, such as standing, walking, and pedaling in able-bodied and disabled persons.


**★ 13497 ★ U.S. Department of Veterans Affairs**
**Rehabilitation Research and Development Center**
**Design Development**
**Laboratory of Neuromuscular Electrophysiology**
3801 Miranda Ave.
Palo Alto, CA 94304-1200
**Phone:** (650)493-5000        **Fax:** (650)493-4919
Christopher Jacobs, Dir.

**Activities/Fields:** Human neuromuscular electrophysiology data. Laboratory activities center around devices used to stimulate and record from both nerve and muscle tissue, and the associated computer peripheral devices to collect, analyze, and record this data.


**★ 13498 ★ U.S. Department of Veterans Affairs**
**Veterans Health Administration**
**Office of Research and Development**
U.S. Department of Veterans Affairs
810 Vermont Ave., NW
Washington, DC 20420
**Phone:** (202)273-8284        **Fax:** (202)273-6526
**Email:** david.thomas@mnil.va.gov
**Website:** http://www.va.gov/resdev/
John R. Feussner, MD, Chf. Res. Off.

**Activities/Fields:** Provides funding for intramural research performed by individual investigators at VA medical centers throughout the United States. These investigators are staff at the medical centers (physicians, basic scientists, nurses, dentists, psychologists, etc.) who apply for research funds from the Central Office of Research and Development through the medical centers' research and development committees. **Pub:** *Journal of Rehabilitation*, semimonthly.


**★ 13499 ★ U.S. Department of Veterans Affairs**
**Veterans Health Administration**
**Office of Research and Development**
**Health Services Research and Development Service**
**(Service Directed Research Program)**
810 Vermont Ave. NW
Washington, DC 20240
**Fax:** (202)273-6526

**Activities/Fields:** Addresses health care issues relating to the veteran population, the VA's system of health care networks, and the nation as a whole. Research projects are conducted in response to mandates and requests from a variety of constituencies, including Congress, federal agencies, the Secretary of Veterans Affairs and other VA administrators.


**★ 13500 ★ U.S. Department of Veterans Affairs**
**Veterans Health Administration**
**Office of Research and Development**
**Health Services Research and Development Service**
**(Investigator Initiated Research Program)**
810 Vermont Ave. NW
Washington, DC 20240
**Fax:** (202)273-6526

**Activities/Fields:** Supports VA-funded health services research projects related to health care outcomes, access to care, cost and cost-effectiveness, assessment and assurance of quality, alternative organizational and delivery models, and development of new research methods and measurement tools.


**★ 13501 ★ U.S. Department of Veterans Affairs**
**Veterans Health Administration**
**Office of Research and Development**
**Health Services Research and Development Service**
**(Management Decision and Research Center)**
VA Medical Center (152M)
150 S Huntington Ave.
Boston, MA 02130
**Phone:** (617)278-4433        **Fax:** (617)278-4438
**Email:** MDRC.Boston@med.va.gov
Martin P. Charns, DBA, Dir.

**Activities/Fields:** Research associated with the organization and management of healthcare services.


**★ 13502 ★ U.S. Department of Veterans Affairs**
**Veterans Health Administration**
**Office of Research and Development**
**Health Services Research and Development Service**
**(Center for the Study of Healthcare Provider Behavior)**
Sepulveda Campus/VA Greater Los Angeles Healthcare System
16111 Plummer St. (152)
Sepulveda, CA 91343
**Phone:** (818)895-9449        **Fax:** (818)895-9559
**Email:** lisar@rand.org
Lisa V. Rubenstein, MD, Dir.

**Activities/Fields:** Research on provider behavior and practice patterns, health care quality and outcomes, quality improvement, clinical practice guideline implementation, and primary care/managed care evaluation.

**★ 13503 ★ U.S. Department of Veterans Affairs**
**Veterans Health Administration**
**Office of Research and Development**
**Health Services Research and Development Service**
**(Northwest Center for Outcomes Research in Older Adults)**
VA Puget Sound Health Care System
1660 S Columbia Way
Seattle, WA 98108
**Phone:** (206)764-2430    **Fax:** (206)764-2935
**Email:** sfihn@u.washington.edu
**Website:** http://www.hrsd.seattle.med.va.gov
Stephan D. Fihn, MD, Contact
**Activities/Fields:** Research on the care of the aging, veteran, ambulatory care, outcome research, and disease prevention/health promotion.

**★ 13504 ★ U.S. Department of Veterans Affairs**
**Veterans Health Administration**
**Office of Research and Development**
**Health Services Research and Development Service**
**(Center for Chronic Disease Outcomes Research)**
VA Medical Center (152/2E)
1 Veterans Dr.
Minneapolis, MN 55417
**Phone:** (612)725-1979    **Fax:** (612)727-5699
**Email:** joanne.karvonen@med.va.gov
Dr. Hanna B. Rubins, MD, MP, Dir.
**Activities/Fields:** Research on the delivery and accessibility of high quality, cost-effective health care for veterans with chronic disease, including health care interventions that improve outcomes for persons with chronic illnesses, evidence-based practice for improved outcomes in chronic disease, and innovative models for managing chronic disease within an integrated service network.

**★ 13505 ★ U.S. Department of Veterans Affairs**
**Veterans Health Administration**
**Office of Research and Development**
**Health Services Research and Development Service**
**(Center for Mental Healthcare and Outcomes Research)**
Central Arkansas Veteran's Health Care System
2200 Fort Roots Dr.
North Little Rock, AR 72114
**Phone:** (501)257-1710    **Fax:** (501)257-1707
**Email:** owenrichardr@uams.edu
Dr. Richard R. Owen, Dir.
**Activities/Fields:** Research on improving mental health care through the development, implementation, and dissemination of policy-relevant and clinically-relevant health services research, including cognitive impairment, cormobidity, depression, schizophrenia, and substance abuse.

**★ 13506 ★ U.S. Department of Veterans Affairs**
**Veterans Health Administration**
**Office of Research and Development**
**Health Services Research and Development Service**
**(Center for Health Services Research in Primary Care)**
VA Medical Center (152)
508 Fulton St.
Durham, NC 27705-3897
**Phone:** (919)286-6936    **Fax:** (919)416-5836
**Email:** Oddone.Eugene@durham.va.gov
**Website:** http://hsrd.durham.med.va.gov/hsr&d/default.htm
Eugene Z. Oddone, MD, Dir.

**Activities/Fields:** Research on strategies that enhance the delivery, quality, and efficiency of primary care for veterans, including ambulatory care, women's health, geriatrics, and epidemiology of chronic diseases.

**★ 13507 ★ U.S. Department of Veterans Affairs**
**Veterans Health Administration**
**Office of Research and Development**
**Medical Research Service**
**(Environmental Hazards Research Center )**
VA Medical Center, 116B-4
150 S Huntington Ave.
Boston, MA 02130
**Phone:** (617)278-4517    **Fax:** (617)278-4448
**Email:** rwhite@bu.edu
Roberta F. White, PhD, Dir.
**Activities/Fields:** Research on behavioral toxicology.

**★ 13508 ★ U.S. Department of Veterans Affairs**
**Veterans Health Administration**
**Office of Research and Development**
**Medical Research Service**
**(Alcoholism Research Center )**
VA Connecticut Health Care System
950 Campbell Ave.
West Haven, CT 06516
**Phone:** (203)937-4790    **Fax:** (203)937-3468
John Harrison Krystal, MD, Dir.
**Activities/Fields:** Research on the neurobiology, genetics, and pharmacology of alcoholism.

**★ 13509 ★ U.S. Department of Veterans Affairs**
**Veterans Health Administration**
**Office of Research and Development**
**Medical Research Service**
**(AIDS Research Center )**
VA San Diego Health Care System
3350 La Jolla Village Dr.
San Diego, CA 92161
**Phone:** (858)552-7439    **Fax:** (858)552-7445
**Email:** drichman@ucsd.edu
Douglas Richman, MD, Dir.
**Activities/Fields:** Research on the molecular pathogenesis of HIV, as well as vaccines and chemotherapy.

**★ 13510 ★ U.S. Department of Veterans Affairs**
**Veterans Health Administration**
**Office of Research and Development**
**Medical Research Service**
**(AIDS Research Center )**
VA Medical Center
508 Fulton St.
Durham, NC 27705
**Phone:** (919)286-0411    **Fax:** (919)286-0441
Dr. John Hamilton, MD, Contact
**Activities/Fields:** Molecular and cellular characterization of HIV and related pathogens, including vaccine development, HIV gene regulation, virulence factors and common opportunistic infections in HIV-infected persons.

**★ 13511 ★ U.S. Department of Veterans Affairs**
**Veterans Health Administration**
**Office of Research and Development**
**Medical Research Service**
**(Schizophrenia Research Center)**
Brockton VA Medical Center
940 Belmont St.
Brockton, MA 02301-5568
**Phone:** (508)583-4500    **Fax:** (508)586-0894

**Email:** robert.mccarley@med.va.gov
Dr. Robert McCarley, MD, Dir.
**Activities/Fields:** Research directed toward understanding the pathophysiology, clinical characteristics, and treatment of schizophrenia, including the role stress plays in the pathophysiology of schizophrenia, brain tissues studies to evaluate glutamatergic transmission in schizophrenics, the efficacy of dycyloserine on treating the symptoms of schizophrenia, and Magnetic Resonance Imaging (MRI) projects to evaluate activity in the brain.

**★ 13512 ★ U.S. Department of Veterans Affairs**
**Veterans Health Administration**
**Office of Research and Development**
**Medical Research Service**
**(Schizophrenia Research Center)**
VA Connecticut Health Care System
950 Campbell Ave.
West Haven, CT 06516
**Fax:** (203)937-3878
Robert Innis, PhD, Dir.
**Activities/Fields:** Research on the clinical study of antipsychotic drugs in schizophrenia, including schizophrenia pathophysiology, abnormal chemical transmission in the brain, cellular neuroscience, neuroimaging, and clinical drug trials aimed at improving treatment for patients with schizophrenia.

**★ 13513 ★ U.S. Department of Veterans Affairs**
**Veterans Health Administration**
**Office of Research and Development**
**Rehabilitation and Development Service**
**(Center for Rehabilitative Auditory Research)**
VA Medical Center
3710 SW U.S. Veterans Hosp. Rd.
R&D-NCPAR
Portland, OR 97207
**Phone:** (503)220-8262    **Fax:** (503)220-3439
**Email:** stephen.fausti@med.va.gov
**Website:** http://www.ncrar.gov
Stephen A. Fausti, PhD, ACCE & Dir.
**Activities/Fields:** Research on alleviating the communicative, social, and economic problems caused by auditory system impairment. **Pub:** *The Hearing Journal.* • *Journal Rehabilitation Research and Development (JRRD).* • *Journal of the International Neurophysical Society.* • *Journal of Speech and Hearing Research.* • *Newsletter*, quarterly. **Frmly:** (2000) Center for Rehabilitative Auditory Research.

**★ 13514 ★ U.S. Department of Veterans Affairs**
**Veterans Health Administration**
**Office of Research and Development**
**Rehabilitation and Development Service**
**(Center for Mobility)**
3801 Miranda Ave., MS-153
Rehabilitation Research & Development Center
Palo Alto, CA 94304
**Phone:** (650)493-5000    **Fax:** (650)493-4919
**Email:** cjacobs@roses.stanford.edu
**Website:** http://guide.stanford.edu
Christopher R. Jacobs, PhD, Dir.
**Activities/Fields:** The Clinical Emphasis of the Center is to improve mobility, either ambulation or manipulation, in individuals with Neurologic Impairments or Orthopaedic Impairments. We specifically target four conditions that cause significant loss of mobility to veterans and non-veterans alike: Stroke, Spinal Cord Injury, Arthritis, and Osteoporosis.

**★ 13515 ★ U.S. Department of Veterans Affairs**
**Veterans Health Administration**
**Office of Research and Development**
**Rehabilitation and Development Service**
**(Center for Healthy Aging with Disabilities)**
VA Medical Center (39B)
2002 Holcombe Blvd.
Houston, TX 77030
**Phone:** (713)794-7254　　**Fax:** (713)794-7623
**Email:** ams@bcm.tmc.edu
**Website:** http://VARehab.bcm.tmc.edu
Arthur M. Sherwood, PhD, Dir.

**Activities/Fields:** The Center of Excellence on Healthy Aging with Disabilities (CHAD) has as its mission the understanding of the process of aging with disabilities in the design, implementation and evaluation of strategies to enhance health, functioning and well-being of veterans aging with disabilities.

**★ 13516 ★ U.S. Department of Veterans Affairs**
**Veterans Health Administration**
**Office of Research and Development**
**Rehabilitation and Development Service**
**(Center for Functional Electric Stimulation)**
11000 Cedar Ave., Ste. 230
Cleveland, OH 44106-3052
**Phone:** (216)231-3257　　**Fax:** (216)231-3258
**Email:** info@fesc.org
**Website:** http://www.fesc.org
P. Hunter Peckham, PhD, Dir.

**Activities/Fields:** Research on Functional Electrical Stimulation (FES), a technology that relies on controlled electric current to activate paralyzed muscles and plays a critical role in returning full or partial physical function to disabled persons.

**★ 13517 ★ Veterans Research Foundation**
921 NE 13th St.
Oklahoma City, OK 73104-5028
**Phone:** (405)270-5170　　**Fax:** (405)297-5911
**Activities/Fields:** Biomedical research for veterans.

## Federal Government Agencies

★ **13518** ★ **U.S. Department of Health and Human Services**
**National Institutes of Health (NIH)**
**National Institute of Arthritis and Musculoskeletal and Skin Diseases (NIAMS)**
9000 Rockville Pike
Bethesda, MD 20892
**Phone:** (301)496-4353
**Website:** http://www.nih.gov/niams/
Steven I. Katz, MD, Director
**Desc:** The Institute supports research into the causes, treatment, and prevention of arthritis and musculoskeletal and skin diseases; the training of basic and clinical scientists to carry out this research; and the dissemination of information on research progress in these diseases.

## Foundations & Other Funding Organizations

### Private Foundations

**Nora Eccles Treadwell Foundation**
*See:* Entry 4919

**RGK Foundation**
*See:* Entry 613

★ **13519** ★ **Robert W. Wilson Foundation**
520 83rd St., Ste. 3R
Brooklyn, NY 11209
**Phone:** (718)748-6113
**Email:** jhampton@rgkfoundation.org
**Website:** http://www.rgkfoundation.org
Robert Wilson, Trustee
**Fnded:** 1992. **Priorities:** *Arts & Humanities:* 15%. Supports museums, libraries, music, and art foundations. *Education:* 1%. *International:* 4%. Medical research and deafness receive funding. *Note:* Total contributions made in 1999. **Typ. Recipients:** Arthritis, Clinics/Medical Centers, Emergency/Ambulance Services, Health-General, Medical Research, Mental Health, Multiple Sclerosis, People with Disabilities, Single-Disease Health Associations, Speech & Hearing, Substance Abuse. **Geo. Dist:** Washington, DC; Bronx, NY; New York, NY; Roseburg, OR; Arlington, VA.

## Corporate Foundations

**Bandai Foundation**
*See:* Entry 11694

**Boswell Foundation, Inc.**
*See:* Entry 897

★ **13520** ★ **Copolymer Foundation**
PO Box 2591
Baton Rouge, LA 70821
**Phone:** (225)267-3400          **Fax:** (225)267-3623
Larry Powell, Chairman, President & Chief Executive Of
**Priorities:** *Arts & Humanities:* 15%. Primarily for arts funds, symphonies, and public broadcasting. *Civic & Public Affairs:* 11%. Community foundations. *Education:* 26%. Colleges, universities, and scholarship funds. *Environment:* 42%. Focus on United Way. *International:* 6%. Primarily supports single-disease health associations. *Note:* Total contributions in fiscal 1999. **Typ. Recipients:** Arthritis, Cancer, Child Abuse, Domestic Violence, Hospices, Medical Research, Single-Disease Health Associations. **Geo. Dist:** LA.

**Dickson Foundation**
*See:* Entry 998

## Other Funding Organizations

★ **13521** ★ **Amyotrophic Lateral Sclerosis Association (ALSA)**
27001 Agoura Rd. Ste. 150
Calabasas Hills, CA 91301-5104
**Phone:** (818)880-9007          **Free:** 800-782-4747
**Fax:** (818)880-9006
**Email:** alsinfo@alsa-national.org
**Website:** http://www.alsa.org
Michael W. Havlicek, Pres. /CEO
**Desc:** Patients; relatives and friends of patients; doctors, neurologists, physical therapists, nurses, and professional organizations dedicated to finding the cause, prevention, and cure for amyotrophic lateral sclerosis (ALS). Offers help and information to ALS patients and their families. Funds ALS-specific research at major medical institutions. Works with other agencies, including the government, to increase their involvement on a priority basis in ALS research. Conducts patient meetings. **Awards:** Grant (annual) for ALS research.

★ **13522** ★ **Benign Essential Blepharospasm Research Foundation (BEBRF)**
PO Box 12468
Beaumont, TX 77726-2468
**Phone:** (409)832-0788          **Fax:** (409)832-0890
**Email:** bebrf@ih2000.net
**Website:** http://www.blepharospasm.org/
Bob Campbell, Contact
**Desc:** Victims of benign essential blepharospasm (BEB), a rare disorder of unknown cause characterized by an involuntary forcible closure of the eyelids. Purpose is to undertake, promote, and develop research into the cause and cure of BEB and related disorders and infirmities of the facial musculature, such as Meige's Syndrome (involving muscle spasms of the eyes, lower face, mouth, tongue, throat, and respiratory system). Seeks to foster public awareness of the disorder in order to guarantee detection at the onset of symptoms. Encourages continuity and cooperation among neurologists, neuro-ophthalmologists, ophthalmologists, plastic surgeons, psychologists, psychiatrists, and other medical professionals in rendering correct diagnoses, implementing effective treatment, improving surgical procedure, and discovering a cure. Organizes seminars, clinical studies, and other programs in continuing education; sponsors fundraising activities. Endeavors to locate sufferers of the disorder and to compile data in order to determine the incidence of BEB and to advise on available treatment. Carries out research activities in areas such as brain tissue collection and experimental treatments. **Awards:** Grant (annual) for research.

**Dystonia Medical Research Foundation**
*See:* Entry 13870

★ **13523** ★ **Facioscapulohumeral (FSH) Society**
3 Westwood Rd.
Lexington, MA 02420
**Phone:** (781)860-0501          **Fax:** (781)860-0599
**Email:** info@fshsociety.org
**Website:** http://www.fshsociety.org
Daniel Paul Perez, Pres.
**Desc:** Individuals, families, and medical and business professionals interested in Facioscapulohumeral Muscular Dystrophy. (FSHD is an inheritable disease that causes a progressive loss of skeletal muscle with weakness of facial, scapular, and upper arm muscles.) Promotes research, solicits contributions and grants, and disperses information on FSHD. Offers support groups, acts as clearinghouse for researchers, clinicians and patients to facilitate participation in FSHD studies. Funds Research on FSHD. **Awards:** Marjorie Bronfman Grant (semiannual) FSHD research; 1 Delta Railroad Construction Fellowship (annual) FSHD Research.

★ **13524** ★ **Forward Face**
317 E 34th St.. Ste. 901A
New York, NY 10016
**Phone:** (212)684-5860          **Free:** 800-FWD-FACE
**Fax:** (212)684-5864
**Website:** http://www.forwardface.org/
Pam D'Elia, Admin. Coor.
**Desc:** Individuals with craniofacial disorders, their families and friends, and health care professionals. Provides medical, psychological, and financial support services. Facilitates communication and cooperation between patients and health care professionals; operates referral service. Offers workshops; conducts

networking activities and children's services; Also includes a support group, Inner Faces, specifically for teenagers and young adults; activities include communications workshops theatre productions and social functions. Operates family assistance fund to assist families with expenses not covered by insurance, such as lodging and transportation. **Awards:** Forward Face (annual) for members; The John McNeil Burns Scholarship (annual) for educational purposes.

### ★ 13525 ★ Foundation for Hand Research and Education
8501 Harcourt Rd.
PO Box 80434
Indianapolis, IN 46280-0434
**Phone:** (317)471-4340          **Free:** 800-888-HAND
**Fax:** (317)876-0462
**Email:** information@indianahandcenter.com
**Website:** http://www.indianahandcenter.com
Elaine Skopelja, MALS, Fnd. Mgr.

**Desc:** Promotes the advancement of hand surgery and research. Aims to improve the quality of life of persons with injuries or disorders of the hands and upper extremities. Conducts educational programs. **Awards:** Research Grant (annual) board certified hand surgeons engaged in research.

### ★ 13526 ★ Myasthenia Gravis Foundation of America
5841 Cedar Lake Rd., Ste. 204
Minneapolis, MN 55416
**Phone:** (952)545-9438          **Free:** 800-541-5454
**Fax:** (952)545-6073
**Email:** myastheniagravis@msn.com
**Website:** http://www.myasthenia.org
Debora K. Boelz, CEO

**Desc:** Persons suffering from myasthenia gravis; their families, doctors, and nurses; others dedicated to the detection, treatment, and cure of MG. Raises funds for research and for professional and public education programs. Provides literature. Lay and professional materials available upon request. **Awards:** Henry R. Viets Students Medical Students Fellowships (annual); Nurse's Fellowship (annual) for research related to myasthenia gravis; Postdoctural Research Grants (annual).

### ★ 13527 ★ National Association for Pseudoxanthoma Elasticum (NAPE)
8764 Manchester Rd., Ste. 200
Saint Louis, MO 63144
**Phone:** (314)962-0100          **Fax:** (314)962-0100
**Email:** pxenape@estreet.com
**Website:** http://www.pxenape.org
Frances Benham, PhD, Board Chair

**Desc:** People who have Pseudoxanthoma Elasticum (PXE), as well as interested others(Pseudoxanthoma elasticum is a rare connective tissue disorder that can affect eyes, skin, and organs). Provides educational information about PXE. Compiles statistics. Serves to unite PXE patients with professionals who treat the disease and others who have the disease. Maintains database of patients with PXE. **Awards:** Grant to scientists studying PXE; monetary to finance low-vision devices for affected members.

### ★ 13528 ★ National Marfan Foundation (NMF)
382 Main St.
Port Washington, NY 11050
**Phone:** (516)883-8712          **Free:** 800-862-7326
**Fax:** (516)883-8040
**Email:** support@marfan.org
**Website:** http://www.marfan.org
Karen Wolk, CSW, Dir. Support Svcs.

**Desc:** Persons affected with the Marfan syndrome and related connective tissue disorders; families of affected persons; genetic counselors; cardiologists, ophthalmologists, orthopedists, and other medical professionals. (Marfan syndrome is a heritable disorder of the connective tissue affecting the skeleton, lungs, eyes, heart, and blood vessels.) Objectives are to: dissemi-

nate accurate and timely information on Marfan syndrome; act as support network and provide a means for patients and relatives to share experiences; improve medical care. Supports and fosters research. **Awards:** NMF Research Grant (annual) for basic and clinical research on Marfan Syndrome and related connective tissue disorders.

### ★ 13529 ★ North American Spine Society (NASS)
22 Calendar Ct., 2nd Fl.
La Grange, IL 60525
**Phone:** (708)588-8080          **Free:** 877-SPI-NEDR
**Fax:** (708)588-1080
**Email:** info@spine.org
**Website:** http://www.spine.org
Eric J. Muehlbauer, Exec. Dir.

**Desc:** Organization of physicians, osteopaths, orthopedists, neurosurgeons, physiatrists, radiologists, and other professionals that advances quality spine care through education, research and advocacy. Works to improve the quality of scientific practice in spinal disorders; exchange ideas and disseminate scientific information about clinical techniques; investigate and propagate methods by which malfunction of the spine can be corrected. Makes inquiries into practice characteristics, language usage and terminology, and treatment methods. **Awards:** Research Grant (annual) quality research on spinal care.

### ★ 13530 ★ OsteoArthritis Research Society International (OARSI)
2025 M St., Ste.800
Washington, DC 20036
**Phone:** (202)367-1177          **Fax:** (202)367-2177
**Email:** oarsi@orsi.org
**Website:** http://www.oarsi.org

**Desc:** Researchers and health care professionals with an interest in osteoarthritis. Seeks to promote and encourage fundamental and applied research on osteoarthritis and its treatment. Gathers and disseminates information on osteoarthritis and related research; sponsors educational programs. **Awards:** OARSI Award in Osteoarthritis Research (annual); Student Scholarship (periodic).

### ★ 13531 ★ Pain Management and Sclerotherapy
5002 E Woodmill Dr.
Wilmington, DE 19808
**Phone:** (302)996-0300          **Free:** 800-471-6114
**Fax:** (302)996-5300
Linda Pavina, Exec. Sec.

**Desc:** Dedicated to improving the practice of and disseminating knowledge about sclerotherapy. (The academy defines sclerotherapy as the stimulation of the formation of fibrous-connective tissues by the body, in a specific location, by the specific application of a sclerosing modality.) The most frequently used modality is the injection of certain medications, known as sclerosants. Primary studies involve the treatment of: unstable joints, venous abnormalities, and tendeno-osseous points of hyper-irritability. Supports research program; maintains speakers' bureau. **Awards:** Scholarship (annual) bestowed to an osteopathic medical student submitting best paper on sclerotherapy; student is invited to present paper at academy convention.

### ★ 13532 ★ PXE International
c/o Sharon F. Terry
23 Mountain St.
Sharon, MA 02067-2234
**Phone:** (781)784-3817          **Fax:** (781)784-6672
**Email:** pxe@pxe.org
**Website:** http://www.pxe.org
Sharon F. Terry, Exec. Dir.

**Desc:** Dedicated to supporting those affected by Pseudoxanthomas elasticum (PXE) and to research into its causes, treatments, and cure. (Pseudoxanthomas elasticum is a heritable connective tissue disorder causing calcification of connective tissue, potentially

affecting the skin, arteries, gastro-intestinal tissue, and the retina.) Provides information and support to patients, their families, and clinicians on diagnosis, effects, and treatment. Through a consortium of researchers worldwide, supports research by providing to researchers monetary grants and samples from its confidential Blood and Tissue Bank. Initiates and conducts epidemiological studies and other research. **Awards:** Excellence in PXE Research (annual) for special contributions to PXE research; grant (periodic).

### ★ 13533 ★ Scleroderma Foundation (SF)
12 Kent Way, Ste. 101
Byfield, MA 01922
**Phone:** (978)463-5843          **Free:** 800-722-4673
**Fax:** (978)463-5809
**Email:** sfinfo@sclerdoma.org
**Website:** http://www.scleroderma.org
Peter Giusti, Exec. Dir.

**Desc:** Scleroderma organizations. Promotes medical research to find a cure for scleroderma, a chronic systemic disease affecting all organs resulting from uncontrolled growth of connective tissue. Seeks to foster an understanding of the disease through media and outreach programs; raises funds. Provides patients with educational materials and referrals to local organizations and medical specialists. Offers encouragement and consultation services towards the formation and development of local support groups. Acts as a clearinghouse for information about scleroderma research, drugs, and therapies. Conducts accredited programs for professionals. Maintains speakers' bureau; compiles statistics. Funds one million dollars a year in new research. **Awards:** Grant (annual) for medical research.

### ★ 13534 ★ Scleroderma Research Foundation (SRF)
2320 Bath St., Ste. 315
Santa Barbara, CA 93105
**Phone:** (805)563-9133          **Free:** 800-441-CURE
**Fax:** (805)563-2402
**Email:** srfcure@srfcure.org
**Website:** http://www.srfcure.org/
Sharon Monsky, Chm.

**Desc:** Seeks to find a cure for scleroderma, a life-threatening and degenerative illness. Funds and facilitates research and public awareness. **Awards:** Thomas Jefferson University Grant for research projects.

### ★ 13535 ★ Sjogren's Syndrome Foundation (SSF)
8120 Woodmont Ave., No. 530
Bethesda, MD 20814
**Phone:** (301)718-0300          **Free:** 800-475-6473
**Fax:** (301)718-0322
**Email:** ssf@sjorgrens.org
**Website:** http://www.sjogrens.com
Author Grayzel, MD, Pres.

**Desc:** Individuals who have Sjogren's Syndrome, xerostomia (dry mouth), or keratoconjunctivitis sicca (dry eyes); specialists, internists, immunologists, rheumatologists, otolaryngologists, opthalmologists, gynecologists, gastroenterologists, pulmonologists, dermatologists, neurologists, urologists, pharmaceutical companies, and dentists. (Sjogren's Syndrome is a disorder marked by dryness of all mucous membranes, resulting from deficient secretion of the glands, particularly the lacrimal and salivary glands, those of the upper respiratory tract, the sweat glands, and the vaginal area. Approximately 50% of Sjogren's Syndrome patients also have rheumatoid arthritis, lupus, or scleroderma.) Objectives are to increase public awareness and medical knowledge about Sjogren's Syndrome, educate patients and their families, and allow patients to share information on coping with the syndrome. Supports research. Sponsors support groups with meetings in which doctors speak on aspects of the syndrome. Compiles statistics. **Awards:** Research Fellowship (annual) for research in the field; Research Grant (periodic).

## Society of Otorhinolaryngology and Head/ Neck Nurses (SOHN)
*See:* Entry 14939

### ★ 13536 ★ Tourette Syndrome Association (TSA)
42-40 Bell Blvd.
Bayside, NY 11361-2820
**Phone:** (718)224-2999      **Fax:** (718)279-9596
**Email:** ts@tsa-usa.com
**Website:** http://www.tsa-usa.org/
Fred Cook, VP

**Desc:** People with Tourette Syndrome (TS) and their families and friends; physicians, nurses, teachers, psychologists, social workers, and other professionals; organizations such as mental health agencies. (TS is characterized by involuntary muscular movements and utterances of sounds or words, and is often undiagnosed or misdiagnosed.) Develops and disseminates educational materials to families, professionals, and agencies involved in health care, education, and governments. Schedules meetings and seminars for professionals and families to explore the latest information on TS. Stimulates support for research into the nature and causes of the disorder. Apprises members of rights, services, and benefits provided by the government and other organizations. Provides lists of doctors experienced in treating the disorder. Operates support groups and other services to help persons with TS and their families. Maintains sources for advocacy referral services in the areas of education, employment, and housing. **Awards:** Permanent Research Fund Award (annual) for research.

## National & International Organizations

### Acoustic Neuroma Association of Canada (ANAC)
*See:* Entry 13884

### ★ 13537 ★ African League Against Rheumatism (ALAR)
Hopital Mongi Slim
2046 La Marsa, Tunisia
**Phone:** 216 1 759360      **Fax:** 216 1 765118
**Email:** anac@compusmart.ab.ca
**Website:** http://www.anac.ca

**Lang(s):** Arabic, English, French. **Desc:** Health care professionals specializing in the treatment of rheumatic diseases. Seeks to improve the diagnosis and treatment of rheumatic disorders. Serves as a forum for the exchange of information among members; sponsors continuing professional development courses; makes available health care services.

### ★ 13538 ★ ALS Diagnostic Support Group
**(Vereniging Spierziekten Nederland — VSN)**
van Heutxzlaan 6
NL-3743 JN Baarn, Netherlands
**Phone:** 31 33 4802016
**Email:** vsn@vsn.nl
**Website:** http://www.vsn.nl

**Fnded:** 1967. **Reg. Groups:** 10. **Desc:** Individuals in The Netherlands affected by Amyotrophic Lateral Sclerosis (ALS), a muscle wasting condition. Provides a forum for support and exchange of information.

### ★ 13539 ★ ALS Support Group - Belgium
**(ALS Zelfhulpgroep Belgie)**
Oulde Gentweg 105
B-8000 Brugge, Belgium
**Phone:** 32 81 655885      **Fax:** 32 81 655885
**Email:** andre.carpels@unicall.be

**Fnded:** 1994. **Desc:** Individuals in Belgium affected by Amyotrophic Lateral Sclerosis (ALS), a muscle wasting condition. Provides a forum for support and exchange of information. **Pub:** Newsletter, periodic.

### ★ 13540 ★ American Autoimmune Related Diseases Association
22100 Gratiot Ave.
East Detroit, MI 48021-2227
**Phone:** (586)776-3900      **Free:** 800-598-4668
**Fax:** (810)776-3903
**Email:** aarda@aol.com
**Website:** http://www.aarda.org
Virginia Ladd, Exec. Dir.

**Fnded:** 1991. **Desc:** Promotes national focus and collaborative efforts among state and national volunteer health groups on autoimmunity, the major cause of serious chronic diseases. Offers research and educational programs; maintains speakers' bureau. **Pub:** *InFocus*, quarterly. Newsletter. *Price:* $24/year.

### ★ 13541 ★ American Back Society (ABS)
2647 International Blvd., Ste. 401
Oakland, CA 94601
**Phone:** (510)536-9929      **Fax:** (510)536-1812
**Email:** info@americanback.org
**Website:**      http://www.americanbacksoc.org/contact.html

**Desc:** Orthopedic and neurological surgeons, physical therapists, chiropractors, and other health care professionals with an interest back and spinal health. Promotes continuing professional development of members; seeks to advance the prevention, diagnosis, and treatment of back and spinal disorders. Serves as a clearinghouse on spinal health; sponsors research and educational programs; facilitates exchange of information among members.

### ★ 13542 ★ American Behcet's Disease Association (ABDA)
PO Box 15247
Chattanooga, TN 37415-0240
**Free:** 800-723-4238
**Email:** shrinkrap2@aol.com
**Website:** http://www.behcets.com
Bettina Bailey, Pres.

**Fnded:** 1986. **Mem:** 1,000. **Local Groups:** 25. **Desc:** Gathers statistics on people with Behcet's syndrome; educates the public and medical community about the disease. (Behcet's syndrome is characterized by painful oral ulcers which often resolve spontaneously, but recur at unpredictable intervals. Other symptons include recurring genital lesions, skin lesions, blurred vision, pain and redness of the eyes, and nervous system abnormalities. The disease is most common among young adults, and methods of treatment are varied and controversial.) Conducts educational programs; maintains speakers' bureau. **Pub:** *ABDA Flame*, biennial. Newsletter. Contains news on research projects, treatments, patients, and organizational activities. *Price:* $35. • *Behcet's Disease and Your Eyes.* Brochure. • *Behcet's Disease and Your Nervous System.* Brochure. • *Behcet's Disease: What You Should Know.* Brochure. • *Only Hope.* Brochure. **Frmly:** (1995) American Behcet's Association.

### ★ 13543 ★ American College of Rheumatology (ACR)
1800 Century Pl., Ste. 250
Atlanta, GA 30345
**Phone:** (404)633-3777      **Fax:** (404)633-1870
**Email:** acr@rheumatology.org
Mark Andrejeski, Exec. VP

**Fnded:** 1934. **Mem:** 8,200. **Desc:** Rheumatologists and rheumatology health professionals. Provides unified leadership in research, education, and the care of people with rheumatic diseases. **Pub:** *ACR Membership Directory*, annual. Membership Directory. *Price:* $10/copy for members; $35/copy for nonmembers. • *ACR Scientific Program*, annual. • *Arthritis and Rheumatism*, monthly. Journal. Covers research and trends in the treatment and investigation in the field. Includes

book reviews, calendar of events, and employment opportunities. *Price:* $90/year for individuals; $115/year for institutions; $45/year for students Agency subscription rates are:; $103.50/year for institutions. • *Arthritis Care and Research*, quarterly. Journal. For health professionals interested in the rheumatic diseases. *Price:* $115 institutions; $60 individuals. **Frmly:** (1989) American Rheumatism Association.

### ★ 13544 ★ American Fibromyalgia Syndrome Association (AFSA)
6380 E Tanque Verde, Ste. D
Tucson, AZ 85715
**Phone:** (520)733-1570
**Website:** http://www.afsafund.org/
Kristin Thorson, Pres.

**Fnded:** 1994. **Desc:** Dedicated to research, education and patient advocacy for fibromyalgia syndrome (FMS) and chronic fatigue syndrome (CFS). Provides phone service "warm line" for patients and physicians. Sponsors information booths at major medical conferences. **Pub:** *AFSA Update*.

### ★ 13545 ★ American Juvenile Arthritis Organization (AJAO)
1330 W Peachtree St.
Atlanta, GA 30309
**Phone:** (404)872-7100      **Free:** 800-283-7800
**Fax:** (404)872-9559
**Website:**      http://24.104.35.17/communities/about_ajao.asp
Stephen Pitts, Contact

**Fnded:** 1980. **Mem:** 3,000. **State Groups:** 58. **Desc:** Parents, health care professionals, and others interested in the problems of juvenile arthritis. Serves as advocate for the needs of those affected by juvenile arthritis. A council of the Arthritis Foundation. **Pub:** *Arthritis in Children*. Brochure. • *Decision Making for Teens*. Brochure. • *Educational Rights for Children with Arthritis: A Manual for Parents*. Manual. • *Kids Get Arthritis, Too*, bimonthly. Newsletter. Covers AJAO activities, current research, legislative topics, and medical and scientific updates. *Price:* $25 for nonmembers; Free, for members. • *When Your Student*. Brochure.

### ★ 13546 ★ American Society for Bone and Mineral Research (ASBMR)
2025 M St. NW, Ste. 800
Washington, DC 20036-3309
**Phone:** (202)367-1161      **Fax:** (202)367-2161
**Email:** asbmr@dc.sba.com
**Website:** http://www.asbmr.org
Joan R. Goldberg, Exec. Dir.

**Fnded:** 1977. **Mem:** 3,100. **Desc:** Physicians, dentists, veterinarians, clinical investigators, and researchers interested in bone and mineral metabolism. Provides placement service. Is a member of FASEB. **Pub:** *Journal of Bone and Mineral Research*, monthly. Journal. • *Primer on the Metabolic Bone Diseases and Disorders of Mineral Metabolism*. • Membership Directory, annual.

### ★ 13547 ★ Arthritis Care (AC)
18 Stephenson Way
London NW1 2HD, United Kingdom
**Phone:** 44 207 3806500      **Fax:** 44 207 3806505
**Email:** lizziee@arthritiscare.org.uk
**Website:** http://www.arthritiscare.org.uk

**Fnded:** 1948. **Mem:** 44,000. **Nat'l Groups:** 3. **Reg. Groups:** 4. **Local Groups:** 620. **Lang(s):** English. **Desc:** Individuals with arthritis and concerned others. Seeks to: increase awareness of the problems associated with rheumatic diseases; disseminate information; establish a nationwide network of branches; improve welfare facilities; provide information, advice and practical aid. Maintains hotels. Provides home-visiting service. **Pub:** *Arthritis News*, bimonthly. Magazine. **Frmly:** British Rheumatism and Arthritis Association.

## ★ 13548 ★ Arthritis Foundation (AF)

PO Box 7669
Atlanta, GA 30357-0669
**Phone:** (404)872-7100 **Free:** 800-283-7800
**Fax:** (404)872-0457
**Website:** http://www.arthritis.org
Mr. Tino Mantello, CEO/Pres.
**Fnded:** 1948. **Mem:** 700,000. **Local Groups:** 71. **Desc:** Seeks to: discover the cause and improve the methods for the treatment and prevention of arthritis and other rheumatic diseases; increase the number of scientists investigating rheumatic diseases; provide training in rheumatic diseases for more doctors; extend knowledge of arthritis and other rheumatic diseases to the lay public, emphasizing the socioeconomic as well as medical aspects of these diseases. **Pub:** *Arthritis Today*, bimonthly. Magazine. Includes research reports and selfhelp tips from readers. *Price:* Included in membership dues. • *Bulletin on the Rheumatic Diseases*, bimonthly. Bulletin. Contains articles on developments in research and management of rheumatic diseases; geared for the nonrheumatologist. *Price:* Free. • *Index of Rheumatology*, annual. **Frmly:** Arthritis and Rheumatism Foundation.

## ★ 13549 ★ Arthritis and Rheumatism Natural Therapy Research Association

Cracoe House Cottage
Cracoe
Skipton BD23 6LB, United Kingdom
**Phone:** 44 1756 730240 **Fax:** 44 1756 730240
**Email:** renewnham@aol.com
**Fnded:** 1994. **Mem:** 220. **Desc:** Seeks to educate people about arthritic diseases. Conducts research into the causes and cures of arthritis. **Pub:** *Arthritis Without Drugs*. Book. • Newsletter, quarterly.

## ★ 13550 ★ Arthritis Society

393 University Ave., Ste. 1700
Toronto, ON, Canada M5G 1E6
**Phone:** (416)979-7228 **Free:** 800-321-1433
**Fax:** (416)979-8366
**Email:** info@arthritis.ca
**Website:** http://www.arthritis.ca/
**Reg. Groups:** 1000. **Desc:** Committed to funding and promoting arthritis research, programs, education, and patient care. Sponsors awareness and fundraising events. Celebrates Arthritis Month every September to increase awareness of the impact of arthritis. **Pub:** *Arthritis News*. Magazine.

## ★ 13551 ★ Arthritis Society of Ireland (ASI)

1 Clanwilliam Sq.
Grand Canal Quay
Dublin 2, Ireland
**Phone:** 353 1 6618188 **Fax:** 353 1 6618261
**Lang(s):** English, Irish. **Desc:** Individuals and organizations with an interest in arthritis. Seeks to improve the quality of life of people with arthritis; promotes advancement in the diagnosis and treatment of arthritis. Serves as a clearinghouse on arthritis, its treatment, and services available to people with arthritis; makes available aids and appliance to make life easier for people with arthritis; conducts educational programs; sponsors children's services; provides financial support to arthritis research programs. **Pub:** *Arthritis News*, quarterly. Newsletter.

## ★ 13552 ★ Arthritis Trust of America (ATA)

7376 Walker Rd.
Fairview, TN 37062-8141
**Phone:** (615)799-1002 **Fax:** (615)799-1002
**Email:** administration@arthritistrust.org
**Website:** http://www.arthritistrust.org
Perry A. Chapdelaine, Sr., Contact
**Fnded:** 1982. **Mem:** 30,000. **Desc:** Seeks to eradicate rheumatoid diseases, numbering about 100. Promotes research, physician referral list, publications, website, and explanation of true causes of the diseases, including osteoarthritis and related diseases. **Pub:**
*Arthritis*. Book. • *The Arthritis Trust Newsletter*, quarterly. Newsletter. **AKA:** Rheumatoid Disease Foundation.

## ★ 13553 ★ Asia Pacific League of Associations for Rheumatism (APLAR)

Department of Medicine
Prince of Wales Hospital
Chinese University of Hong Kong
Hong Kong, People's Republic of China
**Lang(s):** Chinese, English. **Desc:** Health care professionals with an interest in rheumatism. Seeks to advance the prevention, diagnosis, and treatment of rheumatism and related disorders. Serves as a clearinghouse on rheumatism; facilitates exchange of information among members; conducts research and continuing professional development programs.

## ★ 13554 ★ Asian Academy of Craniomandibular Disorders (AACD)

Seungwon Bldg. 5F, Apt. 1699-2
Seocho-Dong
Seocho-ku
Seoul 137-070, Republic of Korea
**Lang(s):** English, Korean. **Desc:** Health care professionals with an interest in craniomandibular disorders. Seeks to advance the prevention, diagnosis, and treatment of craniomandibular maladies. Serves as a clearinghouse on craniomandibular abnormailities and diseases; sponsors research and continuing professional development programs.

## ★ 13555 ★ Asian Association for Dynamic Osteosynthesis (AADO)

c/o Orthopedic Learning Centre
1/F Li Ka Shing Specialist Clinics
Prince of Wales Hospital
Shatin
Hong Kong, People's Republic of China
**Phone:** 852 26323482 **Fax:** 852 26477432
**Email:** secretariat@aado.org
**Website:** http://www.aado.org
**Lang(s):** Chinese, English. **Desc:** Health care professionals with an interest in osteosynthesis. Seeks to advance the study, teaching, and practice of dynamic osteosynthesis; promotes professional development of members. Serves as a clearinghouse on osteosynthesis; sponsors research and educational programs.

## ★ 13556 ★ Asociacion Distrofia Muscular

Cordoba 5824
1414 Buenos Aires, Argentina
**Phone:** 54 11 7731714 **Fax:** 54 11 9561471
**Email:** dubro@interactive.com.ar
**Desc:** Individuals in Argentina who work toward the dissemination of information and research concerning muscular dystrophy, a hereditary disease characterized by progressive deterioration of muscles.

## ★ 13557 ★ Asociacion Espanola de Esclerosis Lateral Amiotrofica (ADELA)

C/Hierbabuena No. 12 Bajo
E-28039 Madrid, Spain
**Email:** adlea@readysoft.es
**Website:** http://advernet.es/adela
**Fnded:** 1990. **Reg. Groups:** 3. **Desc:** Individuals in Spain affected by Amyotrophic Lateral Sclerosis (ALS), a muscle wasting condition. Offers home care services. Provides a forum for support and exchange of information.

## ★ 13558 ★ Asociacion Espanola de Esclerosis Multiple (AEDEM)

c/o Francisco Delgado Valcarcel
Modesto Lafuente
8-1 Centro Derecha
E-28010 Madrid, Spain
**Phone:** 34 914 481 261 **Fax:** 34 914 481 261
**Email:** aedem26884@teleline.es
**Fnded:** 1984. **Reg. Groups:** 30. **Desc:** MS patients, families and professionals. Seeks to improve the quality of life for persons with multiple sclerosis and their families.

## ★ 13559 ★ Asociacion Mexicana Contra Esclerosis Multiple

c/o Ian Thomas
Calzada de Tlalpan 4515
14050 Toriello, DF, Mexico
**Phone:** 52 5 550 9987 **Fax:** 52 5616 4509
**Email:** thomasi@infosel.net.mx
**Fnded:** 1984. **Reg. Groups:** 3. **Desc:** MS patients, families and professionals. Seeks to improve the quality of life for persons with multiple sclerosis and their families.

## ★ 13560 ★ Associacao Brasileira de Esclerose Multipla (ABEM)

c/o Collete Levy
Rua Demostenes, 283
04614-011 Sao Paulo, Brazil
**Phone:** 55 11 533 0582 **Fax:** 55 11 533 3542
**Email:** abem@abem.org.br
**Fnded:** 1984. **Mem:** 4,000. **Reg. Groups:** 5. **Desc:** MS patients, families and professionals. Seeks to improve the quality of life for persons with multiple sclerosis and their families; provides social care.

## ★ 13561 ★ Association of Neuromuscular Disorders

Hatboyu cad. No. 12
Yesilkoy
34800 Istanbul, Turkey
**Phone:** 90 212 5730975 **Fax:** 90 212 6630168
**Email:** personalcoskunoz@superonline.com
**Website:** http://www.kashastaliklari.org.tr
**Fnded:** 1978. **Mem:** 1,000. **Reg. Groups:** 5. **Lang(s):** English. **Desc:** Promotes study and research of neurological muscle diseases. Works as a support group for individuals suffering with muscle disorders. Conducts educational programs. **Pub:** *Hope and Life*, quarterly. Journal. Provides information about neuromuscular disorders and activities. • Pamphlets.

## ★ 13562 ★ Association of Rheumatology Health Professionals (ARHP)

1800 Century Pl. Ste. 250
Atlanta, GA 30345
**Phone:** (404)633-3777 **Fax:** (404)633-1870
**Email:** arhp@rheumtalogy.org
**Website:** http://www.rheumatology.org/arhp/
Mark Andrejeski, Exec. VP
**Fnded:** 1965. **Mem:** 1,000. **Nat'l Groups:** 1. **Desc:** Advanced practice nurses, physician assistants, nurses, occupational and physical therapists, social workers, psychologists, vocational counselors, pharmacists, and other health professionals concerned with the practice, education, and research of rheumatic diseases. Seeks to establish a scientific base of knowledge to improve the quality and provision of health services to individuals with rheumatic diseases. Disseminates information regarding the study and treatment of rheumatic diseases. Develops and implements medical and scientific programs in the field of rheumatology. A division of the American College of Rheumatology. **Pub:** *ARHP News*, 4/year. Newsletter. *Price:* Included in membership dues. • *Arthritis Care and Research*, bimonthly. Journal. • *Book for Clinicians*, periodic. Book. Includes research updates. *Price:* Included in membership dues. • *Clinical Care in the Rheumatic Diseases*, periodic. Book. **Frmly:** (1993) Arthritis Health Professions Association.

## ★ 13563 ★ Association Suisse Romande et Italienne Cantre les Myopathies (ASRIM)

Chemin de la Traverse 12
PO Box 179
Aubonne, Switzerland
**Phone:** 41 21 8087411 **Fax:** 41 21 8088111

Email: asrm@planet.ch
Fnded: 1977. Desc: Individuals in Switzerland affected by neuromuscular disorders. Provides a forum for support and exchange of information. Makes available research funding and other financial support.

★ 13564 ★ Associazione Italian Sclerosi
Laterale Amiotrofica (AISLA)
Via Andrea Cost 2/A
I-28100 Novara, Italy
Phone: 39 321 392861　　　Fax: 39 321 392861
Email: segreteria@aisla.it
Website: http://www.aisla.it
Fnded: 1983. Reg. Groups: 11. Desc: Individuals in Italy affected by Amyotrophic Lateral Sclerosis (ALS), a muscle wasting condition. Provides a forum for support and exchange of information. Funds research. Pub: Notiziario AILSA, quarterly. Bulletin.

★ 13565 ★ Associazione Italiana Sclerosi
Multipla (AISM)
c/o Dr. Mario Alberto Battaglia
Vico Chiuso Paggi 3
I-16128 Genova, Italy
Phone: 39 10 27131　　　Fax: 39 10 2470226
Email: aism@aism.it
Website: http://aism.it
Fnded: 1968. Reg. Groups: 86. Desc: MS patients, families and professionals. Seeks to improve the quality of life for persons with multiple sclerosis and their families.

★ 13566 ★ Ataxia-Telangiectasia Society
IACR - Rothamsted
Harpenden AL5 2JQ, United Kingdom
Phone: 44 582 760733　　　Fax: 44 582 760162
Email: atcharity@aol.com
Website: http://www.atsociety.org.uk
Fnded: 1989. Mem: 110. Desc: Seeks to alleviate the suffering caused by Ataxia-Telangiectasia by supporting families, raising awareness of the disease and funding research. Conducts fund-raising activities. Pub: A-T Society News, semiannual. Newsletter.

★ 13567 ★ Australian Rheumatology
Association (ARA)
145 Macquarie St
Sydney, NSW 2000, Australia
Website: http://www.medeserv.com.au/ara/
Lang(s): English. Desc: Physicians who specialize in the assessment and management of musculoskeletal and inflammatory diseases. Promotes rheumatology as a state-of-the-art, evidenced-based discipline and advances research in the field. Supports grant allocating bodies.

Avenues, National Support Group for
Arthrogryposis Multiplex Congenita
See: Entry 4877

★ 13568 ★ Bones Society
6300 N River Rd., Ste. 727
Rosemont, IL 60018-4226
Free: 800-247-9699　　　Fax: (847)823-4921
Email: bones@aaos.org
Website: http://www.bonessociety.org
Fnded: 1969. Mem: 1,400. Desc: Solo practitioners, private group practices and university-affiliated groups of all sizes. Dedicated to the professional development of the orthopaedic practice administrator through educational and research programs and peer interaction.

★ 13569 ★ Brazilian Association of
Amyotrophic Lateral Sclerosis
(Associacao Brasileira de Esclerose
Lateral Amiotrofica)
Rua Pedro de Toledo 377
Sao Paulo, SP, Brazil
Phone: 55 11 8184002　　　Fax: 55 11 8184909
Email: capovila@sup.br
Desc: Individuals in Brazil affected by Amyotrophic Lateral Sclerosis (ALS), a muscle wasting condition. Provides a forum for support and exchange of information. Conducts research into development of multimedia communication systems for patients with severe motor and speech impairments.

★ 13570 ★ British Institute of
Musculoskeletal Medicine
34 The Ave.
Watford WD17 4AH, United Kingdom
Phone: 44 1923 220999　　　Fax: 44 1923 249037
Email: info@bimm.org.uk
Website: http://www.bimm.org.uk
Fnded: 1992. Mem: 360. Desc: Doctors involved in musculoskeletal medicine. Concerned with the furtherance of knowledge and expertise in musculoskeletal medicine which includes treatment of sports injuries, backpain and other conditions of the locomotor system. By osteopathy, injections and other physical modalities. Pub: Journal of Orthopaedic Medicine, quarterly. Journal.

★ 13571 ★ British League Against
Rheumatism (BLAR)
41 Eagle St.
London WC1R 4AR, United Kingdom
Phone: 44 20 72423313　　　Fax: 44 20 72423277
Email: blar@rheumatology.org.uk
Website: http://www.rheumatology.org.uk/dimiral/blar.htm
Fnded: 1972. Mem: 23. Reg. Groups: 15. Desc: Umbrella organization of national societies concerned with rheumatic and musculoskeletal diseases. Has developed patient-centered standards for the care of individuals with arthritis. Conducts audits of current levels of support and care. Aims to raise awareness of the need for high quality services for those with rheumatic and musculoskeletal diseases. Promotes the development of prevention, treatment, rehabilitation, and relief from the disease. Fosters cooperation, understanding, and mutual support between individuals and organizations concerned with rheumatic diseases. Provides a forum for the exchange of ideas and information. Pub: BLAR Purchaser's Pack. Contains guidelines for providing the best service for people with rheumatic diseases. • Disability & Arthritis. Report. Discusses the impact of osteoarthritis and rheumatoid arthritis on quality of life.

★ 13572 ★ Brittle Bone Society
30 Guthrie St.
Dundee DD1 5BS, United Kingdom
Phone: 44 1382 204446　　　Free: 8000 282459
Fax: 44 1382 206771
Email: bbs@brittlebone.org
Website: http://www.brittlebone.org
Fnded: 1971. Mem: 2,000. Nat'l Groups: 1. Desc: Supports research into osteogenesis imperfecta and related conditions. Supplies or identifies alternative sources of accurate information on genetics and other medical issues associated with OI. Pub: Newsletter, quarterly.

★ 13573 ★ Bulgarian Neuromuscular
Disease Association
90 Pilska St., Entr. 2, App. 4
7004 Rousse, Bulgaria
Phone: 359 82 237045　　　Fax: 359 82 452055
Desc: Individuals in Bulgaria affected by Amyotrophic Lateral Sclerosis (ALS), a muscle wasting condition. Provides a forum for support and exchange of information.

★ 13574 ★ Canadian Association of
Friedreich's Ataxia (ACAF)
(Association Canadienne de l'Ataxie de
Friedreich — ACAF)
5620, rue C.A. Jobin
Montreal, QC, Canada H1P 1H8
Phone: (514)321-8684　　　Free: 800-222-3968
Fax: (514)321-2957
Email: acaf@cam.org
Website: http://www.cam.org/~acaf
Fnded: 1972. Mem: 1,500. Local Groups: 2. Lang(s): English, French. Desc: Individuals with Friedreich's Ataxia (a muscular disorder which results in an inability to coordinate voluntary muscular movements). Encourages exchange between families of ataxic persons. Raises funds for medical research; offers social services to victims; recruits volunteer support. Facilitates contact with medical specialists and disseminates information about the disease. Pub: Eldorado, quarterly. Newsletter.

★ 13575 ★ Canadian Ehlers Danlos
Association (CEDA)
86 De Rose Ave.
Bolton, ON, Canada L7E 1A8
Phone: (416)334-2102
Email: office@ceda.ca
Website: http://www.ceda.ca
Fnded: 1996. Reg. Groups: 6. Lang(s): English. Desc: People who suffer from Ehlers-Danlos Syndrome (EDS), their families, and other interested individuals. Works to enhance the lives of all persons affected by EDS. Increases public awareness, provides information resources, works to establish EDS self-help groups. Pub: Newsletter, quarterly.

Canadian Marfan Association (CMA)
See: Entry 9305

★ 13576 ★ Canadian Rheumatology
Association (CRA)
(La Societe Canadienne de Rhumatologie
— SCR)
1560 Sherbrooke St. E
Montreal, QC, Canada H2L 4K8
Phone: (514)876-7131　　　Fax: (514)876-6630
Email: info@marfan.ca
Website: http://www.marfan.ca
Lang(s): English, French. Desc: Rheumatologists, people with rheumatic diseases, and other individuals with an interest in rheumatology. Seeks to advance rheumatological study and practice. Serves as a clearinghouse on rheumatology; sponsors research and educational programs.

★ 13577 ★ Chronic Granulomatous
Disease Association
c/o Mary Hurley
2616 Monterey Rd.
San Marino, CA 91108-1646
Phone: (626)441-4118
Email: cgda@socal.rt.com
Website: http://www.cgdassociation.org
Mary Hurley, Pres.
Fnded: 1982. Desc: Seeks to improve the quality of life of people with chronic granulomatous disease (CGD) and their families (CGD is chracterized by the presence of multiple granulomas, or nodular inflammatory lesions). Provides support and services to people with CGD; assists in the formation of support networks for people with CGD; maintains international registry of CGD patients; compiles statistics. Pub: Newsletter, semiannual. • Brochures.

Coalition For Heritable Disorders Of
Connective Tissue
See: Entry 9311

## ★ 13578 ★ Council of Musculoskeletal Special Societies (COMSS)

c/o Richard B. Welch, MD
6300 N River Rd., Ste. 727
Rosemont, IL 60018-4226
**Phone:** (847)698-1629    **Fax:** (847)823-8125
**Email:** jones@aaos.org
**Website:** http://www.aaos.org/
Richard B. Welch, MD, Ch.

**Desc:** Advocates the interests of its orthopedic specialty societies while promoting and encouraging orthopedic unity among the specialty societies and the American Academy of Orthopedic Surgeons and the American Association of Orthopedic Surgeons.

## ★ 13579 ★ Cyprus Multiple Sclerosis Association

c/o Clelia Petridou
PO Box 26749
Nicosia 1647, Cyprus
**Phone:** 357 2 525053    **Fax:** 357 2 524287
**Email:** multips@logos.cy.net

**Fnded:** 1986. **Mem:** 200. **Reg. Groups:** 1. **Desc:** MS patients, families and professionals. Seeks to improve the quality of life for persons with multiple sclerosis and their families. Provides financial assistance, employment assistance, and organizes support groups. **Pub:** *Is Multiple Sclerosis your Problem?*.

## ★ 13580 ★ Czech Multiple Sclerosis Society

c/o Jaroslav Zika
PO Box 38
CS-120 00 Prague, Czech Republic
**Phone:** 42 2 472 8619    **Fax:** 42 2 667 12511
**Email:** roska@roska-czmss.cz

**Fnded:** 1992. **Reg. Groups:** 30. **Desc:** MS patients, families and professionals. Seeks to improve the quality of life for persons with multiple sclerosis and their families.

## ★ 13581 ★ Danish Multiple Sclerosis Society

c/o Ole A. Busck
Mosedalvej 15
Valby
DK-2500 Copenhagen, Denmark
**Phone:** 45 364 63646    **Fax:** 45 364 63677
**Email:** info@skleroseforeningen.dk

**Fnded:** 1957. **Reg. Groups:** 15. **Local Groups:** 33. **Desc:** MS patients, families and professionals. Seeks to improve the quality of life for persons with multiple sclerosis and their families.

## ★ 13582 ★ Deutsche Gesellschaft fur Muskelkranke

Im Moos 4
D-79112 Freiburg, Germany
**Phone:** 49 7665 94470    **Fax:** 49 7665 944720
**Email:** dgm_bgs@t-online.de
**Website:** http://www.dgm.org

**Fnded:** 1865. **Reg. Groups:** 18. **Desc:** Individuals in Germany affected by Amyotrophic Lateral Sclerosis (ALS), a muscle wasting condition. Provides a forum for support and exchange of information.

## ★ 13583 ★ Deutsche Multiple Sklerose Gesellschaft (DMSG)

c/o Gottfried Milde Staatsminister
Vahrenwalderstr. 205-207
D-30165 Hannover, Germany
**Phone:** 49 511 96 83 40  **Fax:** 49 511 96 83 450
**Email:** dmsg@dmsg.de

**Fnded:** 1952. **Reg. Groups:** 855. **Desc:** MS patients, families and professionals. Seeks to improve the quality of life for persons with multiple sclerosis and their families.

## ★ 13584 ★ Ehlers Danlos National Foundation (EDNF)

6399 Wilshire Blvd., Ste. 203
Los Angeles, CA 90048
**Phone:** (323)651-3038    **Free:** 800-956-2902
**Fax:** (323)651-1366
**Email:** ednfboard@aol.com
**Website:** http://www.ednf.org
Linda Neumann-Potash, Exec. Dir.

**Fnded:** 1985. **Mem:** 1,400. **Local Groups:** 25. **Desc:** Individuals who are affected with Ehlers Danlos Syndrome (EDS); medical professionals involved in the treatment of EDS. (Ehlers Danlos Syndrome, which is named after dermatologists Edward L. Ehlers (1863-1937) and Henri A. Danlos (1844-1912), is an inheritable connective tissue disorder characterized by fragile skin, hypermobile joints, and poor wound healing.) Provides networking among members for communication and support. Local branches and support groups throughout the U.S. provide support, educational material and public awareness to people affected by EDS, their families and health care professionals. **Pub:** *The Facts about Ehlers Danlos Syndrome.* Brochures. Includes the types of Ehlers Danlos Syndrome and Genetic Inheritance Pattern to Ehlers Danlos Syndrome. • *Loose Connections*, quarterly. Newsletter. Includes medical updates on EDS, personal interest stories, local branch information. *Price:* Included in membership dues. • *The Types of Ehlers Danlos Syndrome.* Pamphlets.

## ★ 13585 ★ Esclerosis Multiple Argentina

c/o Vernon R. Dougall
Uriarte 1465/69
1414 Buenos Aires, Argentina
**Phone:** 54 114 831 6617  **Fax:** 54 114 831 6786
**Email:** emarg@dacas.com.ar

**Fnded:** 1968. **Mem:** 950. **Reg. Groups:** 2. **Desc:** MS patients, families and professionals. Seeks to improve the quality of life for persons with multiple sclerosis and their families. Provides self-help groups, physiotherapy, occupational therapy, and home visits.

## ★ 13586 ★ European Alliance of Neuromuscular Disorders Associations (EANDA)

7-11 Prescott Pl.
London SW4 6BS, United Kingdom
**Phone:** 44 171 7208055

**Fnded:** 1971. **Mem:** 33. **Lang(s):** English. **Desc:** Organizations representing people with neurmuscular disorders and health care professionals with an interest in neurological maladies. Seeks to improve the quality of life of people with neuromuscular disorders; promotes advances in the prevention, diagnosis, and treatment of neurological diseases. Facilitates exchange of information among members; serves as a clearinghouse on neuromuscular disorders; sponsors research and educational programs.

## ★ 13587 ★ European Committee for Treatment and Research in Multiple Sclerosis

Vanheylenstr 16
B-1910 Melsbroek, Belgium
**Fax:** 32 2 7518030

## ★ 13588 ★ European Dystonia Federation

69 East King St.
Helensburgh G84 7RE, United Kingdom
**Phone:** 44 143 6678799    **Fax:** 44 143 6678799
**Email:** alanlehg@dystonia.org.uk
**Website:** http://www.dystonia-europe.org

**Fnded:** 1994. **Nat'l Groups:** 12. **Desc:** National dystonia patient support groups of individual countries in Europe.

## ★ 13589 ★ European League Against Rheumatism (EULAR) (Ligue Europeenne Contre le Rhumatisme)

Witikonerstrasse 15
CH-8032 Zurich, Switzerland
**Phone:** 41 1 3839690    **Fax:** 41 1 3839810
**Email:** secretariat@eular.org
**Website:** http://www.eular.org

**Fnded:** 1947. **Mem:** 12,000. **Reg. Groups:** 4. **State Groups:** 3. **Lang(s):** English, French, German. **Desc:** Members of social and scientific organizations and pharmaceutical firms in 40 countries. Maintains small collection of rheumatology journals. **Pub:** *Annals of the Rheumatic Diseases*, monthly. Journal.

## ★ 13590 ★ Evans Syndrome Research and Support Group

c/o Lou Addington
PO Box 290203
Port Orange, FL 32119
**Phone:** (386)322-2656    **Fax:** (386)760-5583
**Email:** lnalou@aol.com
**Website:** http://www.legalnurseassociates.com
Lou Addington, Contact

**Fnded:** 1992. **Desc:** Provides mutual support and ongoing research for parents and concerned friends and caregivers of children with Evans Syndrome. (Evans Syndrome is a rare autoimmune disease.) Facilitates networking and exchange of information. Distributes literature. Developing a group of interested physicians in immunology, genetics, and hematology/oncology. Works to formulate questions for caregivers/patients to ask their doctors.

## ★ 13591 ★ Facioscapulohumeral (FSH) Society

3 Westwood Rd.
Lexington, MA 02420
**Phone:** (781)860-0501    **Fax:** (781)860-0599
**Email:** info@fshsociety.org
**Website:** http://www.fshsociety.org
Daniel Paul Perez, Pres.

**Fnded:** 1992. **Mem:** 1,000. **Reg. Groups:** 6. **Desc:** Individuals, families, and medical and business professionals interested in Facioscapulohumeral Muscular Dystrophy. (FSHD is an inheritable disease that causes a progressive loss of skeletal muscle with weakness of facial, scapular, and upper arm muscles.) Promotes research, solicits contributions and grants, and disperses information on FSHD. Offers support groups, acts as clearinghouse for researchers, clinicians and patients to facilitate participation in FSHD studies. Funds Research on FSHD. **Pub:** *FSH WATCH*, semiannual. Newsletter. Contains updates on FSHD Internationally and cites current research articles. • Also publishes a patient brochure.

## Families of S.M.A. (FSMA)

*See:* Entry 14005

## ★ 13592 ★ Fibromyalgia Association - U.S.A.

PO Box 20408
Columbus, OH 43220
**Email:** fibroUSA@Fibromyalgiaaassnusa.org
**Website:** http://www.fsma.org

**Desc:** Provides the latest research, information about pain management, and other topics about Fibromyalgia (FM). National telephone network, support group network, legal and medical advice, and information on diet and exercise are available to members. **Pub:** Newsletter, quarterly.

## ★ 13593 ★ Finnish MS Society

c/o Anssi Kemppi
Box 15
SF-21251 Masku, Finland
**Phone:** 358 2 439 2111    **Fax:** 358 2 439 2133
**Email:** ms-liitto@ms-liitto.fi

**Mem:** 10,000. **Local Groups:** 70. **Desc:** MS patients, families and professionals. Seeks to improve the quality of life for persons with multiple sclerosis and their families; promotes social justice and equality for members; strives to assist patients to maintain functional capacity in order to live independently. Established the MS Foundation to encourage research in medial and nursing sciences of MS and rare neurological diseases in Finland. **Pub:** *Avain - The Key*, 7/year. Newsletter. • Brochures. Contain information on disease and advice to overcome a handicap.

**★ 13594 ★ Finnish Muscular Diseases Association (FMD)**
Lantinen Pitkakatu 35
SF-2100 Turku, Finland
**Phone:** 358 2 2739700      **Fax:** 358 2 2739701
**Email:** eila.ahokas@lihastautiliitto.fi
**Website:** http://www.lihastautiliitto.fi
**Fnded:** 1972. **Reg. Groups:** 12. **Desc:** Individuals in Finland affected by Amyotrophic Lateral Sclerosis (ALS), a muscle wasting condition. Provides a forum for support and exchange of information. Offers educational programs.

**★ 13595 ★ Foundation for Hand Research and Education**
8501 Harcourt Rd.
PO Box 80434
Indianapolis, IN 46280-0434
**Phone:** (317)471-4340      **Free:** 800-888-HAND
**Fax:** (317)876-0462
**Email:** information@indianahandcenter.com
**Website:** http://www.indianahandcenter.com
Elaine Skopelja, MALS, Fnd. Mgr.
**Fnded:** 1988. **Desc:** Promotes the advancement of hand surgery and research. Aims to improve the quality of life of persons with injuries or disorders of the hands and upper extremities. Conducts educational programs. **Pub:** *Indiana Hand Center Newsletter*, 3/year. Newsletter. Full color descriptions of hand surgery and rehabilitation. *Price:* $75/year. **Frmly:** Indiana Foundation for Hand Surgical Research.

**★ 13596 ★ Greek Multiple Sclerosis Society**
c/o Yiannis Kotsirilos
Vouliagmenis Ave.
GR-16777 Hellenikon, Greece
**Phone:** 30 1 964 4166      **Fax:** 30 1 963 3383
**Email:** mssoc@hol.gr
**Fnded:** 1993. **Mem:** 1,700. **Reg. Groups:** 3. **Desc:** MS patients, families and professionals. Seeks to improve the quality of life for persons with multiple sclerosis and their families. Provides telephone consultations, social advice, psychological treatment, home visits, and physiotherapy.

**★ 13597 ★ Hong Kong Society of Rheumatalogy**
c/o Dr. Emily Kun
Department of Medicine
7A1 PO Hospital
Tai Po
Hong Kong, People's Republic of China
**Phone:** 852 26076907
**Email:** kunwl@ha.org.hk
**Website:** http://www.fmshk.com.hk/hksr
**Fnded:** 1987. **Mem:** 89. **Desc:** Promotes interest in and understanding of rheumatology in Hong Kong. Conduct research in prevention, treatment, and patient care.

**★ 13598 ★ Hungarian Multiple Sclerosis Society**
c/o Central Hospital of County
Fejer Department of Neurology
Seregelyesi ut. 3
H-8001 Szekesfehervar, Hungary
**Phone:** 36 22 316001      **Fax:** 36 22 314198

**Fnded:** 1984. **Mem:** 2,400. **Reg. Groups:** 22. **Desc:** MS patients, families and professionals. Seeks to improve the quality of life for persons with multiple sclerosis and their families. Provides home services.

**★ 13599 ★ International Association of ALS/MND Associations**
PO Box 246
Northampton NN1 2PR, United Kingdom
**Phone:** 44 1604 250505      **Fax:** 44 1604 611852
**Email:** alliance@alsmndalliance.org
**Fnded:** 1992. **Desc:** Umbrella organization for Amyotrophic Lateral Sclerosis (ALS) and Motor Neruone Disease (MND) associations. ALS and MND are muscle-wasting conditions. Provides a forum for support and exchange of information for ALS and MND associations worldwide. **Pub:** Directory.

**International Association of Oral and Maxillofacial Surgeons (IAOMS)**
*See:* Entry 19563

**★ 13600 ★ International Federation of Manual/Musculoskeletal Medicine**
c/o Dr. Michel Dedee
Their Saive 49
B-4608 Warsage, Belgium
**Phone:** 32 4 3766438      **Fax:** 32 4 3766528
**Email:** michel.dedee@skynet.be
**Website:** http://www.fimm-online.org
**Fnded:** 1965. **Mem:** 26. **Nat'l Groups:** 26. **Lang(s):** English, French, German. **Desc:** National organizations of musculoskeletal medicine from countries throughout the world. Promotes scientific research in the field of musculoskeletal medicine. Provides including quality management, education, legal representation in dealing with official authorities.

**International Fibrodysplasia Ossificans Progressiva Association (IFOPA)**
*See:* Entry 9336

**★ 13601 ★ International MS Support Foundation (IMSSF)**
9420 E Golf Links Rd., No. 291
Tucson, AZ 85720-1340
**Email:** together@ifopa.org
**Website:** http://www.msnews.org/
**Desc:** Dedicated to providing support, education and resources to individuals, families and friends of those suffering from Multiple Sclerosis.

**★ 13602 ★ International Myopain Society (IMS)**
c/o Barbara Runnels
PO Box 690402
San Antonio, TX 78269
**Phone:** (210)567-4661      **Fax:** (210)567-6669
**Email:** russell@uthscsa.edu
**Website:** http://www.myopain.org/
Robert M. Bennett, MD, Pres.
**Desc:** Research scientists, physicians, other health care professionals, individuals in training toward a health-related career, institutions, foundations, and commercial companies. Promotes information exchange, research, and education about soft tissue pain syndrome such as myofascial pain syndrome and fibromyalgia syndrome. **Pub:** *Journal of Musculoskeletal Pain*, quarterly. Journal. Devoted to the topic of soft tissue pain.

**International Research Council of Neuromuscular Disorders (IRCND)**
*See:* Entry 14037

**International Skeletal Society (ISS)**
*See:* Entry 18145

**★ 13603 ★ Irish Raynaud's and Scleroderma Society (IRSS)**
PO Box 2958
Foxrock
Dublin 18, Ireland
**Phone:** 353 1 2350900      **Fax:** 353 1 2350900
**Email:** irss@indigo.ie
**Website:** http://www.mdimedia.com/irss
**Fnded:** 1988. **Mem:** 400. **Nat'l Groups:** 1. **State Groups:** 1. **Lang(s):** English, Irish. **Desc:** Individuals and organizations. Seeks to improve the quality of life of people with Raynaud's disease or scleroderma and their families. Promotes better physician-patient communication. Makes available support and services; conducts educational and advocacy campaigns. **Pub:** Newsletter, semiannual.

**★ 13604 ★ Israel Multiple Sclerosis Society**
c/o Michael Sela
75 Yehuda Halevi St.
65796 Tel Aviv, Israel
**Phone:** 972 3 560 9222      **Fax:** 972 3 560 9224
**Fnded:** 1976. **Nat'l Groups:** 1. **Desc:** MS patients, families and professionals. Seeks to improve the quality of life for persons with multiple sclerosis and their families.

**★ 13605 ★ Japan Multiple Sclerosis Society**
c/o Kiyoaki Kikuchi
4-1-2 Kotobuki
Taito-Ku
Tokyo, Japan
**Phone:** 81 3 3847 3504      **Fax:** 81 3 3842 0289
**Fnded:** 1977. **Mem:** 31. **Reg. Groups:** 1. **Desc:** MS patients, families and professionals. Seeks to improve the quality of life for persons with multiple sclerosis and their families. **Pub:** *Seeking your Understanding of and Co-operation with the Japan MS Society (2000)*. • Newsletter.

**★ 13606 ★ Jaw Joints and Allied Musculo-Skeletal Disorders Foundation (JJAMD)**
The Forsyth Institute
140 Fenway
Boston, MA 02115-3799
**Phone:** (617)266-2550      **Fax:** (617)267-9020
**Email:** tmjoints@aol.com
**Website:** http://www.tmjoints.org
Renee Glass; Co-Founder/Pres.
**Fnded:** 1982. **Desc:** Promotes public awareness of temporomandibular joint disorder (TMJ) and related musculoskeletal disorders. Provides information on prevention, treatment, and responsible diagnosis. Conducts research and educational programs; monitors legislative activities. Provides advocacy, networking, patients, professionals, governmental agencies, healthcare, academic, research communities, insurance providers, and support group activities. **Pub:** *Plain Talk Guide to TMJ; with Self-Help Tips to Keep Your Jaw Joints Healthy*. Pamphlet.

**★ 13607 ★ Jennifer Trust for Spinal Muscular Atrophy (JTSMA)**
Elta House
Birmingham Rd.
Stratford-Upon-Avon CV37 0AQ, United Kingdom
**Phone:** 44 1789 267520      **Fax:** 44 1789 268371
**Email:** jennifer@jtsma.org.uk
**Website:** http://www.jtsma.org.uk
**Fnded:** 1985. **Mem:** 1,500. **Lang(s):** English. **Desc:** Offers support information and advice to all those whose lives have been affected by spinal muscular atrophy (SMA).

★ **13608** ★ **Klippel-Trenaunay Support Group (KTSG)**
5404 Dundee Rd.
Edina, MN 55436
**Phone:** (952)925-2596          **Fax:** (612)925-4708
**Email:** contactkt@hotmail.com
**Website:** http://www.k-t.org/
Judy Vessey, Dir.
**Fnded:** 1986. **Mem:** 600. **Desc:** Support group for individuals affected by Klippel-Trenaunay Syndrome and their families. (Klippel-Trenaunay Syndrome is a congenital malformation of the extremities and is characterized by birth marks the color of port wine, excessive growth of the soft tissue and bone, and varicose veins. The cause is presently unknown but believed to be either genetic or the result of an intrauterine insult occuring between the third and sixth week of gestation.) Acts as a clearinghouse of information and correspondence between members. **Pub:** *K-T Newsletter*, quarterly. **AKA:** K-T Support Group.

★ **13609** ★ **L. E. Support Club (LESC)**
8039 Nova Ct.
North Charleston, SC 29420
**Phone:** (843)764-1769          **Fax:** (843)572-9909
**Email:** hbmesic@knology.net
**Website:** http://www.galaxymall.com/commerce/lupus/
Harriet B. Mesic, Dir. & Editor
**Fnded:** 1984. **Desc:** Individuals suffering from lupus erythematosus and other autoimmune diseases; friends and families of patients. Offers emotional support and selfhelp education to lupus patients through newsletters and personal correspondence; provides information on nutrition and medication. **Pub:** *Lupus Beacon*, 5/year. Newsletter. *Price:* Included in membership dues.

★ **13610** ★ **Latvijas Multiplas Sklerozes Asociacijas**
c/o Valerijs Ulmanis
Melidas Str 10
LV-1015 Riga, Latvia
**Phone:** 371 734 0349          **Fax:** 371 734 0341
**Fnded:** 1995. **Mem:** 917. **Reg. Groups:** 5. **Desc:** MS patients, families and professionals. Seeks to improve the quality of life for persons with multiple sclerosis and their families. **Pub:** Newsletter.

★ **13611** ★ **Ligue Francaise Contre la Sclerose en Plaques**
c/o Rene Marteau
40 rue Duranton
F-75015 Paris, France
**Phone:** 33 1 53989880          **Fax:** 33 1 53989888
**Email:** info@lfsep.asso.fr
**Fnded:** 1986. **Mem:** 4,500. **Reg. Groups:** 102. **Desc:** MS patients, families and professionals. Seeks to improve the quality of life for persons with multiple sclerosis and their families.

★ **13612** ★ **Ligue Luxembourgeoise de la Sclerose en Plaques**
c/o Pierre Wagner
Boite Postale 1444
L-1014 Luxembourg, Luxembourg
**Phone:** 352 40 08 44          **Fax:** 352 40 08 04
**Fnded:** 1980. **Mem:** 1,500. **Desc:** MS patients, families and professionals. Seeks to improve the quality of life for persons with multiple sclerosis and their families; offers occupational therapy and gymnastics.

★ **13613** ★ **Ligue Nationale Belge de la Sclerose en Plaques**
av. Eugene Plaskylaan, 173/11
B-1030 Brussels, Belgium
**Phone:** 32 2 736 16 38          **Fax:** 32 2 732 39 59
**Email:** ms.sep@ms-sep.be
**Website:** http://www.ms-sep.be

**Desc:** MS patients, families and professionals. Seeks to improve the quality of life for persons with multiple sclerosis and their families.

★ **13614** ★ **Lupus Foundation of America**
1300 Piccard Dr., Ste. 200
Rockville, MD 20850-4303
**Phone:** (301)670-9292          **Free:** 800-558-0121
**Fax:** (301)670-9486
**Email:** lupusinfo@aol.com
**Website:** http://www.lupus.org
Kathleen Hurley, VP, Finance & Operations
**Fnded:** 1977. **Local Groups:** 94. **Desc:** Works to increase knowledge and public awareness of lupus erythematosus, a noncontagious disease that may affect the skin alone or may manifest itself as a chronic, systemic, and inflammatory disease of the connective tissues. Assists lupus patients and their families, through chapters and patient support groups, to cope with the daily problems associated with lupus. Collects and distributes funds for research. Works to bring lupus to the attention of the public by encouraging the publication of articles on the disease by syndicated medical writers, national magazines, and newspapers, and by obtaining radio and television coverage. Has successfully worked for the establishment of an annual Lupus Awareness Month. Chapters hold patient meetings and occasional medical seminars. **Pub:** *Lupus Erythematosus.* Pamphlet. • *Lupus News*, quarterly. Newsletter. Reports current research both directly and indirectly related to lupus. *Price:* Free. For members only. • Also publishes other informational materials in Braille and Spanish.

★ **13615** ★ **Lupus Information Network (LIN)**
230 Ranch Dr.
Bridgeport, CT 06606-1747
**Phone:** (203)372-5795
**Website:** http://www.lupusinformationnetwork.org
Linda J. Rosinsky, Pres.
**Fnded:** 1985. **Desc:** Educators, medical professionals, and individuals suffering from systemic lupus erythematosus. (Systemic lupus erythematosus is a chronic inflammatory disease of the connective tissue that affects the skin, joints, kidneys, nervous system, and mucous membranes.) Seeks to foster better understanding of the disease among patients, educators, and professionals through the distribution of information, both orthodox and alternative. **Pub:** *Introduction to Lupus.* Brochure. • Pamphlets. • Reprints. **Frmly:** (2001) Lupus Network.

★ **13616** ★ **Lyme Disease Foundation (LDF)**
1 Financial Plaza, 18th Fl.
Hartford, CT 06103
**Phone:** (860)525-2000          **Free:** 800-886-LYME
**Fax:** (860)525-8425
**Email:** lymefnd@aol.com
**Website:** http://www.lyme.org
Karen Vanderhoof-Forschner, Chm. & Pres.
**Fnded:** 1988. **Local Groups:** 200. **Desc:** Seeks to educate medical professionals and the public about Lyme Borreliosis (Lyme disease), which is spread to humans by ticks with symptoms including rashes, joint swelling and pain, fever, severe headaches, and heart arrhythmia. Provides treatment protocols, diagnostic guidelines, and photographic case histories. Assists in the formation of support groups; offers referral service; maintains speakers' bureau. Sponsors medical seminars; provides videotape and slide programs; conducts research. Maintains registry of infected pregnant women and congenital cases. Works in cooperation with Congress, Centers for Disease Control, and National Institutes of Health. **Pub:** *Journal of Spirochetal and Tick Bourne Disease*, quarterly. Journal. *Price:* $75/year. • *Lymelight*, quarterly. Newsletter. *Price:* $30/year. • *Monthly Update. Price:* $50/year. • Pamphlets. **Frmly:** (1992) Lyme Borreliosis Foundation.

★ **13617** ★ **Malignant Hyperthermia Association (MHA)**
Toronto General Hospital
200 Elizabeth St., CCRW-2, Rm. 834
Toronto, ON, Canada M5G 2C4
**Phone:** (416)340-3238          **Fax:** (416)340-4960
**Email:** mha@mhassn.com
**Website:** http://www.mhassn.com
**Fnded:** 1979. **Mem:** 2,000. **Lang(s):** English, French. **Desc:** Individuals with malignant hyperthermia (high fever and muscle rigidity, usually brought on by a reaction to certain anesthetics, to which some individuals are genetically predisposed), their families, and interested health care professionals. Seeks to advance the prevention and treatment of malignant hyperthermia. Conducts research; operates charitable programs; maintains support groups. **Pub:** *Hotline*, semiannual. Newsletter.

★ **13618** ★ **MHE Coalition**
c/o Susan Wynn
8838 Holly Lane
Olmsted Falls, OH 44138
**Phone:** (440)235-6325          **Fax:** (440)427-9032
**Email:** mheandme@yahoo.com
**Website:** http://www.geocities.com/mhecoalition
Chele Zelina, Pres.
**Mem:** 275. **Desc:** Support group for individuals and families affected by Multiple Hereditary Exostoses, encouraging research and services. **Pub:** *MHE Coalition Newsletter*, quarterly. Newsletter.

★ **13619** ★ **Moldavian Myopathy Association**
Str. Bulgar 24
MD-2001 Kishinev, Moldova
**Phone:** 373 2 272687
**Email:** vtonu@mednet.md
**Fnded:** 1996. **Reg. Groups:** 4. **Desc:** Individuals in Moldova affected by neuromuscular disorders. Provides a forum for support and exchange of information.

★ **13620** ★ **Movement Disorder Society**
611 E Wells St.
Milwaukee, WI 53202
**Phone:** (414)276-2145          **Fax:** (414)276-3349
**Email:** info@movementdisorders.org
**Website:** http://www.movementdisorders.org
Caley A. Kleczka, Dir. /Admin.
**Fnded:** 1988. **Desc:** Provides international forums and research to disseminate information on recent advances in clinical and basic science pertinent to movement disorders, enhance education of physicians and public, and enrich the quality of care to patients.

★ **13621** ★ **MS Felag Islands**
c/o Gyda Olafsdottir
Slettluvegur 5
IS-103 Reykjavik, Iceland
**Phone:** 354 568 8620          **Fax:** 354 568 8688
**Email:** msfelag@mmedia.is
**Fnded:** 1968. **Mem:** 600. **Reg. Groups:** 2. **Desc:** MS patients, families and professionals. Seeks to improve the quality of life for persons with multiple sclerosis and their families.

★ **13622** ★ **Multipel Sklerose Forbundet I Norge**
c/o Gerd Hagen
Sorkedalsveien 3
N-0369 Oslo, Norway
**Phone:** 47 22 604960          **Fax:** 47 22 567695
**Email:** msfnorge@c2i.net
**Fnded:** 1966. **Mem:** 4,500. **Reg. Groups:** 45. **Desc:** MS patients, families and professionals. Seeks to improve the quality of life for persons with multiple sclerosis and their families; provides education to persons with MS. Sponsors MS Day. **Pub:** *MS Bladet 2001.* • *MS-En Veiledning For Helsepersonell.*

**★ 13623 ★ Multiple Sclerose Vereniging Nederland (MSVN)**
c/o Nina van 't Hof-Mennink
Bronovolaan Id
Postbus 30470
NL-2500 GL The Hague, Netherlands
**Phone:** 31 70 374 7777   **Fax:** 31 70 374 7770
**Email:** info@msvn.nl
**Website:** http://www.msweb.nl

**Fnded:** 1963. **Mem:** 12,000. **Reg. Groups:** 23. **Desc:** MS patients, families and professionals. Seeks to improve the quality of life for persons with multiple sclerosis and their families.

**★ 13624 ★ Multiple Sclerosis Society of Canada**
250 Bloor St. E, Ste. 1000
Toronto, Canada M4W 3P9
**Phone:** (416)922-6065   **Free:** 800-268-7582
**Fax:** (416)922-7538
**Email:** info@mssociety.ca
**Website:** http://www.mssociety.ca

**Desc:** Seeks to improve the quality of life for persons with multiple sclerosis and their families.

**★ 13625 ★ Multiple Sclerosis Society of India**
c/o N.S. Rao
Samata Sadan, 2nd Fl.
SH. Paralkar Rd.
Shivaji Park
Dadar
Bombay 400 028, India
**Phone:** 91 22 4442067   **Fax:** 91 22 4442067
**Email:** mssindia@bom8.vsnl.net.in

**Fnded:** 1985. **Mem:** 1,005. **Reg. Groups:** 7. **Desc:** MS patients, families and professionals. Seeks to improve the quality of life for persons with multiple sclerosis and their families. Provides counseling services and home visits.

**★ 13626 ★ Multiple Sclerosis Society of Malta**
c/o Leslie N. Agius
PO Box 209
Valletta, Malta
**Phone:** 356 418066   **Fax:** 356 230 538

**Fnded:** 1997. **Desc:** MS patients, families and professionals. Seeks to improve the quality of life for persons with multiple sclerosis and their families. Conducts fund raisers and public awareness campaigns. **Pub:** Bulletin, quarterly.

**★ 13627 ★ Multiple Sclerosis Society of New Zealand (MSSNZ)**
c/o Peter Old
PO Box 2627
Wellington, New Zealand
**Phone:** 64 4 499 4677   **Fax:** 64 4 499 4675
**Email:** mssnz@clear.net.nz

**Fnded:** 1968. **Reg. Groups:** 18. **Desc:** MS patients, families and professionals. Seeks to improve the quality of life for persons with multiple sclerosis and their families. Offers national support services program, national carers support network, MS support network, training video, and an education fund for children with MS. Hosts fundraisers, including Four Leaf Clover Raffle, Readathon, and the Great NZ Horse Ride.

**★ 13628 ★ Muscular Dystrophy Ireland (MDI)**
c/o Coleraine House
Coleraine St.
Dublin 7, Ireland
**Phone:** 353 1 8721501   **Fax:** 353 1 8724482
**Email:** info@mdi.ie
**Website:** http://www.mdi.ie

**Fnded:** 1972. **Mem:** 500. **Reg. Groups:** 5. **Lang(s):** English. **Desc:** Individuals and organizations. Seeks to improve the quality of life of people with muscular dystrophy and their families. Makes available support and services; conducts educational and advocacy campaigns. **Pub:** MDI Update, quarterly. Magazine.

**★ 13629 ★ Muskelsvindfonden**
Kongsvang Alle' 23
DK-8000 Arhus, Denmark
**Phone:** 45 89482222   **Fax:** 45 89482212
**Email:** msfoplys@post1.tele.dk
**Website:** http://www.muskelsvindfonden.dk

**Desc:** Promotes the research of muscular diseases affecting individuals in Denmark. Fosters communication among members. Offers supportive services to patients and their families.

**★ 13630 ★ Myositis Association of America**
755 Cantrell Ave., Ste. C
Harrisonburg, VA 22801
**Phone:** (540)433-7686   **Free:** 800-821-7356
**Fax:** (540)432-0206
**Email:** maa@myositis.org
**Website:** http://www.myositis.org
Nancy Armentrout, CEO

**Fnded:** 1986. **Mem:** 1,000. **Reg. Groups:** 22. **Desc:** Seeks to educate members in ways to avoid future degeneration process of myositis, give emotional support, investigate the different causes of the disease, act as a clearinghouse to physicians and scientists, and disseminate information to patients to inform on some of the known causes, pursue additional funding for research, investigate the most effective medical treatments available that have the least side effects and, most important, research a cure into these debilitating diseases. **Pub:** Newsletter for Myositis, quarterly. Newsletter. Price: $4 for past Newsletters. Frmly: (2000) National Myositis Association.

**★ 13631 ★ National Arthritis Foundation**
336 Smith St., Ste. 6-302
New Bridge Centre
Singapore 050336, Singapore
**Phone:** 65 2279726   **Fax:** 65 2270257
**Email:** nafsin@pacific.net.sg

**Fnded:** 1984. **Desc:** Aims to improve quality of life for arthritis suffers. Offers educational programs. Conducts research; disseminates information. **Pub:** Newsletter, periodic.

**★ 13632 ★ National Association for Pseudoxanthoma Elasticum (NAPE)**
8764 Manchester Rd., Ste. 200
Saint Louis, MO 63144
**Phone:** (314)962-0100   **Fax:** (314)962-0100
**Email:** pxenape@estreet.com
**Website:** http://www.pxenape.org
Frances Benham, PhD, Board Chair

**Fnded:** 1989. **Mem:** 625. **Nat'l Groups:** 1. **Desc:** People who have Pseudoxanthoma Elasticum (PXE), as well as interested others(Pseudoxanthoma elasticum is a rare connective tissue disorder that can affect eyes, skin, and organs). Provides educational information about PXE. Compiles statistics. Serves to unite PXE patients with professionals who treat the disease and others who have the disease. Maintains database of patients with PXE. **Pub:** PXE Awareness, quarterly. Newsletter. Current treatment, research and legislative information. Price: $3/printed copy; $5/taped copy. Frmly: (1999) NAPE, Inc.

**★ 13633 ★ National CFIDS Foundation**
103 Althea Rd.
Needham, MA 02492
**Phone:** (781)449-3535   **Fax:** (781)449-8606
**Email:** info@ncf-net.com
**Website:** http://www.ncf-net.org
Gail R. Kansky, Pres.

**Fnded:** 1996. **Mem:** 4,000. **Desc:** Provides education, advocacy and fundraising for research. **Pub:** The National Forum, quarterly. Journal.

**★ 13634 ★ National Fibromyalgia Research Association (FNRA)**
PO Box 500
Salem, OR 97308
**Website:** http://www.nfra.net/

**Fnded:** 1992. **Desc:** Dedicated to education, treatment and finding a cure for fibromyalgia. Produces a Fibromyalgia Awareness Pin to raise public awareness and research dollars.

**★ 13635 ★ National Institute of Arthritis and Musculoskeletal and Skin Diseases Information Clearinghouse**
c/o National Institutes of Health
1 AMS Cir.
Bethesda, MD 20892-3675
**Phone:** (301)495-4484   **Free:** 877-226-4267
**Fax:** (301)718-6366
**Email:** niamsweb@mail.nih.gov
**Website:** http://www.niams.nih.gov
Kelly Collins, Project Mgr.

**Desc:** Collects, publishes, and disseminates professional and public educational materials for persons concerned with arthritis and musculoskeletal and skin diseases. **Pub:** Reports. **Frmly:** (1999) National Arthritis and Musculoskeletal and Skin Diseases Information Clearinghouse (NAMSIC).

**★ 13636 ★ National Marfan Foundation (NMF)**
382 Main St.
Port Washington, NY 11050
**Phone:** (516)883-8712   **Free:** 800-862-7326
**Fax:** (516)883-8040
**Email:** support@marfan.org
**Website:** http://www.marfan.org
Karen Wolk, CSW, Dir. Support Svcs.

**Fnded:** 1981. **Mem:** 25,000. **State Groups:** 15. **Local Groups:** 60. **Desc:** Persons affected with the Marfan syndrome and related connective tissue disorders; families of affected persons; genetic counselors; cardiologists, ophthalmologists, orthopedists, and other medical professionals. (Marfan syndrome is a heritable disorder of the connective tissue affecting the skeleton, lungs, eyes, heart, and blood vessels.) Objectives are to: disseminate accurate and timely information on Marfan syndrome; act as support network and provide a means for patients and relatives to share experiences; improve medical care. Supports and fosters research. **Pub:** Cardiac Concerns, Ocular Concerns, Pediatric Concerns, Orthopedic Concerns. Brochures. Overview of related disorders, physical activity guidelines. • Connective Issues, quarterly. Newsletter. Includes research reports, chapter news, and legislative reports. Price: Included in membership dues. • How Do Your Genes Fit?. Video. Explains about genetic disorders, especially, Marfan Syndrome. Contains information for middle school students, families and support groups. • The Marfan Syndrome. Booklet. • The Marfan Syndrome: A Booklet for Teachers. Booklet. • The Marfan Syndrome: A Booklet for Teenagers. Booklet.

**★ 13637 ★ National Multiple Sclerosis Society of Australia**
c/o Trevor Farrell
34 Jackson St.
Toorak, VIC A-3142, Australia
**Phone:** 61 3 982 87222   **Fax:** 61 3 982 69054
**Email:** public@mssociety.com.au
**Website:** http://www.mssociety.com.au

**Desc:** MS patients, families and professionals. Seeks to improve the quality of life for persons with multiple sclerosis and their families.

**★ 13638 ★ National Osteoporosis Foundation (NOF)**
1232 22nd St., NW
Washington, DC 20037-1292
**Phone:** (202)223-2226   **Fax:** (202)223-2237
**Email:** nofmail@nof.org

**Website:** http://www.nof.org
Sandra C. Raymond, Exec. Dir.

**Fnded:** 1984. **Mem:** 300,000. **Desc:** A national voluntary health organization dedicated to reducing the widespread prevalence of osteoporosis. (Osteoporosis is an excessive loss of bone tissue which often results in fractures of the hip, spine, and wrist.) Seeks to: increase public awareness and knowledge about osteoporosis; provide information about osteoporosis to sufferers and their families; educate physicians and allied health professionals; advocate for increased governmental support for research on osteoporosis; and support basic biomedical, epidemiological, clinical, behavioral, and social research and research training. Sponsors Research Grant program; conducts public and professional education programs. **Pub:** *Boning Up on Osteoporosis. Price:* $3 each; $2.75/101 or more. • *Facts About Osteoporosis, Arthritis and Osteoarthritis. Price:* $.30 each; $.25/500 copies or more. • *Falls and Related Fractures. Price:* $.75 each; $.70/500 or more. • *How Strong Are Your Bones, periodic. Price:* $.70 each; $.60/500 or more. • *Living with Osteoporosis. Price:* $.35 each; $.30/500 copies or more. • *Medications and Bone Loss. Price:* $.75 each; $.70/500 or more. • *Osteoporosis Education Kit. Price:* $65 each. • *Osteoporosis Report,* quarterly. Newsletter. Includes current medical journal references and listing of consumer publications and recent articles related to the subject of osteoporosis. *Price:* Included in membership dues. • *Stand Up to Osteoporosis. Price:* $.45 each; $.40/500 copies or more. **Frmly:** (1985) The Osteoporosis Foundation.

★ 13639 ★ **National Osteoporosis Society**
Camerton
Bath BA2 0PJ, United Kingdom
**Phone:** 44 1761 471771     **Fax:** 44 1761 471104
**Email:** info@nos.org.uk
**Website:** http://www.nos.org.uk

**Fnded:** 1986. **Mem:** 27,000. **Desc:** National charity dedicated to improving the diagnosis, prevention, and treatment of osteoporosis. Works with health care professionals to facilitate greater understanding of the needs of individuals with the disease. Offers support to people with osteoporosis and their families through a range of detailed information booklets, a national telephone helpline and a network of regional support groups throughout the UK. Raises funds for research to increase understanding of the disease and improve treatment options and patient care. Raises awareness of the disease and campaigns to promote bone health.

★ 13640 ★ **National RSD Assistance Center**
PO Box 1261
Knightdale, NC 27545
**Email:** rsdac@bellsouth.net
**Website:** http://www.rsdac.org/

**Fnded:** 1999. **Desc:** Individuals suffering from Reflex Sympathetic Dystrophy. Offers assistance for medications and utilities treatment, as well as food or utility bills if needed. Provides other contact resources for further assistance. Collects and disseminates information about the disease. RSD is a medical condition resulting from an injury to a nerve or soft tissue (e.g., broken bone, or even a sliver) that does not heal properly.

★ 13641 ★ **National Scoliosis Foundation (NSF)**
5 Cabot Pl.
Stoughton, MA 02072-4624
**Phone:** (781)341-6333     **Free:** 800-673-6922
**Fax:** (781)341-8333
**Email:** NSF@scoliosis.org
**Website:** http://www.scoliosis.org

**Fnded:** 1976. **Mem:** 25,000. **State Groups:** 3. **Desc:** Supporters are businesses, organizations, and individuals concerned with the early detection and prevention of progressing scoliosis, kyphosis, and structural lordosis. Purposes are to promote programs and activities leading to the elimination of the crippling effects of scoliosis and to educate the public about all abnormal

spinal curvatures. Assists local groups in identifying available medical resources and personnel to help conduct volunteer screening programs; encourages legislation requiring scoliosis screening for each student in the 5th through 10th grades throughout the U.S. Maintains resource center for individuals or schools seeking information on abnormal spinal curvatures; provides information on how to promote and assist in spinal screening programs; sponsors multimedia educational exhibits and programs for adults and children. Maintains speakers' bureau. **Pub:** *Spinal Connection,* biennial. Newsletter. Membership activities newsletter. *Price:* Free. • Booklets. • Brochures. • Manuals. • Also publishes resource lists and produces school audiovisual materials.

**National Sjogren's Syndrome Association (NSSA)**
*See:* Entry 3226

★ 13642 ★ **Neurologiskt Handikappades Riksforbund**
c/o Monika Paulin
Box 32 84
S-103 65 Stockholm, Sweden
**Phone:** 46 8 6777010     **Fax:** 46 8 241315
**Email:** nhr@nhr.se
**Website:** http://www.nhr.se

**Fnded:** 1957. **Reg. Groups:** 119. **Desc:** MS patients, families and professionals. Seeks to improve the quality of life for persons with multiple sclerosis and their families.

★ 13643 ★ **Neuromuscular Diseases Association of Romania**
Institute of Neurology
C.P. 44-12
RO-75128 Bucharest, Romania
**Phone:** 40 1 3306273     **Fax:** 40 1 3213964

**Desc:** Promotes interest in neuromuscular diseases research among medical and scientific communities and the public in Romania. Disseminates information about the diseases.

★ 13644 ★ **Nordic Audiological Society (Nordisk Audiologisk Selskab — NAS)**
Frankrigsgade 4
DK- 2300 Copenhagen, Denmark
**Email:** nasbc@vip.cybercity.dk
**Website:** http://www.nas.dk

**Fnded:** 1960.

★ 13645 ★ **Nordic Spine Deformity Society**
Arhus University Hospital
DK-8000 Arhus, Denmark
**Phone:** 45 89493333     **Fax:** 45 89494120
**Email:** estender@dadlnet.dk

**Fnded:** 1974. **Desc:** Fosters research and treatment of scoliosis and all diseases of the back that may lead to spinal deformity.

★ 13646 ★ **Norwegian Fibromyalgia Patients' Association (NFP) (Norges Fibromyalgi Forbund — NFF)**
Sollivn. 55
N-1366 Lysaker, Norway
**Phone:** 47 67583067     **Fax:** 47 67583158
**Email:** fm-medl@os.felia.no

**Fnded:** 1985. **Mem:** 8,000. **Local Groups:** 67. **Lang(s):** English, Norwegian. **Desc:** Persons in Norway suffering from fibrositis or fibromyalgia (rheumatic disorders involving fibrous tissues). Funds research into the cause and cure of fibrositis or fibromyalgia. Promotes understanding of the disease; disseminates information. Conducts educational programs. **Pub:** *Fibromyalgi,* quarterly. Magazine. **Frmly:** Norges Fibromyalgi Forbund.

★ 13647 ★ **Ollier's/Maffucci Self-Help Group**
430 Palmetto Dr.
Venice, FL 34293-5943
**Email:** olliers@aol.com
**Website:** http://www.ollier-maffucci.org
Bonnie Schmid-Hatch, Pres. /Founder

**Fnded:** 1987. **Mem:** 500. **Nat'l Groups:** 5. **State Groups:** 1. **Local Groups:** 1. **Desc:** Self-help group for persons with Ollier's disease, Maffacci and MHE or any diseases with enchodromas. (Ollier's disease is a rare, nongenetic bone disorder.) Aims to find as many patients as possible to support research program objectives. **Pub:** *Olliers News,* quarterly. Newsletter. *Price:* Donations. **Frmly:** (1998) Ollier's Disease Self-Help Group.

★ 13648 ★ **OsteoArthritis Research Society International (OARSI)**
2025 M St., Ste.800
Washington, DC 20036
**Phone:** (202)367-1177     **Fax:** (202)367-2177
**Email:** oarsi@orsi.org
**Website:** http://www.oarsi.org

**Desc:** Researchers and health care professionals with an interest in osteoarthritis. Seeks to promote and encourage fundamental and applied research on osteoarthritis and its treatment. Gathers and disseminates information on osteoarthritis and related research; sponsors educational programs. **Pub:** *Membership Directory,* annual. Directory. • *OA Today,* quarterly. Newsletter. • *Osteoarthritis and Cartilage,* bimonthly. Journal.

**Osteogenesis Imperfecta Foundation (OIF)**
*See:* Entry 9357

★ 13649 ★ **Osteoporosis Society of Canada (La Societe de l'Osteoporose du Canada)**
33 Laird Dr.
Toronto, ON, Canada M4G 3S9
**Phone:** (416)696-2663     **Free:** 800-463-6842
**Fax:** (416)696-2673
**Email:** osc@osteoporosis.ca
**Website:** http://www.osteoporosis.ca

**Fnded:** 1982. **Reg. Groups:** 9. **Lang(s):** English, French. **Desc:** Individuals and organizations interested in the prevention, diagnosis, and treatment of osteoporosis. Supports research programs that seek to improve the quality of life for women with osteoporosis. Promotes education about osteoporosis among professional health practitioners. Disseminates informational materials to individuals with osteoporosis, physicians, and the public. Offers audio visual programs; participates in public forums. **Pub:** *Osteoblast.* Newsletter. A donor newsletter. • *Osteoporosis Update,* quarterly. Newsletter.

★ 13650 ★ **Osterreichische Multiple Sklerose Gessellschaft**
c/o Universitatsklinik f.
Neurologie
Waehringer Guertel 18-20
A-1090 Vienna, Austria
**Phone:** 43 1 404003121     **Fax:** 43 1 404003141
**Email:** msgs@akh-wien.ac.at

**Fnded:** 1965. **Reg. Groups:** 25. **Desc:** MS patients, families and professionals. Seeks to improve the quality of life for persons with multiple sclerosis and their families.

★ 13651 ★ **Paget Foundation for Paget's Disease of Bone and Related Disorders (PFPDBRD)**
120 Wall St., Ste. 1602
New York, NY 10005-4001
**Phone:** (212)509-5335     **Free:** 800-23-PAGET
**Fax:** (212)509-8492
**Email:** pagetfdn@aol.com

**Website:** http://www.paget.org
Charlene Waldman, Exec. Dir.

**Fnded:** 1978. **Desc:** Patients and their families and friends; physicians; paramedical professionals interested in improving health care of persons suffering from Paget's disease, a chronic disorder which may result in enlarged, deformed, and fragile bones in one or more regions of the skeleton, fibrous dysplasia, and primary hyperparathyroidism (PHPT). Also addresses related bone disorders such as fibrous dysplasia and both breast, prostate cancer hetastatic to bone. Conducts educational programs for patients, health care professionals, and the public; provides patient assistance and research advocacy; maintains referral service for patients seeking physicians who specialize in treating Paget's disease and PHPT. **Pub:** *A Patient's Guide to Paget's Disease of Bone.* Brochures. • *Paget's Disease of Bone: Clinical Assessment, Present and Future Therapy.* • *Questions and Answers.* • *Update,* 3/year. Newsletter. *Price:* Free. • Bibliography. • Reprints. • Please see enclosed for a listing of all publications. **Frmly:** (1992) Paget's Disease Foundation.

**★ 13652 ★ Pan American League of Associations for Rhuematology (PANLAR)**
c/o Dr. Abraham Garcia-Kutzbach
Clinicas Hospital Herrera Llerandi Norte
6a Avenida 7-55, Zona 10
Ala Norte 2o Piso
Guatemala City, Guatemala
**Phone:** 502 3343859          **Fax:** 502 3343859
**Email:** agarciak@ufm.edu.gt
**Fnded:** 1942. **Mem:** 10,000. **Reg. Groups:** 22. **Lang(s):** English, French, Portuguese, Spanish. **Desc:** Physicians and other professionals devoted to the prevention and treatment of rheumatic diseases. Seeks to educate health professionals. Conducts biomedical and epidemiological research. Offers assistance in the coordination of national, professional, and social agencies. Makes available professional publications. **Pub:** *PANLAR Bulletin,* biennial. Bulletin. **Frmly:** (2000) Pan American League Against Rhuematism.

**★ 13653 ★ Polskie Towarzystwo Stwardnienia Rozsianego**
c/o Hotel Marriott
Al Jerozolimskie 65/79
PL-00-697 Warsaw, Poland
**Phone:** 48 22 630 7220          **Fax:** 48 22 630 7220
**Email:** rgptsr@plearn.edu.pl
**Desc:** MS patients, families and professionals. Seeks to improve the quality of life for persons with multiple sclerosis and their families.

**★ 13654 ★ Psoriatric Arthropathy Alliance (PAA)**
PO Box 111
Saint Albans AL2 3JQ, United Kingdom
**Phone:** 44 870 703212          **Fax:** 44 870 703212
**Email:** info@paalliance.org
**Website:** http://www.paalliance.org
**Fnded:** 1993. **Lang(s):** English. **Desc:** Individuals with psoriatic arthritis and its associated skin disorder, psoriasis. Seeks to "protect, serve, and respect the interests and rights of people who have or might become susceptible to psoriatic arthritis." Conducts educational programs to raise public awareness of psoriatic arthritis and related disorders; provides support and assistance to people with psoriatic arthritis and their families; sponsors advocacy programs benefiting members. **Pub:** *Psoriatic Care Fact File.* • *Skin 'N' Bones Connection.* Pamphlets.

**★ 13655 ★ PXE International**
c/o Sharon F. Terry
23 Mountain St.
Sharon, MA 02067-2234
**Phone:** (781)784-3817          **Fax:** (781)784-6672
**Email:** pxe@pxe.org

**Website:** http://www.pxe.org
Sharon F. Terry, Exec. Dir.

**Fnded:** 1995. **Mem:** 4,000. **Nat'l Groups:** 22. **Reg. Groups:** 20. **Desc:** Dedicated to supporting those affected by Pseudoxanthomas elasticum (PXE) and to research into its causes, treatments, and cure. (Pseudoxanthomas elasticum is a heritable connective tissue disorder causing calcification of connective tissue, potentially affecting the skin, arteries, gastrointestinal tissue, and the retina.) Provides information and support to patients, their families, and clinicians on diagnosis, effects, and treatment. Through a consortium of researchers worldwide, supports research by providing to researchers monetary grants and samples from its confidential Blood and Tissue Bank. Initiates and conducts epidemiological studies and other research. **Pub:** *MemberGram,* quarterly. Newsletter. Contains information on PXE; patient group and organization activities; research updates; profiles of patients, volunteers, and researchers. • Bulletin, periodic.

**★ 13656 ★ Restless Legs Syndrome Foundation (RLS)**
PO Box 7050, Department WWW
Rochester, MN 55902-2985
**Phone:** (507)287-6465          **Fax:** (507)287-6312
**Email:** rlsfoundation@rls.org
**Website:** http://www.rls.org
Allan O'Bryan, Acting Exec. Dir.
**Fnded:** 1990. **Mem:** 10,000. **Desc:** Sufferers of restless leg syndrome and other interested people. Supports research of effective treatments and a cure. Acts as and develops support groups for sufferers and their friends and families. Educates physicians, patients and the public to increase awareness.

**★ 13657 ★ Roger Wyburn-Mason and Jack M. Blount Foundation for the Eradication of Rheumatoid Disease (RDF)**
7111 Sweetgum Dr., No. A
Fairview, TN 37062-9384
**Phone:** (615)799-1002          **Fax:** (615)799-1002
**Email:** admin@arthritistrust.org
**Website:** http://www.arthritistrust.org
Perry A. Chapdelaine, Exec. Dir. & Sec.
**Fnded:** 1982. **Mem:** 60,000. **Nat'l Groups:** 2. **Desc:** Seeks to eradicate rheumatoid disease. Promotes professional university research and supplies free information to physicians and disease victims on Dr. Roger Wyburn-Mason's treatment protocol as modified by other physicians. (Such treatment includes oral medications, intraneural injections, and dietary control and, according to the foundation, has been successful in 80% of patients treated.) Conducts educational programs for the public and physicians; sponsors medical seminars; provides physician referrals and speakers' bureau. Emphasizes complementary, alternative, and holistic treatments especially for forms of arthritides. **Pub:** *The Art of Getting Well.* Book. Includes recommended primary treatments plus important complementary treatments. *Price:* $5. • *Arthritis: Little Known Treatments.* Book. Contains a collection of alternative, complementary, and holistic treatments. *Price:* 5. • *Away with Arthritis.* Book. *Price:* $15 15. • *The Causation of Rheumatoid Disease and Many Human Cancers – A New Concept in Medicine.* Pamphlet. *Price:* $10. • *Cell Wall Deficient Forms: Stealth Pathogens.* Book. *Price:* $65 65. • *Dr. Braly's Food Allergy & Nutrition - Revolution.* Book. *Price:* $20 20. • *Flax Oil as a True Aid Against Arthritis, Heart Infarction, Cancer and Other Diseases.* Book. *Price:* $10. • *Healing Dimensions of Herbal Medicine.* Book. *Price:* $12. • *Home Remedies.* Book. *Price:* $15. • *Intraneural Injections for Rheumatoid Arthritis and Osteoarthritis and The Control of Pain in Arthritis of the Knee.* Pamphlet. Explains a new concept on treating the pain of arthritis. *Price:* $9.95. • *Nourishing Traditions.* Book. Cookbook. *Price:* $25. • *Pain,Pain Go Away.* Book. *Price:* $18 18. • *Why Arthritis?.* Book. *Price:* $20. • Books. • Newsletter, quarterly. • Also publishes several journals, papers, and articles on

topics related to arthritis. **AKA:** Rheumatoid Disease Foundation; The Arthritis Trust of America.

**★ 13658 ★ RSDHope Group (RSDS)**
PO Box 875
Harrison, ME 04040
**Website:** http://www.rsdhope.org/
**Desc:** Patients suffering from Reflex Sympathetic Dystrophy Syndrome, Chronic Pain, their parents and friends. Dedicated to increasing the awareness of Reflex Sympathetic Dystrophy Syndrome (RSDS), chronic pain. **Pub:** Newsletter.

**★ 13659 ★ Schweizerische Multiple Sklerose Gesellschaft**
c/o Pascal Couchepin
Brinerstrasse 1
Postfach
CH-8036 Zurich, Switzerland
**Phone:** 41 1 466 6999          **Fax:** 41 1 466 6990
**Email:** info@multiplesklero.se.ch
**Fnded:** 1959. **Reg. Groups:** 39. **Desc:** MS patients, families and professionals. Seeks to improve the quality of life for persons with multiple sclerosis and their families.

**★ 13660 ★ Scleroderma Foundation (SF)**
12 Kent Way, Ste. 101
Byfield, MA 01922
**Phone:** (978)463-5843          **Free:** 800-722-4673
**Fax:** (978)463-5809
**Email:** sfinfo@scleroderma.org
**Website:** http://www.scleroderma.org
Peter Giusti, Exec. Dir.
**Fnded:** 1983. **Mem:** 16,000. **Reg. Groups:** 75. **Desc:** Scleroderma organizations. Promotes medical research to find a cure for scleroderma, a chronic systemic disease affecting all organs resulting from uncontrolled growth of connective tissue. Seeks to foster an understanding of the disease through media and outreach programs; raises funds. Provides patients with educational materials and referrals to local organizations and medical specialists. Offers encouragement and consultation services towards the formation and development of local support groups. Acts as a clearinghouse for information about scleroderma research, drugs, and therapies. Conducts accredited programs for professionals. Maintains speakers' bureau; compiles statistics. Funds one million dollars a year in new research. **Pub:** *About Scleroderma.* Brochure. • *Helpful Hints for Living with Scleroderma.* • *Newsline,* quarterly. Price: Included in membership. • *Understanding and Managing Scleroderma.* Booklet. **Frmly:** (1984) International Scleroderma Federation; (1998) Scleroderma Federation.

**★ 13661 ★ Scleroderma Research Foundation (SRF)**
2320 Bath St., Ste. 315
Santa Barbara, CA 93105
**Phone:** (805)563-9133          **Free:** 800-441-CURE
**Fax:** (805)563-2402
**Email:** srfcure@srfcure.org
**Website:** http://www.srfcure.org/
Sharon Monsky, Chm.
**Fnded:** 1978. **Reg. Groups:** 1. **Desc:** Seeks to find a cure for scleroderma, a life-threatening and degenerative illness. Funds and facilitates research and public awareness. **Pub:** *Scleroderma Handbook & Resource Guide.* Handbook. • *Scleroderma Research Foundation Newsletter,* semiannual. Newsletter. *Price:* Included in membership dues.

**Scleroderma Support Group (SSG)**
*See:* Entry 6845

**★ 13662 ★ Scoliosis Association (SAI)**
PO Box 811705
Boca Raton, FL 33481-1705

**Phone:** (561)994-4435 **Free:** 800-800-0669
**Fax:** (561)994-2455
**Email:** normlipin@aol.com
**Website:** http://www.scoliosis-assoc.org
Stanley Sacks, CEO

**Fnded:** 1976. **Mem:** 5,000. **Local Groups:** 52. **Desc:** Individuals or families involved or interested in scoliosis (lateral or sidewards curvature of the spine). Educates the public about scoliosis and other spinal deviations. Encourages and supports spinal screening programs in schools throughout the U.S. and Canada. Sponsors the formation of scoliosis chapters throughout the country which serve as support groups for the scoliosis patient and his or her family. Aids the patient in attaining a positive social and emotional adjustment during treatment of scoliosis. Plans to compile statistics; works with researchers in scoliosis. Raises funds for scoliosis research. Has sponsored scoliosis spinal conferences with several hospitals and leading spinal orthopaedists. **Pub:** *Backtalk*, periodic. Newsletter. Contains research and chapter news, article reprints, book reviews, and listings of publications. *Price:* $30 for individuals outside the U.S.; $40 for institutions; $40. • *Scoliosis, An Adult Perspective*. Video. *Price:* $19.95. • Bibliography.Lists books, articles, pamphlets, and papers on scoliosis. *Price:* $6 for part one; $3 for part two; $8 for parts one and two. • Brochure. • Also issues posters.

★ **13663** ★ **Scoliosis Association (SAUK)**
2 Ivebury Ct.
323-327 Latimer Rd.
London W10 6RA, United Kingdom
**Phone:** 44 20 89645343 **Fax:** 44 20 89645343
**Email:** sauk@sauk.org.uk
**Website:** http://www.sauk.org.uk

**Fnded:** 1981. **Mem:** 2,700. **Local Groups:** 29. **Lang(s):** English. **Desc:** Individuals affected by scoliosis; their parents and families. Seeks to increase knowledge and understanding of scoliosis (a lateral curvature of the spine) and emphasize the importance of early detection. Encourages contact between members; disseminates information to members and the public. **Pub:** *A Twist of Fate*. The psychological problems of coping with Scoliosis - especially for young people. • *Newsletter*, 2/year. Newsletter. • *Newsletter Index*. Lists and cross-references SAUK's newsletters. • *Schools Fact Sheet*. Contains information on scoliosis for parents of school-age children. • *Scoliosis: An Information Booklet*. Booklet. • *Shona's Story*. A teenagers' account of her operations and the care she received.

★ **13664** ★ **Scoliosis Research Society (SRSO)**
611 E Wells St.
Milwaukee, WI 53202
**Phone:** (414)289-9107 **Fax:** (414)276-3349
**Email:** tgoulding@execinc.com
**Website:** http://www.srs.org
Tressa Goulding, Exec. Dir.

**Fnded:** 1966. **Mem:** 760. **Desc:** Orthopedic surgeons and physicians. Furthers research and education in spinal deformities, particularly scoliosis, a twisting of the spine to one side. Most cases are of unknown cause, though scoliosis can result from a birth defect, polio, or spinal injury and usually develops in children during the growth spurt between ages ten and 15. Early detection followed with use of a brace and exercise can halt the curvature and prevent deformity.

★ **13665** ★ **Sjogren's Syndrome Foundation (SSF)**
8120 Woodmont Ave., No. 530
Bethesda, MD 20814
**Phone:** (301)718-0300 **Free:** 800-475-6473
**Fax:** (301)718-0322
**Email:** ssf@sjorgens.com
**Website:** http://www.sjogrens.com
Author Grayzel, MD, Pres.

**Fnded:** 1983. **Mem:** 6,750. **Local Groups:** 80. **Desc:** Individuals who have Sjogren's Syndrome, xerostomia (dry mouth), or keratoconjunctivitis sicca (dry eyes);

specialists, internists, immunologists, rheumatologists, otolaryngologists, opthalmologists, gynecologists, gastroenterologists, pulmonologists, dermatologists, neurologists, urologists, pharmaceutical companies, and dentists. (Sjogren's Syndrome is a disorder marked by dryness of all mucous membranes, resulting from deficient secretion of the glands, particularly the lacrimal and salivary glands, those of the upper respiratory tract, the sweat glands, and the vaginal area. Approximately 50% of Sjogren's Syndrome patients also have rheumatoid arthritis, lupus, or scleroderma.) Objectives are to increase public awareness and medical knowledge about Sjogren's Syndrome, educate patients and their families, and allow patients to share information on coping with the syndrome. Supports research. Sponsors support groups with meetings in which doctors speak on aspects of the syndrome. Compiles statistics. **Pub:** *Moisture Seekers Newsletter*, 9/year. Newsletter. Covers information on new products, treatments, and developments, status of research, and discussion by specialists. *Price:* Included in membership dues. • *The New Sjogren's Syndrome Handbook*. • Articles. • Brochure. **Frmly:** (1985) Moisture Seekers.

★ **13666** ★ **Slovensky zvaz Sclerosis Multiplex**
c/o Milan Surgos
Culenova 12
917 00 Trnava, Slovakia
**Phone:** 421 33 5513 009 **Fax:** 421 33 5513 009
**Fnded:** 1990. **Mem:** 530. **Reg. Groups:** 16. **Desc:** MS patients, families and professionals. Seeks to improve the quality of life for persons with multiple sclerosis and their families.

★ **13667** ★ **Sociedade Portuguesa de Esclerose Multipla (SPEM)**
c/o Manuela Martins, MD
Rua Tomas Alcaide 63C
P-1900 Lisbon, Portugal
**Phone:** 351 21 837 6610 **Fax:** 351 21 837 6610
**Email:** spem@clix.pt
**Fnded:** 1984. **Mem:** 1,100. **Desc:** MS patients, families and professionals. Seeks to improve the quality of life for persons with multiple sclerosis and their families.

★ **13668** ★ **South African National Multiple Sclerosis Society**
c/o David Phillimore
PO Box 9177
Auckland Park
Johannesburg 2006, Republic of South Africa
**Phone:** 27 41 581 2900 **Fax:** 27 41 581 5705
**Email:** sanmss@jhb.lia.net
**Fnded:** 1962. **Mem:** 1,900. **Reg. Groups:** 33. **Desc:** MS patients, families and professionals. Seeks to improve the quality of life for persons with multiple sclerosis and their families.

★ **13669** ★ **Spondylitis Association of America (SAA)**
14827 Ventura Blvd., No. 222
PO Box 5872
Sherman Oaks, CA 91403
**Phone:** (818)981-1616 **Free:** 800-777-8189
**Email:** info@spondylitis.org
**Website:** http://www.spondylitis.org
Jane Bruckel, Exec. Dir.

**Fnded:** 1983. **Mem:** 4,000. **Desc:** Individuals affected by Ankylosing Spondylitis, psoriatic arthritis, and Reiter's Syndrome; and their families and friends; health care professionals; scientific researchers. (Ankylosing Spondylitis is a condition most often affecting those between 17-40 years of age and characterized by pain or stiffness in the back. Although the cause and cure are not known, the condition may be contained through a program of anti-inflammatory drugs, posture awareness, and regular, therapeutic exercise; it is believed to be a hereditary condition.) Disseminates information; promotes public awareness and research;

conducts educational programs. **Pub:** *A Family of Related Diseases*. Booklet. • *Back in Action*. Videos. • *Guidebook for Patients*. • *Juvenile AS*. Booklet. • *Physical Therapy Exercises*. Audiotapes. • *Spondylitis Plus*, quarterly. Newsletter. Includes information on treatment, research, and coping with the condition. *Price:* Included in membership dues. • *Straight Talk on Spondylitis*. Book. • *The Water Workout*. Video. **Frmly:** (1993) Ankylosing Spondylitis Association.

★ **13670** ★ **Taiwan Motor Neuron Disease Association**
Neurological Service
Veterans General Hospital
201 Shih-pai Rd., Sec. 11
Taipei 11217, Taiwan
**Phone:** 886 2 28743815 **Fax:** 886 2 28743814
**Email:** mnda2874@ms39.hinet.net
**Website:** http://www.mnda.org.tw
**Fnded:** 1996. **Desc:** Individuals in Taiwan affected by neuromuscular diseases. Provides a forum for support and exchange of information. Works to raise awareness of the benefits of home care. **Pub:** Magazine, semiannual.

★ **13671** ★ **TMJ Association (TMJA)**
PO Box 26770
Milwaukee, WI 53226
**Fax:** (414)259-8112
**Email:** info@tmj.org
**Website:** http://www.tmj.org
**Desc:** Offers support to those suffering from pain and dysfunction resulting from temporomandibular joint diseases (TMJ). Promotes awareness of TMJ problems; advocates research, safe and effective diagnostic treatments, and reimbursement for health care costs. Advocates for a registry for TMJ implant patients. Conducts surveys and support groups.

★ **13672** ★ **Tuberous Sclerosis Association**
c/o Mrs. Janet Medcalf
PO Box 9644
Bromsgrove B61 0FP, United Kingdom
**Phone:** 44 1527 871898 **Fax:** 44 1527 579452
**Email:** support@tuberous-sclerosis.org
**Website:** http://www.tuberous-sclerosis.org
**Fnded:** 1977. **Mem:** 1,450. **Desc:** Supports families and individuals affected by tuberous sclerosis. Raises awareness of the condition and to educate professionals, sufferers and the general public.

★ **13673** ★ **Turkiye Multipl Skleroz Dernegi**
c/o Sule Ozkaner
Buyukdere Caddesi
Hukukcular Sitesi No. 24/21
Mecidiyekoy
Istanbul, Turkey
**Phone:** 90 212 275 2296 **Fax:** 90 212 265 9420
**Fnded:** 1989. **Mem:** 750. **Reg. Groups:** 5. **Desc:** MS patients, families and professionals. Seeks to improve the quality of life for persons with multiple sclerosis and their families.

★ **13674** ★ **Union of Muscular Dystrophy Societies of Croatia**
Nova Ves 44
10000 Zagreb, Croatia
**Phone:** 385 1 4666849 **Fax:** 385 1 4673172
**Email:** marija.sostarko@zg.tel.hr
**Desc:** Works as a communication network for muscular dystrophy support and discussion groups. Encourages the medical and scientific communities to continue researching muscular dystrophy. Strives to heighten community awareness about the disease.

★ **13675** ★ **USA Fibromyalgia Association**
PO Box 1483
Dublin, OH 43017

**Phone:** (614)851-9177
**Desc:** Promotes awareness of fibrositis and fibromyalgia.

**World Alliance of Neuromuscular
Disorder Associations (WANDA)**
*See:* Entry 14132

**★ 13676 ★ Yugoslav MND Association**
Dr. Subotica br.6
YU-11000 Belgrade, Serbia
**Phone:** 381 11 684355        **Fax:** 381 11 684577
**Email:** zsmndyu@hotmail.com
**Website:** http://www.w-a-n-d-a.org
**Fnded:** 1977. **Desc:** Individuals in Yugoslavia affected by Motor Neruone Disease (MND), a muscle wasting condition. Participates in clinical trials of new medications. Provides a forum for support and exchange of information.

**★ 13677 ★ Zdruzenje Multiple Sklerose
Slovenie (ZMSS)**
c/o Alojz Jeselnik
Maroltova 14-16
SLO-1113 Ljubljana, Slovenia
**Phone:** 386 1 568 7299        **Fax:** 386 1 568 7279
**Email:** zmss@yahoo.com
**Fnded:** 1973. **Reg. Groups:** 28. **Desc:** MS patients, families and professionals. Seeks to improve the quality of life for persons with multiple sclerosis and their families.

# Research Centers

**★ 13678 ★ American Society for Bone
and Mineral Research**
2025 M St., NW, Ste. 800
Washington, DC 20036-3309
**Phone:** (202)367-1161        **Fax:** (202)367-2161
**Email:** asbmr@dc.sba.com
**Website:** http://www.asbmr.org
Joan Goldberg, Exec. Dir.
**Activities/Fields:** Bone, and mineral diseases, focusing on the prevention of osteoporosis. **Pub:** *Journal of Bone and Mineal Research.* • *Primer on Metabolic Bone Diseases and Disorders of Mineral Metabolism.*

**★ 13679 ★ Arthritis Foundation**
Atlanta, GA 30357-0669
**Phone:** (404)872-7100        **Free:** 800-283-7800
**Fax:** (404)872-0457
**Email:** mscott@arthritis.org
**Website:** http://www.arthritis.org/
M. Scott, Contact
**Activities/Fields:** Causes, cures, and prevention of the various forms of arthritis and improved medical care and services for Americans affected by arthritis. **Pub:** *Bulletin on the Rheumatic Diseases*, semimonthly. • *Primer on the Rheumatic Diseases*, quinquenially.

**★ 13680 ★ Arthritis and Immune
Disorder Research Centre (AIDRC)**
Ontario Cancer Institute/Princess Margaret Hospital
610 University Ave., 16th Fl.
Toronto, ON, Canada M5G 2M9
**Phone:** (416)946-2924        **Fax:** (416)946-2291
**Email:** aarc@oci.utoronto.ca
**Website:** http://www.whri.on.ca/index.html
Dr. Edward Keystone, Contact
**Activities/Fields:** Arthritis and immune disorders, including musculoskeletal and rheumatic diseases, immunology, endocrine disorders, clinical epidemiology, therapeutic endoscopy, vascular diseases, and community health programs.

**★ 13681 ★ Arthritis and Immune
Disorder Research Centre
Arthritis Community Research and
Evaluation Unit (ACREU)**
Ontario Cancer Institute/Princess Margaret Hospital
610 University Ave., 16th Fl.
Toronto, ON, Canada M5G 2M9
**Phone:** (416)946-2902        **Fax:** (416)946-2291
Linda Rothman, Contact
**Activities/Fields:** Impact of arthritis on people with arthritis in Ontario; identify gaps and needs in services; and develop and evaluate programs for support, care, and health promotion for people with arthritis and their families. **Pub:** *Working papers.*

**★ 13682 ★ Benign Essential
Blepharospasm Research Foundation,
Inc. (BEBRF)**
Baptist Hospital Doctors Bldg.
637 N 7th St.
PO Box 12468
Beaumont, TX 77726-2468
**Phone:** (409)832-0788        **Fax:** (409)832-0890
**Email:** bebrf@ih2000.net
**Website:** http://www.blepharospasm.org/
Mary Lou Thompson, Pres.
**Activities/Fields:** Benign Essential Blepharospasm/Meige (BEB/M) Syndrome and related disorders and infirmities of the facial musculature. BEB/M is an involuntary, uncontrollable spastic contraction of the eyelids and other facial musculature. **Pub:** *Newsletter*, bimonthly.

**Boston University
Neuromuscular Research Center
Electromyography Laboratory**
*See:* Entry 14153

**Boston University
Neuromuscular Research Center
Injury Analysis and Prevention
Laboratory**
*See:* Entry 14155

**Boston University
Neuromuscular Research Center
Motor Control Laboratory**
*See:* Entry 14157

**Boston University
Neuromuscular Research Center
Signal Processing Laboratory**
*See:* Entry 14160

**★ 13683 ★ Brigham and Women's
Hospital
Robert B. Brigham Multipurpose Arthritis
and Musculoskeletal Diseases Center**
75 Francis St.
Boston, MA 02115
**Phone:** (617)732-5356        **Fax:** (617)732-5505
**Email:** mhliang@partners.org
**Website:** http://nmrc.bu.edu
Dr. Matthew H. Liang, Dir.
**Activities/Fields:** Rheumatic disease, including technology assessment, policy studies, the relationship between clinical practice, outcome, and efficiency, and psychological, social, and economic factors. Also studies clinimetrics and epidemiology of rheumatic disease, Lyme disease, Carpal Tunnel Syndrome, spinal stenosis, doctor-patient communication, and SLE risk factors.

**Bucknell University
Immunobiology Research Laboratory**
*See:* Entry 3240

**★ 13684 ★ Case Western Reserve
University
Northeast Ohio Multipurpose Arthritis
Center**
University Hospitals of Cleveland
11100 Euclid Ave.
Cleveland, OH 44106-5076
**Phone:** (216)844-3168        **Fax:** (216)844-5172
**Email:** rwm3@po.cwru.edu
**Website:** http://www.bucknell.edu
Dr. Roland W. Moskowitz, Dir.
**Activities/Fields:** The causes, diagnosis, and treatment of arthritis, including biochemistry and pathophysiology of joints in osteoarthritis, models of degenerative joint disease and inflammatory arthritis, immunologic disorders such as systemic lupus erythematosus and rheumatoid arthritis, disorders of the spine, genetic control of arthritis disorders, and juvenile arthritis. Orthopedic studies include bioengineering, joint replacement, transplant surgery, and bone metabolism. Also investigates community health systems, including self care needs of the elderly, legal needs of patients with chronic illness such as rheumatoid arthritis, and patients' perceived needs for community services.

**★ 13685 ★ Case Western Reserve
University
Skeletal Research Center**
Department of Biology
2080 Adelbert Rd.
Cleveland, OH 44106-7080
**Phone:** (216)368-3562        **Fax:** (216)368-4077
Arnold I. Caplan, PhD, Dir.
**Activities/Fields:** Tissue engineered regeneration and clinical aspects of skeletal tissue, includi cartilage, bones, tendons, and ligaments.

**Center for Intelligent Biomedical Devices
and Musculoskeletal Systems**
*See:* Entry 4628

**★ 13686 ★ Christine M. Kleinert Institute
for Hand and Microsurgery, Inc.**
225 Abraham Flexner Way, Ste. 850
Louisville, KY 40202
**Phone:** (502)562-0312        **Fax:** (502)562-0326
**Email:** fellowship@cmki.org
**Website:** http://www.cmki.org
Tina McMongal, Coord.
**Activities/Fields:** Upper extremity care, including nerve compression conditions and carpal tunnel syndrome; nerve regeneration; biomechanical studies; replanted and transplanted tissue and the most effective ways of increasing survival and function; and hand and microsurgery techniques, including anatomical studies.

**★ 13687 ★ Harrington Arthritis Research
Center**
300 N 18 St.
Phoenix, AZ 85006
**Phone:** (602)254-0377        **Fax:** (602)253-4817
**Email:** lcooper@harcaz.org
**Website:** http://www.harcaz.org
Lisa R. Cooper, Dir. of Oper.
**Activities/Fields:** Arthritis, including microbial involvement; and Alzheimer's disease.

**★ 13688 ★ Helen Hayes Hospital
Regional Bone Center**
Rte. 9W
West Haverstraw, NY 10993
**Phone:** (845)786-4839        **Free:** 888-707-3422
**Fax:** (845)786-4878
**Email:** dempster@helenhayeshosp.org
**Website:** http://www.helenhayeshospital.org/research.htmregional
David W. Dempster, PhD, Dir.

**Activities/Fields:** Bone and calcium metabolism, including pathophysiology of bone and clinical research on the pathogenesis and treatment of diseases such as osteoporosis, primary hyperparathyroidism, and Paget's disease. Conducts calciotropic hormone assays, bone biopsies and histomorphometry.

**Hospital for Joint Diseases**
**Orthopaedic Institute**
**Cartilage and Bone Research Center**
*See:* Entry 16947

**★ 13689 ★ Hospital for Joint Diseases**
**Orthopaedic Institute**
**Musculoskeletal Research Center**
301 E 17th St., 15th Fl.
New York, NY 10003
**Phone:** (212)598-6567     **Fax:** (212)598-6096
**Email:** pedicesare@aol.com
**Website:** http://www.msnyuhealth.org/hospitals/hja/
html/body_ortho_cart_bone_res.html
Paul Di Cesare, MD, Dir.

**Activities/Fields:** Prevention and treatment of musculoskeletal diseases, including basic studies of biological and synthetic biomaterials, biomechanics, kinematics, mathematical modeling, arthritis, and cartilage repair, and gene therapy.

**Hospital for Special Surgery**
**Research Division**
*See:* Entry 16950

**Hospital for Special Surgery**
**Research Division**
**Laboratory for Soft Tissues Research**
*See:* Entry 16951

**★ 13690 ★ Hospital for Special Surgery**
**Research Division**
**Mineralized Tissues Research Section**
535 E 70th St.
New York, NY 10021
**Phone:** (212)606-1459     **Fax:** (212)472-5331
**Email:** boskeya@hss.edu
**Website:** http://www.hss.edu
Adele L. Boskey, PhD, Sect. Hd.

**Activities/Fields:** Mechanisms of calcification and mineralized tissue remodeling, calcium handling by cells, cell and molecular biology of diseases of calcified tissues (including osteoporosis and osteogenesis imperfecta), and the genetics of bone density and IR imaging of connective tissues.

**★ 13691 ★ Indiana University-Purdue**
**University at Indianapolis**
**Multipurpose Arthritis and**
**Musculoskeletal Diseases Center**
541 Clinical Dr., Rm. 492
Indianapolis, IN 46202-5103
**Phone:** (317)274-4225     **Fax:** (317)274-7792
Dr. Kenneth D. Brandt, Dir.

**Activities/Fields:** Basic and clinical research related to rheumatic diseases. Activities are structured in two major areas: a Biomedical Component and an Epidemiology, Education, and Health Services Research Component. **Pub:** *Newsletter,* 3/year. **Frmly:** Specialized Center of Research in Osteoarthritis.

**Indiana University-Purdue University at**
**Indianapolis**
**Oral Health Research Institute**
**Bioresearch Facility**
*See:* Entry 4649

**International Research Council of**
**Neuromuscular Disorders**
*See:* Entry 14210

**Johns Hopkins University**
**Adolescent Idiopathic Scoliosis**
**Laboratory (AIS)**
*See:* Entry 9405

**★ 13692 ★ Johns Hopkins University**
**Kathryn and Alan C. Greenberg Center**
**for Skeletal Dysplasias**
Blalock 1012
600 N Wolfe St.
Baltimore, MD 21287-4922
**Phone:** (410)614-0977     **Fax:** (410)614-2522
**Email:** bmarosy@jhmi.edu
**Website:** http://www.med.jhu.edu/Greenberg.Center/
Greenbrg.htm
Victor McKusick, MD, Dir.

**Activities/Fields:** Skeletal dysplasias, especially dwarfism.

**★ 13693 ★ Kuzell Institute for Arthritis**
**and Infectious Diseases**
California Pacific Medical Center
2200 Webster St., 3rd Fl.
San Francisco, CA 94115
**Phone:** (415)561-1734     **Fax:** (415)441-8548
**Email:** kiaid@cooper.cpmc.org
Dr. Lowell S. Young, Dir.

**Activities/Fields:** Arthritis and related diseases and infectious diseases. In the area of arthritis, the Institute conducts fundamental investigations on the biology, biochemistry, and pharmacology of tissues and cellular inflammatory reactions, and studies of autoimmune diseases, including systematic lupus erthymatosus (SLE), the biology of neutrophils, replacement of joints, and pharmacology of steroidal and nonsteroidal anti-inflammatory agents. Infectious disease research emphasizes host defense against opportunistic pathogens and includes development of monoclonal antibodies against virulence factors of gram negative bacteria, evaluation of new antimicrobial agents, and the pathogenesis and treatment of atypical mycobacterial infections, particularly as they occur in AIDS.

**★ 13694 ★ Little People's Research**
**Fund, Inc.**
80 Sister Pierre Dr.
Towson, MD 21204-7534
**Phone:** (410)494-0055     **Free:** 800-232-5773
**Fax:** (410)494-0062
**Email:** lprf@lprf.org
**Website:** http://www.lprf.org
Dr. Steven Kopits, Med. Dir.

**Activities/Fields:** Orthopedic disabilities associated with skeletal dysplasia (also known as dwarfism), including child development from adolescence and into adulthood and new surgical procedures. **Pub:** *Newsletter,* semiannually.

**★ 13695 ★ McGill University**
**Montreal Neurological Institute**
**Neuromuscular Research Group**
3801 University St.
Montreal, QC, Canada H3A 2B4
**Phone:** (514)398-6644     **Fax:** (514)398-8310
**Email:** mcgk@musica.mcgill.ca
**Website:** http://www.mcgill.ca/mni/index.html
Dr. George Karpati, Coord.

**Activities/Fields:** Neuromuscular research, including molecular genetics, muscle biochemistry, muscle metabolism, neurotoxicology, neuropathology, neurophysiology, cytochemistry, and magnetic resonance spectroscopy. Research focuses on gene therapy for muscle and motor neurons, coordinated expression of genes coding for myofibrillar molecules during differentiation and denervation, use of transgenic mice, cell adhesion molecules and molecular mechanisms of myoblast fusion in vitro, molecular biology of muscle mitochondria (especially in mitochondrial diseases), microscopic and biochemical cytoskeletal alterations in neurons pertaining to diseases such as amyotrophic lateral sclerosis and toxic neuropathies, in vivo magnetic resonance spectroscopy of neuromuscular diseases, comprehensive multidisciplinary investigation of complex neuromuscular diseases, and gene therapy for dystrophin deficiency states, and malignant brain tumors.

**★ 13696 ★ MCP Hahnemann University**
**of the Health Sciences**
**Allegheny Orthopaedic Institute**
221 N Broad St., 1st Fl.
Philadelphia, PA 19107
**Phone:** (215)762-8500     **Fax:** (215)564-2825
Dr. Norman Johanson, Dir.

**Activities/Fields:** Arthritis.

**★ 13697 ★ Medical Research Council**
**Protein Structure and Function Group**
Department of Biochemistry
University of Alberta
Edmonton, AB, Canada T6G 2H7
**Phone:** (780)492-5460     **Fax:** (780)492-0886
**Email:** bds@fossil.biochem.ualberta.ca
Dr. Brian D. Sykes, Dir.

**Activities/Fields:** Muscle protein structure and function, enzyme structure and function, protein-nucleic acid interactions, and phosphorylation-dephosphorylation of proteins. Performs X-ray diffraction, CD, flourescence, amino acid analysis and sequence analysis, peptide synthesis, nuclear magnetic resonance (NMR) and molecular biology.

**★ 13698 ★ Medical University of South**
**Carolina**
**Arthritis Clinical and Research Center**
171 Ashley Ave.
Charleston, SC 29425
**Phone:** (843)792-3484
**Email:** silverr@musc.edu
Richard M. Silver, MD, Dir.

**Activities/Fields:** Molecular mechanisms of connective tissue diseases, microvascular investigations, alterations in gene expression in fibroblasts, adhesion and nonadhesion molecular interactions in cell behavior, rheumatic disorders, immunologic investigations in rheumatic disease (such as the function of T-cell subsets), cell culture, and other clinical investigations, especially in Raynaud's, scleroderma, undifferentiated connective tissue syndromes (UCTS) and SLE. Research is undertaken in an effort to investigate the underlying mechanisms and the nature of rheumatic and connective tissue diseases, to expand education and training opportunities in the management of musculoskeletal diseases, and to develop patient care and community programs which increase the awareness of arthritis and improve access to quality rheumatologic care. **Frmly:** Multipurpose Arthritis Center.

**★ 13699 ★ Michigan State University**
**Laboratory for Comparative Orthopaedic**
**Research (LCOR)**
Department of Small Animal Clinical Sciences
G-387 Veterinary Medical Center
East Lansing, MI 48824-1314
**Phone:** (517)353-8964     **Fax:** (517)353-8980
**Email:** arnoczky@cvm.msu.edu
**Website:** http://www.cvm.msu.edu/lcor/descript.htm
Dr. Steven P. Arnoczky, Dir.

**Activities/Fields:** Musculoskeletal system of humans and animals. The laboratory focuses its research on sports related injuries such as the repair and reconstruction of ligamentous and meniscal injuries of the knee. **Pub:** *Newsletter.*

**★ 13700 ★ Ohio Valley Tissue and Skin**
**Center**
2939 Vernon Pl.
Cincinnati, OH 45219-2430
**Phone:** (513)558-6400     **Free:** 800-558-5004
**Fax:** (513)558-6440
**Website:** http://www.ovtsc.org
Edward C. Robb, Exec. Dir.

**Activities/Fields:** Human tissue, skin and bones.

**★ 13701 ★ Oklahoma Medical Research Foundation**
**Arthritis/Immunology Research Program**
825 NE 13th St.
Oklahoma City, OK 73104
**Phone:** (405)271-7766 **Fax:** (405)271-4110
**Email:** john-harley@omrf.ouhsc.edu
John Harley, MD, Ch.
**Activities/Fields:** Molecular aspects of systemic auto-immunity.

**Palo Alto Institute of Molecular Medicine**
*See:* Entry 4673

**Parkinson's and Movement Disorder Institute (PMDI)**
*See:* Entry 14261

**★ 13702 ★ Polytechnical School of Montreal**
**Research Group in Biomechanics and Biomaterials**
Institut de genie biomedical
PO Box 6079, Downtown Sta.
Montreal, QC, Canada H3C 3A7
**Phone:** (514)340-4378 **Fax:** (514)340-4611
**Email:** yahia@grbb.polymtl.ca
**Website:** http://www.grbb.polymtl.ca
L'Hocine Yahia, Dir.
**Activities/Fields:** Biomechanical behavior of the musculoskeletal system, including the following: modelling of the behavior of human joints and biological tissues; graphic representation of biological structures; biomechanics and microstructure of biological tissues and artificial substitutes; computer-aided design and manufacturing of orthopedic and rehabilitation devices; and stress analysis of knee implants.

**★ 13703 ★ Queen's University at Kingston**
**Human Mobility Research Centre**
Syl & Molly Apps Research Centre
Kingston General Hospital
Kingston, ON, Canada K7L 3N6
**Phone:** (613)548-2430 **Fax:** (613)549-2529
**Email:** alden@post.queensu.ca
**Website:** http://http://conn.me.quennsu.ca/~webcem/
Dr. Marg Alden, Dir.
**Activities/Fields:** Mechanism of musculoskeletal diseases and disorders i.e. the causes, the prevention, and the treatment of bone and joint disorders caused by arthritis, osteoporosis, and injury. **Frmly:** Clinical Mechanics Group.

**★ 13704 ★ Rush University**
**Rush Arthritis and Orthopedics Institute**
1725 W Harrison St., Ste. 1055
Chicago, IL 60612
**Phone:** (312)563-2420 **Fax:** (312)243-7707
**Email:** arth-orth-institute@rush.edu
**Website:** http://www.rush.edu/arthritis/
Dr. Jorge O. Galante, Dir.
**Activities/Fields:** Osteoarthritis and cartilage physiology, inflammatory joint disease, joint replacement, low back pain, orthopedic oncology (musculoskeletal tumors), sports medicine, and scoliosis.

**★ 13705 ★ Rush University**
**Rush Arthritis and Orthopedics Institute Center for Clinical Studies**
1725 W Harrison St., Ste. 1017
Chicago, IL 60612-3824
**Phone:** (312)942-2167 **Fax:** (312)563-2267
**Email:** ccs@rush.edu
**Website:** http://www.rush.edu
Dr. Joel A. Block, Dir.

**Activities/Fields:** Evaluating new treatments and therapies for arthritis and related conditions, including problems associated with wound healing.

**★ 13706 ★ Shriners Hospital for Children (Portland, OR)**
**Research Center**
3101 SW Sam Jackson Pk. Rd.
Portland, OR 97201
**Phone:** (503)221-1537 **Fax:** (503)221-3451
**Email:** wah@shcc.org
**Website:** http://shcc.org/research
Dr. William A. Horton, Dir. of Res.
**Activities/Fields:** Connective tissues, matrix biology, skeletal development.

**Shriners Hospital for Children (St. Louis, MO)**
**Center for Metabolic Bone Disease and Molecular Research**
*See:* Entry 8764

**★ 13707 ★ State University of New York Health Science Center at Stony Brook**
**Osteoporosis Center**
26 Research Way, Technology Park
Belle Meade Rd.
Setauket, NY 11733
**Phone:** (631)444-2663
**Email:** mwhyte@shrinenet.org
**Website:** http://www.informatics.sunysb.edu/internalmed/osteo/osteo.html
Barry L. Gruber, MD, Dir.
**Activities/Fields:** Osteoporosis, particularly bone biology.

**★ 13708 ★ Thomas Jefferson University Lupus Center**
1015 Chestnut St., Ste. 1520
Philadelphia, PA 19107
**Phone:** (215)955-8430 **Fax:** (215)923-5828
**Email:** raphaeldehoratius@mail.tju.edu
Raphael J. DeHoratius, MD, Dir.
**Activities/Fields:** Systemic lupus erthematosus and autoimmune diseases, including reproductive immunology.

**★ 13709 ★ Thomas Jefferson University Scleroderma and Arthritis Research Center**
233 S 10th St.
Philadelphia, PA 19107
**Phone:** (215)503-5042 **Fax:** (215)923-4649
**Email:** sergio.jimenez@mail.tju.edu
Dr. Sergio A. Jimenez, Dir.
**Activities/Fields:** Molecular biology and biochemistry of the connective tissue, pathogenesis of scleroderma and other fibrotic diseases, biological functions of the immune system in health and disease, molecular biology of articular cartilage matrix and heritable diseases of articular cartilage, and identification of gene mutations in human connective tissue diseases and animal models of disease. **Pub:** *Scientific Research Articles/Scientific Reviews.* **Frmly:** Arthritis Clinical Research Center.

**U.S. Department of Health and Human Services**
**Centers for Disease Control and Prevention**
**National Institute for Occupational Safety and Health**
**National Occupational Research Agenda (Musculoskeletal Disorders of the Upper Extremities)**
*See:* Entry 16810

**★ 13710 ★ U.S. Department of Health and Human Services**
**National Institute of Arthritis and Musculoskeletal and Skin Diseases**
NIH Bldg. 31, Rm. 4C32
31 Center Dr., MSC 2350
Bethesda, MD 20892
**Phone:** (301)496-4353 **Fax:** (301)480-6069
**Email:** katz@mail.nih.gov
**Website:** http://www.niams.nih.gov
Dr. Stephen I. Katz, PhD, Dir.
**Activities/Fields:** Large number of diverse diseases, including rheumatoid arthritis, osteoarthritis, systemic lupus erythematosus, muscle diseases, osteoporosis, Paget's disease, back disorders, osteogenesis imperfecta, psoriasis, acne, ichthyosis, epidermolysis bullosa, and vitiligo. The Institute's Intramural Research Program conducts basic research studies in immunology, biophysics, biochemistry, molecular biology, structural biology, pathology and histochemistry, and pharmacology. Through its Arthritis and Rheumatism Branch, the Institute leads basic and clinical research and treatment programs in lupus erythematosus, rheumatoid arthritis, and other connective tissue diseases. The Institute's Extramural Activities Program is organized in five branches: Rheumatic Diseases Branch, Musculoskeletal Diseases Branch, Bone Biology and Bone Diseases Branch, Muscle Biology Branch, and Skin Diseases Branch. Other extramural programs include the Centers Program. The Institute supports basic and clinical research through investigator-initiated research grants, research center grants, individual and institutional research training awards, career development awards, and contracts to public and private research institutions and organizations.

**★ 13711 ★ U.S. Department of Health and Human Services**
**National Institute of Arthritis and Musculoskeletal and Skin Diseases**
**Extramural Activities Program**
**Centers Program**
45 Center Dr., MSC 6500
Bethesda, MD 20892
**Phone:** (301)594-5052 **Fax:** (301)480-4543
**Email:** freemanb@exchange.nih.gov
**Website:** http://www.niams.nih.gov/rtac/funding/grants/centers_programs.htmP30
Julia B. Freeman, PhD, Dir.
**Activities/Fields:** Operates Multidisciplinary Clinical Research Centers (MCRC)s in Arthritis, Musculoskeletal and Skin Diseases. The goal of the Multidisciplinary Clinical Research Center (MCRC) program is to assess and improve outcomes for patients with arthritis and rheumatic diseases; musculoskeletal disorders including orthopedic and bone diseases; muscle diseases; and skin diseases. Maintains Specialized Centers of Research (SCORs) in rheumatoid arthritis, lupus, osteoarthritis, scleroderma, and osteoporosis. Sponsors Core Centers with programs in skin and rheumatic diseases and musculoskeletal disorders. **Frmly:** Multipurpose Arthritis Centers Program.

**★ 13712 ★ U.S. Department of Health and Human Services**
**National Institute of Arthritis and Musculoskeletal and Skin Diseases**
**Extramural Activities Program**
**Muscle Biology Program**
Bldg. 45, Rm 5AS-49E
45 Center Dr., MSC 6500
Bethesda, MD 20892-6500
**Phone:** (301)594-5128 **Fax:** (301)480-4543
**Email:** lymnr@mail.nih.gov
**Website:** http://www.niams.nih.gov/rtac/index.htm
Richard W. Lymn, PhD, Dir.
**Activities/Fields:** Skeletal muscle development and function in normal disease conditions, including studies on the structure and function of muscle, development and regeneration of muscle, normal and abnormal muscle metabolism, and selected diseases and disorders of skeletal muscle.

**★ 13713 ★ U.S. Department of Health and Human Services**
**National Institute of Arthritis and Musculoskeletal and Skin Diseases**
**Extramural Activities Program**
**Musculoskeletal Diseases Branch**
Bldg. 31., Rm. 4-C-02
Bethesda, MD 20892
**Phone:** (301)495-4484　　　**Fax:** (301)480-2814
**Activities/Fields:** Understanding of the structure, function, formation, metabolism, and biomechanics of bones, joints, and skeletal support structures. Research activity focuses on: osteoporosis and other metabolic diseases; joint replacement methods and materials; developmental disorders, including scoliosis, bone immunology, and transplantation; inherited connective tissue disorders; back disorders; and exercise pathophysiology.

**★ 13714 ★ U.S. Department of Health and Human Services**
**National Institute of Arthritis and Musculoskeletal and Skin Diseases**
**Intramural Research Program**
**Arthritis and Rheumatism Branch**
NIH Bldg. 10, Rm. 9N244
10 Center Dr., MSC 1820
Bethesda, MD 20892
**Phone:** (301)496-1474　　　**Fax:** (301)402-0012
**Email:** plotzp@mail.nih.gov
**Website:** http://www.niams.nih.gov/rtbc/arbintro.htm
Dr. Paul Plotz, Chf.
**Activities/Fields:** Arthritis, connective tissue diseases, and related areas, including immunology. Activities involve: disease-related studies on the etiology, pathology, and therapy of connective tissue disorders, with special emphasis on systemic lupus erythematosus, polymyositis, and rheumatoid arthritis (both human disease and animal models of these diseases are studied); and fundamental studies on immune regulation, with special emphasis on autoimmunity and mechanisms of immune responses at the cellular and molecular level. **Pub:** *Proceedings.*

**★ 13715 ★ U.S. Department of Health and Human Services**
**National Institute of Arthritis and Musculoskeletal and Skin Diseases (NIAMS)**
**Intramural Research Program (IRP)**
**Laboratory of Physical Biology (LPB)**
NIH Bldg. 50, Rm. 1140
900 Rockville Pike MSC 8024
Bethesda, MD 20892-8024
**Phone:** (301)496-5880　　　**Fax:** (301)402-0009
**Email:** wang@helix.nih.gov
Dr. Kuan Wang, PhD, Dir.
**Activities/Fields:** Mechanism of muscle contraction in intact cells and simplified preparations using time-resolved X-ray diffraction in conjunction with mechanochemical techniques. Electron microscopy is used with a wide variety of preparations, and digital image processing techniques are used to enhance resolution.

**★ 13716 ★ U.S. Department of Health and Human Services**
**National Institute of Arthritis and Musculoskeletal and Skin Diseases**
**Intramural Research Program**
**Laboratory of Skin Biology**
NIH Bldg. 50 Room 1523
9000 Rockville Pike
Bethesda, MD 20892-8023
**Phone:** (301)496-1578　　　**Fax:** (301)402-2886
Peter Steinert, Chf.
**Activities/Fields:** Structural, molecular, and cellular biology and genetics of skin proteins.

**U.S. Department of Health and Human Services**
**National Institutes of Health**
**National Institute of Child Health and Human Development**
**Division of Intramural Research (Heritable Disorders Branch)**
*See:* Entry 9468

**U.S. Department of Health and Human Services**
**National Institutes of Health**
**National Institute of Dental and Craniofacial Research**
**Division of Intramural Research**
*See:* Entry 6629

**U.S. Department of Veterans Affairs**
**Veterans Health Administration**
**Office of Research and Development**
**Rehabilitation and Development Service (Center for Mobility)**
*See:* Entry 13514

**★ 13717 ★ University of Alabama at Birmingham**
**Arthritis and Musculoskeletal Center**
Tinsley Harrison Tower, Rm. 429
1900 University Blvd.
Birmingham, AL 35294-0006
**Phone:** (205)934-5306　　　**Fax:** (205)934-1564
**Email:** Robert.Kimberly@ccc.uab.edu
**Website:** http://info.dom.uab.edu/rheum/centers/arthritis.htm
Dr. Robert P. Kimberly, Dir.
**Activities/Fields:** Arthritis and related rheumatic disorders, including investigations into cause, diagnosis, control, and treatment of arthritis and complications resulting from arthritis and related musculoskeletal disorders. **Pub:** *Arthritis Today Newsletter,* biennially.

**★ 13718 ★ University of British Columbia**
**Biomechanics Laboratory**
War Memorial Gymnasium
29 6081 University Blvd.
Vancouver, BC, Canada V6T 1Z1
**Phone:** (604)822-9192　　　**Fax:** (604)822-6842
**Email:** david.sanderson@ubc.ca
**Website:** http://www.hkin.educ.ubc.ca/biomech/hometop.htm
David J. Sanderson, PhD, Dir.
**Activities/Fields:** Human motions which are cyclical in nature such as cycling, walking, running and wheelchair propulsion, encompassing amputee, spinal cord injured, and non-injured individuals. The similarities in these movements across individuals reflect the mechanical properties of the musculoskeletal system and that forms the backdrop of the lab's work.

**University of Calgary**
**Joint Injury and Arthritis Research Group**
*See:* Entry 20356

**University of California, Davis**
**Rehabilitation Research and Training Center in Neuromuscular Diseases**
*See:* Entry 14393

**★ 13719 ★ University of California, Los Angeles**
**Duchenne Muscular Dystrophy Research Center (DMDRC)**
5833 Life Science Bldg.
Los Angeles, CA 90095
**Fax:** (310)825-8489
**Email:** dmdrc@physci.ucla.edu
**Website:** http://www.physci.ucla.edu/DMD/
Dr. James Tidball, Dir.
**Activities/Fields:** Development of treatments for Duchenne muscular dystrophy. Researchers are most interested in understanding the role the immune system plays in this condition.

**★ 13720 ★ University of California, San Diego**
**Cartilage Tissue Engineering Laboratory**
Department of Bioengineering, Mail Code 0412
9500 Gilman Dr.
La Jolla, CA 92093-0412
**Phone:** (858)534-0821　　　**Fax:** (858)534-6896
**Email:** rsah@ucsd.edu
**Website:** http://www-bioeng.ucsd.edu/research/research_groups/cte/
Robert L. Sah, MD, Prin. Investigator
**Activities/Fields:** Biological processes of cartilage growth, aging, degeneration, and repair by examining the relationships between tissue with the ultimate goal of improving clinical treatment, diagnosis, and prevention.

**★ 13721 ★ University of California, San Diego**
**Multipurpose Arthritis and Musculoskeletal Diseases Center**
Department of Med.
9500 Gilman Dr.
La Jolla, CA 92093-0635
**Phone:** (858)534-2033
**Email:** hbluestein@ucsd.edu
Harry G. Bluestein, Dir.
**Activities/Fields:** Causes and treatment of arthritis.

**★ 13722 ★ University of California, San Francisco**
**Rosalind Russell Medical Research Center for Arthritis**
350 Parnassus Ave., Ste. 600
San Francisco, CA 94117
**Phone:** (415)476-1141　　　**Fax:** (415)476-3526
**Website:** http://medicine.ucsf.edu/rheum/russell.shtml
Dr. William Seaman, Contact
**Activities/Fields:** Arthritis and its probable causes, focusing on on immunology, immunogenetics, and inflammation. Examines health services and policy and educational approaches and methods for arthritis patients and health professionals.

**★ 13723 ★ University of Chicago**
**Gwen Knapp Center for Lupus and Immunology Research**
924 E 57th St.
Chicago, IL 60637
**Fax:** (773)702-1576
**Activities/Fields:** Immunological and molecular biological research on the cause and treatment of systemic lupus erythematosus.

**★ 13724 ★ University of Cincinnati**
**Cincinnati Rheumatic Disease Study Group**
231 Bethesda Ave., Mail Location 563
Cincinnati, OH 45267
**Phone:** (513)558-4701　　　**Fax:** (513)558-3799
**Email:** ffinkelman@mem.po.com
Fred Finkelman, Dir.
**Activities/Fields:** Rheumatic and allergic diseases, including abnormalities in systemic lupus erythematosus, immunogenetics of connective tissue disease, mechanisms of tolerance and immunomodulation, and asthma pathogenesis autoimmune disease.

**University Hospital of Quebec**
**Pavilion CHUL Research Center**
**Rheumatology and Immunology Research**
**Center**
*See:* Entry 3302

**★ 13725 ★ University of Iowa**
**Orthopaedic Biochemistry and Cell**
**Biology Laboratory**
Orthopaedic Surgery, 1182 ML
Iowa City, IA 52242
**Phone:** (319)335-2595
**Email:** joseph-buckwalter@uiowa.edu
**Website:** http://www.uiowa.edu/~vpr/research/organize/orthchem.htm
Joseph A. Buckwalter, Dir.

**Activities/Fields:** Biochemistry and cell biology of the musculoskeletal system, including proteoglycan biochemistry, age related changes in articular cartilage and intervertebral disc, degeneration and repair of articular cartilage, and synthesis of selected bone proteins.

**★ 13726 ★ University of Iowa**
**Orthopaedic Biomechanics Laboratory**
Orthopedic Surgery
2181 Westlawn Bldg.
Iowa City, IA 52242
**Phone:** (319)335-7528          **Fax:** (319)335-7530
**Email:** tom-brown@uiowa.edu
**Website:** http://www.uiowa.edu/~vpr/research/organize/orthmech.htm
Thomas D. Brown, Dir.

**Activities/Fields:** Mechanics of the musculoskeletal system, including articular joint pathology and estimating forces and stresses in bones, cartilage, muscles, and ligaments, mechanical devices for clinical application in orthopedic surgery, and the relationship between the mechanical environment and tissue and cell responses and their mechanisms.

**★ 13727 ★ University of Manitoba**
**Rheumatic Diseases Research Laboratory**
805 John Buhler Research Centre
715 McDermot Ave.
Winnipeg, MB, Canada R3E 3P4
**Phone:** (204)789-3835          **Fax:** (204)789-3987
**Email:** jwilkin@cc.umanitoba.ca
Dr. John Wilkins, Sci. Dir.

**Activities/Fields:** Immunoregulatory abnormalities and inflammation in rheumatic diseases.

**University of Maryland**
**Center for Alternative Medicine Research**
**on Arthritis**
*See:* Entry 4343

**University of Medicine and Dentistry of**
**New Jersey**
**Institute for Disability Prevention and**
**Wellness**
*See:* Entry 14430

**★ 13728 ★ University of Medicine and**
**Dentistry of New Jersey**
**Lyme Disease Center**
Medical Education Bldg., 484
1 Robert Wood Johnson Pl.
New Brunswick, NJ 08901
**Phone:** (732)235-7702          **Fax:** (732)235-7238
**Email:** sigallh@umdnj.edu
**Website:** http://www.compmed.ummc.umaryland.edu
Leonard H. Sigal, MD, Dir.

**Activities/Fields:** Lyme disease, including epidemiology and clinical manifestations, immunopathogenesis, and the molecular biology of neurologic manifestations.

**★ 13729 ★ University of Michigan**
**Center for Biorestoration of Oral Health**
3310 School of Dentistry, Rm. 3310
1101 N University Ave.
Ann Arbor, MI 48109-1078
**Phone:** (734)763-3388          **Fax:** (734)763-5503
**Email:** ppglab@umich.edu
**Website:** http://www.umich.edu/~cboh
Martha Somerman, Contact

**Activities/Fields:** Connective tissue formation and repair, focusing on identifying and characterizing proteins and genes and establishing their function during development, wound healing, and aging; the role of stem cells to bone cell function and the role of bone environment in cell metastasis. **Frmly:** Laboratories for Connective Tissue Research.

**★ 13730 ★ University of Michigan**
**Multipurpose Arthritis and**
**Musculoskeletal Diseases Center**
3918 Taubman Center, Box 0358
1500 E Medical Center Dr.
Ann Arbor, MI 48109-0358
**Phone:** (734)936-5566          **Fax:** (734)763-1253
**Email:** dcox@umich.edu
**Website:** http://www.med.umich.edu/intmed/rheumatology/mac/mac.htm
David A. Fox, MD, Dir.

**Activities/Fields:** HLA-DRB1 allele-specific signaling aberration in rheumatoid arthritis, role of apoptosis in supraspinatus tendinosis, biomarkers of osteoarthritis and their epidemiology, cognitive and neurochemical function in fibromyalgia. Research focuses on biostatistics, flow cytometry, hydridoma, protein and carbohydate strcuture, transgenic animals, biomechanics and image processing, and DNA sequencing. **Pub:** *MAC Mainline Newsletter*, monthly.

**University of Michigan**
**Orthopaedic Research Laboratories**
*See:* Entry 16961

**★ 13731 ★ University of Minnesota**
**Center for Muscle and Muscle Disorders**
Medical School, MMC 295
420 Delaware St. SE
Minneapolis, MN 55455-0374
**Phone:** (612)625-6180          **Fax:** (612)625-7950
**Email:** johnday@umn.edu
**Website:** http://www1.umn.edu/cmmd/
John Day, MD, Co-Dir.

**Activities/Fields:** Muscle function and disorders.

**★ 13732 ★ University of Missouri—**
**Columbia**
**Missouri Arthritis Rehabilitation Research**
**and Training Center (MARRTC)**
Department of Medicine
1 Hospital Dr.
Columbia, MO 65212
**Phone:** (573)882-6826          **Free:** 877-882-6826
**Fax:** (573)884-3020
**Email:** marrtc@health.missouri.edu
**Website:** http://www.muhealth.org/~arthritis/
Jerry C. Parker, PhD, Dir.

**Activities/Fields:** Arthritis and arthritis rehabilitation, including management of depression and disability in rheumatoid arthritis. **Pub:** *Newsletter "Arthritis Newsbreak"*, quarterly.

**★ 13733 ★ University of North Carolina**
**at Chapel Hill**
**Thurston Arthritis Research Center**
CB 7280
3330 Thurston Bldg.
Chapel Hill, NC 27599-7280
**Phone:** (919)966-0552          **Fax:** (919)966-1739
**Email:** john_winfield@med.unc.edu
**Website:** http://www.med.unc.edu/mac/
John B. Winfield, MD, Dir.

**Activities/Fields:** Arthritis and autoimmune disease. Laboratory research focuses on immunogenetics, immunoregulation, molecular biology, animal models, and complement studies. Non-laboratory research emphasizes social, behavioral, epidemiology, health services research, and educational aspects of chronic arthritis. **Frmly:** Multipurpose Arthritis Center.

**★ 13734 ★ University of North Texas**
**Health Science Center at Fort Worth**
**Center for Osteoporosis Prevention and**
**Treatment (COPT)**
855 Montgomery
Fort Worth, TX 76107
**Phone:** (817)735-2661
Prof. Bernard Rubin, DO, Contact

**Activities/Fields:** Treatment and prevention of post-menopausal osteoporosis, treatment of steroid-induced osteoporosis, and epidemiology of osteoporosis among various ethnic groups.

**★ 13735 ★ University of Pennsylvania**
**Pennsylvania Muscle Institute**
D700 Richards Bldg.
Sch. of Medicine
3700 Hamilton Walk
Philadelphia, PA 19104-6083
**Phone:** (215)898-4017          **Fax:** (215)898-2653
**Email:** goldmany@mail.med.upenn.edu
**Website:** http://www.uphs.upenn.edu/~pmi
Dr. Yale E. Goldman, Dir.

**Activities/Fields:** Studies muscle tissue as it relates to heart disease using specialized techniques developed by the Institute, including rapid spectroscopic methods for measurement of cytoplasmic ions, electron energy loss analysis, and electron probe X-ray analysis for obtaining compositional information about cells. Serves as a regional interdisciplinary center for collaborative studies on development, molecular organization, and function of contractile and regulatory proteins and on mechanics, energetics, excitation/contraction coupling mechanism, and intracellular ion movements in cardiac, smooth, and skeletal muscle.

**★ 13736 ★ University of Texas**
**Southwestern Medical Center at Dallas**
**Harold C. Simmons Arthritis Research**
**Center**
5323 Harry Hines Blvd.
Dallas, TX 75390-8884
**Phone:** (214)648-9110          **Fax:** (214)648-7995
**Email:** david.karp@utsouthwestern.edu
**Website:** http://www.swmed.edu/home_pages/rheumatology
David R. Karp, MD, Interim Dir.

**Activities/Fields:** Inflammatory arthritis, autoimmune disease.

**★ 13737 ★ University of Vermont**
**McClure Musculoskeletal Research Center**
Stafford Hall, 4th Fl.
Department of Orthopaedic and Rehabilitation
Burlington, VT 05405-0084
**Phone:** (802)656-2250          **Fax:** (802)656-4247
**Email:** bruce.beymon@uvm.edu
**Website:** http://www.uvm.edu/~ortho
Bruce D. Beynnon, PhD, Dir.

**Activities/Fields:** Occupational and sports injuries and nontraumatic and congenital disorders, including how musculoskeletal structures are injured and how they heal. Research focuses on lower back pain, including studies of vehicle vibration, exercise, and different low back pain treatments; sports medicine, including knee, shoulder, and ankle injuries; scoliosis, including the etiology of idiopathic scoliosis and growth asymmetry research; osteoarthritis; and joint replacement studies.

# State & Regional Organizations

## Arthritis

*Listed below are chapters of the Arthritis Founda-tion, 1330 W Peachtree St., Atlanta, GA 30309, (800)283-7800, http://www.arthritis.org/.*

### Alabama

**★ 13738 ★ Arthritis Foundation**
**Alabama Chapter**
300 Vestavia Pkwy., Ste. 3500
Birmingham, AL 35216
**Phone:** (205)979-5700          **Free:** 800-879-7896
**Fax:** (205)979-4172
**Email:** info.al@arthritis.org
**Website:** http://www.arthritis.org/communities/chap-ters/Chapter.asp?Chapid=8
Dixie Kuykendall, President

### Arizona

**★ 13739 ★ Arthritis Foundation**
**Greater Southwest Chapter**
1313 E Osborn Rd., Ste. 200
Phoenix, AZ 85014
**Phone:** (602)264-7679          **Free:** 800-477-7679
**Fax:** (602)264-0563
**Email:** info.caz@arthritis.org
**Website:** http://www.arthritis.org/communities/chap-ters/Chapter.asp?Chapid=64
Carol Chamberlin, President
**Remarks:** Serves Arizona, New Mexico, and El Paso, Texas.

### Arkansas

**★ 13740 ★ Arthritis Foundation**
**Arkansas Chapter**
6213 Father Tribou St.
Little Rock, AR 72205
**Phone:** (501)664-7242          **Free:** 800-482-8858
**Fax:** (501)664-6588
**Email:** info.ar@arthritis.org
**Website:** http://www.arthritis.org/communities/chap-ters/Chapter.asp?Chapid=9
Diane Stephenson, President

### California

**★ 13741 ★ Arthritis Foundation**
**Northeastern California Chapter**
3040 Explorer Dr., Ste. 1
Sacramento, CA 95827
**Phone:** (916)368-5599          **Free:** 800-571-3456
**Fax:** (916)368-5596
**Email:** info.neca@arthritis.org
**Website:** http://www.arthritis.org/communities/chap-ters/Chapter.asp?Chapid=35
Joan Stevie, President
**Remarks:** Also serves northern Nevada.

**★ 13742 ★ Arthritis Foundation**
**Northern California Chapter**
657 Mission St., Ste. 603
San Francisco, CA 94105-4120
**Phone:** (415)356-1230          **Free:** 800-464-6240
**Fax:** (415)356-1240
**Email:** info.nca@arthritis.org
**Website:** http://www.arthritis.org/communities/chap-ters/Chapter.asp?Chapid=33
Judith E. McAbee, President

**★ 13743 ★ Arthritis Foundation**
**San Diego Area Chapter**
9089 Clairemont Mesa Blvd., Ste. 104
San Diego, CA 92123-1288
**Phone:** (858)492-1090          **Free:** 800-422-8885
**Fax:** (858)492-9248
**Email:** info.sd@arthritis.org
**Website:** http://www.arthritis.org/communities/chap-ters/Chapter.asp?Chapid=50
Kathy Woodland, Director

**★ 13744 ★ Arthritis Foundation**
**Southern California Chapter**
4311 Wilshire Blvd., Ste. 530
Los Angeles, CA 90010-3775
**Phone:** (323)954-5750          **Free:** 800-954-2873
**Fax:** (323)954-5790
**Email:** info.sca@arthritis.org
**Website:** http://www.arthritis.org/communities/chap-ters/Chapter.asp?Chapid=49
**Remarks:** Also serves Hawaii and southern Nevada.

### Colorado

**★ 13745 ★ Arthritis Foundation**
**Rocky Mountain Chapter**
2280 S Albion St.
Denver, CO 80222-4906
**Phone:** (303)756-8622          **Free:** 800-475-6447
**Fax:** (303)759-4349
**Email:** info.rm@arthritis.org
**Website:** http://www.arthritis.org/communities/chap-ters/Chapter.asp?Chapid=80
Ted Zerwin, President
**Remarks:** Serves Colorado and Wyoming.

### Connecticut

**★ 13746 ★ Arthritis Foundation**
**Southern New England Chapter**
35 Cold Spring Rd., Ste. 411
Rocky Hill, CT 06067
**Phone:** (860)563-1177          **Free:** 800-541-8350
**Fax:** (860)563-6018
**Email:** info.sne@arthritis.org
**Website:** http://www.arthritis.org/communities/chap-ters/Chapter.asp?Chapid=66
Leslie Kotke, President
**Remarks:** Serves Connecticut and Rhode Island.

### Delaware

**★ 13747 ★ Arthritis Foundation**
**Delaware Chapter**
100 W 10th St., Ste. 1105
Wilmington, DE 19801-1663
**Phone:** (302)777-1212          **Free:** 800-292-9599
**Fax:** (302)777-1841
**Email:** info.de@arthritis.org
**Website:** http://www.arthritis.org/communities/chap-ters/Chapter.asp?Chapid=15
Martha M. Buccino, President

### District of Columbia

**★ 13748 ★ Arthritis Foundation**
**Metropolitan Washington Chapter**
4455 Connecticut Ave. NW, Ste. 300
Washington, DC 20008
**Phone:** (202)537-6800          **Fax:** (202)537-6859
**Email:** info.mwa@arthritis.org
**Website:** http://www.arthritis.org/communities/chap-ters/Chapter.asp?Chapid=32
**Remarks:** Serves Washington DC, Maryland, and Virginia.

### Florida

**★ 13749 ★ Arthritis Foundation**
**Florida Chapter**
400 Hibiscus St., Ste. 200
West Palm Beach, FL 33401
**Phone:** (561)655-4970          **Free:** 800-672-0882
**Fax:** (561)655-2780
**Email:** info.fl@arthritis.org
**Website:** http://www.arthritis.org/communities/chap-ters/Chapter.asp?Chapid=61

### Georgia

**★ 13750 ★ Arthritis Foundation**
**Georgia Chapter**
550 Pharr Rd., Ste. 550
Atlanta, GA 30305
**Phone:** (404)237-8771          **Free:** 800-933-7023
**Fax:** (404)237-8153
**Email:** info.ga@arthritis.org
**Website:** http://www.arthritis.org/communities/chap-ters/Chapter.asp?Chapid=19
Elizabeth A. Martin, President

### Hawaii

**★ 13751 ★ Arthritis Foundation**
**Soutern California Chapter**
**Hawaii Office**
615 Piikoi St., Ste. 1812
Honolulu, HI 96814
**Phone:** (808)596-2900          **Free:** 800-954-2873
**Fax:** (808)596-2904
**Email:** info.sca.hib@arthritis.org
**Website:** http://www.arthritis.org

### Illinois

**★ 13752 ★ Arthritis Foundation**
**Greater Chicago Chapter**
303 E Wacker Dr., Ste. 300
Chicago, IL 60601-5206
**Phone:** (312)616-3470          **Free:** 800-735-0096
**Fax:** (312)616-9281
**Email:** info.gc@arthritis.org
**Website:** http://www.arthritis.org/communities/chap-ters/Chapter.asp?Chapid=11

**★ 13753 ★ Arthritis Foundation**
**Greater Illinois Chapter**
2621 N Knoxville Ave.
Peoria, IL 61604
**Phone:** (309)682-6600          **Free:** 800-795-9115
**Fax:** (309)682-6732
**Email:** info.gil@arthritis.org
**Website:** http://www.arthritis.org/communities/chap-ters/Chapter.asp?Chapid=20
Gary Dutro, President

### Indiana

**★ 13754 ★ Arthritis Foundation**
**Indiana Chapter**
8660 Guion Rd.
Indianapolis, IN 46268
**Phone:** (317)879-0321          **Free:** 800-783-2342
**Fax:** (317)876-5608
**Email:** info.in@arthritis.org
**Website:** http://www.arthritis.org/communities/chap-ters/Chapter.asp?Chapid=22
Marva Cobb, President

### Iowa

**★ 13755 ★ Arthritis Foundation**
**Iowa Chapter**
2600 72nd St., Ste. D
Des Moines, IA 50322-4724
**Phone:** (515)278-0636          **Free:** (866)378-0636
**Fax:** (515)278-2603
**Email:** info.ia@arthritis.org

**Website:** http://www.arthritis.org/communities/chapters/Chapter.asp?Chapid=21
Amy L. Selene, President

**Remarks:** Also serves Rock Island County, Illinois.

## Kansas

★ **13756** ★ **Arthritis Foundation**
**Kansas Chapter**
1602 E Waterman
Wichita, KS 67211-1878
**Phone:** (316)263-0116      **Free:** 800-362-1108
**Fax:** (316)263-3260
**Email:** info.ks@arthritis.org
**Website:** http://www.arthritis.org/communities/chapters/Chapter.asp?Chapid=23
Doris E. Newman, President

## Kentucky

★ **13757** ★ **Arthritis Foundation**
**Kentucky Chapter**
2908 Brownsboro Rd., Ste. 100
Louisville, KY 40206-3506
**Phone:** (502)585-1866      **Free:** 800-633-5335
**Fax:** (502)585-1657
**Email:** info.ky@arthritis.org
**Website:** http://www.arthritis.org/communities/chapters/Chapter.asp?Chapid=24
Cynthia A. Harbin, President

**Remarks:** Also serves southern Indiana.

## Louisiana

★ **13758** ★ **Arthritis Foundation**
**Louisiana Chapter**
15254 Old Hammond Hwy., Ste. A4
Baton Rouge, LA 70816
**Phone:** (225)275-1119      **Free:** 800-673-7508
**Fax:** (225)275-1172
**Email:** info.la@arthritis.org
**Website:** http://www.arthritis.org/communities/chapters/Chapter.asp?Chapid=25
Debbie Goss, President

## Maryland

★ **13759** ★ **Arthritis Foundation**
**Maryland Chapter**
1777 Reisterstown Rd., Ste. 150
Baltimore, MD 21208
**Phone:** (410)602-0160      **Free:** 800-365-3811
**Fax:** (410)602-0420
**Email:** info.md@arthritis.org
**Website:** http://www.arthritis.org/communities/chapters/Chapter.asp?Chapid=28
Jan Thompson, President

**Remarks:** Also serves eastern West Virginia.

## Massachusetts

★ **13760** ★ **Arthritis Foundation**
**Massachusetts Chapter**
29 Crafts St., Ste. 450
Newton, MA 02458-1287
**Phone:** (617)244-1800      **Free:** 800-766-9449
**Fax:** (617)558-7686
**Email:** info.ma@arthritis.org
**Website:** http://www.arthritis.org/communities/chapters/Chapter.asp?Chapid=27
Joanne R. Donoghue, President

## Michigan

★ **13761** ★ **Arthritis Foundation**
**Michigan Chapter**
17117 W 9 Mile Rd., Ste. 950
Southfield, MI 48075-4508
**Phone:** (248)424-9001      **Free:** 800-968-3030
**Fax:** (248)424-9005
**Email:** info.mi@arthritis.org

**Website:** http://www.arthritis.org/communities/chapters/Chapter.asp?Chapid=29
Michelle R.B. Glazier, President

## Minnesota

★ **13762** ★ **Arthritis Foundation**
**North Central Chapter**
1902 Minnehaha Ave. W
Saint Paul, MN 55104
**Phone:** (651)644-4108      **Free:** 800-333-1380
**Fax:** (651)644-4219
**Email:** info.mn@arthritis.org
**Website:** http://www.arthritis.org/communities/chapters/Chapter.asp?Chapid=30

**Remarks:** Serves Minnesota, North Dakota, and South Dakota.

## Mississippi

★ **13763** ★ **Arthritis Foundation**
**Mississippi Chapter**
350 N Mart Plaza
PO Box 9185
Jackson, MS 39286-9185
**Phone:** (601)362-6283      **Free:** 800-844-8400
**Fax:** (601)362-6469
**Email:** info.ms@arthritis.org
**Website:** http://www.arthritis.org/communities/chapters/Chapter.asp?Chapid=31
T.J. McSparrin, President

## Missouri

★ **13764** ★ **Arthritis Foundation**
**Eastern Missouri Chapter**
8390 Delmar Blvd.
Saint Louis, MO 63124
**Phone:** (314)991-9333      **Free:** 800-406-2491
**Fax:** (314)991-4020
**Email:** info.emo@arthritis.org
**Website:** http://www.arthritis.org/communities/chapters/Chapter.asp?Chapid=16
Brenda Susan Van Slyck, President

★ **13765** ★ **Arthritis Foundation**
**Western Missouri/Greater Kansas City Chapter**
3420 Broadway, Ste. 105
Kansas City, MO 64111
**Phone:** (816)753-2220      **Free:** 888-719-5670
**Fax:** (816)753-2227
**Email:** info.wmo@arthritis.org
**Website:** http://www.arthritis.org/communities/chapters/Chapter.asp?Chapid=58
Brad Ziegler, President

## Montana

★ **13766** ★ **Arthritis Foundation**
**Rocky Mountain Chapter**
**Montana Branch**
1643 Lewis Ave., Ste. 3
Billings, MT 59102-4151
**Phone:** (406)245-0231      **Free:** 888-245-0231
**Fax:** (406)245-0397
**Email:** info.rm.mb@arthritis.org
**Website:** http://www.arthritis.org

## Nebraska

★ **13767** ★ **Arthritis Foundation**
**Nebraska Chapter**
7101 Newport Ave., Ste. 304
Omaha, NE 68152
**Phone:** (402)572-3040      **Free:** 800-642-5292
**Fax:** (402)572-3048
**Email:** info.ne@arthritis.org
**Website:** http://www.arthritis.org/communities/chapters/Chapter.asp?Chapid=34
Anne Hellbusch, Exec Director

**Remarks:** Also serves Iowa.

## Nevada

★ **13768** ★ **Arthritis Foundation**
**Southern California Chapter**
**Las Vegas Branch**
2450 Chandler Ave., Ste. 17
Las Vegas, NV 89120-4059
**Phone:** (702)367-1626      **Free:** 800-954-2873
**Fax:** (702)367-6381
**Email:** info.sca.lvb@arthritis.org
**Website:** http://www.arthritis.org

## New Hampshire

★ **13769** ★ **Arthritis Foundation**
**Northern New England Chapter**
**New Hampshire Regional Office**
6 Chenell Dr., Ste. 260
Concord, NH 03301
**Phone:** (603)224-9322      **Free:** 800-639-2113
**Fax:** (603)224-3778
**Email:** info.nne@arthritis.org
**Website:** http://www.arthritis.org

## New Jersey

★ **13770** ★ **Arthritis Foundation**
**New Jersey Chapter**
200 Middlesex Tpke.
Iselin, NJ 08830
**Phone:** (732)283-4300      **Free:** 888-467-3112
**Fax:** (732)283-4633
**Email:** info.nj@arthritis.org
**Website:** http://www.arthritis.org/communities/chapters/Chapter.asp?Chapid=38
Dennis Hirschfelder, President

## New York

★ **13771** ★ **Arthritis Foundation**
**Central New York Chapter**
5858 E Molloy Rd., Ste. 123
Syracuse, NY 13211
**Phone:** (315)455-8553      **Free:** 800-870-1771
**Fax:** (315)455-8714
**Email:** info.cny@arthritis.org
**Website:** http://www.arthritis.org/communities/chapters/Chapter.asp?Chapid=12

★ **13772** ★ **Arthritis Foundation**
**Long Island Chapter**
501 Walt Whitman Rd.
Melville, NY 11747
**Phone:** (631)427-8272      **Fax:** (631)427-3546
**Email:** info.li@arthritis.org
**Website:** http://www.arthritis.org/communities/chapters/Chapter.asp?Chapid=26
Patrick T. McAsey, President

★ **13773** ★ **Arthritis Foundation**
**New York Chapter**
122 E 42nd St., 18th Fl.
New York, NY 10168
**Phone:** (212)984-8700      **Fax:** (212)878-5960
**Email:** info.ny@arthritis.org
**Website:** http://www.arthritis.org/communities/chapters/Chapter.asp?Chapid=43

★ **13774** ★ **Arthritis Foundation**
**Northeastern New York Chapter**
1717 Central Ave., Ste. 105
Albany, NY 12205
**Phone:** (518)456-1203      **Free:** 800-420-5554
**Fax:** (518)869-3123
**Email:** rloy@arthritis.org
**Website:** http://www.arthritis.org/communities/chapters/Chapter.asp?Chapid=36
Ronald K. Loy, President

## North Carolina *(Upstate New York continued)*

**★ 13775 ★ Arthritis Foundation**
**Upstate New York Chapter**
3300 Monroe Ave., Ste. 319
Rochester, NY 14618
**Phone:** (585)264-1480 **Fax:** (585)264-1517
**Email:** info.uny@arthritis.org
**Website:** http://www.arthritis.org/communities/chapters/Chapter.asp?Chapid=59
Carol Anne DeMoulin, President

### North Carolina

**★ 13776 ★ Arthritis Foundation**
**Carolinas Chapter**
5019 Nations Crossing, Ste. 217
Charlotte, NC 28217
**Phone:** (704)529-5166 **Free:** 800-883-8806
**Fax:** (704)529-0626
**Email:** info.car@arthritis.org
**Website:** http://www.arthritis.org/communities/chapters/Chapter.asp?Chapid=54
Jim Batten, President
**Remarks:** Serves North Carolina and South Carolina.

### Ohio

**★ 13777 ★ Arthritis Foundation**
**Central Ohio Chapter**
3740 Ridge Mill Dr.
Hilliard, OH 43026
**Phone:** (614)876-8200 **Free:** 888-382-4673
**Fax:** (614)876-8363
**Email:** info.coh@arthritis.org
**Website:** http://www.arthritis.org/communities/chapters/Chapter.asp?Chapid=13
Irene Baird, President

**★ 13778 ★ Arthritis Foundation**
**Northeastern Ohio Chapter**
Chagrin Plaza E, Ste. 210
23811 Chagrin Blvd.
Cleveland, OH 44122-5525
**Phone:** (216)831-7000 **Free:** 800-245-2275
**Fax:** (216)831-1764
**Email:** info.neoh@arthritis.org
**Website:** http://www.arthritis.org/communities/chapters/Chapter.asp?Chapid=37
Susan S. Loessin, President

**★ 13779 ★ Arthritis Foundation**
**Northwestern Ohio Chapter**
309 N Reynolds Rd., Ste. F
Toledo, OH 43615
**Phone:** (419)537-0888 **Free:** 800-551-PALS
**Fax:** (419)537-6553
**Email:** info.nwoh@arthritis.org
**Website:** http://www.arthritis.org/communities/chapters/Chapter.asp?Chapid=78
Cherie Chatreau-Grifo, Director

**★ 13780 ★ Arthritis Foundation**
**Ohio River Valley Chapter**
7811 Laurel Ave.
Cincinnati, OH 45243
**Phone:** (513)271-4545 **Free:** 800-383-6843
**Fax:** (513)271-4703
**Email:** info.orv@arthritis.org
**Website:** http://www.arthritis.org/communities/chapters/Chapter.asp?Chapid=65
Sidney Wittenberg, President
**Remarks:** Serves Kentucky, Ohio, and West Virginia.

### Oklahoma

**★ 13781 ★ Arthritis Foundation**
**Eastern Oklahoma Chapter**
4520 S Harvard, Ste. 100
Tulsa, OK 74135-2932
**Phone:** (918)743-4526 **Free:** 800-400-4526
**Fax:** (918)743-6910
**Email:** info.eok@arthritis.org

**Website:** http://www.arthritis.org/communities/Chapter.asp?Chapid=17
Hope Sutherland, President

**★ 13782 ★ Arthritis Foundation**
**Oklahoma Chapter**
500 N Broadway, Ste. 200
Oklahoma City, OK 73102
**Phone:** (405)236-3399 **Free:** 800-627-5486
**Fax:** (405)236-3393
**Email:** info.ok@arthritis.org
**Website:** http://www.arthritis.org/communities/chapters/Chapter.asp?Chapid=44
Suzi White, President

### Oregon

**★ 13783 ★ Arthritis Foundation**
**Oregon Chapter**
4412 SW Barbur Blvd., Ste. 220
Portland, OR 97239-4004
**Phone:** (503)222-7246 **Free:** 800-283-3004
**Fax:** (503)222-5542
**Email:** info.or@arthritis.org
**Website:** http://www.arthritis.org/communities/chapters/Chapter.asp?Chapid=45

### Pennsylvania

**★ 13784 ★ Arthritis Foundation**
**Central Pennsylvania Chapter**
17 S 19th St.
PO Box 668
Camp Hill, PA 17011
**Phone:** (717)763-0900 **Free:** 800-776-0746
**Fax:** (717)763-0903
**Email:** info.cpa@arthritis.org
**Website:** http://www.arthritis.org/communities/chapters/Chapter.asp?Chapid=14

**★ 13785 ★ Arthritis Foundation**
**Eastern Pennsylvania Chapter**
219 N Broad St., 2nd Fl.
Philadelphia, PA 19107
**Phone:** (215)564-9800 **Free:** 800-355-9040
**Fax:** (215)564-6599
**Email:** info.epa@arthritis.org
**Website:** http://www.arthritis.org/communities/chapters/Chapter.asp?Chapid=18
Lyn Boocock-Taylor, President

**★ 13786 ★ Arthritis Foundation**
**Western Pennsylvania Chapter**
Warner Center, 5th Fl.
332 5th Ave.
Pittsburgh, PA 15222
**Phone:** (412)566-1645 **Free:** 800-522-9900
**Fax:** (412)391-1677
**Email:** info.wpa@arthritis.org
**Website:** http://www.arthritis.org/communities/chapters/Chapter.asp?Chapid=60
Jerry Ellis, President

### Rhode Island

**★ 13787 ★ Arthritis Foundation**
**Southern New England Chapter**
**Rhode Island Office**
Airport Office Park
2348 Post Rd., Ste. 104
Warwick, RI 02886
**Phone:** (401)739-3773 **Fax:** (401)739-8990
**Email:** info.sne.rio@arthritis.org
**Website:** http://www.arthritis.org

### South Carolina

**★ 13788 ★ Arthritis Foundation**
**Carolinas Chapter**
**Coastal Region Office**
1156 Bowman Rd., Ste. 225
Mount Pleasant, SC 29464
**Phone:** (843)416-1174 **Free:** 800-883-8806
**Fax:** (843)416-1173
**Email:** clebaron@arthritis.org
**Website:** http://www.arthritis.org

### Tennessee

**★ 13789 ★ Arthritis Foundation**
**Tennessee Chapter**
1 Vantage Way, Ste. D-220
Nashville, TN 37228
**Phone:** (615)254-6795 **Free:** 800-454-4662
**Fax:** (615)254-8316
**Email:** info.tn@arthritis.org
**Website:** http://www.arthritis.org/communities/chapters/Chapter.asp?Chapid=53
Charles P. Taylor, President

### Texas

**★ 13790 ★ Arthritis Foundation**
**North Texas Chapter**
2824 Swiss Ave.
Dallas, TX 75204
**Phone:** (214)826-4361 **Free:** 800-442-6653
**Fax:** (214)824-5842
**Email:** info.ntx@arthritis.org
**Website:** http://www.arthritis.org/communities/chapters/Chapter.asp?Chapid=40

**★ 13791 ★ Arthritis Foundation**
**Northwest Texas Chapter**
3001 W 5th St.
Fort Worth, TX 76107
**Phone:** (817)820-0635 **Free:** 800-283-7733
**Fax:** (817)820-0642
**Email:** info.nwtx@arthritis.org
**Website:** http://www.arthritis.org/communities/chapters/Chapter.asp?Chapid=42
Debra Phelan, President

**★ 13792 ★ Arthritis Foundation**
**South Texas Chapter**
3701 Kirby Dr., Ste. 1230
Houston, TX 77098
**Phone:** (713)529-0800 **Free:** 800-364-8000
**Fax:** (713)529-6622
**Email:** info.stx@arthritis.org
**Website:** http://www.arthritis.org/communities/chapters/Chapter.asp?Chapid=52

### Utah

**★ 13793 ★ Arthritis Foundation**
**Utah/Idaho Chapter**
448 East 400 South, Ste. 103
Salt Lake City, UT 84111
**Phone:** (801)536-0990 **Free:** 800-444-4993
**Fax:** (801)536-0991
**Email:** info.utid@arthritis.org
**Website:** http://www.arthritis.org/communities/chapters/Chapter.asp?Chapid=62
Lisa B. Fall, President

### Vermont

**★ 13794 ★ Arthritis Foundation**
**Northern New England Chapter**
257 S Union St.
Burlington, VT 05401
**Phone:** (802)864-4988 **Free:** 800-639-2113
**Fax:** (802)864-5339
**Email:** info.nne@arthritis.org

**Website:** http://www.arthritis.org/communities/chapters/Chapter.asp?Chapid=39
**Remarks:** Serves Maine, New Hampshire, and Vermont.

## Virginia

**★ 13795 ★ Arthritis Foundation**
**Virginia Chapter**
3805 Cutshaw Ave., Ste. 200
Richmond, VA 23230
**Phone:** (804)359-1700          **Free:** 800-456-4687
**Fax:** (804)359-4900
**Email:** info.va@arthritis.org
**Website:** http://www.arthritis.org/communities/chapters/Chapter.asp?Chapid=55
C. Annie Magnant, President

## Washington

**★ 13796 ★ Arthritis Foundation**
**Washington/Alaska Chapter**
3876 Bridge Way N, Ste. 300
Seattle, WA 98103
**Phone:** (206)547-2707          **Free:** 800-542-0295
**Fax:** (206)547-2805
**Email:** info.wa@arthritis.org
**Website:** http://www.arthritis.org/communities/chapters/Chapter.asp?Chapid=56
Karen Smith, President

## Wisconsin

**★ 13797 ★ Arthritis Foundation**
**Wisconsin Chapter**
8556 W National Ave.
West Allis, WI 53227
**Phone:** (414)321-3933          **Free:** 800-242-9945
**Fax:** (414)321-0365
**Email:** info.wi@arthritis.org
**Website:** http://www.arthritis.org/communities/chapters/Chapter.asp?Chapid=57

# Lupus Erythematosus

*The following are constituent chapters of the Lupus Foundation of America, 1300 Piccard Dr., Ste. 200, Rockville, MD 20850-4303, (800)558-0121, http://www.lupus.org/.*

## Alaska

**★ 13798 ★ Lupus Foundation of America**
**Alaska Chapter**
PO Box 240628
Anchorage, AK 99524-0268
**Phone:** (907)338-6332          **Free:** 800-307-5878
**Email:** LFA_Alaska@hotmail.com
**Website:** http://members.xoom.com/LFA_Alaska/index.html

## Arkansas

**★ 13799 ★ Lupus Foundation of America**
**Arkansas Chapter**
220 Mockingbird
Hot Springs, AR 71913
**Phone:** (501)525-9380          **Free:** 800-294-8878
**Email:** lupusarkhs@cs.com

## California

**★ 13800 ★ Lupus Foundation of America**
**Northern California Chapter**
2775 Cottage Way, Ste. 5
Sacramento, CA 95825
**Phone:** (916)973-0776
**Email:** saclupus@excite.com
**Website:** http://www.saclupus.org

**★ 13801 ★ Lupus Foundation of America**
**San Diego Chapter**
3914 Murphy Canyon Rd., Ste. A132
San Diego, CA 92123
**Phone:** (858)278-2788

## Connecticut

**★ 13802 ★ Lupus Foundation of America**
**Connecticut Chapter**
97 South St., Ste. 110
West Hartford, CT 06110-1960
**Phone:** (860)953-0387
**Email:** CTLFA@aol.com
**Website:** http://www.lupusct.org

## Delaware

**★ 13803 ★ Lupus Foundation of America**
**Delaware Chapter**
100 W 10th St., Ste. 1015
Wilmington, DE 19801
**Phone:** (302)622-8700          **Free:** 800-880-8686

## Florida

**★ 13804 ★ Lupus Foundation of America**
**Greater Florida Chapter**
300 S Duncan Ave., Ste. 235-B
Clearwater, FL 33755
**Phone:** (727)447-7075          **Free:** 800-684-9276
**Email:** Greaterfla@aol.com
**Website:** http://www.lupusflorida.org

**★ 13805 ★ Lupus Foundation of America**
**Northwest Florida Chapter**
PO Box 17841
Pensacola, FL 32522-7841
**Phone:** (850)478-8107          **Free:** 800-458-8211
**Email:** info@lupus.pensacola.com
**Website:** http://www.lupus.pensacola.com

**★ 13806 ★ Lupus Foundation of America**
**Southeast Florida Chapter**
75 NE 6th Ave., Ste. 223
Delray Beach, FL 33483
**Phone:** (561)279-8606          **Free:** 800-339-0586
**Email:** lupusfl@bellsouth.net
**Website:** http://www.lupusfl.com

## Georgia

**★ 13807 ★ Lupus Foundation of America**
**Georgia Chapter**
6425 Powers Ferry Rd. NW, Ste. 275
Atlanta, GA 30339-2920
**Phone:** (770)952-3891          **Free:** 800-800-4LFA
**Email:** lfagac@attglobal.net
**Website:** http://www.lfaga.org

## Hawaii

**★ 13808 ★ Hawaii Lupus Foundation**
1200 College Walk, Ste. 114
Honolulu, HI 96817
**Phone:** (808)538-1522
**Email:** hlf@pixi.com

## Indiana

**★ 13809 ★ Lupus Foundation of America**
**Central Indiana Chapter**
PO Box 51066
Indianapolis, IN 46251-1066
**Phone:** (317)858-9133
**Email:** lupuscentralin@cs.com

**★ 13810 ★ Lupus Foundation of America**
**Northwest Indiana Chapter**
PO Box 2763
Portage, IN 46368
**Phone:** (219)762-6575
**Email:** lupusnwichapter@aol.com

## Iowa

**★ 13811 ★ Lupus Foundation of America**
**Iowa Chapter**
PO Box 13174
Des Moines, IA 50310-0174
**Phone:** (515)279-3048          **Free:** 888-279-3048
**Email:** LupusIAchapter@aol.com

## Kansas

**★ 13812 ★ Lupus Foundation of America**
**Kansas Chapter**
PO Box 12204
Wichita, KS 67277-2204
**Phone:** (316)262-6180
**Email:** lupus@kansaslupus.org
**Website:** http://www.kansaslupus.org

## Louisiana

**★ 13813 ★ Louisiana Lupus Foundation**
7732 Goodwood Blvd., Ste. L
Baton Rouge, LA 70806
**Phone:** (225)927-8052          **Free:** 888-60-LUPUS

## Maryland

**★ 13814 ★ Lupus Foundation of America**
1300 Piccard Dr., Ste. 200
Rockville, MD 20850-4303
**Phone:** (301)670-9292          **Free:** 800-558-0121

## Missouri

**★ 13815 ★ Lupus Foundation of America**
**Kansas City Chapter**
1012-A Main St.
Grandview, MO 64030
**Phone:** (816)761-0850
**Email:** lupuskcm@crn.org
**Website:** http://www.crn.org/lupus/

**★ 13816 ★ Lupus Foundation of America**
**Missouri Chapter**
8390 Delmar Blvd.
Saint Louis, MO 63124
**Phone:** (314)432-0008          **Free:** 800-958-7876
**Email:** information@lupusmo.org
**Website:** http://www.lupusmo.org

## Nevada

**★ 13817 ★ Lupus Foundation of America**
**Northern Nevada Chapter**
1000 Bible Way, Ste. 69
Reno, NV 89502
**Phone:** (775)323-2444

**★ 13818 ★ Lupus Foundation of America**
**Southern Nevada Chapter**
PO Box 34645
Las Vegas, NV 89133-4645
**Phone:** (702)566-1425
**Email:** SNVLupus@aol.com

## New Hampshire

**★ 13819 ★ New Hampshire Lupus**
**Foundation, Inc.**
PO Box 5500
Manchester, NH 03108-5500
**Phone:** (603)424-0111

**Email:** Lupusnh@email.msn.com
**Website:** http://communities.msn.com/Lupusmemorabilia

## New Jersey

★ **13820** ★ **Lupus Foundation of America
New Jersey Chapter**
PO Box 320
Elmwood Park, NJ 07407
**Phone:** (201)791-7868          **Free:** 800-322-5816
**Email:** NJ4lupus@aol.com

★ **13821** ★ **Lupus Foundation of America
South Jersey Chapter**
Business Executive Complexes
1873 Rte. 70 E, Ste. 110F
Cherry Hill, NJ 08003
**Phone:** (856)424-0255          **Free:** 877-475-8787
**Email:** lupssj@cs.com

## New Mexico

★ **13822** ★ **Lupus Foundation of America
New Mexico Chapter**
2917 Carlisle Blvd. NE, Ste. 103
Albuquerque, NM 87110-2850
**Phone:** (505)881-9081
**Email:** lfanm@juno.com
**Website:** http://www.lupusnm.org

## New York

★ **13823** ★ **Lupus Foundation of America
Bronx Chapter**
PO Box 1117
Bronx, NY 10462
**Phone:** (718)822-6542

★ **13824** ★ **Lupus Foundation of America
Central New York Chapter**
Pickard Office Bldg.
5858 E Molloy Rd., Ste. 173
Syracuse, NY 13211
**Phone:** (315)454-9886          **Fax:** (315)454-9887
**Email:** cnylupus@aol.com

★ **13825** ★ **Lupus Foundation of America
Genesee Valley Chapter**
500 Helendale Rd., Ste. 153
Rochester, NY 14609
**Phone:** (585)288-2910
**Email:** lupusgvc@frontiernet.net

★ **13826** ★ **Lupus Foundation of America
Marguerite Curri Chapter**
PO Box 139
Utica, NY 13503
**Phone:** (315)829-4272
**Email:** lupusmcurri@aol.com
**Remarks:** Serves the counties of Herkimer, Jefferson, Lewis, Madison, Oneida, Otsego and St. Lawrence.

★ **13827** ★ **Lupus Foundation of America
Northeastern New York Chapter**
790 Watervliet-Shaker Rd.
Latham, NY 12110
**Phone:** (518)786-9698          **Free:** 888-749-0100
**Email:** NENYLFA@aol.com
**Website:** http://nenylfa.tripod.com

## North Carolina

★ **13828** ★ **Lupus Foundation of America
Harnett County/Fayetteville/Raleigh
  Branch**
PO Box 1622
Coats, NC 27521
**Phone:** (910)897-8917

**Email:** rbenson@intrastar.net
**Website:** http://www.ncneighbors.com/1090

★ **13829** ★ **Lupus Foundation of America
Piedmont Chapter**
1235-E East Blvd., No. 226
Charlotte, NC 28203
**Phone:** (704)375-8787
**Email:** lupuslinks@aol.com
**Website:** http://www.lupuslinks.org

★ **13830** ★ **Lupus Foundation of America
Winston—Triad Lupus Chapter NCLF**
2841 Foxwood Lane
Winston-Salem, NC 27103
**Phone:** (336)768-1493
**Email:** lfawinston-t.nclf@juno.com

## Ohio

★ **13831** ★ **Lupus Foundation of America
Akron Area Chapter**
2769 Front St.
Cuyahoga Falls, OH 44221
**Phone:** (330)945-6767
**Email:** lupusakron@aol.com
**Website:** http://www.lupusohio.org

★ **13832** ★ **Lupus Foundation of America
Columbus, Marcy Zitron Chapter**
6161 Busch Blvd., Ste. 76
Columbus, OH 43229
**Phone:** (614)221-0811
**Email:** columbus@lupusohio.org
**Website:** http://www.lupusohio.org

★ **13833** ★ **Lupus Foundation of America
Greater Cleveland Chapter**
12930 Chippewa Rd., Ste. 6
Rt. 82 at Riverview
Brecksville, OH 44141
**Phone:** (440)717-0183
**Email:** lupuscleveland@aol.com
**Website:** http://www.lupuscleveland.org

★ **13834** ★ **Lupus Foundation of America
Northwest Ohio Lupus Chapter**
337 S Main St., Rm. 14
Findlay, OH 45840
**Phone:** (419)423-9313          **Free:** 888-33-LUPUS
**Fax:** (419)423-5959
**Email:** lupusnwo@juno.com
**Website:** http://www.lupusohio.org

## Oklahoma

★ **13835** ★ **Oklahoma Lupus Foundation**
3131 N MacArthur, Ste. 106-B
Oklahoma City, OK 73122
**Phone:** (405)495-8787          **Free:** 800-725-6445
**Email:** oklupus@flash.net

## Pennsylvania

★ **13836** ★ **Lupus Foundation of America
Southeastern Pennsylvania Chapter**
25 Washington Ln., Ste. 39LL
Wyncote, PA 19095
**Phone:** (215)517-5070
**Email:** info@lupus-sepa.org
**Website:** http://www.lupus-sepa.org

★ **13837** ★ **Lupus Foundation of
  Pennsylvania
Erie Branch**
3711 W 12th St., Unit 7
Erie, PA 16505
**Phone:** (814)838-0713          **Free:** 800-800-5776
**Website:** http://www.lupuspa.org

★ **13838** ★ **Lupus Foundation of
  Pennsylvania
Harrisburg Branch**
5405 Jonestown Rd., Ste. 110
Harrisburg, PA 17112
**Phone:** (717)671-9515          **Free:** 888-215-8787
**Fax:** (717)671-9532
**Email:** cplclfa@aol.com
**Website:** http://www.lupuspa.org

★ **13839** ★ **Lupus Foundation of
  Pennsylvania
Pittsburgh Branch**
Landmarks Bldg.
One Station Square Dr., Ste. 575
Pittsburgh, PA 15219
**Phone:** (412)261-5886          **Free:** 800-800-5776
**Fax:** (412)261-5365
**Email:** info@lupuspa.org
**Website:** http://www.lupuspa.org

★ **13840** ★ **Lupus Foundation of
  Pennsylvania
Pocono/Northeast Branch**
Keystone College
One College Green
La Plume, PA 18440-0200
**Phone:** (570)945-5118          **Free:** 888-995-8787
**Fax:** (570)945-5119
**Email:** LUPUSNEPA@aol.com
**Website:** http://www.lupuspa.org

## Rhode Island

★ **13841** ★ **Lupus Foundation of America
Rhode Island Chapter**
8 Fallon Ave.
Providence, RI 02908
**Phone:** (401)421-7227

## South Carolina

★ **13842** ★ **Lupus Foundation of America
South Carolina Chapter**
PO Box 1427
Easley, SC 29641-1427
**Phone:** (864)269-2887          **Free:** 877-895-8787
**Fax:** (864)220-1009
**Email:** lupuslfasc@juno.com
**Website:** http://www.midnet.sc.edu/Lupus/Lupus.htm

## Tennessee

★ **13843** ★ **Lupus Foundation of America
East Tennessee Chapter**
10409 Lovell Center Dr.
Knoxville, TN 37922
**Phone:** (865)692-9825          **Free:** 888-59-LUPUS
**Fax:** (865)692-9826
**Email:** lupusTN1@aol.com

★ **13844** ★ **Lupus Foundation of America
Memphis Area Chapter**
3181 Poplar Ave., Ste. 100
Memphis, TN 38111
**Phone:** (901)458-5302
**Email:** MemLupusFund@aol.com
**Website:** http://hometown.aol.com/tdhood69/myhomepage/business.html

★ **13845** ★ **Lupus Foundation of America
Nashville Area Chapter**
4004 Hillsboro Rd., Ste. 223-B
Nashville, TN 37215
**Phone:** (615)298-2273
**Email:** lupustn@usit.com
**Website:** http://www.lupusnashville.org

## Texas

**★ 13846 ★ Lupus Foundation of America**
**El Paso Area Branch**
1401 Montana Ave., Ste. N
El Paso, TX 79902
**Phone:** (915)542-0330　　　**Fax:** (915)542-0012
**Email:** butterfly_hugs@cs.com

**★ 13847 ★ Lupus Foundation of America**
**North Texas Chapter**
PO Box 810310
Dallas, TX 75381-0310
**Phone:** (972)345-4824　　　**Free:** 800-285-2369
**Website:** http://www.lupus-northtexas.org

**★ 13848 ★ Lupus Foundation of America**
**South Central Texas Chapter, Inc.**
3308 Broadway, Stes. 209-210
San Antonio, TX 78209
**Phone:** (210)651-9480　　　**Free:** 800-809-3953
**Email:** lupustx@sbcglobal.net
**Website:** http://www.lupusstx.org

**★ 13849 ★ Lupus Foundation of America**
**Texas Gulf Coast Chapter**
3730 Kirby Dr., Ste. 720
Houston, TX 77098
**Phone:** (713)529-0126　　　**Free:** 800-458-7870

**Email:** LFA@lupustexas.org
**Website:** http://www.lupustexas.org

**★ 13850 ★ Lupus Foundation of America**
**West Texas Chapter**
1717 Ave. K, Ste. 224
Lubbock, TX 79401
**Phone:** (806)744-6666　　　**Free:** 800-580-5878
**Email:** lfawesttx@juno.com

## Utah

**★ 13851 ★ Lupus Foundation of America**
**Utah Chapter, Inc.**
455 E 500 S, Lower Level No. 2
Salt Lake City, UT 84111
**Phone:** (801)364-0366　　　**Free:** 800-657-6398
**Email:** LFAUtah1@mcleodusa.net
**Website:** http://lupuswest.topcities.com
**Remarks:** Also serves Idaho, Montana and Wyoming.

## Vermont

**★ 13852 ★ Lupus Foundation of America**
**Vermont Chapter**
PO Box 115
Waterbury, VT 05676
**Phone:** (802)244-5988
**Email:** LupusVT@aol.com

## Virginia

**★ 13853 ★ Lupus Foundation of America**
**Eastern Virginia Chapter**
Pembroke One
281 Independence Blvd., Ste. 434
Virginia Beach, VA 23462
**Phone:** (757)490-2793　　　**Fax:** (757)490-1086
**Email:** evalupus@yahoo.com

## Washington

**★ 13854 ★ Lupus Foundation of America**
**Pacific Northwest Chapter**
17962 Midvale Ave. N, Ste. 208
Shoreline, WA 98133
**Phone:** (206)546-6785　　　**Free:** 877-774-2992
**Email:** lupuspncwa@earthlink.net
**Remarks:** Serves Washington, Oregon and Idaho.

## Wisconsin

**★ 13855 ★ Lupus Foundation of America**
**Wisconsin Chapter, Inc.**
8544 W National Ave., Ste. 22-24
West Allis, WI 53227
**Phone:** (414)541-3033
**Email:** lupuswi@aol.com

# Foundations & Other Funding Organizations

## Private Foundations

**Clara and Spencer Werner Foundation**
*See:* Entry 2888

**Corbett Foundation**
*See:* Entry 17782

**★ 13856 ★ Esther A. and Joseph Klingenstein Fund, Inc.**
787 Seventh Ave., 6th Floor
New York, NY 10019-6016
**Phone:** (212)492-6181 **Fax:** (212)492-7007
**Email:** cswernerf@tigerpaw.com
John Klingenstein, President
**Fnded:** 1946. **Philosophy:** The Fund's major interests are in two program areas: neuroscience and independent secondary education. The primary focus of the neuroscience program is the annual fellowship awards to young investigators (up to ten a year) doing basic research in neuroscience, specifically related to the etiology of epilepsy. In independent secondary education, major support is for the development of faculty members and administrators through programs at the Klingenstein Center for Independent Education at Teachers College, Columbia University. Grants are also made to organizations concerned with the separation of church and state; animal-based research for the advancement of medicine; and prevention of teenage pregnancy. The directors continue to support institutions in which they are personally involved. **Priorities:** *Education:* 61%. Support independent secondary education and the Klingenstein Fellowships. *Environment:* 1%. *International:* 17%. Support for neuroscience/epilepsy research and animal-based medical research. **Typ. Recipients:** Adolescent Health Issues, Cancer, Children's Health/Hospitals, Clinics/Medical Centers, Family Planning, Hospitals, Hospitals (University Affiliated), Medical Education, Medical Research, Mental Health, People with Disabilities, Preventive Medicine/Wellness Organizations, Public Health, Research/Studies Institutes, Single-Disease Health Associations. **Geo. Dist:** nationally.

**★ 13857 ★ Oberkotter Foundation**
1600 Market St., Ste. 3600
Philadelphia, PA 19103
**Phone:** (215)751-2601
**Email:** George_Nofer@SHSL.com
George Nofer, Co-Trustee and Executive Director
**Fnded:** 1992. **Priorities:** *Education:* 67%. Funds schools for the deaf and medical schools. *International:* 33%. Supports hospitals, medical research, and hearing foundations. *Note:* Total contributions made in 2000. **Typ. Recipients:** Alzheimers Disease, Cancer, Children's Health/Hospitals, Clinics/Medical Centers, Diabetes, Hospitals, Medical Education, Medical Re-

search, People with Disabilities, Public Health, Research/Studies Institutes, Speech & Hearing.

**Oxford Foundation**
*See:* Entry 574

**Valley Foundation**
*See:* Entry 734

## Corporate Foundations

**FBW Foundation**
*See:* Entry 7878

**Robbins and Myers Foundation**
*See:* Entry 8554

**★ 13858 ★ US West Foundation**
1801 California St., Ste. 1360
Denver, CO 80202-2658
**Phone:** (303)896-1266 **Fax:** (303)896-4982
**Email:** Lnash@uswest.com
**Website:** http://www.valley.org
Larry Nash, Director, Administration
**Priorities:** *Arts & Humanities:* 6%. Supports a wide range of cultural and artistic expression. Major interests include culturally diverse works that extend access to other audiences through electronic communications. Extends cultural opportunities by sponsoring performances, exhibits, outreach, or other access through communications technologies, especially in rural areas. *Civic & Public Affairs:* 3%. Interested in programs and organizations that advance economic development and small business support. Provides information access and technical assistance to enhance and grow small business. Encourages strategic planning surrounding economic development connections between communities. Attempts to educate citizens of diverse cultural backgrounds to value the strength and to build leadership within the cultural fabric of their communities. *Education:* 64%. Primary focus of the foundation. Looks for opportunities to improve education and to provide equity in education for all students. Interested in developing partnerships such as those including universities and K-12 educators and those involving business, social service agencies, and school systems. Specifically, major interests include early childhood education, diversity and greater sensitivity to difference, and expansion of interdisciplinary technology in the classroom. *Environment:* 26%. Primary support for the United Way. *Religion:* 1%. Supports science centers. *Note:* Total contributions made in 1998. **Typ. Recipients:** Alzheimers Disease, Emergency/Ambulance Services. **Geo. Dist:** 14 western states served by company.

## Other Funding Organizations

**A-T Medical Research Foundation**
*See:* Entry 9272

**★ 13859 ★ Alzheimer's Association**
919 N Michigan Ave., Ste. 1100
Chicago, IL 60611-1676
**Phone:** (312)335-8700 **Free:** 800-272-3900
**Fax:** (312)335-1110
**Email:** info@alz.org
**Website:** http://www.alz.org
Patricia Pinkowski, Dir. Library
**Desc:** Alzheimer's disease is a progressive, degenerative brain disease in which changes occur in the central nervous system and regions of the brain causing memory loss and other changes in thought, personality, and behavior. Promotes research to find the cause, treatment, and cure for the disease; provides educational programs for the public, media, and health care and medical professionals; represents the continuing care needs of the affected population before government and social service agencies. Seeks to destroy the myth that what were once called "senile behaviors" are a natural part of aging. Works to develop family support systems for relatives of victims of the disease. Sponsors educational forums; operates speakers' bureau. Compiles statistics. Library available. **Awards:** Grant for research.

**★ 13860 ★ American Academy of Neurology (AAN)**
1080 Montreal Ave.
Saint Paul, MN 55116-2325
**Phone:** (651)695-1940 **Free:** 800-879-1960
**Email:** web@aan.com
**Website:** http://www.aan.com
Catherine M. Rydell, Exec. Dir.
**Desc:** Professional society of medical doctors specializing in brain and nervous system diseases. Maintains placement service. Sponsors research and educational programs. Compiles statistics. Publishes scientific journal. **Awards:** Bruce S. Schoenberg International Award and Lecture in Neuroepidemiology (annual) for a young investigator from a developing country; Founder's Award (annual) for a junior member who is the senior author of a research-based manuscript; John Jay Dystel Prize (annual) for multiple sclerosis research; Lawrence C. McHenry Award (annual) for excellence in research in the history of neurology; Medical Student Essay Awards (annual); Potamkin Prize (annual) for research in Pick's, Alzheimer's, and related diseases; S. Weir Mitchell Award (annual) for research by a junior member.

**★ 13861 ★ American Brain Tumor Association (ABTA)**
2720 River Rd., Ste. 146
Des Plaines, IL 60018
**Phone:** (847)827-9910 **Free:** 800-886-2282
**Fax:** (847)827-9918
**Email:** info@abta.org
**Website:** http://www.abta.org
Naomi Berkowitz, Exec. Dir.
**Desc:** Seeks to eliminate brain tumors through research and meet the needs of brain tumor patients and their families. **Awards:** Grant (annual) for post-doctorates conducting brain tumor research; Research Awards for Post-Doctorates (annual) for post-doctoral

candidates whose intent is to pursue a career in brain tumor research.

### ★ 13862 ★ American Headache Society (AHS)

19 Mantua Rd.
Mount Royal, NJ 08061
**Phone:** (856)423-0043     **Fax:** (856)423-0082
**Email:** ahshq@talley.com
**Website:** http://www.ahsnet.org
Linda McGillicuddy, Exec. Dir.

**Desc:** Professional society of health care providers dedicated to the study and treatment of headache and face pain. Objectives are to promote the exchange of information and ideas concerning the causes and treatments of headache and related painful disorders, to educate physicians, health professionals and the public, and to encourage research. **Awards:** AASH/Eli Lilly Headache and Depression Research Award (annual); AASH/Glaxo Wellcome (annual); AASH/Glaxo Wellcome Headache Research Award (annual); AASH/Merck US Human Health Clinical Fellowship Stipend (annual); AASH/Merck US Human Health Migraine & Women's Health Research Award (annual); AASH/Pfizer Headache Research Award (annual); Behavioral Poster Award (annual); Harold G. Wolff Lecture Award (annual); Kaplan Award for Chronic Daily Headache (annual); Poster Award (annual); Resident/Fellow Travel Award (annual).

### ★ 13863 ★ American Neurotology Society (ANS)

c/o Paul Lambert, MD, Chairman
Medical University of South Carolina
Box 250582
Charleston, SC 29425
**Phone:** (843)792-7161     **Fax:** (843)792-0546
**Email:** lambert@muse.edu
**Website:** http://itsa.ucsf.edu/~ajo/ANS/ANS.html
Stephen G. Harner, MD, Pres.

**Desc:** Physicians and audiologists interested in the diagnosis and treatment of hearing and balance disorders. Promotes education and research in the field of neurotology. **Awards:** Monetary (annual).

### ★ 13864 ★ American Society of Electroneurodiagnostic Technologists (ASET)

204 W 7th St.
Carroll, IA 51401-2317
**Phone:** (712)792-2978     **Fax:** (712)792-6962
**Email:** info@aset.org
**Website:** http://www.aset.org
Debra Jester Carson, Pres.

**Desc:** Persons engaged in clinical electroencephalographic (EEG) technology, evoked potential responses, nerve conduction studies, and polysomnography (sleep studies). Objective is the advancement of electroneurodiagnostic technology education and practice standards. **Awards:** Maureen Berkeley Memorial Award (annual) for the best article by an EEG technologist published in the *American Journal of Electroneurodiagnostic Technology*; scholarship (quarterly) for members for expenses in attending the annual meeting and short courses.

### ★ 13865 ★ American Spinal Injury Association (ASIA)

345 E Superior, Rm. 1436
Chicago, IL 60611
**Phone:** (312)238-1242     **Fax:** (312)238-0869
**Email:** mars@northwestern.edu
**Website:** http://www.asia-spinalinjury.org
Marianne G. Kaplan, Exec. Sec.

**Desc:** Medical doctors and Allied Health Care professionals who have been trained in the care of spinal injury patients and who are either actively engaged in the field and acknowledged to be competent by their peers or who have made a significant contribution to the advancement of the basic sciences or one of the clinical fields of practice as they are applicable to the treatment of spinal cord injury. Purposes are to: develop knowledge and investigation of the causes, cure, and prevention of spinal injury and related trauma; pursue excellence in spinal injury patient care; promote and exchange ideas between professionals in the field; standardize medical terminology in spinal cord injury; foster and encourage basic research in the field; develop teaching and educational material; foster education of the medical profession and laity in the prevention and proper management of spinal injury, including the necessity for specialized regional spinal injury centers, provision for educational and vocational training, removal of architectural barriers, and promotion of a society more sensitive to the physically inconvenienced individual, including adequate housing and transportation; establish criteria for centers and/or systems of spinal injury management so as to provide optimal care of the spinal injured person. Conducts annual scientific sessions. Sponsors G. Heiner Sell Distinguished Lectureship. **Awards:** G. Heiner Sell Educational Award (annual).

### ★ 13866 ★ Associated Professional Sleep Societies (APSS)

6301 Bandel Rd. NW, Ste. 101
Rochester, MN 55901
**Phone:** (507)287-6006     **Fax:** (507)287-6008
**Email:** info@aasmet.org
**Website:** http://www.apss.org
Jerry Barrett, Exec. Dir.

**Desc:** Members are the Sleep Research Society and American Academy of Sleep Medicine . Works to facilitate sleep research and development of sleep disorder s medicine by encouraging cooperation and exchange of information among members. **Awards:** Dement/Kleitman/Hatfield (annual) academic achievement/distinguished service/public policy.

### ★ 13867 ★ Batten Disease Support and Research Association (BDSRA)

120 Humphries Dr., Ste. 2
Reynoldsburg, OH 43068
**Phone:** (740)927-4298     **Free:** 800-448-4570
**Email:** bdsra1@bdsra.org
**Website:** http://www.bdsra.org
Lance W. Johnson, Exec. Dir.

**Desc:** Families of children afflicted with Batten Disease; health care professionals; interested others. (Batten Disease, is a degenerative neurological disease affecting children, causing seizures, dementia, loss of motor skills, and blindness.) Represents the interest of individuals with Batten; seeks to educate the public and professional community concerning the needs of Battens Disease patients. Provides information and referral services. Conducts support group activities. Maintains registry. **Awards:** Batten Disease Research (annual) for pertinent research.

### ★ 13868 ★ Brain Injury Association of America

105 N Alfred St.
Alexandria, VA 22314
**Phone:** (703)236-6000     **Free:** 800-444-6443
**Fax:** (703)236-6001
**Email:** PublicRelations@biausa.org
**Website:** http://www.biausa.org
Allan I. Bergman, Pres. & CEO

**Desc:** National organization working for and with people with brain injury and their families. Seeks to create a better future through brain injury prevention, research, education and advocacy. **Awards:** Founders Award (annual) for outstanding contributions in building and strengthening the BIA, enabling it to fulfill its mission; Jim and Sarah Brady Public Service Award (annual) for an individual who has enhanced the understanding of brain injury through public service and education at the national level; Sheldon Berrol Clinical Service Award (annual) for individual who, through clinical service, has made outstanding contributions to improving quality of care, professional training, and/or education; Silvio O. Conte Award (annual) for outstanding contributions in affecting national policy as it relates to brain injury; William Fields Caveness Award (annual) for individual who, through research, has made outstanding contributions toward bettering the lives of persons who have sustained traumatic brain injuries; a cash award of $2,000 is given to further the work of the recipient; Young Investigator Award (annual) for an individual within five years of completing professional training.

### ★ 13869 ★ The Brain Tumor Society (TBTS)

124 Watertown St., Ste. 3-H
Watertown, MA 02472
**Phone:** (617)924-9997     **Free:** 800-770-8287
**Fax:** (617)924-9998
**Email:** info@tbts.org
**Website:** http://www.tbts.org
Lawrence Z. Pizzi, Exec. Dir.

**Desc:** Strives to improve the quality of life of brain tumor patients by providing support for them and their families. Raises funds for research in order to find a cure for brain tumors. **Awards:** Grant (annual) for scientific research.

### Children's Brain Tumor Foundation (CBTF)

*See:* Entry 5593

### Dysautonomia Foundation

*See:* Entry 9277

### ★ 13870 ★ Dystonia Medical Research Foundation

1 E Wacker Dr., Ste. 2430
Chicago, IL 60601-2001
**Phone:** (312)755-0198     **Free:** 800-377-DYST
**Fax:** (312)803-0138
**Email:** dystonia@dystonia-foundation.org
**Website:** http://www.dystonia-foundation.org
Valerie F. Levitin, PhD., Exec. Dir.

**Desc:** Dystonia patients and their families; medical personnel; health agencies; interested individuals. Promotes and funds research and encourages increased public awareness of dystonia, a neurologic muscular disorder causing muscles to jerk and contract into abnormal positions. Disseminates information concerning dystonia. Sponsors patient and family support groups. **Awards:** Research Grant (annual) Dystonia research.

### ★ 13871 ★ Epilepsy Foundation

4351 Garden City Dr.
Landover, MD 20785
**Phone:** (301)459-3700     **Free:** 800-332-1000
**Fax:** (301)577-4941
**Email:** info@efa.org
**Website:** http://www.efa.org
Eric R. Hargis, Pres. /CEO

**Desc:** National voluntary health agency which serves as the "focal point for the fight against epilepsy in the United States." Augmented by 64 affiliates in the U.S. committed to preventing and controlling epilepsy and improving the lives of those who have it. Provides federal government liaison. The foundation supports medical, social, rehabilitational, legal, employment, and information, education, and advocacy programs. Sponsors research in causes of epilepsy, prevention, psychosocial needs, and improved methods of treatment. Provides research and training grants and fellowships to students and professionals. Assistance and counseling to epilepsy patients and their families is provided through local organizations and the National Information Center on Epilepsy. Annual projects include National Epilepsy Month (November), School Alert (a national educational program for schools), selection of the Epilepsy Poster Child, and a continuing professional and public education and information program. Maintains a resource center. Provides members with access to mail order pharmacy program. Compiles statistics; maintains placement program. **Awards:** Grant (annual) for epilepsy research.

**Gazette International Networking Institute (GINI)**
*See:* Entry 12003

**★ 13872 ★ Huntington's Disease Society of America (HDSA)**
158 W 29th St., 7th Fl.
New York, NY 10001-5300
**Phone:** (212)242-1968      **Free:** 800-345-4372
**Fax:** (212)239-3430
**Email:** hdsainfo@hdsa.org
**Website:** http://www.hdsa.org
Barbara Boyle, Exec. Dir.
**Desc:** Individuals and groups of volunteers concerned with Huntington's disease, an inherited and terminal neurological condition causing progressive brain and nerve deterioration. Goals are to: identify HD families; educate the public and professionals, with emphasis on increasing consumer awareness of HD; promote and support basic and clinical research into the causes and cure of HD; maintain patient services program, coordinated with various community services, to assist families in meeting the social, economic, and emotional problems resulting from HD. Is working to change the attitude of the working community toward the HD patient, enhance the HD patient's lifestyle, and promote better health care and treatment, both in the community and in facilities. Has launched nationwide campaign in support of federal and state legislation establishing clinics, genetic counseling and screening centers, and diagnostic and treatment centers for HD patients and those suffering from other chronic, debilitating diseases. Actively cooperates with researchers in ongoing studies; co-sponsors and supports workshops and symposia; provides grants to individual researchers; sponsors brain donor program. Crisis intervention and other support services are available. **Awards:** Grant (periodic) Researchers investigating a treatment or cure for Huntington's Disease.

**★ 13873 ★ Hydrocephalus Association (HA)**
870 Market St., Ste. 705
San Francisco, CA 94102
**Phone:** (415)732-7040      **Free:** 888-598-3789
**Fax:** (415)732-7044
**Email:** hydroassoc@aol.com
**Website:** http://www.hydroassoc.org
Emily Fudge, Exec. Dir.
**Desc:** People with hydrocephalus and their families, health care professionals with an interest in hydrocephalus, and interested businesses and foundations. Works to improve the quality of life of people with hydrocephalus through education. Conducts training for families of people with hydrocephalus; sponsors social gatherings; facilitates networking among families of people with hydrocephalus and between organizations representing people with hydrocephalus. **Awards:** Gerard Fudge Memorial Scholarship (3/year) for a person ages 18 to 30 with hydrocephalus.

**International Society for Neuroimmunomodulation**
*See:* Entry 3180

**★ 13874 ★ International Society of Neurovirology**
c/o Brian Wigdahl, Dept. of Microbiology and Immunology Penn State College of Medicine
500 University Dr.
PO Box 850
Hershey, PA 17033
**Phone:** (717)531-8258      **Fax:** (717)531-5580
**Email:** bwigdahl@psu.edu
**Website:** http://www.isnv.org
Brian Wigdahl, PhD, Pres.
**Desc:** Neurovirologists. **Awards:** Pioneer Award (annual) for outstanding contribution to the field of neurovirology.

**★ 13875 ★ Muscular Dystrophy Association (MDA)**
3300 E Sunrise Dr.
Tucson, AZ 85718
**Phone:** (520)529-2000      **Free:** 800-572-1717
**Fax:** (520)529-5300
**Email:** mda@mdausa.org
**Website:** http://www.mdausa.org
Bob Mackle, Dir. Public Information
**Desc:** National voluntary health agency fostering research into the cause and cure of neuromuscular diseases in the following 8 categories. Muscular dystrophies: Becker; congenital; distal; Duchenne (pseudohypertrophic); Emery-Dreifuss; facioscapulohumeral (Landouzy-Dejerine); limb-girdle; myotonic (Steinert's disease); oculopharyngeal. Motor Neuron Diseases: adult spinal muscular atrophy (Aran-Duchenne type); amyotrophic lateral sclerosis (ALS); infantile progressive spinal muscular atrophy (type 1, Werdnig-Hoffmann disease); intermediate spinal muscular atrophy (type 2); juvenile spinal muscular atrophy (type 3, Kugelberg-Welander disease); Spinal Bulbar Muscular Atrophy (SBMA). Inflammatory Myopathies: dermatomyositis; polymyositis; inclusion body myositis. Diseases of Neuromuscular Junction: Eaton-Lambert (myasthenic) syndrome;congenital myasthenic syndrome; myasthenia gravis. Diseases of the Peripheral Nerve: Dejerine-Sottas disease; Friedreich's ataxia; Charcot-Marie-Tooth disease (peroneal muscular atrophy). Metabolic Diseases of Muscle: acid maltase deficiency (Pompe's disease); carnitine deficiency; carnitine palmityl transferase deficiency; Debrancher enzyme deficiency (Cori'sor Forbes' disease); lactate dehydrogenase deficiency; mitochondrial myopathy; myoadenylate deaminase deficiency; phosphofructokinase deficiency (Tarui's disease); phosphoglycerate kinase deficiency; phosphoglycerate mutase deficiency; phosphorylase deficiency (McArdle's disease). Myopathies due to Endocrine Abnormalities: hyperthyroid myopathy; hypothyroid myopathy. Other myopathies: central core disease; myotonia congenita; myotubular myopathy; nemaline myopathy; paramyotonia congenita; periodic paralysis. Supports international programs of some 350 research awards, major university-based neuromuscular disease research/clinical centers, and 230 outpatient clinics in hospitals in the U.S. and Puerto Rico. Awards grants for neuromuscular disease research to individual scientific investigators. Renders services to patients locally through its chapters, including: diagnostic examinations; follow-up medical evaluations; wheelchairs; leg braces; physical therapy; flu shots; summer camps. **Awards:** Neuromuscular disease research grants (semiannual) must meet eligibility requirements set by MDA.

**National Ataxia Foundation (NAF)**
*See:* Entry 9284

**★ 13876 ★ National Brain Tumor Foundation (NBTF)**
414 13th St., No. 700
Oakland, CA 94612-2603
**Phone:** (510)839-9777      **Free:** 800-934-CURE
**Fax:** (510)839-9779
**Email:** nbtf@braintumor.org
**Website:** http://www.braintumor.org
Janis Brewer, Exec. Dir.
**Desc:** Medical researchers, doctors, brain tumor patients, and relatives working together to improve the quality of life for brain tumor patients and their families and find a cure through research. Raises funds for brain tumor research; offers patient services such as educational materials, a toll-free brain tumor information line, a quarterly newsletter, information about support groups and patient networks, and national and regional conferences. **Awards:** Grant (annual) for research.

**National Neurofibromatosis Foundation (NNFF)**
*See:* Entry 9286

**★ 13877 ★ National Neurotrauma Society**
c/o Linda Garcia
PO Box 143060
Gainesville, FL 32608
**Phone:** (352)271-1169      **Fax:** (352)271-3060
**Email:** lindahou@aol.com
**Website:** http://www.neurotrauma.org
Linda Garcia, Contact
**Desc:** Conducts scientific research in neurotrauma field. **Awards:** Student Travel Award (annual).

**★ 13878 ★ National Parkinson Foundation (NPF)**
1501 NW 9th Ave.
Bob Hope Parkinson's Research Center
Miami, FL 33136-1494
**Phone:** (305)547-6666      **Free:** 800-327-4545
**Fax:** (305)548-4403
**Email:** mailbox@npf.med.miami.edu
**Website:** http://www.parkinson.org
Herbert C. Zemel, Pres.
**Desc:** Doctors, nurses, scientists, pharmacologists, and therapists who research, diagnose, and treat Parkinsonism. Supports basic and clinical research for Parkinsonism and related neurological disorders and provides physical, speech, and occupational therapy. NPF is associated with the University of Miami School of Medicine, and supports the National Parkinson Institute, which provides diagnosis, treatment, care, and rehabilitation. Conducts educational programs. Distributes literature to medical libraries, nurses training schools, health clinics, physicians, and patients. Sponsors regional patient self-support groups where problems are discussed and experiences are exchanged under guidance of physicians, social workers, and psychologists. Maintains offices at 122 E. 42nd St., New York, NY 10017 and 4929 Wilshire Blvd., Los Angeles, CA 90010. **Awards:** Research Grants (annual).

**★ 13879 ★ National Stroke Association (NSA)**
9707 E Easter Ln.
Englewood, CO 80112-3747
**Phone:** (303)649-9299      **Free:** 800-STR-OKES
**Fax:** (303)649-1328
**Email:** info@stroke.org
**Website:** http://www.stroke.org
Patti Shwayder, Exec. Dir. /CEO
**Desc:** Stroke survivors and their families; health care professionals and institutions; the lay community. Seeks to reduce the incidence and impact of stroke by promoting research, educating the public, and providing a network for stroke survivors and concerned persons. Serves as an information referral clearinghouse on stroke; makes available educational materials on stroke prevention, treatment, rehabilitation, resocialization, and research. Offers guidance in the development of stroke support groups and clubs. Maintains speakers' bureau and Stroke Information and Referral Center; compiles statistics. Conducts educational symposiums/meetings. **Awards:** Community Education Award (annual) for medical facilities and community Organization; Research Fellowship Award in Cerebrovascular Disease (annual) for doctors dedicated to the field of stroke as a career.

**Neurofibromatosis (NF)**
*See:* Entry 9288

**★ 13880 ★ Neuropathy Association**
Lincoln Bldg.
60 E 42nd St., Ste. 942
New York, NY 10165
**Phone:** (212)692-0662      **Free:** 800-247-6968
**Fax:** (212)692-0668
**Email:** info@neuropahty.org
**Website:** http://www.neuropathy.org
Catherine Law, CFO
**Desc:** Offers support to persons suffering from disorders affecting the peripheral nerves; provides patient support and education, advocates for patients' inter-

ests, promotes research into the causes and cure for peripheral neuropathies. **Awards:** Grant (periodic).

★ **13881** ★ **Reflex Sympathetic Dystrophy Association of America**
PO Box 502
Milford, CT 06460
**Phone:** (203)877-3790          **Free:** 877-662-7737
**Fax:** (203)882-8362
**Email:** jwbroatch@aol.com
**Website:** http://www.rsds.org
James Broaich, MSW, Exec. Dir.
**Desc:** People with Reflex Sympathetic Dystrophy Syndrome, also known as Complex Regional Pain Syndrome Type I and Type II; health care professionals treating RSDS patients. (RSDS is a disorder of the autonomic nervous system whose onset is usually preceded by a minor trauma such as a muscle sprain; symptoms of RSDS include severe pain, loss of muscle motion and use, swelling, skin and nail changes, and softening of the bones in affected areas.) Promotes increased awareness of RSDS among health care professionals and the public; conducts media campaigns; maintains national network of physicians involved in RSDS treatment and research. Encourages and supports RSDS research; has a national data bank for the coordination of RSDS research and treatment information. Aids in the formation of support groups for people with RSDS; develops in-service programs and seminars for use at hospitals and educational institutions. Makes available referral services. Conducts educational programs; maintains speakers' bureau; compiles statistics, funds research, has published clinical practice guidelines for diagnosis, treatment, and management of RSDS/CRPS. **Awards:** RSDSA Fellowship Grant (annual) for research.

★ **13882** ★ **Sturge-Weber Foundation (SWF)**
PO Box 418
Mount Freedom, NJ 07970-0418
**Phone:** (973)895-4445          **Free:** 800-627-5482
**Fax:** (973)895-4846
**Email:** swf@sturge-weber.com
**Website:** http://www.sturge-weber.com
Karen L. Ball, CEO
**Desc:** Persons with Sturge-Weber syndrome and their families; concerned professionals and supporters. Serves as an information clearinghouse on Sturge-Weber syndrome, port-wine stains, and Klippel-Trenaunay Weber syndrome. (Sturge-Weber syndrome is a congenital neurological disorder characterized by facial port-wine stains, seizures, glaucoma, and loss of motor control, accompanied in rare cases by internal organ irregularities.) Disseminates information; offers support to afflicted persons. Maintains speakers' bureau; compiles statistics. Funds research. **Awards:** Grant (annual) for research into port wine stains, glaucoma, and Sturge-Weber.

★ **13883** ★ **World Federation of Neurosurgical Societies (WFNS)**
c/o Dr. Edward Laws
University of Virginia Health Systems
Department of Neuro-Societies
PO Box 800212
Charlottesville, VA 22908
**Phone:** (804)924-2650          **Fax:** (804)924-5894
**Website:** http://www.wfns.org
Dr. Edward Laws, Sec.
**Desc:** National neurosurgical societies representing approximately 17,400 neurosurgeons. Works for the advancement of neurological surgery. **Awards:** Gold Medal of Honor (quadrennial) for excellence in neurosurgery; Scoville Award (quadrennial) for excellence in nuerosurgery; Young Neurosurgeons Award (quadrennial) for excellence in neurosurgery.

## National & International Organizations

★ **13884** ★ **Acoustic Neuroma Association of Canada (ANAC)**
PO Box 369
Edmonton, AB, Canada T5J 2J6
**Phone:** (780)428-3384          **Free:** 800-561-2622
**Email:** anac@compusmart.ab.ca
**Website:** http://www.anac.ca
**Fnded:** 1983. **Mem:** 451. **Lang(s):** English, French. **Desc:** For people with acoustic neuroma, Bell's Palsy, and other neuromuscular disorders, their families, health care professionals, and other interested individuals. Seeks to improve the quality of life of people with neuromuscular diseases; promotes research into the causes and treatment of acoustic neuroma. Conducts charitable programs; provides support and services to people with neuromuscular disorders; maintains speakers' bureau. **Pub:** *Connection*, quarterly. Newsletter.

**ALS Diagnostic Support Group (Vereniging Spierziekten Nederland — VSN)**
*See:* Entry 13538

**ALS Support Group - Belgium (ALS Zelfhulpgroep Belgie)**
*See:* Entry 13539

★ **13885** ★ **Alzheimer Angehorige Austria (AAA)**
Obere Augartenstrasse 26-28
A-1020 Vienna, Austria
**Phone:** 43 1 3325166          **Fax:** 43 1 3342141
**Email:** andre.carpels@unicall.be
**Website:** http://www.vsn.nl
**Lang(s):** English, German. **Desc:** Individuals and organizations. Seeks to improve the quality of life of people with Alzheimer's disease and their families. Makes available support and services; facilitates research on Alzheimer's disease and related disorders; conducts educational programs.

★ **13886** ★ **Alzheimer Europe (AE)**
145 Route de Thionville
L-2611 Luxembourg, Luxembourg
**Phone:** 352 297970          **Fax:** 352 297972
**Email:** info@alzheimer-europe.org
**Website:** http://www.alzheimer-europe.org
**Fnded:** 1990. **Mem:** 27. **Lang(s):** English, French, German. **Desc:** Health care providers and other individuals and organizations with an interest in Alzheimer's disease. Promotes improvement in the diagnosis, prevention, and treatment of Alzheimer's disease; seeks to improve the quality of life of people with Alzheimer's disease and their families. Makes available health care and nursing services; sponsors research and educational programs.

★ **13887** ★ **Alzheimer Keskuslitto (AK)**
Luotsikatu 4E
SF-00160 Helsinki, Finland
**Phone:** 358 9 6226200          **Fax:** 358 9 62262020
**Email:** varpu.kettunen@alzheimer.fi
**Website:** http://www.alzheimer.fi
**Lang(s):** English, Finnish. **Desc:** Individuals and organizations. Seeks to improve the quality of life of people with Alzheimer's disease and their families. Makes available support and services; facilitates research on Alzheimer's disease and related disorders; conducts educational programs.

★ **13888** ★ **Alzheimer Scotland-Action on Dementia (ASAD)**
22 Drumsheugh Gardens
Edinburgh EH3 7RN, United Kingdom
**Phone:** 44 131 2431453          **Fax:** 44 131 2431450
**Email:** alzheimer@alzscot.org
**Website:** http://www.alzscot.org
**Fnded:** 1994. **Mem:** 1,400. **Reg. Groups:** 47. **Lang(s):** English. **Desc:** Individuals and organizations. Seeks to improve the quality of life of people with Alzheimer's disease and their families. Makes available support and services; facilitates research on Alzheimer's disease and related disorders; conducts educational programs.

**Alzheimer Society of Canada (ASC)**
*See:* Entry 2915

★ **13889** ★ **Alzheimer Society of Ireland (ASI)**
Alzheimer House
43 Northumberland Ave.
Dublin, Ireland
**Phone:** 353 1 2846616          **Fax:** 353 1 2846030
**Email:** info@alzheimer.ie
**Website:** http://www.alzheimer.ie
**Fnded:** 1982. **Mem:** 5,000. **Reg. Groups:** 8. **Local Groups:** 30. **Lang(s):** English, Irish. **Desc:** Individuals and organizations. Seeks to improve the quality of life of people with Alzheimer's disease and their families; promotes advancement in the diagnosis and treatment of Alzheimer's disease. Makes available home support and day care service to people with Alzheimer's disease and their families; maintains respite home; serves as a clearinghouse on Alzheimer's disease and services available to people with the disease. **Pub:** *Alheimer Society of Ireland Newsletter*, quarterly. Newsletter.

★ **13890** ★ **Alzheimer Society Romania (SA) (Societatea Alzheimer)**
Bd. Mihail Kgalniceanu 95A
Sc. A et. 1 apt. 8 sector 5
70603 Bucharest, Romania
**Phone:** 40 1 6863470          **Fax:** 40 1 3113471
**Email:** aftudose@fx.ro
**Website:** http://www.alzheimer-europe.org/Romania
**Fnded:** 1992. **Mem:** 900. **Nat'l Groups:** 6. **Lang(s):** English, Romanian. **Desc:** Individuals and organizations. Seeks to improve the quality of life of people with Alzheimer's disease and their families. Makes available support and services; facilitates research on Alzheimer's disease and related disorders; conducts educational programs. **Pub:** Newsletter, quarterly.

★ **13891** ★ **Alzheimerforeningen**
Skt. Lukas Vej 6
DK-2900 Hellerup, Denmark
**Phone:** 45 39400488          **Fax:** 45 39616669
**Email:** post@alzheimer.dk
**Website:** http://www.alzheimer.dk
**Fnded:** 1969. **Mem:** 3,000. **Nat'l Groups:** 1. **Local Groups:** 16. **Lang(s):** Danish, English. **Desc:** Individuals and organizations. Seeks to improve the quality of life of people with Alzheimer's disease and their families. Makes available support and services; facilitates research on Alzheimer's disease and related disorders; conducts educational programs.

★ **13892** ★ **Alzheimerforeningen I Sverige (AIS)**
PO Box 4109
SE-227 22 Lund, Sweden
**Phone:** 46 46 147318          **Fax:** 46 46 188978
**Email:** info@alzheimerforeningen.nu
**Website:** http://www.alzheimerforeningen.nu
**Fnded:** 1986. **Mem:** 4,000. **Lang(s):** English, Swedish. **Desc:** Individuals and organizations. Seeks to improve the quality of life of people with Alzheimer's disease and their families. Makes available support

and services; facilitates research on Alzheimer's disease and related disorders; conducts educational programs. **Pub:** *Alzheimer Foreningen.* Newsletter.

**★ 13893 ★ Alzheimer's Association**
919 N Michigan Ave., Ste. 1100
Chicago, IL 60611-1676
**Phone:** (312)335-8700 **Free:** 800-272-3900
**Fax:** (312)335-1110
**Email:** info@alz.org
**Website:** http://www.alz.org
Patricia Pinkowski, Dir. Library
**Fnded:** 1980. **Local Groups:** 154. **Desc:** Alzheimer's disease is a progressive, degenerative brain disease in which changes occur in the central nervous system and regions of the brain causing memory loss and other changes in thought, personality, and behavior. Promotes research to find the cause, treatment, and cure for the disease; provides educational programs for the public, media, and health care and medical professionals; represents the continuing care needs of the affected population before government and social service agencies. Seeks to destroy the myth that what were once called "senile behaviors" are a natural part of aging. Works to develop family support systems for relatives of victims of the disease. Sponsors educational forums; operates speakers' bureau. Compiles statistics. Library available. **Pub:** *Advances,* quarterly. Newsletter. Covers stories and developments of interest to patients with Alzheimer's disease and related disorders, and their families and friends. *Price:* Free. • Brochures. • Also publishes a variety of fact sheets, video kits, and patient care publications. **Frmly:** (1989) Alzheimer's Disease and Related Disorders Association.

**★ 13894 ★ Alzheimer's Association of Australia**
PO Box 108
Higgins, ACT 2615, Australia
**Phone:** 61 2 62544233 **Fax:** 61 2 62787225
**Email:** secretariat@alzheimers.org.au
**Website:** http://www.alzheimers.org.au
**Lang(s):** English. **Desc:** Represents member interests on all matters relating to dementia and caregiver issues.

**★ 13895 ★ Alzheimer's Association NSW**
PO Box 6042
North Ryde, NSW 1670, Australia
**Fax:** 61 2 98051665
**Email:** library@alznsw.asn.au
**Website:** http://www.alznsw.asn.au
**Fnded:** 1982. **Lang(s):** English. **Desc:** Provides support to people with dementia and their families and works to raise community awareness in New South Wales about Alzheimer's disease and other dementias. **Pub:** Handbooks. HelpNotes covering dementia.

**★ 13896 ★ Alzheimer's Disease International (ADI)**
45/46 Lower Marsh
London SE1 7RG, United Kingdom
**Phone:** 44 207 6203011 **Fax:** 44 207 4017351
**Email:** info@alz.co.uk
**Website:** http://www.alz.co.uk
**Fnded:** 1984. **Mem:** 57. **Lang(s):** English. **Desc:** Umbrella organization of 57 national Alzheimer associations worldwide. Main goal is to build and strengthen these associations so that they are better able to meet the needs of people with dementia and their carers. **Pub:** *Global Perspective,* quarterly. Newsletter. Booklets

**★ 13897 ★ Alzheimer's Society (AS)**
Gordon House
10 Greencoat Pl.
London SW1P 1PH, United Kingdom
**Phone:** 44 20 73060606 **Fax:** 44 20 73060808
**Email:** info@alzheimers.org.uk
**Website:** http://www.alzheimers.org.uk

**Fnded:** 1979. **Mem:** 22,000. **Reg. Groups:** 12. **Lang(s):** English. **Desc:** Individuals and organizations. Seeks to improve the quality of life of people with Alzheimer's disease and their families. Makes available support and services; facilitates research on Alzheimer's disease and related disorders; conducts educational programs. **Frmly:** (1999) Alzheimer's Disease Society.

**★ 13898 ★ Alzheimerstichting**
Postbus 183
NL-3980 CD Bunnik, Netherlands
**Phone:** 31 30 6596285 **Fax:** 31 30 6596283
**Email:** info@alzheimer-ned.nl
**Website:** http://www.alzheimer-ned.nl
**Lang(s):** Dutch, English. **Desc:** Individuals and organizations. Seeks to improve the quality of life of people with Alzheimer's disease and their families. Makes available support and services; facilitates research on Alzheimer's disease and related disorders; conducts educational programs.

**★ 13899 ★ American Academy for Cerebral Palsy and Developmental Medicine (AACPDM)**
6300 N River Rd., Ste. 727
Rosemont, IL 60018
**Phone:** (847)698-1635 **Fax:** (847)823-0536
**Email:** king@aaos.org
**Website:** http://www.aacpdm.org
Sheril King, Exec. Dir.
**Fnded:** 1947. **Mem:** 1,600. **Desc:** Professional organization of physicians, Ph.D.s, and allied health care individuals concerned with dignosis, care, treatment, and research of cerebral palsy and developmental disorders. **Pub:** *AACPDM News,* biennial. Newsletter. Includes academy news. *Price:* Included in membership dues. • *Journal of Developmental Medicine and Child Neurology,* monthly. • *Membership Roster,* annual. **Frmly:** (1976) American Academy for Cerebral Palsy.

**★ 13900 ★ American Academy of Clinical Neurophysiology**
104 13th St.
Hudson, WI 54016
**Phone:** (715)381-3440 **Fax:** (715)381-3442
**Email:** dtjorneh@pressenter.com
**Website:** http://www.pressenter.com/~dtjorneh/
Dan Tjornehoj, Exec. Dir.
**Fnded:** 1985. **Mem:** 800. **Desc:** Clinical neurophysiologists. Fosters an understanding of the function of the nervous system among health professionals, scientists, and the public by serving as a forum for interaction and the communication of new developments. Offers educational programs.

**American Academy of Neurological and Orthopaedic Surgeons (AANOS)**
*See:* Entry 19462

**American Academy of Neurological Surgery**
*See:* Entry 19463

**★ 13901 ★ American Academy of Neurology (AAN)**
1080 Montreal Ave.
Saint Paul, MN 55116-2325
**Phone:** (651)695-1940 **Free:** 800-879-1960
**Email:** web@aan.com
**Website:** http://www.aan.com
Catherine M. Rydell, Exec. Dir.
**Fnded:** 1948. **Mem:** 17,200. **Desc:** Professional society of medical doctors specializing in brain and nervous system diseases. Maintains placement service. Sponsors research and educational programs. Compiles statistics. Publishes scientific journal. **Pub:** *AAN Governmental Report,* bimonthly. Newsletter. Includes news on legislative affairs. • *AANews,* month-

ly. Newsletter. General information and placement publication. • *American Academy of Neurology Membership Directory,* annual. Membership Directory. • *ICD-9-CM for Neurologists.* Booklet. To aid users of ICD-9 diagnostic codes. • *Medical Specialty of Neurology.* Brochure. Discusses neurology as a career. • *Neurologist.* Brochure. For patients. • *Neurology,* monthly. Journal. Includes research reports. • *Patient Information Guide for Neurology.* Handbook for patients to find educational information about disorders.

**★ 13902 ★ American Academy of Pain Medicine (AAPM)**
4700 W Lake Ave.
Glenview, IL 60025-1485
**Phone:** (847)375-4731 **Fax:** 877-734-8750
**Email:** aapm@amctec.com
**Website:** http://www.painmed.org
Jeffrey W. Engle, Exec. Dir.
**Fnded:** 1983. **Mem:** 1,200. **Desc:** Anesthesiologists, internists, neurologists, neurosurgeons, orthopedic surgeons, physiatrists, and psychiatrists. Promotes a socioeconomic and political climate conducive to the effective and efficient practice of pain medicine. Ensures quality medical care by physicians specializing in pain medicine. Participates in networking and liaison activities with other organizations dealing in pain medicine. Conducts educational programs. Holds a seat in the American Medical Association House of Delegates. **Pub:** *A Guide to Pain Medicine.* Brochure. • *AAPM Membership Directory,* annual. Membership Directory. Lists primary care and specialty physicians with an interest in pain medicine. • *Pain Medicine,* quarterly. Journal. Contains clinical articles, research information, articles concerning socioeconomic issues, and news. *Price:* Included in membership dues. • *Pain Medicine Network,* quarterly. Newsletter. Covers news about the academy and its members. **Frmly:** American Academy of Algology.

**★ 13903 ★ American Academy of Sleep Medicine (AASM)**
One Westbrook Corp. Ctr., Ste. 920
Westchester, IL 60154
**Phone:** (708)492-0930 **Fax:** (708)492-0943
**Email:** info@aasmet.org
**Website:** http://www.aasmnet.org/
Jerry Barrett, Exec. Dir.
**Fnded:** 1975. **Mem:** 2,900. **Desc:** Sleep disorders centers and individuals united to provide full diagnostic and treatment services and to improve the quality of care for patients with all types of sleep disorders. Fosters educational activities at medical schools and in continuing medical education programs; conducts site visits to assure minimum standards at member centers; trains and evaluates the competence of individuals who care for patients with sleep disorders. Conducts research programs, including a cooperative case study series on all patients seen by sleep disorders centers throughout the country. **Pub:** *ASDA News,* quarterly. Newsletter. • *SLEEP,* 9/year. Journal. *Price:* $129 individual; $185 institutional. • Also publishes a roster of centers. **Frmly:** American Association of Sleep Disorders Centers; (1987) Association of Sleep Disorders Centers; (2000) American Association of Sleep Disorders.

**★ 13904 ★ American Academy of Somnology (AAS)**
PO Box 27077
Las Vegas, NV 89126
**Phone:** (702)371-0159 **Free:** 800-513-2757
**Fax:** (702)458-5833
**Email:** somnology@aol.com
**Website:** http://www.hopperinstitute.com/aas_intro.html
Dr. David L. Hopper, PhD, Founder & Pres.
**Fnded:** 1986. **Mem:** 75. **Desc:** Clinicians, researchers, and students in the field of somnology; interested individuals. Promotes advancement of somnology as a health care specialty. (Somnology is the study of sleep and sleep disorders.) Advocates standardization of university programs in somnology and a multidisciplin-

ary approach to the study and treatment of sleep disorders; conducts continuing education program. Sponsors American Board of Somnology to evaluate qualifications of applicants, administer examinations, and confer diplomate status on qualified individuals. Provides a forum for somnology clinicians and researchers to present findings and exchange ideas. Maintains speakers' bureau. **Pub:** *AAS Membership Directory*, annual. Membership Directory. • *Certification Handbook*, periodic. • *Journal of Somnology*, annual. Journal. • *The Somnologist*, quarterly. • Also publishes constitution, ethical standards, and bylaws.

**American Association of Neurological Surgeons (AANS)**
*See:* Entry 19469

**American Association of Neuropathologists (AANP)**
*See:* Entry 17124

**American Association of Neuroscience Nurses (AANN)**
*See:* Entry 15640

**American Association of Spinal Cord Injury Psychologists and Social Workers (AASCIPSW)**
*See:* Entry 12344

**American Board of Neurological Surgery (ABNS)**
*See:* Entry 19476

**American Board of Neuroscience Nursing (ABNN)**
*See:* Entry 15645

**★ 13905 ★ American Board of Pain Medicine**
4700 W Lake Ave.
Glenview, IL 60025-1485
**Phone:** (847)375-4726          **Fax:** (847)375-4777
**Email:** info@abpm.org
**Website:** http://www.abpm.org
Jeffrey W. Engle, Exec. Dir.
**Fnded:** 1991. **Mem:** 1,335. **Desc:** Develops and administers practice-related examinations in the field of pain medicine. Awards certification to physicians successfully completing the examination and credentialing process. **Frmly:** American College of Pain Medicine.

**★ 13906 ★ American Board of Professional Neuropsychology**
John Heinz Institute of Rehabilitation Medicine
150 Mundy St.
Wilkes-Barre Township, PA 18702
**Phone:** (570)826-3771          **Fax:** (570)826-3898
**Website:** http://abpn.net
Michael J. Raymond, PhD., Exec. Sec.
**Desc:** Professional neuropsychologists.

**American Board of Psychiatry and Neurology (ABPN)**
*See:* Entry 12348

**★ 13907 ★ American Board of Registration of EEG and EP Technologists (ABRET)**
1904 Croyden Dr.
Springfield, IL 62703
**Phone:** (217)553-3758          **Fax:** (217)585-6663
**Email:** abreteo@aol.com
**Website:** http://www.abret.org
Janice Walbert, Exec. Sec.

**Fnded:** 1961. **Desc:** Determines the competency of electroneurodiagnostic technologists through administration of written and oral examinations. **Frmly:** (1992) American Board of Registration of EEG Technologists.

**★ 13908 ★ American Board of Sleep Medicine**
6301 Bandel Rd. NW, Ste. 101
Rochester, MN 55901
**Phone:** (507)285-4377          **Fax:** (507)287-6008
**Email:** info@aasmet.org
**Website:** http://www.absm.org/
Nicole Jabs, Exam. Coord.
**Fnded:** 1991. **Desc:** Works to encourage the study and elevate the standards of sleep medicine. Offers certification in sleep medicine to licensed physicians and individuals with Ph.D.s in health related fields. **Pub:** Brochure.Contains information for applicants.

**★ 13909 ★ American Brain Tumor Association (ABTA)**
2720 River Rd., Ste. 146
Des Plaines, IL 60018
**Phone:** (847)827-9910          **Free:** 800-886-2282
**Fax:** (847)827-9918
**Email:** info@abta.org
**Website:** http://www.abta.org
Naomi Berkowitz, Exec. Dir.
**Fnded:** 1973. **Desc:** Seeks to eliminate brain tumors through research and meet the needs of brain tumor patients and their families. **Pub:** *Building Knowledge Series*. Pamphlets. A Brain Tumor-Sharing Hope (also in Spanish); Dictionary for Brain Tumor patients; Living with a Brain Tumor; A Primer of Brain Tumors. *Price:* Free. • *Connections - A Pen Pal Program*. Pamphlet. • *Focusing on Treatment Series*. Pamphlets. Pamphlet titles include: Gene Therapy; Radiation Therapy of Brain Tumors: A Basic Guide; Stereotactic Radiosurgery. • *Focusing on Tumors Series*. Pamphlets. Ependymoma; Glioblastoma Multiforme & Anaplastic Astrocytoma; Medullobblastoma; Meningioma; Metastatic Brain Tumors; Oligodendroglioma. • *For & About Children Series*. Pamphlets. Titles include: Alex's Journey: The Story of a Child with a Brain Tumor for ages 9-13, video and booklet format; When Your Child Returns to School. • *Listing of Bereavement (Grief) Support Groups by State*. Pamphlet. • *Listing of Brain Tumor Support Groups by State*. Pamphlet. • *Messageline*, 3/year. Newsletter. • *Mini-Medical School*. Pamphlet. • *Organizing a Support Group, A 'How To' Pamphlet*. Pamphlet. • *Physician Resource Lists*. Pamphlet. • *Physicians Offering Clinical Trials for Brain Tumors in ADULTS*. Pamphlet. • *Physicians Offering Clinical Trials for Brain Tumors in CHILDREN*. Pamphlet. • *Sharing Knowledge Series*. Pamphlets. • *Sharing Resources Series*. Pamphlets. • *Support Group Leader Mentorship Program*. Pamphlet. **Frmly:** (1992) Association for Brain Tumor Research.

**★ 13910 ★ American Chronic Pain Association (ACPA)**
PO Box 850
Rocklin, CA 95677
**Phone:** (916)632-0922          **Fax:** (916)632-3208
**Email:** acpa@pacbell.net
**Website:** http://www.theacpa.org
Penney Cowan, Exec. Dir.
**Fnded:** 1980. **Nat'l Groups:** 450. **Desc:** Individuals suffering from chronic pain; health care professionals. Mutual support organization that works to help individuals suffering from chronic pain (pain lasting more than six months) learn positive ways to deal with pain and become involved in their own recovery. Fosters the managing of pain through methods such as exercise, assertiveness, self-awareness, and relaxation techniques. Consults with health care facilities in developing and upgrading pain management units; disseminates guidelines for selecting pain management facilities. (The organization stresses that it provides no medical advice or treatment.) Operates speakers' bureau; conducts charitable program. **Pub:** *ACPA Chronicle*, quarterly. Newsletter. • *ACPA Facilitation Guide*, periodic. Directory. Features

how-tos for ACPA group development and ongoing resources. • *Family Manual*. A handbook for caregivers. • *From Patient to Person: First Steps*, periodic. • *Reflections of You*. A daily meditation and personal journal. • *Staying Well: Advanced Pain Management for Members Workbook*. Handbook.

**★ 13911 ★ American Clinical Neurophysiology Society**
PO Box 30
Bloomfield, CT 06002
**Phone:** (860)243-3977          **Fax:** (860)286-0787
**Email:** acns@ssmgt.com
**Website:** http://www.acns.org/
Jacquelyn T. Coleman, Exec. Dir.
**Fnded:** 1946. **Mem:** 1,450. **Desc:** Professional society of electroencephalographers and neurophysiologists. Offers clinical course annually. **Pub:** *Joural of Critical Neurophysiology*, bimonthly. Journal. **Frmly:** (1997) American Electroencephalographic Society.

**American College of Neuropsychiatrists (ACN)**
*See:* Entry 16988

**★ 13912 ★ American Council for Headache Education (ACHE)**
19 Mantua Rd.
Mount Royal, NJ 08061
**Phone:** (856)423-0258          **Free:** 800-255-ACHE
**Fax:** (856)423-0082
**Email:** achehq@talley.com
**Website:** http://www.achenet.org
Linda McGillicuddy, Exec. Dir.
**Fnded:** 1990. **Mem:** 5,000. **Desc:** Headache sufferers and physicians dedicated to advancing treatment and management of headache; promotes public awareness. **Pub:** *Headache*, quarterly. Newsletter. Provides current information on new treatments and management strategies. *Price:* Included in membership dues.

**★ 13913 ★ American Epilepsy Society (AES)**
342 N Main St.
West Hartford, CT 06117-2507
**Phone:** (860)586-7505          **Fax:** (860)586-7550
**Email:** info@aesnet.org
**Website:** http://www.aesnet.org
M. Suzanne C. Berry, CAE, Exec. Dir.
**Fnded:** 1946. **Mem:** 3,000. **Desc:** Clinicians, scientists investigating basic and clinical aspects of epilepsy, and related professional workers with an active interest in seizure disorders. Seeks to promote interdisciplinary communication, scientific investigation and exchange of clinical information about epilepsy. Works to prevent and treat epilepsy. **Pub:** *Epilepsia*, monthly. Journal. Published in conjunction with the International League Against Epilepsy. *Price:* Included in membership fee. • Also publishes Epilepsy Research incorporating the Journal of Epilepsy **Frmly:** (1959) American League Against Epilepsy.

**★ 13914 ★ American Headache Society (AHS)**
19 Mantua Rd.
Mount Royal, NJ 08061
**Phone:** (856)423-0043          **Fax:** (856)423-0082
**Email:** ahshq@talley.com
**Website:** http://www.ahsnet.org
Linda McGillicuddy, Exec. Dir.
**Fnded:** 1959. **Mem:** 2,500. **Desc:** Professional society of health care providers dedicated to the study and treatment of headache and face pain. Objectives are to promote the exchange of information and ideas concerning the causes and treatments of headache and related painful disorders, to educate physicians, health professionals and the public, and to encourage research. **Pub:** *Headache: The Journal of Head and Face Pain*, 10/year. Journal. Presents papers concerning basic research and clinical studies. Includes book reviews. *Price:* Included in membership dues;

$40/year for medical students, interns, and residents; $95/year for U.S. nonmembers; $110/year for nonmembers outside U.S. **Frmly:** (2001) American Association for the Study of Headache.

**★ 13915 ★ American Neurological Association (ANA)**
5841 Cedar Lake Rd. S, Ste. 204
Minneapolis, MN 55416-1491
**Phone:** (952)545-6284          **Fax:** (952)545-6073
**Email:** lindawilkerson@msn.com
**Website:** http://www.aneuroa.org
Linda J. Wilkerson, Exec. Dir.

**Fnded:** 1875. **Mem:** 960. **Desc:** Physicians and scientists interested in the form, functioning, and disorders of the nervous system. Conducts research programs. **Pub:** *Annals of Neurology*, monthly. Journal. Includes book reviews. *Price:* Included in membership dues; $68/year for nonmembers; $84/year for institutions; $52.50/year for students.

**★ 13916 ★ American Neuromodulation Society**
6287 Chesshire Ln. N
Osseo, MN 55311-4245
**Phone:** (763)559-4108          **Fax:** (763)559-4161
**Email:** american@neuromodulation.org
**Website:** http://www.neuromodulation.org/
Samuel J. Hassenbusch, MD, Pres.

**Desc:** Dedicated to advancing the field of neuromodulation therapies through clinical research, education and print material within the U.S.; aims to increase avenues of development for members through professional networking systems, ongoing communication and other opportunities. **Pub:** *Economic Newsletter*. Newsletter. Contains topics such as coding, reimbursement rates (RVU), payor coverage, and hospital topics. • *Neuromodulation*, quarterly. Journal.

**American Neuropsychiatric Association (ANPA)**
*See:* Entry 12357

**★ 13917 ★ American Pain Society (APS)**
4700 W Lake Ave.
Glenview, IL 60025
**Phone:** 877-734-8758          **Fax:** (847)375-6315
**Email:** info@ampainsoc.org
**Website:** http://www.ampainsoc.org
Christine Miaskowski, Pres.

**Fnded:** 1977. **Mem:** 3,500. **Reg. Groups:** 6. **Desc:** Physicians, dentists, psychologists, nurses, and other health professionals interested in the study and treatment of pain. Purposes are to: promote control, management, and understanding of pain through scientific meetings and research activities; develop standards for training and ethical management of pain patients. Conducts scientific conferences. **Pub:** *APS Bulletin*, bimonthly. Newsletter. • *Guideline for the Management of Aeute & Chronic Pain in Sickle Cell Disease.* • *Pain Facilities Directory*. Directory. • *The Pain Journal*, quarterly. Journal. • *Principles of Analgesic Use in the Treatment of Acute Pain and Cancer Pain (4th edition)*, periodic.

**★ 13918 ★ American Paraplegia Society (APS)**
75-20 Astoria Blvd.
Jackson Heights, NY 11372
**Phone:** (718)803-3782          **Fax:** (718)803-0414
**Email:** aps@epva.org
**Website:** http://www.apssci.org
DrPH Vivian Beyda, Associate Exec. Dir.

**Fnded:** 1954. **Mem:** 550. **Desc:** Physicians and researchers in the spinal cord injury field. Purpose is to advance and foster improved health care of spinal cord injury patients, and develop and promote education and research in the neuroscience fields. Sponsors seminars; maintains library. Conducts annual educational program. **Pub:** *Journal of Spinal Cord Medicine*, quarterly. Journal.

**★ 13919 ★ American Parkinson's Disease Association (APDA)**
1250 Hylan Blvd., Ste. 4B
Staten Island, NY 10305-1946
**Phone:** (718)981-8001          **Free:** 800-223-2732
**Fax:** (718)981-4399
**Website:** http://www.apdaparkinson.com
Joel Gerstel, Exec. Dir.

**Fnded:** 1961. **Mem:** 2,000. **Reg. Groups:** 90. **Local Groups:** 400. **Desc:** Works to find the cure for Parkinson's disease and to alleviate the suffering of its victims by subsidizing information and referral centers and providing funds for research. Offers counseling services to patients and their families. Maintains 51 information and referral centers and more than 800 support groups. Conducts symposia. **Pub:** *American Parkinson Disease Association–Newsletter*, quarterly. Newsletter. Includes association and research news, and calendar of events. *Price:* Free. • *Be Active! A Suggested Exercise Program for People with Parkinson's Disease*. Booklet. • *Be Independent! To Help the Patient with Parkinson's Disease in the Activities of Daily Living*. Booklet. • *Coping With Parkinson's Disease*. Booklet. • *Let's Communicate: Speech Problems and Swallowing Problems in Parkinson's Disease*. Booklet. • *Parkinson's Disease Handbook*. Booklet. • Annual Report. • Also publishes educational supplements.

**★ 13920 ★ American Sleep Apnea Association (ASAA)**
1424 K St. NW, Ste. 302
Washington, DC 20005
**Phone:** (202)293-3650          **Fax:** (202)293-3656
**Email:** asaa@sleepapnea.org
**Website:** http://www.sleepapnea.org
Christin Engelhardt, Exec. Dir.

**Fnded:** 1990. **Mem:** 5,000. **Local Groups:** 225. **Desc:** Individuals affected by sleep apnea; health care professionals. Promotes public awareness of sleep apnea; encourages research on the causes and treatments of breathing abnormalities during sleep. Sponsors educational programs and support groups through the A.W.A.K.E. Network. Serves as an advocate for people with sleep apnea. . **Pub:** *Get the Facts about Sleep Apnea*. Brochure. • *Wake Up Call The Wellness Letter for Snoring and Apnea*, bimonthly. Newsletter. Articles of interest to people affected by sleep apnea. *Price:* With membership. • Choosing a CPAP, Choosing a Mask and Headgear, Sleep and the Internet, Sleep Apnea and Driving, Reprints of newsletter articles.

**★ 13921 ★ American Society for Clinical Evoked Potentials (ASCEP)**
c/o Mrs. S. Moss
14 Soundview Ave., No. 51
White Plains, NY 10606
**Phone:** (914)761-4713
Mrs. S. Moss, Exec. Sec.

**Fnded:** 1981. **Mem:** 410. **Desc:** Physicians in physical medicine and rehabilitation, neurology, neurosurgery, ophthalmology, and anesthesiology. Purpose is to study the central nervous system's transmissions and to teach electrodiagnostic reading of evoked potentials. (Evoked potential is the sum of the stimulus-evoked bioelectrical potentials from the peripheral nerve, retina, or cochlear mechanism, from the spinal cord or central conduction pathways, and from cortical and subcortical structures.) Teaches and encourages the practice of and research in the clinical application of evoked potentials for the betterment of patient care. Conducts seminars and workshops; maintains speakers' bureau. **Pub:** Membership Directory, periodic. • Journal.

**★ 13922 ★ American Society of Electroneurodiagnostic Technologists (ASET)**
204 W 7th St.
Carroll, IA 51401-2317
**Phone:** (712)792-2978          **Fax:** (712)792-6962
**Email:** info@aset.org

**Website:** http://www.aset.org
Debra Jester Carson, Pres.

**Fnded:** 1959. **Mem:** 2,650. **Desc:** Persons engaged in clinical electroencephalographic (EEG) technology, evoked potential responses, nerve conduction studies, and polysomnography (sleep studies). Objective is the advancement of electroneurodiagnostic technology education and practice standards. **Pub:** *American Journal of Electroneurodiagnostic Technology*, quarterly. Journal. Covers EEG, evoked potentials, polysomnography, nerve conduction, and related electroneurodiagnostics. *Price:* Included in membership dues; $40/year for nonmembers in U.S.; $55/year for nonmembers outside U.S.; $80/year for institutions in U.S. • *ASET Newsletter*, quarterly. Newsletter. Includes calendar of events, local, state, and regional society news and workshop and seminar news. *Price:* Included in membership dues. • *Who's Who in Electroneurodiagnostics–Membership Directory*, annual. Membership Directory. Provides product listings for suppliers. Member listings are arranged alphabetically and geographically. *Price:* Included in membership dues. • Monographs.Provides information on selected END technology and related management subjects. • Books. • Also publishes study materials and guides. **Frmly:** (1985) American Society of Electroencephalographic Technologists.

**★ 13923 ★ American Society for Experimental Neuro Therapeutics (ASENT)**
611 E Wells St.
Milwaukee, WI 53202
**Phone:** (414)273-8290          **Fax:** (414)276-3349
**Email:** info@asent.org
**Website:** http://www.asent.org
Kay Whalen, Exec. Dir.

**Fnded:** 1997. **Mem:** 225. **Desc:** Neurologists and other medical professionals with an interest in experimental neuro therapeutics. Seeks to advance the development of improved therapies for diseases and disorders of the nervous system; promotes professional advancement of members. Serves as a forum for the exchange of information among those concerned with the development of neuro therapeutics; works to maintain friendly and cooperative relationships between members and government agencies and industries with an interest in neurology; assists in the formulation of public policies affecting experimental neuro therapeutics; provides support to health care professionals and research scientists pursuing careers in neuro therapeutics. **Pub:** *ASENT Membership Directory*, annual. Directory.

**American Society of Neuroimaging (ASN)**
*See:* Entry 18115

**American Society of Neuroradiology (ASNR)**
*See:* Entry 18116

**★ 13924 ★ American Society of Neurorehabilitation**
5841 Cedar Lk. Rd., Ste. 204
Minneapolis, MN 55416
**Phone:** (952)545-6324          **Fax:** (952)545-6073
**Email:** todd@toddtroost.com
**Website:** http://www.asnr.com
Lori Anderson, Exec. Dir.

**Fnded:** 1990. **Mem:** 700. **Desc:** Neurologists, neurosurgeons, psychiatrists, pediatricians, and other medical professionals interested in disorders of the nervous system. Rehabilitates and monitors patients with neurological disabilities. Acts as an advocate for patients; liases with other neurological organizations. Promotes research. **Pub:** *Neurorehabilitation and Neural Repair*, quarterly. Journal. • Newsletter, semiannual.

**American Society of Pain Management Nurses**
*See:* Entry 15656

**American Society of Pediatric Neuroradiology**
*See:* Entry 5615

★ **13925** ★ **American Spinal Injury Association (ASIA)**
345 E Superior, Rm. 1436
Chicago, IL 60611
**Phone:** (312)238-1242          **Fax:** (312)238-0869
**Email:** mars@northwestern.edu
**Website:** http://www.asia-spinalinjury.org
Marianne G. Kaplan, Exec. Sec.
**Fnded:** 1973. **Mem:** 500. **Desc:** Medical doctors and Allied Health Care professionals who have been trained in the care of spinal injury patients and who are either actively engaged in the field and acknowledged to be competent by their peers or who have made a significant contribution to the advancement of the basic sciences or one of the clinical fields of practice as they are applicable to the treatment of spinal cord injury. Purposes are to: develop knowledge and investigation of the causes, cure, and prevention of spinal injury and related trauma; pursue excellence in spinal injury patient care; promote and exchange ideas between professionals in the field; standardize medical terminology in spinal cord injury; foster and encourage basic research in the field; develop teaching and educational material; foster education of the medical profession and laity in the prevention and proper management of spinal injury, including the necessity for specialized regional spinal injury centers, provision for educational and vocational training, removal of architectural barriers, and promotion of a society more sensitive to the physically inconvenienced individual, including adequate housing and transportation; establish criteria for centers and/or systems of total spinal injury management so as to provide optimal care of the spinal injured person. Conducts annual scientific sessions. Sponsors G. Heiner Sell Distinguished Lectureship. **Pub:** *ASIA Meeting Abstracts*, annual. Proceedings. • *International Standards of Neurological Classification of Spinal Injuries*. A teaching package which includes videos and manuals. • *Task Force Report on Durable Medical Equipment*. Reports. • Bulletin, semiannual.

★ **13926** ★ **American Syringomyelia Alliance Project (ASAP)**
PO Box 1586
Longview, TX 75606-1586
**Phone:** (903)236-7079          **Free:** 800-ASAP-282
**Fax:** (903)757-7456
**Email:** syringo@syringo.org
**Website:** http://www.syringo.org
Don White, Co. -Founder/Chair.
**Fnded:** 1988. **Mem:** 1,500. **Nat'l Groups:** 1. **Desc:** Seeks to increase awareness of and promote research on syringomyelia, a rare spinal disorder. Conducts fundraising activities and children's services. **Pub:** *Syringomyelia Connections*, bimonthly. Newsletter. *Price:* $20. • *What Is Syringomyelia*. Brochure.

★ **13927** ★ **Amyotrophic Lateral Sclerosis Association (ALSA)**
27001 Agoura Rd. Ste. 150
Calabasas Hills, CA 91301-5104
**Phone:** (818)880-9007          **Free:** 800-782-4747
**Fax:** (818)880-9006
**Email:** alsinfo@alsa-national.org
**Website:** http://www.alsa.org
Michael W. Havlicek, Pres. /CEO
**Fnded:** 1985. **Mem:** 250,000. **Reg. Groups:** 135. **Desc:** Patients; relatives and friends of patients; doctors, neurologists, physical therapists, nurses, and professional organizations dedicated to finding the cause, prevention, and cure for amyotrophic lateral sclerosis (ALS). Offers help and information to ALS patients and their families. Funds ALS-specific research at major medical institutions. Works with other agencies, including the government, to increase their involvement on a priority basis in ALS research. Conducts patient meetings. **Pub:** *Amyotrophic Lateral Sclerosis Association–Link*, quarterly. Newspaper. Includes book reviews and research and chapter news. *Price:* Free. • Also publishes fact sheets and pamphlets on ALS and patient care. **AKA:** ALS Association.

★ **13928** ★ **Amyotrophic Lateral Sclerosis Society of Canada (ALSSC) (Societe Canadienne de la Sclerose Laterale Amyotrophique — SCSLA)**
265 Yorkland Blvd., Ste. 300
Toronto, ON, Canada M2J 1S5
**Phone:** (416)497-2267          **Free:** 800-267-4257
**Fax:** (416)497-1256
**Email:** alscanada@als.ca
**Website:** http://www.als.ca
**Fnded:** 1977. **Nat'l Groups:** 1. **Reg. Groups:** 11. **Lang(s):** English, French. **Desc:** Health care professionals; individuals with amyotrophic lateral sclerosis (ALS) and their families. Promotes advancement in the diagnosis of ALS and seeks to find a cure for the disease; works to improve the quality of life for people with ALS and their families. Provides support and services to people with ALS and their families: sponsors research and educational programs. **Pub:** *Coast to Coast*, bimonthly. Newsletter. Contains items of interest to the ALS Canada Network.

★ **13929** ★ **ASEAN Neurological Association**
Clinical Neuroscience Society - Singapore
c/o Department of Neurology
Singapore General Hospital
Outram Rd.
Singapore 169606, Singapore
**Phone:** 65 2223322          **Fax:** 65 2203321
**Website:** http://www.asean-neurology.org
**Lang(s):** Chinese, English. **Desc:** Health care professionals with an interest in neurology. Seeks to advance neurological study, teaching, and practice. Facilitates exchange of information among members; sponsors research and continuing professional development programs. **Frmly:** (2001) ASEAN Neurological Society.

**Asian-Australasian Society of Neurological Surgeons (AASNS)**
*See:* Entry 19507

★ **13930** ★ **Asian - Australasian Society of Neurological Surgeons (AASNS)**
23 Bharath Dasan Rd.
Teynampet
Chennai 600018, India
**Email:** kganap@usnl.com
**Website:** http://aasns.com
**Fnded:** 1964. **Mem:** 5,000. **Nat'l Groups:** 16. **Lang(s):** English. **Desc:** Neurosurgeons seeking to advance neurosurgical studies and promote understanding between members from different countries. Conducts educational programs. **Pub:** Newsletter, annual.

★ **13931** ★ **Asian and Oceanian Epilepsy Organization (AOEO)**
All India Institute of Medical Sciences
New Delhi 110 029, India
**Phone:** 91 11 6594210          **Fax:** 91 6521086
**Email:** satjain55@atshotmail.com
**Fnded:** 1991.

★ **13932** ★ **Asian and Pacific Cerebral Palsy Association (APCPA)**
APCPA Secretariat
DEB Services
PO Box 315
Manly, NSW 2095, Australia
**Phone:** 61 2 99763595          **Fax:** 61 2 99778238
**Lang(s):** English. **Desc:** Physicians and other health care personnel with an interest in cerebral palsy; people with cerebral palsy and their families. Seeks to prevent cerebral palsy and to improve the quality of life of people with the disease. Serves as a clearinghouse on cerebral palsy; provides support and services to people with cerebral palsy and their families; sponsors research and educational programs.

★ **13933** ★ **Asian Pacific Neural Network Assembly (APNNA)**
University of Otago
PO Box 56
Dunedin, New Zealand
**Phone:** 64 3 4798319          **Fax:** 64 3 4798311
**Email:** sylee@eekaist.ac.kr
**Website:** http://www.cse.cuhk.edu.hk/~apnna
**Fnded:** 1993. **Lang(s):** Chinese, English, Japanese, Korean. **Desc:** Researchers, scientists, and industry professionals with an interest in neural networks. Promotes more active interaction among members. Serves as a clearinghouse on neural networks; facilitates communication and cooperation among members.

★ **13934** ★ **Asian Pacific Society for Neurochemistry (APSN)**
Clinical Research Center
Royal Brisbane Hospital Federation
Royal Brisbane Hospital
Brisbane, QLD 4029, Australia
**Phone:** 61 7 3620495          **Fax:** 61 7 3620108
**Lang(s):** English. **Desc:** Neurologists and chemists with an interest in neurology. Seeks to advance the study, teaching, and practice of neurochemistry. Gathers and disseminates information on neurochemistry; sponsors research and educational programs.

**Asian Society for Stereotactic Functional and Computer Assisted Neurosurgery**
*See:* Entry 19511

**Asociacion Espanola de Esclerosis Lateral Amiotrofica (ADELA)**
*See:* Entry 13557

★ **13935** ★ **Associacao Portuguesa de Miastenia Gravis e Doencas Neuromusculares (APMG-DNM)**
Hospital de Santa Maria
P-1649-035 Lisbon, Portugal
**Phone:** 351 21 7805320          **Fax:** 351 21 7805630
**Email:** info@apmg-dnm.rcts.pt
**Website:** http://www.miastenia.co.pt
**Fnded:** 1989. **Mem:** 800. **Lang(s):** English. **Desc:** Promotes interest in neuromuscular diseases research among medical and scientific communities and the public in Portugal. Disseminates information. Provides medical and social support to patients and their families. **Pub:** *Boletim Informative*, quarterly. Journal. Contains news about neuromuscular dystrophy and information for patients.

★ **13936** ★ **Associated Professional Sleep Societies (APSS)**
6301 Bandel Rd. NW, Ste. 101
Rochester, MN 55901
**Phone:** (507)287-6006          **Fax:** (507)287-6008
**Email:** info@aasmet.org
**Website:** http://www.apss.org
Jerry Barrett, Exec. Dir.
**Fnded:** 1985. **Desc:** Members are the Sleep Research Society and American Academy of Sleep Medicine . Works to facilitate sleep research and development of sleep disorder s medicine by encouraging cooperation and exchange of information among members. **Pub:** *SLEEP*, 8/year. Journal. *Price:* $129/year for individuals; $185/year for institutions; $159/year for foreign individuals; $220/year for foreign institutions. **Frmly:** Association of Professional Sleep Societies.

**★ 13937 ★ Association Alzheimer Suisse (ALZ)**
Rue des Pecheurs 8
CH-1400 Yverdon-les-Bains, Switzerland
**Phone:** 41 24 4262000 **Fax:** 41 24 4262167
**Email:** alz@bluewin.ch
**Website:** http://www.alz.ch
**Fnded:** 1988. **Mem:** 5,500. **Nat'l Groups:** 1. **State Groups:** 18. **Local Groups:** 82. **Lang(s):** English, French, German, Italian. **Desc:** Individuals and organizations. Seeks to improve the quality of life of people with Alzheimer's disease and their families. Makes available support and services; facilitates research on Alzheimer's disease and related disorders; conducts educational programs. **Pub:** *Alzheimer Info*, 3/year. Magazine.

**★ 13938 ★ Association of British Neurologists**
Ormond House, 4th Fl.
27 Boswell St.
London WC1N 3JZ, United Kingdom
**Phone:** 44 207 4054060 **Fax:** 44 207 4054070
**Email:** abn@abnoffice.demon.co.uk
**Website:** http://www.theabn.org
**Fnded:** 1933. **Mem:** 1,000. **Desc:** Trainee and consultant in the neurological sciences. To promote the advancement of the neurological sciences, including the practice of neurology in the British Isles. **Pub:** Newsletter, quarterly.

**★ 13939 ★ Association for Comprehensive NeuroTherapy (ACN)**
c/o Latitudes
PO Box 210848
Royal Palm Beach, FL 33421-0848
**Phone:** (561)798-0472 **Fax:** (561)798-9820
**Email:** acn@latitudes.org
**Website:** http://www.latitudes.org
**Desc:** Practitioners and lay persons. Dedicated to exploring advanced and complementary treatments for neurological conditions, focusing on autism, Tourette syndrome, attention deficit disorder/hyperactivity, learning disabilities, and exploding child. Articles, editorials, and letters, as well as a survey on Tourette Syndrome, are available through their website. **Pub:** *Latitudes*. Newsletter. Contains articles, research updates, and clinical findings about autism, Tourette syndrome, attention disorders and learning problems.

**★ 13940 ★ Association France Alzheimer (AFA)**
21, boulevard Montmartre
F-75002 Paris, France
**Phone:** 33 1 42975241 **Fax:** 33 1 42960470
**Email:** cd.fralzheimer@wanadoo.fr
**Website:** http://www.maladie-alzheimer.com
**Lang(s):** English, French. **Desc:** Individuals and organizations. Seeks to improve the quality of life of people with Alzheimer's disease and their families. Makes available support and services; facilitates research on Alzheimer's disease and related disorders; conducts educational programs.

**★ 13941 ★ Association Luxembourg Alzheimer (ALA)**
Boite Postale 5021
L-1050 Luxembourg, Luxembourg
**Phone:** 352 4216761 **Fax:** 352 42167630
**Email:** ala@sl.lu
**Website:** http://www.alzheimer-europe.org/luxembourg
**Lang(s):** English, French, German. **Desc:** Individuals and organizations. Seeks to improve the quality of life of people with Alzheimer's disease and their families. Makes available support and services; facilitates research on Alzheimer's disease and related disorders; conducts educational programs.

**★ 13942 ★ Association of Multiple Sclerosis Therapy Centres - Scotland (AMSTCS)**
MS Therapy Centre
1 Burnett Rd.
Inverness IV1 1FT, United Kingdom
**Phone:** 44 1463 240365
**Fnded:** 1992. **Mem:** 12. **Lang(s):** English. **Desc:** Multiple sclerosis therapy centers. Seeks to advance the treatment of multiple sclerosis; promotes an improved quality of life for people with multiple sclerosis and their families. Facilitates communication and cooperation among members; conducts research and educational programs; participates in charitable activities; compiles statistics.

**★ 13943 ★ Association for the Neurologically Disabled of Canada (AND)**
**(Association Canadienne pour les Handicapes Neurologiques — ACHN)**
59 Clement Rd.
Etobicoke, ON, Canada M9R 1Y5
**Phone:** (416)244-1992 **Free:** 800-561-1497
**Fax:** (416)244-4099
**Email:** info@and.ca
**Website:** http://www.and.ca
**Fnded:** 1983. **Mem:** 150. **Desc:** Individuals with neurological disabilities and their families; health care professionals working with people with neurological disabilities. Seeks to improve the quality of life of people with neurological disabilities and their families; promotes advancement in the treatment of neurological disabilities. Provides support and services to people with neurological disabilities and their families. **Pub:** *AND...Now*, quarterly. Newsletter.

**★ 13944 ★ Association des Neurologues Liberaux de Langue Francaise (ANLLF)**
39, blvd. du Roi
F-78000 Versailles, France
**Phone:** 33 1 39532064 **Fax:** 33 1 39519244
**Fnded:** 1987. **Mem:** 560. **Reg. Groups:** 3. **Local Groups:** 3. **Lang(s):** English, French. **Desc:** French-speaking clinical neurologists working in the private sector. Provides for information exchange and organizes post-university teaching adapted to meet the needs of members. Makes arrangements for follow-up treatment of patients who have relocated. **Pub:** *Journal Faxe de Neurologie*, weekly. Journal. • *Neurologie Liberale*, quarterly. Journal.

**Association of Neuromuscular Disorders**
*See:* Entry 13561

**★ 13945 ★ Association of Neuroscience Departments and Programs (ANDP)**
9650 Rockville Pike
Bethesda, MD 20814
**Phone:** (301)530-7120
**Email:** personalcoskunoz@superonline.com
**Website:** http://www.andp.org
**Desc:** Association of neuroscience departments and programs; sponsors training fellows program. **Pub:** *Survey Report*. Report.

**★ 13946 ★ Association of Neurosurgical Physician Assistants (ANSPA)**
PO Box 559
Bernardsville, NJ 07924
**Free:** 888-94A-NSPA **Fax:** (732)805-9582
**Email:** TheANSPA@aol.com
**Website:** http://www.anspa.org
Susan Lusty, Exec. Dir.
**Fnded:** 1990. **Mem:** 250. **Desc:** Physicians assistants active in the field of neurosurgery; students enrolled in accredited physicians assistant education programs. Promotes professional advancement of members. Represents members before medical organizations; conducts continuing professional development and educational and training programs. **Pub:** *Surgical Physician Assistant*, periodic. Journal. **Price:** $110/year.

**★ 13947 ★ Association of Polysomnographic Technologists (APT)**
PO Box 14861
Lenexa, KS 66285-1991
**Phone:** (913)541-1991 **Fax:** (913)541-0156
**Email:** soneal@goamp.com
**Website:** http://www.aptweb.org
Sheila O'Neal, Exec. Dir.
**Fnded:** 1978. **Mem:** 1,600. **Desc:** Individuals who practice polysomnography in research or clinical settings. (Polysomnographic technology deals with the measurement and recording of multiple physiological activity, such as eye movement and heart rate, during sleep.) Seeks to establish standards for polysomnographic technology and provide education and training for people entering in the field. Acts as a forum for communication among members. **Pub:** *A2ZZZ Newsletter*, quarterly. Newsletter.

**★ 13948 ★ Association pour la Recherche sur la Sclerose Laterale Amyotrophique (ARS)**
24, rue Lacharriere
F-75011 Paris, France
**Phone:** 33 1 43389989 **Fax:** 33 1 43383159
**Email:** a.r.s.@wanadoo.fr
**Fnded:** 1985. **Mem:** 4,000. **Nat'l Groups:** 1. **Reg. Groups:** 19. **State Groups:** 1. **Local Groups:** 43. **Desc:** Promotes interest in amyotropic lateral sclerosis or ALS (a rare progressive degenerative disease of the motor neurons, characterized by atrophy of the muscles of the hands, forearms, and legs spreading to involve most of the body; also called Lou Gehrig's Disease) research among medical and scientific communities and the public. Faciliates exchange of information with ALS patients, researchers, clinics, and discussion/support groups. **Pub:** Booklets. • Magazine, annual. • Newsletter, quarterly. • Reports.

**Association for the Rehabilitation of the Brain Injured (ARBI)**
*See:* Entry 20103

**Association for Repetitive Motion Syndromes (ARMS)**
*See:* Entry 16763

**Association for Research in Nervous and Mental Disease (ARNMD)**
*See:* Entry 12401

**Association Suisse Romande et Italienne Cantre les Myopathies (ASRIM)**
*See:* Entry 13563

**Associazione Italian Sclerosi Laterale Amiotrofica (AISLA)**
*See:* Entry 13564

**Ataxia-Telangiectasia Society**
*See:* Entry 13566

**★ 13949 ★ Ataxia - UK**
10 Winchester House
Kennington Park
Cranmer Rd.
London SW9 6EJ, United Kingdom
**Phone:** 44 207 5821444 **Fax:** 44 207 5829444
**Email:** office@ataxia.org.uk
**Website:** http://www.ataxia.org.uk
**Fnded:** 1965. **Mem:** 2,700. **Lang(s):** English. **Desc:** Fundraising organization supporting research into Friedreich's, Cerebellar, and other ataxias (hereditary

spinal diseases which cause the loss of muscular coordination). Offers support services for ataxia sufferers and their families. **Pub:** *Ataxian*, quarterly. Magazine. • *Fax/Ataxian*, periodic. Audiotapes. • Brochures, periodic. • Newsletter, quarterly.

★ **13950** ★ **Australian Association of Neurologists**
AAN Secretariat
145 Macquarie St.
Sydney, NSW 2000, Australia
**Phone:** 61 2 92565443          **Fax:** 61 2 92518174
**Email:** aansyd@hotkey.net.au
**Website:** http://www.medeserv.com.au/aan/index.cfm
**Fnded:** 1950. **Mem:** 450. **Lang(s):** English. **Desc:** Neurologists and researchers and scientists with an interest in neurology. Seeks to "ensure that high standards of clinical neurology are practised in Australia." Develops standards of neurological training and practice; conducts research and continuing professional development programs; functions as a clearinghouse on neurology. **Pub:** Newsletter, 3/year.

★ **13951** ★ **Austrian Neuroscience Association (ANA) (Osterreichische Gesellschaft fur Neurowissenschaften)**
Division of Neurochemistry
Department of Psychiatry
Anichstr. 35
A-6020 Innsbruck, Austria
**Phone:** 43 512 5043710          **Fax:** 43 512 5043716
**Email:** alois.saria@uibk.ac.at
**Website:**          http://www.univie.ac.at/ANA/ANAHn-Top.html
**Fnded:** 1993. **Desc:** Promotes neuroscience in Austria. **Pub:** *OGN-Newsletter*. Newsletter.

**Avenues, National Support Group for Arthrogryposis Multiplex Congenita**
*See:* Entry 4877

**Back Association of Canada (BAC)**
*See:* Entry 20106

★ **13952** ★ **BackCare, The National Organisation for Healthy Backs**
16 Elmtree Rd.
Teddington TW11 8ST, United Kingdom
**Phone:** 44 208 9775474          **Fax:** 44 208 9435318
**Email:** back_pain@compuserve.com
**Website:** http://www.backpain.org
**Fnded:** 1968. **Mem:** 6,000. **Local Groups:** 50. **Lang(s):** English. **Desc:** Back pain sufferers, osteopaths, chiropractors, medical doctors, and safety and training officers in 12 countries. Sponsors research on the causes and treatment of back pain. Teaches individuals to use their bodies sensibly in order to prevent spinal damage. Promotes the formation of local branches. Keeps back pain sufferers informed on current developments in research, education, treatment and equipment. **Pub:** *A Carer's Guide to Moving and Handling Patients*. Manual. • *Guide to the Handling of Patients*. Fourth edition. • *Lifting and Handling - An Ergonomic Approach*. Manual. • *Safer Handling of People in the Community*. Manual. • *TalkBack*, quarterly. Magazine. **Frmly:** (2000) National Back Pain Association.

★ **13953** ★ **Batten Disease Support and Research Association (BDSRA)**
120 Humphries Dr., Ste. 2
Reynoldsburg, OH 43068
**Phone:** (740)927-4298          **Free:** 800-448-4570
**Email:** bdsra1@bdsra.org
**Website:** http://www.bdsra.org
Lance W. Johnson, Exec. Dir.
**Fnded:** 1987. **Mem:** 900. **State Groups:** 18. **Desc:** Families of children afflicted with Batten Disease; health care professionals; interested others. (Batten

Disease, is a degenerative neurological disease affecting children, causing seizures, dementia, loss of motor skills, and blindness.) Represents the interest of individuals with Batten; seeks to educate the public and professional community concerning the needs of Battens Disease patients. Provides information and referral services. Conducts support group activities. Maintains registry. **Pub:** *Family Directory*, annual. Directory. *Price:* Free; available to member families only. • *Illuminator*, quarterly. Newsletter. Provides information on research, education, meetings, and other topics of interest. *Price:* Free.

★ **13954** ★ **Benign Essential Blepharospasm Research Foundation (BEBRF)**
PO Box 12468
Beaumont, TX 77726-2468
**Phone:** (409)832-0788          **Fax:** (409)832-0890
**Email:** bebrf@ih2000.net
**Website:** http://www.blepharospasm.org/
Bob Campbell, Contact
**Fnded:** 1981. **Mem:** 8,900. **Reg. Groups:** 4. **State Groups:** 50. **Local Groups:** 170. **Desc:** Victims of benign essential blepharospasm (BEB), a rare disorder of unknown cause characterized by an involuntary forcible closure of the eyelids. Purpose is to undertake, promote, and develop research into the cause and cure of BEB and related disorders and infirmities of the facial musculature, such as Meige's Syndrome (involving muscle spasms of the eyes, lower face, mouth, tongue, throat, and respiratory system). Seeks to foster public awareness of the disorder in order to guarantee detection at the onset of symptoms. Encourages continuity and cooperation among neurologists, neuro-ophthalmologists, ophthalmologists, plastic surgeons, psychologists, psychiatrists, and other medical professionals in rendering correct diagnoses, implementing effective treatment, improving surgical procedure, and discovering a cure. Organizes seminars, clinical studies, and other programs in continuing education; sponsors fundraising activities. Endeavors to locate sufferers of the disorder and to compile data in order to determine the incidence of BEB and to advise on available treatment. Carries out research activities in areas such as brain tissue collection and experimental treatments. **Pub:** *BEBRF Newsletter*, bimonthly. Newsletter. Includes research reports and statistics, medical articles, patient stories. *Price:* $15/year. • *Blepharospasm and Related Disorders*. *Price:* $16. • *Physician Reprint Articles*. Articles. • Pamphlets.

★ **13955** ★ **Brain Injury Association of America**
105 N Alfred St.
Alexandria, VA 22314
**Phone:** (703)236-6000          **Free:** 800-444-6443
**Fax:** (703)236-6001
**Email:** PublicRelations@biausa.org
**Website:** http://www.biausa.org
Allan I. Bergman, Pres. & CEO
**Fnded:** 1980. **Mem:** 45. **State Groups:** 47. **Desc:** National organization working for and with people with brain injury and their families. Seeks to create a better future through brain injury prevention, research, education and advocacy. **Pub:** *Brain Injury Association CER Catalogue of Educational Resources*, annual. Catalog. Includes listings of books, articles, videotapes, audiocassette tapes, booklets, and other materials on head injury available through BIA. *Price:* Free. • *Brain Injury Awareness Presentation Kit*. Handbook. *Price:* $175. • *The Brain Injury Source*, quarterly. Magazine. *Price:* $32 annually. • *National Directory of Rehabilitation Services*, annual. Directory. *Price:* $16. • *TBI Challenge!*, bimonthly. Newsletter. *Price:* $25/year. **Frmly:** National Head Injury Foundation; (2002) Brain Injury Association.

★ **13956** ★ **Brain Research Society of Finland (BRSF)**
c/o Prof. Esa R. Korpi
University of Turku

Department of Pharmacology & Clinical Pharmacology
Kiinamyllynkatu 10
FIN-20520 Turku, Finland
**Email:** esa.korpi@utu.fi
**Website:** http://brain.utu.fi/
**Mem:** 200. **Desc:** Basic and clinical neuroscientists. Promotes basic and clinical research into the neurosciences.

★ **13957** ★ **The Brain Tumor Society (TBTS)**
124 Watertown St., Ste. 3-H
Watertown, MA 02472
**Phone:** (617)924-9997          **Free:** 800-770-8287
**Fax:** (617)924-9998
**Email:** info@tbts.org
**Website:** http://www.tbts.org
Lawrence Z. Pizzi, Exec. Dir.
**Fnded:** 1989. **Desc:** Strives to improve the quality of life of brain tumor patients by providing support for them and their families. Raises funds for research in order to find a cure for brain tumors. **Pub:** *Color Me Hope*. A Resource Guide for patients and families. *Price:* Free.

★ **13958** ★ **Brainwave - The Irish Epilepsy Association (BIEA)**
249 Crumlin Rd.
Dublin 12, Ireland
**Phone:** 353 1 4557500
**Email:** info@epilepsy.ie
**Website:** http://www.epilepsy.ie
**Lang(s):** English, Irish. **Desc:** Individuals and organizations. Seeks to improve the quality of life of people with epilepsy; promotes advancement in the diagnosis and treatment of epilepsy. Serves as a clearinghouse on epilepsy; provides support and assistance to people with epilepsy and their families and caregivers working with people with epilepsy.

**Brazilian Association of Amyotrophic Lateral Sclerosis (Associacao Brasileira de Esclerose Lateral Amiotrofica)**
*See:* Entry 13569

★ **13959** ★ **Brazilian Muscular Dystrophy Association (Associacao Brasileira de Distrofia Muscular)**
715 Engenheiro Teixeira Soares St.
Butanta
05505-030 Sao Paulo, SP, Brazil
**Phone:** 55 11 38148562          **Fax:** 55 11 38148562
**Email:** abdim@sili.com.br
**Website:** http://www.abdim.org.br
**Fnded:** 1981. **Desc:** Promotes interest in muscular dystrophy research among medical and scientific communities and the public in Brazil. Disseminates information. **Pub:** *Revista da ABDIM*, every 3 months. Magazine. Contains Muscular Dystrophy interests like researches, treatments, and work with children and adolescents from Brazil.

**British Association of Neuroscience Nurses**
*See:* Entry 15675

★ **13960** ★ **British Epilepsy Association**
New Anstey House
Gate Way Dr.
Yeadon
Leeds LS19 7XY, United Kingdom
**Phone:** 44 113 2108800          **Fax:** 44 113 3910300
**Email:** epilepsy@bea.org.uk
**Website:** http://www.epilepsy.org.uk
**Fnded:** 1950. **Mem:** 20,000. **Reg. Groups:** 140. **Desc:** Association is owned by its members. Provides

care in the community for the country's estimated 420,000 people with epilepsy. Publications on all aspects of epilepsy counselling, advice, information and support and the National Epilepsy Helpline. Around 140 regional groups and branch - regional office in Belfast. National information centre provides extensive service to public and professionals. **Pub:** *Epilepsy Today*, quarterly. Magazine. • *Seizure*, quarterly. Journal.

**★ 13961 ★ British Neuroscience Association (BNA)**
BNA Conference Office
New Medical School
Liverpool L69 3GE, United Kingdom
**Phone:** 44 151 7945449    **Fax:** 44 151 7945517
**Email:** bna@liv.ac.uk
**Website:** http://www.bna.org.uk/
**Desc:** Promotes study of the structure and functions of the nervous system.

**★ 13962 ★ British Society for Clinical Neurophysiology**
Department of Clinical Neurophysiology
Middlesex Hospital
Mortimer St.
London W1N 8AA, United Kingdom
**Email:** secretariat@bscn.org.uk
**Website:** http://www.bscn.org.uk
**Fnded:** 1942. **Mem:** 350. **Desc:** Medical practitioners, scientists and technologists. Medical and scientific study of electrical activity which can be recorded from the nervous system. **Pub:** Papers. Presents abstracts of scientific papers. **Frmly:** (1992) EEG Society.

**Bulgarian Neuromuscular Disease Association**
*See:* Entry 13573

**★ 13963 ★ Cajal Club (CC)**
c/o Henry J. Ralston, MD
Department of Anatomy
University of California
San Francisco, CA 94143-0452
**Phone:** (415)476-1861
**Email:** hjr@phy.ucsf.edu
**Website:** http://www.anatomy.org/
Dr. Henry J. Ralston, MD, Contact
**Fnded:** 1947. **Mem:** 450. **Desc:** Neuroanatomists who meet for discussion and the presentation of papers on prospective research, technique, and history of neurology. (Club is named after Sr. Don Santiago Ramon y Cajal, a founder of and Nobel laureate for the science of neuroanatomy.) **Pub:** *History of Cajal Club*, quinquennial. • Proceedings, periodic.

**Canadian Association for Child Neurology (CACN)**
**(Association Canadienne de Neurologie Pediatrique — ACNP)**
*See:* Entry 5638

**★ 13964 ★ Canadian Association of Neuropathologists (CAND)**
**(Association Canadienne de Neuropathologistes — ACN)**
c/o Department of Pathology & Lab Medicine
University of Alberta Hospital
8440-12th St.
Edmonton, AB, Canada T6G 2B7
**Phone:** (780)407-8952    **Fax:** (780)407-3009
**Email:** edwardj@ualberta.ca
**Website:** http://canp.medical.org
**Fnded:** 1960. **Mem:** 100. **Lang(s):** English, French. **Desc:** Neuropathologists and other health care professionals with an interest in the field. Promotes professional development of members; seeks to advance the practice of neuropathology. Facilitates exchange of information among members; conducts continuing professional education programs.

**★ 13965 ★ Canadian Association of Neuroscience Nurses (CANN)**
**(Association Canadienne des Infirmieres en Sciences Neurologiques — ACISN)**
1818 W 6th Ave., Ste. 205
Vancouver, BC, Canada V6J 1R6
**Email:** birwin@cw.bc.ca
**Website:** http://www.cann.ca
**Lang(s):** English, French. **Desc:** Neuroscience nurses. Seeks to advance the practice of neuroscience nursing; promotes professional development of members. Facilitates exchange of information among members; conducts continuing professional development courses.

**★ 13966 ★ Canadian Board of Registration of Electroencephalograph Technologists**
The Moncton Hosptial
Electrodiagnostic Department
135 MacBeth Ave.
Moncton, NB, Canada E1C 6Z8
**Phone:** (506)875-4111
**Email:** ahopkins@sehcc.health.nb.ca
**Fnded:** 1972. **Lang(s):** English, French. **Desc:** Registered electroencephalograph technologists. Promotes professional development of members; seeks to advance the practice of electroencephalography. Serves as a forum for the exchange of information among members; represents members within the health care industry; nationally registers EEG technologists.

**★ 13967 ★ Canadian Brain Injury Coalition (CBIC)**
1 Donald Rd.
Winnipeg, MB, Canada R1A 2T2
**Phone:** (204)757-7102    **Fax:** (204)757-7103
**Lang(s):** English, French. **Desc:** Individuals with brain injuries; health care professionals with an interest in the treatment of brain injuries. Seeks to improve the quality of life of people with brain injuries; promotes advancement in the treatment of brain injuries. Provides support and services to people with brain injuries; conducts continuing professional development courses for health care professionals.

**★ 13968 ★ Canadian Brain Tissue Bank (CBTB)**
**(Banque Canadienne de Tissue du Cerveau — BCTC)**
c/o Bantin Institute
399 Bathurst St., Fell Wing 5-222
Toronto, ON, Canada M5T 2S8
**Phone:** (416)978-5490    **Fax:** (416)978-7935
**Email:** cbtb@uhn.on.ca
**Lang(s):** English, French. **Desc:** Neurologists, psychiatrists, and other individuals with an interest in the structure and function of the brain. Seeks to advance understanding of the brain and its function; promotes professional development of members. Maintains brain tissue bank for research and study; provides support and assistance to brain research programs; conducts educational programs.

**★ 13969 ★ Canadian Congress of Neurological Sciences (CCNS)**
**(Societe Canadienne de Neurologie — SCN)**
PO Box 5456, Sta. A
Calgary, AB, Canada T2H 2X8
**Phone:** (403)229-9544    **Fax:** (403)229-1661
**Email:** brains@ccns.org
**Website:** http://www.ccns.org
**Fnded:** 1989. **Mem:** 560. **Lang(s):** English, French. **Desc:** Neurologists, scientists, and other individuals with an interest in neurology and related fields. Seeks to advance the study and practice of the neurological sciences; promotes professional development of members. Facilitates exchange of information among members; sponsors research and educational pro-grams. **Pub:** *Canadian Journal of Neurological Sciences*, quarterly. Journal.

**★ 13970 ★ Canadian Epilepsy Consortium (CEC)**
55 Queen St. E
9th Fl., Ste. 921
Toronto, ON, Canada M5C 1R6
**Phone:** (416)864-5506    **Fax:** (416)864-5636
**Email:** cec-hq@egroups.com
**Website:** http://www.epilepsyconsortium.ca
**Fnded:** 1996. **Mem:** 40. **Lang(s):** English. **Desc:** Licensed neurologists residing in Canada who specialize in treating and/or researching pediatric and/or adult patients with epilepsy. Works to develop and promote multi-centre epilepsy research projects in Canada. Partners with industry to evaluate and execute clinical trials of new agents.

**Canadian Neurosurgery Society (CNS)**
**(Societe Canadienne de Neurochirurgie — SCN)**
*See:* Entry 19538

**★ 13971 ★ Canadian Society for Brain, Behaviour and Cognitive Science (CSBBCS)**
**(Societe Canadienne des Sciences du Cerveau, du Comportement et de la Cognition — SCSCCC)**
Department of Psychology
McMaster University
1280 Main St. W
Hamilton, ON, Canada L8S 4K1
**Email:** bbcs@mcmaster.ca
**Website:** http://psych.mcmaster.ca/bbcs/index.html
**Lang(s):** English, French. **Desc:** Canadian scientists actively engaged in brain, behaviour, and cognitive science research. Promotes Canadian research in experimental psychology and behavioral neuroscience. Works with federal and provincial funding agencies and science ministries with a view to influencing science policy and funding.

**★ 13972 ★ Canadian Society of Clinical Neurophysiologists (CSCN)**
**(Societe Canadienne de Neurophysiologistes Cliniques — SCNC)**
c/o Canadian Congress of Neurological Sciences
709 7015 Macleod Tr. SW
Calgary, AB, Canada T2H 2K6
**Phone:** (403)229-9544    **Fax:** (403)229-1661
**Email:** brains@ccns.org
**Website:** http://www.ccns.org/cscnpage.htm
**Lang(s):** English, French. **Desc:** Neurophysiologists and other individuals with an interest in the field. Seeks to advance the study and practice of neurophysiology. Facilitates exchange of information among members; sponsors research and educational pro-grams.

**★ 13973 ★ Cervical Spine Research Society (CSRS)**
c/o Peggy Wlezien
6300 N River Rd., Ste. 727
Rosemont, IL 60018-4226
**Phone:** (847)698-1628    **Fax:** (847)823-0536
**Email:** wlezien@aaos.org
**Website:** http://www.csrs.org/navbar.html
Peggy Wlezien, Mgr.
**Fnded:** 1973. **Desc:** Promotes the exchange and development of ideas and philosophy regarding the diagnosis and treatment of cervical spine injury and disease.

**★ 13974 ★ Charcot-Marie-Tooth Association (CMTA)**
2700 Chestnut St.
Chester, PA 19013
**Phone:** (610)499-9264     **Free:** 800-606-CMTA
**Fax:** (610)499-9267
**Email:** cmtassoc@aol.com
**Website:** http://www.charcot-marie-tooth.org
Pat Dreibelbis, Dir. of Program Services
**Fnded:** 1983. **Mem:** 14,000. **Nat'l Groups:** 1. **Reg. Groups:** 25. **Desc:** Charcot-Marie-Tooth patients and their families, medical professionals treating the disorder, and interested individuals. (Charcot-Marie-Tooth Disease, also known as peroneal muscular atrophy or hereditary motor sensory neuropathy, is a progressive neurological disorder beginning in childhood or adult life with weakness and muscle wasting in feet, legs, hands, and arms.) Works to inform and educate patients and their families, the medical community, and the public about medical treatment for CMT. Offers support groups for patients and their families; disseminates educational materials; encourages and funds research; sponsors lay and professional symposia. Makes available videotapes; maintains speakers' bureau. **Pub:** *A Physician's Guide to CMT Disorder.* Handbook. *Price:* $20. • *Charcot-Marie-Tooth Disorders.* Pamphlets. • *CMT Facts I*, periodic. Booklets. *Price:* $3. • *CMT-Facts II*, periodic. Booklets. *Price:* $5. • *CMT Facts III*, periodic. Booklets. Containing articles on CMT topics, research news, patient profiles, and meeting and program announcements. *Price:* $5 with membership. • *CMT-Facts IV*, periodic. Booklets. *Price:* $8. • *CMTA Report*, bimonthly. Newsletter. Containing articles on CMT topics, research news, patient profiles, and meeting and program announcements. *Price:* With membership. **Frmly:** (1990) National Foundation for Peroneal Muscular Atrophy.

**★ 13975 ★ Chemotherapy Foundation (CF)**
183 Madison Ave., Rm. 403
New York, NY 10016
**Phone:** (212)213-9292     **Fax:** (212)213-3831
**Website:** http://www.chemotherapyfoundation.com
Shirley Cox, Exec. Dir.
**Fnded:** 1968. **Mem:** 3,500. **Desc:** Supports laboratory and clinical research for the control, cure, and prevention of cancer through innovative medical therapies; conducts professional symposia to enable oncologists to incorporate advances in cancer treatment into the care of their patients; distributes free educational literature. Grant allocations currently include six major metropolitan medical centers. **Pub:** *The Breast Cancer Epidemic in the United States - How 15,000 More Lives Can Be Saved Each Year.* Booklet. Provides educational information for patients and the public. *Price:* Free. • *Chemotherapy - Your Weapon Against Cancer.* Booklet. Contains educational material for patients and the public. *Price:* Free. • *Major Research Achievements of the Chemotherapy Foundation Grant Programs 1968-1999.* Booklet. *Price:* Free. • *Souvenir Journal*, annual. Book. Updates status of chemotherapy, foundation activities, and studies being conducted by its research recipients. • *Symposium Abstracts*, annual, For medical oncologists.Booklet. *Price:* $15 per copy. • *What Every Man Should Know About Prostate Cancer.* Booklet. Contains educational material for patients and the public. *Price:* Free. • *What Every Woman and Her Doctor Should Discuss About Ovarian Cancer.* Booklet. Contains educational material for patients and the public. *Price:* Free. • Newsletter, semiannual. Includes research reports and membership activities.

**Child Neurology Society (CNS)**
*See:* Entry 5653

**★ 13976 ★ Children and Adults With Attention Deficit/Hyperactivity Disorder (CHADD)**
8181 Professional Pl., Ste.201
Landover, MD 20785
**Phone:** (301)306-7070     **Free:** 800-233-4050
**Fax:** (301)306-7090
**Email:** national@chadd.org
**Website:** http://www.chadd.org
E. Clarke Ross, D.P.A., CEO
**Fnded:** 1987. **Mem:** 22,000. **Local Groups:** 300. **Desc:** Parents, adults, and professionals with an interest in attention-deficit disorders. (ADD is a neurologically-based disorder which affects an individual's behavior and learning. The disorder is characterized by deficits in attention span and impulse control, and is often accompanied by hyperactivity.) Goals are to: maintain a support group for parents of children with ADD; provide a forum for continuing education for parents and professionals about ADD; act as a resource for information about ADD; assure that the best educational opportunities are available to children with ADD so that their specific difficulties will be recognized and appropriately managed within educational settings. Operates speakers' bureau. **Pub:** *ATTENTION*, bimonthly. Magazine. • *Inside Chadd*, quarterly. Newsletter. • Booklets. • Brochures. • Also publishes fact sheets. **Frmly:** (1993) Children with Attention-Deficit Disorders; (2001) Children and Adults With Attention Deficit Disorder.

**★ 13977 ★ Christopher Reeve Paralysis Foundation**
500 Morris Ave.
Springfield, NJ 07081
**Phone:** (973)379-2690     **Free:** 800-225-0292
**Fax:** (973)912-9433
**Website:** http://www.christopherreeve.org
David R. Landrey, Chair/Exec. Committee
**Fnded:** 1982. **Nat'l Groups:** 1. **Reg. Groups:** 1. **Desc:** Seeks to encourage and support research to find a cure for paralysis caused by spinal cord injury and other central nervous system disorders. **Pub:** *American Paralysis Association Progress in Research*, semiannual. Newsletter. • *Annual Review*. • *Progress in Research*, 2-3/year. • *Walking Tomorrow*, semiannual. Newsletter. **Frmly:** (1981) Kent Waldrep International Spinal Cord Research Foundation; (2002) American Paralysis Association.

**★ 13978 ★ Collegium Internationale Neuro-Psychopharmacologicum (CINP)**
c/o Oakley Ray, PhD
2014 Broadway, Ste. 250
Nashville, TN 37203
**Phone:** (615)343-2068     **Fax:** (615)343-2069
**Email:** oray@cinp.org
**Website:** http://www.cinp.org
Oakley Ray, PhD, Intl. Coor.
**Fnded:** 1957. **Mem:** 1,000. **Desc:** Individuals engaged in experimental and clinical neuropsychopharmacological research and teachers in this field. Purposes are to advance the experimental and clinical aspects of the neuropsychopharmacological sciences; facilitate international relations between branches of the neuropsychopharmacological disciplines; further the international exchange of information and promote personal relations; consider the medico-social problems of psychopharmacology. **Pub:** *Mailings*, periodic. Journal. • Proceedings.Covers symposia and congresses. • Reports. • Also publishes abstracts.

**★ 13979 ★ Coma Recovery Association (CRA)**
807 Carman Ave.
Westbury, NY 11590-6429
**Phone:** (516)997-1826     **Fax:** (516)997-1613
**Email:** office@comarecovery.org
**Website:** http://www.comarecovery.org
Florence Manginaro, Pres.
**Fnded:** 1980. **Mem:** 1,056. **Reg. Groups:** 1. **State Groups:** 2. **Local Groups:** 1. **Desc:** Coma and head injury survivors and their families; medical professionals; interested persons. Goal is to provide support to and assist families of coma and head injury survivors. Provides information and referrals regarding treatment, rehabilitation, and socialization options. Represents the common needs of families and patients before legislative bodies. Offers Medicaid case management services. **Pub:** *Coma Recovery Association Newsletter*, quarterly. Newsletter. *Price:* Included in membership dues.

**★ 13980 ★ Confederacion Espanola de Familiares de Enfermos de Alzheimer y Otras Demencias (CEAFA)**
Pintor Maezt, 2 bajo
E-31008 Pamplona, Spain
**Phone:** 34 948 174517     **Fax:** 34 948 265739
**Email:** alzheimer@cin.es
**Website:** http://www.ceafa.org
**Fnded:** 1990. **Mem:** 35,000. **Lang(s):** English, Spanish. **Desc:** Individuals and organizations. Seeks to improve the quality of life of people with Alzheimer's disease and their families. Makes available support and services; facilitates research on Alzheimer's disease and related disorders; conducts educational programs.

**Congress of Neurological Surgeons (CNS)**
*See:* Entry 19543

**★ 13981 ★ Danish Epilepsy Society (Dansk Epilepsiforening)**
Kettegard Alle 30
DK-2650 Hvidovre, Denmark
**Phone:** 45 36323632     **Fax:** 45 31473941
**Email:** info@1cns.org
**Website:** http://www.neurosurgery.org
**Fnded:** 1970.

**★ 13982 ★ Danish Society for Neuroscience (DSfN) (Dansk Selskab for Neurovidenskab — DSfN)**
c/o Dr. Aase Frandsen
Institut for Farmakologi
Farmaceutisk Hojskole
Universitetsparken 2
DK-2100 Copenhagen, Denmark
**Phone:** 45 35306000     **Fax:** 45 35374457
**Email:** aaf@mail.dfh.dk
**Website:** http://www.dsfn.dk/
**Desc:** Promotes basic research in the field of neuroscience; provides educational activities.

**★ 13983 ★ Deutsche Alzheimer Gesellschaft (DAG)**
Friedrichstrasse 236
D-10969 Berlin, Germany
**Phone:** 49 30 31505733     **Fax:** 49 30 31505735
**Email:** info@deutsche-alzheimer.de
**Website:** http://www.deutsche-alzheimer.de
**Lang(s):** English, German. **Desc:** Individuals and organizations. Seeks to improve the quality of life of people with Alzheimer's disease and their families. Makes available support and services; facilitates research on Alzheimer's disease and related disorders; conducts educational programs.

**Deutsche Gesellschaft fur Muskelkranke**
*See:* Entry 13582

**★ 13984 ★ Dysautonomia Foundation**
633 3rd Ave., 12th Fl.
New York, NY 10017
**Phone:** (212)949-6644     **Fax:** (212)682-7625
**Email:** dys212@aol.com
**Website:** http://www.familialdysautonomia.org/
Lenore F. Roseman, Exec. Dir.
**Fnded:** 1954. **Mem:** 14,000. **Desc:** Parents, relatives, friends, and benefactors of children afflicted with Familial dysautonomia, a Jewish genetic disease of the autonomic nervous system. Now that the FD Gene has been located and there is a carrier available, we must now fund research into discovering the function

the gene plays within the body. **Pub:** *DYS/COURSE*, semiannual. Newsletter. Includes research updates. *Price:* Free. • *Dysautonomia Foundation–Journal*, annual. Journal. *Price:* Free upon ad of $300 or more.

★ **13985** ★ **Dystonia Medical Research Foundation**
1 E Wacker Dr., Ste. 2430
Chicago, IL 60601-2001
**Phone:** (312)755-0198    **Free:** 800-377-DYST
**Fax:** (312)803-0138
**Email:** dystonia@dystonia-foundation.org
**Website:** http://www.dystonia-foundation.org
Valerie F. Levitin, PhD., Exec. Dir.
**Fnded:** 1977. **Mem:** 25,000. **Nat'l Groups:** 5. **Reg. Groups:** 8. **State Groups:** 100. **Local Groups:** 2. **Desc:** Dystonia patients and their families; medical personnel; health agencies; interested individuals. Promotes and funds research and encourages increased public awareness of dystonia, a neurologic muscular disorder causing muscles to jerk and contract into abnormal positions. Disseminates information concerning dystonia. Sponsors patient and family support groups. **Pub:** *Dystonia Dialogue*, 3/year. Newsletter. Includes foundation and chapter news and research updates. *Price:* Free. • Brochures.

★ **13986** ★ **Electrophysiological Technologists' Association (EPTA)**
Staffordshire General Hopital
Weston Rd.
Stafford ST16 3SA, United Kingdom
**Phone:** 44 171 6018859
**Fnded:** 1950. **Mem:** 600. **Lang(s):** English. **Desc:** Neurophysiology technicians; medical staff working in neurophysiology; individuals from commercial firms dealing with neurophysiology equipment. Promotes understanding of neurophysiology through preparation and presentation of scientific papers; oversees training of electrophysiology technology students. **Pub:** *Journal of Electrophysiological Technology*, 3/year. Journal. • *Newsletter*, periodic. Newsletter.

★ **13987** ★ **Epilepsy Action Scotland (EAS)**
48 Govan Rd.
Glasgow G51 1JL, United Kingdom
**Phone:** 44 141 4274911    **Fax:** 44 141 4191709
**Email:** enquiries@epilepsyscotland.org.uk
**Website:** http://www.epilepsyscotland.org.uk
**Fnded:** 1954. **Mem:** 600. **Reg. Groups:** 10. **Local Groups:** 6. **Lang(s):** English. **Desc:** Individuals and organizations with an interest in epilepsy. Seeks to improve the quality of life of people with epilepsy; promotes advancement in the diagnosis and treatment of epilepsy. Provides information, and support to people with epilepsy; conducts educational programs to raise public awareness of epilepsy; sponsors training courses for various personnel working with people with epilepsy; makes available advocacy services on behalf of people with epilepsy and their families; lobbies local and national government agencies on legislation affecting people with epilepsy; offers a helpline, literature, and website to members. to members. **Pub:** *Epilepsy News*, semiannual. Newsletter. • Booklets. **Frmly:** Epilepsy Association of Scotland.

★ **13988** ★ **Epilepsy Canada (EC)**
1470 Peel St., Ste. 745
Montreal, QC, Canada H3A 1T1
**Phone:** (514)845-7855    **Fax:** (514)845-7866
**Email:** epilepsy@epilepsy.ca
**Website:** http://www.epilepsy.ca
**Fnded:** 1966. **Lang(s):** English, French. **Desc:** People with epilepsy and their families; health care professionals with an interest in epilepsy and related disorders. Seeks to improve the quality of life of people affected by epilepsy through promotion and support of research. Offers education and awareness initiatives that build understanding and acceptance of epilepsy. **Pub:** *Lumina*, semiannual. Newsletter. • Brochure.

★ **13989** ★ **Epilepsy Foundation**
4351 Garden City Dr.
Landover, MD 20785
**Phone:** (301)459-3700    **Free:** 800-332-1000
**Fax:** (301)577-4941
**Email:** info@efa.org
**Website:** http://www.efa.org
Eric R. Hargis, Pres. /CEO
**Fnded:** 1967. **Mem:** 16,000. **Desc:** National voluntary health agency which serves as the "focal point for the fight against epilepsy in the United States." Augmented by 64 affiliates in the U.S. committed to preventing and controlling epilepsy and improving the lives of those who have it. Provides federal government liaison. The foundation supports medical, social, rehabilitational, legal, employment, and information, education, and advocacy programs. Sponsors research in causes of epilepsy, prevention, psychosocial needs, and improved methods of treatment. Provides research and training grants and fellowships to students and professionals. Assistance and counseling for epilepsy patients and their families is provided through local organizations and the National Information Center on Epilepsy. Annual projects include National Epilepsy Month (November), School Alert (a national educational program for schools), selection of the Epilepsy Poster Child, and a continuing professional and public education and information program. Maintains a resource center. Provides members with access to mail order pharmacy program. Compiles statistics; maintains placement program. **Pub:** *Between Us*, bimonthly. Magazine. Magazine for women. • *Epilepsy USA*, 8/year. Newspaper. Provides information on national legislation and administrative political decisions that affect the disabled, people with epilepsy, and others. • *EpilepsyUSA*, bimonthly. Magazine. News magazine. • *In Touch*, quarterly. Newsletter. For adults with epilepsy. *Price:* Free. • *Kids News*, quarterly. Magazine. Magazine for children. • Also publishes pamphlets and makes available audiovisual material and informational/educational pieces for diversified audiences.

★ **13990** ★ **Epilepsy Support Foundation**
No. 3 Crocket Rd.
PO Box A104
Avondale
Harare, Zimbabwe
**Phone:** 263 4 724071
**Fnded:** 1990. **Mem:** 1,205. **Reg. Groups:** 3. **Lang(s):** English, Shona. **Desc:** Seeks to improve the quality of life for persons with epilepsy. Raises public awareness about epilepsy and its effects. Disseminates information. Makes available counseling services; maintains support groups; conducts rural outreach programs. **Pub:** *Epilepsy Back Up*, monthly. Newsletter. • Pamphlets, periodic. Contains information on epilepsy for patients, service providers, medical personnel, and various professionals.

★ **13991** ★ **Esther A. and Joseph Klingenstein Fund**
787 7th Ave., 6th Fl.
New York, NY 10019-6016
**Phone:** (212)492-6181    **Fax:** (212)492-7007
John Klingenstein, Pres.
**Fnded:** 1945. **Desc:** Works to support neuroscience research, especially in the area of epilepsy, independent school education, separation of Church and State, and animal-based research.

**European Alliance of Neuromuscular Disorders Associations (EANDA)**
*See:* Entry 13586

**European Association for NeuroOncology (EANO)**
*See:* Entry 10161

★ **13992** ★ **European Association of Neurosurgical Societies (EANS)**
60 Cobden Ave.
Southampton SO18 1FT, United Kingdom
**Phone:** 44 23 80585115    **Fax:** 44 23 80585115
**Email:** stephanie.garfield@virgin.net
**Website:** http://www.eans.org
**Fnded:** 1971. **Mem:** 8,000. **Lang(s):** English. **Desc:** National European neurological societies in 32 countries. Sponsors two training courses per year and various other activities and research projects. **Pub:** *Acta Neurochirurgica*, 3-4/year. Journal. • *EANS Bulletin*, semiannual. Bulletin. • Directory, annual. • Directory, annual.

★ **13993** ★ **European Brain and Behaviour Society (EBBS)**
c/o Dr. Susan J. Sara
Institut des Neurosciences
9 quai St. Bernard
F-75005 Paris, France
**Phone:** 33 1 44273460    **Fax:** 33 1 44273251
**Email:** ebbs@snv.jussieu.fr
**Website:** http://www.ebbs-science.org/
**Fnded:** 1966. **Mem:** 550. **Lang(s):** Dutch, English, French. **Desc:** Scientists with an interest in the study of the brain and behavior. Promotes and facilitates exchange of information among members and between members and others working in related fields. Conducts research and and educational programs. **Pub:** Books, biennial. • Newsletter, periodic.

★ **13994** ★ **European Brain Injury Society (EBIS)**
17, rue de Londres
B-1050 Brussels, Belgium
**Phone:** 32 2 5022046    **Fax:** 32 2 5023488
**Email:** ebis@euronet.be
**Fnded:** 1989.

★ **13995** ★ **European College of Neuropsychopharmacology**
Department of Psychiatry
Frederiksborg General Hospital
DK-3400 Hillerod, Denmark
**Phone:** 45 42261500    **Fax:** 45 86600244
**Fnded:** 1985.

★ **13996** ★ **European Federation of Child Neurology Societies (EFCNS)**
10 Av Hippocrate
1200 Brussels, Belgium
**Phone:** 32 2 7645231    **Fax:** 32 2 7641303
**Fnded:** 1970.

★ **13997** ★ **European Federation of Neurological Societies (EFNS)**
c/o Neurological Hospital
Rosenhuegel Riedelgasse 5
A-1130 Vienna, Austria
**Phone:** 43 1 88000270    **Fax:** 43 1 8892581
**Email:** headoffice@efns.org
**Website:** http://www.efns.org
**Fnded:** 1991. **Mem:** 38. **Desc:** Promotes the advancement of neurological sciences, including the practice of neurology, in Europe.

★ **13998** ★ **European Neurofibromatosis**
82 London Rd.
Kingston Upon Thames KT2 6PX, United Kingdom
**Phone:** 44 208 5471636    **Fax:** 44 208 9745601
**Email:** nfa@zetnet.co.uk
**Website:** http://www.nfa.zetnet.co.uk
**Fnded:** 1981. **Mem:** 1,870. **Reg. Groups:** 36. **Desc:** Seeks to establish and maintain a network of family support workers who are able to support and offer practical help and advice to those affected by Neurofibromatosis and their families. Neurofibromatosis is a genetic disorder of the nerve tissue, the characteristics

of which include six or more coffee colored marks on the skin in the first two years of life and nodules on or just below the surface of the skin, or tumors on both acoustical nerves. Fosters research; disseminates information. **Pub:** Newsletter, quarterly. • Annual Report.

**★ 13999 ★ European Neurological Society (ENS)**
78, rue du General Leclerc
F-94275 Le Kremlin-Bicetre, France
**Phone:** 33 1 45212618     **Fax:** 33 1 46700931
**Website:** http://www.ensinfo.com

**★ 14000 ★ European Pediatric Neurology Society**
48, bd Serrurier
F-75019 Paris, France
**Phone:** 33 1 40034773     **Fax:** 33 1 40034774
**Fnded:** 1970. **Desc:** Promotes development of knowledge in child neurology.

**★ 14001 ★ European Sleep Research Society (ESRS)**
c/o Dr. Porkka-Heiskanen
Institute of Biomedicine
Biomedicum
PO Box 63
FIN-00014 Helsinki, Finland
**Phone:** 358 9191 25317     **Fax:** 358 9191 25302
**Email:** porkka@cc.helsinki-fi
**Website:** http://www.esrs.org
**Fnded:** 1972. **Mem:** 700. **Desc:** Those interested in sleep research. Promotes research on sleeping and other related disorders and to assist in the care of patients with sleeping disorders. Provides continuing education of all professional groups involved with this research and disseminates information regarding the disorder.

**★ 14002 ★ European Society for Neurochemistry (ESN)**
Department of Neurobiology
Weizmann Institute of Science
IL-76100 Rehovot, Israel
**Phone:** 972 8 9343095
**Email:** bnyavin@weizmann.weizmann.ac.il
**Fnded:** 1976. **Mem:** 685. **Lang(s):** English. **Desc:** Researchers in 33 countries working in neurochemistry, neurology, molecular neurobiology, molecular neuropharmacology, and psychiatry. Works toward a greater understanding of the biochemical foundations of nervous activity and insight into neural and mental diseases. Conducts seminars and workshops. **Pub:** *ESN Directory*, periodic. Directory. • *Newsletter*, periodic. Newsletter. • *Proceedings of Biennial General Meetings.*

**European Society of Neurogastroenterology and Gastrointestinal Motility**
*See:* Entry 9121

**★ 14003 ★ European Society of Neuroradiology (ESNR)**
c/o MGR Congress Division
Via Altura 3
I-40139 Bologna, Italy
**Phone:** 39 2 6225520     **Fax:** 39 2 6225785
**Email:** marco.leonardi@centauro.it
**Website:** http://www.esnr.org
**Fnded:** 1969. **Mem:** 650. **Lang(s):** English. **Desc:** Mission is accomplish the following: to promote neuroradiology in all its fields; to coordinate work and documents in neuroradiology and to ensure the circulation throughout Europe; to coordinate relations with general radiology and the clinical specialties concerning the nervous system; to contribute to the development of unified methods of teaching neuroradiology and unified standards for training and certification in

neuroradiology; to promote and coordinate relations among the existing European national neuroradiological societies or national sections of the ESNR in countries where there are no existing societies; to form European research teams to deal with specific neuroradiological issues. **Pub:** *Neuroradiology*, monthly. Journal. • Directory, periodic.

**Facioscapulohumeral (FSH) Society**
*See:* Entry 13591

**★ 14004 ★ Familiares y Amigos de Enfermos de la Neurona Motora (FYADENMAC)**
Maestro Rural Num. 74
Col. Un Hogar para Nostros
11330 Mexico City, DF, Mexico
**Phone:** 52 5 3411595
**Email:** fyadermac@yahoo.com
**Website:** http://www.fshsociety.org
**Fnded:** 1982. **Mem:** 34. **Lang(s):** English, German. **Desc:** Promotes interest in motor neurone disease (MND) research among medical and scientific communities and the public in Mexico. Offers support services to MND sufferers and their families. Disseminates information about the disease.

**★ 14005 ★ Families of S.M.A. (FSMA)**
PO Box 196
Libertyville, IL 60048-0196
**Phone:** (847)367-7620     **Free:** 800-886-1762
**Fax:** (847)367-7623
**Email:** sma@fsma.org
**Website:** http://www.fsma.org
Audrey Lewis, Dir.
**Fnded:** 1985. **Mem:** 3,500. **Reg. Groups:** 1. **State Groups:** 21. **Local Groups:** 22. **Desc:** Individuals with Spinal Muscular Atrophy; their families; medical professionals; and interested others. Major funder of SMA research. Promotes public awareness. SMA diseases include: Infantile Progressive SMA (Werdnig-Hoffman Disease), Juvenile Progressive SMA (Kugelberg-Welander Disease) and Adult Progressive SMA (Aran-Duchenne Type). Offers support to families. **Pub:** *Direction*, quarterly. Newsletter. Includes research updates and information network. **Price:** $25/year for families in U.S.; $35/year for professionals in U.S.; $40/year outside U.S. • *Living with SMA*. Video. • *Understanding Muscular Atrophy.*

**★ 14006 ★ Federation of European Neuroscience Societys (FENS)**
c/o Prof./Dr. Monica Di Luca
University Milan
Institute for Pharmacological Sciences
via Balzaretti 9
I-20133 Milan, Italy
**Phone:** 39 2 20488374     **Fax:** 39 2 29404961
**Email:** monica.diluca@unimi.it
**Website:** http://www.fens.org/
**Desc:** Neuroscience societies and those in the field of neurosciences. Promotes the neurosciences in Europe. Organizes Winter and Summer Schools.

**★ 14007 ★ Federazione Alzheimer Italia (FAI)**
Via T. Marino 7
I-20121 Milan, Italy
**Phone:** 39 2 809767     **Fax:** 39 2 875781
**Email:** alzit@tin.it
**Website:** http://www.alzheimer.it
**Lang(s):** English, Italian. **Desc:** Individuals and organizations. Seeks to improve the quality of life of people with Alzheimer's disease and their families. Makes available support and services; facilitates research on Alzheimer's disease and related disorders; conducts educational programs.

**Finnish Muscular Diseases Association (FMD)**
*See:* Entry 13594

**★ 14008 ★ Forbes Norris MDA-ALS Research Center (ALSNRF)**
c/o California Pacific Medical Center
2324 Sacramento St., Ste. 150
San Francisco, CA 94115
**Phone:** (415)923-3604     **Fax:** (415)673-5184
**Email:** eila.ahokas@lihastautiliitto.fi
**Website:** http://www.lihastautiliitto.fi
Giovanna Kushner, Contact
**Fnded:** 1981. **Local Groups:** 3. **Desc:** Serves as clearinghouse for laboratory and clinical research into neuromuscular diseases, primarily Amyotrophic Lateral Sclerosis (Lou Gehrig's Disease). ALS is a paralytic and usually fatal disease of the motor neurons, nerves which innervate the muscles to allow movement. Although patients maintain their full intellectual capacities, they gradually lose their ability to move, talk, and breathe. Sponsors the ALS Research Center at the California Pacific Medical Center in San Francisco, CA and maintains an extensive bank of ALS patient information. Offers educational programs and a speakers' bureau. speakers' bureau. **Pub:** *Forbes Norris Research Center–Support Group Newsletter*, monthly. Newsletter. **Price:** Free. • Newsletter, semiannual. **Frmly:** (1994) ALS and Neuromuscular Research Foundation; (1999) ALS Forbes Norris Research Center.

**French-Language Neuro-Anesthetic-Resuscitation Association (Association de Neuro-Anesthesie-Reanimation de Langue Francaise)**
*See:* Entry 4460

**★ 14009 ★ French-Speaking Neuropsychological Society (Societe de Neuropsychologie de Langue Francaise)**
Hopital Purpan
F- 31059 Toulouse, France
**Phone:** 33 5 61779505     **Fax:** 33 5 61499524
**Email:** agniel@purpan.inserm.fr
**Fnded:** 1977.

**★ 14010 ★ Friedreichs Ataxia Society of Ireland (FASI)**
San Martino
Mart Ln.
Foxrock
Dublin 18, Ireland
**Phone:** 353 1 2894788     **Fax:** 353 1 2894788
**Email:** fasi@tinet.ie
**Website:** http://www.fasi.ie
**Fnded:** 1980. **Mem:** 250. **Nat'l Groups:** 1. **Lang(s):** English. **Desc:** Individuals and organizations. Seeks to improve the quality of life of people with Friedreich's ataxia and their families. Makes available support and services; conducts educational and advocacy campaigns. **Pub:** *FASI Newsletter*. Newsletter.

**★ 14011 ★ Fundacion Alzheimer Espana (AAE)**
Rafael Salgado, 7-1o dcha
E-28036 Madrid, Spain
**Phone:** 34 91 3448130     **Fax:** 34 91 4579542
**Email:** alzheuro@lander.es
**Website:** http://www.solitel.es/alzheimer
**Fnded:** 1991. **Lang(s):** English, Spanish. **Desc:** Individuals and organizations. Seeks to improve the quality of life of people with Alzheimer's disease and their families. Makes available support and services; facilitates research on Alzheimer's disease and related disorders; conducts educational programs.

**★ 14012 ★ German Neuroscience Society (Neurowissenschaftliche Gesellschaft e.V.)**
c/o Meino Alexandra Gibson
Max Delbruck Center for Moleculare Medizin
Robert Rossle Str. 10
D-13122 Berlin, Germany
**Phone:** 49 30 94063133      **Fax:** 49 30 94063819
**Email:** gibson@mdc-berlin.de

**Desc:** Supports research and education in the field of neuroscience; establishes political concepts; partners with industry; offers methodological courses and educational programs for teachers. **Pub:** *Neuroforum*, quarterly. Journal. Contains review articles, book reviews, historical and methodological articles, information on grants programs, prizes and more.

**★ 14013 ★ Greek Alzheimer's Association (GAA)**
Macri 16
Sikies
GR-56625 Thessaloniki, Greece

**Lang(s):** English, Greek. **Desc:** Individuals and organizations. Seeks to improve the quality of life of people with Alzheimer's disease and their families. Makes available support and services; facilitates research on Alzheimer's disease and related disorders; conducts educational programs.

**★ 14014 ★ Guardians of Hydrocephalus Research Foundation (GHRF)**
2618 Ave. Z
Brooklyn, NY 11235-2023
**Phone:** (718)743-4473      **Fax:** (718)743-1171
**Email:** ghrf2618@aol.com
Katherine Soriano, VP

**Fnded:** 1977. **Mem:** 5,000. **State Groups:** 11. **Local Groups:** 2. **Desc:** Hydrocephalics and their families, health care professionals, and other concerned individuals. Seeks to find the cause and cure of hydrocephalus. (Hydrocephalus is the buildup of cerebrospinal fluid in the brain cavity, which can cause brain damage or death if untreated.) Disseminates information on hydrocephalus; conducts public awareness and fundraising projects. Plans to conduct research and educational programs, and to operate computerized services. **Pub:** *An Introduction to Hydrocephalus.* • *Journal Ad Book*, annual. Journal. • Newsletter, quarterly. Includes news briefs and fundraising and project information. *Price:* Included in membership dues. • Makes available documentary film.

**★ 14015 ★ Guillain-Barre Syndrome Foundation International (GBSFI)**
PO Box 262
Wynnewood, PA 19096
**Phone:** (610)667-0131      **Fax:** (610)667-7036
**Email:** gbint@ix.netcom.com
**Website:** http://www.webmast.com/gbs/
Estelle L. Benson, Exec. Dir.

**Fnded:** 1980. **Mem:** 15,000. **Reg. Groups:** 148. **Desc:** Individuals concerned with Guillain-Barre syndrome (Acute Idiopathic Polyneuritis), a rare, paralyzing, potentially catastrophic disorder of the peripheral nerves. Objectives are to: educate the public and medical community about the availability of support groups and maintain their awareness of the disorder; foster research on cause, prevention, and treatment; encourage financial support for research; develop nationwide support groups. Arranges for recovered or recovering patients to visit patients in acute care and rehabilitation hospitals; assists patients in dealing with disabilities should complete recovery not occur. Maintains steering committee of physicians, some of who have had the disorder. **Pub:** *Communicator*, quarterly. Newsletter. • *Guide for Caregivers.* Handbook. • *Guillain-Barre Syndrome, an Overview for the Layperson.* Booklet. **Frmly:** (1988) Guillain-Barre Syndrome Support Group; (1990) Guillain-Barre Syndrome Support Group International.

**★ 14016 ★ Head Injury Hotline (PP)**
c/o Constance Miller
212 Pioneer Bldg.
Seattle, WA 98104-2221
**Phone:** (206)621-8558      **Fax:** (206)624-4961
**Email:** brain@headinjury.com
**Website:** http://www.headinjury.com
Constance Miller, Contact

**Fnded:** 1985. **Desc:** A non profit clearinghouse founded and operated by head injury activists since 1985. It is a place where visitors can get information, join a discussion group, build advocacy skills, and self-care skills. The site integrates resources from diverse organizations including support groups, rehabilitation, and research sites, as well as lay and professional journals and more. Maintains speakers' bureau. **Pub:** *From the Ashes: A Head Injury Self-Advocacy Guide*, periodic. Contains worksheets to assist in locating and assessing doctors and therapists; self-assessment inventories; glossary of commonly-used phrases. *Price:* $20/copy; $5 shipping and handling. **Frmly:** (1993) Phoenix Project.

**★ 14017 ★ Headway Ireland - National Head Injuries Association (HINHIA)**
Baggot St. Hospital
18 Upper Baggot St.
Dublin 4, Ireland
**Phone:** 353 1 6689893      **Fax:** 353 1 6689892
**Email:** headwave@aonad.iol.ie

**Fnded:** 1993. **Mem:** 800. **Reg. Groups:** 8. **Lang(s):** English, Irish. **Desc:** Individuals and organizations. Seeks to improve the quality of life of people with head injuries and their families. Makes available support and services; conducts educational and advocacy campaigns; sponsors training programs for providers of care and services to people with head injuries.

**★ 14018 ★ Huntington Society of Canada (HSC)**
22 Antares Dr., Ste. 102
Nepean, ON, Canada K2E 7Z6
**Phone:** (613)228-3155      **Free:** 800-998-7398
**Fax:** (613)228-3242
**Email:** info@hsc-ca.org
**Website:** http://www.hsc-ca.org

**Fnded:** 1973. **Mem:** 8,000. **Nat'l Groups:** 1. **Reg. Groups:** 60. **Lang(s):** English, French. **Desc:** Individuals with Huntington disease (a hereditary neurological disorder) and their families; health care professionals and others with an interest in Huntington disease and related disorders. Seeks to identify the cause and find a cure for Huntington disease; promotes an improved quality of life for people with Huntington disease. Serves as a clearinghouse on Huntington disease; conducts educational programs; funds research; maintains speakers' bureau. **Pub:** *Horizon*, quarterly. Newsletter.

**★ 14019 ★ Huntington's Disease Association (HDA)**
108 Battersea High St.
London SW11 3HP, United Kingdom
**Phone:** 44 207 2237000      **Fax:** 44 207 2239489
**Email:** info@hda.org.uk
**Website:** http://www.hda.org.uk

**Fnded:** 1971. **Mem:** 5,700. **Local Groups:** 40. **Lang(s):** English. **Desc:** Individuals united to provide assistance, treatment, and information on the effects of Huntington's Disease, a hereditary nervous disorder causing terminal physical and mental disability. Services include: counseling program designed for families and involved professionals; network of regional advisers and local groups throughout the country; confidential telephone and correspondence service; financial assistance; aid to patients undergoing presymptomatic tests or brain tissue donations. Encourages research on the medical and social effects of Huntington's Disease; raises funds. **Pub:** *Facing Huntington's Disease*, periodic. Booklet. • Newsletter, semiannual. • Pamphlets, periodic. **Frmly:** (1991) Association to Combat Huntington's Disease.

**★ 14020 ★ Huntington's Disease Association of Ireland (HDAI)**
Carmichael House
N Brunswick St.
Dublin 7, Ireland
**Phone:** 353 1 8721303      **Fax:** 353 1 8729931
**Email:** hdai@indigo.ie
**Website:** http://indigo.ie/~hdai

**Lang(s):** English, Irish. **Desc:** Individuals and organizations. Seeks to improve the quality of life of people with Huntington's disease and their families. Makes available support and services; conducts educational and advocacy campaigns; serves as a clearinghouse on Huntington's disease.

**★ 14021 ★ Huntington's Disease Society of America (HDSA)**
158 W 29th St., 7th Fl.
New York, NY 10001-5300
**Phone:** (212)242-1968      **Free:** 800-345-4372
**Fax:** (212)239-3430
**Email:** hdsainfo@hdsa.org
**Website:** http://www.hdsa.org
Barbara Boyle, Exec. Dir.

**Fnded:** 1986. **Mem:** 50,000. **Reg. Groups:** 34. **Local Groups:** 3331. **Desc:** Individuals and groups of volunteers concerned with Huntington's disease, an inherited and terminal neurological condition causing progressive brain and nerve deterioration. Goals are to: identify HD families; educate the public and professionals, with emphasis on increasing consumer awareness of HD; promote and support basic and clinical research into the causes and cure of HD; maintain patient services program, coordinated with various community services, to assist families in meeting the social, economic, and emotional problems resulting from HD. Is working to change the attitude of the working community toward the HD patient, enhance the HD patient's lifestyle, and promote better health care and treatment, both in the community and in facilities. Has launched nationwide campaign in support of federal and state legislation establishing clinics, genetic counseling and screening centers, and diagnostic and treatment centers for HD patients and those suffering from other chronic, debilitating diseases. Actively cooperates with researchers in ongoing studies; cosponsors and supports workshops and symposia; provides grants to individual researchers; sponsors brain donor program. Crisis intervention and other support services are available. **Pub:** *Huntington's Disease Society of America-The Marker*, semiannual. Magazine. *Price:* Free. • *Toward A Cure*, semiannual. Newsletter. • Booklets. • Pamphlets. • Videos.

**★ 14022 ★ Hydrocephalus Association (HA)**
870 Market St., Ste. 705
San Francisco, CA 94102
**Phone:** (415)732-7040      **Free:** 888-598-3789
**Fax:** (415)732-7044
**Email:** hydroassoc@aol.com
**Website:** http://www.hydroassoc.org
Emily Fudge, Exec. Dir.

**Fnded:** 1983. **Mem:** 2,000. **Desc:** People with hydrocephalus and their families, health care professionals with an interest in hydrocephalus, and interested businesses and foundations. Works to improve the quality of life of people with hydrocephalus through education. Conducts training for families of people with hydrocephalus; sponsors social gatherings; facilitates networking among families of people with hydrocephalus and between organizations representing people with hydrocephalus. **Pub:** *About Hydrocephalus - A Book for Parents.* Booklet. • *About Normal Pressure Hydrocephalus-A book for Adults and their families.* Booklet. • *Directory of Hydrocephalus Support Groups*, periodic. Directory. • *Directory of Pediatric Neurosurgeons.* Directory. Lists 130 neurosurgeons geographically and alphabetically. • *Fact Sheet 12 Different Topics.* Pamphlet. • *Prenatal Hydrocephalus A Book for Parents.* Booklet. • *Quarterly Newsletter*, quarterly. Newsletter. • *Resource Guide.* Bibliography.

## ★ 14023 ★ Indian Brain Research Association

35 Ballygunge Circular Rd.
Calcutta 700 019, India
**Fnded:** 1964.


## ★ 14024 ★ Indian Muscular Dystrophy Association (IMDA)

MIG 72
APHB Colony
Machilipatnam 521 001, India
**Phone:** 91 8 6722817

**Fnded:** 1982. **Mem:** 850. **Nat'l Groups:** 3. **State Groups:** 7. **Lang(s):** English. **Desc:** Individuals in India who work toward the dissemination of information and research concerning muscular dystrophy, a hereditary disease characterized by progressive deterioration of muscles. **Pub:** *Bridge*, quarterly. Newsletter. • *Varadhi*.


## International Academy for Child Brain Development (IACBD)

*See:* Entry 5689


## ★ 14025 ★ International Aphasia Association (IAA) (Association Internationale Aphasie — AIA)

Ave. des Heros 50
B-1160 Brussels, Belgium
**Phone:** 32 2 6724051      **Fax:** 32 2 6751245
**Email:** institutes@iahp.org
**Website:** http://www.iahp.org

**Lang(s):** English, French. **Desc:** Individuals with aphasia; therapists health care professionals with an interest in speech disorders. Promotes more effective treatment of aphasia; seeks to improve the quality of life of people with aphasia. Provides therapy and other services to people with aphasia; conducts training courses for speech therapists.


## International Association of ALS/MND Associations

*See:* Entry 13599


## ★ 14026 ★ International Association for the Study of Pain (IASP)

909 NE 43rd St., Ste. 306
Seattle, WA 98105-6020
**Phone:** (206)547-6409      **Fax:** (206)547-1703
**Email:** iaspdesk@juno.com
**Website:** http://www.iasp-pain.org
Louisa E. Jones, Exec. Off.

**Fnded:** 1973. **Mem:** 7,000. **Nat'l Groups:** 57. **Reg. Groups:** 57. **Desc:** Scientists, physicians, and other health professionals interested in pain research and therapy. Encourages research on pain mechanisms and syndromes; seeks to improve management of patients with acute and chronic pain. Promotes education and training in the field of pain; informs the public of results of current research. Fosters development of an international data bank, adoption of a uniform classification and definition regarding pain and pain syndromes, and creation of a uniform records system on information relating to pain mechanisms, syndromes, and management. Promotes the formation of national associations for the study and treatment of pain. **Pub:** *A Virtual Pocket Dictionary of Pain Terms.* Online only. • *Abstracts - 9th World Congress on Pain.* Book. • *Acute and Procedure Pain in Infants and Children.* Book. • *Assessment and Treatment of Cancer Pain - 1998.* Book. • *The Child With Headache: Diagnosis and Treatment.* Book. • *Chronic and Recurrent Pain in Children and Adolescents.* Book. • *Classification of Chronic Pain, 2nd ed. 1994.* Book. • *Complex Regional Pain Syndrome.* Book. • *Curriculum on Pain for Students in Psychology.* • *Desirable Characteristics for Pain Treatment Facilities.* • *Epidemiology of Pain.* Book. • *Ethical Guidelines for Investigations of Experimental Pain in Conscious Animals.* •

*Ethical Guidelines for Pain Research in Humans.* • *IASP Pain Terminology.* • *Manual de Farmacoes Utilizados en el Tratamiento del Dolor Cronico.* Book. • *Measurement of Pain in Infants and Children.* Book. • *Molecular Neurobiology of Pain.* Book. • *Neuropathic Pain: Pathophysiology and Treatment.* Book. • *Opiod Sensitivity of Chronic Noncancer Pain.* Book. • *Outline Curriculum on Pain for Medical Schools.* • *Outline Curriculum on Pain for Schools of Nursing.* • *Outline Curriculum on Pain for Schools of Occupational Therapy and Physical Therapy.* • *Outline Curriculum on Pain for Schools of Pharmacy.* • *Pain*, 15/year. Journal. • *Pain and Suffering.* Book. • *Pain: Clinical Updates*, quarterly. Newsletter. • *Pain Imaging.* Book. • *Pain in the Elderly.* Book. • *Pain 1999 - An Updated Review (Refresher Course Syllabus) 1999.* Book. • *Pain Treatment Centers at a Crossroads: A Practical and Conceptual Reappraisal.* Book. • *Pharmacological Approaches to the Treatment of Chronic Pain.* Book. • *Proceedings.*


## International Behavioural and Neural Genetics Society (IBANGS)

*See:* Entry 9335


## ★ 14027 ★ International Brain Research Organization (IBRO) (Organisation Internationale de Recherche sur le Cerveau)

51, Blvd. de Montmorency
F-75016 Paris, France
**Phone:** 33 1 46479292      **Fax:** 33 1 45206006
**Email:** admin@ibro.org
**Website:** http://www.ibro.org

**Fnded:** 1960. **Mem:** 50,000. **Lang(s):** English, French. **Desc:** Scientists working in neuroanatomy, neuroendocrinology, the behavioral sciences, neurocommunications and biophysics, brain pathology, and clinical and health-related sciences. Works to promote international cooperation in research on the nervous system. Sponsors fellowships, exchange of scientific workers, and traveling teams of instructors to supplement local teachings. Organizes international neuroscience symposia and workshops. **Pub:** *Directory of Members*, periodic. Directory. • *Neuroscience*, bimonthly. • *News*, annual.


## ★ 14028 ★ International Bureau for Epilepsy (IBE) (Bureau International pour l'Epilepsie)

PO Box 21
NL-2100 AA Heemstede, Netherlands
**Phone:** 31 23 5291019      **Fax:** 31 23 5470119
**Email:** ibe@xs4all.nl
**Website:** http://www.ibe-epilepsy.org

**Fnded:** 1961. **Mem:** 90. **Nat'l Groups:** 55. **Lang(s):** English. **Desc:** National organizations and individuals interested in the medical, social, and scientific aspects of epilepsy. Focuses on aspects of daily life with epilepsy. Facilitates exchange of information and experience regarding the care of persons with epilepsy. Provides material on how to organize and finance non-medical societies. Organizes training sessions. Works to build an international film library on epilepsy. **Pub:** *A Manual for Epilepsy Self-Help Groups.* Manual. • *Employing People with Epilepsy: Principles for Good Practice.* Handbook. • *Epilepsy Education Manual.* Manual. • *Epilepsy in Focus*, biennial. Report. Catalogue of audiovisual materials. • *International Epilepsy News*, quarterly. Magazine. Contains information on epilepsy.


## ★ 14029 ★ International Federation of Clinical Neurophysiology (Federation Internationale de Neurophysiologie Clinique)

c/o IFCN Secretariat
42 Canham Rd.
London W3 7SR, United Kingdom
**Phone:** 44 208 7433106      **Fax:** 44 208 7431010
**Email:** ifcn@concorde-uk.com
**Website:** http://www.ifcn.info

**Lang(s):** English, Japanese. **Desc:** Neurologists, physiologists, and other medical professionals; scientists and researchers. Seeks to advance knowledge in clinical neurophysiology and related fields; promotes development of more effective neurological diagnostic and surgical procedures. Serves as a clearinghouse on neurophysiology; conducts educational, training, and continuing professional development courses.


## ★ 14030 ★ International Federation for Hydrocephalus and Spina Bifida (IFHSB)

Cellebroersstr 16
B-1000 Brussels, Belgium
**Phone:** 32 2 5020413      **Fax:** 32 2 5021129
**Email:** if@wanadoo.be
**Website:** http://www.ifglobal.org

**Fnded:** 1981. **Desc:** Disseminates information and expertise throughout the world to families, individuals, professionals and volunteers involved in the Hydrocephalus and Spina Bifida field, stimulates research; encourages cooperation between organizations; stimulates international discussion on ethics.


## ★ 14031 ★ International Huntington Association (IHA)

Callunahof 8
NL-7217 ST Harfsen, Netherlands
**Phone:** 31 573 431595      **Fax:** 31 573 431719
**Email:** iha@huntington-assoc.com
**Website:** http://www.huntington-assoc.com

**Fnded:** 1974. **Mem:** 52. **Nat'l Groups:** 41. **Lang(s):** Dutch, English. **Desc:** National health agencies concerned about Huntington's disease. (Huntington's disease is an inherited neurological disorder causing physical, emotional, and cognitive deterioration.) Promotes international cooperation in efforts to find a cure for Huntington's disease. Serves as a clearinghouse on Huntington's disease and related research. Maintains liaison with scientists and scientific organizations engaged in work pertaining to Huntington's disease worldwide. Assists in the establishment of new Huntington's disease associations and in the establishment of international collaborative research efforts to find a cure for the disease. Provides support and services to people with Huntington's disease and their families; conducts educational programs for health care professionals treating people with Huntington's disease and the public. **Pub:** *Living With HD Your Guide to Effective Eating and Diet.* Brochures. • *Nutrition and Huntington's Disease.* Books.


## ★ 14032 ★ International Joseph Disease Foundation (IJDF)

PO Box 2550
Livermore, CA 94551-2550
**Fax:** (925)371-1288
**Email:** bashor@ijdf.net
**Website:** http://www.ijdf.net
Rose Marie Silva, Exec. Dir.

**Fnded:** 1977. **Mem:** 1,500. **Desc:** Geneticists, neurologists, patients and their families, and individuals interested in Joseph disease. (Joseph disease is a neurological genetic disorder of the motor system affecting all races and many ethnic groups, which is often misdiagnosed as multiple sclerosis, or Parkinson's disease.) Locates families throughout the world affected by the disease. Educates the medical profession and the public on Joseph disease in an effort to promote more accurate diagnosis and better treatment. Diagnostic marker to identify carriers of the disorder is now available. **Pub:** *IJDF Newsletter*, quarterly. Newsletter. Includes research developments.


## ★ 14033 ★ International League Against Epilepsy (ILAE)

Ave. Marcel Thiry 204
B-1200 Brussels, Belgium
**Phone:** 32 2 7749547      **Fax:** 32 2 7749690
**Email:** njejerman@iname.com
**Website:** http://www.ilae-epilepsy.org

**Fnded:** 1909. **Mem:** 72. **Nat'l Groups:** 72. **Lang(s):** English, French, German, Spanish. **Desc:** National organizations united to encourage scientific research on epilepsy, and to promote optimal treatment and rehabilitation of epileptic patients. Fosters development of and cooperation among associations with common interests. **Pub:** *Epigraph*, 2/year. Newsletter. • *Epilepsia*, monthly. Journal. Contains scientific papers and meeting abstracts for professional researchers in the field of epilepsy. Includes book reviews and research reports.

★ **14034** ★ **International Medical Society of Paraplegia**
c/o National Spinal Injuries Centre
Stoke Mandeville Hospital
Aylesbury HP21 8AL, United Kingdom
**Phone:** 44 1296 315866 **Fax:** 44 1296 315870
**Email:** imsop@bucks.net
**Website:** http://www.imsop.org.uk

**Fnded:** 1961. **Mem:** 1,820. **Desc:** Qualified medical practitioners with an interest and activity in research or treatment and rehabilitation of spinal cord afflictions. To study all problems concerning traumatic and non-traumatic problems of the spinal cord. To advance research, treatment and prevention; social integration of paraplegics - encourage medical services throughout the world especially in developing countries. To sponsor young specialists to attend annual scientific meetings and undertake research work. **Pub:** *Spinal Cord*, monthly. Newsletter.

★ **14035** ★ **International Neural Network Society (INNS)**
19 Mantua Rd.
Mount Royal, NJ 08061
**Phone:** (856)423-0162 **Fax:** (856)423-3420
**Email:** innshq@talley.com
**Website:** http://www.inns.org
Tom Sims, Exec. Dir.

**Fnded:** 1987. **Mem:** 1,000. **Desc:** Individuals interested in theoretical and computational understanding of the brain. Provides a forum for neurocomputing and theoretical approaches to neuroscience. Promotes research on behavioral processes and models of the brain. Encourages development of computing applications which use neural modeling concepts. **Pub:** *INNS Newsletter*, 9/year. Newsletter. Includes calendar of events and special interest group information. • *Neural Networks*, bimonthly. Journal.

★ **14036** ★ **International Neuromodulation Society**
c/o Tia Sofatzis
2000 Van Ness Ave., Ste. 402
San Francisco, CA 94109
**Phone:** (415)567-1219 **Fax:** (415)567-2534
**Email:** tiasofatzis@aol.com
**Website:** http://www.neuromodulation.com
Sherri Kae Calkins, Contact

**Fnded:** 1994. **Mem:** 250. **Nat'l Groups:** 1. **Desc:** Individuals with an interest in implantable technologies that impact on the nervous system. Promotes advancement of neuromodulation technologies and techniques; encourages continuing professional development of members. Serves as a forum for the exchange of scientific information on neuromodulation; conducts research and educational programs. **Pub:** *Neuromodulation*, quarterly. Journal.

★ **14037** ★ **International Research Council of Neuromuscular Disorders (IRCND)**
1434 Pleasantville Rd.
Lancaster, OH 43130
**Phone:** (740)653-1098 **Fax:** (740)653-3121
James R. Grilliot, D.C., Exec. Dir.

**Fnded:** 1982. **Mem:** 82. **Desc:** Health professionals interested in neuromuscular diseases of the human body. Purpose is to advance and disseminate information on the causes, effects, occurrence, cure, and prevention of neuromuscular disorders and associated

topics related to the human spine. Coordinates and encourages basic research and the exchange of ideas and related materials between professionals in the field. Prepares teaching and educational materials. Compiles statistics for distribution; sponsors seminars and speakers' bureau. Is currently developing a library. **Pub:** *Information/Newsletter*, annual. Newsletter.

**International Rett Syndrome Association (IRSA)**
*See:* Entry 5699

**International Society for Minimal Intervention in Spinal Surgery**
*See:* Entry 19573

★ **14038** ★ **International Society for Neuroimmunomodulation**
c/o Craig C. Smith
National Institute of Health
36 Convent Dr., Rm. 1A23/MSC 4020
Bethesda, MD 20892-4020
**Phone:** (301)496-4561 **Fax:** (301)496-6095
**Email:** ccs@codon.nih.gov
**Website:** http://www.isnim.org
Craig C. Smith, Exec. Dir.

**Fnded:** 1986. **Mem:** 150. **Desc:** Professional society for scientists involved in interdisciplinary research in the molecular and cellular aspects of neurobiology, neuroendocrinology, immunology, and the behavioral sciences. Interests focus on discerning the integrative elements underlying communication and modulation between the central nervous, endocrine, and immune systems, and upon related disease states. **Pub:** *NeuroImmunoModulation*. Journal.

**International Society of Neuropathology (Societe Internationale de Neuropathologie)**
*See:* Entry 17144

★ **14039** ★ **International Society of Neurovirology**
c/o Brian Wigdahl, Dept. of Microbiology and Immunology Penn State College of Medicine
500 University Dr.
PO Box 850
Hershey, PA 17033
**Phone:** (717)531-8258 **Fax:** (717)531-5580
**Email:** bwigdahl@psu.edu
**Website:** http://www.isnv.org
Brian Wigdahl, PhD, Pres.

**Fnded:** 1998. **Mem:** 200. **Nat'l Groups:** 1. **Desc:** Neurovirologists. **Pub:** *Journal of NeuroVirology*, bimonthly. Journal.

★ **14040** ★ **International Society for the Study of the Lumbar Spine**
2075 Bayview Ave., Room MG323
Toronto, ON, Canada M4N 3M5
**Phone:** (416)480-4833 **Fax:** (416)480-6055
**Email:** shirley.fitzgerald@swchsc.on.ca
**Website:** http://www.issls.org/main.html

**Fnded:** 1974. **Mem:** 346. **Desc:** Aims to bring together those individuals throughout the world, who, by their contributions and activities both in the area of research and clinical study, have, or are indicating interest in the lumbar spine in health and in disease.

★ **14041** ★ **International Tremor Foundation (ITF)**
7046 W 105th St.
Overland Park, KS 66212-1803
**Phone:** (913)341-3880 **Free:** 888-387-3667
**Fax:** (913)341-1296
**Email:** staff@essentialtremor.org
**Website:** http://www.essentialtremor.org
Catherine S. Rice, Exec. Dir.

**Fnded:** 1988. **Mem:** 25,000. **State Groups:** 54. **Desc:** Provides services, support, research, funds, and education to families, friends, and individuals suffering from Benign Essential Tremor. Current treatment includes drug therapy and surgical intervention. Provides patient information and referrals to physicians who specialize in Essential Tremor. **Pub:** Newsletter, quarterly. Includes research reports and networking information. *Price:* Included in membership dues.

★ **14042** ★ **Irish Motor Neurone Disease Association**
Coleraine House
Coleraine St.
Dublin 7, Ireland
**Phone:** 353 1 8730422 **Fax:** 353 1 8735283
**Email:** info@imnda.ie

**Fnded:** 1985. **Desc:** Promotes interest in motor neurone disease (MND) research among medical and scientific communities and the public in Ireland. Offers support services to MND sufferers and their families. Disseminates information about the disease. **Pub:** *IMNDA Newsletter*, quarterly. Newsletter.

★ **14043** ★ **Israel Society for Neurosciences**
c/o Prof. Israel Silman
PO Box 66
75706 Rishon Le Zion, Israel
**Phone:** 972 8 9694126 **Fax:** 972 3 9660841
**Email:** ayg@inter.net.il
**Website:** http://isfn.org.il

**Lang(s):** English. **Desc:** Promotes neuroscience in Israel.

★ **14044** ★ **Japan ALS Association**
7-103 Nando-cho
Shinjuku
Tokyo 162-0837, Japan
**Phone:** 81 3 32676942 **Fax:** 81 3 32674123
**Email:** jalsa@jade.dti.ne.jp
**Website:** http://www.jade.dti.ne.jp/~jalsa

**Desc:** Individuals interested in amyotropic lateral sclerosis or ALS (also known as Lou Gehrig's Disease). Works to: heighten public awareness and understanding of the disease; encourage research among medical and scientific communities.

★ **14045** ★ **Korean Society for the Cerebral Palsied (KSCP)**
771 Sanggye, 6-dong
Nowon-ku
Seoul 139-831, Republic of Korea
**Phone:** 82 2 9324292 **Fax:** 82 2 9324413
**Email:** kscpw@hitel.net
**Website:** http://www.kscp.net

**Fnded:** 1978. **Mem:** 155. **Local Groups:** 2. **Lang(s):** English, Korean. **Desc:** People who have a professional interest in rehabilitation for the people with cerebral palsy and their families. Promotes high quality care for people with cerebral palsy. Acts as a national coordinating body, provides guidance and seeking to achieve the optimal use of resources, acts as a vehicle for the exchange of information. Aims to provide rehabilitation services for people with cerebral palsy. **Pub:** *Newsletter of KSCP*, monthly. Newsletter.

★ **14046** ★ **Korean Society for Clinical Neurophysiology**
c/o Kwang-Woo Lee
Department of Neurology
College of Medicine
Seoul National University
28 Yongon-Dong, Chongno-Gu
Seoul 110-744, Republic of Korea
**Phone:** 82 2 7603215 **Fax:** 82 2 7441785

**Fnded:** 1996. **Reg. Groups:** 14. **Desc:** Fosters research and conducts patho-physiological experiments.

**Latin American Club of Neuro Ophthalmology (Club Latinoamericano de Neuroftalmologia — CLAN)**
*See:* Entry 21014


**Middle East Neurosurgical Society (Societe de Neurochirurgie du Moyen Orient)**
*See:* Entry 19579


★ 14047 ★ **Migraine Action Association**
Oakley Hay Lodge Business Park, Unit 6
Great Folds Rd.
Great Oakley NN18 9AS, United Kingdom
**Phone:** 44 1536 461333     **Fax:** 44 1536 461444
**Email:** info@migraine.org.uk
**Fnded:** 1958. **Mem:** 17,000. **Desc:** Migraine sufferers, their families and friends, or anyone else who is interested, including medical professionals. Support for research into aspects of migraine, grants, information, understanding and encouragement to migraine sufferers. **Pub:** *Migraine Action News*, quarterly. Newsletter. • *The Migraine Handbook.* Handbook. **Frmly:** (1997) British Migraine Association.


★ 14048 ★ **Migraine Association of Canada (MAC)**
365 Bloor St. E, Ste. 1912
Toronto, ON, Canada M4W 3L4
**Phone:** (416)920-4916     **Free:** 800-663-3557
**Fax:** (416)920-3677
**Email:** support@migraine.ca
**Website:** http://www.migraine.ca
**Fnded:** 1974. **Mem:** 7,000. **Local Groups:** 2. **Lang(s):** English, French. **Desc:** Individuals who experience migraine headaches. Promotes "empowerment of migraine sufferers to obtain relief." Serves as a clearinghouse on migraine headaches and their prevention and treatment. Conducts educational programs; participates in charitable activities. **Pub:** *Headlines*, quarterly.


★ 14049 ★ **Migrane Awareness Group: A National Understanding for "Migraineurs" (MAGNUM)**
113 S Saint Asaph, Ste. 300
Alexandria, VA 22314
**Phone:** (703)739-9384     **Fax:** (703)739-2432
**Email:** magnumnonprofit@hotmail.com
**Website:** http://www.migraines.org
Michael John Coleman, Exec. V. P.
**Fnded:** 1994. **Desc:** Works to bring public and governmental awareness to the medical seriousness of the migraine disease. Provides information and support to migraine sufferers and their families.


**Moldavian Myopathy Association**
*See:* Entry 13619


★ 14050 ★ **Motor Neurone Disease Association**
PO Box 246
Northampton NN1 2PR, United Kingdom
**Phone:** 44 1604 250505     **Fax:** 44 1604 638289
**Email:** enquiries@mndassociation.org
**Website:** http://www.mndassociation.org
**Fnded:** 1979. **Mem:** 6,500. **Local Groups:** 95. **Desc:** Raises awareness of motor neurone disease (MND). Provides care and support for people with MND and their families, and funds vital research into causes, treatments, and a cure for the disease. **Pub:** *Annual Review.* Booklets. Information leaflets. • *Thumbprint*, quarterly. Magazine.


★ 14051 ★ **Motor Neurone Disease Association of Australia**
PO Box 23
Canterbury, VIC 3126, Australia
**Phone:** 61 3 98302122     **Fax:** 61 3 98302228
**Email:** mmiller@mndaa.asn.au
**Website:** http://home.vicnet.net.au/~mndaust
**Fnded:** 1991. **Mem:** 7. **Nat'l Groups:** 2. **State Groups:** 7. **Desc:** Promotes interests in motor neurone disease (MND) research among medical and scientific communities and the public in Australia. Offers support services to MND sufferers and their families. Disseminates information about the disease.


★ 14052 ★ **Motor Neurone Disease Association of India**
40 Kologarh Rd.
St. No. 5
Rajendra Nagar 248 001, Delhi, India
**Phone:** 91 135 754487     **Fax:** 91 135 754487
**Email:** lbhagat@nae.vsnl.net.in
**Fnded:** 1993. **Mem:** 260. **Nat'l Groups:** 1. **Reg. Groups:** 2. **Local Groups:** 2. **Lang(s):** English, Hindi. **Desc:** Promotes interest in motor neurone disease (MND) research among medical and scientific communities and the public in India. Works as a support group to further the interests of MND sufferers and their families throughout the country. Disseminates information about the disease. **Pub:** *MND Newsletter*, biennial. Newsletter. Fundraising brochure containing comprehensive and general information on MND/ALS. **Frmly:** (1994) The MND Support Group of India.


★ 14053 ★ **Motor Neurone Disease Association of New Zealand**
PO Box 2129
Wellington, New Zealand
**Phone:** 64 4 4735555     **Fax:** 64 4 4735626
**Email:** mndanz@xtra.co.nz
**Fnded:** 1985. **Local Groups:** 5. **Desc:** Supports people living with Motor Neurone Disease by providing emotional, social and practical support, advocacy, information, and by raising awareness. **Pub:** *MND Newsletter*, quarterly. Newsletter.


★ 14054 ★ **Motor Neurone Disease Association of South Africa**
PO Box 781880
Sandton
Guateng 2146, Republic of South Africa
**Phone:** 27 11 7064883     **Fax:** 27 11 4636855
**Email:** dianeh@iafrica.com
**Fnded:** 1991. **Reg. Groups:** 3. **Desc:** Promotes interests in motor neurone disease (MND) research among medical and scientific communities and the public in South Africa. Offers support services to MND sufferers and their families. Disseminates information about the disease.


★ 14055 ★ **Motor Neurone Disease and Esclerosis Lateral Amiotrofica in Uruguay (MONDELA)**
Av. Italia 3318
Montevideo, Uruguay
**Phone:** 598 2 4871616     **Fax:** 598 2 475461
**Fnded:** 1991. **Mem:** 30. **Reg. Groups:** 3. **Local Groups:** 4. **Lang(s):** English, French, Italian. **Desc:** Promotes interest in motor neurone disease (MND) and amyotrophic lateral sclerosis (ALS) research among medical and scientific communities and the public in Uruguay. Offers support services to MND sufferers and their families. Disseminates information about the disease. **Pub:** *A Downstream Event in the Spinal Cord Slice: A Model of Early Excitotoxic Injury*, monthly. Report. • *Fisioterapia para las Enfermedades Neuromusculares.* Report. • *Mioterapia Oro Faringo Facial.* Report. **Frmly:** (1992) Asociacion de Enfermedades Motoneuronales y Esclerosis Lateral Amiotrofica del Uruguay (MON DELA).


★ 14056 ★ **Motor Neurone Disease Research Institute of Australia**
PO Box 23
Canterbury 3161, Australia
**Phone:** 61 3 98302122     **Fax:** 61 3 98302228
**Email:** mndria@vicnet.net.au
**Website:** http://home.vicnet.net.au/~mndri/
**Desc:** Promotes interest in motor neurone disease (MND) and amyotrophic lateral sclerosis (ALS) research among medical and scientific communities and the public in Australia. Offers support services to MND sufferers and their families. Disseminates information about the disease.


★ 14057 ★ **Multiple Sclerosis Association of America (MSAA)**
706 Haddonfield Rd.
Cherry Hill, NJ 08002-2652
**Phone:** (609)488-4500     **Free:** 800-532-7667
**Fax:** (856)661-9797
**Email:** msaa@msaa.com
**Website:** http://www.msaa.com
Douglas G. Franklin, Pres.
**Fnded:** 1970. **Mem:** 31,000. **Reg. Groups:** 5. **Desc:** Works to fulfill the daily needs of multiple sclerosis patients. Provides patient support, counseling, local transportation, therapeutic equipment, MRI scans for initial diagnosis and barrier-free housing. Conducts public education programs and symptom relief therapy research. **Pub:** *The Motivator*, bimonthly. Newsletter. *Price:* Free.


★ 14058 ★ **Multiple Sclerosis Care Centre**
Bushy Park House
65 Bushy Park Rd.
Rathgar
Dublin 6, Ireland
**Phone:** 353 1 1906234     **Fax:** 353 1 4906724
**Email:** msc@iol.ie
**Fnded:** 1989. **Desc:** Provides short-term respite care to people with Multiple Sclerosis and other neurological conditions. Assists people in dealing with disability and maintaining independence.


★ 14059 ★ **Multiple Sclerosis Foundation (MSF)**
6350 N Andrews Ave.
Fort Lauderdale, FL 33309-2130
**Phone:** (954)776-6805     **Free:** 888-673-6287
**Fax:** (954)938-8708
**Email:** support@msfocus.org
**Website:** http://www.msfocus.org
Jules Kuperberg, National Dir.
**Fnded:** 1986. **Desc:** Dedicated to helping create "A Brighter Tomorrow" for those with MS, the foundation offers a wide array of free services, including: information and referral, subsidized home care and outreach, educational programs, free publications, a quarterly news magazine, and more to improve the quality of life for those affected by MS. **Pub:** *MS Fact Sheets.* Booklets. • *MSFocus Magazine*, quarterly. Magazine. • *MSFYi*, monthly. Newsletter. Internet newsletter. • *Multiple Sclerosis: Helpful Information for Patients and Families.* Booklet.


★ 14060 ★ **Multiple Sclerosis International Federation**
3rd. Fl., Skyline House
200 Union St.
London SE1 0LY, United Kingdom
**Phone:** 44 207 6201911     **Fax:** 44 207 6201922
**Email:** info@msif.org
**Website:** http://www.ifmss.org.uk
**Fnded:** 1967. **Mem:** 36. **Lang(s):** English, French. **Desc:** Key aims are to stimulate scientific research at a global scale, disseminate information internationally, assist the development of national MS societies, and encourage full integration and participation of all people affected by MS. **Pub:** *Annual Report*, annual. Magazine. • *Federation Updates*, biennial. • *MS*

*Management.* • *MS Research in Progress.* • *MS Therapeutic Claims.* Frmly: (2001) International Federation of Multiple Sclerosis Societies.

### ★ 14061 ★ Multiple Sclerosis Society of Great Britain and Northern Ireland

MS National Centre
372 Edgware Rd.
London NW2 6ND, United Kingdom
**Phone:** 44 208 4380700　**Fax:** 44 208 4380701
**Email:** info@mssociety.org.uk
**Website:** http://www.mssociety.org.uk
**Fnded:** 1953. **Mem:** 60,000. **Reg. Groups:** 400. **Desc:** Persons with an interest in multiple sclerosis. Promoting and funding research to find the cause and cure of multiple sclerosis and the provision of a welfare and support service for anyone affected by MS. **Pub:** *MS Matters,* bimonthly. Magazine. Additional information on MS and living with Ms available upon request.

### ★ 14062 ★ Multiple Sclerosis Society of Ireland (MSSI)

The Royal Hospital Donnybrook
Bloomfield Ave.
Morehampton Rd.
Dublin 4, Ireland
**Phone:** 353 1 2694599
**Email:** info@ms-society.ie
**Website:** http://www.ms-society.ie
**Fnded:** 1961. **Mem:** 5,000. **Nat'l Groups:** 1. **Reg. Groups:** 8. **Local Groups:** 40. **Lang(s):** English, Irish. **Desc:** Individuals and organizations. Seeks to improve the quality of life of people with multiple sclerosis and their families. Makes available support and services; conducts educational and advocacy campaigns. **Pub:** *MS News,* quarterly. Magazine.

### ★ 14063 ★ Multiple Sclerosis Society of Zimbabwe

PO Box BE1234
Belvedere
Harare, Zimbabwe
**Phone:** 263 4 740472　**Fax:** 264 4 740472
**Email:** pwmsic@ifmss.org.uk
**Website:** http://www.ifmss.org.uk
**Fnded:** 1972. **Mem:** 50. **Nat'l Groups:** 1. **State Groups:** 9. **Desc:** Works to alleviate the suffering of persons with multiple sclerosis. Supports research to discover the cause of and cure for the disease. Offers financial assistance and counseling to individuals suffering from the disease. The society has just completed the constuction of a daycare/rehabilitation which will be geared to rehabilitate pwms, offer sympton management, carer & family training as well as support. **Pub:** *Missive,* monthly. Newsletter.

### ★ 14064 ★ Muscular Dystrophy Association (MDA)

3300 E Sunrise Dr.
Tucson, AZ 85718
**Phone:** (520)529-2000　**Free:** 800-572-1717
**Fax:** (520)529-5300
**Email:** mda@mdausa.org
**Website:** http://www.mdausa.org
Bob Mackle, Dir. Public Information
**Fnded:** 1950. **Local Groups:** 157. **Desc:** National voluntary health agency fostering research into the cause and cure of neuromuscular diseases in the following 8 categories. Muscular dystrophies: Becker; congenital; distal; Duchenne (pseudohypertrophic); Emery-Dreifuss; facioscapulohumeral (Landouzy-Dejerine); limb-girdle; myotonic (Steinert's disease); oculopharyngeal. Motor Neuron Diseases: adult spinal muscular atrophy (Aran-Duchenne type); amyotrophic lateral sclerosis (ALS); infantile progressive spinal muscular atrophy (type 1, Werdnig-Hoffmann disease); intermediate spinal muscular atrophy (type 2); juvenile spinal muscular atrophy (type 3, Kugelberg-Welander disease), Spinal Bulbar Muscular Atrophy (SBMA). Inflammatory Myopathies: dermatomyositis; polymyositis; inclusion body myositis. Diseases of Neuromuscular Junction: Eaton-Lambert (myasthenic)

syndrome;congenital myasthenic syndrome; myasthenia gravis. Diseases of the Peripheral Nerve: Dejerine-Sottas disease; Friedreich's ataxia; Charcot-Marie-Tooth disease (peroneal muscular atrophy). Metabolic Diseases of Muscle: acid maltase deficiency (Pompe's disease); carnitine deficiency; carnitine palmityl transferase deficiency; Debrancher enzyme deficiency (Cori'sor Forbes' disease); lactate dehydrogenase deficiency; mitochondrial myopathy; myoadenylate deaminase deficiency; phosphofructokinase deficiency (Tarui's disease); phosphoglycerate kinase deficiency; phosphoglycerate mutase deficiency; phosphorylase deficiency (McArdle's disease). Myopathies due to Endocrine Abnormalities: hyperthyroid myopathy; hypothyroid myopathy. Other myopathies: central core disease; myotonia congenita; myotubular myopathy; nemaline myopathy; paramyotonia congenita; periodic paralysis. Supports international programs of some 350 research awards, major university-based neuromuscular disease research/clinical centers, and 230 outpatient clinics in hospitals in the U.S. and Puerto Rico. Awards grants for neuromuscular disease research to individual scientific investigators. Renders services to patients locally through its chapters, including: diagnostic examinations; follow-up medical evaluations; wheelchairs; leg braces; physical therapy; flu shots; summer camps. **Pub:** *Annual Report,* annual. Annual Report. • *Quest,* bimonthly. Magazine. Contains stories, research updates, etc. of concern to those w/neuromuscular diseases. *Price:* Free to individuals served by MDA. • Also publishes general and technical literature on muscular dystrophy and other neuromuscular diseases.

### Muscular Dystrophy Ireland (MDI)
*See:* Entry 13628

### ★ 14065 ★ Myasthenia Gravis Association

Keynes House
Chester Pk.
Alfreton Rd.
Derby DE21 4AS, United Kingdom
**Phone:** 44 1332 290219　**Fax:** 44 1332 293641
**Email:** mg@mgaderby.fsnet.co.uk
**Website:** http://www.mgauk.org
**Fnded:** 1976. **Mem:** 1,125. **Reg. Groups:** 41. **Desc:** Supports research into the management and cure of Myasthenia.

### ★ 14066 ★ Myasthenia Gravis Foundation of America

5841 Cedar Lake Rd., Ste. 204
Minneapolis, MN 55416
**Phone:** (952)545-9438　**Free:** 800-541-5454
**Fax:** (952)545-6073
**Email:** myastheniagravis@msn.com
**Website:** http://www.myasthenia.org
Debora K. Boelz, CEO
**Fnded:** 1952. **Mem:** 30,000. **State Groups:** 36. **Desc:** Persons suffering from myasthenia gravis; their families, doctors, and nurses; others dedicated to the detection, treatment, and cure of MG. Raises funds for research and for professional and public education programs. Provides literature. Lay and professional materials available upon request. **Pub:** Brochures, annual. • Handbooks.For sales. • Manuals.For physicians and nurses. • Pamphlets. **Frmly:** (1998) Myasthenia Gracis Foundation.

### ★ 14067 ★ Narcolepsy Association United Kingdom (UKAN)

Craven House, 1st Floor
121 Kingsway
London WC2B 6PA, United Kingdom
**Phone:** 44 20 77218904　**Fax:** 44 1322 863056
**Email:** info@narcolepsy.org.uk
**Website:** http://www.narcolepsy.org.uk
**Fnded:** 1981. **Mem:** 700. **Reg. Groups:** 12. **Lang(s):** English. **Desc:** Narcoleptics, their relatives, and others interested in improving the lives of those afflicted with narcolepsy. Promotes awareness of narcolepsy and

provides authoritative information about it to narcoleptics, the medical profession, and to the public. Supports the establishment of local self-help groups; encourages research; co-operates with narcolepsy associations overseas. **Pub:** *Catnap,* quarterly. Newsletter. Reports national and international developments in cause and treatment of narcolepsy.

### ★ 14068 ★ Narcolepsy Network

10921 Reed Hartman Highway
Cincinnati, OH 45242
**Phone:** (513)891-3522　**Fax:** (513)891-3836
**Email:** narnet@aol.com
**Website:** http://www.websciences.org/narnet
Robert L. Cloud, Exec. Dir.
**Fnded:** 1986. **Local Groups:** 60. **Desc:** Individuals with narcolepsy, their friends and families, sleep professionals, and interested others. Seeks to improve the quality of life of individuals who have narcolepsy. Works to educate members and the general public about narcolepsy. Fosters communication among members. Offers referral service. Supports research; disseminates information. **Pub:** *Narcolepsy: A Guide to Understanding.* • *The Network,* quarterly. Newsletter.

### ★ 14069 ★ National Academy of Neuropsychology (NAN)

2121 S Oneida St., Ste. 550
Denver, CO 80224-2594
**Phone:** (303)691-3694　**Fax:** (303)691-5983
**Email:** office@nanonline.org
**Website:** http://www.NANonline.org
Josette G. Harris, PhD, Exec. Dir.
**Fnded:** 1975. **Mem:** 3,024. **Desc:** Clinical neuropsychologists and others interested in brain-behavior relationships. Works to preserve and advance knowledge regarding the assessment and remediation of neuropsychological disorders. Promotes the development of neuropsychology as a science and profession; develops standards of practice and training guidelines for the field; fosters communication between members; represents the professional interests of members; serves as an information resource; facilitates the exchange of information among related organizations. Offers continuing education programs; conducts research. **Pub:** *Archives of Clinical Neuropsychology,* bimonthly. Journal. *Price:* Included in membership dues; $185/year for nonmember institutions. • *Bulletin of the National Academy of Neuropsychologists,* quarterly. Bulletin. *Price:* Included in membership dues. • Membership Directory, biennial.

### ★ 14070 ★ National Ataxia Foundation (NAF)

2600 Fernbrook Ln. N, No. 119
Minneapolis, MN 55447
**Phone:** (763)553-0020　**Fax:** (763)553-0167
**Email:** naf@mail.ataxia.org
**Website:** http://www.ataxia.org
Donna Gruetzmacher, Exec. Dir.
**Fnded:** 1957. **Mem:** 2,000. **Local Groups:** 58. **Desc:** Membership is open to any individual who wishes to contribute to the eradication of ataxia (a genetic disease characterized by the degeneration of the nerves of the spinal cord and the cerebellum, causing a loss of coordination and disturbance in gait and related conditions such as peroneal muscular atrophy, hereditary spastic paraplegia, and hereditary tremor. Ataxia may be inherited as a recessive or dominant trait and may strike persons from a very early age up to and even beyond 50 years of age. Ataxia is very similar to multiple sclerosis; however, multiple sclerosis is not inherited and has a different origin.) Objectives are: to make an early diagnosis of ataxia by locating all potential victims and encouraging them to have an examination; to educate the public and the helping professions about ataxia; to initiate basic research and coordinate efforts of worldwide research centers. Emphasis is on locating and understanding the genes responsible. Provides services and information to ataxia victims and their families. **Pub:** *Generations,* quarterly. Newsletter. Includes foundation news,

calendar of events, and research updates. *Price:* Free to members and those who suffer from ataxia. • *Together - There is Hope.* Video. • Brochures. • Also publishes Together. . .(video) and brochures.

**★ 14071 ★ National Attention Deficit Disorder Association (ADDA)**
1788 Second St., Ste. 200
Highland Park, IL 60035
**Phone:** (847)432-2332          **Fax:** (847)432-5874
**Email:** mail@add.org
**Website:** http://www.add.org
Nancy Ratey, Pres.

**Fnded:** 1989. **Desc:** Seeks to: promote a greater public awareness of the multiple needs of individuals with ADD and their families; address their educational, psychological, and social needs; encourage more responsiveness with regard to ADD in the academic and health care communities. Maintains database of support groups throughout the country. **Pub:** *Addalog.* Catalog. Lists books, brochures, monographs, and other materials available for purchasing. • *Focus.* Newsletter. • Monographs. • Pamphlets. **Frmly:** (1992) Attention-Deficit Disorder Association.

**★ 14072 ★ National Brachial Plexus-Erb's Palsy Association**
PO Box 23
Larsen, WI 54947-0023
**Phone:** (920)836-3843
**Email:** erbspalsy@usa.net
**Website:** http://www.nbpepa.org/
Brenda Copeland-Moore, Contact

**Fnded:** 1995. **Mem:** 1,000. **Desc:** Serves as a resource, information, and support center for the disease Brachial Plexus-Erb's Palsy. **Pub:** *BPI News,* quarterly. Newsletter.

**★ 14073 ★ National Coalition for Research in Neurological Disorders (NCR)**
1250 24th St. NW, Ste. 300
Washington, DC 20037
**Phone:** (202)293-5453          **Fax:** (202)466-0585
**Email:** info@brainnet.org
**Website:** http://www.brainnet.org
Dominick P. Purpura, MD, Chair

**Fnded:** 1952. **Mem:** 57. **Desc:** Represents voluntary health agencies and professional societies concerned with obtaining funds for neurological research. Seeks to stimulate public information regarding the field of neurological disorders. Lobbies for increased funding for training and research in neurological disorders. **Pub:** *NCR News,* quarterly. **Frmly:** National Committee for Research in Neurological Disorders; (1988) National Committee for Research in Neruological and Communicative Disorders; (1989) National Coalition for Research in Neurological and Communicative Disorders.

**★ 14074 ★ National Disability Sports Alliance (NDSA)**
25 W Independence Way
Kingston, RI 02881-1124
**Phone:** (401)792-7130          **Fax:** (401)792-7132
**Email:** info@ndsaonline.org
**Website:** http://www.ndsaonline.org
Jerry McCole, Exec. Dir.

**Fnded:** 1986. **Mem:** 3,000. **Reg. Groups:** 30. **State Groups:** 15. **Local Groups:** 100. **Desc:** Athletes with cerebral palsy, athletic officials including coaches and administrators, health care professionals, and other interested individuals. Seeks to offer competitive athletic opportunities for athletes with cerebral palsy or traumatic brain injury and stroke survivors; provides support and training assistance to athletes with varying degrees of disability. Organizes multi-sport competitions at the local, regional, national, and international levels; maintains 8-level classification system to ensure that competition is based on the functional level of participants rather than their neurological capability. Selects athletes to represent the U.S. in the Paralym-

pic Games and other international competitions. Provides referral service to assist members in obtaining support for local sports programs; develops fundraising programs. Operates Youth Sports Program, which provides guidelines and assistance to young people with special needs who wish to learn a sport. Conducts educational clinics and seminars. Compiles statistics; maintains speakers' bureau and library. Plans to make available to members liability insurance and reduced rates on special sports equipment. **Pub:** *Update,* quarterly. Newsletter. • *USCPAA Classification and Rules Manual.* **Frmly:** (2002) United States Cerebral Palsy Athletic Association.

**★ 14075 ★ National Headache Foundation (NHF)**
428 W Saint James Pl., 2nd Fl.
Chicago, IL 60614-2750
**Phone:** (773)388-6399          **Free:** 888-NHF-5552
**Fax:** (773)525-7357
**Email:** info@headaches.org
**Website:** http://www.headaches.org
Seymore Diamond, MD, Exec. Dir.

**Fnded:** 1970. **Mem:** 20,000. **Desc:** Headache sufferers, physicians, health care professionals. Serves as an information resource to headache sufferers, their families, and the physicians who treat them. Promotes research into potential headache causes and treatments. Educates the public to the fact that headaches are a legitimate biological disease and sufferers need understanding and continuity of care. Disseminates free information on headache causes and treatments. Funds research. Operates network of local support groups. **Pub:** *About Headaches.* Pamphlet. • *The Headache Handbook.* Brochure. • *How to Talk to Your Doctor About Headaches.* Brochure. • *NHF Head Lines,* bimonthly. Newsletter. Includes information on headache causes and treatments, foundation news, book reviews, research reports, support group updates, and reader Q&A. *Price:* Included in membership dues. • Headache: A Guide to Prevention & Treatment/A Patient's Guide to Migraine Prevention & Treatment/Headache Q & A. **Frmly:** (1986) National Migraine Foundation.

**★ 14076 ★ National Multiple Sclerosis Society (NMSS)**
733 3rd Ave.
New York, NY 10017
**Phone:** (212)986-3240          **Free:** 800-FIGHT-MS
**Fax:** (212)986-7981
**Email:** info@nmss.org
**Website:** http://www.nmss.org
Michael J. Duggan, Pres.

**Fnded:** 1946. **Mem:** 470,000. **State Groups:** 93. **Desc:** Stimulates, supports, and coordinates research into the cause, treatment, and cure of multiple sclerosis; provides services for persons with MS and related diseases and their families; aids in establishing MS clinics and therapy centers. Conducts Creative Will, biennial competition for artists with MS. Maintains numerous committees including international and research and medical programs, and services. Maintains speakers' bureau; compiles statistics. **Pub:** *Inside MS,* 4/year. Magazine. Contains book reviews, research updates, legislative updates, and annual report. *Price:* Included in membership dues. **Frmly:** (1947) Association for Advancementof Research on Multiple Sclerosis.

**★ 14077 ★ National Neurofibromatosis Foundation (NNFF)**
95 Pine St., 16th Fl.
New York, NY 10005
**Phone:** (212)344-6633          **Free:** 800-323-7938
**Fax:** (212)747-0004
**Email:** nnff@nf.org
**Website:** http://www.nf.org/
Michelle Messinger, Dir. of Public Education

**Fnded:** 1978. **Mem:** 1,700. **State Groups:** 37. **Desc:** The leading resource on neurofibromatosis, a genetic disorder that causes tumors to grow along nerves throughout the body. Provides direct services to

children and adults with NF, as well as information and resources to the public and medical professionals via a toll-free number and a website. **Pub:** *Neurofibromatosis News,* quarterly. Newsletter. *Price:* Free for members.

**★ 14078 ★ National Neurotrauma Society**
c/o Linda Garcia
PO Box 143060
Gainesville, FL 32608
**Phone:** (352)271-1169          **Fax:** (352)271-3060
**Email:** lindahou@aol.com
**Website:** http://www.neurotrauma.org
Linda Garcia, Contact

**Mem:** 500. **Desc:** Conducts scientific research in neurotrauma field.

**★ 14079 ★ National Parkinson Foundation (NPF)**
1501 NW 9th Ave.
Bob Hope Parkinson's Research Center
Miami, FL 33136-1494
**Phone:** (305)547-6666          **Free:** 800-327-4545
**Fax:** (305)548-4403
**Email:** mailbox@npf.med.miami.edu
**Website:** http://www.parkinson.org
Herbert C. Zemel, Pres.

**Fnded:** 1957. **Desc:** Doctors, nurses, scientists, pharmacologists, and therapists who research, diagnose, and treat Parkinsonism. Supports basic and clinical research for Parkinsonism and related neurological disorders and provides physical, speech, and occupational therapy. NPF is associated with the University of Miami School of Medicine, and supports the National Parkinson Institute, which provides diagnosis, treatment, care, and rehabilitation. Conducts educational programs. Distributes literature to medical libraries, nurses training schools, health clinics, physicians, and patients. Sponsors regional patient self-support groups where problems are discussed and experiences are exchanged under guidance of physicians, social workers, and psychologists. Maintains offices at 122 E. 42nd St., New York, NY 10017 and 4929 Wilshire Blvd., Los Angeles, CA 90010. **Pub:** *How to Start and Run a Support Group.* • *Membership List,* periodic. • *The Parkinson Handbook.* • *Parkinson Report,* quarterly. Newsletter. Contains research reports. *Price:* Included in membership dues; Available free of charge to others upon request. • Also publishes other books and brochures.

**★ 14080 ★ National Sleep Foundation**
1522 K St., NW, Ste. 500
Washington, DC 20005
**Phone:** (202)347-3471          **Fax:** (202)347-3472
**Email:** nsf@sleepfoundation.org
**Website:** http://www.sleepfoundation.org
Richard L. Gelula, Exec. Dir.

**Fnded:** 1990. **Desc:** Works to improve the quality of life of people suffering from sleep disorders and to prevent accidents related to sleep disorders. (Sleep disorders include: insomnia, narcolepsy, sleep apnea syndrome, sudden infant death syndrome, stroke, epilepsy, and other disorders of sleep and daytime alertness.) Educates health care professionals and the public about the existance and treatment of sleep disorders. Promotes the development of patient services, community resources, and support groups for individuals affected by sleep disorders. Sponsors educational and research programs. **Pub:** *Sleepmatters.* Magazine. • Brochures.

**★ 14081 ★ National Society for Epilepsy**
Chesham Ln.
Chalfont St. Peter
Gerrards Cross SL9 0RJ, United Kingdom
**Phone:** 44 1494 601300     **Fax:** 44 1494 871927
**Email:** cathyb@epilepsynse.co.uk
**Website:** http://www.epilepsynse.org.uk

**Fnded:** 1892. **Mem:** 2,000. **Desc:** Individuals with an interest in epilepsy who wish to support epilepsy education and research. Provides assessment, treatment, rehabilitation, long term and respite care for adults with epilepsy. The education department provides support and information, produces educational resources and runs conferences and seminars. Coordinates a national network of trained volunteers offering information services.


★ **14082** ★ **National Spasmodic Dysphonia Association (NSDA)**
1 E Wacker Dr., Ste. 2430
Chicago, IL 60601-1905
**Free:** 800-795-6732          **Fax:** (312)803-0138
**Email:** nsda@dysphonia.org
**Website:** http://www.dystonia.org/
Robert O. McAlister, PhD, Exec. Dir.
**Fnded:** 1990. **Mem:** 8,200. **Nat'l Groups:** 45. **Desc:** Individuals diagnosed with spasmodic dysphonia; doctors and scientists providing treatment and conducting research on the disease; interested others. Promotes public awareness of spasmodic dysphonia and the care, welfare, and rehabilitation of those with the disease. (Spasmodic dysphonia is a neurological movement disorder affecting muscular control of the vocal cords, often resulting in an abnormally raspy, breathy, or choppy speech pattern.) Makes information on the disease available to patients, their families, and the public. Encourages research to uncover the causes and treatments of spasmodic dysphonia; offers referral information on specialists administering the botulinum toxin presently used in many cases to temporarily treat the disease. Assists in the formation of local support groups to assist patients. **Pub:** *NSDA Newsletter*, biennial. Newsletter.


★ **14083** ★ **National Spasmodic Torticollis Association (NSTA)**
9920 Talbert Ave., Ste. 233
Fountain Valley, CA 92708
**Phone:** (714)378-7837          **Free:** 800-HUR-TFUL
**Fax:** (714)378-7830
**Email:** nstamail@aol.com
**Website:** http://www.torticollis.org
Jim Ruetz, Pres.
**Fnded:** 1980. **Mem:** 3,400. **Reg. Groups:** 74. **Local Groups:** 48. **Desc:** Persons afflicted with spasmodic torticollis (ST), a syndrome in which the muscles on one side of the neck contract and pull the head to the side, sometimes pushing the chin up or down. ST usually occurs in adults and can sometimes be treated successfully with medication and physical therapy. Educates the public on ST so that persons with early symptoms know to seek proper medical help from a neurologist or neurosurgeon. Provides forum for discussion among ST sufferers and their families in order to share information and experiences and diminish feelings of alienation and self-consciousness. **Pub:** *NSTA News Magazine*, quarterly. Magazine. Includes medical advisor's column. *Price:* Included in membership dues. • *P.T. In-Home Videotape.* Video. *Price:* $21.95. • *Physicians Referral Directory*, annual. Directory. Lists neurologists who treat spasmodic torticollis. *Price:* Free. • *Relaxation/Affirmation Audiotape.* Audiotape. *Price:* $5.95. • *Series of "Helpful Hints" Letters.* • *What is NSTA?.* • Also publishes fact sheet. **Frmly:** Project S.T.


★ **14084** ★ **National Spinal Cord Injury Association (NSCIA)**
6701 Democracy Blvd., Ste. 300-9
Bethesda, MD 20817
**Phone:** (301)588-6959          **Free:** 800-962-9629
**Fax:** (301)588-9414
**Email:** nscia2@aol.com
**Website:** http://www.spinalcord.org
Marcie Roth, Exec. Dir.
**Fnded:** 1948. **Mem:** 5,000. **Local Groups:** 50. **Desc:** Seeks to inform and educate the medical and allied professions, persons with spinal cord injury or disease, their families, and the public on spinal cord injury. Carries out activities in 3 major fields: support of research toward a cure for paralysis from spinal cord injury; public and professional prevention and education programs and services; assistance to individuals

to reach their personal goals. Sponsors In Touch With Kids, a network for parents of children with spinal cord injury or disease. Conducts recreation, advocacy, support group, and peer counseling programs. Maintains placement service; offers information and referral service. referral service. **Pub:** *Options: Spinal Cord Injury and the Future.* • *Spinal Cord Injury Life*, quarterly. Journal. Provides news and articles concerning persons with spinal cord injuries caused by trauma or disease. Includes book reviews. *Price:* Included in membership dues; $40/year subscription. • Also publishes fact sheets on research, sexuality and other topics. **Frmly:** National Spinal Cord Injury Foundation; (1979) National Paraplegia Foundation.


★ **14085** ★ **National Stroke Association (NSA)**
9707 E Easter Ln.
Englewood, CO 80112-3747
**Phone:** (303)649-9299          **Free:** 800-STR-OKES
**Fax:** (303)649-1328
**Email:** info@stroke.org
**Website:** http://www.stroke.org
Patti Shwayder, Exec. Dir. /CEO
**Fnded:** 1984. **Mem:** 7,500. **State Groups:** 16. **Local Groups:** 1200. **Desc:** Stroke survivors and their families; health care professionals and institutions; the lay community. Seeks to reduce the incidence and impact of stroke by promoting research, educating the public, and providing a network for stroke survivors and concerned persons. Serves as an information referral clearinghouse on stroke; makes available educational materials on stroke prevention, treatment, rehabilitation, resocialization, and research. Offers guidance in the development of stroke support groups and clubs. Maintains speakers' bureau and Stroke Information and Referral Center; compiles statistics. Conducts educational symposiums/meetings. **Pub:** *Be Stroke Smart*, bimonthly. Magazine. *Price:* Free. • *Hope: the Stroke Recovery Guide.* Book. • *Journal of Stroke and Cerebravascular Diseases*, quarterly. Journal. *Price:* $129/year for individual; $204/year for institution. • *State Listing of Stroke Clubs*, periodic. Directory. • *Stroke: Clinical Updates*, bimonthly. Newsletter. Professional newsletter with available slides. *Price:* Free with professional membership.


**National Tay-Sachs and Allied Diseases Association (NTSAD)**
*See:* Entry 8726


★ **14086** ★ **Nationale Alzheimer Liga (NAL)**
c/o Mr. Van Daele
39 Watertorenlaan
B-1831 Mechelen, Belgium
**Email:** ntsad-boston@att.net
**Website:** http://www.ntsad.org
**Lang(s):** English, French. **Desc:** Individuals and organizations. Seeks to improve the quality of life of people with Alzheimer's disease and their families. Makes available support and services; facilitates research on Alzheimer's disease and related disorders; conducts educational programs.


**Neuro-developmental Treatment Association (NDTA)**
*See:* Entry 20161


★ **14087** ★ **Neurofibromatosis (NF)**
8855 Annapolis Rd., Ste. 110
Lanham, MD 20706-2924
**Phone:** (301)918-4600          **Free:** 800-942-6825
**Fax:** (301)918-0009
**Email:** nfinc1@aol.com
**Website:** http://www.nfinc.org
John C. Vickerman, CMP, Exec. Dir.
**Fnded:** 1988. **Reg. Groups:** 9. **Desc:** Organizations providing support for individuals with neurofibromatosis (NF) and their families, physicians, and other health care providers. (NF is a genetic neurological

disorder that can cause tumors to form on nerves and is linked to learning disabilities, hearing loss, vision impairment, epilepsy, and cancer.) Increases public awareness of NF through information dissemination; informs federal, state, and local legislators of the needs of NF families. Promotes, supports, and funds medical, clinical, educational, and sociological research that addresses the need to diagnose, treat, cure, and prevent NF. Identifies local NF support and peer counseling groups; offers referrals to medical resources and scientifically-evaluated research. Participates in networking of voluntary health organizations. **Pub:** *Neurofibromatosis Ink*, semiannual. Newsletter. Includes research summaries, reports, chapter news, and symposia information, bibliography, fundraising activities. • *Understanding Neurofibromatosis: An Introduction for Patients and Parents.* Booklets. *Price:* $3 for each multiple copy.


★ **14088** ★ **Neurofibromatosis Association of Ireland (NAI)**
Carmichael Center
North Brunswick St.
Dublin 7, Ireland
**Phone:** 353 1 8726338          **Fax:** 353 1 8735737
**Email:** nfaireland@eircom.net
**Website:** http://www.nfaireland.ie
**Fnded:** 1985. **Mem:** 280. **Lang(s):** English, Irish. **Desc:** Individuals and organizations. Seeks to improve the quality of life of people with neurofibromatosis and their families; promotes increased awareness of neurofibromatosis among health care providers and the public. Makes available support and services; conducts educational and advocacy campaigns; sponsors research.


**Neuromuscular Diseases Association of Romania**
*See:* Entry 13643


★ **14089** ★ **Neuropathy Association**
Lincoln Bldg.
60 E 42nd St., Ste. 942
New York, NY 10165
**Phone:** (212)692-0662          **Free:** 800-247-6968
**Fax:** (212)692-0668
**Email:** info@neuropahty.org
**Website:** http://www.neuropathy.org
Catherine Law, CFO
**Fnded:** 1995. **Mem:** 50,000. **Local Groups:** 200. **Desc:** Offers support to persons suffering from disorders affecting the peripheral nerves; provides patient support and education, advocates for patients' interests, promotes research into the causes and cure for peripheral neuropathies. **Pub:** *A Guide to the Peripheral Neuropathies.* Booklet. • *Exercising with Neuropathy.* Booklet. • *Explaining Peripheral Neuropathy.* Booklet. • *Neuropathy News.* Newsletter.


★ **14090** ★ **Neurosurgical Society of Australasia**
Verdun St.
Nedlands
Perth, WA 6009, Australia
**Phone:** 61 8 93463333          **Fax:** 61 8 93463824
**Website:** http://www.nsa.on.net
**Fnded:** 1940.


★ **14091** ★ **New Zealand Pain Society (NZPS)**
PO Box 5303
Wellington, New Zealand
**Phone:** 64 4 4995957          **Fax:** 64 4 4995953
**Email:** info@nzps.org.nz
**Website:** http://www.nzps.org.nz
**Fnded:** 1983. **Mem:** 250. **Lang(s):** English. **Desc:** Health professionals and scientists interested in pain research and management. Works to improve the management of pain. Encourages research into pain mechanisms and pain syndromes; recommends the adoption of a uniform classification, nomenclature, and

definition of pain and pain syndromes; advises national and regional agencies on standards relating to the use of drugs, appliances, and procedures in the therapy of pain; promotes education and training in pain management; facilitates information dissemination. Conducts lectures and workshops. Formerly a section of the Australasian Pain Society. **Pub:** *Directory*, annual. Directory. • *New Zealand Pain Society Newsletter*, quarterly. Newsletter.

### ★ 14092 ★ North American Skull Base Society (NASBS)

c/o Lawrence H. Leong
4815 Rugby Ave., Ste. 203
Bethesda, MD 20814
**Phone:** (301)654-6802          **Fax:** (301)718-8692
**Email:** info@nasbs.org
**Website:** http://www.nabss.org
Lawrence H. Leong, Exec. Dir.

**Fnded:** 1989. **Mem:** 500. **Desc:** Neurosurgeons, otolaryngologists, and others with an interest in diseases associated with the skull base. Promotes advancement of medical practice relating to diseases of the skull base. Conducts continuing professional education programs. **Pub:** *Skull Base*, quarterly. Journal.

### ★ 14093 ★ North American Spine Society (NASS)

22 Calendar Ct., 2nd Fl.
La Grange, IL 60525
**Phone:** (708)588-8080          **Free:** 877-SPI-NEDR
**Fax:** (708)588-1080
**Email:** info@spine.org
**Website:** http://www.spine.org
Eric J. Muehlbauer, Exec. Dir.

**Fnded:** 1985. **Mem:** 3,100. **Desc:** Organization of physicians, osteopaths, orthopedists, neurosurgeons, physiatrists, radiologists, and other professionals that advances quality spine care through education, research and advocacy. Works to improve the quality of scientific practice in spinal disorders; exchange ideas and disseminate scientific information about clinical techniques; investigate and propagate methods by which malfunction of the spine can be corrected. Makes inquiries into practice characteristics, language usage and terminology, and treatment methods. **Pub:** *Common Coding Scenarios for Comprehensive Spine Care*, annual. Book. • *Common Cuding Scenarios for Spine Procedures and Injection Techniques*, annual. Book. *Price:* Available for purchase. • *Contemporary Concepts in Spine Care*. Paper. • *The Spine Journal*, bimonthly. Journal. • *Spine Line*, bimonthly. Magazine. Contains news on association activities, peer-reviewed research topics.

### ★ 14094 ★ Norwegian Epilepsy Association (NEA) (Norsk Epilepsiforbund — NEF)

Storgaten 39
N-0192 Oslo, Norway
**Phone:** 47 22 206021          **Fax:** 47 23353101
**Email:** nef@epilepsi.no

**Fnded:** 1974. **Mem:** 5,300. **Reg. Groups:** 7. **Local Groups:** 39. **Lang(s):** English, Norwegian. **Desc:** Disseminates information to individuals with epilepsy and their families, health care centers, hospitals, and schools. Collaborates with related groups. **Pub:** *The Epilepsy Handbook*. Handbook. • *Epilepsy News*, quarterly. Magazine. Also publishes brochures (in Norwegian).

### ★ 14095 ★ Norwegian Multiple Sclerosis Society (NMSS) (Multipel Sklerose Forbundet i Norge — MSFN)

Sorkedalsveien 3
N-0369 Oslo, Norway
**Phone:** 47 22 604960          **Fax:** 47 22 567695
**Email:** msfnorge@c2i.net
**Website:** http://www.msf.no

**Fnded:** 1966. **Mem:** 4,300. **Reg. Groups:** 37. **Lang(s):** English. **Desc:** Promotes interest in multiple sclerosis research among medical and scientific communities and the public in Norway. Facilitates exchange of information among members. **Pub:** *MS-bladet*, 5/year. Magazine. • *MS - En veiledning for helsepersonell*. Books. • Pamphlets.

### ★ 14096 ★ Norwegian Neuroscience Society (NNS)

PO Box 83
Grefsen
N-0409 Oslo, Norway
**Website:** http://folk.uio.no/terjesa/nns/

**Fnded:** 1998. **Desc:** Promotes information exchange between European neuroscientists; provides educational courses.

### ★ 14097 ★ Norwegian Parkinson Association (NPA) (Norges Parkinsonforbund — NPF)

Schweigaardsgt 34, F.2
N-0191 Oslo, Norway
**Phone:** 47 22 175861          **Fax:** 47 22 175862
**Email:** parkinson@ai.net
**Website:** http://www.parkinson.no

**Fnded:** 1984. **Mem:** 4,000. **Nat'l Groups:** 1. **Reg. Groups:** 17. **Local Groups:** 15. **Lang(s):** English. **Desc:** Parkinson patients and their relatives. Teaches patients about their disease and how to deal with the related problems. Represents members' interests in matters of social and health politics. Supports research efforts; conducts educational seminars. Offers lectures. **Pub:** *Parkinsonposten*, quarterly. Newsletter.

### ★ 14098 ★ Pain Society

9 Bedford Sq.
London WC1B 3RE, United Kingdom
**Phone:** 44 20 76318870          **Fax:** 44 20 73232015
**Email:** info@painsociety.org
**Website:** http://www.painsociety.org

**Fnded:** 1967. **Mem:** 1,400. **Desc:** Professional body representing healthcare professionals working in chronic and acute pain. Aims to relieve the suffering of pain by the promotion of education, training and research. Supplies general information and a list of pain clinics by county. **Pub:** *Pain Society Newsletter*, quarterly. Newsletter.

### ★ 14099 ★ Pan-African Association of Neurological Sciences (PAANS) (Association Pan-Africaine des Sciences Neurologiques — PAANS)

PO Box 20413
Nairobi, Kenya
**Phone:** 254 2 722487          **Fax:** 254 2 725776
**Email:** ruberti@africaonline.co.ke
**Website:** http://www.paans.nu.ac.za/

**Fnded:** 1972. **Mem:** 250. **Lang(s):** English, French. **Desc:** African neurologists specializing in neurosurgery, neuroradiology, neuropathology, neurophysiology, neurobiochemistry, and other branches of neuroscience; non-African neurologists maintaining connections with Africa. Furthers neurological sciences and encourages the exchange of ideas and information among neurologists in Africa and worldwide. Strives to acquaint the public and interested laymen with current developments in neuroscience. Conducts epidemiological research. **Pub:** *African Journal of Neurological Sciences*, semiannual. Journal. Contains information on neurology, neurosurgery, and neurosciencec. • *Pan African Association of Neurological Sciences Rules*.

### ★ 14100 ★ Parkinson Foundation of Canada (PFC)

4211 Yonge St., Ste. 316
Toronto, ON, Canada M2P 2A9
**Phone:** (416)227-9700          **Free:** 800-565-3000
**Fax:** (416)227-9600
**Email:** general.info@parkinson.ca
**Website:** http://www.parkinson.ca

**Fnded:** 1965. **Mem:** 16,000. **Reg. Groups:** 5. **Local Groups:** 100. **Lang(s):** English, French. **Desc:** Provides services to people with Parkinson's or related disorders, their families, and interested health care professionals. Seeks to publicize the nature and availability of treatment and assistance programs available to people with Parkinson's. Promotes research into the cause and cure of Parkinson's. Conducts fundraising activities; maintains support groups; makes available referral services. Sponsors research and educational programs. **Pub:** *Network*, quarterly. Newsletter. Current information on Parkinson's and The Parkinson Foundation of Canada.

### ★ 14101 ★ Parkinson's Disease Society of the United Kingdom

215 Vauxhall Bridge Rd.
London SV1W 1EJ, United Kingdom
**Phone:** 44 20 79318080          **Fax:** 44 20 72339908
**Email:** enquiries@parkinsons.org.uk
**Website:** http://www.parkinsons.org.uk

**Fnded:** 1969. **Mem:** 26,000. **Reg. Groups:** 250. **Local Groups:** 250. **Desc:** Promotes awareness of Parkinson's disease.

### ★ 14102 ★ Polish Alzheimer's Association (PAA)

Ul. Hoza 54/1
PL-00-682 Warsaw, Poland
**Phone:** 48 22 6221122          **Fax:** 48 22 6221122
**Email:** alzheimer_pl@hotmail.com
**Website:** http://www.alzheimer.pl

**Fnded:** 1992. **Mem:** 500. **Nat'l Groups:** 1. **Local Groups:** 24. **Lang(s):** English, Polish. **Desc:** Individuals and organizations. Seeks to improve the quality of life of people with Alzheimer's disease and their families. Makes available support and services; facilitates research on Alzheimer's disease and related disorders; conducts educational programs. **Pub:** *Blizej Alzheimera*, quarterly. Newsletter. Contains information for the caregiver.

### ★ 14103 ★ Polish Association of People Suffering From Epilepsy (PAPSE)

Fabryczna Str. 57
PL-15-482 Bialystok, Poland
**Phone:** 48 85 6754420          **Fax:** 48 85 6754420
**Email:** epi99@2n.pl
**Website:** http://www.padaczka.bialystok.org.pl

**Fnded:** 1985. **Mem:** 400,000. **Reg. Groups:** 6. **Lang(s):** English, Polish. **Desc:** Nongovernmental organizations, foundations, funds, and individuals with an interest in people with epilepsy. Promotes an improved quality of life for people with epilepsy. Represents the rights and interests of people with epilepsy before government agencies; makes available international exchange program; identifies and seeks to acquire and distribute emerging technologies and equipment for the diagnosis and treatment of epilepsy. **Pub:** *Padaezki - Pytania I Odpowidzi*. Book.

### ★ 14104 ★ Reflex Sympathetic Dystrophy Association of America

PO Box 502
Milford, CT 06460
**Phone:** (203)877-3790          **Free:** 877-662-7737
**Fax:** (203)882-8362
**Email:** jwbroatch@aol.com
**Website:** http://www.rsds.org
James Broaich, MSW, Exec. Dir.

**Fnded:** 1984. **Mem:** 4,500. **Local Groups:** 100. **Desc:** People with Reflex Sympathetic Dystrophy Syndrome, also known as Complex Regional Pain Syndrome Type I and Type II; health care professionals treating RSDS patients. (RSDS is a disorder of the autonomic nervous system whose onset is usually preceded by a minor trauma such as a muscle sprain; symptoms of RSDS include severe pain, loss of muscle motion and use, swelling, skin and nail changes, and softening of the bones in affected areas.) Promotes increased awareness of RSDS among health care professionals and the public;

conducts media campaigns; maintains national network of physicians involved in RSDS treatment and research. Encourages and supports RSDS research; has a national data bank for the coordination of RSDS research and treatment information. Aids in the formation of support groups for people with RSDS; develops in-service programs and seminars for use at hospitals and educational institutions. Makes available referral services. Conducts educational programs; maintains speakers' bureau; compiles statistics, funds research, has published clinical practice guidelines for diagnosis, treatment, and management of RSDS/CRPS. **Pub:** *Clinical Practice Guidelines for Diagnosis, Treatment, and Management of RSD/CRPS.* • *RSDSA Review*, quarterly. Newsletter. *Price:* Included in membership dues. • Also publishes fact sheets. **Frmly:** (1998) Reflex Sympathetic Dystrophy Association.

### ★ 14105 ★ Research Center Against Meningitis and Schistosomiasis (Centre de Recherches sur les Meningites et les Schistosomiases)

Boite Postale 10887
Niamey, Niger
**Phone:** 227 752045 **Fax:** 227 753180
**Email:** cermes@ird.ne
**Website:** http://www.mpl.ird.fr/cermes
**Fnded:** 1978. **Lang(s):** English, French. **Desc:** Health care professionals and researchers. Promotes development of improved diagnostic techniques and treatments for meningitis and schistosomiasis. Conducts research; gathers and disseminates information; makes available health services.

### ★ 14106 ★ Scandinavian Neurological Association (SNA) (Nordisk Neurologisk Forening — NNF)

Department of Neurology
University of Helsinki
FIN-00290 Helsinki, Finland
**Phone:** 358 9 4712261 **Fax:** 358 9 4714009
**Email:** jorma.palo@helsinki.fi
**Fnded:** 1922. **Mem:** 5. **Lang(s):** Danish, English, Finnish, Icelandic, Norwegian, Swedish. **Desc:** Scandinavian national societies representing 900 neurologists and other specialists with an interest in neuroscience. Promotes neurological research and cooperation among Scandinavian neurologists. Provides educational counseling. **Pub:** *Congress Abstracts*, biennial. Proceedings.

### ★ 14107 ★ Scandinavian Neurosurgical Society (SNS) (Nordisk Neurokirurgisk Forening — NNF)

Institute of Clinical Neuroscience
Department of Neurosurgery
Karolinska Hospital
S-171 76 Stockholm, Sweden
**Phone:** 46 8 51770000 **Fax:** 46 31 416719
**Email:** tiitmathiesen@neuro.ks.se
**Fnded:** 1945. **Mem:** 160. **Lang(s):** English. **Desc:** Scandinavian neurosurgeons and neurosurgical residents; practicing neurosurgeons outside of Scandinavia. Works to facilitate collaboration among Scandinavian neurosurgeons.

### Scientific Society of Psychosomatic Medicine
*See:* Entry 12632

### ★ 14108 ★ Scottish Motor Neurone Disease Association

76 Firhill Rd.
Glasgow G20 7BA, United Kingdom
**Phone:** 44 141 9451077 **Fax:** 44 141 9452578
**Email:** info@scotmnd.sol.co.uk
**Website:** http://www.scotmnd.org.uk
**Fnded:** 1981. **Mem:** 500. **Lang(s):** English. **Desc:** Promotes interest in motor neurone disease (MND) research among medical and scientific communities

and the public in Scotland. Offers care and support services to MND patients in Scotland, and their families. Disseminates information about the disease. **Pub:** *Aware*, quarterly. Newsletter.

### ★ 14109 ★ Shingles Support Society

c/o Marian Nicholson, Dir.
41 North Rd.
London N7 9DP, United Kingdom
**Phone:** 44 20 76079661
**Email:** marian@herpes.org.uk
**Website:** http://www.herpes.org.uk
**Fnded:** 1985. **Lang(s):** English. **Desc:** Individuals suffering from post-herpetic neuralgia and their families. Offers advice on self-help for post-herpetic neuralgia which can follow shingles. Provides information for primary care doctors by a consultant neurologist regarding drug treatment with dosage information.

### ★ 14110 ★ Sleep Research Society (SRS)

6301 Bandel Rd., Ste. 101
Rochester, MN 55901
**Phone:** (507)287-0846 **Fax:** (507)287-6006
**Email:** lbrink@aasmnet.org
**Website:** http://www.sleepresearchsociety.org
Dr. David Dinges, Pres.
**Fnded:** 1961. **Mem:** 850. **Desc:** Physiologists, psychologists, and physicians with research interests in the study of sleep. Disseminates scientific papers on the physiological and psychological aspects of sleep. Facilitates communication among research workers in this field, but does not sponsor research investigations on its own. **Pub:** *Sleep*, 9/year. Journal. Includes book reviews and bibliography of recent literature. *Price:* $129/year for nonmembers, US funds; $185/year to institutions, US funds; $159/year for nonmembers - foreign. • *Sleep Research Society–Sleep Research*, annual. Monograph. Series containing author and keyword-in-context index. *Price:* $220/year to institutions - foreign; Included in membership dues. **Frmly:** (1983) Association for the Psychophysiological Study of Sleep.

### ★ 14111 ★ Slovak Society of Neurology

c/o Neurological Clinic
Hospital Ruzinov
Ruzinovska 6
SK-826 06 Bratislava, Slovakia
**Phone:** 42 7 43333148 **Fax:** 42 7 43336433
**Email:** lisy@ivzba.sk
**Fnded:** 1953. **Mem:** 652. **Lang(s):** English, Slovak. **Desc:** Neurologists. Works to improve the diagnostics and treatment neurological disease and to advance the professional standing of members. Represents members' interests. **Pub:** *Spravodaj Slovenskej neurologickej spoloonosti*, quarterly.

### ★ 14112 ★ Sociedad Argentina de Ciencias Neurologicas, Psiquitricas y Neuroquirzrgicas

Santa Fe 1171
1059 Buenos Aires, Argentina
**Phone:** 54 1 411633
**Fnded:** 1920.

### Society for Behavioral Neuroendocrinology (SBN)
*See:* Entry 8734

### ★ 14113 ★ Society of Neurological Surgeons (SNS)

200 1st St. SW
Rochester, MN 55905
**Phone:** (507)284-2254 **Fax:** (507)284-5206
**Email:** ras5@mailhub.cc.colmbia.edu
**Website:** http://www.societyns.org
David Piepgras, MD, Sec.
**Fnded:** 1920. **Mem:** 344. **Desc:** Neurological surgeons interested in and contributing to education.

### Society of Neurosurgical Anesthesia and Critical Care (SNACC)
*See:* Entry 4471

### ★ 14114 ★ Society for Progressive Supranuclear Palsy (SPSP)

1838 Greene Tree Rd.
Baltimore, MD 21208
**Phone:** (410)486-3330 **Free:** 800-457-4777
**Fax:** (410)486-4283
**Email:** epkatz@psp.org
**Website:** http://www.psp.org
Ellen Katz, Dir.
**Fnded:** 1990. **Mem:** 19,000. **Nat'l Groups:** 1. **Reg. Groups:** 75. **Desc:** Works to provide help and support to persons with progressive supranuclear palsy (PSP), a degenerative brain disorder related to Parkinson's Disease. Sponsors medical research; educates physicians, persons with PSP and their families on the disease and care; provides advocacy and support, support groups, symposiums and videos. **Pub:** *The PSP Advocate*, quarterly. Newsletter.

### Society for Research into Hydrocephalus and Spina Bifida (SRHSB)
*See:* Entry 4895

### ★ 14115 ★ Spanish AIS Association (ADELA) (Association Espanola de ELA)

Hierbabuena No. 12
E-28039 Madrid, Spain
**Phone:** 34 902 142142 **Fax:** 34 902 118369
**Email:** adela@readysoft.es
**Website:** http://advernet.es/adela
**Fnded:** 1990. **Mem:** 1,500. **Nat'l Groups:** 1. **State Groups:** 10. **Local Groups:** 20. **Lang(s):** Spanish. **Desc:** Promotes interest in amyotrophic lateral sclerosis or ALS (also called Lou Gehrig's disease) research among medical and scientific communities and the public in Spain. Offers support services to ALS sufferers and their families. Disseminates information about the disease. **Pub:** *Adela Informa*, quarterly. Bulletin. Contains general information about ALS. • *Adela Informa, Suplemento Cientifico*.

### ★ 14116 ★ Spinal Cord Society (SCS)

19051 County Hwy. 1
Fergus Falls, MN 56537-7609
**Phone:** (218)739-5252 **Fax:** (218)739-5262
**Website:** http://members.aol.com/scsweb/
Dr. Chase E. Carson, Pres.
**Fnded:** 1978. **Mem:** 9,000. **Local Groups:** 170. **Desc:** Spinal cord injury victims and their friends and families; physicians, nurses, physical and rehabilitation therapists, and other medical professionals. Purposes are to promote research and increase public awareness concerning the potential for a cure of paralysis due to spinal cord injury. Focuses on the cure rather than rehabilitation for paralysis due to spinal injury. Promotes funding of reversal-oriented pure and applied medical research; encourages establishment of spinal injury centers in conjunction with existing hospitals and medical centers; maintains data bank of chronic spinal cord injury case histories, continuously monitored and upgraded for improving treatment, guiding research, and screening patients for referral to other physician s or to a spinal injury center. Through concentration on research, data, and treatment, seeks to provide a base of information, statistical analysis, and experience, with accelerated progress and minimal duplication of effort. Maintains medical center in Minneapolis, MN that applies state-of-art treatment to paralysis victims. **Pub:** *Spinal Cord Society Newsletter*, monthly. Newsletter. Includes convention news, letters, and information on services. *Price:* $30/year.

### ★ 14117 ★ Spinal Injuries Action Association (SIAA)

National Rehabilitation Hospital
Rochestown Ave.
Dun Laoghaire, Dublin, Ireland
**Phone:** 353 1 2854777      **Fax:** 353 1 2350955
**Email:** siaairl@eircom.net

**Fnded:** 1993. **Mem:** 1,200. **Nat'l Groups:** 1. **Lang(s):** English, Irish. **Desc:** Individuals and organizations. Seeks to improve the quality of life of people with spinal injuries and their families. Makes available support and services; conducts educational and advocacy campaigns. **Pub:** *Spinal News*, quarterly. Newsletter.

### ★ 14118 ★ Spinal Injuries Association (SIA)

76 St. James's Ln.
London N1O 3DF, United Kingdom
**Phone:** 44 181 4442121      **Fax:** 44 181 4443761
**Email:** sia@spinal.co.uk
**Website:** http://www.spinal.co.uk

**Fnded:** 1974. **Mem:** 6,500. **Local Groups:** 10. **Lang(s):** English. **Desc:** National organisation for individuals with spinal cord injuries. Provides assistance through: an information service that answers member queries on all aspects of daily living including specialist holiday and travel information; a personal assistance service which provides short term, emergency cover; a solicitors referral scheme, a counseling service; publications and bi-monthly newsletter. **Pub:** *Sexuality Booklets*. Booklets. Covers sexuality, including heterosexual men, heterosexual women, gay men, and lesbians. • *Spinal Cord Injuries: Guidance for General Practitioners*.

### ★ 14119 ★ Stichting ALS Onderzoekfonds

Joos van Clevelaan 8
NL-3723 PG Bilthoven, Netherlands
**Phone:** 31 30 2533591      **Fax:** 31 30 2533665
**Email:** etrietsch@ktu.nl

**Fnded:** 1981. **Desc:** Individuals interested in amyotropic lateral sclerosis or ALS (also known as Lou Gehrig's Disease). Works to: heighten public awareness and understanding of the disease; encourage research among medical and scientific communities. Sponsors researchers.

### ★ 14120 ★ Stroke Clubs, International (SCI)

805 12th St.
Galveston, TX 77550
**Phone:** (409)762-1022
**Email:** strokeclub@aol.com
Ellis Williamson, CPA, Pres.

**Fnded:** 1968. **Mem:** 12,000. **Desc:** Active members are stroke victims; associate members are individuals interested in the problems of stroke victims. To unite stroke victims for the purpose of aiding each other; to instruct them and their families regarding the nature of stroke and the means for overcoming the resulting handicaps; to aid them in finding employment; and to give the stroke victim hope and encouragement. At monthly meetings, qualified speakers discuss the medical aspects of strokes and member stroke victims discuss their progress and problems. Maintains list of over 900 clubs throughout the U.S. **Pub:** *Stroke Club International Bulletin*, annual. Bulletin. Includes book and cassette recommendations. **Frmly:** (1973) The Stroke Club; (1978) Stroke Club of America.

### ★ 14121 ★ Sturge-Weber Foundation (SWF)

PO Box 418
Mount Freedom, NJ 07970-0418
**Phone:** (973)895-4445      **Free:** 800-627-5482
**Fax:** (973)895-4846
**Email:** swf@sturge-weber.com
**Website:** http://www.sturge-weber.com
Karen L. Ball, CEO

**Fnded:** 1986. **Mem:** 1,500. **Reg. Groups:** 21. **Desc:** Persons with Sturge-Weber syndrome and their families; concerned professionals and supporters. Serves as an information clearinghouse on Sturge-Weber syndrome, port-wine stains, and Klippel-Trenaunay Weber syndrome. (Sturge-Weber syndrome is a congenital neurological disorder characterized by facial port-wine stains, seizures, glaucoma, and loss of motor control, accompanied in rare cases by internal organ irregularities.) Disseminates information; offers support to afflicted persons. Maintains speakers' bureau; compiles statistics. Funds research. **Pub:** *Branching Out Newsletter*, quarterly. Newsletter. *Price:* $30/year; $40/year outside U.S. • Brochures.

### ★ 14122 ★ Swedish Association of Neurologically Disabled (Neurologiskt Handikappades Riksforbund — NHR)

Box 3284
S-103 65 Stockholm, Sweden
**Phone:** 46 8 6777010      **Fax:** 46 8 241315
**Email:** nhr@nhr.se
**Website:** http://www.nhr.se

**Fnded:** 1957. **Mem:** 15,500. **Reg. Groups:** 26. **Local Groups:** 90. **Desc:** Promotes the interests of disabled individuals affected by neurological diseases living in Sweden. Works to offer support services. **Pub:** *Handikapp-Reflex*, bimonthly.

### Taiwan Motor Neuron Disease Association

*See:* Entry 13670

### ★ 14123 ★ Tourette Syndrome Association (TSA)

42-40 Bell Blvd.
Bayside, NY 11361-2820
**Phone:** (718)224-2999      **Fax:** (718)279-9596
**Email:** ts@tsa-usa.com
**Website:** http://www.tsa-usa.org/
Fred Cook, VP

**Fnded:** 1972. **Mem:** 30,000. **Reg. Groups:** 5. **State Groups:** 50. **Local Groups:** 300. **Desc:** People with Tourette Syndrome (TS) and their families and friends; physicians, nurses, teachers, psychologists, social workers, and other professionals; organizations such as mental health agencies. (TS is characterized by involuntary muscular movements and utterances of sounds or words, and is often undiagnosed or misdiagnosed.) Develops and disseminates educational materials to families, professionals, and agencies involved in health care, education, and governments. Schedules meetings and seminars for professionals and families to explore the latest information on TS. Stimulates support for research into the nature and causes of the disorder. Apprises members of rights, services, and benefits provided by the government and other organizations. Provides lists of doctors experienced in treating the disorder. Operates support groups and other services to help persons with TS and their families. Maintains sources for advocacy referral services in the areas of education, employment, and housing. **Pub:** *Leadership Bulletins*, 4/year. Bulletin. *Price:* Free. • *Medical Letter: Summary of the Recent Literature*, annual. • *Tourette Syndrome Association Newsletter*, quarterly. Newsletter. Includes book reviews. *Price:* Included in membership dues. **Frmly:** Gilles de la Tourette Syndrome Association.

### ★ 14124 ★ Tourette Syndrome (UK) Association

c/o Mr. Roy Hilliard
PO Box 26149
Dunfermline KY12 9WT, United Kingdom
**Phone:** 44 1892669151      **Fax:** 44 1892669151
**Email:** enquiries@tha.org.uk

**Fnded:** 1981. **Mem:** 995. **Desc:** Aims to provide relief to people suffering from the neurological disorder known as gilles de la tourette syndrome.

### Toxoplasmosis Trust (TTT)

*See:* Entry 5768

### ★ 14125 ★ Trigeminal Neuralgia Association (TNA)

2801 SW Archer Rd., Ste. C
Gainesville, FL 32608
**Phone:** (352)376-9955      **Fax:** (352)376-8688
**Email:** tnnational@tna-support.org
**Website:** http://www.tna-support.org
Claire W. Patterson, Pres.

**Fnded:** 1990. **Mem:** 20,000. **Nat'l Groups:** 3. **Local Groups:** 50. **Desc:** Individuals with trigeminal neuralgia, a neurological disorder characterized by sudden attacks of pain along the distribution of one or more branches of the trigeminal nerve in the face and head. Works to increase public and professional awareness and understanding of the disorder. Provides a forum for discussion among individuals with trigeminal neuralgia in order to share information and experiences and offer support to patients and their families. Offers physician referrals. Conducts educational programs. **Pub:** *Striking Back.* Book. Comprehensive guide for the layperson about TN. *Price:* $14 plus shipping. • *TNAlert*, quarterly. Newsletter. *Price:* Free. • *Trigeminal Neuralgia - An Overview for Patients and Their Families*.

### ★ 14126 ★ Turkish Neuroscience Society

Ege University School of Medicine
Department of Physiology
TR-35100 Ismir, Turkey
**Phone:** 90 232 3883868      **Fax:** 90 232 3746597
**Email:** nhariri@alpha.med.ege.edu.tr
**Website:** http://www.med.ege.edu.tr/%7Etns/

**Desc:** Promotes research and study in the field of Neuroscience. Conducts educational programs.

### ★ 14127 ★ United Cerebral Palsy Associations (UCP)

1660 L St. NW, Ste. 700
Washington, DC 20036
**Phone:** (202)776-0406      **Free:** 800-USA-5UCP
**Fax:** (202)776-0414
**Email:** national@ucp.org
**Website:** http://www.ucp.org
Kristen A. Nyrop, Exec. Dir.

**Fnded:** 1948. **Mem:** 111. **Desc:** Voluntary national federation of state and local affiliates aiding persons with cerebral palsy and other disabilities, and their families. Goals are to prevent cerebral palsy, minimize its effects, and improve the quality of life for persons with cerebral palsy and other disabilities, and their families. Supports research and traineeships for medical and allied personnel; sponsors professional and public education in the prevention and management of cerebral palsy; cooperates with governmental and other agencies concerned with the welfare of persons with disabilities; acts as an advocate on the federal, state, and local levels for the civil rights of people with cerebral palsy and other disabilities, and their families. Establishes standards and promotes national accreditation of UCP affiliates; undertakes demonstration projects to establish models of exemplary community services for persons with cerebral palsy and other disabilities. Services provided by local and state affiliates include: medical, therapeutic, and social services for people with cerebral palsy and individuals with similar service needs; career development training; special education programs; recreational opportunities for children and adults; early intervention and assistive technology programs; family counseling services for parents of children with disabilities; personal assistance services; accessible and supported housing facilities where people with disabilities may live independently. **Pub:** *Family Support Bulletin*, quarterly. Bulletin. *Price:* Free. • *The Networker*, quarterly. *Price:* $12. • *Washington Watch*, biweekly. Newsletter. Electronic Newsletter. • *Word from Washington*, bimonthly. Newsletter. Covers federal legislation, programs, and policy affecting persons with developmental disabilities. *Price:* $55/year; $25 for persons with disabilities or their families. **Frmly:** (1949) National Foundation for Cerebral Palsy.

★ **14128** ★ **United Cerebral Palsy Research and Educational Foundation (UCPREF)**
1660 L St. NW, Ste. 700
Washington, DC 20036-5602
**Phone:** (202)776-0406     **Free:** 800-USA-5UCP
**Fax:** (202)776-0414
**Email:** national@ucp.org
**Website:** http://www.ucp.org
Murray Goldstein, DO, Med. Dir.
**Fnded:** 1955. **Desc:** Sponsors research directly related to the prevention of cerebral palsy and to improvement in the quality of life of persons with cerebral palsy and related developmental disorders. **Pub:** *Research Fact Sheets*, monthly. • Also publishes medical directors' reports and a foundation brochure.

★ **14129** ★ **United Leukodystrophy Foundation (ULF)**
2304 Highland Dr.
Sycamore, IL 60178
**Phone:** (815)895-3211     **Free:** 800-728-5483
**Fax:** (815)895-2432
**Email:** ulf@tbcnet.com
**Website:** http://www.ulf.org
Ron Brazeal, Exec. Dir.
**Fnded:** 1982. **Mem:** 3,000. **Desc:** Leukodystrophy patients, their families, and medical care professionals. (Leukodystrophy refers to a group of disorders which affect the brain, spinal cord, and peripheral nerves by damaging the insulating sheath around nerve strands, interfering with the flow of electrical impulses.) Provides information on leukodystrophy to patients, their families, and the general public; assists in identifying sources of medical care, social services, and counseling; coordinates a communication network among affected families. Promotes and supports research into the causes, treatment, and prevention of white matter disorders. Coordinates cooperation between donor and government agencies, scientific programs, and the private sector. Conducts educational and research programs. Offers second opinion program for those with undiagnosed white matter disorders. **Pub:** *The Facts About Leukodystrophy.* Brochures. • *ULF News*, quarterly. Newsletter. *Price:* Included in membership dues. • *What to Expect When the Diagnosis is a Neurodegenerative Disease.* Booklet.

★ **14130** ★ **United Parkinson Foundation**
833 W Washington Blvd.
Chicago, IL 60607
**Phone:** (312)733-1893     **Fax:** (312)664-2344
**Desc:** Provides supportive services to patients with Parkinson's disease and their families; funds research to find a cure for this progressive, neurological condition. **Pub:** *The Patient Experience.* • Newsletter, quarterly.

★ **14131** ★ **Vereniging Spierziekten Nederland**
Lt. Gen. van Heutszlaan 6
NL-3743 JN Baarn, Netherlands
**Phone:** 31 35 5480480     **Fax:** 31 35 5480499
**Email:** vsn@vsn.nl
**Website:** http://www.vsn.nl
**Fnded:** 1967. **Mem:** 8,500. **Desc:** Works as a support group for individuals suffering from neuromuscular diseases, among others amyotrophic lateral sclerosis or ALS (also known as Lou Gehrig's Disease) and muscular dystrophy (e.g., Duchenne Musc. Dyst.) in the Netherlands. Strives to: heighten public awareness and understanding of the diseases; encourage research among medical and scientific communities; and improve the rehabilitation and professional care for the patients.

★ **14132** ★ **World Alliance of Neuromuscular Disorder Associations (WANDA)**
GPO Box 414
Adelaide, SA 5001, Australia
**Phone:** 61 8 82345266     **Fax:** 61 8 82345866
**Email:** info@mdasa.org.au
**Website:** http://www.w-a-n-d-a.org
**Fnded:** 1990.

★ **14133** ★ **World Federation of Neurology (WFN)**
12 Chandos St.
London W1G 9DR, United Kingdom
**Phone:** 44 207 3234011     **Fax:** 44 207 3234012
**Email:** wfnlondon@aol.com
**Website:** http://www.wfneurology.org/wfn/
**Fnded:** 1955. **Mem:** 23,000. **Nat'l Groups:** 86. **Reg. Groups:** 6. **Lang(s):** English. **Desc:** Neurologists and neuroscientists dedicated to improving the care of neurological patients and to preventing diseases of the nervous system. Disseminates information in the field of neurology. Organizes research groups on disease topics; compiles statistics. Maintains speakers' bureau. Conducts educational and research programs. **Pub:** *Journal of Neurological Sciences*, bimonthly. Contains research papers. • *World Neurology*, quarterly.

**World Federation of Neurosurgical Societies (WFNS)**
*See:* Entry 19611

**World Society for Stereotactic and Functional Neurosurgery (WSSFN)**
*See:* Entry 19612

★ **14134** ★ **World Society for Stereotactic and Functional Neurosurgery (WSSFN)**
59, bd Pinel
F-69003 Lyon, France
**Phone:** 33 4 72118901     **Fax:** 33 4 72357365
**Email:** marc.sindou@chu-lyon.fr
**Website:** http://www.wssfn.org
**Fnded:** 1963.

**Yugoslav MND Association**
*See:* Entry 13676

# Research Centers

★ **14135** ★ **ALS Forbes Norris Research Center**
2324 Sacramento St., Ste. 150
San Francisco, CA 94115
**Phone:** (415)923-3604     **Fax:** (415)673-5184
**Email:** zsmndyu@hotmail.com
Robert G. Miller, MD, Contact
**Activities/Fields:** Neuromuscular diseases, including Amyotrophic Lateral Sclerosis (Lou Gehrig's Disease).

**Alzheimer Treatment Research Center**
*See:* Entry 3042

★ **14136** ★ **American Brain Tumor Association**
2720 River Rd., Ste. 146
Des Plaines, IL 60018
**Phone:** (847)827-9910     **Free:** 800-886-2282
**Fax:** (847)827-9918
**Email:** info@abta.org
**Website:** http://www.abta.org
Naomi Berkowitz, Exec. Dir.

**Activities/Fields:** Elimination of brain tumors and meeting the needs of brain tumor patients and their families. **Pub:** *The Message Line Newsletter*, 3/year.

★ **14137** ★ **American Headache Society (AHS)**
19 Mantua Rd.
Mount Royal, NJ 08061
**Phone:** (856)423-0043     **Fax:** (856)423-0082
**Email:** ahshq@talley.com
**Website:** http://www.ahsnet.org
Linda McGillicuddy, Contact

**Activities/Fields:** Headache and head pain. **Pub:** *Headache - The Journal of Head and Face Pain*, 10/year. **Frmly:** American Association for the Study of Headache.

★ **14138** ★ **Andrews-Reiter Epilepsy Research Program**
1103 Sonoma Ave.
Santa Rosa, CA 95405-4517
**Phone:** (707)578-8985     **Fax:** (707)528-1086
**Email:** djandrews@neteze.com
**Website:** http://andrewsreiter.com
Donna J. Andrews, PhD, Dir.

**Activities/Fields:** Behavioral approach to self-control of seizures; adjunctive therapy and medications. **Pub:** *Books, papers.*

★ **14139** ★ **Arthur M. Fishberg Research Center in Neurobiology**
Mt. Sinai School of Medicine, Box 1065
1 Gustave Levy Pl.
New York, NY 10029
**Phone:** (212)659-5985     **Fax:** (212)849-2510
**Email:** john.morrison@mssm.edu
**Website:** http://www.mssm.edu/neurobio/
John H. Morrison, PhD, Co-Dir.

**Activities/Fields:** Neurobiological systems in humans and mammals, emphasizing aging research. Specific interests include the neuroendocrinology of stress, reproduction and metabolism, the molecular biology of Alzheimer's disease, schizophrenia, and other neurological/psychiatric diseases, and growth factors and growth factor receptor gene expression in the central nervous system.

★ **14140** ★ **Association for Research in Nervous and Mental Disease**
Box 23
Columbia College of Physicians & Surgeons
630 W 168th St.
New York, NY 10032
**Phone:** (212)740-7608     **Fax:** (212)305-4548
**Email:** arnmd@arnmd.org
Jack D. Barchas, MD, Ch.

**Activities/Fields:** Neurology, neurosurgery, and psychiatry.

★ **14141** ★ **Axion Research Foundation, Inc.**
100 Deepwood Dr.
Hamden, CT 06517
**Phone:** (203)773-9300     **Fax:** (203)776-2893
**Email:** bus.manager@axion.org
Dr. D.E. Redmond, Jr., Dir.

**Activities/Fields:** Neural transplantation, neural imaging, Parkinson's disease, and primate visual development.

★ **14142** ★ **Baltimore Headache Institute**
Johns Hopkins at Green Spring Station
Foxleigh Bldg., Ste. 165
2330 W Joppa Rd.
Lutherville, MD 21093
**Phone:** (410)583-7171     **Fax:** (410)583-7173
**Email:** bmondell@jhmi.edu
Dr. Brian Mondell, Med. Dir.

**Activities/Fields:** Treatment of migraine, muscle contraction, and cluster headaches.

## ★ 14143 ★ Barrow Neurological Institute
St. Joseph's Hospital & Medical Center
350 W Thomas Rd.
Phoenix, AZ 85013
**Phone:** (602)406-3000          **Fax:** (602)406-7167
**Email:** mholt@chw.edu
**Website:** http://www.thebni.com
Michael Holt, Contact
**Activities/Fields:** Neurosciences.


## Baylor College of Medicine
## Center for Cell and Gene Therapy
*See:* Entry 9372


## ★ 14144 ★ Baylor College of Medicine Epilepsy Research Center
1 Baylor Plz.
Houston, TX 77030
**Phone:** (713)790-3109          **Fax:** (713)793-1574
**Email:** pierson@bcm.tmc.edu
**Website:**      http://www.bcm.tmc.edu/catalog/center_for_cell_and_gene_thera.html
Dr. Peter Kellaway, Dir.

**Activities/Fields:** Epilepsy research (as related to human patients) in the following areas: clinical research on neurophysiological, pharmacological, and ontogenetic aspects of epilepsy; design and application of computer-based systems to improve EEG detection, characterization, and quantification of the epileptic process in the brain; fundamental studies employing in-vitro brain slice technique to the elucidation of membrane and synaptic mechanisms in epileptogenesis and the mechanisms of action of anticonvulsant and convulsant agents; and developmental neurogenetics of epilepsy.


## ★ 14145 ★ Baylor College of Medicine Jerry Lewis Neuromuscular Disease Research Center
6501 Fannin St., Ste. NB302
Houston, TX 77030
**Phone:** (713)798-4072          **Fax:** (713)798-3854
**Email:** sappel@bcm.tmc.edu
**Website:** http://public.bcm.tmc.edu/researcher-centers.html
Stanley H. Appel, MD, Dir.

**Activities/Fields:** Biochemistry, molecular genetics, and physiology of skeletal muscle and motor nerves, including biochemical, physiological, morphological, and genetic techniques to define and compare basic properties of skeletal muscle and neuromuscular disorders. Applies these approaches to animal models of human neuromuscular disease and to cultured muscle and nerve cells from normal and affected people.


## ★ 14146 ★ Baylor College of Medicine Sleep Disorders and Research Center
2002 Holcombe Blvd., 116A
Houston, TX 77030
**Phone:** (713)794-7563          **Fax:** (713)794-7558
**Email:** maxh@bcm.tmc.edu
Max Hirshkowitz, Dir.

**Activities/Fields:** Neuropsychopharmacology of sleep, sleep disorders and erectile dysfunction.


## ★ 14147 ★ Bernard W. Gimbel Multiple Sclerosis Comprehensive Care Center (MSCCC)
Holy Name Hospital
718 Teaneck Rd.
Teaneck, NJ 07666
**Phone:** (201)837-0727          **Fax:** (201)837-8504
Mary Ann Picone, MD, Dir.

**Activities/Fields:** Treatment and modalities for the relief of symptoms associated with multiple sclerosis, as well as improvement in overall functioning, prevention of worsening of the disease, and promotion of maximal independence. **Pub:** *MSCC Centerpiece Newsletter*, quarterly. Newsletter.


## ★ 14148 ★ Blanchette Rockefeller Neurosciences Institute
PO Box 9301
Morgantown, WV 26506
**Phone:** (304)293-3962
**Website:** http://www.brni.org/body.htm
Dr. Fred Butcher, Interim Exec. Dir.

**Activities/Fields:** Neurodegenerative diseases and other cognitive disorders, particularly those involving learning and memory; mood disorders, such as depression, anxiety, and schizophrenia; epilepsy; central nervous system injury; post-traumatic stress disorder; and other areas of fundamental neuroscience and neural disorders, including auditory and visual processing, particularly in relation to language development.


## ★ 14149 ★ Boston University Harold Goodglass Aphasia Research Center
Sch. of Med.
DVAMC, 12A
150 S Huntington Ave.
Boston, MA 02130-4817
**Phone:** (617)232-9500          **Fax:** (617)522-4786
**Email:** malbert@bu.edu
**Website:** http://www.bu.edu/aphasia
Dr. Martin L. Albert, Dir.

**Activities/Fields:** Cognitive and language impairment following brain damage and closely related topics in psycholinguistics, cognitive science, and behavioral neuroscience. **Frmly:** Aphasia Research Center.


## ★ 14150 ★ Boston University Laboratory of Neuropsychology
715 Albany St., L-815
Boston, MA 02118
**Phone:** (617)638-4803          **Fax:** (617)638-4806
**Email:** hcr@acs.bu.edu
Prof. Marlene Oscar Berman, PhD, Ch.

**Activities/Fields:** Alcoholism, aphasia, apraxia, dementia, memory disorders, autism, schizophrenia, dyslexia, normal brain function and behavior, and psychopharmacology. Projects emphasize the relationship between brain structure and brain function, especially as related to human neurological disorders. **Pub:** *Bostonia Magazine*, quarterly. • *News & Notes*, monthly. • *Research Reports Quarterly*.


## ★ 14151 ★ Boston University Neuromuscular Research Center
19 Deerfield St., 4th Fl.
Boston, MA 02215
**Phone:** (617)353-9757          **Fax:** (617)353-5737
**Email:** ddwong@bu.edu
**Website:** http://nmrc.bu.edu
Dr. Carlo J. De Luca, Dir.

**Activities/Fields:** Motor control, including motor unit firing during sustained isometric contractions, synchronization evaluation, synchronization across muscles, and modeling of force production in the muscle; low back pain, including normative database study of back muscle function, EMG parameters of lumbar back muscles, development of test protocols related to the behavior of back mucles, and muscle performance in the back analysis system compared to lifting tasks; posture and movement, etc. The center is organized into the following components: Motor Unit Lab, Muscle Fatigue Lab, Injury Analysis and Prevention Lab, Motion Analysis Lab, Motor Control Lab, Electrophysiology Lab, Electromyography Lab, Signal Processing Lab and Design Lab. **Pub:** *Annual Activity Report.*


## ★ 14152 ★ Boston University Neuromuscular Research Center Design Laboratory
19 Deerfield St., 4th Fl.
Boston, MA 02215
**Phone:** (617)358-0724          **Fax:** (617)353-5737
**Email:** dgilmore@bu.edu


**Website:** http://nmrc.bu.edu/labs/dl
L. Donald Gilmore, Supv.

**Activities/Fields:** Develops instrumentation for other NMRC laboratories. Electronic hardware and software technologies, used in the investigation of neuromuscular performance, are designed for eventual implementation into the clinical environment. Several devices, including specialized electrodes for detecting and anlyzing the surface electromyographic signal, have been developed here.


## ★ 14153 ★ Boston University Neuromuscular Research Center Electromyography Laboratory
19 Deerfield St., 4th Fl.
Boston, MA 02215
**Phone:** (617)353-9757          **Fax:** (617)353-5737
**Email:** webmaster@nmrc.edu
**Website:** http://nmrc.bu.edu
Dr. Carlo J. DeLuca, Dir.

**Activities/Fields:** Techniques for the detection and analysis of EMG data such as study of the use of innovative electrodes' geometry and comparison of their performance to assess functional activities in ergonomics and risk factors.


## ★ 14154 ★ Boston University NeuroMuscular Research Center Electrophysiology Laboratory
19 Deerfield St., 4th Fl.
Boston, MA 02215
**Phone:** (617)358-0718          **Fax:** (617)353-5737
**Email:** sroy@bu.edu
**Website:** http://nmrc.bu.edu/labs/epl
Dr. Serge Roy, Supv.

**Activities/Fields:** In vitro studies of isolated muscles of rats to compare muscle physiology/morphology to the electrical signals produced during muscle contraction. Aims to further the development of surface electromyography (EMG) as a means of assessing human muscle function and fatigue.


## ★ 14155 ★ Boston University Neuromuscular Research Center Injury Analysis and Prevention Laboratory
19 Deerfield St., 4th Fl.
Boston, MA 02215
**Phone:** (617)353-9638          **Fax:** (617)353-5737
**Email:** loddsson@bu.edu
**Website:** http://nmrc.bu.edu
Dr. Lars I.E. Oddsson, Supvr.

**Activities/Fields:** Injury mechanism related to postural control during slips and falls, as well as lifting and other types of manual load handling. Biomechanical, neurophysiological, electrophysiological, and epidemiological tools are used to develop a better understanding of mechanisms causing injury, thus increasing the possibility of developing successful preventive measures.


## ★ 14156 ★ Boston University Neuromuscular Research Center Motion Analysis Laboratory
19 Deerfield St., 4th Fl.
Boston, MA 02215
**Phone:** (617)353-9635          **Fax:** (617)353-5737
**Email:** pbonato@bu.edu
**Website:** http://nmrc.bu.edu/labs/mal
Prof. Paolo Bonato, Contact

**Activities/Fields:** Explores the full range of human movement, including dynamics and kinematics, with emphasis on the neural control and biomechanics of posture and locomotion.


## ★ 14157 ★ Boston University Neuromuscular Research Center Motor Control Laboratory
19 Deerfield St., 4th Fl.
Boston, MA 02215

**Phone:** (617)358-0719          **Fax:** (617)353-5737
**Email:** webmaster@nmrc.edu
**Website:** http://nmrc.bu.edu
Dr. Gerald L. Gottlieb, Supvr.

**Activities/Fields:** Voluntary control of human limbs, particularly the determinants of movement which are higher motor centers, reflex mechanism, and muscle properties. Both normal motor control and the behavior of patients with diverse movement disorders are explored.


**★ 14158 ★ Boston University**
**NeuroMuscular Research Center**
**Motor Unit Laboratory**
19 Deerfield St., 4th Fl.
Boston, MA 02215
**Phone:** (617)353-9756          **Fax:** (617)353-5737
**Email:** cjd@bu.edu
**Website:** http://nmrc.bu.edu/labs/mul
Dr. Carlo J. De Luca, Dir.

**Activities/Fields:** Investigates how the brain and spinal cord control the activation of muscle cells to produce muscle force. Seeks to examine muscle fiber discharge history in detail, to better understand the physiological rules that regulate muscle contractions, and to improve the ability of the neurologist to categorize and quantify neurological dysfunction.


**★ 14159 ★ Boston University**
**NeuroMuscular Research Center**
**Muscle Fatigue Laboratory**
19 Deerfield St., 4th Fl.
Boston, MA 02215
**Phone:** (617)353-9633          **Fax:** (617)353-5737
**Email:** sroy@bu.edu
**Website:** http://nmrc.bu.edu/labs/mfl
Dr. Serge Roy, Supv.

**Activities/Fields:** Use of advanced signal processing techniques for the analysis of electromyographic signals, especially techniques for the analysis of nonstationary surface EMG data, to estimate localized muscle fatigue during static and dynamic contractions.


**★ 14160 ★ Boston University**
**Neuromuscular Research Center**
**Signal Processing Laboratory**
19 Deerfield St., 4th Fl.
Boston, MA 02215
**Phone:** (617)358-0715          **Fax:** (617)353-5737
**Email:** webmaster@nmrc.bu.edu
**Website:** http://nmrc.bu.edu
Prof. Paolo Bonato, Res. Asst.

**Activities/Fields:** Use of advanced signal processing techniques for the analysis of electromyographic signals, especially the development of techniques for the analysis of nonstationary surface EMG data.


**★ 14161 ★ Brain Research Foundation**
120 S LaSalle St., Ste. 1300
Chicago, IL 60603
**Phone:** (312)759-5150          **Fax:** (312)759-5151
**Email:** info@brainresearchfdn.org
**Website:** http://www.brainresearchfdn.org
Cathy Stein, Actg. Exec. Dir.

**Activities/Fields:** Provides support for research projects, new equipment, and scientific education in neurology, psychiatry, neurobiology, neurosurgery, and pharmacology/physiology at the Brain Research Institute of the University of Chicago. **Pub:** *Annual Audit.* • *Annual Report.* • *Brain Waves Newsletter,* quarterly.


**★ 14162 ★ Brigham and Women's**
**Hospital**
**Center for Neurologic Diseases**
77 Ave., Louis Pasteur HIM 730
Boston, MA 02115-5817
**Phone:** (617)525-5300          **Fax:** (617)525-5252
**Email:** weiner@cnd.bwh.harvard.edu
Dr. Howard L. Weiner, Co-Dir.

**Activities/Fields:** Human autoimmune diseases, including T-cell immunology, T-cell interactions and regulations by cytokines. Also studies immunoregulatory T-cell abnormalities in multiple sclerosis and other autoimmune diseases, and investigations of mechanisms of immunologic tolerance in humans.


**★ 14163 ★ Brown University**
**Center for Neural Sciences**
Department of Neurosciences
PO Box 1953
Providence, RI 02912
**Phone:** (401)863-3548          **Fax:** (401)863-1074
**Email:** mary-ellen_flinn@brown.edu
Mary Ellen Flinn, Contact

**Activities/Fields:** Brain and cerebral cortex, including models and mechanisms of learning, memory, and plasticity.


**★ 14164 ★ Brown University**
**Institute for Brain and Neural Systems**
**(IBNS)**
PO Box 1843
Providence, RI 02912
**Phone:** (401)863-2585          **Fax:** (401)863-3494
**Email:** info@cns.brown.edu
**Website:** http://www.cns.brown.edu/ibns/
Leon N. Cooper, Dir.

**Activities/Fields:** Brain function and neural systems.


**★ 14165 ★ Carleton University**
**Centre for Memory Assessment and**
**Research (CMAR)**
B531 Loeb
1125 Colonel By Dr.
Ottawa, ON, Canada K1S 5B6
**Phone:** (613)520-2659
**Email:** tom_tombaugh@carleton.ca
Tommy N. Tombaugh, Dir.

**Activities/Fields:** Testing and assessment for anyone experiencing memory problems due to illness, aging, injury, or neurological damage; encourages and facilitates research, as well as develops tests for assessing memory and intellectual abilities; and serves as an educational facility and research center focusing on memory illnesses and cognitive rehabilitation.


**★ 14166 ★ Case Western Reserve**
**University**
**Applied Neural Control Laboratory**
Charles B. Bolton Bldg., Rm. 3480
Cleveland, OH 44106-4912
**Phone:** (216)368-2960          **Fax:** (216)368-4872
**Email:** jtm3@po.cwru.edu
J. Thomas Mortimer, PhD, Dir.

**Activities/Fields:** Development of technology based on the electrical excitability of nerve tissue for use in electrically controlling bodily organs or systems. Applications include restoration of paralyzed upper and lower extremities, restoration of diaphragm and bladder function, and stimulation of the central nervous system in epilepsy treatment.


**Case Western Reserve University**
**Neural Engineering Center**
*See:* Entry 4521


**★ 14167 ★ Case Western Reserve**
**University**
**University Memory and Aging Center**
Fairhill Center
12200 Fairhill Rd.
Cleveland, OH 44120
**Phone:** (216)844-6400          **Free:** 800-252-5048
**Fax:** (216)844-6446
**Email:** kxh26@po.cwru.edu
**Website:** http://www.ohioalzcenter.org
Karl Herrup, PhD, Dir.

**Activities/Fields:** Long term studies of persons with memory problems, Alzheimer's disease, caregiver studies, and clinical studies to develop effective treatments for memory disorders. Research focuses on animal models, mechanisms of nerve cell death in dementia and the role of inflammation in neurodegenerative disease. **Pub:** *ADAD Newsletter,* quarterly.
**Frmly:** University Alzheimer Center.


**★ 14168 ★ Center for Biological Timing**
Gilmer Hall, Rm. 285
Department of Biology
University of Virginia
PO Box 400328
Charlottesville, VA 22904-4328
**Phone:** (434)982-4501          **Fax:** (434)982-5626
**Email:** clock@virginia.edu
**Website:** http://www.cbt.virginia.edu
Dr. Gene D. Block, Dir.

**Activities/Fields:** Problems of biological timing within the nervous and endocrine systems. Specific studies include cellular mechanisms within the neuroendocrine system, environmental control of reproductive cycles, neural basis of rhythmic motor behaviors, and circadian rhythmicity. **Frmly:** Biodynamics Institute.


**★ 14169 ★ Center for Neurochemistry**
Nathan S Kline Institute for Psychiatric Research
140 Old Orangeburg Rd.
Orangeburg, NY 10962
**Phone:** (845)398-5530          **Fax:** (845)398-5531
**Email:** Lajtha@nki.rfmh.org
Laura Berlanga, Contact

**Activities/Fields:** Brain protein and peptide metabolism, chronic drug effects, properties of brain receptors, blood-brain barrier, and effects of addictive drugs. **Frmly:** New York State Research Institute for Neurochemistry & Drug Addiction.


**★ 14170 ★ Center for**
**Neurodevelopmental Studies, Inc.**
5430 W Glenn Dr.
Glendale, AZ 85301-2628
**Phone:** (623)915-0345          **Fax:** (623)937-5425
**Email:** cns@netwrx.com
**Website:** http://web1.cirs.org/homepage/cns
Lorna Jean King, Dir.

**Activities/Fields:** Effective treatment methods for autism and developmental disabilities and standardizing measures for evaluating adult sensory/motor functions (the Stepping Test, Vertical Writing Test, and Object Manipulation Speed Test). Collects data on specific responses of developmentally delayed children to various types of sensory stimulation. Evaluates the effectiveness of senory-integrative intervention for pre-school children at risk for learning disabilities.


**★ 14171 ★ Center for Neurologic Study**
9850 Genesee Ave., Ste. 320
La Jolla, CA 92037
**Phone:** (858)455-5463          **Fax:** (858)455-1713
**Email:** cns@cts.com
**Website:** http://www.cnsonline.org
Richard A. Smith, MD, Dir.

**Activities/Fields:** Neuropharmacology and experimental treatment of neurologic diseases. **Pub:** *Handbook of Amyotrophic Lateral Sclerosis.*


**★ 14172 ★ Cerebral Blood Flow**
**Laboratories (CBF Labs)**
Veterans Administration Medical Center, Bldg. 110, Rm. 225
2002 Holcombe Blvd.
Houston, TX 77030
**Phone:** (713)795-5807          **Fax:** (713)794-7583
**Email:** jmeyer@bcm.tmc.edu
John S. Meyer, MD, Dir.

**Activities/Fields:** Measurement of CT morphological changes and cerebral blood flow; cerebrovascular disorders; aging, Alzheimer's and ischemic vascular dementias and responses to medical, surgical, pharmacological, and behavioral treatment; prevention, diagnosis, and treatment of stroke and migraine; cerebral blood flow control and cerebral metabolism; neuropharmacology and physiology; aging; dementia; transient ischemic attacks; and risk factors for stroke. **Pub:** *Books, monographs.* • *Peer-reviewed journal articles.* **Frmly:** Baylor Center for Cerebrovascular Research.

★ **14173** ★ **Chicago Institute of**
　**Neurosurgery and Neuroresearch**
430 W Deming, No. 1
Chicago, IL 60614
**Phone:** (773)388-7860　　　　**Fax:** (773)388-7866
**Email:** j-moskal@nwu.edu
Joseph R. Moskal, PhD, Dir. of Res.

**Activities/Fields:** Molecular glycobiology of brain tumors, glycosyltransferase, molecular biology, and ddrt-pcr-based gene discovery.

★ **14174** ★ **City of Hope**
**National Medical Center and Beckman**
　**Research Institute**
**Division of Neurosciences**
1450 E Duarte Rd.
Duarte, CA 91010
**Phone:** (626)301-8188　　　　**Fax:** (626)301-8948
**Email:** mbarish@coh.org
**Website:** http://bricoh.coh.org
Dr. Michael E. Barish, Ch.

**Activities/Fields:** The Division is composed of 12 research sections studying cell biology, cellular neurochemistry, cellular neurophysiology, developmental neurobiology, membrane biochemistry, molecular biology and genetics, neuroanatomy and ultrastructure, neurobiochemistry, neuroendocrinology, neuropharmacology, neurophysiology, and receptor physiology. Specific studies include the embryonic development of spinal cord neurons; identification, localization, and functions of neuroactive peptides; molecular and functional studies of transmembrane ion channels; the functional relationship between molecular chemical events and electrical excitability of neuronal elements; interactions between neurotransmitter receptor molecules of the membrane with synaptic proteins; developmental and molecular biological processes involved in the function of cholinergic neurons in normal and animal models of Alzheimer's disease; mechanisms of solute transport localized membranes and the effect of lipid components on operation of transport systems; developmental specificity of the formation of neuronal connections; and molecular genetic studies of Alzheimer's disease, schizophrenia, and manic depressive disorder.

★ **14175** ★ **College of Staten Island of**
　**City University of New York**
**Program in Neuroscience**
2800 Victory Blvd., 6S229
Staten Island, NY 10314
**Phone:** (718)982-3950　　　　**Fax:** (718)982-3953
Dr. Ekkehart Trenkner, Mng. Dir.

**Activities/Fields:** Developmental neurobiology and neurochemistry, and synaptic plasticity, focusing on the regulation and adaptation of neural function, utilizing brain slices, neural cell lines, primary CNS neurons grown in culture, aging and development and neuropathological processes (Alzheimer's and genetic diseases). **Frmly:** Center for Developmental Neuroscience and Developmental Disabilities.

★ **14176** ★ **Colorado Neurological**
　**Institute (CNI)**
701 E Hampden Ave., Ste. 330
Englewood, CO 80110
**Phone:** (303)788-4010　　　　**Fax:** (303)788-5469
**Email:** jbriles@thecni.org
**Website:** http://thecni.org/research.htm
Gary D. VanderArk, MD, Pres.

**Activities/Fields:** Neurological diseases, including Parkinson's disease, Huntington's disease and other movement disorders, epilepsy, brain tumors, spinal

cord injuries, head trauma, hearing disorders, stroke, Lou Gehrig's disease, sleep disorders, migraines, neuromuscular disorders.

**Colorado Neurological Institute**
**CNI Brain Tumor Program**
*See:* Entry 10312

★ **14177** ★ **Colorado State University**
**Program in Molecular, Cellular, and**
　**Integrative Neurosciences**
Anatomy/Zoology Bldg.
Anatomy and Neurobiology Department 1670
Fort Collins, CO 80523-1670
**Phone:** (970)491-0425　　　　**Fax:** (970)491-7907
**Email:** gpickard@lamar.colostate.edu
**Website:** http://cvmbs.colostate.edu/mcin
Dr. Gary E. Pickard, Dir.

**Activities/Fields:** Cellular, molecular and integrative approaches to neuroscience, focusing on basic components of the nervous system's development repair, and function largely through studies of cultured neurons, brain slices, and animals. Also investigation of the role of amino acid neurotransmitters in development and aging, structure and function of voltage and ligand gated ion channels, mechanisms of taste reception, basis of circadian rhythms, mechanisms of synaptic function, and regulation of gene expression in early development.

★ **14178** ★ **Columbia-Presbyterian**
　**Medical Center**
**Gertrude H. Sergievsky Center**
630 W 168 St.
New York, NY 10032
**Phone:** (212)305-2515　　　　**Fax:** (212)305-2426
**Email:** rpm2@columbia.edu
**Website:** http://cpmcnet.columbia.edu/dept/sergievsky
Richard Mayeux, MD, Dir.

**Activities/Fields:** Developmental disorders of the nervous system that affect humans from conception until death, including epilepsy, Parkinson's Disease, essential tremor, and Alzheimer's Disease and other age-related brain diseases.

★ **14179** ★ **Columbia-Presbyterian**
　**Medical Center**
**Neurological Institute**
710 W 168th St.
New York, NY 10032-3784
**Phone:** (212)305-6489　　　　**Fax:** (212)305-6978
**Email:** tap2@columbia.edu
**Website:** http://www.neuroinstitute.org
Timothy A. Pedley, MD, Chm., Neurology Dept.

**Activities/Fields:** Neurology, neuropathology, neurophysiology, neurological surgery, dystonia, Parkinson's and Alzheimer's diseases, muscular dystrophy, amyotrophic lateral sclerosis (Lou Gehrig's disease), multiple sclerosis, and epilepsy, including basic and clinical studies on function and disease of the nervous system and treatment of nervous diseases and surgical conditions of the brain and nervous system.

★ **14180** ★ **Columbia University**
**Center for Parkinson's Disease and Other**
　**Movement Disorders**
Neurological Institute
710 W 168th St.
New York, NY 10032
**Phone:** (212)305-5779　　　　**Fax:** (212)305-1304
**Email:** fahn@movdis.cis.columbia.edu
Stanley Fahn, MD, Dir.

**Activities/Fields:** Phenomenology, pharmacology, treatment, and genetics of Parkinson's disease and other movement disorders. Research activities focus on dystonia, Parkinsonism, tremor, dyskinesia, chorea, myoclonus, and tics. **Frmly:** Dystonia Clinical Research Center.

★ **14181** ★ **Columbia University**
**Clinical Research Center for Muscular**
　**Dystrophy**
Department of Neurology, 4-420
College of Physicians & Surgeons
630 W 168th St.
New York, NY 10032
**Phone:** (212)305-1664　　　　**Fax:** (212)305-3986
**Email:** sd12@columbia.edu
Salvatore DiMauro, MD, Co-Dir.

**Activities/Fields:** Molecular genetics and hereditary neuromuscular diseases, particularly metabolic myopathies. Conducts molecular genetic, biochemical, and morphological studies of muscle.

★ **14182** ★ **Columbia University**
**Taub Institute for Research on**
　**Alzheimer's Disease and the Aging**
　**Brain**
College of Physicians & Surgeons
630 W 168th St., P&S Box 16
New York, NY 10032
**Phone:** (212)305-1818　　　　**Fax:** (212)342-2849
**Email:** taubinstitute@columbia.edu
**Website:** http://www.alzheimercenter.org
Michael L. Shelanski, MD, Co-Dir.

**Activities/Fields:** Alzheimer's disease and elderly care. Serves as a resource for tissue, cells, and DNA from Alzheimer's disease and control patients. Areas of research include epidemiology, cell biology, genetics, and aging. **Pub:** *ADRC Newsletter*, semiannually. **Frmly:** Alzheimer's Disease Research Center.

★ **14183** ★ **Concordia University**
　**(Montreal, QC, Canada)**
**Centre for Studies in Behavioral**
　**Neurobiology**
Department of Psychology
1455 de Maisonneuve Blvd. W
Montreal, QC, Canada H3G 1M8
**Phone:** (514)848-2200　　　　**Fax:** (514)848-2817
**Email:** info@csbn.concordia.ca
**Website:** http://csbn.concordia.ca/
Peter Shizgal, PhD, Dir.

**Activities/Fields:** Research addresses the mechanisms that marshall behavior to meet biological needs. Principal topics of study include the neural, hormonal, and psychological processes that maintain homeostasis and ensure successful reproduction as well as the disruption of these processes that leads to drug dependence, obesity, and sexual dysfunction. Research considers three principal themes: reward, motivation, and plasticity. All three combine behavioral measurement methods with techniques in molecular, cellular, and systems neuroscience.

★ **14184** ★ **Cornell University**
**Brain Trauma Foundation**
523 E 72nd St., 8th Fl.
New York, NY 10021
**Phone:** (212)772-0608　　　　**Fax:** (212)772-0357
**Email:** info@braintrauma.org
**Website:** http://www.braintrauma.org/
Ralph Isham, Chm.

**Activities/Fields:** Investigates the pathophysiology of traumatic brain injury, uses an in vitro human glial cell culture model of injury to study brain derived inflammatory mediators, and performs ventricular cerebrospinal fluid analysis in human patients. Established physiological model for post traumatic raised intracranial preserve analysis. **Frmly:** Aitken Neuroscience Center.

★ **14185** ★ **Cornell University**
**Winifred Masterson Burke Medical**
　**Research Institute, Inc.**
**Dementia Research Service**
785 Mamaroneck Ave.
White Plains, NY 10605
**Phone:** (914)597-2351　　　　**Fax:** (914)597-2757

Email: jpblass@mail.med.cornell.edu
Dr. John P. Blass, Dir.

**Activities/Fields:** Clinical and basic studies in genetic, metabolic and nutritional aspects of degenerative diseases of the nervous system, especially Alzheimer's disease. Also studies of the role of reactive oxygen species.

★ **14186** ★ **Craig Center for Spinal Cord Injury Research (CRES)**
Craig Hospital, Research Department
3425 S Clarkson St.
Englewood, CO 80110
**Phone:** (303)789-8600          **Fax:** (303)789-8567
**Email:** gale@craighospital.org
**Website:** http://www.craighospital.org/C_Research/C4_craigCenterSCIRes.html
Gale Whiteneck, PhD, Dir.

**Activities/Fields:** Spinal cord injuries.

★ **14187** ★ **Crawford Research Institute at Shepherd Center**
2020 Peachtree Rd. NW
Atlanta, GA 30309
**Phone:** (404)350-7595          **Fax:** (404)350-7596
**Email:** mike_jones@shepherd.org
**Website:** http://www.shepherd.org
Michael L. Jones, PhD, Dir.

**Activities/Fields:** Clinical health services and outcomes, acquired brain injury, spinal cord injury, and multiple sclerosis.

★ **14188** ★ **Dartmouth College Sleep Disorders Center**
Dartmouth Hitchcock Medical Center
1 Medical Center Dr.
Lebanon, NH 03756
**Phone:** (603)650-7534          **Fax:** (603)650-7820
**Email:** michael.j.sateia@dartmouth.edu
Dr. Michael Sateia, Dir.

**Activities/Fields:** Sleep disorders, sleep apnea due to obesity, hypersomnolence, parasomnias, and insomnia.

★ **14189** ★ **Duke University Duke Center for the Advanced Study of Epilepsy**
401 Bryan Res. Bldg.
Res. Dr.
Box 3676
Durham, NC 27710
**Phone:** (919)684-4241          **Fax:** (919)684-8219
Dr. James O. McNamara, Dir.

**Activities/Fields:** Clinical and experimental approaches to limbic epilepsy. Current projects include studies of early gene expression in the kindling model of epilepsy, mechanisms of development of Ammon's horn sclerosis, microphysiology of limbic seizures, and role of excitatory amino acids and their receptors in limbic epilepsy.

★ **14190** ★ **Duke University Preuss Laboratory for Brain Tumor Research**
Medical center
Research Dr., 177 MSRB
PO Box 3156
Durham, NC 27710
**Phone:** (919)684-5018          **Fax:** (919)684-6458
**Email:** bigne001@mc.duke.edu
Dr. Darell Bigner, Dir.

**Activities/Fields:** Brain tumors.

★ **14191** ★ **Duke University Udall Parkinson's Disease Research Center of Excellence (PDRCE)**
DUMC Box 2903
Durham, NC 27710
**Phone:** (919)681-5696          **Fax:** (919)681-7894

Email: udall@chg.mc.duke.edu
**Website:** http://wwwchg.mc.duke.edu/udall
Jeffery M. Vance, MD, Dir.

**Activities/Fields:** Cause and cure for Parkinson's disease.

★ **14192** ★ **Duluth Clinic Education and Research Foundation**
400 E 3rd St.
Duluth, MN 55805-1951
**Phone:** (218)725-3139          **Fax:** (218)727-7258
**Email:** jdwyer@smdc.org
**Website:** http://www.smdc.org
James M. Dwyer, Dir.

**Activities/Fields:** Parkinson's disease, cancer, heart, stroke, and other medical issues. **Pub:** *Health Strides*.

★ **14193** ★ **Dystonia Medical Research Foundation**
1 E Wacker Dr., Ste. 2430
Chicago, IL 60601-1905
**Phone:** (312)755-0198          **Free:** 800-377-3978
**Fax:** (312)803-0138
**Email:** dystonia@dystonia-foundation.org
**Website:** http://www.dystonia-foundation.org/
Dr. Mahlon R. DeLong, Sci. Dir.

**Activities/Fields:** Causes and treatment of generalized dystonia, spasmodic torticollis, writer's cramp, blepharospasm, oromandibular dystonia, Meige's disease, and laryngeal dystonia. **Pub:** *Brochures*. • *Manuals*. • *Newsletter*, quarterly.

★ **14194** ★ **Emory University Sleep Research Laboratory**
Emory Sleep Disorder Center
1821 Clifton NE
Atlanta, GA 30329
**Phone:** (404)728-4750          **Fax:** (404)728-4756
Dr. Bliwise, Dir.

**Activities/Fields:** Neurophysiological studies of sleep.

★ **14195** ★ **Florida Atlantic University Center for Complex Systems and Brain Sciences**
777 Glades Rd.
Boca Raton, FL 33431
**Phone:** (561)297-2230          **Fax:** (561)297-3634
**Email:** kelso@walt.ccs.fau.edu
**Website:** http://www.ccs.fau.edu
J.A. Scott Kelso, Dir.

**Activities/Fields:** Multidisciplinary studies of complex biological systems, focusing on coordination between neural processes and their resultant behaviors on cognitive, neural, and biophysical levels. Contains four major research facilities: Human Brain and Behavior Laboratories, including functional magnetic resonance imaging; Theoretical (Computational) Neuroscience Laboratory; Basic Neuroscience Research Laboratories, which includes neural growth and development, neurophysiology, neuroanatomy, and cellular biophysics; Coordination Dynamics Laboratory. Houses National Training Program in Complex Systems and Brain Sciences for pre- and postdoctoral fellows.

★ **14196** ★ **Georgetown University Sleep Disorders Center**
3800 Reservoir Rd. NW
Washington, DC 20007
**Phone:** (202)784-3610          **Fax:** (202)784-2920
Dr. Richard Waldhorn, Jr., Dir.

**Activities/Fields:** Treatment techniques for sleep apnea using nasal continuous positive airway pressure, evaluation of people with nocturnal hypoxia and possible correlates to memory impairment, sleep disturbances in geriatric populations, and psychiatric studies dealing with the presence of depression in people with schizophrenia. Other concentrations include monitoring of epilepsy patients and studies of sudden infant death syndrome.

★ **14197** ★ **Georgia Regional Spinal Cord Injury Care System**
Shepherd Center Inc.
2020 Peachtree Rd. NW
Atlanta, GA 30309-1402
**Phone:** (404)350-2020          **Fax:** (404)355-1826
**Website:** http://www.shepherd.org/shepherdhome-page.nsf/Pages/ProgramsSCI?OpenDocument
Herndon Murray, MD, Contact

**Activities/Fields:** Spinal cord injuries and paralyzing neuromuscular diseases. **Pub:** *MS Review*. • *Shepherd Clinical Review Newsletter*. • *Spinal Column magazine*. • *Spineline*.

**Georgia State University Center for Brain Sciences and Health (CBH)**
*See:* Entry 2497

★ **14198** ★ **Guardians of Hydrocephalus Research Foundation (GHRF)**
2618 Ave. Z
Brooklyn, NY 11235-2023
**Phone:** (718)743-4473          **Fax:** (718)743-1171
**Email:** ghrf2618@aol.com
**Website:** http://ghrf.homestead.com/ghrf.html
Michael Fischetti, Chm.

**Activities/Fields:** Hydrocephalics and their families, health care professionals, and other concerned individuals. Seeks to find the cause and cure of hydrocephalus which is the buildup of cerebrospinal fluid in the brain cavity, and can cause brain damage or death if untreated. **Pub:** *GUARDIANews*, quarterly. Newsletter.

★ **14199** ★ **Harvard Brain Tissue Resource Center**
McLean Hospital
115 Mill St.
Belmont, MA 02478-9106
**Phone:** (617)855-2400          **Free:** 800-272-4622
**Fax:** (617)855-3199
**Email:** btrc@mclean.harvard.edu
**Website:** http://www.brainbank.mclean.org:8080
Francine M. Benes, MD, Dir.

**Activities/Fields:** Provides tissues to the neuroscience community for studies of movement disorders, major psychoses, and dementia. **Frmly:** Brain Tissue Resource Center.

★ **14200** ★ **Harvard Medical School Division of Sleep Medicine**
Brigham & Women's Hospital
Department of Medicine
221 Longwood Ave., Ste. 438A
Boston, MA 02115
**Phone:** (617)732-4013          **Fax:** (617)732-4015
**Email:** caczeisler@hms.harvard.edu
**Website:** http://www.hms.harvard.edu/sleep
Dr. Charles A. Czeisler, Contact

**Activities/Fields:** Sleep medicine, circadian and homeostatic regulation of sleep and of hormone release, sleep-related breathing disorders, neuroendocrinology, mathematical modeling, neurobehavioral performance. **Pub:** *Medical Journals*. • *Scientific Journals*. **Frmly:** Circadian Neuroendocrine and Sleep Disorders Section.

★ **14201** ★ **Harvey W. Peters Research Center for the Study of Parkinson's Disease and Disorders of the Central Nervous System**
137 Davidson Hall
Department of Chemistry
Virginia Polytechnic Institute and State University
Blacksburg, VA 24061-0212
**Phone:** (540)231-8200          **Fax:** (540)231-8890
Prof. James F. Wolfe, Co-Dir.

**Activities/Fields:** Molecular mechanisms of xenobiotic metabolism, and chemically-induced neurodegenerative processes, focusing on Parkinson's disease and epileptic disorders.

**Heart and Stroke Foundation of British Columbia and Yukon**
*See:* Entry 5101

**Heart and Stroke Foundation of Canada**
*See:* Entry 5102

**Heart and Stroke Foundation of Newfoundland and Labrador**
*See:* Entry 5103

**Heart and Stroke Foundation of Nova Scotia**
*See:* Entry 5104

**★ 14202 ★ Helen Hayes Hospital Center for Neural Recovery and Rehabilitation Research**
Rte. 9W
West Haverstraw, NY 10993-1195
**Phone:** (845)786-4859          **Fax:** (845)786-4875
**Email:** scharfmanh@helenhayeshosp.org
**Website:** http://ww2.heartandstroke.ca/
Helen E. Scharfman, PhD, Dir.
**Activities/Fields:** Epilepsy, brain injury, neuroendocrinology, spinal cord injury, neurobiology. Degenerative neurological disorders such as Huntington's and Alzheimer's diseases are also investigated. **Pub:** *Scientific Journals*, 3/year. **Frmly:** Neurology Research Center.

**★ 14203 ★ Huntington Medical Research Institutes**
734 Fairmount Ave.
Pasadena, CA 91105
**Phone:** (626)397-5436          **Fax:** (626)397-5801
**Email:** opelw@hmri.org
**Website:** http://www.hmri.org
William Opel, PhD, Exec. Dir.
**Activities/Fields:** Electronic neural prosthetic device development; biology of nitric oxide; prostate and breast cancer; cell biology; moleculor genetics; neural proteomics; drug development; medical applications of magnetic resonance using protons, phosphorous, fluorine, and nitrogen; magnetoencephalography and brain mapping in epilespy. **Pub:** *Newsletter*, quarterly.

**★ 14204 ★ Huntington's Disease Center Without Walls**
Molecular Neurogenetics Unit
Massachusetts General Hospital East, Bldg. 149, Rm. 6214
13th St.
Charlestown, MA 02129
**Phone:** (617)726-5724          **Fax:** (617)726-5735
**Email:** gusella@helix.mgh.harvard.edu
**Website:** http://www.mgh.harvard.edu/depts/molneur/mnu.htm
Dr. James F. Gusella, Prog. Dir.
**Activities/Fields:** Huntington's Disease (HD), including protein abnormalities in the HD brain and their relationship to neuronal loss, neuropathological examination of autopsy brain sections, location and measurement of chemical messengers, neuropsychological tests evaluating deficits in memory and cognitive functioning, social and pyschological impact of HD on families, medications increasing levels of chemical messengers in the brain, DNA studies to determine the HD gene, and peptide localization in the nerve cells.

**Illinois Institute of Technology Pritzker Institute of Medical Engineering**
*See:* Entry 4526

**Illinois Institute of Technology Research Laboratory in Human Biomechanics**
*See:* Entry 4527

**★ 14205 ★ Indiana University Center for Alzheimer's Disease and Related Disorders**
550 N University Blvd., Ste. 3124
Indianapolis, IN 46202
**Phone:** (317)274-4333          **Fax:** (317)274-1497
**Email:** meade@iit.edu
**Website:**          http://www.indiana.edu/~rugs/ctrdir/cadrnd.html
Hugh C. Hendrie, MD, Co-Dir.
**Activities/Fields:** Alzheimer Disease and related neuropsychiatric disorders characterized by memory loss and mood disorders in the older adult. **Frmly:** Alzheimer Disease Center and Related Neuropsychiatric Disorders.

**★ 14206 ★ Indiana University Neuropsychology Research Section**
702 Barnhill Dr., Rm. 3751
Indianapolis, IN 46202
**Phone:** (317)274-7327          **Fax:** (317)274-1337
**Email:** dkareken@iupui.edu
Dr. David A. Kareken, Dir.
**Activities/Fields:** Brain-behavior relationships as measured by functional brain imaging and neuropsychological measurement and as affected by neurologic disease and pharmacologic therapies.

**★ 14207 ★ Institute of Developmental Neuroscience and Aging**
301 University Blvd., UTMB
Galveston, TX 77555-0652
**Phone:** (409)772-3667          **Fax:** (409)772-8028
**Email:** regino.perez-polo@utmb.edu
Dr. Regino Perez-Polo, Pres.
**Activities/Fields:** Developmental neuroscience and aging, focusing on establishing neuroscience programs in developing and third world countries.

**★ 14208 ★ Institutes for Achievement of Human Potential**
8801 Stenton Ave.
Wyndmoor, PA 19038-8397
**Phone:** (215)233-2050          **Fax:** (215)233-9312
**Email:** institutes@iahp.org
**Website:** http://www.iahp.org
Janet Doman, Dir.
**Activities/Fields:** Methods of treating severely brain-injured children, including investigations of effects of programs of sensory inputs individually designed according to each child's growth, as well as functional gains and effects of nutrition in enhancing children's response to therapeutic programs. Studies effects of applying similar environmental enrichment and neurological organization programs to non-disabled children of preschool age. **Pub:** *The Institute Report*, quarterly. **Frmly:** Rehabilitation Center of Philadelphia.

**★ 14209 ★ International Association for the Study of Pain**
909 NE 43rd St., Ste. 306
Seattle, WA 98105-6020
**Phone:** (206)547-6409          **Fax:** (206)547-1703
**Email:** iasp@locke.hs.washington.edu
**Website:** http://www.iasp-pain.org
Louisa E. Jones, Exec. Off.
**Activities/Fields:** Pain mechanisms and syndromes, focusing on patients with acute and chronic pain. **Pub:** *Clinical newsletter*, 3/year. • *Newsletter*, bimonthly. • *PAIN Journal*, monthly.

**★ 14210 ★ International Research Council of Neuromuscular Disorders**
1434 Pleasantville Rd.
Lancaster, OH 43130
**Phone:** (740)653-1098          **Fax:** (740)687-5003
James R. Grilliot, Contact
**Activities/Fields:** Neuromuscular diseases, focusing on cure, prevention, causes, effects, and occurrences.

**★ 14211 ★ John P. Robarts Research Institute Stroke and Aging Group Neurobiology Group**
81 Research Dr.
PO Box 5015
Scarborough, ME 04074
**Phone:** (207)885-8200          **Fax:** (207)885-8179
**Email:** verdiJ@mmc.org
Prof. Joseph M. Verdi, Grp. Ldr.
**Activities/Fields:** Stem cells and regenerative medicine. Stem cells are defined as multipotent, self-renewing undifferentiated cells capable of differentiating into numerous cell lineages. A great deal of interest has focused on the numerous cell lineages. A great deal of interest has focused on the potential therapeutic application of such stem cell populations, not only to repair or replace damaged tissues, but as model systems to understand basic developmental process leading to normal and abnormal cellular development. The system biology and regenrative medicine program that I direct is currently comprised of four investigators including myself which were chosen in the field of stem cell biology and areas of interest include: (i) The role of Notch signaling in self renewal, (ii) the role of wnt signaling in lineage specification of mesodermal stem cells, (iii) the roles of VEGF and FGF in lymphogenesis, (iv) transdifferntation of human stem cells and (v) the intergration of signaling pathways underlying notrla cellular development. Program expansion by 2004 will include the recruitment of six investigators with genetic, cellular, and molecular expertise to address mechanistic based questions in the general areas of (i) hedgehog signaling events in lineage specification, (ii) Stem cell plasticity, (iii) transplantation biology, (iv) non-murine models of development, (v) cellular physiology and molecular pharmacology, and (vi) genomics and proteomics. **Frmly:** Neurodegeneration Research Group.

**★ 14212 ★ Johns Hopkins University Alzheimer's Disease Research Center**
558 Ross Research Bldg.
School of Medicine
720 Rutland Ave.
Baltimore, MD 21205-2196
**Phone:** (410)955-5632          **Fax:** (410)955-9777
**Email:** adrc@jhmi.edu
**Website:** http://www.alzresearch.org
Dr. Donald L. Price, Dir.
**Activities/Fields:** Alzheimer's disease, including basic and applied studies of cognitive symptons and psychiatric problems. **Pub:** *Family Guidelines Series*.

**★ 14213 ★ Johns Hopkins University Baltimore Huntington's Disease Center**
Meyer, 2-181
Johns Hopkins Hospital
600 N Wolfe St.
Baltimore, MD 21287
**Phone:** (410)955-2398          **Fax:** (410)955-8233
Dr. Christopher A. Ross, Dir.
**Activities/Fields:** Huntington's Disease (HD), a hereditary brain disorder and the gene which carries it. Both clinical and basic research programs are conducted by faculty from Johns Hopkins Medical Institutions, Departments of Psychiatry, Neurology, Pathology, Biomedical Engineering, Neuroradiology, Pharmacology, Neuroscience, Biostatistics, and Genetics. **Pub:** *A Physicians Guide to the Management of Huntington's Disease.*

**★ 14214 ★ Johns Hopkins University**
**Center for Inherited Neurovascular**
**Diseases (CIND)**
Meyer 5-181
Johns Hopkins Hospital
600 N Wolfe St.
Baltimore, MD 21287
**Phone:** (410)955-1099          **Fax:** (410)955-9126
**Email:** hrich@jhmi.edu
**Website:** http://www.cind.org
Heather Rich, Contact

**Activities/Fields:** Genetic forms of neurovascular diseases, especially determining which genes are responsible for selected forms of neurovascular disease.


**★ 14215 ★ Johns Hopkins University**
**Epilepsy Research Laboratory (ERL)**
Meyer 2-147
Department of Neurology
School of Medicine
600 N Wolfe St.
Baltimore, MD 21287
**Website:** http://erl.neuro.jhmi.edu
Prof. Piotr J. Franaszczuk, PhD, Contact

**Activities/Fields:** Epilepsy, including the localization of seizure onset in patients, analysis of dynamics of seizure spread in time and space, modeling of seizure dynamics and propagation, and detection of nonstationary signals.


**★ 14216 ★ Johns Hopkins University**
**Laboratory for Computational Motor**
**Control**
416 Traylor Bldg.
Department of Biomedical Engineering
School of Medicine
720 Rutland Ave.
Baltimore, MD 21205-2195
**Phone:** (410)614-3424          **Fax:** (410)614-9890
**Email:** reza@bme.jhu.edu
**Website:** http://www.bme.jhu.edu/~reza/research_page.html
Dr. Reza Shadmehr, PhD, Contact

**Activities/Fields:** The brain and how it controls movements of the arm, particularly how does the brain learn this control; how is the information represented; what parts of the brain are involved in storing the representation and does this change with time; and can damage to the brain affect the ability to learn control. **Frmly:** Laboratory for Human Motor Learning.


**Johns Hopkins University**
**Research and Training Center for Hearing**
**and Balance**
**Auditory Neurophysiology Laboratory**
*See:* Entry 6152


**★ 14217 ★ Johns Hopkins University**
**Research and Training Center for Hearing**
**and Balance**
**Laboratory of Vestibular Neurophysiology**
Johns Hopkins Outpatient Center, Rm. 6253
601 N Caroline St.
Baltimore, MD 21287-0910
**Phone:** (410)955-3403          **Fax:** (410)955-0035
**Email:** lminor@jhmi.edu
**Website:** http://www.bme.jhu.edu/labs/chb/labs/neurophys.html
Dr. Lloyd B. Minor, Dir.

**Activities/Fields:** Neurophysiological mechanisms that control vestibulo-ocular reflexes; development of new diagnostic and treatment modalities applicable to patients with vestibular disorders. **Pub:** *Working papers.*


**Johns Hopkins University**
**Research and Training Center for Hearing**
**and Balance**
**Neural Encoding Laboratory**
*See:* Entry 6153


**★ 14218 ★ Johns Hopkins University**
**Sleep Disorders Center**
Asthma & Allergy Center
Johns Hopkins Bayview Medical Center
5501 Hopkins Bayview Cir.
Baltimore, MD 21224
**Phone:** (410)550-0571          **Fax:** (410)550-2612
**Email:** p.l.smith@welch.jhu.edu
**Website:** http://www.bme.jhu.edu/labs/chb/labs/neural_enc.html
Philip L. Smith, MD, Dir.

**Activities/Fields:** Sleep-related disorders. Studies focus on disorders of daytime hypersomnolence, including narcolepsy, periodic leg movements, psychiatric illness, and sleep apnea; disorder-causing insomnia, psychiatric illness, shift work, and sleep apnea; and disruptive sleep patterns, loud snoring, nocturnal seizures, nocturnal terrors, and sleep walking. Also investigates male erectile impotence, using sleep recordings as a diagnostic tool.


**★ 14219 ★ Johns Hopkins University**
**Zanvyl Krieger Mind/Brain Institute**
Krieger Bldg., Rm. 338
3400 N Charles St.
Baltimore, MD 21218-2685
**Phone:** (410)516-8640          **Fax:** (410)516-8648
**Email:** kenneth.johnson@jhu.edu
**Website:** http://www.mb.jhu.edu
Dr. Kenneth Johnson, MD, Dir.

**Activities/Fields:** Fundamental activities of the human mind, including learning and the use of language, initiation of action and perception, and nervous system plasticity and regeneration. Attempts to address the basic questions of how consciousness is possible and how mind and brain are related.


**★ 14220 ★ Kennedy Krieger Institute**
**Blood-Brain Barrier Laboratory**
707 N Broadway
Baltimore, MD 21205
**Phone:** (410)502-9483          **Free:** 888-554-2080
**Fax:** (410)502-9524
**Email:** goldstein@kennedykrieger.org
Dr. Gary W. Goldstein, Dir.

**Activities/Fields:** Molecular aspects of brain microvessel differentiation, cell-cell signaling, second messengers, and transport systems. Investigates the effects of lead poisoning.


**★ 14221 ★ Laboratory for Research on**
**the Neuroscience of Autism (RNA)**
8110 La Jolla Shores Dr., Ste. 201
La Jolla, CA 92037
**Phone:** (858)551-7925          **Fax:** (858)551-7931
**Email:** ecourchesne@ucsd.edu
**Website:** http://nodulus.extern.ucsd.edu
Eric Courchesne, PhD, Dir.

**Activities/Fields:** Neurophysiological and neuroanatomical basis for autism, including the functional role of the cerebellum in cognition, the brain bases of selective attention, and the neuropsychological consequences of stroke. **Frmly:** Autism and Brain Development Research Laboratory.


**Laval University**
**Robert Giffard Research Centre**
*See:* Entry 12693


**★ 14222 ★ Loma Linda VA Medical**
**Center**
**Sleep Disorders Center**
11201 Benton St., 111P Sleep
Loma Linda, CA 92357
**Phone:** (909)422-3130          **Fax:** (909)777-3214
**Email:** ralph.downey@med.va.gov
Dr. Ralph Downey, III, Dir.

**Activities/Fields:** Sleep disorders, including sleep apnea, insomnia, and narcolepsy.


**★ 14223 ★ Louisiana State University**
**Medical Center**
**Neuroscience Center of Excellence**
2020 Gravier St., Ste. D
New Orleans, LA 70112
**Phone:** (504)599-0909          **Fax:** (504)568-5801
**Email:** nbazan@lsumc.edu
**Website:** http://www.neuroscience.lsumc.edu
Dr. Nicolas G. Bazan, Dir.

**Activities/Fields:** Interdisciplinary unit studying clinical and basic neuroscience.


**Mailman Research Center**
*See:* Entry 4655


**★ 14224 ★ Massachusetts Alzheimer's**
**Disease Research Center**
WAC 830
Massachusetts General Hospital
15 Parkman St.
Boston, MA 02114
**Phone:** (617)726-3987          **Fax:** (617)726-7718
**Email:** growdon@helix.mgh.edu
**Website:** http://spauldingrehab.mgh.harvard.edu/adrc_home/main.html
John H. Growdon, MD, Dir.

**Activities/Fields:** Coordinates research on Alzheimer's disease, including memory loss, dementia, neuropathology, neuropsychology, neurochemistry, and investigational drug studies. Projects focus on biochemical studies on the abnormal proteins that accumulate in the brains of Alzheimer's patients, possible genetic markers or familial traits, anatomical and neurotransmitter abnormalities, and clinical studies of behavior and neuropharmacology.


**★ 14225 ★ Massachusetts Institute of**
**Technology**
**Center for Biological and Computational**
**Learning**
Department of Brain & Cognitive Science
45 Carleton St.
Cambridge, MA 02142
**Phone:** (617)253-5230          **Fax:** (617)253-2964
**Email:** tp@ai.mit.edu
**Website:** http://www.ai.mit.edu/projects/cbcl/web-homepage/web-homepage.html
Tomaso Poggio, PhD, Co-Dir.

**Activities/Fields:** Investigates mathematics of statistical learning, its engineering applications and the mechanisms of biological information processing. Studies focus on machine and human learning, vision, object recognition, bioinformatics, information search and retrieval.


**★ 14226 ★ Massachusetts Institute of**
**Technology**
**Laboratory of Neuroendocrine Regulation**
Bldg. E25-604
Cambridge, MA 02139
**Phone:** (617)253-6731          **Fax:** (617)253-6882
**Email:** dick@mit.edu
Dr. Richard J. Wurtman, Dir.

**Activities/Fields:** Pineal gland and effects of drugs, nutrients, and hormones on brain neurotransmitters and behavior. Specific studies include utilization of choline for acetylcholine and membrane phosphatidylcholine synthesis in cultured neuroblastoma cells and in rat brain; neurotransmitter receptors and second messengers that modulate these two syntheses; interactions of precursor availability (tyrosine and tryptophan) and firing frequency in controlling neurotransmitter (catecholamines and serotonin) release from superfused rat brain slices; effects of tyrosine on catecholamine release from isolated retina; effects of supplemental tyrosine on capacity to withstand stress, sustain motor activity, and perform complex tasks; control of melatonin secretion in rats; mechanisms by which melatonin acts on neurons and induces sleep; aberrant patterns of melatonin secretion in aging and human diseases; effects of macronutrients (carbohydrates and proteins) on brain serotonin synthesis; involvement of serotoninergic neurons in appetite, mood, pain sensitivity, and various appetitive diseases; selective effects of serotoninergic drugs on nutrient selection; Alzheimer's disease; control of APP metabolism by neurotransmitters; and brain phospholipid synthesis; production and maintenance of sleep in humans by melatonin; use of CDP-Choline to treat brain injury or stroke.

★ 14227 ★ **McGill University**
**Centre for Research in Neuroscience**
Montreal General Hospital Research Institute
1650 Cedar Ave.
Montreal, QC, Canada H3G 1A4
**Phone:** (514)937-6011　　　　**Fax:** (514)934-8250
**Email:** info@uro.mcgill.ca
**Website:** http://www.mcgill.ca/mgh/
Dr. Albert J. Aguayo, Dir.

**Activities/Fields:** Studies in neuroscience, particularly in cellular and molecular approaches to the nervous system with emphasis on neural development, regeneration, and neuroendocrine function. Research methodologies include recombinant DNA and classical neuroanatomical and electrophysiological techniques.

★ 14228 ★ **McGill University**
**Laboratory of Neurotoxicology**
Montreal Neurological Institute
3801 University St.
Montreal, QC, Canada H3A 2B4
**Phone:** (514)398-8509　　　**Fax:** (514)398-1509
**Email:** mddm@musica.mcgill.ca
Dr. Heather Durham, Contact

**Activities/Fields:** Neurodegenerative diseases, neurotoxicology, and neurobiology; the biological basis of motor neuron diseases; cell culture models of motor neuron diseases, including amyotrophic lateral sclerosis and toxic neuropathies; and therapy of motor neuron diseases.

★ 14229 ★ **McGill University**
**McConnell Brain Imaging Centre**
3801 University St.
Montreal, QC, Canada H3A 2B4
**Phone:** (514)398-8925　　　　**Fax:** (514)398-8948
**Email:** alan@bic.mni.mcgill.ca
**Website:** http://www.bic.mni.mcgill.ca/bic_welcome.html
Alan C. Evans, PhD, Coord.

**Activities/Fields:** Investigates cerebral function using positron emission tomography (PET) and magnetic resonance imaging (MRI) on healthy volunteers and patients with brain tumors, epilepsy, movement disorders, and other acute and chronic neurological illnesses. Research areas include radiochemistry, imaging physics, mapping of cognitive functions in the brain, kinetic analysis, and modeling of biological systems. **Pub:** *NeuroPIL Bulletin*, monthly.

★ 14230 ★ **McGill University**
**Montreal Neurological Institute**
3801 University St., Rm. 636
Montreal, QC, Canada H3A 2B4
**Phone:** (514)398-1903　　　　**Fax:** (514)398-8248
**Email:** director@mni.lan.mcgill.ca
**Website:** http://www.mcgill.ca/mni
Dr. Richard Murphy, Dir.

**Activities/Fields:** Organic aspects of the nervous system, including studies in molecular neurobiology, neuroanatomy, cerebrovascular disease, neurochemistry, epilepsy, neurogenetics, neuroimaging, neuroimmunology, movement disorders, neuromuscular research, neuro-oncology, neuropharmacology, and neuropsychology. **Pub:** *Annual Report.* • *Neuro Magazine.*

**McGill University**
**Montreal Neurological Institute**
**Brain Tumour Research Centre**
*See:* Entry 10372

★ 14231 ★ **McGill University**
**Montreal Neurological Institute**
**Complex Neural Systems**
3801 University St.
Montreal, QC, Canada H3A 2B4
**Phone:** (514)398-1913　　　　**Fax:** (514)398-5871
**Website:** http://www.mni.mcgill.ca/brain.htm
Dr. B.E. Jones, Coord.

**Activities/Fields:** Neurobiology. **Frmly:** Neurobiology Unit.

★ 14232 ★ **McGill University**
**Spinal Cord Research Group**
McIntyre Medical Sciences Bldg., Rm. 1242
3655 Drummond St.
Montreal, QC, Canada H3G 1Y6
**Email:** ydk@pinalcord.mcgill.ca
**Website:** http://www.spinalcord.mcgill.ca/
Yves De Koninck, PhD, Prin. Investigator

**Activities/Fields:** Structural and functional aspects of the dorsal horn of the mammalian spinal cord. Research interests include neurotrophic factor therapy, neuronal plasticity in basic pharmacology and biophysics of synaptic transmission.

★ 14233 ★ **MCP Hahnemann University**
**of the Health Sciences**
**Center for Neurobiology**
3300 Henry Ave.
Philadelphia, PA 19129
**Phone:** (215)842-4600
Dr. Donald S. Faber, Dir.

**Activities/Fields:** Biological bases of neurological disorders. Research encompasses development, systems and behavioral neurobiology, neuronal degeneration and synaptic plasticity, motor disorders, and the biology of substance abuse.

★ 14234 ★ **MCP Hahnemann University**
**of the Health Sciences**
**Center for Neurosciences Research**
Allegheny General Hospital, South Tower, 8th Fl.
320 E North Ave.
Pittsburgh, PA 15212
**Phone:** (412)359-3235　　　　**Fax:** (412)359-4499
**Email:** rubin@wpahs.org
Robert T. Rubin, MD, Dir.

**Activities/Fields:** Psychobiology of depression. **Frmly:** Neurosciences Research Center.

★ 14235 ★ **MCP Hahnemann University**
**of the Health Sciences**
**Computer Vision Center for Vertebrate**
**Brain Mapping**
Department of Biology and Anatomy
2900 Queen Ln.
Philadelphia, PA 19104
**Phone:** (215)991-8410　　　　**Fax:** (215)843-9367
Dr. Jonathan Nissanov, Dir.

**Activities/Fields:** Algorithms for use in basic biological research with emphasis on the methodological needs of nurobiology, with the overall emphasis on quantitative imaging. Current research projects include artificial intelligence techniques for pattern recognition and automated parcellation of brain structures; quantificaion techniques for analysis of microautoradiograms; correction methods for the differential H-3 quenching between white- and gray-matter; and development of new quantitative descriptors of distribution. **Frmly:** Autoradiographic Image Processing Center.

★ 14236 ★ **MCP Hahnemann University**
**of the Health Sciences**
**Mid Atlantic Regional Epilepsy Center**
3300 Henry Ave.
Philadelphia, PA 19129
**Phone:** (215)842-7706　　　　**Fax:** (215)848-2035
**Email:** mercedes.jacobson@drexel.edu
Dr. Mercedes Jacobson, Dir.

**Activities/Fields:** Epileptic seizure detection, including seizure detection apparatus studies.

★ 14237 ★ **MCP Hahnemann University**
**of the Health Sciences**
**Movement Disorders Center**
Mail Stop 423
Neurology Department
Broad & Vine St.
Philadelphia, PA 19102
**Phone:** (215)762-1350　　　　**Fax:** (215)762-3161
**Email:** sa34@drexel.edu
Dr. Azizi, Med. Advisor

**Activities/Fields:** Huntington's disease (HD), a hereditary brain disorder, including neuropsychological and electrophysiological studies, psychological problems in HD families, cultured fibroblasts in HD, and miscellaneous chemical studies in HD. Acts as a focal point for the development and support of various regional research projects concerned with Huntington's disease and other genetically determined disorders of the nervous system. **Frmly:** Allegheny University of the Health Sciences; Huntington's Disease Diagnostic and Referral Center.

★ 14238 ★ **Medical College of Georgia**
**Alzheimer's Research Center for Clinical**
**and Basic Research**
Department of Pharmacology & Toxicology
Augusta, GA 30912-2300
**Phone:** (706)721-6355　　　　**Fax:** (706)721-9861
**Email:** jbuccafu@mail.mcg.edu
**Website:** http://www.mcg.edu/centers/alz
Dr. Jerry J. Buccafusco, Dir.

**Activities/Fields:** Multidisciplinary research on all aspects of Alzheimer's disease, including new therapeutic approaches, diagnostic procedures, and basic studies of etiology.

★ 14239 ★ **Monell Chemical Senses**
**Center**
3500 Market St.
Philadelphia, PA 19104-3308
**Phone:** (215)898-6666　　　　**Fax:** (215)898-2084
**Email:** beauchamp@monell.org
**Website:** http://www.monell.org
Dr. Gary K. Beauchamp, Dir.

**Activities/Fields:** Mechanisms and functions of the chemical senses (taste, smell) and chemesthesis, chemical irritation, including studies in the areas of biochemistry, biophysics, endocrinology, physiology, ethology, neurology, behavior, genetics, psychophysics, nutrition, organic chemistry, chemical ecology, and zoology. Research relates to solutions of problems in nutrition, environmental odors, reproduction, disease diagnosis, expansion of world food supply, and alternative means of vertebrate pest control. Projects focus on biochemistry of receptor mechanisms, sensory qualities of food, role of early diet in shaping food preferences, relationship between chemosensory function and nutritional and disease states, role of body volatiles in disease diagnosis, methods of altering salt preference, role of taste and smell in food utilization, effect of aging on taste and smell, information processing in taste and smell, diagnosis and treatment of taste and smell disorders, and genetic influence on production and detection of chemostimulants. **Pub:** *The Monell Connection Newsletter.*

★ 14240 ★ **Monell-Jefferson Taste and Smell Research Center**
925 Chestnut St., 6th Fl.
Philadelphia, PA 19107
**Phone:** (215)955-5652      **Fax:** (215)923-4532
**Email:** info@monell.org
**Website:** http://www.monell.org
Beverly J. Cowart, PhD, Clin. Dir.

**Activities/Fields:** Smell and taste disorders using a multidisciplinary approach (psychophysical, biophysical, medical, and dental).

★ 14241 ★ **Mount Sinai School of Medicine of City University of New York**
**Alzheimer's Disease Research Center**
Department of Psychiatry, Box 1230
1 Gustave Levy Pl.
New York, NY 10029
**Phone:** (212)241-8329      **Fax:** (212)996-0987
**Email:** adriana.dimatteo@mssm.edu
Adriana Dimatteo, Contact

**Activities/Fields:** Etiology, diagnosis, and treatment of Alzheimer's disease and related dementias. Clinical studies include trials of new drugs and biological markers and longitudinal follow-up studies. An active autopsy network obtains brain material from Alzheimer patients.

★ 14242 ★ **Mount Sinai School of Medicine of City University of New York**
**Computational Neurobiology and Imaging Center (CNIC)**
1 Gustave L. Levy Pl.
New York, NY 10029
**Phone:** (212)241-5018
**Email:** scott.henderson@mssm.edu
**Website:** http://www.mssm.edu/cnic/
Scott Henderson, PhD, Contact

**Activities/Fields:** Relationships between neural function and structure at levels ranging from the molecular and cellular, through network organization of the brain.

★ 14243 ★ **Mount Sinai Spinal Cord Injury Model System**
1 Gustave Levy Pl., Box 1240
New York, NY 10029-6574
**Phone:** (212)659-9369      **Fax:** (212)348-5901
**Email:** marcel.dijkers@mssm.edu
**Website:** http://www.mssm.edu/rehab/spinal/
Marcel Dijkers, PhD, Dir. of Res.

**Activities/Fields:** Spinal cord injuries.

★ 14244 ★ **National Coalition for Research in Neurological Disorders**
1250 24th St. NW, Ste. 300
Washington, DC 20037
**Phone:** (202)293-5453      **Fax:** (202)466-0585
**Email:** hoffheimer@aol.com
**Website:** http://www.brainnet.org
Lawrence S. Hoffheimer, Dir.

**Activities/Fields:** Neurological research, focusing on funding. Also lobbies for increased funding for training and research.

★ 14245 ★ **National Science Foundation Directorate for Biological Sciences Division of Integrative Biology and Neuroscience**
**Developmental Neuroscience Program**
4201 Wilson Blvd., Rm. 685
Arlington, VA 22230
**Phone:** (703)292-8423      **Fax:** (703)292-9153
**Email:** hvaessin@nsf.gov
**Website:** http://www.nsf.gov/bio/ibn/ibnneuro.htmde
Elizabeth B. Bell, Prog. and Tech. Anal.

**Activities/Fields:** Supports research on the factors that influence the formation, growth, and aging of the nervous system; how neurons and glia differentiate and regenerate; how connections between neurons are formed and maintained; and the interactions of environmental and genetic factors in neural development.

★ 14246 ★ **National Science Foundation Directorate for Biological Sciences Division of Integrative Biology and Neuroscience**
**Neuroscience Program**
4201 Wilson Blvd., Rm. 685
Arlington, VA 22230
**Phone:** (703)292-8420      **Fax:** (703)292-9153
Dr. Soq Siang, Dir.

**Activities/Fields:** Neuroscience.

★ 14247 ★ **Neuropsychiatric Research Institute**
700 1st Ave. S
Fargo, ND 58103
**Phone:** (701)293-1335      **Fax:** (701)293-3226
**Email:** mail@nrifargo.com
**Website:** http://www.nrifargo.com/
James E. Mitchell, MD, Pres.

**Activities/Fields:** Basic and clinical studies of the central nervous system. Specific applications include eating disorders and stroke. **Pub:** *Newsletter (semiannual).*

★ 14248 ★ **The Neurosciences Institute**
10640 John Jay Hopkins Dr.
San Diego, CA 92121
**Phone:** (858)626-2000      **Fax:** (858)626-2099
**Email:** info@nsi.edu
**Website:** http://www.nsi.edu
W. Einar Gall, Res. Dir.

**Activities/Fields:** Promotes conceptual and theoretical progress in understanding the function of the nervous system at all levels, particularly higher functions of the brain (perception, memory, sensation) and their implications in understanding human behavior. A research program for resident Institute Fellows in theoretical neurobiology provides training in methods used to construct neural theories and develops theoretical models of neural systems that are biologically sound and experimentally testable at synaptic, cellular, and network levels. The Institute also conducts a research program in experimental neurobiology. The Institute provides opportunities for visiting scientists to interact in modes that would not ordinarily be possible in their home laboratories. Visiting in small groups or individually for periods from several days to several months, scientists design experiments, discuss research questions with experts in other fields, and share information about recent findings. **Pub:** *Edited Volumes.* • *Monographs Series.*

★ 14249 ★ **New England Medical Center Hospitals, Inc.**
**Electromyography Laboratory**
Neurology Department EMG, Box 314
750 Washington St.
Boston, MA 02111
**Phone:** (617)636-5848      **Fax:** (617)636-8199
Dr. William Brown, Dir.

**Activities/Fields:** Electrical studies of nerves and muscles to aid in the research and diagnosis of muscular dystrophy, amyotrophic lateral sclerosis, and other polyneuropathies.

**New York State Psychiatric Institute**
*See:* Entry 12705

★ 14250 ★ **New York University Center for Neural Science**
4 Washington Pl., Rm. 809
New York, NY 10003
**Phone:** (212)998-7780      **Fax:** (212)995-4011
**Email:** sanes@nyu.edu
**Website:** http://www.cns.nyu.edu
Dan Sanes, Dir.

**Activities/Fields:** Neural science studies, ranging from molecular and cellular aspects to fully integrated systems and cognitive approaches. Specific research includes cell biological mechanisms underlying plasticity and stability of neurons; new sprout formation by adult mammalian neurons; drive and hedonic mechanisms in the brain and how they interact; use of image analysis procedures to study the functional anatomy of sensorimotor integration in the rat brain; neural processes that generate movements; genetic and molecular manipulations in the fruit fly to study the interplay between plasticity and programming in the nervous system; amino acid regulation of dopamine utilization under basal and stress conditions using a variety of techniques, including in vivo microdialysis; individual neurons in visual perception; magnetic fields accompanying the flow of currents within the brain's neurons; effects of developmental visual disorders on the structure and function of the visual system; problems of color vision using both psychophysical and electrophysical techniques; modeling of the human visual system; identification of the neural systems and cellular mechanisms used by the brain to assign emotional significance to sensory stimuli; the acquisition of color information, fusion of visual information from multiple sources, signal detection theory, and visual calibration; analysis of functional properties of neurons; and mathematical and computational models of complex behaviors.

★ 14251 ★ **New York University Jerry Lewis Neuromuscular Disease Center**
Department of Rehabilitation Medicine
400 E 34th St., Rm. RG 29
New York, NY 10016
**Phone:** (212)263-6350      **Fax:** (212)263-5499
Dr. Mathew Lee, Chm.

**Activities/Fields:** Diagnosis and clinical care of patients disabled by neuromuscular disease.

**New York University Medical Center Head Trauma Program**
*See:* Entry 20198

★ 14252 ★ **New York University Medical Center**
**Nathan Kline Institute for Psychiatric Research**
**Center for Alzheimer's Disease Research**
140 Old Orangeburg Rd.
Orangeburg, NY 10962
**Phone:** (845)398-5423      **Fax:** (845)398-5422
**Email:** nixon@nki.rfmh.org
**Website:** http://www.rfmh.org/nki
Dr. Ralph Nixon, Dir.

**Activities/Fields:** Molecular neuroscience and aging, including molecular neurobiology of proteases, signal transduction, neurodegenerative disease, protein/peptide analytical techniques, molecular genetics, vesicle biology, transgenic modeling.

★ 14253 ★ **Northern California Regional Spinal Cord Injury System**
Santa Clara Valley Medical Center
950 S Bascom Ave., Ste. 2011
San Jose, CA 95128
**Phone:** (408)295-9896      **Free:** 800-352-1956
**Fax:** (408)295-9913
**Email:** tamara@tbi-sci.org
**Website:** http://www.tbi-sci.org/
Dr. Tamara Bushnik, Prin. Investigator

**Activities/Fields:** Spinal cord injuries. **Pub:** *InterAct newsletter.*

**★ 14254 ★ Northern New Jersey Spinal Cord Injury System (NNJSCIS)**
Kessler Medical Rehabilitation Research & Education Corp.
1199 Pleasant Valley Way
West Orange, NJ 07052
**Phone:** (973)243-6849      **Free:** 800-248-3221
**Fax:** (973)324-3527
**Email:** dtulsky@kmrrec.org
**Website:** http://www.kmrrec.org/nnjscis
David Tulsky, Contact
**Activities/Fields:** Spinal cord injuries.


**★ 14255 ★ Northwestern University Institute for Neuroscience**
320 E Superior St.
Chicago, IL 60611
**Phone:** (312)503-4300      **Fax:** (312)503-7345
**Email:** e-mugnaini@northwestern.edu
**Website:** http://www.northwestern.edu/nuin/
Dr. Enrico Mugnaini, Dir.
**Activities/Fields:** Sensory neurobiology and psychophysics, neuroendocrinology, biological rhythms, neurobiology of disease, cytoskeleton, motor control mechanisms, cognitive and computational neuroscience, neural development and plasticity, electrophysiology and pharmacology of excitable membranes, and neuroimmunology and virology. **Pub:** *Newsletter*, annually.


**Ohio State University Laboratory of Psychobiology**
*See:* Entry 12707


**★ 14256 ★ Ohio State University Sleep Disorders Center**
Rhodes Hall, Rm. S1039
410 W 10th
Columbus, OH 43210
**Phone:** (614)293-8822      **Fax:** (614)293-4506
**Email:** pollak.7@osu.edu
Dr. Charles Pollak, Dir.
**Activities/Fields:** Diagnosis of impotence, applications of pharmaceutical agents in depression and other psychiatric disorders in adults, and disorders of sleep and arousal. Techniques include psychometric laboratory evaluation, monitoring sleep/awake disorders by all-night polysomnographic recordings, penile tumescence studies, multiple sleep latency studies, and electronic pupillometry. **Frmly:** Psychiatry and Sleep Disorders Center.


**★ 14257 ★ Oregon Health and Science University Neurological Sciences Institute**
West Campus
505 NW 185th Ave.
Beaverton, OR 97006
**Phone:** (503)418-2500      **Fax:** (503)418-2501
**Website:** http://www.ohsu.edu/nsi/
Paul J. Cordo, PhD, Dir.
**Activities/Fields:** Structure and function of the nervous system, from the level of the molecule to the level of the brain and sensory organs. Research focuses on balance and dizziness disorders, Alzheimer's and Parkinson's diseases, stroke, memory loss, multiple sclerosis, blindness, as well as a number of other neurological disorders. **Pub:** *Annual Report.* • *NSI Newsletter.*


**★ 14258 ★ Oregon Health and Science University**
**Oregon Aging and Alzheimer's Disease Center (OADC)**
Department of Neurology, CR 131
3181 SW Sam Jackson Park Rd.
Portland, OR 97201-3098
**Phone:** (503)494-6976
**Email:** kaye@ohsu.edu

**Website:** http://www.ohsu.edu/som-alzheimers/
Jeffrey Kaye, MD, Co-Dir.
**Activities/Fields:** Aging and neurodegenerative diseases.


**Oregon Health and Science University**
**Oregon Center for Complementary and Alternative Medicine Research in Neurological Disorders**
*See:* Entry 4334


**★ 14259 ★ Paralyzed Veterans of America**
**Spinal Cord Research Foundation (SCRF)**
801 18th St. NW
Washington, DC 20006-3517
**Phone:** (202)416-7651      **Free:** 800-424-8200
**Fax:** (202)416-7641
**Email:** scrf@pva.org
**Website:** http://www.pva.org
**Activities/Fields:** Clinical, psychosocial, and technological aspects of spinal cord injury or dysfunction.


**★ 14260 ★ Parkinson's Institute**
1170 Morse Ave.
Sunnyvale, CA 94089-1605
**Phone:** (408)734-2800      **Free:** 800-786-2958
**Fax:** (408)734-8522
**Website:** http://www.parkinsonsinstitute.org
Dr. J. William Langston, CEO
**Activities/Fields:** Cause and cure of movement disorders, identification of better treatment and diagnostic tools, and development of prevention strategies.


**★ 14261 ★ Parkinson's and Movement Disorder Institute (PMDI)**
9940 Talbert Ave., Ste. 204
Fountain Valley, CA 92708
**Phone:** (714)378-5062      **Fax:** (714)378-5061
**Email:** dtruong@pmdi.org
**Website:** http://www.pmdi.org/pmdi.html
Dr. Daniel D. Truong, Contact
**Activities/Fields:** Parkinson's disease and movement disorders such as dystonia, myoclonus, tremor, and chorea.


**★ 14262 ★ Princeton University Cutaneous Communication Laboratory**
Green Hall
Psychology Department
Princeton, NJ 08544-1010
**Phone:** (609)258-5277      **Fax:** (609)258-1113
**Email:** rcholewi@princeton.edu
**Website:** http://www.princeton.edu/~pucclabs
Dr. Roger W. Cholewiak, Prin. Investigator
**Activities/Fields:** Sensory psychophysiology and experimental psychology, including experimental investigations in all phases of cutaneous sensitivity with special reference to utilization of data in communication systems, under conditions of sensory handicap, or when other sensory modalities are overloaded. Research includes studies of pattern recognition and discrimination with psychophysical procedures and scaling techniques, including multidimensional designs; more elementary dimensions of tactile experience; and the interrelations of various dimensions of touch. **Pub:** *Reports of Princeton Cutaneous Research Project*, semiannually.


**★ 14263 ★ Rehabilitation Institute of Toronto**
**Sleep Research Laboratory**
550 University Ave.
Toronto, ON, Canada M5G 2A2
**Phone:** (416)597-3078      **Fax:** (416)597-8959
Dr. T. Douglas Bradley, Dir.
**Activities/Fields:** Disturbances of breathing during sleep, including the mechanisms underlying sleep apnea disorders and possible treatments. Projects

include research on breathing and oxygenation during sleep in patients with congestive heart failure in whom heart failure may be related to, or aggravated by, nocturnal ventilatory disturbances. The effects of treating nocturnal ventilatory disturbances on heart function are being tested.


**★ 14264 ★ Research and Training Center on Community Integration of Individuals With Traumatic Brain Injury**
Mount Sinai Medical Center
1 Gustave L Levy Pl., Box 1240
New York, NY 10029
**Phone:** (212)241-5152      **Free:** 888-241-5752
**Fax:** (212)348-5901
**Email:** teresa_ashman@mssm.edu
**Website:** http://academic.mssm.edu/tbinet/
Dr. Wayne Gordon, Prin. Investigator
**Activities/Fields:** Community integration of traumatic brain injury (TBI) survivors, including increasing understanding of how TBI affects community integration, developing new models of community integration, and treating cognitive/behavioral disorders that most affect the TBI survivor's functioning within the community. **Pub:** *Consumer reports.* • *TBI-NET.* • *Tools for Community Living: A Handbook for Survivors of Traumatic Brain Injury.*


**★ 14265 ★ Rockefeller University Fisher Center for Research on Alzheimer's Disease**
1230 York Ave.
New York, NY 10021
**Phone:** (212)327-7746      **Fax:** (212)327-7746
**Email:** greengd@mail.rockefeller.edu
**Website:** http://www.rockefeller.edu/graduate/cenzach.htm
Prof. Paul Greengard, Dir.
**Activities/Fields:** Alzheimer's disease, including how brain cells process the amyloid precursor phosphoprotein (APP) leading to the production of b-amlyoid, a major component of the plaques that are a hallmark of Alzheimer's disease.


**★ 14266 ★ Rockefeller University Laboratory of Neuroendocrinology**
1230 York Ave.
PO Box 165
New York, NY 10021-6399
**Phone:** (212)327-8624      **Fax:** (212)327-8634
**Email:** mcewen@rockvax.rockefeller.edu
Dr. Bruce S. McEwen, Hd.
**Activities/Fields:** Seeks to locate brain sites and understand the mechanisms by which hormones promote neural plasticity and thereby alter endocrine function, behavior, neurological states, and mood. Also studies the influence of gonadal and adrenal hormones on aging in the brain.


**★ 14267 ★ Rush University Biological Rhythms Research Laboratory**
Rush-Presbyterian-St. Luke's Medical Center
1645 W Jackson Blvd., Ste. 425
Chicago, IL 60612
**Phone:** (312)850-7788      **Fax:** (312)850-7707
**Email:** ceastman@rush.edu
Charmane Eastman, PhD, Dir.
**Activities/Fields:** Human circadian rhythms, focusing on the use of bright light, and melatonin for adaptation to night shift work, and jet-lag.


**★ 14268 ★ Rush University Multiple Sclerosis Center**
1725 W Harrison St., Ste. 309
Chicago, IL 60612
**Phone:** (312)942-8011      **Fax:** (312)942-2253
Dusan Stefoski, MD, Dir.
**Activities/Fields:** Multiple sclerosis, including understanding of nerve impulse conduction in both normal and pathologic states and pathophysiology of conduc-

tion in multiple sclerosis and allied demyelinating conditions, improving conduction in diseased nerves by pharmacologic therapy, and development of a detailed molecular model of the organization of the ion-specific channels of the nerve membrane. Patient studies include programs in neuroactive drugs, thermolability phenomena, analysis of individual's psychological stresses and the resulting coping mechanisms, and the effect of disease on children of patients and the overall family unit.


**★ 14269 ★ Rush University**
**Rush Alzheimer's Disease Center**
8 North
710 S Paulina
Chicago, IL 60612
**Phone:** (312)942-4463　　**Fax:** (312)942-4154
**Email:** jfox@neuro.rush.edu
Dr. Jacob H. Fox, Co-Dir.

**Activities/Fields:** Alzheimer's disease, including causes, treatment, and cure. Conducts clinical trials of new drug treatments and analyzes potential risk factors in the development of Alzheimer's disease.


**★ 14270 ★ Rush University**
**Rush Neuroscience Institute**
Rush-Presbyterian-St. Luke's Medical Center
1725 W Harrison St.
Chicago, IL 60612
**Phone:** (312)942-8729　　**Fax:** (312)942-2380
**Email:** jfox@rush.edu
Dr. Jacob H. Fox, Chm.

**Activities/Fields:** Alzheimer's disease, Parkinson's disease, and stroke, including community-based studies, clinical investigations, and laboratory investigations using brain tissue and animal experimentation. Studies also focus on development of new drugs to improve symptoms of multiple sclerosis.


**★ 14271 ★ Rutgers University**
**Center for Molecular and Behavioral**
**Neuroscience**
197 University Ave.
Newark, NJ 07102
**Phone:** (973)353-1080　　**Fax:** (973)353-1760
**Email:** tallal@axon.rutgers.edu
**Website:** http://www.cmbn.rutgers.edu/cmbn/cmbn-home.html
Dr. Paula Tallal, Co-Dir.

**Activities/Fields:** Molecular and behavioral neuroscience research for applications to behavioral dysfunctions in humans. Serves as a technology transfer unit between the University and industry.


**★ 14272 ★ Salk Institute for Biological**
**Studies**
**Computational Neurobiology Laboratory**
**(CNL)**
10010 N Torrey Pines Rd.
La Jolla, CA 92037
**Phone:** (858)453-4100
**Email:** terry@salk.edu
**Website:** http://www.cnl.salk.edu/
Dr. Terrence Sejnowski, Contact

**Activities/Fields:** Computational resources of the brain from the biophysical to the systems levels. The central issues being addressed are how dendrites integrate synaptic signals in neurons, how networks of neurons generate dynamical patterns of activity, how sensory information is represented in the cerebral cortex, how memory representations are formed and consolidated during sleep and how visuo-motor transformations are adaptively organized. **Pub:** *Annual report.* • *Papers.*


**Scripps Research Institute**
**Department of Neuropharmacology**
*See:* Entry 17372


**★ 14273 ★ Solomon Park Research**
**Institute**
12815 NE 124th St., Ste. L
Kirkland, WA 98034-8313
**Phone:** (425)650-2020　　**Fax:** (425)650-2028
**Email:** pclapshaw@solomon.org
**Website:** http://www.solomon.org
Patric A. Clapshaw, PhD, Dir.

**Activities/Fields:** Amyotrophic lateral sclerosis (ALS), also known as Lou Gehrig's Disease.


**★ 14274 ★ Southern Illinois University at**
**Carbondale**
**Center for Alzheimer Disease and Related**
**Disorders (CADRD)**
PO Box 19643
Springfield, IL 62794-9643
**Phone:** (217)545-8249　　**Fax:** (217)545-1903
**Email:** neuro@siumed.edu
**Website:** http://www.siumed.edu/neuro/cadrd.html
Rodger J. Elble, PhD, Dir.

**Activities/Fields:** Aging, Alzheimer's Disease, Parkinson's Disease, vascular dementia, and gait disturbances in the elderly.


**★ 14275 ★ Stanford University**
**Center for Research on Sleep and**
**Circadian Rhythm**
701 Welch Rd., Ste. 2226
Palo Alto, CA 94304
**Phone:** (650)723-8134　　**Fax:** (650)725-7341
**Website:** http://www.sleepquest.com
Dr. William C. Dement, Dir.

**Activities/Fields:** Sleep, including brain mechanisms which control transitions between sleep and wakefulness, transitions between sleep states, and the circadian timing between those various states.


**★ 14276 ★ Stanford University**
**Stanford Pain Management Service**
300 Pasteur Dr., Rm. A408
Stanford, CA 94305
**Phone:** (650)723-6238　　**Fax:** (650)725-7743
**Email:** gaeta@stanford.edu
**Website:** http://paincenter.stanford.edu/main.html
Raymond Gaeta, MD, Dir.

**Activities/Fields:** Pain mechanisms, actions of analgesic substances, and pharmacokinetic and pharmacodynamic modeling.


**★ 14277 ★ State University of New York**
**at Albany**
**Center for Neuroscience Research**
Biology 121
1400 Washington Ave.
Albany, NY 12222
**Phone:** (518)442-4309　　**Fax:** (518)442-4767
**Email:** js213@cnsunix.albany.edu
**Website:** http://www.albany.edu/neuron/center/
John T. Schmidt, Dir.

**Activities/Fields:** Nervous system, particularly neuroplasticity, including the development and plasticity of the nervous system and factors that underlie and influence neurodegeneration and/or behavior. The center investigates the formation of synaptic connections in many different animals and examines how neurons make connections, how excess connections are removed, how neurons recover from damage, and how such neural connections modulate or control behavior. These research approaches are relevant for such problems as Alzheimer's Disease, epilepsy, strabismus, amblyopia, amyotrophic lateral sclerosis, Parkinson's disease and jet lag.


**★ 14278 ★ State University of New York**
**Health Science Center at Brooklyn**
**Neurodynamic Laboratory**
Department of Psychiatry
450 Clarkson Ave., Box 1203
Brooklyn, NY 11203

**Phone:** (718)270-2024　　**Fax:** (718)270-4081
**Email:** hb@cns.hscbklyn.edu
Dr. Henri Begleiter, Dir.

**Activities/Fields:** Use of evoked brain potentials to assess central nervous system changes due to alcoholism and drug addiction. **Frmly:** Evoked Potential Laboratory.


**★ 14279 ★ Sun Health Research Institute**
**Christopher Center for Parkinson's**
**Research**
10515 W Santa Fe
Sun City, AZ 85351
**Phone:** (623)876-5439　　**Fax:** (623)876-5695
**Email:** jeffrey.joyce@sunhealth.org
**Website:** http://www.shri.org/parkinson/index.html
Jeffrey N. Joyce, PhD, Sr. Sci.

**Activities/Fields:** Parkinson's disease, focusing on treatment strategies and basic research on causes.


**★ 14280 ★ Sun Health Research Institute**
**L.J. Roberts Center for Alzheimer's**
**Research**
PO Box 1278
Sun City, AZ 85372
**Phone:** (623)876-5328　　**Fax:** (623)876-5461
**Website:** http://www.shri.org/robertalz/index1.html
Dr. Joseph Rogers, Sr. Sci.

**Activities/Fields:** Alzheimer's disease causes and prevention. **Frmly:** Alzheimer's Center.


**★ 14281 ★ Syracuse University**
**Institute for Sensory Research**
621 Skytop Rd.
Syracuse, NY 13244-5290
**Phone:** (315)443-4164　　**Fax:** (315)443-1184
**Email:** bob_smith@isr.syr.edu
Dr. Robert L. Smith, Dir.

**Activities/Fields:** Sensory processes (hearing, vision, and touch) and orofacial biomechanics, using an interdisciplinary approach, including psychophysics, neurophysiology, neurochemistry, anatomy, cell biology, physiology, biosimulation, biomaterials, and orofacial biomechanics. **Frmly:** Bioacoustics Laboratory; Laboratory of Sensory Communication.


**★ 14282 ★ Temple University**
**Center for Neurovirology and Cancer**
**Biology**
BioLife Sciences Bldg.
College of Science & Technology
1900 N 12th St.
Philadelphia, PA 19122
**Phone:** (215)204-0678　　**Fax:** (215)204-0679
**Email:** k.khalili@astro.temple.edu
**Website:** http://www.temple.edu/cnvcb
Dr. Kamel Khalili, Dir.

**Activities/Fields:** Neurologic disorders. **Pub:** *Journal of NeuroVirology.*


**★ 14283 ★ Temple University**
**Center for Neurovirology and Cancer**
**Biology**
**Laboratory of AIDS Pathogenesis and**
**Molecular Therapeutics**
BioLife Sciences Bldg.
College of Science & Technology
1900 N 12th St.
Philadelphia, PA 19122
**Phone:** (215)204-0605　　**Fax:** (215)204-0679
**Email:** jayrapp@astro.temple.edu
**Website:** http://www.temple.edu/cnvcb
Dr. Jay F. Rappaport, Prin. Investigator

**Activities/Fields:** Treatment of viral-induced neurological disorders and brain tumors using a molecular therapeutic strategy featuring RNA and DNA molecules, the molecular pathogenesis of HIV-1 induced neurological disorders, and HIV vaccine development.

**★ 14284 ★ Temple University**
**Center for Neurovirology and Cancer**
**Biology**
**Laboratory of Immunobiology**
BioLife Sciences Bldg.
College of Science & Technology
1900 N 12th St.
Philadelphia, PA 19122
**Phone:** (215)204-0608    **Fax:** (215)204-0679
**Email:** d.kozbor@astro.temple.edu
Dr. Danuta Kozbor, Prin. Investigator

**Activities/Fields:** Induction of protective immune responses to human immunodeficiency virus (HIV) by orally delivered genetic vaccines.


**★ 14285 ★ Temple University**
**Center for Neurovirology and Cancer**
**Biology**
**Laboratory of Neuro-Immunology (LNI)**
Mail Stop 406
Broad & Vine Sts.
Philadelphia, PA 19102-1192
**Phone:** (215)762-1898    **Fax:** (215)762-3241

**Activities/Fields:** Molecular pathogenesis of multiple sclerosis.


**Temple University**
**Center for Neurovirology and Cancer**
**Biology**
**Laboratory of NeuroAIDS and Gene**
**Therapy**
*See:* Entry 11880


**★ 14286 ★ Temple University**
**Center for Neurovirology and Cancer**
**Biology**
**Laboratory of Neuropathology (LNP)**
BioLife Sciences Bldg.
College of Science & Technology
1900 N 12th St.
Philadelphia, PA 19122
**Phone:** (215)204-0635    **Fax:** (215)204-0679
**Email:** s.croul@astro.temple.edu
Sidney Croul, MD, Prin. Investigator

**Activities/Fields:** Viral infection of the brain and the effect of pathobiological alternatives.


**★ 14287 ★ Temple University**
**Center for Neurovirology and Cancer**
**Biology**
**Laboratory of Neurovirology and Neuro-**
**oncology**
BioLife Sciences Bldg.
College of Science & Technology
1900 N 12th St.
Philadelphia, PA 19122
**Phone:** (215)204-0678    **Fax:** (215)204-0679
**Email:** k.khalili@astro.temple.edu
Dr. Kamel Khalili, Dir.

**Activities/Fields:** Molecular basis for the involvement of the blood-brain barrier in trafficking of inflammatory cells and neurotropic viruses (HIV-1, MHV-4) in the central nervous system, and identification of central nervous system endothelial specific compounds mediating viral infection of the brain.


**Texas Health Research Institute (THRI)**
*See:* Entry 4550


**Texas Scottish Rite Hospital for Children**
**Research Department**
*See:* Entry 5814


**★ 14288 ★ Texas Tech University**
**Tarbox Parkinson's Disease Institute**
Health Science Center
3601 4th St., Rm. 3A105
Lubbock, TX 79430
**Phone:** (806)743-2391    **Fax:** (806)743-5687
**Email:** richb@tsrh.org
**Website:**    http://www.ttuhsc.edu/pages/neuro/
neupsy1.htm

**Activities/Fields:** Neurophysical and neuropharmacological studies of the central nervous system of vertebrates as they relate to Parkinson's disease and other neurological disorders.


**★ 14289 ★ Thomas Jefferson University**
**Neurosurgery Research Laboratories**
909 Walnut St., 3rd Fl.
Philadelphia, PA 19107
**Phone:** (215)955-1010    **Fax:** (215)955-1015
**Email:** fasimeone@mailcity.com
Frederick A. Simeone, MD, Ch.

**Activities/Fields:** Basic mechanisms involved in stroke and trauma including cytokine production, adhesion molecules, infartt size and edema formatiom in vitro and in vivo. Clinical influence of circadian rhythms and identification of hibernation triggers. Genetic identification and molecular basis of glioma tumors. Computer program design for assisting neurosurgical techniques and treatments. Cerebral serotonin alteration with anti-obesity treatments. Molecular basis of epilepsy and vasospasm.


**Thomas Jefferson University**
**Regional Spinal Cord Injury System of**
**Delaware Valley**
*See:* Entry 20204


**★ 14290 ★ Thomas Jefferson University**
**Sleep Disorders Center**
Jefferson Medical College
1015 Walnut St., Ste. 316
Philadelphia, PA 19107
**Phone:** (215)955-6175    **Fax:** (215)955-9783
**Email:** karl.doghramji@mail.tju.edu
**Website:**    http://www.jeffersonhospital.org/psych/
e3front.dll?durki=4263&site=336&return=6680
Karl Doghramji, MD, Dir.

**Activities/Fields:** Hypnotics, wake-promoting agents, antidepressants, sleep/wake disorders or disorders which may have characteristic sleep markers. Also studies seasonal affective disorder; phototherapy for circadian rhythm disorders; and human sexuality, particularly erectile impotence; sleep apnea syndrome, narcolepsy insomnia, and daytime hypersomnia. Research studies are developed in connection with clinical services and with subject groups recruited for special projects. **Frmly:** Center for the Study of Sleep.


**★ 14291 ★ Toronto Rehabilitation**
**Institute**
**Stroke Rehabilitation Unit**
550 University Ave.
Toronto, ON, Canada M5G 2A2
**Phone:** (416)597-3422    **Fax:** (416)597-1977
**Email:** hajek@sprint.ca
Dr. V.E. Hajek, Contact

**Activities/Fields:** Monitors and evaluates aspects of the rehabilitation experience on the Stroke Unit, including patients' response and progress to different therapies and treatments, and to orthotic devices and aids. Also participates in a study of mood disorders and cognitive impairment resulting from stroke.


**Tulane University Health Sciences Center**
**U.S.-Japan Biomedical Research**
**Laboratories**
*See:* Entry 8766


**★ 14292 ★ U.S. Department of Defense**
**Army Medical Research and Materiel**
**Command**
**Walter Reed Army Institute of Research**
**Division of Neurosciences**
503 Robert Grant Ave.
Silver Spring, MD 20910
**Phone:** (301)319-9324    **Fax:** (301)319-9905
**Email:** michael.russo@na.amedd.army.mil
Lt. Col. Michael Russo, Dir.

**Activities/Fields:** Pertinent aspects of military medicine that involve the central nervous system. Research is performed to improve neuroprotection and treatment for combat casualty care, operational stress, infectious disease, and defense against biological and chemical threats.


**U.S. Department of Health and Human**
**Services**
**National Institute on Aging (NIA)**
**Laboratory of Neurosciences**
*See:* Entry 3083


**U.S. Department of Health and Human**
**Services**
**National Institute on Aging**
**Neuroscience and Neuropsychology of**
**Aging Program**
*See:* Entry 3085


**U.S. Department of Health and Human**
**Services**
**National Institute on Alcohol Abuse and**
**Alcoholism**
**Basic Research Division**
**Neurosciences and Behavioral Research**
**Branch**
*See:* Entry 19367


**U.S. Department of Health and Human**
**Services**
**National Institute of Dental Research**
**Division of Intramural Research**
**Neurobiology and Anesthesiology Branch**
*See:* Entry 6624


**U.S. Department of Health and Human**
**Services**
**National Institute of Mental Health**
**Intramural Research Programs Division**
**Experimental Therapeutic Branch**
*See:* Entry 12727


**U.S. Department of Health and Human**
**Services**
**National Institute of Mental Health**
**Intramural Research Programs Division**
**(Basic Research)**
**Cerebral Metabolism Laboratory**
*See:* Entry 12730


**U.S. Department of Health and Human**
**Services**
**National Institute of Mental Health**
**Intramural Research Programs Division**
**(Clinical Research)**
**Clinical Neuroendocrinology Branch**
*See:* Entry 12735

**U.S. Department of Health and Human Services**
**National Institute of Mental Health**
**Intramural Research Programs Division (Clinical Research)**
**Neurophsiology Laboratory**
*See:* Entry 12739

**U.S. Department of Health and Human Services**
**National Institute of Mental Health**
**Intramural Research Programs Division (Clinical Research)**
**Neuropsychology Laboratory**
*See:* Entry 12740

**U.S. Department of Health and Human Services**
**National Institute of Mental Health**
**Intramural Research Programs Division (Neuropsychiatric Research at Saint Elizabeth's Hospital)**
**Biochemical Genetics Laboratory**
*See:* Entry 12742

**U.S. Department of Health and Human Services**
**National Institute of Mental Health**
**Neuroscience and Behavioral Sciences Division**
**Molecular and Cellular Neuroscience Research Branch**
*See:* Entry 12746

**★ 14293 ★ U.S. Department of Health and Human Services**
**National Institute of Neurological Disorders and Stroke**
Bldg. 31, Rm. 8-A52
Bethesda, MD 20892-2540
**Phone:** (301)496-9746          **Fax:** (301)496-0296
**Email:** penna@ninds.nih.gov
**Website:** http://www.ninds.nih.gov
Audrey S. Penn, MD, Actg. Dir.
**Activities/Fields:** Causes, prevention, diagnosis, and treatment of neurological disorders and stroke. The Institute conducts, fosters, and supports research and research training in neurological and muscle disorders through: intramural, collaborative, and field research in its own laboratories, branches, and clinics, and through contracts; research grants to scientific institutions and to individuals; individual and institutional research training awards to increase trained professional research manpower in neurological fields; and cooperation with various agencies in collecting and disseminating educational and informational material related to neurological disorders and stroke. The Institute is organized into: a division of extramural research, which plans and directs initiatives for grant and contract support for research, training, and career development; and a division of intramural research, which conducts basic and clinical research in neurological disorders and related disciplines.

**★ 14294 ★ U.S. Department of Health and Human Services**
**National Institute of Neurological Disorders and Stroke**
**Division of Convulsive, Infectious, and Immune Disorders**
**Epilepsy Branch**
NSC/2113
Bethesda, MD 20892
**Phone:** (301)496-1917          **Fax:** (301)496-2424
**Website:** http://www.ninds.nih.gov
Margaret Jacobs, Dir.
**Activities/Fields:** Epilepsy research. Goals are to promote research into the basic mechanisms, etiologies, prevention, diagnosis, and treatment of epilepsies. Branch implements its program through grant- and contract-supported research programs, with emphasis on: basic research (primarily grant-supported), identification of gap areas, and support of state-of-the-art monographs and international symposia; development of anticonvulsant drugs in conjunction with the Epilepsy Therapeutics Research Program (ETRP) conducted by the National Institute of Neurological Disorders and Stroke; and the development of clinical research centers in epilepsy. The ETRP Program comprises preclinical studies and clinical evaluations. Branch also supports comprehensive epilepsy programs for clinical and laboratory research in the diagnosis, treatment, prognosis, and prevention of epilepsy. These programs facilitate applied research and coordinate research and teaching with health care services. **Pub:** *Annual Report*.

**★ 14295 ★ U.S. Department of Health and Human Services**
**National Institute of Neurological Disorders and Stroke**
**Division of Demyelinating, Atrophic, and Dementing Disorders**
Federal Bldg., Rm. 810
7550 Wisconsin Ave.
Bethesda, MD 20892
**Phone:** (301)496-5679          **Fax:** (301)480-1080
Dr. Michael D. Walker, MD, Dir.
**Activities/Fields:** Understanding, diagnosis, treatment, and prevention of a broad scope of neurological disorders of adults and the aged. These diseases include Alzheimer's disease and other dementias, Parkinson's disease, Huntington's disease, and amyotrophic lateral sclerosis, as well as demyelinating disorders such as multiple sclerosis. In addition, research is funded on infectious diseases, including "slow" virus diseases, encephalitis, meningitis, and neurological aspects of AIDS. Biological research emphasizing neuroendocrinology and the neurological basis of pain is also supported. Research activities include studies of the physiology, biochemistry, pharmacology, anatomy, pathology, genetics, and epidemiology of these diseases and related conditions in humans and animal models.

**★ 14296 ★ U.S. Department of Health and Human Services**
**National Institute of Neurological Disorders and Stroke**
**Division of Demyelinating, Atrophic, and Dementing Disorders**
**Huntington's Disease Research Roster**
Department of Medical Genetics, Medical Research and Library
Indiana University Medical Center
975 W Walnut St.
Indianapolis, IN 46202-5251
**Phone:** (317)274-2245          **Fax:** (317)274-2387
**Website:** http://www.iupui.edu/~medgen
Dr. P. Michael Conneally, Prin. Invest.
**Activities/Fields:** To compile a registry of families with, or at risk for, Huntington's Disease (HD) that can be used as a resource for HD research. The Roster contains 133,163 records of individuals in 2730 families located in all 50 states as well as in other countries. **Pub:** *National Huntington's Disease Research Roster for Patients and Families.*

**★ 14297 ★ U.S. Department of Health and Human Services**
**National Institute of Neurological Disorders and Stroke**
**Division of Extramural Activities**
6002 Executive Blvd., Rm. 3309
Bethesda, MD 20892
**Phone:** (301)402-9248          **Fax:** (301)402-4370
**Email:** atwellc@ninds.nih.gov
**Website:** http://www.ninds.nih.gov/about_ninds/organization.htmextramural
Contance W. Atwell, PhD, Dir.
**Activities/Fields:** Provides administrative support and coordination for the Institute's research grant, research training, and research contract activities. Division directs and carries out scientific and technical merit review of proposals for research contracts, program projects, clinical research centers, special research grants such as multi-institutional clinical trials, and career development and research training. Management services for research grant and contract activities are also provided. Division also coordinates training and career development of young investigators and research opportunities for minority scientists and minority institutions. Opportunities include institutional and individual training awards as well as support through new investigator research awards, research career development awards, and clinical investigator development awards. **Frmly:** (2000) Division of Extramural Activities.

**★ 14298 ★ U.S. Department of Health and Human Services**
**National Institute of Neurological Disorders and Stroke (NINDS)**
**Division of Intramural Research (DIR)**
Bldg. 36, Rm.5A-05
36 Convent Dr.
MSC 4150
Bethesda, MD 20892-4150
**Phone:** (301)435-2232          **Fax:** (301)480-5634
**Email:** landiss@ninds.nih.gov
Dr. Story Landis, PhD, Dir., Facilities Strategic Mgmt.
**Activities/Fields:** Neurological sciences and relevant disciplines, including drug therapies for debilitating neurological diseases such as Parkinsonism, new techniques to help scientists better understand how the brain and nervous system function, and major research advances in neurovirology, neurochemistry, and other fields. Current interests include central nervous system disorders, such as Creutzfeldt-Jakob disease, that appear to be slow infections caused by transmissible virus-like agents; Inherited disorders of lipid metabolism, such as Gaucher's disease, Niemann-Pick disease, Fabry's disease, Krabbe's disease, and Tay-Sachs disease. Studies with the PET scanner, which have shown a relationship between glucose uptake and brain tumor growth, allow scientists to obtain axial transverse or coronal images of the brain. Intramural research is organized in two program areas: Basic Neurosciences and Clinical Neurosciences. **Pub:** *Conference Proceedings.* • *Research Reports.*

**★ 14299 ★ U.S. Department of Health and Human Services**
**National Institute of Neurological Disorders and Stroke**
**Division of Intramural Research (Basic Neurosciences Program)**
Bldg. 36, Rm. 4-D04
9000 Rockville Pike
Bethesda, MD 20892
**Phone:** (301)496-6719          **Fax:** (301)402-1339
**Email:** gainerh@ninds.nih.gov
**Website:** http://intra.ninds.nih.gov
Dr. Harold Gainer, PhD, Lab. Chf.
**Activities/Fields:** Cell biology of neuropeptide and catecholamine cell-specific gene expression, biosynthesis and secretion.

**★ 14300 ★ U.S. Department of Health and Human Services**
**National Institute of Neurological Disorders and Stroke**
**Division of Intramural Research (Basic Neurosciences Program)**
**Laboratory of Central Nervous System Studies**
NIH Bldg. 36, Rm. 4A-05
36 Convent Dr., MSC4122
Bethesda, MD 20892
**Phone:** (301)496-4821          **Fax:** (301)496-9946

**Email:** gibbs@codon.nih.gov
Dr. Clarence J. Gibbs, Jr., Chf.

**Activities/Fields:** Medical surveillance of disease patterns in many primitive and isolated populations; slow, latent, and temperate virus infections, particularly chronic degenerative neurologic diseases and their pathogenesis and mechanisms of virus persistence. Also studies configuration and change resulting in conversion of normal host precursors to infectious proteins in the transmissible amyloidoses of the brain. In addition, aging of the brain, Alzheimer's, Pick's, Parkinson's, and Huntington's diseases, multiple sclerosis, amyotrophic lateral sclerosis, chronic epilepsies, and other diseases are studied in microbiological, immunologic, genetic, and biochemical laboratories and clinics and in foci of high incidence throughout the world. Worldwide study of hemorrhagic fever with renal syndrome is conducted with isolation and molecular and virulence characterization of the hantavirus serotypes. HIV and HTLV I and II genetic variation, and involvement of the nervous system are studied worldwide.

★ 14301 ★ **U.S. Department of Health and Human Services**
**National Institute of Neurological Disorders and Stroke**
**Division of Intramural Research (Basic Neurosciences Program)**
**Laboratory of Developmental Neurogenetics**
NIH Bldg. 36, Rm. 5D06
9000 Rockville Pike
Bethesda, MD 20892
**Phone:** (301)496-9106          **Fax:** (301)496-0899
Dr. Lynn Hudson, Actg. Chf.

**Activities/Fields:** Molecular events that occur in the replication and expression of genetic materials in mammalian cells and their viruses. Genetic, biochemical, and recombinant DNA techniques are used to study gene replication and transcription. Post-transcriptional modification and translation of ribonucleic acids are also examined. The biological systems studied include: measles virus and vesicular stomatitis virus, two members of the negative strand RNA virus family, and glial cells of the central and peripheral nervous system, especially glial cell differentiation and development, with emphasis on the genes involved in myelin synthesis and maintenance. **Frmly:** Molecular Genetics Laboratory.

★ 14302 ★ **U.S. Department of Health and Human Services**
**National Institute of Neurological Disorders and Stroke**
**Division of Intramural Research (Basic Neurosciences Program)**
**Laboratory of Molecular and Cellular Neurobiology**
9000 Rockville Pike, Bldg. 49, Rm. 2A10
Bethesda, MD 20892
**Phone:** (301)496-6647          **Fax:** (301)496-8244
**Email:** quarlesr@ninds.nih.gov
Dr. Richard Quarles, Chf.

**Activities/Fields:** Molecular and cellular neurobiology, myelination, and cell surface receptors.

★ 14303 ★ **U.S. Department of Health and Human Services**
**National Institute of Neurological Disorders and Stroke**
**Division of Intramural Research (Basic Neurosciences Program)**
**Laboratory of Neural Control**
Bldg. 49, Rm. 3A50
49 Convent Dr., MSC 4455
Bethesda, MD 20892-4455
**Phone:** (301)496-4305          **Fax:** (301)402-4836
**Email:** reburke@helix.nih.gov
**Website:** http://intra.ninds.nih.gov/
Dr. Robert E. Burke, Chf.

**Activities/Fields:** Properties of mammalian nerve cells and the organization of neural circuits in the mammalian central nervous system, with particular reference to studies of the control of movement. Current experimental studies involve five main areas: the neurobiology of spinal cord motorneurons and motor units; the organization of interneuron circuits in the spinal cord; the development of motor systems in the embryonic avian and neonatal rodent spinal cord; and the generation of respiratory rhythms. Such studies utilize established as well as newly developed techniques for electrophysiologic recording from single neurons, but other methods, such as those of neuroanatomy and computer simulations, are also used as appropriate. The laboratory has facilities for the development of specialized experimental equipment and for computer-oriented data analysis and model building. **Pub:** *Conference Proceedings.* • *Monographs.*

★ 14304 ★ **U.S. Department of Health and Human Services**
**National Institute of Neurological Disorders and Stroke**
**Division of Intramural Research (Basic Neurosciences Program)**
**Laboratory of Neurobiology**
NIH Bldg. 36, Rm. 2A21
36 Convent Dr., MSC 4157
Bethesda, MD 20892
**Phone:** (301)496-1296          **Fax:** (301)480-1485
**Email:** reeset@ninds.nih.gov
**Website:** http://www.ninds.nih.gov/about_ninds/organization.htmintramural
Dr. Thomas S. Reese, Chf.

**Activities/Fields:** Structural research on the organization of the nervous system. Specific areas of interest are: synaptic transmission, neural membranes, the intracellular sequestration of ions, the blood-brain barrier, and axonal transport. Structural tools used include electron microscopy, X-ray spectroscopy, immunocytochemistry, cryotechniques, and computer processed imaging of light microscopy and electron microscopic images.

★ 14305 ★ **U.S. Department of Health and Human Services**
**National Institute of Neurological Disorders and Stroke**
**Division of Intramural Research (Basic Neurosciences Program)**
**Laboratory of Neurochemistry**
NIH Bldg. 36, Rm. 4D04
9000 Rockville Pike
Bethesda, MD 20892-4130
**Phone:** (301)496-1671          **Fax:** (301)496-1339
**Email:** gainerh@ninds.nih.gov
Dr. Harold Gainer, Chf.

**Activities/Fields:** Molecular events that underlie both the normal functioning of the developing and mature nervous system and the derangements that occur in neurological disease. Areas of study include: mechanisms of active ion transport, protein phosphorylaton, neuronal development and regeneration, gene expression of neuropeptides and their receptors, and neuronal cytoskeletal proteins.

★ 14306 ★ **U.S. Department of Health and Human Services**
**National Institute of Neurological Disorders and Stroke**
**Division of Intramural Research (Basic Neurosciences Program)**
**Laboratory of Neurophysiology**
NIH Bldg. 36, Rm. 4A21
9000 Rockville Pike
Bethesda, MD 20892
**Phone:** (301)496-2414          **Fax:** (301)402-1565
**Email:** barkerj@ninds.nih.gov
**Website:** http://intra.ninds.nih.gov/Lab.asp?Org_ID-91
Jeffery L. Barker, MD, Chf.

**Activities/Fields:** Physiological correlates and determinants of mammalian central nervous development, especially in the cortical, hippocampal and spinal cord regions. Methods are multidisciplinary, and include flow cytometry, imaging with physiological indicator dyes, electrophysiology, and immunocytochemistry. Flow cytometry in conjunction with surface phenotyping and indicator dyes has been used to provide a comprehensive account of physiologically relevant properties emerging during neuronal and glial lineage progressions. The absence of epitopes indicative of commitment or apoptosis has been used to sort uncommitted cells, which can be expanded in vitro and induced to differentiate into neuronal or glial phenotypes. Similar physiological properties emerge among the progeny of these cells with the self-renewing and multi-potential characteristics of neural stem cells as arise in vivo. This novel strategy directly accesses physiological correlates and determinants of cell lineage progression. Two neurotransmitters (acetylcholine and GABA) play key roles during expansion and tissue histogenesis and form the primary focus of ongoing studies. **Pub:** *Annual Report.*

★ 14307 ★ **U.S. Department of Health and Human Services**
**National Institute of Neurological Disorders and Stroke**
**Division of Intramural Research (Basic Neurosciences Program)**
**Neuroepidemiology Branch**
NIH Campus
10 Center Dr.
Bldg. 10 Room 5-S-220
Bethesda, MD 20892-1447
**Phone:** (301)496-1714          **Fax:** (301)496-2358
Cecilia Blutstein, Off. Mgr.

**Activities/Fields:** Neuroepidemiology, the epidemiologic investigation of neurologic disorders, which requires a thorough knowledge of both clinical neurology and epidemiologic methods. The program focuses on research, education, and consultation in neuroepidemiology.

★ 14308 ★ **U.S. Department of Health and Human Services**
**National Institute of Neurological Disorders and Stroke**
**Division of Intramural Research (Clinical Neurosciences Program)**
NIH Bldg. 10, Rm. 5N234
10 Center Dr., MSC 1428
Bethesda, MD 20892-1428
**Phone:** (301)496-1561          **Fax:** (301)402-1007
**Email:** mcfarlandh@ninds.nih.gov
**Website:** http://neuroscience.nih.gov/study_areas.asp
Henry McFarland, MD, Dir.

**Activities/Fields:** Problems important in Clinical Neurology and Neurosurgery. The Office of the Clinical Director provides clinical neurological services to investigators within the Institute and other NIH institutes. Activities include clinical neurophysiological laboratory investigations, neurology consultations, and neuropathology. Principal branches include Biostatics, Developmental and Metabolic Neurology, Developmental and Metabolic Neurology, Epilepsy Research, Experimental Therapeutics, Medical Neurology, Neuroepidemiology, Neurogenetics, Neuroimmunology, Stroke, and Surgical Neurology, Clinical Neurocardiology, Cognitive Assistant Neurosciences, Neuromuscular Diseases.

**★ 14309 ★ U.S. Department of Health and Human Services**
**National Institute of Neurological Disorders and Stroke**
**Division of Intramural Research (Clinical Neurosciences Program)**
**Clinical Neurosciences Branch**
NIH Bldg. 10, Rm. 6N252
10 Center Dr., MSC 1620
Bethesda, MD 20892
**Phone:** (301)496-2103          **Fax:** (301)402-0180
**Email:** goldsteind@ninds.nih.gov
David S. Goldstein, Chf.

**Activities/Fields:** Neurosciences.

**★ 14310 ★ U.S. Department of Health and Human Services**
**National Institute of Neurological Disorders and Stroke**
**Division of Intramural Research (Clinical Neurosciences Program)**
**Developmental and Metabolic Neurology Branch**
NIH Bldg. 10, Rm. 3D04
10 Center Dr. MSC 1260
Bethesda, MD 20892-1260
**Phone:** (301)496-3285          **Fax:** (301)496-9480
**Email:** bradyr@ninds.nih.gov
**Website:** http://www.ninds.nih.gov/about_ninds/organization.htmintramurl
Dr. Roscoe O. Brady, Chf.

**Activities/Fields:** Genetic disorders of metabolism, demyelinating disorders, biochemistry of cell membranes, and signal transduction mechanisms in normal and neoplastic tissues. Principal areas of interest are biochemistry, genetics, neurochemistry, neuroimmunology, molecular genetics, and adult and pediatric neurology.

**★ 14311 ★ U.S. Department of Health and Human Services**
**National Institute of Neurological Disorders and Stroke**
**Division of Intramural Research (Clinical Neurosciences Program)**
**Experimental Therapeutics Branch**
NIH Bldg. 10, Rm. 5C103
10 Center Dr., MSC 1406
Bethesda, MD 20892-1406
**Phone:** (301)496-7993          **Fax:** (301)496-6609
**Email:** zawalich@ninds.nih.gov
Dr. Thomas N. Chase, Chf.

**Activities/Fields:** Improved pharmacotherapies for neurologic disease. The Branch operates a vertically integrated program of research, extending from basic molecular biology to clinical trials, focusing on neurodegenerative diseases such as Alzheimer's disease and Parkinson's disease. Current operating components are the Molecular Pharmacology Section which characterizes central transmitter receptors and information transduction processes; the Genetic Pharmacology Unit investigates pharmaceutical approaches to the selective regulation of gene expression; the Neurophysiology Pharmacology Section studies basal ganglia function in relation to transmitter system interactions; and Clinical Pharmacology Section works clinically and in animal models to elucidate pathophysiologic mechanisms and evaluate novel pharmacologic interventions. **Pub:** *Proceedings.* • *Research Reports.*

**★ 14312 ★ U.S. Department of Health and Human Services**
**National Institute of Neurological Disorders and Stroke**
**Division of Intramural Research (Clinical Neurosciences Program)**
**Laboratory of Molecular Medicine and Neuroscience**
NIH Bldg. 36
36 Convent Dr.
Bethesda, MD 20892-4164
**Phone:** (301)496-1635          **Fax:** (301)594-5799
**Email:** eomajor@codon.nih.gov
Dr. Eugene Major, Chf.

**Activities/Fields:** Neurologic diseases at the clinical, biological, and molecular levels. Experimental emphasis is on the pathogenesis of diseases involving cellular dysfunctions caused by neurotropic viruses, toxic cytokines, or possible genetic alterations.

**★ 14313 ★ U.S. Department of Health and Human Services**
**National Institute of Neurological Disorders and Stroke**
**Division of Intramural Research (Clinical Neurosciences Program)**
**Medical Neurology Branch**
NIH Bldg. 10, Rm. 5N226
10 Center Dr., MSC 1428
Bethesda, MD 20892-1428
**Phone:** (301)496-9526          **Fax:** (301)480-2286
**Email:** hallettm@ninds.nih.gov
**Website:** http://www..ninds.nih.gov/Lab.asp?Org_ID=72
Mark Hallett, MD, Chf.

**Activities/Fields:** Basic and clinical aspects of a variety of neurologic disorders, including: pathophysiological mechanisms and treatment of movement disorders; pathophysiology of speech and language disorders; brain plasticity and rehabilitation.

**★ 14314 ★ U.S. Department of Health and Human Services**
**National Institute of Neurological Disorders and Stroke**
**Division of Intramural Research (Clinical Neurosciences Program)**
**Neuroimmunology Branch**
NIH Bldg. 10, Rm. 5B-16
10 Center Dr., MSC 1400
Bethesda, MD 20892-1400
**Phone:** (301)496-1801          **Fax:** (301)402-0373
Dr. Henry F. McFarland, Chf.

**Activities/Fields:** Activities of the Neuroimmunology Branch include basic and clinical investigations related to multiple sclerosis (MS) and other possible immunological-based diseases. Studies focus on examining basic or fundamental immunological questions, including a study of experimental animal models and the cellular immune response to potential antigens in the nervous system. Research studies also examine the role of human retroviruses, including HTLV-I and HTLV-II in diseases of the nervous system. Clinical studies focus on examining the natural history of MS using magnetic resonance imaging and assessing new innovative therapies in MS.

**★ 14315 ★ U.S. Department of Health and Human Services**
**National Institute of Neurological Disorders and Stroke**
**Division of Intramural Research (Clinical Neurosciences Program)**
**Surgical Neurology Branch**
NIH Bldg. 10, Rm. 5D37
10 Center Dr., MSC 1414
Bethesda, MD 20892-1414
**Phone:** (301)496-5728          **Fax:** (301)402-0380
**Email:** oldfield@box-o.nih.gov
Dr. Edward H. Oldfield, Chf.

**Activities/Fields:** Current areas of research, most of which integrate basic science, applied laboratory science, animal experimentation, and human studies include new therapeutic approaches (genetically-engineered immunotoxins, genetically-engineered viral vectors, new drug delivery techniques) for brain tumors and pituitary tumors, mechanisms of brain edema associated with brain tumors, mechanisms of tumor-associated angiogenesis, mechanisms of the beneficial recovery after cerebral implants or neurotrophic factors for Parkinson's disease, studies of certain types of cerebrovascular disease (vasospasm, regulation of cerebral blood flow, spinal arteriovenous malformations), von Hippel-Lindau syndrome, and functional neurosurgery (seizure surgery, development of implanted prosthesis for blindness).

**★ 14316 ★ U.S. Department of Health and Human Services**
**National Institute of Neurological Disorders and Stroke**
**Division of Stroke, Trauma, and Neurodegenerative Disorders**
7550 Wisconsin Ave.
Federal Bldg., 810
Bethesda, MD 20892
**Phone:** (301)496-2581          **Fax:** (301)480-1080
Dr. Michael Walker, Dir.

**Activities/Fields:** Stroke and central nervous system trauma, including support for basic, applied, and clinical research. This includes support for multidisciplinary cerebrovascular clinical research centers, a comprehensive stroke center program, spinal cord injury centers, a comprehensive CNS trauma center program, and head injury centers, as well as larger numbers of individual, investigator-initiated research grants. Program supports training of young investigators through formal institutional and individual training awards; support is also provided through new investigator research awards, research career development awards, and clinical teacher investigator development awards. In addition, Division administers grants to exploit the research opportunities presented by positron emission tomography (PET). Principal areas of research interest are: cerebrovascular disease (including stroke and its consequences); trauma to the brain, spinal cord, and peripheral nervous system; central nervous system regeneration; primary and metastatic tumors of the brain and/or spinal cord; headache; chronic pain; positron emission tomography; and manipulative therapy.

**★ 14317 ★ U.S. Department of Health and Human Services**
**National Institute of Neurological Disorders and Stroke**
**Division of Stroke, Trauma, and Neurodegenerative Disorders**
**Neural Prosthesis Program**
7550 Wisconsin Ave., Rm. 916
Bethesda, MD 20892
**Phone:** (301)496-5746          **Fax:** (301)402-1501
**Email:** fh2@cu.nih.gov
Dr. Frederick Terry Hambrecht, Hd.

**Activities/Fields:** Development of aids for the neurologically disabled based on direct interfaces with neural tissue. Principal areas of research interest are cochlear implants and cochlear nucleus implants for the deaf; visual prostheses for the blind; and motor prostheses for the paralyzed. Research is carried out under contract and through grants at universities and commercial research laboratories. **Pub:** *Proceedings.* • *Progress reports from contractors*, quarterly. • *Research Reports.*

## ★ 14318 ★ U.S. Department of Health and Human Services
**National Institute of Neurological Disorders and Stroke**
**Small Business Innovation Research Program**
Federal Bldg. 1016
Bethesda, MD 20892
**Phone:** (301)496-4188          **Fax:** (301)402-4370
**Website:** http://www.ninds.nih.gov
Sonny Kreitman, Dir.

**Activities/Fields:** Comprises awards for three phases of research: the objective of Phase I is to establish the technical merit and feasibility of proposed research efforts that may ultimately lead to commercial products or services; the objective of Phase II is to continue the research and development efforts initiated in Phase I that are likely to result in commercial products or services; and the objective of Phase III, where appropriate, is for the small business to pursue, with non-federal funds, the commercialization of the results of the research and development funded in Phases I and II. Recent areas of interest include: development of novel antiepileptic drugs; devices for automated seizure detection; research and development of magnetoencephalography (MEG); development of applications for evoked potentials; development of a portable EEG device; and development of instrumentation for monitoring autonomic nervous system (ANS) function.

**U.S. Department of Health and Human Services**
**National Institutes of Health (NIH)**
**National Institute on Aging**
**Intramural Research Programs**
**(Brain Physiology and Metabolism Section)**
*See:* Entry 3088

## ★ 14319 ★ U.S. Department of Health and Human Services
**National Institutes of Health**
**National Institute of Child Health and Human Development**
**Division of Intramural Research**
**(Laboratory of Developmental Neurobiology)**
Bldg. 49, Rm. 5A38
49 Convent Dr., MSC 4480
Bethesda, MD 20892-4480
**Phone:** (301)496-1463          **Fax:** (301)496-9939
**Email:** sir@helix.nih.gov
**Website:** http://dir.nichd.nih.gov/Ldn/LDNHP.html
Dr. Phillip G. Nelson, Ch.

**Activities/Fields:** Molecular and cellular mechanisms coupling electrical activity in neurons and muscle cells to development of the nervous system.

## ★ 14320 ★ U.S. Department of Health and Human Services
**National Institutes of Health**
**National Institute of Child Health and Human Development**
**Division of Intramural Research**
**(Laboratory of Cellular and Molecular Neurophysiology)**
Bldg. 36, Rm. 2B28
Bethesda, MD 20892
**Phone:** (301)496-9346
**Email:** mlm@helix.nih.gov
**Website:** http://dirz.nichd.nih.gov/labs/lab.php3??
Dr. Mark Mayer, Ch.

**Activities/Fields:** Neurotransmitter receptors and ion channels and the cellular processes they control using patch clamp, imaging, molecular biological, biochemical, structural and neuroanatomical techniques applied to preparations, including transgenic mice, brain slices, cell cultures, in vitro expression systems including Xenopus oocytes and transiently transfected 293 cells, and proteins over-expressed in bacteria. **Pub:** *Papers.*

## ★ 14321 ★ U.S. Department of Health and Human Services
**National Institutes of Health**
**National Institute of Dental and Craniofacial Research**
**Division of Intramural Research**
**(Immunopathology Section)**
Bldg. 30, Rm. 325
30 Convent Dr., MSC 4352
Bethesda, MD 20892-4352
**Phone:** (301)496-9219          **Fax:** (301)402-1064
**Email:** larry.wahl@nih.gov
**Website:** http://wwwdir.nidcr.nih.gov/dirweb/cores/is/is.asp
Larry M. Wahl, PhD, Ch.

**Activities/Fields:** Factors and signal transduction pathways in the modulation of the immune response focusing on human moncytes.

## ★ 14322 ★ U.S. Department of Health and Human Services
**National Institutes of Health**
**National Institute of Dental and Craniofacial Research**
**Division of Intramural Research**
**(Cellular Neuroscience Section)**
Bldg. 49, Rm. 1A11
30 Convent Dr., MSC 4410
Bethesda, MD 20892-4410
**Phone:** (301)402-4980          **Fax:** (301)402-0667
**Email:** maryann.ruda@nih.gov
**Website:** http://wwwdir.nidcr.nih.gov/dirweb/pnmb/cmms.asp
Dr. M.A. Ruda, Ch.

**Activities/Fields:** Neuronal response to peripheral inflammation and hyperalgesia or nerve injury, representing neuronal plasticity at the level of the spinal cord and dorsal root ganglia, focused on the question of nociception.

**U.S. Department of Health and Human Services**
**National Institutes of Health**
**National Institute of Diabetes and Digestive and Kidney Diseases**
**Division of Diabetes, Endocrinology, and Metabolic Diseases**
**(Neuroendocrinology Program)**
*See:* Entry 8798

## ★ 14323 ★ U.S. Department of Health and Human Services
**National Institutes of Health**
**National Institute of Diabetes and Digestive and Kidney Diseases**
**Division of Diabetes, Endocrinology, and Metabolic Diseases**
**(Nuclear Hormone Superfamily Program)**
MSC 5460
6707 Democracy Blvd., Rm. 6107
Bethesda, MD 20892-5460
**Phone:** (301)594-8819          **Fax:** (301)480-6047
**Email:** margolisr@extra.niddk.nih.gov
**Website:** http://www.niddk.nih.gov/fund/program/MRlist.htm
Ronald Margolis, PhD, Sr. Adv.

**Activities/Fields:** Basic and clinical research on members of the steroid hormone superfamily (also known as the nuclear receptor superfamily), including structure/function studies and the role in signal transduction and regulation of gene expression of the steroid hormones including glucocorticoids, mineralocorticoids, progesterone, estrogens, androgens (testosterone, DHEA) and the nuclear receptors including thyroid hormone, vitamin D, retinoids (RAR, RXR, vitamin A), PPARs, and orphan receptors (LXR, Nur77, COUP-TF, and others).

## ★ 14324 ★ U.S. Department of Health and Human Services
**National Institutes of Health**
**National Institute of Diabetes and Digestive and Kidney Diseases**
**Division of Diabetes, Endocrinology, and Metabolic Diseases**
**(Intracellular Signal Transduction Research Program)**
2 Democracy Pl., Rm. 607
Bethesda, MD 20892
**Phone:** (301)594-8817
**Email:** abrahamk@extra.niddk.nih.gov
**Website:** http://www.niddk.nih.gov/fund/program/FLlist.htm
Kristin Abraham, PhD, Dir.

**Activities/Fields:** Understanding the structure and function of intracellular signal transducing molecules. Specific areas of support include (1) intracellular kinases, phosphatases, and anchoring proteins; (2) signaling mechanisms that have altered activity in response to protein phosphorylation, Ca2+ and cAMP; (3) approaches to solving the three-dimensional structure of signaling proteins including crystallography and NMR; (4) functional analysis of these proteins including comparison of wild-type and naturally occurring or synthetic, mutant proteins or expression of dominant-negative forms of the proteins; (5) microscopic techniques to localize these proteins within cells; (6) identification of substrates for these signaling proteins; and (7) analysis of crosstalk among distinct signal transduction pathways.

**U.S. Department of Health and Human Services**
**National Institutes of Health**
**National Institute of Diabetes and Digestive and Kidney Diseases**
**Division of Digestive Diseases and Nutrition**
**(Gastrointestinal Neuroendocrinology Research Program)**
*See:* Entry 9175

## ★ 14325 ★ U.S. Department of Health and Human Services
**National Institutes of Health**
**National Institute of Environmental Health Sciences**
**Division of Extramural Research and Training**
**(Organs and Systems Toxicology Branch)**
PO Box 12233
Research Triangle Park, NC 27709
**Phone:** (919)541-5327          **Fax:** (919)541-5064
**Email:** mcclure@niehs.nih.gov
**Website:** http://www.niehs.nih.gov/dert/dertostb/ostbmisn.htm
Dr. Michael McClure, Dir.

**Activities/Fields:** Neurotoxicology, immunotoxicology, pulmonary/cardiovascular toxicology, and reproductive and developmental toxicology.

## ★ 14326 ★ U.S. Department of Health and Human Services
**National Institutes of Health**
**National Institute of Environmental Health Sciences**
**Laboratory of Signal Transduction**
**(Inositol Signaling Group)**
PO Box 12233
Research Triangle Park, NC 27709
**Phone:** (919)541-0793          **Fax:** (919)541-1898
**Email:** shears@niehs.nih.gov

**Website:** http://dir.niehs.nih.gov/dirlst/groups/shears.htm
Dr. Stephen B. Shears, Hd.
**Activities/Fields:** Inositol derivatives as regulators of cellular physiology.


★ **14327** ★ **U.S. Department of Health and Human Services**
**National Institutes of Health**
**National Institute of Environmental Health Sciences**
**Laboratory of Signal Transduction**
**(Ion Channel Physiology Group)**
PO Box 12233
Research Triangle Park, NC 27709
**Email:** yakel@niehs.nih.gov
**Website:** http://dir.niehs.nih.gov/dirlst/groups/yakel.htm
Dr. Jerrel L. Yakel, Hd.
**Activities/Fields:** 5-HT3 subtype of serotonin receptor; modulation of voltage-dependent calcium channels.


★ **14328** ★ **U.S. Department of Health and Human Services**
**National Institutes of Health**
**National Institute of Environmental Health Sciences**
**Laboratory of Signal Transduction**
**(Calcium Signaling Group)**
PO Box 12233
Research Triangle Park, NC 27709
**Phone:** (919)541-1420          **Fax:** (919)541-1898
**Email:** putney@niehs.nih.gov
**Website:** http://dir.niehs.nih.gov/dirlst/groups/putney.htm
Dr. James W. Putney, Jr., Hd.
**Activities/Fields:** Cellular calcium regulation; neurotransmitter utilization of calcium.


★ **14329** ★ **U.S. Department of Health and Human Services**
**National Institutes of Health**
**National Institute of Mental Health**
**Biological Psychiatry Branch**
**(Section on Molecular Neurobiology)**
MSC 1381
Bldg. 10, Rm. 4n222
Bethesda, MD 20892-1381
**Phone:** (301)496-4183          **Fax:** (301)480-8348
**Email:** nimhinfo@nih.gov
**Website:** http://intramural.nimh.nih.gov/research/bpb/smn.htm
De-Maw Chuang, PhD, Ch.
**Activities/Fields:** Molecular mechanisms underlying programmed cell death (apoptosis) of neurons and its implication for central nervous system (CNS) development, as well as the pathogenesis of neuropsychiatric and neurodegenerative disorders.


★ **14330** ★ **U.S. Department of Health and Human Services**
**National Institutes of Health**
**National Institute of Mental Health**
**Experimental Therapeutics Branch**
**(Section on Functional Imaging Methods)**
MSC 1148
Bldg. 10, Rm. 1D80B
10 Center Dr.
Bethesda, MD 20892-1148
**Phone:** (301)402-1333          **Fax:** (301)402-1370
**Email:** nimhinfo@nih.gov
**Website:** http://fim.nimh.nih.gov/
Peter Bandettini, PhD, Ch.
**Activities/Fields:** Aims to increase the utility and interpretability of functional magnetic resonance imaging (fMRI), involving characterization of the neuronal, physiologic, and biophysical processes that contribute to blood oxygenation level dependent (BOLD) and perfusion-based contrast in fMRI; tailoring specific neuroscience questions to unique characteristics of fMRI processing and acquistion; development of pulse sequences, hardware, and processing techniques toward the direction of increased fMRI utility; exploration of measurement and quantification of previously unmeasured neuronal or physiological processes by MRI. **Pub:** *Papers.*


★ **14331** ★ **U.S. Department of Health and Human Services**
**National Institutes of Health**
**National Institute of Mental Health**
**Experimental Therapeutics Branch**
**(Section on Cognitive Neuropsychology)**
MSC 1366
10 Center Dr., Rm. 4C104
Bethesda, MD 20892-1366
**Phone:** (301)435-4931          **Fax:** (301)402-0921
**Email:** alex@codon.nih.gov
**Website:** http://lbc.nimh.nih.gov/research.htmlSection%20on%20Cognitive
Alex Martin, PhD, Ch.
**Activities/Fields:** Human cognitive systems through the study of how these systems break down in patients with brain injury or disease.


★ **14332** ★ **U.S. Department of Health and Human Services**
**National Institutes of Health**
**National Institute of Mental Health**
**Experimental Therapeutics Branch**
**(Section on Clinical and Experimental Neurospsychology)**
MSC 1366
10 Center Dr., Rm. 4C104
9000 Rockville Pike
Bethesda, MD 20892
**Phone:** (301)496-2551          **Fax:** (301)594-5142
**Email:** nimhinfo@nih.gov
**Website:** http://lbc.nimh.nih.gov/research.html
Allan F. Mirsky, PhD, Ch.
**Activities/Fields:** Central nervous system (CNS) factors underlying normal and abnormal behavioral states, particularly on the interaction between environmental and genetic effects.


★ **14333** ★ **U.S. Department of Health and Human Services**
**National Institutes of Health**
**National Institute of Mental Health**
**Experimental Therapeutics Branch**
**(Section on Neurocircuitry)**
MSC 1366
10 Center Dr., Rm. 4C104
Bethesda, MD 20892-1366
**Phone:** (301)435-4932          **Fax:** (301)402-0921
**Email:** nimhinfo@nih.gov
**Website:** http://lbc.nimh.nih.gov/research.html
Leslie G. Ungerleider, PhD, Ch.
**Activities/Fields:** Understanding the role of the visual association cortex in perception and memory.


★ **14334** ★ **U.S. Department of Health and Human Services**
**National Institutes of Health**
**National Institute of Mental Health**
**Experimental Therapeutics Branch**
**(Laboratory of Brain and Cognition)**
MSC 1366
10 Center Dr., Rm. 4C104
Bethesda, MD 20892-1366
**Phone:** (301)435-4932          **Fax:** (301)402-0921
**Email:** nimhinfo@nih.gov
**Website:** http://lbc.nimh.nih.gov/
Leslie Ungerleider, Ch.
**Activities/Fields:** Basic and clinical research on normal and impaired attention, learning, memory and perception in humans, and on the underlying anatomical, genetic, neurophysiologic, and psychophysiologic mechanisms.


★ **14335** ★ **U.S. Department of Health and Human Services**
**National Institutes of Health**
**National Institute of Mental Health**
**Experimental Therapeutics Branch**
**(Section on Fuctional Brain Imaging)**
MSC 1366
10 Center Dr., Rm. 4C104
Bethesda, MD 20892-1366
**Phone:** (301)435-4925          **Fax:** (301)402-0921
**Email:** nimhinfo@nih.gov
**Website:** http://lbc.nimh.nih.gov/research.html
James V. Haxby, PhD, Ch.
**Activities/Fields:** Functional organization of intact human brain using functional brain imaging to measure local changes in cerebral blood flow associated with perceptual, cognitive, and mnemonic functions.


★ **14336** ★ **U.S. Department of Health and Human Services**
**National Institutes of Health**
**National Institute of Mental Health**
**Experimental Therapeutics Branch**
**(Section on PET Radiopharmaceutical Sciences)**
Bldg. 1, Rm. 3B310
1 Center Dr.
Bethesda, MD 20892-0135
**Phone:** (301)594-1089          **Fax:** (301)480-3610
**Email:** pikev@intra.nimh.nih.gov
**Website:** http://intramural.nimh.nih.gov/research/mib
Victor Pike, PhD, Ch.
**Activities/Fields:** Development and implementation of radioligands and radiotracers for selective PET (positron emission tomography) imaging of molecular targets in animal and human brain in order to understand causes of mental illness and of the mechanisms and efficacies of existing or proposed treatments.


★ **14337** ★ **U.S. Department of Health and Human Services**
**National Institutes of Health**
**National Institute of Mental Health**
**Experimental Therapeutics Branch**
**(Section on PET Neuroimaging Sciences)**
Bldg. 1, Rm. 3B310
1 Center Dr.
Bethesda, MD 20892-0135
**Phone:** (301)594-1089          **Fax:** (301)480-3610
**Email:** innisr@.intra.nimh.nih.gov
**Website:** http://intramural.nimh.nih.gov/research/mib/
Robert B. Innis, MD, Ch.
**Activities/Fields:** PET (positron emission tomography) tracers as molecular probes of physiology and pathophysiology in animals and humans; probes of intracellular signals transduction and gene expression as well as traditional receptor targets.


★ **14338** ★ **U.S. Department of Health and Human Services**
**National Institutes of Health**
**National Institute of Mental Health**
**Experimental Therapeutics Branch**
**(Section on Neuroimaging)**
Bldg. 1, Rm. 3B310
1 Center Dr.
Bethesda, MD 20892-0135
**Phone:** (301)594-1089          **Fax:** (301)480-3610
**Email:** drevetsw@intra.nimh.nih.gov
**Website:** http://intramural.nimh.nih.gov/research/mib/
Wayne Drevets, MD, Ch.
**Activities/Fields:** Functional and structural neuroimaging measures to investigate biological mechanisms of normal and pathological emotional states.

**★ 14339 ★ U.S. Department of Health and Human Services**
National Institutes of Health
National Institute of Mental Health
Experimental Therapeutics Branch
(Molecular Imaging Branch)
Bldg. 1, Rm. 3B310
1 Center Dr.
Bethesda, MD 20892-0135
**Phone:** (301)594-1089     **Fax:** (301)480-3610
**Email:** innisr@intra.nimh.nih.gov
**Website:** http://intramural.nimh.nih.gov/research/mib/
Robert B. Innis, MD, Ch.

**Activities/Fields:** Neuroimaging techniques to explore molecular and chemical mechanisms associated with neural function in health and disease, investigates pathophysiological mechanisms associated with mental illnesses in order to enhance available treatments.

**★ 14340 ★ U.S. Department of Health and Human Services**
National Institutes of Health
National Institute of Mental Health
Experimental Therapeutics Branch
(Section on Neuroendocrine Immunology and Behavior)
Bldg. 10, Rm. 2D46
9000 Rockville Pike
Bethesda, MD 20892
**Phone:** (301)496-1891     **Fax:** (301)402-1561
**Email:** nimhinfo@nih.gov
**Website:** http://intramural.nimh.nih.gov/research/cne/
Esther M. Sternberg, MD, Contact

**Activities/Fields:** Bi-directional communication between the immune system and the central nervous system (CNS), whose genetic, infectious, toxic, or pharmacological dysregulation confers susceptibility to inflammatory and affective disorders; clinical studies in early inflammatory disease, depression, and fatigue states.

**★ 14341 ★ U.S. Department of Health and Human Services**
National Institutes of Health
National Institute of Mental Health
Experimental Therapeutics Branch
(Clinical Neuroendocrinology Branch)
Bldg. 10, Rm. 2D46
9000 Rockville Pike
Bethesda, MD 20892
**Phone:** (301)496-1891     **Fax:** (301)402-1561
**Email:** nimhinfo@nih.gov
**Website:** http://intramural.nimh.nih.gov/research/cne/
Philip W. Gold, MD, Ch.

**Activities/Fields:** Committed to advancing knowledge to improve the diagnosis, treatment and overall health of patients suffering from depression.

**U.S. Department of Health and Human Services**
National Institutes of Health
National Institute of Mental Health
Experimental Therapeutics Branch
(Section on Neuropathology)
*See:* Entry 12748

**★ 14342 ★ U.S. Department of Health and Human Services**
National Institutes of Health
National Institute of Mental Health
Experimental Therapeutics Branch
(Section on Clinical Studies)
Bldg. 10, Rm. 3n212
9000 Rockville Pike
Bethesda, MD 20892
**Phone:** (301)496-4805     **Fax:** (301)402-0052
**Email:** nimhinfo@nih.gov

**Website:** http://intramural.nimh.nih.gov/research/cbdb/
Daniel R. Weinberger, MD, Ch.

**Activities/Fields:** Neuropsychiatric disorders, especially schizophrenia, Tourette's syndrome, and dementia.

**★ 14343 ★ U.S. Department of Health and Human Services**
National Institutes of Health
National Institute of Mental Health
Experimental Therapeutics Branch
(Unit on Reproduction Endocrine Studies)
MSC 1276
Bldg. 10, Rm. 3N238
Bethesda, MD 20892-1276
**Phone:** (301)496-9576     **Fax:** (301)496-2588
**Email:** nimhinfo@nih.gov
**Website:** http://intramural.nimh.nih.gov/research/beb/
index2.htm
Peter Schmidt, MD, Ch.

**Activities/Fields:** Role of gonadal steroids in the regulation of neurophysiology and affective state in humans. Studies focus on the evaluation and treatment of mood disorders linked to the perimenopause and midlife, as well as, the psychotropic effects of gonadal steroids such as estradiol, testosterone, and dehydroepiandrosterone (DHEA).

**★ 14344 ★ U.S. Department of Health and Human Services**
National Institutes of Health
National Institute of Mental Health
Experimental Therapeutics Branch
(Section on Development and Affective Neuroscience)
MSC 1381
Bldg. 10, Rm. 4n222
Bethesda, MD 20892-1381
**Phone:** (301)496-4183     **Fax:** (301)480-8348
**Email:** nimhinfo@nih.gov
**Website:** http://intramural.nimh.nih.gov/research/etpb
Daniel S. Pine, MD, Ch.

**Activities/Fields:** Brain development, emotion regulation, and risk for mood and anxiety disorders in children and adolescents.

**★ 14345 ★ U.S. Department of Health and Human Services**
National Institutes of Health
National Institute of Mental Health
Experimental Therapeutics Branch
(Experimental Therapeutics and Pathophysiology Branch)
MSC 1381
Bldg. 10, Rm. 4n222
Bethesda, MD 20892-1381
**Phone:** (301)496-4183     **Fax:** (301)480-8348
**Email:** nimhinfo@nih.gov
**Website:** http://intramural.nimh.nih.gov/research/etpb
Dennis S. Charney, MD, Ch.

**Activities/Fields:** Pathophysiology, etiology, and treatment of mood and anxiety disorders of children, adolescents, and adults; identification of neural circuits and neurochemicals.

**★ 14346 ★ U.S. Department of Health and Human Services**
National Institutes of Health
National Institute of Mental Health
Experimental Therapeutics Branch
(Section on Behavioral Neuropharmacology)
MSC 1380
10 Center Dr., Rm. 4D11
Bethesda, MD 20892-1375
**Phone:** (301)496-7855     **Fax:** (301)480-1164
**Email:** nimhinfo@nih.gov

**Website:** http://intramural.nimh.nih.gov/research/etb/
sbn/
Jacqueline N. Crawley, PhD, Ch.

**Activities/Fields:** Investigates behavior actions of brain neurotransmitters using rodent models of symptoms of neuropsychiatric diseases, including behavior neuopharmacology and behavioral genetics.

**★ 14347 ★ U.S. Department of Health and Human Services**
National Institutes of Health
National Institute of Mental Health
Laboratory of Biochemical Genetics
Bldg. 10, Rm. 2D54
10 Center Dr.
Bethesda, MD 20892
**Phone:** (301)435-3582
**Email:** nimhinfo@nih.gov
**Website:** http://intramural.nimh.nih.gov/research/lbg/
index2.htm
Carl Merril, Ch.

**Activities/Fields:** Molecular variations in the central nervous system (CNS) in normal, aging and disease states, including proteome and the mitochondrial genome.

**★ 14348 ★ U.S. Department of Health and Human Services**
National Institutes of Health
National Institute of Mental Health
Laboratory of Cellular and Molecular Regulation
(Section on Molecular Neuroscience)
Bldg. 36, Rm. 2A-11
9000 Rockville Pike
Bethesda, MD 20892
**Phone:** (301)496-8287     **Fax:** (301)402-1748
**Email:** eiden@codon.nih.gov
**Website:** http://intramural.nimh.nih.gov/lcmr/smn/
Lee Eiden, PhD, Chf.

**Activities/Fields:** Molecular basis of cell-specific expression of neuropeptide, secretory protein and vesicular transporter genes responsible for chemically coded neurotransmission in the central and peripheral autonomic nervous systems.

**★ 14349 ★ U.S. Department of Health and Human Services**
National Institutes of Health
National Institute of Mental Health
Laboratory of Cellular and Molecular Regulation
(Section on Neural Gene Expression)
Bldg. 10, Rm. 2D06
9000 Rockville Pike
Bethesda, MD 20892
**Phone:** (301)496-8767
**Email:** scott@codon.nih.gov
**Website:** http://intramural.nimh.nih.gov/lcmr/snge/
Dr. W. Scott Young, III, Ch.

**Activities/Fields:** Regulation of genes in the central nervous system, particularly on those expressed within the paraventricular and supraoptic nuclei of the hypothalamus.

**★ 14350 ★ U.S. Department of Health and Human Services**
National Institutes of Health
National Institute of Mental Health
Laboratory of Cellular and Molecular Regulation
(Section on Functional Neuroanatomy)
Bldg. 36, Rm. 2D15
9000 Rockville Pike
Bethesda, MD 20892
**Phone:** (301)496-8287
**Email:** milesh@codon.nih.gov
**Website:** http://intramural.nimh.nih.gov/lcmr/sfn/
Miles A. Herkenham, PhD, Ch.

**Activities/Fields:** Investigates dynamic aspects of nervous system function in order to define and map regulatory events that occur in animals when they respond and adapt to immune challenges, repeated drug administration, or chronic stress.

**★ 14351 ★ U.S. Department of Health and Human Services**
National Institutes of Health
National Institute of Mental Health
Laboratory of Cellular and Molecular Regulation
Bldg. 10, Rm. 2A11
9000 Rockville Pike
Bethesda, MD 20892
**Phone:** (301)496-5590　　　　**Fax:** (301)402-1748
**Email:** zatz@codon.nih.gov
**Website:**　　　　http://intramural.nimh.nih.gov/lcmr/index2.html
Martin Zats, MD, Ch.

**Activities/Fields:** Anatomical, cellular, physiological, pharmacological, biochemical and molecular bases of the expression and regulation of brain functions.

**★ 14352 ★ U.S. Department of Health and Human Services**
National Institutes of Health
National Institute of Mental Health
Laboratory of Cellular and Molecular Regulation
**(Section on Biochemical Pharmacology)**
Bldg. 10, Rm. 3S231
9000 Rockville Pike
Bethesda, MD 20892
**Phone:** (301)496-5590　　　　**Fax:** (301)402-1748
**Email:** zatz@codon.nih.gov
**Website:** http://intramural.nimh.nih.gov/research/lcmr
Martin Zatz, MD, Ch.

**Activities/Fields:** Cellular and biochemical mechanisms involved in the generation of circadian rhythms, their regulation by light, neurotransmitters, drugs, and their expression as behavioral and physiologic cycles. Relevant anatomic systems consist of pineal gland, supra chiasmatic nucleus of the hypothalamus, and the retina. Related research areas include regulation of photoreceptors, vitamin A, and phototransduction; receptors and second messenger systems; iorn transport and fluxes; enzyme induction, hormone synthesis, and release.

**★ 14353 ★ U.S. Department of Health and Human Services**
National Institutes of Health
National Institute of Mental Health
Laboratory of Cerebral Metabolism
**(Unit on Neurobiology)**
Bldg. 10, Rm. 3S231
9000 Rockville Pike
Bethesda, MD 20892
**Phone:** (301)496-1371
**Email:** nimhinfo@nih.gov
**Website:** http://intramural.nimh.nih.gov/research/lcm
Carolyn B. Smith, Ch.

**Activities/Fields:** Understanding of the biochemical events associated with development, plasticity, and involution of the nervous system.

**★ 14354 ★ U.S. Department of Health and Human Services**
National Institutes of Health
National Institute of Mental Health
Laboratory of Cerebral Metabolism
**(Section on Developmental Neurochemistry)**
Bldg. 10, Rm. 3S231
9000 Rockville Pike
Bethesda, MD 20892
**Phone:** (301)496-1371　　　　**Fax:** (301)480-1668
**Email:** nimhinfo@nih.gov

**Website:** http://intramural.nimh.nih.gov/research/lcm
Louis Sokoloff, MD, Ch.

**Activities/Fields:** Development and application of methods that quantitatively measure the rates of physiological and biochemical processes in the individual structures of the nervous systems of conscious and behaving animals and humans, including cerebral blood flow, local cerebral glucose utilization, and local cerebral protein synthesis.

**★ 14355 ★ U.S. Department of Health and Human Services**
National Institutes of Health
National Institute of Mental Health
Laboratory of Cerebral Metabolism
Bldg. 10, Rm. 3S231
9000 Rockville Pike
Bethesda, MD 20892
**Phone:** (301)496-1371　　　　**Fax:** (301)480-1668
**Email:** nimhinfo@nih.gov
**Website:** http://intramural.nimh.nih.gov/research/lcm
Louis Sokoloff, MD, Ch.

**Activities/Fields:** Biochemical aspects of growth, development, maturation, and regulation of metabolism in the central nervous system (CNS).

**★ 14356 ★ U.S. Department of Health and Human Services**
National Institutes of Health
National Institute of Mental Health
Laboratory of Clinical Sciences
**(Section on Clinical Neuropharmacology)**
Bldg. 10, Rm. 3D41
9000 Rockville Pike
Bethesda, MD 20892-1264
**Phone:** (301)496-3421　　　　**Fax:** (301)402-0188
**Email:** theresad@codon.nih.gov
**Website:** http://intramural.nimh.nih.gov/research/lcs/index2.html
Dennis Murphy, MD, Ch.

**Activities/Fields:** Development of critical analysis of strategies and techniques for use in evaluating functional status of the brain, serotonergic neurotransmitter system, including genes and drugs and neuropepticle systems that affect it in normal behavior, including the dimensions of personality that may be relevant to psychopathology.

**★ 14357 ★ U.S. Department of Health and Human Services**
National Institutes of Health
National Institute of Mental Health
Laboratory of Genetics
**(Unit on Cell Biology)**
Bldg. 36, Rm. 3A31
9000 Rockville Pike
Bethesda, MD 20892
**Phone:** (301)496-5351
**Email:** nimhinfo@nih.gov
**Website:** http://intramural.nimh.nih.gov/research/log/
Ted Usdin, PhD, Ch.

**Activities/Fields:** Endogenous factors that modulate neuronal function, including pain perception and pituitary hormone secretion.

**★ 14358 ★ U.S. Department of Health and Human Services**
National Institutes of Health
National Institute of Mental Health
Laboratory of Neurochemistry
Bldg. 36, Rm. 3D32
9000 Rockville Pike
Bethesda, MD 20892
**Phone:** (301)496-3579　　　　**Fax:** (301)480-9284
**Email:** nimhinfo@nih.gov
**Website:** http://intramural.nimh.nih.gov/research/lnc/
John Giovanelli, Contact

**Activities/Fields:** Regulation of synthesis of dopamine, norepinerine, serotonin, and the endothelium-derived relaxing factor nitric oxide, including the

characterization of phenylalanine, tyrosine, and tryptophan hydroxylases (the enzymes that catalyze the rate-limiting steps in the biosynthesis of these neurotransmitters).

**★ 14359 ★ U.S. Department of Health and Human Services**
National Institutes of Health
National Institute of Mental Health
Laboratory of Neurotoxicology
**(Unit on Neuroimmunology)**
10 Center Dr., Rm. 3D42
Bethesda, MD 20892-1262
**Phone:** (301)496-4022
**Email:** nimhinfo@nih.gov
Melvyn P. Heyes, PhD, Hd.

**Activities/Fields:** Clinical studies of patient groups with neurologic, genetic, or chronic inflammation disorders as well as patients with HIV.

**★ 14360 ★ U.S. Department of Health and Human Services**
National Institutes of Health
National Institute of Mental Health
Laboratory of Neurotoxicology
10 Center Dr., Rm. 3D42
Bethesda, MD 20892-1262
**Phone:** (301)496-4022　　　　**Fax:** (301)451-5780
**Email:** nimhinfo@nih.gov
**Website:** http://intramural.nimh.nih.gov/research/lnt/index2.html
Dr. Sanford P. Markey, PhD, Ch.

**Activities/Fields:** Biochemical events that cause neuronal injury and degeneration produced by genetic disease, inflammation, trauma, and exposure to neurotoxic substances.

**★ 14361 ★ U.S. Department of Health and Human Services**
National Institutes of Health
National Institute of Mental Health
Laboratory of System Neuroscience
**(Unit of Neural Network Physiology)**
Bldg. 36, Rm. 2D30
Bethesda, MD 20892
**Phone:** (301)402-2249　　　　**Fax:** (301)402-8960
**Email:** dplenz@codon.nih.gov
**Website:** http://intramural.nimh.nih.gov/lsn/NeuralNetworkPhys/NNP_Homepage.htm
Dietmar Plenz, PhD, Ch.

**Activities/Fields:** Cortex-basal ganglia (Cx-BG) circuits, including reconstruction and analysis of Cx-BG systems in vitro using organotypic cultures from rats and mice.

**★ 14362 ★ U.S. Department of Health and Human Services**
National Institutes of Health
National Institute of Mental Health
Laboratory of System Neuroscience
**(Section on Neuroanatomy)**
Bldg. 36, Rm. 2D30
9000 Rockville Pike
Bethesda, MD 20892
**Phone:** (301)496-4341　　　　**Fax:** (301)402-8960
**Email:** gerfen@helix.nih.gov
**Website:**　　　　http://intramural.nimh.nih.gov/lsn/neuroanatomy/na_homepage.htm
Charles R. Gerfen, PhD, Ch.

**Activities/Fields:** Understanding the role of basal ganglia in the frontal cortical function, using in situ hybridization histochemical techniques to quantify, at the cellular level, neurotransmitter receptor mediated changes in messenger RNAs encoding proteins or other substances that are utilized by striatal neurons, in connectionally identified subsets of neuron populations, particularly regulation of striatal neurons expressing D1 and D2 dopamine receptor subtypes.

## ★ 14363 ★ U.S. Department of Health and Human Services
**National Institutes of Health**
**National Institute of Mental Health**
**Laboratory of System Neuroscience**
Bldg. 36, Rm. 2D30
9000 Rockville Pike
Bethesda, MD 20892
**Phone:** (301)496-4341          **Fax:** (301)402-8960
**Email:** gerfen@codon.nih.gov
**Website:** http://intramural.nimh.nih.gov/lsn/
Charles R. Gerfen, PhD, Ch.

**Activities/Fields:** Neurobiology of higher brain function, including physiologic organization of primate motor cortex other parts of the frontal lobe as well as mechanisms of regulating information flow into and within the cortex.

## ★ 14364 ★ U.S. Department of Health and Human Services
**National Institutes of Health**
**National Institute of Mental Health**
**Laboratory of System Neuroscience**
**(Section on Neurophysiology)**
MS Code 4401
Bldg. 36, Rm. 2D30
9000 Rockville Pike
Bethesda, MD 20892
**Phone:** (301)402-5452          **Fax:** (301)402-5441
**Email:** nimhinfo@nih.gov
**Website:** http://nihac.info.nih.gov/
Steven P. Wise, PhD, Ch.

**Activities/Fields:** Functional organization of the primate frontal cortex; monitors activity of single neurons in awake, behaving monkeys.

## ★ 14365 ★ U.S. Department of Health and Human Services
**National Institutes of Health**
**National Institute of Mental Health**
**Section on Developmental Neurobiology**
Bldg. 31, Rm. 8A-52
9000 Rockville Pike
Bethesda, MD 20892
**Phone:** (301)443-4513
**Email:** nimhinfo@nih.gov
**Website:** http://intramural.nimh.nih.gov/research/sdn

**Activities/Fields:** Biochemical and molecular mechanisms involved in the development and function of chemical synapses; major focus in on trophic factors that promote differentiation and survival of nerve cells and the targets they innervate.

**U.S. Department of Health and Human Services**
**National Institutes of Health**
**National Institute of Neurological Disorders and Stroke**
**Division of Extramural Research**
**(Neurogenetics Program)**
*See:* Entry 9491

## ★ 14366 ★ U.S. Department of Health and Human Services
**National Institutes of Health**
**National Institute of Neurological Disorders and Stroke**
**Division of Extramural Research**
**(Clinical Trials Program)**
NSC/2216
6001 Executive Blvd.
Bethesda, MD 20892-9531
**Phone:** (301)496-9520          **Fax:** (301)480-1080
**Email:** jm137f@nih.gov
**Website:** http://www.ninds.nih.gov/about_ninds/clusters/clinical_trials.htm
John Marler, MD, Assoc. Dir.

**Activities/Fields:** Neurological diseases, including stroke and managing the symptoms of stroke.

## ★ 14367 ★ U.S. Department of Health and Human Services
**National Institutes of Health (NIH)**
**National Institute of Neurological Disorders and Stroke**
**Division of Extramural Research**
**(Systems and Cognitive Neuroscience Cluster)**
NSC/2109
6601 Executive Blvd.
Bethesda, MD 20892-9531
**Phone:** (301)496-9964          **Fax:** (301)402-2060
**Email:** ee48r@nih.gov
**Website:** http://ninds.nih.gov/about_ninds/clusters/systems_and_cognitive_neuroscience.htm
Emmeline Edwards, PhD, Dir.

**Activities/Fields:** Neurobiology of higher cognitive functions and complex behaviors; advances understanding of neuronal circuits underlying specific cognitive and motor functions.

## ★ 14368 ★ U.S. Department of Health and Human Services
**National Institutes of Health**
**National Institute of Neurological Disorders and Stroke**
**Division of Extramural Research**
**(Channels, Synapses and Circuits Cluster)**
NSC/2110B
6001 Executive Blvd.
Bethesda, MD 20892-9523
**Phone:** (301)496-1917          **Fax:** (301)480-2424
**Email:** yl5o@nih.gov
**Website:** http://www.ninds.nih.gov/about_ninds/clusters/channels_synapses_and_circuits.htm
Yuan Liu, PhD, Dir.

**Activities/Fields:** Channels, synapses, and neural circuits that underlie normal brain functions and dysfunctions related to neurological disorders, such as epilepsy.

## ★ 14369 ★ U.S. Department of Health and Human Services
**National Institutes of Health**
**National Institute of Neurological Disorders and Stroke**
**Division of Extramural Research**
**(Neurodegeneration Cluster Program)**
NSC/2223
6001 Executive Blvd.
Bethesda, MD 20892
**Phone:** (301)496-5680          **Fax:** (301)480-1080
**Email:** dm152o@nih.gov
**Website:** http://www.ninds.nih.gov/about_ninds/clusters/neurodegeneration.htm
Dr. Diane Murphy, PhD, Co-Dir.

**Activities/Fields:** Understanding neuronal cell death, including Parkinson's disease, Alzheimer's disease, amyotrophic lateral sclerosis, Huntington's disease, Pick's disease, brain cell death.

## ★ 14370 ★ U.S. Department of Health and Human Services
**National Institutes of Health (NIH)**
**National Institute of Neurological Disorders and Stroke**
**Division of Extramural Research**
**(Repair and Plasticity Program)**
NSC/2206
6001 Executive Blvd.
Bethesda, MD 20892-9525
**Phone:** (301)496-1447          **Fax:** (301)480-1080
**Email:** mm108w@nih.gov
**Website:** http://www.ninds.nih.gov/about_ninds/clusters/repair_and_plasticity.htm
Mary Ellen Cheung, PhD, Dir.

**Activities/Fields:** Traumatic brain injury (TBI), including mechanisms of injury in the acute and chronic stages, clinical trail design for traumatic brain injury, and possible use of imaging technology to assess cognitive/behavioral changes after TBI.

## ★ 14371 ★ U.S. Department of Health and Human Services
**National Institutes of Health**
**National Institute of Neurological Disorders and Stroke**
**Division of Extramural Research**
**(Neural Environment Cluster Program)**
NSC/2110
6001 Executive Blvd.
Bethesda, MD 20892-9521
**Phone:** (301)496-1431          **Fax:** (301)480-2424
**Email:** tb72z@nih.gov
**Website:** http://www.ninds.nih.gov/about_ninds/clusters/neural_environment.htm
Toby Behar, PhD, Dir.

**Activities/Fields:** Strives to reduce the burden of neurological diseases by increasing knowledge of glial and cerebrovascular cell function in normal and pathological states, as well as immune cell function and infectious agents in diseased nervous systems.

## ★ 14372 ★ U.S. Department of Health and Human Services
**National Institutes of Health (NIH)**
**National Institute of Neurological Disorders and Stroke**
**Division of Extramural Research**
**(Office of Minority Health and Research)**
NSC/2150
6601 Executive Blvd.
Bethesda, MD 20892-9531
**Phone:** (301)496-3102          **Fax:** (301)594-5929
**Email:** gj62v@nih.gov
**Website:** http://www.ninds.nih.gov/about_ninds/clusters/special_programs_in_neuroscience.htm
Gayathri Jeyarasasingam, PhD, Dir.

**Activities/Fields:** Provides grants which support research groups aiming to reduce disease disparity of populations historically at increased risk for diseases and disorders of the brain, spinal cord, and peripheral nervous system.

## ★ 14373 ★ U.S. Department of Health and Human Services
**National Institutes of Health (NIH)**
**National Institute of Neurological Disorders and Stroke**
**Division of Intramural Research**
**(Behavioral Neuroscience Unit)**
Bldg. 36, Rm. B205
36 Convent Dr., MSC 4124
Bethesda, MD 20892-4124
**Phone:** (301)496-3906          **Fax:** (301)402-2281
**Email:** schreurs@codon.nih.gov
**Website:** http://www.ninds.nih.gov/about_ninds/labs/archive/14.htm
Bernard G. Schreurs, PhD, Investigator

**Activities/Fields:** Behavior laws, or understanding what happens in the brain when learning occurs; aims to identify physiological basis of classical conditioning, an associative form of learning and memory.

## ★ 14374 ★ U.S. Department of Health and Human Services
**National Institutes of Health (NIH)**
**National Institute of Neurological Disorders and Stroke**
**Division of Intramural Research**
**(Cognitive Neuroscience Section)**
Bldg. 10, Rm. 5C205
10 Center Dr., MSC 1440
Bethesda, MD 20892-1440
**Phone:** (301)496-0220          **Fax:** (301)480-2909
**Email:** grafmanj@ninds.nih.gov
**Website:** http://www.ninds.nih.gov/about_ninds/labs/83.htm
Jordan Grafman, PhD, Sr. Investigator

**Activities/Fields:** Studies the underlying cognitive architecture and number of circumscribed prefrontal cortex brain sectors subserving specific cognitive operations and/or knowledge; understanding types of information binding that occur in the human brain.


**★ 14375 ★ U.S. Department of Health and Human Services**
**National Institutes of Health (NIH)**
**National Institute of Neurological Disorders and Stroke**
**Division of Intramural Research (Analytical Cell Biology)**
Bldg. 36, Rm. 2A21
36 Convent Dr., MSC 4062
Bethesda, MD 20892-4062
**Phone:** (301)435-2796     **Fax:** (301)480-1485
**Email:** sba@helix.nih.gov
**Website:** http://www.ninds.nih.gov/about_ninds/labs/38.htm
S. Brian Andrews, PhD, Sr. Investigator

**Activities/Fields:** Cell biology and physiology of neurons, especially the function of intracellular domains that regulate calcium (Ca) signaling following from synaptic activity; development of technologies for quantitative and molecular electron microscopy.


**★ 14376 ★ U.S. Department of Health and Human Services**
**National Institutes of Health (NIH)**
**National Institute of Neurological Disorders and Stroke**
**Division of Intramural Research (Clinical Neurocardiology Section)**
Bldg. 10, Rm. 6N252
10 Center Dr., MSC 1620
Bethesda, MD 20892-1620
**Phone:** (301)496-2103     **Fax:** (301)402-0180
**Email:** daveg@box-d.nih.gov
**Website:** http://www.ninds.nih.gov/about_ninds/labs/82.htm
David S. Goldstein, MD, Sr. Investigator

**Activities/Fields:** Clinical neurocardiology research about disorders of neuroendocrine regulation of the cardiovascular system, with emphasis on diseases where the symptomatic nervous system or catecholamines play important pathogenic roles, such as autonomic failures syndromes, pheochromocytoma, and neurogenetic conditions featuring abnormal catecholamine synthesis or metabolism.


**★ 14377 ★ U.S. Department of Health and Human Services**
**National Institutes of Health (NIH)**
**National Institute of Neurological Disorders and Stroke**
**Division of Intramural Research (Clinical Epilepsy Section)**
Bldg. 10, Rm. 5N250
10 Center Dr., MSC 1408
Bethesda, MD 20892-1408
**Phone:** (301)496-1505     **Fax:** (301)402-2871
**Email:** theodorw@ninds.nih.gov
**Website:** http://www.ninds.nih.gov/about_ninds/labs/63.htm
William H. Theodore, MD, Sr. Investigator

**Activities/Fields:** Evaluation and treatment of uncontrolled epilepsy, emphasizing non-invasive approaches to localization of epileptic foci and cognitive mapping, using video-EEG monitoring, transcranial magnetic stimulation (TMS), positron emission tomography (PET), and magnetic resonance imaging (MRI), including functional MRI and MR spectroscopy.


**★ 14378 ★ U.S. Department of Health and Human Services**
**National Institutes of Health**
**National Institute of Neurological Disorders and Stroke**
**Division of Intramural Research (Brain Stimulation Unit)**
Bldg. 10, Rm. 5N230
10 Center Dr., MSC 1430
Bethesda, MD 20892-1430
**Phone:** (301)496-0151     **Fax:** (301)402-1007
**Email:** ewass@codon.nih.gov
**Website:** http://www.ninds.nih.gov/about_ninds/labs/104.htm
Eric Wassermann, MD, Chf.

**Activities/Fields:** Transcranial stimulation as a means of assessing and altering brain function in patients with neurological and psychiatric disorders, as well as, healthy individuals. Studies include measures of axonal excitability and synaptic influences on output cells of the motor cortex, and experimental treatments that alter these measures.


**★ 14379 ★ U.S. Department of Health and Human Services**
**National Institutes of Health (NIH)**
**National Institute of Neurological Disorders and Stroke**
**Division of Intramural Research (Cellular Immunology Section)**
Bldg. 10, Rm. 5B16
10 Center Dr., MSC 1400
Bethesda, MD 20892-1400
**Phone:** (301)402-4488     **Fax:** (301)402-0373
**Email:** martinr@ninds.nih.gov
**Website:** http://www.ninds.nih.gov/about_ninds/labs/98.htm
Roland Martin, MD, Investigator

**Activities/Fields:** Understanding how the cellular immune system in multiple sclerosis (MS) patients reacts to autoantigens of the central nervous system. Research includes studies on molecular mechanisms of T-cell recognition.


**★ 14380 ★ U.S. Department of Health and Human Services**
**National Institutes of Health (NIH)**
**National Institute of Neurological Disorders and Stroke**
**Division of Intramural Research (Biochemistry Section)**
Bldg. 10, Rm. 5D37
10 Center Dr., MSC 1414
Bethesda, MD 20892-1414
**Phone:** (301)496-6628     **Fax:** (301)402-0380
**Email:** youle@helix.nih.gov
**Website:** http://www.ninds.nih.gov/about_ninds/labs/81.htm
Richard J. Youle, PhD, Sr. Investigator

**Activities/Fields:** Immunotoxins, including protein toxins and chemeric toxins; understanding molecular basis of cell death.


**U.S. Department of Health and Human Services**
**National Institutes of Health (NIH)**
**National Institute of Neurological Disorders and Stroke**
**Division of Intramural Research (Advanced MRI Section)**
*See:* Entry 4844


**U.S. Department of Veterans Affairs**
**Rehabilitation Research and Development Center**
**Design Development**
**Laboratory of Neuromuscular Biomechanics**
*See:* Entry 13496


**U.S. Department of Veterans Affairs**
**Rehabilitation Research and Development Center**
**Design Development**
**Laboratory of Neuromuscular Electrophysiology**
*See:* Entry 13497


**★ 14381 ★ U.S. Department of Veterans Affairs**
**Rehabilitation Research and Development Service**
**Center for Excellence in Functional Recovery in Chronic Spinal Cord Injury**
Rehab R&D Center (128)
Miami VA Medical Center
1201 NW 16th St.
Miami, FL 33125
**Phone:** (305)324-3363
**Email:** marca.sipskialexander@med.va.gov
**Website:** http://www.vard.org/cent/miami.htm
Marca L. Sipski, MD, Dir.

**Activities/Fields:** Spasticity, pain management, recovery of motor and sensory function, and other areas of critical importance to spinal cord injury patients seeking to regain their independence.


**★ 14382 ★ U.S. Department of Veterans Affairs**
**Rehabilitation Research and Development Service**
**Center of Excellence on Restoration of Function in Spinal Cord Injury and Multiple Sclerosis**
VA Connecticut Health Care System
950 Campbell Ave.
West Haven, CT 06516
**Phone:** (203)932-3802
**Email:** stephen.waxman@yale.edu
**Website:** http://www.vard.yale.edu/
Stephen G. Waxman, MD, Dir.

**Activities/Fields:** Understanding the molecular, cellular and physiological basis of abnormal impulse conduction, and applying this understanding to the development of strategies to restore function in people with spinal cord injury and multiple sclerosis. **Pub:** *Journal articles.*


**★ 14383 ★ U.S. Department of Veterans Affairs**
**Veterans Affairs Medical Center (West Los Angeles, CA)**
**Human Brain and Spinal Fluid Resource Center**
Neurology Research (127A)
West Los Angeles Healthcare Center
11301 Wilshire Blvd.
Los Angeles, CA 90073
**Phone:** (310)268-3536     **Fax:** (310)268-4768
**Email:** brainbnk@ucla.edu
**Website:** http://www.loni.ucla.edu/~nnrsb/nnrsb
Dr. W.W. Tourtellotte, Dir.

**Activities/Fields:** Serves as a resource bank for cryopreserved human brain, spinal fluid, serum, and other tissue. Provides specimens to research community, particularly in the area of neurological and psychiatric diseases, including Huntington's disease, Alzheimer's disease, Down's syndrome, multiple sclerosis, and epilepsy. **Frmly:** National Neurological Research Specimen Bank.


**★ 14384 ★ University of Alabama at Birmingham**
**Center for Neuroimmunology**
Department of Neurology
625 19th St. S
Birmingham, AL 35233
**Phone:** (205)934-2402     **Fax:** (205)975-6030
**Email:** jwhitaker@email.neuro.uab.edu

**Website:** http://main.uab.edu/show.asp?durki=11026
John Whitaker, MD, Co-Dir.

**Activities/Fields:** Multiple sclerosis, myasthenia gravis, glia, paraneoplastic syndromes, and idiotypes. **Frmly:** Multiple Sclerosis Research Center.


★ **14385** ★ **University of Alabama at Birmingham**
**Kirklin Pain Treatment Center**
UAB Medical Ctr.
2000 6th Ave. S, 3rd Fl.
Birmingham, AL 35233
**Phone:** (205)801-8250          **Fax:** (205)801-8253
Dr. Judy McDanal, Med. Dir.

**Activities/Fields:** Chronic pain and the management of chronic pain from benign or malignant sources. Also conducts studies on the effectiveness of group outpatient therapy for pain patients and their families and prior physical and/or sexual trauma and its relation to pain. Multimodal therapeutic regimes include behavior therapy, nerve blocks, hypnotherapy, stimulation produced analgesia (transcutaneous electrical nerve stimulation, acupuncture, and deep brain stimulation), biofeedback, and neuroablation. Affiliated with numerous departments and research centers at the University, which allows for patients to be treated according to their specific needs.


★ **14386** ★ **University of Alabama at Birmingham**
**Parkinson's Disease Center**
Jefferson Tower, Rm. 1225
Birmingham, AL 35294-7340
**Phone:** (205)934-9100          **Fax:** (205)934-0928
**Email:** tony@email.neuro.uab.edu
**Website:** http://main.uab.edu/show.asp?durki=11026
Paul Atchison, MD, Co-Dir.

**Activities/Fields:** Investigates Parkinson's disease, catecholamine receptors, genetics, and basal ganglion; and conducts related drug studies.


★ **14387** ★ **University of Alberta**
**Neurochemical Research Unit**
MacKenzie Centre
Department of Psychiatry
Edmonton, AB, Canada T6G 2B7
**Phone:** (780)492-7604          **Fax:** (780)492-6841
**Email:** glen.baker@ualberta.ca
**Website:** http://www.med.ualberta.ca/psychiatry/research.htmNeurochemical
Prof. G.B. Baker, Co-Dir.

**Activities/Fields:** Biochemical basis of depression, anxiety disorders and stroke; studies on the mechanisms of action of antidepressants and neuroleptics; neurochemical bases of reward; mechanisms of brain cell death; synthesis and pharmacological testing of potential antidepressants, anxiolytics and neuroprotective drugs; roles of amino acids and neuroactive steroids in the etiology and pharmacotherapy of anxiety disorders; drug metabolism and drug-drug interactions involving cytochrome P450 enzymes.


★ **14388** ★ **University of Arizona**
**Sleep Disorders Center**
University Medical Center, Rm. 1338
College of Medicine
Tucson, AZ 85724
**Phone:** (520)694-6112          **Fax:** (520)694-2515
**Email:** squan@sneeze.resp-sci.arizona.edu
Stuart F. Quan, MD, Dir.

**Activities/Fields:** Sleep disorders guided by studies in neurology, psychology, pulmonology, and pediatrics. Research efforts concentrate on sleep apnea, sudden infant death syndrome, nocturnal penile tumescence, male sexual dysfunction, seizure disorders, insomnia, narcolepsy, and restless leg syndrome.


★ **14389** ★ **University of British Columbia**
**Brain Research Centre**
2211 Wesbrook Mall
Vancouver, BC, Canada V6T 2B5
**Phone:** (604)822-7246          **Fax:** (604)822-0361
**Email:** info@brain.ubc.ca
**Website:** http://www.brain.ubc.ca
Dr. Max S. Cynader, Dir.

**Activities/Fields:** Neuroscience, especially neurodegeneration, multiple sclerosis, schizophrenia and mood disorders, stroke, neurotrauma, and vision.


★ **14390** ★ **University of British Columbia**
**Kinsmen Laboratory of Neurological Research**
2255 Wesbrook Mall
Vancouver, BC, Canada V6T 1Z3
**Phone:** (604)822-7375          **Fax:** (604)822-7981
**Email:** neurosci@interchange.ubc.ca
**Website:** http://www.interchg.ubc.ca/neurosci/
Dr. Steven Vincent, Hd.

**Activities/Fields:** Neurological sciences, including studies on behavioral effects of specific brain lesions and/or drugs, central nervous system histochemistry and electron microscopy, Parkinsonism, epilepsy, Alzheimer's disease, dystonia, neurotransmitter systems and behavior, chorea, muscular dystrophy, psychopharmacology, and in vivo brain microdialysis and voltammetry.


★ **14391** ★ **University of British Columbia**
**Laboratories of Neurophysiology**
Copp Bldg.
Department of Physiology
2146 Health Science Mall
Vancouver, BC, Canada V6T 1Z3
**Phone:** (604)822-2494          **Fax:** (604)822-6048
**Email:** info@physiology.ubc.ca
**Website:** http://www.physiology.ubc.ca
Dr. Kenneth Baimbridge, Dir.

**Activities/Fields:** Neurophysiology, including studies of basal ganglia, limbic forebrain, spinal cord, mechanisms of synaptic transmission in central nervous system, and amino acids.


★ **14392** ★ **University of Calgary**
**Neuroscience Research Group**
3330 Hospital Dr. NW
Calgary, AB, Canada T2N 4N1
**Phone:** (403)220-4472          **Fax:** (403)270-2700
**Email:** neuro@ucalgary.ca
**Website:** http://www.acs.ucalgary.ca/~neuro/
Dr. Keith Sharkey, Chm.

**Activities/Fields:** Multidisciplinary group of independently funded researchers investigating various aspects of the nervous system, including hypothalamic mechanisms of thermoregulation, endocrine and autonomic control, axonal transport, nerve regeneration, actions of anesthetics, developmental neurobiology, synaptic circuitry, molluscan neurobiology, neurotransmitter/peptide pharmacology, structure and function of visual system, neuropathological disorders, molecular neurobiology, molecular biology of neurodegenerative disorders, sensory and motor physiology, cerebellar structure and function, and restorative neurology.


★ **14393** ★ **University of California, Davis**
**Rehabilitation Research and Training Center in Neuromuscular Diseases**
Department of Physical Medicine & Rehabilitation, TB 191
School of Medicine
Davis, CA 95616
**Phone:** (530)752-2903          **Fax:** (530)752-3468
**Email:** NMDinfo@ucdavis.edu
**Website:** http://www.rehabinfo.net
Craig McDonald, MD, Dir.

**Activities/Fields:** Increase of functional capacity, quality of life, and community integration of persons with neuromuscular diseases. Twelve research and/or training projects are organized into four cores: Interventions to Preserve Functional Capacity; Genetic Information and Research; Interventions to Enhance Community Integration; and Training and Information Services. The projects include Management of Muscle Wasting in Neuromuscular Disease; Exercise and Dietary Intervention in Slowly Progressive Neuromuscular Disease; Nutritional Assessment and Intervention in Duchenne Muscular Dystrophy; Exercise-Related Fatigue and Injury in an Animal Model of Muscular Dystrophy; Pain in Neuromuscular Disease: Incidence, Severity and Relationship to Physical Impairment and Disability; Outcome of Lower-Limb Orthotic Intervention in Hereditary and Acquired Neuromuscular Disease; Role of Personal Strivings in the Quality of life and Community Integration of Individuals with Neuromuscular Disorders; Stress and Coping in Children and Adolescents Living with Muscular Dystrophy and other Neuromuscular Diseases; Enhancing Medical Students' Attitudes and Knowledge about Those Who Live with Disabilities; Meeting Information Needs to Enhance the Community Integration of Individuals with Neuromuscular Disease; Risks and Benefits of Genetic Testing in Persons with Hereditary Neuromuscular Disease; and National Clearinghouse of Information on Neuromuscular Disease. **Pub:** *RRTC Newsletter*.


★ **14394** ★ **University of California, Irvine**
**Herklotz Research Facility**
**Center for the Neurobiology of Learning and Memory**
320 Qureshey Research Laboratory
Irvine, CA 92697-3800
**Phone:** (949)824-5193          **Fax:** (949)824-8439
**Email:** jlmcgaug@uci.edu
**Website:** http://www.memory.uci.edu
Dr. James L. McGaugh, Dir.

**Activities/Fields:** Neurobiology of learning and memory, including biochemical mechanisms, systems neurophysiology, modulation of memory, cognitive neuropsychology, and neural modeling. **Pub:** *Annual Report.* • *Conference Proceedings*.


★ **14395** ★ **University of California, Irvine**
**Memory Disorders Clinic**
Department of Neurology
Irvine, CA 92697
**Phone:** (949)824-6088          **Fax:** (949)824-2132
**Email:** astarr@uci.edu
Arnold Starr, MD, Dir.

**Activities/Fields:** Multidisciplinary approach to diagnosis and treatment of memory disorders, including the development and testing of memory enhancement programs.


★ **14396** ★ **University of California, Irvine**
**Reeve-Irvine Research Center**
1105 Gillespie Neuroscience Research Facility
Irvine, CA 92697-4292
**Phone:** (949)824-3993          **Fax:** (949)824-2625
**Email:** osteward@uci.edu
**Website:** http://www.reeve.uci.edu
Oswald Steward, PhD, Dir.

**Activities/Fields:** Injuries to and diseases of the spinal cord that result in paralysis or other loss of neurologic function, with the goal of finding a cure. **Pub:** *Newsletter.* • *Research manuscripts*.


★ **14397** ★ **University of California, Los Angeles**
**Alzheimer's Disease Center (ADC)**
710 Westwood Plz., Rm. 2238
Los Angeles, CA 90095-1769
**Phone:** (310)206-5238          **Fax:** (310)206-5287
**Email:** adc@ucla.edu
**Website:** http://www.adc.ucla.edu
Donna Masterman, MD, Dir.

**Activities/Fields:** Diagnosis, pathophysiology, and treatment of dementing illnesses, such as Alzheimer's disease. **Pub:** *Newsletter*, annually.

**★ 14398 ★ University of California, Los Angeles**
**Brain Research Institute (BRI)**
Gonda Goldschmied Neuroscience & Genetics
Research Center
Los Angeles, CA 90095-1761
**Phone:** (310)825-5061          **Fax:** (310)206-5855
**Website:** http://www.bri.ucla.edu
Allan Tobin, Dir.

**Activities/Fields:** Brain and central nervous system, including interdisciplinary studies in developmental neurobiology, molecular neurobiology, neuroanatomy, neurobiophysics, neurochemistry, neurocytology, neuroendocrinology, neuroimaging, neuromuscular physiology, neuropathology, neuropharmacology, neurophysiology, behavior, neuroimmunology, and experimental epilepsy. Also conducts research on aging, Alzheimer's Disease, alcohol effects on the central nervous system, cellular neurobiology, neuroendocrinology, and neuromuscular plasticity. **Pub:** *Neuroscience News.*

**★ 14399 ★ University of California, Los Angeles**
**Laboratory of Neuro Imaging Resource**
Department of Neurology
School of Medicine
710 Westwood Plz., Rm. 4238
Los Angeles, CA 90095-1769
**Phone:** (310)206-2101          **Fax:** (310)206-5518
**Email:** toga@loni.ucla.edu
**Website:** http://www.loni.ucla.edu/
Arthur W. Toga, PhD, Prin. Investigator
**Activities/Fields:** Brain structure and function.

**University of California, Los Angeles Neuropsychiatric Institute**
*See:* Entry 12754

**★ 14400 ★ University of California, Los Angeles**
**Reed Neurological Research Center**
**Laboratory of Neuro Imaging**
710 Westwood Plz., Rm. 4-238
Los Angeles, CA 90095
**Phone:** (310)206-2101          **Fax:** (310)206-5518
**Email:** toga@loni.ucla.edu
**Website:** http://www.loni.ucla.edu
Arthur W. Toga, PhD, Contact
**Activities/Fields:** Neuroanatomy, neuroimaging, neurophysiology, and neurological diseases.

**★ 14401 ★ University of California, San Diego**
**Alzheimer's Disease Research Center**
9500 Gilman Dr.
La Jolla, CA 92093-0948
**Phone:** (858)622-5800          **Fax:** (858)622-1017
**Email:** adrc@ucsd.edu
**Website:** http://adrc.ucsd.edu
Dr. Leon Thal, Prin. Investigator
**Activities/Fields:** Longitudinal research on the clinical and cognitive changes associated with Alzheimer's disease and other dementing illnesses by obtaining epidemiological data, medical histories, analysis of blood and sera, administration of batteries of neuropsychological tests, and neurological examinations of patients. Performs clinical drug trials, research on electrophysiology and neuroimaging studies, evaluations of the effects of caregiving stress on the caregivers, studies of memory and language dysfunction, and the possibility of a genetic or metabolic basis for Alzheimer's disease. Also conducts olfaction studies.

**★ 14402 ★ University of California, San Francisco**
**Brain Tumor Research Center**
PO Box 0520
San Francisco, CA 94143-0520
**Phone:** (415)476-4590          **Fax:** (415)476-9687
**Website:** http://www.som.ucsf.edu/neuros/research/
BTRC.htm
Mitchel S. Berger, MD, Dir.
**Activities/Fields:** Cytotoxic therapies, radiation therapy, and chemotherapy; elucidates the difference between normal brain cells and brain tumor cells; molecular biology of brain tumors.

**★ 14403 ★ University of California, San Francisco**
**Gladstone Institute of Neurological Disease (GIND)**
PO Box 419100
San Francisco, CA 94141-9100
**Phone:** (415)695-3819          **Fax:** (415)826-6541
**Website:** http://gladstone.ucsf.edu/gind/
Lennart Mucke, MD, Dir.
**Activities/Fields:** Understanding the central nervous system so that rational strategies can be developed to more effectively treat Alzheimer's disease, Huntington's disease, HIV-associated dementia, and stroke.

**★ 14404 ★ University of California, San Francisco**
**Keck Center for Integrative Neurosciences**
513 Parnassus Ave., Rm. HSE-802
PO Box 0444
San Francisco, CA 94143-0444
**Phone:** (415)502-4975          **Fax:** (415)502-4848
**Email:** keck-info@phy.ucsf.edu
**Website:** http://www.keck.ucsf.edu/keck/
Dr. Steve Lisberger, Dir.
**Activities/Fields:** Neurochemistry of pain modulatory systems in the brainstem and spinal cord, using in vivo microdialysis, cytochemistry and high pressure liquid chromotography.

**★ 14405 ★ University of California, San Francisco**
**Pain Clinical Research Center (PCRC)**
1701 Divisadero, Ste. 480
San Francisco, CA 94117
**Phone:** (415)885-7899
**Email:** mcrwind@itsa.ucsf.edu
**Website:** http://itsa.ucsf.edu/~pcrc/general.html
Amir Lachman, Contact
**Activities/Fields:** Neuropathic pain, which is pain from damage to nerves that has occurred from disease processes, viruses, or injury.

**★ 14406 ★ University of California, San Francisco**
**Wheeler Center for the Neurobiology of Addiction**
Box 0453
San Francisco, CA 94143-0453
**Phone:** (415)502-4140          **Fax:** (415)476-9386
**Email:** ucsfcna@itsa.ucsf.edu
**Website:** http://www.ucsf.edu/cnba/Center
Dr. Howard Fields, Dir.
**Activities/Fields:** Identification of the neural circuits, molecular targets, and biochemical actions that help drugs of abuse take command of the brain. **Pub:** *Wheeler Center Newsletter.*

**★ 14407 ★ University of California, Santa Barbara**
**Autism Research Center**
Phelps Hall, Rm. 1180
Research Office
Graduate School of Education
Santa Barbara, CA 93106-9490
**Phone:** (805)893-2416          **Fax:** (805)893-5923
**Email:** koegel@education.ucsb.edu
**Website:** http://www.education.ucsb.edu/~autism/
Robert Koegel, PhD, Dir.
**Activities/Fields:** Autism, especially education for autistic children; the effect of treatment programs on the child, the child's family and the integration of the child in the school setting and the community; and the development and use of non-aversive treatment for severe problems such as self-injury and aggression, as often seen in autistic children.

**★ 14408 ★ University of Chicago**
**Brain Research Institute**
MC 3026
Department of Surgery
5841 S Maryland Ave.
Chicago, IL 60637-0026
**Phone:** (773)702-2123          **Fax:** (773)702-3518
**Email:** dtorrey@surgery.bsd.uchicago.edu
Bryce Weir, MD, Dir.
**Activities/Fields:** Alzheimer's disease, amyotrophic lateral sclerosis, myasthenia gravis, AIDS, sleep and sleep disorders, dyslexia, hyperkinesia, epilepsy and epileptoid disorders, mental retardation, mental illness, and brain and nervous system disorders such as multiple sclerosis, muscular dystrophy, cerebral palsy, encephalitis, Parkinson's disease, stroke, cerebral hemorrhage, aneurysm tumor, head injury, and intractable pain. Conducts basic research in neurophysiology, neuropharmacology, neuroanatomy, molecular biology, neuroimmunology, and virology.

**★ 14409 ★ University of Cincinnati**
**Headache Center**
Aring Neurology Department
222 Piedmont Ave., Ste. 2300
Cincinnati, OH 45219
**Phone:** (513)475-8730          **Fax:** (513)475-8033
Dr. Joseph Nicolas, Co-Dir.
**Activities/Fields:** Migraine headaches.

**★ 14410 ★ University of Colorado—Denver**
**Rocky Mountain Taste and Smell Center**
Campus Box B-205
4200 E 9th Ave.
Denver, CO 80262-0205
**Phone:** (303)315-6600          **Fax:** (303)315-8787
**Email:** bruce.jafek@uchsc.edu
Bruce W. Jafek, MD, Med. Dir.
**Activities/Fields:** Taste and smell dysfunction, using animal and human models, including ultrastructural change in the sense of smell during post viral states, head trauma, aging and taste dysfunction due to radiation therapy, and drugs.

**★ 14411 ★ University of Connecticut**
**Center for Neurological Sciences**
University of Connecticut Health Center
263 Farmington Ave., Rm. L4071A
Farmington, CT 06030-3401
**Phone:** (860)679-2645          **Fax:** (860)679-8766
**Email:** kent@neuron.uchc.edu
**Website:** http://www3.uchc.edu/~nsinfo/
D. Kent Morest, MD, Dir.
**Activities/Fields:** Normal functions and disorders of the nervous system. expression and membrane biogenesis in neurons and glia; gene expression, release, and physiological roles of endogenous opioids; electrophysiology of excitable tissue at the cellular and systems level; development of the heart and the autonomic nervous system; cell culture of neural tissue and neural crest development; stimulus coding, synaptic organization, and development of sensory systems; communicative sciences; structure and function of auditory and gustatory systems; mathematical modeling of neural systems; central nervous system trauma; biology of multiple sclerosis; regeneration and transplantation; biology of epilepsy; and neurobiology of Alzheimer's.

## ★ 14412 ★ University of Connecticut Connecticut Chemosensory Clinical Research Center

University of Connecticut Health Center
263 Farmington Ave.
Farmington, CT 06030
**Phone:** (860)679-1000 **Fax:** (860)679-1856
**Email:** raisz@nso.uchc.edu
Dr. Lawrence G. Raisz, Dir.

**Activities/Fields:** Taste and smell disorders of various etiologies, plus independent research projects studying chemosensory function.

## ★ 14413 ★ University of Florida Center for Neurobiological Sciences

Med. Sci. Bldg.
Medical Science, PO Box 100244
Gainesville, FL 32610-0244
**Phone:** (352)392-3383 **Fax:** (352)392-8347
**Email:** vierck@ufbi.ufl.edu
Dr. Charles Vierck, Jr., Dir.

**Activities/Fields:** Neurobiological sciences, including neuroanatomy, neurology, neuropsychology, neurophysiology, neurochemistry, neuropharmacology, and neuroendocrinology. Centralizes interdisciplinary communication and research training in neurobiological sciences and coordinates graduate student, postdoctoral, and faculty research in this area at the University.

## ★ 14414 ★ University of Florida Center for Neurobiology of Aging

College of Pharmacy
Box 100487, JHMHC
Gainesville, FL 32610
**Phone:** (352)392-8509 **Fax:** (352)392-9364
**Email:** meyerlab@grove.ufl.edu
**Website:** http://www.cop.ufl.edu/centers/cna/cna.htm
Edwin M. Meyer, PhD, Dir.

**Activities/Fields:** Alzheimer's disease studies, including evaluation of gene expression in Alzheimer's patients and evaluation of complex behaviors, especially memory.

## ★ 14415 ★ University of Florida McKnight Brain Institute

PO Box 100015
Gainesville, FL 32610-0015
**Phone:** (352)392-0490 **Fax:** (352)846-0185
**Email:** ufbi@ufbi.ufl.edu
**Website:** http://www.mbi.ufl.edu/
William G. Luttge, PhD, Exec. Dir.

**Activities/Fields:** Peripheral Nerve Trauma Research Program, including biomaterials research, peripheral nerve regeneration, and mechanisms and control of pain associated with peripheral nerve trauma; Head Injury Research Program, including injury- and/or stroke-induced problems with memory, language, attention, emotion, motor skills, and epilepsy; molecular, cellular, and immunological mechanisms involved in nerve cell death and injury following stroke or closed head injury; Neurodegenerative Diseases Program, including molecular biologic studies of genetic bases of a variety of neurologic dysfunctions, including neurodegenerative movement disorders, cell biological studies on Batten's disease, and cell biological and MRI studies of laboratory animal models of multiple sclerosis. Additional studies include the underlying causes of Alzheimer's disease; the neurobiological consequences of alcohol and cocaine abuse in both adults and fetuses; and the molecular and cellular mechanisms and the behavioral and neurologic consequences of such viral-induced neurodegenerative diseases as AIDS, polio, and measles.

## ★ 14416 ★ University of Illinois at Chicago Consultation Clinic for Epilepsy

912 S Wood St., Rm. 156
Chicago, IL 60612
**Phone:** (312)996-7360 **Fax:** (312)413-7704
**Email:** neuro@uic.edu
**Website:** http://www.uic.edu/depts/mcne
Dr. Daniel B. Hier, Dir.

**Activities/Fields:** Neurophysiology and neuropharmacology in the convulsive state, including studies on surgery for intractable psychomotor epilepsy, epidemiology of epilepsy, and side effects of various anticonvulsants. Also evaluates various new anticonvulsants.

## ★ 14417 ★ University of Illinois at Chicago Electroencephalography Laboratory

MC 722
Department of Neurology
1740 W Taylor, 5th Fl., Rm. 530
Chicago, IL 60612
**Phone:** (312)996-3865 **Fax:** (312)413-8540
**Email:** jhughes@uic.edu
Dr. John R. Hughes, Hd.

**Activities/Fields:** Psychophysiology, including studies on clinical correlates of electroencephalic abnormalities, epilepsy, and organic brain disease.

## ★ 14418 ★ University of Iowa Alzheimer's Disease Research Center

Department of Neurology
College of Medicine
200 Hawkins Dr.
Iowa City, IA 52242
**Phone:** (319)356-4296 **Fax:** (319)356-4505
**Email:** antonio_damasio@uiowa.edu
Antonio Damasio, Dir.

**Activities/Fields:** Alzheimer's disease and related conditions. Departments with participating specialists include anatomy, radiology, pathology, ophthalmology and psychology.

## ★ 14419 ★ University of Iowa Iowa Spine Research Center

Biomedical Engineering, 1202 EB
Iowa City, IA 52242
**Phone:** (319)384-0504 **Fax:** (319)353-7139
**Email:** malcolm-pope@uiowa.edu
**Website:** http://www.uiowa.edu/~vpr/research/organize/spine.htm
Malcolm H. Pope, Dir.

**Activities/Fields:** Causes, prevention, treatment, and rehabilitation of low back pain and other spinal disorders, including ergonomics, biomechanics, outcomes research, and epidemiology.

## University of Kansas Alzheimer's Disease Center (ADC)

See: Entry 12759

## ★ 14420 ★ University of Kansas Center for Neurobiology and Immunology Research (CNIR)

Higuchi Biosciences Center
2099 Constant Ave.
Lawrence, KS 66047-2535
**Phone:** (785)864-7339 **Fax:** (785)864-5738
**Email:** emichaelis@ku.edu
**Website:** http://www.hbc.ukans.edu/
Dr. Elias K. Michaelis, Dir.

**Activities/Fields:** Neurobiology and immunology, focusing on the problems of chronic, neurodegenerative diseases and immunological disorders. Specific interests include the development of new analytical methods for monitoring nerve cell activity in the brain, exploratory research in the mechanisms of neurodegeneration and the development of new therapeutic strategies based on the use of proteins or oligonucleotides as drug treatments, studies of the regulation of antibody production by immune system cells and the development of new screening procedures for immunotherapeutic agents, designing of new peptide drugs for the control of immune rejection reactions, and new molecular biological tools for recombinant DNA research. **Pub:** *HBC Newsletter*, 3/year.

## ★ 14421 ★ University of Kansas Neurobiology Research Laboratory

VA Medical Center
4801 Linwood Blvd.
Kansas City, MO 64128
**Phone:** (816)861-4700 **Fax:** (816)922-3375
**Email:** bfestoff@kumc.edu
**Website:** http://www.kumc.edu/kcvamc/research/nbrl
Barry W. Festoff, MD, Dir.

**Activities/Fields:** Development, plasticity, and diseases of the nervous system. Studies focus on synaptic formation and metabolism; roles of serine proteases and inhibitors (serpins); regulation of amyloid precursor protein processing in Alzheimer's disease; and biological markers in head injuries.

## ★ 14422 ★ University of Kentucky Center for Sensor Technology (CenSeT)

306 Davis Mills Bldg.
800 Rose St.
Lexington, KY 40536-0098
**Phone:** (859)323-4531 **Fax:** (859)257-5310
**Email:** censet@pop.uky.edu
**Website:** http://www.mc.uky.edu/censet/
Greg Gerhardt, PhD, Dir.

**Activities/Fields:** Design and construction of computer-based microsensor techniques to directly monitor biological signaling of the intact brain in real time. The long-term goal is to develop methods leading to improved health care for individuals with brain disorders.

## ★ 14423 ★ University of Kentucky Sanders-Brown Center on Aging Alzheimer's Disease Research Center

101 Sanders-Brown Bldg.
800 S Limestone
Lexington, KY 40536-0230
**Phone:** (859)323-6040 **Fax:** (859)323-2866
**Email:** wmarkesbery@aging.coa.uky.edu
**Website:** http://www.coa.uky.edu
William R. Markesbery, MD, Dir.

**Activities/Fields:** Alzheimer's disease, focusing on the cause, treatment, and eventual cure. **Pub:** *ADRC Update*, quarterly. Newsletter. • *Alzheimer's Disease Review*. Journal.

## ★ 14424 ★ University of Kentucky Spinal Cord and Brain Injury Research Center (SCoBIRC)

226 Sanders-Brown Bldg.
Chandler Medical Center
800 S Limestone
Lexington, KY 40536-0230
**Phone:** (859)257-1412 **Fax:** (859)323-2866
**Email:** jgeddes@uky.edu
**Website:** http://www.mc.uky.edu/scobirc/default.asp
James W. Geddes, PhD, Dir.

**Activities/Fields:** Injuries to the spinal cord and brain that result in paralysis or other loss of neurologic function.

## ★ 14425 ★ University of Manitoba Spinal Cord Research Centre (SCRC)

Faculty of Medicine
436 Basic Medical Science Bldg.
730 William Ave.
Winnipeg, MB, Canada R3E 3J7
**Phone:** (204)789-3761 **Fax:** (204)789-3930
**Email:** info@scrc.umanitoba.ca
**Website:** http://www.scrc.umanitoba.ca/scrc/about.html
Prof. Larry M. Jordan, PhD, Dir.

**Activities/Fields:** Mechanisms controlling major functional systems in the brain and spinal cord and development of clinical tools for the treatment of injury and diseases affecting these systems.

**★ 14426 ★ University of Maryland**
**Maryland Center for Multiple Sclerosis**
Neurology Department, N4W49
22 S Greene St.
Baltimore, MD 21201
**Phone:** (410)328-5605          **Fax:** (410)328-5425
**Email:** scoates@mdcms.org
**Website:** http://www.mdcms.org
Kenneth P. Johnson, MD, Dir.

**Activities/Fields:** Immunologic and virologic research in multiple sclerosis. Also conducts clinical trials of new treatment for multiple sclerosis.


**★ 14427 ★ University of Maryland**
**Maryland Stroke Center**
655 Baltimore St., Rm. 12-006
Baltimore, MD 21201-1559
**Phone:** (410)706-0414          **Fax:** (410)706-0816
**Email:** skittner@umaryland.edu
Dr. Steven Kittner, Dir.

**Activities/Fields:** Cerebrovascular disease, including stroke, computer modelling of stroke, use of artificial intelligence in stroke patient care, aphasia recovery in stroke patients, and development of prognostics for stroke patient care, criteria of diagnosis of embolic stroke, drug use/abuse as a cause of stroke, stroke in the young, and progressing ischemic stroke. Activities are carried out through the Stroke Epidemiology Unit, Systolic Hypertension in the Elderly Project, Cardiovascular Health Study. **Pub:** *Newsletter*, quarterly. **Frmly:** Clinical Stroke Research Center; Center for the Study of Cerebrovascular Disease and Stroke.


**★ 14428 ★ University of Maryland at**
**College Park**
**Neuroscience and Cognitive Science**
**Program**
College of Life Science
College Park, MD 20742
**Phone:** (301)405-8910          **Fax:** (301)314-9358
**Email:** sd136@umail.umd.edu
**Website:** http://www.life.umd.edu/nacs
Dr. Arthur Popper, Dir.

**Activities/Fields:** Coordinates and integrates neurosciences and cognitive studies.


**★ 14429 ★ University of Massachusetts**
**at Amherst**
**Center for Neuroendocrine Studies (CNS)**
Tobin Hall
Neuroscience & Behavior Program
135 Hicks Way
Amherst, MA 01003-7720
**Phone:** (413)545-1524          **Fax:** (413)545-0769
**Email:** blaustein@cns.umass.edu
**Website:** http://www.umass.edu/cns/
Prof. Jeffrey D. Blaustein, Dir.

**Activities/Fields:** Relationships among hormones, the brain, physiology, and behavior, including the relationship of environmental pollutants to reproduction and hormonal response, sexual differentiation of the nervous system and behavior, neuroendocrine control of circadian rhythms, and hormonal regulation of behaviors.


**★ 14430 ★ University of Medicine and**
**Dentistry of New Jersey**
**Institute for Disability Prevention and**
**Wellness**
1 Medical Center Dr., Ste. 146
Stratford, NJ 08084
**Phone:** (856)566-6247          **Fax:** (856)566-6397
**Email:** cjd@bu.edu
Dr. Carlo J. Deluca, Dir.

**Activities/Fields:** Rehabilitation and neuromuscular disorders and wellness. **Frmly:** Neuromusculoskeletel Institute.


**★ 14431 ★ University of Miami**
**Center for Neurological Diseases**
1501 NW 9th Ave.
PO Box 016960
Miami, FL 33136-6960
**Phone:** (305)243-6732          **Free:** 800-707-5589
**Fax:** (305)243-3321
Noble David, MD, Contact

**Activities/Fields:** Neuroscience, including physiological, neurochemical, anatomical, metabolic, neuropharmacological and vascular mechanisms that account for normal brain function, and the changes in these which underlie neurological diseases such as stroke, senile dementia, epilepsy, Parkinson's syndrome, Alzheimer's disease, multiple sclerosis, amyotrophic lateral sclerosis (ALS), and other neurological dysfunctions.


**★ 14432 ★ University of Miami**
**Cerebral Vascular Disease Research**
**Center**
Department of Neurology, D4-5
PO Box 016960
Miami, FL 33101-6960
**Phone:** (305)243-6449          **Fax:** (305)243-5830
**Email:** mdginsberg@stroke.med.miami.edu
Dr. Myron D. Ginsberg, Dir.

**Activities/Fields:** Cerebrovascular physiology, brain metabolism, and pathophysiology of cerebral ischemia/hypoxia, focusing on animal models of focal and global ischemia.


**★ 14433 ★ University of Miami**
**Miami Project to Cure Paralysis**
Mail Locator R-48
School of Medicine
PO Box 016960
Miami, FL 33101-6960
**Phone:** (305)243-7108          **Free:** 800-782-6387
**Fax:** (305)243-3913
**Email:** mpinfo@miamiproject.miami.edu
**Website:** http://www.themiamiproject.org
Maria Amador, Dir.

**Activities/Fields:** Spinal cord injury (SCI), emphasizing characterization of SCI (magnetic resonance imaging, electron microscopy, experimental models, and electrophysiology); design of effective treatments (molecular neurobiology, cell therapy, and tissue transplantation); and maximization of function (body weight support gait training, functional electrical stimulation, sexual function/male fertility, and motor-evoked potentials). **Pub:** *The Project Newsletter*, 3/year.


**★ 14434 ★ University of Miami**
**Touch Research Institutes**
Department of Pediatrics
Sch. of Medicine
PO Box 016820
Miami, FL 33101-6820
**Phone:** (305)243-6781          **Fax:** (305)243-6488
**Email:** tfield@med.miami.edu
**Website:** http://www.miami.edu/touch-research
Dr. Tiffany M. Field, Dir.

**Activities/Fields:** Sense of touch, including the biology of touch in health and development, and the role of touch therapy in medicine and the treatment of disease. Specific research areas include the use of massage in enhancing immune function in AIDS and cancer patients, massage effects on growth in premature infants, underlying mechanism responsible for the relationship between touch and physical growth and emotional development in infants and children, the role of massage in sports medicine and wound healing, the effects of touch therapy on addictive personalities, pain reduction during invasive medical procedures, and alleviation of skin disorders such as eczema and psoriasis. Studies the effects of touch on persons of all ages. **Pub:** *Touch Research Series.* • *Touchpoints Newsletter*.


**University of Michigan**
**Biomechanics Research Laboratory (BRL)**
*See:* Entry 3109


**★ 14435 ★ University of Michigan**
**Center for Neural Communication**
**Technology**
Electrical Engineering & Computer Science
1301 Beal Ave.
Ann Arbor, MI 48109
**Phone:** (734)764-5252          **Fax:** (734)763-8041
**Email:** dja@eecs.umich.edu
**Website:** http://www.engin.umich.edu/facility/cnct/
Prof. David J. Anderson, PhD, Dir.

**Activities/Fields:** Design of silicon substrate multichannel microelectrodes for use in electrophysiology and clinical applications; device fabrication and post processing technologies such as coatings and packaging; use technology such as delivery systems, signal processing, and data handling.


**★ 14436 ★ University of Michigan**
**Michigan Alzheimer's Disease Research**
**Center**
Department of Neurology, TC 1914
1500 E Medical Center Dr.
Ann Arbor, MI 48109-0489
**Phone:** (734)764-2190          **Fax:** (734)763-5059
**Email:** sgilman@umich.edu
**Website:** http://www.med.umich.edu/madrc/
Sid Gilman, MD, Ch.

**Activities/Fields:** Alzheimer's disease and other neurodegenerative diseases associated with dementia, including Dementia with lewy bodies, Parkinson's disease, multiple system atrophy, progressive supranuclear palsy, and olivopontocerebellar atrophy. The effects on the health of caregivers of Alzheimer's disease patients is also studies. **Pub:** *Bridges Newsletter*, 3/year. Newsletter.


**★ 14437 ★ University of Michigan**
**Neurobiology Laboratory**
6223 School of Dentistry
1101 N University Ave.
Ann Arbor, MI 48109-1078
**Phone:** (734)763-1080          **Fax:** (734)764-2110
**Email:** rmbrad@umich.edu
Prof. Robert M. Bradley, Contact

**Activities/Fields:** Sensory and motor circuits, taste sensation, and associated reflexes, including salivation. Specific areas of study include the sense of taste, focusing on the cellular factors that regulate functional differentiation of salt taste pathways; interrelations between afferent taste input and brainstem control of salivary gland reflexes; and regeneration of peripheral taste nerves through micro-electrode arrays to develop a system from chronic, in vivo study of regenerated sensory nerve fibers.


**★ 14438 ★ University of Michigan**
**Neurosurgery Laboratory**
Kresge Medical Research Bldg.
Ann Arbor, MI 48109
**Phone:** (734)764-1207          **Fax:** (734)763-7322
**Email:** jhoff@umich.edu
Dr. J.T. Hoff, Dir.

**Activities/Fields:** Cerebral ischemia, edema, structure and function of central nervous system and its ability to sustain trauma, vascular insufficiency, and brain tumor oncogenesis.


**★ 14439 ★ University of Michigan**
**University of Michigan Model Spinal Cord**
**Injury Care System**
University of Michigan Health System
Department of Physical Medicine & Rehabilitation
300 N Ingalls, Rm. NI2A09
Ann Arbor, MI 48109-0491
**Phone:** (734)763-0971          **Fax:** (734)936-5492
**Email:** model_sci@umich.edu

**Website:** http://www.med.umich.edu/pmr/model_sci/
David R. Gater, MD, Co-Dir.
**Activities/Fields:** Spinal cord injuries. **Pub:** *SCI ACCESS Newsletter*, semiannually.


★ **14440** ★ **University of Minnesota**
**Barin Sciences Center**
Veterans Affairs Medical Center, 11B
1 Veterans Dr.
Minneapolis, MN 55417
**Phone:** (612)725-2282          **Fax:** (612)725-2291
**Email:** omega@maroon.tc.umn.edu
Apostolos P. Georgopoulos, MD, Dir.
**Activities/Fields:** Brain physiology, cognitive psychology, .and motor control.


★ **14441** ★ **University of Missouri—**
**Columbia**
**Missouri Model Spinal Cord Injury**
**System (MOMSCIS)**
Department of Health Psychology
1 Hospital Dr., DC046.00
Columbia, MO 65212
**Phone:** (573)884-7972          **Free:** 800-720-6286
**Fax:** (573)884-2902
**Email:** willettjm@health.missouri.edu
**Website:** http://www.hsc.missouri.edu/~momscis/
Joanne Willett, Contact
**Activities/Fields:** Spinal cord injuries. **Pub:** *Spinal Series Newsletter*.


★ **14442** ★ **University of Missouri—St.**
**Louis**
**Center for Neurodynamics**
8001 Natural Bridge Rd.
Saint Louis, MO 63121
**Phone:** (314)516-5015          **Fax:** (314)516-6152
**Email:** mossf@umsl.edu
**Website:** http://www.umsl.edu/~neurodyn/intro.html
Dr. Frank Moss, Dir.
**Activities/Fields:** Study of the dynamical properties of neurons in the central nervous system.


★ **14443** ★ **University of Montreal**
**Experimental Neuropsychology Research**
**Group**
PO Box 6128, Downtown Sta.
Montreal, QC, Canada H3C 3J7
**Phone:** (514)343-2341          **Fax:** (514)343-5787
**Email:** franco.lepore@umontreal.ca
Dr. Franco Lepore, Dir.
**Activities/Fields:** Neural substrates of sensory-motor integration in animals and humans, focusing on the functional organization of sensory systems (vision, somesthesis, audition) in several animal species, especially monkeys and cats. Behavioral evaluation of humans with normal sensory-motor function (visual perception, visuomotor functions, audition), music perception, and humans with congenital or acquired cerebral damage (agenesis of the corpus callosum, hemispherectomies, and Alzheimer). Also studies various higher level cognition functions, such as language and memory both in normal subjects and neurologically or functionally anamolous subjects.


★ **14444** ★ **University of Montreal**
**Neurological Sciences Research Centre**
C.P. 6128, succ.
centre-ville
Montreal, QC, Canada H3C 3J7
**Phone:** (514)343-6366          **Fax:** (514)343-6113
**Email:** crsn@physio.umontreal.ca
**Website:** http://www.crsn.umontreal.ca
Dr. Serge Rossignol, Dir.
**Activities/Fields:** Functions of the nervous system, including sensory motor functions, and the cortical and subcortical control of rhythmical movements of the limbs and voluntary movements of the arm and the hand; the sensory motor system; sensory mechanisms concerning pain and plasticity; functional properties

and localization of cell ensembles defined by their neurotransmitter in various regions of the brain; and functions of sleep, speech, and aging.


★ **14445** ★ **University of Montreal**
**Research Group on the Autonomic**
**Nervous System**
Department of Physiology/Faculty of Medicine
2900 blvd. Edouard-Montpetit
PO Box 6128, Downtown Sta.
Montreal, QC, Canada H3C 3J7
**Phone:** (514)343-7562          **Fax:** (514)343-2257
**Email:** grsna@ere.umontreal.ca
Dr. Jacques de Champlain, Dir.
**Activities/Fields:** Studies of the autonomic nervous system, focusing on cell and molecular biology of sympathetic neurotransmission, receptors, second messengers, cardiovascular regulation, and clinical research projects in hypertension and cardiac dysfunctions. **Pub:** *Annual Report.* Annual report.


★ **14446** ★ **University of Nebraska**
**Medical Center**
**Center for Neurovirology and**
**Neurodegenerative Disorders (CNND)**
985215 Nebraska Medical Center
Omaha, NE 68198-5215
**Phone:** (402)559-2797
**Email:** hegendel@unmc.edu
**Website:** http://www.unmc.edu/cnnd/
Howard E. Gendelman, MD, Dir.
**Activities/Fields:** Neurodegenerative disorders, especially focusing on the concept that the pathophysiological basis for neurodegenerative disorders revolves around brain inflammation and the production of neurotoxic factors by glial cells.


**University of Nebraska Medical Center**
**Signal Transduction Laboratory**
*See:* Entry 9512


★ **14447** ★ **University of North Carolina**
**at Chapel Hill**
**Neuroscience Center**
CB 7250
Neurosciences Research Bldg.
103 Mason Farm Rd.
Chapel Hill, NC 27599-7250
**Phone:** (919)843-8623          **Fax:** (919)966-1844
**Email:** wsnider@med.unc.edu
**Website:** http://www.neuroscience.unc.edu
William D. Snider, MD, Dir.
**Activities/Fields:** Prevention, diagnosis, and treatment of mental retardation and related aspects of human development utilizing a single disciplinary or interdisciplinary approach. Basic research is targeted at obtaining new knowledge of structure and function of the developing nervous system to be applied to other neurological and psychiatric illness. Studies include childhood autism, childhood hyperactivity with learning disabilities, genetic disorders associated with mental retardation, children whose nervous systems have been damaged by metallic environmental pollutants, and mentally retarded children whose aggressive stereotypic and self-injurious behavior requires that they be institutionalized. **Frmly:** Biological Sciences Research Center; Brain and Development Research Center.


★ **14448** ★ **University of Oregon**
**Institute of Neuroscience (ION)**
Huestis Hall
Eugene, OR 97403
**Phone:** (541)686-4556          **Fax:** (541)686-4548
**Email:** morrow@uoneuro.uoregon.edu
**Website:** http://www.neuro.uoregon.edu
Dr. William Roberts, Dir.
**Activities/Fields:** Interdisciplinary approaches to basic questions in neuroscience, with particular emphasis on behavior, neurochemistry, neurophysiology,

developmental neurobiology, and sensory systems. The Institute is composed of faculty members from the Departments of Biology, Computer Science, Psychology, and Physical Education. **Pub:** *Graduate Studies at the Institute of Neuroscience.*


★ **14449** ★ **University of Ottawa**
**Neurosciences Research Institute**
451 Smyth Rd.
Ottawa, ON, Canada K2H 8M5
**Phone:** (613)562-5800          **Fax:** (613)562-5403
**Email:** kchaundy@uottawa.ca
**Website:** http://www.nri.on.ca
K. Chaundy, Contact
**Activities/Fields:** Neuroprotection, neuronal regeneration and recovery, mechanisms of cell injury, stroke, depression, schizophrenia, and axotomy.


★ **14450** ★ **University of Pennsylvania**
**Brain Behavior Laboratory**
10 Gates Pavilion
Neuropsychiatry Section
Department of Psychiatry
3400 Spruce St.
Philadelphia, PA 19104-4283
**Phone:** (215)662-2826          **Fax:** (215)662-7903
**Email:** gur@bbl.med.penn.edu
**Website:** http://www.uphs.upenn.edu/bbl/
Ruben Gur, PhD, Dir.
**Activities/Fields:** New techniques for measuring regional brain function in relationship to behavior including cerebral blood flow, and metabolism using positron emmission tomography (PET); and functional MRI (FMRI); anatomic measures using magnetic resonance imaging (MRI), and neuropsychological testing for studying brain behavior relationships. Populations studied include normals (average and talented), psychiatric (schizophrenic, major depression, anxiety disorders, and dementia), and neurologic (stroke or cerebrovascular disease, epilepsy and parkinsonism).


★ **14451** ★ **University of Pennsylvania**
**Center for Neurodegenerative Disease**
**Research (CNDR)**
Maloney Bldg., 3rd Fl.
Department of Pathology & Laboratory Medicine
3600 Spruce St.
Philadelphia, PA 19104
**Phone:** (215)662-4708          **Fax:** (215)349-5909
**Email:** viale@mail.med.upenn.edu
**Website:** http://www.uphs.upenn.edu/cndr/
Virginia M.-Y. Lee, PhD, Co-Dir.
**Activities/Fields:** Causes and mechanisms leading to brain dysfunction and degeneration in Alzheimer's disease, Parkinson's disease, motor neuron disease and other less common neurodegenerative disorders that also occur more frequently with advancing age.


★ **14452** ★ **University of Pennsylvania**
**Cerebrovascular Research Center**
Stemmler Hall, Rm. 415
3450 Hamilton Walk
Philadelphia, PA 19104-6063
**Phone:** (215)662-2632          **Fax:** (215)349-5629
**Email:** reivich@cvrc.med.upenn.edu
Dr. Martin Reivich, Dir.
**Activities/Fields:** Cerebrovascular research with an emphasis on cerebral circulation and metabolism. Conducts PET, SPECT, MRI, neuropsychologic, and neurologic studies on various brain disorders, including acute stroke, brain tumor, epilepsy, dementia,Parkinson's disease,and schizophrenia. Studies include measurements of regional cerebral blood flow, glucose and oxygen metabolism, blood volume, and neuroreceptor number and affinity. Also conducts basic animal research, including development of blood flow agents for the brain, research on animal models of stroke, and studies on treatment modalities for acute stroke in animal models.

**★ 14453 ★ University of Pennsylvania**
**David Mahoney Institute of Neurological**
**Sciences**
Stemmler Hall, Rm. 467
Philadelphia, PA 19104-6074
**Phone:** (215)898-8048          **Fax:** (215)573-2015
**Email:** dichter@mail.med.upenn.edu
**Website:** http://www.med.upenn.edu/ins/
Prof. Marc A. Dichter, MD, Dir.

**Activities/Fields:** Nervous system, including neuro-anatomy, neurobiology, neurochemistry, neuroem-bryology, neurophysiology, neuropharmacology, physiological psychology, computational neuroscience, cognitive neuroscience, pathophysiology of neurological, and psychiatric diseases. **Pub:** *Newsletter.*

**★ 14454 ★ University of Pennsylvania**
**Smell and Taste Center**
5 Ravdin Bldg.
3400 Spruce St.
Philadelphia, PA 19104
**Phone:** (215)662-6580          **Fax:** (215)349-5266
**Email:** doty@mail.med.upenn.edu
Dr. Richard L. Doty, Dir.

**Activities/Fields:** Identifies and treats disorders of taste and smell. Develops clinical smell and taste tests, investigates nasal airflow parameters, examines gustatory glucose sensitivity in diabetes and depression, studies MRI-based measures of brain volume changes in olfactory disorders, studies neuroendo-crine relations with chemosensory function, conducts behavioral and neurophysiological studies of olfactory and trigeminal function, and studies the pathophysiology of oral sensory abnormalities.

**University of Pittsburgh**
**Center for Injury Research and Control**
   **(CIRCL)**
*See:* Entry 2715

**★ 14455 ★ University of Pittsburgh**
**Center for Neuroscience**
Biomedical Science Tower, E1440
Pittsburgh, PA 15261
**Phone:** (412)648-9537          **Fax:** (412)648-1441
**Email:** plevitt@pitt.edu
**Website:** http://cnup.neurobio.pitt.edu/
Pat Levitt, Co-Dir.

**Activities/Fields:** Neuroscience and neural diseases.

**★ 14456 ★ University of Quebec at**
   **Montreal**
**Cognitive Neuroscience Centre**
PO Box 8888
Montreal, QC, Canada H3C 3P8
**Phone:** (514)987-7002          **Fax:** (514)987-8952
**Email:** cnc@uqam.ca
Francois Richer, PhD, Dir.

**Activities/Fields:** Cognitive neuroscience, including frontal dysfunction, movement disorders and cerebral bases of speech, language, attention, and memory. Also performs fMRi, evoked potential modeling and quantitative speech analysis.

**University of Rochester**
**Center for Visual Science**
*See:* Entry 21180

**★ 14457 ★ University of Saskatchewan**
**Cameco MS Neuroscience Research**
   **Centre**
Saskatoon City Hospital, Rm. 5800
701 Queen St.
Saskatoon, SK, Canada S7K 0M7
**Email:** david@cvs.rochester.edu
**Website:** http://www.usask.ca/healthsci/cmsnrc
David J. Schreyer, Dir.

**Activities/Fields:** Treatment and cure of multiple sclerosis and other neurological disorders.

**★ 14458 ★ University of South Florida**
**Roskamp Institute for Research into**
   **Neurodegenerative Diseases**
3515 E Fletcher Ave.
Tampa, FL 33613
**Phone:** (813)974-3722          **Fax:** (813)974-3915
**Email:** roskamp@hsc.usf.edu
**Website:** http://roskamp.hsc.usf.edu/body_index.html
Michael Mullan, MD, Dir.

**Activities/Fields:** Cause of and potential therapies for Alzheimer's disease.

**★ 14459 ★ University of Tennessee**
**Center for Neuroscience**
875 Monroe Ave., Rm. 422
Memphis, TN 38163-2194
**Phone:** (901)448-5956          **Fax:** (901)448-4685
**Email:** skitai@utmem1.edu
**Website:** http://cns.utmem.edu/home.html
Dr. Stephen T. Kitai, Dir.

**Activities/Fields:** General neurosciences, including epilepsy studies; movement disorders (Parkinson's disease, Huntington's disease, and muscular dystrophy); vision studies (retinal disease and central visual pathways malfunction); developmental neurobiology (tissue culture and transplant in the basal ganglia, development of neural circuitry in the central visual system, neurological mutants and chimeras, development of cerebral and cerebellar cortical cytoarchitechtonics, and development of synapses in the retina); neuroendocrinology (control of brain neurotransmitters, temperature regulation in host defense response to infectious agents, and hormonal regulation of neuroeffector mechanisms); neurotransmitter action in the brain (biochemical analysis of neurotransmitters and hormone action, second messenger systems and effect of psychiatric medicine on these systems, and neuropeptide systems involved in pain and stress); and central nervous system control of the cardiovascular system (hypertension and temperature regulation); and sleep mechanisms.

**★ 14460 ★ University of Texas at Austin**
**Laboratory for Artificial Neural Systems**
ACES 3.118
Department of Electrical & Computer Engineering
Austin, TX 78712-1084
**Phone:** (512)471-8980          **Fax:** (512)471-2893
**Email:** ghosh@ece.utexas.edu
**Website:** http://www.lans.ece.utexas.edu/
Prof. Joydeep Ghosh, Dir.

**Activities/Fields:** Artificial neural systems.

**★ 14461 ★ University of Texas—Houston**
   **Health Science Center**
**Neuroscience Research Center (NRC)**
Medical School Bldg. 7.046
6431 Fannin
Houston, TX 77030
**Phone:** (713)500-5540          **Fax:** (713)500-0623
**Email:** nba-nrc@uth.tmc.edu
**Website:** http://nba19.med.uth.tmc.edu/nrc/
John H. Byrne, PhD, Dir.

**Activities/Fields:** Neurobehavioral sciences, particularly understanding, preventing, and treating various neural and behavioral disorders such as: dementias resulting from Alzheimer's Disease and stroke; mental retardation and learning and developmental disabilities; mental illnesses, including schizophrenia and manic-depressive illness; alcoholism and other substance abuse problems; and loss of cognitive functions due to factors such as the aging process and head trauma. **Pub:** *Newsletter.*

**★ 14462 ★ University of Texas**
   **Southwestern Medical Center at Dallas**
**Alzheimer's Disease Center**
Department of Psychiatry
5323 Harry Hines Blvd.
Dallas, TX 75390-8898
**Phone:** (214)648-3353          **Fax:** (214)648-2450

**Email:** munro.cullum@utsouthwestern.edu
Dr. Munro Cullum, Dir., Neuropsychology

**Activities/Fields:** Alzheimer's disease and aging in the brain, focusing on loss of cognitive functions and test measurements including IQ, problem solving, abstract thinking, spatial and dexterity skills, attention and concentration, language function, and memory.

**★ 14463 ★ University of Texas**
   **Southwestern Medical Center at Dallas**
**Center for Basic Neuroscience**
5323 Harry Hines Blvd.
Dallas, TX 75390-9111
**Phone:** (214)648-1876          **Fax:** (214)648-1879
**Email:** tsudho@mednet.swmed.edu
**Website:** http://www2.swmed.edu/cbn/
Prof. Thomas C. Süumldhof, MD, Dir.

**Activities/Fields:** Brain functions in health and disease, ranging from the development of the nervous system over studies on fundamental mechanisms of synaptic transmission to investigations of vision and olfaction.

**★ 14464 ★ University of Texas**
   **Southwestern Medical Center at Dallas**
**Neuromuscular Treatment Center**
Department of Neurology
5323 Harry Hines Blvd.
Dallas, TX 75390-8897
**Phone:** (214)648-6419          **Fax:** (214)648-9311
**Email:** gil.wolfe@utsouthwestern.edu
**Website:** http://neurology.swmed.edu
Gil Wolfe, MD, Dir.

**Activities/Fields:** Immune-mediated neuromuscular disorders, including myasthenia gravis, inflammatory neuropathy, amyotrophic lateral sclerosis (Lou Gehrig's Disease), spinal muscular atrophy. Activities include clinical therapeutic trials.

**University of Texas Southwestern Medical**
   **Center at Dallas**
**Sleep Disorders Center for Children**
*See:* Entry 5833

**★ 14465 ★ University of Texas**
   **Southwestern Medical Center at Dallas**
**Sleep Study Unit**
Department of Psychiatry
5323 Harry Hines Blvd.
Dallas, TX 75390-9070
**Phone:** (214)648-7350          **Fax:** (214)648-7359
Roseanne Armitage, PhD, Dir.

**Activities/Fields:** Sleep/wake studies, including insomnia, depression, narcolepsy, schizophrenia and normal sleep, as well as basic sleep neurophysiology. **Pub:** *Biological Psychiatry.* • *Neuropsychopharmacology.* • *Psychiatry Research.* • *Sleep.*

**★ 14466 ★ University of Toronto**
**Centre for Research in Neurodegenerative**
   **Diseases**
Tanz Neuroscience Bldg.
6 Queen's Park Cres. W
Toronto, ON, Canada M5S 3H2
**Phone:** (416)978-7461          **Fax:** (416)978-1878
**Email:** crnd.info@utoronto.ca
**Website:** http://www.utoronto.ca/crnd
Dr. Peter St. George-Hyslop, Int. Dir.

**Activities/Fields:** Neurodegenerative diseases of the human brain, focusing on the causes of Alzheimer's disease, Amyotrophic Lateral Sclerosis, and other nerve cell defects, the development of effective treatment for patient care, and clinical trials. Specific areas of study include genetic mutation of chromosome 21, protein degeneration of synapses and synaptic vesicles, identification and characterization of the molecular development of the nervous systems, collaborative studies on the aluminum hypothesis for Alzheimer's disease, and the study of motor control and the mechanisms that result in nerve cell degeneration in both the brain and the spinal cord.

**★ 14467 ★ University of Toronto**
**Toronto Western Research Institute**
**University Health Network**
399 Bathurst St.
Toronto, ON, Canada M5T 2S8
**Phone:** (416)603-5030          **Fax:** (416)603-5745
**Email:** chris.wallace@uhn.on.ca
Dr. M. Christopher Wallace, Dir.

**Activities/Fields:** Cell and membrane neurobiology, molecular neurobiology, neuroprotection, cognitive and neurophysiological aspects of normal and abnormal limb movement control, normal and pathological eye movement control and visual processing, neuropharmacology, spinal cord injury, neuro-oncology, epilepsy and cerebrovascular disease. **Frmly:** Toronto Hospital Research Institute; Playfair Neuroscience Unit.

**★ 14468 ★ University of Vermont**
**Clinical Neuroscience Research Unit**
**(CNRU)**
Arnold 6
1 S Prospect St.
Burlington, VT 05401-1195
**Phone:** (802)847-4560          **Fax:** (802)847-7889
**Email:** paul.newhouse@uvm.edu
**Website:** http://www.uvm.edu/~cnru/cnru.htm
Paul Newhouse, MD, Dir.

**Activities/Fields:** Mechanisms, treatment, and amelioration of complex neuropsychiatric disorders. Disorders of particular interest include those that have a behavioral and cognitive component, such as Alzheimer's disease and Parkinson's disease. The center also studies complex neuropsychiatric disorders function after menopause; new pharmaceutical agents for Alzheimer's disease; and depression, post-traumatic stress disorder and anxiety disorders in young and elderly populations.

**★ 14469 ★ University of Virginia**
**Center for the Study of**
**Neurodegenerative Diseases (CSND)**
Charlottesville, VA 22908
**Phone:** (434)924-8374          **Fax:** (434)924-0370
**Email:** bennett@virginia.edu
Dr. James P. Bennett, Jr., Dir.

**Activities/Fields:** Abnormal mitochondrial function and its role in causing neurodegenerative brain diseases. The major hypothesis being examined is that individuals with sporadic forms of Parkinson's and Alzheimer's diseases inherit mitochondria with mutations in the mitochondrial DNA. These mutations lead to reduced activities of enzyme complexes in the electron transport chain and an increased susceptibility to programmed cell death.

**★ 14470 ★ University of Virginia**
**Neuromuscular Center**
Department of Neurology
UVA Medical Center
PO Box 800394
Charlottesville, VA 22908
**Phone:** (434)924-5361          **Fax:** (434)924-9068
Dr. Larry H. Phillips, II, Co-Dir.

**Activities/Fields:** Electrophysiology of dystrophy skeletal muscle fibers, biochemical studies of the properties of normal and dystrophic cells in culture, structure and chromosome linkage of human muscle genes, genetic heterogeneity among the hereditary motor sensory neuropathies, long chain fatty acids in Olivo-Ponto-cerebellar atrophy, the axonal cytoskeleton following IDPN administration, biochemical differences in shrimp claw muscle protein, membrane enzymes involved in muscle regulation, safety margin of neuromuscular transmission in normal and diseased muscle, and the humoral hypothesis in the Eaton-Lambert syndrome. Also conducts clinical research in such neuromuscular diseases as myasthe-

nia gravis, Eaton-Lambert syndrome, Charcot-Marie-tooth disease, and diabetic polyneuropathy.

**★ 14471 ★ University of Washington**
**Alzheimer's Disease Research Center**
1660 S Columbian Way (116 MIRECC)
Seattle, WA 98108
**Phone:** (206)782-1010          **Free:** 800-317-5382
**Fax:** (206)768-5456
**Email:** mwalt@u.washington.edu
**Website:** http://depts.washington.edu/adrcweb/
Marie Walters, Contact

**Activities/Fields:** Basic mechanisms underlying the development of adult dementing disorders, with particular attention to heritable susceptibility factors underlying Alzheimer's disease. **Pub:** *Dimensions Newsletter*, quarterly.

**★ 14472 ★ University of Washington**
**Northwest Regional Spinal Cord Injury**
**System**
School of Medicine
Department of Rehabilitation Medicine
Box 356490
Seattle, WA 98195-6490
**Phone:** (206)543-3600          **Fax:** (206)685-3244
**Email:** rehab@u.washington.edu
**Website:** http://depts.washington.edu/rehab/sci/
Dr. Diana D. Cardenas, MD, Proj. Dir.

**Activities/Fields:** Spinal cord injuries. **Pub:** *Spinal Cord Injury Update Newsletter*, 3/year. Newsletter. • *Staying Healthy After a Spinal Cord Injury (Series of 10 brochures)*. Brochure. .

**University of Washington**
**Pediatric Epilepsy Research Center**
**(PERC)**
*See:* Entry 5837

**University of Western Ontario**
**Dementia Study Group**
*See:* Entry 3117

**★ 14473 ★ University of Wisconsin—**
**Madison**
**Neuropsychology Laboratory**
600 N Highland Ave.
Madison, WI 53792-6180
**Phone:** (608)263-5430          **Fax:** (608)265-0172
**Email:** hermann@neurology.wisc.edu
**Website:** http://depts.washington.edu/perc/
Dr. Bruce Hermann, Dir.

**Activities/Fields:** Clinical neuropsychology in neuropsychological correlates of epilepsy, cognitive and affective changes in aging, and differential diagnosis of dementia with a view toward cognitive and memory remediation.

**★ 14474 ★ Vanderbilt University**
**Neuromagnetic Pain Management Project**
407 Godchaux Hall
461 21st Ave. S
Nashville, TN 37240
**Phone:** (615)322-2783          **Fax:** (615)343-3998
**Email:** sharon.jones@mcmail.vanderbilt.edu
Sharon Jones, Contact

**Activities/Fields:** Pain, especially the mechanisms underlying painful conditions and techniques for interrupting pain by altering pain pathways. **Frmly:** Center for Pain Research and Neuromagnetics.

**★ 14475 ★ Veterans Health**
**Administration**
**Office of Research and Development**
**Rehabilitation Outcomes Research Center**
**for Veterans with Central Nervous**
**System Damage**
North Florida/South Georgia Veterans Health
  System Research
Gainesville, FL 32608
**Phone:** (352)376-1611          **Fax:** (352)379-2332
**Email:** rorc@med.va.gov
**Website:** http://www.stroketoolbox.com/rorc/index.htm
Pamela W. Duncan, PhD, Dir.

**Activities/Fields:** Structure, process, and outcomes of rehabilitation services for patients with central nervous system damage; emerging therapies and technologies for these same patients.

**★ 14476 ★ Virginia Commonwealth**
**University**
**Neurosciences Center**
1200 E Broad St.
PO Box 980317
Richmond, VA 23298-0317
**Phone:** (434)828-6370          **Fax:** (434)828-2501
**Website:** http://stealth.nsc.vcu.edu/nsc
John D. Ward, MD, Dir.

**Activities/Fields:** Neurosciences, particularly neuroimaging, neurochemistry, and molecular neurobiology.

**★ 14477 ★ Virginia Commonwealth**
**University**
**Virginia Commonwealth Regional Spinal**
**Cord Injury System**
Medical College of Virginia
Department of Physical Medicine & Rehabilitation
Box 980677
1233 E Marshall St., 4th Fl.
Richmond, VA 23298-0677
**Phone:** (434)828-4230          **Fax:** (434)828-6340
**Email:** wmckinle@hsc.vcu.edu
**Website:** http://www.pmr.vcu.edu/department/faculty/clinical/wmckinley.html
Dr. William O. McKinley, Dir.

**Activities/Fields:** Spinal cord injuries, including exploration of clinical pathway outcomes across the continuum of care; evaluation of innovative medical issues related to spinal cord injuries; delineation of the incidence of and formulation of management strategies for the rehabilitation of persons with dual diagnosis of spinal cord injuries and traumatic brain injury; and identification of incidences and treatment strategies for individuals with spinal cord injuries and substance abuse.

**★ 14478 ★ Wake Forest University**
**Center for Investigative Neuroscience**
**(CIN)**
School of Medicine
Medical Center Blvd.
Winston Salem, NC 27157
**Phone:** (336)716-0083          **Fax:** (336)716-0237
**Email:** bestein@wfubmc.edu
**Website:** http://www.wfubmc.edu/CIN/
Barry E. Stein, PhD, Interim Dir.

**Activities/Fields:** Diseases of the central nervous system.

**★ 14479 ★ Wake Forest University**
**Cerebrovascular Research Center**
Department of Neurology
Medical Center Blvd.
Winston Salem, NC 27157-1068
**Phone:** (336)716-2336          **Fax:** (336)716-5477
**Email:** jtoole@wfubmc.edu
Dr. James F. Toole, Dir.

**Activities/Fields:** Cerebrovascular research, including ultrasound, neurological diseases, coronary studies, biostatistics, transient ischemic attack (TIA), comparative medicine in atherosclerosis, neuropsychological evaluation, cerebral circulation, and anatomy/physiology. **Pub:** *Stroke Monitor Newsletter*, quarterly.

**★ 14480 ★ Wake Forest University Comprehensive Epilepsy Center**
Department of Neurology
School of Medicine
Medical Center Blvd.
Winston Salem, NC 27157
**Phone:** (336)716-0488        **Fax:** (336)716-7548
**Email:** wbell@wfubmc.edu
**Website:** http://www.wfubmc.edu/neurology/epilepsy/
William L. Bell, MD, Dir.

**Activities/Fields:** Epilepsy, especially methods for detecting seizures, epilepsy surgery, psychosocial issues, antiepileptic drugs, etc.

**★ 14481 ★ Wake Forest University Epilepsy Education Information Service**
Medical Center Blvd.
Winston Salem, NC 27157-1078
**Phone:** (336)716-2321        **Free:** 800-642-0500
**Fax:** (336)716-9489
**Email:** pgibson@wfubmc.edu
Patricia Gibson, Dir.

**Activities/Fields:** Social and psychological aspects of epilepsy and clinical trials of anti-epileptic medication.

**★ 14482 ★ Wakefulness Sleep Education and Research Foundation, Inc.**
1442 Santa Luisa Dr.
Solana Beach, CA 92075
**Phone:** (858)457-4233        **Fax:** (858)657-0559
**Email:** mitter@scripps.edu
Merrill M. Mitler, PhD, Dir.

**Activities/Fields:** Clinical sleep studies including narcolepsy, drug development, and sleep apnea.

**★ 14483 ★ Washington University in St. Louis Alzheimer's Disease Research Center**
4488 Forest Park Ave., Ste. 130
Saint Louis, MO 63108
**Phone:** (314)286-2881        **Fax:** (314)286-2763
**Email:** adrc@neuro.wustl.edu
**Website:** http://www.adrc.wustl.edu
Eugene M. Johnson, PhD, Dir.

**Activities/Fields:** Aging and dementia, neurobiology of aging and cognition, Alzheimer's disease and related disorders, and the impact of dementia on the family or caregiver and the community. Studies include clinical research, clinical drug trials, neuropathological (autopsy) studies, genetic and other medical studies of persons with dementia, bench studies, behavioral/social research, and psychometric studies. **Pub:** *Horizons Newsletter*.

**★ 14484 ★ Wayne State University Laura S. Nye Surgical Research Fund for Desmoid Tumors**
Harper Hospital
Department of Surgery
3990 John R
Detroit, MI 48201
**Phone:** (313)745-8778        **Fax:** (313)745-1873
**Email:** dfsurg@aol.com
David Fromm, MD, Ch.

**Activities/Fields:** Desmoid tumor treatment, including photodynamic therapy after excision of tumor.

**★ 14485 ★ William T. Gossett Parkinson's Disease Center**
Department of Neurology
Henry Ford Hospital
2799 W Grand Blvd.
Detroit, MI 48202
**Phone:** (313)916-7323        **Fax:** (313)916-3014

**Email:** gorell@neuro.hfh.edu
Jay M. Gorell, MD, Dir.

**Activities/Fields:** Parkinson's disease and its causes and treatments, including risk factors, cognitive and motor deficits, new medication trials, animal nerve cell investigations, and disordered brain chemistry measurements.

**★ 14486 ★ Yale University PVA/EPVA Center for Neuroscience and Regeneration Research**
Medical Center, Bldg. 34, 127A
West Haven, CT 06516
**Phone:** (203)937-3802        **Fax:** (203)937-3801
**Email:** stephen_waxman@qm.yale.edu
**Website:** http://info.med.yale.edu/neurol/pva-epva-center
Dr. Stephen G. Waxman, Dir.

**Activities/Fields:** Basic mechanisms of central nervous system development, function, injury, and functional recovery with a major emphasis on spinal cord dysfunction. Concerns include molecular basis for neurological disorders, nerve cell growth and regeneration, pathophysiology of conduction in injured nerve fibers, regeneration of the central nervous system in mammalian species, and multiple sclerosis as a model for understanding how demyelinated nerve fibers regain their ability to effectively transmit electrical impulses. Areas of expertise of scientific staff include neurocytology, experimental neuropathology, immunology, developmental neuroscience, electrophysiology, biophysics, and molecular biology.

# State & Regional Organizations

## Alzheimer's Disease

*State chapters of the Alzheimer's Association are listed below. The national office is located at 919 N Michigan Ave., Ste. 1100, Chicago, Illinois 60611-1676. Additional information can be obtained by calling the national office at (800) 272-3900, or by consulting their web site at http://www.alz.org.*

### Arizona

**★ 14487 ★ Alzheimer's Association Desert Southwest Chapter**
1028 E McDowell Rd.
Phoenix, AZ 85005
**Phone:** (602)528-0545        **Free:** 800-392-0022
**Fax:** (602)528-0546
**Email:** Scott.Gardner@alz.org
**Website:** http://www.alzaz.org
Scott Gardner, Exec Director

**Remarks:** Serves Arizona and Nevada.

### California

**★ 14488 ★ Alzheimer's Association California Central Coast Chapter**
2024 De La Vina, Ste. B
Santa Barbara, CA 93105
**Phone:** (805)563-0020        **Free:** 800-660-1993
**Fax:** (805)682-1811
**Website:** http://www.centralcoastz.org

**★ 14489 ★ Alzheimer's Association Los Angeles, Riverside, and San Bernardino Counties Chapter**
5900 Wilshire Blvd., Ste. 1700
Los Angeles, CA 90036
**Phone:** (323)938-3379        **Free:** 800-660-1993
**Fax:** (323)938-1036
**Website:** http://www.alzla.org/

**★ 14490 ★ Alzheimer's Association Northern California and Northern Nevada Chapter**
2065 W El Camino Real, Ste. C
Mountain View, CA 94040
**Phone:** (650)962-8111        **Free:** 800-660-1993
**Fax:** (650)962-9644
**Website:** http://www.alznorcal.org
Bill Fisher, EDIR, Contact

**★ 14491 ★ Alzheimer's Association Orange County Chapter**
2540 N Santiago Blvd.
Orange, CA 92867
**Phone:** (714)283-1111        **Free:** 800-660-1993
**Fax:** (714)283-1240
**Website:** http://www.alzoc.org/

**★ 14492 ★ Alzheimer's Association San Diego Chapter**
8514 Commerce Ave.
San Diego, CA 92121
**Phone:** (858)537-5040        **Free:** 800-660-1993
**Fax:** (858)537-5045
**Email:** info@sanalz.org
**Website:** http://www.sanalz.org

### Colorado

**★ 14493 ★ Alzheimer's Association Rocky Mountain Chapter**
789 Sherman St., Ste. 500
Denver, CO 80203
**Phone:** (303)813-1669        **Free:** 800-864-4404
**Fax:** (303)813-1670
**Email:** cheryl.dunaway@alz.org
**Website:** http://www.alzrockymtn.org
Linda Mitchell, Exec Director

**★ 14494 ★ Alzheimer's Association Rocky Mountain Chapter/Grand Junction Office**
761 Rood Ave.
Grand Junction, CO 81501
**Phone:** (970)256-1274        **Free:** 800-864-4404
**Fax:** (970)243-6924
**Email:** maria.williams@alz.org
**Website:** http://www.alz.org

### Connecticut

**★ 14495 ★ Alzheimer's Association Northern Connecticut Chapter**
96 Oak St.
Hartford, CT 06106
**Phone:** (860)956-9560        **Free:** 800-356-5502
**Fax:** (860)956-9590
**Website:** http://www.alzct.org

**★ 14496 ★ Alzheimer's Association Southern Connecticut Chapter**
2911 Dixwell Ave.
Hamden, CT 06518
**Phone:** (203)230-1777        **Fax:** (203)230-1712
**Website:** http://www.ctalz.org

### Florida

**★ 14497 ★ Alzheimer's Association Central and North Florida Chapter**
2010 Mizell Ave.
Winter Park, FL 32792
**Phone:** (407)629-1997        **Fax:** (407)629-2042
**Email:** annette.kelly@alz.org
**Website:** http://www.alzorlando.org/
Annette Kelly, Exec Director

**★ 14498 ★ Alzheimer's Association**
**Florida Gulf Coast Chapter**
9365 U.S. Hwy. 19 N, Ste. B
Pinellas Park, FL 33782
**Phone:** (727)578-2558          **Free:** 800-772-8672
**Fax:** (727)578-2286
**Email:** info@alz-tbc.org
**Website:** http://www.alz-tbc.org

**★ 14499 ★ Alzheimer's Association**
**South Florida Chapter**
1175 NE 125th St., Ste. 600
Miami, FL 33161
**Phone:** (305)891-6228          **Fax:** (305)892-0355

**★ 14500 ★ Alzheimer's Association**
**Southeast Florida Chapter**
8333 W McNab Rd., Ste. 210
Fort Lauderdale, FL 33321
**Phone:** (954)726-0002          **Free:** 800-861-7826
**Fax:** (954)726-0055
**Website:** http://www.alzsefc.org

### Georgia

**★ 14501 ★ Alzheimer's Association**
**Georgia Chapter**
1925 Century Blvd., Ste. 10
Atlanta, GA 30345-3315
**Phone:** (404)728-1181          **Free:** 888-649-7800
**Fax:** (404)636-9768
**Email:** memoryga@bellsouth.net
**Website:** http://www.alzga.org
Jan Bequeath, Exec Director

### Hawaii

**★ 14502 ★ Alzheimer's Association**
**Aloha Chapter**
1050 Ala Moana Blvd., Bldg. D
Honolulu, HI 96814
**Phone:** (808)591-2771          **Fax:** (808)591-9071

### Illinois

**★ 14503 ★ Alzheimer's Association**
**Central Illinois Chapter**
606 W Glen Ave.
Peoria, IL 61614
**Phone:** (309)681-1100          **Free:** 800-681-1181
**Fax:** (309)681-1101
**Email:** marlene.rush@alz.org
**Website:** http://www.alzillinois.org/
Marlene Rush, Exec Director

**★ 14504 ★ Alzheimer's Association**
**Greater Illinois Chapter**
4709 Golf Rd., Ste. 1015
Skokie, IL 60076
**Phone:** (847)933-2413          **Free:** 800-272-3900
**Fax:** (847)933-2417
**Website:** http://www.alzheimers-illinois.org

### Indiana

**★ 14505 ★ Alzheimer's Association**
**Central Indiana Chapter**
9135 N Meridian St., Ste. B-4
Indianapolis, IN 46260
**Phone:** (317)575-9620          **Free:** 888-575-9624
**Fax:** (317)582-0669
**Email:** Heather.Hershberger@alz.org
**Website:** http://www.standbyyou.org/
Heather Allen Hershberger, Exec Director

**★ 14506 ★ Alzheimer's Association**
**Northern Indiana Chapter**
108 N Main St., Ste. 707
South Bend, IN 46601

**Phone:** (574)232-4121          **Free:** 888-303-0180
**Fax:** (574)232-4235
**Email:** alznic@sbt.infi.net
**Website:** http://www.alz-nic.org/

### Iowa

**★ 14507 ★ Alzheimer's Association**
**Big Sioux Chapter**
Mercy Medical Bldg.
522 4th St., Lower Level
PO Box 3716
Sioux City, IA 51101
**Phone:** (712)279-5802          **Free:** 800-426-6512
**Fax:** (712)277-8076
**Email:** help@alz-sioux.org
**Website:** http://www.alz-sioux.org
**Remarks:** Serves Iowa, Nebraska, and South Dakota.

**★ 14508 ★ Alzheimer's Association**
**East Central Iowa Chapter**
1642 42nd St. NE
Cedar Rapids, IA 52402
**Phone:** (319)294-9699          **Free:** 888-397-9635
**Fax:** (319)294-0068
**Email:** kelly.hauer@alz.org
**Website:** http://www.alzeci.org/

**★ 14509 ★ Alzheimer's Association**
**Greater Iowa Chapter**
Iowa Lutheran Hospital
700 E University, Level B
Des Moines, IA 50316
**Phone:** (515)263-2464          **Free:** 800-738-8071
**Fax:** (515)263-2466
**Website:** http://www.alz.org/greateriowa
**Remarks:** Serves Iowa and Illinois.

**★ 14510 ★ Alzheimer's Association**
**Waterloo Branch Office**
2101 Kimball Ave., Ste. 125
Waterloo, IA 50702
**Phone:** (319)272-2300          **Free:** 888-397-9635
**Fax:** (319)272-2109
**Email:** kristi.kajewski@alz.org
**Website:** http://www.alz.org

### Kansas

**★ 14511 ★ Alzheimer's Association**
**Heart of America Chapter**
3846 W 75th St.
Prairie Village, KS 66208
**Phone:** (913)831-3888          **Free:** 800-733-1981
**Fax:** (913)831-1916
**Email:** kim.collins@alz.org
**Website:** http://www.alz.org/kcalz.org
**Remarks:** Serves Kansas and Missouri.

**★ 14512 ★ Alzheimer's Association**
**Sunflower Chapter**
347 S Laura
Wichita, KS 67211
**Phone:** (316)267-7333          **Free:** 877-267-7333
**Fax:** (316)267-6369
**Website:** http://www.alzheimerskansas.org

### Kentucky

**★ 14513 ★ Alzheimer's Association**
**Greater Kentucky and Southern Indiana**
**Chapter**
3703 Taylorsville Rd., Ste. 102
Louisville, KY 40220
**Phone:** (502)451-4266          **Free:** 800-221-1277
**Fax:** (502)456-2701
**Website:** http://www.alzinky.org/

### Louisiana

**★ 14514 ★ Alzheimer's Association**
**Greater New Orleans Chapter**
1040 Calhoun St.
New Orleans, LA 70118
**Phone:** (504)895-6223          **Free:** 800-459-3528
**Fax:** (504)895-0493

**★ 14515 ★ Alzheimer's Association**
**Northeast/Central Louisiana Chapter**
PO Box 2471
Monroe, LA 71207
**Phone:** (318)322-2828          **Free:** 888-202-2828
**Fax:** (318)327-6301

### Maine

**★ 14516 ★ Alzheimer's Association**
**Maine Chapter**
163 Lancaster St., Ste. 160B
Portland, ME 04101-2406
**Phone:** (207)772-0115          **Free:** 800-660-2871
**Fax:** (207)772-0354
**Email:** eleanor.goldberg@alz.org
**Website:** http://www.mainealz.org
Eleanor Goldberg, Exec Director

### Maryland

**★ 14517 ★ Alzheimer's Association**
**Greater Maryland Chapter**
1850 York Rd., Ste. D
Lutherville Timonium, MD 21093
**Phone:** (410)561-9099          **Free:** 800-443-2273
**Fax:** (410)561-3433
**Website:** http://www.alzgmd.org

### Massachusetts

**★ 14518 ★ Alzheimer's Association**
**Massachusetts Chapter**
36 Cameron Ave.
Cambridge, MA 02140
**Phone:** (617)868-6718          **Free:** 800-548-2111
**Fax:** (978)868-6720
**Email:** elaine.cohen@alz.org
**Website:** http://www.alzmass.org/
James Wessler, Exec Director
**Alt. Contact:** Spanish speaker's line: (617) 868-8599.

### Michigan

**★ 14519 ★ Alzheimer's Association**
**Greater Michigan Chapter**
17220 W 12 Mile Rd., Ste. 100
Southfield, MI 48076
**Phone:** (248)557-8277          **Free:** 800-337-3827
**Fax:** (248)557-4642

**★ 14520 ★ Alzheimer's Association**
**Michigan Great Lakes Chapter**
107 Aprill Dr., Ste. 1
Ann Arbor, MI 48103
**Phone:** (734)677-3081          **Free:** 800-337-3827
**Fax:** (734)677-3091
**Website:** http://www.alzmigreatlakes.org

**★ 14521 ★ Alzheimer's Association**
**North/West Michigan Chapter**
225 W 30th St.
Holland, MI 49423
**Phone:** (616)392-8365          **Free:** 800-893-8365
**Fax:** (616)392-1712
**Email:** janet.magennis@alz.org
**Website:** http://www.nwmialz.org
Janet Magennis, Exec Director

## Minnesota

**★ 14522 ★ Alzheimer's Association**
**Minnesota-Dakotas Chapter**
4550 W 77th St., Ste. 200
Minneapolis, MN 55435
**Phone:** (952)830-0512          **Free:** 800-232-0851
**Fax:** (952)830-0513
**Email:** john.kemp@alz.org
**Website:** http://www.alzmndak.org
John Kemp, Exec Director
**Remarks:** Serves Minnesota, North Dakota, and South Dakota.

## Mississippi

**★ 14523 ★ Alzheimer's Association**
**Mississippi Chapter**
1900 Dunbarton Dr., Ste. I
Jackson, MS 39216
**Phone:** (601)987-0020          **Free:** 877-525-HELP
**Fax:** (601)987-9020

## Missouri

**★ 14524 ★ Alzheimer's Association**
**Mid-Missouri Chapter**
1121 Business Loop 70 E, Ste. 2B
Columbia, MO 65201
**Phone:** (573)443-8665          **Free:** 800-693-8665
**Fax:** (573)499-9701
**Email:** penny.braun@alz.org
**Website:** http://www.alz.org/chapters/template/mid-mo/default.htm

**★ 14525 ★ Alzheimer's Association**
**Saint Louis Chapter**
9374 Olive Blvd.
Saint Louis, MO 63132
**Phone:** (314)432-3422          **Free:** 800-980-9080
**Fax:** (314)432-3824
**Email:** info@alzstl.org
**Website:** http://www.alzstl.org
**Remarks:** Also serves Illinois.

**★ 14526 ★ Alzheimer's Association**
**Southwest Missouri Chapter**
Glen Isle Ctr.
1500 S Glenstone
Springfield, MO 65804
**Phone:** (417)886-2199          **Free:** 800-487-0747
**Fax:** (417)886-0337
**Website:** http://www.alz-swmo.org/

## Montana

**★ 14527 ★ Alzheimer's Association**
**Montana Chapter**
2900 12th Ave., Ste. 4E
Billings, MT 59101
**Phone:** (406)252-3053          **Fax:** (406)237-4285
**Website:** http://www.alz-mt.org

## Nebraska

**★ 14528 ★ Alzheimer's Association**
**Great Plains Chapter**
5601 S 27th St., Ste. 201
Lincoln, NE 68512
**Phone:** (402)420-2540          **Free:** 888-487-2585
**Fax:** (402)420-2541
**Website:** http://www.alznebraska.org
**Remarks:** Serves Nebraska and Wyoming.

**★ 14529 ★ Alzheimer's Association**
**Midlands Chapter**
7101 Newport Ave., Ste. 305
Omaha, NE 68152
**Phone:** (402)572-3059          **Free:** 800-309-2112
**Fax:** (402)572-3038

**Email:** alz@infobridge.com
**Website:** http://www.omaha-cb-alz.org/
Connie Kudlacek, Exec Director
**Remarks:** Serves Iowa and eastern Nebraska.

## New Jersey

**★ 14530 ★ Alzheimer's Association**
**Greater New Jersey Chapter**
400 Morris Ave., Ste. 251
Denville, NJ 07834
**Phone:** (973)586-4300          **Free:** 800-883-1180
**Fax:** (973)586-4342
**Email:** jean.gallo@alz.org
**Website:** http://www.alz.org/gnj

## New Mexico

**★ 14531 ★ Alzheimer's Association**
**New Mexico Chapter**
8100 Mountain Rd. NE, Ste. 201
Albuquerque, NM 87110
**Phone:** (505)266-4473          **Free:** 800-777-8155
**Fax:** (505)266-0108
**Email:** info@nm-alzheimers.org
**Website:** http://www.nm-alzheimers.org/

## New York

**★ 14532 ★ Alzheimer's Association**
**Central New York Chapter**
441 W Kirkpatrick St.
Syracuse, NY 13204-1361
**Phone:** (315)472-4201          **Free:** 800-339-4177
**Fax:** (315)472-4206
**Website:** http://www.alzcny.org

**★ 14533 ★ Alzheimer's Association**
**Hudson Valley/Rockland/Westchester, NY Chapter**
2 Jefferson Plaza, Ste. 203
Poughkeepsie, NY 12601
**Phone:** (845)471-2655          **Free:** 800-872-0994
**Fax:** (845)471-8960
**Email:** elaine.sproat@alz.org
**Website:** http://www.alz.org/midhudson/

**★ 14534 ★ Alzheimer's Association**
**Long Island Chapter**
3281 Veterans Memorial Hwy., Ste. E-13
Ronkonkoma, NY 11779
**Phone:** (631)580-5100          **Fax:** (631)580-3100
**Website:** http://www.alzheimersli.org
Fred M. Kadin, Exec Director

**★ 14535 ★ Alzheimer's Association**
**New York City Chapter**
360 Lexington Ave., 5th Fl.
New York, NY 10017
**Phone:** (212)983-0700          **Fax:** (212)697-6158
**Email:** Jed.Levine@alz.org
**Website:** http://www.alzheimernyc.org/

**★ 14536 ★ Alzheimer's Association**
**Northeastern New York Chapter**
85 Watervliet Ave.
Albany, NY 12206
**Phone:** (518)438-2217          **Free:** 800-303-2218
**Fax:** (518)438-2219
**Email:** alzneny@crisny.org
**Website:** http://www.alzneny.org/

**★ 14537 ★ Alzheimer's Association**
**Rochester Chapter**
435 E Henrietta Rd.
Rochester, NY 14620
**Phone:** (585)760-5400          **Free:** 800-724-0587
**Fax:** (585)760-5401
**Email:** alzroch@servtech.org

**Website:** http://www.alz-rochesterny.org

**★ 14538 ★ Alzheimer's Association**
**Western New York Chapter**
1284 French Rd.
Depew, NY 14043-4882
**Phone:** (716)656-8448          **Free:** 800-273-6737
**Fax:** (716)656-8525
**Email:** info@alzwny.org
**Website:** http://www.alzwny.org/

## North Carolina

**★ 14539 ★ Alzheimer's Association**
**Eastern North Carolina Chapter**
400 Oberlin Rd., Ste. 208
Raleigh, NC 27605-1351
**Phone:** (919)832-3732          **Free:** 800-228-8738
**Fax:** (919)832-7989

**★ 14540 ★ Alzheimer's Association**
**Western Carolina Chapter**
3800 Shamrock Dr.
Charlotte, NC 28215
**Phone:** (704)532-7392          **Free:** 800-888-6671
**Fax:** (704)532-5421
**Email:** alz@perigree.net
**Website:** http://www.perigee.net/~alz/

## Ohio

**★ 14541 ★ Alzheimer's Association**
**Central Ohio Chapter**
3380 Tremont Rd.
Columbus, OH 43221
**Phone:** (614)457-6003          **Free:** 800-735-6751
**Fax:** (614)457-6634
**Email:** cclark@alzheimerscentralohio.org
**Website:** http://www.alzheimerscentralohio.org/

**★ 14542 ★ Alzheimer's Association**
**Cleveland Area Chapter**
12200 Fairhill Rd.
Cleveland, OH 44120-1013
**Phone:** (216)721-8457          **Free:** 800-441-3322
**Fax:** (216)721-1629
**Email:** webinfo@alzclv.org
**Website:** http://www.alzclv.org/
Rimas J. Jasinevicius, Exec Director

**★ 14543 ★ Alzheimer's Association**
**East Central Ohio Chapter**
126 W Church St.
Newark, OH 43055
**Phone:** (740)345-5102          **Free:** 800-441-3322
**Fax:** (740)345-5099

**★ 14544 ★ Alzheimer's Association**
**Greater Cincinnati Chapter**
644 Linn St., Ste. 1026
Cincinnati, OH 45203
**Phone:** (513)721-4284          **Free:** 800-441-3322
**Fax:** (513)345-8446
**Website:** http://www.alz.org/grtrcinc
**Remarks:** Also serves Indiana and Kentucky.

**★ 14545 ★ Alzheimer's Association**
**Greater East Ohio Area Chapter**
1815 W Market St., Ste. 301
Akron, OH 44313
**Phone:** (330)864-5646          **Free:** 800-441-3322
**Fax:** (330)864-7336
**Email:** pamschuellerman@alz.org
**Website:** http://www.tricountyalz.org/
Pamela Schuellerman, Exec Director
**Remarks:** Also serves Pennsylvania.

**★ 14546 ★ Alzheimer's Association**
**Miami Valley Chapter**
The Laurelwood
3797 Summit Glen Dr., Ste. G100
Dayton, OH 45449
**Phone:** (937)291-3332　　　**Free:** 800-441-3322
**Fax:** (937)291-0463
**Website:** http://www.miamivalleycare.org/alzheimer

**★ 14547 ★ Alzheimer's Association**
**Northwest Ohio Chapter**
2500 N Reynolds Rd.
Toledo, OH 43615-2820
**Phone:** (419)537-1999　　　**Free:** 800-441-3322
**Fax:** (419)536-5591
**Website:** http://www.nwoalz.org

### Oklahoma

**★ 14548 ★ Alzheimer's Association**
**Oklahoma/Western Arkansas Chapter**
6465 S Yale, Ste. 206
Tulsa, OK 74136-7810
**Phone:** (918)481-7741　　　**Free:** 800-493-1411
**Fax:** (918)481-7745
**Website:** http://www.alzokar.org

### Oregon

**★ 14549 ★ Alzheimer's Association**
**Oregon-Greater Idaho Chapter**
1311 NW 21st Ave.
Portland, OR 97209
**Phone:** (503)413-7115　　　**Free:** 800-733-0402
**Fax:** (503)413-6909
**Email:** andi.miller@alz-or.org
**Website:** http://www.alz.org/oregon
Liz McKinney, Exec Director
**Remarks:** Also serves Washington.

### Pennsylvania

**★ 14550 ★ Alzheimer's Association**
**Delaware Valley Chapter**
100 N 17th St., 2nd Fl.
Philadelphia, PA 19103
**Phone:** (215)561-2919　　　**Free:** 800-272-3900
**Fax:** (215)561-4663
**Website:** http://www.alz-delawarevalley.org
**Remarks:** Serves Delaware, New Jersey, and Pennsylvania.

**★ 14551 ★ Alzheimer's Association**
**Greater Pennsylvania Chapter**
2001 N Front St., Ste. 321, Bldg. 2
Harrisburg, PA 17102
**Phone:** (717)232-3580　　　**Free:** 800-975-8848
**Fax:** (717)232-3609

### Rhode Island

**★ 14552 ★ Alzheimer's Association**
**Rhode Island Chapter**
245 Waterman St., Ste. 306
Providence, RI 02906
**Phone:** (401)421-0008　　　**Free:** 800-244-1428
**Fax:** (401)421-0115
**Website:** http://www.alz-ri.org

### South Carolina

**★ 14553 ★ Alzheimer's Association**
**Palmetto Chapter**
PO Box 7044
Columbia, SC 29202
**Phone:** (803)772-3346　　　**Free:** 800-636-3346
**Fax:** (803)772-3349
**Email:** paul.jeter@alz.org
**Website:** http://www.midnet.sc.edu/alz/alz.htm
Paul Jeter, Exec Director

**★ 14554 ★ Alzheimer's Association**
**Upstate South Carolina Chapter**
521 N McDuffie St.
Anderson, SC 29621
**Phone:** (864)224-3045　　　**Free:** 800-273-2555
**Fax:** (864)225-1387
**Email:** alz@carol.net
**Website:** http://www.upstatescalz.org

### Tennessee

**★ 14555 ★ Alzheimer's Association**
**Eastern Tennessee Chapter**
Portland Bldg., Ste. H-102
2200 Sutherland Ave.
Knoxville, TN 37919
**Phone:** (865)544-6288　　　**Fax:** (865)544-6249
**Email:** corinne.patrick@alz.org
**Website:** http://www.tnalz.org

**★ 14556 ★ Alzheimer's Association**
**Mid South Chapter**
4004 Hillsboro Rd., Ste. 219B
Nashville, TN 37215
**Phone:** (615)292-4938　　　**Fax:** (615)386-9768
**Website:** http://www.alztn.org
**Remarks:** Serves Alabama, Arkansas, and Tennessee.

**★ 14557 ★ Alzheimer's Association**
**Northeast Tennessee Chapter**
207 N Boone St., Ste. 1500
Johnson City, TN 37604
**Phone:** (423)928-4080　　　**Fax:** (423)928-1152
**Remarks:** Also serves Virginia.

**★ 14558 ★ Alzheimer's Association**
**Southeast Tennessee Chapter**
735 Broad St., Ste. 300
Chattanooga, TN 37402
**Phone:** (423)265-3600　　　**Free:** 800-616-1922
**Fax:** (423)265-3611

### Texas

**★ 14559 ★ Alzheimer's Association**
**Greater Austin Chapter**
3420 Executive Ctr. Dr., Ste. 301
Austin, TX 78731
**Phone:** (512)241-0420　　　**Free:** 800-367-2132
**Fax:** (512)241-0430
**Email:** alz@alz-austin.org
**Website:** http://www.alz-austin.org/
Gail Harmon, Exec Director

**★ 14560 ★ Alzheimer's Association**
**Greater Dallas Chapter**
7610 N Stemmons Fwy., Ste. 600
Dallas, TX 75247-4228
**Phone:** (214)827-0062　　　**Free:** 800-515-8201
**Fax:** (214)827-2064
**Email:** dawn.mckinney@alz.org
**Website:** http://www.alzdallas.org/

**★ 14561 ★ Alzheimer's Association**
**North Central Texas Chapter**
PO Box 9709
Fort Worth, TX 76147
**Phone:** (817)336-4949　　　**Free:** 800-471-4422
**Fax:** (817)336-4966
**Email:** theresa.hocker@alz.org
**Website:** http://www.alz.org/ncc
Theresa Hocker, Exec Director

**★ 14562 ★ Alzheimer's Association**
**STAR Chapter**
4400 N Mesa, Ste. 9
El Paso, TX 79902

**Phone:** (915)544-1799　　　**Free:** 877-544-1799
**Fax:** (915)544-8746

### Utah

**★ 14563 ★ Alzheimer's Association**
**Utah Chapter**
1414 East 4500 South, Ste. 2
Salt Lake City, UT 84117
**Phone:** (801)274-1944　　　**Free:** 800-371-6694
**Fax:** (801)274-1226
**Website:** http://www.alzutah.org
**Remarks:** Also serves Idaho.

### Vermont

**★ 14564 ★ Alzheimer's Association**
**Vermont and New Hampshire Chapter**
PO Box 1139
Montpelier, VT 05601
**Phone:** (802)229-1022　　　**Free:** 800-698-1022
**Fax:** (802)229-5231
**Email:** susan.gordon@alz.org
**Website:** http://www.alz.org/vermont

### Virginia

**★ 14565 ★ Alzheimer's Association**
**Central and Western Virginia Chapter**
PO Box 4634
Charlottesville, VA 22905
**Phone:** (434)973-6122　　　**Free:** 888-809-7383
**Fax:** (434)973-4224
**Email:** kitter@cstone.net
**Website:** http://monticello.avenue.org/alzheimers/
Elizabeth Seabrook, Exec Director

**★ 14566 ★ Alzheimer's Association**
**Greater Richmond Chapter**
4600 Cox Rd., Ste. 130
Glen Allen, VA 23060
**Phone:** (804)967-2580　　　**Free:** 800-598-4673
**Fax:** (804)967-2588
**Email:** sherry.peterson@alz.org
**Website:** http://www.richmondalzheimers.org/
Sherry E. Peterson, Exec Director

**★ 14567 ★ Alzheimer's Association**
**National Capital Area Chapter**
11240 Waples Mill Rd., Ste. 402
Fairfax, VA 22030
**Phone:** (866)259-0042　　　**Free:** (866)259-0042
**Fax:** (703)359-4441
**Website:** http://www.alz-nca.org
**Remarks:** Serves Maryland, Virginia, and Washington DC.

**★ 14568 ★ Alzheimer's Association**
**Southeastern Virginia Chapter**
20 Interstate Corporate Ctr., Ste. 233
Norfolk, VA 23502
**Phone:** (757)459-2405　　　**Free:** 800-755-1129
**Fax:** (757)461-7902
**Website:** http://www.alz.org/chapters/template/hamptrds/welcome.html

### Washington

**★ 14569 ★ Alzheimer's Association**
**Inland Northwest Chapter**
601 W Maxwell, No. 4
Spokane, WA 99201
**Phone:** (509)483-8456　　　**Free:** 800-256-6659
**Fax:** (509)483-6067
**Website:** http://www.inwalz.org
**Remarks:** Serves Idaho and Washington.

★ 14570 ★ **Alzheimer's Association**
**Western and Central Washington State**
   **Chapter**
12721 30th Ave. NE, Ste. 101
Seattle, WA 98125
**Phone:** (206)363-5500       **Free:** 800-848-7097
**Fax:** (206)363-5700
**Website:** http://www.alzwa.org/

## West Virginia

★ 14571 ★ **Alzheimer's Association**
**West Virginia Chapter**
1111 Lee St. E
Charleston, WV 25301
**Phone:** (304)343-2717       **Free:** 800-491-2717
**Fax:** (304)343-2723
**Website:** http://wvalz.org
**Remarks:** Also serves Ohio and Virginia.

## Wisconsin

★ 14572 ★ **Alzheimer's Association**
**Greater Wisconsin Chapter**
2900 Curry Ln., Ste. A
Green Bay, WI 54311
**Phone:** (920)469-2110       **Free:** 800-360-2110
**Fax:** (920)469-2131
**Remarks:** Serves Minnesota and Wisconsin.

★ 14573 ★ **Alzheimer's Association**
**South Central Wisconsin Chapter**
517 N Segoe Rd., Ste. 301
Madison, WI 53705
**Phone:** (608)232-3400       **Free:** 800-428-9280
**Fax:** (608)232-3407
**Email:** paul.rusk@alzwisc.org
**Website:** http://www.alzwisc.org/
Paul Rusk, Exec Director

★ 14574 ★ **Alzheimer's Association**
**Southeastern Wisconsin Chapter**
6130 W National Ave., Ste. 200
Milwaukee, WI 53214
**Phone:** (414)479-8800       **Free:** 800-922-2413
**Fax:** (414)479-8819
**Email:** info@alzheimers-sewi.org
**Website:** http://www.alzheimers-sewi.org/
Sig Tomkalski, Exec Director

## <u>Amyotrophic Lateral Sclerosis</u>

*State chapters of the ALS Association are listed below. The national office is located at 27001 Agoura Rd., Ste. 150, Calabasas Hills, CA 91301-5104. Additional information can be obtained by calling the national office at (800) 782-4747, or by consulting their web site at http://www.alsa.org.*

## Arizona

★ 14575 ★ **ALS Association**
**Arizona Chapter**
5040 E Shea Blvd., Ste. 151
Scottsdale, AZ 85254
**Phone:** (480)609-3888       **Fax:** (480)556-9927
**Email:** sue@alsaz.org
**Website:** http://alsaz.org

## California

★ 14576 ★ **ALS Association**
**Bay Area Chapter**
140 Geary St., 4th Fl.
San Francisco, CA 94108-5611
**Phone:** (415)392-2572       **Fax:** (415)438-3972
**Email:** fightals@alsabayarea.com
**Website:** http://www.alsabayarea.com

★ 14577 ★ **ALS Association**
**Greater Los Angeles Chapter**
PO Box 565
Agoura Hills, CA 91376
**Phone:** (818)865-8067       **Fax:** (818)865-8066
**Email:** ALSAGLAC@aol.com
**Website:** http://www.alsa.org/serving/la_chapter.cfm

★ 14578 ★ **ALS Association**
**Greater Sacramento Chapter**
2717 Cottage Way, Ste. 15
Sacramento, CA 95825
**Phone:** (916)979-9265       **Fax:** (916)979-9271
**Email:** alssacramento@netzero.com
**Alt. Contact:** PO Box 190, Sacramento, CA 95812.

★ 14579 ★ **ALS Association**
**Orange County Chapter**
2230 W Chapman Ste. 123
Orange, CA 92868
**Phone:** (714)938-1080       **Fax:** (714)938-1299
**Email:** alsaoc@hotmail.com
**Website:** http://www.alsa.org/serving/orange_chapter.cfm
Cheryl Holt, Exec Director

## Colorado

★ 14580 ★ **ALS Association**
**Rocky Mountain Chapter**
PO Box 7964
Boulder, CO 80306
**Phone:** (720)890-8311       **Fax:** (970)532-1225
**Email:** sbaum@idcomm.com
Patti Abendroth, Exec Director

## Connecticut

★ 14581 ★ **ALS Association**
**Connecticut Chapter**
The Westport Gallery
125 Main St.
Westport, CT 06880
**Phone:** (203)226-6619       **Fax:** (203)222-8470
**Email:** als.assoc@snet.net
**Website:** http://www.alsact.org
Bob O'Brien, Exec Director

## Florida

★ 14582 ★ **ALS Association**
**Florida Chapter**
Gateway Corporate Center
9887 Fourth St. North
Saint Petersburg, FL 33702
**Email:** Hwalker@als-florida.org
**Website:** http://www.als-florida.org

★ 14583 ★ **ALS Association**
**Florida East Coast Regional Office**
1998 SW Taurus Ln.
Port Saint Lucie, FL 34984
**Phone:** (561)871-2453       **Fax:** (561)871-2223
**Email:** dotburk@aol.com
**Website:** http://www.alsa.org/serving/florida_goldcoast_chapter.cfm
Dottie Burkett, Exec Director

★ 14584 ★ **ALS Association**
**Southern Florida Chapter**
4631 NW 31st Ave., No. 166
Fort Lauderdale, FL 33309
**Phone:** (954)977-6815
**Email:** southflals@aol.com
Lillian Moskowitz, President

★ 14585 ★ **ALS Association**
**Tampa Bay Chapter**
3641 W Kennedy Blvd., Ste. C
Tampa, FL 33609
**Phone:** (813)879-7999       **Free:** 888-257-1717
**Fax:** (813)874-2088
**Email:** weplan4u@gte.net
**Website:** http://www.als-tampabay.org
David Smith, President

## Georgia

★ 14586 ★ **ALS Association**
**Georgia Chapter**
1955 Monroe Dr. NE
PO Box 13427
Atlanta, GA 30327
**Phone:** (404)870-4424       **Fax:** (404)875-7060
**Email:** susan@constantine.com
**Website:** http://www.alsaga.org
Susan Constantine, Exec Director

## Indiana

★ 14587 ★ **ALS Association**
**Indiana Chapter**
1980 E 116th St., Ste. 105
Carmel, IN 46032
**Free:** 888-508-3232
**Email:** alsa.in@juno.com
Brooke Billingsley, Exec Director

## Kansas

★ 14588 ★ **ALS Association**
**Keith Worthington Chapter**
8340 Mission Rd., Ste. B4
Prairie Village, KS 66206
**Phone:** (913)648-2062       **Fax:** (913)642-2431
**Email:** bcooper@alsa-midwest.org
**Website:** http://www.alsa-midwest.org
Beckie Cooper, Exec Director

★ 14589 ★ **ALS Association**
**Keith Worthington Chapter**
**Central/Western Kansas - Branch Office**
5920 E Central, Ste. 102
Wichita, KS 67208
**Phone:** (316)612-0188       **Fax:** (316)612-8768
**Website:** http://www.alsa-midwest.org

## Kentucky

★ 14590 ★ **ALS Association**
**Kentucky CIO**
PO Box 910130
Lexington, KY 40591
**Phone:** (859)225-0251
**Email:** LCCenters@aol.com

## Maryland

★ 14591 ★ **ALS Association**
**National Capital Area Chapter**
615 South Frederick Ave.
Ste. 308
Gaithersburg, MD 20877
**Phone:** (301)977-9855       **Fax:** (301)978-7654
**Email:** pfreiberg@alsa-ncac.org
**Website:** http://www.alsa-ncac.org

## Massachusetts

★ 14592 ★ **ALS Association**
**Massachusetts Chapter**
75 McNeil Way
Ste. 201
Dedham, MA 02026
**Phone:** (781)326-8884       **Fax:** (781)326-4940
**Email:** alsama@msn.com
**Website:** http://www.als-ma.org

**★ 14593 ★ ALS Association**
**Massachusetts Chapter - Wakefield Office**
7 Lincoln St.
Wakefield, MA 01880
**Free:** 800-258-3323
**Email:** alsma@msn.com
**Website:** http://www.als-ma.org
Donna Jordan, Exec Director

## Michigan

**★ 14594 ★ ALS Association**
**ALS of Michigan Inc.**
8521 Lyndon St., Ste. 2000
Detroit, MI 48238
**Free:** 800-882-5764                **Fax:** (313)933-8721
**Email:** ALSofMI@alsofmi.org
**Website:** http://www.alsofmi.org

**★ 14595 ★ ALS Association**
**West Michigan Chapter**
678 Front St. NW, Ste. 232
Grand Rapids, MI 49504
**Free:** 800-387-7121                **Fax:** (616)459-4522
**Email:** alsawmc@aol.com
**Website:** http://www.alsa.org/serving/westmi_chapter.cfm

## Minnesota

**★ 14596 ★ ALS Association**
**Minnesota Chapter**
528 Hennepin Ave., Ste. 610
Minneapolis, MN 55403-1802
**Phone:** (612)672-0484            **Free:** 800-672-0484
**Fax:** (612)672-9110
**Email:** info@alsmn.com
**Website:** http://www.alsamn.com
Marlin Possehl, Exec Director

## Missouri

**★ 14597 ★ ALS Association**
**Greater Saint Louis Chapter**
3945 W Pine Blvd.
Saint Louis, MO 63108
**Phone:** (314)534-0610            **Fax:** (314)534-4258
**Email:** alsstl@inetmail.att.net
**Website:** http://www.alsa.org/serving/stlouis_chapter.cfm
David Busker, President
Sharon Gacki, Exec Director

**★ 14598 ★ ALS Association**
**Keith Worthington Chapter**
**Central Missouri Branch Office**
1447 F South Enterprise
Springfield, MO 65803
**Phone:** (417)886-5003            **Fax:** (417)886-5058
**Website:** http://www.alsa-midwest.org

**★ 14599 ★ ALS Association**
**St. Louis Regional Chapter**
5616 Pershing Ave., Ste. 20
Saint Louis, MO 63112
**Phone:** (314)534-0610            **Fax:** (314)361-3019
**Email:** info@alsastl.org
**Website:** http://www.alsa.org/serving/stlouis_chapter.cfm

## Nevada

**★ 14600 ★ ALS Association**
**Nevada Chapter**
2101 S Jones, Ste. 120
Las Vegas, NV 89146
**Phone:** (702)248-4507            **Fax:** (702)248-8070
**Email:** alsanv@nevp.com
**Website:** http://www.alsnevada.com

## New Mexico

**★ 14601 ★ ALS Association**
**New Mexico CIO**
PO Box 16495
Albuquerque, NM 87191-6495
**Phone:** (505)323-6348
**Email:** cborgman@wans.net
**Website:** http://www.alsa-nm.org

## New York

**★ 14602 ★ ALS Association**
**Greater New York Chapter**
116 John St., Ste. 1304
New York, NY 10038
**Phone:** (212)619-7409            **Free:** 800-672-8857
**Fax:** (212)619-7409
**Email:** als@als-ny.org
**Website:** http://www.als-ny.org
Lauri Norvick, Exec Director

## North Carolina

**★ 14603 ★ ALS Association**
**North Carolina Chapter**
6512 Six Forks Rd., Ste. 602A
Raleigh, NC 27615
**Free:** 877-568-4347            **Fax:** (919)844-4295
**Email:** carolinaschapter@aol.com
**Website:** http://www.ncalsa.org

## Ohio

**★ 14604 ★ ALS Association**
**Northeast Ohio Chapter**
2500 E 22nd St., Ste. 101
Cleveland, OH 44115
**Phone:** (216)592-2572            **Fax:** (216)592-2575
**Email:** mjarmst216@aol.com
**Website:** http://www.alsaohio.org
Judy Post, Administrator

**★ 14605 ★ ALS Association**
**Western Ohio Chapter**
1810 MacKenzie Dr.
Ste. 120
Columbus, OH 43202
**Phone:** (614)273-2572            **Fax:** (614)273-2573
**Email:** edalsawo@.msn.com
**Website:** http://www.alsohio.org
Marlin Seymour, Exec Director

## Pennsylvania

**★ 14606 ★ ALS Association**
**Greater Philadelphia Chapter**
500 Office Center Dr., Ste. 340
Fort Washington, PA 19034
**Phone:** (215)643-5434            **Fax:** (215)643-9307
**Email:** alsassoc@philadelphia.org
**Website:** http://www.als-phila.org
Mary Connell, President

**★ 14607 ★ ALS Association**
**Western Pennsylvania Chapter**
1323 Forbes Ave., Ste. 200
Pittsburgh, PA 15219
**Free:** 800-967-9296            **Fax:** (412)471-2722
**Email:** ALSAWPA@aol.com
**Website:** http://www.alsa.org
Cathy Easter, Exec Director

## Rhode Island

**★ 14608 ★ ALS Association**
**Rhode Island Chapter**
2845 Post Rd., Ste. 110
Warwick, RI 02886-3145
**Phone:** (401)732-1609            **Fax:** (401)732-2577
**Email:** alsarinf@aol.com

**Website:** http://www.alsari.org
Nancy Feroldi, Exec Director

## Tennessee

**★ 14609 ★ ALS Association**
**Central Tennessee Chapter**
2625 Critz Ln.
Thompsons Station, TN 37179
**Phone:** (615)794-4010            **Fax:** (615)302-2680

## Texas

**★ 14610 ★ ALS Association**
**North Texas Chapter**
2100 Highway 360
Ste. 190
Grand Prairie, TX 75050
**Phone:** (817)226-4257
**Email:** hope@alsanorthtexas.org
**Website:** http://www.alsanorthtexas.org
**Remarks:** The mission of the Dallas/Ft. Worth Chapter of the ALS Association is to help those living with ALS and their caregivers and to support research to find a cure. **Program(s):** Support groups, advocacy, education, and loaning of equipment and reading materials.

**★ 14611 ★ ALS Association**
**South Texas Chapter**
6800 Park Ten Blvd., Ste. 220N
San Antonio, TX 78213
**Phone:** (210)733-5204            **Fax:** (210)733-5206
**Email:** alsasotex@stic.net
**Website:** http://www.alsa-south-tx.org
April Coldsmith, Exec Director

## Vermont

**★ 14612 ★ ALS Association**
**Northern New England CIO**
80 Colchester Ave.
Burlington, VT 05401
**Phone:** (802)862-8882            **Free:** 888-257-7733
**Fax:** (802)862-2138
**Email:** krusinsk@salus.med.uvm.edu

## Washington

**★ 14613 ★ ALS Association**
**Evergreen Chapter**
6627 S 191st Place
Ste. F-106
Kent, WA 98032
**Phone:** (425)656-1650            **Fax:** (425)656-1649
**Email:** info@asla-ec.org
**Website:** http://www.alsa-ec.org

## Wisconsin

**★ 14614 ★ ALS Association**
**Southeast Wisconsin Chapter**
6909 W North Ave.
Wauwatosa, WI 53213
**Phone:** (414)771-9400            **Fax:** (414)771-9503
**Email:** gehrigse@execpc.com
**Website:** http://www.se-wis-als.org

## Cerebral Palsy

*State chapters of the United Cerebral Palsy Association are listed below. The national office is located at 1660 L St. NW, Ste. 700, Washington, DC 20036. Additional informational can be obtained by calling the national office at (800) 872-5827, or by consulting their web site at http://www.ucpa.org/.*

## Alabama

**★ 14615 ★ United Cerebral Palsy Association**
**Alabama Chapter**
c/o East Central Alabama Chapter
301 EA. Darden Dr.
Box 694
Anniston, AL 36202
**Phone:** (256)237-8203          **Fax:** (256)235-2388
**Email:** ucpofeca@hiwaay.net

**★ 14616 ★ United Cerebral Palsy Association**
**East Central Alabama Chapter**
301 E A. Darden Dr.
Box 694
Anniston, AL 36202
**Phone:** (256)237-8203          **Fax:** (256)235-2388
**Email:** linda@ecaucp.org
**Website:** http://www.ecaucp.org

**★ 14617 ★ United Cerebral Palsy Association**
**Greater Birmingham Chapter**
120 Oslo Cir.
Birmingham, AL 35211
**Phone:** (205)944-3900          **Fax:** (205)944-3933
**Email:** lindab@ucpbham.com
**Website:** http://www.ucpbham.com

**★ 14618 ★ United Cerebral Palsy Association**
**Huntsville and Tennessee Valley Chapter**
2075 Max Luther Dr.
Huntsville, AL 35810
**Phone:** (256)852-5600          **Fax:** (256)852-6722
**Email:** therapy@ucphuntsville.org

**★ 14619 ★ United Cerebral Palsy Association**
**Mobile Chapter**
3058 Dauphin Sq. Connector
Mobile, AL 36607
**Phone:** (251)479-4900          **Fax:** (251)479-4998
**Email:** gharger1947@aol.com

**★ 14620 ★ United Cerebral Palsy Association**
**Northwest Alabama Chapter**
4212 Jackson Hwy.
Sheffield, AL 35660
**Phone:** (256)381-4310          **Fax:** (256)381-3478
**Email:** ucpofnwa@hiwaay.net

**★ 14621 ★ United Cerebral Palsy Association**
**West Alabama Chapter**
1100 UCP Pkwy.
Northport, AL 35476
**Phone:** (205)345-3031          **Fax:** (205)345-3035
**Email:** toniucpwa@comcast.net

## Alaska

**★ 14622 ★ United Cerebral Palsy Association**
**Alaska Chapter/PARENTS, Inc.**
4743 Northern Lights Blvd.
Anchorage, AK 99508
**Phone:** (907)337-7678          **Fax:** (907)337-7671
**Email:** parents@parentsinc.org
**Website:** http://www.parentsinc.org

## Arizona

**★ 14623 ★ United Cerebral Palsy Association**
**Southern Arizona Chapter**
3941 E 29th St., Ste. 601-604
Tucson, AZ 85711
**Phone:** (520)795-3108          **Fax:** (520)795-3196
**Email:** staff@ucpsa.org
**Website:** http://www.ucpsa.org

**★ 14624 ★ United Cerebral Palsy Association of Central Arizona, Inc.**
321 W Hatcher St., Ste. 102
Phoenix, AZ 85021
**Phone:** (602)943-5472          **Fax:** (602)943-4936
**Email:** info@ucpofaz.com
**Website:** http://www.ucpofaz.com

## Arkansas

**★ 14625 ★ United Cerebral Palsy Association**
**Central Arkansas Chapter**
9720 N Rodney Parham Rd.
Little Rock, AR 72227
**Phone:** (501)224-6067          **Fax:** (501)227-5591
**Email:** info@ucpcark.org
**Website:** http://www.ucpcark.org

**★ 14626 ★ United Cerebral Palsy Association**
**South Arkansas Chapter**
714 W Grove
El Dorado, AR 71730
**Phone:** (870)863-8194          **Fax:** (870)881-4600

## California

**★ 14627 ★ United Cerebral Palsy Association**
**Central California Chapter**
4224 N Cedar Ave.
Fresno, CA 93726-3700
**Phone:** (559)221-8272          **Fax:** (559)221-9347
**Email:** melishah@ccucp.org
**Website:** http://www.ccupc.org

**★ 14628 ★ United Cerebral Palsy Association**
**Golden Gate Chapter**
1970 Broadway, Ste. 600
Oakland, CA 94612
**Phone:** (510)832-7430          **Fax:** (510)839-1329
**Email:** info@ucpgg.org
**Website:** http://www.ucpgg.org

**★ 14629 ★ United Cerebral Palsy Association**
**Greater Sacramento Chapter**
191 Lathrop Way, Ste. N
Sacramento, CA 95815
**Phone:** (916)565-7700          **Fax:** (916)565-7773
**Email:** ucp@ucpsacto.org
**Website:** http://www.ucpsacto.org

**★ 14630 ★ United Cerebral Palsy Association**
**Inland Empire Chapter**
35325 Date Palm Dr., Ste. 136
Cathedral City, CA 92234
**Phone:** (760)321-8184          **Fax:** (760)321-8284
**Email:** ucpaie@aol.com

**★ 14631 ★ United Cerebral Palsy Association**
**Los Angeles and Ventura Counties Chapter**
6430 Independence Ave.
Woodland Hills, CA 91367
**Phone:** (818)782-2211          **Fax:** (818)909-9106
**Email:** ucpla@aol.com

**★ 14632 ★ United Cerebral Palsy Association**
**North Bay Chapter**
PO Box 7788
Santa Rosa, CA 95407-0788
**Phone:** (707)566-8647          **Fax:** (707)586-3279
**Email:** ucpnb@sonic.net

**★ 14633 ★ United Cerebral Palsy Association**
**Orange County Chapter**
3010 W Harvard St.
Santa Ana, CA 92704
**Phone:** (714)557-1291          **Fax:** (714)546-0943
**Email:** jminer@ucpaoc.org
**Website:** http://www.ucpaoc.org

**★ 14634 ★ United Cerebral Palsy Association**
**San Diego County Chapter**
8525 Gibbs Dr., Ste. 100
San Diego, CA 92123
**Phone:** (858)571-7803          **Fax:** (858)571-0919
**Email:** ucpsd@pacbell.net
**Website:** http://www.san.rr.com/ucpsd/

**★ 14635 ★ United Cerebral Palsy Association**
**San Joaquin, Calaveras, and Amador Counties Chapter**
333 W Benjamin Holt Dr., Ste. 1
Stockton, CA 95207
**Phone:** (209)956-0290          **Fax:** (209)956-0294
**Email:** jschumacher@ucpsj.org
**Website:** http://www.ucpsj.org

**★ 14636 ★ United Cerebral Palsy Association**
**San Luis Obispo Chapter**
3620 Sacramento Dr., Ste. 201-C
San Luis Obispo, CA 93401
**Phone:** (805)543-2039          **Fax:** (805)543-2045
**Email:** ucpslo@fix.net
**Website:** http://www.ucp-slo.org

**★ 14637 ★ United Cerebral Palsy Association**
**Santa Barbara County Chapter**
423 W Victoria St.
Santa Barbara, CA 93101
**Phone:** (805)966-1112          **Fax:** (805)962-7201
**Email:** ucpla@aol.com

**★ 14638 ★ United Cerebral Palsy Association**
**Santa Clara and San Mateo Counties Chapter**
480 San Antonio Rd., Ste. 215
Mountain View, CA 94040-1218
**Phone:** (650)917-6900          **Fax:** (650)948-8503
**Email:** ucp@ucpscsm.org
**Website:** http://www.ucpscsm.org

**★ 14639 ★ United Cerebral Palsy Association**
**Stanislaus County Chapter**
1213 13th St.
Modesto, CA 95354

**Phone:** (209)577-2122          **Fax:** (209)577-2392
**Email:** joanb30@hotmail.com

## Connecticut

★ 14640 ★ **United Cerebral Palsy Association**
**Eastern Connecticut Chapter**
Shaw's Cove 6, Ste. 101
New London, CT 06320
**Phone:** (860)447-3889          **Fax:** (860)447-3789
**Email:** united.cerebra.palsy@snet.net

★ 14641 ★ **United Cerebral Palsy Association**
**Greater Hartford Chapter**
80 Whitney St.
Hartford, CT 06105
**Phone:** (860)236-6201          **Fax:** (860)236-6205
**Email:** ucpgh@netscape.net

★ 14642 ★ **United Cerebral Palsy Association**
**Southern Connecticut Chapter**
105C S Elm St.
Wallingford, CT 06492
**Phone:** (203)269-3511          **Fax:** (203)269-7411
**Email:** ucpasouthernct@yahoo.com

## Delaware

★ 14643 ★ **United Cerebral Palsy Association**
**Delaware Chapter**
700A River Rd.
Wilmington, DE 19809-2746
**Phone:** (302)764-2400          **Fax:** (302)764-8713
**Email:** williammccool@juno.com

## District of Columbia

★ 14644 ★ **United Cerebral Palsy Association**
**Washington DC and Northern Virginia Chapter**
3135 8th St. NE
Washington, DC 20017
**Phone:** (202)269-1500          **Fax:** (202)526-0519
**Email:** webmaster@ucpdc.org
**Website:** http://www.ucpdcnova.org

## Florida

★ 14645 ★ **United Cerebral Palsy Association**
**Child Development Centers**
3305 S Orange Ave.
Orlando, FL 32806
**Phone:** (407)852-3300          **Fax:** (407)852-3301
**Email:** mbetts@ucpcdc.org
**Website:** http://www.ucpcdc.org

★ 14646 ★ **United Cerebral Palsy Association**
**Kentucky Chapter**
c/o Sunrise Group
9040 Sunset Dr.
Miami, FL 33173
**Phone:** (305)596-9040          **Fax:** (305)598-8240
**Email:** lleech@sunrisegroup.org
**Website:** http://www.sunrisegroup.org

★ 14647 ★ **United Cerebral Palsy Association**
**North Florida Chapter/Tender Love and Care**
1241-B East Ave.
Panama City, FL 32401
**Phone:** (850)769-7960          **Fax:** (850)769-1060

**Email:** kdrugachmc@aol.com

★ 14648 ★ **United Cerebral Palsy Association**
**Northeast Florida Chapter**
3311 Beach Blvd.
Jacksonville, FL 32207
**Phone:** (904)396-1462          **Fax:** (904)396-1199
**Email:** cpnefagency@hotmail.com

★ 14649 ★ **United Cerebral Palsy Association**
**Northwest Florida Chapter**
2912 N East St.
Pensacola, FL 32501-1324
**Phone:** (850)432-1596          **Fax:** (850)432-1930
**Email:** ucpnwfl@aol.com

★ 14650 ★ **United Cerebral Palsy Association**
**Sarasota-Manatee Chapter**
1090 S Tamiami Trail
Sarasota, FL 34236
**Phone:** (941)957-3599          **Fax:** (941)957-3499
**Email:** ucpsmi@gte.net

★ 14651 ★ **United Cerebral Palsy Association**
**South Florida Chapter**
1411 NW 14th Ave.
Miami, FL 33125
**Phone:** (305)325-1080          **Fax:** (305)325-1313
**Email:** info@ucpsouthflorida.org
**Website:** http://www.ucpsouthflorida.org

★ 14652 ★ **United Cerebral Palsy Association**
**Tallahassee Chapter**
1830 Buford Ct.
Tallahassee, FL 32308
**Phone:** (850)922-5630          **Fax:** (850)922-1258
**Email:** gator1@nettally.com
**Website:** http://www.nettally.com/ucp

★ 14653 ★ **United Cerebral Palsy Association**
**Tampa Bay Chapter**
2215 E Henry Ave.
Tampa, FL 33610
**Phone:** (813)239-1179          **Fax:** (813)237-3091
**Email:** kryals@ucptampa.org
**Website:** http://www.ucptampa.org

★ 14654 ★ **United Cerebral Palsy Association of Florida, Inc.**
1830 Buford Ct.
Tallahassee, FL 32308
**Phone:** (850)878-2141          **Fax:** (850)922-1258
**Email:** ucpadm@nettally.com

## Georgia

★ 14655 ★ **United Cerebral Palsy Association**
**Georgia Chapter**
3300 Northeast Expy., Bldg. 9
Atlanta, GA 30341
**Phone:** (770)676-2000          **Fax:** (770)455-8040
**Email:** info@ucpga.org
**Website:** http://www.ucpga.org

## Hawaii

★ 14656 ★ **United Cerebral Palsy Association**
**Hawaii Chapter**
414 Kuwili St., Ste. 105
Honolulu, HI 96817-5050

**Phone:** (808)532-6744          **Fax:** (808)532-6747
**Email:** ucpa@diverseabilities.org
**Website:** http://www.diverseabilities.org

## Idaho

★ 14657 ★ **United Cerebral Palsy Association**
**Idaho Chapter**
5420 W Franklin Rd., Ste. A
Boise, ID 83705
**Phone:** (208)377-8070          **Fax:** (208)322-7133
**Email:** ucpidaho@aol.com

## Illinois

★ 14658 ★ **Easter Seals/United Cerebral Palsy Association**
507 E Armstrong
Peoria, IL 61603
**Phone:** (309)686-1177          **Fax:** (309)686-2035
**Email:** sthompson@easterseals-ucp.org
**Website:** http://www.easterseals-ucp.org

★ 14659 ★ **United Cerebral Palsy Association**
**East Central Illinois Chapter**
2715 N 27th St.
Decatur, IL 62526-2126
**Phone:** (217)428-5033          **Fax:** (217)428-5094
**Email:** ucpeci@msn.com

★ 14660 ★ **United Cerebral Palsy Association**
**Greater Chicago Chapter**
160 N Wacker Dr.
Chicago, IL 60606
**Phone:** (312)368-0380          **Fax:** (312)368-0018
**Email:** pdulle@ucpnet.org
**Website:** http://www.ucpnet.org

★ 14661 ★ **United Cerebral Palsy Association**
**Illinois Chapter**
312 E Adams
Springfield, IL 62701
**Phone:** (217)528-9681          **Fax:** (217)528-9739
**Email:** ucpil@aol.com

★ 14662 ★ **United Cerebral Palsy Association**
**Land of Lincoln Chapter**
130 N 16th St.
Springfield, IL 62703
**Phone:** (217)525-6522          **Fax:** (217)525-9017
**Email:** ucpll@hotmail.com

★ 14663 ★ **United Cerebral Palsy Association**
**Land of Lincoln Chapter**
130 N 16th St.
Springfield, IL 62703
**Phone:** (217)525-6522          **Fax:** (217)525-9017
**Email:** ucpll@hotmail.com

★ 14664 ★ **United Cerebral Palsy Association**
**Southern Illinois Chapter**
9 Cusumano Professional Plaza Dr.
Mount Vernon, IL 62864
**Phone:** (618)244-2505          **Fax:** (618)244-3568
**Email:** ucpsi@onemain.com

★ 14665 ★ **United Cerebral Palsy Association**
**Will County Chapter**
311 S Reed St.
Joliet, IL 60436

Phone: (815)744-3500
Fax: (815)744-3504
Email: ucpwill@ucpwill.org
Website: http://www.ucpwill.org

## Indiana

★ 14666 ★ United Cerebral Palsy
Association
**Greater Indiana Chapter**
615 N Alabama St., Ste. 322
Indianapolis, IN 46204-1484
Phone: (317)632-3561
Fax: (317)632-3338
Email: donnar@ucpaindy.org

★ 14667 ★ United Cerebral Palsy
Association
**Wabash Valley Chapter**
621 Poplar St.
Terre Haute, IN 47804
Phone: (812)232-6305
Fax: (812)234-3683
Email: ucp.wv@verizon.net

## Kansas

★ 14668 ★ United Cerebral Palsy
Association
**Kansas Chapter**
5111 E 21st St.
Wichita, KS 67208
Phone: (316)688-1888
Fax: (316)688-5687
Email: davej@cprf.org
Website: http://www.cprf.org

## Louisiana

★ 14669 ★ United Cerebral Palsy
Association
**Baton Rouge Chapter**
1805 College Dr.
Baton Rouge, LA 70808
Phone: (225)923-3420
Fax: (225)922-9316
Email: jketcham@ucpbr.org
Website: http://www.ucpbr.org

★ 14670 ★ United Cerebral Palsy
Association
**Greater New Orleans Chapter**
1000 Leonidas St. and Leake Ave.
New Orleans, LA 70118
Phone: (504)865-0003
Fax: (504)865-0300
Email: info@ucpgno.com
Website: http://www.ucpgno.org

## Maine

★ 14671 ★ United Cerebral Palsy
Association
**Northeastern Maine Chapter**
700 Mt. Hope Ave., Ste. 320
Bangor, ME 04401
Phone: (207)941-2952
Fax: (207)941-2955
Email: ucp2@midmaine.com

## Maryland

★ 14672 ★ United Cerebral Palsy
Association
**Central Maryland Chapter**
1700 Reisterstown Rd., Ste. 226
Baltimore, MD 21208-2935
Phone: (410)484-4540
Free: 800-451-2452
Fax: (410)484-1807
Email: info@ucp-cm.org
Website: http://www.ucp-cm.org

★ 14673 ★ United Cerebral Palsy
Association
**Prince Georges and Montgomery
Counties Chapter**
3901 Woodhaven Ln.
Bowie, MD 20715
Phone: (301)262-4993
Fax: (301)262-4982
Email: ucppgmc@aol.com

★ 14674 ★ United Cerebral Palsy
Association
**Southern Maryland Chapter**
211 Chinquapin Round Rd.
Annapolis, MD 21401
Phone: (410)280-2003
Fax: (410)269-5757
Email: ucpinfo@ucpsm.org
Website: http://www.ucpsm.org

## Massachusetts

★ 14675 ★ United Cerebral Palsy
Association
**Berkshire County Chapter**
141 North St.
Pittsfield, MA 01201
Phone: (413)442-1562
Fax: (413)499-4077
Email: ucp@netconnx.net

★ 14676 ★ United Cerebral Palsy
Association
**Metro Boston Chapter**
71 Arsenal St.
Watertown, MA 02472
Phone: (617)926-5480
Fax: (617)926-3059
Email: ucpbost@aol.com

## Michigan

★ 14677 ★ United Cerebral Palsy
Association
**Metropolitan Detroit Chapter**
23077 Greenfield, Ste. 205
Southfield, MI 48075
Phone: (248)557-5070
Fax: (248)557-4456
Email: main@ucpdetroit.org
Website: http://www.ucpdetroit.org

★ 14678 ★ United Cerebral Palsy
Association
**Michigan Chapter**
3401 E Saginaw, Ste. 216
Lansing, MI 48912
Phone: (517)203-1200
Free: 800-828-2714
Fax: (517)203-1203
Email: ucp@ucpmichigan.org
Website: http://www.ucpmichigan.org

## Minnesota

★ 14679 ★ United Cerebral Palsy
Association
**Central Minnesota Chapter**
510 25th Ave. N
Saint Cloud, MN 56303-3255
Phone: (320)253-0765
Fax: (320)253-6753
Email: info@ucpcentralmn.org
Website: http://www.ucpcentralmn.org

★ 14680 ★ United Cerebral Palsy
Association
**Minnesota Chapter**
1821 University Ave. W, Ste. 219 S
Saint Paul, MN 55104-2892
Phone: (651)646-7588
Fax: (651)646-3045
Email: ucpmn@cpinternet.com

## Missouri

★ 14681 ★ United Cerebral Palsy
Association
**Greater Kansas City Chapter**
1044 Main St., Ste. 600
Kansas City, MO 64105
Phone: (816)531-4454
Fax: (816)531-3383
Email: bscott@ucpkc.org
Remarks: Also serves Kansas City, Kansas.

★ 14682 ★ United Cerebral Palsy
Association
**Greater Saint Louis Chapter**
8645 Old Bonhomme Rd.
Saint Louis, MO 63132-3999
Phone: (314)994-1600
Fax: (314)994-0179
Email: forkoshr@ucpstl.org
Website: http://www.ucpstl.org

★ 14683 ★ United Cerebral Palsy
Association
**Missouri Chapter**
8645 Old Bonhomme Rd.
Saint Louis, MO 63132-3999
Phone: (314)994-1600
Fax: (314)994-0179

★ 14684 ★ United Cerebral Palsy
Association
**Northwest Missouri Chapter**
3303 Frederick Ave.
Saint Joseph, MO 64506
Phone: (816)364-3836
Fax: (816)390-8546
Email: ucpnwmo@ccp.com

## Nebraska

★ 14685 ★ United Cerebral Palsy
Association
**Nebraska Chapter**
7101 Newport Ave., Ste. 309
Omaha, NE 68152
Phone: (402)572-3686
Free: 800-729-2556
Fax: (402)572-3002
Email: ucpofne@aol.com

## Nevada

★ 14686 ★ United Cerebral Palsy
Association
**Northern Nevada Chapter**
4068 S McCarran Blvd., Ste. B
Reno, NV 89502-7532
Phone: (775)331-3323
Fax: (775)331-7913
Email: ucpnn@ucpnn.org
Website: http://www.ucpnn.org

## New Jersey

★ 14687 ★ United Cerebral Palsy
Association
**Hudson County Chapter**
8814 Kennedy Blvd.
North Bergen, NJ 07047
Phone: (201)662-0080
Fax: (201)861-4605
Email: hudsonucp@aol.com

★ 14688 ★ United Cerebral Palsy
Association
**Morris-Somerset Chapter**
245 Main St., Ste. 113
Chester, NJ 07930
Phone: (908)879-2243
Fax: (908)879-8363
Email: info@ucpmsnj.com
Website: http://www.ucpmsnj.com

## New York

**★ 14689 ★ United Cerebral Palsy Association**
**Center for the Disabled**
314 S Manning Blvd.
Albany, NY 12208
**Phone:** (518)437-5602     **Fax:** (518)437-5667
**Email:** krafchin@cftd.org
**Website:** http://www.cftd.org

**★ 14690 ★ United Cerebral Palsy Association**
**Greater Suffolk Chapter**
250 Marcus Blvd.
PO Box 18045
Hauppauge, NY 11788
**Phone:** (631)232-0011     **Fax:** (631)232-4422
**Email:** info@ucp-suffolk.org
**Website:** http://www.ucp-suffolk.org

**★ 14691 ★ United Cerebral Palsy Association**
**Nassau County Chapter**
380 Washington Ave.
Roosevelt, NY 11575
**Phone:** (516)378-2000     **Fax:** (516)378-0357
**Email:** info@ucpn.org
**Website:** http://www.ucpn.org

**★ 14692 ★ United Cerebral Palsy Association**
**New York City Chapter**
80 Maiden Ln., 8th Fl.
New York, NY 10038-4811
**Phone:** (212)683-6700     **Fax:** (212)685-8394
**Email:** info@ucpnyc.org
**Website:** http://www.ucpnyc.org

**★ 14693 ★ United Cerebral Palsy Association**
**Western New York Chapter**
7 Community Dr.
Buffalo, NY 14225
**Phone:** (716)505-5500     **Fax:** (716)894-8257
**Email:** info@ucpwny.org
**Website:** http://www.ucpwny.org

## North Carolina

**★ 14694 ★ United Cerebral Palsy Association**
**North Carolina Chapter**
PO Box 27707
Raleigh, NC 27611-7707
**Phone:** (919)832-3787     **Fax:** (919)832-5928
**Email:** soneal@ucpnc.org
**Website:** http://www.ucpnc.com
**Remarks:** Also serves South Carolina.

## Ohio

**★ 14695 ★ United Cerebral Palsy Association**
**Central Ohio Chapter**
440 Industrial Mile Rd.
Columbus, OH 43228-2411
**Phone:** (614)279-0109     **Fax:** (614)279-2527
**Email:** ucpoco@mindspring.com

**★ 14696 ★ United Cerebral Palsy Association**
**Cincinnati Chapter**
3601 Victory Pkwy.
Cincinnati, OH 45229
**Phone:** (513)221-4606     **Fax:** (513)872-5262
**Email:** ucpcrend@one.net
**Remarks:** Also serves Kentucky.

**★ 14697 ★ United Cerebral Palsy Association**
**Greater Cleveland Chapter**
10011 Euclid Ave.
Cleveland, OH 44106
**Phone:** (216)791-8363     **Fax:** (216)721-3372
**Email:** sdean@ucpcleveland.org
**Website:** http://www.ucpcleveland.org

## Oklahoma

**★ 14698 ★ United Cerebral Palsy Association**
**Oklahoma Chapter**
5208 W Reno, Ste. 275
Oklahoma City, OK 73127
**Phone:** (405)917-7080     **Fax:** (405)917-7082
**Email:** oklahoma@ucpok.org
**Website:** http://www.ucpok.org

## Oregon

**★ 14699 ★ United Cerebral Palsy Association**
**Oregon and Southwest Washington Chapter**
7830 SE Foster Rd.
Portland, OR 97206
**Phone:** (503)777-4166     **Free:** 800-473-4581
**Fax:** (503)771-8048
**Email:** ucpa@ucpaorwa.org
**Website:** http://www.ucpaorwa.org

## Pennsylvania

**★ 14700 ★ United Cerebral Palsy Association**
**Beaver, Butler and Lawrence Counties Chapter**
114 Skyline Dr.
Butler, PA 16001
**Phone:** (724)283-3198     **Fax:** (724)283-5945
**Email:** ucpbbl@nauticom.net

**★ 14701 ★ United Cerebral Palsy Association**
**Central Pennsylvania Chapter**
44 S 38th St.
Camp Hill, PA 17011
**Phone:** (717)975-0611     **Fax:** (717)975-0839
**Email:** kidscenter@ucpcentralpa.org
**Website:** http://www.ucpcentralpa.org

**★ 14702 ★ United Cerebral Palsy Association**
**MECA Chapter**
3745 W 12th St.
Erie, PA 16505
**Phone:** (814)836-9113     **Fax:** (814)833-3919
**Email:** leaton@erie.net

**★ 14703 ★ United Cerebral Palsy Association**
**Pennsylvania Chapter**
1902 Market St.
Camp Hill, PA 17011
**Phone:** (717)761-6129     **Fax:** (717)761-2534
**Email:** info@ucpofpa.org
**Website:** http://www.ucpofpa.org

**★ 14704 ★ United Cerebral Palsy Association**
**Philadelphia and Vicinity Chapter**
102 E Mermaid Ln.
Philadelphia, PA 19118
**Phone:** (215)242-4200     **Fax:** (215)247-4229
**Email:** ucpkravitz@aol.com

**★ 14705 ★ United Cerebral Palsy Association**
**Pittsburgh Chapter**
4638 Centre Ave.
Pittsburgh, PA 15213
**Phone:** (412)683-7100     **Fax:** (412)683-4160
**Email:** info@ucppittsburgh.org
**Website:** http://trfn.clpgh.org/ucp/

**★ 14706 ★ United Cerebral Palsy Association**
**South Central Pennsylvania Chapter**
788 Cherrytree Ct.
Hanover, PA 17331
**Phone:** (717)632-5552     **Fax:** (717)632-2315
**Email:** sroberts@ucpsouthcentral.org

**★ 14707 ★ United Cerebral Palsy Association**
**Southern Alleghenies Region Chapter**
616 Somerset St.
Johnstown, PA 15901
**Phone:** (814)535-7708     **Fax:** (814)536-8833
**Email:** ucpsar@yahoo.com

**★ 14708 ★ United Cerebral Palsy Association**
**Southwestern Pennsylvania Chapter**
Washington Federal Sq.
190 N Main St., Ste. 306
Washington, PA 15301
**Phone:** (724)229-0851     **Fax:** (724)229-9252
**Email:** info@ucpswpa.org
**Website:** http://www.ucpswpa.org/
**Remarks:** Also serves West Virginia.

**★ 14709 ★ United Cerebral Palsy Association**
**Western Pennsylvania Chapter**
1 Corporate Cir., Ste. 2000
Greensburg, PA 15601
**Phone:** (724)832-8272     **Fax:** (724)837-8278
**Email:** gbg@ucpwpa.org
**Website:** http://www.ucpwpa.org

## Rhode Island

**★ 14710 ★ United Cerebral Palsy Association**
**Rhode Island Chapter**
200 Main St., Ste. 210
PO Box 36
Pawtucket, RI 02862
**Phone:** (401)728-1800     **Fax:** (401)728-0182
**Email:** all@ucpri.org
**Website:** http://www.ucpri.org

## Tennessee

**★ 14711 ★ United Cerebral Palsy Association**
**Mid-South Chapter**
4189 Leroy
Memphis, TN 38108
**Phone:** (901)761-4277     **Fax:** (901)761-7876
**Email:** ucp@ucpmemphis.org
**Website:** http://www.ucpmemphis.org
**Remarks:** Also serves Mississippi.

**★ 14712 ★ United Cerebral Palsy Association**
**Middle Tennessee Chapter**
209 10th Ave. S, Ste. 154
Nashville, TN 37203
**Phone:** (615)242-4091     **Fax:** (615)242-3582
**Email:** info@ucpnashville.org
**Website:** http://www.nashville.net/~ucp/index.html

## Texas

**★ 14713 ★ United Cerebral Palsy Association**
**Greater Houston Chapter**
4500 Bissonnet, Ste. 340
Bellaire, TX 77401
**Phone:** (713)838-9050      **Fax:** (713)838-9098
**Email:** swaldner@ucphouston.org
**Website:** http://www.ucphouston.org

**★ 14714 ★ United Cerebral Palsy Association**
**Metropolitan Dallas Chapter**
8802 Harry Hines Blvd.
Dallas, TX 75235
**Phone:** (214)351-2500      **Free:** 800-999-1898
**Fax:** (214)351-2610
**Email:** eddyherrera@ucpdallas.org
**Website:** http://www.ucpdallas.org

**★ 14715 ★ United Cerebral Palsy Association**
**Tarrant County Chapter**
1555 Merrimac Cir., Ste. 102
Fort Worth, TX 76107
**Phone:** (817)332-7171      **Fax:** (817)332-7601
**Email:** info@ucptc.org
**Website:** http://www.ucptc.org

**★ 14716 ★ United Cerebral Palsy Association**
**Texas Chapter**
5555 N Lamar St., Ste. L139
Austin, TX 78751
**Phone:** (512)472-8696      **Free:** 800-798-1492
**Fax:** (512)472-8026
**Email:** ucptx@onr.com
**Website:** http://www.main.org/ucpa

## Utah

**★ 14717 ★ United Cerebral Palsy Association**
**Utah Chapter**
3550 South 700 West
South Salt Lake, UT 84119
**Phone:** (801)266-1805      **Fax:** (801)266-2404
**Email:** shellyp@ucputah.org
**Website:** http://www.ucputah.org

## Washington

**★ 14718 ★ United Cerebral Palsy Association**
**South Puget Sound Chapter**
6315 S 19th St., No. 25
Tacoma, WA 98466-6217
**Phone:** (253)565-1463      **Fax:** (253)565-0153
**Email:** info@ucp-sps.org
**Website:** http://www.ucp-sps.org

## Wisconsin

**★ 14719 ★ United Cerebral Palsy Association**
**Greater Dane County Chapter**
1502 Greenway Cross
Madison, WI 53713
**Phone:** (608)273-4434      **Fax:** (608)273-3426
**Email:** ucpgdc@itis.com

**★ 14720 ★ United Cerebral Palsy Association**
**North Central Wisconsin Chapter**
740 N 3rd St.
Wausau, WI 54403
**Phone:** (715)842-8700      **Free:** 800-472-4408
**Fax:** (715)848-3511

**Email:** glamping@ucp-wausau.org
**Website:** http://www.ucp-wausau.org

**★ 14721 ★ United Cerebral Palsy Association**
**Southeastern Wisconsin Chapter**
7519 W Oklahoma Ave.
Milwaukee, WI 53219
**Phone:** (414)329-4500      **Free:** 888-482-7739
**Fax:** (414)329-4510
**Email:** ucpofsew@execpc.com
**Website:** http://www.ucp.org/ucp_local.cfm/155

**★ 14722 ★ United Cerebral Palsy Association**
**West Central Wisconsin Chapter**
206 Water St.
Eau Claire, WI 54703
**Phone:** (715)832-1782      **Fax:** (715)832-8203
**Email:** ucpwcw@aol.com

**★ 14723 ★ United Cerebral Palsy Association**
**Wisconsin Chapter**
206 Water St.
Eau Claire, WI 54703
**Phone:** (715)832-1782      **Free:** 800-261-1895
**Fax:** (715)832-8203
**Email:** ucpwcw@aol.com

## Chronic Pain

*State chapters of the American Pain Society are listed below. The national office is located at 4700 W Lake Ave., Glenview, IL 60025. Additional information can be obtained by calling the national office at (847) 375-4715, or by consulting their web site at http://www.ampainsoc.org/.*

### California

**★ 14724 ★ American Pain Society**
**Western USA Pain Society**
8700 Beverly Blvd.
Los Angeles, CA 90048
**Phone:** (310)855-8030      **Fax:** (310)659-3928
**Website:** Cedars-Sinai Comprehensive Cancer Center
Corinne Manetto, PhD, President

### Illinois

**★ 14725 ★ American Pain Society**
**Midwest Pain Society**
4700 W Lake Ave.
Glenview, IL 60025
**Phone:** (847)375-4730      **Fax:** (847)375-4777
**Email:** jkokkines@amctec.com
Jim Kokkines, Contact

### North Carolina

**★ 14726 ★ American Pain Society**
**Southern Pain Society**
PO Box 5033
Cary, NC 27512
**Phone:** (919)303-0045      **Fax:** (919)303-9666
**Email:** lori@southernpain.org
**Website:** http://www.southernpain.org
Lori H. Postal, Contact

### Pennsylvania

**★ 14727 ★ American Pain Society**
**Greater Philadelphia Pain Society**
Park Towne Place, Ste. 108 N
2200 Ben Franklin Parkway
Philadelphia, PA 19130
**Phone:** (215)557-9705      **Fax:** (215)557-9683
Ed White, Contact

## Virginia

**★ 14728 ★ American Pain Society**
**Eastern Pain Association**
PO Box 11086
Richmond, VA 23230-1086
**Phone:** (804)282-0063      **Fax:** (804)282-0090
**Email:** kay@societyhq.com
Kay Holmes, Contact

**★ 14729 ★ American Pain Society**
**New England Pain Association**
2209 Dickens Rd.
Richmond, VA 23230-1086
**Phone:** (804)282-4011      **Fax:** (804)282-0090
**Email:** nepa@societyhq
**Website:** http://www.ampainsoc.org/member/nepa/index.htm
Stewart Hinckley, Contact
Paul Arnstein, PhD, President

## Epilepsy

*The following are state affiliates of the Epilepsy Foundation of America, 4351 Garden City Dr., Landover, MD 20785, (800)EFA-1000, http://www.efa.org/.*

### Alabama

**★ 14730 ★ Epilepsy Foundation of North and Central Alabama**
701 37th St. S, Ste. 2
Birmingham, AL 35222-3222
**Phone:** (205)324-4222      **Free:** 800-950-6662
**Website:** http://www.epilepsyfoundation.org/ncalabama

**★ 14731 ★ Epilepsy Foundation of South Alabama**
951 Government St., Ste. 201
Mobile, AL 36604-2425
**Phone:** (251)432-0970      **Free:** 800-626-1582
**Website:** http://www.epilepsyfoundation.org/SouthAlabama

### Arizona

**★ 14732 ★ Epilepsy Foundation of Arizona**
PO Box 25084
Phoenix, AZ 85002-5084
**Phone:** (602)406-3581      **Free:** 888-768-2690
**Website:** http://www.epilepsyfoundation.org/arizona

**★ 14733 ★ Epilepsy Foundation of Arizona**
PO Box 25084
Phoenix, AZ 85002-5084
**Phone:** (602)406-3581      **Free:** 888-768-2690
**Website:** http://www.epilepsyfoundation.org/arizona

### California

**★ 14734 ★ Epilepsy Foundation of Los Angeles, Orange, San Bernardino & Ventura Counties**
5777 W Century Blvd.
Los Angeles, CA 90045-5600
**Phone:** (310)670-2870      **Free:** 800-564-0445
**Website:** http://www.epilepsy-socalif.org

**★ 14735 ★ Epilepsy Foundation of Northern California**
1624 Franklin St., Ste. 900
Oakland, CA 94612-2824
**Phone:** (510)893-6272      **Free:** 800-632-3532
**Website:** http://www.epilepsyfoundation.org/norcal

★ **14736** ★ **Epilepsy Foundation of San Diego County**
2055 El Cajon Blvd.
San Diego, CA 92104-1091
**Phone:** (619)296-0161   **Free:** 800-408-4322
**Website:** http://www.epilepsysandiego.org

## Colorado

★ **14737** ★ **Epilepsy Foundation of Colorado, Inc.**
234 Columbine St., Ste. 333
Denver, CO 80206-4711
**Phone:** (303)377-9774   **Free:** 888-378-9779
**Website:** http://www.epilepsycolorado.org

## Connecticut

★ **14738** ★ **Epilepsy Foundation of Connecticut, Inc.**
386 Main St.
Middletown, CT 06457-3360
**Phone:** (860)346-1924   **Free:** 800-899-3745
**Website:** http://www.epilepsyfoundation.org/connecticut

## Delaware

★ **14739** ★ **Epilepsy Foundation of Delaware**
Tower Office Park
Newport, DE 19804-3167
**Phone:** (302)999-9313   **Free:** 800-422-3653
**Website:** http://www.epilepsyfoundation.org/delaware

## Florida

★ **14740** ★ **Epilepsy Foundation of Northeast Florida, Inc.**
5209 San Jose Blvd., Ste. 101
Jacksonville, FL 32207-7663
**Phone:** (904)731-3752   **Free:** 888-897-8579
**Website:** http://www.efnef.org

★ **14741** ★ **Epilepsy Foundation of South Florida, Inc.**
Chase Federal Bldg., Ste. 700
7300 N Kendall Dr.
Miami, FL 33156-7840
**Phone:** (305)670-4949
**Website:** http://www.epilepsyofla.org

## Georgia

★ **14742** ★ **Epilepsy Foundation of Georgia**
100 Edgewood Ave. NE, Ste. 1200
Atlanta, GA 30303-3069
**Phone:** (404)527-7155   **Free:** 800-527-7105
**Website:** http://www.epilepsyga.org/

## Hawaii

★ **14743** ★ **Epilepsy Foundation of Hawaii, Inc.**
245 N Kukui St., Ste. 207
Honolulu, HI 96817-3921
**Phone:** (808)528-3058
**Website:** http://www.hawaiiepilepsy.com/efh

## Idaho

★ **14744** ★ **Epilepsy Foundation of Idaho**
310 W Idaho St.
Boise, ID 83702-6039
**Phone:** (208)344-4340   **Free:** 800-237-6676
**Website:** http://www.epilepsyidaho.org

## Illinois

★ **14745** ★ **Epilepsy Foundation of Greater Chicago**
20 E Jackson Blvd., 13th Fl.
Chicago, IL 60604-2200
**Phone:** (312)939-8622   **Free:** 800-273-6027
**Website:** http://www.epilepsyfoundation.org/chicago

★ **14746** ★ **Epilepsy Foundation of North/Central Illinois**
321 W State St., Ste. 208
Rockford, IL 61101-1119
**Phone:** (815)964-2689   **Free:** 800-221-2689
**Website:** http://www.epilepsyfoundation.org/ncillinois
**Remarks:** Also serves Iowa.

★ **14747** ★ **Epilepsy Foundation of Southwestern Illinois**
1931 W Main St.
Belleville, IL 62226-7479
**Phone:** (618)236-2181
**Website:** http://www.neuro.wustl.edu/easwi

## Kentucky

★ **14748** ★ **Epilepsy Foundation Kentuckiana**
501 E Broadway, Ste. 110
Louisville, KY 40202-1797
**Phone:** (502)584-8817
**Website:** http://www.efky.org
**Remarks:** Serves Indiana and Kentucky.

## Louisiana

★ **14749** ★ **Epilepsy Foundation of Southeast Louisiana**
3701 Canal St., Ste. H
New Orleans, LA 70119-6101
**Phone:** (504)486-6326   **Free:** 800-960-0587
**Website:** http://www.laepilepsy.org

## Maryland

★ **14750** ★ **Epilepsy Foundation of the Chesapeake Region**
Hampton Plaza
300 E Joppa Rd., Ste. 1103
Towson, MD 21286-3012
**Phone:** (410)828-7700   **Free:** 800-492-2523
**Website:** http://www.abilitiesnetwork.org
**Remarks:** This affiliate serves Maryland, the District of Columbia, and Alexandria, Arlington, Fairfax, Falls Church, Loudoun, and Prince William counties in Virginia.

## Massachusetts

★ **14751** ★ **Epilepsy Foundation of Massachusetts and Rhode Island**
540 Gallivan Blvd.
Boston, MA 02124-5401
**Phone:** (617)506-6041   **Free:** 888-576-9996
**Website:** http://www.epilepsyfoundation.org/massri

## Michigan

★ **14752** ★ **Epilepsy Foundation of Michigan**
26211 Central Park Blvd., Ste. 100
Southfield, MI 48076-4154
**Phone:** (248)351-7979   **Free:** 800-377-6226
**Website:** http://www.epilepsyfoundation.org/michigan

★ **14753** ★ **Epilepsy Foundation of Michigan**
26211 Central Park Blvd., Ste. 100
Southfield, MI 48076-4154
**Phone:** (248)351-7979   **Free:** 800-377-6226
**Website:** http://www.epilepsyfoundation.org/michigan

## Minnesota

★ **14754** ★ **Epilepsy Foundation of Minnesota**
2356 University Ave W, No. 405
Saint Paul, MN 55114-1850
**Phone:** (651)646-1771   **Free:** 800-779-0777
**Website:** http://www.efmn.org
**Remarks:** This affiliate also serves Barnes, Cass, Cavalier, Grand Forks, Griggs, Nelson, Pembina, Ramsey, Ransom, Richland, Sargent, Steele, and Walsh counties in North Dakota.

## Mississippi

★ **14755** ★ **Epilepsy Foundation of Mississippi**
PO Box 16232
Jackson, MS 39236-6232
**Phone:** (601)362-2761   **Free:** 800-898-0291

## Missouri

★ **14756** ★ **Epilepsy Foundation of Kansas & Western Missouri**
6550 Troost Ave., Ste. B
Kansas City, MO 64131-1266
**Phone:** (816)444-2800   **Free:** 800-972-5163
**Website:** http://www.efha.org

★ **14757** ★ **Epilepsy Foundation of the Saint Louis Region**
7100 Oakland Ave.
Saint Louis, MO 63117-1813
**Phone:** (314)645-6969   **Free:** 800-264-6970
**Website:** http://www.epilepsyfoundation.org/stlouis
**Remarks:** Also serves Illinois.

## New Jersey

★ **14758** ★ **Epilepsy Foundation of New Jersey**
429 River View Plaza
Trenton, NJ 08611-3420
**Phone:** (609)392-4900   **Free:** 800-336-5843
**Website:** http://www.efnj.com

## New York

★ **14759** ★ **Epilepsy Foundation of Long Island, Inc.**
506 Stewart Ave.
Garden City, NY 11530-4706
**Phone:** (516)739-7733   **Free:** 888-672-7154
**Website:** http://www.epilepsyfoundation.org/longisland

★ **14760** ★ **Epilepsy Foundation of New York City**
305 7th Ave., 12th Fl.
New York, NY 10001-6008
**Phone:** (212)633-2930
**Website:** http://www.epilepsyfoundation.org/nyc

★ **14761** ★ **Epilepsy Foundation of Northeastern New York**
3 Washington Sq.
Albany, NY 12205-5523
**Phone:** (518)456-7501   **Free:** 800-894-3223
**Website:** http://www.epilepsyfoundation.org/efneny

★ **14762** ★ **Epilepsy Foundation of Rochester-Syracuse-Binghamton**
1000 Elmwood Ave., Ste. 800
Rochester, NY 14620-3042
**Phone:** (716)442-4430   **Free:** 800-724-7930

Website: http://www.epilepsyfoundation.org/rochester

**★ 14763 ★ Epilepsy Foundation of Southern New York, Inc.**
1 Blue Hill Plaza, No. 1745
Pearl River, NY 10965-3104
Phone: (845)627-0627      Free: 800-640-0371
Website: http://www.epiinfo.org

## North Carolina

**★ 14764 ★ Epilepsy Foundation of North Carolina, Inc.**
3001 Spring Forest Rd.
Raleigh, NC 27616-2817
Phone: (919)876-7788      Free: 800-451-0694
Website: http://www.supportnetworks.org/info/efnc.htm

## Ohio

**★ 14765 ★ Epilepsy Foundation of Central Ohio**
454 E Main St., Ste. 250
Columbus, OH 43215-5354
Phone: (614)228-4401      Free: 800-878-3226
Website: http://www.epilepsy-ohio.org

**★ 14766 ★ Epilepsy Foundation of Greater Cincinnati, Inc.**
895 Central Ave., Ste. 550
Cincinnati, OH 45202-5757
Phone: (513)721-2905
Website: http://www.epilepsyfoundation.org/cincinnati
Remarks: This affiliate serves Clark and Floyd counties in Indiana as well as the majority of Kentucky.

**★ 14767 ★ Epilepsy Foundation of Northeast Ohio**
2800 Euclid Ave., Rm. 450
Cleveland, OH 44115-2418
Phone: (216)579-1330
Website: http://www.efneo.org

**★ 14768 ★ Epilepsy Foundation of Northwest Ohio**
1251 S Reynolds Rd., PMB 323
Toledo, OH 43615-3938
Phone: (419)351-7979      Free: 800-377-6226

**★ 14769 ★ Epilepsy Foundation of Western Ohio**
7523 Brandt Pike
Dayton, OH 45424-2337
Phone: (937)233-2500      Free: 800-360-3296
Website: http://www.epilepsyfoundation.org/western-ohio

## Oregon

**★ 14770 ★ Epilepsy Foundation of Oregon**
619 SW 11th Ave., Ste. 225
Portland, OR 97205-2646
Phone: (503)228-7651      Free: 888-828-7651
Website: http://www.epilepsyfoundation.org/oregon
Remarks: This affiliate also serves Clark County in Washington.

## Pennsylvania

**★ 14771 ★ Epilepsy Foundation of Eastern Pennsylvania**
7 Benjamin Franklin Pkwy.
Philadelphia, PA 19103-1208
Phone: (215)523-9180      Free: 800-887-7165
Website: http://www.efsepa.org

**★ 14772 ★ Epilepsy Foundation of Western and Central Pennsylvania**
Vocational Rehab Center
1323 Forbes Ave., No. 102
Pittsburgh, PA 15219-4725
Phone: (412)261-5880      Free: 800-361-5885
Website: http://www.efwp.org

## Puerto Rico

**★ 14773 ★ Sociedad Puertorriquena de Epilepsia**
Hospital Ruiz Soler
Bayamon, PR 00959
Phone: (787)782-6200      Fax: (787)782-6262
Website: http://www.sociedadepilepsiapr.org

## South Carolina

**★ 14774 ★ Epilepsy Foundation of South Carolina**
652 Bush River Rd., Ste. 211
Columbia, SC 29210-7537
Phone: (803)798-8502
Website: http://www.epilepsysc.org

## Tennessee

**★ 14775 ★ Epilepsy Foundation of East Tennessee**
PO Box 3156
Knoxville, TN 37927-3156
Phone: (865)522-4991      Free: 800-522-4991
Website: http://www.efeasttn.org

**★ 14776 ★ Epilepsy Foundation of Middle Tennessee**
2002 Richard Jones Rd., Ste. C202
Nashville, TN 37215-2809
Phone: (615)269-7091      Free: 800-244-0768
Website: http://efmt.citysearch.com

**★ 14777 ★ Epilepsy Foundation of Southeast Tennessee**
744 McCallie Ave., Ste. 301
Chattanooga, TN 37403-2511
Phone: (423)756-1771
Website: http://www.epilepsy-setn.org
Remarks: This affiliate also serves Catoosa, Dade, and Walker counties in Georgia.

**★ 14778 ★ Epilepsy Foundation of West Tennessee**
70 Timber Creek Dr., No. 1
Cordova, TN 38018-4285
Phone: (901)624-7148
Remarks: This affiliate also serves DeSoto County, Mississippi.

## Texas

**★ 14779 ★ Epilepsy Foundation of Central and South Texas**
10615 Perrin Beitel Rd., Ste. 602
San Antonio, TX 78217-3142
Phone: (210)653-5353      Free: 888-606-5353
Website: http://www.epilepsyfoundation.org/efcst

**★ 14780 ★ Epilepsy Foundation of Greater North Texas**
2906 Swiss Ave.
Dallas, TX 75204-5929
Phone: (214)823-8809      Free: 800-447-7778
Website: http://www.efgnt.org

**★ 14781 ★ Epilepsy Foundation of Southeast Texas**
2650 Fountain View Dr., Ste. 316
Houston, TX 77057-7619
Phone: (713)789-6295      Free: 888-548-9716
Website: http://www.epilepsyfoundation.org/setexas

## Vermont

**★ 14782 ★ Epilepsy Foundation of Vermont**
PO Box 6292
Rutland, VT 05702-6292
Phone: (802)775-1686

## Virginia

**★ 14783 ★ Epilepsy Foundation of Virginia**
UVA Health Services Ctr.
Charlottesville, VA 22908-0001
Phone: (434)924-8669
Website: http://www.efva.org/

## Washington

**★ 14784 ★ Epilepsy Foundation Washington**
3800 Aurora Ave. N, No. 370
Seattle, WA 98103-8721
Phone: (206)547-4551      Free: 800-752-3509
Website: http://www.epilepsyfoundation.org/washington

## Wisconsin

**★ 14785 ★ Epilepsy Foundation of Central and Northeast Wisconsin**
1004 1st St., Ste. 5
Stevens Point, WI 54481-2627
Phone: (715)341-5811      Free: 800-924-9932

**★ 14786 ★ Epilepsy Foundation South Central Wisconsin**
7617 Mineral Point Rd.
Madison, WI 53717-1623
Phone: (608)833-8888      Free: 800-657-4929
Website: http://www.epilepsyfoundation.org/socentralwisc

**★ 14787 ★ Epilepsy Foundation of Southeast Wisconsin**
735 N Water St., Ste. 701
Milwaukee, WI 53202-4104
Phone: (414)271-0110
Website: http://www.epilepsyfoundationsewi.org

**★ 14788 ★ Epilepsy Foundation of Southern Wisconsin, Inc.**
205 N Main St., Ste. 106
Janesville, WI 53545-3062
Phone: (608)755-1821      Free: 800-693-2287
Website: http://www.epilepsyfoundation.org/southwisc

**★ 14789 ★ Epilepsy Foundation of Western Wisconsin**
1812 Brackett Ave., Ste. 5
Eau Claire, WI 54701-4677
Phone: (715)834-4455      Free: 800-924-2105
Website: http://www.epilepsyfoundation.org/westernwisc

## Multiple Sclerosis

*State chapters of the Multiple Sclerosis Association of America are listed below. The national office is located at 706 Haddonfield Rd., Cherry Hill, NJ 08002. Additional information can be obtained by calling the* national office at (800) LEARN-MS, or by consulting their web site at http://www.msaa.com/.

## Arkansas

★ 14790 ★ **Multiple Sclerosis Association of America**
**Mid-South Regional Office**
107 Avonshire Terrace, Diamonhead
Hot Springs, AR 71913
**Phone:** (501)262-9380    **Free:** 877-MS-SOUTH
**Fax:** (501)262-9381
**Email:** midsouth@msaa.com
**Website:** http://www.msaa.com/regionms.htm
Adam Roberts, Director
Judith Harper-Bennie, Client Services Coordinator

## Montana

★ 14791 ★ **Multiple Sclerosis Association of America**
**NorthwWestern Regional Office**
600 Central Ave., Ste. 13
Great Falls, MT 59401
**Phone:** (406)454-2758    **Free:** 800-565-6722
**Fax:** (406)454-2767
**Email:** northwest@msaa.com
**Website:** http://www.msaa.com
Sue Pencoske, Director

## New Jersey

★ 14792 ★ **Multiple Sclerosis Association of America**
**Northeastern Regional Office**
706 Haddonfield Rd.
Cherry Hill, NJ 08002
**Phone:** (856)488-4500    **Free:** 800-532-7667
**Fax:** (856)488-8257
**Email:** sfreund@msaa.com
**Website:** http://www.msaa.com
Susan Freund, Director

## Ohio

★ 14793 ★ **Multiple Sclerosis Association of America**
**Mid-Western Regional Office**
1873 E Aurora Rd.
Twinsburg, OH 44087
**Phone:** (330)405-9055    **Free:** 800-589-7962
**Fax:** (330)405-9052
**Email:** midwest@msaa.com
**Website:** http://www.msaa.com/regionmw.htm
Renee Williams, Director

## Myasthenia Gravis

*State chapters of the Myasthenia Foundation are listed below. The national office is located at 5841 Cedar Lake Rd., Ste. 204, Minneapolis, MN 55416. Additional information can be obtained by calling the national office at (800) 541-5454, or by consulting their web site at http://www.myasthenia.org/.*

## Alabama

★ 14794 ★ **Myasthenia Gravis Foundation of America**
**Alabama Chapter**
200 Office Park Cir., Ste. 312
Birmingham, AL 35223
**Phone:** (205)868-1210    **Free:** (866)749-0844
**Email:** alchaptermgfa@aol.com

## Arizona

★ 14795 ★ **Myasthenia Gravis Foundation of America**
**Jim L. Walker, Arizona Chapter**
935 E Main St., Ste. 206
Mesa, AZ 85203
**Phone:** (480)464-9648    **Fax:** (480)464-9754
**Email:** azmgfa@cox.net
**Website:** http://www.geocities.com/azmgfa
Trevor Lloyd, Chairman of the Board

## Arkansas

★ 14796 ★ **Myasthenia Gravis Foundation of America**
**Arkansas Chapter**
PO Box 388
Mabelvale, AR 72103
**Phone:** (501)455-4448    **Fax:** (501)455-4055
**Email:** bktuck50@aol.com

## Connecticut

★ 14797 ★ **Myasthenia Gravis Foundation of America**
**Connecticut "Nutmeg" State Chapter**
7 Dobson Dr.
East Hartford, CT 06118
**Phone:** (860)568-0657    **Free:** (866)329-8784
**Email:** RSpeaotMG@cs.com
**Website:** http://pages.cthome.net/ctnutmeg
**Remarks:** Serves Connecticut, Maine, Rhode Island, and Vermont.

## Florida

★ 14798 ★ **Myasthenia Gravis Foundation of America**
**East Central Florida Chapter**
PO Box 623
Ormond Beach, FL 32175-0623
**Phone:** (386)672-2635    **Free:** 888-291-5067
**Email:** jimburkemgfa@cfl.rr.com
**Website:** http://www.myasthenia.org/chapters/E_Florida/

★ 14799 ★ **Myasthenia Gravis Foundation of America**
**South Florida Gold Coast Chapter**
2077 NE 21st Terr.
Jensen Beach, FL 34957
**Phone:** (727)334-9579
**Email:** lou_cor@bellsouth.net

★ 14800 ★ **Myasthenia Gravis Foundation of America**
**West Central Florida Chapter**
13540 Andova Dr.
Largo, FL 33774
**Phone:** (727)596-1491
**Email:** mpetersfl@aol.com

## Georgia

★ 14801 ★ **Myasthenia Gravis Foundation of America**
**Georgia State Chapter**
PO Box 93604
Atlanta, GA 30318
**Phone:** (770)973-3269    **Free:** 800-743-4339
**Fax:** (770)319-3848
**Email:** gachapter_mgfa@hotmail.com
**Website:** http://members.tripod.com/~gcmgfa/
**Remarks:** Serves Georgia, Louisiana, Mississippi, and Tennessee.

## Illinois

★ 14802 ★ **Myasthenia Gravis Foundation of America**
**Illinois Chapter**
2411 New St.
Blue Island, IL 60406
**Phone:** (708)385-3888    **Fax:** (708)385-0447
**Email:** myasthenialLL@aol.com
**Website:** http://www.myastheniagravis.org

## Indiana

★ 14803 ★ **Myasthenia Gravis Foundation of America**
**Greater Indianapolis Chapter**
8922 Haverstick Rd.
Indianapolis, IN 46240
**Phone:** (317)846-1462
**Email:** spynke@aol.com

## Kentucky

★ 14804 ★ **Myasthenia Gravis Foundation of America**
**Kentucky Chapter**
8510 Eastland Dr.
Spottsville, KY 42458
**Phone:** (270)826-1312
**Email:** heatherhagan@hotmail.com

## Maryland

★ 14805 ★ **Myasthenia Gravis Foundation of America**
**Maryland/DC/Delaware Chapter**
PO Box 186
Pasadena, MD 21123-0186
**Phone:** (410)437-2881    **Free:** 800-803-5775
**Email:** maryland@myasthenia.org
**Website:** http://www.myasthenia.org/chapters/maryland

## Massachusetts

★ 14806 ★ **Myasthenia Gravis Foundation of America**
**Massachusetts/New Hampshire Chapter**
PO Box 192
Shelburne Falls, MA 01370
**Phone:** (508)435-3808
**Email:** sba-mb@mindspring.com

## Michigan

★ 14807 ★ **Myasthenia Gravis Foundation of America**
**Detroit Chapter**
17117 W 9 Mile Rd., Ste. 1745
Southfield, MI 48075
**Phone:** (248)423-9700    **Free:** 800-227-1763
**Fax:** (248)423-9705
**Email:** mgadetroit@mich.com
**Website:** http://www.mgadetroit.org

★ 14808 ★ **Myasthenia Gravis Foundation of America**
**Great Lakes Chapter**
2680 Horizon Dr. SE, Ste. C-9
Grand Rapids, MI 49546-7500
**Phone:** (616)956-0622    **Fax:** (616)956-9234
**Email:** office@greatlakesmgf.org
**Website:** http://www.greatlakesmgf.org

## Minnesota

**★ 14809 ★ Myasthenia Gravis Foundation of America**
**Minnesota Chapter**
1001 S Lake Ave.
Duluth, MN 55802
**Phone:** (218)727-6064
**Email:** mgfamn@aol.com
**Remarks:** Serves Minnesota, Nebraska, North Dakota, and South Dakota.

## Missouri

**★ 14810 ★ Myasthenia Gravis Foundation of America**
**Greater Saint Louis Chapter**
7514 Forrest View Dr.
Saint Louis, MO 63121
**Phone:** (314)382-7490
**Email:** MGFAStl@aol.com
**Website:** http://www.myathenia.org/chapters/St_Louis

## New Jersey

**★ 14811 ★ Myasthenia Gravis Foundation of America**
**Garden State Chapter**
PO Box 4258
Wayne, NJ 07474
**Phone:** (973)628-6034　　　**Free:** 800-437-4949
**Fax:** (973)628-6035
**Email:** khaughey@mgnj.org
**Website:** http://www.mgnj.org

## New Mexico

**★ 14812 ★ Myasthenia Gravis Foundation of America**
**New Mexico Chapter**
PO Box 26873
Albuquerque, NM 87125
**Phone:** (505)897-0932
**Email:** myasgrav@cybermesa.com
**Website:** http://www.myasthenia.org/chapters/New_Mexico
**Remarks:** Also serves Colorado.

## New York

**★ 14813 ★ Myasthenia Gravis Foundation of America**
**Metro New York Chapter**
116 Goldie Ave.
North Bellmore, NY 11710
**Phone:** (631)409-8420　　　**Free:** 800-667-9807
**Email:** metronymgfa@yahoo.com
**Website:** http://mgfametrony.homestead.com/nymgmgfa.html

## North Carolina

**★ 14814 ★ Myasthenia Gravis Foundation of America**
**Carolinas Chapter**
506 E Forest Hills Blvd.
Durham, NC 27707
**Phone:** (919)490-2937　　　**Free:** 800-842-8711
**Fax:** (919)489-7564
**Email:** carolinasmgfa@nc.rr.com
**Remarks:** Serves North Carolina and South Carolina.

## Ohio

**★ 14815 ★ Myasthenia Gravis Foundation of America**
**Mahoning-Shenango Valley Chapter**
PO Box 282
Girard, OH 44420

**Phone:** (330)539-7582　　　**Fax:** (330)539-7582

**★ 14816 ★ Myasthenia Gravis Foundation of America**
**Ohio Chapter**
2907 Lincoln Way E, Unit B
Massillon, OH 44646
**Phone:** (330)834-9066
**Email:** ohiochaptermgf@nci2000.net
**Website:** http://ohiochaptermgf.org

## Oklahoma

**★ 14817 ★ Myasthenia Gravis Foundation of America**
**Oklahoma Chapter**
6465 S Yale Ave., Ste. 623
Tulsa, OK 74136-7811
**Phone:** (918)494-4951
**Email:** okmgf@valornet.com
**Website:** http://www.myasthenia.org/chapters/oklahoma
Peggy Foust, Exec Director

## Pennsylvania

**★ 14818 ★ Myasthenia Gravis Foundation of America**
**Pennsylvania Chapter**
2665 Pinewood Rd.
Lancaster, PA 17601
**Phone:** (866)7PA-MGFA
**Email:** pennamgfa@aol.com

## Texas

**★ 14819 ★ Myasthenia Gravis Foundation of America**
**Greater Dallas/Fort Worth Chapter**
2022 Sage Valley Dr.
Richardson, TX 75080
**Phone:** (972)690-1302　　　**Fax:** (972)699-8698
**Email:** dfwmgf@hotmail.com

**★ 14820 ★ Myasthenia Gravis Foundation of America**
**Greater South Texas Chapter**
10592-A Fuqua St., Ste. 313
Houston, TX 77089-1402
**Phone:** (281)987-9393　　　**Fax:** (281)328-2430
**Email:** gowens@accesscomm.net

**★ 14821 ★ Myasthenia Gravis Foundation of America**
**Northwest Texas Chapter**
281 County Rd. 135
Ovalo, TX 79541
**Phone:** (915)554-7038　　　**Fax:** (915)554-7044
**Email:** nwtc@camalott.com

## Utah

**★ 14822 ★ Myasthenia Gravis Foundation of America**
**Utah State Intermountain Chapter**
8717 South 910 East
Sandy, UT 84094
**Phone:** (801)816-2204

## Virginia

**★ 14823 ★ Myasthenia Gravis Foundation of America**
**Virginia Chapter**
2304 Angus
Charlottesville, VA 22901
**Phone:** (434)295-9861　　　**Free:** 800-728-4405
**Fax:** (434)295-1909
**Email:** pma8n@cstone.net

**Website:** http://www.geocities.com/HotSprings/Spa/9948/
**Remarks:** Serves Virginia and West Virginia.

## Washington

**★ 14824 ★ Myasthenia Gravis Foundation of America**
**Pacific Northwest Chapter**
18115 116th Ave. SE
Renton, WA 98058-6562
**Phone:** (425)235-1435　　　**Free:** 877-252-0677
**Fax:** (425)204-2070
**Email:** nwmg@cs.com
**Remarks:** Serves Alaska, Hawaii, Idaho, Montana, Nevada, Oregon, Washington, and Wyoming.

## Wisconsin

**★ 14825 ★ Myasthenia Gravis Foundation of America**
**Wisconsin Chapter**
6644 W Revere Pl.
West Allis, WI 53219
**Phone:** (262)938-9800
**Email:** wiscmg@yahoo.com

## Neurofibromatosis

*State chapters of the National Neurofibromatosis Foundation are listed below. The national office is located at 95 Pine St., 16th Fl., New York, NY 10005. Additional information can be obtained by calling the national office at (800) 323-7938, or by consulting their web site at http://neurofibromatosis.org/.*

## California

**★ 14826 ★ National Neurofibromatosis Foundation**
**California Chapter**
2365 Westwood Blvd., Ste. 21
Los Angeles, CA 90064
**Phone:** (310)470-3888　　　**Free:** 888-314-6633
**Fax:** (310)441-1601
**Email:** NFCAL@aol.com
**Website:** http://www.neurofibromatosis.org/california
Stuart J. Rogoff, Vice President

## Colorado

**★ 14827 ★ National Neurofibromatosis Foundation**
**Colorado Chapter**
11776 Glencoe St.
Thornton, CO 80233
**Phone:** (303)460-8313
**Email:** bkhnn1@aol.com
**Website:** http://www.neurofibromatosis.org/colorado
Kent Draper, President

## Florida

**★ 14828 ★ National Neurofibromatosis Foundation**
**Florida Chapter**
735 36th Ave. N
Saint Petersburg, FL 33704
**Free:** 800-540-5721
**Email:** ssuzearle@aol.com
**Website:** http://www.neurofibromatosis.org/florida
Suzanne Earle, President

## Georgia

**★ 14829 ★ National Neurofibromatosis Foundation**
**Georgia Chapter**
PO Box 1948
Hiram, GA 30141-1742
**Phone:** (770)445-4224

**Email:** ChikNMama1@aol.com
Rhonda Bridges, President

## Illinois

★ 14830 ★ **National Neurofibromatosis
Foundation**
**Illinois Chapter**
3224 Heather Glen Dr.
Aurora, IL 60504
**Phone:** (630)236-7356        **Free:** 800-500-6633
**Email:** donwojonf@aol.com
**Website:** http://www.neurofibromatosis.org/illinois
Don Wojtnyek, President

## Iowa

★ 14831 ★ **National Neurofibromatosis
Foundation**
**Iowa Chapter**
321 Glenview Dr.
Des Moines, IA 50312
**Phone:** (515)277-8494
**Email:** Drev@aol.com
**Website:** http://www.neurofibromatosis.org/iowa
Sheila Drevyanko, President

## Louisiana

★ 14832 ★ **National Neurofibromatosis
Foundation**
**Louisiana Chapter**
PO Box 499
Baton Rouge, LA 70821
**Phone:** (225)665-3547
**Email:** nflouisiana1@cox.net
**Website:** http://www.neurofibromatosis.org/louisiana
Debbie Bouy, President

## Maryland

★ 14833 ★ **National Neurofibromatosis
Foundation**
**Mid-Atlantic Region Chapter**
3357 Garrison Cir.
Abingdon, MD 21009
**Phone:** (410)887-5576
**Email:** NNFF@nf.org
**Website:** http://www.nf.org
Mike Daughaday, President

## Massachusetts

★ 14834 ★ **National Neurofibromatosis
Foundation**
**Massachusetts Chapter**
31 Springhill Ave.
Marlborough, MA 01752
**Phone:** (508)624-4533        **Free:** 888-585-5316
**Fax:** (508)624-7553
**Email:** nfma2000@aol.com
**Website:** http://www.neurofibromatosis.org/massa-chusetts
Matthew LaBarre, Vice President

## Michigan

★ 14835 ★ **National Neurofibromatosis
Foundation**
**Michigan Chapter**
6069 Brynthrop
Shelby Township, MI 48316
**Phone:** (810)731-7811
**Email:** hawkeyenf@aol.com
**Website:** http://www.neurofibromatosis.org/michigan
Peter Dingeman, President

## Missouri

★ 14836 ★ **National Neurofibromatosis
Foundation**
**Missouri Chapter**
1015 Locust St., Ste. 1032
Saint Louis, MO 63101
**Phone:** (314)436-6877        **Free:** 888-848-NNFF
**Fax:** (314)436-0524
**Email:** NFMissouri@aol.com
**Website:** http://www.neurofibromatosis.org/missouri
Rebecca Sastry, Exec Director

## Nebraska

★ 14837 ★ **National Neurofibromatosis
Foundation**
**Northern Plains Chapter**
PO Box 540843
Omaha, NE 68154-0843
**Phone:** (402)362-7279        **Free:** 877-449-7979
**Email:** NFNebraska@hotmail.com
Amy Hayes, President
**Remarks:** Serves Nebraska, North Dakota, and South Dakota.

## New York

★ 14838 ★ **National Neurofibromatosis
Foundation**
**New York/New Jersey Chapter**
95 Pine St., 16th Fl.
New York, NY 10005
**Phone:** (212)344-NNFF        **Fax:** (212)747-0004
**Website:** http://www.neurofibromatosis.org/ny_nj
Pamela Linton, Exec Director

## Oregon

★ 14839 ★ **National Neurofibromatosis
Foundation**
**Oregon Chapter**
**Patient Information and Support**
1717 SW Park Ave., Apt. 1108
Portland, OR 97201
**Phone:** (503)412-6599
**Email:** walktours1@aol.com
**Website:** http://www.neurofibromatosis.org/oregon
Terri Wardell, Contact

## South Carolina

★ 14840 ★ **National Neurofibromatosis
Foundation**
**South Carolina Chapter**
PO Box 358
Cordova, SC 29039
**Phone:** (803)534-0962
**Email:** rudestu@bellsouth.net
Stu Wright, President

## Tennessee

★ 14841 ★ **National Neurofibromatosis
Foundation**
**Tennessee Chapter**
9025 Old Smyrna Rd.
Brentwood, TN 37027
**Phone:** (615)252-2360
**Email:** gbulso@bccb.com
Gino Bulso, President

## Utah

★ 14842 ★ **National Neurofibromatosis
Foundation**
**Utah Chapter**
1746 South 300 East
Kaysville, UT 84037
**Phone:** (801)451-0383        **Fax:** (801)968-0981

**Email:** bloomerjc@earthlink.net
Cherilyn Bloomer, President

## Washington

★ 14843 ★ **National Neurofibromatosis
Foundation**
**Washington State Chapter**
6628 212th St. SW, Ste. 100
Lynnwood, WA 98036
**Phone:** (425)672-9610        **Fax:** (425)672-9518
**Email:** NF@nnffwa.org
**Website:** http://www.neurofibromatosis.org/washington
Susan Blalock, Exec Director

## Wisconsin

★ 14844 ★ **National Neurofibromatosis
Foundation**
**Wisconsin Chapter**
Milwaukee, WI
**Phone:** (414)438-0985
**Email:** Epankownf@aol.com
Elaine Pankow, President

## Wyoming

★ 14845 ★ **National Neurofibromatosis
Foundation**
**Wyoming Chapter**
2434 Coulter Dr.
Casper, WY 82604
**Phone:** (307)473-7723
**Email:** n13good@aol.com
Norma Good, Contact

## Parkinson's Disease

*State chapters of the American Parkinson Disease Association are listed below. The national office is located at 1250 Hylan Blvd., Ste. 4B, Staten Island, NY 10305-1946. Additional information can be obtained by calling the national office at (800) 223-2732, or by consulting their web site at http://apdaparkinson.com/.*

## Alabama

★ 14846 ★ **American Parkinson Disease
Association**
**Birmingham Chapter**
800 Jeffery Ln.
Birmingham, AL 35235
**Phone:** (205)833-4940
**Email:** Parkinson@pell.net
Paul E. Hayes, President

★ 14847 ★ **American Parkinson Disease
Association**
**North Alabama Chapter**
1910 Crapemyrtle Green SE
Huntsville, AL 35802
**Phone:** (256)883-2835
Jean Smith, President

★ 14848 ★ **American Parkinson Disease
Association**
**Tuscaloosa Chapter**
1515 19th Ave. E, Apt. 813
Tuscaloosa, AL 35404
**Phone:** (205)556-5327
Verna Patterson, President

## Arizona

**★ 14849 ★ American Parkinson Disease Association**
**Arizona Chapter**
616 N Country Club Rd., Ste. C
Tucson, AZ 85716
**Phone:** (520)326-5400     **Free:** 800-541-4960
**Email:** holmes@u.arizona.edu
Bob Dolezal, President

## Arkansas

**★ 14850 ★ American Parkinson Disease Association**
**Arkansas Chapter**
200 Scottwood
Hot Springs, AR 71901
**Phone:** (501)321-1539
**Email:** urmilgupta@aol.com
Urmil Gupta, President

## California

**★ 14851 ★ American Parkinson Disease Association**
**Greater Los Angeles Chapter**
c/o First Charter Bank
9454 Wilshire Blvd.
Beverly Hills, CA 90212
**Phone:** (310)248-2109
**Email:** sblock@firstcharterbank.com
Steve Block, President

**★ 14852 ★ American Parkinson Disease Association**
**San Diego Chapter**
8555 Aero Dr., Ste. 205
San Diego, CA 92123-1745
**Phone:** (858)273-6763
**Email:** info@sd-pc.com
**Website:** http://www.sd-pc.com
William M. Stilwell, President

## Connecticut

**★ 14853 ★ American Parkinson Disease Association**
**Connecticut Chapter**
27 Allendale Dr.
North Haven, CT 06473
**Phone:** (203)288-0546
**Email:** gladkt@hotmail.com
**Website:** http://www.ctapda.com
Gladys Tiedemann, President

## Florida

**★ 14854 ★ American Parkinson Disease Association**
**South Florida Chapter**
10100 NW 2nd St.
Coral Springs, FL 33071
**Phone:** (954)786-2305
David Levy, President

**★ 14855 ★ American Parkinson Disease Association**
**Sun Coast Parkinson Chapter**
9937 87th St.
Largo, FL 33777
**Phone:** (727)391-8214
**Email:** vgbw@aol.com
Ginny Bernard, President

## Georgia

**★ 14856 ★ American Parkinson Disease Association**
**Atlanta Chapter**
PO Box 49416
Atlanta, GA 30359
**Phone:** (770)979-3495
**Email:** bergatlapda@juno.com
Barbara Berger, RN, Contact

## Idaho

**★ 14857 ★ American Parkinson Disease Association**
**Middle Snake Idaho Chapter**
5567 Willowlawn Way
Boise, ID 83714
**Phone:** (208)376-4401
**Email:** dojem@rmci.net
Don Mills, President

## Illinois

**★ 14858 ★ American Parkinson Disease Association**
**Midwest Chapter**
2050 Pfingsten Rd., Ste. 127
Glenview, IL 60025
**Phone:** (847)724-7087
**Email:** cacapda@aol.com
Maxine Dust, President

## Louisiana

**★ 14859 ★ American Parkinson Disease Association**
**Bayou Chapter**
PO Box 405
Thibodaux, LA 70302
**Phone:** (504)447-9043
**Email:** RWarch@mobiletel.com
Richard G. Weimer, President

## Maine

**★ 14860 ★ American Parkinson Disease Association**
**Maine State Chapter**
107 Woodville Rd.
Falmouth, ME 04105
**Phone:** (207)781-3070
**Email:** cnbarker@maine.rr.com
Carl Barker, President

## Maryland

**★ 14861 ★ American Parkinson Disease Association**
**Anne Arundel County Chapter**
PO Box 893
Severna Park, MD 21146
**Phone:** (410)729-3461
Tom Mislan, President

**★ 14862 ★ American Parkinson Disease Association**
**Central Maryland Parkinson Outreach Chapter**
PO Box 3153
Frederick, MD 21705
**Phone:** (301)682-9009
**Email:** bruff1terp@aol.com
Bill Ruff, President

**★ 14863 ★ American Parkinson Disease Association**
**Delmarva Parkinson's Chapter/Support Group**
4049 Oakland School Rd. at Trace Hollow Run
Salisbury, MD 21801
**Phone:** (410)543-0110
**Email:** johnston@intercom.net
Will Johnston, President

**★ 14864 ★ American Parkinson Disease Association**
**Howard County Chapter**
5625 Waterloo Rd.
Ellicott City, MD 21043
**Phone:** (410)465-2825     **Fax:** (410)465-2825
**Email:** pdmd@starpower.net
**Website:** http://www.apdaparkinson.com/howard_county.htm
Thomas Collins, President

**★ 14865 ★ American Parkinson Disease Association**
**Western Maryland Chapter**
13555 Donnybrook Dr.
Hagerstown, MD 21742
**Phone:** (301)790-2044
**Email:** nittanylion57@prodigy.net
Don and Pat Zilch, President
Peggy Barron, President

**★ 14866 ★ American Parkinson Disease Association**
**Young Parkinson's Chapter of Maryland**
601 N Caroline St., Ste. 5065
Baltimore, MD 21287-0875
**Phone:** (410)955-8795
**Email:** tcsc56@cs.com
Sandy Pollock, President

## Massachusetts

**★ 14867 ★ American Parkinson Disease Association**
**Massachusetts Chapter**
203 Brimbal Ave.
Beverly, MA 01915
**Phone:** (978)922-1473
**Email:** apdafay@aol.com
**Website:** http://www.apdama.org
Fay Winson, President

## Missouri

**★ 14868 ★ American Parkinson Disease Association**
**Greater Saint Louis Chapter**
660 S Euclid Ave.
Campus Box 8111
Saint Louis, MO 63110
**Phone:** (314)362-3299
**Email:** levins@neuro.wustl.edu
**Website:** http://www.geocities.com/parkinson_disease_saint_louis/
Joseph Marchbein, CPA, President

## Montana

**★ 14869 ★ American Parkinson Disease Association**
**Great Falls Chapter**
2101 6th Ave. S
Great Falls, MT 59405
**Phone:** (406)761-6086
Ethel Stump, Contact

★ 14870 ★ **American Parkinson Disease Association**
**Missoula Branch Chapter**
2415 57th St.
Missoula, MT 59803
**Phone:** (406)251-5338
**Email:** mtcookies@msn.com
Carole Kamrath, President

## Nebraska

★ 14871 ★ **American Parkinson Disease Association**
**Nebraska Chapter**
7701 Pacific St., Ste. 122
Omaha, NE 68114-5480
**Phone:** (402)397-2766
Sandy Woods-Kreifels, President

## Nevada

★ 14872 ★ **American Parkinson Disease Association**
**Southern Nevada Chapter**
c/o University of Nevada School of Medicine
1707 W Charleston Blvd., Ste. 220
1001 Shadow Ln.
Las Vegas, NV 89102-2353
**Phone:** (702)464-3132
Julia Bernick, President

## New Hampshire

★ 14873 ★ **American Parkinson Disease Association**
**Granite State Chapter**
61 Dublin Ave.
Nashua, NH 03063-2045
**Phone:** (603)889-3251
**Email:** gmchugh@ma.ultranet.com
George McHugh, President

## New Jersey

★ 14874 ★ **American Parkinson Disease Association**
**New Jersey Chapter**
601 Hillside Ave.
Point Pleasant, NJ 08742
**Phone:** (732)714-0475
**Email:** hwl351@aol.com
Jack McMillian, Contact

## New Mexico

★ 14875 ★ **American Parkinson Disease Association**
**El Paso Chapter**
112 Lisa
Box 107
Chaparral, NM 88021
**Phone:** (505)824-4306
**Email:** timotea@angelfire.com
Thomas Arellanes, President

★ 14876 ★ **American Parkinson Disease Association**
**New Mexico Chapter**
10817 Griffith Park NE
Albuquerque, NM 87123
**Phone:** (505)292-3844   **Free:** 800-278-5386
**Email:** tasec@cs.com
Bobby Dunagan, President

## New York

★ 14877 ★ **American Parkinson Disease Association**
**Faye Springer Memorial Rockaway Chapter**
33 Point Breeze Ave.
Breezy Point, NY 11697
Marion Manley, President

★ 14878 ★ **American Parkinson Disease Association**
**Nassau County Chapter**
18 Wren Dr.
Woodbury, NY 11797
**Phone:** (516)798-8375
Sebastian Moschitto, President
Jim Hall, President

★ 14879 ★ **American Parkinson Disease Association**
**New York Young Professionals Chapter**
c/o Bear Stearns
383 Madison Ave., 5th Fl.
New York, NY 10179
**Phone:** (212)272-8280
**Email:** sschefrin@bear.com
Scott Schefrin, President

★ 14880 ★ **American Parkinson Disease Association**
**Salvatore and Elena Esposito Chapter**
18 St. Julian's Pl.
Staten Island, NY 10301
**Phone:** (718)727-2713
**Email:** winshear@pronetisp.net
Sophia Maestrone, President

★ 14881 ★ **American Parkinson Disease Association**
**Southern Tier Chapter**
PO Box 72
Binghamton, NY 13903
**Phone:** (607)723-7167
Winslow Shearman, Contact

★ 14882 ★ **American Parkinson Disease Association**
**Suffolk County Chapter**
c/o St. Catherine of Sienna Hospital
50 Rte. 25A
Smithtown, NY 11787
**Phone:** (631)862-3560
**Email:** newslady@obtonline.net
**Website:** http://www.suffolkapda.org/
Virginia Cravotta, President

## North Carolina

★ 14883 ★ **American Parkinson Disease Association**
**Asheville Chapter**
C/O Robin Fox, R.N
Thomas Rehabilitation Hospital
68 Sweeton Creek Rd.
Asheville, NC 28803
**Phone:** (828)692-7623
Shirley Jankowski, Contact

## Ohio

★ 14884 ★ **American Parkinson Disease Association**
**Cincinnati Tri-State Chapter**
125 W Galbraith Rd., Ste 218
Cincinnati, OH 45216
**Phone:** (513)984-1100   **Free:** 800-840-2732
**Email:** info@parkinsonswellness.org

**Website:** http://www.parkinsonswellness.org
Debbie Mills, President

## Oklahoma

★ 14885 ★ **American Parkinson Disease Association**
**Muskogee Area Chapter**
9601 Taft Rd.
Muskogee, OK 74401
**Phone:** (918)687-4519
Roleen Bishop, President

★ 14886 ★ **American Parkinson Disease Association**
**Oklahoma PD Chapter**
19125 Park St.
Claremore, OK 74017
**Phone:** (918)341-5097
Dan Moore, President

★ 14887 ★ **American Parkinson Disease Association**
**Owasso Area Chapter**
12600 E 73rd St. N
Owasso, OK 74055
**Phone:** (918)834-2441
Donna Norris, President

★ 14888 ★ **American Parkinson Disease Association**
**Ponca City Area Chapter**
PO Box 743
Ponca City, OK 74602
Bill Hill, President

★ 14889 ★ **American Parkinson Disease Association**
**Tulsa Area Chapter**
PO Box 521165
Tulsa, OK 74152
**Phone:** (918)747-9320
**Email:** prairiec@swbell.net
Christine Kennedy, President

## Pennsylvania

★ 14890 ★ **American Parkinson Disease Association**
**Greater Delaware Valley Chapter**
c/o APDA Information & Resource Center
Crozer-Chester Medical Center
1 Medical Center Blvd.
Upland, PA 19013
**Phone:** (610)447-2911
Robert Hurka, President

★ 14891 ★ **American Parkinson Disease Association**
**J. Louis Blumberg Chapter**
6700 Eastwood St.
Philadelphia, PA 19149
**Phone:** (215)342-6689
Belle Englander, President

★ 14892 ★ **American Parkinson Disease Association**
**Pittsburgh Area Chapter**
420 E North Ave., Ste. 206
Pittsburgh, PA 15212
**Phone:** (412)441-4100
**Email:** mallen@wpahs.org
Catherine Birk, MD, President

### Rhode Island

**★ 14893 ★ American Parkinson Disease Association**
**Rhode Island Chapter**
PO Box 41659
Providence, RI 02940-1659
**Phone:** (401)823-5700    **Free:** 800-498-2732
**Email:** RIchapAPDA@aol.com
**Website:**     http://www.parkinsondisease-rhodeisland.org
Athol Cochrane, President

### Tennessee

**★ 14894 ★ American Parkinson Disease Association**
**Middle Tennessee Chapter**
c/o Information and Resource Center
2300 Patterson St.
Nashville, TN 37203
**Phone:** (615)329-9955
**Email:** asapmac@mindspring.com
**Website:**     http://www.apdaparkinson.com/tn_chapter.htm
Meredith Car, President

### Texas

**★ 14895 ★ American Parkinson Disease Association**
**Central Texas Parkinson's Chapter**
PO Box 153
Brownwood, TX 76804
**Phone:** (915)641-0020
**Email:** mamadunk@hotmail.com
Linda Duncan, President

**★ 14896 ★ American Parkinson Disease Association**
**Hill Country Kerrville Chapter**
145 Village Dr.
Kerrville, TX 78028
**Phone:** (830)895-2431
**Email:** beshaw@ktc.com
Fred Kleis, President

**★ 14897 ★ American Parkinson Disease Association**
**Northeast Texas Chapter**
1400 Preston Rd., Ste. 200
Plano, TX 75093
**Phone:** (214)345-4224
**Email:** bjwells@flash.net
Jerry Wells, Esq., President

**★ 14898 ★ American Parkinson Disease Association**
**Parkinson's Caring, Sharing & Comparing Chapter of Central Texas**
2809 Arroyo Ct. N
College Station, TX 77845
**Phone:** (979)696-6966
**Email:** b.erwin2@verizon.net
Bill Erwin, President

**★ 14899 ★ American Parkinson Disease Association**
**San Antonio Chapter/Alamo Area Parkinson's Disease Support Group**
8507 Chesam
San Antonio, TX 78250
**Email:** joanieduval@earthlink.net
Joan Duval, President

**★ 14900 ★ American Parkinson Disease Association**
**West Texas Parkinsonism Society Chapter**
5805 Duke Ave.
Lubbock, TX 79416
**Phone:** (806)793-3691
Steve Swain, President

### Utah

**★ 14901 ★ American Parkinson Disease Association**
**Northern Chapter of Utah**
c/o APDA Information & Resource Center
University of Utah School of Medicine
Department of Neurology
50 N Medical Dr., Rm. 3R144
Salt Lake City, UT 84132
**Phone:** (801)585-2354
**Email:** mmkearns@worldnett.att.net
Miriam Kearns, President

### Vermont

**★ 14902 ★ American Parkinson Disease Association**
**Vermont Chapter**
70 Hurdle Rd.
Moretown, VT 05660
**Phone:** (802)626-3707    **Free:** 888-763-3366
**Email:** advnture@sover.net
Bruce Talbot, President

### Virginia

**★ 14903 ★ American Parkinson Disease Association**
**Richmond Metro Chapter**
PO Box 70283
Richmond, VA 23255
**Phone:** (804)740-6806
**Email:** Kathy_morton@wescanric.org
Kathy Morton, President

**★ 14904 ★ American Parkinson Disease Association**
**Virginia Beach Chapter**
Our Lady of Perpetual Help
4560 Princess Anne Rd.
Virginia Beach, VA 23462
**Phone:** (757)495-3062
**Email:** tcmedlc@tc.cc.va.us
Christine Medlin, Contact

### Washington

**★ 14905 ★ American Parkinson Disease Association**
**Washington State Chapter**
PO Box 75169
Seattle, WA 98125-0169
**Phone:** (425)881-3116
**Email:** matulinde@aol.com
Maria Linde, President

### West Virginia

**★ 14906 ★ American Parkinson Disease Association**
**North Central West Virginia Chapter**
107 C'Anna Sq.
Fairmont, WV 26554
**Phone:** (304)363-1028
**Email:** tracey_robertson@att.net
Tracey Robertson, President
Larry Policano, President

### Wyoming

**★ 14907 ★ American Parkinson Disease Association**
**Bighorn Basin Parkinson Chapter**
PO Box 221
Powell, WY 82435
**Phone:** (307)754-2130
Dean Schultz, President

# Chapter 42
# Nursing

## Federal Government Agencies

**★ 14908 ★ U.S. Department of Health and Human Services (NIH)**
**National Institutes of Health (NINR)**
**National Institute of Nursing Research**
9000 Rockville Pike
Bethesda, MD 20892
**Phone:** (301)496-0207
**Website:** http://www.nih.gov.ninr/
Patricia A. Grady, Director

**Desc:** The Institute provides leadership for nursing research, supports and conducts research and training, and disseminates information to build a scientific base for nursing practice and patient care and to promote health and ameliorate the effects of illness on the American people.

## Foundations & Other Funding Organizations

### Private Foundations

**★ 14909 ★ Alletta Morris McBean Charitable Trust**
400 S El Camino Real, Ste. 777
San Mateo, CA 94402
**Phone:** (650)558-8480            **Fax:** (650)558-8481
**Email:** mcbeancharitabletrust@att.net
**Fnded:** 1986. **Philosophy:** The trustees give special attention to organizations whose charitable activities are focused on the City of Newport, Rhode Island, and Aquidneck Island, Rhode Island, and are designed to enhance the quality of life in and to perpetuate the history of the City of Newport and Aquidneck Island. **Priorities:** *Arts & Humanities:* 31%. Focuses funding on historic preservation projects. *Civic & Public Affairs:* 9%. Funds community foundations and commissions. *Education:* 8%. Supports a university. *Environment:* 6%. Supports youth organizations. *International:* 19%. Funds donor banks and nursing services. *Note:* Total contributions made in 1999. **Typ. Recipients:** Emergency/Ambulance Services, Health-General, Home-Care Services, Hospices, Hospitals, Nursing Services. **Geo. Dist:** Aquidneck Island, RI; Newport, RI.

**Caleb C. and Julia W. Dula Educational and Charitable Foundation**
*See:* Entry 11369

**★ 14910 ★ Charlotte R. Schmidlapp Fund**
MD 00864
Cincinnati, OH 45263
**Phone:** (513)579-6034            **Fax:** (513)744-6997
Dr. Lawra Baumann, Foundation Officer

**Fnded:** 1907. **Philosophy:** The primary focus of the fund is to support programs aimed at helping young women establish themselves in life. The fund has begun a program of grants for women in the study of math and science. To help increase the number of role models for young women, grants are made to female teachers of math and science. The fund also supports critically needed day care for the children of female high school and college students. Although the challenges today are different from when Mr. Schmidlapp established the fund, it continues to help women in significant ways. **Priorities:** *Arts & Humanities:* 3%. Supports museums and art associations. *Civic & Public Affairs:* 16%. Funds urban and women's centers. *Education:* 19%. Focus on women's and children's education. *Environment:* 24%. Funds child welfare and youth organizations. *International:* 38%. Hospitals and pediatric health. *Note:* Total contributions made in fiscal 1998. **Typ. Recipients:** Cancer, Children's Health/Hospitals, Nursing Services, Public Health. **Geo. Dist:** IN; KY; Cincinnati, OH.

**★ 14911 ★ Helene Fuld Health Trust**
50 E 42nd St. 19th floor
New York, NY 10017
**Phone:** (212)681-1237            **Fax:** (212)681-1335
**Email:** jpaik@fuldtrust.org
**Website:** http://www.fuldtrust.org
Jina Paik, Grants Manager

**Fnded:** 1969. **Philosophy:** The Trust concentrates its grant making in the following three areas: "Curriculum and Faculty Development in Community-based Care... Grants will be given to establish and improve nursing program curricula and clinical training experience related to community-based health care, and to support faculty to practice and be better prepared to teach in these areas." "Education Mobility... The Trust will promote educational mobility by making grants for targeted financial aid to students pursuing higher degrees in nursing. Grants will also support activities which will improve the facilitation and articulation among the different levels of nursing programs." "Leadership Development... The Trust will continue to sponsor the Fuld Fellowship Program for associate degree and baccalaureate nursing students, with some modifications, in order to recognize outstanding students and promote their leadership development. Also, the Trust will solicit creative, meaningful 'leadership-oriented' proposals for grants from nonprofit nursing-related organizations." **Priorities:** *Education:* 100%. Primarily supports colleges and universities for nursing education. *Note:* Contributions made in fiscal 2000. **Typ. Recipients:** Children's Health/Hospitals, Clinics/Medical Centers, Health Organizations, Health-General, Hospitals, Medical Education, Medical Research, Nursing Services. **Geo. Dist:** nationally.

**James M. Johnston Trust for Charitable and Educational Purposes**
*See:* Entry 400

**Kohler Foundation**
*See:* Entry 18212

**★ 14912 ★ Lettie Pate Evans Foundation**
50 Hurt Plaza, Ste. 1200
Atlanta, GA 30303
**Phone:** (404)522-6755            **Fax:** (404)522-7026
**Email:** fdns@woodruff.org
**Website:** http://www.lpevans.org
Charles McTier, President

**Fnded:** 1945. **Philosophy:** The foundation's primary interests are education and the arts. **Priorities:** *Arts & Humanities:* 10%. Cultural organizations, historical preservation, museums, and performing arts. *Civic & Public Affairs:* 14%. Community foundation. *Education:* 29%. Colleges and universities and religion education. *Environment:* 5%. Human Services. *International:* 38%. Children's health care. *Note:* Total contributions made in 1999. **Typ. Recipients:** Cancer, Health Organizations, Hospitals, Nursing Services, Public Health. **Geo. Dist:** GA, emphasis on Atlanta; VA.

**The Louis and Rachel Rudin Foundation, Inc.**
*See:* Entry 481

**Marshall L. and Perrine D. McCune Charitable Foundation**
*See:* Entry 5558

**Mary J. Hutchins Foundation**
*See:* Entry 11407

**Mericos Foundation**
*See:* Entry 541

**★ 14913 ★ Nicholas H. Noyes, Jr. Memorial Foundation**
1950 E Greyhound Pass, Ste. 18-356
Carmel, IN 46033-7730
**Phone:** (317)844-8009            **Fax:** (317)844-8099
**Email:** admin@noyesfoundation.org
**Website:** http://www.noyesfoundation.org
Nany Ayres, President

**Fnded:** 1951. **Philosophy:** The foundation distributes its giving to a variety of interests. Educational funding favors secondary schools and private academies. Social service recipients include united funds, housing, work centers, and day care. Most of the support for the arts is centered on the performing arts in Indianapolis. Health care favors nursing and hospitals. Other interests include zoos, conservation, and religion. **Priorities:** *Arts & Humanities:* 20%. Funds museums, music, and art centers. *Civic & Public Affairs:* 3%. Includes zoos and economic development. *Education:* 37%. Funds colleges, universities, precollege education, and education funds. *Environment:* 28%. Supports youth groups, united funds, and family services. *International:* 7%. Contributes to hospitals and medical centers. *Note:* Total contributions made in 1999. **Typ. Recipients:** Cancer, Children's Health/Hospitals, Clinics/Medical Centers, Diabetes, Emergency/Ambulance Services, Family Planning,

Hospitals, Medical Rehabilitation, Medical Research, Nursing Services, People with Disabilities, Single-Disease Health Associations, Substance Abuse. **Geo. Dist:** Indianapolis, IN.

## Corporate Foundations

**Bank of New York Co., Inc.**
*See:* Entry 868

### ★ 14914 ★ Bausch & Lomb Foundation, Inc.
One Bausch & Lomb Place
Rochester, NY 14604-2701
**Phone:** (716)338-6000        **Fax:** (716)338-6007
Barbara Kelley, Vice President
**Priorities:** *Arts & Humanities:* 11%. Supports historical sites. *Civic & Public Affairs:* 55%. Funds a zoological society and the UNCGR Foundation. *Education:* 12%. Supports higher education institutions and a children's center. *Environment:* (Health and Social Welfare) 22%. Under this program area, the foundation funds a career development center, a park, and a veterans outreach program. *Note:* Total contributions made in 2000. **Typ. Recipients:** Clinics/Medical Centers, Geriatric Health, Nursing Services, People with Disabilities. **Geo. Dist:** Rochester, NY.

**BD**
*See:* Entry 879

**Briggs & Stratton Corp. Foundation**
*See:* Entry 903

**Fabri-Kal Foundation**
*See:* Entry 1037

**Guardian Life Insurance Co. of America**
*See:* Entry 1103

**Gulfstream Aerospace Corp.**
*See:* Entry 5473

**Northern Indiana Public Service Co.**
*See:* Entry 1276

**Teleflex Foundation**
*See:* Entry 1427

**UPS Foundation**
*See:* Entry 1466

## Other Funding Organizations

### ★ 14915 ★ Alpha Tau Delta (ATD)
150 Cruickshank Dr.
Folsom, CA 95630
**Phone:** (916)984-9150
**Email:** kerrik@atdnursing.org
**Website:** http://www.atdnursing.org
Kerri L. Kaye, Pres.
**Desc:** Professional fraternity - nursing. Seeks to further educational standards for the nursing profession. Maintains scholarship program for members only. **Awards:** Miriam Furlong Grant (annual) for member students; National Advisor of the Year (annual); National Member of Year (annual); PRN Grant (annual) for alummni members.

**American Holistic Nurses Association (AHNA)**
*See:* Entry 3328

### ★ 14916 ★ American Nurses' Foundation (ANF)
600 Maryland Ave. SW, Ste. 100W
Washington, DC 20024-2571
**Phone:** (202)651-7227        **Fax:** (202)651-7354
**Email:** anf@ana.org
**Website:** http://www.nursingworld.org/anf
Leo Schargorodski, Dir.
**Desc:** Research, education, and charitable arm of the American Nurses' Association. Promotes nursing and consumers wherever nurses practice. Mission accomplished through four major functions: fundraising, Nursing Research Grants, grant development and management, and American Nurses Publishing. **Awards:** Distinguished Contribution to Nursing Science Award (semiannual); grant for nurse researchers.

### ★ 14917 ★ American Organization of Nurse Executives (AONE)
325 Seventh St. NW
Washington, DC 20004
**Phone:** (202)626-2240        **Fax:** (202)638-5499
**Email:** aone@aha.org
**Website:** http://www.aone.org
Pamela Thompson, RN, Exec. Dir.
**Desc:** Provides leadership, professional development, advocacy, and research to advance nursing practice and patient care, promote nursing leadership and excellence, and shape healthcare public policy. Supports and enhances the management, leadership, educational, and professional development of nursing leaders. Offers placement service through Career Development and Referral Center. **Awards:** Research Award (annual); scholarship.

### ★ 14918 ★ American Radiological Nurses Association (ARNA)
820 Jorie Blvd.
Oak Brook, IL 60523
**Phone:** (630)571-9072        **Fax:** (630)571-7837
**Email:** arna@rsna.org
**Website:** http://www.arna.net
Betty Rohr, Account Executive
**Desc:** Radiological nurses. Seeks to provide, promote, and maintain continuity of quality patient care through education, standards of care, professional growth, and collaboration with other health care providers. **Awards:** Dorothy Budnek Scholarship (annual).

### ★ 14919 ★ American Society of Plastic Surgical Nurses (ASPSN)
E Holly Ave.
Box 56
Pitman, NJ 08071
**Phone:** (856)256-2340        **Fax:** (856)589-7463
**Email:** asprsn@ajj.com
Rick Grimes, Exec. Dir.
**Desc:** Registered nurses, licensed practical nurses, and licensed vocational nurses working with plastic surgeons or interested in plastic and reconstructive nursing. Objectives are: to enhance leadership qualities of nurses in the field of plastic surgery; to increase the skills, knowledge, and understanding of personnel in plastic surgery nursing through continuing education; to study existing practices and new developments in the field; to encourage participation and interest in professional organizations; to cooperate with others in the profession. **Awards:** Grant (annual).

### ★ 14920 ★ Association of Rehabilitation Nurses (ARN)
4700 W Lake Ave.
Glenview, IL 60025-1485
**Phone:** (847)375-4710        **Free:** 800-229-7530
**Fax:** 877-734-9384
**Email:** info@rehabnurse.org
**Website:** http://www.rehabnurse.org
Donna Williams, Pres.
**Desc:** Registered nurses concerned with or actively engaged in the practice of rehabilitation nursing; others interested in rehabilitation. Works to advance the quality of rehabilitation nursing practice through educational opportunities and to facilitate the exchange of ideas. Committees involve members in issues of organizational, local, and national importance and provide an avenue to effect change. Has formed the Rehabilitation Nursing Foundation to promote, develop, and engage in scientific research in the rehabilitation field. **Awards:** MaryAnn Mikulic Scholarship (annual); RNF Research Grant (annual).

### ★ 14921 ★ Chi Eta Phi Sorority
3029 13th St. NW
Washington, DC 20009
**Phone:** (202)232-3858        **Fax:** (202)232-3460
**Email:** chietaphi@erols.com
**Website:** http://www.chietaphi.com
Carolyn Mosley, Pres.
**Desc:** Professional sorority - registered and student nurses. Objectives are to: encourage continuing education; stimulate friendship among members; develop working relationships with other professional groups for the improvement and delivery of health care services. Sponsors leadership training seminars every two years and holds additional seminars at the local, regional, and national levels. Offers educational programs for entrance into nursing and allied health fields. Maintains health screening and consumer health education programs; volunteers assistance to senior citizens; sponsors recruitment and retention programs for minority students in nursing. Operates speakers' bureau on health education. **Awards:** Scholarship students.

**Emergency Nurses Association (ENA)**
*See:* Entry 8561

### ★ 14922 ★ Frontier Nursing Service (FNS)
132 FNS Dr.
Wendover, KY 41775
**Phone:** (606)672-2317        **Fax:** (606)672-3022
**Email:** gvelianoff@ena.org
**Website:** http://www.frontiernursing.org
Deanna Severance, CEO
**Desc:** Provides health care to persons in approximately 1000 square miles of eastern Kentucky using a 40-bed hospital, two primary care centers, three rural health clinics, and a home health agency. Operates Frontier School of Midwifery and Family Nursing. Provides social and ancillary services; conducts research on health services; compiles statistics; offers educational programs. Maintains a hall of fame and museum. **Awards:** Scholarship for nurses in higher education.

### ★ 14923 ★ Helene Fuld Health Trust
452 Fifth Ave., 17th Fl.
New York, NY 10018
**Phone:** (212)525-2418        **Fax:** (212)681-1335
**Email:** www.mail@fuldtrust.org
**Website:** http://www.fuldtrust.org
Jina Piak, Grants Mgr.
**Desc:** Strives to support the improvement of the health, welfare, and education of student nurses. **Awards:** Grant.

### ★ 14924 ★ International Nurses Society on Addictions (NNSA)
1500 Sunday Dr., No. 102
Raleigh, NC 27607
**Phone:** (919)783-5871        **Fax:** (919)787-4916
**Email:** nnsa@mercury.interpath.com
**Website:** http://www.intnsa.org
**Desc:** Promotes quality nursing care for persons addicted to alcohol and other drugs, and their families. Fosters continuing education and development of skills among nurses involved in the field; works to enhance the professional image of addictions nurses.

Participates in public policy and social issues related to alcohol or chemical abuse. Serves as liaison between members and professional groups with common goals. Represents members' interests before national organizations. Regional groups sponsor workshops. Provides certification program. **Awards:** Grant (periodic).

★ 14925 ★ **International Society of Psychiatric Mental Health Nurses (ISPN)**
1211 Locust St.
Philadelphia, PA 19107
**Phone:** (215)545-2843          **Free:** 800-826-2950
**Fax:** (215)545-8107
**Email:** ispn@nursecominc.com
**Website:** http://www.ispn-psych.org
Kenneth Cleveland, Acct. Exec.

**Desc:** Psychiatric and mental health nurses. Seeks to advance the study, teaching, and practice of psychiatric and mental health nursing. Represents members' professional and economic interests. **Awards:** Robert O. Gilbert Foundation Research Award (annual).

★ 14926 ★ **International Transplant Nurses Society (ITNS)**
1739 E Carson St., No. 351
Pittsburgh, PA 15203-1700
**Phone:** (412)488-0240          **Fax:** (412)431-5911
**Email:** itns@msn.com
**Website:** http://www.itns.org
Beth A. Kassalen, MBA, Exec. Dir.

**Desc:** Nurses, LVNs, LPNs, and others involved in patient care for organ transplantation. Works to encourage cooperation among all medical disciplines involved in transplantation, disseminate information, and establish certification for this nursing specialty. **Awards:** Nursing Research (annual) grant proposal.

★ 14927 ★ **National Association of Clinical Nurse Specialists**
3969 Green St.
Harrisburg, PA 17110
**Phone:** (717)234-6799          **Fax:** (717)375-4777
**Email:** info@nacns.org
**Website:** http://www.nacns.org
Christine Carson Filipovich, Exec. Dir.

**Desc:** Clinical Nurse Specialists. **Awards:** CNS of the Year (annual) per jury of peers; Graduate Student Scholarship (annual) based on manuscript submission.

**National Association of Directors of Nursing Administration in Long Term Care (NADONA/LTC)**
*See:* Entry 9596

★ 14928 ★ **National Association of Hispanic Nurses (NAHN)**
1501 Sixteenth St. NW
Washington, DC 20036
**Phone:** (202)387-2477          **Fax:** (202)483-7183
**Email:** info@nahnhq.org
**Website:** http://www.thehispanicnurses.org/
Dr. Carmen J. Portillo, Pres.

**Desc:** Nurses on all educational levels, from all Hispanic subgroups; non-Hispanic nurses concerned about the health delivery needs of the Hispanic community; nursing students. Serves the nursing and health care delivery needs of the Hispanic community and the professional needs of Hispanic nurses. Provides a forum in which Hispanic nurses can analyze, research, and evaluate the health care needs of the Hispanic community. Disseminates findings of that research to local, state, and federal agencies so as to affect policy-making and resource allocation. Aims to ensure that Hispanic nurses have equal access to educational, professional, and economic opportunities. Identifies Hispanic nurses throughout the nation to determine the size of the work force available to provide culturally sensitive nursing care to Hispanics.

**Awards:** Henrietta Villaescusa Award; Ildaura Murillo-Rhode Awards; scholarship.

★ 14929 ★ **National Association of Pediatric Nurse Practitioners (NAPNAP)**
20 Brace Rd., Ste. 200
Cherry Hill, NJ 08034
**Phone:** (856)857-9700          **Fax:** (856)857-1600
**Email:** info@napnap.org
**Website:** http://www.napnap.org
Robert A. Hall, MED, Exec. Dir.

**Desc:** Pediatric, school, and family nurse practitioners and interested persons. Seeks to improve the quality of infant, child, and adolescent health care by making health care services accessible and providing a forum for continuing education of members. Facilitates and supports legislation designed to promote the role of pediatric nurse practitioners and associates; promotes salary ranges commensurate with practitioners' and associates' responsibilities; facilitates exchange of information between prospective employers and job seekers in the field. Participates in the implementation of certification and certification maintenance of practitioners and associates, in cooperation with the National Certification Board of Pediatric Nurse Practitioners and Nurses. Supports research programs; compiles statistics. **Awards:** NAPNAP/McNeil Scholarship (semiannual) for students entering pediatric nurse practitioner programs; recognition.

★ 14930 ★ **National Association of Physician Nurses (NAPN)**
900 S Washington St., No. G-13
Falls Church, VA 22046
**Phone:** (703)237-8616          **Fax:** (703)533-1153
Susan Young, Dir.

**Desc:** Physicians' nurses united to bring added stature and purpose to their profession and to create for themselves the benefits normally limited to members of specialized professional and fraternal groups. **Awards:** Scholarship.

★ 14931 ★ **National Federation for Specialty Nursing Organizations (NFSNO)**
E Holly Ave., Box 56
Pitman, NJ 08071
**Phone:** (856)256-2333          **Fax:** (856)589-7463
**Email:** nfsno@ajj.com
**Website:** http://www.inurse.com/nfsno/about/
Sheila Haas, Pres.

**Desc:** Nursing specialty organizations representing approximately 400,000 individuals. Provides a forum for the discussion of issues of mutual concern to members; attempts to gain more input in the establishment of nursing standards. Sponsors Nurse in Washington Internship. **Awards:** Nurse In Washington Internship Scholarship (annual).

★ 14932 ★ **National Gerontological Nursing Association**
7794 Grow Dr.
Pensacola, FL 32514
**Phone:** (850)473-1174          **Free:** 800-723-0560
**Fax:** (850)484-8762
**Email:** ngna@puetzamc.com
**Website:** http://www.ngna.org
Belinda E. Puetz, RN,PHD, Contact

**Desc:** Gerontological nurses. Seeks to effectively improve the care and well-being of older adults. Provides a forum in which gerontological nursing issues are identified and explored. Develops and supports educational programs for nurses, health providers, and the general public. Disseminates information. **Awards:** Innovations in Practice Award (annual); Judith V. Braun Research Award (annual); Mary Opal Wolanin Scholarship (annual).

★ 14933 ★ **National Nursing Staff Development Organization**
7794 Grow Dr.
Pensacola, FL 32514
**Phone:** (850)474-0995          **Free:** 800-489-1995
**Fax:** (850)484-8762
**Email:** nnsdo@puetzamc.com
**Website:** http://www.nnsdo.org
Belinda E. Puetz, Ph.d.,,, Contact

**Desc:** Advances the specialty practice of staff development for the enhancement of quality healthcare outcomes. Staff development, as a specialty of nursing practice, is defined by standards, based on research critical to quality patient and organizational outcomes. Provides a forum for networking among staff development educators. **Awards:** Affiliate Excellence in Quality Programs Awards (annual); Belinda E. Puetz Award (annual); Excellence Awards (quarterly); grant (annual).

★ 14934 ★ **National Organization for Associate Degree Nursing (N-OADN)**
11250 Roger Bacon Dr., Ste. 8
Reston, VA 20190-5202
**Phone:** (703)437-4377          **Fax:** (703)435-4390
**Email:** noadn@aol.com
**Website:** http://www.noadn.org
Maureen Thompson, Exec. Dir.

**Desc:** Individuals interested in retaining current competency level examinations and endorsement of RN licensure from state to state for associate degree nursing graduates. Represents and advances the status of associate degree nursing education and practice. Provides networking among members to facilitate the exchange of legislative information and support. Offers clearinghouse for interpretation of legal issues and liability insurance. **Awards:** Naomi Brack (annual) student.

★ 14935 ★ **National Organization of Nurse Practitioners Faculties**
1522 K St., NW, Ste. 702
Washington, DC 20005
**Phone:** (202)289-8044          **Fax:** (202)289-8046
**Email:** nonpf@nonpf.org
**Website:** http://www.nonpf.com
Lucy Marion, PhD RN, Pres.

**Desc:** Works to promote public health by developing and implementing nurse practitioner education. Disseminates research related to nurse practitioner education; provides a forum for the exchange of information; works to influence policy affecting nurse practitioners; and develops national guidelins for nurse practitioner educational programs. **Awards:** Achievement in Research Award (annual); Outstanding Group Faculty Practice Award (annual); Outstanding Nurse Practitioner Educator Award (annual); Small Grant Research Award (annual).

★ 14936 ★ **National Student Nurses' Association (NSNA)**
45 Main St., Ste. 606
Brooklyn, NY 11201
**Phone:** (718)210-0705          **Fax:** (718)210-0710
**Email:** nsna@nsna.org
**Website:** http://www.nsna.org
Diane J. Mancino, Ed.D., RN CAE, Exec. Dir.

**Desc:** Students enrolled in state-approved schools for the preparation of registered nurses. Seeks to aid in the development of the individual nursing student and to urge students of nursing, as future health professionals, to be aware of and to contribute to improving the health care of all people. Encourages programs and activities in state groups concerning nursing, health, and the community. Provides assistance for state board review, as well as materials for preparation for state RN licensing examination. Cooperates with nursing organizations in recruitment of nurses and in professional, community, and civic programs. Sponsors Foundation of the National Student Nurses' Association in memory of Frances Tompkins to award scholarships to student nurses. **Awards:** Scholarship (annual).

**★ 14937 ★ Nurses Educational Funds (NEF)**
555 W 57th St., 13th Fl., Ste. 1327
New York, NY 10019
**Phone:** (212)399-1428          **Fax:** (212)581-2368
**Email:** bbnef@aol.com
Barbara Butler, Exec. Dir.
**Desc:** Seeks to establish, maintain, and administer funds to provide financial assistance to registered nurses studying for advanced degrees; masters/doctoral level only formulate policies for the administration of such funds; collect and manage all funds contributed to it. Masters study must be full-time only GRE/MAT scores are required. **Awards:** Scholarship for RN, member of professional nursing, full-time student at Master's Level, full or part-time at doctoral level, U.S. Citizen, enrolled in or applying to NLNAC or CCNE accredited nursing masters program or at doctoral level; for academic and service leader.

**Pediatric Endocrinology Nursing Society (PENS)**
*See:* Entry 8664

**★ 14938 ★ Preventive Cardiovascular Nurses Association (PCNA)**
7611 Elmwood Ave., Ste. 202
Middleton, WI 53562-3161
**Phone:** (608)831-5683          **Fax:** (608)831-5122
**Email:** info@pcna.net
**Website:** http://www.pcna.net
Carol Mason, RN, ANP, Pres.
**Desc:** Works to develop and promote the role of nurses in managing of patients with lipid disorders. Defines a certification process; disseminates information to increase consumer awareness; funds a training grant; seeks to have lipid nursing designated a nursing specialty. **Awards:** Grant.

**★ 14939 ★ Society of Otorhinolaryngology and Head/Neck Nurses (SOHN)**
116 Canal St., Ste. A
New Smyrna Beach, FL 32168
**Phone:** (904)428-1695          **Fax:** (904)423-7566
**Email:** sohnnet@aol.com
**Website:** http://www.sohnnurse.com/
Sandra Schwartz, R.N., Exec. Dir.
**Desc:** Registered nurses specializing in otorhinolaryngology (the study of the ear, nose, and throat) and the head and neck. Seeks to: promote awareness of professional techniques and new developments in the field; enhance professional standards; create a channel for the exchange of ideas, concerns, and information; develop interaction with similar groups. Offers programs and seminars that have been approved for continuing education credits by the American Nurses' Association. **Awards:** Recognition; scholarship.

**★ 14940 ★ Society of Pediatric Nurses (SPN)**
7794 Grow Dr.
Pensacola, FL 32514
**Phone:** (850)494-9467          **Free:** 800-723-2902
**Fax:** (850)484-8762
**Email:** spn@puetzamc.com
**Website:** http://www.pedsnurses.org
Belinda E. Puetz, PhD RN, Contact
**Desc:** Registered pediatric nurses are regular members; nursing students and other professionals with an interest in pediatric nursing are associate members. Promotes quality health and nursing care of children. Conducts advocacy campaigns to improve access to affordable care for children; works to advance techniques of pediatric nursing and health care. Sponsors research and educational programs for members; formulates standards of practice and ethics; fosters collaboration between members and other health care professionals, child health care advocates, and related organizations. **Awards:** Corinne J. Barnes Research Grant (annual); Educational Scholarship Award (annual); Excellence in Advanced Practice Award (annual);

Excellence in Clinical Practice Award (annual); Excellence in Education Award (annual); Excellence in Research Award (annual).

**★ 14941 ★ Society for Vascular Nursing (SVN)**
7794 Grow Dr.
Pensacola, FL 32514
**Phone:** (850)474-6963          **Free:** 888-536-4SVN
**Fax:** (850)484-8762
**Email:** svn@puetzamc.com
**Website:** http://www.svnnet.org
Belinda Puetz, PhD, RN , Exec. Dir.
**Desc:** Nurses and other health care professionals interested in providing comprehensive care for persons with vascular disease. Seeks to educate public about prevention of PVD. Provides educational programs; conducts research. Operates speakers' bureau. **Awards:** Distinguished Service Award (annual); scholarship (annual).

**★ 14942 ★ Wound, Ostomy and Continence Nurses Society: An Association of E.T. Nurses (WOCN)**
4700 W Lake Ave.
Glenview, IL 60025
**Phone:** (847)375-6730          **Free:** 888-224-9626
**Email:** membership@wocn.org
**Website:** http://www.wocn.org
Maureen O'Connor, Senior Mgr.
**Desc:** Enterostomal therapy (ET) nurses, wound, ostomy and continence care nurses in 10 countries trained in WOCN accredited schools; individuals interested in objectives of the association who hold a valid license in medicine or nursing; health-related firms. Seeks to support ET, wound, ostomy, and continence nurses by promoting educational, clinical, and research opportunities and to guide the delivery of expert health care to individuals with wounds, ostomies, and incontinence. **Awards:** ET/WOC Nursing Education Programs and Advanced Degree Scholarships (quarterly).

# Medical & Allied Health Schools

## Nursing

*The institutions listed below offer programs in nursing. For more information, contact the National League for Nursing, 61 Broadway, New York, NY 10006, (800)669-1656, http://www.nln.org/.*

### Alabama

**★ 14943 ★ Auburn University, Montgomery School of Nursing**
PO Box 244023
Montgomery, AL 36124-4023
**Phone:** (334)244-3863          **Fax:** (334)244-3243
**Email:** lstutheit@mickey.aum.edu
**Website:** http://www.aum.edu
Lorinda B. Stutheit, Contact
**Fnded:** 1967. **Degrees Offered:** BSN.

**★ 14944 ★ Jacksonville State University College of Nursing and Health Sciences**
Graduate Studies
700 Pelham Rd. N
Jacksonville, AL 36265-1602
**Phone:** (256)782-5431          **Fax:** (256)782-5406
**Email:** bhembree@jsucc.jsu.edu
**Website:** http://www.jsu.edu/
Dr. Beth Hembree, Contact
**Fnded:** 1883. **Degrees Offered:** BSN, MSN.

**★ 14945 ★ Samford University Ida V. Moffett School of Nursing**
800 Lakeshore Dr.
Birmingham, AL 35229
**Phone:** (205)726-2047          **Fax:** (205)726-2219
**Email:** jsmarting@samford.edu
**Website:** http://www.samford.edu
Dr. Jane Martin, Contact
**Fnded:** 1841. **Degrees Offered:** BSN, MSN, MSN/MBA.

**★ 14946 ★ Spring Hill College Division of Nursing**
4000 Dauphin St.
Mobile, AL 36608
**Phone:** (334)380-4492          **Fax:** (334)380-4495
**Email:** charrison@shc.edu
**Website:** http://www.shc.edu
Dr. Carol Harrison, Contact
**Fnded:** 1830. **Degrees Offered:** BSN.

**★ 14947 ★ Troy State University School of Nursing**
305 S Ripley St.
Montgomery, AL 36104
**Phone:** (334)834-2320          **Fax:** (334)262-4167
**Website:** http://www.troyst.edu
Dr. Charlene Schwab, Contact
**Fnded:** 1887. **Degrees Offered:** BSN, MSN.

**★ 14948 ★ Tuskegee University Program in Nursing**
Basil O'Connor Hall, Rm. 209
Tuskegee Institute, AL 36088
**Phone:** (334)727-8382          **Fax:** (334)727-5461
**Email:** dholeman@acd.tusk.edu
**Website:** http://www.tusk.edu
Dr. Doris S. Holeman, Contact
**Fnded:** 1881. **Degrees Offered:** BSN.

**★ 14949 ★ University of Alabama Capstone College of Nursing**
Nursing Student Services
PO Box 870358
Tuscaloosa, AL 35487-0358
**Phone:** (205)348-6640          **Fax:** (205)348-5559
**Email:** tbuttram@nursing.ua.edu
**Website:** http://www.ua.edu
Dr. Tom Buttram, Contact
**Fnded:** 1831. **Degrees Offered:** BSN, MSN.

**★ 14950 ★ University of Alabama, Birmingham School of Nursing**
1530 3rd Ave., S, NB 108
Birmingham, AL 35294-1210
**Phone:** (205)934-6787          **Fax:** (205)975-6142
**Email:** harrisol@admin.son.uab.edu
**Website:** http://www.uab.edu/son/sonintr2.htm/
Dr. Lynda Harrison, Contact
**Fnded:** 1969. **Degrees Offered:** BSN, MSN, MSN/MPH, PhD.

**★ 14951 ★ University of Alabama, Huntsville College of Nursing**
Nursing Student Affairs
Huntsville, AL 35899
**Phone:** (256)824-6742          **Fax:** (256)824-6026
**Email:** mcgeel@email.uah.edu
**Website:** http://www.uah.edu/colleges/nursing/
Laura McGee, Contact
**Fnded:** 1950. **Degrees Offered:** BSN, MSN.

**★ 14952 ★ University of Mobile School of Nursing**
PO Box 13220
Mobile, AL 36663-0220

**Phone:** (334)442-2227 **Fax:** (334)442-2520
**Email:** rosemaryadams@free.umobile.edu
**Website:** http://www.umobile.edu/
Dr. Rosemary Adams, Contact
**Fnded:** 1961. **Degrees Offered:** BSN, MSN.


★ **14953** ★ **University of North Alabama**
**College of Nursing**
Florence, AL
**Phone:** (256)765-4311 **Fax:** (256)765-4935
**Website:** http://www.una.edu/
**Fnded:** 1830. **Degrees Offered:** BSN.


★ **14954** ★ **University of South Alabama**
**College of Nursing**
University of South Alabama
Mobile, AL 36688-0002
**Phone:** (334)434-3410 **Fax:** (334)434-3413
**Email:** rrhodes@usamail.usouthal.edu
**Website:** http://www.southalabama.edu
Dr. Rosemary S. Rhodes, Contact
**Fnded:** 1963. **Degrees Offered:** BSN, MSN.


## Alaska

★ **14955** ★ **University of Alaska,**
**Anchorage**
**School of Nursing**
3211 Providence Dr.
Anchorage, AK 99508-8030
**Phone:** (907)786-4571 **Fax:** (907)786-4558
**Email:** aftdd@uaa.alaska.edu
**Website:** http://www.son.uaa.alaska.edu
Dr. Tina Delapp, Contact
**Fnded:** 1954 **Degrees Offered:** BS, MS.


★ **14956** ★ **University of Alaska,**
**Anchorage**
**School of Nursing**
3211 Providence Dr.
Anchorage, AK 99508-8030
**Phone:** (907)786-4571 **Fax:** (907)786-4558
**Email:** aftdd@uaa.alaska.edu
**Website:** http://www.uaa.alaska.edu/
Dr. Tina D. Lapp, Contact
**Fnded:** 1954 **Degrees Offered:** BSN.


## Alberta

★ **14957** ★ **Athabasca University**
**Centre for Nursing and Health Sciences**
1 University Dr.
Athabasca, AB, Canada T9S 3A3
**Free:** 800-788-9041 **Fax:** (780)675-6468
**Email:** marge@athabascau.ca
**Website:** http://www.athabascau.ca
Dr. Margaret Edwards, Contact
**Fnded:** 1970. **Degrees Offered:** BN, MHS.


★ **14958** ★ **University of Alberta**
**Faculty of Nursing**
Edmonton, AB, Canada
**Phone:** (780)492-6251 **Fax:** (780)492-6029
**Email:** elaine.carswell@ualberta.ca
**Website:** http://www.us-nursing.ualberta.ca/
Elaine Carswell, Contact
**Fnded:** 1906. **Degrees Offered:** BSCN, MA, PhD


★ **14959** ★ **University of Calgary**
**Faculty of Nursing**
2500 University Dr. NW
Calgary, AB, Canada T2N 1N4
**Phone:** (403)220-6241 **Fax:** (403)284-4803
**Email:** pjolly@ucalgary.ca
**Website:** http://www.nursing.ucalgary.ca/
Pat Jolly, Contact
**Fnded:** 1945. **Degrees Offered:** BN, MN, PhD.


★ **14960** ★ **The University of Lethbridge**
**School of Health Sciences**
4401 University Dr.
Lethbridge, AB, Canada T1K 3M4
**Phone:** (403)329-2121
**Email:** schrage@uleth.ca
**Website:** http://www.uleth.ca/
Kathy Schrage, Contact
**Fnded:** 1967. **Degrees Offered:** BN, M SC.


## Arizona

★ **14961** ★ **Arizona State University**
**College of Nursing**
Office of Student Services
Box 872602
Tempe, AZ 85287-2602
**Phone:** (480)965-2987 **Fax:** (480)965-8468
**Email:** maurine.lee@asu.edu
**Website:** http://www.asu.edu
Maurine Lee, Contact
**Fnded:** 1885. **Degrees Offered:** BSN, MS, MS/MHA


★ **14962** ★ **Grand Canyon University**
**Samaritan College of Nursing**
3300 W Camelback Rd.
Phoenix, AZ 85017
**Phone:** (501)589-2431 **Fax:** (602)589-2098
**Email:** crussell@grand-canyon.edu
**Website:** http://www.grand-canyon.edu
Dr. Cynthia A. Russell, Contact
**Fnded:** 1949. **Degrees Offered:** BSN.


★ **14963** ★ **Northern Arizona University**
**Department of Nursing**
PO Box 15035
Flagstaff, AZ 86011
**Phone:** (520)523-6711 **Fax:** (520)523-7171
**Email:** ruth.nicholls@nau.edu
**Website:** http://www.nau.edu/~hp/dept/nurse/programs.html
Ruth Nicholls, Contact
**Fnded:** 1899. **Degrees Offered:** BSN, MS.


★ **14964** ★ **University of Arizona**
**College of Nursing**
1305 N Martin St.
PO Box 210203
Tucson, AZ 85721-0203
**Phone:** (520)626-6154 **Fax:** (520)626-6425
**Email:** thompson@nursing.arizona.edu
**Website:** http://www.arizona.edu
Gloria Thompson, Contact
**Fnded:** 1855. **Degrees Offered:** BSN, MS, PhD.


★ **14965** ★ **University of Phoenix,**
**Phoenix Campus**
**College of Nursing and Health Care**
**Sciences**
Phoenix, AZ
**Website:** http://www.phoenix.edu/
**Fnded:** 1976. **Degrees Offered:** BSN, MSN, MSN/MBA.


★ **14966** ★ **University of Phoenix,**
**Southern Arizona Campus**
**College of Nursing and Health Care**
**Sciences**
5099 E Grant Rd.
Tucson, AZ 85712
**Phone:** (520)881-6512
**Email:** monica.castillo@apollogrp.edu
**Website:** http://www.phoenix.edu/
Monica Castillo, Contact
**Degrees Offered:** BSN, MSN.


## Arkansas

★ **14967** ★ **Arkansas State University**
**Department of Nursing**
PO Box 910
State University, AR 72467-0069
**Phone:** (870)972-3074 **Fax:** (870)972-2954
**Email:** estokes@crow.astate.edu
**Website:** http://www.astate.edu/
Dr. Elizabeth Stokes, Contact
**Fnded:** 1909. **Degrees Offered:** BSN, MSN


★ **14968** ★ **Arkansas Tech University**
**Program in Nursing**
224 G Dean Hall
Russellville, AR 72801
**Phone:** (501)968-0437 **Fax:** (501)968-0219
**Email:** Rebecca.burris@mail.atu.edu
**Website:** http://www.atu.edu
Rebecca Francis Burris, Contact
**Fnded:** 1909. **Degrees Offered:** BSN.


★ **14969** ★ **Harding University**
**School of Nursing**
PO Box 12265
Searcy, AR 72149-0001
**Phone:** (501)279-4682 **Fax:** (501)305-8902
**Email:** dkemper@harding.edu
**Website:** http://www.harding.edu
Deborah G. Kemper, Contact
**Fnded:** 1924. **Degrees Offered:** BSN, MSN.


★ **14970** ★ **Henderson State University**
**Department of Nursing**
PO Box 7803
1100 Henderson St.
Arkadelphia, AR 71999-0001
**Phone:** (870)230-5015 **Fax:** (870)230-5390
**Email:** festal@hsu.edu
**Website:** http://www.hsu.edu
Dr. Laura Festa, Contact
**Fnded:** 1890. **Degrees Offered:** BSN.


★ **14971** ★ **University of Arkansas,**
**Fayetteville**
**Eleanor Mann School of Nursing**
217 Ozark Hall
Fayetteville, AR 72701
**Phone:** (501)575-3907 **Fax:** (501)575-3218
**Email:** bsconrad@comp.uark.edu
**Website:** http://www.uark.edu
Dr. Barbara Conrad, Contact
**Fnded:** 1871. **Degrees Offered:** BSN.


★ **14972** ★ **University of Arkansas for**
**Medical Sciences**
**College of Nursing**
4301 W Markham, Slot 529
Little Rock, AR 72205-7199
**Phone:** (501)686-5390 **Fax:** (501)686-8350
**Email:** bellpeggel@.uams.edu
**Website:** http://www.uams.edu/
Dr. Pegge Bell, Contact
**Fnded:** 1879. **Degrees Offered:** BSN, MN SC, PhD


★ **14973** ★ **University of Arkansas,**
**Monticello**
**Division of Nursing**
PO Box 3606
Monticello, AR 71656
**Phone:** (870)460-1069 **Fax:** (870)460-1969
**Email:** mitchellbr@aumont.edu
**Website:** http://uamont.edu
Dr. Brenda Mitchell, Contact
**Fnded:** 1909. **Degrees Offered:** BSN.

**★ 14974 ★ University of Arkansas, Pine Bluff**
**Department of Nursing**
1200 N University Dr.
Box 4973
Pine Bluff, AR 71611
**Phone:** (870)543-8220          **Fax:** (870)543-8229
**Email:** henderson_i@vx4500.uapb.edu
Dr. Irene T. Henderson, Contact
**Fnded:** 1873. **Degrees Offered:** BSN.

**★ 14975 ★ University of Central Arkansas**
**Department of Nursing**
201 Donaghey Ave.
Conway, AR 72035
**Phone:** (501)450-3119          **Fax:** (501)450-5560
**Email:** beckyl@mail.uca.edu
**Website:** http://www.uca.edu/chas/nursing.html
Dr. Rebecca Lancaster, Contact
**Fnded:** 1907. **Degrees Offered:** BSN, MSN.

### British Columbia

**★ 14976 ★ British Columbia Institute of Technology**
**School of Health Sciences**
Burnaby, BC, Canada
**Phone:** (604)432-8884          **Fax:** (604)432-1816
**Email:** loreen_martin@bcit.ca
**Website:** http://www.bcit.ca/
Loreen Martin, Contact
**Fnded:** 1964. **Degrees Offered:** BS.

**★ 14977 ★ Kwantlen University College**
**Faculty of Community and Health Sciences**
Surrey, BC, Canada
**Phone:** (604)599-2234
**Email:** heatherm@kwantlen.bc.ca
**Website:** http://www.kwantlen.bc.ca/
Heather McMann, Contact
**Degrees Offered:** BSN.

**★ 14978 ★ Malaspin University-College**
**Department of Nursing**
900 Fifth St.
Nanaimo, BC, Canada
**Phone:** (250)751-2494
**Website:** http://www.mala.bc.ca/
**Fnded:** 1969. **Degrees Offered:** BSCN.

**★ 14979 ★ Okanagan University College**
**Nursing Department**
Kelowna, BC, Canada
**Phone:** (250)762-5445          **Fax:** (250)762-5461
**Email:** dcallaghan@okanagan.bc.ca
**Website:** http://www.ouc.bc.ca/
Doris Callaghan, Contact
**Degrees Offered:** BSN.

**★ 14980 ★ Trinity Western University**
**Department of Nursing**
7600 Glover Rd.
Langley, BC, Canada V2Y 1Y1
**Phone:** (604)888-7511          **Fax:** (604)513-2018
**Email:** emblen@twu.ca
**Website:** http://www.twu.ca/
Dr. Julie Dianne Emblen, Contact
**Fnded:** 1962. **Degrees Offered:** BSCN.

**★ 14981 ★ University of British Columbia**
**School of Nursing**
T201-2211, Westbrook Mall
Vancouver, BC, Canada V6T 2B5
**Phone:** (604)822-7498          **Fax:** (604)822-7466
**Email:** hilton@nursing.ubc.ca

**Website:** http://www.ubc.ca/
Ann Hilton, Contact
**Fnded:** 1915. **Degrees Offered:** BSN, MSN, PhD.

**★ 14982 ★ University College of the Cariboo**
**School of Nursing**
PO Box 3010
900 College Dr.
Kamloops, BC, Canada V2C 5N3
**Phone:** (250)828-5435          **Fax:** (250)828-5450
**Email:** zawaduk@cariboo.bc.ca
**Website:** http://www.caribou.bc.ca/
Cheryl Zawaduk, Contact
**Fnded:** 1970. **Degrees Offered:** BSN.

**★ 14983 ★ University of Northern British Columbia**
**Nursing Programme**
3333 University Way
Prince George, BC, Canada V2N 4Z9
**Phone:** (250)960-5645          **Fax:** (250)960-5744
**Email:** fayled@unbc.ca
**Website:** http://www.unbc.ca/
Deanna Fayle, Contact
**Degrees Offered:** BSCN.

**★ 14984 ★ University of Victoria**
**School of Nursing**
PO Box 1700
Victoria, BC, Canada V8W 2Y2
**Phone:** (250)721-7955          **Fax:** (250)721-6231
**Email:** dwalton@uvic.ca
**Website:** http://www.uvic.ca/
Diana Walton, Contact
**Fnded:** 1963. **Degrees Offered:** BSN, MN.

### California

**★ 14985 ★ Azusa Pacific University**
**School of Nursing**
901 E Alosta Ave.
Azusa, CA 91702
**Phone:** (626)815-5386          **Fax:** (626)815-5414
**Email:** bbarthelmess@apunet.apu.edu
**Website:** http://www.apu.edu
Barb Barthelmess, Contact
**Fnded:** 1899. **Degrees Offered:** BSN, MSN.

**★ 14986 ★ Biola University**
**Department of Nursing**
13800 Biola Ave.
La Mirada, CA 90639
**Phone:** (562)903-4850          **Fax:** (562)903-4803
**Email:** anne_gewe@peter.biola.edu
**Website:** http://www.biola.edu/
Anne L. Gewe, Contact
**Fnded:** 1908. **Degrees Offered:** BS

**★ 14987 ★ California State University, Bakersfield**
**Program in Nursing**
9001 Stockdale Hwy.
Bakersfield, CA 93311-1099
**Phone:** (661)664-3108          **Fax:** (661)665-6903
**Email:** bmikhail@csub.edu
**Website:** http://www.csub.edu/nursing/masters.htm
Dr. Blanche Mikhail, Contact
**Fnded:** 1970. **Degrees Offered:** BSN, MSN.

**★ 14988 ★ California State University, Chico**
**School of Nursing**
Chico, CA 95929-0200
**Phone:** (530)898-6207          **Fax:** (530)898-4363
**Email:** syoung@facultypo.csuchico.edu
**Website:** http://www.csuchico.edu/
Shelley Young, Contact

**Fnded:** 1887. **Degrees Offered:** BSN, MSN.

**★ 14989 ★ California State University, Dominguez Hills**
**Program in Nursing**
Student Advising Center
Carson, CA 90747
**Free:** 800-344-5484          **Fax:** (310)516-3542
**Email:** sohadvising@soh.csudh.edu
**Website:** http://www.csudh.edu
**Fnded:** 1960. **Degrees Offered:** BSN, MSN.

**★ 14990 ★ California State University, Fresno**
**Department of Nursing**
2345 E San Ramon Ave.
Fresno, CA 93740-8031
**Phone:** (559)278-2041          **Fax:** (559)278-6360
**Email:** michael_russler@csufresno.edu
**Website:** http://www.csufresno.edu
Mike Russler, Contact
**Fnded:** 1911. **Degrees Offered:** BSN, MSN.

**★ 14991 ★ California State University, Fullerton**
**Department of Nursing**
PO Box 6868
Fullerton, CA 92834-6868
**Phone:** (714)278-3336          **Fax:** (714)278-3338
**Email:** lliu@fullerton.edu
**Website:** http://hdcs.fullerton.edu/
Leanne Liu, Contact
**Fnded:** 1957.

**★ 14992 ★ California State University, Hayward**
**Department of Nursing and Health Sciences**
25800 Carlos Bee Blvd.
Hayward, CA 94542
**Phone:** (510)885-2797          **Fax:** (510)885-2156
**Email:** bfelton@scuhayward.edu
**Website:** http://www.csuhayward.edu/
Dr. Bette Felton, Contact
**Fnded:** 1957. **Degrees Offered:** BSN, MSN, MSN/MHA.

**★ 14993 ★ California State University, Long Beach**
**Department of Nursing**
1250 Bellflower Blvd.
Long Beach, CA 90840-0119
**Phone:** (562)985-4469          **Fax:** (562)985-2382
**Email:** amsty@umbsky.cc.umb.edu
**Website:** http://www.csulb.edu/
Dr. Judy Smith, Contact
**Fnded:** 1949. **Degrees Offered:** BSN, MSN, MSN/MPH.

**★ 14994 ★ California State University, Los Angeles**
**Department of Nursing**
5151 State University Dr.
Los Angeles, CA 90032
**Phone:** (323)343-4700          **Fax:** (323)343-6454
**Email:** jpapen@calstatela.edu
**Website:** http://www.calstatela.edu/
Dr. Judith Papenhausen, Contact
**Fnded:** 1947. **Degrees Offered:** BS, MS.

**★ 14995 ★ California State University, Northridge**
**Nursing Program**
18111 Nordhoff St.
Northridge, CA 91330-8285
**Phone:** (818)677-2423          **Fax:** (818)677-2045
**Email:** ellen.mcfadden@csun.edu

**Website:** http://www.csun.edu
Dr. Ellen McFadden, Contact
**Fnded:** 1958. **Degrees Offered:** BSN.


**★ 14996 ★ California State University,
Sacramento
Division of Nursing**
6000 J St.
Sacramento, CA 95819-6096
**Phone:** (916)278-6525       **Fax:** (916)278-6311
**Email:** ackermanpl@csus.edu
**Website:** http://www.csus.edu/
Dr. Patricia Ackerman, Contact
**Fnded:** 1947. **Degrees Offered:** BS, MS.


**★ 14997 ★ California State University,
San Bernardino
Department of Nursing**
5500 University Pkwy.
San Bernardino, CA 92407
**Phone:** (909)880-5380       **Fax:** (909)880-7089
**Email:** slloyd@csub.edu
**Website:** http://www.csusb.edu/
Dr. Susan Lloyd, Contact
**Fnded:** 1965. **Degrees Offered:** BSN, MSN.


**★ 14998 ★ California State University,
Stanislaus
Department of Nursing**
801 Monte Vista Ave.
Turlock, CA 95382
**Phone:** (209)667-3141       **Fax:** (209)667-3690
**Email:** iworthington@stan.csustan.edu
**Website:** http://www.csustan.edu
Ilene M. Worthington, Contact
**Fnded:** 1957. **Degrees Offered:** BSN.


**★ 14999 ★ Dominican University of
California
School of Health Sciences**
50 Acacia Ave.
San Rafael, CA 94901-2298
**Phone:** (415)485-1344       **Fax:** (415)257-0120
**Email:** jossens@dominican.edu
**Website:** http://www.dominican.edu//
Marilyn Jossens, Contact
**Fnded:** 1890. **Degrees Offered:** BSN, MSN.


**★ 15000 ★ Holy Names College
Department of Nursing**
3500 Mountain Blvd.
Oakland, CA 94619-1699
**Phone:** (510)436-1648
**Email:** melms@hnc.edu
**Website:** http://www.hnc.edu
Danita Melms, Contact
**Fnded:** 1868. **Degrees Offered:** BSN, MSN.


**★ 15001 ★ Humboldt State University
Department of Nursing**
1 Harpst St.
Arcata, CA 95521
**Phone:** (707)826-3215       **Fax:** (707)826-5141
**Email:** nurs@axe.humboldt.edu
**Website:** http://www.humboldt.edu
Dr. Wendy Woodward, Contact
**Fnded:** 1913. **Degrees Offered:** BSN.


**★ 15002 ★ Loma Linda University
School of Nursing**
Loma Linda, CA 92350
**Phone:** (909)478-8061       **Fax:** (909)478-4134
**Website:** http://www.llu.edu
Joyce Bates, Contact
**Fnded:** 1905. **Degrees Offered:** BS, MS, MSN/MA,
MSN/MPH.


**★ 15003 ★ Mount St. Mary's College
Department of Nursing**
12001 Chalon Rd.
Los Angeles, CA 90049-1599
**Phone:** (310)954-4233       **Fax:** (310)954-4229
**Email:** mmccarty@msmc.la.edu
**Website:** http://msmc.la.edu
Meg McCarty, Contact
**Fnded:** 1925. **Degrees Offered:** BSN.


**★ 15004 ★ National University
Department of Nursing**
11255 N Torrey Pines Rd.
La Jolla, CA 92037-1011
**Phone:** (858)642-8361       **Fax:** (858)642-8715
**Email:** mhazzard@nu.edu
**Website:** http://www.nu.edu
Dr. Mary Hazzard, Contact
**Fnded:** 1971. **Degrees Offered:** BSN, MSN.


**★ 15005 ★ Pacific Union College
Department of Nursing**
One Angwin Ave.
Angwin, CA 94508
**Phone:** (707)965-7262       **Free:** 800-965-6499
**Fax:** (707)965-6499
**Email:** jlpearce@puc.edu
**Website:** http://www.puc.edu
Dr. Julia Pearce, Contact
**Fnded:** 1882. **Degrees Offered:** BSN.


**★ 15006 ★ Point Loma Nazarene
University
Department of Nursing**
3900 Lomaland Dr.
San Diego, CA 92106-2899
**Phone:** (619)849-2236       **Fax:** (619)849-2672
**Email:** dcrummy@ptloma.edu
**Website:** http://www.ptloma.edu
Dottie E. Crummy, Contact
**Fnded:** 1902. **Degrees Offered:** BSN.


**★ 15007 ★ St. Mary's College of
California
Department of Nursing**
Moraga, CA 94575
**Phone:** (510)869-4000       **Fax:** (510)869-6077
**Email:** asargent@samuelmerritt.edu
**Website:** http://www.stmarys-ca.edu
Arlene Sargent, Contact
**Fnded:** 1863. **Degrees Offered:** BSN, MSN.


**★ 15008 ★ Samuel Merritt College
Department of Nursing**
370 Hawthorne Ave.
Oakland, CA 94609
**Phone:** (510)869-6727       **Fax:** (510)869-6525
**Email:** jgartens@samuelmerritt.edu
**Website:** http://www.samuelmerritt.edu
John Garten-Shuman, Contact
**Fnded:** 1909. **Degrees Offered:** BSN, MSN.


**★ 15009 ★ San Diego State University
School of Nursing**
5500 Campanile Dr.
San Diego, CA 92182-4158
**Phone:** (619)594-2540       **Fax:** (619)594-2765
**Email:** lsaarman@mail.sdsu.edu
**Website:** http://www.sdsu.edu/
Dr. Lembi Saarmann, Contact
**Fnded:** 1897. **Degrees Offered:** BSN, MSN.


**★ 15010 ★ San Francisco State
University
School of Nursing**
San Francisco, CA 94132-4161
**Phone:** (415)338-1802       **Fax:** (415)338-0555
**Email:** femc@sfsu.edu


**Website:** http://www.sfsu.edu/
Frank McLaughlin, Contact
**Fnded:** 1899. **Degrees Offered:** BSN, MSN.


**★ 15011 ★ San Jose State University
School of Nursing**
1 Washington Sq.
San Jose, CA 95192
**Phone:** (408)924-1325       **Fax:** (408)924-3135
**Email:** jmcohen@email.sjsu.edu
**Website:** http://www.sjsu.edu
Dr. Jayne Cohen, Contact
**Fnded:** 1857. **Degrees Offered:** BS, MS.


**★ 15012 ★ Sonoma State University
Department of Nursing**
1801 E Cotati Ave.
Rohnert Park, CA 94928
**Phone:** (707)664-2465       **Fax:** (707)664-2465
**Email:** cohen@sonoma.edu
**Website:** http://www.sonoma.edu/
Becky Schroeder Cohen, Contact
**Fnded:** 1960. **Degrees Offered:** BSN, MSN


**★ 15013 ★ University of California, Los
Angeles
School of Nursing**
Box 951702
Los Angeles, CA 90095-1702
**Phone:** (310)825-7181       **Fax:** (310)206-7433
**Email:** sonsaff@ucla.edu
**Website:** http://www.nursing.ucla.edu/
Kathy Scriver, Contact
**Fnded:** 1919. **Degrees Offered:** BS, MSN, MSN/
MBA, PhD.


**★ 15014 ★ University of California, San
Francisco
School of Nursing**
2 Kirkham St., Rm. N319X
San Francisco, CA 94143-0602
**Phone:** (415)476-1435       **Fax:** (415)476-9707
**Email:** jeff.kilmer@nursing.ucsf.edu
**Website:** http://www.ucsf.edu/
Jeff Kilmer, Contact
**Fnded:** 1864. **Degrees Offered:** MS, PhD.


**★ 15015 ★ University of Phoenix,
Northern California Campus
College of Nursing and Health Care
Sciences**
Pleasanton, CA
**Phone:** 877—4-STUDENT
**Email:** Heather.Cornell@apollogrp.edu
**Website:** http://www.phoenix.edu/
Heather Cornell, Contact
**Degrees Offered:** BSN, MSN.


**★ 15016 ★ University of Phoenix,
Sacramento Campus
College of Nursing and Health Care
Sciences**
Sacramento, CA
**Free:** 800-266-2107
**Email:** Teresa.Brink@appollogrp.edu
**Website:** http://www.phoenix.edu/
Teresa Brink, Contact
**Degrees Offered:** BSN, MSN.


**★ 15017 ★ University of Phoenix, San
Diego Campus
College of Nursing and Health Care
Sciences**
San Diego, CA
**Email:** Brett.Ericson@apollogrp.edu
**Website:** http://www.phoenix.edu/
Brett Ericson, Contact

**Degrees Offered:** BSN, MSN.

★ **15018** ★ **University of Phoenix,
    Southern California Campus**
**College of Nursing and Health Care
    Sciences**
10540 Talbert Ave.
West Tower, Ste. 120
Fountain Valley, CA 92708
**Free:** 800-468-6867
**Email:** Anthony.Mercado@apollogrp.edu
**Website:** http://www.phoenix.edu/
Anthony Mercado, Contact
**Degrees Offered:** BSN, MSN.

★ **15019** ★ **University of San Diego**
**Hahn School of Nursing and Health
    Sciences**
Student Services
5998 Alcala Pk.
San Diego, CA 92110-2492
**Phone:** (619)260-4548        **Fax:** (619)260-6814
**Email:** cmm@acusd.edu
**Website:** http://www.sandiego.edu
Cathleen Mumper, Contact
**Fnded:** 1949. **Degrees Offered:** BSN, MSN, MSN/
MBA, PhD.

★ **15020** ★ **University of San Francisco**
**School of Nursing**
2130 Fulton St.
Cowell Hall 110
San Francisco, CA 94117-1080
**Phone:** (415)422-2961        **Fax:** (415)422-6877
**Email:** reedr@usfca.edu
**Website:** http://www.usfca.edu/
Robert J. Reed, Contact
**Fnded:** 1855. **Degrees Offered:** BSN, MSN, MSN/
MBA.

★ **15021** ★ **University of Southern
    California**
**Department of Nursing**
CHP 222
1540 E Alcazar St.
Los Angeles, CA 90089-9012
**Phone:** (323)442-2001        **Fax:** (323)442-2090
**Website:** http://www.usc.edu/
Lynette Merriman, Contact
**Fnded:** 1880. **Degrees Offered:** BSN, MSN, MSN/
MBA.

### Colorado

★ **15022** ★ **Mesa State College**
**Department of Nursing and Radiologic
    Sciences**
PO Box 2647
1175 Texas Ave.
Grand Junction, CO 81501
**Phone:** (970)248-1774        **Fax:** (970)248-1133
**Website:** http://www.mesastate.edu/
Judy Goodhart, Contact
**Fnded:** 1925. **Degrees Offered:** BSN.

★ **15023** ★ **Metropolitan State College of
    Denver**
**Department of Health Professions**
Campus Box 33
PO Box 173362
Denver, CO 80217-3362
**Phone:** (303)556-3130        **Fax:** (303)556-3439
**Website:** http://www.mscd.edu
**Fnded:** 1963. **Degrees Offered:** BS.

★ **15024** ★ **Regis University**
**Department of Nursing**
3333 Regis Blvd.
Denver, CO 80221-1099
**Phone:** (303)458-4927        **Fax:** (303)964-5533
**Email:** bmetzger@regis.edu
**Website:** http://www.regis.edu
Brent Metzger, Contact
**Fnded:** 1877. **Degrees Offered:** BSN, MSN.

★ **15025** ★ **University of Colorado**
**Health Sciences Center**
**School of Nursing**
4200 E 9th Ave., Box C 288
Denver, CO 80262
**Phone:** (303)315-5592        **Fax:** (303)315-8660
**Email:** mary.lepley@uchsc.edu
**Website:** http://www.uchsc.edu/
Mary M. Lepley, Contact
**Fnded:** 1883. **Degrees Offered:** BS, MS, MSN/MBA,
PhD.

★ **15026** ★ **University of Colorado,
    Colorado Springs**
**Beth El College of Nursing and Health
    Sciences**
1420 Austin Bluffs Pkwy.
PO Box 7150
Colorado Springs, CO 80933-7150
**Phone:** (719)262-4422        **Fax:** (719)262-3383
**Email:** bnagata@mail.uccs.edu
**Website:** http://www.uccs.edu/
Dr. Barbara Joyce Nagata, Contact
**Fnded:** 1965. **Degrees Offered:** BSN, MSN.

★ **15027** ★ **University of Northern
    Colorado**
**School of Nursing**
Box 125
Greeley, CO 80639
**Phone:** (303)351-2663        **Fax:** (303)351-1707
**Email:** jrichter@unco.edu
**Website:** http://www.unco.edu
Dr. Judy Richter, Contact
**Fnded:** 1890. **Degrees Offered:** BS, MS.

★ **15028** ★ **University of Phoenix,
    Colorado Campus**
**College of Nursing and Health Care
    Sciences**
10004 Park Meadow Dr.
Lone Tree, CO 80124-9909
**Phone:** (303)600-1307
**Email:** mike.true@apollogrp.edu
**Website:** http://www.phoenix.edu/
Mike True, Contact
**Degrees Offered:** BSN, MSN.

★ **15029** ★ **University of Southern
    Colorado**
**Department of Nursing**
2200 Bonforte Blvd.
Pueblo, CO 81001
**Phone:** (719)549-2100        **Fax:** (719)549-2732
**Email:** steen@uscolo.edu
**Website:** http://www.uscolo.edu
Dr. Melva J. Steen, Contact
**Fnded:** 1933. **Degrees Offered:** BSN.

### Connecticut

★ **15030** ★ **Central Connecticut State
    University**
**Department of Health and Human Service
    Professions**
1615 Stanley St.
New Britain, CT 06050-4010
**Phone:** (860)832-2154        **Fax:** (860)832-2188

**Email:** williamsmj@ccsu.edu
**Website:** http://www.ccsu.edu
Dr. Mary Jane Williams, Contact
**Fnded:** 1849. **Degrees Offered:** BSN.

★ **15031** ★ **Fairfield University**
**School of Nursing**
N Benson Rd.
Fairfield, CT 06430-5195
**Phone:** (203)254-4150        **Fax:** (203)254-4126
**Email:** kwheeler@fair1.fairfield.edu
**Website:** http://www.fairfield.edu
Dr. Kathleen Wheeler, Contact
**Fnded:** 1942. **Degrees Offered:** BS, MSN.

★ **15032** ★ **Quinnipiac College**
**Department of Nursing**
275 Mount Carmel Ave.
Hamden, CT 06518
**Phone:** (203)582-8672        **Fax:** (203)582-3443
**Email:** graduate@quinnipiac.edu
**Website:** http://www.quinnipiac.edu
Scott Farber, Contact
**Fnded:** 1929. **Degrees Offered:** BS, MSN.

★ **15033** ★ **Sacred Heart University**
**Program in Nursing**
5151 Park Ave.
Fairfield, CT 06432
**Phone:** (203)371-7715        **Fax:** (203)365-7662
**Email:** sullivand@sacredheart.edu
**Website:** http://www.sacredheart.edu
Dr. Dori Taylor Sullivan, Contact
**Fnded:** 1963. **Degrees Offered:** BS, MSN, MSN/
MBA.

★ **15034** ★ **Saint Joseph College**
**Department of Nursing**
1678 Asylum Ave.
West Hartford, CT 06117-2700
**Phone:** (860)231-5316        **Fax:** (860)231-8396
**Email:** ndrew@mercy.sjc.edu
**Website:** http://www.sjc.edu
Dr. Nancy Drew, Contact
**Fnded:** 1932. **Degrees Offered:** BS, MSN.

★ **15035** ★ **Southern Connecticut State
    University**
**Department of Nursing**
501 Crescent St.
New Haven, CT 06515
**Phone:** (203)392-6482        **Fax:** (203)392-6493
**Email:** killion@scsu.ctstateu.edu
**Website:** http://southernct.edu
Dr. Susan Killion, Contact
**Fnded:** 1893. **Degrees Offered:** BSN, MSN.

★ **15036** ★ **University of Connecticut**
**School of Nursing**
Academic Advisory Center
231 Glenbrook Rd.
Unit 2026
Storrs, CT 06269-2026
**Phone:** (860)486-4730        **Fax:** (860)486-0906
**Email:** nuradmo02@uconnvm.uconn.edu
**Website:** http://www.uconn.edu
Eva Gorbants, Contact
**Fnded:** 1881. **Degrees Offered:** BS, MS, MSN/MBA,
MSN/MPH, PhD.

★ **15037** ★ **University of Hartford**
**College of Education, Nursing, and
    Health Professions**
200 Bloomfield Ave.
West Hartford, CT 06117-1599
**Phone:** (860)768-5116        **Fax:** (860)768-5346
**Email:** mhall@mail.hartford.edu

**Website:** http://www.hartford.edu/
Marlene J. Hall, Contact
**Fnded:** 1877. **Degrees Offered:** BSN, MSN, MSN/MSOB.


★ 15038 ★ **Western Connecticut State University**
**Department of Nursing**
181 White St.
Danbury, CT 06810
**Phone:** (203)837-8564     **Fax:** (203)837-8526
**Website:** http://www.wcsu.edu
**Fnded:** 1903. **Degrees Offered:** BSN, MSN.


★ 15039 ★ **Yale University**
**School of Nursing**
100 Church St. S
PO Box 9740
New Haven, CT 06536-0740
**Phone:** (203)737-2557     **Fax:** (203)737-5409
**Email:** sharon.sanderson@yale.edu
**Website:** http://info.mea.yale.edu/nursing
Sharon Sanderson, Contact
**Fnded:** 1701. **Degrees Offered:** DN SC, MSN, MSN/MBA, MSN/MPH.


## Delaware

★ 15040 ★ **Delaware State University**
**Department of Nursing**
Office of Admissions
Dover, DE 19901-2277
**Phone:** (302)857-6353
**Website:** http://www.dsc.edu
**Fnded:** 1891. **Degrees Offered:** BSN.


★ 15041 ★ **University of Delaware**
**Department of Nursing**
357 McDowell Hall
Newark, DE 19716
**Phone:** (302)831-2193     **Fax:** (302)831-2382
**Email:** selekman@udel.edu
**Website:** http://www.udel.edu/nursing/udnursing.html
Dr. Janice Selekman, Contact
**Fnded:** 1743. **Degrees Offered:** BSN, MSN.


★ 15042 ★ **Wesley College**
**Division of Nursing**
120 N State St.
Dover, DE 19901
**Phone:** (302)736-2512     **Fax:** (302)736-2548
**Email:** gambarlu@mail.Wesley.edu
**Website:** http://www.wesley.edu
Dr. Lucille Gambardella, Contact
**Fnded:** 1873. **Degrees Offered:** MSN.


★ 15043 ★ **Wilmington College**
**Division of Nursing**
320 DuPont Hwy.
New Castle, DE 19720
**Phone:** (302)328-9407     **Fax:** (302)328-5902
**Email:** bwils@wilmcoll.edu
**Website:** http://www.wilmcoll.edu/
Barbara Wilson, Contact
**Fnded:** 1967. **Degrees Offered:** BSN, MSN.


## District of Columbia

★ 15044 ★ **Catholic University of America**
**School of Nursing**
116 Gowan Hall
Washington, DC 20064
**Phone:** (202)319-5403     **Fax:** (202)319-6485
**Email:** brooks@cua.edu
**Website:** http://nursing.cua.edu/www/NUR/welcome.htm
Dr. Anne Marie Brooks, Contact

**Fnded:** 1887. **Degrees Offered:** BSN, DN SC, MA/MSM, MSN.


★ 15045 ★ **Georgetown University**
**School of Nursing and Health Sciences**
3700 Reservoir Rd. NW
Washington, DC 20007
**Phone:** (202)687-8439     **Fax:** (202)687-5553
**Email:** ATW4@georgetown.edu
**Website:** http://www.georgetown.edu/
Amy Windisch, Contact
**Fnded:** 1789. **Degrees Offered:** BSN, MS.


★ 15046 ★ **Howard University**
**Division of Nursing**
501 Bryant St. NW
Washington, DC 20059
**Phone:** (202)806-7460     **Fax:** (202)806-5958
**Email:** bkelly@howard.edu
**Website:** http://www.howard.edu/
Dr. Beatrice Adderley-Kelly, Contact
**Fnded:** 1867. **Degrees Offered:** BSN, MSN.


★ 15047 ★ **University of the District of Columbia**
**Nursing Education Program**
4200 Connecticut Ave. NW
Washington, DC 20008
**Phone:** (202)274-5899     **Fax:** (202)274-5952
**Email:** cwebster@udc.edu
**Website:** http://www.udc.edu
Dr. Connie Marie Webster, Contact
**Fnded:** 1976. **Degrees Offered:** BSN.


## Florida

★ 15048 ★ **Barry University**
**School of Nursing**
11300 2nd Ave. NE
Miami Shores, FL 33161-6695
**Phone:** (305)899-3800     **Fax:** (305)899-3831
**Email:** jdyer@mail.barry.edu
**Website:** http://www.barry.edu
Dr. Janice Dyer, Contact
**Fnded:** 1940. **Degrees Offered:** BSN, MSN, MSN/MBA, PhD.


★ 15049 ★ **Bethune-Cookman College**
**Division of Nursing**
640 Dr. Mary McLeod Bethune Blvd.
Daytona Beach, FL 32114
**Phone:** (904)323-2031     **Fax:** (904)257-5338
**Email:** dixona@cookman.edu
**Website:** http://www.bethune.cookman.edu/
Sr. Alma Dixon, Contact
**Fnded:** 1904. **Degrees Offered:** BSN.


★ 15050 ★ **Florida Agricultural and Mechanical University**
**School of Nursing**
PO Box 136
Tallahassee, FL 32307
**Phone:** (850)599-3017     **Fax:** (850)599-3849
**Email:** mlewis@famu.edu
**Website:** http://www.famu.edu
Dr. Margaret Lewis, Contact
**Fnded:** 1887. **Degrees Offered:** BSN MSN.


★ 15051 ★ **Florida Atlantic University**
**College of Nursing**
777 Glades Rd.
PO Box 3091
Boca Raton, FL 33431-0991
**Phone:** (561)297-3384     **Fax:** (561)297-0088
**Email:** idunphy@fau.edu
**Website:** http://www.fau.edu/divdept/nursing/
Dr. Lynn M. Youngkin, Contact
**Fnded:** 1961. **Degrees Offered:** BSN, MS.


★ 15052 ★ **Florida Gulf Coast University**
**School of Nursing**
10501 FGCU Boulevard South
Fort Myers Beach, FL 33931
**Phone:** (941)590-7512     **Fax:** (941)590-7474
**Email:** kmiles@fgcu.edu
**Website:** http://www.fgcu.edu/
Dr. Karen Miles, Contact
**Fnded:** 1991. **Degrees Offered:** BSN, MSN.


★ 15053 ★ **Florida International University**
**Department of Nursing**
3000 NE 151st St., ACII-230
North Miami, FL 33181
**Phone:** (305)919-5845     **Fax:** (305)919-5395
**Email:** porterl@fiu.edu
**Website:** http://www.fiu.edu/~wellness
Dr. Luz Porter, Contact
**Fnded:** 1965. **Degrees Offered:** BSN, MSN.


★ 15054 ★ **Florida State University**
**School of Nursing**
103 Vivian M. Duxbury Hall
Tallahassee, FL 32306-4310
**Phone:** (850)644-5626     **Fax:** (850)644-7660
**Email:** jflanner@mailer.fsu.edu
**Website:** http://www.fsu.edu
Dr. Jeanne Flannery, Contact
**Fnded:** 1857. **Degrees Offered:** BSN, MSN.


★ 15055 ★ **Jacksonville University**
**School of Nursing**
2800 University Blvd. N
Jacksonville, FL 32211
**Phone:** (904)745-7286     **Fax:** (904)745-7287
**Email:** jmcdani@ju.edu
**Website:** http://www.ju.edu
Becky Cromwell, Contact
**Fnded:** 1934. **Degrees Offered:** BSN, MSN.


★ 15056 ★ **University of Central Florida**
**School of Nursing**
PO Box 162210
Orlando, FL 32816-2210
**Phone:** (407)823-2744     **Fax:** (407)823-5675
**Email:** estullen@pegasus.cc.ucf.edu
**Website:** http://www.ucf.edu/
Dr. Elizabeth Stullenbarger, Contact
**Fnded:** 1963. **Degrees Offered:** BSN, MSN.


★ 15057 ★ **University of Florida**
**College of Nursing**
PO Box 100197
Gainesville, FL 32610-0197
**Phone:** (352)392-3518     **Fax:** (352)392-8100
**Email:** bivenpm.ufcon@shands.ufl.edu
**Website:** http://con.ufl.edu/
Patricia M. Bivens, Contact
**Fnded:** 1853. **Degrees Offered:** BSN, MSN, PhD.


★ 15058 ★ **University of Miami**
**School of Nursing**
5801 Red Rd.
Coral Gables, FL 33124-2343
**Phone:** (305)284-4325     **Fax:** (305)284-4827
**Email:** knguyen@miami.edu
**Website:** http://www.miami.edu
Kim Nguyen, Contact
**Fnded:** 1925. **Degrees Offered:** BSN, MSN, PhD.


★ 15059 ★ **University of North Florida**
**Department of Nursing**
College of Health Advising Office
Room 3025A, Bldg. 39
Jacksonville, FL 32224-2673
**Phone:** (904)620-2812     **Fax:** (904)620-2848
**Website:** http://www.unf.edu

Fnded: 1965. Degrees Offered: BSN, MSN.

★ 15060 ★ **University of Phoenix, Butler Pointe Campus**
**College of Nursing and Health Care Sciences**
4500 Salisbury Rd.
Ste. 200
Jacksonville, FL 32216
Phone: (904)636-6645
Email: Mary.Young@apollogrp.edu
Degrees Offered: BSN, MSN.

★ 15061 ★ **University of Phoenix, Fort Lauderdale Campus**
**College of Nursing and Health Care Sciences**
Jacksonville, FL
Phone: (954)382-5303
Email: Brooks.Meseroll@apollogrp.edu
Website: http://www.phoenix.edu/
Brooks Meseroll, Contact
Degrees Offered: BSN, MSN.

★ 15062 ★ **University of Phoenix, Orlando Campus**
**College of Nursing and Health Care Sciences**
Maitland, FL 32751
Email: Kimberly.Drager@apollogrp.edu
Website: http://www.phoenix.edu/
Degrees Offered: BSN, MSN.

★ 15063 ★ **University of Phoenix, Tampa Campus**
**College of Nursing and Health Care Sciences**
Tampa, FL
Phone: (813)626-7911
Email: Chad.Bandy@apollogrp.edu
Website: http://www.phoenix.edu/
Chad Bandy, Contact
Degrees Offered: BSN, MSN.

★ 15064 ★ **University of South Florida**
**College of Nursing**
12901 Bruce Downs Blvd.
MDC Box 22
Tampa, FL 33612-4766
Phone: (813)974-9305        Fax: (813)974-5418
Email: pmartini@hsc.usf.edu
Website:     http://www.med.usf.edu/PUBAFF/bsc/nursing1.html
Dr. Patricia Martini Clark, Contact
Fnded: 1956. Degrees Offered: BSN, MSN.

★ 15065 ★ **University of Tampa**
**Department of Nursing**
401 W Kennedy Blvd.
Tampa, FL 33606-1490
Phone: (813)253-6223        Fax: (813)258-7214
Email: nross@alpha.utampa.edu
Website: http://www.utampa.edu
Dr. Nancy Ross, Contact
Fnded: 1931. Degrees Offered: BSN, MSN, MSN/MBA.

★ 15066 ★ **University of West Florida**
**Department of Nursing**
Office of Admissions
11000 University Pkwy.
Pensacola, FL 32514
Phone: (850)474-2884        Fax: (850)474-3360
Email: admissions@uwf.edu
Website: http://www.uwf.edu
Fnded: 1963. Degrees Offered: BSN.

# Georgia

★ 15067 ★ **Albany State University**
**College of Health Professions**
504 College Dr.
Albany, GA 31705
Phone: (912)430-4727        Fax: (912)430-3937
Email: lgrimsl@asurams.edu
Website: http://www.alsnet.peachnet.edu
Linda Grimsley, RN, Contact
Fnded: 1903. Degrees Offered: BSN, MSN.

★ 15068 ★ **Armstrong Atlantic State University**
**Program in Nursing**
11935 Abercorn St.
Savannah, GA 31419-1997
Phone: (912)927-5311        Fax: (912)920-6579
Email: youngsue@mail.armstrong.edu
Website: http://www.armstrong.edu/
Dr. Sue Young, Contact
Fnded: 1935. Degrees Offered: BSN, MN/MHSA, MSN.

★ 15069 ★ **Brenau University**
**School of Health and Science**
1 Centennial Circle
Gainesville, GA 30501
Phone: (770)534-6162
Website: http://www.brenau.edu
Cathy Cobb, Contact
Fnded: 1878. Degrees Offered: BSN, MSN.

★ 15070 ★ **Clayton College & State University**
**Department of Nursing**
5900 North Lee St.
Morrow, GA 30260
Phone: (770)961-3484        Fax: (770)961-3639
Email: lydiamcallister@mail.clayton.edu
Website: http://www.clayton.edu/
Dr. Lydia McAllister, Contact
Fnded: 1969. Degrees Offered: BSN.

★ 15071 ★ **Columbus State University**
**Baccalaureate Degree Nursing Program**
4225 University Ave.
Columbus, GA 31907-2079
Phone: (706)568-2243
Email: mitchell-tibbsmarlene@colstate.edu
Website: http://www.colstate.edu
Dr. Marlene Mitchell-Tibbs, Contact
Fnded: 1958. Degrees Offered: BSN.

★ 15072 ★ **Emory University**
**Nell Hodgson Woodruff School of Nursing**
1520 Clifton Rd. NE
Atlanta, GA 30322
Phone: (404)727-7980        Fax: (404)727-8509
Email: admit@nurse.emory.edu
Website: http://www.nurse.emory.edu
Amanda Leach, Contact
Fnded: 1836. Degrees Offered: BSN, MSN, MSN/MPH, PhD.

★ 15073 ★ **Georgia Baptist College of Nursing of Mercer University**
**Department of Nursing**
274 Boulevard NE
Atlanta, GA 30312
Phone: (678)547-6700        Fax: (678)547-6796
Email: kim.wagner@gbhcs.org
Website: http://www.nursing.mercer.edu/
Kim Hays, Contact
Fnded: 1988. Degrees Offered: BSN.

★ 15074 ★ **Georgia College and State University**
**School of Health Sciences**
CBX 64
231 W Hancock St.
Milledgeville, GA 31061
Phone: (478)445-2633        Fax: (478)445-1913
Email: ckish@mail.gcsu.edu
Website: http://www.gcsu.edu/
Dr. Cheryl Kish, Contact
Fnded: 1889. Degrees Offered: BSN, MSN, MSN/MBA.

★ 15075 ★ **Georgia Southern University**
**Department of Nursing**
PO Box 8158
Statesboro, GA 30460-8158
Phone: (912)681-5056        Fax: (912)681-0536
Email: dhodnicki@gsvms2.cc.gasou.edu
Website: http://www2.gasou.edu/nursing
Dr. Donna Hodnicki, Contact
Fnded: 1906. Degrees Offered: BSN, MSN.

★ 15076 ★ **Georgia Southwestern State University**
**School of Nursing**
800 Wheatley St.
Americus, GA 31709
Phone: (229)931-2275        Fax: (229)931-2288
Email: jmm@canes.gsw.edu
Website: http://www.gsw.edu
Dr. Judith Malchowski, Contact
Fnded: 1906. Degrees Offered: BSN.

★ 15077 ★ **Georgia State University**
**School of Nursing**
University Plaza
Atlanta, GA 30303
Phone: (404)651-3064        Fax: (404)651-4871
Email: bbsmith@gsu.edu
Website: http://www.gsu.edu/
Barbara Smith, Contact
Fnded: 1913. Degrees Offered: BS, MS, PhD.

★ 15078 ★ **Kennesaw State University**
**Department of Baccalaureate Degree Nursing**
1000 Chastain Rd.
Kennesaw, GA 30144
Phone: (770)423-6061        Fax: (770)423-6627
Email: gdorman@ksu.mail.kennesaw.edu
Website: http://www.kennesaw.edu
Dr. Regina Dorman, Contact
Fnded: 1963. Degrees Offered: BSN, MSN.

★ 15079 ★ **LaGrange College**
**Department of Nursing**
601 Broad St.
LaGrange, GA 30240-2999
Phone: (706)880-8220        Fax: (706)880-8029
Email: msauter@lgc.edu
Website: http://www.lgc.edu
Dr. Maranah A. Sauter, Contact
Fnded: 1831. Degrees Offered: BSN.

★ 15080 ★ **Medical College of Georgia**
**School of Nursing**
AA-170-Kelly Bldg.
Augusta, GA 30912
Phone: (706)721-2725        Fax: (706)721-0186
Email: gradadm@mail.mcg.edu
Website: http://www.mcg.edu/
Fnded: 1828. Degrees Offered: BSN, MSN, PhD.

**★ 15081 ★ North Georgia College and State University**
**Department of Nursing**
Rte. 60
Dahlonega, GA 30597
**Phone:** (706)864-1930  **Fax:** (706)864-1845
**Email:** tbarnett@ngcsu.edu
**Website:** http://www.ngcsu.edu
Toni Barnett, Contact
**Fnded:** 1873. **Degrees Offered:** BSN, MSN.

**★ 15082 ★ State University of West Georgia**
**Department of Nursing**
1601 Maple St.
Carrollton, GA 30118
**Phone:** (770)836-6552  **Fax:** (770)836-4409
**Email:** kgrams@westga.edu
**Website:** http://www.westga.edu/
Dr. Kathryn Mary Grams, Contact
**Fnded:** 1933. **Degrees Offered:** BSN.

**★ 15083 ★ Thomas University**
**Division of Nursing**
1501 Millpond Rd.
Thomasville, GA 31792-7490
**Free:** 800-538-9784  **Fax:** (229)226-1653
**Email:** cdaniel@thomasu.edu
**Website:** http://www.thomasu.edu
Crystal Daniel, Contact
**Fnded:** 1950. **Degrees Offered:** BSN.

**★ 15084 ★ Valdosta State University**
**College of Nursing**
1300 N Patterson St.
Valdosta, GA 31698-0130
**Phone:** (229)333-5959  **Fax:** (229)333-7300
**Email:** mreichen@valdosta.edu
**Website:** http://www.valdosta.edu
Dr. MaryAnn Reichenbach, Contact
**Fnded:** 1906. **Degrees Offered:** BSN, MSN.

### Guam

**★ 15085 ★ University of Guam**
**College of Nursing and Health Sciences**
Office of Admissions and Records
UOG Station
Mangilao, GU 96923
**Phone:** (671)735-2210  **Fax:** (671)734-4245
**Email:** admitme@uog9.uog.edu
**Website:** http://uog.edu
Dr. Catalina G. Taijeron, Contact
**Fnded:** 1952. **Degrees Offered:** BSN.

### Hawaii

**★ 15086 ★ Hawaii Pacific University**
**Division of Nursing**
45-045 Kamehameha Highway
Kaneohe, HI 96744-5297
**Phone:** (808)236-3552  **Fax:** (808)236-5818
**Email:** plangeot@hpu.edu
**Website:** http://www.hpu.edu/
Patricia Lange-Otsuka, Contact
**Fnded:** 1965. **Degrees Offered:** BSN, MSN, MSN/MBA.

**★ 15087 ★ University of Hawaii, Hilo**
**Department of Nursing**
200 W Kawili St.
College Hall 8
Hilo, HI 96720
**Phone:** (808)974-7761  **Fax:** (808)974-7665
**Email:** cmukai@hawaii.edu
**Website:** http://www.uhh.hawaii.edu/
Dr. Cecilia Mukai, Contact
**Fnded:** 1970. **Degrees Offered:** BSN.

**★ 15088 ★ University of Hawaii, Manoa**
**School of Nursing and Dental Hygiene**
2528 McCarty Mall
Honolulu, HI 96822
**Phone:** (808)956-5326  **Fax:** (808)956-5296
**Email:** jinouye@hawaii.edu
**Website:** http://www.uhm.hawaii.edu/
Dr. Jillian Inouye, Contact
**Fnded:** 1907. **Degrees Offered:** BS, MS, PhD.

**★ 15089 ★ University of Phoenix, Hawaii Campus**
**College of Nursing and Health Care Sciences**
Honolulu, HI 96801
**Phone:** (808)236-7655
**Email:** Teddy.Sotelo@apollogrp.edu
**Website:** http://www.phoenix.edu/
Teddy Sotelo, Contact
**Degrees Offered:** BSN, MSN.

### Idaho

**★ 15090 ★ Boise State University**
**Department of Nursing**
1910 University Dr.
Boise, ID 83725-0399
**Phone:** (208)426-3783  **Fax:** (208)426-1370
**Email:** ptaylor@boisestate.edu
**Website:** http://www.boisestate.edu
Pat Taylor, Contact
**Fnded:** 1932. **Degrees Offered:** BSN.

**★ 15091 ★ Idaho State University**
**Department of Nursing**
Box 8101
Pocatello, ID 83209-8101
**Phone:** (208)282-3798  **Fax:** (208)282-4476
**Email:** robikris@isu.edu
**Website:** http://www.isu.edu/departments/nursing
Dr. Kris Robinson, Contact
**Fnded:** 1901. **Degrees Offered:** BSN.

**★ 15092 ★ Lewis-Clark State College**
**Division of Nursing**
500 8th Ave.
Lewiston, ID 83501
**Phone:** (208)792-2250  **Fax:** (208)702-2062
**Email:** dblum@lcsc.edu
**Website:** http://www.lcsc.edu/
Dianne Blum, Contact
**Fnded:** 1893. **Degrees Offered:** BSN.

### Illinois

**★ 15093 ★ Aurora University**
**School of Nursing**
347 S Gladstone Ave.
Aurora, IL 60506-4892
**Phone:** (630)844-5130  **Fax:** (630)844-7822
**Email:** mlocklin@aurora.edu
**Website:** http://www.aurora.edu
Dr. Maryanne Locklin, Contact
**Fnded:** 1893. **Degrees Offered:** BSN.

**★ 15094 ★ Benedictine University**
**Department of Nursing**
5700 College Rd.
Lisle, IL 60532
**Phone:** (630)829-6583  **Fax:** (630)829-6551
**Email:** eragland@ben.edu
**Website:** http://www.ben.edu/
Dr. Ethel C. Ragland, Contact
**Fnded:** 1887. **Degrees Offered:** BSN.

**★ 15095 ★ Blessing-Rieman College of Nursing**
**School of Nursing**
Broadway at 11th St.
Box 7005
Quincy, IL 62305-7005
**Phone:** (217)228-5520  **Fax:** (217)223-4661
**Email:** cmgee@blessinghospital.com
**Website:** http://www.brcn.edu/
Connie McGee, Contact
Heather Tourney, Contact
**Degrees Offered:** BS.

**★ 15096 ★ Bradley University**
**Department of Nursing**
Peoria, IL 61625
**Phone:** (309)677-2530  **Fax:** (309)677-2527
**Email:** mmiller@bradley.edu
**Website:** http://www.bradley.edu/
Marilyn Miller, Contact
**Fnded:** 1897. **Degrees Offered:** BSN, MSN.

**★ 15097 ★ Chicago State University**
**College of Nursing and Allied Health Professions**
9501 S Martin Luther King Dr.
Chicago, IL 60628
**Phone:** (773)995-3992  **Fax:** (773)821-2438
**Website:** http://www.csu.edu
Miss Stony McCoy, Contact
**Fnded:** 1867. **Degrees Offered:** BSN.

**★ 15098 ★ Concordia University and West Suburban College of Nursing**
**College of Nursing**
3 Erie Ct.
Oak Park, IL 60302
**Phone:** (708)763-6538  **Fax:** (708)763-1531
**Email:** gpgale77@yahoo.com
Greg Gale, Contact
**Degrees Offered:** BSN.

**★ 15099 ★ DePaul University**
**Department of Nursing**
900 W Fullerton Ave.
Chicago, IL 60614
**Phone:** (773)325-7280  **Fax:** (773)325-7282
**Email:** cwerdric@wppost.depaul.edu
**Website:** http://www.depaul.edu/
Ms. Christine Werdrick, Contact
**Fnded:** 1898. **Degrees Offered:** BS, MS.

**★ 15100 ★ Elmhurst College**
**Deicke Center for Nursing Education**
Elmhurst, IL
**Phone:** (630)617-3344  **Fax:** (630)617-3237
**Email:** lindan@elmhurst.edu
**Website:** http://www.elmhurst.edu/
Dr. Linda Niedringhaus, Contact
**Fnded:** 1871. **Degrees Offered:** BSN.

**★ 15101 ★ Governors State University**
**Division of Nursing and Health Science**
University Park, IL 60466
**Phone:** (708)235-2133  **Fax:** (708)235-2197
**Email:** j-krawcz@govst.edu
**Website:** http://www.govst.edu/
Dr. June Krawczak, Contact
**Fnded:** 1969. **Degrees Offered:** BS, MS.

**★ 15102 ★ Illinois State University**
**Mennonite College of Nursing**
5810 Edwards Hall
Normal, IL 61790-5810
**Phone:** (309)438-2365  **Fax:** (309)438-2620
**Email:** dbkrona@ilstu.edu
**Website:** http://www.mcn.ilstu.edu/
Dr. Donna Konradi, Contact

**Fnded:** 1919. **Degrees Offered:** BSN, MSN.

★ 15103 ★ **Illinois Wesleyan University**
**School of Nursing**
PO Box 2900
Bloomington, IL 61702-2900
**Phone:** (309)556-3051        **Fax:** (309)556-3043
**Email:** dhartweg@titan.iwu.edu
**Website:** http://www.iwu.edu/
Dr. Donna L. Hartweg, Contact
**Fnded:** 1850. **Degrees Offered:** BSN.

★ 15104 ★ **Lakeview College of Nursing**
903 N Logan Ave.
Danville, IL 61832
**Phone:** (217)443-5238        **Fax:** (217)442-2279
**Email:** kholden@lakeviewcol.edu
Kelly Holden, Contact
**Fnded:** 1987. **Degrees Offered:** BSN.

★ 15105 ★ **Lewis University**
**College of Nursing**
One University Parkway
Romeoville, IL 60446
**Phone:** (815)836-5355        **Fax:** (815)838-8306
**Email:** stephelo@lewisu.edu
**Website:** http://www.lewisu.edu
Lois Stephens, Contact
**Fnded:** 1932. **Degrees Offered:** BSN, MSN, MSN/
MBA.

★ 15106 ★ **Loyola University, Chicago**
**Marcella Niehoff School of Nursing**
6525 N Sheridan Rd.
Chicago, IL 60626
**Phone:** (773)508-3261        **Fax:** (773)508-3241
**Email:** mmaurer@luc.edu
**Website:** http://www.luc.edu/
Dr. Marcia C. Maurer, Contact
**Fnded:** 1870. **Degrees Offered:** BSN, MSN, MSN/
MBA, PhD.

★ 15107 ★ **MacMurray College**
**Department of Nursing**
447 E College Ave.
Jacksonville, IL 62650
**Phone:** (217)479-7083        **Fax:** (217)479-7086
**Email:** macbsn@fgi.net
**Website:** http://www.mac.edu/
Tammy L. Reeves, Contact
**Fnded:** 1846. **Degrees Offered:** BSN.

★ 15108 ★ **McKendree College**
**Division of Nursing**
701 College Rd.
Lebanon, IL 62254
**Phone:** (618)537-6943        **Fax:** (618)537-6259
**Email:** pchamber@atlas.mckendree.edu
**Website:** http://www.mckendree.edu/
Pamela Chambers, Contact
**Fnded:** 1828. **Degrees Offered:** BSN.

★ 15109 ★ **Millikin University**
**School of Nursing**
1184 W Main St.
Decatur, IL 62522
**Phone:** (217)424-6348        **Fax:** (217)424-3993
**Email:** ncreason@mail.millikin.edu
**Website:** http://www.millikin.edu
Dr. Nancy Creason, Contact
**Fnded:** 1901. **Degrees Offered:** BSN.

★ 15110 ★ **North Park University**
**School of Nursing**
Chicago, IL
**Phone:** (773)244-5508
**Email:** tjames@northpark.edu

**Website:** http://www.northpark.edu/
Trevor James, Contact
**Fnded:** 1891. **Degrees Offered:** BSN, MS, MSN/
MBA.

★ 15111 ★ **Northern Illinois University**
**School of Nursing**
1240 Normal Rd.
DeKalb, IL 60115-2864
**Phone:** (815)753-6557        **Fax:** (815)753-0814
**Email:** gkruse@niu.edu
**Website:** http://www.niu.edu/
Gayle Kruse, Contact
**Fnded:** 1895. **Degrees Offered:** MS, MSN/MPH.

★ 15112 ★ **Olivet Nazarene University**
**Division of Nursing**
One University Ave.
Bourbonnais, IL 60914
**Phone:** (815)939-5186        **Fax:** (815)935-4991
**Email:** linda.westerberg@apollogrp.edu
**Website:** http://www.olivet.edu/
Linda Westerberg, Contact
**Fnded:** 1907. **Degrees Offered:** BS, MSN.

★ 15113 ★ **Rockford College**
**Department of Nursing**
5050 E State St.
Rockford, IL 61108
**Phone:** (815)226-4050        **Fax:** (815)226-2822
**Email:** stephanie_meiera@rockford.edu
**Website:** http://www.rockford.edu/
Stephanie Meier, Contact
**Fnded:** 1847. **Degrees Offered:** BSN.

★ 15114 ★ **Rush University**
**College of Nursing**
Armour Academic Center
600 S Paulina St., Ste. 440 AR
Chicago, IL 60612
**Phone:** (312)942-7100        **Fax:** (312)942-2219
**Email:** ruadmissions@rushu.rush.edu
**Website:** http://www.rushu.rush.edu/nursing
**Fnded:** 1969. **Degrees Offered:** BSN, DC SC, MSN,
MSN/MM.

★ 15115 ★ **Saint Anthony College of**
**Nursing**
5658 E State St.
Rockford, IL 61108-2468
**Phone:** (815)395-5100        **Fax:** (815)395-2275
**Email:** nancysanders@sacn.edu
**Website:** http://www.sacn.edu/
Nancy Sanders, Contact
**Fnded:** 1915. **Degrees Offered:** BSN.

★ 15116 ★ **Saint Francis Medical Center**
**College of Nursing**
**Baccalaureate Nursing Program**
511 NE Greenleaf Ave.
Peoria, IL 61603-3783
**Phone:** (309)655-2596        **Fax:** (309)624-8973
**Email:** janice.farquharson@osfhealthcare.org
**Website:** http://www.sfmccon.edu
Janice E. Farquharson, Contact
**Fnded:** 1986. **Degrees Offered:** BSN.

★ 15117 ★ **Saint John's College**
**Department of Nursing**
421 N 9th St.
Springfield, IL 62702
**Phone:** (217)525-5628        **Fax:** (217)757-6870
**Email:** bbeasley@.st-johns.org
**Website:** http://www.st-johns.org/collegeofnursing/
Beth Beasley, Contact
**Fnded:** 1886. **Degrees Offered:** BSN.

★ 15118 ★ **Saint Xavier University**
**School of Nursing**
3700 W 103rd St.
Chicago, IL 60655
**Phone:** (773)298-3708        **Fax:** (773)298-3704
**Email:** filipski@sxu.edu
**Website:** http://www.sxu.edu/
Dr. Ann Filipski, Contact
**Fnded:** 1847. **Degrees Offered:** BS, MS, MS/MBA.

★ 15119 ★ **Southern Illinois University,**
**Edwardsville**
**School of Nursing**
Alumni Hall, Rm. 2107
Edwardsville, IL 62026-1066
**Phone:** (618)650-3930        **Fax:** (618)650-3854
**Email:** bstorer@siue.edu
**Website:** http://www.siue.edu/
Bev Storer, Contact
**Fnded:** 1957. **Degrees Offered:** BS, MS.

★ 15120 ★ **Trinity Christian College**
**Department of Nursing**
6601 W College Dr.
Palos Heights, IL 60463
**Free:** 800-748-0085        **Fax:** (708)385-5665
**Email:** admissions@trnty.edu
**Website:** http://www.trnty.edu/
**Fnded:** 1959. **Degrees Offered:** BSN.

★ 15121 ★ **University of Illinois, Chicago**
**College of Nursing**
845 S Damen Ave.
Chicago, IL 60612-7350
**Phone:** (312)996-2184        **Fax:** (312)413-8066
**Email:** leahb@uic.edu
**Website:** http://www.uic.edu/grad
Leah C. Beckwith, Contact
**Fnded:** 1946. **Degrees Offered:** BSN, MS, PhD.

★ 15122 ★ **University of St. Francis**
**Saint Joseph College of Nursing and**
**Allied Health**
500 Wilcox St.
Joliet, IL
**Phone:** (815)740-3395        **Fax:** (815)740-3537
**Email:** drakoski@stfrancis.edu
**Website:** http://www.stfrancis.edu/
Donna Rakoski, Contact
**Fnded:** 1920. **Degrees Offered:** BSN, MSN.

### Indiana

★ 15123 ★ **Anderson University**
**Department of Nursing**
1100 E 5th St.
Anderson, IN 46012
**Phone:** (765)641-4390        **Fax:** (765)641-3851
**Email:** sdailey@anderson.edu
**Website:** http://www.anderson.edu
Sharon Dailey, Contact
**Fnded:** 1917. **Degrees Offered:** BSN

★ 15124 ★ **Ball State University**
**School of Nursing**
Muncie, IN 47306
**Phone:** (765)285-5764        **Fax:** (765)285-2169
**Email:** mryan@bsgw.bsu.edu
**Website:** http://www.bsu.edu
Dr. Marilyn Ryan, RN, Contact
**Fnded:** 1918. **Degrees Offered:** BS, MS.

★ 15125 ★ **Bethel College**
**Department of Nursing**
1001 W McKinley St.
Mishawaka, IN 46545
**Phone:** (219)257-2594        **Fax:** (219)257-3326
**Email:** davidhr@bethel-in.edu

**Website:** http://www.bethel-in.edu/
Dr. Ruth E. Davidhizar, Contact
**Fnded:** 1947. **Degrees Offered:** BSN.


★ **15126** ★ **Goshen College**
**Department of Nursing**
1700 S Main St.
Goshen, IN 46526
**Phone:** (219)535-7535　　　**Fax:** (219)535-7609
**Email:** admissions@goshen.edu
**Website:** http://www.goshen.edu/
**Fnded:** 1894. **Degrees Offered:** BSN.


★ **15127** ★ **Indiana State University**
**School of Nursing**
Terre Haute, IN 47809
**Phone:** (812)237-2317　　　**Fax:** (812)237-4300
**Email:** nulink@befac.indstate.edu
**Website:** http://web.indstate.edu
Sylvia Cruz Link, Contact
**Fnded:** 1865. **Degrees Offered:** BS, MS.


★ **15128** ★ **Indiana University,**
　**Bloomington**
**Department of Nursing**
Sycamore Hall, Rm. 401
Bloomington, IN 47405
**Phone:** (812)855-2592　　　**Fax:** (812)855-6986
**Email:** lwrasse@indiana.edu
**Website:** http://www.indiana.edu/
Lisa Wrasse, Contact
**Fnded:** 1820. **Degrees Offered:** BSN.


★ **15129** ★ **Indiana University, East**
**Division of Nursing**
2325 Chester Blvd.
Richmond, IN 47374-1289
**Phone:** (765)973-8257　　　**Fax:** (765)973-8220
**Email:** jrains@indiana.edu
**Website:** http://www.iue.indiana.edu
Jan Robey Marker, Contact
**Fnded:** 1971. **Degrees Offered:** BSN.


★ **15130** ★ **Indiana University, Kokomo**
**Division of Nursing**
2300 S Washington St.
PO Box 9003
Kokomo, IN 46904-9003
**Phone:** (765)455-9384　　　**Fax:** (765)455-9421
**Email:** lseaman@iuk.edu
**Website:** http://www.iuk.Indiana.edu/
Lori A. Seaman, Contact
**Fnded:** 1945. **Degrees Offered:** BSN.


★ **15131** ★ **Indiana University, Northwest**
**Division of Nursing**
3400 Broadway
Gary, IN 46408
**Phone:** (219)980-6549　　　**Fax:** (219)980-6578
**Email:** lgraves@iun.edu
**Website:** http://www.indiana.edu/
Ms. Laura J. Graves, Contact
**Fnded:** 1959. **Degrees Offered:** BSN.


★ **15132** ★ **Indiana University, Purdue**
　**University, Fort Wayne**
**Department of Nursing**
2010 E Coliseum Blvd.
Fort Wayne, IN 46805
**Phone:** (219)481-5446　　　**Fax:** (219)481-5767
**Email:** leinbach@ipfw.edu
**Website:** http://www.ipfw.edu/
Nancy Leinbach, Contact
**Fnded:** 1917. **Degrees Offered:** BSN, MS.


★ **15133** ★ **Indiana University, Purdue**
　**University, Indianapolis**
**School of Nursing**
1111 Middle Dr., NU 136
Indianapolis, IN 46202
**Phone:** (317)274-3115　　　**Fax:** (317)274-2996
**Email:** smorriss@iupui.edu
**Website:** http://www.iupui.edu/~nursing/index.html
Dr. Sue Morrissey, Contact
**Fnded:** 1969. **Degrees Offered:** BSN, MSN, MSN/MPH, PhD.


★ **15134** ★ **Indiana University, South**
　**Bend**
**School of Nursing and Health**
　**Professions**
1700 Mishawaka
PO Box 7111
South Bend, IN 46634-7111
**Phone:** (219)237-4571　　　**Fax:** (219)237-4461
**Email:** nursing@iusb.edu
**Website:** http://www.iusb.edu
**Fnded:** 1922. **Degrees Offered:** BSN.


★ **15135** ★ **Indiana University, Southeast**
**Division of Nursing**
4201 Grant Line Rd., LF-102
New Albany, IN 47150
**Phone:** (812)941-2283　　　**Fax:** (812)941-2687
**Email:** bhackett@ius.edu
**Website:** http://www.ius.indiana.edu/
Brenda Hackett, Contact
**Fnded:** 1941. **Degrees Offered:** BSN.


★ **15136** ★ **Indiana Wesleyan University**
**Division of Nursing Education**
4201 S Washington St.
Marion, IN 46953
**Phone:** (765)677-2266　　　**Fax:** (765)677-2284
**Email:** sstranah@indwes.edu
**Website:** http://www.indwes.edu/
Dr. Susan D. Stranahan, Contact
**Fnded:** 1920. **Degrees Offered:** BS, MS.


★ **15137** ★ **Marian College**
**Department of Nursing and Nutritional**
　**Science**
3200 Cold Spring Rd.
Indianapolis, IN 46222-1997
**Phone:** (317)955-6157　　　**Fax:** (317)955-6448
**Email:** bhart@marian.edu
**Website:** http://www.marian.edu/
Barbara Hart, RN,BSN, Contact
**Fnded:** 1851. **Degrees Offered:** BSN.


★ **15138** ★ **Purdue University**
**School of Nursing**
1337 Johnson Hall of Nursing
West Lafayette, IN 47907
**Phone:** (765)494-4030　　　**Fax:** (765)494-6339
**Email:** pcrogers@nursing.purdue.edu
**Website:** http://www.purdue.edu/
Dr. Patricia Coyle-Rogers, Contact
**Fnded:** 1869. **Degrees Offered:** BS.


★ **15139** ★ **Purdue University, Calumet**
**School of Nursing**
2200 169th St.
Hammond, IN 46323-2094
**Phone:** (219)989-2815　　　**Fax:** (219)989-2848
**Email:** psgerard@calumet.purdue.edu
**Website:** http://www.calumet.purdue.edu
Dr. Peggy Gerard, Contact
**Fnded:** 1951. **Degrees Offered:** BS, MS.


★ **15140** ★ **Saint Mary's College**
**Department of Nursing**
120A LeMans
Notre Dame, IN 46556
**Phone:** (219)284-4587　　　**Fax:** (219)284-4716
**Email:** jfreze@saintmarys.edu
**Website:** http://www.saintmarys.edu
Jenny Freeze, Contact
**Fnded:** 1844. **Degrees Offered:** BS.


★ **15141** ★ **University of Evansville**
**Department of Nursing**
1800 Lincoln Ave.
Evansville, IN 47722
**Phone:** (812)479-2550　　　**Fax:** (812)479-2717
**Email:** rb7@cedars.evansville.edu
**Website:** http://www.evansville.edu
Dr. Rita S. Behnke, Contact
**Fnded:** 1854. **Degrees Offered:** BSN.


★ **15142** ★ **University of Indianapolis**
**School of Nursing**
1400 E Hanna Ave.
Indianapolis, IN 46227-3697
**Phone:** (317)788-3471　　　**Fax:** (317)788-3542
**Email:** siccardi@uindy.edu
**Website:** http://www.uindy.edu/
Anita Siccardi, Contact
**Fnded:** 1902. **Degrees Offered:** BSN, MSN, MSN/MBA.


★ **15143** ★ **University of Saint Francis**
**Department of Nursing**
2701 Spring St.
Fort Wayne, IN 46808
**Phone:** (219)434-3284　　　**Fax:** (219)434-7404
**Email:** ngillespie@sf.edu
**Website:** http://www.sf.edu
Dr. Nancy Gillespie, Contact
**Fnded:** 1890. **Degrees Offered:** BSN, MSN.


★ **15144** ★ **University of Southern**
　**Indiana**
**School of Nursing and Health**
　**Professions**
8600 University Blvd.
Evansville, IN 47712
**Phone:** (812)465-1171　　　**Fax:** (812)465-7092
**Email:** mvandeve@usi.edu
**Website:** http://www.usi.edu
Dr. Melissa Vandeveer, Contact
**Fnded:** 1965. **Degrees Offered:** BSN, MSN.


★ **15145** ★ **Valparaiso University**
**College of Nursing**
Valparaiso, IN 46383-6493
**Phone:** (219)464-5289　　　**Fax:** (219)464-5425
**Email:** janet.brown@valpo.edu
**Website:** http://www.valpo.edu/
Dr. Janet M. Brown, Contact
**Fnded:** 1859. **Degrees Offered:** BSN, MSN.

### Iowa

★ **15146** ★ **Allen College**
**Nursing Program**
1825 Logan Ave.
Waterloo, IA 50703
**Phone:** (319)226-2002
**Website:** http://www.allencollege.edu
Barb Sieble, Contact
**Fnded:** 1989. **Degrees Offered:** BSN, MSN.


★ **15147** ★ **Briar Cliff College**
**Department of Nursing**
3303 Rebecca St.
Sioux City, IA 51104
**Phone:** (712)279-5458　　　**Fax:** (712)279-1698

**Email:** daumer@briarcliff.edu
**Website:** http://www.briarcliff.edu
Ruth Daumer, Contact
**Fnded:** 1930. **Degrees Offered:** BSN.


★ 15148 ★ **Clarke College**
**Department of Nursing and Health**
1550 Clark Dr.
Dubuque, IA 52001-3198
**Phone:** (319)588-6361
**Email:** mmooney@clarke.edu
**Website:** http://www.clarke.edu
Dr. Mary Margaret Mooney, Contact
**Fnded:** 1843. **Degrees Offered:** BS, MSN.


★ 15149 ★ **Coe College**
**Department of Nursing**
1220 1st Ave. NE
Cedar Rapids, IA 52402
**Phone:** (319)369-8120          **Fax:** (319)399-8121
**Email:** johrt@coe.edu
**Website:** http://www.coe.edu/
H. Jule Ohrt, Contact
**Fnded:** 1851. **Degrees Offered:** BSN.


★ 15150 ★ **Grand View College**
**Division of Nursing**
1200 Grandview Ave.
Des Moines, IA 50316-1599
**Phone:** (515)263-6091          **Fax:** (515)263-6077
**Email:** dkonopka@gvc.edu
**Website:** http://www.gvc.edu
Del Konopka, Contact
**Fnded:** 1896. **Degrees Offered:** BSN.


★ 15151 ★ **Iowa Wesleyan College**
**Division of Nursing**
601 N Main St.
Mount Pleasant, IA 52641
**Free:** 800-582-2383          **Fax:** (319)385-6296
**Email:** jlynes@iwc.edu
**Website:** http://www.iwc.edu/
Jim Lynes, Contact
**Fnded:** 1842. **Degrees Offered:** BSN.


★ 15152 ★ **Luther College**
**Department of Nursing**
700 College Dr.
Decorah, IA 52101
**Phone:** (319)387-1057          **Fax:** (319)387-2149
**Email:** greenru@luther.edu
**Website:** http://www.luther.edu
Ruth Green, Contact
**Fnded:** 1861. **Degrees Offered:** BA.


★ 15153 ★ **Marycrest International**
**University**
**Department of Nursing**
1607 W 12th St.
Davenport, IA 52804-4096
**Phone:** (319)326-9278          **Fax:** (319)326-9473
**Email:** lhintze@mcrest.edu
**Website:** http://www.mcrest.edu
Dr. Louise Hintze, Contact
**Fnded:** 1939. **Degrees Offered:** BSN.


★ 15154 ★ **Morningside College**
**Department of Nursing Education**
1501 Morningside Ave.
Sioux City, IA 51106
**Phone:** (712)274-5239          **Fax:** (712)274-5101
**Email:** rap002@morningside.edu
**Website:** http://www.morningside.edu/
Richard A. Petersen, Contact
**Fnded:** 1894. **Degrees Offered:** BSN.


★ 15155 ★ **Mount Mercy College**
**Department of Nursing**
1330 Elmhurst Dr. NE
Cedar Rapids, IA 52402-4749
**Free:** 800-248-4504
**Email:** mtarbox@mmc.mtmercy.edu
**Website:** http://www.mtmercy.edu
Dr. Mary P. Tarbox, Contact
**Fnded:** 1928. **Degrees Offered:** BS.


★ 15156 ★ **University of Iowa**
**College of Nursing**
444 Nursing Bldg.
Iowa City, IA 52242
**Phone:** (319)334-4667          **Fax:** (319)335-9990
**Email:** tracy-middleton@uiowa.edu
**Website:** http://www.nursing.uiowa.edu/
Tracy Middleton, Contact
**Fnded:** 1847. **Degrees Offered:** BSN, MSN, MSN/
MBA, PhD.


## Kansas

★ 15157 ★ **Baker University**
**School of Nursing**
1500 SW 10th St.
Topeka, KS 66604-1353
**Phone:** (785)354-5829          **Fax:** (785)354-5832
**Website:** http://www.bakeru.edu
Peggy Geier, Contact
**Fnded:** 1858. **Degrees Offered:** BSN.


★ 15158 ★ **Bethel College**
**Department of Nursing**
300 E 27th St.
North Newton, KS 67117
**Phone:** (316)283-2500          **Fax:** (316)284-5286
**Email:** moore@bethelks.edu
**Website:** http://www.bethelks.edu/
Dr. Carol Moore, Contact
**Fnded:** 1887. **Degrees Offered:** BSN.


★ 15159 ★ **Emporia State University**
**Newman Division of Nursing**
1127 Chestnut St.
Emporia, KS 66801-2523
**Phone:** (316)343-6800          **Fax:** (316)341-7871
**Email:** calhounj@emporia.edu
**Website:** http://www.emporia.edu/
Dr. Judith E. Calhoun, Contact
**Fnded:** 1863. **Degrees Offered:** BSN.


★ 15160 ★ **Fort Hays State University**
**Department of Nursing**
600 Park St.
Stroup Hall 122 A
Hays, KS 67601-4099
**Phone:** (785)628-4327          **Fax:** (785)628-4080
**Email:** ecurl@fhsu.edu
**Website:** http://www.fhsu.edu/
Dr. Eileen Deges Curl, Contact
**Fnded:** 1902. **Degrees Offered:** BSN, MSN.


★ 15161 ★ **Kansas Wesleyan University**
**Department of Nursing Education**
100 E Claflin Ave.
Salina, KS 67401
**Phone:** (785)827-5541          **Fax:** (785)827-0927
**Email:** pbrown@kwu.edu
**Website:** http://www.kwu.edu
Dr. Patricia L. Brown, Contact
**Fnded:** 1886. **Degrees Offered:** BSN.


★ 15162 ★ **MidAmerican Nazarene**
**University**
**Division of Nursing**
2030 E College Way
Olathe, KS 66062-1899
**Phone:** (913)782-3750          **Fax:** (913)791-3408
**Email:** psmith@mnu.edu
**Website:** http://www.mnu.edu
Dr. Palma Lenn Smith, Contact
**Fnded:** 1966. **Degrees Offered:** BSN.


★ 15163 ★ **Newman University**
**Division of Nursing**
3100 McCormick Ave.
Wichita, KS 67213
**Phone:** (316)942-4291          **Fax:** (316)942-4483
**Email:** jeffersj@newmanu.edu
**Website:** http://www.newmanu.edu
Dr. Jeanette Jeffers, Contact
**Fnded:** 1933. **Degrees Offered:** BSN, MSN.


★ 15164 ★ **Pittsburg State University**
**Department of Nursing**
1701 S Broadway
Pittsburg, KS 66762
**Phone:** (316)235-4431          **Fax:** (316)235-4449
**Email:** ckeil@pittstate.edu
**Website:** http://www.pittstate.edu/
Dr. Carolyn Keil, Contact
**Fnded:** 1903. **Degrees Offered:** BSN, MSN


★ 15165 ★ **Southwestern College**
**Nursing Program**
Winfield, KS
**Phone:** (316)221-8306          **Fax:** (316)229-2713
**Email:** mbutler@sckans.edu
**Website:** http://www.sckans.edu/
Dr. Martha R. Butler, Contact
**Fnded:** 1885. **Degrees Offered:** BSN.


★ 15166 ★ **University of Kansas**
**School of Nursing**
3901 Rainbow Blvd.
Kansas City, KS 66160-7501
**Phone:** (913)588-1619          **Fax:** (913)588-1615
**Email:** soninfo@kumc.edu
**Website:** http://www.kumc.edu/instruction/nursing/de-
grees.htm
Dr. Rita Clifford, Contact
**Fnded:** 1866. **Degrees Offered:** BSN, MS, MS/
MSHA, PhD.


★ 15167 ★ **Washburn University of**
**Topeka**
**School of Nursing**
1700 Southwest College Ave.
Topeka, KS 66621
**Phone:** (785)231-1032          **Fax:** (785)231-1032
**Email:** zzalle@washburn.edu
**Website:** http://www.washburn.edu/
Mary V. Allen, Contact
**Fnded:** 1865. **Degrees Offered:** BSN.


★ 15168 ★ **Wichita State University**
**School of Nursing**
1845 Farmount
Wichita, KS 67260-0041
**Phone:** (316)978-3610          **Fax:** (316)978-3094
**Email:** huckstad@chp.twsu.edu
**Website:** http://www.twsu.edu
Dr. Alicia Huckstadt, Contact
**Fnded:** 1895. **Degrees Offered:** BSN, MSN, MSN/
MBA.


## Kentucky

★ 15169 ★ **Bellarmine College**
**Allan and Donna Lansing School of**
**Nursing and Health Sciences**
2001 Newburg Rd.
Louisville, KY 40205-0671
**Phone:** (502)452-8414          **Fax:** (502)452-8058
**Email:** maggie.miller@bellarmine.edu

**Website:** http://www.bellarmine.edu
Dr. Margaret E. Miller, Contact
**Fnded:** 1950. **Degrees Offered:** BSN, MSN, MSN/MBA.

**★ 15170 ★ Berea College**
**Department of Nursing**
CPO 1794
Berea, KY 40404
**Phone:** (859)985-3384     **Fax:** (859)985-3917
**Email:** pam_farley@berea.edu
**Website:** http://www.berea.edu
Dr. Pam Farley, Contact
**Fnded:** 1855. **Degrees Offered:** BS.

**★ 15171 ★ Eastern Kentucky University**
**Department of Baccalaureate and**
**    Graduate Nursing**
223 Rowlett Bldg.
Richmond, KY 40475
**Phone:** (606)622-1971     **Fax:** (606)622-1972
**Email:** bsnbaugh@acs.eku.edu
**Website:** http://www.eku.edu/
Dr. Carol Baugh, Contact
**Fnded:** 1906. **Degrees Offered:** BSN, MSN.

**★ 15172 ★ Midway College**
**Program in Nursing (Baccalaureate)**
512 E Stephens St.
Midway, KY 40347
**Phone:** (606)846-5743
**Email:** dweaver@midway.edu
**Website:** http://www.midway.edu
Dr. Diana Weaver, Contact
**Fnded:** 1847. **Degrees Offered:** BSN.

**★ 15173 ★ Morehead State University**
**Department of Nursing and Allied Health**
**    Sciences**
UPO 715
Morehead, KY 40351
**Phone:** (606)783-5173     **Fax:** (606)783-5039
**Email:** j.gross@morehead/st.edu
**Website:** http://www.moreheadstate.edu
Dr. Janet J. Gross, Contact
**Fnded:** 1922. **Degrees Offered:** BSN.

**★ 15174 ★ Murray State University**
**Department of Nursing**
PO Box 9
120 Mason Hall
Murray, KY 42071-0009
**Phone:** (270)762-6671     **Fax:** (502)762-6662
**Email:** nancey.france@murraystate.edu
**Website:** http://www.murraystate.edu
Dr. Nancey E. M. France, Contact
**Fnded:** 1922. **Degrees Offered:** BSN, MSN.

**★ 15175 ★ Northern Kentucky University**
**Department of Nursing**
Highland Heights, KY 41076
**Phone:** (859)572-5178     **Fax:** (859)572-6098
**Email:** robinson@nku.edu
**Website:** http://www.nku.edu/
Dr. Denise Robinson, Contact
**Fnded:** 1968. **Degrees Offered:** BSN, MSN.

**★ 15176 ★ Spalding University**
**School of Nursing and Health Sciences**
851 S 4th St.
Louisville, KY 40203-2188
**Phone:** (502)585-7125     **Fax:** (502)588-7175
**Email:** ccrabtree@spalding.edu
**Website:** http://www.spalding.edu/
Dr. Cynthia R. Crabtree, Contact
**Fnded:** 1814. **Degrees Offered:** BSN, MSN.

**★ 15177 ★ Thomas More College**
**Program in Nursing**
Crestview Hills, KY 41017
**Phone:** (859)344-3508     **Fax:** (859)344-3345
**Website:** http://www.thomasmore.edu/
**Fnded:** 1921. **Degrees Offered:** BSN.

**★ 15178 ★ University of Kentucky**
**College of Nursing**
Rm. 309 CON/HSLC
Lexington, KY 40536-0232
**Phone:** (606)323-5108     **Fax:** (606)323-1057
**Email:** conss@pop.uky.edu
**Website:** http://www.uky.edu/
**Fnded:** 1865. **Degrees Offered:** BSN, MSN, PhD.

**★ 15179 ★ University of Louisville**
**School of Nursing**
555 S Floyd St.
Louisville, KY 40292
**Phone:** (502)852-5366     **Fax:** (502)852-8783
**Email:** cammccu01@gwise.louisville.edu
**Website:** http://www.louisville.edu/nursing/
Dr. Cynthia McCurren, Contact
**Fnded:** 1798. **Degrees Offered:** BSN, MSN.

**★ 15180 ★ Western Kentucky University**
**Department of Nursing**
1 Big Red Way
Bowling Green, KY 42101-3576
**Phone:** (270)745-3490     **Fax:** (502)745-3392
**Email:** beverly.siegrist@wku.edu
**Website:** http://www.wku.edu
Dr. Beverly C. Siegrist, Contact
**Fnded:** 1906. **Degrees Offered:** BSN, MS.

### Louisiana

**★ 15181 ★ Dillard University**
**Division of Nursing**
2601 Gentilly Blvd.
New Orleans, LA 70122
**Phone:** (504)286-4717     **Fax:** (504)286-4861
**Fnded:** 1869. **Degrees Offered:** BSN.

**★ 15182 ★ Grambling State University**
**School of Nursing**
PO Box 1192
Grambling, LA 71245
**Phone:** (318)274-2897     **Fax:** (318)274-3491
Rhonda Hensley, Contact
**Fnded:** 1901. **Degrees Offered:** BSN, MSN.

**★ 15183 ★ Louisiana College**
**Department of Nursing**
PO Box 556
Pineville, LA 71359-0556
**Phone:** (318)487-7127     **Fax:** (318)487-7488
**Website:** http://www.lacollege.edu
**Fnded:** 1906. **Degrees Offered:** BSN.

**★ 15184 ★ Louisiana State University**
**    Health Sciences Center**
**School of Nursing**
1900 Gravier St.
New Orleans, LA 70112
**Phone:** (504)568-4107     **Fax:** (504)568-5853
**Email:** ahufft@lsuhc.edu
**Website:** http://www.lsumc.edu/
Dr. Anita Hufft, Contact
**Fnded:** 1931. **Degrees Offered:** BSN, DNS, MN.

**★ 15185 ★ Loyola University, New**
**    Orleans**
**Program in Nursing**
6363 St. Charles Ave.
New Orleans, LA 70118
**Phone:** (504)865-3142     **Fax:** (504)865-3254
**Email:** bwilson@loyno.edu
**Website:** http://www.loyno.edu/
Dr. Billie Ann Wilson, Contact
**Fnded:** 1912. **Degrees Offered:** BSN.

**★ 15186 ★ McNeese State University**
**College of Nursing**
PO Box 90415
Lake Charles, LA 70609-0415
**Phone:** (318)475-5733     **Fax:** (318)475-5702
**Email:** pwolfe@acc.mcneese.edu
**Website:** http://www.mcneese.edu
Dr. Peggy Wolfe, Contact
**Fnded:** 1939. **Degrees Offered:** BSN, MSN.

**★ 15187 ★ Nicholls State University**
**Department of Nursing**
PO Box 2143
Thibodaux, LA 70310
**Phone:** (504)448-4696     **Fax:** (504)448-4923
**Email:** nurs-tjs@mail.nich.edu
**Website:** http://www.nicholls.edu
Dr. Thomas Smith, Contact
**Fnded:** 1948. **Degrees Offered:** BSN.

**★ 15188 ★ Northwestern State University**
**    of Louisiana**
**Division of Nursing**
1800 Line Ave.
Shreveport, LA 71101
**Phone:** (318)677-3100     **Fax:** (318)677-3127
**Website:** http://www.nsula.edu/
Norann Planchock, Contact
**Fnded:** 1884. **Degrees Offered:** BSN.

**★ 15189 ★ Our Lady of Holy Cross**
**    College**
**Division of Nursing**
4123 Woodland Dr.
New Orleans, LA 70131
**Phone:** (504)394-7744     **Fax:** (504)391-2421
**Email:** smcneely@olhcc.edu
**Website:** http://www.olhcc.edu/
Stanton McNeeley, Contact
**Fnded:** 1916. **Degrees Offered:** BSN.

**★ 15190 ★ Southeastern Louisiana**
**    University**
**School of Nursing**
4849 Essen Lane
Baton Rouge, LA 70808
**Phone:** (504)765-2324
**Email:** sthornhill@selu.edu
**Website:** http://www.selu.edu/Academics/Nursing/
Dr. Kay Thornhill, Contact
**Fnded:** 1925. **Degrees Offered:** BSN.

**★ 15191 ★ Southern University and A&M**
**    College**
**School of Nursing**
PO Box 11784
Baton Rouge, LA 70813
**Phone:** (225)771-2663     **Fax:** (225)771-3547
**Email:** sandrabrown@suson.subr.edu
**Website:** http://www.subr.edu
Dr. Sandra C. Brown, Contact
**Fnded:** 1880. **Degrees Offered:** BSN, MSN, PhD.

**★ 15192 ★ University of Louisiana,**
**    Lafayette**
**College of Nursing**
PO Box 43810
Lafayette, LA 70504-3810
**Phone:** (337)482-5617     **Fax:** (337)482-5053
**Email:** carolyn@louisiana.edu
**Website:** http://www.louisiana.edu
Dr. Carolyn Delahoussaye, Contact

**Fnded:** 1898. **Degrees Offered:** BSN, MSN.


★ **15193** ★ **University of Louisiana,**
  **Monroe**
**School of Nursing**
700 University Ave.
Monroe, LA 71209-0460
**Phone:** (318)342-1460          **Fax:** (318)342-1567
**Email:** nucorder@ulm.edu
**Website:** http://www.nlu.edu
Dr. Jan B. Corder, Contact
**Fnded:** 1931. **Degrees Offered:** BS.


★ **15194** ★ **University of Phoenix,**
  **Louisiana Campus**
**College of Nursing and Health Care**
  **Sciences**
Metairie, LA
**Phone:** (225)927-4443
**Email:** Brent.Fitch@apollogrp.edu
**Website:** http://www.phoenix.edu/
Brent Fitch, Contact
**Degrees Offered:** BSN, MSN.

## Maine

★ **15195** ★ **Husson College**
**School of Nursing**
1 College Cir.
Bangor, ME 04401-2999
**Phone:** (207)941-7065          **Fax:** (207)941-7883
**Email:** sheam@husson.edu/
**Website:** http://www.husson.edu
Mary L. Shea, Contact
**Fnded:** 1898. **Degrees Offered:** BSN, MSN.


★ **15196** ★ **Saint Joseph's College**
**Department of Nursing**
278 Whites Bridge Rd.
Standish, ME 04084-5263
**Phone:** (207)893-7957          **Fax:** (207)892-7423
**Email:** lconover@sjcme.edu
**Website:** http://www.sjcme.edu/
Dr. Linda Conover, Contact
**Fnded:** 1912. **Degrees Offered:** BSN, MSN.


★ **15197** ★ **University of Maine**
**School of Nursing**
218 Dunn Hall
Orono, ME 04469
**Phone:** (207)581-2605          **Fax:** (207)581-2585
**Email:** cwood@maine.edu
**Website:** http://www.ume.maine.edu/~graduate/
Dr. Carol Wood, Contact
**Fnded:** 1865. **Degrees Offered:** BSN, MSN.


★ **15198** ★ **University of Maine, Fort Kent**
**Department of Nursing**
25 Pleasant St.
Fort Kent, ME 04743-1292
**Phone:** (207)834-7582          **Fax:** (207)834-7577
**Email:** pcaron@maine.edu
**Website:** http://www.umfk.maine.edu/
Pam Caron, Contact
**Fnded:** 1878. **Degrees Offered:** BSN.


★ **15199** ★ **University of New England**
**Department of Nursing**
11 Hills Beach Rd.
Biddeford, ME 04005
**Phone:** (207)283-0171          **Fax:** (207)282-6379
**Email:** cspirito@mailbox.une.edu
**Website:** http://www.une.edu/
Dr. Carl Spirito, Contact
**Fnded:** 1831. **Degrees Offered:** BSN, MSN.


★ **15200** ★ **University of Southern Maine**
**College of Nursing and Health**
  **Professions**
PO Box 9300
Portland, ME 04104-9300
**Phone:** (207)780-4136          **Fax:** (207)780-4997
**Email:** phealy@usm.maine.edu
**Website:** http://www.usm.maine.edu/con/
Dr. Phyllis Healy, Contact
**Fnded:** 1878. **Degrees Offered:** BS, MS.

## Manitoba

★ **15201** ★ **Brandon University**
**School of Health Studies**
270 18th St.
Brandon, MB, Canada R7A 6A9
**Phone:** (204)727-7403          **Fax:** (204)728-7292
**Email:** demas@brandonu.ca
**Website:** http://www.brandonu.ca/
Cathy Demas, Contact
**Fnded:** 1899. **Degrees Offered:** BSCN.


★ **15202** ★ **University of Manitoba**
**Faculty of Nursing**
Helen Glass Centre for Nursing
Winnipeg, MB, Canada R3T 2N2
**Phone:** (204)474-9317          **Fax:** (204)474-7682
**Email:** karen_chalmers@umanitoba.ca
**Website:** http://www.umanitoba.ca/
Dr. Karen Chalmers, Contact
**Fnded:** 1877. **Degrees Offered:** BN, MN.

## Maryland

★ **15203** ★ **Bowie State University**
**Program in Nursing**
14000 Jericho Park Rd.
Bowie, MD 20715
**Phone:** (301)860-3202          **Fax:** (301)860-3222
**Email:** ncoleman@bowiestate.edu
**Website:** http://www.bowiestate.edu
Nethelyne Coleman, Contact
**Fnded:** 1865. **Degrees Offered:** BSN, MSN.


★ **15204** ★ **College of Notre Dame of**
  **Maryland**
**Department of Nursing**
4701 N Charles St.
Baltimore, MD 21210-2476
**Phone:** (410)532-5500
**Email:** wec@ndm.edu
**Website:** http://www.ndm.edu/
**Fnded:** 1873. **Degrees Offered:** BSN.


★ **15205** ★ **Columbia Union College**
**Nursing Department**
7600 Flower Ave.
Takoma Park, MD 20912
**Phone:** (301)891-4144          **Fax:** (301)891-4191
**Email:** jessex@cuc.edu
**Website:** http://www.cuc.edu/
Joy Essex, Contact
**Fnded:** 1904. **Degrees Offered:** BSN.


★ **15206** ★ **Coppin State College**
**Helene Fuld School of Nursing**
2500 W North Ave.
Baltimore, MD 21215-3698
**Phone:** (410)383-5740          **Fax:** (410)462-3032
**Email:** dboyd@wye.coppin.edu
**Website:** http://www.coppin.edu/
Darryl A. Boyd, Contact
**Fnded:** 1900. **Degrees Offered:** BSN.


★ **15207** ★ **Johns Hopkins University**
**School of Nursing**
525 N Wolfe St.
Baltimore, MD 21205-2110
**Phone:** (410)955-7548          **Fax:** (410)614-7086
**Email:** orourke@son.jhmi.edu
**Website:** http://www.son.jhmi.edu/
Mary O'Rourke, Contact
**Fnded:** 1876. **Degrees Offered:** BS, MSN, MSN/
MBA, MSN/MPH, PhD.


★ **15208** ★ **Salisbury State University**
**Program in Nursing**
1101 Camden Ave.
Salisbury, MD 21801
**Phone:** (410)543-6420          **Fax:** (410)548-3313
**Email:** rmcarroll@ssu.edu
**Website:**   http://www.ssu.edu/Schools/Henson/De-
grees.html
Dr. Ruth M. Carroll, Contact
**Fnded:** 1925. **Degrees Offered:** BS, MS.


★ **15209** ★ **Towson University**
**Department of Nursing**
8000 York Rd.
Towson, MD 21252-0001
**Phone:** (410)704-4212          **Fax:** (410)704-4325
**Email:** ckielinen@towson.edu
**Website:** http://www.towson.edu
Dr. Cynthia E. Kielinen, Contact
**Fnded:** 1866. **Degrees Offered:** BS, MS.


★ **15210** ★ **University of Maryland**
**School of Nursing**
655 W Lombard St., Rm. 102
Baltimore, MD 21201-1579
**Phone:** (410)706-0489          **Fax:** (410)706-7238
**Email:** moore@son.umaryland.edu
**Website:** http://www.umaryland.edu/
Cassandra Smith Moore, Contact
**Fnded:** 1807. **Degrees Offered:** BSN, MS, MS/MBA,
PhD.


★ **15211** ★ **Villa Julie College**
**Nursing**
1525 Greenspring Valley Rd.
Stevenson, MD 21153-0641
**Fax:** (410)486-3552
**Email:** fac-feus@mail.vjc.edu
**Website:** http://www.vjc.edu/
Dr. Judith A. Feustle, Contact
**Fnded:** 1952. **Degrees Offered:** BS.

## Massachusetts

★ **15212** ★ **American International**
  **College**
**Divison of Nursing**
1000 State St.
Springfield, MA 01109
**Phone:** (413)205-3800          **Fax:** (413)205-3943
**Website:** http://www.aic.edu
Dr. Peter J. Miller, Contact
**Fnded:** 1885. **Degrees Offered:** BSN


★ **15213** ★ **Anna Maria College**
**Department of Nursing**
10 Sunset Ln.
Paxton, MA 01612-1198
**Phone:** (508)829-3316          **Fax:** (508)849-3362
**Email:** asilveri@annamaria.edu
**Website:** http://www.annamaria.edu
Audrey Marie Silveri, RN, Contact
**Fnded:** 1946. **Degrees Offered:** BSN

**★ 15214 ★ Atlantic Union College**
**Department of Nursing**
BS Coordinator
338 Main St.
South Lancaster, MA 01561
**Phone:** (978)368-2402     **Fax:** (978)368-2015
**Email:** mrittenhouse@atlanticuc.edu
**Website:** http://www.atlanticuc.edu
**Fnded:** 1882. **Degrees Offered:** BS.

**★ 15215 ★ Boston College**
**School of Nursing**
140 Commonwealth Ave.
Chestnut Hill, MA 02467-3812
**Phone:** (617)552-4059     **Fax:** (617)552-0745
**Email:** andrea.alexander@bc.edu
**Website:** http://www.bc.edu/nursing/
Andrea Alexander, Contact
**Fnded:** 1863. **Degrees Offered:** BS, MS, MS/MHA, MS/MBA, PhD.

**★ 15216 ★ College of Our Lady of the Elms**
**Division of Nursing**
291 Springfield St.
Chicopee, MA 01013
**Phone:** (413)594-2761     **Fax:** (413)594-2761
**Email:** childersm@elms.edu
**Website:** http://www.elms.edu
Dr. Marjorie S. Childers, Contact
**Fnded:** 1928. **Degrees Offered:** BS

**★ 15217 ★ Curry College**
**Division of Nursing and Health Sciences**
1071 Blue Hill Ave.
Milton, MA 02186
**Free:** 800-669-0686     **Fax:** (617)333-2114
**Email:** mpoll@curry.edu
**Website:** http://www.curry.edu/
Michael Poll, Contact
**Fnded:** 1879. **Degrees Offered:** BS.

**★ 15218 ★ Emmanuel College**
**Department of Nursing**
400 The Fenway
Boston, MA 02115
**Phone:** (617)735-9935     **Fax:** (617)735-9797
**Email:** riley@emmanuel.edu
**Website:** http://www.emmanuel.edu/
Dr. Joan Riley, Contact
**Fnded:** 1919. **Degrees Offered:** BSN.

**★ 15219 ★ Endicott College**
**Program in Nursing**
376 Hale St.
Beverly, MA 01915
**Phone:** (978)921-1000
**Email:** admissio@endicott.edu
**Website:** http://www.endicott.edu/
**Fnded:** 1939. **Degrees Offered:** BS.

**★ 15220 ★ Fitchburg State College**
**Department of Nursing**
160 Pearl St.
Fitchburg, MA 01420-2697
**Phone:** (978)665-3181     **Fax:** (978)665-3658
**Email:** awallen@fsc.edu
**Website:** http://www.fsc.edu/
Dr. Andrea J. Wallen, Contact
**Fnded:** 1894. **Degrees Offered:** BSN,MS.

**★ 15221 ★ Framingham State College**
**Department of Nursing**
100 State St.
Framingham, MA 01701
**Phone:** (508)626-4715     **Fax:** (508)626-4746
**Email:** dtorti@frc.mass.edu
**Website:** http://www.framingham.edu/
Dr. Dolores Rojas Torti, Contact
**Fnded:** 1839. **Degrees Offered:** BS.

**★ 15222 ★ Massachusetts College of Pharmacy and Health Sciences**
**Division of Nursing**
179 Longwood Ave.
Boston, MA 02115-5896
**Phone:** (617)732-2882     **Fax:** (617)732-2236
**Email:** sgibson@mcp.edu
**Website:** http://www.mcp.edu/
Dr. Sandra Gibson, Contact
**Fnded:** 1823. **Degrees Offered:** BSN, MSN.

**★ 15223 ★ MGH Institute of Health Professions**
**Program in Nursing**
101 Merrimac St.
Boston, MA 02114
**Phone:** (617)726-3140     **Fax:** (617)726-8010
**Website:** http://www.mghihp.edu
**Fnded:** 1977. **Degrees Offered:** MSN.

**★ 15224 ★ Northeastern University**
**School of Nursing**
203 Mugar Hall
360 Huntington Ave.
Boston, MA 02115
**Phone:** (617)373-3829     **Fax:** (617)373-4701
**Email:** w.purnell@neu.edu
**Website:** http://www.neu.edu
Bill Purnell, Contact
**Fnded:** 1898. **Degrees Offered:** BSN, MS, MSN/MBA.

**★ 15225 ★ Regis College**
**Division of Nursing**
235 Wellesley St.
Weston, MA 02493
**Phone:** (781)768-7188     **Fax:** (781)768-7089
**Email:** patricia.andaloro@regiscollege.edu
**Website:** http://www.regiscollege.edu/
Patricia Andaloro, Contact
**Fnded:** 1927. **Degrees Offered:** BS, MS.

**★ 15226 ★ Salem State College**
**Nursing Department**
352 Lafayette St.
Salem, MA 01970
**Phone:** (978)542-6310     **Fax:** (978)542-7215
**Email:** susan.anderson@salem.mass.edu
**Website:** http://www.salem.mass.edu/
Dr. Susan Anderson, Contact
**Fnded:** 1854. **Degrees Offered:** BSN, MSN, MSN/MBA.

**★ 15227 ★ Simmons College**
**Department of Nursing**
300 The Fenway
Boston, MA 02115
**Phone:** (617)521-2139     **Fax:** (617)521-3045
**Email:** judy.beal@simmons.edu
**Website:** http://www.simmons.edu/
Dr. Judith Beal, Contact
**Fnded:** 1899. **Degrees Offered:** BS, MS.

**★ 15228 ★ University of Massachusetts, Amherst**
**School of Nursing**
Arnold House
715 N Pleasant St.
Amherst, MA 01003-9304
**Phone:** (413)545-5091     **Fax:** (413)577-2550
**Email:** youngmason@nursing.umass.edu
**Website:** http://www.umass.edu/
Dr. Jeanine Young-Mason, Contact
**Fnded:** 1863. **Degrees Offered:** BS, MS, PhD.

**★ 15229 ★ University of Massachusetts, Boston**
**College of Nursing**
100 Morrissey Blvd.
Boston, MA 02125
**Phone:** (617)287-6000     **Fax:** (617)287-7173
**Email:** enrollment.information@umb.edu
**Website:** http://www.umb.edu/
Jon Hutton, Contact
**Fnded:** 1964. **Degrees Offered:** BS, MS, MSN/MBA, PhD.

**★ 15230 ★ University of Massachusetts, Dartmouth**
**College of Nursing**
285 Old Westport Rd.
North Dartmouth, MA 02747-2300
**Phone:** (508)999-8159     **Fax:** (508)999-9127
**Email:** ndluhy@umassd.edu
**Website:** http://www.umassd.edu/
Dr. Nancy Dluhy, Contact
**Fnded:** 1895. **Degrees Offered:** BSN, MS.

**★ 15231 ★ University of Massachusetts, Lowell**
**Department of Nursing**
Lowell, MA 01854-2881
**Phone:** (978)934-4467     **Fax:** (978)934-3006
**Email:** may_futrell@uml.edu
**Website:** http://www.uml.edu/
Dr. May Futrell, Contact
**Fnded:** 1894. **Degrees Offered:** BS, MS, PhD.

**★ 15232 ★ University of Massachusetts, Worcester**
**Graduate School of Nursing**
55 Lake Ave. N
Worcester, MA 01655-0115
**Phone:** (508)856-5801     **Fax:** (508)856-6552
**Email:** elizabeth.flodin@umassmed.edu
**Website:** http://www.umassmed.edu/gsn/
Elizabeth Flodin, Contact
**Fnded:** 1962. **Degrees Offered:** MS, PhD.

**★ 15233 ★ Worcester State College**
**Department of Nursing**
486 Chandler St.
Worcester, MA 01602
**Phone:** (508)929-8758     **Fax:** (508)929-8183
**Email:** pantonino@worcester.edu
**Website:** http://www.worcester.edu/
Patricia Antonino, Contact
**Fnded:** 1874. **Degrees Offered:** BSs

### Michigan

**★ 15234 ★ Andrews University**
**Department of Nursing**
Berrien Springs, MI 49104
**Phone:** (616)471-3192     **Fax:** (616)471-3454
**Email:** francesj@andrews.edu
**Website:** http://www.andrews.edu
Dr. Frances Johnson, Contact
**Fnded:** 1874. **Degrees Offered:** BS, MS

**★ 15235 ★ Eastern Michigan University**
**Department of Nursing**
301 Marshall Bldg.
Ypsilanti, MI 48197
**Phone:** (734)487-3274     **Fax:** (734)487-6946
**Website:** http://www.emich.edu
Dr. Lorraine Wilson, Contact
**Fnded:** 1849. **Degrees Offered:** BSN, MSN

**★ 15236 ★ Ferris State University**
**Department of Nursing**
Big Rapids, MI 49307
**Phone:** (231)591-2267     **Fax:** (231)591-2325

**Email:** johnsons@ferris.edu
**Website:** http://www.ferris.edu/
Dr. Sally K. Johnson, Contact
**Fnded:** 1884. **Degrees Offered:** BSN.


★ 15237 ★ **Grand Valley State University**
**Russell B. Kirkhof School of Nursing**
206 Henry Hall
Allendale, MI 49401-9403
**Phone:** (616)895-3558    **Fax:** (616)895-2510
**Email:** bondl@gvsu.edu
**Website:** http://www.gvsu.edu/nursing/
Dr. Linda Bond, Contact
**Fnded:** 1960. **Degrees Offered:** BSN, MSN, MSN/
MBA.


★ 15238 ★ **Hope-Calvin Nursing Program**
105 E 14th St.
Holland, MI 49423
**Phone:** (616)957-6255
**Email:** cfeenstr@calvin.edu
**Website:** http://www.hope.edu
Dr. Cheryl J. Feenstra, Contact
**Degrees Offered:** BSN.


★ 15239 ★ **Lake Superior State**
**University**
**Department of Nursing**
650 W Easterday Ave.
Sault Sainte Marie, MI 49783
**Phone:** (906)635-2446    **Fax:** (906)635-2266
**Email:** lconklin@gw.lssu.edu
**Website:** http://www.lssu.edu
Dr. Lynn Conklin, Contact
**Fnded:** 1946. **Degrees Offered:** BSN.


★ 15240 ★ **Madonna University**
**College of Nursing and Health**
36600 Schoolcraft Rd.
Livonia, MI 48150-1173
**Phone:** (734)432-5461    **Fax:** (734)432-5463
**Email:** braunste@smtp.munet.edu
**Website:** http://www.munet.edu/
Dr. Millie Braunstein, Contact
**Fnded:** 1947. **Degrees Offered:** BSN, MSN, MSN/
MSBA.


★ 15241 ★ **Michigan State University**
**College of Nursing**
A-230 Life Sciences Bldg.
East Lansing, MI 48824
**Phone:** (517)353-4827    **Fax:** (517)353-9553
**Email:** nuro7@msu.edu
**Website:** http://www.msu.edu/unit/nurse/
Renee B. Canady, Contact
**Fnded:** 1855. **Degrees Offered:** BSN, MSN, PhD.


★ 15242 ★ **Northern Michigan University**
**College of Nursing and Allied Health**
**Science**
2407 New Science Facility
Marquette, MI 49855
**Phone:** (906)227-2486    **Fax:** (906)227-1658
**Email:** jschor@nmu.edu
**Website:** http://www.nmu.edu/
Dr. Julie K. Schorr, Contact
**Fnded:** 1899. **Degrees Offered:** BSN, MSN.


★ 15243 ★ **Oakland University**
**School of Nursing**
445 O'Dowd Hall
Rochester, MI 48309-4401
**Phone:** (248)370-4082    **Fax:** (248)370-2996
**Email:** mullin@oakland.edu
**Website:** http://www.oakland.edu/
Sarah Mullin, Contact
**Fnded:** 1957. **Degrees Offered:** BSN, MSN.


★ 15244 ★ **Saginaw Valley State**
**University**
**College of Nursing**
120 Wickes Hall
7400 Bay Rd.
University Center, MI 48710-0001
**Phone:** (517)249-1696    **Fax:** (517)790-0180
**Website:** http://www.svsu.edu/
**Fnded:** 1963. **Degrees Offered:** BSN.


★ 15245 ★ **University of Detroit Mercy**
**McAuley School of Nursing**
PO Box 19900
Detroit, MI 48219-0900
**Phone:** (313)993-6177    **Fax:** (313)993-6175
**Website:** http://www.udmercy.edu/
Lynn Vitale, Contact
**Fnded:** 1877. **Degrees Offered:** BSN, MS.


★ 15246 ★ **University of Michigan**
**School of Nursing**
400 N Ingalls Bldg., Rm. 1160
Ann Arbor, MI 48109-0482
**Phone:** (734)647-0109    **Fax:** (734)647-1419
**Email:** ceheiser@umich.edu
**Website:** http://www.umich.edu/~nursing/
Dr. Carol E. Heiser, Contact
**Fnded:** 1817. **Degrees Offered:** BSN, MS, MSN/
MBA, PhD.


★ 15247 ★ **University of Michigan, Flint**
**Department of Nursing**
516 French Hall
303 E Kearsley
Flint, MI 48502-1950
**Phone:** (810)766-6760    **Fax:** (810)766-6851
**Email:** chanlon@flint.umich.edu
**Website:** http://www.flint.umich.edu/
Charlene Hanlon, Contact
**Fnded:** 1956. **Degrees Offered:** BSN, MSN.


★ 15248 ★ **University of Phoenix, Grand**
**Rapids Campus**
**College of Nursing and Health Care**
**Sciences**
Grand Rapids, MI
**Email:** patrick.king@apollogrp.edu
**Website:** http://www.phoenix.edu/
**Degrees Offered:** BSN, MSN.


★ 15249 ★ **University of Phoenix, Metro**
**Detroit Campus**
**College of Nursing and Health Care**
**Sciences**
5480 Corporate Dr.
Ste. 240
Troy, MI 48098-9729
**Free:** 800-834-2438
**Email:** denise.vernon@apollogrp.edu
**Website:** http://www.phoenix.edu/
Denise Vernon, Contact
**Degrees Offered:** BSN, MSN.


★ 15250 ★ **Wayne State University**
**College of Nursing**
10 Cohn Bldg.
5557 Cass Ave.
Detroit, MI 48202
**Phone:** (313)577-4082    **Fax:** (313)577-6949
**Email:** Vickie.radoye@wayne.edu
**Website:** http://www.wayne.edu/
Vickie Radoye, Contact
**Fnded:** 1868. **Degrees Offered:** BSN, MSN, PhD.


★ 15251 ★ **Western Michigan University**
**College of Health and Human Services**
Kalamazoo, MI 49008

**Phone:** (616)387-8150    **Fax:** (616)387-8170
**Email:** marsha.mahan@wmich.edu
**Website:** http://www.wmich.edu/
Marsha Ann Mahan, Contact
**Fnded:** 1903. **Degrees Offered:** BS.


## Minnesota

★ 15252 ★ **Augsburg College**
**Program in Nursing**
2211 Riverside Ave. S
Minneapolis, MN 55454
**Phone:** (612)330-1204    **Fax:** (612)330-1649
**Email:** watson@augsburg.edu
**Website:** http://www.augsburg.edu
Luann Watson, Contact
**Fnded:** 1869. **Degrees Offered:** BS, MA.


★ 15253 ★ **Bemidji State University**
**Department of Nursing**
Bemidji, MN 56601
**Phone:** (218)755-3892    **Fax:** (218)755-4402
**Email:** rscheela@bemidji.edu
**Website:** http://www.bemidji.msus.edu
Dr. Rochelle A. Scheela, Contact
**Fnded:** 1919. **Degrees Offered:** BS.


★ 15254 ★ **Bethel College**
**Department of Nursing**
3900 Bethel Dr.
Saint Paul, MN 55112
**Phone:** (651)638-6336    **Fax:** (651)638-6001
**Email:** m-schaffer@bethel.edu
**Website:** http://www.bethel.edu/cgcs/
Dr. Marjorie Schaffer, Contact
**Fnded:** 1871. **Degrees Offered:** BSN,MA.


★ 15255 ★ **College of Saint Benedict**
**Department of Nursing**
37 College Ave., S
Saint Joseph, MN 56374
**Phone:** (320)363-5404    **Fax:** (320)363-6099
**Email:** ktwohy@csbsju.edu
**Website:** http://www.csbsju.edu/
Dr. Kathleen M. Twohy, Contact
**Fnded:** 1887. **Degrees Offered:** BS.


★ 15256 ★ **College of St. Catherine**
**Department of Nursing**
2004 Randolph Ave.
F-22
Saint Paul, MN 55105
**Phone:** (651)690-6588    **Fax:** (651)690-6941
**Email:** gmvarecka@stkate.edu
**Website:** http://www.stkate.edu/
Dr. Gay Maureen Varecka, Contact
**Fnded:** 1905. **Degrees Offered:** BS, MA.


★ 15257 ★ **College of St. Scholastica**
**Program in Nursing**
1200 Kenwood Ave.
Duluth, MN 55811
**Phone:** (218)723-6452    **Fax:** (218)723-6472
**Email:** cmaynard@css.edu
**Website:**    http://www.css.edu/depts/grad/grad-
page.html
Dr. Carleen Maynard, Contact
**Fnded:** 1912. **Degrees Offered:** BA, MS.


★ 15258 ★ **Concordia College**
**Department of Nursing**
901 S 8th St.
Moorhead, MN 56562
**Phone:** (218)299-3883    **Fax:** (218)299-4308
**Email:** lnelson@cord.edu
**Website:** http://www.cord.edu/
Dr. Lois F. Nelson, Contact
**Fnded:** 1891. **Degrees Offered:** BA.

**★ 15259 ★ Gustavus Adolphus College**
**Department of Nursing**
Saint Peter, MN 56082
Phone: (507)933-6094 Fax: (507)933-6153
Email: jcwc@gustavus.edu
Website: http://www.gustavus.edu/
Jane Walgenbasch, Contact
Fnded: 1862. Degrees Offered: BA.


**★ 15260 ★ Metropolitan State University**
**School of Nursing**
700 E 7th St.
Saint Paul, MN 55106-5000
Phone: (651)772-3798 Fax: (651)772-6130
Email: lynda.zimmerman@metrostate.edu
Website: http://www.metrostate.edu
Lynda Zimmerman, Contact

Fnded: 1971. Degrees Offered: BSN, MSN.


**★ 15261 ★ Minnesota State University,**
**Mankato**
**School of Nursing**
360 Wissink Hall, MSU 27
Mankato, MN 56001
Phone: (507)389-1317 Fax: (507)389-6516
Email: Sharon.aadalen@mankato.msus.edu
Website: http://www.mankato.msus.edu/
Dr. Sharon P. Aadalen, Contact
Fnded: 1868. Degrees Offered: BS, MSN.


**★ 15262 ★ Minnesota State University,**
**Moorhead**
**Nursing Department**
1104 7th Ave., S
Moorhead, MN 56563
Phone: (218)236-4696 Fax: (218)299-5990
Email: vellenga@mnstate.edu
Website: http://www.moorhead.msus.edu/
Dr. Barbara Vellenga, Contact
Fnded: 1885. Degrees Offered: BSN.


**★ 15263 ★ Saint Olaf College**
**Department of Nursing**
1520 St. Olaf Ave.
Northfield, MN 55057-1098
Phone: (507)646-3265 Fax: (507)646-3733
Email: glazebro@stolaf.edu
Website: http://www.stolaf.edu/
Dr. Rita S. Glazebrook, Contact
Fnded: 1874. Degrees Offered: BA.


**★ 15264 ★ University of Minnesota, Twin**
**Cities**
**School of Nursing**
5-160 Weaver-Densford Hall
308 Harvard St. SE
Minneapolis, MN 55455-0213
Phone: (612)625-5965 Fax: (612)624-3174
Email: rosan003@tc.umn.edu
Website: http://www.nursing.umn.edu/
Jennifer Rosand, Contact
Fnded: 1851. Degrees Offered: BSN, MS, MS/MPH, PhD.


**★ 15265 ★ Winona State University**
**College of Nursing**
859 SE 30th Ave.
Rochester, MN 55904
Phone: (507)285-7489 Fax: (507)292-5127
Email: wmcbreen@winona.msus.edu
Website: http://www.winona.msus.edu/
Dr. William McBreen, Contact
Fnded: 1858. Degrees Offered: BSN, MS.


## Mississippi

**★ 15266 ★ Alcorn State University**
**School of Nursing**
15 Campus Dr.
Natchez, MS 39120
Phone: (601)442-3901 Fax: (601)446-5942
Email: stiner@lorman.alcorn.edu
Website: http://www.alcorn.edu/
Dr. Evelyn Stiner, Contact
Fnded: 1871. Degrees Offered: BSN,MSN.


**★ 15267 ★ Delta State University**
**School of Nursing**
PO Box 3343
Cleveland, MS 38733
Phone: (662)846-4255 Fax: (662)846-4267
Email: dlamar@dsu.deltast.edu
Website: http://www.deltast.edu/
Dr. Dana Lamar, Contact
Fnded: 1924. Degrees Offered: BSN, MSN.


**★ 15268 ★ Mississippi College**
**School of Nursing**
Box 4037
200 S Capitol St.
Clinton, MS 39058
Phone: (601)925-3278 Fax: (601)925-3379
Email: padgett@mc.edu
Dr. Mary Jean Padgett, Contact
Fnded: 1826. Degrees Offered: BSN.


**★ 15269 ★ Mississippi University for**
**Women**
**Division of Nursing**
Box W-910
15th St., N
Columbus, MS 39701
Phone: (662)329-7323 Fax: (662)329-7372
Email: mcurtis@muw.edu
Website: http://www.muw.edu/nursing/
Dr. Mary Pat Curtis, Contact
Fnded: 1884. Degrees Offered: BSN, MSN.


**★ 15270 ★ University of Mississippi**
**Medical Center**
**School of Nursing**
2500 N State St.
Jackson, MS 39216-4505
Phone: (601)984-6256 Fax: (601)815-5957
Email: oallen@son.umsmed.edu
Website: http://umc.edu/
Dr. Ola Allen, Contact
Fnded: 1955. Degrees Offered: BSN, MNS, PhD.


**★ 15271 ★ University of Southern**
**Mississippi**
**College of Nursing**
Southern Station, Box 5095
Hattiesburg, MS 39406-5095
Phone: (601)266-5639 Fax: (601)266-5927
Email: bonnie.harbaugh@usm.edu
Website: http://www.nursing.usm.edu/
Dr. Bonnie Lee Harbaugh, Contact
Fnded: 1910. Degrees Offered: BSN, MSN, PhD.


**★ 15272 ★ William Carey College**
**School of Nursing**
498 Tuscan Ave.
Hattiesburg, MS 39401
Phone: (601)582-6147 Fax: (601)582-6446
Email: mware@wmcarey.edu
Website: http://www.wmcarey.edu/
Dr. Mary A. Ware, Contact
Fnded: 1906. Degrees Offered: BSN.


## Missouri

**★ 15273 ★ Avila College**
**Department of Nursing**
Office of Admissions
11901 Wornall Rd.
Kansas City, MO 64145
Phone: (816)942-8400 Fax: (816)501-2453
Email: admissions@mail.avila.edu
Website: http://www.avila.edu/
Fnded: 1916. Degrees Offered: BSN.


**★ 15274 ★ Central Missouri State**
**University**
**Department of Nursing**
Hum 410
Warrensburg, MO 64093
Phone: (660)543-4621
Email: perrin@cmsu1.cmsu.edu
Website: http://www.cmsu.edu/
Dr. Novella Perrin, Contact
Fnded: 1871. Degrees Offered: BS, MS.


**★ 15275 ★ Culver-Stockton College**
**Blessing-Rieman College of Nursing**
Canton, MO
Website: http://www/culver.edu/
Fnded: 1853.


**★ 15276 ★ Deaconess College of**
**Nursing**
6150 Oakland Ave.
Saint Louis, MO 63139
Phone: (314)768-5617 Fax: (314)768-5673
Email: peggy.hudson@tenethealth.com
Website: http://www.deaconess.edu
Peggy Hudson, Contact
Fnded: 1889. Degrees Offered: BSN.


**★ 15277 ★ Graceland University**
**Division of Health Care Professions**
1401 West Truman Rd.
Independence, MO 64050-3434
Phone: (816)833-0524 Fax: (816)833-2990
Email: karenf@graceland.edu
Website: http://www.graceland.edu
Karen Fernengel, Contact
Fnded: 1895. Degrees Offered: BSN, MSN


**★ 15278 ★ Jewish Hospital College of**
**Nursing and Allied Health**
**Program in Nursing**
306 S Kingshighway Blvd.
Saint Louis, MO 63116
Phone: (314)454-8416 Fax: (314)454-5239
Email: sjb@bjcmail.carenet.org
Dr. Elizabeth A. Buck, Contact
Fnded: 1902. Degrees Offered: BSN, MSN


**★ 15279 ★ Maryville University, Saint**
**Louis**
**School of Health Professions**
**Nursing Program**
13550 Conway Rd.
Saint Louis, MO 63141-7299
Phone: (314)529-9435 Fax: (314)529-9139
Email: sstopke@maryville.edu
Website: http://www.maryville.edu/
Sherry Stopke, Contact
Fnded: 1872. Degrees Offered: BSN, MSN.


**★ 15280 ★ Missouri Southern State**
**College**
**Department of Nursing**
3950 E Newman Rd.
Joplin, MO 64801-1595
Phone: (417)625-9322 Fax: (417)625-3186

**Email:** box-b@mail.mssc.edu
**Website:** http://www.mssc.edu/
Dr. Barbara J. Box, Contact
**Fnded:** 1937. **Degrees Offered:** BSN.


★ 15281 ★ **Missouri Western State College**
**Department of Nursing**
4525 Downs Dr.
Saint Joseph, MO 64507
**Phone:** (816)271-4415     **Fax:** (816)271-5849
**Email:** nursing@griffon.mwsc.edu
**Website:** http://www.mwsc.edu/
**Fnded:** 1915. **Degrees Offered:** BSN.


★ 15282 ★ **Research College of Nursing**
2316 E Meyer Blvd.
Kansas City, MO 64132-1199
**Phone:** (816)276-4733     **Fax:** (816)276-3526
**Email:** lamendenhall@healthmidwest.org
Leslie Mendenhall, Contact
**Fnded:** 1980. **Degrees Offered:** BSN, MSN.


★ 15283 ★ **Saint Louis University**
**School of Nursing**
3525 Caroline Mall
Saint Louis, MO 63104
**Phone:** (314)577-8970     **Fax:** (314)577-8949
**Email:** ruchalpl@slu.edu
**Website:** http://imagine.slue.edu/
Dr. Patsy Ruchala, Contact
**Fnded:** 1818. **Degrees Offered:** BSN, MSN, MSN/MPH, PhD.


★ 15284 ★ **Saint Luke's College**
**Nursing College**
4426 Wornall Rd.
Kansas City, MO 64111
**Phone:** (816)932-2073     **Fax:** (816)932-3831
**Email:** mjthomas@saint-lukes.org
**Website:** http://www.saint-lukes.org/
Marsha Thomas, Contact
**Fnded:** 1903. **Degrees Offered:** BSN.


★ 15285 ★ **Southeast Missouri State University**
**Department of Nursing**
1 University Plaza, MS8300
Cape Girardeau, MO 63701-4799
**Phone:** (573)651-2871     **Fax:** (573)651-2142
**Email:** ejackson@semovm.semo.edu
**Website:** http://www.semo.edu/
Dr. Elaine Jackson, Contact
**Fnded:** 1873. **Degrees Offered:** BSN.


★ 15286 ★ **Southwest Missouri State University**
**Department of Nursing**
901 S National
Springfield, MO 65804
**Phone:** (417)836-5310     **Fax:** (417)836-5484
**Email:** kathrynhope@mail.smsu.edu
**Website:** http://www.smsu.edu/academic/acad/chhs/nursdept.html
Dr. Kathryn L. Hope, Contact
**Fnded:** 1905. **Degrees Offered:** BSN, MSN.


★ 15287 ★ **Truman State University**
**Program in Nursing**
Barnett Hall 223
100 E Normal St.
Kirksville, MO 63501
**Phone:** (660)785-4557     **Fax:** (660)785-7424
**Email:** cayers@truman.edu
**Website:** http://www.truman.edu/
Dr. Constance J. Ayers, Contact
**Fnded:** 1867. **Degrees Offered:** BSN.


★ 15288 ★ **University of Missouri, Columbia**
**School of Nursing**
S235 School of Nursing
Columbia, MO 65211
**Phone:** (573)882-0277     **Fax:** (573)884-4544
**Email:** johnsonn@missouri.edu
Nancy Lee Johnson, Contact
**Fnded:** 1839. **Degrees Offered:** BSN, MS, PhD.


★ 15289 ★ **University of Missouri, Kansas City**
**School of Nursing**
2220 Holmes St.
Kansas City, MO 64108
**Phone:** (816)235-1740     **Fax:** (816)235-1701
**Email:** jellisonj@umkc.edu
**Website:** http://www.umkc.edu/
Judy A. Jellison, Contact
**Fnded:** 1929. **Degrees Offered:** BSN, MSN, PhD.


★ 15290 ★ **University of Missouri, Saint Louis**
**College of Nursing**
8001 Natural Bridge Rd.
Saint Louis, MO 63121-4499
**Phone:** (314)516-7087     **Fax:** (314)516-7519
**Email:** canda@umsl.edu
**Website:** http://www.umsl.edu/divisions/nursing/
Kathern Canda, Contact
**Fnded:** 1963. **Degrees Offered:** BSN, MSN, PhD.


★ 15291 ★ **Webster University**
**Department of Nursing**
470 E Lockwood Ave.
Saint Louis, MO 63119
**Phone:** (314)968-7483     **Fax:** (314)963-6101
**Email:** headysa@websteruniv.edu
**Website:** http://www.webster.edu/depts/aasci/nursing/nursing.html
Dr. Susan Heady, Contact
**Fnded:** 1915. **Degrees Offered:** BSN, MSN.


★ 15292 ★ **William Jewell College**
**Department of Nursing**
500 College Hill
Liberty, MO 64068
**Phone:** (816)781-7700     **Fax:** (816)415-5024
**Email:** kerstenj@william.jewell.edu
**Website:** http://www.jewell.edu/
Dr. Joanne W. Kersten, Contact
**Fnded:** 1849. **Degrees Offered:** BS.


## Montana

★ 15293 ★ **Carroll College**
**Department of Nursing**
Helena, MT 59625
**Phone:** (406)447-4382     **Fax:** (406)447-4533
**Email:** sknicker@carroll.edu
**Website:** http://www.carroll.edu/
Scott Knickerbocker, Contact
**Fnded:** 1909. **Degrees Offered:** BA.


★ 15294 ★ **Montana State University, Bozeman**
**College of Nursing**
PO Box 173560
Bozeman, MT 59717-3560
**Phone:** (406)994-3784     **Fax:** (406)994-6020
**Email:** gmcneely@montana.edu
**Website:** http://www.montana.edu/wwwnu/
Dr. A. Gretchen McNeely, Contact
**Fnded:** 1893. **Degrees Offered:** BSN, MSN.


★ 15295 ★ **Montana State University, Northern**
**Department of Nursing**
2100 16th Ave., S
PO Box 6010
Great Falls, MT 59406
**Free:** 800-662-6132
**Email:** elossing@msun.msun.edu
**Website:** http://www.msun.edu/
Emily Mayer Lossing, Contact
**Fnded:** 1929. **Degrees Offered:** BSN.


## Nebraska

★ 15296 ★ **Clarkson College**
**Department of Nursing**
101 S 42nd St.
Omaha, NE 68131-2739
**Free:** 800-647-5500     **Fax:** (402)552-6057
**Email:** damewood@clrkcol.crhsnet.edu
**Website:** http://www.clarksoncollege.edu/
Tony Damewood, Contact
**Fnded:** 1888. **Degrees Offered:** BSN, MSN.


★ 15297 ★ **College of Saint Mary**
**School of Health Care Professions**
1901 S 72nd St.
Omaha, NE 68124
**Phone:** (402)399-2653     **Fax:** (402)399-2654
**Email:** mpartusch@csm.edu
**Website:** http://www.csm.edu/
Dr. Mary E. Partusch, Contact
**Fnded:** 1923. **Degrees Offered:** BSN.


★ 15298 ★ **Creighton University**
**School of Nursing**
2500 California Plaza
Omaha, NE 68178
**Phone:** (402)280-2041     **Fax:** (402)280-2045
**Email:** bbevans@creighton.edu
**Website:** http://nursing.creighton.edu/
Dr. Brenda Bergman-Evans, Contact
**Fnded:** 1878. **Degrees Offered:** BSN, MS


★ 15299 ★ **Midland Lutheran College**
**Department of Nursing**
900 N Clarkson
Fremont, NE 68025
**Phone:** (402)721-5480     **Fax:** (402)941-6279
**Email:** harms@admin.mlc.edu
**Website:** http://www.mlc.edu
Dr. Nancy A. Harris, Contact
**Fnded:** 1883. **Degrees Offered:** BSN.


★ 15300 ★ **Nebraska Methodist College**
**Department of Nursing**
8501 W Dodge Rd.
Omaha, NE 68114-3426
**Phone:** (402)354-4981     **Fax:** (402)354-8875
**Email:** nmockel@nmhs.org
**Website:** http://www.methodistcollege.edu/
Nancy Mockelstrom, Contact
**Fnded:** 1891. **Degrees Offered:** BSN, MSN.


★ 15301 ★ **Nebraska Wesleyan University**
**Department of Nursing**
5000 St. Paul Ave.
Lincoln, NE 68504
**Phone:** (402)465-2334     **Fax:** (402)465-2179
**Email:** pjm@nebrwesleyan.edu
**Website:** http://www.nebrwesleyan.edu/
Dr. Patricia Jean Morin, Contact
**Fnded:** 1887. **Degrees Offered:** BSN, MSN.


★ 15302 ★ **Union College**
**Division of Health Sciences**
3800 S 48 St.
Lincoln, NE 68506

Phone: (402)486-2524　　Fax: (402)486-2559
Email: kaminear@ucollege.edu
Website: http://www.ucollege.edu/
Karen W. Minear, Contact
Fnded: 1891. Degrees Offered: BSN.

★ 15303 ★ University of Nebraska
Medical Center
College of Nursing
985330 Nebraska Medical Center
Omaha, NE 68198-5330
Phone: (402)559-7457　　Fax: (402)559-4303
Email: mwilson@unmc.edu
Website: http://www.unmc.edu/
Dr. Margaret Wilson, Contact
Fnded: 1869. Degrees Offered: BSN, MSN, PhD.

### Nevada

★ 15304 ★ University of Nevada, Las
Vegas
Department of Nursing
4505 Maryland Pkwy.
Las Vegas, NV 89154
Phone: (702)895-3360　　Fax: (702)895-4807
Website: http://www.unlv.edu/
Dr. Margaret Louis, Contact
Fnded: 1957. Degrees Offered: BSN, MSN.

★ 15305 ★ University of Nevada, Reno
Orvis School of Nursing
Mail Stop No. 134
Reno, NV 89557
Phone: (775)784-6841　　Fax: (775)784-4262
Email: jaynem@unr.edu
Website: http://www.unr.edu
Jayne Moore, Contact
Fnded: 1874. Degrees Offered: BS, MS.

### New Brunswick

★ 15306 ★ Universite de Moncton
School of Nursing
Pavillon Leopold Taillon
Moncton, NB, Canada E1A 3E9
Phone: (506)858-4443　　Fax: (506)858-4544
Email: bordely@umoncton.ca
Website: http://www.umoncton.ca/
Yoland Bordeleau, Contact
Degrees Offered: BSCN, M SC N. Cnt: 1963.

★ 15307 ★ University of New Brunswick
Faculty of Nursing
PO Box 4400
Fredericton, NB, Canada E3B 5A3
Phone: (506)458-7630　　Fax: (506)447-3374
Email: mdupuis@unb.ca
Website: http://www.unb.ca/
Dr. Mary Dupuis, Contact
Fnded: 1785. Degrees Offered: BN, MN.

### New Hampshire

★ 15308 ★ Colby-Sawyer College
Department of Nursing
100 Main St.
New London, NH 03257-4648
Phone: (603)526-3646　　Fax: (603)526-3452
Email: kthies@colby-sawyer.edu
Website: http://www.colby-sawyer.edu/
Dr. Kathleen M. Thies, Contact
Fnded: 1837. Degrees Offered: BS.

★ 15309 ★ Rivier College
Department of Nursing and Health
Sciences
420 Main St.
Nashua, NH 03060-5086
Phone: (603)897-8529　　Fax: (603)897-8884

Email: kbaranowski@rivier.edu
Website: http://www.rivier.edu/
Dr. Karen L. Baranowski, Contact
Fnded: 1933. Degrees Offered: BS, MS.

★ 15310 ★ Saint Anselm College
Department of Nursing
100 St. Anselm Dr.
Manchester, NH 03102-1310
Phone: (603)656-6199　　Fax: (603)641-7550
Email: ntessier@anselm.edu
Website: http://www.anselm.edu/
Nancy Tessier, Contact
Fnded: 1889. Degrees Offered: BS.

★ 15311 ★ University of New Hampshire
Department of Nursing
Hewitt Hall
4 Library Way
Durham, NH 03824-3563
Phone: (603)862-2260　　Fax: (603)862-4771
Email: geh@christa.unh.edu
Website: http://www.unh.edu/nursing/
Gene Harkless, Contact
Fnded: 1866. Degrees Offered: BS, MS.

### New Jersey

★ 15312 ★ Bloomfield College
Division of Nursing
1 Park Pl.
Bloomfield, NJ 07003
Phone: (973)748-9000　　Fax: (973)748-0916
Email: frank_nash@bloomfield.edu
Website: http://www.bloomfield.edu
Frank Nash, Contact
Fnded: 1868. Degrees Offered: BSN.

★ 15313 ★ College of New Jersey
School of Nursing
PO Box 7718
2000 Pennington Rd.
Ewing, NJ 08628-0718
Phone: (609)771-2591　　Fax: (609)637-5159
Email: lindberg@tcnj.edu
Website: http://www.tcnj.edu
Dr. Claire Lindberg, Contact
Fnded: 1855. Degrees Offered: BSN, MSN.

★ 15314 ★ College of Saint Elizabeth
Department of Nursing
2 Convent Rd.
Morristown, NJ 07960-6989
Phone: (973)290-4056　　Fax: (973)290-4177
Email: jlehmann@liza.st-elizabeth.edu
Website: http://www.st-elizabeth.edu/
Sr. Janet Lehmann, Contact
Fnded: 1899. Degrees Offered: BSN.

★ 15315 ★ Fairleigh Dickinson University
Teaneck-Hackensack Campus
Henry P. Becton School of Nursing and
Allied Health
Dickinson Hall-444A
1000 River Rd.
Teaneck, NJ 07666
Phone: (201)692-2888　　Fax: (201)692-2388
Email: swarren@mailbox.fdu.edu
Website: http://www.fdu.edu/
Dr. Susan Warren, Contact
Fnded: 1942. Degrees Offered: BSN.

★ 15316 ★ Felician College
Department of Professional Nursing-BSN
262 S Main St.
Lodi, NJ 07644
Phone: (201)559-6000
Email: navaroo@inet.felican.edu

Website: http://www.felician.edu/
Omar X. Navarro, Contact
Fnded: 1942. Degrees Offered: BSN, MSN.

★ 15317 ★ Kean University
Department of Nursing
PO Box 411
Union, NJ 07083-0411
Phone: (908)527-3147　　Fax: (908)352-6427
Email: dulafp@aol.com
Website: http://www.kean.edu/
Dr. Dula Pacquiao, Contact
Fnded: 1855. Degrees Offered: BSN, MSN, MSN/
MPA.

★ 15318 ★ Monmouth University
Marjorie K. Unterberg School of Nursing
West Long Branch, NJ 07764
Phone: (732)571-3443　　Fax: (732)263-5131
Email: mahoney@monmouth.edu
Website: http://www.monmouth.edu/
Dr. Janet Mahoney, Contact
Fnded: 1933. Degrees Offered: BSN, MSN.

★ 15319 ★ New Jersey City University
Department of Nursing
2039 Kennedy Blvd.
Jersey City, NJ 07305
Phone: (201)200-3240　　Fax: (201)200-3141
Email: gboseman@njcu.edu
Website: http://www.njcu.edu/core.htm
Dr. Gloria Boseman, Contact
Fnded: 1927. Degrees Offered: BSN, MS.

★ 15320 ★ Richard Stockton College of
New Jersey
Program in Nursing
Office of Enrollment Management
PO Box 195
Pomona, NJ 08240
Phone: (609)652-4837
Email: admissions@stockton.edu
Website: http://www.stockton.edu/
Fnded: 1969. Degrees Offered: BSN. MSN.

★ 15321 ★ Rutgers, the State University
of New Jersey
Camden College of Arts and Sciences
Department of Nursing
Armitage Hall
311 N 5th St.
Camden, NJ 08102
Phone: (856)225-6526　　Fax: (856)225-6541
Email: greipp@crab.rutgers.edu
Website: http://www.rutgers.edu/
Marie O'Toole, Contact
Fnded: 1927. Degrees Offered: BS, MS.

★ 15322 ★ Rutgers, the State University
of New Jersey
College of Nursing
Newark Admission Office
180 University Ave.
Newark, NJ 07102-1803
Phone: (973)353-5295　　Fax: (973)353-1277
Email: dolinsky@nightingale.rutgers.edu
Website: http://www.rutgers.edu/
Dr. Elaine Dolinsky, Contact
Fnded: 1956. Degrees Offered: BS, MS, PhD.

★ 15323 ★ Saint Peter's College
Nursing Program
Hudson Terrace
Englewood Cliffs, NJ 07632
Phone: (201)586-5208　　Fax: (201)569-1254
Email: yam_m@spcvxa.spc.edu
Website: http://www.spc.edu
Dr. Marylou Yam, Contact

**Fnded:** 1872. **Degrees Offered:** BSN, MSN.

★ 15324 ★ **Seton Hall University**
**College of Nursing**
400 S Orange Ave.
South Orange, NJ 07079-2693
**Phone:** (973)761-9285      **Fax:** (973)761-9607
**Email:** bugelmar@shu.edu
**Website:** http://www.shu.edu/
Mary Jo Bugel, Contact
**Fnded:** 1856. **Degrees Offered:** BSN, MSN, MSN/MA, MSN/MBA.

★ 15325 ★ **Thomas Edison State College**
**Program in Nursing**
101 W State St.
Trenton, NJ 08625
**Phone:** (609)633-6460      **Fax:** (609)777-3003
**Email:** sobrien@tesc.edu
**Website:** http://www.tesc.edu/
Dr. Susan O'Brien, Contact
**Fnded:** 1972. **Degrees Offered:** BSN.

★ 15326 ★ **University of Medicine and**
    **Dentistry of New Jersey**
**School of Nursing**
65 Bergen St., Rm. 1126
Newark, NJ 07107-3001
**Phone:** (973)972-5336      **Fax:** (973)972-7453
**Email:** shields@umdnj.edu
**Website:** http://www.umdnj.edu/
Joan Z. Shields, Contact
**Fnded:** 1954. **Degrees Offered:** BSN,MSN.

★ 15327 ★ **William Paterson University of**
    **New Jersey**
**Department of Nursing**
300 Pompton Rd., W240
Wayne, NJ 07470
**Phone:** (973)720-3495      **Fax:** (973)720-3517
**Email:** baredfordc@wpunj.edu
**Website:** http://www.wpunj.edu
Dr. Connie Geim Bareford, Contact
**Fnded:** 1855. **Degrees Offered:** BSN, MSN.

## New Mexico

★ 15328 ★ **Eastern New Mexico**
    **University**
**Department of Allied Health-Nursing**
Station Ste. 12
Portales, NM 88130
**Phone:** (505)562-2403      **Fax:** (505)562-2293
**Email:** ellen.bral@enmu.edu
**Website:** http://www.enmu.edu/
Dr. Ellen E. Bral, Contact
**Fnded:** 1934. **Degrees Offered:** BSN.

★ 15329 ★ **New Mexico State University**
**Department of Nursing**
Department 3185
PO Box 30001
Las Cruces, NM 88003-8001
**Phone:** (505)646-1919      **Fax:** (505)646-2167
**Email:** mpase@nmsu.edu
**Website:** http://www.nmsu.edu/~nursing/
Marilyn Pase, Contact
**Fnded:** 1888. **Degrees Offered:** BSN, MSN.

★ 15330 ★ **University of New Mexico**
**College of Nursing**
NRPH Bldg.
2502 Marble, NE
Albuquerque, NM 87131-5688
**Phone:** (505)272-0849      **Fax:** (505)272-3970
**Email:** amorgan@salud.unm.edu
**Website:** http://www.unm.edu/consg/index.html
Alan Morgan, Contact

**Fnded:** 1889. **Degrees Offered:** BSN, MS/MPH, MSN.

★ 15331 ★ **University of Phoenix, New**
    **Mexico Campus**
**College of Nursing and Health Care**
    **Sciences**
Albuquerque, NM
**Phone:** (505)821-4800
**Email:** Tammy.Fernandez@apollogrp.edu
**Website:** http://www.phoenix.edu/
Tammy Fernandez, Contact
**Degrees Offered:** BSN.

## New York

★ 15332 ★ **Adelphi University**
**School of Nursing**
Levermore Hall
South Ave.
Garden City, NY 11530
**Phone:** (516)877-3052      **Fax:** (516)877-3039
**Email:** posillic@adelphi.edu
**Website:** http://www.adelphi.edu
Joseph Posillico, Contact
**Fnded:** 1896. **Degrees Offered:** BS, MS, MS/MBA.

★ 15333 ★ **College of Mount Saint**
    **Vincent**
**Division of Nursing**
6301 Riverdale Ave.
Riverdale, NY 10471-1093
**Phone:** (718)405-3354      **Fax:** (718)405-3286
**Website:** http://www.cmsv.edu
Dr. Susan Apold, Contact
**Fnded:** 1911. **Degrees Offered:** BS, MS.

★ 15334 ★ **College of New Rochelle**
**School of Nursing**
New Rochelle, NY 10805-2308
**Phone:** (914)654-5813      **Fax:** (914)654-5994
**Email:** bjoyce@cnr.edu
**Website:** http://cnr.edu/
Dr. Barbara Joyce, Contact
**Fnded:** 1904. **Degrees Offered:** BSN, MS.

★ 15335 ★ **College of Staten Island of**
    **the City University of New York**
**Department of Nursing**
2800 Victory Blvd.
Staten Island, NY 10314
**Phone:** (718)982-3845      **Fax:** (718)982-3813
**Email:** lunney@postbox.csi.cuny.edu
**Website:** http://www.csi.cuny.edu/
Dr. Margaret Lunney, Contact
**Fnded:** 1955. **Degrees Offered:** BS, MS.

★ 15336 ★ **Columbia University**
**School of Nursing**
630 W 168th St.
Box 6
New York, NY 10032
**Phone:** (212)305-5756      **Fax:** (212)305-3680
**Email:** pk360@columbia.edu
**Website:** http://www.columbia.edu/
Paulette Linson Keegan, Contact
**Fnded:** 1754. **Degrees Offered:** BS, DN SC, MN/MPH, MS, MSN/MBA.

★ 15337 ★ **Columbia University,**
    **Teacher's College**
**Department of Organization and**
    **Leadership**
525 W 120th St.
Box 150
New York, NY 10027
**Phone:** (212)678-3421      **Fax:** (212)678-3950
**Email:** rh89@columbia.edu

**Website:** http://www.tc.columbia.edu/
Rosemarie Horgan, Contact
**Fnded:** 1887. **Degrees Offered:** EDD, MA.

★ 15338 ★ **Daemen College**
**Department of Nursing**
4380 Main St.
Amherst, NY 14226
**Phone:** (716)839-8408      **Fax:** (716)839-8516
**Email:** dwydysh@daemen.edu
**Website:** http://www.daemen.edu/
Deborah Wydysh, Contact
**Fnded:** 1947. **Degrees Offered:** BS, MS.

★ 15339 ★ **Dominican College of Blauvelt**
**Division of Nursing**
Orangeburg, NY 10962-1210
**Phone:** (845)359-7800      **Fax:** (845)398-4999
**Website:** http://www.dc.edu/
Lynne Weisman, Contact
**Fnded:** 1952. **Degrees Offered:** BSN, MS.

★ 15340 ★ **D'Youville College**
**Department of Nursing**
320 Porter Ave.
Buffalo, NY 14201
**Phone:** (716)881-6506      **Fax:** (716)881-8159
**Email:** snell@dyc.edu
**Website:** http://www.dyc.edu/
Dr. Linda Snell, Contact
**Fnded:** 1908. **Degrees Offered:** BS, MS.

★ 15341 ★ **Elmira College**
**Program in Nursing Education**
1 Park Pl.
Elmira, NY 14901
**Phone:** (607)735-1724      **Fax:** (607)735-1718
**Email:** bneal@elmira.edu
**Website:** http://www.elmira.edu/
William S. Neal, Contact
**Fnded:** 1855. **Degrees Offered:** BS.

★ 15342 ★ **Excelsior College**
**Program in Nursing**
7 Columbia Cir.
Albany, NY 12203
**Phone:** (518)464-8500      **Fax:** (518)465-8577
**Email:** msn@regents.edu
**Website:** http://www.regents.edu/
Deborah L. Sopczyk, Contact
**Fnded:** 1970. **Degrees Offered:** BSN, MS.

★ 15343 ★ **Hartwick College**
**Department of Nursing**
Oneonta, NY 13820
**Phone:** (607)431-4789      **Fax:** (607)431-4850
**Email:** seloverl@hartwick.edu
**Website:** http://www.hartwick.edu/
Lynda Ann Selover, Contact
**Fnded:** 1797. **Degrees Offered:** BS.

★ 15344 ★ **Hunter College of the City**
    **University of New York**
**Hunter-Bellevue School of Nursing**
425 E 25th St.
New York, NY 10010
**Phone:** (212)481-4465      **Fax:** (212)481-4427
**Email:** mramshor@hejira.hunter.cuny.edu
**Website:** http://www.hunter.cuny.edu/
Dr. Mary T. Ramshorn, Contact
**Fnded:** 1870. **Degrees Offered:** BS, MS, MSN/MPH.

★ 15345 ★ **Keuka College**
**Division of Nursing**
PO Box 98
Keuka Park, NY 14478-0098
**Phone:** (315)536-5273      **Fax:** (315)536-5660

**Email:** lrrossi@mail.keuka.edu
**Website:** http://www.keuka.edu/
Dr. Linda Rossi, Contact
**Fnded:** 1890. **Degrees Offered:** BS.


★ **15346** ★ **Lehman College of the City University of New York**
**Department of Nursing**
250 Bedford Park Blvd., W
Bronx, NY 10468
**Phone:** (718)960-8374          **Fax:** (718)960-8488
**Website:** http://www.lehman.cuny.edu/
**Fnded:** 1931. **Degrees Offered:** BS, MS.


★ **15347** ★ **Long Island University C.W. Post Campus**
**Program in Nursing**
Rm. 270
720 Northern Blvd.
Brookville, NY 11548-1300
**Phone:** (516)299-2320          **Fax:** (516)299-2527
**Email:** lknapp@hornet.liunet.edu
**Website:**        http://www.cwpost.liunet.edu/cwis/cwp/post.html
Dr. Lori Knapp, Contact
**Fnded:** 1954. **Degrees Offered:** BS, MS.


★ **15348** ★ **Long Island University, Brooklyn Campus**
**School of Nursing**
1 University Plaza
Brooklyn, NY 11201
**Phone:** (718)488-1059          **Fax:** (718)780-4019
**Email:** cpk1217@aol.com
**Website:**        http://www.brooklyn.liunet.edu/cwis/bklyn/bklyn.html
Dawn F. Kilts, Contact
**Fnded:** 1926. **Degrees Offered:** BS, MS.


★ **15349** ★ **Medgar Evers College of the City University of New York**
**Department of Nursing**
Admissions Office
1650 Bedford Ave.
Brooklyn, NY 11225
**Phone:** (718)270-6024          **Fax:** (718)270-6496
**Website:** http://www.mec.cuny.edu/
**Fnded:** 1969. **Degrees Offered:** BS.


★ **15350** ★ **Mercy College**
**Department of Nursing**
555 Broadway
Dobbs Ferry, NY 10522
**Phone:** (914)674-9331          **Fax:** (914)674-9457
**Email:** clansberry@mercynet.edu
**Website:** http://www.mercynet.edu/
Dr. Carolyn R. Lansberry, Contact
**Fnded:** 1951. **Degrees Offered:** BS, MS.


★ **15351** ★ **Molloy College**
**Department of Nursing**
1000 Hempstead Ave.
PO Box 5002
Rockville Centre, NY 11570-5002
**Phone:** (516)256-2218          **Fax:** (516)678-9718
**Email:** cclifford@molloy.edu
**Website:** http://www.molloy.edu/
Dr. Carol A. Clifford, Contact
**Fnded:** 1955. **Degrees Offered:** BS, MS.


★ **15352** ★ **Mount Saint Mary College**
**Division of Nursing**
330 Powell Ave.
Newburgh, NY 12550
**Phone:** (914)569-3138          **Fax:** (914)562-6762
**Email:** deboer@msmc.edu
**Website:** http://www.msmc.edu/
Sr. Leona DeBoer, Contact

**Fnded:** 1960. **Degrees Offered:** BS, MS.


★ **15353** ★ **Nazareth College of Rochester**
**Department of Nursing**
4245 East Ave.
Rochester, NY 14618-3790
**Phone:** (716)389-2711          **Fax:** (716)389-2714
**Email:** pahanson@naz.edu
**Website:** http://www.naz.edu/
Dr. Patricia A. Hanson, Contact
**Fnded:** 1924. **Degrees Offered:** BS, MS.


★ **15354** ★ **New York University**
**Division of Nursing**
246 Greene St.
New York, NY 10003
**Phone:** (212)992-9418          **Fax:** (212)995-4302
**Email:** nursing.programs@nyu.edu
**Website:** http://www.education.nyu.edu/nursing/
Vida Samuel-Wheeler, Contact
**Fnded:** 1831. **Degrees Offered:** BS, MA, MS/MA, PhD.


★ **15355** ★ **Pace University, New York City Campus**
**Lienhard School of Nursing**
861 Bedford Rd.
Pleasantville, NY 10570
**Phone:** (914)773-3555          **Fax:** (914)773-3345
**Email:** kkeith@pace.edu
**Website:** http://www.pace.edu/
Dr. Karen Keith, Contact
**Fnded:** 1906. **Degrees Offered:** BS, MS.


★ **15356** ★ **Pace University, Pleasantville/ Briarcliff Campus**
**Lienhard School of Nursing**
861 Bedford Rd.
Pleasantville, NY 10570
**Phone:** (914)773-3553          **Fax:** (914)773-3345
**Email:** kkeith@pace.edu
**Website:** http://www.pace.edu/
Dr. Karen Keith, Contact
**Degrees Offered:** BS, MS.


★ **15357** ★ **Roberts Wesleyan College**
**Division of Nursing**
2301 Westside Dr.
Rochester, NY 14624
**Phone:** (716)594-6400          **Fax:** (716)594-6371
**Email:** admissions@roberts.edu
**Website:** http://www.roberts.edu/
Linda Kurtz, Contact
**Fnded:** 1866. **Degrees Offered:** BS.


★ **15358** ★ **Russell Sage College**
**Division of Nursing**
Troy, NY 12180
**Phone:** (518)244-2384
**Email:** kelmag@sage.edu
**Website:** http://www.sage.edu/html/rsc/welcome.html
Dr. Glenda Kelman, Contact
**Fnded:** 1916. **Degrees Offered:** BS, MS.


★ **15359** ★ **Sage Graduate School**
**Division of Nursing**
Troy, NY 12180-4115
**Phone:** (518)244-2384          **Fax:** (518)244-2009
**Email:** kelmag@sage.edu
**Website:** http://www.sage.edu
Dr. Glenda Kelman, Contact
**Fnded:** 1949. **Degrees Offered:** MS, MSN/MBA.


★ **15360** ★ **St. John Fisher College**
**Nursing Program**
3690 East Ave.
Rochester, NY 14618
**Phone:** (716)385-8471          **Fax:** (716)385-8466
**Email:** mccloskey@sjfc.edu
**Website:** http://www.sjfc.edu/
Dr. Cynthia McCloskey, Contact
**Fnded:** 1948. **Degrees Offered:** BS, MS.


★ **15361** ★ **Saint Joseph's College, New York**
**Department of Nursing**
245 Clinton Ave.
Brooklyn, NY 11205-3688
**Phone:** (718)399-0185          **Fax:** (718)638-8839
**Email:** bsands@sjcny.edu
**Website:** http://www.sjcny.edu/
Dr. Barbara L. Sands, Contact
**Fnded:** 1916. **Degrees Offered:** BSN.


★ **15362** ★ **State University of New York Upstate Medical University**
**College of Nursing**
750 E Adams St.
Syracuse, NY 13210
**Phone:** (315)464-4276          **Fax:** (315)464-5168
**Email:** gavanc@upstate.edu
**Website:** http://www.upstate.edu
Dr. Carol Gavan, Contact
**Fnded:** 1950. **Degrees Offered:** BS, MS.


★ **15363** ★ **State University of New York, Binghamton**
**School of Nursing**
PO Box 6000
Binghamton, NY 13902-6000
**Phone:** (607)777-4964          **Fax:** (607)777-4440
**Email:** jferrari@binghamton.edu
**Website:** http://dson.binghamton.edu
Joyce Ferrario, Contact
**Fnded:** 1946. **Degrees Offered:** BS, MS, PhD.


★ **15364** ★ **State University of New York, Buffalo**
**School of Nursing**
1020 Kimball Tower
Buffalo, NY 14214-3079
**Phone:** (716)829-2537          **Fax:** (716)829-2021
**Email:** nurse-studentaffairs@buffalo.edu
**Website:** http://wings.buffalo.edu/nursing/
Dr. Elaine R. Cusker, Contact
**Fnded:** 1846. **Degrees Offered:** BS, DNS, MS,


★ **15365** ★ **State University of New York College, Brockport**
**Department of Nursing**
350 New Campus Dr.
Brockport, NY 14420-2988
**Phone:** (716)395-5320          **Fax:** (716)395-5312
**Email:** ctorres@brockport.edu
**Website:** http://www.brockport.edu
Dr. Charlotte Torres, Contact
**Fnded:** 1867. **Degrees Offered:** BSN, MS.


★ **15366** ★ **State University of New York Health Science Center, Brooklyn**
**College of Nursing**
450 Clarkson Ave.
Box 60A
Brooklyn, NY 11203-2098
**Phone:** (718)270-7605          **Fax:** (718)270-7636
**Email:** lsedhom@netmail.hscbklyn.edu
**Website:** http://www.downstate.edu
Dr. Laila N. Sedhom, Contact
**Fnded:** 1858. **Degrees Offered:** BS, MS.

**★ 15367 ★ State University of New York Institute of Technology, Utica/Rome**
**School of Nursing**
PO Box 3050
Utica, NY 13504-3050
**Phone:** (315)792-7295    **Fax:** (315)792-7555
**Email:** snlr@sunyit.edu
**Website:** http://www.sunyit.edu/SUNY/acad_prog/nurs_info/nursing.html
Nancy Rickard, Contact
**Fnded:** 1966. **Degrees Offered:** BS, MS.

**★ 15368 ★ State University of New York, New Paltz**
**Department of Nursing**
VLC 205
New Paltz, NY 12561
**Phone:** (845)257-2961    **Fax:** (845)257-2926
**Website:** http://www.newpaltz.edu/
Dr. Eleanor Richards, Contact
**Fnded:** 1828. **Degrees Offered:** BSN, MSN.

**★ 15369 ★ State University of New York, Plattsburgh**
**Department of Nursing**
101 Broad St.
Hawkins Hall 209B
Plattsburgh, NY 12901
**Phone:** (518)564-4225    **Fax:** (518)564-3100
**Email:** gretchen.beebe@plattsburgh.edu
**Website:** http://www.plattsburgh.edu/
Dr. Gretchen Crawford Beebe, Contact
**Fnded:** 1889. **Degrees Offered:** BS.

**★ 15370 ★ State University of New York, Stony Brook**
**School of Nursing**
Stony Brook, NY 11794-8240
**Phone:** (631)444-3200    **Fax:** (631)444-6628
**Website:** http://www.uhmc.sunysb.edu/nursing/
**Fnded:** 1957. **Degrees Offered:** BSN, MSN.

**★ 15371 ★ Syracuse University**
**College of Nursing**
426 Ostrom Ave.
Syracuse, NY 13244-3240
**Phone:** (315)443-1094    **Fax:** (315)443-2164
**Website:** http://sumweb.syr.edu/nursing/index.htm
Linda Littlejohn, Contact
**Fnded:** 1870. **Degrees Offered:** BS, MS.

**★ 15372 ★ University of Rochester**
**School of Nursing**
Box SON
601 Elmwood St.
Rochester, NY 14642
**Phone:** (716)275-2375    **Fax:** (716)756-8299
**Email:** son_admissions@urmc.rochester.edu
**Website:** http://www.urmc.rochester.edu/son
Elaine M. Andolina, Contact
**Fnded:** 1850. **Degrees Offered:** BS, MS, MS/MBA, PhD.

**★ 15373 ★ Utica College of Syracuse**
**Department of Nursing**
1600 Burrstone Rd.
Utica, NY 13502
**Phone:** (315)792-3006    **Fax:** (315)792-3003
**Email:** lnorth@utica.ucsu.edu
**Website:** http://www.utica.edu
Leslie B. North, Contact
**Fnded:** 1946. **Degrees Offered:** BS.

**★ 15374 ★ Wagner College**
**Department of Nursing**
Staten Island, NY
**Phone:** (718)390-3444    **Fax:** (718)420-4009
**Email:** ahren@wagner.edu
**Website:** http://www.wagner.edu/
Dr. Kathleen Ahern, Contact
**Fnded:** 1883. **Degrees Offered:** BS, MS.

**★ 15375 ★ York College of the City University of New York**
**Program in Nursing**
94-20 Guy R. Brewer Blvd.
Jamaica, NY 11451
**Phone:** (718)262-2165
**Website:** http://www.york.cuny.edu/
**Fnded:** 1967. **Degrees Offered:** BS.

## Newfoundland

**★ 15376 ★ Memorial University of Newfoundland**
**School of Nursing**
Health Science Centre
Prince Philip Pkwy.
Saint John's, NF, Canada A1B 3V6
**Phone:** (709)737-6679    **Fax:** (709)737-7037
**Email:** slefort@morgan.ucs.mun.ca
**Website:** http://www.mun.ca/sgs/prospectus
Dr. Sandra LeFort, Contact
**Fnded:** 1925. **Degrees Offered:** BN, MN.

## North Carolina

**★ 15377 ★ Barton College**
**Department of Nursing**
PO Box 5000
Wilson, NC 27893-7000
**Phone:** (252)399-6400    **Fax:** (252)399-6416
**Email:** ppruden@barton.edu
**Website:** http://www.barton.edu
Dr. Pet S. Pruden, Contact
**Fnded:** 1902. **Degrees Offered:** BSN.

**★ 15378 ★ Duke University**
**School of Nursing**
Box 3322 Medical Center
Durham, NC 27710
**Phone:** (919)415-3853    **Fax:** (919)681-8899
**Email:** admissions@mc.duke.edu/
**Website:** http://son3.mc.duke.edu
Jennifer Avery, Contact
**Fnded:** 1838. **Degrees Offered:** MSN, MSN/MBA, MSN/MCM.

**★ 15379 ★ East Carolina University**
**School of Nursing**
Rivers Bldg.
Greenville, NC 27858-4353
**Phone:** (252)328-4302    **Fax:** (252)328-4300
**Email:** turnerp@mail.ecu.edu
**Website:** http://www.ecu.edu/
Dr. Phyllis S. Tuner, Contact
**Fnded:** 1907. **Degrees Offered:** BSN, MSN.

**★ 15380 ★ Gardner-Webb University**
**School of Nursing**
PO Box 7268
Boiling Springs, NC 28017
**Phone:** (704)406-4360    **Fax:** (704)406-3919
**Email:** stoney@gardner-webb.edu
**Website:** http://www.gardner-webb.edu/
Dr. Shirley P. Toney, Contact
**Fnded:** 1905. **Degrees Offered:** BSN, MSN, MSN/MBA.

**★ 15381 ★ Lenoir-Rhyne College**
**Department of Nursing**
PO Box 7292
Hickory, NC 28603
**Phone:** (828)328-7282    **Fax:** (828)328-7284
**Email:** reecel@lrc.edu
**Website:** http://www.lrc.edu/
Dr. Linda W. Reece, Contact
**Fnded:** 1891. **Degrees Offered:** BS.

**★ 15382 ★ North Carolina Agricultural and Technical State University**
**School of Nursing**
1601 E Market St.
Greensboro, NC 27411
**Phone:** (336)334-7752    **Fax:** (336)334-7752
**Email:** daviss@ncat.edu
**Website:** http://www.ncat.edu/
Sophia Davis, Contact
**Fnded:** 1891. **Degrees Offered:** BSN.

**★ 15383 ★ North Carolina Central University**
**Department of Nursing**
PO Box 19798
Durham, NC 27707
**Phone:** (919)560-6431    **Fax:** (919)560-5343
**Email:** bpdennis@wpo.nccu.edu
**Website:** http://www.nccu.edu/
Dr. Betty Pierce Dennis, Contact
**Fnded:** 1910. **Degrees Offered:** BSN.

**★ 15384 ★ Queens College**
**Division of Nursing**
1900 Selwyn Ave.
Charlotte, NC 28274
**Phone:** (704)337-2363    **Fax:** (704)337-2477
**Email:** martink@queens.edu
**Website:** http://www.queens.edu/
Dr. Karen J. Martin, Contact
**Fnded:** 1857. **Degrees Offered:** BSN, MSN, MSN/MBA.

**★ 15385 ★ Southeastern North Carolina Nursing Consortium**
PO Box 1510
Pembroke, NC 28372
**Phone:** (910)521-6522    **Fax:** (910)521-6178
**Email:** lockt@nat.uncp.edu
Tonya Locklear, Contact
**Degrees Offered:** BSN.

**★ 15386 ★ University of North Carolina, Chapel Hill**
**School of Nursing**
301 Carrington Hall
College Box 7460
Chapel Hill, NC 27599-7460
**Phone:** (919)966-4260    **Fax:** (919)966-3540
**Email:** kmoore@unc.edu
**Website:** http://www.unc.edu/depts/nursing
Katherine Moore, Contact
**Fnded:** 1789. **Degrees Offered:** BSN, MSN, PhD.

**★ 15387 ★ University of North Carolina, Charlotte**
**College of Nursing and Health Professions**
9201 University City Blvd.
Charlotte, NC 28223-0001
**Phone:** (704)687-4684    **Fax:** (704)687-3180
**Email:** bkhemlst@email.uncc.edu
**Website:** http://www.uncc.edu/gradmiss
Brenna Helmstutler, Contact
**Fnded:** 1946. **Degrees Offered:** BSN, MSN.

**★ 15388 ★ University of North Carolina, Greensboro**
**School of Nursing**
PO Box 26172
Greensboro, NC 27402-6172
**Phone:** (336)334-5561    **Fax:** (336)334-3628
**Email:** eileen_kohlenberg@uncg.edu

**Website:** http://www.uncg.edu/nur/
Eileen Kohlenberg, Contact
**Fnded:** 1891. **Degrees Offered:** BSN, MSN, MSN/
MBA.


★ **15389** ★ **University of North Carolina,
Wilmington**
**School of Nursing**
601 S College Rd.
Wilmington, NC 28403-3297
**Phone:** (910)962-3208     **Fax:** (910)962-3723
**Email:** nursing@uncwil.edu
**Website:** http://www.uncwil.edu/
Nancy L. McLemore, Contact
**Fnded:** 1947. **Degrees Offered:** BS, MSN.


★ **15390** ★ **Western Carolina University**
**Department of Nursing**
Cullowhee, NC 28723
**Phone:** (828)227-7467     **Fax:** (828)227-7071
**Email:** grenwicki@wcu.edu
**Website:** http://www.wcu.edu/
Dr. Sandra Grenieiicki, Contact
**Fnded:** 1889. **Degrees Offered:** BSN, MSN.


★ **15391** ★ **Winston-Salem State
University**
**Department of Nursing**
601 Martin Luther King Jr. Dr.
Winston-Salem, NC 27110
**Phone:** (336)750-2560     **Fax:** (336)750-2599
**Email:** McInnis@wssu.edu
**Website:** http://www.wssu.edu
Nancy McInnis, Contact
**Fnded:** 1892. **Degrees Offered:** BSN.


## North Dakota


★ **15392** ★ **Dickinson State University**
**Department of Nursing**
291 Campus Dr.
Dickinson, ND 58601-4896
**Phone:** (701)483-2516     **Fax:** (701)483-2524
**Website:** http://www.dsu.nodak.edu/
Mary Ann Marsh, Contact
**Fnded:** 1918. **Degrees Offered:** BSN.


★ **15393** ★ **Jamestown College**
**Department of Nursing**
Admissions Department
6081 College Ln.
Jamestown, ND 58405
**Phone:** (701)252-3467     **Fax:** (701)253-4318
**Website:** http://www.jc.edu/
**Fnded:** 1883. **Degrees Offered:** BSN.


★ **15394** ★ **Medcenter One College of
Nursing**
512 North 7th St.
Bismarck, ND 58501
**Phone:** (701)323-6271     **Fax:** (701)323-6967
**Email:** msmith@mohs.org
**Website:** http://www.medcenterone.com/nursing/
nursing.htm/
Mary Smith, Contact
**Fnded:** 1988. **Degrees Offered:** BSN.


★ **15395** ★ **Minot State University**
**College of Nursing**
500 University Ave., W
Minot, ND 58707-0002
**Phone:** (701)858-3101     **Fax:** (701)858-4309
**Email:** petterse@misu.nodak.edu
**Website:** http://www.misu.nodak.edu/
Linda Pettersen, Contact
**Fnded:** 1913. **Degrees Offered:** BSN.


★ **15396** ★ **North Dakota State University**
**Department of Nursing**
136 Sudro Hall
Fargo, ND 58105
**Phone:** (701)231-7772     **Fax:** (701)231-7606
**Email:** lois_nelson@ndsu.nodak.edu
**Website:** http://www.ndsu.edu/
Dr. Lois F. Nelson, Contact
**Fnded:** 1890. **Degrees Offered:** BSN.


★ **15397** ★ **University of Mary**
**Division of Nursing**
7500 University Dr.
Bismarck, ND 58504
**Phone:** (701)255-7500     **Fax:** (701)255-7687
**Website:** http://www.umary.edu/nursing/
**Fnded:** 1959. **Degrees Offered:** BSN, MSN.


★ **15398** ★ **University of North Dakota**
**College of Nursing**
Box 9025
Grand Forks, ND 58202-9025
**Phone:** (701)777-4552     **Fax:** (701)777-4096
**Email:** ginny_guido@mail.und.nodak.edu
**Website:** http://www.und.nodak.edu/dept/nursing/
Dr. Ginny W. Guido, Contact
**Fnded:** 1883. **Degrees Offered:** BSN, MS.


## Nova Scotia


★ **15399** ★ **Dalhousie University**
**School of Nursing**
5869 University Ave.
Halifax, NS, Canada B3H 3J5
**Phone:** (902)494-2143     **Fax:** (902)494-3487
**Email:** donna.meagher-stewart@dal.ca
**Website:** http://is.dal.ca/~son/main/nursing.htm
Donna Meagher-Stewart, Contact
**Fnded:** 1818. **Degrees Offered:** BSCN, MN.


★ **15400** ★ **St. Francis Xavier University**
**Department of Nursing**
PO Box 5000
Antigonish, NS, Canada B2G 2W5
**Phone:** (902)867-3923     **Fax:** (902)867-5154
**Email:** rsepton@stfx.ca
**Website:** http://www.stfx.ca/
Mary Coyle, Contact
**Fnded:** 1853. **Degrees Offered:** BSCN.


## Ohio


★ **15401** ★ **Ashland University**
**Department of Nursing**
Ashland, OH 44805
**Phone:** (419)289-5242     **Fax:** (419)258-5989
**Email:** dstitzlein@ashland.edu
**Website:** http://www.ashland.edu
Dr. Dorothy A. Stitzlein, Contact
**Fnded:** 1878. **Degrees Offered:** BSN, MSN, MSN/
MBA.


★ **15402** ★ **Capital University**
**School of Nursing**
Columbus, OH 43209-2394
**Phone:** (614)236-6331     **Fax:** (614)236-6157
**Email:** gglasgow@capital.edu
**Website:** http://www.capital.edu/
Dr. Gretchen Glasgow, Contact
**Fnded:** 1878. **Degrees Offered:** BSN, MSN, MSN/
MBA.


★ **15403** ★ **Case Western Reserve
University**
**Frances Payne Bolton School of Nursing**
10900 Euclid Ave.
Cleveland, OH 44106-4904
**Phone:** (216)368-2016     **Fax:** (216)368-3542
**Email:** rhd3@po.cwru.edu
**Website:** http://fpb.cwru.edu/
Rob Davis, Contact
**Fnded:** 1826. **Degrees Offered:** BSN, MSN, MSN/
MA, MSN/MBA.


★ **15404** ★ **Cedarville University**
**Department of Nursing**
251 N Main St.
Cedarville, OH 45314-0601
**Free:** 800-233-2784     **Fax:** (937)766-2760
**Email:** admissions@cedarville.edu
**Website:** http://www.cedarville.edu
Roscoe Smith, Contact
**Fnded:** 1887. **Degrees Offered:** BSN.


★ **15405** ★ **Cleveland State University**
**Department of Nursing**
1860 E 22nd St. (RT 915)
Cleveland, OH 44115-4435
**Phone:** (216)687-3548     **Fax:** (216)687-3556
**Email:** j.romeo@csuohio.edu
**Website:** http://www.csuohio.edu/
Dr. June Heart Romeo, Contact
**Fnded:** 1964. **Degrees Offered:** BSN, MSN.


★ **15406** ★ **College of Mt. Saint Joseph**
**Department of Nursing**
5701 Delhi Rd.
Cincinnati, OH 45233-1670
**Phone:** (513)244-4511     **Fax:** (513)451-2547
**Email:** darla_vale@mail.msj.edu
**Website:** http://www.msj.edu/
Dr. Darla Vale, Contact
**Fnded:** 1920. **Degrees Offered:** BSN.


★ **15407** ★ **Franciscan University,
Steubenville**
**Department of Nursing**
Steubenville, OH 43952
**Phone:** (740)284-7245     **Fax:** (740)284-6449
**Email:** jdavis@franuniv.edu
**Website:** http://www.franuniv.edu/
Dr. Joan Davis, Contact
**Fnded:** 1946. **Degrees Offered:** BSN, MSN.


★ **15408** ★ **Kent State University**
**College of Nursing**
PO Box 5190
Kent, OH 44242-0001
**Phone:** (330)672-2234     **Fax:** (330)672-2433
**Email:** dbiordi@kent.edu
**Website:** http://www.kent.edu/
Diana Biordi, Contact
**Fnded:** 1910. **Degrees Offered:** BSN, MSN, MSN/
MBA, MSN/MPA.


★ **15409** ★ **Lourdes College**
**Department of Nursing**
6832 Convent Blvd.
Sylvania, OH 43560
**Phone:** (419)824-3780     **Fax:** (419)824-3513
**Email:** pwelter@lourdes.edu
**Website:** http://www.lourdes.edu
Pam Welter, Contact
**Fnded:** 1958. **Degrees Offered:** BSN.


★ **15410** ★ **Malone College**
**Department of Nursing**
515 25th St. NW
Canton, OH 44709
**Phone:** (330)471-8145     **Fax:** (330)454-6977
**Email:** admissions@malone.edu
**Website:** http://www.malone.edu
John Chopka, Contact
**Fnded:** 1892. **Degrees Offered:** BSN.

**★ 15411 ★ Medical College of Ohio**
**School of Nursing**
3015 Arlington Ave.
Toledo, OH 43614-5803
**Phone:** (419)383-5892 **Fax:** (419)383-5894
**Email:** jrobinson@mco.edu
**Website:** http://www.mco.edu
Dr. Janet H. Robinson, Contact
**Fnded:** 1964. **Degrees Offered:** BSN, MSN.

**★ 15412 ★ Miami University**
**Department of Nursing**
1601 Peck Blvd.
Hamilton, OH 45011
**Phone:** (513)785-3280 **Fax:** (513)785-3284
**Email:** millsem@muohio.edu
**Website:** http://www.sas.muohio.edu/nsg/welcome-frame.html
Dr. Eugenia M. Mills, Contact
**Fnded:** 1809. **Degrees Offered:** BSN.

**★ 15413 ★ Mount Carmel College of**
**Nursing**
**Baccalaureate Nursing Program**
127 South Davis St.
Columbus, OH 43222
**Phone:** (614)234-5144 **Fax:** (614)234-2875
**Email:** mmenfield@mchs.com
Merchel Menefield, Contact
**Degrees Offered:** BSN.

**★ 15414 ★ Ohio State University**
**College of Nursing**
1585 Neil Ave.
Columbus, OH 43210-1289
**Phone:** (614)292-8962 **Fax:** (614)292-4948
**Email:** frazier.7@osu.edu
**Website:** http://www.osu.edu
Katherine Frazier, Contact
**Fnded:** 1870. **Degrees Offered:** BSN, MS, MS/MHA, MS/MPH, PhD.

**★ 15415 ★ Ohio University**
**School of Nursing**
312 McCracken Hall
Athens, OH 45701
**Phone:** (740)593-4494 **Fax:** (740)593-0286
**Email:** grippa@ohio.edu
**Website:** http://www.ohiou.edu
Dr. Kathleen M. Rose-Grippa, Contact
**Fnded:** 1804. **Degrees Offered:** BSN.

**★ 15416 ★ Otterbein College**
**Program in Nursing**
155 W Main St.
Westerville, OH 43081
**Phone:** (614)823-1894 **Fax:** (614)823-3131
**Email:** emikolaj@otterbein.edu
**Website:** http://www.otterbein.edu/
Dr. Eda Mikolaj, Contact
**Fnded:** 1847. **Degrees Offered:** BSN, MSN.

**★ 15417 ★ University of Akron**
**College of Nursing**
209 Carroll St.
Akron, OH 44325-3701
**Phone:** (330)972-7555 **Fax:** (330)972-5737
**Email:** kr1@uakron.edu
**Website:** http://odin.chemistry.uakron.edu/nursing
Dr. Kathy Ross-Alaolmolki, Contact
**Fnded:** 1870. **Degrees Offered:** BSN, MSN, PhD.

**★ 15418 ★ University of Cincinnati**
**College of Nursing**
PO Box 210038
Cincinnati, OH 45221-0038
**Phone:** (513)558-5072 **Fax:** (513)558-7523
**Email:** loren.carter@uc.edu
**Website:** http://www.uc.edu
Loren Carter, Contact
**Fnded:** 1819. **Degrees Offered:** BSN, MSN, MSN/MBA, PhD.

**★ 15419 ★ Ursuline College**
**The Breen School of Nursing**
2550 Lander Rd.
Pepper Pike, OH 44124
**Phone:** (440)449-3425 **Fax:** (440)449-4267
**Email:** cwaggoner@ursuline.edu
**Website:** http://www.ursuline.edu
Dr. Carol Waggoner, Contact
**Fnded:** 1871. **Degrees Offered:** BSN, MSN.

**★ 15420 ★ Walsh University**
**Department of Nursing**
2020 Easton St. NW
North Canton, OH 44720
**Phone:** (330)490-7250 **Fax:** (330)490-7206
**Email:** mmeeker@walsh.edu
**Website:** http://www.walsh.edu
Dr. Mary E. Meeker, Contact
**Fnded:** 1958. **Degrees Offered:** BSN.

**★ 15421 ★ Wright State University**
**College of Nursing and Health**
3640 Colonel Glenn Highway
Dayton, OH 45435
**Phone:** (937)775-3132 **Fax:** (937)775-4571
**Email:** theresa.haghnazarian@wright.edu
**Website:** http://www.nursing.wright.edu/
Theresa Haghnazarian, Contact
**Fnded:** 1964. **Degrees Offered:** BSN, MS, MS/MBA.

**★ 15422 ★ Xavier University**
**Department of Nursing**
3800 Victory Pkwy.
Cincinnati, OH 45207-7351
**Phone:** (513)745-4392 **Fax:** (513)745-1087
**Email:** gomez@admin.xu.edu
**Website:** http://www.xu.edu/
Marilyn Volk Gomez, Contact
**Fnded:** 1831. **Degrees Offered:** BSN, MSN, MSN/MBA.

**★ 15423 ★ Youngstown State University**
**Department of Nursing**
1 University Plaza
Youngstown, OH 44555
**Phone:** (330)742-1796 **Fax:** (330)742-2309
**Website:** http://www.ysu.edu
Dr. Sharon Shipton, Contact
**Fnded:** 1908. **Degrees Offered:** BSN, MSN.

## Oklahoma

**★ 15424 ★ East Central University**
**Department of Nursing**
1100 E 14th St.
Ada, OK 74820
**Phone:** (580)310-5434 **Fax:** (580)310-5785
**Email:** eschmlng@mailclerk.ecok.edu
**Website:** http://www.ecok.edu
Dr. Elizabeth Schmelling, Contact
**Fnded:** 1909. **Degrees Offered:** BS.

**★ 15425 ★ Langston University**
**School of Nursing and Health Profession**
302 University Women Bldg.
Langston, OK 73050
**Phone:** (405)466-3411 **Fax:** (405)466-2195
**Email:** tigriffin@lunet.edu
**Website:** http://www.lunet.edu
Tanara Griffin, Contact
**Fnded:** 1897. **Degrees Offered:** BSN.

**★ 15426 ★ Northeastern State University**
**Department of Nursing**
705 N Grand
Tahlequah, OK 74464-2300
**Phone:** (918)458-2087 **Fax:** (918)458-2349
**Email:** vannostr@nsuok.edu
**Website:** http://www.nsuok.edu/
Dr. Joyce A. Van Nostrand, Contact
**Fnded:** 1846. **Degrees Offered:** BSN.

**★ 15427 ★ Northwestern Oklahoma State**
**University**
**School of Nursing**
709 Oklahoma Blvd.
Alva, OK 73717-2799
**Phone:** (580)327-8489 **Fax:** (580)327-8434
**Email:** jestephens@nwosu.edu
**Website:** http://www.nwalva.edu/
Dr. Janice E. Stephens, Contact
**Fnded:** 1897. **Degrees Offered:** BSN.

**★ 15428 ★ Oklahoma Baptist University**
**School of Nursing**
500 West University
Shawnee, OK 74804
**Phone:** (405)878-2081 **Fax:** (405)878-2082
**Email:** lana_bolhouse@mail.okbu.edu
**Website:** http://www.okbu.edu
**Fnded:** 1910. **Degrees Offered:** BSN.

**★ 15429 ★ Oklahoma City University**
**Kramer School of Nursing**
2501 N Blackwelder
Oklahoma City, OK 73106
**Phone:** (405)521-5901 **Fax:** (405)521-5914
**Email:** gkirkham@okcu.edu
**Website:** http://www.okcu.edu
Glenda Kirkham, Contact
**Fnded:** 1904. **Degrees Offered:** BSN.

**★ 15430 ★ Oklahoma Panhandle State**
**University**
**Bachelor of Science in Nursing Program**
PO Box 430
323 West Eagle Blvd.
Goodwell, OK 73939
**Phone:** (580)349-2611 **Fax:** (580)349-2302
**Email:** conniec@opsu.edu
**Website:** http://www.opus.edu
Dr. Connie J. Carpenter, Contact
**Fnded:** 1909. **Degrees Offered:** BSN.

**★ 15431 ★ Oklahoma Wesleyan College**
**Division of Nursing**
2201 Silver Lake Rd.
Bartlesville, OK 74006
**Phone:** (918)335-6254 **Fax:** (918)335-6204
**Email:** tpgiles@bwc.edu
Pamela Ann Giles, RN, Contact
**Fnded:** 1909. **Degrees Offered:** BSN.

**★ 15432 ★ Oral Roberts University**
**Anna Vaughn School of Nursing**
Tulsa, OK 74171
**Phone:** (918)495-6198 **Fax:** (918)495-6020
**Email:** kjezek@oru.edu
**Website:** http://www.oru.edu/
Dr. Kenda Jezek, Contact
**Fnded:** 1963. **Degrees Offered:** BSN.

**★ 15433 ★ Southern Nazarene University**
**School of Nursing**
6729 Northwest 39th Expressway
Bethany, OK 73008
**Phone:** (405)491-6365 **Fax:** (405)491-6264
**Email:** aferguso@snu.edu
**Website:** http://www.snu.edu/
Dr. Ann Ferguson, Contact

**Fnded:** 1899. **Degrees Offered:** BS.

★ **15434** ★ **Southwestern Oklahoma State University**
**Division of Nursing**
100 Campus Dr.
Weatherford, OK 73096-3098
**Phone:** (580)774-3261          **Fax:** (580)774-7075
**Email:** henrikd@swosu.edu
**Website:** http://www.swosu.edu/
Debbie Henriksen, Contact
**Fnded:** 1901. **Degrees Offered:** BSN.

★ **15435** ★ **University of Central Oklahoma**
**Department of Nursing**
100 N University Dr.
Edmond, OK 73034-5209
**Phone:** (405)974-5000          **Fax:** (405)974-3824
**Email:** plagrow@ucok.edu
**Website:** http://www.cwc.cc.wy.us/
Dr. Patricia A. LaGrow, Contact
**Fnded:** 1890. **Degrees Offered:** BS.

★ **15436** ★ **University of Oklahoma Health Sciences Center**
**College of Nursing**
PO Box 26901
Oklahoma City, OK 73190
**Phone:** (405)271-2428          **Fax:** (405)271-3443
**Email:** patti-matney@ouhsc.edu
**Fnded:** 1890. **Degrees Offered:** BSN, MS.

★ **15437** ★ **University of Tulsa**
**School of Nursing**
600 S College Ave.
Tulsa, OK 74104-3189
**Phone:** (918)631-3116          **Fax:** (918)631-2068
**Email:** susan-gaston@utulsa.edu
**Website:** http://www.utulsa.edu/
Dr. Susan Gaston, Contact
**Fnded:** 1894. **Degrees Offered:** BSN.

### Ontario

★ **15438** ★ **Lakehead University**
**School of Nursing**
Thunder Bay, ON, Canada P7B 5E1
**Phone:** (807)343-8395          **Fax:** (807)343-8246
**Email:** lorne.mcdougall@lakeheadu.ca
**Website:** http://www.lakeheadu.ca/
Dr. Lorne McDougall, Contact
**Fnded:** 1965. **Degrees Offered:** BSN.

★ **15439** ★ **Laurentian University**
**School of Nursing**
935 Ramsey Lake Rd.
Sudbury, ON, Canada P3E 2C6
**Phone:** (705)675-6589          **Fax:** (705)675-4861
**Email:** erukholm@nickel.laurentian.ca
**Website:** http://www.laurentian.ca/
Dr. Ellen Rukholm, Contact
**Fnded:** 1960. **Degrees Offered:** BSCN.

★ **15440** ★ **McMaster University**
**School of Nursing**
1200 Main St. W
Rm 3N10
Hamilton, ON, Canada L8N 3Z5
**Phone:** (905)525-9140          **Fax:** (905)546-1129
**Website:** http://www.mcmaster.ca/
**Fnded:** 1887. **Degrees Offered:** BSCN, M SC PhD.

★ **15441** ★ **Queen's University, Kingston**
**School of Nursing**
Cataraqui Bldg.
90 Barrie St.
Kingston, ON, Canada K7L 3N6
**Phone:** (613)533-6000          **Fax:** (613)533-6770
**Email:** kisilevb@post.queensu.ca
**Website:** http://meds-ss10.meds.queensu.ca/nursing/
Dr. Barbara Kisilevsky, Contact
**Fnded:** 1841. **Degrees Offered:** BSCN, M SC.

★ **15442** ★ **Ryerson Polytechnic University**
**Program in Nursing**
350 Victoria St.
Toronto, ON, Canada M5B 2K3
**Phone:** (416)979-5300
**Email:** ncherry@acs.ryerson.ca
**Website:** http://www.ryerson.ca/
Nichole Cherry, Contact
**Fnded:** 1948. **Degrees Offered:** BSCN.

★ **15443** ★ **University of Ottawa**
**School of Nursing**
451 Smyth Rd., Rm. 2009
Ottawa, ON, Canada K1H 8M5
**Phone:** (613)562-5800          **Fax:** (613)562-5470
**Email:** ychenier@uottawa.ca
**Website:** http://www.uottawa.ca/
Yolande Chenier, Contact
**Fnded:** 1848. **Degrees Offered:** BSCN, M SC N.

★ **15444** ★ **University of Toronto**
**Faculty of Nursing**
Student Services Office
50 St. George St.
Toronto, ON, Canada M5S 3H4
**Phone:** (416)978-2863          **Fax:** (416)978-8222
**Email:** inquiry.nursing@utornto.ca
**Website:** http://www.utoronto.ca/uoft.html
**Fnded:** 1827. **Degrees Offered:** BSCN, MN, MN/ MBA, PhD.

★ **15445** ★ **University of Western Ontario**
**Faculty of Nursing**
London, ON, Canada N6A 5C1
**Phone:** (519)661-2111          **Fax:** (519)661-3928
**Email:** sleblan2@julian.uwo.ca
**Website:** http://www.uwo.ca/
Shelley le Blanc, Contact
**Fnded:** 1878. **Degrees Offered:** BSCN, M SC N.

★ **15446** ★ **University of Windsor**
**School of Nursing**
401 Sunset Ave.
Windsor, ON, Canada N9B 3P4
**Phone:** (519)253-3000          **Fax:** (519)973-7084
**Email:** srotond@uwindsor.ca
**Website:** http://www.uwindsor.ca/
Dr. Barbara Thomas, Contact
**Fnded:** 1857. **Degrees Offered:** BSCN, M SC N.

★ **15447** ★ **York University**
**Department of Nursing, Atkinson College**
Atkinson Room 404
4700 Keele St.
Toronto, ON, Canada M3J 1P3
**Phone:** (416)736-5271          **Fax:** (416)736-5714
**Email:** kathem@yorku.ca
**Website:** http://www.yorku.ca/
Dr. Kathleen MacDonald, Contact
**Fnded:** 1959. **Degrees Offered:** BSCN.

### Oregon

★ **15448** ★ **Linfield College**
**School of Nursing, Portland Campus**
2215 NW Northrup St.
Portland, OR 97210
**Phone:** (503)413-8481          **Fax:** (503)413-6283
**Email:** bwoodwar@linfield.edu
**Website:** http://www.linfield.edu/
Beth A. Woodward, Contact
**Fnded:** 1849. **Degrees Offered:** BSN.

★ **15449** ★ **Oregon Health Sciences University**
**School of Nursing**
3181 SW Sam Jackson Park Rd.
Portland, OR 97201-3098
**Phone:** (503)494-3805          **Fax:** (503)494-4350
**Email:** proginfo@ohsu.edu
**Website:** http://www.ohsu.edu/~son/
Gabrielle Pedersen, Contact
**Fnded:** 1974. **Degrees Offered:** BS, MS, PhD.

★ **15450** ★ **University of Portland**
**School of Nursing**
5000 N Willamette Blvd.
Portland, OR 97203-5798
**Phone:** (503)943-7107          **Fax:** (503)943-7399
**Email:** chadwick@up.edu
**Website:** http://www.up.edu/
Dr. Patricia L. Chadwick, Contact
**Fnded:** 1901. **Degrees Offered:** BSN, MS.

★ **15451** ★ **Walla Walla College**
**School of Nursing**
10345 SE Market St.
Portland, OR 97216
**Phone:** (503)251-6115          **Fax:** (503)261-6249
**Email:** whitlo@wwc.edu
**Website:** http://www.wwc.edu/academics/departments/nursing/
Lois Whitchurch, Contact
**Fnded:** 1892. **Degrees Offered:** BS.

### Pennsylvania

★ **15452** ★ **Alvernia College**
**Department of Nursing**
Reading, PA
**Phone:** (610)796-8306          **Fax:** (610)796-8464
**Email:** Karen.thacker@alvernia.edu
**Website:** http://www.alvernia.edu
Karen S. Thacker, Contact
**Fnded:** 1958. **Degrees Offered:** BSN.

★ **15453** ★ **Bloomsburg University of Pennsylvania**
**Department of Nursing**
MCHS 3121
Bloomsburg, PA 17815
**Phone:** (570)389-4602          **Fax:** (570)389-5008
**Email:** haymaker@husky.bloomu.edu
**Website:** http://www.bloomu.edu/
Dr. Sharon Haymaker, Contact
**Fnded:** 1839. **Degrees Offered:** BSN, MSN

★ **15454** ★ **California University of Pennsylvania**
**Department of Nursing**
250 University Ave.
Box 60
California, PA 15419-1394
**Phone:** (724)938-5739          **Fax:** (724)938-1612
**Email:** marcinek@cup.edu
**Website:** http://www.cup.edu/
Dr. Margaret Marcinek, Contact
**Fnded:** 1852. **Degrees Offered:** BSN.

**★ 15455 ★ Carlow College**
**Division of Nursing**
3333 5th Ave.
Pittsburgh, PA 15213
**Phone:** (412)578-6092          **Fax:** (412)578-6321
**Email:** lwaigand@carlow.edu
**Website:** http://www.carlow.edu/
Lee Waigand, Contact
**Fnded:** 1929. **Degrees Offered:** BSN, MSN.

**★ 15456 ★ Cedar Crest College**
**Nursing Department**
100 College Dr.
Allentown, PA 18104-6196
**Phone:** (610)606-4606          **Fax:** (610)606-4615
**Email:** lmurray@cedarcrest.edu
**Website:** http://www.cedarcrest.edu/
Dr. Laurie R. Murray, Contact
**Fnded:** 1867. **Degrees Offered:** BS.

**★ 15457 ★ Clarion University of**
**Pennsylvania**
**School of Nursing**
Strain Behavioral Science Bldg.
Slippery Rock, PA 16057-1326
**Phone:** (724)738-2323          **Fax:** (724)738-2881
**Email:** joyce.white@sru.edu
**Website:** http://www.clarion.edu/academic/nursing/index.htm
Dr. Joyce White, Contact
**Fnded:** 1967. **Degrees Offered:** BSN, MSN.

**★ 15458 ★ College Misericordia**
**Program in Nursing**
301 Lake St.
Dallas, PA 18612
**Phone:** (717)674-6440          **Fax:** (570)674-8902
**Email:** jsteel@miseri.edu
**Website:** http://www.miseri.edu/
Dr. Jean Steelman, Contact
**Fnded:** 1924. **Degrees Offered:** BSN, MSN.

**★ 15459 ★ DeSales University**
**Department of Nursing and Health**
2755 Station Ave.
Center Valley, PA 18034-9568
**Phone:** (610)282-1100          **Fax:** (610)282-2254
**Email:** carol.mest@desales.edu
**Website:** http://www.desales.edu
Carol Mest, Contact
**Fnded:** 1964. **Degrees Offered:** BSN, MSN.

**★ 15460 ★ Duquesne University**
**School of Nursing**
623 College Hall
600 Forbes Ave.
Pittsburgh, PA 15282-1760
**Phone:** (412)396-6536          **Fax:** (412)396-6346
**Email:** gaberson@duq.edu
**Website:** http://www.duq.edu/
Dr. Kathleen Gaberson, Contact
**Fnded:** 1878. **Degrees Offered:** BSN, MSN, MSN/MBA, PhD.

**★ 15461 ★ East Stroudsburg University**
**of Pennsylvania**
**Department of Nursing**
200 Prospect St.
East Stroudsburg, PA 18301-2999
**Phone:** (570)422-3474          **Fax:** (570)422-3848
**Email:** kkarner@esu.edu
**Website:** http://www.esu.edu/
Dr. Karen Johnson Karner, Contact
**Fnded:** 1893. **Degrees Offered:** BS.

**★ 15462 ★ Eastern College**
**Program in Nursing**
1300 Eagle Rd.
Saint Davids, PA 19087
**Phone:** (610)341-5896          **Fax:** (610)225-5016
**Email:** mlacey@eastern.edu
**Website:** http://www.eastern.edu/
Dr. Margaret Lacey, Contact
**Fnded:** 1952. **Degrees Offered:** BSN.

**★ 15463 ★ Edinboro University of**
**Pennsylvania**
**Department of Nursing**
136 Centennial Hall
Edinboro, PA 16444
**Phone:** (814)732-4669          **Fax:** (814)732-2536
**Website:** http://www.edinboro.edu
Dr. Judy Schilling, Contact
**Fnded:** 1857. **Degrees Offered:** BS, MSN.

**★ 15464 ★ Gannon University**
**Villa Maria School of Nursing**
109 University Sq.
Erie, PA 16541-0001
**Phone:** (814)871-5363          **Fax:** (814)871-5662
**Email:** shoemaker001@gannon.edu
**Website:** http://www.gannon.edu/
Ruth Ellen Shoemaker, Contact
**Fnded:** 1925. **Degrees Offered:** BSN, MA/MSM, MSN.

**★ 15465 ★ Gwynedd-Mercy College**
**Program in Nursing**
PO Box 901
Gwynedd Valley, PA 19437
**Phone:** (215)646-7300          **Fax:** (215)641-5517
**Website:** http://www.gmc.edu
Dr. Barbara A. Jones, Contact
**Fnded:** 1948. **Degrees Offered:** BSN, MSN.

**★ 15466 ★ Holy Family College**
**Division of Nursing**
Grant and Frankford Aves.
Philadelphia, PA 19114-2094
**Phone:** (215)637-7700          **Fax:** (215)637-1478
**Email:** schiavo@hfc.edu
**Website:** http://www.hfc.edu/
Dr. Antoinette Schiavo, Contact
**Fnded:** 1954. **Degrees Offered:** BSN, MSN.

**★ 15467 ★ Immaculata College**
**Nursing Department**
1145 King Rd.
Immaculata, PA 19345
**Phone:** (610)647-4400          **Fax:** (610)251-1668
**Email:** jcranmer@immaculata.edu
**Website:** http://www.immaculata.edu/
Dr. Janice Cranmer, Contact
**Fnded:** 1920. **Degrees Offered:** BSN.

**★ 15468 ★ Indiana University of**
**Pennsylvania**
**Department of Nursing**
Rm. 129 Stright Hall
Indiana, PA 15705-1087
**Phone:** (724)357-2222          **Fax:** (724)357-7518
**Email:** jpetersn@grove.iup.edu
**Website:** http://www.iup.edu/
Dr. James Petersen, Contact
**Fnded:** 1875. **Degrees Offered:** BSN, MSN.

**★ 15469 ★ Kutztown University of**
**Pennsylvania**
**Department of Nursing**
Beekey Bldg., Rm. 219
Kutztown, PA 19530
**Phone:** (610)683-4328          **Fax:** (610)683-4708
**Email:** kjohnsto@kutztown.edu

**Website:** http://www.kutztown.edu
Dr. Kimberly Anne Johnston, Contact
**Fnded:** 1866. **Degrees Offered:** BSN.

**★ 15470 ★ La Salle University**
**School of Nursing**
1900 W Olney Ave.
Philadelphia, PA 19141-1199
**Phone:** (215)951-1413          **Fax:** (215)951-1896
**Email:** beitz@lasalle.edu
**Website:** http://www.lasalle.edu
Dr. Janice Beitz, Contact
**Fnded:** 1863. **Degrees Offered:** BSN, MSN, MSN/MBA.

**★ 15471 ★ LaRoche College**
**Department of Nursing and Nursing**
**Management**
9000 Babcock Blvd.
Pittsburgh, PA 15237
**Phone:** (412)536-1262          **Fax:** (412)536-1283
**Email:** kozlowr1@laroche.edu
**Website:** http://www.laroche.edu
Renee A. Kozlowski, Contact
**Fnded:** 1963. **Degrees Offered:** BSN, MSN.

**★ 15472 ★ Mansfield University of**
**Pennsylvania**
**Robert Packer Department of Health**
**Sciences**
Admissions Office
Alumni Hall
Mansfield, PA 16933
**Phone:** (570)622-4243          **Fax:** (570)662-4121
**Email:** admissns@mnsfld.edu
**Website:** http://www.mansfield.edu
**Fnded:** 1857. **Degrees Offered:** BSN.

**★ 15473 ★ Marywood University**
**Department of Nursing**
2300 Adams Ave.
Scranton, PA 18509
**Phone:** (570)348-6211          **Fax:** (570)961-4761
**Email:** golden@ac.marywood.edu
**Website:** http://www.marywood.edu/
Dr. Mary Alice Elizabeth Golden, Contact
**Fnded:** 1915. **Degrees Offered:** BSN, MS.

**★ 15474 ★ MCP Hahnemann University**
**College of Nursing and Health**
**Professions**
245 N 15th St., MS 501
Philadelphia, PA 19102-1192
**Phone:** (215)762-1644          **Fax:** (215)762-1259
**Email:** emb1@drexel.edu
**Website:** http://www.mcphu.edu/
Elizabeth Blunt, Contact
**Fnded:** 1848. **Degrees Offered:** BSN, MSN.

**★ 15475 ★ Messiah College**
**Department of Nursing**
1 College Ave.
Grantham, PA 17027
**Phone:** (717)691-6000          **Fax:** (717)796-5374
**Email:** strausba@messiah.edu
**Website:** http://www.messiah.edu/
William Strausbaugh, Contact
**Fnded:** 1909. **Degrees Offered:** BSN.

**★ 15476 ★ Millersville University of**
**Pennsylvania**
**Department of Nursing**
PO Box 1002
Millersville, PA 17551-0302
**Phone:** (717)871-5276          **Fax:** (717)872-3985
**Email:** barbara.haus@millersv.edu
**Website:** http://www.millersv.edu/
Dr. Barbara E. Haus, Contact

Fnded: 1855. **Degrees Offered:** BSN, MSN.

★ **15477** ★ **Mount Aloysius College**
**Department of Nursing**
7373 Admiral Peary Hwy.
Cresson, PA 16630
**Phone:** (814)886-6393          **Fax:** (814)886-4906
**Email:** cwebb@mtaloy.edu
**Website:** http://www.mtaloy.edu/
Dr. Cheryl Webb, Contact
**Fnded:** 1939. **Degrees Offered:** BSN.

★ **15478** ★ **Neumann College**
**Program in Nursing**
1 Neumann Dr.
Aston, PA 19014-1298
**Free:** 800-963-8626          **Fax:** (610)459-1370
**Email:** nursdiv@neumann.edu
**Website:** http://www.neumann.edu/
**Fnded:** 1965. **Degrees Offered:** BS, MSN.

★ **15479** ★ **Pennsylvania State University,**
**University Park Campus**
**School of Nursing**
203 Health and Human Development, E
University Park, PA 16802
**Phone:** (814)863-2211          **Fax:** (814)865-3779
**Email:** kmh10@psu.edu
**Website:** http://www.psu.edu
Dr. Freida Holt, Contact
**Fnded:** 1855. **Degrees Offered:** BS, MS, PhD.

★ **15480** ★ **Saint Francis University**
**Department of Nursing**
Box 600
Loretto, PA 15940-0060
**Phone:** (814)472-3027          **Fax:** (814)472-3849
**Email:** jsamii@sfcpa.edu
**Website:** http://www.sfcpa.edu/
**Fnded:** 1847. **Degrees Offered:** BSN.

★ **15481** ★ **Slippery Rock University of**
**Pennsylvania**
**Department of Nursing**
115A Behavioral Sciences Bldg.
Slippery Rock, PA 16057
**Phone:** (724)738-2323          **Fax:** (724)738-2881
**Email:** joyce.white@sru.edu
**Website:** http://www.sru.edu
Dr. Joyce White, Contact
**Fnded:** 1889. **Degrees Offered:** BSN, MSN.

★ **15482** ★ **Temple University**
**Department of Nursing**
3307 N Broad St.
Philadelphia, PA 19140
**Phone:** (215)707-4617          **Fax:** (215)707-1599
**Website:** http://www.temple.edu
Dr. Margaret Shepard, Contact
**Fnded:** 1884. **Degrees Offered:** BSN, MSN.

★ **15483** ★ **Thomas Jefferson University**
**Department of Nursing**
130 S 9th St., Ste. 1200
Philadelphia, PA 19107
**Phone:** (215)503-7937          **Fax:** (215)932-1468
**Email:** mary.schaal@mail.tju.edu
**Website:** http://www.tju.edu/
Dr. Mary G. Schaal, Contact
**Fnded:** 1824. **Degrees Offered:** BSN, MSN.

★ **15484** ★ **University of Pennsylvania**
**School of Nursing**
420 Guardian Dr.
Philadelphia, PA 19104-6096
**Phone:** (215)898-3489          **Fax:** (215)573-8439

**Email:**     jcarroll@nursing.upenn.edu/~nursing/in-
dex.html
**Website:** http://dolphin.upenn.edu
Julie Stapleton Carroll, Contact
**Fnded:** 1740. **Degrees Offered:** BSN, MSN, MSN/
MBA, MSN/PhD.

★ **15485** ★ **University of Pittsburgh**
**School of Nursing**
239 Victoria Bldg.
3500 Victoria St.
Pittsburgh, PA 15261
**Phone:** (412)624-9670          **Fax:** (412)624-2409
**Email:** nursao@pitt.edu
**Website:** http://www.nursing.pitt.edu/
Dr. Lynette Jack, Contact
**Fnded:** 1787. **Degrees Offered:** BSN, MSN, PhD.

★ **15486** ★ **University of Pittsburgh,**
**Bradford**
**Department of Nursing**
Admissions Department
300 Campus Dr.
Bradford, PA 16701
**Free:** 800-872-1787
**Website:** http://www.pitt.edu/
**Fnded:** 1963. **Degrees Offered:** BSN.

★ **15487** ★ **University of Scranton**
**Department of Nursing**
McGurrin Hall
Scranton, PA 18510
**Phone:** (570)941-4060          **Fax:** (570)941-7093
**Email:** hansonm2@scranton.edu
**Website:** http://www.uofs.edu/
Dr. Mary Jane Hanson, Contact
**Fnded:** 1888. **Degrees Offered:** BS, MS.

★ **15488** ★ **Villanova University**
**College of Nursing**
Villanova, PA 19085-1690
**Phone:** (610)519-4934          **Fax:** (610)519-7997
**Email:** claire.manfredi@villanova.edu
**Website:** http://www.vill.edu/
Dr. Claire Manfredi, Contact
**Fnded:** 1842. **Degrees Offered:** BSN, MSN.

★ **15489** ★ **Waynesburg College**
**Department of Nursing**
203 Steward Science Hall
Waynesburg, PA 15370-1222
**Phone:** (724)852-3356          **Fax:** (724)627-6416
**Email:** pkraft@waynesburg.edu
**Website:** http://www.waynesburg.edu
Dr. Patty Kraft, Contact
**Fnded:** 1849. **Degrees Offered:** BSN.

★ **15490** ★ **West Chester University of**
**Pennsylvania**
**Department of Nursing**
100 S Church St.
West Chester, PA 19383
**Phone:** (610)436-2258
**Email:** jhickman@wcupa.edu
**Website:** http://www.wcupa.edu
Dr. Janet S. Hickman, Contact
**Fnded:** 1871. **Degrees Offered:** BSN, MSN.

★ **15491** ★ **Widener University**
**School of Nursing**
1 University Pl.
Chester, PA 19013
**Phone:** (610)499-4208          **Fax:** (610)499-4216
**Email:** mary.b.walker@widener.edu
**Website:** http://www.widener.edu/
Dr. Mary Walker, Contact
**Fnded:** 1821. **Degrees Offered:** BSN, DN SC, MSN.

★ **15492** ★ **Wilkes University**
**Department of Nursing**
109 S Franklin St.
Wilkes Barre, PA 18766
**Phone:** (570)408-4076          **Fax:** (570)408-7807
**Email:** telban@wilkes.edu
**Website:** http://www.wilkes.edu/
Dr. Sharon Telban, Contact
**Fnded:** 1933. **Degrees Offered:** BS, MS.

★ **15493** ★ **York College of Pennsylvania**
**Department of Nursing**
York, PA 17405-7199
**Phone:** (717)815-1420          **Fax:** (717)849-1651
**Email:** jharring@ycp.edu
**Website:** http://www.ycp.edu
Dr. Jacquelin H. Harrington, Contact
**Fnded:** 1787. **Degrees Offered:** BS.

## Prince Edward Island

★ **15494** ★ **University of Prince Edward**
**Island**
**School of Nursing**
550 University Ave.
Charlottetown, PE, Canada C1A 4P3
**Phone:** (902)566-0733          **Fax:** (902)566-0777
**Email:** mhines@upei.ca
**Website:** http://upei.ca/
Mary Lou Hines, Contact
**Fnded:** 1834. **Degrees Offered:** BSCN.

## Puerto Rico

★ **15495** ★ **Inter American University of**
**Puerto Rico, Metropolitan Campus**
**Carmen Torres de Tiburcio School of**
**Nursing**
PO Box 191293
San Juan, PR 00919-1293
**Phone:** (787)763-3066          **Fax:** (787)250-1242
**Email:** geortiz@inter.edu
**Website:** http://metro.inter.edu
Dr. Gloria E. Ortiz, Contact
**Fnded:** 1960. **Degrees Offered:** BSN.

★ **15496** ★ **Pontifical Catholic University**
**of Puerto Rico**
**Department of Nursing**
Ave. Las Americas, Station 6
Ponce, PR 00732
**Phone:** (787)841-2000          **Fax:** (787)841-2000
**Email:** mlespier@pcupr.edu
**Website:** http://www.pcupr.edu
Dr. Mildred Lespier, Contact
**Fnded:** 1948. **Degrees Offered:** BSN, MNS.

★ **15497** ★ **Universidad Adventista de las**
**Antillas**
**Department of Nursing**
PO Box 118
Mayaguez, PR 00681-0118
**Phone:** (787)834-9595          **Fax:** (787)834-9597
**Email:** ycancel@uaa.edu
**Website:** http://www.uaa.edu/
Maria L. Cruz, Contact
**Fnded:** 1957. **Degrees Offered:** BSN.

★ **15498** ★ **Universidad Metropolitana**
**Department of Nursing**
PO Box 21150
San Juan, PR 00928-1150
**Phone:** (787)766-1717          **Fax:** (787)769-7663
**Website:** http://umet_mie.suagm.edu/
Evelyn Garcia, Contact
**Fnded:** 1980. **Degrees Offered:** BSN.

**★ 15499 ★ University of Puerto Rico, Arecibo**
**Department of Nursing**
Arecibo, PR
**Phone:** (787)878-2830          **Fax:** (787)880-4972
Luz Santiago, Contact
**Fnded:** 1967. **Degrees Offered:** BSN.


**★ 15500 ★ University of Puerto Rico, Humacao University College**
**Nursing Department**
San Juan, PR 00927
**Phone:** (787)850-0000          **Fax:** (787)850-9411
**Email:** f_rodriquez@cuhac.upr.clu.edu
**Website:** http://cuhwww.upr.clu.edu/indexe.html
**Fnded:** 1962. **Degrees Offered:** BS.


**★ 15501 ★ University of Puerto Rico, Mayaguez Campus**
**Department of Nursing**
PO Box 9015
Mayaguez, PR 00681
**Phone:** (787)263-3482          **Fax:** (787)823-3875
**Email:** z_torres@rumac.uprm.edu
**Website:** http://www.uprm.edu/
Zaida Lina Torres, Contact
**Fnded:** 1911. **Degrees Offered:** BSN.


**★ 15502 ★ University of Puerto Rico, Medical Sciences Campus**
**School of Nursing**
**MSN Department**
San Juan, PR 00936-5067
**Phone:** (787)758-2525          **Fax:** (787)281-0721
**Website:** http://www.rcm.upr.clu.edu/
Dr. Leonor Irizarry, Contact
**Fnded:** 1950. **Degrees Offered:** BSN, MSN.


**★ 15503 ★ University of the Sacred Heart**
**Program in Nursing**
PO Box 12383
Santurce, PR 00914-0383
**Phone:** (787)728-1515          **Fax:** (787)728-1250
**Email:** grivas@sagrado.edu
**Website:** http://www.sagrado.edu/
Gloria Rivas, Contact
**Fnded:** 1935. **Degrees Offered:** BSN, MS.


### Quebec

**★ 15504 ★ McGill University**
**School of Nursing**
Wilson Hall
3506 University St.
Montreal, QC, Canada H3A 2A7
**Phone:** (514)398-4151          **Fax:** (514)398-8455
**Email:** nursing@po-box.mcgill.ca
**Website:** http://www.mcgill.ca/
Anna M. Santandrea, Contact
**Fnded:** 1821. **Degrees Offered:** BSCN, M SC, PhD.


**★ 15505 ★ Universite Laval**
**Faculty of Nursing**
Sainte-Foy, QC, Canada G1K 7P4
**Phone:** (418)656-2131          **Fax:** (418)656-7747
**Email:** helen.provencher@fsi.ulaval.ca
**Website:** http://www.ulaval.ca/fsi/
Lucie Turgeon-Rheault, Contact
**Fnded:** 1852. **Degrees Offered:** BSCN, MSN, PhD.


**★ 15506 ★ Universite de Montreal**
**Faculty of Nursing**
CP 6128
Succursale Centre-Ville
Montreal, QC, Canada H3C 3J7
**Phone:** (514)343-6178          **Fax:** (514)343-2306
**Email:** jacinthe.pepin@umontreal.ca
**Website:** http://www.umontreal.ca/
Jacinthe Pepin, Contact
**Fnded:** 1920. **Degrees Offered:** BSCN, M SC, PhD.


**★ 15507 ★ Universite du Quebec a Chicoutimi**
**Program in Nursing**
555 Blvd. de L'Universite
Chicoutimi, QC, Canada G7H 2B1
**Phone:** (418)545-5011          **Fax:** (418)545-5012
**Email:** francoise_courville@uqac.uquebec.ca
**Website:** http://www.uqac.uquebec.ca/
Francoise Courville, Contact
**Fnded:** 1969. **Degrees Offered:** BSN, MSN.


**★ 15508 ★ Universite du Quebec a Hull**
**Departement des sciences infirmieres**
C-3333
Hull, QC, Canada J8X 3X7
**Phone:** (819)595-3900          **Fax:** (819)595-2384
**Email:** chantal_stpierre@uqah.uquebec.ca
**Website:** http://www.uquebec.ca/
Chantal Saint-Pierre, Contact
**Fnded:** 1981. **Degrees Offered:** BSCN, M SC N.


**★ 15509 ★ Universite du Quebec a Rimouski**
**Program in Nursing**
300 Ave. des Ursulines
Rimouski, QC, Canada G5L 3A1
**Phone:** (418)723-1986          **Fax:** (418)724-1849
**Email:** nicole_ouellet@uqar.uquebec.ca
**Website:** http://www.uquebec.ca/
Nicole Ouellet, Contact
**Fnded:** 1973. **Degrees Offered:** BSCN.


**★ 15510 ★ Universite du Quebec a Trois-Rivieres**
**Program in Nursing**
Casier Postal 500
Trois Rivieres, QC, Canada G9A 5H7
**Phone:** (819)376-5114          **Fax:** (819)376-5218
**Email:** michele_cote@uqtr.uquebec.ca
**Website:** http://www.uqtr.uquebec.ca/
Dr. Michele Cote, Contact
**Fnded:** 1969. **Degrees Offered:** BS.


**★ 15511 ★ Universite du Sherbrooke**
**Department of Nursing**
Sherbrooke, QC, Canada J1H 5N4
**Phone:** (819)564-5358          **Fax:** (819)820-6816
**Email:** dstcyr@courrier.usherb.ca
**Website:** http://www.usherb.ca/
Dr. Denise St. Cyr-Tribble, Contact
**Fnded:** 1954. **Degrees Offered:** BSCN, M SC, PhD.


**★ 15512 ★ University of Quebec en Abitibi-Temiscamingue**
**Department des sciences sociales et de la sante**
445 Boulevard de l'Universite
Rouyn-Noranda, QC, Canada J9X 5E4
**Phone:** (819)762-0971          **Fax:** (819)797-4727
**Email:** renee.charrois@uqat.uquebec.ca
**Website:** http://www.uqat.uquebec.ca
Renee Charrois, Contact
**Fnded:** 1983. **Degrees Offered:** BN.


### Rhode Island

**★ 15513 ★ Rhode Island College**
**Department of Nursing**
600 Mt. Pleasant Ave.
Providence, RI 02908-1991
**Phone:** (401)456-8013          **Fax:** (401)456-8206
**Email:** jwilliams@ric.edu
**Website:** http://www.ric.edu
Dr. Jane Williams, Contact
**Fnded:** 1854. **Degrees Offered:** BS.


**★ 15514 ★ Salve Regina University**
**Department of Nursing**
100 Ochre Point Ave.
Newport, RI 02840-4192
**Free:** 888-467-2583          **Fax:** (401)848-2823
**Email:** sruadmis@salve.edu
**Website:** http://www.salve.edu/
Laura E. McPhie-Oliveira, Contact
**Fnded:** 1934. **Degrees Offered:** BS.


**★ 15515 ★ University of Rhode Island**
**College of Nursing**
White Hall
Kingston, RI 02881
**Phone:** (401)874-2766          **Fax:** (401)874-2061
**Email:** dsb@uri.edu
**Website:** http://www.uri.edu
Dr. Donna Schwartz-Barcott, Contact
**Fnded:** 1892. **Degrees Offered:** BS, MS, PhD.


### Saskatchewan

**★ 15516 ★ University of Saskatchewan**
**College of Nursing**
A102 Health Sciences Bldg.
Saskatoon, SK, Canada S7N 5E5
**Phone:** (306)966-6229          **Fax:** (306)966-6703
**Email:** gail.laing@sask.usask.ca
**Website:** http://www.usask.ca/
Dr. Gail Laing, Contact
**Fnded:** 1907. **Degrees Offered:** BSN, MN.


### South Carolina

**★ 15517 ★ Charleston Southern University**
**Wingo School of Nursing**
PO Box 118087
9200 University Blvd.
Charleston, SC 29423-8087
**Phone:** (843)863-7075          **Fax:** (843)863-7540
**Email:** mlarisey@csuniv.edu
**Website:** http://www.charlestonsouthern.edu/
Dr. Marian M. Larisey, Contact
**Fnded:** 1964. **Degrees Offered:** BSN.


**★ 15518 ★ Clemson University**
**School of Nursing**
Advising Center
309 Edwards Hall
Clemson, SC 29634-0744
**Phone:** (864)656-5495          **Fax:** (864)656-1688
**Email:** mary2@clemson.edu
**Website:** http://www.clemson.edu/
Beth Hearn, Contact
**Fnded:** 1889. **Degrees Offered:** BS, MS.


**★ 15519 ★ Lander University**
**School of Nursing**
Stanley Ave.
Greenwood, SC 29649
**Phone:** (864)388-8307          **Fax:** (864)388-8125
**Email:** jroark@lander.edu
**Website:** http://www.lander.edu
Jackie DeVore Roark, Contact
**Fnded:** 1872. **Degrees Offered:** BSN.


**★ 15520 ★ Medical University of South Carolina**
**College of Nursing**
99 Johnathan Lucas St.
PO Box 250160
Charleston, SC 29425
**Phone:** (843)792-3844          **Fax:** (843)792-9258
**Email:** wohns@musc.edu

**Website:** http://www.musc.edu
Stephanie W. Auwaerter, Contact
**Fnded:** 1824. **Degrees Offered:** BSN, MSN, PhD.

★ **15521** ★ **University of South Carolina**
**College of Nursing**
1601 Greene St.
William Brice Bldg.
Columbia, SC 29208
**Phone:** (803)777-3754     **Fax:** (803)777-0616
**Email:** cyjackso@nrwpo.nurs.sc.edu
**Website:** http://www.sc.edu/nursing/
Cheryl Nelson-Jackson, Contact
**Fnded:** 1801. **Degrees Offered:** BSN, MSN, MSN/
MPH, PhD.

★ **15522** ★ **University of South Carolina,**
**Aiken**
**School of Nursing**
471 University Pkwy.
Aiken, SC 29801
**Phone:** (803)648-6851     **Fax:** (803)641-3362
**Email:** trudyg@aiken.sc.edu
**Website:** http://www.usca.sc.edu
Dr. Trudy G. Groves, Contact
**Fnded:** 1961. **Degrees Offered:** BSN.

★ **15523** ★ **University of South Carolina,**
**Spartanburg**
**Mary Black School of Nursing**
800 University Way
Spartanburg, SC 29303
**Phone:** (864)503-5469     **Fax:** (864)503-5411
**Email:** adavis@gw.uscs.edu
**Website:** http://www.uscs.edu/
Dr. Angie Davis, Contact
**Fnded:** 1967. **Degrees Offered:** BSN.

## South Dakota

★ **15524** ★ **Augustana College**
**Department of Nursing**
2001 S Summit Ave.
Sioux Falls, SD 57197
**Phone:** (605)336-4729     **Fax:** (605)336-4723
**Email:** mnelson@inst.augie.edu
**Website:** http://www.augie.edu
Dr. Margaret Nelson, Contact
**Fnded:** 1860. **Degrees Offered:** BS, MS

★ **15525** ★ **Mount Marty College**
**Nursing Program**
1105 W 8th St.
Yankton, SD 57078-3724
**Phone:** (605)668-1594     **Fax:** (605)668-1607
**Email:** mquintus@mtmc.edu
**Website:** http://www.mtmc.edu
Dr. Marcine Quintus, Contact
**Fnded:** 1936. **Degrees Offered:** BS.

★ **15526** ★ **Presentation College**
**Department of Nursing**
1500 N Main St.
Aberdeen, SD 57401
**Phone:** (605)229-8473     **Fax:** (605)229-8489
**Email:** janicesw@presentation.edu
**Website:** http://www.presentation.edu
Dr. Janice Williams, Contact
**Fnded:** 1951. **Degrees Offered:** BSN.

★ **15527** ★ **South Dakota State University**
**College of Nursing**
Rotunda Lane, NFA 217
Box 2275
Brookings, SD 57007-0098
**Phone:** (605)688-4114     **Fax:** (605)688-6119
**Email:** penny_powers@sdstate.edu
**Website:** http://www.sdstate.edu
Dr. Penny Powers, Contact
**Fnded:** 1881. **Degrees Offered:** BS, MS.

## Tennessee

★ **15528** ★ **Austin Peay State University**
**College of Human Services and Nursing**
PO Box 4658
Clarksville, TN 37044
**Phone:** (931)221-7737     **Fax:** (931)221-7595
**Email:** thompson@apsu.edu
**Website:** http://www.apsu.edu
Dr. Linda W. Thompson, DNS, Contact
**Fnded:** 1927. **Degrees Offered:** BSN.

★ **15529** ★ **Belmont University**
**School of Nursing**
1900 Belmont Blvd.
Nashville, TN 37212-3757
**Phone:** (615)460-6027     **Fax:** (615)460-5644
**Email:** higginsl@mail.belmont.edu
**Website:** http://www.belmont.edu/nursing/graduate_
nursing.html
Dr. Leslie Higgins, Contact
**Fnded:** 1951. **Degrees Offered:** BSN, MSN.

★ **15530** ★ **Carson-Newman College**
**Department of Nursing**
1646 Russell Ave.
Jefferson City, TN 37760
**Phone:** (865)471-3426     **Fax:** (865)471-4574
**Email:** harley@cncacc.cn.edu
**Website:** http://www.cn.edu
Dr. Ann Harley, Contact
**Fnded:** 1851. **Degrees Offered:** BSN, MSN.

★ **15531** ★ **Cumberland University**
**Division of Nursing**
1 Cumberland Sq.
Lebanon, TN 37087-3554
**Phone:** (615)444-2562     **Fax:** (615)443-8427
**Email:** nursing@cumberland.edu
**Website:** http://www.cumberland.edu
Dr. Leanne Busby, Contact
**Fnded:** 1842. **Degrees Offered:** BSN.

★ **15532** ★ **East Tennessee State**
**University**
**College of Nursing**
PO Box 70617
Johnson City, TN 37614-0617
**Phone:** (423)439-4578     **Fax:** (423)439-4522
**Email:** admitnur@etsu.edu
**Website:** http://www.etsu.edu
Steve Robinson, Contact
**Fnded:** 1911. **Degrees Offered:** BSN, MSN.

★ **15533** ★ **Lincoln Memorial University**
**Department of Nursing**
Cumberland Gap Pkwy.
Harrogate, TN 37752
**Phone:** (423)869-6324     **Fax:** (423)869-6244
**Email:** ebarr@inetlmu.lmunet.eud
**Website:** http://www.lmunet.edu/
Dr. Elisa Barr, Contact
**Fnded:** 1897. **Degrees Offered:** BSN.

★ **15534** ★ **Middle Tennessee State**
**University**
**School of Nursing**
1301 E Main St.
Murfreesboro, TN 37132-0001
**Phone:** (615)898-2437     **Fax:** (615)898-5441
**Email:** pgholder@mtsu.edu
**Website:** http://www.mtsu.edu
Dr. Pamela G. Holder, Contact
**Fnded:** 1911. **Degrees Offered:** BSN.

★ **15535** ★ **Southern Adventist University**
**School of Nursing**
Collegedale, TN 37315
**Phone:** (423)238-2940     **Fax:** (423)238-3004
**Email:** lmarlowe@southern.edu
**Website:** http://www.southern.edu/
Linda Marlowe, Contact
**Fnded:** 1892. **Degrees Offered:** BS, MSN, MSN/
MBA.

★ **15536** ★ **Tennessee State University**
**School of Nursing**
3500 John A. Merritt Blvd.
Box 9590
Nashville, TN 37209-1561
**Phone:** (615)963-5261     **Fax:** (615)963-7614
**Email:** bbrown@picard.tnstate.edu
**Website:** http://www.tnstate.edu
Dr. Barbara E. Brown, Contact
**Fnded:** 1912. **Degrees Offered:** BSN, MSN.

★ **15537** ★ **Tennessee Technological**
**University**
**School of Nursing**
PO Box 5001
Cookeville, TN 38505-0001
**Phone:** (931)372-3203     **Fax:** (932)372-6244
**Email:** nursing@tntech.edu
**Website:** http://www.tntech.edu/
Susan Buchanan, Contact
**Fnded:** 1915. **Degrees Offered:** BSN.

★ **15538** ★ **University of Memphis**
**Loewenberg School of Nursing**
105 Newport Hall
Memphis, TN 38152
**Phone:** (901)678-2003     **Fax:** (901)678-4906
**Email:** shall@memphis.edu
**Website:** http://www.memphis.edu/
Sheila Hall, Contact
**Fnded:** 1912. **Degrees Offered:** BSN.

★ **15539** ★ **University of Tennessee**
**College of Nursing**
Student Services Office
1200 Volunteer Blvd.
Knoxville, TN 37996-4180
**Phone:** (865)974-7606     **Fax:** (865)974-3569
**Email:** bbarret@utk.edu
**Website:** http://www.tennessee.edu/
**Fnded:** 1794. **Degrees Offered:** BSN, MSN, PhD.

★ **15540** ★ **University of Tennessee,**
**Chattanooga**
**College of Nursing**
615 Mcallie Ave.
Chattanooga, TN 37403-2598
**Phone:** (423)755-4750     **Fax:** (423)755-4668
**Email:** kay-lindgren@utc.edu
**Website:** http://www.utc.edu/
Dr. Katherine Russell Lindgren, Contact
**Fnded:** 1886. **Degrees Offered:** BSN, MSN.

★ **15541** ★ **University of Tennessee**
**Health Science Center**
**College of Nursing**
877 Madison Ave., Rm. 602
Memphis, TN 38163
**Phone:** (901)448-6118     **Fax:** (901)448-4121
**Email:** mrice@utmem.edu
**Website:** http://www.utmem.edu/
Muriel C. Rice, Contact
**Fnded:** 1911. **Degrees Offered:** DN SC, MSN.

**★ 15542 ★ University of Tennessee, Martin**
Department of Nursing
Gooch Hall 136J
Martin, TN 38238
**Phone:** (901)587-7131    **Fax:** (901)587-7939
**Email:** brendac@utm.edu
**Website:** http://www.utm.edu
Brenda W. Campbell, Contact
**Fnded:** 1900. **Degrees Offered:** BSN.

**★ 15543 ★ Vanderbilt University**
School of Nursing
102 Godchaux Hall
Nashville, TN 37240
**Phone:** (615)322-3800    **Fax:** (615)343-0333
**Email:** paddy.peerman@mcmail.vanderbilt.edu
**Website:** http://www.mc.vanderbilt.edu/nursing/
Patricia Peerman, Contact
**Fnded:** 1873. **Degrees Offered:** MSN, MSN/MBA, PhD.

### Texas

**★ 15544 ★ Abilene Intercollegiate School of Nursing**
2149 Hickory St.
Abilene, TX 79601
**Phone:** (915)672-2441    **Fax:** (915)672-5026
**Email:** aisnadv@abilene.com
Jo Garcia, Contact
**Degrees Offered:** BSN,MSW.

**★ 15545 ★ Angelo State University**
Program in Nursing
PO Box 10902
San Angelo, TX 76909
**Phone:** (915)942-2224    **Fax:** (915)942-2236
**Email:** leslie.mayrand@angelo.edu
**Website:** http://www.angelo.edu/dept/nut/
Dr. Leslie Mayrand, Contact
**Fnded:** 1928. **Degrees Offered:** BSN, MSN

**★ 15546 ★ Baylor University**
School of Nursing
3700 Worth St
Dallas, TX 75246
**Phone:** (214)820-3361    **Fax:** (214)820-4770
**Email:** pauline_Johnson@baylor.edu
**Website:** http://www.baylor.edu
Dr. Pauline Johnson, Contact
**Fnded:** 1845. **Degrees Offered:** BSN, MSN

**★ 15547 ★ East Texas Baptist University**
Department of Nursing
1209 N Grove
Marshall, TX 75670
**Phone:** (903)935-7963    **Fax:** (903)938-9225
**Email:** chammocke@etbu.edu
**Website:** http://www.etbu.edu
Dr. Celeste K. Hammock, Contact
**Fnded:** 1912. **Degrees Offered:** BSN.

**★ 15548 ★ Houston Baptist University**
College of Nursing
7502 Fondren St.
Houston, TX 77074
**Phone:** (281)649-3300    **Fax:** (281)649-3340
**Email:** bbinder@hbu.edu
**Website:** http://www.hbu.edu/
Dr. Brenda Binder, Contact
**Fnded:** 1960. **Degrees Offered:** BSN, MNS.

**★ 15549 ★ Lamar University**
Department of Nursing
PO Box 10081
Beaumont, TX 77710
**Phone:** (409)880-8868    **Fax:** (409)880-1865
**Website:** http://www.lamar.edu/
Chandra Pieret, Contact
**Fnded:** 1923. **Degrees Offered:** BSN, MSN.

**★ 15550 ★ Lubbock Christian University**
Department of Nursing
5601 W 19th St.
Lubbock, TX 79407
**Phone:** (806)796-8800    **Fax:** (806)796-8917
**Email:** bev.byers@lcu.edu
Dr. Beverly Byers, Contact
**Fnded:** 1957. **Degrees Offered:** BSN.

**★ 15551 ★ Midwestern State University**
Nursing Program
3410 Taft Blvd.
Wichita Falls, TX 76308
**Phone:** (940)397-4599    **Fax:** (940)397-4513
**Email:** deborah.garrison@nexus.mwsu.edu
**Website:** http://www.mwsu.edu
Dr. Deborah Garrison, Contact
**Fnded:** 1922. **Degrees Offered:** BSN, MSN.

**★ 15552 ★ Prairie View A&M University**
College of Nursing
6436 Fannian St.
Houston, TX 77030
**Phone:** (713)797-7003    **Fax:** (713)797-7013
**Email:** chloe_gaines@pvamu.edu
**Website:** http://www.pvamu.edu/nursing/index.html
Dr. Chloe Gaines, Contact
**Fnded:** 1878. **Degrees Offered:** BSN, MS.

**★ 15553 ★ Southwestern Adventist University**
Department of Nursing
Keene, TX 76059
**Phone:** (817)645-3921    **Fax:** (817)556-4713
**Email:** moorep@swau.edu
**Website:** http://www.swau.edu/
Dr. Penny Moore, Contact
**Fnded:** 1894. **Degrees Offered:** BS.

**★ 15554 ★ Stephen F. Austin State University**
Division of Nursing
SFA Box 6156
Nacogdoches, TX 75962
**Phone:** (409)468-3604    **Fax:** (409)468-1696
**Website:** http://www.sfasu.edu/
Dr. Glenda C. Walker, Contact
**Fnded:** 1923. **Degrees Offered:** BSN.

**★ 15555 ★ Tarleton State University**
Department of Nursing
Box T-0500
Stephenville, TX 76402
**Phone:** (254)968-9851    **Fax:** (254)968-9716
**Email:** eevans@tarleton.edu
**Website:** http://www.tarleton.edu/
Dr. Elaine Evans, Contact
**Fnded:** 1899. **Degrees Offered:** BSN.

**★ 15556 ★ Texas A&M University**
School of Nursing
5201 University Blvd.
Laredo, TX 78041-1900
**Phone:** (956)326-2450    **Fax:** (956)326-2449
**Email:** sbaker@tamiu.edu
**Website:** http://www.tamiu.edu/
Dr. Susan Scoville Baker, Contact
**Fnded:** 1969. **Degrees Offered:** BSN.

**★ 15557 ★ Texas A&M University, Corpus Christi**
Department of Nursing and Health Sciences
6300 Ocean Dr.
FC152
Corpus Christi, TX 78412
**Phone:** (361)825-3323    **Fax:** (361)825-2484
**Email:** ejoyce@falcon.tamucc.edu
**Website:** http://www.tamucc.edu/
Dr. Esperanza Joyce, Contact
**Fnded:** 1947. **Degrees Offered:** BSN, MSN.

**★ 15558 ★ Texas Christian University**
Harris College of Nursing
TCU Box 298620
2800 West Bowie
Fort Worth, TX 76129
**Phone:** (817)257-7650    **Fax:** (817)257-7944
**Email:** m.austinweeks@tcu.edu
**Website:** http://www.tcu.edu/
Melissa Austin-Weeks, Contact
**Fnded:** 1873. **Degrees Offered:** BSN.

**★ 15559 ★ Texas Tech University Health Sciences Center**
School of Nursing
3601 4th St.
3BC100
Lubbock, TX 79430
**Phone:** (806)743-2737    **Fax:** (806)743-1697
**Email:** sonemj@ttuhsc.edu
**Website:** http://www.nursing.ttuhsc.edu
Exa Mae Jackson, Contact
**Fnded:** 1969. **Degrees Offered:** BSN, MSN, MSN/MBA.

**★ 15560 ★ Texas Woman's University**
College of Nursing
1810 Inwood Rd.
Dallas, TX 75235-7299
**Phone:** (214)689-6551    **Fax:** (214)689-6539
**Email:** cmobley@twu.edu
**Website:** http://www.twu.edu/nursing/
Dr. Caryl Mobley, Contact
**Fnded:** 1901. **Degrees Offered:** BS, MS, PhD.

**★ 15561 ★ University of the Incarnate Word**
Program in Nursing
4301 Broadway
San Antonio, TX 78209
**Phone:** (210)829-3988    **Fax:** (210)829-3174
**Email:** strickla@universe.uiwtx.edu
**Website:** http://www.uiw.edu/
Dr. Sandra Strickland, Contact
**Fnded:** 1881. **Degrees Offered:** BSN, MSN, MSN/MBA.

**★ 15562 ★ University of Mary Hardin-Baylor**
School of Nursing
900 College St.
UMHB Station Box 8015
Belton, TX 76513-2599
**Phone:** (254)295-4662    **Fax:** (254)295-4141
**Website:** http://www.umhb.edu/
Dr. Grace Labaj, Contact
**Fnded:** 1845. **Degrees Offered:** BSN.

**★ 15563 ★ University of Texas, Arlington**
School of Nursing
UTA Box 19407
411 S Nedderman Dr.
Arlington, TX 76019-0407
**Phone:** (817)272-7086    **Fax:** (817)272-5006
**Email:** grove@uta.edu
**Website:** http://www.uta.edu/
Dr. Susan K. Grove, Contact

**Fnded:** 1895. **Degrees Offered:** BSN, MSN, MSN/ MBA, MSN/MPH.

**★ 15564 ★ University of Texas, Austin**
**School of Nursing**
Student Affairs Office, Graduate Admissions
1700 Red River St.
Austin, TX 78701-1499
**Phone:** (512)471-7311        **Fax:** (512)471-4910
**Email:** nugrad@uts.cc.utexas.edu/nursing/
**Website:** http://www.utexas.edu
**Fnded:** 1883. **Degrees Offered:** BSN, MSN, MSN/ MBA, PhD.

**★ 15565 ★ The University of Texas,**
**Brownsville**
**Department of Nursing**
Brownsville, TX
**Phone:** (956)574-6690        **Fax:** (956)544-8881
**Email:** eherriage@utb1.utb.edu
**Website:** http://www.utb.edu/
Dr. Ella Herriage, Contact
**Fnded:** 1973. **Degrees Offered:** BSN, MS.

**★ 15566 ★ University of Texas, El Paso**
**School of Nursing**
1101 N Campbell St.
El Paso, TX 79902
**Phone:** (915)747-7246        **Fax:** (915)747-7207
**Email:** stuppy@miners.utep.edu
**Website:** http://www.utep.edu
Dr. Dorothy Stuppy, Contact
**Fnded:** 1913. **Degrees Offered:** BSN, MSN.

**★ 15567 ★ University of Texas Health**
**Science Center, Houston**
**School of Nursing**
Registrar's Office
1100 Holcombe Blvd., No. 6.100
Houston, TX 77030
**Phone:** (713)500-3361        **Fax:** (713)500-2107
**Email:** uthshro@admin4.hsc.uth.tmc.edu
**Website:** http://son1.nur.uth.tmc.edu/
**Fnded:** 1972. **Degrees Offered:** BSN, DSN, MSN.

**★ 15568 ★ University of Texas Health**
**Science Center, San Antonio**
**School of Nursing**
7703 Floyd Curl Dr.
Mail Code 7945
San Antonio, TX 78229-3900
**Phone:** (210)567-5805        **Fax:** (210)567-3813
**Email:** binzer@uthscsa.edu
Dr. Carol D. Binzer, Contact
**Fnded:** 1976. **Degrees Offered:** BSN, MSN, MSN/ MPH, PhD.

**★ 15569 ★ University of Texas Medical**
**Branch, Galveston**
**School of Nursing**
301 University Blvd.
Galveston, TX 77555-1029
**Phone:** (409)772-7311        **Fax:** (409)747-1519
**Email:** jhartsho@utmb.edu
**Website:** http://www.utmb.edu/
Dr. Jeanette C. Hartshorn, Contact
**Fnded:** 1891. **Degrees Offered:** BSN, MSN, PhD.

**★ 15570 ★ University of Texas, Pan**
**American**
**Department of Nursing**
1201 W University Dr.
Edinburg, TX 78539
**Phone:** (956)316-7082        **Fax:** (956)381-2384
**Email:** btucker@panam.edu
**Website:** http://www.panam.edu
Dr. Barbara Tucker, Contact
**Fnded:** 1927. **Degrees Offered:** BSN, MSN.

**★ 15571 ★ University of Texas, Tyler**
**College of Nursing**
Tyler, TX 75799
**Phone:** (903)565-5534        **Fax:** (903)565-5533
**Email:** kcaufield@mail.uttyler.edu
**Website:** http://www.uttyler.edu/
Kay Caufield, Contact
**Fnded:** 1971. **Degrees Offered:** BSN, MSN, MSN/ MBA.

**★ 15572 ★ West Texas A&M University**
**Division of Nursing**
PO Box 60969
Canyon, TX 79016-0001
**Phone:** (806)651-2634        **Fax:** (806)651-2632
**Email:** lrobinson@mail.wtamu.edu
**Website:** http://www.wtamu.edu
Lynda Robinson, Contact
**Fnded:** 1909. **Degrees Offered:** BSN, MSN.

## Utah

**★ 15573 ★ Brigham Young University**
**College of Nursing**
500 SWKT
PO Box 25426
Provo, UT 84602-5426
**Phone:** (801)378-4142        **Fax:** (801)378-3198
**Email:** denise_gibbons@byu.edu
**Website:** http://www.nurse.byu.edu/
Denise Gibbons Davis, Contact
**Fnded:** 1875. **Degrees Offered:** BS, MS.

**★ 15574 ★ University of Phoenix, Utah**
**Campus**
**College of Nursing and Health Care**
**Sciences**
Salt Lake City, UT
**Phone:** (801)263-1444
**Email:** Scott.Jones@apollogrp.edu
**Website:** http://www.phoenix.edu/
**Degrees Offered:** BSN, MSN.

**★ 15575 ★ University of Utah**
**College of Nursing**
10 S 2000 East Front
Salt Lake City, UT 84112-5880
**Phone:** (801)581-3414        **Fax:** (801)581-4642
**Email:** joyce.rathbun@nurs.utah.edu
**Website:** http://www.utah.edu/
Joyce Rathbun, Contact
**Fnded:** 1850. **Degrees Offered:** BS, MS, PhD.

**★ 15576 ★ Weber State University**
**Nursing Program**
4005 University Circle
Ogden, UT 84408-4005
**Phone:** (801)626-6128        **Fax:** (801)626-8035
**Email:** rholt@weber.edu
**Website:** http://www.weber.edu/
Robert Holt, Contact
**Fnded:** 1889. **Degrees Offered:** BSN.

**★ 15577 ★ Westminster College**
**Saint Mark's-Westminster School of**
**Nursing and Health Sciences**
1840 S 1300 East
Salt Lake City, UT 84105
**Phone:** (801)832-2150        **Fax:** (801)467-8601
**Email:** mpeck@wcslc.edu
**Website:** http://www.wcslc.edu/
Dr. Marj Peck, Contact
**Fnded:** 1875. **Degrees Offered:** BS, MS.

## Vermont

**★ 15578 ★ Norwich University**
**Division of Nursing**
Office of Admissions
Northfield, VT 05663
**Phone:** (802)485-2100        **Fax:** (802)485-2032
**Email:** nuadm@norwich.edu
**Website:** http://www.norwich.edu
**Fnded:** 1819. **Degrees Offered:** BSN.

**★ 15579 ★ Southern Vermont College**
**Department of Nursing**
982 Mansion Dr.
Bennington, VT 05201
**Phone:** (802)447-4661        **Fax:** (802)447-4652
**Email:** kphilpot@svc.edu
**Website:** http://www.svc.edu/
Kay Philpott, Contact
**Fnded:** 1926. **Degrees Offered:** BSN.

**★ 15580 ★ University of Vermont**
**School of Nursing**
Rowell Bldg., Rm. 216
Burlington, VT 05405-0068
**Phone:** (802)656-3830        **Fax:** (802)656-8306
**Email:** jcarr@zoo.uvm.edu
**Website:** http://www.uvm.edu/
Dr. Jeanine Carr, Contact
**Fnded:** 1791. **Degrees Offered:** BS, MS.

## Virgin Islands

**★ 15581 ★ University of the Virgin**
**Islands**
**Division of Nursing**
2 John Brewer's Bay
St Thomas, VI 00802-9990
**Phone:** (340)693-1291        **Fax:** (340)693-1285
**Email:** gcallwo@uvi.edu
**Website:** http://manta.uvi.edu/
Dr. Gloria B. Callwood, Contact
**Fnded:** 1962. **Degrees Offered:** BS.

## Virginia

**★ 15582 ★ Christopher Newport**
**University**
**Department of Nursing**
1 University Pl.
Newport News, VA 23606-2998
**Phone:** (757)594-7252        **Fax:** (757)594-7862
**Email:** mardis@cnu.edu
**Website:** http://www.cnu.edu/
Lisa Ardis, Contact
**Fnded:** 1960. **Degrees Offered:** BSN.

**★ 15583 ★ Community Hospital of**
**Roanoke Valley**
**College of Health Sciences**
**Nursing Education Program**
PO Box 13186
Roanoke, VA 24013
**Phone:** (540)985-8573        **Fax:** (540)985-9773
**Email:** becky@health.chs.edu
**Website:** http://www.chs.edu
Dr. Rebecca Culver Clark, Contact
**Fnded:** 1982. **Degrees Offered:** BSN.

**★ 15584 ★ Eastern Mennonite College**
**Department of Nursing**
1200 Park Rd.
Harrisonburg, VA 22802
**Free:** 800-368-2665        **Fax:** (540)432-4444
**Email:** millereb@emu.edu
**Website:** http://www.emu.edu/
Ellen B. Miller, Contact
**Fnded:** 1917. **Degrees Offered:** BSN.

**★ 15585 ★ George Mason University**
**College of Nursing and Health Sciences**
Mailstop 3C4
4400 University Dr.
Fairfax, VA 22030-4444
**Phone:** (703)993-1913          **Fax:** (703)993-1949
**Email:** jvail@gmu.edu
**Website:** http://www.gmu.edu
Dr. James Vail, Contact
**Fnded:** 1957. **Degrees Offered:** BSN, MSN, MSN/
MBA, PhD.

**★ 15586 ★ Hampton University**
**Department of Nursing**
Hampton, VA 23668
**Phone:** (757)727-5251          **Fax:** (757)727-5423
**Email:** sgore@hamptonu.edu
**Website:** http://www.hamptonu.edu/
Dr. Shirley Gore, Contact
**Fnded:** 1868. **Degrees Offered:** BS, MS, PhD.

**★ 15587 ★ James Madison University**
**Department of Nursing**
MSC 2102
800 S Main St.
Harrisonburg, VA 22807
**Phone:** (540)568-6314          **Fax:** (540)568-7896
**Email:** ketterdb@jmu.edu
**Website:** http://www.jmu.edu/
Donna Jo Ketterman, Contact
**Fnded:** 1908. **Degrees Offered:** BSN.

**★ 15588 ★ Liberty University**
**Department of Nursing**
1971 University Blvd.
Lynchburg, VA 24502
**Phone:** (804)582-2519          **Fax:** (804)582-7035
**Email:** dbritt@liberty.edu
**Website:** http://www.liberty.edu/
Dr. Deanna Britt, Contact
**Fnded:** 1971. **Degrees Offered:** BSN.

**★ 15589 ★ Lynchburg College**
**Department of Nursing**
McMillan Nursing Bldg.
1501 Lakeside Dr.
Lynchburg, VA 24501-3199
**Phone:** (804)544-8324          **Fax:** (804)544-8323
**Email:** whitman_n@mail.lynchburg.edu
**Website:** http://www.lynchburg.edu/
Dr. Nancy I. Whitman, Contact
**Fnded:** 1903. **Degrees Offered:** BS.

**★ 15590 ★ Marymount University**
**School of Health Professions**
Arlington, VA 22207-4299
**Phone:** (703)284-1580          **Fax:** (703)284-3819
**Email:** bmill@marymount.edu
**Website:** http://www.marymount.edu/
Dr. Betty Miller, Contact
**Fnded:** 1950. **Degrees Offered:** BSN, MSN.

**★ 15591 ★ Norfolk State University**
**Department of Nursing**
700 Park Ave., Rm. 420 Robinson
Norfolk, VA 23504-8026
**Phone:** (757)823-9013          **Fax:** (757)823-8241
**Email:** wfwhite-parson@nsu.edu
**Website:** http://www.nsu.edu
Dr. Willar White-Parson, Contact
**Fnded:** 1935. **Degrees Offered:** BSN.

**★ 15592 ★ Old Dominion University**
**School of Nursing**
Norfolk, VA 23529-0500
**Phone:** (757)683-4298          **Fax:** (757)683-5253
**Email:** lgarzon@odu.edu
**Website:** http://odu.edu
Dr. Laurel Garzon, Contact
**Fnded:** 1930. **Degrees Offered:** BSN, MSN.

**★ 15593 ★ Radford University**
**School of Nursing**
Box 6964
RU Station
Waldron Hall
Radford, VA 24142
**Phone:** (540)831-7645          **Fax:** (540)831-7700
**Email:** kgivens@radford.edu
**Website:** http://www.runet.edu/
Dr. Karolyn Givens, Contact
**Fnded:** 1910. **Degrees Offered:** BSN, MSN.

**★ 15594 ★ Shenandoah University**
**Division of Nursing**
1775 North Sector Court
Winchester, VA 22601
**Phone:** (540)665-5508          **Fax:** (540)665-5519
**Email:** mmorrow@su.edu
**Website:** http://www.su.edu
Dr. Martha Morrow, Contact
**Fnded:** 1875. **Degrees Offered:** BSN. MSN.

**★ 15595 ★ University of Virginia**
**School of Nursing**
PO Box 800782
McLeod Hall
Charlottesville, VA 22908
**Free:** 888-283-8703          **Fax:** (804)982-0528
**Email:** nur-osa@virginia.edu
**Website:** http://www.nursing.virginia.edu/
**Fnded:** 1819. **Degrees Offered:** BSN, MSN, MSN/
HSM, MSN/MA, MSN/MBA, MSN, PhD.

**★ 15596 ★ University of Virginia's**
**College, Wise**
**Department of Nursing**
1 College Ave.
Wise, VA 24293-4400
**Phone:** (540)328-0275          **Fax:** (540)328-0247
**Email:** kwh3c@uvawise.edu
**Website:** http://www.uvwise.edu
Dr. Kathleen W. Huttlinger, Contact
**Fnded:** 1954. **Degrees Offered:** BS, MS, PhD.

**★ 15597 ★ Virginia Commonwealth**
**University**
**School of Nursing**
PO Box 567
Richmond, VA 23298-0567
**Phone:** (804)828-5171          **Fax:** (804)828-7743
**Email:** slipp@hsc.vcu.edu
**Website:** http://views.vcu.edu/son/son.html
Susan L. Lipp, Contact
**Fnded:** 1838. **Degrees Offered:** BS, MS, PhD.

## Washington

**★ 15598 ★ Gonzaga University**
**Program in Nursing**
Spokane, WA 99258-0038
**Phone:** (509)323-6643          **Fax:** (509)323-5827
**Email:** tiedt@gu.gonzaga.edu
**Website:** http://www.gu.gonzaga.edu/
Jane Tiedt, Contact
**Fnded:** 1887. **Degrees Offered:** BSN, MSN.

**★ 15599 ★ Intercollegiate Center for**
**Nursing Education**
**Washington State University College of**
**Nursing**
**College of Nursing**
2917 W Fort George Wright Dr.
Spokane, WA 99224-5291
**Phone:** (509)324-7334          **Fax:** (509)324-7336
**Email:** mruby@wsu.edu
Margaret Ruby, Contact
**Degrees Offered:** BSN, MN.

**★ 15600 ★ Pacific Lutheran University**
**School of Nursing**
Tacoma, WA 98447-0003
**Phone:** (253)536-8872          **Fax:** (253)535-7590
**Email:** deforrlt@plu.edu
**Website:** http://www.plu.edu/
Dr. Laura DeForrest, Contact
**Fnded:** 1890. **Degrees Offered:** BSN, MSN.

**★ 15601 ★ Seattle Pacific University**
**School of Health Sciences**
Green Hall
3307 3rd Ave., W
Seattle, WA 98119-1997
**Phone:** (206)281-2649          **Fax:** (206)281-2649
**Email:** dallis@spu.edu
**Website:** http://www.spu.edu/dept/bsc/
Dr. Donna Allis, Contact
**Fnded:** 1891. **Degrees Offered:** BSN, MSN.

**★ 15602 ★ Seattle University**
**School of Nursing**
900 Broadway
Seattle, WA 98122-4460
**Phone:** (206)296-5663          **Fax:** (206)296-5544
**Email:** mpwhitley@seattleu.edu
**Website:** http://www.seattleu.edu/
Dr. Marilyn Whitley, Contact
**Fnded:** 1891. **Degrees Offered:** BSN, MSN.

**★ 15603 ★ University of Washington**
**School of Nursing**
Health Sciences Bldg.
Box 357260
Seattle, WA 98195
**Phone:** (206)543-8736          **Fax:** (206)685-1613
**Email:** egg@u.washington.edu
**Website:** http://www.son.washington.edu
Carolyn Chow, Contact
**Fnded:** 1861. **Degrees Offered:** BSN, MN, MN/MPH,
MSN/MHA, PhD.

## West Virginia

**★ 15604 ★ Alderson-Broaddus College**
**Department of Nursing**
Box 2003
Philippi, WV 26416
**Phone:** (304)457-1700          **Fax:** (304)457-6308
**Email:** boni@ab.edu
**Website:** http://www.ab.edu
Dr. M. Sharon Boni, Contact
**Fnded:** 1871.

**★ 15605 ★ Bluefield State College**
**Program in Nursing**
219 Rock St.
Bluefield, WV 24701
**Phone:** (304)327-4139          **Fax:** (304)327-4219
**Email:** bpritchett@bluefield.wvnet.edu
**Website:** http://www.bluefield.wvnet.edu
Beth Pritchett, Contact
**Fnded:** 1895. **Degrees Offered:** BSN.

**★ 15606 ★ Fairmont State College**
**School of Health Careers**
Fairmont, WV 26554
**Phone:** (304)367-4761          **Fax:** (304)367-4268
**Email:** mmeighen@mail.fscwv.edu
**Website:** http://www.fscwv.edu/
Dr. Mary G. Meighen, Contact
**Degrees Offered:** BSN.

**★ 15607 ★ Marshall University**
**College of Nursing and Health**
**Professions**
400 Hal Greer Blvd.
Huntington, WV 25755-9500
**Phone:** (304)696-2618  **Fax:** (304)696-6739
**Email:** conhp@marshall.edu
**Website:** http://www.marshall.edu/
Dr. Linda Scott, Contact
**Fnded:** 1837. **Degrees Offered:** BSN, MSN.


**★ 15608 ★ Mountain State University**
**Program in Nursing**
PO Box 9003 AG
Beckley, WV 25802-2830
**Phone:** (304)253-7351  **Fax:** (304)253-0789
**Email:** jsharp@cwv.edu
**Website:** http://www.cwv.edu/
Dr. Jessica Sharp, Contact
**Fnded:** 1933. **Degrees Offered:** BSN, MSN.


**★ 15609 ★ Shepherd College**
**Department of Nursing Education**
Shepherdstown, WV 25443
**Phone:** (304)876-5341  **Fax:** (304)876-5169
**Email:** lhanson@shepherd.wvnet.edu
**Website:** http://www.shepherd.edu/
Lynn Ellen Hanson, Contact
**Fnded:** 1871. **Degrees Offered:** BSN.


**★ 15610 ★ University of Charleston**
**Department of Nursing**
2300 MacCorkle Ave., SE
Charleston, WV 25304
**Phone:** (304)357-4750  **Fax:** (304)357-4781
**Email:** admissions@uchaswv.edu
**Website:** http://www.wchaswv.edu
Lynn Jackson, Contact
**Fnded:** 1888. **Degrees Offered:** BSN.


**★ 15611 ★ West Liberty State College**
**Department of Health Sciences**
West Liberty, WV 26074
**Phone:** (304)336-8108  **Fax:** (304)336-5104
**Email:** lukichda@wlsc.wvnet.edu
**Website:** http://www.wlsc.wvnet.edu/
Dr. Donna Lukich, Contact
**Fnded:** 1837. **Degrees Offered:** BSN.


**★ 15612 ★ West Virginia University**
**School of Nursing**
6417 RCB Health Science Center
PO Box 9640
Morgantown, WV 26506-9600
**Phone:** (304)293-4298  **Fax:** (304)293-2784
**Email:** mjsmith@wvu.edu
**Website:** http://www.hsc.wvu.edu/son/
Mary Jane Smith, Contact
**Fnded:** 1867. **Degrees Offered:** BSN, DSN, MSN.


**★ 15613 ★ West Virginia Wesleyan**
**College**
**Department of Nursing**
59 College Ave.
Buckhannon, WV 26201-2995
**Phone:** (304)473-8224  **Fax:** (304)473-8435
**Email:** aurelio_@wvwc.edu
**Website:** http://www.wvwc.edu/
Shauna Lively Aurelio, Contact
**Fnded:** 1890. **Degrees Offered:** BSN.


**★ 15614 ★ Wheeling Jesuit College**
**Department of Nursing**
316 Washington Ave.
Wheeling, WV 26003-6233
**Phone:** (304)243-2344  **Fax:** (304)243-2608
**Email:** ccarroll@wju.edu
**Website:** http://www.wju.edu/
Carol Carroll, Contact
**Fnded:** 1954. **Degrees Offered:** BSN, MSN.


## Wisconsin

**★ 15615 ★ Alverno College**
**Division of Nursing**
3401 S 43rd St.
PO Box 343922
Milwaukee, WI 53234-3922
**Phone:** (414)382-6284  **Fax:** (414)382-6279
**Email:** judeen.schulte@alverno.edu
**Website:** http://www.alverno.edu
Dr. Judeen A. Schulte, Contact
**Fnded:** 1887. **Degrees Offered:** BSN


**★ 15616 ★ Bellin College of Nursing**
**Nursing Program**
725 S Webster Ave.
Green Bay, WI 54301
**Phone:** (920)433-5803  **Fax:** (920)433-7416
**Email:** pcroghan@bcon.edu
**Website:** http://www.bcon.edu
Dr. Peggy Croghan, Contact
**Fnded:** 1909. **Degrees Offered:** BSN.


**★ 15617 ★ Cardinal Stritch University**
**College of Nursing**
6801 N Yates Rd.
Milwaukee, WI 53217-3985
**Phone:** (414)410-4388  **Fax:** (414)410-4239
**Website:** http://www.stritch.edu
Dr. Nancy Cervenansky, Contact
**Fnded:** 1937. **Degrees Offered:** BSN, MSN.


**★ 15618 ★ Columbia College of Nursing**
**College of Nursing**
Office of Admissions
2121 E Newport Ave.
Milwaukee, WI 53211
**Phone:** (414)961-3897  **Fax:** (414)961-4121
**Website:** http://www.ccon.edu/
Dr. Gerald Luecht, Contact
**Fnded:** 1901. **Degrees Offered:** BSN.


**★ 15619 ★ Concordia University,**
**Wisconsin**
**Program in Nursing**
12800 N Lake Shore Dr.
Mequon, WI 53097
**Phone:** (262)243-4452  **Fax:** (262)243-4506
**Email:** ruth.gresley@cuw.edu
**Website:** http://www.cuw.edu/
Dr. Ruth Gresley, Contact
**Fnded:** 1881. **Degrees Offered:** BSN, MSN.


**★ 15620 ★ Edgewood College**
**Program in Nursing**
1000 Edgewood College Dr.
Madison, WI 53711
**Phone:** (608)663-2292  **Fax:** (608)663-2863
**Email:** mkellypowell@edgewood.edu
**Website:** http://www.edgewood.edu/
Dr. Mary L. Kelly-Powell, Contact
**Fnded:** 1927. **Degrees Offered:** BS, MS.


**★ 15621 ★ Marian College of Fond du**
**Lac**
**Division of Nursing**
45 S National Ave.
Fond du Lac, WI 54935
**Phone:** (920)923-8732  **Fax:** (920)923-8770
**Email:** nricketts@mariancollege.edu
**Website:** http://www.mariancollege.edu/
Nancy Ricketts, Contact
**Fnded:** 1936. **Degrees Offered:** BSN.


**★ 15622 ★ Marquette University**
**College of Nursing**
PO Box 1881
Clark Hall
Milwaukee, WI 53201-1881
**Phone:** (414)288-3810  **Fax:** (414)288-1597
**Email:** judith.miller@marquette.edu
**Website:** http://www.marquette.edu/
Dr. Judith F. Miller, Contact
**Fnded:** 1881. **Degrees Offered:** BSN, MSN.


**★ 15623 ★ Milwaukee School of**
**Engineering**
**School of Nursing**
1025 N Broadway St.
Milwaukee, WI 53202-3109
**Phone:** (414)277-4516  **Fax:** (414)277-4540
**Email:** brown@msoe.edu
**Website:** http://www.msoe.edu/
Dr. Mary Louise Brown, Contact
**Fnded:** 1903. **Degrees Offered:** BSN.


**★ 15624 ★ University of Wisconsin, Eau**
**Claire**
**School of Nursing**
Eau Claire, WI 54702-4004
**Phone:** (715)836-5279  **Fax:** (715)836-5925
**Email:** sparskrk@uwec.edu
**Website:** http://www.uwec.edu/
Dr. Rita Kisting Sparks, Contact
**Fnded:** 1916. **Degrees Offered:** BSN, MSN.


**★ 15625 ★ University of Wisconsin,**
**Green Bay**
**Professional Program in Nursing**
2420 Nicolet Dr.
Green Bay, WI 54311-7001
**Phone:** (920)465-2365  **Fax:** (920)465-2854
**Email:** muhlj@uwgb.edu
**Website:** http://www.uwgb.edu/
Dr. V. Jane Muhl, Contact
**Fnded:** 1968. **Degrees Offered:** BSN.


**★ 15626 ★ University of Wisconsin,**
**Milwaukee**
**School of Nursing**
Student Affairs
PO Box 413
Milwaukee, WI 53201
**Phone:** (414)229-5473  **Fax:** (414)229-5554
**Email:** schulgal@uwm.edu
**Website:** http://www.uwm.edu/
Lisa Schulga, Contact
**Fnded:** 1956. **Degrees Offered:** BS, MS, PhD.


**★ 15627 ★ University of Wisconsin,**
**Oshkosh**
**College of Nursing**
800 Algoma Blvd.
Oshkosh, WI 54901-8660
**Phone:** (920)424-2106  **Fax:** (920)424-0123
**Email:** smithr@uwosh.edu
**Website:** http://www.uwosh.edu/colleges/con/umaster.html
Dr. Rosemary Smith, Contact
**Fnded:** 1871. **Degrees Offered:** BSN, MSN.


**★ 15628 ★ Viterbo College**
**School of Nursing**
815 S 9th St.
La Crosse, WI 54601
**Phone:** (608)796-3010  **Fax:** (608)796-3050
**Email:** bjnesbitt@viterbo.edu
**Website:** http://www.viterbo.edu/
Dr. Bonnie Nesbitt, Contact
**Fnded:** 1890. **Degrees Offered:** BSN, MSN.

## Wyoming

### ★ 15629 ★ University of Wyoming School of Nursing
PO Box 3065
Laramie, WY 82071-3065
**Phone:** (307)766-3906          **Fax:** (307)766-4294
**Email:** bjtaheri@uwyo.edu
**Website:** http://marshall.uwyo.edu/nursing/home/welcome.htm
Dr. Beverly L. Taheri-Kennedy, Contact
**Fnded:** 1886. **Degrees Offered:** BSN, MS.

# National & International Organizations

### ★ 15630 ★ Academy of Medical Surgical Nurses (AMSN)
East Holly Ave.
PO Box 56
Pitman, NJ 08071-0056
**Phone:** (856)256-2323          **Fax:** (856)589-7463
**Email:** amsn@ajj.com
**Website:** http://www.medsurgnurse.org/cover.htm
**Desc:** Adult/health, medical-surgical nurses. Promotes standards of nursing. Collaborates with other nursing organizations to provide educational programs, practice guidelines and new ideas for its members. **Pub:** *Certification Review Course Manual*. Manual. Available to educators providing continuing nursing education.

### ★ 15631 ★ Air and Surface Transport Nurses Association (ASTNA)
9101 E Kenyon Ave., Ste. 3000
Denver, CO 80237
**Free:** 800-897-6362          **Fax:** (303)770-1812
**Email:** astna@gwami.com
**Website:** http://www.astna.org
Karen Wojdyla, CAE, Exec. Dir.
**Fnded:** 1981. **Mem:** 1,700. **Reg. Groups:** 10. **Desc:** Transport nurses. Seeks to promote the quality of transport nursing by developing standards for the profession and exploring educational opportunities. Seeks optimum working conditions for members. Provides assistance to hospitals for developing air medical services programs. Maintains speakers' bureau. **Pub:** *Across the Board*, bimonthly. Newsletter. • *Journal of Air Medical Transport*, monthly. Journal. • Also produces educational learning module. **AKA:** (1999) National Flight Nurses Association.

### ★ 15632 ★ Alpha Tau Delta (ATD)
150 Cruickshank Dr.
Folsom, CA 95630
**Phone:** (916)984-9150
**Email:** kerrik@atdnursing.org
**Website:** http://www.atdnursing.org
Kerri L. Kaye, Pres.
**Fnded:** 1921. **Mem:** 6,000. **Nat'l Groups:** 1. **Reg. Groups:** 2. **State Groups:** 12. **Desc:** Professional fraternity - nursing. Seeks to further educational standards for the nursing profession. Maintains scholarship program for members only. **Pub:** *President's Letter*, quarterly. • *The Pulse...A publication of Alpha Tau Delta*, quarterly. Newsletter. Contains reports, member and chapter news, and calendar of events, CEU, interview and nursing news. *Price:* Included in membership dues. • Brochure.

### American Academy of Ambulatory Care Nursing (AAACN)
*See:* Entry 9682

### ★ 15633 ★ American Academy of Hospice and Palliative Medicine (AAHPM)
4700 W Lake Ave.
Glenview, IL 60025-1485
**Phone:** (847)375-4712          **Fax:** 877-734-8671
**Email:** aahpm@aahpm.org
**Website:** http://www.aahpm.org
**Fnded:** 1988. **Desc:** Physicians and other medical professionals dedicated to excellence in palliative medicine and prevention and relief of suffering; fosters research; provides public advocacy. training programs in hospice and palliative care. Educates the public regarding the rights of the dying and other issues affecting hospice and palliative medicine. **Pub:** *Hospice and Palliative Medicine Core Curriculum and Review Syllabus*. • *Position Statements*, periodic. Reports. • *UNIPACs: Hospice/Palliative Care Training for Physicians and other Medical Professionals*. **Frmly:** Academy of Hospice Physicians.

### ★ 15634 ★ American Academy of Nurse Practitioners (AANP)
National Administrative Office
PO Box 12846
Austin, TX 78711
**Phone:** (512)442-4262          **Fax:** (512)442-6469
**Email:** admin@aanp.org
**Website:** http://www.aanp.org
Zo DeMarchi, Dir. of Association Services
**Fnded:** 1985. **Mem:** 13,000. **Desc:** Promotes high standards of health care delivered by nurse practitioners. Acts as a forum to enhance the identity and continuity of nurse practitioners. Addresses national and state legislative issues that affect members; acts as a resource center on legislative activity. Supports continuing education programs. Encourages research in the field. Compiles statistics. **Pub:** *Academy Update*, monthly. Newsletter. • *Journal of the American Academy of Nurse Practitioners*, monthly. Journal. Focuses on clinical practice, management, and education. • Brochures.

### ★ 15635 ★ American Academy of Nursing (AAN)
600 Maryland Ave., NW, Ste. 100 West
Washington, DC 20024-2571
**Phone:** (202)651-7238          **Fax:** (202)554-2641
**Email:** tgaffney@ana.org
**Website:** http://www.nursingworld.org/aan
Terri Gaffney, Dir.
**Fnded:** 1973. **Mem:** 800. **Desc:** Purposes are to: advance new concepts in nursing and health care; identify and explore issues in health, the professions, and society that concern nursing; examine interrelationships among the segments within nursing and the interaction among nurses as these affect the development of the nursing profession; identify and propose resolutions to issues and problems confronting nursing and health, including alternative plans for implementation. Sponsors symposia. **Pub:** *American Academy of Nursing Directory*, biennial. Directory. *Price:* Included in membership dues. • *Differentiating Nursing Practice: Into the 21st Century*. • *Knowledge About Care and Caring: State of the Art and Future Directions*. • *Nursing Outlook*, bimonthly. Journal. Includes calendar of events, obituaries, and research reports. *Price:* Included in membership dues; $25/year for nonmembers. • *Practice and Inquiry for Nursing Administration: Intra- and Interdisciplinary Perspectives*.

### ★ 15636 ★ American Assembly for Men in Nursing (AAMN)
c/o NYSNA
11 Cornell Rd.
Latham, NY 12110-1499
**Phone:** (518)782-9400          **Fax:** (518)782-9530
**Email:** aamn@aamn.org
**Website:** http://www.aamn.org
Gene Tranbarger, Pres.
**Fnded:** 1971. **Mem:** 200. **Reg. Groups:** 5. **State Groups:** 4. **Desc:** Registered nurses. Works to: help eliminate prejudice in nursing; interest men in the nursing profession; provide opportunities for the discussion of common problems; encourage education and promote further professional growth; advise and assist in areas of professional inequity; help develop sensitivities to various social needs; promote the principles and practices of positive health care. Acts as a clearinghouse for information on men in nursing. Conducts educational programs. Promotes education and research about men's health issues. **Pub:** *Interaction*, quarterly. Newsletter. Contains statement of objectives and information on officers, events, and activities. *Price:* Included in membership dues. **Frmly:** (1982) National Male Nurse Association.

### ★ 15637 ★ American Association of Colleges of Nursing (AACN)
1 Dupont Cir. NW, Ste. 530
Washington, DC 20036
**Phone:** (202)463-6930          **Fax:** (202)785-8320
**Email:** webmaster@aacn.nche.edu
**Website:** http://www.aacn.nche.edu
Jennifer Ahearn, Exec. Dir.
**Fnded:** 1969. **Mem:** 555. **Desc:** Institutions offering baccalaureate and/or graduate degrees in nursing. Seeks to advance the practice of professional nursing by improving the quality of baccalaureate and graduate programs, promoting research, and developing academic leaders. Works with other professional nursing organizations and organizations in other health professions to evaluate and improve health care. Conducts educational programs on masters and doctoral nursing education and faculty practice; sponsors executive development series for new and aspiring deans of nursing. **Pub:** *Data Base for Graduate Education in Nursing*. *Price:* $6. • *Enrollment and Graduations in Baccalaureate and Graduate Programs in Nursing*, annual. Report. • *Essentials of College and University Education for Professional Nursing*. *Price:* $2.75 for members; $3.75 for nonmembers. • *Executive Development Series II: The Dean's Role in Organizational Assessment and Development*. *Price:* $26.95 for members; $36.95 for nonmembers. • *Faculty Salaries in Baccalaureate and Graduate Programs in Nursing*, annual. Report. • *Issue Bulletin*, 3/year. Bulletin. Examines issues in nursing education and research. • *Journal of Professional Nursing*, bimonthly. Journal. • *Meet the Press. . .and Succeed: A Handbook for Nurse Educators*. *Price:* $4.75 for members; $5.75 for nonmembers. • *Position Statement on Nursing Research*. *Price:* $3. • *Primary Health Care: Nurses Lead the Way–A Global Perspective*. *Price:* $10 for members; $15 for nonmembers. • *Salaries of Administrative Nursing Faculty in Baccalaureate and Graduate Programs in Nursing*, biennial. Report. • *Salaries of Deans in Baccalaureate and Graduate Programs in Nursing*, annual. Report. *Price:* $28. • *Special Report on Institutional Resources and Budgets in Baccalaureate and Graduate Programs in Nursing*, biennial. Report. *Price:* $25. • *Syllabus*, bimonthly. Newsletter. • *Annual Report*.

### ★ 15638 ★ American Association of Critical-Care Nurses (AACN)
101 Columbia
Aliso Viejo, CA 92656-4109
**Phone:** (949)362-2000          **Free:** 800-899-AACN
**Fax:** (949)362-2020
**Email:** info@aacn.org
**Website:** http://www.aacn.org
Micheal L. Williams, Pres.
**Fnded:** 1969. **Mem:** 65,000. **Local Groups:** 275. **Desc:** Professional critical care nurses. Established to provide continuing education programs for nurses specializing in critical care and to develop standards of nursing care of critically ill patients. Conducts educational programs. Offers certification program for critical care nurses through AACN Certification Corporation. Seeks liaison with other professional nursing organizations and related health agencies. **Pub:** *AACN Clinical Issues*, quarterly. Journal. Contains peer-reviewed articles on clinically relevant topics. *Price:* $49.30/year for members; $58/year for nonmembers; $90/year for institutions. • *American Journal of Critical Care*, bimonthly. Journal. Covers original research in critical

care. Contains directory of educational programs. *Price:* Included in membership dues; $45/year for nonmembers; $110 for institutions. • *Core Curriculum for Critical-Care Nursing.* • *Critical Care Nurse,* bimonthly. Clinical, peer-reviewed magazine focusing on critical care clinical practice. Contains listing of educational programs. *Price:* Included in membership dues; $27/year for nonmembers; $45/year for institutions. **Frmly:** (1970) American Association of Cardiovascular Nurses.

**American Association of Legal Nurse Consultants (AALNC)**
*See:* Entry 12226

**★ 15639 ★ American Association of Managed Care Nurses (AAMCN)**
4435 Waterfront Dr., Ste. 101
PO Box 4975
Glen Allen, VA 23058-4975
**Phone:** (804)747-9698 **Fax:** (804)747-5316
**Email:** rbailey@aamcn.org
**Website:** http://www.aamcn.org
M. Rene Bailey, Exec. Admin.
**Fnded:** 1994. **Mem:** 2,500. **State Groups:** 5. **Desc:** Managed health care professionals, including registered nurses, licensed practical nurses, and nurse practitioners. Seeks to enhance the abilities of members to meet the future needs of the managed health care profession through education. Provides a home study program as a pre-requisite for the Certified Managed Care Nurse (CMCN) exam. **Pub:** *Nurses' Notes,* quarterly. Newsletter. *Price:* Included in membership dues.

**★ 15640 ★ American Association of Neuroscience Nurses (AANN)**
4700 W Lake Ave.
Glenview, IL 60025
**Phone:** (847)375-4733 **Free:** 888-557-2266
**Fax:** (847)375-6333
**Email:** info@aann.org
**Website:** http://www.aann.org
Shelly Johnson, Exec. Dir.
**Fnded:** 1968. **Mem:** 4,000. **State Groups:** 50. **Desc:** Registered nurses engaged in or primarily interested in neurosurgical or neurological nursing. Objectives are to: foster interest, education, and high standards of practice in the field of neuroscience nursing; encourage continuing growth in the field; provide a medium for communication among neuroscience nurses in the U.S. and Canada. Has developed core curriculum for neuroscience nursing practice. **Pub:** *American Association of Neuroscience Nurses Synapse,* bimonthly. Newsletter. Includes calendar of events, continuing education course listings, employment listings, and information on new members and publications. *Price:* Included in membership dues. • *Core Curriculum for Neuroscience Nursing.* • *Journal of Neuroscience Nursing,* bimonthly. Journal. Includes book reviews, pharmacology update, and research reports. *Price:* Included in membership dues; $110/year for nonmembers; $135/year for institutions.

**American Association of Nurse Anesthetists (AANA)**
*See:* Entry 4438

**American Association of Nurse Attorneys (TAANA)**
*See:* Entry 12227

**★ 15641 ★ American Association of Occupational Health Nurses (AAOHN)**
2920 Brandy Wine Rd., Ste. 100
Atlanta, GA 30341
**Phone:** (770)455-7757 **Fax:** (770)455-7271
**Email:** aaohn@aaohn.org
**Website:** http://www.aaohn.org
Susan A. Randolph, VP

**Fnded:** 1942. **Mem:** 12,500. **Reg. Groups:** 1. **State Groups:** 34. **Local Groups:** 138. **Desc:** Registered professional nurses employed by business and industrial firms; nurse educators, nurse editors, nurse writers, and others interested in occupational health nursing. Promotes and sets standards for the profession. Provides and approves continuing education; maintains governmental affairs program; offers placement service. **Pub:** *AAOHN Core Curriculum Study Guide.* Includes guidelines of Occupational Health & Safety Services. • *AAOHN Journal,* monthly. Journal. • *AAOHN News,* monthly. Newsletter. • *SuccessTools: Strategies for Thriving & Surviving in Business.* Includes guidelines for Occupational Health & Safety Services. **Frmly:** (1977) American Association of Industrial Nurses.

**★ 15642 ★ American Association of Office Nurses (AAON)**
109 Kinderkamack Rd.
Montvale, NJ 07645
**Phone:** (201)391-2600 **Free:** 800-457-7504
**Fax:** (201)573-8543
**Email:** aaonmail@aaon.org
**Website:** http://www.aaon.org
Joyce Logan, Exec. Dir.
**Fnded:** 1988. **Mem:** 4,000. **Reg. Groups:** 21. **Desc:** Nurses working primarily in physicians' offices. Promotes improvement of the image of the office nurse. Encourages professional growth and development; facilitates exchange of information among members. Provides continuing education opportunities. Issues publications. **Pub:** *NEON,* quarterly. Newsletter.

**★ 15643 ★ American Association of Spinal Cord Injury Nurses (AASCIN)**
75-20 Astoria Blvd.
East Elmhurst, NY 11370-1177
**Phone:** (718)803-3782 **Fax:** (718)803-0414
**Email:** aascin@epva.org
**Website:** http://www.aascin.org
Sara Lerman, MPH, Prog. Mgr.
**Fnded:** 1983. **Mem:** 1,200. **Desc:** Nurses who care for patients with spinal cord impairment; nurses interested in the field of spinal cord impairment; persons who have provided extraordinary service to improve the quality of life for spinal cord impairment patients. Purposes are to: promote and improve nursing care of spinal cord impairment patients; develop and advance related education and research; recognize nurses whose careers are devoted to the problems of spinal cord impairment; keep medical personnel informed of state-of-the-art techniques. Focuses on topics such as sexuality and spinal cord impairment, care of respiratory dependent spinal cord impairment patients, alcohol and drug dependent spinal cord impairment patients, and planning for care in the community. Monitors and participates in legislative and regulatory activities affecting spinal cord impairment and professional nursing practice. Conducts research and educational programs. **Pub:** *Clinical Practice Guideline: Autonomic Dysreflexia.* Pamphlet. *Price:* $10. • *Education Guide for Spinal Cord Injury Nurses: A Manual for Teaching Patients, Families, and Caregivers, 1990.* *Price:* $5. • *SCI Nursing,* quarterly. Journal. Contains articles on all facets on spinal cord injury patient care and association news. • *Spinal Cord Injury: Education Content for Professional Nursing Practice, 2nd ed. 1996. Price:* $20. • *Standards of Spinal Cord Injury Nursing Practice.* Pamphlet. *Price:* $6.

**★ 15644 ★ American Board of Managed Care Nursing (ABMCN)**
4435 Waterfront Dr., Ste. 101
Glen Allen, VA 23060-3393
**Phone:** (804)527-1905 **Fax:** (804)747-5316
**Email:** rbailey@aamcn.org
**Website:** http://www.abmcn.org
**Fnded:** 1998. **Desc:** Seeks to advance the study, teaching, and practice of managed care nursing. Conducts examinations and bestows certification upon qualified nurses.

**★ 15645 ★ American Board of Neuroscience Nursing (ABNN)**
4700 W Lake Ave.
Glenview, IL 60025
**Phone:** (847)375-4733 **Free:** 888-557-2266
**Fax:** (847)375-6333
**Email:** info@aann.org
**Website:** http://www.AANN.org
Louise S. Miller, Dir. of Certification
**Fnded:** 1978. **Desc:** Certifying body for registered nurses who have passed a written examination demonstrating achievement in neuroscience nursing. Objective is to promote excellence in the field by encouraging professional growth and individual study; granting neuroscience nursing certification; measuring knowledge and level of theory required for certification; establishing certification standards. Administers certifying examination. **Frmly:** (1984) Neurosurgical Nurses.

**★ 15646 ★ American Board of Nursing Specialties (ABNS)**
4035 Running Spgs.
San Antonio, TX 78261
**Phone:** (830)438-4897
**Email:** abns@H-R-S.org
**Website:** http://www.nursingcertification.org
Dr. Maxine Bernreuter, Exec. Dir.
**Fnded:** 1991. **Mem:** 25. **Desc:** National nursing certification boards and nursing organizations concerned with nursing credential issues. National peer review program for specialty nursing certification bodies.

**★ 15647 ★ American Board for Occupational Health Nurses (ABOHN)**
201 E Ogden Ave., Ste. 114
Hinsdale, IL 60521-3652
**Phone:** (630)789-5799 **Free:** 888-842-2646
**Fax:** (630)789-8901
**Email:** info@abohn.org
**Website:** http://www.abohn.org
Sharon D. Kemerer, MSN, Exec. Dir.
**Fnded:** 1972. **Mem:** 6,600. **Desc:** Occupational health nurses. Establishes standards and confers initial and ongoing certification in occupational health nursing. Conducts semiannual certification examination. **Pub:** *The ABOHN Report,* semiannual. Newsletter. • *Directory of Certified Occupational Health Nurses,* annual. Directory. Contains contact information for certified occupational health nurses. • *Reference Guide for Examination Preparation.* • Also publishes position papers on occupational health nursing issues.

**American Board of Peri Anesthesia Nursing Certification (ABPANC)**
*See:* Entry 4440

**American College of Nurse-Midwives (ACNM)**
*See:* Entry 16643

**★ 15648 ★ American College of Nurse Practitioners (ACNP)**
1111 19th St. NW, Ste. 404
Washington, DC 20002
**Phone:** (202)659-2190 **Fax:** (202)659-2191
**Email:** acnp@nurse.org
**Website:** http://www.nurse.org/acnp
Eric G. Scharf, CAE, Exec. Dir.
**Fnded:** 1993. **Mem:** 2,800. **Desc:** Licensed and student nurse practitioners; state and national associations representing nurse practitioners. Seeks to strengthen the voice of nurse practitioners within the medical profession; promotes advancement in the study, teaching, and practice of nursing. ACNP's mission is to unite and represent nurse practitioners on policy and professional issues, in order to ensure an appropriate, prevention-based health care system that meets the needs of individuals, families and communities. ACNP provides advocacy on federal

policy issues, publishes newsletters and continuing education materials, sponsors conferences and symposia and provides a range of professional networking opportunities. **Pub:** *Forum*, quarterly. Newsletter. • *Nurse Practitioner World News*, periodic. Newsletter. • *Washington Word*, monthly. Newsletter.

**American Holistic Nurses Association (AHNA)**
*See:* Entry 4215

★ **15649** ★ **American Licensed Practical Nurses Association (ALPNA)**
1090 Vermont Ave. NW, Ste. 800
Washington, DC 20005
**Phone:** (202)682-9000
**Email:** ahna-flag@flaglink.com
**Website:** http://www.ahna.org
Paul M. Tendler, Exec. Dir.

**Fnded:** 1984. **Mem:** 6,200. **Desc:** Licensed practical nurses. Promotes the practical nursing profession; lobbies and maintains relations with the government on issues and legislation that may have an impact on LPNs. Conducts continuing education classes. Facilitates discussion of issues affecting the nursing and health professions. **Pub:** Pamphlets.Contain information on legislation and nursing standards. • Papers.

★ **15650** ★ **American Nephrology Nurses' Association (ANNA)**
Box 56, E Holly Ave.
Pitman, NJ 08071
**Phone:** (856)256-2320          **Free:** 888-600-2662
**Fax:** (856)589-7463
**Email:** anna@ajj.org
**Website:** http://www.annanurse.org
Mike Cunningham, Exec. Dir.

**Fnded:** 1969. **Mem:** 11,500. **Reg. Groups:** 4. **Local Groups:** 106. **Desc:** Registered nurses; physicians, dietitians, social workers, and technicians. Promotes continuing education of members at national, regional, and local levels. **Pub:** *Building Your Career in Dialysis*. Video. *Price:* $29. • *Contemporary Nephrology Nursing Textbook*. Book. *Price:* $88 members; $103 nonmembers. • *Continuous Quality Improvement: From Concept to Reality*. Manual. *Price:* $30 members; $45 non-members. • *Core Curriculum for Nephrology Nursing*. *Price:* $70 member; $90 non-member. • *Nephrology Nursing: A Guide to Professional Development*. *Price:* $35 member; $50 non-member. • *Nephrology Nursing Certification Review Guide*. *Price:* $20 members; $30 non-members. • *Nephrology Nursing Journal*. *Price:* $32 individual; $47 individual outside USA; $45 institution; $60 institution outside USA. • *RPA Shared Decision-Making in the Appropriate Initiation of and Withdrawal from Dialysis*. *Price:* $10 members. • *Standardized Training Program for the Patient Care Technician in Hemodialysis - Instructor's Guide*. *Price:* $18. • *Standardized Training Program for the Patient Care Technician in Hemodialysis - Learner's Guide*. *Price:* $28. • *Standards and Guidelines of Clinical Practice for Nephrology Nursing*. *Price:* $35 members; $50 non-members. • *Standards of Clinical Practice for Continuous Renal Replacement Therapy*. This publication is included in Standards of Clinical Practice for Nephrology Nursing. *Price:* $10 members; $15 non-members. **Frmly:** (1984) American Association of Nephrology Nurses and Technicians.

★ **15651** ★ **American Nurses Association (ANA)**
600 Maryland Ave. SW, Ste. 100 W
Washington, DC 20024-2571
**Phone:** (202)651-7000          **Free:** 800-274-4262
**Fax:** (202)651-7001
**Email:** anf@ana.org
**Website:** http://www.nursingworld.org
Mary Foley, Pres.

**Fnded:** 1896. **Mem:** 210,000. **State Groups:** 53. **Local Groups:** 860. **Desc:** Membership association representing registered nurses. **Pub:** *The American Nurse*, monthly. Newspaper. Includes employment

listings. *Price:* Included in membership dues; $20/year for nonmembers; $10/year for full-time nursing students. • *Proceedings of the House of Delegates*, periodic. Proceedings. • Catalog, annual. • Also publishes nursing standards and professional literature. **Frmly:** (1911) Nurses Associated Alumnae of United States and Canada.

★ **15652** ★ **American Nurses' Foundation (ANF)**
600 Maryland Ave. SW, Ste. 100W
Washington, DC 20024-2571
**Phone:** (202)651-7227          **Fax:** (202)651-7354
**Email:** anf@ana.org
**Website:** http://www.nursingworld.org/anf
Leo Schargorodski, Dir.

**Fnded:** 1955. **Desc:** Research, education, and charitable arm of the American Nurses' Association. Promotes nursing and consumers wherever nurses practice. Mission accomplished through four major functions: fundraising, Nursing Research Grants, grant development and management, and American Nurses Publishing. **Pub:** Books.

★ **15653** ★ **American Nursing Informatics Association (ANIA)**
PMB 105
10808 Foothill Blvd., Ste. 160
Rancho Cucamonga, CA 91730
**Email:** mbrs@ania.org
**Website:** http://www.ania.org
Angelique Weathersby, MBA,RN, Pres.

**Fnded:** 1992. **Mem:** 350. **Desc:** Licensed nurses, nursing students, and individuals involved with clinical, administrative and educational aspects of healthcare information systems. Provides networking, education, and information resources to members; serves as a forum for the advancement of nursing and nursing professionals in informatics. Makes available discounts on professional program attendance and conference tuition to members. **Pub:** *Input-Output*, periodic. Newsletter. *Price:* Free to members.

**American Organization of Nurse Executives (AONE)**
*See:* Entry 9703

★ **15654** ★ **American Psychiatric Nurses Association (APNA)**
2107 Wilson Blvd., Ste. 300-A
Arlington, VA 22201-3042
**Phone:** (703)243-2443          **Fax:** (703)243-3390
**Email:** info@apna.org
**Website:** http://www.apna.org
Timothy Gordon, Exec. Dir.

**Fnded:** 1987. **Mem:** 3,900. **State Groups:** 28. **Desc:** Provides leadership to advance psychiatric mental health nursing practice, improve mental health care for culturally diverse families, individuals, groups and communities, and shape health policy for the delivery of mental health services. **Pub:** *APNA News*, bimonthly. Newsletter. • *Journal of the American Psychiatric Nurses Association*, bimonthly. Journal.

**American Radiological Nurses Association (ARNA)**
*See:* Entry 18110

★ **15655** ★ **American Society of Ophthalmic Registered Nurses (ASORN)**
PO Box 193030
San Francisco, CA 94119
**Phone:** (415)561-8513          **Fax:** (415)561-8531
**Email:** asorn@aao.org
**Website:** http://www.asorn.org
Sue Brown, Exec. Admin.

**Fnded:** 1976. **Mem:** 1,200. **Local Groups:** 27. **Desc:** Registered nurses and other ophthalmic medical personnel specializing in the field of ophthalmology. Promotes excellence in ophthalmic nursing for the

best and safest care of patients with eye disorders or injuries. Facilitates continuing education through the study, discussion, and exchange of knowledge, experience, and ideas in the field. Represents members' interests before governmental agencies, hospitals, industries, research organizations, technical societies, universities, and other professional associations. Conducts educational programs. **Pub:** *Insight, The Journal of the American Society of Ophthalmic Registered Nurses*, quarterly. Journal. Covers trends in ophthalmology, standards of care, and legislative issues. Includes society news, calendar of events, and chapter news. *Price:* Included in membership dues; $48 nonmember; $64.20 Canada; $60 outside U.S. and Canada. • Ophthalmic Procedures, A Nursing Perspective Volumes I, II, & III. Core curriculum for Ophthalmic Nursing; Care & Handling of Ophthalmic Microsurgical Instruments; Standards of Ophthalmic Clinical Nursing Practice.

★ **15656** ★ **American Society of Pain Management Nurses**
7794 Grow Dr.
Pensacola, FL 32514
**Phone:** (850)473-0233          **Free:** 888-342-7766
**Fax:** (850)484-8762
**Email:** aspmn@puetzamc.com
**Website:** http://www.aspmn.org

**Fnded:** 1990. **Mem:** 1,600. **State Groups:** 20. **Desc:** Professional nurses. Dedicated to promoting and providing optimal care of patients with pain. **Pub:** *Pain Management*, quarterly. Journal. • *Pathways*, bimonthly. Newsletter.

★ **15657** ★ **American Society of PeriAnesthesia Nurses (ASPAN)**
10 Melrose Ave., Ste. 110
Cherry Hill, NJ 08003-3696
**Phone:** (856)616-9600          **Free:** 877-737-9696
**Fax:** (856)616-9601
**Email:** aspan@aspan.org
**Website:** http://www.aspan.org
Kevin Dill, CEO

**Fnded:** 1980. **Mem:** 10,000. **Nat'l Groups:** 3. **Reg. Groups:** 40. **Local Groups:** 100. **Desc:** Nurses practicing in all phases of ambulatory surgery, preanesthesia and post anesthesia care. Promotes quality and cost effective care for patients, their families, and the community through public and professional education, research and standards of practice. Offers continuing education programs. **Pub:** *Breathline*, bimonthly. Newsletter. • *The Journal of PeriAnesthesia Nursing*, bimonthly. Journal. • Also publishes a manual of forms and the Core Curriculum for Post Anesthesia Nursing Practice. **Frmly:** (2001) American Society of Post Anesthesia Nurses.

★ **15658** ★ **American Society of Plastic Surgical Nurses (ASPSN)**
E Holly Ave.
Box 56
Pitman, NJ 08071
**Phone:** (856)256-2340          **Fax:** (856)589-7463
**Email:** asprsn@ajj.com
Rick Grimes, Exec. Dir.

**Fnded:** 1975. **Mem:** 1,830. **Reg. Groups:** 4. **State Groups:** 30. **Desc:** Registered nurses, licensed practical nurses, and licensed vocational nurses working with plastic surgeons or interested in plastic and reconstructive nursing. Objectives are: to enhance leadership qualities of nurses in the field of plastic surgery; to increase the skills, knowledge, and understanding of personnel in plastic surgery nursing through continuing education; to study existing practices and new developments in the field; to encourage participation and interest in professional organizations; to cooperate with others in the profession. **Pub:** *ASPRS News*, bimonthly. Newsletter. *Price:* available to members only. • *ASPRSN Membership Directory*, annual. Membership Directory. • *Core Curriculum for Plastic and Reconstructive Surgical Nursing*. • *Plastic Surgical Nursing*, quarterly. Journal. **Frmly:** (2001)

American Society of Plastic and Reconstructive Surgical Nurses.

**★ 15659 ★ Anthroposophical Nurses Association of America**
1923 Geddes Ave.
Ann Arbor, MI 48104
**Phone:** (734)761-5172    **Fax:** (734)761-6617
**Email:** artemisia@anthroposophy.org
**Website:** http://www.artemisia.net/anaa/
Rise Smythe-Freed, Pres.

**Fnded:** 1985. **Mem:** 90. **Desc:** Seeks to further the practice of anthroposophical nursing in the U.S. (Anthroposophy is a 20th century body of knowledge centering on human development.) Encourages nurses to apply their knowledge of humankind to nursing practices. Promotes members' continued education. **Pub:** Newsletter, annual. *Price:* $12.

**Army Nurse Corps Association (ANCA)**
*See:* Entry 13457

**★ 15660 ★ Association of Black Nursing Faculty (ABNF)**
5823 Queens Cove
Lisle, IL 60532
**Phone:** (630)969-3809    **Fax:** (630)969-3895
**Email:** stewarth@wt.net
**Website:** http://abnfinc.org
Bess Stewart, Pres.

**Fnded:** 1987. **Mem:** 127. **State Groups:** 25. **Desc:** Black nursing faculty teaching in nursing programs accredited by the National League for Nursing. Works to promote health-related issues and educational concerns of interest to the black community and ABNF. Serves as a forum for communication and the exchange of information among members; develops strategies for expressing concerns to other individuals, institutions, and communities. Assists members in professional development; develops and sponsors continuing education activities; fosters networking and guidance in employment and recruitment activities. Promotes health-related issues of legislation, government programs, and community activities. Supports black consumer advocacy issues. Encourages research. Maintains speakers' bureau and hall of fame. Offers charitable program and placement services. Compiles statistics. Is establishing a computer-assisted job bank; plans to develop bibliographies related to research groups. **Pub:** *ABNF Journal*, bimonthly. Journal. Includes research reports and scholarly papers. *Price:* $125/year. • *ABNF Newsletter*, quarterly. Newsletter. Includes member profiles and activities, research abstracts, conference information, job opportunities, and fellowship information. *Price:* Included in membership dues; $25/year. • *Membership Directory of the ABNF*, annual. Membership Directory.

**★ 15661 ★ Association of Camp Nurses (ACN)**
8504 Thorsonveien NE
Bemidji, MN 56601
**Phone:** (218)586-2633    **Fax:** (218)586-3661
**Email:** acn@campnurse.org
**Website:** http://www.campnurse.org
Linda Ebner Erceg, RN, Exec. Dir.

**Fnded:** 1990. **Mem:** 450. **Nat'l Groups:** 2. **Reg. Groups:** 9. **Desc:** Works to promote and develop the nursing practice in the camp community. Maintains resource center; provides consulting services; supports camp nursing research; conducts educational programs. **Pub:** *Compass Point*, quarterly. Newsletter.

**★ 15662 ★ Association for Common European Nursing Diagnoses, Interventions and Outcomes (ACENDIO)**
Royal College of Nursing
20 Cavendish Sq.
London W1G 0RN, United Kingdom
**Email:** anne.casey@rcn.org.uk
**Website:** http://www.acendio.net

**Fnded:** 1995. **Lang(s):** English. **Desc:** Nurses and nursing organizations. Network and development of resources towards standards supporting sharing and comparison of data about nursing.

**★ 15663 ★ Association of Community Health Nursing Educators**
7794 Grow Dr.
Pensacola, FL 32514
**Phone:** (850)474-8821    **Fax:** (850)484-8762
**Email:** achne@nysna.org
Belinda E. Puetz, Exec. Dir.

**Mem:** 350. **Reg. Groups:** 5. **Desc:** Nurses and graduate students. Committed to "excellence in community and public health nursing education, research, and practice." **Pub:** Newsletter, quarterly.

**★ 15664 ★ Association of Hong Kong Nursing Staff (AHKNS)**
Hing Wan Commercial Bldg., 3/F
25-27 Parkes St.
Jordan
Kowloon
Hong Kong, People's Republic of China
**Phone:** 852 23146900    **Fax:** 852 27366020
**Email:** info@nurse.org.hk
**Website:** http://www.nurse.org.hk

**Fnded:** 1977. **Mem:** 15,500. **Lang(s):** Chinese, English. **Desc:** Registered, enrolled, and student nurses. Seeks to advance the nursing profession; promotes professional development of members. Represents members' legal and professional interests. Conducts continuing professional education and training courses; makes available to members services including legal advice and travel and merchandise discounts. **Pub:** *AHKNS Newsletter*, quarterly. Newsletter. **Frmly:** (1990) Association of Government Nursing Staff.

**★ 15665 ★ Association of Nursery Training Colleges**
The Chiltern College
16 Peppard Rd.
Caversham
Reading RQ48 JZ, United Kingdom
**Phone:** 44 118 9471847    **Fax:** 44 118 9463218
**Email:** info@chilterncollege.com

**Fnded:** 1931. **Mem:** 5. **Desc:** Private colleges providing nursery nurse training. Aims to foster co-operation between like minded organizations, to exchange information and promote interest in the training of a nursery nurse.

**★ 15666 ★ Association of Nurses in AIDS Care (ANAC)**
80 S Summit St.
500 Courtyard Sq.
Akron, OH 44308
**Phone:** (330)762-5739    **Free:** 800-260-6780
**Fax:** (330)762-5813
**Email:** anac@anacnet.org
**Website:** http://www.anacnet.org/
Adele Webb, Exec. Dir.

**Fnded:** 1987. **Mem:** 2,800. **Reg. Groups:** 2. **State Groups:** 52. **Desc:** Nurses and other health care professionals involved in caring for people who are HIV-infected or have AIDS. Functions as a network and provides leadership and educational services for members. Promotes public awareness of AIDS issues; advocates for HIV-infected individuals. Plans to develop a national standard for care of people with AIDS. **Pub:** *ANACdotes.* Newsletter. • *Journal of the Association of Nurses in AIDS Care*, bimonthly. Journal. • Also publishes position papers.

**Association of Pediatric Oncology Nurses (APON)**
*See:* Entry 5628

**★ 15667 ★ Association of PeriOperative Registered Nurses (AORN)**
2170 S Parker Rd., Ste. 300
Denver, CO 80231-5711
**Phone:** (303)755-6300    **Free:** 800-755-2676
**Fax:** (303)755-4511
**Email:** clindmar@aorn.org
**Website:** http://www.aorn.org/
Tom Cooper, Exec. Dir.

**Fnded:** 1949. **Mem:** 41,000. **Local Groups:** 350. **Desc:** Professional perioperative (operating room) nurses. Provides education, representation, and standards for quality patient care. **Pub:** *AORN Journal*, monthly. Journal. Includes film and book reviews, educational opportunities, employment listings, and legislation. *Price:* Included in membership dues; $80/year for domestic nonmembers; $90/year for foreign nonmembers. • *SSM*, bimonthly. Contains information about trends in management and the surgical environment, changing policies & regulations, clinical practice, and other issues. **Frmly:** (1999) Association of Operating Room Nurses.

**★ 15668 ★ Association of Rehabilitation Nurses (ARN)**
4700 W Lake Ave.
Glenview, IL 60025-1485
**Phone:** (847)375-4710    **Free:** 800-229-7530
**Fax:** 877-734-9384
**Email:** info@rehabnurse.org
**Website:** http://www.rehabnurse.org
Donna Williams, Pres.

**Fnded:** 1974. **Mem:** 9,000. **Local Groups:** 80. **Desc:** Registered nurses concerned with or actively engaged in the practice of rehabilitation nursing; others interested in rehabilitation. Works to advance the quality of rehabilitation nursing practice through educational opportunities and to facilitate the exchange of ideas. Committees involve members in issues of organizational, local, and national importance and provide an avenue to effect change. Has formed the Rehabilitation Nursing Foundation to promote, develop, and engage in scientific research in the rehabilitation field. **Pub:** *ARN Network*, 6/year. Newsletter. • *Rehabilitation Nursing*, bimonthly. Journal. • Membership Directory, annual.

**★ 15669 ★ Association of Women's Health, Obstetric and Neonatal Nurses (AWHONN)**
2000 L St. Nw, Ste. 740
Washington, DC 20036
**Phone:** (202)261-2400    **Free:** 800-673-8499
**Fax:** (202)728-0575
**Email:** gaik@awhonn.org
**Website:** http://www.awhonn.org
Gail Kincaide, Exec. Dir.

**Fnded:** 1969. **Mem:** 22,000. **Reg. Groups:** 10. **State Groups:** 62. **Desc:** Members are registered nurses; associate members are allied health workers with an interest in obstetric, women's health, and neonatal (OGN) nursing. Promotes and establishes the highest standards of OGN nursing practice, education, and research; cooperates with all members of the health team; stimulates interest in OGN nursing. Sponsors educational meetings, audiovisual programs, and continuing education courses. **Pub:** *AWHONN Lifelines*, bimonthly. Magazine. Includes annual index, calendar of events, employment opportunity listings, and legislative news. *Price:* $26/yr. for individuals. • *Journal of Obstetric, Gynecologic, and Neonatal Nursing*, bimonthly. Journal. Includes advertisers' index and annual subject and author index. Contains book reviews, case studies, and employment opportunity listings. *Price:* $50/year for individuals; $170/year for institutions. • Also publishes manual of standards and OGN nursing practice resources. **Frmly:** Nurses Association of the American College of Obstetricians and Gynecologists; (1993) NAACOG: The Organization of Obstetric, Gynecologic, and Neonatal Nurses.

## ★ 15670 ★ Australian College of Occupational Health Nurses (ACOHN)
PO Box 1205
Tullamarine, VIC 3043, Australia
**Phone:** 61 3 93352577     **Fax:** 61 3 93353454
**Email:** admin@acohn.com.au
**Website:** http://www.acohn.com.au
**Fnded:** 1976. **Mem:** 400. **Lang(s):** English. **Desc:** Registered nurses and nurses in training working in occupational health and safety or in a relevant discipline. Promotes occupational health; promotes high standards and encourage excellence in the practice of occupational health; supports education for nurses who practice in occupational health; encourages research by nurses in the field.

## ★ 15671 ★ Australian Nursing Federation (ANF)
Unit 3
PO Box 1995
Woden, ACT 2606, Australia
**Phone:** 61 2 62829455     **Fax:** 61 2 62828447
**Email:** actanf@austarmetro.com.au
**Website:** http://www.anf.org.au
**Fnded:** 1924. **Mem:** 115,000. **Reg. Groups:** 8. **Lang(s):** English. **Desc:** Nurses in both the public and private sectors in Australia. Provides industrial and professional representation of nurses and pursues improved public policy on health and related issues. Participates in the development of policy in nursing, nursing regulation, community services, veterans' affairs, education, training, occupational health and safety, industrial matters, immigration and law reform. **Pub:** *Australian Journal of Advanced Nursing (AJAN)*, quarterly. Journal. Includes peer reviewed research. • *Australian Nursing Journal (ANJ)*, monthly. Journal. Includes clinical articles and latest nursing news.

## ★ 15672 ★ Baromedical Nurses Association (BNA)
5 Richland Medical Pk.
Columbia, SC 29203
**Phone:** (803)434-1221     **Fax:** (803)434-4354
**Email:** wound_nurse@juno.com
**Website:** http://www.hyperbaricnurses.org
Valerie Larson, Pres.
**Fnded:** 1985. **Mem:** 160. **Reg. Groups:** 6. **Desc:** Registered nurses practicing baromedicine (hyperbaric medicine), involved in research related to baromedical nursing, completing basic orientation in baromedicine, or contributing to literature on baromedicine or baromedical nursing. Defines, develops, and promotes the status and standards of baromedical nursing. Facilitates professional activities and continuing education programs. Provides a forum for the exchange of ideas, information, and support; maintains speakers' bureau. **Pub:** *BNA Update*, quarterly. Newsletter. Includes research findings, safety and educational information, and upcoming events. *Price:* Free. For members only. • Membership Directory, periodic.

## ★ 15673 ★ Board of Nephrology Examiners Nursing and Technology (BONENT)
PO Box 15945-282
Lenexa, KS 66285
**Phone:** (913)541-9077     **Fax:** (913)599-5340
**Email:** bonent-info@goamp.co
**Website:** http://www.goamp.com/bonent/
Stacie M. Beckwith, CMP, Exec. Dir.
**Fnded:** 1974. **Mem:** 1,900. **Desc:** Registered nurses, licensed practical nurses, licensed vocational nurses, and dialysis technicians. Provides nephrology nursing and technology certification examinations. Through certification, seeks to ensure: safe, competent practitioners in nephrology nursing and technology; excellence in the quality of care of the nephrology patient; the continued study and advance of the science of nursing and technological fields in nephrology. Compiles statistics. **Pub:** *Bonent Update*, quarterly. Newsletter. *Price:* Included in membership dues. **Frmly:** (2002) Board of Nephrology Examiners - Nursing and Technology.

## ★ 15674 ★ British Association of Dental Nurses
11 Pharos St.
Fleetwood FY7 6BG, United Kingdom
**Phone:** 44 1253 778631     **Fax:** 44 1253 773266
**Email:** admin@badn.org.uk
**Fnded:** 1940. **Lang(s):** English. **Desc:** Professional association representing dental nurses in the UK and overseas as well as other members of the dental industry. Represents members working in specialist areas such as training, orthodontics, special care, and the armed forces. Aims to support, encourage, and provide advice to dental nurses; to develop and maintain nationally recognised standards; to protect the professional status of the dental nurse; and to maintain contact with the necessary bodies to achieve the above. **Pub:** *The British Dental Nurses Journal*, quarterly, always March, June, September, and December. Journal. **Frmly:** (1994) ABDSA.

## ★ 15675 ★ British Association of Neuroscience Nurses
1 Parkhall Rd.
Antrim BT41 1BU, United Kingdom
**Phone:** 44 28 94461203
**Website:** http://www.bann.org.uk
**Fnded:** 1971. **Mem:** 310. **Desc:** Promotes the highest standards of patient care in the Neurosciences field. Provides opportunities for knowledge transfer between neuroscience nurses. Encourages clinical research and promotes interest in the neuroscience area.

## ★ 15676 ★ Canadian Association of Advanced Practice Nurses
c/o Rosemary Kohr
London Health Sciences Centre
E-510-375 South St.
London, ON, Canada N6A 4G5
**Phone:** (519)685-8500
**Email:** rkohr@lhsc.on.ca
**Website:** http://www.caapn.com
**Lang(s):** English, French. **Desc:** Nurses engaged in clinical practice. Promotes professional development of members; seeks to advance the practice of clinical nursing. Facilitates communication and cooperation among members; sponsors continuing professional education courses. **Frmly:** (1999) Canadian Clinical Nurse Specialist Group.

## ★ 15677 ★ Canadian Association of Burn Nurses (CABN)
48 Strath Ln.
Dartmouth, NS, Canada B2X 1Z3
**Lang(s):** English, French. **Desc:** Nurses specializing in the treatment of burns. Promotes professional advancement of members. Facilitates exchange of information among members; conducts continuing professional education programs.

## ★ 15678 ★ Canadian Association of Critical Care Nurses (CACCN)
PO Box 25322
London, ON, Canada N6C 6B1
**Phone:** (519)649-5284     **Fax:** (519)649-1458
**Email:** caccn@caccn.ca
**Website:** http://www.caccn.ca/
**Fnded:** 1985. **Mem:** 1,050. **Reg. Groups:** 10. **Lang(s):** English, French. **Desc:** Critical care nurses. Promotes professional advancement of members and improvement in the practice of critical care nursing. Conducts continuing professional education programs for members. **Pub:** *Dynamics Official Journal of the CACCN*, quarterly. Journal. • *Standards for Critical Care Nursing Practice (2nd Edition).* • *Study Guide for Critical Care Nursing Certification Examination (2nd Edition).*

## ★ 15679 ★ Canadian Association of Nephrology Nurses and Technologists (CANNT)
336 Yonge St., Ste. 322
Barrie, ON, Canada L4N 4C8
**Phone:** (705)720-2819     **Fax:** (705)720-1451
**Email:** cannt@cannt.ca
**Website:** http://www.cannt.ca
**Fnded:** 1984. **Desc:** Nephrology nurses and technicians. Dedicated to quality of care to individuals with renal disease; disseminates information to health care providers; participates in certification exam development activities with the CNA. Established and maintains Standards of Practice. **Pub:** *CANNT Journal*, quarterly. Journal.

## ★ 15680 ★ Canadian Association of Nuclear Medicine (CANM)
774 Echo Dr. Ottawa
Ottawa, ON, Canada K1S 5N8
**Phone:** (613)730-6254     **Fax:** (613)730-1116
**Email:** canm@rcpsc.edu
**Lang(s):** English, French. **Desc:** Physicians and other health care professionals with an interest in nuclear medicine. Seeks to advance the practice of nuclear medicine; promotes professional development of members. Sponsors research; conducts continuing professional education programs.

## ★ 15681 ★ Canadian Association of Nurses in AIDS Care (Association Canadienne des Infirmieres et Infirmiers en Sidologie)
1331 Nelson St., Apt. 6
Vancouver, BC, Canada V6E 1J8
**Phone:** (604)669-1030     **Fax:** (604)669-5975
**Email:** info@canac.org
**Website:** http://www.canac.org
**Lang(s):** English, French. **Desc:** Nurses engaged in the care of people with AIDS and HIV. Seeks to improve the quality of life of people with AIDS and HIV, and to advance the prevention and treatment of autoimmune diseases. Provides support and services to people with AIDS and HIV; makes available continuing professional development programs.

## ★ 15682 ★ Canadian Association of Nurses in Independent Practice (CANIP)
c/o Canadian Nurses Association
50 The Driveway
Ottawa, ON, Canada K2P 1E2
**Phone:** (416)240-2368     **Fax:** (416)242-7241
**Email:** bgourlay@telusplanet.net
**Fnded:** 1985. **Mem:** 130. **State Groups:** 4. **Lang(s):** English, French. **Desc:** Nurses operating independent practices. Encourages establishment of independent nursing practices; promotes professional and commercial advancement of members. Facilitates exchange of information among members; makes available continuing professional development courses. **Pub:** *Visions*, quarterly. Newsletter.

## ★ 15683 ★ Canadian Association of Nurses in Oncology (CANO)
232-329 March Rd., Box 11
Kanata, ON, Canada K2K 2E1
**Phone:** (613)270-0711     **Fax:** (613)599-7027
**Email:** canoacio@igs.net
**Fnded:** 1985. **Mem:** 850. **Lang(s):** English, French. **Desc:** Registered nurses in independent practice. Promotes improved public access to health care; seeks to increase the role of nurses in the delivery of health care services. Develops business and practice guidelines for members. Provides support and assistance to members; conducts educational programs to raise public awareness of nursing and other health care services; sponsors business and continuing professional development courses for members. Conducts lobbying activities; undertakes research

projects; compiles statistics. **Pub:** *Visions*, quarterly. Newsletter. • Brochure. • Directory, periodic.

**Canadian Association of Pediatric Nurses (CAPN)**
*See:* Entry 5640

**★ 15684 ★ Canadian Association of University Schools of Nursing (CAUSN) (Association Canadienne des Ecoles Universitaires de Nursing — ACEUN)**
350 Albert St., Ste. 325
Ottawa, ON, Canada K1R 1B1
**Phone:** (613)235-3150 **Fax:** (613)563-7739
**Email:** info@causn.org
**Website:** http://www.causn.org
**Fnded:** 1942. **Mem:** 65. **Reg. Groups:** 4. **State Groups:** 10. **Lang(s):** English, French. **Desc:** University schools of nursing. Promotes excellence in the study, teaching, and practice of nursing. Facilitates communication and cooperation among members; sponsors research and educational programs.

**★ 15685 ★ Canadian Council of Cardiovascular Nurses (CCCN) (Conseil Canadien des Infirmieres en Nursing Cardiovasculaire — CCINC)**
222 Queen St., Ste. 1402
Ottawa, ON, Canada K1P 5V9
**Phone:** (613)569-4361 **Fax:** (613)569-3278
**Email:** madam@ottawaheart.ca
**Website:** http://www.cardiovascularnurse.com
**Lang(s):** English, French. **Desc:** Nurses specializing in cardiovascular practice. Promotes advancement of cardiovascular nursing; facilitates continuing professional development of members. Serves as a forum for the exchange of information among members; conducts educational and training programs.

**★ 15686 ★ Canadian Federation of Mental Health Nurses (CFMHN)**
631 B 11th St.
Courtrey, BC, Canada V9N 1S9
**Phone:** (250)338-2691 **Fax:** (250)338-1591
**Email:** info@iciweb.com
**Website:** http://www.cfmhn.org
**Lang(s):** English, French. **Desc:** Nurses engaged in mental health practice. Promotes professional development of members; seeks to advance the practice of mental health nursing. Facilitates communication and cooperation among members; sponsors continuing professional education programs.

**★ 15687 ★ Canadian Federation of Nurses Unions (CFNU) (Federation Canadienne des Syndicats d'Infirmieres et Infirmiers — FCSII)**
2841 prom Riverside Dr.
Ottawa, ON, Canada K1V 8X7
**Phone:** (613)526-4661 **Free:** 800-321-9821
**Fax:** (613)526-1023
**Email:** cfnu@nursesunions.ca
**Website:** http://www.nursesunions.ca
**Lang(s):** English, French. **Desc:** Canadian nurses. Promotes nurses and the nursing profession. Lobbies the federal government; represents the profession in dealings with the media; provides information resources.

**★ 15688 ★ Canadian Gerontological Nursing Association (CGNA) (Association Canadienne des Infirmiers et Infirmiers en Gerontologie — ACIG)**
c/o South Granville Business Services
101-1001 W Broadway Department 370
Vancouver, BC, Canada V6H 4E4
**Phone:** (250)769-0664 **Fax:** (604)734-0778
**Email:** cgna@home.com
**Website:** http://www.cgna.net

**Lang(s):** English, French. **Desc:** Nurses specializing in gerontological practice. Promotes professional development of members; seeks to advance the practice of gerontological nursing. Serves as a forum for the exchange of information among members; conducts continuing professional education programs.

**★ 15689 ★ Canadian Holistic Nurses Association (CHNA) (Association Canadienne des Infirmieres en Approches Holistiques de Soins)**
50 Driveway
Ghana, BC, Canada K2P 1E2
**Phone:** (604)237-3520
**Website:** http://mypage.direct.ca/h/hutchings/chna.html
**Fnded:** 1988. **Mem:** 140. **Lang(s):** English, French. **Desc:** Registered nurses are members; health care providers including registered psychiatric nurses, massage therapists, physiotherapists, nursing students, and chiropractors are associate members. Seeks to further the development of the field of holistic nursing. Promotes use of a conceptual framework based on nursing principles and human environmental field theory in the treatment of patients; encourages employment of noninvasive strategies for promoting health and wellness. Promulgates and enforces standards of practice in holistic nursing; provides consulting services and other support to members; interacts with health care consumer and provider organizations to influence health policy formation. **Pub:** Newsletter, semiannual.

**★ 15690 ★ Canadian Intravenous Nurses Association (CINA)**
18 Wynford Dr., No. 516
North York, ON, Canada M3C 3S2
**Phone:** (416)445-4516 **Fax:** (416)445-4513
**Email:** cinacsot@idirect.com
**Website:** http://web.idirect.com/~csotcina/cina.html
**Fnded:** 1975. **Mem:** 725. **Local Groups:** 6. **Lang(s):** English. **Desc:** Registered nurses specializing in intravenous therapy or employed in supervisory, educational, or administrative positions related to intravenous therapy. Works to establish and promote standards of intravenous therapy. Offers educational programs designed to enhance patient care and safety. Facilitates discussion of intravenous therapy issues. **Pub:** *CINA Journal*, annual. Journal. • *CINA Mainliner*, quarterly. Newsletter. • *I.V. Therapy Guidelines*.

**★ 15691 ★ Canadian Nurses Association (CNA) (Association des Infirmieres et Infirmiers du Canada — AIIC)**
50 Driveway
Ottawa, ON, Canada K2P 1E2
**Phone:** (613)237-2133 **Fax:** (613)237-3520
**Email:** dross@cna-nurses.ca
**Website:** http://www.cna-nurses.ca
**Fnded:** 1908. **Mem:** 111,708. **Local Groups:** 11. **Lang(s):** English, French. **Desc:** Works to advance the quality of nursing in the interests of the public. Promotes high standards of nursing practice, education, research, and administration in order to achieve quality nursing care in the public interest. Also promotes uniform and high quality regulatory practices in the public interest and in collaboration with nursing regulatory bodies. Acts in the public interest for Canadian nursing and nurses, providing national and international leadership in nursing and health issues. **Pub:** *Canadian Nurse/Infirmiere Canadienne*, 10/year. Journal. • Monograph, periodic.

**★ 15692 ★ Canadian Nurses Foundation (CNF) (Fondation des Infirmieres et Infirmiers du Canada — FIIC)**
50 Driveway
Ottawa, ON, Canada K2P 1E2
**Phone:** (613)237-2133 **Fax:** (613)237-3520

**Email:** cnf@cnursefdn.ca
**Website:** http://www.canadiannursesfoundation.com
**Fnded:** 1961. **Mem:** 678. **Lang(s):** English, French. **Desc:** Promotes health and patient care in Canada; fosters excellence in nursing through nursing research grants, scholarships, specialty certification, and financial support for other educational purposes. **Pub:** *Foundation Focus*, 3-4/year. Newsletter.

**★ 15693 ★ Canadian Nurses Protective Society (CNPS)**
50 Driveway
Ottawa, ON, Canada K2P 1E2
**Phone:** (613)237-2092 **Free:** 800-267-3390
**Fax:** (613)237-6300
**Email:** info@cnps.ca
**Website:** http://www.cnps.ca
**Fnded:** 1988. **Lang(s):** English, French. **Desc:** Provides legal liability protection related to nursing practice to eligible registered nurses in Canada by providing information, education, and financial and legal assistance. Also offers a group insurance plan.

**★ 15694 ★ Canadian Nurses Respiratory Society (CNRS) (Societe Canadienne des Infirmieres en Sante Respiratoire — SCISR)**
300-3 Raymond St.
Ottawa, ON, Canada K1R 1A3
**Phone:** (613)569-6411 **Fax:** (613)569-8860
**Website:** http://www.lung.ca/resp
**Lang(s):** English, French. **Desc:** Nurses specializing in the treatment of respiratory diseases. Promotes excellence in the practice of nursing; encourages professional development of members. Serves as a forum for the exchange of information among members; sponsors research and educational programs.

**★ 15695 ★ Canadian Occupational Health Nurses Association (COHNA) (Association Canadienne des Infirmieres et Infirmiers en Sante du Travail — ACIST)**
PO Box 383
CBS
Mauels, NF, Canada A1W 1M9
**Phone:** (709)778-1561
**Email:** brenda.greenslade@nf.sympatico.ca
**Fnded:** 1992. **Mem:** 2,000. **Reg. Groups:** 9. **Lang(s):** English, French. **Desc:** Nurses specializing in occupational health. Seeks to advance the study and practice of occupational health nursing. Facilitates communication among members; sponsors research and educational programs on a national basis.

**★ 15696 ★ Canadian Orthopaedic Nurses Association (CONA) (Association Canadienne des Infirmieres et Infirmiers en Orthopedie — ACIO)**
88 Mill Settlement Rd.
Hoyt, NB, Canada E5L 2G6
**Phone:** (506)452-5392
**Email:** knorr@sympatico.ca
**Website:** http://www.cona-nurse.org
**Lang(s):** English, French. **Desc:** Nurses specializing in orthopedic practice. Promotes advancement of the profession of orthopedic nursing. Sponsors continuing professional development courses for members. **Pub:** *Orthoscope*, quarterly. Newsletter.

**★ 15697 ★ Canadian Society of Gastroenterology Nurses and Associates (CSGNA)**
27 Nicholson Dr.
Lakeside, NS, Canada B3T 1B3
**Phone:** (902)473-6541 **Fax:** (902)473-4406
**Email:** ednalang@hotmail.com
**Website:** http://www.csgna.com

**Fnded:** 1985. **Mem:** 510. **Reg. Groups:** 14. **Lang(s):** English, French. **Desc:** Gastroenterology nurses, medical technicians, and sales representatives of medical equipment and pharmaceutical manufacturers. Promotes excellence in the teaching and practice of gastroenterological nursing. Facilitates communication among members; produces patient education materials. Conducts continuing professional education programs; maintains speakers' bureau. **Pub:** *Guiding Light*, 3/year. Newsletter.


★ **15698** ★ **Certification Board Perioperative Nursing (CBPN)**
c/o Shannon Carter
2170 S Parker Rd., Ste. 295
Denver, CO 80231
**Phone:** (303)369-9566          **Free:** 888-257-2667
**Fax:** (303)695-8464
**Email:** webmaster@certboard.org
**Website:** http://www.certboard.org
Shannon S. Carter, Exec. Dir.

**Fnded:** 1979. **Mem:** 30,000. **Desc:** Works to promote surgical services registered nurses. Offers certification programs for nurses practicing in the operating room and assist in surgeries. **Frmly:** (2001) National Certification Board Perioperative Nursing.


★ **15699** ★ **Chi Eta Phi Sorority**
3029 13th St. NW
Washington, DC 20009
**Phone:** (202)232-3858          **Fax:** (202)232-3460
**Email:** chietaphi@erols.com
**Website:** http://www.chietaphi.com
Carolyn Mosley, Pres.

**Fnded:** 1932. **Mem:** 8,000. **Desc:** Professional sorority - registered and student nurses. Objectives are to: encourage continuing education; stimulate friendship among members; develop working relationships with other professional groups for the improvement and delivery of health care services. Sponsors leadership training seminars every two years and holds additional seminars at the local, regional, and national levels. Offers educational programs for entrance into nursing and allied health fields. Maintains health screening and consumer health education programs; volunteers assistance to senior citizens; sponsors recruitment and retention programs for minority students in nursing. Operates speakers' bureau on health education. **Pub:** *Chi Line*, semiannual. Newsletter. Includes membership activities. *Price:* available to members only. • *The Directory*, biennial. Directory. • *Glowing Lamp - Journal of Chi Eta Phi Sorority*, annual. Journal. *Price:* $15. • *History of Chi Eta Phi Sorority, Inc.* • *Mary Eliza Mahoney, America's First Black Professional Nurse.*


★ **15700** ★ **Chinese Nursing Association**
42 Dongsi Xi Da Jie
Beijing 100710, People's Republic of China
**Phone:** 86 10 65265331     **Fax:** 86 10 65123754
**Fnded:** 1909. **Mem:** 240,000. **Lang(s):** English, Japanese. **Desc:** Nurses and nursing attendants in the People's Republic of China. Promotes research and advanced technological developments in the nursing profession; represents members' interests. Conducts educational programs. **Pub:** *Chinese Journal of Nursing*, monthly. Journal.


★ **15701** ★ **Commission on Graduates of Foreign Nursing Schools (CGFNS)**
3600 Market St., Ste. 400
Philadelphia, PA 19104
**Phone:** (215)222-8454          **Fax:** (215)662-0425
**Email:** info@cgfns.org
**Website:** http://www.cgfns.org
Barbara Nichols, RN,MSN, Chief Exec. Officer

**Fnded:** 1977. **Desc:** Established to help ensure safe nursing care for the American public while assisting nurses educated outside the United States in assesing their ability to become licensed, as well as to practice, in the U.S. Offers a certification program with credentials review and exam of nursing knowledge and

English-language proficiency for registered nurses. Provides the CGFNS Credentials Evaluation Service which can evaluate any nurse's academic records in terms of U.S. comparability. Conducts studies and surveys; participates in policy discussions concerning international nursing education, licensure, and practice. **Pub:** *CGFNS Qualifying Exam: Practice English.* Booklet. Includes audiotape. • *Official Study Guide for the CGFNS Qualifying Examination.* Book. Includes study materials and practice exam. • CGFNS Regional Directories of U.S. hospitals, nursing licensure agencies and insurance offices.


★ **15702** ★ **Commonwealth Nurses Federation (CNF)**
c/o International Office
Royal College of Nursing
20 Cavendish Sq.
London W1M 0AB, United Kingdom
**Phone:** 44 20 76473593     **Fax:** 44 20 76473413
**Email:** cnf@rcn.org.uk
**Fnded:** 1973. **Mem:** 54. **Nat'l Groups:** 54. **Reg. Groups:** 6. **Lang(s):** English. **Desc:** Organization of national nurses associations in Commonwealth countries. Strives to further the development of nursing and midwifery for the benefit of the community in Commonwealth nations. Promotes cooperation and coordinated activities among member associations. Liaises with governmental and health agencies to facilitate the delivery of appropriate health services. Disseminates professional information, advice, and assistance. Supports regional and pan-Commonwealth educational nursing projects. **Pub:** *CNF Newsletter*, semiannual. Newsletter. • *Directory of Nursing Associations and Chief Nursing Officers in Countries of the Commonwealth*, periodic. Directory. • *Reports of Workshops*, periodic. Reports.


★ **15703** ★ **Community Health Nurses Association of Canada (CHNAC)**
c/o Donna L. Smith
106 Bellevista Dr.
Dartmouth, NS, Canada B2W 2X7
**Phone:** (902)435-1368
**Fnded:** 1989. **Mem:** 2,500. **Lang(s):** English, French. **Desc:** Community health nurses and provincial organizations. Seeks to advance the practice of community health nursing and enhance members' professional status. Represents members' interests before government agencies and medical associations; provides support, services, and assistance to members. **Pub:** *CHNAC*, quarterly. Newsletter.


**Council on Certification of Nurse Anesthetists (CCNA)**
*See:* Entry 4456


★ **15704** ★ **Dermatology Nurses' Association (DNA)**
E Holly Ave.
PO Box 56
Pitman, NJ 08071
**Phone:** (856)256-2330          **Fax:** (856)589-7463
**Email:** dna@mail.ajj.com
**Website:** http://dna.inurse.com/
Cynthia Nowicki, Exec. Dir.

**Fnded:** 1982. **Mem:** 1,600. **Desc:** Addresses professional issues involving dermatology nurses; develops high standards of dermatologic nursing care; facilitates communication and interdisciplinary cooperation among members. Conducts educational meetings. **Pub:** *DNA Membership Directory*, annual. Directory. • *Product Guide*, annual. • Newsletter, bimonthly.


★ **15705** ★ **Developmental Disabilities Nurses Association**
PMB 1214
1733 H St., Ste. 330
Blaine, WA 98230-5107
**Free:** 800-888-6733
**Email:** ddnahq@aol.com

**Website:** http://www.ddna.org
Randy Bryson, RN, Exec. Dir.
**Fnded:** 1992. **Mem:** 1,100. **Reg. Groups:** 21. **Desc:** Dedicated to serving individuals with developmental disabilities, as well as having a certification program for RN's, and a developing program for LPN/LVN's.


★ **15706** ★ **Emergency Nurses Association (ENA)**
915 Lee St.
Des Plaines, IL 60016
**Phone:** 800-900-9659          **Free:** 800-243-8362
**Fax:** (847)460-4001
**Email:** gvelianoff@ena.org
**Website:** http://www.ena.org
George Velianoff, CEO

**Fnded:** 1970. **Mem:** 23,000. **State Groups:** 50. **Local Groups:** 150. **Desc:** Registered nurses, licensed practical nurses, and licensed vocational nurses; emergency medical technicians or nurses and members of allied health fields engaged or interested in emergency patient care. Objectives are to: promote emergency nursing and to establish standards in the field; to work with other health-related organizations toward the improvement of emergency care; to serve as a resource for emergency nursing education and research. Seeks to identify and address emergency nursing issues. Disseminates educational and research information in the field. Sponsors: Emergency Nursing Core Curriculum; Standards of Emergency Nursing Practice; Emergency Nursing Pediatric Course; Trauma Nursing Core Course; Concepts in Advanced Trauma Nursing Course. **Pub:** *CEN Review Manual.* • *Connection*, 9/year. Newsletter. • *Emergency Nursing Core Curriculum.* • *Emergency Nursing Scope of Practice.* • *International Journal of Trauma Nursing*, quarterly. Journal. • *Journal of Emergency Nursing*, bimonthly. Journal. • *Leadership and Clinical Monograph Series.* • *Standards of Emergency Nursing Practice.* • *Triage: Meeting the Challenge.* **Frmly:** (1974) National Emergency Department Nurses Association; (1984) Emergency Department Nurses Association.


★ **15707** ★ **English National Board for Nursing, Midwifery and Health Visiting**
c/o Victory House
170 Tottenham Court Rd.
London W1P 0HA, United Kingdom
**Phone:** 44 20 73883131     **Fax:** 44 20 73834031
**Email:** link@enb.org.uk
**Website:** http://www.enb.org.uk/
**Fnded:** 1983. **Desc:** The Board consists of 10 members who were appointed by the Secretary of State for Health - 7 non-executive members consisting of a nurse, midwife, and health visitor, and someone currently in education, and 3 executive members. Main purpose is to ensure that the institutions it approves conduct education programmes which equip nurses, midwives and health visitors to meet existing and changing health care needs.


★ **15708** ★ **European Dialysis and Transplant Nurses Association/ European Renal Care Association (EDTNA/ERCA)**
Pilatusstrasse 35
Postfach 3052
CH-6002 Lucerne, Switzerland
**Phone:** 41 4407555          **Fax:** 41 4403962
**Email:** edtna_erca@compuserve.com
**Website:** http://www.edtna-erca.org
**Fnded:** 1972. **Mem:** 5,000. **Nat'l Groups:** 2. **Lang(s):** Dutch, English, French, German, Greek, Italian, Spanish. **Desc:** Nurses working in the field of nephrology, dialysis technicians, paramedical personnel, dietitians, social workers, and companies involved in renal disease research and treatment. Promotes research on renal disease to develop preventive methods and to improve patient care. Organizes educational programs. **Pub:** *Journal of the European Dialysis and Transplant Nurses Association/European Renal Care Association*, quarterly. Journal. Contains selected pre-

sentations made at the annual conference. • *Newsletter*, 4/yr. Newsletter.

#### ★ 15709 ★ European Federation of Nurse Educators

c/o Arne Kolsum
Eggervej 30
DK-2900 Hellerup, Denmark
**Phone:** 45 38 384422 **Fax:** 45 38 384400
**Fnded:** 1992. **Desc:** Promotes the continuing development of excellence of nurse education in Europe. Fosters quality assurance and professionalism in nurse education. Works to influence policy on the national and international levels in the European Union.

#### ★ 15710 ★ European Oncology Nursing Society (EONS)

83 Ave. E Mounier
B-1200 Brussels, Belgium
**Phone:** 32 2 7799923 **Fax:** 32 2 7799937
**Email:** eons@village.uunet.be
**Fnded:** 1987. **Mem:** 175. **Lang(s):** Dutch, English, French. **Desc:** Organizations, institutions, and individuals involved in cancer nursing. Seeks to promote and develop the practice of cancer nursing in Europe. Facilitates exchange of oncology nursing information; participates in European educational and research activities; makes available discounts on professional conference attendance fees to members. **Pub:** *Oncology Nurses Today*, periodic. Newsletter.

#### ★ 15711 ★ Federation for Accessible Nursing Education and Licensure (FANEL)

PO Box 1418
Lewisburg, WV 24901
**Phone:** (304)645-4357 **Fax:** (304)645-4357
**Email:** fedaccnsgedlic@hotmail.com
Twyla Wallace, Pres.
**Fnded:** 1983. **Desc:** Registered nurses, licensed practical nurses, educators, health organizations, schools, and hospital administrators seeking to maintain licensure through current educational programs for RNs and LPNs. **Pub:** Brochures. • Newsletter, biennial.

#### ★ 15712 ★ Federation of Nurses and Health Professionals (FNHP)

555 New Jersey Ave. NW
Washington, DC 20001
**Phone:** (202)879-4491 **Free:** 800-238-1133
**Fax:** (202)879-4597
**Email:** healthcare@aft.org
**Website:** http://www.aft.org/fnhp/index.html
Gary Stevenson, Dir.
**Fnded:** 1978. **Mem:** 54,000. **Nat'l Groups:** 1. **Local Groups:** 95. **Desc:** AFL-CIO. A division of the American Federation of Teachers. Collective bargaining organization of registered nurses, licensed practical nurses, and other professional and technical employees in the health field. Works to improve members' professional standards through promoting continuing education, advancing their economic status, and securing working conditions conducive to optimum performance and the most effective delivery of health care. Seeks to have an impact on legislation affecting national health insurance, cost containment, utilization of manpower resources, consumer health education, health personnel training funds, allocation of health research grants, and other national health issues. Maintains legal defense fund to provide assistance to members whose legal or contractual rights have been violated. **Pub:** *Healthwire*, bimonthly. Newsletter. Includes book reviews. *Price:* Included in membership dues.

#### ★ 15713 ★ Frontier Nursing Service (FNS)

132 FNS Dr.
Wendover, KY 41775
**Phone:** (606)672-2317 **Fax:** (606)672-3022
**Website:** http://www.frontiernursing.org
Deanna Severance, CEO
**Fnded:** 1925. **Mem:** 15. **Desc:** Provides health care to persons in approximately 1000 square miles of eastern Kentucky using a 40-bed hospital, two primary care centers, three rural health clinics, and a home health agency. Operates Frontier School of Midwifery and Family Nursing. Provides social and ancillary services; conducts research on health services; compiles statistics; offers educational programs. Maintains a hall of fame and museum. **Pub:** *Quarterly Bulletin*. Bulletin. *Price:* $5 for individuals; $10 for institutions. • Brochure, annual. For Christmas appeal.

#### ★ 15714 ★ Helene Fuld Health Trust

452 Fifth Ave., 17th Fl.
New York, NY 10018
**Phone:** (212)525-2418 **Fax:** (212)681-1335
**Email:** www.mail@fuldtrust.org
**Website:** http://www.fuldtrust.org
Jina Piak, Grants Mgr.
**Desc:** Strives to support the improvement of the health, welfare, and education of student nurses.

#### ★ 15715 ★ Home Healthcare Nurses Association (HHNA)

228 Seventh St. SE
Washington, DC 20003
**Phone:** (202)546-4754 **Free:** 800-558-4462
**Fax:** (202)547-3540
**Email:** hhna-info@nahc.org
**Website:** http://www.hhna.org
Margaret J. Cushan, Exec. Dir.
**Fnded:** 1999. **Mem:** 800. **Local Groups:** 10. **Desc:** Works to develop and promote the specialty of home healthcare nursing. Provides a forum for members to exchange information; influences public policy affecting the practice; fosters excellence in practice. **Pub:** *Home Healthcare Nurse*, 10/year. Journal. Published by Lippincott.

#### ★ 15716 ★ Hong Kong Society for Nursing Education

PO Box 98898
Tsimshatsui Post Office
Hong Kong, People's Republic of China
**Phone:** 852 28192626 **Fax:** 852 23148550
**Email:** bscheng@hkucc.hku.hk
**Website:** http://www.medicine.org.hk/hksne/home.htm
**Fnded:** 1985. **Mem:** 200. **Lang(s):** Chinese, English. **Desc:** Nurses and nursing educators. Promotes excellence in nursing education; seeks to advance the practice of nursing. Represents the interests of the nursing profession; facilitates communication among nurses and nursing educators; conducts continuing professional development courses; sponsors research; maintains liaison with nursing education organizations worldwide. **Pub:** *Newsletter of the Hong Kong Society for Nursing Education*, monthly. Newsletter.

#### ★ 15717 ★ Hospice and Palliative Nurses Association (HPNA)

Penn Center W One, Ste. 229
Pittsburgh, PA 15276
**Phone:** (412)787-9301 **Fax:** (412)787-9305
**Email:** hpna@hpna.org
**Website:** http://www.hpna.org
Judy Lentz, Exec. Dir.
**Fnded:** 1985. **Mem:** 4,000. **Reg. Groups:** 8. **Desc:** Registered nurses engaged in end of life care in all settings. Promotes excellence in the specialties of hospice and palliative nursing. Conducts education and research programs. Has the only certification boards in hospice and palliative nursing. **Pub:** *Hospice and Palliative Care Clinical Practice Protocol: Dyspnea*. Monographs. • *Hospice and Palliative Care Clinical Practice Protocol: Nausea and Vomiting*. Monograph. • *Hospice and Palliative Care Clinical Practice Protocol: Terminal Restlessness.*. • *Journal of Hospice and Palliative Nursing*, quarterly. Journal. *Price:* $50. • *Study Guide for the Generalist Hospice & Palliative Nurse*. Frmly: (1998) Hospice Nurses Association.

#### ★ 15718 ★ Infection Control Nurses' Association

Freepost
Drumcross Hall
Bathgate EH48 4BR, United Kingdom
**Phone:** 44 1506 811077 **Fax:** 44 1506 811477
**Email:** info@frtwise.co.uk
**Website:** http://www.icna.co.uk
**Fnded:** 1969. **Mem:** 1,079. **Nat'l Groups:** 8. **Reg. Groups:** 11. **Desc:** Infection control nurses and allied professionals. Concerned with the education of public and health care staff in infection. **Pub:** *British Journal of Infection Control*, quarterly. Journal.

#### ★ 15719 ★ Infusion Nurses Society (INS)

220 Norwood Park S
Norwood, MA 02062
**Phone:** (781)440-9408 **Fax:** (781)441-3009
**Email:** chris.hunt@ins1.org
**Website:** http://www.ins1.org
Mary Alexander, CEO
**Fnded:** 1973. **Mem:** 5,300. **Reg. Groups:** 62. **Local Groups:** 62. **Desc:** Registered nurses involved in infusion therapy; licensed practical nurses and pharmacists. Works to promote the education of individuals practicing infusion therapy. Conducts certification program for nurses and advanced studies program in infusion nursing. Maintains speakers' bureau; compiles statistics. **Pub:** *Infusion Nursing Standards of Practice*. • *Infusion Therapy in Clinical Practice*, bimonthly. Newsletter. Includes convention news, legislative network information, chapter agendas, and calendar of events. • *Journal of Infusion Nursing*, bimonthly. Journal. Includes information on meetings, clinical manuscripts, products, and certification and recertification exams. *Price:* Included in membership dues; Year for nonmembers; Year for institutions; Year for students. • *Policies and Procedures for Infusion Nursing*, periodic. • Also publishes news releases and nursing standards. Frmly: (2002) Intravenous Nurses Society.

#### ★ 15720 ★ International Association of Forensic Nurses (IAFN)

PO Box 56, East Holly Ave.
Pitman, NJ 08071-0056
**Phone:** (856)256-2425 **Fax:** (856)589-7463
**Email:** iafn@ajj.com
**Website:** http://www.forensicnurse.org
Kim Marrero, Exec. Sec.
**Fnded:** 1992. **Mem:** 2,050. **State Groups:** 15. **Desc:** The IAFN is a professional association of registered nurses working in the medico-legal arena whose purpose is to develop, promote, and disseminate information about the science of forensic nursing internationally. IAFN works with other nursing organizations to set standards of practice and strives to foster growth and development of forensic nursing as an emerging area of nursing expertise. IAFN also promotes the exchange of ideas and the transmission of developing knowledge among its members and with other interested professionals. **Pub:** *On the Edge*, quarterly. Newsletter. • Membership Directory, annual.

#### ★ 15721 ★ International Committee of Catholic Nurses and Medio-Social Assistants (ICCN) (Comite International Catholique des Infirmieres et Assistantes Medico Sociales — CICIAMS)

43 Sq. Vergote
B-1030 Brussels, Belgium
**Phone:** 32 2 7321050 **Fax:** 32 2 7348460
**Fnded:** 1928. **Mem:** 79. **Reg. Groups:** 5. **Lang(s):** English, French, German. **Desc:** Professional Catholic nursing associations, Catholic nursing and medico-social work schools, and other Catholic groups repre-

senting the nursing profession in 57 countries. Works to encourage the development of members and ensure their technical ability in accordance with Christian moral principles. Promotes development of the nursing profession in general; fosters health and social welfare measures consistent with Christian principles and scientific progress while respecting individual religious convictions. Provides assistance to nursing schools and associations in developing countries; facilitates exchange of statistics between hospital establishments and medico-social organizations. **Pub:** *CICIAMS News*, quarterly. **Frmly:** (1946) International Study Committee of Catholic Nursing Associations.

★ **15722** ★ **International Council of Nurses (ICN)**
**(Conseil International des Infirmieres — CII)**
3, place Jean-Marteau
CH-1201 Geneva, Switzerland
**Phone:** 41 22 9080100          **Fax:** 41 22 9080101
**Email:** icn@icn.ch
**Website:** http://www.icn.ch
**Fnded:** 1899. **Mem:** 124. **Nat'l Groups:** 112. **Lang(s):** English, French, Spanish. **Desc:** Federation of national nurses' associations, representing nurses in more than 120 countries. World's first and widest reaching international organisation for health professionals. Operated by nurses for nurses working to ensure quality nursing care for all, sound health policies globally, the advancement of nursing knowledge, and the presence worldwide of a respected nursing profession and a competent and satisfied nursing workforce. **Pub:** *International Nursing Review*, bimonthly. Journal. Contains information on nursing and health issues. • Brochures, periodic.

**International Nurses Anonymous (INA)**
*See:* Entry 19300

★ **15723** ★ **International Nurses Society on Addictions (NNSA)**
1500 Sunday Dr., No. 102
Raleigh, NC 27607
**Phone:** (919)783-5871          **Fax:** (919)787-4916
**Email:** nnsa@mercury.interpath.com
**Website:** http://www.intnsa.org
**Fnded:** 1975. **Mem:** 800. **Reg. Groups:** 10. **Desc:** Promotes quality nursing care for persons addicted to alcohol and other drugs, and their families. Fosters continuing education and development of skills among nurses involved in the field; works to enhance the professional image of addictions nurses. Participates in public policy and social issues related to alcohol or chemical abuse. Serves as liaison between members and professional groups with common goals. Represents members' interests before national organizations. Regional groups sponsor workshops. Provides certification program. **Pub:** *The Care of Clients with Addictions: Dimensions of Nursing Practice and Standards of Addictions*. Book. • *The Core Curriculum of Addictions Nursing*. Book. • *NNSA Today*, quarterly. Newsletter. Includes articles on clinical and research areas of addictions field. *Price:* Available to members only. • *Nursing Care Planning with the Addicted Client*. Book. • *Nursing Practice with Selected Diagnoses and Criteria*. Book. • Booklets. • Monographs. • Papers. **Frmly:** (1983) National Nurses Society on Alcoholism; (2001) National Nurses Society on Addictions.

★ **15724** ★ **International Society of Nurses in Genetics (ISONG)**
c/o Eileen Rawnsley, RN BSN CGC
7 Haskins Rd.
Hanover, NH 03755
**Phone:** (603)643-5706
**Email:** erawn@valley.net
**Website:** http://nursing.creighton.edu/isong
Eileen Rawnsley, RN BSN, Exec. Dir.
**Mem:** US. **Desc:** Case managers, administrators, coordinators of public and private programs, educators in the field of nursing and/or genetics, genetic counsel-

ors, researchers. Committed to incorporating the knowledge of human genetics into nursing practice, education and research activities. **Pub:** Newsletter. • Membership Directory.

**International Society of Psychiatric Mental Health Nurses (ISPN)**
*See:* Entry 5704

★ **15725** ★ **International Transplant Nurses Society (ITNS)**
1739 E Carson St., No. 351
Pittsburgh, PA 15203-1700
**Phone:** (412)488-0240          **Fax:** (412)431-5911
**Email:** itns@msn.com
**Website:** http://www.itns.org
Beth A. Kassalen, MBA, Exec. Dir.
**Fnded:** 1992. **Mem:** 850. **Reg. Groups:** 16. **Local Groups:** 17. **Desc:** Nurses, LVNs, LPNs, and others involved in patient care for organ transplantation. Works to encourage cooperation among all medical disciplines involved in transplantation, disseminate information, and establish certification for this nursing specialty. **Pub:** *ITNS Newsletter*, quarterly. Newsletter. Contains clinical transplant articles, society updates. *Price:* Included in membership dues. • *Progress in Transplantation*, quarterly. Journal. *Price:* $55 annually.

★ **15726** ★ **Japanese Nursing Association**
5-8-2 Jingu-mae
Shibuya-ku
Tokyo 150-0001, Japan
**Phone:** 81 3 34008331          **Fax:** 81 3 34008767
**Email:** webmaster@nurse.or.jp
**Website:** http://www.nurse.or.jp
**Fnded:** 1946. **Desc:** Promotes the status of nurses in Japan. **Pub:** *Kyokai (Association) News*, monthly. Newsletter.

★ **15727** ★ **NANDA International**
1211 Locust St.
Philadelphia, PA 19107
**Phone:** (215)545-8105          **Free:** 800-647-9002
**Fax:** (215)545-8107
**Email:** nanda@rmpinc.com
**Website:** http://www.nanda.org
Mary Ann Lavin, Pres.
**Fnded:** 1972. **Mem:** 400. **Desc:** Registered nurses; individuals interested in nursing language and informatics. Purpose is to develop, refine, and promote a taxonomy of nursing terminology for use by professional nurses. **Pub:** *NANDA Nursing Diagnoses: Definitions and Classification 2001-2002*, biennial. Book. *Price:* $18.95. • *Nursing Diagnoses and Critical Thinking*. Book. *Price:* $24.95. • *Nursing Diagnosis Journal*, quarterly. Journal. *Price:* $42/year; $54/year for members outside the U.S.; Included in membership. **AKA:** North American Nursing Diagnosis Association.

★ **15728** ★ **National Alliance of Nurse Practitioners (NANP)**
325 Pennsylvania Ave. SE
Washington, DC 20003-1100
**Phone:** (202)675-6350
Mane Eileen O'Neal, Chairperson
**Fnded:** 1985. **Mem:** 25,000. **Nat'l Groups:** 6. **Desc:** Nurse practitioners. Seeks to emphasize the role of Nurse Practitioners in efficient and cost-effective health care services. Promotes continuing education for all health care professionals. Promotes and supports legislation & health policy for NPs.

★ **15729** ★ **National Association of Clinical Nurse Specialists**
3969 Green St.
Harrisburg, PA 17110
**Phone:** (717)234-6799          **Fax:** (717)375-4777
**Email:** info@nacns.org

**Website:** http://www.nacns.org
Christine Carson Filipovich, Exec. Dir.
**Fnded:** 1995. **Mem:** 1,150. **Reg. Groups:** 8. **Desc:** Clinical Nurse Specialists. **Pub:** *Statement on Clinical Nurse Specialist Practice and Education*. Handbook. *Price:* $15/copy for members; $25/copy for nonmembers.

**National Association of Directors of Nursing Administration in Long Term Care (NADONA/LTC)**
*See:* Entry 9749

★ **15730** ★ **National Association of Hispanic Nurses (NAHN)**
1501 Sixteenth St. NW
Washington, DC 20036
**Phone:** (202)387-2477          **Fax:** (202)483-7183
**Email:** info@nahnhq.org
**Website:** http://www.thehispanicnurses.org/
Dr. Carmen J. Portillo, Pres.
**Fnded:** 1976. **Mem:** 1,000. **Nat'l Groups:** 1. **State Groups:** 10. **Local Groups:** 24. **Desc:** Nurses on all educational levels, from all Hispanic subgroups; non-Hispanic nurses concerned about the health delivery needs of the Hispanic community; nursing students. Serves the nursing and health care delivery needs of the Hispanic community and the professional needs of Hispanic nurses. Provides a forum in which Hispanic nurses can analyze, research, and evaluate the health care needs of the Hispanic community. Disseminates findings of that research to local, state, and federal agencies so as to affect policy-making and resource allocation. Aims to ensure that Hispanic nurses have equal access to educational, professional, and economic opportunities. Identifies Hispanic nurses throughout the nation to determine the size of the work force available to provide culturally sensitive nursing care to Hispanics. **Pub:** *First National Hispanic Nurse Symposium Proceedings: Recruitment, Retention, Career Mobility - Strategy for Change*. Proceedings. • *Hispanic Nurse*, quarterly. *Price:* $15. **Frmly:** (1979) National Association of Spanish Speaking-Spanish Surnamed Nurses.

★ **15731** ★ **National Association of Neonatal Nurses (NANN)**
4700 W Lake Ave.
Glenview, IL 60025-1485
**Phone:** (847)375-3660          **Free:** 800-451-3795
**Fax:** 888-477-6266
**Email:** info@nann.org
**Website:** http://www.nann.org
Linda S. Chreno, CAE, Exec. Dir.
**Fnded:** 1984. **Mem:** 11,500. **Reg. Groups:** 60. **Desc:** Nurses currently working in neonatal intensive care units. Promotes professional development of members. Provides educational and networking opportunities. Disseminates legislative information. **Pub:** *Central Lines*, quarterly. Newsletter. • *Position Statements*. • *Practice Guidelines*. • *Technical Bulletins*.

★ **15732** ★ **National Association of Nurse Massage Therapists (NANMT)**
2203 Woodridge Ct.
Grand Island, NE 68801
**Free:** 800-262-4017
**Email:** simpson@nebi.com
**Website:** http://members.aol.com/nanmt1/about.html
Cam Spencer, Pres.
**Fnded:** 1987. **Mem:** 650. **Desc:** Nurses and other healthcare professionals who practice massage therapy. Promotes the integration of massage and other therapeutic forms of bodywork into existing healthcare practice. Promotes Nurse Massage Therapists as specialists within the nursing profession. Establishes standards of professional practice and criteria for national certification of Nurse Massage Therapists. Educates the medical community and the general public about bodywork therapies. Monitors legislation. **Pub:** *NANMT Membership Directory*, annual. Membership Directory. *Price:* Included in membership

dues. • *Nurse's Touch*, quarterly. Magazine. *Price:* Included in membership dues; $20/year for institutions.

**★ 15733 ★ National Association of Nurse Practitioners in Women's Health (NPWH)**
503 Captiol Ct. NE, Ste. 300
Washington, DC 20002
**Phone:** (202)543-9693      **Fax:** (202)543-9858
**Email:** info@npwh.org
**Website:** http://www.npwh.org
Susan Wysocki, Pres.
**Fnded:** 1980. **Mem:** 2,000. **Desc:** Nurse practitioners involved in women's healthcare. Advocates quality healthcare to be inclusive of an individual's physical, emotional, and spiritual needs. Promotes women as decision-makers for their own healthcare. Encourages nurses to participate in continuing education programs. Disseminates information. **Pub:** *The Monthly Cycle*, monthly. Newsletter. *Price:* Available to members only. **Frmly:** (2001) National Association of Nurse Practitioners in Reproductive Health.

**★ 15734 ★ National Association of Orthopaedic Nurses (NAON)**
E Holly Ave.
Box 56
Pitman, NJ 08071-0056
**Phone:** (856)256-2310      **Free:** 800-289-6266
**Fax:** (856)589-7643
**Email:** naon@mail.ajj.com
**Website:** http://naon.inurse.com
Carol L. Baird, Chair
**Fnded:** 1980. **Mem:** 8,300. **Local Groups:** 154. **Desc:** Registered, licensed practical, or licensed vocational nurses involved or knowledgeable in orthopedic nursing. Enhances the personal and professional growth of orthopedic nurses through continuing education programs. Promotes research development and advances in orthopedic nursing; promotes an awareness of patients' rights. Stresses the concept of man's physical, psychological, social, emotional, and spiritual needs in the development of patient care plans. Maintains liaison with and serves as resource to hospitals, universities, industries, and government agencies. Operates special interest groups. Sponsors workshops; maintains speakers' bureau; offers research grants. Makes available audiovisual presentation. **Pub:** *News*, bimonthly. • *Orthopaedic Nursing*, bimonthly. Journal. • Bibliographies. • Monographs. • Proceedings.

**★ 15735 ★ National Association of Pediatric Nurse Practitioners (NAPNAP)**
20 Brace Rd., Ste. 200
Cherry Hill, NJ 08034
**Phone:** (856)857-9700      **Fax:** (856)857-1600
**Email:** info@napnap.org
**Website:** http://www.napnap.org
Robert A. Hall, MED, Exec. Dir.
**Fnded:** 1973. **Mem:** 6,372. **State Groups:** 47. **Desc:** Pediatric, school, and family nurse practitioners and interested persons. Seeks to improve the quality of infant, child, and adolescent health care by making health care services accessible and providing a forum for continuing education of members. Facilitates and supports legislation designed to promote the role of pediatric nurse practitioners and associates; promotes salary ranges commensurate with practitioners' and associates' responsibilities; facilitates exchange of information between prospective employers and job seekers in the field. Participates in the implementation of certification and certification maintenance of practitioners and associates, in cooperation with the National Certification Board of Pediatric Nurse Practitioners and Nurses. Supports research programs; compiles statistics. **Pub:** *Journal of Pediatric Health Care*, bimonthly. Journal. Includes annual index, book reviews, legislative news, literature abstracts, multi-media reviews, and product news. *Price:* $55/year for individuals; $104/year for institutions; $28/year for students. • *Pediatric Nurse Practitioner*, bimonthly.

Newsletter. Contains calendar of events and legislative news. *Price:* Free to members. • Brochures. **Frmly:** (2002) National Association of Pediatric Nurse Associates and Practitioners.

**★ 15736 ★ National Association of Physician Nurses (NAPN)**
900 S Washington St., No. G-13
Falls Church, VA 22046
**Phone:** (703)237-8616      **Fax:** (703)533-1153
Susan Young, Dir.
**Fnded:** 1973. **Mem:** 4,000. **Desc:** Physicians' nurses united to bring added stature and purpose to their profession and to create for themselves the benefits normally limited to members of specialized professional and fraternal groups. **Pub:** *The Nightingale*, monthly. Newsletter. *Price:* $30/year included in membership dues; $15/year for nonmembers. • *Salary Survey Report*, biennial. Report. • Also publishes special reports.

**★ 15737 ★ National Association for Practical Nurse Education and Service (NAPNES)**
8607 Second Ave., Ste. 404-A
Silver Spring, MD 20910-2745
**Phone:** (301)588-2491      **Fax:** (301)588-2839
**Email:** napnes@bellatlantic.net
Helen M. Larsen, Exec. Dir.
**Fnded:** 1941. **Mem:** 30,000. **State Groups:** 20. **Desc:** Licensed practical/vocational nurses, registered nurses, physicians, hospital and nursing home administrators, and interested others. Provides consultation service to advise schools wishing to develop a practical/vocational nursing program on facilities, equipment, policies, curriculum, and staffing. Promotes recruitment of students through preparation and distribution of recruitment materials. Sponsors seminars for directors and instructors in schools of practical/vocational nursing and continuing education programs for LPNs/LVNs; approves continuing education programs and awards contact hours; holds national certification courses in post licensure specialities such as pharmacology, long term care and gerontics. **Pub:** *Journal of Practical Nursing*, quarterly. Journal. Contains news of association activities, nursing law, and pending legislation affecting the nursing profession. *Price:* Included in membership dues; $15/year for nonmembers; $30/year for nonmembers outside the U.S. • *NAPNES Forum*, 8/year. Journal. Supplement to the *Journal of Practical Nusing*. • Also publishes brochures, pamphlets, and reprints.

**★ 15738 ★ National Association of Registered Nurses (NARN)**
11512 Allecingie Pky., Ste. D
Richmond, VA 23235
**Phone:** (804)794-6513      **Free:** 800-383-9826
**Fax:** (804)379-7698
**Email:** fdebondt@aol.com
**Website:** http://www.associationsusa.org
Francis R. deBondt, PhD, Admin.
**Fnded:** 1979. **Mem:** 250. **Desc:** Nurses' associations. Seeks to offer nurses the opportunity to plan and create a financially sound future through financial management programs. Provides financial products, consultation, and services including Individual Retirement Accounts, full investment services, and group life insurance. Conducts educational programs. **Pub:** Brochures, periodic. • Newsletter, periodic.

**★ 15739 ★ National Association of School Nurses (NASN)**
1416 Park St., Ste. A
Castle Rock, CO 80104
**Phone:** (303)663-2329      **Free:** (866)627-6767
**Fax:** (303)663-0403
**Email:** nasn@nasn.org
**Website:** http://www.nasn.org
Judith Robinson, Exec. Dir.
**Fnded:** 1969. **Mem:** 11,000. **State Groups:** 47. **Desc:** Improves health and educational success of children

and youth by developing and providing leadership to advance school nursing practice. **Pub:** *Journal of School Nursing*, bimonthly. Magazine. Includes book reviews, resources, education topics and legislative updates. *Price:* $70/year. • *NASNewsletter*, bimonthly. Newsletter. *Price:* Included in membership dues. • *Postural Screening*. *Price:* $7 members; $11 nonmembers. • *Scope and Standards of Professional School Nursing Practice*. *Price:* $10 members; $15 nonmembers. • *Vision Screening Guidelines for School Nurses*. *Price:* $7 members; $11 nonmembers. • Offers various guides, brochures, manuals, and other publications. **Frmly:** (1977) Department of School Nurses/NEA.

**★ 15740 ★ National Association of State School Nurse Consultants (NASSNC)**
PO Box 708
Kent, OH 44240-0708
**Desc:** Registered nurses employed by state departments of education or health. Promotes development of standards of practice among school nurse consultants; facilitates continuing professional advancement of members. Serves as a forum for the exchange of information among members and between members and related professionals; promotes and supports research activities; formulates nursing standards; sponsors educational programs.

**★ 15741 ★ National Association of Theatre Nurses**
Daisy Ayris House
6 Grove Park Ct.
Harrogate HG1 4DP, United Kingdom
**Phone:** 44 1423 508079      **Fax:** 44 1423 531613
**Email:** hq@natn.org.uk
**Website:** http://www.natn.org.uk
**Fnded:** 1964. **Mem:** 8,000. **Reg. Groups:** 47. **Desc:** Operating theatre nurses. Workshops and study days are organized locally and nationally throughout the year. **Pub:** *British Journal of Perioperitive Nurses*, monthly. Journal.

**★ 15742 ★ National Association of Traveling Nurses (NATN)**
PO Box 35189
Chicago, IL 60707-0189
**Phone:** (708)453-0080      **Fax:** (708)453-0083
**Email:** natn@rentamark.com
**Website:** http://www.travelingnurse.org
L. David Stoller, Chm.
**Fnded:** 1990. **Mem:** 78,,951. **Nat'l Groups:** 1. **Desc:** Members of the medical profession. Provides travel information. Provides information to nurses, health care professionals on traveling assignments and job placement opportunities. Offers substantial discounts for members at major hotels, resorts, and car rental agencies. Provides members with complete list of approved travel industry suppliers, including travel agents, vendors, airlines, cruise ship companies, and hotels. **Pub:** *Journal of Traveling Nurses*, quarterly. Journal. Online journal. *Price:* for members. • *National Online*. Newsletter. National invites authors to submit articles in "WORD" format via email for publication in the national online journal.

**★ 15743 ★ National Black Nurses Association (NBNA)**
8630 Fenton St., Ste. 330
Silver Spring, MD 20910
**Phone:** (301)589-3200      **Fax:** (301)589-3223
**Email:** nbna@erols.com
**Website:** http://www.nbna.org/
Millicent Gorham, Exec. Dir.
**Fnded:** 1971. **Mem:** 5,000. **Nat'l Groups:** 78. **Desc:** Registered nurses, licensed practical nurses, licensed vocational nurses, and student nurses. Functions as a professional support group and as an advocacy group for the black community and their health care. Recruits and assists blacks interested in pursuing nursing as a career. Presents scholarships to student nurses, including the Dr. Lauranne Sams Scholarship. Compiles

statistics; maintains biographical archives. **Pub:** *Journal of Black Nurses Association*, semiannual. Journal. *Price:* Included in membership dues. • *National Black Nurses Association–Book of Reports*, annual. *Price:* available to members only. • *National Black Nurses Association–Proceedings*, periodic. • *NBNA Newsletter*, quarterly. Newsletter. Includes calendar of events, research updates, scholarships, grants, and fellowships. *Price:* Included in membership dues. • Annual Report.

★ **15744** ★ **National Board for Nursing, Midwifery and Health Visiting for Northern Ireland**
Centre House
79 Chichester St.
Belfast BT1 4JE, United Kingdom
**Phone:** 44 28 9023 8152   **Fax:** 44 28 9033 3298
**Email:** enquiries@nbni.n-i.nhs.uk
**Website:** http://www.n-i.nhs.uk/NBNI
**Fnded:** 1979. **Mem:** 9. **Lang(s):** English. **Desc:** Non-executive members appointed by the Head of Department of Health and Social Services for Northern Ireland, executive members ie the Chief Executive, and Director of Finance & Administration of the National Board. The majority of members are registered nurses, midwives or health visitors. To approve institutions in relation to provision of training courses for nurses, midwives and health visitors which meet Central Council standards; to collaborate with Council in the promotion of improved training methods; and such other functions as the Head of the Department of Health may by order prescribe. **Pub:** Annual Report, annual. • Papers.

★ **15745** ★ **National Certification Board of Pediatric Nurse Practitioners and Nurses (NCBPNP/N)**
800 S Frederick Ave., Ste. 104
Gaithersburg, MD 20877-4151
**Phone:** (301)330-2921        **Free:** 888-641-2767
**Fax:** (301)330-1504
**Email:** info@pnpcert.org
**Website:** http://www.pnpcert.org
Janet S. Wyatt, Ph.D., CPNP, Exec. Dir.
**Fnded:** 1976. **Desc:** Participants include physician and nurse representatives from the American Academy of Pediatrics, National Association of Pediatric Nurse Associates and Practitioners, the Association of Faculties of Pediatric Nurse Associate/Practitioner Programs, a consumer representative and certified CPNP and CPN members at large. Seeks to ensure quality child health care. Administers certification, recertification, and self-assessment programs for general and advanced practice pediatric nursing. **Frmly:** (1989) National Board of Pediatric Nurse Practitioners and Associates.

★ **15746** ★ **National Certification Corp. for the Obstetric, Gynecologic and Neonatal Nursing Specialties (NCC)**
645 N Michigan Ave., Ste. 900
Chicago, IL 60611
**Phone:** (312)951-0207
**Website:** http://www.nccnet.org
Betty Burns, CAE, Exec. Dir.
**Fnded:** 1975. **Mem:** 55,000. **Desc:** Promotes quality nursing care by encouraging nurses to demonstrate special knowledge by participating in a voluntary national certification program for obstetric/gynecologic nurse practitioners, inpatient obstetric nurses, neonatal intensive care nurses, neonatal nurse practitioners, low-risk neonatal nurses, electronic fetal monitoring, breastfeeding, menopause, and maternal newborn nurses. **Pub:** *NCC News*, periodic. Newsletter. • *Self Assessment Program*. Brochure. **Frmly:** (1991) NAACOG Certification Corporation.

★ **15747** ★ **National Consortium of Chemical Dependency Nurses (NCCDN)**
PMB 1211
1733 H St., Ste. 330
Blaine, WA 98230
**Phone:** (360)332-9105        **Free:** 800-87-NCCDN
**Fax:** (360)332-2280
Randy Bryson, Exec. Dir.
**Fnded:** 1987. **Mem:** 1,000. **Reg. Groups:** 12. **Desc:** Professional nurses specializing in chemical dependency treatment. Goals are: to increase the effectiveness of nursing services for chemical dependency; to establish a professional standard in chemical dependency nursing through a system of competency-based testing and programs of professional development and certification. Aims to increase public awareness of the need for chemical dependency treatment and nurses specializing in this field. Encourages the growth of knowledge, skills, and competency in chemical dependency nursing. Offers certification exam for nurses with 4000 hours experience in the previous 5 years and 30 hours of chemical dependency coursework; conducts educational programs. Maintains speakers' bureau. **Pub:** *CD Nurse Briefing*, quarterly. Newsletter. Covers issues of interest of NCCDN membership. *Price:* available to members only. • Pamphlets.

★ **15748** ★ **National Council of Maori Nurses (Te Kaunihera O Nga Neehi Maori O Aotearoa)**
40 Second Ave.
Kingsland
Auckland, New Zealand
**Phone:** 64 9 8462253        **Fax:** 64 9 8462258
**Email:** national.council@extra.co.nz
**Website:** http://www.healthsite.co.nz/hauora_maori/ncmn/index.html
**Local Groups:** 6. **Lang(s):** English. **Desc:** Nurses of Maori descent. Promotes continuing professional development and advancement of members; works to ensure accessibility of health care to Maori people; conducts educational and training programs.

★ **15749** ★ **National Council of State Boards of Nursing (NCSBN)**
676 N St. Clair St., Ste. 550
Chicago, IL 60611
**Phone:** (312)787-6555        **Fax:** (312)787-6898
**Email:** info@ncsbn.org
**Website:** http://www.ncsbn.org
**Fnded:** 1978. **Mem:** 61. **Desc:** State boards of nursing. Assists member boards in administering the National Council Licensure Examinations for Registered Nurses and Practical Nurses and works to insure relevancy of the exams to current nursing practice. Aids boards in the collection and analysis of information pertaining to the licensure and discipline of nurses. Provides consultative services, conducts research, develops model nursing legislation and administrative regulations, and sponsors educational programs. **Pub:** *Council Connector*, monthly. Newsletter. Newsletter for member boards. • *NCLEX Exam Test Plans*, annual. Booklets. Educational booklets. • Also publishes research results and monographs.

★ **15750** ★ **National Federation of Licensed Practical Nurses (NFLPN)**
893 US Highway 70 W, Ste. 202
Garner, NC 27529
**Phone:** (919)779-0046        **Free:** 800-948-2511
**Fax:** (919)779-5642
**Email:** cbarbour@mgmt4u.com
**Website:** http://www.nflpn.org
Charlene Barbour, Exec. Dir.
**Fnded:** 1949. **Mem:** 5,000. **State Groups:** 22. **Desc:** Federation of state associations of licensed practical and vocational nurses. Aims to: preserve and foster the ideal of comprehensive nursing care for the ill and aged; improve standards of practice; secure recognition and effective utilization of LPNs; further continued improvement in the education of LPNs. Acts as clearinghouse for information on practical nursing and cooperates with other groups concerned with better patient care. Maintains loan program. **Pub:** *Licensed Practical Nurse*, quarterly. Journal. Includes state and legislative news and list of new members. *Price:* Included in membership dues. • *LPN*, quarterly. Magazine.

★ **15751** ★ **National Federation for Specialty Nursing Organizations (NFSNO)**
E Holly Ave., Box 56
Pitman, NJ 08071
**Phone:** (856)256-2333        **Fax:** (856)589-7463
**Email:** nfsno@ajj.com
**Website:** http://www.inurse.com/nfsno/about/
Sheila Haas, Pres.
**Fnded:** 1972. **Mem:** 36. **Desc:** Nursing specialty organizations representing approximately 400,000 individuals. Provides a forum for the discussion of issues of mutual concern to members; attempts to gain more input in the establishment of nursing standards. Sponsors Nurse in Washington Internship. **Pub:** *NFSNO Focus on the Federation*, quarterly. Newsletter. **Frmly:** (1981) Federation of Specialty Nursing Organizations and the American Nurses Association.

★ **15752** ★ **National Gerontological Nursing Association**
7794 Grow Dr.
Pensacola, FL 32514
**Phone:** (850)473-1174        **Free:** 800-723-0560
**Fax:** (850)484-8762
**Email:** ngna@puetzamc.com
**Website:** http://www.ngna.org
Belinda E. Puetz, RN,PHD, Contact
**Fnded:** 1984. **Mem:** 1,489. **Local Groups:** 13. **Desc:** Gerontological nurses. Seeks to effectively improve the care and well-being of older adults. Provides a forum in which gerontological nursing issues are identified and explored. Develops and supports educational programs for nurses, health providers, and the general public. Disseminates information. **Pub:** *Geriatric Nursing*, bimonthly. Journal. • *SIGN*, bimonthly. Newsletter.

★ **15753** ★ **National League for Nursing (NLN)**
61 Broadway 33rd Fl.
New York, NY 10006-2701
**Phone:** (212)363-5555        **Free:** 800-669-1656
**Fax:** (212)812-0393
**Email:** rcorcor@nln.org
**Website:** http://www.nln.org
Ruth Corcoran, EdD RN, CEO
**Fnded:** 1893. **Mem:** 7,500. **State Groups:** 45. **Desc:** Champions the pursuit of quality nursing education. A professional association of nursing faculty, education agencies, healthcare agencies, allied/public agencies, and public members whose mission is to advance quality nursing education that prepares the nursing workforce to meet the needs of diverse populations in an ever-changing health care environment. Serves as the primary source of information about every type of nursing education, from the LVN and LPN to the EDD and PHD. There are 38 affiliated constituent leagues that provide a local forum for members. The National League for Nursing Accrediting Commission is an independent corporate affiliate of the NLN, responsible for providing accreditation services to all levels of nursing education. NLN's bimonthly update is available free of charge on the website and by email. **Pub:** *Nursing Data Review*, annual. • *Nursing Education Perspectives*, bimonthly. Journal. Contains news, legislative updates, education, service analyses, and editorials. • *State Approved Schools of Nursing - LPN*, annual. • *State Approved Schools of Nursing - RN*, annual. • Books.Covers health policy, administration, management, and education. • Manuals. • Reports. • Videos.Covers nursing theory, curriculum, home care, and recruitment.

**★ 15754 ★ National Nurses Association of Kenya (NNAK)**
PO Box 49422
Nairobi, Kenya
**Phone:** 254 2 229083 **Fax:** 254 2 335438
**Fnded:** 1958. **Local Groups:** 19. **Lang(s):** English.
**Desc:** Nurses in Kenya. Promotes primary health care; facilitates exchange and cooperation between members; upholds ethics of the profession and encourages high standards. Represents members' interests before the government; provides help for members in times of difficulty; offers scholarships and operates trust fund. Operates foster child program. Works in conjunction with the National Council of Women in Kenya. Conducts workshops and seminars. **Pub:** *Kenya Nurses Newsletter*, quarterly. Newsletter. • *Kenya Nursing Journal*, semiannual. Journal.

**★ 15755 ★ National Nursing Staff Development Organization**
7794 Grow Dr.
Pensacola, FL 32514
**Phone:** (850)474-0995 **Free:** 800-489-1995
**Fax:** (850)484-8762
**Email:** nnsdo@puetzamc.com
**Website:** http://www.nnsdo.org
Belinda E. Puetz, Ph.d.,, Contact
**Fnded:** 1989. **Mem:** 2,232. **Local Groups:** 39. **Desc:** Advances the specialty practice of staff development for the enhancement of quality healthcare outcomes. Staff development, as a specialty of nursing practice, is defined by standards, based on research critical to quality patient and organizational outcomes. Provides a forum for networking among staff development educators. **Pub:** *Journal for Nurses in Staff Development*, periodic. Journal. • *Trendlines*, bimonthly. Newsletter.

**★ 15756 ★ National Organization for Associate Degree Nursing (N-OADN)**
11250 Roger Bacon Dr., Ste. 8
Reston, VA 20190-5202
**Phone:** (703)437-4377 **Fax:** (703)435-4390
**Email:** noadn@aol.com
**Website:** http://www.noadn.org
Maureen Thompson, Exec. Dir.
**Fnded:** 1986. **Mem:** 750. **State Groups:** 10. **Desc:** Individuals interested in retaining current competency level examinations and endorsement of RN licensure from state to state for associate degree nursing graduates. Represents and advances the status of associate degree nursing education and practice. Provides networking among members to facilitate the exchange of legislative information and support. Offers clearinghouse for interpretation of legal issues and liability insurance. **Pub:** *NOADN Newsletter*, quarterly. • Newsletter, quarterly. Includes national and state association news, activities, and information. • Also issues position papers. **Frmly:** (1986) National Organization for Advancement of Associate Degree Nursing.

**★ 15757 ★ National Organization of Nurse Practitioners Faculties**
1522 K St., NW, Ste. 702
Washington, DC 20005
**Phone:** (202)289-8044 **Fax:** (202)289-8046
**Email:** nonpf@nonpf.org
**Website:** http://www.nonpf.org
Lucy Marion, PhD RN, Pres.
**Fnded:** 1981. **Mem:** 1,000. **Desc:** Works to promote public health by developing and implementing nurse practitioner education. Disseminates research related to nurse practitioner education; provides a forum for the exchange of information; works to influence policy affecting nurse practitioners; and develops national guidelins and criteria for nurse practitioner educational programs. **Pub:** *National Directory of NP Programs*, biennial. Directory. • *NONPF Quarterly Newsletter*, quarterly. Newsletter. • Brochure. **Frmly:** (1998) National Organization of Nursing Pratitioners.

**★ 15758 ★ National Student Nurses' Association (NSNA)**
45 Main St., Ste. 606
Brooklyn, NY 11201
**Phone:** (718)210-0705 **Fax:** (718)210-0710
**Email:** nsna@nsna.org
**Website:** http://www.nsna.org
Diane J. Mancino, Ed.D., RN CAE, Exec. Dir.
**Fnded:** 1952. **Mem:** 26,000. **State Groups:** 48. **Local Groups:** 500. **Desc:** Students enrolled in state-approved schools for the preparation of registered nurses. Seeks to aid in the development of the individual nursing student and to urge students of nursing, as future health professionals, to be aware of and to contribute to improving the health care of all people. Encourages programs and activities in state groups concerning nursing, health, and the community. Provides assistance for state board review, as well as materials for preparation for state RN licensing examination. Cooperates with nursing organizations in recruitment of nurses and in professional, community, and civic programs. Sponsors Foundation of the National Student Nurses' Association in memory of Frances Tompkins to award scholarships to student nurses. **Pub:** *Convention News*. • *Dean's Notes*, 5/year. • *Imprint*, 5/year. Magazine. • *NSNA News*, 2/year. • Manuals.

**★ 15759 ★ New Zealand Nurses Organization (NZNO)**
PO Box 2128
Wellington, New Zealand
**Phone:** 64 4 3850847 **Fax:** 64 4 3829993
**Email:** nurses@nzno.org.nz
**Website:** http://www.nzno.org.nz
**Fnded:** 1909. **Mem:** 26,500. **Reg. Groups:** 11. **Desc:** Nurses, nurses' aids and medical radiation technologist. Represents and promotes nurses' interests and concerns on health issues through participation in health and social policy development. Conducts research on health issues. Offers health education programs. **Pub:** *New Zealand Nursing Journal*, 11/year. Journal.

**★ 15760 ★ Nurse Healers Professional Associates International (NH-PAI)**
3760 Highland Dr., No. 429
Salt Lake City, UT 84106
**Phone:** (801)273-3399 **Fax:** (801)693-3537
**Email:** nh-pai@therapeutice-touch.org
**Website:** http://www.therapeutic-touch.org
Rebecca M. Good, MA, RN, LPC, Coor.
**Fnded:** 1977. **Mem:** 700. **Desc:** Official organization for Therapeutic Touch (TT). Healthcare professionals and lay persons united to promote a holistic approach to healing and health maintenance and nontraditional healing methods. Disseminates information on therapeutic touch. Maintains speakers' bureau; conducts research and educational programs for Therapeutic Touch. Sets standards and scope of practice for TT and recognition program for Qualified Therapeutic Touch teachers and practitioners. **Pub:** *Cooperative Connection*, quarterly. Newsletter. Cooperative connection newsletter of the Nurse Healers Professonal Associate International, Inc (NH-PAI). *Price:* $20/year in U.S.; $28/year outside U.S. **Frmly:** (2002) Nurse Healers Professional Associates.

**★ 15761 ★ Nurses Educational Funds (NEF)**
555 W 57th St., 13th Fl., Ste. 1327
New York, NY 10019
**Phone:** (212)399-1428 **Fax:** (212)581-2368
**Email:** bbnef@aol.com
Barbara Butler, Exec. Dir.
**Fnded:** 1954. **Mem:** 30. **Desc:** Seeks to establish, maintain, and administer funds to provide financial assistance to registered nurses studying for advanced degrees; masters/doctoral level only formulate policies for the administration of such funds; collect and manage all funds contributed to it. Masters study must be full-time only GRE/or MAT scores are required. **Pub:** *Nurses Educational Funds Annual Report*, annual. Annual Report. Includes NEF activity highlights and financial summary for the fiscal year. *Price:* Available to members and donors only. **Frmly:** (1954) Isabel Hampton Robb Memorial Fund.

**★ 15762 ★ Nurses' House**
2113 Western Ave., Ste. 2
Guilderland, NY 12084-9559
**Phone:** (518)456-7858 **Fax:** (518)452-3760
**Email:** mail@nurseshouse.org
**Website:** http://www.nurseshouse.org
Cathryne A. Welch, Exec. Dir.
**Fnded:** 1925. **Mem:** 1,100. **Reg. Groups:** 6. **Desc:** Registered nurses and interested individuals united to assist registered nurses in financial and other crises. Provides short-term financial aid for shelter, food, and utilities until nurses obtain entitlements or jobs. Offers counseling and referrals. Encourages homebound or retired nurses through a volunteer corps. **Pub:** *Appeal*, annual. Newsletter. • *The Dolphin*, semiannual. Newsletter. • Also publishes promotional flyer.

**★ 15763 ★ Nurses Organization of Veterans Affairs (NOVA)**
1726 M St. NW, Ste. 1101
Washington, DC 20036
**Phone:** (202)296-0888 **Fax:** (202)833-1577
**Email:** nova@vanurse.org
**Website:** http://www.vanurse.org
Deborah Beck, Exec. Dir.
**Fnded:** 1980. **Mem:** 2,782. **Reg. Groups:** 99. **Desc:** Voluntary, nonprofit professional society of Department of Veterans Affairs registered nurses. Objective is to provide VA nurses with the opportunity to preserve and improve quality care and professionalism through legislative influence. Conducts competitions, seminars, and educational programs. **Pub:** *News From NOVA*, quarterly. Newsletter. *Price:* $40/year for nonmembers. • Also publishes Legislatively Speakings. **Frmly:** (1989) Nurses Organization of the Veterans Administration.

**★ 15764 ★ Nursing Touch and Massage Therapy Association International (NTMTAI)**
1438 Shortcut, Ste. E
Slidell, LA 70458
**Phone:** (504)893-8002 **Fax:** (504)892-3493
**Email:** ntmta@aol.com
**Website:** http://members.aol.com/ntmta
**Desc:** Massage therapists. Seeks to advance the study and practice of therapeutic massage. Conducts research, educational, and promotional activities.

**★ 15765 ★ Oncology Nursing Society (ONS)**
501 Holiday Dr.
Pittsburgh, PA 15220
**Phone:** (412)921-7373 **Fax:** (412)921-6565
**Email:** customer.service@ons.org
**Website:** http://www.ons.org
Pearl Moore, CEO
**Fnded:** 1975. **Mem:** 29,000. **Local Groups:** 207. **Desc:** Registered nurses and other health care professionals with an interest in oncology. Seeks to: promote high professional standards in oncology nursing; provide a network for the exchange of information, resources, and peer support; encourage nurses to specialize in oncology; promote and develop educational programs in oncology nursing extending through the graduate level; identify, encourage, and foster nursing research in improving the quality of patient care. Conducts instructional and abstract sessions. Compiles statistics. **Pub:** *Clinical Journal of Oncology Nursing*, bimonthly. Journal. *Price:* $95/year. • *Oncology Nursing Forum*, 10/year. Journal. Contains advertisers' index, calendar of events, information on new products, employment opportunity listings, chapter directory, and promotion news. *Price:* $115 for one-year subscription; $215 for two-year subscription; $95/year for institutions. • *ONS News*, monthly. Newsletter. Contains Washington, DC, news, calendar of events,

employment opportunity listings, member news, and chapter news. *Price:* Included in membership dues.

★ **15766** ★ **Pediatric Endocrinology Nursing Society (PENS)**
PO Box 2933
Gaithersburg, MD 20886-2933
**Website:** http://www.pens.org
**Fnded:** 1986. **Mem:** 325. **Desc:** Pediatric endocrine nurses. Promotes professional responsibility, accountability, ethics and respect; dedicated to the advancement of the art and science of pediatric endocrine nursing; establishes and maintains standards of practice; enhances nursing research, clinical expertise and recognition of excellence in nursing. **Pub:** *PENS Manual.* Manual. Contains individual chapters authored by nurses in the field of pediatric endocrinology. • *PENS Reporter*, quarterly. Newsletter. Includes society news, committee reports, deadlines, articles with focus on endocrine disorders and nursing research, lay organization information.

★ **15767** ★ **Preventive Cardiovascular Nurses Association (PCNA)**
7611 Elmwood Ave., Ste. 202
Middleton, WI 53562-3161
**Phone:** (608)831-5683          **Fax:** (608)831-5122
**Email:** info@pcna.net
**Website:** http://www.pcna.net
Carol Mason, RN,ANP, Pres.
**Fnded:** 1991. **Mem:** 500. **Desc:** Works to develop and promote the role of nurses in managing of patients with lipid disorders. Defines a certification process; disseminates information to increase consumer awareness; funds a training grant; seeks to have lipid nursing designated a nursing specialty. **Pub:** *The Bulletin*, quarterly. Newsletter. • Membership Directory. **Frmly:** (2001) Lipid Nurse Task Force.

★ **15768** ★ **Professional Association of Nursery Nurses**
c/o Professional Association Teachers
2 St. James' Ct.
Friar Gate
Derby DE1 1BT, United Kingdom
**Phone:** 44 1332 372337     **Fax:** 44 1332 290310
**Email:** pann@pat.org.uk
**Website:** http://www.pat.org.uk
**Fnded:** 1982. **Mem:** 5,000. **Local Groups:** 11. **Lang(s):** English. **Desc:** Qualified and experienced child care practitioners within education, social services, the health service, the private sector (including nannies). Represents the interests of qualified and student nursery nurses, nannies, and other child care workers throughout the UK. Promotes professionalism at all times. **Pub:** *All You Need to Know About Working as a Nanny.* Book. • *Professionalism in Practice*, quarterly. Journal. Also publishes booklets, fact sheets, and information packs.

★ **15769** ★ **Psychiatric Nurses Association of Ireland**
2 Gardiner Pl.
Dublin 1, Ireland
**Phone:** 353 1 8746793       **Fax:** 353 1 8740315
**Fnded:** 1971. **Mem:** 4,700. **Reg. Groups:** 7. **Local Groups:** 32. **Desc:** Psychiatric nurses in Ireland. Seeks to advance the study and practice of psychiatric nursing. Encourages professional advancement for psychiatric nurses. Liaises with the Department of Health, Department of Environment, Health Boards, and Hospitals. **Pub:** *Psychiatric Nursing*, 3/year. Journal.

★ **15770** ★ **Respiratory Nursing Society (RNS)**
c/o NYSNA
11 Cornell Rd.
Latham, NY 12110
**Phone:** (518)782-9400
**Email:** ms@nysna.org

**Website:** http://www.respiratorynursingsociety.org/
Donna Wood, Pres.
**Fnded:** 1990. **Mem:** 400. **Local Groups:** 2. **Desc:** Nurses who care for clients with pulmonary dysfunction, and who are interested in the promotion of pulmonary health. Fosters the personal and professional development of respiratory nurses, and quality care of their clients. Provides educational opportunities and promotes research in the field. **Pub:** *Respiratory Exchange*, quarterly. Newsletter.

★ **15771** ★ **Royal College of Nursing - Australia**
1 Napier Close
Deakin, VIC 2600, Australia
**Phone:** 61 6 2825633          **Fax:** 61 6 2823565
**Fnded:** 1949.

★ **15772** ★ **Royal College of Nursing of the United Kingdom**
20 Cavendish Sq.
London W1G 0RN, United Kingdom
**Phone:** 44 207 4093333     **Fax:** 44 207 6473435
**Email:** webteam@rcn.org.uk
**Website:** http://www.rcn.org.uk
**Fnded:** 1916. **Mem:** 310,000. **Desc:** Nurses, midwives and health visitors. Represents nurses working at all levels of responsibility and in a wide variety of settings, from the NHS to the independent sector and from local government to private industry. **Pub:** *Nursing Standard*, weekly. Journal.

★ **15773** ★ **Sigma Theta Tau International (STTI)**
550 W North St.
Indianapolis, IN 46202
**Phone:** (317)634-8171          **Free:** 888-634-7575
**Fax:** (317)634-8188
**Email:** stti@stti.iupui.edu
**Website:** http://www.nursingsociety.org
Nancy Dickenson-Hazard, CEO
**Fnded:** 1922. **Mem:** 120,000. **Local Groups:** 406. **Desc:** One of the lsargest and most prestigious nursing organizations in the world. Committed to fostering nursing excellence, scholarship and leadership to improve health care worldwide, its members promote research-based practice by making resources available to all interested people and institutions. Sigma Theta Tau International is comprised of chapter honor societies that are locasted on more than 500 colleges and university campuses in all 50 states, Puerto Rico, Canada, South Korea, Taiwan, Australia, Pakistan and Hong Kong. Members are active in 94 countries and territories. **Pub:** *Directory of Nurse Researchers*. Directory. *Price:* $60 print; $25 compact disc. • *Journal of Nursing Scholarship*, quarterly. Journal. Includes manuscripts, books reviews, and opinion pieces. *Price:* $34/year; $56/2 years. • *The Online Journal of Knowledge Synthesis for Nursing (Full-Text Electronic Journal)*. Journal. *Price:* $90/year for members; $105/year for non-members; $75/year for small institution; $350/year for large institution. • *Reflections on Nursing Leadership*, quarterly. Magazine. Includes President's message, executive update, inside the society, feature articles, people and announcements. *Price:* $20/2years. **Frmly:** (1985) Sigma Theta Tau.

**Society of Nursery Nursing (SNN)**
*See:* Entry 5757

★ **15774** ★ **Society of Otorhinolaryngology and Head/Neck Nurses (SOHN)**
116 Canal St., Ste. A
New Smyrna Beach, FL 32168
**Phone:** (904)428-1695          **Fax:** (904)423-7566
**Email:** sohnnet@aol.com
**Website:** http://www.sohnnurse.com/
Sandra Schwartz, R.N., Exec. Dir.

**Fnded:** 1976. **Mem:** 1,200. **Local Groups:** 15. **Desc:** Registered nurses specializing in otorhinolaryngology (the study of the ear, nose, and throat) and the head and neck. Seeks to: promote awareness of professional techniques and new developments in the field; enhance professional standards; create a channel for the exchange of ideas, concerns, and information; develop interaction with similar groups. Offers programs and seminars that have been approved for continuing education credits by the American Nurses' Association. **Pub:** *ORL-Head and Neck Nursing*, quarterly. Includes book reviews and current trends in nursing. *Price:* Included in membership dues; $30/year for nonmembers. • *Society of Otorhinolaryngology and Head-Neck Nurses–Update*, quarterly. Newsletter. Includes employment opportunity listings. *Price:* Included in membership dues.

★ **15775** ★ **Society of Pediatric Nurses (SPN)**
7794 Grow Dr.
Pensacola, FL 32514
**Phone:** (850)494-9467          **Free:** 800-723-2902
**Fax:** (850)484-8762
**Email:** spn@puetzamc.com
**Website:** http://www.pedsnurses.org
Belinda E. Puetz, PhD RN, Contact
**Fnded:** 1990. **Mem:** 1,550. **Local Groups:** 31. **Desc:** Registered pediatric nurses are regular members; nursing students and other professionals with an interest in pediatric nursing are associate members. Promotes quality health and nursing care of children. Conducts advocacy campaigns to improve access to affordable care for children; works to advance techniques of pediatric nursing and health care. Sponsors research and educational programs for members; formulates standards of practice and ethics; fosters collaboration between members and other health care professionals, child health care advocates, and related organizations. **Pub:** *Journal of Pediatric Nursing*, bimonthly. Journal. • *SPN News*, quarterly. Newsletter.

★ **15776** ★ **Society of Trauma Nurses (STN)**
PMB 193
2743 S Veterans Pkwy
Springfield, IL 62704-6536
**Phone:** (217)787-3281          **Fax:** (217)787-3285
**Email:** stnexecdir@aol.com
**Website:** http://www.traumanursesoc.org
Katheen Martin, Pres.
**Fnded:** 1989. **Mem:** 650. **Nat'l Groups:** 1. **Reg. Groups:** 7. **Desc:** Nurses involved in all facets of trauma care. Seeks to communicate trauma nursing information and recognize excellence and innovation in trauma nursing. Addresses legislative issues; assists in the development of standards. Facilitates research. **Pub:** *Journal of Trauma Nursing*, quarterly. Journal. *Price:* Included in membership dues; $70/year for nonmembers; $85 outside U.S.

★ **15777** ★ **Society of Urologic Nurses and Associates (SUNA)**
c/o Richard P. Grimes
E Holly Ave.
PO Box 56
Pitman, NJ 08071-0056
**Phone:** (856)256-2335          **Free:** 888-827-7862
**Fax:** (856)589-7463
**Email:** suna@ajj.com
**Website:** http://www.suna.org
Richard P. Grimes, Exec. Dir.
**Fnded:** 1972. **Mem:** 2,600. **Reg. Groups:** 4. **Local Groups:** 30. **Desc:** Nurses and other health care providers working in the field of urology. Promotes excellence in urological education; establishes standards of care for urology patients. Conducts educational programs; holds examinations and bestows professional certification; facilitates communication among members. **Pub:** *Uro-Gram*, bimonthly. Newsletter.

**★ 15778 ★ Society for Vascular Nursing (SVN)**
7794 Grow Dr.
Pensacola, FL 32514
**Phone:** (850)474-6963        **Free:** 888-536-4SVN
**Fax:** (850)484-8762
**Email:** svn@puetzamc.com
**Website:** http://www.svnnet.org
Belinda Puetz, PhD, RN , Exec. Dir.
**Fnded:** 1982. **Mem:** 750. **State Groups:** 9. **Desc:** Nurses and other health care professionals interested in providing comprehensive care for persons with vascular disease. Seeks to educate public about prevention of PVD. Provides educational programs; conducts research. Operates speakers' bureau. **Pub:** *Journal of Vascular Nursing*, quarterly. Journal. *Price:* Included in membership dues. • *SVN...prn.* Newsletter. • Also publishes patient educational materials. **Frmly:** (1992) Society for Peripheral Vascular Nursing.

**★ 15779 ★ Visiting Nurse Associations of America (VNAA)**
c/o Carolyn S. Markey
11 Beacon St. Ste. 910
Boston, MA 02108
**Phone:** (617)523-4042        **Free:** 800-426-2547
**Fax:** (617)227-4843
**Email:** vnaa@vnaa.org
**Website:** http://www.vnaa.org
Carolyn S. Markey, Pres. /CEO
**Fnded:** 1982. **Mem:** 210. **Desc:** Voluntary, nonprofit home health care agencies. Develops competitive strength among community-based nonprofit visiting nurse organizations; works to strengthen business resources and economic programs through contracting, marketing, governmental affairs and publications. **Pub:** *Nursing Procedure Manual*, monthly. Manual. *Price:* Free for members' CEOs. • *VNAA Spectrum*, monthly. *Price:* Free for members' CEOs. **Frmly:** (1985) American Affiliation of Visiting Nurses Associations and Services.

**Wound, Ostomy and Continence Nurses Society: An Association of E.T. Nurses (WOCN)**
*See:* Entry 20188

# Research Centers

**★ 15780 ★ City of Hope**
**National Medical Center and Beckman Research Institute**
**Department of Nursing Research and Education**
1500 E Duarte Rd.
Duarte, CA 91010
**Phone:** (626)301-2346        **Fax:** (626)301-8941
**Email:** mgrant@coh.org
**Website:** http://www.wocn.org
Marcia Grant, Dir.
**Activities/Fields:** Clinical nursing, including nursing administration, nursing education, delivery of nursing services, nursing organization, and the relationship of patient problems to nursing. Research focuses on quality of life, pain and symptom management, improving nursing attitudes and skills in caring for patients and their families, and reducing complications and side effects of therapy and patient psychological distresses associated with therapeutic and diagnostic procedures.

**★ 15781 ★ East Carolina University**
**Office of Research and Evaluation**
Rivers Bldg., Rm. 105
School of Nursing
Greenville, NC 27858-4353
**Phone:** (252)328-4325        **Fax:** (252)328-2168
**Email:** engelkem@mail.ecu.edu

**Website:** http://www.ecu.edu
Dr. Martha Engelke, Inerim Assoc. Dean, Res. & Eval.
**Activities/Fields:** Basic and applied nursing research, including symptom management, women's health care, rural health, and family health. **Pub:** *Research Pulsations Newsletter*, bimonthly.

**★ 15782 ★ Medical College of Georgia**
**Center for Nursing Research**
Jennings Wing, EB-201
School of Nursing
Augusta, GA 30912
**Phone:** (706)721-3676        **Fax:** (706)721-7049
**Email:** sbunting@mail.mcg.edu
**Website:** http://www.mcg.edu/son/resources1.html
Dr. Sheila Bunting, Actg. Sr. Sci.
**Activities/Fields:** Cognitive functioning and control in institutionalized elderly; asthma; family, health risk, and lifestyle change; learning with computer-aided education (CAE) equipment, and computer-aided instruction (CAI); and cancer and rehabilitation nursing, rural health, self-esteem, and abuse and homeless issues. **Pub:** *Informer.*

**★ 15783 ★ State University of New York at Binghamton**
**Roger L. Kresge Center for Nursing Research**
Decker School of Nursing
PO Box 6000
Binghamton, NY 13902-6000
**Email:** gspencer@binghamton.edu
**Website:** http://dson.binghamton.edu/kresge.htm
Prof. Gale A. Spencer, PhD, Dir.
**Activities/Fields:** Health care and nursing science. **Pub:** *Newsletter.*

**★ 15784 ★ U.S. Department of Health and Human Services**
**National Institute of Nursing Research**
NIH Bldg. 31, Rm. 5B-10
31 Center Dr.
Bethesda, MD 20892-2178
**Phone:** (301)496-0207        **Fax:** (301)480-0045
**Email:** info@ninr.nih.gov
**Website:** http://www.nih.gov/ninr
Dr. Patricia A. Grady, Dir.
**Activities/Fields:** Basic and clinical nursing research, training, and other programs in patient care research and information dissemination. The research programs of the Institute address actual and potential health problems. These programs focus on health promotion and disease prevention, understanding and mitigating the effects of acute and chronic illnesses and disabilities, and the delivery of nursing services. Nursing research examines the biological, biomedical, and behavioral processes in health care and its environment. Its purpose is to accomplish both short-and long-term improvements in nursing practice, patient health, and recovery from illness.

**★ 15785 ★ U.S. Department of Health and Human Services**
**National Institute of Nursing Research**
**Division of Extramural Activities**
Bldg. 31, Rm. 5B05
Bethesda, MD 20892-6300
**Phone:** (301)594-5963        **Fax:** (301)594-3405
**Email:** mleveck@exchange.nih.gov
**Website:** http://www.nih.gov/ninr/research/dea.html
Dr. Mary D. Leveck, Dep. Dir.
**Activities/Fields:** Human responses to illness and disability throughout the life span. Focus is on the biological, behavioral, and psychosocial factors that contribute to these conditions and on methods to improve responses or alleviate the effects of the illness or disease. Research topics of acute illness range from sleep-wake patterns of pre-term infants in the neonatal intensive care unit to the biobehavioral factors affecting recovery following a myocardial infarction. Research involving nursing care of patients

with chronic illness addresses symptom management for conditions such as arthritis, diabetes, AIDS, and cancer. Additional research includes the assessment and management of pain, stress, cognitive impairment and urinary incontinence.

**★ 15786 ★ U.S. Department of Health and Human Services**
**National Institute of Nursing Research**
**Intramural Research Division**
**Clinical Therapeutics Laboratory**
Bldg. 10, Rm. 10C 103 (MSC1851)
9000 Rockville Pike
Bethesda, MD 20892-1851
**Phone:** (301)402-1833        **Fax:** (301)496-7184
Christine Grady, Chf.
**Activities/Fields:** Symptom management with emphasis on two primary groups: HIV-infected adults and the elderly.

**★ 15787 ★ U.S. Department of Health and Human Services**
**National Institute of Nursing Research**
**Intramural Research Division**
**Laboratory for the Study of Human Responses to Health and Illness**
Bldg. 9 Room 1-W-125
9 Central Dr.
Bethesda, MD 20892-0967
**Phone:** (301)594-3752        **Fax:** (301)480-0726
**Email:** annette_wysocki@nih.gov
Dr. Annette B. Wysocki, PhD, Dir.
**Activities/Fields:** Research in wound healing.

**★ 15788 ★ University of Akron**
**Center for Nursing**
209 Caroll St.
Akron, OH 44325
**Phone:** (330)972-6968        **Fax:** (330)972-5883
**Email:** ekinion@uakron.edu
Dr. Elizabeth Kinion, Dir.
**Activities/Fields:** Nursing outcomes, education and research and the relationship between family influences and health behaviors. Offers health care services to vulnerable individuals and families and provides a clinical laboratory for faculty and students to address patient care and response to care.

**★ 15789 ★ University of Iowa**
**Center for Nursing Classification**
407 Nursing Bldg.
College of Nursing
Iowa City, IA 52242
**Phone:** (319)335-7051        **Fax:** (319)335-7082
**Email:** joanne-dochterman@uiowa.edu
**Website:** http://ncvhs.hhs.gov/970416w6.htm
Joanne McCloskey Dochterman, Dir.
**Activities/Fields:** Nursing language classifications. **Pub:** *NIC/NOC Classifications.* • *NIC/NOC Letter*, semiannually.

**University of Iowa**
**Gerontological Nursing Interventions Research Center**
*See:* Entry 3106

**★ 15790 ★ University of Manitoba**
**Manitoba Nursing Research Institute**
Helen Glass Centre, Room 302
Winnipeg, MB, Canada R3T 2N2
**Phone:** (204)474-9080        **Fax:** (204)474-7683
**Email:** nursing_research@umanitoba.ca
**Website:** http://www.umanitoba.ca/nursing/research/mnri
Prof. Lorna Guse, PhD, Dir.
**Activities/Fields:** Health outcomes, and surveys of nurses.

**★ 15791 ★ University of Miami**
**Institute for the Study of Culture and**
**Nursing**
School of Nursing
5801 Red Rd.
Coral Gables, FL 33143
**Phone:** (305)284-1553          **Fax:** (305)284-5686
**Email:** swalsh@miami.edu
Dr. S. Walsh, Dir.
**Activities/Fields:** Clinical nursing, focusing on serving multicultural populations and managing multicultural organizations.

**★ 15792 ★ University of Texas at**
**Arlington**
Center for Nursing Research
PO Box 19407
Arlington, TX 76019
**Phone:** (817)272-2776          **Fax:** (817)272-5006
**Email:** clcason@uta.edu
Dr. Carolyn L. Cason, Dir.
**Activities/Fields:** Hispanic health needs, health promotion and prevention of illness, palliative care, rural health care, nursing care outcomes, and economics of health care delivery.

# State Government Agencies

## <u>Nursing Boards</u>

**★ 15793 ★ Alabama Board of Nursing**
RSA Plaza
770 Washington Ave., Ste. 250
PO Box 3900
Montgomery, AL 36130-3900
**Phone:** (205)242-4060          **Fax:** (205)242-4360
**Email:** abn@abn.state.al.us
**Website:** http://www.abn.state.al.us/

**★ 15794 ★ Alaska Board of Nursing**
**Licensing**
PO Box 110806
Juneau, AK 99811-0806
**Phone:** (907)269-8161          **Fax:** (907)269-8196
**Email:** dorothy_fulton@dced.state.ak.us
**Website:** http://www.dced.state.ak.us/occ/pnur.htm
Dorothy Fulton, Contact

**★ 15795 ★ Arizona Board of Nursing**
1651 E Morten Ave., Ste. 150
Phoenix, AZ 85020-4313
**Phone:** (602)331-8111          **Fax:** (602)906-9365
**Email:** arizona@azbn.org
**Website:** http://www.state.az.us/bn

**★ 15796 ★ Arkansas State Board of**
**Nursing**
University Tower Bldg.
1123 S University, Ste. 800
Little Rock, AR 72204-1619
**Phone:** (501)686-2700          **Fax:** (501)686-2714
**Website:** http://www.state.ar.us/nurse/

**★ 15797 ★ Board of Nurse Examiners for**
**the State of Texas**
333 Guadalupe Ste. 3-460
PO Box 430
Austin, TX 78767
**Phone:** (512)305-7400          **Fax:** (512)305-7401
**Email:** webmaster@bne.state.tx.us
**Website:** http://www.bne.state.tx.us/
Katherine A. Thomas, Director

**★ 15798 ★ California Board of**
**Registered Nursing**
400 R St., Ste 4030
PO Box 944210
Sacramento, CA 94244-2100
**Phone:** (916)322-3350          **Fax:** (916)327-4402
**Email:** webmasterbrn@dca.ca.gov
**Website:** http://www.rn.ca.gov/

**★ 15799 ★ California Board of**
**Registered Nursing**
400 R St., Ste. 4030
PO Box 944210
Sacramento, CA 94244-2100
**Phone:** (916)322-3350          **Fax:** (916)327-4402
**Website:** http://www.rn.ca.gov/

**★ 15800 ★ Colorado Board of Nursing**
1560 Broadway, Ste. 880
Denver, CO 80202
**Phone:** (303)894-2430
**Email:** Webmaster@dora.state.co.us
**Website:** http://www.dora.state.co.us/nursing/
Patricia F. Uris, PhD, 180ChiropractChiropractic

**★ 15801 ★ Commonwealth of Puerto**
**Rico**
**Board of Nurse Examiners**
800 Roberto H. Todd Ave.
Room 202, Stop 18
Santurce, PR 00908
**Phone:** (787)725-7506          **Fax:** (787)725-7903
Magda Bouet, Contact

**★ 15802 ★ Delaware Board of Nursing**
Cannon Bldg., Ste. 203
861 Silver Lake Blvd.
PO Box 1401
Dover, DE 19903-1401
**Phone:** (302)739-4522          **Fax:** (302)739-2711

**★ 15803 ★ DHS Connecticut Board of**
**Examiners for Nursing**
410 Capitol Ave. MS No. 12APP
PO Box 340308
Hartford, CT 06134
**Phone:** (860)509-7624          **Fax:** (860)509-7553
**Email:** donna.winiarski@po.state.ct.us
**Website:** http://www.state.ct.us/dph/
Dorothy Pacyna, RN, Contact

**★ 15804 ★ District of Columbia Board of**
**Nursing**
825 N Capitol St, NE, 2nd Fl.
Washington, DC 20002
**Phone:** (202)442-4776          **Fax:** (202)442-9431
**Website:** http://www.dchealth.com/

**★ 15805 ★ Florida State Board of**
**Nursing**
4052 Bald Cypress Way, BIN CO2
Tallahassee, FL 32399
**Phone:** (850)488-0595          **Fax:** (850)245-4172
**Email:** MQA_Nursing@doh.state.fl.us
**Website:**      http://www.doh.state.fl.us/mqa/nursing/
rnhome.htm
Ruth R. Stiehl, PhD, Director

**★ 15806 ★ Georgia Board of Nursing**
237 Coliseum Dr.
Macon, GA 31217-3858
**Phone:** (478)207-1620          **Fax:** (478)207-1633
**Email:** sacamp@sos.state.ga.us
**Website:** http://www.sos.state.ga.us/ebd-rn/
Shirley A. Camp, RN, Director

**★ 15807 ★ Georgia State Board of**
**Licensed Practical Nurses**
237 Coliseum Dr.
Macon, GA 31217-3858
**Email:** rtmathis@sos.state.ga.us
**Website:** http://www.sos.state.ga.us/ebd-lpn/
Jacqueline Hightower, Director

**★ 15808 ★ Guam Board of Nurse**
**Examiners**
PO Box 2816
Agana, GU 96910
**Phone:** (671)475-0251          **Fax:** (671)477-4733
Margarita Bautista-Gay, Director

**★ 15809 ★ Idaho Board of Nursing**
280 N 8th St., Ste. 210
PO Box 83720
Boise, ID 83720
**Phone:** (208)334-3110          **Fax:** (208)334-3262
**Email:** lcoley@ibn.state.id.us
**Website:** http://www2.state.id.us/ibn/ibnhome.htm

**★ 15810 ★ Illinois Department of**
**Professional Regulation**
**Board of Nursing**
320 W Washington St.
Springfield, IL 62786
**Phone:** (217)785-0800          **Fax:** (217)782-7645
**Website:** http://www.dpr.state.il.us/WHO/nurs.cfm

**★ 15811 ★ Indiana State Board of**
**Nursing**
**State Board of Nursing**
402 W Washington St., Rm. W041
Indianapolis, IN 46204
**Phone:** (317)234-2043
**Email:** dlafollette@hpb.state.in.us
**Website:** http://www.state.in.us/hpb/isbn/
Kristen Kelley, Director

**★ 15812 ★ Iowa Board of Nursing**
River Point Business Park
400 SW 8th St., Ste. B
Des Moines, IA 50309-4685
**Phone:** (515)281-3255          **Fax:** (515)281-4825
**Website:** http://www.iowaccess.org/nursing/

**★ 15813 ★ Kansas State Board of**
**Nursing**
Landon State Office Bldg.
900 SW Jackson, Rm. 551-S
Topeka, KS 66612-1230
**Phone:** (785)296-4929          **Fax:** (785)296-3929
**Email:** mary.blubaugh@ksbn.state.ks.us
**Website:** http://www.ksbn.org/
Mary Blubaugh, R.N., Contact

**★ 15814 ★ Kentucky State Board of**
**Nursing**
312 Wittington Parkway, Ste. 300
Louisville, KY 40222-5172
**Phone:** (502)329-7000          **Free:** 800-305-2042
**Fax:** (502)329-7011
**Email:** KBNWebmaster@mail.state.ky.us
**Website:** http://www.kbn.state.ky.us/

**★ 15815 ★ Louisiana State Board of**
**Nursing**
3510 N Causeway Blvd., Ste. 501
Metairie, LA 70002
**Phone:** (504)838-5332          **Fax:** (504)838-5349
**Email:** morvantb@lsbn.state.la.us
**Website:** http://www.dhh.state.la.us/boards.HTM
Barbara Morvent, Director

**★ 15816 ★ Louisiana State Board of Practical Nurse Examiners**
3421 N Causeway Blvd., Ste. 203
Metairie, LA 70002
**Phone:** (504)838-5791 **Fax:** (504)838-5279
**Email:** claire@lsbpne.com
**Website:** http://www.dhh.state.la.us/boards.htm
Claire Doody Glavilano, RN, Contact

**★ 15817 ★ Maine State Board of Nursing**
24 Stone St.
158 State House Station
Augusta, ME 04333
**Phone:** (207)287-1133 **Fax:** (207)287-1149
**Email:** myra.a.broadway@state.me.us
**Website:** http://www.state.me.us/nursingbd/

**★ 15818 ★ Maryland Board of Nursing**
4140 Patterson Ave.
Baltimore, MD 21215-2299
**Phone:** (410)585-1900 **Free:** 888-202-9861
**Email:** wayne48@erols.com
**Website:** http://www.dhmh.state.md.us/mbn/

**★ 15819 ★ Massachusetts Board of Registration in Nursing**
239 Causeway St., Ste. 500
Boston, MA 02114
**Phone:** (617)727-9961
**Email:** gerald.galvin@state.ma.us
**Website:** http://www.state.ma.us/reg/boards/rn/default.htm
Theresa Bonanno, Director

**★ 15820 ★ Michigan Board of Nursing**
PO Box 30670
Lansing, MI 48909-8170
**Phone:** (517)335-0918 **Fax:** (517)373-2179
**Email:** bhserinfo@cis.state.mi.us
**Website:** http://www.cis.state.mi.us/bhser/lic/boards/bdnurse.htm
Margaret Hedlund, Contact

**★ 15821 ★ Minnesota Board of Nursing**
2829 University Ave. SE, Ste. 500
Minneapolis, MN 55414-3253
**Phone:** (612)617-2270 **Free:** 888-234-2690
**Fax:** (612)617-2190
**Email:** nursing.board@state.mn.us
**Website:** http://www.nursingboard.state.mn.us/

**★ 15822 ★ Mississippi Board of Nursing**
1935 Lakeland Dr., Ste. B
Jackson, MS 39216
**Phone:** (601)987-4188 **Fax:** (601)364-2352
**Email:** info@msbn.state.ms.us
**Website:** http://www.msbn.state.ms.us/webtest/

**★ 15823 ★ Missouri State Board of Nursing**
3605 Missouri Blvd.
PO Box 656
Jefferson City, MO 65102
**Phone:** (573)751-0681 **Fax:** (573)751-0075
**Email:** nursing@mail.state.mo.us
**Website:** http://www.ecodev.state.mo.us/pr/nursing
Calvina Thomas, PhD, Director

**★ 15824 ★ Montana State Board of Nursing**
301 S Park Ave. 4th Fl.
PO Box 200513
Helena, MT 59620-0513
**Phone:** (406)841-2340 **Fax:** (406)841-2343
**Email:** compolnur@state.mt.us
**Website:** http://commerce.state.mt.us/LICENSE/pol/pol_boards/nur_board/board_page.htm
Barb Swehla, Director

**★ 15825 ★ Nebraska Board of Nursing Bureau of Examining Boards**
301 Centennial Mall South
PO Box 94986
Lincoln, NE 68509-4986
**Phone:** (402)471-4376 **Fax:** (402)471-3577
**Email:** Charlene.Kelly@hhss.state.ne.us
**Website:** http://www.hhs.state.ne.us/crl/crlindex.htm
Charlene Kelly, Contact

**★ 15826 ★ Nevada State Board of Nursing**
1755 E Plumb Ln., Ste. 260
Reno, NV 89502
**Phone:** (775)688-2620 **Free:** 800-746-3980
**Fax:** (775)688-2628
**Email:** nsbnreno@govmail.state.nv.us
**Website:** http://www.state.nv.us/boards/nsbn/

**★ 15827 ★ New Hampshire Board of Nursing**
79 Regional Dr., Bldg. B
Concord, NH 03302-3898
**Phone:** (603)271-6599
**Website:** http://www.state.nh.us/nursing/
Cynthia Gray, R.N., Contact

**★ 15828 ★ New Jersey Board of Nursing**
124 Halsey St., 6th Fl.
PO Box 45010
Newark, NJ 07101
**Phone:** (973)504-6430
**Email:** askconsumeraffairs@smtp.lps.state.nj.us
**Website:** http://www.state.nj.us/lps/ca/medical.htmnur6
Patricia A. Polansky, Director

**★ 15829 ★ New Mexico Board of Nursing**
4206 Louisiana NE, Ste. A
Albuquerque, NM 87109
**Phone:** (505)841-8340 **Fax:** (505)841-8347
**Email:** boardofnursing@state.nm.us
**Website:** http://www.state.nm.us/nursing/

**★ 15830 ★ New York State Board of Nursing**
Office of the Professions
State Education Bldg., 2nd Fl.
89 Washington Ave.
Albany, NY 12234
**Phone:** (518)474-3817
**Email:** op4info@mail.nysed.gov
**Website:** http://www.op.nysed.gov/nurse.htm
Barbara Zittel, Contact

**★ 15831 ★ North Carolina Board of Nursing**
PO Box 2129
3724 National Dr., Ste. 201
Raleigh, NC 27602-2129
**Phone:** (919)782-3211 **Fax:** (919)781-9461
**Email:** email@ncbon.com
**Website:** http://www.ncbon.com/

**★ 15832 ★ North Dakota Board of Nursing**
919 S 7th St., Ste. 504
Bismarck, ND 58504-5881
**Phone:** (701)328-9778 **Fax:** (701)328-9785
**Email:** ckalanek@ndbon.org
**Website:** http://www.ndbon.org/
Constance B. Kalanek, Contact

**★ 15833 ★ Ohio Board of Nursing**
77 S High St., Ste. 400
Columbus, OH 43215-3412
**Phone:** (614)466-3947
**Email:** board@nur.state.oh.us
**Website:** http://www.state.oh.us/nur/

**★ 15834 ★ Oklahoma Board of Nursing Registration and Education**
2915 N Classen Blvd., Ste. 524
Oklahoma City, OK 73106
**Phone:** (405)962-1800 **Fax:** (405)962-1821
**Email:** obnwebmaster@nursing.state.ok.us
**Website:** http://www.youroklahoma.com/nursing/
Kim Glazier, Director

**★ 15835 ★ Oregon State Board of Nursing**
800 NE Oregon St., Ste. 465
Portland, OR 97232-2162
**Phone:** (503)731-4745 **Fax:** (503)731-4755
**Email:** oregon.bn.info@state.or.us
**Website:** http://www.osbn.state.or.us/

**★ 15836 ★ Pennsylvania State Board of Nursing**
PO Box 2649
124 Pine St.
Harrisburg, PA 17105-2649
**Phone:** (717)783-7142 **Fax:** (717)783-0822
**Email:** nursing@pados.dos.state.pa.us
**Website:** http://www.dos.state.pa.us/bpoa/nurbd/mainpage.htm
Joan Bouchard, Contact

**★ 15837 ★ Rhode Island Board of Nursing**
105 Cannon Health Bldg.
3 Capitol Hill, Rm. 105
Providence, RI 02908
**Phone:** (401)222-5700 **Fax:** (401)222-3352
**Email:** CharlieA@doh.state.ri.us
**Website:** http://www.health.state.ri.us/hsr/nurses.htm
Charles Alexandre, Director

**★ 15838 ★ South Dakota Board of Nursing**
4300 S Louise Ave., Ste. C1
Sioux Falls, SD 57106
**Phone:** (605)362-2760 **Fax:** (605)362-2768
**Email:** carey.duffy@state.sd.us
**Website:** http://www.state.sd.us/dcr/nursing/nurshom.htm
Diana Vander Woude, Contact

**★ 15839 ★ State Board of Nursing for South Carolina**
Koger Office Park
Kingstree Bldg.
110 Centerview Dr., Ste. 202
PO Box 12367
Columbia, SC 29210
**Phone:** (803)896-4550 **Fax:** (803)896-4525
**Email:** spiresp@mail.llr.state.sc.us
**Website:** http://www.llr.state.sc.us/POL/Nursing/Default.htm
Pam Spires, Contact

**★ 15840 ★ State of Hawaii Board of Nursing**
PO Box 3469
DCCA-PVL
Honolulu, HI 96801
**Phone:** (808)586-2695 **Fax:** (808)586-2689
**Email:** nursing@dcca.state.hi.us
**Website:** http://www.state.hi.us/dcca/pvl/areas_nurse.html
Kathleen Yokouchi-Tokumoto, Contact

**★ 15841 ★ Tennessee State Board of Nursing**
Cordell Hull Bldg., 3rd Fl.
425 Fifth Ave. N
Nashville, TN 37247
**Phone:** (615)532-3202 **Free:** 888-310-4650
**Email:** DDenton@state.tn.us

**Website:** http://www2.state.tn.us/health/Boards/Nursing/index.htm
Elizabeth Cole, Contact


★ **15842** ★ **Texas Board of Vocational Nurse Examiners**
333 Guadalupe St., Ste. 3-400
Austin, TX 78701
**Phone:** (512)305-8100 **Free:** 800-821-3205
**Fax:** (512)305-8101
**Email:** info@bvne.state.tx.us
**Website:** http://www.bvne.state.tx.us/
Geneva Harvey, Director


★ **15843** ★ **Utah Department of Occupational and Professional Licensing**
**Utah State Board of Nursing**
160 E 300 South, 4th floor
Salt Lake City, UT 84111
**Phone:** (801)530-6628 **Fax:** (801)530-6511
**Email:** lduke@br.state.ut.us
**Website:** http://www.dopl.utah.gov/licensing/nurse.html
Laura Poe, Director


★ **15844** ★ **Vermont State Board of Nursing**
109 State St.
Montpelier, VT 05609-1106
**Phone:** (802)828-2396 **Fax:** (802)828-2484
**Email:** aristau@sec.state.vt.us
**Website:** http://www.vtprofessionals.org/opr1/nurses/
Anita Ristau, Director


★ **15845** ★ **Virgin Islands Board of Nurse Licensure**
Plot No. 3, Kongens Gade
Veterans Dr. Sta.
St Thomas, VI 00803
**Phone:** (340)776-7397 **Fax:** (340)777-4003
Winifred Garfield, Contact


★ **15846** ★ **Virginia State Board of Nursing**
6606 W Broad St., 4th Fl.
Richmond, VA 23230-1717
**Phone:** (804)662-9909 **Fax:** (804)662-9512
**Email:** nursebd@dhp.state.va.us
**Website:** http://www.dhp.state.va.us/nursing/default.htm
Nancy K. Durrett, Director


★ **15847** ★ **Washington State Health Care Professions Quality Assurance**
**Nursing Care Quality Commission**
1300 SE Quince St.
PO Box 1099
Olympia, WA 98504-7864
**Phone:** (360)236-4700 **Fax:** (360)236-4738
**Email:** hpqa.csc@doh.wa.gov
**Website:** http://www.doh.wa.gov/Nursing
Paula Meyer, Director


★ **15848** ★ **West Virginia Board of Examiners for Licensed Practical Nurses**
101 Dee Dr.
Charleston, WV 25311
**Phone:** (304)558-3572 **Free:** 877-558-LPNS
**Fax:** (304)558-4367
**Email:** lpnboard@state.wv.us
**Website:** http://www.lpnboard.state.wv.us/
Lanette Anderson, Contact


★ **15849** ★ **West Virginia Board of Examiners for Registered Nurses**
101 Dee Dr.
Charleston, WV 25311
**Phone:** (304)558-3596 **Fax:** (304)558-3666
**Email:** westvirginiarn@ncsbn.org
**Website:** http://www.state.wv.us/nurses/rn/
Laura Rhodes, Director


★ **15850** ★ **Wisconsin Board of Nursing**
1400 E Washington Ave.
PO Box 8935
Madison, WI 53708-8935
**Phone:** (608)266-0145 **Fax:** (608)261-7083
**Email:** web@drl.state.wi.us
**Website:** http://www.drl.state.wi.us/
Kimberly Nania, Director


★ **15851** ★ **Wyoming State Board of Nursing**
2020 Carey Ave., Ste. 110
Cheyenne, WY 82001
**Phone:** (307)777-7601 **Fax:** (307)777-3519
**Email:** ckoski@state.wy.us
**Website:** http://nursing.state.wy.us/
Cheryl L. Koski, Contact


# State & Regional Organizations

## Nursing

*The following state organizations are affiliates of the American Nurses Association, 600 Maryland Ave. SW, Ste. 100 West, Washington, DC 20024, (800)274-4ANA, http://www.nursingworld.org/.*

### Alabama

★ **15852** ★ **Alabama State Nurses' Association**
360 N Hull St.
Montgomery, AL 36104-3658
**Phone:** (334)262-8321 **Fax:** (334)262-8578
**Email:** alabamasna@mindspring.com
**Website:** http://www.nursingworld.org/snas/al
Karen L. Pakkala, RN, Exec Director

### Alaska

★ **15853** ★ **Alaska Nurses Association**
2207 E Tudor Rd., Ste. 34
Anchorage, AK 99507-1069
**Phone:** (907)274-0827 **Fax:** (907)272-0292
**Email:** aknurse@aknurse.org
**Website:** http://www.aknurse.org
Camille Soleil, Exec Director

### Arizona

★ **15854** ★ **Arizona Nurses Association**
1850 E Southern Ave., Ste. 1
Tempe, AZ 85282
**Phone:** (480)831-0404 **Fax:** (480)839-4780
**Email:** info@aznurse.org
**Website:** http://www.aznurse.org
Marla Weston, RN, MS, Exec Director

### Arkansas

★ **15855** ★ **Arkansas Nurses Association**
804 N University
Little Rock, AR 72205
**Phone:** (501)664-5853 **Fax:** (501)664-5859
**Email:** arna@prodigy.net
**Website:** http://www.arna.org
David Eubanks, RN, Contact

### California

★ **15856** ★ **ANA/California**
1121 L St., Ste. 409
Sacramento, CA 95814
**Phone:** (916)447-0225 **Fax:** (916)447-5568
**Email:** anacalif@pacbell.net
**Website:** http://www.anacalifornia.org
Tricia Hunter, RN, Contact

### Colorado

★ **15857** ★ **Colorado Nurses Association**
950 S Cherry, Ste. 508
Denver, CO 80246
**Phone:** (303)757-7483 **Fax:** (303)758-0190
**Email:** cna@nurses-co.org
**Website:** http://www.nurses-co.org/cna
Linda Metzner, RN, JD, Exec Director

### Connecticut

★ **15858** ★ **Connecticut Nurses Association**
Meritech Business Park
377 Research Pkwy., Ste. 2D
Meriden, CT 06450
**Phone:** (203)238-1207 **Fax:** (203)238-3437
**Email:** polly@ctnurses.org
**Website:** http://www.nursingworld.org/snas/ct
Polly T. Barey, MS, RN, Exec Director

### Delaware

★ **15859** ★ **Delaware Nurses Association**
2644 Capitol Trail, Ste. 330
Newark, DE 19711
**Phone:** (302)368-2333 **Fax:** (302)366-1775
**Email:** delnurse@erols.com
**Website:** http://www.nursingworld.org/snas/de/
Ruth Bashford, MN, RN, Exec Director

### District of Columbia

★ **15860** ★ **American Nurses Association**
600 Maryland Ave. SW, Ste. 100W
Washington, DC 20024-2571
**Phone:** (202)651-7000 **Free:** 800-274-4ANA
**Fax:** (202)651-7001
**Email:** lstierle@ana.org
**Website:** http://www.nursingworld.org/
Linda J. Stierle, MSN, CEO


★ **15861** ★ **District of Columbia Nurses Association, Inc.**
5100 Wisconsin Ave. NW, Ste. 306
Washington, DC 20016
**Phone:** (202)244-2705 **Fax:** (202)362-8285
**Email:** dcnurses1@aol.com
**Website:** http://dcnaonline.com
Tom Wachter, Contact


★ **15862** ★ **Federal Nurses Association (FedNA)**
600 Maryland Ave. SW, Ste. 100W
Washington, DC 20024
**Phone:** (202)651-7333 **Fax:** (202)651-7355
**Email:** FedNA@ana.org
**Website:** http://www.nursingworld.org/FedNA
Pamela C. Hagan, MSN, Contact

### Florida

★ **15863** ★ **Florida Nurses Association**
PO Box 536985
Orlando, FL 32853-6985
**Phone:** (407)896-3261 **Fax:** (407)896-9042
**Email:** info@floridanurse.org
**Website:** http://www.floridanurse.org
Paula Massey, MN, RN, Exec Director

## Georgia

**★ 15864 ★ Georgia Nurses Association**
3032 Briarcliff Rd. NE
Atlanta, GA 30329-2655
**Phone:** (404)325-5536        **Fax:** (404)325-0407
**Email:** gna-ceo@mindspring.com
**Website:** http://www.georgianurses.org
Deborah Hackman, CEO

## Guam

**★ 15865 ★ Guam Nurses Association**
PO Box CG
Hagatna, GU 96932
**Phone:** (671)477-6877        **Fax:** (671)477-6877
**Email:** guamnurse@ite.net
Glynis S. Almonte, RN, Exec Director

## Hawaii

**★ 15866 ★ Hawaii Nurses Association**
677 Ala Moana Blvd., Ste. 301
Honolulu, HI 96813
**Phone:** (808)531-1628        **Fax:** (808)524-2760
**Email:** nancy@hawaiinurses.org
**Website:** http://www.hawaiinurses.org
Nancy McGukin, Exec Director

## Idaho

**★ 15867 ★ Idaho Nurses Association**
200 N 4th St., Ste. 20
Boise, ID 83702-6001
**Phone:** (208)345-0500        **Fax:** (208)385-0166
**Email:** idahonursesassn@hotmail.com
**Website:** http://www.nursingworld.org/snas/id
Judy Murray, PhD,RN, Exec Director

## Illinois

**★ 15868 ★ Illinois Nurses Association**
105 W Adams St., Ste. 2101
Chicago, IL 60603
**Phone:** (312)419-2900        **Fax:** (312)419-2920
**Email:** cholmgren@illinoisnurses.com
**Website:** http://www.illinoisnurses.com
Cathy Holmgren, RN, Exec Director

## Indiana

**★ 15869 ★ Indiana State Nurses Association**
2915 N High School Rd.
Indianapolis, IN 46224
**Phone:** (317)299-4575        **Fax:** (317)297-3525
**Email:** isnarn@prodigy.net
**Website:** http://www.indiananurses.org
Ernest C. Klein, Jr., RN, Exec Director

## Iowa

**★ 15870 ★ Iowa Nurses Association**
1501 42nd St., Ste. 471
West Des Moines, IA 50266
**Phone:** (515)225-0495        **Fax:** (515)225-2201
**Email:** iowanurses@aol.com
**Website:** http://www.iowanurses.org
Linda Goeldner, MA,CHE, Exec Director

## Kansas

**★ 15871 ★ Kansas State Nurses Association**
1208 SW Tyler
Topeka, KS 66612-1735
**Phone:** (785)233-8638        **Fax:** (785)233-5222
**Email:** troberts@echo.sound.net
**Website:** http://www.nursingworld.org/snas/ks
Terri R. Roberts, JD, RN, Exec Director

## Kentucky

**★ 15872 ★ Kentucky Nurses Association**
1400 S 1st St.
PO Box 2616
Louisville, KY 40201-2616
**Phone:** (502)637-2546        **Fax:** (502)637-8236
**Email:** mkeenan@kentucky-nurses.org
**Website:** http://www.kentucky-nurses.org
Maureen Keenen, JD, Contact

## Louisiana

**★ 15873 ★ Louisiana State Nurses Association**
5700 Florida Blvd., Ste. 720
Baton Rouge, LA 70806
**Phone:** (225)201-0993        **Free:** 800-457-6378
**Fax:** (225)201-0971
**Email:** lsna@lsna.org
**Website:** http://www.lsna.org
Tawna Pounders, RN, Exec Director

## Maine

**★ 15874 ★ American Nurses Association-Maine (ANA-Maine)**
PO Box 254
Auburn, ME 04212-0254
**Phone:** (207)667-0260
**Email:** josephn@acadia.net
**Website:** http://www.anamaine.org

## Maryland

**★ 15875 ★ Maryland Nurses Association**
849 International Dr.
Airport Sq. 21, Ste. 255
Linthicum, MD 21090
**Phone:** (410)859-3000        **Fax:** (410)859-3001
**Email:** marylandnursesassociation@erols.com
**Website:** http://www.nursingworld.org/snas/md
Kathryn V. Hall, MS, RN, Exec Director

## Massachusetts

**★ 15876 ★ Massachusetts Association of Registered Nurses, Inc.**
PO Box 70668
Quinsigamond Village Station
345 Greenwood St.
Worcester, MA 01607
**Phone:** (781)344-6926        **Fax:** (781)341-8495
**Email:** info@marnonline.org
**Website:** http://www.nursingworld.org/cmas/ma
Karen Daley, RN, President

## Michigan

**★ 15877 ★ Michigan Nurses Association**
2310 Jolly Oak Rd.
Okemos, MI 48864-4599
**Phone:** (517)349-5640        **Fax:** (517)349-5818
**Email:** tom.renkes@minurses.org
**Website:** http://www.minurses.org
Tom Renkes, MS, RN, Exec Director

## Minnesota

**★ 15878 ★ Minnesota Nurses Association**
1625 Energy Park Dr.
Saint Paul, MN 55108
**Phone:** (651)646-4807        **Free:** 800-536-4662
**Fax:** (651)647-5301
**Email:** emurphy@mnnurses.org
**Website:** http://www.mnnurses.org
Erin Murphy, RN, Exec Director

## Mississippi

**★ 15879 ★ Mississippi Nurses Association**
31 Woodgreen Pl.
Madison, MS 39110
**Phone:** (601)898-0670        **Fax:** (601)898-0190
**Email:** mna@msnurses.org
**Website:** http://www.msnurses.org
Betty R. Dickson, Exec Director

## Missouri

**★ 15880 ★ Missouri Nurses Association**
1904 Bubba Lane
PO Box 105228
Jefferson City, MO 65110-5228
**Phone:** (573)636-4623        **Free:** 888-662-MONA
**Fax:** (573)636-9576
**Email:** belinda@missourinurses.org
**Website:** http://www.missourinurses.org
Belinda Heimericks, RN, Exec Director

## Montana

**★ 15881 ★ Montana Nurses Association**
104 Broadway, Ste. G-2
Helena, MT 59601
**Phone:** (406)442-6710        **Fax:** (406)442-1841
**Email:** info@mtnurses.org
**Website:** http://www.nursingworld.org/snas/mt/
Sami Butler, RN, Exec Director

## Nebraska

**★ 15882 ★ Nebraska Nurses Association**
715 S 14th St.
Lincoln, NE 68508
**Phone:** (402)475-3859        **Fax:** (402)475-3961
**Email:** ne.nurses@prodigy.net
**Website:** http://www.nursingworld.org/snas/ne/index.htm
Chuck Stepanek, Exec Director

## Nevada

**★ 15883 ★ Nevada Nurses Association**
PO Box 530399
Henderson, NV 89053-0399
**Phone:** (702)260-7886        **Fax:** (702)260-7052
**Email:** nvnurses@aol.com
**Website:** http://www.nvnurses.org
Richard Schlegel, CAE, Exec Director

## New Hampshire

**★ 15884 ★ New Hampshire Nurses Association**
48 West St.
Concord, NH 03301-3595
**Phone:** (603)225-3783        **Fax:** (603)228-6672
**Email:** nh_nurses@compuserve.com
**Website:** http://www.nhnurses.myassociation.com
Robert Best, BSE, Exec Director

## New Jersey

**★ 15885 ★ New Jersey State Nurses Association**
1479 Pennington Rd.
Trenton, NJ 08618-2661
**Phone:** (609)883-5335        **Fax:** (609)883-5343
**Email:** njsna@njsna.org
**Website:** http://www.njsna.org
Andrea Aughenbaugh, RN, CS, CEO

## New Mexico

**★ 15886 ★ New Mexico Nurses Association**
PO Box 80300
Albuquerque, NM 87198

**Phone:** (505)268-7744          **Fax:** (505)268-7711
**Email:** nmnurses@hotmail.com
**Website:** http://www.nursingworld.org/snas/nm
Carrie Roberts, RN, Exec Director

## New York

★ 15887 ★ **New York State Nurses Association**
11 Cornell Rd.
Latham, NY 12110
**Phone:** (518)782-9400          **Fax:** (518)782-9530
**Email:** martha.orr@nysna.org
**Website:** http://www.nysna.org
Martha L. Orr, MN, RN, Exec Director

## North Carolina

★ 15888 ★ **North Carolina Nurses Association**
103 Enterprise St.
Box 12025
Raleigh, NC 27605
**Phone:** (919)821-4250          **Fax:** (919)829-5807
**Email:** rns@ncnurses.org
**Website:** http://www.ncnurses.org
Sindy Barker, CAE, Exec Director

## North Dakota

★ 15889 ★ **North Dakota Nurses Association**
531 Airport Rd., Ste. D
Bismarck, ND 58504-6107
**Phone:** (701)223-1385          **Fax:** (701)223-0575
**Email:** ndna@prodigy.net
Sharon Moos, RN, Contact

## Ohio

★ 15890 ★ **Ohio Nurses Association**
4000 E Main St.
Columbus, OH 43213-2983
**Phone:** (614)237-5414          **Fax:** (614)237-6081
**Email:** gharsheymeade@ohnurses.org
**Website:** http://www.ohnurses.org
Gingy Harshey-Meade, RN, CEO

## Oklahoma

★ 15891 ★ **Oklahoma Nurses Association**
6414 N Santa Fe, Ste. A
Oklahoma City, OK 73116
**Phone:** (405)840-3476          **Fax:** (405)840-3013
**Email:** ona@oknurses.com
**Website:** http://www.oknurses.com
Jane Nelson, CAE, Exec Director

## Oregon

★ 15892 ★ **Oregon Nurses Association**
9600 SW Oak, Ste. 550
Portland, OR 97223
**Phone:** (503)293-0011          **Fax:** (503)293-0013
**Email:** ona@oregonrn.org
**Website:** http://www.oregonrn.org
Susan E. King, MS, RN, Contact
Ken Fitzsimon, JD, Director

## Pennsylvania

★ 15893 ★ **Pennsylvania State Nurses Association**
PO Box 68525
Harrisburg, PA 17106-8525

**Phone:** (717)657-1222          **Free:** 888-707-7762
**Fax:** (717)657-3796
**Email:** psna@psna.org
**Website:** http://www.psna.org
Michele P. Campbell, RN, Contact

## Rhode Island

★ 15894 ★ **Rhode Island State Nurses Association**
550 S Water St., Unit 540B
Providence, RI 02903-4344
**Phone:** (401)421-9703          **Fax:** (401)421-6793
**Email:** risna@prodigy.net
**Website:** http://www.risnarn.org
Pamela L. McCue, MSN, Exec Director

## South Carolina

★ 15895 ★ **South Carolina Nurses Association**
1821 Gadsden St.
Columbia, SC 29201
**Phone:** (803)252-4781          **Fax:** (803)779-3870
**Email:** scna@prodigy.net
**Website:** http://www.scnurses.org
Judith C. Thompson, Exec Director

## South Dakota

★ 15896 ★ **South Dakota Nurses Association**
PO Box 1015
Pierre, SD 57501-1015
**Phone:** (605)945-4265          **Fax:** (605)945-4266
**Email:** sdnurse1@dtgnet.com
**Website:** http://www.nursingworld.org/snas/sd/
Ed Jacobson, Exec Director

## Tennessee

★ 15897 ★ **Tennessee Nurses Association**
545 Mainstream Dr., Ste. 405
Nashville, TN 37228-1201
**Phone:** (615)254-0350          **Fax:** (615)254-0303
**Email:** lbrowntna@aol.com
**Website:** http://www.tnaonline.org
Louise Browning, CAE, Exec Director

## Texas

★ 15898 ★ **Texas Nurses Association**
7600 Burnet Rd., Ste. 440
Austin, TX 78757-1292
**Phone:** (512)452-0645          **Fax:** (512)452-0648
**Email:** memberinfo@texasnurses.org
**Website:** http://www.texasnurses.org
Clair B. Jordan, RN, Exec Director

## Utah

★ 15899 ★ **Utah Nurses Association**
3761 S 700 E, No. 201
Salt Lake City, UT 84106
**Phone:** (801)293-8351          **Free:** 800-236-1617
**Fax:** (801)293-8458
**Email:** una@xmission.com
**Website:** http://www.utahnurses.org
Bill Sartain, Exec Director

## Vermont

★ 15900 ★ **Vermont State Nurses Association**
100 Dorset St., Ste. 13
South Burlington, VT 05403-6241
**Phone:** (802)651-8886          **Fax:** (802)651-8998
**Email:** vtnurse@prodigy.net
**Website:** http://www.nesna.org
Margaret M. Sharpe, RN, Exec Director

## Virgin Islands

★ 15901 ★ **Virgin Islands State Nurses Association**
PO Box 583
Christiansted, VI 00821-0583
**Phone:** (809)773-1261
**Email:** vcgvina@viaccess.net
Verna Christian-Garcia, RN, Exec Director

## Virginia

★ 15902 ★ **Virginia Nurses Association**
7113 Three Chopt Rd., Ste. 204
Richmond, VA 23226
**Phone:** (804)282-1808          **Fax:** (804)282-4916
**Email:** vnajmj@aol.com
**Website:** http://www.virginianurses.com
Jan Marshall Johnson, MS, RN, Exec Director

## Washington

★ 15903 ★ **Washington State Nurses Association**
575 Andover Park W, Ste. 101
Seattle, WA 98188-3321
**Phone:** (206)575-7979          **Fax:** (206)575-1908
**Email:** wsna@wsna.org
**Website:** http://www.wsna.org
Judith A. Huntington, MN, RN, Exec Director

## West Virginia

★ 15904 ★ **West Virginia Nurses Association**
100 Capitol St., Ste. 1009
PO 1946
Charleston, WV 25301
**Phone:** (304)342-1169          **Free:** 800-400-1226
**Fax:** (304)346-1861
**Email:** centraloffice@wvnurses.org
**Website:** http://www.wvnurses.org
Cheri Heflin, Exec Director

## Wisconsin

★ 15905 ★ **Wisconsin Nurses Association**
6117 Monona Dr.
Madison, WI 53716
**Phone:** (608)221-0383          **Fax:** (608)221-2788
**Email:** wna@execpc.com
**Website:** http://www.wisconsinnurses.com
Gina Dennik-Champion, RN, Contact

## Wyoming

★ 15906 ★ **Wyoming Nurses Association**
Majestic Bldg., Rm. 305
1603 Capitol Ave.
Cheyenne, WY 82001
**Phone:** (307)635-3955          **Fax:** (307)635-2173
**Email:** wyonurse@aol.com
Beverly McDermott, MS, RN, Exec Director

# Chapter 43
# Nursing Homes

## Foundations & Other Funding Organizations

### Private Foundations

**Alletta Morris McBean Charitable Trust**
*See:* Entry 14909

**Bat Hanadiv Foundation No. 3**
*See:* Entry 11366

**Bingham Trust**
*See:* Entry 10040

**★ 15907 ★ McMahon Foundation**
PO Box 2156
Lawton, OK 73502
**Phone:** (580)355-4622     **Fax:** (580)357-3248
**Email:** mcbeancharitabletrust@att.net
James Wood, Director
**Fnded:** 1940. **Philosophy:** The foundation makes grants primarily for education (including scholarship funds), the arts, youth, the handicapped, and community funds for local projects. Past contributions in Lawton went to an auditorium, a museum devoted to the history of the Great Plains, a city/county health center, a nursing home for the elderly, a mental health center, a public library, a recreational park, and a boys' club gymnasium. Support for other civic and arts organizations has been provided as well. **Priorities:** *Arts & Humanities:* 5%. Supports arts and humanities. *Civic & Public Affairs:* 41%. Supports community development. *Education:* 49%. Supports schools and universities. *Environment:* 3%. Funds the United Way and rehabilitation services. *Note:* Total contributions made in fiscal 1999. **Typ. Recipients:** Emergency/Ambulance Services, Hospices, Nursing Services, Substance Abuse. **Geo. Dist:** OK, Comanche County; OK, only Oklahoma; Lawton, OK.

**Orville D. and Ruth A. Merillat Foundation**
*See:* Entry 571

**Paul Stock Foundation**
*See:* Entry 578

**Philip L. Van Every Foundation**
*See:* Entry 590

**Sapirstein-Stone-Weiss Foundation**
*See:* Entry 660

**Surdna Foundation**
*See:* Entry 712

**Walton Family Foundation**
*See:* Entry 10057

### Corporate Foundations

**ASARCO Foundation**
*See:* Entry 7875

**Boler Co. Foundation**
*See:* Entry 10061

**Bourns Foundation**
*See:* Entry 898

**Century 21 Associates Foundation**
*See:* Entry 11425

**Habig Foundation**
*See:* Entry 11434

**★ 15908 ★ IMMI Word and Deed Foundation**
PO Box 408
Westfield, IN 46074
**Phone:** (317)896-9531     **Fax:** (317)867-0311
**Email:** dboyle@imminet.com
**Website:** http://www.imminet.com
Donald Boyle, Director
**Fnded:** 1991. **Priorities:** *Note:* Total contributions in fiscal 1999. **Typ. Recipients:** Health Organizations, Long-Term Care.

**Lowe's Charitable and Educational Foundation**
*See:* Entry 1212

**Schurz Communications Foundation**
*See:* Entry 1377

**Springs Industries, Inc.**
*See:* Entry 1402

**Stonecutter Foundation**
*See:* Entry 1413

**Teleflex Foundation**
*See:* Entry 1427

**Wachtell, Lipton, Rosen & Katz Foundation**
*See:* Entry 2894

## Other Funding Organizations

**★ 15909 ★ Hospice Foundation of America (HFA)**
2001 S St. NW, Ste. 300
Washington, DC 20009
**Free:** 800-854-3402     **Fax:** (202)638-5312
**Email:** david@hospicefoundation.org
**Website:** http://www.hospicefoundation.org
David Abrams, Pres.
**Desc:** Works to promote the philosophy and application of hospice care for terminally ill people and improve the American health system. Advocates the hospice concept of care; offers professional development and educational programs; sponsors research on ethical issues; participates in public policy initiatives; provides technical assistance to hospices
**Awards:** Grant.

## National & International Organizations

**★ 15910 ★ Academy of Hospice and Palliative Medicine (AAHPM)**
4700 W Lake Ave.
Glenview, IL 60025-1485
**Phone:** (847)375-4712     **Free:** 877-734-8671
**Website:** http://www.aahpm.org
Carla Alexander, MD, Pres.
**Fnded:** 1988. **Desc:** Physicians. Committed to improvement of care of the dying.

**★ 15911 ★ America Association for Homecare**
625 Slaters Ln., Ste. 200
Alexandria, VA 22314-1171
**Phone:** (703)836-6263     **Fax:** (703)836-6730
**Email:** info@aahomecare.org
**Website:** http://www.aahomecare.org
**Mem:** 1,000. **Desc:** Home care providers. Advocate for quality medical care at home to the extent technically feasible. **Pub:** *HME Answer Book*, quarterly. Manual. Provides information and guidance on Medicare coverage, billing and payment rules for DMEPOS claims processing under DMERCs.

**★ 15912 ★ American Academy of Home Care Physicians (AAHCP)**
PO Box 1037
Edgewood, MD 21040-0337
**Phone:** (410)676-7966     **Fax:** (410)676-7980
**Email:** aahcp@mindspring.com
**Website:** http://www.aahcp.org
Constance F. Row, Exec. Dir.
**Desc:** Physicians, home care professionals and agencies, and student affiliates and corporate sponsors-members. Patient referral services.

**American College of Health Care Administrators (ACHCA)**
*See:* Entry 9693

**American Disabled for Attendant Program Today (ADAPT)**
*See:* Entry 2921

**★ 15913 ★ American Health Care Association (AHCA)**
1201 L St. NW
Washington, DC 20005
**Phone:** (202)842-4444　　　**Fax:** (202)842-3860
**Email:** national@adapt.org
**Website:** http://www.ahca.org
Dr. Charles H. Roadman, II, CEO
**Fnded:** 1949. **Mem:** 12,000. **State Groups:** 50. **Desc:** Federation of state associations of long-term health care facilities. Promotes standards for professionals in long-term health care delivery and quality care for patients and residents in a safe environment. Focuses on issues of availability, quality, affordability, and fair payment. Operates as liaison with governmental agencies, Congress, and professional associations. Compiles statistics. **Pub:** *AHCA Notes*, monthly. Newsletter. Covers legislation and regulations. *Price:* Included in membership dues. • *Provider: For Long Term Care Professionals*, monthly. Magazine. Includes buyers' guide, news reports, advertisers' index, a listing of new products and services, and calendar of events. *Price:* Free to long-term health care professionals; $48/year for nonmembers and libraries. • Also produces audiovisual aids. **Frmly:** (1975) American Nursing Home Association.

**★ 15914 ★ American Medical Directors Association (AMDA)**
10480 Little Patuxent Pky., Ste. 760
Columbia, MD 21044
**Phone:** (410)740-9743　　　**Free:** 800-876-2632
**Fax:** (410)740-4572
**Email:** info@amda.com
**Website:** http://www.amda.com
Lorraine Tarnove, Exec. Dir.
**Fnded:** 1975. **Mem:** 8,000. **State Groups:** 35. **Desc:** Physicians providing care in long-term facilities including nursing homes. Sponsors continuing medical education in geriatrics and medical administration. Promotes improved long term care. **Pub:** *AMDA Reports*, bimonthly. Newsletter. Includes calendar of events, reviews of articles, publications, and other resources. *Price:* available to members only. • *Nursing Home Medicine: The Annals of Long Term Care*, 10/year. Journal. *Price:* Free for members; $2/single issue. • Audiotapes.Related to medical direction. • Videos.Related to long term care issues such as restraints, CPT coding, and advance directions.

**American Society of Consultant Pharmacists (ASCP)**
*See:* Entry 17511

**Association of Jewish Aging Services (AJAS)**
*See:* Entry 2930

**★ 15915 ★ Canadian Association for Community Care (CACC)**
**(Association Canadienne de Soins et Services Communautaires — ACSSC)**
1 Nicholas St. Ste. 712
Ottawa, ON, Canada K1N 7B7
**Phone:** (613)241-7510　　　**Fax:** (613)241-5923
**Email:** info@cacc-acssc.com
**Website:** http://www.cacc-acssc.com
**Fnded:** 1980. **Lang(s):** English, French. **Desc:** Home health care services and long-term care facilities. Promotes development of a "range of high-quality, flexible, responsive and accessible community care services" in Canada. Serves as a clearinghouse

on community care services; conducts public advocacy on behalf of members, consumers, and researchers; develops standards of practice and facilities in community care; serves as liaison between members and government, consumers, and related organizations. **Frmly:** HomeSupport Canada; Canadian Long Term Care Association.

**★ 15916 ★ Continuing Care at Home Association**
Churchview
Sunningwell Willage
Abingdon OX13 6RD, United Kingdom
**Phone:** 44 1865 326595
**Website:** http://www.concah.demon.co.uk/
**Fnded:** 1992. **Desc:** Health and social service professionals. To improve the relief at home of those people suffering from chronic illness and disability, and to advance the learning and understanding of those caring for such persons

**★ 15917 ★ Hospice Association of America (HAA)**
228 Seventh St., SE
Washington, DC 20003
**Phone:** (202)547-7424　　　**Fax:** (202)547-3540
**Email:** exec@nahc.org
**Website:** http://www.nahc.org
**Desc:** Home care, hospice and home care aide services. Working to heighten the public visibility of hospice services, to affect legislative and regulatory processes impinging on hospice services. To promote hospice care as a viable component of the health care delivery system. To provide an organized and unified voice for hospice providers, to disseminate information and provide for the exchange of information, to collaborate with state organizations representing hospice interests and initiate, sponsor and promote research related to hospice services.

**★ 15918 ★ Mutual Help Home Association (MHHA)**
**(Association d'Entraide vive Chez Nous — AECN)**
84 rue Principale
Saint Fidele, QC, Canada G0T 1T0
**Phone:** (418)434-2561
**Lang(s):** English, French. **Desc:** Individuals and organizations. Seeks to improve the quality of lives of elderly people living in nursing homes. Monitors conditions in nursing homes; provides support and services to the elderly.

**★ 15919 ★ National Association of Boards of Examiners of Long Term Care Administrators (NABE)**
1444 I St. NW, Ste. 700
Washington, DC 20005-2210
**Phone:** (202)712-9040　　　**Fax:** (202)216-9646
**Email:** nab@bostromdc.com
**Website:** http://www.nabweb.org
Randy Lindner, CAE, Exec. Dir.
**Fnded:** 1972. **Mem:** 550. **Desc:** State boards responsible for licensing nursing homes administrators. Produces exam to test the competence of nursing home adminstrators; operates continuing education review service; disseminates information and educational materials on nursing home administration. **Pub:** *NAB Study Guide: How To Prepare For the Nursing Home Administrators Examination*. The third edition. *Price:* $65.00. • *RC/AL Study Guide: How to Prepare for the Residential Care/Assisted Living Administrators Examination*, annual. *Price:* $34. **Frmly:** National Association of Boards of Examiners of Nursing Home Administrators.

**★ 15920 ★ National Association for Home Care (NAHC)**
228 7th St. SE
Washington, DC 20003
**Phone:** (202)547-7424　　　**Fax:** (202)547-3540

**Email:** exec@nahc.org
**Website:** http://www.nahc.org
Val J. Halamandaris, Pres.
**Fnded:** 1982. **Mem:** 6,000. **Desc:** Providers of home health care, hospice, and homemaker-home health aide services; interested individuals and organizations. Develops and promotes high standards of patient care in home care services. Seeks to affect legislative and regulatory processes concerning home care services; gathers and disseminates home care industry data; develops public relations strategies; works to increase political visibility of home care services. Interprets home care services to governmental and private sector bodies affecting the delivery and financing of such services. Provides legal and accounting consulting services; conducts market research and compiles statistics. Offers members insurance discounts. Sponsors educational programs for organizations and individuals concerned with home care services. **Pub:** *Caring*, monthly. Magazine. *Price:* Included in membership dues; $45/year in U.S.; $65/year outside U.S. • *Homecare News*, monthly. Tabloid covering association news; serves as an information exchange between state associations and providers/suppliers to the industry. *Price:* Included in membership dues; $18/year for nonmembers. • *Hospice Forum*, biweekly. Newsletter. Covers legislative and research news. *Price:* Included in membership dues; $105/year for nonmembers. • *NAHC Report*, weekly. Newsletter. Covers legislative and regulatory issues related to the home health care industry. Contains employment opportunity listings. *Price:* Included in membership dues; $325/year for nonmembers. • *National Home Care and Hospice Directory*, annual. Directory.

**★ 15921 ★ National Association for the Support of Long Term Care (NASL)**
1321 Duke St., Ste. 304
Alexandria, VA 22314
**Phone:** (703)549-8500　　　**Fax:** (703)549-8342
**Email:** member@nasl.org
**Website:** http://www.nasl.org
Peter Clendenin, Exec. VP.
**Fnded:** 1989. **Desc:** Long term care executives and businesses. Dedicated to providing a national communication forum and legislative and regulatory representation for the long term care industry.

**★ 15922 ★ National Care Homes Association**
45/49 Leather Ln.
4th Fl.
London EC1N 7TJ, United Kingdom
**Phone:** 44 20 78317090　　　**Fax:** 44 20 78317040
**Email:** ncha@btclick.com
**Website:** http://www.ncha.gb.com
**Fnded:** 1981. **Mem:** 3,000. **Lang(s):** English. **Desc:** Independent sector care and nursing homes. Serves as a trade association representing members' interests. **Pub:** *Newsletter*, monthly. Newsletter.

**★ 15923 ★ National Family Caregivers Association (NFCA)**
10400 Connecticut Ave., Ste. 500
Kensington, MD 20895-3944
**Phone:** (301)942-6430　　　**Free:** 800-896-3650
**Fax:** (301)942-2302
**Email:** info@nfcacares.org
**Website:** http://www.nfcacares.org
Suzanne Geffen Mintz, Pres.
**Fnded:** 1992. **Mem:** 10,000. **Desc:** Individual caregivers, family friends, professionals, affiliated organizations, healthcare providers. Works to meet the needs of family caregivers and improve the caregiver's quality of life. Offers educational materials for caregivers and health professionals; advocates for respite assistance and other resources for caregivers. Provides information and referrals. **Pub:** *Take Care!*, quarterly. Newsletter. *Price:* Free with membership. • Brochure. • The Resourceful Caregiver

**★ 15924 ★ Registered Nursing Home Association**
Calthorpe House
Hagley Rd.
Edgbaston
Birmingham B16 8QY, United Kingdom
**Phone:** 44 121 4542511    **Fax:** 44 121 4540932
**Email:** rnhao@aol.com
**Website:** http://www.rnha.co.uk
**Fnded:** 1968. **Mem:** 1,600. **Reg. Groups:** 33. **Desc:** Nursing Home Owners. **Pub:** *Nursing Home News*, monthly. Newsletter. • *RNHA Guide*, annual. Book. A reference book on nursing homes in U.K.

**★ 15925 ★ United Kingdom Home Care Association**
42B Banstead Rd.
Carshalton Beeches SM5 3NW, United Kingdom
**Phone:** 44 20 82881551    **Fax:** 44 20 82881550
**Email:** enquiries@ukhca.demon.co.uk
**Website:** http://www.ukhca.co.uk
**Fnded:** 1988. **Mem:** 1,300. **Lang(s):** English. **Desc:** Represents independent home care organizations providing home care and nursing care to people in their own homes. Identifies and promotes the highest standards of home care. **Pub:** *Home Care Workers Handbook*. Handbook. • *The Homecarer*, bimonthly. Newsletter.

## Research Centers

**★ 15926 ★ Aging Research Institute**
217 SE 8th St.
Topeka, KS 66603-3906
**Phone:** (785)233-0585    **Fax:** (785)233-9471
**Email:** jrgrace@kahsa.org
**Website:** http://www.kahsa.org
John R. Grace, Dir.
**Activities/Fields:** Managed care and nursing facilities, staff recruitment and retention, worker safety in nursing homes.

**★ 15927 ★ Maryland Long-Term Care Project**
Department of Epidemiology & Preventive Medicine
University of Maryland
660 W Redwood St., Ste. 200
Baltimore, MD 21201
**Phone:** (410)706-3553    **Fax:** (410)706-4433
**Email:** jmagazine@epi.umaryland.edu
**Website:** http://gerontology.umaryland.edu/long-term.html
Jay Magaziner, PhD, Prin. Investigator
**Activities/Fields:** Research focuses on nursing home acquired infections, the incidence of antibiotic use, the beliefs underlying caregivers' decision to institutionalize a family member, the prevalence of dementia, the relationship of dementia to health, the provision of special care to residents with dementia, the relationship between the structure and process of care to health outcomes for all residents, the prevalence of osteoporosis and its relationship to subsequent fractures; and the educational/training needs of nursing home personnel.

## State Government Agencies

### Nursing Home Administrator Examining Boards

**★ 15928 ★ Alabama State Board of Examiners for Nursing Home Administrators**
4156 Carmichael Rd.
Montgomery, AL 36106
**Phone:** (334)271-6214
**Email:** KMagdon@anha.org
**Website:** http://www.alboenha.state.al.us/

**★ 15929 ★ Alaska Board of Nursing Home Administrators**
PO Box 110806
Juneau, AK 99811-0806
**Phone:** (907)465-2695    **Fax:** (907)465-2974
**Email:** p.j._gingras@dced.state.ak.us
**Website:** http://www.dced.state.ak.us/occ/pnha.htm

**★ 15930 ★ Arizona Board of Examiners for Nursing Care Institution Administrators**
1400 W Washington, Ste. 230
Phoenix, AZ 85007
**Phone:** (602)542-3095    **Fax:** (602)542-3093
**Website:** http://www.revenue.state.az.us/609/nursing-care.htm
Frances Goetzinger-Amendt, Contact

**★ 15931 ★ Arkansas Department of Human Services**
**Medical Services Division**
**Long Term Care Office**
**Nursing Home Certification and Licensure Section**
PO Box 1437, Slot 1100
Little Rock, AR 72203-1437
**Phone:** (501)682-8424    **Fax:** (501)682-6171
**Email:** OLTC.@mail.state.ar.us
**Website:** http://www.medicaid.state.ar.us/Arkansas-Medicaid/DMSUnits/OLTC/LTCmain.htm

**★ 15932 ★ California Board of Examiners of Nursing Home Administrators**
1800 Third St., Ste. 162
PO Box 942732
Sacramento, CA 94234-7320
**Phone:** (916)323-6838    **Free:** 800-236-9747
**Website:** http://www.dca.ca.gov/r_r/nurseho1.htm

**★ 15933 ★ Colorado Board of Examiners of Nursing Home Administrators**
1560 Broadwawy, Ste. 1310
Denver, CO 80202
**Phone:** (303)894-7760    **Fax:** (303)894-7764
**Email:** NHA@dora.state.co.us
**Website:** http://www.dora.state.co.us/Nursing-Home-Administrators/

**★ 15934 ★ Connecticut Department of Public Health**
**Regulatory Services Bureau**
**Health Systems Regulation Division**
410 Capitol Ave.
PO Box 340308
Hartford, CT 06134-0308
**Phone:** (860)509-7406    **Fax:** (860)509-7539
**Email:** webmaster.dph@po.state.ct.us
**Website:** http://www.state.ct.us/dph/DPH_Main/About_DPH/brs/brs.htm
Cynthia Denne, Director

**★ 15935 ★ Delaware State Board of Examiners of Nursing Home Administrators**
Cannon Bldg, Ste. 203
861 Silver Lake Blvd.
Dover, DE 19904-2467
**Phone:** (302)739-4505    **Fax:** (302)739-2711
**Email:** dspruill@state.de.us
**Website:** http://professionallicensing.state.de.us/boards/nursinghomeadmin/index.shtm
Dana Spruill, Contact

**★ 15936 ★ District of Columbia Health Regulation Administration**
**Health Care Facilities Division**
825 N Capitol St. NE
Washington, DC 20002
**Phone:** (202)442-5888
**Website:** http://www.dchealth.com/hra/services.htm

**★ 15937 ★ Florida Board of Nursing Home Administrators**
4052 Bald Cypress Way, Bin C-04
PO Box 6330
Tallahassee, FL 32399-3254
**Phone:** (850)245-4292
**Email:** nqa_nursinghomeadmin@doh.state.fl.us
**Website:** http://www.doh.state.fl.us/mqa/nurshome/nha_home.html

**★ 15938 ★ Georgia State Professional Licensing Boards Division**
**Board of Examiners for Nursing Home Administrators**
237 Coliseum Dr.
Macon, GA 31217-3858
**Phone:** (478)207-1670    **Fax:** (478)207-1676
**Website:** http://www.sos.state.ga.us/plb/contact.htm/

**★ 15939 ★ Hawaii Board of Examiners of Nursing Home Administrators**
1010 Richards St.
DCCA-PVL, Attn NHA
PO Box 3469
Honolulu, HI 96801
**Phone:** (808)586-3000
**Email:** nursing_home@dcca.state.hi.us
**Website:** http://www.state.hi.us/dcca/pvl/areas_nursing_home.html
Kathleen Yokouchi-Tokumoto, Contact

**★ 15940 ★ Idaho Bureau of Occupational Licenses**
**Nursing Home Administrator Examining Board**
Owyhee Plaza, 2nd Fl.
1109 Main St., Ste. 220
Boise, ID 83702-5642
**Phone:** (208)334-3233    **Fax:** (208)334-3945
**Email:** bhetrick@ibol.state.id.us
**Website:** http://www2.state.id.us/ibol/nha.htm
Budd Hetrick, Contact

**★ 15941 ★ Illinois Department of Professional Regulation**
**Nursing Home Administrators Licensing and Disciplinary Board**
320 W Washington St.
Springfield, IL 62786
**Phone:** (217)785-0800    **Fax:** (217)782-7645
**Website:** http://www.dpr.state.il.us
Leonard Sherman, Director

**★ 15942 ★ Indiana Health Professions Bureau**
**Board of Health Facility Administrators**
402 W Washington, Rm. 041
Indianapolis, IN 46204
**Phone:** (317)232-2960    **Fax:** (317)234-2051
**Email:** hpb6@hpb.state.in.us
**Website:** http://www.in.gov/hpb/
Tonja Thompson, Director

**★ 15943 ★ Iowa State Board of Examiners for Nursing Home Administrators**
Lucas State Office Bldg, 5th floor
321 E 12th St.
Des Moines, IA 50319-0075
**Phone:** (515)242-6385    **Fax:** (515)281-3121
**Email:** sdozier@idph.state.ia.us

**Website:** http://www.iowaccess.org/idph_pl/nursing_home/index.html

★ **15944** ★ **Kansas Health Occupations Credentialing**
**Board of Adult Care Home Administrators**
1000 SW Jackson, Ste. 330
Topeka, KS 66612-1365
**Phone:** (785)296-0061    **Fax:** (785)296-3075
**Email:** bnesbitt@kdhe.state.ks.us
**Website:** http://www.kdhe.state.ks.us/hoc/index.html
Brenda Nesbitt, Contact

★ **15945** ★ **Kentucky Board of Licensure for Nursing Home Administrators**
PO Box 1360
Frankfort, KY 40602
**Phone:** (502)564-3296    **Fax:** (502)564-4818
**Email:** Barbara.Sudduth@mail.state.ky.us
**Website:** http://www.state.ky.us/agencies/finance/occupations/nursinghomeadmin
Barbara Sudduth, Contact

★ **15946** ★ **Louisiana State Board of Examiners for Nursing Facility Administrators**
5615 Corporate Blvd., Ste. 8D
Baton Rouge, LA 70808
**Phone:** (225)922-0009    **Fax:** (225)922-0006
**Email:** 103736.1436@compuserve.com
**Website:** http://www.dhh.state.la.us/boards.HTM
C. Kemp Wright, Director

★ **15947** ★ **Maine Nursing Home Administrator Licensing Board**
35 State House Station
Augusta, ME 04333-0035
**Phone:** (207)624-8420    **Fax:** (207)624-8637
**Email:** elaine.m.thibodeau@state.me.us
**Website:** http://www.state.me.us/pfr/olr/categories/cat27.htm
Elaine Thibodeau, Contact

★ **15948** ★ **Maryland Board of Examiners for Nursing Home Administrators**
4201 Patterson Ave.
Baltimore, MD 21215-2299
**Phone:** (410)764-4750    **Fax:** (410)358-9187
**Email:** hannigap@dhmh.state.md.us
**Website:** http://www.dhmh.state.md.us/bonha/

★ **15949** ★ **Massachusetts Board of Registration for Nursing Home Administrators**
239 Causeway St., Ste. 500
Boston, MA 02114
**Phone:** (617)727-9925    **Fax:** (617)727-2197
**Email:** stephen.j.nemmers@state.ma.us
**Website:** http://www.state.ma.us/reg/boards/nh/default.htm
Stephen Nemmers, PhD, Director

★ **15950** ★ **Michigan Bureau of Health Services**
**Board of Nursing Home Administrators**
PO Box 30670
Lansing, MI 48909
**Phone:** (517)335-0918    **Fax:** (517)373-2179
**Email:** bhserinfo@cis.state.mi.us
**Website:** http://www.cis.state.mi.us/bcs/nha/home.htm

★ **15951** ★ **Minnesota Board of Examiners for Nursing Home Administrators**
2829 University Ave. SE, Ste. 440
Minneapolis, MN 55414-3245

**Phone:** (612)617-2117    **Fax:** (612)617-2119
**Email:** BENHA@state.mn.us
**Website:** http://www.benha.state.mn.us/
Randy Snyder, Director

★ **15952** ★ **Mississippi State Board of Nursing Home Administrators**
1400 Lakeover Rd., Ste. 120
Jackson, MS 39213
**Phone:** (601)364-2310    **Fax:** (601)364-2306
**Email:** cwalker@bnha.state.ms.us
**Website:** http://www.bnha.state.ms.us/
Cathy Walker, Director

★ **15953** ★ **Montana Board of Nursing Home Administrators**
Arcade Bldg, Lower Level
111 North Jackson
PO Box 200513
Helena, MT 59620
**Phone:** (406)444-3561    **Fax:** (406)444-1667
Pamela Bragg, Contact

★ **15954** ★ **Nebraska Health and Human Services Regulation and Licensing Credentialing Division**
**Board of Examiners of Nursing Home Administration**
301 Centennial Mall South, 3rd floor
PO Box 94986
Lincoln, NE 68509-4986
**Phone:** (402)471-2115    **Fax:** (402)471-3577
**Email:** marie.mcclatchey@hhss.state.ne.us
**Website:** http://www.hhs.state.ne.us/crl/crlindex.htm
Helen Meeks, Contact

★ **15955** ★ **New Jersey Department of Health and Senior Services**
**Long Term Care Systems**
**New Jersey Nursing Home Administrators Licensing Board**
PO Box 367
120 S Stockton St.
Trenton, NJ 08625-0367
**Phone:** (609)633-9051    **Fax:** (609)633-9087
**Email:** ltc@doh.state.nj.us
**Website:** http://www.state.nj.us/health/ltc/nhalb.htm

★ **15956** ★ **New Mexico Board of Nursing Home Administrators**
2055 Pacheco St., Ste. 400
Santa Fe, NM 87504
**Phone:** (505)476-7122    **Fax:** (505)827-7095
**Email:** NursingHomeAdminBd@state.nm.us
**Website:** http://www.rld.state.nm.us/b&c/nhab/index.htm
Carmen E. Payne, Contact

★ **15957** ★ **New York State Department of Health - Office of Continuing Care**
**Bureau of Professional Credentialing**
**Board of Examiners of Nursing Home Administrators**
161 Delaware Ave.
Delmar, NY 12054
**Phone:** (518)478-1060    **Fax:** (518)478-1058
**Email:** nyhealth@health.state.ny.us
**Website:** http://www.health.state.ny.us/nysdoh/provider/nhadmin/instructions.htm

★ **15958** ★ **North Carolina State Board of Examiners for Nursing Home Administrators**
3733 National Dr., Ste. 228
Raleigh, NC 27612
**Phone:** (919)571-4164    **Fax:** (919)571-4166
**Email:** ncbenha@mindspring.com
**Website:** http://www.ncbenha.org/
Jane A. Baker, Director

★ **15959** ★ **North Dakota Board of Examiners for Nursing Home Administrators**
1900 N 11th St.
Bismarck, ND 58501-1914
**Phone:** (701)222-4867    **Fax:** (701)223-0977
**Email:** hermanb@btigate.com
**Website:** http://www.governor.state.nd.us/boards/boards-query.asp?Board_ID=73
Bev Herman, Contact

★ **15960** ★ **Ohio Board of Examiners for Nursing Home Administrators**
246 N High St, 1st floor
PO Box 118
Columbus, OH 43216-0118
**Phone:** (614)466-5114    **Fax:** (614)466-0271
**Email:** dandrews@gw.odh.state.oh.us
**Website:** http://www.ohiobenha.org/
Douglas R. Andrews, Contact

★ **15961** ★ **Oklahoma State Department of Health**
**Home Care Administrator Registry**
1000 NE 10th, Rm. 1109
Oklahoma City, OK 73117
**Phone:** (405)271-4093
**Website:** http://www.health.state.ok.us/PROGRAM/hcar/index.html

★ **15962** ★ **Oregon Board of Examiners of Nursing Home Administrators**
Portland State Office Bldg., Ste. 407C
800 NE Oregon, Ste. 21
Portland, OR 97232
**Phone:** (503)731-4046    **Fax:** (503)731-4207
**Email:** barbara.orazio@state.or.us
Barbara Orazio, Contact

★ **15963** ★ **Pennsylvania State Board of Examiners of Nursing Home Administrators**
PO Box 2649
Harrisburg, PA 17105-2649
**Phone:** (717)783-7155    **Fax:** (717)787-7769
**Email:** nha@pados.dos.state.pa.us
**Website:** http://www.dos.state.pa.us/bpoa/cwp/view.asp?a=1104&q=432855

★ **15964** ★ **Rhode Island Health Services Regulation Division**
**Board of Examiners for Nursing Home Administrators**
3 Capitol Hill, Rm 105
Providence, RI 02908-5097
**Phone:** (401)222-5888    **Fax:** (401)222-3352
**Email:** PaulaM@doh.state.ri.us
**Website:** http://www.health.state.ri.us/hsr/nh_admin.htm
Paula Morrissey, Contact

★ **15965** ★ **South Carolina Board of Long Term Health Care Administrators**
Koger Office Park
Kingstree Bldg.
110 Centerview Dr., Ste. 202
PO Box 11329
Columbia, SC 29211-1329
**Phone:** (803)896-4544    **Fax:** (803)896-4555
**Email:** welbornd@mail.llr.state.sc.edu
**Website:** http://www.llr.state.sc.us/POL/LongTermHealthCare/Default.htm
Dana Welborn, Contact

★ **15966** ★ **South Dakota Board of Examiners for Nursing Home Administrators**
PO Box 632
Sioux Falls, SD 57101-0632

**Phone:** (605)331-5040       **Fax:** (605)331-2043
**Email:** sdnha@uswestmail.net
**Website:** http://www.state.sd.us/dcr/nursinghome/nu-rhom-h.htm
Joyce Vos, Contact

★ 15967 ★ **Tennessee Board of Examiners for Nursing Home Administrators**
Cordell Hull Bldg., 1st Fl.
425 Fifth Ave. N
Nashville, TN 37247-1010
**Phone:** (615)532-5155      **Free:** 888-310-4650
**Fax:** (615)532-5369
**Website:** http://www2.state.tn.us/health/Boards/NHA/index.htm
Harold Walker, Contact

★ 15968 ★ **Texas Department of Human Services**
**Nursing Facility Administrator Advisory Committee**
701 W 51st St.
PO Box 149030
Austin, TX 78714
**Free:** 888-834-7406
**Email:** credential@dhs.state.tx.us
**Website:** http://www.dhs.state.tx.us/programs/ltc/credentialing/

★ 15969 ★ **Utah Board of Nursing Home Administrator Licensure**
160 E 300 S, 4th Fl.
PO Box 146741
Salt Lake City, UT 84114-6741
**Phone:** (801)530-6254      **Free:** (866)275-3675
**Fax:** (801)530-6511
**Website:** http://www.dopl.utah.gov/

★ 15970 ★ **Vermont Board of Examiners of Nursing Home Administrators**
26 Terrace St.
Drawer 09
Montpelier, VT 05609-1101
**Phone:** (802)828-2453      **Fax:** (802)828-2496
**Email:** bashford@sec.state.vt.us
**Website:** http://vtprofessionals.org/opr1/nursing_homes/
Bob Ashford, Contact

★ 15971 ★ **Virginia Board of Nursing Home Administrators**
6606 W Broad St., 4th Fl.
Richmond, VA 23230-1717
**Phone:** (804)662-7457      **Free:** 800-533-1560
**Fax:** (804)662-7246
**Email:** denbd@dhp.state.va.us
**Website:** http://www.dhp.state.va.us/nha/default.htm
Sandra Reen, Director

★ 15972 ★ **Washington State Department of Health**
**Health Professions Quality Assurance Board for Nursing Home Administrators**
1300 SE Quince St.
PO Box 47860
Olympia, WA 98504-7860
**Phone:** (360)236-4700      **Fax:** (360)236-4818
**Email:** hpqa.csc@doh.wa.gov
**Website:** https://wws2.wa.gov/doh/hpqa-licensing/HPS3/Nursing_Home_Admin/default.htm

★ 15973 ★ **West Virginia Nursing Home Administrator Board**
5303 Kensington Dr.
Cross Lanes, WV 25313
**Phone:** (304)759-0722
**Website:** http://www.state.wv.us/bep/lmi/license/LICOCCMS.HTMnursing home administrator

★ 15974 ★ **Wisconsin Regulation and Licensing Department**
**Nursing Home Administrators Examining Board**
1400 East Washington Ave.
PO Box 8935
Madison, WI 53708-8935
**Phone:** (608)266-5511      **Fax:** (608)267-3816
**Email:** web@drl.state.wi.us
**Website:** http://www.drl.state.wi.us/Regulation/applicant_information/dod036.html

★ 15975 ★ **Wyoming State Board of Nursing Home Administrators**
1116 Logan Ave., Rm. 106
Cheyenne, WY 82002
**Phone:** (307)432-0465      **Fax:** (307)432-0492
**Email:** vspire@state.wy.us
**Website:** http://soswy.state.wy.us/director/ag-bd/n-home.htm
Vicki L. Spires, Contact

# State & Regional Organizations

## Health Care

*The following are state affiliates of the American Health Care Association (1201 L St. NW, Washington, DC 20005, (202)842-4444, http://www.ahca.org/), a national organization representing long term health care facilities.*

### Alabama

★ 15976 ★ **Alabama Nursing Home Association**
4156 Carmichael Rd.
Montgomery, AL 36106
**Phone:** (334)271-6214      **Fax:** (334)244-6509
**Email:** anha@anha.org
**Website:** http://www.anha.org
Nancy Thomas, Contact

### Alaska

★ 15977 ★ **Alaska State Hospital and Nursing Home Association**
426 Main St.
Juneau, AK 99801
**Phone:** (907)586-1790      **Fax:** (907)463-3573
**Email:** ldashnha@eagle.ptialaska.net
**Website:** http://www.ashnha.com
Linda Fink, Contact

### Arizona

★ 15978 ★ **Arizona Health Care Association**
5020 N 8th Pl., Ste. A
Phoenix, AZ 85014
**Phone:** (602)265-5331      **Fax:** (602)265-4401
**Email:** azhca@goodnet.com
**Website:** http://www.azhca.org
Kathleen Collins Pagels, Contact

### Arkansas

★ 15979 ★ **Arkansas Health Care Association**
1401 W Capitol, Ste. 180
Little Rock, AR 72201
**Phone:** (501)374-4422      **Fax:** (501)374-1077
**Email:** arkhca@aol.com
**Website:** http://arhealthcare.com
Randy Wyatt, Director

### California

★ 15980 ★ **California Association of Health Facilities**
California Center for Assisted Living
PO Box 537004
2201 K St.
Sacramento, CA 95853
**Phone:** (916)441-6400      **Fax:** (916)441-6441
**Email:** gmacomber@cahf.mailport.com
**Website:** http://www.cahf.org
Peggy Goldstein, Contact

### Colorado

★ 15981 ★ **Colorado Health Care Association**
225 E 16th Ave., Ste. 1100
Denver, CO 80203
**Phone:** (303)861-8228      **Fax:** (303)839-8068
**Email:** amiles@cohca.org
**Website:** http://www.cohca.org
Arlene Miles, Director

### Connecticut

★ 15982 ★ **Connecticut Association of Health Care Facilities**
Connecticut Center for Assisted Living
99 E River Dr., 8th Fl.
East Hartford, CT 06108
**Phone:** (860)290-9424      **Fax:** (860)290-9478
**Website:** http://www.cahcf.org
Toni Fatone, Vice President

### Delaware

★ 15983 ★ **Delaware Health Care Facilities Association**
726 Loveville Rd., Ste. 3000
Hockessin, DE 19707
**Phone:** (302)235-6895      **Fax:** (302)235-6899
Yrene E. Waldron, Director

### District of Columbia

★ 15984 ★ **District of Columbia Health Care Association**
1250 H St. NW, Ste. 555
Washington, DC 20005
**Phone:** (202)393-5712      **Fax:** (202)393-7180
**Email:** dbeck@ppsv.com
David Beck, Director

### Florida

★ 15985 ★ **Florida Health Care Association**
Florida Center for Assisted Living
307 W Park Ave.
Tallahassee, FL 32301
**Phone:** (850)224-3907      **Fax:** (850)681-2075
**Email:** wphelan@fhca.org
**Website:** http://www.fhca.org
William Phelan, Director

### Georgia

★ 15986 ★ **Georgia Nursing Home Association**
160 Country Club Dr.
Stockbridge, GA 30281
**Phone:** (678)289-6555      **Fax:** (678)289-6400
**Email:** fwatson@gnha.org
**Website:** http://www.gnha.org/
Fred Watson, President

## Hawaii

**★ 15987 ★ Healthcare Association of Hawaii**
932 Ward Ave., Ste. 430
Honolulu, HI 96814
**Phone:** (808)521-8961　　　**Fax:** (808)599-2879
**Email:** jwhite@hah.org
**Website:** http://www.hah.org
Terri J. Byers, Contact

## Idaho

**★ 15988 ★ Idaho Health Care Association**
Idaho Center for Assisted Living
802 W Bannock, Ste. 304
PO Box 2623
Boise, ID 83701
**Phone:** (208)343-9735　　　**Fax:** (208)343-6891
**Email:** scott@ihca-net.org
**Website:** http://www.ihca-net.org
Robert Van de Merwe, Contact

## Illinois

**★ 15989 ★ Illinois Health Care Association**
1029 S 4th St.
Springfield, IL 62703
**Phone:** (217)528-6455　　　**Fax:** (217)528-0452
**Email:** info@ihca.com
**Website:** http://www.ihca.com
William Kempiners, Director

## Indiana

**★ 15990 ★ Indiana Health Care Association**
Indiana Center for Assisted Living
1 N Capitol, Ste. 1115
Indianapolis, IN 46204
**Phone:** (317)636-6406　　　**Fax:** (317)638-3749
**Email:** info@ihca.org
**Website:** http://www.ihca.org
Arthur L. Logsdon, J.D., President

## Iowa

**★ 15991 ★ Iowa Health Care Association**
6750 Westown Pkwy., Ste. 100
West Des Moines, IA 50266
**Phone:** (515)327-5020　　　**Fax:** (515)327-5019
**Email:** promans@netins.net
**Website:** http://www.iowahealthcare.org
Steve Ackerson, Vice President

## Kansas

**★ 15992 ★ Kansas Health Care Association**
221 SW 33rd St.
Topeka, KS 66611
**Phone:** (785)267-6003　　　**Fax:** (785)267-0833
**Email:** khca@cjnetworks.com
John Kiefhaber, Vice President

## Kentucky

**★ 15993 ★ Kentucky Association of Health Care Facilities**
9403 Mill Brook Rd.
Louisville, KY 40223
**Phone:** (502)425-5000　　　**Fax:** (502)425-3431
**Email:** kyhealthcare@worldnet.att.net
**Website:** http://www.kahcf.org
Rich Miller, President

## Maine

**★ 15994 ★ Maine Health Care Association**
317 State St.
Augusta, ME 04330
**Phone:** (207)623-1146　　　**Fax:** (207)623-4080
**Website:** http://www.mehca.org
Richard Erb, Contact

## Maryland

**★ 15995 ★ Health Facilities Association of Maryland**
7060 Oakland Mills Rd., Ste. M
Columbia, MD 21046
**Phone:** (410)792-4390　　　**Fax:** (410)792-4617
**Website:** http://www.hfam.org/
Adele Wilzack, President

## Massachusetts

**★ 15996 ★ Massachusetts Extended Care Federation**
2310 Washington St., Ste. 300
Newton Lower Falls, MA 02462
**Phone:** (617)558-0202　　　**Fax:** (617)558-3546
**Website:** http://www.mecf.org
Ned Morse, President

## Michigan

**★ 15997 ★ Health Care Association of Michigan**
c/o Michigan Center for Assisted Living
PO Box 80050
Lansing, MI 48908
**Phone:** (517)627-1561　　　**Fax:** (517)627-3016
**Website:** http://www.hcam.org
Reginald Carter, Vice President

## Minnesota

**★ 15998 ★ Care Providers of Minnesota**
2850 Metro Dr., Ste. 200
Bloomington, MN 55425
**Phone:** (952)854-2844　　　**Fax:** (952)854-6214
**Email:** rcarter@careproviders.org
**Website:** http://www.careproviders.org
Rick Carter, President

## Mississippi

**★ 15999 ★ Mississippi Health Care Association**
114 Marketridge Dr.
Ridgeland, MS 39157
**Phone:** (601)956-3472　　　**Fax:** (601)977-0273
**Website:** http://www.mshca.org
Martha Carole Jones, Director

## Missouri

**★ 16000 ★ Missouri Health Care Association**
236 Metro Dr.
Jefferson City, MO 65109
**Phone:** (573)893-2060　　　**Fax:** (573)893-5248
Earl Carlson, Director

## Nebraska

**★ 16001 ★ Nebraska Health Care Association**
Nebraska Assisted Living Association
421 S 9th St., Ste. 137
Lincoln, NE 68508
**Phone:** (402)435-3551　　　**Fax:** (402)435-4829
**Email:** pats@nhca.org
**Website:** http://www.nhca.org
Patricia Snyder, Director

## Nevada

**★ 16002 ★ Nevada Health Care Association**
4425 S Jones Blvd., Ste. 4
Las Vegas, NV 89103
**Phone:** (702)434-2273　　　**Fax:** (702)434-3974
**Email:** nevitc@msn.com
Charles Perry, Contact

## New Hampshire

**★ 16003 ★ New Hampshire Health Care Association**
125 Airport Rd.
Concord, NH 03301
**Phone:** (603)226-4900　　　**Fax:** (603)226-3376
**Website:** http://www.nhhca.org
John Poirier, Director

## New Jersey

**★ 16004 ★ Health Care Association of New Jersey**
2131 Rte. 33
Hamilton, NJ 08690
**Phone:** (609)890-8700　　　**Fax:** (609)584-1047
**Email:** raatnjahcf@aol.com
**Website:** http://www.hcanj.org
Paul Langevin, Contact

## New Mexico

**★ 16005 ★ New Mexico Health Care Association**
New Mexico Center for Assisted Living
4411 McLeod NE, Ste. G
Albuquerque, NM 87109
**Phone:** (505)880-1088　　　**Fax:** (505)880-1157
**Website:** http://www.nmhca.org
Linda Sechovec, Director

## New York

**★ 16006 ★ New York State Health Facilities Association**
33 Elk St., Ste. 300
Albany, NY 12207
**Phone:** (518)462-4800　　　**Fax:** (518)426-4051
**Email:** estafford@nyshfa.org
**Website:** http://www.nyshfa.org
Richard Herrick, Contact

## North Carolina

**★ 16007 ★ North Carolina Health Care Facilities Association**
5109 Bur Oak Cir.
Raleigh, NC 27612
**Phone:** (919)782-3827　　　**Fax:** (919)787-8418
**Email:** nchcfa@nchcfa.net
**Website:** http://www.nchcfa.org
J. Craig Souza, President

## North Dakota

**★ 16008 ★ North Dakota Long Term Care Association**
1900 N 11th St.
Bismarck, ND 58501
**Phone:** (701)222-0660　　　**Fax:** (701)223-0977
**Email:** ndltca@btigate.com
**Website:** http://www.ndltca.org
Shelly Peterson, President

## Ohio

**★ 16009 ★ Ohio Health Care Association**
Ohio Centers for Assisted Living
55 Green Meadows Dr. S
Lewis Center, OH 43035
**Phone:** (614)436-4154　　　**Fax:** (614)436-0939

**Email:** scochran@ohca.org
**Website:** http://www.ohca.org
Peter van Runkle, Vice President

## Oregon

**★ 16010 ★ Oregon Health Care Association**
Oregon Center for Assisted Living
8995 SW Miley Rd., Ste. 205
Wilsonville, OR 97070
**Phone:** (503)694-6580        **Fax:** (503)694-6587
**Email:** JCatOHCA@aol.com
**Website:** http://www.ohca.com
Jim Carlson, Director

## Pennsylvania

**★ 16011 ★ Pennsylvania Health Care Association**
Center for Assisted Living Management
315 N 2nd St.
Harrisburg, PA 17101
**Phone:** (717)221-1800        **Fax:** (717)221-8690
**Email:** rmoran@phca.org
**Website:** http://www.phca.org
Alan Rosenbloom, Contact

## Rhode Island

**★ 16012 ★ Rhode Island Health Care Association**
57 Kilvert St., Ste. 200
Warwick, RI 02886
**Phone:** (401)732-9333        **Fax:** (401)739-3103
**Email:** rihca@msn.com
**Website:** http://www.rihca.com
Alfred Santos, Vice President

## South Carolina

**★ 16013 ★ South Carolina Health Care Association**
176 Laurelhurst Dr.
Columbia, SC 29210
**Phone:** (803)772-7511        **Fax:** (803)772-7943
**Website:** http://www.schca.org
J. Randall Lee, Vice President

## South Dakota

**★ 16014 ★ South Dakota Health Care Association**
804 N Western Ave.
Sioux Falls, SD 57104
**Phone:** (605)339-2071        **Fax:** (605)339-1354
**Email:** sdhca@worldnet.att.net
**Website:** http://www.sdhca.org
Mark Deak, Director

## Tennessee

**★ 16015 ★ Tennessee Health Care Association**
2809 Foster Ave.
PO Box 100129
Nashville, TN 37224
**Phone:** (615)834-6520        **Fax:** (615)834-2502
**Website:** http://www.thca.org
Richard Sadler, Director

## Texas

**★ 16016 ★ Texas Health Care Association**
4214 Medical Pkwy., 3rd Fl.
Austin, TX 78756
**Phone:** (512)458-1257        **Fax:** (512)467-9575
**Email:** thca@jump.net
**Website:** http://www.txhca.org
Tim Graves, Director

## Utah

**★ 16017 ★ Utah Health Care Association**
275 E South Temple, Ste. 200
Salt Lake City, UT 84111
**Phone:** (801)994-3990        **Fax:** (801)994-3994
**Email:** uhca@vii.com
**Website:** http://www.vii.com/~uhca/
Joan Gallegos, Director

## Vermont

**★ 16018 ★ Vermont Health Care Association**
617 Comstock Rd., Ste. 8
Montpelier, VT 05602
**Phone:** (802)229-5700        **Fax:** (802)223-4826
**Email:** vhca@aol.com
**Website:** http://www.virtualvermont.com/healthcare/vhca
Mary Shriver, Director

## Virginia

**★ 16019 ★ Virginia Health Care Association**
Virginia Center for Assisted Living
2112 W Laburnum Ave., Ste. 206
Richmond, VA 23227
**Phone:** (804)353-9101        **Fax:** (804)353-3098
**Email:** steve.morrisette@vhca.org
**Website:** http://www.vhca.org
Steve Morrisette, President

## Washington

**★ 16020 ★ Washington Health Care Association**
2120 State St. NE, Ste. 102
Olympia, WA 98506
**Phone:** (360)352-3304        **Fax:** (360)754-2412
**Email:** jerryreilly@whca.org
**Website:** http://www.whca.org
Brendan Williams, Contact

## West Virginia

**★ 16021 ★ West Virginia Health Care Association**
8 Capitol St., Ste. 700
Charleston, WV 25301
**Phone:** (304)346-4575        **Fax:** (304)342-0519
**Email:** wvhca@citynet.net
**Website:** http://www.wvhca.org
P. John Alfano, CEO

## Wisconsin

**★ 16022 ★ Wisconsin Health Care Association**
121 S Pinckney St., Ste. 500
Madison, WI 53703
**Phone:** (608)257-0125        **Fax:** (608)257-0025
**Website:** http://www.whca.com
Thomas Moore, Director

## Wyoming

**★ 16023 ★ Wyoming Health Care Association**
PO Box 2270
Cheyenne, WY 82003
**Phone:** (307)635-0178        **Fax:** (307)635-1911
Tom Jones, Contact

# Chapter 44
# Nutrition

## Federal Government Agencies

★ 16024 ★ **U.S. Department of Agriculture**
**Agricultural Research Service (ARS)**
5601 Sunnyside Ave., Rm. 1-2250
Beltsville, MD 20705-5128
**Phone:** (301)504-1638          **Fax:** (301)504-1648
**Website:** http://www.usda.gov
**Desc:** The Agricultural Research Service conducts research to develop and transfer solutions to agricultural problems of high national priority. It provides information access and dissemination to ensue high-quality, safe food and other agricultural products; assess the nutritional needs of Americans; sustain a competitive agricultural economy; enhance the natural resource base and the environment; and provide economic opportunities for rural citizens, communities, and society as a whole.

★ 16025 ★ **U.S. Department of Agriculture**
**Center for Nutrition Policy and Promotion**
1120 20th St. NW, Ste. 200
Washington, DC 20036-3406
**Phone:** (202)418-2312          **Fax:** (202)208-2321
**Website:** http://www.cnpp.usda.gov
**Desc:** The Center for Nutrition Policy and Promotion coordinates nutrition policy in the USDA and provides overall leadership in nutrition education for the American public. It also coordinates with the Department of Health and Human Services in the review, revision, and dissemination of the *Dietary Guidelines for Americans,* the federal government's statement of nutrition policy formed by a consensus of scientific and medical professionals.

★ 16026 ★ **U.S. Department of Agriculture**
**Food and Nutrition Service**
3101 Park Center Dr.
Alexandria, VA 22302
**Phone:** (703)305-2286          **Fax:** (703)305-2420
**Website:** http://www.usda.gov/fns.htm
**Desc:** The Food and Nutrition Service, operated in cooperation with states and local governments, administers programs to make food assistance available to people in need. In particular, the service administers Special Nutrition Programs designed to improve the nutrition of children, particularly those from low income families.

**U.S. Department of Health and Human Services**
**Food and Drug Administration**
**Center for Food Safety and Applied Nutrition**
*See:* Entry 17864

## Foundations & Other Funding Organizations

### Private Foundations

**Beneficia Foundation**
*See:* Entry 73

**Mary Reynolds Babcock Foundation**
*See:* Entry 5559

### Corporate Foundations

**Campbell Soup Foundation**
*See:* Entry 915

★ 16027 ★ **Conoco, Inc.**
Box 2197
Houston, TX 77252
**Phone:** (281)293-5778          **Fax:** (281)293-2767
**Email:** info@mrbf.org
**Website:** http://www.mrbf.org
Mary Jane Mudd, Director, Corp. Community Affairs
**Priorities:** *Arts & Humanities:* 25%. Supports cultural and arts institutions in directly pursuing their traditional missions. Company often sponsors culturally-diverse programs. *Civic & Public Affairs:* 25%. Focus is on neighborhood revitalization, safety issues, and other community improvement activities. Support reflects the cultural diversity of the metropolitan Houston area. *Education:* 25%. Grants are made to selected colleges and universities to improve academic resources. Also supports higher education funds for academicresearch on a technical, social, or economic level. Other interests include summer scholarship and co-op programs, and opportunities for minorities in engineering, business, and geoscience. Precollege interests include reduction of absenteeism and drop-out rates, with an emphasis on programs developing critical thinking skills, math, and science. Also supports employee matching gift program and funding for the education of employee family members. *International:* 25%. Focus is on preventive programs with direct benefit to the community and the disadvantaged, as opposed to medical research or the treatment of individuals. Also makes large donations to the United Way on an annual basis. *Note:* Total contributions made in 1998. **Typ. Recipients:** Nutrition. **Geo. Dist:** geographical areas where facilities and employees are located.

**Hasbro Children's Foundation**
*See:* Entry 11435

**Hershey Foods Corp.**
*See:* Entry 11437

**Lipton Foundation**
*See:* Entry 1206

**McCormick & Co. Inc.**
*See:* Entry 18222

★ 16028 ★ **Novartis US Foundation**
564 Morris Ave.
A-2081
Summit, NJ 07901
**Phone:** (908)277-5850          **Fax:** (908)277-4680
**Email:** david.s1-french@pharma.novartis.com
**Website:** http://www.hersheys.com
David French, Director
**Priorities:** *Arts & Humanities:* 20%. Provide funding for national and community based organizations such as the National Black Arts Festival, and community arts councils. *Civic & Public Affairs:* 20%. Supports Chambers of Commerce. *Education:* 20%. Supports the character Education Program, AgriScience computer laboratory, the Reading Connections Literacy program, the SEED Program, the South Louisiana School-to-Work Initiative, and scholarships and internships in the sciences. *International:* 20%. **Typ. Recipients:** Nutrition. **Geo. Dist:** principally near operating locations and to national organizations.

**Toyota U.S.A. Foundation**
*See:* Entry 1444

### Other Funding Organizations

★ 16029 ★ **American Dietetic Association (ADA)**
216 W Jackson Blvd.
Chicago, IL 60606-6995
**Phone:** (312)899-0040          **Free:** 800-877-1600
**Fax:** (312)899-1979
**Email:** membrshp@eatright.org
**Website:** http://www.eatright.org
Ronald Moen, CEO
**Desc:** Food and nutrition professionals. Promotes nutrition, health and well-being. **Awards:** Recognition; scholarship.

★ 16030 ★ **American Society for Parenteral and Enteral Nutrition (ASPEN)**
8630 Fenton Ste., No. 412
Silver Spring, MD 20910-3805
**Phone:** (301)587-6315          **Fax:** (301)587-2365
**Email:** aspen@nutr.org
**Website:** http://www.nutritioncare.org
Robin Kriegel, Exec. Dir.
**Desc:** Physicians, dietitians, nurses, pharmacists, and members of the industry. Works to promote quality patient care, education, and research in the field of nutrition and metabolic support in all health care settings. Educates health care professionals. Conducts postgraduate courses and research programs; compiles statistics. **Awards:** Discipline Research

Awards (annual) for research by nurse, dietitian, and pharmacist members of ASPEN; Dudrick Research Scholar Award (annual) for past research accomplishments of a young investigator in the field of nutrition support; RHOADS Foundation Research Award (annual) for nutrition researchers in the early stages of their careers, to encourage research in the fields of nutrition and metabolic support and related areas of clinical nutrition; Vars Award (annual) for best research by a young investigator at each Clincial Congress.

★ 16031 ★ **Consultant Dietitians in Health Care Facilities (CDHCF)**
2219 Cardinal Dr.
Waterloo, IA 50701
**Phone:** (319)235-0991　　**Fax:** (319)235-7224
**Email:** cdhcf@cdhcf.org
**Website:** http://www.cdhcf.org
Marolyn Steffani, RD, LD, Chm.
**Desc:** A special interest group of the American Dietetic Association. Dietitians employed in extended care facilities, nursing homes, homecare, and a variety of food service operations. Disseminates information; assists in solving their problems in the field. Conducts workshops; offers networking opportunities for professionals. **Awards:** CDHCF Horizon Award (annual); CDHCF Scholarship Award (annual); Gaynold Jenson Education Stipend (annual).

★ 16032 ★ **International Union of Nutritional Sciences (IUNS)**
c/o Prof. Osman M. Galal
UCLA School of Public Health
International Health Program
PO Box 951772
Los Angeles, CA 90095-1772
**Phone:** (310)206-9639　　**Fax:** (310)794-1805
**Email:** ogalal@ucla.edu
**Website:** http://www.iuns.org
Prof. O.M. Galal, Contact
**Desc:** National nutritional societies. Promotes international cooperation in the scientific study of nutrition and its applications. Encourages research and the exchange of scientific information. Cooperates with the Food and Agriculture Organization of the United Nations, the United Nations Educational, Scientific and Cultural Organization, and the World Health Organization. Maintains 24 committees. **Awards:** IUNS Award (quadrennial); IUNS Fellow (quadrennial).

★ 16033 ★ **Lifegain Institute (LI)**
115 Dunder Rd.
Burlington, VT 05401
**Phone:** (802)862-8855　　**Fax:** (802)862-6389
**Email:** info@healthyculture.com
**Website:** http://www.healthyculture.com
Judd Allen, PhD, Pres.
**Desc:** People who work with health promotion programs in hospitals, corporations, colleges, and communities. Promotes healthy practices such as exercise, nutrition, safety, and the reduction or curtailment of smoking and alcohol consumption through health promotion programs that provide a supportive environment. Maintains speakers' bureau. Compiles data on improvements cultural support nationwide. **Awards:** Robert F. Symbol of HOPE Award (annual) for health promotion contribution to underserved populations.

# Medical & Allied Health Schools

## Dietetics

*Listed below are coordinated dietetic programs accredited by the Commission on Accreditation/ Approval for Dietetics Education of the American Dietetic Association. These programs offer academic preparation and clinical experience at the bachelor and master's levels. The Association also accredits post-baccalaureate dietetic internships and pre-professional practice programs and approves didactic programs in dietetics, as well as dietetic technician programs. For information on these, as well as advanced degree programs in nutrition and related areas, contact the American Dietetic Association, 216 W Jackson Blvd., Chicago, IL 60606-6995, (312)899-0040, http://www.eatright.org/.*

## Alabama

★ 16034 ★ **Alabama A & M University Division of Family and Consumer Services Nutrition and Hospitality Management**
PO Box 639
Normal, AL 35762-0639
**Phone:** (256)858-4103　　**Fax:** (256)851-5433
**Email:** awarren@asnaam.edu
Ann P. Warren, Director

★ 16035 ★ **Auburn University Nutrition and Food Science Dietetics-Didactic Program**
328 Spidle Hall
Auburn, AL 36849-5605
**Phone:** (334)844-4261　　**Fax:** (334)844-3268
**Email:** rfellers@humsci.auburn.edu
**Website:** http://www.humsci.auburn.edu/
Robin B. Fellers, PhD, Director

★ 16036 ★ **Jacksonville State University Family and Consumer Sciences Dietetics-Didactic Program**
Mason Hall
Jacksonville, AL 36265
**Phone:** (205)782-5054　　**Fax:** (205)782-5916
**Email:** dgoodwin@jsucc_jsu.edu
Debra K. Goodwin, Director

★ 16037 ★ **Oakwood College Family and Consumer Science Dietetics-Preprofessional Practice Program**
Oakwood Rd.
Huntsville, AL 35896
**Phone:** (256)726-7228　　**Fax:** (256)726-7233
**Email:** calcock@oakwood.edu
Claudia S. Alcock, Director

★ 16038 ★ **Oakwood College Family and Consumer Sciences Dietetics-Didactic Program**
7000 Adventist Blvd.
Huntsville, AL 35896
**Phone:** (256)726-7230　　**Fax:** (256)726-7233
**Email:** dsmith@oakwood.edu
**Website:** http://www.oakwood.edu/fcs/
Donna A. Smith, Director

★ 16039 ★ **Samford University Family and Consumer Education Dietetics-Didactic Program**
800 Lakeshore Dr.
Birmingham, AL 35229-2239
**Phone:** (205)726-2930　　**Fax:** (205)726-2068
**Email:** pchart@samford.edu
**Website:** http://www.samford.edu/
Patricia C. Hart, PhD, Director

★ 16040 ★ **Tuskegee University Food and Nutrition Sciences**
204 Campbell Hall
Tuskegee, AL 36083
**Phone:** (334)727-8326　　**Fax:** (334)727-8493
**Email:** ghebwp@tusk.edu
Beatrice W. Phillips, EdD, Director

★ 16041 ★ **University of Alabama Department of Human Nutrition and Hospitality Management**
PO Box 870158
Tuscaloosa, AL 35487-0158
**Phone:** (205)348-8130　　**Fax:** (205)348-3789
**Email:** dmorriso@ches.ua.edu
Debra W. Morrison, Director

★ 16042 ★ **University of Alabama Department of Human Nutrition and Hospitality Management Dietetics-Didactic Program**
PO Box 870158
Tuscaloosa, AL 35487-0158
**Phone:** (205)348-4710　　**Fax:** (205)348-3789
**Email:** shancock@ches.ua.edu
**Website:** http://www.ches.ua.edu
Shelley R. Hancock, Director
Debra W. Morrison, Contact

★ 16043 ★ **University of Alabama, Birmingham Department of Nutritional Sciences Dietetic Internship Program**
1675 University Blvd.
Webb Bldg., Rm. 212
Birmingham, AL 35294
**Phone:** (205)934-3006　　**Fax:** (205)934-7049
**Email:** canfield@uab.edu
Gayl J. Canfield, PhD, Director

★ 16044 ★ **University of Montevallo Family and Consumer Sciences Dietetics-Didactic Program**
Station 6385
Bloch Hall
Montevallo, AL 35115-6000
**Phone:** (205)665-6385　　**Fax:** (205)665-6387
**Email:** andrews@um.montevallo.edu
**Website:** http://www.montevallo.edu/
Frances E. Andrews, PhD, Director

## Alaska

★ 16045 ★ **University of Alaska, Anchorage Dietetics-Preprofessional Practice Program**
3211 Providence Dr.
Anchorage, AK 99508
**Phone:** (907)786-1362　　**Fax:** (907)786-1402
**Email:** annok@uaa.alaska.edu
Nancy Overpeck, EdD, Director

## Arizona

★ 16046 ★ **Arizona State University East Department of Nutrition Dietetic Internship Program**
7001 E Williams Field Rd., Bldg. 20
Mesa, AZ 85212
**Phone:** (480)727-1722　　**Fax:** (480)727-1064
**Email:** rose.martin@asu.edu
Rose L. Martin, Director

★ 16047 ★ **Arizona State University East Department of Nutrition Dietetics-Didactic Program**
7001 E Williams Field Rd.
Mesa, AZ 85212
**Phone:** (480)727-1722
**Email:** linda.vaughan@asu.edu
Linda A. Vaughan, PhD, Director

**★ 16048 ★ Carondelet Saint Mary's Hospital**
**Dietetic Internship Program**
1601 W St. Mary's Rd.
Tucson, AZ 85745
**Phone:** (520)740-6109　　　**Fax:** (520)740-6108
**Email:** kyee@carondelet.org
Kelli Jo Yee, Director

**★ 16049 ★ Focus on Nutrition**
**Dietetics-Preprofessional Practice Program**
3923 E Thunderbird Rd., Stes. 26-113
Phoenix, AZ 85032
**Phone:** (602)788-7096　　　**Fax:** (602)404-8596
**Email:** kwardrd@aol.com
Kimberly A. Ward, Director

**★ 16050 ★ Maricopa County Department of Public Health**
**Office of Nutrition Services**
**Dietetics-Preprofessional Practice Program**
1414 W Broadway, Ste. 237
Tempe, AZ 85282
**Phone:** (480)966-3090　　　**Fax:** (480)966-3233
**Email:** shirleystrembel@mail.maricopa.gov
Shirley K. Strembel, Director

**★ 16051 ★ Northern Arizona University**
**Food and Nutrition Science**
**Dietetics-Didactic Program**
NAU Box 15095
Flagstaff, AZ 86011-5095
**Phone:** (520)523-6164　　　**Fax:** (520)523-0148
**Email:** njc3@jan.ucc.nau.edu
Nancy J. Cahill, Director

**★ 16052 ★ Paradise Valley Unified School District**
**Dietetics-Preprofessional Practice Program**
20621 N 32nd St.
Phoenix, AZ 85050
**Phone:** (602)493-6330　　　**Fax:** (602)493-6334
**Email:** kglindmeier@pvusd.k12.az.us
Kathleen M. Glindmeier, Director

**★ 16053 ★ University of Arizona**
**Department of Nutritional Sciences**
**Dietetics-Didactic Program**
Tucson, AZ 85721-0038
**Phone:** (520)621-1619　　　**Fax:** (520)621-9446
**Email:** whhowell@ag.arizona.edu
**Website:** http://ag.arizona.edu/NSC/nschome.htm
Wanda Hain Howell, PhD, Director

**★ 16054 ★ University of Arizona**
**Support Services**
**Dietetic Internship Program**
1501 N Campbell Ave.
Tucson, AZ 85724-5088
**Phone:** (520)694-7563　　　**Fax:** (520)694-6617
**Email:** sbristol@umcaz.edu
Susan E. Bristol, Director

**★ 16055 ★ Yavapai County Health Department**
**Dietetic Internship Program**
930 Division St.
Prescott, AZ 86301
**Phone:** (520)771-3138　　　**Fax:** (520)771-3369
**Email:** wic1300@hs.state.az.us
Judy S. Lee-Norris, Director

## Arkansas

**★ 16056 ★ Harding University**
**Department of Family and Consumer Sciences**
**Dietetics-Didactic Program**
Box 12233
900 E Center Ave.
Searcy, AR 72149-0001
**Phone:** (501)279-4472　　　**Fax:** (501)279-4098
**Email:** lritchie@harding.edu
Lisa Ritchie, Director

**★ 16057 ★ Henderson State University**
**Department of Family and Consumer Sciences**
**Dietetics-Didactic Program**
PO Box 7510
Arkadelphia, AR 71999-0001
**Phone:** (870)230-5542　　　**Fax:** (870)230-5455
**Email:** lockwol@hsu.edu
Laura P. Lockwood, Director

**★ 16058 ★ Ouachita Baptist University**
**Department of Biology**
**Dietetics-Didactic Program**
PO Box 3769
Arkadelphia, AR 71998-0001
**Phone:** (870)245-5542　　　**Fax:** (870)245-5500
**Email:** freemans@alpha.obu.edu
**Website:** http://www.obu.edu/biology/program_in_dietetics.htm
Stacy L. Freeman, Director

**★ 16059 ★ University of Arkansas**
**School of Human Environmental Sciences**
**Dietetics-Didactic Program**
118 HOEC
Fayetteville, AR 72701
**Phone:** (501)575-4306　　　**Fax:** (501)575-7171
**Email:** mfitch@comp.uark.edu
**Website:** http://www.uark.edu/depts/hesweb/index.html
Marjorie E. Fitch-Hilgenberg, PhD, Director

**★ 16060 ★ University of Arkansas for Medical Sciences**
**Veterans Affairs Medical Center**
**Dietetic Internship Program**
4301 W Markham St., Slot 627
Little Rock, AR 72205-7199
**Phone:** (501)686-5714　　　**Fax:** (501)686-5716
**Email:** carrollpollya@exchange.uams.edu
Polly A. Carroll, Director

**★ 16061 ★ University of Arkansas, Pine Bluff**
**Department of Home Economics**
**Dietetics-Didactic Program**
PO Box 4971
Pine Bluff, AR 71611
**Phone:** (870)543-8817　　　**Fax:** (870)543-8823
**Email:** neal_e@vx4500.uapb.edu
**Website:** http://www.uapb.edu/safhs/index.html
Lucille Meadows, Director

**★ 16062 ★ University of Central Arkansas**
**Family and Consumer Sciences**
**Dietetic Internship Program**
McAlister Hall
Conway, AR 72035
**Phone:** (501)450-5950　　　**Fax:** (501)450-5958
**Email:** lizc@mail.uca.edu
Elizabeth L. Coffman, Director

**★ 16063 ★ University of Central Arkansas**
**Family and Consumer Sciences**
**Dietetics-Didactic Program**
McAlister Hall, Rm. 100
Conway, AR 72035
**Phone:** (501)450-5950　　　**Fax:** (501)450-5958
**Email:** maryh@mail.uca.edu
**Website:** http://www.UCA.EDU/CHAS/diet
Mary H. Harlan, EdD, Director

## California

**★ 16064 ★ California Polytechnic State University**
**Food Science & Nutrition Department**
**Dietetics-Didactic Program**
San Luis Obispo, CA 93407
**Phone:** (805)756-6126　　　**Fax:** (805)756-1146
**Email:** kmcburne@calpoly.edu
**Website:** http://www.calpoly.edu/~fsn/
Kathleen A. McBurney, PhD, Director

**★ 16065 ★ California State Polytechnic University**
**Foods and Nutrition Department**
**Dietetic-Didactic Program**
3801 W Temple Ave.
Pomona, CA 91768-2557
**Phone:** (909)869-2163　　　**Fax:** (909)869-5078
**Email:** macaudill@cusupomona.edu
**Website:** http://www.csupomona.edu/macaudill
Marie A. Caudill, PhD, Director

**★ 16066 ★ California State Polytechnic University**
**Foods and Nutrition/Home Economics**
3801 W Temple Ave.
Pomona, CA 91768-2557
**Phone:** (909)869-2163　　　**Fax:** (909)869-5078
**Email:** kcaldwellfre@csupomona.edu
Kara Caldwell-Freeman, PhD, Director

**★ 16067 ★ California State University, Chico**
**Department of Biological Sciences**
**Dietetics-Didactic Program**
Tehama Hall 124
Chico, CA 95929-0515
**Phone:** (530)898-6805　　　**Fax:** (530)898-4363
**Email:** fjohnson@csuchico.edu
Faye C. Johnson, EdD, Director

**★ 16068 ★ California State University, Chico**
**Nutrition and Food Sciences**
**Department of Biological Sciences**
**Dietetic Internship Program**
Chico, CA 95929-0002
**Phone:** (530)898-6805　　　**Fax:** (530)898-4757
**Email:** bkirks@csuchico.edu
Barbara A. Kirks, EdD, Director

**★ 16069 ★ California State University, Fresno**
**Department of Enology, Food Science and Nutrition**
5300 N Campus Dr., MS FF17
Fresno, CA 93740-8019
**Phone:** (559)278-8009　　　**Fax:** (559)278-7623
**Email:** mollie_smith@csufresno.edu
Mollie M. Smith, Director

**★ 16070 ★ California State University, Fresno**
**Ecology, Food Science and Nutrition**
**Dietetics-Didactic Program**
5300 N Campus Dr.
Fresno, CA 93740-8019
**Phone:** (559)278-2043     **Fax:** (559)278-7623
**Email:** sandra_witte@csufresno.edu
**Website:** http://www.csufresno.edu/fsn
Sandra S. Witte, PhD, Director

**★ 16071 ★ California State University, Long Beach**
**Family and Consumer Sciences**
**Dietetic Internship Program**
1250 N Bellflower Blvd.
Long Beach, CA 90840-0501
**Phone:** (562)985-4494     **Fax:** (562)985-4414
**Email:** gcfrank@csulb.edu
Gail C. Frank, DrPH, Director

**★ 16072 ★ California State University, Long Beach**
**Family and Consumer Sciences**
**Dietetics-Didactic Program**
1250 Bellflower Blvd.
Long Beach, CA 90840-0501
**Phone:** (562)985-4545     **Fax:** (562)985-4414
**Email:** jjlee@csulb.edu
**Website:** http://www.csulb.edu
Jacqueline D. Lee, PhD, Director

**★ 16073 ★ California State University, Los Angeles**
**Health and Nutritional Sciences**
**Coordinated Program in Dietetics**
5151 State University Dr.
Los Angeles, CA 90032-8172
**Phone:** (323)343-5439     **Fax:** (323)343-5016
**Email:** lcalder@jupiter.calstatela.edu
Laura L. Calderon, DrPH, Director

**★ 16074 ★ California State University, Los Angeles**
**Health and Nutritional Sciences**
**Dietetics-Didactic Program**
5151 State University Dr.
Los Angeles, CA 90032-8172
**Phone:** (323)343-5439     **Fax:** (323)343-5016
**Email:** jgota@calstatela.edu
**Website:** http://www.calstatela.edu/dept/hnut_sci/dept_pro.htm
Joyce Y. Gota, Director
Laura Calderon, DrPH, Contact

**★ 16075 ★ California State University, Northridge**
**Family Environmental Sciences**
**Dietetic Internship Program**
18111 Nordhoff St.
Northridge, CA 91330-8308
**Phone:** (818)677-3051
**Email:** elaine.blyler@csun.edu
**Website:** http://www.csun.edu/~hffes003
Elaine M. Blyler, Director

**★ 16076 ★ California State University, Northridge**
**Family Environmental Sciences**
**Dietetics-Didactic Program**
18111 Nordhoff St.
Northridge, CA 91330-8308
**Phone:** (818)677-3051     **Fax:** (818)677-4778
**Email:** christine.smith@csun.edu
Christine H. Smith, PhD, Director

**★ 16077 ★ California State University, Sacramento**
**Human Environmental Sciences**
**Dietetics-Didactic Program**
6000 J St.
Sacramento, CA 95819-6053
**Phone:** (916)278-4271     **Fax:** (916)278-7520
**Email:** salgeert@csus.edu
**Website:** http://www.csus.edu/facs
Susan J. Algert, Director

**★ 16078 ★ California State University, San Bernardino**
**Health Science and Human Ecology**
**Dietetics-Didactic Program**
5500 University Pkwy.
San Bernardino, CA 92407-2318
**Phone:** (909)880-5340     **Fax:** (909)880-7037
**Email:** dchen@csusb.edu
Dorothy C. Chen-Maynard, PhD, Director

**★ 16079 ★ Charles R. Drew University of Medicine and Science**
**College of Allied Health**
**Coordinated Program in Dietetics**
1731 E 120th St.
Los Angeles, CA 90059-3025
**Phone:** (323)563-4811     **Fax:** (323)563-4923
**Email:** madike@cdrewu.edu
Margie R. Bray-Dike, PhD, Director

**★ 16080 ★ Children's Hospital of Los Angeles**
**Child Development and Development Disorders**
**Dietetic Internship Program**
Mailstop 53
PO Box 54700
Los Angeles, CA 90054-0700
**Phone:** (323)669-2300     **Fax:** (323)953-0439
**Email:** aharris@chla.usc.edu
Anne Bradford Harris, Director

**★ 16081 ★ Glendale Memorial Hospital and Health Center**
**Food and Nutrition Services**
**Dietetic Internship Program**
1420 S Central Ave.
Glendale, CA 91204-2594
**Phone:** (818)502-2248     **Fax:** (818)507-4665
**Email:** ncarvalh@mail.unihealth.org
Nicole K. Carvalho, Director

**★ 16082 ★ Loma Linda University**
**Department of Nutrition and Dietetics**
**School of Allied Health Professions**
**Coordinated Program in Dietetics**
Loma Linda, CA 92350
**Phone:** (909)558-4593     **Fax:** (909)558-4291
**Email:** bert-connell@sahp.llu.edu
**Website:** http://www.llu.edu/llu/nutrition
Bert Connell, PhD, Director

**★ 16083 ★ Loma Linda University**
**School of Public Health**
**Nutrition Department**
**Coordinated Program in Dietetics**
Nichol Hall, Rm. 1102
Loma Linda, CA 92350
**Phone:** (909)558-4598     **Fax:** (909)558-4095
**Email:** ehaddad@sph.llu.edu
**Website:** http://www.llu.edu/llu/nutrition/
Ella H. Haddad, DrPH, Director

**★ 16084 ★ Los Angeles County/USC Medical Center**
**Dietetic Internship Program**
1200 N State St., Rm. 1506
Los Angeles, CA 90033-4525
**Phone:** (323)226-6901     **Fax:** (323)222-3422
**Email:** emalacusc@juno.com
Elizabeth H. Ma, Director

**★ 16085 ★ Napa State Hospital**
**Dietetic Internship Program**
2100 Napa Vallejo Hwy.
Napa, CA 94558-6293
**Phone:** (707)253-5428     **Fax:** (707)254-2422
Wen F. Pao, Director

**★ 16086 ★ Olive View/UCLA Medical Center**
**Department of Food and Nutrition**
**Dietetic Internship Program**
14445 Olive View Dr., Rm. 1C112
Sylmar, CA 91342-1438
**Phone:** (818)364-4220     **Fax:** (818)364-3998
**Email:** robmmck@cs.com
Robin M. McKelvey, Director

**★ 16087 ★ Pacific Union College**
**Family and Consumer Sciences**
**Dietetics-Didactic Program**
1 Angwin Ave.
Angwin, CA 94508-6694
**Phone:** (707)965-6694     **Fax:** (707)965-6390
**Email:** kjames@puc.edu
**Website:** http://www.puc.edu
Kenneth D. James, PhD, Director

**★ 16088 ★ Patton State Hospital**
**Dietetic Internship Program**
3102 E Highland Ave.
Patton, CA 92369
**Phone:** (909)425-7575     **Fax:** (909)425-7069
**Email:** asimoran@dmhspsh.state.ca.us
Anneke G. Simorangkir, Director

**★ 16089 ★ Pepperdine University**
**Natural Science Division**
**Dietetics-Didactic Program**
24255 Pacific Coast Hwy.
Malibu, CA 90263-4325
**Phone:** (310)456-4325     **Fax:** (310)456-4785
**Email:** shelm@pepperdine.edu
**Website:** http://www.pepperdine.edu/
Susan E. Helm, PhD, Director

**★ 16090 ★ Porterville Development Center**
**Dietetic Internship Program**
PO Box 2000
Porterville, CA 93258-2000
**Phone:** (559)782-2753     **Fax:** (559)782-2756
**Email:** addintern@ocsnet.net
Christine N. Hahesy, Director

**★ 16091 ★ Public Health Foundation Enterprises**
**WIC Program**
**Dietetic Internship Program**
12781 Schabarum Ave.
Irwindale, CA 91706
**Phone:** (626)856-6618     **Fax:** (626)813-9390
**Email:** robin@phfewic.org
Robin B. Evans, Director

**★ 16092 ★ San Diego State University**
**Exercise and Nutritional Sciences**
**Dietetic Internship Program**
5500 Campanile Dr.
San Diego, CA 92182-7251

**Phone:** (619)594-1341    **Fax:** (619)594-6553
**Email:** cswann@mail.sdsu.edu
Cynthia L. Swann, Director

**★ 16093 ★ San Diego State University**
**Exercise and Nutritional Sciences**
**Dietetics-Didactic Program**
San Diego, CA 92182-7251
**Phone:** (619)594-3045    **Fax:** (619)594-6553
**Email:** spindler@mail.sdsu.edu
**Website:** http://www.sdsu.edu/
Audrey A. Spindler, PhD, Director

**★ 16094 ★ San Francisco State**
**University**
**Consumer and Family Studies/Dietetics**
**Dietetic Internship Program**
1600 Holloway Ave.
San Francisco, CA 94132
**Phone:** (415)338-1219    **Fax:** (415)338-0947
**Email:** ajrigby@sfsu.edu
Alison J. Rigby-Mathews, Director

**★ 16095 ★ San Francisco State**
**University**
**Consumer and Family Studies/Dietetics**
**Dietetics-Didactic Program**
1600 Holloway Ave.
San Francisco, CA 94132-1722
**Phone:** (415)338-1219    **Fax:** (415)338-0947
**Email:** vijay@sfsu.edu
**Website:** http://www.sfsu.edu/
Vijay Ganji, PhD, Director

**★ 16096 ★ San Jose State University**
**Nutrition, Food and Science**
**Dietetic Internship Program**
1 Washington Sq.
San Jose, CA 95192-0058
**Phone:** (408)924-3104    **Fax:** (408)924-3114
Kathryn P. Sucher, ScD, Director

**★ 16097 ★ San Jose State University**
**Nutrition and Food Science**
**Dietetics-Didactic Program**
San Jose, CA 95192-0058
**Phone:** (408)924-3109    **Fax:** (408)924-3114
**Email:** nancyclu@email.sjsu.edu
Nancy C. Lu, PhD, Director

**★ 16098 ★ Univeristy of California—San**
**Francisco**
**Department of Nutrition and Dietetics**
**Dietetic Internship Program**
Medical Center, Box 0212, Rm. M-294
San Francisco, CA 94143-0212
**Phone:** (415)353-1355    **Fax:** (415)476-3181
**Email:** patricia.booth@ucsfmedctr.org
Patricia A. Booth, Director

**★ 16099 ★ University of California,**
**Berkeley**
**Department of Nutritional Sciences**
**Dietetics-Didactic Program**
119 Morgan Hall
Berkeley, CA 94720
**Phone:** (510)642-4090    **Fax:** (510)642-0535
**Email:** hudson@nature.berkeley.edu
**Website:** http://nature.berkeley.edu/departments/nut/
Nancy R. Hudson, Director

**★ 16100 ★ University of California,**
**Berkeley**
**School of Public Health**
**Dietetic Internship Program**
129 Morgan Hall-3104
Berkeley, CA 94720-3104

**Phone:** (510)642-0980    **Fax:** (510)642-0535
**Email:** mmead@nature.berkeley.edu
Mary Mead, Director

**★ 16101 ★ University of California, Davis**
**Department of Nutrition**
**Dietetics-Didactic Program**
1 Shields Ave.
Davis, CA 95616-8669
**Phone:** (530)752-0160    **Fax:** (530)752-8966
**Email:** frmsteinberg@ucdavis.edu
**Website:** http://www.nutrition.ucdavis.edu
Francene M. Steinberg, PhD, Director

**★ 16102 ★ VA San Diego Healthcare**
**System**
**Dietetic Internship Program**
Dietetics and Clinical Nutrition Services 120
3350 La Jolla Village Dr.
San Diego, CA 92161-0002
**Phone:** (858)552-8585    **Fax:** (858)552-4340
**Email:** teresa.bush-zurn@med.va.gov
Teresa Bush-Zurn, Director

**★ 16103 ★ Veterans Affairs Medical**
**Center—West Los Angeles**
**Dietetic Internship Program**
Nutrition and Food Department 120
11301 Wilshire Blvd.
Los Angeles, CA 90073
**Phone:** (310)268-3120    **Fax:** (310)268-4787
**Email:** jenna.mason@med.va.gov
Jenna Mason, Director

**Colorado**

**★ 16104 ★ Centura Health/Penrose-St.**
**Francis Health Services**
**Nutrition Services**
**Dietetic Internship Program**
PO Box 7021
Colorado Springs, CO 80933-7021
**Phone:** (719)776-5863    **Fax:** (719)776-2500
**Email:** yvonnesteinhour@centura.org
Yvonne Steinhour, Director

**★ 16105 ★ Colorado State University**
**Department of Food Science and Human**
**Nutrition**
**Dietetics-Didactic Program or Dietetic**
**Internship Program**
Gifford Bldg., Rm. 205
Fort Collins, CO 80523-1571
**Phone:** (970)491-7462    **Fax:** (970)491-7252
**Email:** harris@lamar.colostate.edu
**Website:** http://www.colostate.edu/Dept/FSHN/
Mary A. Harris, PhD, Director

**★ 16106 ★ Tri-County Health Department**
**Nutrition Services**
**Dietetic Internship Program**
4857 S Broadway
Englewood, CO 80110-6894
**Phone:** (303)761-1340    **Fax:** (303)761-1528
Anne E. Bennett, Director

**★ 16107 ★ University of Northern**
**Colorado**
**Community, Health and Nutrition**
**Dietetic Internship Program**
Gunter 2050
Greeley, CO 80639
**Phone:** (970)351-1769    **Fax:** (970)351-1489
**Email:** nbenell@hhs.unco.edu
Naomi Benell, Director

**★ 16108 ★ University of Northern**
**Colorado**
**Department of Community Health and**
**Nutrition**
**Dietetics-Didactic Program**
Gunter 2320
Greeley, CO 80639
**Phone:** (970)351-1706    **Fax:** (970)351-1489
**Email:** jerskine@hhs.unco.edu
**Website:** http://www.hhs.unco.edu/Diet.htm
Jamie M. Erskine, PhD, Director

**Connecticut**

**★ 16109 ★ Danbury Hospital**
**Preprofessional Practice Program in**
**Dietetics**
24 Hospital Ave.
Danbury, CT 06810-6099
**Phone:** (203)797-7418    **Fax:** (203)797-7619
**Email:** nancy.massari@danhosp.org
Nancy E. Massari, Director

**★ 16110 ★ Saint Joseph College**
**Department of Nutrition and Family**
**Studies**
**Dietetics-Didactic Program**
1678 Asylum Ave.
West Hartford, CT 06117-2700
**Phone:** (860)231-5388    **Fax:** (860)231-8396
**Email:** mlawrence@sjc.edu
Margery L. Lawrence, PhD, Director
Margaret E. Gaughan, PhD, Contact

**★ 16111 ★ Saint Joseph College**
**Nutrition and Family Studies**
**Coordinated Program in Dietetics**
1678 Asylum Ave.
West Hartford, CT 06117-2700
**Phone:** (860)231-5234    **Fax:** (860)231-8396
**Email:** mgaughan@mercy.sjc.edu
Margaret E. Gaughan, PhD, Director

**★ 16112 ★ Saint Joseph College**
**Nutrition and Family Studies**
**Dietetic Internship Program**
1678 Asylum Ave.
West Hartford, CT 06117-2700
**Phone:** (860)232-5254    **Fax:** (860)231-8396
**Email:** dcorcora@sjc.edu
Donna W. Corcoran, Director

**★ 16113 ★ University of Connecticut**
**Dietetics-Didactic Program**
Nutritional Sciences U-17
3624 Horsebarn Rd. Extension
Storrs, CT 06269
**Phone:** (860)486-0119    **Fax:** (860)486-3674
**Email:** eshanley@canrl.cag.uconn.edu
**Website:** http://www.alliedhealth.uconn.edu/acad110.html
Ellen Rosa Shanley, Director

**★ 16114 ★ University of Connecticut**
**School of Allied Health**
**Coordinated Program in Dietetics or**
**Dietetic Internship Program**
358 Mansfield Rd., U-101
Storrs, CT 06269-2101
**Phone:** (860)486-0116    **Fax:** (860)486-1588
**Email:** martha.ludemann@uconn.edu
**Website:** http://www.canr.uconn.edu/nusci/
Martha Ludemann, Director

**★ 16115 ★ University of New Haven**
**School of Hotel/Restaurant/Dietetics and**
 **Tourism Administration**
**Dietetics-Didactic Program**
300 Orange Ave.
West Haven, CT 06516-1916
**Phone:** (203)932-7413          **Fax:** (203)932-7083
**Email:** shrtda@charger.newhaven.edu
**Website:** http://www.newhaven.edu
Beverly A. Bentivegna, MEd, Director

**★ 16116 ★ Yale-New Haven Hospital**
**Food & Nutrition**
**Dietetic Internship Program**
20 York St., GBB
New Haven, CT 06504
**Phone:** (203)785-5074          **Fax:** (203)688-2412
**Email:** ford@gwpo.ynhh.com
Deborah F. Flanel, Director

### Delaware

**★ 16117 ★ Delaware State University**
**Department of Family and Consumer**
 **Sciences**
**Dietetics-Didactic Program**
1200 N Dupont Highway
Dover, DE 19901-2277
**Phone:** (302)857-6440          **Fax:** (302)857-6441
**Email:** mclause@dsc.edu
**Website:** http://www.dsc.edu
Maggie R. Clausell, PhD, Director

**★ 16118 ★ University of Delaware**
**Department of Nutrition and Dietetics**
**Dietetics-Didactic Program**
234A Alison Hall
Newark, DE 19716-3301
**Phone:** (302)831-8976          **Fax:** (302)831-4186
**Email:** mfk@udel.edu
**Website:** http://www.UDEL.EDU
Marie T. Fanelli Kuczmarski, PhD, Director

**★ 16119 ★ University of Delaware**
**Nutrition and Dietetics**
**Dietetic Internship Program**
315 Alison Hall
Newark, DE 19716
**Phone:** (302)831-1677          **Fax:** (302)831-4186
**Email:** hamilton@udel.edu
Charlene Hamilton, PhD, Director

### District of Columbia

**★ 16120 ★ Howard University**
**Department of Nutritional Sciences**
**Dietetics-Didactic Program**
Sixth and Bryant Sts. NW
Annex I
Washington, DC 20059
**Phone:** (202)806-5648          **Fax:** (202)806-9233
**Email:** tbaker@fac.howard.edu
Thelma B. Baker, PhD, Director

**★ 16121 ★ University of the District of**
 **Columbia**
**Department of Biological and**
 **Environmental Sciences**
**Dietetics-Didactic Program**
4200 Connecticut Ave. NW
Bldg. 44, Rm. 200-02
Washington, DC 20008-1173
**Phone:** (202)274-5516          **Fax:** (202)274-5952
**Email:** pganganna@udc.edu
Prema Ganganna, PhD, Director

**★ 16122 ★ Walter Reed Army Medical**
 **Center**
**Nutrition Care Directorate**
**Dietetic Internship Program**
6900 Georgia Ave. NW
Washington, DC 20307-5001
**Phone:** (202)782-6333          **Fax:** (202)782-9289
**Email:** brenda.ellison@NA.Amedd.army.mil
Melanie J. Craig, Director

### Florida

**★ 16123 ★ Florida International**
 **University**
**Department of Dietetics and Nutrition**
**Coordinated Program in Dietetics**
University Park
Health Bldg. Rm. 201
Miami, FL 33199
**Phone:** (305)348-2878          **Fax:** (305)348-1996
**Email:** dixonz@fiu.edu
Zisca R. Dixon, PhD, Director

**★ 16124 ★ Florida International**
 **University**
**Department of Dietetics and Nutrition**
**Dietetic Internship Program**
University Park
Health Bldg. Rm 206
Miami, FL 33199
**Phone:** (305)348-2878          **Fax:** (305)348-1996
Amy Jaffe, Director

**★ 16125 ★ Florida International**
 **University**
**Department of Dietetics and Nutrition**
**Dietetics-Didactic Program**
University Park CH201
Miami, FL 33199
**Phone:** (305)348-2878          **Fax:** (305)348-1996
**Email:** castellv@fiu.edu
**Website:** http://www.fiu.edu/orgs/dietetic/
Victoria A. Hammer Castellanos, PhD, Director
Zisca R. Dixon, PhD, Director

**★ 16126 ★ Florida State University**
**Department of Nutrition, Food and**
 **Exercise Sciences**
436 Sandels Bldg.
Tallahassee, FL 32306-1493
**Phone:** (850)644-4794          **Fax:** (850)645-5000
**Email:** jdorsey@mailer.fsu.edu
**Website:** http://www.fsu.edu/~human/
Jodee L. Dorsey, PhD, Director

**★ 16127 ★ Florida State University**
**Department of Nutrition, Food and**
 **Exercise Sciences**
**Dietetic Internship Program**
400 Sandels Bldg.
Tallahassee, FL 32306-1493
**Phone:** (850)644-1828          **Fax:** (850)644-5000
**Email:** lcook@mailer.fsu.edu
Laura R. Cook, PhD, Director

**★ 16128 ★ James A. Haley Veterans**
 **Hospital**
**Dietetic Internship Program**
13000 N Bruce B. Downs Blvd.
Tampa, FL 33612-4745
**Phone:** (813)972-2000          **Fax:** (813)978-5838
**Email:** anne.brezina@med.va.gov
Anne E. Brezina, Director

**★ 16129 ★ Pasco County Health**
 **Department**
**Nutrition Division**
**Dietetic Internship Program**
10841 Little Rd.
New Port Richey, FL 34654-2533
**Phone:** (727)869-3900          **Fax:** (727)863-9734
**Email:** clara_lawhead@def.state.fl.us
Clara R. Lawhead, Director

**★ 16130 ★ St. Luke's Hospital/Mayo**
 **Clinic Jacksonville**
**Dietetic Internship Program**
4201 Belfort Rd.
Jacksonville, FL 32216-1431
**Phone:** (904)296-3733          **Fax:** (904)296-5268
**Email:** robinson.nell@mayo.edu
Nell E. Robinson, Director

**★ 16131 ★ Sarasota District Schools**
**Food and Nutrition Services**
**Dietetic Internship Program**
101 Old Venice Rd.
Osprey, FL 34229-9023
**Phone:** (941)486-2199          **Fax:** (941)486-2021
Beverly L. Girard, Director

**★ 16132 ★ Sarasota Memorial Hospital**
**Food and Nutrition Services**
**Dietetic Internship Program**
1700 S Tamiami Trail
Sarasota, FL 34239-3555
**Phone:** (941)917-1080          **Fax:** (941)917-6169
Jana L. Boston, PhD, Director

**★ 16133 ★ University of Florida**
**Food Science and Human Nutrition**
 **Department**
**Dietetic Internship Program**
359 FSB
PO Box 110370
Gainesville, FL 32611
**Phone:** (352)392-1991          **Fax:** (352)392-9467
**Email:** gpk@gnv.ifas.ufl.edu
Gail Abbott Kauwell, PhD, Director

**★ 16134 ★ University of Florida**
**Food Science and Human Nutrition**
 **Department**
**Dietetics-Didactic Program**
PO Box 110370
Gainesville, FL 32611-0370
**Phone:** (352)392-1512          **Fax:** (352)392-9467
**Email:** psm@gnv.ifas.ufl.edu
**Website:** http://fshn.ifas.ufl.edu/
Pamela J. McMahon, PhD, Director

**★ 16135 ★ University of North Florida**
**College of Health**
**Dietetics-Didactic Program**
4567 St. Johns Bluff Rd. S
Jacksonville, FL 32224-2645
**Phone:** (904)620-2840          **Fax:** (904)620-2848
**Email:** jrodrigu@unf.edu
**Website:** http://www.unf.edu/
Judith C. Rodriguez, PhD, Director

**★ 16136 ★ University of North Florida**
**Department of Health Science**
**Dietetic Internship Program**
4567 St. Johns Bluff Rd. S
Jacksonville, FL 32224-2646
**Phone:** (904)620-2840          **Fax:** (904)620-2848
**Email:** llockett@unf.edu
Linda L. Brown, Director

## Georgia

**★ 16137 ★ Emory University Hospital**
**Food and Nutrition Services**
**Dietetic Internship Program**
1364 Clifton Rd. NE
Atlanta, GA 30322
**Phone:** (404)712-4178 **Fax:** (404)712-7452
**Email:** maureen_mcandrews@emory.org
Maureen C. McAndrews, Director

**★ 16138 ★ Fort Valley State University**
**Department of Family and Consumer**
**Sciences**
**Dietetics-Didactic Program**
805 State College Dr.
Fort Valley, GA 31030-3242
**Phone:** (912)825-6234 **Fax:** (912)825-6078
**Email:** hunts@fvsu.edu
Sharon K. Hunt, Director

**★ 16139 ★ Georgia Southern University**
**Department of Family and Consumer**
**Sciences**
**Dietetics-Didactic Program**
Box 8034
Statesboro, GA 30460
**Phone:** (912)681-5345 **Fax:** (912)681-0276
**Email:** fbrown2@gsaix2.cc.gasou.edu
Elfrieda F. Brown, Director

**★ 16140 ★ Georgia State University**
**Department of Nutrition and Dietetics**
**Dietetic Internship Program**
University Plaza
Atlanta, GA 30303-3083
**Phone:** (404)651-1082 **Fax:** (404)651-1235
**Email:** bhopkins@gsu.edu
Barbara L. Hopkins, Director

**★ 16141 ★ Georgia State University**
**Department of Nutrition and Dietetics**
**Dietetics-Didactic Program**
University Plaza
PO Box 873
Atlanta, GA 30303-3083
**Phone:** (404)651-1108 **Fax:** (404)651-1235
**Email:** naddhb@panther.gsu.edu
**Website:** http://www.gsu.edu/~wwwntr/
Delia H. Baxter, PhD, Director

**★ 16142 ★ Life University**
**Department of Nutrition**
**Dietetics-Didactic Program**
1269 Barclay Circle
Marietta, GA 30060-2903
**Phone:** (770)426-2736 **Fax:** (770)426-2698
**Email:** tbrigman@life.edu
Tracey B. Brigman, Director

**★ 16143 ★ Southern Regional Medical**
**Center**
**Dietetic Internship Program**
11 Upper Riverdale Rd. SW
Riverdale, GA 30274-2600
**Phone:** (770)991-8033 **Fax:** (770)991-8690
**Email:** scrocker@srmc.org
Stephanie L. Crocker, Director

**★ 16144 ★ University of Georgia**
**Department of Foods and Nutrition**
**Dietetic Internship Program**
Dawson Hall
Athens, GA 30602
**Phone:** (706)542-4908 **Fax:** (706)542-5059
**Email:** bgrossman@fcs.uga.edu
Barbara M. Grossman, PhD, Director

**★ 16145 ★ University of Georgia**
**Department of Foods and Nutrition**
**Dietetics-Didactic Program**
Dawson Hall
Athens, GA 30602
**Phone:** (706)542-7983 **Fax:** (706)542-5059
**Email:** jfischer@fcs.uga.edu
Joan G. Fischer, PhD, Director

## Hawaii

**★ 16146 ★ University of Hawaii, Manoa**
**Department of Food Science and Human**
**Nutrition**
**Dietetics-Didactic Program**
2515 Campus Rd., Miller Hall 12B
Honolulu, HI 96822-2218
**Phone:** (808)956-3847 **Fax:** (808)956-4024
**Email:** amybrown@hawaii.edu
**Website:** http://www.hawaii.edu/dietetics
Amy Brown, PhD, Director

**★ 16147 ★ University of Hawaii, Manoa**
**School of Public Health**
**Dietetic Internship Program**
1960 East-West Rd., D-104J
Honolulu, HI 96822-2319
**Phone:** (808)956-5745 **Fax:** (808)956-4585
**Email:** cwaslien@hawaii.edu
Carol I. Waslien, PhD, Director

## Idaho

**★ 16148 ★ Idaho State University**
**Department Health and Nutrition Sciences**
**Dietetics-Didactic Program or Dietetic**
**Internship Program**
Campus Box 8109
Pocatello, ID 83209-8109
**Phone:** (208)282-2352 **Fax:** (208)282-4903
**Email:** dundmary@isu.edu
Mary L. Dundas, PhD, Director

**★ 16149 ★ University of Idaho**
**College of Agriculture**
**School of Family and Consumer**
**Sciences**
**Coordinated Program in Dietetics**
Moscow, ID 83844-3183
**Phone:** (208)885-6026 **Fax:** (208)885-5751
**Email:** kgabel@uidaho.edu
**Website:** http://www.uidaho.edu/fcs
Kathleen A. Gabel, PhD, Director

## Illinois

**★ 16150 ★ Benedictine University**
**Department of Biological Sciences**
**Dietetics-Didactic Program**
5700 College Rd.
Lisle, IL 60532-0900
**Phone:** (630)829-6534 **Fax:** (630)829-6551
**Email:** cstein@ben.edu
**Website:** http://alt.ben.edu/departments/nutrition/
nutrprog.htm
Catherine L. Stein, Director

**★ 16151 ★ Benedictine University**
**Department of Nutrition**
**Dietetic Internship Program**
5700 College Rd.
Lisle, IL 60532-0900
**Phone:** (630)829-6548 **Fax:** (630)829-6551
**Email:** jmoreschi-mason@ben.edu
Julie Moreschi-Mason, Director

**★ 16152 ★ Bradley University**
**Family and Consumer Sciences**
**Department**
**Dietetics-Didactic Program**
1501 W Bradley Ave.
Peoria, IL 61625
**Phone:** (309)677-2436 **Fax:** (309)677-3813
**Email:** jad@bumail.bradley.edu
**Website:** http://www.bradley.edu/
Jeannette Davidson, PhD, Director

**★ 16153 ★ Dominican University**
**Department of Nutrition Sciences**
**Dietetics-Didactic Program**
7900 W Division St.
River Forest, IL 60305-1066
**Phone:** (708)524-6906 **Fax:** (708)366-5360
**Email:** judybeto@email.dom.edu
**Website:** http://www.dom.edu
Judith A. Beto, PhD, Director

**★ 16154 ★ Eastern Illinois University**
**School of Family and Consumer**
**Sciences**
**Dietetics-Didactic Program or Dietetic**
**Internship Program**
600 Lincoln Ave.
Klehm Hall 109-B
Charleston, IL 61920-3099
**Phone:** (217)581-6680 **Fax:** (217)581-6090
**Email:** cfmdt1@eiu.edu
**Website:** http://www.eiu.edu/~famsci/
Melanie T. Burns, PhD, Director

**★ 16155 ★ Edward Hines Jr. VA Hospital**
**Dietetic Internship Program**
Nutrition and Food Service (120D)
Hines, IL 60141
**Phone:** (708)216-2343 **Fax:** (708)202-2252
**Email:** foley.sharon@hines.va.gov
Sharon Foley, Director

**★ 16156 ★ Illinois State University**
**Department of Family and Consumer**
**Sciences**
**Dietetic Internship Program**
Campus Box 5060
Normal, IL 61790-5060
**Phone:** (309)438-7031 **Fax:** (309)438-5659
**Email:** mawilson@isstu.edu
Mardell A. Wilson, EdD, Director

**★ 16157 ★ Illinois State University**
**Department of Family and Consumer**
**Sciences**
**Dietetics-Didactic Program**
Campus Box 5060
Normal, IL 61790-5060
**Phone:** (309)438-8850 **Fax:** (309)438-5659
**Email:** rcullen@ilstu.edu
**Website:** http://www.cast.ilstu.edu/fcs/fcshome.htm
Robert W. Cullen, PhD, Director

**★ 16158 ★ Ingalls Memorial Hospital**
**Dietetic Internship Program**
1 Ingalls Dr.
Harvey, IL 60426
**Phone:** (708)915-5723 **Fax:** (708)210-3110
**Email:** mvaughn@ingalls.org
Mary Keith Vaughn, Director

**★ 16159 ★ Loyola University, Chicago**
**Department of Food and Nutrition**
**Dietetic Internship Program**
6525 N Sheridan Rd.
Chicago, IL 60626-5311
**Phone:** (773)508-8298 **Fax:** (773)508-8296

Email: jkouba@luc.edu
Joanne Kouba, Director


**★ 16160 ★ Loyola University, Chicago**
**Department of Food and Nutrition**
**Dietetics-Didactic Program**
6525 N Sheridan Rd.
Chicago, IL 60626-5311
Phone: (773)508-8299      Fax: (773)508-8296
Email: tcarlyl@wpo.it.luc.edu
Website: http://www.luc.edu/depts/nutrition
Tracey L. Carlyle, Director


**★ 16161 ★ Northern Illinois University**
**School of Family, Consumer and**
**Nutritional Sciences**
**Dietetic Internship Program**
DeKalb, IL 60115-2854
Phone: (815)753-6384      Fax: (815)753-1321
Email: joanquinn@niu.edu
Website: http://www.niu.edu
Joan E. Quinn, MEd, Director


**★ 16162 ★ Northern Illinois University**
**School of Family, Consumer and**
**Nutritional Sciences**
**Dietetics-Didactic Program**
DeKalb, IL 60115-2854
Phone: (815)753-6384      Fax: (815)753-1321
Email: joanquinn@niu.edu
Joan E. Quinn, Director


**★ 16163 ★ Olivet Nazarene University**
**Department of Family and Consumer**
**Sciences**
**Dietetics-Didactic Program**
1 University Dr.
Kankakee, IL 60901
Phone: (815)939-5398      Fax: (815)935-4990
Email: canstrom@olivet.edu
Website: http://web.olivet.edu/facs/
Cantherine N. Anstrom, Director


**★ 16164 ★ OSF St. Francis Medical**
**Center**
**Dietetic Internship Program**
530 NE Glen Oak Ave.
Peoria, IL 61637-0001
Phone: (309)655-3707      Fax: (309)655-4022
Email: mei-ling.lin@osfhealthcare.org
Mei-Ling Lin, Director


**★ 16165 ★ Rush Presbyterian-St. Luke's**
**Medical Center**
**Dietetic Internship Program**
1653 W Congress Pkwy.
Chicago, IL 60612-3864
Phone: (312)942-3349      Fax: (312)942-5203
Email: askipper@rush.edu
Annalynn Skipper, Director


**★ 16166 ★ St. John's Hospital**
**Dietetic Internship Program**
800 E Carpenter St.
Springfield, IL 62769
Phone: (217)544-6464      Fax: (217)757-6871
Email: slopinsk@st-johns.org
Sara A. Lopinski, Director


**★ 16167 ★ Southern Illinois University,**
**Carbondale**
**Animal Science, Food and Nutrition**
**Dietetics-Didactic Program**
Mail Code 4417
Carbondale, IL 62901-4317
Phone: (618)453-5193      Fax: (618)453-7517
Email: banz@siu.edu

Website: http://www.siu.edu/cwis
William J. Banz, PhD, Director


**★ 16168 ★ Southern Illinois University,**
**Carbondale**
**Food and Nutrition**
**Dietetic Internship Program**
Mail Code 4317
Carbondale, IL 62901-4317
Phone: (618)453-5192      Fax: (618)453-7517
Email: fnms01@siu.edu
Janet Sundberg, Director


**★ 16169 ★ University of Illinois, Chicago**
**College of Health and Human**
**Development Sciences**
**Department of Human Nutrition and**
**Dietetics**
**Coordinated Program in Dietetics**
1919 W Taylor St.
M/C 517
Chicago, IL 60612-7256
Phone: (312)996-8055      Fax: (312)413-0319
Email: braunsch@uic.edu
Carol L. Braunschweig, PhD, Director


**★ 16170 ★ University of Illinois, Urbana,**
**Champaign**
**Department of Food Science and Human**
**Nutrition**
**Dietetic Internship Program**
345 Bevier Hall
905 S Goodwin Ave.
Urbana, IL 61801-3852
Phone: (217)333-2987      Fax: (217)265-0925
Email: tappende@uiuc.edu
Kelly A. Tappenden, PhD, Director


**★ 16171 ★ University of Illinois, Urbana,**
**Champaign**
**Department of Food Science and Human**
**Nutrition**
**Dietetics-Didactic Program**
345 Bevier Hall
905 S Goodwin Ave.
Urbana, IL 61801-3852
Phone: (217)244-2884      Fax: (217)265-0925
Email: plawecki@uiuc.edu
Website: http://www.aces.uiuc.edu/~fshn
Karen L. Plawecki, Director


**★ 16172 ★ Western Illinois University**
**Department of Family and Consumer**
**Sciences**
**Dietetics-Didactic Program**
Macomb, IL 61455
Phone: (309)298-1581      Fax: (309)298-2688
Email: karen_greathouse@ccmail.wiu.edu
Website: http://www.wiu.edu/users/mifcs
Karen R. Greathouse, PhD, Director

### Indiana

**★ 16173 ★ Ball State University**
**Department of Family and Consumer**
**Sciences**
**Dietetics-Didactic Program**
Muncie, IN 47306-0250
Phone: (765)285-5931      Fax: (765)285-2314
Email: 00jblowe@bsu.edu
Website: http://www.bsu.edu/cast/fcs
Judith B. Lowe, Director


**★ 16174 ★ Ball State University**
**Family and Consumer Sciences**
**Dietetic Internship Program**
150 Applied Technology Bldg.
Muncie, IN 47306

Phone: (765)285-5940      Fax: (765)285-2314
Email: mkurtz@bsu.edu
Marla Kurtz, Director


**★ 16175 ★ Indiana State University**
**Department of Family and Consumer**
**Sciences**
**Coordinated Program in Dietetics**
Terre Haute, IN 47809
Phone: (812)237-3309      Fax: (812)237-3304
Email: j-byrne@indstate.edu
Judith C. Byrne, EdD, Director


**★ 16176 ★ Indiana University**
**School of Allied Health**
**Nutrition/Dietetics Program**
**Dietetic Internship Program**
Coleman Hall 316
Indianapolis, IN 46202-5119
Phone: (317)278-0933      Fax: (317)278-3940
Email: jopalka@iupui.edu
Jacquelynn O'Palka, PhD, Director


**★ 16177 ★ Indiana University,**
**Bloomington**
**Department of Applied Health Science**
**Dietetics-Didactic Program**
HPER 116
1025 E Seventh St.
Bloomington, IN 47405-7109
Phone: (812)855-1531      Fax: (812)855-3936
Email: lindema@indiana.edu
Victoria M. Getty, MEd, Director


**★ 16178 ★ Marian College**
**Department of Nursing and Nutritional**
**Sciences**
**Dietetics-Didactic Program or Coordinated**
**Program in Dietetics**
3200 Cold Springs Rd.
Indianapolis, IN 46222-1997
Phone: (317)955-6346      Fax: (317)955-6448
Email: raosborn@marian.edu
Website: http://www.marian.edu/
Robyn A. Osborn, Director


**★ 16179 ★ Purdue University**
**Department of Foods and Nutrition**
**Coordinated Program in Dietetics**
1264 Stone Hall
West Lafayette, IN 47907-1264
Phone: (765)496-6569      Fax: (765)494-0674
Email: bousheyc@cfs.purdue.edu
Carol J. Boushey, PhD, Director


**★ 16180 ★ Purdue University**
**Department of Foods and Nutrition**
**Dietetics-Didactic Program**
1264 Stone Hall
West Lafayette, IN 47907-1264
Phone: (765)494-8238      Fax: (765)494-0674
Email: woodo@cfs.purdue.edu
Website: http://www.cfs.purdue.edu/fdsnutr
Olivia B. Wood, Director
Carol J. Boushey, Contact


**★ 16181 ★ Purdue University, Calumet**
**Department of Behavioral Sciences**
**Preprofessional Practice Program in**
**Dietetics**
2200 169th St.
Hammond, IN 46323-2094
Phone: (219)989-2940      Fax: (219)989-2008
Email: fields@calumet.purdue.edu
Rita A. Fields, Director

## Iowa

**★ 16182 ★ Iowa State University**
**Department of Food Science and Human Nutrition**
**Dietetic Internship Program**
1127 HNS Bldg.
Ames, IA 50011
Phone: (515)294-7316          Fax: (515)294-6193
Email: janderso@iastate.edu
Jean Anderson, Director

**★ 16183 ★ Iowa State University**
**Department of Food Science and Human Nutrition**
**Dietetics-Didactic Program**
1104 Human Nutrition Center
Ames, IA 50011-1120
Phone: (515)294-2321          Fax: (515)294-6193
Email: moakland@iastate.edu
Website: http://www.public.iastate.edu/~dietetics/
Mary Jane Oakland, PhD, Director

**★ 16184 ★ University of Iowa Hospitals and Clinics**
**Dietetic Internship Program**
200 Hawkins Dr.
W146GH
Iowa City, IA 52242-1051
Phone: (319)356-2692          Fax: (319)356-8674
Email: laurie-kroymann@uiowa.edu
Laurie L. Parks, Director

**★ 16185 ★ University of Northern Iowa**
**Department of Design, Family and Consumer Sciences**
**Dietetics-Didactic Program**
1227 W 27th St.
Cedar Falls, IA 50614-0332
Phone: (319)273-2418          Fax: (319)273-7096
Email: hattie.middleton@uni.edu
Website: http://csbsnt.csbs.uni.edu/dept/dfcs/index.html
Hattie M. Middleton, PhD, Director

## Kansas

**★ 16186 ★ Kansas State University**
**Department of Hotel, Restaurant, Institution Management and Dietetics**
**Dietetics-Didactic Program or Coordinated Program in Dietetics**
Justin Hall, Rm. 103
Manhattan, KS 66506-1404
Phone: (785)532-2207          Fax: (785)532-5522
Email: gould@humec.ksu.edu
Website: http://www.ksu.edu/humec/hrimd
Rebecca A. Gould, PhD, Director
Deborah Canter, PhD, Contact

**★ 16187 ★ University of Kansas Medical Center**
**Department of Dietetics and Nutrition**
**Dietetic Internship Program**
3901 Rainbow Blvd.
Kansas City, KS 66160-7250
Phone: (913)588-7683          Fax: (913)588-8946
Email: rbarkley@kumc.edu
Rachel Barkley, Director

## Kentucky

**★ 16188 ★ Berea College**
**Department of Child and Family Studies**
**Dietetics-Didactic Program**
CPO 2192
Berea, KY 40404
Phone: (859)986-3000          Fax: (859)985-3917
Email: janice_blythe@berea.edu

Website:          http://www.berea.edu/CFS/
CFS.home.htmlfaculty
Janice B. Blythe, PhD, Director

**★ 16189 ★ Eastern Kentucky University**
**Human Environmental Sciences**
**Dietetics-Didactic Program or Dietetic Internship Program**
102 Burrier Bldg.
Richmond, KY 40475-3107
Phone: (606)622-3445          Fax: (606)622-1163
Email: hecsutto@acs.eku.edu
Website: http://www.fcs.eku.edu
Sara W. Sutton, Director

**★ 16190 ★ Morehead State University**
**College of Science and Technology**
**Dietetics-Didactic Program or Dietetic Internship Program**
Reed Hall 246
UPO 721
Morehead, KY 40351-1689
Phone: (606)783-2023          Fax: (606)783-5007
Email: m.sampley@morehead-st.edu
Marilyn T. Sampley, PhD, Director

**★ 16191 ★ Murray State University**
**Food Service Systems Management**
**Dietetics-Didactic Program or Dietetic Internship Program**
Applied Sciences Bldg.
200 N Oakley
Murray, KY 42071-3345
Phone: (270)762-6991          Fax: (270)762-6950
Email: kathy.timmons@murraystate.edu
Website: http://www.murraystate.edu/cit/fcs
Kathryn L. Timmons, Director

**★ 16192 ★ Spalding University**
**Dietetic Internship Program**
851 S Fourth St.
Louisville, KY 40203-2115
Phone: (502)585-9911          Fax: (502)588-7175
Email: krapp@spalding.edu
Kathy Rapp, Director

**★ 16193 ★ University of Kentucky**
**Chandler Medical Center**
**Dietetic Internship Program**
800 Rose St.
H-36 Department of Dietetics and Nutrition
Lexington, KY 40536-0293
Phone: (606)323-5154          Fax: (606)257-3287
Email: jlaitk2@pop.uky.edu
Jackie L. Aitkin, Director

**★ 16194 ★ University of Kentucky**
**Department of Nutrition and Food Sciences**
**Dietetics-Didactic Program**
204 Funkhouser Bldg.
Lexington, KY 40506-0054
Phone: (606)257-3800          Fax: (606)257-3707
Email: lgaetke@pop.uky.edu
Website: http://www.uky.edu/
Lisa M. Gaetke, PhD, Director
Hazel W. Forsythe, PhD, Contact

**★ 16195 ★ University of Kentucky**
**Human Environmental Sciences**
**Nutrition and Food Science Department**
204 Funkhouser Bldg.
Lexington, KY 40506-0054
Phone: (606)257-3800          Fax: (606)257-3707
Email: vabl@pop.uky.edu
Hazel W. Forsythe, PhD, Director

**★ 16196 ★ Western Kentucky University**
**Department of Consumer and Family Sciences**
**Dietetics-Didactic Program**
Academic Complex 302F
1 Big Red Way
Bowling Green, KY 42101-3576
Phone: (270)745-4352          Fax: (270)745-2084
Email: Danita.Kelley@wku.edu
Website: http://www.wku.edu/dietetics
Danita M. Saxon Kelley, PhD, Director

## Louisiana

**★ 16197 ★ Louisiana State University**
**School of Human Ecology**
**Dietetics-Didactic Program**
Baton Rouge, LA 70803-4300
Phone: (225)388-2400          Fax: (225)388-2697
Email: ceoneil@unixl.sncc.lsu.edu
Website: http://sun.huec.lsu.edu/
Carol E. O'Neill, Director

**★ 16198 ★ Louisiana State University and A&M College**
**School of Human Ecology**
**Dietetic Internship Program**
125 Human Ecology Bldg.
Baton Rouge, LA 70803-4301
Phone: (225)388-2406          Fax: (225)504-2697
Email: ecross@unixl.sncc.lsu.edu
Evelina Cross, PhD, Director

**★ 16199 ★ Louisiana Tech University**
**College of Human Ecology**
**Dietetics-Didactic Program**
PO Box 3167
Ruston, LA 71272
Phone: (318)257-2607          Fax: (318)257-4014
Email: hunt@hec.latech.edu
Website: http://www.ans.latech.edu/humaneco-index.html
Elaine F. Molaison, PhD, Director

**★ 16200 ★ McNeese State University**
**Dietetic Internship Program**
PO Box 92820 MSU
Lake Charles, LA 70609-2820
Phone: (318)475-5970          Fax: (318)475-5249
Email: dholl205@aol.com
Debra Hollingsworth, PhD, Director

**★ 16201 ★ McNeese State University**
**Dietetics-Didactic Program**
PO Box 92820
Lake Charles, LA 70609
Phone: (337)475-5970          Fax: (337)475-5681
Email: bfontrd@aol.com
Carol B. Fontenot, Director

**★ 16202 ★ Nicholls State University**
**Department of Family and Consumer Sciences**
**Dietetics-Didactic Program**
Box 2014
Thibodaux, LA 70310
Phone: (504)448-4690          Fax: (504)449-7073
Email: facs-cgl@mail.nich.edu
Colette G. Leistner, PhD, Director

**★ 16203 ★ Southern University and A&M College**
**College of Agriculture and Home Economics**
**Dietetics-Didactic Program or Dietetic Internship Program**
PO Box 11342
Baton Rouge, LA 70813-1342

**Phone:** (225)771-4660          **Fax:** (225)771-3107
**Email:** bmcgee@subr.edu
Bernestine B. McGee, PhD, Director


★ 16204 ★ **Touro Infirmary School of Medical Technology**
**Dietetic Internship Program**
1401 Foucher St.
New Orleans, LA 70115-3515
**Phone:** (504)897-8034          **Fax:** (504)897-8093
**Email:** fitzpatrick.pat.rd@worldnet.att.net
Patricia Fitzpatrick, Director


★ 16205 ★ **Tulane University**
**Public Health and Tropical Medicine**
**Dietetic Internship Program**
1430 Tulane Ave.
New Orleans, LA 70112-2699
**Phone:** (504)584-2673          **Fax:** (504)584-3540
**Email:** catkins@mailhost.tcs.tulane.edu
Cheryl L. Atkinson, DrPH, Director


★ 16206 ★ **University of Louisiana, Lafayette**
**College of Applied Life Sciences**
**School of Human Resources**
**Dietetics-Didactic Program or Dietetic Internship Program**
PO Box 40399
Lafayette, LA 70504-0399
**Phone:** (337)482-6577          **Fax:** (337)482-5395
**Email:** boa5197@usl.edu
Bernice O. Adeleye, PhD, Director


## Maine

★ 16207 ★ **University of Maine, Orono**
**Department of Food Science and Human Nutrition**
**Dietetic Internship Program**
5749 Merrill Hall, Rm. 23
Orono, ME 04469-5749
**Phone:** (207)581-3134          **Fax:** (207)581-3111
**Email:** awhite@umenfa.maine.edu
Adrienne A. White, PhD, Director


★ 16208 ★ **University of Maine, Orono**
**Department of Food Science and Human Nutrition**
**Dietetics-Didactic Program**
5749 Merrill Hall, Rm. 24
Orono, ME 04469-5749
**Phone:** (207)581-3130          **Fax:** (207)581-3111
**Email:** susan_sullivan@umenfa.maine.edu
**Website:** http://www.ume.maine.edu/~nfa/fsn/
Susan S. Sullivan, DSc, Director


## Maryland

★ 16209 ★ **Johns Hopkins Bayview Medical Center**
**Clinical Nutrition Department**
**Dietetic Internship Program**
4940 Eastern Ave.
Baltimore, MD 21224-2735
**Phone:** (410)550-1319          **Fax:** (410)550-0650
**Email:** ckoch@jhmi.edu
Cheryl Koch, Director


★ 16210 ★ **Malcolm Grow USAF Medical Center**
**Dietetic Internship Program**
89th Medical Diagnostics and Therapeutics Squadron/S6SD
1050 W Perimeter Rd.
Andrews AFB, MD 20762-6600
**Phone:** (240)857-3154          **Fax:** (240)857-6858
**Email:** molnae@mgmc.af.mil
Edward P. Molnar, Director


★ 16211 ★ **Morgan State University**
**Department of Human Ecology**
**Dietetics-Didactic Program**
1700 E Cold Spring Ln.
Key Hall G-55
Baltimore, MD 21251
**Phone:** (443)885-3905          **Fax:** (443)319-3787
**Email:** iforand@morgan.edu
**Website:** http://www.morgan.edu/
Ivis T. Forrester-Anderson, PhD, Director


★ 16212 ★ **National Institutes of Health**
**Clinic Center Nutrition Department**
**Dietetic Internship Program**
Bldg. Rm. BIS-234
10 Center Dr., MSC 1078
Bethesda, MD 20892-1078
**Phone:** (301)496-3311          **Fax:** (301)496-0622
**Email:** dford@nih.gov
Denise Ford, Director


★ 16213 ★ **University of Maryland, College Park**
**Department of Nutrition and Food Sciences**
**Dietetics-Didactic Program**
College Park, MD 20742-7521
**Phone:** (301)405-4532          **Fax:** (301)314-9327
**Email:** sc49@umail.umd.edu
**Website:** http://www.agnr.umd.edu/
Suzanne R. Curtis, PhD, Director


★ 16214 ★ **University of Maryland, Eastern Shore**
**Department of Human Ecology**
**Dietetics-Didactic Program or Dietetics-Preprofessional Practice Program**
Princess Anne, MD 21853-1299
**Phone:** (410)651-6066          **Fax:** (410)651-6207
**Email:** bblakely@mail.umes.edu
**Website:** http://www.umes.edu/
Bettie Wright Blakely, Director


★ 16215 ★ **University of Maryland Medical System**
**Food and Nutrition Services**
**Dietetic Internship Program**
22 S Greene St.
Baltimore, MD 21201-1595
**Phone:** (410)328-2561          **Fax:** (410)328-1000
**Email:** lwohlber@itg.ummc.umaryland.edu
Laura K. Wohlberg, Director


## Massachusetts

★ 16216 ★ **Beth Israel Deaconess Medical Center**
**Dietetic Internship Program**
330 Brookline Ave.
Boston, MA 02215-5491
**Phone:** (617)667-2565          **Fax:** (617)667-7555
**Email:** psamour@caregroup.harvard.edu
Patricia Queen Samour, Director


★ 16217 ★ **Boston University**
**Sargent College**
**Graduate Nutrition Division**
**Dietetic Internship Program**
635 Commonwealth Ave.
Boston, MA 02215-1605
**Phone:** (617)353-7470          **Fax:** (617)353-7567
**Email:** charland@bu.edu
Joan Salge Blake, Director


★ 16218 ★ **Boston University/Sargent College**
**Dietetics-Didactic Program**
635 Commonwealth Ave.
Boston, MA 02215-1605
**Phone:** (617)353-7488          **Fax:** (617)353-7567
**Email:** rdurschl@bu.edu
**Website:** http://www.bu.edu/sargent/HS
Roberta P. Durschlag, PhD, Director


★ 16219 ★ **Framingham State College**
**Department of Family and Consumer Sciences**
**Dietetics-Didactic Program or Coordinated Program in Dietetics**
100 State St.
Framingham, MA 01701-9101
**Phone:** (508)626-4757          **Fax:** (508)626-4003
**Email:** maberne@frc.mass.edu
**Website:** http://www.framingham.edu
Marilyn M. Abernethy, DrPH, Director
Suzanne H. Neubauer, Contact


★ 16220 ★ **Simmons College**
**Department of Nutrition**
**Dietetic Internship Program**
300 The Fenway
Boston, MA 02115
**Phone:** (617)521-2711          **Fax:** (617)521-3137
Nancie Harvey Herbold, EdD, Director


★ 16221 ★ **Simmons College**
**Department of Nutrition**
**Dietetics-Didactic Program**
300 The Fenway
Boston, MA 02115-5898
**Phone:** (617)521-2708          **Fax:** (617)521-3137
**Email:** khendricks@simmons.edu
**Website:** http://www.simmons.edu/
Elizabeth S. Metallinos-Katsaras, PhD, Director


★ 16222 ★ **University of Massachusetts, Amherst**
**Department of Nutrition**
**Dietetics-Didactic Program**
Box 31420
Chenoweth Laboratory
Amherst, MA 01003-1420
**Phone:** (413)545-0740          **Fax:** (413)545-1074
**Website:** http://www.umass.edu
Samantha Logan, PhD, Director


★ 16223 ★ **University of Massachusetts, Amherst**
**Division of Continuing Education**
**Dietetic Internship Program**
UMass Box 31650
Amherst, MA 01003-1650
**Phone:** (413)545-2484          **Fax:** (413)545-3351
**Email:** aszlosek@admin.umass.edu
Alice E. Szlosek, Director


## Michigan

★ 16224 ★ **Andrews University**
**Department of Nutrition**
**Dietetics-Didactic Program or Dietetics-Preprofessional Practice Program**
Berrien Springs, MI 49104-0210
**Phone:** (616)471-3370          **Fax:** (616)471-3485
**Email:** wcraig@andrews.edu
**Website:** http://www.andrews.edu/NUFS
Winston Craig, PhD, Director

★ 16225 ★ **Central Michigan University**
**Human Environmental Studies**
**Dietetics-Didactic Program or Dietetic**
**Internship Program**
Wightman Hall 205
Mount Pleasant, MI 48859
**Phone:** (517)774-2004    **Fax:** (517)774-2435
**Email:** jack.logomarsino@cmich.edu
**Website:** http://www.cmich.edu
John V. Logomarsino, PhD, Director


★ 16226 ★ **Eastern Michigan University**
**Coordinated Program in Dietetics**
206 Roosevelt Hall
Ypsilanti, MI 48197
**Phone:** (734)487-7862    **Fax:** (734)487-7087
**Email:** judi.brooks@emich.edu
**Website:** http://www.emich.edu
Judith T. Brooks, PhD, Director


★ 16227 ★ **Grand Valley State University**
**Occupational Therapy Program**
322 Henry Hall
1 Campus Dr.
Allendale, MI 49401-9403
**Phone:** (616)895-3356    **Fax:** (616)895-3350
**Email:** grapczyc@gvsu.edu
**Website:** http://www4.gvsu.edu/otp
Cynthia Grapczynski, EdD, Director


★ 16228 ★ **Madonna University**
**Family and Consumer Resources**
**Dietetics-Didactic Program**
36600 Schoolcraft Rd.
Livonia, MI 48150-1173
**Phone:** (734)432-5534    **Fax:** (734)432-5393
**Email:** schmitz@smtp.munet.edu
**Website:** http://www.munet.edu
Karen J. Schmitz, PhD, Director


★ 16229 ★ **Marygrove College**
**Department of Human Nutrition and**
**Foods**
8425 W McNichols Rd.
Detroit, MI 48221
**Phone:** (313)927-1322    **Fax:** (313)927-1345
**Email:** mnettles@marygrove.edu
Ethel M. Nettles, PhD, Director


★ 16230 ★ **Michigan State University**
**Department of Food Science and Human**
**Nutrition**
**Dietetic Internship Program**
2100 Anthony Hall
East Lansing, MI 48824-1225
**Phone:** (517)355-7713    **Fax:** (517)353-1676
**Email:** hord@pilot.msu.edu
Norman G. Hord, PhD, Director


★ 16231 ★ **Michigan State University**
**Department of Food Science and Human**
**Nutrition**
**Dietetics-Didactic Program**
2112 Anthony Hall
East Lansing, MI 48824-1030
**Phone:** (517)355-6483    **Fax:** (517)353-1676
**Email:** shcash@msu.edu
**Website:** http://www.msu.edu/unit/fshn
Stella H. Cash, Director


★ 16232 ★ **Northern Michigan University**
**Department of Health, Physical Education**
**and Recreation**
**Dietetics-Didactic Program**
Marquette, MI 49855
**Phone:** (906)227-2366    **Fax:** (906)227-2181
**Email:** mmowafy@nmu.edu
Mohey A. Mowafy, PhD, Director


★ 16233 ★ **University of Michigan**
**Human Nutrition Program**
**Dietetics-Didactic Program**
1420 Washington Heights
Ann Arbor, MI 48109-2029
**Phone:** (734)764-3277    **Fax:** (734)764-5233
**Email:** dlown@umich.edu
Deborah A. Lown, Director


★ 16234 ★ **University of Michigan**
**Medical Center**
**Dietetic Internship Program**
UH2C227/0056
1500 E Medical Center Dr.
Ann Arbor, MI 48109-0056
**Phone:** (734)936-5199    **Fax:** (734)936-5195
**Email:** joyceks@umich.edu
Joyce Kerestes-Smith, Director


★ 16235 ★ **University of Michigan**
**Medical Center**
**Preprofessional Practice Program in**
**Dietetics**
C333 Medinn Bldg. Box 0832
1500 E Medical Center Dr.
Ann Arbor, MI 48105-0832
**Phone:** (734)763-6170    **Fax:** (734)763-6426
**Email:** apfdir@umich.edu
Andrea Lasichak, Director


★ 16236 ★ **Wayne State University**
**Department of Nutrition and Food**
**Sciences**
**Coordinated Program in Dietetics**
3009 Science Hall
Detroit, MI 48202
**Phone:** (313)577-2500    **Fax:** (313)577-8616
**Email:** treinha@lifesci.wayne.edu
**Website:** http://www.science.wayne.edu/~nfs/dietetics.htm
Tonia Reinhard, Director


★ 16237 ★ **Western Michigan University**
**Department of Family and Consumer**
**Sciences**
**Dietetics-Didactic Program**
3024 Kohrman Hall
Kalamazoo, MI 49008
**Phone:** (616)387-3706    **Fax:** (616)387-3353
**Email:** rojhani@wmich.edu
**Website:** http://www.wmich.edu
Arezoo Rojhani, PhD, Director


★ 16238 ★ **Western Michigan University**
**Family and Consumer Sciences**
**Dietetic Internship Program**
3025 Kohrman Hall
Kalamazoo, MI 49008-5067
**Phone:** (616)387-3710    **Fax:** (616)387-3353
**Email:** petersons@wmich.edu
Maija Peterson, PhD, Director


## Minnesota

★ 16239 ★ **College of Saint Catherine**
**Family, Consumer and Nutritional**
**Sciences**
**Dietetics-Didactic Program**
2004 Randolph Ave.
Saint Paul, MN 55105-1750
**Phone:** (651)690-6204    **Fax:** (651)690-6958
**Email:** peode@stkate.edu
Patricia J. Ode, Director


★ 16240 ★ **College of Saint Scholastica**
**Department of Dietetics**
**Dietetics-Didactic Program**
1200 Kenwood Ave.
Duluth, MN 55811
**Phone:** (218)723-6103    **Fax:** (218)723-6472
**Email:** sbodin@css.edu
**Website:** http://www.css.edu/depts/dietetics.html
Susan Kumsha-Bodin, Director


★ 16241 ★ **Concordia College—**
**Moorehead**
**Department of Family and Nutrition**
**Sciences**
**Dietetics-Didactic Program**
Moorhead, MN 56562
**Phone:** (218)299-3748    **Fax:** (218)299-4308
**Email:** blarson@gloria.cord.edu
**Website:** http://www.cord.edu
Betty J. Larson, EdD, Director


★ 16242 ★ **Concordia College—Moorhead**
**Department of Family and Nutrition**
**Sciences**
**Dietetic Internship Program**
901 S Eighth St.
Moorhead, MN 56562
**Phone:** (218)299-4443    **Fax:** (218)299-4308
**Email:** rusness@cord.edu
Barbara A. Rusness, PhD, Director


★ 16243 ★ **Fairview, University Medical**
**Center**
**Dietetic Internship Program**
Nutrition Services Box 84
420 Delaware St. SE
Minneapolis, MN 55455
**Phone:** (612)273-5004    **Fax:** (612)273-5039
**Email:** tchampol@fairview.org
Teri L. Burgess-Champoux, Director


★ 16244 ★ **Minnesota State University,**
**Mankato**
**Family Consumer Sciences Department**
**Dietetics-Didactic Program**
102 Wiecking Center
Mankato, MN 56001
**Phone:** (507)389-5293    **Fax:** (507)389-2411
**Email:** joye.bond@mankato.msus.edu
**Website:** http://www.mankato.msus.edu/
Joye M. Bond, PhD, Director


★ 16245 ★ **Saint John's University**
**College of Saint Benedict**
**Nutrition Department**
**Coordinated Program in Dietetics**
37 S College Ave.
Saint Joseph, MN 56374-2099
**Phone:** (320)363-5034    **Fax:** (320)363-5582
**Email:** pmarincic@csbsju.edu
**Website:** http://www.CSBSJU.edu/index.html
Patricia Z. Marincic, PhD, Director


★ 16246 ★ **St. Mary's Hospital/Mayo**
**Medical Center**
**Dietetic Internship Program**
1216 Second St. SW
Rochester, MN 55902-1906
**Phone:** (507)255-5221    **Fax:** (507)255-7379
**Email:** jones.rita@mayo.edu
Rita Kay Jones, Director


★ 16247 ★ **University of Minnesota**
**Coordinated Program in Dietetics**
269 Food Science and Nutrition
1334 Eckles Ave.
Saint Paul, MN 55108-6099
**Phone:** (612)624-9278    **Fax:** (612)625-5272

**Email:** mhanson@che2.che.umn.edu
Madge N. Hanson, Director

★ 16248 ★ **University of Minnesota**
**Department of Food Science and**
**Nutrition**
**Dietetic Internship Program or Dietetics-**
**Didactic Program**
269 Food Science and Nutrition
1334 Eckles Ave.
Saint Paul, MN 55108-6099
**Phone:** (612)624-3255          **Fax:** (612)264-5272
**Email:** lmullan@che2.umn.edu
**Website:** http://www.fscn.che.umn.edu
Louise M. Mullan, Director

## Mississippi

★ 16249 ★ **Alcorn State University**
**Department of Family and Consumer**
**Sciences**
**Dietetics-Didactic Program**
1000 ASU Dr., Ste. 839
Lorman, MS 39096-7500
**Phone:** (601)877-6258          **Fax:** (601)927-1345
**Email:** mrasco@lorman.alcorn.edu
Mattie R. Rasco, Director

★ 16250 ★ **Delta State University**
**Division of Family and Consumer**
**Sciences**
**Coordinated Program in Dietetics**
PO Box 3273
Cleveland, MS 38733
**Phone:** (662)846-4317          **Fax:** (662)434-3873
**Email:** awelch@dsu.deltast.edu
Anne S. Welch, PhD, Director

★ 16251 ★ **Mississippi State University**
**School of Human Sciences**
**Dietetics-Didactic Program**
PO Box 9745
Mississippi State, MS 39762-9745
**Phone:** (662)325-7702          **Fax:** (662)325-8188
**Email:** cmalone@humansci.msstate.edu
Carolyn Malone, Director

★ 16252 ★ **University of Mississippi**
**Department of Family and Consumer**
**Sciences**
**Dietetics-Didactic Program**
110 Meek Hall
PO Box 1848
University, MS 38677-1848
**Phone:** (662)915-7371          **Fax:** (662)915-7039
**Email:** smithd@olemiss.edu
Erskine R. Smith, PhD, Director

★ 16253 ★ **University of Southern**
**Mississippi**
**Dietetic Internship Program**
Southern Station
PO Box 5035
Hattiesburg, MS 39406-5053
**Phone:** (601)924-9769          **Fax:** (601)924-1119
**Email:** rabroome@netdoor.com
Ruth Ann Broome, Director

★ 16254 ★ **University of Southern**
**Mississippi**
**Family and Consumer Sciences**
**Dietetics-Didactic Program or Dietetic**
**Internship Program**
2609 W Fourth St.
Hattiesburg, MS 39406
**Phone:** (601)266-4679          **Fax:** (601)266-4680
**Email:** mary.nettles@usm.edu

**Website:** http://www.usm.edu/
Mary F. Nettles, PhD, Director

## Missouri

★ 16255 ★ **Central Missouri State**
**University**
**Department of Human Environmental**
**Sciences**
**Dietetics-Didactic Program**
Grinstead 235
Warrensburg, MO 64093
**Phone:** (660)543-4217          **Fax:** (660)543-8295
**Email:** drake@cmsu1.cmsu.edu
**Website:** http://www.cmsu.edu/csm
Mary Anne Drake, PhD, Director

★ 16256 ★ **College of the Ozarks**
**Dietetics and Nutrition Education**
**Dietetics-Didactic Program**
Point Lookout, MO 65726-0017
**Phone:** (417)334-6411          **Fax:** (417)335-2618
**Email:** smartin@cofo.edu
Suzanne G. Martin, PhD, Director

★ 16257 ★ **Fontbonne College**
**Department of Human Environmental**
**Sciences**
**Dietetics-Didactic Program**
6800 Wydown Blvd.
Saint Louis, MO 63105-3098
**Phone:** (314)889-1415          **Fax:** (314)889-1451
**Email:** chouston@fontbonne.edu
Cheryl A. Houston, Director

★ 16258 ★ **Jewish Hospital-College of**
**Nursing/Allied Health**
**Dietetic Internship Program**
306 S Kingshighway
Saint Louis, MO 63110
**Phone:** (314)454-5307          **Fax:** (314)454-5239
Mary P. Fuhrman, Director

★ 16259 ★ **Northwest Missouri State**
**University**
**College of Education and Human**
**Services**
**Department of Human Environmental**
**Sciences**
**Dietetics-Didactic Program**
Administration Bldg., Rm. 309
Maryville, MO 64468-6001
**Phone:** (660)562-1167          **Fax:** (660)562-1900
**Email:** jciak@mail.nwmissouri.edu
**Website:** http://www.nwmissouri.edu
Jenell D. Ciak, PhD, Director

★ 16260 ★ **Saint Louis University**
**School of Allied Health Professions**
**Department of Nutrition and Dietetics**
**Dietetics-Didactic Program or Dietetic**
**Internship Program**
3437 Caroline St.
Saint Louis, MO 63104-1111
**Phone:** (314)577-8523          **Fax:** (314)577-8520
**Email:** mensecg@slu.edu
**Website:** http://www.slu.edu/colleges/AH/
Cynthia Gurdian Mense, Director

★ 16261 ★ **Southeast Missouri State**
**University**
**Department of Human Environmental**
**Studies**
**Dietetic Internship Program**
1 University Plaza
Cape Girardeau, MO 63701-4799
**Phone:** (573)651-2733          **Fax:** (573)651-2949

**Email:** abmarietta@semovm.semo.edu
Ann B. Marietta, PhD, Director

★ 16262 ★ **Southeast Missouri State**
**University**
**Department of Human Environmental**
**Studies**
**Dietetics-Didactic Program**
Cape Girardeau, MO 63701-4799
**Phone:** (573)651-2109          **Fax:** (573)651-2949
**Email:** gsyler@semovm.semo.edu
**Website:** http://www2.semo.edu/mnelms
Georganne P. Syler, PhD, Director

★ 16263 ★ **Southwest Missouri State**
**University**
**Department of Biomedical Sciences**
**Dietetics-Didactic Program**
Springfield, MO 65804
**Phone:** (417)836-5321          **Fax:** (417)836-5588
**Email:** hcr678f@mail.smsu.edu
**Website:** http://www.smsu.edu/
Helen C. Reid, PhD, Director

★ 16264 ★ **University of Missouri,**
**Columbia**
**Coordinated Program in Dietetics**
318 Clark Hall
Columbia, MO 65211
**Phone:** (573)882-4136          **Fax:** (573)884-4885
**Email:** petersonca@missouri.edu
**Website:** http://www.missouri.edu/~nutsci/
Catherine A. Peterson, PhD, Director

## Montana

★ 16265 ★ **Montana State University**
**Department of Health and Human**
**Development**
**Dietetics-Didactic Program**
201 Romney
Bozeman, MT 59717
**Phone:** (406)994-6338          **Fax:** (406)994-6314
**Email:** pharris@montana.edu
**Website:** http://www.montana.edu/nutrition
Pamela R. Harris, Director

## Nebraska

★ 16266 ★ **University of Nebraska,**
**Kearney**
**Department of Family and Consumer**
**Sciences**
**Dietetics-Didactic Program**
Otto Olsen Bldg., Rm. 205C
00-905 W 25th St.
Kearney, NE 68849-2130
**Phone:** (308)865-8229          **Fax:** (308)865-8040
**Email:** daviss@unk.edu
**Website:** http://www.unk.edu/
Sharon L. Davis, Director

★ 16267 ★ **University of Nebraska,**
**Lincoln**
**Department of Nutritional Science and**
**Dietetics**
**Dietetics-Didactic Program**
202 Ruth Leverton Hall
Lincoln, NE 68583-0806
**Phone:** (402)472-2925          **Fax:** (402)472-1587
**Email:** lyoung3@unl.edu
**Website:** http://www.unl.edu/unlpub/index.shtml
Linda O. Young, Director

★ 16268 ★ **University of Nebraska**
**Medical Center**
**Dietetic Internship Program**
981200 Nebraska Medical Center
Omaha, NE 68198-1200

**Phone:** (402)559-7365    **Fax:** (402)559-6010
**Email:** gwoscyna@unmc.edu
Glenda R. Woscyna, Director

## Nevada

### ★ 16269 ★ University of Nevada, Reno
**Department of Nutrition**
**Dietetic Internship Program**
Mail Stop 142
Reno, NV 89557-0132
**Phone:** (775)784-6442    **Fax:** (775)784-6449
**Email:** dswilson@unr.edu
David S. Wilson, PhD, Director

### ★ 16270 ★ University of Nevada, Reno
**Department of Nutrition**
**Dietetics-Didactic Program**
Mail Stop 142
Reno, NV 89557-0132
**Phone:** (775)784-6446    **Fax:** (775)784-6449
**Email:** read@scs.unr.edu
Marsha H. Read, PhD, Director

## New Hampshire

### ★ 16271 ★ Keene State College
**Home Economics/Human Services**
**Dietetic Internship Program or Dietetics-**
  **Didactic Program**
229 Main St.
Joslin House Rm. 207
Keene, NH 03431
**Phone:** (603)358-2860    **Fax:** (603)358-2892
**Email:** psmithos@keene.edu
**Website:** http://www.keene.edu/
Pamela J. Smith, EdD, Director

### ★ 16272 ★ University of New Hampshire
**Department of Animal and Nutritional**
  **Sciences**
**Human Nutrition Center**
**Dietetics-Didactic Program or Dietetic**
  **Internship Program**
Colovos Rd.
Durham, NH 03824
**Phone:** (603)862-1723    **Fax:** (603)862-0308
**Email:** chjs@hopper.unh.edu
**Website:** http://arethusa.unh.edu/colsa/ansci/ans.htm
Colette Janson-Sand, PhD, Director

## New Jersey

### ★ 16273 ★ College of Saint Elizabeth
**Department of Foods and Nutrition**
**Dietetics-Didactic Program or Dietetic**
  **Internship Program**
2 Convent Rd.
Morristown, NJ 07960-6989
**Phone:** (973)290-4045    **Fax:** (973)290-4676
**Email:** mboyle@liza.st-elizabeth.edu
**Website:** http://www.st-elizabeth.edu
Marie B. Struble, PhD, Director

### ★ 16274 ★ Montclair State University
**Department of Home Ecology**
**Preprofessional Practice Program in**
  **Dietetics**
Upper Montclair, NJ 07043
**Phone:** (973)655-4375    **Fax:** (973)655-4399
Carol A. Sokolik, Director

### ★ 16275 ★ Montclair State University
**Department of Human Ecology**
**Dietetics-Didactic Program**
111 Finley
Upper Montclair, NJ 07043
**Phone:** (973)655-7155    **Fax:** (973)655-4399
**Email:** bauerk@mail.montclair.edu
**Website:** http://www.montclair.edu/pages/HECO/
Food-Dietetics.html
Kathleen D. Bauer, PhD, Director

### ★ 16276 ★ Rutgers, the State University
  of New Jersey
**Department of Nutritional Sciences**
**Dietetics-Didactic Program**
2298 Davison Hall
26 Nichol Ave.
New Brunswick, NJ 08901-2882
**Phone:** (732)932-9570    **Fax:** (732)932-6522
**Email:** bltangel@rci.rutgers.edu
**Website:** http://aesop.rutgers.edu/~nutrition
Barbara L. Tangel, Director

### ★ 16277 ★ University of Medicine and
  Dentistry of New Jersey
**School of Health Related Professions**
**Coordinated Program in Dietetics**
65 Bergen St.
Newark, NJ 07107-3001
**Phone:** (973)972-6245    **Fax:** (973)972-7403
**Email:** maillet@umdnj.edu
**Website:** http://www.umdnj.edu/shrp
Julie O. Maillet, PhD, Director

### ★ 16278 ★ University of Medicine and
  Dentistry of New Jersey
**School of Health Related Professions**
**Dietetic Internship Program**
1776 Raritan Rd.
Scotch Plains, NJ 07076
**Phone:** (908)889-2488    **Fax:** (908)889-2487
**Email:** mckayge@umdnj.edu
M. Geraldine McKay, Director

## New Mexico

### ★ 16279 ★ New Mexico State University
**Department of Home Economics**
**Dietetics-Didactic Program**
Box 30003/MSC 3470
Las Cruces, NM 88003-8003
**Phone:** (505)646-1178    **Fax:** (505)646-1889
**Email:** abock@nmsuvm1.nmsu.edu
**Website:** http://www.nmsu.edu/~famcom
Margaret Ann Bock, PhD, Director

### ★ 16280 ★ University of New Mexico
**Individual, Family and Community**
  **Education**
**Dietetic Internship Program**
Education Office Bldg. 204
Albuquerque, NM 87131-1231
**Phone:** (505)277-6434    **Fax:** (505)277-4362
Donna W. Lockner, PhD, Director

### ★ 16281 ★ University of New Mexico
**Individual, Family and Community**
  **Education**
**Dietetics-Didactic Program**
215 College of Education
Albuquerque, NM 87131-1231
**Phone:** (505)277-6434    **Fax:** (505)277-4362
**Email:** kheller@unm.edu
Karen E. Heller, PhD, Director

## New York

### ★ 16282 ★ City University of New York
**Brooklyn College**
**Department of Health and Nutrition**
  **Sciences**
**Dietetics-Didactic Program or**
  **Preprofessional Practice Program in**
  **Dietetics**
2900 Bedford Ave.
Brooklyn, NY 11210-2889

**Phone:** (718)951-5541    **Fax:** (718)951-4670
**Email:** ahlawson@brooklyn.cuny.edu
**Website:** http://academic.brooklyn.cuny.edu/hns/
Annie S. Hauck-Lawson, PhD, Director

### ★ 16283 ★ City University of New York
**Herbert H. Lehman College**
**Department of Health Services, Dietetics,**
  **Food and Nutrition**
**Dietetics-Didactic Program**
Bedford Park Blvd. W
Bronx, NY 10468-1589
**Phone:** (718)960-8775    **Fax:** (718)960-8908
**Website:** http://www.lehman.cuny.edu
Alice Tobias, EdD, Director

### ★ 16284 ★ City University of New York
**Hunter College**
**Dietetics-Didactic Program**
Brookdale Health Science Center
425 E 25th St.
New York, NY 10010-2590
**Phone:** (212)481-5118    **Fax:** (212)481-5260
**Email:** knavder@hunter.cuny.edu
Khursheed P. Navder, PhD, Director

### ★ 16285 ★ City University of New York
**Herbert H. Lehman College**
**Department of Health Services**
**Dietetic Internship Program**
250 Bedford Park Blvd. W
Bronx, NY 10468-1589
**Phone:** (718)960-8796    **Fax:** (718)960-8908
**Email:** aboyar@alpha.lehman.cuny.edu
Andrea P. Boyar, PhD, Director

### ★ 16286 ★ City University of New York,
  Queens College
**Department of Family, Nutrition and**
  **Exercise Sciences**
**Dietetics-Didactic Program or Dietetic**
  **Internship Program**
65-30 Kissena Blvd.
Flushing, NY 11367-1597
**Phone:** (718)997-4152    **Fax:** (718)997-4163
**Email:** marcia_miller@qc1.qc.edu
**Website:** http://www.qc.edu/
Marcia C. Miller, EdD, Director

### ★ 16287 ★ Columbia University Teachers
  College
**Health and Behavior Studies**
**Dietetic Internship Program**
525 W 120th St., Box 137
New York, NY 10027-6625
**Phone:** (212)678-3950    **Fax:** (212)678-4048
**Email:** cg180@columbia.edu
M. Joanne Rudolph, EdD, Director

### ★ 16288 ★ Cornell University
**Division of Nutritional Sciences**
**Dietetics-Didactic Program or Dietetic**
  **Internship Program**
373 MVR Hall
Ithaca, NY 14853-4401
**Phone:** (607)255-2638    **Fax:** (607)255-0178
**Email:** myk1@cornell.edu
**Website:** http://www.nutrition.cornell.edu/diet.html
Marie Y. Kamp, Director

### ★ 16289 ★ Cornell University
**School of Hotel Administration**
**Dietetics-Didactic Program**
252 Statler Hall
Ithaca, NY 14853
**Phone:** (607)255-3458    **Fax:** (607)255-4179
**Email:** tabacchi@courier1.sha.cornell.edu
Mary H. Tabacchi, PhD, Director

**★ 16290 ★ D'Youville College**
**Coordinated Program in Dietetics**
320 Porter Ave.
Buffalo, NY 14201-1084
**Phone:** (716)881-7752   **Fax:** (716)881-7790
**Email:** baumgartc@dyc.edu
**Website:** http://www.dyc.edu
Charlotte W. Baumgart, PhD, Director

**★ 16291 ★ Long Island University, C W**
**Post Campus**
**Department of Nutrition**
**Dietetics-Didactic Program or Dietetic**
**Internship Program**
720 Northern Blvd.
Brookville, NY 11548
**Phone:** (516)299-2690   **Fax:** (516)299-3106
**Email:** fgizis@liu.edu
**Website:** http://www.liu.edu/nutrit
Frances C. Gizis, PhD, Director

**★ 16292 ★ Marymount College**
**Department of Human Ecology**
**Dietetics-Didactic Program or Dietetic**
**Internship Program**
100 Marymount Ave.
Tarrytown, NY 10591
**Phone:** (914)332-6559   **Fax:** (914)631-8586
**Email:** gezo@mmc.marymt.edu
**Website:** http://www.marymt.edu
Evelyn Gezo, Director

**★ 16293 ★ New York Institute of**
**Technology**
**Department of Nutrition and Food**
**Studies**
**Dietetics-Didactic Program**
35 W Fourth St., 10th Fl.
New York, NY 10012-1172
**Phone:** (212)998-5580   **Fax:** (212)995-4194
**Email:** judith.gilbride@nyu.edu
**Website:** http://www.nyit.edu/
Judith A. Gilbride, PhD, Director

**★ 16294 ★ New York Institute of**
**Technology**
**Dietetic Internship Program**
NYCOM II, Rm. 334
Old Westbury, NY 11568-8000
**Phone:** (516)686-3827   **Fax:** (516)686-3795
**Email:** jpmeyer@iris.nyit.edu
Jennifer Meyer, Director

**★ 16295 ★ New York University**
**Department of Nutrition and Food**
**Studies**
**Dietetics-Didactic Program**
Education Bldg.
35 W Fourth St., 10th Fl.
New York, NY 10012-1172
**Phone:** (212)998-5580   **Fax:** (212)995-4194
**Email:** judith.gilbride@nyu.edu
**Website:** http://www.nyu.edu/education/nutrition/
Judith A. Gilbride, PhD, Director

**★ 16296 ★ Rochester Institute of**
**Technology**
**School of Food, Hotel and Tourism**
**Management**
**Coordinated Program in Dietetics**
14 Lomb Memorial Dr.
Rochester, NY 14623-5604
**Phone:** (716)475-2357   **Fax:** (716)475-5099
**Email:** eakism@rit.isc.edu
Elizabeth A. Kmiecinski, Director

**★ 16297 ★ Rochester Institute of**
**Technology**
**School of Food, Hotel and Tourism**
**Management**
**Dietetics-Didactic Program**
14 Lomb Memorial Dr.
Rochester, NY 14623-5604
**Phone:** (716)475-2352   **Fax:** (716)475-5099
**Email:** bxcism@ritvax.isc.rit.edu
**Website:** http://www.rit.edu
Barbara Cerio, Director
Elizabeth A. Kmiecinski, Contact

**★ 16298 ★ Russell Sage College**
**Nutrition Science Department**
**Dietetics-Didactic Program**
Ackerman Hall
Troy, NY 12180-4115
**Phone:** (518)244-2048   **Fax:** (518)244-2009
**Email:** cummia@Sage.edu
**Website:** http://www.sage.edu
Ann Rogan, PhD, Director

**★ 16299 ★ Sage Graduate School**
**Dietetic Internship Program**
45 Ferry St.
Troy, NY 12180-4115
**Phone:** (518)244-2396   **Fax:** (518)244-2009
**Email:** preaw1234@aol.com
Melodie Bell-Cavallino, Director

**★ 16300 ★ State University of New York**
**Buffalo State College**
**Nutrition, Hospitality and Fashion**
**Department**
**Dietetics-Didactic Program**
1300 Elmwood Ave.
Buffalo, NY 14222-1095
**Phone:** (716)878-4333   **Fax:** (716)878-5834
**Email:** raot@buffalostate.edu
Tejaswini Rao, PhD, Director
Donna M. Hayes, Contact

**★ 16301 ★ State University of New York,**
**Buffalo**
**Dietetic Internship Program**
15 Farber Hall
3435 Main St.
Buffalo, NY 14214
**Phone:** (716)829-3680   **Fax:** (716)829-3700
**Email:** platek@buffalo.edu
Mary E. Platek, Director

**★ 16302 ★ State University of New York**
**College, Buffalo**
**Nutrition, Hospitality and Fashion**
**Department**
**Coordinated Program in Dietetics**
1300 Elmwood Ave.
Buffalo, NY 14222-1095
**Phone:** (716)878-5634   **Fax:** (716)878-5834
**Email:** hayesdm@buffalostate.edu
Donna M. Hayes, Director

**★ 16303 ★ State University of New York**
**College, Oneonta**
**Department of Human Ecology**
**Dietetics-Didactic Program or Dietetic**
**Internship Program**
201 Human Ecology
Oneonta, NY 13820-4015
**Phone:** (607)436-2705   **Fax:** (607)436-2051
**Email:** haessicj@oneonta.edu
**Website:** http://www.ONEONTA.EDU
Carolyn J. Haessig, PhD, Director

**★ 16304 ★ State University of New York,**
**Plattsburgh**
**Nutrition and Food Studies**
**Dietetics-Didactic Program**
101 Broad St.
Plattsburgh, NY 12901-2681
**Phone:** (518)564-4222   **Fax:** (518)564-3100
**Email:** coatesja@splava.cc.plattsburgh.edu
Jean A. Ostasz-Coates, PhD, Director

**★ 16305 ★ State University of New York,**
**Stony Brook**
**Department of Family Medicine**
**Dietetic Internship Program**
Health Sciences Center Level 4
Stony Brook, NY 11794-8461
**Phone:** (516)444-8246   **Fax:** (516)444-7552
**Email:** jconnoll@fammed.som.sunysb.edu
Josephine Connolly Schoonen, Director

**★ 16306 ★ Syracuse University**
**Department of Nutrition and Foodservice**
**Management**
**Dietetics-Didactic Program or Dietetic**
**Internship Program or Coordinated**
**Program in Dietetics**
034 Slocum Hall
Syracuse, NY 13244-1250
**Phone:** (315)443-2386   **Fax:** (315)443-2562
**Email:** thoracek@mailbox.syr.edu
**Website:** http://chd.syr.edu/Majors/DIET/diet_de-
scription.html
Tanya M. Horacek, PhD, Director
Kay Stearns Bruening, PhD, Contact

## North Carolina

**★ 16307 ★ Appalachian State University**
**Department of Family and Consumer**
**Sciences**
**Dietetics-Didactic Program**
Boone, NC 28608-2630
**Phone:** (828)262-2698   **Fax:** (828)265-8620
**Email:** proulxwr@appstate.edu
**Website:** http://www.appstate.edu/
William R. Proulx, PhD, Director

**★ 16308 ★ Appalachian State University**
**Family and Consumer Sciences**
**Dietetic Internship Program**
PO Box 32056
Boone, NC 28608-2056
**Phone:** (828)262-2631   **Fax:** (828)265-8620
**Email:** bogardussl@appstate.edu
Susan L. Bogardus, PhD, Director

**★ 16309 ★ Bennett College**
**Home Economics Department**
**Dietetics-Didactic Program**
900 E Washington St.
Greensboro, NC 27401-3239
**Phone:** (336)370-8793   **Fax:** (336)378-0511
**Email:** bjones@bennett1.bennett.edu
Beth P. Jones, Director

**★ 16310 ★ East Carolina University**
**School of Human Environmental Sciences**
**Department of Nutrition and Hospitality**
**Management**
**Dietetics-Didactic Program or Dietetic**
**Internship Program**
Greenville, NC 27858-4353
**Phone:** (252)328-6917   **Fax:** (252)328-4276
**Email:** escottstumps@mail.ecu.edu
**Website:** http://www.ecu.edu/hes/NUHMnutri-
tionBS.htm
Sylvia Escott-Stump, Director

★ 16311 ★ **Meredith College**
**Department of Human Environmental**
**Sciences**
**Dietetics-Didactic Program or Dietetic**
**Internship Program**
3800 Hillsborough St.
Raleigh, NC 27607-5298
**Phone:** (919)760-8079     **Fax:** (919)760-2819
**Email:** munroes@meredith.edu
Susan G. Munroe, PhD, Director


★ 16312 ★ **North Carolina A & T State**
**University**
**Department of Home Economics**
**Dietetics-Didactic Program**
102 Benbow Hall
Greensboro, NC 27411-1064
**Phone:** (336)334-7850     **Fax:** (336)334-7265
Karen W. Bennett, PhD, Director


★ 16313 ★ **North Carolina Central**
**University**
**Department of Human Sciences**
**Dietetics-Didactic Program or Dietetic**
**Internship Program**
PO Box 19615
Durham, NC 27707-0099
**Phone:** (919)530-7439     **Fax:** (919)530-7983
**Email:** eokeiyi@wpo.nccu.edu
Esther Okeiyi, PhD, Director


★ 16314 ★ **University of North Carolina,**
**Chapel Hill**
**Department of Nutrition**
**Dietetics-Didactic Program or Coordinated**
**Program in Dietetics**
McGavran-Greenburg Hall
CB 7400
Chapel Hill, NC 27599-7400
**Phone:** (919)966-7214     **Fax:** (919)966-7216
**Email:** carolyn_barrett@unc.edu
**Website:** http://www.unc.edu/nutr
Carolyn H. Barrett, Director


★ 16315 ★ **University of North Carolina,**
**Greensboro**
**Food, Nutrition and Foodservice**
**Management**
**Dietetic Internship Program**
318 Stone Bldg.
PO Box 26170
Greensboro, NC 27402-6170
**Phone:** (336)334-5313     **Fax:** (336)334-4129
**Email:** marth_taylor@ncg.edu
Martha L. Taylor, PhD, Director


★ 16316 ★ **University of North Carolina,**
**Greensboro**
**Nutrition and Foodservice Systems**
**Dietetics-Didactic Program**
PO Box 26170
Greensboro, NC 27402-6170
**Phone:** (336)334-5313     **Fax:** (336)334-4129
**Email:** cheryl_lovelady@uncg.edu
**Website:** http://www.uncg.edu/fns
Cheryl A. Lovelady, PhD, Director


★ 16317 ★ **Western Carolina University**
**Department of Health Sciences**
**Dietetics-Didactic Program**
Cullowhee, NC 28723
**Phone:** (828)227-7113     **Fax:** (828)227-7071
**Email:** hosig@wpoff.wcu.edu
Kathryn W. Hosig, PhD, Director


## North Dakota

★ 16318 ★ **North Dakota State University**
**Department of Food and Nutrition**
**Coordinated Program in Dietetics**
EML Hall 351
Fargo, ND 58105-5057
**Phone:** (701)231-7480     **Fax:** (701)231-7174
**Email:** lymoore@prairie.nodak.edu
**Website:** http://www.ndsu.nodak.edu/instruct/grossn-
ic/FoodNutr
Lynette S. Winters, Director


★ 16319 ★ **North Dakota State University**
**Department of Food and Nutrition**
**Dietetics-Didactic Program**
Human Development and Education, Box 5057
Fargo, ND 58105
**Phone:** (701)231-7479     **Fax:** (701)231-7174
**Email:** north@plains.nodak.edu
Barbara B. North, Director


★ 16320 ★ **North Dakota State University**
**Dietetic Internship Program**
EML Hall 351H
PO Box 5057
Fargo, ND 58105-5057
**Phone:** (701)231-7479     **Fax:** (701)231-7174
**Email:** north@plains.nodak.edu
**Website:** http://www.ndsu.edu/instruct/north/north/
Barbara B. North, Director


★ 16321 ★ **University of North Dakota**
**Department of Nutrition and Dietetics**
**Coordinated Program in Dietetics**
PO Box 8237
Centennial Dr.
Grand Forks, ND 58202-8237
**Phone:** (701)777-2539     **Fax:** (701)777-3650
**Email:** n_and_d@sage.und.nodak.edu
**Website:** http://www.und.edu/academics/departments
Judith Hall, Director


## Ohio

★ 16322 ★ **Bluffton College**
**Family and Consumer Sciences**
**Dietetics-Didactic Program**
280 W College Ave.
Box 896
Bluffton, OH 45817-1196
**Phone:** (419)358-3233     **Fax:** (419)358-3323
**Email:** solteszk@bluffton.edu
**Website:** http://www.bluffton.edu/dept/fcs
Kay Soltesz, PhD, Director


★ 16323 ★ **Bowling Green State**
**University**
**Department of Family and Consumer**
**Sciences**
**Dietetics-Didactic Program**
206 Johnston Hall
Bowling Green, OH 43403-0254
**Phone:** (419)372-2026     **Fax:** (419)372-7854
**Email:** ykim@bgnet.bgsu.edu
**Website:** http://www.bgsu.edu/colleges/edhd/FCS
Younghee Kim, PhD, Director


★ 16324 ★ **Case Western Reserve**
**University**
**Department of Nutrition**
**Dietetics-Didactic Program**
10900 Euclid Ave
Cleveland, OH 44106-4906
**Phone:** (216)368-2442     **Fax:** (216)368-6644
**Email:** mmc3@po.cwru.edu
**Website:**     http://www.cwru.edu/med/nutrition/
home.html
Margaret M. Cicirella, Director


★ 16325 ★ **Case Western Reserve**
**University**
**School of Medicine**
**Department of Nutrition**
**Dietetic Internship Program**
10900 Euclid Ave.
Cleveland, OH 44106-1712
**Phone:** (216)368-6626     **Fax:** (216)368-6644
**Email:** imp@po.cwru.edu
Isabel M. Parraga, PhD, Director


★ 16326 ★ **Kent State University**
**School of Family and Consumer Studies**
**Dietetics-Didactic Program**
Nixson Hall/Nutrition and Dietetics
Kent, OH 44242
**Phone:** (330)672-2197     **Fax:** (330)672-2194
**Email:** klowry@kent.edu
**Website:** http://www.kent.edu/f&cs
Karen R. Gordon, PhD, Director


★ 16327 ★ **Miami University**
**Department of Physical Education, Health**
**and Sports Studies**
**Dietetics-Didactic Program**
150 Phillips Hall
Oxford, OH 45056
**Phone:** (513)529-5036     **Fax:** (513)529-5006
**Email:** rudgesj@muohio.edu
Susan J. Rudge, PhD, Director


★ 16328 ★ **Mount Carmel College of**
**Nursing**
**Dietetic Internship Program**
127 S Davis Ave.
Columbus, OH 43222-1504
**Phone:** (614)234-5439     **Fax:** (614)234-2875
**Email:** kblancha@mchs.com
Kathleen M. Blanchard, Director


★ 16329 ★ **Notre Dame College**
**Dietetics-Didactic Program**
4545 College Rd.
South Euclid, OH 44121-4293
**Phone:** (216)381-1680     **Fax:** (216)381-3227
**Email:** mcullis@ndc.edu
**Website:** http://www.ndc.edu
Margaret A. Cullis, Director


★ 16330 ★ **Ohio State University**
**Department of Human Nutrition and Food**
**Management**
**Dietetics-Didactic Program or Dietetic**
**Internship Program**
1787 Neil Ave
Columbus, OH 43210-1220
**Phone:** (614)292-0715     **Fax:** (614)292-8880
**Email:** smith.23@osu.edu
Anne M. Smith, PhD, Director


★ 16331 ★ **Ohio State University**
**School of Allied Medical Professions**
**Medical Dietetics Division**
**Dietetic Internship Program**
1583 Perry St.
Columbus, OH 43210-1234
**Phone:** (614)292-0635     **Fax:** (614)292-0210
**Email:** schiller.1@osu.edu
**Website:** http://www.amp.ohio-state.edu/
M. Rosita Schiller, PhD, Director


★ 16332 ★ **Ohio University**
**School of Human and Consumer**
**Sciences**
**Dietetics-Didactic Program**
101-A Tupper Hall
Athens, OH 45701-2979
**Phone:** (740)593-2874     **Fax:** (740)593-0289

**Email:** hagerman@ohio.edu
Marjorie T. Hagerman, Director

**★ 16333 ★ University of Akron**
**Home Economics and Family Ecology**
**Coordinated Program in Dietetics**
215 Schrank Hall S
Akron, OH 44325-6103
**Phone:** (330)972-8842　　　**Fax:** (330)972-4934
**Email:** eston@uakron.edu
Eston B. Brown, Director

**★ 16334 ★ University of Akron**
**Home Economics and Family Ecology**
**Dietetics-Didactic Program**
215 Schrank Hall S
Akron, OH 44325-6103
**Phone:** (330)972-8088　　　**Fax:** (330)972-4934
**Email:** vmremig@uakron.edu
**Website:** http://www.uakron.edu/hefe/hefepage.html
Valentina M. Remig, PhD, Director
Eston B. Brown, Contact

**★ 16335 ★ University of Cincinnati**
**Department of Health Sciences**
**Dietetics-Didactic Program**
364 Hastings and William French Bldg.
Cincinnati, OH 45267-0394
**Phone:** (513)558-7506　　　**Fax:** (513)558-7500
**Email:** rita.smith@uc.edu
**Website:** http://oz.uc.edu/chrp/food/under.htm
Rita R. Smith, Director

**★ 16336 ★ University of Dayton**
**Health and Sports Science Department**
**Dietetics-Didactic Program**
300 College Park Ave.
Dayton, OH 45469-1210
**Phone:** (937)229-4203　　　**Fax:** (937)229-4244
**Email:** patricia.dolan@notes.udayton.edu
**Website:** http://homepages.udayton.edu/~dolanp
Patricia Dolan, Director

**★ 16337 ★ University Hospitals of**
**　Cleveland**
**Dietetic Internship Program**
11100 Euclid Ave.
Lakeside 5021
Cleveland, OH 44106-5000
**Phone:** (216)844-1310　　　**Fax:** (216)844-8188
**Email:** bonnie.rigutto@uhhs.com
Sharon K. Schwartz, Director

**★ 16338 ★ Youngstown State University**
**Coordinated Program in Dietetics**
1 University Plaza
Youngstown, OH 44555-0001
**Phone:** (330)742-3344　　　**Fax:** (330)742-2309
**Email:** jhassell@cc.ysu.edu
Jean Hassell, Director

**★ 16339 ★ Youngstown State University**
**Department of Human Ecology**
**Dietetics-Didactic Program**
1 University Plaza
Youngstown, OH 44555-0001
**Phone:** (330)742-3345　　　**Fax:** (330)742-2309
**Email:** mrshayes@cc.ysu.edu
**Website:** http://www.ysu.edu
Mohammad R. Shayesteh, PhD, Director
Jean H. Hassel, Contact

## Oklahoma

**★ 16340 ★ Langston University**
**Department of Human Ecology**
**Dietetics-Didactic Program**
308/304 Jones Hall
Langston, OK 73050
**Phone:** (405)466-3337　　　**Fax:** (405)466-3364
**Email:** ssangiah@lunet.edu
Saigeetha Sangiah, PhD, Director

**★ 16341 ★ Northeastern State University**
**College of Business and Industry**
**Dietetics-Didactic Program**
600 N Grand, 210A PA Bldg.
Tahlequah, OK 74464-2399
**Phone:** (918)456-5511　　　**Fax:** (918)458-2337
**Email:** millerak@nsuok.edu
**Website:** http://www.nsuok.edu
Alexandria R. Miller, PhD, Director

**★ 16342 ★ Oklahoma State University**
**Department of Nutritional Sciences**
**Dietetics-Didactic Program**
HES 425
Stillwater, OK 74078-6141
**Phone:** (405)744-5041　　　**Fax:** (405)744-7113
**Email:** nutrsci-i@okstate.edu
**Website:** http://www.okstate.edu/hes/nsci/
Kathryn S. Keim, PhD, Director

**★ 16343 ★ University of Central**
**　Oklahoma**
**College of Education**
**Department of Human Environmental**
**　Sciences**
**Dietetics-Didactic Program**
Edmond, OK 73034
**Phone:** (405)974-5805　　　**Fax:** (405)974-3850
**Email:** mwaters@ucok.edu
**Website:** http://204.154.115.1/
Marilyn S. Waters-Seig, PhD, Director

**★ 16344 ★ University of Central**
**　Oklahoma**
**Human Environmental Sciences**
**Dietetic Internship Program**
100 N University Dr.
Edmond, OK 73034
**Phone:** (405)974-5369　　　**Fax:** (405)974-3850
**Email:** kmeyers@ucok.edu
Karen D. Meyers, Director

**★ 16345 ★ University of Oklahoma**
**Health Sciences Center**
**College of Allied Health, Nutritional**
**　Sciences Department**
**Dietetics-Didactic Program**
PO Box 26901
Oklahoma City, OK 73190
**Phone:** (405)271-2113　　　**Fax:** (405)271-1560
**Email:** stephen-glore@ouhsc.edu
**Website:** http://w3.ouhsc.edu/ahealth/ns.htm
Stephen R. Glore, PhD, Director

**★ 16346 ★ University of Oklahoma**
**Health Sciences Center**
**Department of Nutritional Sciences**
**Coordinated Program in Dietetics**
PO Box 26901
Oklahoma City, OK 73190
**Phone:** (405)271-2113　　　**Fax:** (405)271-1560
**Email:** marinell-guild@ouhsc.edu
**Website:** http://moon.ouhsc.edu/mguild
Marinell F. Guild, Director

## Oregon

**★ 16347 ★ Oregon Health Sciences**
**　University**
**Dietetic Internship Program**
VAMC EJH-10
3181 SW Sam Jackson Park Rd.
Portland, OR 97201
**Phone:** (503)494-7596　　　**Fax:** (503)494-4496
**Email:** hagand@ohsu.edu
Dorothy W. Hagan, PhD, Director

**★ 16348 ★ Oregon State University**
**Nutrition and Food Management**
**Dietetics-Didactic Program**
14B Milam Hall
Corvallis, OR 97331-5103
**Phone:** (541)737-0960　　　**Fax:** (541)737-6914
**Email:** cluskeym@orst.edu
**Website:** http://www.orst.edu
Mary M. Cluskey, PhD, Director

## Pennsylvania

**★ 16349 ★ Cedar Crest College**
**Dietetics-Didactic Program**
100 College Dr.
Allentown, PA 18104-6132
**Phone:** (610)437-4471　　　**Fax:** (610)606-4624
**Email:** kadrummo@cedarcrest.edu
**Website:** http://www.cedarcrest.edu/academic/ntr/
Karen A. Drummond, EdD, Director

**★ 16350 ★ Drexel University**
**Nutrition and Food Sciences**
**Dietetics-Didactic Program**
3141 Chestnut St.
Philadelphia, PA 19104-2875
**Phone:** (215)895-2788　　　**Fax:** (215)895-1273
**Email:** mckinney@drexel.edu
**Website:** http://www.sciences.drexel.edu/
Shortie McKinney, PhD, Director

**★ 16351 ★ Edinboro University of**
**　Pennsylvania**
**Department of Biology and Health**
**　Services**
**Coordinated Program in Dietetics**
Edinboro, PA 16444
**Phone:** (814)732-2458　　　**Fax:** (814)732-2422
**Email:** lanz@edinboro.edu
Sally J. Lanz, Director

**★ 16352 ★ Gannon University**
**College of Sciences, Engineering and**
**　Health Sciences**
**Coordinated Program in Dietetics**
109 University Square
Erie, PA 16541-0001
**Phone:** (814)871-5452　　　**Fax:** (814)871-5662
**Email:** mugha1001@gannon.edu
Dawna T. Mughal, PhD, Director

**★ 16353 ★ Immaculata College**
**Department of Fashion, Foods and**
**　Nutrition**
**Dietetics-Didactic Program**
Box 722
Immaculata, PA 19345-0722
**Phone:** (610)647-4400　　　**Fax:** (610)251-1668
**Email:** pthibau2@immaculata.edu
Marion Jeanne Bell, Director

**★ 16354 ★ Immaculata College**
**Nutrition Education**
**Dietetic Internship Program**
Box 500-Graduate Division
Immaculata, PA 19345-0901

**Phone:** (610)647-4400          **Fax:** (610)993-8550
**Email:** sjohnst2@immaculata.edu
Susan Johnston, Director


**★ 16355 ★ Indiana University of Pennsylvania**
**Department of Food and Nutrition**
**Dietetics-Didactic Program or Dietetic Internship Program**
10 Ackerman Hall
911 South Dr.
Indiana, PA 15705-1087
**Phone:** (724)357-4440          **Fax:** (724)357-7582
**Email:** jsteiner@grove.iup.edu
**Website:** http://www.hhs.iup.edu/
Joanne B. Steiner, PhD, Director


**★ 16356 ★ La Salle University**
**Dietetics-Didactic Program**
1900 W Olney Ave.
Philadelphia, PA 19141-1108
**Phone:** (215)951-1258          **Fax:** (215)951-1772
**Email:** henstenb@lasalle.edu
**Website:** http://www.lasalle.edu/academ/bio/nutrition
Jule Anne D. Henstenburg, Director


**★ 16357 ★ Mansfield University**
**Department of Health Sciences**
**Dietetics-Didactic Program**
203C Elliott Hall
Mansfield, PA 16933
**Phone:** (570)662-4628          **Fax:** (570)662-4111
**Email:** kwright@mnsfld.edu
**Website:** http://www.mnsfld.edu/~health/index.htm
Kathy J. Wright, Director


**★ 16358 ★ Marywood University**
**Department of Nutrition and Dietetics**
**Coordinated Program in Dietetics and Dietetic Internship Program**
2300 Adams Ave.
Scranton, PA 18509
**Phone:** (570)348-6277          **Fax:** (570)348-6029
**Email:** nutrition@ac.marywood.edu
Marianne E. Borja, EdD, Director


**★ 16359 ★ Marywood University**
**Department of Nutrition and Dietetics**
**Dietetics-Didactic Program**
2300 Adams Ave.
Scranton, PA 18509-1514
**Phone:** (570)348-6277          **Fax:** (570)348-6029
**Email:** nutrition@ac.marywood.edu
**Website:** http://www.marywood.edu
Gina Pazzaglia, PhD, Director
Marianne E. Borja, EdD, Contact


**★ 16360 ★ Mercyhurst College**
**Department of Human Ecology**
**Coordinated Program in Dietetics**
501 E 38th St.
Erie, PA 16546
**Phone:** (814)824-2462          **Fax:** (814)824-3053
**Email:** cglispy@mercyhurst.edu
**Website:** http://www.mercyhurst.edu/
Charlene Glispy, Director


**★ 16361 ★ Messiah College**
**Department of Natural Sciences**
**Dietetics-Didactic Program**
Grantham, PA 17027
**Phone:** (717)766-2511          **Fax:** (717)691-6046
**Email:** mmihok@messiah.edu
Mary Ann Mihok, Director


**★ 16362 ★ Pennsylvania State University**
**College of Health and Human Development**
**Nutrition Department**
**Dietetics-Didactic Program**
University Park, PA 16802-6500
**Phone:** (814)863-2923          **Fax:** (814)863-6103
**Email:** pmk3@psu.edu
**Website:** http://nutrition.psu.edu
Penny Kris-Etherton, PhD, Director


**★ 16363 ★ Seton Hill College**
**Division of Family and Consumer Sciences**
**Coordinated Program in Dietetics**
Greensburg, PA 15601-1599
**Phone:** (724)830-1045          **Fax:** (724)830-4611
**Email:** sandrick@setonhill.edu
**Website:** http://www.setonhill.edu
Janice G. Sandrick, PhD, Director


**★ 16364 ★ University of Pittsburgh**
**School of Health and Rehabilitation Sciences**
**Dietetics-Didactic Program or Coordinated Program in Dietetics**
4044 Forbes Tower
Pittsburgh, PA 15260-1802
**Phone:** (412)647-1212          **Fax:** (412)647-6216
**Email:** rmonda@pitt.edu
Regina M. Onda, PhD, Director


**★ 16365 ★ University of Pittsburgh Medical Center**
**Dietetic Internship Program**
5230 Centre Ave.
Pittsburgh, PA 15232-1304
**Phone:** (412)623-2114          **Fax:** (412)623-2429
**Email:** scottsmithjl@msx.upmc.edu
Joyce L. Scott-Smith, Director


**★ 16366 ★ West Chester University**
**Sturzebecker Health Sciences Center**
**Department of Health**
**Dietetics-Didactic Program**
H302 Department of Health
West Chester, PA 19383
**Phone:** (610)436-2655          **Fax:** (610)436-2860
**Email:** jharris@wcupa.edu
**Website:** http://www.wcupa.edu/
Jeffrey E. Harris, Director


### Puerto Rico

**★ 16367 ★ University of Puerto Rico**
**College of Health Related Professions**
**Dietetic Internship Program**
Medical Sciences Campus
PO Box 365067
San Juan, PR 00936-5067
**Phone:** (787)758-2525          **Fax:** (787)759-3645
**Email:** ritalucca@cprs.tcm.upr.edu
Rita L. Delgado, Director


**★ 16368 ★ University of Puerto Rico**
**Rio Piedras Campus**
**Dietetics-Didactic Program**
Box 23347, UPR Station
San Juan, PR 00931-3347
**Phone:** (787)764-0000          **Fax:** (787)772-1422
**Email:** ihernan1@rrpac.upr.clu.edu
Iris Z. Hernandez, Director


### Rhode Island

**★ 16369 ★ Johnson and Wales University**
**College of Culinary Arts**
**Dietetics-Didactic Program**
1 Washington Ave.
Providence, RI 02905
**Phone:** (401)598-1881          **Fax:** (401)598-1161
**Email:** suevieira@aol.com
**Website:** http://www.uab.edu/nutrition
Suzanne P. Vieira, Director


**★ 16370 ★ University of Rhode Island**
**Department of Food Science and Nutrition**
**Dietetics-Didactic Program**
17 Woodward Hall
Kingston, RI 02881-0804
**Phone:** (401)874-5869          **Fax:** (401)874-4017
**Email:** cathy@uri.edu
**Website:** http://www.uri.edu
Catherine English, PhD, Director


### South Carolina

**★ 16371 ★ Clemson University**
**Department of Food Science**
**Dietetics-Didactic Program**
223 Poole, Agricultural Center
Clemson, SC 29634-0371
**Phone:** (864)656-5690          **Fax:** (864)656-0331
**Email:** bkunkel@clemson.edu
**Website:** http://hubcap.clemson.edu/foodscience/
Mary E. Kunkel, PhD, Director


**★ 16372 ★ Medical University of South Carolina**
**Dietetic Internship Program**
96 Jonathan Lucas St., Ste. 219K
PO Box 250602
Charleston, SC 29425
**Phone:** (843)792-1454          **Fax:** (843)792-6486
**Email:** milkerjr@musc.edu
Joanne Milkereit, Director


**★ 16373 ★ South Carolina State University**
**Dietetics-Didactic Program**
Staley Hall
PO Box 7084
300 College St. NE
Orangeburg, SC 29117-0001
**Phone:** (803)536-8620          **Fax:** (803)533-3628
**Email:** zs_bowensj@alpha2.scsu.edu
Juanita Bowens, PhD, Director


**★ 16374 ★ Winthrop University**
**Department of Human Nutrition**
**Dietetics-Didactic Program**
Rock Hill, SC 29733
**Phone:** (803)323-4520          **Fax:** (803)323-2254
**Email:** wolmanp@winthrop.edu
**Website:** http://www.winthrop.edu/nutrition
Patricia G. Wolman, EdD, Director


### South Dakota

**★ 16375 ★ Mount Marty College**
**Department of Nutrition and Food Science**
**Dietetics-Didactic Program or Coordinated Program in Dietetics**
1105 W Eighth St.
Yankton, SD 57078-3724
**Phone:** (605)668-1520          **Fax:** (605)668-1607
**Email:** tholzbauer@mtmc.edu
**Website:** http://www.mtmc.edu
Sister Thecla M. Holzbauer, Director

## ★ 16376 ★ South Dakota State University
**College of Family and Consumer Sciences**
**Dietetics-Didactic Program**
PO Box 2275A
Brookings, SD 57007-0497
**Phone:** (605)688-4045 **Fax:** (605)688-4439
**Email:** kendra_kattelmann@sdstate.edu
**Website:** http://www.sdstate.edu/fcs/NFSH/cours-es.htm
Kendra Kattelmann, PhD, Director

## ★ 16377 ★ University of South Dakota
**School of Medicine**
**Preprofessional Practice Program in Dietetics**
414 E Clark St.
Vermillion, SD 57069-2390
**Phone:** (605)677-5311 **Fax:** (605)677-6274
**Email:** gjohanns@usd.edu
Gail Johannsen, Director

### Tennessee

## ★ 16378 ★ Carson-Newman College
**Dietetics-Didactic Program**
Box 71881
Jefferson City, TN 37760-7001
**Phone:** (865)471-3295 **Fax:** (865)471-3502
**Email:** coffey@cncacc.cn.edu
**Website:** http://www.cn.edu/
Kitty R. Coffey, PhD, Director

## ★ 16379 ★ David Lipscomb University
**Department of Family and Consumer Sciences**
**Dietetics-Didactic Program**
3901 Granny White Pike
Nashville, TN 37204-3951
**Phone:** (615)269-1000 **Fax:** (615)269-1808
**Email:** nancy.hunt@lipscomb.edu
Nancy Hunt, Director

## ★ 16380 ★ East Tennessee State University
**Department of Applied Human Sciences**
**Dietetics-Didactic Program**
PO Box 70671
Johnson City, TN 37614-0671
**Phone:** (423)439-7532 **Fax:** (423)439-7539
**Email:** verheggr@etsu.edu
**Website:** http://www.etsu.edu/
Ruth D. Verhegge, Director

## ★ 16381 ★ Middle Tennessee State University
**Department of Human Sciences**
**Dietetics-Didactic Program**
PO Box 86
Murfreesboro, TN 37132
**Phone:** (615)898-2091 **Fax:** (615)898-5130
**Email:** dewalker@frank.mtsu.edu
**Website:** http://www.mtsu.edu
Dellmar Walker, PhD, Director

## ★ 16382 ★ Tennessee State University
**Department of Family and Consumer Sciences**
**Dietetics-Didactic Program**
PO Box 9538
3500 John A. Merritt Blvd.
Nashville, TN 37209-1561
**Phone:** (615)963-5619 **Fax:** (615)963-5033
**Email:** godwin@acad.tnstate.edu
**Website:** http://www.tnstate.edu
Sandria L. Godwin, PhD, Director

## ★ 16383 ★ Tennessee Technological University
**School of Home Economics**
**Dietetics-Didactic Program**
Box 5035
Cookeville, TN 38505
**Phone:** (931)372-3865 **Fax:** (931)372-3150
**Email:** abrunt@tntech.edu
**Website:** http://iweb.tntech.edu/abrunt
Ardith R. Brunt, PhD, Director

## ★ 16384 ★ University of Memphis
**Consumer Science and Education**
**Dietetic Internship Program**
Manning Hall, Rm. 4006G
Memphis, TN 38125
**Phone:** (901)678-3108 **Fax:** (901)678-5324
**Email:** LHClemens@cc.memphis.edu
Linda H. Clemens, EdD, Director

## ★ 16385 ★ University of Memphis
**Department of Consumer Science and Education**
**Dietetics-Didactic Program**
Memphis, TN 38152
**Phone:** (901)678-3110 **Fax:** (901)678-5324
**Email:** roach.robin@coe.memphis.edu
**Website:** http://www.coe.memphis.edu
Robin Roach, EdD, Director

## ★ 16386 ★ University of Tennessee, Chattanooga
**Department of Human Ecology**
**Dietetics-Didactic Program**
202 Hunter Hall
Chattanooga, TN 37403
**Phone:** (423)755-4792 **Fax:** (423)755-4479
**Email:** patricia-garrett@utc.edu
Patricia M. Garrett, Director

## ★ 16387 ★ University of Tennessee, Knoxville
**College of Human Ecology**
**Department of Nutrition**
**Dietetics-Didactic Program**
1215 Cumberland Ave., Rm. 229
Knoxville, TN 37996-1900
**Phone:** (865)974-6244 **Fax:** (865)974-3491
**Email:** skinner@utk.edu
Jean Skinner, PhD, Director

## ★ 16388 ★ University of Tennessee, Martin
**Department of Human Environmental Sciences**
**Dietetic Internship Program or Dietetics-Didactic Program**
330E Gooch Hall
Martin, TN 38238-5045
**Phone:** (901)587-7101 **Fax:** (901)587-7106
**Email:** kowalsky@utm.edu
**Website:** http://www.utm.edu/
Leigh A. Kowalsky, Director

## ★ 16389 ★ Vanderbilt University Medical Center
**Dietetic Internship Program**
B-802TVC
Nashville, TN 37232-5510
**Phone:** (615)322-0062 **Fax:** (615)343-8810
**Email:** cynthia.broadhurst@mcmail.vanderbilt.edu
Cynthia B. Broadhurst, Director

### Texas

## ★ 16390 ★ Abilene Christian University
**Department of Family and Consumer Sciences**
**Dietetics-Didactic Program**
ACU Box 28155
Abilene, TX 79699
**Phone:** (915)674-2089 **Fax:** (915)674-2086
**Email:** joness@nicanor.acu.edu
**Website:** http://www.acu.edu/academics/fcs
Sheila Jones, Director

## ★ 16391 ★ Baylor University
**Department of Family and Consumer Sciences**
**Dietetics-Didactic Program**
BU Box 97346
Waco, TX 76798-7346
**Phone:** (254)710-6258 **Fax:** (254)710-3629
**Email:** LuAnn_Soliah@baylor.edu
LuAnn Soliah, PhD, Director

## ★ 16392 ★ Baylor University Medical Center
**Dietetic Internship Program**
3500 Gaston Ave.
Dallas, TX 75246-2045
**Phone:** (214)820-4019 **Fax:** (214)820-2263
**Email:** ja.grim@baylordallas.edu
Julie A. Grim, Director

## ★ 16393 ★ Lamar Institute of Technology
**Department of Family and Consumer Sciences**
**Dietetics-Didactic Program**
PO Box 10035
Beaumont, TX 77710-0035
**Phone:** (409)880-8663 **Fax:** (409)880-8666
**Email:** elliffcj@hal.lamar.edu
**Website:** http://www.lamar.edu
Connie Ruiz, Director

## ★ 16394 ★ Lamar Institute of Technology
**Family and Consumer Sciences**
**Preprofessional Practice Program in Dietetics**
PO Box 10035
Beaumont, TX 77710-0035
**Phone:** (409)880-8663 **Fax:** (409)880-8666
**Email:** pembertoar@hal.lamar.edu
Amy Pemberton, PhD, Director

## ★ 16395 ★ Prairie View A&M University
**Department of Human Sciences**
**Dietetics-Didactic Program or Dietetic Internship Program**
PO Box 4329
Prairie View, TX 77446-4329
**Phone:** (409)857-4417 **Fax:** (409)857-4441
**Email:** sharon_mcwhinney@pvamu.edu
**Website:** http://www.pvamu.edu
Sharon McWhinney, PhD, Director

## ★ 16396 ★ Sam Houston State University
**Food Science and Nutrition**
**Dietetics-Didactic Program**
SHSU Box 2177
Huntsville, TX 77341
**Fax:** (409)294-4204
**Email:** hec_zak@shsu.edu
**Website:** http://www.shsu.edu/~hec_www/
Zaheer Kirmani, PhD, Director

**★ 16397 ★ Southwest Texas State University**
**Department of Family and Consumer Sciences**
**Dietetics-Didactic Program or Dietetic Internship Program**
601 University Dr.
San Marcos, TX 78666-4616
**Phone:** (512)245-2482      **Fax:** (512)245-3829
**Email:** sh07@swt.edu
**Website:**      http://www.fcs.swt.edu/fcs_dept/nutrition.html
Sylvia L. Crixell, PhD, Director


**★ 16398 ★ Stephen F. Austin State University**
**Department of Human Sciences**
**Dietetics-Didactic Program**
SFA Station 13014
Nacogdoches, TX 75962-3014
**Phone:** (936)468-4502      **Fax:** (936)468-2140
**Email:** sweems@sfasu.edu
**Website:** http://www.SFASU.EDU
Mary K. Suzy-Weems, PhD, Director


**★ 16399 ★ Stephen F. Austin State University**
**Preprofessional Practice Program in Dietetics**
SFA Station 13014
Nacogdoches, TX 75962-3014
**Phone:** (409)468-4502      **Fax:** (409)468-2140
**Email:** dhunt@sfasu.edu
Donna-Jean Hunt, PhD, Director


**★ 16400 ★ Tarleton State University**
**Department of Human Sciences**
**Dietetics-Didactic Program**
Box T-0380
Stephenville, TX 76402
**Phone:** (254)968-9196      **Fax:** (254)968-9728
**Email:** arichmond@tarleton.edu
**Website:** http://www.tarleton.edu/
Annemarie Richmond, PhD, Director


**★ 16401 ★ Texas A&M University**
**Human Nutrition Section**
**Dietetics-Didactic Program or Dietetic Internship Program**
218 Kleburg
College Station, TX 77843-2471
**Phone:** (979)845-2142      **Fax:** (979)862-2378
**Email:** karen-beathard@ansc.tamu.edu
**Website:** http://www.tamu.edu
Karen Beathard, Director


**★ 16402 ★ Texas A&M University, Kingsville**
**Department of Human Sciences**
**Dietetics-Didactic Program or Dietetic Internship Program**
Campus Box 168
Kingsville, TX 78363
**Phone:** (361)593-2211      **Fax:** (361)593-2230
**Email:** l_appelt@tamuk.edu
**Website:** http://www.TAMUK.edu
Lisa C. Appelt, PhD, Director


**★ 16403 ★ Texas Christian University**
**Department of Nutrition and Dietetics**
**Coordinated Program in Dietetics**
TCU Box 298600
Fort Worth, TX 76129
**Phone:** (817)257-7309      **Fax:** (817)257-5849
**Email:** a.vanbeber@tcu.edu
**Website:** http://www.tcu.edu
Anne D. VanBeber, PhD, Director
Marla D. Murphy, PhD, Contact


**★ 16404 ★ Texas Christian University**
**Department of Nutrition and Dietetics**
**Dietetics-Didactic Program**
Box 298600
Fort Worth, TX 76129
**Phone:** (817)257-6321      **Fax:** (817)257-5849
**Email:** m.murphy@tcu.edu
Marla D. Murphy, PhD, Director


**★ 16405 ★ Texas Southern University**
**Department of Human Services and Consumer Sciences**
**Dietetics-Didactic Program**
3100 Cleburne Ave.
Houston, TX 77004-4575
**Phone:** (713)313-7699      **Fax:** (713)313-7228
Oddis C. Turner, DrPH, Director


**★ 16406 ★ Texas Tech University**
**Health Sciences Center**
**Department of Education, Nutrition and Restaurant-Hotel Management**
**Dietetics-Didactic Program or Dietetic Internship Program**
PO Box 41162
Lubbock, TX 79409-1162
**Phone:** (806)742-3068      **Fax:** (806)742-3042
**Email:** mboylan@hs.ttu.edu
Lee M. Boylan, PhD, Director


**★ 16407 ★ Texas Woman's University**
**Department of Nutrition and Food Sciences**
**Dietetics-Didactic Program**
304 Administration Dr., Clock Tower
Denton, TX 76201
**Phone:** (940)898-2636      **Fax:** (940)898-2634
**Email:** v_imrhan@twu.edu
**Website:** http://www.twu.edu/hs/nfs/nfs.htm
Victoria L. Imrhan, PhD, Director


**★ 16408 ★ Texas Woman's University**
**Dietetic Internship Program**
1130 M D Anderson Blvd.
Houston, TX 77030-2897
**Phone:** (713)794-2371      **Fax:** (713)794-2374
**Email:** nfs_houston@twu.edu
Rose M. Bush, Director


**★ 16409 ★ Texas Woman's University**
**Nutrition and Food Sciences**
**Dietetic Internship Program**
PO Box 425888
Denton, TX 76204-3888
**Phone:** (940)898-2657      **Fax:** (940)898-2634
**Email:** mrew@twu.edu
Martha L. Rew, Director


**★ 16410 ★ University of Houston**
**Department of Human Development and Consumer Sciences**
**Dietetics-Didactic Program or Dietetic Internship Program**
4800 Calhoun Rd.
Houston, TX 77204-6861
**Phone:** (713)743-4120      **Fax:** (713)743-4033
**Email:** scoscio@bayou.uh.edu
**Website:** http://www.tech.uh.edu/hdcs/hnf.htm
Stacey A. Coscio, Director


**★ 16411 ★ University of the Incarnate Word**
**Dietetic Internship Program**
4301 Broadway, Box 73
San Antonio, TX 78209
**Phone:** (210)829-3152      **Fax:** (210)829-3153
**Email:** josephb@universe.uiwtx.edu
Joseph C. Bonilla, PhD, Director


**★ 16412 ★ University of the Incarnate Word**
**Dietetics-Didactic Program**
4301 Broadway St.
San Antonio, TX 78209-6318
**Phone:** (210)829-3167      **Fax:** (210)829-3153
**Email:** morse@universe.uiwtx.edu
Mary Kaye Sawyer-Morse, Director


**★ 16413 ★ University of Texas, Austin**
**Department of Human Ecology**
**Coordinated Program in Dietetics**
A2700
Austin, TX 78712-1097
**Phone:** (512)471-4934      **Fax:** (512)471-5630
**Email:** cpd@mail.utexas.edu
**Website:**      http://www.utexas.edu/depts/he/nutr_science/dietetics/
Beth Gillham, PhD, Director


**★ 16414 ★ University of Texas, Austin**
**Department of Human Ecology**
**Dietetics-Didactic Program**
GEA 117
Austin, TX 78712
**Phone:** (512)471-7639      **Fax:** (512)471-5630
**Email:** cpd@mail.utexas.edu
**Website:** http://www.utexas.edu/depts/he/
Jane F. Tillman, Director


**★ 16415 ★ University of Texas Health Science Center, Houston**
**School of Public Health**
**Dietetic Internship Program**
1200 Herman Pressler Dr.
E619 RAS Bldg.
Houston, TX 77030
**Phone:** (713)500-9347      **Fax:** (713)500-9329
**Email:** jmartin@utsph.sph.uth.tmc.edu
Jeanne Martin, PhD, Director


**★ 16416 ★ University of Texas, Pan American**
**College of Health and Human Services**
**Coordinated Program in Dietetics**
1201 W University Dr.
Edinburg, TX 78539-2909
**Phone:** (956)318-5264      **Fax:** (956)318-5265
**Email:** ebriones@panam.edu
**Website:** http://www.panam.edu/
Esperanza R. Briones, PhD, Director


**★ 16417 ★ University of Texas Southwestern Medical Center, Dallas**
**Department of Clinical Nutrition**
**Coordinated Program in Dietetics**
5323 Harry Hines Blvd.
Dallas, TX 75235-8877
**Phone:** (214)648-1520      **Fax:** (214)648-1514
**Email:** clindiet@email.swmed.edu
**Website:** http://www.swmed.edu/home_pages/clinnut
Joyce P. Barnett, Director


## Utah

**★ 16418 ★ Brigham Young University**
**Food Science and Nutrition Department**
**Dietetics-Didactic Program or Dietetic Internship Program**
S219 ESC
PO Box 24620
Provo, UT 84602-4620
**Phone:** (801)378-6676      **Fax:** (801)378-8714
**Email:** nora_nyland@byu.edu
**Website:** http://bioag.byu.edu/fsn/fsn.htm
Nora Nyland, PhD, Director

**★ 16419 ★ University of Utah**
Division of Foods and Nutrition
Coordinated Program in Dietetics
Dietetic Internship Program
250 S 1850 E, No. 239
Salt Lake City, UT 84112
**Phone:** (801)581-6730 **Fax:** (801)585-3874
**Email:** jean.zancanella@health.utah.edu
**Website:** http://www.fdnu.utah.edu/
Jean Zancanella, Director

**★ 16420 ★ Utah State University**
Department of Nutrition and Food
 Sciences
Dietetics-Didactic Program or Coordinated
 Program in Dietetics
8700 Old Main Hall
Logan, UT 84322-8700
**Phone:** (435)797-2105 **Fax:** (435)797-2379
**Email:** noreens@cc.usu.edu
**Website:** http://www.usu.edu/~dietetic
Noreen B. Schvaneveldt, Director

**★ 16421 ★ Utah State University**
 Extension
Dietetic Internship Program
PO Box 160485
Clearfield, UT 84016-0485
**Phone:** (801)728-7665 **Fax:** (801)774-7674
**Email:** annmil@ext.usu.edu
Ann Martin Mildenhall, Director

### Vermont

**★ 16422 ★ University of Vermont**
Department of Nutritional Sciences
Dietetics-Didactic Program
Terrill Hall
Burlington, VT 05405
**Phone:** (802)656-0539 **Fax:** (802)656-0407
**Email:** jross@zoo.uvm.edu
**Website:** http://nutrition.uvm.edu/
Jane K. Ross, PhD, Director

### Virginia

**★ 16423 ★ James Madison University**
Department of Health Sciences
Dietetics-Didactic Program
MSC 1202
Moody Hall 213A
Harrisonburg, VA 22807
**Phone:** (540)568-6362 **Fax:** (540)568-8166
**Email:** brevarpb@jmu.edu
**Website:** http://www.jmu.edu/
Patricia B. Brevard, PhD, Director

**★ 16424 ★ James Madison University**
Dietetic Internship Program
MSC 4301
800 S Main St.
Harrisonburg, VA 22807
**Phone:** (540)568-7084 **Fax:** (540)568-8166
**Email:** gloeckjw@jmu.edu
Janet W. Gloeckner, PhD, Director

**★ 16425 ★ Norfolk State University**
Food Science and Nutrition/Chemistry
Dietetics-Didactic Program
700 Park Ave.
Norfolk, VA 23504-3992
**Phone:** (757)823-9532 **Fax:** (757)823-2909
**Email:** lallen@vger.nsu.edu
**Website:** http://www.sci.nsu.edu
Mary Linda Allen, Director

**★ 16426 ★ Radford University**
Department of Health Services
Dietetics-Didactic Program
PO Box 6962
Radford, VA 24142-5826
**Phone:** (540)831-7680 **Fax:** (540)831-6719
**Email:** m-miller@radford.edu
**Website:** http://www.radford.edu/~fdsn-web/
Mary J. Miller, Director

**★ 16427 ★ Radford University**
Foods and Nutrition Program
Dietetic Internship Program
PO Box 6962
Radford, VA 24142-6962
**Phone:** (540)831-6794 **Fax:** (540)831-6719
**Email:** sfclark@radford.edu
Susan F. Clark, PhD, Director

**★ 16428 ★ University of Virginia Health**
 Sciences Center
Dietetic Internship Program
Box 800673
Charlottesville, VA 22908
**Phone:** (804)924-2286 **Fax:** (804)982-3957
**Email:** ara6t@virginia.edu
Ana Abad Sinden, Director

**★ 16429 ★ Virginia Commonwealth**
 University/Medical College of Virginia
Dietetic Internship Program
PO Box 980294
Richmond, VA 23298-0294
**Phone:** (804)828-9108 **Fax:** (804)828-2499
**Email:** aerobbin@hsc.vcu.edu
Ann E. Robbins, Director

**★ 16430 ★ Virginia Polytechnic Institute**
 and State University
College of Human Resources and
 Education
Department of Human Nutrition, Foods
 and Exercise
Dietetics-Didactic Program or Dietetic
 Internship Program
Blacksburg, VA 24061-0430
**Phone:** (540)231-5778 **Fax:** (540)231-3916
**Email:** schlenkr@vt.edu
**Website:** http://www.chre.vt.edu
Eleanor D. Schlenker, PhD, Director

**★ 16431 ★ Virginia State University**
Department of Human Ecology
Dietetics-Didactic Program or Dietetic
 Internship Program
Box 9211
Petersburg, VA 23806
**Phone:** (804)524-5502 **Fax:** (804)524-5561
**Email:** gyoung@vsu.edu
**Website:** http://www.vsu.edu
Gloria Young, EdD, Director

### Washington

**★ 16432 ★ Bastyr University**
Nutrition Program
Dietetic Internship Program
14500 Juanita Dr. NE
Bothell, WA 98011-4966
**Phone:** (425)602-3124 **Fax:** (425)823-6222
**Email:** smyer@bastyr.edu
Suzzanne Nelson Myers, Director

**★ 16433 ★ Central Washington University**
Department of Family and Consumer
 Sciences
Dietetics-Didactic Program or Dietetic
 Internship Program
400 E Eighth Ave.
Ellensburg, WA 98926-7565
**Phone:** (509)963-2366 **Fax:** (509)963-2787
**Email:** bergmane@cwu.edu
**Website:** http://www.cwu.edu
Ellen A. Bergman, PhD, Director

**★ 16434 ★ Sea Mar Community Health**
 Center
Dietetic Internship Program
8720 14th Ave. S
Seattle, WA 98108-4807
**Phone:** (206)764-4726 **Fax:** (206)762-5642
**Email:** lead101w@wonder.em.cdc.gov
Debra A. Boutin, Director

**★ 16435 ★ Seattle Pacific University**
Department of Family and Consumer
 Sciences
Dietetics-Didactic Program
3307 Third Ave. W
Seattle, WA 98119-1997
**Phone:** (206)281-2708 **Fax:** (206)281-2035
**Email:** ehackman@paul.spu.edu
**Website:** http://www.spu.edu
Evette M. Hackman, PhD, Director

**★ 16436 ★ University of Washington**
Dietetic Internship Program
Box 353410
305 Raitt Hall
Seattle, WA 98195-3410
**Phone:** (206)646-7362 **Fax:** (206)685-1696
**Email:** brochure@u.washington.edu
**Website:** http://depts.washington.edu/~brochure/diet-eticp.html
Barbara A. Bruemmer, PhD, Director

**★ 16437 ★ Washington State University**
Department of Food Science and Human
 Nutrition
Dietetics-Didactic Program or Coordinated
 Program in Dietetics
106F Bldg.
PO Box 646376
Pullman, WA 99164-6376
**Phone:** (509)335-8448 **Fax:** (509)335-4815
**Email:** peckl@wsu.edu
**Website:** http://avfshn.wsu.edu/
Louise W. Peck, PhD, Director

**★ 16438 ★ Washington State University**
Food Science and Human Nutrition
Dietetic Internship Program
601 W First Ave.
Spokane, WA 99201-3899
**Phone:** (509)358-7562 **Fax:** (509)358-7505
**Email:** msandall@mail.wsu.edu
Janet K. Beary, PhD, Director

### West Virginia

**★ 16439 ★ Marshall University**
Family and Consumer Sciences
Dietetics-Didactic Program or Dietetic
 Internship Program
400 Hal Greer Blvd.
203 Corbly Hall
Huntington, WV 25755-9521
**Phone:** (304)696-4336 **Fax:** (304)696-3177
**Email:** williamsk@marshall.edu
Kelli J. Williams, Director

**★ 16440 ★ West Virginia University**
**College of Agriculture and Forestry**
**Dietetics-Didactic Program or Dietetic**
   **Internship Program**
PO Box 6124
702 Allen Hall
Morgantown, WV 26506-6124
**Phone:** (304)293-3402          **Fax:** (304)293-2750
**Email:** bforbes3@wvu.edu
**Website:** http://www.caf.wvu.edu/
Betty J. Forbes, Director


**★ 16441 ★ West Virginia University**
   **Hospitals**
**Department of Nutrition and**
   **Environmental Services**
**Dietetic Internship Program**
Medical Center Dr.
Morgantown, WV 26506-8016
**Phone:** (304)598-4105          **Fax:** (304)598-4119
**Email:** arnolds@rcbhsc.wvu.edu
Susan J. Arnold, Director


**★ 16442 ★ West Virginia Wesleyan**
   **College**
**Department of Human Ecology**
**Dietetics-Didactic Program**
Haymond Hall 113
PO Box 15
Buckhannon, WV 26201-0015
**Phone:** (304)473-8566          **Fax:** (304)473-8187
**Email:** halverson@wvwc.edu
Lillian S. Halverson, PhD, 483Dietetic Dietetic Disorders


## Wisconsin

**★ 16443 ★ Mount Mary College**
**Graduate Program in Dietetics**
**Dietetic Internship Program or**
   **Coordinated Program in Dietetics**
2900 N Menomonee River Pkwy.
Milwaukee, WI 53222-4597
**Phone:** (414)256-1216          **Fax:** (414)256-1224
**Email:** starkl@mtmary.edu
Lisa Stark, Director


**★ 16444 ★ University of Wisconsin,**
   **Green Bay**
**Department of Human Biology**
**Dietetic Internship Program or Dietetics-**
   **Didactic Program**
2420 Nicolet Dr.
ES 301
Green Bay, WI 54311-7001
**Phone:** (920)465-2332          **Fax:** (920)465-2769
**Email:** laceyk@uwgb.edu
**Website:** http://www.uwgb.edu/humbio/nutri.htm
Karen Lacey, Director


**★ 16445 ★ University of Wisconsin**
   **Hospitals and Clinics**
**Dietetic Internship Program**
Food and Nutrition Services F4/120
600 Highland Ave.
Madison, WI 53792-1510
**Phone:** (608)263-8237          **Fax:** (608)263-0343
**Email:** me.morgan@uwmsg.hosp.wisc.edu
Marjorie U. Morgan, Director


**★ 16446 ★ University of Wisconsin,**
   **Madison**
**Department of Nutritional Sciences**
**Coordinated Program in Dietetics**
1415 Linden Dr.
Madison, WI 53706-1571
**Phone:** (608)262-5847          **Fax:** (608)262-5860
**Email:** karls@nutrisci.wisc.edu
Lynette M. Karls, Director


**★ 16447 ★ University of Wisconsin,**
   **Madison**
**Department of Nutritional Sciences**
**Dietetics-Didactic Program**
1415 Linden Dr.
Madison, WI 53706-1571
**Phone:** (608)262-2727          **Fax:** (608)262-5860
**Email:** ney@nutrisci.wisc.edu
**Website:** http://wiscinfo.doit.wisc.edu/nutrisci/
Denise M. Ney, PhD, Director
Lynette M. Karls, Contact


**★ 16448 ★ University of Wisconsin,**
   **Stevens Point**
**School of Health Promotion and Human**
   **Development**
**Dietetics-Didactic Program**
Stevens Point, WI 54481
**Phone:** (715)346-4087          **Fax:** (715)346-3751
**Email:** jchithar@uwsp.edu
**Website:** http://www.uwsp.edu/acad/hphd/
Jayne S. Chitharanjan, Director


**★ 16449 ★ University of Wisconsin,**
   **Stout**
**College of Human Development**
**Dietetics-Didactic Program**
Menomonie, WI 54751
**Fax:** (715)232-2366
**Email:** seabornc@uwstout.edu
**Website:** http://www.uwstout.edu/programs/
Carol D. Seaborn, PhD, Director


**★ 16450 ★ University of Wisconsin,**
   **Stout**
**Department of Food and Nutrition**
**Dietetic Internship Program**
220 Home Economics Bldg.
Menomonie, WI 54751
**Phone:** (715)232-1994          **Fax:** (715)232-2366
**Email:** knousb@uwstout.edu
Barbara L. Knous, PhD, Director


**★ 16451 ★ Viterbo College**
**Nutrition and Dietetics Department**
**Coordinated Program in Dietetics or**
   **Dietetic Internship Program**
815 S Ninth St.
La Crosse, WI 54601-4797
**Phone:** (608)796-3660          **Fax:** (608)796-3050
**Email:** lclewis@mail.viterbo.edu
**Website:** http://www.viterbo.edu/academic/ug/sls/majors/Dietetics
Lorraine C. Lewis, Director


## Wyoming

**★ 16452 ★ University of Wyoming**
**Department of Family and Consumer**
   **Sciences**
**Dietetics-Didactic Program**
Laramie, WY 82071-3354
**Phone:** (307)766-4145          **Fax:** (307)766-3379
**Email:** schantz@uwyo.edu
Rhoda M. Schantz, PhD, Director


# National & International Organizations

**★ 16453 ★ Africa Council for Food and**
   **Nutrition Sciences (ACFNS)**
c/o TFNC
PO Box 977
Dar es Salaam, United Republic of Tanzania
**Phone:** 255 51 29621          **Fax:** 255 51 44029

**Lang(s):** English. **Desc:** Food and nutrition scientists and health care professionals. Seeks to advance the study, teaching, and practice of the food and nutrition sciences. Serves as a forum for the exchange of information among members; sponsors research and educational programs.


**★ 16454 ★ African-American Natural**
   **Foods Association (AANFA)**
c/o Cheryl A. Simms
PO Box 497336
Chicago, IL 60649
**Phone:** (773)363-3939
Cheryl A. Simms, Pres.

**Fnded:** 1990. **Desc:** Natural and health food retailers, health practitioners, manufacturers, and distributors; interested individuals. Works to increase awareness of natural foods and the nutritional industry in minority communities. Sponsors seminars and workshops; maintains library and speakers' bureau. Plans to establish a natural food resource and information center.


**American Academy of Veterinary**
   **Nutrition (AAVN)**
*See:* Entry 20532


**★ 16455 ★ American Association of**
   **Nutritional Consultants (AANC)**
400 Oak Hill Dr.
Winona Lake, IN 46590
**Phone:** 888-828-2262          **Fax:** (219)269-4060
**Email:** registrar@aanc.net
**Website:** http://www.aanc.net
Wilma Johnson, Asst. Admin.

**Fnded:** 1980. **Mem:** 5,000. **Desc:** Professional nutritional consultants. Seeks to create a forum for exchange of nutritional information. Offers benefits such as car rental and laboratory discounts. **Pub:** *Health-Keepers Journal*, quarterly. Journal. Focuses on innovation in the field of professional nutritional counseling, and vitamin, mineral, and food therapies. Includes nutrition digest. *Price:* Available to members only. • Membership Directory.


**★ 16456 ★ American Board of Nutrition**
   **(ABN)**
University of Alabama at Birmingham
1675 University Blvd./WEBB 232
Department of Nutrition Sciences
Birmingham, AL 35294-3360
**Phone:** (205)975-5564          **Fax:** (205)934-7049
**Email:** joness@shrp.uab.edu
**Website:** http://www.uab.edu/nusc/abn.htm
Donna Swaggerty, Contact

**Fnded:** 1948. **Mem:** 524. **Desc:** Physicians qualified to treat nutritional and metabolic disorders; doctoral recipients working on problems of human nutrition and nutrient requirements. Establishes standards for qualification of persons as specialists in the field of clinical human nutrition; holds examinations and certifies those who meet its qualifications. **Pub:** *Directory of Diplomates in Human Nutrition and Clinical Nutrition*, biennial. Directory. *Price:* Free.


**★ 16457 ★ American College of Nutrition**
   **(ACN)**
300 S Duncan Ave., Ste. 225
Clearwater, FL 33755
**Phone:** (727)446-6086          **Fax:** (727)446-6202
**Email:** office@am-coll-nutr.org
**Website:** http://www.am-coll-nutr.org
Stanley Wallach, MD, Exec. Dir.

**Fnded:** 1959. **Mem:** 1,170. **Nat'l Groups:** 1. **Desc:** Physicians, research scientists, nutritionists, dietitians, allied health personnel, and postbaccalaureate students and trainees in these fields. Provides education on clinical, scientific, and experimental developments in the field of nutrition. Stimulates the exchange of information between nutrition scientists and physicians interested in applying research findings to the care of patients; encourages nutrition education in medical schools; provides for continuing education of physicians and other scientists on nutritional subjects. Sponsors a postgraduate course on nutritional problems. Advises physicians on nutrition developments of clinical importance. Certifies credentials of professional nutritionists, including by formal examination. **Pub:** *ACN Newsletter*, quarterly. Newsletter. • *Journal of the American College of Nutrition*, bimonthly. Journal. Contains peer-reviewed articles. *Price:* Included in membership dues; $70/year for U.S. nonmembers; $160/year for U.S. institutions; $100/year for nonmembers outside the U.S.

### ★ 16458 ★ American Council of Applied Clinical Nutrition (ACACN)

PO Box 509
Florissant, MO 63032
**Phone:** (314)921-3997      **Free:** 800-826-5366
**Fax:** (314)921-8485
Clarence T. Smith, PhD, Pres.

**Fnded:** 1974. **Mem:** 500. **Desc:** Clinical nutrition specialists. Offers structured academic course and certification; conducts research.

### ★ 16459 ★ American Dietetic Association (ADA)

216 W Jackson Blvd.
Chicago, IL 60606-6995
**Phone:** (312)899-0040      **Free:** 800-877-1600
**Fax:** (312)899-1979
**Email:** membrshp@eatright.org
**Website:** http://www.eatright.org
Ronald Moen, CEO

**Fnded:** 1917. **Mem:** 64,000. **State Groups:** 52. **Desc:** Food and nutrition professionals. Promotes nutrition, health and well-being. **Pub:** *Journal of the American Dietetic Association*, monthly. Journal. Contains research and practice articles, association news, literature abstracts, and a list of new publications. *Price:* Included in membership dues; $98/year for nonmembers.

### ★ 16460 ★ American Society for Clinical Nutrition (ASCN)

9650 Rockville Pike
Bethesda, MD 20814-3998
**Phone:** (301)530-7110      **Fax:** (301)571-1863
**Email:** ambocus@ascn.faseb.org
**Website:** http://www.faseb.org/ascn
Ann Marie Bocus, Admin. Asst.

**Fnded:** 1959. **Mem:** 1,565. **Desc:** Physicians and scientists actively engaged in clinical nutrition research. Promotes teaching, research, and reporting of progress in clinical nutrition. Offers annual postgraduate course. **Pub:** *The American Journal of Clinical Nutrition*, monthly. Journal. Contains original research findings. Includes book reviews, commentaries, letters to the editor, and editorials. *Price:* $60/year for members; $120/year for nonmembers in U.S.; $140/year for nonmembers outside U.S.; $50/year for students. • Publishes 6-8 supplements per year. **Frmly:** (1997) American Institute of Nutrition.

### ★ 16461 ★ American Society for Nutritional Sciences (ASNS)

9650 Rockville Pke.
Bethesda, MD 20814-3990
**Phone:** (301)530-7050      **Fax:** (301)571-1892
**Email:** sec@asns.faseb.org
**Website:** http://www.faseb.org/asns/
Richard G. Allison, PhD, Exec. Off.

**Fnded:** 1928. **Mem:** 3,100. **Desc:** Professional society of nutrition research scientists from universities, government, and industry. **Pub:** *Journal of Nutrition*, monthly. Journal. Peer-reviewed research papers covering all aspects of experimental nutrition, critical reviews, biographies, and commentaries on controversial issues. *Price:* Included in membership dues; $105/year for nonmembers; $125/year outside the U.S.; $25/ year for students. • *Nutrition Notes*, quarterly. Newsletter. Provides information about the Institute's activities as well as topical national and international issues in nutrition. *Price:* Included in membership dues; $30/year for nonmembers. **Frmly:** (1997) American Institute of Nutrition.

### ★ 16462 ★ American Society for Parenteral and Enteral Nutrition (ASPEN)

8630 Fenton Ste., No. 412
Silver Spring, MD 20910-3805
**Phone:** (301)587-6315      **Fax:** (301)587-2365
**Email:** aspen@nutr.org
**Website:** http://www.nutritioncare.org
Robin Kriegel, Exec. Dir.

**Fnded:** 1975. **Mem:** 6,000. **State Groups:** 49. **Desc:** Physicians, dietitians, nurses, pharmacists, and members of the industry. Works to promote quality patient care, education, and research in the field of nutrition and metabolic support in all health care settings. Educates health care professionals. Conducts postgraduate courses and research programs; compiles statistics. **Pub:** *Journal of Parenteral and Enteral Nutrition*, bimonthly. Journal. Includes current research, book reviews, case reports, and citations from world literature. *Price:* Included in membership dues; $45/year for students; $151 for institutions; $90 for individuals. • *Nutrition in Clinical Practice*, bimonthly. Journal. Contains abstracts of literature in the field from other publications, ASPEN news, case reports, legislative news, and a list of new products. *Price:* Included in membership dues; $25/year for students; $88 for institutions; $42 for individuals. • *Nutrition Support Practice Manual*. Manual. Covers product resources. • Monographs. • Also publishes course syllabi on a variety of clinical nutrition topics, self-assessment programs, and reference anthologies.

### ★ 16463 ★ Asia Pacific Clinical Nutrition Society (APCNS)

c/o Asia Pacific Health and Nutrition Centre
PO Box 11A
Monash University
Clayton, VIC 3800, Australia
**Phone:** 61 3 99058145      **Fax:** 61 3 99058146
**Email:** mark.wahlqvist@med.monash.edu.au

**Lang(s):** English. **Desc:** Nutritionists and other health care professionals with an interest in nutrition. Seeks to advance the study, teaching, and practice of nutrition. Serves as a clearinghouse on nutrition; sponsors research and continuing professional development programs.

### ★ 16464 ★ Asia-Pacific Network for Food and Nutrition (APNFN)

c/o RCFSAP
FAO Regional Office for Asia and the Pacific
Maliwan Mansion
Phra Atit Rd.
Bangkok 10200, Thailand
**Phone:** 66 2 2817844      **Fax:** 66 2 2800445

**Lang(s):** English, Thai. **Desc:** Academics and health care professionals with an interest in food and nutrition. Seeks to advance the study, teaching, and practice of nutrition counseling. Serves as a clearinghouse on food and nutrition; sponsors research and educational programs.

### ★ 16465 ★ Asia Pacific Public Health Nutrition Association (APPHNA)

Public Health Nutrition Program
421 Warren Hall
University of California
Berkeley, CA 94720-7360
**Phone:** (510)642-3852      **Fax:** (510)643-6981
**Email:** zaksabry@socrates.berkeley.edu
**Website:** http://www.monash.edu.au/APPHNA/
Zak Sabry, Contact

**Desc:** Public health practitioners and nutritionists. Promotes nutrition as a vital component of good health. Develops and implements national and international public health nutrition strategies; sponsors research and educational programs.

### Asian Pan-Pacific Society for Paediatric Gastroenterology and Nutrition

*See:* Entry 5619

### BODYWHYS: Help, Support, Understanding for Anorexia and Bulimia Nervosa

*See:* Entry 12420

### ★ 16466 ★ British Dietetic Association (BDA)

Charles House, 5th Fl.
148/9 Great Charles St. Queensway
Birmingham B3 3HT, United Kingdom
**Phone:** 44 121 2008080      **Fax:** 44 121 2008081
**Email:** info@bda.uk.com
**Website:** http://www.bda.uk.com

**Fnded:** 1936. **Mem:** 4,000. **Local Groups:** 11. **Lang(s):** English. **Desc:** Professional registered dietitians. Promotes advancement of the science and practice of dietetics and related subjects. Sponsors training and educational programs. Arranges meetings, refresher courses, and study conferences. Provides liaison between dietitians in the United Kingdom and other countries. **Pub:** *Adviser Magazine*, quarterly. • *Journal of Human Nutrition and Dietetics*, bimonthly. • *Members' Newsletter*, monthly. Newsletter.

### ★ 16467 ★ British Nutrition Foundation

High Holborn House
52-54 High Holborn
London WC1V 6RQ, United Kingdom
**Phone:** 44 207 4046504      **Fax:** 44 207 4046747
**Email:** postbox@nutrition.org.uk
**Website:** http://www.nutrition.org.uk

**Fnded:** 1967. **Mem:** 41. **Desc:** No individual members. Corporate membership open to any organisation, company or corporation (except trade associations) interested or concerned in achieving the objectives of the Foundation (which are listed in the Annual Report). Provides reliable information and scientifically based advice on nutrition and related health matters. Aims to help individuals understand how they may best match their diet with their lifestyle. Produces a wide range of publications on many aspects of diet and health. **Pub:** *BNF Bulletin*, 3/year. Bulletin. • *Food: A Fact of Life*. Nutrition program for schools. • *Proceedings of Annual Conference*, annual. • Papers. Briefing papers.

### ★ 16468 ★ Canadian Foundation for Dietetic Research (CFDR) (La Fondation Canadienne de la Recherche en Dietetique — FCRD)

480 University, Ste. 604
Toronto, ON, Canada M5G 1V2
**Phone:** (416)596-1294      **Fax:** (416)596-0603
**Email:** cfdr@dietitians.ca
**Website:** http://www.dietitians.ca/cfdr

**Fnded:** 1991. **Lang(s):** English, French. **Desc:** Dietitians and other individuals with an interest in nutrition. Seeks to advance dietetic research. Provides support and assistance to nutrition research projects; conducts educational programs. **Pub:** Report, annual.

### ★ 16469 ★ Canadian Society for Nutritional Sciences (CSNS) (Societe Canadienne des Sciences de la Nutrition — SCSN)

c/o School of Dieticians and Human Nutrition
MacDonald Campus
McGill University
21111 Lakeshore
Ste.-Anne-de-Bellevue, QC, Canada H9X 3V9
**Phone:** (514)398-7547      **Fax:** (514)398-7739

**Lang(s):** English, French. **Desc:** Dieticians and other scientists and health care professionals with an interest in nutrition. Seeks to advance the study and practice of the nutritional sciences. Serves as a forum for the exchange of information among members; sponsors research and educational programs.

**★ 16470 ★ Chinese Nutrition Society**
29 Nanwei Rd.
Beijing 100050, People's Republic of China
**Phone:** 852 10 63043472   **Fax:** 852 10 63011875

**★ 16471 ★ Consultant Dietitians in Health Care Facilities (CDHCF)**
2219 Cardinal Dr.
Waterloo, IA 50701
**Phone:** (319)235-0991        **Fax:** (319)235-7224
**Email:** cdhcf@cdhcf.org
**Website:** http://www.cdhcf.org
Marolyn Steffani, RD, LD, Chm.
**Fnded:** 1975. **Mem:** 6,100. **Reg. Groups:** 7. **State Groups:** 50. **Desc:** A special interest group of the American Dietetic Association. Dietitians employed in extended care facilities, nursing homes, homecare, and a variety of food service operations. Disseminates information; assists in solving their problems in the field. Conducts workshops; offers networking opportunities for professionals. **Pub:** *The Consultant Dietitian*, quarterly. Newsletter. *Price:* $25/year. • *Dining Skills.* • *Inservice Manual.* • *Pocket Resource for Nutrition Assessment.* • *Tool Box (Adults with Developmental Disabilities).* • *Video Tapes on Dining Skills.* **Frmly:** Consultant Dieticians Special Interest Group.

**Council on Health Information and Education (CHIE)**
*See:* Entry 12079

**★ 16472 ★ Council for Responsible Nutrition (CRN)**
1875 Eye St. NW, Ste. 400
Washington, DC 20036-5409
**Phone:** (202)872-1488        **Fax:** (202)872-9594
**Email:** webmaster@crnusa.org
**Website:** http://www.crnusa.org
John Cordaro, Pres. /CEO
**Fnded:** 1973. **Mem:** 100. **Desc:** Manufacturers, distributors, and other companies involved in the production and sale of nutritional supplements, including vitamins, minerals and herbal products. Seeks an improvement in the general health of the U.S. population through responsible nutrition, including the appropriate use of nutritional supplements. Acts as a liaison between vitamin and mineral products manufacturers and government regulatory agencies, such as the Food and Drug Administration, the Federal Trade Commission, and the U.S. Congress. Keeps members informed of relevant legislative developments. Provides a forum to review governmental actions and evaluate current nutrition information. Acts as a clearinghouse to keep members informed of new scientific developments in nutrient safety, health, and nutrition. **Pub:** *CRN News*, monthly. Newsletter. *Price:* For members only.

**★ 16473 ★ Dietary Managers Association (DMA)**
406 Surrey Woods Dr.
Saint Charles, IL 60174
**Phone:** (630)587-6336        **Free:** 800-323-1908
**Fax:** (630)587-6308
**Email:** info@dmaonline.com
**Website:** http://www.dmaonline.org
Jackie Dewitt, CDM, Chair
**Fnded:** 1960. **Mem:** 14,000. **State Groups:** 50. **Desc:** Dietary managers united to maintain a high level of competency and quality in dietary departments through continuing education. Provides educational programs and placement service. **Pub:** *Diet Therapy for the Dietary Manager*. Book. *Price:* $47.50 for nonmembers. • *Dietary Manager*, bimonthly. Magazine. *Price:* $24/year. • *Managing Foodservice Operations*. Book. • *Professional Procurement Practices*. Book. **Frmly:** Hospital, Institution and Educational Food Service Society.

**★ 16474 ★ Dietitians Association of Australia (DAA)**
1/8 Phipps Pl.
Deakin, ACT 2600, Australia
**Phone:** 61 2 62829555        **Fax:** 61 2 62829888
**Email:** national@daa.asn.au
**Website:** http://www.daa.asn.au
**Fnded:** 1976. **Mem:** 2,200. **Nat'l Groups:** 1. **State Groups:** 18. **Lang(s):** English. **Desc:** Accredited dietitians, students, and other individuals with an interest in nutrition. Works to improve public health through establishment of healthier eating habits. Seeks to enhance the professional standing of members. Serves as a liaison linking members to related professional, governmental, industrial, and educational organizations. Provides technical and professional support to members; lobbies government agencies responsible for food and nutrition. **Pub:** *Australian Journal of Nutrition and Dietetics*, quarterly. Journal. • *Vision and Strategic Direction Statement*. Brochure. • Annual Report. • Handbooks. • Newsletter, periodic. • Pamphlets. • Papers. • Proceedings.

**★ 16475 ★ Dietitians of Canada (DC)**
480 University Ave., Ste. 604
Toronto, ON, Canada M5G 1V2
**Phone:** (416)596-0857        **Fax:** (416)596-0603
**Email:** centralinfo@dietitians.ca
**Website:** http://www.dietitians.ca
**Fnded:** 1935. **Mem:** 5,000. **Lang(s):** English, French. **Desc:** Leads and supports members to promote health and well being through expertise in food and nutrition. **Pub:** *Canadian Journal of Dietetic Research and Practice*, quarterly. Journal.

**Eating Disorders Northern Ireland**
*See:* Entry 12462

**European Association for Nutrition and Child Development Studies (Association Europeene pour l'Etude de l'Alimentation et du Developpement de l'Enfant)**
*See:* Entry 5673

**★ 16476 ★ European Association for Studies on Nutrition and Child Development (ADE) (Association Europeenne pour l'Etude de l'Alimentation et du Developpement de l'Enfant — ADE)**
4, Place du Breteuil
F-75015 Paris, France
**Phone:** 33 1 44736739        **Fax:** 33 1 44736739
**Email:** ade.paris@wanadoo.fr
**Fnded:** 1976. **Mem:** 120. **Nat'l Groups:** 4. **Lang(s):** English, French, German. **Desc:** Medical doctors, nutritionists, biologists, statisticians, and others working in related fields. Conducts surveys and research in nutrition and early childhood development; holds training sessions. Provides children's services. Humanitarian actions for children in distress, (orphans of war, street children). Ergotherapy by arts. Works in Sudan, Uganda, Poland, Russia, Georgia, China, and Albania. **Pub:** *Civil War: Children in International Conflict*, periodic. Book.

**European Council on Eating Disorders (ECED)**
*See:* Entry 12469

**★ 16477 ★ European Federation of the Associations of Dietitians (EFAD) (Federation Europeenne des Associations de Dieteticiens — FEAD)**
Ziegeleiweg 4
D-46446 Emerich, Germany
**Phone:** 49 2822 63867        **Fax:** 49 2822 68358
**Email:** secretariat@efad.org

**Website:** http://www.efad.org/
**Fnded:** 1978. **Mem:** 22. **Lang(s):** English, French. **Desc:** National association of dietitians. Furthers dietetics as a scientific discipline and a profession. Objectives are: to improve the nutritional practices of European populations; to advance education in dietetics; to harmonize professional qualification criteria. Evaluates opportunities in the field.

**★ 16478 ★ Feingold Association of the United States (FAUS)**
127 East Main St., Ste. 106
Riverhead, NY 11901
**Phone:** (516)369-9340        **Free:** 800-321-3287
**Fax:** (516)369-2988
**Email:** help@feingold.org
**Website:** http://www.feingold.org
Jane Hersey, Dir.
**Fnded:** 1976. **Mem:** 30,000. **Reg. Groups:** 7. **Local Groups:** 30. **Desc:** Individuals who believe overactivity, aggression, Attention Deficit Disorder, sleep disturbances, and learning disabilities are often alleviated by adherence to a program developed by Ben F. Feingold, M.D. which eliminates synthetic colors, synthetic flavors, and BHA, BHT, and TBHQ (preservatives) from the diet. Goals are: to support the dietary management schedule known as the Feingold Program; to gather and disseminate information on food supply and to support public availability of such information. **Pub:** *Impossible Kids? Possible Answers*. Video. • *Pure Facts*, 10/year. Newsletter. *Price:* Included in membership dues; $28/year for nonmembers. • *Why Can't My Child Behave?*. Book. *Price:* $38. • Pamphlet.

**★ 16479 ★ Food and Nutrition Board (FNB)**
2101 Constitution Ave. NW
Washington, DC 20418
**Phone:** (202)334-1732        **Fax:** (202)334-2316
**Email:** fnb@nas.edu
Allison Yates, Dir
**Fnded:** 1940. **Mem:** 13. **Desc:** Division of National Academy of Sciences - Institute of Medicine. Evaluates and offers advice to the federal government concerning the relationship between food consumption, nutritional status, and public health. **Pub:** Booklets. • Monographs.Covers nutrition, public health and food safety. • Report.

**★ 16480 ★ French-Language Society of Nutrition and Dietetics (Societe de Nutrition et de Dietetique de Langue Francaise — SNDLF)**
Hopital Bichat
F-75877 Paris, France
**Phone:** 33 1 40257200        **Fax:** 33 1 40258783
**Fnded:** 1963.

**★ 16481 ★ German Association of Dietitians (AGD) (Verband der Diatassistenten - Deutscher Bundesverband — VDDe.v.)**
Postfach 10 51 12
D-40042 Dusseldorf, Germany
**Phone:** 49 211 162175        **Fax:** 49 211 357389
**Email:** vdd-duesseldorf@t-online.de
**Website:** http://www.vdd.de
**Fnded:** 1957. **Mem:** 3,800. **Lang(s):** English, German. **Desc:** Dietitians in Germany working to improve nutritional practices. Represents interests of members. Provides a forum for information exchange among dieticians, doctors, and other medical workers. Supports training of dietitians. Affiliated with the European Federation of the Associations of Dietitians (EFAD) and with the International Confederation of Dietetic Associations (ICDA). **Pub:** *Diet & Information*, bimonthly. Journal. • *Ernahrungs Umschau*, annual. Journal.

**Gerson Institute (GI)**
*See:* Entry 4262


★ **16482** ★ **Greek Dietetic Association**
Erythrou Stavrou 8-10 St.
GR-115 26 Athens, Greece
**Phone:** 30 1 6984400          **Fax:** 30 1 6984400
**Email:** nutritio@otenet.gr
**Website:** http://www.hda.gr
**Fnded:** 1969. **Mem:** 250. **Lang(s):** Greek. **Desc:**
Professional dietitians. Promotes advancement in the
study and application of dietetics; advises government
agencies and the public regarding a healthy diet.
Conducts research and educational programs. **Pub:**
*Journal of Nutrition and Dietetics*, quarterly. Journal.


★ **16483** ★ **Greek Society of Nutrition
and Foods**
c/o Department of Epidemiology
School of Medicine
University of Athens
M. Asias 75
GR-115 27 Athens, Greece
**Phone:** 30 1 7488042          **Fax:** 30 1 7488902
**Email:** afeamtzi@mut.uoa.gz
**Fnded:** 1981. **Mem:** 146. **Lang(s):** Greek. **Desc:**
Physicians and nutritionists in Greece. Promotes
education in nutrition. Conducts research; compiles
statistics. Maintains speakers' bureau. Sponsors semi-
nars. **Pub:** *Statitute*, periodic. Also publishes confer-
ence proceedings and pamphlets.


**HELP - Institute for Body Chemistry
(HELP)**
*See:* Entry 8705


★ **16484** ★ **Hungarian Society of
Nutrition (HSN)
(Magyar Taplalkozastudomanyi Tarsasag
— MTT)**
c/o Prof. Dr. Barna Maria
Gyali ut. 3/a
H-1085 Horanszky, Hungary
**Phone:** 36 1 3382855          **Fax:** 36 1 3382043
**Email:** drbarnam@hotmail.com
**Website:** http://home.earthlink.net/~ekrimmel2
**Fnded:** 1966. **Mem:** 270. **Lang(s):** Hungarian. **Desc:**
Promotes the study of general and clinical nutrition.
Researches medical aspects of food production and
consumption. Conducts periodic discussion groups on
nutrition related issues and problems; offers postgrad-
uate training courses. **Pub:** *Taplalkozasallergia, dieta*,
bimonthly. Journal. Contains reviews, experimental
studies, and information on scientific meetings. Comes
with English summary. **Frmly:** Hungarian Society of
Nutritional Sciences.


★ **16485** ★ **Indian Society for Parenteral
and Enteral Nutrition (ISPEN)**
C-13 Qutab Institutional Area
New Delhi 110 016, Delhi, India
**Email:** crnss@hotmail.com
**Fnded:** 1994. **Desc:** Promotes advancement in the
study and application of parenteral and enteral nutri-
tion.


★ **16486** ★ **Institute of Nutrition of
Central America and Panama (INCAP)
(Instituto de Nutricion de Centro America
y Panama — INCAP)**
Calzada Roosevelt, Zoha 11
Apartado Postal 1188
01901 Guatemala City, Guatemala
**Phone:** 502 2 4715655          **Fax:** 502 2 4756529
**Email:** hdelgado@incap.org.gt
**Website:** http://www.incap.org.gt
**Fnded:** 1949. **Nat'l Groups:** 7. **Lang(s):** English,
Spanish. **Desc:** Representatives of Belize, Costa
Rica, El Salvador, Guatemala, Honduras, Nicaragua,

and Panama. Advises members on policies concerning nutrition in their countries. Encourages technical
cooperation by coordinating available resources and
promoting exchange of information and personnel in
areas such as food and nutrition surveillance, mater-
nal-infant nutrition, food aid programs, food and nutrition in school programs, improvement of basic grains,
development of food resources, and nutritional fortification of foods. Conducts research in the areas of food
sciences, food technology, and agro-industrial activities. Provides specialized training courses for professional, technical, and auxiliary personnel. Sponsors
tutorial training programs for all levels in related fields;
offers postgraduate courses in food and nutrition,
health, and food sciences and technology. Conducts
periodic conferences, seminars, and workshops. Compiles statistics. Administered by the Pan American
Health Organization.


★ **16487** ★ **International and American
Association of Clinical Nutritionists
(IAACN)**
16775 Addison Rd., Ste. 102
Addison, TX 75001
**Phone:** (972)407-9089          **Fax:** (972)250-0233
**Email:** ccnl990ccn@msn.com
**Website:** http://www.iaacn.org
Winna C. Henry, Exec. Dir.
**Fnded:** 1971. **Mem:** 400. **Desc:** Physicians (medical,
osteopathic, chiropractic), dentists, veterinarians, clini-
cal nutritionists, pharmacists, nurses and scientists.
Practitioners hold accredited undergraduatiate, graduate or professional degrees in science and/or nutrition,
or in fields related to nutrition with the addition of
required core courses. IAACN sponsors the Certified
Clinical Nutritionist (CCN) credential under the responsibility of the Clinical Nutrition Certicication Board
(CNCB). Members work in the U.S. and other countries to stimulate and encourage research in the
nutritional aspects of disease, promote the science
and study of nutrition and complementary therapies in
medical and dental schools, hospitals, colleges and
research institutions. Provides a referral service for
people seeking nutrition/preventive health care providers. Holds an annual scientific symposium with world-
class faculty. **Pub:** *International Academy of Nutrition
and Preventive Medicine Membership Directory*, annual. Directory. *Price:* Included in membership dues;
$15/copy for nonmembers. • *Journal of Applied Nutri-
tion*, quarterly. Journal. *Price:* Included in membership
dues; $85/year for nonmembers and institutions; $40/
year for students; $110/year outside U.S. • *Your
Health*, bimonthly. Newsletter. Includes information on
nutrition and preventative medicine applied to a variety
of health issues. *Price:* Included in membership dues.
**Frmly:** (1998) International Academy of Nutrition and
Preventitive Medicine.


★ **16488** ★ **International Life Sciences
Institute, European Branch (ILSI Europ)**
Av E Mounier 83
1200 Brussels, Belgium
**Phone:** 32 2 7620044          **Fax:** 32 2 7710014
**Email:** rmarquet@ilsieurope.be
**Website:** http://www.ilsi.org
**Fnded:** 1986. **Desc:** Supports research on nutritional
quality and safety of the food supply.


**International Life Sciences Institute -
North America (ILSINA)**
*See:* Entry 17344


★ **16489** ★ **International Union of
Nutritional Sciences (IUNS)**
c/o Prof. Osman M. Galal
UCLA School of Public Health
International Health Program
PO Box 951772
Los Angeles, CA 90095-1772
**Phone:** (310)206-9639          **Fax:** (310)794-1805
**Email:** ogalal@ucla.edu

**Website:** http://www.iuns.org
Prof. O.M. Galal, Contact
**Fnded:** 1946. **Mem:** 65. **Desc:** National nutritional
societies. Promotes international cooperation in the
scientific study of nutrition and its applications. Encourages research and the exchange of scientific
information. Cooperates with the Food and Agriculture
Organization of the United Nations, the United Nations
Educational, Scientific and Cultural Organization, and
the World Health Organization. Maintains 24 committees. **Pub:** *Annual Report.* • *Directory*, quadrennial.
Directory. • *Newsletter*, 1-2/year. Newsletter.


★ **16490** ★ **International Vitamin A
Consultative Group (IVACG)**
c/o ILSI Human Nutrition Institute
One Thomas Cir. NW, 9th Fl.
Washington, DC 20005
**Phone:** (202)659-9024          **Fax:** (202)659-3617
**Email:** hni@ilsi.org
**Website:** http://www.ilsi.org
Veronica Triana, MPH, Project Mgr.
**Fnded:** 1974. **Desc:** Participants from 60 countries
interested in international activities aimed at reducing
the incidence of vitamin A deficiency in humans.
Offers consultation and guidance to operating and
donor agencies that are seeking to reduce vitamin A
deficiencies. Prepares guidelines and recommendations for assessing the regional distribution and magnitude of vitamin A deficiency, developing intervention
methods and strategies against the deficiency, evaluating the effectiveness of implemented programs, and
conducting research needed to support the assessment of intervention. Holds international meeting every
18 months. Publishes and distributes technical references which are used globally; conducts task forces.
**Pub:** *A Brief Guide to Current Methods of Assessing
Vitamin A Status. Price:* $4. • *The Bioavailability of
Dietary Carotenoids: Current Concepts. Price:* $4. •
*Biochemical Methodology for the Assessment of Vita-
min A Status, and Reprints of Selected Methods for
the Analysis of Vitamin A and Carotenoids.* Book. •
*Combining Vitamin A Distribution with EPI Contacts.
Price:* $4. • *Delivery of Vitamin A Supplements with
DPT/Polio and Measles Immunization. Price:* $4. •
*IVACG Meeting Reports.* Report. *Price:* Free. • *IVACG
Policy Statement on Vitamin A, Diarrhea and Measles.
Price:* $4. • *IVACG Policy Statement on Vitamin A
Status and Childhood Mortality. Price:* $4. • *IVACG
Statement on Clustering of Xerophthalmia and Vitamin
A Deficiency Within Communities and Families. Price:*
$4. • *IVACG Statement on Maternal Night Blindness:
Extent and Associated Risk Factors. Price:* $4. •
*IVACG Statement on Safe Doses of Vitamin A During
Pregnancy and Lactation. Price:* $4. • *IVACG State-
ment on Vitamin A and Iron Interactions. Price:* $4. •
*Nutrition Communications in Vitamin A Programs: A
Resource Book. Price:* $4. • *The Safe Use of Vitamin
A. Price:* $4. • *The Safe Uses of Vitamin A by Women
During the Reproductive Years. Price:* $4. • *Status of
the Studies on Vitamin A and Human Immunodeficien-
cy Virus Infection. Price:* $4. • *Strategic Placement of
IVACG in the Evolving Micronutrient Field. Price:* Free.
• *Vitamin A Conversions to SI. Price:* Free. • *Vitamin A
Supplements: A Guide to their Use in the Treatment
and Prevention of Vitamin A Deficiency and Xero-
phthalmia. Price:* $4. • Also publishes monographs,
guidelines, and books.


★ **16491** ★ **Irish Nutrition and Dietetic
Institute (INDI)**
Ashgrove House
Kill Ave.
Dun Laoghaire, Dublin, Ireland
**Phone:** 353 1 2804839          **Fax:** 353 1 2804299
**Email:** info@indi.ie
**Website:** http://www.indi.ie
**Fnded:** 1968. **Mem:** 350. **Lang(s):** English. **Desc:**
Professional dietitians. Promotes growth in the num-
ber of dietary and nutrition-related positions in the
Republic of Ireland. Represents the interests of mem-
bers. **Pub:** Papers. Contain information on diet, health,
and food for sport.

**★ 16492 ★ Italian Association of Dietitians**
c/o Mrs. Novella Dell'Orto
via Stefano 38B
I-40125 Bologna, Italy
**Phone:** 39 51 237014　　**Fax:** 39 51 237014
**Fnded:** 1985. **Mem:** 700. **State Groups:** 16. **Lang(s):** Italian. **Desc:** Professional dietitians. Promotes advancement in the study and application of dietetics; advises government agencies and the public regarding a healthy diet. Conducts research and educational programs. **Pub:** *ANDID Notizie*, quarterly. Journal. Provides information about association activities; publishes original and translated scientific articles.

**★ 16493 ★ Latin American Federation of Societies of Obesity (FLASO)**
**(Federacion Latinoamericana de Sociedades de Obesidad)**
JE Uriburu, 1312 Pta Baja A
Buenos Aires, Argentina
**Phone:** 54 11 49013272　　**Fax:** 54 11 49013272
**Email:** jcmontero@ciudad.com.ar
**Website:** http://www.iotf.org/oonet/flaso.htm
**Fnded:** 1990.

**★ 16494 ★ Latin American Society of Nutrition (SLAN)**
**(Sociedad Latinoamericana de Nutricion)**
B De Irigoyen 240
1071 Buenos Aires, Argentina
**Phone:** 54 1 43341545　　**Fax:** 54 1 43456011
**Email:** cesni@datamarkets.com.ar
**Fnded:** 1964.

**Latin American Society for Pediatric Gastroenterology and Nutrition**
**(Sociedad Latinoamericana de Gastroenterologia Pediatrica y Nutricion — SLAGPN)**
*See:* Entry 9143

**★ 16495 ★ Luxembourg Dietetic Association**
**(Association Nationale des Dieteticiens du Luxembourg)**
Boite Postale 62
L-7201 Walferdange, Luxembourg
**Phone:** 352 26552728　　**Fax:** 352 367684
**Email:** slagpn@mandic.com.br
**Website:** http://www.andp.pu
**Mem:** 50. **Lang(s):** English, French, German. **Desc:** Professional dietitians. Promotes advancement in the study and application of dietetics; advises government agencies and the public regarding a healthy diet.

**★ 16496 ★ National Institute of Nutrition (NIN)**
265 Carling Ave., Ste. 302
Ottawa, ON, Canada K1S 2E1
**Phone:** (613)235-3355　　**Fax:** (613)235-7032
**Email:** nin@nin.ca
**Website:** http://www.nin.ca
**Fnded:** 1983. **Lang(s):** English, French. **Desc:** Promotes the nutritional health of Canadians through research and education. Moves the nutrition agenda forward by encouraging exchange on key public policy issues. Conducts research that supports decision making across many sectors. **Pub:** *Healthy Bites*, quarterly. • *NIN Review*, annual. Report. • *Rapport*, quarterly. Newsletter. • Annual Report, annual.

**National Meals on Wheels Foundation**
*See:* Entry 3017

**North American Society for Pediatric Gastroenterology, Hepatology and Nutrition (NASPGHAN)**
*See:* Entry 5737

**★ 16497 ★ Norwegian Dietetics Association**
**(Norsk Forening for Ernaering og Dietetikk)**
Postboks 9202
Grenland
0134 Oslo, Norway
**Phone:** 47 21013600　　**Fax:** 47 21013660
**Email:** nfed@kfo.no
**Website:** http://www.nfed.no
**Fnded:** 1948. **Mem:** 1,450. **Local Groups:** 18. **Lang(s):** Norwegian. **Desc:** Professional dietitians. Promotes advancement in the study and application of dietetics; advises government agencies and the public regarding a healthy diet. Conducts research and educational programs. **Pub:** *Kigkkenskriveren*, 8/year. Magazine.

**★ 16498 ★ Nutrition Foundation of the Philippines (NFP)**
c/o Azucena B. Limbo
107 E Rodriguez, Sr. Blvd.
Quezon City, Metro Manila 1102, Philippines
**Phone:** 63 2 7121474　　**Fax:** 63 2 7113980
**Website:**　　http://www.nutrition-foundation.it/la_fnnf.html
**Fnded:** 1959. **Mem:** 350. **Lang(s):** English. **Desc:** Nutritionists, educators, medical doctors, scientists, midwives, and food companies in the Philippines. Promotes public awareness and practice of sound nutritional principles. Conducts nutrition education campaigns primarily directed toward those most vulnerable to malnutrition. Trains individuals to participate in community nutrition programs and offers continuing educational opportunities for health care professionals. Provides technical assistance to public and private agencies working to improve nutrition in the Philippines, consulting services for program planning and implementation, and diet counseling program. Undertakes nutrition research and aids institutions conducting studies in the field; offers reference service. Operates speakers' bureau and placement and children's services. **Pub:** *Bulletin of the NFP*, bimonthly. Newsletter. Current trends in foods, nutrition, and dietetics. • *Low-Fat, Low-Cholesterol Cookbook*. Book. • *Monograp Series*. Book. Kitchen tested recipes for preschoolers.

**★ 16499 ★ Nutrition Institute of America (NIA)**
1524 Crystal St.
Kansas City, MO 64126
**Phone:** (816)241-8315　　**Fax:** (816)231-6423
George Coulas, Pres.
**Fnded:** 1974. **Mem:** 6. **Desc:** Sponsors original research in nutrition and other areas that may affect our physical and emotional well-being. Sponsors lectures, symposia, adult education programs, and special tutor programs in nutrition; maintains extensive research library; compiles statistics. Presently inactive.

**★ 16500 ★ Nutrition for Optimal Health Association (NOHA)**
PO Box 380
Winnetka, IL 60093
**Phone:** (847)604-3258
**Email:** nohainfo@aol.com
**Website:** http://www.nutrition4health.org
Neil Levin, Pres.
**Fnded:** 1972. **Mem:** 300. **Desc:** Physicians and others interested in making informed health decisions through better nutrition. Promotes good nutrition as a means of achieving and maintaining optimal health; advances and disseminates scientifically based information on the practical application of sound nutritional principles to daily living. Offers cooking classes and

workshops; conducts nutrition education programs and seminars. Maintains speakers' bureau. **Pub:** *Enjoy Nutritious Variety*. • *NOHA News*, quarterly. Newsletter. Includes association news and book reviews. *Price:* Included in membership dues; $10/year for nonmembers. • Membership Directory, annual.

**★ 16501 ★ Nutrition Society (NS)**
10 Cambridge Ct.
210 Shepherds Bush Rd.
London W6 7NJ, United Kingdom
**Phone:** 44 20 760203228　　**Fax:** 44 20 76021756
**Email:** office@nutsoc.org.uk
**Website:** http://www.nutsoc.org.uk
**Fnded:** 1941. **Mem:** 1,850. **Lang(s):** English. **Desc:** Persons involved in nutrition research or in health maintenance organized to promote the scientific study of nutrition. Maintains special interest groups; disseminates information. **Pub:** *British Journal of Nutrition*, monthly. • *Gazette*, periodic. Magazine. • *Nutrition Research Reviews*. Report. • *Proceedings of the Nutrition Society*, 3/year. Proceedings.

**★ 16502 ★ Oley Foundation for Home Parenteral and Enteral Nutrition**
214 Hun Memorial, A-28
Albany Medical Center
Albany, NY 12208
**Phone:** (518)262-5079　　**Free:** 800-776-OLEY
**Fax:** (518)262-5528
**Email:** bishopj@mail.amc.edu
**Website:** http://www.oley.org
Joan Bishop, Exec. Dir.
**Fnded:** 1983. **Mem:** 5,000. **Reg. Groups:** 70. **Desc:** The Oley Foundation, a national non-profit organization, provides information and psycho-social support for home nutrition support patients, their families, caregivers and professionals. Programs include: bimonthly newsletter, national network of volunteers providing patient support, annual summer conference, regional meetings, toll-free patient-to-patient networking and information clearinghouse. Visit www.oley.org and/or call (800) 776-6539 for additional information. Seeks to enrich and enhance the lives of those requiring home nutrition support through an outreach system of patient volunteers, educational meetings and clearinghouse activities. **Pub:** *LifelineLetter*, bimonthly. Newsletter. *Price:* $40/year for others. • Brochures.

**★ 16503 ★ Organization for Nutrition Education (ONE)**
Woodlawn Postal Outlet
PO Box 25
Guelph, ON, Canada N1H 8H6
**Phone:** (306)966-5836　　**Fax:** (306)966-6377
**Email:** lwadswor@stfx.ca
**Website:**　　http://www.stfx.ca/academic/human-nutrition/organization/main.html
**Fnded:** 1980. **Mem:** 200. **Lang(s):** English, French. **Desc:** Nutrition professionals and organizations and other individuals and corporations with an interest in nutrition and related fields. **Pub:** *National Membership Roster*, annual. Directory. • *O.N.E. Annual Report*, annual. • *O.N.E. Bulletin*, 3/year. Newsletter. • *O.N.E. Report*. Annual Report.

**★ 16504 ★ Price-Pottenger Nutrition Foundation (PPNF)**
7890 Broadway
Lemon Grove, CA 91945
**Phone:** (619)462-7600　　**Free:** 800-366-3748
**Fax:** (619)433-3136
**Email:** info@price-pottenger.org
**Website:** http://www.price-pottenger.org
Ed Bennet, BS, Pres.
**Fnded:** 1952. **Mem:** 2,000. **Desc:** Seeks to increase awareness of natural health, organic gardening, nutrition and ecology. Disseminates information to the medical and dental professions, as well as to the public, through publications, seminars, classes, study groups, and scientific exhibits. Stresses the benefits of

chemically-untreated "whole" foods. Named in honor of Weston A. Price, DDS and Francis M. Pottenger, Jr., M.D., known for their work in nutrition research. **Pub:** *Nutrition and Physical Degeneration*. Book. • *Pottenger's Cats: A Study in Nutrition*. Book. • *PPNF Health Journal: Health and Healing Wisdom*, quarterly. Journal. Contains articles on health, book reviews, recipes, and a calendar. *Price:* $35/yr; $100/yr for professional. **Frmly:** (1954) Santa Barbara Medical Research Foundation; (1965) Weston A. Price Memorial Foundation; (1973) Price-Pottenger Foundation.

★ **16505** ★ **Protein Foods and Nutrition Development Association of India (PFNDAI)**
Mahalaxmi Chambers
22 Bhulabhai Desai Rd.
Bombay 400 026, Maharashtra, India
**Phone:** 91 22 4928858          **Fax:** 91 22 4938998
**Email:** pfndai@vsnl.com
**Website:** http://www.pfndai.com
**Fnded:** 1968. **Mem:** 58. **Nat'l Groups:** 48. **Reg. Groups:** 1. **State Groups:** 7. **Local Groups:** 2. **Lang(s):** English. **Desc:** Indian food industries. Collects, analyzes, and disseminates information on nutrition and food science and technology. Promotes balanced nutrition; identifies nutrient needs and food preferences through surveys; offers consultive services to national and international agencies for the development of low-cost nutritional supplements; offers project consultive services to the food industry. Assists government agencies in formulating food standards, regulations, and legislation; compiles statistics. Provides job placement assistance for food scientists. Conducts research. **Pub:** *Pfndai Bulletin*, monthly. Bulletin. Contains news items connected with food science and nutrition. • Papers. Contains research reports and proceedings. • Videos.

★ **16506** ★ **Scientific Society of Nutrition and Dietetics**
Department of hygiene, ecology and occupat. diseases
15 boul. D.Nestorov
BG-1527 Sofia, Bulgaria
**Phone:** 359 2 5940611          **Fax:** 359 2 595106
**Fnded:** 1986. **Mem:** 101. **Lang(s):** English, Russian.
**Desc:** Fosters research in apiotherapy.

★ **16507** ★ **Society for Nutrition Education (SNE)**
9202 N Meridian, Ste. 200
Indianapolis, IN 46260
**Phone:** (317)571-5618          **Fax:** (317)571-5603
**Email:** info@sne.org
**Website:** http://www.sne.org
Marilyn Briggs, Pres.
**Fnded:** 1967. **Mem:** 1,800. **Reg. Groups:** 15. **Desc:** Nutrition educators from the fields of dietetics, public health, home economics, medicine, industry, and education (elementary, secondary, college, university, and consumer affairs). Vision of SNE is healthy people in healthy communities. **Pub:** *Journal of Nutrition Education*, bimonthly. Journal. For educators, practitioners, and researchers on nutrition education. Includes book reviews and employment opportunity listings. *Price:* Included in membership dues; $119/year for individuals; $170/year for institutions; $60/year for individuals in training. • Also publishes journal supplements.

★ **16508** ★ **Swedish Association of Dietitians (SAD) (Svensk Dietistforening — SD)**
St. Eriksgatan 26
Box 12069
S-102 22 Stockholm, Sweden
**Phone:** 46 31 852369          **Fax:** 46 31 198003
**Fnded:** 1921. **Mem:** 1,200. **Local Groups:** 20. **Lang(s):** English. **Desc:** Professional dietitians. Promotes the study and practice of dietetics and dietetics

science in Sweden. **Pub:** *Dietisten*, annual. Journal. A journal of dietetics and catering.

★ **16509** ★ **Swiss Dietetic Association (Schweizerischer Verband Diplomierter Ernarnrungsberaterinnen — SVERB/ASDD)**
Geschaftsstelle
Oberstadt 8
CH-6204 Sempach-Stadt, Switzerland
**Phone:** 41 41 4627066          **Fax:** 41 41 4627061
**Email:** service@sverb-asdd.ch
**Website:** http://www.sverb-asdd.ch
**Fnded:** 1942. **Mem:** 811. **Reg. Groups:** 8. **Desc:** Professional dietitians. Promotes advancement in the study and application of dietetics; advises government agencies and the public regarding a healthy diet. Conducts research and educational programs. **Pub:** *Ernahrungs Info*, bimonthly. Magazine.

★ **16510** ★ **Veris Research Information Service**
5325 S 9th Ave.
La Grange, IL 60525-3602
**Phone:** (952)927-7104          **Free:** 800-554-1708
**Fax:** (952)927-6406
**Email:** slandvik@aol.com
**Website:** http://www.veris-online.org
Sharon Landvik, Exec. Officer
**Desc:** Acts as an information clearinghouse on antioxidants, including vitamin E, caroteroids, and alpha-lipoic acid for health care professionals, researchers, and nutrition and health communicators. **Pub:** *VERIS*, quarterly. Newsletter. Reports on current research. • Also publishes research summaries. **Frmly:** (1998) Vitamin E Research and Information Service.

★ **16511** ★ **Weight Watchers International (WWI)**
175 Crossways Park West
Woodbury, NY 11797-2055
**Phone:** (516)390-1632          **Fax:** (516)390-1795
**Email:** media@weightwatchers.com
**Website:** http://www.weightwatchers.com
Linda Huett, Pres. /CEO/Dir.
**Fnded:** 1963. **Desc:** The Weight Watchers Program includes a balanced diet, exercise and behavior modification. At weekly meetings, Weight Watchers members learn how to modify their current eating and exercise habits. Operates centers worldwide.

# Research Centers

★ **16512** ★ **Columbia University Institute of Human Nutrition**
College of Physicians & Surgeons
630 W 168th St., PH 15E, Rm. 1512
New York, NY 10032
**Phone:** (212)305-4808          **Fax:** (212)305-3079
**Email:** rjd20@columbia.edu
**Website:** http://cpmcnet.columbia.edu/dept/ihn/
Richard J. Deckelbaum, MD, Dir.
**Activities/Fields:** Atherosclerosis; lipoprotein-receptor-cell interaction; lipid emulsion metabolism; free fatty acids and cell lipid metabolism; basic retinoid and vitamin A physiology, biochemistry, and molecular biology; food and nutrition policy and law; intestinal ion transport mechanisms; enteric nervous system; human lipoprotein metabolism; lipolytic enzymes and endothelial cell biology; atherosclerosis; mineral metabolism and toxicology; carbohydrate and lipid metabolism, obesity, diabetes mellitus, food intake regulation; calcium metabolism; vascular cell biology; pathogenesis of thrombosis; regulation of intracellular cholesterol metabolism; endocytic pathways in macrophages; cholestryl ester transfer; protein structure/function and mutagenesis; regulation of gene expression; molecular nutrition; molecular mechanisms of carcinogenesis. **Frmly:** Institute of Nutrition Sciences.

★ **16513** ★ **Indiana University-Purdue University at Indianapolis Mead Johnson Mass Spectrometry Laboratory**
RR 208
Indianapolis, IN 46202
**Phone:** (317)274-4715          **Fax:** (317)274-2065
**Email:** sdenne@iupui.edu
**Website:**          http://www.indiana.edu/~rugs/ctrdir/mjmsl.html
Scott C. Denne, MD, Dir.
**Activities/Fields:** Nutrition and metabolism, including fetal, neonatal, and adult protein and glucose metabolism; infant and adult energy expenditure and body composition; human muscle metabolism and exercise; and diabetes.

★ **16514** ★ **Johns Hopkins University Center for Human Nutrition**
School of Hygiene and Public Health
615 N Wolfe St.
Baltimore, MD 21205
**Phone:** (410)614-4070          **Fax:** (410)955-0196
**Email:** bcaballe@jhsph.edu
**Website:** http://www.jhsph.edu/Research/Centers/Nutrition
Dr. Benjamin Caballero, Dir.
**Activities/Fields:** The role of nutrition in health and disease and the development of new ways to apply that knowledge to improve the health of people, including maternal and child nutrition, obesity and chronic diseases, micronutrient deficiencies, and nutrient metabolism.

★ **16515** ★ **King James Medical Laboratory/Omegatech**
24700 Center Ridge Rd.
Cleveland, OH 44145
**Phone:** (440)835-2150          **Free:** 800-437-1404
**Fax:** (440)835-2177
**Email:** headquarters@kingjamesomegatech-lab.com
**Website:** http://www.kingjamesomegatech-lab.com
Dr. Raymond J. Shamberger, Dir.
**Activities/Fields:** Nutrition and trace elements, including role of dietary thiamine, serum enzyme activities, synthesis and utilization of creatine, effect of zinc supplement, and sorption from the gut. **Frmly:** Preventive Medicine Research Center of Cleveland.

★ **16516** ★ **Laval University Human Nutrition Research Group**
Pavillon Paul-Comtois
Sainte Foy, QC, Canada G1K 7P4
**Phone:** (418)656-2131          **Fax:** (418)656-3353
**Email:** helene.jacques@aln.ulaval.ca
Helene Jacques, Dir.
**Activities/Fields:** Nutrient bioavailability: mechanisms and metabolic impact.

★ **16517** ★ **Laval University Joseph Rheaume Laboratory**
Pavillon Paul-Comtois
Quebec, QC, Canada G1K 7P4
**Phone:** (418)656-2315          **Fax:** (418)656-3353
**Email:** laurent.savoie@nhc.ulaval.ca
Laurent Savoie, Dir.
**Activities/Fields:** Nutrient bioavailability, the effect of food proteins on mineral bioavailability in vitro and in vivo, and kinetics and forms of amino acids at various levels of blood circulation.

★ **16518** ★ **McGill University McGill Nutrition and Food Science Centre**
Royal Victoria Hospital
687 Pine Ave. W, Rm. H6.61
Montreal, QC, Canada H3A 1A1
**Phone:** (514)843-1665          **Fax:** (514)843-1706
**Email:** errol.marliss@muhc.mcgill.ca
Dr. Errol B. Marliss, Dir.

**Activities/Fields:** Promotes clinical and basic research in nutrition and food science.

**Northwestern University
Center for Endocrinology, Metabolism and Molecular Medicine**
*See:* Entry 8762

**U.S. Department of Defense
Army Medical Research and Materiel Command
Army Research Institute of Environmental Medicine
Military Nutrition and Biochemistry Division**
*See:* Entry 13475

**U.S. Department of Health and Human Services
Food and Drug Administration
Center for Food Safety and Applied Nutrition**
*See:* Entry 18003

**★ 16519 ★ U.S. Department of Health and Human Services
Food and Drug Administration
Center for Food Safety and Applied Nutrition
Office of Plant and Diary Foods and Beverages**
Rm. 4827, HFS-300
5100 Paint Branch Pkway
College Park, MD 20740
**Phone:** (301)436-1700     **Fax:** (301)436-2632
**Email:** ttroxell@cfsan.fda.gov
**Website:**     http://www.fda.gov/oc/orgcharts/orgchart.html
Dr. Terry C. Troxell, PhD, Dir.
**Activities/Fields:** Safety and quality of foods derived from plants, milk, eggs, and game foods, including studies on detection of inorganic and organic contaminants, pesticides and natural toxins; identification of virulence factors associated with foodborne pathogens; impact of foodborne pathogens on immune response; natural product chemistry of herbal products; and food processing and packaging; and risk assessment of harmful substances in foods. **Pub:** *Annual Pesticide Residue Monitoring Report.* • *Pesticide Analytical Manual.*

**U.S. Department of Health and Human Services
National Cancer Institute
Memorial Sloan-Kettering Cancer Center
Institute for Cancer Research
(Clinical Nutrition Research Unit)**
*See:* Entry 10499

**★ 16520 ★ U.S. Department of Health and Human Services
National Institute of Diabetes and Digestive and Kidney Diseases
Division of Digestive Diseases and Nutrition
Nutritional Sciences Branch**
45 Center Dr. MSC 6600
Bethesda, MD 20892-6600
**Phone:** (301)594-8883     **Fax:** (301)480-8300
Dr. Van S. Hubbard, Ch. -Nutritional Sciences Branch
**Activities/Fields:** Basic, clinical, and behavioral research and training directed toward the improvement of human health. Priority areas of research are: human nutrition requirements, including environmental and host factors that may affect requirements, such as nutrient imbalance, drugs, disease, stress, and activity levels; physiological function of essential nutrients in health and disease, with emphasis on amino acids, calcium, magnesium, trace elements, and vitamins; and significance of proportion and amount of macronutrients (dietary proteins, fats, and carbohydrates) in metabolism. Studies are also conducted on the health significance of dietary fiber; prevention and control of obesity, including the relationship among genetic predisposition, induced metabolic change, and social, environmental, physiological, and behavioral factors; supportive nutrition of hospitalized patients; and assessment of nutritional status and dietary intake. Principal Branch components are the: Clinical Nutrition Research Units; Nutrient Metabolism Program; Obesity and Eating Disorders Program; and U.S.-Japan Malnutrition Panel. **Frmly:** Nutrition Program.

**U.S. Department of Health and Human Services
National Institute of Diabetes and Digestive and Kidney Diseases
Division of Intramural Research
Molecular, Cellular, and Nutritional Endocrinology Branch**
*See:* Entry 8784

**U.S. Department of Health and Human Services
National Institutes of Health
National Cancer Institute
Division of Cancer Epidemiology and Genetics
(Nutritional Epidemiology Branch)**
*See:* Entry 10554

**★ 16521 ★ University of California, Davis
Clinical Nutrition Research Unit**
Division of Clinical Nutrition & Metabolism
TB 156 School of Medicine
Davis, CA 95616
**Phone:** (530)752-6778     **Fax:** (530)752-3470
**Email:** chhalsted@ucdavis.edu
**Website:** http://dceg.cancer.gov/ebp/neb/index.html
Dr. Charles Halsted, MD, Dir.
**Activities/Fields:** Human nutrition in health and disease. Studies focus on the relationship of diet to disease, energy metabolism, and development.

**University of California, Davis
Gastroenterology and Nutrition Center**
*See:* Entry 9183

**★ 16522 ★ University of Chicago
Clinical Nutrition Research Unit**
MC 4080
5841 S Maryland Ave.
Chicago, IL 60637
**Phone:** (773)702-6741     **Fax:** (773)702-6972
**Email:** msitrin@medicine.bsd.uchicago.edu
**Website:** http://www.ucdmc.ucdavis.edu
Dr. Michael D. Sitrin, MD, Dir.
**Activities/Fields:** Human and clinical nutritional biology, particularly in relation to pregnancy, growth retardation, digestive and cardiovascular diseases, diabetes, and cancer. Conducts vitamin metabolism, lipoprotein, lipid, stable isotope, trace metal, and radioimmunoassay analyses.

**University of Chicago
Liver Study Unit**
*See:* Entry 9188

**University of Colorado
B.F. Stolinsky Research Laboratories**
*See:* Entry 6906

**★ 16523 ★ University of Maryland
Nutrition Laboratory**
Henson Center, Rm. 2101
Department of Human Ecology
Princess Anne, MD 21853
**Phone:** (410)651-6056     **Fax:** (410)651-6207
**Email:** bwblakely@mail.umes.edu
Dr. Bettie Blakely, Contact
**Activities/Fields:** Nutrition and metabolism.

**★ 16524 ★ University of Nevada, Reno
Nutrition Education and Research Program**
Redfield Bldg., Mail Stop 153
Sch. of Medicine
Reno, NV 89557
**Phone:** (775)784-4474     **Fax:** (775)784-4468
**Email:** sach@unr.edu
Dr. Sachiko T. St. Jeor, Dir.
**Activities/Fields:** Clinical nutrition.

**★ 16525 ★ University of Texas
Southwestern Medical Center at Dallas
Center for Human Nutrition**
5323 Harry Hines Blvd.
Dallas, TX 75235-9052
**Phone:** (214)648-2890     **Fax:** (214)648-4837
**Email:** scott.grundy@utsouthwestern.edu
Dr. Scott M. Grundy, Dir.
**Activities/Fields:** Human nutrition. Investigates the preventive effects of vitamins C and E on atherosclerosis.

**★ 16526 ★ University of Washington
Clinical Nutrition Research Unit**
Division of Metabolism
Department of Medicine
PO Box 356426
Seattle, WA 98195-6426
**Phone:** (206)543-6166     **Fax:** (206)685-8346
**Website:** http://depts.washington.edu/uwcnru/
Prof. Alan Chait, MD, Prin. Investigator
**Activities/Fields:** Human nutrition in health and disease, including nutritional health maintenance, improved nutritional support of the acutely and chronically ill, assessment of nutritional status, effects of diseased states on nutritional needs, and effects of nutrition on disease states. Conducts research with human subjects and populations. Also basic and animal research.

**★ 16527 ★ USDA Agricultural Research Service
Grand Forks Human Nutrition Research Center**
2420 2nd Ave. N
PO Box 9034
Grand Forks, ND 58202-9034
**Phone:** (701)795-8353     **Fax:** (701)795-8395
**Email:** fnielsen@gfhnrc.ars.usda.gov
**Website:** http://www.gfhnrc.ars.usda.gov
Forrest Nielsen, PhD, Dir.
**Activities/Fields:** Role of mineral elements (including magnesium, copper, manganese, iron, boron, selenium, chromium and zinc) in nutrition; bone, cardiovascular, and brain development, maintenance, and function; body composition; and neurological response; and other mechanisms by which these elements sustain life and promote growth in humans.

**USDA Human Nutrition Research Center on Aging**
*See:* Entry 3118

**★ 16528 ★ Vanderbilt University
Clinical Nutrition Research Unit**
C2104 Medical Center
21st & Garland Ave.
Nashville, TN 37232-2279

**Phone:** (615)322-7740      **Fax:** (615)343-6229
**Email:** raymond.burk@mcmail.vanderbilt.edu
**Website:** http://www.mc.vanderbilt.edu/nutrition/
Raymond F. Burk, MD, Dir.

**Activities/Fields:** Mechanisms of body weight and regulation, focusing on exercise and energy expenditure. Metabolism of amino acids, carbohydrates, lipids, minerals, and trace elements. Research also includes molecular nutrition.

# State & Regional Organizations

## Dietetic Disorders

*State chapters of the American Dietetic Association are listed below. The national office is located at 216 W Jackson Blvd., Chicago, IL 60606-6995. Additional information can be obtained by calling the national office at (312) 899-0040, or by consulting their web site at http://www.eatright.org/. Another source of information is the National Eating Disorders Association, at 603 Stewart St., Ste. 803, Seattle, WA 98101. Their phone number is (206) 382-3587, and their web site is http://www.nationaleatingdisorders.org/.*

### Alabama

★ **16529** ★ **Alabama Dietetic Association**
PO Box 11594
Montgomery, AL 36111-0594
**Phone:** (334)260-7970      **Fax:** (334)272-7128
**Website:** http://www.eatrightalabama.org
Larry A. Vinson, Contact

### Alaska

★ **16530** ★ **Alaska Dietetic Association**
10140 Kasilof Blvd.
Anchorage, AK 99516
**Email:** hullma@aol.com
**Website:** http://www.eatrightalaska.org
Alison Hull, President

### Arizona

★ **16531** ★ **Arizona Dietetic Association**
Document Development Services
PO Box 10344
Phoenix, AZ 85064
**Phone:** (602)955-4451      **Fax:** (602)957-4532
**Email:** azdietetic@aol.com
**Website:** http://www.eatrightarizona.org
Patty Williams, Exec Director

### Arkansas

★ **16532** ★ **Arkansas Dietetic Association**
PO Box 55234
Little Rock, AR 72215-5234
**Phone:** (501)374-3300      **Fax:** (501)778-9050
**Email:** arda@up-link.net
**Website:** http://www.arkansasdietetics.org/
Otty Newcomb, Contact

### California

★ **16533** ★ **California Dietetic Association**
7740 Manchester Ave., Ste. 102
Playa del Rey, CA 90293-8499
**Phone:** (310)822-0177      **Fax:** (310)823-0264
**Email:** cdaep@aol.com
**Website:** http://www.dietitian.org/
Pat Smith, Contact

### Colorado

★ **16534** ★ **Colorado Dietetic Association**
PO Box 1775
Estes Park, CO 80517
**Phone:** (970)577-8777      **Fax:** (970)577-0823
**Email:** codietassoc@aol.com
**Website:** http://www.eatrightcolorado.org/
Lorinda Sipe, Exec Director

### Connecticut

★ **16535** ★ **Connecticut Dietetic Association**
138 Oakridge Rd.
Unionville, CT 06085
**Phone:** (860)673-2520      **Fax:** (860)673-6438
**Email:** cda@worldnett.att.net
**Website:** http://www.eatrightct.org
Vikki Allen, Contact

### Delaware

★ **16536** ★ **Delaware Dietetic Association**
2621 Drayton Dr.
Wilmington, DE 19808
**Email:** lindbrugler@chi-east.org
**Website:** http://www.dedietassn.org
Linda Brugler, President

### District of Columbia

★ **16537** ★ **District of Columbia Dietetic Association**
DC Hospital Association
1250 I St. NW, No. 700
Washington, DC 20005-3922
**Phone:** (202)289-4215      **Fax:** (202)371-8151
Toni Brown, Contact

### Florida

★ **16538** ★ **Florida Dietetic Association**
PO Box 12608
Tallahassee, FL 32317-2608
**Phone:** (850)386-8850      **Fax:** (850)386-7918
**Email:** DIETNUTR@aol.com
**Website:** http://www.fldieteticassn.org
Christine Stapell, RD, Exec Director

### Georgia

★ **16539** ★ **Georgia Dietetic Association**
1260 Winchester Pkwy., Ste. 205
Smyrna, GA 30080
**Phone:** (770)433-9044      **Fax:** (770)433-2907
**Email:** gdahpam@aol.com
**Website:** http://www.gda-online.org
Christen Smith, Contact

### Hawaii

★ **16540** ★ **Hawaii Dietetic Association**
64-5252 Kalae Place
Kamuela, HI 96743
**Phone:** (808)885-1996      **Fax:** (808)881-4855
**Email:** bunomc@msn.com
**Website:** http://www.nutritionhawaii.org
Corazon Buno, P, Contact

### Idaho

★ **16541** ★ **Idaho Dietetic Association**
700 S Main St.
Moscow, ID 83843
**Phone:** (208)883-6341      **Fax:** (208)883-2239
**Email:** ekuren@gritman.org
**Website:** http://www.eatrightidaho.org
Nancy Kure, President

### Illinois

★ **16542** ★ **Illinois Dietetic Association**
PO Box 234
Sparland, IL 61565
**Phone:** (309)274-9969      **Fax:** (309)274-9970
**Email:** tdmforida@yahoo.com
**Website:** http://www.eatrightillinois.org
Terri McBride, Exec Director

### Indiana

★ **16543** ★ **Indiana Dietetic Association**
150 N Illinois St.
Elberfeld, IN 47613
**Phone:** (812)983-9911      **Fax:** (812)983-9911
**Email:** dsdenton@aol.com
**Website:** http://www.dietetics.com/ida
Debra Denton, Contact

### Iowa

★ **16544** ★ **Iowa Dietetic Association**
27924 Butler Center Rd.
Clarksville, IA 50619
**Phone:** (319)885-6557      **Fax:** (319)885-6558
**Email:** lursen@netins.net
**Website:** http://www.eatrightiowa.org
Monica Lursen, RD, Contact

### Kansas

★ **16545** ★ **Kansas Dietetic Association**
Kansas State University
Dept. of Hotel, Restaurant, Institution Mgmt. and Dietetics
103 Justin Hall
Manhattan, KS 66506-1404
**Phone:** (785)532-2206      **Fax:** (785)532-5522
**Email:** shanklin@humec.ksu.edu
**Website:**      http://www2.kumc.edu/sah/dietetics/kda/kdahome.htm
Carol Shanklin, Contact

### Kentucky

★ **16546** ★ **Kentucky Dietetic Association**
1501 Twilight Tr.
Frankfort, KY 40601
**Phone:** (502)223-4937      **Fax:** (502)223-4937
Tom Underwood, Contact

### Louisiana

★ **16547** ★ **Louisiana Dietetic Association**
8550 United Plaza Blvd., Ste. 1001
Baton Rouge, LA 70809
**Phone:** (225)922-4570      **Fax:** (225)922-4611
**Email:** LDA@pncpa.com
**Website:** http://www.eatrightlda.org
Bland O'Connor, Exec Director

### Maine

★ **16548** ★ **Maine Dietetic Association**
RR 1, Box 5030
Athens, ME 04912
**Email:** gcalbert@tdstelme.net
**Website:** http://www.eatrightmaine.org
Georgia Clark-Albert, President

### Maryland

★ **16549** ★ **Maryland Dietetic Association**
11319 Glen Arm Rd.
Glen Arm, MD 21057
**Email:** mariedemarco@hotmail.com
**Website:** http://www.eatwellmd.org
Marie DeMarco, President

## Massachusetts

**★ 16550 ★ Massachusetts Dietetic Association**
92 Woodlands Dr.
Falmouth, MA 04105
**Phone:** (617)501-7083
**Email:** mdadirector@aol.com
**Website:** http://www.massnutrition.org
Carol M. Coughlin, RD, Exec Director

## Michigan

**★ 16551 ★ Michigan Dietetic Association**
Association Management Professionals, Inc.
3319 Greenfield Rd., No. 321
Dearborn, MI 48120
**Phone:** (313)271-7543      **Fax:** (313)271-1102
**Email:** ampteam@comcast.net
**Website:** http://www.eatrightmich.org
David Kasunic, CAE, Contact

## Minnesota

**★ 16552 ★ Minnesota Dietetic Association**
1910 W County Rd., B Ste. 212
Saint Paul, MN 55113-5448
**Phone:** (651)628-9250      **Fax:** (651)628-0023
**Email:** mda@eatrightmn.org
**Website:** http://www.eatrightmn.org
D'ann Brosnahan, CAE, Contact

## Mississippi

**★ 16553 ★ Mississippi Dietetic Association**
330 N Mart Plaza
Jackson, MS 39206
**Phone:** (601)981-0740      **Fax:** (601)362-9544
**Email:** msdietetic@yahoo.com
**Website:** http://www.eatrightmississippi.org
Gordon Haydel, Exec Director

## Missouri

**★ 16554 ★ Missouri Dietetic Association**
PO Box 1225
Jefferson City, MO 65102-1225
**Phone:** (573)636-2822      **Fax:** (573)636-9749
**Email:** Broling@socket.net
**Website:** http://www.eatrightmissouri.org
Brenda Roling, Director

## Montana

**★ 16555 ★ Montana Dietetic Association**
3225 3rd Ave. N
Great Falls, MT 59401
**Phone:** (406)454-2791      **Fax:** (406)771-3067
**Email:** jmistevens@msn.com
Marni Stevens, Contact

## Nebraska

**★ 16556 ★ Nebraska Dietetic Association**
4101 SW 2nd St.
Lincoln, NE 68522
**Phone:** (402)421-6236
**Email:** serowan@aol.com
**Website:** http://ianrwww.unl.edu/nda/index.htm
Sharon Rowan, Contact

## Nevada

**★ 16557 ★ Nevada Dietetic Association**
8710 White Fir Dr.
Reno, NV 89523
**Phone:** (775)746-4774
**Email:** holzog@aol.com
Holly Herzog, RD, Contact

## New Hampshire

**★ 16558 ★ New Hampshire Dietetic Association**
8 Nottingham Circle
Lebanon, NH 03766
**Phone:** (603)650-6289      **Fax:** (603)650-6289
**Email:** Jil.Shangraw@hitchock.org
**Website:** http://www.eatrightnh.org
Jil Shangraw, President

## New Jersey

**★ 16559 ★ New Jersey Dietetic Association**
Professional Management Associates
203 Towne Centre Dr.
Hillsborough, NJ 08844
**Phone:** (908)359-1184      **Fax:** (908)359-7619
**Email:** marlene@profmgmt.com
**Website:** http://www.eatrightnj.org
Marlene Reardon, Contact

## New Mexico

**★ 16560 ★ New Mexico Dietetic Association**
11301 Anaheim Ave.
Albuquerque, NM 87122
**Email:** mmartine@phs.org
**Website:** http://www.phs.org
Mary Martinez, President

## New York

**★ 16561 ★ New York State Dietetic Association**
PO Box 30953
New York, NY 10011-0109
**Phone:** (212)691-7906      **Fax:** (212)741-9334
**Email:** fredtripp@prodigy.net
**Website:** http://www.eatrightny.org
Fred Tripp, MS, RD, Exec Director

## North Carolina

**★ 16562 ★ North Carolina Dietetic Association**
Management Concepts, Inc.
893 US Hwy 70 W, Ste. 202
PO Box 1818
Garner, NC 27529
**Phone:** (919)779-6010      **Free:** 800-849-2799
**Fax:** (919)779-5642
**Email:** cbarbour@mgmt4u.com
**Website:** http://www.eatrightnc.org
Charlene Barbour, Contact

## North Dakota

**★ 16563 ★ North Dakota Dietetic Association**
2603 Olive St.
Grand Forks, ND 58201
**Phone:** (701)777-2539      **Fax:** (701)777-3650
**Email:** Sandy_Walen@mail.und.nodak.edu
**Website:** http://www.ndsu.nodak.edu/ndda
Sandy Walen, Contact

## Ohio

**★ 16564 ★ Ohio Dietetic Association**
Blendonview Office Park
5008-05 Pine Creek Dr.
Westerville, OH 43081-4899
**Phone:** (614)895-1253      **Fax:** (614)895-3466
**Email:** oda@eatrightohio.org
**Website:** http://www.eatrightohio.org
Marlisa Bannister, Exec Director

## Oklahoma

**★ 16565 ★ Oklahoma Dietetic Association**
125 HES
Stillwater, OK 74078-6116
**Phone:** (405)744-7469      **Free:** 877-OK-NUTRI
**Fax:** (405)744-6843
**Email:** o-d-a@okstate.edu
**Website:** http://www.oknutrition.org
Carol Beier, MS, RD, Exec Director

## Oregon

**★ 16566 ★ Oregon Dietetic Association**
5811 SE Salmon St.
Portland, OR 97215-2738
**Phone:** (503)408-6448      **Fax:** (503)408-6448
**Email:** shelleyb@pop.nwlint.com
**Website:** http://www.eatrightoregon.org
Shelley Banfe, Contact

## Pennsylvania

**★ 16567 ★ Pennsylvania Dietetic Association**
PO Box 60870
Harrisburg, PA 17106-0870
**Phone:** (717)236-1220      **Fax:** (717)233-2790
**Email:** mccann@epix.net
**Website:** http://www.eatrightpa.org
Colleen McCann, MPH, Contact

## Puerto Rico

**★ 16568 ★ Puerto Rico Dietetic Association**
PO Box 360915
San Juan, PR 00936-0915
**Phone:** (787)753-7144      **Fax:** (787)767-7880
Minerva Martinez, Contact

## Rhode Island

**★ 16569 ★ Rhode Island Dietetic Association**
PO Box 6892
Providence, RI 02904-6892
**Phone:** (401)729-4701
Tricia Harrington, Contact

## South Carolina

**★ 16570 ★ South Carolina Dietetic Association**
1345 Garner Ln., Ste. 103A
Columbia, SC 29210
**Free:** 800-344-7232      **Fax:** (803)794-7378
**Email:** cnc@netside.com
**Website:** http://www.eatrightsc.org
Edna Cox, Contact

## Tennessee

**★ 16571 ★ Tennessee Dietetic Association**
2706 Greystone Rd.
Nashville, TN 37204
**Phone:** (615)463-7944      **Fax:** (615)297-9799
**Email:** allisona@juno.com
**Website:** http://www.eatright-tn.org
Nan Allison, MS, RD, Contact

## Texas

**★ 16572 ★ Texas Dietetic Association**
2695 Villa Creek Dr., Ste. 260
Dallas, TX 75234
**Phone:** (972)755-2530      **Fax:** (972)755-2561
**Email:** tda@challenge-management.com
**Website:** http://www.nutrition4texas.org
John Swinburn, CAE, Exec Director

## Utah

**★ 16573 ★ Utah Dietetic Association**
1497 Sweetwater Ln.
Farmington, UT 84025-3074
**Phone:** (801)451-2221
**Email:** shortedmond@cs.com
Lynda Short, Contact

## Vermont

**★ 16574 ★ Vermont Dietetic Association**
1902 Bland Farm Dr.
East Thetford, VT 05043
**Phone:** (802)847-8913　　**Fax:** (802)847-3401
**Email:** julie.martin@vtmednet.org
**Website:** http://www.eatrightvt.org
Julie Martin, President

## Virginia

**★ 16575 ★ Virginia Dietetic Association**
PO Box 439
Centreville, VA 20122
**Phone:** (703)815-8293　　**Fax:** (703)815-8293
**Email:** vdahdqtrs@aol.com
**Website:** http://www.eatright-va.org
Jackie Darling, RD, Contact

## Washington

**★ 16576 ★ Washington State Dietetic Association**
PO Box 2016
Edmonds, WA 98020-9516
**Phone:** (425)778-6162　　**Fax:** (425)771-9588
**Email:** wsda@melbycameronhull.com
**Website:** http://www.nutritionwsda.org
Kendra Wanzenried, Exec Director

## West Virginia

**★ 16577 ★ West Virginia Dietetic Association**
859 Sherwood Rd.
Charleston, WV 25314
**Email:** stclair859@charter.net
**Website:** http://www.wvda.org
Linda St. Clair, President

## Wisconsin

**★ 16578 ★ Wisconsin Dietetic Association**
1411 W Montgomery St.
Sparta, WI 54656-1003
**Phone:** (608)269-0042　　**Free:** 888-232-8631
**Fax:** (608)269-0043
**Email:** wda@centurytel.net
**Website:** http://www.eatrightwisc.org
Lynn Lawler, RD, CD, Contact

## Wyoming

**★ 16579 ★ Wyoming Dietetic Association**
Department of Family and Consumer Science
PO Box 3354
Laramie, WY 82071
**Phone:** (307)766-5669
**Email:** gupton@wyo.edu
Mona Gupton, Contact

# Chapter 45
# Obstetrics & Gynecology

## Federal Government Agencies

**U.S. Department of Health and Human Services**
**Health Resources and Services Administration**
**Maternal and Child Health Bureau**
*See:* Entry 9

## Foundations & Other Funding Organizations

### Private Foundations

**★ 16580 ★ Koch Foundation, Inc.**
2830 Northwest 41st St., Ste. H
Gainesville, FL 32606
**Phone:** (352)373-7491          **Fax:** (352)337-1548
**Website:** http://mchb.hrsa.gov/
Michael Marconi, Executive Director
**Fnded:** 1979. **Philosophy:** "The Koch Foundation goals are to strengthen and propagate the Catholic Faith by providing grant support for a wide variety of evangelical work. We are dedicated to being of service to those who tend the gardens Spirit wherever they are to be found. In considering applications, major emphasis is placed on sound but financially needy evangelical programs. The foundation is international in scope." **Priorities:** *Arts & Humanities:* 4%. Funds Catholic mass media. *Civic & Public Affairs:* 3%. Emphasis on capital projects. *Education:* 11%. Supports Catholic schools. *Environment:* Primarily for community service programs. *Note:* Total giving in 1999. **Typ. Recipients:** Prenatal Health Issues. **Geo. Dist:** internationally; nationally.

**Schumann Fund for New Jersey**
*See:* Entry 666

**Wenner-Gren Foundation for Anthropological Research**
*See:* Entry 11693

### Corporate Foundations

**CIGNA Foundation**
*See:* Entry 940

**IBP Foundation**
*See:* Entry 11441

**J.D. Edwards Foundation**
*See:* Entry 1154

## Other Funding Organizations

**★ 16581 ★ American Association of Gynecological Laparoscopists (AAGL)**
13021 E Florence Ave.
Santa Fe Springs, CA 90670-4505
**Phone:** (562)946-8774          **Free:** 800-554-2245
**Fax:** (562)946-0073
**Email:** generalmail@aagl.com
**Website:** http://www.aagl.com
Jordan M. Phillips, MD, Bd. Chm.
**Desc:** Physicians who specialize in obstetrics and gynecology and who are interested in gynecological endoscopic procedures. Purposes are to: teach; demonstrate; exchange ideas; distribute literature; stimulate interest in gynecological laparoscopy; maintain and improve medical standards in medical schools and hospitals regarding gynecological laparoscopy; maintain and improve the ethics, practice, and efficiency of the medical practice pertaining to obstetrics and laparoscopy. Conducts seminars and workshops. **Awards:** Circon ACMI Golden Hysteroscope Award (annual) presented to best submitted paper on hysteroscopy by a physician; Olympus Golden Laparoscope Award (annual) presented to best submitted surgical video/film on gynecologic endoscopy by a physician.; Postgraduate Prize Paper (annual) presented to best submitted paper on gynecologic endoscopy by a resident or fellow physician. Must have proof of training status.

**★ 16582 ★ American College of Osteopathic Obstetricians and Gynecologists (ACOOG)**
900 Auburn Rd.
Pontiac, MI 48342-3365
**Phone:** (248)332-6360          **Free:** 800-875-6360
**Fax:** (248)332-4607
**Email:** acoog@acoog.com
**Website:** http://www.acoog.com
Jaki K. Holzer, Admin.
**Desc:** Osteopathic physicians and surgeons specializing in obstetrics and gynecology. Conducts educational programs, and reviews osteopathic obstetric and gynecologic residency training programs. Holds annual postgraduate course and annual convention. **Awards:** Annual ORTHO-ACOOG Resident Thesis Competition (annual) for research papers.

**★ 16583 ★ Association of Women's Health, Obstetric and Neonatal Nurses (AWHONN)**
2000 L St. Nw, Ste. 740
Washington, DC 20036
**Phone:** (202)261-2400          **Free:** 800-673-8499
**Fax:** (202)728-0575
**Email:** gailk@awhonn.org
**Website:** http://www.awhonn.org
Gail Kincaide, Exec. Dir.
**Desc:** Members are registered nurses; associate members are allied health workers with an interest in obstetric, women's health, and neonatal (OGN) nursing. Promotes and establishes the highest standards of OGN nursing practice, education, and research; cooperates with all members of the health team; stimulates interest in OGN nursing. Sponsors educational meetings, audiovisual programs, and continuing education courses. **Awards:** Research Award (periodic).

**★ 16584 ★ Lamaze International**
2025 M St., NW, Ste. 800
Washington, DC 20036
**Phone:** (202)367-1128          **Free:** 800-368-4404
**Fax:** (202)367-2128
**Email:** lamaze@dc.sba.com
**Website:** http://www.lamaze-childbirth.com
Linda Harmon, Exec. Dir.
**Desc:** Physicians, nurses, nurse-midwives, certified teachers of psychoprophylatic (Lamaze) method of childbirth, other professionals, parents, and others interested in Lamaze childbirth preparation and family-centered maternity care. Disseminates information about the theory and practical application of psychoprophylaxis in obstetrics; administers teacher training courses and certifies qualified Lamaze teachers; provides educational lectures, public forums, films, and written materials; maintains national and local teacher and physician referral service. Also presents materials to prospective parents concerning the demands of childrearing. National office serves as information clearinghouse. **Awards:** Elisabeth Bing Award (annual) for members enrolled in Lamaze Childbirth Educator Program who demonstrate financial need; Lamaze Childbirth Educator Program Scholarship (annual) for members enrolled in Lamaze Childbirth Educator Program who demonstrate financial need; Marjorie Karmel Award (annual); President's Award (annual).

**★ 16585 ★ Maternity Center Association (MCA)**
281 Park Ave. S, 5th Fl.
New York, NY 10010
**Phone:** (212)777-5000          **Fax:** (212)777-9320
**Email:** info@maternitywise.org
**Website:** http://www.maternity.org
Maureen Corry, Exec. Dir.
**Desc:** Laypersons, physicians, nurses, nurse-midwives, childbirth educators, and public health workers interested in improvement of maternity care, maternal and infant health, and family life. A national nonprofit health organization for over 800 years, MCA's goals are to expand access to family-centered maternity care through collaborative practice, education, publications, consultation services, public policy initiatives and demonstration programs. Sponsors research; administers nurse-midwifery student assistance fund. Co-sponsors community-based Nurse-Midwifery Education Program. **Awards:** Hazel Corbin Grant (annual) open to individuals who are enrolled in ACNM accredited certification programs.

**National Ovarian Cancer Coalition (NOCC)**
*See:* Entry 10090

**★ 16586 ★ National Perinatal Association (NPA)**
3500 E Fletcher Ave., Ste. 205
Tampa, FL 33613
**Phone:** (813)971-1008     **Free:** 888-971-3295
**Fax:** (813)971-9306
**Email:** npa@nationalperinatal.org
**Website:** http://www.nationalperinatal.org
Shelia S. Sorkin, Exec. Dir.
**Desc:** Organizations and individuals interested in perinatal health care. Purpose is to promote improved patient care, education, research, advocacy and delivery systems for perinatal health. **Awards:** National Perinatal Association Award (annual) for contribution to maternal/child health; Stanley N. Graven Leadership Award (annual); State Initiative (annual).

**★ 16587 ★ Polycystic Ovarian Syndrome Association**
PO Box 80517
Portland, OR 97280
**Phone:** (303)814-0297     **Free:** 877-775-PCOS
**Fax:** (413)751-4866
**Email:** info@pcosupport.org
**Website:** http://www.pcosupport.org
Kristin Rencher, Exec. Dir.
**Desc:** Chapters worldwide provide support, education and advocacy for women suffering from polycystic ovary syndrome (PCOS). Host educational events combining lectures with support sessions. Advocate for women with PCOS in the media and medical community by attending and speaking at professional meetings as well as hosting exhibit booths. **Awards:** Chair's Award (annual) for outstanding service of an individual volunteer; Director's Award (annual) for outstanding service of an individual volunteer; Founder's Award (annual) for outstanding service of an individual volunteer; scholarship (periodic) given to those who indicate need.

**★ 16588 ★ Read Natural Childbirth Foundation (RNCF)**
PO Box 150956
San Rafael, CA 94915-0956
Margaret B. Farley, P. T. Pres.
**Desc:** Doctors, nurses, childbirth instructors, and parents. Promotes and teaches expectant parents the philosophies of natural childbirth pioneered by Grantly Dick-Read, a British doctor who began writing in 1932 about the then extremely controversial concept of natural childbirth and advocated relaxation as the key to comfortable labor. Techniques include abdominal and rib cage breathing and alleviation of fear, and thus pain, through knowledge. Acts as resource agency for the International Childbirth Education Association. Conducts charitable programs. Offers speakers' bureau. **Awards:** Scholarship for couples and single mothers.

**★ 16589 ★ Society for Gynecologic Investigation (SGI)**
409 12th St. SW
Washington, DC 20024-2188
**Phone:** (202)863-2544     **Fax:** (202)863-0739
**Email:** sgiava@aol.com
**Website:** http://www.socgyninv.org
Ava A. Tayman, Exec. Dir.
**Desc:** Present and former faculty members of institutions interested or engaged in fundamental gynecologic research. Purpose is to stimulate, encourage, assist, and conduct gynecologic research. **Awards:** Solvay/Joseph Mortoln Research Grant (annual).

**★ 16590 ★ Society for Maternal Fetal Medicine (SMFM)**
409 12th St. SW
Washington, DC 20024-2188
**Phone:** (202)863-2476     **Fax:** (202)554-1132
**Email:** info@smfm.org
**Website:** http://www.smfm.org
Pat Stahr, Exec. Dir.
**Desc:** Obstetricians specializing in maternal-fetal medicine. Works to improve perinatal care through promotion and expansion of education in obstetrical perinatology. Provides a forum for exchange between members. **Awards:** SMFM Scholarship Award (annual) for research.

**★ 16591 ★ Society for Menstrual Cycle Research (SMCR)**
10559 N 104th Pl.
Scottsdale, AZ 85258
**Phone:** (480)451-9731     **Fax:** (480)451-9731
**Email:** maryannafriederich@msn.com
**Website:** http://www.pop.psu.edu/smcr
Mary Anna Friederich, MD, Sec. -Treas.
**Desc:** Physicians, nurses, endocrinologists, geneticists, physiologists, psychologists, sociologists, researchers, educators, students, and others interested in the health needs of women as related to the menstrual cycle. Goals are: to identify research priorities, recommend research strategies, and promote interdisciplinary research on the menstrual cycle; to establish a communication network for facilitating interdisciplinary dialogue on menstrual cycle events; to disseminate information and promote discussion of issues among public groups. **Awards:** Linda McKeever Student Prize (biennial) for student who presents paper at meeting.

**★ 16592 ★ Society for Obstetric Anesthesia and Perinatology (SOAP)**
1910 Byrd Ave., Ste. 100
PO Box 11086
Richmond, VA 23230-1086
**Phone:** (804)282-5051     **Fax:** (804)282-0090
**Email:** soap@societyhq.com
**Website:** http://www.soap.org
Joy L. Hawkins, MD, Pres.
**Desc:** Physicians and scientists interested in perinatal health care. Purpose is to improve the health care of pregnant women and their unborn children. Conducts specialized education programs; compiles statistics. **Awards:** OAPEF/SOAP Research Starter Grant for young members who wish to launch an academic career in obstetric anesthesia.

# Medical & Allied Health Schools

## Nurse-Midwifery

*The following are certificate and graduate nurse-midwifery programs accredited by the Division of Accreditation of the American College of Nurse-Midwives, 818 Connecticut Ave. NW, Ste. 900, Washington, DC 20006, (202)728-9860, http://www.acnm.org/.*

## California

**★ 16593 ★ Charles R. Drew University of Medicine and Science**
**College of Allied Health Sciences**
**Nurse-Midwifery Certificate Education Program**
1621 E 120th St.
Mail Point 22
Los Angeles, CA 90059
**Phone:** (323)563-4951
**Email:** frcushen@cdrewu.edu
**Website:** http://www.cdrewu.edu
H. Frances Hayes-Cushenberry, JD, Director

**★ 16594 ★ San Diego State University/ University of California, San Diego**
**USCD Division of Graduate Nursing Education**
**Nurse-Midwifery Graduate Program**
9500 Gilman Dr.
Department 0809
La Jolla, CA 92093-0809
**Phone:** (619)543-5480
Lauren Hunter, Director

**★ 16595 ★ University of California, Los Angeles**
**UCLA School of Nursing**
**Nurse-Midwifery Graduate Program**
Factor Bldg., Rm. 5934-A
Box 956819
Los Angeles, CA 90095-6919
**Phone:** (310)794-4434
**Email:** shuser@sonnet.ucla.edu
**Website:** http://www.nursing.ucla.edu/son
Susan Huser, Director

**★ 16596 ★ University of California, San Francisco/San Francisco General Hospital**
**Interdepartmental Nurse-Midwifery Graduate Education Program**
San Francisco General Hospital, Ward 6D, Rm. 21
1001 Potrero Ave.
San Francisco, CA 94110
**Phone:** (415)206-5106
**Email:** linda@ob.ucsf.edu
**Website:** http://nurseweb.ucsf.edu/www/speclist.htm
Linda Ennis, Director

**★ 16597 ★ University of Southern California**
**Nurse-Midwifery Graduate Program**
1540 Alcazar St., CHP 222
Los Angeles, CA 90033
**Phone:** (323)442-2001
**Email:** bjsnell@hsc.usc.edu
**Website:** http://uscnurse.usc.edu
B.J. Snell, PhD, Director

## Colorado

**★ 16598 ★ University of Colorado**
**Health Sciences Center**
**School of Nursing**
**Nurse-Midwifery Graduate Program**
4200 E 9th Ave.
Box C288-14
Denver, CO 80262
**Phone:** (303)724-1183
**Email:** marie.hastings-tolsma@uchsc.edu
**Website:** http://freenet.uchsc.edu/son
Marie Hastings-Tolsma, PhD, Director

## Connecticut

**★ 16599 ★ Yale University**
**School of Nursing**
**Nurse-Midwifery Graduate Program**
100 Church St. S
PO Box 9740
New Haven, CT 06536-0740
**Phone:** (203)785-2389     **Fax:** (203)785-6455
**Email:** lynette.ament@yale.edu
**Website:** http://info.med.yale.edu/nursing
Lynette Ament, PhD, Director

## District of Columbia

**★ 16600 ★ Georgetown University**
**School of Nursing and Health Studies**
**Graduate Program in Nurse-Midwifery**
3700 Reservoir Rd. NW
PO Box 571107
Washington, DC 20007
**Phone:** (202)687-4772 **Fax:** (202)687-5553
**Email:** midwife@gunet.georgetown.edu
**Website:** http://www.dml.georgetown.edu/schnurs/
midwife1.html
Ann Silvonek, Director

## Florida

**★ 16601 ★ University of Florida**
**UFHSC-J College of Nursing**
**Nurse-Midwifery Graduate Program**
653 W 8th St., Bldg. 1, 2nd Fl.
Jacksonville, FL 32209-6561
**Phone:** (904)244-5174
**Email:** poeah@nursing.ufl.edu
**Website:** http://con.ufl.edu
Alice H. Poe, Director

**★ 16602 ★ University of Miami**
**School of Nursing**
**Nurse-Midwifery Graduate Program**
5801 Red Rd.
PO Box 248153
Coral Gables, FL 33124-3850
**Phone:** (305)284-6256
**Email:** jgottlieb@miami.edu
**Website:** http://www.miami.edu/nur/net20/graduate/
midwife.htm
Jeanne Gottlieb, Director

## Georgia

**★ 16603 ★ Emory University**
**Neil Hodgson Woodruff School of**
**Nursing**
**Nurse-Midwifery Graduate Program**
Atlanta, GA 30322
**Phone:** (404)727-6961 **Fax:** (404)727-0536
**Email:** makelle@nurse.emory.edu
**Website:** http://www.nurse.emory.edu
Maureen Kelley, PhD, Director

## Illinois

**★ 16604 ★ University of Illinois, Chicago**
**College of Nursing M/C 802**
**Nurse-Midwifery Graduate Program**
845 S Damen Ave.
Chicago, IL 60612
**Phone:** (312)996-1867 **Fax:** (312)996-8871
**Email:** engstrom@uic.edu
**Website:** http://www.nurs.uic.edu
Janet Engstrom, PhD, Director

## Kansas

**★ 16605 ★ University of Kansas**
**Nurse-Midwifery Graduate Program**
3901 Rainbow Blvd.
Kansas City, KS 66160-7502
**Phone:** (913)588-1683 **Fax:** (913)588-8299
**Email:** gbreedlove@kumc.edu
**Website:** http://www2.kumc.edu/midwife
Ginger Breedlove, PhD, Director

## Kentucky

**★ 16606 ★ Frontier School of Midwifery**
**and Family Nursing**
**Community-Based Nurse-Midwifery**
**Certificate Education Program (CNEP)**
195 School St.
PO Box 528
Hyden, KY 41749
**Phone:** (606)672-2312 **Fax:** (606)672-3776
**Email:** CNEP@midwives.org
**Website:** http://www.midwives.org
Susan Ulrich, PhD, Director

## Maryland

**★ 16607 ★ University of Maryland**
**School of Nursing**
**Nurse-Midwifery Graduate Program**
655 W Lombard St., Ste. 575
Baltimore, MD 21201
**Phone:** (410)706-8625
**Email:** stom@son.umaryland.edu
**Website:** http://nursing.umaryland.edu
Sally Tom, Director

## Massachusetts

**★ 16608 ★ Baystate Medical Center**
**Midwifery Certificate Education Program**
689 Chestnut St.
Springfield, MA 01199
**Phone:** (413)794-4448 **Fax:** (413)794-8770
**Email:** barbara.graves@bhs.org
**Website:** http://www.baystatehealth.com/baystatem-
idwifery
Barbara W. Graves, Director

**★ 16609 ★ Boston University**
**School of Public Health**
**Department of Maternal and Child Health**
**Nurse-Midwifery Graduate Education**
**Program T-5W**
715 Albany St.
Boston, MA 02118
**Phone:** (617)638-5012
**Email:** mbarger@bu.edu
**Website:** http://www.bumc.bu.edu/shp/mc
Mary Barger, Director

## Michigan

**★ 16610 ★ University of Michigan**
**School of Nursing**
**Nurse-Midwifery Graduate Program**
400 N Ingalls, Rm. 3320
Ann Arbor, MI 48109-0482
**Phone:** (313)763-3710 **Fax:** (313)647-0351
**Email:** dswalker@umich.edu
**Website:** http://www-personal.umich.edu/~dswalker/
umhome.html
Deborah Walker, DNSc, Director

## Minnesota

**★ 16611 ★ University of Minnesota**
**School of Nursing**
**Nurse-Midwifery Graduate Program**
6-101 Weaver-Densford Hall
308 Harvard St. SE
Minneapolis, MN 55455
**Phone:** (612)624-6494
**Email:** avery003@tc.umn.edu
**Website:** http://www.nursing.umn.edu/MS/MSmidwif-
ery.html
Melissa Avery, PhD, Director

## Missouri

**★ 16612 ★ University of Missouri,**
**Columbia**
**Sinclair School of Nursing**
**Nurse-Midwifery Graduate Program**
Columbia, MO 65211
**Phone:** (573)882-0235
**Email:** chelinik@health.missouri.edu
**Website:** http://www.muhealth.org/~son/docs/midwif-
ery.html
Katherine Chelini, Director

## New Jersey

**★ 16613 ★ University of Medicine and**
**Dentistry of New Jersey**
**School of Health Related Professions**
**Nurse-Midwifery Certificate Program**
65 Bergen St.
Newark, NJ 07107-3001
**Phone:** (973)972-4298
**Email:** diegmaek@umdnj.edu
**Website:** http://www.umdnj.edu/shrpweb/programs/
midwife
Elaine Diegmann, N.D., Director

## New Mexico

**★ 16614 ★ University of New Mexico**
**College of Nursing**
**Nurse-Midwifery Graduate Program**
Nursing/Pharmacy Bldg.
Albuquerque, NM 87131-1061
**Phone:** (505)272-1184 **Fax:** (505)272-8901
**Email:** midwyfe@unm.edu
**Website:** http://hsc.unm.edu/consg/msn_midw.html
Julie Gorwoda, Director

## New York

**★ 16615 ★ Columbia University**
**School of Nursing**
**Graduate Program in Midwifery**
630 W 168th St.
Box 49
New York, NY 10032
**Phone:** (212)305-5236 **Fax:** (212)305-3680
**Email:** jed19@columbia.edu
**Website:** http://cpmcnet.columbia.edu/dept/nursing
Jennifer Dohrn, Director

**★ 16616 ★ New York University**
**Nurse-Midwifery Graduate Education**
**Program**
246 Greene St.
New York, NY 10003-6677
**Phone:** (212)998-5895
**Email:** patricia.burkhardt@nyu.edu
**Website:** http://www.nyu.edu/education/nursing
Patricia Burkhardt, DrPH, Director

**★ 16617 ★ State University of New York,**
**Brooklyn**
**Health Sciences Center**
**College of Health Related Professions**
**Nurse-Midwifery Graduate Education**
**Program**
450 Clarkson Ave.
Box 1227
Brooklyn, NY 11203
**Phone:** (718)270-7740 **Fax:** (718)270-7634
**Email:** lhsia@downstate.edu
**Website:** http://www.hscbklyn.edu/CHRP/Midwif
Lily Hsia, Director

**★ 16618 ★ State University of New York, Stony Brook**
**School of Nursing**
**Nurse-Midwifery Graduate Program**
Health Sciences Center
Stony Brook, NY 11794-8240
**Phone:** (516)444-2867
**Email:** peter.johnson@stonybrook.edu
**Website:** http://www.pathwaystomidwifery.org
Peter Johnson, PhD, Director

## North Carolina

**★ 16619 ★ East Carolina University**
**School of Nursing**
**Nurse-Midwifery Graduate Program**
Greenville, NC 27858-1818
**Phone:** (252)328-4303          **Fax:** (252)328-2332
**Email:** mossn@mail.ecu.edu
**Website:** http://www.ecu.edu/nursing
Nancy Moss, PhD, Director

## Ohio

**★ 16620 ★ Case Western Reserve University**
**Frances Payne Bolton School of Nursing**
**Nurse-Midwifery Graduate Program**
10900 Euclid Ave.
Cleveland, OH 44106-1712
**Phone:** (216)368-2532
**Email:** ggm@po.cwru.edu
**Website:** http://cwru4.nurs.cwru.edu
Gretchen Mettler, Director

**★ 16621 ★ Ohio State University**
**College of Nursing**
**Nurse-Midwifery Graduate Program**
1585 Neil Ave.
Columbus, OH 43210-1289
**Phone:** (614)292-4041          **Fax:** (614)494-3878
**Email:** nursing@osu.edu
**Website:** http://www.con.ohio-state.edu
Nancy K. Lowe, PhD, Director

**★ 16622 ★ University of Cincinnati**
**College of Nursing and Health**
**Nurse-Midwifery Graduate Program**
PO Box 210038
Cincinnati, OH 45221-0038
**Phone:** (513)558-5282
**Email:** mary.akers@uc.edu
**Website:** http://www.uc.edu/www/nursing
Mary Carol Akers, Director

## Oregon

**★ 16623 ★ Oregon Health Sciences University**
**School of Nursing**
**Nurse-Midwifery Graduate Program**
3181 SW Sam Jackson Park Rd.
Portland, OR 97201
**Phone:** (503)494-3822
**Email:** howec@ohsu.edu
**Website:** http://www.ohsu.edu/son-primcare/indexnmwh.html
Carol Howe, DNSc, Director

## Pennsylvania

**★ 16624 ★ Institute of Midwifery, Women and Health**
**Midwifery Certificate Program**
Hayward Hall, Rm. 222
Schoolhouse Lane and Henry Ave.
Philadelphia, PA 19144
**Phone:** (215)951-2525          **Fax:** (215)951-2526
**Email:** instituteofmidwifery@philau.edu
**Website:** http://www.instituteofmidwifery.org
Jerrilyn Hobdy, Director

**★ 16625 ★ University of Pennsylvania**
**School of Nursing**
**Graduate Program in Nurse-Midwifery**
Nursing Education Bldg.
420 Guardian Dr.
Philadelphia, PA 19104-6096
**Phone:** (215)898-4335
**Email:** mccoolwf@nursing.upenn.edu
**Website:** http://www.nursing.upenn.edu/midwifery
William F. McCool, PhD, Director

## Puerto Rico

**★ 16626 ★ University of Puerto Rico**
**Graduate School of Public Health**
**Nurse-Midwifery Graduate Program**
Medical Sciences Campus
PO Box 5067
San Juan, PR 00936-5067
**Phone:** (787)281-7355
**Website:** http://www.upr.edu/upri
Irene dela Torre, Director

## Rhode Island

**★ 16627 ★ University of Rhode Island**
**College of Nursing**
**Graduate Program in Nurse-Midwifery**
White Hall
Kingston, RI 02881-0814
**Phone:** (401)874-5327
**Email:** jmercer@uri.edu
**Website:** http://www.uri.edu/nursing/programs/msmidwife.html
Judith Mercer, Director

## South Carolina

**★ 16628 ★ Medical University of South Carolina**
**College of Nursing**
**Nurse-Midwifery Graduate Program**
99 Jonathan Lucas St.
Charleston, SC 29403
**Phone:** (843)792-4642          **Fax:** (843)792-1741
**Email:** hickeym@musc.edu
**Website:** http://www.musc.edu
Marcella Hickey, Director

## Tennessee

**★ 16629 ★ Vanderbilt University**
**School of Nursing**
**Nurse-Midwifery Graduate Program**
102 Godchaux Hall
21st Ave. S
Nashville, TN 37240-0008
**Phone:** (615)322-3800
**Email:** vusn_admissions@mcmail.vanderbilt.edu
**Website:** http://www.mc.vanderbilt.edu/nursing
Barbara Petersen, EdD, Director

## Texas

**★ 16630 ★ Baylor College of Medicine**
**Nurse-Midwifery Graduate Program**
6550 Fannin, Ste. 954
Houston, TX 77030
**Phone:** (713)793-8895          **Fax:** (713)793-8647
**Email:** sbarry@bcm.tmc.edu
**Website:** http://www.bcm.tmc.edu/midwifery
Susan E. Barry, Director

**★ 16631 ★ University of Texas, El Paso/Texas Tech University**
**Department of OB/GYN**
**Nurse-Midwifery Graduate Program**
Texas Tech University Health Sciences Center
4800 Alberta Ave.
El Paso, TX 79905
**Phone:** (915)545-6490
**Email:** midwifery@ttmcelp.ttuhsc.edu
**Website:** http://www.nurse.utep.edu/nursing/degree.programs/midwife.htm
Carlene Nelson, PhD, Director

**★ 16632 ★ University of Texas Medical Branch, Galveston**
**School of Nursing**
**Collaborative Nurse-Midwifery Graduate Education Program**
1100 Mechanic
Galveston, TX 77555-1029
**Phone:** (409)772-8347
**Email:** bcamune@utmb.edu
**Website:** http://www.utmb.edu
Barbara Camune, Director

**★ 16633 ★ University of Texas Southwestern Medical Center, Dallas/Parkland Memorial Hospital**
**Parkland School of Nurse-Midwifery**
**Nurse-Midwifery Certificate Program**
5201 Harry Hines Blvd.
MS 6107A
Dallas, TX 75235
**Phone:** (214)590-2580          **Fax:** (214)590-0436
**Email:** mbruck@parknet.pmh.org
**Website:** http://www.swmed.edu/home_pages/parkland/midwifery/midwifehome.html
Mary C. Brucker, Director

## Utah

**★ 16634 ★ University of Utah**
**College of Nursing**
**Nurse-Midwifery Graduate Program**
10 South 2000 East Front
Salt Lake City, UT 84112-5880
**Phone:** (801)581-8274
**Email:** jane.dyer@nurse.utah.edu
**Website:** http://medstat.med.utah.edu/nmw
Jane Dyer, Director

## Virginia

**★ 16635 ★ Shenandoah University**
**Division of Nursing**
**Nurse-Midwifery Graduate Program**
1775 N Sector Ct.
Winchester, VA 22601
**Phone:** (540)678-4382
**Email:** jfehr@su.edu
**Website:** http://www.su.edu/nursing/mas_mid.html
Juliana Fehr, PhD, Director

## Washington

**★ 16636 ★ University of Washington**
**School of Nursing**
**Nurse-Midwifery Graduate Program**
Box 357262
Seattle, WA 98195-7262
**Phone:** (206)543-8241
**Email:** midwife@u.washington.edu
**Website:** http://www.son.washington.edu/departments/fcn/midwifery
Aileen Macharen, PhD, Director

## Wisconsin

**★ 16637 ★ Marquette University**
**College of Nursing**
**Graduate Program in Nurse-Midwifery**
PO Box 1881
Milwaukee, WI 53201-1881
**Phone:** (414)288-3842
**Email:** leona.vandevusse@marquette.edu
**Website:** http://www.mu.edu
Leona VandeVusse, PhD, Director

# National & International Organizations

## ★ 16638 ★ American Academy of Husband-Coached Childbirth (AAHCC)

PO Box 5224
Sherman Oaks, CA 91413-5224
**Phone:** (818)788-6662          **Free:** 800-4-A-BIRTH
**Fax:** (818)788-1580
**Website:** http://www.bradleybirth.com
Marjie Hathaway, Exec. Dir.

**Fnded:** 1970. **Mem:** 1,200. **Desc:** Trains instructors in the Bradley method of natural childbirth. Provides referals to Bradley teachers. **Pub:** *Directory of Instructors*, 2-3/year. *Price:* Free. • *Fetal Advocate*, periodic.

## ★ 16639 ★ American Association of Gynecological Laparoscopists (AAGL)

13021 E Florence Ave.
Santa Fe Springs, CA 90670-4505
**Phone:** (562)946-8774          **Free:** 800-554-2245
**Fax:** (562)946-0073
**Email:** generalmail@aagl.com
**Website:** http://www.aagl.com
Jordan M. Phillips, MD, Bd. Chm.

**Fnded:** 1972. **Mem:** 7,200. **Desc:** Physicians who specialize in obstetrics and gynecology and who are interested in gynecological endoscopic procedures. Purposes are to: teach; demonstrate; exchange ideas; distribute literature; stimulate interest in gynecological laparoscopy; maintain and improve medical standards in medical schools and hospitals regarding gynecological laparoscopy; maintain and improve the ethics, practice, and efficiency of the medical practice pertaining to obstetrics and laparoscopy. Conducts seminars and workshops. **Pub:** *Endoscopic Female Sterilization*. Book. Covers methods, complications, legal implications, and comparisions of endoscopic female tubal stevailization. *Price:* $35. • *Endoscopy in Gynecology*. Book. *Price:* $45. • *Hysteroscopy: Principles and Practice*. Book. Covers many aspects of hysteroscopy. *Price:* $50. • *Manual of Endoscopy*. Book. *Price:* $90. • *Microsurgery in Gynecology*. Book. Contains proceedings from the AAGL First Seminar in Laparoscopy and Tubal Reconstsruction by Microsurgery. *Price:* $35. • *Microsurgery in Gynecology II*. Book. *Price:* $45.

## ★ 16640 ★ American Board of Obstetrics and Gynecology (ABOG)

2915 Vine St.
Dallas, TX 75204
**Phone:** (214)871-1619          **Fax:** (214)871-1943
**Email:** info@abog.org
**Website:** http://www.abog.org
Norman F. Gant, MD, Exec. Dir.

**Fnded:** 1927. **Mem:** 15. **Desc:** Certification board to establish qualifications, conduct examinations, and certify as diplomates those doctors whom the board finds qualified to specialize in obstetrics and gynecology. **Pub:** Bulletin, annual.

## ★ 16641 ★ American College of Domiciliary Midwives (ACDM)

3889 Middlefield Rd.
Palo Alto, CA 94303-4718
**Phone:** (650)328-8491          **Fax:** (650)328-8491
**Email:** info@collegeofmidwives.org
**Website:** http://www.collegeofmidwives.org
Faith Gibson, Exec. Dir.

**Fnded:** 1993. **Mem:** 75. **State Groups:** 2. **Desc:** Strives to preserve lawful access to home-based maternity care as provided by community midwives and family-practice physicians. **Pub:** *International Journal of Domiciliary Midwifery*, quarterly. Journal. Includes historical and contemporary articles on the history, politics, and practice of independent midwifery. *Price:* Free.

## ★ 16642 ★ American College of Home Obstetrics (ACHO)

2821 Rose St.
Franklin Park, IL 60131
**Phone:** (847)455-2030
Gregory White, MD, Pres.

**Fnded:** 1978. **Mem:** 30. **Desc:** Physicians interested in cooperating with families who wish to give birth in the home. Objective is to accumulate and exchange data on home birth. Maintains speakers' bureau; compiles statistics. Plans to conduct research. **Pub:** Newsletter, periodic. • Also publishes statement of purpose.

## ★ 16643 ★ American College of Nurse-Midwives (ACNM)

818 Connecticut Ave., Ste. 900
Washington, DC 20006
**Phone:** (202)728-9860          **Fax:** (202)289-9897
**Email:** info@acnm.org
**Website:** http://www.midwife.org
Deanne Williams, Exec. Dir.

**Fnded:** 1955. **Mem:** 6,200. **Reg. Groups:** 6. **Local Groups:** 53. **Desc:** Seeks to develop and support the profession of certified nurse-midwives in order to promote the health and well-being of women and infants within their families and communities. A CNM is a licensed health care practitioner educated in the two disciplines of nursing and midwifery. Provides gynecological services and care of mothers and babies throughout the maternity cycle; members have completed an ACNM accredited program of study and clinical experience in midwifery and passed a national certification exam. Cooperates with allied groups to enable nurse-midwives to concentrate their efforts in the improvement of services for mothers and newborn babies. Seeks to identify areas of nurse-midwifery practices as they relate to the total service and educational aspects of maternal and newborn care. Studies and evaluates activities of nurse-midwives in order to establish qualifications; cooperates in planning and developing educational programs. conducts research and continuing education workshops. sponsors research. Compiles statistics. Maintains speakers' bureau and archives; offers placement service. **Pub:** *American College of Nurse-Midwives Membership Directory Supplement*, annual. Directory. *Price:* Included in membership dues. • *Directory of Nurse-Midwifery Practices*, annual. Directory. Computer listing of certified nurse-midwives by state. *Price:* Included in membership dues; $10 for nonmembers. • *Journal of Nurse-Midwifery*, bimonthly. Journal. Covers topics relevant to maternal and newborn health, obstetrics, well-woman gynecology, family planning, and midwifery education. *Price:* Included in membership dues; $48/year for nonmembers; $69/year for institutions. • *Quickening*, bimonthly. Newsletter. Includes activities, calendar of events, employment listings, and legislative updates. *Price:* Included in membership dues. • Also publishes pamphlets and brochures. **Frmly:** (1969) American College of Nurse-Midwifery.

## ★ 16644 ★ American College of Obstetricians and Gynecologists (ACOG)

409 12th St. SW
PO Box 96920
Washington, DC 20090-6920
**Phone:** (202)638-5577          **Fax:** (202)484-8107
**Email:** mgraves@acog.org
**Website:** http://www.acog.org
Ralph Hale, MD, Exec. VP

**Fnded:** 1951. **Mem:** 41,000. **Reg. Groups:** 10. **State Groups:** 50. **Desc:** Physicians specializing in childbirth and the diseases of women. Sponsors continuing professional development program. **Pub:** *ACOG Newsletter*, monthly. Newsletter. • *Committee Opinions, Educational Bulletins, Practice Bulletins, and Criteria sets* ., periodic. Bulletin. Includes technical information. • *Obstetrics and Gynecology*, monthly. Journal. *Price:* $70 med. students/residents; $160 personal; $255 libraries. • Manuals. **Frmly:** (1956) American Academy of Obstetrics and Gynecology.

## American College of Osteopathic Obstetricians and Gynecologists (ACOOG)

*See:* Entry 16992

## ★ 16645 ★ American Foundation for Maternal and Child Health (AFMCH)

439 E 51st St., 8th Fl.
New York, NY 10022
**Phone:** (212)759-5510          **Fax:** (212)935-0191
**Email:** acoog@acoog.com
**Website:** http://www.acoog.com
Doris Haire, Pres.

**Fnded:** 1972. **Desc:** Serves as a clearinghouse for interdisciplinary research on maternal and child health; focuses on the perinatal or birth period and its effect on infant development. Sponsors medical research designed to improve application of technology in maternal and child health; conducts educational programs; compiles statistics. Operates extensive reference library.

## ★ 16646 ★ American Gynecological and Obstetrical Society (AGOS)

University of Utah
50 N Medical Dr.
Salt Lake City, UT 84132
**Phone:** (801)581-5501          **Fax:** (801)581-7199
Paul B. Underwood, Jr., Sec.

**Fnded:** 1981. **Mem:** 243. **Desc:** Works to cultivate and promote knowledge concerning obstetrics and gynecology. **Pub:** *Transactions*, annual.

## ★ 16647 ★ American Rights Coalition

3335 Ringgold Rd.
Chattanooga, TN 37401
**Phone:** (423)698-7960          **Free:** 800-634-2224
**Fax:** (423)698-7893
**Website:** http://www.jericho.org/~jericho/_carc.html

**Desc:** "ARC helps women who are having physical and emotional problems after an abortion. ARC strongly believes that those who have injured these women should be sued for malpractice." Offers referrals to medical, legal, and emotional services within the woman's local area.

## ★ 16648 ★ American Society of Breast Disease

PO Box 140186
Dallas, TX 75214
**Phone:** (214)368-6836          **Fax:** (214)368-5719
**Email:** asbd1@aol.com
**Website:** http://www.asbd.org
Andrew D. Seidman, MD, Contact

**Fnded:** 1976. **Mem:** 650. **Desc:** Physicians and nurses, primarily those engaged in the fields of obstetrics and gynecology, surgery, radiology, family practice, and medical and radiation oncology. Seeks to further the study of diseases of the breast and to inform physicians and other health care professionals of developments in the diagnosis and treatment of breast cancer and benign diseases of the breast. Serves as a forum for discussion among members. Encourages research pertaining to breast disease. **Pub:** *ASBD Advisor*, quarterly. Newsletter. • *The Breast Journal*, bimonthly. **Frmly:** (1994) Society for the Study of Breast Disease.

## ★ 16649 ★ American Society of Childbirth Educators (ASCE)

PO Box 2282
Sedona, AZ 86339
**Phone:** (928)284-9897          **Fax:** (928)284-9897
**Email:** jsasmor@sedona.net
Dr. James C. Sasmor, Corporate Sec.

**Fnded:** 1972. **Desc:** Seeks to provide a medium for the exchange and dissemination of information relating to prepared childbirth as a shared family experience and disseminate information to qualified professionals regarding standards, techniques, and skills relevant to the concept of prepared birth. Presently inactive.

### ★ 16650 ★ American Society for Colposcopy and Cervical Pathology (ASCCP)

20 W Washington St., Ste. 1
Hagerstown, MD 21740
**Phone:** (301)733-3640     **Free:** 800-787-7227
**Fax:** (301)733-5775
**Website:** http://www.asccp.org
Kathleen Poole, Admin. Dir.

**Fnded:** 1964. **Mem:** 3,800. **Desc:** Gynecologists, family physicians, pathologists, nurses, and other individuals interested in promoting the accurate and ethical application of colposcopy (the examination of the lower genital tract by means of a colposcope). Organizes and approves training programs and audio visual materials in the diagnosis and management of lower genital tract disease. Conducts accredited postgraduate courses. **Pub:** *ASCCP Videoguide to Colposcopy.* Video. 30-minute videotape on colposcopy, LGSIL, HGSIL, and cancer. *Price:* $20 in U.S.; $35 outside U.S. • *Comprehensive Colposcopy Review. Price:* $150 for members; $180 for non-members. • *Home Study Program,* quarterly. *Price:* $160/year. • *Journal of Lower Genital Tract Disease,* quarterly. *Price:* $85/year. **Frmly:** American Society for Colposcopy and Colpomicroscopy.

### ★ 16651 ★ Asia and Oceania Federation of Obstetrics and Gynecology (AOFOG)

National University Hospital
Department of Obstetrics and Gynaecology
Lower Kent Ridge Rd.
Singapore 119074, Singapore

**Lang(s):** Chinese, English. **Desc:** Obstetricians and gynecologists. Seeks to advance the study, teaching, and practice of obstetrics and gynecology; promotes professional development of members. Serves as a forum for the exchange of information among members; sponsors research and educational programs.

### Asociacion Nacional Contra el Cancer (ANCEC)

*See:* Entry 10117

### ★ 16652 ★ Association for Childbirth at Home, International (ACHI)

14140 Magnolia Blvd.
Sherman Oaks, CA 91423
**Phone:** (818)386-1082     **Fax:** (818)386-9374
**Email:** nbwc@ix.netcom.com
**Website:** http://www.panamatravel.com/ancec.htm
Tonya Brooks, Founder & Pres.

**Fnded:** 1972. **Mem:** 30,000. **Reg. Groups:** 9. **State Groups:** 40. **Local Groups:** 120. **Desc:** Parents, midwives, doctors, childbirth educators, other professionals, and interested individuals, all of whom support childbirth at home. Purposes are to bring accurate information and competent support to parents seeking home birth and safe hospital birth; to identify and implement correct obstetrical and pediatric practice. Offers parent education classes, leader training programs, international resource and referral service, and professional education seminars and programs; instructs parents, childbirth educators, midwives, and physicians in safe home birth and noninterventive alternative techniques. Conducts research; compiles statistics. Maintains speakers' bureau. **Pub:** *Birth Notes,* quarterly. Newsletter. *Price:* $25/year. • *Founders Letter,* 6/year. • *Giving Birth at Home.* Handbook. • Brochures. **Frmly:** Association for Childbirth at Home.

### Association of Maternal and Child Health Programs (AMCHP)

*See:* Entry 5625

### ★ 16653 ★ Association of Professors of Gynecology and Obstetrics (APGO)

2130 Priest Bridge Dr., Ste. 7
Crofton, MD 21114
**Phone:** (410)451-9560     **Fax:** (410)451-9568
**Email:** djohnson@apgo.org
**Website:** http://www.apgo.org
Donna Wachter, Exec. Dir.

**Fnded:** 1962. **Mem:** 1,500. **Desc:** Departments of obstetrics and gynecology in approved medical schools in the U.S. and Canada, and in non-university teaching hospitals with active educational program for undergraduate medical students in OB/GYN. Works to consider problems relating to the departments of obstetrics and gynecology; to advance and improve the study of gynecology and obstetrics; to provide a means of exchanging information relating to the programs of study, teaching methods, and research activities of such departments. Compiles statistics. **Pub:** *Academic Position Report,* 3/year. Report. Job openings in the academic OB/GYN community. *Price:* $5. • *APGO Membership Directory,* annual. Membership Directory. *Price:* $20. • *The APGO Reporter.* Newsletter. • *Exploring Issues in Obstetric and Gynecologic Medical Ethics. Price:* $30. • *Medical Student Educational Objectives. Price:* $20 per copy; $17.50 2-49 copies.

### ★ 16654 ★ Association of Radical Midwives (ARM)

62 Greetby Hill
Ormskirk L39 2DT, United Kingdom
**Phone:** 44 1695 572776     **Fax:** 44 1695 572776
**Email:** arm@radmid.demon.co.uk
**Website:** http://www.radmid.demon.co.uk

**Fnded:** 1976. **Mem:** 1,700. **Local Groups:** 50. **Lang(s):** English. **Desc:** Midwives, mothers, health professionals, and interested individuals. Supports the interests of midwives. Provides supportive services and information to women experiencing difficulty in securing adequate and sympathetic maternity care. **Pub:** *Choices in Childbirth.* Booklet. • *Midwifery Matters,* quarterly. Magazine. "What is a Midwife?" Leaflet in English, sponsored. No further advertising. Free single distribution, bulk orders for postage costs only.

### Association of Women's Health, Obstetric and Neonatal Nurses (AWHONN)

*See:* Entry 15669

### ★ 16655 ★ Australasian Menopause Society (AMS)

PO Box 876
Kingsford, NSW 2032, Australia
**Phone:** 61 2 93826732     **Fax:** 61 2 93826728
**Email:** ams@netlink.com.au
**Website:** http://www.menopause.org.au

**Lang(s):** English. **Desc:** Doctors, nurses, paramedical and community workers, and those with an interest in menopause. Seeks to improve the quality of life of women during and after menopause.

### ★ 16656 ★ Australian College of Obstetricians and Gynaecologists (ACOG)

8 La Trobe St.
Melbourne, VIC 3000, Australia
**Fnded:** 1978.

### ★ 16657 ★ Boston Women's Health Book Collective

c/o BU School of Public Health
715 Albany St., W-1, Rm. 120
Boston, MA 02118
**Phone:** (617)414-1230     **Fax:** (617)414-1233
**Email:** office@bwhbc.org
**Website:** http://www.ourbodiesourselves.org
Judy Norsigian, Exec. Dir.

**Fnded:** 1969. **Desc:** Promotes increased awareness of women's health issues among health care professional and the public. Gathers and disseminates information on health topics of concern to women. Maintains speakers' bureau. **Pub:** *Nuestros Cuevpos, Nuestras Videas.* Book. Our Bodies Ourselves adapted for Latinas. *Price:* $24. • *Our Bodies, Ourselves for the New Century.* Book. Contains comprehensive information regarding women's health. *Price:* $24. **Frmly:** BWHBC.

### Breast Cancer Care

*See:* Entry 10128

### Bulgarian Society for Immunology of Reproduction (IBIR-BAN)

*See:* Entry 3204

### ★ 16658 ★ C/SEC

22 Forest Rd.
Framingham, MA 01701
**Phone:** (508)877-8266
**Email:** bcc@breastcancercare.org.uk
**Website:** http://www.breastcancercare.org.uk
Norma Shulman, Dir.

**Fnded:** 1972. **Mem:** 2,000. **Desc:** Childbirth groups, doctors, laypersons, and nurses. Established out of concern for the lack of resources available to couples who anticipate or have had a cesarean delivery. Goals are to: improve the cesarean childbirth experience and make the cesarean delivery a good and meaningful childbirth experience for each couple; provide information and promote education on cesarean prevention and vaginal birth after cesarean; change attitudes and policies that affect the cesarean childbirth experience. Offers support for cesarean couples through informal discussion meetings, telephone contact, and personal reply to letters. Provides information on many aspects of cesarean childbirth in order to make couples aware of exactly what the procedure entails and what options are available. Works with doctors, hospitals, childbirth educators, and others in the medical community to effect policy changes and to promote family-centered maternity care for cesarean couples. Conducts in-service programs for hospital staffs and has spoken at conventions and workshops on childbirth. Acronym C/SEC stands for Cesareans/Support, Education and Concern. **Pub:** *Frankly Speaking.* Book. Discussion of cesarean birth. *Price:* $4. • *Preventing Unnecessary Cesareans: A Guide to Labor Management and Detailed Bibliography.* Pamphlet. Outlines avoidable factors which may lead to preventable cesareans. *Price:* $2. **Frmly:** (1976) C/SEC (Cesarean Sections: Education and Concern).

### ★ 16659 ★ Canadian Pelvic Inflammatory Disease Society

PO Box 33804, Sta. D
Vancouver, BC, Canada V6J 4L6
**Phone:** (604)684-5704

**Fnded:** 1985. **Mem:** 300. **Lang(s):** English, French. **Desc:** Women with Pelvic Inflammatory Disease (PID), medical professionals, health care organizations, and interested individuals. (PID is an infection or inflammation of a women's pelvic organs which can result in scarring and adhesion of the reproductive organs, infertility, recurring or chronic infection, ectopic pregnancy, chronic abdominal pain, and miscarriage.) Provides information and support to women with PID and their families. Promotes public education and the prevention of PID; produces and distributes educational materials; supports research on prevention of PID. Maintains speakers' bureau. **Pub:** *Fact Sheet for Men about PID,* periodic. • *News Coverage of PID.* Video. • *Pelvic Inflammatory Disease (PID).* Booklet. • *PID Brochure.* Brochure. • *PID True/False Public Education Questionnaire.* Bulletin. • *Royal Commission Briefs on PID.* Bulletin.

**★ 16660 ★ Center for Humane Options in Childbirth Experiences (CHOICE)**
3474 N High St.
Columbus, OH 43214
**Phone:** (614)263-2229     **Fax:** (614)449-0140
**Website:** http://www.birthchoice.org/
Abby Kinne, Dir.
**Fnded:** 1977. **Mem:** 1,200. **Local Groups:** 1. **Desc:** Medical professionals, paraprofessionals, and interested individuals. Purpose is to teach and encourage parents, parents-to-be, groups, and interested individuals working in family-oriented childbirth in hospital birth centers and out-of-hospital situations. Trains and certifies attendants to attend or coach births. Acts as consumer advocate for hospital births. Services include medical referrals, childbirth education classes, and supplementary prenatal care. Sponsors community educational programs; operates speakers' bureau; compiles statistics.

**Center for Study of Multiple Birth (CSMB)**
*See:* Entry 18259

**★ 16661 ★ Childbirth Without Pain Education Association (CWPEA)**
20134 Snowden
Detroit, MI 48235
**Phone:** (313)341-3816
**Email:** cat-flora@juno.com
**Website:** http://www.multiplebirth.com
Flora Hommel, Exec. Dir. /Founder
**Fnded:** 1958. **Mem:** 2,000. **Nat'l Groups:** 8. **Reg. Groups:** 3. **State Groups:** 3. **Local Groups:** 1. **Desc:** Former and current students of the Lamaze-Pavlov (psychoprophylactic) method of painless childbirth; physicians, nurses, midwifes, students, former students and interested individuals. Sponsors classes and films for women with or without partners, nurses, midwifes and medical and lay groups about the method, which is based on conditioned reflexes to help prevent pain, thus allowing for normal, usually drug- and intervention free childbirth. Works to provide a method-trained person (monitrice) in attendance at the birth where possible. Collects data for further development of the method; surveys maternity services. Sponsors childbirth teacher and monitrice training and certification nationally with workshops. Provides teen pregnancy programs. Offers some referral service. **Pub:** *Childbirth Without Pain Education Association Memo*, bimonthly. Newsletter. Includes association news and book reviews, and current practices and research. *Price:* Included in membership dues; $50/year for physicians; $35/year for nurses and nonmembers; $16/year for alumni. **AKA:** Lamaze Birth Without Pain Education Association.

**★ 16662 ★ Chilean Society of Obstetrics and Gynecology (Sociedad Chilena de Obstetricia y Ginecologia)**
Roman Diaz 205, Of 205, Providencia
Santiago, Chile
**Phone:** 56 2 2359133     **Fax:** 56 2 2351294
**Fnded:** 1935.

**★ 16663 ★ Colombian Society of Obstetrics and Gynecology (SCOG)**
Apdo Aereo 34188
Santa Fe de Bogota, Colombia
**Phone:** 57 1 2681485
**Fnded:** 1943.

**★ 16664 ★ Council on Resident Education in Obstetrics and Gynecology (CREOG)**
PO Box 96920
Washington, DC 20090-6920
**Phone:** (202)863-2554     **Fax:** (202)863-4994
**Email:** creog@acog.org
DeAnne Nehra, Assoc. Dir.
**Fnded:** 1967. **Mem:** 450. **Desc:** A semiautonomous nonregulatory organization founded by the American College of Obstetricians and Gynecologists and comprised of national specialty organizations. Works to promote and maintain high standards of resident training in obstetrics and gynecology. Services include: consultative site visits to residency programs; clearinghouse for residency positions; conferences; a resident data bank; national in-training examination. **Pub:** *A Design for Resident Education in Obstetrics and Gynecology.* • *Basic Science Monographs in Obstetrics and Gynecology*, periodic. Monograph. Covers metabolism, genetics, maternal physiology, pharmacology, microbiology, and other aspects of reproductive health. *Price:* $10 for members; $15 for nonmembers. • *Council on Resident Education in Obstetrics and Gynecology–Council News*, 3/year. Newsletter. Contains membership activities and *CREOG Directory of Obstetric and Gynecologic Residency Programs* update. • *CREOG Directory of Obstetric and Gynecologic Residency Programs and Directors*, annual. Directory. Lists accredited residency programs in the U.S. and Canada. *Price:* $10. • *Educational Objectives for Residents in Obstetrics and Gynecology.*

**★ 16665 ★ Danish Society for Obstetrics and Gynecology (Dansk Selskab for Obstetrik og Gynaekologi)**
Brendstrupgaardsvej
DK-8200 Arhus, Denmark
**Phone:** 45 89496458     **Fax:** 45 89496460
**Fnded:** 1898.

**DES Action Canada**
*See:* Entry 18268

**★ 16666 ★ DES Action, U.S.A.**
610 16th St., Ste. 301
Oakland, CA 94612
**Phone:** (510)465-4011     **Free:** 800-DES-9288
**Fax:** (510)465-4815
**Email:** desaction@earthlink.net
**Website:** http://www.desaction.org
Nora Cody, Exec. Dir.
**Fnded:** 1977. **Mem:** 3,000. **Reg. Groups:** 20. **Desc:** DES-exposed persons and others "working to try to ameliorate the problems caused by DES." DES (diethylstilbestrol) is a synthetic estrogen in use since 1938 and often prescribed for prevention of miscarriage, diabetes during pregnancy, difficulty in conceiving, staining during pregnancy, and cessation of premature labor. It has since been found that, in some cases, daughters born to women taking DES in the first five months of pregnancy have developed cervical and vaginal abnormalities, a very small percentage of which have resulted in cancer, and a greater number of DES daughters experience problems with pregnancies, including seven times the rate of tubal pregnancy and twice the rate of miscarriage. DES mothers have a higher risk of breast cancer. Goal is to reach DES-exposed persons and to stress to them the need for medical attention and monitoring; to educate professionals and the public. **Pub:** *DES Action Voice: A Focus on Diethylstilbestrol Exposure*, quarterly. Newsletter. Includes medical question and answer column; book reviews; legislation and litigation news; conference reports. *Price:* $35/year. • *Fertility and Pregnancy Guide for DES Daughters and Sons. Price:* $6. Also publishes fact sheets, booklets and doctor referral sheet. **Frmly:** (1986) DES Action, National.

**★ 16667 ★ Doulas of North America (DONA)**
PO Box 626
Jasper, IN 47547-0626
**Email:** doula@dona.org
**Website:** http://www.dona.org
Kristi Ridd-Young, Admin. Dir.
**Fnded:** 1992. **Mem:** 3,500. **Reg. Groups:** 9. **State Groups:** 50. **Desc:** Seeks to help doulas provide quality labor support to birthing women. Offers certification program for doulas; provides continuing education opportrinties; establishes standards of practice and code of ethics; compiles statistics. **Pub:** *DONA Referral Directory.* Directory. • *The International Doula*, quarterly. Newsletter. • *The International Doula Trainer*, quarterly. Newsletter. • *Introducing the Doula.* Video. *Price:* $15 for members; $25 for non-members.

**★ 16668 ★ Elliot Institute**
PO Box 7348
Springfield, IL 62791-7348
**Phone:** (217)525-8202     **Fax:** (217)525-8212
**Email:** elliotinst@afterabortion.org
David C. Reardon, PhD, Dir.
**Fnded:** 1988. **Desc:** Seeks to promote post abortion healing and reconciliation through research and education on the after affects of abortion on women, men, children and society. Conducts educational and research programs; compiles statistics; maintains speakers' bureau. **Pub:** *The Post-Abortion Review*, quarterly. Newsletter. Original articles reporting on post-abortion research of trends in post-abortion healing & advocacy. *Price:* $20/yr. **AKA:** (1999) Elliot Institute for Social Sciences Research.

**★ 16669 ★ Endometriosis Association (EA)**
8585 N 76th Pl.
Milwaukee, WI 53223
**Phone:** (414)355-2200     **Free:** 800-992-3636
**Fax:** (414)355-6065
**Email:** endo@endometriosisassn.org
**Website:** http://www.endometriosisassn.org
Mary Lou Ballweg, Exec. Dir.
**Fnded:** 1980. **Mem:** 10,000. **Reg. Groups:** 200. **Desc:** Provides help and support to those affected by endometriosis; educates public and medical community about the disease. promotes research. **Pub:** *Are You a Teenager?*. Brochure. *Price:* Free. • *Endometriosis Association Newsletter*, bimonthly. Newsletter. Includes news, tips, reviews, and research reports; also covers association and chapter news and activities. *Price:* Included in membership dues. • *The Endometriosis Sourcebook.* Book. • *Endometriosis: The Inside Story.* Video. • *Overcoming Endometriosis.* Book. • *Teens Speak Out on Endometriosis.* Video. • *Teensource*, quarterly. Newsletter. • *What is Endometriosis.* Brochure. In 28 languages. • *You're Not Alone.* Video. • *You're Not Alone: Understanding Endometriosis.* Video. In 27 languages.

**★ 16670 ★ European Association of Perinatal Medicine (EAPM)**
c/o Ricardo N. Laurini
Department of Obstetrics and Gynecology
University Hospital San Joao
4200 Porto, Portugal
**Phone:** 351 22 5094958     **Fax:** 351 22 5505870
**Email:** rlaurini@hotmail.com
**Website:** http://www.krenet.it/A/EAPM/welcome.htm
**Fnded:** 1968. **Mem:** 900. **Lang(s):** English. **Desc:** Pediatricians, obstetricians, anesthesiologists, medical doctors, students, and nurses interested in perinatal medicine. Works to advance information and interest in perinatal medicine. **Pub:** *Perinatal Medicine*, biennial.

**★ 16671 ★ European Board and College of Obstetrics and Gynecology (EBCOG)**
Herestr 49
B-3000 Leuven, Belgium
**Phone:** 32 1 6344205     **Fax:** 32 1 6344208
**Email:** charlotte.mercer@btinternet.com
**Website:** http://www.ebcog.org
No Change 020501 European Board and College of Obstetrics and Gynecolog, y, Contact
**Desc:** Enhances the health of women and their babies by promoting the highest possible standards of care in all European countries.

**★ 16672 ★ European Midwives Liaison Committee (EMLC)**
**(Comite de Liaison des Sages-Femmes Europeennes)**
c/o Marianne Mead
Postbus 18
NL-3720 AA Bilthoven, Netherlands
**Phone:** 31 30 2294299    **Fax:** 31 30 2294162
**Email:** info@noverl.nl
**Fnded:** 1968. **Mem:** 16. **Nat'l Groups:** 16. **Lang(s):** English, French. **Desc:** Representatives of associations of midwives in the European Union. Promotes the interests of midwives; represents midwife associations before the Commission of the European Communities and other organizations. Also publishes Responsibilities and Independence of Midwives within the European Union - 1996. **Frmly:** EEC Midwives Liaison Committee.

**★ 16673 ★ European Society of Gynaecological Oncology (ESGO)**
Gynecologic Institute
University of Padova
3 via Giustiniani
I-35128 Padova, Italy
**Phone:** 39 0698213410    **Fax:** 39 0498750860
**Email:** simga@unipd.it
**Fnded:** 1983. **Mem:** 600. **Desc:** Promotes international communication in order to promote the improvement the standard of care in Gynecologic Oncology. Promotes clinical and basic research in Gynecologic Oncology.

**★ 16674 ★ European Society for Gynecological Endoscopy (ESGE)**
4, bd Charles de Gaulle
F-63003 Clermont-Ferrand, France
**Fax:** 33 4 73931706
**Fnded:** 1991. **Desc:** Promotes study of gynecological surgical techniques using endoscopy; recommends standards of training in gynecological endoscopy.

**★ 16675 ★ European Society for Infectious Diseases in Obstetrics and Gynaecology (ESIDOG)**
Klinikum Grosshadern Frauenklinik
Postf. 702027
D-81320 Munich, Germany
**Phone:** 49 89 70954730    **Fax:** 49 89 70958884
**Email:** contact@europeansociety100g.de
**Fnded:** 1985. **Mem:** 500. **Lang(s):** English. **Desc:** Promotes the study of infectious diseases in obstetrics and gynaecology.

**★ 16676 ★ Federation of Asia-Oceania Perinatal Societies**
246 Clayton Rd.
Clayton, VIC 3168, Australia
**Phone:** 61 3 95945191    **Fax:** 61 3 95946115
**Fnded:** 1980. **Desc:** Promotes the science and art of perinatology, maternal, fetal, and neonatal welfare; encourages cooperation with international bodies; provides expert advice to governmental and other bodies.

**★ 16677 ★ Federation of French-Language Gynecologists and Obstetricians**
**(Federation des Gynecologues et Obstetriciens de Langue Francaise — FGOLF)**
c/o Prof. Jean Rene Zorn
Clinique Universitaire Baudelocque
123, blvd. de Port-Royal
F-75674 Paris Cedex 14, France
**Phone:** 33 1 42341143    **Fax:** 33 1 42341231
**Fnded:** 1950. **Mem:** 700. **Lang(s):** French. **Desc:** French-speaking gynecologists and obstetricians. Purpose is to promote scientific study in the French language of all aspects of the biology of human reproduction. Conducts training sessions and travel and exchange programs. Maintains permanent committees to deal with special topics. **Pub:** *Journal de Gynecologie Obstetrique et Biologie de la Reproduction*, bimonthly. Journal.

**★ 16678 ★ Federation of Obstetric and Gynecological Societies of India**
31/C Dr. NA. Purandare Marg
Bombay 400 007, India
**Phone:** 91 22 3614011
**Fnded:** 1950.

**★ 16679 ★ Group B Strep Association**
PO Box 16515
Chapel Hill, NC 27516
**Phone:** (919)932-5344    **Fax:** (919)932-5344
**Website:** http://www.groupbstrep.org
Gina Burns, Pres.
**Fnded:** 1990. **Mem:** 3,000. **Nat'l Groups:** 1. **Desc:** Seeks to educate the public about Group B Strep (GBS) infections during pregnancy. Promotes screening of mothers and the development of a vaccine. Seeks to control the disease which is a leading cause of life-threatening infections in newborns. Acts as a support group; provides educational programs. **Pub:** *GBSA Public Education Packet.* • Also provides GBSA Public Education Packet, medical contacts and legislation information.

**Gynecologic Oncology Group (GOG)**
*See:* Entry 10175

**★ 16680 ★ Gynecologic Surgery Society (GSS)**
c/o Debi Maines
6900 Grove Rd.
Thorofare, NJ 08086-9431
**Phone:** (856)293-2046    **Fax:** (856)848-5274
**Email:** information@gynecologicsurgerysociety.org
**Website:** http://www.gynecologicsurgerysociety.org
John Marlow, Pres.
**Fnded:** 1979. **Mem:** 700. **Desc:** Individuals interested in gynecologic surgery. Facilitates communication among members. Conducts educational programs and demonstrations of new surgical techniques. **Pub:** *Journal of Gynecologic Surgery*, periodic. Journal. • Newsletter, periodic.

**★ 16681 ★ Hong Kong Gynaecological Endoscopy Society (HKGES)**
Department of Obstetrics and Gynaecology
Prince of Wales Hospital
30-32 Ngan Shing St.
Hong Kong, People's Republic of China
**Phone:** 852 26322810    **Fax:** 852 26360008
**Email:** pmyuen@cuhk.edu.hk
**Website:** http://www.fmshk.com.hk/hkges
**Fnded:** 1994. **Mem:** 60. **Lang(s):** Chinese, English. **Desc:** Gynecological endoscopists and other health care professionals. Promotes advancement of the practice of gynecological endoscopy. Conducts continuing professional education programs. **Pub:** *Endovision*, quarterly. Newsletter.

**★ 16682 ★ Hysterectomy Educational Resources and Services Foundation (HERS)**
422 Bryn Mawr Ave.
Bala Cynwyd, PA 19004
**Phone:** (610)667-7757    **Free:** 888-750-HERS
**Fax:** (610)667-8096
**Email:** hersfdn@aol.com
**Website:** http://www.uterinearteryembolization.com
Nora W. Coffey, Pres.
**Fnded:** 1982. **Desc:** Helps women make informed decisions regarding hysterectomy and alternatives to surgery. Provides medical journal articles and other educational materials concerning hysterectomy and alternative procedures, networking with other women on a one to one basis, referral to physicians and telephone counseling by appointment. **Pub:** *HERS Annual Hysterectomy Conference Proceedings*. Proceedings. • *HERS Newsletter*, quarterly. Newsletter. Contains book reviews, medical and scientific literature reviews, writer's chronicle of journal, and letters from readers. *Price:* $20/year. • *Hysterectomy Pamphlet.* Pamphlet. • Reprints. • Also makes available reading list and copies of medical journal articles; distributes audio cassettes and other related materials. **AKA:** HERS Foundation.

**★ 16683 ★ Independent Midwives Association**
1 The Great Quarry
Guildford
Surrey GU1 3XN, United Kingdom
**Phone:** 44 1483 821104
**Email:** info@independentmidwives.org.uk
**Website:** http://www.independentmidwives.org.uk
**Fnded:** 1982. **Mem:** 60. **Lang(s):** English. **Desc:** Midwives practicing in England. Promotes the involvement of midwives in childbirth. Promotes education in midwifery. Represents members' interests.

**★ 16684 ★ Indonesian Society for Perinatology (PERINASIA)**
**(Perkumpulan Perinatologi Indonesia — PERINASIA)**
Jalan Tebet Utara IA/22
12820 Jakarta, Indonesia
**Phone:** 62 21 8281243    **Fax:** 62 21 8281243
**Email:** perinasi@centrin.net.id
**Fnded:** 1981. **Mem:** 1,104. **Local Groups:** 19. **Lang(s):** English, Indonesian. **Desc:** Obstetricians, gynecologists, pediatricians, midwives, and interested others. Strives to reduce the perinatal mortality rate; works to improve prenatal, natal, and postnatal health care; seeks improved medical facilities. Holds workshops, congresses, seminars, and symposia on perinatal health care and related subjects. Advocates research in safe birth practices; promotes the use of preventive medicine in prenatal care. Encourages community participation in health care improvement programs. Offers technical assistance to government authorities. Cooperates with similar international organizations. Conducts surveys. Disseminates information. **Pub:** *Perinasia Bulletin*, quarterly. Bulletin. • Proceedings, periodic.

**★ 16685 ★ Informed Homebirth/Informed Birth and Parenting (IH/IBP)**
PO Box 1733
Fair Oaks, CA 95628
**Phone:** (916)961-6923    **Fax:** (916)961-6923
**Email:** ihibp@aol.com
Rahima Baldwin Dancy, Pres.
**Fnded:** 1977. **Desc:** Expectant and new parents, childbirth educators, midwives, nurses, preschool and elementary school teachers, and others interested in safe childbirth alternatives. Seeks to provide information on alternatives in childbirth methods, parenting, and developmental education. Childbirth Educator Training Program leading to certification as Childbirth Educator; Childbirth Assistant Training emphasizing practical skills to help the birthing woman and the primary caregiver. **Frmly:** (1981) Informed Homebirth.

**★ 16686 ★ Integral Health for Women (Salud Integral para la Mujer — SIPAM)**
Vista Hermosa 89
Col. Portales
C.P. 03300
Mexico City, DF, Mexico
**Phone:** 52 55 55398703    **Fax:** 52 55 55398703
**Email:** sipam@laneta.apc.org
**Fnded:** 1987. **Lang(s):** English, Spanish. **Desc:** Feminist and citizens' organization that contributes to the full and pleasant exercise of women's sexuality and the enjoyment of their sexual and reproductive health as axles for the personal, cultural, and political trans-

formation of Mexican society. Made up of women from various backgrounds and professional fields. Promotes the knowledge and exercise of women's sexual and reproductive rights. Makes conceptual and methodological proposals and influences public policies to create favorable conditions for the exercise of these rights. Contributes to strengthen organized civil society and the public projection of its proposals and promotes the citizens' participation of women and contributes to the construction of a democratic civil society with equality and respect for plurality and diversity from a gender perspective. Aims to achieve its objectives through communicative efforts and actions to influence the public opinion, research and systemization, education and training, and the design and development of proposals for public policies.

**★ 16687 ★ International Association for Maternal and Neonatal Health (IAMENEH)**
c/o Mrs. Gerda M. Santschi
Blavenstrasse 47
CH-4054 Basel, Switzerland
**Phone:** 41 61 3024548　　**Fax:** 41 61 3039508
**Email:** iamaneh_schweiz@compuserve.com
**Website:** http://www.medicusmundi.ch/iamaneh/francais/iamaneh.htm
**Fnded:** 1977. **Mem:** 4,500. **Nat'l Groups:** 39. **Lang(s):** English, French. **Desc:** Medical professionals and individuals interested in improving maternal and neonatal care throughout the world, especially at the primary health care level. Objectives are to: promote basic and applied research in the field of human reproduction and publish and distribute the findings; improve the standards of medical and paramedical care in the field of obstetrics and gynecology; foster research programs on social problems related to maternal and perinatal health; purpose curriculum on improving maternal and perinatal health to higher education institutions; disseminate scientific information concerning women, mothers, fetuses, newborns, and children. **Pub:** *High Risk Mothers and Newborns - Detection, Management and Prevention.* Book. • *Maternal and Child Care in Developing Countries - Assessment, Promotion and Implementation.* Book. • *Maternal and Infant Mortality.* Book. • *Primary Maternal and Neonatal Health - A Global Concern.* Book. **Frmly:** (1994) Mother and Child International.

**★ 16688 ★ International Association of Parents and Professionals for Safe Alternatives in Childbirth (NAPSAC)**
Rte. 4, Box 646
Marble Hill, MO 63764-9418
**Phone:** (573)238-2010　　**Fax:** (573)238-2010
**Email:** napsac@clas.net
**Website:** http://www.napsac.org
Lee Stewart, Pres.
**Fnded:** 1975. **Mem:** 1,000. **Nat'l Groups:** 20. **Local Groups:** 20. **Desc:** Parents, midwives, physicians, nurses, health officials, social workers, and childbirth educators in 10 countries who are "dedicated to exploring, examining, implementing, and establishing family-centered childbirth programs which meet the needs of families as well as provide the safe aspects of medical science." Promotes education concerning the principles of natural childbirth; facilitates communication and cooperation among parents, medical professionals, and childbirth educators; assists in the establishment of maternity and childbearing centers. Provides educational opportunities to parents and parents-to-be, enabling them to assume more personal responsibility for pregnancy, childbirth, infant care, and child rearing. **Pub:** *Childbirth Activitists Handbook.* Book. *Price:* $15.95. • *Emergency Childbirth. Price:* $12.95. • *Five Standards for Safe Childbearing.* • *NAPSAC Directory of Alternative Birth Services and Consumer Guide,* biennial. Directory. Lists midwives, birth centers, noninterventive physicians, and educators for safe alternatives in childbirth. *Price:* $7.95/copy. • *NAPSAC News,* quarterly. Newsletter. Includes association news, book reviews, and calendar of events. *Price:* Included in membership dues. • *Safe Alternatives in Childbirth. Price:* $9.95. • *Transitions.*

*Price:* $10.95. • *21st Century Obstetrics Now. Price:* $14.95/2 vol. **Frmly:** (1979) National Association of Parents and Professionals for Safe Alternatives in Childbirth.

**★ 16689 ★ International Cesarean Awareness Network (ICAN)**
PO Box 3894
Topeka, KS 66604-6894
**Phone:** (785)542-6400　　**Fax:** (785)542-5368
**Email:** info@ican-online.org
**Website:** http://www.ican-online.org
Connie Banack, Pres.
**Fnded:** 1982. **Mem:** 600. **Reg. Groups:** 15. **Desc:** Men and women and birth professionals concerned with the increasing rate of cesarean births. Objectives are: to oppose and lower through education the high cesarean rate currently prevalent and to offer encouragement, information and support to those women who wish to have a vaginal birth after previous cesarean(s) or VBAC. ICAN shall endeavor to share information about the prevention of unnecessary cesareans and to encourage vaginal birth; to encourage positive birthing assistance that is non-interventive in nature; to refer mothers desiring a VBAC to birth attndants who will assist them; to inform the public as to VBAC option; and to offer direct encouragement, counseling and support to women pursuing a VBAC. ICAN shall assist and encourage the establishment of local associations, committees, and support groups to further the purposes outlined above. Promote the sasfety of vaginal birth vs. cesarean section through printed and other media nationwide. Provide information on cesarean and VBAC issus via our website asnd through printed media. Active ICAN chapters throughout the US sand Internationally. **Pub:** *The Clarion,* quarterly. Newsletter. Includes research and informational articles, book reviews and chapter news. *Price:* Included in membership dues; One free copy for nonmembers. **Frmly:** (1992) Cesarean Prevention Movement.

**★ 16690 ★ International Childbirth Education Association (ICEA)**
PO Box 20048
Minneapolis, MN 55420-0048
**Phone:** (952)854-8660　　**Fax:** (952)854-8772
**Email:** info@icea.org
**Website:** http://www.icea.org/
Pat Turner RN, ICLE, ICD, Pres.
**Fnded:** 1960. **Mem:** 12,000. **Local Groups:** 275. **Desc:** Purposes are: to further the educational, physical, and emotional preparation of expectant parents for childbearing and breastfeeding; to increase public awareness on current issues related to childbearing; to cooperate with physicians, nurses, physical therapists, hospitals, health, education, and welfare agencies, and other individuals and groups interested in furthering parental participation and minimal obstetric intervention in uncomplicated labors; to promote development of safe, low-cost alternatives in childbirth that recognize the rights and responsibilities of those involved. Develops, publishes, and distributes literature pertaining to family-centered maternity care. Offers a teacher certifi cation program for childbirth educat ors. Conducts workshops. Operates mail order book store in Minneapolis, MN which makes available literature on all aspects of childbirth education and family-centered maternity care. **Pub:** *ICEA Bookmarks,* 4/year. • *International Journal of Childbirth Education,* 4/year. Journal. • *Membership Directory,* annual. • Also publishes pamphlets.

**★ 16691 ★ International Confederation of Midwives (ICM)**
**(Confederation Internationale des Sages-Femmes — CISF)**
Eisenhowerlaan 138
NL-2517 KN The Hague, Netherlands
**Phone:** 31 70 3060520　　**Fax:** 31 70 3555651
**Email:** intlmidwives@compuserve.com
**Fnded:** 1919. **Mem:** 82. **Reg. Groups:** 4. **Lang(s):** English, French, Spanish. **Desc:** National midwives'

associations in 66 countries. Seeks to improve the standard of care provided to mothers, babies, and the family by promoting midwifery education and disseminating information about the art and science of midwifery. **Pub:** *A Birthday for Midwives - Seventy Five Years of International Collaboration.* Book. • *International Code of Ethics for Midwives, 1993.* Book. • *International Midwifery Matters,* semiannual. Newsletter. • *Planning for Action for Midwives.*

**★ 16692 ★ International Correspondence Society of Obstetricians and Gynecologists (ICSOG)**
12693 Tamiami Tr. E, No. 213
Naples, FL 34113
**Fax:** (941)417-2780
**Email:** dmlassoc@mediaone.net
Dean M. Laux, Exec. Sec.
**Fnded:** 1960. **Mem:** 2,600. **Desc:** Physicians concerned with obstetrics and gynecology and related surgery; medical schools and libraries; civilian and military hospitals; others with research or clinical interests. **Pub:** *The Collected Letters,* monthly. Newsletter. *Price:* $119.

**★ 16693 ★ International Federation for Cervical Pathology and Colposcopy (IFCPC)**
**(Federacion Internacional de Patologia Cervical y Colposcopia)**
c/o Giuseppe De Palo, M.D.
Instituto Nazionale Tumori
Via Venezian, 1
I-20133 Milan, Italy
**Phone:** 39 2 2390324　　**Fax:** 39 2 2367430
**Email:** instituto@tuimori.mi.it
**Website:** http://www.ifcpc.org
**Fnded:** 1972. **Mem:** 34. **Nat'l Groups:** 34. **Lang(s):** English, French, German, Spanish. **Desc:** Federation of national societies encouraging basic and applied research and the dissemination of information concerning uterine cervical pathology and colposcopy. **Pub:** *IFCPC Newsletter,* 6 monthly. Newsletter.

**★ 16694 ★ International Federation of Gynecology and Obstetrics (FIGO)**
**(Federation Internationale de Gynecologie et d'Obstetrique — FIGO)**
70 Wimpole St.
London W1G 8AX, United Kingdom
**Phone:** 44 207 2243270　　**Fax:** 44 207 9350736
**Email:** figo@figo.org
**Website:** http://www.figo.org
**Fnded:** 1954. **Mem:** 100. **Lang(s):** English, French, Spanish. **Desc:** Objectives are to: promote and assist in the development of scientific and research work relating to all facets of gynecology and obstetrics; improve the physical and mental health of women, mothers, and their children; provide an exchange of information and ideas; improve teaching standards; promote international cooperation among medical bodies. Acts as liaison with World Health Organization and other international organizations. **Pub:** *Figo Annual Report on the Results of Treatment of Gynecologic Cancer,* annual. Annual Report. Provides results of treatment in gynecological cancer. • *Figo Newsletter,* 3/year. Newsletter. • *International Journal of Gynecology and Obstetrics,* monthly. Journal.

**International Federation of Infantile and Juvenile Gynecology (IFIJG)**
**(Federation Internationale de Gynecologie Infantile et Juvenile — FIGIJ)**
*See:* Entry 5694

**★ 16695 ★ International Menopause Society**
c/o Monique Boulet chez Maitre M. Steyaert
3/1 Av. des Cattleyas
B-1150 Brussels, Belgium

**Phone:** 32 2 7722183          **Fax:** 32 2 7624295
**Email:** imsociety@filink.net
**Website:** http://www.imsociety.org
**Fnded:** 1978. **Mem:** 800. **Nat'l Groups:** 30. **Lang(s):** English. **Desc:** Medical doctors, sociologists, psychologists, anthropologists, and others in 42 countries interested in basic research and clinical work in the field of menopause and climacteric. Objectives are to promote study of medical, sociological, and psychological aspects of the climacteric, or menopausal, stage in men and women and to advance international exchange of information and research plans. Studies subjects such as anatomy, gynecology, biochemistry, cardiology, etc. and psychology as they relate to the aging process; examines methods of management, preventive measures, and therapeutic problems related to aging. **Pub:** *Climacteric*, quarterly. Journal. • *Newsletter*, 4/year. Newsletter. • *Proceedings of World Congress*, triennial.


★ **16696** ★ **International SOC of Ultrasound in Obstetrics and Gynecology**
c/o Sarah Johnson
Academic Department of Obstetrics & Gynecology
Lanesborough Wing, 3rd Fl.
St. George's Hospital Medical School
Crammer Terr.
London SW17 0RE, United Kingdom
**Phone:** 44 20 87252505          **Fax:** 44 20 87250212
**Email:** johnson@sghms.ac.uk
**Website:**          http://obg.med.wayne.edu/ISUOG/home.htm
**Fnded:** 1991. **Mem:** 2,000. **Desc:** Healthcare practitioners in the field of ultrasound in obstetrics and gynecology. Fosters scientific and educational advancements in ultrasound technology in obstetrics and gynecology. Conducts training programs. **Pub:** *Ultrasound in Obstetrics and Gynecology*, monthly. Journal. • Newsletter, semiannual.


★ **16697** ★ **International Society for Gynecologic Endoscopy**
c/o ISGE Secretariat
Spaarne Hospital
PO Box 1644
2003 BR Haarlem, Netherlands
**Email:** isgeoff@euronet.nl
**Website:** http://isge.org
**Desc:** Aims to establish an international forum for the timely exchange of information and new ideas between gynecologic endoscopists of all nations.


★ **16698** ★ **La Leche League (LLL) (Ligue La Leche — LLL)**
12 rue Quintal
Charlemagne, QC, Canada J5Z 1V9
**Phone:** (514)990-8917          **Fax:** (450)582-3536
**Email:** information@allaitement.ca
**Website:** http://www.allaitement.ca
**Fnded:** 1960. **Mem:** 802. **Lang(s):** French. **Desc:** French-speaking Canadians with an interest in breast-feeding. Promotes breastfeeding as the most healthy method of nourishing infants. Provides support and services to women wishing to breastfeed. Conducts charitable programs. **Pub:** *La Voie Lactee*, bimonthly. Magazine.


★ **16699** ★ **Lamaze International**
2025 M St., NW, Ste. 800
Washington, DC 20036
**Phone:** (202)367-1128          **Free:** 800-368-4404
**Fax:** (202)367-2128
**Email:** lamaze@dc.sba.com
**Website:** http://www.lamaze-childbirth.com
Linda Harmon, Exec. Dir.
**Fnded:** 1960. **Mem:** 5,000. **Local Groups:** 25. **Desc:** Physicians, nurses, nurse-midwives, certified teachers of psychoprophylatic (Lamaze) method of childbirth, other professionals, parents, and others interested in Lamaze childbirth preparation and family-centered maternity care. Disseminates information about the theory and practical application of psychoprophylaxis in obstetrics; administers teacher training courses and certifies qualified Lamaze teachers; provides educational lectures, public forums, films, and written materials; maintains national and local teacher and physician referral service. Also presents materials to prospective parents concerning the demands of childrearing. National office serves as information clearinghouse. **Pub:** *Genesis*, quarterly. Newsletter. Contains book and film reviews and calendar of events. *Price:* Included in membership dues. • *Journal of Perinatal Education*, quarterly. Journal. *Price:* Free for members; $55 for individual; $155 for institution. **Frmly:** (1998) American Society for Psychoprophylaxis in Obstetrics.


**Legal Action for Women (LAW)**
*See:* Entry 12240


★ **16700** ★ **Maternity Alliance - England (MA)**
45 Beech St.
London EC2P 2LX, United Kingdom
**Phone:** 44 207 5588583          **Fax:** 44 207 5888584
**Email:** info@maternityalliance.org.uk
**Website:** http://www.maternityalliance.org
**Fnded:** 1980. **Mem:** 70. **Lang(s):** English. **Desc:** Individuals and organizations concerned with rights and services for parents and babies. Campaigns for improvements in rights and services for mothers, fathers, and babies. Concerns include: improvement in health care before conception and the first year of life; financial support for low income families; protection of working mothers' rights; and availability of transportation and housing. Conducts research programs. **Pub:** *Getting Fit for Pregnancy*. • *Maternity Action*, periodic. Bulletin. • *Money for Mothers and Babies*, periodic. • *Pregnant at Work 2000*, annual. • *Thinking About a Baby - A Man's Guide to Pre-Pregnancy Health*, periodic.


★ **16701** ★ **Maternity Center Association (MCA)**
281 Park Ave. S, 5th Fl.
New York, NY 10010
**Phone:** (212)777-5000          **Fax:** (212)777-9320
**Email:** info@maternitywise.org
**Website:** http://www.maternity.org
Maureen Corry, Exec. Dir.
**Fnded:** 1918. **Desc:** Laypersons, physicians, nurses, nurse-midwives, childbirth educators, and public health workers interested in improvement of maternity care, maternal and infant health, and family life. A national nonprofit health organization for over 800 years, MCA's goals are to expand access to family-centered maternity care through collaborative practice, education, publications, consultation services, public policy initiatives and demonstration programs. Sponsors research; administers nurse-midwifery student assistance fund. Co-sponsors community-based Nurse-Midwifery Education Program. **Pub:** *Birth Atlas*. Book. Instructional Aide. • *Growing Uterus Chart Series*. • *Journey to Parenthood*. Booklets. • *Publications Catalog*, annual. Catalog. *Price:* Free. • Books. • Pamphlets. • Videos. • Also publishes teaching aids for health professionals, charts, and slides.


★ **16702** ★ **Maternity Coalition**
PO Box 73
Brunswick South, VIC 3055, Australia
**Phone:** 61 3 93802863          **Fax:** 61 3 93811362
**Website:** http://www.maternitycoalition.org.au
**Fnded:** 1989. **Mem:** 250. **State Groups:** 3. **Lang(s):** English. **Desc:** Midwives, educators and researchers in the area of childbirth and women's health, mothers and other interested individuals. Acts as an umbrella organization to bring together support groups and individuals for effective lobbying, information sharing, networking and support in maternity services. Works for the rights of mothers and seeks to improve maternity care for women during pregnancy, birth and beyond. Provides consumer information on choices for childbirth. **Pub:** *Birth Matters*, quarterly. Journal.


★ **16703** ★ **Menopauze: Clinic**
University Hospital Gasthuisberg
Department of Obstetrics and Gynecology
Herestraat 49
B-3000 Louvain, Belgium
**Phone:** 32 16 344202          **Fax:** 32 16 344238
**Fnded:** 1968. **Mem:** 8. **Lang(s):** Dutch, English, French. **Desc:** Promotes the study of menopause. Supports theories of psychosomatic menopause. Conducts clinical training and teaching programs in psychosomatic gynecology. Offers marriage and family therapy sessions. Conducts sexological research.


★ **16704** ★ **Midwest Parentcraft Center (MPC)**
5525 W Henderson
Chicago, IL 60641
**Phone:** (773)725-7767
Margaret Gamper, R.N., Exec. Dir.
**Fnded:** 1950. **Desc:** Prenatal instructors, parents, and professionals involved in parenting and pregnancy. To instruct and educate expectant mothers and others in the Gamper Method of childbirth. (The Gamper Method, based on the teachings of several 19th century physicians and developed by Margaret Gamper in 1946, is designed to prepare the prospective mother for childbirth by instilling self-determination and confidence in her ability to work with the physiological changes of her body during pregnancy, labor, and delivery.) Conducts prenatal and grandparenting classes and workshops; operates in-service programs for hospitals and clinics; sponsors programs on topics such as grieving and history of birth procedures. Disseminates teaching aids including slides, films, records, and tapes. Grants childbirth educator certificates to qualified applicants who have taught Gamper Method classes under the supervision of an instructor. Operates charitable program and speakers' bureau; maintains library of 6000 volumes on childbirth, midwifery, marriage, sex, and childcare. The center's activities are currently concentrated in Ohio, Illinois, Indiana, Wisconsin, and Michigan. **Pub:** *Heir Raising News*, quarterly. • *Preparation for the Heir Minded*.


★ **16705** ★ **Midwives Alliance of North America (MANA)**
4805 Lawrenceville Hwy., No. 116-279
Lilburn, GA 30047
**Free:** 888-923-6262          **Fax:** (801)720-3026
**Email:** info@mana.org
**Website:** http://www.mana.org
Diane Holzer, Pres.
**Fnded:** 1982. **Mem:** 1,000. **Reg. Groups:** 10. **Desc:** Midwives, student/apprentice midwives, and persons supportive of midwifery. Seeks to expand communication and support among midwives. Works to promote basic competency in midwives; develops and encourages guidelines for their education. Offers legal, legislative, and political information and resource referrals; conducts networking on local, state, and regional bases; compiles statistics. **Pub:** *MANA News*, bimonthly. • Brochures. • Also publishes information packets.


★ **16706** ★ **Midwives Information and Resource Services (MIDIRS)**
9 Elmdale Rd.
Clifton
Bristol BS8 1SL, United Kingdom
**Phone:** 44 117 9251791          **Fax:** 44 117 9251792
**Website:** http://www.midirs.org
**Fnded:** 1983. **Mem:** 14,000. **Lang(s):** English. **Desc:** Provides information for midwives and nurses who want to keep up-to-date with contemporary knowledge and thinking in the world of midwifery care, women's health, and care of new borns. Offers articles, books, and other information concerning midwifery. Conducts educational programs. **Pub:** *Directory of Maternity Organisations*, periodic. Directory. • *MIDIRS Midwifery Digest*, quarterly.

**Miscarriage Association**
*See:* Entry 18334

**★ 16707 ★ Museum of Menstruation**
　　**(MUM)**
PO Box 2398
Landover Hills Branch
Hyattsville, MD 20784-2398
**Phone:** (301)459-4450　　　**Fax:** (301)577-2913
**Email:** hfinley@mum.org
**Website:** http://www.mum.org
Harry Finley, Founder & Dir.

**Fnded:** 1994. **Mem:** 310. **Desc:** Seeks to educate the public on the cultural history of menstruation. Conducts research and statistical studies. Offers assistance to individuals conducting patent and advertising research, and scholarly work, musuem displays of advertising history and menstrual devices.

**★ 16708 ★ National Association of**
　　**Childbearing Centers (NACC)**
3123 Gottschall Rd.
Perkiomenville, PA 18074
**Phone:** (215)234-8068　　　**Fax:** (215)234-8829
**Email:** reachnacc@birthcenters.org
**Website:** http://www.birthcenters.org
Kate Bauer, Exec. Dir.

**Fnded:** 1983. **Mem:** 600. **Reg. Groups:** 6. **State Groups:** 2. **Desc:** Working on public and policy levels in government, industry and the health professions, NACC is dedicated to developing quality, holistic services for childbearing families that promote self-reliance and confidence in birth and parenting. Collects and disseminates information on birth centers. Sets national standards for birth center operation, promotes state regulation for licensure, and national accreditation by the Commission for the Accreditation of Birth Centers. Provides a Parent Information Service for consumers looking for birth centers. Provides information on birth center. **Pub:** *Birth Center Information Packet.* Articles. Covers growth and development, regulation, costs, reimbursement, research, and selected issues of NACC News. *Price:* $30. • *Continuous Quality Improvement Manual.* Manual. Contains forms and instructions for implementing a continuous quality improvement/risk management program in birth centers. *Price:* $100 for members; $150 for nonmembers. • *Marketing the Birth Center.* • *NACC Fact Folder.* Designed to communicate the birth center concept. Includes information on the proven quality, improved access and reduced cost of birth centers. *Price:* $4 members; $4.50 nonmembers. • *NACC Membership Directory,* annual. Membership Directory. *Price:* Included in membership dues. • *NACC News,* quarterly. • *NACC Uniform Data Set. Price:* $299 members; $599 nonmembers. • *National Birth Center Study.* Reprint. *Price:* $1. • *Sample Birth Center Policy and Procedure Manual.* Manual. Contains sample policies and procedures of an accredited birth center. Includes diskettes for customization. *Price:* $200 members; $300 nonmembers. • *Standards for Birth Centers. Price:* $15 for members; $30 for non-members. • *Survey Report of Birth Center Experience. Price:* $10 members; $20 nonmembers. • *"The Birth Center" Brochure.* Brochure. Contains information describing freestanding birth centers. Designed for public education and promotion of the concept of birth centers. *Price:* $49/100 brochures. • *"The Birth Center" Video.* Video. Designed to increase public awareness of the presence of birth centers. *Price:* $39.95.

**National Association of Neonatal Nurses**
　　**(NANN)**
*See:* Entry 15731

**★ 16709 ★ National Association for**
　　**Premenstrual Syndrome**
7 Swifts Ct.
High St.
Seal
Sevenoaks TN15 0EG, United Kingdom
**Phone:** 44 1732 760011　　**Fax:** 44 1732 760011

**Email:** contact@pms.org.uk
**Website:** http://www.pms.org.uk
**Fnded:** 1983. **Mem:** 1,000. **Reg. Groups:** 8. **Desc:** Provides help, information and support to PMS sufferers and their families; promotes a better understanding of PMS and its treatment by the medical profession. **Pub:** *NAPS News,* monthly. Newsletter.

**National Certification Corp. for the**
　　**Obstetric, Gynecologic and Neonatal**
　　**Nursing Specialties (NCC)**
*See:* Entry 15746

**★ 16710 ★ National Coalition of Abortion**
　　**Providers (NCAP)**
c/o Ron Fitzsimmons
206 King St.
Alexandria, VA 22314
**Phone:** (703)684-0055　　**Fax:** (703)684-5051
**Email:** ron@ncap.com
**Website:** http://www.ncap.com
Ron Fitzsimmons, Exec. Dir.

**Desc:** Abortion providers.

**★ 16711 ★ National Council on Women's**
　　**Health**
1300 York Ave.
PO Box 52
New York, NY 10021
**Phone:** (212)746-6967　　**Fax:** (212)746-8691
**Email:** sdb2002@mail.med.cornell.edu
**Website:** http://www.ncwh.org
Roberta G. Rubin, MD, Pres.

**Fnded:** 1979. **Mem:** 500. **Desc:** Working partnership of health professionals and consumers whose mission is to educate the public and policy-makers on women's health issues and empower women to make informed healthcare choices. Open to everyone concerned with furthering the goals of the Council, fostering better quality health care, increased availability of information to patients, and improving doctor-patient relationship. The goals of the organization are accomplished through a variety of educational efforts including forums and conferences for the general public, publications for professionals and the public, and networking with a wide range of organizations concerned with women's health. **Pub:** Newsletter, quarterly.

**★ 16712 ★ National Endometriosis**
　　**Society**
Ste. 50
Westminster Place Gardens
1-7 Artillery Row
London SW1P 1RL, United Kingdom
**Phone:** 44 207 222 2781　**Fax:** 44 207 222 2786
**Email:** endoinfo@compuserve.com
**Website:** http://www.endo.org.uk
**Fnded:** 1982. **Mem:** 3,500. **Reg. Groups:** 60. **Lang(s):** English. **Desc:** Women with personal experience of endometriosis and clinicians. Funds research into endometriosis and raises public awareness of it among medical professionals and the public. **Pub:** *Endolink,* quarterly. Newsletter.

**National Healthy Mothers, Healthy Babies**
　　**Coalition**
*See:* Entry 5727

**★ 16713 ★ National Perinatal Association**
　　**(NPA)**
3500 E Fletcher Ave., Ste. 205
Tampa, FL 33613
**Phone:** (813)971-1008　　　**Free:** 888-971-3295
**Fax:** (813)971-9306
**Email:** npa@nationalperinatal.org
**Website:** http://www.nationalperinatal.org
Shelia S. Sorkin, Exec. Dir.

**Fnded:** 1976. **Mem:** 1,500. **Nat'l Groups:** 20. **Reg. Groups:** 1. **State Groups:** 27. **Desc:** Organizations and individuals interested in perinatal health care.

Purpose is to promote improved patient care, education, research, advocacy and delivery systems for perinatal health. **Pub:** *Journal of Perinatology,* bimonthly. Journal. Examines all facets of perinatology/neonatology from a variety of perspectives. *Price:* Included in membership dues; $40/year for nonmembers. • *National Perinatal Association Bulletin,* quarterly. Newsletter. Includes article reviews and legislative news. *Price:* Included in membership dues. • Proceedings.

**★ 16714 ★ National Women's Health**
　　**Resource Center (NWHRC)**
120 Albany St., Ste. 820
New Brunswick, NJ 08901
**Free:** 877-986-9472　　　**Fax:** (732)249-4671
**Email:** info@healthywomen.org
**Website:** http://www.healthywomen.org/
Amy R. Niles, Exec. Dir.

**Fnded:** 1988. **Desc:** Disseminates information about women's health. Serves as the national clearinghouse for women's health information. Provides comprehensive, unbiased health information. **Pub:** *National Women's Health Report,* bimonthly. Newsletter. Information on current women's health issues. *Price:* $25 for individuals; $75 for organizations and institutions.

**★ 16715 ★ New Zealand College of**
　　**Midwives**
PO Box 21-106
217 Bealey Ave.
Christchurch, New Zealand
**Phone:** 64 3 3772732　　　**Fax:** 64 3 3775662
**Email:** nzcom@clear.net.nz
**Website:** http://www.midwife.org.nz
**Fnded:** 1990. **Mem:** 2,000. **Reg. Groups:** 10. **Lang(s):** English. **Desc:** Midwives, consumer groups, and interested individuals. Promotes midwifery services and education, and represents the interests of midwives to governmental bodies and the public. Prescribes and monitors standards for the practice and education of midwifery. Acts as a consultant for governmental agencies; engages in the negotiation of government funding for community and independent midwifery services. Offers courses jointly with colleges and universities. **Pub:** *New Zealand College of Midwives,* semiannual. Journal. Contains articles on midwifery. • *New Zealand College of Midwives National Newsletter,* quarterly. Newsletter.

**★ 16716 ★ New Zealand Endometriosis**
　　**Foundation**
PO Box 1683
Palmerston North, New Zealand
**Phone:** 64 6 3592613　　　**Fax:** 64 6 3592613
**Email:** nzendo@xtra.co.nz
**Website:** http://www.nzendo.co.nz
**Fnded:** 1986. **Mem:** 500. **Local Groups:** 16. **Lang(s):** English. **Desc:** Offers education, information and support for girls and women with endometriosis and others interested in the disease. The Foundation fosters research and works with gynecologists and other health professionals in New Zealand and around the world. **Pub:** Newsletter, quarterly.

**★ 16717 ★ Nordic Federation of**
　　**Societies of Obstetrics and Gynecology**
　　**(Nordisk Forening for Obstetrik och**
　　**Gynekologi)**
Department of OB & GYN
Karolinska Hospital
S-171 76 Stockholm, Sweden
**Email:** viveca.odlind@ks.se
**Website:** http://www.nfog.org

**Fnded:** 1933. **Mem:** 4,000. **Nat'l Groups:** 5. **Lang(s):** Swedish. **Desc:** Gynecologists and obstetricians from five Nordic countries. Conducts education programs; sponsors competitions and holds Nordic Congress for Obstetricians and Gynecologists every other year. **Pub:** *Acta Obstetrica Gynecologica Scandinavica,* 10/year. Journal. Includes supplements. • *Bulletin,* quarterly. Newsletter. **Frmly:** Scandinavian Association of

Obstetrics and Gynecology; (1999) Federation of Scandinavian Societies of Obstetrics and Gynecology.

### ★ 16718 ★ North American Menopause Society (NAMS)

PO Box 94527
Cleveland, OH 44101
**Phone:** (440)442-7550     **Fax:** (440)442-2660
**Email:** info@menopause.org
**Website:** http://www.menopause.org
Wulf H. Utian, MD,PhD, Exec. Dir.

**Fnded:** 1989. **Mem:** 2,500. **Desc:** Physicians, scientists, research and clinical personnel, and other health care professionals are active members; student or physicians serving residencies or fellowships are associate members. Promotes understanding of menopause in women. Advances the exchange of research plans and experience between members. Offers educational programs. **Pub:** *Flashes*, 3/year. Newsletter. • *Menopause Management*, bimonthly. A review publication. • *Menopause: The Journal of the North American Menopause Society*, bimonthly. Journal.

### ★ 16719 ★ Obstetrical and Gynaecological Society of Hong Kong

Duke of Windsor Social Service Bldg., 4/F
15 Hennessy Rd.
Hong Kong, People's Republic of China
**Phone:** 852 25278898     **Fax:** 852 28650345
**Website:** http://www.medicine.org.hk/ogshk/home.htm

**Fnded:** 1961. **Mem:** 330. **Lang(s):** Chinese, English. **Desc:** Obstetricians and gynecologists; medical students with an interest in the field. Seeks to advance the study and practice of obstetrics and gynecology. Conducts continuing professional development courses for members. **Pub:** *Hong Kong Journal of Gynecology, Obstetrics & Midwifery*, periodic. Journal.

### ★ 16720 ★ Organisation Gestosis - Society for the Study of Pathophysiology of Pregnancy (OG) (Geburtshilfe und Gynakologie FMH)

Geburtshilfe und Gynakologie FMH
Gerbergasse 14
CH-4051 Basel, Switzerland
**Phone:** 41 61 2615555     **Fax:** 41 61 2615934

**Fnded:** 1969. **Mem:** 4,500. **Reg. Groups:** 11. **Lang(s):** English, German. **Desc:** Obstetricians, gynecologists, neonatologists, nephrologists, epidemiologists, pathologists, geneticists, immunologists, physiologists, and health officials in 75 countries in the field of EPH-Gestosis. EPH-Gestosis is a term adopted by the society to describe a malady that may occur during pregnancy wherein a woman exhibits excessive accumulation of body water, protein in the urine, and/or abnormal elevation of blood pressure; EPH is derived from the terms for 3 conditions: edema, proteinuria, and hypertension; gestosis is derived from the word gestation and the suffix -osis which means disturbance. The condition is prevalent in socioeconomically depressed areas where poor hygiene and malnutrition aggravate the effects of inadeq uate prenatal care. The society reports that EPH-Gestosis occurs in 10% of world population births, is responsible for as much as 50% of perinatal/fetal death, and is the cause of up to 33% of maternal mortality. Objectives are to: disseminate information to medical and lay personnel and the public; foster research, preventive health care, and therapy; internationalize nomenclature, classification, and definitions in the field of EPH-Gestosis for diagnosis, therapy, and comparative techniques; standardize methods of investigation; serve as documentation center; foster exchange of scientists. Conducts discussion groups and study groups on topics such as edema, proteinuria, cytology, serumprotein, and hypertension. Suggests alterations of definitions of EPH-Gestosis as offered by International Classification of Diseases of the World Health Organization. Makes recommendations for the most modern and successful measures of prevention and treatment of EPH-Gestosis. Collects and publishes papers submitted by researchers worldwide. Sponsors symposia and workshops; conducts surveys. worldwide. Sponsors symposia and workshops; conducts surveys. **Pub:** *Instruction Bulletin*, periodic. Bulletin. • *International Journal of Feto-Maternal Medicine*, periodic. Journal. • *OG News*, periodic. • Proceedings.

### ★ 16721 ★ Perinatal Society of New Zealand (PSNZ)

c/o Christ Church Women's Hospital
Department of Obstetrics and Gynecology
Private Bag 4711
Christchurch, New Zealand
**Phone:** 64 3 3644630     **Fax:** 64 3 3644634

**Fnded:** 1979. **Mem:** 120. **Local Groups:** 12. **Lang(s):** English. **Desc:** Pediatricians, obstetricians, neo-natal and obstetric nurses, scientists, dietitians, radiologists, physiotherapists and other paediatric specialists and midwives in New Zealand. Aims to foster continued improvement in the standards of perinatal medicine and nursing. Works to increase public understanding of the activities in and the objectives of perinatology. Sponsors continuing education programs in perinatology. Promotes collaboration and open discussion among members. **Frmly:** (1990) New Zealand Perinatal Society.

### ★ 16722 ★ Polycystic Ovarian Syndrome Association

PO Box 80517
Portland, OR 97280
**Phone:** (303)814-0297     **Free:** 877-775-PCOS
**Fax:** (413)751-4866
**Email:** info@pcosupport.org
**Website:** http://www.pcosupport.org
Kristin Rencher, Exec. Dir.

**Fnded:** 1997. **Mem:** 2,500. **Nat'l Groups:** 1. **Local Groups:** 12. **Desc:** Chapters worldwide provide support, education and advocacy for women suffering from polycystic ovary syndrome (PCOS). Host educational events combining lectures with support sessions. Advocate for women with PCOS in the media and medical community by attending and speaking at professional meetings as well as hosting exhibit booths. **Pub:** *PCOS Bulletin*, quarterly. Newsletter. • *PCOS Record*, monthly. Newsletter.

### ★ 16723 ★ Postpartum Adjustment Services - Canada (PASS-CAN)

Unit 3 460 Woody Rd.
PO Box 7282, Sta. Main
Oakville, ON, Canada L6K 3T6
**Phone:** (905)844-9009     **Free:** 800-897-6660
**Fax:** (905)844-5973
**Email:** info@passcan.ca
**Website:** http://www.passcan.ca

**Fnded:** 1972. **Mem:** 500. **Lang(s):** English, French. **Desc:** Health care and mental health professionals; parents of preschool children. Seeks to "ease the transition to parenthood for families of infants or preschoolers" and to "reduce the stigma of postpartum depression or anxiety." Serves as the national clearinghouse on postpartum depression. Conducts advocacy, networking, and educational activities; maintains discussion and support groups for mothers experiencing postpartum anxiety or depression. Participates in charitable activities; maintains speakers' bureau. **Pub:** *ComPass*, periodic. Newsletter. • *Passwords*, periodic. Newsletter. • *Ups and Downs - A New Mother's Guide*. Booklet.

### Pre-Eclamptic Toxaemia Society

*See:* Entry 18360

### ★ 16724 ★ Pregnancy Counseling Services

PO Box 669
Cambridge, New Zealand
**Phone:** 64 7 8274482     **Fax:** 64 7 8274495
**Email:** royrodgers@tra.co.nz
**Website:** http://www.dawnjames.clara.net

**Fnded:** 1980. **Mem:** 300. **Local Groups:** 22. **Lang(s):** English. **Desc:** Provides counseling and support to pregnant women in New Zealand. Works to ensure maternal and child health; conducts educational programs. Offers post abortion counseling. **Pub:** *Diary Notes*, semiannual. Provides information to supporters and pro life groups. • Annual Report.

### ★ 16725 ★ Professional Midwives Association of Germany (Bund Freiberuflicher Hebammen Deutschlands eV)

Am Alten Nordkanal 10
D-41748 Viersen, Germany
**Phone:** 49 2162 352149     **Fax:** 49 2162 358592
**Email:** geschaeftsstelle@bfhd.de
**Website:** http://www.bfhd.de

**Fnded:** 1984. **Mem:** 800. **Reg. Groups:** 12. **Lang(s):** English, Spanish. **Desc:** Midwives in Germany. Represents the interests of midwives. Informs and contributes to the health education of the population. Promotes continuing education for midwives in the interests of mother and child. **Pub:** *Hebammen Info*, semimonthly. Newsletter. Contains articles about midwifery.

### ★ 16726 ★ Read Natural Childbirth Foundation (RNCF)

PO Box 150956
San Rafael, CA 94915-0956
Margaret B. Farley, P. T. Pres.

**Fnded:** 1978. **Mem:** 30. **State Groups:** 3. **Desc:** Doctors, nurses, childbirth instructors, and parents. Promotes and teaches expectant parents the philosophies of natural childbirth pioneered by Grantly Dick-Read, a British doctor who began writing in 1932 about the then extremely controversial concept of natural childbirth and advocated relaxation as the key to comfortable labor. Techniques include abdominal and rib cage breathing and alleviation of fear, and thus pain, through knowledge. Acts as resource agency for the International Childbirth Education Association. Conducts charitable programs. Offers speakers' bureau. **Pub:** *A Time to Be Born*. Video. • *Preparation for Childbirth: Handbook for Use in Exercise Classes for Expectant Parents*. Handbook.

### ★ 16727 ★ Royal College of Midwives

15 Mansfield St.
London W1G 9NH, United Kingdom
**Phone:** 44 20 73123535     **Fax:** 44 20 73123536
**Email:** info@rcm.org.uk

**Fnded:** 1881. **Mem:** 36,000. **Nat'l Groups:** 4. **Local Groups:** 230. **Lang(s):** English. **Desc:** Promotes the practice of midwifery, and works to maintain high standards in the field. Provides educational programs to midwives in the areas of maternity, child care, and personal development. Represents worker rights of midwives to national legal and political authorities. Encourages and supports research. **Pub:** *Midwives*. Magazine. • *RCM Midwives Journal*, monthly. Journal.

### ★ 16728 ★ Society for Gynecologic Investigation (SGI)

409 12th St. SW
Washington, DC 20024-2188
**Phone:** (202)863-2544     **Fax:** (202)863-0739
**Email:** sgiava@aol.com
**Website:** http://www.socgyninv.org
Ava A. Tayman, Exec. Dir.

**Fnded:** 1953. **Mem:** 963. **Desc:** Present and former faculty members of institutions interested or engaged in fundamental gynecologic research. Purpose is to stimulate, encourage, assist, and conduct gynecologic research. **Pub:** *Journal of the Society for Gynecologic Investigation*, bimonthly. Journal. Published by Elsevier Sciences.

### Society of Gynecologic Oncologists (SGO)

*See:* Entry 10251

**★ 16729 ★ Society for Maternal Fetal Medicine (SMFM)**
409 12th St. SW
Washington, DC 20024-2188
**Phone:** (202)863-2476 **Fax:** (202)554-1132
**Email:** info@smfm.org
**Website:** http://www.smfm.org
Pat Stahr, Exec. Dir.
**Fnded:** 1977. **Mem:** 1,900. **Desc:** Obstetricians specializing in maternal-fetal medicine. Works to improve perinatal care through promotion and expansion of education in obstetrical perinatology. Provides a forum for exchange between members. **Pub:** *American Journal of Obstetrics and Gynecology*, periodic. Journal. **Frmly:** (1999) Society of Perinatal Obstetricians.

**★ 16730 ★ Society for Menstrual Cycle Research (SMCR)**
10559 N 104th Pl.
Scottsdale, AZ 85258
**Phone:** (480)451-9731 **Fax:** (480)451-9731
**Email:** maryannafriederich@msn.com
**Website:** http://www.pop.psu.edu/smcr
Mary Anna Friederich, MD, Sec. -Treas.
**Fnded:** 1979. **Mem:** 100. **Desc:** Physicians, nurses, endocrinologists, geneticists, physiologists, psychologists, sociologists, researchers, educators, students, and others interested in the health needs of women as related to the menstrual cycle. Goals are: to identify research priorities, recommend research strategies, and promote interdisciplinary research on the menstrual cycle; to establish a communication network for facilitating interdisciplinary dialogue on menstrual cycle events; to disseminate information and promote discussion of issues among public groups. **Pub:** *Changing Perspectives on Menopause.* Book. • *Culture, Society and Menstruation.* Book. • *Membership Roster*, annual. Membership Directory. • *Menarche: The Transition from Girl to Woman.* Book. • *The Menstrual Cycle, Volume 1: A Synthesis of Interdisciplinary Research.* • *The Menstrual Cycle, Volume 2: Research and Implications for Women's Health.* • *Menstrual Health in Women's Lives.* • *Menstruation, Health, and Illness.* • *Mind-Body Rhythmicity, A Menstrual Cycle Prospective.* Book. • *Proceedings 8th Conference Society for Menstrual Cycle Research.* Proceedings. • Newsletter, quarterly.

**★ 16731 ★ Society for Obstetric Anesthesia and Perinatology (SOAP)**
1910 Byrd Ave., Ste. 100
PO Box 11086
Richmond, VA 23230-1086
**Phone:** (804)282-5051 **Fax:** (804)282-0090
**Email:** soap@societyhq.com
**Website:** http://www.soap.org
Joy L. Hawkins, MD, Pres.
**Fnded:** 1969. **Mem:** 1,000. **Desc:** Physicians and scientists interested in perinatal health care. Purpose is to improve the health care of pregnant women and their unborn children. Conducts specialized education programs; compiles statistics. **Pub:** *Society for Obstetric Anesthesia and Perinatology Newsletter*, quarterly. Newsletter. **Price:** Included in membership dues.

**Society for Prevention of Infertility (SPI)**
*See:* Entry 18377

**★ 16732 ★ Vulval Pain Society**
PO Box 514
Slough SL1 2BP, United Kingdom
**Email:** frbaby@msn.com
**Website:** http://www.vul-pain.dircon.co.uk
**Fnded:** 1996. **Mem:** 500. **Local Groups:** 2. **Desc:** Provides information and support to women who suffer from Vulval pain and discomfort.

**★ 16733 ★ Vulvar Pain Foundation**
PO Drawer 177
Graham, NC 27253
**Phone:** (336)226-0704 **Fax:** (336)226-8518
**Website:** http://www.vulvarpainfoundation.org
Joanne J. Yount, Exec. Dir.
**Fnded:** 1992. **Mem:** 7,000. **Reg. Groups:** 17. **Desc:** Women who have vulvar pain and related disorders (fibromyalgia, interstitial cystitis, irritable bowel), family members, and interested health care professionals. Educates patients, physicians, and the public about successful treatment and current research. Identifies interested health care professionals, promotes scientific research, coordinates support networks and groups. **Pub:** *The Low Oxalate Cookbook.* Book. Contains dietary guidelines, recipes, and other related information. *Price:* $30. • *VPF.* Brochure. Describes the purposes, activities, and membership benefits of the foundation. *Price:* Free. • *The Vulvar Pain Newsletter.* Newsletter. **AKA:** The VP Foundation.

**★ 16734 ★ Woman to Woman Support Network**
Airport Plz., Unit 5
1341 W Main Rd.
Middletown, RI 02842
**Phone:** (401)841-9211
**Email:** jmartellino@home.com
**Website:** http://www.thombs.com/woman2woman/
**Desc:** Provides free support and referals to women experiencing a problem pregnancy.

**Women's Health**
*See:* Entry 2439

**Y-ME National Breast Cancer Organization (Y-ME)**
*See:* Entry 10262

# Research Centers

**★ 16735 ★ Baylor College of Medicine Maternal Fetal Medicine**
Smith Plz., Ste. 901
6550 Fannin
Houston, TX 77030
**Phone:** (713)798-7593 **Fax:** (713)798-6956
**Email:** ymeone@aol.com
**Website:** http://www.y-me.org
Dr. Isabelle Wilkins, Dir.
**Activities/Fields:** Prenatal diagnosis by ultrasonography, amniocentesis, and fetal blood sampling, chorionic villi sampling, longitudinal fetal growth, and pre/post-conceptual counseling. Conducts evaluation of intrauterine growth retardation in at-risk patients on prospective basis. **Pub:** *Annual Report of Department of Obstetrics/Gynecology.* **Frmly:** Prenatal Diagnostic Center.

**★ 16736 ★ Center for Study of Multiple Birth**
333 E Superior St., Ste. 464
Chicago, IL 60611
**Phone:** (312)908-7532 **Fax:** (312)908-8500
**Email:** lgk395@nwu.edu
**Website:** http://www.multiplebirth.com
Louis Keith, Contact
**Activities/Fields:** Multiple birth, twin gestation, twin pregnancy diagnosis, and twin care. Research is aimed at decreasing the high infant mortality rate involved in multiple births.

**★ 16737 ★ Institute for the Study and Treatment of Endometriosis**
2425 W 22nd St., Ste. 102
Oak Brook, IL 60523
**Phone:** (630)954-0054 **Fax:** (630)954-0064
**Email:** wpdmowski@oakbrookfertility.com
**Website:** http://www.endometriosisinstitute.com
W. Paul Dmowski, MD, Dir.
**Activities/Fields:** Elucidation of pathophysiology of endometriosis, identification of new diagnostic tests and development of new treatment methods.

**Jeanette Kennelly Kroch Center for Twin Studies**
*See:* Entry 9404

**★ 16738 ★ Joint Division of Newborn Medicine**
Medical Center
600 S 42nd St.
Omaha, NE 68198-1205
**Phone:** (402)559-6750 **Fax:** (402)559-7341
**Email:** pleusche@unmc.edu
Pat Leuschen, Res. Dir.
**Activities/Fields:** Cell and molecular basis of cerebral ischemia, ontogency of C3 complement in human lung, and physiologic and pharmacodynamic evaluation of infants on ECMO therapy. Conducts clinical trials of two types of high frequency ventilation. Participating in clinical trials of Infasurf, a fetal calf surfactant. **Frmly:** Neonatology Research Laboratory.

**★ 16739 ★ Lawson Health Research Institute**
St. Joseph's Healthe Centre
University of Western Ontario
268 Grosvenor St.
London, ON, Canada N6A 4V2
**Phone:** (519)646-6100 **Fax:** (519)646-6110
**Email:** dhill@lri.sjhc.london.on.ca
**Website:** http://www.lhrionhealth.ca
Dr. David J. Hill, Sci. Dir.,VP,Res.
**Activities/Fields:** Maternal and newborn health issues, including prematurity and low birth weight; imaging, particularly the improvement of medical diagnosis through use of imaging techniques and understanding the effects of magnetic fields; molecular medicine, especially regarding diabetes and lung biology; musculoskeletal system, including muscles, joints, and wounds; rehabilitation and geriatrics, especially unique approaches to all aspects of management of spinal cord injury and physical mental health of the elderlu; urology; and gastroenterology, vascular biology, transplant, neuroscience, advanced surgical techniques, mental health. **Pub:** *Probe Newsletter*, bimonthly. Newsletter. **Frmly:** Lawson Research Institute.

**Melpomene Institute for Women's Health Research**
*See:* Entry 19186

**New England Medical Center Hospitals, Inc.**
**Gynecologic Oncology Group (GOG)**
*See:* Entry 10384

**Northwestern University**
**John I. Brewer Trophoblastic Disease Center**
*See:* Entry 10390

**★ 16740 ★ University of Alabama at Birmingham**
**Ob/Gyn Infectious Disease Research Laboratory**
Department of Ob/Gyn
619 19th St. S
Birmingham, AL 35249-7333
**Phone:** (205)934-5271 **Fax:** (205)975-4375
**Email:** bandrews@uab.campus.mci.net
**Website:** http://www.nemc.org
Dr. William W. Andrews, Dir.
**Activities/Fields:** Infectious etiologies of preterm labor, premature rupture of membranes, markers for preterm birth, new antimicrobial therapies for postpartum endometritis, the relationship between maternal

infection and subsequent neonatal sepsis, and sexually transmitted diseases.

**★ 16741 ★ University of Chicago**
**Perinatal Center**
MC 2001
5841 S Maryland Ave.
Chicago, IL 60637
**Phone:** (773)702-3733     **Fax:** (773)702-1085
**Email:** amoawad@babies.bsd.uchicago.edu
Atef H. Moawad, MD, Co-Dir.
**Activities/Fields:** Fetal-maternal medicine, neonatology, and morbidity and mortality within perinatal medicine.

**★ 16742 ★ University of Montreal**
**Sainte-Justine Hospital Research Centre**
3175 Chemin de la Cote-Sainte-Catherine
Montreal, QC, Canada H3T 1C5
**Phone:** (514)345-4691     **Fax:** (514)345-4698
**Email:** levye@justine.umontreal.ca
Emile Levy, Dir.
**Activities/Fields:** Basic and clinical research in the field of diseases of the mother and child, including cardiology and pulmonary medicine, endocrinology, gastroenterology, nutrition, orthopedics, and epidemiology. Studies also include hematology-oncology, immunology, microbiology, virology, medical genetics, nephrology, and obstetrics. **Pub:** *Annual Report.*

**★ 16743 ★ University of Saskatchewan**
**Reproductive Biology Research Unit**
Royal University Hospital
Department of Obstetrics & Gynecology
College of Medicine
103 Hospital Dr.
Saskatoon, SK, Canada S7N 0W8
**Phone:** (306)966-8033     **Fax:** (306)966-8040
**Email:** pierson@erato.usask.ca
Dr. Roger A. Pierson, Dir.
**Activities/Fields:** Mammalian reproduction, emphasizing human reproductive biology, fertility, infertility, contraception, and embryo transfer. Emphasizes basic and applied ovarian physiology, including superovulation. Also studies reproductive ultrasonography, three-dimensional ultrasonography, and computerized image processing. **Pub:** *Annual Report.*

**★ 16744 ★ University of Southern**
**California**
**Neonatology Research Units**
1240 Mission Rd., Rm. L919
Los Angeles, CA 90033
**Phone:** (323)226-3409     **Fax:** (213)226-3440
**Email:** ramanath@hsc.usc.edu
Dr. Rangasamy Ramanathan, Dir.
**Activities/Fields:** Clinical problems of the newborn and premature infant, including studies on neonatal jaundice, phototherapy, nutrition and energy metabolism, body composition, renal function, pulmonary function and assisted ventilation, circulation, Sudden Infant Death Syndrome, biophysical monitoring of neonates, and follow-up of motor/mental performance of high risk infants. Operates in conjunction with the Hospital's newborn service, which delivers and cares for 18,000 infants yearly; investigation of research problems is integrated with clinical care of infants and training program for physicians.

# State Government Agencies

## Maternal & Child Health

**Alabama Department of Public Health**
**Family Health Services Bureau**
*See:* Entry 5844

**Alaska Department of Health and Social**
**Services**
**Public Health Division**
**Maternal and Child Family Health Section**
*See:* Entry 5845

**Arizona Department of Health Services**
**Family Health and Community Services**
**Division**
**Women and Children's Health Office**
*See:* Entry 5846

**California Health and Welfare Agency**
**Health Services Department**
**Maternal and Child Health Branch**
*See:* Entry 5847

**Colorado Public Health and Environment**
**Department**
**Health Office**
**Division of Prevention and Intervention**
**Services for Children and Youth**
*See:* Entry 5848

**Connecticut Department of Public Health**
**Community Health Bureau**
**Child Adolescent Health Division**
*See:* Entry 5849

**Delaware Department of Health and**
**Social Services**
**Public Health Division**
**Family Health Services**
*See:* Entry 5850

**District of Columbia Department of**
**Health**
**Office of Maternal and Child Health**
*See:* Entry 5851

**Georgia Department of Community Health**
**Division of Medical Assistance**
**Maternal and Child Health Division**
*See:* Entry 5852

**Hawaii Department of Health**
**Health Resources Administration**
**Family Health Services Division**
**Maternal and Child Health Branch**
*See:* Entry 5853

**Idaho Department of Health and Welfare**
**Health Division**
**Maternal and Child Health Bureau**
*See:* Entry 5854

**Indiana Department of Health**
**Maternal and Child Health Services**
**Division**
*See:* Entry 5855

**Iowa Department of Public Health**
**Family and Community Health Division**
**Maternal and Child Health Section**
*See:* Entry 5856

**Kansas Department of Health and**
**Environment**
**Health Division**
**Family Health Bureau**
*See:* Entry 5857

**Kentucky Health Services Cabinet**
**Health Services Department**
**Maternal and Child Health Services**
**Division**
*See:* Entry 5858

**Louisiana Department of Health and**
**Hospitals**
**Public Health Office**
**Health Services Programs**
**Maternal and Child Health Section**
*See:* Entry 5859

**Maine Department of Human Services**
**Health Bureau**
**Maternal and Child Health Division**
*See:* Entry 5860

**Massachusetts Executive Office of Health**
**and Human Services**
**Public Health Department**
**Family Health Services Division**
*See:* Entry 5861

**Minnesota Department of Health**
**Maternal and Child Health Section**
*See:* Entry 5862

**Mississippi Department of Health**
**Health Services Bureau**
**WIC Services**
*See:* Entry 5863

**Missouri Department of Health**
**Maternal, Child and Family Health**
**Division**
*See:* Entry 5864

**Montana Department of Public Health and**
**Human Services**
**Child and Family Services Division**
*See:* Entry 5865

**Nebraska Department of Health and**
**Human Services**
**Health Promotion and Disease Prevention**
**Office of Family Health**
*See:* Entry 5866

**Nevada Department of Human Resources**
**Health Division**
**Family Health Service**
*See:* Entry 5867

**New Hampshire Department of Health**
**and Human Services**
**Public Health Services Division**
**Maternal and Child Health Bureau**
*See:* Entry 5868

**New Jersey Department of Health**
**Family Health Services Division**
**Maternal and Child Health Services**
*See:* Entry 5869

**New Mexico Department of Health**
**Public Health Division**
**Maternal and Child Health Bureau**
*See:* Entry 5870

**North Carolina Department of Health, and Human Services**
**Public Health Division**
**Women's and Children's Health**
*See:* Entry 5871

**North Dakota Department of Health**
**Preventive Health Section**
**Maternal and Child Health Division**
*See:* Entry 5872

**Oklahoma Department of Health**
**Personal Health Services**
**Maternal and Child Health Services**
*See:* Entry 5873

**Oregon Department of Human Resources**
**Health Division**
**Child and Family Health Center**
*See:* Entry 5874

**Rhode Island Department of Health**
**Family Health Office**
*See:* Entry 5875

**South Carolina Department of Health and Environmental Control**
**Health Services Office**
**Maternal and Child Health Bureau**
*See:* Entry 5876

**South Dakota Department of Health**
**Maternal and Child Health Program**
*See:* Entry 5877

**Tennessee Department of Health**
**Health Services Bureau**
**Maternal and Children's Health Section**
*See:* Entry 5878

**Vermont Agency of Human Services**
**Health Department**
**Maternal and Child Health Bureau**
*See:* Entry 5879

**Virginia Office of Health and Human Resources**
**Health Department**
**Women and Infants Health Division**
*See:* Entry 5880

**Washington Department of Health**
**Community and Family Health Services Division**
*See:* Entry 5881

**West Virginia Department of Health and Human Resources**
**Public Health Bureau**
**Bureau for Children and Families**
*See:* Entry 5882

**Wisconsin Department of Health and Family Services**
**Division of Public Health**
**Family Health Program**
**Maternal and Child Health Section**
*See:* Entry 5883

**Wyoming Department of Health**
**Public Health Division**
**Maternal and Child Health Services**
*See:* Entry 5884

# Chapter 46
# Occupational Health & Medicine

## Federal Government Agencies

**★ 16745 ★ Federal Mine Safety and Health Review Commission**
1730 K St. NW, Ste. 6000
Washington, DC 20006-3867
**Phone:** (202)653-5625 **Fax:** (202)653-5030
**Email:** info@fmshrc.gov
**Website:** http://www.fmshrc.gov
Mary Lu Jordan, Chairman of the Board
**Desc:** The Commission ensures compliance with occupational safety and health standards in the Nation's surface and underground coal, metal, and nonmetal mines.

**★ 16746 ★ Occupational Safety and Health Review Commission**
1120 20th St. NW
Washington, DC 20036-3419
**Phone:** (202)606-5100 **Fax:** (202)606-5050
**Website:** http://www.oshrc.gov/
Thomasina V. Rogers, Chairman of the Board
**Desc:** The Commission works to ensure the timely and fair resolution of cases involving the alleged exposure of American workers to unsafe or unhealthy working conditions.

**★ 16747 ★ U.S. Department of Commerce**
**National Institute of Standards and Technology**
**Office of the Director of Administration**
**Occupational Health and Safety Division**
Washington, DC 20230
**Phone:** (301)975-6478 **Fax:** (301)926-1630
**Email:** inquiries@nist.gov
**Website:** http://www.nist.gov/

**★ 16748 ★ U.S. Department of Health and Human Services**
**Centers for Disease Control and Prevention (CDCP)**
**National Institute for Occupational Safety and Health (NIOSH)**
1600 Clifton Rd. NE
Atlanta, GA 30333
**Phone:** (404)639-3311
**Website:** http://www.cdc.gov/niosh/homepage.html
**Desc:** NIOSH is the primary federal agency engaged in research to eliminate on-the-job hazards to health and safety. Institute is responsible for identifying occupational safety and health hazards, for determining methods to control them, and for recommending federal standards to limit the hazards. Institute is also responsible for administering the X-ray surveillance program for coal miners, and testing and certifying respirators and hazard measuring devices.

**★ 16749 ★ U.S. Department of Labor**
**Bureau of Labor Statistics**
**Office of Compensation and Working Conditions**
**Office of Safety, Health, and Working Conditions**
2 Massachusetts Ave. NW
Washington, DC 20212
**Phone:** (202)691-5200
**Desc:** Office compiles occupational safety and health statistics; and makes grants to states and other local agencies to assist in the development and administration of programs dealing with occupational safety and health statistics. Office maintains the nationwide employer record keeping system on job-related injuries and illnesses, conducts the annual survey based on these records, analyzes the results, and compiles supplementary statistics from other sources. Office also implements the Supplementary Data System (SDS), by which states provide additional information on occupational accidents and exposures from workers' compensation records in order to give a more accurate definition of occupational safety and health problems, associated characteristics, and possible action indicators. In addition, Office examines selected types of work injuries in order to develop a detailed profile of characteristics associated with data from questionnaires completed by injured workers.

**★ 16750 ★ U.S. Department of Labor**
**Mine Safety and Health Administration (MSHA)**
4015 Wilson Blvd., Ste. 601
Arlington, VA 22203
**Phone:** (703)235-1452 **Fax:** (703)235-1563
**Desc:** The Mine Safety and Health Administration develops and promulgates mandatory safety and health standards; ensures compliance with such standards; assesses civil penalties for violations; investigates accidents; cooperates with and provides assistance to the states in the development of effective state mine safety and health programs; improves and expands training programs in cooperation with the states and the mining industry; and in coordination with the Department of Health and Human Services and the Department of the Interior, contributes to the improvement and expansion of mine safety and health research and development. All of these activities are aimed at preventing and reducing mine accidents and occupational diseases in the mining industry.

**★ 16751 ★ U.S. Department of Labor**
**Occupational Safety and Health Administration (OSHA)**
200 Constitution Ave. NW
Washington, DC 20210
**Phone:** (202)693-1999
**Desc:** The Occupational Safety and Health Administration sets and enforces workplace safety and health standards and assists employers in complying with these standards. The Administration has a four-fold focus: firm and fair enforcement of safety and health rules; partnership with States running their own OSHA-approved programs and with employers and employees interested in developing effective workplace safety and health programs; efficient promulgation of new rules that are clear and easy to understand and follow; and increased outreach and training to help employers and employees eliminate safety and health standards.

## Foundations & Other Funding Organizations

### Other Funding Organizations

**★ 16752 ★ American Board for Occupational Health Nurses (ABOHN)**
201 E Ogden Ave., Ste. 114
Hinsdale, IL 60521-3652
**Phone:** (630)789-5799 **Free:** 888-842-2646
**Fax:** (630)789-8901
**Email:** info@abohn.org
**Website:** http://www.abohn.org
Sharon D. Kemerer, MSN, Exec. Dir.
**Desc:** Occupational health nurses. Establishes standards and confers initial and ongoing certification in occupational health nursing. Conducts semiannual certification examination. **Awards:** ABOHN Employer Award (annual) for firms that promote certification of occupational health nurses; ABOHN Research Award (annual) for research related to occupational health; Marguerite Ahern Graff Excellence Award (annual) for the Candidate Receiving the highest score on the COHN certification exam; Mayrose Snyder Excellence Award (annual) for the candidate receiving the highest score on the COHN-S certification exam.

**★ 16753 ★ American Occupational Therapy Association (AOTA)**
4720 Montgomery Ln.
PO Box 31220
Bethesda, MD 20824-1220
**Phone:** (301)652-2682 **Free:** 800-377-8555
**Fax:** (301)652-7711
**Email:** praota@aota.org
**Website:** http://www.aota.org
Joseph C. Isaacs, Exec. Dir.
**Desc:** Occupational therapists and occupational therapy assistants who provide services to people whose lives have been disrupted by physical injury or illness, developmental problems, the aging process, or social or psychological difficulties. Occupational therapy focuses on the active involvement of the patient in specially designed therapeutic tasks and activities to improve function, performance capacity, and the ability to cope with demands of daily living. **Awards:** Scholarship (annual) awardee must be accepted in an occupational therapy education program.

**Association of Occupational and Environmental Clinics (AOEC)**
*See:* Entry 8880

**Vocational Evaluation and Work Adjustment Association (VEWAA)**
*See:* Entry 7896

# National & International Organizations

**★ 16754 ★ American Academy of Physician Assistants in Occupational Medicine (AAPA-OM)**
950 N Washington St.
Alexandria, VA 22314-1552
**Free:** 800-596-4398          **Fax:** (703)684-1924
**Email:** aapaom@aapa.org
**Website:** http://www.aapa.org/paom.html
**Fnded:** 1981. **Desc:** Physicians, physician assistants, students and graduates of PA programs. Designed for an exchange of information and ideas within occupational health field. Endorses the code of ethical conduct established by the American College of Occupational Medicine. **Pub:** *AAPA-OM Membership Directory.* Directory. • *AAPA-OM Newsletter,* quarterly. Newsletter.

**American Association of Occupational Health Nurses (AAOHN)**
*See:* Entry 15641

**★ 16755 ★ American Board of Industrial Hygiene (ABIH)**
6015 W St. Joseph, Ste. 102
Lansing, MI 48917-3980
**Phone:** (517)321-2638          **Fax:** (517)321-4624
**Email:** abih@abih.org
**Website:** http://www.abih.org/
Lynn C. O'Donnell, CIH, Exec. Dir.
**Fnded:** 1960. **Mem:** 19. **Desc:** Certifies industrial hygienists and promotes high standards within the profession. Maintains a record of holders of certificates. **Pub:** *ABIH Candidate Handbook.* • *ABIH News,* Biannual. Newsletter. • *Roster of the American Board of Industrial Hygiene,* annual.

**American Board for Occupational Health Nurses (ABOHN)**
*See:* Entry 15647

**★ 16756 ★ American College of Occupational and Environmental Medicine (ACOEM)**
1114 N Arlington Hts. Rd.
Arlington Heights, IL 60004-4770
**Phone:** (847)818-1800          **Fax:** (847)818-9266
**Email:** acoeminfo@acoem.org
**Website:** http://www.acoem.org
Barry S. Eisenberg, Exec. Dir.
**Fnded:** 1916. **Mem:** 7,000. **Reg. Groups:** 31. **Desc:** Physicians specializing in occupational and environmental medicine. Promotes maintenance and improvement of the health of workers; works to increase awareness of occupational medicine as a medical specialty. Sponsors educational programs; maintains placement service. **Pub:** *ACOEM Report,* monthly. Newsletter. Covers Occupational Safety and Health Administration rulings. *Price:* Included in membership dues. • *American College of Occupational and Environmental Medicine–Membership Directory,* annual. Membership Directory. Arranged alphabetically, geographically, and by affiliation. *Price:* Included in membership dues; $150/copy for nonmembers. • *Journal of Occupational and Environmental Medicine,* monthly. Journal. Contains book reviews, calendar of events, and employment listings. • *MRO Update,* 10/year. Newsletter. Designed for medical review officers and provides latest information on alcohol and drug testing. *Price:* $200 members; $225 nonmembers. **Frmly:** (1992) American College of Occupational Medicine.

**★ 16757 ★ American Conference of Governmental Industrial Hygienists (ACGIH)**
1330 Kemper Meadow Dr., Ste. 600
Cincinnati, OH 45240
**Phone:** (513)742-2020          **Fax:** (513)742-3355
**Email:** mail@acgih.org
**Website:** http://www.acgih.org
A. Anthony Rizzuto, Exec. Dir.
**Fnded:** 1938. **Mem:** 5,500. **Desc:** Professional society of occupational and environmental safety and health professionals. Devoted to the development of administrative and technical aspects of worker health protection. Functions mainly as a medium for the exchange of ideas and the promotion of standards and techniques in industrial health. Compiles statistics; conducts educational programs. **Pub:** *Air Sampling Instruments.* • *Applied Occupational and Environmental Hygiene,* monthly. Journal. Includes book reviews, peer-reviewed scientific/technical articles and columns, employment listings and information on new products and literature. *Price:* Included in membership dues; $118/year for nonmembers; $204 for institutions. • *Guidelines for the Assessment of Bioaerosols in the Indoor Environment.* • *Industrial Ventilation–A Manual of Recommended Practice.* • *Threshold Limit Values and Biological Exposure Indices.* • *Ventilation System Testing.* • Also publishes other manuals, guides, and studies. **Frmly:** (1945) National Conference of Governmental Industrial Hygienists.

**★ 16758 ★ American Industrial Hygiene Association (AIHA)**
2700 Prosperity Ave., Ste. 250
Fairfax, VA 22031
**Phone:** (703)849-8888          **Fax:** (703)207-3561
**Email:** infonet@aiha.org
**Website:** http://www.aiha.org
O. Gordon Banks, Exec. Dir.
**Fnded:** 1939. **Mem:** 12,500. **Local Groups:** 70. **Desc:** Professional society of industrial hygienists. Promotes the study and control of environmental factors affecting the health and well-being of workers. Sponsors continuing education courses in industrial hygiene, government affairs program, and public relations. Accredits laboratories. Maintains 40 technical committees and a foundation. Operates placement service. Conducts educational and research programs. **Pub:** *The AIHA Journal,* bimonthly. Journal. Includes peer-reviewed technical and scientific articles. • *The Synergist,* monthly, update online. Includes news magazine covering occupational and environmental health and safety issues. *Price:* $65/year in U.S.; $90/year international. • *Who's Who in Industrial Hygiene,* annual. Directory. • Books. • Manuals. • Videos.

**★ 16759 ★ American Occupational Therapy Foundation (AOTF)**
4720 Montgomery Lane
PO Box 31220
Bethesda, MD 20824-1220
**Phone:** (301)652-2682          **Fax:** (301)656-3620
**Email:** aotf@aotf.org
**Website:** http://www.aotf.org
**Fnded:** 1965. **Desc:** Encourages practice, research and scholarship in occupation and occupational therapy. Educates the public and professionals about occupation and occupational therapy. **Pub:** *The Occupational Therapy Journal of Research,* quarterly. Journal.

**★ 16760 ★ Asian Association of Occupational Health (AAOH)**
c/o Society of Occupational and Environmental Medicine
Malaysian Medical Association
124 Jalan Pahang
53000 Kuala Lumpur, Malaysia
**Phone:** 60 3 4420617          **Fax:** 60 3 4418187
**Lang(s):** English, Malay. **Desc:** Health care professionals and occupational health organizations. Promotes improved workplace safety; seeks to advance occupational health scholarship and practice. Serves as a clearinghouse on occupational health; provides consulting services to public health agencies; sponsors research and educational programs.

**★ 16761 ★ Association of Occupational and Environmental Clinics (AOEC)**
1010 Vermont Ave. NW, Ste. 513
Washington, DC 20005-1503
**Phone:** (202)347-4976          **Fax:** (202)347-4950
**Email:** aoec@aoec.org
**Website:** http://www.aoec.org
Katherine H. Kirkland, Exec. Dir.
**Fnded:** 1987. **Mem:** 324. **Desc:** Seeks to enhance the practice of occupational and environmental medicine. Shares information. Provides educational and research programs. **Pub:** *AOEC News,* quarterly. Newsletter.

**★ 16762 ★ Association of Occupational Health Professionals in Healthcare (AOHP)**
500 Commonwealth Dr.
Warrendale, PA 15086
**Free:** 800-362-4347          **Fax:** (724)772-8349
**Email:** aohp1@aol.com
**Website:** http://www.podi.com/aohp/
MaryAnne Gruden, Exec. Pres.
**Desc:** Occupational health professionals. **Pub:** *The Journal,* quarterly.

**★ 16763 ★ Association for Repetitive Motion Syndromes (ARMS)**
PO Box 471973
Aurora, CO 80047-1973
**Phone:** (303)369-0803
**Email:** arms@lightspeed.net
**Website:** http://www.certifiedpst.com/arms
Stephanie M. Barnes, Exec. Dir.
**Fnded:** 1990. **Nat'l Groups:** 1. **Reg. Groups:** 1. **State Groups:** 1. **Desc:** Individuals suffering from repetitive motion injuries; other interested individuals and organizations. Promotes the welfare of persons at risk of developing repetitive motion injuries. Works to increase public awareness of repetitive motion injuries and prevention and treatment. Develops and implements occupational safety standards and educational programs. Compiles, analyzes, and disseminates data; conducts research programs; and clearinghouse. **Pub:** *ARMS News,* quarterly. Newsletter. *Price:* $20 individual; $75 professional; $150 organization membership.

**★ 16764 ★ Australian Association of Occupational Therapists (AAOT)**
97 Grange Rd.
Alphington, VIC 3078, Australia
**Fnded:** 1945.

**Australian College of Occupational Health Nurses (ACOHN)**
*See:* Entry 15670

**★ 16765 ★ British Association and College of Occupational Therapists**
106-114 Borough High St.
London SE1 1HL, United Kingdom
**Phone:** 44 207 3576480          **Fax:** 44 207 4502299
**Email:** beryl.steeden@cot.co.uk
**Website:** http://www.cot.org.uk
**Fnded:** 1932. **Mem:** 23,000. **Reg. Groups:** 20. **Desc:** State registered Occupational Therapists, Occupational Therapy Helpers and Technical Instructors. Acts as a professional association in the field of rehabilitative medicine; promotion of occupational therapy education; honourable practice, repression of malpractice and to provide the facilities for the advancement of the science of occupational therapy. BAOT is also the Trade Union for the members. **Pub:** *British Journal of Occupational Therapy,* monthly. Journal. Contains

articles on clinical, educational, research, and management aspects of occupational therapy. • *Occupational Therapy News*, monthly. Magazine.

★ 16766 ★ **British Association of Occupational Therapists**
106-114 Borough High St.
Southwark
London SE1 1LB, United Kingdom
**Phone:** 44 207 3576480　　**Fax:** 44 207 4502299
**Email:** cot@cot.co.uk
**Website:** http://www.cot.co.uk
**Fnded:** 1974. **Mem:** 21,000. **Reg. Groups:** 20. **Desc:** Promotes high standards among occupational therapists. Supports the provision of efficient, reliable, and effective services that benefit all users of occupational therapy. Encourages personal and intellectual development of occupational therapists and support staff.

★ 16767 ★ **British Institute of Industrial Therapy**
243 Shelley Rd.
Wellingborough NN8 3EN, United Kingdom
**Phone:** 44 1933 675327　　**Fax:** 44 1933 675327
**Fnded:** 1970. **Mem:** 59. **Desc:** Directors and managers of services and units providing industrial therapy for those working in the mental health field. Provides information regarding developments in industrial therapy and work schemes as appropriate to those working in the field of training people who are suffering or recovering from mental illness so that they may remain in sheltered or open employment. **Pub:** *Focus*, monthly.

★ 16768 ★ **British Occupational Hygiene Society (BOHS)**
Georgian House, Ste. 2
Great Northern Rd.
Derby DE1 1LT, United Kingdom
**Phone:** 44 1332 298101　　**Fax:** 44 1332 298099
**Email:** admin@bohs.org
**Website:** http://www.bohs.org/
**Fnded:** 1953. **Mem:** 1,000. **Local Groups:** 7. **Lang(s):** English. **Desc:** Individuals and companies. Promotes public and professional awareness of occupational and environmental hygiene practices and standards. Encourages research. **Pub:** *Annals of Occupational Hygiene*, 8/year. Journal. • *Directory*, annual. Directory. • *Occupational Hygiene Newsletter*, quarterly. Newsletter.

★ 16769 ★ **Canadian Association of Occupational Therapists (CAOT) (Association Canadienne des Ergotherapeutes — ACE)**
CTTC Bldg.
1125 Colonel By Dr., Ste. 3400
Ottawa, ON, Canada K1S 5R1
**Phone:** (613)523-2268　　**Fax:** (613)523-2552
**Website:** http://www.caot.ca
**Fnded:** 1926. **Mem:** 6,400. **Lang(s):** English, French. **Desc:** Occupational therapists. Promotes professional development of members; seeks to advance the practice of occupational therapy. Facilitates communication among members; makes available continuing professional development programs.

★ 16770 ★ **Canadian Council on Rehabilitation and Work (CCRW) (Conseil Canadien de la Readaptation et du Travail — CCRT)**
500 University Ave., Ste. 302
Toronto, ON, Canada M5G 1V7
**Phone:** (416)260-3060　　**Free:** 800-664-0925
**Fax:** (416)260-3093
**Email:** info@ccrw.org
**Website:** http://www.ccrw.org
**Fnded:** 1976. **Lang(s):** English, French. **Desc:** Promotes and supports the meaningful employment of persons with disabilities. **Pub:** *Ability & Enterprise*, every 6-8 weeks. Newsletter.

**Canadian Occupational Health Nurses Association (COHNA) (Association Canadienne des Infirmieres et Infirmiers en Sante du Travail — ACIST)**
*See:* Entry 15695

★ 16771 ★ **Center for the Well Being of Health Professionals**
21 W Colony Pl., Ste. 150
Durham, NC 27705-5589
**Phone:** (919)489-9167　　**Fax:** (919)419-0011
**Email:** cpwb@mindspring.com
**Website:** http://www.cpwb.org
John-Henry Pfifferling, PhD, Founder & Dir.
**Desc:** Offers presentations on all areas relevant to professional well-being. Works to find a balance between personal and professional lives.

★ 16772 ★ **Council for Accreditation in Occupational Hearing Conservation (CAOHC)**
611 E Wells St.
Milwaukee, WI 53202
**Phone:** (414)276-5338　　**Fax:** (414)276-2146
**Email:** info@caohc.org
**Website:** http://www.caohc.org
Barbara L. Lechner, Exec. Dir.
**Fnded:** 1973. **Mem:** 22,000. **Desc:** To establish and maintain standards for the training of audiometric technicians (persons certified to conduct pure tone air conduction hearing tests and related duties as part of an occupational hearing conservation program). Approves courses in occupational hearing conservation and certifies those who pass these courses. Council members represent professional associations in the hearing conservation field. **Pub:** *CABLE*, semiannual. Newsletter. Newsletter to course directors. • *Occupational Hearing Conservation Manual*. Manual. Contains information on the hearing conservationist's mission, training, and role; and federal and state regulations. *Price:* $40/each. • *The Update*, quarterly. Newsletter.

★ 16773 ★ **Council of Occupational Therapists for the European Countries (COTEC)**
106-114 Borough High St.
London SE1 1LB, United Kingdom
**Phone:** 44 171 3576480　　**Fax:** 44 171 4502349
**Email:** berylsteeden@cot.co.uk
**Website:** http://216.87.175.20
**Fnded:** 1986. **Mem:** 20. **Lang(s):** English. **Desc:** European national organizations representing occupational therapists. Seeks to improve the standard of practice in occupational therapy and create career opportunities for occupational therapists. Serves as a clearinghouse on developments in occupational therapy; provides advice and technical assistance to members; conducts continuing professional development courses. Makes available student exchange programs. **Pub:** *COTEC Newsletter*, semiannual. Newsletter. Contains short news from member associations.

★ 16774 ★ **Faculty of Occupational Medicine**
c/o Royal College of Physicians
6 St. Andrews Pl.
Regent's Park
London NW1 4LB, United Kingdom
**Phone:** 44 207 3175890　　**Fax:** 44 207 3175899
**Website:** http://www.facoccmed.ac.uk/

★ 16775 ★ **Hong Kong Occupational Therapy Association (HKOTA)**
c/o Department of Rehabilitation Sciences
Hong Kong Polytechnic University
Hong Kong, People's Republic of China
**Phone:** 852 27666727　　**Fax:** 852 23308656
**Email:** samuelycchan@ctimail3.com
**Website:** http://www.fmshk.com.hk/hkota/home.htm
**Fnded:** 1987. **Mem:** 300. **Lang(s):** Chinese, English. **Desc:** Occupational therapists and students. Seeks to insure high standards of practice in the field of occupational therapy. Serves as a forum for exchange of information among members; represents members' interests; conducts continuing professional development programs. **Pub:** *Hong Kong Journal of Occupational Therapy*, annual. Journal. • *Hong Kong Occupational Therapy Newsletter*, 3/year.

★ 16776 ★ **Institute for Labor and Mental Health (ILMH)**
3137 Telegraph Ave.
Oakland, CA 94609
**Phone:** (510)653-6166
Dr. Richard Epstein, Dir.
**Fnded:** 1977. **Mem:** 50. **Desc:** Purpose is to help working people with problems related to the workplace. Seeks to identify conditions at work that cause stress; believes that education and communication about common work problems are the first steps in dealing with job stress. Assists unions in handling grievances and stress-related disabilities; provides counseling to union members and their families; offers legal and worker compensation assistance to working people. Provides consultation to government and businesses on ways to reduce stress. Develops ongoing stress programs; operates summer institute on occupational stress. **Pub:** *Occupational Stress*, bimonthly. Newsletter. • *Occupational Stress: A Union Based Approach.* • *Occupational Stress: The Inside Story.* • *Surplus Powerlessness.* Book. • *Directory*, periodic.

★ 16777 ★ **Institute of Occupational Medicine (IOM)**
8 Roxburgh Pl.
Edinburgh EH8 9SU, United Kingdom
**Phone:** 44 131 6675131　　**Fax:** 44 131 6670136
**Email:** iom@iomhq.org.uk
**Website:** http://www.iom-world.org
**Fnded:** 1969. **Desc:** Major independent centre of scientific excellence in the fields of occupational and environmental health, hygiene and safety. We aim to provide quality research, consultancy and training to help ensure that peoples health is not damaged by conditions at work or in the environment. **Pub:** *COSHH - A Helpful Guide.* • *COSHH - Making an Assessment.* • *NORSE - A Helpful Guide.* • *Technical Memoranda*, 10/year. Reports. • *Thermal Environment.*

★ 16778 ★ **International Association of Agricultural Medicine and Rural Health (IAAMRH) (Association Internationale de Medecine Agricole et de Sante Rurale)**
Stonnictwo Konserwatywno
Ludowe, 62-800
Targowa 24
00-608 Warsaw, Poland
**Phone:** 48 22 8258513　　**Fax:** 48 22 8258513
**Email:** dg@krus.gov.pl
**Website:** http://www.iaamrh.org
**Fnded:** 1961. **Mem:** 450. **Nat'l Groups:** 4. **Reg. Groups:** 3. **Lang(s):** English, French, German, Polish, Russian. **Desc:** Independent association for agricultural and rural professionals in over 40 countries. Studies agricultural medicine and rural health around the world. Strives to improve the health of rural communities and to protect the health of agricultural workers. Studies agricultural and rural health in association with other sciences and provides scientific information and advice. Cooperates with other

branches of medicine, health, agricultural, environmental and other related sciences. Studies the effects of social, physical and environmental conditions on human health. **Pub:** *Agricultural Medicine and Rural Health*, semiannual. Journal.


★ **16779** ★ **International Commission on Occupational Health (Commission Internationale de la Sante au Travail)**
c/o Prof. J. Jeyaratnam
Department of Community, Occupational, and Family Medicine
National University of Singapore
Lower Kent Ridge Rd.
Singapore 0511, Singapore
**Phone:** 65 7749300          **Fax:** 65 7791489
**Website:** http://www.who.int/ina-ngo/ngo/ngo043.htm
**Lang(s):** Chinese, English. **Desc:** Physicians specializing in occupational medicine and other individuals with an interest in occupation safety and health. Seeks to advance the study, teaching, and practice of occupational medicine. Serves as a forum for the exchange of information among members; sponsors research and educational programs.


**International Ergophthalmological Society (Societas Ergophthalmologica Internationalis — SEI)**
*See:* Entry 20987


★ **16780** ★ **International Healthcare Safety Professional Certification Board (IHSPCB)**
8009 Carita Ct.
Bethesda, MD 20817
**Phone:** (301)469-0648
**Email:** info@chcm-chsp.org
**Website:** http://www.chcm-chsp.org
Harold M. Gordon, Exec. Dir.
**Fnded:** 1978. **Desc:** Individuals working or consulting in hospitals or healthcare facilities who are responsible for the handling and control of hazardous materials. Areas of concern include: emergency and disaster planning; biological, chemical, and physical hazards; ventilation; fire prevention and protection; maintenance and engineering; personal protective equipment; sanitation; life safety code. Grants affiliate, associate, and executive level distinctions for the title of Certified Healthcare Safety Professional. Encourages exchange of ideas and technology to improve performance. Sponsors HSP Academy, which conducts professional development activities. **Pub:** *Directory of Certified Healthcare Safety Professionals*, annual. Directory. • Brochure.


★ **16781** ★ **Nordic Institute for Advanced Training in Occupational Health (NIATOH) (Nordisk Arbetsmiljoutbildning)**
Topeliuksenkatu 41a A
FIN-00250 Helsinki, Finland
**Phone:** 358 9 47471          **Fax:** 358 9 47472497
**Email:** niva@occuphealth.fi
**Website:** http://www.occuphealth.fi/niva
**Fnded:** 1982. **Lang(s):** Danish, English, Finnish, Norwegian, Swedish. **Desc:** Occupational health service personnel, doctoral students, and researchers. Provides courses in occupational health and working life questions. **Pub:** Catalog, annual. **Frmly:** (1989) Nordic Institute of Advanced Occupational Environment Studies.


★ **16782** ★ **Occupational and Environmental Medical Association of Canada (OEMAC)**
54 Forward Ave.
London, ON, Canada N6H 1B7
**Phone:** (519)439-7970          **Fax:** (519)439-8840
**Email:** oemac@esc.net

**Website:** http://www.oemac.org
**Fnded:** 1985. **Mem:** 400. **Lang(s):** English, French. **Desc:** Health care professionals with an active interest in occupational and environmental medicine. Promotes improved standards of education and practice in the field. Serves as a unified voice for Canadian occupational and environmental medicine; acts as a forum for exchange of scientific and professional information. Conducts continuing professional education programs. **Pub:** *Liaison*, quarterly. Newsletter. Contains information about the association's activities. • Directory, annual.


★ **16783** ★ **Scientific Society of Hygiene**
c/o Medical University
Department of Hygiene, Ecology & Occupational Health
D.Nestorov 15
BG-1431 Sofia, Bulgaria
**Phone:** 359 2 594061          **Fax:** 359 2 595106
**Fnded:** 1922. **Mem:** 200. **Reg. Groups:** 10. **Lang(s):** English, French, Russian. **Desc:** Fosters research in occupational medicine, occupational diseases, environmental health, toxicology, military hygiene, ergonomics, hygiene of residental areas, nutrition, child and adolescent hygiene. **Pub:** *Journal of Hygiene and Public Health*, bimonthly. Journal. **Frmly:** (1996) Scientific Society of Sanitation.


**Self-Help Association for the Electrically Sensitive (Selbsthilfeverein fuer Elektrosensible)**
*See:* Entry 8928


★ **16784** ★ **Society for Occupational and Environmental Health (SOEH)**
6728 Old McLean Village Dr.
Mc Lean, VA 22101
**Phone:** (703)556-9222          **Fax:** (703)556-8729
**Email:** soeh@degnon.org
**Website:** http://www.soeh.org
Ana Maria Osorio, MD, Contact
**Fnded:** 1972. **Mem:** 350. **Desc:** Scientists, academicians, and industry and labor representatives. Seeks to improve the quality of both working and living places by operating as a neutral forum for conferences involving all aspects of occupational health. Focuses public attention on scientific, social, and regulatory problems; studies specific categories of hazards, methods for assessment of health effects, and diseases associated with particular jobs. Identifies hazards in the occupational and general environment and proposes actions to reduce their danger. **Pub:** *Archives of Environmental Health*. Journal. *Price:* Included in membership dues. • *Society for Occupational and Environmental Health–Bulletin*, quarterly. Newsletter. *Price:* Free, for members only.


★ **16785** ★ **Society of Occupational Medicine**
6 St. Andrew's Pl.
Regent's Park
London NW1 4LB, United Kingdom
**Phone:** 44 207 4862641     **Fax:** 44 207 4860028
**Email:** som@sococcmed.demon.co.uk
**Website:** http://www.som.org.uk/
**Fnded:** 1935. **Mem:** 2,000. **Desc:** Doctors working in occupational medicine. Many of the members have specialist qualifications in occupational medicine but others may be family practitioners connected with or holding part-time appointments in the specialty. Concerned with protecting the health of people at work and the prevention and management of occupational diseases and injuries. Seeks to interest and inform members through publications and scientific meetings, organised regionally and nationally. Stimulates research and education in occupational medicine and actively liaises with professional organisations relevant to occupational health. **Pub:** *Newsletter Periodical*, quarterly. Newsletter. • *Occupational Medicine Journal*, bimonthly. Journal. • Papers.

**Swedish Association for the Electrosensitive**
*See:* Entry 8929


# Research Centers


★ **16786** ★ **Deep South Center for Occupational Health and Safety**
School of Public Health
University of Alabama at Birmingham
1530 3rd Ave. S
Birmingham, AL 35294-0022
**Phone:** (205)934-7178          **Fax:** (205)975-7179
**Email:** dsc@uab.edu
**Website:** http://www.uab.edu/dsc
R. Kent Oestenstad, PhD, Dir.
**Activities/Fields:** Health and safety of workers.


★ **16787** ★ **Duke University Occupational Mental Health Programs**
Medical Center
PO Box 3834
Durham, NC 27712
**Phone:** (919)286-1244          **Free:** 800-336-3853
**Fax:** (919)286-1121
Dr. Judith Holder, Dir.
**Activities/Fields:** Occupational mental health, including managed mental health care, employee assistance programs, and mental health outcome research. **Frmly:** Career Assessment and Development Laboratory.


**Environmental and Occupational Health Sciences Institute (EOHSI)**
*See:* Entry 8940


★ **16788** ★ **Harvard University Harvard Education and Research Center**
Occupational Health Program
School of Public Health
665 Huntington Ave.
Boston, MA 02115
**Phone:** (617)432-1260          **Fax:** (617)432-3441
**Email:** dchris@hohp.harvard.edu
**Website:** http://www.hsph.harvard.edu/erc/
David C. Christiani, Dir.
**Activities/Fields:** Cause and prevention of the leading work-related safety and health problems.


★ **16789** ★ **Institute for Work and Health**
250 Bloor St. E, Ste. 702
Toronto, ON, Canada M4W 1E6
**Phone:** (416)927-2027          **Fax:** (416)927-4167
**Email:** info@iwh.on.ca
**Website:** http://www.iwh.on.ca/
J. Fraser Mustard, Hd.
**Activities/Fields:** Underlying factors contributing to workplace health and disability, evaluation of designated Ontario rehabilitation facilities, and provision of pertinent and timely information on workplace health and rehabilitation to health care workers and stakeholders. **Pub:** *Newsletter.*


★ **16790** ★ **Iowa's Center for Agricultural Safety and Health (ICASH)**
124 IREH
Oakdale Campus
University of Iowa
Iowa City, IA 52242-5000
**Phone:** (319)335-4190          **Fax:** (319)335-4225
**Email:** kelley-donham@uiowa.edu
**Website:** http://www.public-health.uiowa.edu/ICASH/index.html
Kelley J. Donham, DVM, Dir.
**Activities/Fields:** Health and safety of Iowa's farm families, farm workers, and the agricultural community. Priority areas include provision of agricultural health

and safety services, prevention of tractor injuries, prevention of injuries and illnesses in farm youth, prevention of illnesses among producers working in livestock confinement operations, and surveillance of farm injuries and illnesses. **Pub:** *Annual report.* • *Newsletter*, quarterly.

**★ 16791 ★ Johns Hopkins University**
**Center for Information Technology and**
**Health Research**
School of Hygiene & Public Health
615 N Wolfe St., Rm. 4028
Baltimore, MD 21205
**Phone:** (410)955-3608　　**Fax:** (410)955-9334
**Email:** pbreysse@jhsph.edu
Dr. Patrick N. Breysse, Dir.

**Activities/Fields:** Health effects of information technology with an emphasis on children and the aging. **Frmly:** Center for VDT and Health Research.

**★ 16792 ★ Johns Hopkins University**
**Education and Research Center for**
**Occupational Safety and Health**
Bloomberg School of Public Health
615 N Wolfe St., Rm. W7041
Baltimore, MD 21205-2179
**Phone:** (410)955-0423　　**Fax:** (410)614-4986
**Email:** dzerbe@jhsph.edu
**Website:** http://www.jhsph.edu/~c-erc/
Diane Zerbe, Dir.

**Activities/Fields:** Occupational and environmental safety and health.

**★ 16793 ★ McMaster University**
**Health Information Research Unit**
1200 Main St. W, Rm. 3H7
Hamilton, ON, Canada L8N 3Z5
**Phone:** (905)525-9140　　**Fax:** (905)546-0401
**Website:** http://hiru.mcmaster.ca/main.htm
Dr. Alex Jadad, Ch.

**Activities/Fields:** Workplace disability, particularly the factors that contribue to it; disability treatment, and ways to ensure optimal recovery and a safe return to work. **Pub:** *Newsletter*.

**★ 16794 ★ National Farm Medicine**
**Center**
1000 N Oak Ave.
Marshfield, WI 54449-5790
**Free:** 800-662-6900　　**Fax:** (715)389-4950
**Email:** gunderp@mfldclin.edu
**Website:** http://www.marshfieldclinic.org/nfmc/
Barbara Lee, PhD, Dir.

**Activities/Fields:** Agriculture-related health problems, including injury, respiratory diseases, noise-induced hearing loss, migrant health, and cancer. **Pub:** *Progress Report*.

**★ 16795 ★ New York/New Jersey**
**Occupational Safety and Health**
**Education and Research Center**
Department of Community & Preventive Medicine
Mt. Sinai School of Medicine
1 Gustave L. Levy Pl.
PO Box 1057
New York, NY 10029-6574
**Phone:** (212)241-4804　　**Fax:** (212)996-0407
**Email:** phil.landrigan@mssm.edu
**Website:** http://www.nynjerc.org/
Philip J. Landrigan, MD, Dir.

**Activities/Fields:** Occupational health and safety.

**NYCAMH**
*See:* Entry 8951

**★ 16796 ★ Oregon Health and Science**
**University**
**Center for Research on Occupational and**
**Environmental Toxicology (CROET)**
3181 SW Sam Jackson Pk. Rd., L606
Portland, OR 97201-3098
**Phone:** (503)494-4273　　**Fax:** (503)494-4278
**Email:** spencer@ohsu.edu
**Website:** http://www.ohsu.edu/croet
Dr. Peter S. Spencer, Dir.

**Activities/Fields:** Adverse effects of occupational and environmental chemicals on the human nervous system; region-specific surveillance of the use, dissemination and release of occupational chemicals and identification, analysis and categorization of all types of chemicals that may perturb normal neurological function; collaborative research on the exposure pathways and chemical fate of environmental pollutants, and their contact, entry and distribution in human subjects; field-based investigations epidemiological studies on human populations at risk for cancer, neurodegenerative diseases and stress-related disorders that impair workplace performance; studies on the health impact of xenobiotics incorporating, when possible, biological markers of susceptibility exposure and effect, including neurobehavioral (and other) screening batteries for the detection of early, reversible abnormalities in brain function; development of wild-type and transgenic animals as models to investigate the consequences of an environmental-chemical induced genomic and proteomic change and cytotoxicity in the central and peripheral nervous system; studies on the molecular and cellular mechanisms underlying the adverse effects of chemicals on the nervous system during development, in the adult and the aged; development of models to assess the physiological and morphology of neural circuits, including signal transduction, and their responses to chemical attack; investigations into the chronic and delayed actions of chemical substances, the genetic basis for susceptibility to chemical toxicity, and the role of occupational and environmental chemical outreach activities to disseminate information regarding the effects of exposure to occupational and environmental chemicals and current research at the center.

**★ 16797 ★ OSHTECH Inc.**
400 York St., Ste. 100
London, ON, Canada N6B 3N2
**Phone:** (519)642-1122　　**Fax:** (519)542-0331
**Email:** oshtech@oshtechinc.com
**Website:** http://www.oshtechinc.com
Dr. Peter Pityn, Contact

**Activities/Fields:** Occupational health and safety, residential and office air quality, ergonomics, inhalational studies, and occupational hygiene, analytical methods development. **Pub:** *Reports*. **Frmly:** Occupational Health and Safety Resource Centre.

**★ 16798 ★ Productive Rehabilitation**
**Institute of Dallas for Ergonomics**
**(PRIDE)**
5701 Maple, Ste. 100
Dallas, TX 75235
**Phone:** (214)351-6600　　**Fax:** (214)351-6453
**Email:** prode@airmail.net
**Website:** http://www.pridedallas.com
Robert J. Gatchel, PhD, Dir.

**Activities/Fields:** Ergonomics. Projects focus on utilizing physical exercise for rehabilitating chronic back problems. Patients use gym and spa equipment, participate in aerobics, and mimic job-related conditions such as crawling through pipes, moving equipment on assembly lines, driving four-wheelers, crawling around on building skeletons, and jumping up and onto a moving platform. **Pub:** *Functional Restoration*, quarterly.

**★ 16799 ★ Texas A&M University**
**Occupational Health and Safety Institute**
Department of Nuclear Engineering
College Station, TX 77843-3133
**Phone:** (979)862-4409　　**Fax:** (979)845-6443
**Email:** j-rock@tamu.edu
Dr. James C. Rock, Dir.

**Activities/Fields:** Occupational health and safety, with a goal of safe use and disposal of essential hazardous materials and processes. Areas of study include industrial hygiene, health physics, safety engineering, aerosol science, occupational epidemiology, fire protection engineering, product safety engineering, occupational exposure assessment, industrial ventilation, indoor air quality, noise and vibration control, material substitution, electrofiltration, separation sciences, indoor bioaerosols, electrostatic separation for hazardous waste streams, and low toxicity product substitution.

**U.S. Department of Defense**
**Army Medical Research and Materiel**
**Command**
**Army Research Institute of Environmental**
**Medicine**
**Occupational Health and Performance**
**Directorate**
*See:* Entry 13476

**U.S. Department of Health and Human**
**Services**
**Centers for Disease Control and**
**Prevention**
**National Institute for Occupational Safety**
**and Health**
**Division of Respiratory Disease Studies**
*See:* Entry 18762

**★ 16800 ★ U.S. Department of Health**
**and Human Services**
**Centers for Disease Control and**
**Prevention**
**National Institute for Occupational Safety**
**and Health**
**Division of Safety Research**
1095 Willowdale Rd.
Morgantown, WV 26505-2888
**Phone:** (304)285-5894　　**Free:** 800-356-4676
**Email:** richard.johnson@na.amedd.army.mil
**Website:** http://www.cdc.gov/niosh/im-dsr.html
Nancy Stout, EdD, Dir.

**Activities/Fields:** Occupational injury. Programs are organized around the public health approach to occupational injury prevention, including surveillance, analytic epidemiology, safety and human factors engineering, and health communication.

**★ 16801 ★ U.S. Department of Health**
**and Human Services**
**Centers for Disease Control and**
**Prevention**
**National Institute for Occupational Safety**
**and Health**
**Health Effects Laboratory Division**
1095 Willowdale Rd.
Morgantown, WV 26505
**Phone:** (304)285-6121　　**Free:** 800-356-4676
**Website:** http://www.cdc.gov/niosh/im-held.html
Albert E. Munson, PhD, Dir.

**Activities/Fields:** Workplace health and safety. Research involves causes, mechanisms, prevention and control of adverse health effects from workplace hazards, including ergonomics and toxins.

**★ 16802 ★ U.S. Department of Health and Human Services**
**Centers for Disease Control and Prevention**
**National Institute for Occupational Safety and Health**
**National Occupational Research Agenda (Traumatic Injuries)**
Division of Safety Research
1095 Willowdale Rd.
Morgantown, WV 26505
**Phone:** (304)285-5894        **Free:** 800-356-4676
**Fax:** (304)285-6046
**Email:** nas5@cdc.gov
**Website:** http://www.cdc.gov/niosh/nrtram.html
Nancy Stout, EdD, Ch.

**Activities/Fields:** Reducing the incidence and toll of traumatic injuries at work through research and collaboration. **Pub:** *Reports.*


**★ 16803 ★ U.S. Department of Health and Human Services**
**Centers for Disease Control and Prevention**
**National Institute for Occupational Safety and Health**
**National Occupational Research Agenda (Special Populations at Risk)**
4676 Columbia Pkwy.
Cincinnati, OH 45226
**Phone:** (513)458-7159        **Free:** 800-356-4676
**Email:** slb8@cdc.gov
**Website:** http://www.cdc.gov/niosh/nrspop.html
Sherry Baron, Team Ldr.

**Activities/Fields:** Special populations of workers, overlooked in the past, who may be at risk of injury and illness in the workplace. These populations are defined by biologic, social, and/or economic characteristics, including: age, gender, race, genetic susceptibility, disability, education, language, literacy, culture, lifestyle/lifework, low income, nationality, citizenship, and political vulnerability. **Pub:** *Reports.*


**★ 16804 ★ U.S. Department of Health and Human Services**
**Centers for Disease Control and Prevention**
**National Institute for Occupational Safety and Health**
**National Occupational Research Agenda (Surveillance Research Methods)**
Surveillance Branch
4676 Columbia Pkwy.
Cincinnati, OH 45226
**Phone:** (513)841-4303        **Free:** 800-356-4676
**Fax:** (513)841-4489
**Email:** jps4@cdc.gov
**Website:** http://www.cdc.gov/niosh/nrsurv.html
John P. Sestito, Team Ldr.

**Activities/Fields:** Surveillance systems, which describe where occupational injuries or illnesses are occurring, how frequent they are, whether they are increasing or decreasing, and whether prevention methods have been effective. **Pub:** *Papers, charts.*


**★ 16805 ★ U.S. Department of Health and Human Services**
**Centers for Disease Control and Prevention**
**National Institute for Occupational Safety and Health**
**National Occupational Research Agenda (Social and Economic Consequences of Workplace Illness and Injury)**
1095 Willowdale Rd.
Morgantown, WV 26501
**Phone:** (304)285-6015        **Free:** 800-356-4676
**Email:** egb6@cdc.gov
**Website:** http://www.cdc.gov/niosh/nrsoce.html
Elyce Biddle, Contact

**Activities/Fields:** Social and economic consequences of workplace illness and injury.


**★ 16806 ★ U.S. Department of Health and Human Services**
**Centers for Disease Control and Prevention**
**National Institute for Occupational Safety and Health**
**National Occupational Research Agenda (Organization of Work)**
4676 Columbia Pkwy.
Cincinnati, OH 45226
**Phone:** (513)533-8383        **Free:** 800-356-4676
**Email:** sls4@cdc.gov
**Website:** http://www.cdc.gov/niosh/nrworg.html
Steven L. Sauter, Team Ldr.

**Activities/Fields:** Organization of work refers to the way work processes are structured and managed. In addition to job stress associated with aspects of work organization, studies are now identifying its contributions to other diverse health problems, including musculoskeletal disorders and cardiovascular diseases. Research areas include: surveillance, and etiologic studies of risk factors and intervention strategies to mitigate adverse work organization factors and outcomes.


**★ 16807 ★ U.S. Department of Health and Human Services**
**Centers for Disease Control and Prevention**
**National Institute for Occupational Safety and Health**
**National Occupational Research Agenda (Risk Assessment Methods)**
Risk Evaluation Branch
4676 Columbia Pkwy., C15
Cincinnati, OH 45226
**Phone:** (513)533-8365        **Free:** 800-356-4676
**Fax:** (513)533-8224
**Email:** lts2@cdc.gov
**Website:** http://www.cdc.gov/niosh/nrram.html
Leslie Stayner, PhD, Team Ldr.

**Activities/Fields:** To promote the development of new methods that will improve ability to accurately predict the risks associated with occupational exposure, which will facilitate the development of policies to protect workers.


**★ 16808 ★ U.S. Department of Health and Human Services**
**Centers for Disease Control and Prevention**
**National Institute for Occupational Safety and Health**
**National Occupational Research Agenda (Mixed Exposures)**
MS 4020
1095 Willowdale Rd.
Morgantown, WV 26505
**Phone:** (304)285-6121        **Free:** 800-356-4676
**Fax:** (304)285-6126
**Email:** fjh1@cdc.gov
**Website:** http://www2.cdc.gov/NORA/noratopic-temp.asp?rschearea=me
Frank J. Hearl, D. E. Team Ldr.

**Activities/Fields:** Identify the effects of the exposure to combinations of chemicals or physical agents to agricultural, industrial, and other workers.


**★ 16809 ★ U.S. Department of Health and Human Services**
**Centers for Disease Control and Prevention**
**National Institute for Occupational Safety and Health**
**National Occupational Research Agenda (Low Back Disorders)**
MS R-12
4676 Columbia Pkwy.
Cincinnati, OH 45226
**Phone:** (513)841-4428        **Free:** 800-356-4676
**Email:** ljf4@cdc.gov
**Website:** http://www.cdc.gov/niosh/nrlowbck.html
Lawrence J. Fine, Team Ldr.

**Activities/Fields:** Identify work activities and awkward postures that contribute to the causes of low back disorders.


**★ 16810 ★ U.S. Department of Health and Human Services**
**Centers for Disease Control and Prevention**
**National Institute for Occupational Safety and Health**
**National Occupational Research Agenda (Musculoskeletal Disorders of the Upper Extremities)**
MS R-12
4676 Columbia Pkwy.
Cincinnati, OH 45226
**Phone:** (513)841-4428        **Free:** 800-356-4676
**Email:** ljf4@cdc.gov
**Website:** http://www.cdc.gov/niosh/nrmusc.html
Lawrence J. Fine, MD, Dir.

**Activities/Fields:** Work-related musculoskeletal disorders (MSD), such as low back pain, tendonitis, hand-arm vibration syndrome, and carpel tunnel syndrome.


**★ 16811 ★ U.S. Department of Health and Human Services**
**Centers for Disease Control and Prevention**
**National Institute for Occupational Safety and Health**
**National Occupational Research Agenda (Intervention Effectiveness Research)**
4686 Columbia Pkwy.
Cincinnati, OH 45226
**Phone:** (513)841-4493        **Free:** 800-356-4676
**Email:** lyg9@cdc.gov
**Website:** http://www.cdc.gov/niosh/nriefr.html
Linda M. Goldenhar, Team Ldr.

**Activities/Fields:** Occupational disease and injury intervention, including safety and health training programs; health communications; changes in work environment or practices; control technologies (e.g., engineering techniques, recommending the use of protective equipment, and specific work practices); and regulatory and voluntary safety and health standards. **Pub:** *Evaluation Manual for Occupational Health & Safety Professionals.*


**★ 16812 ★ U.S. Department of Health and Human Services**
**Centers for Disease Control and Prevention**
**National Institute for Occupational Safety and Health**
**National Occupational Research Agenda (Infectious Diseases)**
1095 Willowdale Rd.
Morgantown, WV 26505
**Phone:** (304)285-5943        **Free:** 800-356-4676
**Email:** thh1@cdc.gov
**Website:** http://www.cdc.gov/niosh/nrinfc.html
Thomas K. Hodous, MD, Team Ldr.

**Activities/Fields:** Research to determine the extent of occupational transmission of infectious diseases, to understand the barriers to the use of safe work practices and vaccines, and develop and evaluate new control methods.

**★ 16813 ★ U.S. Department of Health and Human Services**
**Centers for Disease Control and Prevention**
**National Institute for Occupational Safety and Health**
**National Occupational Research Agenda (Indoor Environment)**
4676 Columbia Pkwy., R-16
Cincinnati, OH 45226
**Phone:** (513)841-4445      **Free:** 800-356-4676
**Fax:** (513)841-4486
**Email:** mfm0@cdc.gov
**Website:** http://www.cdc.gov/niosh/nrinev.html
Mark J. Mendell, PhD, Contact
**Activities/Fields:** Non-industrial workplace safety and health, including allergic and infectious diseases to non-specific symptoms such as headaches and eye irritation. **Pub:** *Articles.*

**★ 16814 ★ U.S. Department of Health and Human Services**
**Centers for Disease Control and Prevention**
**National Institute for Occupational Safety and Health**
**National Occupational Research Agenda (Hearing Loss)**
Robert A. Taft Laboratories
4756 Columbia Pkwy., MS C-27
Cincinnati, OH 45226
**Phone:** (513)533-8482      **Free:** 800-356-4676
**Fax:** (513)533-8139
**Email:** jrf3@cdc.gov
**Website:** http://www.cdc.gov/niosh/nrhear.html
John R. Franks, PhD, Team Ldr.
**Activities/Fields:** Occupational hearing loss as a result of chronic exposure to ototraumatic (damaging to the ear or hearing process) agents, including noise, solvents, metals, asphyxiants (e.g. carbon monoxide), and heat. **Pub:** *Papers.*

**U.S. Department of Health and Human Services**
**Centers for Disease Control and Prevention**
**National Institute for Occupational Safety and Health**
**National Occupational Research Agenda (Fertility and Pregnancy Abnormalities)**
*See:* Entry 18408

**★ 16815 ★ U.S. Department of Health and Human Services**
**Centers for Disease Control and Prevention**
**National Institute for Occupational Safety and Health**
**National Occupational Research Agenda (Health Services Research)**
Centers for Disease Control & Prevention
1600 Clifton Rd. NE, D40
Atlanta, GA 30333
**Phone:** (404)639-1534      **Free:** 800-356-4676
**Fax:** (404)639-2170
**Email:** sed2@cdc.gov
**Website:** http://www2.cdc.gov/NORA/noratopic-temp.asp?rscharea=hsr
Scott Deitchman, MD, Dep. Dir.
**Activities/Fields:** Identify priority topics for occupational health services; identify priority topics to develop tools and methodology for occupational health services research; promote the study of occupational health to researchers in the field; and disseminate the results of occupational health services research in

order to improve occupational health care. **Pub:** *Papers.*

**★ 16816 ★ U.S. Department of Health and Human Services**
**Centers for Disease Control and Prevention**
**National Institute for Occupational Safety and Health**
**National Occupational Research Agenda (Control Technology and Personal Protective Equipment)**
Engineering Control Technology Branch
Division of Physical Sciences & Engineering
MS-R5
4676 Columbia Pkwy.
Cincinnati, OH 45226
**Phone:** (513)841-4221      **Free:** 800-356-4676
**Fax:** (513)841-4506
**Email:** ler3@cdc.gov
**Website:** http://www.cdc.gov/niosh/nrppe.html
Larry Reed, Team Ldr.
**Activities/Fields:** Reduction of worker exposures to occupational hazards by various methods, including design changes to equipment, modifications to training efforts, or the use of personal protective equipment.

**★ 16817 ★ U.S. Department of Health and Human Services**
**Centers for Disease Control and Prevention**
**National Institute for Occupational Safety and Health**
**National Occupational Research Agenda (Exposure Assessment Methods Research)**
4676 Columbia Pkwy.
Cincinnati, OH 45226
**Phone:** (513)533-8465      **Free:** 800-356-4676
**Email:** mlw2@cdc.gov
**Website:** http://www.cdc.gov/niosh/nrexpo.html
Mary Lynn Woebkenberg, Team Ldr.
**Activities/Fields:** Reduction of workplace exposures. Research includes defining exposure-response relationships in epidemiologic studies in order to better identify at-risk workers, develop cost-effective control and intervention strategies and improved baseline data for standard setting and risk management.

**U.S. Department of Health and Human Services**
**Centers for Disease Control and Prevention**
**National Institute for Occupational Safety and Health**
**National Occupational Research Agenda (Cancer Research Methods)**
*See:* Entry 10430

**U.S. Department of Health and Human Services**
**Centers for Disease Control and Prevention**
**National Institute for Occupational Safety and Health**
**National Occupational Research Agenda (Occupational Asthma and Chronic Obstructive Pulmonary Disease)**
*See:* Entry 18763

**U.S. Department of Health and Human Services**
**Centers for Disease Control and Prevention**
**National Institute for Occupational Safety and Health**
**National Occupational Research Agenda (Allergic and Irritant Dermatitis)**
*See:* Entry 6855

**★ 16818 ★ U.S. Department of Health and Human Services**
**Centers for Disease Control and Prevention**
**National Institute for Occupational Safety and Health**
**National Occupational Research Agenda**
Hubert H. Humphrey Bldg.
200 Independence Ave. SW, Rm. 715H
Washington, DC 20201
**Phone:** (202)401-6977      **Free:** 800-356-4676
**Email:** bdtl@cdc.gov
**Website:** http://www.cdc.gov/niosh/nora
Kathleen M. Rest, Actg. Dir.
**Activities/Fields:** Occupational safety and health. **Pub:** *NORA News.*

**★ 16819 ★ U.S. Department of Health and Human Services**
**Centers for Disease Control and Prevention—National Institute for Occupational Safety and Health**
**National Farm Medicine Center**
**Midwest Center for Agricultural Disease and Injury Research, Education, and Prevention**
1000 N Oak Ave.
Marshfield, WI 54449-5790
**Free:** 800-662-6900      **Fax:** (715)389-3808
**Email:** nfmcsh@mfldclin.edu
**Website:** http://www.marshfieldclinic.org/nfmc/projects/default.htm
Dr. Anne Greenlee, Prin. Investigator
**Activities/Fields:** Investigating agricultural exposures, host susceptibility factors and risk of parkinson's disease; agromedicine training programs; safety education and prevention/intervention programs promoting sustained health of agricultural workers and families.

**★ 16820 ★ U.S. Department of Health and Human Services**
**National Institute for Occupational Safety and Health**
Hubert H. Humphrey Bldg., Rm. 715 H
Centers for Disease Control & Prevention
200 Independence Ave. SW
Washington, DC 20201
**Phone:** (202)401-6997      **Free:** 800-356-4674
**Fax:** (202)260-4464
**Email:** pubstaff@cdc.gov
**Website:** http://www.cdc.gov/niosh/homepage.html
Linda Rosenstock, MDM, Dir.
**Activities/Fields:** Research to eliminate on-the-job hazards to health and safety. Institute is responsible for identifying occupational safety and health hazards, for determining methods to control them, and for recommending federal standards to limit the hazards. Institute is also responsible for administering the x-ray surveillance program for coal miners and for testing and certifying respirators and hazard measuring devices. In addition to research done in laboratories, NIOSH conducts health hazard evaluations in all types of workplaces (including mines), assists other agencies to investigate potentially hazardous situations, and supports research and training programs through extramural grants. To focus research efforts and resources, the Institute has identified ten leading work-related diseases and injuries and has developed a proposed prevention strategy for each. The Institute, in

partnership with its stakeholders, developed a national Occupational Research Agenda (NORA) with 21 research areas. The Institute is working with other groups, both local and national, to establish a comprehensive national surveillance system for occupational disease and injuries. NIOSH recommendations are transmitted to the Department of Labor, which is responsible for setting and enforcing occupational standards. NIOSH laboratory research is conducted at the Robert A. Taft Laboratory and the Alice Hamilton Laboratory for Occupational Safety and Health in Cincinnati, OH, and at the Appalachian Laboratory for Occupational Safety and Health in Morgantown, WV, the Pittsburgh Research Laboratory in Burceto, PA and the Spokane research Laboratory in Spokane, WA. Data Base NIOSH maintains the Registry of Toxic Effects of Chemical Substances (RTECS) and the NIOSHTIC database with 144,000 entries; both are available in a variety of formats. **Pub:** *Proceedings.* • *Research Reports.* • *Technical and research reports*, periodically.

### ★ 16821 ★ U.S. Department of Health and Human Services
**National Institute for Occupational Safety and Health**
**Appalachian Laboratory for Occupational Safety and Health**
1095 Willowdale Rd.
Morgantown, WV 26505-2888
**Phone:** (304)285-5704          **Fax:** (304)285-5820
Charlotte Dalton, Management Oper. Off.

**Activities/Fields:** Occupational safety and health, focusing on safe working environments, occupational-related respiratory diseases, cross-sectional prospective morbidity and mortality studies, and performance records of respirators and hazard measuring instruments. Maintains a national surveillance data system for the early detection and monitoring of occupational accidents and injuries, and NIOSHTIC database and microfiche collection.

### ★ 16822 ★ U.S. Department of Health and Human Services
**National Institute for Occupational Safety and Health**
**Biomedical and Behavioral Science Division**
**Applied Biology Branch**
Robert A. Taft Laboratories
4676 Columbia Pkwy.
Cincinnati, OH 45226-1998
**Phone:** (513)533-8433          **Fax:** (513)533-8494
Gayle DeBord, PhD, Chf.

**Activities/Fields:** Biological monitoring and immunochemistry/immunotoxicology studies, inhalation toxicology, animal husbandry, and pathology.

### ★ 16823 ★ U.S. Department of Health and Human Services
**National Institute for Occupational Safety and Health**
**Biomedical and Behavioral Science Division**
**Applied Psychology and Ergonomics Branch**
Robert A. Taft Laboratories
4676 Columbia Pkwy. M.S C-24
Cincinnati, OH 45226-1998
**Phone:** (513)533-8291          **Fax:** (513)533-8596
**Email:** sls4@cdc.gov
Steve Sauter, Chf.

**Activities/Fields:** Occupational stress and ergonomics.

### ★ 16824 ★ U.S. Department of Health and Human Services
**National Institute for Occupational Safety and Health**
**Biomedical and Behavioral Science Division**
**Experimental Toxicology Branch**
Robert A. Taft Laboratories
Mail Stop C-23
4676 Columbia Pkwy.
Cincinnati, OH 45226
**Phone:** (513)533-8392          **Fax:** (513)533-8510
Dr. Russell Savage, Chf.

**Activities/Fields:** Toxicity of industrial chemicals. Activities involve investigations of carcinogenesis, mutagenesis, toxicity to the male and female reproductive systems, developmental toxicity, cardiovascular disease, pulmonary toxicology, dermatotoxicology, and biological monitoring and metabolism of xenobiotics. **Pub:** *Proceedings.*

### ★ 16825 ★ U.S. Department of Health and Human Services
**National Institute for Occupational Safety and Health**
**Biomedical and Behavioral Science Division**
**Physical Agents Effects Branch**
Robert A. Taft Laboratories, MS C-27
4676 Columbia Pkwy.
Cincinnati, OH 45226-1998
**Phone:** (513)533-8153          **Fax:** (513)533-8139
**Email:** wlotz@cdc.gov
**Website:** http://www.cdc.gov/niosh/homepage.html
W. Gregory Lotz, PhD, Sect. Chf.

**Activities/Fields:** Health effects of non-ionizing radiation and noise in the workplace.

### ★ 16826 ★ U.S. Department of Health and Human Services
**National Institute for Occupational Safety and Health**
**Education and Information Division**
**Information Resources Branch**
Robert A. Taft Laboratories
4676 Columbia Pkwy.
Cincinnati, OH 45226-1998
**Phone:** (513)533-8319          **Free:** 800-356-4674
**Fax:** (513)533-8347
**Email:** vep1@cdc.gov
**Website:** http://www.cdc.gov/niosh/im-eid.html
Vern Anderson, Chf.

**Activities/Fields:** Provides technical information support for NIOSH research programs. Its activities include collecting, organizing, and retrieving published and unpublished technical literature related to the field of occupational safety and health. **Pub:** *Audiovisual Catalog*, periodically. • *New Publication List*, periodically.

### ★ 16827 ★ U.S. Department of Health and Human Services
**National Institute for Occupational Safety and Health**
**Physical Sciences and Engineering Division**
**Engineering Control Technology Branch**
Robert A. Taft Laboratories
Mail Stop R-5
4676 Columbia Pkwy.
Cincinnati, OH 45226-1998
**Phone:** (513)841-4221          **Fax:** (513)841-4506
Robert Kurimo, Actg. Chf.

**Activities/Fields:** Planning and conducting worksite and laboratory research to identify and evaluate engineering control technology that will prevent worker exposure to toxic substances and harmful physical agents; promoting the transfer and widespread application of effective preventive engineering control measures for safeguarding worker health; providing engineering expertise in formulating effective and credible workplace standards; and providing technical consultation to other elements of the National Institute for Occupational Safety and Health and the Department of Labor in the application of new and improved techniques for hazard prevention and engineering controls. Branch comprises sections for chemical industry, minerals, materials processing, and general industry.

### ★ 16828 ★ U.S. Department of Health and Human Services
**National Institute for Occupational Safety and Health**
**Physical Sciences and Engineering Division**
**Methods Research Branch**
Robert A. Taft Laboratories
Mail Stop R-7
4676 Columbia Pkwy.
Cincinnati, OH 45226-1998
**Phone:** (513)841-4241          **Fax:** (513)841-4500
**Email:** erk1@cdc.gov
**Website:** http://www.cdc.gov/niosh/homepage.html
Dr. Eugene Kennedy, Chf.

**Activities/Fields:** Research that develops, improves and evaluates analytical methods for the evaluation of levels of toxic materials found in the work environment, and in industrial materials; providing expert consultation for the development of occupational health criteria and standards on methods for chemical analytical procedures; providing special consultation to the National Institute for Occupational Safety and Health and other government agencies; and providing validated NIOSH procedures for sampling and analytical methods. Branch comprises one section for special analyses for laboratory methods development. **Pub:** *NIOSH Manual of Analytical Methods*, biennially.

### ★ 16829 ★ U.S. Department of Health and Human Services
**National Institute for Occupational Safety and Health**
**Physical Sciences and Engineering Division**
**Quality Assurance and Statistics Activity**
Robert A. Taft Laboratories
4676 Columbia Pkwy. MS R-3
Cincinnati, OH 45226-1998
**Phone:** (513)841-4200          **Fax:** (513)841-4500
**Email:** pcs1@cdc.gov
Paul Schlecht, Chf.

**Activities/Fields:** Quality of NIOSH industrial hygiene laboratory services; conduct with the American Industrial Hygiene Association (AIHA) a proficiency testing program for industrial hygiene laboratories (the Proficiency Analytical Testing Program, covering a variety of metal and organic analyses, silica, and asbestos analyses); conduct with the U.S. Environmental Protection Agency and AIHA a proficiency testing program for environmental labs, including the Environmental Lead Proficiency Analytical Testing Program, which covers lead analyses in paint chips, soil, and dust wipes; and provide statistical support for NIOSH industrial hygiene chemistry and engineering control research. **Pub:** *NIOSH Manual of Analytical Methods.* **Frmly:** (1991) Monitoring and Control Research Branch; (2000) Physical Sciences and Engineering Division; Quality Assurance and Statistics Activity.

### ★ 16830 ★ U.S. Department of Health and Human Services
**National Institute for Occupational Safety and Health**
**Surveillance, Hazard Evaluations, and Field Studies Division**
Mail Stop R-12
Robert A. Taft Laboratories
4676 Columbia Pkwy.
Cincinnati, OH 45226-1998
**Phone:** (513)841-4428          **Fax:** (513)929-2653
**Email:** kjm3@cdc.gov

**Website:** http://www.cdc.gov/niosh/im-dshe.html
Kathy Masterson, Sec.

**Activities/Fields:** Epidemiologic field research and national surveillance in occupational health. Activities are carried out in three branches: Hazard Evaluations and Technical Assistance, Industrywide Studies, and Surveillance. A fourth branch, Support Services, provides medical, computer, and statistical services. **Pub:** *Proceedings.* • *Research Reports.*

**★ 16831 ★ U.S. Department of Health and Human Services**
**National Institute for Occupational Safety and Health**
**Surveillance, Hazard Evaluations, and Field Studies Division**
**Hazard Evaluations and Technical Assistance Branch**
Robert A. Taft Laboratories
Mail Stop R-9
4676 Columbia Pkwy.
Cincinnati, OH 45226-4382
**Phone:** (513)841-4505　　　**Fax:** (513)841-4483
**Email:** dss2@nioshe1.em.cdc.gov
**Website:** http://www.cdc.gov/niosh/im-dshe.html
Mr. Dave Sundin, Dep. Dir.

**Activities/Fields:** General industry requests for assistance in evaluating potential health hazard situations, including requests from employers, employees, employee representatives, other federal agencies, and state and local agencies. Branch evaluates whether or not chemical, biological, or physical agents are hazardous as used or found in the workplace and makes recommendations for control procedures, improved work practices, and medical screening to reduce exposure levels and subsequent health effects. Branch comprises sections for industrial hygiene and medical studies.

**★ 16832 ★ U.S. Department of Health and Human Services**
**National Institute for Occupational Safety and Health**
**Surveillance, Hazard Evaluations, and Field Studies Division**
**Industrywide Studies Branch**
Robert A. Taft Laboratories
4676 Columbia Pkwy., Rm. 13
Cincinnati, OH 45226-1998
**Phone:** (513)841-4203　　　**Fax:** (513)841-4486
**Email:** dz7k@nih.gov
**Website:**　　　http://www.cdc.gov/brances/itb/itb_index.html
Teresa Schnorr, Chf.

**Activities/Fields:** Industrywide studies, through record studies and clinical/environmental studies, to: identify occupational causes of disease in the working population and their offspring; determine the incidence and prevalence of acute and chronic effects from work-related exposures to toxic and hazardous substances; and provide information needed to develop standards to control occupational health hazards. Branch comprises sections for industrial hygiene and epidemiology.

**★ 16833 ★ U.S. Department of Health and Human Services**
**National Institute for Occupational Safety and Health**
**Surveillance, Hazard Evaluations, and Field Studies Division**
**Surveillance Branch**
Robert A. Taft Laboratories
4676 Columbia Pkwy., ML-R19
Cincinnati, OH 45226-1998
**Phone:** (513)841-4208　　　**Fax:** (513)841-4483
**Email:** jps4@cdc.gov
**Website:** http://www.cdc.gov/niosh/im-dshe.html
John Sestito, Ch. Surveillance Branch

**Activities/Fields:** Surveillance system of the nation's work force and its environs and to make an early detection and continuous assessment of the magnitude and extent of job-related illnesses, exposures, and hazardous agents. Branch comprises sections for medical activity, hazards, and illness effects.

**U.S. Department of Health and Human Services**
**National Institutes of Health**
**National Cancer Institute**
**Division of Cancer Epidemiology and Genetics**
**(Occupational Epidemiology Branch)**
*See:* Entry 10551

**U.S. Department of Transportation**
**Coast Guard**
**Office of Health and Safety**
**Safety and Environmental Health Division**
*See:* Entry 8973

**★ 16834 ★ University of California at Berkeley**
**Center for Occupational and Environmental Health**
School of Public Health
Berkeley, CA 94720-7360
**Phone:** (510)642-0761　　　**Fax:** (510)642-5815
**Email:** llew@uclink4.berkeley.edu
**Website:** http://coeh.berkeley.edu/
Dr. John R. Balmes, Dir.

**Activities/Fields:** Occupational medicine, toxicology, industrial hygiene, epidemiology, occupational health nursing, and ergonomics. Specific research includes studies on the causes, diagnosis, and prevention of occupational and environmental injuries and illnesses. **Pub:** *Center for Occupational and Environmental Health Newsletter,* quarterly. **Frmly:** Northern California Occupational Health Center.

**★ 16835 ★ University of California, Los Angeles**
**California Education and Research Center-Southern**
School of Public Health
650 Charles E Young Dr., S
CHS 56-071
Los Angeles, CA 90095-1772
**Phone:** (310)825-7152　　　**Fax:** (310)206-9903
**Email:** whinds@ucla.edu
**Website:** http://www.ph.ucla.edu/erc
William C. Hinds, ScD, Dir.

**Activities/Fields:** Occupational and environmental health issues. **Pub:** *Newsletter,* quarterly.

**★ 16836 ★ University of Cincinnati**
**Education and Research Center (ERC)**
3223 Eden Ave., ML No. 0056
Cincinnati, OH 45267-0056
**Phone:** (513)558-1749　　　**Fax:** (513)556-4999
**Email:** clarkcs@uc.edu
**Website:** http://www.uc.edu/erc/about_us.htm
Dr. Scott Clark, Dir.

**Activities/Fields:** Occupational safety and health.

**★ 16837 ★ University of Iowa**
**Great Plains Center for Agricultural Health**
Institute for Rural and Environmental Health
Iowa City, IA 52242-5000
**Phone:** (319)385-4887　　　**Free:** 877-611-4971
**Fax:** (319)335-4225
**Email:** gpch@mail.public-health.uiowa.edu
**Website:**　　　http://www.public-health.uiowa.edu/GPCAH/
Dr. Stephen Reynolds, Dir.

**Activities/Fields:** Training of agricultural health professionals; farm safety chapter development; education of health professionals; production of materials; industrial hygiene, including respirator evaluation, anhydrous ammonia, pesticide exposure, composting exposure, and dust reduction studies; toxicology, including organic dust induced lung inflammation, molecular biology methods for bioaerosol exposure assessment, and inhalation toxicology models; ergonomics, including etiology and prevention of carpal tunnel syndrome, and evaluation of assistive technologies; and rural health, including respiratory disease, dermatologic and allergic disease, hearing loss, neurologic disease and mental health, reproductive health outcomes, and the determinants of these disease outcomes in a random sample of farm, rural non-farm and town households in the Keokuk County, Iowa. **Frmly:** Center for Agricultural Disease and Injury Research, Education, and Prevention.

**★ 16838 ★ University of Iowa**
**Institute for Rural and Environmental Health**
Department of Occupational & Environmental Health
IREH, Oakdale Campus
Iowa City, IA 52242-5000
**Phone:** (319)335-4415　　　**Fax:** (319)335-4225
**Email:** craig-zwerling@uiowa.edu
Dr. Craig Zwerling, Dir.

**Activities/Fields:** Occupational injury and disease research and prevention and environmental health among farmers, those living in rural areas, and general industry. Conducts multidisciplinary studies of health effects due to modern agricultural and industrial practices, particularly in the areas of agricultural medicine, occupational medicine, industrial hygiene, environmental health, and environmental chemistry. **Frmly:** Institute of Agricultural Medicine and Occupational Health.

**★ 16839 ★ University of Maryland**
**Center for the Study of Human Performance in Dentistry**
Dental School
Baltimore College of Dental Surgery
666 W Baltimore St.
Baltimore, MD 21201-1586
**Phone:** (410)706-7342　　　**Fax:** (410)706-3028
**Email:** mmb001@dental.umaryland.edu
Michael M. Belenky, Dir.

**Activities/Fields:** Physical posture and ergonomic process for practicing dentistry, human-centered ergonomics for preclinical psychomotor education, and psychomotor skill applications to patient dental care. Studies optimal proprioceptive posture for peak performance, patient support, aseptic performance process, facility design, performance logic, performance simulation, psychomotor education, and the reduction/elimination of back, neck, and shoulder pain.

**★ 16840 ★ University of Michigan—Flint**
**Physical Therapy Cumulative Trauma Disorders Laboratory**
LS&A Bldg., Rm. 101
Physical Therapy Department
School of Health Professions & Studies
Flint, MI 48502
**Phone:** (810)762-3373　　　**Fax:** (810)766-6668
**Email:** cpfalzer@umich.edu
**Website:** http://www.flint.umich.edu/departments/pt
Lucinda Pfalzer, PhD, Dir.

**Activities/Fields:** Cumulative trauma disorders in the workplace, particularly carpal tunnel syndrome. Also studies the biomechanical, lifestyle, psychosocial, and economic factors involved in injury prevention in the work place. **Pub:** *Instructional Video.* • *Practice Video and Booklet.*

**★ 16841 ★ University of Minnesota**
**Midwest Center for Occupational Health and Safety**
School of Public Health
420 Delaware St. SE
Minneapolis, MN 55455

**Phone:** (612)626-0900  **Fax:** (612)626-4837
**Website:** http://www1.umn.edu/mcohs/
Ian A. Greaves, MD, Dir.

**Activities/Fields:** Occupational health and safety.

★ **16842** ★ **University of Montreal**
**Centre for Occupational Stress and**
**Health**
Sch. of Industrial Relations
Montreal, QC, Canada H3C 3J7
**Phone:** (514)343-7320  **Fax:** (514)343-5764
Dr. Shimon L. Dolan, Dir.

**Activities/Fields:** Diagnosis and intervention in the field of occupational stress, focusing on stress in police officers, social workers, hospital workers, executive personnel, and workers in other stressful occupations.

★ **16843** ★ **University of North Alabama**
**Occupational and Environmental Health**
**Laboratory**
UNA Box 5049
Department of Chemistry & Industrial Hygiene
Florence, AL 35632-0001
**Phone:** (205)765-4474  **Fax:** (205)765-4329
**Email:** mmoeller@unanov.una.edu
Dr. Michael Moeller, Contact

**Activities/Fields:** Conducts research in the areas of environmental health, industrial hygiene, and risk assessment.

★ **16844** ★ **University of North Carolina**
**at Chapel Hill**
**North Carolina Occupational Safety and**
**Health Education and Research Center**
**(NCERC)**
3300 Hwy. 54 West
Chapel Hill, NC 27516-8264
**Phone:** (919)962-2101  **Free:** 888-235-3320
**Fax:** (919)966-7579
**Email:** oshercww@sph.unc.edu
**Website:** http://www.sph.unc.edu/osherc/
David S. Abrams, Pres.

**Activities/Fields:** Occupational health and safety.

★ **16845** ★ **University of Quebec at**
**Montreal**
**Centre for Study of Biological**
**Interactions Between Environment and**
**Health**
PO Box 8888, Downtown Sta.
Montreal, QC, Canada H3C 3P8
**Phone:** (514)987-3915  **Fax:** (514)987-6183
**Email:** leduc.johanne@uqam.ca
**Website:** http://www.unites.uqam.ca/cinbiose/
Johanne Leduc, Contact

**Activities/Fields:** Occupational health, ergonomics.

★ **16846** ★ **University of Saskatchewan**
**Centre for Agricultural Medicine**
Royal University Hospital,
PO Box 120
103 Hospital Dr.
Saskatoon, SK, Canada S7N 0W8
**Phone:** (306)966-8286  **Fax:** (306)966-8799
**Email:** dosman@sask.usask.ca
**Website:** http://www.usask.ca/medicine/agmedicine
James A. Dosman, MD, Dir.

**Activities/Fields:** Agricultural health problems, including farm accidents, lung disease, cancer, stress, skin problems, and hearing loss.

★ **16847** ★ **University of South Florida**
**Sunshine Education and Research Center**
College of Public Health
13201 Bruce B. Downs Blvd., MDC 56
Tampa, FL 33612-3805
**Phone:** (813)974-6624  **Fax:** (813)974-7857

**Email:** dmcclusk@hsc.usf.edu
**Website:** http://www.hsc.usf.edu/erc/
Dr. Stuart M. Brooks, Dir.

**Activities/Fields:** Health in the workplace, including prevention of occupational asthma, analysis of repetitive motion injuries and ergonomic controls, management of indoor air quality, function and use of personal protective equipment, occupational infectious diseases including blood-borne pathogens, strategies that integrate the principles of risk analysis and assessment, and cost and quality issues of managed care for workers' compensation programs.

★ **16848** ★ **University of Utah**
**Rocky Mountain Center for Occupational**
**and Environmental Health**
75 South 2000 East
Salt Lake City, UT 84112
**Phone:** (801)581-8719  **Fax:** (801)581-7224
**Email:** rmoser@rmcoeh.utah.edu
**Website:** http://www.rmcoeh.utah.edu/
Dr. Royce Moser, Dir.

**Activities/Fields:** Occupational and environmental health and safety with emphasis on exposure assessment, environmental epidemiology, asbestos-related health problems, musculoskeletal and other injury evaluation and prevention, and ergonomic aspects of the work environment.

**University of Vermont**
**McClure Musculoskeletal Research Center**
*See:* Entry 13737

★ **16849** ★ **University of Virginia**
**International Health Care Worker Safety**
**Center**
PO Box 800764
Charlottesville, VA 22903
**Phone:** (434)924-5159  **Fax:** (434)982-0821
**Email:** bruce.beymon@uvm.edu
**Website:**  http://www.med.virginia.edu/~epinet/
center2.html
Janine Jagger, PhD, Dir.

**Activities/Fields:** Reduction of occupational exposures to and transmission of bloodborne pathogens to health care workers worldwide. **Pub:** *Advances in Exposure Prevention*, bimonthly.

★ **16850** ★ **University of Washington**
**Northwest Center for Occupational Health**
**and Safety**
Department of Environmental Health, Box 357234
School of Public Health
Seattle, WA 98195-7234
**Phone:** (206)685-3250  **Fax:** (206)616-2687
**Email:** mmorgan@u.washington.edu
Prof. Michael Morgan, Dir.

**Activities/Fields:** Occupational health and safety.

★ **16851** ★ **University of Wisconsin—**
**Madison**
**Wisconsin Occupational Health**
**Laboratory**
2601 Agriculture Dr.
PO Box 7996
Madison, WI 53703-7996
**Free:** 800-446-0403  **Fax:** (608)224-6213
**Email:** wohldirector@mail.slh.wisc.edu
**Website:** http://www.slh.wisc.edu/wohl/

**Activities/Fields:** Industrial hygiene. **Pub:** *Reactions Newsletter.* Newsletter.

★ **16852** ★ **Virginia Commonwealth**
**University**
**Rehabilitation Research and Training**
**Center on Workplace Supports**
1314 W Main St.
PO Box 842011
Richmond, VA 23284-2011

**Phone:** (434)828-1851  **Fax:** (434)828-2193
**Website:** http://www.worksupport.com/
John Kregel, Contact

**Activities/Fields:** Return to work strategies for persons who become disabled while employed; key components of effective disability management programs; financial tax credits to encourage hiring, retention, and advancement of the disabled; the impact of work support interventions on employment and advancement; employer perceptions of obstacles to hiring and retaining the disabled; and the significance of structural changes in the American economy on people with disabilities. **Pub:** *Newsletter.*

**Wayne State University**
**Institute of Environmental Health**
**Sciences**
*See:* Entry 17409

★ **16853** ★ **West Virginia University**
**Institute of Occupational and**
**Environmental Health**
3801 HSC
Sch. of Medicine
PO Box 9190
Morgantown, WV 26506-9190
**Phone:** (304)293-3693  **Fax:** (304)293-2629
**Email:** cmartin@hsc.wvu.edu
**Website:** http://www.hsc.wvu.edu/ioeh
Edward Doyle, MD, Dir.

**Activities/Fields:** Occupational and environmental health, including occupational medicine and environmental toxicology. **Pub:** *Occupational Health.*

**Western Michigan University**
**Occupational Therapy Teaching Research**
**Clinic**
*See:* Entry 20214

---

# State Government Agencies

## Occupational Health

★ **16854** ★ **Alabama Department of Labor**
**Occupational Injury Statistics and Fatality**
**Data Division**
100 N Union St.
Montgomery, AL 36130
**Phone:** (334)242-3460  **Fax:** (334)240-3417
**Email:** jbarnhart@email.state.al.us
**Website:** http://www.alalabor.state.al.us/
James Barnhart, Director

★ **16855** ★ **Alaska Department of Labor**
**Labor Standards and Safety Division**
**Occupational Safety and Health Section**
PO Box 21149
Juneau, AK 99802-1149
**Phone:** (907)465-4855  **Fax:** (907)465-3584
**Website:**  http://www.labor.state.ak.us/lss/osh-home.htm

★ **16856** ★ **Arizona Industrial**
**Commission**
**Occupational Safety and Health Division**
800 W Washington, 2nd Fl.
Phoenix, AZ 85007
**Phone:** (602)542-5795  **Fax:** (602)542-1614
**Email:** webmaster@ica.state.az.us
**Website:** http://www.ica.state.az.us/
Darin Perkins, Contact

**★ 16857 ★ Arkansas Department of Labor**
Safety Division
10421 W Markham
Little Rock, AR 72205
**Phone:** (501)682-4522          **Fax:** (501)682-4535
**Email:** clark.thomas@osha.gov
**Website:** http://www.accessarkansas.org/labor/divisions/safety_p1.html
Clark Thomas, Contact

**★ 16858 ★ California Department of Industrial Relations**
Occupational Safety and Health Division
455 Golden Gate Ave., 10th Fl.
San Francisco, CA 94102
**Phone:** (415)703-5100          **Fax:** (415)703-5135
**Email:** InfoCons@dir.ca.gov
**Website:** http://www.dir.ca.gov/dosh/dosh1.html

**★ 16859 ★ Colorado Department of Personnel**
General Support Services
Risk Management Division
1313 Sherman St, Rm 114
Denver, CO 80203
**Phone:** (303)866-3848          **Free:** 800-268-8092
**Fax:** (303)894-2409
**Email:** benefits.risk@state.co.us
**Website:** http://www.state.co.us/gov_dir/gss/hr/risk/riskindex.htm

**★ 16860 ★ Connecticut Department of Labor**
Occupational Safety and Health Division
38 Wolcott Hill Rd.
Wethersfield, CT 06109
**Phone:** (860)566-4550          **Fax:** (860)566-6916
**Website:** http://www.ctdol.state.ct.us/osha/osha.htm
Donald A. Heckler, Director

**★ 16861 ★ Delaware Department of Labor**
Industrial Affairs Division
Occupational Safety and Health Administration
4425 N Market St, 3rd floor
PO Box 8902
Wilmington, DE 19802
**Phone:** (302)761-8200
**Email:** ttrznadel@state.de.us
**Website:** http://www.delawareworks.com/divisions/industaffairs/occu.safety.html
Traci Trznadel, Contact

**★ 16862 ★ District of Columbia Department of Employment Services**
Labor Standards Office
Occupational Safety and Health Office
77 P St. NE
Washington, DC 20002
**Phone:** (202)671-1800
**Website:** http://does.ci.washington.dc.us/home/contact.shtm

**★ 16863 ★ Hawaii Department of Labor and Industrial Relations**
Occupational Safety and Health Branch
Keelikolani Bldg.
830 Punchbowl St., Rm. 423
Honolulu, HI 96813
**Phone:** (808)586-9100          **Fax:** (808)586-9104
**Website:** http://www.state.hi.us/dlir/hiosh/

**★ 16864 ★ Idaho Department of Labor and Industrial Services**
Safety Division
317 W Main St.
Boise, ID 83735-0060
**Phone:** (208)334-3570          **Fax:** (208)334-6300
**Email:** WWW@labor.state.id.us
**Website:** http://www.labor.state.id.us/

**★ 16865 ★ Illinois Department of Labor**
Public Safety Division
1 W Old State Capitol Plaza, Rm. 300
Springfield, IL 62701-1293
**Phone:** (217)782-9386
**Website:** http://www.state.il.us/agency/idol/
Robert M. Healey, Director

**★ 16866 ★ Indiana Department of Labor**
Safety, Education and Training Bureau
402 W Washington, Rm. W195
Indianapolis, IN 46204
**Phone:** (317)232-2688          **Fax:** (317)233-3790
**Email:** mstillman@dol.state.in.us
**Website:** http://www.state.in.us/labor/busets/buset.html

**★ 16867 ★ Kansas Department of Human Resources**
Labor-Management Relations and Employment Standards Division
Industrial Safety and Health Section
800 SW Jackson, Ste. 600
Topeka, KS 66612-1227
**Phone:** (785)296-4386          **Free:** 800-332-0353
**Email:** astanton@hr.state.ks.us
**Website:** http://www.hr.state.ks.us/wc/html/wcish.htm

**★ 16868 ★ Kentucky Labor Cabinet**
Occupational Safety and Health Review Commission
4 Mill Creek Pk.
Milville Rd.
Frankfort, KY 40601-9427
**Phone:** (502)573-6892          **Fax:** (502)573-4619
**Email:** george.kilbourne@mail.state.ky.us
**Website:** http://www.state.ky.us/agencies/labor/rchome.htm

**★ 16869 ★ Louisiana Department of Labor**
Worker's Compensation Office
Health and Safety Division
1001 N 23 St.
PO Box 94094
Baton Rouge, LA 70804-9094
**Phone:** (225)342-3111
**Email:** os@ldol.state.la.us
**Website:** http://www.ldol.state.la.us/

**★ 16870 ★ Maine Department of Labor**
Labor Standards Bureau
Safety Division
45 State House Station
Augusta, ME 04333-0045
**Phone:** (207)624-6400          **Fax:** (207)624-6449
**Email:** dave.e.wacker@state.me.us
**Website:** http://janus.state.me.us/labor/worksafe.htm
Michael V. Frett, Director

**★ 16871 ★ Maryland Department of Licensing and Regulation**
Labor and Industry Division
Occupational Safety and Health Section
1100 N Eutaw St., Rm. 208
Baltimore, MD 21201
**Phone:** (410)767-7233          **Fax:** (410)767-2003
**Email:** dli@dllr.state.md.us
**Website:** http://www.dllr.state.md.us/labor/mosh.html

**★ 16872 ★ Massachusetts Department of Labor and Workforce Development**
Division of Occupational Safety
OSHA Consultation Division
1001 Watertown St.
West Newton, MA 02465
**Phone:** (617)969-7177          **Fax:** (617)727-4581
**Email:** joe.lamalva@state.ma.us
**Website:** http://www.state.ma.us/dos/Consult/Consult.htm

**★ 16873 ★ Michigan Department of Consumer and Industry Services**
Bureau of Safety and Regulation
Occupational Health Division
7150 Harris Dr.
PO Box 30649
Lansing, MI 48909-8149
**Phone:** (517)322-1608          **Free:** 800-866-4674
**Email:** bsrinfo@cis.state.mi.us
**Website:** http://www.cis.state.mi.us/bsr/divisions/occ/home.htm

**★ 16874 ★ Minnesota Department of Labor and Industry**
Work Place Services Division
OSHA Consultation Unit
443 Lafayette Rd. N
Saint Paul, MN 55155
**Phone:** (651)284-5050          **Free:** 877-470-6742
**Email:** OSHA.Compliance@state.mn.us
**Website:** http://www.doli.state.mn.us/mnosha.html

**★ 16875 ★ Mississippi Department of Health**
Occupational Safety and Health Compliance
Mississippi State Univ.
Center for Safety and Health
106 Crosspark Dr., Suite C
Pearl, MS 39208
**Phone:** (601)939-2047          **Fax:** (601)939-6742
**Email:** kelly.tucker@ms-c-jackson.osha.gov
**Website:** http://www.msstate.edu/dept/csh/

**★ 16876 ★ Missouri Department of Labor and Industrial Relations**
Labor Standards Division
On-site Safety and Health Consultation Program
3315 W Truman Blvd.
PO Box 449
Jefferson City, MO 65102-0504
**Phone:** (573)751-3403          **Free:** 800-475-2130
**Fax:** (573)751-3721
**Email:** RSimmons@dolir.state.mo.us
**Website:** http://www.dolir.state.mo.us/ls/onsite/index.html
Robert Simmons, Director

**★ 16877 ★ Montana Department of Labor and Industry**
Employment Relations Division
Safety Bureau
PO Box 1728
Helena, MT 59624
**Phone:** (406)444-6401          **Fax:** (406)444-4140
**Email:** jmaloney@mt.gov
**Website:** http://erd.dli.state.mt.us/SB/page2.html

**★ 16878 ★ Nebraska Department of Labor**
Safety Division
301 Centennial Mall S
PO Box 95024
Lincoln, NE 68509-5024
**Phone:** (402)471-2239          **Free:** 800-582-7076

**Website:** http://www.dol.state.ne.us/nwd/center.cfm?PRICAT=1&SUBCAT=1D
Gary I. Hirsh, Director

**★ 16879 ★ Nevada Department of Business and Industry**
**Industrial Relations Division**
**Occupational Safety and Health Enforcement Section**
1301 N Green Valley Pkwy., Ste. 200
Henderson, NV 89014
**Phone:** (702)486-9044 **Fax:** (702)990-0358
**Email:** jwiles@govmail.state.nv.us
**Website:** http://dirweb.state.nv.us/oshes.htm
L. Tom Czehowski, Director

**★ 16880 ★ New Hampshire Department of Labor**
**Inspection Division**
**Safety Office**
95 Pleasant St.
PO Box 2230
Concord, NH 03301-3836
**Phone:** (603)271-6850
**Website:** http://www.state.nh.us/dol/dol-st/index.html
Cynthia Flynn, Contact

**★ 16881 ★ New Jersey Department of Health**
**Environmental and Occupational Health Services**
**Occupational Health Services Office**
PO Box 360
John Fitch Plaza
Trenton, NJ 08625-0369
**Phone:** (609)984-1863 **Fax:** (609)984-2779
**Email:** koleary@doh.state.nj.us
**Website:** http://www.state.nj.us/health/eoh/odisweb/
Kathleen O'Leary, Contact

**★ 16882 ★ New Mexico Department Environment**
**Environmental Protection Division**
**Occupational Health and Safety Bureau**
Harold S Runnels Bldg
1190 St. Francis Dr.
Santa Fe, NM 87502-0110
**Phone:** (505)827-2855 **Free:** 800-219-6157
**Email:** melanie_montoya@nmenv.state.nm.us
**Website:** http://www.nmenv.state.nm.us/Ohsb/osha-home.htm

**★ 16883 ★ New York State Department of Labor**
**Occupational Safety and Health Division**
W Averill Harriman Campus
Rm. 522 Bldg. 12
Albany, NY 12240
**Phone:** (518)457-1125 **Fax:** (518)457-1167
**Website:** http://www.labor.state.ny.us/business_ny/employer_responsibilities/safety/shdists.htm
Richard Cucolo, Director

**★ 16884 ★ North Carolina Department of Labor**
**Occupational Safety and Health Review Board**
4 W Edenton St., Ste. 105
Raleigh, NC 27603-3432
**Phone:** (919)733-3589
**Email:** lkafel@mail.dol.state.nc.us
**Website:** http://www.dol.state.nc.us/osha/osh.htm

**★ 16885 ★ North Dakota Department of Loss Prevention**
**Worker's Compensation Bureau**
500 E Front Ave.
Bismarck, ND 58504-5685

**Phone:** (701)328-3800 **Free:** 800-777-5033
**Email:** ndworkerscomp@wcb.state.nd.us
**Website:** http://www.ndworkerscomp.com/

**★ 16886 ★ Ohio Department of Health**
**Prevention Division**
**Bureau of Health Promotion and Risk Reduction**
246 N High St.
PO Box 118
Columbus, OH 43216
**Phone:** (614)466-2144
**Email:** webmaster@gw.odh.state.oh.us
**Website:** http://www.odh.state.oh.us/
Frank Bright, Director

**★ 16887 ★ Oklahoma Department of Labor**
**OSHA Consultation Division**
4001 N Lincoln Blvd.
Oklahoma City, OK 73105-5212
**Phone:** (405)528-1500 **Free:** 888-269-5353
**Fax:** (405)528-5751
**Email:** labor.info@oklaosf.state.ok.us
**Website:** http://www.state.ok.us/~okdol/osha/index.htm

**★ 16888 ★ Oregon Consumer and Business Services Department**
**Occupational Safety and Health Division**
350 Winter St., NE
Rm. 430
Salem, OR 97301-3882
**Phone:** (503)378-3272 **Free:** 800-922-2689
**Fax:** (503)947-7461
**Email:** tia.m.howell@state.or.us
**Website:** http://www.cbs.state.or.us/osha/

**★ 16889 ★ Pennsylvania Department of Labor and Industry**
**Occupational and Industrial Safety Bureau**
Labor and Industry Bldg.
7th & Forster St.
Harrisburg, PA 17121
**Phone:** (717)787-3323 **Fax:** (717)783-5225
**Website:** http://www.li.state.pa.us/bois/index.html

**★ 16890 ★ Rhode Island Department of Labor and Training**
**Workforce Regulation and Safety Division**
**Occupational Safety and Health Administration**
Center General Complex
1511 Pontiac Ave.
Cranston, RI 02910
**Phone:** (401)462-8580
**Email:** mmadonna@dlt.state.ri.us
**Website:** http://www.dlt.state.ri.us/

**★ 16891 ★ South Carolina Department of Labor, Licensing, and Regulation**
**Occupational Safety and Health Division**
110 Centerview Dr.
Columbia, SC 29210
**Phone:** (803)734-9599 **Fax:** (803)734-9741
**Email:** scovp@mail.llr.state.sc.us
**Website:** http://www.llr.state.sc.us/scovp/index.asp?file=ovpform.htm

**★ 16892 ★ South Dakota Department of Health**
**Health Systems Development and Regulation Division**
600 E Capitol
Pierre, SD 57501-2536
**Phone:** (605)773-3364 **Free:** 800-738-2301
**Email:** DOH.INFO@state.sd.us

**Website:** http://www.state.sd.us/doh/programs.htm

**★ 16893 ★ Tennessee Department of Labor**
**Occupational Safety and Health Division**
Andrew Johnson Tower, 3rd floor
710 James Robertson Pkwy.
Nashville, TN 37243
**Phone:** (615)741-2793 **Free:** 800-249-8510
**Fax:** (615)253-1623
**Email:** steve.hawkins@state.tn.us
**Website:** http://www.state.tn.us/labor-wfd/tosha.html
John Winkler, Contact

**★ 16894 ★ Texas Department of Health**
**Toxic Substances Control Division**
**Industrial Hygiene Branch**
1100 W 49th St.
Austin, TX 78756
**Phone:** (512)834-6600 **Fax:** (512)834-6644
**Email:** ih@tdh.state.tx.us
**Website:** http://www.tdh.state.tx.us/beh/ih/

**★ 16895 ★ USF Safety Florida Consultation Program**
**Safety Division**
4003 East Fowler Ave
Tampa, FL 33617
**Phone:** (813)974-9962
**Email:** cvespi@hsc.usf.edu
**Website:** http://www.safetyflorida.usf.edu/
Charlene Vespi, Contact

**★ 16896 ★ Utah Labor Commission**
**OSHA Division**
160 E 300 S, 3rd Fl.
PO Box 146600
Salt Lake City, UT 84114-6600
**Phone:** (801)530-6901
**Email:** nanderson@utah.gov
**Website:** http://www.uosh.utah.gov/
Larry Patrick, Contact

**★ 16897 ★ Vermont Department of Labor and Industry**
**Occupational Safety and Health Administration**
National Life Bldg.
Drawer 20
Montpelier, VT 05620-3401
**Phone:** (802)828-2765 **Fax:** (802)828-2195
**Email:** voshainfo@labind.state.vt.us
**Website:** http://www.state.vt.us/labind/vosha.htm
Robert McLeod, Director

**★ 16898 ★ Virginia Department of Labor and Industry**
**Occupational Health Compliance Division**
Powers Taylor Bldg.
13 S 13th St.
Richmond, VA 23219
**Phone:** (804)786-0574
**Email:** hcompliance@doli.state.va.us
**Website:** http://www.dli.state.va.us/programs/safety.htm

**★ 16899 ★ Washington Department of Labor and Industries**
**Consultation and Compliance Services Division**
PO Box 44648
Olympia, WA 98504
**Phone:** (360)902-5588
**Website:** http://www.wa.gov/lni/scs/

**★ 16900 ★ West Virginia Department of Health and Human Resources**
**Public Health Bureau**
**Environmental Health Office**
**Radiation, Toxic, and Indoor Air Quality Division**
815 Quarrier St., Ste. 418
Charleston, WV 25301
**Phone:** (304)558-2981          **Fax:** (304)558-1289
**Email:** rcurtis@wvdhhr.org
**Website:** http://www.wvdhhr.org/oehs/rtia.html
Randy C. Curtis, Director

**★ 16901 ★ Wisconsin Department of Commerce**
**Safety and Buildings Division**
201 W Washington Ave.
4th floor
Madison, WI 53703
**Phone:** (608)266-3151
**Email:** ttaylor@commerce.state.wi.us
**Website:** http://www.commerce.state.wi.us/SB/SB-HomePage.html

**★ 16902 ★ Wyoming Department of Employment**
**Workers Safety and Compensation Division**
1510 E Pershing Blvd.
122 W 25th St.
Cheyenne, WY 82002
**Phone:** (307)777-7159          **Fax:** (307)777-5946
**Email:** kmckin1@state.wy.us
**Website:** http://wydoe.state.wy.us/doe.asp?ID=9
Kathleen McKinna, Contact

# Chapter 47
# Orthopedics

## Foundations & Other Funding Organizations

### Other Funding Organizations

**American College of Chiropractic Orthopedists (ACCO)**
*See:* Entry 5886

**★ 16903 ★ American Orthopaedic Foot and Ankle Society (AOFAS)**
2517 Eastlake Ave. E, Ste. 200
Seattle, WA 98102
**Phone:** (206)223-1120     **Free:** 800-235-4855
**Fax:** (206)223-1178
**Email:** aofas@aofas.org
**Website:** http://www.aofas.org
Richard Cantrall, Exec. Dir.

**Desc:** Members of American Academy of Orthopaedic Surgeons (see separate entry) interested in research on, education in, and care of the foot and ankle. Sponsors continuing medical education courses. **Awards:** Goldner Award (annual); Kenneth Johnson MD Memorial Lectureship (annual); Roger Mann MD Award (annual).

**★ 16904 ★ American Orthopaedic Society for Sports Medicine (AOSSM)**
6300 N River Rd., Ste. 200
Rosemont, IL 60018
**Phone:** (847)292-4900     **Free:** 877-321-3500
**Fax:** (847)292-4905
**Email:** irv@aossm.org
**Website:** http://www.sportsmed.org
Irvin E. Bomberger, Exec. Dir.

**Desc:** Promotes sports medicine education, research, communication and fellowship; disseminates information to orthopaedic surgeons working in sports medicine. **Awards:** Excellence in Research (annual).

**★ 16905 ★ Association of Bone and Joint Surgeons (ABJS)**
6300 N River Rd., Ste. 727
Rosemont, IL 60018-4226
**Phone:** (847)698-1636     **Fax:** (847)823-0536
**Email:** jones@aaos.org
**Website:** http://www.abjs.org
Colette Hohimer, Soc. Dir.

**Desc:** Orthopedic surgeons interested in clinical aspects of orthopedics and in training of leaders in the specialty. **Awards:** Marshall R. Urist Award; Nicolas Andry Award (annual).

**★ 16906 ★ Pediatric Orthopaedic Society of North America (POSNA)**
6300 N River Rd., Ste. 727
Rosemont, IL 60018-4226
**Phone:** (847)698-1692     **Fax:** (847)823-0536
**Email:** goldberg@aaos.org

**Website:** http://www.posna.org
Sharon Goldberg, Exec. Dir.

**Desc:** Pediatric orthopedic surgeons. Purpose is to provide continuing education to members. Conducts tutorial programs. **Awards:** Huene Award (annual) for past and future research in pediatric orthodpaedics - publishable material.

**★ 16907 ★ Ruth Jackson Orthopaedic Society (RJOS)**
c/o Mary Gebhardt
6300 N River Rd., Ste. 727
Rosemont, IL 60018
**Fax:** (847)823-0536
**Email:** gebhardt@aaos.org
Mary Gebhardt, Contact

**Desc:** Women orthopaedic surgeons, residents, fellows, and medical students. Seeks to advance the science of orthopaedic surgery and to provide support for women orthopaedic surgeons. Named for practicing orthopaedic surgeon Dr. Ruth Jackson (1902-94), the first woman certified by the American Board of Orthopaedic Surgery and the first female member of the American Academy of Orthopaedic Surgeons. Conducts educational programs; operates placement service and speakers' bureau, holds biennial meeting, sponsors mentoring program, offers traveling fellowship and resident research award. **Awards:** Resident Research Award (annual); RJOS Traveling Fellowship (annual) for interest in promoting the general cause of women in orthopaedics.

**★ 16908 ★ Scoliosis Research Society (SRSO)**
611 E Wells St.
Milwaukee, WI 53202
**Phone:** (414)289-9107     **Fax:** (414)276-3349
**Email:** tgoulding@execinc.com
**Website:** http://www.srs.org
Tressa Goulding, Exec. Dir.

**Desc:** Orthopedic surgeons and physicians. Furthers research and education in spinal deformities, particularly scoliosis, a twisting of the spine to one side. Most cases are of unknown cause, though scoliosis can result from a birth defect, polio, or spinal injury and usually develops in children during the growth spurt between ages ten and 15. Early detection followed with use of a brace and exercise can halt the curvature and prevent deformity. **Awards:** Grant (periodic).

## National & International Organizations

**★ 16909 ★ Academic Orthopaedic Society (AOS)**
6300 N River Rd., Ste. 727
Rosemont, IL 60018-4226
**Phone:** (847)698-1694     **Fax:** (847)823-0536
**Email:** wlezien@aaos.org/swift@aaos.org

**Website:** http://www.a-o-s.org
Peggy Wlezien, Mgr.

**Fnded:** 1971. **Desc:** Chairpersons and faculty members of orthopedic departments and divisions of medical schools; directors of orthopedic residency programs; fellowship directors. Provides forum for discussion of administrative and departmental problems concerning undergraduate and graduate orthopedics education in medical schools. Coordinates and plans activities requiring cooperation between orthopedic departments and residencies. Acts as liaison between orthopedic organizations and organizations interested in medical education. **Pub:** *Presidential Newsletter*, semiannual. Newsletter. • Directory, annual. **Frmly:** (1989) Association of Orthopaedic Chairmen; (1991) American Orthopaedic Society.

**American Academy of Neurological and Orthopaedic Surgeons (AANOS)**
*See:* Entry 19462

**American Academy of Orthopaedic Surgeons (AAOS)**
*See:* Entry 19464

**★ 16910 ★ American Association of Orthopedic Medicine (AAOM)**
30897 CR 356-3
PO Box 4997
Buena Vista, CO 81211-4997
**Phone:** (719)475-0032     **Free:** 800-992-2063
**Fax:** (719)395-5615
**Email:** orthopaedic@aaomed.org
**Website:** http://www.aaomed.org
Jeff Peterson, DO, Contact

**Fnded:** 1982. **Mem:** 450. **Desc:** Physicians and allied health professionals interested in the advancement of knowledge, diagnosis, and nonsurgical treatment of musculoskeletal and related disorders. Seeks to: advance the standards of practice and quality of service in the field of orthopedic medicine; unite the common interests and skills of medicine and osteopathy; serve as a forum of learning for all of the specialties that deal with pain and dysfunction in the neural, muscular, skeletal, and vascular systems. Encourages research and the dissemination of results. Provides training and continuing medical education in orthopedic medicine; conducts regional seminars every two to three months. **Pub:** *AAOM Membership Directory*, annual. Membership Directory. • *AAOM News*, quarterly. • *The Journal of Orthopaedic Medicine*, 3/year. Journal. Contains scientific papers and articles, editorials, and book reviews. *Price:* Included in membership dues.

**American Board of Orthopaedic Surgery (ABOS)**
*See:* Entry 19478

**★ 16911 ★ American College of Chiropractic Orthopedists (ACCO)**
c/o Dr. Jesse Rothenberger
1030 Broadway, Ste. 101
El Centro, CA 92243
**Phone:** (760)370-9106
**Website:** http://www.accoweb.org
Dr. Jesse Rothenberger, Pres.
**Fnded:** 1964. **Mem:** 730. **Desc:** Certified (426) and noncertified (304) chiropractic orthopedists; students enrolled in a postgraduate chiropractic orthopedic program (100). Seeks to establish and maintain optimal educational and clinical standards within the field of chiropractic orthopedics. Sponsors educational programs. **Pub:** *Journal of the American College of Chiropractic Orthopedists*, semiannual. Journal. *Price:* available to members only. • Membership Directory, annual. • Also publishes orthopedic and neurologic tests booklets. **AKA:** American College of Chiropractic Specialists.

**American College of Foot and Ankle Orthopedics and Medicine (ACFAOM)**
*See:* Entry 17705

**★ 16912 ★ American Orthopaedic Association (AOA)**
6300 N River Rd., Ste. 505
Rosemont, IL 60018-4263
**Phone:** (847)318-7330      **Fax:** (847)318-7339
**Email:** info@aoassn.org
**Website:** http://www.aoassn.org
Thomas E. Stautzenbach, Exec. Dir.
**Fnded:** 1887. **Mem:** 10,000. **Desc:** Professional society of bone and joint surgeons. Seeks to further knowledge in the diagnosis and treatment of crippling diseases. **Pub:** *American Orthopedic Association–Newsletter*, 3/year. Journal. • *Journal on Bone and Joint Surgery*, 8/year. Journal.

**★ 16913 ★ American Orthopaedic Foot and Ankle Society (AOFAS)**
2517 Eastlake Ave. E, Ste. 200
Seattle, WA 98102
**Phone:** (206)223-1120      **Free:** 800-235-4855
**Fax:** (206)223-1178
**Email:** aofas@aofas.org
**Website:** http://www.aofas.org
Richard Cantrall, Exec. Dir.
**Fnded:** 1969. **Mem:** 1,800. **Desc:** Members of American Academy of Orthopaedic Surgeons interested in research on, education in, and care of the foot and ankle. Sponsors continuing medical education courses. **Pub:** *A Guide to Children's Shoes.* Pamphlet. • *The Adult Foot.* Pamphlet. • *The Child's Foot.* Pamphlet. • *The Diabetic Foot.* Pamphlet. • *Foot and Ankle International*, monthly. Journal. *Price:* Included in membership dues; $149/year for nonmembers; $180/year for institutions; $11/copy. • *Getting in Step with Arthritis.* Pamphlet. • *How to Select Sport Shoes.* Pamphlet. • *Ten Points of Shoe Fit.* Pamphlet. **Frmly:** (1983) American Orthopaedic Foot Society.

**★ 16914 ★ American Orthopaedic Society for Sports Medicine (AOSSM)**
6300 N River Rd., Ste. 200
Rosemont, IL 60018
**Phone:** (847)292-4900      **Free:** 877-321-3500
**Fax:** (847)292-4905
**Email:** irv@aossm.org
**Website:** http://www.sportsmed.org
Irvin E. Bomberger, Exec. Dir.
**Fnded:** 1972. **Mem:** 1,600. **Desc:** Promotes sports medicine education, research, communication and fellowship; disseminates information to orthopaedic surgeons working in sports medicine. **Pub:** *American Journal of Sports Medicine*, bimonthly. Journal. Reports on the diagnosis, treatment, prevention, and rehabilitation of sports-related injury and disease; also includes society news and book reviews. *Price:* $80/year for individuals; $100/year for institutions; $30/year students.

**American Shoulder and Elbow Surgeons (ASES)**
*See:* Entry 19487

**★ 16915 ★ American Society of Orthopaedic Physician's Assistants (ASOPA)**
6300 N River Rd., Ste. 727
Rosemont, IL 60018-4226
**Free:** 800-998-6022      **Fax:** (847)823-0536
**Email:** asopa@aaos.org
**Website:** http://www.asopa.org
**Desc:** Physician's assistants who specialize in orthopaedic board-certified surgery. Aims to enhance the quality of medical treatment of orthopaedic patients. Provides information on advances in the field through continuing education, certification, publications and meetings.

**★ 16916 ★ Argentine Orthopedic and Traumatology Association (A.A.O.T.) (Asociacion Argentina de Ortopedia y Traumatologia)**
Vicente Lopez 1878
1128 Buenos Aires, Argentina
**Phone:** 54 1 48012320      **Fax:** 54 1 48017703
**Fnded:** 1936.

**Arthroscopy Association of North America (AANA)**
*See:* Entry 19504

**★ 16917 ★ ASEAN Orthopedic Association**
Orthopaedic Clinic
Mt. Elizabeth Medical Centre 05-07
3 Mt. Elizabeth
Singapore 228510, Singapore
**Phone:** 65 7342244      **Fax:** 65 7331485
**Email:** shannongoh@pacific.net.sg
**Website:** http://www.aana.org
**Lang(s):** Chinese, English. **Desc:** Orthopedists and other health care professionals with an interest in orthopedics. Seeks to advance orthopedic study, teaching, and practice. Facilitates exchange of information among members; sponsors continuing professional development courses.

**★ 16918 ★ Asia Pacific Orthopaedic Association (APOA)**
c/o APOA Business Centre
68 Greenhill Rd.
Wayville, SA 5034, Australia
**Phone:** 61 8 82746060      **Fax:** 61 8 82746000
**Email:** apoa@sapmea.asn.au
**Website:** http://www.asiapacificoa.com
**Fnded:** 1962. **Mem:** 1,602. **Reg. Groups:** 12. **Lang(s):** English. **Desc:** Orthopedic surgeons in 16 Asia countries. Facilitates the exchange of ideas and discuss new developments and methods relating to orthopedic surgery. Sponsors the Zimmer-WPOA Travelling Fellowship which enables young orthopedic surgeons to travel to academic training centers in the Asia Pacific region. **Pub:** *Journal of Orthopaedic Surgery*, 3/year. Journal. • *Newsletter of the Western Pacific Orthopaedic Association*, quarterly.

**Asian Association for Dynamic Osteosynthesis (AADO)**
*See:* Entry 13555

**★ 16919 ★ Association of Bone and Joint Surgeons (ABJS)**
6300 N River Rd., Ste. 727
Rosemont, IL 60018-4226
**Phone:** (847)698-1636      **Fax:** (847)823-0536
**Email:** jones@aaos.org

**Website:** http://www.abjs.org
Colette Hohimer, Soc. Dir.
**Fnded:** 1947. **Mem:** 265. **Desc:** Orthopedic surgeons interested in clinical aspects of orthopedics and in training of leaders in the specialty. **Pub:** *Clinical Orthopaedics and Related Research*, monthly. Journal. **Frmly:** ABJS.

**★ 16920 ★ Australian Orthopedic Association**
229 Macquarie St
Sydney, NSW 2000, Australia
**Phone:** 61 2 2333018      **Fax:** 61 2 2218301
**Fnded:** 1936.

**Bones Society**
*See:* Entry 13568

**★ 16921 ★ British Orthopaedic Association**
c/o Royal College of Surgeons
35-43 Lincoln's Inn Fields
London WC2A 3PN, United Kingdom
**Phone:** 44 207 4056507      **Fax:** 44 207 8312676
**Email:** secretary@boa.ac.uk
**Website:** http://www.boa.ac.uk
**Fnded:** 1918. **Mem:** 2,700. **Desc:** Practising orthopaedic surgeons, orthopaedic surgeons in training, retired orthopaedic surgeons, orthopaedic surgeons resident abroad who have done all or part training in the United Kingdom. Concerned with the advancement of the science, art and practice of orthopaedic surgery with the aim of bringing relief to patients of all ages suffering from the effects of injury or disease to the musculo-skeletal system. **Pub:** *British Orthopaedic News*, semiannual.

**British Society for Surgery of the Hand**
*See:* Entry 19533

**★ 16922 ★ Canadian Orthopaedic Association (COA) (Association Canadienne d'Orthopedie — ACO)**
1440 St. Catherine St. W, Ste. 718
Montreal, QC, Canada H3G 1R8
**Phone:** (514)874-9003      **Fax:** (514)874-0464
**Email:** info@coa-aco.org
**Website:** http://www.coa-aco.org
**Fnded:** 1945. **Mem:** 1,100. **Lang(s):** English, French. **Desc:** Orthopedic surgeons. Seeks to advance the study and practice of orthopedics. Facilitates exchange of information among members; sponsors research and educational programs. **Pub:** *COA Bulletin*, quarterly. Magazine.

**★ 16923 ★ Canadian Orthopaedic Foundation (COF)**
1033 McNicoll Ave., 2nd Fl.
Toronto, ON, Canada M1W 3W6
**Phone:** (416)492-3341      **Free:** 800-461-3639
**Email:** mailbox@canorth.org
**Website:** http://www.canorth.org
**Lang(s):** English, French. **Desc:** Health care professionals specializing in orthopedics. Seeks to advance orthopedic research, study, and practice. Serves as a clearinghouse on orthopedices; provides support and assistance to medical students; sponsors educational programs.

**Canadian Orthopaedic Nurses Association (CONA) (Association Canadienne des Infirmieres et Infirmiers en Orthopedie — ACIO)**
*See:* Entry 15696

**★ 16924 ★ Canadian Society of Orthopaedic Technologists (CSOT) (Societe Canadienne des Technologistes en Orthopedie — SCTO)**
18 Wynford Dr., No. 516
North York, ON, Canada M3C 3S2
**Phone:** (416)445-4516 **Fax:** (416)445-4513
**Email:** cinacsot@idirect.com
**Website:** http://www.csotcina.com
**Fnded:** 1972. **Mem:** 325. **Reg. Groups:** 7. **Lang(s):** English. **Desc:** Individuals employed in the application of plaster casts and traction assemblies; associate members are persons working in related fields; industrial members are those engaged in the manufacture or sale of orthopedic equipment or supplies. Promotes and develops uniform training programs and examinations that contribute to the science of medicine. Facilitates cooperation between orthopedic technologists and the medical profession. **Pub:** *Body Cast*, quarterly. Journal. • *News Cast*, quarterly.

**★ 16925 ★ Clinical Orthopaedic Society (COS)**
PO Box 531823
Indianapolis, IN 46253-1823
**Phone:** (317)388-0329 **Free:** 800-843-9735
**Fax:** (317)388-8984
**Email:** clinicalorthosoc@aol.com
**Website:** http://www.cosociety.org
Stephen K. Bubb, Pres.
**Fnded:** 1912. **Mem:** 700. **Desc:** Orthopedic surgeons practicing in cities of the Midwest. **Pub:** Directory, annual.

**★ 16926 ★ Conservative Orthopedics International Association (COIA)**
2547 Monroe St.
Dearborn, MI 48124
**Phone:** (313)563-0360 **Fax:** (248)669-0636
Dr. Stephen R. Castor, Pres.
**Fnded:** 1982. **Mem:** 4,222. **Desc:** Medical doctors, osteopaths, chiropractors, orthopedists, psychiatrists, and physical therapists. Promotes continuing education, research, and practice of conservative orthopedics. (Conservative orthopedics concentrates on nonoperative, nonradical, preventive and rehabilitative treatment of musculoskeletal disorders.) Seeks to advance the science and art of conservative orthopedics as they relate to the whole person. Operates charitable program; compiles statistics. Maintains speakers' bureau; offers educational and research programs. Sponsors hall of fame. **Pub:** *Conservative Orthopedics International Bulletin*, annual. Bulletin. • *Updates*, periodic. • Membership Directory, periodic. • Newsletter, quarterly.

**Council on Chiropractic Orthopedics (CCO)**
*See:* Entry 5924

**★ 16927 ★ Danish Orthopedic Society (Dansk Ortopaedisk Selskab — DOS)**
Blegdamsvej
DK-2100 Copenhagen, Denmark
**Email:** dok@dadlnet.dk
**Website:** http://www.ortopaedi.dk
**Fnded:** 1946.

**★ 16928 ★ Egyptian Orthopaedic Association (EOA)**
c/o Hasan Elzaher Hassan, Pres.
Sharia Houda Shaarawi
Cairo 11111, Egypt
**Phone:** 20 2 3930013 **Fax:** 20 2 3930054
**Email:** eoa@starnet.com
**Website:** http://www.eoa.org.eg
**Fnded:** 1948. **Mem:** 2,000. **Lang(s):** English. **Desc:** Seeks to improve the knowledge of its members. Offers courses in orthopedics.

**★ 16929 ★ European Pediatric Orthopaedic Society (EPOS)**
Weligerveld 1
3212 Pellenberg, Belgium
**Phone:** 32 1 6338803 **Fax:** 32 1 6338800
**Email:** guy.fabry@uz.kuleuven.ac.be
**Fnded:** 1982. **Desc:** Promotes the advancement of pediatric orthopedics, particularly in the practice, scientific research and teaching of effects on the locomotor system during growth and of understanding of the bone pathology of the child.

**★ 16930 ★ European Society for Movement Analysis in Adults and Children (ESMAC)**
Tayside Orthopaedic and Rehabilitation Technology Centre
Ninewells Hospital and Medical School
Dundee DD1 9SY, United Kingdom
**Phone:** 44 1382 496286 **Fax:** 44 1382 496322
**Email:** j.r.linskell@dundee.ac.uk
**Website:** http://www.dundee.ac.uk/orthopaedics/esmac/
**Fnded:** 1992. **Lang(s):** English. **Desc:** Orthopedists and other health care professionals, researchers, and scientists with an interest in human gait and posture and their impact on overall health. Works to advance scientific knowledge in the field of movement analysis; promotes continuing professional development of members. Facilitates communication and cooperation among members; conducts educational programs and courses.

**★ 16931 ★ French Society of Manual Medicine, Orthopedic and Osteopathics (Societe Francaise de Medecine Manuelle Orthopedique et Osteopathique — SOFMMOO)**
56, av Joseph Giordan
F-06200 Nice, France
**Phone:** 33 4 93211043 **Fax:** 33 4 93216547
**Fnded:** 1968. **Desc:** Promotes and teaches orthopedic medicine and manual medicine.

**★ 16932 ★ International College of Cranio-Mandibular Orthopedics**
c/o Hallie Truswell
619 N 35th St., Ste. 307
Seattle, WA 98103
**Phone:** (206)633-4355 **Free:** 800-446-1763
**Fax:** (206)633-4352
**Email:** hallie@tmj-iccmo.org
**Website:** http://tmj-iccmo.org
Hallie Truswell, Exec. Dir.
**Fnded:** 1979. **Mem:** 550. **Desc:** Cranio-mandibular orthopedists. Seeks to advance the study and practice of cranio-mandibular orthopedics. Conducts continuing professional development courses for members. **Pub:** *ICCMO Newsletter*, 3/year. Newsletter. • *Journal of Craniomandibular Orthopedics*, 3/year. Journal.

**International Society of Arthroscopy, Knee Surgery and Orthopaedic Sports Medicine (ISAKOS)**
*See:* Entry 19570

**★ 16933 ★ International Society of Orthopaedic Surgery and Traumatology (Societe Internationale de Chirurgie Orthopedique et de Traumatologie — SICOT)**
40, rue Washington, bte. 9
B-1050 Brussels, Belgium
**Phone:** 32 2 6486823 **Fax:** 32 2 6498601
**Email:** hq@sicot.org
**Website:** http://www.sicot.org
**Fnded:** 1929. **Mem:** 3,000. **Nat'l Groups:** 108. **Lang(s):** English, French. **Desc:** Orthopaedic surgeons in 108 countries united to contribute to the progress of science by conducting studies related to orthopedic surgery and traumatology. **Pub:** *International Orthopedics*, bimonthly. Journal. Includes Newsletter.

**National Association of Orthopaedic Nurses (NAON)**
*See:* Entry 15734

**★ 16934 ★ National Association of Orthopaedic Technologists (NAOT)**
2950 Buskirk Ave., Ste. 170
Walnut Creek, CA 94596
**Phone:** (925)472-5822 **Fax:** (925)472-5901
**Email:** naot@hp-assoc.com
**Website:** http://naot.org
Kent Lindeman, Exec. Dir.
**Fnded:** 1982. **Mem:** 1,100. **Reg. Groups:** 4. **Local Groups:** 23. **Desc:** Allied health assistants working with orthopedic patients. Promotes continued professional education of members and other orthopedic health care providers; administers certification examination. Seeks to enhance public understanding of orthopedics. Conducts seminars; compiles statistics. **Pub:** *OnLine: Advancements in Orthopaedic Technology*, bimonthly. Newsletter. Includes orthopaedic articles, meeting updates, and technology tips.

**★ 16935 ★ National Board for Certification of Orthopaedic Technologists (NBCOT)**
PMB No. 166
4736 Onondaga Blvd.
Syracuse, NY 13219
**Free:** (866)466-2268 **Fax:** (866)466-2268
**Email:** gonbcot@aol.com
**Website:** http://www.nbcot.net
Jeffrey Virgo, Chairman
**Fnded:** 1983. **Mem:** 1,386. **Desc:** Determines educational standards for certification in orthopedics. Provides educational programs for recertification. Offers telephone referral service.

**Orthopaedic Section, American Physical Therapy Association**
*See:* Entry 20164

**★ 16936 ★ Orthopaedic Trauma Association (OTA)**
6300 N River Rd., Ste. 727
Rosemont, IL 60018-4226
**Phone:** (847)698-1631 **Free:** 800-346-2267
**Fax:** (847)823-0536
**Email:** franzon@aaos.org
**Website:** http://www.ota.org
Nancy E. Franzon, Exec. Dir.
**Fnded:** 1983. **Mem:** 450. **Desc:** Physicians and other health care professionals with an interest in orthopedic trauma. Seeks to advance research and education in the practice of orthopedics; promotes development of improved orthopedic trauma treatment techniques; works to educate the public regarding safety issues in motor vehicle accidents. Serves as a clearinghouse on orthopedic trauma; conducts continuing professional development courses. **Pub:** *Fracture Lines*, periodic. Newsletter. *Price:* For members only. • *Journal of Orthopaedic Trauma*, periodic. Journal. • Abstracts of lectures given at annual meeting in JBJS and on-line.

**★ 16937 ★ Orthopaedics Overseas (OO)**
PO Box 65157
Washington, DC 20035-5157
**Phone:** (202)296-0928 **Fax:** (202)296-8018
**Email:** info@hvousa.org
**Website:** http://www.hvousa.org
Nancy Kelly, Exec. Dir.
**Fnded:** 1959. **Mem:** 775. **Desc:** Orthopedic surgeons interested in volunteering as consultants in developing countries. Trains physicians in developing countries in diagnostic, conservative, and operative management

techniques. Addresses chronic and acute orthopedic problems and crippling diseases such as polio and arthritis. Operates programs in Cambodia, Bhutan, Nepal, Malawi, Kenya, St. Lucia, South Africa, Uganda, Vietnam, and Ethiopia. Formerly a project of CARE, the group is a division of Health Volunteers Overseas. HVO also sponsors Anesthesia Overseas, Dentistry Overseas, Nursing Overseas, Oral and Maxillofacial Surgery Overseas, and Pediatrics Overseas, Internal Medicine Overseas, Nurse Anesthesia Overseas, and Physical Therapy Overseas.

★ 16938 ★ **Orthopedic Research Society (ORS)**
6300 N River Rd., Ste. 727
Rosemont, IL 60018-4226
**Phone:** (847)384-4240          **Fax:** (847)823-4921
**Email:** ors@aaos.org
**Website:** http://www.ors.org
Brenda Welborn, Exec. Dir.

**Fnded:** 1954. **Mem:** 1,870. **Desc:** Orthopedic surgeons and other investigators who are elected as active members on the basis of previous scientific activity, continued participation in the field of research, and accomplishments in orthopedic surgery. Promotes orthopedic research and provides a meeting place for presentation and discussion of orthopedic research activities. **Pub:** *Journal of Orthopedic Research*, quarterly. Published for Musculoskeletal investigators. *Price:* $164 in U.S.; $190 elsewhere. • *Transactions of Annual Meeting*. Proceedings. *Price:* $45.

**Pediatric Orthopaedic Society of North America (POSNA)**
*See:* Entry 5743

★ 16939 ★ **Physicians Association for Orthopedics
(Berufsverband der Arzte fur Orthopadie)**
Am Lindenbaum 6-8
D-60433 Frankfurt, Germany
**Phone:** 49 69 520095          **Fax:** 49 69 532083
**Email:** goldberg@aaos.org
**Website:** http://www.posna.org

**Fnded:** 1951. **Mem:** 6,300. **Desc:** Orthopedic physicians in Germany. Promotes the practice of orthopedics. **Pub:** *Informationen*, bimonthly. Newsletter.

★ 16940 ★ **Ruth Jackson Orthopaedic Society (RJOS)**
c/o Mary Gebhardt
6300 N River Rd., Ste. 727
Rosemont, IL 60018
**Fax:** (847)823-0536
**Email:** gebhardt@aaos.org
Mary Gebhardt, Contact

**Fnded:** 1983. **Mem:** 469. **Desc:** Women orthopaedic surgeons, residents, fellows, and medical students. Seeks to advance the science of orthopaedic surgery and to provide support for women orthopaedic surgeons. Named for practicing orthopaedic surgeon Dr. Ruth Jackson (1902-94), the first woman certified by the American Board of Orthopaedic Surgery and the first female member of the American Academy of Orthopaedic Surgeons. Conducts educational programs; operates placement service and speakers' bureau, holds biennial meeting, sponsors mentoring program, offers traveling fellowship and resident research award. **Pub:** *Membership List*, periodic. Newsletter. *Price:* $150. • *Ruth Jackson Society Newsletter*, semiannual. Newsletter. Includes articles on international members and careers and personal life; also contains calendar of events, upcoming meetings and courses. *Price:* Free. **Frmly:** (1991) Ruth Jackson Society.

★ 16941 ★ **Society of Military Orthopaedic Surgeons (SOMOS)**
810 North St.
Belgium, WI 53004-9531
**Phone:** (262)285-4280          **Fax:** (262)285-4231

**Email:** yolich@email.msn.com
**Website:** http://www.somos.org/
Ellen M. Yolich, Exec. Sec.

**Fnded:** 1958. **Mem:** 750. **Desc:** Orthopedic surgeons who have served in the active or reserve military. Objectives are to: stimulate scholarly contribution by military medical residents; act as clearinghouse; provide opportunities for consultation with and contributions of surgeons who are retired from the military; further the continuing education of orthopedic surgeons and residents. Presents scientific papers at annual meeting.

★ 16942 ★ **South African Orthopaedic Association (SAOA)
(Suid-Afrikaanse Ortopediese Vereniging — SAOV)**
PO Box 12918
Brandhof 9324, Republic of South Africa
**Phone:** 27 51 4303280          **Fax:** 27 51 4303284
**Email:** saoa@megaweb.co.za
**Website:** http://www.saoa.org.za/

**Fnded:** 1942. **Mem:** 850. **Lang(s):** Afrikaans, English. **Desc:** Works to advance the science and art of orthopedic surgery and to protect the professional, financial, and educational interests of members. Provides orthopedic services to neighboring regions without orthopedic facilities. Promotes research in the field. **Pub:** *Journal of Bone and Joint Surgery*, monthly. Journal. • *Membership Directory*, annual. Directory. • *SA Orthopaedic Bulletin*, quarterly. Bulletin.

★ 16943 ★ **Turkish Association of Orthopaedics and Traumatology (TAOT)
(Turk Ortopedi ve Travmatoloji Dernegi — TOTD)**
I.U. Istanbul Tip Fakultesi
Ortopedi ve Travmatoloji
Anabilim Dali
Capa
TR-34390 Istanbul, Turkey
**Phone:** 90 212 5241053          **Fax:** 90 212 6352835
**Email:** info@aott.org.tr

**Fnded:** 1939. **Mem:** 1,300. **Lang(s):** English, Turkish. **Desc:** Medical professionals specializing in orthodics and trauma care. Conducts seminars on orthopedic surgery. Offers postgraduate educational courses; conducts research. **Pub:** *Acta Orthopaedica et Traumatologica Turcica*, 5/year. Journal. Includes abstracts in English. • Books.

## Research Centers

★ 16944 ★ **Anderson Orthopaedic Research Institute**
PO Box 7088
Alexandria, VA 22307
**Phone:** (703)619-4411          **Fax:** (703)799-5982
**Email:** research@aori.org
**Website:** http://www.aori.org
Dr. Charles A. Engh, Sr., Med. Dir.

**Activities/Fields:** Orthopaedics, focusing on total joint replacements.

★ 16945 ★ **Center for Hip and Knee Surgery**
Orthopaedic Research Foundation, Inc.
Kendrick Memorial Hospital
1199 Hadley Rd.
Mooresville, IN 46158
**Phone:** (317)831-2273          **Fax:** (317)831-9347
**Email:** pegbal@aol.com
**Website:** http://www.hipandkneesurgery.com
Marjorie J. Albohm, Dir.

**Activities/Fields:** Total joint replacement surgery, arthritis surgery, reconstructive joint surgery, sports medicine, physical therapy, and foot, ankle, and shoulder surgery.

**Cincinnati Sports Medicine Research and Education Foundation**
*See:* Entry 19176

★ 16946 ★ **Foundation for Hand Research and Education**
8501 Harcourt Rd.
PO Box 80434
Indianapolis, IN 46280-0434
**Phone:** (317)471-4340          **Fax:** (317)876-0462
**Email:** eskopelja@indianahandcenter.com
**Website:** http://www.indianahandcenter.com
Elaine Skopelja, Mgr.

**Activities/Fields:** Upper extremity surgery and rehabilitation. **Pub:** *Indiana Hand Center Newsletter*, quarterly.

★ 16947 ★ **Hospital for Joint Diseases Orthopaedic Institute
Cartilage and Bone Research Center**
301 E 17th St.
New York, NY 10003
**Phone:** (212)598-6567          **Fax:** (212)598-6096
**Email:** pedicesare@aol.com
**Website:** http://www.msnyuhealth.org/hospitals/hja/html/body_ortho_cart_bone_res.html
Paul Di Cesare, MD, Contact

**Activities/Fields:** Role of noncollagenous matrix in human rheumatoid and osteoarthritis and the role of the inflammatory phase in demineralized bone osteoinduction.

★ 16948 ★ **Hospital for Joint Diseases Orthopaedic Institute
Geriatric Hip Fracture Research Group**
301 E 17th St.
New York, NY 10003
**Phone:** (212)598-6106          **Fax:** (212)598-6793
**Email:** gina.aharonoff@med.nyu.edu
Joseph D. Zuckerman, MD, Dir.

**Activities/Fields:** Hip fracture patients and their recovery after surgery.

★ 16949 ★ **Hospital for Joint Diseases Orthopaedic Institute
Shoulder Institute and Research Group**
301 E 17th St.
New York, NY 10003
**Phone:** (212)598-6498          **Fax:** (212)598-6096
**Website:** http://www.msnyuhealth.org/hospitals/hjd/html/orthopaedics.html
Frances Cuomo, MD, Dir.

**Activities/Fields:** Shoulder disorders, including the effect of osteoarthritis and instability on proprioceptive ability, strength recovery following rotator cuff repair, operative vs. nonoperative treatment of type II distal clavicle fractures, and recovery of strength and propriaception after two different capsulorrhaphy procedures.

★ 16950 ★ **Hospital for Special Surgery Research Division**
535 E 70th St.
New York, NY 10021
**Phone:** (212)606-1453          **Fax:** (212)717-1192
**Email:** boskeya@hss.edu
**Website:** http://www.hss.edu
Adele L. Boskey, PhD, Dir. of Res.

**Activities/Fields:** Orthopedics and rheumatic diseases, including studies on bone, cartilage, connective tissues, immune system, and related areas of musculoskeletal disease. **Frmly:** Philip D. Wilson Research Foundation.

**Hospital for Special Surgery Research Division
Biomechanics and Biomaterials Section**
*See:* Entry 4647

**★ 16951 ★ Hospital for Special Surgery
Research Division
Laboratory for Soft Tissues Research**
535 E 70th St.
New York, NY 10021
**Phone:** (212)606-1178    **Fax:** (212)772-6389
**Email:** warrenr@hss.edu
**Website:** http://www.hss.edu/
Russell F. Warren, MD, Sect. Hd.
**Activities/Fields:** Connective soft tissues related to orthopedics and rheumatology.


**★ 16952 ★ Johns Hopkins University
Biomechanics Research Laboratory**
Department of Orthopaedic Surgery
5601 Loch Raven Blvd., 4N
Baltimore, MD 21239
**Phone:** (410)532-4486    **Fax:** (410)532-4488
**Email:** echao@jhmi.edu
**Website:** http://www.biomech.jhu.edu
Dr. Edmund Y.S. Chao, Contact
**Activities/Fields:** Orthopedic concerns and the application of engineering principles to the better treatment and care of patients.


**Little People's Research Fund, Inc.**
*See:* Entry 13694


**★ 16953 ★ National Orthotic and
Prosthetic Research Institute**
PO Box 491
New York, NY 10021
**Phone:** (212)755-3366
**Email:** lprf@lprf.org
**Website:** http://www.lprf.org
Ralph Florio, Pres.
**Activities/Fields:** Fabrication of aluminum into canes, crutches, and walkers.


**★ 16954 ★ Northwestern University
Prosthetics Research Laboratory**
345 E Superior St., Rm. 1441
Chicago, IL 60611-4496
**Phone:** (312)238-6502    **Fax:** (312)238-6510
**Email:** d-childress@northwestern.edu
**Website:** http://www.repoc.northwestern.edu/
Dr. Dudley S. Childress, Dir.
**Activities/Fields:** Improvement of prostheses and orthoses, fitting and manufacturing processes for such devices, and basic understanding of human interactions with systems of these types. **Pub:** *Resource Guide of Prosthetics and Orthotics.*


**★ 16955 ★ Northwestern University
Rehabilitation Engineering Research
Center in Prosthetics and Orthotics**
Rehabilitation Institute of Chicago
345 E Superior St., Rm. 1441
Chicago, IL 60611-4496
**Phone:** (312)238-6500    **Fax:** (312)238-6510
**Email:** d-childress@northwestern.edu
Dr. Dudley S. Childress, Dir.
**Activities/Fields:** Improvement of prostheses and orthoses, improved fitting and manufacturing processes for prothesis/orthosis systems, and improved basic understanding of human interactions with these systems. **Pub:** *Reports.* • *Resource Guide of Prosthetics and Orthotics.*


**★ 16956 ★ Orthopedic Biomechanics
Institute**
5848 South 300 East
Murray, UT 84107-6121
**Phone:** (801)314-4030    **Fax:** (801)314-4015
E. Paul France, PhD, Dir.
**Activities/Fields:** Orthopedic biomechanics and sports injuries.


**★ 16957 ★ Orthopedic Research Institute**
929 N St. Francis
Wichita, KS 67214-3882
**Phone:** (316)268-5454    **Fax:** (316)291-4998
**Email:** ori@via-christi.org
**Website:** http://www.via-christi.org/ori/
David A. McQueen, Pres.
**Activities/Fields:** Design, development, and testing of orthopaedic implants, materials, and instruments. Specific areas of research include artificial replacement joints, absorbable pins and rods for surgically stabilizing bone fractures, devices for the fusion of severely compromised knees, applying a metal foam to orthopaedic implants for tissue attachment, improving external frames for controlling grossly unstable fractures of the pelvis, and combining absorbable glass fibers and plastics for composite implants in the human body. **Pub:** *Orthopaedic Technology Brief,* occasionally.


**★ 16958 ★ Orthopedic Research Society**
6300 N River Rd., Ste. 727
Rosemont, IL 60018-4226
**Phone:** (847)698-1625    **Fax:** (847)823-4921
**Email:** ors@aaos.org
**Website:** http://www.ors.org
Colette Hohimer, Dir.
**Activities/Fields:** Orthopedic surgery and research.


**★ 16959 ★ Pennsylvania State University
Center for Locomotion Studies**
Recreation Bldg., Rm. 29
University Park, PA 16802-2002
**Phone:** (814)865-1972    **Fax:** (814)863-4755
**Email:** prc@psu.edu
**Website:** http://www.celos.psu.edu
Peter R. Cavanagh, PhD, Dir.
**Activities/Fields:** Gait analysis and foot mechanics with particular emphasis on diabetic patients, children with cerebral palsy, and the elderly; elucidation of the pathogenesis of osteoporosis, including genetic control, and development of preventative interventions; development of computer modeling tools for selection of cerebral palsy patients who are likely to benefit from specific interventions and providing rationales for new measures to correct the mechanics of walking disrupted by cerebral palsy; the nature and causes of locomotor pathologies. **Pub:** *The Foot in Diabetes: A Bibliography.*


**★ 16960 ★ Ranawat Orthopedic Research
Foundation, Inc.**
Lenox Hill Hospital
130 E 77th St.
New York, NY 10021-1803
**Phone:** (212)434-4700    **Fax:** (212)628-4782
**Email:** csranawat@mindspring.com
**Website:** http://www.totaljoint.com
Chitranjan S. Ranawat, MD, Dir.
**Activities/Fields:** Materials and methods related to total hip and knee replacement surgery.


**Texas Health Research Institute (THRI)**
*See:* Entry 4550


**Texas Scottish Rite Hospital for Children
Research Department**
*See:* Entry 5814


**★ 16961 ★ University of Michigan
Orthopaedic Research Laboratories**
400 N Ingalls Bldg.
Ann Arbor, MI 48109-0486
**Phone:** (734)763-9674    **Fax:** (734)647-0003
**Email:** richb@tsrh.edu
**Website:** http://www.orl.med.umich.edu/orl/orl.html
Dr. S.A. Goldstein, Dir.
**Activities/Fields:** Applies principles of engineering to understand the musculoskeletal system, investigates orthopedic clinical problems, and develops prosthetic devices for treatment of arthritis. **Frmly:** Biomechanics Trauma and Sports Medicine Laboratory.


**Wayne State University
Bioengineering Center**
*See:* Entry 4576

## Foundations & Other Funding Organizations

### Other Funding Organizations

**★ 16962 ★ American Association of Colleges of Osteopathic Medicine (AACOM)**
5550 Friendship Blvd., Ste. 310
Chevy Chase, MD 20815-7231
**Phone:** (301)968-4100 **Fax:** (301)968-4101
**Email:** dwood@aacom.org
**Website:** http://www.aacom.org
Douglas L. Wood, DO, Pres.
**Desc:** Osteopathic medical colleges. Operates centralized application service; monitors and works with Congress and other government agencies in the planning of health care programs. Gathers statistics on osteopathic medical students, on innovations in medical education, faculty, administers federal contract, develops national communication programs on behalf of member colleges. **Awards:** Sherry R. Arnstein Minority Student Scholarship (annual) qualifying current or incoming minority student at a U.S. collegeof osteopathic medicine.

**★ 16963 ★ American Osteopathic Association (AOA)**
142 E Ontario St.
Chicago, IL 60611
**Free:** 800-621-1773 **Fax:** (312)202-8200
**Email:** info@aoa-net.org
**Website:** http://www.aoa-net.org
John B. Crosby, Exec. Dir.
**Desc:** Osteopathic physicians, surgeons, and graduates of approved colleges of osteopathic medicine. Associate members include teaching, research, administrative, and executive employees of approved colleges, hospitals, divisional societies, and affiliated organizations. Forms (with its affiliates) an officially recognized structure of the osteopathic profession. Promotes the public health, to encourage scientific research, and to maintain and improve high standards of medical education in osteopathic colleges. Inspects and accredits colleges and hospitals; conducts a specialty certification program; sponsors a national examining board satisfactory to state licensing agencies; maintains mandatory program of continuing medical education for members. Compiles statistics on location and type of practice of osteopathic physicians. Sponsors research activities through Bureau of Research in osteopathic colleges and hospitals. Maintains Physician Placement Service. Produces public service radio and television programs; maintains 2000 item library and biographical archives on osteopathic medicine and history. Offers speakers' bureau. **Awards:** Grant; scholarship.

**★ 16964 ★ American Osteopathic Foundation (AOF)**
c/o Leda Hanin
142 East Ontario
Chicago, IL 60611
**Phone:** (312)202-8234 **Fax:** (312)202-8216
**Email:** Sdowney@aoa-net.org
**Website:** http://www.osteopathic.org
Eugene A. Oliveri, Chair
**Desc:** Osteopathic physicians and laypersons interested in raising and administering funds for osteopathic medical education, research, colleges, and hospitals. Functions as philanthropic affiliate of the American Osteopathic Association; seeks to foster understanding of osteopathic principles and practice. **Awards:** Bristol-Myers Squibb Outstanding Resident Award (annual) for a 2nd or 3rd yr. osteopathic medical resident in Family Practice, Internal Medicine, or Pediatrics; Donna Jones Moritsugu Award (annual) for a spouse of a fourth-year osteopathic medical student; Russell C. McCaughan Education Fund Scholarship (annual) for a rising second-year student at each of the osteopathic colleges; Zeneca Pharmaceuticals Underserved Healthcare Grant (annual) for one or two student in the colleges of osteopathic medicine, demonstrating commitment to practice in underserved or minority populations.

**★ 16965 ★ Auxiliary to the American Osteopathic Association (AAOA)**
142 E Ontario St.
Chicago, IL 60611
**Fax:** (312)202-8218
**Email:** bprice@aoa-net.org
**Website:** http://www.aux-aoa.org
Bridget Price, Exec. Dir.
**Desc:** Immediate family members of osteopathic physicians; spouses of students of osteopathic medicine. Promotes public health education; provides funds for scholarships for the training of osteopathic physicians and surgeons, and for research and other activities at osteopathic colleges; encourages establishment and continuation of volunteer service organizations in nonprofit osteopathic hospitals; participates in national and community health programs. Sponsors summer seminars. **Awards:** Scholarship (annual) for sophomores attending an accredited osteopathic college.

## Medical & Allied Health Schools

### Osteopathic Medicine

*The following schools of osteopathic medicine are accredited by the American Osteopathic Association, Bureau of Professional Education. Professional associations to contact for general information on osteopathic medical education are the American Osteopathic Association (142 E Ontario St., Chicago, IL 60611, (800)621-1773, http://www.aoa-net.org/) and the American Association of Colleges of Osteopathic Medicine (5550 Friendship Blvd., Ste. 310, Chevy Chase, MD 20815-7231, (301)968-4100, http://www.aacom.org/).*

### Arizona

**★ 16966 ★ Arizona College of Osteopathic Medicine (AZCOM)**
19555 N 59th Ave.
Glendale, AZ 85308
**Phone:** (623)572-3215 **Free:** 888-247-9277
**Website:** http://www.midwestern.edu/Pages/AZCOM.html

### California

**★ 16967 ★ Touro University College of Osteopathic Medicine (TUCOM)**
Mare Island, Quarters C
832 Walnut Ave.
Vallejo, CA 94592
**Phone:** (707)562-5100
**Website:** http://www.tucom.edu

**★ 16968 ★ Western University of Health Sciences**
**College of Osteopathic Medicine of the Pacific (COMP)**
309 E 2nd St. and College Plaza
Pomona, CA 91766-1889
**Phone:** (909)623-6116
**Website:** http://www.westernu.edu/comp.html

### Florida

**★ 16969 ★ Nova Southeastern University College of Osteopathic Medicine (NSU-COM)**
3200 S University Dr.
Fort Lauderdale, FL 33328
**Phone:** (954)262-1407 **Free:** 800-356-0026
**Fax:** (954)262-2250
**Website:** http://medicine.nova.edu

### Illinois

**★ 16970 ★ Midwestern University**
**Chicago College of Osteopathic Medicine (CCOM)**
555 31st St.
Downers Grove, IL 60515
**Phone:** (630)515-6171 **Free:** 800-458-6253
**Website:** http://www.midwestern.edu/Pages/CCOM.html

## Iowa

**★ 16971 ★ Des Moines University**
**College of Osteopathic Medicine and**
**Surgery**
3200 Grand Ave.
Des Moines, IA 50312
**Phone:** (515)271-1450
**Website:** http://www.uomhs.edu

## Kentucky

**★ 16972 ★ Pikeville College**
**School of Osteopathic Medicine (PCSOM)**
147 Sycamore St.
Pikeville, KY 41501
**Phone:** (606)218-5250
**Website:** http://pcsom.pc.edu

## Maine

**★ 16973 ★ University of New England**
**College of Osteopathic Medicine (UNE/**
**COM)**
11 Hills Beach Rd.
Biddeford, ME 04005
**Free:** 800-477-4863
**Website:** http://www.une.edu/com/main.html

## Michigan

**★ 16974 ★ Michigan State University**
**College of Osteopathic Medicine (MSU/**
**COM)**
E Fee Hall, A-309
East Lansing, MI 48824
**Phone:** (517)353-7740
**Website:** http://www.com.msu.edu

## Missouri

**★ 16975 ★ Kirksville College of**
**Osteopathic Medicine (KCOM)**
800 W Jefferson St.
Kirksville, MO 63501
**Phone:** (660)626-2237
**Website:** http://www.kcom.edu

**★ 16976 ★ University of Health Sciences**
**College of Osteopathic Medicine (UHS-**
**COM)**
1750 Independence Ave.
Kansas City, MO 64106
**Free:** 800-234-4847
**Website:** http://www.uhs.edu

## New Jersey

**★ 16977 ★ University of Medicine and**
**Dentistry of New Jersey**
**School of Osteopathic Medicine (UMDNJ-**
**SOM)**
Academic Center
1 Medical Center Dr.
Stratford, NJ 08084
**Phone:** (856)566-6000
**Website:** http://som.umdnj.edu

## New York

**★ 16978 ★ New York Institute of**
**Technology**
**New York College of Osteopathic**
**Medicine (NYCOM)**
PO Box 8000
Old Westbury, NY 11568
**Phone:** (516)626-6947
**Website:** http://www.nyit.edu

## Ohio

**★ 16979 ★ Ohio University**
**College of Osteopathic Medicine**
**(OUCOM)**
Grosvenor and Irvine Halls
Athens, OH 45701
**Free:** 800-345-1560
**Website:** http://www.tcom.ohiou.edu/oucom

## Oklahoma

**★ 16980 ★ Oklahoma State University**
**College of Osteopathic Medicine**
**(OSUCOM)**
1111 W 17th St.
Tulsa, OK 74107
**Free:** 800-677-1972
**Website:** http://osu.com.okstate.edu/osucom.html

## Pennsylvania

**★ 16981 ★ Lake Erie College of**
**Osteopathic Medicine (LECOM)**
1858 W Grandview Blvd.
Erie, PA 16509
**Phone:** (814)866-6641
**Website:** http://www.lecom.edu

**★ 16982 ★ Philadelphia College of**
**Osteopathic Medicine (PCOM)**
4170 City Ave.
Philadelphia, PA 19131
**Phone:** (215)871-6701     **Free:** 800-999-6998
**Website:** http://www.pcom.edu

## Texas

**★ 16983 ★ University of North Texas,**
**Fort Worth (UNT)**
**Health Science Center (HSCFW)**
**Texas College of Osteopathic Medicine**
**(TCOM)**
3500 Camp Bowie Blvd.
Fort Worth, TX 76107-2970
**Phone:** (817)735-2205
**Website:** http://www.hsc.unt.edu/education/tcom

## West Virginia

**★ 16984 ★ West Virginia School of**
**Osteopathic Medicine (WVSOM)**
400 N Lee St.
Lewisburg, WV 24901
**Phone:** (304)647-6373
**Website:** http://www.wvsom.edu

---

# National & International Organizations

**★ 16985 ★ American Academy of**
**Osteopathy (AAO)**
3500 DePauw Blvd., Ste. 1080
Indianapolis, IN 46268
**Phone:** (317)879-1881     **Fax:** (317)879-0563
**Email:** snoone@academyofosteopathy.org
**Website:** http://www.academyofosteopathy.org
Stephen J. Noone, CAE, Exec. Dir.
**Fnded:** 1937. **Mem:** 4,200. **Reg. Groups:** 14. **Desc:**
Doctors of osteopathy. Seeks to develop and teach
the science and art of osteopathic manipulative treatment and encourage greater proficiency in the use of
osteopathic structural diagnostic and therapeutic procedures. Conducts graduate courses and seminars;
offers structural consultation and treatment service at
meetings. Conducts research. **Pub:** *American Academy of Osteopathy–Quarterly Journal*, quarterly. Jour-

nal. *Price:* $60/year. • *The Clinical Writings of William
L. Johnston, DO, FAAO.* Yearbooks. • *Membership
Directory*, annual. Directory. • *Millennial Edition of
AAO Yearbook (2001).* Yearbook. • Videos. **Frmly:**
(1944) Osteopathic Manipulative Therapeutic and
Clinical Research Association; (1970) Academy of
Applied Osteopathy.

**★ 16986 ★ American Association of**
**Colleges of Osteopathic Medicine**
**(AACOM)**
5550 Friendship Blvd., Ste. 310
Chevy Chase, MD 20815-7231
**Phone:** (301)968-4100     **Fax:** (301)968-4101
**Email:** dwood@aacom.org
**Website:** http://www.aacom.org
Douglas L. Wood, DO, Pres.
**Fnded:** 1898. **Mem:** 19. **Desc:** Osteopathic medical
colleges. Operates centralized application service;
monitors and works with Congress and other government agencies in the planning of health care programs. Gathers statistics on osteopathic medical
students, on innovations in medical education, faculty,
administers federal contract, develops national communication programs on behalf of member colleges.
**Pub:** *AACOM Organizational Guide*, annual. Directory
including lists of members and administrative staff and
faculty at U.S. colleges of osteopathic medicine. *Price:*
Free. • *American Association of Colleges of Osteopathic Medicine–Annual Statistical Report.* Covers
activities of the colleges of osteopathic medicine;
provides information on enrollment , student costs,
and scholarships and loans. *Price:* $18/copy. • *Col-
lege Information.* Book. • *Debts and Career Plans of
Osteopathic Medical Students*, annual. Report describing financial debt and career plans of freshmen
and seniors in osteopathic colleges. Contains statistics
on debts. *Price:* $16/copy. **Frmly:** (1970) American
Association of Osteopathic Colleges.

**★ 16987 ★ American Association of**
**Physician Specialists (AAPS)**
2296 Henderson Mill Rd., Ste. 206
Atlanta, GA 30345
**Phone:** (770)939-8555     **Free:** 800-447-9397
**Fax:** (770)939-8559
**Email:** wcarbone@aapsga.org
**Website:** http://www.aapsga.org
William J. Carbone, Exec. Dir.
**Fnded:** 1952. **Mem:** 2,500. **Desc:** 4Represents twelve
major specialties and twelve sub-specialties of medicine. Accepts qualified physicians into membership
with either an allopathic (M.D.) or osteopathic (D.O.)
degree. Official headquarters for 12 academies of
medicine and boards of certification in the following
specialties: anesthesiology, dermatology, emergency
medicine, family practice, internal medicine, geriatric
medicine, neurology/psychiatry, obstetrics/gynecolo-
gy, orthopedic surgery, plastic/reconstructive surgery,
radiology, surgery. **Pub:** *AAPS Directory*, annual.
Directory. Provides alphabetical and geographical list
of members. *Price:* Included in membership dues. •
*The American Journal of Clinical Medicine (AJCM)*,
quarterly. • *Member Notes*, quarterly. Newsletter.
**Frmly:** American Association of Osteopathic Specialists; (1984) American Academy of Osteopathic Surgeons.

**★ 16988 ★ American College of**
**Neuropsychiatrists (ACN)**
28595 Orchard Lake Rd., Ste. 200
Farmington Hills, MI 48334
**Phone:** (248)553-0010     **Fax:** (248)553-0818
**Email:** acn-aconp@msn.com
Louis E. Rentz, Exec. Dir.
**Fnded:** 1937. **Mem:** 420. **Desc:** Psychiatrists, neurologists, physicians in training, and persons in interrelated professions. Promotes study and research in
neurology and psychiatry in the osteopathic profession. Maintains specialized education programs. **Pub:**
*Journal of the American College of Neuropsychiatrists*,
semiannual. Journal. Reports information on medical
developments, case studies, and analysis of political

actions. Includes calendar of events and research updates. *Price:* Included in membership dues. • Directory, annual.

★ 16989 ★ **American College of Osteopathic Emergency Physicians (ACOEP)**
142 E Ontario St., Ste. 550
Chicago, IL 60611
**Phone:** (312)587-3709  **Free:** 800-521-3709
**Fax:** (312)587-9951
**Email:** jwachtler@acoep.org
**Website:** http://www.acoep.org
Janice Wachtler, Exec. Dir.

**Fnded:** 1975. **Mem:** 1,500. **Desc:** Provides and evaluates postdoctoral and continuing education for osteopathic emergency physicians; encourages and implements the training of emergency physicians; promotes the coordination of community emergency care facilities and personnel. Sponsors Emergency Medicine CME Program for Accreditation. Conducts research and educational programs. Maintains speakers' bureau. **Pub:** *ACOEP Newsletter*, quarterly. *Price:* $25 /year for nonmembers. • *Member Directory.* • *Student's Guide to AOA Approved Emergency Medicine Residency Programs.*

★ 16990 ★ **American College of Osteopathic Family Physicians (ACFP)**
330 E Algonquin, Ste. 1
Arlington Heights, IL 60005
**Free:** 800-323-0794  **Fax:** (847)228-9755
**Email:** elained@acofp.org
**Website:** http://www.acofp.org
Kieren P. Kanpp, DO, Pres.

**Fnded:** 1950. **Mem:** 20,000. **State Groups:** 35. **Desc:** Provides information, education and advocacy for osteopathic physicians practicing family medicine. **Pub:** *American College of Osteopathic Family Physicians Membership Directory*, annual. Membership Directory. • *Osteopathic Family Physician News*, monthly. Newsletter. Includes calendar of events and member news. *Price:* Free. **Frmly:** (1993) American College of General Practitioners in Osteopathic Medicine and Surgery.

★ 16991 ★ **American College of Osteopathic Internists (ACOI)**
3 Bethesda Metro Ctr., Ste.508
Bethesda, MD 20814
**Phone:** (301)656-8877  **Free:** 800-327-5183
**Fax:** (301)656-7133
**Email:** bjd@acoi.org
**Website:** http://www.acoi.org
Theresa M. Matzura, DO, Pres.

**Fnded:** 1943. **Mem:** 1,300. **Desc:** Osteopathic doctors who limit their practice to internal medicine and various subspecialties and who intend, through postdoctoral education, to qualify as certified specialists in the field. Aims to provide educational programs and to improve educational standards in the field of osteopathic internal medicine. Sponsors competitions. Compiles statistics; offers placement service. **Pub:** Directory, annual. • Newsletter, monthly.

★ 16992 ★ **American College of Osteopathic Obstetricians and Gynecologists (ACOOG)**
900 Auburn Rd.
Pontiac, MI 48342-3365
**Phone:** (248)332-6360  **Free:** 800-875-6360
**Fax:** (248)332-4607
**Email:** acoog@acoog.com
**Website:** http://www.acoog.com
Jaki K. Holzer, Admin.

**Fnded:** 1934. **Mem:** 1,100. **Desc:** Osteopathic physicians and surgeons specializing in obstetrics and gynecology. Conducts educational programs, and reviews osteopathic obstetric and gynecologic residency training programs. Holds annual postgraduate course and annual convention. **Pub:** *ACOOG Newsletter*, quarterly. Newsletter. Includes legislative news,

calendar of events, employment listings, and lists of residents completing training and newly certified physicians. *Price:* Free. • *American College of Osteopathic Obstetricians and Gynecologists Membership Directory*, annual. Membership Directory. *Price:* Included in membership dues. • Also publishes medical education brochures.

**American College of Osteopathic Pediatricians (ACOP)**
*See:* Entry 5610

★ 16993 ★ **American College of Osteopathic Surgeons (ACOS)**
123 N Henry St.
Alexandria, VA 22314-2903
**Phone:** (703)684-0416  **Fax:** (703)684-3280
**Email:** info@theacos.org
**Website:** http://www.facos.org
Guy D. Beaumont, Jr., Exec. Dir.

**Fnded:** 1927. **Mem:** 1,700. **Desc:** Professional society of osteopathic physicians specializing in surgery and surgical specialties. Maintains placement service; conducts seminars in continuing surgical education. **Pub:** *ACOS News*, monthly. Newsletter. Covers association activities and legislative and regulatory issues affecting osteopathic surgeons. Includes calendar of events. *Price:* Included in membership dues.

★ 16994 ★ **American Fracture Association (AFA)**
20 N Michigan Ave.
Chicago, IL 60602
**Phone:** (312)263-7150  **Fax:** (312)782-0553
**Website:** http://www.afa4docs.org
Barbara J. Dehority, Exec. Dir.

**Fnded:** 1938. **Mem:** 500. **Desc:** Orthopedic, general, industrial, plastic, traumatic, and dental surgeons and physicians interested in the care and treatment of fractures. Seeks to further and create interest in the study of the various accepted types of bone fracture therapy. **Pub:** *Orthopedic Transactions*, annual. • Directory, periodic. **Frmly:** American Ambulatory Fracture Association.

**American Osteopathic Academy of Addiction Medicine**
*See:* Entry 19253

★ 16995 ★ **American Osteopathic Academy of Orthopedics (AOAO)**
PO Box 291690
Davie, FL 33329-1690
**Phone:** (954)262-1700  **Free:** 800-741-2626
**Fax:** (954)262-1748
**Email:** mmorris@noa.edu
**Website:** http://www.aoao.org
Dr. Morton Morris, Exec. Dir.

**Fnded:** 1941. **Mem:** 450. **Desc:** Professional society of osteopathic orthopedic surgeons. **Pub:** *American Osteopathic Academy of Orthopedics–Membership Roster*, annual. Membership Directory. Arranged alphabetically and geographically; also lists resident candidates and AOAO-approved residency programs. *Price:* Free. • *Orthopod*, semiannual. *Price:* Included in membership dues.

★ 16996 ★ **American Osteopathic Academy of Sports Medicine (AOASM)**
7600 Terrace Ave., Ste. 203
Middleton, WI 53562-3174
**Phone:** (608)831-4400  **Fax:** (608)831-5122
**Email:** info@aoasm.org
**Website:** http://www.aoasm.org/
Thomas Miller, Exec. Dir.

**Fnded:** 1975. **Mem:** 500. **Desc:** Members of the American Osteopathic Association and students enrolled in approved colleges of osteopathic medicine. Objectives are to promote education, development of high ethical standards, communication, and research

in the field of sports medicine. Conducts study programs, lectures, forums, and seminars. Encourages publication of articles and dissertations in scientific and professional journals. Sponsors student academy organizations at osteopathic education institutions. Maintains speakers' bureau. **Pub:** *Sport Medicine Today*, quarterly. Newsletter. Reviews research and educational programs in sports medicine. Contains calendar of events. *Price:* Included in membership dues. • Membership Directory, annual.

★ 16997 ★ **American Osteopathic Association (AOA)**
142 E Ontario St.
Chicago, IL 60611
**Free:** 800-621-1773  **Fax:** (312)202-8200
**Email:** info@aoa-net.org
**Website:** http://www.aoa-net.org
John B. Crosby, Exec. Dir.

**Fnded:** 1897. **Mem:** 23,000. **State Groups:** 50. **Desc:** Osteopathic physicians, surgeons, and graduates of approved colleges of osteopathic medicine. Associate members include teaching, research, administrative, and executive employees of approved colleges, hospitals, divisional societies, and affiliated organizations. Forms (with its affiliates) an officially recognized structure of the osteopathic profession. Promotes the public health, to encourage scientific research, and to maintain and improve high standards of medical education in osteopathic colleges. Inspects and accredits colleges and hospitals; conducts a specialty certification program; sponsors a national examining board satisfactory to state licensing agencies; maintains mandatory program of continuing medical education for members. Compiles statistics on location and type of practice of osteopathic physicians. Sponsors research activities through Bureau of Research in osteopathic colleges and hospitals. Maintains Physician Placement Service. Produces public service radio and television programs; maintains 2000 item library and biographical archives on osteopathic medicine and history. Offers speakers' bureau. **Pub:** *American Osteopathic Association Yearbook and Directory.* Directory. • *The D.O.*, monthly. • *Journal of AOA*, monthly. Journal. • Brochures.

★ 16998 ★ **American Osteopathic Board of Emergency Medicine (AOBEM)**
c/o Josette Fleming
142 E Ontario St.
Chicago, IL 60611
**Phone:** (312)335-1065  **Fax:** (312)335-5489
**Website:** http://www.aobem.org
Josette M. Fleming, Admin.

**Fnded:** 1980. **Mem:** 9. **Desc:** Seeks to improve the quality of emergency medical care, to establish and maintain high standards of excellence in the specialty of emergency medicine, to improve medical education and facilities for training emergency physicians, to evaluate specialists in emergency medicine applying for certification and recertification, and to serve the public, physicians, hospitality, and medical schools by furnishing lists of medical schools by furnishing lists of those diplomates certified by the board. **Pub:** *American Osteopathic Association Yearbook and Directory of Osteopathic Physicians.* Directory.

★ 16999 ★ **American Osteopathic Board of Family Physicians (AOBFP)**
330 E Algonquin Rd., Ste. 6
Arlington Heights, IL 60005
**Phone:** (847)640-8477
**Website:** http://www.aobfp.org
Carol A. Thoma, Exec. Dir.

**Fnded:** 1972. **Desc:** Certifying board for osteopathic physicians. Prepares and administers semiannual certification examination and annual recertification exam. **Frmly:** (1993) American Osteopathic Board of General Practice.

**★ 17000 ★ American Osteopathic Board of Pediatrics (AOBP)**
142 E Ontario St., 6th Fl.
Chicago, IL 60645
**Phone:** (312)202-8267
**Email:** rmcclary@aoa-net.org
**Website:** http://www.aobp.org
Robbin McClary, Coord.

**Desc:** Certification board for osteopathic pediatricians. Standards are formulated by the American Osteopathic Association (see separate entry). Certification is conducted by annual examination.

**★ 17001 ★ American Osteopathic College of Anesthesiologists (AOCA)**
17201 E US Hwy. 40, No. 204
Independence, MO 64055
**Phone:** (816)373-4700          **Free:** 800-842-2622
**Fax:** (816)373-1529
David Bitonte, Pres.

**Fnded:** 1952. **Mem:** 500. **Desc:** Members of American Osteopathic Association who are engaged in the practice of anesthesiology. **Pub:** Membership Directory, annual. • Newsletter, 3/year. **Frmly:** (1952) American Osteopathic Society of Anesthesiologists.

**★ 17002 ★ American Osteopathic College of Dermatology (AOCD)**
PO Box 7525
1501 E Illinois St.
Kirksville, MO 63501-7525
**Phone:** (660)665-2184          **Free:** 800-449-2623
**Fax:** (660)627-2623
**Email:** execdirector@aocd.org
**Website:** http://www.aocd.org
Rebecca A. Mansfield, Exec. Dir.

**Fnded:** 1958. **Mem:** 300. **Desc:** Members of the osteopathic profession certified or involved in dermatology. Conducts specialized education programs. **Pub:** *American Osteopathic College of Dermatology Annual Membership Directory*, annual. Directory. *Price:* Free. • Newsletter, quarterly.

**★ 17003 ★ American Osteopathic College of Pathologists (AOCP)**
c/o Joan Gross
12368 NW 13th Ct.
Pembroke Pines, FL 33026-3817
**Phone:** (954)432-9640
**Website:** http://www.aocp.org
Joan Gross, Exec. Dir.

**Fnded:** 1954. **Mem:** 180. **Desc:** Osteopathic physicians who have completed residency training programs in pathology and clinical pathology; candidate members are in residency training in pathology. Establishes guidelines for training programs in pathology and clinical pathology for osteopathic physicians; maintains standards in residency training programs. Offers placement service and mid-year tutorial program. Maintains collection of slide study sets. **Pub:** *American Osteopathic College of Pathologists Directory*, annual. Directory. • *Nova*, monthly. Newsletter. Includes reports on employment opportunities and topics of interest. *Price:* Included in membership dues.

**★ 17004 ★ American Osteopathic College of Physical Medicine and Rehabilitation (AOCPMR)**
314 S Knight Ave.
Park Ridge, IL 60068-3804
**Phone:** (847)825-2515          **Fax:** (847)825-2509
**Email:** Executive.Director@aocpmr.org
**Website:** http://www.aocpmr.org/
Barbara Guerra, Exec. Dir.

**Fnded:** 1954. **Mem:** 125. **Desc:** Osteopathic physicians with a strong interest in physical and rehabilitation medicine as a specialty. Active members are those certified in the specialty by the American Osteopathic Board of Rehabilitation Medicine of the American Osteopathic Association (see separate entry). To stimulate study, extend knowledge, and im-

prove practice in rehabilitation medicine. Cosponsors training programs; sponsors competitive writing for predoctoral osteopathic medical students, interns, and residents. **Pub:** Directory, annual. • Newsletter, periodic. **Frmly:** (1955) American Osteopathic Academy of Physical Medicine and Rehabilitation; (1970) American Osteopathic College of Physical Medicine and Rehabilitation; (2001) American Osteopathic College of Rehabilitation Medicine.

**★ 17005 ★ American Osteopathic College of Preventive Medicine (AOCPM)**
PO Box 2606
Leesburg, VA 20177
**Free:** 800-558-8686          **Fax:** (703)443-0576
**Email:** aocopm@starpower.net
**Website:** http://www.aocpm.org/
James T. Alexander, Sec.

**Fnded:** 1982. **Mem:** 160. **Desc:** Osteopathic doctors. Prepares and educates doctors of osteopathy who wish to specialize in aerospace medicine, occupational/environmental medicine, or public health preventive medicine. Seeks to foster an understanding of these fields of study among osteopathic doctors and the public. Provides consultant services to other physicians. Maintains speakers' bureau. Conducts studies. **Pub:** Directory, annual. • Newsletter, quarterly.

**★ 17006 ★ American Osteopathic College of Proctology (AOCPr)**
9948 State Rte. 682
Athens, OH 45701-5090
**Fax:** (740)594-5090
Dr. Zolton Brody, Exec. Officer

**Mem:** 155. **Desc:** Osteopathic physicians and surgeons specializing in treatment of diseases of the anus, rectum, and colon.

**★ 17007 ★ American Osteopathic College of Radiology (AOCR)**
119 E 2nd St.
Milan, MO 63556
**Phone:** (660)265-4011          **Fax:** (660)265-3494
**Email:** aocr@nemr.net
**Website:** http://www.aocr.org/
Pamela A. Smith, Exec. Dir.

**Fnded:** 1941. **Mem:** 730. **Desc:** Certified radiologists, residents-in-training, and others active in the field of radiology. **Pub:** *Viewbox*, quarterly. Newsletter. • Membership Directory, annual.

**★ 17008 ★ American Osteopathic Colleges of Ophthalmology and Otolaryngology-Head and Neck Surgery (AOCOO-HNS)**
320 W Grand Ave.
Dayton, OH 45405
**Phone:** (937)222-8820          **Free:** 800-455-9404
**Fax:** (937)222-8840
**Email:** dbailey@aocoohns.org
**Website:** http://www.aocoohns.org
Dr. Alvin Dubin, Exec. VP

**Fnded:** 1916. **Mem:** 670. **Desc:** Osteopathic physicians who have completed formal specialty training or are acquiring such training in ophthalmology, otorhinolaryngology, and facial plastic surgery, and those who are certified specialists in one or more of the above named areas. Develops application of osteopathic concepts in this specialty; determines minimum standards of education at undergraduate and postgraduate levels. Sponsors research programs. **Pub:** *American Osteopathic Colleges of Ophthalmology and Otolaryngology Head & Neck Surgery–News Letter*, quarterly. Newsletter. *Price:* Included in membership dues. • *AOCOO-HNS*, annual. Journal. • Directory, periodic. • Also publishes collected papers. **Frmly:** Osteopathic College of Ophthalmology and Otorhinolaryngology.

**★ 17009 ★ American Osteopathic Foundation (AOF)**
c/o Leda Hanin
142 East Ontario
Chicago, IL 60611
**Phone:** (312)202-8234          **Fax:** (312)202-8216
**Email:** Sdowney@aoa-net.org
**Website:** http://www.osteopathic.org
Eugene A. Oliveri, Chair

**Fnded:** 1949. **Mem:** 9,300. **Desc:** Osteopathic physicians and laypersons interested in raising and administering funds for osteopathic medical education, research, colleges, and hospitals. Functions as philanthropic affiliate of the American Osteopathic Association; seeks to foster understanding of osteopathic principles and practice. **Pub:** *AOF In Touch*, triennial. Newsletter. *Price:* Free. For members only. **Frmly:** (1960) Osteopathic Foundation; (1998) National Osteopathic Foundation.

**American Osteopathic Healthcare Association (AOHA)**
*See:* Entry 11478

**★ 17010 ★ Association of Osteopathic State Executive Directors (AOSED)**
c/o American Osteopathic Association
142 East Ontario St.
Chicago, IL 60611
**Free:** 800-621-1773          **Fax:** (312)202-8200
**Email:** aoha@osteohdq.org
**Website:** http://www.aoa-net.org/AffiliatedOrgs/AOSED/aosed.htm
John B. Crosby, JD, Exec. Dir.

**Fnded:** 1919. **Mem:** 75. **Desc:** Divisional and affiliated societies of the American Osteopathic Association. Objectives are: to promote and improve associations and procedures among members; to examine and develop procedures and policies that will bring about an efficient unit of operation within the divisional societies; to disseminate information on the activities of members and foster and participate in the objects of the AOA. **Pub:** *Association of Osteopathic State Executive Directors*. Newsletter. • *Directory of Osteopathic Publications*, biennial. Directory.

**★ 17011 ★ Auxiliary to the American Osteopathic Association (AAOA)**
142 E Ontario St.
Chicago, IL 60611
**Fax:** (312)202-8218
**Email:** bprice@aoa-net.org
**Website:** http://www.aux-aoa.org
Bridget Price, Exec. Dir.

**Fnded:** 1940. **Mem:** 5,000. **Desc:** Immediate family members of osteopathic physicians; spouses of students of osteopathic medicine. Promotes public health education; provides funds for scholarships for the training of osteopathic physicians and surgeons, and for research and other activities at osteopathic colleges; encourages establishment and continuation of volunteer service organizations in nonprofit osteopathic hospitals; participates in national and community health programs. Sponsors summer seminars. **Pub:** *AAOA Accent*, quarterly. Newsletter. Covers osteopathic medicine and related subjects such as safety projects, public health information, and osteopathic college scholarship awards. *Price:* Included in membership dues. • *Newsbriefs*, bimonthly. • *Roster of Affiliates*, annual. • Annual Report. • Also publishes handbooks.

**★ 17012 ★ British Osteopathic Association**
Langham House West
Luton LU1 2NA, United Kingdom
**Phone:** 44 158 2488455     **Fax:** 44 158 2481533
**Email:** enquiries@osteopathy.org
**Website:** http://www.osteopathy.org

**Fnded:** 1911. **Mem:** 100. **Desc:** Medically qualified osteopaths. Professional association protecting the interests of osteopaths. Running a charitable osteopathic clinic. **Pub:** Directory, annual. Membership information.

★ **17013** ★ **Bureau of Professional Education of the American Osteopathic Association (BPEAOA)**
American Osteopathic Association
142 E Ontario St.
Chicago, IL 60611
**Phone:** (312)202-8048        **Free:** 800-621-1773
**Fax:** (312)202-8202
**Email:** kretz@aoa-net.org
**Website:** http://www.aoa-net.org
Konrad C. Miskowicz, PhD, Sec.

**Desc:** Membership comprises American Osteopathic Associations representatives from other AOA affiliates, and public representatives. Approves policy regarding new and/or different intern and residency training programs in approved osteopathic hospitals. Serves as accrediting agency for colleges of osteopathic medicine. Oversees osteopathic continuing medical education activities.

★ **17014** ★ **Canadian Osteopathic Aid Society (COAS)**
**(Societe Canadienne d'Assistance Osteopathique — SCAO)**
575 Waterloo St.
London, ON, Canada N6B 2R2
**Phone:** (519)439-5521        **Fax:** (519)439-2619
**Email:** coas@golden.net
**Lang(s):** English, French. **Desc:** Osteopathic physicians. Seeks to advance the study and practice of osteopathic medicine. Facilitates communication and cooperation among members; provides support and assistance to osteopathic medical students.

★ **17015** ★ **Canadian Osteopathic Association (COA)**
**(Societe Canadienne Osteopathique — SCO)**
575 Waterloo St.
London, ON, Canada N6B 2R2
**Phone:** (519)439-5521        **Fax:** (519)439-2616
**Email:** coas@golden.net
**Lang(s):** English, French. **Desc:** Osteopathic physicians and students of osteopathy. Seeks to advance the study and practice of osteopathic medicine. Serves as a clearinghouse on osteopathy; sponsors research and educational programs.

★ **17016** ★ **College of Osteopathic Healthcare Executives (COHE)**
5550 Friendship Blvd., Ste. 300
Chevy Chase, MD 20815-7201
**Phone:** (301)968-2642        **Fax:** (301)968-4195
David L. Kushner, Pres.

**Fnded:** 1954. **Mem:** 124. **Desc:** Executives and other employees of osteopathic hospitals. To encourage development of hospital administration; to set criteria of competency; to assist in educational programs; to contribute to advancement of efficient hospital administration. **Pub:** *Osteopathic Membership Directory*, annual. Directory. • *Osteopathic Progress*, bimonthly. Newsletter. *Price:* Included in membership dues. **Frmly:** (1986) American College of Osteopathic Hospital Administrators.

★ **17017** ★ **Cranial Academy (CA)**
8202 Clearvista Parkway, No. 9-D
Indianapolis, IN 46256
**Phone:** (317)594-0411        **Fax:** (317)594-9299
**Email:** cranacad@aol.com
**Website:** http://www.cranialacademy.com
Patricia Crampton, Exec. Dir.

**Fnded:** 1947. **Mem:** 1,200. **Desc:** A component society of the American Academy of Osteopathy. Osteopathic physicians interested in study and development of osteopathic cranial concepts and techniques of diagnosis and treatment in structural manip-

ulation of the body; members have taken a Cranial Academy approved basic course in Osteopathy in the cranial field. Promotes research programs. **Pub:** *Clinical Cranial Osteopathy*. Book. *Price:* $45 for members; $50 for nonmembers. • *The Cranial Bowl*. Book. *Price:* $15; $17 for nonmembers. • *The Cranial Bowl*. Brochure. *Price:* $.90 for members; $1 for nonmembers. • *The Cranial Concept*. Brochure. *Price:* $27/100 for members; $30/100 for nonmembers. • *The Cranial Letter*, quarterly. Newsletter. Contains articles related to new developments in cranial osteopathy. *Price:* $60/year. • *Journal of OCA 1948, 49, 54, 57, & 58. Price:* $18 for members; $20 for nonmembers. • *Manual of Cranial Technique*. Book. *Price:* $22.50 for members; $25 for nonmembers. • *Member Information Directory*, annual. Directory. *Price:* Included in membership dues. **Frmly:** (1960) Osteopathic Cranial Association.

★ **17018** ★ **European Liaison Committee for Osteopaths (ELCO)**
**(Comite de Liaison Europeen des Osteopathes — CLEO)**
116 Av. des Chames Elysee's
F-75008 Paris, France
**Phone:** 33 1 44218075
**Fnded:** 1978. **Mem:** 4. **Lang(s):** French. **Desc:** National associations in Belgium, England, France, and Greece. Seeks to protect the rights of osteopaths in the European Economic Community.

★ **17019** ★ **International Academy of Osteopathy**
Barones Ludwina de Borrekenslaan 84
2630 Aartselaar, Belgium
**Website:** http://www.iao.be

★ **17020** ★ **International Cranial Association**
478 Baker St.
Middlesex
Enfield EN1 3QS, United Kingdom
**Phone:** 44 20 83675561        **Fax:** 44 20 82026686
**Fnded:** 1965. **Mem:** 84. **Desc:** Osteopaths, chiropractors, manipulative therapists. Holds a register of members for enquiries from the public; provides a training course each year; holds an annual conference for members and the public; provides a code of ethics. **Pub:** Newsletter, quarterly. **Frmly:** (1999) Cranial Osteopathic Association.

★ **17021** ★ **Israel Society on Calcified Tissues Research**
c/o Metabolic Diseases
Beilison Medical Center
49100 Petah Tikva, Israel
**Phone:** 972 3 376124        **Fax:** 972 3 376143
**Fnded:** 1971. **Mem:** 120. **Lang(s):** English. **Desc:** Physicians and graduate students in Israel engaged in the clinical research on calcified tissues. Seeks to advance knowledge in the field of bone and mineral metabolism.

★ **17022** ★ **Israeli Foundation for Osteoporosis and Bone Diseases**
PO Box 1513
IL-37000 Pazdes Hanna, Israel
**Phone:** 972 4 6274549        **Fax:** 972 4 6274549
**Email:** Ifob@ineznet.zahav.net.il
**Website:** http://www.ifob.too.co.il
**Fnded:** 1998. **Mem:** 4,000. **Nat'l Groups:** 1. **State Groups:** 1. **Local Groups:** 5. **Lang(s):** English. **Desc:** Promotes the education of the medical profession, patients, and the general public on osteoporosis and bone disease. Conducts political lobbying. **Pub:** *Bone-Tone*, quarterly. Newsletter.

★ **17023** ★ **National Board of Osteopathic Medical Examiners (NBOME)**
8765 W Higgins Rd., Ste. 200
Chicago, IL 60631
**Phone:** (773)714-0622        **Fax:** (773)714-0631
**Email:** admin@nbome.org
**Website:** http://www.nbome.org
Joseph F. Smoley, PhD, Exec. Dir.

**Fnded:** 1935. **Mem:** 12. **Desc:** Examining and evaluating board to investigate the qualifications of, and administer examinations and grant diplomate status to osteopathic physicians. **Pub:** *Information Bulletin*, annual. Bulletin. **Frmly:** (1986) National Board of Examiners for Osteopathic Physicians and Surgeons.

★ **17024** ★ **Pain Management and Sclerotherapy**
5002 E Woodmill Dr.
Wilmington, DE 19808
**Phone:** (302)996-0300        **Free:** 800-471-6114
**Fax:** (302)996-5300
Linda Pavina, Exec. Sec.

**Fnded:** 1938. **Mem:** 145. **Nat'l Groups:** 1. **Desc:** Dedicated to improving the practice of and disseminating knowledge about sclerotherapy. (The academy defines sclerotherapy as the stimulation of the formation of fibrous-connective tissues by the body, in a specific location, by the specific application of a sclerosing modality.) The most frequently used modality is the injection of certain medications, known as sclerosants. Primary studies involve the treatment of: unstable joints, venous abnormalities, and tendenoosseous points of hyper-irritability. Supports research program; maintains speakers' bureau. **Pub:** *Get the Point*, semiannual. Newsletter. Reports on the results of studies; evaluates differing sclerotherapeutic treatments. *Price:* Included in membership dues. • Directory, periodic. **Frmly:** (1956) American Osteopathic Academy of Sclerotherapy; (1959) American Academy of Sclerotherapy.

★ **17025** ★ **Student Osteopathic Medical Association (SOMA)**
142 E Ontario St.
Chicago, IL 60611
**Free:** 800-621-1772
**Email:** webmaster@studentdo.com
**Website:** http://www.studentdo.com/
**Fnded:** 1970. **Mem:** 6,000. **Desc:** Seeks to improve the quality of healthcare delivery; contributes to the education of osteopathic medical students, aims to improve awareness of osteopathic medicine, and establish communication between healthcare professionals. **Pub:** *Student DOctor*. Magazine.

## Research Centers

★ **17026** ★ **Johns Hopkins University Center for Osteonecrosis Research and Education**
The Good Samaritan Professional Bldg., Rm. 201
Department of Orthopaedic Surgery
School of Medicine
5601 Loch Raven Blvd.
Baltimore, MD 21239
**Phone:** (410)532-5906        **Fax:** (410)532-5908
**Email:** dhunger@mail.jhmi.edu
**Website:** http://www.med.jhu.edu/avncenter/
Lynne C. Jones, PhD, Dir.

**Activities/Fields:** Etiology, pathogenesis, diagnosis and treatment of osteonecrosis.

★ **17027** ★ **Otosclerosis Study Group**
PO Box 17987
Memphis, TN 38187-0987
Linda Slinkard, MD, Dir.

**Activities/Fields:** Otosclerosis, focusing on the ear and its diseases.

**★ 17028 ★ U.S. Department of Health and Human Services**
**National Institutes of Health**
**National Institute of Diabetes and Digestive and Kidney Diseases**
**Division of Diabetes, Endocrinology, and Metabolic Diseases**
**(Bone and Mineral Research Program)**
2 Democracy Plaza, Rm. 603
Bethesda, MD 20892
**Phone:** (301)451-9871　　**Fax:** (301)480-3503
**Email:** mt270t@extra.niddk.nih.gov
**Website:** http://www.niddk.nih.gov/fund/program/A-Elist.htmb&m
Mehrdad Tondravi, PhD, Dir.
**Activities/Fields:** Basic and clinical research on the hormonal regulation of bone and mineral metabolism in health and disease.

**★ 17029 ★ University of Alabama at Birmingham**
**Center for Metabolic Bone Disease (CMBD)**
509 Lyons-Harrison Research Bldg.
701 S 19th St.
Birmingham, AL 35294-0007
**Phone:** (205)934-6666　　**Fax:** (205)975-9927
**Email:** cmbd@path.uab.edu
**Website:** http://www.path.uab.edu/cmbd
Jay McDonald, MD, Dir.
**Activities/Fields:** Metabolic bone diseases, including osteoporosis. **Pub:** *Newsletter.*

**★ 17030 ★ University of Iowa**
**Bone Healing Research Laboratory**
Orthopaedic Surgery, 1012 RCP
Iowa City, IA 52242
**Phone:** (319)356-2466　　**Fax:** (319)353-8968
**Email:** james-nepola@uiowa.edu
**Website:** http://www.uiowa.edu/~vpr/research/organize/boneheal.htm
James V. Nepola, Co-Dir.
**Activities/Fields:** Bone healing, including effects of pulsed electromagnetic fields, distraction osteogenesis, synthetic bone graft and vertebral disc materials, and the prevention of osteomyelitis.

**★ 17031 ★ University of Maryland at Baltimore**
**Baltimore Hip Studies**
Department of Epidemiology & Preventive Medicine
660 W Redwood St., Ste. 200
Baltimore, MD 21201
**Phone:** (410)706-3553　　**Fax:** (410)706-4433
**Email:** jmagazine@epi.umaryland.edu
**Website:** http://gerontology.umaryland.edu/hipstudy.html
Jay Magaziner, PhD, Prin. Investigator
**Activities/Fields:** Recovery from hip fracture, including changes in functional ability, changes in bone mineral density, examination of markers of bone turnover, and the design and evaluation of interventions to enhance recovery from hip fracture.

# State Government Agencies

## Osteopathic Medical Boards

**★ 17032 ★ Alabama State Board of Medical Examiners**
848 Washington Ave.
PO Box 946
Montgomery, AL 36101-0946
**Phone:** (334)242-4116　　**Fax:** (334)242-4155
**Email:** bmedixon@mindspring.com
**Website:** http://www.albme.org/

**★ 17033 ★ Alaska State Medical Board**
PO Box 110806
Juneau, AK 99811-0806
**Phone:** (907)269-8163　　**Fax:** (907)269-8196
**Email:** leslie_abel@dced.state.ak.us
**Website:** http://www.commerce.state.ak.us/occ/pmed.htm

**★ 17034 ★ Arizona Board of Osteopathic Examiners in Medicine and Surgery**
9535 E Doubletree Ranch Rd.
Scottsdale, AZ 85258
**Phone:** (480)657-7703　　**Fax:** (480)657-7715
**Email:** information@azosteoboard.org
**Website:** http://www.azosteoboard.org/
Ann Marie Berger, Director

**★ 17035 ★ Arkansas State Medical Board**
2100 Riverfront Dr., Ste. 200
Little Rock, AR 72202
**Phone:** (501)296-1802　　**Fax:** (501)296-1805
**Email:** office@armedicalboard.org
**Website:** http://www.armedicalboard.org/

**★ 17036 ★ Colorado State Board of Medical Examiners**
1560 Broadway, Ste. 1300
Denver, CO 80202
**Phone:** (303)894-7690　　**Fax:** (303)894-7692
**Email:** medical@dora.state.co.us
**Website:** http://www.dora.state.co.us/Medical/
Susan Miller, Contact

**★ 17037 ★ Connecticut State Board of Medical Quality Assurance**
410 Capitol Ave.
Hartford, CT 06134
**Phone:** (860)509-7579　　**Fax:** (860)509-8457
**Email:** webmaster.dph@po.state.ct.us
**Website:** http://www.state.ct.us/dph/

**★ 17038 ★ Delaware Board of Medical Practice**
Cannon Bldg, Ste. 203
861 Silver Lake Blvd.
PO Box 1401
Dover, DE 19903
**Phone:** (302)739-4522　　**Fax:** (302)739-2711

**★ 17039 ★ District of Columbia Board of Medicine**
825 North Capital St, NE, 2nd Fl
Washington, DC 20002
**Phone:** (202)442-9200　　**Fax:** (202)442-9431
**Email:** dchealth@dc.gov
**Website:** http://dchealth.dc.gov/index.asp

**★ 17040 ★ Florida Board of Osteopathic Medicine**
4052 Bald Cypress Way, Bin C-06
Tallahassee, FL 32399-1753
**Phone:** (850)245-4161　　**Fax:** (850)487-9874
**Email:** Christy_Robinson@doh.state.fl.us
**Website:** http://www.doh.state.fl.us/mqa/osteopath/oshome.htm
Karen Eaton, Director

**★ 17041 ★ Georgia Composite State Board of Medical Examiners**
2 Peachtree St.,NW, 10th St.
Atlanta, GA 30303
**Phone:** (404)656-3913　　**Fax:** (404)656-9723
**Email:** GCox@dma.state.ga.us
**Website:** http://www.medicalboard.state.ga.us
Karen Mason, Contact

**★ 17042 ★ Idaho State Board of Medicine**
1755 Westgate Dr.
PO Box 83720
Boise, ID 83720
**Phone:** (208)327-7000　　**Fax:** (208)327-7005
**Email:** info@bom.state.id.us
**Website:** http://www.bom.state.id.us/

**★ 17043 ★ Illinois Department of Professional Regulation**
**Medical Licensing Board**
**Board of Osteopathic Medicine**
320 W Washington St.
Springfield, IL 62786
**Phone:** (217)785-0800　　**Fax:** (217)524-2169
**Website:** http://www.dpr.state.il.us/WHO/med.cfm

**★ 17044 ★ Indiana Health Professions Bureau**
**Board of Osteopathic Medicine**
402 W Washington, Rm. 041
Indianapolis, IN 46204
**Phone:** (317)232-2960　　**Fax:** (317)233-4236
**Website:** http://www.in.gov/hpb/contact/index.html

**★ 17045 ★ Iowa State Board of Medical Examiners**
400 SW 8th St., Ste. C
Des Moines, IA 50309-4686
**Phone:** (515)281-5171　　**Fax:** (515)242-5908
**Email:** amowery@bon.state.ia.us
**Website:** http://www.docboard.org/ia/ia_home.htm
Ann E. Mowery, PhD, Director

**★ 17046 ★ Kansas Board of Healing Arts**
235 SW Topeka Blvd.
Topeka, KS 66603-3068
**Phone:** (785)296-7413　　**Fax:** (785)296-0852
**Email:** Healer3@ink.org
**Website:** http://www.ksbha.org/

**★ 17047 ★ Kentucky Board of Medical Licensure**
310 Whittington Pkwy, Ste 1B
310 Whittington Pkwy., Ste 1B
Louisville, KY 40222
**Phone:** (502)429-8046　　**Fax:** (502)429-9923
**Email:** kbml@mail.state.ky.us
**Website:** http://www.state.ky.us/agencies/kbml/

**★ 17048 ★ Louisiana State Board of Medical Examiners**
630 Camp St.
PO Box 30250
New Orleans, LA 70190-0250
**Phone:** (504)568-6820　　**Fax:** (504)599-0503
**Email:** lsbmever@lsbme.org
**Website:** http://www.lsbme.org/

**★ 17049 ★ Maine Board of Osteopathic Licensure**
142 State House Station
2 Bangor St.
Augusta, ME 04333-0142
**Phone:** (207)287-2480
**Email:** susan.e.strout@state.me.us
**Website:** http://www.docboard.org/me-osteo/

**★ 17050 ★ Maryland Board of Physician Quality Assurance**
4201 Patterson Ave.
Baltimore, MD 21215-0095
**Phone:** (410)764-4777　　**Free:** 800-492-6836
**Fax:** (410)358-2252
**Email:** bpqa@erols.com
**Website:** http://www.bpqa.state.md.us/

**★ 17051 ★ Massachusetts Board of Registration in Medicine**
10 West St. 3rd Fl.
Boston, MA 02111
Phone: (617)727-3086    Fax: (617)451-9568
Email: webmaster@massmedboard.org
Website: http://www.massmedboard.org./

**★ 17052 ★ Michigan Board of Osteopathic Medicine and Surgery**
PO Box 30670
Lansing, MI 48909-8170
Phone: (517)335-0918    Fax: (517)373-2179
Email: bhserinfo@cis.state.mi.us
Website: http://www.michigan.gov/cis

**★ 17053 ★ Minnesota Board of Medical Practice**
2829 University Ave. SE
Ste. 400
Minneapolis, MN 55414-3246
Phone: (612)617-2130    Free: 800-657-3709
Fax: (612)617-2166
Email: medical.board@state.mn.us
Website: http://www.bmp.state.mn.us/

**★ 17054 ★ Mississippi State Board of Medical Licensure**
1867 Crane Ridge Dr.
Ste. 200-B
PO Box 9268
Jackson, MS 39286-9268
Phone: (601)987-3079    Fax: (601)987-4159
Email: mboard@msbml.state.ms.us
Website: http://www.msbml.state.ms.us/

**★ 17055 ★ Missouri State Board of Registration for the Healing Arts**
3605 Missouri Blvd.
PO Box 4
Jefferson City, MO 65102
Phone: (573)751-0098    Fax: (573)751-3166
Email: healarts@mail.state.mo.us
Website: http://www.ecodev.state.mo.us/pr/healarts/
Tina Steinman, Director

**★ 17056 ★ Montana Board of Medical Examiners**
301 S Park, 4th Fl.
PO Box 200513
Helena, MT 59620-0513
Phone: (406)841-2360    Fax: (406)841-2363
Email: dlibsdmed@state.mt.us
Website: http://www.discoveringmontana.com/dli/bsd/license/hc_licensing_boards.htm
Jeanne Worsech, Director

**★ 17057 ★ Nebraska Department of Health and Human Services**
State Board of Examiners in Medicine and Surgery
PO Box 94986
Lincoln, NE 68509-4986
Phone: (402)471-2118    Fax: (402)471-3577
Email: Becky.Wisell@hhss.state.ne.us
Website: http://www.hhs.state.ne.us/crl/msh.htm
Becky Wisell, Contact

**★ 17058 ★ Nevada State Board of Osteopathic Medicine**
2860 E Flamingo Rd., Ste. G
Las Vegas, NV 89121
Phone: (702)732-2147    Fax: (702)732-2079
Website: http://www.osteo.state.nv.us
Larry Tarno, Director

**★ 17059 ★ New Hampshire Board of Registration in Medicine**
2 Industrial Park Dr., Ste. 8
Concord, NH 03301-8520
Phone: (603)271-1203    Fax: (603)271-6702
Website: http://webster.state.nh.us/medicine/

**★ 17060 ★ New Jersey State Board of Medical Examiners**
PO Box 183
Trenton, NJ 08625-0183
Phone: (609)826-7100    Fax: (609)826-7117
Website: http://www.state.nj.us/lps/ca/medical.htmbme5
William Roeder, Director

**★ 17061 ★ New Mexico Board of Osteopathic Medical Examiners**
92055 Pacheco St., Ste. 400
PO Box 25101
Santa Fe, NM 87504
Phone: (505)476-7120    Fax: (505)476-7095
Email: OsteoBoard@state.nm.us
Website: http://www.rld.state.nm.us/b&c/osteopathic_examiners_board.htm

**★ 17062 ★ New York State Board for Medicine**
Office of the Professions
State Education Bldg., 2nd Fl.
Albany, NY 12234
Phone: (518)474-3817    Fax: (518)486-4846
Email: medbd@mail.nysed.gov
Website: http://www.op.nysed.gov/med.htm
Thomas J. Monahan, Contact

**★ 17063 ★ North Carolina Board of Medical Examiners**
1201 Front St, Ste. 100
Raleigh, NC 27609-7533
Phone: (919)326-1100    Fax: (919)326-1130
Email: public.affairs@ncmedboard.org
Website: http://www.ncmedboard.org/

**★ 17064 ★ North Dakota State Board of Medical Examiners**
418 E Broadway, Ste. 12
Bismarck, ND 58501
Phone: (701)328-6500    Fax: (701)328-6505
Website: http://www.ndbomex.com/
Rolf P. Sletten, J.D., Contact

**★ 17065 ★ Ohio State Medical Board**
77 S High St., 17th Fl.
Columbus, OH 43215-6127
Phone: (614)466-3934    Free: 800-554-7717
Fax: (614)728-5946
Website: http://www.state.oh.us/med/

**★ 17066 ★ Oklahoma Board of Osteopathic Examiners**
4848 N Lincoln Blvd., Ste. 100
Oklahoma City, OK 73105-3335
Phone: (405)528-8625    Fax: (405)557-0653
Website: http://www.docboard.org/ok/ok.htm
Paul F. Benien, Director

**★ 17067 ★ Oregon Board of Medical Examiners**
1500 SW 1st Ave., Ste. 620
Portland, OR 97201
Phone: (503)229-5770    Free: 877-254-6263
Fax: (503)229-6543
Email: bme.info@state.or.us
Website: http://www.bme.state.or.us

**★ 17068 ★ Osteopathic Medical Board of California**
2720 Gateway Oaks Dr, Ste 350
Sacramento, CA 95833
Phone: (916)263-3100
Linda J. Bergmann, Director

**★ 17069 ★ Pennsylvania State Board of Osteopathic Medicine**
PO Box 2649
Harrisburg, PA 17105-2649
Phone: (717)783-4858    Fax: (717)787-7769
Website: http://www.dos.state.pa.us
Gina K. Bittner, Contact

**★ 17070 ★ Puerto Rico Board of Medical Examiners**
Call Box 13969
San Juan, PR 00908
Phone: (787)792-8949    Fax: (787)792-4436
Pablo Valentin-Torres, Director

**★ 17071 ★ Rhode Island Board of Medical Licensure and Discipline**
3 Capitol Hill, Rm. 205
Providence, RI 02908-5097
Phone: (401)222-3855    Fax: (401)222-2158
Website: http://www.docboard.org/ri/main.htm

**★ 17072 ★ South Carolina Board of Medical Examiners**
Synergy Business Park
Kingstree Bldg.
110 Centerview Dr., Ste. 202
PO Box 11289
Columbia, SC 29211-1289
Phone: (803)896-4500    Fax: (803)896-4515
Email: medboard@mail.llr.state.sc.us
Website: http://www.llr.state.sc.us/POL/Medical/Default.htm

**★ 17073 ★ South Dakota State Board of Medical and Osteopathic Examiners**
1323 S Minnesota Ave.
Sioux Falls, SD 57105
Phone: (605)334-8343    Fax: (605)336-0270
Email: jphalen@sdsma.org
Website: http://www.state.sd.us/dcr/medical/medhom.htm
Paul Jensen, Contact

**★ 17074 ★ Tennessee State Board of Osteopathic Examiners**
Cordell Hull Bldg., 3rd Fl.
425 Fifth Ave. N
Nashville, TN 37247-1010
Phone: (615)532-3202    Free: 888-310-4650
Fax: (615)253-4484
Email: DDenton@mail.state.tn.us
Website: http://www.fsmb.org/
Rosemarie Otto, Contact

**★ 17075 ★ Texas State Board of Medical Examiners**
333 Guadalupe St., Tower 3, Ste. 610
PO Box 2018
Austin, TX 78768-2018
Phone: (512)305-7010    Free: 800-248-4062
Fax: (512)463-9416
Website: http://www.tsbme.state.tx.us/

**★ 17076 ★ Utah Physicians Licensing Board**
Board of Osteopathic Medicine
160 E 300 S, 4th Fl.
PO Box 146741
Salt Lake City, UT 84114
Phone: (801)530-6628    Fax: (801)530-6511
Email: lduke@br.state.ut.us

**Website:** http://www.dopl.utah.gov/
Diana Baker, Contact

**★ 17077 ★ Vermont Board of Osteopathic Physicians and Surgeons**
26 Terrace St.
Drawer 09
Montpelier, VT 05609-1106
**Phone:** (802)828-2373     **Fax:** (802)828-2465
**Email:** patkins@sec.state.vt.us
**Website:** http://www.sec.state.vt.us
Peggy Atkins, Contact

**★ 17078 ★ Virgin Islands Board of Medical Examiners**
Department of Health
48 Sugar Estate
St Thomas, VI 00802
**Phone:** (340)774-0117     **Fax:** (340)777-4001
Lydia Scott, Contact

**★ 17079 ★ Virginia Board of Medicine**
6606 W Broad St., 4th Fl.
Richmond, VA 23230-1717
**Phone:** (804)662-9908     **Free:** 800-533-1560
**Fax:** (804)662-9517
**Email:** medbd@dhp.state.va.us
**Website:** http://www.dhp.state.va.us/medicine/default.htm
William L. Harp, MD, Director

**★ 17080 ★ Washington State Board of Osteopathic Medicine and Surgery**
Department of Health
Health Professions Quality Assurance
1112 SE Quince St.
PO Box 47870
Olympia, WA 98504-7870
**Phone:** (360)236-4943     **Fax:** (360)236-2406
**Email:** hpqa.csc@doh.wa.gov
**Website:** http://www.doh.wa.gov
Robert Nicoloff, Director

**★ 17081 ★ West Virginia Board of Osteopathy**
334 Penco Rd.
Weirton, WV 26062
**Phone:** (304)723-4638     **Fax:** (304)723-6723
**Email:** bdosteo@mail.wvnet.edu
**Website:** http://www.state.wv.us/bdosteo/
Cheryl Schreiber, Contact

**★ 17082 ★ Wisconsin Medical Examining Board**
1400 E Washington Ave., Rm. 178
PO Box 8935
Madison, WI 53708-8935
**Phone:** (608)266-2112     **Fax:** (608)261-7083
**Email:** web@drl.state.wi.us
**Website:** http://www.drl.state.wi.us/
Deanna Zychomski, Director

**★ 17083 ★ Wyoming Medical Examiners Board**
211 W 19th St., 2nd Fl.
Cheyenne, WY 82002
**Phone:** (307)778-7053     **Free:** 800-438-5784
**Fax:** (307)778-2069
**Email:** wyomedical@wyomedicalboard.org
**Website:** http://wyomedboard.state.wy.us/
Carole Shotwell, Contact

---

# State & Regional Organizations

## Osteopathic Medicine

*Listed below are state divisional societies of the American Osteopathic Association, 142 E Ontario St., Chicago, IL 60611, (800)621-1773, http://www.aoa-net.org/.*

### Arizona

**★ 17084 ★ Arizona Osteopathic Medical Association**
5150 N 16th St., No. A122
Phoenix, AZ 85016
**Phone:** (602)266-6699     **Free:** 888-266-6699
**Fax:** (602)266-1393
**Email:** mweaver@az-osteo.org
**Website:** http://www.az-osteo.org
Amanda Weaver, MBA, Exec Director
David J. Wilson, DO, Vice President

### Arkansas

**★ 17085 ★ Arkansas Osteopathic Medical Association**
412 Union Train Station
1400 West Markham
Little Rock, AR 72201
**Phone:** (501)374-8900     **Fax:** (501)374-8959
**Email:** osteomed@ipa.net
**Website:** http://www.arkosteomed.org
Ed Bullington, Exec Director
David Rowe, DO, Treasurer

### California

**★ 17086 ★ Osteopathic Physicians and Surgeons of California**
1900 Point West Way, Ste. 188
Sacramento, CA 95815
**Phone:** (916)561-0724     **Fax:** (916)561-0728
**Email:** opsc@opsc.org
**Website:** www.opsc.org
Ken Young, CAE, Exec Director
Kevin M. Jenkins, DO, Vice President

### Colorado

**★ 17087 ★ Colorado Society of Osteopathic Medicine**
650 S Cherry St., Ste. 440
Denver, CO 80246
**Phone:** (303)322-1752     **Fax:** (303)322-1956
**Email:** info@coloradodo.org
**Website:** http://www.coloradodo.org
Kathleen Brennan, Exec Director
Cynthia Egan, DO, Vice President

### Delaware

**★ 17088 ★ Delaware State Osteopathic Medical Society**
PO Box 8177
Talleyville, DE 19803-8177
**Phone:** (302)764-1198     **Fax:** (302)764-1322
**Email:** dsoms@del.net
**Website:** http://www.deosteopathic.org
Christine Kelly, Contact
James Fierro, DO, Vice President

### Florida

**★ 17089 ★ Florida Osteopathic Medical Association**
2007 Apalachee Pkwy.
Tallahassee, FL 32301
**Phone:** (850)878-7364     **Fax:** (850)942-7538

**Email:** admin@foma.org
**Website:** http://www.foma.org
Stephen R. Winn, Exec Director
Larry Mattingly, DO, Vice President

### Georgia

**★ 17090 ★ Georgia Osteopathic Medical Association**
2160 Idlewood Rd.
Tucker, GA 30084-4815
**Phone:** (770)493-9278     **Fax:** (770)908-3210
**Email:** exdir@goma.org
**Website:** http://www.goma.org
Holly W. Barnwell, Exec Director
Ben Abraham, DO, Vice President

### Idaho

**★ 17091 ★ Idaho Osteopathic Medical Association**
7685 Emerald
Boise, ID 83704
**Phone:** (208)376-2522     **Fax:** (208)375-5860
Ronald Higgenbotham, DO, Secretary

### Illinois

**★ 17092 ★ Illinois Osteopathic Medical Association**
142 E Ontario
Chicago, IL 60611
**Phone:** (312)202-8179     **Free:** 800-621-1773
**Fax:** (312)202-8479
**Email:** ioms@ioms.org
**Website:** http://www.ioms.org
Michael Mallie, Exec Director

**★ 17093 ★ New York State Osteopathic Medical Society, Inc.**
142 E Ontario
Chicago, IL 60611
**Phone:** (312)202-8179     **Free:** 800-841-4131
**Fax:** (312)202-8224
**Email:** nysoms@nysoms.org
**Website:** http://www.nysoms.org
Michael Mallie, Exec Director

### Indiana

**★ 17094 ★ Indiana Osteopathic Association**
3520 Guion Rd., Ste. 202
Indianapolis, IN 46222-1672
**Phone:** (317)926-3009     **Fax:** (317)926-3984
**Email:** mclaphan@aol.com
**Website:** http://www.inosteo.org
Michael H. Claphan, CAE, Exec Director

### Iowa

**★ 17095 ★ Iowa Osteopathic Medical Association**
950 12th St.
Des Moines, IA 50309
**Phone:** (515)283-0002     **Fax:** (515)283-0355
**Email:** leah@ioma.org
**Website:** http://www.ioma.org
Norman Pawlewski, Exec Director

### Kansas

**★ 17096 ★ Kansas Association of Osteopathic Medicine**
1260 SW Topeka Blvd.
Topeka, KS 66612
**Phone:** (785)234-5563     **Fax:** (785)234-5564
**Email:** kansasdo@aol.com
Charles Wheelen, Exec Director

## Kentucky

**★ 17097 ★ Kentucky Osteopathic Medical Association**
1501 Twilight Tr.
Frankfort, KY 40601
**Phone:** (502)223-5322          **Fax:** (502)223-4937
**Email:** info@koma.org
**Website:** http://www.koma.org
Tom Underwood, Exec Director

## Maine

**★ 17098 ★ Maine Osteopathic Association**
693 Western Ave., No. 1
Manchester, ME 04351
**Phone:** (207)623-1101          **Fax:** (207)623-4228
**Email:** info@mainedo.org
**Website:** http://www.mainedo.org
Kellie P. Miller, MS, Exec Director

## Maryland

**★ 17099 ★ Association of Military Osteopathic Physicians and Surgeons**
1796 Severn Hills Lane
Severn, MD 21144-1061
**Phone:** (410)519-8217          **Fax:** (410)519-7657
**Email:** jyonts@amops.org
**Website:** http://www.amops.org
Jim Yonts, Exec Director

**★ 17100 ★ Maryland Association of Osteopathic Physicians**
3603 Southside Ave.
Phoenix, MD 21131
**Phone:** (410)683-8100          **Free:** 888-741-6267
**Fax:** (410)683-8200
**Email:** maops@maops.com
Darleen Won, Exec Director

## Michigan

**★ 17101 ★ Michigan Osteopathic Association**
2445 Woodlake Cir.
Okemos, MI 48864-5941
**Phone:** (517)347-1555          **Fax:** (517)347-1556
**Email:** okemos@moa-do.com
**Website:** http://www.moa-do.com
Dennis M. Paradis, Exec Director

## Mississippi

**★ 17102 ★ Mississippi Osteopathic Medical Association**
PO Box 16890
Jackson, MS 39236
**Phone:** (601)366-3105          **Free:** (866)423-6286
**Fax:** (601)366-2868
**Email:** info@moma-net.org
**Website:** http://www.moma-net.org
Jeffrey J. LeBoeuf, Exec Director

## Montana

**★ 17103 ★ Montana Osteopathic Association**
224 W Main, No. 401
Lewistown, MT 59457
**Phone:** (406)538-7721          **Fax:** (406)538-5201
William J. Munro, DO, Exec Director

## Nevada

**★ 17104 ★ Nevada Osteopathic Medical Association**
2920 N Green Valley Pkwy., No. 527
Henderson, NV 89014-0406

**Phone:** (702)434-7112          **Fax:** (702)434-7110
**Email:** nvoma@aol.com
**Website:** http://www.nevadaosteopathic.com
Denise Selleck-Davis, Exec Director

## New Hampshire

**★ 17105 ★ New Hampshire Osteopathic Association**
7 N State St.
Concord, NH 03301
**Phone:** (603)224-1909
Joy Potter, Contact

## New Jersey

**★ 17106 ★ New Jersey Association of Osteopathic Physicians and Surgeons (NJAOPS)**
1 Distribution Way, Ste. 201
Monmouth Junction, NJ 08852-3001
**Phone:** (732)940-9000          **Fax:** (732)940-8899
**Email:** njaops@njosteo.org
**Website:** http://www.njosteo.com
Frank Cagliari, Exec Director

## North Dakota

**★ 17107 ★ North Dakota State Osteopathic Association**
1600 2nd Ave. SW, Ste. 120
Minot, ND 58701
**Phone:** (701)852-8798          **Free:** 800-437-4010
**Fax:** (701)837-5410
**Website:** http://www.nadk.net
Carmen Christianson Bell, MS, Exec Director

## Ohio

**★ 17108 ★ Ohio Osteopathic Association**
53 W 3rd Ave.
PO Box 8130
Columbus, OH 43201-0130
**Phone:** (614)299-2107          **Fax:** (614)294-0457
**Email:** execdir@ooanet.org
**Website:** http://www.ooanet.org
Jon F. Wills, Exec Director

## Oklahoma

**★ 17109 ★ Oklahoma Osteopathic Association**
4848 N Lincoln Blvd.
Oklahoma City, OK 73105-3335
**Phone:** (405)528-4848          **Free:** 800-522-8379
**Fax:** (405)528-6102
**Email:** lynette@okosteo.org
**Website:** http://www.okosteo.org
Lynette McClain, Exec Director

## Oregon

**★ 17110 ★ Osteopathic Physicians and Surgeons of Oregon**
2121 SW Broadway, Ste. 300
Portland, OR 97201-3146
**Phone:** (503)222-2279          **Free:** 800-533-6776
**Fax:** (503)222-2392
**Email:** edied@opso.org
**Website:** http://www.opso.com
Jeff Heatherington, Exec Director

## Pennsylvania

**★ 17111 ★ Pennsylvania Osteopathic Medical Association**
1330 Eisenhower Blvd.
Harrisburg, PA 17111-2395
**Phone:** (717)939-9318          **Free:** 800-544-POMA
**Fax:** (717)939-7255
**Email:** mlanni@poma.org

**Website:** http://www.poma.org
Mario E. J. Lanni, Exec Director

## South Dakota

**★ 17112 ★ South Dakota Osteopathic Association**
MASSA—Berry Clinic
890 Lazelle St.
Sturgis, SD 57785
**Phone:** (605)347-3616          **Fax:** (605)347-4713
David Lauer, DO, Secretary

## Tennessee

**★ 17113 ★ Tennessee Osteopathic Medical Association**
200 4th Ave. N, Ste. 900
Nashville, TN 37219
**Phone:** (615)242-3032          **Fax:** (615)254-7047
**Email:** dawalker@wmgt.org
**Website:** http://www.wmgt.org
DeeAnn Walker, Exec Director

## Texas

**★ 17114 ★ Texas Osteopathic Medical Association**
1415 Lavaca St.
Austin, TX 78701-1634
**Phone:** (512)708-8662          **Free:** 800-444-8662
**Fax:** (512)708-1415
**Email:** terryb@txosteo.org
**Website:** http://www.txosteo.org/
Terry R. Boucher, MPH, Exec Director

## Vermont

**★ 17115 ★ Vermont State Association of Osteopathic Physicians and Surgeons, Inc.**
72 Barre St.
Montpelier, VT 05602-3508
**Phone:** (802)229-9418          **Free:** 800-454-9663
**Fax:** (802)229-5619
**Email:** nocdos@shore.net
John M. Peterson, DO, Exec Director

## Washington

**★ 17116 ★ Washington Osteopathic Medical Association**
PO Box 16486
Seattle, WA 98116
**Phone:** (206)937-5358          **Fax:** (206)933-6529
**Email:** kathie@woma.org
**Website:** http://www.woma.org
Kathleen S. Itter, Exec Director

## West Virginia

**★ 17117 ★ West Virginia Society of Osteopathic Medicine, Inc.**
PO Box 5266
Charleston, WV 25361-0266
**Phone:** (304)345-9836          **Fax:** (304)345-9865
**Email:** wvdo@wvsominc.org
**Website:** http://www.wvsominc.org
Charlotte Cales Pulliam, Exec Director

## Wisconsin

**★ 17118 ★ Wisconsin Association of Osteopathic Physicians and Surgeons**
34615 Rd. E
Oconomowoc, WI 53066-2543
**Phone:** (262)567-0520          **Fax:** (262)567-0520
Robert J. Finnegan, CAE, Exec Director

## Foundations & Other Funding Organizations

### Other Funding Organizations

**★ 17119 ★ Renal Pathology Society (RPS)**
c/o Guillermo Herrera
Department of Pathology
LSUMC Shreveport
1501 Kings Hwy
Shreveport, LA 71130-3932
**Phone:** (318)675-5878  **Fax:** (318)675-7662
**Email:** gherra@lsumc.edu
**Website:** http://www.renalpathsoc.org
Dr. Guillermo A. Herrerame, Sec. -Treas.
**Desc:** Works to spread and increase knowledge of pathology of the kidney and seeks to develop renal pathology as a subspecialty. Conducts research and educational programs. **Awards:** Jacob Churg Award (annual); Young Investigator Award (biennial).

**★ 17120 ★ Society of Toxicologic Pathologists (STP)**
19 Mantua Rd.
Mount Royal, NJ 08061
**Phone:** (856)423-3610  **Fax:** (856)423-3420
**Email:** stphq@talley.com
**Website:** http://www.toxpath.org
Stephanie Dickinson, Dir.
**Desc:** Promotes the advancement of the Individuals interested in toxicology and toxicologic pathology from industry, academic institutions, and government. **Awards:** Student Invetigator Awards (annual).

**★ 17121 ★ Society for Ultrastructural Pathology**
c/o Joseph M. Harb, PhD
14655 East View Ct.
Brookfield, WI 53005
**Phone:** (414)781-6703
**Email:** khewanl@zappa.ultrakohl.com
**Website:** http://sup.ultrakohl.com/
Joseph Harb, PhD, Treas.
**Desc:** Promotes the art and science of diagnostic electron microscopy. Fosters the application of electron microscopy in the diagnosis and research of human diseases. Also provides an opportunity for the exchange of information, particularly ultrastructural and immunohistochemical, relevant to diagnostic pathology. Relevance of molecular pathology techniques to tumor pathology is also a focus. **Awards:** Pathologist in Training Award (annual) for best poster with ultrastructural study at U.S.-Canadian Academy of Pathology.

**★ 17122 ★ United States and Canadian Academy of Pathology**
3643 Walton Way Extension
Augusta, GA 30909
**Phone:** (706)733-7550  **Fax:** (706)733-8033
**Email:** iap@uscap.org
**Website:** http://www.uscap.org
Fred Silva, MD, Sec. -Treas.
**Desc:** Works for the advancement of pathology teaching, practice, and research. Disseminates information to members. Sponsors educational programs to serve the needs of pathologists of various levels of experience. Presents Maude Abbott Lectureship to a recognized and respected person in contemporary pathology. **Awards:** Benjamin Castleman Award (annual) for a pathologist or pathologist-in-training under 40 years old who has written an outstanding paper on human pathology in English; Council's Distinguished Pathologist Award for an individual who has made a major contribution to pathology over the years; F. K. Mostofi Distinguished Service Award (annual) for a member who has rendered outstanding service to the Academy and the International Academy of Pathology; Stowell-Orbison Awards for Pathologists-in-Training for authors of outstanding papers.

## National & International Organizations

**★ 17123 ★ American Academy of Oral and Maxillofacial Pathology (AAOMP)**
710 E Ogden Ave No. 600
Naperville, IL 60563-8614
**Phone:** (630)369-2406  **Free:** 888-552-2667
**Fax:** (630)369-2488
**Email:** aaomp@b-online.com
**Website:** http://www.aaomp.org
Carl M. Allen, VP
**Fnded:** 1946. **Mem:** 800. **Desc:** Professional society of oral pathologists. **Pub:** *Oral Radiology and Endodontics*. Journal. • *Oral Surgery, Oral Medicine, Oral Pathology*, monthly. **Frmly:** (1994) American Academy Oral Pathology.

**★ 17124 ★ American Association of Neuropathologists (AANP)**
c/o J.E. Parisi, MD
Department Lab Med & Pathology
Mayo Clinic
200 First St. SW
Rochester, MN 55905
**Phone:** (507)284-3394  **Fax:** (507)284-1599
**Email:** aanp@mayo.edu
**Website:** http://www.aanp-jnen.com
Dr. Joseph Parisi, Sec. -Treas.
**Fnded:** 1959. **Mem:** 800. **Desc:** Promotes neuropathology, especially the study of diverse aspects of diseases of the nervous system including changes at tissue, cellular, subcellular, and molecular levels with consideration of etiology and pathophysiology, genetics, epidemiology and clinical manifestations of such diseases. **Pub:** *Journal of Neuropathology and Experimental Neurology*, monthly. Journal. • Membership Directory, annual. **Frmly:** (1932) Club of Neuropathologists.

**★ 17125 ★ American Association of Pathologists' Assistants (AAPA)**
Rosewood Office Plaza
1711 W County Rd. B, Ste. 300 N
Roseville, MN 55113-4036
**Phone:** (651)697-9264  **Free:** 800-532-AAPA
**Fax:** (651)635-0307
**Email:** oei@mn.state.net
**Website:** http://www.pathologistsassistants.org
Tom Reilly, Pres.
**Fnded:** 1972. **Mem:** 600. **Desc:** Pathologists' assistants and individuals qualified by academic and practical training to provide service in anatomic pathology under the direction of a qualified pathologist who is responsible for the performance of the assistant. Promotes the mutual association of trained pathologists' assistants and informs the public and the medical profession concerning the goals of this profession. Compiles statistics on salaries, geographic distribution, and duties of pathologists' assistants. Sponsors a continuing medical education program; offers placement services for members only. **Pub:** *AAPA Newsletter*, quarterly. Newsletter. Includes employment and educational opportunity listings. *Price:* Included in membership dues. • Membership Directory, biennial.

**★ 17126 ★ American Board of Oral and Maxillofacial Pathology**
625 N Michigan Ave., No. 1820
Chicago, IL 60611
**Phone:** (312)642-0070  **Fax:** (312)642-8584
**Email:** cefilas@aboms.org
**Website:** http://www.aboms.org/
Clarita Wendrich, Exec. Sec.
**Fnded:** 1948. **Mem:** 260. **Desc:** Works to encourage the study of and promote and improve the practice of oral pathology; arrange, conduct, and control examinations to determine the competence of applicants; grant and issue certificates. **Frmly:** American Board of Oral Pathology.

**★ 17127 ★ American Board of Pathology (ABP)**
PO Box 25915
Tampa, FL 33622-5915
**Phone:** (813)286-2444  **Fax:** (813)289-5279
**Website:** http://www.abpath.org/
William H. Hartmann, MD, Exec. VP
**Fnded:** 1936. **Mem:** 12. **Desc:** Seeks to: encourage study of pathology; maintain profesional standards and advance practice in the field; maintain registry of certified pathologists; participate in the evaluation and review of graduate medical education programs in pathology. Examines doctors of medicine or osteopathy who have had three to five years postgraduate training in laboratory medicine and pathology. Certifies qualified and successful applicants as specialists in pathology. **Pub:** *The American Board of Pathology*, 2-3/year. Newsletter. • *Information Booklet*, annual. Booklet.

**American College of Veterinary Pathologists (ACVP)**
*See:* Entry 20562


★ **17128** ★ **American Pathology Foundation (APF)**
1202 Allanson Rd.
Mundelein, IL 60060
**Phone:** (847)949-6055    **Fax:** (847)566-4580
**Email:** mbuckley2@covad.net
**Website:** http://americanpathologyfoundation.org
Edward J. Stygar, Jr., Exec. Dir.

**Fnded:** 1959. **Mem:** 750. **Desc:** Board-certified pathologists. Objectives are: to promote the practice of pathology in private laboratories; to provide for exchange of information that will improve anatomic and clinical pathology; to cooperate in the development of the art and sciences of medicine and pathology. Compiles statistics. **Pub:** Directory, annual. • Newsletter, quarterly. **Frmly:** Private Practitioners of Pathology Foundation.


★ **17129** ★ **American Registry of Pathology (ARP)**
c/o Armed Forces Institute of Pathology
14th St. & Alaska Ave. NW
Washington, DC 20306-6000
**Phone:** (202)782-2143    **Fax:** (202)782-4567
**Website:** http://www.afip.org/ARP/arp.html
John Duckworth, Pres.

**Fnded:** 1976. **Desc:** Engages in cooperative enterprises in medical research and education with the Armed Forces Institute of Pathology. Functions as a fiscal agent in the management of research grants and monies derived from tuition fees, publications, and contributions. Serves as a link between, and encourages cooperation among, the military and civilian medical, dental, and veterinary communities for the mutual benefit of military and civilian medicine. Provides personnel and other services in support of research. Offers 38 continuing medical education courses annually. Bestows annual John Hill Brinton Award in recognition of outstanding young researcher, John Shaw Billings Lifetime Achievement Award to senior AFIP staff member, Callender-Binford fellowships.


**American Society for Clinical Pathology (ASCP)**
*See:* Entry 12193


**American Society of Dermatopathology (ASDP)**
*See:* Entry 6794


★ **17130** ★ **American Society for Investigative Pathology (ASIP)**
9650 Rockville Pke.
Bethesda, MD 20814-3993
**Phone:** (301)530-7130    **Fax:** (301)571-1879
**Email:** asip@pathol.faseb.org
**Website:** http://asip.uthscsa.edu
Mark E. Sobel, MD,PhD, Exec. Officer

**Fnded:** 1976. **Mem:** 1,700. **Desc:** Experimental research pathologists who have made significant contributions to the knowledge of disease. **Pub:** *The American Journal of Pathology*, monthly. Journal. Research papers in experimental pathology. Covers cell injury and death, inflammatory reactions, disturbances in circulation, and neoplastic growth. *Price:* Included in membership dues; $195/year for nonmembers; $350/year for institutions. • *ASIP Newsletter*, bimonthly. Newsletter. Contains articles on public policy issues and research opportunities. Includes new members and personnel promotions and appointments. *Price:* Included in membership dues. • *The Journal of Molecular Diagnostics*, quarterly. Journal. Research papers in experimental pathology. Covers cell injury and death, inflammatory reactions, disturbances in circulation, and neoplastic growth. *Price:* Included in membership dues; $195/year for nonmem-

bers; $350/year for institutions. • Membership Directory, annual. **Frmly:** (1992) American Association of Pathologists.


★ **17131** ★ **Armed Forces Institute of Pathology (AFIP)**
6825 16th St. NW
Washington, DC 20306-6000
**Phone:** (202)782-2111    **Fax:** (202)782-9376
**Email:** wagner@afip.osd.mil
**Website:** http://www.afip.org/
Captain Glenn N. Wagner, Dir.

**Fnded:** 1862. **Mem:** 842. **Desc:** Chartered by the Department of Defense to: maintain a consultation service for the diagnosis of pathologic material; conduct experimental, statistical, and morphological research in pathology; provide instruction in advanced pathology and related subjects; prepare, procure, and duplicate teaching aids; operate the AFIP Repository and Research Services; maintain the National Museum of Health and Medicine of the AFIP and a Visual Information Service for the collection, preparation, duplication, reference, and filing of medical illustrative material. Sponsors a series of courses. **Pub:** *AFIP Letter*, bimonthly. Newsletter. Third series, containing 30 separate fascicles, with international distribution. • *Atlas of Tumor Pathology*. **Frmly:** (1949) Army Medical Museum.


★ **17132** ★ **Asia Pacific Association of Societies of Pathologists (APASP)**
Department of Pathology
Beijing Medical University
Beijing 100083, People's Republic of China

**Lang(s):** Chinese, English. **Desc:** Professional associations representing pathologists. Seeks to advance the study, teaching, and practice of pathology. Facilitates exchange of information among members; sponsors research and continuing professional development programs.


★ **17133** ★ **Association of Clinical Pathologists (ACP)**
189 Dyke Rd.
Hove BN3 1TL, United Kingdom
**Phone:** 44 1273 775700    **Fax:** 44 1273 773303
**Website:** http://www.pathologists.org.uk

**Fnded:** 1927. **Mem:** 2,000. **Reg. Groups:** 12. **Lang(s):** English. **Desc:** Promotes the study and practice of clinical pathology. Offers courses. **Pub:** *ACP News*, quarterly. Newsletter. • *ACP Yearbook*. Directory. Includes transcripts of speeches delivered at the annual meeting. • *Journal of Clinical Pathology*, monthly. Journal.


★ **17134** ★ **Association for Molecular Pathology (AMP)**
9650 Rockville Pike
Bethesda, MD 20814-3993
**Phone:** (301)634-7939    **Fax:** (301)571-1879
**Email:** amp@pathol.faseb.org
**Website:** http://www.ampweb.org/
Frances A. Pitlick, PhD, Exec. Officer

**Fnded:** 1995. **Mem:** 750. **Desc:** Individuals interested in, or engaged in the practice of, molecular pathology. Promotes clinical practice, basic research, and education in the field. Represents members' interests within the health care industry. Develops and maintains liaison with other organizations and agencies concerned with molecular pathology; serves as a forum for the exchange of ideas and information among members. Participates in the development of regulatory and credentialing policies applied to molecular pathology; promulgates guidlines for molecular pathology training programs. Conducts educational programs to increase public awareness of molecular pathology. **Pub:** *AMP Membership Directory*, annual. Directory. • Newsletter, periodic.

★ **17135** ★ **Association of Pathology Chairs (APC)**
c/o Dr. Frances A. Pitlick
9650 Rockville Pike
Bethesda, MD 20814-3993
**Phone:** (301)571-1880    **Fax:** (301)571-1879
**Email:** apc@pathol.faseb.org
**Website:** http://www.apcprods.org/
Abbott Julian Garvin, MD, Pres.

**Fnded:** 1967. **Mem:** 152. **Reg. Groups:** 4. **Desc:** Chairs of medical school departments of pathology. Acts as a communications center for exchange of information and for workshops on innovations for teaching and resident training, department administration, and relationships with governmental and other nonuniversity agencies. Compiles statistics. **Pub:** Newsletter, quarterly. *Price:* available to members only. **Frmly:** (1970) American Association of Chairmen of Medical School Departments of Pathology; (1993) Association of Pathology Chairmen.


★ **17136** ★ **British Association in Forensic Medicine**
Department of Forensic Medicine and Science
University of Glasgow
Glasgow G12 8QQ, United Kingdom
**Phone:** 44 141 3304574    **Fax:** 44 141 3304602
**Email:** j.clark@formed.gla.ac.uk
**Website:** http://www.shef.ac.uk/~bafm

**Fnded:** 1950. **Mem:** 200. **Desc:** Promotes the specialty of forensic pathology. Represents members' interests.


**Canadian Association of Neuropathologists (CAND) (Association Canadienne de Neuropathologistes — ACN)**
*See:* Entry 13964


★ **17137** ★ **Canadian Association of Pathologists (CAP) (Association Canadienne des Pathologistes — ACP)**
774 Echo Dr.
Ottawa, ON, Canada K1S 5N8
**Phone:** (613)730-6230    **Free:** 800-668-3740
**Fax:** (613)730-0260
**Email:** cap@rcpsc.edu
**Website:** http://cap.medical.org

**Lang(s):** English, French. **Desc:** Pathologists and other health care professionals with an interest in pathology. Promotes professional development of members; seeks to advance the study and practice of pathology. Facilitates communication and cooperation among members; conducts continuing professional education programs.


★ **17138** ★ **Clinical Cytometry Society (CCS)**
PO Box 25456
Colorado Springs, CO 80936
**Phone:** (719)836-2025    **Fax:** (719)836-2122
**Email:** admin@cytometry.org
**Website:** http://www.cytometry.org/

**Desc:** Fosters the development and implementation of cytometry in relation to human pathology. **Pub:** *Communications in Clinical Cytometry*, semiannual. Journal. • Newsletter.


**College of American Pathologists (CAP)**
*See:* Entry 12201


★ **17139** ★ **European Society for Analytical Cellular Pathology (ESACP)**
UFR Pharmacie
51, rue Cognacq-Jay
F-51100 Reims, France
**Phone:** 33 326 913590    **Fax:** 33 326 918015
**Email:** jean.dufer@univ-reims.fr

**Website:** http://www.esacp.org/

**Lang(s):** English, French. **Desc:** Scientists actively engaged in the field of analytical cellular pathology; health care professionals and scientists working in related fields; pharmaceutical manufacturers and biotechnology firms. Seeks to advance the study, teaching, and practice of analytical cellular pathology; promotes development of new technologies relevant to the field. Facilitates exchange of information among members; sponsors research and educational programs; serves as a clearinghouse on analytical cellular pathology. **Pub:** *Journal of Analytical Cellular Pathology*, periodic.


★ 17140 ★ **European Society of Pathology (ESP)**
c/o Prof. John M. Nesland
The Norwegian Radium Hospital and Institute for Cancer Resea
Department of Pathology
Montebello
N-0310 Oslo, Norway
**Phone:** 47 22 935620          **Fax:** 47 22 730164
**Email:** j.m.nesland@labmed.uio.no
**Website:** http://129.240.38.9/esp/
**Fnded:** 1964. **Mem:** 1,352. **Lang(s):** English, French, German, Italian, Russian, Spanish. **Desc:** Pathologists and other medical doctors in 49 countries with an interest in pathology. Fosters communication among pathologists; promotes publication of works on pathology and the development of a European school of pathology. **Pub:** *European Pathology Newsletter*, periodic. • *Pathology Research and Practice*, periodic. Journal. • *Pathology Update*, periodic. Journal.


**European Society of Veterinary Pathology (ESVP)**
*See:* Entry 20611


★ 17141 ★ **Finnish Society for Dermatopathology (FSD) (Suomen Dermatopatologiyhdistys)**
c/o University Central Hospital
Department of Dermatology
Meilahdentie 2
FIN-00250 Helsinki, Finland
**Phone:** 358 9 47186263          **Fax:** 358 9 47186474
**Email:** manfred.reinacher@vetmed.uni-giessen.de
**Website:** http://www.bris.ac.uk/Depts/PathAndMicro/EuroVet/esvp.htm
**Fnded:** 1984. **Mem:** 131. **Lang(s):** English, Finnish. **Desc:** Medical doctors. Promotes the study of dermatopathology.


★ 17142 ★ **Hong Kong Pathology Society**
c/o Dr. Chan Kwok Wah
Department of Pathology
Queen Mary Hospital
Pokfulam Rd.
Hong Kong, People's Republic of China
**Phone:** 852 28554874          **Fax:** 852 28725197
**Fnded:** 1982. **Mem:** 45. **Lang(s):** Chinese, English. **Desc:** Medical doctors in the field of pathology. Seeks to advance the profession of pathology. Serves as a forum for discussion and exchange of information among members. Conducts continuing professional development programs; sponsors research; holds competitions and social functions. **Pub:** Newsletter, quarterly.


★ 17143 ★ **International Academy of Pathology (IAP)**
c/o Florabel G. Mullick
Armed Forces Institute of Pathology
Center for Advanced Pathology
14th St. & Alaska Ave. NW
Washington, DC 20306-6000
**Phone:** (202)782-2550          **Fax:** (202)782-7166
**Email:** mullick@email.afp.osd.mil
**Website:** http://www.afip.org/iap/
Florabel G. Mullick, Sec.

**Fnded:** 1906. **Mem:** 8,300. **Reg. Groups:** 32. **Desc:** Professional society of pathologists and medical scientists. Aim is to improve methods of teaching pathology. Coordinates anatomical pathology, pathologic physiology, and comparative pathology; promotes research in pathology in medical schools, laboratories, hospitals, and medical museums. **Pub:** *International Pathology*, quarterly. Newsletter. *Price:* Included in membership dues. **Frmly:** (1954) International Association of Medical Museums.


**International Association of Oral Pathologists (IAOP)**
*See:* Entry 6545


**International Federation for Cervical Pathology and Colposcopy (IFCPC) (Federacion Internacional de Patologia Cervical y Colposcopia)**
*See:* Entry 16693


★ 17144 ★ **International Society of Neuropathology (Societe Internationale de Neuropathologie)**
c/o Dr. Janice R. Anderson
Department of Histopathology
Addenbrooke's Hospital
Cambridge CB2 2QQ, United Kingdom
**Email:** hkalimo@mailhost.utu.fi
**Website:** http://www.ifcpc.org
**Fnded:** 1972. **Mem:** 2,500. **Lang(s):** English. **Desc:** Members of national societies of neuropathology in 30 countries. Works to foster the formation of national and regional societies of neuropathology and to promote cooperation among these societies. Maintains liaison with international organizations in various fields of neurological sciences. Encourages the exchange of information and persons engaged in neuropathology. Initiates research projects. **Pub:** *Brain Pathology*, quarterly. Journal. • *Membership Directory*, periodic. Directory.


★ 17145 ★ **Intersociety Committee on Pathology Information (ICPI)**
9650 Rockville Pike
Bethesda, MD 20814-3993
**Phone:** (301)571-1880          **Fax:** (301)571-1879
**Email:** icpi@pathol.faseb.org
**Website:** http://www.pathologytraining.org
Frances Pitlick, Info. Counsel

**Fnded:** 1957. **Mem:** 5. **Desc:** One representative from each sponsoring society: American Society for Investigative Pathology; American Society of Clinical Pathologists; Association of Pathology Chairs; College of American Pathologists; U.S. & Canadian Academy of Pathology. Disseminates information about the medical practice and research achievements of pathology. Produces career information. **Pub:** *Directory of Pathology Training Programs: Residencies and Fellowships in US and Canada*, annual. Directory. *Price:* $25; $5 for medical students/residents; Free to medical schools/medical libraries/teaching; Hospital. • *Pathology as a Career in Medicine*. Brochure.


★ 17146 ★ **Permanent International Committee of Congresses of Comparative Pathology (Comite International Permanent des Congres de Pathologie Comparee)**
4 rue Theodule-Ribot
F-75017 Paris, France
**Phone:** 33 1 6225319

**Lang(s):** English, French. **Desc:** Pathologists and other interested individuals. Seeks to advance scholarship and practice in the field of pathology. Serves as a clearinghouse on pathology; facilitates exchange of information among members; sponsors research and educational programs.

**Polish Paediatric Pathology Society (Polski Towarzystwo Patologii Dzieciecej)**
*See:* Entry 5745


★ 17147 ★ **Renal Pathology Society (RPS)**
c/o Guillermo Herrera
Department of Pathology
LSUMC Shreveport
1501 Kings Hwy
Shreveport, LA 71130-3932
**Phone:** (318)675-5878          **Fax:** (318)675-7662
**Email:** gherra@lsumc.edu
**Website:** http://www.renalpathsoc.org
Dr. Guillermo A. Herrerame, Sec. -Treas.

**Fnded:** 1993. **Mem:** 220. **Desc:** Works to spread and increase knowledge of pathology of the kidney and seeks to develop renal pathology as a subspecialty. Conducts research and educational programs. **Pub:** Directory. • Bulletin.


★ 17148 ★ **Royal College of Pathologists of Australasia**
Durham Hall
207 Albion St.
Surry Hills, NSW 2010, Australia
**Fnded:** 1956.


★ 17149 ★ **Scientific Society of Pathology**
Dept. of General and Clinical Pathology and Laboratory of
Cytopathology
Meidcal University of Varna
Marin Drinov str. 55
BG-9002 Varna, Bulgaria
**Phone:** 359 2 522302851          **Fax:** 359 52 302874
**Email:** uni@asclep.muvar.acad.bg
**Fnded:** 1945. **Mem:** 120. **Nat'l Groups:** 2. **Reg. Groups:** 3. **State Groups:** 2. **Lang(s):** English, French, Russian. **Desc:** Fosters research in pathomorphology and cytology. **Pub:** *Cytopathology*, periodic. Journal. • *Savremenna Medicina*, monthly. Journal.


★ 17150 ★ **Sociedad Argentina de Patologia**
Santa Fe 1171
1059 Buenos Aires, Argentina
**Phone:** 54 1 411633
**Fnded:** 1933.


★ 17151 ★ **Society for Pediatric Pathology**
c/o United States & Canadian Academy of Pathology
3643 Walton Way Extension
Augusta, GA 30909
**Phone:** (706)364-3375          **Fax:** (706)733-8033
**Email:** spp@uscap.org
**Website:** http://path.upmc.edu/spp/
Ronald Jaffe, Pres.

**Desc:** Pediatric pathologists. Seeks to advance the science and practice of pediatric pathology. Facilities integration of scientific developments in the field; conducts continuing medical education programs.


★ 17152 ★ **Society of Toxicologic Pathologists (STP)**
19 Mantua Rd.
Mount Royal, NJ 08061
**Phone:** (856)423-3610          **Fax:** (856)423-3420
**Email:** stphq@talley.com
**Website:** http://www.toxpath.org
Stephanie Dickinson, Dir.

**Fnded:** 1971. **Mem:** 700. **Reg. Groups:** 5. **Desc:** Promotes the advancement of the individuals interested in toxicology and toxicologic pathology from industry, academic institutions, and government. **Pub:** *STP*

*Newsletter*, quarterly. Newsletter. *Price:* available to members only. • *Toxicologic Pathology*, bimonthly. Journal. *Price:* $175/year for individuals in the U.S.; $195/year for individuals outside the U.S.; $195/year for institutions in the U.S.; $215/year for institutions outside the U.S.

★ **17153** ★ **Society for Ultrastructural Pathology**
c/o Joseph M. Harb, PhD
14655 East View Ct.
Brookfield, WI 53005
**Phone:** (414)781-6703
**Email:** khewanl@zappa.ultrakohl.com
**Website:** http://sup.ultrakohl.com/
Joseph Harb, PhD, Treas.
**Fnded:** 1986. **Mem:** 185. **Desc:** Promotes the art and science of diagnostic electron microscopy. Fosters the application of electron microscopy in the diagnosis and research of human diseases. Also provides an opportunity for the exchange of information, particularly ultrastructural and immunohistochemical, relevant to diagnostic pathology. Relevance of molecular pathology techniques to tumor pathology is also a focus. **Pub:** *Organelles in Tumor Diagnosis: An Ultrastructural Atlas.* Book. Atlas designed to identify diagnostic cell structures and tumors through the use of electron microscopy. *Price:* $39.50. • *Ultrastructural Pathology with Related Surgical and Molecular Pathology*, bimonthly. Journal. *Price:* $292.

★ **17154** ★ **United States and Canadian Academy of Pathology**
3643 Walton Way Extension
Augusta, GA 30909
**Phone:** (706)733-7550          **Fax:** (706)733-8033
**Email:** iap@uscap.org
**Website:** http://www.uscap.org
Fred Silva, MD, Sec. -Treas.
**Fnded:** 1906. **Mem:** 7,500. **Desc:** Works for the advancement of pathology teaching, practice, and research. Disseminates information to members. Sponsors educational programs to serve the needs of pathologists of various levels of experience. Presents Maude Abbott Lectureship to a recognized and respected person in contemporary pathology. **Pub:** *Directory of Members*, annual. Membership Directory. *Price:* Free to members. • *Laboratory Investigation*, monthly. Journal. Focuses on significant advances in research dealing with human and experimental diseases. *Price:* Free to members. • *Modern Pathology*, bimonthly. Journal. Concentrates on the practice of diagnostic human pathology. *Price:* Free to members.

★ **17155** ★ **Universities Associated for Research and Education in Pathology (UAREP)**
9650 Rockville Pike
Bethesda, MD 20814-3993
**Phone:** (301)571-1880          **Fax:** (301)571-1879
**Website:** http://www.pathol.org/
Vinay Kumar, MD, Pres.
**Fnded:** 1964. **Mem:** 25. **Desc:** University pathology departments, including faculty members, residents, and research fellows. Provides core material in convenient form for updating and enriching teaching and researching of pathology, with special emphasis on toxicology and chemical carcinogens. Encourages biomedical projects; administers contracts. Has developed guidelines for the National Highway Safety Bureau for use in scientific investigations in accidents. Operates the Registry of Comparative Pathology which provides news of progress in the experimental study of disease from animal models. **Pub:** *Atlas of Tumor Pathology.* Book. • Monographs.

★ **17156** ★ **World Association of Societies of Pathology - Anatomic and Clinical (WASP)**
**(Association Mondiale des Societes de Pathologie - Anatomique et Clinique)**
c/o Dr. Kenneth D. McClatchey
WASP Administrative Office
Sakura-Sugamo Bldg. 7F
Sugamo 2-11-1
Tokyo 170-0002, Japan
**Phone:** 81 3 39496168          **Fax:** 81 3 39496168
**Email:** ncp_d@ja2.so-net.or.jp
**Fnded:** 1947. **Mem:** 54. **Lang(s):** English. **Desc:** National societies of anatomic and clinical pathology in 40 countries united to foster cooperation between members and improve standards in anatomic and clinical pathology. Maintains a variety of committees and educational programs. **Pub:** *Directory*, biennial. Directory. • *News Bulletin of the World Association of Societies of Pathology/Commission on World Standards*, quarterly. Bulletin. **Frmly:** (1969) International Society of Clinical Pathology.

# Research Centers

★ **17157** ★ **Case Western Reserve University**
**Institute of Pathology**
2085 Adelbert Rd.
Cleveland, OH 44106
**Phone:** (216)368-2480          **Fax:** (216)368-0495
**Email:** gxp7@po.cwru.edu
**Website:** http://www.cwru.edu/med/pathology
Dr. George Perry, Interim Ch.
**Activities/Fields:** Immunology, immunopathology, aging, cell biology, neurodegenerative disease, and oncology.

★ **17158** ★ **Institute for Clinical Science, Inc.**
301 S East St., Ste. 3A
Philadelphia, PA 19106
**Phone:** (215)829-7068          **Fax:** (215)829-3094
**Email:** sundermansr@aol.com
Dr. F. William Sunderman, Pres. /Dir.
**Activities/Fields:** Anatomic and clinical pathology, including studies in metal carcinogenesis and toxicology. **Pub:** *Annals of Clinical and Laboratory Science.* • *Procedures Manual for the Institute's Applied Seminars.*

★ **17159** ★ **Mallory Institute of Pathology Foundation**
784 Massachusetts Ave.
Boston, MA 02118
**Phone:** (617)414-5314          **Fax:** (617)414-5315
Dr. Leonard S. Gottlieb, Dir.
**Activities/Fields:** Experimental medicine and pathology, with particular reference to cardiovascular diseases, gastrointestinal diseases, liver and kidney diseases, pulmonary diseases, hematopathology, nutritional pathology, immunopathology, environmental pathology, and oncology.

**South Carolina Health and Environmental Control Department**
**Health Services Division**
**Bureau of Laboratories**
**Division of Clinical Cytology**
*See:* Entry 12222

**U.S. Department of Health and Human Services**
**Food and Drug Administration**
**National Center for Toxicological Research**
**Pathology Associates**
*See:* Entry 17382

**U.S. Department of Health and Human Services**
**National Institute of Allergy and Infectious Diseases**
**Laboratory of Immunopathology**
*See:* Entry 3285

★ **17160** ★ **Universities Associated for Research and Education in Pathology, Inc.**
9650 Rockville Pke.
Bethesda, MD 20814-3993
**Phone:** (301)571-1880          **Fax:** (301)571-1879
**Email:** uarep@pathol.faseb.org
**Website:** http://www.pathologytraining.org
Frances A. Pitlick, PhD, Exec. Off.
**Activities/Fields:** Administers and coordinates educational and research activities in human pathology, including studies on environmental factors in human diseases, environmental pathology, safety of food additives, health effects attributed to unregulated toxic waste disposal sites, accident and forensic pathology, and environmental health policies. Provides core material for pathology instruction to medical students and residents and for web-based educational materials. Supports the development of new directions in pathology, most recently by fostering the initiation and growth of two societies: API - the Association of Pathology Informatics, and ISBER - the International Society for Biological and Environmental Repositories. **Pub:** *Atlas of Tumor Pathology.*

★ **17161** ★ **University of Southern California**
**Lung Disease, Cancer, and Environmental Pathobiology**
2011 Zonal Ave., HMR 201
Los Angeles, CA 90033
**Phone:** (323)257-3599          **Fax:** (323)224-5252
**Email:** sherwin@hsc.usc.edu
Dr. Russell P. Sherwin, Hd.
**Activities/Fields:** Environmental and oncologic pathology, lung disease, cancer, lymphocytes, macrophages, air toxicants, general pathobiology, histochemistry, histopathology, radioisotopes, tissue culture, and electron microscopy, including studies on pathogenesis of lung and breast cancer, pathogenesis and pathologic diagnosis of pulmonary emphysema, biologic effects of air pollution, and computer-assisted image analysis.

★ **17162** ★ **University of Washington**
**Glomerular Disease Research Group**
Division of Nephrology
University of Washington Medical Center
Seattle, WA 98195
**Phone:** (206)543-3695
**Email:** wgc@u.washington.edu
**Website:** http://faculty.washington.edu/uwrenal/
Dr. William G. Couser, Co-Prin. Investigator
**Activities/Fields:** Pathogenesis of glomerular and interstitial diseases using experimental models and cellular and molecular technology.

# Chapter 50
# Pharmacology & Toxicology

## Federal Government Agencies

★ 17163 ★ **U.S. Department of Health and Human Services**
**Food and Drug Administration**
**National Center for Toxicological Research**
3900 NC.T.R. Rd.
Jefferson, AR 72079-9502
**Phone:** (870)543-7130
**Website:** http://www.fda.gov/nctr
Bernard A. Schwetz, Director
**Desc:** The Center conducts peer-reviewed scientific research which supports and anticipates FDA current and future regulatory needs. This involves fundamental and applied research specifically designed to define mechanisms of action underlying the toxicity of products regulated by the FDA. The research is aimed at understanding critical biological events in the expression of toxicity and at development methods to improve assessment of human exposure, susceptibility and risk.

## Foundations & Other Funding Organizations

### Other Funding Organizations

**American Board of Veterinary Toxicology (ABVT)**
*See:* Entry 20484

★ 17164 ★ **American College of Medical Toxicology (ACMT)**
777 E Park Dr.
PO Box 8820
Harrisburg, PA 17105-8820
**Phone:** (717)558-7846      **Free:** 888-633-5784
**Fax:** (717)558-7841
**Email:** hmiller@pamedsoc.org
**Website:** http://www.acmt.net
Heather S. Miller, Exec. Dir.
**Desc:** Seeks to advance the science, study and practice of medical toxicology by fostering the development of medical toxicology in its provision of emergency, consultation, forensic, legal, community and industrial services; and by otherwise striving to advance and elevate the science, study and practice of medical toxicology. **Awards:** ACMT Research Award (annual).

★ 17165 ★ **American Society of Clinical Psychopharmacology (ASCP)**
PO Box 2257
New York, NY 10116
**Phone:** (212)696-1088      **Free:** 800-248-4344
**Fax:** (212)696-0563
**Website:** http://www.ascpp.org
J. Craig Nelson, MD, Pres.
**Desc:** Works to encourage clinical research in psychopharmacology and provide continuing education for members. Sponsors research; facilitates exchange of information; conducts professional educational programs and; provides educational programs on the treatment of psychiatric disorders for patients and families; develops relationships with mental health advocacy groups; advocates public policies which promote research and the delivery of high quality care. **Awards:** Residency Travel Award (annual) goes to 4 outstanding psychiatry residents.

★ 17166 ★ **Universities Associated for Research and Education in Pathology (UAREP)**
9650 Rockville Pike
Bethesda, MD 20814-3993
**Phone:** (301)571-1880      **Fax:** (301)571-1879
**Website:** http://www.pathol.org/
Vinay Kumar, MD, Pres.
**Desc:** University pathology departments, including faculty members, residents, and research fellows. Provides core material in convenient form for updating and enriching teaching and researching of pathology, with special emphasis on toxicology and chemical carcinogens. Encourages biomedical projects; administers contracts. Has developed guidelines for the National Highway Safety Bureau for use in scientific investigations in accidents. Operates the Registry of Comparative Pathology which provides news of progress in the experimental study of disease from animal models. **Awards:** Grant.

## Medical & Allied Health Schools

### Pharmacology

*Listed below are schools of medicine, schools of osteopathic medicine, schools of pharmacy, and schools of veterinary medicine that offer programs in pharmacology. To obtain general information on these programs, including specialties offered, contact the American Society for Pharmacology and Experimental Therapeutics, 9650 Rockville Pike, Bethesda, MD 20814-3995, (301)530-7060, http://www.aspet.org.*

### Alabama

★ 17167 ★ **Auburn University**
**College of Veterinary Medicine**
**Department of Anatomy, Physiology, and Pharmacology**
**Graduate Program in Pharmacology**
Hargis Hall
Auburn, AL 36849
**Phone:** (334)844-4425      **Fax:** (334)884-5388
**Email:** gradadm@mail.auburn.edu
**Website:** http://www.vetmed.auburn.edu/anatphys/

★ 17168 ★ **Auburn University**
**School of Pharmacy**
**Department of Pharmacal Sciences**
**Graduate Study in Pharmaceutical Sciences**
Office of Academic and Student Affairs
209 Pharmacy Bldg.
Auburn, AL 36849-5501
**Phone:** (334)844-8358      **Fax:** (334)844-8353
**Email:** raviswr@mail.auburn.edu

★ 17169 ★ **University of Alabama, Birmingham**
**Graduate School**
**Department of Pharmacology**
1400 University Blvd., Ste. 511
Birmingham, AL 35294-1150
**Phone:** (205)934-8227      **Fax:** (205)934-8413
**Email:** inquire@gradschool.huc.uab.edu
**Website:** http://main.uab.edu/show.asp?durki=26060

★ 17170 ★ **University of South Alabama**
**College of Medicine**
**Pharmacology and Toxicology Department**
251 CSAB
Mobile, AL 36688-0002
**Phone:** (334)460-6153
**Email:** jayling@jaguar1.usouthal.edu
**Website:** http://www.southalabama.edu/pharmacology/index.html

### Arkansas

★ 17171 ★ **University of Arkansas for Medical Sciences**
**Department of Pharmacology and Toxicology**
Biomedical Research Ctr.
4301 W Markham St., Slot 611
Little Rock, AR 72205
**Phone:** (501)686-8895      **Fax:** (501)686-5521
**Email:** mayeuxphilipr@exchange.uams.edu
**Website:** http://www.uams.edu/pharmtox/pharmtox.htm

## California

**★ 17172 ★ Alliant International University**
**California School of Professional**
**Psychology**
**Clinical Psychopharmacology Program**
1005 Atlantic Ave.
Alameda, CA 94501
**Free:** 800-457-1273          **Fax:** (415)931-8322
**Website:** http://www.alliant.edu/

**★ 17173 ★ Loma Linda University**
**Graduate School of Medicine**
**Department of Physiology and**
**Pharmacology**
Graduate School Admissions
Office of the Dean
Loma Linda, CA 92354-9965
**Phone:** (909)558-1800          **Free:** 800-422-4558
**Fax:** (909)558-4859
**Email:** gradschool@univ.llu.edu
**Website:**       http://www.llu.edu/llu/medicine/bulletin/
phys.htm

**★ 17174 ★ Stanford University**
**School of Medicine**
**Department of Molecular Pharmacology**
Graduate Admissions Office
Room 137, Old Union
Stanford, CA 94305
**Phone:** (650)723-4291
**Website:** http://www.stanford.edu/dept/molepharm/

**★ 17175 ★ University of California, Davis**
**School of Medicine**
**Department of Medical Pharmacology and**
**Toxicology**
4138 Meyer Hall
1 Shields Ave.
Davis, CA 95616-8588
**Phone:** (530)752-4516          **Fax:** (530)752-3394
**Email:** cdwinter@envtox.ucdavis.edu
**Website:** http://etx.ucdavis.edu/ptx

**★ 17176 ★ University of California, Irvine**
**College of Medicine**
**Department of Pharmacology**
360 Med Surge II
Irvine, CA 92697
**Phone:** (949)824-6761          **Fax:** (949)824-2095
**Email:** pharm@uci.edu
**Website:** http://www.ucihs.uci.edu/pharmaco/

**★ 17177 ★ University of California, Los**
**Angeles**
**School of Medicine**
**Department of Molecular and Medical**
**Pharmacology**
10833 Le Conte Ave.
Los Angeles, CA 90095-1735
**Phone:** (310)794-7726
**Email:** gradinfo@pharm.medsch.ucla.edu
**Website:** http://www.nuc.ucla.edu/

**★ 17178 ★ University of California, San**
**Francisco**
**Department of Pharmaceutical Sciences**
**and Pharmacogenomics**
513 Parnassus, Room S945
San Francisco, CA 94143-0446
**Phone:** (415)502-7788          **Fax:** (415)514-0502
**Email:** pspg@itsa.ucsf.edu
**Website:**       http://www.pharmchem.ucsf.edu/grad-
page.html

**★ 17179 ★ University of the Pacific**
**School of Pharmacy**
**Department of Pharmaceutical Sciences**
3601 Pacific Ave.
Stockton, CA 95211
**Phone:** (209)946-2261          **Fax:** (209)946-2858
**Email:** gradschool@uop.edu
**Website:** http://www.uop.edu/uop.nsf/

**★ 17180 ★ University of Southern**
**California**
**School of Medicine**
**Programs in Biomedical and Biological**
**Sciences**
Office of Academic and Scientific Affairs
1975 Zonal Ave.
KAM-110
Los Angeles, CA 90033
**Phone:** (323)442-1609          **Fax:** (323)442-1610
**Email:** acadsci@hsc.usc.edu
**Website:** http://www.usc.edu/medicine/pibbs

**★ 17181 ★ University of Southern**
**California**
**School of Pharmacy**
**Department of Molecular Pharmacology**
**and Toxicology**
Stouffer Pharmaceutical Sciences Center 207
1985 Zonal Ave.
Los Angeles, CA 90033
**Phone:** (213)342-1474
**Email:** gradapp@enroll1.usc.edu
**Website:** http://www.usc.edu/hsc/pharmacy/

## Colorado

**★ 17182 ★ University of Colorado**
**Health Sciences Center**
**Department of Pharmacology**
Campus Box C-236
4200 E 9th St.
Denver, CO 80262
**Phone:** (303)315-8120          **Fax:** (303)315-7097
**Email:** judy.deboer@uchsc.edu
**Website:** http://prosche.uchsc.edu/pharm/

## Connecticut

**★ 17183 ★ University of Connecticut**
**School of Pharmacy**
**Department of Pharmaceutical Science**
372 Fairfield Rd., U-92
PO Box U-92
Storrs, CT 06269-2092
**Phone:** (860)486-2493
**Email:** Phrmacy8@uconnvm.uconn.edu
**Website:** http://pharmacy.uconn.edu/

**★ 17184 ★ University of Connecticut**
**Health Center**
**Graduate School**
**Department of Cellular and Molecular**
**Pharmacology**
263 Farmington Ave., MC-3906
Farmington, CT 06030
**Phone:** (860)679-4306          **Fax:** (860)679-1899
**Email:** robertson@nso2.uchc.edu
**Website:** http://grad.uchc.edu

**★ 17185 ★ Yale University**
**Graduate School of Arts and Sciences**
**Department of Pharmacology**
PO Box 208084
New Haven, CT 06520-8084
**Phone:** (203)785-3735
**Email:** bbs@yale.edu
**Website:** http://info.med.yale.edu/bbs/

## District of Columbia

**★ 17186 ★ George Washington University**
**Columbian School of Arts and Sciences**
**Department of Biomedical Sciences**
Phillips Hall, Rm. 107
801 22nd St. NW
Washington, DC 20052
**Phone:** (202)994-6211          **Fax:** (202)994-6213
**Email:** csasgrad@gwu.edu
**Website:** http://www.gwu.edu/~gwibs/

**★ 17187 ★ Georgetown University**
**Medical Center**
**School of Medicine**
**Pharmacological Sciences Training**
**Program**
3900 Reservoir Rd. NW
Medical Dental Bldg. SE-404
Washington, DC 20007
**Phone:** (202)687-6939          **Fax:** (202)687-4872
**Email:** bwolfe01@georgetown.edu
**Website:** http://www.dml.georgetown.edu/depts/phar-
macology/

**★ 17188 ★ Howard University**
**Graduate School of Arts and Sciences**
**Department of Pharmacology**
Office of Admissions
Fourth and College Sts. NW
Washington, DC 20059
**Phone:** (202)806-5805          **Fax:** (202)462-4053
**Email:** hugsadmission@howard.edu
**Website:** http://www.hucmlrc.howard.edu/Pharmacol-
ogy/default.htm

## Florida

**★ 17189 ★ Florida A&M University**
**Division of Graduate Studies, Research,**
**and Continuing Education**
**Pharmacology and Toxicology Program**
Graduate Admission Office
G-9 Foote-Hilyer Administration Bldg.
Tallahassee, FL 32307
**Phone:** (850)599-3796          **Fax:** (850)599-3952
**Email:** admissions@famu.edu
**Website:**    http://www.famu2.famu.edu/acad/colleges/
copps/

**★ 17190 ★ University of Florida**
**College of Medicine**
**Department of Physiology and**
**Pharmacology**
PO Box 100215
Gainesville, FL 32610-0215
**Phone:** (352)392-0740
**Email:** stevens@phys.med.ufl.edu
**Website:** http://rgp.ufl.edu/education/

**★ 17191 ★ University of Miami**
**School of Medicine**
**Department of Biochemistry and**
**Molecular Biology**
PO Box 016029
1600 NW 10th Ave.
Coral Gables, FL 33114
**Phone:** (305)243-6265          **Fax:** (305)243-5665
**Email:** rwerner@miami.edu

**★ 17192 ★ University of South Florida**
**College of Medicine**
**Department of Pharmacology and**
**Therapeutics**
MDC Box 9
12901 Bruce B. Downs Blvd.
Tampa, FL 33612-4799
**Phone:** (813)974-9922          **Fax:** (813)974-3081
**Website:** http://www.med.usf.edu/PHD/

## Georgia

**★ 17193 ★ Emory University**
**Graduate Division of Biological and**
   **Biomedical Sciences**
**Program in Molecular and Systems**
   **Pharmacology**
1462 Clifton Rd., Ste. 314
Atlanta, GA 30322
**Phone:** (404)727-2545     **Fax:** (404)727-3322
**Website:** http://www.biomed.emory.edu/program_
msp.html

**★ 17194 ★ Morehouse School of**
   **Medicine**
**Office of Graduate Education in the**
   **Biomedical Sciences**
**Doctoral Program in Biomedical Sciences**
720 Westview Dr.
Atlanta, GA 30310
**Phone:** (404)752-1755     **Fax:** (404)752-1164
**Email:** doec@msm.edu

**★ 17195 ★ University of Georgia**
**College of Pharmacy**
**Department of Pharmaceutical and**
   **Biomedical Science**
Athens, GA 30602
**Phone:** (706)542-5403     **Fax:** (706)542-5358
**Email:** jwilson@rx.uga.edu
**Website:** http://www.gradsch.uga.edu/

## Hawaii

**★ 17196 ★ University of Hawaii, Manoa**
**Department of Pharmacology**
Graduate Division Admissions Office
2540 Maile Way
Honolulu, HI 96822
**Phone:** (808)956-8544
**Email:** admissions@admin.grad.hawaii.edu

## Idaho

**★ 17197 ★ Idaho State University**
**College of Pharmacy**
**Department of Pharmaceutical Sciences**
Campus Box 8334
Pocatello, ID 83209
**Phone:** (208)282-2682     **Fax:** (208)282-4482
**Email:** btaylor@otc.isu.edu
**Website:** http://rx.isu.edu/

## Illinois

**★ 17198 ★ Finch University of Health**
   **Sciences**
**School of Graduate and Postdoctoral**
   **Studies**
**Department of Pharmacology and**
   **Molecular Biology**
Office of Graduate Admissions
3333 Green Bay Rd.
North Chicago, IL 60064
**Phone:** (847)578-3271

**★ 17199 ★ Illinois State University**
**Department of Biological Sciences**
Campus Box 4120
Normal, IL 61790-4120
**Phone:** (309)438-3664     **Fax:** (309)438-3722
**Email:** cawinch@ilstu.edu
**Website:** http://www.bio.ilstu.edu/

**★ 17200 ★ Loyola University/Chicago**
   **Medical Center**
**Biomedical Sciences Department**
**Pharmacology and Experimental**
   **Therapeutics**
2160 S 1st Ave.
Bldg. 102, Rm. 3621
Maywood, IL 60153
**Phone:** (708)216-6594     **Fax:** (708)216-6596
**Email:** lroeder@luc.edu
**Website:** http://www.meddean.luc.edu/lumen/Dept-
Webs/PHARM/Index.htm

**★ 17201 ★ Northwestern University**
   **Medical School**
**Integrated Graduate Program in the Life**
   **Sciences**
303 E Chicago Ave.
Ward 12-373/W150
Chicago, IL 60611-3008
**Free:** 800-255-4166     **Fax:** (312)908-5253
**Email:** igp@northwestern.edu
**Website:** http://www.nums.northwestern.edu/igp/

**★ 17202 ★ Rush University**
**The Graduate College**
**Department of Pharmacology**
2242 W Harrison St.
Chicago, IL 60612
**Phone:** (312)942-6247     **Fax:** (312)942-8112
**Email:** ruinfo@rushu.rush.edu
**Website:** http://www.rushu.rush.edu/pharm/dept/

**★ 17203 ★ Southern Illinois University**
**Graduate School**
**Department of Pharmacology**
Carbondale, IL 62901-4716
**Phone:** (618)536-7791
**Email:** gradschl@siu.edu

**★ 17204 ★ Southern Illinois University**
**School of Medicine**
**Department of Pharmacology**
PO Box 19629
Springfield, IL 62794-9629
**Phone:** (217)785-2191     **Fax:** (217)524-0145
**Email:** pscott@siumed.edu
**Website:** http://www.siumed.edu/pharm/home.html

**★ 17205 ★ University of Chicago**
**Division of the Biological Sciences**
**Department of Neurobiology,**
   **Pharmacology, and Physiology**
947 E 58th St.
MC0926
Chicago, IL 60637-5416
**Phone:** (773)702-6371     **Fax:** (773)702-1216

**★ 17206 ★ University of Illinois, Chicago**
**College of Medicine**
**Department of Pharmacology**
835 S Wolcott Ave.
M/C 868
Chicago, IL 60612-7243
**Phone:** (312)996-7635     **Fax:** (312)413-0185
**Email:** gradcoll@uic.edu
**Website:** http://www.uic.edu/depts/mcph/

**★ 17207 ★ University of Illinois, Chicago**
**Department of Pharmacognosy**
833 S Wood
M/C 877
Chicago, IL 60612-7231
**Phone:** (312)996-7253     **Fax:** (312)413-0185
**Email:** gradcoll@uic.edu
**Website:** http://www.uic.edu/pharmacy/

## Indiana

**★ 17208 ★ Butler University**
**College of Pharmacy**
**Graduate Pharmacology Program**
Indianapolis, IN 46208
**Phone:** (317)940-9969     **Free:** 800-368-6852
**Fax:** (317)940-6172
**Email:** admission@butler.edu

**★ 17209 ★ Indiana University**
**Graduate School, IUPI Campus**
**Department of Pharmacology and**
   **Toxicology**
Van Nuys Medical Science Bldg.
635 Barnhill Dr.
Indianapolis, IN 46202
**Phone:** (317)274-7844     **Fax:** (317)274-7714
**Email:** besch@indiana.edu
**Website:** http://www.iupui.edu/~iuphtx/home1.html
Dr. Henry R. Besch, Jr., Chairman of the Board

**★ 17210 ★ Indiana University**
**School of Medicine**
**Medical Sciences Program**
**Graduate Pharmacology Programs**
105 Jordan Hall
Bloomington, IN 47405
**Phone:** (812)855-8118
**Email:** bevhill@indiana.edu
**Website:** http://www.indiana.edu/~medsci/

**★ 17211 ★ Purdue University**
**School of Pharmacy and Pharmacal**
   **Sciences**
**Department of Medicinal Chemistry and**
   **Molecular Pharmacology**
1333 Pharmacy Bldg.
West Lafayette, IN 47907-1330
**Phone:** (765)494-5968     **Fax:** (765)494-7880
**Email:** gradprog@pharmacy.purdue.edu
**Website:** http://www.pharmacy.purdue.edu/~mcmp/

**★ 17212 ★ Purdue University**
**School of Veterinary Medicine**
**Department of Basic Medical Sciences**
**Pharmacology Program**
School of Veterinary Medicine
Department of Basic Medical Sciences
West Lafayette, IN 47907-1246
**Phone:** (317)494-8632     **Fax:** (317)494-0781
**Email:** gradinfo@purdue.edu

## Iowa

**★ 17213 ★ University of Iowa**
**College of Medicine**
**Department of Pharmacology**
BSB 2-532
Iowa City, IA 52242-1109
**Phone:** (319)335-7965     **Fax:** (319)335-8930
**Email:** pharmacology@uiowa.edu

## Kansas

**★ 17214 ★ University of Kansas**
   **Medical Center**
**Department of Pharmacology, Toxicology,**
   **and Therapeutics**
3901 Rainbow Blvd.
Kansas City, KS 66160-7417
**Phone:** (913)588-7140     **Fax:** (913)588-7501
**Email:** pharmgrd@kumc.edu
**Website:** http://www.kumc.edu/research/medicine/
pharmacology/dhp.html

**★ 17215 ★ University of Kansas**
**School of Pharmacy**
**Department of Pharmacology and**
**Toxicology**
300 Strong Hall
Lawrence, KS 66045-1729
**Phone:** (785)864-4141　**Fax:** (785)864-4555
**Email:** graduate@raven.cc.ukans.edu
**Website:** http://www.pharm.ukans.edu/pharmtox/index.html

### Kentucky

**★ 17216 ★ University of Kentucky**
**College of Medicine**
**Department of Biomedical Pharmacology**
**Graduate Program in Cell and Molecular**
**Biology**
800 Rose St.
A.B. Chandler Medical Center, MS 305
Lexington, KY 40536
**Phone:** (859)323-6085　**Fax:** (859)323-1981
**Email:** dturner@pop.uky.edu
**Website:** http://www.mc.uky.edu/pharmacology/default.asp

**★ 17217 ★ University of Louisville**
**Graduate School**
**Department of Pharmacology and**
**Toxicology**
Office of Research and Graduate Programs
Louisville, KY 40292
**Phone:** (502)852-6495
**Email:** admitme@louisville.edu
**Website:** http://www.louisville.edu/medschool/pharmacology/

### Louisiana

**★ 17218 ★ Louisiana State University**
**Health Sciences Center**
**Department of Pharmacology and**
**Experimental Therapeutics**
1901 Perdido St.
New Orleans, LA 70112
**Phone:** (504)568-4740　**Fax:** (504)568-2361
**Email:** emize@lsuhsc.edu
**Website:** http://www.medschool.lsuhsc.edu/phar/

**★ 17219 ★ Louisiana State University**
**School of Medicine**
**Department of Pharmacology and**
**Therapeutics**
Health Service Center
PO Box 33932
Shreveport, LA 71130-3932
**Phone:** (318)675-4803　**Fax:** (318)675-7857
**Email:** kmcmar@lsumc.edu
**Website:** http://gradsch.shreveport.lsumc.edu/Pharm/Pharm.html

**★ 17220 ★ Tulane University**
**Graduate School of Arts and Sciences**
**Department of Pharmacology**
Gibson Hall, Room 324
New Orleans, LA 70118
**Phone:** (504)865-5100　**Free:** 800-347-5935
**Email:** graduate.school@tulane.edu
**Website:** http://www.tmc.tulane.edu/departments/pharmacology/

**★ 17221 ★ Tulane University**
**School of Medicine**
**Department of Pharmacology**
Office of Graduate Studies
1430 Tulane Ave. (SL 00)
New Orleans, LA 70112-9962
**Phone:** (504)588-5187　**Fax:** (504)588-3721
**Email:** medsch@tmcpop.tmc.tulane.edu

**Website:** http://www1.omi.tulane.edu/departments/pharmacology/pharm.html

### Maryland

**★ 17222 ★ Johns Hopkins University**
**School of Medicine**
**Department of Pharmacology and**
**Molecular Sciences**
**Graduate Program in Pharmacology and**
**Molecular Sciences**
725 N Wolfe St.
Baltimore, MD 21205
**Email:** mguercio@bs.jhmi.edu
**Website:** http://www.med.jhu.edu/pharmacology/

**★ 17223 ★ Uniformed Services University**
**of the Health Sciences**
**Graduate Education Office**
**Pharmacology Department**
4301 Jones Bridge Rd.
Bethesda, MD 20814-4799
**Phone:** (301)295-9474　**Free:** 800-772-1747
**Fax:** (301)295-6772
**Website:** http://www.usuhs.mil/geo/gradpgm_index.html

**★ 17224 ★ University of Maryland**
**School of Medicine**
**Department of Pharmacology and**
**Experimental Therapeutics**
Graduate Program Coordinator
20 N Pine St.
Baltimore, MD 21201
**Phone:** (410)706-7131　**Fax:** (410)706-3473
**Email:** gradinfo@umaryland.edu
**Website:** http://som1.umaryland.edu/~smPharm/pharm.html

### Massachusetts

**★ 17225 ★ Massachusetts College of**
**Pharmacy and Allied Health Sciences**
**Department of Pharmaceutical Sciences**
Coordinator of Graduate Admissions
179 Longwood Ave.
Boston, MA 02115
**Phone:** (617)732-2850　**Fax:** (617)732-2801
**Email:** admissions@mcp.edu
**Website:** http://www.mcp.edu/ps/pharms.htm

**★ 17226 ★ Northeastern University**
**Bouve College of Pharmacy and Health**
**Sciences**
**Pharmacology Program**
203 Mugar Life Sciences Bldg.
360 Huntington Ave.
Boston, MA 02115
**Phone:** (617)373-2708　**Fax:** (617)373-3216
**Email:** w.purnell@nunet.neu.edu
**Website:** http://www.bouve.neu.edu/department/phar/pharmsci/bms.html

**★ 17227 ★ Tufts University**
**Sackler School of Graduate Biomedical**
**Sciences**
**Department of Pharmacology and**
**Experimental Therapeutics**
136 Harrison Ave.
Boston, MA 02111
**Phone:** (617)636-7000　**Fax:** (617)636-0309
**Email:** sschool@infonet.tufts.edu
**Website:** http://www.tufts.edu/sackler/pharmacology/

**★ 17228 ★ University of Massachusetts**
**Medical Center at Worcester**
**Department of Biochemistry and**
**Molecular Pharmacology**
55 Lake Ave. N
Worcester, MA 01655-0122
**Phone:** (508)856-2405　**Fax:** (508)856-5080
**Email:** kendall.knight@ummed.edu
**Website:** http://www.umassmed.edu/pharmacology/

### Michigan

**★ 17229 ★ Michigan State University**
**College of Human Medicine**
**Department of Pharmacology and**
**Toxicology**
B440 Life Sciences Bldg.
East Lansing, MI 48824
**Phone:** (517)353-7146
**Email:** hummeld@pilot.msu.edu
**Website:** http://www.phmtox.msu.edu/

**★ 17230 ★ University of Michigan**
**Medical School**
**Department of Pharmacology**
1301 MSRB III
Ann Arbor, MI 48109-0632
**Phone:** (734)764-8166　**Fax:** (734)763-4450
**Email:** effergie@umich.edu
**Website:** http://www.med.umich.edu/pharm/homepage.html

**★ 17231 ★ Wayne State University**
**School of Medicine**
**Department of Pharmacology**
6374 Scott Hall
Detroit, MI 48202
**Phone:** (313)577-6737　**Fax:** (313)577-6739
**Email:** s.r.terlecky@wayne.edu
**Website:** http://www.med.wayne.edu/pharm/home.htm

### Minnesota

**★ 17232 ★ Mayo Graduate School**
**Department of Pharmacology**
200 First St. SW
Rochester, MN 55905
**Phone:** (507)284-2747　**Fax:** (507)284-9111
**Email:** schwerman.debbie@mayo.edu
**Website:** http://www.mayo.edu/research/mpet/

**★ 17233 ★ University of Minnesota**
**Medical School**
**Department of Pharmacology**
6-120 Jackson Hall
321 Church St. SE
Minneapolis, MN 55455
**Phone:** (612)625-9997　**Fax:** (612)625-8408
**Email:** campb034@umn.edu
**Website:** http://www.pharmacology.med.umn.edu/

### Mississippi

**★ 17234 ★ University of Mississippi**
**School of Medicine**
**Graduate Programs in the Basic Medical**
**Sciences**
**Department of Pharmacology and**
**Toxicology**
Division of Student Services and Records
2500 N State St.
Jackson, MS 39216-4505
**Phone:** (601)984-5010
**Website:** http://pharmacology.umc.edu/

★ **17235** ★ **University of Mississippi**
**School of Pharmacy**
**Department of Pharmacology**
303A Faser
University, MS 38677
**Phone:** (662)915-7330 **Fax:** (662)915-5118
**Email:** dfeller@olemiss.edu
**Website:** http://www.olemiss.edu/depts/pharmacology

### Missouri

★ **17236** ★ **Saint Louis University**
**Department of Pharmacological and**
**Physiological Science**
1402 S Grand Blvd. (M228)
Saint Louis, MO 63104
**Phone:** (314)577-8418 **Fax:** (314)268-5396
**Email:** grequest@slu.edu
**Website:** http://www.slu.edu/departments/pharm_
phys/

★ **17237** ★ **University of Missouri,**
**Columbia**
**School of Medicine**
**Department of Pharmacology**
M-517B Medical Sciences Bldg.
Columbia, MO 65212
**Phone:** (573)882-7188 **Fax:** (573)884-4558
**Email:** burgessp@missouri.edu
**Website:** http://www.muhealth.org/~pharmacology/
gradprog.html

★ **17238** ★ **University of Missouri,**
**Kansas City**
**School of Pharmacy**
**Department of Pharmaceutical Science**
5100 Rockhill Rd.
Kansas City, MO 64110-2499
**Phone:** (816)235-1111 **Fax:** (816)235-1717
**Email:** admit@umkc.edu
**Website:** http://www.umkc.edu/pharm/PHARMS-
CI.HTML

### Nebraska

★ **17239** ★ **Creighton University**
**Graduate School**
**Department of Pharmacology**
2500 California Plaza
Omaha, NE 68178
**Phone:** (402)280-2870
**Email:** gradsch@creighton.edu
**Website:** http://spahp.creighton.edu/

★ **17240** ★ **University of Nebraska**
**Medical Center**
**Eppley Institute for Research in Cancer**
**and Allied Diseases**
**Cancer Research Training Program**
986805 Nebraska Medical Center
Omaha, NE 68198-6805
**Phone:** (402)559-4401 **Fax:** (402)559-4651
**Email:** dbulling@unmc.edu
**Website:** http://www.unmc.edu/Eppley/crtp.htm

★ **17241** ★ **University of Nebraska,**
**Omaha**
**University of Nebraska Medical Center**
**Biomedical Research Training Program**
**Department of Pharmacology**
Office of the Dean for Graduate Studies and
Research
986810 Nebraska Medical Center
Omaha, NE 68198-6810
**Phone:** (402)559-6531 **Free:** 800-626-8431
**Fax:** (402)559-7845
**Email:** dbulling@unmc.edu
**Website:** http://www.unmc.edu/Pharmacology/

### Nevada

★ **17242** ★ **University of Nevada, Reno**
**School of Medicine**
**Department of Cell and Molecular**
**Pharmacology and Physiology**
Graduate School, Rm. 326
Reno, NV 89557-0035
**Phone:** (775)784-6869 **Fax:** (775)784-6064
**Email:** gradadmissions@unr.edu

### New Hampshire

★ **17243** ★ **Dartmouth College**
**Medical School**
**Department of Pharmacology and**
**Toxicology**
Office of Admissions
7650 Remsen, Rm. 522
Hanover, NH 03755-3833
**Phone:** (603)650-1667
**Email:** pharmacology.and.toxicology@dartmouth.edu
**Website:** http://www.dartmouth.edu/dms/pharmtox/

### New Jersey

★ **17244** ★ **Rutgers, the State University**
**of New Jersey**
**Division of Life Sciences**
**Doctorate Programs in Molecular**
**Biosciences**
**Graduate Program in Pharmacology**
Nelson Biological Laboratory, Rm. A102
Piscataway, NJ 08854
**Phone:** (732)445-3430 **Fax:** (732)445-6370
**Email:** ambrose@biology.rutgers.edu
**Website:** http://lifesci.rutgers.edu/~molbiosci/

★ **17245** ★ **Rutgers, the State University**
**of New Jersey**
**Graduate School**
**Department of Cellular and Molecular**
**Pharmacology**
Office of Graduate and Professional Admissions
Van Nest Hall
PO Box 5053
New Brunswick, NJ 08903-5053
**Phone:** (732)932-1766 **Fax:** (732)932-8231
**Email:** mcnamame@umdnj.edu
**Website:** http://pharmacy.rutgers.edu/graduate-pro-
grams.htm

★ **17246** ★ **University of Medicine and**
**Dentistry of New Jersey**
**Graduate School of Biomedical Sciences,**
**Newark**
**Department of Pharmacology and**
**Physiology**
30 Bergen St.
ADMC 110
Newark, NJ 07107-3000
**Phone:** (973)972-4511
**Email:** gsbsnadm@umdnj.edu
**Website:** http://www.umdnj.edu/~physio/home.html

★ **17247** ★ **University of Medicine and**
**Dentistry of New Jersey**
**Graduate School of Biomedical Sciences,**
**Piscataway**
**Department of Cellular and Molecular**
**Pharmacology**
675 Hoes Lane
Piscataway, NJ 08854-5635
**Phone:** (732)235-5016
**Email:** gsbspisc@umdnj.edu
**Website:** http://www2.umdnj.edu/~pharm/
gradphrm.htm

### New Mexico

★ **17248** ★ **University of New Mexico**
**School of Medicine**
**Biomedical Sciences Graduate Program**
Box 520
Albuquerque, NM 87131-5196
**Phone:** (505)272-1887 **Fax:** (505)272-8738
**Email:** bsgp@salud.unm.edu
**Website:** http://hsc.unm.edu/som/bsgs/info.html

### New York

★ **17249** ★ **Albany Medical College**
**Department of Vascular Biology**
Graduate Studies Program Office
47 New Scotland Ave., MC-16
Albany, NY 12208-3479
**Phone:** (518)262-5253 **Fax:** (518)262-5183
**Email:** graduate-studies@ccgateway.amc.edu
**Website:** http://www.amc.edu/Academic/GradStu-
dies/gradstudies.htm

★ **17250** ★ **Albany Medical College**
**Neuropharmacology and Neuroscience**
**Program**
47 New Scotland Ave., MC-16
Albany, NY 12208
**Phone:** (518)262-5253 **Fax:** (518)262-5183
**Email:** graduate-studies@mail.amc.edu
**Website:** http://www.amc.edu/Academic/GradStu-
dies/gradstudies.htm

★ **17251** ★ **Columbia University**
**College of Physicians and Surgeons**
**Department of Pharmacology**
630 W 168th St.
New York, NY 10032
**Phone:** (212)305-8058 **Fax:** (212)305-1031
**Email:** GSASatPandS@columbia.edu
**Website:** http://cpmcnet.columbia.edu/dept/gsas

★ **17252** ★ **Cornell University**
**Graduate School**
**College of Veterinary Medicine**
**Department of Pharmacology**
S3 016 Schurman Hall
Ithaca, NY 14853-6401
**Phone:** (607)253-3276 **Fax:** (607)253-3756
**Email:** vetgradpgms@cornell.edu
**Website:** http://web.vet.cornell.edu/public/research/
graded/index.html

★ **17253** ★ **Long Island University,**
**Brooklyn**
**Arnold and Marie Schwartz College of**
**Pharmacy and Health Sciences**
**Division of Pharmacology, Toxicology,**
**and Medicinal Chemistry**
1 University Plaza
Brooklyn, NY 11201
**Phone:** (718)488-1062 **Fax:** (718)797-2399
**Email:** attend@liu.edu

★ **17254** ★ **Mount Sinai School of**
**Medicine**
**Graduate Program in the Biomedical**
**Sciences**
**Department of Pharmacology**
PO Box 1022
1 Gustave L. Levy Pl.
New York, NY 10029-6574
**Phone:** (212)241-6546 **Fax:** (212)241-0651
**Email:** grads@smtplink.mssm.edu
**Website:** http://www.mssm.edu/gradschool/

★ 17255 ★ **New York Medical College**
**Graduate School of Basic Medical Sciences**
**Department of Pharmacology**
Director of Admissions
95 Grasslands Rd.
Valhalla, NY 10595
**Phone:** (914)594-4110    **Fax:** (914)594-4944
**Email:** GSBMS_apply@nymc.edu

★ 17256 ★ **New York University**
**Sackler Institute of Graduate Biomedical Sciences**
**Program in Molecular Pharmacology and Signal Transduction**
550 1st Ave.
New York, NY 10016
**Phone:** (212)263-5648    **Fax:** (212)263-7600
**Email:** sackler-info@nyumed.med.nyu.edu
**Website:** http://www.med.nyu.edu/Sackler/Home-Page.html

★ 17257 ★ **State University of New York, Buffalo**
**School of Medicine**
**Department of Pharmacology and Toxicology**
Buffalo, NY 14214-3000
**Phone:** (716)829-2800    **Fax:** (716)829-2801
**Email:** harbison@acsu.buffalo.edu

★ 17258 ★ **State University of New York, Buffalo**
**School of Pharmacy**
**Department of Pharmaceutics**
517 Hochstetter Hall
Buffalo, NY 14260-1200
**Phone:** (716)645-2842    **Fax:** (716)645-3693
**Email:** hlfung@acsu.buffalo.edu

★ 17259 ★ **State University of New York, Stony Brook**
**Department of Pharmacological Sciences**
**Molecular and Cellular Pharmacology**
BST 8-196 Z=8651
Stony Brook, NY 11794-8651
**Phone:** (631)444-3057    **Fax:** (631)444-3218
**Email:** grad@pharm.sunysb.edu
**Website:** http://www.pharm.sunysb.edu/

★ 17260 ★ **State University of New York Upstate Medical Center**
**College of Graduate Studies**
**Department of Pharmacology**
SUNY Health Science Center
750 E Adams St.
Syracuse, NY 13210
**Phone:** (315)464-4538    **Fax:** (315)464-4544
**Email:** gradstud@hscsyr.edu

★ 17261 ★ **University of Buffalo**
**Roswell Park Cancer Institute**
**Department of Molecular Pharmacology and Cancer Therapeutics**
RPCI, Elm and Carlton Sts.
Buffalo, NY 14263
**Phone:** (716)845-8225    **Fax:** (716)845-8857
**Email:** gradapp@roswellpark.org
**Website:** http://www.roswellpark.org/gradeducation/

★ 17262 ★ **University of Rochester**
**School of Medicine and Dentistry**
**Department of Pharmacology and Physiology**
601 Elmwood Ave.
PO Box 711
Rochester, NY 14642-8711
**Phone:** (716)275-1679    **Fax:** (716)244-9283
**Website:** http://www.urmc.rochester.edu/phph/

★ 17263 ★ **Yeshiva University**
**Albert Einstein College of Medicine**
**Department of Molecular Pharmacology**
1300 Morris Park Ave.
Bronx, NY 10461-1602
**Phone:** (718)430-2505
**Email:** rubin@aecom.yu.edu

## North Carolina

★ 17264 ★ **Duke University Medical Center**
**Department of Pharmacology and Cancer Biology**
**Pharmacology and Cancer Biology Graduate Program**
Box 3813
Durham, NC 27710
**Phone:** (919)613-8650
**Website:** http://pharmacology.mc.duke.edu/

★ 17265 ★ **East Carolina University**
**School of Medicine**
**Department of Pharmacology**
Greenville, NC 27858-4353
**Phone:** (252)816-2758
**Email:** tschetterp@mail.ecu.edu
**Website:** http://www.research2.ecu.edu/grad/

★ 17266 ★ **University of North Carolina, Chapel Hill**
**School of Medicine**
**Department of Pharmacology**
1106 Mary Ellen Jones Bldg.
CB 7365
Chapel Hill, NC 27599
**Phone:** (919)966-4383    **Fax:** (919)966-5640
**Email:** phcograd@med.unc.edu
**Website:** http://www.med.unc.edu/pharm/

★ 17267 ★ **Wake Forest University**
**Bowman Gray School of Medicine**
**Department of Pharmacology**
Dean of the Graduate School
Medical Center Blvd.
Winston-Salem, NC 27199-0603
**Phone:** (910)716-4303    **Free:** 800-438-4723
**Fax:** (910)716-4204
**Email:** bggrad@wfubmc.edu
**Website:** http://isnet.is.wfu.edu/physpharm/home-page.html

## North Dakota

★ 17268 ★ **University of North Dakota**
**Graduate School**
**Department of Pharmacology and Toxicology**
501 N Columbia Rd.
Grand Forks, ND 58202-9037
**Phone:** (701)777-3975    **Fax:** (701)777-4490
**Email:** pharmphys@medicine.nodak.edu
**Website:** http://www.med.und.nodak.edu

## Ohio

★ 17269 ★ **Case Western Reserve University**
**School of Medicine**
**Biomedical Sciences Training Program**
10900 Euclid Ave. (WG46)
Cleveland, OH 44106-4934
**Phone:** (216)368-3347    **Fax:** (216)368-0795
**Email:** bstp@po.cwru.edu
**Website:** http://www.cwru.edu/med/bstp/info.html

★ 17270 ★ **Case Western Reserve University**
**School of Medicine**
**Department of Pharmacology**
Office of Graduate Admissions
10900 Euclid Ave.
Cleveland, OH 44106-7027
**Fax:** (216)368-3395
**Email:** rak5@po.cwru.edu
**Website:** http://www.cwru.edu/med/bstp/info.html

★ 17271 ★ **Medical College of Ohio**
**Department of Pharmacology**
3035 Arlington Ave.
Toledo, OH 43614
**Phone:** (419)383-4182    **Fax:** (419)383-2871
**Email:** mheck@mco.edu

★ 17272 ★ **Medical College of Ohio**
**Graduate School**
**Department of Molecular and Cellular Biology**
3000 Arlington Ave.
Toledo, OH 43614
**Phone:** (419)383-4918    **Fax:** (419)383-3089
**Email:** rruch@mco.edu

★ 17273 ★ **Northeastern Ohio Universities**
**College of Medicine**
**Psychopharmacology Program**
PO Box 95
Rootstown, OH 44272-0095
**Phone:** (216)325-2511    **Fax:** (330)325-8372

★ 17274 ★ **Ohio State University**
**College of Pharmacy**
500 W 12th St.
Columbus, OH 43210-1291
**Phone:** (614)292-2266    **Fax:** (614)292-2588
**Email:** gadmbrks@dendrite.pharmacy.ohio-state.edu
**Website:** http://www.pharmacy.ohio-state.edu/

★ 17275 ★ **Ohio State University**
**Integrated Biomedical Science Graduate Program**
**Pharmacology Program**
Graves Hall, Room 1190
333 W 10th Ave.
Columbus, OH 43210
**Phone:** (614)292-0857    **Fax:** (614)292-6226
**Email:** yates.1@osu.edu
**Website:** http://www.ibgp.org/

★ 17276 ★ **University of Cincinnati**
**College of Medicine**
**Department of Pharmacology and Cell Biophysics**
231 Bethesda Ave.
PO Box 670555
Cincinnati, OH 45267-0575
**Phone:** (513)558-2366    **Fax:** (513)558-1169
**Website:** http://www.med.us.edu/pharmacology/

★ 17277 ★ **University of Cincinnati**
**College of Pharmacy**
**Pharmacology and Toxicology Program**
3223 Eden Ave.
PO Box 670004
Cincinnati, OH 45267-0004
**Phone:** (513)558-3784    **Fax:** (513)558-4372
**Email:** marcia.sedam@uc.edu

**★ 17278 ★ Wright State University**
**School of Medicine**
**Department of Pharmacology and**
**Toxicology**
Dayton, OH 45435
**Phone:** (937)775-2159 **Fax:** (937)775-7221
**Email:** robert.grubbs@wright.edu
**Website:** http://www.med.wright.edu/som/academic/
pharm/pharm.html

## Oklahoma

**★ 17279 ★ University of Oklahoma**
**Health Sciences Center**
**Graduate College**
**Department of Cell Biology**
PO Box 26901
Oklahoma City, OK 73190
**Phone:** (405)271-2406 **Fax:** (405)271-3548
**Email:** Brenda-callahan@ouhsc.edu

## Pennsylvania

**★ 17280 ★ Duquesne University**
**Graduate School of Pharmaceutical**
**Sciences**
**Pharmacy Department**
449 Mellon Hall of Science
Pittsburgh, PA 15282
**Phone:** (412)396-5662 **Fax:** (412)396-5593
**Email:** gsps-adm@duq.edu

**★ 17281 ★ MCP Hahnemann University**
**Department of Pharmacology and**
**Physiology**
**Pharmacology and Physiology Program**
**Pharmacology Program**
245 N 15th St.
Philadelphia, PA 19102
**Phone:** (215)762-2383 **Fax:** (215)762-2299
**Email:** Robert.Nichols@drexel.edu

**★ 17282 ★ MCP Hahnemann University**
**School of Medicine**
**Department of Pharmacology and**
**Physiology**
Office of Biomedical Graduate Study
2900 Queen Ln.
Philadelphia, PA 19129
**Phone:** (215)991-8570
**Email:** MCPHU.MedAdmissions@drexel.edu

**★ 17283 ★ Pennsylvania State University**
**College of Medicine**
**Department of Pharmacology**
Department of Pharmacology H-078
500 University Dr.
Hershey, PA 17033
**Phone:** (717)531-8285 **Fax:** (717)531-5013
**Email:** pharm-grad-hmc@psu.edu
**Website:** http://www.hmc.psu.edu/pharmacology_
program/index.html

**★ 17284 ★ Temple University**
**School of Medicine**
**Department of Pharmacology**
3400 N Broad St.
Philadelphia, PA 19140-9630
**Phone:** (215)204-1380
**Email:** tu_grad@blue.temple.edu
**Website:** http://www.temple.edu/pharmacology/

**★ 17285 ★ Thomas Jefferson University**
**College of Graduate Studies**
**Department of Pharmacology**
1020 Locust St., M-46
Philadelphia, PA 19107-6799
**Phone:** (215)503-4400 **Fax:** (215)503-3433
**Email:** cgs-info@mail.tju.edu

**★ 17286 ★ University of Pennsylvania**
**School of Medicine**
**Department of Pharmacological Sciences**
Philadelphia, PA 19104
**Phone:** (215)898-8025
**Email:** leroy@pharm.med.upenn.edu

**★ 17287 ★ University of Pittsburgh**
**School of Medicine**
**Department of Molecular Pharmacology**
INTBP, 322 Scaife Hall
3550 Terrace St.
Pittsburgh, PA 15261
**Phone:** (412)648-8957 **Fax:** (412)648-1236
**Email:** biomed_phd@fs1.dean-med.pitt.edu

**★ 17288 ★ University of the Sciences in**
**Philadelphia**
**Graduate School**
**Department of Pharmacology and**
**Toxicology**
600 S 43rd St.
Philadelphia, PA 19104
**Phone:** (215)596-8937 **Fax:** (215)895-1185
**Email:** Graduate@usip.edu
**Website:** http://www.usip.edu/graduate/pharmacolo-
gy_toxicology.htm

## Puerto Rico

**★ 17289 ★ University of Puerto Rico**
**School of Medicine**
**Department of Pharmacology and**
**Toxicology**
Medical Sciences Campus
GPO 5067
San Juan, PR 00936
**Phone:** (787)724-1006 **Fax:** (787)282-0568
**Email:** scorey@neurobio.upr.clu.edu

## Rhode Island

**★ 17290 ★ Brown University**
**Division of Biology and Medicine**
**Graduate Program in Molecular**
**Pharmacology and Physiology**
Box G-B3
Providence, RI 02912
**Phone:** (401)863-2574
**Email:** Cheryl_Pariseau@brown.edu

**★ 17291 ★ University of Rhode Island**
**College of Pharmacy**
**Department of Pharmacology**
117 Fogarty Hall
Kingston, RI 02881-0809
**Phone:** (401)874-5842
**Email:** urigrad@uriacc.uri.edu

## South Carolina

**★ 17292 ★ Medical University of South**
**Carolina**
**College of Graduate Studies**
**Department of Cell and Molecular**
**Pharmacology**
41 Bee St.
PO Box 250203
Charleston, SC 29425
**Phone:** (843)792-8710 **Fax:** (843)792-6615
**Email:** oes-web@musc.edu

## South Dakota

**★ 17293 ★ University of South Dakota**
**School of Medicine**
**Department of Pharmacology**
414 E Clark St.
Vermillion, SD 57069-2390

**Phone:** (605)677-5254 **Fax:** (605)677-6381
**Email:** biomed@usd.edu

## Tennessee

**★ 17294 ★ East Tennessee State**
**University**
**James H. Quillen College of Medicine**
**Department of Pharmacology**
PO Box 70720
Johnson City, TN 37614-0720
**Phone:** (615)929-6241
**Email:** gradsch@etsu.edu
**Website:** http://www.etsu.edu/gradstud/index.htm

**★ 17295 ★ University of Tennessee,**
**Memphis**
**College of Graduate Health Sciences**
**Department of Pharmacology**
894 Union Ave.
Memphis, TN 38163
**Phone:** (901)448-4465 **Fax:** (901)448-7126
**Email:** schneide@Physio1.utmem.edu
**Website:** http://www.utmem.edu/grad/PROGRAMS/
program_pharmacol.html

**★ 17296 ★ Vanderbilt University**
**The Graduate School**
**Department of Pharmacology**
411 Kirkland Hall
Nashville, TN 37240
**Phone:** (615)343-2573 **Free:** 800-810-8993
**Fax:** (615)322-3827
**Email:** vugs@nwfs1.gs.vanderbilt.edu

## Texas

**★ 17297 ★ Baylor College of Medicine**
**Department of Pharmacology**
One Baylor Plaza
Houston, TX 77030
**Phone:** (713)798-7902 **Fax:** (713)798-3145
**Email:** pchan@bcm.tmc.edu

**★ 17298 ★ Texas A&M University**
**College of Medicine**
**Department of Medical Pharmacology and**
**Toxicology**
Reynolds Medical Bldg.
Mail Stop 1114
College Station, TX 77843-1114
**Phone:** (409)845-2888 **Fax:** (409)845-0699
**Email:** gdfrye@medicine.tamu.edu

**★ 17299 ★ Texas A&M University**
**Health Science Center**
**College of Medicine**
**Graduate Program in Medical Sciences**
TAMU Health Science Center
College Station, TX 77843-1114
**Phone:** (409)845-0370 **Fax:** (409)845-6509
**Email:** gradofficehsc@medicine.tamu.edu

**★ 17300 ★ Texas Tech University**
**Health Sciences Center**
**Graduate School of Biomedical Sciences**
**Department of Pharmacology**
3601 4th St.
Lubbock, TX 79430
**Phone:** (806)743-2556 **Free:** 800-528-5391
**Fax:** (806)743-2656
**Email:** acagsbs@ttuhsc.edu
**Website:** http://www2.ttuhsc.edu/pages/grad/de-
fault.htm

**★ 17301 ★ University of Houston**
**College of Pharmacy**
**Department of Pharmacological and**
**Pharmaceutical Sciences**
141 Science & Research Bldg. 2
Houston, TX 77204-5000
**Phone:** (713)743-1222    **Fax:** (713)743-1229
**Email:** vigreen@uh.edu

**★ 17302 ★ University of North Texas**
**Health Science Center**
**Graduate School of Biomedical Sciences**
**Department of Pharmacology**
3500 Camp Bowie Blvd.
Fort Worth, TX 76107
**Phone:** (817)735-2560    **Fax:** (817)735-0243
**Website:** http://www.hsc.unt.edu/education/gsbs/

**★ 17303 ★ University of Texas, Austin**
**College of Pharmacy**
**Department of Pharmacology and**
**Toxicology**
Division of Pharmacology/Toxicology
College of Pharmacy
Austin, TX 78712-1074
**Phone:** (512)471-1737
**Email:** KehrerJim@mail.utexas.edu

**★ 17304 ★ University of Texas Health**
**Science Center, San Antonio**
**Graduate School of Biomedical Sciences**
**Department of Pharmacology**
7703 Floyd Curl Dr.
Mail Code 7764
San Antonio, TX 78229-3900
**Phone:** (210)567-4220    **Fax:** (210)567-4303
**Email:** pharmgrad@uthscsa.edu
**Website:** http://pharmacology.uthscsa.edu/

**★ 17305 ★ University of Texas, Houston**
**Graduate School of Biomedical Sciences**
**Department of Pharmacology**
PO Box 20334
Houston, TX 77225-0334
**Free:** 800-UTH-GSBS    **Fax:** (713)500-9877

**★ 17306 ★ University of Texas Medical**
**Branch, Galveston**
**Graduate School of Biomedical Sciences**
**Department of Pharmacology and**
**Toxicology**
5106 Administration Bldg.
301 University Blvd.
Galveston, TX 77555-0132
**Phone:** (409)772-2665    **Fax:** (409)772-0772
**Email:** grad.school@utmb.edu

**★ 17307 ★ University of Texas**
**Southwestern Medical Center, Dallas**
**Graduate School of Biomedical Sciences**
**Division of Cell and Molecular Biology**
**Department of Pharmacology**
5323 Harry Hines Blvd.
Dallas, TX 75390-9004
**Phone:** (214)648-8099    **Fax:** (214)648-2978
**Email:** dcmbinfo@utsouthwestern.edu
**Website:** http://swnt240.swmed.edu/gradschool/web-pages/dcmbhpg.htm

### Utah

**★ 17308 ★ University of Utah**
**College of Pharmacy**
**Department of Pharmacology and**
**Toxicology**
30 S 2000 E, Rm. 201
Salt Lake City, UT 84112
**Phone:** (801)581-6447    **Fax:** (801)581-4049

**Email:** gradapplicants@deans.pharm.utah.edu

### Vermont

**★ 17309 ★ University of Vermont**
**College of Medicine**
**Department of Pharmacology**
Given Medical Bldg.
Burlington, VT 05405
**Phone:** (802)656-2500    **Fax:** (802)656-4523
**Email:** jhayes@zoo.uvm.edu

### Virginia

**★ 17310 ★ University of Virginia**
**Graduate School of Arts and Sciences**
**Department of Pharmacology**
437 Cabell Hall
Charlottesville, VA 22903
**Phone:** (804)924-7184    **Fax:** (804)924-6737
**Email:** grad-a-s@virginia.edu

**★ 17311 ★ Virginia Commonwealth**
**University**
**School of Medicine**
**Department of Pharmacology and**
**Toxicology**
PO Box 980613
Richmond, VA 23298
**Phone:** (804)828-8400    **Fax:** (804)828-1532
**Email:** ssawyer@hsc.vcu.edu
**Website:** http://www.vcu.edu/gradweb/programs/pfmed.htmphar

### Washington

**★ 17312 ★ University of Washington**
**School of Medicine**
**Department of Pharmacology**
PO Box 357280
Seattle, WA 98195-7280
**Phone:** (206)685-9252    **Fax:** (206)685-3822
**Email:** uwgrad@u.washington.edu

**★ 17313 ★ Washington State University**
**College of Pharmacy**
**Department of Pharmaceutical Sciences**
**Graduate Program in Pharmacology and**
**Toxicology**
PO Box 646534
Pullman, WA 99164-6534
**Phone:** (509)335-7598    **Fax:** (509)335-5902
**Email:** pharmtox@wsu.edu

### West Virginia

**★ 17314 ★ Marshall University**
**School of Medicine**
**Department of Biomedical Sciences**
Office of Research and Graduate Education
1542 Spring Valley Dr.
Huntington, WV 25704
**Phone:** (304)696-7326    **Fax:** (304)696-7171
**Email:** gruettem@marshall.edu
**Website:** http://meb.marshall.edu/graduate/course.htm

**★ 17315 ★ West Virginia University**
**School of Medicine**
**Department of Pharmacology and**
**Toxicology**
PO Box 9024
Morgantown, WV 26506-9024
**Phone:** (304)293-7116    **Fax:** (304)293-7038
**Email:** cnoel@hsc.wvu.edu

### Wisconsin

**★ 17316 ★ University of Wisconsin,**
**Madison**
**Medical School**
**Department of Pharmacology**
3750 Medical Sciences Center
1300 University Ave.
Madison, WI 53706
**Phone:** (608)262-9826    **Fax:** (608)262-1257
**Email:** lsquire@facstaff.wisc.edu

# National & International Organizations

**★ 17317 ★ Alliance for the Prudent Use**
**of Antibiotics (APUA)**
75 Kneeland St.
Boston, MA 02111-1901
**Phone:** (617)636-0966    **Fax:** (617)636-3999
**Email:** jane_s.rogers@tufts.edu
**Website:** http://www.apua.org
Kathleen T. Young, Exec. Dir.

**Fnded:** 1981. **Mem:** 1,000. **Nat'l Groups:** 24. **Desc:** International membership of physicians, scientists, and medical and public health personnel; other individuals supporting prudent use of antibiotics. (Believes that extensive use of antibiotics leads to development of resistant strains of pathogenic and common, nonpathogenic bacteria with resistance traits transferable from one bacterium to others. These resistant strains are no longer susceptible to antibiotics and therefore can undermine treatment of infectious bacterial diseases.) Advocates and defines "good usage" of antibiotics; informs and educates the public about the dangers of misusing and overusing antibiotics and other antimicrobial agents; provides data to individuals and organizations interested in preventing antibiotic misuse and overuse. Informs and educates medical and paramedical personnel worldwide about the defined and specific action of antibiotics and the necessity of controlling their dispensation and prescription. Supports research projects. Maintains speakers' bureau. **Pub:** *APUA Newsletter,* quarterly. Newsletter. Includes pharmacology reviews. *Price:* Included in membership dues.

**★ 17318 ★ American Academy of Clinical**
**Toxicology (AACT)**
777 E Park Dr.
PO Box 8820
Harrisburg, PA 17105-8820
**Phone:** (717)558-7750    **Free:** 888-633-5784
**Fax:** (717)558-7845
**Email:** ashambaugh@pamedsoc.org
**Website:** http://www.clintox.org
Anne Shambaugh, Exec. Dir.

**Fnded:** 1968. **Mem:** 600. **Desc:** Physicians, veterinarians, pharmacists, nurses research scientists, and analytical chemists. Objectives are to: unite medical scientists and facilitate the exchange of information; encourage the development of therapeutic methods and technology; Conducts professional training in poison information and emergency service personnel. **Pub:** *Journal of Toxicology-Clinical Toxicology,* 7/year. Journal. *Price:* Included in membership dues. • Current Awareness-Publication of Contemporary References in clinical toxicology and AACTion-organization newsletter.

**★ 17319 ★ American Academy of**
**Pharmaceutical Physicians Education**
**Foundation**
c/o Anne G. Arella, Executive Director
1031 Pemberton Hill Rd., Ste. 101
Apex, NC 27502
**Phone:** (919)355-1000    **Fax:** (919)355-1010
**Email:** office@aapp.org

**Website:** http://www.aapp.org
Anne G. Arella, Exec. Dir.
**Fnded:** 1993. **Mem:** 1,200. **Reg. Groups:** 9. **Desc:** Physicians dedicated to pharmaceutical medicine, research, education and practice who spend 50% of their professional time practicing pharmaceutical medicine. **Pub:** *AAPP...Rx*, quarterly. Newsletter.


**American Academy of Veterinary and Comparative Toxicology (AAVCT)**
*See:* Entry 20531


**American Academy of Veterinary Pharmacology and Therapeutics (AAVPT)**
*See:* Entry 20533


★ **17320** ★ **American Association of Pharmacy Technicians (AAPT)**
PO Box 1447
Greensboro, NC 27402
**Free:** 877-368-4771                    **Fax:** (336)275-7222
**Email:** felt@pulse.net
**Website:** http://www.pharmacytechnician.com/
Kim Felt, Pres.

**Desc:** Pharmacy technicians. Promotes professional advancement of members. Represents members before health care and public organizations; conducts continuing professional development courses; publicizes the role of the pharmacy technician as an "integral part of the patient care team."


★ **17321** ★ **American Association of Poison Control Centers (AAPCC)**
3201 New Mexico Ave. NW, Ste. 310
Washington, DC 20016
**Phone:** (202)362-7217
**Email:** aapcc@poison.org
**Website:** http://www.aapcc.org
Alan Woolf, MD, Pres.

**Fnded:** 1958. **Mem:** 1,400. **Reg. Groups:** 70. **Desc:** ""–4 Individuals and organizations engaged in operation of poison control centers and/or interested in poison prevention. Has established standards for poison information, control centers and specialists in poison information. Compiles statistics about poison exposures in the United States. **Pub:** *Annual Report of the American Association of Poison Control Centers Toxic Exposure Surveillance System*, annual. Annual Report. Contains a summary of poison exposures. *Price:* $10 reprint. • Membership Directory, annual.


**American Board of Veterinary Toxicology (ABVT)**
*See:* Entry 20554


★ **17322** ★ **American College of Clinical Pharmacology (ACCP)**
3 Ellinwood Ct.
New Hartford, NY 13413-1105
**Phone:** (315)768-6117                    **Fax:** (315)768-6119
**Email:** accp1ssu@aol.com
**Website:** http://www.accp1.org
Susan S. Ulrich, Exec. Dir.

**Fnded:** 1969. **Mem:** 1,000. **Local Groups:** 8. **Desc:** Strives to be the premier professional society with the size, influence, and diversity of membership consistent with the breadth of the discipline of clinical pharmacology. Provides educational programs and forum for membership, health professionals, students, and the public. Assists in the development and dissemination of basic and clinical knowledge to improve rational drug use and patient outcomes. Serves as a forum for active public debate to influence scientific, regulatory, and public health policy issues. Provides opportunities to influence future directions of the College. Supports and encourages the discovery and development efforts designed to provide improved therapeutic modalities. **Pub:** *ACCP Newsletter*, 3/year. Newsletter. *Price:* Free for members. • *American College of Clinical*

*Pharmacology–Directory*, annual. Membership Directory. *Price:* Included in membership dues. • *Journal of Clinical Pharmacology*, monthly. Journal. *Price:* Included in membership dues; $238 for nonmembers in the U.S.; $299 for nonmembers outside the U.S.


★ **17323** ★ **American College of Medical Toxicology (ACMT)**
777 E Park Dr.
PO Box 8820
Harrisburg, PA 17105-8820
**Phone:** (717)558-7846                    **Free:** 888-633-5784
**Fax:** (717)558-7841
**Email:** hmiller@pamedsoc.org
**Website:** http://www.acmt.net
Heather S. Miller, Exec. Dir.

**Fnded:** 1993. **Mem:** 282. **Desc:** Seeks to advance the science, study and practice of medical toxicology by fostering the development of medical toxicology in its provision of emergency, consultation, forensic, legal, community and industrial services; and by otherwise striving to advance and elevate the science, study and practice of medical toxicology. **Pub:** *Internet Journal of Medical Toxicology*. Journal. • Newsletter, 3/year. *Price:* for members only. **Frmly:** American Board of Medical Toxicology.


★ **17324** ★ **American College of Neuropsychopharmacology (ACNP)**
2014 Broadway, Ste. 320
Nashville, TN 37203
**Phone:** (615)322-2075                    **Fax:** (615)343-0662
**Email:** acnp@acnp.org
**Website:** http://www.acnp.org
Oakley Ray, PhD, Exec. Sec.

**Fnded:** 1961. **Mem:** 735. **Desc:** Experienced investigators whose work is related to neuropsychopharmacology. Promotes and encourages the scientific study and application of neuropsychopharmacology. Conducts study groups and plenary sessions. **Pub:** *Mailings*, monthly. Journal. • *Neuropsychopharmacology*, monthly. Journal. Focuses on clinical and basic science contributions to neuropharmacology. *Price:* Included in membership dues. • *Roster*, annual.


★ **17325** ★ **American Society for Clinical Pharmacology and Therapeutics (ASCPT)**
528 N Washington St.
Alexandria, VA 22314-2314
**Phone:** (703)836-6981                    **Fax:** (703)836-5223
**Email:** info@ascpt.org
**Website:** http://www.ascpt.org
Sharon J. Swan, Exec. Dir.

**Fnded:** 1900. **Mem:** 2,150. **Desc:** Works to "promote and advance the science of human pharmacology and therapeutics and in so doing to maintain the highest standards of research, education, and exchange of scientific information." Provides a Medical Education Program of Continuing Education for practicing physicians. **Pub:** *Clinical Pharmacology and Therapeutics*, monthly. Journal. *Price:* Included in membership dues.


★ **17326** ★ **American Society of Clinical Psychopharmacology (ASCP)**
PO Box 2257
New York, NY 10116
**Phone:** (212)696-1088                    **Free:** 800-248-4344
**Fax:** (212)696-0563
**Website:** http://www.ascpp.org
J. Craig Nelson, MD, Pres.

**Fnded:** 1992. **Mem:** 1,200. **Nat'l Groups:** 1. **Desc:** Works to encourage clinical research in psychopharmacology and provide continuing education for members. Sponsors research; facilitates exchange of information; conducts professional educational programs and; provides educational programs on the treatment of psychiatric disorders for patients and families; develops relationships with mental health advocacy groups; advocates public policies which promote research and the delivery of high quality care. **Pub:**

*ASCP Update*, quarterly. Newsletter. *Price:* Free for members. • *Progress Notes*, quarterly. Newsletter.


★ **17327** ★ **American Society of Pharmacognosy (ASP)**
c/o R.J. Krueger, Treas.
College of Pharmacy
901 S State St.
Big Rapids, MI 49307
**Phone:** (616)592-2236                    **Fax:** (616)592-3829
**Email:** kruegerr@ferris.edu
**Website:** http://www.phcog.org
S. William Pellefier, Pres.

**Fnded:** 1959. **Mem:** 1,200. **Desc:** Professional society of pharmacognosists (persons engaged in the study of drugs from a natural origin) and others interested in the plant sciences and natural products. **Pub:** *Journal of Natural Products*, monthly. Journal. • Newsletter, quarterly.


★ **17328** ★ **American Society for Pharmacology and Experimental Therapeutics (ASPET)**
9650 Rockville Pike
Bethesda, MD 20814-3995
**Phone:** (301)530-7060                    **Fax:** (301)530-7061
**Email:** info@aspet.org
**Website:** http://www.aspet.org
Christine K. Carrico, PhD, Exec. Officer

**Fnded:** 1908. **Mem:** 4,400. **Desc:** Scientific society of investigators in pharmacology and toxicology interested in research and promotion of pharmacological knowledge and its use among scientists and the public. **Pub:** *Clinical Pharmacology and Therapeutics*, monthly. • *Drug Metabolism and Disposition*, monthly. • *Journal of Pharmacology and Experimental Therapeutics*, monthly. Journal. • *Molecular Pharmacology*, monthly. • *Pharmacological Reviews*, quarterly. • *Pharmacologist*, quarterly. • Brochures. • Also distributes listings of schools of medicine and pharmacy.


★ **17329** ★ **Association of Clinical Research Professionals (ACRP)**
1012 14th St. NW, Ste. 807
Washington, DC 20005
**Phone:** (202)737-8100                    **Fax:** (202)737-8101
**Email:** office@acrpnet.org
**Website:** http://www.acrpnet.org
Sherrin H. Baky, CEO

**Fnded:** 1976. **Mem:** 12,000. **Desc:** Individuals engaged in clinical pharmacology and other related research professions, including clinical monitors and research associates, nurses, pharmacists, pharmacologists, physicians, and regulatory professionals. Promotes professional growth in the field through the dissemination of information, the exchange of ideas, and the development of educational programs. Provides continuing education credits to pharmacy and nursing professionals through the American Council on Pharmaceutical Education and the American Nurses Association. **Pub:** *ACRP Membership Directory*, annual. Membership Directory. *Price:* Free. For members only. • *Monitor*, quarterly. Magazine. Includes activities information and committee reports, industry news, calendar of events, clinical research articles. *Price:* Free. For members only. **Frmly:** (1999) Associates of Clinical Pharmacology.


**Australasian Society of Oral Medicine and Toxicology (ASOMAT)**
*See:* Entry 6472


★ **17330** ★ **Behavioral Toxicology Society (BTS)**
c/o Chris Newland
Auburn University
Department of Psychology
Auburn, AL 36849
**Phone:** (919)541-5075                    **Fax:** (919)541-4849
**Email:** newlamc@auburn.edu

**Website:** http://www.behavioraltoxicology.org
Chris Newland, PhD, Pres.

**Fnded:** 1982. **Desc:** Promotes scientific research into the effects of toxic agents on behavior and the nervous system; provides a forum for presentation and discussion of research; provides education in neurotoxicology. **Pub:** *Neurotoxicology and Teratology*. Journal. A joint publication of BTS and the Neurobehavioral Teratology Society.


★ **17331** ★ **British Association for Psychopharmacology (BAP)**
c/o Susan Chandler
36 Cambridge Pl.
Hills Rd.
Cambridge CB2 1NS, United Kingdom
**Phone:** 44 1223 358395     **Fax:** 44 1223 321268
**Email:** susan@bap.org.uk
**Website:** http://www.bap.org.uk
**Fnded:** 1974. **Mem:** 900. **Lang(s):** English. **Desc:** Psychopharmacologists, psychiatrists, neuropharmacologists, psychologists, and neurochemists. Brings together scientists working in academic, clinical, and industrial applications of psychopharmacology. Arranges scientific meetings, study groups, and seminars; encourages basic research and pharmaceutical development. Offers professional guidance to the public on matters related to psychopharmacology. **Pub:** *Journal of Psychopharmacology*, bimonthly. Journal. • Monographs, periodic.


★ **17332** ★ **British Pharmacological Society**
16, Angel Gate
City Rd.
London EC1V 2SG, United Kingdom
**Phone:** 44 171 4170113     **Fax:** 44 171 4170114
**Email:** admin@bps.ac.uk
**Website:** http://cbl.leeds.ac.uk/raven/pha/bpstxt.html
**Fnded:** 1931. **Mem:** 2,400. **Lang(s):** English. **Desc:** Pharmacologists and clinical pharmacologists in academia and industry in 20 countries. Conducts educational symposia and lectures; makes available travel bursaries. **Pub:** *British Journal of Clinical Pharmacology*, monthly. Journal. • *British Journal of Pharmacology*, 2x/mo. Journal.


**Business Alliance for Commerce in Hemp (IASPA)**
**(Associazione Italiana Informatori Scientifici del Farmaco — AIISF)**
*See:* Entry 2017


★ **17333** ★ **Canadian Society for Clinical Pharmacology (CSCP)**
76 Grenville St., Ste. 947
Toronto, ON, Canada M5S 1B2
**Phone:** (416)323-7552     **Fax:** (416)323-7553
**Email:** c.vandergiessen@utoronto.ca
**Lang(s):** English, French. **Desc:** Clinical pharmacologists and other health care professionals and scientists with and interest in pharmacy. Seeks to advance the study, teaching, and practice of clinical pharmacology. Serves as a network linking members; sponsors research and educational programs.


★ **17334** ★ **Chinese Pharmacological Society**
1 Xian Nong Tan St.
Beijing 100050, People's Republic of China
**Phone:** 86 10 3013366     **Fax:** 86 10 3017757
**Email:** cnphars@cnphars.org
**Website:** http://www.cnphars.org
**Fnded:** 1985. **Mem:** 3,303. **Lang(s):** English, Japanese. **Desc:** Pharmacologists and interested individuals in the People's Republic of China. Promotes the study of pharmacology. Conducts research programs. Fosters exchange among members and pharmacologists in other countries. Provides consulting services. **Pub:** *China Journal of Pharmacology and Toxicology,*

periodic. Journal. • *Chinese Pharmacological Bulletin*. Newsletter. • *Chinese Pharmacology and Clinical Application*, periodic. Journal. • *Pharmacologica Sinica*, periodic. Journal. • *Pharmacology and Clinics of Chinese Materia Medica*. Directory.


**Collegium Internationale Neuro-Psychopharmacologicum (CINP)**
*See:* Entry 13978


★ **17335** ★ **European Association of Poisons Centres and Clinical Toxicologists (EAPCCT)**
**(Association Europeenne des Centres Anti-Poisons et de Toxicologie Clinique)**
Service de Reanimation Medicale et Centre Anti-Poisons
Hopitalix Universitaires de Strasbourg
Hopital Civil, BP426
1 Place del' Hopital
67091 Strasbourg, France
**Phone:** 33 3 88373737     **Fax:** 33 3 88116377
**Email:** oray@cinp.org
**Website:** http://www.eapcct.org/
**Fnded:** 1964. **Mem:** 300. **Lang(s):** English. **Desc:** Physicians and scientists working in clinical toxicology and related fields. Association works to improve contacts between clinical toxicologists and poisons information specialists. Regularly organizes joint meetings with the World Health Organization and the European Commission. Is a member of the International Union on Toxicology (IUTOX). **Pub:** *Journal of Toxicology: Clinical Toxicology*, bimonthly. Journal. • *Newsletter*, quarterly. Newsletter. **Frmly:** (1990) European Association of Poison Control Centres.


★ **17336** ★ **European Behavioral Pharmacology Society (EBPS)**
University of Wales
Department of Psychology
Singleton Park
Swansea SA2 8PP, United Kingdom
**Phone:** 44 1792 295844     **Fax:** 44 1792 295679
**Email:** president@ebps.org
**Website:** http://www.ebps.org/main.htm
**Desc:** Seeks to advance the development of behavioral pharmacology; disseminates research to members and non-members; assists practitioners of behavioral pharmacology to obtain knowledge extending into related disciplines.


**European College of Neuropsychopharmacology**
*See:* Entry 13995


★ **17337** ★ **European Society of Biochemical Pharmacology (ESBP)**
c/o Dr. Brian Burchell
University of Dundee
Department of Biochem. Med.
Ninewells Medical School
Dundee DD1 9SY, United Kingdom
**Phone:** 44 1382 632164     **Fax:** 44 1382 633952
**Email:** b.burchell@dundee.ac.uk
**Website:** http://www.mti.uni-jena.de/~iro/esbp.html
**Desc:** Researchers at academic institutions and in the pharmaceutical industry. Promotes advancements in the field of pharmacology.


★ **17338** ★ **European Society for Developmental Pharmacology (ESDP)**
82, av Denfert-Rochereau
F-75674 Paris, France
**Fax:** 33 1 40488328
**Fnded:** 1988. **Desc:** Promotes foetal, perinatal or pediatric pharmacology.

★ **17339** ★ **EUROTOX**
c/o Prof. E. Hietanen
University of Turku
Department of Clinical Physiology
SF-20520 Turku, Finland
**Phone:** 358 2 2612664     **Fax:** 358 2 2611666
**Email:** eino.hietanen@utu.fi
**Website:** http://www.eurotox.com
**Fnded:** 1962. **Mem:** 6,500. **Nat'l Groups:** 30. **Lang(s):** English. **Desc:** Industrial, university, and government toxicology researchers in 50 countries. Purpose is to encourage and advance research in the field of drug toxicity and in other areas of toxicology. Fosters exchange of information concerning problems in toxicology. Topics of interest have included the effects of drugs on the human fetus, toxicological methods and their reliability, toxicity problems of organs such as the liver and the nervous system, carcinogenesis, and sensitization. Sponsors working groups and training courses in toxicology. **Pub:** *EUROTOX*, 3/year. Newsletter. Contains news and views on a variety of toxicological issues. • *EUROTOX Membership Directory*, periodic. Directory. Contains names and addresses of members. • *Proceedings of the Annual Meeting*.


★ **17340** ★ **Indian Pharmacological Society**
c/o Department of Pharmacology and Therapeutics
Patna Medical College
Patna 800 014, Bihar, India
**Desc:** Fosters the science of pharmacology. Promotes research in pharmacology and allied disciplines with reference to current health needs in India and national health policy. Collects, evaluates, and disseminates scientific knowledge about drugs. **Pub:** *IPS Newsletter*, periodic. Newsletter. • Journal, periodic.


★ **17341** ★ **International Academy of Compounding Pharmacists (IACP)**
PO Box 1365
Sugar Land, TX 77487
**Free:** 800-927-4227     **Fax:** (281)495-0602
**Email:** iacpinfo@iacprx.org
**Website:** http://www.iacprx.org
L.D. King, Exec. Dir.
**Fnded:** 1991. **Mem:** 1,600. **Desc:** Pharmacists who compound custom medications to meet unique patient needs. Seeks to "enhance credibility and respect of the compounding pharmacy practice to the health care community and its patients"; promotes empowerment of compounding pharmacists. Develops and enforces codes of ethics and practice for members; facilitates cooperation and exchange of information among members; sponsors research and educational programs. **Pub:** *The Pharmacists Link*, quarterly.


★ **17342** ★ **International Association of Radiopharmacology (IAR)**
c/o Dr. Steve McQuarrie
Faculty of Pharmacy
University of Alberta
Edmonton, AB, Canada T6G 2N8
**Phone:** (780)492-2905     **Fax:** (780)492-1217
**Email:** steve.mcquarrie@ualberta.ca
**Fnded:** 1980. **Desc:** Represents members' interest. **Pub:** *Symposium Proceedings*, biennial.


★ **17343** ★ **International Association of Therapeutic Drug Monitoring and Clinical Toxicology (IATDMCT)**
IATDMCT Business Office
PO Box 1570
4 Cataraqui St., Ste. 310
Kingston, ON, Canada K7L 5C8
**Phone:** (613)531-8166     **Fax:** (613)531-0626
**Email:** iatdmct@eventsmgt.com
**Website:** http://www.iatdmct.org
**Desc:** Professionals with an interest in either therapeutic drug monitoring and clinical toxicology, physicians, clinical chemists, pharmacologists, medical

technologists, toxicologists and environmental analysts. Aims are to promote the knowledge and understanding of clinical drug analysis and interpretation of results. Enhances communication between scientists and physicians of all disciplines involved in therapeutic drug monitoring and clinical toxicology. Encourages the effective application of therapeutic drug monitoring and clinical toxicology.

**★ 17344 ★ International Life Sciences Institute - North America (ILSINA)**
One Thomas Cir. NW, 9th Fl.
Washington, DC 20005
**Phone:** (202)659-0074    **Fax:** (202)659-3859
**Email:** ilsi@ilsi.org
**Website:** http://www.ilsi.org
Morris E. Potter, Exec. Dir.

**Fnded:** 1985. **Mem:** 60. **Desc:** Sponsored by companies within the food, pharmaceutical, chemical, toxicology, and related industries. Promotes basic research and education in the areas of nutrition food safety, toxicology, risk assessment, and the environment through support of research, scientific symposia, workshops, and monographs. Fosters career development of outstanding young scientists. **Pub:** *Nutrition Reviews*, monthly. • *Present Knowledge in Nutrition*, quinquennial. • Also publishes monographs, reprints, scientific reports, and educational materials. **Frmly:** (1991) International Life Sciences Institute - Nutrition Foundation.

**International Society of Cardiovascular Pharmacotherapy (ISCP)**
*See:* Entry 5025

**★ 17345 ★ International Society of Chemotherapy (ISC)**
**(Societe Internationale de Chimiotherapie)**
c/o Dr. Faridah Moosdeen
31 St. Olav's Ct.
City Business Centre
25 Lower Rd.
London SE16 2XB, United Kingdom
**Phone:** 44 20 72312944    **Fax:** 44 20 72312124
**Email:** moosdeen@ischemo.demon.co.uk
**Website:** http://www.ischemo.org

**Fnded:** 1961. **Mem:** 16,000. **Nat'l Groups:** 60. **Reg. Groups:** 5. **Lang(s):** English. **Desc:** Societies or specialized groups within societies that are concerned with chemotherapy; scientists and clinicians working in chemotherapy. (Chemotherapy is the use of chemical agents in the treatment or control of infectious and neoplastic diseases and immunological disorder.) Promotes the development of chemotherapy through scientific and educational means. Encourages cooperation between members and scientists in related fields. Urges formation of new societies in countries where such groups do not exist. Promotes and/or sponsors formation of international working groups and training projects in the field of antimicrobial, antiparasitic, and antineoplastic chemotherapy; coordinates their activities. Appoints commissions for special activities. **Pub:** *Antibiotics Chemotherapy*, quarterly. Newsletter. • *Congress Proceedings*, biennial. • *International Journal of Antimicrobial Agents*, 8/year. Journal.

**★ 17346 ★ International Society for Pharmacoeconomics and Outcomes Research**
3100 Princeton Pke., Bldg 3, Ste. D
Lawrenceville, NJ 08648
**Phone:** (609)219-0773    **Fax:** (609)219-0774
**Email:** info@ispor.org
**Website:** http://www.ispor.org
Marilyn Dix Smith, Exec. Dir.

**Fnded:** 1995. **Mem:** 2,000. **Nat'l Groups:** 13. **Reg. Groups:** 3. **Desc:** Researchers who study the cost effectiveness of treatments. Researchers and users of cost-effectiveness information, health care decision makers. **Pub:** *ISPOR News*, bimonthly. Newsletter. Pharmacoeconomic news articles. • *Value in Health*,

bimonthly. Journal. Provides information on pharmacoeconomic and outcomes research; health policy development. Now indexed in "Index Medicus/Medline". *Price:* $165 per year.

**★ 17347 ★ International Union of Pharmacology (IUPHAR)**
c/o Prof. P.M. Vanhoutte
University of Strathclyde
204 George St.
Glasgow G1 1XW, United Kingdom
**Phone:** 44 141 5524400    **Fax:** 44 141 5522562
**Email:** w.cbowman@strath.ac.uk
**Website:** http://www.who.int/ina-ngo/ngo/ngo136.htm

**Fnded:** 1966. **Mem:** 52. **Nat'l Groups:** 52. **Lang(s):** English. **Desc:** National and international societies in pharmacology and related disciplines representing approximately 30,000 individuals. Purpose is to promote cooperation between pharmacological societies and encourage free international exchange of ideas and research. Acts as a forum for participation between related scientific bodies. Works to standardize the use of drugs worldwide and rationally define the receptors and ion channels on which they act. **Pub:** *Congress Proceedings*, quadrennial. • *Directory of IUPHAR*, annual. • *IUPHAR Newsletter*, semiannual. Newsletter.

**★ 17348 ★ Medical Letter (ML)**
1000 Main St.
New Rochelle, NY 10801
**Phone:** (914)235-0500    **Free:** 800-211-2769
**Fax:** (914)632-1733
**Email:** custserv@themedicalletter.org
**Website:** http://www.medletter.com
Mark Abramowicz, MD, Ed.

**Fnded:** 1959. **Desc:** Gathers and publishes information on the therapeutic and side effects of drugs for the benefit of physicians and other members of the health professions. Emphasis is on new drugs. **Pub:** *Advice for Travelers*, semiannual. Provides quick access to information about specific countries, diseases and travel-related risks. *Price:* $139 20% discount for renewals. • *Handbook of Antimicrobial Therapy*. Handbook. • *Medical Letter: A Searchable Collection on CD-ROM*, annual. Permits users to quickly access, search and print articles. *Price:* $65. • *Medical Letter Handbook of Adverse Drug Interactions*. Handbook. *Price:* $22; $12 for members. • *Medical Letter on Drugs and Therapeutics*, biweekly. Newsletter. Evaluates drugs for physicians. *Price:* $49/year. **Frmly:** Drug and Therapeutic Information.

**★ 17349 ★ Scottish Pharmaceutical Federation**
135 Wellington St.
Glasgow G2 2XD, United Kingdom
**Phone:** 44 141 2211235    **Fax:** 44 141 2265047
**Email:** secretary@spf.netkonect.co.uk

**Fnded:** 1919. **Mem:** 1,050. **Desc:** Independent retail pharmacists in Scotland. Provides legal representation, general insurance, professional indemnity cover, staff training, clearing house and information services for Scotland. **Pub:** Newsletter, periodic.

**★ 17350 ★ Sociedad de Farmacologia de Chile**
Casilla 70000, Correo 7
Santiago, Chile
**Phone:** 56 2 776560    **Fax:** 56 2 2225515
**Fnded:** 1979.

**★ 17351 ★ Society of Environmental Toxicology and Chemistry (SETAC)**
1010 N 12th Ave.
Pensacola, FL 32501-3367
**Phone:** (850)469-1500    **Free:** 888-899-2088
**Fax:** (850)469-9778
**Email:** setac@setac.org
**Website:** http://www.setac.org
Rodney Parrish, Exec. Dir.

**Fnded:** 1979. **Mem:** 5,000. **Reg. Groups:** 16. **Desc:** Professionals in the fields of chemistry, toxicology, biology, and ecology; atmospheric, health, and earth sciences; and environmental engineering. Promotes the use of multidisciplinary approaches to examine the impacts of chemicals and technology on the environment. Strives to balance the interests of academia, business, and government. Conducts workshops and symposia on research topics of interest to members. **Pub:** *Environmental Toxicology and Chemistry*, monthly. Journal. Contains peer-reviewed research papers. *Price:* $640 for institutions. • *Life-Cycle Assessment Data Quality: A Conceptual Framework*. Report. • *Radiotelemetry Applications for Wildlife Toxicology Field Studies*. • *SETAC News*, bimonthly. Newsletter. Highlights environmental topics, SETAC activities, employment activities, and meetings of interest. • *Membership Directory*, annual. Lists addresses and specialties of members. *Price:* available to members only. • Publishes various technical and informal reports.

**★ 17352 ★ Society for Medicinal Plant Research**
**(Gesellschaft fur Arzneipflanzenforschung — GA)**
c/o Dr. B. Frank
Am Grundbach 5
D-97271 Kleinrinderfeld, Germany
**Phone:** 49 931 8002270    **Fax:** 49 931 8002275
**Email:** ga-secretary@t-online.de
**Website:** http://www.ga-online.org

**Fnded:** 1953. **Mem:** 980. **Lang(s):** English, German. **Desc:** Scientists in 70 countries who promote medicinal plant research. Organized to serve as an international focal point for such interests as pharmacognosy, pharmacology, phytochemistry, plant biochemistry and physiology, chemistry of natural products; plant cell culture and application of medicinal plants in medicine. Acts as liaison with governments, pharmacopoeia commissions, and international health organizations on matters pertaining to the medicinal plant field. Serves as forum for international exchange of information on the different aspects of medicinal plant research. **Pub:** *Newsletter*, semiannual. Newsletter. Includes news of the society and congress announcements. • *Planta Medica*, bimonthly. Journal. **Frmly:** (1970) German Society for Medicinal Plant Research.

**Society of Toxicologic Pathologists (STP)**
*See:* Entry 17152

**★ 17353 ★ South African Pharmacology Society (SAPS)**
c/o Prof. WJ du Plooy
Department of Pharmacology
PO Box 225
Medunsa 0204, Republic of South Africa
**Phone:** 27 12 5214145    **Fax:** 27 12 5214123
**Email:** wdplooy@medunsa.ac.za
**Website:** http://www.toxpath.org

**Fnded:** 1966. **Mem:** 265. **Desc:** Pharmacists; pharmacologists; physicians; chemical pathologists; psychiatrists; analytical chemists; statisticians. Promotes work in pharmacology and related fields. **Pub:** Newsletter, biennial.

# Research Centers

**★ 17354 ★ Canadian Network of Toxicology Centres (CNTC)**
Bovey Bldg.
Gordon St.
Guelph, ON, Canada N1G 2W1
**Phone:** (519)837-3320    **Fax:** (519)837-3861
**Email:** lritter@tox.uoguelph.ca
**Website:** http://www.uoguelph.ca/cntc/
Dr. Len Ritter, Exec. Dir.

**Activities/Fields:** Toxicology, including risk assessment and epidemiology, environmental concerns, carcinogenesis and genetics, teratology, metabolism and pharmacokinetics, pathology, and analytical chemistry. **Pub:** *CNTC/RCCT News Brief.* • *Metals in the Environment News.*

★ **17355** ★ **Colorado State University**
**Center for Environmental Toxicology and**
**Technology**
Foothills Campus
Fort Collins, CO 80523-1680
**Phone:** (970)491-8522          **Fax:** (970)491-8304
**Email:** raymond.yang@colostate.edu
**Website:** http://www.cvmbs.colostate.edu/enhealth/cett/
Dr. Raymond S.H. Yang, Dir.
**Activities/Fields:** Hazards associated with environmental exposure to chemical and physical agents, focusing on complex chemical mixtures and chemical-radiation interaction. Also studies growth, reproduction, immune function, physiologically based pharmacokinetics, genetic and molecular markers of disease, and ecotoxicology and bioremediation, focusing on hazardous waste mixtures. **Frmly:** Collaborative Radiological Health Laboratory.

★ **17356** ★ **Cornell University**
**Laboratory of Pediatric Critical Care**
525 68th St., Rm. M508
New York, NY 10021
**Phone:** (212)746-3056          **Fax:** (212)746-8332
**Email:** hmushay@med.cornell.edu
Dr. H. Michael Ushay, Dir.
**Activities/Fields:** Adrenergic receptor pharmacology, including receptor-related events at the cellular and molecular levels, and molecular biology of acute lung injury.

★ **17357** ★ **CTRC Research Foundation**
**Institute for Drug Development**
14960 Omicron Dr.
San Antonio, TX 78245-3217
**Phone:** (210)677-3800          **Fax:** (210)677-0058
**Email:** jcole@saci.org
**Website:** http://www.ctrc.saci.org
John F. Cole, PhD, COO
**Activities/Fields:** Anticancer drug discovery and development. tubulin and topoisomerase I and II; measurement of telomerase activity; growth inhibitory activity of cancer cells from biopsy tissue; and cell cycle distribution in relation to drug-cell interactions, drug resistance, and programmed cell death. Clinical Investigations Section researches new drugs as they are first introduced into humans, and examines the pharmacokinetic profile of new drugs.

**Harvard Thorndike Laboratory**
*See:* Entry 5097

★ **17358** ★ **Hawaii Heptachlor Research**
**and Education Foundation**
250 Ward Ave., Ste. 217
Honolulu, HI 96814-4007
**Phone:** (808)589-2963          **Fax:** (808)589-2964
**Email:** hhref@lava.net
**Website:** http://www.lava.net/~hhref
Dr. Willis Butler, Pres.
**Activities/Fields:** Sponsors and supports medical research and medical treatment programs, including research on the effects of pesticides and other toxic substances on humans, and methods and treatment of medical problems caused by exposure to such substances. Current research projects include a medical monitoring program, which will examine the health effects of chronic exposure of Oahu's residents to Heptachlor in dairy products. Other projects sponsored by the Foundation include Induction of Parkinsonian Syndrome by Heptachlor and a feasibility study on the long-term health effects in women of exposure to chlorinated hydrocarbon insecticides.

★ **17359** ★ **Henry Ford Hospital**
**Sleep Disorders Center**
2799 W Grand Blvd., CFP3
Detroit, MI 48202
**Phone:** (313)916-4417          **Fax:** (313)916-5167
Thomas Roth, PhD, Dir.
**Activities/Fields:** Psychopharmacology of sleep, daytime sleepiness, and sleep disorders, including sleep-related apnea.

★ **17360** ★ **Indiana University-Purdue**
**University at Indianapolis**
**Pharmacology Research Laboratory**
School of Medicine
635 Barnhill Dr.
Indianapolis, IN 46202-5120
**Phone:** (317)274-7844          **Fax:** (317)274-7714
**Email:** besch@iupui.edu
**Website:** http://www.iupui.edu/~iuphtx/home1.html
Dr. Henry R. Besch, Jr., Chm.
**Activities/Fields:** Cardiovascular pharmacology, molecular toxicology, drug metabolism, cyclic AMP, membrane biophysics, cancer chemotherapy and cardiac glycosides, and antiarrythmics, including studies on metabolism of transplanted tumors, structure activity relations of cardiac glycosides, and ryanodine analogs.

**Institute for Clinical Science, Inc.**
*See:* Entry 17158

★ **17361** ★ **Inter-University Centre for**
**Toxicology (CIRTOX)**
Department Biological Sciences
Universite of Quebec at Montreal
PO Box 8888, Downtown Sta.
Montreal, QC, Canada H3C 3P8
**Phone:** (514)987-3000          **Fax:** (514)987-4647
**Email:** chevalier.gaston@uqam.ca
Joseph Zayed, PhD, Dir.
**Activities/Fields:** Biological detection of environmental contaminants in living organisms, characterization of harmful effects of potentially toxic chemicals, and development of diagnostic tests and methods for evaluating toxicity.

★ **17362** ★ **John P. Robarts Research**
**Institute**
**Clinical Pharmacology Group**
100 Perth Dr.
PO Box 5015
London, ON, Canada N6A 5K8
**Phone:** (519)663-5777          **Fax:** (519)663-3789
**Email:** ross.feldman@lhsc.on.ca
Dr. Ross Feldman, Dir.
**Activities/Fields:** Studies cardivasular and immunosuppressive agents, both in vivo and in vitro, and drug analysis and pharmacokinetic and pharmacodynamic studies, as well as in vitro determinations of mechanisms of adverse drug reactions.

**Johns Hopkins University**
**Behavioral Pharmacology Research Unit**
*See:* Entry 19357

★ **17363** ★ **Laval University**
**Research Unit in Nephrology**
Hotel-Dieu de Quebec Research Centre
11, Cote du Palais
Quebec, QC, Canada G1R 2J6
**Phone:** (418)525-4444          **Fax:** (418)691-5562
**Email:** marcel.lebel@crhdq.ulaval.ca
Dr. Marcel Lebel, Dir.
**Activities/Fields:** Pathogenesis of high blood pressure and renal diseases.

**Massachusetts Institute of Technology**
**Laboratory of Neuroendocrine Regulation**
*See:* Entry 14226

★ **17364** ★ **Meadowbrook Medical**
**Education and Research Foundation,**
**Inc.**
2201 Hempstead Tpke.
East Meadow, NY 11554-1859
**Phone:** (516)572-6724          **Fax:** (516)572-5974
**Email:** dick@mit.edu
Alan F. King, Exec. Sec. /Treas.
**Activities/Fields:** Clinical drugs studies.

★ **17365** ★ **Medical Care and Research**
**Foundation**
1420 Ogden
Denver, CO 80218-1910
**Phone:** (303)831-0267          **Fax:** (303)831-4079
Frank B. McGlone, MD, Exec. Dir.
**Activities/Fields:** Drug studies. **Pub:** *Court Visitor Training Manual.* • *New Hope in Board and Care: Guidelines for Establishing and Operating Small Facilities.* • *Providing New Directions.*

★ **17366** ★ **Medical University of South**
**Carolina**
**Interdisciplinary Program in Cell and**
**Molecular Pharmacology and**
**Experimental Therapeutics**
171 Ashley Ave.
Charleston, SC 29425
**Phone:** (843)792-2471          **Fax:** (843)792-2475
**Email:** margolhs@musc.edu
**Website:** http://www2.musc.edu/pharm/pharm.html
Dr. Harry Margolius, Chm.
**Activities/Fields:** Pharmacology, toxicology, molecular genetics and structural biology, including structure-function studies of proteins for primary sequence, posttranslational modifications, and characterization of the binding site of ligands; investigations of molecular design; and studies on cellular and molecular processes that control systemic arterial pressure, especially arachidonate metabolism, neurotransmitters, drug disposition and drug toxicity. Conducts studies of excitation-contraction coupling, excitation-secretion coupling, and water transport and regulation in cells and membrane mechanisms by norepinephrine, arachidonic acid metabolites, kallikrein-kinins, atrial peptides, and antihypertensive drugs. Also conducts studies of isolated cells, cell fragments, and isolated membranes, as well as studies on volunteer patients with hypertension, shock, and other cardiovascular-renal abnormalities.

★ **17367** ★ **Ohio State University**
**Clinical Pharmacology Division**
Graves Hall, Rm. 5084
College of Medicine
333 W 10th Ave.
Columbus, OH 43210-1239
**Phone:** (614)292-8600          **Fax:** (614)292-4253
**Email:** apselosf.l@osu.edu
Dr. Glen Apselosf, Dir.
**Activities/Fields:** Clinical drug studies.

★ **17368** ★ **Oregon Health and Science**
**University**
**DMSO Research Laboratory**
3181 SW Sam Jackson Pk. Rd., L225
Portland, OR 97201
**Phone:** (503)494-8474          **Fax:** (503)494-5352
**Email:** jacobs@ohsu.edu
**Website:** http://www.dmso.org
Stanley W. Jacob, MD, Hd.
**Activities/Fields:** Pharmacological properties of dimethyl sulfoxide (DMSO). Provides staff consultants in clinical and basic research relevant to pharmacological activity of dimethyl sulfoxide.

**★ 17369 ★ Reproductive Toxicology Center**
7831 Woodmont Ave., Ste. 375
Bethesda, MD 20814-6030
**Phone:** (301)620-8690
**Email:** reprotox@reprotox.org
**Website:** http://reprotox.org
Anthony Scialli, MD, Dir.
**Activities/Fields:** Effects of the chemical and physical environment on human fertility, pregnancy, and development.

**★ 17370 ★ Rockefeller University**
**Laboratory of Metabolism-Pharmacology**
1230 York Ave.
New York, NY 10021-6399
**Phone:** (212)327-8494  **Fax:** (212)327-8690
Dr. Attallah Kappas, Hd.
**Activities/Fields:** Regulation of heme biosynthesis and heme catabolism as affected by those genetic and environmental factors that have major influences on the oxidative metabolism of drugs, hormones, and environmental chemicals in liver and other tissues.

**St. Clare's Hospital and Health Center**
**Spellman Center for HIV-Related Disease**
*See:* Entry 11875

**★ 17371 ★ St. Jude Children's Research Hospital**
**Department of Molecular Pharmacology**
332 N Lauderdale
Memphis, TN 38105-2729
**Phone:** (901)495-3440  **Fax:** (901)521-1668
**Email:** peter.haughton@stjude.org
**Website:** http://www.stjude.org/departments/d-molpharm.htm
Dr. Peter Houghton, Chm.
**Activities/Fields:** Human tumor xenografts, experimental chemotherapy, selectivity of drug action in in vivo, cytostasis and cytotoxicity, colon carcinoma and rhabdomyosarcoma, thymidylate synthase, molecular events controlling cell death, and relationships between genes involved in cell cycle control and sensitivity to chemotherapy.

**★ 17372 ★ Scripps Research Institute**
**Department of Neuropharmacology**
10550 N Torrey Pines Rd.
La Jolla, CA 92037
**Phone:** (858)784-9730  **Fax:** (858)784-8851
**Email:** fbloom@scripps.edu
Dr. Floyd E. Bloom, Dir.
**Activities/Fields:** Mechanisms of cellular communication in the nervous and endocrine systems. Primary areas of research include: the molecular identification of chemical messengers (neurotransmitters and hormones) and characterization of the structure and function of the cells that secrete them; establishing the role of these substances in normal physiological regulation; establishing the possible pathophysiological roles in clinical disorders of the brain and endocrine system; employing molecular genetic methods to detect virus-selected pathologic mechanisms; interactions between neurotransmitters, cytokines, neurons, glia, and brain macrophages in virus or neurodegenerative disorders; and mechanisms of actions of addictive drugs.

**★ 17373 ★ Sherbrooke University**
**Institute of Pharmacology of Sherbrooke**
Faculty of Medicine
3001 12 Ave. Nord
Sherbrooke, QC, Canada J1H 5N4
**Phone:** (819)564-5239  **Fax:** (819)564-5400
**Email:** p.sirois@courrier.usherb.ca
**Website:** http://ips.med.usherb.ca/
Prof. Pierre Sirois, Contact
**Activities/Fields:** Cardiovascular and pulmonary pharmacology, including peptides and lipids, prosta-

glandins, leukotrienes, angiotensin, bradykinin, and related compounds.

**Stanford University**
**AIDS Clinical Trials Unit**
*See:* Entry 11876

**Stanford University**
**Laboratory for Transplantation Immunology**
*See:* Entry 20355

**Stanford University**
**Stanford Pain Management Service**
*See:* Entry 14276

**★ 17374 ★ State University of New York at Buffalo**
**Clinical Pharmacokinetics Laboratory**
Cooke Hall 556
School of Pharmacy
Amherst, NY 14260
**Phone:** (716)867-0550  **Fax:** (716)838-0756
**Email:** schentag@buffalo.edu
**Website:** http://www.wings.buffalo.edu/academic/department/pharmacy/cpl/
Dr. Jerome J. Schentag, Dir.
**Activities/Fields:** Pharmacokinetics and pharmacodynamics of drugs in volunteers and hospitalized patients. Major emphasis on geriatric patients, pharmacology, nutrition, cancer, cardiology, metabolism, and infectious disease states. Other research activities include technology transfer using computer software in the critical care unit and influence of disease states on the pharmacokinetics and pharmacodynamics of drugs. **Pub:** *Research Papers.*

**Syracuse Cancer Research Institute**
*See:* Entry 10420

**Texas A&M University**
**Institute of Ocular Pharmacology**
*See:* Entry 21144

**★ 17375 ★ Thomas Jefferson University**
**Occupational and Environmental Health Sciences Division**
Jefferson Medical College
1020 Locust St., Rm. 314-JAH
Philadelphia, PA 19107
**Phone:** (215)955-8381  **Fax:** (215)955-2169
**Email:** lance.simpson@mail.tju.edu
**Website:** http://www.ngen.com/hs-cancer
Dr. Lance Simpson, Dir.
**Activities/Fields:** Mechanisms and actions of toxins at the cellular, subcellular, and molecular levels.

**★ 17376 ★ U.S. Department of Health and Human Services**
**Agency for Toxic Substances and Disease Registry**
**Division of Toxicology**
1600 Clifton Rd., NE
Mail Stop E-29
Atlanta, GA 30333
**Phone:** (404)498-0160  **Fax:** (404)498-0094
**Email:** cderosa@cdc.gov
Dr. Christopher DeRosa, Dir.
**Activities/Fields:** Priority hazardous substances. Sets priorities for research, initiates programs, and identifies data needs for publication of *Toxicological Profiles.* Comprises Research Analysis Branch.

**U.S. Department of Health and Human Services**
**Food and Drug Administration**
**Center for Food Safety and Applied Nutrition**
*See:* Entry 18003

**★ 17377 ★ U.S. Department of Health and Human Services**
**Food and Drug Administration**
**National Center for Toxicological Research**
**Biochemical Toxicology Division**
HFT-110
3900 NCTR Dr.
Jefferson, AR 72079
**Phone:** (870)543-7202  **Fax:** (870)543-7136
Dr. Frederick A. Beland, Dir.
**Activities/Fields:** Biochemical mechanisms of toxicity and chemical carcinogenesis, including research on the metabolic activation of chemical toxicants; identification of cellular constituents modified by activated chemical toxicants; elucidation of biochemical and other mechanisms by which chemical carcinogenicity and mutagenicity are initiated and expressed; determination of critical detoxification pathways; studies on effects of cellular repair mechanisms on toxic response; and research on metabolism routes and rates.

**★ 17378 ★ U.S. Department of Health and Human Services**
**Food and Drug Administration**
**National Center for Toxicological Research**
**Biometry Staff**
NCTR Rd. 3900
Jefferson, AR 72079
**Phone:** (870)543-7008
**Email:** rkodell@nctr.sda.gov
Dr. Ralph Kodell, Dir.
**Activities/Fields:** Statistical design and analysis of toxicological experiments. Principal area of research interest is biostatistics in toxicology, including survival analysis, time to tumor estimation and testing, and extrapolation of effects from high to low doses, and dose-response modeling for developmental defects. Focus is on quantitative risk estimation. **Pub:** *Research Reports.*

**★ 17379 ★ U.S. Department of Health and Human Services**
**Food and Drug Administration**
**National Center for Toxicological Research**
**Chemistry Division**
Bldg. 51, Mail Stop HFT-230
3900 NCTR Rd.
Jefferson, AR 72079
**Phone:** (870)543-7301  **Fax:** (870)543-7686
**Email:** rturesky@nctr.fda.gov
**Website:** http://www.fda.gov/nctr/science/divisions/chemistry.htm
Robert Turesky, PhD, Dir.
**Activities/Fields:** New or improved chemical procedures for the trace analysis of carcinogens, teratogens, mutagens, toxicants, and other biologically-active substrates; state-of-the-art techniques to enhance sensitivity, speed, and accuracy of trace-level analytical chemical determinations; instrument laboratory and conducting studies utilizing highly specialized spectrometric techniques; develops and implements automated chemical data systems; and develops and implements analytical methods to ensure nutritional integrity and absence of deleterious substances in animal diets as they affect bioassay results. Areas of interest also include environmental/occupational surveillance and methods, inductively coupled plasma emission, Fourier transform infrared spectroscopy, and LC-MS and GC-MS.

**★ 17380 ★ U.S. Department of Health and Human Services**
**Food and Drug Administration**
**National Center for Toxicological Research**
**Genetic Toxicology Division**
Bldg. 13
3900 NCTR Dr.
Jefferson, AR 72079
**Phone:** (870)543-7050    **Fax:** (870)543-7393
**Email:** mmmoore@nctr.fda.gov
**Website:** http://www.fda.gov/nctr/science/divisions/genreptox.htm
Martha Moore, PhD, Dir.

**Activities/Fields:** Directs an interdisciplinary toxicological research center emphasizing the use of genomic, proteomic and informatic tools to modify and develop standards that are applicable to The Food and Drug Administration's mission to protect the public health. **Frmly:** Genetic Toxicology Division.


**★ 17381 ★ U.S. Department of Health and Human Services**
**Food and Drug Administration**
**National Center for Toxicological Research**
**Office of Research Support**
3900 NCTR Rd.
Jefferson, AR 72079-9502
**Phone:** (870)543-7130    **Fax:** (870)543-7576
**Email:** vattwood@nctr.fda.gov
**Website:** http://www.fda.gov/oc/orgcharts.html
Victor G. Attwood, Dep. Dir., Mgt.

**Activities/Fields:** Provides support to the NCTR by providing facility maintenance, animal husbandry, computer operations, and pathological services.


**★ 17382 ★ U.S. Department of Health and Human Services**
**Food and Drug Administration**
**National Center for Toxicological Research**
**Pathology Associates**
PO Box 26
3900 NCTR Rd.
Jefferson, AR 72079
**Phone:** (870)543-7027    **Free:** 800-638-3321
**Fax:** (870)543-7030
**Email:** tbucci@nctr.foa.gov
John Latendresse, Prog. Dir.

**Activities/Fields:** Effects of a number of chemicals and their varying dosages for different time intervals of treated animals (including making inferences about the potential effect of the same chemicals upon the health of human beings); and studies on the toxicological effects of nerve agents (in cooperation with the Department of Defense), including standard teratology, delayed neuropathy, dominant-lethal, subchronic, and multigenerational protocols. Program also evaluates techniques required to recognize meaningful deviations from normal at earlier times or promise increased specificity in identifying these. Continuing cross-training of technical staff allows for comprehensive pathology services. **Frmly:** (2000) Pathology Associates.


**★ 17383 ★ U.S. Department of Health and Human Services**
**National Cancer Institute**
**Chemistry of Carcinogenesis Laboratory**
Bldg. 538, Rm. 115
PO Box B
Frederick, MD 21702-1201
**Phone:** (301)846-5852    **Fax:** (301)846-6146
**Email:** moschel@ncifcrf.gov
**Website:** http://web.ncifcrf.gov/research/ccl/default.asp
Dr. Robert Moschel, Ch.

**Activities/Fields:** Strives to improve the understanding of how certain chemicals initiate the process of carcinogenesis, and to use this understanding to help prevent or treat the disease.


**U.S. Department of Health and Human Services**
**National Cancer Institute (NCI)**
**Division of Cancer Treatment and Diagnosis (DCTD)**
**Developmental Therapeutics Program (DTP)**
**(Toxicology and Pharmacology Branch — T&PB)**
*See:* Entry 10450


**U.S. Department of Health and Human Services**
**National Cancer Institute**
**Laboratory of Biological Chemistry**
*See:* Entry 10477


**U.S. Department of Health and Human Services**
**National Cancer Institute**
**Laboratory of Molecular Pharmacology**
*See:* Entry 10493


**U.S. Department of Health and Human Services**
**National Center for Infectious Diseases**
**Division of Parasitic Diseases**
**Entomology Branch**
**(Vector Biology and Toxicology Section)**
*See:* Entry 11892


**U.S. Department of Health and Human Services**
**National Institute of Diabetes and Digestive and Kidney Diseases**
**Laboratory of Bioorganic Chemistry**
*See:* Entry 4728


**U.S. Department of Health and Human Services**
**National Institute of Environmental Health Sciences**
**Division of Intramural Research**
**Environmental Toxicology Program**
*See:* Entry 8967


**U.S. Department of Health and Human Services**
**National Institute of Environmental Health Sciences**
**Environmental Toxicology Program**
**Toxicology Branch**
*See:* Entry 8970


**★ 17384 ★ U.S. Department of Health and Human Services**
**National Institute of General Medical Sciences**
**Pharmacology and Biorelated Chemistry Program**
45 Center Dr., MSC 6200
Bethesda, MD 20892-6200
**Phone:** (301)594-3827    **Fax:** (301)480-2802
**Email:** rogersm@nigms.nih.gov
**Website:** http://www.nigms.nih.gov
Dr. Michael E. Rogers, Dir.

**Activities/Fields:** Supports research and research training aimed at improving the molecular-level understanding of fundamental biological processes and discovering approaches to their control. Research supported by the Division takes a multi-faceted approach to problems in pharmacology, physiology, biochemistry, and biorelated chemistry that are either very basic in nature or that have implications for more than one disease area. The goals of supported research include an improved understanding of drug action and mechanisms of anesthesia; pharmacogenetics and mechanisms underlying individual responses to drugs. The division also supports quantitative new methods and targets for drug discovery; advances in natural products synthesis; an enhanced understanding of biological catalysis; a greater knowledge of metabolic regulation and fundamental physiological processes; and the integration and application of basic physiological, pharmacological, and biochemical research to clinical issues in pharmacology, anesthesia, and trauma and burn injury.


**★ 17385 ★ U.S. Department of Health and Human Services**
**National Institute of General Medical Sciences**
**Pharmacology Research Associate Program**
Bldg. 45, Rm. 2AS-43
Bethesda, MD 20892-6200
**Phone:** (301)594-3583    **Fax:** (301)480-2802
**Email:** prat@nigms.nih.gov
**Website:** http://www.nigms.nih.gov/about_nigms/prat.html
Alison E. Cole, PhD, CoDir.

**Activities/Fields:** Developing leaders in pharmacological research for key positions in academic, industrial, and government research laboratories. Each year 7 recently trained scientists are selected for a two-year period of postdoctoral research in laboratories of the National Institutes of Health. Fellows conduct research under the direction of one of more than 120 senior scientists and may take coursework in areas of their choice, such as applied mathematics, experimental statistics, medicinal chemistry, human biochemical genetics, and molecular biophysics. Since 1978, Program has specifically targeted several positions to clinical pharmacology (considered a shortage area). Applicants for such positions must have an M.D. degree, a minimum of one year of graduate medical training (internship or residency), and a demonstrated interest in a research career in clinical pharmacology.


**U.S. Department of Health and Human Services**
**National Institute of Mental Health**
**Intramural Research Programs Division**
**(Neuropsychiatric Research at Saint Elizabeth's Hospital)**
**Biochemical Genetics Laboratory**
*See:* Entry 12742


**U.S. Department of Health and Human Services**
**National Institute for Occupational Safety and Health**
**Biomedical and Behavioral Science Division**
**Experimental Toxicology Branch**
*See:* Entry 16824


**U.S. Department of Health and Human Services**
**National Institutes of Health**
**National Institute of Environmental Health Sciences**
**Division of Extramural Research and Training**
**(Organs and Systems Toxicology Branch)**
*See:* Entry 14325

**U.S. Department of Health and Human Services**
**National Institutes of Health**
**National Institute of Mental Health**
**Laboratory of Cellular and Molecular Regulation**
**(Section on Biochemical Pharmacology)**
*See:* Entry 14352

**★ 17386 ★ U.S. Department of Health and Human Services**
**National Toxicology Program**
PO Box 12233
Research Triangle Park, NC 27709
**Phone:** (919)541-3201          **Fax:** (919)541-2260
**Email:** hart@niehs.nih.gov
**Website:** http://ntp-server.niehs.nih.gov/
Dr. Kenneth Olden, Dir.

**Activities/Fields:** Reliable series of relatively inexpensive short-term tests and protocols useful for the public health regulation of toxic chemicals, including the development of test batteries to assess genetic, neurobehavioral, and immunological toxicities; expand the toxicological profiles of chemicals tested; increase the rate of testing of chemicals for such toxic effects as carcinogenicity, mutagenicity, and reproductive and developmental effects (NTP also examines the chemicals for neurobehavioral, immunological, and other toxic effects where appropriate) within funding limits; and disseminate results of NTP's testing and methods development programs to government research and regulatory agencies, industry, labor, environmental groups, the scientific community, and the public. Chemicals chosen for testing are those that involve widespread or intense human exposure, or those for which existing data on toxic effects are inadequate. Some chemicals are selected for testing because study of them may tell more about how structurally related chemicals are likely to affect human health. Other criteria include: amount produced, significant physical and chemical properties, interest by regulatory and research agencies, and possible public health significance. The NTP testing strategy is to identify the major toxic effects of each chemical studied (genetic mutations; damage to critical organs such as the lungs, liver, and nervous system; birth defects; or cancer). Chemicals are nominated for testing by a variety of sources, including representatives of the agencies on the NTP Executive Committee; government agencies not represented on the Committee; academic, industry, and labor groups; state and local governments; and individuals. Persons interested in proposing chemicals for testing should give the reasons for their nominations and, when known, include production and usage information, data on human exposures, results of toxicological studies, data on the chemical's reactions in the human body, information concerning the chemical's relationship to structurally similar chemicals about which there are data, and other pertinent information. **Pub:** *DOE and EPA Research Related to Toxicology.* • *NTP Annual Plan.* • *Report on Carcinogens,* annually. • *Review of Current DHHS.* • *Technical reports.*

**U.S. Department of Veterans Affairs**
**Rehabilitation Research and Development Service**
**Center for Anabolic Therapies in Spinal Cord Injury**
*See:* Entry 8203

**★ 17387 ★ University of Arizona**
**Arizona Poison and Drug Information Center**
College of Pharmacy
1501 N Campbell Ave., Rm. 1156
Tucson, AZ 85724
**Phone:** (520)626-6016          **Fax:** (520)626-2720
**Email:** tong@pharmacy.arizona.edu
**Website:** http://www.vard.org/cent/bronx.htm
Dr. Theodore G. Tong, Dir.

**Activities/Fields:** Toxicology and psychopharmacology, including studies of relative efficacy of certain antidotes in treatment of various poisonings. Conducts research in drug information, including patent information services, post-marketing surveillances, and adverse drug reactions. **Pub:** *Newsletter,* quarterly.

**★ 17388 ★ University of Arizona**
**Center for Health Outcomes and PharmacoEconomic Research**
College of Pharmacy
Tucson, AZ 85721
**Phone:** (520)626-4721          **Fax:** (520)626-2023
**Email:** grizzle@pharmacy.arizona.edu
**Website:** http://www.pharmacy.arizona.edu
Amy Grizzle, Asst. Dir.

**Activities/Fields:** Assessment of costs and outcomes associated with the use of pharmaceuticals, including quality of life assessment and pharmacoeconomic analysis (cost-effectiveness and decision analysis). Also focuses on pharmaceutical policy evaluation. **Frmly:** Center for Pharmaceutical Economics.

**University of California, Davis**
**Center for Health and the Environment**
*See:* Entry 8977

**University of California, San Francisco**
**Dermatology Drug Research Unit**
*See:* Entry 6858

**University of California, San Francisco**
**Immunogenetics and Transplantation Laboratory**
*See:* Entry 3299

**University of Florida**
**Center for Environmental and Human Toxicology**
*See:* Entry 8982

**★ 17389 ★ University of Illinois at Chicago**
**Center for Pharmaceutical Biotechnology**
MC 870
Molecular Biology Research Bldg.
College of Pharmacy
900 S Ashland Ave.
Chicago, IL 60607-7313
**Phone:** (312)996-0796          **Fax:** (312)413-9303
**Email:** mjohnson@uic.edu
**Website:** http://www.uic.edu/pharmacy/research/cphb
Dr. Michael E. Johnson, Dir.

**Activities/Fields:** Structural and molecular biology focusing on pharmaceutical applications.

**University of Kansas**
**Center for Drug Delivery Research**
*See:* Entry 4759

**★ 17390 ★ University of Kansas**
**Higuchi Biosciences Center (HBC)**
2099 Constant Ave.
Lawrence, KS 66047-2535
**Phone:** (785)864-5183          **Fax:** (785)864-3738
**Email:** ekm@ku.edu
**Website:** http://www.hbc.ukans.edu
Dr. Elias K. Michaelis, Dir.

**Activities/Fields:** Biomedical problems, bioanalytical chemistry, drug delivery systems, neurological science, immunology, combinatorial chemistry, gene delivery, and related biotechnology. **Pub:** *HBC Newsletter,* 3/year. Newsletter.

**University of Kansas**
**Higuchi Biosciences Center**
**Center for Biomedical Research**
*See:* Entry 4760

**University of Louisiana at Lafayette**
**New Iberia Research Center**
*See:* Entry 2690

**★ 17391 ★ University of Louisiana at Monroe**
**Institute of Toxicology**
Sugar Hall 306
700 University Ave.
Monroe, LA 71209
**Phone:** (318)342-1691          **Fax:** (318)342-1686
**Email:** pymenhendale@ulm.edu
**Website:** http://rxweb.ulm.edu/pharmacy/Mehendale/lithmpg.htm
Dr. Harihara M. Mehendale, Dir.

**Activities/Fields:** Molecular mechanisms by which chemicals (both drugs and environmental agents) cause harmful effects.

**★ 17392 ★ University of Louisiana at Monroe**
**Louisiana Drug and Poison Information Center**
School of Pharmacy, Rm. 152
Monroe, LA 71209
**Phone:** (318)342-3648          **Fax:** (318)342-1744
**Email:** pydick@alpha.nlu.edu
**Website:** http://www.lapcc.org
Dr. Ronald M. Dick, Dir.

**Activities/Fields:** New poison antidotes, efficacy of current poisoning treatments.

**★ 17393 ★ University of Louisville**
**Institute for Molecular Diversity and Drug Design (IMD3)**
Department of Chemistry
Louisville, KY 40292
**Phone:** (502)852-5979          **Fax:** (502)852-3899
**Email:** spatola@louisville.edu
**Website:** http://www.imd3.org/
Dr. Arno F. Spatola, Dir.

**Activities/Fields:** Drug design, focusing on modern methods of rational and combinatorial lead generation, bioassays, structure optimization, including receptor selectivity, biostability, and pharmacokinetics, as well as process development and including bioinfomatics.

**★ 17394 ★ University of Maryland**
**Lamy Center on Drug Therapy and Aging**
506 W Fayette St., Ste. 101
Baltimore, MD 21201
**Phone:** (410)706-2434          **Fax:** (410)706-1488
**Email:** brucestuar@rx.umaryland.edu
**Website:** http://www.pharmacy.umaryland.edu/lamy
Bruce C. Stuart, PhD, Dir.

**Activities/Fields:** Geriatrics and gerontology, focusing on drug use in the elderly and the development of artificial intelligence programs in support of optimal drug use. **Pub:** *Eldercare News,* quarterly. Newsletter. **Frmly:** Center for the Study of Pharmacy and Therapeutics for the Elderly.

**★ 17395 ★ University of Miami**
**Marine and Freshwater Biomedical Sciences Center**
Rosenstiel Sch. of Marine & Atmospheric Science
4600 Rickenbacker Cswy.
Miami, FL 33149-1098
**Phone:** (305)361-4738          **Free:** 888-232-8635
**Fax:** (305)361-4001
**Email:** pwalsh@rsmas.miami.edu
**Website:** http://www.rsmas.miami.edu/groups/niehs
Patrick J. Walsh, PhD, Dir.

Activities/Fields: Neurotoxicology, potent marine metabolites present in seafood, a description of a piscine model for human neurofibromatosis, environmental toxicants, fisheries models for hepatic metabolism, and development of sentinel species for xenobiotic evaluation.


### ★ 17396 ★ University of Michigan Antiviral Laboratory
4222 Sch. of Dentistry
1011 N University Ave.
Ann Arbor, MI 48109
**Phone:** (734)763-5579 **Fax:** (734)764-7406
**Email:** jcdrach@umich.edu
**Website:** http://www.umich.edu/~websvcs/doughb/bms/people/drach.html
Dr. John C. Drach, Hd.

**Activities/Fields:** Antiviral and antineoplastic drugs, including the discovery of new antiviral drugs, how such drugs act at the genetic, cellular and biochemical level, and how they are metabolized in uninfected and virus-infected cells. Areas of research include viruses, herpes, and AIDS.


### ★ 17397 ★ University of Michigan Upjohn Center for Clinical Pharmacology
Sch. of Medicine
3709 Upjohn Center
Ann Arbor, MI 48109-0504
**Phone:** (734)764-9121 **Fax:** (734)763-3438
**Email:** PLF@umich.edu
Dr. William D. Ensminger, Dir.

**Activities/Fields:** Clinical pharmacology.


### ★ 17398 ★ University of Mississippi National Center for Natural Products Research (NCNPR)
Thad Cochran Research Center
School of Pharmacy
PO Box 1848
University, MS 38677
**Phone:** (662)915-1005 **Fax:** (662)915-1006
**Email:** ncnpr@olemiss.edu
**Website:** http://www.olemiss.edu/depts/ncnpr/
Dr. Larry Walker, Interim Dir.

**Activities/Fields:** Discovery and development of natural products for use as pharmaceuticals, dietary supplements, and agrochemicals, and understanding of the biological and chemical properties of medicinal plants. **Pub:** *Newsletter.*


**University of Mississippi**
**Research Institute of Pharmaceutical Sciences**
*See:* Entry 17578


### ★ 17399 ★ University of Montreal Fernand Seguin Research Centre
Hopital Louis-H.-Lafontaine
7331 Rue Hochelaga
Montreal, QC, Canada H1N 3V2
**Phone:** (514)251-4015 **Fax:** (514)251-2617
**Email:** prompre@crfs.umontreal.ca
**Website:** http://www.olemiss.edu/depts/pharm_school/
Dr. Pierre-Paul Rompre, Dir.

**Activities/Fields:** Neurochemistry, including drug mechanisms of action; psychopharmacology, including pharmacodynamics and pharmacokinetics of psychoactive drugs; and psychosocial behavioral and clinical evaluations, including the development of psychotherapeutic methods, evaluation of programs, and societal problems.


**University of Nevada, Reno**
**Allie M. Lee Cancer Research Laboratory**
*See:* Entry 10611

**University of Pennsylvania**
**Mood and Anxiety Disorders Section**
*See:* Entry 12769


### ★ 17400 ★ University of Southern California
**Laboratory of Applied Pharmacokinetics**
Clinical Science Center, Rm. 134-B
Keck School of Medicine
2250 Alcazar St.
Los Angeles, CA 90033
**Phone:** (323)442-1300 **Fax:** (323)442-1302
**Email:** jelliffe@hsc.usc.edu
**Website:** http://www.usc.edu/hsc/lab_apk
Roger W. Jelliffe, MD, Dir.

**Activities/Fields:** Designing systems for pharmacokinetic studies and strategies for optimal therapeutic drug monitoring in patients and optimally individualized adaptive control of drug dosage regimens for patients. Activities include development and testing of computer programs for simulation, parameter identification, parametric and nonparametric population pharmacokinetic and pharmacodynamic modeling,and optimal multiple model adaptive control of drug dosage regimens and pharmacokinetic systems in clinical settings; investigation of process and measurement noise in the clinical therapeutic environment; development of software for making population pharmacokinetic models; software for stochastic adaptive control of drug dosage regimens; and development of clinically reliable interfaces and intelligent automated apparatus for delivering complex drug regimens. **Pub:** *Manuscripts.* • *Technical Reports.*


### ★ 17401 ★ University of Tennessee Center of Excellence in Pediatric Pharmacokinetics and Therapeutics
Pharmacokinetics
St. Jude Children's Research Hospital
332 N Lauderdale
Memphis, TN 38105
**Phone:** (901)495-3663 **Fax:** (901)525-6869
**Email:** william.evans@stjude.org
Dr. William E. Evans, Co-Dir.

**Activities/Fields:** Drug therapy research in children. Seeks to promote and protect children's well-being by minimizing or eliminating pharmaceutical risks. Addresses the child's stage of physical development and rate of metabolism, in addition to body-weight and size, in determining effects of drugs.


### ★ 17402 ★ University of Tennessee Drug Information Center
875 Monroe, Ste. 109
Memphis, TN 38163
**Phone:** (901)448-5555 **Fax:** (901)448-5419
**Email:** utdic@utmem1.utmem.edu
Dr. Linda R. Young, Dir.

**Activities/Fields:** Therapeutic and pharmaceutical drugs. Provides therapeutic and pharmaceutic drug information to health care professionals.


### ★ 17403 ★ University of Texas at Austin Drug Dynamics Institute
College of Pharmacy
Austin, TX 78712-1074
**Phone:** (512)471-4841 **Fax:** (512)471-2746
**Email:** mcginity.jw@mail.utexas.edu
James W. McGinity, Dir.

**Activities/Fields:** Pharmaceutical research, development, and testing, including discovery of new medicinal agents, improvement of drug therapy, mechanisms of drug action, and re-evaluation of marketed products.


### ★ 17404 ★ University of Utah Center for Controlled Chemical Delivery
Biomedical Polymers Research Bldg., Rm. 205
Salt Lake City, UT 84112
**Phone:** (801)581-6654 **Fax:** (801)581-7848

**Email:** rburns@pharm.utah.edu
Dr. Sung Wan Kim, Dir.

**Activities/Fields:** Controlled drug delivery systems. Specific studies include the following: hydrogel and polymer synthesis, including water-soluble, bioactive, and biodegradable polymers; transdermal drug delivery, including skin immunoreaction and sensitization, irritation mechanism, drug interaction with stratum corneum membranes, physicochemical analysis of drug permeation mechanisms, and design of optimum delivery of matrix or rate-controlling membranes; functional polymers for gastrointestinal drug delivery; polymeric prodrugs and chemical modification of drugs for specific organ targeting or long-term delivery of therapeutic agents; and delivery of peptides and protein drugs.


### ★ 17405 ★ University of Utah Center for Human Toxicology
20 South 230 East, Rm. 490
Salt Lake City, UT 84112-9457
**Phone:** (801)581-5117 **Fax:** (801)581-5034
Dennis Crouch, Interim Dir.

**Activities/Fields:** Clinical, forensic, and bioanalytical toxicology, including studies in clinical pharmacology and toxicology, drug metabolism, disposition, adverse interactions, alcohol/drugs and driving, proficiency testing, postmortem toxicology, data interpretation, and new chromatographic and mass spectrometry techniques in toxicology.


**University of Wisconsin—Milwaukee**
**Marine and Freshwater Biomedical Sciences Center**
*See:* Entry 4785


### ★ 17406 ★ Vanderbilt University Center in Molecular Toxicology
Biochemistry Department
23rd Ave. & Pierce
Nashville, TN 37232-0146
**Phone:** (615)322-2261 **Fax:** (615)322-3141
**Email:** info@toxicology.mc.vanderbilt.edu
**Website:** http://www.toxicology.mc.vanderbilt.edu
Dr. F. Peter Guengerich, Dir.

**Activities/Fields:** Biochemical and chemical toxicology and carcinogenesis, including enzymatic oxidation and conjugation, oxidative damage, DNA damage and mutagenesis, regulation of gene expression, and neurotoxicology. Service core facilities include mass spectrometry, NMR, cell biology, protein chemistry, and molecular recognition. **Pub:** *Annual report.*


### ★ 17407 ★ Veterans Affairs Medical Center (Birmingham, AL) Research and Development Service
700 S 19th St.
Birmingham, AL 35233
**Phone:** (205)558-4747 **Fax:** (205)933-4471
**Email:** warren.blackburn@med.va.gov
Dr. Warren D. Blackburn, Jr., Assoc. Ch. of Staff

**Activities/Fields:** Cancer, gastroenterology, rheumatology and arthritis, neurology, and spinal cord injury, repair systems, cordiology, nephrology, pulmonary disease, endocrinology, informatics and health services research.


### ★ 17408 ★ Veterans Health Administration Geriatric Research, Education and Clinical Center-Gainesville
GRECC, 182
1601 Archer Rd.
Gainesville, FL 32608-1197
**Phone:** (352)374-6077 **Fax:** (352)374-6142
**Email:** dlowenth@college.med.ufl.edu
**Website:** http://www.med.ufl.edu/pharm/facdata/GRECC
Dr. David T. Lowenthal, Dir.

**Activities/Fields:** Geropharmacology, including mechanisms of drug action, pharmacokinetics, therapeutic uses, drug abuse, polypharmacy and drug compliance as it applies to geriatric patients. Clinical research is conducted in the areas of exercise in the healthy, frail, and elderly, cardiovascular function, and cognitive disorders in the elderly. Basic research is conducted in pharmacologic mechanisms of temperature regulation, obesity, febril response to infections, immunology, and muscle strength.

**★ 17409 ★ Wayne State University
Institute of Environmental Health
    Sciences**
2727 2nd Ave., Rm. 4000
Detroit, MI 48201
**Phone:** (313)577-0100     **Fax:** (313)577-0082
**Email:** ad5440@wayne.edu
**Website:** http://www.chemtox.org
Dr. Raymond F. Novak, Dir.
**Activities/Fields:** Chemical hazards of the environment and industrial workplace, including toxicology of air pollutants, solvents, and heavy metals. Also studies carcinogenesis, metabolic, and hematologic effects resulting from exposure to toxic agents; and molecular and cellular approaches to examine early events in toxicity. **Frmly:** Institute of Chemical Toxicology.

**★ 17410 ★ World Life Research Institute**
23000 Grand Terrace Rd.
Colton, CA 92324
**Phone:** (909)825-4773     **Fax:** (909)783-3477
**Email:** wlri@earthlink.net
Bruce W. Halstead, MD, Dir.
**Activities/Fields:** Toxicology, medical research, poisonous and venomous marine animals, drugs from the sea, chronic degenerative diseases, marine biotoxicology, and ethnobotany and terrestrial phytochemistry in a search for new drugs from natural resources, especially organic chemical agents derived from plants or animals having application to therapeutic medicine and human nutrition. Maintains extensive foreign contacts in 6,000 regions of the world, particularly underdeveloped areas in Asia and Latin America, in search of new drugs.

# Chapter 51
# Pharmacy

## Foundations & Other Funding Organizations

### Other Funding Organizations

★ 17411 ★ **Academy of Pharmaceutical Research and Science (APRS)**
American Pharmaceutical Association
2215 Constitution Ave. NW
Washington, DC 20037-2985
**Phone:** (202)628-4410 **Free:** 800-237-2742
**Fax:** (202)783-2351
**Email:** sagraves@uic.edu
**Website:** http://www.aphanet.org/about/aprs.html
Arthur H. Kibbe, Pres.

**Desc:** A part of American Pharmaceutical Association. Pharmaceutical scientists from industry and academia. Objective is to serve the profession of pharmacy by developing knowledge and integrating the process of science into the profession. Sponsors national meetings to provide a forum for presentation and discussion of original research, controversial topics, and continuing communication. Provides consultation and advice to: pharmacists on scientific matters as they relate to policy; congressional committees on bills of interest to pharmaceutical scientists; governmental agencies. **Awards:** Best Published Paper in the Economic, Social, and Administrative Sciences (annual); Ebert Prize (annual); Kilmer Prize (annual); Postgraduate Best Paper Awards (annual); Research Achievement Award (annual); Takeru Higuchi Research Prize (triennial).

★ 17412 ★ **American Institute of the History of Pharmacy (AIHP)**
777 Highland Ave.
Madison, WI 53705
**Phone:** (608)262-5378
**Email:** aihp@aihp.org
**Website:** http://www.aihp.org
Gregory J. Higby, Dir.

**Desc:** Pharmacists, firms, and organizations interested in historical and social aspects of the pharmaceutical field. Maintains pharmaceutical Americana collection; conducts research programs. **Awards:** Fischelis Grants; Graduate Study in the History of Pharmacy Grants.

★ 17413 ★ **ASHP Foundation**
7272 Wisconsin Ave.
Bethesda, MD 20814
**Phone:** (301)657-3000 **Fax:** (301)657-8817
**Email:** foundation@ashp.org
**Website:** http://www.ashpfoundation.org
Stephen J. Allen, Exec. VP/CEO

**Desc:** Established for pharmaceutical care and research purposes. Offers research grants, awards; and anticoagulation, asthma, stem cell transplantation, diabetes, pain management, oncology, and traineeships. **Awards:** Fellowship for the study of practice areas such as oncology drug therapy, psychiatric drug therapy, clinical pharmacokinetics, cardiovascular drug therapy, critical care, drug information, and pharmacy nutritional support; grant for research and special projects; recognition (annual) for the most significant contributions to literature in the areas of research and practice.

★ 17414 ★ **Christian Pharmacists Fellowship International (CPFI)**
PO Box 1717
501 5th St.
Bristol, TN 37621-1717
**Phone:** (423)764-6000 **Free:** 888-253-6885
**Fax:** (423)764-4490
**Email:** cpfi@tricon.net
**Website:** http://www.cpfi.org
Allan Sharp, P.D., Admin. Dir.

**Desc:** To promote and maintain fellowship among Christian pharmacists. Establishes clubs and chapters at universities, colleges, schools, hospitals, and in communities; sponsors activities and retreats for Christian pharmacists and their families. Encourages active Christian witness and evangelism; teaches pharmacists how to share and present the Gospel of Jesus Christ in their practice; disseminates information among Christian pharmacists; identifies areas of service for pharmacists in missions worldwide and sponsors missionaries in the field. Provides and promotes Christian pharmacist-speakers. speakers at state and national pharmacy meetings. **Awards:** Scholarship Award (annual).

**Drug Information Association (DIA)**
*See:* Entry 12002

★ 17415 ★ **Multidisciplinary Association for Psychedelic Studies (MAPS)**
2105 Robinson Ave.
Sarasota, FL 34232
**Phone:** (941)924-6277 **Free:** 888-868-6927
**Fax:** (941)924-6265
**Email:** info@maps.org
**Website:** http://www.maps.org
Dr. Rick Doblin, Pres.

**Desc:** Promotes the development of beneficial, socially sanctioned uses of psychedelic drugs and marijuana. Helps researchers design, obtain government approval for, fund, conduct and report on psychedelic research in human volunteers; funds MDMA psychotherapy studies; facilitates research and FDA approval for marijuana to be prescribed for medical uses. **Awards:** Grant.

## Medical & Allied Health Schools

### Pharmacy

*The following colleges and schools of pharmacy offer programs accredited by the American Council on Pharmaceutical Education, 20 N Clark St., Ste. 2500, Chicago, IL 60602-5109, (312)664-3575, http://www.acpe-accredit.org. For additional information on the colleges or pharmacy as a career, contact the American Association of Colleges of Pharmacy, 1426 Prince St., Alexandria, VA 22314, (703)739-2330, http://www.aacp.org/.*

### Alabama

★ 17416 ★ **Auburn University Harrison School of Pharmacy**
217 Walker Bldg.
Auburn University, AL 36849-5501
**Phone:** (334)844-8348 **Fax:** (334)844-8353
**Email:** evansrl@auburn.edu
**Website:** http://pharmacy.auburn.edu
R. Lee Evans, Jr., Director

★ 17417 ★ **Samford University McWhorter School of Pharmacy**
800 Lakeshore Dr.
Birmingham, AL 35229
**Phone:** (205)726-2820 **Fax:** (205)726-2759
**Email:** jodean@samford.edu
**Website:** http://www.samford.edu/schools/pharmacy.html
Joseph O. Dean, Jr., Director

### Arizona

★ 17418 ★ **Midwestern University, Glendale College of Pharmacy**
19555 N 59th Ave.
Glendale, AZ 85308
**Phone:** (623)572-3500 **Fax:** (623)572-3510
**Email:** dslark@arizona.midwestern.edu
**Website:** http://www.midwestern.edu/Pages/CPG.html
David J. Slatkin, PhD, Director

★ 17419 ★ **University of Arizona College of Pharmacy**
1703 E Mabel St.
PO Box 210207
Tucson, AZ 85721
**Phone:** (520)626-1427 **Fax:** (520)626-4063
**Email:** bootman@pharmacy.arizona.edu
**Website:** http://www.pharmacy.arizona.edu
J. Lyle Bootman, PhD, Director

## Arkansas

**★ 17420 ★ University of Arkansas for Medical Sciences**
**College of Pharmacy**
4301 W Markham St., Slot 522
Little Rock, AR 72205
**Phone:** (501)686-5557          **Fax:** (501)686-8315
**Email:** MilneLarryD@uams.edu
**Website:** http://www.uams.edu/cop
L. D. Milne, PhD, Director

## California

**★ 17421 ★ University of California, San Francisco**
**School of Pharmacy**
521 Parnassus Ave., Rm. C-156
Box 0622
San Francisco, CA 94143-0622
**Phone:** (415)476-1225          **Fax:** (415)476-6632
**Email:** makx@itsa.ucsf.edu
**Website:** http://www.sop.ucsf.edu
Mary Anne Koda-Kimble, Director

**★ 17422 ★ University of the Pacific**
**Thomas J. Long School of Pharmacy and Health Sciences**
3601 Pacific Ave.
Stockton, CA 95211
**Phone:** (209)946-2561          **Fax:** (209)946-2410
**Email:** poppenhe@uop.edu
**Website:** http://www.uop.edu/pharmacy/index.html
Phillip R. Oppenheimer, Director

**★ 17423 ★ University of Southern California**
**School of Pharmacy**
1985 Zonal Ave.
Los Angeles, CA 90089-9121
**Phone:** (323)442-1369          **Fax:** (323)442-1681
**Email:** knipe@hsc.usc.edu
**Website:** http://pharmacy.usc.edu
Dr. Timothy M. Chan, Director

**★ 17424 ★ Western University of Health Sciences**
**College of Pharmacy**
309 E 2nd St.
Pomona, CA 91766-1854
**Phone:** (909)469-5500          **Fax:** (909)469-5539
**Email:** mdray@westernu.edu
**Website:** http://www.westernu.edu
Max Ray, PhD, Director

## Colorado

**★ 17425 ★ University of Colorado Health Sciences Center**
**School of Pharmacy**
4200 E 9th Ave., C-238
Denver, CO 80262
**Phone:** (303)315-5055          **Fax:** (303)315-6281
**Email:** louis.diamond@uchsc.edu
**Website:** http://www.uchsc.edu/sp/sp
Louis Diamond, PhD, Director

## Connecticut

**★ 17426 ★ University of Connecticut**
**School of Pharmacy**
372 Fairfield Rd., Unit 2092
Storrs, CT 06269-2092
**Phone:** (860)486-2129          **Fax:** (860)486-1553
**Email:** michael.gerald@uconn.edu
**Website:** http://pharmacy.uconn.edu
Michael C. Gerald, PhD, Director

## District of Columbia

**★ 17427 ★ Howard University**
**College of Pharmacy**
2300 4th St. NW
Washington, DC 20059
**Phone:** (202)806-5431          **Fax:** (202)234-1375
**Email:** plecca@howard.edu
**Website:** http://www.howard.edu
Pedro J. Lecca, PhD, Director

## Florida

**★ 17428 ★ Florida Agricultural and Mechanical (A&M) University**
**College of Pharmacy and Pharmaceutical Sciences**
201 Dyson Pharmacy Bldg.
Tallahassee, FL 32307
**Phone:** (850)559-3301          **Fax:** (850)559-3347
**Email:** henry.lewisiii@famu.edu
**Website:** http://www.famu.edu/copps
Henry Lewis, III, Director

**★ 17429 ★ Nova Southeastern University**
**College of Pharmacy**
3200 S University Dr.
Fort Lauderdale, FL 33328
**Phone:** (954)262-1300          **Fax:** (954)262-2278
**Email:** hardigan@nova.edu
**Website:** http://www.nova.edu/cwis/centers/hdp/pharmacy
William D. Hardigan, PhD, Director

**★ 17430 ★ Palm Beach Atlantic College**
**School of Pharmacy**
901 S Flagler Dr.
PO Box 24708
West Palm Beach, FL 33416-4708
**Phone:** (561)803-2700          **Fax:** (561)803-2703
**Email:** swigarts@pbac.edu
**Website:** http://www.pbac.edu
Scott Swigart, Director

**★ 17431 ★ University of Florida**
**College of Pharmacy**
J. Hillis Miller Health Center
1600 SE Archer Rd., Rm. 454
Box 100484
Gainesville, FL 32610
**Phone:** (352)392-9714          **Fax:** (352)392-3480
**Website:** http://www.cop.ufl.edu
William H. Riffee, PhD, Director

## Georgia

**★ 17432 ★ Mercer University**
**Southern School of Pharmacy**
3001 Mercer University Dr.
Atlanta, GA 30341-4415
**Phone:** (678)547-6304          **Fax:** (678)547-6315
**Email:** matthews_h@mercer.edu
**Website:** http://www.mercer.edu/dean_phm.htm
H. W. Matthews, PhD, Director

**★ 17433 ★ University of Georgia**
**College of Pharmacy**
Athens, GA 30602-2351
**Phone:** (706)542-1914          **Fax:** (706)542-5269
**Email:** soie@mail.rx.uga.edu
**Website:** http://www.rx.uga.edu
Svein Oie, PhD, Director

## Idaho

**★ 17434 ★ Idaho State University**
**College of Pharmacy**
Box 8288
Pocatello, ID 83209
**Phone:** (208)282-2175          **Fax:** (208)282-4482
**Email:** jsteiner@pharmacy.isu.edu
**Website:** http://rx.isu.edu
Joseph F. Steiner, Director

## Illinois

**★ 17435 ★ Midwestern University**
**Chicago College of Pharmacy**
555 31st St.
Downers Grove, IL 60515
**Phone:** (630)971-6417          **Fax:** (630)971-6097
**Email:** mleexx@midwestern.edu
**Website:** http://www.midwestern.edu/Pages/CCP.html
Mary Lee, Director

**★ 17436 ★ University of Illinois, Chicago**
**College of Pharmacy**
833 S Wood St.
M/C 874
Chicago, IL 60612
**Phone:** (312)996-7240          **Fax:** (312)996-3272
**Email:** sagraves@uic.edu
**Website:** http://www.uic.edu/pharmacy
Rosalie Sagraves, Director

## Indiana

**★ 17437 ★ Butler University**
**College of Pharmacy and Health Sciences**
4600 Sunset Ave.
Indianapolis, IN 46208
**Phone:** (317)940-9735          **Fax:** (317)940-6172
**Email:** pchase@butler.edu
**Website:** http://www.butler.edu/www/cophs
Patricia Chase, PhD, Director

**★ 17438 ★ Purdue University**
**School of Pharmacy and Pharmacal Sciences**
1330 Heine Pharmacy Bldg.
West Lafayette, IN 47907
**Phone:** (765)494-1368          **Fax:** (765)494-7880
**Email:** chipr@pharmacy.purdue.edu
**Website:** http://www.pharmacy.purdue.edu/index.html
Charles O. Rutledge, PhD, Director

## Iowa

**★ 17439 ★ Drake University**
**College of Pharmacy and Health Sciences**
25th and University Aves.
Des Moines, IA 50311
**Phone:** (515)271-1814          **Fax:** (515)271-4171
**Email:** stephen.hoag@drake.edu
**Website:** http://www.pharmacy.drake.edu
Stephen G. Hoag, PhD, Director

**★ 17440 ★ University of Iowa**
**College of Pharmacy**
Iowa City, IA 52242
**Phone:** (319)335-8794          **Fax:** (319)335-5594
**Email:** jordan-cohen@uiowa.edu
**Website:** http://www.uiowa.edu/~pharmacy
Jordan Cohen, PhD, Director

## Kansas

**★ 17441 ★ University of Kansas**
**School of Pharmacy**
Malott Hall, Rm. 2056
1251 Wescoe Hall Dr.
Lawrence, KS 66045-2500
**Phone:** (785)864-3591          **Fax:** (785)864-5265
**Email:** jfincham@ku.edu
**Website:** http://www.pharm.ukans.edu/dean/index.htm
Jack E. Fincham, PhD, Director

## Kentucky

**★ 17442 ★ University of Kentucky**
**College of Pharmacy**
907 Rose St., Ste. 327
Lexington, KY 40536-0082
**Phone:** (859)323-7601    **Fax:** (859)257-2128
**Email:** krobe2@pop.uky.edu
**Website:** http://www.uky.edu/Pharmacy
Kenneth B. Roberts, PhD, Director

## Louisiana

**★ 17443 ★ University of Louisiana,**
**Monroe**
**College of Pharmacy**
700 University Ave.
Monroe, LA 71209-0400
**Phone:** (318)342-1600    **Fax:** (318)342-1606
**Email:** pybourn@ulm.edu
**Website:** http://www.ulm.edu
William M. Bourn, PhD, Director

**★ 17444 ★ Xavier University of Louisiana**
**College of Pharmacy**
1 Drexel Dr.
New Orleans, LA 70125
**Phone:** (504)483-7424    **Fax:** (504)485-7930
**Email:** wharris@xula.edu
**Website:** http://www.xula.edu
Wayne T. Harris, PhD, Director

## Maryland

**★ 17445 ★ University of Maryland**
**School of Pharmacy**
20 N Pine St., Rm. 730
Baltimore, MD 21201-1180
**Phone:** (410)706-7651    **Fax:** (410)706-4012
**Email:** dknapp@rx.umaryland.edu
**Website:** http://www.pharmacy.umaryland.edu
David A. Knapp, PhD, Director

## Massachusetts

**★ 17446 ★ Massachusetts College of**
**Pharmacy and Health Sciences, Boston**
179 Longwood Ave.
Boston, MA 02115
**Phone:** (617)732-2108    **Fax:** (617)732-2244
**Email:** abelmonte@mcp.edu
**Website:** http://www.mcp.edu
Albert A. Belmonte, PhD, Director

**★ 17447 ★ Massachusetts College of**
**Pharmacy and Health Sciences,**
**Worcester**
**School of Pharmacy**
19 Foster St.
Worcester, MA 01608
**Phone:** (508)890-8855    **Fax:** (508)890-8515
**Email:** dpisano@mcp.edu
**Website:** http://www.mcp.edu
Douglas Pisano, PhD, Director

**★ 17448 ★ Northeastern University**
**School of Pharmacy**
206 Mugar Hall
Boston, MA 02115
**Phone:** (617)373-8917    **Fax:** (617)373-7655
**Email:** d.robinson@neu.edu
**Website:** http://www.neu.edu/bouve/pharma.html
Daniel C. Robinson, Director

## Michigan

**★ 17449 ★ Ferris State University**
**College of Pharmacy**
220 Ferris Dr.
Big Rapids, MI 49307
**Phone:** (231)591-2254    **Fax:** (231)591-3829
**Email:** Ian_Mathison@ferris.edu
**Website:** http://www.pharmacy.ferris.edu
Ian W. Mathison, PhD, Director

**★ 17450 ★ University of Michigan**
**College of Pharmacy**
428 Church St.
Ann Arbor, MI 48109-1065
**Phone:** (734)764-7312    **Fax:** (734)763-2022
**Email:** gkenyon@umich.edu
**Website:** http://www.umich.edu/~pharmacy
George L. Kenyon, PhD, Director

**★ 17451 ★ Wayne State University**
**Eugene Applebaum College of Pharmacy**
**and Health Sciences**
105 Shapero Hall
Detroit, MI 48202
**Phone:** (313)577-1574    **Fax:** (313)577-0457
**Email:** bschmoll@wizard.pharm.wayne.edu
**Website:** http://wizard.pharm.wayne.edu/wel-come.html
Beverly J. Schmoll, PhD, Director

## Minnesota

**★ 17452 ★ University of Minnesota**
**College of Pharmacy**
308 Harvard St. SE
5-130 Weaver-Densford Hall
Minneapolis, MN 55455-0343
**Phone:** (612)624-1900    **Fax:** (612)624-2974
**Email:** speed001@tc.umn.edu
**Website:** http://www.pharmacy.umn.edu
Marilyn K. Speedie, PhD, Director

## Mississippi

**★ 17453 ★ University of Mississippi**
**School of Pharmacy**
PO Box 1848
University, MS 38677
**Phone:** (662)915-7265    **Fax:** (662)915-5118
**Email:** wells@olemiss.edu
**Website:** http://www.olemiss.edu/depts/pharm_school
Barbara G. Wells, Director

## Missouri

**★ 17454 ★ Saint Louis College of**
**Pharmacy**
4588 Parkview Pl.
Saint Louis, MO 63110
**Phone:** (314)367-8700    **Fax:** (314)367-2784
**Email:** kkirk@stlcop.edu
**Website:** http://www.stlcop.edu
Kenneth W. Kirk, PhD, Director

**★ 17455 ★ University of Missouri,**
**Kansas City**
**School of Pharmacy**
5005 Rockhill Rd.
Kansas City, MO 64110-2499
**Phone:** (816)235-1609    **Fax:** (816)235-5190
**Email:** rpiepho@cctr.umkc.edu
**Website:** http://www.umkc.edu/pharmacy
Robert W. Piepho, PhD, Director

## Montana

**★ 17456 ★ University of Montana**
**School of Pharmacy and Allied Health**
**Sciences**
340 Skaggs Bldg.
Missoula, MT 59812-1512
**Phone:** (406)243-4621    **Fax:** (406)243-4209
**Email:** forbesds@selway.umt.edu
**Website:** http://www.umt.edu/pharmacy
David S. Forbes, PhD, Director

## Nebraska

**★ 17457 ★ Creighton University**
**School of Pharmacy and Allied Health**
**Professions**
2500 California Plaza
Omaha, NE 68178
**Phone:** (402)280-2950    **Fax:** (402)280-5738
**Email:** stohs@creighton.edu
**Website:** http://www.spahp.creighton.edu
Sidney J. Stohs, PhD, Director

**★ 17458 ★ University of Nebraska**
**Medical Center**
**College of Pharmacy**
986000 Nebraska Medical Center
Omaha, NE 68198-6000
**Phone:** (402)559-4333    **Fax:** (402)559-5060
**Email:** cueda@unmc.edu
**Website:** http://www.unmc.edu/Pharmacy/col-lege.html
Clarence T. Ueda, PhD, Director

## New Jersey

**★ 17459 ★ Rutgers, the State University**
**of New Jersey**
**Ernest Mario School of Pharmacy**
William Levine Hall
160 Frelinghuysen Rd.
Piscataway, NJ 08854-8020
**Phone:** (732)445-2675    **Fax:** (732)445-5767
**Email:** jlcolaiz@rci.rutgers.edu
**Website:** http://www.pharmacy.rutgers.edu
John L. Colaizzi, PhD, Director

## New Mexico

**★ 17460 ★ University of New Mexico**
**College of Pharmacy**
2502 Marble NE
Albuquerque, NM 87131-5691
**Phone:** (505)272-3241    **Fax:** (505)272-6749
**Email:** wmhadley@unm.edu
**Website:** http://www.hsc.unm.edu/Pharmacy.html
William Hadley, PhD, Director

## New York

**★ 17461 ★ Albany College of Pharmacy**
106 New Scotland Ave.
Albany, NY 12208
**Phone:** (518)445-7200    **Fax:** (518)445-7294
**Email:** andritzm@acp.edu
**Website:** http://www.acp.edu
Mary H. Andritz, Director

**★ 17462 ★ Long Island University**
**Arnold and Marie Schwartz College of**
**Pharmacy and Health Sciences**
75 DeKalb Ave. at University Plaza
Brooklyn, NY 11201
**Phone:** (718)488-1004    **Fax:** (718)488-0628
**Email:** sgross@liu.edu
**Website:** http://www.liunet.edu
Stephen M. Gross, PhD, Director

**★ 17463 ★ Saint John's University**
**College of Pharmacy and Allied Health**
**Professions**
8000 Utopia Pkwy.
Jamaica, NY 11439
**Phone:** (718)990-6411    **Fax:** (718)990-1871
**Email:** mangionr@stjohns.edu
**Website:** http://www.stjohns.edu
Robert A. Mangione, EdD, Director

**★ 17464 ★ State University of New York/ University of Buffalo**
School of Pharmacy and Pharmaceutical Sciences
126 Cooke Hall
Amherst, NY 14260-1200
**Phone:** (716)645-2823　　　**Fax:** (716)645-3688
**Email:** wka@buffalo.edu
**Website:** http://www.pharmacy.buffalo.edu
Wayne K. Anderson, PhD, Director

## North Carolina

**★ 17465 ★ Campbell University**
School of Pharmacy
Buies Creek, NC 27506
**Phone:** (910)893-1200　　　**Fax:** (910)893-1943
**Email:** maddox@mailcenter.edu
**Website:** http://www.campbell.edu/pharmacy
Ronald W. Maddox, PhD, Director

**★ 17466 ★ University of North Carolina, Chapel Hill**
School of Pharmacy
Beard Hall
Campus Box 7360
Chapel Hill, NC 27599
**Phone:** (919)966-1121　　　**Fax:** (919)966-6919
**Email:** bill_campbell@unc.edu
**Website:** http://www.pharmacy.unc.edu
William H. Campbell, PhD, Director

## North Dakota

**★ 17467 ★ North Dakota State University**
College of Pharmacy
123 Sudro Hall
Fargo, ND 58105-5055
**Phone:** (701)231-7609　　　**Fax:** (701)231-7606
**Email:** charles.peterson@ndsu.nodak.edu
**Website:** http://www.ndsu.nodak.edu/pharmacy
Charles D. Peterson, PhD, Director

## Ohio

**★ 17468 ★ Ohio Northern University**
College of Pharmacy
Ada, OH 45810
**Phone:** (419)772-2277　　　**Fax:** (419)772-2720
**Email:** b-bryant@onu.edu
**Website:** http://www.onu.edu/Pharmacy
Bobby Bryant, Director

**★ 17469 ★ Ohio State University**
College of Pharmacy
500 W 12th Ave.
Columbus, OH 43210
**Phone:** (614)292-5711　　　**Fax:** (614)292-3113
**Email:** cassady.l@osu.edu
**Website:** http://www.pharmacy.ohio-state.edu
John M. Cassady, PhD, Director

**★ 17470 ★ University of Cincinnati**
College of Pharmacy
PO Box 670004
Cincinnati, OH 45267-0004
**Phone:** (513)558-3326　　　**Fax:** (513)558-4372
**Email:** Daniel.Acosta@uc.edu
**Website:** http://www.pharmacy.uc.edu
Daniel Acosta, Jr., P, Director

**★ 17471 ★ University of Toledo**
College of Pharmacy
2801 W Bancroft St.
Toledo, OH 43606-3390
**Phone:** (419)530-1931　　　**Fax:** (419)530-1907
**Email:** johnnie.early@utoledo.edu
**Website:** http://www.utoledo.edu/pharmacy
Johnnie L. Early, II, Ph, Director

## Oklahoma

**★ 17472 ★ Southwestern Oklahoma State University**
School of Pharmacy
100 Campus Dr.
Weatherford, OK 73096
**Phone:** (580)774-3105　　　**Fax:** (580)774-7020
**Email:** bergmad@swosu.edu
**Website:** http://www.swosu.edu/depts/pharmacy/index.html
H. David Bergman, PhD, Director

**★ 17473 ★ University of Oklahoma**
College of Pharmacy
1110 N Stonewall Ave.
PO Box 26901
Oklahoma City, OK 73190
**Phone:** (405)271-6485　　　**Fax:** (405)271-3830
**Email:** carl-buckner@ouhsc.edu
**Website:** http://www.oupharmacy.com
Carl K. Buckner, PhD, Director

## Oregon

**★ 17474 ★ Oregon State University**
College of Pharmacy
203 Pharmacy Bldg.
Corvallis, OR 97331-3507
**Phone:** (541)737-3424　　　**Fax:** (541)737-3999
**Email:** Wayne.Kradjan@orst.edu
**Website:** http://pharmacy.orst.edu
Wayne A. Kradjan, Director

## Pennsylvania

**★ 17475 ★ Duquesne University**
Mylan School of Pharmacy
306 Bayer Learning Ctr.
Pittsburgh, PA 15282-1504
**Phone:** (412)396-6377　　　**Fax:** (412)396-1810
**Email:** vanderveen@duq.edu
**Website:** http://www.duq.edu/pharmacy/pharmacy.htm
R. Pete Vanderveen, PhD, Director

**★ 17476 ★ Lake Erie College of Osteopathic Medicine**
School of Pharmacy
1858 W Grandview Blvd.
Erie, PA 16509
**Phone:** (814)866-6641　　　**Fax:** (814)866-8123
**Email:** dswaffar@lecom.edu
**Website:** http://www.lecom.edu/pharmacy
Diane Swaffar, PhD, Director

**★ 17477 ★ Temple University**
School of Pharmacy
3307 N Broad St.
Philadelphia, PA 19140
**Phone:** (215)707-4990　　　**Fax:** (215)707-3678
**Email:** peter.doukas@temple.edu
**Website:** http://www.temple.edu/pharmacy
Peter H. Doukas, PhD, Director

**★ 17478 ★ University of Pittsburgh**
School of Pharmacy
1104 Salk Hall
3501 Terrace St.
Pittsburgh, PA 15261
**Phone:** (412)624-3270　　　**Fax:** (412)648-1086
**Email:** rjuhl@pitt.edu
**Website:** http://www.pharmacy.pitt.edu
Randy P. Juhl, PhD, Director

**★ 17479 ★ University of the Sciences in Philadelphia**
Philadelphia College of Pharmacy
600 S 43rd St.
Philadelphia, PA 19104-4495
**Phone:** (215)596-8870　　　**Fax:** (215)596-8977
**Email:** gdowns@usip.edu
**Website:** http://www.usip.edu
George E. Downs, PhD, Director

**★ 17480 ★ Wilkes University**
Nesbitt School of Pharmacy
Wilkes-Barre, PA 18766
**Phone:** (570)408-4280　　　**Fax:** (570)408-7828
**Email:** grahamb@wilkes.edu
**Website:** http://www.pharmacy.wilkes.edu
Bernard W. Graham, PhD, Director

## Puerto Rico

**★ 17481 ★ University of Puerto Rico**
Medical Sciences Campus
School of Pharmacy
PO Box 365067
San Juan, PR 00936-5067
**Phone:** (787)758-2525　　　**Fax:** (787)751-5680
**Email:** ioquendo@rcm.upr.edu
**Website:** http://www.upr.clu.edu
Ilia Oquendo, PhD, Director

## Rhode Island

**★ 17482 ★ University of Rhode Island**
College of Pharmacy
41 Lower College Rd.
Kingston, RI 02881
**Phone:** (401)874-2761　　　**Fax:** (401)874-2181
**Email:** del@uri.edu
**Website:** http://www.uri.edu/pharm
Donald E. Letendre, Director

## South Carolina

**★ 17483 ★ Medical University of South Carolina**
College of Pharmacy
280 Calhoun St.
PO Box 250141
Charleston, SC 29425
**Phone:** (843)792-8450　　　**Fax:** (843)792-9081
**Email:** cormierj@musc.edu
**Website:** http://www.musc.edu/pharmacy
John Cormier, Director

**★ 17484 ★ University of South Carolina**
College of Pharmacy
Columbia, SC 29208
**Phone:** (803)777-4151　　　**Fax:** (803)777-4945
**Email:** sadikf@cop.sc.edu
**Website:** http://www.pharm.sc.edu
Farid Sadik, PhD, Director

## South Dakota

**★ 17485 ★ South Dakota State University**
College of Pharmacy
Box 2202-C
Brookings, SD 57007-0099
**Phone:** (605)688-6197　　　**Fax:** (605)688-6232
**Email:** danny-lattin@sdstate.edu
**Website:** http://www3.sdstate.edu/Academics/CollegeOfPharmacy
Danny L. Lattin, PhD, Director

## Tennessee

**★ 17486 ★ University of Tennessee, Memphis**
College of Pharmacy
847 Monroe Ave., Ste. 226
Memphis, TN 38163

**Phone:** (901)448-6036 **Fax:** (901)448-7053
**Email:** dgourley@utmem.edu
**Website:** http://www.pharmacy.utmem.edu
Dick R. Gourley, PhD, Director

## Texas

### ★ 17487 ★ Texas Southern University
**College of Pharmacy and Health Sciences**
3100 Cleburne Ave.
Houston, TX 77004
**Phone:** (713)313-7164 **Fax:** (713)313-1091
**Email:** hayes_be@tsu.edu
**Website:** http://www.tsu.edu
Dick Gourley, Director

### ★ 17488 ★ Texas Tech University
**Health Sciences Center**
**School of Pharmacy**
1300 S Coulter
Amarillo, TX 79106
**Phone:** (806)354-5463 **Fax:** (806)356-4613
**Email:** arthur@cortex.ama.ttuhsc.edu
**Website:** http://www.pharmacy.ama.ttuhsc.edu
Arthur A. Nelson, Jr., P, Director

### ★ 17489 ★ University of Houston
**College of Pharmacy**
141 Sciences and Research 2 Bldg.
Houston, TX 77204-5000
**Phone:** (713)743-1300 **Fax:** (713)743-5678
**Email:** mlokhandwala@uh.edu
**Website:** http://www.pharmacy.uh.edu
Mustafa F. Lokhandwala, PhD, Director

### ★ 17490 ★ University of Texas, Austin
**College of Pharmacy**
Austin, TX 78712-1074
**Phone:** (512)471-1737 **Fax:** (512)471-8783
**Email:** sleslie@mail.utexas.ed
**Website:** http://www.utexas.edu/pharmacy
Steven W. Leslie, PhD, Director

## Utah

### ★ 17491 ★ University of Utah
**College of Pharmacy**
30 South 2000 East, Rm. 201
Salt Lake City, UT 84112-5820
**Phone:** (801)581-6731 **Fax:** (801)581-3716
**Email:** jmauger@deans.pharm.utah.edu
**Website:** http://www.pharmacy.utah.edu
John W. Mauger, PhD, Director

## Virginia

### ★ 17492 ★ Hampton University
**School of Pharmacy**
Hampton, VA 23668
**Phone:** (757)727-5071 **Fax:** (757)727-5840
**Email:** arcelia.johnson-fannin@hamptonu.edu
**Website:** http://www.hamptonu.edu
Arcelia Johnson-Fannin, Director

### ★ 17493 ★ Shenandoah University
**Bernard J. Dunn School of Pharmacy**
1460 University Dr.
Winchester, VA 22601
**Phone:** (540)665-1282 **Fax:** (540)665-1283
**Email:** amckay@su.edu
**Website:** http://www.su.edu/pharmacy
Alan B. McKay, PhD, Director

### ★ 17494 ★ Virginia Commonwealth University
**Medical College of Virginia**
**School of Pharmacy**
410 N 12th St.
MCV Box 980581
Richmond, VA 23298-0581
**Phone:** (804)828-3006 **Fax:** (804)827-0002
**Email:** vayanchi@vcu.edu
**Website:** http://www.pharmacy.vcu.edu
Victor A. Yanchick, PhD, Director

## Washington

### ★ 17495 ★ University of Washington
**School of Pharmacy**
H364 Health Sciences
Box 357631
Seattle, WA 98195-7631
**Phone:** (206)543-2030 **Fax:** (206)685-9297
**Email:** sidnels@u.washington.edu
**Website:** http://www.depts.washington.edu/pha
Sidney D. Nelson, Jr., P, Director

### ★ 17496 ★ Washington State University
**College of Pharmacy**
PO Box 646510
Pullman, WA 99164-6510
**Phone:** (509)335-4750 **Fax:** (509)335-2530
**Email:** fassett@mail.wsu.edu
**Website:** http://www.pharmacy.wsu.edu
William E. Fassett, PhD, Director

## West Virginia

### ★ 17497 ★ West Virginia University
**School of Pharmacy**
1136 Health Sciences Center N
PO Box 9500
Morgantown, WV 26506-9500
**Phone:** (304)293-5101 **Fax:** (304)293-5483
**Email:** gspratto@hsc.wvu.edu
**Website:** http://www.hsc.wvu.edu/sop/index.html
George R. Spratto, PhD, Director

## Wisconsin

### ★ 17498 ★ University of Wisconsin, Madison
**School of Pharmacy**
777 Highland Ave.
Madison, WI 53705-2222
**Phone:** (608)262-1414 **Fax:** (608)262-3397
**Email:** mhw@pharmacy.wisc.edu
**Website:** http://www.wisc.edu/pharmacy
Melvin H. Weinswig, PhD, Director

## Wyoming

### ★ 17499 ★ University of Wyoming
**School of Pharmacy**
Box 3375
Laramie, WY 82071-3375
**Phone:** (307)766-6120 **Fax:** (307)766-2953
**Email:** uwpharmacy@uwyo.edu
**Website:** http://www.uwyo.edu/pharmacy
Paul L. Ranelli, PhD, Director

# National & International Organizations

### ★ 17500 ★ Academy of Managed Care Pharmacy (AMCP)
100 N Pitt St., Ste. 400
Alexandria, VA 22314-2747
**Phone:** (703)683-8416 **Free:** 800-827-2627
**Fax:** (703)683-8417
**Email:** amcp@amcp.org
**Website:** http://www.amcp.org
Judith A. Cahill, Exec. Dir.
**Fnded:** 1989. **Mem:** 4,700. **Desc:** Professional society for pharmacists working for managed care health services. Promotes the "development and application of pharmaceutical care in order to ensure appropriate outcomes for all individuals." Represents the views and interests of managed care pharmacy. Conducts educational courses and continuing professional development programs for members. **Pub:** *AMCP News*, monthly. Newsletter. • *Concept Series in Managed Care Pharmacy*, periodic. Paper. • *JMCP*, bimonthly. Journal. • *Who's Who*, annual. Directory.

### ★ 17501 ★ Academy of Pharmaceutical Research and Science (APRS)
American Pharmaceutical Association
2215 Constitution Ave. NW
Washington, DC 20037-2985
**Phone:** (202)628-4410 **Free:** 800-237-2742
**Fax:** (202)783-2351
**Email:** sagraves@uic.edu
**Website:** http://www.aphanet.org/about/aprs.html
Arthur H. Kibbe, Pres.
**Fnded:** 1965. **Mem:** 3,000. **Desc:** A part of American Pharmaceutical Association. Pharmaceutical scientists from industry and academia. Objective is to serve the profession of pharmacy by developing knowledge and integrating the process of science into the profession. Sponsors national meetings to provide a forum for presentation and discussion of original research, controversial topics, and continuing communication. Provides consultation and advice to: pharmacists on scientific matters as they relate to policy; congressional committees on bills of interest to pharmaceutical scientists; governmental agencies. **Pub:** *Abstracts of Papers*, annual. Published in Journal of the American Pharmaceutical Ass'n. • *Journal of Pharmaceutical Sciences*, monthly. Journal. • Manuals. • Monographs. **Frmly:** (1987) Academy of Pharmaceutical Sciences.

### ★ 17502 ★ Academy of Students of Pharmacy (APhA-ASP)
2215 Constitution Ave., NW
Washington, DC 20037
**Phone:** (202)429-7595 **Free:** 800-237-APHA
**Fax:** (202)783-2351
**Email:** kdm@mail.aphanet.org
**Website:** http://www.aphanet.org/students/students-new.htm
Patrick K. Brady, Pres.
**Fnded:** 1954. **Mem:** 16,000. **Reg. Groups:** 8. **Local Groups:** 79. **Desc:** A program of the American Pharmaceutical Association. Professional society of pharmacy students. Keeps members informed of the affairs of the APhA and the profession. Provides a forum for the expression of student opinion on activities and policies. Seeks to strengthen the program whereby student members, upon graduation, become active members of the APhA. Encourages participation by pharmacy students in interdisciplinary projects that attempt to find solutions to social problems; works in community-oriented drug education programs; supports interdisciplinary clinical training for pharmacists. **Pub:** *Academy of Students of Pharmacy–Chapter Management*, monthly. Newsletter. For chapter presidents only. • *The Pharmacy Student*, quarterly. Magazine. *Price:* Included in membership dues; $25/year for nonmembers. **Frmly:** (1969) American Pharmaceutical Association Student Section; (1988) Student American Pharmaceutical Association.

### ★ 17503 ★ American Association of Colleges of Pharmacy (AACP)
1426 Prince St.
Alexandria, VA 22314
**Phone:** (703)739-2330 **Fax:** (703)836-8982
**Email:** aconnelly@aacp.org
**Website:** http://www.aacp.org
Amy B. Connelly, Mgr.
**Fnded:** 1900. **Mem:** 3,000. **Desc:** College of pharmacy programs accredited by American Council on Pharmaceutical Education; corporations and individu-

als. Compiles statistics. **Pub:** *AACP News*, monthly. Newsletter. Includes information on association activities, employment opportunities, and new members. *Price:* Included in membership dues; $100/year for nonmembers. • *American Association of Colleges of Pharmacy–Graduate Programs in the Pharmaceutical Sciences*, annual. Directory. Lists graduate programs in pharmacy; provides comparative analysis of pharmacy schools and admissions criteria for graduate programs. *Price:* $25/copy. • *American Journal of Pharmaceutical Education*, quarterly. Journal. Includes book reviews, listing of recent publications, and statistics. *Price:* Included in membership dues; $40/year for nonmembers in the U.S. and Canada; $65/year for nonmembers outside the U.S. and Canada; $100/year for libraries. • *Pharmacy School Admission Requirements*, annual. Directory. Lists pharmacy schools arranged by state; provides comparative analysis of pharmacy schools and admissions criteria for professional programs. *Price:* $25/copy. • *Roster of Teaching Personnel in Colleges of Pharmacy*, annual. Includes calendar of events. *Price:* Included in membership dues; $100/copy for nonmembers. **Frmly:** (1925) American Conference of Pharmaceutical Faculties.

★ **17504** ★ **American Chinese Pharmaceutical Association (ACPA)**
PO Box 2623
Cherry Hill, NJ 08034
**Phone:** (609)394-6121
**Email:** clau@chsnj.org
**Website:** http://www.geocities.com/acpa_rx
**Fnded:** NNas. **Mem:** soci,ate. **Desc:** Pharmacists and pharmaceutical scientists. Seeks to advance the professional well being of pharmacists and pharmaceutical scientists of Chinese heritage; encourages exchange of ideas; provides educational opportunities; promotes health-related issues to the Chinese community. Encourages development of pharmacy practice in China, Taiwan, and Hong Kong. **Pub:** Newsletter, quarterly. Contains organization's events, activities and membership news. • Membership Directory.

★ **17505** ★ **American College of Apothecaries (ACA)**
2830 Summer Oaks Dr.
Bartlett, TN 38134-3811
**Phone:** (901)383-8119          **Fax:** (901)383-8882
**Email:** acainfo@acaresourcecenter.org
Dr. D. C. Huffman, Jr., Exec. VP
**Fnded:** 1940. **Mem:** 1,000. **Reg. Groups:** 13. **State Groups:** 24. **Desc:** Professional society of pharmacists owning and operating ethical prescription pharmacies, including hospital pharmacists, pharmacy students, and faculty of colleges of pharmacy. Primary objective is the translation, transformation, and dissemination of knowledge, research data, and recent developments in the pharmaceutical industry and public health. Offers continuing education courses and certificate program. Conducts research programs; sponsors charitable program; compiles statistics; operates speakers' bureau. **Pub:** *American College of Apothecaries–Directory*, annual. Membership Directory. *Price:* Included in membership dues. • *American College of Apothecaries Newsletter*, monthly. Newsletter. Covers membership activities and developments affecting the profession. *Price:* Included in membership dues. • *American College of Apothecaries–Patron's Newsletter*, monthly. Newsletter. Provides tips on health and medications for patrons of member pharmacists. *Price:* Included in membership dues. • *American College of Apothecaries–Physician's Newsletter*, monthly. Newsletter. Provides health tips on the use of drugs and medications. *Price:* Included in membership dues. • *Voice of the Pharmacist*, quarterly. Newsletter. Provides information on issues affecting pharmacy practice, including legislative developments. *Price:* Included in membership dues; $40/year for nonmembers. • Books. • Handbooks. • Also publishes bylaws.

★ **17506** ★ **American College of Clinical Pharmacy (ACCP)**
3101 Broadway, Ste. 650
Kansas City, MO 64111
**Phone:** (816)531-2177          **Fax:** (816)531-4990
**Email:** accp@accp.com
**Website:** http://www.accp.com
Robert M. Elenbaas, Exec. Dir.
**Fnded:** 1979. **Mem:** 6,900. **Reg. Groups:** 16. **Desc:** Clinical pharmacists dedicated to: promoting rational use of drugs in society; advancing the practice of clinical pharmacy and interdisciplinary health care; assuring high quality clinical pharmacy by establishing and maintaining standards in education and training at advanced levels. Encourages research and recognizes excellence in clinical pharmacy. Offers educational programs, symposia, research forums, fellowship training, and college-funded grants through competitions. Maintains placement service. **Pub:** *ACCP Report*, monthly. Newsletter. *Price:* Free. • *Pharmacotherapy: The Journal of Human Pharmacology and Drug Therapy*, monthly. Journal. *Price:* Included in membership dues. • *Residency and Fellowship Programs Offered by ACCP Members*, annual. Directory of training programs in clinical pharmacy. *Price:* Free.

★ **17507** ★ **American Council on Pharmaceutical Education (ACPE)**
20 N Clark St., Ste. 2500
Chicago, IL 60602-5109
**Phone:** (312)664-3575          **Fax:** (312)664-4652
**Email:** pvlasses@acpe-accredit.org
**Website:** http://www.acpe-accredit.org
Peter H. Vlasses, PharmD, Exec. Dir.
**Fnded:** 1932. **Desc:** Accrediting agency for the professional programs of colleges and schools of pharmacy and approval of providers of continuing pharmaceutical education. **Pub:** *Accredited Professional Programs of Colleges and Schools of Pharmacy*, annual. Directory. • *Approved Providers of Continuing Pharmaceutical Education*, annual. Directory.

★ **17508** ★ **American Foundation for Pharmaceutical Education (AFPE)**
1 Church St., Ste. 202
Rockville, MD 20850-4158
**Phone:** (301)738-2160          **Fax:** (301)738-2161
**Email:** afpe@worldnet.att.net
Robert M. Bachman, Pres.
**Fnded:** 1942. **Mem:** 40. **Desc:** Established by pharmaceutical and drug trade associations to improve pharmaceutical education, colleges of pharmacy, and pharmacy student performance. Accepts and administers gifts, legacies, bequests, and funds and makes disbursements for fellowships and the promotion of pharmaceutical education. **Pub:** *Annual Progress Report*, annual. Report. Reports on contributions and programs. *Price:* Free.

★ **17509** ★ **American Institute of the History of Pharmacy (AIHP)**
777 Highland Ave.
Madison, WI 53705
**Phone:** (608)262-5378
**Email:** aihp@aihp.org
**Website:** http://www.aihp.org
Gregory J. Higby, Dir.
**Fnded:** 1941. **Mem:** 1,000. **Desc:** Pharmacists, firms, and organizations interested in historical and social aspects of the pharmaceutical field. Maintains pharmaceutical Americana collection; conducts research programs. **Pub:** *AIHP Notes*, quarterly. Newsletter. *Price:* Included in membership dues. • *Pharmacy in History*, quarterly. Journal. Contains writings on the history of pharmaceutical practice, including drugs and therapeutics and related facets of the medical sciences. *Price:* Included in membership dues. • Booklets.

★ **17510** ★ **American Pharmaceutical Association - Academy of Pharmacy Practice and Management (APHA-APPM)**
c/o Anne Burns
2215 Constitution Ave. NW
Washington, DC 20037-2985
**Phone:** (202)628-4410          **Free:** 800-237-APHA
**Fax:** (202)783-2351
**Email:** apha-appm@mail.aphanet.org
**Website:** http://www.aphanet.org
Anne Burns, Dir., Practice Development and Research
**Fnded:** 1965. **Mem:** 26,000. **Desc:** Pharmacists concerned with rendering professional services directly to the public, without regard for status of employment or environment of practice. Purposes are to provide a forum and mechanism whereby pharmacists may meet to discuss and implement programs and activities relevant and helpful to the practitioner of pharmacy; to recommend programs and courses of action which should be undertaken or implemented by the profession; to coordinate academy efforts so as to be an asset to the progress of the profession. Provides and cosponsors continuing education meetings, seminars, and workshops; produces audiovisual materials. **Frmly:** (1966) General Practice Section of APhA; (1975) Academy of General Practice of Pharmacy; (1987) Academy of Pharmacy Practice; (1995) Academy of Pharmacy Practice and Management.

★ **17511** ★ **American Society of Consultant Pharmacists (ASCP)**
1321 Duke St.
Alexandria, VA 22314-3563
**Phone:** (703)739-1300          **Free:** 800-355-2727
**Fax:** (703)739-1321
**Email:** info@ascp.com
**Website:** http://www.ascp.com
R. Timothy Webster, Exec. Dir.
**Fnded:** 1969. **Mem:** 7,000. **State Groups:** 20. **Desc:** Provides leadership, education, advocacy, and resources to advance the practice of senior care pharmacy practice. welfare. Conducts surveys of long-term care pharmacy operations. Sponsors educational and research programs. Maintains information center, hall of fame, and speakers' bureau; operates placement service; compiles statistics. **Pub:** *UPDATE*, bimonthly. Newsletter. *Price:* Included in membership dues. • Also publishes books and manuals.

★ **17512** ★ **American Society of Health System Pharmacists (ASHP)**
7272 Wisconsin Ave.
Bethesda, MD 20814
**Phone:** (301)657-3000          **Fax:** (301)664-8867
**Email:** foundation@ashp.org
**Website:** http://www.ashp.org
Stephen J. Allen, Exec. VP
**Fnded:** 1942. **Mem:** 30,000. **State Groups:** 50. **Desc:** Professional society of pharmacists employed by hospitals, HMOs, clinics, and other health systems. Provides personnel placement service for members; sponsors professional and personal liability program. Conducts educational and exhibit programs. Has 30 practice interest areas, special sections for home care practitioners and clinical specialists, and research and education subsidiary. **Pub:** *AHFS Drug Information*, annual. *Price:* $163/year. • *American Journal of Health System Pharmacy*, semimonthly. Journal. *Price:* Included in membership dues; $137/year for nonmembers (U.S.). • *ASHP Newsletter*, monthly. Newsletter. Covers developments in pharmacy and health care. Includes information on legislation and regulations and association news. *Price:* Included in membership dues. • *Handbook on Injectable Drugs*, biennial. *Price:* $158. • *International Pharmaceutical Abstracts*, semimonthly. *Price:* $100/year for members; $425/year for nonmembers (U.S.); $450/year for nonmembers (outside U.S.); $20 for single copy. • Books. • Videos. • Also publishes user manuals and aids, and produces software, CD-ROMS, and training programs.

**American Society for Pharmacy Law (ASPL)**
*See:* Entry 12231

**★ 17513 ★ Arab Academy of Pharmacy (AAP)**
2 A Elui St.
PO Box 1848
Cairo 11511, Egypt
**Email:** bobplye@assn-srvs.com
**Website:** http://www.aspl.org
**Lang(s):** Arabic, English. **Desc:** Professional pharmacists and pharmacy educators and students. Seeks to advance the study, teaching, and practice of pharmacy. Functions as a forum for the exchange of information among members; conducts research and educational programs.

**★ 17514 ★ ASHP Foundation**
7272 Wisconsin Ave.
Bethesda, MD 20814
**Phone:** (301)657-3000    **Fax:** (301)657-8817
**Email:** foundation@ashp.org
**Website:** http://www.ashpfoundation.org
Stephen J. Allen, Exec. VP/CEO
**Fnded:** 1968. **Desc:** Established for pharmaceutical care and research purposes. Offers research grants, awards; and anticoagulation, asthma, stem cell transplantation, diabetes, pain management, oncology, and traineeships. **Pub:** *Resource Book on Progressive Pharmaceutical Services.* **AKA:** American Society of Hospital Pharmacists Research and Education Foundation; ASHP Research and Education Foundation.

**★ 17515 ★ Association of Danish Pharmacists**
Rygards Allel
DK-2900 Hellerup, Denmark
**Phone:** 45 39463600    **Fax:** 45 39463639
**Email:** df@pharmaceut.dk
**Website:** http://www.pharmaceut.dk
**Fnded:** 1873. **Mem:** 3,500. **Reg. Groups:** 10. **State Groups:** 5. **Lang(s):** English. **Desc:** Pharmaceutical executives and editors of pharmaceutical journals of Denmark, Finland, Iceland, Norway, and Sweden. Promotes members' interests. Encourages cooperation among members. **Pub:** *Farmaceuten,* every second week. Journal. **Frmly:** Union of Nordic Pharmacists.

**★ 17516 ★ Association of Deans of Pharmacy of Canada (ADPC) (Association des Doyens de Pharmacie du Canada — ADPC)**
School of Pharmacy
Memorial University of Newfoundland
Saint John's, NF, Canada A1B 3V6
**Phone:** (709)737-6571    **Fax:** (709)737-7044
**Email:** cwloomis@morgan.ucs.mun.ca
**Lang(s):** English, French. **Desc:** Deans of pharmacy. Promotes excellence in pharmacy education. Facilitates communication among schools of pharmacy and among members; conducts research and educational programs.

**★ 17517 ★ Association of Democratic Pharmacists (Verein Demokratischer Pharmazeutinnen und Pharmazeuten)**
Fleming-Apotheke
Grindelallee 182
D-20144 Hamburg, Germany
**Phone:** 49 40 458768    **Fax:** 49 40 458768
**Email:** geschaeftsstelle@vdpp.de
**Website:** http://www.vdpp.de
**Fnded:** 1989. **Mem:** 160. **Desc:** Promotes the interests of registered pharmacists in Germany. Concerned with issues focusing on environmental and public health policies. **Pub:** *VDPP-Rundbriet,* bimonthly. Journal.

**Association of the European Self-Medication Industry (AESGP) (Europaischer Fachverband der Arzneimittel-Hersteller)**
*See:* Entry 9957

**★ 17518 ★ Association of Faculties of Pharmacy of Canada (AFPC)**
2609 Eastview
Saskatoon, SK, Canada S7J 3G7
**Phone:** (306)374-6327    **Fax:** (306)374-0555
**Email:** jblackburn@sk.sympatico.ca
**Website:** http://www.pharmacy.ualberta.ca/afpc
**Fnded:** 1944. **Mem:** 250. **Lang(s):** English, French. **Desc:** Educators engaged in postsecondary pharmacy programs. Promotes excellence in pharmacy education; encourages continuing professional development among members. Facilitates exchange of information among members; conducts research and educational programs.

**★ 17519 ★ Australasian Pharmaceutical Science Association (APSA)**
Department of Pharmacy
University of Sydney
Sydney, NSW 2007, Australia
**Phone:** 61 2 93512320    **Fax:** 61 2 93512320
**Fnded:** 1960.

**★ 17520 ★ Australian College of Pharmacy Practice (ACPP)**
PO Box 7007
Canberra Mail Centre
Canberra, ACT 2610, Australia
**Phone:** 61 2 62738989    **Fax:** 61 2 62738988
**Email:** info@acpp.edu.au
**Website:** http://www.acpp.edu.au
**Fnded:** 1983. **Mem:** 1,124. **Lang(s):** English. **Desc:** Provides postgraduate pharmacy educational opportunities for pharmacists throughout Australia. **Pub:** *Pharmacy Risins,* quarterly. Newsletter.

**★ 17521 ★ Australian Self-Medication Industry**
140 Arthur St., Level 4
North Sydney, NSW 2060, Australia
**Phone:** 61 2 99225111    **Fax:** 61 2 99593693
**Email:** juliet@asmi.com.au
**Website:** http://www.asmi.com.au
**Fnded:** 1974. **Mem:** 56. **Desc:** Manufacturers nonprescription medicines, also know as over the counter medicines. Seeks to ensure the safe and effective over the counter medications are readily available at a reasonable to cost. Serves as a source of information on responsible and cost-effective self medication. Represents members before parliament and government and industry organizations. Commissions research. **Frmly:** (2000) Proprietary Medicine Association of Address unknown since 1993 edition.

**★ 17522 ★ Canadian Academy of the History of Pharmacy (CAHP) (Academie Canadienne d'Histoire de la Pharmacie — ACHP)**
Faculty of Pharmacy
University of Toronto
19 Russell St.
Toronto, ON, Canada M5S 2S2
**Phone:** (416)978-2889    **Fax:** (416)978-8511
**Email:** wayne.hindmarsh@utoronto.ca
**Website:** http://www.utoronto.ca
**Lang(s):** English, French. **Desc:** Pharmacists, historians, and other individuals with an interest in the history of pharmacy. Promotes historical research. Provides support and assistance to pharmaceutical historians; conducts educational programs; serves as a clearinghouse on pharmacy history.

**★ 17523 ★ Canadian Association of Pharmacy in Oncology (CAPhO)**
PO Box 32
Don Mills Postal Station
Don Mills, ON, Canada M3C 2R6
**Website:** http://capho.ca
**Lang(s):** English. **Desc:** Pharmacists and other health care professionals interested in the practice of oncology pharmacy in Canada. Represents the professional interests and issues of oncology pharmacy at a national level.

**★ 17524 ★ Canadian Association of Pharmacy Technicians (CAPT)**
PO Box 1271 Station F,
Toronto, ON, Canada M4Y 2V8
**Phone:** (416)410-1142
**Email:** contact@capt.ca
**Website:** http://www.capt.ca
**Fnded:** 1983. **Mem:** 600. **Lang(s):** English. **Desc:** Pharmacy technicians in Canada. Seeks to improve the communication, education, and recognition of pharmacy technicians. **Pub:** Newsletter, bimonthly.

**★ 17525 ★ Canadian Council for Accreditation of Pharmacy Programs (CCAPP) (Le Conseil Canadien de l'Agrement des Programmes de Pharmacie — CCAPP)**
Thorvaldson Bldg., Rm. 123
110 Science Pl.
Saskatoon, SK, Canada S7N 5C9
**Phone:** (306)966-6388    **Fax:** (306)966-6377
**Email:** schnell@sask.usask.ca
**Lang(s):** English, French. **Desc:** Promotes excellence in the study and teaching of pharmacy. Formulates and enforces standards for pharmacy training programs; examines pharmacy programs and bestows accreditation.

**★ 17526 ★ Canadian Council on Continuing Education in Pharmacy (CCCEP)**
3861 Athol St.
Regina, SK, Canada S4S 3J2
**Phone:** (306)584-5703    **Fax:** (306)584-5703
**Email:** nmcbean@accesscomm.ca
**Website:** http://www.accesscomm.ca/users/cccep/
**Lang(s):** English. **Desc:** Pharmacists, educators, and educational institutions. Promotes professional development of pharmacists; seeks to advance the accreditation standards and criteria and accredit continuing professional education courses for pharmacists.

**★ 17527 ★ Canadian Foundation for Pharmacy (CFP) (Fondation Canadienne pour la Pharmacie — FCP)**
15 Sawyer Crescent
Markham, ON, Canada L3P 5V2
**Phone:** (905)201-9559    **Fax:** (905)201-0717
**Email:** da-browns@home.com
**Fnded:** 1947. **Lang(s):** English, French. **Desc:** Pharmacists and other health care personnel. Seeks to advance pharmaceutical practice and research. Provides support and assistance to pharmacy research projects; conducts continuing professional education courses.

**★ 17528 ★ Canadian Pain Society (CPS)**
c/o Sherry Franklin
50 Driveway
Ottawa, ON, Canada K2P 1E2
**Phone:** (613)234-0812    **Fax:** (613)234-9894
**Email:** sfranklin@cna-nurses.ca
**Website:** http://www.medicine.dal.ca/cps
**Fnded:** 1982. **Lang(s):** English, French. **Desc:** Health care professionals and medical and pharamceutical researchers with an interest in pain and its alleviation. Fosters research on the causes of pain; seeks im-

proved methods of pain management. Facilitates communication and cooperation among pain researchers and clinicians; sponsors educational and research programs. **Pub:** *Pain Research and Management*, quarterly. Journal.

**★ 17529 ★ Canadian Pharmacists Association (CPhA)**
**(Association des Pharmaciens du Canada — APhC)**
1785 Alta Vista Dr.
Ottawa, ON, Canada K1G 3Y6
**Phone:** (613)523-7877          **Fax:** (613)523-0445
**Email:** cpha@cdnpharm.ca
**Website:** http://www.cdnpharm.ca
**Fnded:** 1907. **Mem:** 9,000. **Lang(s):** English, French. **Desc:** Pharmacists in Canada. Works to improve the professional image of pharmacists and the quality of pharmacy services and health care in Canada. Monitors government health care policies and legislation; lobbies for the interests of pharmacists. Maintains liaison with government departments, pharmaceutical manufacturers, and health care organizations. Conducts education and research programs. Bestows awards. **Pub:** *Annual Report*, annual. • *Canadian Pharmaceutical Journal*, 10/year. • *Compendium of Pharmaceuticals and Specialties*, annual. **Frmly:** Canadian Pharmaceutical Association.

**★ 17530 ★ Canadian Society of Hospital Pharmacists (CSHP)**
**(Societe Canadienne des pharmaciens d'Hopitaux — SCPH)**
1145 Hunt Club Rd., Ste. 350
Ottawa, ON, Canada K1V 0Y3
**Phone:** (613)736-9733          **Fax:** (613)736-5660
**Email:** halligan@cshp.ca
**Website:** http://www.cshp.ca
**Fnded:** 1947. **Mem:** 2,400. **State Groups:** 8. **Lang(s):** English, French. **Desc:** Hospital pharmacists, graduate pharmacists, and students. Promotes safe and effective drug therapy in organized health care settings. Provides leadership to members in institutional pharmacy practice. Evaluates and accredits postgraduate training programs in hospital pharmacy through the Canadian Hospital Pharmacy Residency Board. Enhances the visibility of hospital pharmacy in the health care field through public relations activities and meetings with government and health care associations. Promotes programs of continuing education; operates the CSHP Research and Educational Foundation. Maintains committees and task forces to recommend development of areas of interest and need to members; promotes funding and research programs. **Pub:** *Canadian Journal of Hospital Pharmacy*, bimonthly. Journal. • *Employment Opportunities Bulletin*, biweekly. Bulletin. • *Pharmascope*, bimonthly. Newsletter.

**★ 17531 ★ Chinese Pharmaceutical Association**
A38 Lishi Rd. N
Beijing 100810, People's Republic of China
**Phone:** 852 10 68316576

**★ 17532 ★ Christian Pharmacists Fellowship International (CPFI)**
PO Box 1717
501 5th St.
Bristol, TN 37621-1717
**Phone:** (423)764-6000          **Free:** 888-253-6885
**Fax:** (423)764-4490
**Email:** cpfi@tricon.net
**Website:** http://www.cpfi.org
Allan Sharp, P.D., Admin. Dir.
**Fnded:** 1984. **Mem:** 1,200. **Reg. Groups:** 3. **State Groups:** 3. **Local Groups:** 7. **Desc:** To promote and maintain fellowship among Christian pharmacists. Establishes clubs and chapters at universities, colleges, schools, hospitals, and in communities; sponsors activities and retreats for Christian pharmacists and their families. Encourages active Christian witness and

evangelism; teaches pharmacists how to share and present the Gospel of Jesus Christ in their practice; disseminates information among Christian pharmacists; identifies areas of service for pharmacists in missions worldwide and sponsors missionaries in the field. Provides and promotes Christian pharmacist-speakers. speakers at state and national pharmacy meetings. **Pub:** *Christian Pharmacists Fellowship International–Newsletter*, bimonthly. Newsletter. Reports on the activities of members and the fellowship, as well as Christian events in pharmacy. Includes book reviews and directory. *Price:* Free. • *Christianity and Pharmacy*. Journal. Official journal of chrisitian Pharmacists Fellowship International. • Membership Directory, biennial.

**★ 17533 ★ Commission for Certification in Geriatric Pharmacy (CCGP)**
1321 Duke St.
Alexandria, VA 22314
**Phone:** (703)535-3038          **Fax:** (703)739-1500
**Email:** info@ccgp.org
**Website:** http://www.ccgp.org
**Fnded:** 1997. **Desc:** Working to promote excellence in Geriatric Health Care through education and certification.

**★ 17534 ★ Commonwealth Pharmaceutical Association (CPA)**
1 Lambeth High St.
London SE1 7JN, United Kingdom
**Phone:** 44 207 7522364          **Fax:** 44 207 7522508
**Email:** bfalconbridge@rpsgb.org.uk
**Fnded:** 1970. **Mem:** 550. **Nat'l Groups:** 39. **Reg. Groups:** 6. **Lang(s):** English. **Desc:** Pharmaceutical organizations in 39 Commonwealth countries; pharmacists. Objectives are to: maintain the honor and traditions of the profession and promote high standards of conduct, practice, and education at all levels; encourage close links among members in the profession and facilitate personal contacts between pharmacists and students; disseminate information about the professional practice of pharmacy and the pharmaceutical sciences. **Pub:** *Newsletter*, quarterly. Newsletter.

**★ 17535 ★ European Association of Hospital Pharmacists (EAHP)**
**(Association Europeene des Pharmaciens des Hopitaux)**
Cornerways
Beechey Ave.
Marston
Oxford OX3 OJU, United Kingdom
**Phone:** 44 1865 202304          **Fax:** 44 1865 202304
**Fnded:** 1972. **Mem:** 9,000. **Lang(s):** English, French, German. **Desc:** Individuals from 16 countries. Promotes and protects the interests of hospital pharmacists; disseminates information. **Pub:** *European Journal of Hospital Pharmacy*, periodic. Journal.

**★ 17536 ★ European Generic Medicines Association (EGA)**
Ave de Cortenbergh 66
1000 Brussels, Belgium
**Phone:** 32 2 7367438          **Fax:** 32 2 7368411
**Email:** info@ecagenerics.com
**Website:** http://www.egagenerics.com
**Fnded:** 1991. **Desc:** Maintains and develops the common scientific and technical interests of the generics branch of the pharmaceutical industry and manufactures of bulk chemicals destined for medicines.

**★ 17537 ★ European Society of Clinical Pharmacy (ESCP)**
Theda Mansholtstraat 5B
NL-2331 JE Leiden, Netherlands
**Phone:** 31 71 5722430          **Fax:** 31 71 5722431
**Email:** office@escp.nl
**Website:** http://www.escp.nl

**Fnded:** 1979. **Mem:** 1,000. **Desc:** Seeks to develop and promote the rational and appropriate use of medicines. Provides a forum for the communication of new knowledge and new developments in clinical pharmacy. Plans, accredits, and develops educational and research programs in clinical pharmacy. Liaises with health care organizations worldwide. **Pub:** *Progress in Clinical Pharmacy*, annual. Proceedings. • Newsletter, bimonthly.

**★ 17538 ★ Foreign Pharmacy Graduate Examination Committee (FPGEC)**
c/o Carmen A. Catizone
National Association of Boards of Pharmacy
700 Busse Hwy.
Park Ridge, IL 60068
**Phone:** (847)698-6227          **Fax:** (847)698-0124
**Website:** http://www.nabp.net
Carmen A. Catizone, Exec. Dir.
**Fnded:** 1982. **Desc:** A committee of the National Association of Boards of Pharmacy. Provides information to foreign pharmacy graduates regarding entry into the U.S. pharmacy profession and health care systems. Evaluates qualifications of foreign pharmacy graduates. Gathers and disseminates data on foreign graduates; maintains information on foreign pharmacy schools in order to produce an examination that measures academic competence with regard to U.S. pharmacy school standards. **Frmly:** (1988) Foreign Pharmacy Graduate Examination Commission.

**HealthCare Compliance Packaging Council (HCPC)**
*See:* Entry 9975

**International Committee of Homeopathic Pharmacists**
**(Comite International des Pharmaciens Homeopathiques — CIPH)**
*See:* Entry 4278

**★ 17539 ★ International Federation of Associations of Pharmaceutical Physicians (IFAPP)**
Rendementsweg 24 E-l
NL-3641 SL Mijdrecht, Netherlands
**Phone:** 31 297 285144          **Fax:** 31 297 256046
**Email:** ifapp@planet.nl
**Website:** http://www.ifapp.org
**Fnded:** 1975. **Mem:** 24. **Nat'l Groups:** 24. **Lang(s):** English. **Desc:** National organizations representing 6000 physicians in 24 countries specializing in pharmaceutical medicine. Encourages contact among members. **Pub:** *International Journal of Pharmaceutical Medicine: IFAPP Section*, bimonthly. Newsletter.

**★ 17540 ★ International Pharmaceutical Federation (IPF)**
**(Federation Internationale Pharmaceutique — FIP)**
PO Box 84200
NL-2508 AE The Hague, Netherlands
**Phone:** 31 70 3021970          **Fax:** 31 70 3021999
**Email:** fip@fip.org
**Website:** http://www.fip.org
**Fnded:** 1912. **Mem:** 4,500. **Lang(s):** English, French, German, Spanish. **Desc:** Worldwide organization of pharmacists and pharmaceutical scientists. Objectives are to: develop pharmacy at the international level in professional and scientific fields; development and standardization of professional standards; extend the role of the pharmacist in the health care field; foster communication among members; act as a clearinghouse; collaborate with efforts to improve pharmaceutical structures in various countries; advocate and support measures to ensure distribution, dispensation, and proper use of medicines. Exchanges opinions on professional and ethical issues; develops research and study programs; fosters cooperation among pharmacists, teachers, research workers, and the practitioners in the field of drug information; improves

methods for assembling, selecting, summarizing, indexing, storing, classifying, and analyzing clinical and social surveys. Subjects studied include biopharmaceutics, pharmacokinetics and drug metabolism, administrative and social pharmacy, pharmacognosy, and the history of pharmacy. Collaborates with World Health Organization. **Pub:** *International Pharmacy Journal*, bimonthly. • *Scientific Congress Proceedings*, biennial. Also publishes abstracts.

**★ 17541 ★ International Study Group for Steroid Hormones (ISGSH)
(Gruppo di Studio Internazionale degli Ormoni Steroidei)**
Dip di Fisipatologia medica
Universita degli Studi
Viale Policlinico
I-00161 Rome, Italy
**Phone:** 39 6 490465        **Fax:** 39 6 49970560
**Fnded:** 1961. **Mem:** 350. **Lang(s):** English. **Desc:** Researchers, physicians, and professors in medical specialties such as endocrinology, urology, oncology, and gynecology, whose main scientific activity concerns steroid hormones; pharmaceutical firms. Strives to encourage and advance steroid hormone studies and research. Promotes education and training in steroid assays. **Pub:** *Abstracts of the Meeting*, biennial. • *Research on Steroids*, biennial. Contains proceeding. • *Steroids*. Journal.

**★ 17542 ★ National Association of Boards of Pharmacy (NABP)**
700 Busse Hwy.
Park Ridge, IL 60068
**Phone:** (847)698-6227        **Fax:** (847)698-0124
**Email:** info@nabp.net
**Website:** http://www.nabp.net
Carmen A. Catizone, Exec. Dir.
**Fnded:** 1904. **Mem:** 67. **Desc:** Pharmacy boards of several states, District of Columbia, Puerto Rico, Virgin Islands, several Canadian provinces, and the states of Victoria, Australia, and New South Wales. Provides for inter-state reciprocity in pharmaceutic licensure based upon a uniform minimum standard of pharmaceutic education and uniform legislation; improves the standards of pharmaceutical education licensure and practice. Provides legislative information; sponsors uniform licensure examination; also provides information on accredited school and college requirements. Maintains pharmacy and drug law statistics. **Pub:** *Annual Meeting Proceedings*, annual. Proceedings. • *NABP Newsletter*, 10/year. Newsletter. Reports on regulation and licensure in the pharmacy profession. Contains information on NABP competency assessment programs. *Price:* $25/year. • *The NAPLEX Candidate's Review Guide*, annual. • *State Board Newsletters*, quarterly. Newsletter. Covers 35 states. • *Survey of Pharmacy Law*, annual. Survey. • Surveys. • Also publishes periodically updated guides and examination manuals.

**★ 17543 ★ National Association of Women Pharmacists (NAWP)**
c/o Office Manager
Royal Pharmaceutical Society of Great Britain
1 Lambeth High St.
London SE1 7JN, United Kingdom
**Email:** enquiries@nawp.org.uk
**Website:** http://www.nawp.org.uk
**Fnded:** 1905. **Mem:** 300. **Reg. Groups:** 3. **Local Groups:** 4. **Lang(s):** English. **Desc:** Women pharmacists. Promotes the careers of women in pharmacy and the role of women pharmacists in public life. Encourages continuing education and career development for women pharmacists. Maintains communication with pharmacists who have left the Register of the Royal Pharmaceutical Society of Great Britain (RPSGB) during a career break. Works with other women's organizations. Conducts courses and lectures, provides mentoring for members. **Pub:** *Careers in Pharmacy*. Book. • *NAWP*, 3/year. Newsletter.

**★ 17544 ★ National Catholic Pharmacists Guild of the United States (NCPG)**
1012 Surrey Hills Dr.
Saint Louis, MO 63117-1438
**Phone:** (314)645-0085
John Paul Winkelmann, Exec. Dir. & Co-Pres.
**Fnded:** 1962. **Mem:** 400. **Nat'l Groups:** 1. **Desc:** Catholic pharmacists, pharmacy graduates, students, and pharmacy technicians. Upholds the principles of the Catholic faith and all laws of church and country, especially those pertaining to the practice of pharmacy; assists ecclesiastical authorities in the diffusion of Catholic pharmacy ethics; promotes donations of funds and supplies to the needy; opposes the sale of pornographic literature, especially that which is being sold in pharmacies; fosters solidarity and goodwill among all pharmacists. Provides pharmaceuticals and funds for people worldwide. **Pub:** *The Catholic Pharmacist*, quarterly. Journal. Includes obituaries, membership and professional news, new member listings, and book reports as well as other reports and issues. *Price:* Included in membership dues; $20/year for members only.

**★ 17545 ★ National Council on Patient Information and Education (NCPIE)**
4915 Saint Elmo Ave., Ste. 505
Bethesda, MD 20814-6082
**Phone:** (301)656-8565        **Fax:** (301)656-4464
**Email:** ncpie@erols.com
**Website:** http://www.talkaboutrx.org
Linda Golodner, Chair
**Fnded:** 1982. **Mem:** 160. **Desc:** Health care professional organizations, pharmaceutical manufacturing organizations, federal agencies, voluntary health agencies, and consumer groups. Increases the availability of information and improves the dialogue between consumers and health care providers about prescription medicines; increases professional awareness of the need to give adequate information on prescription therapy; expands consumers' participation with health professionals on matters of drug therapy. Communicates with health care providers on the importance of giving consumers oral and written information on prescription medicines and encourages consumers to ask questions about medicines and explain factors that may affect their ability to follow prescriptions. **Pub:** *A Parents Guide to Medicine Use By Children*. Brochure. • *The Active Consumer: Getting the Most from Your Medicines*. Brochure. • *Get the Answers*. Brochure. • *Guidelines for Improving Prescription Medicine Use Among Children and Teenagers*. Report. • *Medicine: Before You Take It, Talk About It*. Brochure. • *Medicines: What Every Woman Should Know*. Brochure. • *NCPIE News*, quarterly. Newsletter. • *Talk About Prescriptions: Month Planning Kit*, annual.

**National Council of State Pharmacy Association Executives (NCSPAE)**
*See:* Entry 9757

**National Lupron Victims Network (NLVN)**
*See:* Entry 2300

**★ 17546 ★ National Pharmaceutical Association (NPhA)**
107 Kilmayne Dr., Ste. C
Cary, NC 27511
**Free:** 800-944-NPHA        **Fax:** (919)469-5870
**Email:** tvbbamc@aol.com
**Website:** http://www.npha.net/
Marcelius Grace, Pres.
**Fnded:** 1947. **Mem:** 325. **Desc:** State and local associations of professional minority pharmacists. To provide a means whereby members may "contribute to their common improvement, share their experiences, and contribute to the public good." **Pub:** *Journal of the NPhA*, quarterly. Journal. *Price:* $20/year for individuals (U.S.); $35/year for institutions (U.S.); $30/year for individuals (outside U.S.); $45/year for institutions (outside U.S.).

**Pediatric Pharmacy Advocacy Group (PPAG)**
*See:* Entry 5744

**★ 17547 ★ Pharmaceutical Group of the European Union**
159, rue Belliard
B-1040 Brussels, Belgium
**Phone:** 32 2 2380818        **Fax:** 32 2 2380819
**Email:** pharmacy@pgeu.org
**Website:** http://www.pgeu.org
**Fnded:** 1959. **Mem:** 25. **Lang(s):** English, French. **Desc:** International association representing community pharmacists. **Pub:** *Annual Reports*, annual. **Frmly:** Pharmaceutical Group of the European Community.

**★ 17548 ★ Pharmaceutical Society of Denmark
(Danmarks Farmaceutiske Selskab)**
Universitetsparken 2
DK-2100 Copenhagen, Denmark
**Phone:** 45 31370850
**Fnded:** 1912.

**★ 17549 ★ Pharmaceutical Society of Ghana (PSGh)**
c/o The Hon. General Secretary
PO Box 2133
Accra, Ghana
**Phone:** 233 21 228341        **Fax:** 233 21 239583
**Email:** psgh@ighmail.com
**Fnded:** 1935. **Mem:** 1,200. **Lang(s):** English. **Desc:** Registered pharmacists in Ghana. Promotes and protects pharmacy and pharmacists and safeguards the interests and concerns of government and the public regarding pharmaceutical and related affairs. Encourages and regulates the education and training of pharmacists. **Pub:** *Ghana Pharmaceutical Journal*. Journal.

**★ 17550 ★ Pharmaceutical Society of Northern Ireland**
73 University St.
Belfast BT7 1HL, United Kingdom
**Phone:** 44 2890 326927        **Fax:** 44 2890 439919
**Email:** chief.exec@psni.org.uk
**Fnded:** 1925. **Mem:** 1,707. **Desc:** Registered pharmacists. Acts as a professional and registration body for pharmacists and pharmacies in Northern Ireland.

**★ 17551 ★ Pharmaceutical Society of Singapore (PSS)**
Alumni Medical Centre
2 College Rd.
Singapore 169850, Singapore
**Phone:** 65 2211136        **Fax:** 65 2230969
**Email:** admin@pss.org.sg
**Website:** http://www.pss.org.sg
**Fnded:** 1967. **Mem:** 950. **Lang(s):** English. **Desc:** Seeks to maximize the contribution of pharmacists to health care by enforcing a code of ethics, cooperating with other organizations, and providing educational programs. Sponsors competitions. **Pub:** *Singapore Pharmaceutical Bulletin*, quarterly. Bulletin. **Frmly:** (1967) Malayan Pharmaceutical Association.

**★ 17552 ★ Pharmaceutical Society of South Africa (PSSA)**
26 Juta St.
PO Box 31360
Braamfontein 2017, Republic of South Africa
**Phone:** 27 11 3391752        **Fax:** 27 11 4031309
**Website:** http://www.medisource.co.za/associations/pharmaceutical.htm
**Fnded:** 1946. **Mem:** 5,500. **Lang(s):** Afrikaans, English. **Desc:** Registered pharmacists. Promotes high standards of ethics and practice in pharmacy. Conducts continuing professional education courses; faci-

litates communication among members; maintains museum. **Pub:** *South Africa Pharmaceutical Journal*, monthly. Journal.


★ **17553** ★ **Royal Institute of Public Health and Hygiene (RIPH)**
28 Portland Pl.
London W1B 1DE, United Kingdom
**Phone:** 44 20 75802731   **Fax:** 44 20 75806157
**Email:** info@riph.org.uk
**Website:** http://www.riph.org.uk
**Fnded:** 1897. **Mem:** 500. **Lang(s):** English. **Desc:** Caterers, doctors, environmental health officers, food technologists, laboratory and mortuary technicians, microbiologists, nurses, and teachers promoting the advancement of domestic, industrial, and personal health and hygiene. Encourages the study of hygiene, preventive medicine, and public health. Offers courses; holds seminars. **Pub:** *Handbook of Mortuary Practice and Safety for Anatomical Pathology Technicians.* ● *Health and Hygiene*, quarterly. Journal. ● *Public Health*, bimonthly. Journal. ● *Supervisors Handbook of Food Safety*. HACCP Training Standard, Food Safety Trainers Guide, Hygiene for Care Assistants in Residential Homes for Elderly People.


★ **17554** ★ **Royal Pharmaceutical Society of Great Britain (RPSGB)**
1 Lambeth High St.
London SE1 7JN, United Kingdom
**Phone:** 44 20 7359141   **Fax:** 44 20 75870395
**Email:** enquiries@rpsgb.org.uk
**Website:** http://www.rpsgb.org.uk
**Fnded:** 1841. **Mem:** 40,000. **Lang(s):** English. **Desc:** Pharmacists. Professional, statutory and regulatory body for practicing pharmacists in Great Britain. **Pub:** *The Extra Pharmacopeia*, triennial. Book. ● *Martindale Online Newsletter*, periodic. Newsletter. ● *Martindale Online User Guide*. Handbook. ● *Martindale Thesaurus*. Book.


★ **17555** ★ **Scottish Pharmaceutical General Council**
42 Queen St.
Edinburgh EH2 3NH, United Kingdom
**Phone:** 44 131 4677766   **Fax:** 44 131 4677767
**Email:** enquiries@spgc.org.uk
**Website:** http://www.spgc.org.uk
**Fnded:** 1913. **Desc:** Body recognised by Secretary of State for Scotland as representing the interests of the general body of chemist contractors in Scotland. Concerned with all NHS matters which affect retail pharmacy in Scotland.


**Society of Infectious Diseases Pharmacists (SIDP)**
*See:* Entry 11830


★ **17556** ★ **Society for Medicines Research (SMR)**
c/o Ms. Lilian Attar
Triangle House
Broomhill Rd.
London SW18 4HX, United Kingdom
**Phone:** 44 208 8752431   **Fax:** 44 208 8752424
**Email:** secretariat@socmr.org
**Website:** http://www.socmr.org
**Fnded:** 1966. **Mem:** 526. **Lang(s):** English. **Desc:** Researchers at academic institutions and in the pharmaceutical industry; other concerned individuals. Promotes advancement in the field of medicinal education and research in order to provide the public with proper information on drug usage for relief of sickness. **Pub:** *Proceedings*, periodic. ● Newsletter, 3-4/year. **Frmly:** (1994) Society for Drug Research.


★ **17557** ★ **United States Pharmacopeia**
12601 Twinbrook Pky.
Rockville, MD 20852

**Phone:** (301)881-0666   **Free:** 800-822-8772
**Fax:** (301)816-8299
**Email:** webmaster@usp.org
**Website:** http://www.usp.org
Roger L. Williams, MD, Exec. VP & CEO
**Fnded:** 1820. **Mem:** 400. **Desc:** Dedicated to promoting the public health by establishing and disseminating officially recognized standards of quality and authoritive information for the use of medicines and other health care technologies by health professionals, patients and consumers. Also helps to monitor quality and prevent errors in human and veterinary medicine through national reporting programs. Achieves its goals through the contributions of volunteers representing pharmacy, medicine, and other health care professions, as well as science, academia, the US government, the pharmaceutical industry, and consumer organizations. **Pub:** *Pharmacopeial Forum*, bimonthly. ● *Proceedings of Quinquennial Meetings.* ● *The United States Pharmacopeia and the National Formulary*, quinquennial. Includes semiannual supplement. ● *USAN and USP Dictionary of Drug Names*, annual. ● *USP DI, Volume III, Approved Drug Products and Legal Requirements*, annual. **Frmly:** (1999) U.S. Pharmacopeial Convention.


## Research Centers


★ **17558** ★ **Academy of Pharmaceutical Research and Science**
American Pharmaceutical Association
2215 Constitution Ave. NW
Washington, DC 20037-2985
**Phone:** (202)628-4410   **Free:** 800-237-2742
**Fax:** (202)628-0443
**Email:** llm@mail.aphanet.org
**Website:** http://www.aphanet.org
Lucinda Maine, PhD, Contact
**Activities/Fields:** Pharmaceuticals, focusing on quality measurement, development of practice-based research, and outcomes research in the broadcast sense.


**Alberta Cancer Board**
**Edmonton Radiopharmaceutical Centre**
*See:* Entry 18163


★ **17559** ★ **American College of Apothecaries**
**Research and Education Foundation**
PO Box 341266
Memphis, TN 38184
**Phone:** (901)383-8119   **Fax:** (901)383-8882
**Email:** acainfo@acainfo.org
**Website:** http://www.acainfo.org
D.C. Huffman, Jr., Exec. Dir.
**Activities/Fields:** Three-fold objective of the Foundation is to promote public welfare through development of services in institutions providing health care, encourage and conduct research to improve health care and education, and encourage health care practitioners to improve the quality and availability of their services.


★ **17560** ★ **Georgetown University**
**Center for Drug Development Sciences**
Department of Pharmacology
Georgetown University Medical Center
Med-Dent Bldg., Rm. NE405
3900 Reservoir Rd. NW
Washington, DC 20007
**Phone:** (202)687-1618   **Fax:** (202)687-0193
**Email:** sawlerj@gunet.georgetown.edu
**Website:** http://www.dml.georgetown.edu/depts/pharmacology/cdds/
Carl C. Peck, MD, Dir.
**Activities/Fields:** Improvement of clinical evaluation of drugs in development.

★ **17561** ★ **Massachusetts Institute of Technology**
**Program on the Pharmaceutical Industry (POPI)**
Bldg. E56-390
Sloan Sch. of Management
38 Memorial Dr.
Cambridge, MA 02139-4307
**Phone:** (617)253-5194   **Fax:** (617)253-3033
**Email:** popi-www@mit.edu
**Website:** http://web.mit.edu/popi/
Stan N. Finkelstein, MD, Dir.
**Activities/Fields:** Competitiveness, performance, and productivity in the pharmaceutical field.


★ **17562** ★ **Oklahoma Medical Research Foundation**
**Clinical Pharmacology Research Program**
825 NE 13th St.
Oklahoma City, OK 73104
**Phone:** (405)271-6673   **Fax:** (405)271-3980
**Email:** carl-manion@omrf.ouhsc.edu
**Website:** http://www.omrf.org/OMRF/Research/17/Program.asp
Carl V. Manion, MD, Contact
**Activities/Fields:** Effects of medicines given to treat the heart, lungs and liver.


★ **17563** ★ **Purdue University**
**Center for Pharmaceutical Processing Research (CPPR)**
1336 Robert E Heine Pharmacy Bldg.
Department of Industrial & Physical Pharmacy
West Lafayette, IN 47907-1336
**Phone:** (765)494-1401   **Fax:** (765)494-6545
**Email:** slnail@pharmacy.purdue.edu
**Website:** http://www.pharmacy.purdue.edu/~nsf/
Steven L. Nail, Dir.
**Activities/Fields:** Pharmaceutical processing.


★ **17564** ★ **Research Institute of Kansas**
2600 N Woodlawn
Wichita, KS 67220
**Phone:** (316)858-2598   **Fax:** (316)858-2521
**Email:** kjantz@galichia.com
**Activities/Fields:** Pharmaceutic drug and device studies.


★ **17565** ★ **Tufts Center for the Study of Drug Development**
Tufts University
192 South St., Ste. 550
Boston, MA 02111
**Phone:** (617)636-2185   **Fax:** (617)636-2425
**Email:** peg.hewitt@tufts.edu
**Website:** http://www.tufts.edu/med/csdd
Kenneth I. Kaitin, PhD, Dir.
**Activities/Fields:** Public policy on worldwide drug development and its trends, including study of the impact of drug regulation on pharmaceutical innovation; survey of pharmaceutical firms to determine origin, flow, and fate of new chemical entities (NCEs) and biopharmaceuticals; evaluation of therapeutic significance of marketed drugs; economic analysis of drug development costs; and legal and regulatory issues in drug development and distribution. **Pub:** *Tufts CSDD Impact Report.* **Frmly:** Center for the Study of Drug Development.


**U.S. Department of Health and Human Services**
**Food and Drug Administration**
**Center for Drug Evaluation and Research**
*See:* Entry 18002

**★ 17566 ★ U.S. Department of Health and Human Services**
**Food and Drug Administration**
**Center for Drug Evaluation and Research**
**Division of Over-the-Counter Drug Products**
**(Office of Drug Evaluation)**
9201 Corporate Blvd.
Rockville, MD 20850
**Phone:** (301)827-2241    **Fax:** (301)827-2316
**Email:** ganley@cder.fda.gov
**Website:** http://www.fda.gov/cder/otc/index.htm
Dr. Charles J. Ganley, MD, Dir.

**Activities/Fields:** Reviews over-the-counter (OTC) medications marketed in the United States.

**★ 17567 ★ U.S. Department of Health and Human Services**
**Food and Drug Administration**
**Center for Drug Evaluation and Research**
**Office of Generic Drugs**
**(Bioequivalence Division)**
Metro Park North
7500 Standish Pl.
Rockville, MD 20855
**Phone:** (301)443-1544    **Fax:** (301)594-0181
James Chaney, Dir.

**Activities/Fields:** Bioequivalence and dissolution testing data submitted by pharmaceutical firms in support of abbreviated new drug applications. Principal fields of research include biopharmaceutics, pharmacokinetics, and analytical methods. **Pub:** *Research Reports.* **Frmly:** Office of Drug Standards.

**★ 17568 ★ U.S. Department of Health and Human Services**
**Food and Drug Administration**
**Center for Drug Evaluation and Research**
**Office of Testing and Research**
**(Division of Testing and Applied Analytical Development)**
1114 Market St., Rm. 1002
Saint Louis, MO 63101
**Phone:** (314)539-2134    **Fax:** (314)539-2113
**Email:** layloftt@ddastl.cder.fda.gov
**Website:** http://www.fda.gov/cder/dtaad/
Thomas P. Layloff, Jr., Dir.

**Activities/Fields:** Conducts method validation for new drug applications and analyzes drug substances for abbreviated new drug applications; serves as the FDA collaborating laboratory for the acceptance of reference standards for the United States Pharmacopeia; assists in monitoring the quality of marketed drugs through surveillance and compliance actions; conducts research to establish official laboratory techniques or methods to test drugs for compliance with standards of identity, strength, and purity; develops analytical methods, particularly automated methods adapted to large volumes of samples; and collects data to support bioavailability and bioequivalence reviews of drugs. Laboratory operations include long-range research activities related to analytical methods and analyses related to the FDA's surveillance programs and other aspects of drug monitoring. **Pub:** *Research Reports.* **Frmly:** Office of Research Resources; Drug Analysis Division.

**U.S. Department of Health and Human Services**
**Food and Drug Administration**
**Office of Orphan Products Development**
*See:* Entry 2609

**★ 17569 ★ U.S. Department of Health and Human Services**
**Food and Drug Administration**
**Office of Planning and Evaluation**
**Evaluation and Analysis Staff**
Mail Code HFP-10
5600 Fishers Ln., Rm. 1571
Rockville, MD 20857
**Phone:** (301)827-5252    **Fax:** (301)827-5260
**Email:** kmcevoy@oc.fda.gov
**Website:** http://www.fda.gov/ope/eval.html
John Uzzell, Dir.

**Activities/Fields:** In-house analytical consulting services to the FDA Commissioner and program managers. Activities involve evaluation, data collection, and analysis for all program policies and operations administered by the FDA, including pre-market review of drugs and medical devices.

**U.S. Department of Health and Human Services**
**National Cancer Institute**
**Division of Cancer Treatment and Diagnosis**
**Developmental Therapeutics Program**
**(Grants and Contracts Operations Branch)**
*See:* Entry 10451

**U.S. Department of Health and Human Services**
**National Cancer Institute**
**Division of Cancer Treatment, Diagnosis, and Centers**
**Developmental Therapeutics Program**
**(Drug Synthesis and Chemistry Branch)**
*See:* Entry 10459

**★ 17570 ★ University of Alabama at Birmingham**
**Center for Biophysical Sciences and Engineering (CBSE)**
MCLM 262
1530 3rd Ave. S
Birmingham, AL 35294-0005
**Phone:** (205)934-3841    **Fax:** (205)934-2659
**Email:** woodruff@cmc.uab.edu
**Website:** http://www.cbse.uab.edu/
Lawrence J. DeLucas, PhD, Dir.

**Activities/Fields:** Structure and function of macromolecules as applied to new drug discovery.

**★ 17571 ★ University of Alberta**
**Faculty of Pharmacy and Pharmaceutical Sciences**
**Noujaim Institute for Pharmaceutical Oncology Research**
3118 Dentistry/Pharmacy Bldg.
University of Alberta
Edmonton, AB, Canada T6G 2N8
**Phone:** (780)492-5904    **Fax:** (780)492-8241
**Email:** gmiller@pharmacy.ualberta.ca
**Website:** http://www.pharmacy.ualberta.ca/noujaim/About.html
Gerald G. Miller, PhD, Dir.

**Activities/Fields:** Targeted anticancer therapy and drug delivery.

**★ 17572 ★ University of Florida**
**Center for Drug Discovery**
Pharmaceutics Department
College of Pharmacy
J. Hillis Miller Health Center
PO Box 100497
Gainesville, FL 32610-0496
**Phone:** (352)392-8186    **Fax:** (352)392-8589
**Email:** bodor@cop.ufl.edu
**Website:** http://www.cop.ufl.edu/
Prof. Nicholas Bodor, PhD, Exec. Dir.

**Activities/Fields:** Pharmaceutical research embracing a variety of topics from computer-aided drug design and medicinal chemistry to analytical, pharmacokinetic and pharmacodynamic programs, drug stability and formulation development, and drug metabolism and toxicity. Current projects focus on retrometabolic drug design. **Frmly:** Center for Drug Design and Delivery.

**★ 17573 ★ University of Iowa**
**Center for Advanced Drug Development (CADD)**
100 Oakdale Campus, Rm. 1 PRL
Iowa City, IA 52242
**Phone:** (319)335-4096    **Fax:** (319)335-4120
**Email:** alta-botha@uiowa.edu
**Website:** http://www.uiowa.edu/~vpr/research/units/advdrug.htm
Dr. S. Alta Botha, Lab. Dir.

**Activities/Fields:** New and old drug substances and formulations, particularly regarding stability indication and validation, preformulation studies, in vitro testing of dosage forms, stability studies, testing on active pharmaceutical ingredients.

**★ 17574 ★ University of Iowa**
**Pharmaceutical Service Division**
College of Pharmacy
115 S Grand Ave.
Iowa City, IA 52242
**Phone:** (319)335-8674    **Fax:** (319)335-9418
**Email:** rolland-poust@uiowa.edu
**Website:** http://www.uiowa.edu/~pharmser/
Rolland I. Poust, Dir.

**Activities/Fields:** Drug delivery systems for pharmaceutical investigations, including parenterals, capsules, tablets, liquids, lyophilized products, and dermatologicals, for human clinical trials.

**★ 17575 ★ University of Kentucky**
**Center for Pharmaceutical Science and Technology**
309 Pharmacy Bldg.
907 Rose St.
Lexington, KY 40536-0082
**Phone:** (859)257-5288    **Fax:** (859)323-5985
**Email:** jay@pop.uky.edu
**Website:** http://www.uky.edu/Pharmacy/cpst/
Dr. Michael Jay, Dir.

**Activities/Fields:** Drug product development and evaluation. Provides industrial support through the development and preparation of clinical supplies of drug products under government regulations.

**★ 17576 ★ University of Maryland**
**Center on Drugs and Public Policy**
Sch. of Pharmacy
100 N Greene St., 6th Fl.
Baltimore, MD 21201-1563
**Phone:** (410)706-0133    **Fax:** (410)706-5394
**Email:** fpalumbo@rx.umaryland.edu
Dr. Francis B. Palumbo, JD, Dir.

**Activities/Fields:** Dug policy, legal and regulatory; drug utilization review; outpatient drug benefits under the OBRA 90; cost effective drug therapies; pharmaceutical care services; health outcomes related to drug therapy; pharmacoepidemiology, pharmacy manpower; the pharmaceutical industry; impact of changes in the organization and financing of health care services; and patient compliance with prescribed drug regimen.

**★ 17577 ★ University of Mississippi**
**Pharmaceutical Marketing and Management Research Program**
Waller Lab Complex, Rm. 101
University, MS 38677
**Phone:** (662)915-5948    **Fax:** (662)915-5262
**Email:** mkolassa@olemiss.edu
**Website:** http://www.olemiss.edu/depts/rips/pmmrp/
Dr. Eugene M. (Mick) Kolassa, Interim Coord.

**Activities/Fields:** Proprietary and inhouse marketing and management studies relating to pharmaceutical products, including formulary decision factors, generic substitution, reimbursement issues, medication compliance and consumer preferences. Conducts mail surveys, telephone interviews, focus groups, internet surveys, consumer reaction panels, and surveys of professionals at national and state meetings.

**★ 17578 ★ University of Mississippi Research Institute of Pharmaceutical Sciences**
School of Pharmacy
University, MS 38677-1848
**Phone:** (662)915-7265 **Fax:** (662)915-5704
**Email:** gailcook@olemiss.edu
**Website:** http://www.olemiss.edu/depts/pharm_school/
Dr. Barbara G. Wells, Dean/Exec. Dir.
**Activities/Fields:** Discovery and design of important biologically active natural products; health services, focusing on rural health; toxicology studies on the fate and effects of environmental chemicals; pharmaceutical marketing and management. **Pub:** *Pharmacy Report*, semiannually.

**★ 17579 ★ University of Toledo Center for Applied Pharmacology**
College of Pharmacy
2801 W Bancroft St.
Toledo, OH 43606-3390
**Phone:** (419)530-2010 **Fax:** (419)530-8407
**Email:** kbachma@utnet.utoledo.edu
**Website:** http://www.utoledo.edu/pharmcap/
Kenneth Bachmann, PhD, Contact
**Activities/Fields:** Relationship between drug disposition and drug dynamics, especially pharmacokinetics and pharmacodynamics in normal healthy subjects and in defined patient groups, bioavailability, pharmacokinetic/pharmacodynamic modeling, population kinetics, and drug interactions. **Pub:** *Reports*.

**★ 17580 ★ University of Toledo Center for Drug Design and Development (CD3)**
College of Pharmacy
2801 W Bancroft St.
Toledo, OH 43606-3390
**Phone:** (419)530-4257 **Fax:** (419)530-6110
**Website:** http://www.utoledo.edu/cd3/
**Activities/Fields:** Drug therapies and diagnostics.

**★ 17581 ★ University of Washington Pharmaceutical Outcomes Research and Policy Program (PORPP)**
Box 357630
Health Sciences Bldg., Rm. H375
Department of Pharmacy
Seattle, WA 98195-7630
**Phone:** (206)543-6788 **Fax:** (206)543-3835
**Email:** sdsull@u.washington.edu
**Website:** http://depts.washington.edu/porpp/
Prof. Sean D. Sullivan, PhD, Dir.
**Activities/Fields:** Effects and use of pharmaceuticals in human populations.

# State Government Agencies

## Pharmacy Boards

**★ 17582 ★ Alabama State Board of Pharmacy**
1 Perimeter Park S, Ste. 425 S
Birmingham, AL 35243
**Phone:** (205)967-0130 **Fax:** (205)967-1009
**Email:** jmoore@albop.com

**Website:** http://www.albop.com
Jerry Moore, Director

**★ 17583 ★ Arizona State Board of Pharmacy**
4425 W Olive Ave, Ste 140
Glendale, AZ 85302
**Phone:** (623)463-2727 **Fax:** (623)934-0583
**Email:** vsevilla@azsbp.com
**Website:** http://www.pharmacy.state.az.us/
Llyn. A. Lloyd, Director

**★ 17584 ★ Arkansas State Board of Pharmacy**
101 E Capitol, Ste. 218
Little Rock, AR 72201
**Phone:** (501)682-0190 **Fax:** (501)682-0195
**Email:** Charlie.campbell@mail.state.ar.us
**Website:** http://www.state.ar.us/asbp/
Charles S. Campbell, Director

**★ 17585 ★ California State Board of Pharmacy**
400 R St., Ste. 4070
Sacramento, CA 95814
**Phone:** (916)445-5014 **Fax:** (916)327-6308
**Email:** rxwebmaster@dca.ca.gov
**Website:** http://www.pharmacy.ca.gov/
John Jones, Director

**★ 17586 ★ CareMed Chicago**
322 S Green St. Ste. 300
Chicago, IL 60607
**Phone:** (312)738-8622 **Fax:** (312)738-0317
**Email:** caremed@caremedchicago.com
**Website:** http://www.caremedchicago.com/

**★ 17587 ★ Colorado State Board of Pharmacy**
1560 Broadway, Ste. 1310
Denver, CO 80202
**Phone:** (303)894-7750 **Fax:** (303)894-7764
**Email:** Pharmacy@dora.state.co.us
**Website:** http://www.dora.state.co.us/pharmacy/
Susan L. Warren, Contact

**★ 17588 ★ Delaware Department of Administrative Services Division of Professional Regulation Delaware State Board of Pharmacy**
Jesse Cooper Bldg., Room 205
PO Box 637
Dover, DE 19903
**Phone:** (302)739-4547 **Fax:** (302)739-3071
**Email:** grbunting@state.de.us
**Website:** http://professionallicensing.state.de.us/boards/pharmacy/index.shtml
Gradella Bunting, Contact

**★ 17589 ★ Department of Consumer Protection License Services Division Connecticut Commission of Pharmacy**
165 Capitol Ave.
Hartford, CT 06106
**Phone:** (860)713-6065 **Fax:** (860)713-7239
**Email:** drug.control@po.state.ct.us
**Website:** http://www.dcp.state.ct.us/licensing/drug.htm

**★ 17590 ★ District of Columbia Board of Pharmacy**
825 N Capitol St, NE, room 2224
Washington, DC 20002
**Phone:** (202)442-4775 **Fax:** (202)442-9431
Graphelia Ramseur, Contact

**★ 17591 ★ Georgia State Board of Pharmacy**
237 Coliseum Dr.
Macon, GA 31217-3858
**Phone:** (678)207-1686 **Fax:** (678)207-1363
**Email:** rfthompson@sos.state.ga.us
**Website:** http://www.sos.state.ga.us/plb/
Anita O. Martin, Director

**★ 17592 ★ Hawaii State Board of Pharmacy**
1010 Richards St.
PO Box 3469
DCCA-PVL
ATT: PHAR
Honolulu, HI 96801
**Phone:** (808)586-2694
**Email:** pharmacy@dcca.state.hi.us
**Website:** http://www.state.hi.us/dcca/pvl/areas_pharmacy.html
Lee Ann Teshima, Contact

**★ 17593 ★ Idaho Board of Pharmacy**
3380 Americana Terrace., Ste. 320
PO Box 83720
Boise, ID 83720-0067
**Phone:** (208)334-2356 **Fax:** (208)334-3536
**Website:** http://www.accessidaho.org/bop/contact/contact.html
Richard Mick Markuson, Director

**★ 17594 ★ Illinois Department of Professional Regulation Board of Pharmacy**
320 W Washington St.
Springfield, IL 62786
**Phone:** (217)785-0800 **Fax:** (217)782-7645
**Website:** http://www.dpr.state.il.us/WHO/phar.asp
John Rose, Director

**★ 17595 ★ Indiana Board of Pharmacy Health Professions Bureau**
402 W Washington St., Rm. 041
Indianapolis, IN 46204
**Phone:** (317)232-2960 **Fax:** (317)233-4236
**Email:** mboone@hpb.state.in.us
**Website:** http://www.in.gov/hpb/
888-333-7515 Donna S. Wall, Director

**★ 17596 ★ Iowa Board of Pharmacy Examiners**
400 SW Eighth St., Ste. E
Des Moines, IA 50309-4688
**Phone:** (515)281-5944 **Fax:** (515)281-4609
**Email:** lloyd.jessen@ibpe.state.ia.us
**Website:** http://www.iowaccess.org/ibpe/
Lloyd K. Jessen, Director

**★ 17597 ★ Kansas State Board of Pharmacy**
900 W Jackson, Rm. 513
Topeka, KS 66612-1231
**Phone:** (785)296-4056 **Free:** 888-RX-BOARD
**Fax:** (785)296-8420
**Email:** pharmacy@ink.org
**Website:** http://www.ink.org/public/pharmacy/
Jim Kinderknecht, R.Ph., Contact

**★ 17598 ★ Kentucky Board of Pharmacy**
23 Millcreek Park
Frankfort, KY 40601-9230
**Phone:** (502)573-1580 **Fax:** (502)573-1582
**Website:** http://www.state.ky.us/boards/pharmacy/

**★ 17599 ★ Louisiana Board of Pharmacy**
5615 Corporate Blvd., Ste. 8E
Baton Rouge, LA 70808-2537
**Phone:** (225)925-6496
**Email:** labp@labp.com

**Website:** http://www.labp.com/
Howard B. Bolton, Director

**★ 17600 ★ Maine Board of
  Commissioners of Pharmacy
Department of Professional & Financial
  Regulation
Division of Licensing & Enforcement**
35 State House Station
Augusta, ME 04333
**Phone:** (207)624-8500          **Fax:** (207)624-8690
**Email:** jeri.l.betts@state.me.us
**Website:** http://www.state.me.us/pfr/olr/index.htm
Jeri L. Betts, Contact

**★ 17601 ★ Maryland Board of Pharmacy**
4201 Patterson Ave.
Baltimore, MD 21215-2299
**Phone:** (410)764-4755          **Free:** 800-542-4964
**Fax:** (410)358-6207
**Email:** md_pharmacy_board@yahoo.com
**Website:** http://www.dhmh.state.md.us/pharmacy-board/
LaVerne G. Naesea, Director

**★ 17602 ★ Massachusetts Board of
  Registration in Pharmacy**
239 Causeway St., Ste. 500
Boston, MA 02114
**Phone:** (617)727-3074          **Fax:** (617)727-2197
**Email:** charles.r.young@state.ma.us
**Website:** http://www.state.ma.us/reg/boards/ph/default.htm
Charles Young, Director

**★ 17603 ★ Michigan Board of Pharmacy**
PO Box 30670
Lansing, MI 48909-8170
**Phone:** (517)335-0918          **Fax:** (517)373-2179
**Email:** bhserinfo@cis.state.mi.us
**Website:** http://www.cis.state.mi.us/bhser/lic/boards/bdpharm.htm

**★ 17604 ★ Minnesota Board of Pharmacy**
2829 University Ave. SE, Ste. 530
Minneapolis, MN 55414
**Phone:** (612)617-2201          **Fax:** (612)617-2212
**Email:** David.Holmstrom@state.mn.us
**Website:** http://www.phcybrd.state.mn.us/mn_home.htm
David E. Holmstrom, Director

**★ 17605 ★ Mississippi State Board of
  Pharmacy**
PO Box 24507
Jackson, MS 39225-4507
**Phone:** (601)354-6750          **Fax:** (601)354-6071
**Email:** cwilliams@mbp.state.ms.us
**Website:** http://www.mbp.state.ms.us/
Leland "Mac" McDivitt, Director

**★ 17606 ★ Missouri Board of Pharmacy**
3605 Missouri Blvd.
PO Box 625
Jefferson City, MO 65102
**Phone:** (573)751-0091          **Fax:** (573)526-3464
**Email:** pharmacy@mail.state.mo.us
**Website:** http://www.ded.state.mo.us/regulatorylicensing/
Kevin E. Kinkade, Director

**★ 17607 ★ Montana Department of Labor
  and Industry
Business Standards Division
Montana Board of Pharmacy**
301 S Park, 4th Fl.
Helena, MT 59602
**Phone:** (406)841-2355          **Fax:** (406)841-2305
**Email:** compolpha@state.mt.us

**Website:** http://www.discoveringmontana.com/dli/bsd/license/bsd_boards/pha_board/board_page.htm
Rebecca Deschamps, Contact

**★ 17608 ★ Nebraska Department of HHS
  Regulation and Licensure
Nebraska Board of Examiners in
  Pharmacy**
PO Box 95007
Lincoln, NE 68509-5007
**Phone:** (402)471-4923
**Email:** hhs_system_information@hhss.state.ne.us
**Website:** http://www.hhs.state.ne.us/crl/crlindex.htm
Helen Meeks, Contact

**★ 17609 ★ Nevada State Board of
  Pharmacy**
555 Double Eagle Court, Ste. 1100
Reno, NV 89511-8991
**Phone:** (775)850-1440          **Free:** 800-364-2081
**Fax:** (775)850-1444
**Email:** pharmacy@govmail.state.nv.us
**Website:** http://glsuitewww.glsuite.com/nvbopweb/
Larry Pinson, Director

**★ 17610 ★ New Hampshire Board of
  Pharmacy**
57 Regional Dr.
Concord, NH 03301-8518
**Phone:** (603)271-2350          **Fax:** (603)271-2856
**Email:** nhpharmacy@nhsa.state.nh.us
**Website:** http://www.state.nh.us/pharmacy/
Paul G. Boisseau, Contact

**★ 17611 ★ New Jersey State Board of
  Pharmacy**
PO Box 45013
Newark, NJ 07101
**Phone:** (973)504-6450
**Email:** askconsumeraffairs@dca.lps.state.nj.us
**Website:** http://www.state.nj.us/lps/ca/medical.htmpharm11
Debra Whipple, Director

**★ 17612 ★ New Mexico Board of
  Pharmacy**
1650 University Blvd. NE, Ste. 400B
Albuquerque, NM 87102
**Phone:** (505)841-9102          **Free:** 800-565-9102
**Fax:** (505)841-9113
**Email:** pharmacy.board@state.nm.us
**Website:** http://www.state.nm.us/pharmacy/
Jerry Montoya, Director

**★ 17613 ★ New York Board of Pharmacy**
State Education Bldg.
Office of the Professions, 2nd Fl.
89 Washington Ave.
Albany, NY 12234
**Phone:** (518)474-3817          **Fax:** (518)473-6995
**Email:** pharmbd@mail.nysed.gov
**Website:** http://www.op.nysed.gov/pharm.htm
Lawrence H. Mokhiber, Contact

**★ 17614 ★ North Carolina Board of
  Pharmacy**
Carrboro Plaza
PO Box 459
Carrboro, NC 27510
**Phone:** (919)942-4454          **Fax:** (919)967-5757
**Email:** drw@ncbop.org
**Website:** http://www.ncbop.org/
David R. Work, Director

**★ 17615 ★ North Dakota State Board of
  Pharmacy**
405 E Broadway Ave., Rm. 300
PO Box 1354
Bismarck, ND 58502-1354

**Phone:** (701)328-9535          **Fax:** (701)328-9312
**Email:** ndboph@btinet.com
**Website:** http://www.governor.state.nd.us/boards/boards-query.asp?Board_ID=81
Howard C. Anderson, R.Ph, Director

**★ 17616 ★ Ohio State Board of
  Pharmacy**
77 S High St., 17th Fl.
Columbus, OH 43215-6126
**Phone:** (614)466-4143          **Free:** 800-750-0750
**Fax:** (614)752-4836
**Email:** exec@bop.state.oh.us
**Website:** http://www.state.oh.us/pharmacy
William T. Winsley, Director

**★ 17617 ★ Oklahoma State Board of
  Pharmacy**
4545 Lincoln Blvd., Ste. 112
Oklahoma City, OK 73105-3488
**Phone:** (405)521-3815          **Fax:** (405)521-3758
**Email:** pharmacy@oklaosf.state.ok.us
**Website:** http://www.state.ok.us/~pharmacy/
Bryan H. Potter, D.Ph., Director

**★ 17618 ★ Oregon State Board of
  Pharmacy**
State Office Bldg., Ste. 425
800 NE Oregon St., No. 9
Portland, OR 97232
**Phone:** (503)731-4032          **Fax:** (503)731-4067
**Email:** gary.a.schnabel@state.or.us
**Website:** http://www.pharmacy.state.or.us/
Gary A. Schnabel, Director

**★ 17619 ★ Pennsylvania State Board of
  Pharmacy**
PO Box 2649
Harrisburg, PA 17105-2649
**Phone:** (717)783-7156          **Fax:** (717)787-7769
**Email:** pharmacy@pados.dos.state.pa.us
**Website:** http://www.dos.state.pa.us/bpoa/cwp/view.asp?a=1104&q=432995

**★ 17620 ★ Puerto Rico Board of
  Pharmacy
Department of Health
Board of Pharmacy**
800 Avenida Robert T. Todd
Office No. 201, Stop No. 18
Call Box 10200
Santurce, PR 00908
**Phone:** (787)725-8161
Magda Bouet, Director

**★ 17621 ★ Rhode Island Board of
  Pharmacy
Department of Health
Division of Drug Control**
3 Capitol Hill, Rm. 205
Providence, RI 02908-5097
**Phone:** (401)222-2837          **Fax:** (401)222-2158
**Email:** dianet@doh.state.ri.us
**Website:** http://www.health.state.ri.us/hsr/pharmacy.htm
Diane Tellier, Contact

**★ 17622 ★ South Carolina Board of
  Pharmacy**
PO Box 11927
Columbia, SC 29211-1927
**Phone:** (803)896-4700          **Fax:** (803)896-4596
**Email:** funderbm@mail.llr.state.sc.us
**Website:** http://www.llr.state.sc.us/POL/Pharmacy/Default.htm
Lee Ann Bundrick, Contact

★ **17623** ★ **South Dakota State Board of Pharmacy**
4305 S Louise Ave., Ste. 104
Sioux Falls, SD 57106
**Phone:** (605)362-2737　　　**Fax:** (605)362-2738
**Email:** dennis.jones@state.sd.us
**Website:** http://www.state.sd.us/dcr/pharmacy/pharm-ho.htm
David L. Volk, Secretary

★ **17624** ★ **Tennessee Board of Pharmacy**
Davy Crockett Tower
500 James Robertson Pkwy., 2nd Fl.
Nashville, TN 37243-1149
**Phone:** (615)741-2718　　　**Fax:** (615)741-2722
**Email:** klynch@mail.state.tn.us
**Website:** http://www.state.tn.us/commerce/pharmacy/index.htm
Kendall M. Lynch, Director

★ **17625** ★ **Texas State Board of Pharmacy**
333 Guadalupe St., Tower 3, Ste. 600
Austin, TX 78701-3942
**Phone:** (512)305-8000　　　**Fax:** (512)305-8082
**Email:** geninfo@tsbp.state.tx.us
**Website:** http://www.tsbp.state.tx.us/
Gay Dodson, Director

★ **17626** ★ **Utah Board of Pharmacy**
160 E 300 S, 4th Fl.
PO Box 146741
Salt Lake City, UT 84145-0805
**Phone:** (801)530-6633　　　**Fax:** (801)530-6511
**Email:** dtjones@br.state.ut.us

★ **17627** ★ **Vermont Board of Pharmacy**
**Office of Professional Regulation**
109 State St.
Montpelier, VT 05609-1106
**Phone:** (802)828-2875
**Email:** cpreston@sec.state.vt.us
**Website:** http://www.vtprofessionals.org/pharmacists/
Carla Preston, Secretary

★ **17628** ★ **Virgin Islands Board of Pharmacy**
**Department of Health**
Roy L. Schneider Hospital
48 Sugar Estate
St Thomas, VI 00802
**Phone:** (340)774-0117　　　**Fax:** (340)777-4001
Lydia T. Scott, Director

★ **17629** ★ **Virginia Board of Pharmacy**
6606 W Broad St., 4th Fl.
Richmond, VA 23230-1717
**Phone:** (804)662-9911　　　**Free:** 800-533-1560
**Fax:** (804)662-9313
**Email:** pharmbd@dhp.state.va.us
**Website:** http://www.dhp.state.va.us/pharmacy/default.htm
Elizabeth Scott Russell, Director

★ **17630** ★ **Washington State Board of Pharmacy**
1300 SE Quince St.
PO Box 47863
Olympia, WA 98504-7863
**Phone:** (360)236-4825　　　**Fax:** (360)586-4359
**Website:** http://www.doh.wa.gov/Pharmacy/default.htm
Donald H. Williams, Director

★ **17631** ★ **West Virginia Board of Pharmacy**
232 Capitol St.
Charleston, WV 25301
**Phone:** (304)558-0558　　　**Fax:** (304)558-0572
**Email:** bpayne@wvbop.com
**Website:** http://www.wvbop.com/wvbop/25301/default.htm
William T. Douglas, Jr., Contact

★ **17632** ★ **Wisconsin Pharmacy Examining Board**
1400 E Washington Ave.
PO Box 8935
Madison, WI 53708-8935
**Phone:** (608)266-2811　　　**Fax:** (608)267-0644
**Email:** dorl@drl.state.wi.us
**Website:** http://badger.state.wi.us/agencies/drl/Regulation/applicant_information/dod270.html

★ **17633** ★ **Wyoming State Board of Pharmacy**
1720 S Poplar St., Ste. 4
Casper, WY 82601
**Phone:** (307)234-0294　　　**Fax:** (307)234-7226
**Email:** wypharmbd@wercs.com
**Website:** http://pharmacyboard.state.wy.us/
James T. Carder, Contact

# State & Regional Organizations

## Pharmacy

*Listed below are state pharmacy associations. The national organization is the National Council of State Pharmacy Association Executives, c/o Iowa Pharmacy Association, 8515 Douglas Ave., Ste. 16, Des Moines, IA 50322, (515)270-0713, http://www.ncspae.org.*

### Alabama

★ **17634** ★ **Alabama Pharmacy Association**
1211 Carmichael Way
Montgomery, AL 36106-3672
**Phone:** (334)271-4222　　　**Fax:** (334)271-5423
**Email:** weley@aparx.org
**Website:** http://www.aparx.org
William Eley, II, Exec Director

### Alaska

★ **17635** ★ **Alaska Pharmaceutical Association**
Box 10-1185
Anchorage, AK 99510-1185
**Phone:** (907)563-8880　　　**Fax:** (907)573-7880
**Email:** akphrmcy@alaska.net
**Website:** http://www.alaskapharmacy.org
Erin Byrne, Exec Director

### Arizona

★ **17636** ★ **Arizona Pharmacy Association**
1845 E Southern Ave.
Tempe, AZ 85282-5831
**Phone:** (480)838-3385　　　**Fax:** (480)838-3557
**Email:** azpa@azpharmacy.org
**Website:** http://www.azpharmacy.org
Kathy Boyle, Exec Director

### Arkansas

★ **17637** ★ **Arkansas Pharmacists Association**
417 S Victory
Little Rock, AR 72201
**Phone:** (501)372-5250　　　**Fax:** (501)372-0546

**Email:** rbeck@arpharmacists.org
**Website:** http://www.arpharmacists.org
Richard Beck, PD,CAE, CEO

### California

★ **17638** ★ **California Pharmacists Association**
1112 I St., Ste. 300
Sacramento, CA 95814
**Phone:** (916)444-7811　　　**Fax:** (916)444-7929
**Email:** cmichelotti@cpha.com
**Website:** http://www.cpha.com
Carlo Michelotti, RPh, CEO

### Colorado

★ **17639** ★ **Colorado Pharmacists Society**
5150 E Yale Cir., Ste. 304
Denver, CO 80222
**Phone:** (303)756-3069　　　**Fax:** (303)756-3649
**Email:** valkalnins@interfold.com
**Website:** http://www.coloradopharmacy.org
Val Kalnins, R.Ph., Exec Director

### Connecticut

★ **17640** ★ **Connecticut Pharmacists Association**
35 Cold Spring Rd., Ste. 125
Rocky Hill, CT 06067
**Phone:** (860)563-4619　　　**Fax:** (860)257-8241
**Email:** marghiecpa@aol.com
**Website:** http://www.ctpharmacists.org
Marghie Giuliano, R.Ph., Exec VP

### Delaware

★ **17641** ★ **Delaware Pharmacists Society**
PO Box 454
Smyrna, DE 19977-0454
**Phone:** (302)659-3088　　　**Fax:** (302)659-3089
**Email:** patsgrants@aol.com
**Website:** http://www.depharmacy.org
Pat Carroll-Grant, RPh, Exec Director

### Florida

★ **17642** ★ **Florida Pharmacy Association**
610 N Adams St.
Tallahassee, FL 32301
**Phone:** (850)222-2400　　　**Fax:** (850)561-6758
**Email:** mjackson@pharmview.com
**Website:** http://www.pharmview.com
Michael Jackson, R.Ph., Exec VP

### Georgia

★ **17643** ★ **Georgia Pharmacy Association, Inc.**
50 Lenox Pointe NE
Atlanta, GA 30324
**Phone:** (404)231-5074　　　**Fax:** (404)237-8435
**Email:** bharden@gpha.org
**Website:** http://www.gpha.org
Buddy Harden, Jr., R.Ph., Exec VP

### Hawaii

★ **17644** ★ **Hawaii Pharmacists Association**
PO Box 22472
Honolulu, HI 96823-2472
**Phone:** (808)432-5536　　　**Fax:** (808)432-5535
**Email:** amtanigu@lava.net
Ronald Taniguchi, PharmD, Contact

## Idaho

**★ 17645 ★ Idaho State Pharmacy Association**
PO Box 140117
305 W Jefferson St.
Boise, ID 83714-0117
**Phone:** (208)424-1107     **Fax:** (208)424-1102
**Email:** condie2@mindspring.com
**Website:** http://www.idahopharmacy.org
JoAn Condie, Exec Director

## Illinois

**★ 17646 ★ Illinois Pharmacists Association**
204 W Cook St.
Springfield, IL 62704-2526
**Phone:** (217)522-7300     **Fax:** (217)522-7349
**Email:** terrim@ipha.org
**Website:** http://www.ipha.org
Terri McEntaffer, R.Ph., Exec Director

## Indiana

**★ 17647 ★ Indiana Pharmacists Alliance**
729 N Pennsylvania St.
Indianapolis, IN 46204-1171
**Phone:** (317)634-4968     **Fax:** (317)632-1219
**Email:** ipalary@indianapharmacists.org
**Website:** http://www.indianapharmacists.org
Lawrence Sage, Exec VP
**Frmly:** Indiana Pharmacists Association.

## Iowa

**★ 17648 ★ Iowa Pharmacy Association**
8515 Douglas Ave., Ste. 16
Des Moines, IA 50322
**Phone:** (515)270-0713     **Fax:** (515)270-2979
**Email:** ttemple@iarx.org
**Website:** http://www.iarx.org
Thomas Temple, R.Ph., CEO

## Kansas

**★ 17649 ★ Kansas Pharmacists Association**
1020 SW Fairlawn Rd.
Topeka, KS 66604-2019
**Phone:** (785)228-2327     **Fax:** (785)228-9147
**Email:** bob@kansaspharmacy.org
**Website:** http://www.kansaspharmacy.org
Robert Williams, CAE, Exec Director

## Kentucky

**★ 17650 ★ Kentucky Pharmacists Association**
1228 U.S. 127 S
Frankfort, KY 40601
**Phone:** (502)227-2303     **Fax:** (502)227-2258
**Email:** kyphassoc@aol.com
Mike Mayes, FACHE, Exec Director

## Louisiana

**★ 17651 ★ Louisiana Pharmacists Association**
4744 Jamestown, Ste. 101
Baton Rouge, LA 70808
**Phone:** (225)926-2666     **Fax:** (225)926-1020
**Email:** lpa2000@tlxnet.net
**Website:** http://www.louisianapharmacists.org

## Maine

**★ 17652 ★ Maine Pharmacy Association**
PMB 323
11 Bangor Mall Blvd., Ste. D
Bangor, ME 04401
**Free:** 800-639-1609     **Fax:** (207)989-6743
**Email:** mpa@mparx.com
**Website:** http://www.mainepharmacyassoc.com
Bob Morrisette, President

## Maryland

**★ 17653 ★ Maryland Pharmacists Association**
650 W Lombard St.
Baltimore, MD 21201-1572
**Phone:** (410)727-0746     **Fax:** (410)727-2253
**Email:** mpha@erols.com
**Website:** http://www.rxstat.com/mpha/
Howard Schiff, Exec Director

**★ 17654 ★ Washington, DC Pharmaceutical Association**
908 Caddington Ave.
Silver Spring, MD 20901-1109
**Phone:** (301)593-3292     **Fax:** (301)593-7215
**Email:** midpharm@aol.com
Herb Kwash, Exec Director

## Massachusetts

**★ 17655 ★ Massachusetts Pharmacists Association**
681 Main St., Ste. 3-32
Waltham, MA 02451
**Phone:** (781)736-0101     **Fax:** (781)736-0080
**Email:** carmelo@masspharmacists.org
**Website:** http://www.masspharmacists.org
Carmelo Cinquenonce, Exec VP

## Michigan

**★ 17656 ★ Michigan Pharmacists Association**
815 N Washington Ave.
Lansing, MI 48906-5198
**Phone:** (517)484-1466     **Fax:** (517)484-4893
**Email:** larry@michiganpharmacists.org
**Website:** http://www.michiganpharmacists.org
Larry Wagenknecht, R.Ph., CEO

## Minnesota

**★ 17657 ★ Minnesota Pharmacists Association**
1935 W County Rd. B-2
Roseville, MN 55113-2722
**Phone:** (651)697-1771     **Fax:** (651)697-1776
**Email:** julie@mpha.org
**Website:** http://www.mpha.org
Julie Johnson, R.Ph., Exec VP

## Mississippi

**★ 17658 ★ Mississippi Pharmacists Association**
341 Edgewood Terrace Dr.
Jackson, MS 39206-6299
**Phone:** (601)981-0416     **Fax:** (601)981-0451
**Email:** mpha@bellsouth.net
S.E. "Bo" Dalton, R.Ph., Exec Director

## Missouri

**★ 17659 ★ Missouri Pharmacy Association**
211 E Capitol Ave.
Jefferson City, MO 65101-3001
**Phone:** (573)636-7522     **Fax:** (573)636-7485
**Email:** jim@morx.com
**Website:** http://www.morx.com
Jim Frederich, R.Ph., Contact

## Montana

**★ 17660 ★ Montana Pharmacy Association**
34 W 6th St., 1C
Helena, MT 59601
**Phone:** (406)449-3843     **Fax:** (406)443-1592
**Email:** jimesmith@qwest.net
**Website:** http://www.rxmt.org
Jim Smith, Exec Director

## Nebraska

**★ 17661 ★ Nebraska Pharmacists Association**
6221 S 58th St., Ste. A
Lincoln, NE 68516
**Phone:** (402)420-1500     **Fax:** (402)420-1406
**Email:** gary@npharm.org
**Website:** http://www.npharm.org
Gary J. Cheloha, R.Ph., Exec VP

## Nevada

**★ 17662 ★ Nevada Pharmacy Alliance**
PO Box 95277
Las Vegas, NV 89193
**Phone:** (702)433-7133     **Fax:** (702)435-2177
**Email:** nvphall@lvdi.net
Mary Grear, R.Ph., Exec VP

## New Hampshire

**★ 17663 ★ New Hampshire Pharmacists Association**
2 Eagle Sq., Ste. 400
Concord, NH 03301-4956
**Phone:** (603)229-0292     **Fax:** (603)224-7769
Elizabeth Gower, RPh, Exec Director

## New Jersey

**★ 17664 ★ New Jersey Pharmacists Association**
760 Alexander Rd.
PO Box 1
Princeton, NJ 08543-0001
**Phone:** (609)275-4246     **Fax:** (609)275-4066
**Email:** njpharm@aol.com
**Website:** http://www.njpha.com
Joe Morris, CEO

## New Mexico

**★ 17665 ★ New Mexico Pharmaceutical Association**
4800 Zuni SE
Albuquerque, NM 87108
**Phone:** (505)265-8729     **Fax:** (505)255-8476
**Email:** d_tinker@nm-pharmacy.com
**Website:** http://www.NM-pharmacy.com
R. Dale Tinker, Exec Director

## New York

**★ 17666 ★ Pharmacists Society of the State of New York**
201 Washington Ave. Ext.
Albany, NY 12203
**Free:** 800-632-8822     **Fax:** (518)464-0618
**Email:** craigb@pssny.org
**Website:** http://www.pssny.org
Craig Burridge, CAE, Exec Director
**Frmly:** Pharmaceutical Society of the State of New York.

## North Carolina

**★ 17667 ★ North Carolina Association of Pharmacists**
109 Church St.
Chapel Hill, NC 27516
**Phone:** (919)962-2237     **Fax:** (919)968-9430
**Email:** fred@ncpharmacists.org
**Website:** http://www.ncpharmacists.org
Fred Eckel, R.Ph., Contact
**Frmly:** North Carolina Pharmaceutical Association.

## North Dakota

**★ 17668 ★ North Dakota Pharmaceutical Association**
1906 E Broadway Ave.
Bismarck, ND 58501-4700
**Phone:** (701)258-4968     **Fax:** (701)258-9312
**Email:** ndpha@nodakpharmacy.com
**Website:** http://www.nodakpharmacy.com
Galen Jordre, R.Ph., Exec VP

## Ohio

**★ 17669 ★ Ohio Pharmacists Association**
6037 Frantz Rd., Ste. 106
Dublin, OH 43017
**Phone:** (614)798-0037     **Fax:** (614)798-0978
**Email:** eboyd@ohiopharmacists.org
**Website:** http://www.ohiopharmacists.org
Ernest Boyd, PD,CAE, Exec Director

## Oklahoma

**★ 17670 ★ Oklahoma Pharmacists Association**
Box 18731
45 NE 52nd St.
Oklahoma City, OK 73154
**Phone:** (405)528-3338     **Fax:** (405)528-1417
**Email:** pwoodward@opha.com
**Website:** http://www.opha.com
Phil Woodward, Exec Director
**Frmly:** Oklahoma Pharmaceutical Association.

## Oregon

**★ 17671 ★ Oregon State Pharmacists Association**
29702-B SW Town Center Loop
Wilsonville, OR 97070
**Phone:** (503)582-9055     **Fax:** (503)582-9046
**Email:** tomh@oregonpharmacists.com
**Website:** http://www.oregonpharmacists.com
Tom Holt, Exec Director

## Pennsylvania

**★ 17672 ★ Pennsylvania Pharmacists Association**
508 N 3rd St.
Harrisburg, PA 17101-1199
**Phone:** (717)234-6151     **Fax:** (717)236-1618
**Email:** ppa@papharmacists.com
**Website:** http://www.papharmacists.com
Carmen DiCello, R.Ph., Exec Director

## Puerto Rico

**★ 17673 ★ Colegio de Farmaceuticos de Puerto Rico**
PO Box 360206
San Juan, PR 00936-0206
**Phone:** (787)753-7157     **Fax:** (787)759-9793
**Email:** cfpr2000@coqui.net
Milagros Morales, R.Ph., Exec Director

## Rhode Island

**★ 17674 ★ Rhode Island Pharmacists Association**
500 Prospect St.
Pawtucket, RI 02860
**Phone:** (401)725-4141     **Fax:** (401)725-9960
**Email:** ripharm@aol.com
**Website:** http://www.ripharm.com

## South Carolina

**★ 17675 ★ South Carolina Pharmacy Association**
1350 Browning Rd.
Columbia, SC 29210
**Phone:** (803)354-9977     **Fax:** (803)354-9207
**Email:** jbracewell@scpharmacyassociation.org
**Website:** http://www.scpharmacyassociation.org
Jim Bracewell, Exec VP

## South Dakota

**★ 17676 ★ South Dakota Pharmacists Association**
514 W Elizabeth
Pierre, SD 57501-0518
**Phone:** (605)224-2338     **Fax:** (605)224-1280
**Email:** director2@sdpha.org
**Website:** http://www.sdpha.org
Bob Coolidge, Exec Director
**Frmly:** South Dakota Pharmaceutical Association.

## Tennessee

**★ 17677 ★ Tennessee Pharmacists Association**
226 Capitol Blvd., Ste. 810
Nashville, TN 37219-1893
**Phone:** (615)256-3023     **Fax:** (615)255-3528
**Email:** bblack@tnpharm.org
**Website:** http://www.tnpharm.org
Baeteena Black, D.Ph., Exec Director

## Texas

**★ 17678 ★ Texas Pharmacy Association**
PO Box 14709
Austin, TX 78761-4709
**Phone:** (512)836-8350     **Fax:** (512)836-0308
**Email:** jmartin@txpharmacy.com
**Website:** http://www.txpharmacy.com
Jim Martin, R.Ph., Exec Director

## Utah

**★ 17679 ★ Utah Pharmaceutical Association**
1850 S Columbia Ln.
Orem, UT 84097-8036
**Phone:** (801)762-0452     **Fax:** (801)762-0454
**Email:** upha@upha.com
**Website:** http://www.upha.com
Reid L. Barker, Exec Director

## Vermont

**★ 17680 ★ Vermont Pharmacists Association**
PO Box 790
Richmond, VT 05477-0790
**Phone:** (802)434-3001     **Fax:** (802)434-4803
**Email:** vpaorg@aol.com
**Website:** http://www.vtpharmacists.org
Fred Dobson, PhD, Exec Director

## Virginia

**★ 17681 ★ Virginia Pharmacists Association**
5501 Patterson Ave., Ste. 200
Richmond, VA 23226
**Phone:** (804)285-4145     **Fax:** (804)285-4227
**Email:** rrsnead@erols.com
**Website:** http://pharmacy.su.edu/vpha
Rebecca Snead, R.Ph., Exec Director

## Washington

**★ 17682 ★ Washington State Pharmacists Association**
1501 Taylor Ave. SW
Renton, WA 98055-3139
**Phone:** (425)228-7171     **Fax:** (425)277-3897
**Email:** rshafer@u.washington.edu
**Website:** http://www.pharmcare.org
Rod Shafer, R.Ph., CEO

## West Virginia

**★ 17683 ★ West Virginia Pharmacists Association**
2003 Quarrier St.
Charleston, WV 25311-2212
**Phone:** (304)344-5302     **Fax:** (304)344-5316
**Email:** wvrds@aol.com
Richard Stevens, Exec Director

## Wisconsin

**★ 17684 ★ Pharmacy Society of Wisconsin**
701 Heartland Tr.
Madison, WI 53717
**Phone:** (608)827-9200     **Fax:** (608)827-9292
**Email:** cdecker@pswi.org
**Website:** http://www.pswi.org
Christopher Decker, R.Ph., CEO
**Frmly:** Wisconsin Pharmacists Association.

## Wyoming

**★ 17685 ★ Wyoming Pharmacists Association**
PO Box 2109
Glenrock, WY 82637
**Phone:** (307)436-8001     **Fax:** (307)436-8002
**Email:** wpha@juno.com
**Website:** http://www.wpha.net
Robert Smith, R.Ph., Exec Director

## Foundations & Other Funding Organizations

### Other Funding Organizations

**★ 17686 ★ American Association for Women Podiatrists (AAWP)**
c/o Rachel Wood
1207 S Park Victoria Dr.
Milpitas, CA 95035
**Phone:** (408)263-8141      **Fax:** (408)263-4746
**Email:** rwoodfoot@aol.com
**Website:** http://www.aawpinc.com
Dr. Corinne Kauderer, Pres.
**Desc:** Promotes the advancement of the educational, political, financial and social well-being of members. Provides networking opportunities, consulting and financial assistance to student members. Maintains speakers' bureau **Awards:** Founders Scholarship (annual) Female student member of AAWP.

**American College of Foot and Ankle Surgeons (ACFAS)**
*See:* Entry 19439

**★ 17687 ★ American Podiatric Medical Writers Association (APMWA)**
PO Box 750129
Forest Hills, NY 11375
**Phone:** (718)897-9700      **Fax:** (718)896-5747
**Email:** bblock@prodigy.net
**Website:** http://www.acfas.org/
Dr. Barry H. Block, Exec. Dir.
**Desc:** Podiatric medical writers. Promotes the improvement of writing on podiatric topics. **Awards:** Elizabeth H. Roberts Award (annual); Golden Quill Award (annual); Student Writers Award (annual).

**★ 17688 ★ American Society of Podiatric Dermatology (ASPD)**
c/o Dr. Steven Berlin
1901 Sulfer Spring Rd.
Baltimore, MD 21227-0378
**Fax:** (410)247-7329
Dr. Richard Chase, Contact
**Desc:** Doctors of podiatric medicine with demonstrated expertise in foot dermatology (100); candidates for D.P.M. degrees in colleges of podiatric medicine (400). Fosters research in podiatric dermatology; supports college-affiliated study groups; conducts semiannual continuing education programs; sponsors student affiliates. Maintains speakers' bureau; conducts research programs; sponsors competitions. **Awards:** Ortho Pharmaceutical Award (annual) for best paper on podiatric dermatology by a podiatric resident or medical student.

**★ 17689 ★ American Society of Podiatric Medical Assistants (ASPMA)**
2124 S Austin Blvd.
Cicero, IL 60804
**Phone:** (708)863-6303      **Free:** 888-88ASPMA
**Fax:** (708)863-5375
**Email:** SandraPMAC@aol.com
**Website:** http://www.aspma.org
Sandra Lohrentz, PMAC, Exec. Dir.
**Desc:** Podiatric assistants. Purposes are to hold educational seminars and to administer certification examinations. **Awards:** Scholarship; Zelda W. Vicha Memorial Scholarship Fund financial need and academic standing.

**★ 17690 ★ Fund for Podiatric Medical Education (FPME)**
9312 Old Georgetown Rd.
Bethesda, MD 20814
**Phone:** (301)581-9200      **Fax:** (301)530-2752
**Email:** mpgaujean@apma.org
**Website:** http://www.apma.org/fpme/fundmain.htm
Steven J. Berlin, Pres.
**Desc:** Open to all People who wish to join. Offers financial support to third and fourth year podiatric medical students. Awards scholarships. **Awards:** Scholarship (annual) offers financial support to third and fourth year podiatric medical students with highest financial and academic qualifications.

## Medical & Allied Health Schools

### Podiatry

*The following colleges of podiatric medicine are accredited by the Council on Podiatric Medical Education. For further information, contact the Council, or the American Podiatric Medical Association, at 9312 Old Georgetown Rd., Bethesda, MD 20814-1698, (301)571-9200, http://www.apma.org.*

### California

**★ 17691 ★ California College of Podiatric Medicine**
100 Corporate Pl., Ste. C
Vallejo, CA 94590
**Phone:** (707)558-1333      **Free:** 800-443-2276
**Website:** http://www.ccpm.edu
Clyde Taylor, President
Jeffrey C. Page, Director

### Florida

**★ 17692 ★ Barry University School of Graduate Medical Sciences College of Podiatric Medicine**
11300 NE 2nd Ave.
Miami Shores, FL 33161
**Phone:** (305)899-3249
**Website:** http://www2.barry.edu/vpaa-gms/podiatry.html
Jeanne O'Laughlin, PhD, Director
Chester A. Evans, Director

### Illinois

**★ 17693 ★ Finch University Dr. William M. Scholl College of Podiatric Medicine**
1001 N Dearborn St.
Chicago, IL 60610
**Phone:** (312)280-2880
**Website:** http://www.scholl.edu
Terence B. Albright, DPM, Director

### Iowa

**★ 17694 ★ Des Moines University College of Podiatric Medicine**
3200 Grand Ave.
Des Moines, IA 50312
**Phone:** (515)271-1464
**Website:** http://www.uomhs.edu/cpms/index.html
Robert T. Yoho, DPM, Director

### New York

**★ 17695 ★ New York College of Podiatric Medicine**
1800 Park Ave.
New York, NY 10035
**Phone:** (212)410-8000
**Website:** http://www.nycpm.edu
Louis L. Levine, Director
Michael J. Trepal, DPM, Director

### Ohio

**★ 17696 ★ Ohio College of Podiatric Medicine**
10515 Carnegie Ave.
Cleveland, OH 44106
**Phone:** (216)231-3300
**Website:** http://www.ocpm.edu
Thomas V. Melillo, DPM, Director
Vincent J. Hetherington, DPM, Director

### Pennsylvania

**★ 17697 ★ Temple University School of Podiatric Medicine**
8th at Race St.
Philadelphia, PA 19107

**Phone:** (215)625-5400
**Website:** http://www.pcpm.edu
John A. Mattiacci, Director

# National & International Organizations

★ **17698** ★ **Academy of Ambulatory Foot and Ankle Surgery (AAFS)**
1601 Walnut, Ste. 1005
Philadelphia, PA 19102
**Phone:** (215)569-3303      **Free:** 800-433-4892
Dr. Harriet Waloss, Program Coordinator
**Fnded:** 1972. **Mem:** 1,500. **Desc:** Podiatric physicians who advocate performing foot surgery in their offices or on an outpatient basis, thereby keeping patients ambulatory and able to function normally, and lowering the patients' medical costs. Promotes the advancement of podiatric surgical procedures that can eliminate the necessity of hospital admission. Sponsors national and regional continuing medical education seminars and semiannual research program. Compiles statistics. **Pub:** *Action Letter*, bimonthly. Newsletter. • *Journal of the Academy of Ambulatory Foot Surgery*, periodic. Journal. • Directory, periodic.

**American Academy of Podiatric Practice Management**
*See:* Entry 9685

★ **17699** ★ **American Association of Colleges of Podiatric Medicine (AACPM)**
1350 Piccard Dr., Ste. 322
Rockville, MD 20850
**Phone:** (301)990-7400      **Free:** 800-922-9266
**Fax:** (301)990-2807
**Email:** aacpmas@aacpm.org
**Website:** http://www.aacpm.org
Moraith G. North, Exec. Dir.
**Fnded:** 1932. **Mem:** 6. **Desc:** Professional organization of administrators, faculty, practitioners, students, and other individuals associated with podiatric medical education. Provides vocational guidance material for secondary schools and colleges. Conducts public affairs activities and legislative advocacy. Compiles statistics. **Frmly:** American Association of Colleges of Chiropody; (1970) American Association of Colleges of Podiatry.

★ **17700** ★ **American Association of Hospital Podiatrists (AAHP)**
8508 18th Ave.
Brooklyn, NY 11214
**Phone:** (718)259-1822      **Fax:** (718)259-4002
Frank Rinaldi, Exec. Dir.
**Fnded:** 1950. **Mem:** 800. **Desc:** A general specialty group of the American Podiatric Medical Association. Podiatrists (trained and certified persons dealing in the care and diseases of the foot) who are affiliated with hospitals. Seeks to: elevate the standards of podiatry practices in hospitals and health institutions; standardize hospital podiatry procedures, charting, recording forms, and methods; promote understanding among personnel in podiatry, medicine, and allied health professions; aid podiatrists in attaining institutional affiliations; assist in the educational and teaching programs of health institutions and hospitals; foster the development of podiatric internships and residencies in hospitals and institutions. Compiles statistics. **Pub:** *The Hospital Podiatrist*, annual. • Newsletter, annual.

★ **17701** ★ **American Association of Podiatric Physicians and Surgeons (AAPPS)**
1328 Southern Ave. SE, Ste. 200
Washington, DC 20032
**Phone:** (202)562-2777      **Fax:** (202)562-5351

**Email:** rsbenjamin@aol.com
**Website:** http://www.theaapps.com
Richard S. Benjamin, DPM, Exec. Sec.
**Fnded:** 1979. **Mem:** 1,500. **State Groups:** 14. **Desc:** Podiatrists. Seeks to represent members' interests and educate podiatrists and the public. Provides training and certification for podiatry and podiatric surgery. Offers accreditation to agencies providing podiatric services, education, or training; also provides podiatric peer review. Operates speakers' bureau and placement service; compiles statistics. **Pub:** *AAPPS Newsletter*, annual. Newsletter.

★ **17702** ★ **American Association for Women Podiatrists (AAWP)**
c/o Rachel Wood
1207 S Park Victoria Dr.
Milpitas, CA 95035
**Phone:** (408)263-8141      **Fax:** (408)263-4746
**Email:** rwoodfoot@aol.com
**Website:** http://www.aawpinc.com
Dr. Corinne Kauderer, Pres.
**Fnded:** 1965. **Mem:** 997. **Reg. Groups:** 14. **Desc:** Promotes the advancement of the educational, political, financial and social well-being of members. Provides networking opportunities, consulting and financial assistance to student members. Maintains speakers' bureau **Pub:** *AAWP Newsletter*, quarterly. Newsletter. *Price:* Included in membership dues; Free to students.

★ **17703** ★ **American Board of Podiatric Orthopedics and Primary Medicine (ABPOPPM)**
22910 Crenshaw Blvd., Ste. B
Torrance, CA 90505
**Phone:** (310)891-0100      **Fax:** (310)891-0500
**Email:** admin@abpoppm.org
**Website:** http://www.abpoppm.org/
Gerald A. Weber, DPM, Pres.
**Fnded:** 1975. **Mem:** 3,000. **Desc:** Podiatrists who have taken a competency exam prepared by the board. Offers certifying examinations in podiatric orthopedics and primary podiatric medicine aims at improving public health by encouraging and elevating standards for practicing podiatrics. **Pub:** *ABPOPPM Newsletter*, semiannual. Newsletter. *Price:* Free w/ membership. • *Directory of Diplomates*, annual. Membership Directory. Includes alphabetical and geographical listing of members. *Price:* Free. **Frmly:** American Board of Podiatric Orthopedics.

★ **17704** ★ **American Board of Podiatric Surgery (ABPS)**
3330 Mission St.
San Francisco, CA 94110-5009
**Phone:** (415)826-3200      **Fax:** (415)826-4640
**Email:** info@abps.org
**Website:** http://www.abps.org
James A. Lamb, Exec. Dir.
**Fnded:** 1975. **Mem:** 4,200. **Desc:** Podiatrists certified as diplomates. Objectives are: to protect and improve public health by advancing the science of foot surgery and by encouraging the study and evaluation of standards of foot surgery; to act upon application for certification of legally licensed podiatrists to ascertain their competency in foot surgery; to grant certificates to candidates who have met all qualifications.

★ **17705** ★ **American College of Foot and Ankle Orthopedics and Medicine (ACFAOM)**
3525 Ellicott Mills Dr., Ste. N
Ellicott City, MD 21042
**Free:** 800-265-8263      **Fax:** (410)418-4805
**Email:** info@acfaom.org
**Website:** http://www.acfaom.org/
Bret Ribotsky, DPM, Pres.
**Fnded:** 1949. **Mem:** 1,300. **Desc:** Professional society of podiatrists sanctioned as specialists to practice foot orthopedics (deformities and diseases of bones,

joints, and muscles of the foot) and primary podiatric medicine. **Pub:** *ACFAOM News*, quarterly. Newsletter. *Price:* $5 for nonmembers. **Frmly:** (1993) American CLG of Foot Orthopedists.

★ **17706** ★ **American College of Foot and Ankle Pediatrics (ACFAP)**
6477 College Park Sq.
Virginia Beach, VA 23464
**Phone:** (757)523-0414      **Fax:** (757)523-2047
Patrick Agnew, DPM, Pres.
**Fnded:** 1977. **Mem:** 200. **Desc:** Podiatric physicians and surgeons, general physicians and surgeons, psychologists, and physical therapists. Seeks to bring together all professionals interested in children's foot health. Goals are to: disseminate information; consider all forms of therapy of value in foot and ankle pediatrics; bring to all those interested the most advanced and valuable forms of therapy through publications, seminars, and research sessions; establish teaching courses on foot and ankle pediatrics so that more podiatric students will consider specializing in the field. Encourages individual research projects; maintains speakers' bureau. **Pub:** *ACP Abstracts*, bimonthly. Newsletter. • Newsletter, annual. **Frmly:** (1993) American College of Podopediatrics.

**American College of Foot and Ankle Surgeons (ACFAS)**
*See:* Entry 19482

★ **17707** ★ **American College of Podiatric Medical Review (ACPMR)**
c/o Dr. Craig Gastwirth, Secretary
3800 Woodward Ave., Ste. 318
Detroit, MI 48201
**Phone:** (313)833-3090
**Email:** drpod1215@aol.com
**Website:** http://www.acpmr.org
Douglas Stoker, DPM, Pres.
**Fnded:** 1190. **Mem:** 65. **Desc:** Licensed podiatric professionals. Works to elevate standards, improve education, standardize guidelines, develop universal methods for peer and claims review. Clearinghouse and liaison for the podiatric medical profession, the public and government agencies.

★ **17708** ★ **American College of Podiatric Radiologists (ACPR)**
VA Medical Ctr.
Rte. 9
Martinsburg, WV 25401
Irving H. Block, D.P.M., Sec. -Treas.
**Fnded:** 1944. **Mem:** 80. **Desc:** Professional society of podiatrists interested in the use and interpretation of X-rays in treating ailments of the lower extremities. Sponsors postgraduate seminars on podiatric radiology; supports research. Makes available 1400 volume archives to members. Maintains speakers' bureau. **Pub:** *Post Convention Reports*, 1-2/year. • Newsletter, 2-4/year. **Frmly:** (1962) American College of Chiropodial Roentgenologists; (1974) American College of Foot Roentgenologists.

★ **17709** ★ **American Council of Certified Podiatric Physicians and Surgeons**
6421 Inkster Rd., Ste. 102
Bloomfield Hills, MI 48301
**Phone:** (248)855-7740      **Fax:** (248)855-7743
**Email:** accpps@juno.com
**Website:** http://www.accpps.com
Howard L. Lazar, DPM,JD, Exec. Dir.
**Fnded:** 1982. **Mem:** 650. **Desc:** Promotes the profession of podiatric medicine and surgery. Gains equal acceptance for all podiatrists by hospitals and managed care organizations.

**★ 17710 ★ American Podiatric Medical Association (APMA)**
9312 Old Georgetown Rd.
Bethesda, MD 20814-1621
**Phone:** (301)581-9200 **Free:** 800-ASK-APMA
**Fax:** (301)530-2752
**Email:** askapma@apma.org
**Website:** http://www.apma.org
Glenn B. Gastwirth, DPM

**Fnded:** 1912. **Mem:** 10,500. **State Groups:** 53. **Desc:** Professional society of doctors of podiatric medicine. **Pub:** *APMA News*, monthly. Magazine. Includes calendar of events, research updates, and statistics. *Price:* Included in membership dues; $50/year for nonmembers. • *Desk Reference of the APMA*, annual. • *Journal of the American Podiatric Medical Association*, monthly. Journal. *Price:* Included in membership dues; $90 for non-members. • Also publishes foot health literature. **Frmly:** (1958) National Association of Chiropodists; (1984) American Podiatry Association.

**★ 17711 ★ American Podiatric Medical Students Association (APMSA)**
9312 Old Georgetown Rd.
Bethesda, MD 20814
**Phone:** (301)493-9667
**Website:** http://www.apmsa.org/
Jennifer Wiggins, Exec. Dir.

**Fnded:** 1954. **Mem:** 2,000. **Desc:** Podiatric medical students enrolled at seven podiatric schools in the U.S. Purpose is to represent the interests of podiatric medical students in legislative, professional, and educational programs. Cosponsors seminars and writing contests. Compiles statistics. **Pub:** *First Step*, quarterly. Newsletter. • *Graduation Handbook*, annual. Reference guide. **Frmly:** American Podiatric Students Association.

**American Podiatric Medical Writers Association (APMWA)**
*See:* Entry 12067

**★ 17712 ★ American Society of Podiatric Dermatology (ASPD)**
c/o Dr. Steven Berlin
1901 Sulfer Spring Rd.
Baltimore, MD 21227-0378
**Fax:** (410)247-7329
**Email:** bblock@prodigy.net
Dr. Richard Chase, Contact

**Fnded:** 1914. **Mem:** 260. **Desc:** Doctors of podiatric medicine with demonstrated expertise in foot dermatology (100); candidates for D.P.M. degrees in colleges of podiatric medicine (400). Fosters research in podiatric dermatology; supports college-affiliated study groups; conducts semiannual continuing education programs; sponsors student affiliates. Maintains speakers' bureau; conducts research programs; sponsors competitions. **Pub:** Monographs. • Newsletter, quarterly. Includes book reviews, information on new products, and obituaries. *Price:* Free. **Frmly:** (1973) American Board of Chiropodical Dermatology.

**★ 17713 ★ American Society of Podiatric Medical Assistants (ASPMA)**
2124 S Austin Blvd.
Cicero, IL 60804
**Phone:** (708)863-6303 **Free:** 888-88ASPMA
**Fax:** (708)863-5375
**Email:** SandraPMAC@aol.com
**Website:** http://www.aspma.org
Sandra Lohrentz, PMAC, Exec. Dir.

**Fnded:** 1964. **Mem:** 1,350. **Nat'l Groups:** 1. **Reg. Groups:** 14. **Desc:** Podiatric assistants. Purposes are to hold educational seminars and to administer certification examinations. **Pub:** Journal, quarterly. *Price:* Free to members.

**★ 17714 ★ American Society of Podiatric Medicine (ASPM)**
c/o Dr. Warren L. Simmonds
1111 Kane Concourse Ste. 111
Miami, FL 33154-2039
Dr. Warren L. Simmonds, Sec.

**Fnded:** 1944. **Mem:** 110. **Desc:** Promotes research in podiatry. Sponsors postgraduate courses and presents scientific programs at annual meeting. Focuses on aging and diabetes. Maintains collection of material presented by candidates for fellowship. Maintains speakers' bureau; conducts research programs. **Frmly:** American Academy of Chiropody.

**★ 17715 ★ American Society of Podiatrists and Chiropractors (ASPC)**
PO Box 35189
Chicago, IL 60707-0189
**Phone:** (708)453-0080 **Fax:** (708)453-0083
**Email:** aspc@rentamark.com
**Website:** http://www.rentamark.com/aspc/
L. Stroller, Contact

**Fnded:** 1975. **Mem:** 58,989. **Nat'l Groups:** 1. **Desc:** Podiatrists and chiropractors. Seeks to increase members' public visibility and professional influence. Provides trademark licensing and product and service endorcement services to support members' activities. A platform to network Podiatrists and Chiropractors with patients on the net. **Pub:** *ASPC Journal*. Journal. Online journal.

**★ 17716 ★ Board for Certification in Pedorthics (BCP)**
7150 Columbia Gateway Dr., Ste. G
Columbia, MD 21046-1151
**Phone:** (410)381-5729 **Free:** 800-560-2025
**Fax:** (410)381-1167
**Email:** info@cpeds.org
**Website:** http://www.cpeds.org
William Boettge, Exec. Dir.

**Fnded:** 1958. **Mem:** 1,332. **Desc:** Certified Pedorthists. (Pedorthists fit and provide prescription footwear, footwear modifications and foot orthoses to clients referred by physicians.) Sponsors certification program; sets standards of practice in pedorthics and requires continuing education of certificants to maintain certification. **Pub:** *Pedorthic Candidate's Handbook*, annual. • *Study Guide for Pedorthic Skills Examination*.

**★ 17717 ★ Canadian Podiatric Medical Association (CPMA) (Association Medicale Podiatrique Canadienne — AMPC)**
45 Sheppard Ave. E, Ste. 900
Toronto, ON, Canada M2N 5W9
**Phone:** (416)927-9111 **Free:** 888-220-3668
**Fax:** (416)733-2491
**Email:** info@podiatrycanada.org
**Website:** http://podiatrycanada.org

**Fnded:** 1924. **Mem:** 250. **Nat'l Groups:** 1. **Reg. Groups:** 4. **Lang(s):** English, French. **Desc:** Podiatrists recognized by the DPM designation. Seek to advance the study, teaching, and practice of podiatric medicine. Facilitates communication and cooperation among members; formulates and enforces standards of ethics and practice for the field of podiatry; sponsors continuing professional development programs.

**★ 17718 ★ Council on Podiatric Medical Education (CPME)**
9312 Old Georgetown Rd.
Bethesda, MD 20814-1621
**Phone:** (301)571-9200 **Free:** 800-275-2762
**Fax:** (301)530-2752
**Email:** askapma@apma.org
**Website:** http://www.apma.org
Richard B. Viehe, Pres.

**Fnded:** 1918. **Mem:** 11. **Desc:** Accrediting agency for colleges of podiatric medicine, podiatric residency programs and continuing education programs in podiatry. Conducts in-service training programs for members engaged in accrediting activities. **Pub:** *Council on Podiatric Medical Education–Annual Report*. Annual Report. • *Standards and Requirements for Accreditation*. • Also publishes lists of accredited institutions and approved programs. **Frmly:** (1984) Council on Podiatry Education.

**★ 17719 ★ Federation of Podiatric Medical Boards (FPMB)**
c/o Larry Shane, Exec. Dir.
PO Box 880187
Boca Raton, FL 33488-0187
**Phone:** (561)477-3060
**Website:** http://www.fpmb.org/
Larry I. Shane, Exec. Dir.

**Fnded:** 1936. **Mem:** 45. **State Groups:** 52. **Desc:** State boards of podiatry examiners. Goals are to: serve as a repository for information relating to common problems among boards of podiatry examiners; promote competency examinations with national standards to be utilized by examining boards; monitor and catalog legislation pertaining to podiatry. Conducts business sessions and educational programs on topics concerning the licensure and regulation of health professions. Compiles statistics. **Pub:** *Disciplinary Data Reports*, semiannual. • *Federation News*, quarterly. Bulletin. *Price:* Included in membership dues. **Frmly:** (1985) Federation of Podiatry Boards; (1986) Federation of Podiatry Medical Boards.

**★ 17720 ★ Fund for Podiatric Medical Education (FPME)**
9312 Old Georgetown Rd.
Bethesda, MD 20814
**Phone:** (301)581-9200 **Fax:** (301)530-2752
**Email:** mpgaujean@apma.org
**Website:** http://www.apma.org/fpme/fundmain.htm
Steven J. Berlin, Pres.

**Fnded:** 1959. **Desc:** Open to all People who wish to join. Offers financial support to third and fourth year podiatric medical students. Awards scholarships.

**★ 17721 ★ Institute of Chiropodists and Podiatrists**
27 Wright St.
Southport PR9 0TL, United Kingdom
**Phone:** 44 1704 546141 **Fax:** 44 1704 500477
**Email:** editor@inst-chiropodist.org.uk
**Website:** http://www.inst-chiropodist.org.uk

**Fnded:** 1938. **Mem:** 2,500. **Local Groups:** 31. **Desc:** State registered and non-state registered chiropodists. Members governed by strict code of ethics. Third party surgery risks insurance provided for members. **Pub:** *Chiropody Review*, bimonthly. Journal. Journal for chiropodists and podiatrists. **Frmly:** (1997) Institute of Chiropodists.

**★ 17722 ★ National Board of Podiatric Medical Examiners (NBPME)**
PO Box 510
Bellefonte, PA 16823
**Phone:** (814)357-0487 **Fax:** (814)357-0581
**Email:** nbpmeofc@aol.com
Charles W. Gibley, Exec. Dir.

**Fnded:** 1956. **Mem:** 12. **Desc:** Professional podiatrists. Purpose is to prepare and administer examinations for podiatry students seeking state licensure. Monitors test validity and reliability. **Pub:** Annual Report. • Bulletin, annual. • Membership Directory, annual. **Frmly:** (1985) National Board of Podiatry Examiners.

**★ 17723 ★ National College of Foot Surgeons (NCFS)**
c/o Dr. Albert Apkarian
PO Box 264
Woodland, CA 95776-0264
**Phone:** (818)340-0616
Dr. Albert Apkarian, Sec.

**Fnded:** 1960. **Desc:** Doctors of surgical podiatry. Certifies foot surgeons as fellows and associates of the college. Holds seminars and courses; conducts research programs. Maintains speakers' bureau and hall of fame. **Pub:** Journal, annual.

### ★ 17724 ★ National Podiatric Medical Association (NPMA)

c/o Raymond E. Lee, D.P.M.
1706 E 87th St.
Chicago, IL 60617
**Phone:** (773)374-1616　　　**Fax:** (773)374-5860
**Email:** npmadebby1@aol.com
Dr. Johndelle Jenkins, D.P.M., Contact

**Fnded:** 1971. **Mem:** 200. **Desc:** Minority podiatrists, predominately black. Promotes the science and art of podiatry. Seeks to: improve public health; raise the standards of the podiatric profession and education; stimulate a favorable relationship between all podiatrists; nurture growth and diffusion of podiatric information; stimulate public education concerning public health and features of podiatric medicine. Sponsors proposal of podiatric laws; works to eliminate religious and racial discrimination and segregation in American medical institutions. **Pub:** *Annual Seminar Ad Book.* • *National Podiatric Medical Association–Newsletter*, annual. Newsletter. Includes calendar of events and news from student-affiliated associations. *Price:* Included in membership dues. **Frmly:** (1987) National Podiatry Association.

### ★ 17725 ★ Society of Chiropodists and Podiatrists

1 Fellmongers Path, Tower Bridge Rd.
London SE1 3LY, United Kingdom
**Phone:** 44 207 2348620　　　**Fax:** 44 207 2348621
**Email:** enq@scpod.org
**Website:** http://www.feetforlife.org

**Fnded:** 1945. **Mem:** 7,800. **Lang(s):** English. **Desc:** State registered chiropodists. The principal activities are to fulfill both a pre-registration and post-registration education function, to act as a trade union for its members employed in the National Health Service, to monitor the professional and ethical conduct and standards of its members, to publish professional journals, and to fulfil a public relations role. **Pub:** *The Journal of British Podiatric Medicine*, quarterly. Journal. Features articles on podiatric research. • *Podiatry Now*, monthly. Journal.

## Research Centers

### ★ 17726 ★ Temple University Gait Study Center

School of Podiatric Medicine
8th & Race Sts.
Philadelphia, PA 19107
**Phone:** (215)625-5366　　　**Fax:** (215)629-0278
**Email:** hhillstrom@tuspm.temple.edu
**Website:** http://podiatry.temple.edu/gaitlab/index2.htm
Dr. Howard Hillstrom, Dir.

**Activities/Fields:** Posture and locomotion studies, focusing on the causes of abnormal gait conditions. Conducts basic and clinical research in biomechanics and biomedical engineering with special emphasis on the lower extremities. Areas of interest include the functional role of in-shoe orthoses and insoles; the role of conservative realignment and innovative therapies to treat osteoarthritis; the etiology and management of neuropathic ulcers in the diabetic foot; and optimization of foot and ankle surgeries and related fixation parameters.

## State Government Agencies

### Podiatry Boards

### ★ 17727 ★ Alabama State Board of Podiatric Medicine

13 Innisbrook Ln
Birmingham, AL 35242
**Phone:** (205)995-8537　　　**Fax:** (205)595-8537
**Email:** AlPodBoard@aol.com
**Website:** http://members.aol.com/alpodboard/index.html
Gail Clark, Contact

### ★ 17728 ★ Alaska State Medical Board

PO Box 110806
Juneau, AK 99811-0806
**Phone:** (907)269-8163　　　**Fax:** (907)269-8196
**Email:** leslie_gallant@dced.state.ak.us
**Website:** http://www.dced.state.ak.us/occ/pmed.htm
Leslie A. Gallant, Contact

### ★ 17729 ★ Arizona State Board of Podiatry Examiners

1400 W Washington, Ste. 230
Phoenix, AZ 85007
**Phone:** (602)542-3095
**Website:** http://www.revenue.state.az.us/609/licensingguide.htmPROFESSION

### ★ 17730 ★ Arkansas State Podiatry Examining Board

2001 Georgia Ave.
Little Rock, AR 72207-5014
**Phone:** (501)664-3668

### ★ 17731 ★ California Board of Podiatric Medicine

1420 Howe Ave., Ste. 8
Sacramento, CA 95825-3229
**Phone:** (916)263-2647　　　**Fax:** (916)263-2651
**Email:** bpm@dca.ca.gov
**Website:** http://www.dca.ca.gov/bpm/index.html
James Rathlesberger, Contact

### ★ 17732 ★ Colorado Podiatry Board

1560 Broadway, Ste. 1545
Denver, CO 80202
**Phone:** (303)894-2464　　　**Fax:** (303)894-7885
**Email:** podiatrists@dora.state.co.us
**Website:** http://www.dora.state.co.us/Podiatrists/
Kevin D. Heupel, Contact

### ★ 17733 ★ Connecticut Board of Podiatry Licensure

410 Capitol Ave.
PO Box 340308
Hartford, CT 06134-0308
**Phone:** (860)509-7562
**Website:** http://www.ct-clic.com/detail.asp?code=1763

### ★ 17734 ★ District of Columbia Board of Podiatry

825 N Capital St NE, 2nd floor
Washington, DC 20002
**Phone:** (202)442-4778　　　**Fax:** (202)442-9431
**Website:** http://dchealth.dc.gov/prof_license/services/boards_main.asp

### ★ 17735 ★ Florida Board of Podiatric Medicine

4052 Bald Cypress Way, Bin C-07
Tallahassee, FL 32399-3257
**Phone:** (850)245-4355　　　**Fax:** (850)922-8876
**Email:** mqa_podiatry@doh.state.fl.us
**Website:** http://www.doh.state.fl.us/mqa/index.html
Joe Baker, Jr., DIR

### ★ 17736 ★ Georgia State Board of Podiatry

237 Coliseum Dr.
Macon, GA 31217-3858
**Phone:** (478)207-1686　　　**Fax:** (478)207-1363
**Email:** rfthompson@sos.state.ga.us
**Website:** http://www.sos.state.ga.us/plb/
Anita O. Martin, Director

### ★ 17737 ★ Hawaii Board of Podiatric Medicine

DCCA-PVL
PO Box 3469
Honolulu, HI 96801
**Phone:** (808)586-2708
**Email:** medical@dcca.state.hi.us
**Website:** http://www.state.hi.us/dcca/pvl/areas_medical.html
Constance Cabral-Makanani, Director

### ★ 17738 ★ Idaho State Board of Podiatry Bureau of Occupational Licenses

1109 Main St., Ste. 220
Boise, ID 83702-5642
**Phone:** (208)334-3233　　　**Fax:** (208)334-3945
**Email:** csimpson@ibol.state.id.us
**Website:** http://www2.state.id.us/ibol/pod.htm

### ★ 17739 ★ Illinois Department of Professional Regulation Podiatry Examining Committee

320 W Washington St.
Springfield, IL 62786
**Phone:** (217)785-0800　　　**Fax:** (217)782-7645
**Website:** http://www.dpr.state.il.us

### ★ 17740 ★ Indiana Health Professions Bureau Board Podiatric Medicine

402 W Washington, Rm. W041
Indianapolis, IN 46204-2739
**Phone:** (317)234-2064
**Email:** hpb5@hpb.state.in.us
**Website:** http://www.in.gov/hpb/boards/bpm/
Wade A. Lowhorn, Director

### ★ 17741 ★ Iowa Bureau of Professional Licensing Iowa Board of Podiatry Examiners

Lucas State Office Bldg., 5th Fl.
321 E 12th St.
Des Moines, IA 50319-0075
**Phone:** (515)242-6385　　　**Fax:** (515)281-3121
**Email:** jmanning@idph.state.ia.us
**Website:** http://www.iowaccess.org/idph_pl/podiatry/index.html

### ★ 17742 ★ Kansas Board of Healing Arts

235 SW Topeka Blvd.
Topeka, KS 66603-3068
**Phone:** (785)296-7413　　　**Fax:** (785)296-0852
**Email:** Healer3@ink.org
**Website:** http://www.ksbha.org/

### ★ 17743 ★ Kentucky Board of Podiatry

906B S 12th St.
Murray, KY 42071-2947
**Phone:** (270)759-0007

### ★ 17744 ★ Louisiana State Board of Medical Examiners

630 Camp St.
PO Box 30250
New Orleans, LA 70190-0250
**Phone:** (504)568-6820　　　**Fax:** (504)599-0503

**Email:** lsbmever@lsbme.org
**Website:** http://www.lsbme.org/

★ 17745 ★ **Maine Office of Licensing and Registration**
**Board of Podiatric Examiners**
35 State House Station
Augusta, ME 04333-0035
**Phone:** (207)624-8626      **Fax:** (207)624-8637
**Email:** diane.l.staples@state.me.us
**Website:** http://www.state.me.us/pfr/olr/categories/cat33.htm

★ 17746 ★ **Maryland Board of Podiatric Medicine Examiners**
4201 Patterson Ave.
Baltimore, MD 21215-2299
**Phone:** (301)764-4785      **Fax:** (410)740-8692
**Website:** http://www.cmeonline.com/state/maryland.html

★ 17747 ★ **Massachusetts Board of Examiners in Podiatry**
239 Causeway St., Ste. 500
Boston, MA 02114
**Phone:** (617)727-4499      **Fax:** (617)727-2197
**Email:** hansy.noel@state.ma.us
**Website:** http://www.magnet.state.ma.us/reg/boards/pd/default.htm

★ 17748 ★ **Michigan Consumer and Industry Services**
**Bureau of Health**
**Board of Podiatric Medicine and Surgery**
PO Box 30670
Lansing, MI 48909-8170
**Phone:** (517)335-0918      **Fax:** (517)373-2179
**Email:** bhserinfo@cis.state.mi.us
**Website:** http://www.michigan.gov/cis/

★ 17749 ★ **Minnesota Board of Podiatric Medicine**
2829 University Ave. SE, Ste. 430
Minneapolis, MN 55414-3246
**Phone:** (612)617-2200
**Website:** http://www.mnworkforcecenter.org/lmi/lic_occ/podiatri.htm
Joan Benesh, Director

★ 17750 ★ **Mississippi State Board of Medical Licensure**
PO Box 9268
Jackson, MS 39286-9268
**Phone:** (601)987-3079      **Fax:** (601)987-4159
**Email:** mboard@msbml.state.ms.us
**Website:** http://www.msbml.state.ms.us/

★ 17751 ★ **Missouri State Board of Podiatric Medicine**
3605 Missouri Blvd.
PO Box 423
Jefferson City, MO 65102
**Phone:** (573)751-0873      **Fax:** (573)751-1155
**Email:** podiatry@mail.state.mo.us
**Website:** http://www.ecodev.state.mo.us/pr/podiatry/
Patricia A. Handly, Director

★ 17752 ★ **Montana Department of Labor and Industry**
**Business Standards Division**
**Health Care Licensing Bureau**
301 S Park
Room 430
Helena, MT 59602
**Phone:** (406)841-2300      **Fax:** (406)841-2305
**Email:** vmanuel@state.mt.us
**Website:** http://www.discoveringmontana.com/dli/bsd/license/licensing_boards.htm

★ 17753 ★ **Nebraska Department of Health and Human Services**
**Regulation and Licensure**
**Credentialing Division**
PO Box 94986
Lincoln, NE 68509-4986
**Phone:** (402)471-2115      **Fax:** (402)471-3577
**Email:** marie.mcclatchey@hhs.state.ne.us
**Website:** http://www.hhs.state.ne.us/reg/regindex.htm

★ 17754 ★ **Nevada State Board of Podiatric Medicine**
PO Box 12215
Reno, NV 89510-2215
**Phone:** (775)789-2605
**Website:** http://podiatry.state.nv.us/

★ 17755 ★ **New Hampshire Board of Registration in Podiatry**
2 Industrial Park Dr.
Ste. 8
Concord, NH 03301
**Phone:** (603)271-1203      **Fax:** (603)271-6702
**Website:** http://webster.state.nh.us/podiatry/
Brian Fradette, Director

★ 17756 ★ **New Jersey State Board of Medical Examiners**
PO Box 183
Trenton, NJ 08625-0183
**Phone:** (609)826-7100
**Website:** www.state.nj.us/lps/ca/medical.htmbme5
William Roeder, Director

★ 17757 ★ **New Mexico Board of Podiatric Medicine**
2055 Pacheco St., Ste. 300
Santa Fe, NM 87504
**Phone:** (505)476-7096
**Email:** PodiatryBoard@state.nm.us
**Website:** http://www.rld.state.nm.us/b&c/podiatry_board.htm

★ 17758 ★ **New York State Board of Podiatry**
Office of the Professions
State Education Bldg., 2nd Fl.
Albany, NY 12234
**Phone:** (518)474-3817      **Fax:** (518)474-1449
**Email:** podbd@mail.nysed.gov
**Website:** http://www.op.nysed.gov/pod.htm

★ 17759 ★ **North Carolina Board of Podiatry Examiners**
1500 Sunday Dr.
Ste. 102
Raleigh, NC 27607
**Phone:** (919)561-5583      **Fax:** (919)787-4916
**Email:** info@ncbpe.org
**Website:** http://www.ncbpe.org/

★ 17760 ★ **North Dakota Board of Registry in Podiatry**
PO Box 400
Bismarck, ND 58502-0400
**Phone:** (701)223-2890      **Fax:** (701)223-7865
**Website:** http://www.governor.state.nd.us/boards/boards_query.asp?Board_id=84
Gary R. Thune, Director

★ 17761 ★ **Ohio State Medical Board**
77 S High St., 17th Fl.
Columbus, OH 43266-0315
**Phone:** (614)466-3934      **Free:** 800-554-7717
**Fax:** (614)728-5946
**Website:** http://www.state.oh.us/med/

★ 17762 ★ **Oklahoma Board of Medical Licensure and Supervision**
**Board of Podiatry**
5104 N Francis, Ste. C
PO Box 18256
Oklahoma City, OK 73154-0256
**Phone:** (405)848-6841      **Fax:** (405)848-8240

★ 17763 ★ **Oregon Board of Medical Examiners**
1500 SW 1st Ave., Ste. 620
Portland, OR 97201
**Phone:** (503)229-5770      **Free:** 877-254-6263
**Fax:** (503)229-6543
**Email:** bme.info@state.or.us
**Website:** http://www.bme.state.or.us

★ 17764 ★ **Pennsylvania State Board of Podiatry**
PO Box 2649
Harrisburg, PA 17105-2649
**Phone:** (717)783-4858      **Fax:** (717)787-7769
**Email:** podiatry@pados.state.pa.us
**Website:** http://www.dos.state.pa.us/bpoa/site/default.asp

★ 17765 ★ **Puerto Rico Board of Podiatry Examiners**
Call Box 10200
San Juan, PR 00908-0200
**Phone:** (787)725-8161      **Fax:** (787)725-7903

★ 17766 ★ **Rhode Island Podiatry Board**
3 Capitol Hill, Rm. 104
Providence, RI 02908
**Phone:** (401)222-2827      **Fax:** (401)222-1272
**Email:** RussellS@doh.state.ri.us
**Website:** http://www.healthri.org/hsr/professions/podiat.htm
Russell Spaight, Contact

★ 17767 ★ **South Carolina Board of Podiatric Medicine**
Synergy Business Park
Kingstree Bldg.
110 Centerview Dr, suite 202
PO Box 11289
Columbia, SC 29211-1289
**Phone:** (803)896-4685      **Fax:** (803)896-4515
**Email:** podiatry@mail.llr.state.sc.us
**Website:** http://www.llr.state.sc.us/POL/Podiatry/Default.htm
John Volmer, Contact

★ 17768 ★ **South Dakota Board of Podiatry**
135 E Illinois, Ste. 214
Spearfish, SD 57783
**Phone:** (605)642-1600      **Fax:** (605)642-1756
**Email:** proflic@rushmore.com
**Website:** http://www.state.sd.us/dcr/podiatry/podhome.htm
Carol Tellinghuisen, Contact

★ 17769 ★ **Tennessee State Board of Registration in Podiatry**
Cordell Hull Bldg., 1st Fl.
425 Fifth Ave. N
Nashville, TN 37247-1010
**Phone:** (615)532-3202
**Website:** http://www.tennesseeanytime.org

★ 17770 ★ **Texas State Board of Podiatric Medical Examiners**
333 Guadalupe St., Ste 2-320
PO Box 12216
Austin, TX 78711-2216
**Phone:** (512)305-7000      **Fax:** (512)305-7003
**Email:** allen.hymans@foot.tx.state.us

**Website:** http://www.foot.state.tx.us/
Allen Hymans, Contact

**★ 17771 ★ Utah Division of Occupational
and Professional Licensing**
160 E 300 S, 4th Fl.
PO Box 146741
Salt Lake City, UT 84114-6741
**Phone:** (801)530-6628          **Fax:** (801)530-6511
**Website:** http://www.dopl.utah.gov/directory.html

**★ 17772 ★ Vermont Board of Medical
Practice**
109 State St.
Montpelier, VT 05609-1106
**Phone:** (802)828-2673          **Fax:** (802)828-5450
**Email:** gloria.hurd@medbd.state.vt.us
**Website:** http://www.docboard.org/vt/vermont.htm
Gloria Hurd, Director

**★ 17773 ★ Virginia Department of Health
Professions**
**Virginia Board of Medicine**
6606 W Broad St., 4th Fl.
Richmond, VA 23230-1717

**Phone:** (804)662-9908          **Fax:** (804)662-9517
**Email:** medbd@dhp.state.va.us
**Website:** http://www.dhp.state.va.us/medicine/default.htm/
William L. Harp, MD, Director

**★ 17774 ★ Washington State Department
of Health**
**Health Professions Quality Assurance**
**Washington State Podiatric Medical
Board**
1300 SE Quince St.
PO Box 47860
Olympia, WA 98504-7860
**Phone:** (360)236-4700          **Fax:** (360)236-4818
**Email:** hpqa.csc@doh.wa.gov
**Website:** https://wws2.wa.gov/doh/hpqa-licensing/HPS7/Podiatry/default.htm

**★ 17775 ★ West Virginia State Board of
Medicine**
101 Dee Dr.
Charleston, WV 25311
**Phone:** (304)558-2921          **Fax:** (304)558-2084
**Email:** ronaldwalton@wvdhhr.org

**Website:** http://www.wvdhhr.org/wvbom/
Ronald D. Walton, Director

**★ 17776 ★ Wisconsin Department of
Regulation and Licensing**
**Wisconsin Podiatry Examining Board**
1400 E Washington Ave.
PO Box 8935
Madison, WI 53708-8935
**Phone:** (608)266-2811
**Email:** web@drl.state.wi.us
**Website:** http://badger.state.wi.us/agencies/drl/Regulation/applicant_information/dod135.html

**★ 17777 ★ Wyoming Board of
Registration in Podiatry**
2020 Carey Ave., Ste. 201
Cheyenne, WY 82002
**Phone:** (307)777-3507          **Fax:** (307)777-3508
**Website:** http://www.state.wy.us/governor/boards/bdlist.asp
Nanette M. Brown, Contact

# Chapter 53
# Preventive Medicine

## Federal Government Agencies

★ 17778 ★ **U.S. Department of Health and Human Services**
**Centers for Disease Control and Prevention**
**National Center for Chronic Disease Prevention and Health Promotion**
1600 Clifton Rd. NE
Atlanta, GA 30333
**Phone:** (404)639-3311
**Website:** http://www.cdc.gov/nccdphp/index.htm

★ 17779 ★ **U.S. Department of Health and Human Services**
**Centers for Disease Control and Prevention**
**National Center for Injury Prevention and Control**
1600 Clifton Rd. NE
Atlanta, GA 30333
**Phone:** (404)639-3311
**Website:** http://www.cdc.gov/ncipc/ncipchm.htm

## Foundations & Other Funding Organizations

### Private Foundations

★ 17780 ★ **Bullitt Foundation**
1212 Minor Ave.
Seattle, WA 98101-2825
**Phone:** (206)343-0807      **Fax:** (206)343-0822
**Email:** info@bullitt.org
**Website:** http://www.bullitt.org
Marilyn Fike, Administrator
**Fnded:** 1952. **Philosophy:** The purpose of the Bullitt Foundation is to protect and restore the natural physical environment. During the past year the foundation has given grants solely to environmental causes. Gifts are confined to the Pacific Northwest. The foundation has seven specific priorities among environmental issues. *Energy and Climate Change.* "The foundation will promote a swift transition toward the efficient use of energy sources that are safe, sustainable, and environmentally attractive." *Forests and Land Ecosystems.* "The foundation seeks to maintain species endemic to the Northwest, and the ecosystems on which they depend, and to safeguard the beauty, natural wealth, and recreational activities of the region." *Growth Management and Transportation.* "The foundation supports efforts to promote land-use policies and practices that protect environmentally sensitive areas; accommodate agriculture, fisheries, and forestry; and promote communities in which residential, commercial, industrial, and civic functions are integrated." *Public Outreach, Education, and Capacity Building.* "The foundation supports projects that educate the public, promote stewardship, ensure adequate funding and support for quality environmental education in schools, and encourage more informed and active voters." *Rivers, Wetlands, and Estuaries.* "The foundation strives to protect aquatic resources, from the pure water of mountain streams to the productive richness of marine environments." *Sustainable Agriculture.* "The foundation supports efforts that preserve farmlands, conserve biodiversity, and foster sustainable agricultural policies and practices." *Toxic Substances, Mining, and Radioactive Waste.* "The foundation supports efforts to advance policies and practices that reduce toxic substance use, eliminate the release of toxic substances, reform destructive mining practices, and clean up areas already contaminated by toxic substances." The foundation will also consider environmental proposals that do not fall within the seven priority areas, but that do fall within its geographic area and overall mission. Bullitt Foundation Annual Report **Priorities:** *Civic & Public Affairs:* 4%. *Environment:* 2%. *Note:* Contributions made in fiscal 2000. **Typ. Recipients:** Preventive Medicine/Wellness Organizations. **Geo. Dist:** AK, Coastal Rainforests; ID; MT, Western part of state; OR; WA; BC.

★ 17781 ★ **Castle Rock Foundation**
4100 East Mississippi Ave., Ste. 1850
Denver, CO 80246
**Phone:** (303)388-1636      **Fax:** (303)388-1684
**Email:** generalinfo@castlerockfdn.org
Sally Rippey, Contact
**Fnded:** 1993. **Philosophy:** "The mission of the Castle Rock Foundation is to: promote a better understanding of the free enterprise system; preserve the principles upon which our democracy was founded, to help ensure a limited role for government and the protection of individual rights as provided for in the Constitution; encourage personal responsibility and leadership; and to uphold traditional Judeo-Christian values." **Priorities:** *Arts & Humanities:* 7%. Supports museums and historical preservation. *Civic & Public Affairs:* 38%. Supports civic and public affairs, civil rights, and law and justice. *Education:* 33%. Supports educational institutions programs, leadership training, economics education, and colleges. *International:* 8%. Supports cancer research and treatment. *Note:* Total contributions were made in fiscal 2000. **Typ. Recipients:** Cancer, Clinics/Medical Centers, Health Policy/Cost Containment, Medical Research, Preventive Medicine/Wellness Organizations. **Geo. Dist:** nationally.

★ 17782 ★ **Corbett Foundation**
127 West 9th St., Ste. 3
Cincinnati, OH 45202
**Phone:** (513)241-3320      **Fax:** (513)723-4422
Karen McKim, Executive Director
**Fnded:** 1958. **Philosophy:** "Grants are generally restricted to the field of cultural arts and education and community projects; however, to the extent the funds are available, grants may be made for other purposes." In recent years, the foundation has made major grants to the University of Cincinnati College Conservatory of Music for capital improvements. **Priorities:** *Arts & Humanities:* About 17%. Focus is primarily in the Cincinnati area. *Civic & Public Affairs:* 14%. Supports festivals and a city park. *Education:* 68%. Includes $1,000,000 grant to the University of Cincinnati. *Note:* Total contributions made in fiscal 1999. **Typ. Recipients:** Alzheimers Disease, Nutrition, Preventive Medicine/Wellness Organizations, Substance Abuse. **Geo. Dist:** Cincinnati, OH.

**Louise Taft Semple Foundation**
*See:* Entry 7872

**Turner Foundation**
*See:* Entry 733

## Corporate Foundations

★ 17783 ★ **Medtronic Foundation**
7000 Central Ave., NE
Minneapolis, MN 55432
**Phone:** (612)514-3029      **Fax:** (612)514-3464
**Website:** http://www.medtronic.com/foundation
Penny Hunt, Executive Director, Community Affairs
**Priorities:** *Civic & Public Affairs:* 27%. Community grants are made to strengthen communities and specifically to improve the lives of people who are socio-economically disadvantaged through grants to selected human service, arts and culture, and civic programs. United Ways are supported by Medtronic employees through employee campaigns. Supports human service programs that benefit disadvantaged children and youth and their families; programs of arts organizations that increase access to the arts by people who are disadvantaged; civic organizations that address the needs of the disadvantaged; and cultural organizations that make significant contributions to the life of the community. *Education:* 30%. Supports K-12 education, with focus on kindergarten through grade 12 science education programs under STAR (Science and Technology Are Rewarding), a grant initiative designed to stimulate and sustain the interest of young people in science. Limited funding is available for creative programs that have a lasting impact on children. Post-secondary education is supported with grants in programs that benefit those traditionally underrepresented in science, technology, engineering or health, socio-economically disadvantaged students and women. Local education in operating communities is also supported. *International:* 43%. Grants are provided under the Medtronic Healthy Tomorrows Programs to programs and projects that directly impact the lives of community members who are most in need. Supports projects that: serve economically disadvantaged people, cultural communities, and those most vulnerable in operating communities; address the need to strengthen the capacity of communities, violence, access to health care, and developing and maintaining healthy lifestyles; involve the people most affected by the problem in defining and then delivering the solutions; emphasize prevention of health problems, including outreach efforts,

support groups, health education, and supportive services; and include partnerships and collaborations in the sponsorship of programs. Special consideration is given to projects that focus on diseases or conditions that are addressed by Medtronic as a business, including: heart disease, neurological disorders, incontinence, sleep apnea, and chronic pain. The Full Life Patient Partnership engages patients, providers, and policymakers to improve the quality of health care for people with chronic disease through three national programs: Patient Link, Health Leadership Grants, and HeartRescue. Medtronic also supports the Healthy Countries initiative, providing funding for disease prevention and treatment in parts of China, India, Mexico, and Eastern Europe. *Voluntarism:* Supports the Medtronic Volunteer Program (MVP) and the Time N Talent Fund. *Note:* Total contributions made in fiscal 2001. **Typ. Recipients:** Adolescent Health Issues, Cancer, Children's Health/Hospitals, Clinics/Medical Centers, Emergency/Ambulance Services, Geriatric Health, Health Organizations, Health Policy/Cost Containment, Health-General, Heart, Hospitals, Long-Term Care, Medical Education, Medical Education, Nursing Services, Preventive Medicine/Wellness Organizations, Public Health, Trauma Treatment. **Geo. Dist:** internationally in Medtronic plant communities; nationally in Medtronic plant communities; Minneapolis, MN, metropolitan area; St. Paul, MN, metropolitan area.

★ **17784** ★ **Pheonix Foundation**
2090 Palm Beach Lakes Boulevard, Ste. 700
West Palm Beach, FL 33409
**Phone:** (561)640-5898
Maria Ornelas, Director

**Fnded:** 1957. **Priorities:** *Arts & Humanities:* 29%. Primarily supports museums and art centers. *Civic & Public Affairs:* 30%. Supports justice and community foundations. *Environment:* 16%. Supports Boy Scouts and United Way. *Note:* Total contributions made in 1999. **Typ. Recipients:** Preventive Medicine/Wellness Organizations, Public Health. **Geo. Dist:** FL.

**Scripps Howard Foundation**
*See:* Entry 8555

★ **17785** ★ **Weyerhaeuser Co. Foundation**
CH1 L32
PO Box 9777
Federal Way, WA 98063-9777
**Phone:** (253)924-3159 **Fax:** (253)924-3658
**Email:** cottingham@scripps.com
**Website:** http://www.weyerhauser.com/community/
Elizabeth Crossman, Vice President

**Priorities:** *Arts & Humanities:* 9%. Special emphasis is placed on projects promoting rural access to the arts. *Civic & Public Affairs:* 16%. Housing component promotes low-income and affordable housing, primarily to further public/private partnerships. Some awards are also made for projects that will have a significant impact on housing policies. The civic and community initiatives and facilities segment is limited to Weyerhaeuser's major communities, with emphasis on Seattle-Tacoma, WA area. In most cases, the foundation will not consider requests that are in excess of 10% of the project's cost. *Education:* 40%. One-time grants to colleges and universities in Weyerhaeuser operating locations for research, curriculum, and for issues related to the forest products industry. Also supports curriculum improvement and scholarships to community colleges, usually in disciplines related to careers in the forest products industry. Elementary and secondary schools receive support for efforts leading to district-wide improvements in public schools. Two scholarship programs are offered for children of employees. Mississippi, Oklahoma, North Carolina, and Arkansas are current priorities. *Environment:* 20%. Housing, United Way, family services, and youth organizations. *International:* 3%. Supports preventive healthcare services that show a reasonable promise of reducing costs. Grants for facilities are normally considered only in key Weyerhaeuser locales where no other services are available. No awards are made to national-level organizations. The foundation sup-

ports the United Way as the primary means for helping with critical human services. *Religion:* 1%. *Note:* Total contributions made in 1999. **Typ. Recipients:** Children's Health/Hospitals, Clinics/Medical Centers, Emergency/Ambulance Services, Hospices, Hospitals, People with Disabilities, Public Health, Substance Abuse. **Geo. Dist:** nationally, with emphasis on communities, particularly remote communities, in which company has significant numbers of employees; AL; AR; MS; NC; OK; OR; WA.

## Other Funding Organizations

**Lifegain Institute (LI)**
*See:* Entry 16033

★ **17786** ★ **National Wellness Institute**
PO Box 827
Stevens Point, WI 54481-0827
**Phone:** (715)342-2969 **Free:** 800-244-8922
**Fax:** (715)342-2979
**Email:** nwi@nationalwellness.org
**Website:** http://www.nationalwellness.org
Anne Helmke, Dir. Member Services

**Desc:** Purposes are to provide national leadership in the wellness movement; to assist professionals working in health and wellness promotion in all types of settings; and organizations with planning, development, implementation, and evaluation of wellness programs; and to assist in the development of high quality wellness products and services. Acts as clearinghouse on wellness information. Provides consultations; offers professional development conferences. Sponsors National Wellness Association. **Awards:** National Wellness Institute Research Merit Award (annual) for original research in health and wellness not yet published.

## National & International Organizations

★ **17787** ★ **Aerobics and Fitness Association of America (AFAA)**
15250 Ventura Blvd., Ste. 200
Sherman Oaks, CA 91403
**Phone:** 800-446-2322 **Free:** 877-968-7263
**Fax:** (818)788-6301
**Email:** contactafaa@afaa.com
**Website:** http://www.afaa.com
Linda D. Pfeffer, R.N., Pres.

**Fnded:** 1983. **Mem:** 145,000. **Desc:** Promotes safety and excellence in exercise instruction. World's largest fitness educator offering certifications in Aerobics, Personal Training, Weightroom, Step, KickBoxing, Emergency Response and the AFAA Fitness Practioner. **Pub:** *American Fitness*, bimonthly. Magazine. Features exercise trends, research, interviews, products, health, and nutrition. *Price:* $27 /year for nonmembers. • *Fitness Theory and Practice.* Book.

**American Association for Health Freedom**
*See:* Entry 4205

★ **17788** ★ **American Board of Preventive Medicine (ABPM)**
330 S Wells St., Ste. 1018
Chicago, IL 60606
**Phone:** (312)939-2276 **Fax:** (312)939-2218
**Email:** abpm@abprevmed.org
**Website:** http://www.abprevmed.org
James M. Vanderploeg, MD,MPH, Exec. Dir.

**Fnded:** 1948. **Mem:** 16. **Desc:** Determines requirements, administers examinations, and certifies qualified physicians in the specialty areas of public health and general preventive medicine, aerospace medicine, and occupational medicine. **Pub:** *ABPM Booklet of Information.* Booklet. Covers board requirements. *Price:* Free. • *Study Guide.* Includes outlines of

examinations. **Frmly:** (1952) American Board of Preventive Medicine and Public Health.

★ **17789** ★ **American College for Advancement in Medicine (ACAM)**
23121 Verdugo Dr., Ste. 204
Laguna Hills, CA 92653
**Phone:** (949)583-7666 **Fax:** (949)455-9679
**Email:** acam@acam.org
**Website:** http://www.acam.org
Edward A. Shaw, PhD, Exec. Officer

**Fnded:** 1973. **Mem:** 535. **Desc:** Physicians organized for the promotion of preventive medicine throughout the world. Conducts research and educational programs in the fields of chelation therapy, nutritional medicine, and other preventive modalities. Maintains physician referrals. Offers specialized education program; compiles statistics. **Pub:** *ACAM Update*, monthly. Newsletter. Contains abstracts on issues and developments in preventive medicine. Includes book reviews and calendar of events. *Price:* Included in membership dues. • *Journal of Advancement in Medicine*, quarterly. Journal. Covers research and clinical applications pertaining to preventive and nutritional medicine. *Price:* Included in membership dues. • Membership Directory, annual. **Frmly:** (1987) American Academy of Medical Preventics.

★ **17790** ★ **American College of Preventive Medicine (ACPM)**
1307 New York Ave. NW, No. 200
Washington, DC 20005
**Phone:** (202)466-2044 **Fax:** (202)466-2662
**Email:** info@acpm.org
**Website:** http://www.acpm.org
Dorothy Lane, MD, Pres.

**Fnded:** 1954. **Mem:** 2,200. **Desc:** Professional society of medical doctors specializing in preventive medicine, public health, aerospace medicine, and occupational medicine. Sponsors educational programs. **Pub:** *ACPM News*, quarterly. Newsletter. Reports on continuing medical education, legislative activities, and programs of the college. Includes calendar of events and research updates. *Price:* Included in membership dues; $25/year for nonmembers. • *American Journal of Preventive Medicine*, bimonthly. Journal. • *Careers in Preventive Medicine.* • *Directory of Residency Programs*, periodic. Directory.

★ **17791** ★ **American Council on Exercise (ACE)**
4851 Paramount Dr.
San Diego, CA 92123-1449
**Phone:** (858)535-8227 **Free:** 800-825-3636
**Fax:** (858)535-1778
**Email:** acemail@acefitness.org
**Website:** http://www.acefitness.org
Jean Walcher, PR Dir.

**Fnded:** 1985. **Desc:** Certifies fitness professionals and non-profit organization. Keeps them aware of new information in the health and fitness industry. Offers continuing education programs. Sponsors children's services. Provides consumers with health and fitness research and information. **Pub:** *ACE Certified News*, bimonthly. Newsletter. For ACE-certified fitness professional. • *ACE Faculty Network.* • *Ace Fitness/Matters*, bimonthly. Magazine. *Price:* $25/year; $60/3 years; $33/year in North America; $49 outside North America.

★ **17792** ★ **American Health Foundation (AHF)**
300 E 42nd St.
New York, NY 10017-5947
**Phone:** (212)953-1900 **Fax:** (212)687-2339
**Email:** Vbaker60@yahoo.com
**Website:** http://www.ahf.org
Dr. Daniel Nixon, Pres.

**Fnded:** 1969. **Desc:** Devoted to promoting preventive medicine, emphasizing four major fields: research (nutrition, environmental carcinogenesis, molecular biology, experimental pathology, and epidemiology); clinical research and service for children (through screening and intervention); public health action (educating laymen and medical and government personnel in the principles of preventive medicine); health economics research (investigating direct and indirect costs of major diseases and comparing them with preventive approaches). in New York City. in New York City. **Pub:** *Preventive Medicine*, monthly. Journal. Contains scientific, preventive medicine and public health information. *Price:* $264 institutional subscription; $132 personal subscription. **Frmly:** (1968) Environmental Health Foundation.


**★ 17793 ★ American Institute for Preventive Medicine**
30445 Northwestern Hwy., Ste. 350
Farmington Hills, MI 48334
**Phone:** (248)539-1800     **Free:** 800-345-2476
**Fax:** (248)539-1808
**Email:** aipm@healthy.net
**Website:** http://www.healthylife.com
Dr. Don R. Powell, Pres.

**Fnded:** 1983. **Desc:** Not an association. Consulting firm.Conducts educational programs. Maintains speakers' bureau. **Pub:** *A Year of Health Hints - 365 Practical Ways to Feel Better and Live Longer. Price:* $23.95. • *Being a Wise Healthcare Consumer.* • *Guide to Mental Fitness.* • *Guide to Self Care.* • *Health at Home: Your Complete Guide to Symptoms, Solutions, and Self Love.* Book. *Price:* $17.95. • *Healthy Self: The Guide to Self Care and Wise Consumers.* Book. *Price:* $7.95. • *Hotlines to Health Directory,* annual. Directory. *Price:* $2.95. • *Self Care: Your Family Guide to Symptoms and How to Treat Them.* Book. *Price:* $14.95. • *Seniors Health at Home.* Book. *Price:* $19.95.


**★ 17794 ★ American Osteopathic College of Occupational and Preventive Medicine (AOCOPM)**
PO Box 2606
Leesburg, VA 20177
**Free:** 800-558-8686     **Fax:** (703)443-0567
**Email:** aocopm@starpower.net
**Website:** http://www.aocopm.org/homepage.htm
**Fnded:** 1995. **Desc:** Designed to promote the public health and practice of preventive medicine in order to create a better understanding of the relationship of health and prevention in regard to the wellness of the population. Provides a three-part basic course in occupational/environmental medicine.


**★ 17795 ★ American Society of Preventive Oncology (ASPO)**
c/o Dr. Richard R. Love
256 WARF Bldg.
610 Walnut St.
Madison, WI 53705
**Phone:** (608)263-9515     **Fax:** (608)263-4497
**Email:** hasahel@facstaff.wisc.edu
**Website:** http://www.aspo.org
Heidi Sahel, Exec. Dir.

**Fnded:** 1976. **Mem:** 400. **Desc:** Professionals in clinical, educational, or research disciplines concerned with the field of cancer prevention. Promotes the exchange of information and ideas relating to cancer prevention and the causes of human cancer, including environmental exposures and lifestyles; encourages research. Works to implement programs for the prevention and early detection of cancer. Evaluates programs intended to reduce cancer incidence, mortality, and morbidity. Encourages professional and public education regarding cancer prevention. Maintains communication and liaison with other oncological societies. Provides expert advice to scientific, public health, and governmental organizations and agencies. **Pub:** *Cancer Epidemiology, Biomarkers, and Prevention*, monthly. Journal.


**Asian Academy of Preventive Dentistry (AAPD)**
*See:* Entry 6463


**★ 17796 ★ Asian Committee for Standardization of Physical Fitness Tests (ACSPFT)**
Seijo Haimu
3-11-2-404 Soshigaya
Setagaya-ku
Tokyo 157, Japan
**Phone:** 81 3 4848915
**Email:** sakaio1@college.fdcnet.ac.jp

**Lang(s):** English, Japanese. **Desc:** Physical fitness agencies and organizations. Promotes formulation and use of standardized tests for determining an individual's physical fitness. Serves as a forum for the discussion of mutual interest to members; develops model physical fitness tests.


**★ 17797 ★ Association of Teachers of Preventive Medicine (ATPM)**
1660 L St. NW, Ste. 206
Washington, DC 20036
**Phone:** (202)463-0550     **Free:** (866)474-ATPM
**Fax:** (202)463-0555
**Email:** info@atpm.org
**Website:** http://www.atpm.org
Barbara J. Calkins, MA, Exec. Dir.

**Fnded:** 1942. **Mem:** 900. **Desc:** Dedicated to advancing individual and community health promotion and disease prevention in the education of physicians and other health professionals. Individual members are teachers, researchers, practitioners, administrators, residents and students. Institutional members include preventive medicine and related departments in medical schools, schools and graduate programs in public health and preventive medicine, other health professions schools and various health agencies. **Pub:** *American Journal of Preventive Medicine*, bimonthly. Journal. • *ATPM News Now!*, weekly. Newsletter. An electronic newsletter. • *ATPM Quarterly*, quarterly. Newsletter. • *Directory and Profile of Academic Units in Preventive Medicine*, periodic. Directory. **Frmly:** (1955) Conference of Professors of Preventive Medicine.


**★ 17798 ★ Canadian Fitness and Lifestyle Research Institute (CFLRI) (Institute Canadien de la Recherche sur la Condition Physique et le Mode de Vie — ICRCP)**
185 Somerset St. W, Ste. 201
Ottawa, ON, Canada K2P 0J2
**Phone:** (613)233-5528     **Fax:** (613)233-5536
**Email:** info@cflri.ca
**Website:** http://www.cflri.ca
**Fnded:** 1980. **Mem:** 8. **Lang(s):** English, French. **Desc:** Conducts research on physical activities in Canada and distributes information about physical activity. **Pub:** *The Research File*, 4/year. Contains summaries of research on physical activity.


**Cancer Control Society (CCS)**
*See:* Entry 10143


**★ 17799 ★ Cooper Institute for Aerobics Research**
12330 Preston Rd.
Dallas, TX 75230
**Phone:** (972)341-3200     **Free:** 800-635-7050
**Fax:** (972)341-3227
**Email:** courses@cooperinst.org
**Website:** http://www.cooperinst.org
Mark Donovan, Controller

**Fnded:** 1970. **Desc:** Goals are to promote understanding of the relationship between living habits and health, to provide leadership in enhancing the physical and emotional well-being of individuals, and to promote participation in aerobics. Seeks to increase the

quality and quantity of fitness programs within major institutions. Conducts innovative studies on health and living habits and methods of facilitating changes in living habits; promotes the awareness and skills needed to develop a positive life-style. Sponsors workshops and seminars; conducts weekly training course and certification testing of fitness leaders in education, government, human services, and corporate sectors. **Frmly:** (2000) Institute for Aerobics Research.


**★ 17800 ★ Estonian Health Protection Association (Eesti Tervikaitse Selts)**
Mardit.3
EE-10146 Tallinn, Estonia
**Phone:** 372 2 6607026     **Fax:** 372 2 6607870
**Email:** h.tkt@neti.ee

**Fnded:** 1967. **Mem:** 200. **Local Groups:** 20. **Lang(s):** English, German. **Desc:** Promotes better health care for people living in Estonia. **Pub:** *Estonian Health Protection Association 1967-1992.* Brochure. Contains information on 25 years of the association.


**European Cancer Prevention Organization (ECP)**
*See:* Entry 10162


**★ 17801 ★ Exercise Safety Association (ESA)**
PO Box 3340
Spring Hill, FL 34611-3340
**Phone:** (352)683-5246     **Fax:** (352)666-7862
**Email:** askesa@aol.com
**Website:** http://www.exercisesafety.com
Sharon Foy, Dir.

**Fnded:** 1978. **Mem:** 20,000. **Local Groups:** 150. **Desc:** Fitness instructors, personal trainers, health spas, YMCAs, community recreation departments, and hospital wellness programs. Purposes are: to improve the qualifications of exercise instructors; to train instructors to develop safe exercise programs that will help people avoid injury while exercising; to prepare instructors for national certification. Offers training in aerobics and exercise and on the physiological aspects of exercise. Conducts exercise safety and research programs. Sponsors charitable program; maintains speakers' bureau. Offers instructor placement services. **Pub:** *ESA Member Directory*, annual. Membership Directory. • *Exercise Safety Association Newsletter*, bimonthly. Newsletter. Provides exercise information based on current scientific research. Includes schedule of upcoming programs. *Price:* Included in membership dues. **Frmly:** Exer-Safety Association; (1985) International Exer-Safety Association.


**★ 17802 ★ Fitness Industry Association**
115 Eastbourne Mews
London W2 6LQ, United Kingdom
**Phone:** 44 207 2986730     **Fax:** 44 207 2986731
**Email:** info@fia.org.uk
**Website:** http://www.fia.org.uk

**Fnded:** 1989. **Mem:** 1,400. **Desc:** Operators, suppliers, educational establishments, and professionals in the fitness industry. Aims to raise standards across the industry via the publicising of the Code of Practice. **Pub:** *Club Business International*, monthly. Magazine. Provides health club indstry news. • *Health Club Management*, monthly. • *Leisure Management Magazine*, monthly. Magazine. • *Leisure Opportunities.*


**★ 17803 ★ Fitness Motivation Institute of America Association (FMIAA)**
428 Airport Blvd.
Watsonville, CA 95076
**Phone:** (831)761-9898     **Free:** 800-538-7790
**Fax:** (831)761-9899
**Email:** info@fmia.com
**Website:** http://www.fmia.com
C. Travis Watkins, Pres.

**Fnded:** 1971. **Desc:** Persons involved with health and physical fitness. Works to motivate, educate, activate, and evaluate individuals in the area of physical fitness. Program is based on four parameters: why the body needs exercise; what a fit body is; methods of getting fit; motivation to stay fit. Offers quarterly training session. **Pub:** *Fitfacts Journal*, quarterly. Journal. Provides new ideas on using Isorobics exercise programs. *Price:* $25/year. • *Fitness Motivation Institute of America Association–Newsletter*, bimonthly. Newsletter. Reports on the fitness industry. *Price:* available to members only.

### ★ 17804 ★ Harvard Injury Control Research Center (HICRC)

Harvard School of Public Health
677 Huntington Ave., 3rd Fl.
Boston, MA 02115
**Phone:** (617)432-3420          **Fax:** (617)432-3699
**Email:** hicrc@hsph.harvard.edu
**Website:** http://www.hsph.harvard.edu/hicrc
David Hemenway, PhD, Dir.

**Fnded:** 1998. **Desc:** A comprehensive CDC-funded Center. Primary activity is the interdisciplinary study of the causes and etiology of injury among vulnerable populations and applications for primary prevention and intervention strategies and policy. Areas of focus are violence - primarily youth and family violence - and cross-cutting issues - including alcohol and drug use, firearm use and treatment setting. Also offers graduate courses, internships, conferences, trainings, grand rounds, and a Seminar Series, and provides technical assistance to State Health Departments and Regional Networks. **Frmly:** (1998) Injury Control Center; (2001) Injury Control Research Center.

### Hong Kong Anti-Cancer SOC (HKACS)
*See:* Entry 10178

### ★ 17805 ★ IDEA, The Health and Fitness Source

6190 Cornerstone Ct. E, Ste. 204
San Diego, CA 92121-3773
**Phone:** (619)535-8979          **Free:** 800-999-IDEA
**Fax:** (858)535-8234
**Email:** member@ideafit.com
**Website:** http://www.ideafit.com
Kathie Davis, Exec. Dir.

**Fnded:** 1982. **Mem:** 23,000. **Desc:** Provides continuing education for fitness professionals including; fitness instructors, personal trainers, program directors, and club/studio owners. Offers workshops for continuing education credits. **Pub:** *Gearing Up: How to Evaluate and puchase Quality Home Exercise Equipment*. Brochure. • *Get Active: How to Make Activity A Habit and Change Your Life*. Brochure. • *Get Real: A Personal Guide to Real-Life Weight Management*. Book. Contains information on weight management. • *Get Real: 8 Keys to Healthy Sensible Weight Management*. Brochure. • *IDEA Fitness Manager*, 5/yr.Newsletter. • *IDEA Health & Fitness Source*, 10/year. Magazine. Includes articles on exercise science, teaching techniques, and business management. Also includes annual index to articles and calendar of events. *Price:* Included in membership dues. • *IDEA Personal Trainer*, 10/year. Magazine. Includes marketing client relationship and business information. • *Personal Best: How to Choose the Personal Trainer Who's Right For You*. Brochure. • *Young At Heart: How to Preserve Your Health with Active Living at any Age!*. Brochure. • Brochures. • Pamphlets. • Videos. **Frmly:** (1982) IDEA: International Dance Exercise Association; (1989) IDEA: The Association for Fitness Professionals; (1997) Idea, The Health & Fitness Source.

### International and American Association of Clinical Nutritionists (IAACN)
*See:* Entry 16487

### International College for Health Cooperation in Developing Countries - Italy
### (CUAMM - Medici con l'Africa)
*See:* Entry 17947

### ★ 17806 ★ International Council for Physical Activity and Fitness Research (ICPAFR)

Faculty of Physical Education & Physiotherapy
Katholieke Universitet Leuven
Tervuursevest 101
B-3001 Leuven, Belgium
**Phone:** 32 16 329083          **Fax:** 32 16 329197
**Email:** albrecht.claessens@flok.kuleuven.ac.be
**Website:**          http://www.padovanet.it/associazioni/cuamm/casa.htm

**Fnded:** 1964. **Mem:** 140. **Nat'l Groups:** 36. **Lang(s):** English. **Desc:** Medical doctors, physiologists, anthropologists, biochemists, physical educators, and psychologists in 30 countries who have done substantial research on physical fitness. Promotes international comparative studies on the effect of physical fitness upon the welfare of children, adults, and the aged. Works toward establishing standardized physical fitness assessment and measurement procedures. Operates speakers' bureau. Maintains advisory committees for the establishment of a sports research center and for the facilitation of scientific cooperation in the preparation, execution, and publication of comparative studies. **Pub:** *Nutrition and Physical Activity*. • *Physical Fitness and the Ages of Man*. • *Physical Fitness Assessment: Principles, Practices and Application*. **Frmly:** (1978) International Committee on Physical Fitness Research; (1992) International Council for Physical Fitness Research.

### International Society for Preventive Oncology (ISPO)
*See:* Entry 10200

### ★ 17807 ★ Lifegain Institute (LI)
115 Dunder Rd.
Burlington, VT 05401
**Phone:** (802)862-8855          **Fax:** (802)862-6389
**Email:** info@healthyculture.com
**Website:** http://www.healthyculture.com
Judd Allen, PhD, Pres.

**Fnded:** 1977. **Mem:** 600. **Desc:** People who work with health promotion programs in hospitals, corporations, colleges, and communities. Promotes healthy practices such as exercise, nutrition, safety, and the reduction or curtailment of smoking and alcohol consumption through health promotion programs that provide a supportive environment. Maintains speakers' bureau. Compiles data on improvements cultural support nationwide. **Pub:** *American Journal of Health Promotion*, quarterly. Journal. • *Lifegain: A Culture-Based Approach to Positive Health*. Book. • *Lifegain Healthy Communities System*. • Articles. • Also publishes support materials. **AKA:** Human Resources Institute.

### ★ 17808 ★ Medical Fitness Association
PO Box 73103
Richmond, VA 23235-8026
**Phone:** (804)327-0330          **Free:** 888-675-2211
**Fax:** (804)327-1630
**Email:** mfacomm@aol.com
**Website:** http://medicalfitness.org
Cary Wing, EdD, Exec. Dir.

**Fnded:** 1991. **Mem:** 450. **Desc:** Hospitals, organizations, and medically based fitness and wellness center professionals. Seeks to reduce community health care costs through preventive care. Promotes strengthened operations and standards in fitness centers maintained by hospitals and organizations; works to improve the financial viability of fitness facilities. Serves as a network linking fitness professionals and facilities. Conducts research and educational programs; compiles statistics. **Pub:** *Medical Fitness Centers, 4th Edition*, biennial. Directory. Comprehensive Listing/Profile of Medical Fitness Centers In North America. *Price:* $295. • *Re:Source, Journal of the Medical Fitness Association*, quarterly. Journal. Contains industry news, center profiles, and programming ideas. **Frmly:** (1998) Association of Hospital Health and Fitness.

### ★ 17809 ★ National Association for Health and Fitness
401 W Michigan St.
Indianapolis, IN 46202-3233
**Phone:** (317)237-5630          **Fax:** (317)237-5632
**Email:** info@physicalfitness.org
**Website:** http://www.physicalfitness.org
Cindy Porteous, Exec. Dir.

**Fnded:** 1979. **Mem:** 200. **Reg. Groups:** 4. **State Groups:** 40. **Desc:** State governor's fitness councils. Works with state government to establish and maintain governor's councils on physical fitness and health. Seeks to promote the quality of life for individuals in the U.S. through physical fitness, sports, and healthy lifestyles. **Pub:** *NAGCPFS*, quarterly. Newsletter. *Price:* Free. **Frmly:** (2000) National Association of Governor's Councils on Physical Fitness and Sport.

### ★ 17810 ★ National Register of Personal Trainers (NRPT)
16 Borough High St.
London SE1 9QG, United Kingdom
**Phone:** 44 20 74079223          **Fax:** 44 20 74079225
**Email:** sarah@nrpt.co.uk
**Website:** http://www.nrpt.co.uk

**Fnded:** 1992. **Mem:** 1,000. **Desc:** Qualified fitness instructors available for one to one personal training throughout the UK. Representative and advisory body for personal fitness trainers in UK. Acts as a referral service for the general public when looking for a personal trainer; provides networking and secures the best possible services and products for personal trainers to enhance their professionalism. **Pub:** *NRPT News*, bimonthly. Newsletter. **Frmly:** (2001) National Register of Personal Fitness Trainers.

### ★ 17811 ★ National Wellness Institute
PO Box 827
Stevens Point, WI 54481-0827
**Phone:** (715)342-2969          **Free:** 800-244-8922
**Fax:** (715)342-2979
**Email:** nwi@nationalwellness.org
**Website:** http://www.nationalwellness.org
Anne Helmke, Dir. Member Services

**Fnded:** 1977. **Mem:** 2,000. **Desc:** Purposes are to provide national leadership in the wellness movement; to assist professionals working in health and wellness promotion in all types of settings; and organizations with planning, development, implementation, and evaluation of wellness programs; and to assist in the development of high quality wellness products and services. Acts as clearinghouse on wellness information. Provides consultations; offers professional development conferences. Sponsors National Wellness Association. **Pub:** *American Journal of Health Promotion*, bimonthly. Journal. • *Health Issues Update/Resource News*, bimonthly. Newsletter. An E-newsletter. *Price:* Included in membership dues. • *Health Promotion Practitioner*, bimonthly. Newsletter. An E-newsletter. • *Testwell Assessment Series*. • *Wellness Management*, quarterly. Newsletter. An e-newsletter. *Price:* Included in membership dues. • *Wellness Resource Directory*. Directory. • Brochures.

### ★ 17812 ★ SMARTRISK
790 Bay St.
Toronto, ON, Canada M5G 1N8
**Phone:** (416)977-7350          **Fax:** (416)596-2700
**Website:** http://www.smartrisk.ca

**Lang(s):** English, French. **Desc:** Works to reduce the number of injuries in Canada. Sponsors campaigns to raise public awareness of preventable causes of injury in automobiles, the home, and the workplace. **Frmly:** (2001) Canadian Injury Prevention Foundation.

**★ 17813 ★ Wellness Associates**
PO Box 8422
Asheville, NC 28814
**Phone:** (828)251-5594
**Email:** info@thewellspring.com
**Website:** http://www.thewellspring.com
John W. Travis, MD, Dir.
**Fnded:** 1975. **Desc:** Provides high quality resource materials for lifestyle improvement integrating the major components of wellness: self-responsibility, stress management, nutrition, and physical awareness. Expands wellness education into the fields of emotional and psychological health. Recognizes spiritual growth and the search for meaning to be essential elements in the experience of wellness. Offers wellness publications and resources for helping professionals to assist them in realizing the principles of wellness in their own lives and to help their clients experience their own capacity for good health and well-being. Provides consultation for wellness centers, individuals, universities, agencies, hospitals, and government groups. **Pub:** *A Change of Heart: The Global Wellness Inventory.* Book. *Price:* $8. • *Simply Well: Choices for a Healthy Life.* Book. *Price:* $9.95. • *Wellness for Helping Professionals.* Book. *Price:* $39. • *Wellness Index.* Booklet. *Price:* $4.95. • *Wellness Inventory.* Booklet. *Price:* $2.95. • *Wellness Workbook.* Book. *Price:* $19.95. **Frmly:** (1979) Wellness Resource Center.

**★ 17814 ★ Wellness Center (AWCI)**
145 W 28th St., Rm. 9R
New York, NY 10001
**Phone:** (212)465-8062
**Website:** http://wellness.ucdavis.edu/
Howard Moscow, Contact
**Fnded:** 1979. **Mem:** 1,500. **Desc:** Individuals concerned with wellness and preventive health care; firms, institutions, and organizations with wellness centers or employee assistance programs. Educates health practitioners and the public on methods of developing healthier lifestyles through the prevention and treatment of degenerative diseases and other health disorders. Provides professional training workshops in wellness counseling, an approach that integrates many scientific and medical disciplines, to assist members with problems related to weight control, stress, alcoholism, personal relationships, drug addiction, and other physical, mental, or social problems. Conducts individual and group counseling sessions and support groups. Provides speakers on topics such as wellness, lifestyle changes, longevity, diseases and alternative therapies. **Pub:** *Bibliographical Essay,* periodic. • *Directory of Members,* annual. Membership Directory. • *Life-Style for Wellness,* quarterly. Journal. Includes research reports, book reviews, and listings of employment opportunities. *Price:* $50/year. • *Mailing List,* periodic.

## Research Centers

**★ 17815 ★ American Health Foundation**
**Naylor Dana Institute for Disease Prevention**
1 Dana Rd.
Valhalla, NY 10595
**Phone:** (914)592-2600    **Fax:** (914)592-2317
**Website:** http://www.ahf.org
Joanne Braley, Libn.
**Activities/Fields:** Medicine, science, and social science, focusing on cancer, smoking and health, nutrition, and biology and chemistry.

**★ 17816 ★ American University**
**National Center for Health Fitness**
Nebraska Hall, Lower Level
4400 Massachusetts Ave. NW
Washington, DC 20016-8037
**Phone:** (202)885-6275    **Fax:** (202)885-6288
**Email:** dhfaa@american.edu

**Website:** http://www.healthy.american.edu
Robert C. Karch, Exec. Dir.
**Activities/Fields:** Worksite health promotion programs, focusing on costs, benefits, and cost-effectiveness, and including international health promotion and special populations. Consulting activities include health promotion program design, implementation, and management.

**★ 17817 ★ Arizona Health Services Department**
**Public Health Services**
**Office of Prevention and Health Promotion**
2700 N 3rd St., Ste. 4050
Phoenix, AZ 85004
**Phone:** (602)542-7200    **Fax:** (602)542-7520
**Email:** dcooper@hs.state.az.us
**Website:** http://www.hs.state.az.us/phs/ophp/
Dorothy Cooper, Contact
**Activities/Fields:** Health.

**★ 17818 ★ Canadian Fitness and Lifestyle Research Institute**
201-185 Somerset W
Ottawa, ON, Canada K2P 0J2
**Phone:** (613)233-5528    **Fax:** (613)233-5536
**Email:** info@cflri.ca
**Website:** http://www.cflri.ca/
**Activities/Fields:** Population fitness levels, recreation habits, and link between physical activity and other life-style patterns of Canadians; benefits and costs of a physically active lifestyle. **Pub:** *The Research File,* 3/year. **Frmly:** Canada Fitness Survey.

**Colorado State University**
**Colorado Injury Control Research Center (CICRC)**
*See:* Entry 20190

**★ 17819 ★ Columbia University**
**Harlem Center for Health Promotion and Disease Prevention**
Harlem Hospital Center
506 Lenox Ave., NNR 524
New York, NY 10037
**Phone:** (212)939-4150    **Fax:** (212)939-4144
**Email:** nr9@columbia.edu
**Website:** http://www.cvmbs.colostate.edu/EnHealth/CICRC
Dr. Alwyn Cohall, Dir.
**Activities/Fields:** Assessment of health status and examination of risk factors in the Harlem community, to reduce excess mortality and morbidity.

**★ 17820 ★ Cooper Institute for Aerobics Research**
12330 Preston Rd.
Dallas, TX 75230
**Phone:** (214)341-3200    **Free:** 800-635-7050
**Fax:** (214)341-3224
**Email:** csterling@cooperinst.org
**Website:** http://www.cooperinst.org
Dr. Charles L. Sterling, Exec. Dir.
**Activities/Fields:** Cardiovascular disease, stress management, women's health, exercise physiology, health promotion, nutrition, youth fitness, hypertension, aging, and epidemiology. Using data from the affiliated Cooper Clinic, the Institute conducts the Aerobics Center Longitudinal Study, which monitors 25,000 subjects over their lifetime to study the effects of exercise and health habits on death and disability rates from chronic diseases.

**Johns Hopkins University**
**Center for Adolescent Health Promotion and Disease Prevention**
*See:* Entry 5797

**★ 17821 ★ Johns Hopkins University**
**Johns Hopkins Center for Injury Research and Policy**
Department of Health Policy & Management
Bloomberg School of Public Health
624 N Broadway
Baltimore, MD 21205
**Phone:** (410)502-8671    **Fax:** (410)614-2797
**Email:** sdefranc@jhsph.edu
**Website:** http://www.jhsph.edu/Research/Centers/CIRP
Susan DeFrancesco, Asst. Scientist
**Activities/Fields:** Adolescent drowning and poisoning, alcohol related injuries, aviation safety, childhood injuries, fall injuries in nursing homes, financing trauma care and rehabilitation, homicide and suicide, injuries from firearms, injuries in developing countries, injury sequelae and rehabilitation, injury severity scoring, injury surveillance systems, mathematical models of response to impact, motor vehicle related injuries, occupational injuries, and elderly and highway safety. Develops injury interventions, evaluates legal interventions, examines preventive measures, and evaluates trauma care. **Frmly:** Injury Prevention Center.

**Johns Hopkins University**
**Welch Center for Prevention, Epidemiology, and Clinical Research**
*See:* Entry 9051

**★ 17822 ★ Methodist Health Care System**
**Sid W. Richardson Institute for Preventive Medicine**
6550 Fannin St., SM583
Houston, TX 77030
**Phone:** (713)790-6450    **Fax:** (713)793-1269
**Email:** cathyeaster@tmh.tmc.edu
**Website:** http://www.methodisthealth.com/ipm
Cathy Easter DeBrusk, Contact
**Activities/Fields:** Analyzes health insurance claims and employee absentee data to evaluate various preventive medicine programs, evaluates the effect of smoking cessation on the occurrence of chronic lung disease, compares different program approaches taken in cardiac rehabilitation (exercise versus comprehensive approaches), and studies depression in patients with heart disease and their spouses. **Pub:** *The Journal.*

**★ 17823 ★ Oakland University**
**Meadowbrook Health Enhancement Institute**
Rochester, MI 48309-4401
**Phone:** (248)370-3198    **Fax:** (248)370-4522
**Email:** fwstrans@oakland.edu
**Website:** http://www.oakland.edu/mbhei
Dr. Fred W. Stransky, Dir.
**Activities/Fields:** Exercise physiology and the health profile enhancement of residents in internal medicine. **Pub:** *Way of Life Newsletter,* quarterly. Newsletter.

**★ 17824 ★ Preventive Medicine Institute**
428 E 72nd St.
New York, NY 10021-4601
**Phone:** (212)794-4900    **Fax:** (212)794-4959
**Email:** osborne@strang.org
**Website:** http://www.strang.org
Dr. Michael P. Osborne, Dir.
**Activities/Fields:** Breast, colon, prostate, and other cancers and nutrition.

**★ 17825 ★ Preventive Medicine Research Institute**
900 Bridgeway, Ste. 1
Sausalito, CA 94965
**Phone:** (415)332-2525    **Fax:** (415)332-5730
**Email:** ebpett@aol.com
**Website:** http://www.pmri.org
Dean Ornish, MD, Pres.

**Activities/Fields:** Prevention and treatment of heart disease and other chronic diseases and lifestyle risk factors through modification of diet, exercise, and relaxation techniques such as yoga, meditation, and visualization.

★ **17826** ★ **Stanford University**
**Center for Research in Disease**
**Prevention**
School of Medicine
1000 Welch Rd.
Palo Alto, CA 94304-1825
**Phone:** (650)723-6145        **Fax:** (650)725-6906
**Email:** fortmann@stanford.edu
**Website:** http://prevention.stanford.edu
Stephen P. Fortmann, MD, Dir.
**Activities/Fields:** Prevention and control of chronic disease, alcohol and drug abuse, and injury and death. Stresses a public health or community approach to disease prevention and health promotion and seeks methods to improve the overall level of community health by favorably modifying the environmental and personal factors known to influence chronic disease incidence, including blood pressure, blood cholesterol, cigarette use, nutrition, obesity, physical activity, and stress. **Pub:** *Catalogue available for health promotion materials.* **Frmly:** Stanford Heart Disease Prevention Program.

**Strang Cancer Prevention Center**
*See:* Entry 10417

**Trauma Foundation**
*See:* Entry 8609

**U.S. Department of Defense**
**Army Medical Research and Materiel**
**Command**
**Walter Reed Army Institute of Research**
**(WRAIR)**
**Preventive Medicine Division**
*See:* Entry 13484

★ **17827** ★ **U.S. Department of Health**
**and Human Services**
**National Center for Chronic Disease**
**Prevention and Health Promotion**
Mail Stop
4770 Buford Hwy., NE
Atlanta, GA 30341-3717
**Phone:** (770)488-5080        **Fax:** (770)488-5969
**Email:** ccdinfo@cdc.gov
**Website:** http://www.cdc.gov/nccdphp
Dr. James S. Marks, Dir.
**Activities/Fields:** Prevention of chronic diseases such as cardiovascular disease, diabetes, and cancer. Translates research findings into community programs and healthier lifestyles. Supports programs to improve nutrition, reproductive health, and exercise, and to discourage destructive behaviors, such as alcohol abuse and smoking. NCCDPHP's major organization units are: Office on Smoking and Health, the Division of Reproductive Health, the Division of Nutrition and Physical Activity, the Division of Adolescent and School Health, the Division of Diabetes Translation, the Division of Adult and Community Health, and the Division of Oral Health. **Frmly:** Center for Health Promotion and Education; (1991) Center for Chronic Disease Prevention and Health Promotion.

★ **17828** ★ **U.S. Department of Health**
**and Human Services**
**National Center for Injury Prevention and**
**Control**
4770 Buford Hwy. NE, MS K65
Atlanta, GA 30341-3724
**Phone:** (770)488-1506        **Fax:** (770)488-1667
**Email:** ema0@cdc.gov
**Website:** http://www.cdc.gov/ncipc
Elfrieda Alston, Contact

**Activities/Fields:** Specific injury control research designed to: yield results directly applicable to identifying interventions to prevent injury occurrence or minimize disability; apply and evaluate the effect of known interventions on injury morbidity, mortality, disability, and costs; or elucidate the etiology and mechanisms of injuries. **Pub:** *Proceedings.* • *Research Reports.* **Frmly:** (1993) Injury Control Division; (1991) Injury Epidemiology and Control Division.

★ **17829** ★ **U.S. Department of Health**
**and Human Services**
**National Center for Prevention Services**
**Sexually Transmitted Disease / HIV**
**Prevention Division (NCHSTP)**
**Behavioral and Prevention Research**
**Branch**
Mail Stop E-44
1600 Clifton Rd., NE
Atlanta, GA 30333
**Phone:** (404)639-8376        **Fax:** (404)639-8622
**Email:** n2s4@odc.gov
Janet S. St. Lawrence, PhD, Chf.
**Activities/Fields:** Individual and group behavior patterns as they affect STD and HIV occurrence and transmission. Undertakes studies to evaluate new methods of prevention and intervention of HIV and STDs, and conducts surveys, studies, and methodological research on the sexual and drug-using behavior. Performs intervention research to prevent HIV/STD transmission. **Pub:** *MMWR.* • *Professional Journals.* **Frmly:** Epidemiology Research Branch; (2000) Sexually Transmitted Disease/HIV Prevention Division; Behavioral and Prevention Research Branch.

**U.S. Department of Health and Human**
**Services**
**National Heart, Lung, and Blood Institute**
**Division of Epidemiology and Clinical**
**Applications**
**Clinical Applications and Prevention**
**Program**
*See:* Entry 5148

**U.S. Department of Health and Human**
**Services**
**National Institute on Alcohol Abuse and**
**Alcoholism**
**Prevention Research Center**
*See:* Entry 19373

**U.S. Department of Health and Human**
**Services**
**National Institute of Mental Health**
**Epidemiology and Services Research**
**Division**
**Prevention Research Branch**
*See:* Entry 12724

**U.S. Department of Health and Human**
**Services**
**National Institutes of Health**
**National Cancer Institute**
**Division of Cancer Control and**
**Population Sciences (DCCPS)**
**((Behavioral Research Program)**
**Helath Promotion Research Branch —**
**HPRB)**
*See:* Entry 10537

**U.S. Department of Health and Human**
**Services**
**National Institutes of Health**
**National Cancer Institute**
**Division of Cancer Control and**
**Population Sciences (DCCPS)**
**(Behavioral Research Program)**
*See:* Entry 10547

**U.S. Department of Health and Human**
**Services**
**National Institutes of Health**
**National Institute of Child Health and**
**Human Development**
**Division of Intramural Research**
**(Division of Epidemiology, Statistics and**
**Prevention Research)**
*See:* Entry 9065

★ **17830** ★ **U.S. Department of Health**
**and Human Services**
**National Institutes of Health**
**National Institute of Child Health and**
**Human Development**
**Division of Intramural Research**
**((Division of Epidemiology, Statistics and**
**Prevention Research)**
**Biometry and Mathematical Statistics**
**Branch)**
Bldg. 6100, Rm. 7B05
9000 Rockville Pike
Bethesda, MD 20892-7510
**Phone:** (301)496-6813        **Fax:** (301)402-2084
**Email:** mk90h@nih.gov
**Website:**        http://www.nichd.nih.gov/about/despr/bio.htm
Kai F. Yu, PhD, Ch.
**Activities/Fields:** Statistical theory and methodology relevant to problems under investigation in areas of maternal and child health.

★ **17831** ★ **U.S. Department of Health**
**and Human Services**
**National Institutes of Health**
**National Institute of Dental and**
**Craniofacial Research**
31 Center Dr., MSC 2290
Bldg. 31, Rm. 2C39
Bethesda, MD 20892-2290
**Phone:** (301)496-3571        **Fax:** (301)402-2185
**Email:** lawrence.tabak@nih.gov
**Website:** http://www.nidcr.nih.gov
Lawrence A. Tabak, DDS,Ph, Dir.
**Activities/Fields:** Oral, dental, and craniofacial health, as well as prevention of those diseases and conditions; also develops new diagnostics and therapeutics.

**U.S. Department of Health and Human**
**Services**
**National Institutes of Health**
**National Institute of Dental and**
**Craniofacial Research**
**Division of Extramural Research**
**(Clinical Trials Program)**
*See:* Entry 6628

**U.S. Department of Health and Human**
**Services**
**National Institutes of Health**
**National Institute of Diabetes and**
**Digestive and Kidney Diseases**
**Division of Diabetes, Endocrinology, and**
**Metabolic Diseases**
**(Type 2 Diabetes in the Pediatric**
**Population Program)**
*See:* Entry 8789

**★ 17832 ★ U.S. Department of Health and Human Services**
**National Institutes of Health**
**National Institute of Environmental Health Sciences**
**Division of Extramural Research and Training**
**(Centers for Children's Environmental Health and Disease Prevention)**
PO Box 12233
Research Triangle Park, NC 27709
**Phone:** (919)541-3254 **Fax:** (919)316-4606
**Email:** dearry@niehs.nih.gov
**Website:** http://www.niehs.nih.gov/dert/programs/translat/children/children.htm
Allen Dearry, PhD, Ch.

**Activities/Fields:** Applied intervention and prevention methods in connection with community-based prevention research; supports studies on the causes and mechanisms of children's disorders having an environmental etiology, identifies environmental exposures, intervenes to reduce hazardous exposures and their adverse health effects. Strives to decrease the prevalence, morbidity and mortality of environmentally related childhood diseases.

**★ 17833 ★ U.S. Department of Health and Human Services**
**Office of Disease Prevention and Health Promotion**
Humphrey Bldg.
200 Independence Ave. SW, Rm. 738G
Washington, DC 20201
**Phone:** (202)401-6295 **Fax:** (202)205-9478
**Website:** http://nhic-nt.health.org
Linda Meyers, Actg. Dir.

**Activities/Fields:** Develops and manages the National Health Goals and Objectives (known as Healthy People 2000) for the National Health Information Center. Coordinates policy and program for the Public Health Service.

**U.S. Department of Veterans Affairs**
**Veterans Health Administration**
**Office of Research and Development**
**Rehabilitation and Development Service**
**(Center for Healthy Aging with Disabilities)**
*See:* Entry 13515

**★ 17834 ★ University of Alabama at Birmingham**
**Center for Health Promotion**
School of Public Health
1665 University Blvd., Ste. 227 Royals
Birmingham, AL 35294
**Phone:** (205)934-6020 **Fax:** (205)934-9325
**Email:** jrac@uab.edu
**Website:** http://VARehab.bcm.tmc.edu
Dr. Jim Raczynski, Dir.

**Activities/Fields:** Health promotion and disease prevention for underserved population. The center is divided into several components, including the Community Care, Project Assessment Care, Survey Research Unit, Surveillance Data Unit, Behavioral Assessment and Intervention Care, Health Communications Unit, and Biopsychosocial Laboratory.

**★ 17835 ★ University of Alabama at Birmingham**
**Injury Control Research Center**
933 19th St. S, Ste. 403
CHSB-19
Birmingham, AL 35294-2041
**Phone:** (205)934-7845 **Fax:** (205)975-8143
**Email:** rfine@uab.edu
**Website:** http://www.uab.edu/icrc
Russ Fine, PhD, Dir.

**Activities/Fields:** Rehabilitation and occupationally-related injuries, spinal cord injuries, and traumatic brain injuries, focusing on improving rehabilitation practices and processes to help persons with injuries achieve maximum rehabilitation potential; stimulating local faculty development of prevention, acute-care, rehabilitation, epidemiology, and biomechanics research projects; training health care workers and other practitioners, scientists, and students in the discipline of injury prevention and control; providing technical assistance and disseminate information in support of the nation's injury control agenda; and promoting the explicit incorporation of injury prevention initiatives targeting high-risk populations. Center also conducts multidisciplinary research involving faculty from other areas of the University. **Pub:** *Newsletter.* • *Report,* biennially.

**★ 17836 ★ University of California, Irvine**
**Health Promotion Center**
School of Social Ecology
Irvine, CA 92697
**Phone:** (949)824-5047 **Fax:** (949)824-8566
**Email:** ucihpc@uci.edu
**Website:** http://www.healthpromotioncenter.uci.edu/
Daniel Stokols, PhD, Co-Dir.

**Activities/Fields:** Health promotion. Research focuses on comprehensive, integrated approaches to health promotion, especially on workplace-based health promotion. **Pub:** *Wellness Programming Guides.* • *Technical reports.* • *Newsletter.*

**★ 17837 ★ University of California, Los Angeles**
**Southern California Injury Prevention Research Center**
School of Public Health
10911 Weyburn Ave., Ste. 200
Los Angeles, CA 90024-2884
**Phone:** (310)794-2706 **Fax:** (310)794-0787
**Email:** jfkraus@ucla.edu
**Website:** http://www.ph.ucla.edu/sciprc
Jess F. Kraus, PhD, Dir.

**Activities/Fields:** Intentional and unintentional injuries in the socioeconomically disadvantaged, underserved, and ethnically diverse populations in the Southern California region. Research projects include: work-related injuries in high-risk occupations; risk of motor vehicle crash; injuries to children; injuries and deaths; injuries in the elderly; worksite intervention to reduce work-related assault; earthquake injury and preparedness; expanding methods in injury epidemiology; long-term consequences of brain and spinal cord injuries; violence in contemporary American film; marital and youth violence.

**★ 17838 ★ University of California, San Francisco**
**Center for AIDS Prevention Studies (CAPS)**
AIDS Research Institute
74 New Montgomery St., Ste. 600
San Francisco, CA 94105
**Phone:** (415)597-9100 **Fax:** (415)597-9213
**Email:** tcoates@psg.ucsf.edu
**Website:** http://www.caps.ucsf.edu/capsweb
Thomas J. Coates, PhD, Dir.

**Activities/Fields:** Methods to change AIDS high risk behavior. Activities include developing and testing AIDS prevention strategies for at-risk populations, promoting multidisciplinary research on the prevention of HIV disease, funding pilot studies on minority issues in AIDS, and operating the CAPS International Visiting Scholars Program, which brings scholars from Africa, Asia, Eastern Europe, and Latin America to work with CAPS scientists in developing AIDS prevention research protocols. **Pub:** *CAPS Bibliography.* • *Prevention Fact Sheets.*

**★ 17839 ★ University of California, San Francisco**
**Center for Health Improvement and Prevention Studies (CHIPS)**
Division of Behavioral Sciences
601 Montgomery St., Ste. 810
San Francisco, CA 94111
**Phone:** (415)502-7283 **Fax:** (415)502-7314
**Email:** chips@itsa.ucsf.edu
**Website:** http://itsa.ucsf.edu/~chips/
Barbara Gerbert, PhD, Res. Dir.

**Activities/Fields:** Behavioral risks and patient, provider, and systemic barriers to optimal health care delivery.

**★ 17840 ★ University of California, San Francisco**
**San Francisco Injury Center**
San Francisco General Hospital
Department of Surgery, Ward 3A, Box 0807
1001 Potrero Ave.
San Francisco, CA 94110
**Phone:** (415)206-4623 **Fax:** (415)206-5950
**Email:** pknudson@sfghsurg.ucsf.edu
**Website:** http://www.surgery.ucsf.edu/sfic
M. Margaret Knudson, MD, Dir.

**Activities/Fields:** Acute trauma care, injury prevention and surveillance.

**★ 17841 ★ University of Iowa**
**Injury Prevention Research Center**
College of Public Health
100 Oakdale Campus, No. 158 IREH
Iowa City, IA 52242-5000
**Phone:** (319)335-4458 **Fax:** (319)335-4631
**Email:** john-lundell@uiowa.edu
**Website:** http://www.public-health.uiowa.edu/iprc
Dr. Craig Zwerling, Dir.

**Activities/Fields:** Control and prevention of rural injuries in these high risk populations through research, education and training, and public policy targeting especially rural motor vehicle injuries and farm and other occupational injuries. The specific aims of the research projects include examining the rates and risk factors of farm-related injuries among Iowa farmers; evaluating the effectiveness of trauma care in Iowa; and examining driving avoidance behavior in drivers with traumatic brain injuries.

**★ 17842 ★ University of Louisville**
**Health Promotion and Wellness Center**
Crawford Gym
Louisville, KY 40292
**Phone:** (502)852-5711 **Fax:** (502)852-4534
**Email:** bryant@louisville.edu
Bryant A. Stamford, PhD, Dir.

**Activities/Fields:** Performs fitness analyses for county police departments, fire fighters, and commonwealth police. Also studies exercise routines.

**★ 17843 ★ University of Maryland at Baltimore**
**Organized Research Center in Health Promotion and Disease Prevention**
Department of Epidemiology & Preventive Medicine
Howard Hall, Ste. 109
660 W Redwood St.
Baltimore, MD 21201
**Phone:** (410)706-3450
**Email:** shavas@epi.umaryland.edu
**Website:** http://medschool.umaryland.edu/Epidemiology/hp_dp.html
Dr. Stephen Havas, Co-Dir.

**Activities/Fields:** Health promotion and disease prevention, especially prevention of cancer, heart disease, and stroke.

**University of Michigan—Flint**
**Physical Therapy Cumulative Trauma**
 **Disorders Laboratory**
*See:* Entry 16840


**University of Montreal**
**Clinical Research Institute of Montreal**
**Multidisciplinary Research Group on**
 **Hypertension**
*See:* Entry 5191


**★ 17844 ★ University of North Carolina**
 **at Chapel Hill**
**Center for Health Promotion and Disease**
 **Prevention**
CB 7400
255 Rosenau Hall
Chapel Hill, NC 27599-7400
**Phone:** (919)966-6035 **Fax:** (919)966-6264
**Email:** across@unc.edu
**Website:** http://www.flint.umich.edu/departments/pt
Dr. Alan W. Cross, Dir.

**Activities/Fields:** Health promotion and disease prevention at state, regional, and national levels, focusing
on women and minority health, children's health,
tobaco and health promotion in the workplace.


**★ 17845 ★ University of North Carolina**
 **at Chapel Hill**
**Injury Prevention Research Center**
Chase Hill, CB 7505
Chapel Hill, NC 27599-7505
**Phone:** (919)966-2251 **Fax:** (919)966-0466
**Email:** iprc@unc.edu
**Website:** http://www.sph.unc.edu/iprc/
Carol W. Runyan, PhD, Dir.

**Activities/Fields:** Studies the epidemiology, prevention, acute care, and rehabilitation aspects of injuries,
including workplace injury, road safety, violence, childhood injury, and program development and evaluation.
**Pub:** *IPRC News.*


**★ 17846 ★ University of Pennsylvania**
**Center for Urban Health Research**
School of Nursing
Nursing Education Bldg.
420 Guardian Dr.
Philadelphia, PA 19104
**Phone:** (215)898-6313 **Fax:** (215)573-9193
**Email:** jemmott@nursing.upenn.edu
**Website:** http://www.nursing.upenn.edu/urban/
Dr. Loretta Sweet Jemmott, Dir.

**Activities/Fields:** Identification of factors that influence health risk-related behaviors and the design of
culturally tailored interventions to promote healthy
lifestyles, with a focus on AIDS, pregnancy, and
violence prevention.


**★ 17847 ★ University of South Carolina**
 **at Columbia**
**Center for Health Promotion and Risk**
 **Reduction in Special Populations**
Williams-Brice Bldg., No. 56
College of Nursing
Columbia, SC 29208
**Phone:** (803)777-2868
**Email:** carolyn.murdaugh@sc.edu
**Website:** http://www.sc.edu/nursing/center/index.htm
Carolyn Murdaugh, PhD, Dir.

**Activities/Fields:** Health promotion and health risk
reduction in special populations. **Pub:** *Newsletter.*


**★ 17848 ★ University of South Florida**
**Florida Prevention Research Center**
 **(FPRC)**
4809 E Busch Blvd.
Tampa, FL 33617
**Phone:** (813)971-2119 **Fax:** (813)971-2280
**Email:** rmcdermo@com1.med.usf.edu
**Website:** http://www.hsc.usf.edu/prc/index.html
Robert J. McDermott, PhD, Dir.

**Activities/Fields:** Sustained disease prevention and
health promotion, through community-based prevention marketing.


**★ 17849 ★ University of Southern**
 **California**
**Institute for Health Promotion and**
 **Disease Prevention Research**
1000 S Fremont Ave.
Alhambra, CA 91803
**Phone:** (626)457-6600 **Fax:** (626)457-4012
**Email:** lisath@hsc.usc.edu
**Website:** http://www.usc.edu/go/ipr
C. Anderson Johnson, PhD, Dir.

**Activities/Fields:** Chronic disease prevention, behavioral epidemiology, obesity prevention, patient compliance, HIV/AIDS, and tobacco, alcohol, and other and
drug abuse. Activities focus on research in health
promotion and disease prevention, with young people
as the principal target. **Pub:** *Technical Reports.*
**Frmly:** Health Behavior Research Institute.


**★ 17850 ★ University of Texas—Houston**
 **Health Science Center**
**Center for Health Promotion and**
 **Prevention Research**
School of Public Health
7000 Fannin, 25th Fl.
Houston, TX 77030
**Phone:** (713)500-9609 **Fax:** (713)500-9602
**Email:** chppr@sph.uth.tmc.edu
**Website:** http://www.sph.uth.tmc.edu/chppr
Dr. Stephen H. Kelder, Acting Dir.

**Activities/Fields:** Health promotion research and
development, with emphasis on institutional settings
(worksites, medical care facilities, schools, and communities). Studies include the interaction of educational, economic, and environmental influences on health
promotion, testing interventions directed toward institutions and individuals, and the innovation, diffusion,
and maintenance of health promotion programs. Conducts survey research for monitoring and surveillance
of health knowledge, attitudes, opinion, and behavior;
evaluates methods and strategies for health care
adapted to select populations; provides technical
assistance, consultation, and collaboration with agencies, industries, institutions, media, and universities
throughout Texas; and helps develop educational
materials. **Pub:** *Prevention Research News,* semiannually. Newsletter. **Frmly:** Center for Health Promotion Research and Development.


**★ 17851 ★ University of Toronto**
**Research Services Unit**
Department of Public Health Sciences
Faculty of Medicine
401B McMurruch Blvd.
Toronto, ON, Canada M5S 1A8
**Phone:** (416)978-5351 **Fax:** (416)978-8299
**Email:** vartouhi.jazmaji@utoronto.ca
Vartouhi Jazmaji, Dir.

**Activities/Fields:** Design and analysis of clinical trials
and epidemiological studies, including biostatistics,
demography, and data management and analysis.


**★ 17852 ★ University of Vermont**
**Office of Health Promotion Research**
1 S Prospect St.
Burlington, VT 05401
**Phone:** (802)656-4187 **Fax:** (802)656-8826
**Email:** bflynn@zoo.uvm.edu
**Website:** http://www.uvm.edu/~ohpr
Dr. Brian S. Flynn, Dir.

**Activities/Fields:** Health education, smoking prevention (primarily with youth), smoking cessation, particularly with women of child-bearing age; breast screening promotion, breast self-exam education, behavioral/
lifestyle change, and alcohol-use prevention in adolescents. **Frmly:** Vermont Lung Center.


**★ 17853 ★ University of Virginia**
**Vascular Medicine and Preventive**
 **Cardiology Unit**
UVA Health System, Box 800146
Charlottesville, VA 22908-0146
**Phone:** (434)924-2765 **Fax:** (434)924-9604
**Email:** cra2e@virginia.edu
**Website:** http://www.hsc.virginia.edu/heart
Carlos R. Ayers, MD, Hd.

**Activities/Fields:** Cardiovascular problems, including
hypertension, hyperlipidemia, renal blood flow, xenon
washout technique, renin-angiotension-aldosterone
metabolism, catecholamine metabolism, plethysmog-
raphy, peripheral vascular physiology and disease,
and cardiovascular risk reduction. **Frmly:** Virginia
Heart Laboratory; Hypertension/Atherosclerosis Unit.


**★ 17854 ★ University of Washington**
**Harborview Injury Prevention and**
 **Research Center**
325 9th Ave.
PO Box 359960
Seattle, WA 98104
**Phone:** (206)521-1520 **Fax:** (206)521-1562
**Email:** navajo@u.washington.edu
**Website:** http://depts.washington.edu/hiprc/
David C. Grossman, MD, Dir.

**Activities/Fields:** Injury prevention and the causes,
effects and treatment of injuries, including studies in
epidemiology, health education, psychology, acute
care, biomechanics, rehabilitation.


**★ 17855 ★ University of Washington**
**Health Promotion Research Center**
 **(HPRC)**
School of Public Health & Community Medicine,
 Box 358852
146 N Canal St., Ste. 110
Seattle, WA 98103
**Phone:** (206)543-2891 **Fax:** (206)543-8841
**Email:** logerfo@u.washington.edu
**Website:** http://depts.washington.edu/hprc/
James P. LoGerfo, MD, Dir.

**Activities/Fields:** Promotion of the health and well-
being of Washington state residents, with a focus on
older adults.

## Federal Government Agencies

**★ 17856 ★ Consumer Product Safety Commission**
East-West Towers
4330 East-West Hwy.
Bethesda, MD 20814
**Phone:** (301)504-0580      **Free:** 800-638-CPSC
**Website:** http://www.cpsc.gov/
Ann Brown, Chairman of the Board
**Desc:** The purpose of the Consumer Product Safety Commission is to protect the public against unreasonable risks of injury from consumer products; to assist consumers in evaluating the comparative safety of consumer products; to develop uniform safety standards for consumer products and minimize conflicting state and local regulations; and to promote research and investigation into the causes and prevention of product-related deaths, illnesses, and injuries.

**★ 17857 ★ Nuclear Regulatory Commission (NRC)**
11555 Rockville Pike
Washington, DC 20555
**Phone:** (301)415-7000
**Website:** http://www.nrc.gov/
Richard A. Meserve, Chairman of the Board
**Desc:** The Nuclear Regulatory Commission licenses and regulates the civilian uses of nuclear energy to protect public health and safety and the environment.

**★ 17858 ★ U.S. Department of Agriculture**
**Food Safety and Inspection Service**
14th St. & Independence Ave. SW
Washington, DC 20250
**Phone:** (202)720-7943      **Fax:** (202)720-1843
**Website:** http://www.usda.gov/agency/fsis/home-page.htm
**Desc:** The service is responsible for ensuring that meat and poultry products moving in interstate and foreign commerce for human consumption are safe, wholesome, and accurately labeled.

**★ 17859 ★ U.S. Department of Health and Human Services**
**Centers for Disease Control and Prevention (CDCP)**
1600 Clifton Rd. NE
Atlanta, GA 30333
**Phone:** (404)639-3311
**Website:** http://www.cdc.gov/
Dr. Julie L. Gerberding, Director
**Desc:** The Centers for Disease Control is charged with protecting the public health of the Nation by providing leadership and direction in the prevention and control of diseases and other preventable conditions and responding to public health emergencies.

**★ 17860 ★ U.S. Department of Health and Human Services**
**Centers for Disease Control and Prevention**
**Public Health Practice Program Office**
1600 Clifton Rd. NE
Atlanta, GA 30333
**Phone:** (404)639-3311
**Website:** http://www.phppo.cdc.gov/

**★ 17861 ★ U.S. Department of Health and Human Services**
**Food and Drug Administration (FDA)**
5600 Fishers Ln.
Rockville, MD 20857
**Phone:** (301)443-1544
**Website:** http://www.fda.gov/
**Desc:** The mission of the Food and Drug Administration is to ensure that food is safe, pure, and wholesome; human and animal drugs, biological products, and medical devices are safe and effective; and electronic products that emit radiation ar safe. The Administration's major operating components are: (1) the Center for Biologics Evaluation and Research, (2) the Center for Devices and Radiological Health, (3) the Center for Drug Evaluation and Research, (4) the Center for Food Safety and Applied Nutrition, (5) the Center for Veterinary Medicine, and (6) the National Center for Toxicological Research.

**★ 17862 ★ U.S. Department of Health and Human Services**
**Food and Drug Administration**
**Center for Biologics Evaluation and Research**
1401 Rockville Pike, Ste. 200N
Rockville, MD 20852-1448
**Phone:** (301)827-1800      **Free:** 800-835-4709
**Website:** http://www.fda.gov/cber
Kathryn C. Zoon, PhD, Director
**Desc:** The Center regulates biological products, plans and conducts research on both new and old biological products, inspects manufacturers' facilities for compliance with standards, tests products submitted for release, establishes written and physical standards, and approves licensing of manufacturers to produce biological products. The Center plans and conducts research on the preparation, preservation, and safety of blood and blood products, the methods of testing safety, purity, potency, and efficacy of such products for therapeutic use, and the immunological problems concerned with products, testing, and use of diagnostic reagents employed in grouping and typing blood.

**U.S. Department of Health and Human Services**
**Food and Drug Administration**
**Center for Devices and Radiological Health**
*See:* Entry 18088

**★ 17863 ★ U.S. Department of Health and Human Services**
**Food and Drug Administration**
**Center for Drug Evaluation and Research**
5600 Fishers Ln.
Rockville, MD 20857
**Phone:** (301)827-4573
**Website:** http://www.fda.gov/cder
Janet Woodcock, MD, Director
**Desc:** Center develops FDA policy with regard to the safety, effectiveness, and labeling of all drugs for human use; reviews and evaluates new drug applications and investigates new drug applications; develops and implements standards for the safety and effectiveness of all over-the-counter drugs; and monitors the quality of marketed drugs through product testing, surveillance, and compliance programs.

**★ 17864 ★ U.S. Department of Health and Human Services**
**Food and Drug Administration**
**Center for Food Safety and Applied Nutrition**
5100 Paint Branch Parkway
College Park, MD 20740-3835
**Free:** 888-463-6332
**Website:** http://www.cfsan.fda.gov/
Joseph A. Levitt, Director
**Desc:** The Center conducts research and develops standards on the composition, quality, nutrition, and safety of foods, food additives, colors, and cosmetics; conducts research designed to improve the detection, prevention, and control of contamination that may be responsible for illness or injury conveyed by foods, colors, and cosmetics; coordinates and evaluates FDA's surveillance and compliance programs relating to foods, color, and cosmetics.

**★ 17865 ★ U.S. Department of Health and Human Services**
**Office of Public Health and Science (OPHS)**
5600 Fishers Ln.
Rockville, MD 20857
**Phone:** (301)443-3921
**Desc:** The Office ensures that the Department conducts broad-based public health assessments designed to anticipate future public health issues and problems and devises and implements appropriate interventions and evaluations to maintain, sustain, and improve the health of the Nation; provides assistance in managing the implementation and coordination of Secretarial decisions for PHS operating divisions and coordination of population-based health, clinical prevention services, and science initiatives that cut across operating divisions; provides presentations to foreign governments and multilateral agencies on international health issues; and provides direction and policy oversight, through the Surgeon General, for the Public Health Service Commissioned Corps.

## ★ 17866 ★ U.S. Department of Health and Human Services
**Office of Public Health and Science**
**Office of the Assistant Secretary for Health and Surgeon General**
200 Independence Ave. SW
Washington, DC 20201
**Phone:** (202)619-0257
**Website:** http://www.dhhs.gov
Eve E. Slater, MD, Assistant Secretary for Health
**Desc:** The Office consists of general and special staff offices that support the Assistant Secretary for Health in planning and directing the activities of the Public Health Service. Components include the Office of the Surgeon General, the Office of Disease Prevention and Health Promotion, the Office of Health Communications, the Office of Health Operations, the Office of Health Planning and Evaluation, the Office of Intergovernmental Affairs, and the Office of Population Affairs. Also under the administration of the Assistant Secretary for Health are the President's Council on Physical Fitness and Sports and a major operating center, the Agency for Health Care Policy and Research.

# Foundations & Other Funding Organizations

## Private Foundations

**Courtney S. Turner Charitable Trust**
*See:* Entry 147

## ★ 17867 ★ Foundation for Deep Ecology
1062 Fort Cronkhite
Sausalito, CA 94965
**Phone:** (415)229-9339          **Fax:** (415)229-9340
**Email:** info@deepecology.org
**Website:** http://www.deepecology.org
Jerry Mander, Megatechnology & Globalization Program O
**Fnded:** 1991. **Philosophy:** The Foundation for Deep Ecology concentrates on supporting fundamental ecological issues with certain general goals: to articulate the root causes of today's problems; to support activism that reverses or quells the present drives of society; and to protect forest lands, habitats, and other places around the world. Grant making is divided into three broad categories: Wilderness and Biodiversity, which concerns itself with the decimation of the world's tropical and temperate forests, habitats and biodiversity; Sustainable Agriculture, which supports programs retarding or reversing the destruction of the world's forests and new thinking and alternative models for agriculture; and Megatechnology and Economic Globalization, which seeks proposals for effective analysis, organization, and action on issues related to the industrialization of agriculture and forestry. **Priorities:** *Civic & Public Affairs:* 5%. Supports public policy organizations and community foundations. *Note:* Total contributions made in fiscal 1999. **Typ. Recipients:** Public Health. **Geo. Dist:** internationally; nationally.

**Henry Luce Foundation**
*See:* Entry 339

**Horizons Foundation**
*See:* Entry 358

**James L. Stamps Foundation**
*See:* Entry 8540

**John Ernest Bamberger and Ruth Eleanor Bamberger Memorial Foundation**
*See:* Entry 417

**Louis and Sandra Berkman Foundation**
*See:* Entry 10048

**Loyola Foundation, Inc.**
*See:* Entry 10049

**Maclellan Foundation**
*See:* Entry 18214

**Marion I. and Henry J. Knott Foundation**
*See:* Entry 504

**The Meadows Foundation**
*See:* Entry 538

## ★ 17868 ★ New World Foundation
666 West End Ave.
New York, NY 10025
**Phone:** (212)249-1023          **Fax:** (212)472-0508
**Email:** cgreer@newwf.org
**Website:** http://www.newwf.org
Mr. Colin Greer, President
**Fnded:** 1954. **Philosophy:** Due to the recent decrease in availability of federal funding, the New World Foundation has decided to provide support to community and public institutions. The foundation seeks to implement connections between activists and policymakers, and decrease future levels of poverty, homelessness, and chronic unemployment. Other interests are race, gender, and class issues as well as a variety of causes, largely progressive in nature. The foundation supports programs from the local to the national level. The following principal areas of giving are Equal Rights and Opportunities: those programs which promote participation of all groups in all aspects of American life; Education and Youth: those projects that use community resources to enhance the quality of public education; Public Health: programs to raise public and personal health standards, including health needs of the disadvantaged, as well as environmental and occupational health and safety; and Community Initiatives: those projects that encourage citizen efforts in equal justice and opportunity, improve quality of community life, enhance delivery systems, and meet local needs in a variety of other areas **Priorities:** *Civic & Public Affairs:* 28%. Primarily supports community institutions that promote equal opportunities and encourage citizens to participate in society. *Education:* 6%. Supports educational associations and literary assistance. *Environment:* 38%. Funds food banks and shelters. *Note:* Total contributions made in fiscal 2000. **Typ. Recipients:** Health Organizations, People with Disabilities. **Geo. Dist:** nationally.

## ★ 17869 ★ Public Welfare Foundation
1200 U St. NW
Washington, DC 20009
**Phone:** (202)965-1800          **Fax:** (202)265-8852
**Email:** general@publicwelfare.org
**Website:** http://www.publicwelfare.org
Larry Kressley, Executive Director
**Fnded:** 1947. **Philosophy:** "The Public Welfare Foundation is dedicated to supporting organizations that provide services to disadvantaged populations, and to those working for lasting improvements in the delivery of services that meet basic human needs. Our funding is focused in nine program areas: Criminal Justice, Human Rights and Global Security, Disadvantaged Elderly, Disadvantaged Youth, Environment, Health, Community Economic Development and Security, Population & Reproductive Health, and Community Support. The Foundation is willing to allocate seed money and to take risks to helping organizations with little else but dedication to a sound idea, a reasonable plan for carrying it out, and a strong base in and commitment to their communities. An important factor in the Foundation's grantmaking decisions is identifying specific, short-term financial needs our support would address. A grant should not create a long-term dependency or function simply as a contribution. An organization's ability to demonstrate community sup-

port, whether in the form of grants or in-kind contributions, is an additional factor. Our funding has no geographic restrictions. Grants outside the U.S. are generally made to organizations with offices both in the U.S. and in the region where the program is operating, although the foundation has increased its efforts to directly fund organizations in other countries. Regardless, the involvement of the local or regional community is always an important consideration." **Priorities:** *Civic & Public Affairs:* 23%. Supports philanthropic and grantmaking organizations, community justice system and high crime-rate neighborhoods, community economic development and participation, housing, public policy, womens affairs, and employment/jobtraining & welfare reform. *Environment:* 17%. Funds programs for disadvantaged elderly and youth, family planning services, family services, daycare and homeless. *International:* 30%. Funds programs that target prevention, mental health care, nutrition, and occupational and environmental factors; supports reproductive rights, education, and health; health policy, health Funds, AIDS, and health reform. *Note:* Total contributions made in fiscal 1998. **Typ. Recipients:** Adolescent Health Issues, AIDS/HIV, Children's Health/Hospitals, Clinics/Medical Centers, Domestic Violence, Emergency/Ambulance Services, Family Planning, Geriatric Health, Health Organizations, Health Policy/Cost Containment, Hospitals, Hospitals (University Affiliated), Medical Research, Mental Health, Nutrition, People with Disabilities, Prenatal Health Issues, Public Health. **Geo. Dist:** nationally.

## ★ 17870 ★ Rockefeller Family Fund
437 Madison Ave., 37th Floor
New York, NY 10022
**Phone:** (212)812-4252          **Fax:** (212)812-4299
**Email:** mmccarthy@rffund.org
**Website:** http://www.rffund.org
Mr. Lee Wasserman, Director
**Fnded:** 1967. **Philosophy:** The Rockefeller Family Fund makes grants in five program areas: Citizen Participation and Government Accountability, increasing voter participation and structural improvement to systems of government; Economic Justice for Women, enhancing the economic status of women by providing them with equitable employment opportunities and improving their work lives; The Environment, emphasizing the reduction of military pollution, the conservation of natural resources and the protection of health as affected by the environment; Institutional Responsiveness, supporting projects to influence public opinion and private institutions on issues of social concern; and Self-Sufficiency, which helps groups working within the fund's program areas to increase their income by obtaining funds from new sources or improving their ability to raise money from current sources. **Priorities:** *Civic & Public Affairs:* 68%. Program areas include citizen education and participation, economic justice for women, institutional responsiveness, and self-sufficiency. *Note:* Total contributions made in 2000. **Typ. Recipients:** Health Policy/Cost Containment, Health-General, People with Disabilities, Public Health. **Geo. Dist:** nationally; the fund does not generally consider projects which pertain to one city or state, unless the project could serve as a national model.

**Wieboldt Foundation**
*See:* Entry 19634

## Corporate Foundations

**CIGNA Foundation**
*See:* Entry 940

## ★ 17871 ★ Edison Family Foundation
PO Box 16940
Saint Louis, MO 63105
**Phone:** (314)727-6400          **Fax:** (314)727-1030
**Email:** deborah.veney-robinson@cigna.com
**Website:** http://www.cigna.com/general/about/community/index.html
Andrew Newman, President

**Fnded:** 1956. **Priorities:** *Civic & Public Affairs:* 32%. Supports community organizations. *Education:* 68%. Supports high schools and educational programs. *Note:* Total contributions made in fiscal 1999. **Typ. Recipients:** Public Health, Substance Abuse. **Geo. Dist:** MO, primarily St. Louis.

**FINA Foundation**
*See:* Entry 1046

**Harley-Davidson Foundation**
*See:* Entry 5575

**Hewlett-Packard Co. Foundation**
*See:* Entry 1127

**Oshkosh Truck Foundation**
*See:* Entry 10067

**The Reebok Human Rights Foundation**
*See:* Entry 1346

**Sunoco Inc.**
*See:* Entry 11465

**Teleflex Foundation**
*See:* Entry 1427

**Van Leer U.S. Foundation**
*See:* Entry 1475

**Varian Medical Systems, Inc.**
*See:* Entry 1477

**Wausau Paper Mills Foundation**
*See:* Entry 11471

**★ 17872 ★ Western Resources Foundation**
818 South Kansas Ave.
Topeka, KS 66612
**Phone:** (785)575-1927          **Fax:** (785)575-6399
**Email:** geri.noonan@reebok.com
**Website:** http://www.wr.com
Kimberly Groninger, President
**Fnded:** 1991. **Priorities:** *Arts & Humanities:* 17%. Funds museums, theater, music, and festivals. *Civic & Public Affairs:* 3%. Supports local public affairs and employment programs. *Education:* 56%. Funds colleges and universities; major support for scholarships through matching funds. *Environment:* 18%. United Way and youth programs, especially those dealing with employment opportunity enhancement. Also contributes to groups dealing with the problems of aging. *International:* 3%. Supports hospitals, hospice, and emergency relief. *Voluntarism:* Community Partners is a voluntary program for active and retired Western Resources employees. *Note:* Total contributions made in 2000. **Typ. Recipients:** Public Health. **Geo. Dist:** headquarters and operating communities.

**Yellow Corp. Foundation**
*See:* Entry 1516

# Medical & Allied Health Schools

## Public Health

*The following graduate schools of public health are members of the Association of Schools of Public Health (1101 15th St. NW, Ste. 910, Washington,* DC 20005, (202)296-1099, http://www.asph.org/) *and are accredited by the Council on Education for Public Health, 800 Eye St., NW, Ste. 202, Washington, DC 20001-3710, (202)789-1050, http://www.ceph.org/.*

### Alabama

**★ 17873 ★ University of Alabama, Birmingham**
**School of Public Health**
1665 University Blvd.
120 Ryals Bldg.
Birmingham, AL 35294-0022
**Phone:** (205)934-4993
**Website:** http://www.uab.edu/PublicHealth/

### California

**★ 17874 ★ Loma Linda University**
**School of Public Health**
Loma Linda, CA 92350
**Phone:** (909)824-4694          **Free:** 800-422-4558
**Fax:** (909)824-4087
**Website:** http://www.llu.edu/llu/grad/grad.html

**★ 17875 ★ San Diego State University**
**College of Health & Human Services**
**Graduate School of Public Health**
5500 Campanile Dr.
San Diego, CA 92182-4162
**Phone:** (619)594-6317          **Fax:** (619)594-6112
**Website:** http://www-rohan.edu/dept/gsphsdsu/web/gsph.html

**★ 17876 ★ University of California, Berkeley**
**School of Public Health**
19 Earl Warren Hall
Berkeley, CA 94720
**Phone:** (510)643-0881
**Website:** http://ist_socrates.berkeley.edu/~sph/

**★ 17877 ★ University of California, Los Angeles**
**School of Public Health**
Center for Health Sciences, Rm. 16-071
Box 951722
Los Angeles, CA 90095
**Phone:** (310)825-5516          **Fax:** (310)825-8440
**Website:** http://www.ph.ucla.edu

### Connecticut

**★ 17878 ★ University of Connecticut Health Center**
**Graduate Program in Public Health**
236 Farmington Ave.
Farmington, CT 06030-1910
**Phone:** (860)679-3351          **Fax:** (860)679-2374
**Email:** mph@nso.uchc.edu
**Website:** http://grad.uchc.edu/

**★ 17879 ★ Yale University**
**School of Medicine**
**Department of Epidemiology and Public Health**
60 College St., Rm. 208
New Haven, CT 06520-8034
**Phone:** (203)785-2844          **Fax:** (203)785-7296
**Website:** http://info.med.yale.edu/eph/

### District of Columbia

**★ 17880 ★ George Washington University**
**School of Public Health and Health Services**
2300 Eye St. NW, Rm. 719
Washington, DC 20037
**Phone:** (202)994-0248
**Website:** http://www.gwumc.edu/sphhs

### Florida

**★ 17881 ★ University of South Florida**
**College of Public Health**
13201 Bruce B. Downs Blvd.
MDC-56
Tampa, FL 33612-3805
**Phone:** (813)974-3623          **Fax:** (813)974-4718
**Website:** http://com1.med.usf.edu/pubhealth/coph1.html

### Georgia

**★ 17882 ★ Emory University**
**Rollins School of Public Health**
1518 Clifton Rd. NE
Atlanta, GA 30322
**Phone:** (404)727-3956          **Fax:** (404)727-3996
**Website:** http://www.sph.emory.edu

### Hawaii

**★ 17883 ★ University of Hawaii**
**School of Public Health**
1960 East-West Rd.
Honolulu, HI 96822
**Phone:** (808)956-8267          **Fax:** (808)956-4585
**Website:** http://www2.hawaii.edu/~sphdean

### Illinois

**★ 17884 ★ University of Illinois, Chicago**
**School of Public Health**
2121 W Taylor St.
Chicago, IL 60612
**Phone:** (312)996-6625          **Fax:** (312)996-1374
**Website:** http://www.uic.edu/sph/

### Indiana

**★ 17885 ★ Indiana University**
**Committee for the School of Public Health**
Robert Long Hospital, LO-211
1110 W Michigan St.
Indianapolis, IN 46202-5102
**Phone:** (317)278-0377
**Email:** skeough@indiana.edu
**Website:** http://www.indiana.edu/~aphs/phed.html
Dr. Mohammad R. Torabi, Contact

### Iowa

**★ 17886 ★ University of Iowa**
**Department of Preventive Medicine and Environmental Health**
**Public Health Program**
2800 Steindler Bldg.
Iowa City, IA 52242-1008
**Phone:** (319)335-8992          **Free:** 800-553-IOWA
**Fax:** (319)335-9200
**Email:** program-director@mail.public-health.uiowa.edu
**Website:** http://www.public-health.uiowa.edu/

### Louisiana

**★ 17887 ★ Tulane University**
**School of Public Health and Tropical Medicine**
1430 Tulane Ave.
New Orleans, LA 70112
**Phone:** (504)588-5387          **Fax:** (504)588-5718
**Website:** http://www.sph.tulane.edu

## Maryland

**★ 17888 ★ Johns Hopkins University School of Hygiene and Public Health**
615 N Wolfe St.
Baltimore, MD 21205-2179
**Phone:** (410)955-3543   **Fax:** (410)955-0121
**Website:** http://www.jhsph.edu

## Massachusetts

**★ 17889 ★ Boston University School of Public Health**
80 E Concord St., A-403
Boston, MA 02118-2394
**Phone:** (617)638-4640   **Fax:** (617)638-5299
**Website:** http://www-busph.bu.edu

**★ 17890 ★ Harvard University School of Public Health**
677 Huntington Ave., Rm. G-4
Boston, MA 02115
**Phone:** (617)432-1031   **Fax:** (617)277-5320
**Website:** http://www.hsph.harvard.edu/

**★ 17891 ★ University of Massachusetts School of Public Health**
101 Arnold House
Amherst, MA 01003-0037
**Phone:** (413)545-1303   **Fax:** (413)545-1264
**Website:** http://www.umass.edu/soph/

## Michigan

**★ 17892 ★ University of Michigan School of Public Health**
109 S Observatory St.
Ann Arbor, MI 48109-2029
**Phone:** (734)764-5425   **Fax:** (734)763-5455
**Website:** http://www.sph.umich.edu/

## Minnesota

**★ 17893 ★ University of Minnesota School of Public Health**
420 Delaware St. SE
Box 197 Mayo
Minneapolis, MN 55455
**Phone:** (612)626-3500   **Free:** 800-774-8636
**Fax:** (612)626-6931
**Website:** http://www.sph.umn.edu/

## Missouri

**★ 17894 ★ Saint Louis University School of Public Health**
3663 Lindell Ave.
Saint Louis, MO 63108-3342
**Phone:** (314)977-8144   **Fax:** (314)977-8150
**Website:** http://www.slu.edu/colleges/sph/slusph/Default.htm

## New Jersey

**★ 17895 ★ University of Medicine and Dentistry of New Jersey / Rutgers, the State University of New Jersey / New Jersey Institute of Technology Public Health Program**
675 Hoes Ln.
Piscataway, NJ 08854-5635
**Phone:** (732)235-4549   **Fax:** (732)235-4569
**Email:** rmcintyr@umdnj.edu
**Website:** http://www2.umdnj.edu/ethicweb/
Russell L. McIntyre, Contact

## New York

**★ 17896 ★ Columbia University School of Public Health**
600 W 168th St.
New York, NY 10032
**Phone:** (212)305-3927   **Fax:** (212)305-1460
**Website:** http://cpmcnet.columbia.edu/dept/sph/

**★ 17897 ★ State University of New York, Albany School of Public Health**
1 University Pl.
Rensselaer, NY 12144-3456
**Phone:** (518)402-0300   **Fax:** (518)485-5565
**Website:** http://www.albany.edu/sph/

## North Carolina

**★ 17898 ★ University of North Carolina, Chapel Hill School of Public Health**
Campus Box 7400
Chapel Hill, NC 27599-7400
**Phone:** (919)966-7676   **Fax:** (919)966-7678
**Website:** http://www.sph.unc.edu

## Ohio

**★ 17899 ★ Ohio State University School of Public Health**
320 W 10th Ave.
M120 Starling-Loving Hall
Columbus, OH 43210-1240
**Phone:** (614)293-3907
**Website:** http://medicine.osu.edu/

## Oklahoma

**★ 17900 ★ University of Oklahoma College of Public Health**
Health Sciences Center, CHB 139
PO Box 26901
Oklahoma City, OK 73190
**Phone:** (405)271-2308   **Fax:** (405)271-3039
**Website:** http://www.ouhsc.edu

## Pennsylvania

**★ 17901 ★ MCP Hahnemann University School of Public Health**
Broad & Vine Sts.
Bellet Bldg., 11th Fl.
Mail Stop 660
Philadelphia, PA 19102-1192
**Phone:** (215)762-8288   **Fax:** (215)246-5347
**Email:** enroll@mcphu.edu
**Website:** http://www.drexel.edu/pubhealth
**Frmly:** Allegheny University of the Health Sciences

**★ 17902 ★ University of Pittsburgh Graduate School of Public Health**
114 Parran Hall
Pittsburgh, PA 15261
**Phone:** (412)624-3002   **Fax:** (412)624-3309
**Website:** http://www.pitt.edu/~gsphhome/

## Puerto Rico

**★ 17903 ★ University of Puerto Rico School of Public Health**
Health Sciences Center
GPO Box 365067
San Juan, PR 00936-5067
**Phone:** (787)764-5975
**Website:** http://wwwrcm.upr.clu.edu

## South Carolina

**★ 17904 ★ University of South Carolina School of Public Health**
Health Sciences Bldg.
Columbia, SC 29208
**Phone:** (803)777-5031   **Fax:** (803)777-4783
**Website:** http://www.sph.sc.edu

## Tennessee

**★ 17905 ★ University of Tennessee, Memphis School of Public Health**
66 N Pauline St., Ste. 633
Memphis, TN 38163
**Phone:** (901)448-5826
**Website:** http://www.utmem.edu/

## Texas

**★ 17906 ★ Texas A&M University School of Rural Public Health**
Health Science Center
260 Centeq Bldg.
TAMU 1266
College Station, TX 77843-1266
**Phone:** (409)845-2387
**Website:** http://hsc.tamu.edu/SRPH/

**★ 17907 ★ University of North Texas Department of Public Health and Preventive Medicine**
Health Science Center
3500 Camp Bowie Blvd.
Fort Worth, TX 76107-2699
**Phone:** (817)735-2204   **Free:** 800-535-TCOM
**Fax:** (817)735-2225
**Email:** studaffr@hsc.unt.edu
**Website:** http://www.hsc.unt.edu/

**★ 17908 ★ University of Texas Health Sciences Center at Houston School of Public Health**
PO Box 20186
Houston, TX 77225
**Phone:** (713)500-9100   **Fax:** (713)791-1369
**Website:** http://www.sph.uth.tmc.edu

## Washington

**★ 17909 ★ University of Washington School of Public Health and Community Medicine**
Box 357230
Seattle, WA 98195-7230
**Phone:** (206)543-1144   **Fax:** (206)543-3813
**Website:** http://weber.u.washington.edu/~sphcm/sphcm.html

# National & International Organizations

**★ 17910 ★ African Medical & Research Foundation (AMREF USA)**
19 W 44th St., Ste. 710
New York, NY 10036
**Phone:** (212)768-2440   **Fax:** (212)768-4230
**Email:** amrefusa@amrefusa.org
**Website:** http://www.amref.org
Priscilla S. Goldfarb, Contact
**Fnded:** 1957. **Reg. Groups:** 11. **Desc:** U.S. branch of the African Medical & Research Foundation. Voluntary organization providing medical services to aid and augment health programs in developing nations and in rural areas of East Africa. Attempts to reach isolated peoples and outlying medical facilities through a

network of 100 two-way radios, clinic-equipped mobile units, and a "Flying Doctor Service." Undertakes research programs in the field of medicine and general health surveys. Designs and implements primary health care projects. Provides health education courses through its training center to train health educators and is implementing a program of continuing education for health workers. health workers. **Pub:** *AFYA*, bimonthly. Journal. • *Defender: Health Journal for Africa*, bimonthly. Journal. • *Rural Health Series*, periodic. **Frmly:** African Research Foundation; (1973) African Medical and Research Foundation; (1981) International Medical and Research Foundation.

**★ 17911 ★ African Medical and Research Foundation - Canada (AMREF Cana)**
489 College St., Ste. 407
Toronto, ON, Canada M6G 1A2
**Phone:** (416)961-6981          **Fax:** (416)961-6984
**Email:** amref.canada@amref.org
**Website:** http://www.amref.org/canada.html
**Fnded:** 1973. **Lang(s):** English, French. **Desc:** Medical and public health professionals in Africa. Seeks to identify and address health needs in rural areas of Africa. Develops, implements, and evaluates public health programs and services; encourages enhancement of local administrative capabilities through training, education, and community participation; facilitates increased participation by women in community development. Conducts outreach and fundraising activities. **Pub:** Newsletter, 3/year. • Brochure, periodic.

**African Medical and Research Foundation - Denmark (AMRFD)**
*See:* Entry 1852

**African Medical and Research Foundation - France (AMRFF)**
*See:* Entry 1853

**★ 17912 ★ African Medical and Research Foundation - Uganda (AMREF/Ugan)**
PO Box 10663
Kampala, Uganda
**Phone:** 256 41 250319          **Fax:** 256 41 344565
**Email:** amrefug@imul.com
**Website:** http://www.amref.org
**Fnded:** 1957. **Desc:** Purpose is to improve the health of people living in Uganda. Focus is on public heath education, sanitation, medical auxilaries, preventive medicine, health care teams, and clinics.

**★ 17913 ★ American Association of Public Health Dentistry (AAPHD)**
3760 SW Lyle Ct.
Portland, OR 97221
**Phone:** (503)242-0712          **Fax:** (503)242-0721
**Email:** natoff@aol.com
**Website:** http://www.aaphd.org
Dr. Rebecca King, Pres.
**Fnded:** 1937. **Mem:** 900. **Desc:** Professional society of dentists, dental hygienists, health educators, and others actively engaged in dental public health. Sponsors competitions. **Pub:** *American Association of Public Health Dentistry–Communique*, quarterly. Newsletter. *Price:* Included in membership dues; $20/year for nonmembers. • *Journal of Public Health Dentistry*, quarterly. Journal. Covers fluoridation, sealants, demographics, and utilization of dental services. Includes research reports and book reviews. *Price:* Included in membership dues; $100/year for nonmembers in U.S.; $100/year for nonmembers outside U.S.; $135/year airmail. **Frmly:** (1983) American Association of Public Health Dentists.

**★ 17914 ★ American Association of Public Health Physicians (AAPHP)**
MSC No. 1720
PO Box 2430
Pensacola, FL 32513-2430
**Phone:** (630)604-3256          **Fax:** (630)604-3256
**Email:** aaphp@iname.com
**Website:** http://www.aaphp.org
David Cuncliff, MD, Pres.
**Fnded:** 1954. **Mem:** 200. **Desc:** Physicians actively engaged in public health. Promotes leadership in the field of public health; speaks for its membership on proposed health legislation at various levels; supports coordination of public health responsibilities in a variety of agencies. Conducts or cosponsors educational seminars. **Pub:** *American Association of Public Health Physicians–Bulletin*, quarterly. Newsletter. *Price:* Included in membership dues.

**★ 17915 ★ American Board of Dental Public Health (ABDPH)**
c/o Stanley Lotzkar, D.D.S.
1321 NW 47th Ter.
Gainesville, FL 32605
**Phone:** (352)378-6301          **Fax:** (352)367-8430
**Email:** slotzkar@yahoo.com
**Website:** http://www.pitt.edu/
Dr. Caswell Evans, Jr., Pres.
**Fnded:** 1950. **Mem:** 5. **Desc:** Board whose purpose is to investigate the qualifications of, administer examinations to, and certify as diplomates, dentists specializing in dental public health. Sponsored by American Association of Public Health Dentistry. **Pub:** *ABDPH Membership Directory*, triennial. Directory. • Newsletter, annual.

**★ 17916 ★ American Council on Science and Health (ACSH)**
1995 Broadway, 2nd Fl.
New York, NY 10023-5860
**Phone:** (212)362-7044          **Fax:** (212)362-4919
**Email:** acsh@acsh.org
**Website:** http://www.acsh.org
Dr. Elizabeth M. Whelan, Pres.
**Fnded:** 1978. **Mem:** 2,000. **Desc:** Provides consumers with scientifically balanced evaluations of food, chemicals, the environment, and human health. Council personnel participate in government regulatory proceedings, congressional hearings, appear on radio and television programs, and public debates and forums. **Pub:** *Cigarettes: What the Warning Label Doesn't Tell You.* • *Directory of Scientific Advisors*, triennial. Directory. • *Media Update*, semiannual. • *News From ACSH*, semiannual. • *Priorities*, quarterly. Magazine. Health and environmental reports for consumers. *Price:* $6.25 single copy; $25 annual subscription. • Papers. • Reports.On health risks and benefits associated with public health and environmental issues.

**American Osteopathic College of Occupational and Preventive Medicine (AOCOPM)**
*See:* Entry 17794

**★ 17917 ★ American Public Health Association (APHA)**
800 I St., NW
Washington, DC 20001-3710
**Phone:** (202)777-2742          **Fax:** (202)777-2534
**Email:** comments@apha.org
**Website:** http://www.apha.org
Mohammad Akhter, MD, Exec. Dir.
**Fnded:** 1872. **Mem:** 32,000. **Desc:** Professional organization of physicians, nurses, educators, academicians, environmentalists, epidemiologists, new professionals, social workers, health administrators, optometrists, podiatrists, pharmacists, dentists, nutritionists, health planners, other community and mental health specialists, and interested consumers. Seeks to protect and promote personal, mental, and environmental health. Services include: promulgation of standards; establishment of uniform practices and procedures; development of the etiology of communicable diseases; research in public health; exploration of medical care programs and their relationships to public health. Sponsors job placement service. **Pub:** *Ameri-*

*can Journal of Public Health*, monthly. Journal. Includes news briefs and annual leadership directory. *Price:* Included in membership dues; $125/year for nonmembers. • *The Nation's Health*, 11/year. Reports on current and proposed legislation, regulations, and policy issues affecting public health; includes reports on current health issues. *Price:* Included in membership dues; $25/year for nonmembers. • Also publishes books, manuals, and pamphlets; maintains publications service.

**Andean Rural Health Care (ARHC)**
*See:* Entry 1933

**★ 17918 ★ Ars Medica pro Humanitate International (AMHI)**
Ave. Abbe Huyberechts 14
B-1340 Ottignies, Belgium
**Email:** sarale@haywood.main.nc.us
**Lang(s):** English, French. **Desc:** Physicians and public health organizations. Seeks to advance medical research and the study and practice of medicine. Serves as a clearinghouse on medical research; makes available health services; sponsors research and educational programs.

**★ 17919 ★ Asian Health Institute (AHI)**
987-30 Minamiyama
Komenogi
Nisshin, Aichi 470-0111, Japan
**Phone:** 81 5617 31950          **Fax:** 81 5617 31990
**Email:** ahi@jca.apc.org
**Website:** http://www.jca.apc.org/ahi/
**Fnded:** 1980. **Mem:** 7,500. **Lang(s):** English, Japanese. **Desc:** Promotes improved public health, particularly in Asia. Conducts public educational campaigns to create indigenous leadership for public health initiatives in the region. **Pub:** *Ajia no Kenko*, bimonthly. Magazine. Member Newsletter. • *Ajia no Kodomo*, semiannual. Magazine. Children's magazine on the lives of children in Asian countries. • *Asian Health Institute*, quarterly. Newsletter. Forum for training course alumni, grassroots health workers. Occasional reports on study tours, special research projects, retrospectives, and so on.

**★ 17920 ★ Asian and Pacific Islander American Health Forum**
c/o Marnelle Marasigan
942 Market St. Ste 200
San Francisco, CA 94102
**Phone:** (415)954-9988          **Fax:** (415)954-9999
**Email:** hforum@apiahf.org
**Website:** http://www.apiahf.org
Tessie Guillermo, Exec. Dir.
**Fnded:** 1986. **Mem:** 350. **Desc:** Promotes policy, program, and research efforts for the improvement of health status of all Asian and Pacific Islander Americans. Examines and review the distribution of factors associated with health problems and issues facing Asian and Pacific Islander Americans, including infectious diseases, diabetes, hypertension, cancer, HIV/AIDS, substance abuse, and mental health disorders. Compiles statistics. Conducts research programs. **Pub:** *APIAHF Focus*, quarterly. Newsletter. • *APITEN Newsletter*. Newsletter. • *Confronting Critical Health Issues of Asian and Pacific Islander Americans*. Book.

**Association of Community Health Nursing Educators**
*See:* Entry 15663

**★ 17921 ★ Association of Local Public Health Agencies (ALOPA)**
425 University Ave., Ste. 502
Toronto, ON, Canada M5G 1T6
**Phone:** (416)595-0006          **Fax:** (416)595-0030
**Email:** mail@alphaweb.org
**Website:** http://www.alphaweb.org

**Lang(s):** English, French. **Desc:** Local public health agencies. Promotes increased availability and effectiveness of public health programs. Lobbies for improved legislation governing public health; facilitates communication and cooperation among members; publicizes public health programs. **Frmly:** (1997) Association of Local Official Health Agencies.

**★ 17922 ★ Association of Public Health Laboratories (APHL)**
2025 M St. NW, Ste. 550
Washington, DC 20036-3320
**Phone:** (202)822-5227          **Fax:** (202)887-5098
**Email:** info@aphl.org
**Website:** http://www.aphl.org
Scott J. Becker, Exec. Dir.

**Fnded:** 1989. **Mem:** 320. **Desc:** Represents national, state and local public health laboratories. Collaborates with partners in private and public sectors, advocating and formulating sound public health and partners in private and public sectors advocating and formulating sound public health and environmental health policies, and providing technical assistance and training. **Pub:** *APHL Washington Bulletin*, monthly. Report. Features legislation update.

**★ 17923 ★ Association of Schools of Public Health (ASPH)**
1101 15th St. NW, Ste. 910
Washington, DC 20005
**Phone:** (202)296-1099          **Fax:** (202)296-1252
**Email:** info@asph.org
**Website:** http://www.asph.org
Susan Scrimshaw, Chair

**Fnded:** 1941. **Mem:** 28. **Desc:** Accredited graduate schools of public health. Provides focus for the enhancement of academic public health programs. Serves as an information center for governmental and private groups, and individuals whose concerns overlap those of higher education for public health. **Pub:** *Gerontology Programs and Curricula in U.S. Schools of Public Health.* • *Public Health Career Information.* • *Reach.*

**★ 17924 ★ Association of Schools of Public Health in the European Region (ASPHER)**
**(Association des Ecoles de Sante Publique de la Regional Europeenne)**
c/o Marie Cardon, Sec.
14, rue du val d'Onse
F-94415 Saint Maurice Cedex, France
**Phone:** 33 1 43966459     **Fax:** 33 1 43966463
**Email:** aspher@aspher.ensp.fr
**Website:** http://www.ensp.fr/aspher

**Fnded:** 1966. **Mem:** 57. **Lang(s):** English, French, German, Spanish. **Desc:** Schools of public health and other institutions offering graduate instruction in public health. Promotes the study and development of education in public health and health services. Conducts workshops and seminars. Organizes exchange of students and staff between member schools. **Pub:** Newsletter, monthly. Contains information about the association's activities.

**★ 17925 ★ Association of State Drinking Water Administrators (ASDWA)**
1025 Connecticut Ave. NW, Ste. 903
Washington, DC 20036-3902
**Phone:** (202)293-7655          **Fax:** (202)293-7656
**Email:** asdwa@erols.com
**Website:** http://www.asdwa.org
Vanessa M. Leiby, Exec. Dir.

**Fnded:** 1984. **Mem:** 56. **Desc:** Managers of state and territorial drinking water programs; state regulatory personnel. Works to meet communication and coordination needs of state drinking water program managers; facilitates the exchange of information and experience among state drinking water agents. Acts as a collective voice for the protection of public health through assurance of high quality drinking water; oversees the implementation of the Safe Drinking Water Act. Liaises with Congress and the Environmental Protection Agency. Holds training sessions. **Pub:** *ASDWA Update*, bimonthly. Newsletter. For state drinking water administrators, water industry personnel, and all others interested in the latest issues related to drinking water. *Price:* Included in membership dues; $40/year for nonmembers.

**★ 17926 ★ Association of State and Territorial Directors of Public Health Education (ASTDHPPHE)**
1101 5th St., NW, Ste. 601
Washington, DC 20005
**Phone:** (202)659-2230          **Fax:** (202)659-2339
**Email:** director@astdhpphe.org
**Website:** http://www.astdhpphe.org
Rose Marie Matulionis, Exec. Dir.

**Fnded:** 1946. **Mem:** 175. **Desc:** Directors of public health education in state and territorial departments of health and Indian health service areas. Seeks to improve the quality of public health education practice; promote information exchange and advocacy. Develops practice guidelines and supports collection and dissemination of data and information relevant to public health education. **Pub:** *Conference Call*, quarterly. Newsletter. • *Roster of Members*, quarterly. • Proceedings, annual. **Frmly:** (1989) Conference of State and Territorial Directors of Public Health Education.

**★ 17927 ★ Brazilian Association for the Promotion of Appropriate Technology in Health Care**
**(Associacao Brasileira de Tecnologia Alternativa na Promocao da Saude — TAPS)**
Caixa Postal 20396
04041-990 Sao Paulo, SP, Brazil
**Phone:** 55 11 55720466     **Fax:** 55 11 55720465
**Email:** info@taps.org.br
**Website:** http://www.taps.org.br

**Fnded:** 1981. **Mem:** 40. **Lang(s):** Portuguese. **Desc:** Promotes health and domestic development in Brazil with emphasis on improving health care through appropriate technology. Functional in the following areas: health and nutrition; technical assistance; training and publications.

**★ 17928 ★ Canadian Association of Poison Control Centres**
Foot Hills Hospital
1403 29th St. NW
Calgary, AB, Canada T2N 2T9
**Phone:** (403)670-1414     **Free:** 800-332-1414
**Fax:** (403)813-7489
**Email:** ingridvicis@calgaryhealthregion.ca

**Fnded:** 1981. **Lang(s):** English, French. **Desc:** Poison control centers. Promotes increased public awareness of poisoning prevention and the steps to take in case of poisoning. Facilitates communication and cooperation among members; conducts educational and promotional programs.

**Canadian Association of Public Health Dentistry**
**(L'Association Canadienne des Dentistes en Sante Communautaire)**
*See:* Entry 6491

**★ 17929 ★ Canadian Council on Multicultural Health (CCMH)**
**(Conseil Canadien de la Sante Multiculturelle — CCSM)**
1017 Wilson Ave., Ste. 400
Downsview, ON, Canada M3K 1Z1
**Phone:** (416)630-8835          **Fax:** (416)638-6076
**Email:** ccmh@inforamp.net
**Website:** http://www.caphd-acsdp.org

**Lang(s):** English, French. **Desc:** Health care professionals and other individuals with an interest in public health. Promotes increased availability of health care services among previously underserved populations. Serves as a clearinghouse on multicultural health and related issues; makes available support and assistance to health care services.

**★ 17930 ★ Canadian Institute of Public Health Inspectors (CIPHI)**
**(Institut Canadien des Inspecteurs en Hygiene Publique — ICIHP)**
PO Box 75264
White Rock Postal Outlet
White Rock, BC, Canada V8B 5L4
**Free:** 888-245-8180          **Fax:** (604)543-0936
**Email:** president@ciphi.ca
**Website:** http://www.ciphi.ca

**Fnded:** 1934. **Mem:** 1,000. **Lang(s):** English, French. **Desc:** Public health inspectors. Seeks to advance the profession of public health inspection; promotes adherence to high standards of ethics and practice among members. Conducts advocacy campaigns to increase public appreciation of the role of public health inspectors; sponsors educational and training programs.

**★ 17931 ★ Canadian Public Health Association**
Ste. 400
1565 Carling Ave.
Ottawa, ON, Canada K1Z 8R1
**Phone:** (613)725-3769          **Fax:** (613)725-9826
**Email:** info@cpha.ca
**Website:** http://www.cpha.ca

**Fnded:** 1912. **Mem:** 1,600. **Lang(s):** English, French. **Desc:** Works to mobilize national charitable and volunteer resources to address public health concerns worldwide. Conducts immunization, maternal and child health, and HIV/AIDS programs in at-risk areas.

**★ 17932 ★ Canadian Society for International Health (SCIH)**
**(Societe Canadienne de Sante Internationale — SCSI)**
1 Nichols St., Ste. 1105
Ottawa, ON, Canada K1N 7B7
**Phone:** (613)241-5785          **Fax:** (613)541-3845
**Email:** csih@csih.org
**Website:** http://www.csih.org

**Fnded:** 1977. **Mem:** 600. **Lang(s):** English, French. **Desc:** Health care services and individuals and organizations with an interest in global public health. Promotes increased availability and quality of health services in previously underserved areas worldwide. Advocates for health policy and programming that contributes to global objectives of health for all; equity, and social justice through partnership building with Canadian and other institutions and organizations. **Pub:** *Online Synergy*, weekly. Newsletter. • *PAHO News*, weekly.

**★ 17933 ★ CityMatch**
c/o Magda G. Peck
University of Nebraska Medical Center
Department of Pediatrics
982170 Nebraska Medical Center
Omaha, NE 68198-2170
**Phone:** (402)561-7500          **Fax:** (402)561-7525
**Email:** citymch@unmc.edu
**Website:** http://www.citymatch.org/
Magda G. Peck, SC.D., Exec. Dir. /CEO

**Fnded:** 1989. **Mem:** 142. **Nat'l Groups:** 11. **Reg. Groups:** 10. **Local Groups:** 11. **Desc:** City and county health departments, leaders representing urban communities in the United States, and interested others. Seeks to provide optimal health care for children and families in urban areas. Gives particular attention to increasing racial disparities in infant mortality, inadequate access to prenatal care, substance abuse in pregnancy, and interpersonal violence. Provides children's services; compiles statistics. **Pub:** *CityLights*, quarterly. Newsletter. • *Technical Reports.* • *What Works: 1990 Urban MCH Programs*. Directory.

Maternal and Child health programs in major urban health departments.

**Clinical Directors Network (CDN)**
*See:* Entry 2061

**ComCARE Alliance**
*See:* Entry 8577

★ 17934 ★ **Commissioned Officers Association of the United States Public Health Service (COA)**
8201 Corporate Dr., Ste. 560
Landover, MD 20785
**Phone:** (301)731-9080　　　**Fax:** (301)731-9084
**Email:** gfarrell@coausphs.org
**Website:** http://www.coausphs.org
Jerry Farrell, Exec. Dir.
**Fnded:** 1910. **Mem:** 6,700. **Local Groups:** 52. **Desc:** Commissioned officers of the U.S. Public Health Service; includes career active duty, retired, and inactive reserve officers who are physicians, dentists, scientists, engineers, pharmacists, nurses, and other types of professional personnel. Acts as an official spokesperson for the Commissioned Corps, as an information center for its members, and "as a sounding board where views and concerns of the Corps may be brought to the proper authorities for official action." **Pub:** *Frontline*, 10/year. Bulletin. • *Proceedings of Annual Meeting*. Proceedings.

★ 17935 ★ **Community Systems Foundation (CSF)**
1310 Hill St.
Ann Arbor, MI 48104
**Phone:** (734)761-1357　　　**Fax:** (734)761-1356
**Email:** williamddrake@cs.com
**Website:** http://www-personal.umich.edu/~wddrake/csf/
William D. Drake, Pres.
**Fnded:** 1963. **Mem:** 10. **Desc:** Organization committed to improving the quality of life through applied research and direct assistance to communities, governmental agencies, and service-oriented entities in the private sector. Focuses on community learning and encourages citizen involvement. Is working to develop systems for evaluating, monitoring, and implementing programs of nutrition and family planning such as UNICEF's ChildInfo System. **Pub:** *Research Reports*. Reports.

★ 17936 ★ **Consumer's Health Forum of Australia (CHF)**
PO Box 170
Curtin, ACT 2605, Australia
**Phone:** 61 2 6281 0811　　　**Fax:** 61 2 6281 0959
**Email:** info@chf.org.au
**Website:** http://www.chf.org.au
**Fnded:** 1987. **Mem:** 250. **Desc:** Health organizations. Promotes public and preventative health perspective; encourages development of health services; promotes consumer rights in the area of health care. **Pub:** Annual Report.

★ 17937 ★ **Council on Education for Public Health (CEPH)**
800 Eye St., NW Ste. 202
Washington, DC 20001-3710
**Phone:** (202)789-1050　　　**Fax:** (202)789-1895
**Email:** patevans@ceph.org
**Website:** http://www.ceph.org
Patricia P. Evans, Exec. Dir.
**Fnded:** 1974. **Mem:** 2. **Desc:** Participants are professional associations representing public health practice (American Public Health Association) and public health education (Association of Schools of Public Health). Seeks to strengthen educational programs in schools of public health and graduate public health programs through accreditation, consultation, research, and other appropriate services; and to encourage the development of experimental and innovative programs which will ensure educational quality. **Pub:** *Manuals for Accreditation of Graduate Schools of Public Health and Graduate Public Health Programs*. Manuals.

★ 17938 ★ **Delta Omega**
c/o Judy Peterson/Marsha Reinking
1101 15th St. NW, Ste. 910
Washington, DC 20005
**Phone:** (612)624-6669　　　**Free:** 800-774-8636
**Fax:** (612)626-3500
**Email:** ajf@asph.org
**Website:** http://www.deltaomega.org
Leonard Schuman, MD, Contact
**Fnded:** 1924. **Mem:** 4,000. **Reg. Groups:** 18. **Local Groups:** 18. **Desc:** Honorary society - men and women, public health. Promotes research and scholarly attainment; sponsors lectures.

★ 17939 ★ **DKT International - Vietnam (DKTIVN)**
8 Trang Thi St., Glass House No. 13-15
Hanoi, Vietnam
**Phone:** 84 4 8260043　　　**Fax:** 84 4 8260262
**Email:** larry@dktinternational.org
**Website:** http://www.dktinternational.org
**Fnded:** 1993. **Lang(s):** English, French, Vietnamese. **Desc:** Population and public health programs operating in Vietnam. Seeks to increase availability of primary health care and family planning services. Makes available health services; conducts educational programs to raise public awareness of population issues.

★ 17940 ★ **Estonian Centre for Health Education and Promotion (Eesti Tervisekasvatuse Keskus)**
Ruutli St. 24
EE-0001 Tallinn, Estonia
**Phone:** 372 6 279280　　　**Fax:** 372 6 440800
**Email:** kadi@tervis.ee
**Fnded:** 1993. **State Groups:** 15. **Lang(s):** English, Finnish, Russian. **Desc:** Conducts health promotion and evaluation activities in Estonia to prevent disease. **Pub:** *Tervist*, monthly. Newsletter.

★ 17941 ★ **European Public Health Alliance**
33, rue de Pascale
B-1040 Brussels, Belgium
**Phone:** 32 2 2303056　　　**Fax:** 32 2 2333880
**Email:** genon@epha.org
**Website:** http://www.epha.org
**Fnded:** 1993. **Mem:** 82. **Lang(s):** Dutch, English, French, German, Italian, Spanish. **Desc:** Strives to improve public health in Europe through policy monitoring and development. Works to heighten public awareness on current public health reforms. Communicates with other organizations with similar interests. **Pub:** *Commercial Sponsorship and NGOs*. Booklet. Discusses the potential advantages and disadvantages of commercial sponsorship and NGOs. • *Creating a Citizen-centered EU Health Policy*. Paper. Position paper on the health strategy for the European union. • *European Health Directory*. Directory. Contains contact details of major European health stakeholders (NGOs and other not-for-profit associations). • *European Public Health Update*. Newsletter. • *Public Health and the EU - an Overview*. Book. Thirteen chapters introducing a range of health related EU policies. • *Research Priorities for Public Health in Europe*. The final report of a major EPHA conference held in Brussels, Belgium in July 1993.

★ 17942 ★ **Faculty of Public Health Medicine**
4 St Andrew's Pl.
London NW1 4LB, United Kingdom
**Phone:** 44 171 9350243　　　**Fax:** 44 171 2246973
**Email:** enquiries@fphm.org.uk
**Website:** http://www.fphm.org.uk
**Fnded:** 1972. **Mem:** 2,500. **Desc:** Principally trainees and consultants in public health medicine. To promote, for the public benefit, the advancement of education in the field of public health medicine; and to develop public health medicine with a view to maintaining the highest possible standards of professional competence and practice, and act as an authoritative body for the purpose of consultation in matters of education or public interest concerning public health medicine. **Pub:** *HFA 2000 News*, quarterly. • *Journal of Public Health Medicine*, quarterly. Journal. • *Public Health Physician*, quarterly. • Reports.

**Food and Nutrition Board (FNB)**
*See:* Entry 16479

★ 17943 ★ **Foundation for Revitalization of Local Health (FRLHT)**
50 MSH Layout, 2nd Stage, 3rd Main
Anandnagar
Bangalore 560 024, Karnataka, India
**Phone:** 91 80 3336909　　　**Fax:** 91 80 3334167
**Email:** root@frlht.ernet.in
**Fnded:** 1991. **Lang(s):** English, Hindi. **Desc:** Promotes traditional medicine as an integral part of public health programs in developing areas. Facilitates international cooperation in understanding the theoretical foundation and epistemology of traditional medical practices; works to preserve the biodiversity upon which traditional medicine depends. Gathers and disseminates information on medicinal plants. Promotes development of traditional medical centers. **Pub:** *Amruth*, bimonthly. Magazine.

★ 17944 ★ **General Association of Municipal Health and Technical Experts (GAMHTE) (Association Generale des Hygienistes et Techniciens Municipaux — AGHTM)**
83 Av. Foch
BP 3916
F-75761 Paris cedex 16, France
**Phone:** 33 1 53701353　　　**Fax:** 33 1 53701340
**Email:** aghtm@aghtm.org
**Website:** http://www.aghtm.org
**Fnded:** 1905. **Mem:** 3,500. **Local Groups:** 5. **Lang(s):** French. **Desc:** Engineers, engineering consultants, technicians, architects, scientists, administrators, and municipal and private services in 32 countries. Objectives are to: stimulate fundamental and applied research on urban and rural public hygiene; disseminate findings of such research; encourage the exchange of information and ideas among members. Areas of interest include city planning, energy management, traffic problems, and pollution prevention. Operates information service; organizes field tours. **Pub:** *Techniques Sciences-Methodes*, monthly. Also publishes monographs. **Frmly:** Association Generale des Ingenieurs, Architectes et Hygienistes Municipaux de France, Algerie, Tunisie, Belgique, Suisse et Luxembourg.

**Global Human Research Foundation (GHR)**
*See:* Entry 11775

★ 17945 ★ **Health Education Foundation (HEF)**
2600 Virginia Ave. NW, Ste. 502
Washington, DC 20037
**Phone:** (202)338-3501　　　**Fax:** (202)965-6520
**Email:** hefmona@erols.com
Morris E. Chafetz, MD, Pres.
**Fnded:** 1975. **Desc:** Seeks to develop cost-effective health promotion programs for government, industry, and the business community; helps people make informed decisions about their physical and mental health; participates in research for analysis and development of standards and programs to meet public health needs. **Pub:** *Conference Proceedings*, periodic.

Proceedings. • *Health Fact Tips*, semiannual. • *HEF News: Perspectives on Health, Behavior, and Lifestyle*, quarterly. Newsletter. *Price:* $15/year. • Monograph. • Pamphlets.

**★ 17946 ★ Indian Public Health Association**
110 Chittaranjan Av
Calcutta 700 073, India

**★ 17947 ★ International College for Health Cooperation in Developing Countries - Italy**
**(CUAMM - Medici con l'Africa)**
Via San Francesco 126
I-35100 Padua, Italy
**Phone:** 39 49 8751649　　**Fax:** 39 49 8574738
**Email:** cuamm@cuamm.org
**Website:** http://www.padovanet.it/associazioni/cuamm/casa.htm
**Fnded:** 1950. **Mem:** 324. **Lang(s):** English, Italian. **Desc:** Works to improve public health and increase the availability of health care services and preventive medical programs in developing countries. Facilitates cooperation among international development agencies with health-related programs. Conducts educational and training programs in health related areas including community development and water supply and sanitation. Makes available emergency medical relief services. **Pub:** *CUAMM Notizie - Salute E Sviluppo*, quarterly. Journal.

**★ 17948 ★ International Institute of Concern for Public Health (IICPH)**
517 College St., Ste. 233
Toronto, ON, Canada M6G 4A2
**Phone:** (416)929-9808　　**Fax:** (416)260-3404
**Email:** info@iicph.org
**Website:** http://www.iicph.org
**Fnded:** 1984. **Mem:** 80. **Lang(s):** English, French, Spanish. **Desc:** Promotes dissemination of information on public health and related topics including environmental and occupational health and human rights. Serves as a clearinghouse on international public health and related issues; assists in the development of model health-related human rights legislation. Conducts research and educational programs; compiles statistics; maintains speakers' bureau. Provides support and assistance to communities wishing to maintain their own public health databases. **Pub:** *International Perspectives in Public Health*, annual. Journal. • Newsletter, bimonthly. Contains articles relating to the environment, work and health.

**★ 17949 ★ International Medical Services for Health (INMED)**
45449 Severn Way, Ste. 161
Sterling, VA 20166
**Phone:** (703)444-4477　　**Free:** 800-521-1175
**Fax:** (703)444-4471
**Email:** contact@inmed.org
**Website:** http://www.inmed.org
Linda Pfeiffer, PhD, Pres.
**Fnded:** 1986. **Desc:** Works to help disadvantaged people worldwide to improve the health of their families and communities. Assists community based programs in 98 countries to achieve lasting changes for better health. Operates MotherNet America, a lay home visiting program to reduce infant mortality, low birthweight, child abuse and neglect and other risks facing disadvantaged families; conducts the Children as Agents of Change treatment and education program; links businesses and non-profit organizations in strategic alliances; provides access to medicine for non-profit organizations; offers technical assistance and training. **Pub:** *InScope*, quarterly. Newsletter.

**★ 17950 ★ International Network for the History of Public Health (INHPH)**
c/o Marie C. Nelson
The Tema Institute

Linkoping University
S-58183 Linkoping, Sweden
**Phone:** 46 13 282808　　**Fax:** 46 13 281843
**Email:** marne@tema.liu.se
**Website:** http://www.tema.liu.se/inhph
**Fnded:** 1992. **Mem:** 294. **Lang(s):** English. **Desc:** Scholars throughout the world who are interested in history of public health. Promotes the study of the history of the collective efforts for the improvement of the health of populations from antiquity to modern times. Seeks to improve communication among scholars in the field and promotes comparative research efforts.

**★ 17951 ★ Josiah Macy, Jr. Foundation**
44 E 64th St.
New York, NY 10021
**Free:** 800-521-0600
**Website:** http://www.josiahmacyfoundation.org
June E. Osborn, MD, Pres.
**Desc:** Strives to promote public health awareness. **Pub:** *Chairman's Summary of the Conference, Education for More Synergistic Practice of Medicine and Public Health.* Proceedings. Contains information on conference.

**★ 17952 ★ MAP International - Kenya**
3rd Fl. Studio House
Intersection of Argwings Kohdek and Chaka Rds.
PO Box 21663
Nairobi, Kenya
**Phone:** 254 2 727586　　**Fax:** 254 2 714422
**Email:** mapesa@map.org
**Website:** http://www.map.org
**Mem:** 10. **Desc:** Provides training, consultancy, and health education services. Disseminates information about AIDS and other health issues. Provides a forum for the exchange of information. **Pub:** *A Pastoral Counselling Manual for AIDS.* Booklet. • *AIDS in Africa, the Churches Opportunity.* Booklet. • *AIDS in Your Community.* Booklet. • *Community Balanced Development.* Booklet. • *Facts and Feelings About AIDS.* Booklet. • *Giving and Getting AIDS.* Booklet. • *Growing Together.* Booklet. • *Helpers for a Healing Community.* Booklet. • *Patterns for Life.* Booklet. • *Springs of Life.* Video. Educational AIDS video for church leaders.

**★ 17953 ★ Medicine in the Public Interest (MIPI)**
192 South St., Ste. 500
Boston, MA 02111
**Phone:** (617)728-7977　　**Fax:** (617)728-9135
Michael R. Sonnenreich, Pres.
**Fnded:** 1973. **Desc:** Professionals in medicine, law, and the social sciences. Promotes and funds research into medicine and related social, legal, and ethical issues; disseminates research findings and proposals. Encourages the development of long-range public health, welfare, and social planning at the federal, state, and local levels. Cooperates with governmental representatives in analyzing and developing legislation and programs designed to serve the public health and welfare. **Pub:** *Intellectual Property Rights and Their Special Impact on Biotechnology.* Booklet. Contains conference proceedings. *Price:* $10. • *The Net DTC Conference.* Booklet. *Price:* $10. • Reports.

**★ 17954 ★ National Association of County and City Health Officials (NACCHO)**
1100 17th St. NW 2nd Fl.
Washington, DC 20036-4631
**Phone:** (202)783-5550　　**Fax:** (202)783-1583
**Email:** info@naccho.org
**Website:** http://www.naccho.org
Thomas Milne, Exec. Dir.
**Fnded:** 1965. **Mem:** 1,000. **Desc:** County and city (local) health officials. Purposes are to stimulate and contribute to the improvement of local health programs and public health practices throughout the U.S.; disseminate information on local health programs and

practices; participate in the formulation of the policies of the National Association of Counties. Is developing self-assessment instrument for use by local health officials. Operates Primary Care Project which helps to strengthen the link between local health departments and community health centers. Provides educational workshops for local health officials. **Pub:** *Membership Monthly*, monthly. Information guide for members. *Price:* Included in membership dues. • *NACCHO News*, bimonthly. *Price:* Included in membership dues. • Annual Report. **Frmly:** National Association of County Health Officials; (1975) National Association of County Health Officers.

**National Association of Public Health Service Dentists**
**(Bundesverband der Zahnarzte des Offentlichen Gesundheitsdienstes)**
*See:* Entry 6564

**★ 17955 ★ National Association for Public Health Statistics and Information Systems (NAPHSIS)**
1220 19th St., NW, Ste. 802
Washington, DC 20036
**Phone:** (202)463-8851　　**Fax:** (202)463-4870
**Email:** hq@naphsis.org
**Website:** http://www.NAPHSIS.org
Delton Atkinson, Contact
**Fnded:** 1933. **Mem:** 250. **Desc:** Advocates, creates, and maintains comprehensive public health information systems that integrate vital records registration, public health statistics, and other health information. **Pub:** *The Journal*, bimonthly. Journal.

**National Association of Public Hospitals and Health Systems (NAPH)**
*See:* Entry 11503

**★ 17956 ★ National Pediculosis Association (NPA)**
PO Box 610189
Newton, MA 02458
**Phone:** (781)449-6487　　**Free:** 800-446-4NPA
**Fax:** (781)449-8129
**Email:** npa@headlice.org
**Website:** http://www.headlice.org
Deborah Z. Altschuler, Pres.
**Fnded:** 1983. **Desc:** Parents, physicians, school nurses, and individuals representing hospitals and county health departments. Works to eliminate the incidence, particularly among children, of pediculosis (head lice). Conducts public education campaign to make pediculosis control a public health priority; acts as consumer advocate to ensure the quality and safety of products for treating pediculosis and scabies; encourages scientific research to discover methods of treatment that minimize the use of pesticides, which may harm pregnant and nursing women as well as infants and children. Disseminates information on identifying, treating, and preventing pediculosis, with emphasis on finding and removing nits (louse eggs) in the hair. Provides consultations to schools, camps, and other organizations. Maintains speakers' bureau and creates exhibits for professional meetings and conferences. Operates lending library of audiovisual aids; makes available other educational tools including posters and pamphlets. Sponsors National Pediculosis Prevention Month in September. Sponsors scientific advisory board of experts in such fields as entomology, dermatology, toxicology, pediatrics, parasitology, and pharmacology. **Pub:** *Keep Your Wits Not Your Nits.* • *Latest Greatest Coloring Book About Lice.*

**★ 17957 ★ National Restaurant Association Quality Assurance Study Group**
c/o National Restaurant Association
1200 17th St. NW
Washington, DC 20036

**Phone:** (202)331-5900     **Free:** 800-424-5156
**Fax:** (202)331-2429
**Email:** ga@lists.restaurant.org
**Website:** http://www.restaurant.org/ga/index.cfm
Rosemary Y. Curtis, Admin. Asst.

**Mem:** 208. **Desc:** Professional quality assurance and quality control personnel sanitarians from the National Restaurant Association working in foodservice facilities. Provides members with the opportunity to share common goals, concerns, ideas, and problems. Conducts research and educational programs and semiannual study group meeting.

★ **17958** ★ **People's Health Centre (PHC) (Gonoshasthaya Kendra — GK)**
Nayarhat
Dhaka 1350, Bangladesh
**Phone:** 880 2 9332245     **Fax:** 880 2 863567
**Email:** gk.mail@drik.bgd.toolnet.org

**Fnded:** 1971. **Mem:** 1,500. **Lang(s):** Bangla, English. **Desc:** Health care professionals and other individuals with an interest in public health, nutrition, civil and human rights issues, and agricultural development. Seeks to insure a higher standard of living for people living in rural areas of southern Asia. Provides primary health care services; manufactures and distributes vaccines and other medications. Conducts leadership training courses for women; sponsors educational and vocational training programs. Facilitates the establishment of incomegenerating microenterprises. **Pub:** Monthly Gonoshasthaya, monthly. Magazine.

★ **17959** ★ **Public Citizen Health Research Group (PCHRG)**
1600 20th St. NW
Washington, DC 20009
**Phone:** (202)588-1000     **Fax:** (202)588-7796
**Email:** member@citizen.org
**Website:** http://www.citizen.org/
Joan Claybrook, Pres.

**Fnded:** 1971. **Desc:** Works on issues of health care delivery, workplace safety and health, drug regulation, food additives, medical device safety, and environmental influences on health. Petitions or sues federal agencies on consumers' behalf, testifies before Congress on health matters, and monitors the enforcement of health and safety legislation. Publicizes important health findings; makes available to the public a broad spectrum of research and consumer action materials in the form of books and reports. **Pub:** Health Letter, monthly. Consumer newsletter reporting on health and health policy issues. **Price:** $18/year. • Health Research Group List of Publications, annual. • Worst Pills, Best Pills News, monthly. Newsletter. Consumer newsletter reporting an drug safety issues. **Price:** $20/year.

★ **17960** ★ **Public Health Association**
58 Langdale Rd.
Manchester M14 5PN, United Kingdom
**Email:** info@dukpha.org.uk

**Fnded:** 1989. **Mem:** 1,000. **Reg. Groups:** 4. **State Groups:** 3. **Desc:** Aims to promote public health, by bringing people together across UK, especially tackling inequalities.

★ **17961** ★ **Public Health Association of Australia (PHAA)**
20 Napier Close
Deakin, ACT 2600, Australia
**Phone:** 61 2 62852373     **Fax:** 61 2 62825438
**Email:** phaa@phaa.net.au
**Website:** http://www.phaa.net.au

**Fnded:** 1990. **Mem:** 1,800. **State Groups:** 7. **Lang(s):** English. **Desc:** Individuals, corporations, government agencies, and community-based organizations from more than 40 public health related disciplines. Provides a forum for the exchange of ideas, knowledge, and information on public health. Advocates for public health policy, development, research, and training. **Pub:** Australian and New Zealand Journal of Public Health, bimonthly. Journal.

★ **17962** ★ **Public Health Committee of the Council of Europe**
Council of Europe
F-67075 Strasbourg Cedex, France
**Phone:** 33 3 88412176
**Email:** peter.baum@coe.int
**Website:** http://www.coe.fr/soc-sp

**Desc:** A steering committee of the Council of Europe. Representatives of national ministries of health. Coordinates activities of the committees of experts assembled by CE under the Partial Agreement in the Social and Pubic Health Field. The goal of the Agreement is to assist in the development of uniform legislation in participating countries in the areas of public health and consumer protection.

★ **17963** ★ **Royal Institute of Health and Hygiene and Society of Public Health**
28 Portland Place
London W1N 4DE, United Kingdom
**Phone:** 44 171 5802731
**Website:** http://www.riph.org.uk

**Fnded:** 1856. **Mem:** 1,700. **Nat'l Groups:** 12. **Lang(s):** English. **Desc:** Medical practitioners, dental practitioners, and environmental health officers from 19 countries. Seeks to advance public health and integrated health services. Provides a forum for information exchange among specialists. Reviews existing methodologies and proposes new practices. Serves as an advisory body to governmental and other organizations. Assists in developing continuing professional training for specialists in public health and preventive medicine. Conducts research. **Pub:** Health & Hygiene, quarterly. Journal. Features articles on health hygiene. • Public Health, bimonthly. Journal. Contains articles submitted on public health matters worldwide. **Frmly:** Society of Public Health; (1856) Society of Medical Officers of Health; (1973) Society of Community Medicine.

★ **17964** ★ **SEAMEO Regional Centre for Public Health**
c/o College of Public Health
625 Pedro Gil St.
Ermita
Manila, Philippines
**Phone:** 63 2 5242703     **Fax:** 63 2 5211394
**Email:** vchan@cph.upm.edu.ph

**Fnded:** 1927. **Mem:** 59. **Desc:** A project of the Southeast Asian Ministers of Education Organization. Encourages excellence in public health education programs in southeast Asia. Conducts training programs.

★ **17965** ★ **Singapore Medical Association (SMA)**
Alumni Medical Centre
2 College Rd., Level 2
Singapore 169850, Singapore
**Phone:** 65 2231264     **Fax:** 65 2247827
**Email:** sma@sma.org.sg
**Website:** http://www.sma.org.sg

**Fnded:** 1959. **Mem:** 3,200. **Lang(s):** English. **Desc:** Promotes medicine and allied sciences in Singapore. Maintains the honour and interests of the medical profession. Represents the medical profession before government and other organizations. Maintains standards of medical ethics and conduct. Provides a forum for social, cultural, and professional contact among members. Organizes public health educational programs; offers CPR training; administers a training programme for health care assistants. **Pub:** Singapore Medical Association, monthly. Newsletter. News article, classified ads. • Singapore Medical Journal, monthly. Journal. Includes scientific papers.

★ **17966** ★ **Society of Health Education and Health Promotion Specialists (SHEPS)**
c/o The Membership Sec.
64 Terregles Ave.
Glasgow G41 4LX, United Kingdom

**Phone:** 44 141 2014774     **Fax:** 44 141 2019801
**Email:** stewart.maclennar@glasgow-hb.scot.nhs.uk
**Website:** http://www.hj-web.co.uk/sheps/

**Fnded:** 1980. **Mem:** 500. **Reg. Groups:** 10. **Lang(s):** English. **Desc:** Provides a voice for health promotion theory and practice within the broader context of public health. **Frmly:** (2001) Society of Health Education and Promotion Specialists.

**Society for Nutrition Education (SNE)**
See: Entry 16507

★ **17967** ★ **Society for Public Health Education (SOPHE)**
750 First St. NE, Ste. 910
Washington, DC 20002-4242
**Phone:** (202)408-9804     **Fax:** (202)408-9815
**Email:** info@sophe.org
**Website:** http://www.sophe.org
Elaine Auld, Exec. Dir.

**Fnded:** 1950. **Mem:** 1,900. **Local Groups:** 20. **Desc:** Researchers and practitioners in health education/ health promotion concerned with personal and community health problems. Seeks to promote, encourage, and contribute to the advancement of health of all people by encouraging research, improving health practices, elevating standards of achievement in public health education, and advocating for public health policies. **Pub:** Health Education & Behavior, bimonthly. Journal. Research and practice in social/behavioral sciences and health education. **Price:** Included in membership. • News and Views, bimonthly. Newsletter. • SOPHE Membership Directory & Buyer's Guide. Membership Directory. **Frmly:** Society of Public Health Educators.

★ **17968** ★ **U.S.-Mexico Border Health Association (USMBHA)**
5400 Suncrest Dr., Ste. C-5
El Paso, TX 79912-5615
**Phone:** (915)833-6450     **Fax:** (915)833-7840
**Email:** mail@usmbha.org
**Website:** http://www.usmbha.org
Alfonso Ruiz, Exec. Dir.

**Fnded:** 1943. **Mem:** 500. **Desc:** Physicians, public health administrators, nurses, sanitary engineers, veterinarians, scientists, laboratory workers, and other health officers from the 4 American and 6 Mexican states bordering the two countries. Seeks to make easier and more efficient the improvement of public health along both sides of the border; provides for exchange of experiences, discussion of mutual problems in human and animal diseases, and development of personal and professional contacts necessary for carrying out health projects. Sponsors seminars and workshops covering topics such as: food handling; rabies; tuberculosis; epidemiological principles; sexually transmitted diseases. Compiles statistics. **Pub:** Journal of Border Health, quarterly. Journal. Contains articles on U.S.-Mexico border health issues. **Price:** $5/issue. • Report of Activities, annual. • U.S.-Mexico Border Health Association–News/Noticias, quarterly. **Frmly:** (1975) United States-Mexico Border Health Association.

★ **17969** ★ **Women's International Public Health Network (WIPHN)**
7100 Oak Forest Ln.
Bethesda, MD 20817
**Phone:** (301)469-9210     **Fax:** (301)469-8423
**Email:** wiphn@erols.com
Dr. Naomi Baumslag, Pres.

**Fnded:** 1987. **Mem:** 12,500. **Desc:** Individuals and organizations with an interest in women's health issues. Promotes adoption of public health policies and programs providing greater access to health care for women. Conducts educational programs. **Pub:** WIPHN News, 3/year. Newsletter. **Price:** $35 for individuals; $50/yr for organizations.

**★ 17970 ★ World Federation of Public Health Associations (WFPHA)**
c/o Amer. Public Health Assn.
800 I St., NW
Washington, DC 20001-3710
**Phone:** (202)777-2486          **Fax:** (202)777-2534
**Email:** allen.jones@apha.org
**Website:** http://www.wfpha.org
Mohammad N. Akhter, Exec. Dir.
**Fnded:** 1967. **Mem:** 61. **Nat'l Groups:** 61. **Reg. Groups:** 5. **Desc:** National public health associations united "to strengthen the public health profession and to improve community health throughout the world." Encourages formation of national public health associations. Organizes projects; conducts special studies; offers lectures; compiles reports; sponsors triennial world congress. **Pub:** *Reports of Triennial International Congresses.* Reports. • *WFPHA Report,* quarterly. Report.

**★ 17971 ★ World Health Organization - Regional Office for the Western Pacific (WPRO)**
PO Box 2932
Manila 1000, Philippines
**Phone:** 63 2 5288001          **Fax:** 63 2 5211036
**Email:** postmaster@who.org.ph
**Website:** http://www.wpro.who.int
**Desc:** Regional branch of the World Health Organization. Works to ensure that WHO programs effectively meet the particular public health needs of the western Pacific; serves as a liaison between national and local public health agencies and the WHO.

**★ 17972 ★ World Health Organization - Zimbabwe (WHOZ)**
PO Box 773
Harare, Zimbabwe
**Phone:** 263 4 703580          **Fax:** 263 479 0146
**Email:** regafro@whoafr/org
**Website:** http://www.who.int
**Lang(s):** English. **Desc:** National branch of the international organization. Public health services and programs. Seeks to ensure that programs of the World Health Organization effectively meet the particular needs of people in Zimbabwe. Serves as a liaison between local public health programs and agencies and the WHO

## Research Centers

**★ 17973 ★ Arizona Health Services Department**
**Public Health Services**
**State Laboratory Services**
1520 W Adams
Phoenix, AZ 85007-2698
**Phone:** (602)542-1188          **Fax:** (602)542-1169
Wesley Press, Contact
**Activities/Fields:** State health laboratory.

**★ 17974 ★ Arizona Health Services Department**
**Public Health Services**
**State Laboratory Services**
**Flagstaff Regional Laboratory**
2500 N Fort Valley Rd.
Flagstaff, AZ 86001
**Phone:** (520)226-1154          **Fax:** (520)774-9419
Leva Jensen, Mgr.
**Activities/Fields:** Public health laboratory.

**★ 17975 ★ Arizona Health Services Department**
**Public Health Services**
**State Laboratory Services**
**Tucson Regional Laboratory**
416 W Congress St., Ste. 119
Tucson, AZ 85701
**Phone:** (520)628-6360          **Fax:** (520)628-6356
Judy Fordyce, Mgr.
**Activities/Fields:** Public health regional lab.

**★ 17976 ★ Ball State University**
**Public Health Entomology Laboratory**
2000 University Ave.
Muncie, IN 47306
**Phone:** (765)285-1504          **Fax:** (765)285-3210
**Email:** rpinger@bsu.edu
**Website:**          http://www.bsu.edu/physiology-health/phel.html
Dr. Robert R. Pinger, Dir.
**Activities/Fields:** Ticks and tick-borne diseases in Indiana, and other insects affecting human and animal health. Projects include a Rocky Mountain spotted fever and lyme disease tick testing program funded by the Indiana State Department of Health. Provides identification of insects of public health importance. **Pub:** *Pamphlets.*

**★ 17977 ★ Battelle Memorial Institute**
**Centers for Public Health Research and Evaluation (CPHRE)**
505 King Ave.
Columbus, OH 43201
**Phone:** (614)424-6424
**Email:** solutions@battelle.org
**Website:** http://www.battelle.org/cphre/
**Activities/Fields:** Health and its determinants, particularly social and behavioral risk assessment and environmental and occupational risk assessment.

**★ 17978 ★ Center for the Study of Rochester's Health**
University of Rochester
601 Elmwood Ave., Box 644
Rochester, NY 14642
**Phone:** (716)275-6423          **Fax:** (716)756-7761
**Email:** cfre@son.rochester.edu
**Website:** http://www.urmc.rochester.edu/URMC/csrh/
Dr. Nancy M. Bennett, Dir.
**Activities/Fields:** Analysis of community-level data to determine opportunities for intervention, evaluation of community interventions and identification of effective community health practices and multidisciplinary collaborative medicine and public health projects.

**★ 17979 ★ Consumer Product Safety Commission**
**Epidemiology and Health Sciences Directorate**
4330 East-West Hwy.
Bethesda, MD 20814-4408
**Phone:** (301)504-0957          **Fax:** (301)504-0124
**Website:** http://www.cpsc.gov
Dr. Mary Ann Danello, Dir.
**Activities/Fields:** Determines exposure to hazardous chemicals from consumer products. This includes investigation of children's products; pollutant emissions (both chemical and biological) from structural materials, consumer products, and indoor combustion sources and their impact on indoor air quality; bioavailability and potential for consumer exposure to carcinogenic and other chemical hazard-containing commercial substances; and acute and chemical toxicity of various household products to determine proper precautionary and first aid labeling. Directorate is also responsible for implementation of the Poison Prevention Packaging Act with respect to hazardous household substances, including drugs; and processing requests for exemption from regulations under this Act. Also studies design and effectiveness of child

resistant packaging and supports work on physiological modeling and other injury behavior.

**★ 17980 ★ Consumer Product Safety Commission**
**Epidemiology and Health Sciences Directorate**
**Hazard Analysis Division**
4330 East-West Hwy.
Bethesda, MD 20814
**Phone:** (301)504-0470          **Fax:** (301)504-0081
**Email:** rroegner@cpsc.gov
**Website:** http://cpsc.gov
Russ Roegner, PhD, Dir.
**Activities/Fields:** Analyses of product-related injury data to the Commission and other organizations to guide and support remedial strategy development and decision-making. As a part of this function, Division analysts and statisticians participate in the selection and planning of projects; develop guidelines for investigations and surveys and monitor their progress; compile and analyze data and information available from established Commission projects, other health and safety-oriented organizations, and computer searches of medical, scientific, and technical literature databases; prepare issue-oriented data summaries, reports, and memoranda describing the frequency and severity of injuries and major hazard patterns related to specific types of products; participate in oral briefings of the Commission on the nature and scope of injuries to be addressed by each remedial option considered; participate in the identification of injury reductions related to past Commission actions; and identify emerging hazards through continuous monitoring of injury trends. **Pub:** *Division's Hazard Analyses.* • *Special Reports.*

**★ 17981 ★ Georgia Southern University**
**Center for Rural Health and Research**
PO Box 8148
Statesboro, GA 30460-8148
**Phone:** (912)681-0260          **Fax:** (912)486-7553
**Email:** k_guion@gsvms2.cc.gasou.edu
W. Kent Guion, MD, Dir.
**Activities/Fields:** Rural health in Georgia. Currently conducting a census of programs promoting well-being of children and families in the state and a study of the impact of social suport on the well being of HIV/AIDS patients.

**★ 17982 ★ Harvard University**
**Prevention Research Center on Nutrition and Physical Activity**
677 Huntington Ave.
Boston, MA 02115
**Phone:** (617)432-1135          **Fax:** (617)432-3755
**Email:** sgortmak@hsph.harvard.edu
**Website:** http://www.cdc.gov/prc/centers-harvard.htm
Steven Gortmaker, Prin. Investigator
**Activities/Fields:** Public health issues, especially behaviors that place Americans at risk for chronic diseases and conditions. Of particular concern is the improvement in quality of life for special populations, including the young, elderly, racial ethnic populations, and the underserved.

**★ 17983 ★ Health Research, Inc.**
1 University Pl.
Rensselaer, NY 12144-3455
**Phone:** (518)431-1200          **Fax:** (518)431-1234
**Website:** http://www.hrinet.org
Dawn Cox, Dir.
**Activities/Fields:** Public health and cancer, including basic and clinical research in cause and treatment of cancer and related malignancies; environmental studies to determine long-range health hazards of pesticides, industrial discharge, and radioactive and sewage wastes; and detection and prevention of infectious diseases, including AIDS and tuberculosis. Also studies rehabilitation, biology, immunology, hematology, virology, chemistry, toxicology, and environment.

**★ 17984 ★ Indiana University-Purdue University at Indianapolis**
**Institute of Action Research for Community Health**
1111 Middle Dr., Rm. 236
Indianapolis, IN 46202
**Phone:** (317)274-3319　　**Fax:** (317)274-2285
**Email:** citynet@iupui.edu
**Website:** http://www.iupui.edu/~citynet/cnet.html
Dr. Beverly Flynn, Dir.

**Activities/Fields:** Community health issues in Indiana as well as nationally and internationally.


**★ 17985 ★ Marshall University**
**Robert C. Byrd Center for Rural Health**
School of Medicine
Huntington, WV 25701
**Phone:** (304)691-1198　　**Fax:** (304)691-1183
**Email:** rwalker@marshall.edu
**Website:** http://crh.marshall.edu/
Robert Walker, MD, Dir.

**Activities/Fields:** Rural health problems. Also guides predoctoral and postdoctoral research on rural health, rural geriatrics, and prevention in rural populations.


**★ 17986 ★ Michigan Public Health Institute (MPHI)**
2436 Woodlake Cir., Ste. 300
Okemos, MI 48864
**Phone:** (517)324-8301　　**Fax:** (517)381-0260
**Email:** central@mphi.org
**Website:** http://www.mphi.org/
Jeffrey R. Taylor, PhD, Exec. Dir.

**Activities/Fields:** Public health issues, including disease prevention.


**★ 17987 ★ Morehouse College**
**Prevention Research Center**
Center for Public Health Practice
School of Medicine
777 Cleveland Ave., Ste. 410
Atlanta, GA 30310
**Phone:** (404)752-1624　　**Fax:** (404)752-1160
**Email:** danielb@msm.edu
**Website:**　　http://www.cdc.gov/prc/centers-morehouse.htm
Daniel Blumenthal, MD, Prin. Investigator

**Activities/Fields:** Public health issues, especially behaviors that place Americans at risk for chronic diseases and conditions. Of particular concern is the improvement in quality of life for special populations, including the young, elderly, racial ethnic populations, and the underserved.


**★ 17988 ★ New York State Department of Health**
**Wadsworth Center**
PO Box 509
Albany, NY 12201-0509
**Phone:** (518)474-7592　　**Fax:** (518)474-3439
**Email:** sturman@wadsworth.org
**Website:** http://www.wadsworth.org
Lawrence S. Sturman, PhD, Dir.

**Activities/Fields:** Biomedical and environmental sciences. Investigators study cell and molecular structure, including molecular assemblies, protein and glycoprotein structure and function, and chromosome dynamics; also, genetics, development and cancer, with studies of developmental and human genetics, developmental neuroscience, genetic factors involved in cancer causation, mechanisms of tumor formation, and development of more effective cancer therapies. Researchers also investigate microbial genomics and pathogenesis, including HIV, nucleic acid dynamics, infectious disease epidemiology, environmental chemistry, and molecular toxicology. Emphasis is placed on emerging scientific disciplines, especially genomics, bioinformatics and nanobiotechnology.


**★ 17989 ★ Pacific Institute for Research and Evaluation**
**PIRE Chapel Hill Center**
1229 E Franklin St., 2nd Fl.
Chapel Hill, NC 27514
**Phone:** (919)967-8998　　**Fax:** (919)968-1498
**Email:** jester@pire.org
**Website:** http://www.pire.org/centers/ChapelHill.htm
Janet Jester, Contact

**Activities/Fields:** Design and implementation of innovative program evaluation and needs assessment studies, and epidemiological research relating to public health issues.


**★ 17990 ★ Pennsylvania Department of Health**
**Bureau of Laboratories**
110 Pickering Way
Lionville, PA 19353
**Phone:** (610)280-3464　　**Fax:** (610)436-3346
**Email:** bkleger@state.pa.us
**Website:** http://www.health.state.pa.us
Bruce Kleger, Dir.

**Activities/Fields:** Public health issues.


**★ 17991 ★ Pennsylvania Department of Health**
**Public Health Assessment Epidemiology Bureau**
Health & Welfare Bldg., Rm. 933
PO Box 90
Harrisburg, PA 17108
**Phone:** (717)783-4677　　**Fax:** (717)772-6975
Joel Hersh, Dir.

**Activities/Fields:** Disease control and incidences in populations for the purposes of intervention. Specific programs include: communicable disease epidemiology, environmental health assessment, HIV/AIDS epidemiology, cancer epidemiology, and chronic disease epidemiology.


**★ 17992 ★ Public Citizen Health Research Group**
1600 20th St. NW
Washington, DC 20009
**Phone:** (202)588-1000　　**Fax:** (202)588-7796
**Website:** http://www.citizen.org
Sidney M. Wolfe, MD, Dir.

**Activities/Fields:** Health care delivery, workplace safety and health, drug regulation, food additives, medical device safety, and environmental influences on health. Conducts consumer advocacy and lobbying on health matters and monitors the enforcement of health and safety legislation. **Pub:** *Best Pills News.* • *Health Letter*, monthly. • *Health Research Group List of Publications*, annually. • *Worst Pills.*


**★ 17993 ★ Public Health Centre**
2400 D'Estimauville St.
Beauport, QC, Canada G1E 7G9
**Phone:** (418)666-7000　　**Fax:** (418)666-2776
Michel Vezina, Dir.

**Activities/Fields:** Operational research, including effectiveness of interventions of sexual behavior of seropositive individuals; psychological stress of homosexual AIDS patients; and studies on organochlorinated contaminants.


**★ 17994 ★ Public Health Institute**
2001 Addison St., 2nd Fl.
Berkeley, CA 94704-1103
**Phone:** (510)644-8200　　**Fax:** (510)644-9319
**Email:** dssofaer@phi.org
**Website:** http://www.phi.org
Joseph M. Hafey, Pres. /CEO

**Activities/Fields:** Conducts research on a broad range of public health issues, including drug and alcohol problems, occupational health, diet and nutrition, maternal and child health, violence, reproductive

health, genetics, and lead poisoning prevention. **Frmly:** California Public Health Foundation.


**★ 17995 ★ St. Louis University**
**Prevention Research Center**
School of Public Health
3663 Lindell Blvd.
Saint Louis, MO 63108
**Phone:** (314)977-8110　　**Fax:** (314)977-3234
**Email:** brownson@slu.edu
**Website:** http://www.cdc.gov/prc/centers-stlouis.htm
Ross C. Brownson, PhD, Prin. Investigator

**Activities/Fields:** Public health issues, especially behaviors that place Americans at risk for chronic diseases and conditions. Of particular concern is the improvement in quality of life for special populations, including the young, elderly, racial ethnic populations, and the underserved.


**★ 17996 ★ Tennessee State University**
**Institute of Government**
330 10th Ave. N
Nashville, TN 37203-3401
**Phone:** (615)963-7241　　**Fax:** (615)963-7245
**Email:** arizzo@tnstate.edu
**Website:** http://www.tsu.edu
Dr. Ann-Marie Rizzo, Dir.

**Activities/Fields:** Public administration and public services. **Pub:** *The Public Servant*, 3/year. Newsletter.


**★ 17997 ★ Texas A&M University**
**Center for Urban and Structural Entomology**
Department of Entomology
College Station, TX 77843-2475
**Phone:** (979)845-5855　　**Fax:** (979)845-5926
Dr. Roger Gold, Dir.

**Activities/Fields:** Urban and public health entomology, focusing on investigations of the parasites and predators of cockroaches.


**★ 17998 ★ Tulane University**
**Environmental Diseases Prevention Research Center**
School of Public Health & Tropical Medicine
Tulane Medical Center, TW-43
1430 Tulane Ave.
New Orleans, LA 70112
**Phone:** (504)584-1774　　**Fax:** (504)587-7352
**Email:** lawhite@mailhost.tcs.tulane.edu
**Website:** http://www.cdc.gov/prc/centers-tulane.htm
William R. Hartley, Prin. Investigator

**Activities/Fields:** Public health issues, especially behaviors that place Americans at risk for chronic diseases and conditions. Of particular concern is the improvement in quality of life for special populations, including the young, elderly, racial ethnic populations, and the underserved.


**★ 17999 ★ U.S. Department of Health and Human Services**
**Centers for Disease Control and Prevention**
1600 Clifton Rd., NE
Atlanta, GA 30333
**Phone:** (404)639-3311　　**Fax:** (404)639-7111
**Email:** netinfo@cdc.gov
**Website:** http://www.cdc.gov
Dr. David W. Fleming, MD, Actg. Dir.

**Activities/Fields:** Responsible for protecting the public health of the nation by preventing disease, disability, and premature death and promoting healthy lifestyles for all Americans. Specifically, CDC research focuses on the prevention of infectious diseases, chronic diseases, injury or disease associated with environmental, home, and workplace hazards, and controllable risk factors such as poor nutrition, smoking, lack of exercise, high blood pressure, and lack of appropriate immunizations. **Pub:** *Chronic Disease Notes and Reports.* • *Health United States.* • *Morbidity* *and Mortality Weekly Report series.* • *NCHS Monthly Vital Statistics Report.* • *Vital and Health Statistics series.*

**U.S. Department of Health and Human Services**
**Centers for Disease Control and Prevention**
**Epidemiology Program Office**
*See:* Entry 9059

**★ 18000 ★ U.S. Department of Health and Human Services**
**Food and Drug Administration**
Rm. 1471
5600 Fishers Ln.
Rockville, MD 20857
**Phone:** (301)827-2410          **Fax:** (301)443-3100
**Email:** crawford@oc.fda.gov
**Website:** http://www.fda.gov
Lester Crawford, DVM, Dep. Commnr.

**Activities/Fields:** Public health of the nation as it may be impaired by foods, drugs, biological products, cosmetics, medical devices, ionizing and nonionizing radiation-emitting products and substances, poisons, pesticides, and food additives. FDA's functions are to ensure that: foods are safe, pure, and wholesome; drugs, medical devices, and biological products are safe and effective; cosmetics are harmless; that all of the above are honestly and informatively packaged; and that exposure to potentially injurious radiation is minimized. The principal components of FDA are the Center for Biologics Evaluation and Research; Center for Devices and Radiological Health; Center for Drug Evaluation and Research; Center for Food Safety and Applied Nutrition; Center for Veterinary Medicine; the National Center for Toxicological Research; and the Office of Regulatory Affairs, which directs FDA's field operations. Research activities are also carried out in field laboratories and research centers located throughout the country–see entries that follow under FDA Regional Research Centers.

**★ 18001 ★ U.S. Department of Health and Human Services**
**Food and Drug Administration**
**Center for Devices and Radiological Health**
9200 Corporate Blvd., Rm. 100
Rockville, MD 20850
**Phone:** (301)443-4690          **Fax:** (301)594-1320
**Website:** http://www.fda.gov/cdhr
David W. Feigal, Jr., M, Dir.

**Activities/Fields:** Develops and carries out a national program designed to control unnecessary exposures of humans to and assure the safe and efficacious use of ionizing and nonionizing radiation-emitting electronic products; and develops and carries out a national program to assure the safety, effectiveness, and proper labeling of medical devices for human use.

**★ 18002 ★ U.S. Department of Health and Human Services**
**Food and Drug Administration**
**Center for Drug Evaluation and Research**
1451 Rockville Pike, Rm. 6027
Rockville, MD 20852
**Phone:** (301)594-5400          **Fax:** (301)594-6197
**Website:** http://www.fda.gov/cder/
Janet Woodcock, Dir.

**Activities/Fields:** Develops FDA policy with regard to the safety, effectiveness, and labeling of all drugs for human use; reviews and evaluates new drug applications and notices of claimed investigational exemption of new drugs; develops and implements standards for the safety and effectiveness of all over-the-counter drugs; monitors the quality of marketed drugs through product testing, surveillance, and compliance programs; develops guidelines on current Good Manufacturing Practices for use by the drug industry; develops and disseminates information and educational materi-

al on drugs to the medical community and the public; conducts research and develops scientific standards on the composition, quality, safety, and efficacy of human drugs; collects and evaluates information on the effects and use trends of marketed drugs; monitors prescription drug advertising and promotional labeling to assure their accuracy and integrity; analyzes data on accidental poisonings; and disseminates toxicity and treatment information on medicines. Principal Center components are the Office of Compliance, Office of +Drug Evaluation I, Office of +Drug Evaluation II, Office of +Drug Standards, Office of Epidemiology and Biostatistics, and Office of Research Resources.

**★ 18003 ★ U.S. Department of Health and Human Services**
**Food and Drug Administration**
**Center for Food Safety and Applied Nutrition**
5100 Paint Branch Pkwy.
College Park, MD 20740
**Phone:** (301)436-1600          **Fax:** (301)436-2668
Joseph Levitt, Dir.

**Activities/Fields:** Principal goals are to gather, analyze, and monitor published and unpublished information pertinent to the consumption, quality, and safety of foods and cosmetics; determine the nutritional needs of various population groups and develop strategies to improve the nutritional status of those at risk; isolate, purify, and identify potentially hazardous food and cosmetic constituents and adulterants, including biological, microbial, and chemical contaminants; develop, validate, and apply quantitative methods of analysis for potentially hazardous constituents, adulterants, and contaminants of foods and cosmetics, including environmental contaminants, animal drugs, and metabolites of microbial origin; develop, improve, and validate biological tests for various forms of human toxicity, including chronic toxicity, fetal and neonatal toxicity, behavioral and immunotoxicity, and dermal and ocular toxicity; apply toxicity tests and epidemiological studies to determine the adverse effects (hazards) of food constituents and contaminants and of cosmetics ingredients, singly or in combination; improve the accuracy of methods used to assess potential risks to human health associated with the constituents and contaminants of foods and cosmetics; develop practical control technologies necessary to detect or prevent hazards resulting from the storage or processing of foods or cosmetics; and assess social, economic, and environmental determinants and impacts of Center actions. Research activities are primarily carried out in units of the Center's Office of Plant, Dairy Foods and Beverages, Office of Food Labeling, Office of Special Nutritionals, Office of Seafood, and Office of Special Research Skills.

**★ 18004 ★ U.S. Department of Health and Human Services**
**National Institutes of Health**
**Office of Medical Applications of Research**
Bldg. 31, Rm. 1B03
31 Center Dr., MSC-2082
Bethesda, MD 20892
**Phone:** (301)496-5641          **Free:** 888-644-2667
**Fax:** (301)402-0420
**Email:** bk76p@nih.gov
**Website:** http://consensus.nih.gov
Barnett S. Kramer, MD, MP, Dir.

**Activities/Fields:** Translation of results of biomedical research pertinent to health care into knowledge that can effectively be employed in the practice of medicine and public health. The Office facilitates and coordinates technical consensus development activities at the National Institutes of Health through the implementation of consensus conferences. These conferences bring together biomedical research scientists, practicing physicians, consumers, and others in an effort to reach general agreement on whether a given medical technology is safe and effective. OMAR works with NIH institutes to promote the effective dissemination of information derived from the consensus development

process to the biomedical research and health care communities, the public, and other federal agencies. Principal area of research interest is health care technologies assessment, including drugs, devices, and medical and surgical procedures.

**★ 18005 ★ University of Arizona**
**Southwest Center for Community Health Promotion**
1145 N Campbell
PO Box 210028
Tucson, AZ 85721-0028
**Phone:** (520)318-7270          **Fax:** (520)326-0435
**Email:** mlebowit@u.arizona.edu
**Website:** http://www.cdc.gov/prc/centers-uaz.htm
Michael Lebowitz, PhD, Dir.

**Activities/Fields:** Public health issues, especially behaviors that place Americans at risk for chronic diseases and conditions. Of particular concern is the improvement in quality of life for special populations, including the young, elderly, racial ethnic populations, and the underserved.

**★ 18006 ★ University of California, Los Angeles**
**Program on Global Health and Education**
11290 Bunche Hall, MC 148703
Los Angeles, CA 90095-1487
**Phone:** (310)206-8984          **Fax:** (310)206-4018
**Email:** djamison@isop.ucla.edu
**Website:** http://www.international.ucla.edu/gh
Dean T. Jamison, Dir.

**Activities/Fields:** Health and education on a world scale.

**★ 18007 ★ University of California, Los Angeles**
**UCLA/RAND Center for Adolescent Health Promotion**
Department of Pediatrics, 12-466 MDCC
Box 951752
10833 Le Conte Ave.
Los Angeles, CA 90095-1752
**Phone:** (310)206-1954          **Fax:** (310)206-4855
**Email:** schuster@rand.org
**Website:** http://www.cdc.gov/prc/centers-ucla.htm
Mark A. Schuster, MD, Dir.

**Activities/Fields:** Public health issues, especially behaviors that place Americans at risk for chronic diseases and conditions. Of particular concern is the improvement in quality of life for special populations, including the young, elderly, racial ethnic populations, and the underserved.

**★ 18008 ★ University of Colorado**
**Rocky Mountain Prevention Research Center**
Department of Preventive Medicine & Biometrics, C-245
4200 E 9th Ave.
Denver, CO 80262
**Phone:** (303)315-6863          **Fax:** (303)315-3183
**Email:** richard.hamman@uchsc.edu
**Website:**          http://www.cdc.gov/prc/centers-00directory.htm
Richard F. Hamman, MD, Dir.

**Activities/Fields:** Public health issues, especially behaviors that place Americans at risk for chronic diseases and conditions. Of particular concern is the improvement in quality of life for special populations, including the young, elderly, racial ethnic populations, and the underserved.

**★ 18009 ★ University of Connecticut Health Center**
**Center for International Community Health Studies**
263 Farmington Ave.
Farmington, CT 06030-6330
**Phone:** (860)679-1570          **Fax:** (860)679-1581

**Email:** cichs@nso2.uchc.edu
**Website:** http://www.commed.uchc.edu/cichs/cichs.htm
Stephen L. Schensul, PhD, Dir.

**Activities/Fields:** The health of underprivileged people in the U.S. and abroad, emphasizing international primary health care and community health, including international health policy, urban health in developing and developed countries, maternal and child health, health programs and problems in Peru, Sri Lanka, Kenya, Mauritius, and Connecticut, effects of economic development on health, and the role of the hospital in the developing world. Facilitates international health research for faculty and graduate students through consultation on grant proposals, networking with international contacts, advocating for researchers within international agencies, and establishing foreign research and educational placements. **Pub:** *Annual Training Program Catalogue.* • *CICHS Connections Newsletter.*

★ **18010 ★ University of Illinois at Chicago**
**Illinois Prevention Research Center**
M/C 275
850 W Jackson Blvd., Ste. 400
Chicago, IL 60607
**Phone:** (312)996-1167     **Fax:** (312)996-2703
**Email:** slevy@uic.edu
**Website:** http://www.cdc.gov/prc/centers-illinois.htm
Susan R. Levy, PhD, Prin. Investigator

**Activities/Fields:** Public health issues, especially behaviors that place Americans at risk for chronic diseases and conditions. Of particular concern is the improvement in quality of life for special populations, including the young, elderly, racial ethnic populations, and the underserved.

**University of Iowa**
**Center for International Rural and Environmental Health (CIREH)**
*See:* Entry 8984

★ **18011 ★ University of Iowa**
**State Hygienic Laboratory**
102 Oakdale Campus, H101 OH
Iowa City, IA 52242-5002
**Phone:** (319)335-4500     **Fax:** (319)335-4600
**Email:** director@uhl.uiowa.edu
**Website:** http://www.uhl.uiowa.edu
Mary J.R. Gilchrist, PhD, Dir.

**Activities/Fields:** Virolology, limnology, industrial hygiene, neonatal metabolic and prenatal diseases detection, microbiology, and organic, inorganic, and radiation chemistry. Conducts research and service in all areas relating to the environment and public health, including rapid diagnosis of disease agents by molecular methods and enzyme immunoassay, and monitoring immune status by flow cytometry. Studies the epidemiology of infectious diseases, food quality control, surface and/or groundwater contaminants, radioisotopes in groundwater, airborne contaminants and various contaminants in soil. The Laboratory develops and evaluates test methods for a wide variety of analyses and sample matrices, often to provide data as an aid to the decision and rule making process. **Pub:** *Annual Report.* • *Lab Hotline,* monthly.

★ **18012 ★ University of Kentucky**
**Prevention Research Center**
Markey Cancer Center
2365 Harrodsburg Rd., Ste. B100
Lexington, KY 40504-3381
**Phone:** (859)219-0771     **Fax:** (859)219-0557
**Email:** swyatt@kcp.uky.edu
**Website:** http://www.cdc.gov/prc/centers-kentucky.htm
Stephen A. Wyatt, MD, Prin. Investigator

**Activities/Fields:** Public health issues, especially behaviors that place Americans at risk for chronic diseases and conditions. Of particular concern is the improvement in quality of life for special populations,

including the young, elderly, racial ethnic populations, and the underserved.

**University of Maryland at Baltimore**
**Center for Vaccine Development (CVD)**
*See:* Entry 11949

★ **18013 ★ University of Maryland at College Park**
**Minority Health Research Laboratory (MHRL)**
HHP Bldg., Rm. 1241
College Park, MD 20742
**Phone:** (301)405-2467     **Fax:** (301)314-9167
**Email:** ac166@umail.umd.edu
**Website:** http://medschool.umaryland.edu/CVD/
Dr. Aria Crump, Dir.

**Activities/Fields:** Promotes health and disease prevention among poorly served, underserved, and never served populations in the U.S., by researching issues that impact diverse populations.

★ **18014 ★ University of Michigan**
**Prevention Research Center of Michigan**
School of Public Health
109 Observatory
Ann Arbor, MI 48109-2029
**Phone:** (734)763-5454     **Fax:** (734)763-5455
**Email:** nmclark@umich.edu
**Website:** http://www.cdc.gov/prc/centers-mich.htm
Noreen Clark, PhD, Prin. Investigator

**Activities/Fields:** Public health issues, especially behaviors that place Americans at risk for chronic diseases and conditions. Of particular concern is the improvement in quality of life for special populations, including the young, elderly, racial ethnic populations, and the underserved.

★ **18015 ★ University of Minnesota**
**National Teen Pregnancy Prevention Research Center**
University Gateway
200 Oak St. SE, Ste. 260
Minneapolis, MN 55455-2002
**Phone:** (612)624-9111     **Fax:** (612)626-2134
**Email:** resni001@tc.umn.edu
**Website:** http://www.cdc.gov/prc/centers-minn.htm
Michael Resnick, PhD, Dir.

**Activities/Fields:** Public health issues, especially behaviors that place Americans at risk for chronic diseases and conditions. Of particular concern is the improvement in quality of life for special populations, including the young, elderly, racial ethnic populations, and the underserved.

★ **18016 ★ University of Montreal**
**Interdisciplinary Health Research Group**
CP 6128 Succursale Centre-Ville
Montreal, QC, Canada H3C 3J7
**Phone:** (514)343-6185     **Fax:** (514)343-2207
**Email:** gris@umontreal.ca
**Website:** http://www.medsp.umontreal.ca
Paul Lamarche, Dir.

**Activities/Fields:** Health services, including analysis of health care system, evaluation of interventions, studies of determinants of health in populations, and investigations of methodological and conceptual developments in the field of health services research. Specific projects conducted in areas of curative and preventive practices, global health care, behavior of professionals and organizations, health education, health promotion, and maternal and child health. **Pub:** *RUPTURES,* semiannually.

★ **18017 ★ University of New Mexico**
**Center for Health Promotion and Disease Prevention**
Surge Bldg., Rm. 251
Health Sciences Center

2701 Frontier NE
Albuquerque, NM 87131-5311
**Phone:** (505)272-4462     **Fax:** (505)272-4857
**Email:** smdavis@unm.edu
**Website:** http://www.cdc.gov/prc/centers-newmexico.htm
Sally Davis, PhD, Prin. Investigator

**Activities/Fields:** Public health issues, especially behaviors that place Americans at risk for chronic diseases and conditions. Of particular concern is the improvement in quality of life for special populations, including the young, elderly, racial ethnic populations, and the underserved.

★ **18018 ★ University of North Dakota**
**Center for Rural Health**
School of Medicine & Health Sciences
PO Box 9037
Grand Forks, ND 58202-9037
**Phone:** (701)777-3848     **Fax:** (701)777-2389
**Email:** bgibbens@medicine.nodak.edu
Brad Gibbens, Assoc. Dir.

**Activities/Fields:** Rural health issues. **Pub:** *Focus on Rural Health.* • *State Rural Health Watch.*

★ **18019 ★ University of Oklahoma**
**Native American Prevention Research Center**
Rogers Bldg., Rm. 532
Health Sciences Center
College of Public Health
800 NE 15th St.
Oklahoma City, OK 73104
**Phone:** (405)271-2330     **Fax:** (405)271-6285
**Email:** everett-rhoades@ouhsc.edu
**Website:** http://www.cdc.gov/prc/centers-oklahoma.htm
Everett R. Rhoades, MD, Prin. Investigator

**Activities/Fields:** Public health issues, especially behaviors that place Americans at risk for chronic diseases and conditions. Of particular concern is the improvement in quality of life for special populations, including the young, elderly, racial ethnic populations, and the underserved.

★ **18020 ★ University of South Carolina**
**Prevention Research Center**
School of Public Health
800 Sumter St.
Columbia, SC 29208
**Phone:** (803)777-4253     **Fax:** (803)777-9007
**Email:** bainsworth@sph.sc.edu
**Website:** http://www.cdc.gov/prc/centers-southcarolina.htm
Barbara Ainsworth, PhD, Prin. Investigator

**Activities/Fields:** Public health issues, especially behaviors that place Americans at risk for chronic diseases and conditions. Of particular concern is the improvement in quality of life for special populations, including the young, elderly, racial ethnic populations, and the underserved.

★ **18021 ★ University of South Florida**
**Center for Community-Based Prevention Marketing**
Department of Community & Family Health, MDC 56
College of Public Health
13201 Bruce B. Downs Blvd.
Tampa, FL 33612-3805
**Phone:** (813)974-4867     **Fax:** (813)974-5172
**Email:** rmcdermo@hsc.usf.edu
**Website:** http://www.cdc.gov/prc/centers-southfla.htm
Robert J. McDermott, PhD, Prin. Investigator

**Activities/Fields:** Public health issues, especially behaviors that place Americans at risk for chronic diseases and conditions. Of particular concern is the improvement in quality of life for special populations, including the young, elderly, racial ethnic populations, and the underserved.

**★ 18022 ★ University of Texas Health Science Center at Houston**
**Center for Society and Population Health**
1200 Herman Pressler, RAS E-901
Houston, TX 77030
**Phone:** (713)500-9485　　　**Fax:** (713)500-9493
**Email:** david.low@uth.tmc.edu
**Website:** http://www.sph.uth.tmc.edu:8052/csph/
M. David Low, MD, Dir.

**Activities/Fields:** Improvement in the health of all people, particularly those living in Texas.

**★ 18023 ★ University of Washington**
**Northwest Prevention Effectiveness Center**
146 N Canal St., Ste. 110
Seattle, WA 98103-8652
**Phone:** (206)543-2590　　　**Fax:** (206)543-8841
**Email:** logerfo@u.washington.edu
**Website:** http://www.cdc.gov/prc/centers-washington.htm
James P. LoGerfo, MD, Prin. Investigator

**Activities/Fields:** Public health issues, especially behaviors that place Americans at risk for chronic diseases and conditions. Of particular concern is the improvement in quality of life for special populations, including the young, elderly, racial ethnic populations, and the underserved.

**★ 18024 ★ University of Wisconsin—Madison**
**State Laboratory of Hygiene**
465 Henry Mall
Madison, WI 53706
**Phone:** (608)262-0322　　　**Free:** 888-494-4324
**Fax:** (608)262-3257
**Email:** rhl@mail.slh.wisc.edu
**Website:** http://www.slh.wisc.edu
Dr. R.H. Laessig, Dir.

**Activities/Fields:** Bacteriology, cancer cytology, cytogenetics, immunology, industrial hygiene, environmental health, pathology, clinical chemistry, toxicology, and virology, including respiratory and enterovirus infections, a survey of zoonosis in Wisconsin, especially California encephalitis virus, and chromosomal studies in congenital anomalies. **Pub:** *Results*, quarterly. • *Wisconsin State Laboratory of Hygiene Research, Teaching and Outreach Activity Report*, annually.

**★ 18025 ★ University of Wisconsin—Madison**
**State Laboratory of Hygiene**
**General Bacteriology Unit**
465 Henry Mall
Madison, WI 53706
**Fax:** (608)262-3257
**Email:** babs@mail.slh.wisc.edu
**Website:** http://www.slh.wisc.edu
Dr. R.H. Laessig, Dir.

**Activities/Fields:** Antimicrobial susceptibility studies, enteric serotyping, and culture and identification of fastidious and unusual pathogens. Provides bacteriology laboratory support for outbreak management.

**★ 18026 ★ West Virginia University**
**Prevention Research Center**
Robert C. Byrd Health Sciences Center
PO Box 9190
Morgantown, WV 26506-9190
**Phone:** (304)293-8612　　　**Fax:** (304)293-8624
**Email:** gdino@hsc.wvu.edu
**Website:** http://www.cdc.gov/prc/centers-westvirginia.htm
Geri A. Dino, PhD, Prin. Investigator

**Activities/Fields:** Public health issues, especially behaviors that place Americans at risk for chronic diseases and conditions. Of particular concern is the improvement in quality of life for special populations, including the young, elderly, racial ethnic populations, and the underserved.

**★ 18027 ★ Yale University**
**Yale University-Griffin Hospital Prevention Research Center**
Department of Epidemiology & Public Health
School of Medicine
60 College St.
PO Box 208034
New Haven, CT 06520-8034
**Phone:** (203)785-2867　　　**Fax:** (203)785-6103
**Email:** michael.merson@yale.edu
**Website:** http://www.cdc.gov/prc/centers-yale.htm
Michael H. Merson, MD, Prin. Investigator

**Activities/Fields:** Public health issues, especially behaviors that place Americans at risk for chronic diseases and conditions. Of particular concern is the improvement in quality of life for special populations, including the young, elderly, racial ethnic populations, and the underserved.

# State Government Agencies

## Public Health

**★ 18028 ★ Arizona Department of Health Services**
1740 W Adams St.
Phoenix, AZ 85007
**Phone:** (602)542-1001　　　**Fax:** (602)542-0883
**Email:** webmaster@hs.state.az.us
**Website:** http://www.hs.state.az.us/
Catherine Eden, Director

**★ 18029 ★ Arkansas Department of Health**
4815 W Markham
PO Box 3278
Little Rock, AR 72205
**Phone:** (501)661-2000　　　**Fax:** (501)671-1450
**Website:** http://www.healthyarkansas.com
Fay Boozman, Director
**Alt. Contact:** Second office location: 5800 W. 10th St., Little Rock, AR 72204.

**★ 18030 ★ California Department of Health Services**
**Office of Public Affairs**
714 P St, Room 1350
Sacramento, CA 95814
**Phone:** (916)445-4171　　　**Fax:** (916)657-0240
**Website:** http://www.dhs.cahwnet.gov/

**★ 18031 ★ Colorado Public Health and Environment Department**
**Health Office**
4300 Cherry Creek Dr. S
Denver, CO 80246-1530
**Phone:** (303)692-2100　　　**Fax:** (303)782-0095
**Email:** cdphe.information@state.co.us
**Website:** http://www.cdphe.state.co.us/health-h.asp

**★ 18032 ★ Connecticut Department of Public Health**
410 Capitol Ave.
PO Box 340308
Hartford, CT 06134-0308
**Phone:** (860)509-8000　　　**Fax:** (860)509-7227
**Email:** webmaster.dph@po.state.ct.us
**Website:** http://www.state.ct.us/dph/
Joxel Garcia, MD, Contact

**★ 18033 ★ Delaware Department of Health and Social Services**
**Public Health Division**
Jesse Cooper Bldg.
Federal & Water Sts.
PO Box 637
Dover, DE 19903
**Phone:** (302)739-4701　　　**Fax:** (302)739-6659
**Email:** dhssinfo@state.de.us
**Website:** http://www.state.de.us/dhss/dph/dphhome.htm
Dr. Ulder Jane Tillman, Director

**★ 18034 ★ District of Columbia Department of Health**
Office of the Director
825 N Capitol St. NE
Washington, DC 20002
**Phone:** (202)442-5999　　　**Fax:** (202)442-4788
**Website:** http://www.dchealth.dc.gov

**★ 18035 ★ Florida Department of Health**
4052 Bald Cypress Way, Bin A00
Tallahassee, FL 32399-1701
**Phone:** (850)245-4443
**Email:** health@doh.state.fl.us
**Website:** http://www.doh.state.fl.us/

**★ 18036 ★ Georgia Department of Human Resources**
**Division of Public Health**
2 Peachtree St. NW
Atlanta, GA 30303-3186
**Phone:** (404)657-2700
**Email:** gdphinfo@dhr.state.ga.us
**Website:** http://health.state.ga.us/

**★ 18037 ★ Hawaii Department of Health**
1250 Punchbowl St.
Honolulu, HI 96813
**Phone:** (808)586-4400　　　**Fax:** (808)586-4444
**Email:** webmail@mail.health.state.hi.us
**Website:** http://www.state.hi.us/health/
Bruce Anderson, PhD, Director

**★ 18038 ★ Idaho Department of Health and Welfare**
**Health Division**
Pete T. Cenarrusa Bldg. 4th Fl.
450 W State St.
PO Box 83720
Boise, ID 83720-0036
**Phone:** (208)334-5945
**Email:** dhwinfor@idhw.state.id.us
**Website:** http://www2.state.id.us/dhw/index.htm
Richard H. Schultz, Contact

**★ 18039 ★ Illinois Department of Public Health**
535 W Jefferson St.
Springfield, IL 62761
**Phone:** (217)782-4977　　　**Fax:** (217)782-3987
**Email:** mailus@idph.state.il.us
**Website:** http://www.idph.state.il.us/
John R. Lumpkin, MD, Director

**★ 18040 ★ Indiana State Department of Health**
2 N Meridian St.
Indianapolis, IN 46204
**Phone:** (317)233-1325
**Email:** webmaster@ai.org
**Website:** http://www.state.in.us/doh/
Gregory A. Wilson, MD, Director

**★ 18041 ★ Iowa Department of Public Health**
Lucas State Office Bldg.
321 E 12th St.
Des Moines, IA 50319-0075
**Phone:** (515)281-5787
**Email:** webmaster@idph.state.ia.us
**Website:** http://idph.state.ia.us/
Stephen C. Gleason, Director

**★ 18042 ★ Kansas Department of Health and Environment**
**Health Division**
1000 SW Jackson, ste.300
Topeka, KS 66612-1365
**Phone:** (785)296-1343      **Fax:** (785)296-1562
**Website:** http://www.kdhe.state.ks.us/health/
Michael Moser, MD, Director

**★ 18043 ★ Kentucky Health Services Cabinet**
**Department for Public Health**
275 E Main St.
Frankfort, KY 40621
**Phone:** (502)564-3970      **Fax:** (502)564-9377
**Email:** dphwebsite@mail.state.ky.us
**Website:** http://publichealth.state.ky.us/
Rice C. Leach, MD, Director

**★ 18044 ★ Louisiana Department of Health and Hospitals**
**Public Health Services Office**
**Metropolitan Regional Office**
1001 Howard Ave., Ste. 100A
New Orleans, LA 70113
**Phone:** (504)599-0100      **Free:** 800-256-4609
**Fax:** (504)599-0200
**Website:** http://www.dhh.state.la.us/OPH/Regions/reg1.htm

**★ 18045 ★ Louisiana Public Health Agency**
**Acadian Regional Office**
Brandywine III, Ste. 100
825 Kaliste Saloom Rd.
Lafayette, LA 70508
**Phone:** (318)262-5311      **Fax:** (318)262-5237
**Website:** http://www.dhh.state.la.us/OPH/Regions/reg4.htm

**★ 18046 ★ Louisiana Public Health Agency**
**Capitol Regional Office**
1772 Wooddale Blvd.
Baton Rouge, LA 70806
**Phone:** (504)925-7200      **Fax:** (504)925-7245
**Website:** http://www.dhh.state.la.us/OPH/Regions/reg2.htm

**★ 18047 ★ Louisiana Public Health Agency**
**Region III Office**
206 E 3rd
Thibodaux, LA 70301
**Phone:** (504)447-0916      **Fax:** (504)447-0920
**Website:** http://www.dhh.state.la.us/OPH/Regions/reg3.htm

**★ 18048 ★ Louisiana Public Health Authority**
**Central Regional Office**
1500 Lee St.
PO Box 8199
Alexandria, LA 71306-1199
**Phone:** (318)487-5262      **Fax:** (318)487-5338
**Website:** http://www.dhh.state.la.us/OPH/Regions/reg6.htm

**★ 18049 ★ Louisiana Public Health Authority**
**Northeast Regional Office**
2913 Betin St.
PO Box 6118
Monroe, LA 71211-6118
**Phone:** (318)362-5211      **Fax:** (318)362-3163
**Website:** http://www.dhh.state.la.us/OPH/Regions/reg8.htm

**★ 18050 ★ Louisiana Public Health Authority**
**Northwest Regional Office**
1525 Fairfield Ave., Rm. 569
Shreveport, LA 71101-4388
**Phone:** (318)676-7489      **Fax:** (318)676-7560
**Website:** http://www.dhh.state.la.us/OPH/Regions/reg7.htm

**★ 18051 ★ Louisiana Public Health Authority**
**Southeast Regional Office**
520 Old Spanish Tr., Ste. 100
Slidell, LA 70458
**Phone:** (504)646-6459      **Fax:** (504)646-6476
**Website:** http://www.dhh.state.la.us/OPH/Regions/reg9.htm

**★ 18052 ★ Lousiana Public Health Authority**
**Southwest Regional Office**
4240 Senator J. Bennett Johnston Ave.
Lake Charles, LA 70615
**Phone:** (318)491-2040      **Fax:** (318)491-2041
**Website:** http://www.dhh.state.la.us/OPH/Regions/reg5.htm

**★ 18053 ★ Maine Bureau of Health**
11 State House Station
157 Capitol St.
Augusta, ME 04333
**Phone:** (207)287-8016
**Email:** marcie.sanders@state.me.us
**Website:** http://www.state.me.us/dhs/boh/index.htm
Lani Graham, MD, Director

**★ 18054 ★ Maine Department of Human Services**
**Health Bureau**
11 State House Station
157 Capitol St.
Augusta, ME 04333
**Phone:** (207)287-8016
**Email:** kerry.bagley@state.me.us
**Website:** http://janus.state.me.us/dhs/boh/index.htm
Marcie Sanders, MD, Contact

**★ 18055 ★ Maryland Department of Health and Mental Hygiene**
**Community and Public Health Administration**
201 W Preston St., 3rd Fl.
Baltimore, MD 21201
**Phone:** (410)767-5300
**Email:** webmaster@dhmh.state.md.us
**Website:** http://mdpublichealth.org/
Georges C. Benjamin, Contact

**★ 18056 ★ Massachusetts Department of Public Health**
250 Washington St.
Boston, MA 02108-4619
**Phone:** (617)624-6000
**Email:** dph.info@state.ma.us
**Website:** http://www.state.ma.us/dph/
Howard Koh, MD, Director

**★ 18057 ★ Michigan Department of Community Health**
Lewis Cass Bldg., 6th Fl.
320 S Walnut St.
Lansing, MI 48913
**Phone:** (517)373-3500      **Fax:** (517)335-3090
**Email:** arias@state.mi.us
**Website:** http://www.mdch.state.mi.us/

**★ 18058 ★ Minnesota Department of Health**
717 Delaware St. SE
PO Box 64975
Minneapolis, MN 55440-9441
**Phone:** (651)215-5800      **Fax:** (651)623-5043
**Email:** library@health.state.mn.us
**Website:** http://www.health.state.mn.us/

**★ 18059 ★ Mississippi State Department of Health**
State Board of Health Bldg.
570 E Woodrow Wilson
PO Box 1700
Jackson, MS 39215-1700
**Phone:** (601)576-7400      **Fax:** (601)576-7364
**Email:** info@msdh.state.ms.us
**Website:** http://www.msdh.state.ms.us/

**★ 18060 ★ Mississippi State Department of Health**
**Public Health Statistics**
571 Stadium Dr.
PO Box 1700
Jackson, MS 39215-1700
**Phone:** (601)576-7960      **Fax:** (601)576-7505
**Website:** http://www.msdh.state.ms.us/phs/index.htm

**★ 18061 ★ Missouri Department of Health**
920-930 Wildwood Dr.
PO Box 570
Jefferson City, MO 65102-0570
**Phone:** (573)751-6400      **Fax:** (573)751-6010
**Email:** info@mail.health.state.mo.us
**Website:** http://www.health.state.mo.us/
Maureen Dempsey, MD, Director

**★ 18062 ★ Montana Department of Public Health and Human Services**
**Health Policy and Services Division**
Cogswell Bldg.
1400 Broadway
PO Box 202951
Helena, MT 59620
**Phone:** (406)444-4540      **Fax:** (406)444-1861
**Email:** nellery@state.mt.gov
**Website:** http://www.dphhs.state.mt.us/divisions/hps/hps_phone.htm
Maggie Bullock, Contact

**★ 18063 ★ Nebraska Department of Health and Human Services**
**Department of Services**
PO Box 95044
Lincoln, NE 68509-5044
**Phone:** (402)471-2306
**Email:** hhsinfo@hhs.state.ne.us
**Website:** http://www.hhs.state.ne.us/svc/svcindex.htm
Ron Ross, Director

**★ 18064 ★ Nevada State Health Division**
**Administrative Office**
505 E King St., Rm. 201
Carson City, NV 89701
**Phone:** (775)684-4200      **Fax:** (775)684-4211
**Website:** http://www.state.nv.us/health/

**★ 18065 ★ New Hampshire Department of Health and Human Services**
**Office of Administration**
129 Pleasant St.
Concord, NH 03301-3857
**Phone:** (603)271-4814      **Fax:** (603)271-5590
**Website:** http://www.dhhs.state.nh.us/

**★ 18066 ★ New Jersey Department of Health and Senior Services**
John Fitch Plaza
PO Box 360
Trenton, NJ 08625-0360
**Phone:** (609)292-7837
**Website:** http://www.state.nj.us/health/
Christine Grant, Director

**★ 18067 ★ New Mexico Department of Health**
**Public Health Division**
Harold Runnels Bldg.
1190 St. Francis Dr.
Santa Fe, NM 87504
**Phone:** (505)827-2613
**Website:** http://www.health.state.nm.us/

**★ 18068 ★ New York State Department of Health**
Corning Tower
Empire State Plaza
Albany, NY 12237
**Phone:** (518)474-2011
**Email:** nyhealth@health.state.ny.us
**Website:** http://www.health.state.ny.us/
Maryellen Jacobson, Secretary

**★ 18069 ★ North Carolina Department of Health and Human Services**
**Health Director's Office**
Adams Bldg.
101 Blair Dr.
2001 Mail Service Ctr.
Raleigh, NC 27699-2001
**Phone:** (919)733-4534    **Free:** 800-662-7030
**Fax:** (919)715-4645
**Website:** http://www.dhhs.state.nc.us/docs/divinfo/secretary.htm
Carmen Hooker Odom, MD, Secretary

**★ 18070 ★ North Dakota Department of Health**
600 E Boulevard Ave.
Bismarck, ND 58505-0200
**Phone:** (701)328-2372    **Fax:** (701)328-4727
**Email:** ajohnson@state.nd.us
**Website:** http://www.health.state.nd.us/
Terry Dwelle, Director

**★ 18071 ★ Ohio Department of Health**
246 N High St.
PO Box 118
Columbus, OH 43215
**Phone:** (614)466-3543    **Fax:** (614)644-0085
**Website:** http://www.odh.state.oh.us/
J. Nick Baird, Director

**★ 18072 ★ Oklahoma State Department of Health**
1000 NE 10th St.
Oklahoma City, OK 73117
**Phone:** (405)271-5600
**Email:** webmaster@health.state.ok.us
**Website:** http://www.health.state.ok.us/
Leslie M. Beitsch, MD, Director

**★ 18073 ★ Oregon Department of Human Resources**
**Health Division**
Portland State Office Bldg.
800 NE Oregon St., No. 21
Portland, OR 97232
**Phone:** (503)731-4000
**Email:** ohd.info@state.or.us
**Website:** http://www.ohd.hr.state.or.us/
Martin Wasserman, Director

**★ 18074 ★ Pennsylvania Department of Health**
Health and Welfare Bldg.
PO Box 90
Harrisburg, PA 17108
**Phone:** (717)787-6436
**Email:** webmaster@health.state.pa.us
**Website:** http://www.health.state.pa.us/
Robert Zimmerman, Director

**★ 18075 ★ Rhode Island Department of Health**
3 Capitol Hill
Providence, RI 02908
**Phone:** (401)222-2231    **Free:** 800-745-5555
**Fax:** (401)222-6548
**Email:** library@health.state.ri.us
**Website:** http://www.health.state.ri.us/
Patricia A. Nolan, MD, Director

**★ 18076 ★ South Carolina Department of Health and Environmental Control**
**Health Services Office**
2600 Bull St.
PO Box 101106
Columbia, SC 29211-0106
**Phone:** (803)898-3432
**Website:** http://www.scdhec.net/hs/

**★ 18077 ★ South Dakota Department of Health**
Health Bldg.
600 E Capitol
Pierre, SD 57501-2536
**Phone:** (605)773-3361    **Free:** 800-738-2301
**Email:** DOH.INFO@state.sd.us
**Website:** http://www.state.sd.us/doh/
Doneen Hollingsworth, Secretary

**★ 18078 ★ Tennessee Department of Health**
**Health Statistics and Information**
Cordell Hull Bldg., 4th Fl.
425 5th Ave. N
Nashville, TN 37247-5262
**Phone:** (615)741-1954    **Fax:** (615)532-7904
**Email:** DDenton@mail.state.tn.us
**Website:** http://www.state.tn.us/health/statistics/

**★ 18079 ★ Texas Department of Health**
1100 W 49th St.
Austin, TX 78756-3199
**Phone:** (512)458-7111    **Free:** 888-963-7111
**Email:** webmaster@tdh.state.tx.us
**Website:** http://www.tdh.texas.gov/

**★ 18080 ★ Utah Department of Health**
PO Box 1010
Salt Lake City, UT 84114-1010
**Phone:** (801)538-6101

**Email:** pwightma@doh.state.ut.us
**Website:** http://www.health.state.ut.us/

**★ 18081 ★ Vermont Department of Health**
108 Cherry St.
PO Box 70
Burlington, VT 05402-0070
**Phone:** (802)863-7200    **Fax:** (802)865-7754
**Email:** webkeeper@vdh.state.vt.us
**Website:** http://www.healthyvermonters.info/

**★ 18082 ★ Virgin Islands Department of Health**
St. Thomas Hospital
48 Sugar Estate
Charlotte Amalie, VI 00802
**Phone:** (340)774-0117    **Fax:** (340)777-4001
**Website:** http://www.usvi.org/health/index.html

**★ 18083 ★ Virginia Office of Health and Human Resources**
**Health Department**
Main St. Station
1500 E Main St., Ste. 214
Richmond, VA 23219
**Phone:** (804)786-3561
**Email:** rnash@vdh.state.va.us
**Website:** http://www.vdh.state.va.us/
Robert B. Stroube, MD, Director

**★ 18084 ★ Washington State Department of Health**
1112 SE Quince St.
PO Box 47890
Olympia, WA 98504-7890
**Phone:** (360)236-4010    **Free:** 800-525-0127
**Email:** doh.webmaster@doh.wa.gov
**Website:** http://www.doh.wa.gov/
Mary Selecky, Director

**★ 18085 ★ West Virginia Department of Health and Human Resources**
**Public Health Bureau**
350 Capitol St., Rm. 702
Charleston, WV 25301-3712
**Phone:** (304)558-2971    **Fax:** (304)558-1035
**Website:** http://www.wvdhhr.org/bph/
Henry G. Taylor, MD, Director

**★ 18086 ★ Wisconsin Department of Health and Family Services**
**Public Health Division**
PO Box 2659
Madison, WI 53701-2659
**Phone:** (608)266-1251    **Fax:** (608)267-2832
**Email:** webmaster@dhfs.state.wi.us
**Website:** http://www.dhfs.state.wi.us/aboutdhfs/dph/dphservs.htm
John Chapin, Director

**★ 18087 ★ Wyoming Department of Health**
**Public Health Division**
117 Hathaway Bldg.
Cheyenne, WY 82002
**Phone:** (307)777-7656    **Fax:** (307)777-7327
**Email:** wdh@state.wy.us
**Website:** http://wdhfs.state.wy.us/WDH/
Garry L. McKee, PhD, Director

# Chapter 55
# Radiological Health

## Federal Government Agencies

★ **18088** ★ **U.S. Department of Health and Human Services**
**Food and Drug Administration**
**Center for Devices and Radiological Health**
1350 Piccard Dr., HFZ-210
Rockville, MD 20850
**Phone:** (301)827-3990 **Free:** 888-463-6332
**Website:** http://www.fda.gov/cdrh
David W. Feigal, MD, Director
**Desc:** The Center develops and carries out a national program designed to control unnecessary exposure of humans to potentially hazardous ionizing and non-ionizing radiation and ensure its safe use. It develops policy and priorities regarding FDA programs relating to the safety, effectiveness, and labeling of medical devises for human use; conducts and electronic product radiation control program; develops regulations, standards, and criteria and recommends changes in FDA legislative authority necessary to protect the public health; and provides scientific and technical support to other components within the FDA and other agencies on matters relating to radiological health and medical devices.

## Foundations & Other Funding Organizations

### Other Funding Organizations

**American Radiological Nurses Association (ARNA)**
*See:* Entry 14918

## National & International Organizations

**British Society for Dental and Maxillofacial Radiology**
*See:* Entry 6482

**Cardiovascular and Interventional Radiological Society of Europe (CIRSE)**
*See:* Entry 4991

★ **18089** ★ **Clinical Magnetic Resonance Society (CMRS)**
4550 Post Oak Pl., Ste. 342
Houston, TX 77027
**Phone:** (713)623-8336 **Free:** 877-841-2522
**Fax:** (713)960-0488
**Email:** cmrs@one.net
**Website:** http://www.cmrs.com
Darcee Brown, Acct. Exec.
**Fnded:** 1995. **Mem:** 1,000. **Desc:** Offers experience-based credentialing for physicians who practice MRI. Provides a forum for networking among members. Defines procedure protocols and safety information. **Pub:** *CMRS Vision*, quarterly. Newsletter. Contains information on new developments in magnetic resonance imaging.

★ **18090** ★ **Professional Board for Radiography and Clinical Technology**
533 Vermeulen St.
Arcadia
PO Box 205
Pretoria 0083, Republic of South Africa
**Phone:** 27 12 3286680 **Fax:** 27 12 3285120
**Email:** hpcsa@hpcsa.co.za
**Fnded:** 1974. **Mem:** 3,997. **Lang(s):** Afrikaans, English. **Desc:** Works to maintain professional standards of education and conduct of radiographers; strives to prevent the admission of unqualified individuals into the radiography profession. Cooperates with the Health Professions Council of South Africa in approving training courses in radiography. Investigates reports of unprofessional conduct. Represents interests of the public. Disseminates information; compiles statistics. **Pub:** *HPCSA Bulletin*, quarterly. Bulletin. • *Technical Journal*, periodic. Journal. **Frmly:** (2000) Professional Board for Radiography.

★ **18091** ★ **Society for Computer Applications in Radiology (SCAR)**
10105 Cottesmore Ct.
Great Falls, VA 22066-3540
**Phone:** (703)757-0054 **Fax:** (703)757-0454
**Email:** info@scarnet.org
**Website:** http://www.scarnet.org
Anna Marie Mason, Exec. Dir.
**Fnded:** 1980. **Mem:** 1,600. **Desc:** Individuals, corporations, and health facilities with an interest in medical imaging organized to promote and advance through study research, design and testing, the development and application of advanced technology information systems that will improve the delivery of medical imaging services. **Pub:** *Journal of Digital Imaging*, quarterly. Journal. • *SCAR News*, quarterly. Newsletter. • *SCAR University Primer 1: Security Issues in the Digital Medical Enterprise.* • *SCAR University Primer 3: QA: Meeting the Challenge of the Digital Medical Enterprise.* Handbook. • *SCAR University Primer 2: Achiving Issues in the Digital Medical Enterprise.* Handbook. • *Understanding Image Compression 1997.* Handbook. • *Understanding Teleradiology 1994.* Handbook.

## Research Centers

**Albert Einstein Center for Synchrotron Biosciences**
*See:* Entry 4614

★ **18092** ★ **McGill University**
**Medical Physics Unit**
Montreal General Hospital
1650 Cedar Ave., Rm. L5-109
Montreal, QC, Canada H3G 1A4
**Phone:** (514)934-8052 **Fax:** (514)934-8229
**Email:** epodgorsak@medphys.mcgill.ca
**Website:** http://www.medphys.mcgill.ca
Prof. Ervin B. Podgorsak, Dir.
**Activities/Fields:** Medical imaging, including resonant cavity imaging, filter functions (computer tomography), positron emission tomography, nuclear magnetic resonance imaging, and electronic processing. Other studies include physical aspects of radiation oncology and radiation dosimetry, radiosurgery, radiation hazards and protection, physical aspects of nuclear cardiology, and dosimetry in diagnostic radiology.

★ **18093** ★ **University of Chicago**
**Kurt Rossmann Laboratories for Radiologic Image Research**
Department of Radiology
5841 S Maryland Ave., M/C 2026
Chicago, IL 60637
**Phone:** (773)702-6154 **Fax:** (773)702-0371
**Email:** k-doi@uchicago.edu
**Website:** http://xray.bsd.uchicago.edu/krl/
Kunio Doi, PhD, Dir.
**Activities/Fields:** Diagnostic accuracy of radiological imaging techniques and minimization of patient exposure incurred during radiographic examinations.

★ **18094** ★ **University of Texas Health Science Center at San Antonio**
**Center for Environmental Radiation Toxicology**
MSC 7889
7703 Floyd Curl Dr.
San Antonio, TX 78229-3900
**Phone:** (210)567-5560 **Fax:** (210)567-3446
**Email:** meltz@uthscsa.edu
Martin Meltz, PhD, Dir.
**Activities/Fields:** Effects of individual and combined exposures to microwave radiation, ionizing radiation, UV light and chemicals on biological systems. Current investigations focus on a variety of normal and cancerous in vitro cell lines, and human peripheral blood lymphocytes. The endpoints studied include signal transduction mechanisms, protein and protooncogene induction, primary DNA damage and repair, and chromosome damage. Also conducts hyperthermia investigations. **Frmly:** Center for Basic Research in Radiation Bioeffects.

★ **18095** ★ **University of Utah Radiobiology Laboratory**
729 Arapeen Dr., Ste. 2334
Salt Lake City, UT 84102-1218
**Phone:** (801)581-6600     **Fax:** (801)581-7008

**Email:** scott.miller@hsc.utah.edu
**Website:** http://www.utah.edu/radiobiology
Dr. Scott C. Miller, Dir.

**Activities/Fields:** Chemistry, physics, biochemistry, bone sciences, and veterinary aspects and pathology of long-term physiological and biochemical effects of internally deposited radioisotopes. **Pub:** *Research in Radiobiology*, annually. Report.

# Chapter 56
# Radiology

## Foundations & Other Funding Organizations

### Other Funding Organizations

**American Academy of Oral and Maxillofacial Radiology (AAOMR)**
*See:* Entry 6329

★ **18096** ★ **American Roentgen Ray Society (ARRS)**
44211 Slatestone Ct.
Leesburg, VA 20176-5109
**Phone:** (703)729-3353    **Free:** 800-438-2777
**Fax:** (703)729-4839
**Email:** rdunnick@umich.edu
**Website:** http://www.arrs.org
N. Reed Dunnick, Pres.

**Desc:** Trade association for radiologists worldwide. Offers many educational programs. **Awards:** ARRS Scholar (annual) for a practicing radiologist.

★ **18097** ★ **International Society for Magnetic Resonance in Medicine**
2118 Milvia St., Ste. 201
Berkeley, CA 94704
**Phone:** (510)841-1899    **Fax:** (510)841-2340
**Email:** info@ismrm.org
**Website:** http://www.ismrm.org
Jane Tiemann, Exec. Dir.

**Desc:** Devoted to furthering the development and application of MRI and its techniques in medicine and biology. Sponsors educational and research programs. **Awards:** Yound Investigator's Award/Student Stipends (annual).

★ **18098** ★ **North American Society for Cardiac Imaging (NASCI)**
930 Edgecliff Way
Redwood City, CA 94061
**Phone:** (650)216-6621    **Fax:** (650)556-1678
**Email:** info@nasci.org
**Website:** http://www.nasci.org
Joan Oefner, CAE, Exec. Dir.

**Desc:** Approved individuals engaged in the practice and advancement of cardiac and vascular imaging are active members; medical students, other individuals, and corporations with an interest in cardiac imaging are sponsors. Seeks to advance the practice of cardiac imaging and to develop improved medical imaging technologies. Serves as a forum for the exchange of information among individuals and corporations with an interest in cardiac imaging; sponsors educational programs; maintains NASCI Research and Education Fund. **Awards:** AHA Council of Cardiovascular Radiology (annual); Berlex Poster Awards (annual); Young Investigator's Awards (annual).

★ **18099** ★ **Radiological Society of North America (RSNA)**
820 Jorie Blvd.
Oak Brook, IL 60523-2251
**Phone:** (630)571-2670    **Fax:** (630)571-7837
**Email:** informat@rsna.org
**Website:** http://www.rsna.org
David Fellers, CAE, Exec. Dir.

**Desc:** Radiologists and scientists in fields closely related to radiology. Promotes study and practical application of radiology, radium, electricity, and other branches of physics related to medical science. **Awards:** Grant (annual); Research and Education Fund (annual); RSNA Gold Medal (annual) for outstanding contribution in radiology field.

★ **18100** ★ **Society of Cardiovascular and Interventional Radiology (SCVIR)**
10201 Lee Hwy., Ste. 500
Fairfax, VA 22030
**Phone:** (703)691-1805    **Free:** 800-488-7284
**Fax:** (703)691-1855
**Email:** info@scvir.org
**Website:** http://www.scvir.org
Paul Pomerantz, Exec. Dir.

**Desc:** Physicians who are leaders in the field of cardiovascular and interventional radiology. Facilitates exchange of new ideas and techniques and provides educational courses for all physicians working in the field. Conducts annual postgraduate course. Conducts Interventional Radiology Political Action. **Awards:** Young Investigator Award (annual).

## National & International Organizations

★ **18101** ★ **Alliance for Lung Cancer Advocacy, Support and Education (ALCASE)**
PO Box 849
500 W 8th St., Ste. 240
Vancouver, WA 98666
**Phone:** (360)696-2436    **Free:** 800-298-2436
**Fax:** (360)735-1305
**Email:** info@alcase.org
**Website:** http://www.alcase.org
Betty Layne, Interim Co-Exec. Dir.

**Fnded:** 1995. **Mem:** 35,000. **Desc:** Dedicated to helping people living with or at risk of lung cancer on a worldwide basis. **Pub:** *Information for the Asking.* Booklet. Designed to increase communication between survivors and their healthcare team. *Price:* Free. • *The Lung Cancer Manual.* Manual. Contains information on lung cancer treatments, diagnosis and staging , complementary medicine, financial issues, and end-of-life issues. *Price:* Free. • *Lung Cancer Resource Guide.* Booklet. Includes list of organizations, programs, and other services for people living with lung cancer. *Price:* Free. • *Spirit and Breath*, quarterly. Newsletter. Provides information on new treatments, patient profiles, symptom management and advocacy issues. *Price:* Free. **Frmly:** (1998) Spirit and Breath.

★ **18102** ★ **American Association for Women Radiologists (AAWR)**
4550 Post Oak Pl., Ste. 342
Houston, TX 77027
**Phone:** (713)623-8335    **Fax:** (713)960-0488
**Email:** admin@aawr.org
**Website:** http://www.aawr.org
Lise Swanson, Acct. Exec.

**Fnded:** 1981. **Mem:** 1,400. **Local Groups:** 3. **Desc:** Physicians involved in diagnostic or therapeutic radiology, nuclear medicine, or radiologic physics. Facilitates exchange of knowledge and information as it relates to women in radiology; encourages publication of materials on radiology and medicine by members; supports women who are training in the field and encourages women at all levels to participate in radiological societies. Maintains ad hoc committees on affirmative action, radiation therapists, and policy on pregnancy. **Pub:** *AAWR Focus*, quarterly. Newsletter. *Price:* Free, to members only. • *AAWR Membership Directory*, annual. Membership Directory. *Price:* Free, to members only. • *Survival Guide for Women Radiologists: The AAWR Pocket Mentor. Price:* Free; available to members only. **Frmly:** (1991) American Association of Women Radiologists.

★ **18103** ★ **American Board of Nuclear Medicine (ABNM)**
900 Veteran Ave., Rm. 13-152
Los Angeles, CA 90024-2703
**Phone:** (310)825-6787    **Fax:** (310)794-4821
**Email:** abnmweb@hotmail.com
**Website:** http://www.abnm.org
Andrew T. Taylor, MD, Chair

**Fnded:** 1971. **Mem:** 12. **Desc:** A primary medical specialty board and member of the American Board of Medical Specialties. Provides educational standards and evaluates the competence of physicians in nuclear medicine; establishes requirements for certification. Conducts examinations and issues certification. Maintains registry of certificate holders. Aids in the assessment and accreditation of nuclear medicine programs in hospitals and institutions offering graduate training. **Pub:** *American Board of Nuclear Medicine Information, Policies and Procedures*, annual. Brochure. Provides information on the annual certifying examination. *Price:* Free.

★ **18104** ★ **American Board of Radiology (ABR)**
5255 E Williams Cir., Ste. 200
Tucson, AZ 85711-7401
**Phone:** (520)790-2900    **Fax:** (520)790-3200
**Email:** info@theabr.org
**Website:** http://www.theabr.org/
M. Paul Capp, MD, Exec. Dir.

**Fnded:** 1934. **Mem:** 23. **Desc:** Certification board to establish qualifications, conduct examinations, and certify physicians in the specialty of radiology and physicists in radiological physics and related branches (science dealing with X-rays or rays from radioactive substances for medical use). **Pub:** Booklets.On examinations in diagnostic radiology, radiological physics, radiation oncology, and special competence in nuclear radiology.

**American Chiropractic College of Radiology (ACCR)**
*See:* Entry 5909

**American Chiropractic Registry of Radiologic Technologists (ACRRT)**
*See:* Entry 5910

**American College of Medical Physics**
*See:* Entry 4587

★ 18105 ★ **American College of Nuclear Medicine (ACNM)**
PO Box 175
Landisville, PA 17538
**Phone:** (717)898-5008          **Fax:** (717)898-2555
**Email:** rpowell2248@aol.com
**Website:** http://www.acnucmed.org/
Robert Powell, Contact

**Fnded:** 1972. **Mem:** 500. **Desc:** Physicians and medical scientists in nuclear medicine united to: advance the science of nuclear medicine; improve its benefits to patients; study the socioeconomic aspects of the practice of nuclear medicine; encourage improved and continuing education for practitioners in this and allied fields. **Pub:** *ACNM Directory*, biennial. Directory. • *ACNM Report*, bimonthly. Newsletter.

★ 18106 ★ **American College of Nuclear Physicians (ACNP)**
1850 Samuel Morse Dr.
Reston, VA 20190-5316
**Phone:** (703)326-1190          **Fax:** (703)708-9015
**Email:** peter@acnp.com
**Website:** http://www.acnponline.org/
Virginia Pappas, Acting Exec. Dir.

**Fnded:** 1974. **Mem:** 1,600. **Desc:** Nuclear medicine physicians, scientists, and corporations. Objectives are: to foster the highest standards of nuclear medicine service and consultation to the public, hospitals, and referring physicians; to advance the science of nuclear medicine and improve nuclear medicine consultation and service through study, education, and improvement of the socioeconomic aspects of the practice of nuclear medicine; to promote the continuing competence of practitioners of nuclear medicine. Problem-solving areas include: unnecessary and costly regulations and restrictions; public fear, lack of understanding, and misinformation; complex state and federal legislation; transportation difficulties involving nuclear medicine supplies; previous lack of cohesive effort in attacking such problems. Conducts educational seminars and continuing education program; maintains speakers' bureau. **Pub:** *Scanner*, 10/year. • Directory, annual.

**American College of Podiatric Radiologists (ACPR)**
*See:* Entry 17708

★ 18107 ★ **American College of Radiation Oncology (ACRO)**
820 Jorie Blvd.
Oak Brook, IL 60523-1860
**Phone:** (630)368-3733          **Fax:** (630)571-7837
**Email:** acro@rsna.org
**Website:** http://www.acro.org
Catherine Carey, Contact

**Fnded:** 1989. **Mem:** 1,500. **Desc:** Radiation oncologists, physicists, and administrators. Seeks to ensure that regulatory legislation is fair to radiation oncologists. Lobbies on behalf of radiation oncology physi-

cians. Represents physicians in fee disputes with Medicare. **Pub:** *ACRO Bulletin*, quarterly. Newsletter. *Price:* Included in membership dues.

★ 18108 ★ **American College of Radiology (ACR)**
1891 Preston White Dr.
Reston, VA 20191-4397
**Phone:** (703)648-8900          **Free:** 800-ACR-LINE
**Fax:** (703)295-6773
**Email:** info@acr.org
**Website:** http://www.acr.org
John J. Curry, Exec. Dir.

**Fnded:** 1923. **Mem:** 32,000. **State Groups:** 53. **Desc:** Principal organization serving radiologists with programs which focus on the practice of radiology and the delivery of comprehensive radiological health services. These programs in medical sciences, education, and in practice management, serve the public interest and the interests of the medical community in which radiologists serve in both diagnostic and therapeutic roles. Seeks to "advance the science of radiology, improve radiologic service to the patient, study the economic aspects of the practice of radiology, and encourage imroved and continuing education for radiologists and allied professional fields". **Pub:** Booklets. • Books. • Bulletin, monthly. • Directory, annual. • Pamphlets. • Also publishes textbooks, reprints, kits, and slides.

**American College of Veterinary Radiology (ACVR)**
*See:* Entry 20563

**American Healthcare Radiology Administrators (AHRA)**
*See:* Entry 9701

★ 18109 ★ **American Institute of Ultrasound in Medicine (AIUM)**
14750 Sweitzer Ln., Ste. 100
Laurel, MD 20707-5906
**Phone:** (301)498-4100          **Free:** 800-638-5352
**Fax:** (301)498-4450
**Email:** admin@aium.org
**Website:** http://www.aium.org
Carmine M. Valente, PhDCAE, CEO

**Fnded:** 1951. **Mem:** 9,500. **Desc:** A multidisciplinary organization dedicated to advancing the art and science of ultrasound in medicine through its educational, scientific, literary and professional activities. Membership comprises professionals from many medical specialties, as well as basic scientists, engineers, manufacturers, nurses, physicists, radiologic technologists, sonographers and veterinarians involved with diagnostic medical ultrasound. **Pub:** *AIUM Sound Waves*, monthly. Newsletter. Covers institute activities and developments in diagnostic ultrasound. Includes listing of continuing education courses and employment opportunities. *Price:* Included in membership dues. • *Journal of Ultrasound in Medicine*, monthly. Journal. Contains research papers and case reports covering all aspects of diagnostic ultrasound, advances in instrumentation, and biological effects. *Price:* Included in membership dues; $145/year for nonmembers; $190/year for institutions. • Videos. • *AIUM Annual Convention Proceedings. Price:* $12/copy for members; $22/copy for nonmembers.

**American Osteopathic College of Radiology (AOCR)**
*See:* Entry 17007

★ 18110 ★ **American Radiological Nurses Association (ARNA)**
820 Jorie Blvd.
Oak Brook, IL 60523
**Phone:** (630)571-9072          **Fax:** (630)571-7837
**Email:** arna@rsna.org

**Website:** http://www.arna.net
Betty Rohr, Account Executive

**Fnded:** 1981. **Mem:** 1,547. **State Groups:** 23. **Desc:** Radiological nurses. Seeks to provide, promote, and maintain continuity of quality patient care through education, standards of care, professional growth, and collaboration with other health care providers. **Pub:** *Images*, quarterly. Journal. Conveys news related to developments in practice, technology, and research. Prints timely papers. *Price:* Free to members; $15/copy; $50/year. • *RN News*, quarterly. Newsletter. Conveys news of the association. *Price:* Free to members.

★ 18111 ★ **American Registry of Diagnostic Medical Sonographers (ARDMS)**
600 Jefferson Plz., Ste. 360
Rockville, MD 20852-1150
**Phone:** (301)738-8401          **Free:** 800-541-9754
**Fax:** (301)738-0312
**Email:** administration@ardms.org
**Website:** http://www.ardms.org
Dale R. Cyr, MBA, Exec. Dir.

**Fnded:** 1975. **Mem:** 40,000. **Desc:** Administers examinations in the field of diagnostic medical sonography and vascular technology throughout the U.S. and Canada and registers candidates passing those exams in the specialties of their expertise. Maintains central office for administering examination plans and schedules and assisting registered candidates and those interested in becoming registered. **Pub:** *American Registry of Diagnostic Medical Sonographers Directory*, annual. Directory. *Price:* Free. • *Continuing Competency Requirements.* Brochure. • *Examination Information and Application Booklet.* Booklet. • *Informational Brochure*, annual. Brochure. • *Mailing List Brochure.* Brochure.

★ 18112 ★ **American Registry of Radiologic Technologists (ARRT)**
1255 Northland Dr.
Saint Paul, MN 55120-1155
**Phone:** (651)687-0048
**Website:** http://www.arrt.org
Jerry B. Reid, Exec. Dir.

**Fnded:** 1922. **Mem:** 223,000. **Desc:** Radiologic technologist certification board that administers examinations, issues certificates of registration to radiographers, nuclear medicine technologists, and radiation therapists, and investigates the qualifications of practicing radiologic technologists. Governed by trustees appointed from American College of Radiology and American Society of Radiologic Technologists. **Pub:** *ARRT Annual Report.* Annual Report. • *Educator Update*, 2/year. Newsletter. **Frmly:** American Registry of X-Ray Technicians; (1936) American Registry of Radiological Technicians.

★ 18113 ★ **American Roentgen Ray Society (ARRS)**
44211 Slatestone Ct.
Leesburg, VA 20176-5109
**Phone:** (703)729-3353          **Free:** 800-438-2777
**Fax:** (703)729-4839
**Email:** rdunnick@umich.edu
**Website:** http://www.arrs.org
N. Reed Dunnick, Pres.

**Fnded:** 1900. **Mem:** 14,000. **Desc:** Trade association for radiologists worldwide. Offers many educational programs. **Pub:** *American Journal of Roentgenology*, monthly, Peer reviewed.Journal. *Price:* $210/year. • *ARRS Memo*, quarterly. Newsletter. • *Categorical Course Syllabi.* **Frmly:** (1906) Roentgen Society of the U.S.

★ 18114 ★ **American Society of Echocardiography (ASE)**
1500 Sunday Dr., Ste. 102
Raleigh, NC 27607
**Phone:** (919)787-5181          **Fax:** (919)787-4916
**Email:** rbarry@asecho.org

**Website:** http://www.asecho.org
Robin L. Barry, Exec. Dir.

**Fnded:** 1976. **Mem:** 7,000. **Desc:** Physicians and sonographers specializing in ultrasound heart imaging and diagnosis. Promotes excellence in the ultrasonic examination of the heart and assists in establishing standards for education of physicians and cardiac-sonographers in echocardiography. Sponsors educational activities including distribution of self-testing materials, continuing education calendar, and annual scientific sessions. Maintains liaison with governmental agencies and other professional groups. **Pub:** *American Society of Echocardiography Standards Documents*, periodic. • *ASE Membership Directory*, biennial. Membership Directory. • *Journal of the American Society of Echocardiography*, monthly. Journal. For physicians and sonographers covering echocardiography. Includes legislative and membership updates. • Also publishes standards documents and number news briefs.

### American Society for Laser Medicine and Surgery (ASLMS)
*See:* Entry 19495

### ★ 18115 ★ American Society of Neuroimaging (ASN)
c/o B. Todd Troost, MD
Department of Neurology
Wake Forest University School of Medicine
Medical Center Blvd.
Winston Salem, NC 27157
**Phone:** (336)716-3429          **Fax:** (336)716-9489
**Email:** todd@toddtroost.com
**Website:** http://www.asnweb.org
Todd Troost, VP

**Fnded:** 1977. **Mem:** 800. **Desc:** Neurologists, neurosurgeons, neuroradiologists, and scientists. Promotes the development of computerized tomography (CT scanning), magnetic resonanace imaging (MRI), neurosonology, and other neurodiagnostic techniques for clinical service, teaching, and research. Encourages the collaboration of members to improve techniques through educational programs and scientific research. Holds annual certification exam in MRI and neurosonology. **Pub:** *Journal of Neuroimaging*, quarterly. Journal. • Newsletter, semiannual. **Frmly:** (1980) Society for Computerized Tomography and Neuroimaging.

### ★ 18116 ★ American Society of Neuroradiology (ASNR)
2210 Midwest Rd., Ste. 207
Oak Brook, IL 60521
**Phone:** (630)574-0220          **Fax:** (630)574-0661
**Email:** jgantenberg@asnr.org
**Website:** http://www.asnr.org
James B. Gantenberg, Exec. Dir. /CEO

**Fnded:** 1962. **Mem:** 2,905. **Desc:** Neuroradiologists who spend at least half of their time practicing neuroradiology. Fosters education, basic science research, and communication in neuroradiology. **Pub:** *American Journal of Neuroradiology*, 10/year. Journal. *Price:* Included in membership dues; $210/year for nonmembers; $270/year for nonmembers outside the U.S.; $90 in training. • *Membership Roll*, annual.

### American Society of Pediatric Neuroradiology
*See:* Entry 5615

### ★ 18117 ★ American Society of Radiologic Technologists (ASRT)
15000 Central Ave. SE
Albuquerque, NM 87123
**Phone:** (505)298-4500          **Free:** 800-444-2778
**Fax:** (505)298-5063
**Email:** customerservices@asrt.org
**Website:** http://www.asrt.org
Joan Parsons, Exec. VP, Operations

**Fnded:** 1920. **Mem:** 94,000. **Reg. Groups:** 10. **State Groups:** 50. **Desc:** Professional society of diagnostic radiography, radiation therapy, ultrasound, and nuclear medicine technologists. Advances the science of radiologic technology; establishes and maintains high standards of education; evaluates the quality of patient care; improves the welfare and socioeconomics of radiologic technologists. Operates ASRT Education and Research Foundation, which provides educational materials to radiologic technologists. **Pub:** *ASRT Scanner*, monthly. Magazine. Includes calendar of events, member profiles, state affiliate news, educational opportunities, and research updates. *Price:* Included in membership dues. • *Radiation Therapist*, semiannual. Journal. *Price:* Included in membership dues; $25/year for nonmembership in U.S.; $50/year for nonmembers outside U.S. • *Radiologic Technology*, bimonthly. Journal. Includes advertisers and cumulative annual author and title indexes, book reviews, literature abstracts, and calendar of events. *Price:* Included in membership dues; $49/year for nonmembers; $75/year for nonmembers outside the U.S.; $29.50/year for students. **Frmly:** (1934) American Society of Radiographers; (1964) American Society of X-Ray Technicians.

### ★ 18118 ★ American Society of Spine Radiology (ASSR)
2210 Midwest Rd., Ste. 207
Oak Brook, IL 60523
**Phone:** (630)574-0220          **Fax:** (630)574-0661
**Website:** http://www.asnr.org

**Fnded:** 1993. **Mem:** 500. **Desc:** Radiologists. Provide support and exchange ideas and information concerning spine radiology. Hold meetings, lectures and discussions.

### ★ 18119 ★ American Society for Therapeutic Radiology and Oncology (ASTRO)
12500 Fair Lakes Cir., Ste. 375
Fairfax, VA 22033-3882
**Phone:** (703)502-1550          **Free:** 800-962-7876
**Fax:** (703)502-7852
**Email:** webmaster@astro.org
**Website:** http://www.astro.org
Tom Nelson, Exec. Dir.

**Fnded:** 1958. **Mem:** 5,800. **Desc:** Physicians who limit their practice to radiation therapy; associate members are scientists and health care personnel who have a major interest "in furthering the aims of the society"; junior members are residents who have completed one year of training in radiation therapy. Aim is "to extend the benefits of radiation therapy to patients with cancer or other disorders, to advance its scientific basis, and to provide for the education and professional fellowship of its members." **Pub:** *ASTRO News*, bimonthly. Magazine. *Price:* Included in membership dues. • *The International Journal of Radiation Oncology, Biology, and Physics*, 13/year. Journal. **Frmly:** (1983) American Society of Therapeutic Radiologists.

### ★ 18120 ★ ASEAN Association of Radiology
Department of Radiological Sciences
Santa Tomas University Hospital
Espana
Manila, Philippines
**Phone:** 63 2 7313001

**Lang(s):** English, Filipino. **Desc:** Radiologists and health care facilities in southeastern Asia. Seeks to advance the study, teaching, and practice of radiology; promotes professional advancement of radiologists. Serves as a clearinghouse on radiology; conducts research and educational programs.

### ★ 18121 ★ Asian Federation of Societies for Ultrasound in Medicine and Biology (AFSUMB)
Department of Obstetrics and Gynecology
National Taiwan University Hospital
1 Chang-Fe St.
Taipei 10016, Taiwan
**Phone:** 886 2 3816939
**Email:** watanabe@amuom.meiji-u.ac.jp

**Fnded:** 1985. **Mem:** 17,,352. **Nat'l Groups:** 13. **Lang(s):** Chinese, English. **Desc:** Ultrasonographers and other medical professionals with an interest in ultrasound technology. Promotes application of ultrasonography in a variety of medical and biological specialties; seeks to advance the practice of ultrasonography. Serves as a clearinghouse on ultrasound technology and its uses; sponsors research and educational programs. **Pub:** *Journal of Medical Ultrasound*, quarterly. Journal.

### ★ 18122 ★ Asian and Oceanian Society of Neuroradiology and Head and Neck Radiolog y (AOSNHNR)
Taipei Veterans General Hospital
Department of Radiology
201 Section 2
Shih-Pai Rd.
Taipei, Taiwan
**Phone:** 886 2 8757357          **Fax:** 886 2 8733643

**Lang(s):** Chinese, English. **Desc:** Radiologists, neurologists, and otorhinolaryngologists. Seeks to advance the practice of neuroradiology and head and neck radiology. Facilitates exchange of information among members; sponsors research and continuing professional development programs.

### ★ 18123 ★ Asian-Pacific Society of Cardiovascular and Interventional Radiology (APSCIR)
c/o Royal Melbourne Hospital
Department of Radiology
Grattan St.
Parkville, VIC 34052, Australia

**Lang(s):** English. **Desc:** Cardiovascular and interventional radiologists. Seeks to advance the study, teaching, and practice of radiology. Serves as a forum for the exchange of information among members; sponsors research and continuing professional development programs.

### ★ 18124 ★ Association of Freestanding Radiation Oncology Centers (AFROC)
1875 Eye St. NW, 12th Fl.
Washington, DC 20006
**Free:** 888-334-4542          **Fax:** (949)376-3456
**Email:** info@AFROC.org
**Website:** http://www.tampabay2002.com:130/news
Howard Adler, Exec. Dir.

**Fnded:** 1986. **Mem:** 200. **Desc:** Freestanding radiation oncology center employees; radiologists; oncologists; physicists; radiation therapists; laboratory clinicians. Promotes the interests of freestanding radiation oncology centers to insure high quality care for patients. Upgrades management services offered. Represents members in legal matters and to other associations. **Pub:** Directory, annual.

### ★ 18125 ★ Association of Program Directors in Radiology (APDR)
820 Jorie Blvd.
Oak Brook, IL 60523
**Phone:** (630)368-3737          **Fax:** (630)571-7837
**Email:** apdr@rsna.org
**Website:** http://www.apdr.org
Josette Szalko, Acct. Exec.

**Fnded:** 1993. **Mem:** 402. **Desc:** Directors, associate directors, assistant directors, and coordinators of medical residency and fellowship programs in radiology. Promotes the "advancement of the art and science of radiology." Facilitates communication and cooperation among members; sponsors research and educational programs.

## ★ 18126 ★ Association of Residents in Radiation Oncology (ARRO)

12500 Fair Lakes Circle, Ste. 375
Fairfax, VA 22033
**Phone:** (703)502-1550    **Free:** 800-962-7876
**Fax:** (703)502-7852
**Email:** arro@astro.org
**Website:** http://www.arro.org/
Meredith Christiansen, Coord.

**Fnded:** 1983. **Mem:** 441. **Desc:** Medical residents in the field of radiation oncology. Seeks to "formalize resident input into professional organizations affecting radiation oncology residents." Serves as a clearing-house on radiation oncology; fosters communication and cooperation among members.

## ★ 18127 ★ Association of University Radiologists (AUR)

820 Jurie Blvd.
Oak Brook, IL 60523
**Phone:** (630)368-3730    **Fax:** (630)571-7837
**Email:** aur@rsna.org
**Website:** http://www.aur.org/
Josette Szalko, Exec.

**Fnded:** 1953. **Mem:** 1,600. **Desc:** Physician and non-physician scientists who have been appointed to a university faculty. Seeks to: encourage excellence in laboratory and clinical investigation, teaching, and clinical practice; stimulate interest in academic radiology as a medical career; advance radiology as a medical science; provide a forum for university based radiologists to present and discuss results of research, teaching, and administrative issues. **Pub:** *Academic Radiology*, monthly. Journal. • Also publishes award and scientific papers.

## ★ 18128 ★ Association of Vascular and Interventional Radiographers

820 Jorie Blvd.
Oak Brook, IL 60523
**Phone:** (630)571-2266    **Fax:** (630)571-7837
**Email:** avir@rsna.org
**Website:** http://www.avir.org
Betty Rohr, Exec. Sec.

**Fnded:** 1988. **Mem:** 1,100. **Desc:** Cardiovascular and interventional radiographers and allied health care professionals. **Pub:** *AVIR Interventional Informer*, quarterly. Newsletter. *Price:* $35 for nonmembers.

## ★ 18129 ★ Australian Institute of Radiography (AIR)

PO Box 1169
Collingwood, VIC 3066, Australia
**Phone:** 61 3 94193336    **Fax:** 61 3 94160783
**Email:** air@a-i-r.com.au
**Website:** http://www.a-i-r.com.au

**Fnded:** 1950. **Mem:** 3,800. **Lang(s):** English. **Desc:** Diagnostic radiographers, radiation therapists, and sonographers in Australia. Fosters cooperation and exchange of information between members. Conducts educational and research projects; prepares guide-lines and policies for the practice of radiography in Australia. Encourages high professional standards. Disseminates information; offers educational pro-grams and seminars. **Pub:** *Radiographer*, 3/year, April, August, December. Journal. • *Spectrum*, 10/yr. **Frmly:** Australasian Institute of Radiography.

## ★ 18130 ★ British Institute of Radiology (BIR)

c/o Mary-Anne Piggott
36 Portland Pl.
London W1B 1AT, United Kingdom
**Phone:** 44 207 3071400    **Fax:** 44 207 3071414
**Email:** admin@bir.org.uk
**Website:** http://www.bir.org.uk

**Fnded:** 1897. **Mem:** 2,000. **Reg. Groups:** 1. **Local Groups:** 4. **Lang(s):** English. **Desc:** Medical radiologists, scientists, and allied professionals in 55 coun-tries. Conducts seminars; bestows awards. **Pub:** *British Journal of Radiology*, monthly. Journal. Multi-disciplinary research. • Membership Directory, period-ic. **Frmly:** (1924) British Association for the Advance-ment of Radiology and Physiotherapy.

## ★ 18131 ★ British Medical Ultrasound Society (BMUS)

36 Portland Pl.
London W1B 1LS, United Kingdom
**Phone:** 44 207 6363714    **Fax:** 44 107 3232175
**Email:** secretariat@bmus.org
**Website:** http://www.bmus.org

**Fnded:** 1969. **Mem:** 2,230. **Lang(s):** English. **Desc:** Medical practitioners, physicists/scientists, sonogra-phers radiographers, veterinarians, and manufacturers of sonographic equipment. Seeks to advance the science and technology of ultrasound and to improve education in the field. **Pub:** *BMUS Bulletin*, quarterly. Newsletter. • *BMUS Membership Register*, triennial. • *Proceedings of Annual Meeting*, annual. Published in the British Journal of Radiology. **Frmly:** (1984) British Medical Ultrasound Group.

## ★ 18132 ★ Canadian Academy of Oral and Maxillofacial Radiology (Academie Canadienne de Radiologie Buccale et Maxillofaciale)

124 Edward St.
Faculty of Dentistry
University of Toronto
Toronto, ON, Canada M5G 1G6
**Phone:** (416)979-4900    **Fax:** (416)979-4936
**Email:** rbohay@julian.uwo.ca

**Lang(s):** English, French. **Desc:** Oral radiologists. Seeks to advance the study, teaching, and practice of oral radiology. Conducts research; makes available continuing professional education courses. **Frmly:** (2000) Canadian Academy of Oral Radiology.

## ★ 18133 ★ Canadian Association of Medical Radiation Technologists (CAMRT) (Association Canadienne des Technologues en Radiation Medicale — ACTRM)

130 Albert St., Ste. 1510
Ottawa, ON, Canada K1P 5G4
**Phone:** (613)234-0012    **Fax:** (613)234-1097
**Email:** skamble@camrt.ca
**Website:** http://www.camrt.ca

**Fnded:** 1942. **Mem:** 10,100. **Lang(s):** English, French. **Desc:** Certifies medical radiation technolo-gists in the fields of radiography, radiation therapy, nuclear medicine, and magnetic resonance imaging. Provides standards in the training and certification of members; promotes and maintains code of ethics. Participates in the accreditation of medical radiation technologist training programs; organizes continuing education programs. Advises private and governmen-tal organizations involved in the fields of health and education. Provides placement assistance, profes-sional liability insurance and numerous other member benefits. **Pub:** *CAMRT News*, quarterly. Newsletter. Contains activity information and education pro-grammes. • *Canadian Journal of Medical Radiation Technology*, quarterly. Journal.

## Canadian Association of Radiation Oncologists (CARO)

*See:* Entry 10134

## ★ 18134 ★ Canadian Association of Radiologists (CAR) (Association Canadienne des Radiologistes — ACR)

1740 Cote Vertu Blvd.
St.-Laurent, QC, Canada H4L 2A4
**Phone:** (514)738-3111    **Fax:** (514)738-5199
**Email:** info@car.ca
**Website:** http://www.car.ca

**Fnded:** 1937. **Mem:** 1,300. **Lang(s):** English, French. **Desc:** Physicians specializing in radiology and medi-cal imaging. Seeks to advance the practice of radiolo-gy; promotes continuing professional development of members. Represents the medical, scientific, and economic interests of radiologists; sponsors research and educational programs.

## ★ 18135 ★ Computerized Medical Imaging Society (CMIS)

c/o Natl. Biomedical Research Foundation
Georgetown Univ. Med. Center
3900 Reservoir Rd. NW
Washington, DC 20007
**Phone:** (202)687-2121    **Fax:** (202)687-1662
**Email:** ledlex@nbrf.georgetown.edu
Robert S. Ledley, Editor-in-Chief

**Fnded:** 1976. **Mem:** 350. **Desc:** Physicians and other medical personnel concerned with computerized to-mography (a diagnostic technique using X-ray photo-graphs in which the shadows of structures before and behind the section under scrutiny do not show), and other radiological diagnostic procedures. Provides a forum for the exchange of information concerning the medical use of computerized tomography in radiologi-cal diagnosis. **Pub:** *Computerized Medical Imaging and Graphics*, bimonthly. **Frmly:** (1983) Computerized Tomography Society; (1988) Computerized Radiology Society.

## ★ 18136 ★ Council on Diagnostic Imaging

PO Box 567
Wake Forest, NC 27588
**Phone:** (919)562-6570    **Fax:** (919)705-1178
**Email:** dacbrnc@aol.com
Dr. Kathy Thorn, Sec. -Treas.

**Fnded:** 1936. **Mem:** 2,000. **Desc:** Professional soci-ety of chiropractic roentgenologists, educators, stu-dents, and chiropractors interested in roentgenology. **Pub:** *Topics in Diagnostic Radiology and Advanced Imaging*, quarterly. Journal. Covers diagnostic radiolo-gy, advanced imaging, thermology, and case studies. *Price:* $50; $75 only in U.S.A.; $100 outside of U.S.A. **Frmly:** (1963) National Council of Chiropractic Roent-genologists; (1968) American Council on Chiropractic Roentgenology; (1970) American Chiropractic Council on Roentgenology; (1983) Council on Roentgeneology to the American Chiropractic Association.

## ★ 18137 ★ Czech Radiological Society (CRS) (Ceska Radiologicka Spolecnost — CRS)

c/o Dept. of Radiology
University
Hospital Brno, Bohunce
Jihlavska
CZ-63900 Brno 100, Czech Republic
**Phone:** 42 5 43193007    **Fax:** 42 5 47192383
**Email:** vlvalek@med.muni.cz
**Website:** http://www.crs.cz

**Fnded:** 1929. **Mem:** 340. **Nat'l Groups:** 1. **State Groups:** 1. **Local Groups:** 1. **Lang(s):** Czech. **Desc:** Diagnostic and interventional radiologists in the Czech Republic. Disseminates information on developments in diagnostic and interventional radiology. Acts as a forum for discussion among professionals. **Pub:** *Ces-ka Radiologie*, bimonthly. Journal. Covers all fields of interest in diagnostic radiology, radio-therapy and nuclear medicine. **Frmly:** (1993) Czechoslovak Radio-logical Society.

## ★ 18138 ★ European Association of Radiology

Inselspital
CH-3010 Bern, Switzerland
**Phone:** 41 31 6322435    **Fax:** 41 31 6324874
**Email:** peter.vock@insel.ch
**Website:** http://www.ecr.org

**Fnded:** 1962. **Mem:** 34. **Lang(s):** English, French, German. **Desc:** National European societies of radiol-ogy representing 20,000 radiologists. Objectives are to: promote radiology as a unified scientific and clinical discipline; further and monitor the application of radiology in biology and medicine; investigate the theoretical and technical problems connected with different applications of radiation; coordinate study and examination programs in the field of radiology in member countries; standardize training for radiologists and nonmedical assistants; encourage a constructive rapport with scientific, professional, and industrial organizations; promote international exchange of medical and paramedical personnel. **Pub:** *European Radiology*, bimonthly. Newsletter. **Frmly:** (2001) Institute for Diagnostic Radiology.

★ 18139 ★ **European Federation of Societies of Ultrasound in Medicine and Biology (EFSUMB)**
Carpenters Court
4a Lewes Rd.
Bromley BR1 2RN, United Kingdom
**Phone:** 44 20 84028973      **Fax:** 44 20 84029344
**Email:** efsumb@compuserve.com
**Website:** http://www.efsumb.org/
**Fnded:** 1972. **Mem:** 13,500. **Nat'l Groups:** 26. **Lang(s):** English. **Desc:** Interdisciplinary national organizations and subgroups of bodies representing 26 countries. Members promote the application of ultrasound in biology and medicine or engage in research and development in the field. Proposes standards for ultrasound use and interpretation; arranges congresses and study and development meetings; promotes the exchange of information on ultrasound as applied to biology and medicine. Represents the European national societies in the World Federation of Societies for Ultrasound in Medicine and Biology. **Pub:** *European Journal of Ultrasound*, quarterly. Journal.

★ 18140 ★ **European Society of Head and Neck Radiology (ESHNR)**
Hopital de Hautepierre
F-67098 Strasbourg, France
**Fnded:** 1987. **Desc:** Promotes knowledge in the field of head and neck diagnostic radiology, interventional radiology and diagnostic imaging; fosters research in head and neck radiology; improves methods of teaching radiologic diagnosis of diseases of the head and neck area.

★ 18141 ★ **European Society of Paediatric Radiology (ESPR)**
c/o Freddy Avni, Gen.Sec.
Radiologie Pediatrique
Hospital Universitaire des Enfants Reine Fabiola
Ave. JJ Crocq, 15
B-1020 Brussels, Belgium
**Phone:** 32 2 4773220      **Fax:** 32 2 4785439
**Email:** f.e.anvi@huderf.be
**Website:** http://users.skynet.be/espr
**Fnded:** 1963. **Mem:** 471. **Lang(s):** English. **Desc:** Radiologists involved or interested in pediatric radiology. Seeks to contribute to the advancement of the clinical and scientific aspects of pediatric radiology in European countries through educational activities. Conducts Annual postgraduate courses; sponsors research programs. **Pub:** *Paediatric Radiology*, annual. • *Pediakic Radiology*, annual. Includes proceedings. • Bulletin, semiannual.

**European Society for Therapeutic Radiology and Oncology (ESTRO)**
*See:* Entry 10167

★ 18142 ★ **European Society of Thoracic Imaging (ESTI)**
Herestr 49
3000 Leuven, Belgium
**Phone:** 32 1 6343769      **Fax:** 32 1 6343782
**Email:** johny.verschakelen@uz.kuleuven.ac.be
**Website:** http://www.esti-Society.org/
**Fnded:** 1993. **Desc:** Stimulates training and research in this radiology sub-specialty.

★ 18143 ★ **Foundation for Blood Irradiation (FFBI)**
1315 Apple Ave.
Silver Spring, MD 20910
**Phone:** (301)587-8686      **Fax:** (301)587-8688
**Email:** uv@uvbi.com
Dr. Carl Schleicher, Exec. Officer
**Fnded:** 1964. **Mem:** 175. **Desc:** Persons concerned with the research and development of ultraviolet blood irradiation therapy (intravenously applied ultraviolet energy administered to increase the body's natural ability to fight infection and resist disease). Conducts training programs. Compiles statistics and sponsors charitable programs. **Pub:** *Clinic Results of Ultraviolet Blood Irradiation*, annual. Bulletin. *Price:* $29/copy. • Monographs. • Proceedings, periodic.

★ 18144 ★ **Hong Kong College of Radiologists**
Rm. 909, 9/F Hong Kong Academy of Medicine
Jockey Club Bldg.
99 Wong Chuk Hang Rd.
Aberdeen
Hong Kong, People's Republic of China
**Phone:** 852 28718788      **Fax:** 852 25540739
**Email:** hkcr@netvigator.com
**Website:** http://www.hkcr.org
**Fnded:** 1991. **Mem:** 325. **Desc:** Encourages the study and advancement of the science and practice of diagnostic and therapeutic radiology in Hong Kong. Seeks to develop and maintain high professional standards of competence and ethical integrity. **Pub:** *Journal of the Honk Kong College of Radiologists*, quarterly. Journal. • Newsletter, quarterly.

**International Association of Cancer Victors and Friends (IACVF)**
*See:* Entry 10187

**International Association of Radiopharmacology (IAR)**
*See:* Entry 17342

★ 18145 ★ **International Skeletal Society (ISS)**
c/o Harry K. Genant, M.D.
University of California San Francisco
San Francisco, CA 94143-0628
**Phone:** (415)476-4864      **Fax:** (415)476-8550
**Email:** harry.genant@oarg.ucsf.edu
**Website:** http://www.intskelsoc.com
Michael J. Pitt, MD, Pres.
**Fnded:** 1973. **Mem:** 500. **Desc:** Physicians and scientists interested in skeletal muscle disease. Seeks to advance the science of skeletal radiology; brings together radiologists and individuals in related disciplines; provides continuing education courses. **Pub:** *Skeletal Radiology*, 8/year. Journal. Contains scientific articles and case reports. *Price:* Included in membership dues. • Membership Directory, annual. • Newsletter, semiannual.

★ 18146 ★ **International Society for Magnetic Resonance in Medicine**
2118 Milvia St., Ste. 201
Berkeley, CA 94704
**Phone:** (510)841-1899      **Fax:** (510)841-2340
**Email:** info@ismrm.org
**Website:** http://www.ismrm.org
Jane Tiemann, Exec. Dir.
**Fnded:** 1981. **Mem:** 5,000. **Reg. Groups:** 2. **Desc:** Devoted to furthering the development and application of MRI and its techniques in medicine and biology. Sponsors educational and research programs. **Pub:** *Journal of Magnetic Resonance Imaging*, monthly. Journal. • *Magnetic Resonance in Medicine*, monthly. Journal. • Brochure. • Directory. **Frmly:** (1995) Society for Magnetic Resonance.

★ 18147 ★ **International Society of Radiographers and Radiological Technologists (ISRRT)** **(Societe Internationale des Radiographes et Techniciens de Radiologie)**
170 W The Donway, Ste. 404
Don Mills, ON, Canada M3C 2G3
**Phone:** (416)510-0805      **Fax:** (416)445-4268
**Email:** isrrt@compuserve.com
**Website:** http://www.isrrt.org
**Fnded:** 1959. **Mem:** 72. **Nat'l Groups:** 68. **Reg. Groups:** 3. **Lang(s):** English. **Desc:** National radiographic societies and other organizations having radiographers as members. Objectives are to: advance the science and practice of radiography, radiotherapy, and allied subjects by promoting improved standards of training and research in technical aspects of radiation medicine and protection; make results of research and experience available to practitioners; raise funds to further these objectives. Compiles statistics and maintains museum. Has established educational trust fund. Conducts teachers' seminars. **Pub:** *Health and Safety Manual*, periodic. Proceedings. • *Quality Control Handbook*. **Frmly:** International Society of Radiographers and Radiological Technicians.

★ 18148 ★ **International Society of Radiology (ISR)**
7910 Woodmont Ave., Ste. 800
Bethesda, MD 20814
**Phone:** (301)657-2652      **Fax:** (301)907-8768
**Email:** isr@isradiology.org
**Website:** http://www.his.com/~isr/
O.W. Linton, MSJ, Exec. Dir.
**Fnded:** 1953. **Mem:** 69. **Nat'l Groups:** 69. **Reg. Groups:** 4. **Desc:** National radiological associations. Seeks to promote medical radiology worldwide through the work of its sections and international commissions. Undertakes business referred to it by member societies. Provides financial support for the work of its commissions. **Pub:** *Congress Programs*, biennial. • *Reports of Commissions of ISR*, periodic. • Newsletter, semiannual.

★ 18149 ★ **Latin American Group of Angiography and Phacoemulsification (GLADAOF)** **(Grupo Latino Americano de Angeografia Ocular y Facoemulsificacion)**
Ayacucho 307, 1B
1025 Buenos Aires, Argentina
**Phone:** 54 11 48011486      **Fax:** 54 11 49536801

★ 18150 ★ **Malaysian Society of Radiographers (MSR)** **(Persatuan Juru X-Ray Malaysia — PJXM)**
General Hospital
Department of Radiology
50586 Jalan Pahang
Kuala Lumpur, Malaysia
**Phone:** 60 3 2906674      **Fax:** 60 3 2989845
**Email:** packya@mailcity.com
**Website:** http://www.angelfire.com/ms2/msr/
**Fnded:** 1968. **Mem:** 400. **Lang(s):** English, Malay. **Desc:** Radiographers working in diagnostic and radiotherapeutic specialties. Represents the interests of radiographers and allied practitioners through professional and social activities. Works to foster interest in radiography and radiotherapeutic technique and to improve the standards of practice. Operates a research program in radiation protection. Sponsors weekend lectures, technical sessions, seminars, symposia, workshops, and conferences. **Pub:** *Journal Majuray*, annual. Journal. Features writing pertaining to radiology. • *Newsletter*, quarterly. Newsletter.

★ 18151 ★ **Nuclear Medicine Technology Certification Board (NMTCB)**
2970 Clairmont Rd., Ste. 935
Atlanta, GA 30329

**Phone:** (404)315-1739    **Fax:** (404)315-6502
**Email:** board@nmtcb.org
**Website:** http://www.nmtcb.org
Bhaskar R. Dawadi, PhD, Exec. Dir.

**Fnded:** 1977. **Mem:** 19,500. **Desc:** Purposes are to provide for the certification of nuclear medical technologists and to develop, assess, and administer an examination relevant to nuclear medicine technology. Compiles statistics. **Pub:** *NMTCB Examination Report*, annual. *Price:* Free. • *NMTCB News*, semiannual. *Price:* Free to members. • Brochures.

**Radiation Therapy Oncology Group (RTOG)**
*See:* Entry 10244

★ **18152** ★ **Radiological Society of North America (RSNA)**
820 Jorie Blvd.
Oak Brook, IL 60523-2251
**Phone:** (630)571-2670    **Fax:** (630)571-7837
**Email:** informat@rsna.org
**Website:** http://www.rsna.org
David Fellers, CAE, Exec. Dir.

**Fnded:** 1915. **Mem:** 35,000. **Desc:** Radiologists and scientists in fields closely related to radiology. Promotes study and practical application of radiology, radium, electricity, and other branches of physics related to medical science. **Pub:** *Radiographics*, bimonthly. Features pictorial presentations of selected scientific exhibits from the society's annual meeting. Includes case studies. • *Radiology*, monthly. Journal. Covers diagnostic radiology, neuroradiology, nuclear medicine, pediatric radiology, therapeutic radiology, cardiovascular radiology, and ultrasound. • *RSNA Educational Materials*, annual. Catalog. Lists video/slide set series for CME credits. • Membership Directory, annual. **Frmly:** (1918) Western Roentgen Society.

**Radiology Business Management Association (RBMA)**
*See:* Entry 9762

★ **18153** ★ **Royal Australasian College of Radiologists**
51 Druitt St.
Sydney, NSW 2000, Australia
**Phone:** 61 2 92643555    **Fax:** 61 2 92647799
**Email:** info@rbma.org
**Website:** http://www.rbma.org
**Fnded:** 1935.

★ **18154** ★ **Royal College of Radiologists (RCR)**
38 Portland Pl.
London W1N 4JQ, United Kingdom
**Phone:** 44 171 6364432    **Fax:** 44 171 3233100
**Email:** enquiries@rcr.ac.uk
**Website:** http://www.rcr.ac.uk/

**Fnded:** 1939. **Mem:** 5,679. **Lang(s):** English. **Desc:** Diagnostic and interventional radiologists, nuclear medicine specialists, oncologists, radiotherapists, and ultrasound specialists. Works to advance the science and practice of radiological technology. Offers courses to further the education of practitioners. Establishes qualifications and examinations for fellowships and diplomas. **Pub:** *Clinical Oncology*, bimonthly. Journal. • *Clinical Radiology*, monthly. Journal. • *Members' Handbook*, biennial. Handbook. • *Newsletter*, quarterly. Newsletter. **Frmly:** (1975) Faculty of Radiologists.

★ **18155** ★ **Society of Cardiovascular and Interventional Radiology (SCVIR)**
10201 Lee Hwy., Ste. 500
Fairfax, VA 22030
**Phone:** (703)691-1805    **Free:** 800-488-7284
**Fax:** (703)691-1855
**Email:** info@scvir.org

**Website:** http://www.scvir.org
Paul Pomerantz, Exec. Dir.

**Fnded:** 1973. **Mem:** 2,190. **Desc:** Physicians who are leaders in the field of cardiovascular and interventional radiology. Facilitates exchange of new ideas and techniques and provides educational courses for all physicians working in the field. Conducts annual postgraduate course. Conducts Interventional Radiology Political Action. **Pub:** *Directory of Angiography and Interventional Radiology Fellowship Programs*. Directory. • *Journal of Vascular and Interventional Radiology*, bimonthly. Journal. • *SCVIR Membership Directory*, annual. Membership Directory. • *SCVIR Newsletter*, bimonthly. Newsletter. **Frmly:** (1983) Society of Cardiovascular Radiology.

★ **18156** ★ **Society of Chairman of Academic Radiology Departments (SCARD)**
c/o Josette Szalko
820 Jorie Blvd.
Oak Brook, IL 60523
**Phone:** (630)368-3731    **Fax:** (630)571-7837
**Email:** scard@rsna.org
**Website:** http://www.aur.org/scard/
Josette Szalko, Acct. Exec.

**Desc:** Radiology department chairpersons. Dedicated to the advancement of the art and science of radiology; promotes medical education, research and patient care, the development of methods of teaching in radiology; provides a forum for problem solving and mutual interests.

★ **18157** ★ **Society of Computed Body Tomography and Magnetic Resonance (SCBT/MR)**
c/o Matrix Meetings
PO Box 1026
Rochester, MN 55903-1026
**Phone:** (507)288-5620    **Fax:** (507)288-0014
**Email:** matrix@sparc.isl.net
**Website:** http://www.scbtmr.org
Barbara McLeod, Exec. Dir.

**Fnded:** 1977. **Mem:** 100. **Desc:** Radiologists. Provides continuing medical educational courses on computed tomography and magnetic resonance imaging of the body. Course syllabus. **Frmly:** (1991) Society of Computed Body Tomography.

★ **18158** ★ **Society of Nuclear Medicine (SNM)**
1850 Samuel Morse Dr.
Reston, VA 20190-5316
**Phone:** (703)708-9000    **Fax:** (703)708-9015
**Email:** bhaines@snm.org
**Website:** http://www.snm.org
Becky Haines, Dir.

**Fnded:** 1954. **Mem:** 14,000. **Reg. Groups:** 15. **Desc:** Professional society of physicians, physicists, chemists, radiopharmacists, nuclear medicine technologists, and others interested in nuclear medicine, nuclear magnetic resonance, and the use of radioactive isotopes in clinical practice, research, and teaching. Disseminates information concerning the utilization of nuclear phenomena in the diagnosis and treatment of disease. Oversees the Technologist Section of the Society of Nuclear Medicine. **Pub:** *The Journal of Nuclear Medicine*, monthly. Journal. Includes advertisers' index, case reports, technical notes, book reviews, calendar of events and information on new products. *Price:* Included in membership dues; $120/year for nonmembers; $130/year for nonmembers in Canada and Mexico; $160/year for nonmembers outside North America. • *Journal of Nuclear Medicine Technology*, quarterly. Journal. Includes teaching editorials, commentaries, continuing education, and technologist news. Contains advertisers' index and calendar of events. *Price:* Included in membership dues; $70/year for nonmembers; $75/year for nonmembers in Canada and Mexico; $80/year for nonmembers outside North America. • *Society of Nuclear Medicine Membership Directory*, semiannual. Directory. Arranged geographically and alphabetically.

*Price:* Included in membership dues; $100/issue for nonmembers. • Also publishes other books and patient pamphlets; produces audiovisual materials.

★ **18159** ★ **Society for Pediatric Radiology (SPR)**
4550 Post Oak Pl., Ste. 342
Houston, TX 77027
**Phone:** (713)965-0566    **Fax:** (713)960-0488
**Email:** spr@meetingmanagers.com
**Website:** http://www.pedrad.org
Jennifer Boylan, Exec. Dir.

**Fnded:** 1958. **Mem:** 800. **Desc:** Physicians working in the field of pediatric radiology. Seeks to advance knowledge in pediatric imaging and improve medical care of infants and children. **Pub:** Membership Directory, annual.

**Society for Radiation Oncology Administrators (SROA)**
*See:* Entry 9764

★ **18160** ★ **Society of Radiographers of South Africa (SORSA) (Vereniging van Radiograwe van Suid-Afrika — VRSA)**
PO Box 6014
Cape Town 8012, Republic of South Africa
**Phone:** 27 21 4194857    **Fax:** 27 21 212566
**Email:** smltsa@iafrica.com
**Website:** http://www.sroa.org/

**Fnded:** 1951. **Mem:** 1,500. **Lang(s):** English. **Desc:** Radiographers in South Africa. Strives for the establishment and maintenance of professional standards in the training and practice of radiography. Cooperates with governmental bodies in order to improve working conditions, salaries, and benefits. Represents members' interests nationally and internationally. Communicates with relevant authorities on educational and employment matters. Maintains liaisons with similar national and international organizations. Sponsors seminars and workshops. **Pub:** *The South African Radiographer*, 3/year. Journal. • Newsletter, quarterly.

★ **18161** ★ **Society of Thoracic Radiology (STR)**
820 Jorie Blvd.
Oak Brook, IL 60523-2251
**Phone:** (630)368-3779    **Fax:** (630)571-7837
**Email:** str@thoracicrad.org
**Website:** http://www.thoracicrad.org
Dr. Gordon Gomsu, Pres.

**Fnded:** 1983. **Mem:** 200. **Desc:** Radiologists. Provides for continuing medical education.

★ **18162** ★ **Technologist Section of the Society of Nuclear Medicine (TSSNM)**
1850 Samuel Morse Dr.
Reston, VA 20190
**Phone:** (703)708-9000    **Fax:** (703)708-9015
**Email:** salexand@snm.org
**Website:** http://www.snm.org/about/new_tech_1.html
Mickey T. Clarke, Pres.

**Fnded:** 1970. **Mem:** 7,000. **Reg. Groups:** 15. **Desc:** Members of the Society of Nuclear Medicine who have received formal training in nuclear medicine technology. Purposes are to: promote the continued development and improvement of nuclear medicine technology; enhance the development of nuclear medicine technologists; stimulate continuing education; develop a forum for the exchange of ideas and information. Serves as the central source of information for those interested and involved in the field of nuclear medicine technology. Represents the field in areas of licensure, accreditation, and certification. Sponsors training sessions. Conducts surveys; compiles statistics. **Pub:** *Journal of Nuclear Medicine Technology*, quarterly. Journal. *Price:* Included in membership dues. • Books. • Membership Directory, biennial. • Videos.

# Research Centers

## ★ 18163 ★ Alberta Cancer Board
**Edmonton Radiopharmaceutical Centre**
11560 University Ave.
Edmonton, AB, Canada T6G 1Z2
**Phone:** (780)432-8970 **Fax:** (780)432-8411
J.R. Scott, Dir.

**Activities/Fields:** Radiopharmaceutical development, including brain blood flow tracers and tumor markers.

## ★ 18164 ★ Baylor College of Medicine
**Herbert J. Frensley Center for Imaging Research**
1 Baylor Plz.
Department of Radiology
Houston, TX 77030
**Phone:** (713)798-5146 **Fax:** (713)798-5745
**Email:** lhayman@bcm.tmc.edu
**Website:** http://www.bcm.tmc.edu/imaging/
Dr. L. Anne Hayman, Dir.

**Activities/Fields:** Magnetic resonance imaging and spectroscopy of brain and muscle in normal and altered states (human experimental animal models, excised samples), the development of novel diagnostic imaging applications, and functional magnetic resonance imaging of normal cognitive function following brain injury in psychiatric conditions.

**Center for Radiation Therapy**
*See:* Entry 10303

## ★ 18165 ★ Columbia University
**Center for Radiological Research**
630 W 168th St.
New York, NY 10032
**Phone:** (212)305-5660 **Fax:** (212)305-3229
**Email:** ejh1@columbia.edu
Dr. Eric J. Hall, Dir.

**Activities/Fields:** Human and rodent cell transformation assay systems at the cellular and molecular levels.

## ★ 18166 ★ Lawrence Berkeley National Laboratory
**Center for Functional Imaging**
Mail Stop 55-121
1 Cyclotron Rd.
Berkeley, CA 94720
**Phone:** (510)486-4062 **Fax:** (510)486-4768
**Email:** tfbudinger@lbl.gov
**Website:** http://cfi.lbl.gov
Dr. Thomas F. Budinger, Hd.

**Activities/Fields:** Researches medicine and radiation biophysics, emphasizing imaging instrumentation and radiopharmaceuticals development, and the diagnosis of human diseases. Develops imaging instrumentation and computer programs for the study of brain and heart disease in conjunction with new pharmaceuticals. **Pub:** *Annual Report.* • *Progress Reports.*

## ★ 18167 ★ Long Island Jewish Medical Center
**Nuclear Medicine Division**
270-05 76th Ave.
New Hyde Park, NY 11040
**Phone:** (718)470-7080 **Fax:** (718)470-9247
**Email:** palestro@lij.edu
Christopher Palestro, MD, Dir.

**Activities/Fields:** Applications of radioisotopes to clinical medicine. The Division is especially concerned with research on new applications, including instrumentation, and in use of isotopes in study of metabolic processes and infection.

**Massachusetts Institute of Technology Biotechnology Resource Center for Research in Lasers and Medicine**
*See:* Entry 4532

## ★ 18168 ★ Massachusetts Institute of Technology
**Center for Magnetic Resonance**
**Francis Bitter Magnet Laboratory**
170 Albany St., NW14-3218
Cambridge, MA 02139
**Phone:** (617)253-5478 **Fax:** (617)253-5405
**Email:** cahavers@mit.edu
Cindy Haverstock, Admin. Off.

**Activities/Fields:** Biological molecules (liquid- or solid-state), viral particles, cells, intact tissues, etc. Research includes natural and model membrane structure, dynamics, function, phase diagrams, phase transitions, and solid-state studies of amino acids, peptides, and bone; protein conformation and interactions, e.g., insulin, NMR microscopy; dynamics of energy metabolism in tumors, skeletal muscle, cells, animal brain and heart, and human eye lens; and DNA structure and dynamics.

## ★ 18169 ★ Massachusetts Institute of Technology
**Laser Biomedical Research Center**
77 Massachusetts Ave.
Cambridge, MA 02139
**Phone:** (617)253-7700 **Fax:** (617)253-4513
**Email:** msfeld@mit.edu
**Website:** http://web.mit.edu/spectroscopy/www/Facilieslbrc.html
Dr. Michael S. Feld, Dir.

**Activities/Fields:** Lasers, medicine, and diagnosis of disease. Development of new methods for real-time spectroscopic identification of tissue types and conditions from the studies of fluorescence, scattering and reflection. Raman spectroscopy studies yield biochemical composition of the tissue. Interferometry and phase dispersion microscopy can detect sub-wavelength changes. Conducts time-resolved picosecond studies in tissue and other biological systems. Pursues collaborative research with researchers from outside institutions and provides facilities to outside scientists and physicians nationwide. **Pub:** *Annual report.* • *The Spectrograph Newsletter.*

**Mayo Biomedical Imaging Resource**
*See:* Entry 4534

## ★ 18170 ★ Medical College of Wisconsin
**Biophysics Research Institute**
8701 Watertown Plank Rd.
Milwaukee, WI 53226-0509
**Phone:** (414)456-4000 **Fax:** (414)456-6512
**Email:** cfelix@mcw.edu
**Website:** http://www.biophysics.mcw.edu/
Dr. Balaraman Kalyanaraman, Dir.

**Activities/Fields:** Biophysics, with emphasis on functional magnetic resonance imaging and electron spin resonance.

## ★ 18171 ★ Radiation Oncology Research and Development Center
3990 John R
Detroit, MI 48201
**Phone:** (313)966-9745 **Fax:** (313)966-9747
**Email:** foremanu@karmanos.org
**Website:** http://www.roc.wayne.edu
Dr. Jeffery Forman, Dir.

**Activities/Fields:** Radiation therapy, cancer research, medical information systems, three-dimensional imaging, neutron therapy, radiosurgery, brachytherapy, clinical protocols, and unsealed source therapy.

## ★ 18172 ★ Sherbrooke University
**Group of the Canadian Institutes of Health in the Radiation Sciences**
Faculty of Med.
3001 12th Ave North
Sherbrooke, QC, Canada J1H 5N4
**Phone:** (819)346-1110 **Fax:** (819)564-5442
**Email:** lsanche@courrier.usherb.ca
**Website:** http://www.mednuc.usherb.ca
Dr. Leon Sanche, Dir.

**Activities/Fields:** Identification of the complex sequences of events initiated by the absorption of energy from ionizing radiation in biological material (which ultimately result in transformations at the cellular level), and the development of new types of drugs to enhance the therapeutic and diagnostic efficiency of radiation for the purpose of improving the treatment of human cancer with radio- and phototherapy. **Pub:** *Cahiers de radiobiologie: Aspects physiques, chimiques et biologiques*, 3/year. **Frmly:** MRC Group in the Radiation Sciences.

## ★ 18173 ★ U.S. Department of Energy
**Department of Energy Program Offices— Environment, Safety and Health**
**Office of Biological and Environmental Research**
**((Medical Sciences Division)**
**Radiopharmaceutical Development Research Program)**
19901 Germantown Rd., SC-73
Germantown, MD 20874-1290
**Phone:** (301)903-4071
**Email:** prem.srivastava@science.doe.gov
**Website:** http://www.sc.doe.gov/production/ober/msd_rad_pharm.html
Prem C. Srivastava, Prog. Mgr.

**Activities/Fields:** Radiochemistry and radiolabeling synthesis for attaching radioisotopes to organic structures, including positron emission tomography (PET) research.

## ★ 18174 ★ U.S. Department of Energy
**Department of Energy Program Offices— Environment, Safety and Health**
**Office of Biological and Environmental Research**
**((Medical Sciences Division)**
**Molecular Nuclear Medicine)**
19901 Germantown Rd., SC-73
Germantown, MD 20874-1290
**Phone:** (301)903-4071
**Email:** prem.srivastava@science.doe.gov
**Website:** http://www.sc.doe.gov/production/ober/msd_mol_med.html
Prem C. Srivastava, PhD, Prog. Mgr.

**Activities/Fields:** Biochemical dysfunctions and the mechanisms of dysfunctions associated with pathological states including development of new radiotracer/radiopharmaceutical tools and advanced medical imaging technologies for identification and detection of biomedical dysfunctions as early signs of disease (including cancer, brain diseases, and mental disorders), for molecular correction of biochemical defect and the treatment of disease and disorder.

**U.S. Department of Health and Human Services**
**Food and Drug Administration**
**Center for Devices and Radiological Health**
*See:* Entry 18001

**★ 18175 ★ U.S. Department of Health and Human Services**
**Food and Drug Administration**
**Center for Devices and Radiological Health**
**Biometric Sciences Division**
**(Office of Surveillance and Biometrics)**
Mail Code HFZ-540
5600 Fishers Ln.
Rockville, MD 20857
**Phone:** (301)443-7120          **Fax:** (301)443-0097
**Website:** http://www.fda.gov/cdhr

**Activities/Fields:** Statistical and epidemiologic review; medical devices evaluation, including risk assessment of post marketing long- and intermediate-term epidemiological effects; and review of pre-market approvals and post-market surveillance studies. Activities primarily involve epidemiological and experimental data collection, analysis, and interpretation; statistical methodology development; and statistical modeling of risk/benefit. Division comprises epidemiology, statistics, and post-market surveillance studies branches. **Pub:** *Proceedings.* • *Research Reports.*

**★ 18176 ★ U.S. Department of Health and Human Services**
**Food and Drug Administration**
**Center for Devices and Radiological Health**
**Office of Device Evaluation**
9200 Corporate Blvd.
Rockville, MD 20850
**Phone:** (301)594-2022          **Fax:** (301)594-2510
**Website:** http://www.fda.gov/cdrh
Bernanrd E. Statland, Dir.

**Activities/Fields:** Responsible for the evaluation of clinical and non-clinical data to establish the safety and effectiveness of medical devices and their marketability in the U.S.; and regulatory control of clinical trials involving medical devices. Principal areas of interest are health and physical sciences. **Pub:** *Research reports.*

**★ 18177 ★ U.S. Department of Health and Human Services**
**Food and Drug Administration**
**Center for Devices and Radiological Health**
**Office of Science and Technology**
9200 Corporate Blvd.
HFZ-100
Rockville, MD 20850
**Phone:** (301)827-4777          **Fax:** (301)827-4787
**Email:** dem@cdrh.fda.gov
Donald Marlowe, Dir.

**Activities/Fields:** Pysical, life, and engineering sciences. Specific activities involve: conducting research on the human health effects of radiation and medical devices and on existing and emerging health technologies; providing the Center and other units with laboratory support; and managing the research, development, and product testing engineering programs of the Center. Office comprises divisions for electronics and computer science, life sciences, mechanics and materials science, and physical sciences.

**★ 18178 ★ U.S. Department of Health and Human Services**
**Food and Drug Administration**
**Center for Devices and Radiological Health**
**Office of Surveillance and Biometrics**
**(Division of Biostatistics)**
Mail Code HFZ-542
1350 Piccard Dr.
Rockville, MD 20857
**Phone:** (301)594-0616          **Fax:** (301)443-8559
**Email:** gxc@cdrh.fda.gov
Gregory Campbell, PhD, Dir.

**Activities/Fields:** Statistical aspects of clinical trials submitted to the Center for Devices and Radiological Health (CDRH) as medical device applications. The division also performs statistical research and risk/benefit analyses on the safety, effectiveness, and use of medical devices and the risks of radiation. **Frmly:** Ionizing Radiation and Statistics Branch; Biometric Sciences Division, Statistics Branch.

**U.S. Department of Health and Human Services**
**National Cancer Institute**
**Division of Cancer Treatment, Diagnosis, and Centers**
**Clinical Oncology Program**
**(Radiation Oncology Branch)**
*See:* Entry 10455

**U.S. Department of Health and Human Services**
**National Cancer Institute (NCI)**
**Division of Cancer Treatment, Diagnosis, and Centers**
**Diagnostic Imaging Program**
*See:* Entry 10460

**U.S. Department of Health and Human Services**
**National Cancer Institute**
**Division of Cancer Treatment, Diagnosis, and Centers**
**Radiation Research Program**
**(Radiotherapy Development Branch)**
*See:* Entry 10461

**U.S. Department of Health and Human Services**
**National Cancer Institute**
**Division of Cancer Treatment, Diagnosis, and Centers**
**Radiation Research Program**
*See:* Entry 10462

**★ 18179 ★ University of California, Irvine**
**Beckman Laser Institute and Medical Clinic**
1002 Health Sciences Rd. E
Irvine, CA 92612
**Phone:** (949)824-4713          **Fax:** (949)824-8413
**Email:** mberns@bli.uci.edu
**Website:** http://www.bli.uci.edu
Dr. Michael W. Berns, Dir.

**Activities/Fields:** Basic research includes genetics, cell biology, spectroscopy, and biophysics. Conducts basic laser studies of cellular functions, including genetic expression, cell motility, and cell membrane behavior; and biophysical studies of thermal, fluorescence, acoustic/mechanical, photochemical, and ionization effects of radiation on biological material. Conducts applied research in cancer detection and treatment; reshaping of cornea with excimer laser, diagnosis (imaging) and treatment of portwine stain birthmarks; application of lasers to women's health problems; and development of medical laser devices. **Pub:** *Beckman Laser Institute News,* quarterly. Newsletter.

**★ 18180 ★ University of California, Irvine**
**Brain Imaging Center**
109 Irvine Hall
College of Medicine
Irvine, CA 92697-3960
**Phone:** (949)824-7872          **Fax:** (949)824-2230
**Email:** jcwu@uci.edu
Joseph C. Wu, MD, Clin. Dir.

**Activities/Fields:** PET scan analysis of brain functions focusing on mental illness, brain tumors, Al-

zheimer's disease, near drowning, traumatic brain injury, and aberrant behavior.

**★ 18181 ★ University of California, Irvine**
**Laser Microbeam and Medical Program (LAMMP)**
Beckman Laser Institute Medical Clinic
1002 Health Sciences Rd. E
Irvine, CA 92612
**Phone:** (949)824-8367          **Fax:** (949)824-6969
**Email:** tromberg@bli.uci.edu
**Website:** http://www.bli.uci.edu/lammp/index.html
Dr. Bruce J. Tromberg, Dir.

**Activities/Fields:** Combines sophisticated methods of microscopy, computational methods, and laser spectroscopy to investigate cellular, genetic, and developmental problems that are related to cancer, heart disease, neurobiology, and other health problems. Focuses on basic and translational research, particularly in the areas of laser-tissue interactions, tissue optics, photodynamic therapy, and functional imaging.

**★ 18182 ★ University of California, Los Angeles**
**Leo G. Rigler Center for Radiological Research**
Center for Health Science, Rm. BV-135
Department of Radiology
UCLA Medical Center
Los Angeles, CA 90024
**Phone:** (310)825-6561
**Email:** radiology/riglercenter@medmail3.mednet.ucla.edu
John Robert, Res. Assoc.

**Activities/Fields:** Radiological science and its application to diagnosis and treatment of catastrophic diseases, involving such techniques as magnetic resonance imaging (MRI), internal radiation management of carcinomatous lesions, vascular occlusion with ferrosilicone in tumor management, and cobalt source gamma irradiation of brain tumors.

**University of California, Los Angeles**
**UCLA-DOE Laboratory of Structural Biology and Molecular Medicine**
*See:* Entry 4743

**★ 18183 ★ University of California, San Francisco**
**Radiation Oncology Research Laboratory**
1855 Folsom, Rm. MCB 200
San Francisco, CA 94103
**Phone:** (415)476-2461          **Fax:** (415)476-9069
**Email:** dewey@rorl.ucsf.edu
**Website:** http://www.ucsf.edu/cvtl/index.html
Dr. Wm. Dewey, Prof.

**Activities/Fields:** Effects of ionizing radiation and hyperthermia in killing mammalian cells and interfering with cell cycle progression, with emphasis on applying basic concepts to radiation oncology.

**★ 18184 ★ University of Florida**
**Radiation Oncology Clinic**
Shands Cancer Center
PO Box 100385
Gainesville, FL 32610-0385
**Phone:** (352)265-0287          **Fax:** (352)265-0546
**Email:** mendenan@shands.ufl.edu
Dr. Nancy Mendenhall, Dept. Ch.

**Activities/Fields:** Cancer and radiation therapy and treatment.

**★ 18185 ★ University of Iowa**
**Free Radical and Radiation Biology Program**
Medical Laboratories, Rm. B180
Iowa City, IA 52242
**Phone:** (319)335-8019          **Fax:** (319)335-8039
**Email:** larry-oberley@uiowa.edu

**Website:** http://www.radiology.uiowa.edu/FRRB
Larry W. Oberley, PhD, Dir.

**Activities/Fields:** Radiation biology, free radical biology, antioxidant enzymes, gene expression, and gene therapy. **Frmly:** Radiation Research Laboratory.


**★ 18186 ★ University of Kentucky**
**Radiation Therapy Oncology Center**
UK Medical Center
800 Rose St.
Lexington, KY 40536
**Phone:** (859)323-6486          **Fax:** (859)257-4931
**Email:** mohmohi@pop.uky.edu
Mohammed Mohiuddin, MD, Dir.

**Activities/Fields:** Radiation oncology research, participates in national cooperative group studies, RTOG, SWOG, NSABP, and GOG. Studies brain, bowel, head and neck cancer, and chemotherapy. Conducts research on radiation therapy, cancer treatment using radiation, hyperthermia, and chemotherapy.


**★ 18187 ★ University of Maryland,**
**Baltimore County**
**Remote Sensing Signal and Image**
**Processing Laboratory (RSSIPL)**
ECS Bldg., Rm. 335
1000 Hilltop Cir.
Baltimore, MD 21250
**Phone:** (410)455-6583          **Fax:** (410)455-3969
**Email:** cchang@umbc.edu
**Website:** http://www.umbc.edu/rssipl/homepage.html
Dr. Chein-I Chang, Dir.

**Activities/Fields:** Remote sensing image processing, which includes target detection and classification; identification and quantification analysis; medical imaging, which includes breast cancer detection; MRI classification; enhancement and restoration of text and video images including low resolution expansion; text detection and tracking in video frames and automatic pattern recognition, which includes handwritten character recognition and shape analysis. **Pub:** *Journal articles.* • *Conference papers.*


**★ 18188 ★ University of Michigan**
**Division of Nuclear Medicine**
University Hospital
1500 E Medical Center Dr., B1G412
Ann Arbor, MI 48109-0028
**Phone:** (734)936-5388          **Fax:** (734)936-8182
**Email:** dkuhl@umich.edu
Dr. David E. Kuhl, Contact

**Activities/Fields:** Diagnosis and treatment of disease using radionuclides and radionuclide-labeled compounds. Develops methods of nuclear medicine procedures.


**★ 18189 ★ University of Missouri—**
**Columbia**
**Radiation Oncology Program**
Ellis Fischel Cancer Center
115 Business Loop 70 W
Columbia, MO 65203
**Phone:** (573)882-8644          **Fax:** (573)882-8817
**Email:** westgates@health.missouri.edu
Steven Westgate, Contact

**Activities/Fields:** Clinical protocols; national multi-institutional studies for cancer problems.


**★ 18190 ★ University of New Mexico**
**Clinical and Magnetic Resonance**
**Research Center**
1201 Yale Blvd. NE
Albuquerque, NM 87131-5021
**Phone:** (505)272-0760          **Fax:** (505)272-4056
**Email:** cford@salud.unm.edu
**Website:** http://cmrrc.unm.edu
Dr. Corey C. Ford, Contact

**Activities/Fields:** Magnetic resonance imaging and spectroscopy, neurology, multiple sclerosis, stroke, traumatic brain surgery, lupus, and schizophrenia. **Frmly:** Center for Non-Invasive Diagnosis.


**★ 18191 ★ University of Pennsylvania**
**Metabolic Magnetic Resonance Research**
**and Computing Center**
Stellar-Chance Laboratories, B1
Department of Radiology
Philadelphia, PA 19104-6100
**Phone:** (215)898-2044          **Fax:** (215)573-2113
**Email:** jack@mail.mmrrcc.upenn.edu
**Website:** http://www.mmrrcc.upenn.edu
John S. Leigh, PhD, Dir.

**Activities/Fields:** Performs in vivo monitoring of specific metabolites in localized regions of tissues and organs in humans utilizing multinuclear magnetic resonance spectroscopy and metabolic imaging; develops targeted magnetite-based contrast agents for gene therapy and diagnosis; and develops techniques for near infrared optical imaging and spectroscopy in humans. **Pub:** *Newsletter.*


**★ 18192 ★ University of Rochester**
**Rochester Center for Biomedical**
**Ultrasound**
203 Hopeman Engineering Bldg.
PO Box 270127
Rochester, NY 14627-0127
**Phone:** (716)275-9542          **Fax:** (716)273-4919
**Email:** rcbu@ece.rochester.edu
**Website:** http://henry.ee.rochester.edu:8080/users/rcbu/
Prof. Kevin J. Parker, Dir.

**Activities/Fields:** Ultrasonic diagnosis, including imaging and Doppler ultrasound; ultrasonic treatment, including diathermy and the treatment of glaucoma and kidney and gall stones ultrasonic biophysics, including acoustic cavitation, generation and detection of ultrasound, tissue characterization, attenuation and scattering, shock fields, and nonlinear sound propagation; and biological effects of ultrasound. Also conducts research to establish safety limits for the use of ultrasound and to discover new applications, including new contrast agents. **Pub:** *Annual report.*


**★ 18193 ★ University of Texas**
**Southwestern Medical Center at Dallas**
**Mary Nell and Ralph B. Rogers Magnetic**
**Resonance Center**
5801 Forest Park Rd.
Dallas, TX 75235-9085
**Phone:** (214)648-5886          **Fax:** (214)648-5881
**Email:** cmallo@mednet.swmed.edu
**Website:** http://www2.swmed.edu/rogersmr/
Dr. Craig R. Malloy, Dir.

**Activities/Fields:** Nuclear magnetic resonance (NMR) spectroscopy and imaging for the analysis of metabolism in various small animal and tissue culture models, including high energy phosphate metabolism, intracellular cations, intermediary metabolism, and perfusion. **Frmly:** Biomedical Magnetic Resonance Center.


**★ 18194 ★ University of Texas**
**Southwestern Medical Center at Dallas**
**Southwestern Magnetic Resonance**
**Facility**
**Mary Nell and Ralph B. Rogers Magnetic**
**Resonance Center**
MC-9085
5801 Forest Park Dr.
Dallas, TX 75235-9085
**Phone:** (214)648-5886          **Fax:** (214)648-5881
**Email:** jthach@mednet.swmed.edu
**Website:** http://www2.utsouthwestern.edu/rogersmr/
Dr. Craig R. Malloy, Dir.

**Activities/Fields:** Magnetic resonance imaging and spectroscopy of analytical samples, perfused organs, and small animals.


**★ 18195 ★ University of Utah**
**Dixon Laser Institute**
155 South 1452 East, No. 220
Salt Lake City, UT 84112-8906
**Phone:** (801)581-8201          **Fax:** (801)585-3098
R. Kim Davis, MD, Dir.

**Activities/Fields:** Laser research, including applications of lasers in medicine, industry, and the military. Biomedical studies focus on gastroenterology, cardiology, otolaryngology, obstetrics-gynecology, urology, genetics, microsurgery, dentistry, and photodynamic therapy. In association with the Vanderbildt University Free Electron Laser Lab, the Institute is investigating the development and application of free electron laser technology in medicine and materials science.


**★ 18196 ★ University of Washington**
**Diagnostic Imaging Sciences Center**
HSB AA048
Box 357115
1959 Pacific Ave.
Seattle, WA 98195
**Phone:** (206)685-3530          **Fax:** (206)543-6317
**Email:** aamoss@u.washington.edu
Albert A. Moss, MD, Dir.

**Activities/Fields:** Diagnostic imaging, including PET, NMR spectroscopy and imaging, nucle ar medicine imaging and therapy, x-ray physics, ultrasound imaging, physiology, including angio-intervention techniques, image processing, and contrast media testing.


**★ 18197 ★ University of Wisconsin—**
**Madison**
**National Magnetic Resonance Facility**
Biochemistry Addition Bldg., Room 171
Department of Biochemistry
433 Babcock Dr.
Madison, WI 53706-1544
**Phone:** (608)262-3173          **Fax:** (608)262-3759
**Email:** markley@nmrfam.wisc.edu
**Website:** http://www.nmrfam.wisc.edu
John L. Markley, Hd.

**Activities/Fields:** Structural and conformational analysis of proteins, nucleic acids, carbohydrates, lipids, and other biomolecules; structure-function studies of macromolecular assemblies; noninvasive analysis of the biochemistry or intact cells, tissue, or organs; in vivo investigations of the biochemistry of rats or other small animals; nuclear magnetic resonance (NMR) imaging of small objects. Current core and collaborative projects include: strategies for assigning NMR spectra of proteins; determination of three dimensional (3-D) structures of small proteins and nucleic acids from NMR data; preparation of stable-isotope labeled amino acids and proteins; uses of stable isotopes in multi-dimensional (NMR) studies of proteins; applications of NMR to protein engineering; elucidation of enzyme mechanisms and protein-ligand interactions; application of 2-D and 3-D NMR methodology to the study of cellular biochemistry; computer-aided design of NMR experiments; post-acquisition processing of NMR data; and semi-automated analysis of NMR data from proteins.


**★ 18198 ★ Washington University in St.**
**Louis**
**Mallinckrodt Institute of Radiology**
510 S Kingshighway Blvd.
Saint Louis, MO 63110
**Phone:** (314)362-8436          **Fax:** (314)362-8399
**Email:** welchm@mir.wustl.edu
**Website:** http://www.mir.wustl.edu
Dr. Michael Welch, Contact

**Activities/Fields:** Radiological diagnostic, treatment, research, and training center including nuclear medicine, radiation oncology, radiation sciences, and diagnostic radiology. The diagnostic radiology division is comprised of seven sections: abdominal, cardiac, chest, computer, musculoskeletal, pediatric, and neuroradiology. Maintains laboratories for research in digital image processing, computer sciences, nuclear medicine, radiation oncology, cancer biology, diagnostic radiology, and magnetic resonance imaging. **Pub:** *Focal Spot*, 3/year.

**★ 18199 ★ Washington University in St. Louis**
**Mallinckrodt Institute of Radiology**
**Hyperthermia Service**
Radiation Oncology Center
4939 Children's Pl., Ste. 5500
Saint Louis, MO 63110
**Phone:** (314)362-8503    **Fax:** (314)362-8521
**Email:** myerson@radonc.wustl.edu
Robert J. Myerson, MD, Ch.
**Activities/Fields:** Hyperthermia treatment of cancer, simultaneous thermoradiotherapy, and bioassay of predictors of hyperthermic response.

**★ 18200 ★ Wayne State University**
**MR Center**
Harper Hospital
3990 John R
Detroit, MI 48201
**Phone:** (313)745-1395    **Fax:** (313)993-0233
**Email:** evelhoch@mednet.wayne.edu
Dr. Jeffrey L. Evelhoch, Dir.
**Activities/Fields:** Evaluates the potential for NMR (nuclear magnetic resonance) spectroscopy and imaging to provide predictors of response to chemotherapeutic drugs.

## Foundations & Other Funding Organizations

### Private Foundations

**A. V. Hunter Trust, Inc.**
*See:* Entry 18

★ **18201** ★ **Albert A. List Foundation**
180 W 80th St., Ste. 213
New York, NY 10024-6310
**Fax:** (212)799-1160
**Website:** http://www.avhuntertrust.org
Vikki List, President
**Fnded:** 1953. **Philosophy:** The foundation supports three general focus areas: Democracy and Citizen Participation, Freedom of Expression; and New Problems/New Solutions. The Democracy and Citizen Participation program supports campaign finance reform, voter education and participation, confrontation of anti-democratic objectives, and projects that provide or encourage alternative visions for justice and democracy. The Freedom of Expression program supports organizations that protect the right of inquiry and expression or support strategies to ensure those freedoms. The New Problems/New Solutions program is meant to support groups working for social change that seek to address new challenges. **Priorities:** *Arts & Humanities:* 21% Supports museums, art organizations, public broadcasting, and the performing arts. *Civic & Public Affairs:* 51%. Supports "Democracy and Citizen Participation," with grants funding public policy, civil rights, women's groups, legal and justice issues, minority affairs, and media watchdog groups. *Education:* 4%. Funds education initiatives. *Environment:* 6%. Primarily supports family planning. *Note:* Total contributions made in 2000. **Typ. Recipients:** Clinics/Medical Centers, Family Planning, Long-Term Care, Public Health. **Geo. Dist:** national and regional organizations.

**Andrew W. Mellon Foundation**
*See:* Entry 44

**Arthur S. DeMoss Foundation**
*See:* Entry 19633

**Blumenthal Foundation**
*See:* Entry 82

★ **18202** ★ **Buffett Foundation**
209 Kiewit Plaza
Omaha, NE 68131
**Phone:** (402)345-9168
**Email:** philipb@vnet.net
**Website:** http://www.blumenthalfoundation.org
Allen Greenberg, Executive Director
**Fnded:** 1964. **Philosophy:** The Buffet Foundation makes most of its grants to social service organizations focusing on planned parenthood and international population growth. The foundation also sponsors several scholarships and an outstanding teacher award program (restricted to Omaha public school teachers only). **Priorities:** *Civic & Public Affairs:* 15%. Supports human rights, womens affairs, and law and justice issues. *Education:* 17%. Supports scholarships and fellowships for higher education. *Environment:* 16%. Major support is awarded to family planning services. Also supports United Way and youth programs. *International:* 2%. Supports medical research and reproductive health issues. *Note:* Total contributions made in fiscal 2000. **Typ. Recipients:** Clinics/Medical Centers, Family Planning, Health-General, Hospitals, Hospitals (University Affiliated), Medical Education, Medical Research, Public Health. **Geo. Dist:** no geographic restrictions.

★ **18203** ★ **Burdine Johnson Foundation**
PO Box 1230
Buda, TX 78610-1230
**Phone:** (512)312-1336          **Fax:** (512)295-4773
Robert Giberson, Trustee
**Fnded:** 1960. **Philosophy:** The Burdine Johnson Foundation primarily supports religious, private, and secondary education. Other interests include the performing arts, family planning, and civic affairs. **Priorities:** *Arts & Humanities:* 45%. Supports foundation for performing arts and preservation associations. *Education:* 36%. Supports public and private schools, religious education, and universities. *Environment:* 8%. Supports community center, seniors, and family planning. *International:* 4%. Supports children's hospitals, cancer centers, and the American. *Note:* Total contributions made in 1998. **Typ. Recipients:** Cancer, Children's Health/Hospitals, Domestic Violence, Emergency/Ambulance Services, Family Planning, Medical Education, Medical Research, Sexual Abuse, Single-Disease Health Associations, Substance Abuse, Transplant Networks/Donor Banks. **Geo. Dist:** TX.

**California Wellness Foundation**
*See:* Entry 5547

★ **18204** ★ **Cameron Baird Foundation**
Box 564
Hamburg, NY 14075
**Phone:** (716)845-6000
**Website:** http://www.tcwf.org
Brian Baird, Trustee
**Fnded:** 1960. **Philosophy:** The Cameron Baird Foundation makes most of its grants in the areas of the arts, civic affairs, and education. Arts funding favors musical performances in Buffalo, NY. Funding for civic affairs emphasizes the environment. Educational giving focuses on minority scholarships. The foundation funds a variety of other interests, such as family planning and youth organizations. **Priorities:** *Arts & Humanities:* 57%. Primary support for orchestras, arts institutes, opera, and arts associations. *Civic & Public Affairs:* 2%. Women's affairs and housing. *Education:* 11%. Supports private secondary schools and colleges. *Environment:* 15%. Funds family planning, youth organizations, child welfare, and community services. *International:* 2%. Hospitals, children's health, hospices, and single-disease health associations. *Note:* Total contributions were made in 1997. **Typ. Recipients:** Children's Health/Hospitals, Family Planning, Hospices, Multiple Sclerosis, People with Disabilities, Public Health. **Geo. Dist:** Buffalo, NY.

**Camp Airy and Camp Louise Foundation**
*See:* Entry 104

★ **18205** ★ **Cecil B. Day Foundation**
4725 Peachtree Corners Circle, Ste. 300
Norcross, GA 30092
**Phone:** (770)446-1500          **Fax:** (770)446-2527
**Email:** airlou@airylouise.org
**Website:** http://www.airylouise.org
Edward White, Jr., President
**Fnded:** 1968. **Philosophy:** The primary purpose of the foundation is to "assist local churches in their Christian Mission of sharing the gospel of Jesus Christ New England and the Atlanta, GA regions." The foundation hopes to function as a catalyst to bring the evangelical community closer together, and to fund institutions or ministers who lack denominational means of assistance. Priority is given to groups without other means of obtaining financial support. **Priorities:** *Environment:* 15%. Youth programs and sporting events. *International:* 2%. *Note:* Contributions made in 1998. **Typ. Recipients:** AIDS/HIV, Cancer, Family Planning, Medical Education, Public Health. **Geo. Dist:** New England; Atlanta, GA, including statewide.

**Chichester duPont Foundation**
*See:* Entry 122

**Crestlea Foundation**
*See:* Entry 150

**Educational Foundation of America**
*See:* Entry 197

★ **18206** ★ **Erik E. and Edith H. Bergstrom Foundation**
PO Box 520
Palo Alto, CA 94302-0520
**Phone:** (650)323-0596          **Fax:** (650)324-4596
**Email:** ebergstrom@msn.com
Erik Bergstrom, President
**Fnded:** 1981. **Philosophy:** "All women should have access to the education and means to limit their family size to the number of children they can financially and emotionally sustain. This foundation supports family planning programs because they promote health and well being not only for women, but also for their families and for the entire world." **Priorities:** *Civic & Public Affairs:* 9%. Public Policy. *Education:* 3%. *Environment:* 24%. Planned parenthood services. *Note:* Total contributions made in fiscal 1999. **Typ. Recipients:** Family Planning, Health Organizations.

**Geo. Dist:** U.S.-based organizations operating in Latin America.

★ **18207** ★ **Gardner and Florence Call Cowles Foundation**
715 Locust St.
Des Moines, IA 50309
**Phone:** (515)284-8117          **Fax:** (515)699-7035
Charles Edwards, President & Trustee
**Fnded:** 1934. **Philosophy:** The foundation's grant-giving activities are confined to Iowa. Grants are made primarily to four-year private colleges. The foundation also supports various cultural institutions and selected social agencies, and is planning to focus more on human services. **Priorities:** *Arts & Humanities:* 9%. Supports performing arts and art centers. *Civic & Public Affairs:* 3%. Funds community development and zoos. *Education:* 60%. Supports four-year private colleges and universities. *Environment:* 23%. Supports family planning and YWCA. *Note:* Total contributions made in 1999. **Typ. Recipients:** Family Planning. **Geo. Dist:** IA.

★ **18208** ★ **General Service Foundation**
557 N Mill St., Ste. 201
Aspen, CO 81611
**Phone:** (970)920-6834          **Fax:** (970)920-4578
**Email:** info@generalservice.org
**Website:** http://www.generalservice.org
Lani Shaw, Executive Director
**Fnded:** 1946. **Philosophy:** The current interests of the foundation are international peace, reproductive health and rights, and Western Water. Under the International Peace Program the foundation seeks to address the root causes of conflict and to promote peaceful and stable communities, primarily in Mexico, Central America, and the Caribbean. The foundation considers programs and projects which address the following issues, as well as their interrelationships: political rights and civil freedoms; international law and relations; and economic, environmental, and development causes. Funding is given principally for education and policy analysis and formation, rather than for research. The foundation also may make contributions to organizations working to accomplish the following objectives: develop leadership and participation in the non-governmental organization community; further communication and collaborative efforts among non-governmental organizations; and strengthen interregional organizations, both governmental and non-governmental. The Reproductive Health and Rights Program is dedicated to improving access to comprehensive reproductive health care, including abortion, for women and adolescents; and to supporting education efforts which increase awareness and action around issues of reproductive health, sexuality, and reproductive choices. Priority is given to organizations working with underserved communities and populations whose reproductive health and rights are most impacted by poverty. The Discretionary Arts Program does not contribute through unsolicited proposals, but through a small discretionary program. The funds are distributed only at the request of the board of directors. The Education Program's mission is to fund educational projects within targeted communities as well as Native American youth education programs. Proposals in this program are considered only at the request and initiation of members of the Education Committee. **Priorities:** *International:* About 33%. Primary support for reproductive health and rights. (grants may also be categorized under civic and public affairs.) **Typ. Recipients:** Family Planning, Health-General, Public Health. **Geo. Dist:** national organizations west of the Mississippi River; the Caribbean.

**Geraldine R. Dodge Foundation**
*See:* Entry 289

★ **18209** ★ **Harriet Ford Dickenson Foundation**
c/o Morgan Guaranty Trust, Trustee
3450 Park Ave.
New York, NY 10154

**Phone:** (212)464-1937
**Email:** info@grdodge.org
**Website:** http://www.grdodge.org
James Largey, Contact
**Fnded:** 1958. **Priorities:** *Arts & Humanities:* 47%. Supports opera, museums, ballet, orchestras, libraries, public broadcasting, historic preservation, and music programs. *Civic & Public Affairs:* 11%. Funds botanical gardens, parks, civic groups, legal aid, affordable housing programs, and professional organizations. *Education:* 2%. Gives to colleges and universities. *Environment:* 15%. Supports the United Way, family planning organizations, youth groups, youth services, and camps and recreation programs. *International:* 10%. Hospitals and single-disease health associations receive support. *Note:* Total contributions made in 2000. **Typ. Recipients:** Family Planning, Hospitals, People with Disabilities. **Geo. Dist:** NY, Broome County.

**Hartford Courant Foundation**
*See:* Entry 11689

★ **18210** ★ **Huber Foundation**
PO Box 277
Rumson, NJ 07760
**Phone:** (732)933-7700
**Email:** hcfoundation@courant.com
**Website:** http://www.hartfordcourantfoundation.org
Lorraine Barnhart, Executive Director
**Fnded:** 1949. **Philosophy:** The foundation focuses its grant making on "the issues of Reproductive Freedom, Population Education, and Family Planning." The Huber Foundation 2000 Annual Report. **Priorities:** *Civic & Public Affairs:* 54%. Funds legal defense, women's rights, and reproductive rights groups. *Education:* 2%. College civil liberties programs. *Environment:* 36%. Family planning organizations. *International:* 1%. Supports women's health. *Note:* Total contributions made in 1999. **Typ. Recipients:** Clinics/Medical Centers, Family Planning, Health Organizations, Hospitals, Public Health. **Geo. Dist:** nationally.

★ **18211** ★ **Jessie Smith Noyes Foundation**
6 East 39th St., 12th Fl.
New York, NY 10016
**Phone:** (212)684-6577          **Fax:** (212)689-6549
**Email:** noyes@noyes.org
**Website:** http://www.noyes.org
Victor DeLuca, President
**Fnded:** 1947. **Philosophy:** The foundation is committed to "protecting and restoring Earth's natural systems and promoting a sustainable society by strengthening individuals, institutions and communities pledged to pursuing those goals." As opportunities and needs suggest new directions and areas of emphasis, the foundation continues to modify its program to assure its relevance to contemporary society and to a sustainable future. Currently, the foundation funds projects that promote environmentally sound approaches to development, and that address toxins, sustainable agriculture, reproductive rights, sustainable communities, New York metropolitan area environment, and related interests. The foundation favors programs that deal with the connections between these problems, especially activities that have a potentially widespread impact. Priorities include supporting individuals and organizations in implementing programs that respect the inter-connectedness of human and natural communities. The toxins program's objective is to reduce threats posed by toxins to the environment and human health. The reproductive rights program seeks to promote quality reproductive health care as a human right. Priorities are to broaden the base and agenda of the reproductive rights movement and to influence legislation, policy, and reform initiatives. Reproductive rights in the United States are a focus, especially programs assisting women of color. The foundation's Metro-New York program seeks to promotes an environmentally sound metropolitan New York through an active, informed, and empowered local citizenry. It accomplishes this

objective by strengthening organizations working on environmental issues; by improving public policies and responsiveness of public agencies; and by developing effective coalitions and networks among different organizations, both within the environmental movement and between environmental groups and others. In addition to the programs described above, the foundation makes annual membership contributions and grants to specific charities designated by Charles F. Noyes. Small programs addressing redefining fiduciary responsibility and environmental justice are also implemented by the foundation. The directors give grants from a discretionary fund to organizations outside the foundation's current program areas. Issues of social justice and the environment are a key consideration throughout the grant decision-making process. The foundation does not accept applications for discretionary grants. **Priorities:** *Civic & Public Affairs:* 19%. Primarily supporting public policy organizations, women's affairs, and the metro New York environment. *Environment:* 22%. Reproductive rights. *Note:* Total contributions made in 2000. In addition to its program grants, the foundation also makes annual contributions to pre-selected charities, discretionary grants, and membership contributions. **Typ. Recipients:** AIDS/HIV, Alzheimers Disease, Emergency/Ambulance Services, Family Planning, Health Organizations, Health Policy/Cost Containment, Hospitals, Medical Education, Medical Research, Public Health. **Geo. Dist:** nationally.

**John D. and Catherine T. MacArthur Foundation**
*See:* Entry 12274

★ **18212** ★ **Kohler Foundation**
725 Woodlake Rd., Ste. X
Kohler, WI 53044
**Phone:** (920)458-1972          **Fax:** (920)458-4280
**Email:** 4answers@macfdn.org
**Website:** http://www.macfound.org
Terri Yohoi, Executive Director
**Fnded:** 1940. **Philosophy:** The foundation makes grants primarily for education and cultural programs in Wisconsin. The foundation also funds a scholarship program for higher education of Sheboygan County, WI, residents studying the arts. **Priorities:** *Arts & Humanities:* 95%. Supports performing arts, art galleries, and cultural programs. *Education:* 5%. Support for scholarships. Also funds colleges and universities, public schools, and enrichment programs. *Note:* Total contributions made in 1998. **Typ. Recipients:** Child Abuse, Children's Health/Hospitals, Family Planning, Medical Education, Medical Rehabilitation, Nursing Services, People with Disabilities. **Geo. Dist:** WI.

★ **18213** ★ **Lilly Endowment**
program Office
PO Box 88068
Indianapolis, IN 46208-0068
**Phone:** (317)924-5471          **Fax:** (317)926-4431
**Website:** http://www.lilly.com/about/community/foundation/endowment.html
**Fnded:** 1937. **Philosophy:** "The Endowment affords special emphasis to projects that benefit young people and that promote leadership education and financial self-sufficiency," and considers proposals in three major programming areas: Community Development Division: focus is on "stengthening the civic vitality of Hoosier communities through the GIFT initiative for community foundations... The constant goal is to help Indianapolis be an inviting place to visit and call home." Education Divison: supports projects which raise the "educational attainment level of Indiana citizens" through a scholarship program, student recruitment and placement. Religion Division: "efforts are aimed, in one way or another, at helping as many congregations as possible be strong and vital. Concentrates on efforts to rebuild and environment in which congregations, colleges, theological schools, denominations, and many other religious institutions and agencies can draw upon each others' energies and contribute their own gifts to the work of strengthening the ministry and religious life in the nation." 2000

Annual Report **Priorities:** *Arts & Humanities:* 3%. Funds music and arts centers. *Civic & Public Affairs:* 11%. Community development grants. *Education:* 56%. Leadership education grants and fellowships. *Environment:* 16%. Supports youth services and the United Way. *Note:* Total contributions made in 2000. **Typ. Recipients:** Emergency/Ambulance Services, Family Planning, People with Disabilities, Substance Abuse. **Geo. Dist:** nationally; IN, statewide; Indianopolis, IN.

**Louise Manoogian Simone Foundation**
*See:* Entry 483

**Lynn R. and Karl E. Prickett Fund**
*See:* Entry 489

**★ 18214 ★ Maclellan Foundation**
Provident Bldg., Ste. 501
One Fountain Square
Chattanooga, TN 37402
**Phone:** (423)755-1366          **Fax:** (423)755-1640
**Email:** hugh@maclellan.net
**Website:** http://www.maclellan.net
Hugh Maclellan, Jr., President, Treasurer & Trustee
**Fnded:** 1945. **Philosophy:** The foundation's primary mission is to serve strategic international and national organizations committed to furthering the Kingdom of Christ and select local organizations which foster the spiritual welfare of the Chattanooga area. **Typ. Recipients:** Family Planning, Public Health, Substance Abuse. **Geo. Dist:** internationally; nationally; Chattanooga, TN.

**Mary Reynolds Babcock Foundation**
*See:* Entry 5559

**★ 18215 ★ Nathan Cummings Foundation**
475 10th Ave., 14th Floor
New York, NY 10018
**Phone:** (212)787-7300          **Fax:** (212)787-7377
**Email:** info@cummings.ncf.org
**Website:** http://www.ncf.org
**Fnded:** 1949. **Philosophy:** "The Nathan Cummings Foundation is a national grant-making organization rooted in the Jewish tradition and committed to democratic values, including fairness, diversity, and community. By promoting innovative solutions to major social problems, we seek to build a society that values nature and protects ecological balance for future generations; promotes humane health care; and fosters arts to enrich communities." "The foundation's approach to grant making embodies some basic themes in all of its programs: concern for the poor, disadvantaged, and underserved;respect for diversity; promotion of understanding across cultures; empowerment of communities in need." "We make efforts to document the outcomes of our projects and to share the results of our work and the work of our grantees. Our focus is on grants in the United States." "The foundation is committed to a variety of educational strategies in its programs. We are also interested in leadership development, applications of new technologies, and innovations in communication. We seek to work with partners in the public, private, and nonprofit sectors." In the arts, community-based education programs that support at-risk youth and strengthening community arts will be stressed. For the environment, the focus will be on transportation issues, economics and fiscal policy, campus activities, and spirit, values, and ethics. The health program will stress health among pregnant women and young children and quality of life at the end of life. Programs under the Jewish life focus will enhance the spiritual dimension of Jewish life, improve Jewish education, develop social justice organizations, and build alliances between Jews and non-Jews. The foundation's Interprogram will support democratic values that stress tolerance and pluralism, protect First Amendment rights, and resist challenges to these values; contemplative practice programs that support efforts to explore the benefits of contemplative practice and raise public

awareness; and programs to protect nonprofit advocacy and strengthen the sector. **Priorities:** *Arts & Humanities:* 14%. Supports public broadcasting and theatre. *Civic & Public Affairs:* 15%. Supports public policy institutions. *Education:* 11%. Supports religious education, college and universities. *Environment:* 9%. Supports family services and youth programs. *International:* 8%. Supports medical center and health associations. *Note:* Total contributions made in 1998. **Typ. Recipients:** AIDS/HIV, Cancer, Children's Health/Hospitals, Clinics/Medical Centers, Family Planning, Geriatric Health, Health Organizations, Health Policy/Cost Containment, Hospitals, Long-Term Care, Medical Education, Medical Research, Mental Health, People with Disabilities, Prenatal Health Issues, Preventive Medicine/Wellness Organizations, Public Health, Trauma Treatment. **Geo. Dist:** internationally; nationally.

**★ 18216 ★ Powell Family Foundation**
4350 Shawnee Mission Parkway, Ste. 280
Fairway, KS 66205
**Phone:** (913)236-0003          **Fax:** (913)262-0058
Carrie Hoelscher, Secretary to the Board
**Fnded:** 1969. **Philosophy:** The foundation primarily serves the Kansas City area through grants in education, community support, religion, and youth programs. Camps are strongly supported, with funding allocated to resident and day camps both for facilities and camperships. Grants in education provide scholarships as well as support for innovative educational programs, including projects to use the arts and the outdoors to motivate students. In particular, the foundation supports the Powell Gardens near Lone Jack, MO, a complex established to encourage research and education in horticulture and natural resources. Grants to religious organizations are made primarily to Christian Science churches and religious welfare programs. Occasional grants may be awarded to other denominational groups that provide social services in the Kansas City community. **Priorities:** *Civic & Public Affairs:* About 94%. Supports the Powell Gardens and women's affairs. *Education:* 6%. *Note:* Total contributions made in 1998. **Typ. Recipients:** Cancer, Family Planning. **Geo. Dist:** Kansas City, MO, metropolitan area.

**Powell Foundation**
*See:* Entry 5469

**Prospect Hill Foundation**
*See:* Entry 598

**★ 18217 ★ Robert Sterling Clark Foundation**
135 East 64th St.
New York, NY 10021
**Phone:** (212)288-8900          **Fax:** (212)288-1033
**Email:** nanpmoore@aol.com
**Website:** http://www.fdncenter.org/grantmaker/prospecthill
Ms. Margaret Ayers, Executive Director
**Fnded:** 1952. **Philosophy:** The foundation concentrates its funding in three fields. Interest in improving the performance of public institutions is premised on the belief that a foundation can play an important role by working with government agencies, and by supporting organizations that monitor government actions. The foundation favors initiatives to monitor and improve human services delivery programs and the public school system, to protect the environment in accordance with federal and state mandates, to promote affordable housing and encourage the development of New York's economic base, and to improve the effectiveness and accountability of local and state agencies. To strengthen the management of cultural organizations in New York City, the foundation encourages arts organizations to manage their resources effectively. The foundation also supports projects designed to improve management, encourage resource sharing, increase earned income, and attract private support. The foundation has expanded its arts program to include support for advocacy efforts at the

national level with a focus on freedom of expression in the arts. The third area of foundation interest is reproductive rights. It primarily funds organizations working at the national level to ensure continued access to family planning services. The foundation has stated that it has begun to make grants to pro-choice organizations working in selected states in addition to its support for national pro-choice organizations. **Priorities:** *Arts & Humanities:* 21%. Supports theatre, museums, historic preservation, music, and dance. *Civic & Public Affairs:* 40%. Supports botanical gardens/parks, civil rights, economic development, economic policy, and job training. *Education:* 9%. Supports schools, educational programs, and education funds. *Environment:* 19%. Supports youth organizations, child welfare, family planning, and food distribution. *International:* 3%. Primarily supports single-disease health associations. *Note:* Total contributions made in 1999. **Typ. Recipients:** Domestic Violence, Family Planning, Health Organizations, Health-General, Long-Term Care, Mental Health, Public Health. **Geo. Dist:** nationally; NY, especially northern New York; New York, NY.

**★ 18218 ★ Scherman Foundation**
16 East 52nd St., Ste. 601
New York, NY 10022-5306
**Phone:** (212)832-3086          **Fax:** (212)838-0154
**Website:** http://www.scherman.org
Sandra Silverman, President & Executive Director
**Fnded:** 1943. **Philosophy:** The foundation's main interests are conservation and the environment, disarmament and peace, family planning, human rights and liberties, social welfare, and the arts. Social welfare grants focus on New York City organizations concerned with social justice, housing, public affairs, and community self-help. The foundation emphasizes general support grants, as it is assumed that nonprofit organizations with strong leadership are better able than donors to decide on the most effective use of funds. **Priorities:** *Arts & Humanities:* 16%. Supports theaters, public broadcasting, dance, music, museum, opera, and arts festivals. *Civic & Public Affairs:* 25%. Funds public policy organizations in the fields Disarmament and Peace, Human Rights and Liberties, Reproductive Rights and Services. *Environment:* 31%. Under the category of Social Welfare, the foundation supports violence prevention, housing initiatives, youth organizations, and women's affairs. *Note:* Total contributions made in 2000. **Typ. Recipients:** AIDS/HIV, Domestic Violence, Family Planning, Family Planning, Health Organizations, Outpatient Health Care. **Geo. Dist:** nationally; New York, NY, emphasis on metropolitan New York City for the arts and social welfare.

**★ 18219 ★ Sunnen Foundation**
7910 Manchester Ave.
Saint Louis, MO 63143
**Phone:** (314)781-2100          **Fax:** (314)781-1533
**Website:** http://www.sunnen.com
Kurt Kallous, President
**Fnded:** 1953. **Philosophy:** Available funds are confined to specific, goal-oriented projects that protect First Amendment rights and reproductive freedom. Grant giving in St. Louis focuses on local social service agencies and programs. The foundation also supports educational opportunities for the economically or physically disadvantaged, and youth and family programs. **Priorities:** *Arts & Humanities:* 11%. Supports historical societies and museums. *Civic & Public Affairs:* 6%. Funds public policy organizations. *Education:* 17%. Supports colleges, universities, Junior Achievement, and primary education. *Environment:* 62%. Contributions include Planned Parenthood, youth groups, and family services. *Note:* Total contributions made in 2000. **Typ. Recipients:** Cancer, Children's Health/Hospitals, Clinics/Medical Centers, Domestic Violence, Emergency/Ambulance Services, Family Planning, Health Organizations, Health Policy/Cost Containment, Medical Education, People with Disabilities, Single-Disease Health Associations, Speech & Hearing, Substance Abuse, Transplant Networks/Donor Banks. **Geo. Dist:** St. Louis, MO, metropolitan area & statewide.

**Taconic Foundation**
*See:* Entry 5563

**★ 18220 ★ Tinker Foundation**
55 East 59th St.
New York, NY 10022
**Phone:** (212)421-6858        **Fax:** (212)223-3326
**Email:** tinker@tinker.org
**Website:** http://fdncenter.org/grantmaker/tinker
Renate Rennie, President
**Fnded:** 1959. **Philosophy:** Tinker Foundation grants are awarded to organizations and institutions that promote the interchange and exchange of information within the community of those concerned with the affairs of Spain, Portugal, Ibero-America and Antarctica. (Ibero-America is defined here as the Spanish- and Portuguese-speaking countries of the Western Hemisphere.) Emphasis is placed on those activities that have strong public policy implications, offer innovative solutions to many of the problems facing these regions today, and incorporate new mechanisms for addressing environmental, economic and governance issues. Such activities may include, but are not limited to, research projects, conferences and short-term training workshops related to the Foundation's areas of interest. The Foundation encourages collaboration between organizations in the United States and Iberia or Latin America and among institutions in those regions. **Priorities:** *Civic & Public Affairs:* 12%. Funds foundations and public policy organizations. *Education:* 18%. Colleges and universities, projects and research. *Religion:* 2%. Supports the Woods Hole Research Center. *Note:* Total contributions made in 1999. **Typ. Recipients:** Family Planning. **Geo. Dist:** internationally; nationally.

**Turner Foundation**
*See:* Entry 733

**Victoria Foundation**
*See:* Entry 5566

**Wallace Alexander Gerbode Foundation**
*See:* Entry 745

**★ 18221 ★ Weeden Foundation**
747 Third Ave., 34th Floor
New York, NY 10017
**Phone:** (212)888-1672        **Fax:** (212)888-1354
**Email:** weedenfdn@weedenfdn.org
**Website:** http://www.weedenfdn.org
James Sheldon, Executive Director
**Fnded:** 1963. **Philosophy:** "Prior to his death in 1984, Frank Weeden, the Foundation's founder and chief benefactor, asked that the resources of the Weeden Foundation be used to address the adverse impact of growing human populations and overuse of natural resources on the biological fabric of the planet. From its inception in 1963, the Foundation embraced the protection of biodiversity as its main priority. Population growth, particularly in the United States, has also evolved into a major program interest. Organizations supported to date range from those that protect ecosystems and wildlife to those that raise the status of women and increase awareness about family planning. The Foundation financed the first debt-for-nature swap protecting the Beni Biosphere Reserve in Bolivia and is particularly interested in new and innovative efforts that help to develop sustainable models for conservation action. Projects that serve as catalysts inducing others to lend support receive priority consideration." **Priorities:** *Note:* Contributions made in fiscal 1998. **Typ. Recipients:** Family Planning, Health Funds. **Geo. Dist:** nationally.

**William and Flora Hewlett Foundation**
*See:* Entry 766

**William Penn Foundation**
*See:* Entry 773

**Zemurray Foundation**
*See:* Entry 792

## Corporate Foundations

**Ameritech Michigan**
*See:* Entry 2893

**Berwind Group**
*See:* Entry 885

**Boswell Foundation, Inc.**
*See:* Entry 897

**Citizens Bank-Flint**
*See:* Entry 945

**Corning Inc. Foundation**
*See:* Entry 11427

**H&R Block Foundation**
*See:* Entry 1111

**IBP Foundation**
*See:* Entry 11441

**Lennox Foundation**
*See:* Entry 1199

**Lotus Development Philanthropy Program**
*See:* Entry 1210

**★ 18222 ★ McCormick & Co. Inc.**
18 Loveton Circle
Sparks, MD 21152-6000
**Phone:** (410)771-7310        **Fax:** (410)527-8289
**Email:** mlarue@berwind.com
**Website:** http://www.corning.com/inside_corning/foundation.asp
Allen Barrett, Jr., Vice President, Corporate Communications
**Priorities:** *Arts & Humanities:* Limited support goes to museums, historic preservation, and public broadcasting. *Civic & Public Affairs:* Supports professional and trade associations and programs promoting economic development and the free enterprise system. *Education:* Primary support is given to colleges and universities, with an emphasis on business education programs. Supports scholarship programs. *Environment:* The highest priority, with an emphasis on united fund drives and volunteer service programs. Also supports family and community service organizations and youth activities. **Typ. Recipients:** Family Planning, Health Organizations, Medical Research, Nutrition. **Geo. Dist:** headquarters and operating communities.

**Mid-American Foundation**
*See:* Entry 5582

**★ 18223 ★ Patagonia Inc.**
PO Box 150
Ventura, CA 93002-0150
**Phone:** (805)643-8616
**Email:** jil_zilligen@patagonia.com
Jil Zilligen, Environmental Programs Director
**Priorities:** *Civic & Public Affairs:* 10%. *Note:* Contributions made in fiscal 2000. **Typ. Recipients:** Family Planning. **Geo. Dist:** nationally; Europe.

**Publix Supermarkets Charities**
*See:* Entry 11462

**Reily Foundation**
*See:* Entry 1348

**★ 18224 ★ Salomon Smith Barney**
7 World Trade Center
New York, NY 10048
**Phone:** (212)816-6000        **Fax:** (212)783-4262
**Website:** http://www.smithbarney.com/abt_sb/community/index.html
Jane Heffner, Vice President, Corporate Contributions
**Priorities:** *Arts & Humanities:* 27%. Supports the Old Station House Association. *Civic & Public Affairs:* 1%. Grants were given to The Fulbright Foundation and the Japan Society. *Education:* 6%. Awards given to the Capital Partners for Education and The Inner City Scholarship Foundation. *Environment:* 12%. Funds given to the YMCA of Greater New York, and the National Committee to Prevent Child Abuse. *International:* 6% Grant given to The Hartford Hospital. *Note:* Total contributions made in 1997. Contributions were made by the Traveler's Foundation. The company now gives directly through the Salomon Smith Barney Community Investment Program. **Typ. Recipients:** Family Planning, Hospitals, Medical Research, Single-Disease Health Associations, Substance Abuse. **Geo. Dist:** headquarters and operating communities; nationally. **Frmly:** Salomon Foundation Traveler's Group Foundation Traveler's Foundation.

**Star Tribune Foundation**
*See:* Entry 5475

**Target Foundation**
*See:* Entry 1425

**Van Leer U.S. Foundation**
*See:* Entry 1475

**Wells Fargo Bank Nebraska, N.A.**
*See:* Entry 1496

## Other Funding Organizations

**Society for Maternal Fetal Medicine (SMFM)**
*See:* Entry 16590

**Society of Reproductive Surgeons (SRS)**
*See:* Entry 19454

## National & International Organizations

**★ 18225 ★ Advocates for Youth**
1025 Vermont Ave. NW, Ste. 200
Washington, DC 20005
**Phone:** (202)347-5700        **Fax:** (202)347-2263
**Email:** info@advocatesforyouth.org
**Website:** http://www.advocatesforyouth.org
James Wagoner, Exec. Dir. & Pres.
**Fnded:** 1980. **Desc:** Mission is to create programs and promote policies that help young people make informed and responsible decisions about their sexual and reproductive health. Provides information, training and advocacy to youth-serving Organizations, youth leaders, policymakers, and the media in the US and developing countries. Implements numerous programs and promotes evidence-based policies on effective pregnancy and HIV/STI prevention for youth; sexuality education; gay, lesbian, bisexual and transgender youth issues, in addition to forming online communities for sexual health activists. The Resource Center online offers journal databases of information on youth sexual health, as well as model programs in developing countries. **Pub:** *Linkx*, quarterly. Newsletter. Details school-based health care. • *Options*, quarterly. Newsletter. • *Passages*, quarterly. • Reports. • Also publishes fact sheets, resource guides, and life plan-

ning education curricula. **Frmly:** Center for Population Options.

**★ 18226 ★ Alan Guttmacher Institute (AGI)**
120 Wall St., 21st Fl.
New York, NY 10005
**Phone:** (212)248-1111        **Fax:** (212)248-1951
**Email:** info@agi-usa.org
**Website:** http://www.guttmacher.org
Sara Seims, Pres.

**Fnded:** 1968. **Desc:** The Alan Guttmacher Institute (AGI) is a non-profit organization focused on reproductive health research, policy analysis and public education. The Institute's mission is to protect the reproductive choices of all women and men in the United States and throughout the world. It is to support their ability to obtain the information and services needed to achieve their full human rights, safeguard their health and exercise their individual responsibilities in regard to sexual behavior, reproduction and family information. **Pub:** *Fulfilling the Promise: Public Policy and U.S. Family Planning Clinics.* Report. • *The Guttmacher Report on Public Policy,* bimonthly. Journal. • *In Their Own Right: Addressing the Sexual and Reproductive Health Needs of American Men.* Report. • *International Family Planning Perspectives,* quarterly. Journal. • *Perspectives on Sexual and Reproductive Health,* bimonthly. Journal. **Frmly:** (1975) Center for Family Planning Program Development; (1977) Research and Development Division of Planned Parenthood Federation of America.

**★ 18227 ★ American Samoa Planned Parenthood Association**
PO Box 1043
Pago Pago, American Samoa

**Lang(s):** English. **Desc:** Promotes responsible parenthood and family planning as a means to improve the quality of life for people living in American Samoa. Advocates family planning as a basic human right. Sponsors programs in sex education, family planning, and health. Provides contraceptive and health care services.

**★ 18228 ★ American Society of Andrology (ASA)**
2950 Buskirk Ave., No. 170
Walnut Creek, CA 94596
**Phone:** (415)764-4823        **Fax:** (925)472-5901
**Email:** asa@hp-assoc.com
**Website:** http://www.andrologysociety.com
Kent Lindeman, Contact

**Fnded:** 1975. **Mem:** 800. **Desc:** Individuals interested in andrology, the science and medicine of the male reproductive system. Promotes advancement of knowledge of the male reproductive system and its diseases. Fosters interdisciplinary communication within the field of andrology; cooperates with other organizations holding similar interests. Conducts educational programs. **Pub:** *Handbook of Andrology,* periodic. Handbook. • *Journal of Andrology,* periodic. Journal.

**★ 18229 ★ American Society for Reproductive Medicine (ASRM)**
1209 Montgomery Hwy.
Birmingham, AL 35216-2809
**Phone:** (205)978-5000        **Fax:** (205)978-5005
**Email:** asrm@asrm.com
**Website:** http://www.asrm.com/
Dr. Benjamin Younger, MD, Exec. Dir.

**Fnded:** 1944. **Mem:** 10,500. **Desc:** Gynecologists, obstetricians, urologists, reproductive endocrinologists, veterinarians, research workers, and others interested in reproductive health in humans and animals. Seeks to extend knowledge of all aspects of fertility and problems of infertility and mammalian reproduction; provides a rostrum for the presentation of scientific studies dealing with these subjects. Offers patient resource information and placement service. **Pub:** *American Fertility Society–Membership Directo-*

ry, biennial. Membership Directory. Arranged alphabetically and geographically. *Price:* Included in membership dues. • *Fertility and Sterility,* monthly. Journal. Includes book reviews and announcements of meetings, courses, services, and employment opportunities. *Price:* Included in membership dues; $135/year nonmembers; $220/year institutions. • *Fertility News,* quarterly. Newsletter. Includes new member and regional postgraduate course listings. *Price:* Included in membership dues. • Also publishes syllabi used for postgraduate courses. **Frmly:** American Fertility Society; (1966) American Society for the Study of Sterility.

**★ 18230 ★ Antigua Planned Parenthood Association (APPA)**
Bishopgate St.
PO Box 419
Saint Johns, Antigua-Barbuda
**Phone:** (268)462-1187        **Fax:** (268)560-2297
**Email:** appa@candw.ag
**Website:**        http://www.ippfahr.org/whoweare/affiliate.html

**Fnded:** 1970. **Mem:** 52. **Lang(s):** English. **Desc:** Promotes family planning and maternal and infant health care as a way to improve the quality of life for individuals living in Antigua Barbuda. Seeks to reduce the number of unwanted pregnancies and abortions. Provides contraceptive services for men and women. Sponsors programs on family planning and sex education. Acts as an advocate for family planning on the national level. Conducts research. **Pub:** *Family Fare.* Newsletter. Covers reproductive health issues, family planning and family life education issues.

**★ 18231 ★ Asia-Pacific Society of Impotence Research (APSIR)**
c/o Dr. Tan Huimeng
c/o Subang Jaya Medical Centre
1, JLN ss 12/1A
47500 Suban Jaya, Malaysia
**Email:** aspirmal@tm.net.my
**Website:** http://www.aspir.org

**Fnded:** 1987. **Mem:** 500. **Nat'l Groups:** 730. **Reg. Groups:** 78. **Lang(s):** English. **Desc:** Health care professionals with an interest in impotence. Seeks to advance the diagnosis and treatment of impotence. Serves as a forum for the exchange of information among members; sponsors research and continuing professional development programs. **Pub:** *AMSIR Book on ED.* Book. • Newsletter, monthly.

**★ 18232 ★ Asociacion Argentina de Proteccion Familiar (AAPF)**
Aguero 1355/59
Capital Federal
1425 Buenos Aires, Argentina
**Phone:** 54 11 48261216        **Fax:** 54 11 48248416
**Email:** info@aapf.com.ar
**Website:** http://www.aapf.com.ar

**Fnded:** 1966. **Mem:** 160. **Nat'l Groups:** 1. **Reg. Groups:** 6. **State Groups:** 154. **Local Groups:** 1. **Lang(s):** Spanish. Does not correspond in English. **Desc:** Works to improve the quality of family life in Argentina. Supports and promotes reproductive rights and equal parenting duties. Operates family planning centers; conducts research and educational programs on subjects including the importance of the father figure; sexual health and the transmission of STDs, and birth control methods. Offers training for health and professionals and social workers. Maintains speakers bureau. **Pub:** *Comunicaciones.*

**★ 18233 ★ Asociacion Demografica Costarricense (ADC)**
La Uruca 300 metros al Norte y 100 metros al Este de la Fabrica de Galletas Pozuelo
Apartado Postal 10203
San Jose, Costa Rica
**Phone:** 506 2314430        **Fax:** 506 2314430
**Email:** adc@adc.or.cr
**Website:** http://www.adc.or.cr

**Lang(s):** Spanish. **Desc:** Advocates responsible parenthood and family planning in Costa Rica. Seeks to reduce the number of unwanted pregnancies and abortions. Encourages public awareness of contraception and methods of family planning. Offers contraceptive services. Sponsors programs in family planning, sex education, and awareness of sexually transmitted diseases, especially AIDS. Conducts research.

**★ 18234 ★ Asociacion Demografica Salvadorena (ADS)**
Edificio Profamilia
25 Av. Norte No. 583
Apartado Postal 1338
San Salvador, El Salvador
**Phone:** 503 2250588        **Fax:** 503 2250879
**Email:** info@ads.org.sv
**Website:** http://www.ads.org.sv

**Fnded:** 1962. **Mem:** 220. **Lang(s):** Spanish. **Desc:** Promotes responsible parenthood and family planning. Encourages public knowledge of contraception, family planning, AIDS, and other sexually transmitted diseases. Promotes family planning as a basic human right. Sponsors educational programs on family planning for teens and adults. **Pub:** *Anniversary Magazine,* annual. Magazine. Provides summary of covering and institutional goals. • *Informative News - Carta Informativa,* quarterly. • *Memoria de Labores,* annual. Annual Report. • *National Family Health Survey,* quinquennial.

**★ 18235 ★ Asociacion Hondurena de Planificacion de Familia (ASHONPLAFA)**
Calle Principal, entre: Colonias Alameda y Ruben Dario
Apartado Postal 625
Tegucigalpa, Honduras
**Phone:** 504 323235        **Fax:** 504 325140
**Email:** central@ashonplafa.com
**Website:** http://www.bdzv.de

**Fnded:** 1963. **Mem:** 40. **Lang(s):** Spanish. **Desc:** Works to enhance the quality of life of people living in Honduras through the promotion of responsible parenthood and family planning. Advocates family planning as a basic human right. Seeks to reduce the number of unwanted pregnancies and abortions. Provides programs in family planning, sex education, and health.

**★ 18236 ★ Asociacion Pro-Bienestar de la Familia Colombiana (PROFAMILIA)**
Calle 34, Numero 14-52
Bogota, Colombia
**Phone:** 57 1 3390900        **Fax:** 57 1 2875530
**Email:** info@profamilia.org.co
**Website:** http://www.profamilia.org.co/

**Fnded:** 1965. **Mem:** 917. **State Groups:** 40. **Lang(s):** English, Spanish. **Desc:** Promotes sexual health and reproductive rights in Colombia. Seeks to: improve maternal and child health by increasing the time between pregnancies; foster awareness of the possible effects of demographics on the socio-economic development of Colombia. Operates 35 family planning clinics in Colombia offering legal, medical, and educational services. Has established the Population Management Training Centre for staff employed at the clinics. Provides continuing education programs for gynecologists, obstetricians, and other doctors. Conducts studies and surveys; sponsors lectures, seminars, and workshops. **Pub:** *Annual Report,* annual. Pamphlet. Lists accomplishments of previous year. • *Disfunciones Sexuales.* Booklet.

**★ 18237 ★ Asociacion Pro-Bienestar de la Familia Ecuatoriana (APROFE)**
Letamendi No. 602 y Noguchi
Apartado Postal 5954
Guayaquil, Ecuador
**Phone:** 593 4 2402991        **Fax:** 593 4 419667
**Email:** pmarango@aprofe.org.ec

**Fnded:** 1965. **Mem:** 20. **Lang(s):** Spanish. **Desc:** Works to enhance the quality of life for people living in Ecuador through the promotion of responsible parenthood and family planning. Encourages public knowledge of family planning, contraception, AIDS, and other sexually transmitted diseases. Provides contraceptive and health care services. Sponsors educational programs. Conducts research. **Pub:** *Family Planning in Ecuador*. Reports. Features the history of Aprofe and information on family planning in Eucador.


★ 18238 ★ **Asociacion Pro-Bienestar de la Familia de Guatemala (APROFAM)**
9a Calle 0-57, Zona 1
Apartado Postal 1004
Guatemala City, Guatemala
**Phone:** 502 2 305488　　　　**Fax:** 502 2 514017
**Email:** info@aprofam.org.gt
**Website:** http://www.aprofam.org.gt
**Fnded:** 1964. **Mem:** 90. **Nat'l Groups:** 34. **Reg. Groups:** 1. **Local Groups:** 11. **Lang(s):** Spanish. **Desc:** Educators, doctors, social workers, and others interested in improving the quality of life through the promotion of family planning. Advocates family planning as a basic human right. Conducts family development program that stresses self-sufficiency and offers help in how to improve family income and health. Works to educate the public on family planning, contraception, AIDS, and other sexually transmitted diseases. Operates a clinic for women from which it provides contraceptive and health care services such as instruction in pre- and post-natal care; tests and treatment for infertility; tests to detect cervical and uterine cancer; coloscopies; and ultrasound. Conducts research. **Pub:** *Calendario Demagrafico*, annual. Journal. Contains information on demographics and the environment. • *Calendario Demografico*, annual.


★ 18239 ★ **Associacao Mozambicana para o Desenvolvimento da Familia (AMODEFA)**
Av. Da Tanzania no. 40
50-Amodefa
PO Box 1535
Maputo, Mozambique
**Phone:** 258 1 405107　　　　**Fax:** 258 1 402161
**Fnded:** 1989. **Lang(s):** Portuguese. **Desc:** Works to improve the quality of life for individuals living in Mozambique by promoting responsible parenthood and family planning. Attempts to stop the spread of AIDS and other sexually transmitted diseases. Offers programs in family planning, sex education, and health. Provides contraceptive and health care services. Acts as an advocate for family planning on a national level. Conducts research. **Pub:** *Crescer*, monthly. Magazine.


★ 18240 ★ **Association Ivoirienne de Bien-Etre Familial (AIBEF)**
Treichville
Bd. Giscard d'Estaing
BP 5315
Abidjan 01, Cote d'Ivoire
**Phone:** 225 251811　　　　**Fax:** 225 251868
**Fnded:** 1979. **Mem:** 650. **Lang(s):** French. **Desc:** Promotes advances in women's health care and family planning programs.


★ 18241 ★ **Association of Reproductive Health Professionals (ARHP)**
2401 Pennsylvania Ave. NW, Ste. 350
Washington, DC 20037-1718
**Phone:** (202)466-3825　　　　**Fax:** (202)466-3826
**Email:** arhp@arhp.org
**Website:** http://www.arhp.org
Wayne C. Shields, Pres.
**Fnded:** 1963. **Mem:** 2,000. **Desc:** Professionals in reproductive health, including obstetricians, gynecologists, family practitioners, pediatricians, nurse clinicians, researchers, educators, counselors, and administrators. Interested in contraception, sexually transmitted diseases, HIV/AIDS, menopause, urogenital

disorders, sexuality, cancer prevention/detection, abortion and infertility. Maintains speakers' bureau; sponsors clinical and public educational programs. **Pub:** *Clinical Proceedings*. Proceedings. • *Health and Sexuality*, quarterly. Newsletter. • Journal, bimonthly. • Journals. • Videos. **Frmly:** (1973) American Association of Parenthood Physicians; (1982) Association of Planned Parenthood Physicians; (1987) Association of Planned Parenthood Professionals.


★ 18242 ★ **Association of Supervisors of Midwives**
c/o James Paget Hospital
Corporate Services
Lowestoft Rd.
Gorleston
Great Yarmouth NR31 6LA, United Kingdom
**Phone:** 44 1493 452269　　**Fax:** 44 1493 452078
**Email:** elayne.guest@jpager-tr.anglox.nhs.uk
**Fnded:** 1910. **Mem:** 350. **Desc:** Qualified midwives nominated as Supervisors of Midwives. Promotes a high standard of Supervision of Midwives in the practice and teaching of midwifery. Offers support to members and represents the interests of Supervisors of Midwives at national and international levels. **Pub:** *Risk Management in Midwifery Practice*. • *Teaching Package About Midwifery Supervisor*. • Annual Report, annual.


★ 18243 ★ **Association Tunisienne du Planning Familial (ATPF)**
9, rue Essoyouti
El Menzah
TN-1004 Tunis, Tunisia
**Phone:** 216 1 232419　　　　**Fax:** 216 1 767263
**Email:** atpf@planet.tn
**Fnded:** 1968. **Mem:** 1,200. **Nat'l Groups:** 23. **Reg. Groups:** 450. **State Groups:** 104. **Local Groups:** 1500. **Lang(s):** Arabic, French. **Desc:** Advocates family planning as a basic human right. Works to reduce the number of unwanted pregnancies and abortions. Attempts to stop the spread of AIDS and other sexually transmitted diseases. Offers programs in sex education, family planning, and health. Provides contraceptive and health care services. Acts as an advocate for family planning on the national level. **Pub:** *Bulletin de l'Association*, quarterly. Newsletter.


★ 18244 ★ **Association for Voluntary Surgical Contraception International (AVSC)**
Box 57964
Nairobi, Kenya
**Phone:** 254 2 444922　　　**Fax:** 254 2 441771
**Website:** http://www.engenderhealth.org
**Fnded:** 1945. **Lang(s):** English. **Desc:** Promotes family planning and quality reproductive health services through provision of voluntary sterilization services and technical assistance to partners and governments; seeks to raise public awareness of surgical contraception. Makes available technical assistance for local family planning agencies; trains physicians and nurses in performing surgical contraception and quality improvement methods.


★ 18245 ★ **Australasian College of Sexual Health Physicians**
GPO Box 1614
Sydney, NSW 2001, Australia
**Phone:** 61 2 93827457　　　**Fax:** 61 2 93827475
**Email:** secretariat@acshp.org.au
**Website:** http://www.acshp.org.au/college/
**Fnded:** 1988. **Mem:** 202. **Reg. Groups:** 6. **Lang(s):** English. **Desc:** Physicians engaged in the practice of reproductive medicine and other specialties related to sexual health. Seeks to advance the study, teaching, and practice of sexual health medicine; promotes the prevention and control of sexually transmitted diseases. Establishes standards for sexual health medicine training and practice; holds examinations and accredits qualifying sexual health physicians; con-

ducts continuing professional development courses for members. Makes available consulting services.


★ 18246 ★ **Australian Society for Reproductive Biology**
Department of Biology Science
University of Newcastle
Newcastle, NSW 2308, Australia
**Phone:** 61 49 685511
**Fnded:** 1969.


★ 18247 ★ **Barbados Family Planning Association (BFPA)**
Bay St.
Bridgetown, Barbados
**Phone:** (246)426-2027　　　**Fax:** (246)427-6611
**Email:** bfpa@mail.sunbeach.net
**Website:**　　http://www.cariblife.com/pub/familyplan/home.htm
**Fnded:** 1954. **Lang(s):** English. **Desc:** Promotes family planning as a basic human right. Encourages family planning activities in Barbados. Offers educational programs in family planning, sexually transmitted diseases, and health care. Provides contraceptive services. Acts as an advocate for family planning on a national level. **Pub:** *Annual Report*, annual, always May. • *Family*, semiannual. Newsletter.


★ 18248 ★ **Belize Family Life Association (BFLA)**
127 Barrack Rd.
PO Box 529
Belize City, Belize
**Phone:** 501 2 31018　　　　**Fax:** 501 2 32667
**Email:** bfla@btl.net
**Fnded:** 1985. **Mem:** 5,000. **Lang(s):** English. **Desc:** Works to enhance the quality of life in Belize through promotion of family planning and maternal and infant health care. Encourages public awareness of methods of contraception. Offers educational programs in family planning, sex education, and health care. Conducts AIDS education and counselling. Provides contraceptive services. Also provides diagnosis and treatment of STDs, testing for cervical cancer, and counselling and support (including pre-natal education and post-natal services) for young parents. **Pub:** *Annual Report*, annual. Report. • *Information Sheets*. • *Journey*, quarterly. Newsletter. • Brochures.


★ 18249 ★ **British Andrology Society**
Glaxo-Welcom Research
Immunology Department
Gunnelswood Rd.
Stevenage SG1 2NY, United Kingdom
**Phone:** 44 143 8764418　　**Fax:** 44 143 8763232
**Website:** http://www.repromed.org.uk/bas/index.htm
**Fnded:** 1977. **Desc:** Scientists and clinicians working in the fields of human and mammalian reproduction with an interest in the male. Promotes the interests of members. Research is an important activity in the organization.


★ 18250 ★ **British Fertility Society**
The Old Chapel
Shadwell Lane
Moortown
Leeds LS17 6DR, United Kingdom
**Phone:** 44 113 3931009　　**Fax:** 44 113 3930965
**Email:** bfs@sinclairmason.co.uk
**Website:** http://www.britishfertilitysociety.org.uk
**Fnded:** 1973. **Mem:** 800. **Desc:** Promotes the practice, training, education and research in the field of infertility and reproductive medicine.


★ 18251 ★ **British In-Vitro Diagnostics Association (BIVDA)**
1 Queen Anne's Gate
London SW1H 9BT, United Kingdom
**Phone:** 44 207 9574633　　**Fax:** 44 207 9574644
**Email:** bivda@compuserve.com

**Website:** http://www.bivda.co.uk

**Fnded:** 1992. **Mem:** 98. **Desc:** National trade association for companies with major involvement and interest in the In-Vitro Diagnostics industry.

★ 18252 ★ **Brooks Advisory Centres**
421 Highgate Studios
53-79 Highate Rd.
London WCIX 8UD, United Kingdom
**Phone:** 44 20 72846040    **Fax:** 44 20 72846050
**Email:** administration@brookcentres.org.uk

**Fnded:** 1964. **Lang(s):** English. **Desc:** Seeks to decrease the incidence of unwanted pregnancy among young women. Conducts educational programs in matters of sex, contraception, and reproductive and social responsibility.

★ 18253 ★ **Bulgarian Family Planning and Sexual Health Association (BFPA)**
67, Dondoukou Blvd.
BG-1504 Sofia, Bulgaria
**Phone:** 359 2 9433052    **Fax:** 359 2 9433710
**Email:** bfpa@online.bg
**Website:** http://www.bfpa-bg.org

**Fnded:** 1986. **Mem:** 450. **Desc:** Sponsors reproductive health projects and health and sexuality education for various groups including young people, health and helping professions professionals, minority groups, special needs groups, and young offenders. Promotes training for all aspect of NGO and other management and training programs for trainers. Fosters research in parenting and family development.

★ 18254 ★ **Caesarean Support Network**
55 Cooil Dr.
Douglas
Isle of Man IM2 2HF, United Kingdom
**Phone:** 44 1624 661269

**Desc:** Provides support and information on caesarean birth. Promotes improved maternal and child health-care services.

★ 18255 ★ **Cameroon National Association for Family Welfare (CAMNAFAW)**
BP 11994
Yaounde, Cameroon
**Phone:** 237 236230    **Fax:** 237 236230
**Email:** camnafaw@iccnet.cm

**Fnded:** 1987. **Mem:** 2,000. **Reg. Groups:** 7. **Lang(s):** English, French. **Desc:** Those involved in the domain of reproductive health. Encourages public awareness of family planning and responsible parenthood through youth programs in Cameroon. Works to reduce the number of unwanted pregnancies and abortions and STI/HIV/AIDS. Advocates family planning as a basic human right. Sponsors programs in sex education, family planning, and health. Provides contraceptive services. **Pub:** *CAMNAFAW - The Road so Far*, periodic. Brochure. Containing information on youth and planning issues. • *Youth and Sexuality*. Booklet. • *Youth Prepare for Responsible Parenthood*. Booklet.

★ 18256 ★ **Canadian Fertility and Andrology Society**
2065 Alexandre-de-Seve. Ste. 409
Montreal, QC, Canada H2L 2W5
**Phone:** (514)524-9009    **Fax:** (514)524-2163
**Email:** execdirector@cfas.ca
**Website:** http://www.cfas.ca

**Fnded:** 1954. **Mem:** 530. **Desc:** Medical professionals, scientists, and others with an interest in human fertility and andrology. Serves as a forum for exchange of information.

★ 18257 ★ **Caribbean Family Planning Affiliation (CFPA)**
PO Box 3386
Saint Johns, Antigua-Barbuda
**Phone:** (268)462-4171    **Fax:** (268)462-1187

**Email:** cfpa@candw.ag

**Fnded:** 1971. **Mem:** 18. **Lang(s):** English. **Desc:** Family planning associations in Caribbean countries. Works to increase awareness and acceptance of family planning in the region. Advocates family planning as a basic human right and assists member governments in incorporating family planning into maternal and child health care services. Develops training programs for adolescents and young mothers. Studies demographic, sociological, and health issues. Offers training to teachers, family planning workers, and clinicians. Produces and distributes audiovisual educational materials. Compiles statistics. Offers research programs; sponsors competitive. Operates Documentation Centre for students, teachers, and researchers. Offers educational programs.

**Center Perzent**
*See:* Entry 8909

★ 18258 ★ **Center for Reproductive and Family Health**
C12 Bai Cat Linh
Dong Da
Hanoi, Vietnam
**Phone:** 84 4 8234288    **Fax:** 84 4 8234288
**Email:** rafh@hn.vnn.vn
**Website:** http://www.rafh-vie.org

**Fnded:** 1993. **Mem:** 12. **Nat'l Groups:** 1. **Reg. Groups:** 2. **Local Groups:** 1. **Lang(s):** English, French, Vietnamese. **Desc:** Promotes availability of family planning and reproductive health services throughout Vietnam, and particularly in rural areas. Does both research and intervention on reproductive health, disadvantaged women, and children. Increases awareness and knowledge of community people on gender equality, sexuality, and reproductive rights. Provides assistance to rural development programs operating in Vietnam; works to integrate population control and family planning activities into development programs. **Pub:** *Midwife*. Booklet. • *Reproductive Health*, quarterly. Magazine. • *Women's health Rain Drops - STDs Prevention What's cannot poured out*, annual. Video. Also publishes leaflets and posters. **Frmly:** (2001) Center for Reproductive Health and Family Health.

★ 18259 ★ **Center for Study of Multiple Birth (CSMB)**
333 E Superior St., Ste. 464
Chicago, IL 60611
**Phone:** (312)908-7532    **Fax:** (312)908-8500
**Email:** lgk395@nwu.edu
**Website:** http://www.multiplebirth.com
Louis Keith, MD, Pres.

**Fnded:** 1977. **Desc:** Medical research foundation concerned with the study of multiple birth and the care of multiple birth children. Disseminates information on the medical risks of multiple birth. Encourages funding for the support of medical and social research. Serves as resource center for the media and the public through informative website. **Frmly:** (1981) Center for Study of Multiple Gestation.

★ 18260 ★ **Centre for African Family Studies (CAFS)**
**(Centre d'Etudes de la Famille Africaine — CEFA)**
Pamstech House
Woodvale Grove
Westlands
PO Box 60054
Nairobi, Kenya
**Phone:** 254 2 448618    **Fax:** 254 2 448621
**Email:** info@cafs.org
**Website:** http://www.cafs.org

**Fnded:** 1975. **Lang(s):** English, French. **Desc:** Works to raise public awareness about family planning and reproductive health promotes the significance of family planning in national development. Provides technical assistance to family planning associations; organizes training course for managers, supervisors, and other

personnel employed in family planning programs and organizations. Conducts research; compiles information; compiles statistics. **Pub:** *CAFS Information Brochure*, annual. Brochure. • *CAFS News*, semiannual. Newsletter. Includes family planning issues. • *Programme of Activities*, annual. • *Research Reports*, periodic. Reports. • Annual Report.

★ 18261 ★ **Centre for Development and Population Activities - Egypt (CEDPA)**
53 Manial St., Ste. 500
Cairo 11451, Egypt
**Phone:** 20 2 3654565    **Fax:** 20 2 3654568
**Email:** cedpa@intouch.com

**Fnded:** 1975. **Lang(s):** Arabic, English. **Desc:** Seeks to enhance the managerial and technical capabilities of family planning, health, and development professionals. Conducts reproductive health programs focusing on the need of women and youth. Facilitates creation of primary health care services in rural and developing areas; makes available financial assistance to local health and development initiatives. Sponsors training programs for health and development personnel.

★ 18262 ★ **Centre for Development and Population Activities - India (CEDPA)**
50-M Shanti Path, Gate No. 3
Chanakyapuri
New Delhi 110 021, Delhi, India
**Phone:** 91 11 4672154    **Fax:** 91 11 6885850

**Fnded:** 1975. **Lang(s):** English, Hindi. **Desc:** Health and development professionals from developing countries. Seeks to improve family planning and reproduction health programs worldwide; promotes increased availability of reproductive health services in previously underserved areas. Provides managerial training, technical assistance, and financial support to grass roots population and family planning programs. Conducts training courses for reproduction health and family planning service personnel; sponsors training of women to operate and administer health clinics. Gathers and disseminates information on reproductive health and family planning. Main forces of organization is in empowering women to become full partners in development and helping the girl child to have better options in their lives.

★ 18263 ★ **Centre for Development and Population Activities - Nigeria (CEDPAN)**
18 Temple Rd.
Ikayi, Lagos, Nigeria
**Phone:** 234 1 2670360    **Fax:** 234 1 2600022
**Email:** cedpa@usaid.gov

**Fnded:** 1996. **Local Groups:** 34. **Lang(s):** English. **Desc:** National branch of the international organization. Seeks to improve the technical and managerial capacities of indigenous planning, health, and development professionals. Promotes empowerment of women. Provides training and technical assistance to development, reproductive health, family planning, and environmental protection programs. Conducts educational programs to raise public awareness of population, reproductive health, and development issues. **Pub:** *Democracy & Goverance Training Manual*. • *Small Doctors*. Booklet. • *Women on the Move*, periodic. Journal. • *Women Politicians on the Move*. Produces videotapes.

★ 18264 ★ **China Family Planning Association (CFPA)**
No. 1 Shenggu Beili
Yinghuayuan Xijie
Beijing 100029, People's Republic of China
**Phone:** 86 10 64413375    **Fax:** 86 10 64417612
**Email:** cfpa@public.fhnet.cn.net

**Fnded:** 1980. **Reg. Groups:** 29. **Lang(s):** Chinese, English. **Desc:** Works to enhance the quality of life for individuals living in China by promoting family planning. Works to reduce the number of unwanted pregnancies and abortions. Provides contraceptive and health care services. Sponsors programs in family planning, sex education, and health. **Pub:** *Life*, monthly. Magazine.

**★ 18265 ★ CHOICE**
1233 Locust St., Ste. 301
Philadelphia, PA 19107
**Phone:** (215)985-3355    **Fax:** (215)985-2838
**Email:** info@choice-phila.org
**Website:** http://www.choice-phila.org
Trina Johnston, Exec. Dir.

**Fnded:** 1971. **Mem:** 1,500. **Desc:** CHOICE is a nonprofit healthcare education and advocacy organization dedicted to helping people make informed sexual healthcare decisions. CHOICE has free and anonymous hotlines staffed by trained, professional counselors who provide short-term counseling and referrals for reproductive healthcare, child care, and HIV/AIDS. CHOICE also provides educational programs and workshops designed to raise awareness about sexually transmitted diseases, self-esteem, intimacy, and other sexual healthcare issues. **Pub:** *The Choice is Yours*, periodic. Directory. Directory of HIV testing services. • *Where to Find*, periodic. Directory. Lists family planning services. *Price:* Free. **AKA:** Concern for Health Options - Information, Care and Education.

**Clayton Fund**
*See:* Entry 5665

**★ 18266 ★ Cook Islands Family Welfare Association (CIFWA)**
PO Box 109
Rarotonga, Cook Islands
**Phone:** 682 23420    **Fax:** 682 23421
**Email:** cifwa@oyster.net.ck
**Website:** http://www.usmarshalls.org/injured.html

**Lang(s):** English. **Desc:** Works to enhance the quality of life for individuals living in the Cook Islands by promoting responsible parenthood and family planning. Advocates family planning as a basic human right. Sponsors programs in sex education, family planning, and health. Provides contraceptive and health care services.

**★ 18267 ★ Czech Association for Family Planning and Sex Education (CAFPSE)**
PO Box 399
1 Panska, Czech Republic
**Phone:** 42 2 24232552    **Fax:** 42 2 24232553
**Fnded:** 1990. **Lang(s):** Czech, English. **Desc:** Health care professionals and other individuals and organizations with an interest in reproductive health, family planning, and population control. Promotes increased availability of family planning services and improved access to sex education. Makes available reproductive health care services; conducts educational programs to raise public awareness of population issues; lobbies for improved public policies governing reproductive health, sex education, and family planning services.

**★ 18268 ★ DES Action Canada**
5890 Monkland Ave., Ste. 203
Montreal, QC, Canada H4A 1G2
**Phone:** (514)482-3204    **Free:** 800-4821-DES
**Fax:** (514)482-1445
**Email:** desact@web.net
**Website:** http://www.web.net/~desact

**Fnded:** 1982. **Mem:** 1,000. **Reg. Groups:** 10. **Lang(s):** English, French. **Desc:** Persons who have been exposed to the drug DES (diethylstilbestrol) and/ or concerned individuals. Seeks to detect, instruct, support, and defend the rights of people endangered by DES. Seeks to prevent health problems caused by DES and similar health concerns, especially in the field of reproductive health care. Provides informative written material as well as audio-visual aids for the general public and for health professionals. Offers physician referrals and peer counseling. **Pub:** *A New Look at Breast Cancer*. Booklet. A guide for women in need of Information about breast cancer and treat-

ments related to it. • *Bulletin DES*, quarterly. Bulletin. • *DES Action Canada Newsletter*, quarterly. Newsletter. • *DES-General Info.* Pamphlet. • *DES-The Wonder Drug You Should Wonder About A Pamphlet for Sons*. Pamphlet. • *Direct-to-Consumer Prescription Drug Advertising*. Pamphlet. • *Fertility Issues Associates With DES-Exposure*. Booklet. • *How Safe Are Our Medicines?*. Pamphlet. • *Nursing Curriculum Unit*. Pamphlet.

**★ 18269 ★ Dominica Planned Parenthood Association (DPPA)**
64 King George V St.
PO Box 247
Roseau, Dominica
**Phone:** (809)448-4043    **Fax:** (809)448-0991
**Email:** dppa@tod.dm

**Lang(s):** English. **Desc:** Works to improve the quality of life of individuals living in Dominica by promoting responsible parenthood and family planning. Offers educational programs on family planning and contraception to teens and adults. Encourages public awareness of AIDS and other sexually transmitted diseases. Seeks to decrease the number of unwanted pregnancies and abortions.

**★ 18270 ★ Dutch Association of Abortion Doctors (Nederlands Genootschap van Abortusartsen — NGvA)**
Gustav Stresemann Str. 26
NL-1111 KL Diemen, Netherlands
**Fax:** 31 20 6993428
**Email:** jansen@anon.at
**Website:** http://www.ngva.net

**Fnded:** 1991. **Mem:** 60. **Lang(s):** Dutch, English, French, German. **Desc:** Physicians united to ensure the reproductive rights and health of women in the Netherlands. Conducts research and educational programs on the health, social, and psychological impact of abortion. **Pub:** Handbook, annual.

**★ 18271 ★ Egyptian Population Services Society (EPSS)**
12 Sayem El Dahr St.
Rod El Faraq
Shoubra
Cairo, Egypt
**Phone:** 20 2 2033703

**Fnded:** 1989. **Mem:** 15. **Lang(s):** Arabic, English. **Desc:** Health care professionals and other individuals with an interest in family planning and related health services. Promotes increased availability primary health care in previously underserved areas. Makes available family planning, reproductive health, and pediatric health care services. Conducts surveys to determine medical needs of underserved communities.

**★ 18272 ★ EngenderHealth**
440 9th Ave.
New York, NY 10001
**Phone:** (212)561-8000    **Fax:** (212)561-8067
**Email:** info@engenderhealth.org
**Website:** http://www.engenderhealth.org
Dr. Amy E. Pollack, Pres.

**Fnded:** 1943. **Mem:** 8,000. **Desc:** Seeks to provide women and men with access to voluntary and safe contraception. Helps countries and institutions develop, improve, and expand systems for the provision of clinic-based contraception services. Special expertise in female sterilization and vasectomy. **Pub:** *AVSC News*, quarterly. Newsletter. *Price:* Free. For members only and family planning community. • Brochures. • Also publishes clinical guides and resources for family planning professionals. **Frmly:** (1985) Association for Voluntary Sterilization; (1994) Association for Voluntary Surgical Contraception; (2001) AVSC International.

**English National Board for Nursing, Midwifery and Health Visiting**
*See:* Entry 15707

**★ 18273 ★ European Embryo Transfer Association**
INRA-PRMD
F-37380 Nouzilly, France
**Phone:** 33 2 47427918    **Fax:** 33 2 47427743
**Email:** maugie@tours.inra.fr
**Website:** http://www.tours.inra.fr/aete/aeteeng.htm

**Desc:** Facilitates the diffusion and application of knowledge of embryo transfer in mammals.

**★ 18274 ★ European Menopause Society (EMS)**
15, rue Daru
F-75008 Paris, France
**Phone:** 33 1 42677747    **Fax:** 33 1 46222072

**★ 18275 ★ European Society ofHuman Reproduction and Embryology (ESHRE)**
ESHRE Central Office
Van Akenstraat 41
B-1850 Grimbergen, Belgium
**Phone:** 32 2 2690969    **Fax:** 32 2 2695600
**Email:** herman.merckx1@pandora.be
**Website:** http://www.eshre.com

**Fnded:** 1985. **Mem:** 3,839. **Desc:** Facilitates the study and discussion of all aspects of reproduction and embryology from before conception until the birth.

**★ 18276 ★ Family of the Future Health Care (Banja la Mtsogolo)**
PO Box 3008
Blantyre, Malawi
**Phone:** 265 677671    **Fax:** 265 677859
**Email:** banja@malawi.net

**Fnded:** 1987. **Lang(s):** English. **Desc:** Promotes population control, family planning, and reproductive health. Makes available reproductive health care services in urban areas; conducts campaigns encouraging male factory workers to participate in family planning and population control programs.

**★ 18277 ★ Family Health International (FHI)**
PO Box 13950
Durham, NC 27709
**Phone:** (919)544-7040    **Fax:** (919)544-7261
**Email:** services@fhi.org
**Website:** http://www.fhi.org
Albert J. Siemens, CEO

**Fnded:** 1971. **Mem:** 300. **Desc:** Biomedical researchers and technical assistants. Promotes increased availability, safety, effectiveness, acceptability, and ease of using family planning methods. Works to improve the delivery of voluntary fertility planning and primary health care services, and reduce the spread of sexually transmitted diseases, especially HIV infection. Conducts, analyzes, and disseminates research on contraception and distribution of family planning services. Supports a program of contraceptive safety and health records. Maintains library of 8000 monographs, journals, and reports. Operates computerized services. **Pub:** *Family Health International–Network*, quarterly. Bulletin. Covers reproductive health and family planning for health care personnel and policymakers in developing countries. *Price:* Free. **Frmly:** (1982) International Fertility Research Program.

**★ 18278 ★ Family Life Association of Swaziland (FLAS)**
PO Box 1051
Manzini, Swaziland
**Phone:** 268 53586    **Fax:** 268 53191
**Email:** khetsiwe@org.sz
**Website:** http://www.flas.org.sz

**Fnded:** 1979. **Mem:** 200. **Lang(s):** English, SiSwati. **Desc:** Promotes family planning programs in Swaziland. Works for the improvement of maternal, child, and family health. **Pub:** Newsletter, bimonthly.

★ **18279** ★ **Family Planning Association of Albania**
c/o Bulevardi Zhan d'Ark
palletet e Lanes
Pall 1
Shk1 Ap. 1
Tirana, Albania
**Phone:** 355 42 24269          **Fax:** 355 42 24269
**Email:** afpa@albaniaonline.net
**Fnded:** 1992. **Mem:** 254. **Local Groups:** 15. **Lang(s):** English. **Desc:** Works on issues of reproductive health and rights. **Pub:** *Reproductive Health*, quarterly. Newsletter.

★ **18280** ★ **Family Planning Association of Cyprus (FPA)**
25 Bouboulina St.
Nicosia 1061, Cyprus
**Phone:** 357 22 751093          **Fax:** 357 22 757495
**Email:** famplan@spidernet.com.cy
**Fnded:** 1971. **Mem:** 300. **Lang(s):** English, Greek. **Desc:** Promotes the sexual and reproductive rights of women, men, and young people, including the right to family planning, sex education and access to affordable and high quality services. Provides medical and counseling services to the public. Runs information and awareness campaigns on sexual and reproductive health issues. **Pub:** *Family Law in Cyprus*. Booklet. A series of sex education leaflets in Greek; booklets on contraception and reproductive rights, some information material is also in English.

★ **18281** ★ **Family Planning Association of Estonia (FPA)**
Kooli 7
10133 Tallinn, Estonia
**Phone:** 372 6 446656          **Fax:** 372 6 313934
**Email:** amor@amor.tartu.ee
**Website:** http://www.amor.ee
**Fnded:** 1994. **Mem:** 117. **Lang(s):** English, Estonian, Finnish, Russian. **Desc:** Works to improve reproductive health and family planning services and to increase the availability of such services. Conducts research and educational programs; organizes youth services. **Pub:** *Bulletin of FPA of Estonia*, biennial. Bulletin. Covers important areas of sexuality, health and education. Educational materials for youth on sexual and reproductive health.

★ **18282** ★ **Family Planning Association of Hong Kong**
Southorn Centre, 10/F
130 Hennessy Rd.
Hong Kong, People's Republic of China
**Phone:** 852 25754477          **Fax:** 852 28346767
**Email:** fpahk@famplan.org.hk
**Website:** http://www.famplan.org.hk
**Fnded:** 1950. **Mem:** 1,000. **Lang(s):** Chinese, English. **Desc:** To advocate, promote and provide information, education and services in sexual and reproductive health and responsible parenthood for the community. **Pub:** *Contraceptive Methods*. Video. • *Family Life Education Handbook for Teachers*. Book. • *Marriage: Crisis and Future in the Modern World*. Book. • *Puberty News*. Video. Appendix.

★ **18283** ★ **Family Planning Association of India (FPAI)**
Bajaj Bhavan
Nariman Point
Bombay 400 021, Maharashtra, India
**Phone:** 91 22 2029080          **Fax:** 91 22 2029038
**Email:** fpai@giasbm01.vsnl.net.in
**Website:** http://www.fpaindia.com
**Fnded:** 1949. **Mem:** 2,979. **Lang(s):** English, Hindi Suriname Hindustanti. **Desc:** Works to improve the quality of life for people living in India by promoting family planning and responsible parenthood. Advocates family planning as a basic human right. Works to reduce the number of unwanted pregnancies and abortions. Provides contraceptive and health care services including maternal and child health services. Offers programmes in family life and sexuality education and counselling. Conducts research and training of health professionals, NGOs and other categories of personnel.

★ **18284** ★ **Family Planning Association of Kenya (FPAK)**
PO Box 30581
Nairobi, Kenya
**Phone:** 254 2 603923          **Fax:** 254 2 603928
**Email:** info@fpak.org
**Website:** http://www.fpak.org
**Fnded:** 1961. **Mem:** 6,000. **Lang(s):** English. **Desc:** Seeks to help all Kenyans, especially young people, live quality healthy lives. Provides leadership and plays a pioneering role in offering sustainable, innovative and holistic services in response to health and socio-economic needs of all Kenyans. Aims at being a regional centre of excellence that assists in capacity building for other organizations serving young people. Particularly committed to championing sexual and reproductive health and other rights and the empowerment of Kenya's young people. Believes in upholding human rights to good health and social development through providing high quality gender sensitive services and information, advocating for freedom of choice, access to quality, appropriate and acceptable services, and promoting dialogue with key stake holders and beneficiaries.

★ **18285** ★ **Family Planning Association of Sri Lanka (FPASL)**
37/27, Bullers Ln.
Colombo 7, Sri Lanka
**Phone:** 94 1 584157          **Fax:** 94 1 580915
**Email:** dayafpas@slt.lk
**Fnded:** 1953. **Mem:** 350. **Local Groups:** 17. **Lang(s):** Sinhalese, Tamil. **Desc:** Advocates family planning as a basic human right and as a means to enhance the quality of life for individuals living in Sri Lanka. Works to reduce the number of unwanted pregnancies and abortions. Offers programs in sex education, family planning, and health. Provides contraceptive and health care services. Conducts research. Promotes the empowerment of women and gender equality and reproductive and sexual health for youth. **Pub:** *Annual Report*, annual. Magazine. Contains reports of the year's activities.

★ **18286** ★ **Family Planning Association of Trinidad and Tobago (FPATT)**
79 Oxford St.
Port of Spain, Trinidad and Tobago
**Phone:** (868)623-4764          **Fax:** (868)625-2256
**Email:** fpattrep@wow.net
**Website:** http://www.fpatt.org
**Fnded:** 1956. **Mem:** 15. **Reg. Groups:** 2. **Lang(s):** English. **Desc:** Works toward the following goals: to respond to the need for improved sexual and reproductive health among the underserved population with particular emphasis on young people; to further develop the financial and human resources of the association to boost its efforts; to advocate responsible sexual and reproductive health practices as a catalyst for the improvement of living standards. **Pub:** *Myths, Perceptions, Mistakes. A Study of Trinidadian Adolsecents*. Survey. Identifies the problems of pregnancy, child caring, and attitudes among teenagers in Trinidad. • *The Sexual Health Needs of Youth in Tobago*. Surveys. Assesses the social, economic and political factors that impact the lives and sexual health of youth in Tobago. • *Teenage Sexuality, Perceptions, and Attitudes of the Youth of Tobago*. Survey. Identifies the problems of pregnancy and child bearing among teenagers in Tobago. • *Trinidad and Tobago Demographic and Health Survey*. Survey. Provides detailed information about fertility, family planning, and child health for use in program planning and evaluaton.

★ **18287** ★ **Family Planning Association of Turkey (Turkiye Aile Planlamasi Dernegi)**
Atac Sokak 73/3
TR-06420 Ankara, Turkey
**Phone:** 90 312 4318355          **Fax:** 90 312 4342946
**Email:** tapd@adanet.tr
**Fnded:** 1963. **Mem:** 1,500. **Lang(s):** English. **Desc:** Promotes enhanced awareness of family planning rights and services throughout Turkey. Advocates reproductive health including family planning as a basic human right. Disseminates information. Works for the advancement of women's studies, health, and rights. **Pub:** *Islam and Family Planning*. Booklet. • Books. • Newsletters. • Brochures. Additional publications available on request.

★ **18288** ★ **Family Planning Australia (FPA)**
Ste. 4, Level 1
Construction House
217 Northbourne Ave.
Turner, ACT 2612, Australia
**Phone:** 61 2 62305255          **Fax:** 61 2 62305344
**Email:** fpa@fpa.net.au
**Website:** http://www.fpa.net.au
**Mem:** 7. **State Groups:** 7. **Lang(s):** English. **Desc:** Seeks to heighten governmental and public awareness of the population problems of local communities and the world. Believes that the availability and use of contraceptives is a basic human right. Makes available sexual and reproductive health services; conducts educational programs for the public and for health care providers. **Frmly:** (1992) Family Planning Federation of Australia.

★ **18289** ★ **Family Planning International Assistance - Kenya (FPIA)**
Box 53538
Nairobi, Kenya
**Phone:** 254 2 521855          **Fax:** 254 2 520028
**Email:** fpia@form-net.com
**Fnded:** 1971. **Lang(s):** English, French, Kiswahili. **Desc:** Family planning organization that works to improve reproductive health in developing countries.

★ **18290** ★ **Family Planning International Assistance - Thailand (FPIA)**
37 Soi 15 Petchburi Rd.
56 Silom Rd.
Bangkok 10400, Thailand
**Phone:** 66 2 2548955          **Fax:** 66 2 2548956
**Email:** fpia@mozart.inet.co.th
**Website:** http://www.plannedparenthood.org
**Lang(s):** English, Thai. **Desc:** Health care professionals, family planning and population organizations, and other interested individuals. Promotes increased availability of family planning services. Conducts educational programs to raise public awareness of population issues and family planning services; provides support and assistance to reproductive health and family planning clinics.

★ **18291** ★ **Family Planning International Assistance - USA (FPIA)**
c/o Planned Parenthood Federation of America
810 7th Ave.
New York, NY 10019
**Phone:** (212)541-7800          **Fax:** (212)247-6274
**Email:** fpia@ppfa.org
**Website:** http://www.plannedparenthood.org/fpia
Allie Stickney, Contact
**Fnded:** 1971. **Desc:** Provides financial, technical, and commodity assistance to organizations in developing countries interested in reproductive health programs.

**★ 18292 ★ Family Planning Organization
of the Philippines (FPOP)**
50 Dona M. Hemady St.
New Manilla
Quezon City, Metro Manila 1112, Philippines
**Phone:** 63 2 7217302        **Fax:** 63 2 7214067
**Email:** fpop@fastmail.i-next.net
**Lang(s):** English, Filipino. **Desc:** Advocates family
planning and responsible parenthood as a basic
human right and a means to enhance the quality of life
for individuals living in the Philippines. Attempts to
stop the spread of AIDS and other sexually transmitted
diseases through education and contraceptive services. Provides programs in family planning and health
care. Conducts research.

**★ 18293 ★ Family Planning and Sexual
Health Association (FPSHA)**
58 Saltoniskiu
2600 Vilnius, Lithuania
**Phone:** 370 2 790319        **Fax:** 370 2 790319
**Email:** lithfpa@puni.osf.lt
**Fnded:** 1995. **Mem:** 250. **Local Groups:** 5. **Lang(s):**
English, Lithuanian, Russian. **Desc:** Health care professionals with an interest in reproductive medicine;
individuals interested in family planning and sexual
health. Seeks to avoid unwanted pregnancies and to
eliminate the spread of sexually transmitted diseases.
Promotes increased availability of reproductive health
services; facilitates advancement of reproductive medicine. Serves as a clearinghouse on family planning
and sexual health; conducts public education programs; sponsors continuing professional development
courses; lobbies for improved public policies dealing
with reproductive health issues. **Pub:** Newsletter,
quarterly. • Brochure. • Bulletin.

**★ 18294 ★ Federation of Family Planning
Associations of Malaysia (FFPAM)**
81-B Jalan SS 15/5A
Subang Jaya
47500 Petaling Jaya, Malaysia
**Phone:** 60 3 7337514        **Fax:** 60 3 7346638
**Email:** ffeam@po.jaring.mg
**Website:** http://www.ffpam.org.my
**Lang(s):** Malay. **Desc:** Promotes and advocates
family health including family planning, women's development, family life education, youth sexuality, AIDS
and sexually transmitted disease prevention, through
service, research training and activities. Thus, improving the quality of life of individuals living in Malaysia.

**★ 18295 ★ Federation Laique de Centres
de Planning Familial**
34, rue de la Tulipe
B-1050 Brussels, Belgium
**Phone:** 32 2 5028203        **Fax:** 32 2 5025613
**Email:** g-international@tiscalinet.be
**Fnded:** 1963. **Mem:** 37. **Lang(s):** French. **Desc:**
Advocates family planning as a basic human right.
Works to reduce the number of unwanted pregnancies
and abortions. Attempts to stop the spread of AIDS
and other sexually transmitted diseases through education and contraceptive services. Sponsors programs
in family planning and health. Acts as an advocate for
family planning on a national and international level.
**Pub:** *En Question*, semiannual. Newsletter. **Frmly:**
(2000) Federation Francophone Belge pour le Planning Familial et l'Education Sexuelle.

**★ 18296 ★ Fertility Research Foundation
(FRF)**
877 Park Ave.
New York, NY 10021
**Phone:** (212)744-5500        **Fax:** (212)744-6536
**Email:** info@frfbaby.com
**Website:** http://www.frfbaby.com
Masood A. Khatamee, MD, Exec. Dir.
**Fnded:** 1962. **Nat'l Groups:** 1. **Desc:** Specializes in
human reproduction. Provides therapeutic, diagnostic,
and consultation service for childless couples. Con-

ducts comprehensive infertility surveys which include:
endoscopy, sperm antibodies determination, bacterio-
logical assessment, endocrine studies, laboratory facilities for complete hormone assays, surgical correction of genital diseases, artificial donor insemination,
and ovulation induction. Maintains research projects in
human reproduction pertaining to: the study of influence of mycoplasma on infertility; the relationship of
prostaglandins and infertility; the study of genetic
defects and dermatoglyphics; immunology research;
sperm physiology and migration; ovum transplantation. Conducts educational programs for practicing
physicians, residents, and medical students in infertility and education of the public about the human
reproductive processes. **Frmly:** (1967) New York
Fertility Institute; (1981) New York Fertility Research
Foundation.

**★ 18297 ★ Foundation for Promotion of
Responsible Parenthood - Aruba
(FPRP)**
PO Box 2256
San Nicolas, Aruba
**Phone:** 297 8 48833        **Fax:** 297 8 41107
**Email:** arfamplar@setarnet.aw
**Fnded:** 1970. **Lang(s):** Dutch. **Desc:** Works to im-
prove the quality of life of people living in Aruba
through promotion of family planning and maternal and
infant health care. Sponsors programs in family plan-
ning, sex education, and basic health care. Offers
contraceptive services. Conducts research.

**★ 18298 ★ Foundation for the Promotion
of Responsible Parenthood -
Netherlands Antilles (FPRP)
(Fundashon Famia Plania)**
PO Box 308
Curacao, Netherlands Antilles
**Phone:** 599 9 4611323        **Fax:** 599 9 4611024
**Mem:** 11. **Lang(s):** Dutch. **Desc:** Advocates sexual
and reproductive health, responsible parenthood and
family planning. Seeks to reduce the number of
unwanted pregnancies and abortions. Encourages
public knowledge of AIDS and other sexually transmitted diseases. Offers educational programs on sexual
and reproductive health, family planning and maternal
and infant health care.

**★ 18299 ★ FPA - England**
2-12 Pentonville Rd.
London N1 9FP, United Kingdom
**Phone:** 44 171 8375432        **Fax:** 44 171 8373042
**Website:** http://www.fpa.org.uk
**Fnded:** 1936. **Lang(s):** English. **Desc:** Promotes
family planning and sexual health in England. Con-
ducts public education programs; conducts research.
Provides helpline and reference library. **Pub:** *Contra-
ceptive Education Bulletin*, quarterly. Newsletter.
**Frmly:** (2001) Family Planning Association.

**Global Alliance for Women's Health**
*See:* Entry 2130

**★ 18300 ★ Grenada Planned Parenthood
Association (GPPA)**
Deponthieu St.
PO Box 127
Saint George's, Grenada
**Phone:** (809)440-3341        **Fax:** (809)440-8071
**Email:** gppa@caribsurf.com
**Website:** http://www.gawh.org
**Fnded:** 1964. **Mem:** 26. **Lang(s):** English. **Desc:**
Advocates responsible parenthood and family plan-
ning. Promotes family planning as a basic human
right. Encourages public awareness of contraception,
family planning, and sexually transmitted diseases.
Provides contraceptive health care services. Sponsors
educational programs. Conducts research. **Pub:** An-
nual Report.

**★ 18301 ★ Home Birth Association of
Ireland**
36 Springlawn Ct.
Blanchardstown 15, Dublin, Ireland
**Phone:** 353 1 8206940
**Email:** hba@iol.ie
**Website:** http://www.iol.ie/~hba
**Fnded:** 1982. **Mem:** 120. **Reg. Groups:** 22. **Lang(s):**
English, Galician, Irish. **Desc:** Those interested in
homebirthing. Seeks to increase the awareness of
birth as a normal physiological process, while incorporating homebirthing into mainstream maternity services. Produces information booklets, midwives' directory, and holds conferences and support group meetings. **Pub:** Newsletter, quarterly.

**★ 18302 ★ Hong Kong PHAB
Association**
75 Pokfulam Reservoir Rd.
Hong Kong, People's Republic of China
**Phone:** 852 25514161        **Fax:** 852 28751401
**Email:** hkphab@netvigator.com
**Website:** http://www.hkphab.org.hk
**Fnded:** 1972. **Mem:** 6,000. **Lang(s):** Chinese, English. **Desc:** Works to integrate people with and
without disabilities of all ages in the community
through social, recreational, educational and developmental programs. **Pub:** *PHAB News*, 3/year. Newsletter.

**★ 18303 ★ Hong Kong Sex Education
Association (HKSEA)**
PO Box 50419
Sai Ying Pun
Hong Kong, People's Republic of China
**Phone:** 852 28554488        **Fax:** 852 28551345
**Email:** hksea@glink.net.hk
**Website:** http://www.glink.net.hk/~hksea/
**Fnded:** 1985. **Mem:** 100. **Lang(s):** Chinese, English.
**Desc:** Individuals working in the fields of sex educa-
tion, family planning, social work, psychology, and
medicine; students. Promotes availability of quality
educational programs dealing with sexuality, which the
group defines as "those aspects of the human body
that relate specifically to being male or female."
Conducts research and educational programs; gathers
and disseminates information. **Pub:** *Sex Forum*, semiannual. Newsletter. • Bulletin.

**★ 18304 ★ Indonesian Planned
Parenthood Association (IPPA)**
Jalan Hang Jebat III/F3
PO Box 6017
Kebayoran Baru
12120 Jakarta, Indonesia
**Phone:** 62 21 7394123        **Fax:** 62 21 7253172
**Email:** pkbinet@link.net.id
**Fnded:** 1957. **Mem:** 1,500. **Nat'l Groups:** 1. **Reg.
Groups:** 24. **Local Groups:** 150. **Lang(s):** English,
Indonesian. **Desc:** Works to improve the quality of life
for individuals living in Indonesia through responsible
parenthood and family planning. Advocates family
planning as a basic human right. Offers programs in
family planning, sex education, and reproductive and
family health care. Provides contraceptive and reproductive and general care services. Conducts research.
**Pub:** *IPPA's News Letter*, semiannual. Newsletter. •
*Kabar*, quarterly. Magazine. • Brochures.

**★ 18305 ★ Infertility Awareness
Association of Canada (IAAC)
(Association Canadienne de
Sensibilisation a l'Infertilite)**
406-One Nicholas St.
Ottawa, ON, Canada K1N 7B7
**Phone:** (613)244-7222        **Fax:** (613)244-8908
**Email:** iaac@fox.nstn.ca
**Website:** http://www.iaac.ca
**Fnded:** 1990. **Mem:** 600. **Reg. Groups:** 5. **Lang(s):**
English, French. **Desc:** Individuals and organizations
working to increase the awareness and understanding

of the causes, treatments, and the emotional impact of infertility. Represents the interests of those with infertility concerns. Collaborates with infertility support groups to advance the organization's agenda. Disseminates information through media interviews, seminars, and educational materials. Maintains resource center and speakers' bureau. **Pub:** *Infertility Awareness*, bimonthly. Newsletter.

**★ 18306 ★ Institute for Female Alternative Medicine**
1500 S Central Ave., Ste. 214
Glendale, CA 91204
**Phone:** (818)956-3391　　**Free:** 800-505-4326
**Fax:** (818)956-0545
**Email:** doctor@drdeljuncojr.com
**Website:** http://www.drdeljuncojr.com
Dr. Tirso del Junco, Jr., Medical Dir.

**Desc:** Focusing on alternative surgical procedures for the treatment of benign female pathologies, ie: fibroids, ovarian cystic disease, endometriosis. Philosophy is "reconstructive" with extensive use of lasers, not removal of pelvic organs. **Pub:** *Women's Health quarterly*, quarterly. **Frmly:** (1998) Institute for Reproductive Health.

**★ 18307 ★ Instituto Peruano de Paternidad Responsable (INPPARES)**
Gregorio Escobedo 115
Casilla Postal 2191
Lima 11, Peru
**Phone:** 51 14 2612620　　**Fax:** 51 14 2617885
**Email:** daspilcu@inppares.org
**Website:** http://www.inppares.org.pe

**Fnded:** 1976. **Mem:** 140. **State Groups:** 14. **Local Groups:** 5. **Lang(s):** Spanish. **Desc:** Works to improve the quality of life for people living in Peru through the promotion of information and services related to sexual and reproductive health. Maintains programs in 14 cities. Works with local governments and community leaders to promote gender equality, the empowerment of women, prevention of unsafe abortions, and the prevention and control of sexually transmitted diseases, especially HIV and AIDS. **Pub:** *Information Bulletin*, periodic. Newsletter.

**★ 18308 ★ International Association of Hydatidology (Asociacion Internacional de Hidatologie)**
Florida 460, 3o piso
1005 Buenos Aires, Argentina
**Phone:** 54 11 43244700　　**Fax:** 54 11 43258231
**Website:** http://www.who.int/ina-ngo/ngo/ngo032.htm
**Lang(s):** English, Spanish. **Desc:** Physicians and other health care professionals. Seeks to increase understanding of the hydatid and its diseases. (The hydatid is a vestigal organ present in both the male and female reproductive systems.) Promotes exchange of information on the hydatid; sponsors research and educational programs.

**★ 18309 ★ International Dalkon Shield Victims Education Association (IDEA)**
212 Pioneer Bldg.
Seattle, WA 98104
**Phone:** (206)329-1371　　**Fax:** (206)624-4961
Constance Miller, Treas.

**Fnded:** 1986. **Mem:** 2,000. **State Groups:** 2. **Desc:** Women who have contracted illnesses and/or been disabled through use of the Dalkon Shield intrauterine contraceptive device; their supporters. Promotes public education about the dangers of using the Dalkon Shield. Disseminates information regarding Dalkon Shield injuries, claim resolution, and related topics. Offers seminars. Maintains speakers' bureau.

**★ 18310 ★ International Federation of Fertility Societies (IFFS)**
c/o Bernard Hedon, Sec.Gen.
CSI

337 rue de la Combe Caude
F-34090 Montpellier, France
**Phone:** 33 4 67585903　　**Fax:** 33 4 67583160
**Email:** algcsi@mnet.fr
**Website:** http://www.mnet.fr/webprofessionnel/i/iffs/
**Fnded:** 1953. **Lang(s):** English. **Desc:** National fertility and sterility societies. Conducts congresses to study human reproduction and problems relating to fertility and sterility in humans and animals. **Pub:** *International Journal of Fertility*, quarterly. Journal.

**★ 18311 ★ International Planned Parenthood Federation - Africa Regional Office**
Madison Insurance House
Upper Hill Rd./Ngong Rd.
Nairobi, Kenya
**Phone:** 254 2 720280　　**Fax:** 254 2 726596
**Email:** info@ippfaro.org
**Website:** http://www.ippf.org
**Fnded:** 1971. **Lang(s):** English, French. **Desc:** Coordinates activities of Planned Parenthood member associations operating in sub-Saharan Africa. Advocates family planning as a basic human right. Works to heighten governmental and public awareness of the population problems of local communities in Africa. Seeks to extend and improve family and sexual and reproductive health planning services. Conducts research on human fertility and contraception. **Pub:** *Adam & Eve and the Serpent*. Book. • *Africa Link*, semiannual. Magazine. Reports on sexual and reproductive health programmes of family planning associations in the region and provides related information on global events. • *Contraceptive Update: A Handbook for Health Workers*. Handbook. • *Legal and Policy Barriers Affecting Sexual and Reproductive Health Service in: Burkina Faso, Senegal, Swaziland, Zambia*. • *Regional Conference of Women, Islam and Family Planning, Niamey, Niger*. Report.

**★ 18312 ★ International Planned Parenthood Federation East and South East Asia and Oceania Regional Office**
246 Jalan Ampang
50450 Kuala Lumpur, Mayotte
**Phone:** 603 4256 6122　　**Fax:** 603 4256 6383
**Email:** rk@ippf.po.my
**Fnded:** 1961. **Mem:** 25. **Lang(s):** Malay. **Desc:** Works to co-ordinate activities for Planned Parenthood offices operating in the Asia and Oceania region. Advocates family planning as a basic human right. Works to increase governmental and public awareness of population problems in local regions. Promotes effective family planning programs. Conducts research on human fertility and contraception. **Pub:** *People and Development Challenges*, semiannual. Magazine.

**★ 18313 ★ International Planned Parenthood Federation - Swaziland (IPPF)**
PO Box 1051
Manzini, Swaziland
**Phone:** 268 53586　　**Fax:** 268 5053191
**Email:** flas@iafrica.sz
**Desc:** Promotes family planning and population reduction measures in Swaziland. Operates information campaigns and family planning clinics. Advocates population concerns.

**★ 18314 ★ International Planned Parenthood Federation - Tunis**
Arab World Regional Office
2, Place Virgile
Notre Dame
TN-1082 Tunis, Tunisia
**Phone:** 216 1 847344　　**Fax:** 216 1 788661
**Email:** awro@ippf.intl.tn
**Lang(s):** Arabic, French. **Desc:** Advocates family planning as a basic human right. Works to increase governmental and public awareness of population

problems. Promotes effective family planning services. Conducts research on human fertility and contraception.

**★ 18315 ★ International Planned Parenthood Federation - United Kingdom (IPPF) (Federation Internationale pour la Planification Familiale — IPPF)**
Regent's College
Inner Circle
Regent's Park
London NW1 4NS, United Kingdom
**Phone:** 44 20 74877900　　**Fax:** 44 20 74877950
**Email:** info@ippf.org
**Website:** http://www.ippf.org
**Fnded:** 1952. **Mem:** 139. **Nat'l Groups:** 180. **Reg. Groups:** 6. **Lang(s):** Arabic, English, French, Spanish. **Desc:** Intiates and supports worldwide sexual and reproductive health searvices, including family planning, HIV prevention and care and support programs. **Pub:** *Family Planning Handbook for Doctors*, periodic. Handbook. • *IPPF Annual Report*. Annual Report. • *IPPF Directory of Hormonal Contraceptives*, periodic. Booklet. • *IPPF Medical Bulletin*, bimonthly. Bulletin.

**★ 18316 ★ International Planned Parenthood Federation, Western Hemisphere Region (IPPF/WHR)**
120 Wallstreet, 9th Fl.
New York, NY 10005
**Phone:** (212)248-6400　　**Fax:** (212)248-4221
**Email:** info@ippfwhr.org
**Website:** http://www.ippfwhr.org
Sharon Allison, Pres.
**Fnded:** 1952. **Mem:** 44. **Desc:** A division of the International Planned Parenthood Federation. Provides more than 9 million sexual and reproductive health services and information each year to men, women and youth throughout North and Latin America, and the Caribbean. **Pub:** *Forum*, quarterly. Magazine. Includes calendar of events. Distributed primarily to affiliated family planning programs. • Annual Report. • Also publishes occasional monographs, studies, and position papers.

**★ 18317 ★ International Society of Andrology (ISA)**
Department of Medicine (DO2)
University of Sydney
Sydney, NSW 2006, Australia
**Phone:** 61 2 95157150　　**Fax:** 61 2 93514560
**Email:** djh@med.usyd.edu.au
**Website:** http://www.upmc.edu/isa/
**Fnded:** 1981. **Desc:** Disseminates knowledge of andrology, which is defined as the branches of science and medicine dealing with the male reproductive organs in animals and in men and with diseases of these organs; promotes the development of basic and clinical research in andrology.

**★ 18318 ★ International Society of Endocrinology (ISA)**
Buenos Aires Children's Hospital
Grallo
1425 Buenos Aires, Argentina
**Phone:** 54 11 49635931　　**Fax:** 54 11 49635930
**Email:** president@andrology.org
**Website:** http://andrology.org
**Fnded:** 1981. **Mem:** 8,000. **Desc:** Aims to serve Andrology and andrologists world-wide through its Newsletter.

**★ 18319 ★ International Society of Reproductive Medicine (ISRM)**
c/o Donald C. McEwen, M.D.
336 W Main St.
Bound Brook, NJ 08805-1840
Donald C. McEwen, MD, Sec.

**Fnded:** 1968. **Mem:** 300. **Desc:** Research specialists in reproductive medicine, obstetrics/gynecology, and endocrinology; associate members are laypersons interested in world population problems. Encourages basic and clinical research on the physiology of reproduction with special emphasis on the normal reproductive process, methods for enhancement of fertility, conception control, the pharmacology of steroids and polypeptides, and the immunology of reproduction. Fosters discussion and evaluation of new concepts, controversies in management of patients with reproductive disorders, and clinical relevance of advances in reproductive biology. Disseminates information and promotes continuing education for physicians and scientists. **Pub:** *Annual Proceedings.* **Frmly:** (1970) Family Planning Association of the Americas; (1980) International Family Planning Research Association.

★ **18320** ★ **International Society for Twin Studies (ISTS)**
**(Societe Internationale d'Etudes Gemellaires)**
c/o Jaakko Kaprio, Sec.
Department of Health
Univ. of Helsinki
PO Box 41
SF-00014 Helsinki, Finland
**Website:** http://www.ists.qimr.edu.au
**Fnded:** 1974. **Mem:** 251. **Desc:** Professionals and lay persons interested in twin research; national or large local organizations of twins or mothers of twins. Purposes are to advance twin research as applied to a variety of biomedical and psychological disciplines and to promote high standards of medical and psychosocial management of twin pregnancy and development. Assists researchers in contacting twins through twin clubs and mothers of twins clubs; advises and assists lay organizations conducting surveys or research about twins. Holds workshops. Plans to bestow awards; compiles statistics. **Pub:** *Acta Geneticae Medicae et Gemellologiae/Twin Research*, quarterly. • *Twins*, 1-2/year. Newsletter.

★ **18321** ★ **International Women's Health Coalition (IWHC)**
24 E 21st St.
New York, NY 10010
**Phone:** (212)979-8500          **Fax:** (212)979-9009
**Email:** info@iwhc.org
**Website:** http://www.iwhc.org
Adrienne Germain, Pres.
**Fnded:** 1980. **Desc:** Seeks to promote and provide high quality reproductive health care for women in the Southern countries. Provides technical assistance, supports innovative health care projects and policy-oriented field research in Africa, Asia and Latin America. Produces public education materials. **Pub:** *The Sexuality Connection in Reproductive Health.* Report. Explores the importance of the study of sexuality and gender-based power relations to reproductive health policies and programs. • *Special Challenges in Third World Women's Health: Reproductive Tract Infections, Cervical Cancer, and Contraceptive Safety.* Report. • *Women's Political Action and Population Policy in Three Developing Countries.* Report. • Reports. **Frmly:** (1980) National Women's Health Coalition.

★ **18322** ★ **Irish Family Planning Association (IFPA)**
16-17 Solomons House
42A Pearse St.
Dublin 2, Ireland
**Phone:** 353 1 4740944          **Fax:** 353 1 4740945
**Email:** post@ifpa.ie
**Website:** http://www.ifpa.ie
**Fnded:** 1969. **Nat'l Groups:** 1. **Lang(s):** English. **Desc:** Works to improve the quality of life for individuals living in Ireland by promoting family planning and responsible parenthood. Advocates family planning as a basic human right. Offers programs in sex educa-

tion, family planning, and health. Provides contraceptive and health care services. Conducts research.

★ **18323** ★ **Israel Family Planning Association**
9 Rambam St.
65601 Tel Aviv, Israel
**Phone:** 972 3 5101511          **Fax:** 972 3 5102589
**Email:** ippf@post.com
**Mem:** 250. **Lang(s):** Arabic, Hebrew. **Desc:** Promotes healthy and responsible sexual behavior as a means to enhance the quality of life for individuals living in Israel. Works to stop the spread of AIDS and other sexually transmitted diseases through education and contraceptive services. Advocates women's empowerment through programs enhancing their self image. Operates 14 "Open-Door" sexual counseling clinics. Offers programs in sex education, family planning, and health. Acts as an advocate for family planning on the national level.

★ **18324** ★ **Issue the National Fertility Association**
114 Lichfield St.
West Midlands
Walsall WS1 1SZ, United Kingdom
**Phone:** 44 1922 722888          **Fax:** 44 1922 640070
**Email:** webmaster@issue.co.uk
**Website:** http://www.issue.co.uk
**Fnded:** 1976. **Mem:** 6,000. **Lang(s):** English. **Desc:** Infertile women and men. Disseminates information and provides support and offers telephone counseling to infertile individuals on all aspects of infertility. **Pub:** *ISSUE*, quarterly. Magazine.

★ **18325** ★ **IUD Claims Information Source (ICIS)**
PO Box 84151
Seattle, WA 98104
**Phone:** (206)329-1371          **Fax:** (206)624-4961
Constance Miller, Mng. Dir.
**Fnded:** 1989. **Desc:** Provides information and referrals to women filing lawsuits because of injuries sustained through use of an intrauterine contraceptive device (IUD). Offers professional seminars in claims filing and resolution. Maintains speakers' bureau. **Pub:** *Dalkon Shield Claims Guidebook.* • *Dalkon Shield Legal Guide.*

★ **18326** ★ **Jamaica Family Planning Association (JFPA)**
14 King St.
Kingston, Jamaica
**Phone:** (876)972-2515          **Fax:** (876)972-2224
**Email:** famplan@cwjamaica.com
**Website:** http://www.jamaica-kidz.com/famplan.htm
**Fnded:** 1975. **Mem:** 250. **Lang(s):** English. **Desc:** National affiliate of the International Family Planning Federation. Promotes availability of family planning services; advocates on behalf of family planning. Maintains clinics; conducts educational programs. **Pub:** Newsletter, quarterly. **Frmly:** (1990) Famplan Jamaica.

★ **18327** ★ **Japanese Organization for International Cooperation in Family Planning (JOICFP)**
Hoken Kaikan Shinkan Bldg.
1-10 Ichigaya Tamachi
Shinjuku-ku
Tokyo 162-0843, Japan
**Phone:** 81 3 32685875          **Fax:** 81 3 32357090
**Email:** info@joicfp.or.jp
**Website:** http://www.joicfp.or.jp
**Fnded:** 1968. **Mem:** 307. **Lang(s):** English, Japanese. **Desc:** Provides assistance to reproductive health and family planning programs in 12 countries worldwide. Works closely with Japanese government agencies and international development organizations including UNFPA and IPPF to devise projects and train staff. Promotes the use of videotapes and films in reproduc-

tive health/family planning education programs. **Pub:** *Adolescent Women - Voices Unheard, Marian's Monolog.* Film. • *JOICFP News*, monthly. Newsletter. • *Sekaito Jinko*, monthly. Magazine. • Monographs.

★ **18328** ★ **Jordanian Association for Family Planning and Protection (JAFPP)**
Al Madina Area-Zomokhshary Str.
PO Box 8066
Amman, Jordan
**Phone:** 962 6 5160999          **Fax:** 962 6 5161020
**Email:** jafpp@nol.com.jo
**Fnded:** 1964. **Mem:** 200. **Local Groups:** 3. **Lang(s):** Arabic, English. **Desc:** Social workers and health care professionals in Jordan. Advocates responsible parenthood and family planning in Jordan. Operates family planning clinics and mobile units for rural areas. Offers advice to paretns on issues such as child spacing, marital problems, and child rearing; encourages couples to plan children according to financial means. Provides medical assistance to couples with infertility problems and helps them to overcome the social stigma attached to infertility through counseling services. Conducts annual family planning week. Organizes family planning courses for social workers and volunteers, lectures, workshops, siminar for targeting youth and women on the fields of reproductive health, commmunication skills, sexual health, population issues. Advocacy targeting decision makers. **Pub:** *Selected Lectures in Family Planning.* • Brochures, periodic.

★ **18329** ★ **Latvia's Family Planning and Sexual Health Association**
Valnu Str. 3
LV-10503 Riga, Latvia
**Phone:** 371 7 242700          **Fax:** 371 7 821227
**Email:** lfpa@mailbox.riga.lv
**Website:** http://www.iclub.lv/lfpa
**Fnded:** 1994. **Mem:** 380. **Lang(s):** English, Latvian. **Desc:** Promotes family planning. Gathers and disseminates family planning information; conducts family planning education courses for health care professionals, educators, and social workers. **Pub:** *Abortion.* Brochure. • *Contraception.* Brochure. • *Happy Relations.* Brochure. • *Papardes Lapa*, semiannual. Newsletter. • *STD.* Brochure.

★ **18330** ★ **Lebanon Family Planning Association (LFPA)**
Corniche Mazraa, Al Maskan Bldg.
PO Box 118240
Beirut, Lebanon
**Phone:** 961 1 311978
**Email:** lfpa@dm.net.lb
**Website:** http://ippfnet.ippf.org
**Lang(s):** Arabic. **Desc:** Works to improve the quality of life for individuals living in Lebanon by promoting responsible parenthood and family planning. Advocates family planning as a basic human right. Offers programs in sex education, family planning, and health. Provides contraceptive and health care services. Conducts research.

★ **18331** ★ **Marie Stopes International (MSI)**
153 Cleveland St.
London W1P 5GP, United Kingdom
**Phone:** 44 171 5747400          **Fax:** 44 171 5747417
**Email:** services@stopes.org.uk
**Website:** http://www.mariestopes.org.uk
**Fnded:** 1975. **Desc:** Provides a wide range of maternal health and family planning services. Programs conducted include: contraceptive social marketing; male oriented services. Specializes in working with indigenous personnel to develop clinical family planning services and social marketing programs.

**★ 18332 ★ Marie Stopes International - Vietnam (MSIVN)**
Solday F2 No 1
Phuong, Bach Khoa
Hanoi, Vietnam
**Phone:** 84 4 8694356
**Email:** msihanoi@netnam.org.vn
**Website:** http://www.mariestopes.org.uk/viet_nam.html

**Lang(s):** English, French, Vietnamese. **Desc:** Maternal and child health organizations, health care providers, and other interested individuals. Seeks to increase access to health and family planning services among previously underserved populations. Conducts social marketing of contraceptives; sponsors male-oriented family planning campaigns. Develops locally administered family planning services and social marketing programs.

**★ 18333 ★ Mexican Family Planning Association (MEXFAM) (Fundacion Mexicaca para la Planeacion Familiar)**
Juarez 208 Col.
Tlalpan
14000 Mexico City, DF, Mexico
**Phone:** 52 5 5737100     **Fax:** 52 5 5732318
**Email:** mexinfo@mexfam.org.mx
**Website:** http://www.mexfam.org.mx

**Lang(s):** Spanish. **Desc:** Promotes responsible parenthood and family planning. Advocates family planning as a basic human right. Works to reduce the number of unwanted pregnancies and abortions. Encourages public awareness of family planning, contraception, and sexually transmitted diseases. Offers educational programs for teens and adults. Acts as an advocate for family planning on a national level. Conducts research.

**★ 18334 ★ Miscarriage Association**
c/o Clayton Hospital
Northgate
Wakefield WF1 3JS, United Kingdom
**Phone:** 44 1924 200799     **Fax:** 44 1924 298834
**Email:** miscarriageassociation@care4free.net
**Website:** http://www.miscarriageassociation.org.uk

**Fnded:** 1982. **Mem:** 1,400. **Reg. Groups:** 50. **Lang(s):** English. **Desc:** Provides support and information for all on the subject of pregnancy loss. Gathers information about causes and treatments and promote good practice in the wa y pregnancy loss is managed in hospitals and in the community. **Pub:** Newsletter, quarterly.

**★ 18335 ★ Miscarriage Infant Death Stillbirth Support Group (MIDS)**
c/o Janet Tischler
16 Crescent Dr.
Parsippany, NJ 07054-1605
**Phone:** (973)263-6730     **Fax:** (973)263-0091
**Email:** mids1982@yahoo.com
**Website:** http://www.kumc.edu/gec/support/miscarri.html
Janet Tischler, Founder/Pres.

**Fnded:** 1982. **Mem:** 700. **State Groups:** 2. **Local Groups:** 4. **Desc:** Offers friendship and support to parents who have experienced miscarriage, infant death, or stillbirth. Provides monthly meetings, friendships, in-hospital visits, workshops, and speakers. **Pub:** MIDS Newsletter, 4/year. Newsletter. **Price:** $18/year. • Brochure.

**★ 18336 ★ Moldova Family Planning Association (MFPA)**
Armeneasca str. 47, office 68
MD-2005 Chisinau, Moldova
**Phone:** 373 2 541207     **Fax:** 373 2 541208
**Email:** fpam@cni.md
**Fnded:** 1992. **Lang(s):** English, Russian. **Desc:** Promotes population control through family planning.

Gathers and disseminates information on family planning and reproductive health.

**★ 18337 ★ Mouvement Francais pour le Planning Familial (MFPF)**
4, sq. St. Irenee
F-75011 Paris, France
**Phone:** 33 1 48072910     **Fax:** 33 1 47007977
**Email:** planfami@club-internet.fr

**Fnded:** 1956. **Mem:** 8,000. **Reg. Groups:** 20. **Local Groups:** 70. **Lang(s):** French. **Desc:** Works to enhance the quality of life for individuals living in France by promoting responsible parenthood and family planning. Advocates family planning as a basic human right and defends women's rights to contraception and abortion. Attempts to stop the spread of AIDS and other sexually transmitted diseases. Sponsors programs in sex education, family planning, and health. Provides contraceptive and health care services. Acts as an advocate for family planning on a national level. Conducts research.

**★ 18338 ★ Mozambique Association for Family Development (MAFD) (Asociacao Mocambicana para o Desenvolvimento da Familia — AMODEFA)**
PO Box 1535
Maputo, Mozambique
**Phone:** 258 1 405107     **Fax:** 258 1 405146
**Email:** amodefa@virconn.com
**Website:** http://www.amodefa.org.mz

**Fnded:** 1989. **Mem:** 300. **Nat'l Groups:** 25. **Reg. Groups:** 4. **State Groups:** 19. **Local Groups:** 25. **Lang(s):** English, Portuguese. **Desc:** Promotes an improved quality of life for families. Sponsors reproductive health and family planning programs and services. Conducts public education campaigns; advocates on behalf of more effective public health policies. **Pub:** Newsletter, monthly. For youth.

**★ 18339 ★ National Abortion Federation (NAF)**
1755 Massachusetts Ave. NW Ste 600
Washington, DC 20036
**Phone:** (202)667-5881     **Fax:** (202)667-5890
**Email:** naf@prochoice.org
**Website:** http://www.prochoice.org
Vicki Saporta, Exec. Dir.

**Fnded:** 1977. **Mem:** 400. **Desc:** Abortion service providers (physician offices, clinics, feminist health centers, Planned Parenthood affiliates) and others committed to making safe, legal abortions accessible to all women. Unites abortion service providers into a professional community dedicated to health care; upgrades abortion services by providing continuing medical education, standards, and guidelines; serves as clearinghouse of information on variety and quality of services offered; keeps abreast of educational, legislative, and public policy developments in reproductive health care. Provides referrals. **Pub:** A Clinician's Guide to Medical and Surgical Abortion. Book. • Clinical Training Curriculum in Abortion Practice. Curriculum for residency training, medical reference. **Price:** $130. • Unsure About Your Pregnancy? A Guide to Making the Right Decision for You. Bulletins. • Also publishes fact sheets, bulletins, and position papers on abortion, and resource materials for abortion praviders.

**★ 18340 ★ National Abortion Rights Action League (NARAL)**
1156 15th St. NW, Ste. 700
Washington, DC 20005
**Phone:** (202)973-3000     **Fax:** (202)973-3096
**Email:** comments@naral.org
**Website:** http://www.naral.org
Kate Michelman, Pres.

**Desc:** Politically involved in the pro-choice movement. Outspoken advocate of reproductive freedom and choice. Protects and preserves the right to choose.

Promotes policies and programs to improve women's health. Seeks to make abortion less necessary.

**★ 18341 ★ National Association of Ovulation Method Instructors UK**
Oakfield
Wineham Lane
Bolney
Haywards Heath RH17 5SD, United Kingdom
**Phone:** 44 1444 881744     **Fax:** 44 1444 881744

**Fnded:** 1977. **Lang(s):** English. **Desc:** Provides information on the Billings Ovulation Method of natural family planning; provides training for instructors. **Pub:** Resource List.

**★ 18342 ★ National Association of Postpartum Care Services**
c/o Peter Neuberg
800 Detroit St.
Denver, CO 80206
**Free:** 800-45-DOULA     **Fax:** (303)321-4058
**Email:** doulacare@aol.com
**Website:** http://www.napcs.org/
Peter Neuberg, Contact

**Desc:** Provides care services for women suffering from postpartum depression.

**National Board for Nursing, Midwifery and Health Visiting for Northern Ireland**
See: Entry 15744

**National Center for Education in Maternal and Child Health (NCEMCH)**
See: Entry 5720

**★ 18343 ★ National Commission on Human Life, Reproduction and Rhythm (NCHLRR)**
PO Box 101501
Pittsburgh, PA 15237
**Phone:** (724)444-8013     **Fax:** (412)369-4550
**Email:** info@ncemch.org
**Website:** http://www.ncemch.org
Dr. Brain W. Donnelly, MD, Sec. -Treas.

**Fnded:** 1967. **Mem:** 25. **Desc:** Physicians united to strengthen the family unit and support traditional concepts of marriage, sex, and life. Encourages physicians to place more emphasis on personal attention to patients and less emphasis on the prescribing of medication; promotes pro-life values. Conducts scientific meetings dealing with subjects including: the role of the mother, particularly during her child's first three years; sex education; natural family planning; obstetric delivery; breastfeeding; abortion. Sponsors public meetings. **Pub:** Child and Family, quarterly. Journal. Contains scientific and philosophical articles in support of the traditional family. Consists primarily of reprinted material. **Price:** $12/year; $16/year outside U.S. • Also publishes reprint booklets.

**★ 18344 ★ National Family Planning and Reproductive Health Association (NFPRHA)**
1627 K St. NW, 12th Fl.
Washington, DC 20006
**Phone:** (202)293-3114     **Fax:** (202)293-1990
**Email:** info@nfprha.org
**Website:** http://www.nfprha.org
Judith M. DeSarno, Pres.

**Fnded:** 1971. **Mem:** 1,000. **Desc:** Hospitals, state and city departments of health, health care providers, private nonprofit clinics, and consumers concerned with the maintenance and improvement of family planning and reproductive health services. Serves as a national communications network and advocacy organization. Maintains contact with Congress and government agencies in order to monitor government policy and regulations. **Pub:** NFPRHA Quart., quarterly. • NFPRHA Report. Reports on public policy affecting family planning and reproductive health. **Price:**

$200 for nonmembers. • Also publishes professional papers and educational materials. **Frmly:** (1979) National Family Planning Forum.

**★ 18345 ★ National Organization on Adolescent Pregnancy, Parenting and Prevention (NOAPP)**
2401 Pennsylvania Ave. NW, Ste. 350
Washington, DC 20037
**Phone:** (202)293-8370 **Fax:** (202)293-8805
**Email:** noappp@noappp.org
**Website:** http://www.noappp.org
Mary Martha Wilson, Acting Exec. Dir.
**Fnded:** 1979. **Mem:** 2,000. **Desc:** Professionals, policy makers, community and state leaders, and other concerned individuals and organizations. Promotes comprehensive and coordinated services designed for the prevention and resolution of problems associated with adolescent pregnancy, parenthood and prevention. Supports families in expanding their capability of nurturing children and setting standards that encourage their healthy development through loving, stable relationships. Programs include: providing advocacy services at local, state, and national levels for adolescent pregnancy issues; sharing information and promoting public awareness; conducting conferences, training institutes and workshops to encourage the establishment of effective programs; coalition building assistance. **Pub:** *NOAPPP Network Newsletter*, quarterly. Newsletter. Contains resource and research reviews, state highlights, legislative focus, and successful program models. **Frmly:** (1993) National Organization of Adolescent Pregnancy and Parenting.

**National Perinatal Information Center**
*See:* Entry 11504

**★ 18346 ★ New Zealand Family Planning Association (FPA)**
PO Box 11515
Wellington, New Zealand
**Phone:** 64 4 3844549 **Fax:** 64 4 3828356
**Email:** library@fpanz.org.nz
**Website:** http://www.fpanz.org.nz
**Fnded:** 1936. **Mem:** 300. **Nat'l Groups:** 1. **Reg. Groups:** 3. **State Groups:** 33. **Local Groups:** 12. **Lang(s):** English. **Desc:** Promotes a positive view of sexuality to enable people to make informed choices about their sexual health. Works to reduce the number of unintended pregnancies and abortions. Attempts to stop the spread of AIDS and other sexually transmitted diseases through education and contraceptive services. **Pub:** *Forum*, quarterly. Newsletter.

**★ 18347 ★ Nordic Association for Andrology (NAFA)**
c/o Aleksander Giwercman
University Department of Urology
Malmo University Hospital
SE 205 02 Malmo, Sweden
**Phone:** 46 40337904 **Fax:** 46 13282995
**Email:** aleksander.giwercman@kir.mas.lu.se
**Website:** http://www.ki.se/org/nafa/
**Desc:** Membership is for all physicians and researchers interested in Andrology. Provides a meeting place for Nordic researchers and physicians interested in Andrology. Activities include annual meetings, and courses.

**★ 18348 ★ Obstetrician Family Center (Centro Obstetrico Familiar — COF-Ecuado)**
Pasaje Trivino E4-261
AV. 12, de Octubre
Apartado 17-12434 CCNU
Pichincha
Quito, Ecuador
**Phone:** 593 2 226515 **Fax:** 593 2 226515
**Email:** cofqsld@ecnet.ec
**Fnded:** 1984. **Mem:** 79. **Nat'l Groups:** 13. **Local Groups:** 6. **Lang(s):** Spanish. **Desc:** Works to in-

crease public awareness of all aspects of sexuality and family life. Conducts educational and orientational programs for adolescents and parents on family planning, reproduction, sexuality, and family issues. Trains health care workers and family planning service providers. Investigates relevant topics and disseminates information. **Pub:** *Informe Anual*, annual. • *Manual del Promotor Juvenil Voluntario*. • *Manual Metodos Anticonceptivos*. Manual. • *Revista Boletin Informativo Bi Mensual*. **Frmly:** Centro Obstetrico Familiar COF.

**★ 18349 ★ Osterreichische Gesellschaft fur Familienplanung (OGF)**
Ignaz-Semmelweis-Frauenklinik
Bastiengasse 36-38
A-1180 Vienna, Austria
**Phone:** 43 1 4785242 **Fax:** 43 1 4708970
**Email:** e.pracht@oegf.at
**Website:** http://www.oegf.at
**Fnded:** 1966. **Mem:** 107. **Lang(s):** German. **Desc:** Works to improve the quality of life for individuals living in Austria by promoting family planning and responsible parenthood. Works to reduce the number of unwanted pregnancies and abortions and stop the spread of sexually transmitted diseases, especially AIDS. Provides programs in family planning, sex education, and health. Provides contraceptive services. Advocates for international aspects of reproductive and sexual health and rights among politicians and government officials. **Pub:** *Newsletter OEGF*, semiannual. Newsletter.

**★ 18350 ★ Panamanian Association for Planned Parenthood (Asociacion Panamena para el Planeamiento de la Familia — APLAFA)**
Apartado Postal Ste. 4637
Panama 5, Panama
**Phone:** 507 3170431 **Fax:** 507 2362979
**Email:** aplafa@orbi.net
**Fnded:** 1965. **Mem:** 100. **Reg. Groups:** 7. **Desc:** Fosters family values that include responsible parenting; educates the public about birth control options; conducts programs on health, children's concerns, and women in development.

**★ 18351 ★ Pathfinder International (PI)**
9 Galen St., Ste. 217
Watertown, MA 02472
**Phone:** (617)924-7200 **Fax:** (617)924-3833
**Email:** information@pathfind.org
**Website:** http://www.pathfind.org
Daniel E. Pellegrom, Pres.
**Fnded:** 1957. **Desc:** Established to find, demonstrate, and promote new and more efficient family planning programs in developing countries. Objectives are to introduce and expand the availability of effective family planning services; improve the welfare of families in developing countries; assist developing countries in implementing population policies favorable to national development. Conducts activities with a concern for upholding human rights, enhancing the status and role of women, and respecting the views of family planning clients. **Pub:** *Pathways*, semiannual. Newsletter. Provides information on programs and updates on services. • Annual Report, annual. **AKA:** PF.

**★ 18352 ★ Pathfinder International - Brazil (PI)**
Avenida Tancredo Neves 3343
Centro Empresarial Previnor
Torre B, Salas 606 a 609
41940-650 Salvador, Bahia, Brazil
**Phone:** 55 71 3413022
**Email:** claudari@pathfind.org
**Website:** http://www.pathfind.org/html/Worldwide/brazil_2.htm
**Lang(s):** Portuguese, Spanish. **Desc:** Makes available low- and no-cost family planning services to the needy. Promotes population control through educational programs involving youth; trains indigenous

people to sustain family planning services in their local areas.

**★ 18353 ★ Planned Parenthood Association of Sierra Leone (PPASL)**
45 Adelaide St.
PO Box 1094
Freetown, Sierra Leone
**Phone:** 232 22 22774 **Fax:** 232 22 22774
**Email:** ppasl@sierratel.sl
**Website:** http://www.popiu.org
**Fnded:** 1959. **Mem:** 750. **Lang(s):** English. **Desc:** Works to enhance the standard of living for individuals living in Sierra Leone by promoting family planning. Advocates family planning as a basic human right. Attempts to stop the spread of sexually transmitted diseases, especially AIDS. Offers programs in sex education, family planning, and health. Provides contraceptive and health care services. **Pub:** *PPASL News Letter*, semiannual. Newsletter. • Annual Report. • Reports. From baseline studies.

**★ 18354 ★ Planned Parenthood Association of South Africa (PPASA)**
PPASA National Office
31 Plantation Rd.
Auckland Park, Republic of South Africa
**Phone:** 27 11 4824601 **Fax:** 27 11 4824602
**Email:** ppasa@ppasa.org.za
**Website:** http://www.ppasa.org.za
**Fnded:** 1930. **Mem:** 180. **Reg. Groups:** 5. **Lang(s):** Afrikaans, English, Sotho, Tswana, Xhosa, Zulu. **Desc:** Encourages family planning activities in South Africa and promotes family planning as a basic human right. Works to: improve maternal and child health; reduce the incidence of unwanted pregnancy and abortion; address issues related to adolescent sexuality and teen pregnancy; increase public knowledge of the prevention of AIDS and other sexually transmitted diseases; increase societal awareness of the relationship between population growth, natural resource consumption, and the conservation of the environment. Coordinates information, education, and training programs on sexual responsibility and reproductive health. Conducts research. **Pub:** *Aids Scan*, quarterly. Also publishes *Responsible Teenage Sexuality* (book).

**★ 18355 ★ Planned Parenthood Association of Thailand (PPAT)**
8 Soi Vibhavadi-Rangsit 44
Vibhavadi-Rangsit Super Hwy.
Lard-Yao, Chatuchak
Bangkok 19000, Thailand
**Phone:** 66 2 9412320 **Fax:** 66 2 9412338
**Email:** ppat@samart.co.th
**Fnded:** 1970. **Mem:** 655. **Lang(s):** Thai. **Desc:** Works to improve the quality of life for people living in Thailand by promoting responsible parenthood and family planning. Attempts to reduce the number of unwanted pregnancies and abortions. Offers programs in sex education, family planning, and health. Provides contraceptive and health care services. Conducts research. **Pub:** *PPAT News/Sarn Samphan Newsletter*, bimonthly. Newsletter. Explains PPAT activities.

**★ 18356 ★ Planned Parenthood Federation of America (PPFA)**
810 7th Ave.
New York, NY 10019
**Phone:** (212)541-7800 **Fax:** (212)245-1845
**Email:** communications@ppfa.org
**Website:** http://www.plannedparenthood.org/
Gloria Feldt, Pres.
**Fnded:** 1916. **Reg. Groups:** 169. **Desc:** Organizations providing leadership in making effective means of voluntary fertility regulation, including contraception, abortion, sterilization, and infertility services, available and fully accessible to all as a central element of reproductive health; stimulating and sponsoring relevant biomedical, socioeconomic, and demographic

research; developing appropriate information, education, and training programs to increase knowledge about human reproduction and sexuality. Supports and assists efforts to achieve similar goals worldwide. Operates more than 900 centers that provide medically supervised reproductive health services and educational programs. **Pub:** Annual Report. • Books. • Pamphlets. **AKA:** Planned Parenthood; Planned Parenthood/World Population. **Frmly:** (1939) American Birth Control League.

★ **18357 ★ Planned Parenthood Federation of Canada (PPFC) (Federation pour le planning des naissances du Canada — FPNC)**
1 Nicholas St., Ste. 430
Ottawa, ON, Canada K1N 7B7
**Phone:** (613)241-4474          **Fax:** (613)241-7550
**Email:** admin@ppfc.ca
**Website:** http://www.ppfc.ca
**Fnded:** 1964. **Mem:** 26. **State Groups:** 6. **Local Groups:** 63. **Lang(s):** English, French. **Desc:** Promotes family planning and responsible parenthood. Encourages public awareness of contraceptive methods and the need for family planning. Works to reduce the number of unwanted pregnancies and abortions. Sponsors programs in family planning, sex education, and sexually transmitted diseases, especially AIDS. Provides contraceptive services. Acts as an advocate for family planning issues on a national level. Conducts research. **Pub:** *Beyond the Basics: A Sourcebook for Sexual and Reproductive Health Education.* Book. • *Youth Talk Back: Sex, Sexuality and Media Literacy.* Book. High school textbook that explores sociological issues related to sex, sexuality in the context of media literacy.

★ **18358 ★ Planned Parenthood Federation - Korea (PPFK)**
121-146 Dangsandong 6-GA
Youngdeungpo-Ku
Seoul 150-650, Republic of Korea
**Phone:** 82 2 6348211          **Fax:** 82 2 4678217
**Email:** ppkf@unitel.co.kr
**Fnded:** 1961. **Local Groups:** 12. **Lang(s):** English, Korean. **Desc:** Family planning professionals in the Republic of Korea. Seeks to enhance the quality of life of Koreans by promoting family planning and improving maternal and infant health care. Encourages "culturally, economically, and socially healthy" families. Conducts educational programs for military personnel, industrial workers, students, and other groups; disseminates family planning information through mass media. Operates clinics, audio visual materials development center, and 10 sections. **Pub:** *Happy Home*, monthly. Magazine. • *PPFK Annual Report.*

★ **18359 ★ Planned Parenthood Federation of Nigeria (PPFN)**
224 Ikorodu Rd.
Palmgrove
Somolu
PMB 12657
Lagos, Lagos, Nigeria
**Phone:** 234 1 820945          **Fax:** 234 1 7595580
**Email:** ppfn@rcl.nig.com
**Website:** http://www.ippf.org
**Fnded:** 1964. **Mem:** 3,000. **Nat'l Groups:** 1. **State Groups:** 30. **Local Groups:** 80. **Lang(s):** English. **Desc:** Works to improve the quality of life for individuals living in Nigeria by promoting responsible parenthood and family planning. Advocates family planning as a basic human right. Attempts to stop the spread of AIDS and other sexually transmitted diseases. Offers programs in sex education, family planning, and health. Provides contraceptive and health care services. **Pub:** *Planned News*, semiannual. Newsletter. **Frmly:** (1979) Family Planning Council of Nigeria.

★ **18360 ★ Pre-Eclamptic Toxaemia Society**
c/o Dawn James
Rhianfa
Caernarfon LLS4 7RL, United Kingdom
**Phone:** 44 1286 882685
**Email:** dawnjames@clara.co.uk
**Website:** http://www.dawnjames.clara.net
**Fnded:** 1981. **Mem:** 500. **Desc:** Provides self help and support groups for those suffering or having suffered from pre-eclampsia.

★ **18361 ★ Pro Familia: Deutsche Gesellschaft fur Familienplanung, Sexualpadagogik und Sexualberatung**
Stresemannallee 3
D-60596 Frankfurt am Main, Germany
**Phone:** 49 69 639002          **Fax:** 49 69 639852
**Email:** info@profamilia.de
**Website:** http://www.profamilia.de
**Fnded:** 1952. **Mem:** 5,800. **Nat'l Groups:** 1. **Reg. Groups:** 16. **Local Groups:** 150. **Lang(s):** German. **Desc:** Promotes family planning as a basic human right. Works to reduce the number of unwanted pregnancies and abortions. Attempts to stop the spread of AIDS and other sexually transmitted diseases through education and contraceptive services. Sponsors programs in family planning, sex education, and health. Conducts research.

★ **18362 ★ Pro Familia Hungarian Scientific Society (HSSFWW)**
Keleti Karoly utca 5-7
H-1024 Budapest, Hungary
**Phone:** 36 1 3165517          **Fax:** 36 1 3165517
**Email:** mcsnt@mataynet.hu
**Website:** http://www.szexinfo.hu
**Fnded:** 1975. **Mem:** 900. **Lang(s):** English, French, Hungarian. **Desc:** Advocates family planning as a basic human right. Encourages public awareness of family planning and responsible parenthood. Works to reduce the number of unwanted pregnancies and abortions. Offers programs in sex education, family planning, and health care.

★ **18363 ★ Pro-Choice Defense League (PCDL)**
1324 Motor Pky.
Hauppauge, NY 11788-5226
**Phone:** (516)538-2626
Bill Baird, Dir.
**Fnded:** 1984. **Mem:** 300. **Desc:** Individuals seeking to protect reproductive freedom of choice. Serves as forum for information on reproductive rights. Sponsors public education programs and workshops; conducts training sessions for abortion clinic operators on methods of securing facilities against violence and harassment. **Pub:** Newsletter, periodic. • Also publishes pamphlets.

★ **18364 ★ Religious Coalition for Abortion Rights (RCAR)**
100 Maryland Ave.,NE, Ste. 307
Washington, DC 20002
**Website:** http://www.holysmoke.org/fem/fem0288.htm
**Fnded:** 1973. **Desc:** Coalition of varying faith groups committed to the preservation of religious liberty in relation to reproductive freedom. Advocates that the abortion decision must ultimately remain with the individual. Strives to preserve reproductive and religious freedom through state affiliation, communications, women of color partnership, and legislation.

★ **18365 ★ Reproductive Health Programme - Asia (RHPA)**
Bagdat Cadessi 225/6
Ciftehavuzlar
Istanbul, Turkey
**Phone:** 90 216 3551173          **Fax:** 90 216 3635961

**Lang(s):** English, Turkish. **Desc:** Health care and development organizations. Promotes increased access to quality reproductive health care for previously underserved populations. Makes available health services; provides support and assistance to vocational training, nutrition, and public health programs.

★ **18366 ★ Reproductive Health Programme - Vietnam (RHPV)**
138 A Giang Vo St.
Hanoi, Vietnam
**Phone:** 84 4 430283          **Fax:** 84 4 430487
**Lang(s):** English, French, Vietnamese. **Desc:** Health care and development organizations. Promotes increased access to quality reproductive health care for previously underserved populations. Makes available health services; provides support and assistance to vocational training, nutrition, and public health programs.

**Reproductive Toxicology Center (RTC)**
*See:* Entry 8926

★ **18367 ★ Resolve, The National Infertility Association**
1310 Broadway
Somerville, MA 02144-1779
**Phone:** (617)623-1156          **Free:** 888-623-0744
**Fax:** (617)623-0252
**Email:** info@resolve.org
**Website:** http://www.resolve.org
Joan Bowen, Exec. Dir.
**Fnded:** 1974. **Mem:** 15,000. **Local Groups:** 56. **Desc:** Persons with problems of infertility and associated professionals who work with infertile couples such as adoption workers, physicians, and counselors. Seeks to provide "timely, compassionate support and information to people who are experiencing infertility, and to increase awareness of infertility issues." Offers information, referral, and support to persons with problems of infertility; conducts issue advocacy and public education programs. **Pub:** *Resolve National Newsletter*, quarterly. Newsletter. Provides information on medical, emotional, and legislative issues, and upcoming conferences. Includes book reviews, research reports, and letters. *Price:* Included in membership dues; $4/issue for nonmembers. • *Resolving Infertility*. Book. • Bibliography. • Brochure. • Also publishes fact sheets and briefs. **Frmly:** (1999) RESOLVE.

★ **18368 ★ Royal College of Obstetricians and Gynaecologists**
27 Sussex Pl.
Regent's Park
London NW1 4RG, United Kingdom
**Fax:** 44 207 7230575
**Email:** pbarnett@rcog.org.uk
**Website:** http://www.rcog.org.uk
**Fnded:** 1929. **Mem:** 10,324. **Desc:** Obstetricians and gynecologists, having completed a period of training recognised by the College and passed all components of the MRCOG examination. The encouragement of the study and the improvement of the practice of obstetrics and gynaecology. This is achieved by running examinations, postgraduate meetings, publications, committees and working parties. **Pub:** *British Journal of Obstetrics and Gynaecology*, monthly. Journal. • *Journal for Continuing Professional Development from the Royal College of Obstetricians and Gynaecologists*. Journal. • *The Obstetrician and Gynaecologist*, quarterly.

★ **18369 ★ Russian Family Planning Association**
18/20 Vadkovsky Per.
101479 Moscow, Russia
**Phone:** 7 95 9731559          **Fax:** 7 95 9731917
**Email:** rfpa@dol.ru
**Website:** http://www.family-planning.ru

**Fnded:** 1991. **Mem:** 4,000. **Lang(s):** Russian. **Desc:** Advocates family planning and responsible parenthood as a basic human right and as a means to enhance the quality of life. Works to reduce the number of unwanted pregnancies and abortions. Attempts to stop the spread of AIDS and other sexually transmitted diseases. Offers programs in sex education, family planning, and health. Provides contraceptive and health care services. Conducts research. **Pub:** *Family Planning*, quarterly. Magazine. Provides information on family planning, contraception, and sex education. Also publishes books, brochures, booklets, and posters.

★ **18370** ★ **St. Lucia Planned Parenthood Association (SLPPA)**
83 Chaussee Rd.
Castries, St. Lucia
**Phone:** (758)452-4335     **Fax:** (758)453-7284
**Email:** parenthood@candw.lc
**Website:** http://www.ippfwhr.org/
**Fnded:** 1967. **Mem:** 6. **Lang(s):** English. **Desc:** Encourages responsible parenthood and family planning as a means to improve quality of life for people in St. Lucia. Advocates family planning as a basic human right. Provides health care and contraceptive services. Conducts research.

★ **18371** ★ **Sidelines National High-Risk Pregnancy Support Network**
PO Box 1808
Laguna Beach, CA 92652
**Phone:** (949)497-2265     **Free:** 888-447-4754
**Fax:** (949)497-5598
**Email:** sidelines@sidelines.org
**Website:** http://www.sidelines.org
Candace Hurley, Exec. Dir.
**Fnded:** 1992. **Mem:** 20,000. **Reg. Groups:** 32. **Desc:** Former high-risk mothers dedicated to supporting women and their families experiencing a complicated or high-risk pregnancy. A pregnancy is termed "complicated" when the life or health of the mother and/or baby may be at risk. Committed to helping women overcome the risks of preterm birth, low birthweight, and other serious consequences of high risk pregnancies. Operates the One-On-One program where a mother and her family are paired with a trained "Phone Friend" who has previously been through a complicated pregnancy. Offers prenatal care information and grief and loss counseling. Provides the families with resources and referrals to local businesses, agencies, and services that can assist them. **Pub:** *Left Side Lines*, annual. Magazine. *Price:* $3.50 for hospitals, physicians and patients. • *Sidelines Parent Pack.* Book. *Price:* $15. • *That's What Friends Are For.* Guide for helping the bedresting mom and her family. • *When Pregnancy Isn't Perfect. Price:* $12. **Frmly:** (2002) Sidelines National Support Network.

★ **18372** ★ **Singapore Planned Parenthood Association (SPPA)**
Blk. 3A Holland Close
No. 01-55
Singapore 272003, Singapore
**Phone:** 65 7758981     **Fax:** 65 7768296
**Email:** sppassn@singnet.com.sg
**Fnded:** 1949. **Mem:** 154. **Lang(s):** English. **Desc:** Promotes family planning as a basic human right and as a means to improve the quality of life for people living in Singapore. Works to reduce the number of unwanted pregnancies and abortions. Offers programs in sex education, family planning, and health. Provides contraceptive services. Acts as an advocate for family planning on a national level. **Pub:** *Monthly News Bulletin*, bimonthly. • Report, annual. • Newsletter, biweekly. **Frmly:** (1986) Family Planning Association of Singapore.

★ **18373** ★ **Slovak Society for Family Planning and Parenthood Education (SSPRVR)**
Ruzinovska 1
SK-82102 Bratislava, Slovakia
**Phone:** 42 17 43423880     **Fax:** 42 17 43423880
**Email:** ssprv@nextra.sk
**Website:** http://www.rodicovstvo.sk
**Fnded:** 1990. **Mem:** 310. **Lang(s):** English, Slovak. **Desc:** National branch of the International Planned Parenthood Federation. Promotes family planning and facilitates access to reproductive health services; works to ensure responsible parenthood. Conducts educational programs on population control, family planning, parenthood, and reproductive health. Operates family planning center. **Pub:** *Empatia*, quarterly. Journal.

★ **18374** ★ **Societatea de Educatie Contraceptiva si Sexuala (SECS)**
Calea 13 Septembrie 85
B1.77c, sc1, et8, ap75, Sector 5
R-76100 Bucharest, Romania
**Phone:** 40 1 41011081     **Fax:** 40 1 4101097
**Email:** secs@starnets.ro
**Fnded:** 1990. **Mem:** 1,027. **Reg. Groups:** 32. **Lang(s):** Romanian. **Desc:** Works to improve the quality of life for individuals living in Romania by promoting responsible parenthood and family planning. Attempts to reduce the number of unwanted pregnancies and abortions. Offers programs in family planning, sex education, and health. Acts as an advocate for family planning on a national level. **Pub:** *Newsletter*, quarterly. Newsletter.

★ **18375** ★ **Society for Assisted Reproductive Technology (SART)**
c/o American Society for Reproductive Medicine
1209 Montgomery Ave.
Birmingham, AL 35216-2809
**Phone:** (205)978-5000     **Fax:** (205)978-5015
**Email:** jzeitz@asrm.org
**Website:** http://www.sart.org
Joyce Zeitz, Exec. Admin.
**Fnded:** 1987. **Mem:** 370. **Desc:** Institutions conducting assisted reproductive procedures. Works to extend knowledge of human in vitro fertilization techniques. Conducts educational programs; gathers and disseminates information and outcome statistics on art.

★ **18376** ★ **Society for Education on Contraception and Sexuality (SECS)**
str. Paleologu 4, PO 20
R-70273 Bucharest, Romania
**Phone:** 40 1 3126693     **Fax:** 40 1 3127088
**Fnded:** 1990. **Lang(s):** English, Romanian. **Desc:** Family planning organizations and health care personnel. Promotes universal access to family planning services. Serves as liaison linking members with government agencies responsible for public reproductive health and population programs; conducts continuing professional education courses for health care practitioners.

★ **18377** ★ **Society for Prevention of Infertility (SPI)**
877 Park Ave.
New York, NY 10021
**Phone:** (212)288-3737     **Free:** 888-373-2229
**Fax:** (212)744-6536
**Email:** frfbaby@msn.com
**Website:** http://www.frfbaby.com
Masood A. Khatamee, Exec. Dir.
**Fnded:** 1990. **Mem:** 500. **Desc:** Physicians specializing in obstetrics and gynecology; scientists representing public and private teaching hospitals, medical school faculties, and university research departments; practitioners who work with infertile men and women. Objectives are to: study sexually transmitted infectious diseases (STDs) and their effects on human fertility; reduce the incidence of infection and the possibility of

resulting infertility. Coordinates and encourages research that can lead to successful forms of treatment and control of STDs, thus enhancing the opportunities for childless couples to achieve intrauterine pregnancies and bear healthy children. Encourages the exchange of information among those involved in research on and treatment of STDs. Designs educational and informational strategies intended for the prevention of infertility. **Frmly:** (1991) International Society of Infectious Diseases and Human Infertility.

★ **18378** ★ **Society for Reproductive Endocrinology and Infertility**
c/o American Society for Reproductive Medicine
1209 Montgomery Hwy.
Birmingham, AL 35216-2809
**Phone:** (205)978-5000     **Fax:** (205)978-5005
**Email:** apitman@asrm.org
**Website:** http://www.socrei.org
Angelia Pitman, Admin.
**Fnded:** 1984. **Mem:** 810. **Desc:** Medical doctors with American Board of Obstetrics and Gynecology subspecialty certification as reproductive endocrinologists. Works to extend knowledge of human reproduction and endocrinology; makes available to members continuing education programs. Conducts seminars. **Pub:** *SREI Feedback*, quarterly. Newsletter. Includes Information for members on SREI activities.

**Society of Reproductive Surgeons (SRS)**
*See:* Entry 19601

★ **18379** ★ **Society for the Study of Reproduction (SSR)**
1619 Monroe St.
Madison, WI 53711-2021
**Phone:** (608)256-2777     **Fax:** (608)256-4610
**Email:** ssr@ssr.org
**Website:** http://www.ssr.org
Geula Gibori, Pres.
**Fnded:** 1967. **Mem:** 2,400. **Desc:** Researchers in obstetrics and gynecology, urology, zoology, animal husbandry, and physiology; clinicians in human and veterinary medicine. Purposes are to promote the study of reproduction by fostering interdisciplinary communication within the science. **Pub:** *Biology of Reproduction*, monthly, plus one supplement per year. Journal. Includes peer-reviewed scientific research in the field of reproductive biology. *Price:* $400 U.S.; $435 non U.S. • *Biology of Reproduction Monograph Series 1: Equine Reproduction VI.* Monograph.

★ **18380** ★ **Solomon Islands Planned Parenthood Association (SIPPA)**
PO Box 554
Lombi Cress
Honiara, Solomon Islands
**Phone:** 677 22991     **Fax:** 677 23653
**Fnded:** 1981. **Mem:** 9. **Lang(s):** English. **Desc:** Advocates family planning as a basic human right and as a means to enhance the standard of living for individuals living in the Solomon Islands. Work to stop the spread of sexually transmitted diseases such as AIDS. Offers programs in sex education, family planning, and health. Provides contraceptive services. Conducts research. **Pub:** Video.

★ **18381** ★ **Swedish Association for Sexuality Education (RFSU) (Riksforbundet for Sexuell Upplysning)**
PO Box 121 28
SE-102 24 Stockholm, Sweden
**Phone:** 46 8 6920700     **Fax:** 46 8 6530823
**Email:** staffan.uddeholt@rfsu.se
**Website:** http://www.rfsu.se
**Fnded:** 1933. **Lang(s):** Swedish. **Desc:** Promotes family planning as a basic human right. Works to reduce the number of unwanted pregnancies and abortions. Attempts to stop the spread of AIDS and other sexually transmitted diseases. Offers programs in sex education, youth sexuality, sexual and repro-

ductive health. Provides contraceptive and health care services. Conducts research.

**★ 18382 ★ Swiss Foundation for Sexual and Reproductive Health**
9, avenue de Beaulieu
case postale 313
CH-1000 Lausanne 9, Switzerland
**Phone:** 41 21 6612233      **Fax:** 41 21 6612234
**Email:** info@plan-s.ch
**Website:** http://www.plan-s.ch
**Fnded:** 1993. **Mem:** 200. **Lang(s):** French, German. **Desc:** Promotes family planning and responsible parenthood as a means to improve the quality of life for individuals in Switzerland. Advocates family planning as a basic human right. Works to reduce the number of unwanted pregnancies and abortions. Coordinates members' activities; conducts research. **Pub:** *Info-Bulletin*, periodic. Newsletter.

**★ 18383 ★ Tonga Family Planning Association (TFPA)**
PO Box 1142
Nuku'alofa, Tonga
**Phone:** 676 21209      **Fax:** 676 23766
**Email:** fpatonga@kailanet.to
**Lang(s):** English, Tongan. **Desc:** Advocates family planning and responsible parenthood as a means to enhance the quality of life for individuals living in Tonga. Promotes family planning as a basic human right. Works to stop the spread of AIDS and other sexually transmitted diseases. Offers programs in sex education, family planning, and health. Provides contraceptive and health care services. Conducts research.

**★ 18384 ★ Vietnam Family Planning Association (VINAFPA)**
138A Giang Vo
Hanoi, Vietnam
**Phone:** 84 4 247231      **Fax:** 84 4 247232
**Email:** vinafpa@netnam.org.vn
**Fnded:** 1993. **Mem:** 16,469. **Local Groups:** 42. **Lang(s):** English, French, Vietnamese. **Desc:** National affiliate of the International Planned Parenthood Federation. Provides counseling, services and training programs to complement the activities of existing family planning and reproductive health services; facilitates local control of ongoing family planning initiatives. **Pub:** *Family*, biweekly. Magazine.

**★ 18385 ★ Women With Disabilities - Australia**
PO Box 605
Rosny Park, TAS 7018, Australia
**Phone:** 61 3 62448288      **Fax:** 61 3 62448255
**Email:** wwda@ozemail.com.au
**Website:** http://www.wwda.org.au
**Fnded:** 1995. **Mem:** 1,700. **Nat'l Groups:** 1. **State Groups:** 7. **Desc:** Works for equality in participation and opportunity for disabled women. **Pub:** *WWDA News*, quarterly. Newsletter. Reports and information resources.

**Women's Health**
*See:* Entry 2439

**★ 18386 ★ World Organisation Ovulation Method Billings (WOOMB)**
27 Alexandra Parade
North Fitzroy, VIC 3068, Australia
**Phone:** 61 3 94811722      **Fax:** 61 3 94824208
**Email:** billings@ozemail.com.au
**Website:** http://www.woomb.org
**Desc:** Works to research, study, and evaluate the female ovulation cycle and its direct relation to reproductive medicine. Disseminates information on natural family planning. **Pub:** Bulletin, quarterly.

**★ 18387 ★ Yemen Family Care Association (YFCA)**
PO Box 795
Sana'a, Yemen
**Phone:** 967 1 288145      **Fax:** 967 1 270948
**Email:** yfca@y.net.ye
**Fnded:** 1976. **Mem:** 500. **Lang(s):** Arabic, English. **Desc:** Volunteer association which provides services for the mother, the child, and in the field of family planning, especially in poor under-served areas. Works to spread reproductive health culture within the society, especially among women and young people. In addition, the association works to increase the number of volunteers and to improve the quality of services and the expertise of staff and volunteers. **Pub:** *Al Osra*, bimonthly. Newsletter.

**★ 18388 ★ Zimbabwe National Family Planning Council (ZNFPC)**
c/o Harare Hospital Grounds
Spilhaus Centre
Harare Hospital Grounds
CNR Highfield Rd., Swiss Way
PO Box 220, Southerton
Harare, Zimbabwe
**Phone:** 263 4 620281      **Fax:** 263 4 620280
**Email:** znfpc@internet.co.zw
**Fnded:** 1957. **Lang(s):** English. **Desc:** Promotes family planning and responsible parenthood as a means to improve the quality of life for individuals living in Zimbabwe. Advocates family planning as a basic human right. Works to reduce the number of unwanted pregnancies and abortions. Offers programs in family planning, sex education and health. Provides contraceptive and health care services. Conducts research. **Pub:** *ZNFPC Newsletter*. Annual Report. Also publishes a variety of materials for the general public, clients, service providers, and policy makers. **Frmly:** (1985) Child Spacing and Fertility Association.

# Research Centers

**★ 18389 ★ Baylor College of Medicine Center for Population Research and Studies in Reproduction**
Department of Cell Biology
Houston, TX 77030
**Phone:** (713)798-6200      **Fax:** (713)790-1275
Dr. Bert W. O'Malley, Chm.
**Activities/Fields:** Human reproduction, including studies on mechanism of hormone action, male reproduction, steroid regulation and protein synthesis, spermatogenesis, reproductive endocrinology, nucleic acid chemistry and genetic expression, steroid hormonal receptors, physical chemistry, cell proliferation and regulation, biochemistry of chromatin, ribonucleic acid, deoxyribonucleic acid, and cell biology.

**★ 18390 ★ Center for Biomedical Research**
Population Council
1230 York Ave.
New York, NY 10021
**Phone:** (212)327-8717      **Fax:** (212)327-7678
**Email:** e-johansson@popcbr.rockefeller.edu
Dr. Elof Johansson, Contact
**Activities/Fields:** Physiology of human reproduction, especially the male reproductive system, including studies on gametogenesis, sperm ultrastructure, steroid receptors, hormone action, and testicular function. Contraceptive development includes studies on subdermal implants, the contraceptive ring, the levonorgestrel-releasing intrauterine device, and a male hormonal contraceptive. Health issues research relates to current and potential contraceptive methods, hormone replacement therapy, and microbicides that prevent sexually transmitted diseases.

**★ 18391 ★ Center for Research on Population and Security**
PO Box 13067
Research Triangle Park, NC 27709
**Phone:** (919)933-7491      **Fax:** (919)933-0348
**Email:** smumford@mindspring.com
**Website:** http://www.population-security.org
Stephen D. Mumford, Pres.
**Activities/Fields:** Population growth control, contraceptive method research, including international clinical trial technical support, and the relationship between population growth and national and global security.

**★ 18392 ★ Collaborative Center for Reproduction**
Walter Martin Research Bldg., RB-1
1124 W Carson St.
Torrance, CA 90509
**Phone:** (310)222-1867      **Fax:** (310)533-0627
**Email:** swerdloff@gcrc.rei.edu
Dr. Ronald S. Swerdloff, Dir.
**Activities/Fields:** Overpopulation, infertility, and aging through analysis of endocrinology, physiology, pathology, and molecular biology of the reproductive system.

**★ 18393 ★ Contraceptive Research and Development Program (CONRAD)**
1611 N Kent St., Ste. 806
Arlington, VA 22209
**Phone:** (703)524-4744      **Fax:** (703)524-4770
**Email:** info@conrad.org
**Website:** http://www.conrad.org
Henry L. Gabelnick, PhD, Dir.
**Activities/Fields:** Improvement of contraception methods and reproductive health, especially for use in developing countries; further development of contraceptive choices for women and men and to help prevent the transmission of HIV/AIDS and other sexually transmitted diseases (STDs).

**★ 18394 ★ Cornell University Pregnancy and Newborn Research Laboratory**
T9-020 Veterinary Research Tower
Ithaca, NY 14853
**Phone:** (607)253-3082      **Fax:** (607)253-3455
**Email:** pwn1@cornell.edu
Peter W. Nathanielsz, Dir.
**Activities/Fields:** Development of the animal fetus and newborn for application in human development. **Pub:** *Five-year report*.

**★ 18395 ★ Family Health International (FHI)**
PO Box 13950
Research Triangle Park, NC 27709
**Phone:** (919)544-7040      **Fax:** (919)544-7261
**Email:** brobinson@fhi.org
**Website:** http://www.fhi.org
Dr. Willard Cates, Jr., Pres.
**Activities/Fields:** New contraceptive technology, contraceptive acceptability, contraceptive effectiveness and safety, breast-feeding practices, maternal/child health, demography, interventions to reduce the transmission of sexually transmitted diseases and AIDS, economics of family planning and financing of AIDS programming. Operates the Implementing AIDS Prevention and Care (IMPACT) Project, which seeks to support the local capacity of developing countries to prevent and control HIV. **Pub:** *IMPACT on HIV Journal*, semiannually. • *Network Newsletter*, quarterly.

**★ 18396 ★ Fertility Research Foundation**
877 Park Ave.
New York, NY 10021
**Phone:** (212)744-5500      **Fax:** (212)744-6536
**Email:** frfbaby@msn.com

**Website:** http://www.frfbaby.com
Dr. Masood Khatamee, Exec. Dir.

**Activities/Fields:** Fertility and human reproduction, including studies on microsurgery, fertilization, fallopian tube transplant, artificial embryonation, education and prevention of human infertility, in vitro fertilization gender planning, therapeutic donor insemination, and counselling. **Pub:** *Infertility Journal.*

★ 18397 ★ **Georgetown University**
**Institute for Reproductive Health (IRH)**
3PHC, Rm. 3004
3800 Reservoir Rd. NW
Washington, DC 20007
**Phone:** (202)687-1392          **Fax:** (202)687-6846
**Website:** http://www.irh.org/
Victoria H. Jennings, PhD, Prin. Investigator

**Activities/Fields:** Reproductive health care, especially natural family planning (NFP) and fertility awareness (FA) practices.

★ 18398 ★ **Jones Institute for**
**Reproductive Medicine**
601 Colley Ave.
Norfolk, VA 23507
**Phone:** (757)446-7100          **Fax:** (757)876-6317
**Website:** http://www.jonesinstitute.org
Dr. William Gibbons, Chm.

**Activities/Fields:** Human reproduction, including studies of reproductive physiology during the hours and days surrounding fertilization, fertilization process, gametogenesis, neuroendocrinology, ovarian follicular development, gene expression, reproductive toxicology, endocrine control of menstrual cycle, andrology, reproductive immunology, and cancer.

★ 18399 ★ **Laval University**
**Research Centre on the Biology of**
**Reproduction**
Cite Universite
Sainte Foy, QC, Canada G1K 7P4
**Phone:** (418)656-5229          **Fax:** (418)654-3766
**Website:** http://www.crbr.ulaval.ca
Marc-Andre Sirard, PhD, Dir.

**Activities/Fields:** Physiological, cellular, and molecular factors leading to the production of viable embryos, male infertility and contraception, sexual differentiation, implantation and the maintenance of pregnancy. Focuses on the development and applications of new reproductive techniques for domestic animals and humans. **Frmly:** Ontogeny and Reproduction Research Group.

★ 18400 ★ **Laval University**
**Saint-Francois-d'Assise Hospital Research**
**Centre**
10, Rue de l'Espinay
Quebec, QC, Canada G1L 3L5
**Phone:** (418)525-4461          **Fax:** (418)525-4481
**Email:** Jean-Claude.Forest@bcx.ulaval.ca
**Website:** http://www.crsfa.ulaval.ca
Dr. Jean-Claude Forest, Dir.

**Activities/Fields:** Reproductive endocrinology, perinatalogy, human genetics, biomaterials, magnetic resonance, and biotechnology.

★ 18401 ★ **Laval University**
**Saint-Francois-d'Assise Hospital Research**
**Centre**
**Reproductive Endocrinology Unit**
10, Rue de l'Espinay
Quebec, QC, Canada G1L 3L5
**Phone:** (418)525-4461          **Fax:** (418)525-4481
**Email:** andre.lemay@ogy.ulaval.ca
**Website:** http://www.crsfa.ulaval.ca
Dr. André Lemay, Ch.

**Activities/Fields:** New medical treatments of acne and hirstism (polycystic ovarian diseaese PCO), new modalities of hormonal replacement therapy for meno-

pause, and basic research on growth and immune factors implicated in endometriosis.

**Massachusetts General Hospital**
**Reproductive Endocrine Unit**
*See:* Entry 8757

★ 18402 ★ **McGill University**
**McGill Centre for the Study of**
**Reproduction**
Department of Obstetrics & Gynecology
Woman's Pavilion, Royal Victoria Hospital
687 Pine Ave. W
Montreal, QC, Canada H3A 1A1
**Phone:** (514)842-1231          **Fax:** (514)843-1662
**Email:** beryl.rodrigues@muhc.mcgill.ca
**Website:** http://www.go-testing.com
Beryl Rodriguez, Exec. Sec.

**Activities/Fields:** Reproduction, including gametogenesis, fertilization, fetal development, pregnancy, parturition, and structure and function of the brain/pituitary/gonadal axis andbrain/pituitary/testicular/epididymal axis. Activities include studies of oogenesis, assisted reproductive technology (IVF), follicle development, genomic imprinting, testicular and epididmal physiology, reproductive toxicology, fetal growth, reproductive neuroscience. **Pub:** *Annual Report.*

★ 18403 ★ **Northwestern University**
**Center for Reproductive Science**
2-171 Hogan Hall
2153 N Campus Dr.
Evanston, IL 60208-3520
**Phone:** (847)491-4464          **Fax:** (847)491-5211
**Email:** n-schwartz@northwestern.edu
**Website:** http://www.northwestern.edu/center-for-reproductive-science
Neena B. Schwartz, Dir.

**Activities/Fields:** Reproductive biology, focusing on the regulation of ovarian synthesis and secretion of steroid and peptide hormones on the metabolic pathways and messengers within ovarian structures; regulation of testicular development, secretion of spermatogenesis, and the regulation of synthesis and secretion of the pituitary gonadotropic hormones and prolactin, as well as their actions on the brain, gonads, and breast tissue; and interactions of neural tissue in the brain and spinal cord with the pituitary-gonadal axis.

★ 18404 ★ **Pope Paul VI Institute for the**
**Study of Human Reproduction, Inc.**
6901 Mercy Rd.
Omaha, NE 68106-2604
**Phone:** (402)390-6600          **Fax:** (402)390-9851
**Email:** popepaul@mitec.net
**Website:** http://www.popepaulvi.com
Dr. Thomas W. Hilgers, Dir.

**Activities/Fields:** Human reproduction and Down's Syndrome.

★ 18405 ★ **Population Council**
1 Dag Hammarskjold Plz.
New York, NY 10017
**Phone:** (212)339-0500          **Fax:** (212)755-6052
**Email:** pubinfo@popcouncil.org
**Website:** http://www.popcouncil.org
Linda G. Martin, Pres.

**Activities/Fields:** Biomedical, social science, and public health research. Analyzes demographic trends; conducts biomedical research to understand human reproductive physiology more fully, leading to development of new contraceptives and reproductive health products; works with public and private agencies to promote client-centered reproductive health services of high quality; helps governments design and implement population and development policies; communicates the results of research in the population field; and helps build research capacities in developing countries. **Pub:** *Annual report.* • *Fact books,* quarterly. • *Newsletter,* bimonthly. • *Population and Develop-*

*ment Review,* quarterly. • *Studies in Family Planning,* bimonthly.

**Reproductive Toxicology Center**
*See:* Entry 17369

★ 18406 ★ **Society for Menstrual Cycle**
**Research**
10559 N 104th Pl.
Scottsdale, AZ 85258
**Phone:** (480)451-9731          **Fax:** (480)451-9731
**Email:** fmanna@qwest.net
**Website:** http://www.pop.psu.edu/smcr
Mary Anna Friederich, MD, Contact

**Activities/Fields:** Women's menstrual cycles, including endocrinology, genetics, physiology, psychology, medicine, sociology, and research, focusing on menstrual cycle networking and the health needs of women. **Pub:** *Newsletter,* semiannually. • *Proceedings,* biennially.

★ 18407 ★ **Society for the Study of**
**Reproduction**
1619 Monroe St.
Madison, WI 53711-2063
**Phone:** (608)256-2777          **Fax:** (608)256-4610
**Email:** ssr@ssr.org
**Website:** http://www.ssr.org
Geula Gibori, Pres.

**Activities/Fields:** Reproduction, focusing on interdisciplinary communication within the science. **Pub:** *Biology of Reproduction (13/year).* • *Biology of Reproduction Monograph.*

★ 18408 ★ **U.S. Department of Health**
**and Human Services**
**Centers for Disease Control and**
**Prevention**
**National Institute for Occupational Safety**
**and Health**
**National Occupational Research Agenda**
**(Fertility and Pregnancy Abnormalities)**
4676 Columbia Pkwy.
Cincinnati, OH 45226
**Free:** 800-356-4676
**Email:** ths1@cdc.gov
**Website:** http://www.cdc.gov/niosh/nrpreg.html
Teresa Schnorr, Contact

**Activities/Fields:** Physical and biological agents in the workplace that may affect fertility and pregnancy outcomes.

**U.S. Department of Health and Human**
**Services**
**National Institutes of Health**
**National Institute of Child Health and**
**Human Development**
**Division of Intramural Research**
**((Division of Epidemiology, Statistics and**
**Prevention Research)**
**Biometry and Mathematical Statistics**
**Branch)**
*See:* Entry 17830

**U.S. Department of Health and Human**
**Services**
**National Institutes of Health**
**National Institute of Child Health and**
**Human Development**
**Division of Intramural Research**
**(Division of Epidemiology, Statistics and**
**Prevention Research)**
*See:* Entry 9065

**U.S. Department of Health and Human Services**
**National Institutes of Health**
**National Institute of Child Health and Human Development**
**Division of Intramural Research**
**(Pediatric and Reproductive Endocrinology Branch)**
*See:* Entry 8785

**U.S. Department of Health and Human Services**
**National Institutes of Health**
**National Institute of Diabetes and Digestive and Kidney Diseases**
**Division of Diabetes, Endocrinology, and Metabolic Diseases**
**(Reproductive Endocrinology Program)**
*See:* Entry 8793

**U.S. Department of Health and Human Services**
**National Institutes of Health**
**National Institute of Environmental Health Sciences**
**Division of Extramural Research and Training**
**(Organs and Systems Toxicology Branch)**
*See:* Entry 14325

**U.S. Department of Health and Human Services**
**National Institutes of Health**
**National Institute of Mental Health**
**Experimental Therapeutics Branch**
**(Unit on Reproduction Endocrine Studies)**
*See:* Entry 14343

**★ 18409 ★ U.S. Department of Health and Human Services**
**Public Health Service**
**Office of Adolescent Pregnancy Programs**
4350 East-West Hwy., ste. 200W
Bethesda, MD 20814
**Phone:** (301)594-4004　　　**Fax:** (301)594-5980
**Email:** opa@osophs.dhhs.gov
**Website:** http://opa.osophs.dhhs.gov/titlexx/oapp.html
Dr. Mireille B. Kanda, Actg. Dir. of OPA

**Activities/Fields:** Supports care demonstration projects to help pregnant teenagers and their children and families; and prevention demonstration projects to reach teenagers before they become sexually active. Programs include the award of research and evaluation grants and contracts for studies on the causes and consequences of adolescent sexual behavior, contraceptive use, and early childbearing; and evaluation of service delivery.

**University of Alberta**
**Perinatal Research Centre (PRC)**
*See:* Entry 5815

**University of California, San Francisco**
**Center for Reproductive Sciences**
*See:* Entry 8815

**★ 18410 ★ University of Kentucky**
**Center for Reproductive Medicine**
Department of OB/GYN
College of Medicine
800 Rose St.
Lexington, KY 40536
**Phone:** (859)323-6166　　　**Fax:** (859)323-1931
**Email:** tecurry@pop.uky.edu
**Website:** http://www.mc.uky.edu/obg/
Prof. Thomas Curry, Dir.

**Activities/Fields:** Reproductive medicine, including artificial insemination; in-vitro fertilization; interfallopian tube transfer; ovulation; and follicular development.

**★ 18411 ★ University of Maryland at Baltimore**
**Center for Studies in Reproduction**
Bressler Research Laboratory, Rm. 11-019
655 W Baltimore St.
Baltimore, MD 21201
**Phone:** (410)706-3391　　　**Fax:** (410)706-5747
**Email:** ealbrech@umaryland.edu
**Website:** http://csr.umaryland.edu/
Dr. Eugene D. Albrecht, Dir.

**Activities/Fields:** Reproductive biology, including reproductive neuroendocrinology and cellular reproductive endocrinology, cellular endocrinology, perinatal endocrinology, fetal-placental development, uterine and ovarian physiology and biochemistry, steroid regulation of cancer, ovarian embryology and physiology, neuroendocrine regulation of peptidergic neurons, neuroendocrinology of prolactin secretion, neuroendocrinology of aging, and cancer research.

**★ 18412 ★ University of Michigan**
**Reproductive Sciences Program**
300 N Ingalls Bldg., 11th Fl.
Ann Arbor, MI 48109-0404
**Phone:** (734)763-0247　　　**Fax:** (734)936-8620
**Email:** dlfoster@umich.edu
**Website:** http://www.umich.edu/~rspwww/
Douglas Foster, Chm.

**Activities/Fields:** Biological and behavioral aspects of reproduction, including clinical medicine relating to endocrinological disorders; neuroendocrine regulation of reproduction; morphological and functional studies on the hypothalmic-pituitary-gonadal axis; development of novel, nonradioactive analytical techniques; biosensors and on-line feedback control systems; biological signalling and chronobiology; neuroendocrine physiology and psychology; biochemical endrocrinology relevant to steroidogenesis and hormone action; molecular biology and gene expression; reproductive pharmacology; neurophysiological and sensory regulation of behavior; growth regulation; physical activity and its relationship to neuroendocrine function; biochemical, biological, and behavioral correlates of pregnancy; chemistry and immunology of hormones; synthesis, processing, and secretion of cellular products, including gonadotropins and extracellular matrix; calcium/calmodulin actions; and infertility research.

**University of North Carolina at Greensboro**
**Institute for Health, Science, and Society (IHSS)**
*See:* Entry 3112

**★ 18413 ★ University of Pennsylvania**
**Center for Research on Reproduction and Women's Health**
1355 Biomedical Research Bldg. II/III
University of Pennsylvania Medical Center
Philadelphia, PA 19104-6142
**Phone:** (215)898-0147　　　**Fax:** (215)573-5408
**Email:** jfs3@mail.med.upenn.edu
**Website:** http://www.med.upenn.edu/~crrwh/
Dr. Jerome F. Strauss, III, Dir.

**Activities/Fields:** Human reproduction as it relates to fertility regulation and the diagnosis and treatment of male and female infertility and health issues specific to women.

**University of Pittsburgh**
**Center for Research in Reproductive Physiology**
*See:* Entry 20691

**University of Saskatchewan**
**Reproductive Biology Research Unit**
*See:* Entry 16743

**★ 18414 ★ University of Texas**
**Southwestern Medical Center at Dallas**
**Cecil H. and Ida Green Center for Reproductive Biology Science**
5323 Harry Hines Blvd.
Dallas, TX 75235-9051
**Phone:** (214)648-6498　　　**Fax:** (214)648-5087
**Email:** david.garbers@email.swmed.edu
**Website:** http://greencenter.swmed.edu
Dr. David Garbers, Dir.

**Activities/Fields:** Reproductive biology: gametogenesis, fertilization and nuclear transplantation/reprogramming. Provides a link between research in gamete development, fertilization, and reprogramming of the somatic cell nucleus.

**★ 18415 ★ University of Virginia**
**Center for Research in Contraceptive and Reproductive Health**
University of Virginia Health System
PO Box 800732
Charlottesville, VA 22908
**Phone:** (434)924-1202　　　**Fax:** (434)982-3912
**Email:** jch7k@virginia.edu
**Website:** http://hsc.virginia.edu/medicine/basic-sci/cellbio/crgcv/
John Herr, Dir.

**Activities/Fields:** Human contraceptive vaccine based upon recombinant DNA techniques for both males and females, male contraceptives based on regulation of spermatogenesis. **Frmly:** Center for Recombinant Gamete Contraceptive Vaccinogens.

**★ 18416 ★ University of Virginia**
**Center for Research in Reproduction**
UVA Health Sciences Center
PO Box 800391
Charlottesville, VA 22908
**Phone:** (434)924-1807　　　**Fax:** (434)982-0701
**Website:** http://www.med.virginia.edu/medcntr/centers/crr/
Dr. John C. Marshall, Dir.

**Activities/Fields:** Human reproduction.

# Chapter 58
# Respiratory Diseases

## Federal Government Agencies

**U.S. Department of Health and Human Services**
**National Institutes of Health (NIH)**
**National Heart, Lung, and Blood Institute (NHLBI)**
*See:* Entry 4916

## Foundations & Other Funding Organizations

### Private Foundations

**E and M Charities**
*See:* Entry 189

**Francis Families Foundation**
*See:* Entry 256

**Town Creek Foundation**
*See:* Entry 8544

### Corporate Foundations

**Wausau Paper Mills Foundation**
*See:* Entry 11471

### Other Funding Organizations

**American Academy of Allergy, Asthma and Immunology (AAAAI)**
*See:* Entry 3174

★ 18417 ★ **American Broncho-Esophagological Associat ion (ABEA)**
K4/714 Clinical Science Ctr.
600 Highland Ave.
Madison, WI 53792-7375
**Phone:** (608)263-0192     **Fax:** (608)265-9255
**Email:** peak.woo@mountsinai.org
**Website:** http://www.abea.net/
Peak Woo, Pres.

**Desc:** Professional society of otolaryngologists, chest specialists, thoracic surgeons, and gastroenterologists engaged in the practice of broncho-esophagology (diseases and injuries of the respiratory system and upper digestive tract). Conducts program on study of foreign bodies. **Awards:** Broyles-Maloney Award (annual) for outstanding manuscripts, a thesis, or accomplishments in endoscopy, bronchology, esophagology, laryngology, and related science; Resident Essay

Award (annual) for the best original paper on research in clinical bronchoesophagology, physiology, or pathology of the larynx, tracheobronchial tree, or esophagus written by a resident or fellow in training; Seymour R. Cohen Award (annual) for the resident, fellow, or practicing physician who submits the best original paper in either basic research or clinical investigation in pediatric laryngology and bronchoesophagology.

**American College of Chest Physicians (ACCP)**
*See:* Entry 4924

**Asthma and Allergy Foundation of America (AAFA)**
*See:* Entry 3176

## Medical & Allied Health Schools

### Respiratory Therapy

*Listed below are respiratory therapist educational programs accredited by the Commission on Accreditation of Allied Health Education Programs (35 E Wacker Dr., Ste. 1970, Chicago, IL 60601-2208, (312)553-9355, http://www.caahep.org/) in collaboration with the Committee on Accreditation for Respiratory Care (CoARC). Information on accredited respiratory therapy technician programs may be obtained by contacting CoARC at 1248 Harwood Rd., Bedford, TX 76021-4244, (817)283-2835, http://www.coarc.com/.*

#### Alabama

★ 18418 ★ **George C. Wallace Community College**
**Advanced Respiratory Therapist Program**
Rte. 6
PO Box 62
Dothan, AL 36303
**Phone:** (334)983-3521     **Fax:** (334)983-3600
**Email:** dodom@wcc.cc.al.us
**Website:** http://www.wallace.edu/wccpages/index.html
Drayton Odom, Director

★ 18419 ★ **Shelton State Community College**
**Advanced Respiratory Therapist Program**
3401 Martin Luther King Jr. Blvd.
Tuscaloosa, AL 35401
**Phone:** (205)391-2641     **Fax:** (205)391-2658
**Email:** bspruell@shelton.cc.al.us
**Website:** http://207.157.109.131/
Bruce E. Spruell, Director

★ 18420 ★ **University of Alabama, Birmingham**
**Advanced Respiratory Therapist Program**
1714 Ninth Ave. S, LRC Rm. 317
Birmingham, AL 35294-1270
**Phone:** (205)934-3783     **Fax:** (205)975-7302
**Email:** grangerw@uab.edu
**Website:** http://main.uab.edu/show.asp?durki=3418
Wesley M. Granger, PhD, Director

★ 18421 ★ **University of South Alabama**
**Advanced Respiratory Therapist Program**
1504 Springhill Ave., Rm. 2545
Mobile, AL 36604
**Phone:** (334)434-3405     **Fax:** (334)434-3941
**Email:** wwojciec@jaguar1.usouthal.edu
**Website:** http://www.southalabama.edu/usa/allhealth/crc.htm
William V. Wojciechowski, Director

★ 18422 ★ **Wallace State Community College**
**Advanced Respiratory Therapist Program**
PO Box 2000
Hanceville, AL 35077-2000
**Phone:** (205)352-8310     **Fax:** (205)352-8320
**Website:** http://www.wallacestatehanceville.edu/
Paul D. Taylor, Director

#### Arizona

★ 18423 ★ **Apollo College**
**Mesa Campus**
**Advanced Respiratory Therapist Program**
630 W Southern Ave.
Mesa, AZ 85210
**Phone:** (480)831-6585     **Fax:** (480)827-0022
**Website:** http://www.apollocollege.com/
Valerie S. Spear, Director

★ 18424 ★ **Apollo College, Phoenix Campus**
**Advanced Respiratory Therapist Program**
8503 N 27th Ave.
Phoenix, AZ 85051
**Phone:** (602)864-1571     **Fax:** (602)864-8207
**Website:** http://www.apollocollege.com/rt.htm
Eduardo Yngelmo, Director

★ 18425 ★ **Gateway Community College**
**Advanced Respiratory Therapist Program**
108 N 40th St.
Phoenix, AZ 85034
**Phone:** (602)392-5234     **Fax:** (602)392-5300
**Email:** rodriguez@gwc.maricopa.edu
**Website:** http://www.gwc.maricopa.edu/aop/resp.html
Toni L. Rodriguez, EdD, Director

**★ 18426 ★ Long Technical College**
**Advanced Respiratory Therapist Program**
13450 N Black Canyon Hwy., No. 104
Phoenix, AZ 85029
**Email:** lmidhx2@dancris.edom
Ronda D. Anderson, Director

**★ 18427 ★ Pima Community College**
**Advanced Respiratory Therapist Program**
2202 W Anklam Rd.
HRP 220
Tucson, AZ 85709-0080
**Phone:** (520)206-6916    **Fax:** (520)206-6632
**Email:** rpatze@pimacc.pima.edu
**Website:** http://www.pimacc.pima.edu/~curonline/cat-curr/RTH-P.HTM
Richard A. Patze, Jr., Director

**★ 18428 ★ Pima Medical Institute—Mesa**
**Advanced Respiratory Therapist Program**
957 S Dobson Rd.
Mesa, AZ 85202
**Phone:** (602)345-7777    **Fax:** (602)649-5249
**Website:** http://pimamedical.com/
Cynthia Smathers, Director

**★ 18429 ★ Pima Medical Institute-Tucson**
**Advanced Respiratory Therapist Program**
3350 E Grant Rd.
Tucson, AZ 85716
**Phone:** (520)326-1600    **Fax:** (520)795-3463
**Email:** leanna@flash.net
**Website:** http://pimamedical.com/
Leanna Konechne, Director

## Arkansas

**★ 18430 ★ University of Arkansas for**
**Medical Sciences**
**Advanced Respiratory Therapist Program**
AHEC-SW/PO Box 2871
300 E Sixth St.
Texarkana, AR 71854
**Phone:** (870)779-6033    **Fax:** (870)779-6045
**Email:** p_evans@ahersw.uams.edu
Patrick Evans, Director

**★ 18431 ★ University of Arkansas for**
**Medical Sciences**
**College of Health Related Professions**
**Advanced Respiratory Therapist Program**
4301 W Markham, Slot 704 (148/NLR)
Little Rock, AR 72205
**Phone:** (501)257-2343    **Fax:** (501)257-2349
**Email:** booneernal@exchange.uams.edu
**Website:** http://www.uams.edu/ahec/ahec12.htm
Erna Boone, Director

## California

**★ 18432 ★ American River College**
**Advanced Respiratory Therapist Program**
4700 College Oak Dr.
Sacramento, CA 95841
**Phone:** (916)484-8876    **Fax:** (916)484-8030
**Email:** warmanj@arc.losrios.cc.ca.us
**Website:** http://www.arc.losrios.cc.ca.us/scihlth/resp-care.html
James L. Warman, PhD, Director

**★ 18433 ★ Butte Community College**
**Advanced Respiratory Therapist Program**
3536 Butte Campus Dr.
Oroville, CA 95965
**Phone:** (916)895-2423    **Fax:** (916)895-2472
**Email:** solomonda@butte.cc.ca.us
**Website:** http://www.butte.cc.ca.us/catalog_htmls/RT.html
Daniel J. Solomon, Director

**★ 18434 ★ California College for Health**
**Sciences**
**Advanced Respiratory Therapist Program**
222 W 24th St.
National City, CA 91950
**Phone:** (619)477-4800    **Fax:** (619)477-4360
**Email:** jwelsh@cchs.edu
**Website:** http://www.cchs.edu/bachelors/respcare/
Jeffrey Welsh, PhD, Director

**★ 18435 ★ California Paramedical and**
**Technical College—Riverside**
**Advanced Respiratory Therapist Program**
4550 La Sierra Ave.
Riverside, CA 92505
**Phone:** (909)687-9006    **Fax:** (909)687-9739
**Website:** http://www.pe.net/~compcptc/Respth.htm
Jon Keillipuleole, Director

**★ 18436 ★ College of the Desert**
**Advanced Respiratory Therapist Program**
43-500 Monterey Ave.
Palm Desert, CA 92260
**Phone:** (760)346-8041    **Fax:** (760)776-7414
Ronald Sneider, MD, Director

**★ 18437 ★ Crafton Hills College**
**Advanced Respiratory Therapist Program**
11711 Sand Canyon Rd.
Yucaipa, CA 92399
**Phone:** (909)389-3284    **Fax:** (909)794-0423
**Email:** kbryson@crafton.sbccd.cc.ca.us
**Website:** http://www.sbccd.cc.ca.us/chc/index.htm
Kenneth R. Bryson, Director

**★ 18438 ★ East Los Angeles College**
**Advanced Respiratory Therapist Program**
1301 Avenida Cesar Chavez
Monterey Park, CA 91754
**Phone:** (323)265-8612    **Fax:** (213)265-8684
**Email:** Mcarr89774@aol.com
**Website:** http://www.elac.cc.ca.us/respiratorycat.htm
Michael R. Carr, Director

**★ 18439 ★ El Camino College**
**Advanced Respiratory Therapist Program**
16007 S Crenshaw Blvd.
Torrance, CA 90506
**Phone:** (310)660-3248    **Fax:** (310)660-3378
**Email:** sinopoli@instruction.com
**Website:** http://www.elcamino.cc.ca.us/respiratory-care/default.htm
Louis M. Sinopoli, EdD, Director

**★ 18440 ★ Foothill College**
**Advanced Respiratory Therapist Program**
12345 El Monte Rd.
Los Altos Hills, CA 94022
**Phone:** (650)949-7292    **Fax:** (650)949-7375
**Email:** treanor@admin.fhda.edu
**Website:** http://www.foothill.fhda.edu/bio/programs/respther/
Shirley Treanor, EdD, Director

**★ 18441 ★ Fresno City College**
**Advanced Respiratory Therapist Program**
1101 E University Ave.
Fresno, CA 93741
**Phone:** (559)244-2604    **Fax:** (559)244-2626
**Email:** steven.boyd@do1.scccd.cc.ca.us
**Website:** http://www.fcc.cc.ca.us/healthsci/hsdivi-sion.htmlrcp
Steven L. Boyd, Director

**★ 18442 ★ Grossmont College**
**Advanced Respiratory Therapist Program**
8800 Grossmont College Dr.
El Cajon, CA 92020-1799
**Phone:** (619)644-7448    **Fax:** (619)644-7961
**Email:** lorenda.seibold-phalan@gcccd.net
**Website:** http://grossmont.gcccd.cc.ca.us/healthpro-fessions/RTWebPage/Default.htm
Lorenda Seibold-Phalan, Director

**★ 18443 ★ Loma Linda University**
**Advanced Respiratory Therapist Program**
Nichol Hall, Rm. 1926
Loma Linda, CA 92350
**Phone:** (909)558-4932    **Fax:** (909)558-4701
**Email:** dstanton@sahp.llu.edu
**Website:** http://www.llu.edu/llu/sahp/resp.htmlanchor401949
David Stanton, Director

**★ 18444 ★ Los Angeles Valley College**
**Advanced Respiratory Therapist Program**
5800 Fulton Ave.
Van Nuys, CA 91401-4096
**Phone:** (818)947-2600    **Fax:** (818)947-2610
**Email:** ettingvm@laccd.ca.us.ed
**Website:** http://www.lavc.cc.ca.us/catalog/rt.html
Virginia M. Ettinger, Director

**★ 18445 ★ Modesto Junior College**
**Advanced Respiratory Therapist Program**
435 College Ave.
Modesto, CA 95350
**Phone:** (209)575-6388    **Fax:** (209)575-6593
**Email:** lylet@yosemite.cc.ca.us
**Website:** http://virtual.yosemite.cc.ca.us/catalog/pro-grams/respcarepgm.htm
Terry P. Lyle, Director

**★ 18446 ★ Mount San Antonio College**
**Advanced Respiratory Therapist Program**
1100 N Grand Ave.
Walnut, CA 91789
**Phone:** (909)594-5611    **Fax:** (909)468-3938
**Email:** zin@earthlink.net
**Website:** http://www.mtsac.edu/instruction/dept686.html
Terrance M. Krider, Director

**★ 18447 ★ Napa Valley College**
**Advanced Respiratory Therapist Program**
2277 Napa Vallejo Hwy.
Napa, CA 94558
**Phone:** (707)253-3147    **Fax:** (707)259-8068
**Email:** rchudnofsky@campus.nvc.cc.ca.us
**Website:** http://www.nvc.cc.ca.us/html/repiratory_therapy.html
Robert S. Chudnofsky, Director

**★ 18448 ★ Ohlone College**
**Advanced Respiratory Therapist Program**
43600 Mission Blvd.
PO BOX 3909
Fremont, CA 94539
**Phone:** (510)659-6029    **Fax:** (510)659-6070
**Email:** CmcNamee-Cole@Ohlone.cc.ca.us
**Website:** http://www.ohlone.cc.ca.us/instr/resp_ther/
Carol McNamee-Cole, Director

**★ 18449 ★ Orange Coast College**
**Advanced Respiratory Therapist Program**
2701 Fairview Rd.
PO Box 5005
Costa Mesa, CA 92626
**Phone:** (714)432-5541    **Fax:** (714)432-5534
**Email:** dadelman@cccd.edu
**Website:** http://www.occ.cccd.edu/departments/alh/respcinfo.html
Daniel S. Adelmann, Director

**★ 18450 ★ San Joaquin Valley College**
**Advanced Respiratory Therapist Program**
8400 W Mineral King
Visalia, CA 93291
**Phone:** (559)651-2500    **Fax:** (559)651-3645
**Email:** barryw@sjvc.com
**Website:** http://www.sjvc.com/
Barry Westling, Director

**★ 18451 ★ San Joaquin Valley College**
**Advanced Respiratory Therapist Program**
201 New Stine Rd.
Bakersfield, CA 93309
**Phone:** (661)834-0126
**Email:** jeffreyc@sjvc.com
**Website:** http://www.sjvc.com/
Jeffrey E. Cox, Director

**★ 18452 ★ Skyline College**
**Advanced Respiratory Therapist Program**
3300 College Dr.
San Bruno, CA 94066
**Phone:** (650)738-4382    **Fax:** (650)738-4299
**Email:** williamsonm@smcccd.cc.ca.us
**Website:** http://www.smcccd.cc.ca.us/smcccd/sky-
line/smt/rpth.htmlanchor242942
Michael Williamson, Director

**★ 18453 ★ Victor Valley College**
**Advanced Respiratory Therapist Program**
18422 Bear Valley Rd.
Victorville, CA 92392-9699
**Phone:** (760)245-4271
**Email:** rflome@victor.cc.ca.us
**Website:** http://www.vvcconline.com/allhealth/index_
rt.htm
Robert C. Flome, Director

### Colorado

**★ 18454 ★ Front Range Community**
**College**
**Advanced Respiratory Therapist Program**
3645 W 112th Ave.
Westminster, CO 80030
**Phone:** (303)404-5217    **Fax:** (303)404-2178
**Website:** http://frcc.cc.co.us/about/pubs/cat/pro-
grams/respiratory_care.html
Bob Davis, Director

**★ 18455 ★ Pima Medical Institute—**
**Denver**
**Advanced Respiratory Therapist Program**
1701 W 72nd Ave.
Denver, CO 80221
**Phone:** (303)426-1800    **Fax:** (303)430-4048
**Email:** denverpima@aol.com
**Website:** http://pimamedical.com/
C. Allen Wentworth, Director

**★ 18456 ★ Pueblo Community College**
**Advanced Respiratory Therapist Program**
900 W Orman Ave.
Pueblo, CO 81004
**Phone:** (719)549-3265    **Fax:** (719)549-3381
**Email:** delia.lechtenberg@pcc.cccoes.edu
**Website:** http://www.pcc.cccoes.edu/resp_care/wel-
come.htm
Delia Lechtenberg, Director

**★ 18457 ★ T. H. Pickens Technical**
**Center**
**Advanced Respiratory Therapist Program**
500 Airport Blvd.
Aurora, CO 80011-9307
**Phone:** (303)344-4910    **Fax:** (303)326-1277
**Email:** garys@pickens.aps.k12.co.us
**Website:** http://www.pickenstech.org/Programs/pro-
grams.respiratory.care.tech.html
Gary Schroeder, Director

### Connecticut

**★ 18458 ★ Manchester Community**
**College**
**Advanced Respiratory Therapist Program**
Great Path
PO Box 1046
Manchester, CT 06045-1046
**Phone:** (860)647-6193    **Fax:** (860)647-6370
**Email:** ma_milikowsk@commnet.edu
**Website:** http://www.mcc.commnet.edu/programs/
healthcareers/RespCare/home.html
Karen A. Milikowski, Director

**★ 18459 ★ Norwalk Hospital/Norwalk**
**Community Technical College**
**Advanced Respiratory Therapist Program**
24 Maple St.
Norwalk, CT 06856
**Phone:** (203)852-2479    **Fax:** (203)852-2738
**Email:** edward.reardon@norwalkhealth.org
**Website:** http://www.nctc.commnet.edu/pages/de-
gree/programs/resp-p.htm
Edward A. Reardon, Director

**★ 18460 ★ Quinnipiac College**
**Advanced Respiratory Therapist Program**
Mt. Carmel Ave.
Hamden, CT 06518
**Phone:** (203)582-8682    **Fax:** (203)582-8706
**Email:** Ronald.Beckett@quinnipiac.edu
**Website:** http://www.quinnipiac.edu/academics/de-
partment.asp?School=HS&Dept=115
Ronald G. Beckett, PhD, Director

**★ 18461 ★ University of Hartford**
**Advanced Respiratory Therapist Program**
200 Bloomfield Ave.
West Hartford, CT 06117-1599
**Phone:** (860)768-4823    **Fax:** (860)768-5706
**Email:** pkennedy@mail.hartford.edu
**Website:** http://uhavax.hartford.edu/~healthpro/rt.html
Peter W. Kennedy, PhD, Director

### Delaware

**★ 18462 ★ Delaware Technical and**
**Community College—Owens Campus**
**Advanced Respiratory Therapist Program**
PO Box 610
Georgetown, DE 19947
**Phone:** (302)856-5400    **Fax:** (302)856-5773
**Email:** jlittle@outland.dtcc.edu
**Website:** http://www.dtcc.edu/
James G. Little, Director

**★ 18463 ★ Delaware Technical and**
**Community College—Wilmington**
**Advanced Respiratory Therapist Program**
333 Shipley St.
Wilmington, DE 19801
**Phone:** (302)428-2678    **Fax:** (302)428-2691
**Email:** rlang@christiancare.org
**Website:** http://www.dtcc.edu/
Robert M. Lang, Director

### District of Columbia

**★ 18464 ★ University of the District of**
**Columbia**
**Advanced Respiratory Therapist Program**
4200 Connecticut Ave. NW
Washington, DC 20008
**Phone:** (202)274-5925    **Fax:** (202)274-5952
**Email:** slockwood@udc.edu
**Website:** http://udc2.org
Susan D. Lockwood, Director

### Florida

**★ 18465 ★ ATI Health Education Centers**
**(LB)**
**Advanced Respiratory Therapist Program**
1395 NW 167 St., Ste. 200
Miami, FL 33169
**Phone:** (305)628-1000    **Fax:** (305)628-1461
**Email:** jclavan@aol.com
**Website:** http://www.aticareertraining.com/
Jules Clavan, Director

**★ 18466 ★ Brevard Community College**
**Advanced Respiratory Therapist Program**
1519 Clearlake Rd.
Cocoa, FL 32922
**Phone:** (407)632-1111    **Fax:** (407)634-3731
**Email:** szewczykc@brevard.cc.fl.us
**Website:** http://www.brevard.cc.fl.us/alliedhealth/res-
piratory.html
Carol Szewczyk, Director

**★ 18467 ★ Broward Community College**
**Advanced Respiratory Therapist Program**
1000 Coconut Creek Blvd.
Coconut Creek, FL 33066
**Phone:** (954)969-2082    **Fax:** (954)973-2348
**Email:** jprince@broward.cc.fl.us
**Website:** http://fs.broward.cc.fl.us/~jprince/index.htm
John Prince, Director

**★ 18468 ★ Daytona Beach Community**
**College**
**Advanced Respiratory Therapist Program**
1200 W International Speedway Blvd.
PO Box 2811
Daytona Beach, FL 32114
**Phone:** (904)255-8131    **Fax:** (904)254-4491
**Email:** mccumbm@dbcc.cc.fl.us
**Website:** http://www.dbcc.cc.fl.us/
Michael R. McCumber, EdD, Director

**★ 18469 ★ Edison Community College**
**Advanced Respiratory Therapist Program**
8099 College Pkwy. SW
PO Box 60210
Fort Myers, FL 33906-6210
**Phone:** (941)489-9252    **Fax:** (941)489-9037
**Email:** spilbeam@edison.edu
**Website:** http://www.edison.edu/departments/health-
science/respiratory.htm
Susan P. Pilbeam, Director

**★ 18470 ★ Florida A&M University (LB)**
**Advanced Respiratory Therapist Program**
Ware-Rhaney Bldg., Ste. 223-F
Tallahassee, FL 32307
**Phone:** (904)561-2186    **Fax:** (904)561-2457
**Email:** pjohnson@mailer.fsu.edu
**Website:** http://famu2.famu.edu/acad/colleges/
ahs/rt.html
Alphonso Baldwin, PhD, Director

**★ 18471 ★ Florida Community College—**
**Jacksonville**
**Advanced Respiratory Therapist Program**
North Campus
4501 Capper Rd.
Jacksonville, FL 32218
**Phone:** (904)766-6513    **Fax:** (904)766-6654
**Email:** btabor@fccj.org
**Website:** http://www.fccj.cc.fl.us/catalog/pos/as/Res-
piratoryCare-22440.html
Beverly L.T. Tabor, Director

★ **18472** ★ **Hillsborough Community College**
**Advanced Respiratory Therapist Program**
4001 Tampa Bay Blvd.
PO Box 30030
Tampa, FL 33630-3030
**Phone:** (813)253-7318          **Fax:** (813)253-7491
**Email:** marjiewilk@aol.com
Marjorie Wilkins, Director

★ **18473** ★ **Indian River Community College (LB)**
**Advanced Respiratory Therapist Program**
3209 Virginia Ave.
Fort Pierce, FL 34981-5599
**Phone:** (561)462-4358          **Fax:** (561)462-4900
**Email:** grosenfe@ircc.cc.fl.us
**Website:** http://www.ircc.cc.fl.us/index.htm
Georgette Rosenfeld, Director

★ **18474** ★ **Manatee Community College**
**Advanced Respiratory Therapist Program**
5840 26th St. W
PO Box 1849
Bradenton, FL 34206
**Phone:** (941)755-1511
**Email:** hainesl@bc.mcc.cc.fl.us
**Website:**          http://www.mcc.cc.fl.us/Courses/as-frame.htm
J. Lynn Haines, Director

★ **18475** ★ **Miami-Dade Community College (LB)**
**Advanced Respiratory Therapist Program**
Medical Center Campus
950 NW 20th St.
Miami, FL 33127
**Phone:** (305)237-4031          **Fax:** (305)237-4278
**Email:** millec@mdcc.edu
**Website:** http://www.mdcc.edu/medical/
Carol J. Miller, EdD, Director

★ **18476** ★ **Palm Beach Community College, Gardens Campus**
**Advanced Respiratory Therapist Program**
3160 PGA Blvd.
Palm Beach Gardens, FL 33410-2893
**Phone:** (561)625-2588          **Fax:** (561)625-2305
**Email:** rogersj@pbcc.cc.fl.us
**Website:** http://www.pbcc.cc.fl.us/
Jacqueline Rogers, Director

★ **18477** ★ **Pensacola Junior College**
**Advanced Respiratory Therapist Program**
5555 W Hwy. 98
Pensacola, FL 32507
**Phone:** (850)484-2356          **Fax:** (850)484-2364
**Email:** rwanderson@pjc.cc.fl.us
**Website:** http://www.dept.pjc.cc.fl.us/drs/
Randall W. Anderson, Director

★ **18478** ★ **Saint Petersburg Junior College**
**Advanced Respiratory Therapist Program**
PO Box 13489
Pinellas Park, FL 33780
**Phone:** (727)341-3627          **Fax:** (727)341-3744
**Email:** mikless@spjc.edu
**Website:**          http://www.spjc.cc.fl.us/webcentral/acad/respcare.htm
Stephen P. Mikles, Director

★ **18479** ★ **Santa Fe Community College**
**Advanced Respiratory Therapist Program**
3000 NW 83rd St.
Gainesville, FL 32606-6200
**Phone:** (352)395-5703          **Fax:** (352)395-5711
**Email:** dave.yonutas@santafe.cc.fl.us

**Website:** http://inst.santafe.cc.fl.us/~health/respcare/
David N. Yonutas, Director

★ **18480** ★ **Seminole Community College (LB)**
**Advanced Respiratory Therapist Program**
100 Weldon Blvd.
Sanford, FL 32773
**Phone:** (407)328-2293          **Fax:** (407)328-2470
**Email:** shideles@mail.seminole.cc.fl.us
**Website:** http://www.seminole.cc.fl.us/Respiratory/
Steve Shideler, Director

★ **18481** ★ **Tallahassee Community College**
**Advanced Respiratory Therapist Program**
444 Appleyard Dr.
Tallahassee, FL 32304
**Phone:** (850)922-8103          **Fax:** (850)922-9312
**Email:** streemd@mail.tallahassee.cc.fl.us
**Website:** http://www.tallahassee.cc.fl.us/generalinfo/asrespiratory.htmBridge
Dewey Streetman, Director

★ **18482** ★ **University of Central Florida Department of Health Professions and Physical Therapy**
**Advanced Physical Therapist Program**
Orlando, FL 32816
**Phone:** (407)823-2214          **Fax:** (407)823-6138
**Email:** worrell@pegasus.cc.ucf.edu
**Website:**          http://www.ucf.edu/catalog/9798/Degree_Programs/cardiopulmonary_sciences.ht ml
L. Timothy Worrell, Director

★ **18483** ★ **Valencia Community College**
**Advanced Respiratory Therapist Program**
PO Box 3028
Orlando, FL 32802-9961
**Phone:** (407)299-5000          **Fax:** (407)292-2730
**Email:** lcpraun@valencia.cc.fl.us
**Website:** http://faculty.valencia.cc.fl.us/rescare/
Lynn W. Capraun, Director

## Georgia

★ **18484** ★ **Armstrong Atlantic State University (LB)**
**Advanced Respiratory Therapist Program**
11935 Abercorn St.
Savannah, GA 31419
**Phone:** (912)921-7446          **Fax:** (912)921-5585
**Email:** bowersro@mail.armstrong.edu
**Website:** http://www.rt.armstrong.edu/rcp.html
Ross L. Bowers, III, Director

★ **18485** ★ **Athens Area Technical Institute (LB)**
**Advanced Respiratory Therapist Program**
806 US Hwy. 29 N
Athens, GA 30601-0399
**Phone:** (706)355-5084          **Fax:** (706)355-5181
**Email:** ott@admin1.athens.tcc.ga.us
**Website:** http://admin1.athens.tec.ga.us/rtweb.html
Bruce A. Ott, EdD, Director

★ **18486** ★ **Augusta Technical Institute**
**Advanced Respiratory Therapist Program**
3116 Deans Bridge Rd.
Augusta, GA 30906
**Phone:** (706)771-4194          **Fax:** (706)771-4181
**Email:** rwaller@augusta.tec.ga.us
**Website:**          http://www.augusta.tec.ga.us/academic/A_rtt.htm
Rita Waller, Director

★ **18487** ★ **Darton College**
**Advanced Respiratory Therapist Program**
2400 Gillionville Rd.
Albany, GA 31707
**Phone:** (912)430-6900          **Fax:** (912)430-6910
**Email:** thomasw@dmail.dartnet.peachnet.edu
**Website:** http://www.dartnet.peachnet.edu/Programs/AlliedHealth/respcare.htm
William F. Thomas, Director

★ **18488** ★ **Georgia State University (LB)**
**Advanced Respiratory Therapist Program**
University Plaza
Atlanta, GA 30303
**Phone:** (404)651-3037          **Fax:** (404)651-1531
**Email:** jrau@gsu.edu
**Website:** http://www.gsu.edu/~wwwchs/dept/card/index.htm
Joseph L. Rau, Jr., PhD, Director

★ **18489** ★ **Gwinnett Technical Institute**
**Advanced Respiratory Therapist Program**
5150 Sugarloaf Pkwy.
PO Box 1505
Lawrenceville, GA 30046-1505
**Phone:** (770)962-7580
**Email:** bdelorme@gwinnett.tec.ga.us
**Website:** http://www.gwinnett-tech.org/programs/respiratory_therapist_aatd.html
Robert P. DeLorme, Director

★ **18490** ★ **Macon State College**
**Advanced Respiratory Therapist Program**
100 College Station Dr.
Macon, GA 31297
**Phone:** (912)471-5386          **Fax:** (912)471-2787
**Email:** bbrown@cennet.peachnet.edu
**Website:** http://www.maconstate.edu/
Charles R. Matson, Director

★ **18491** ★ **Medical College of Georgia (LB)**
**Advanced Respiratory Therapist Program**
815 St. Sebastian Way, Rm. HM-143
Augusta, GA 30912
**Phone:** (706)721-3554          **Fax:** (706)721-0495
**Email:** smishoe@mail.mcg.edu
**Website:**          http://www.mcg.edu/SAH/respther/index.html
Shelley C. Mishoe, PhD, Director

★ **18492** ★ **Southwest Georgia Technical College**
**Advanced Respiratory Therapist Program**
15689 US Hwy. 19 N
Thomasville, GA 31792
**Phone:** (912)225-5094          **Fax:** (912)225-5289
**Email:** tmiller@thomas.tec.ga.us
**Website:** http://www.thomas.tec.ga.us/
Tammy A. Miller, Director

## Hawaii

★ **18493** ★ **Kapiolani Community College / University of Hawaii**
**Advanced Respiratory Therapist Program**
4303 Diamond Head Rd.
Honolulu, HI 96816
**Phone:** (808)734-9243          **Fax:** (808)734-9126
**Email:** wehrman@hawaii.edu
**Website:** http://www.kcc.hawaii.edu/academics/catalog/programs/health/index.htm
Stephen F. Wehrman, Director

## Idaho

**★ 18494 ★ Boise State University (LB)**
**College of Health Sciences**
**Advanced Respiratory Therapist Program**
1910 University Dr.
Room HSR 116
Boise, ID 83725
**Phone:** (208)426-3383          **Fax:** (208)426-4093
**Email:** lashwor@boisestate.edu
**Website:** http://selland.boisestate.edu/academic_divisions/heal_serv/resp_ther.htm
Lonny J. Ashworth, Director

## Illinois

**★ 18495 ★ College of DuPage**
**Advanced Respiratory Therapist Program**
425 22nd St.
Glen Ellyn, IL 60137-6599
**Phone:** (630)942-2518          **Fax:** (630)858-9399
**Email:** bretlk@cdnet.cod.edu
**Website:** http://www.cod.edu/Academic/AcadProg/Occ_Voc/RespCare.htm
Kenneth M. Bretl, Director

**★ 18496 ★ ICC/BHC Partnership (LB)**
**Advanced Respiratory Therapist Program**
201 SW Adams St.
Peoria, IL 61635-0001
**Phone:** (309)999-4663          **Fax:** (309)673-9626
**Website:** http://www.icc.cc.il.us/haps/HCprgms4.htmtherapist
Carole K. Crawford-Jones, Director

**★ 18497 ★ Kankakee Community College**
**Advanced Respiratory Therapist Program**
PO Box 888
River Rd.
Kankakee, IL 60901
**Phone:** (815)933-0276          **Fax:** (815)933-0217
**Email:** nfrey@kcc.cc.il.us
**Website:** http://www.kcc.cc.il.us/
Nichola Frey, Director

**★ 18498 ★ Lincoln Land Community College**
**Advanced Respiratory Therapist Program**
5250 Shepherd Rd.
Springfield, IL 62794-9256
**Phone:** (217)786-2814          **Fax:** (217)786-2824
**Email:** randy.prather@llcc.cc.il.us
**Website:** http://www.llcc.cc.il.us/ahp/rcp.htm
Randel A. Prather, Director

**★ 18499 ★ Moraine Valley Community College**
**Advanced Respiratory Therapist Program**
10900 S 88th Ave.
Palos Hills, IL 60465
**Phone:** (708)974-5380          **Fax:** (708)974-1184
**Email:** lehner@moraine.cc.il.us
**Website:** http://www.moraine.cc.il.us/aca_info/health.html
Raymond F. Lehner, Director

**★ 18500 ★ National-Louis University**
**Advanced Respiratory Therapist Program**
2840 N Sheridan Rd.
Evanston, IL 60201
**Phone:** (847)256-5150          **Fax:** (847)256-1057
**Email:** stho@evan1.nl.edu
**Website:** http://www.nl.edu/nlu_cas/divisions/hhs/undergraduate/allied_health/index.h tml
Stephen L. Thompson, PhD, Director

**★ 18501 ★ Parkland College**
**Advanced Respiratory Therapist Program**
2400 W Bradley Ave.
Champaign, IL 61821
**Phone:** (217)351-2224          **Fax:** (217)351-2581
**Email:** tdesjardins@parkland.cc.il.us
**Website:** http://www.parkland.cc.il.us/hp/rc/rtweb.html
Terry Des Jardins, Director

**★ 18502 ★ Rock Valley College**
**Advanced Respiratory Therapist Program**
3301 N Mulford Rd.
Rockford, IL 61114-5699
**Phone:** (815)654-4413          **Fax:** (815)654-4408
**Email:** fahe3js@rvcux1.rvc.cc.il.us
**Website:** http://www.rvc.cc.il.us/classes/helthser/pages/health.htmrespiratory
James R. Sills, Director

**★ 18503 ★ Southern Illinois University, Carbondale**
**Health Care Professions**
**Advanced Respiratory Therapist Program**
Carbondale, IL 62901-6615
**Phone:** (618)453-7221          **Fax:** (618)453-7020
**Email:** stanman@siu.edu
**Website:** http://www.siu.edu/~hcp/
Stanley M. Pearson, II, Director

**★ 18504 ★ Triton College**
**Advanced Respiratory Therapist Program**
2000 N Fifth Ave.
River Grove, IL 60171
**Phone:** (708)456-0300          **Fax:** (708)583-3121
**Email:** kanderso@triton.cc.il.us
**Website:** http://www.triton.cc.il.us/faculty/kanderson/
Kristine Anderson, Director

## Indiana

**★ 18505 ★ Indiana University**
**Advanced Respiratory Therapist Program**
1140 W Michigan St.
Coleman Hall, Rm. 224
Indianapolis, IN 46202
**Phone:** (317)274-7381          **Fax:** (317)278-7383
**Email:** dcullen@iupui.edu
**Website:** http://www.iupui.edu/it/iusahs/bulletin/97-99/prog/resp/
Deborah L. Cullen, EdD, Director

**★ 18506 ★ Indiana University, Northwest (LB)**
**Advanced Respiratory Therapist Program**
Hawthorne Hall
3400 Broadway NW Campus
Gary, IN 46408
**Phone:** (219)980-6955          **Fax:** (219)980-6649
**Email:** copnsko@iunhaw1.iun.indiana.edu
**Website:** http://www.iun.edu/~ahealth/resp.htm
Cheryl Oprisko, JD, Director

**★ 18507 ★ Ivy Tech State College— Central Indiana (LB)**
**Advanced Respiratory Therapist Program**
1 W 26th St, PO BOX 1763
Indianapolis, IN 46206-1763
**Phone:** (317)921-4402          **Fax:** (317)921-4753
**Email:** klee@ivy.tec.in.us
Kathleen F. Lee, Director

**★ 18508 ★ Ivy Tech State College— Lafayette**
**Advanced Respiratory Therapist Program**
3208 Ross Rd.
PO Box 6299
Lafayette, IN 47903
**Phone:** (765)772-9207          **Fax:** (765)772-9214
**Email:** pjames@ivy.tec.in.us

**Website:** http://www.laf.ivy.tec.in.us/degree_programs/health/respiratory.html
Peggy James, Director
**Frmly:** Indiana Vocational Technical College.

**★ 18509 ★ Ivy Tech State college NE— Fort Wayne**
**Advanced Respiratory Therapist Program**
3800 N Anthony Blvd.
Fort Wayne, IN 46805
**Phone:** (219)482-9171          **Fax:** (219)480-4149
**Email:** cschlade@ivy.tec.in.us
**Website:** http://www.ivy.tec.in.us/FortWayne/
Candace Schladenhauffen, Director
**Frmly:** Indiana Vocational Technical College.

**★ 18510 ★ University of Southern Indiana**
**Advanced Respiratory Therapist Program**
8600 University Blvd.
Evansville, IN 47712
**Phone:** (812)464-1702          **Fax:** (812)465-7092
**Email:** rhooper@usl.edu
Robert Hooper, Director

**★ 18511 ★ Vincennes University (LB)**
**Advanced Respiratory Therapist Program**
1002 N First St.
Vincennes, IN 47591
**Phone:** (812)888-4421          **Fax:** (812)888-4550
**Email:** twood@indian.vinu.edu
**Website:** http://www.vinu.edu/resp_th.htm
Everett Wood, Jr., Director

## Iowa

**★ 18512 ★ Des Moines Area Community College (LB)**
**Advanced Respiratory Therapist Program**
2006 Ankeny Blvd.
Ankeny, IA 50021
**Phone:** (515)964-6298          **Fax:** (515)964-6327
**Email:** kegeorge@dmacc.cc.ia.us
**Website:** http://www.dmacc.cc.ia.us/
Kerry E. George, Director

**★ 18513 ★ Kirkwood Community College**
**Advanced Respiratory Therapist Program**
6301 Kirkwood Blvd. SW
PO Box 2068
Cedar Rapids, IA 52406-9973
**Phone:** (319)398-5411          **Fax:** (319)398-1293
**Email:** kbronh@kirkwood.cc.ia.us
**Website:** http://www.kirkwood.cc.ia.us/healthscience/rt.html
H. Kenneth Bronkhorst, Director

**★ 18514 ★ Northeast Iowa Community College**
**Advanced Respiratory Therapist Program**
10250 Sundown Rd.
Peosta, IA 52068
**Phone:** (319)556-5110          **Fax:** (319)556-5058
**Email:** wheelocw@nicc.cc.ia.us
**Website:** http://www.nicc.cc.ia.us/peo_tech.html35
Wendy Wheelock, Director

## Kansas

**★ 18515 ★ Bethany Medical Center / Kansas City Kansas Community College**
**Advanced Respiratory Therapist Program**
7250 State Ave.
Kansas City, KS 66112
**Phone:** (913)334-1100          **Fax:** (913)596-9649
**Email:** mparrett@toto.net
**Website:** http://www.kckcc.cc.ks.us/rtp/index.htm
C. Michael Parrett, Director

**★ 18516 ★ Johnson County Community College**
**Advanced Respiratory Therapist Program**
12345 College Blvd.
Overland Park, KS 66210
**Phone:** (913)469-8500      **Fax:** (913)469-2315
**Email:** ccraig@jccc.net
**Website:** http://www.jccc.net/acad/resp/
Clarissa M. Craig, Director

**★ 18517 ★ Labette Community College**
**Advanced Respiratory Therapist Program**
200 S 14th St.
Parsons, KS 67357
**Phone:** (316)421-6700      **Fax:** (316)421-2786
**Email:** conniec@labette.cc.ks.us
**Website:**      http://www.labette.cc.ks.us/dept/resp-care.htm
Connie S. Crooks, Director

**★ 18518 ★ Newman University**
**Advanced Respiratory Therapist Program**
3100 McCormick Ave.
Wichita, KS 67213-2097
**Phone:** (316)942-4291      **Fax:** (316)942-4483
**Email:** trumppm@newmanu.edu
**Website:**      http://www.ksnewman.edu/depts.htmRESPIRATORY CARE
Margaret L. Trumpp, Director

**★ 18519 ★ Seward County Community College**
**Advanced Respiratory Therapist Program**
PO Box 1137
Liberal, KS 67901-1137
**Phone:** (316)626-3080      **Fax:** (316)626-3040
**Email:** eanderso@sccc.net
**Website:** http://www.sccc.cc.ks.us/RT.html
Edward B. Anderson, Director

**★ 18520 ★ University of Kansas Medical Center (LB)**
**Advanced Respiratory Therapist Program**
3901 Rainbow Blvd.
4006 Delp
Kansas City, KS 66160-7606
**Phone:** (913)588-4630      **Fax:** (913)588-4631
**Email:** bludwig@kumc.edu
**Website:** http://www.kumc.edu/SAH/resp_care/
Barbara A. Ludwig, Director

**★ 18521 ★ Washburn University of Topeka**
**Advanced Respiratory Therapist Program**
1700 College Ave. SW
Topeka, KS 66621
**Phone:** (785)231-1010      **Fax:** (785)231-1027
**Email:** zzmunz@washburn.edu
**Website:**      http://www.washburn.edu/sas/ah/rt/index.html
Patricia M. Munzer, Director

### Kentucky

**★ 18522 ★ Cumberland Valley—Southeast Community College Consortium**
**Advanced Respiratory Therapist Program**
US Rte. 25 East S
PO Box 187
Pineville, KY 40977
**Phone:** (606)337-3106      **Fax:** (606)337-5662
**Email:** mike.good@kctcs.net
**Website:**      http://www.uky.edu/CommunityColleges/Sou/respiratory.html
Michael Good, Director

**★ 18523 ★ Jefferson Community College**
**Advanced Respiratory Therapist Program**
109 E Broadway
Louisville, KY 40202
**Phone:** (502)213-2197      **Fax:** (502)213-2491
**Email:** joan.kruse@kctcs.edu
**Website:** http://www.jcc.uky.edu/dt/Campus_Information/Academic_Programs/Career_Prog/ Respiratory_Care/default.htm
Joan Kruse, Director

**★ 18524 ★ Lexington Community College (LB)**
**University of Kentucky**
**Advanced Respiratory Therapist Program**
Cooper Dr.
Oswald Bldg., Rm. 330
Lexington, KY 40506-0235
**Phone:** (606)257-4872      **Fax:** (606)257-9580
**Email:** jkmatc1@uky.edu
**Website:** http://www.uky.edu/LCC/RCP/
James K. Matchuny, Director

**★ 18525 ★ Northern Kentucky University (LB)**
**Advanced Respiratory Therapist Program**
Nunn Dr., AHC-225
Highland Heights, KY 41076
**Phone:** (606)572-5557      **Fax:** (606)572-6592
**Email:** langenderfer@nku.edu
**Website:**      http://www.nku.edu/~ahhssw/respiratory-care.htmlx
Robert Langenderfer, Director

**★ 18526 ★ University of Louisville (LB)**
**Advanced Respiratory Therapist Program**
K Bldg., Fourth Fl., Rm. 4044
Louisville, KY 40292
**Phone:** (502)852-8280      **Fax:** (502)852-4597
**Email:** jfwalk01@gwise.louisville.edu
**Website:** http://www.louisville.edu/sahs/
Jerome Walker, EdD, Director

**★ 18527 ★ West Kentucky Technical College**
**Advanced Respiratory Therapist Program**
5200 Blandville Rd.
PO Box 7408
Paducah, KY 42002-7408
**Phone:** (270)554-6244      **Fax:** (270)554-6227
**Email:** ruth.thompson@kctcs.net
**Website:** http://www.wkytech.com/respir.html
Ruth Thompson, Director

### Louisiana

**★ 18528 ★ Bossier Parish Community College**
**Advanced Respiratory Therapist Program**
2719 Airline Dr.
Bossier City, LA 71111
**Phone:** (318)675-6814      **Fax:** (318)675-6937
**Email:** dmeren@lsume.edu
**Website:** http://www.bpcc.cc.la.us/asrt.htmlTOP
Diana Merendino, Director

**★ 18529 ★ Delgado Community College**
**Advanced Respiratory Therapist Program**
615 City Park Ave.
New Orleans, LA 70119
**Phone:** (504)483-4114      **Fax:** (504)483-4609
**Email:** dolsen@pop3.dcc.edu
**Website:** http://www.dcc.edu/ahealth/respcare.htm
Diane M. Olsen-Rawls, Director

**★ 18530 ★ Louisiana State University Health Sciences Center**
**Advanced Respiratory Therapist Program**
1900 Gravier St.
New Orleans, LA 70112
**Phone:** (504)568-4229      **Fax:** (504)568-4248
**Email:** jcairo@lsumc.edu
**Website:** http://www.lsuhsc.edu/Schools/AlliedHealth/CardiopulmonaryScience/cps1.htm
James M. Cairo, PhD, Director

**★ 18531 ★ Nicholls State University (LB)**
**Department of Allied Health Sciences**
**Advanced Respiratory Therapist Program**
PO Box 2090
Thibodaux, LA 70310
**Phone:** (504)448-4495      **Fax:** (504)448-4923
**Website:**      http://server.nich.edu/acad/bulletin/bltnalhe.htmlresp
Errol J. Champagne, Director

**★ 18532 ★ Our Lady of Holy Cross College**
**Ochsner School of Allied Health Sciences**
**Advanced Respiratory Therapist Program**
1516 Jefferson Hwy.
New Orleans, LA 70121
**Phone:** (504)842-3267      **Fax:** (504)842-9129
**Email:** mlabiche@ochsner.org
**Website:** http://www.ochsner.org/gmeweb/ahs.htm
Mary LaBiche, Director

**★ 18533 ★ Southern University, Shreveport/Bossier City Campus**
**Advanced Respiratory Therapist Program**
3050 Martin Luther King Jr. Dr.
Shreveport, LA 71107
**Phone:** (318)674-3452      **Fax:** (318)676-5307
**Website:** http://www.susbo.edu/science.htm
JoAnn Warren, Director

### Maine

**★ 18534 ★ Kennebec Valley Technical College**
**Advanced Respiratory Therapist Program**
92 Western Ave.
Fairfield, ME 04937-1367
**Phone:** (207)453-5161      **Fax:** (207)453-5194
**Email:** blarsson@kvtc.net
**Website:** http://www.kvtc.mtcs.tec.me.us/rt.htm
Barbara A. Larsson, Director

**★ 18535 ★ Southern Maine Technical College**
**Advanced Respiratory Therapist Program**
2 Fort Rd.
South Portland, ME 04106
**Phone:** (207)767-9592      **Fax:** (207)767-9690
**Email:** wchop@smtc.net
**Website:**      http://www.smtc.net/programs/respiratory.htm
Walter C. Chop, Director

### Maryland

**★ 18536 ★ Allegany College of Maryland**
**Advanced Respiratory Therapist Program**
12401 Willowbrook Rd. SE
Cumberland, MD 21502-2596
**Phone:** (301)784-5522      **Fax:** (301)784-5015
**Email:** brocks@acc7.ac.cc.md.us
**Website:** http://www.ac.cc.md.us/Department/respther.htm
William R. Rocks, Director
**Frmly:** Allegany Community College.

**★ 18537 ★ Columbia Union College**
**Advanced Respiratory Therapist Program**
7600 Flower Ave.
Takoma Park, MD 20912
**Phone:** (301)891-4080 **Fax:** (301)891-4181
**Website:** http://www.cuc.edu/academics/resp_care.html
Alvin R. Tucker, Director

**★ 18538 ★ Community College of**
**Baltimore County—Essex Campus**
**Advanced Respiratory Therapist Program**
7201 Rossville Blvd.
Baltimore, MD 21237
**Phone:** (410)682-8015 **Fax:** (410)682-8249
**Website:** http://www.ccbc.cc.md.us/campuses/essex/academics/career/aas/e_rc.htm
Barbara Schenk, Director

**★ 18539 ★ Frederick Community College**
**(LB)**
**Advanced Respiratory Therapist Program**
7932 Opossumtown Pike
Frederick, MD 21702
**Phone:** (301)846-2528 **Fax:** (301)846-2498
**Email:** mpaugh@fcc.cc.md.us
**Website:** http://www.fcc.cc.md.us/academic_programs/allied_health_wellness.cfmrtp
Mark L. Paugh, PhD, Director

**★ 18540 ★ Prince George's Community**
**College (LB)**
**Advanced Respiratory Therapist Program**
301 Largo Rd.
Largo, MD 20774
**Phone:** (301)322-0740 **Fax:** (301)386-7528
**Email:** smithlai@pg.cc.md.us
**Website:** http://pgweb.pg.cc.md.us/
Linda A. Smith, Director

**★ 18541 ★ Salisbury State University**
**(LB)**
**Advanced Respiratory Therapist Program**
1101 Camden Ave.
Salisbury, MD 21801
**Phone:** (410)543-6365 **Fax:** (410)548-9185
**Email:** srschneider@ssu.edu
**Website:** http://www.ssu.edu/Schools/Henson.html
Sidney R. Schneider, PhD, Director

**Massachusetts**

**★ 18542 ★ Berkshire Community College**
**Advanced Respiratory Therapist Program**
1350 West St.
Pittsfield, MA 01201
**Phone:** (413)499-4660 **Fax:** (413)448-2700
**Email:** tcarey@cc.berkshire.org
**Website:** http://cc.berkshire.org/perl-cgi/showPage.cgi?deptDatarsp
Thomas P. Carey, Jr., Director

**★ 18543 ★ Massachusetts Bay**
**Community College**
**Division of Health Professions**
**Advanced Respiratory Therapist Program**
50 Oakland St.
Wellesley Hills, MA 02481
**Phone:** (781)239-2273 **Fax:** (781)416-1319
**Email:** stanleys@mbcc.mass.edu
**Website:** http://www.mbcc.mass.edu/mbcc/Programs/PROGRAMS.HTMLRespiratory AS
Scott Stanley, Director

**★ 18544 ★ Massasoit Community College**
**(LB)**
**Advanced Respiratory Therapist Program**
1 Massasoit Blvd.
Brockton, MA 02302
**Phone:** (508)588-9100 **Fax:** (508)427-1250
**Email:** mdesilva@massasoit.mass.edu
**Website:** http://www.massasoit.mass.edu/resp.htm
Martha DeSilva, Director

**★ 18545 ★ North Shore Community**
**College (LB)**
**Advanced Respiratory Therapist Program**
1 Ferncroft Rd.
PO Box 3340
Danvers, MA 01923-0840
**Phone:** (978)762-4166 **Fax:** (978)762-4022
**Email:** gtwomey@nscc.mass.edu
**Website:** http://www.nscc.cc.ma.us/
Geraldine Twomey, Director

**★ 18546 ★ Northeastern University**
**Advanced Respiratory Therapist Program**
100 Dockser Hall
360 Huntington Ave.
Boston, MA 02115
**Phone:** (617)373-3667 **Fax:** (617)373-2968
**Email:** t.barnes@nunet.neu.edu
**Website:** http://www.dac.neu.edu/cps/RTPROG.HTM
Thomas A. Barnes, EdD, Director

**★ 18547 ★ Northern Essex Community**
**College**
**Advanced Respiratory Therapist Program**
45 Franklin St.
Lawrence, MA 01841-4911
**Phone:** (978)738-7514 **Fax:** (978)374-3729
**Email:** crowse@necc.mass.edu
**Website:** http://www.necc.mass.edu/acaprds5.htmRESPIRATORY
Christopher Rowse, Director

**★ 18548 ★ Quinsigamond Community**
**College**
**Advanced Respiratory Therapist Program**
670 W Boylston St.
Worcester, MA 01606
**Phone:** (508)854-4398 **Fax:** (508)852-6943
**Website:** http://www.qcc.mass.edu/
Lynda A. Nesbitt, Director

**★ 18549 ★ Springfield Technical**
**Community College**
**Advanced Respiratory Therapist Program**
1 Armory Sq.
Springfield, MA 01105
**Phone:** (413)755-4829 **Fax:** (413)733-0688
**Email:** robinson@stcc.mass.edu
**Website:** http://www.stcc.mass.edu/academics/Descriptions/Respiratory.asp
Lee J. Robinson, Director

**Michigan**

**★ 18550 ★ Delta College**
**Advanced Respiratory Therapist Program**
University Center, MI 48710
**Phone:** (517)686-9489 **Fax:** (517)686-8736
**Email:** ebgregor@alpha.delta.edu
**Website:** http://www.delta.edu/classes/catalog/RT.html
Earl B. Gregory, Director

**★ 18551 ★ Ferris State University (LB)**
**Advanced Respiratory Therapist Program**
200 Ferris Dr., VFS 210A
Big Rapids, MI 49307-2740
**Phone:** (231)591-2267 **Fax:** (231)591-3788
**Email:** easterj@ferris.edu
**Website:** http://www.ferris.edu/htmls/colleges/alliedhe/respirat.htm
Julian F. Easter, Director

**★ 18552 ★ Henry Ford Community**
**College**
**Health Careers Education Center**
**Advanced Respiratory Therapist Program**
5101 Evergreen Rd.
Dearborn, MI 48128-1495
**Phone:** (313)317-6580 **Fax:** (313)317-6569
**Email:** dszyman@hfcc.net
**Website:** http://www.henryford.cc.mi.us/
Debra A. Szymanski, Director

**★ 18553 ★ Kalamazoo Valley Community**
**College**
**Texas Township Campus**
**Advanced Respiratory Therapist Program**
6767 W O Ave.
PO Box 4070
Kalamazoo, MI 49003-4070
**Phone:** (616)372-5288 **Fax:** (616)372-5458
**Email:** amoss@kvcc.edu
**Website:** http://puma.kvcc.edu/respirat/
Albert W. Moss, Director

**★ 18554 ★ Macomb Community College/**
**Detroit Macomb Hospital Corp.**
**Advanced Respiratory Therapist Program**
44575 Garfield Rd.
E Bldg. Rm. 219
Clinton Township, MI 48038-1139
**Phone:** (810)286-2150 **Fax:** (810)286-2098
**Email:** alsteadm@macomb.cc.mi.us
**Website:** http://www.macomb.cc.mi.us/Courses98LibArts/RSP.htm
Mary E. Alstead, Director

**★ 18555 ★ Marygrove College**
**Advanced Respiratory Therapist Program**
8425 W McNichols Rd.
Detroit, MI 48221-2599
**Phone:** (313)927-1421 **Fax:** (313)927-1345
**Email:** kmiller@marygrove.edu
**Website:** http://www.marygrove.edu/respirat%20care.htm
Kathy Miller, Director

**★ 18556 ★ Monroe County Community**
**College**
**Advanced Respiratory Therapist Program**
1555 S Raisinville Rd.
Monroe, MI 48161
**Phone:** (734)384-4268 **Fax:** (734)384-4187
**Email:** bboggs@mail.monroe.cc.mi.us
**Website:** http://www.monroe.cc.mi.us/academicdept/health.htm
Bonnie Boggs-Clothier, Director

**★ 18557 ★ Mott Community College**
**Advanced Respiratory Therapist Program**
1401 E Court St.
Flint, MI 48503
**Phone:** (810)232-6563 **Fax:** (810)762-5619
**Email:** dpanzlau@mcc.edu
**Website:** http://www.programs.mcc.edu/respiratory_therapy/
David L. Panzlau, Director

**★ 18558 ★ Muskegon Community College**
**Advanced Respiratory Therapist Program**
221 S Quarterline Rd.
Muskegon, MI 49442
**Phone:** (616)777-0370 **Fax:** (616)777-0480
**Email:** knued@muskegon.cc.mi.us
**Website:** http://www.muskegon.cc.mi.us/courses/schedule/resp.htm
Daniel B. Knue, Director

**★ 18559 ★ Oakland Community College**
**Advanced Respiratory Therapist Program**
2480 Opdyke Rd.
Bloomfield Hills, MI 48304-2266
**Phone:** (248)233-2919　　**Fax:** (248)233-2924
Kevin M. Chan, MD, Director

**★ 18560 ★ Washtenaw Community College**
**Advanced Respiratory Therapist Program**
4800 E Huron River Dr.
PO Box D-1
Ann Arbor, MI 48106
**Phone:** (734)973-3331　　**Fax:** (734)677-5078
**Email:** mnorwood@orchard.washtenaw.cc.mi.us
**Website:** http://www.washtenaw.cc.mi.us/dept/health/rth/
Mimi Y. Norwood, Director

**★ 18561 ★ Wayne County Community College**
**Advanced Respiratory Therapist Program**
801 W Fort St.
Detroit, MI 48226
**Phone:** (313)496-2798　　**Fax:** (313)962-5097
**Email:** dafdkw@admin.wccc.edu
Debraha Watson, Director

## Minnesota

**★ 18562 ★ College of Saint Catherine—Minneapolis**
**Advanced Respiratory Therapist Program**
601 25th Ave. S
Minneapolis, MN 55454
**Phone:** (651)690-7819　　**Fax:** (651)690-7849
**Email:** jeboatright@stkate.edu
**Website:** http://www.stkate.edu/Admission/
John E. Boatright, Director

**★ 18563 ★ Lake Superior College**
**Advanced Respiratory Therapist Program**
2101 Trinity Rd.
Duluth, MN 55811
**Phone:** (218)733-5925　　**Fax:** (218)723-4921
**Email:** c.annable@lsc.mnscu.edu
**Website:** http://www.lsc.cc.mn.us/programs/rcpmain.htm
Cynthia Annable, Director

**★ 18564 ★ Northwest Technical College—East Grand Forks**
**Advanced Respiratory Therapist Program**
2022 Central Ave. NE
East Grand Forks, MN 56721
**Phone:** (218)773-3441　　**Fax:** (218)773-4502
**Email:** tonysorum@mail.ntc.mnscu.edu
**Website:** http://www.ntc-online.com/ntc/cat/resp_ats.htm
Anthony Sorum, Director

**★ 18565 ★ Rochester Community and Technical College /Mayo Foundation**
**Advanced Respiratory Therapist Program**
1115 Siebens
Rochester, MN 55905
**Phone:** (507)284-0174　　**Fax:** (507)284-0656
**Email:** ward.jeffrey@mayo.edu
**Website:** http://www.mayo.edu/hrs/hrs_rt.htm
Jeffrey J. Ward, Director

**★ 18566 ★ Saint Paul Technical College**
**Advanced Respiratory Therapist Program**
235 Marshall Ave.
Saint Paul, MN 55102
**Phone:** (612)221-1413　　**Fax:** (612)221-1416
**Website:** http://www.sptc.tec.mn.us/programs/health/respitory.asp
Duane R. Peterson, Director

## Mississippi

**★ 18567 ★ Copiah-Lincoln Community College**
**Natchez Campus Vocational-Technical Division**
**Advanced Respiratory Therapist Program**
30 Campus Dr.
Natchez, MS 39120-5398
**Phone:** (601)446-1161　　**Fax:** (601)446-1298
**Website:** http://www.colin.cc.ms.us/Natchez/Default.htm
Gerald J. Millione, Director

**★ 18568 ★ Hinds Community College (LB)**
**Advanced Respiratory Therapist Program**
1750 Chadwick Dr.
Jackson, MS 39204
**Phone:** (601)371-3517　　**Fax:** (601)371-3508
**Email:** dsylvester@hinds.cc.ms.us
**Website:** http://www.hinds.cc.ms.us/
Diane H. Sylvester, Director

**★ 18569 ★ Itawamba Community College**
**Advanced Respiratory Therapist Program**
602 W Hill St.
Fulton, MS 38843
**Phone:** (601)862-3101　　**Fax:** (601)862-7697
**Email:** hjplunkett@icc.cc.ms.us
**Website:** http://www.icc.cc.ms.us/
James Harold Plunkett, Director

**★ 18570 ★ Mississippi Gulf Coast Community College**
**Advanced Respiratory Therapist Program**
PO Box 100
Gautier, MS 39553
**Phone:** (601)497-7711　　**Fax:** (601)497-7670
**Email:** judiescott@mgccc.cc.ms.us
**Website:** http://www.mgc.cc.ms.us/
Judie A. Scott, Director

**★ 18571 ★ Northeast Mississippi Community College**
**Advanced Respiratory Therapist Program**
Cunningham Blvd.
Booneville, MS 38829
**Phone:** (601)720-7387　　**Fax:** (601)728-1165
**Email:** bprince@necc.cc.ms.us
**Website:** http://www.necc.cc.ms.us/
Beverly D. Prince, Director

**★ 18572 ★ Northwest Mississippi Community College (LB)**
**Advanced Respiratory Therapist Program**
5197 WE Ross Pkwy.
Southaven, MS 38671
**Phone:** (601)280-6151　　**Fax:** (601)280-6161
**Email:** r_clark@nwcc.cc.ms.us
**Website:** http://www.necc.cc.ms.us
Regina K. Clark, Director

**★ 18573 ★ Pearl River Community College—Poplarville (LB)**
**Forrest County Vocational-Technical Center**
**Advanced Respiratory Therapist Program**
5448 US Hwy. 49 S
Hattiesburg, MS 39401
**Phone:** (601)554-7722　　**Fax:** (601)554-9148
**Email:** slking@prcc.cc.ms.us
**Website:** http://www.prcc.cc.ms.us/cat-tecp.htmRESPIRATORY CARE TECHNOLOGY
S. Lee King, Director

## Missouri

**★ 18574 ★ ConCorde Career Institute, Inc.**
**Advanced Respiratory Therapist Program**
3239 Broadway
Kansas City, MO 64111
**Phone:** (816)531-5223　　**Fax:** (816)756-3231
**Email:** lbass@concordecolleges.com
**Website:** http://www.concordecareercolleges.com/
Lana C. Bass, Director

**★ 18575 ★ Missouri Southern State College (LB)**
**Advanced Respiratory Therapist Program**
3950 E Newman Rd.
Joplin, MO 64801-1595
**Phone:** (417)659-4423　　**Fax:** (417)659-4408
**Email:** pippin-g@mail.mssc.edu
**Website:** http://www.mssc.edu/catalog99-01/technology/rt/index.htm
Glenda Pippin, Director

**★ 18576 ★ Ozarks Technical Community College**
**Advanced Respiratory Therapist Program**
PO Box 5958
Springfield, MO 65801
**Phone:** (417)895-7127　　**Fax:** (417)895-7057
**Email:** sbishop@otc.cc.mo.us
**Website:** http://www.otc.cc.mo.us/degrees/alldhlth/rt/index.htm
Stephen I. Bishop, PhD, Director

**★ 18577 ★ Saint Louis Community College—Forest Park (LB)**
**Advanced Respiratory Therapist Program**
5600 Oakland Ave.
Saint Louis, MO 63110
**Phone:** (314)644-9079　　**Fax:** (314)644-9752
**Email:** jbrennan@stlcc.cc.mo.us
**Website:** http://www.stlcc.cc.mo.us/fp/respira/
James R. Brennan, Director

**★ 18578 ★ Sanford-Brown College—Hazelwood Campus**
**Advanced Respiratory Therapist Program**
355 Brookes Dr.
Hazelwood, MO 63042
**Phone:** (314)731-3995　　**Fax:** (314)731-7044
Willis M. Mueller, Director

**★ 18579 ★ University of Missouri, Columbia (LB)**
**Advanced Respiratory Therapist Program**
605 Lewis Hall
Columbia, MO 65211
**Phone:** (573)882-8034　　**Fax:** (573)884-1490
**Email:** prewittm@health.missouri.edu
**Website:** http://www.muhealth.org/~shrp/rtwww/docs/rt.html
Michael W. Prewitt, PhD, Director

## Montana

**★ 18580 ★ Montana State University College of Technology**
**Advanced Respiratory Therapist Program**
PO Box 6010
Great Falls, MT 59406-6010
**Phone:** (406)771-4360　　**Fax:** (406)771-4313
**Email:** lbates@msugf.edu
**Website:** http://msucotgf.montana.edu/~msucotgf/programs/respirat.html
Leonard Bates, Director

## Nebraska

**★ 18581 ★ Algent Health/IMC Midland Lutheran College**
**Advanced Respiratory Therapist Program**
6901 N 72nd St.
Omaha, NE 68122
**Phone:** (402)572-2312 **Fax:** (402)572-3157
**Website:** http://www.mlc.edu/acadmenu.html
Steven L. Carper, Director

**★ 18582 ★ Metropolitan Community College**
**Advanced Respiratory Therapist Program**
PO Box 3777
Omaha, NE 68103
**Phone:** (402)738-4653 **Fax:** (402)738-4005
**Email:** jmoss@metropo.mccneb.edu
**Website:** http://www.mccneb.edu/pr/catalog2.htmRCT
Jerald A. Moss, Director

**★ 18583 ★ Nebraska Methodist College of Nursing and Allied Health**
**Advanced Respiratory Therapist Program**
8501 W Dodge Rd.
Omaha, NE 68114
**Phone:** (402)354-4913 **Fax:** (402)354-8875
**Email:** chamil1@nmhs.org
**Website:** http://www.methodistcollege.edu/
Christine Hamilton, Director

**★ 18584 ★ Southeast Community College**
**Advanced Respiratory Therapist Program**
8800 O St.
Lincoln, NE 68520-1299
**Phone:** (402)437-2782 **Fax:** (402)437-2404
**Email:** dchatter@sccm.ne.us
**Website:** http://www.college.sccm.cc.ne.us/2b6.htmRespiratory Care Program
Dhiren K. Chatterji, Director

## New Hampshire

**★ 18585 ★ New Hampshire Community Technical College**
**Advanced Respiratory Therapist Program**
1 College Dr.
Claremont, NH 03743
**Phone:** (603)542-7744 **Fax:** (603)543-1844
**Email:** jmarcley@tec.nh.us
**Website:** http://www.claremont.tec.nh.us/
John Marcley, Director

## New Jersey

**★ 18586 ★ Bergen Community College**
**Advanced Respiratory Therapist Program**
400 Paramus Rd.
Paramus, NJ 07652
**Phone:** (201)447-7944 **Fax:** (201)612-8225
**Email:** rmuller@mailhost.bergen.cc.nj.us
**Website:** http://www.bergen.cc.nj.us/
Robert A. Muller, Director

**★ 18587 ★ Brookdale Community College**
**Advanced Respiratory Therapist Program**
765 Newman Springs Rd.
Lincroft, NJ 07738
**Phone:** (732)224-2606 **Fax:** (732)224-2772
**Email:** pfusaro@brookdale.cc.nj.us
**Website:** http://www2.brookdale.cc.nj.us/brookdale/storiescc/dsaasrtt.htm
Patricia A. Fusaro, Director

**★ 18588 ★ Northwest New Jersey Consortium for Respiratory Care Education**
**Advanced Respiratory Therapist Program**
Saint Clare's Hospital
400 Blackwell St.
Dover, NJ 07801
**Phone:** (973)537-3906 **Fax:** (973)537-3996
**Email:** dadams@saintclares.org
Dianne Adams, Director

**★ 18589 ★ Passaic County Community College**
**Advanced Respiratory Therapist Program**
1 College Blvd.
Paterson, NJ 07505-1179
**Phone:** (973)684-5280 **Fax:** (973)684-5843
**Email:** smccleaster@pccc.cc.nj.us
**Website:** http://www.pccc.cc.nj.us/courses/therapy.html
Sandra McCleaster, Director

**★ 18590 ★ Union County College**
**Advanced Respiratory Therapist Program**
232 E Second St.
Plainfield, NJ 07060
**Phone:** (908)412-3574 **Fax:** (908)754-2798
**Email:** handrews@hawk.ucc.edu
**Website:** http://www.ucc.edu
Harlan Andrews, Director

**★ 18591 ★ University of Medicine and Dentistry of New Jersey**
**School of Health Related Professions**
**Advanced Respiratory Therapist Program**
PO Box 200
Blackwood, NJ 08012
**Phone:** (856)227-7200 **Fax:** (856)374-4891
**Email:** gross@umdnj.edu
**Website:** http://www.umdnj.edu/shrpweb/catalog/Cardiopulmonary_Sciences/rsj-program.h tm
G. Woodard Gross, Director

**★ 18592 ★ University of Medicine and Dentistry of New Jersey**
**School of Health Related Professions**
**Advanced Respiratory Therapist Program**
65 Bergen St.
Newark, NJ 07107-3006
**Phone:** (973)972-5503 **Fax:** (973)972-5258
**Email:** scanlan@umdnj.edu
**Website:** http://www.umdnj.edu/shrpweb/catalog/Cardiopulmonary_Sciences/index-rnj.htm
Craig L. Scanlan, EdD, Director

## New Mexico

**★ 18593 ★ Albuquerque Technical-Vocational Institute**
**Advanced Respiratory Therapist Program**
525 Buena Vista SE
Albuquerque, NM 87106
**Phone:** (505)224-4111 **Fax:** (505)224-4120
**Email:** rgentile@tvi.cc.nm.us
**Website:** http://www.tvi.cc.nm.us/health/resp.html
Richard J. Gentile, Jr., Director

**★ 18594 ★ Dona Ana Branch Community College**
**Advanced Respiratory Therapist Program**
3400 S Espina St.
Box 30001, Department 3DA
Las Cruces, NM 88003-0001
**Phone:** (505)527-7634 **Fax:** (505)527-7515
**Email:** radams@nmsu.edu
**Website:** http://dabcc-www.nmsu.edu/Catalog/respiratory.html
Rene Adams, Director

## New York

**★ 18595 ★ City University of New York, Borough of Manhattan Community College**
**Advanced Respiratory Therapist Program**
199 Chambers St.
New York, NY 10007
**Phone:** (212)346-8731 **Fax:** (212)346-8738
**Email:** bmhltewf@cunyvm.cuny.edu
**Website:** http://www.bmcc.cuny.edu/acaprogs/respprog.htm
Everett W. Flannery, Director

**★ 18596 ★ Erie Community College— North Campus**
**Advanced Respiratory Therapist Program**
6205 Main St.
Williamsville, NY 14221
**Phone:** (716)851-1531 **Fax:** (716)851-1429
**Email:** siegel@ecc.edu
**Website:** http://nstaff.sunyerie.edu/home/crcn/ah.htm
Marlon B. Siegel, Director

**★ 18597 ★ Genesee Community College**
**Advanced Respiratory Therapist Program**
1 College Rd.
Batavia, NY 14020-1519
**Phone:** (716)343-0055 **Fax:** (716)343-0433
**Email:** rmjacobs@sunygenesee.cc.ny.us
**Website:** http://www.sunygenesee.cc.ny.us/dept/health.htm
Ronald M. Jacobs, Director

**★ 18598 ★ Hudson Valley Community College**
**Advanced Respiratory Therapist Program**
80 Vandenburgh Ave.
Troy, NY 12180
**Phone:** (518)624-7454 **Fax:** (518)624-7594
**Email:** hylanpat@hvcc.edu
**Website:** http://www.hvcc.edu/academ/schools/health/res/
Patricia G. Hyland, Director

**★ 18599 ★ Long Island University, Brooklyn Campus (LB)**
**Advanced Respiratory Therapist Program**
University Plaza
Brooklyn, NY 11201
**Phone:** (718)488-1492 **Fax:** (718)488-1432
**Email:** tjohnson@titan.liunet.edu
**Website:** http://www.brooklyn.liunet.edu/cwis/bklyn/health/bsrescar.html
Thomas J. Johnson, Director

**★ 18600 ★ Mohawk Valley Community College**
**Advanced Respiratory Therapist Program**
1101 Sherman Dr.
Utica, NY 13501
**Phone:** (315)792-5664 **Fax:** (315)792-5666
**Email:** lphillips@mvcc.edu
**Website:** http://www.mvcc.edu/catalog/health/resp1.htm
Lorie Phillips, Director

**★ 18601 ★ Molloy College (LB)**
**Advanced Respiratory Therapist Program**
1000 Hempstead Ave.
Rockville Centre, NY 11571
**Phone:** (516)678-5000 **Fax:** (516)256-2252
**Email:** tbarrett@molloy.edu
**Website:** http://www.molloy.edu/academic/allied.htm
Teresa Barrett, PhD, Director

**★ 18602 ★ Nassau Community College**
**Advanced Respiratory Therapist Program**
1 Education Dr.
Garden City, NY 11530
**Phone:** (516)572-7560
**Email:** hostetw@sunynassau.edu
**Website:** http://www.sunynassau.edu/catalog/acaddep/acadep.htm
Warren Hostetter, Director

**★ 18603 ★ New York University (LB)**
**Advanced Respiratory Therapist Program**
11 W 42nd St., Rm. 518
New York, NY 10036
**Phone:** (212)790-1630      **Fax:** (212)790-1669
**Email:** cqs3166@is4.nyu.edu
**Website:** http://www.scps.nyu.edu/dyncon/heac/cour_alli_resp.html
Carole Smith, Director

**★ 18604 ★ Onondaga Community College**
**Advanced Respiratory Therapist Program**
Rte. 173
Syracuse, NY 13215
**Phone:** (315)498-2458      **Fax:** (315)498-2593
**Email:** cleveland@aurora.sunyocc.edu
**Website:** http://www.sunyocc.edu/
Daniel V. Cleveland, Director

**★ 18605 ★ Rockland Community College**
**Advanced Respiratory Therapist Program**
145 College Rd.
Suffern, NY 10901
**Phone:** (914)574-4539      **Fax:** (914)574-4498
**Email:** closejan@ged.net
**Website:** http://www.sunyrockland.edu/respt/allied-h.html
Janice R. Close, Director

**★ 18606 ★ State University of New York**
**Health Science Center, Stony Brook**
**School of Health Technology and**
**Management**
**Advanced Respiratory Therapist Program**
Stony Brook, NY 11794-8203
**Phone:** (631)444-3180      **Fax:** (631)444-7621
**Email:** kaxton@epo.hsc.sunysb.edu
**Website:** http://www.uhmc.sunysb.edu/shtm/rc/rc_homepage.html
Kenneth L. Axton, Jr., Director

**★ 18607 ★ SUNY Upstate Medical**
**University (LB)**
**Advanced Respiratory Therapist Program**
750 E Adams St.
Syracuse, NY 13210
**Phone:** (315)464-5580      **Fax:** (315)464-6876
**Email:** morfeij@upstate.edu
**Website:** http://www.ec.hscsyr.edu/CHRP/resp/Respiratory_Care.html
Joseph J. Morfei, Director

**★ 18608 ★ Westchester Community**
**College**
**Advanced Respiratory Therapist Program**
75 Grasslands Rd.
Health Science Bldg.
Valhalla, NY 10595
**Phone:** (914)785-6883      **Fax:** (914)785-6889
**Email:** jose.quinones@sunywcc.edu
**Website:** http://www.sunywcc.edu/
Jose Quinones, Director

### North Carolina

**★ 18609 ★ Carteret Community College**
**Advanced Respiratory Therapist Program**
3505 Arendell St.
Morehead City, NC 28557
**Phone:** (252)247-6000      **Fax:** (252)247-2514
**Email:** lap@carteret.cc.nc.us
**Website:** http://gofish.carteret.cc.nc.us/
Laurie A. Pratt, Director

**★ 18610 ★ Catawba Valley Community**
**College**
**Advanced Respiratory Therapist Program**
2550 Hwy. 70 SE
Hickory, NC 28602
**Phone:** (828)327-7000      **Fax:** (828)327-7276
**Email:** cbitsche@cvcc.cc.nc.us
**Website:** http://www.cvcc.cc.nc.us/programs/health/RCPAGE.HTM
Catherine A. Bitsche, Director

**★ 18611 ★ Central Piedmont Community**
**College**
**Advanced Respiratory Therapist Program**
PO Box 35009
Charlotte, NC 28235
**Phone:** (704)330-6274      **Fax:** (704)330-5930
**Email:** tom.morris@cpcc.cc.nc.us
**Website:** http://www.cpcc.cc.nc.us/Health_Sciences/Respiratory_Care/
Thomas R. Morris, Director

**★ 18612 ★ Durham Technical Community**
**College**
**Advanced Respiratory Therapist Program**
1637 Lawson St.
PO Drawer 11307
Durham, NC 27703
**Phone:** (919)686-3643      **Fax:** (919)686-3693
**Website:** http://209.86.110.158/career/progstud/rctech/rctech.htm
Richard D. Miller, PhD, Director

**★ 18613 ★ Edgecombe Community**
**College**
**Advanced Respiratory Therapist Program**
225 Tarboro St.
Rocky Mount, NC 27801
**Phone:** (252)446-0436      **Fax:** (252)985-2212
**Email:** webbrd@edgecombe.cc.nc.us
**Website:** http://www.edgecombe.cc.nc.us/RESP-CARE.HTM
Ralph D. Webb, Director

**★ 18614 ★ Fayetteville Technical**
**Community College**
**Advanced Respiratory Therapist Program**
2201 Hull Rd.
Fayetteville, NC 28303
**Phone:** (910)678-8316      **Fax:** (910)484-8254
**Email:** baldwinr@ftccmail.faytech.cc.nc.us
**Website:** http://atlas.faytech.cc.nc.us/edprog/curr/a45720.html
Ruth A. Baldwin, Director

**★ 18615 ★ Forsyth Technical Community**
**College**
**Advanced Respiratory Therapist Program**
2100 Silas Creek Pkwy.
Winston-Salem, NC 27103
**Phone:** (336)723-0371      **Fax:** (336)734-7444
**Email:** psheppar@forsyth.cc.nc.us
**Website:** http://www.forsyth.tec.nc.us/
Perry W. Sheppard, Director

**★ 18616 ★ Pitt Community College**
**Advanced Respiratory Therapist Program**
PO Drawer 7007
Hwy. 11 S
Greenville, NC 27834
**Phone:** (252)321-4378      **Fax:** (252)321-4451
**Email:** bsteinba@pcc.pitt.cc.nc.us
**Website:** http://www.pitt.cc.nc.us/
R. Bruce Steinbach, Director

**★ 18617 ★ Robeson Community College**
**Advanced Respiratory Therapist Program**
PO Box 1420
Lumberton, NC 28359
**Phone:** (910)738-7101      **Fax:** (910)617-4143
**Email:** kheustess@robeson.cc.nc.us
**Website:** http://www.robeson.cc.nc.us/health.htmRespiratory
Kelli Heustess, Director

**★ 18618 ★ Sandhills Community College**
**Advanced Respiratory Therapist Program**
2200 Airport Rd.
Pinehurst, NC 28374
**Phone:** (910)695-3836      **Fax:** (910)692-6918
**Email:** croftb@email.sandhills.cc.nc.us
**Website:** http://www.sandhills.cc.nc.us/rct/rct-index.html
William L. Croft, Contact

**★ 18619 ★ Southwestern Community**
**College**
**Advanced Respiratory Therapist Program**
447 College Dr.
Sylva, NC 28779-9598
**Phone:** (828)586-4091      **Fax:** (828)586-3129
**Email:** shatfield@southwest.cc.nc.us
**Website:** http://www.southwest.cc.nc.us/Acadprog/rsp.htm
Sharon Hatfield, Director

**★ 18620 ★ Stanly Community College**
**Advanced Respiratory Therapist Program**
141 College Dr.
Albemarle, NC 28001
**Phone:** (704)991-0267      **Fax:** (704)991-0110
**Email:** crump@stanly.cc.nc.us
**Website:** http://www.stanly.cc.nc.us/STUSER/CRSCAT/course_schedule/respcare.htm
Tammy P. Crump, Director

### North Dakota

**★ 18621 ★ North Dakota School of**
**Respiratory Care (LB)**
**University of Mary / Saint Alexius**
**Medical Center**
**Advanced Respiratory Therapist Program**
900 E Broadway
PO Box 5510
Bismarck, ND 58502
**Phone:** (701)530-7757      **Fax:** (701)530-7701
**Email:** wbeachey@primecare.org
**Website:** http://www.umary.edu/course/co_respcare.htm
Wilmer D. Beachey, Director

**★ 18622 ★ North Dakota State University**
**/ MeritCare Hospital Consortium**
**Advanced Respiratory Therapist Program**
720 Fourth St. N
Respiratory Care No. 118
Fargo, ND 58122
**Phone:** (701)234-6147      **Fax:** (701)234-6942
**Email:** garybrown@meritcare.com
**Website:** http://www.ndsu.nodak.edu/instruct/poolson/rt/
Gary Brown, Director

### Ohio

**★ 18623 ★ Bowling Green State**
**University**
**Advanced Respiratory Therapist Program**
901 Rye Beach Rd.
Huron, OH 44839-9791
**Phone:** (419)433-5560      **Fax:** (419)433-9696
**Email:** rroark@bgnet.bgsu.edu
**Website:** http://www.firelands.bgsu.edu/as/rt/
Rod C. Roark, Director

★ 18624 ★ **Cincinnati State Technical and Community College**
**Advanced Respiratory Therapist Program**
3520 Central Pkwy.
Cincinnati, OH 45223
**Phone:** (513)569-1659    **Fax:** (513)569-1559
**Email:** lierld@cinstate.cc.oh.us
**Website:** http://www.cinstate.cc.oh.us/htd-rc.htm
Debra Lierl, Director

★ 18625 ★ **Collins Career Center**
**Advanced Respiratory Therapist Program**
11627 State Rte. 243
Chesapeake, OH 45619
**Phone:** (614)867-6641    **Fax:** (614)867-2009
**Email:** katerry@collins-cc.k12.oh.us
**Website:** http://www.collins-cc.k12.oh.us/
Keith Terry, Director

★ 18626 ★ **Columbus State Community College**
**Advanced Respiratory Therapist Program**
550 E Spring St.
Columbus, OH 43215
**Phone:** (614)227-2513    **Fax:** (614)287-5144
**Email:** dwallace@cscc.edu
David U. Wallace, Director

★ 18627 ★ **Cuyahoga Community College (LB)**
**Advanced Respiratory Therapist Program**
11000 Pleasant Valley Rd.
Parma, OH 44130
**Phone:** (216)987-5267    **Fax:** (216)987-5066
**Email:** dave.lucas@tri-c.cc.oh.us
**Website:** http://www.tri-c.cc.oh.us/HEALTH/RCWEB/Frmset1.htm
David A. Lucas, Director

★ 18628 ★ **Jefferson Community College**
**Advanced Respiratory Therapist Program**
4000 Sunset Blvd.
Steubenville, OH 43952
**Phone:** (614)264-5591    **Fax:** (614)264-1338
**Email:** ccarducci@jefferson.cc.oh.us
**Website:** http://ns3.jeffersohncc.org/jcc/programinfo.asp?programid=40
Cynthia Carducci, Director

★ 18629 ★ **Kettering College of Medical Arts (LB)**
**Advanced Respiratory Therapist Program**
3737 Southern Blvd.
Kettering, OH 45429
**Phone:** (937)298-3399    **Fax:** (937)296-4238
**Email:** tom.hill@kmcnetwork.org
**Website:** http://www.kcma.edu/
Thomas V. Hill, PhD, Director

★ 18630 ★ **Lakeland Community College**
**Advanced Respiratory Therapist Program**
7700 Clocktower Dr.
Kirtland, OH 44094-5198
**Phone:** (216)953-7343    **Fax:** (216)975-4733
**Email:** ckenny@lakeland.cc.oh.us
**Website:** http://www.lakeland.cc.oh.us/ACADEMIC/SH/resp/index.htm
Catherine J. Kenny, Director

★ 18631 ★ **Lima Technical College (LB)**
**Advanced Respiratory Therapist Program**
4240 Campus Dr.
Lima, OH 45804
**Phone:** (419)995-8366    **Fax:** (419)995-8818
**Email:** woodfier@ltc.tec.oh.us
**Website:** http://www.ltc.tec.oh.us/academic/health/resp_care.htm
Richard N. Woodfield, Jr., Director

★ 18632 ★ **North Central State College (LB)**
**Advanced Respiratory Therapist Program**
2441 Kenwood Cir.
PO Box 698
Mansfield, OH 44901
**Phone:** (419)755-4800    **Fax:** (419)755-5630
**Email:** rslabod@ncstate.tec.oh.us
**Website:** http://www.nctc.tec.oh.us/pages/respther.html
Robert A. Slabodnick, Director

★ 18633 ★ **Ohio State University**
**Advanced Respiratory Therapist Program**
1583 Perry St.
Columbus, OH 43210
**Phone:** (614)292-8445    **Fax:** (614)292-0210
**Email:** douce.2@osu.edu
**Website:** http://www.amp.ohio-state.edu/!SAMPWEB/rt-1.htm
F. Herbert Douce, Director

★ 18634 ★ **Shawnee State University**
**Advanced Respiratory Therapist Program**
940 Second St.
Portsmouth, OH 45662
**Phone:** (614)355-2235    **Fax:** (614)355-2354
**Email:** dthomas@shawnee.edu
**Website:** http://www.shawnee.edu/prospective/academics/aca%20deptment/health/parts/mi ds/respiratory.htm
Donald L. Thomas, Director

★ 18635 ★ **Sinclair Community College (LB)**
**Advanced Respiratory Therapist Program**
444 W Third St.
Dayton, OH 45402
**Phone:** (937)512-2849    **Fax:** (937)512-2058
**Email:** cbeckett@sinclair.edu
**Website:** http://www.sinclair.edu/departments/ret/
Cynthia A. Beckett, PhD, Director

★ 18636 ★ **Stark State College of Technology**
**Advanced Respiratory Therapist Program**
6200 Frank Ave. NW
Canton, OH 44720-7299
**Phone:** (330)494-6170    **Fax:** (330)966-6586
**Email:** pcastillo@stark.cc.oh.us
**Website:** http://www.stark.cc.oh.us/academic/health/respiratory_care.htm
Peter R. Castillo, Director
**Frmly:** Stark Technical College.

★ 18637 ★ **University of Akron**
**Advanced Respiratory Therapist Program**
302 E Buchtel Ave.
Akron, OH 44325
**Phone:** (330)972-7906    **Fax:** (330)972-2016
**Email:** laverne@uakron.edu
**Website:** http://www.commtech.uakron.edu/commtech/a_health/respcare.htm
LaVerne C. Yousey, MD, Contact

★ 18638 ★ **University of Toledo**
**College of Health and Human Service**
**Advanced Respiratory Therapist Program**
2801 W Bancroft St.
Toledo, OH 43606
**Fax:** (419)530-4451
**Email:** margaret.traban@utoledo.edu
**Website:** http://www.hhs.utoledo.edu/
Margaret F. Traband, Director

★ 18639 ★ **Washington State Community College**
**Advanced Respiratory Therapist Program**
710 Colegate Dr.
Marietta, OH 45750
**Phone:** (614)374-8716    **Fax:** (614)373-7496
**Email:** rkinker@wscc.edu
James R. Kinker, PhD, Director

★ 18640 ★ **Youngstown State University**
**Advanced Respiratory Therapist Program**
1 University Plaza
Youngstown, OH 44555
**Fax:** (330)742-2921
**Email:** lnharris@cc.ysu.edu
**Website:** http://www.ysu.edu/colleges/hhs/healthp/index.htm
Louis N. Harris, EdD, Director

## Oklahoma

★ 18641 ★ **Francis Tuttle Technology Center**
**Oklahoma City Community College**
**Advanced Respiratory Therapist Program**
12777 N Rockwell Ave.
Oklahoma City, OK 73142-2789
**Phone:** (405)717-4269    **Fax:** (405)717-4789
**Email:** lheyland@francistuttle.com
**Website:** http://www.francistuttle.com/index.htm
Lezli Heyland, Director

★ 18642 ★ **Rose State College**
**Advanced Respiratory Therapist Program**
6420 SE 15th St.
Midwest City, OK 73110
**Phone:** (405)733-7571    **Fax:** (405)736-0338
**Email:** nlorance@ms.rose.cc.ok.us
**Website:** http://www.rose.cc.ok.us/hsdiv/programs/resther.htm
Nancy J. Deck Lorance, Director

★ 18643 ★ **Tulsa Community College**
**Advanced Respiratory Therapist Program**
909 S Boston Ave.
Tulsa, OK 74119
**Phone:** (918)595-7016    **Fax:** (918)595-7091
**Email:** lporter@tulsa.cc.ok.us
**Website:** http://www.tulsa.cc.ok.us/respirat.html
Lindel W. Porter, Director

## Oregon

★ 18644 ★ **Lane Community College**
**Advanced Respiratory Therapist Program**
4000 E 30th Ave.
Eugene, OR 97405
**Phone:** (541)747-4501    **Fax:** (541)744-4151
**Email:** hechtr@lanecc.edu
**Website:** http://lanecc.edu/fahealth/rc1.htm
Roger H. Hecht, Director

★ 18645 ★ **Mount Hood Community College**
**Advanced Respiratory Therapist Program**
26000 SE Stark St.
Gresham, OR 97030
**Phone:** (503)491-7172    **Fax:** (503)491-6047
**Email:** hicksg@mhcc.cc.or.us
**Website:** http://www.mhcc.cc.or.us/catalog/programs/respir.htm
George Hicks, Director

★ 18646 ★ **Rogue Community College**
**Advanced Respiratory Therapist Program**
202 S Riverside Ave.
Medford, OR 97501
**Phone:** (541)774-1004    **Fax:** (541)774-4203
**Email:** jhulse@rogue.cc.or.us

**Website:** http://www2.rogue.cc/alliedhealth/Respiratory/home.htm
James L. Hulse, Contact

## Pennsylvania

★ **18647** ★ **Community College of Allegheny County**
**Advanced Respiratory Therapist Program**
Allegheny Campus
808 Ridge Ave.
Pittsburgh, PA 15212
**Phone:** (412)237-2607        **Fax:** (412)237-4521
**Email:** troop@ccac.edu
**Website:** http://www.acd.ccac.edu/allied-health/programs/resphome.htm
Thomas A. Roop, Director

★ **18648** ★ **Community College of Philadelphia**
**Advanced Respiratory Therapist Program**
1700 Spring Garden St.
Philadelphia, PA 19130
**Phone:** (215)751-8423        **Fax:** (215)751-8937
**Website:** http://inet.ccp.cc.pa.us/vpacaff/PROG&CRS/CREDIT/DIVBS&T/resp/
Frank M. Alsis, EdD, Director

★ **18649** ★ **Gannon University**
**Advanced Respiratory Therapist Program**
University Sq.
Erie, PA 16541
**Phone:** (814)871-5637        **Fax:** (814)871-5662
**Email:** cornfiel001@mail1.gannon.edu
**Website:** http://WWW.GANNON.EDU/RESOURCE/DEPT/respcare/index.html
Charles Cornfield, Director

★ **18650** ★ **Gwynedd-Mercy College (LB)**
**Advanced Respiratory Therapist Program**
Sumneytown Pike
Gwynedd Valley, PA 19437
**Phone:** (215)641-5536        **Fax:** (215)641-5559
**Email:** galvin.w@gmc.edu
**Website:** http://www.gmc.edu/academic/schools/alliedhealth/resp_care.htm
William F. Galvin, Director

★ **18651** ★ **Harrisburg Area Community College**
**Advanced Respiratory Therapist Program**
1 HACC Dr.
Harrisburg, PA 17110
**Phone:** (717)780-2315        **Fax:** (717)780-2551
**Email:** baleidic@hacc.edu
**Website:** http://www.hacc.edu/
Bradley A. Leidich, Director

★ **18652** ★ **Indiana University of Pennsylvania (LB)**
**Advanced Respiratory Therapist Program**
4800 Friendship Ave.
Pittsburgh, PA 15224
**Phone:** (412)578-7000        **Fax:** (412)578-4651
**Email:** bmalley@icubed.com
**Website:** http://www.iup.edu/schedu/catalog/hhumsvc/resp.htmlx
William J. Malley, Director

★ **18653** ★ **Lehigh Carbon Community College**
**Advanced Respiratory Therapist Program**
4525 Education Park Dr.
Schnecksville, PA 18078-2598
**Phone:** (610)799-1527        **Fax:** (610)799-1537
**Email:** dmc1@lex.lccc.edu
**Website:** http://www.lccc.edu/offerings.html
Denise B. McCardle, Director

★ **18654** ★ **Mansfield University**
**Health Sciences Department**
**Advanced Respiratory Therapist Program**
Elliott Hall
Mansfield, PA 16933
**Phone:** (570)882-4513        **Fax:** (570)882-4413
**Email:** lvosburg@ghs.guthrie.org
**Website:** http://www.mnsfld.edu/
Larry B. Vosburgh, Director

★ **18655** ★ **Millersville University of Pennsylvania**
**Advanced Respiratory Therapist Program**
Millersville, PA 17551
**Phone:** (717)290-4912        **Fax:** (717)290-5970
**Email:** jhughes@marauder.millersv.edu
**Website:** http://muweb.millersv.edu/~rtp/
John M. Hughes, Director

★ **18656** ★ **Reading Area Community College**
**Advanced Respiratory Therapist Program**
10 S Second St.
PO Box 1706
Reading, PA 19603
**Phone:** (610)372-4721        **Fax:** (610)607-6254
**Email:** rlamme@email.racc.cc.pa.us
**Website:** http://www.racc.cc.pa.us/health.html
Robert D. Lamme, Director

★ **18657** ★ **University of Pittsburgh, Johnstown**
**Advanced Respiratory Therapist Program**
227 Krebs Hall
Johnstown, PA 15904
**Phone:** (814)269-2960        **Fax:** (814)269-7255
**Email:** bcolbert@pitt.edu
**Website:** http://www.pitt.edu/~upjweb/admissions/programs/allied_health_programs.html
Bruce J. Colbert, Director

★ **18658** ★ **West Chester University / Bryn Mawr Hospital (LB)**
**Advanced Respiratory Therapist Program**
Bryn Mawr Hospital
Bryn Mawr, PA 19010
**Phone:** (610)526-3347        **Fax:** (610)526-8545
**Email:** albright@MLHS.org
**Website:** http://www.wcupa.edu/_academics/sch_shs.hea/UNDERGRA.HTM
Douglas Albright, Director

★ **18659** ★ **Western School of Health and Business Careers**
**Advanced Respiratory Therapist Program**
421 Seventh Ave.
Pittsburgh, PA 15219
**Phone:** (412)281-7083        **Fax:** (412)281-0319
**Email:** tomwollett@westernschool.com
**Website:** http://www.westernschool.com/programs/respiratory.html
Kimberly A. Crilley, Director

★ **18660** ★ **York College of Pennsylvania/York Hospital**
**Advanced Respiratory Therapist Program**
York, PA 17405
**Phone:** (717)851-2464        **Fax:** (717)851-2934
**Email:** al_msimmons@yorkhospital.edu
**Website:** http://goose.ycp.edu/department/biology/index.html
Mark Simmons, Director

## Puerto Rico

★ **18661** ★ **Universidad Adventista de las Antillas**
**Advanced Respiratory Therapist Program**
PO Box 118
Mayaguez, PR 00681-0118
**Phone:** (787)834-9595        **Fax:** (787)834-9597
**Website:** http://www.uaa.edu/
Vilma Torres, Director

★ **18662** ★ **Universidad Metropolitana**
**Advanced Respiratory Therapist Program**
PO Box 21150
San Juan, PR 00928
**Phone:** (787)766-1717        **Fax:** (787)759-7663
**Email:** um_ltorres@suagm4.suagm.edu
Leyda Torres de Marin, Director

## Rhode Island

★ **18663** ★ **Community College of Rhode Island**
**Advanced Respiratory Therapist Program**
1762 Louisquisset Pike
Lincoln, RI 02865-4585
**Phone:** (401)333-7024        **Fax:** (401)333-7111
**Email:** jjacobs@ccri.cc.ri.us
**Website:** http://www.ccri.cc.ri.us/FRAMES/box24FR.htm
Joanne Jacobs, Director

## South Carolina

★ **18664** ★ **Florence-Darlington Technical College**
**Advanced Respiratory Therapist Program**
PO Box 100548
Florence, SC 29501-0548
**Phone:** (843)661-8148        **Fax:** (843)661-8306
**Email:** evansj@flo.tec.sc.us
**Website:** http://www.flo.tec.sc.us/
John A. Evans, Director

★ **18665** ★ **Greenville Technical College (LB)**
**Advanced Respiratory Therapist Program**
PO Box 5616
Station B
Greenville, SC 29606
**Phone:** (864)250-8308        **Fax:** (864)250-8462
**Email:** conrylac@gvltec.edu
**Website:** http://www.greenvilletech.com/resptherac.htm
Lisa Conry, Director

★ **18666** ★ **Midlands Technical College**
**Advanced Respiratory Therapist Program**
PO Box 2408
Columbia, SC 29202
**Phone:** (803)822-3433        **Fax:** (803)822-3079
**Email:** ackermanl@mtc.mid.tec.sc.us
**Website:** http://www.mid.tec.sc.us/edu/home.html
Linda Ackerman, Director

★ **18667** ★ **Piedmont Technical College**
**Advanced Respiratory Therapist Program**
Emerald Rd.
PO Box 1467
Greenwood, SC 29646
**Phone:** (864)941-8524        **Fax:** (864)941-8684
**Email:** Pickelsimer@PED.TEC.SC.US
**Website:** http://www.piedmont.tec.sc.us/academic/respcare.htm
Sherri Pickelsimer, Director

**★ 18668 ★ Spartanburg Technical College**
**Advanced Respiratory Therapist Program**
PO Drawer 4386
Spartanburg, SC 29305-4386
**Phone:** (864)591-3869 **Fax:** (864)591-3708
**Email:** splawnj@spt.tec.sc.us
**Website:** http://199.5.204.101/hs_rc_ad.htm
James Splawn, Director

**★ 18669 ★ Trident Technical College**
**Advanced Respiratory Therapist Program**
PO Box 118067
Charleston, SC 29423
**Phone:** (843)574-6101 **Fax:** (843)574-6585
**Email:** moorea@telli.trident.tec.sc.us
**Website:** http://www.trident.tec.sc.us/alliedhealth/respiratory.html
Ann R. Moore, Director

### South Dakota

**★ 18670 ★ Dakota State University**
**Advanced Respiratory Therapist Program**
Science Center
Madison, SD 57042-1799
**Phone:** (605)322-8613 **Fax:** (605)322-6666
**Email:** bruce.feistner@dsu.edu
**Website:** http://www.departments.dsu.edu/sciences/m_respcare.htm
Bruce A. Feistner, Director

### Tennessee

**★ 18671 ★ Baptist Memorial College of Health Science**
**Advanced Respiratory Therapist Program**
1003 Monroe
Memphis, TN 38104
**Phone:** (901)227-6933 **Fax:** (901)227-5533
**Email:** andrew.mazzoli@bchs.edu
Andrew J. Mazzoli, Director

**★ 18672 ★ Chattanooga State Technical Community College**
**Advanced Respiratory Therapist Program**
4501 Amnicola Hwy.
Chattanooga, TN 37406
**Phone:** (423)697-4450 **Fax:** (423)634-3071
**Email:** mrountree@cstcc.cc.tn.us
**Website:** http://www.cstcc.cc.tn.us/www/academics/alliedhealth/index.htm
McIver Rountree, Jr., Director

**★ 18673 ★ Columbia State Community College**
**Advanced Respiratory Therapist Program**
PO Box 1315
Columbia, TN 38402
**Phone:** (931)540-2663 **Fax:** (931)540-2795
**Email:** gandy@coscc.cc.tn.us
**Website:** http://www.coscc.cc.tn.us/academic/83-139.htmrct
Bill R. Gandy, Director

**★ 18674 ★ East Tennessee State University (LB)**
**Advanced Respiratory Therapist Program**
1000 W East St.
ETSU Nave Center
Elizabethton, TN 37643
**Phone:** (423)547-4916 **Fax:** (423)547-4921
**Email:** mackd@access.etsu.edu
**Website:** http://www.etsu.edu/cpah/hrelated/hrelrttr.htm
Delmar Mack, EdD, Director

**★ 18675 ★ Jackson State Community College**
**Advanced Respiratory Therapist Program**
2046 N Parkway St.
Jackson, TN 38301-3797
**Phone:** (901)425-2612 **Fax:** (901)425-9551
**Email:** cgarner@jscc.cc.tn.us
**Website:** http://www.jscc.cc.tn.us/users/allied/
Cathy K. Garner, Director

**★ 18676 ★ Roane State Community College**
**Advanced Respiratory Therapist Program**
276 Patton Ln.
Rte. 8, PO Box 69
Harriman, TN 37748
**Phone:** (423)882-4539 **Fax:** (423)882-4549
**Email:** hill_la@alrscc.cc.tn.us
**Website:** http://www.rscc.cc.tn.us/academic/health-sci/RespTherapy/
Lesha Hill, Director

**★ 18677 ★ Tennessee State University**
**Advanced Respiratory Therapist Program**
3500 John A. Merritt Blvd.
Nashville, TN 37209
**Phone:** (615)963-7431 **Fax:** (615)963-7422
**Email:** tjohn@picard.tnstate.edu
**Website:** http://www.tnstate.edu/alhp/
Thomas John, PhD, Director

**★ 18678 ★ Volunteer State Community College**
**Advanced Respiratory Therapist Program**
1360 Gallatin Pike
Gallatin, TN 37066
**Phone:** (615)452-8600 **Fax:** (615)230-3224
**Website:** http://www.vscc.cc.tn.us/academic/health/resp.html
Emmy L. Wishum, Director

### Texas

**★ 18679 ★ Alvin Community College**
**Advanced Respiratory Therapist Program**
3110 Mustang Rd.
Alvin, TX 77511
**Phone:** (281)388-4695 **Fax:** (281)388-4936
**Email:** dflatlan@alvin.cc.tx.us
**Website:** http://www.alvin.cc.tx.us/DEPT/resp/resp.htm
Diane Flatland, Director

**★ 18680 ★ Amarillo College (LB)**
**Advanced Respiratory Therapist Program**
PO Box 447
Amarillo, TX 79178
**Phone:** (806)354-6058 **Fax:** (806)354-6076
**Email:** wayoung@actx.edu
**Website:** http://www.actx.edu/~respiratory_care/
William A. Young, Director

**★ 18681 ★ Angelina College**
**Advanced Respiratory Therapist Program**
PO Box 1768
Lufkin, TX 75902-1768
**Phone:** (409)639-1301
**Email:** mparks@angelina.cc.tx.us
**Website:** http://eagle.angelina.cc.tx.us/respiratory/index.htm
Michael Parks, Director

**★ 18682 ★ Collin County Community College**
**Advanced Respiratory Therapist Program**
2200 W University Dr.
McKinney, TX 75070
**Phone:** (972)548-6870 **Fax:** (972)548-6722
**Email:** abarbaro@pmail.cccd.edu
**Website:** http://www.cccd.edu/divisions/hpc/RESPTHER.HTM
Allen W. Barbaro, Director

**★ 18683 ★ Del Mar College**
**Advanced Respiratory Therapist Program**
101 Baldwin and Ayers Sts.
Corpus Christi, TX 78404
**Phone:** (361)698-1101 **Fax:** (361)698-1598
**Email:** jwatson@delmar.edu
**Website:** http://www.delmar.edu/rt/rtweb.htm
Jeffrey T. Watson, Director

**★ 18684 ★ El Centro College**
**Advanced Respiratory Therapist Program**
Main and Lamar Sts.
Dallas, TX 75202
**Phone:** (214)860-2279 **Fax:** (214)860-2268
**Email:** glp5547@dcccd.edu
**Website:** http://www.ecc.dcccd.edu/health-ls/respiratory/RCP.HTM
Gary L. Peschka, Director

**★ 18685 ★ El Paso Community College**
**Advanced Respiratory Therapist Program**
PO Box 20500
El Paso, TX 79998
**Phone:** (915)831-4072 **Fax:** (915)831-4114
**Email:** paulan@epcc.edu
**Website:** http://www.epcc.edu/
Paul Andrade, Director

**★ 18686 ★ Houston Community College System**
**Advanced Respiratory Therapist Program**
**Respiratory Therapist Program**
3100 Shenandoah
Houston, TX 77021
**Phone:** (713)718-7378 **Fax:** (713)718-7401
**Email:** bartel_r@hccs.cc.tx.us
**Website:** http://www.hccs.cc.tx.us/SEcollege/RespCareTechnician.html
Ralph E. Bartel, Director

**★ 18687 ★ Kingwood College-NHMCCD**
**Advanced Respiratory Therapist Program**
20000 Kingwood Dr.
Kingwood, TX 77339
**Phone:** (281)312-1608 **Fax:** (281)312-1490
**Email:** kmccowen@kc.nhmccd.cc.tx.us
**Website:** http://kcweb.nhmccd.edu/programs/shas/respcare/respcare.htm
Kenny P. McCowen, Director

**★ 18688 ★ Lamar Institute of Technology (LB)**
**Advanced Respiratory Therapist Program**
PO Box 10061
Beaumont, TX 77710
**Phone:** (409)880-8852 **Fax:** (409)880-8955
**Email:** bronsonpa@hal.lamar.edu
**Website:** http://www.theinstitute.lamar.edu/programs/respiratorycare.htm
Paul A. Bronson, Director

**★ 18689 ★ Midland College**
**Advanced Respiratory Therapist Program**
3600 N Garfield
Midland, TX 79705
**Phone:** (915)685-4601 **Fax:** (915)685-4762
**Email:** rweidmann@midland.cc.tx.us
**Website:** http://www.midland.cc.tx.us/courses/pr.htmlresp care
Robert Weidmann, Director

**★ 18690 ★ Midwestern State University (LB)**
**Advanced Respiratory Therapist Program**
3410 Taft Blvd.
Wichita Falls, TX 76308
**Phone:** (940)397-4652        **Fax:** (940)397-4513
**Email:** william.burke@nexus.mwsu.edu
**Website:** http://www.mwsu.edu/htmldocs/departments/resphom.html
William C. Burke, PhD, Director

**★ 18691 ★ Odessa College**
**Advanced Respiratory Therapist Program**
201 W University Blvd.
Odessa, TX 79764
**Phone:** (915)335-6456        **Fax:** (915)335-6846
**Email:** jsullivan@odessa.edu
**Website:** http://coyote.odessa.edu/
Jacquelyn R. Sullivan, Director

**★ 18692 ★ San Jacinto College**
**Advanced Respiratory Therapist Program**
8060 Spencer Hwy.
PO Box 2007
Pasadena, TX 77505-2007
**Phone:** (281)476-1864        **Fax:** (281)478-2754
**Email:** vandi@central.sjcd.cc.tx.us
**Website:** http://www.sjcd.cc.tx.us/central/resc/index.htm
Larry P. Vandiver, Director

**★ 18693 ★ South Plains College**
**Advanced Respiratory Therapist Program**
1302 Main St.
Lubbock, TX 79401
**Phone:** (806)747-0576        **Fax:** (806)765-2775
**Email:** vstalcup@spc.cc.tx.us
**Website:** http://www.spc.cc.tx.us/
Valorie Stalcup, Director

**★ 18694 ★ Southwest Texas State University**
**Advanced Respiratory Therapist Program**
San Marcos, TX 78666
**Phone:** (512)245-8243        **Fax:** (512)245-7978
**Email:** cho3@swt.edu
**Website:** http://www.health.swt.edu/
Cade J. Harkins, III, Director

**★ 18695 ★ Tarrant County College**
**Advanced Respiratory Therapist Program**
828 Harwood Rd.
Hurst, TX 76054
**Phone:** (817)515-6435        **Fax:** (817)515-6700
**Email:** jhiser@tcjc.cc.tx.us
**Website:** http://www.tcjc.cc.tx.us/campus_ne/resp/
John D. Hiser, Director

**★ 18696 ★ Temple College**
**Advanced Respiratory Therapist Program**
2600 S First St.
Temple, TX 76504
**Phone:** (254)778-4811        **Fax:** (254)771-4528
**Email:** bill.cornel@templejc.edu
**Website:** http://www.templejc.edu/
William M. Cornelius, III, Director

**★ 18697 ★ Texas Southern University**
**Advanced Respiratory Therapist Program**
3100 Cleburne
Houston, TX 77004
**Phone:** (713)313-7265        **Fax:** (713)313-1094
**Email:** a_reginald@hotmail.com
**Website:** http://www.tsu.edu/pharmacy/index.htm
Reginald G. Allen, Director

**★ 18698 ★ Texas Southmost College / University of Texas, Brownsville**
**Advanced Respiratory Therapist Program**
83 Ft. Brown
Brownsville, TX 78520
**Phone:** (956)544-8262        **Fax:** (956)544-8910
**Email:** jmccabe@utb1.utb.edu
**Website:** http://unix.utb.edu/~kgarcia/rthp.htm
John L. McCabe, PhD, Director

**★ 18699 ★ Tyler Junior College (LB)**
**Advanced Respiratory Therapist Program**
PO Box 9020
Tyler, TX 75711
**Phone:** (903)510-2472        **Fax:** (903)510-2592
**Email:** pwes@tjc.tyler.cc.tx.us
**Website:** http://www.tyler.cc.tx.us/
Paul Weskamp, Director

**★ 18700 ★ University of Texas Health Science Center at San Antonio**
**Advanced Respiratory Therapist Program**
7703 Floyd Curl Dr., Mail Code 6248
San Antonio, TX 78229-3900
**Fax:** (210)567-8852
**Email:** shelledy@uthscsa.edu
**Website:** http://www.uthscsa.edu/sah/rc.html
David C. Shelledy, PhD, Director

**★ 18701 ★ University of Texas Medical Branch, Galveston**
**School of Allied Health Sciences**
**Advanced Respiratory Therapist Program**
301 University Blvd.
Galveston, TX 77555-1028
**Phone:** (409)772-5693        **Fax:** (409)772-3014
**Email:** jnilsest@utmb.edu
**Website:** http://www.rc.utmb.edu/
Jon O. Nilsestuen, PhD, Director

**★ 18702 ★ Victoria College (LB)**
**Advanced Respiratory Therapist Program**
2200 E Red River
Victoria, TX 77901
**Phone:** (361)572-6491        **Fax:** (361)582-2542
**Email:** ckallus@vc.cc.tx.us
**Website:** http://www.vc.cc.tx.us/programs/rescare.html
Chris E. Kallus, Director

## Utah

**★ 18703 ★ Weber State University (LB)**
**Advanced Respiratory Therapist Program**
3904 University Cir.
Ogden, UT 84408-3904
**Phone:** (801)626-7071        **Fax:** (801)626-7683
**Email:** gbills@weber.edu
**Website:** http://weber.edu/resptherapy/
Georgine Bills, Director

## Vermont

**★ 18704 ★ Champlain College**
**Advanced Respiratory Therapist Program**
163 S Willard St.
PO Box 670
Burlington, VT 05401
**Phone:** (802)865-6491        **Fax:** (802)860-2750
**Email:** baconf@champlain.edu
**Website:** http://www.champlain.edu/CLnD/respiratory.htm
Faye Bacon, Director

## Virginia

**★ 18705 ★ Community Hospital of Roanoke Valley**
**College of Health Sciences**
**Advanced Respiratory Therapist Program**
920 S Jefferson St.
PO Box 13186
Roanoke, VA 24031
**Phone:** (540)985-8263        **Fax:** (540)985-9773
**Email:** kroe@health.chs.edu
**Website:** http://www.chs.edu/respiratory_care_education.html
Kim E. Roe, Director

**★ 18706 ★ J. Sargeant Reynolds Community College**
**Advanced Respiratory Therapist Program**
PO Box 85622
Richmond, VA 23285-5622
**Phone:** (804)786-1375        **Fax:** (804)786-5298
**Email:** dodonohue@jsr.cc.va.us
**Website:** http://www.jsr.cc.va.us/Catalog/programs/RespiratoryTherapyAAS.htm
Donald K. O'Donohue, Director

**★ 18707 ★ Mountain Empire Community College**
**Advanced Respiratory Therapist Program**
PO Drawer 700
Big Stone Gap, VA 24219
**Phone:** (540)523-2400        **Fax:** (540)523-8220
**Email:** mcook@me.cc.va.us
**Website:** http://www.me.cc.va.us/dept/nurse/respiratory/RESPCARE.HTML
Michael W. Cook, Director

**★ 18708 ★ Northern Virginia Community College (LB)**
**Advanced Respiratory Therapist Program**
8333 Little River Trnpk.
Annandale, VA 22003
**Phone:** (703)323-3435        **Fax:** (703)323-4576
**Email:** nvstonl@nv.cc.va.us
**Website:** http://www.nv.cc.va.us/annandale/health/rth/rthhome.htm
Linda L. Stone, Director

**★ 18709 ★ Shenandoah University**
**Advanced Respiratory Therapist Program**
1775 N Sector Ct.
Winchester, VA 22601-5195
**Phone:** (540)665-5516        **Fax:** (540)665-5519
**Email:** kschultz@su.edu
**Website:** http://www.su.edu/respcare/index.htm
William A. O'Neill, Director

**★ 18710 ★ Southwest Virginia Community College (LB)**
**Advanced Respiratory Therapist Program**
Box SVCC
Richlands, VA 24641-1510
**Phone:** (540)964-7350        **Fax:** (540)964-9307
**Email:** Joe_DiPietro@sw.cc.va.us
**Website:** http://www.sw.cc.va.us/M&NS/HLTECH.html
Joseph S. DiPietro, PhD, Director

**★ 18711 ★ Tidewater Community College**
**Advanced Respiratory Therapist Program**
1700 College Crescent
Virginia Beach, VA 23456
**Phone:** (757)822-7263        **Fax:** (757)427-1338
**Email:** tccrosg@tc.cc.va.us
**Website:** http://www.tc.cc.va.us/vabeach/hstdiv/rth/
Gary Cross, Director

## Washington

**★ 18712 ★ Highline Community College**
**Advanced Respiratory Therapist Program**
2400 S 240th St.
Des Moines, WA 98198-9800
**Phone:** (206)878-3710    **Fax:** (206)870-3780
**Email:** bhirnle@hcc.ctc.edu
**Website:** http://www.highline.ctc.edu/highlinehome/
home.htm
Robert W. Hirnle, Director

**★ 18713 ★ Seattle Central Community**
**College**
**Advanced Respiratory Therapist Program**
1701 Broadway/2BE 3210
Seattle, WA 98122
**Phone:** (206)587-4161    **Fax:** (206)344-4390
**Email:** tmccown@sccd.ctc.edu
**Website:** http://seattlecentral.org/learn/respiratory/
120_resp.html
Thomasa R. McCown, Director

**★ 18714 ★ Spokane Community College**
**Advanced Respiratory Therapist Program**
N 1810 Greene St.
Spokane, WA 99207
**Phone:** (509)533-7307    **Fax:** (509)533-8621
**Email:** darkell@scc.spokane.cc.wa.us
**Website:** http://www.scc.spokane.cc.wa.us/hes/al-
liedh/respcare.htm
Diana K. Arkell, Director

**★ 18715 ★ Tacoma Community College**
**Advanced Respiratory Therapist Program**
6501 S 19th St.
Tacoma, WA 98466
**Phone:** (253)566-5231    **Fax:** (253)566-5273
**Email:** bleffler@tcc.tacoma.ctc.edu
**Website:** http://www.tacoma.ctc.edu/home/bleffler/in-
dex.htm
Bill M. Leffler, Director

## West Virginia

**★ 18716 ★ Carver Career and Technical**
**Education Center**
**Advanced Respiratory Therapist Program**
4799 Midland Dr.
Charleston, WV 25306
**Phone:** (304)348-1965    **Fax:** (304)348-1938
**Email:** kchaffin@access.k12.wv.us
**Website:** http://www.wvonline.com/carver/health/ad-
vresp.htm
Kym Chaffin, Director

**★ 18717 ★ College of West Virginia (LB)**
**Advanced Respiratory Therapist Program**
609 S Kanawha St.
Beckley, WV 25802-2830
**Phone:** (304)253-7351    **Fax:** (304)253-0789
**Email:** smills@cwv.edu
**Website:** http://www.cwv.edu/nhs/resp/index.html
Sandy Mills, Director

**★ 18718 ★ University of Charleston (LB)**
**Advanced Respiratory Therapist Program**
2300 MacCorkle Ave. SE
Charleston, WV 25304
**Phone:** (304)357-4837    **Fax:** (304)357-4965
**Email:** aparkman@uchaswv.edu
**Website:** http://www.uchaswv.edu/dhs/respcare/
Anna W. Parkman, Director

**★ 18719 ★ West Virginia Northern**
**Community College**
**Advanced Respiratory Therapist Program**
College Sq.
Wheeling, WV 26003

**Phone:** (304)233-5900
**Email:** rlucki@northern.wvnet.edu
**Website:** http://techctr1.northern.wvnet.edu/catalog/
respiratory.htm
Ralph C. Lucki, Director

**★ 18720 ★ Wheeling Jesuit University**
**Advanced Respiratory Therapist Program**
316 Washington Ave.
Wheeling, WV 26003
**Phone:** (304)243-2372    **Fax:** (304)243-4441
**Email:** amaran@wjc.edu
**Website:** http://www.wju.edu/academics/depart-
ments/rt/
Allen H. Marangoni, Director

## Wisconsin

**★ 18721 ★ Madison Area Technical**
**College**
**Advanced Respiratory Therapist Program**
3550 Anderson St.
Madison, WI 53704
**Phone:** (608)246-6686    **Fax:** (608)246-6013
**Email:** ghojem@madison.tec.wi.us
**Website:** http://www.madison.tec.wi.us/catalog/
PROG_CRS/PD/PD105151.ssi
Glenn N. Hojem, Director

**★ 18722 ★ Mid-State Technical College**
**Advanced Respiratory Therapist Program**
2600 W Fifth St.
Marshfield, WI 54449
**Phone:** (715)389-7033    **Fax:** (715)389-2864
**Email:** sosborne@midstate.tec.wi.us
**Website:** http://www.midstate.tec.wi.us/respcare.htm
Scott S. Osborne, Director

**★ 18723 ★ Milwaukee Area Technical**
**College**
**Advanced Respiratory Therapist Program**
700 W State St.
Milwaukee, WI 53233
**Phone:** (414)297-7130    **Fax:** (414)297-7990
**Email:** hoffmanm@matc.edu
**Website:** http://www.milwaukee.tec.wi.us/utility/clas/
prog/alli/resp.htm
Mark J. Hoffman, Director

**★ 18724 ★ Northeast Wisconsin**
**Technical College (LB)**
**Advanced Respiratory Therapist Program**
2740 W Mason St.
PO Box 19042
Green Bay, WI 54307
**Phone:** (920)498-5533    **Fax:** (920)498-5673
**Website:** http://www.nwtc.tec.wi.us/DegreesDiplo-
mas/healthcom.htm
Diana Luder, PhD, Director

**★ 18725 ★ Western Wisconsin Technical**
**College**
**Advanced Respiratory Therapist Program**
304 N Sixth St.
PO Box 908
La Crosse, WI 54602-0908
**Phone:** (608)785-9244    **Fax:** (608)785-9194
**Email:** milischr@email.western.tec.wi.us
**Website:** http://www.western.tec.wi.us/
Robert A. Milisch, Director

## Wyoming

**★ 18726 ★ Western Wyoming Community**
**College**
**Advanced Respiratory Therapist Program**
2500 College Dr.
PO Box 428
Rock Springs, WY 82902-0428
**Phone:** (307)382-1799    **Fax:** (307)382-7665

**Email:** brobinso@wwcc.cc.wy.us
**Website:** http://www.wwcc.cc.wy.us/xresp/index.htm
Ken Lizzi, Director

# National & International Organizations

**Allergy/Asthma Information Association**
**(AAIA)**
*See:* Entry 3186

**Allergy and Asthma Network/Mothers of**
**Asthmatics (AAN/MA)**
*See:* Entry 5601

**★ 18727 ★ Alpha 1 National Association**
8120 Penn Ave. S, Ste. 549
Minneapolis, MN 55431-1326
**Phone:** (952)703-3025    **Free:** 800-521-3025
**Fax:** (952)703-9977
**Email:** info@alpha1.org
**Website:** http://www.alpha1.org
Sandra Brandley, Exec. Officer
**Fnded:** 1989. **Mem:** 1,239. **Nat'l Groups:** 81. **State**
**Groups:** 35. **Local Groups:** 2. **Desc:** Individuals with
Alpha 1 Antitrypsin deficiency emphysema. Provides
advocacy and educational programs. **Pub:** *Alpha 1*
*Quarterly Review*, quarterly. Newsletter. *Price:* For
members only. **Frmly:** (1991) Alpha 1 Antitrypsin
Support Group.

**American Academy of Allergy, Asthma**
**and Immunology (AAAAI)**
*See:* Entry 3188

**★ 18728 ★ American Association for**
**Respiratory Care (AARC)**
11030 Ables Ln.
Dallas, TX 75229-4593
**Phone:** (972)243-2272    **Fax:** (972)484-2720
**Email:** info@aarc.org
**Website:** http://www.aarc.org
Michael T. Amato, Chair
**Fnded:** 1947. **Mem:** 35,000. **Nat'l Groups:** 4. **State**
**Groups:** 50. **Desc:** Allied health society of respiratory
therapists and other respiratory caregivers employed
by hospitals, skilled nursing facilities, home care
companies, group practices, educational institutions,
and municipal organizations. Encourages, develops,
and provides educational programs for persons interested in the profession of respiratory care; and
advances the science of respiratory care. **Pub:** *AARC*
*Times: The Magazine for the Respiratory Care Profes-*
*sional*, monthly. Magazine. Includes advertisers' index, calendar of events, employment opportunities,
and legislative update. *Price:* Included in membership
dues; $75/year for nonmembers in the U.S.; $90/year
for nonmembes outside the U.S. • *Respiratory Care*,
monthly. Provides original studies, case reports, and
method/device evaluations in cardiopulmonary clinical
medicine. *Price:* Included in membership dues; $75/
year for nonmembers in the U.S.; $5/copy; $90/year
for nonmembers outside the U.S. **Frmly:** (1954)
Inhalation Therapy Association; (1967) American Association of Inhalation Therapists; (1973) American
Association for Inhalation Therapy; (1986) American
Association for Respiratory Therapy.

**★ 18729 ★ American Broncho-**
**Esophagological Associat ion (ABEA)**
K4/714 Clinical Science Ctr.
600 Highland Ave.
Madison, WI 53792-7375
**Phone:** (608)263-0192    **Fax:** (608)265-9255
**Email:** peak.woo@mountsinai.org
**Website:** http://www.abea.net/
Peak Woo, Pres.

**Fnded:** 1917. **Mem:** 386. **Desc:** Professional society of otolaryngologists, chest specialists, thoracic surgeons, and gastroenterologists engaged in the practice of broncho-esophagology (diseases and injuries of the respiratory system and upper digestive tract). Conducts program on study of foreign bodies. **Pub:** *Annals of Otology, Rhinology and Laryngology.* Proceedings. • *Transactions,* annual. **Frmly:** (1928) American Bronchoscopic Society.

**American College of Allergy, Asthma and Immunology (ACAAI)**
*See:* Entry 3195

**American College of Chest Physicians (ACCP)**
*See:* Entry 4959

★ 18730 ★ **American Laryngeal Papilloma Foundation (ALPF)**
PO Box 6108
Spring Hill, FL 34611-6108
**Phone:** (352)686-8583          **Fax:** (352)684-7191
**Email:** carrie@atlantic.net
**Website:** http://www.alpf.org
William Lazar, Pres.
**Fnded:** 1991. **Mem:** 1,000. **Reg. Groups:** 6. **Desc:** Individuals and families affected by laryngeal papillomatosis (LP), a rare disease in which tumors grow inside the trachea or larynx preventing normal breathing. Also known as recurrent respiratory papillomatosis. Promotes the health and welfare of victims. Seeks to increase public awareness, solicit donations, and support research efforts. Conducts a vitamin program; maintains national register of those afflicted with the disease. Provides children's services and educational programs; compiles statistics. **Pub:** *ALPF,* annual. Brochure. *Price:* Free. • *ALPF National Newsletter,* semiannual. Newsletter. *Price:* Free. **Frmly:** (1992) Christina Lazar Foundation for Juvenile Papillomatosis; (1995) Christina Lazar Foundation for Laryngeal Papillomatosis.

★ 18731 ★ **American Lung Association (ALA)**
1740 Broadway
New York, NY 10019-4374
**Phone:** (212)315-8700          **Free:** 800-LUN-GUSA
**Fax:** (212)315-8872
**Email:** info@lungusa.org
**Website:** http://www.lungusa.org
John L. Kirkwood, CEO
**Fnded:** 1904. **Local Groups:** 78. **Desc:** Federation of state and local associations of physicians, nurses, and laymen interested in the prevention and control of lung disease. Conducts patient education, advocacy, and research; major areas of focus are asthma, tobacco control and environmental health. Makes policy recommendations regarding medical care of lung disease, occupational health, hazards of smoking, and air conservation. American Lung Association is financed by annual Christmas Seal Campaign and other fundraising activities. **Frmly:** (1918) National Association for the Study and Prevention of Tuberculosis; (1968) National Tuberculosis Association; (1973) National Tuberculosis and Respiratory Disease Association.

★ 18732 ★ **American Thoracic Society (ATS)**
1740 Broadway, 15th Fl.
New York, NY 10019-4374
**Phone:** (212)315-6440          **Fax:** (212)315-6455
**Email:** nblack@thoracic.org
**Website:** http://www.thoracic.org
Carl Booberg, Exec. Dir.
**Fnded:** 1905. **Mem:** 13,300. **State Groups:** 43. **Desc:** International Educational and scientific Society for respiratory and critical care medicine. Seeks to prevent and fight respiratory diseases through research, education and patient advocacy. **Pub:** *American Journal of Respiratory and Critical Care Medicine,* semi-

monthly. Journal. Includes society news, book reviews, and case reports. *Price:* Included in membership dues. • *American Journal of Respiratory Cell and Molecular Biology,* monthly. Journal. • *ATS News,* monthly. Newsletter. Includes summary of health legislation and annual index. *Price:* Included in membership dues. • Membership Directory, biennial. **Frmly:** (1939) American Sanatorium Association; (1960) American Trudeau Society.

★ 18733 ★ **Asia-Pacific Association for Respiratory Care (APARC)**
PCMC Bldg.
Quezon City, Philippines
**Lang(s):** English, Filipino. **Desc:** Health care professionals with an interest in respiratory care; people with respiratory diseases and their families. Seeks to advance the prevention, diagnosis, and treatment of respiratory diseases. Makes available support and services to people with respiratory diseases and their families; sponsors research and educational programs; facilitates exchange of information among members.

★ 18734 ★ **Asian Pacific Society of Respirology (APSR)**
Yoshikawa No. 2 Bldg., 2nd Fl.
2-9-8 Hongo
Bunkyo-ku
Tokyo 113, Japan
**Phone:** 81 3 56843370          **Fax:** 81 3 56843382
**Email:** apsrjp@aol.com
**Fnded:** 1985. **Mem:** 943. **Lang(s):** English, Japanese. **Desc:** Physicians specializing in the treatment of respiratory ailments. Seeks to advance the study, teaching, and practice of respirology. Facilitates exchange of information among members; conducts research and educational programs. **Pub:** *Respirology,* quarterly. Journal.

**Asthma and Allergy Foundation of America (AAFA)**
*See:* Entry 3200

★ 18735 ★ **Asthma Society of Canada**
130 Bridgeland Ave., Ste. 425
Toronto, ON, Canada M6A 1Z4
**Phone:** (416)787-4050          **Free:** 800-787-3880
**Fax:** (416)787-5807
**Email:** info@asthma.ca
**Website:** http://www.asthmasociety.com
**Fnded:** 1974. **Desc:** Dedicated to the treatment and prevention of asthma. Conducts educational and research programs; provides counseling. **Pub:** *Helping People Breathe Easier,* quarterly. Newsletter. • *Living Well with Asthma.*

★ 18736 ★ **Asthma Society of Ireland (ASI)**
Eden House
15-17 Eden Quay
Dublin 1, Ireland
**Phone:** 353 1 8788511          **Fax:** 353 1 8788128
**Email:** asthma@indigo.ie
**Website:** http://www.asthmasociety.ie
**Fnded:** 1973. **Mem:** 3,000. **Nat'l Groups:** 1. **State Groups:** 1. **Local Groups:** 5. **Lang(s):** English, Irish. **Desc:** Individuals with asthma; health care personnel and other individuals providing support and services to people with asthma. Seeks to improve the quality of life of people with asthma. Serves as a clearinghouse on asthma and its treatment; supports health professionals treating people with asthma. **Pub:** *Asthma Society News,* 3/year. Magazine. Contains 64 full colour pages highlighting asthma issues.

★ 18737 ★ **British Lung Foundation (BLF)**
242 St. Vincent St.
Glasgow G2 5PA, United Kingdom

**Phone:** 44 141 2044110
**Email:** redballoon@blfscotland.org.uk
**Website:** http://www.lunguk.org/scotland/index.html
**Fnded:** 1984. **Mem:** 75,000. **Lang(s):** English. **Desc:** Individuals and organizations. Seeks to advance the prevention, diagnosis, and treatment of lung diseases. Maintains support groups for people with lung disease; provides financial and other assistance to lung disease research; conducts educational programs; participates in charitable activities; compiles statistics. **Pub:** *Breathe Easy,* quarterly. Newsletter.

★ 18738 ★ **Canadian Lung Association (CLA) (Association Pulmonaire du Canada — APC)**
National Office
3 Raymond st., Ste. 300
Ottawa, ON, Canada K1R 1A3
**Phone:** (613)569-6411          **Fax:** (613)569-8860
**Email:** info@lung.ca
**Website:** http://www.lung.ca
**Lang(s):** English, French. **Desc:** Individuals and organizations with an interest in lung disease. Seeks to raise public awareness of lung disease and its causes; promotes advancement in the diagnosis, prevention, and treatment of lung disease. Sponsors educational programs; conducts fundraising activities; provides support to research and treatment projects.

**Canadian Nurses Respiratory Society (CNRS) (Societe Canadienne des Infirmieres en Sante Respiratoire — SCISR)**
*See:* Entry 15694

★ 18739 ★ **Canadian Society of Respiratory Therapists (CSRT) (Societe Canadienne des Therapeutes Respiratoires — SCTR)**
1785 Alta Vista Dr., Ste. 102
Ottawa, ON, Canada K1G 3Y6
**Phone:** (613)731-3164          **Free:** 800-267-3422
**Fax:** (613)521-4314
**Email:** info@csrt.com
**Website:** http://www.csrt.com
**Fnded:** 1964. **Mem:** 2,700. **Reg. Groups:** 8. **Lang(s):** English, French. **Desc:** Respiratory therapists. Seeks to advance the study and practice of respiratory therapy; promotes ongoing professional development of members. Facilitates exchange of information among members; sponsors training programs. **Pub:** *Canadian Journal of Respiratory Therapy,* 5/year. Journal. Contains research, clinical information, and association news.

★ 18740 ★ **CCHS Family Network**
71 Maple St.
Oneonta, NY 13820
**Phone:** (607)432-8872          **Fax:** (607)431-4351
**Email:** vanderlaanm@hartwick.edu
**Website:** http://www.cchsnetwork.org
Mary Vanderlaan, Founder/Dir.
**Fnded:** 1990. **Mem:** 300. **Desc:** Seeks to provide support to families with a CCHS child. Supports CCHS research; shares information on ventilation methods and technologies and home care issues; collects data on CCHS. **Pub:** *CCHS Family Newsletter,* 3/year. Newsletter. Shares news on research/technology development and family stories. **Frmly:** (1998) CCHS Family Network.

★ 18741 ★ **Committee on Accreditation for Respiratory Care (COARC)**
1248 Harwood Rd.
Bedford, TX 76021-4244
**Phone:** (817)283-2835          **Free:** 800-874-5615
**Fax:** (817)354-8519
**Email:** info@coarc.com

**Website:** http://www.coarc.com
Harold Stevens, MD, Sec.
**Fnded:** 1963. **Mem:** 13. **Desc:** Physicians (6); respiratory therapists (6); public representative (1). Purposes are to develop standards and requirements for accredited educational programs of respiratory therapy for recommendation to the American Medical Association; to conduct evaluations of educational programs that have applied for accreditation of the AMA and to make recommendations to the AMA's Committee on Allied Health Education and Accreditation; to maintain a working liaison with other organizations interested in respiratory therapy education and evaluation. Publishes lists of programs. **Frmly:** (1970) Board of Schools of Inhalation Therapy; (1998) Joint Review Committee for Respiratory Therapy Education.

**★ 18742 ★ Congress of Lung Association Staff (CLAS)**
1726 M St. NW, Ste. 902
Washington, DC 20036-4502
**Phone:** (202)785-3355 **Fax:** (202)452-1805
**Website:** http://www.lungusa.org
Janet Widmer, Exec. Dir.
**Fnded:** 1912. **Mem:** 800. **Desc:** Professional society of executives and staff members of the American Lung Association. Sponsors network opportunities and staff development and training programs. **Pub:** *CLAS Action Report*, quarterly. • Booklets. • Membership Directory, annual. **Frmly:** National Conference of Tuberculosis Secretaries; (1968) National Conference of Tuberculosis Workers; (1973) National Respiratory Disease Conference.

**Cystic Fibrosis Foundation (CFF)**
*See:* Entry 9316

**★ 18743 ★ Emphysema Anonymous (EA)**
PO Box 3224
Seminole, FL 33775-0224
**Email:** info@cff.org
**Website:** http://www.cff.org
William E. Jaeckle, Exec. Dir.
**Fnded:** 1965. **Mem:** 3,000. **Desc:** Interested individuals and persons who suffer from emphysema (a condition affecting breathing capacity). Aims to help victims of emphysema through education, encouragement, and mutual assistance. National office provides nonmedical counseling service for patients and their families. **Pub:** *Batting the Breeze*, bimonthly. Newsletter. *Price:* $15/year.

**★ 18744 ★ European Respiratory Society (ERS)**
1 Blvd. de Grancy
CH-1006 Lausanne, Switzerland
**Phone:** 41 21 6130202 **Fax:** 41 21 6172865
**Email:** info@ersnet.org
**Website:** http://www.ersnet.org
**Mem:** 5,000. **Nat'l Groups:** 81. **Lang(s):** English, Norwegian. **Desc:** Health care professionals and medical researchers with an interest in respiratory medicine. Seeks to advance the prevention, diagnosis, and treatment of respiratory disorders; promotes continuing professional development of members. Coordinates respiratory medical research efforts and facilitates exchange of information among members; conducts educational and training programs. Conducts promotional activities encouraging improved lung health in Europe; lobbies on public health issues including tobacco advertising. Operates European School of Respiratory Medicine. **Pub:** *European Respiratory Journal*, monthly. • Newsletter, periodic.

**Federation of Hungarian Associations for Asthmatic and Allergic Patients (ABOSZ)**
*See:* Entry 3215

**★ 18745 ★ International Association of Asthmology (INTERASMA) (Asociacion Internacional de Asmologia — INTERASMA)**
c/o Gianni Ralzano, Enrico Melillo Foundation
Maladies Respiratoires
82037 Telese Terme, Italy
**Phone:** 39 082 4909111 **Fax:** 39 082 4909614
**Email:** emelillo@fsm.it
**Website:** http://www.asmanet.com/interasma.html
**Fnded:** 1954. **Mem:** 1,200. **Reg. Groups:** 12. **Lang(s):** English, French, German, Russian, Spanish. **Desc:** Doctors and other individuals interested in asthmology. Promotes a broadening of knowledge of bronchial asthma and related diseases, especially with regard to their etiology, pathological mechanisms, patho-physiology, therapy, epidemiology, rehabilitation, and prevention. Sponsors specialized training in allergology. **Pub:** *INTERASMA Membership Directory*, triennial. Directory. • *Journal of Investigational Allergology and Clinical Immunology*, bimonthly. Journal. • *Newsletter of Interasma*, quarterly. Newsletter.

**★ 18746 ★ International Asthma Council (IAC)**
6 Forest Laneway, Ste. 1607
North York, ON, Canada M2N 5X9
**Phone:** (416)224-9221 **Fax:** (416)224-9220
**Email:** asthma@iacouncil.com
**Website:** http://www.iacouncil.com
**Fnded:** 1991. **Mem:** 56. **Lang(s):** English. **Desc:** Represents people with asthma, their families, and health care personnel engaged in asthma education and control. **Pub:** *Journalist's Guide to Asthma*. Book. • Newsletter, semiannual.

**★ 18747 ★ International Bronchoesophagological Society (IBES)**
c/o David R. Sanderson, M.D.
Mayo Clinic Scottsdale
13400 E Shea Blvd.
Scottsdale, AZ 85259
**Phone:** (602)301-8000 **Fax:** (602)301-4869
**Email:** dsanderson@mayo.edu
David R. Sanderson, MD, Exec. Sec. -Treas.
**Fnded:** 1951. **Mem:** 400. **Desc:** Endoscopists from varying disciplines. Fosters advances in laryngology, bronchoscopy, upper gastrointestinal endoscopy, diagnostic techniques, and endoscopic therapy. Encourages exchange of ideas; conducts original investigations and research.

**★ 18748 ★ International Society for Respiratory Protection (ISRP)**
8598 Kingcome Cr.
Sidney, BC, Canada V8L 5C7
**Email:** rwono@cdc.gov
**Fnded:** 1982. **Mem:** 400. **Lang(s):** English. **Desc:** Technical and professional people involved with all aspects of nonmedical occupational respiratory protection. Seeks to advance knowledge of respiratory protection for firefighters, commercial divers, persons working in and around foundries, coke ovens, and mines, and other individuals exposed to airborne particles and other unsuitable breathing conditions. **Pub:** *ISRP Journal*, quarterly. Journal. Includes scientific articles. • *Special Conference Proceedings*, biennial. Proceedings. • Membership Directory, annual.

**★ 18749 ★ International Union Against Tuberculosis and Lung Disease (IUATLD) (Union Internationale Contre la Tuberculose et les Maladies Respiratoires — UICTMR)**
68, blvd. St. Michel
F-75006 Paris, France
**Phone:** 33 1 44320360 **Fax:** 33 1 43299087
**Email:** union@iuatld.org
**Website:** http://www.iuatld.org

**Fnded:** 1920. **Mem:** 4,500. **Reg. Groups:** 6. **Lang(s):** English, French, Spanish. **Desc:** National associations, physicians, and other individuals worldwide dedicated to the fight against tuberculosis and other respiratory diseases. Promotes community health and, within its framework, the delivery of preventive, diagnostic, and therapeutic measures against tuberculosis. Aids governmental efforts to improve health services; helps countries formulate, prepare, and execute national tuberculosis control programs. Provides training, advice, antituberculosis drugs and vaccines, medical equipment, and transportation. Encourages community participation. Activities include: dissemination of scientific knowledge; exchange of experience and conferences; operational and applied research; field projects under the Mutual Assistance Programme. Acts as liaison with the World Health Organization and other organizations. **Pub:** *The International Journal of Tuberculosis and Lung Disease*, monthly. Journal. With summaries in French and Spanish. • *IUATLD Newsletter*, 3/year. Newsletter. Contains news and reports on the activities of the IUATLD and information on conferences and courses. • *Management of the Child with Cough or Difficult Breathing*. • *Tuberculosis Guide for Low Income Countries*. **Frmly:** (1986) International Union Against Tuberculosis.

**Joint Council of Allergy, Asthma and Immunology (JCAAI)**
*See:* Entry 3222

**★ 18750 ★ LAM Foundation**
10105 Beacon Hills Dr.
Cincinnati, OH 45241
**Phone:** (513)777-6899 **Fax:** (513)777-4109
**Email:** lamfoundtn@Juno.com
**Website:** http://lam.uc.edu/
Sue Byrnes, Exec. Dir.
**Fnded:** 1995. **Desc:** Works to find a cure for LAM (lymphangioleimyomatosis), a progressive, fatal lung disease that affects women. Provides information and support; conducts education programs; promotes and funds clinical research; sponsors a tissue bank; supports a national registry of LAM patients.

**★ 18751 ★ National Association for Medical Direction of Respiratory Care (NAMDRC)**
5454 Wisconsin Ave., Ste. 1270
Chevy Chase, MD 20815
**Phone:** (301)718-2975 **Fax:** (301)718-2976
**Email:** namdrc@erols.com
**Website:** http://www.namdrc.org
Phillip Porte, Exec. Dir.
**Fnded:** 1977. **Mem:** 650. **Desc:** Works to provide educational opportunities for pulmonologists and others involved in respiratory care. Interprets and advises on the changing healthcare delivery system and is a successfull advocate on regulatory and legislative issues affecting pulmonary and critical care medicine. Offers educational programs, publications and assistance regarding coding issues and federal reimbursement policies. **Pub:** *Clinical and Management Quarterly*, quarterly. Newsletter. • *Presidential Update*, biennial. • *Washington Watchline*, monthly.

**★ 18752 ★ National Board for Respiratory Care (NBRC)**
8310 Nieman Rd.
Lenexa, KS 66214
**Phone:** (913)599-4200 **Fax:** (913)541-0156
**Email:** nbrc-info@nbrc.org
**Website:** http://www.nbrc.org
Gary A. Smith, Exec. Dir.
**Fnded:** 1960. **Mem:** 16,000. **Desc:** Offers credentialing examinations for respiratory therapists, respiratory therapy technicians, pulmonary technologists, and perinatal/pediatric respiratory care specialists. **Pub:** Directory, annual. • Newsletter, bimonthly. **Frmly:** (1974) American Registry of Inhalation Therapists; (1982) National Board for Respiratory Therapy.

### ★ 18753 ★ National Jewish Medical and Research Center

1400 Jackson St.
Denver, CO 80206
**Phone:** (303)388-4461          **Free:** 800-222-LUNG
**Fax:** (303)270-2165
**Email:** lungline@njc.org
**Website:** http://www.njc.org
Lynn Taussig, Pres.
**Fnded:** 1899. **Desc:** Devoted to treatment, research, and education in chronic respiratory diseases and immunological disorders such as asthma, tuberculosis, cystic fibrosis, chronic bronchitis, emphysema, interstitial lung disease, and systemic lupus erythematosus. Accepts non-sectarian patients of all ages. Disseminates information to the public. Maintains research library of 15,000 volumes. **Pub:** *Lung Line Letter*, quarterly. Newsletter. *Price:* Free. • *National Jewish Medical and Research Center–Annual Report. Price:* Free. • *National Jewish Medical and Research Center–Medical Scientific Update*, monthly. Newsletter. *Price:* Free. • *New Directions*, quarterly. Newsletter. Updates the center's research programs. *Price:* Free. **Frmly:** (1978) National Jewish Hospital/National Asthma Center; (1998) National Jewish Center for Immunology and Respiratory Medicine.

### Nordic Federation of Heart and Lung Associations (NHL)

### (Nordiska Hjart and Lungsjukas Forbund)
*See:* Entry 5050

### Norwegian Cystic Fibrosis Association (NCFA)

### (Norsk Forening for Cystisk Fibrose — NFCF)
*See:* Entry 9355

### Pulmonary Hypertension Association (PHA)
*See:* Entry 5058

### Respiratory Nursing Society (RNS)
*See:* Entry 15770

### ★ 18754 ★ Slovak Society of Physiology and Pathology of Respiration

c/o Dept. of Pathophysiology, Jes. Med. Fac.
Comenius University
26 Sklabinska str.
SK-037 53 Martin, Slovakia
**Phone:** 42 43 4238213          **Fax:** 42 43 4134807
**Email:** tatar@jfmed.uniba.sk
**Website:** http://www.respiratorynursingsociety.org/
**Fnded:** 1968. **Mem:** 160. **Lang(s):** English, Slovak. **Desc:** Health care professionals treating respiratory ailments. Researchers in the field of respiratory (Experimental and Clinical Physiology and Pathophysiology of Respiration). Promotes professional advancement of members; represents members' interests. **Pub:** *Bulletin of the SSPPR*, 3/year. Newsletter.

### Society of Thoracic Radiology (STR)
*See:* Entry 18161

### Society of Thoracic Surgeons (STS)
*See:* Entry 19603

### ★ 18755 ★ United Mitochondrial Disease Foundation (UMDF)

8085 Saltsburg Rd., Ste. 201
Pittsburgh, PA 15239
**Phone:** (412)793-8077          **Fax:** (412)793-6477
**Email:** info@umdf.org
**Website:** http://www.umdf.org
Antoinette Renda Beasley, Fin. Svcs. Coord.
**Fnded:** 1995. **Mem:** 3,000. **Nat'l Groups:** 1. **Reg. Groups:** 20. **State Groups:** 1. **Local Groups:** 1.

**Desc:** Patients, parents or guardians, friends, relatives, medical professionals, hospitals, and other organizations. Promotes research for cures and treatments of mitochondrial disease; provides support to patients and families. Patient registry database includes information from symptoms and treatment to diagnostic methods and specific disorders. **Pub:** Newsletter, 3/year.

## Research Centers

### ★ 18756 ★ Boston University Pulmonary Center

Sch. of Medicine
715 Albany St., R-304
Boston, MA 02118
**Phone:** (617)638-4860          **Fax:** (617)536-8093
**Email:** mwilliams@lung.bumc.bu.edu
**Website:** http://www.bupulmonary.org
Mary C. Williams, PhD, Assoc. Dir.
**Activities/Fields:** Development of an integrated approach to the cell and molecular biology of lung cells.

### Brigham and Women's Hospital Asthma and Allergic Diseases Cooperative Research Center
*See:* Entry 3239

### Case Western Reserve University Cystic Fibrosis and Pediatric Pulmonary Center
*See:* Entry 9378

### Cystic Fibrosis Center (Portland, OR)
*See:* Entry 9390

### Duke University Cystic Fibrosis Research Center
*See:* Entry 9393

### Duke University Pediatric Asthma and Allergic Disease Center
*See:* Entry 3244

### Emory University Cystic Fibrosis Care, Teaching and Research Center
*See:* Entry 9394

### ★ 18757 ★ Gage Occupational and Environmental Health Unit

St. Michael's Hospital
30 Bond St.
Toronto, ON, Canada M5B 1W8
**Phone:** (416)867-7470          **Fax:** (416)867-3673
**Email:** stulacj@smh.toronto.on.ca
**Website:** http://www.utoronto.ca/occmed/
Dr. Linn Holness, Dir.
**Activities/Fields:** Lung problems related to asthma, bronchitis, and occupational and environmental pollution. Areas of interest include development of more effective treatment for adult asthmatics, connection between asthma and air pollution, acute effects of second-hand tobacco smoke on asthmatics and other people, predictability of asthma outcome, occupational asthma, effects of indoor environments on human comfort and health, and environmental sensitivity. Contact dermatitis, areas of interest include causation, workplace studies, deprostic methods and outcomes, particularly related to return to work and quality of life.

### Indiana University-Purdue University at Indianapolis Cystic Fibrosis and Pediatric Pulmonary Clinic
*See:* Entry 9398

### Johns Hopkins University Asthma and Allergy Center
*See:* Entry 3252

### Johns Hopkins University Cystic Fibrosis Research Center
*See:* Entry 9408

### Laval University Hopital Laval Cardiopulmonary Institute
*See:* Entry 5115

### McGill University McGill Centre for Tropical Diseases
*See:* Entry 11865

### ★ 18758 ★ McGill University Meakins-Christie Laboratories

3626 St. Urbain St.
Montreal, QC, Canada H2X 2P2
**Phone:** (514)398-3864          **Fax:** (514)398-7483
**Email:** jmartin@meakins.lan.mcgill.ca
**Website:** http://www.Meakins.McGill.CA/Meakins/
Dr. James G. Martin, Dir.
**Activities/Fields:** Respiratory physiology and physiopathology, including studies on control of breathing, respiratory mechanics, respiratory muscle fatigue, electromyography, lung morphology and biochemistry, airway dynamics, smooth muscle growth and contractive signalling, eicosanoids, T-lymphocytes, allergic inflammation.

### ★ 18759 ★ McGill University Montreal Chest Institute Research Centre

3650 St. Urbain St.
Montreal, QC, Canada H2X 2P4
**Phone:** (514)849-5201          **Fax:** (514)843-2095
Dr. James G. Martin, Dir.
**Activities/Fields:** Respiratory medicine, focusing on chronic obstructive pulmonary diseases (COPD). Research also includes structure-function, physiology, pharmacology, rehabilitation, environment, body surface motion, asthma, cystic fibrosis, and airway hyper-responsiveness.

### Medical College of Wisconsin Cystic Fibrosis Research Center
*See:* Entry 9414

### National Jewish Medical and Research Center
*See:* Entry 3256

### Ohio State University Division of Pulmonary and Critical Care Medicine
*See:* Entry 3257

### Ohio State University Dorothy M. Davis Heart and Lung Research Institute
*See:* Entry 5126

### ★ 18760 ★ Respiratory Pathogens Research Unit

Department of Molecular Virology & Microbiology
Texas Medical Center

1 Baylor Plz., Rm. 205 A
Houston, TX 77030
**Phone:** (713)798-4474        **Fax:** (713)798-7375
**Email:** rcouch@bcm.tmc.edu
**Website:** http://heartlung.osu.edu
Robert B. Couch, MD, Dir.

**Activities/Fields:** Multidisciplinary studies of acute respiratory diseases in humans and animals, including bacteriologic, virologic, and immunologic studies and vaccine and evaluations.

**★ 18761 ★ Rush University**
**Center for SIDS Research and Disorders**
**of Respiratory Control in Infancy and**
**Childhood**
Rush-Presbyterian-St. Luke's Medical Center
1653 W Congress Pky.
Chicago, IL 60612
**Phone:** (312)942-2723        **Fax:** (312)942-3087
**Email:** dweese@rush.edu
Dr. Debra E. Weese-Mayer, Dir.

**Activities/Fields:** Sudden infant death syndrome (SIDS) research, including monitoring high-risk infants for apnea, congenital central hypoventilation syndrome, genetic characterization of congenital central hypoventilation syndrome, and the effect of prenatal cocaine (throughout gestation) on development and function of the autonomic neurosystem.

**Southern Louisiana Cystic Fibrosis**
**Clinical Care and Research Center/**
**Pediatric Pulmonary Center**
See: Entry 9428

**Tufts University**
**Asthma and Allergic Diseases**
**Cooperative Research Center**
See: Entry 3265

**★ 18762 ★ U.S. Department of Health**
**and Human Services**
**Centers for Disease Control and**
**Prevention**
**National Institute for Occupational Safety**
**and Health**
**Division of Respiratory Disease Studies**
1095 Willowdale Rd.
Morgantown, WV 26505
**Phone:** (304)285-5749        **Free:** 800-356-4676
**Fax:** (304)285-5861
**Email:** johman@lifespan.org
**Website:** http://www.cdc.gov/niosh/im-drds.html
Gregory Wagner, MD, Dir.

**Activities/Fields:** Identification, evaluation, and prevention of occupational respiratory diseases, such as asthma, chronic obstructive pulmonary disease, and pneumoconiosis. Administers legislatively mandated medical services for coal miners; tests, evaluates, certifies, monitors, and conducts research on the quality of respiratory protective devices. **Pub:** Reports.

**★ 18763 ★ U.S. Department of Health**
**and Human Services**
**Centers for Disease Control and**
**Prevention**
**National Institute for Occupational Safety**
**and Health**
**National Occupational Research Agenda**
**(Occupational Asthma and Chronic**
**Obstructive Pulmonary Disease)**
NIOSH Field Studies Branch
H2800
1095 Willowdale Rd.
Morgantown, WV 26505
**Phone:** (304)285-5751        **Free:** 800-356-4676
**Email:** pkh0@cdc.gov
**Website:** http://www.cdc.gov/niosh/nrpulm.html
Paul Henneberger, PhD, Team Ldr.

**Activities/Fields:** Clarify the prevalence, risk factors, and exposure-disease relationships to occupationally-related airway diseases, including asthma and chronic obstructive disease (COPD); to refine techniques for monitoring worker health and the job environment; and to develop effective and practical means for preventing work-related airway diseases in at-risk workers. **Pub:** Papers.

**U.S. Department of Health and Human**
**Services**
**Food and Drug Administration**
**Center for Biologics Evaluation and**
**Research**
**Laboratory of Respiratory Viruses**
See: Entry 4721

**U.S. Department of Health and Human**
**Services**
**National Center for Infectious Diseases**
**Division of Bacterial and Mycotic**
**Diseases**
**Childhood and Respirtory Diseases**
**Branch**
See: Entry 11889

**★ 18764 ★ U.S. Department of Health**
**and Human Services**
**National Center for Infectious Diseases**
**Division of Viral and Rickettsial Diseases**
**Respiratory and Enteric Virus Branch**
1600 Clifton Rd., NE
M.S A-34
Atlanta, GA 30333
**Phone:** (404)639-3596        **Fax:** (404)639-1307
Larry Anderson, Chf.

**Activities/Fields:** Respiratory viruses such as adenoviruses and respiratory syncytial virus, polio and other enteroviruses, and viruses causing gastroenteritis.

**U.S. Department of Health and Human**
**Services**
**National Heart, Lung, and Blood Institute**
See: Entry 5146

**U.S. Department of Health and Human**
**Services**
**National Heart, Lung, and Blood Institute**
**Division of Epidemiology and Clinical**
**Applications**
See: Entry 5147

**U.S. Department of Health and Human**
**Services**
**National Heart, Lung, and Blood Institute**
**Division of Epidemiology and Clinical**
**Applications**
**Clinical Applications and Prevention**
**Program**
See: Entry 5148

**U.S. Department of Health and Human**
**Services**
**National Heart, Lung, and Blood Institute**
**Division of Extramural Affairs**
See: Entry 5149

**★ 18765 ★ U.S. Department of Health**
**and Human Services**
**National Heart, Lung, and Blood Institute**
**Division of Intramural Research**
**Pulmonary-Critical Care Medicine Branch**
NIH Bldg. 10, Rm. 6D03
10 Center Dr. MSC-1590
Bethesda, MD 20892-1590

**Phone:** (301)496-1597        **Fax:** (301)496-2363
**Email:** savagep@nhlbi.nih.gov
**Website:** http://www.nhlbi.nih.gov/
Joel Moss, Chf.

**Activities/Fields:** Structure and function of the lung in health and disease through cellular and biochemical methods. Both laboratory and clinical investigations are conducted and techniques of protein chemistry, molecular biology, tissue culture, and immunology are used. Emphasis is on the regulation of the inflammatory and immune processes in the normal and diseased lung. Clinical research is directed toward correlating physiologic, biochemical, immunologic, and morphologic observations in patients with interstitial lung disease, destructive lung disease, hereditary disorders of connective tissue, hypersensitivity lung disease, and other lung disorders with an immunologic basis.

**★ 18766 ★ U.S. Department of Health**
**and Human Services**
**National Heart, Lung, and Blood Institute**
**Division of Lung Diseases**
Two Rockledge Ctr., Ste. 10018
6701 Rockledge Dr. MSC 7952
Bethesda, MD 20892-7952
**Phone:** (301)435-0233        **Fax:** (301)480-3547
**Email:** kileyj@nhlbi.nih.gov
**Website:**        http://www.nhlbi.nih.gov/about/dld/index.htm
Dr. James P. Kiley, PhD, Dir.

**Activities/Fields:** Focal point for planning and coordinating research and research training programs for all diseases of the respiratory system, including chronic obstructive pulmonary diseases; pediatric pulmonary diseases; occupational and immunologic lung diseases; pulmonary vascular diseases; acute lung injury; asthma; critical care; cystic fibrosis; lung cell biology; respiratory neurobiology and sleep; and pulmonary complications of AIDS. **Pub:** and idiopathic pulmonary fibrosis. • Brochures on asthma, chronic obstructive pulmonary disease. • primary pulmonary hypertension. • sarcoidosis.

**★ 18767 ★ U.S. Department of Health**
**and Human Services**
**National Heart, Lung, and Blood Institute**
**Division of Lung Diseases**
**Cell and Developmental Biology Branch**
**(Lung Biology and Disease Program)**
2 Rockledge Center, Ste. 10122
6701 Rockledge Dr., MSC 7952
Bethesda, MD 20892-7952
**Phone:** (301)435-0222        **Fax:** (301)480-3557
**Email:** gaild@nhlbi.nih.gov
**Website:**        http://www.nhlbi.nih.gov/about/dld/index.htm
Dr. Dorothy Gail, PhD, Dir.

**Activities/Fields:** Pediatric pulmonary diseases, lung cell biology, acute lung injury, interstitial lung disease, pulmonary immunology, AIDS-related lung disease, and tuberculosis.

**U.S. Department of Health and Human**
**Services**
**National Heart, Lung, and Blood Institute**
**Laboratory of Biochemical Genetics**
See: Entry 5160

**U.S. Department of Health and Human**
**Services**
**National Heart, Lung, and Blood Institute**
**Laboratory of Biophysical Chemistry**
See: Entry 5161

**U.S. Department of Health and Human**
**Services**
**National Heart, Lung, and Blood Institute**
**(NHLBI)**
**Laboratory of Cell Biology (LCB)**
See: Entry 5163

**U.S. Department of Health and Human Services**
**National Heart, Lung, and Blood Institute**
**Laboratory of Cell Signaling**
*See:* Entry 5164

**U.S. Department of Health and Human Services**
**National Institute of Allergy and Infectious Diseases**
**Asthma and Allergic Diseases Cooperative Research Center (NIAID)**
*See:* Entry 3271

**U.S. Department of Health and Human Services**
**National Institute of Allergy and Infectious Diseases**
**Division of Allergy, Immunology, and Transplantation**
**Asthma, Allergy, and Inflamation Branch**
*See:* Entry 3273

**U.S. Department of Health and Human Services**
**National Institute of Allergy and Infectious Diseases**
**Division of Microbiology and Infectious Diseases**
**Respiratory Diseases Branch**
*See:* Entry 11924

**U.S. Department of Health and Human Services**
**National Institute of Environmental Health Sciences**
**Division of Intramural Researh**
**Laboratory of Pulmonary Pathobiology**
*See:* Entry 8969

**★ 18768 ★ University of Arizona**
**Arizona Respiratory Center**
1501 N Campbell Ave., Ste. 2349
PO Box 245030
Tucson, AZ 85724-5030
**Phone:** (520)626-6387 **Fax:** (520)626-6623
**Email:** inquire@respiratory.arizona.edu
**Website:** http://www.resp-sci.arizona.edu
Fernando D. Martinez, MD, Dir.
**Activities/Fields:** Causes and modes of development of emphysema, chronic bronchitis and asthma. **Pub:** *Newsletter.*

**★ 18769 ★ University of Calgary**
**Respiratory Research Group**
3330 Hospital Dr. NW, Rm. 207
Calgary, AB, Canada T2N 4N1
**Phone:** (403)210-3816 **Fax:** (403)270-8928
**Email:** dproud@ucalgary.ca
Dr. David Proud, Ch.
**Activities/Fields:** Normal and diseased respiratory systems, including mechanics of the respiratory system, muscles of respiration, neural control of breathing, membrane biophysics of smooth muscles. Pathogenesis of asthma and asthma attacks, airway inflammation, Cells of the airway and their response to provocative agents in asthma, lung pathology and occupational lung disease, neonatal lung development and disease, sudden infant death syndrome, surface properties of the alveoli of the lung, and blood flow to, and from, and through the lungs.

**★ 18770 ★ University of California, San Diego**
**Division of Pulmonary and Critical Care Medicine**
9300 Campus Point Dr.
La Jolla, CA 92037-1300
**Phone:** (858)657-7105 **Fax:** (858)657-7144
**Email:** ljrubin@ucsd.edu
**Website:** http://medicine.ucsd.edu/pul
Lewis J. Rubin, MD, Contact
**Activities/Fields:** Chronic obstructive pulmonary disease, tuberculosis, acute respiratory failure, including its pathogenesis and management, pulmonary vascular diseases. **Frmly:** Specialized Center of Research in Acute Respiratory Failure.

**★ 18771 ★ University of California, San Francisco**
**Lung Biology Center**
CB 0854
San Francisco, CA 94143-0854
**Phone:** (415)206-5959 **Fax:** (415)206-4123
**Email:** deans@itsa.ucsf.edu
**Website:** http://dom.ucsf.edu/lbc/
Dean Sheppard, MD, Dir.
**Activities/Fields:** Diseases of the lung and airways.

**University of Illinois at Chicago**
**Institute for Tuberculosis Research**
*See:* Entry 3303

**University of Miami**
**Cystic Fibrosis Research Center**
*See:* Entry 9506

**★ 18772 ★ University of Michigan**
**Pulmonary and Critical Care Medicine Division**
6301 MSRB 111
1150 W Medical Center Dr.
Ann Arbor, MI 48109-0642
**Phone:** (734)936-5010 **Fax:** (734)764-4556
**Email:** gtoews@umich.edu
**Website:** http://www.med.umich.edu/intmed/pulmonary
Dr. Galen B. Toews, Dir.
**Activities/Fields:** Pulmonary diseases and critical care, including cell biology, immunology, and biochemistry of lung and heart.

**University of Minnesota**
**Cystic Fibrosis Center**
*See:* Entry 9508

**University of Missouri—Columbia**
**Cystic Fibrosis Research Center**
*See:* Entry 9510

**University of Nebraska at Omaha**
**Pediatric Pulmonary and Cystic Fibrosis Research Center**
*See:* Entry 9513

**University of North Carolina at Chapel Hill**
**Center for Environmental Medicine and Lung Biology**
*See:* Entry 8991

**University of Oklahoma**
**Pulmonary and Cystic Fibrosis Center**
*See:* Entry 9514

**University of Texas Southwestern Medical Center at Dallas**
**Sleep Disorders Center for Children**
*See:* Entry 5833

**University of Utah**
**Intermountain Cystic Fibrosis Center**
*See:* Entry 9523

**University of Wisconsin—Madison**
**Allergy/Asthma Clinical Research Unit**
*See:* Entry 3313

**University of Wisconsin—Madison**
**Pediatric Pulmonary Center**
*See:* Entry 9526

**★ 18773 ★ University of Wisconsin—Madison**
**Pulmonary and Critical Care Medicine Section**
Department of Medicine
600 Highland Ave., K4/930
Madison, WI 53792-9988
**Phone:** (608)263-3035 **Fax:** (608)263-3746
**Email:** cggreen@facstaff.wisc.edu
**Website:** http://www2.medsch.wisc.edu/children-shosp/ppc/ppchome.html
Dr. James Skatrud, Sect. Hd.
**Activities/Fields:** Pulmonary physiology, occupational lung disease, and mechanisms of acute lung injury.

**Washington University in St. Louis**
**Cystic Fibrosis Center**
*See:* Entry 9528

**Wayne State University**
**Cystic Fibrosis Care, Teaching and Resource Center**
*See:* Entry 9530

---

# State & Regional Organizations

## Asthma & Allergies

*State chapters of the Asthma and Allergy Foundation of America are listed below. The national office is located at 1233 Twentieth St. NW, Ste. 402, Washington, DC 20036. Additional information can be obtained by calling the national office at (800) 7-ASTHMA or by consulting their web site at http://www.aafa.org.*

### Alaska

**Asthma and Allergy Foundation of America**
**Alaska Chapter**
*See:* Entry 3314

### California

**Asthma and Allergy Foundation of America**
**Northern California Chapter**
*See:* Entry 3315

**Asthma and Allergy Foundation of America**
**Southern California Chapter**
*See:* Entry 3316

## Florida

**Asthma and Allergy Foundation of America**
**Florida Chapter**
*See:* Entry 3317

## Maryland

**Asthma and Allergy Foundation of America**
**Maryland-Greater Washington, D.C., Chapter**
*See:* Entry 3318

## Massachusetts

**Asthma and Allergy Foundation of America**
**New England Chapter**
*See:* Entry 3319

## Michigan

**Asthma and Allergy Foundation of America**
**Michigan State Chapter**
*See:* Entry 3320

## Missouri

**Asthma and Allergy Foundation of America**
**Greater Kansas City Chapter**
*See:* Entry 3321

**Asthma and Allergy Foundation of America**
**Saint Louis Chapter**
*See:* Entry 3322

## New Jersey

**Asthma and Allergy Foundation of America**
**Southeastern Pennsylvania Chapter**
*See:* Entry 3323

## Oregon

**Asthma and Allergy Foundation of America**
**Oregon Chapter**
*See:* Entry 3324

## Texas

**Asthma and Allergy Foundation of America**
**North Texas Chapter**
*See:* Entry 3325

## Washington

**Asthma and Allergy Foundation of America**
**Washington State Chapter**
*See:* Entry 3326

## Respiratory Diseases

*The associations listed below are constituents of the American Lung Association, 1740 Broadway, New York, NY 10019, (800)LUNG-USA, http://www.lungusa.org/.*

## Alabama

**★ 18774 ★ American Lung Association of Alabama**
3125 Independence Dr., Ste. 325
Birmingham, AL 35209
**Phone:** (205)933-8821　　**Fax:** (205)930-1717
**Email:** aodom@alabamalung.org
**Website:** http://www.alabamalung.org

## Alaska

**★ 18775 ★ American Lung Association of Alaska**
500 W International Airport Rd., Ste. 1
Anchorage, AK 99518
**Phone:** (907)276-5864　　**Fax:** (907)565-5587
**Email:** christie@aklung.org
**Website:** http://www.aklung.org
Christie McIntire, Contact

## Arizona

**★ 18776 ★ American Lung Association of Arizona/New Mexico**
102 W McDowell Rd.
Phoenix, AZ 85003-1299
**Phone:** (602)258-7505　　**Free:** 800-LUNG-USA
**Fax:** (602)258-7507
**Email:** bpfeifer@lungaz.org
**Website:** http://www.lungaz.org

**★ 18777 ★ American Lung Association of Arizona/New Mexico**
**Northern Arizona Branch**
102 W McDowell Rd.
Phoenix, AZ 85003-1299
**Phone:** (602)258-7505　　**Fax:** (602)258-7507
**Email:** cclees@lungaz.org
**Website:** http://www.lungaz.org

**★ 18778 ★ American Lung Association of Arizona/New Mexico**
**Southern Arizona Branch**
2819 E Broadway
Tucson, AZ 85716
**Phone:** (520)323-1812　　**Fax:** (520)323-1816
**Email:** jjones@lungaz.org
**Website:** http://www.lungaz.org

## Arkansas

**★ 18779 ★ American Lung Association of Arkansas**
211 Natural Resources Dr.
Little Rock, AR 72205-1539
**Phone:** (501)224-5864　　**Fax:** (501)224-5645
**Email:** carogers@aristotle.net
**Website:** http://www.lungark.org

## California

**★ 18780 ★ American Lung Association of California**
424 Pendleton Way
Oakland, CA 94621-2189
**Phone:** (510)638-LUNG　　**Fax:** (510)638-8984
**Email:** contact@californialung.org
**Website:** http://www.californialung.org
Ben Abate, PhD, President

**★ 18781 ★ American Lung Association of California**
**Redwood Empire Branch**
115 Talbot Ave.
Santa Rosa, CA 95404
**Phone:** (707)527-LUNG　　**Fax:** (707)542-6111
**Email:** lungassn@neteze.com

**★ 18782 ★ American Lung Association of California**
**Superior Branch**
1108 Sheridan Ave., Ste. B
Chico, CA 95926
**Phone:** (530)345-5864　　**Fax:** (530)345-6035
**Email:** patty@alacsb.org
**Website:** http://www.lungusa.org/superiorbranch/index.html

**★ 18783 ★ American Lung Association of Central California**
4948 N Arthur
PO Box 9389
Fresno, CA 93794
**Phone:** (559)222-4800　　**Fax:** (559)221-2081
**Email:** info@amerilungcencal.org
**Website:** http://www.amerilungcencal.org

**★ 18784 ★ American Lung Association of the Central Coast**
550 Camino El Estero, Ste. 100
Monterey, CA 93940-3231
**Phone:** (831)373-7306　　**Free:** 800-LUNG-USA
**Fax:** (831)373-5530
**Email:** admin@alaccoast.org
**Website:** http://www.alacoast.org

**★ 18785 ★ American Lung Association of the East Bay**
295 27th St.
Oakland, CA 94612-3894
**Phone:** (510)893-5474　　**Fax:** (510)893-9008
**Email:** eastbaylung@alac.org

**★ 18786 ★ American Lung Association of the Inland Counties**
441 Mac Kay Dr.
San Bernardino, CA 92408-3230
**Phone:** (909)884-5864　　**Fax:** (909)884-6249
**Email:** lungassn@pe.net

**★ 18787 ★ American Lung Association of Los Angeles County**
5858 Wilshire Blvd., No. 300
PO Box 36926
Los Angeles, CA 90036-0926
**Phone:** (323)935-5864　　**Fax:** (323)935-1873
**Email:** lalung@lalung.org
**Website:** http://www.lalung.org

**★ 18788 ★ American Lung Association of Orange County**
1570 E 17th St.
Santa Ana, CA 92705
**Phone:** (714)835-5864　　**Fax:** (714)835-0169
**Email:** alaoc1@aol.com
**Website:** http://www.oclung.org

**★ 18789 ★ American Lung Association of Sacramento-Emigrant Trails**
909 12th St.
Sacramento, CA 95814-2997
**Phone:** (916)444-LUNG　　**Free:** 800-LUNG-USA
**Fax:** (916)444-6661
**Email:** staff@saclung.org
**Website:** http://www.saclung.org

**★ 18790 ★ American Lung Association of San Diego & Imperial Counties**
2750 4th Ave.
PO Box 3879
San Diego, CA 92163-1879
**Phone:** (619)297-3901　　**Fax:** (619)297-8402
**Email:** info@lungsandiego.org
**Website:** http://www.lungsandiego.org

**★ 18791 ★ American Lung Association
of San Francisco and San Mateo
Counties**
2171 Junipero Serra Blvd., Ste. 720
Daly City, CA 94014-1980
**Phone:** (650)994-5864          **Fax:** (650)994-4601
**Email:** lung@alasfsm.org

**★ 18792 ★ American Lung Association
of Santa Barbara and Ventura Counties**
1510 San Andres St.
Santa Barbara, CA 93101-4104
**Phone:** (805)963-1426          **Fax:** (805)962-2843
**Email:** dkweeks@aol.com

**★ 18793 ★ American Lung Association
of Santa Clara-San Benito Counties**
1469 Park Ave.
San Jose, CA 95126-2530
**Phone:** (408)998-5864          **Fax:** (408)998-0578
**Email:** info@lungsrus.org
**Website:** http://www.lungsrus.org

## Colorado

**★ 18794 ★ American Lung Association
of Colorado**
1600 Race St.
Denver, CO 80206-1198
**Phone:** (303)388-4327          **Fax:** (303)377-1102
**Email:** sgoulding@alacolo.org
**Website:** http://www.alacolo.org

**★ 18795 ★ American Lung Association
of Colorado**
**Northern Region**
2601 S Lemay, No. 7-117
Fort Collins, CO 80525
**Phone:** (970)223-6111          **Fax:** (970)223-6111
**Email:** johnalfredwolfe@attbi.com

**★ 18796 ★ American Lung Association
of Colorado**
**Pikes Peak Region**
421 S Tejon, Ste. 100
Colorado Springs, CO 80903
**Phone:** (719)635-3891          **Fax:** (719)635-4057
**Email:** nutz@alacolo.org
**Website:** http://www.alacolo.org

**★ 18797 ★ American Lung Association
of Colorado**
**Southern Region**
409 N Main St., Ste. 314
Pueblo, CO 81003
**Phone:** (719)296-8800          **Fax:** (719)296-8811
**Email:** jbeasley@alacolo.org
**Website:** http://www.alacolo.org

**★ 18798 ★ American Lung Association
of Colorado**
**Western Region**
PO Box 3154
Grand Junction, CO 81502
**Phone:** (970)245-2120          **Fax:** (970)245-2288
**Email:** canderson@alacolo.org
**Website:** http://www.alacolo.org

## Connecticut

**★ 18799 ★ American Lung Association
of Connecticut**
45 Ash St.
East Hartford, CT 06108-3272
**Phone:** (860)289-5401          **Free:** 800-992-2263
**Fax:** (860)289-5405
**Email:** alaofct@alact.org
**Website:** http://www.alact.org

## Delaware

**★ 18800 ★ American Lung Association
of Delaware**
1021 Gilpin Ave., Ste. 202
Wilmington, DE 19806-3280
**Phone:** (302)655-7258          **Fax:** (302)655-8546
**Website:** http://www.alade.org

## District of Columbia

**★ 18801 ★ American Lung Association
of the District of Columbia**
475 H St. NW
Washington, DC 20001-2617
**Phone:** (202)682-5864          **Fax:** (202)682-5874
**Email:** info@aladc.org
**Website:** http://www.aladc.org

## Florida

**★ 18802 ★ American Lung Association
of Central Florida**
1333 W Colonial Dr.
Orlando, FL 32804-7133
**Phone:** (407)425-5864          **Fax:** (407)425-2876
**Email:** alacf@gdi.net

**★ 18803 ★ American Lung Association
of Florida**
5526 Arlington Rd.
Jacksonville, FL 32211-5216
**Phone:** (904)743-2933          **Free:** 800-940-2933
**Fax:** (904)743-2916
**Email:** alaf@lungfla.org
**Website:** http://www.lungfla.org

**★ 18804 ★ American Lung Association
of Florida**
**Northwest Region**
4300 Bayou Blvd., Ste. 2
Pensacola, FL 32503-2677
**Phone:** (850)478-5864          **Fax:** (850)474-6354
**Email:** alafnw@networktel.net

**★ 18805 ★ American Lung Association
of Florida**
**Spaceport Region**
412 S Palmetto Ave.
Daytona Beach, FL 32114-4922
**Phone:** (386)255-6447          **Fax:** (386)253-2410
**Email:** alafsp@bellsouth.net

**★ 18806 ★ American Lung Association
of Gulfcoast Florida**
110 Carillon Pkwy.
Saint Petersburg, FL 33716
**Phone:** (727)347-6133          **Free:** 800-771-5863
**Fax:** (727)345-0287
**Email:** alagf@alagf.org

**★ 18807 ★ American Lung Association
of South Florida, Inc.**
2020 S Andrews Ave.
Fort Lauderdale, FL 33316-3430
**Phone:** (954)524-4657          **Fax:** (954)524-3162
**Email:** carolruggeri@sflung.org
**Website:** http://www.sflung.org

**★ 18808 ★ American Lung Association
of Southeast Florida**
2701 N Australian Ave.
West Palm Beach, FL 33407-4526
**Phone:** (561)659-7644          **Fax:** (561)835-8967
**Email:** amlungsefl@inhaleexhale.org
**Website:** http://www.inhaleexhale.org

**★ 18809 ★ American Lung Association
of The Big Bend Region**
539 Silver Slipper Ln., Ste. A
Tallahassee, FL 32303-4873
**Phone:** (850)386-2065          **Fax:** (850)422-1894
**Email:** alafbbr@earthlink.net

## Georgia

**★ 18810 ★ American Lung Association
of Georgia**
2452 Spring Rd.
Smyrna, GA 30080
**Phone:** (770)434-5864          **Free:** 800-LUNG-USA
**Fax:** (770)319-0349
**Website:** http://www.alaga.org

## Hawaii

**★ 18811 ★ American Lung Association
of Hawaii**
245 N Kukui St., Ste. 100
Honolulu, HI 96817
**Phone:** (808)537-5966          **Fax:** (808)537-5971
**Website:** http://www.ala-hawaii.org

## Idaho

**★ 18812 ★ American Lung Association
of Idaho/Nevada**
**Boise Office**
1111 S Orchard, Ste. 245
Boise, ID 83705-1966
**Phone:** (208)345-5864          **Fax:** (208)345-5896

## Illinois

**★ 18813 ★ American Lung Association
of Illinois**
3000 Kelly Ln.
Springfield, IL 62707
**Phone:** (217)787-5864          **Free:** 800-LUNG-USA
**Fax:** (217)787-5916
**Email:** info@lungil.org
**Website:** http://www.lungil.org
Harold Wimmer, CEO
Lori Younker, Mgr

**★ 18814 ★ American Lung Association
of Metropolitan Chicago**
1440 W Washington Blvd.
Chicago, IL 60607
**Phone:** (312)243-2000          **Fax:** (312)243-3954
**Website:** http://www.lungchicago.org

## Indiana

**★ 18815 ★ American Lung Association
of Indiana**
9445 Delegates Row
Indianapolis, IN 46240
**Phone:** (317)573-3900          **Fax:** (317)573-3909
**Email:** info@lungin.org
**Website:** http://www.lungin.org

## Iowa

**★ 18816 ★ American Lung Association
of Iowa**
5601 Douglas Ave.
Des Moines, IA 50310-1800
**Phone:** (515)278-5864          **Fax:** (515)334-9564
**Email:** tammy@alaia.org
**Website:** http://www.alaia.org

## Kansas

**★ 18817 ★ American Lung Association
of Kansas**
4300 SW Drury Ln.
Topeka, KS 66604-2419

Phone: (785)272-9290      Fax: (785)272-9297
Website: http://www.kslung.org

## Kentucky

**★ 18818 ★ American Lung Association
of Kentucky**
4100 Churchman Ave.
PO Box 9067
Louisville, KY 40209-0067
Phone: (502)363-2652      Fax: (502)363-0222
Email: menisam@kylung.org
Website: http://www.kylung.org

## Louisiana

**★ 18819 ★ American Lung Association
of Louisiana**
2325 Severn Ave., Ste. 8
Metairie, LA 70001-6918
Phone: (504)828-5864      Fax: (504)828-5867
Email: bfont@bellsouth.net
Website: http://www.louisianalung.org

## Maine

**★ 18820 ★ American Lung Association
of Maine**
122 State St.
Augusta, ME 04330
Phone: (207)622-6394      Fax: (639)426-2919
Email: Cgagne@MaineLung.org
Website: http://www.mainelung.org

## Maryland

**★ 18821 ★ American Lung Association
of Maryland**
1840 York Rd., Ste. M
Timonium, MD 21093-5156
Phone: (410)560-2120      Free: 800-LUNG-USA
Fax: (410)560-0829
Email: info@marylandlung.org
Website: http://www.marylandlung.org

## Massachusetts

**★ 18822 ★ American Lung Association
of Greater Norfolk County**
25 Spring St.
Walpole, MA 02081-4302
Phone: (508)668-6729      Fax: (508)668-6796
Email: lungusa2@earthlink.net

**★ 18823 ★ American Lung Association
of Massachusetts**
One Abbey Ln.
Middleboro, MA 02346-3230
Phone: (508)947-7204      Fax: (508)947-7208
Email: alam@gis.net
Carlos Alvarez, Exec Director

**★ 18824 ★ American Lung Association
of Middlesex County**
5 Mountain Rd.
PO Box 265
Burlington, MA 01803
Phone: (781)272-2866      Fax: (781)273-2846
Email: alaofmc@aol.com
David Ales, Exec Director

**★ 18825 ★ American Lung Association
of Western Massachusetts**
393 Maple St.
Springfield, MA 01105
Phone: (413)737-3506      Fax: (413)737-3511

## Michigan

**★ 18826 ★ American Lung Association
of Michigan**
25900 Greenfield, Ste. 401
Oak Park, MI 48237
Phone: (248)784-2000      Free: 800-543-LUNG
Fax: (248)784-2008
Email: alam@alam.org
Website: http://www.alam.org

**★ 18827 ★ American Lung Association
of Michigan
Capital Region**
403 Seymour Ave.
Lansing, MI 48933-1179
Phone: (517)484-4541      Free: 800-678-5864
Fax: (517)484-2118
Email: smspringer@voyager.net

**★ 18828 ★ American Lung Association
of Michigan
Genesee Valley Region**
519 S Saginaw, Ste. 312
Flint, MI 48502
Phone: (810)232-3177      Fax: (810)232-6257
Email: genesee@123.net

**★ 18829 ★ American Lung Association
of Michigan
Grand Valley and Southwest Regions**
2815 Michigan St. NE, Ste. B
Grand Rapids, MI 49506
Phone: (616)942-0513      Fax: (616)942-0650
Email: grandvalleyalam@voyager.net

**★ 18830 ★ American Lung Association
of Michigan
Huron Valley Region**
412 Huron St.
Ann Arbor, MI 48104
Phone: (734)994-0155      Fax: (734)327-2968
Email: huron@123.net

**★ 18831 ★ American Lung Association
of Michigan
Metro Detroit Region**
25900 Greenfield, Ste. 401
Oak Park, MI 48237
Phone: (248)784-2000      Fax: (248)784-2008
Email: MBaumgartner@alam.org
Website: http://www.alam.org

**★ 18832 ★ American Lung Association
of Michigan
Northwest Region**
153-1/2 E Front St., Ste. D
Traverse City, MI 49684-2508
Phone: (231)946-1344      Fax: (231)946-0150
Email: northw@northlink.net

**★ 18833 ★ American Lung Association
of Michigan
Upper Peninsula Region**
227 W Washington St.
Marquette, MI 49855-4321
Phone: (906)228-9833      Fax: (906)228-3430
Email: cjmargrif@lushen.com

## Minnesota

**★ 18834 ★ American Lung Association
of Minnesota**
490 Concordia Ave.
Saint Paul, MN 55103-2441
Phone: (651)227-8014      Fax: (651)227-5459
Website: http://www.alamn.org

## Mississippi

**★ 18835 ★ American Lung Association
of Mississippi**
731 Pear Orchard Rd., Ste. 18
PO Box 2178
Ridgeland, MS 39158
Phone: (601)206-5810      Free: 800-586-4872
Fax: (601)206-5813
Email: ebarber@alams.org
Website: http://www.alams.org
Elizabeth Barber, Director

**★ 18836 ★ American Lung Association
of South Mississippi**
PO Box 8911
Gulfport, MS 39506-8911
Fax: (228)896-2213
Email: mmcgahan@alams.org
Website: http://www.alams.org

## Missouri

**★ 18837 ★ American Lung Association
of Eastern Missouri**
1118 Hampton Ave.
Saint Louis, MO 63139-3196
Phone: (314)645-5505      Fax: (314)645-7128
Email: tyoung@alaem.org
Website: http://www.alaem.org

**★ 18838 ★ American Lung Association
of Western Missouri**
2007 Broadway
Kansas City, MO 64108-2080
Phone: (816)842-5242      Fax: (816)842-5470
Email: kcmo@alawmo.com
Joe Gilman, Director

## Montana

**★ 18839 ★ American Lung Association
of the Northern Rockies**
825 Helena Ave.
Helena, MT 59601-3459
Phone: (406)442-6556      Fax: (406)442-2346
Email: ala-nr@ala-nr.org
Website: http://www.ala-nr.org
Remarks: Serves Montana and Wyoming.

## Nebraska

**★ 18840 ★ American Lung Association
of Nebraska**
Community Health Plaza
7101 Newport Ave., Ste. 303
Omaha, NE 68152
Phone: (402)572-3030      Fax: (402)572-3028
Email: ala@lungnebraska.org
Website: http://www.lungnebraska.org

## Nevada

**★ 18841 ★ American Lung Association
of Idaho/Nevada**
1091 Haskell St.
PO Box 7056
Reno, NV 89510-7056
Phone: (775)829-5864      Fax: (775)829-5850
Email: dszabo@lungs.org
Website: http://www.lungs.org

## New Hampshire

**★ 18842 ★ American Lung Association
of New Hampshire**
9 Cedarwood Dr., Ste. 12
Bedford, NH 03110
Phone: (603)669-2411      Fax: (603)645-6220
Email: info@nhlung.org
Website: http://www.nhlung.org

## New Jersey

**★ 18843 ★ American Lung Association**
**of New Jersey**
1600 Rte. 22 E
Union, NJ 07083-3407
**Phone:** (908)687-9340　　　**Fax:** (908)851-2625
**Email:** info.alanj@verizon.net

**★ 18844 ★ American Lung Association**
**of Northern New Jersey**
333B Rte. 46 W, Ste. 205
Fairfield, NJ 07004
**Phone:** (973)227-7720　　　**Fax:** (973)227-3270

**★ 18845 ★ American Lung Association**
**of Southern New Jersey**
109 S Main St., Ste. 18
Cranbury, NJ 08512
**Phone:** (609)918-0313　　　**Fax:** (609)918-0314

## New Mexico

**★ 18846 ★ American Lung Association**
**of Arizona/New Mexico**
**New Mexico Branch**
216 Truman NE
Albuquerque, NM 87108
**Phone:** (505)265-0732　　　**Fax:** (505)260-1739
**Email:** joem@alanm.org
**Website:** http://www.alanm.org

## New York

**★ 18847 ★ American Lung Association**
**of Central New York**
1620 Burnet Ave.
Syracuse, NY 13206
**Phone:** (315)422-6142　　　**Fax:** (315)422-9710
**Email:** alaofcny@aol.com

**★ 18848 ★ American Lung Association**
**of the City of New York, Inc.**
432 Park Ave. S, 8th Fl.
New York, NY 10016
**Phone:** (212)889-3370　　　**Fax:** (212)889-3375
**Email:** info@alany.org
**Website:** http://www.alany.org

**★ 18849 ★ American Lung Association**
**of the Finger Lakes Region**
1595 Elmwood Ave.
Rochester, NY 14620
**Phone:** (716)442-4260　　　**Fax:** (716)442-4263
**Email:** aladeb@rochester.rr.com
**Website:** http://www.ggw.org/ala-fl/

**★ 18850 ★ American Lung Association**
**of the Hudson Valley**
35 Orchard St.
White Plains, NY 10603-3397
**Phone:** (914)949-2150　　　**Fax:** (914)949-4765
**Email:** info@alahv.org
**Website:** http://www.alahv.org

**★ 18851 ★ American Lung Association**
**of Mid-New York**
587 Main St., Ste. 109
New York Mills, NY 13417
**Phone:** (315)736-6099　　　**Fax:** (315)736-5976
**Email:** ALAMNY@aol.com
John Storey, Exec Director

**★ 18852 ★ American Lung Association**
**of Nassau Suffolk, New York**
225 Wireless Blvd.
Hauppauge, NY 11788-3914
**Phone:** (631)231-5864　　　**Fax:** (631)231-5118

**Email:** postmaster@alans.org

**★ 18853 ★ American Lung Association**
**of New York State, Inc.**
3 Winners Circle, Ste. 300
Albany, NY 12205-1187
**Phone:** (518)453-0172　　　**Fax:** (518)489-5864
**Email:** postmaster@alanys.org
**Website:** http://www.alanys.org

**★ 18854 ★ American Lung Association**
**of Northeastern New York**
3 Winners Circle, Ste. 300
Albany, NY 12205
**Phone:** (518)459-4197　　　**Fax:** (518)489-5864
**Email:** postmaster@alaneny.org
**Website:** http://www.alaneny.org

**★ 18855 ★ American Lung Association**
**of Western New York**
210 John Glenn Dr., No. 3
Buffalo, NY 14228
**Phone:** (716)691-5864　　　**Fax:** (716)691-5012
**Email:** cschweitzer@alawny.org
**Website:** http://www.alawny.org

## North Carolina

**★ 18856 ★ American Lung Association**
**of North Carolina**
1323 Capital Blvd., Ste. 102
PO Box 27985
Raleigh, NC 27611
**Phone:** (919)832-8326　　　**Free:** 800-892-5650
**Fax:** (919)856-8530
**Email:** swillcox@lungnc.org
**Website:** http://www.lungnc.org

## North Dakota

**★ 18857 ★ American Lung Association**
**of North Dakota**
212 N 2nd St.
PO Box 5004
Bismarck, ND 58502-5004
**Phone:** (701)223-5613　　　**Free:** 800-252-6325
**Fax:** (701)223-5727
**Email:** aland@gcentral.com
Susan Kahler, Exec Director

## Ohio

**★ 18858 ★ American Lung Association**
**of Ohio, Columbus**
**State Office**
1950 Arlingate Ln.
Columbus, OH 43228-4102
**Phone:** (614)279-1700　　　**Fax:** (614)279-4940
**Email:** kelsey@ohiolung.org
**Website:** http://www.ohiolung.org

## Oklahoma

**★ 18859 ★ American Lung Association**
**of Oklahoma**
2805 E Skelly Dr., Ste. 806
Tulsa, OK 74105
**Phone:** (918)747-3441　　　**Fax:** (918)747-4629
**Email:** dakin@oklung.org
**Website:** http://www.oklung.org
Darla Akin, Contact

## Oregon

**★ 18860 ★ American Lung Association**
**of Oregon**
7420 SW Bridgeport Rd., Ste. 200
Portland, OR 97224
**Phone:** (503)924-4094　　　**Free:** 800-LUNG-USA
**Fax:** (503)924-4120

**Email:** admin@lungoregon.org
**Website:** http://www.lungoregon.org

## Pennsylvania

**★ 18861 ★ American Lung Association**
**of Pennsylvania**
6041 Linglestown Rd.
Harrisburg, PA 17112-1208
**Phone:** (717)541-5864　　　**Free:** 800-932-0903
**Fax:** (717)541-8828

## Puerto Rico

**★ 18862 ★ American Lung Association**
**of Puerto Rico**
395 Domenech Ave.
PO Box 195247
San Juan, PR 00919-5247
**Phone:** (787)765-5664　　　**Fax:** (787)765-5964
**Email:** info@pulmon.org
**Website:** http://www.pulmon.org
Yolanda Rosario, Director

## Rhode Island

**★ 18863 ★ American Lung Association**
**of Rhode Island**
298 W Exchange St.
Providence, RI 02903-3700
**Phone:** (401)421-6487　　　**Fax:** (401)331-5266
**Email:** alaofri@aol.com

## South Carolina

**★ 18864 ★ American Lung Association**
**of South Carolina**
1817 Gadsden St.
Columbia, SC 29201-2392
**Phone:** (803)779-5864　　　**Free:** 800-849-5864
**Fax:** (803)254-2711
**Email:** alasc@lungsc.org
**Website:** http://www.lungsc.org

**★ 18865 ★ American Lung Association**
**of South Carolina**
**Coastal Region**
1941 Savage Rd., Ste. 200-A
Charleston, SC 29407-4789
**Phone:** (843)556-8451　　　**Fax:** (843)556-3332
**Email:** scatlin@lungsc.org
**Website:** http://www.lungsc.org
Sally Catlin, Director

**★ 18866 ★ American Lung Association**
**of South Carolina**
**Midlands Region**
1817 Gadsden St.
Columbia, SC 29201-2392
**Phone:** (803)779-5864　　　**Fax:** (803)254-2711
**Email:** gsteele@lungsc.org
**Website:** http://www.lungsc.org
Gabrielle Steele, Director

**★ 18867 ★ American Lung Association**
**of South Carolina**
**Piedmont Region**
84 Villa Rd., B-2
Greenville, SC 29615
**Phone:** (864)233-0517　　　**Fax:** (864)233-2124
**Email:** ckinghorn@lungsc.org
**Website:** http://www.lungsc.org
Cynthia Kinghorn, Director

## South Dakota

**★ 18868 ★ American Lung Association**
**of South Dakota**
1212 W Elkhorn, Ste. 1
Sioux Falls, SD 57104-0233

**Phone:** (605)336-7222　　　**Free:** 800-873-5864
**Fax:** (605)336-7227
**Email:** lung@americanlungsd.org
**Website:** http://www.recess.org/

### Tennessee

★ **18869** ★ **American Lung Association
of Tennessee**
One Vantage Way, Ste. C250
Nashville, TN 37228
**Phone:** (615)329-1151　　　**Free:** 800-432-5864
**Fax:** (615)329-1723
**Email:** alastaff@alatn.org
**Website:** http://www.alatn.org

### Texas

★ **18870** ★ **American Lung Association
of Texas**
5926 Balcones Dr., Ste. 100
PO Box 26460
Austin, TX 78755-0460
**Phone:** (512)467-6753　　　**Fax:** (512)467-7621
**Email:** alatexas@texaslung.org
**Website:** http://www.texaslung.org

★ **18871** ★ **American Lung Association
of Texas**
**Alamo and Southern Region**
The Callaghan Bldg.
7475 Callaghan Rd., Ste. 203
San Antonio, TX 78229
**Phone:** (210)308-8978　　　**Fax:** (210)308-8992
**Email:** alasoutx@onr.com

★ **18872** ★ **American Lung Association
of Texas**
**Central Region**
5926 Balcones Dr., Ste. 105
PO Box 26566
Austin, TX 78755-0566
**Phone:** (512)467-2534　　　**Fax:** (512)467-7539
**Email:** alacentx@onr.com
**Website:** http://www.texaslung.org

★ **18873** ★ **American Lung Association
of Texas**
**Dallas Region**
8150 Brookriver Dr., S-102, LB-151
Dallas, TX 75247
**Phone:** (214)631-5864　　　**Fax:** (214)630-8092

**Email:** dallas@texaslung.org
**Website:** http://www.texaslung.org

★ **18874** ★ **American Lung Association
of Texas**
**Fort Worth Region**
2630 W Freeway, Ste. 202
Fort Worth, TX 76102
**Phone:** (817)332-4549　　　**Fax:** (817)332-4961
**Email:** jaustin@texaslung.org
**Website:** http://www.texaslung.org

★ **18875** ★ **American Lung Association
of Texas**
**Houston and Southeast Region**
2425 W Loop S, Ste. 330
PO Box 27396
Houston, TX 77227-7396
**Phone:** (713)629-1600　　　**Fax:** (713)629-5828

★ **18876** ★ **American Lung Association
of Texas**
**Rio Grande Valley Region**
3827 N 10th St., No. 203
McAllen, TX 78501
**Phone:** (956)631-0514　　　**Fax:** (956)668-9615
**Email:** lrunnels@flash.net

★ **18877** ★ **American Lung Association
of Texas**
**Western Region**
444 Executive Center Blvd., Ste. 206
El Paso, TX 79902
**Phone:** (915)532-6776　　　**Fax:** (915)532-7231
**Email:** westreg@flash.net

### Utah

★ **18878** ★ **American Lung Association
of Utah**
1930 South 1100 East
Salt Lake City, UT 84106-2317
**Phone:** (801)484-4456　　　**Fax:** (801)484-5461
**Email:** wldavis@utahlung.org

### Vermont

★ **18879** ★ **American Lung Association
of Vermont**
30 Farrell St.
South Burlington, VT 05403-6196

**Phone:** (802)863-6817　　　**Fax:** (802)863-6818
**Email:** info@vtlung.org
Sharon Wheelock, Contact

### Virgin Islands

★ **18880** ★ **American Lung Association
of the Virgin Islands**
PO Box 974
St Thomas, VI 00804
**Phone:** (340)774-8620　　　**Fax:** (340)774-8620

### Virginia

★ **18881** ★ **American Lung Association
of Virginia**
9221 Forest Hill Ave.
Richmond, VA 23235
**Phone:** (804)267-1900　　　**Fax:** (804)267-5634
**Email:** resourcecenter@lungva.org

### Washington

★ **18882** ★ **American Lung Association
of Washington**
2625 3rd Ave.
Seattle, WA 98121
**Phone:** (206)441-5100　　　**Free:** 800-732-9339
**Fax:** (206)441-3277
**Email:** alaw@alaw.org
**Website:** http://www.alaw.org

### West Virginia

★ **18883** ★ **American Lung Association
of West Virginia**
415 Dickinson St.
PO Box 3980
Charleston, WV 25339-3980
**Phone:** (304)342-6600　　　**Fax:** (304)342-6096
**Email:** chantal@alawv.org
**Website:** http://www.alawv.org

### Wisconsin

★ **18884** ★ **American Lung Association
of Wisconsin**
13100 W Lisbon Rd., Ste. 700
Brookfield, WI 53005-2508
**Phone:** (262)703-4200　　　**Fax:** (262)781-5180
**Email:** amlung@lungwisconsin.org

# Chapter 59
# Sexuality

## Foundations & Other Funding Organizations

### Other Funding Organizations

**Lesbian Health Fund (LHF)**
*See:* Entry 1548

★ **18885** ★ **Society for the Psychological Study of Lesbian, Gay and Bisexual Issues (SPSLGBI)**
c/o American Psychological Association
750 First St. NE
Washington, DC 20002
**Phone:** (202)336-6037     **Free:** 800-374-2721
**Fax:** (202)336-6040
**Email:** canderson@apa.org
**Website:** http://www.apa.org/divisions/div44
Sari H. Dworkin, PhD, Pres.
**Desc:** Psychologists, graduate students in psychology, and others interested in the psychological study of lesbian, gay, and bisexual issues and the delivery of affirmative mental health services to gay, lesbian, and bisexual individuals. Promotes scholarship in the study of psychology as it relates to bisexual, gay, and lesbian issues; provides training for psychologists in the field. Cooperates with other groups sharing similar goals, including other divisions of the American Psychological Association. Conducts scholarly programs. **Awards:** Distinguished Contributions Awards (annual); Malyon-Smith Scholarship Award (annual) for graduate student research.

★ **18886** ★ **Society for the Scientific Study of Sexuality (SSSS)**
c/o David L. Fleming
PO Box 416
Allentown, PA 18105
**Phone:** (610)530-2483     **Fax:** (610)530-2485
**Email:** thesociety@inetmail.att.net
**Website:** http://www.sexscience.org
David L. Fleming, Exec. Dir.
**Desc:** Dedicated to advancing knowledge of sexuality. Support for research, and an interdisciplinary network of collaborating scholars. **Awards:** Student Research Grant (3/year).

## National & International Organizations

★ **18887** ★ **American Association of Sex Educators, Counselors and Therapists (AASECT)**
PO Box 5488
Richmond, VA 23220-0488
**Phone:** (319)895-8407     **Fax:** (319)895-6203
**Email:** aasect@aasect.org
**Website:** http://www.aasect.org
Howard H. Ruppel, Jr., Exec. Dir.
**Fnded:** 1967. **Mem:** 1,700. **Reg. Groups:** 7. **Desc:** Professionals concerned with sex education, counseling, and therapy; students pursuing degrees in the field. Certifies sex educators, counselors, and therapists. Provides educational services. Acts as a referral service for the general public. **Pub:** *Contemporary Sexuality*, monthly. Newsletter. *Price:* $42. • *Journal of Sex Education and Therapy*, quarterly. Journal. *Price:* $40 U.S.; $50 outside U.S. **Frmly:** (1976) American Association of Sex Educators and Counselors.

**Asociacion Pro-Bienestar de la Familia Colombiana (PROFAMILIA)**
*See:* Entry 18236

**Australasian College of Sexual Health Physicians**
*See:* Entry 18245

★ **18888** ★ **Australian Society of Sex Educators, Researchers and Therapists**
172 Old Northern Dr.
Everton Park, QLD 4556, Australia
**Phone:** 61 7 33532422     **Fax:** 61 7 33532273
**Email:** secretariat@acshp.org.au
**Website:** http://www.acshp.org.au/college/
**Mem:** 50. **Desc:** Promotes the professions of sex educators, sex researchers, and sex therapists.

★ **18889** ★ **British Association for Sexual and Relationship Therapy**
PO Box 13686
London SW20 9ZH, United Kingdom
**Email:** info@basrt.org.uk
**Website:** http://www.basrt.org.uk
**Fnded:** 1975. **Mem:** 700. **Desc:** Professional psychosexual therapists/clinicians/medics working in the field of sexual and marital therapy. Aims to advance the education and training of persons engaged in sexual, marital and relationship therapy; to promote research in this field; to advance public education about sexual, marital and relationship therapy. **Pub:** *Sexual and Marital Therapy*, quarterly. Journal. **Frmly:** (2000) British Association for Sexual and Marital Therapy.

★ **18890** ★ **Council for Sex Information and Education (CSIE)**
2272 Colorado Blvd., No. 1228
Los Angeles, CA 90041
Joel Adams, Dir.
**Fnded:** 1977. **Desc:** A national clearinghouse for information on sexuality and related topics. Premise is that adequate knowledge and understanding of sexuality contributes not only to sexual well-being but to physical and emotional well-being and that helpful information should be readily available. **Frmly:** Sex Information Council of America.

★ **18891** ★ **European Federation of Sexology (EFS)**
48 Boulevard Rodocanache
F-13008 Marseille, France
**Phone:** 33 4 91764489     **Fax:** 33 4 91770139
**Fnded:** 1988. **Reg. Groups:** 58. **Lang(s):** English, French, German. **Desc:** Scientific societies. Promotes study, research, and teaching in the field of sexology. Serves as a clearinghouse on sexology; sponsors research and educational programs.

★ **18892** ★ **European Research Organization of Genital Infection and Neoplasia (EUROGIN)**
174, rue de Courcelles
F-75017 Paris, France
**Phone:** 33 1 47660529     **Fax:** 33 1 47667470
**Desc:** Stimulates research in the field of genital infections, pre-cancers and cancers.

★ **18893** ★ **Exodus Trust (ET)**
1523 Franklin St.
San Francisco, CA 94109
**Phone:** (415)928-1133     **Fax:** (415)928-8061
Ted McIlvenna, Pres.
**Fnded:** 1968. **Desc:** Established to: educate and train professionals interested in sex counseling, therapy, education, or research; provide sex education, counseling, and therapy for adults; research human sexuality; produce films, slides, and literature for use in sex counseling, therapy, and education. Conducts continuing education programs for physicians and nurses, and workshops and counseling programs for professional and laypeople in San Francisco, CA and other cities. **Frmly:** (1989) National Sex Forum.

**Family Planning and Sexual Health Association (FPSHA)**
*See:* Entry 18293

★ **18894** ★ **Gay and Lesbian Medical Association**
459 Fulton St., Ste. 107
San Francisco, CA 94102
**Phone:** (415)255-4547     **Free:** (415)255-4784
**Email:** info@glma.org
**Website:** http://www.glma.org
Maureen S. O'Leary, Exec. Dir.
**Fnded:** 1981. **Mem:** 2,000. **Desc:** Physicians and allied health professionals. Seeks elimination of discrimination on the basis of gender identity and sexual orientation in the health professions; promotes unprejudiced medical care for gay and lesbian patients through advocacy and education. Maintains a referral and support program for HIV infected health care workers. Sponsors annual continuing medical education (CME, CEU) symposium on lesbian and gay health issues. Offers support to lesbian, gay, bisexual, and transgendered health care workers; encourages research into the health needs of gays and lesbians. Maintains liaison with medical schools and other

organizations concerning needs of gay patients and professionals; fosters communication and cooperation among members and other groups and individuals supportive of gay and lesbian physicians. Sponsors Lesbian Health Fund for researching lesbian health needs. **Pub:** *GLMA Report*, quarterly. Newsletter. Covers the activities of the association, the medical community, and the public regarding lesbian and gay health issues. *Price:* Included in membership dues. • *Journal of the Gay and Lesbian Medical Association*, quarterly. Journal. **Frmly:** American Association of Physicians for Human Rights.

★ **18895** ★ **German Society for Sex Research (GSSR)**
**(Deutsche Gesellschaft fuer Sexualforschung — DGSF)**
c/o Universitaets-Klinikum Hamburg-Eppendorf
Klinik fur Psychiatrie und Psychotherapie
Abteilung fur Sexualforschung
Martinistr 52
D-20246 Hamburg, Germany
**Phone:** 49 40 428032225     **Fax:** 49 40 428036406
**Email:** hrichter@uke.uni-hamburg.de
**Fnded:** 1952. **Mem:** 250. **Desc:** Conducts research in sexology. **Pub:** *Beitrage zur Sexualforschung*, periodic. Journal. • *Zeitschrift fur Sexualforschung*, quarterly. Journal. Also publishes research findings.

★ **18896** ★ **I-ANON**
119 S Ruth St.
Maryville, TN 37803
**Free:** 800-669-1603
**Email:** info@impotenceworld.org
Eileen V. MacKenzie, Founder and Conslt.
**Fnded:** 1982. **State Groups:** 100. **Local Groups:** 3. **Desc:** Concerned partners of impotent males. Seeks to provide information and group support to members. Refers members to doctors who treat impotence. Supplies patients with information on prosthetic implants, and other forms of treatment. **Pub:** *Answers to the Most Often Asked Questions About Impotence.* • *Impotence Worldwide*, quarterly. • *Its Not All in Your Head: A Couple's Guide to Overcoming Impotance.*

★ **18897** ★ **Impotence Association**
c/o Ann Craig
PO Box 10296
London SW17 9SH, United Kingdom
**Phone:** 44 20 87677791     **Fax:** 44 20 85167725
**Email:** theia@btinternet.com
**Website:** http://www.impotence.org.uk
**Fnded:** 1995. **Mem:** 1,300. **Desc:** Raises awareness among the public and health professionals on impotence. Offers free advice and information via a telephone hotline. Maintains information up to date information on the treatments available for impotence.

★ **18898** ★ **Impotence Institute of America (IIA)**
119 S Ruth St.
Maryville, TN 37803
**Free:** 800-669-1603
**Email:** info@impotenceworld.org
Eileen MacKenzie, Founder & Chm.
**Fnded:** 1983. **Desc:** Urologists, psychiatrists, psychologists, sex therapists and counselors, and plastic surgeons; manufacturers of penile implant devices and other productsused in the treatment of impotence; impotent men and their partners; hospitals and other institutions that offer assistance and meeting facilities for Impotents Anonymous (IA) and I-ANON. Informs and educates the public on the subject of impotence and its causes and treatments. Provides information on various programs and organizations that can assist individuals concerned about impotence. Aids other charitable, educational, and social welfare organizations. Compiles statistics. **Pub:** *Answers to the Most Often Asked Questions about Impotence.* • *It's Not all in Your Head - A Couple's Guide to Overcoming Impotance.*

**Institute for the Advancement of Human Behavior (IAHB)**
*See:* Entry 12495

**Institute of Psychosexual Medicine**
*See:* Entry 12505

**Instituto Peruano de Paternidad Responsable (INPPARES)**
*See:* Entry 18307

★ **18899** ★ **International Professional Surrogates Association (IPSA)**
3428 Motor Ave.
Los Angeles, CA 90034
**Phone:** (323)469-4720
**Email:** ipsa1@aol.com
**Website:** http://members.aol.com/ipsa1/home.html
Vena Blanchard, Pres.
**Fnded:** 1973. **Mem:** 50. **Nat'l Groups:** 1. **Local Groups:** 1. **Desc:** IPSA is non-profit professional organization of Surrogate Partners and Therapists. IPSA provides referrals to therapists seeking trained, ethical professional surrogate partners and referrals to clients seeking therapists with expertise in surrogate partner therapy. IPSA sponsors training for surrogate partners, and provides continuing education to sex therapists, psychotherapists, and surrogate partners, and recently began offering personal enrichment courses for individuals and couples. IPSA's Code of Ethics helped to establish and maintain the highest professional standards within the field of surrogate partner therapy. **Pub:** *Surrogate Partner Therapy.* • Newsletter, semiannual. *Price:* Available to members only.

★ **18900** ★ **International Society for Impotence Research (ISSIR)**
c/o Jo-Els van de Woude
Postbus 97
NL-3950 AD Maarn, Netherlands
**Phone:** 31 343 443888     **Fax:** 31 343 442043
**Email:** issir@statusplus.nl
**Website:** http://www.issir.org
**Fnded:** 1982. **Mem:** 600. **Reg. Groups:** 4. **Lang(s):** English. **Desc:** Seeks to establish a scientific society to benefit the public y encouraging the highest standards of practice, education, and research in the field of human sexuality. Develops scientific methods for the diagnosis, prevention, and treatment of conditions affecting human sexual function.

★ **18901** ★ **International Union against Sexually Transmitted Infections - Australia**
135 Hutt St.
Adelaide, SA 5000, Australia
**Phone:** 61 8 82324511     **Fax:** 61 8 823796145
**Lang(s):** English. **Desc:** Medical and public health professionals and other individuals with an interest in sexually transmitted diseases. Seeks to minimize the incidence of sexually transmitted disease and improve their diagnosis and treatment. Conducts educational programs to raise public awareness of sexually transmitted diseases and their prevention; sponsors training courses for health care workers serving people with sexually transmitted diseases; serves as a clearinghouse on sexually transmitted diseases and their prevention.

★ **18902** ★ **Latin American Union Against Sexually Transmitted Diseases (Union Latinoamericana contra las Enfermedades de Transmision Sexual — ULACETS)**
Rua Joao Obino 111
90470-150 Porto Alegre, Brazil
**Phone:** 55 51 3341126     **Fax:** 55 51 3341126
**Email:** pnaud@netmarket.com.br
**Website:** http://www.ulacets.com.br

★ **18903** ★ **Lesbian Health Fund (LHF)**
459 Fulton St., Ste. 107
San Francisco, CA 94102
**Phone:** (415)255-4547     **Fax:** (415)255-4784
**Email:** info@glma.org
**Website:** http://www.glma.org/
**Fnded:** 1992. **Desc:** Works to recognize the unique healthcare needs of lesbians; seeks to strengthen the health of lesbians and their families through health and medical research grants and education.

★ **18904** ★ **National Association of Lesbian/Gay Addiction Professionals (NALGAP)**
1911 N Fort Myer Dr., Ste. 900
Arlington, VA 22209-1605
**Phone:** (703)465-0539     **Fax:** (703)741-6989
**Email:** clineal@nalgap.org
**Website:** http://www.nalgap.org
Rodger L. Beatty, PhD, Pres.
**Fnded:** 1979. **Mem:** 95. **Nat'l Groups:** 1. **Desc:** Doctors, nurses, social workers, psychologists, certified counselors, and other professionals who work with gay, lesbian, transgendered, and bisexual alcoholics and addicts; drug, alcohol, and gay agencies, organizations, and institutes. Provides a network for support and communication among professionals working with chemically dependent gay, lesbian, and bisexual people. Seeks to educate members of organizations and agencies about gay, lesbian, and bisexual people and addiction; assure that workshops, seminars, conferences, and publications that deal with addiction address the special needs and problems of gay, lesbian, and bisexual people and their families; coordinates services provided by educators and training personnel who are available to help others in the addiction field to better serve gay and lesbian clients. Acts as a clearinghouse for resource and research information in the field of addiction as it pertains to homosexuality; provides referral information about gay, lesbian, and bisexual groups of Alcoholics Anonymous World Services; develops and distributes a list of resource facilities for gay, lesbian, and bisexual alcoholics, addicts and their family and friends. Maintains a training and speakers' bureau. **Pub:** *The NALGAP Annotated Bibliography: Alcoholism, Substance Abuse, and Lesbians/Gay Men.* Book. • *NALGAP Newsletter*, periodic. Newsletter. *Price:* For members only. • *NALGAP Reporter*, semiannual. Newsletter. Includes book reviews. • *National Directory of Facilities and Services for Lesbian and Gay Alcoholics*, periodic. Directory. • Monographs. **Frmly:** (1984) National Association of Gay Alcoholism Professionals; (1997) National Association of Lesbian/Gay Alcoholism Professionals.

★ **18905** ★ **National Association of Research and Therapy of Homosexuality (NARTH)**
16633 Ventura Blvd., Ste. 1340
Encino, CA 91436-1801
**Phone:** (818)789-4440     **Fax:** (818)786-6452
**Email:** narth4@earthlink.com
**Website:** http://www.narth.com
Joseph Battaglia, PhD, Exec. Dir.
**Fnded:** 1991. **Mem:** 1,000. **Desc:** Mental health care providers, religious leaders, educators, and other individuals with an interest in the study of homosexuality. NARTH investigates the causes and treatment of homosexuality, conducts research and educational programs, and maintains referral service for individuals seeking therapy to overcome homosexuality. **Pub:** *Collected Conference Papers*, annual. Proceedings. • *NARTH Bulletin*, 3/year. Journal. • NARTH's "Understanding Homosexuality". Booklet.

★ **18906** ★ **National Association for the Research and Treatment of Homosexuality (NARTH)**
16633 Ventura Blvd., Ste. 1340
Encino, CA 91436
**Phone:** (818)789-4440     **Fax:** (818)789-6452

**Website:** http://www.narth.com
Joseph Nicolosi, PhD, Pres.

**Fnded:** 1992. **Mem:** 1,000. **Desc:** Individuals with an interest in homosexuality. Seeks to increase understanding of the nature, prevention, and treatment of homosexuality. Sponsors research and educational programs; maintains list of therapists who treat dissatisfied homosexuals. **Pub:** *Narth Bulletin*, 3/year. Magazine. *Price:* $5.

**★ 18907 ★ Nordic Association for Clinical Sexology**
Gronhojgardsvej 147
DK-2630 Tastrup, Denmark
**Phone:** 45 43996619     **Fax:** 45 43996619
**Email:** dacs_dk@hotmail.com

**Fnded:** 1979. **Desc:** promotes scientific exchange and practical collaboration in sexology between Denmark, Finland, Iceland, Norway and Sweden; creates and promotes sexological knowledge and information.

**Obstetrician Family Center (Centro Obstetrico Familiar — COF-Ecuado)**
*See:* Entry 18348

**★ 18908 ★ Old Lesbians Organizing for Change (OLOC)**
PO Box 980422
Houston, TX 77098
**Phone:** (713)869-1482     **Fax:** (713)802-2989
**Email:** chardenea@worldnet.att.net
**Website:** http://www.oloc.org
Arden Eversmeyer, Contact

**Fnded:** 1989. **Mem:** 1,000. **Desc:** Lesbians 60 years or older. Serves as a network to reduce ageism. Exchanges information on diversity of races, ethnicities, class backgrounds, and histories of members. Develops and disseminates educational materials on ageism and how to combat discrimination. **Pub:** *Facilitator's Handbook: Confronting Ageism for Lesbians 60 and Over.* Book. *Price:* $25. **AKA:** Old Lesbians Organizing.

**★ 18909 ★ Potency Restored**
8630 Fenton St., Ste. 218
Silver Spring, MD 20910
**Phone:** (301)588-5777     **Free:** 800-588-4170
**Fax:** (301)588-6220
**Email:** info@dr-giulio-scarzella.com
**Website:**   http://www.dr-giulio-scarzella.com/impotence.html
Giulio I. Scarzella, MD, Exec. Dir.

**Fnded:** 1981. **Mem:** 90. **Desc:** Impotent men who have undergone inflatable penile implant (prosthetic) surgery or are considering the operation; partners of impotent men. Provides mutual help, understanding, and emotional support. Encourages members to become informed spokepersons in the field of impotence; presents scientific programs. Plans to start other groups around the country. **Pub:** Newsletter, monthly. **Frmly:** (1982) Impotence Anonymous.

**★ 18910 ★ Sex Information and Education Council of Canada (SIECC)**
850 Coxwell Ave.
Toronto, ON, Canada M4C 5R1
**Phone:** (416)466-5304     **Fax:** (416)778-0785
**Email:** sieccan@web.net
**Website:** http://www.sieccan.org

**Fnded:** 1964. **Mem:** 800. **Lang(s):** English, French. **Desc:** Individuals and organizations in fields including sex education, counselling, reproductive health and

medicine, and rehabilitation and therapy. Fosters public and professional education about human sexuality. Facilitates networking among members. Maintains information service and speakers' bureau; conducts research programs; sponsors educational programs. **Pub:** *The Canadian Journal of Human Sexuality*, quarterly. Journal. • *SIECCAN Newsletter*, 2-3/year. Newsletter.

**★ 18911 ★ Sexuality Information and Education Council of the U.S. (SIECUS)**
130 W 42nd St., Ste. 350
New York, NY 10036-7802
**Phone:** (212)819-9770     **Fax:** (212)819-9776
**Email:** siecus@siecus.org
**Website:** http://www.siecus.org/
Tamara Krenin, Pres.

**Fnded:** 1964. **Desc:** Promotes education about sexuality. Advocates "the rght of individuals to make responsible sexual choices". Disseminates information. **Pub:** *Fact Sheets.* • *SIECUS Report.* Journal. • Manuals. • Pamphlets. • Booklets. • Bibliographies. • Also publishes guidelines for comprehensive sexuality education and position statement. Publications catalog available on request. **Frmly:** (1998) Sex Information and Education Council of the U.S.

**★ 18912 ★ Society for the Psychological Study of Lesbian, Gay and Bisexual Issues (SPSLGBI)**
c/o American Psychological Association
750 First St. NE
Washington, DC 20002
**Phone:** (202)336-6037     **Free:** 800-374-2721
**Fax:** (202)336-6040
**Email:** canderson@apa.org
**Website:** http://www.apa.org/divisions/div44
Sari H. Dworkin, PhD, Pres.

**Fnded:** 1984. **Mem:** 1,600. **Nat'l Groups:** 1. **Desc:** Psychologists, graduate students in psychology, and others interested in the psychological study of lesbian, gay, and bisexual issues and the delivery of affirmative mental health services to gay, lesbian, and bisexual individuals. Promotes scholarship in the study of psychology as it relates to bisexual, gay, and lesbian issues; provides training for psychologists in the field. Cooperates with other groups sharing similar goals, including other divisions of the American Psychological Association. Conducts scholarly programs. **Pub:** *Division 44 Newsletter*, 3/year. Newsletter. • *Psychological Book Series on Lesbian and Gay Issues*, annual. *Price:* Included in membership dues. **Frmly:** (1998) Society for the Psychological Study of Lesbian and Gay Issues.

**★ 18913 ★ Society for the Scientific Study of Sexuality (SSSS)**
c/o David L. Fleming
PO Box 416
Allentown, PA 18105
**Phone:** (610)530-2483     **Fax:** (610)530-2485
**Email:** thesociety@inetmail.att.net
**Website:** http://www.sexscience.org
David L. Fleming, Exec. Dir.

**Fnded:** 1957. **Mem:** 1,200. **Reg. Groups:** 3. **State Groups:** 4. **Desc:** Dedicated to advancing knowledge of sexuality. Support for research, and an interdisciplinary network of collaborating scholars. **Pub:** *Annual Review of Sex Research*, annual. Contains review articles on selected topics in the field of sexology. *Price:* $76/volume. • *Journal of Sex Research*, quarterly. Journal. Contains book reviews and case studies. *Price:* Included in membership dues; $76/year for nonmembers; $120/year for libraries. • *Society for the Scientific Study of Sex–Membership Handbook/Direc-*

*tory.* Membership Directory. *Price:* available to members only. • *Society for the Scientific Study of Sex–Newsletter*, quarterly. Newsletter. Includes calendar of events. *Price:* Included in membership dues; $20/year for nonmembers. • Also publishes research and clinical material. **Frmly:** (1998) Society for the Scientific Study of Sex.

**★ 18914 ★ Society for Sex Therapy and Research (SSTAR)**
409 12th St. SW
PO Box 96920
Washington, DC 20090
**Phone:** (202)863-1646
**Email:** nibonds@acog.org
**Website:** http://www.sstarnet.org/
Nicole Bonds, Contact

**Fnded:** 1974. **Mem:** 200. **Desc:** Professionals in social work, nursing, physiology, gynecology, urology, internal medicine, primate research, psychiatry, and psychology who have clinical or research interests in human sexual concerns. Seeks to facilitate communications among clinicians who treat problems of sexual identity, sexual function, and reproductive life. Provides a forum for exchange of ideas between researchers and patient care providers. **Pub:** Membership Directory, biennial. • Newsletter, 3-4/year. **Frmly:** (1979) Eastern Academy of Sexual Therapy.

## Research Centers

**Baylor College of Medicine Sleep Disorders and Research Center**
*See:* Entry 14146

**★ 18915 ★ Johns Hopkins University National Institute for the Study, Prevention, and Treatment of Sexual Trauma**
104 E Biddle St.
Baltimore, MD 21202
**Phone:** (410)955-4150     **Fax:** (410)539-1664
**Email:** berlinf@aol.com
Dr. Fred S. Berlin, Dir.

**Activities/Fields:** Biological correlates and treatment of sexual disorders, including pedophilia, sadism, transvestism, voyeurism, exhibitionism, compulsive rape, and other psychosexual disorders. Analyzes and evaluates antiandrogenic and counseling treatment of sex offenders, including the effects of the synthetic progestin, Depo-Provera. **Frmly:** Johns Hopkins Hospital Sexual Disorders Clinic.

**Johns Hopkins University Office of Psychohormonal Research**
*See:* Entry 8753

**Johns Hopkins University STD Research Group**
*See:* Entry 11860

**Ohio State University Sleep Disorders Center**
*See:* Entry 14256

**Thomas Jefferson University Sleep Disorders Center**
*See:* Entry 14290

# Chapter 60
# Smoking

## National & International Organizations

**★ 18916 ★ Action on Smoking and Health (ASH)**
2013 H St. NW
Washington, DC 20006
**Phone:** (202)659-4310          **Fax:** (202)833-3921
**Email:** webmaster@ash.org
**Website:** http://www.ash.org
John F. Banzhaf, III, Exec. Dir.
**Fnded:** 1967. **Desc:** Works for the rights of nonsmokers against the problems of smoking. Provides scientific, educational, legal, and advocacy services. Accomplishments include: ban of tobacco ads from radio and television; establishment of no-smoking sections on airplanes, trains, and interstate buses; persuading the National Association of Insurance Commissioners to adopt a resolution urging insurance companies to force smokers to pay their fair share of health insurance costs by charging them higher rates than non smokers; sued the Occupational Safety and Health Administration (OSHA) to ban smoking in all workplaces. **Pub:** *ASH Smoking and Health Review*, bimonthly. Newsletter. Covers medical, legal, regulatory, commercial, institutional, and humorous news related to smoking. *Price:* $25/year. • Also publishes informational handouts on addiction to nicotine, effects of passive smoking, workplace smoking costs, workplace nonsmokers' rights, filing for workers' compensation, and other materials.

**★ 18917 ★ Action on Smoking and Health - England (ASH)**
102 Clifton St.
London EC2A 4HW, United Kingdom
**Phone:** 44 207 7395902     **Fax:** 44 207 6130531
**Email:** action.smoking.health@dial.pipex.com
**Website:** http://www.ash.org.uk
**Fnded:** 1971. **Mem:** 1,000. **Local Groups:** 10. **Lang(s):** English. **Desc:** Publicizes the dangers of smoking. Campaigns for smoke-free public areas and for tobacco control legislation. Liaises with medical charities, health promotion organizations, and private groups. Disseminates information; monitors media, scientific, and trade publications. **Pub:** *ASH Information Bulletin*, bimonthly. Bulletin. Digest of news on smoking and health. • *ASH Supporter News*, quarterly. • *Fact Sheets*.

**★ 18918 ★ Action on Smoking and Health - Northern Ireland (ASH-NI)**
Ulster Cancer Foundation
40-42 Eglantine Ave.
Belfast BT9 6DX, United Kingdom
**Phone:** 44 2890 663281     **Fax:** 44 2890 660081
**Email:** ucf_info@ulstercancer.org
**Website:** http://www.ulstercancer.org
**Fnded:** 1970. **Desc:** Supports cancer research/prevention and care. Individuals united to disseminate information on the dangers of smoking. Seeks to

establish smoke-free public areas and help those addicted to smoking. Works with medical and health groups in support of its aims. Support groups for cancer patients and families, nurses in cancer centres and units, patient advocacy.

**★ 18919 ★ Action on Smoking and Health - Scotland (ASH-S)**
8 Frederick St.
Edinburgh EH2 2HB, United Kingdom
**Phone:** 44 131 2254725     **Fax:** 44 131 2206604
**Email:** ashscotland@ashscotland.org.uk
**Website:** http://www.ashscotland.org.uk
**Fnded:** 1973. **Local Groups:** 1. **Lang(s):** English. **Desc:** National organisation dedicated to campaigning for a tobacco-free Scotland. Aims to: keep the tobacco issue on the public agenda; promote non-smoking as the norm; contribute to the reduction in the uptake of smoking; support stop smoking initiatives. **Pub:** *Unfiltered News*, semiannual. Newsletter. **Frmly:** (1992) Scottish Committee Action on Smoking and Health.

**★ 18920 ★ Air Space Action on Smoking and Health (ASASH)**
6200 McKay Ave.
Box 141-831
Burnaby, BC, Canada V5H 4M9
**Phone:** (604)444-8016
**Email:** rober7@uniserve.com
**Lang(s):** English, French. **Desc:** Individuals and organizations. Seeks to eliminate tobacco smoking. Lobbies for more stringent laws banning smoking in public places; provides assistance to individuals wishing to quit smoking.

**★ 18921 ★ Americans for Nonsmokers' Rights American Nonsmokers' Rights Foundation (ANR)**
2530 San Pablo Ave., Ste. J
Berkeley, CA 94702
**Phone:** (510)841-3032          **Fax:** (510)841-3060
**Email:** anr@no-smoke.org
**Website:** http://www.no-smoke.org
Cynthia Hallett, Exec. Dir.
**Fnded:** 1976. **Mem:** 15,000. **Desc:** Seeks to protect the rights of nonsmokers in the workplace and other public settings. Maintains American Nonsmokers' Rights Foundation, which promotes smoking prevention, educational programs, and public education about secondhand smoke issues. **Pub:** *ANR Materials*. • *ANR Update*, quarterly. Newsletter. Provides information on issues important to nonsmokers. • *Clearing the Air*. Book. • *Secondhand Smoke*. Manual. • *Teens Take Action Guidebook: How to Butt In*. Book. • *Tobacco Smoke and the Non-Smoker*. Brochure. **Frmly:** (1976) California Group Against Smoking Pollution; (1986) Californians for Nonsmokers' Rights; (2001) Americans for Nonsmokers' Rights.

**★ 18922 ★ Ash Ireland - Action on Smoking and Health**
5 Northumberland Rd.
Dublin, Ireland
**Phone:** 353 1 6607044          **Fax:** 353 1 6607955
**Email:** info@ash.ie
**Website:** http://www.ash.ie
**Fnded:** 1992. **Desc:** Acts as a watchdog, promoting control of advertising and sales of tobacco products in Ireland. Seeks to educate the public on the effects of smoking.

**★ 18923 ★ Asia Pacific Association for the Control of Tobacco (APACT)**
12/F-3 No. 57, Fu Hsin N Rd.
Taipei 10559, Taiwan
**Phone:** 886 2 27734308          **Fax:** 886 2 27522455
**Email:** dyenjtfh@ms35.hinet.net
**Website:** http://www.jtf.org.tw
**Fnded:** 1989. **Mem:** 19. **Lang(s):** English, Mandarin. **Desc:** Working to create a "smoke-free Taiwan." Monitors advertising and government policy on tobacco trade. Campaigns for prohibition of cigarette advertising in Taiwan. **Pub:** *Health for All*, monthly. Magazine.

**★ 18924 ★ Canadian Council for Tobacco Control (CCTC)**
75 Albert St., Ste. 508
Ottawa, ON, Canada K1P 5E7
**Phone:** (613)567-3050          **Fax:** (613)567-2730
**Email:** info-services@cctc.ca
**Website:** http://www.cctc.ca
**Fnded:** 1974. **Lang(s):** English, French. **Desc:** Seeks to raise public awareness regarding the dangers of smoking. Lobbies for reduced tobacco use in Canada; assists those wishing to quit smoking. Disseminates information. **Frmly:** Canadian Council on Smoking and Health.

**★ 18925 ★ Chinese Association on Smoking and Health**
Bldg. 12, District 1
Andingmenwai Anhuaxili
Beijing 100011, People's Republic of China
**Phone:** 86 10 64248985     **Fax:** 86 10 64260978
**Email:** cash@mx.cei.gov.cn
**Fnded:** 1990. **Mem:** 50,000. **Nat'l Groups:** 1. **State Groups:** 28. **Local Groups:** 300. **Lang(s):** English. **Desc:** National academic and non-governmental organization in China promoting smoking cessation and tobacco control. Conducts research and educational programs; compiles statistics. Offers consulting services. **Pub:** *Smoking and Health in China*, quarterly. Newsletter.

**★ 18926 ★ Group Against Smokers' Pollution (GASP)**
PO Box 632
College Park, MD 20741-0632

**Email:** gaspamerica@aol.com
Willard K. Morris, Sec.

**Fnded:** 1971. **Mem:** 10,000. **Nat'l Groups:** 1. **State Groups:** 10. **Local Groups:** 100. **Desc:** Nonsmokers who are adversely affected by tobacco smoke united to promote the rights of nonsmokers, educate the public about the problems of second-hand smoke, and regulate smoking in places where nonsmokers are exposed. Supports the establishment and enforcement of laws and other public policy measures which reduce environmental tobacco smoke. Provides information and referral services; distributes educational literature, buttons, posters, and bumper stickers. Helps members find local GASP chapters or establish a chapter. **Pub:** *Nonsmokers' Bill of Rights.* • *The Nonsmokers' Liberation Guide.* Handbook. • Booklets. • Pamphlets. **AKA:** GASP of America.

**National Center for Tobacco-Free Kids**
*See:* Entry 5721

★ 18927 ★ **Quit**
Ground Fl.
211 Old St.
London EC1V 9NR, United Kingdom
**Phone:** 44 20 73885775    **Free:** 44 800002200
**Fax:** 44 20 73885995
**Email:** paula@quit.appeal.dara.co.uk
**Website:** http://www.quit.org.uk

**Fnded:** 1926. **Desc:** Offers information, advice and support to people who want to stop smoking.

★ 18928 ★ **SmokeFree Educational Services**
PO Box 905
New York, NY 10274-0905
**Phone:** (212)912-0960    **Fax:** (212)488-8911
**Email:** smokefree@usa.net

**Website:** http://www.smokefree.org
Joseph Cherner, Pres.

**Fnded:** 1987. **Mem:** 100,000. **Desc:** Mission statement is "to win the right to live and work in a smokefree environment, and to educate people about the unhealthy and socially undesirable consequences of tobacco addiction." Works for: more education for people on the consequences of tobacco addiction; tobacco-free schools; larger health warnings on cigarette ads and cigarette packs; health warnings on cigarettes sold to less developed countries; ending tobacco sponsorship of youth oriented events; eliminating cigarette vending machines; and 100% smoke-free public places. **Pub:** *SmokeFree Air,* quarterly. Newsletter. *Price:* Included in membership dues. **AKA:** Smokefree America.

★ 18929 ★ **Smokenders**
901 NW 133rd St. Ste. A
Vancouver, WA 98665-6445
**Free:** 800-828-4357    **Fax:** (360)546-2518
**Email:** kwillcuts@smokenders.com
**Website:** http://www.smokenders.com
Kay Willcuts, VP

**Desc:** Teaches smokers to quit smoking through seminars or self-help kits.

★ 18930 ★ **Stop Teen-Age Addiction to Tobacco (STAT)**
360 Huntington Ave., Cushing 241
Boston, MA 02115-5005
**Phone:** (617)373-7828    **Fax:** (617)369-0130
**Email:** stat@exit3.com
**Website:** http://www.smokefreeair.org/Org/Org-det.cfm?ID=2559
Judy Sopenski, Dir.

**Fnded:** 1985. **Desc:** Devoted to reducing the use of tobacco by children and teens through grassroots community projects, policy research, public education,

advocacy, communication and counter-advertising. Trains and educates professionals, practitioners, citizen activists and policy-makers on research and activities in tobacco addiction, youth access and prevention. Offers a range of educational courses and consulting services under contract with private and public organizations around the country. **Pub:** *Community Organizer's Manual.* • *60 Years of Deception: An Analysis and Compilation of Cigarette Advertising From 1925-1985.* • *Tobacco-Free Youth.* Catalog.

# Research Centers

**U.S. Department of Health and Human Services**
**National Institutes of Health**
**National Cancer Institute**
**Division of Cancer Control and Population Sciences (DCCPS)**
**((Behavioral Research Program)**
**Tobacco Control Research Branch — TCRB)**
*See:* Entry 10539

★ 18931 ★ **West Virginia University Tobacco Research Center (TRC)**
Mary Babb Randolph Cancer Center
PO Box 9300
Morgantown, WV 26505
**Phone:** (304)293-6988    **Fax:** (304)293-4693
**Email:** eglover@hsc.wvu.edu
**Website:** http://www.hsc.wvu.edu/mbrcc/trc/
Elbert D. Glover, PhD, Dir.

**Activities/Fields:** Safety and efficacy of smoking cessation products or methods.

# Chapter 61
# Social Work



## Medical & Allied Health Schools

### Social Work

*The following institutions offer accredited programs in social work. For information on these programs, contact the Council on Social Work Education, 1725 Duke St., Ste. 500, Alexandria, VA 22314, (703)683-8080, http://www.cswe.org/.*

### Alabama

★ **18932** ★ **Alabama A & M University**
**Graduate Social Work Department**
**Graduate Program in Social Work**
PO Box 302
Normal, AL 35762
**Phone:** (256)851-5478          **Fax:** (256)851-5484
**Email:** swycoff@aamu.edu
**Website:** http://www.aamu.edu
Shelley Ann Wyckoff, Chairman of the Board

★ **18933** ★ **University of Alabama**
**School of Social Work**
**Graduate Program in Social Work**
Box 870314
Tuscaloosa, AL 35487-0314
**Phone:** (205)348-7027          **Fax:** (205)348-9419
**Email:** dean@sw.ua.edu
**Website:**      http://www.ua.edu/academic/colleges/socwork
James P. Adams, Jr., Director

### Alaska

★ **18934** ★ **University of Alaska, Anchorage**
**School of Social Work**
**College of Health, Education, and Social Welfare**
**Graduate Program in Social Work**
3211 Providence Dr.
Anchorage, AK 99508-8230
**Phone:** (907)786-6907          **Fax:** (907)786-6912
**Email:** afeas1@uaa.alaska.edu
**Website:** http://www.uaa.alaska.edu/socwork
Elizabeth A. Sirles, Director

### Arizona

★ **18935** ★ **Arizona State University**
**School of Social Work**
**Graduate Program in Social Work**
Box 871802
Tempe, AZ 85287-1802
**Phone:** (480)965-2795          **Fax:** (480)965-2799
**Email:** kegerdes@asu.edu

**Website:** http://ssw.asu.edu/
Leslie Leighninger, Director

### Arkansas

★ **18936** ★ **University of Arkansas, Little Rock**
**School of Social Work**
**Graduate Program in Social Work**
2801 S University
Little Rock, AR 72204
**Phone:** (501)569-3240          **Fax:** (501)569-3184
**Email:** hmturney@ualr.edu
**Website:** http://www.ualr.edu/~swdept/
Howard M. Turney, Director

### California

★ **18937** ★ **California State University, Fresno**
**Department of Social Work Education**
**Graduate Program in Social Work**
5310 Campus Dr., PH 102
Fresno, CA 93740-8019
**Phone:** (559)278-3992          **Fax:** (559)278-7191
**Email:** jane_middleton@csufresno.edu
**Website:** http://www.csufresno.edu/
E. Jane Middleton, Director

★ **18938** ★ **California State University, Long Beach**
**Department of Social Work**
**Graduate Program in Social Work**
1250 Bellflower Blvd.
Long Beach, CA 90840-0902
**Phone:** (562)985-7774          **Fax:** (562)985-5514
**Email:** joliver@csulb.edu
**Website:** http://www.csulb.edu/~socialwk/
John Oliver, Director

★ **18939** ★ **California State University, Los Angeles**
**Department of Social Work**
**Graduate Program in Social Work**
5151 State University Dr.
Los Angeles, CA 90008
**Phone:** (323)343-4680          **Fax:** (213)343-5009
**Email:** fanders@cslanet.calstatela.edu
**Website:** http://www.calstatela.edu
E. Frederick Anderson, Director

★ **18940** ★ **California State University, Sacramento**
**Division of Social Work**
**Graduate Program in Social Work**
6000 J St.
Sacramento, CA 95819-6090
**Phone:** (916)278-6943          **Fax:** (916)278-7167
**Website:** http://www.hhs.csus.edu/SWRK
Robin Carter, Director

★ **18941** ★ **California State University, San Bernardino**
**Department of Social Work**
**Graduate Program in Social Work**
5500 University Pkwy.
San Bernardino, CA 92407-2397
**Phone:** (909)880-5501          **Fax:** (909)880-7029
**Email:** tmorris@csusb.edu
**Website:** http://socialwork.csusb.edu
Teresa Morris, Director

★ **18942** ★ **California State University, Stanislaus**
**Social Work Department**
**Graduate Program in Social Work**
801 W Monte Vista Ave.
Turlock, CA 95382
**Phone:** (209)667-3091          **Fax:** (209)667-3869
**Email:** edunbar@stan.csustan.edu
**Website:**      http://www.csustan.edu/Social_Work/index.htm
Ellen R. Dunbar, Director

★ **18943** ★ **Loma Linda University**
**Department of Social Work**
**Graduate Program in Social Work**
Griggs Hall
Loma Linda, CA 92350
**Phone:** (909)558-8548          **Fax:** (909)558-0450
**Email:** .bbuckles@univ.llu.edu
**Website:** http://www.llu.edu/llu/
Beverly J. Buckles, Chairman of the Board

★ **18944** ★ **San Diego State University**
**School of Social Work**
**Graduate Program in Social Work**
5500 Campanile Dr.
San Diego, CA 92182-4119
**Phone:** (619)594-6865          **Fax:** (619)594-5991
**Email:** aharbert@mail.sdsu.edu
**Website:**      http://www-rohan.sdsu.edu/dept/chhs/sw/sw.html
Anita S. Harbert, Director

★ **18945** ★ **San Francisco State University**
**School of Social Work**
**Graduate Program in Social Work**
1600 Holloway Ave.
San Francisco, CA 94132
**Phone:** (415)338-1003          **Fax:** (415)338-0591
**Website:** http://www.sfsu.edu/~socwork
Eileen F. Levy, Director

★ **18946** ★ **San Jose State University**
**College of Social Work**
**Graduate Program in Social Work**
1 Washington Sq., Ste. 215
San Jose, CA 95192-0124
**Phone:** (408)924-5800          **Fax:** (408)924-5892

**Website:** http://www.sjsu.edu/depts/SocialWork
Sylvia R. Andrew, Director

**★ 18947 ★ University of California, Berkeley**
**School of Social Welfare**
**Graduate Program in Social Work**
120 Haviland Hall
Berkeley, CA 94720-7400
**Phone:** (510)642-4341 **Fax:** (510)643-6126
**Email:** lmidanik@uclink4.berkeley.edu
**Website:** http://socialwelfare.berkeley.edu
James Midgley, Director

**★ 18948 ★ University of California, Los Angeles**
**School of Public Policy and Social Research**
**Department of Social Welfare**
**Graduate Program in Social Work**
3250 Public Policy Bldg.
PO Box 951656
Los Angeles, CA 90095-1656
**Phone:** (310)825-2892 **Fax:** (310)206-7564
**Email:** swinfor@sppsr.ucla.edu
**Website:** http://www.sppsr.ucla.edu/sw
A. E. Benjamin, Chairman of the Board

**★ 18949 ★ University of Southern California**
**School of Social Work**
**Graduate Program in Social Work**
699 W 34th St.
Montgomery Ross Fisher Bldg., Rm. 214
Los Angeles, CA 90089-0411
**Phone:** (213)740-2711 **Fax:** (213)740-3301
**Email:** mflynn@usc.edu
**Website:** http://www.usc.edu/dept/socialwork/
Marilyn S. Flynn, Director

### Colorado

**★ 18950 ★ Colorado State University**
**School of Social Work**
**Graduate Program in Social Work**
127 Education Bldg.
Fort Collins, CO 80523-1586
**Phone:** (970)491-6612 **Fax:** (970)491-7280
**Email:** granger@.cahs.colostate.edu
**Website:** http://www.cahs.colostate.edu/sw
Ben P. Granger, Director

**★ 18951 ★ University of Denver**
**Graduate School of Social Work**
2148 S High St.
Denver, CO 80208-2886
**Phone:** (303)871-2203 **Fax:** (303)871-2845
**Email:** caalter@du.edu
**Website:** http://www.du.edu
Catherine F. Alter, Director

### Connecticut

**★ 18952 ★ Southern Connecticut State University**
**Department of Social Work**
**Graduate Social Work Program**
101 Farnham Ave.
New Haven, CT 06515
**Phone:** (203)392-6580 **Fax:** (203)392-6580
**Website:** http://www.southernct.edu
Todd William Rofuth, Director

**★ 18953 ★ University of Connecticut**
**School of Social Work**
**Graduate Program in Social Work**
1798 Asylum Ave.
West Hartford, CT 06117
**Phone:** (860)570-9141 **Fax:** (860)570-9264

**Email:** kay.davidson@uconn.edu
**Website:** http://www.socialwork.uconn.edu/
Kay Davidson, Director

### Delaware

**★ 18954 ★ Delaware State University**
**Department of Social Work**
**Graduate Program in Social Work**
1200 N DuPont Hwy.
Dover, DE 19901
**Phone:** (302)857-6770 **Fax:** (302)857-6794
**Email:** jaustin@dsc.edu
**Website:** http://www.dsc.edu/
John N. Austin, Chairman of the Board

### District of Columbia

**★ 18955 ★ Catholic University of America**
**National Catholic School of Social Service**
**Graduate Program in Social Work**
Shahan Hall
Cardinal Station
Washington, DC 20064
**Phone:** (202)319-5454 **Fax:** (202)319-5093
**Website:** http://ncsss.cua.edu
Ann Patrick Conrad, Director

**★ 18956 ★ Gallaudet University**
**Department of Social Work**
**Graduate Program in Social Work**
800 Florida Ave. NE
Washington, DC 20002-3695
**Phone:** (202)651-5160 **Fax:** (202)651-5817
**Email:** janet.pray@gallaudet.edu
**Website:** http://depts.gallaudet.edu/social.work
Barbara J. White, Chairman of the Board

**★ 18957 ★ Howard University**
**School of Social Work**
**Graduate Program in Social Work**
601 Howard Pl. NW
Washington, DC 20059
**Phone:** (202)806-7300 **Fax:** (202)387-4309
**Email:** renglish@howard.edu
**Website:** http://www.socialwork.howard.edu/
Richard A. English, Director

### Florida

**★ 18958 ★ Barry University**
**School of Social Work**
**Graduate Program in Social Work**
11300 NE 2nd Ave.
Miami Shores, FL 33161
**Phone:** (305)899-3900 **Fax:** (305)899-3934
**Website:** http://www2.barry.edu/vpaa-ssw.default.htm
Stephen M. Holloway, Director

**★ 18959 ★ Florida International University**
**School of Social Work**
**Graduate Program in Social Work**
11200 SW 8th St.
ECS 460
Miami, FL 33199
**Phone:** (305)348-5880 **Fax:** (305)348-5313
**Email:** thomlisr@.fiu.edu
**Website:** http://www.fiu.edu/~cupa/social-work.html
Ray Thomlison, Director

**★ 18960 ★ Florida State University**
**School of Social Work**
**Graduate Program in Social Work**
UCC 2505
Tallahassee, FL 32306-2570
**Phone:** (850)644-4751 **Fax:** (850)644-9750

**Website:** http://ssw.fsu.edu/
C. Aaron McNeece, Director

**★ 18961 ★ University of Central Florida**
**School of Social Work**
**Graduate Program in Social Work**
PO Box 163358
Orlando, FL 32828
**Phone:** (407)823-2114 **Fax:** (407)823-5697
**Email:** mvanhook@pegasus.cc.ucf.edu
**Website:** http://www.cohpa.ucf.edu/social/
Mary P. Van Hook, Director

**★ 18962 ★ University of South Florida**
**School of Social Work**
**Graduate Program in Social Work**
4202 E Fowler Ave.
MGY 132
Tampa, FL 33620-8100
**Phone:** (813)974-2063 **Fax:** (813)974-4675
**Email:** amuso@chuma1.cas.usf.edu
**Website:** http://www.cas.usf.edu/social_work/index.html
Jean F. Amuso, Director

### Georgia

**★ 18963 ★ Clark Atlanta University**
**School of Social Work**
**Graduate Program in Social Work**
James P. Brawley Dr. at Fair St. SW
Atlanta, GA 30314-4391
**Phone:** (404)880-8548 **Fax:** (404)880-6434
**Website:** http://www.cau.edu
Dorcas Davis Bowles, Director

**★ 18964 ★ Georgia State University**
**College of Health and Human Sciences**
**School of Social Work**
**Graduate Program in Social Work**
University Plaza
Atlanta, GA 30303-3083
**Phone:** (404)651-3526 **Fax:** (404)651-1863
**Website:** http://chhs.gsu.edu/socialwork
James L. Wolk, Director

**★ 18965 ★ Savannah State University**
**College of Liberal Arts and Social Sciences**
**Master's Department of Social Work**
PO Box 20553
Savannah, GA 31404
**Phone:** (912)356-2410 **Fax:** (912)356-2458
**Email:** bswmsw@tigerpaw.savstate.edu
**Website:** http://www.savstate.edu
James Maury, Chairman of the Board

**★ 18966 ★ University of Georgia**
**School of Social Work**
**Graduate Program in Social Work**
Tucker Hall
Athens, GA 30602-7016
**Phone:** (706)542-5424 **Fax:** (706)542-3282
**Email:** byegidis@arches.uga.edu
**Website:** http://www.ssw.uga.edu/
Bonnie Yegidis, Director

**★ 18967 ★ Valdosta State University**
**Division of Social Work**
**Graduate Program in Social Work**
1500 Patterson St.
Valdosta, GA 31698
**Phone:** (912)249-4864 **Fax:** (912)245-4341
**Email:** marchiba@valdosta.edu
**Website:** http://www.valdosta.peachnet.edu/sowk
Martha M. Giddings, Director

## Hawaii

**★ 18968 ★ University of Hawaii, Manoa**
**School of Social Work**
**Graduate Program in Social Work**
1800 East-West Rd.
Honolulu, HI 96822
**Phone:** (808)956-6300 **Fax:** (808)956-5964
**Email:** jmatsuok@hawaii.edu
**Website:** http://www2.hawaii.edu/sswork/welcome.html
Jon K. Matsuoka, Director

## Idaho

**★ 18969 ★ Boise State University**
**School of Social Work**
**Graduate Program in Social Work**
1910 University Dr.
Boise, ID 83725
**Phone:** (208)426-1568 **Fax:** (208)426-4291
**Email:** mwilson@boisestate.edu
**Website:** http://www.idbsu.edu/socwork/
Martha Wilson, Director

## Illinois

**★ 18970 ★ Aurora University**
**George Williams College**
**School of Social Work**
**Graduate Program in Social Work**
347 S Gladstone Ave.
Aurora, IL 60506-4892
**Phone:** (630)844-5419 **Fax:** (630)844-4923
**Website:** http://www.aurora.edu/
Sandra S. Alcorn, Director

**★ 18971 ★ Loyola University, Chicago**
**School of Social Work**
**Graduate Program in Social Work**
820 N Michigan Ave.
Chicago, IL 60611
**Phone:** (312)915-7005 **Fax:** (312)915-7645
**Email:** jwalsh3@luc.edu
**Website:** http://www.luc.edu/schools/socialwork/
Joseph A. Walsh, Director

**★ 18972 ★ Southern Illinois University, Carbondale**
**School of Social Work**
**Graduate Program in Social Work**
Quigley Hall, Room 4
Mail Code 4329
Carbondale, IL 62901-4329
**Phone:** (618)453-2243 **Fax:** (618)453-4291
**Email:** mnemet@siu.edu
**Website:** http://www.siu.edu/~socwork
Mizanur R. Miah, Director

**★ 18973 ★ University of Chicago**
**School of Social Service Administration**
**Graduate Program in Social Work**
969 E 60th St.
Chicago, IL 60637
**Phone:** (773)702-1250 **Fax:** (773)834-1582
**Email:** e-lawlor@uchicago.edu
**Website:** http://www.ssa.uchicago.edu/
Edward F. Lawlor, Director

**★ 18974 ★ University of Illinois, Chicago**
**Jane Addams College of Social Work**
**Graduate Program in Social Work**
1040 W Harrison St.
Mail Code 309
Chicago, IL 60607-7134
**Phone:** (312)996-3219 **Fax:** (312)996-1802
**Website:** http://www.uic.edu/jaddams/college/
Creasie Finney Hairston, Director

**★ 18975 ★ University of Illinois, Urbana, Champaign**
**School of Social Work**
**Graduate Program in Social Work**
1207 W Oregon St.
Urbana, IL 61801
**Phone:** (217)333-2261 **Fax:** (217)244-5220
**Email:** social@uiuc.edu
**Website:** http://www.social.uiuc.edu/
John Poertner, Director

## Indiana

**★ 18976 ★ Indiana University**
**School of Social Work**
**Graduate Program in Social Work**
902 W New York St., ES 4138
Indianapolis, IN 46202-5156
**Phone:** (317)274-6705 **Fax:** (317)274-8630
**Email:** rbrock@iupui.edu
**Website:** http://iussw.iupui.edu/
Michael A. Patchner, Director

**★ 18977 ★ University of Southern Indiana**
**Social Work Department**
**Graduate Program in Social Work**
8600 University Blvd.
Evansville, IN 47712
**Phone:** (812)464-1843 **Fax:** (812)464-1116
**Website:** http://www.usi.edu/EDU/SOC_WORK/SOCIAL.HTM
David Charles Cousert, Chairman of the Board

## Iowa

**★ 18978 ★ Saint Ambrose University**
**School of Social Work**
518 W Locust St.
Davenport, IA 52803
**Phone:** (563)333-6379 **Fax:** (563)333-6097
**Email:** ksiska@sau.edu
**Website:** http://www.sau.edu/msw
Brenda L. DuBois, Director

**★ 18979 ★ University of Iowa**
**School of Social Work**
**Graduate Program in Social Work**
308 North Hall
Iowa City, IA 52242-1223
**Phone:** (319)335-1250 **Fax:** (319)335-1711
**Email:** salome-raheim@uiowa.edu
**Website:** http://www.uiowa.edu/~socialwk/
Salome Raheim, Director

## Kansas

**★ 18980 ★ University of Kansas**
**School of Social Welfare**
**Graduate Program in Social Work**
1545 Lilac Ln.
Lawrence, KS 66044-3184
**Phone:** (785)864-4720 **Fax:** (785)864-5277
**Email:** annw@ukans.edu
**Website:** http://www.socwel.ukans.edu/
Ann Weick, Director

**★ 18981 ★ Washburn University**
**Department of Social Work**
**Graduate Program in Social Work**
1700 College Ave.
Topeka, KS 66621
**Phone:** (785)231-1010 **Fax:** (785)231-1027
**Email:** zzdpsw@washburn.edu
**Website:** http://www.washburn.edu/sas/social-work/index.html
Mark Kaufman, Director

## Kentucky

**★ 18982 ★ Spalding University**
**School of Social Work**
**Graduate Program in Social Work**
851 S 4th St.
Louisville, KY 40203-2115
**Phone:** (502)585-9911 **Fax:** (502)992-2413
**Website:** http://www.spalding.edu/university/professionalstudies/socialwork/index.ht
Helen Deines, Director

**★ 18983 ★ University of Kentucky**
**College of Social Work**
**Graduate Program in Social Work**
619 Patterson Office Tower
Lexington, KY 40506-0027
**Phone:** (859)257-6654 **Fax:** (859)323-1030
**Email:** khoffma@pop.uky.edu
**Website:** http://www.uky.edu/SocialWork/welcome.html
Kay S. Hoffman, Director

**★ 18984 ★ University of Louisville**
**Raymond A. Kent School of Social Work**
**Graduate School of Social Work**
Oppenheimer Hall
Louisville, KY 40292
**Phone:** (502)852-3944 **Fax:** (502)852-0422
**Email:** terry.singer@louisville.edu
**Website:** http://www.louisville.edu/kent/
Terry L. Singer, Director

## Louisiana

**★ 18985 ★ Grambling State University**
**School of Social Work**
**Graduate Program in Social Work**
PO Box 907
Grambling, LA 71245
**Phone:** (318)274-3305 **Fax:** (318)274-3254
**Website:** http://www.gram.edu/sosw/sosw.htm
Valiyaveetil Thomas Samuel, Director

**★ 18986 ★ Louisiana State University**
**School of Social Work**
**Graduate Program in Social Work**
Huey P. Long Field House
Baton Rouge, LA 70803
**Phone:** (225)578-1351 **Fax:** (225)578-1357
**Email:** socialwork@lsu.edu
**Website:** http://www.socialwork.lsu.edu
Steven R. Rose, Director

**★ 18987 ★ Southern University, New Orleans**
**School of Social Work**
**Graduate Program in Social Work**
6400 Press Dr.
New Orleans, LA 70126
**Phone:** (504)286-5376 **Fax:** (504)286-5387
**Website:** http://www.suno.edu/
Millie M. Charles, Director

**★ 18988 ★ Tulane University**
**School of Social Work**
**Graduate Program in Social Work**
6823 St. Charles Ave.
New Orleans, LA 70118-5672
**Phone:** (504)865-5314 **Fax:** (504)862-8727
**Email:** sengland@mailhost.tcs.tulane.edu
**Website:** http://www.tulane.edu/~tssw/
Ronald Marks, Director

## Maine

**★ 18989 ★ University of Maine**
**School of Social Work**
**Graduate Program in Social Work**
5770 Social Work Bldg.
Orono, ME 04469
**Phone:** (207)581-2389          **Fax:** (207)581-2396
**Email:** gail.werrbach@umit.maine.edu
**Website:** http://www.ume.maine.edu/~soclwork
Gail Werrbach, Director

**★ 18990 ★ University of New England**
**School of Social Work**
**Graduate Program in Social Work**
11 Hills Beach Rd.
Biddeford, ME 04005
**Phone:** (207)797-7261          **Fax:** (207)541-3100
**Email:** jthompson@mailbox.une.edu
**Website:**          http://www.une.edu/chp/socialwork/index.html
Joanne J. Thompson, Director

## Maryland

**★ 18991 ★ University of Maryland, Baltimore**
**School of Social Work**
**Graduate Program in Social Work**
Louis L. Kaplan Hall
525 W Redwood St.
Baltimore, MD 21201-1777
**Phone:** (410)706-7794          **Fax:** (410)706-0273
**Email:** jharris@ssw.umaryland.edu
**Website:** http://ssw.umaryland.edu/
Jesse J. Harris, Director

## Massachusetts

**★ 18992 ★ Boston College**
**Graduate School of Social Work**
McGuinn Hall
140 Commonwealth Ave.
Chestnut Hill, MA 02467-3807
**Phone:** (617)552-4020          **Fax:** (617)552-2374
**Website:** http://www.bc.edu/gssw
Alberto A. Godenzi, Director

**★ 18993 ★ Boston University**
**School of Social Work**
**Graduate Program in Social Work**
264 Bay State Rd.
Boston, MA 02215
**Phone:** (617)353-3750          **Fax:** (617)353-5612
**Email:** wpeebles@bu.edu
**Website:** http://www.bu.edu/ssw/
Wilma Peebles-Wilkins, Director

**★ 18994 ★ Salem State College**
**School of Social Work**
**Graduate Program in Social Work**
352 Lafayette St.
Salem, MA 01970
**Phone:** (978)542-6650          **Fax:** (978)542-6936
**Email:** donald.riley@salem.mass.edu
**Website:** http://www.salemstate.edu/socialwork
Donald P. Riley, Director

**★ 18995 ★ Simmons College**
**Graduate School of Social Work**
51 Commonwealth Ave.
Boston, MA 02116
**Phone:** (617)521-3900          **Fax:** (617)521-3956
**Email:** jregan@simmons.edu
**Website:** http://www.simmons.edu/programs/ssw/
Joseph M. Regan, Director

**★ 18996 ★ Smith College**
**School for Social Work**
**Graduate Program in Social Work**
Lilly Hall
Northampton, MA 01063
**Phone:** (413)585-7952          **Fax:** (413)585-7994
**Website:** http://www.smith.edu/ssw/
Carolyn Jacobs, Director

**★ 18997 ★ Springfield College**
**School of Social Work**
**Graduate Program in Social Work**
263 Alden St.
Springfield, MA 01109-3797
**Phone:** (413)748-3065          **Fax:** (413)748-3069
**Email:** francine_vecchiolla@spfldcol.edu
**Website:** http://www.spfldcol.edu/
Francine J. Vecchiolla, Director

## Michigan

**★ 18998 ★ Andrews University**
**Social Work Department**
**Graduate Program in Social Work**
Nethery Hall
Berrien Springs, MI 49104
**Phone:** (616)471-6135          **Fax:** (616)471-3686
**Email:** spittman@andrews.edu
**Website:** http://www.andrews.edu
Sharon Pittman, Director

**★ 18999 ★ Eastern Michigan University**
**Graduate Program in Social Work**
317 Marshall Bldg.
Ypsilanti, MI 48197
**Phone:** (734)487-4169          **Fax:** (734)487-6832
**Email:** wanda.bracy@emich.edu
**Website:**          http://www.emich.edu/public/swk/swkhome.htm
John Gunther, Director

**★ 19000 ★ Grand Valley State University**
**School of Social Work**
**Graduate Program in Social Work**
De Vos Center, 3rd Fl.
401 W Fulton
Grand Rapids, MI 49504
**Phone:** (616)771-6550          **Fax:** (616)771-6570
**Email:** mulderr@gvsu.edu
**Website:** http://www4.gvsu.edu/ssw
Rodney Mulder, Director

**★ 19001 ★ Michigan State University**
**School of Social Work**
**Graduate Program in Social Work**
254 Baker Hall
East Lansing, MI 48824
**Phone:** (517)353-8632          **Fax:** (517)353-3038
**Email:** social.work@ssc.msu.edu
**Website:** http://www.ssc.msu.edu/~sw/
Gary Anderson, Director

**★ 19002 ★ University of Michigan**
**School of Social Work**
**Graduate Program in Social Work**
1080 S University
Ann Arbor, MI 48109-1106
**Phone:** (734)764-5340          **Fax:** (734)764-9954
**Email:** pameares@umich.edu
**Website:** http://www.ssw.umich.edu/
Paula Allen-Meares, Director

**★ 19003 ★ Wayne State University**
**School of Social Work**
**Graduate Program in Social Work**
201 Thompson Home
4756 Cass Ave.
Detroit, MI 48202
**Phone:** (313)577-4400          **Fax:** (313)577-8770

**Email:** aa8773@wayne.edu
**Website:** http://www.socialwork.wayne.edu
Phyllis Ivory Vroom, Director

**★ 19004 ★ Western Michigan University**
**School of Social Work**
**Graduate Program in Social Work**
1903 Western Ave.
Kalamazoo, MI 49008-5034
**Phone:** (616)387-3170          **Fax:** (616)387-3183
**Email:** mabrey@wmich.edu
**Website:** http://www.wmich.edu/hhs/sw
Earlie M. Washington, Director

## Minnesota

**★ 19005 ★ Augsburg College**
**Department of Social Work**
**Graduate Program in Social Work**
2211 Riverside Ave.
Minneapolis, MN 55454
**Phone:** (612)330-1189          **Fax:** (612)330-1493
**Email:** bosch@augsberg.edu
**Website:** http://www.augsburg.edu
Anthony A. Bibus, Chairman of the Board

**★ 19006 ★ College of Saint Catherine/ University of Saint Thomas**
**School of Social Work**
**Graduate Program in Social Work**
2115 Summit Ave.
Mail LOR 406
Saint Paul, MN 55105
**Phone:** (651)962-5800          **Fax:** (651)962-5819
**Email:** bwshank@stthomas.edu
**Website:**          http://department.stthomas.edu/grad/index.cfm
Barbara W. Shank, Director

**★ 19007 ★ University of Minnesota, Duluth**
**Department of Social Work**
**Graduate Program in Social Work**
220 Bohannon Hall
Duluth, MN 55812-2496
**Phone:** (218)726-7245          **Fax:** (218)726-7185
**Email:** sw@d.umn.edu
**Website:** http://www.d.umn.edu/sw/
Michael Raschick, Director

**★ 19008 ★ University of Minnesota, Twin Cities**
**School of Social Work**
**Graduate Program in Social Work**
1404 Gortner Ave.
Saint Paul, MN 55108
**Phone:** (612)625-1220          **Fax:** (612)624-3744
**Email:** jguam@che1.che.umn.edu
**Website:** http://ssw.che.umn.edu/
Jean K. Quam, Director

## Mississippi

**★ 19009 ★ Jackson State University**
**Graduate Program in Social Work**
3825 Ridgewood Rd., Ste. 9
Jackson, MS 39211
**Phone:** (601)432-6819          **Fax:** (601)432-6827
**Email:** mswprog@ccaix.jsums.edu
**Website:** http://www.jsums.edu/
Gwendolyn Spencer Prater, Director

**★ 19010 ★ University of Southern Mississippi**
**School of Social Work**
**Graduate Program in Social Work**
PO Box 5114
Hattiesburg, MS 39406
**Phone:** (601)266-4163          **Fax:** (601)266-4165

**Website:** http://www-dept.usm.edu/~socwork/
Michael Forster, Director

## Missouri

### ★ 19011 ★ Saint Louis University
**School of Social Service**
**Graduate Program in Social Work**
3550 Lindell Blvd.
Saint Louis, MO 63103
**Phone:** (314)977-2730      **Fax:** (314)977-2731
**Email:** tebbsc@slu.edu
**Website:** http://www.slu.edu/colleges/socsvc/
Susan C. Tebb, Director

### ★ 19012 ★ Southwest Missouri State University
**School of Social Work**
**Graduate Program in Social Work**
Professional Bldg., Ste. 200
901 S National Ave.
Springfield, MO 65804
**Phone:** (417)836-6953      **Fax:** (417)836-7688
**Email:** JOG495@mail.smsu.edu
**Website:** http://www.smsu.edu/swk/
Mary Ann Jennings, Director

### ★ 19013 ★ University of Missouri, Columbia
**School of Social Work**
**Graduate Program in Social Work**
729 Clark Hall
Columbia, MO 65211-4470
**Phone:** (573)882-4447      **Fax:** (573)882-8926
**Email:** cowgerc@missouri.edu
**Website:** http://web.missouri.edu/~sswmain
Charles Cowger, Director

### ★ 19014 ★ Washington University
**George Warren Brown School of Social Work**
**Graduate Program in Social Work**
1 Brookings Dr.
Campus Box 1196
Saint Louis, MO 63130-4899
**Phone:** (314)935-6693      **Fax:** (314)935-8511
**Email:** mswadmis@gwbssw.wustl.edu
**Website:** http://gwbweb.wustl.edu/
Shanti K. Khinduka, Director

## Nebraska

### ★ 19015 ★ University of Nebraska, Omaha
**School of Social Work**
**Graduate Program in Social Work**
60th and Dodge Sts.
Annex 40
Omaha, NE 68182-0293
**Phone:** (402)554-2793      **Fax:** (402)554-3788
**Website:** http://cid.unomaha.edu/~wwwpa/sw/swhome.html
Sunny Andrews, Director

## Nevada

### ★ 19016 ★ University of Nevada, Las Vegas
**School of Social Work**
**Graduate Program in Social Work**
4505 Maryland Pkwy.
Box 455032
Las Vegas, NV 89154-5032
**Phone:** (702)895-4338      **Fax:** (702)895-4079
**Email:** elangston@ccmail.nevada.edu
**Website:** http://www.nscee.edu/unlv/Colleges/Urban
Esther Jones Langston, Director

### ★ 19017 ★ University of Nevada, Reno
**School of Social Work**
**Graduate Program in Social Work**
Business Bldg., Rm. 523
Mail Stop 090
Reno, NV 89557-0068
**Phone:** (775)784-6542      **Fax:** (775)784-4573
**Email:** pierce@unr.edu
**Website:** http://www.unr.edu/hcs/ssw/index.html
Dean Pierce, Director

## New Hampshire

### ★ 19018 ★ University of New Hampshire
**Department of Social Work**
**Graduate Program in Social Work**
Pettee Hall
50 College Rd.
Durham, NH 03824-3596
**Phone:** (603)862-1799      **Fax:** (603)862-4374
**Email:** rej@christa.unh.edu
**Website:** http://www.unh.edu/social-work/index.html
Robert E. Jolley, Chairman of the Board

## New Jersey

### ★ 19019 ★ Kean University
**Department of Social Work**
**Master of Social Work Program**
1000 Morris Ave.
Hutchinson Hall, Rm. 305
Union, NJ 07083-7131
**Phone:** (908)527-2634      **Fax:** (908)289-5633
**Website:** http://www.kean.edu/
Patricia G. Pearson, Chairman of the Board

### ★ 19020 ★ Monmouth University
**Social Work Department**
**Graduate Program in Social Work**
Norwood and Cedar Ave.
West Long Branch, NJ 07764-1898
**Phone:** (732)571-3543      **Fax:** (732)263-5217
**Website:** http://www.monmouth.edu/socialwork
Mark E. Rodgers, Director

### ★ 19021 ★ Rutgers, the State University of New Jersey
**School of Social Work**
**Graduate Program in Social Work**
536 George St.
New Brunswick, NJ 08901-1167
**Phone:** (732)932-7253      **Fax:** (732)932-8915
**Website:** http://www.rutgers.edu
Mary Edna Davidson, Director

## New Mexico

### ★ 19022 ★ New Mexico Highlands University
**School of Social Work**
**Master of Social Work Program**
Las Vegas, NM 87701
**Phone:** (505)454-3563      **Fax:** (505)454-3454
**Email:** a_garcia@nmhu.edu
**Website:** http://www.nmhu.edu/academics/schsocwork
Alfredo A. Garcia, Director

### ★ 19023 ★ New Mexico State University
**School of Social Work**
**Graduate Program in Social Work**
PO Box 30001, MSC 3SW
Las Cruces, NM 88003-8001
**Phone:** (505)646-2143      **Fax:** (505)646-4116
**Email:** socwork@nmsu.edu
**Website:** http://www.nmsu.edu/~socwork
Stephen C. Anderson, Director

## New York

### ★ 19024 ★ Adelphi University
**School of Social Work**
**Graduate Program in Social Work**
South Ave.
Garden City, NY 11530
**Phone:** (516)877-4355      **Fax:** (516)877-4436
**Email:** levin@adlibv.adelphi.edu
**Website:** http://www.adelphi.edu/socialwork/
Brooke E. Spiro, Director

### ★ 19025 ★ Columbia University
**School of Social Work**
**Master of Social Work Program**
622 W 113th St.
New York, NY 10025
**Phone:** (212)854-5189      **Fax:** (212)854-4585
**Email:** rafl@columbia.edu
**Website:** http://www.columbia.edu/cu/ssw/
Sheila B. Kamerman, Director

### ★ 19026 ★ Fordham University
**Graduate School of Social Service**
**Master of Social Work Program**
Lincoln Center Campus
113 W 60th St., Rm. 726
New York, NY 10023-7479
**Phone:** (212)636-6600      **Fax:** (212)636-7876
**Email:** quaranta@mary.fordham.edu
**Website:** http://www.fordham.edu/gss/index.html
Peter B. Vaughan, Director

### ★ 19027 ★ Hunter College of the City University of New York
**School of Social Work**
**Master of Social Work Program**
129 E 79th St.
New York, NY 10021
**Phone:** (212)452-7085      **Fax:** (212)452-7150
**Email:** bleashore@shiva.hunter.cuny.edu
**Website:** http://www.hunter.cuny.edu/socwork/
Bogart R. Leashore, Director

### ★ 19028 ★ New York University
**Shirley M. Ehrenkranz School of Social Work**
**Graduate Program in Social Work**
1 Washington Sq. N
New York, NY 10003
**Phone:** (212)998-5959      **Fax:** (212)995-4172
**Email:** essw.admissions@nyu.edu
**Website:** http://www.nyu.edu/socialwork/
Suzanne E. England, Director

### ★ 19029 ★ Roberts Wesleyan College
**Master of Social Work Program**
2301 Westside Dr.
Rochester, NY 14624-1997
**Phone:** (716)594-6410      **Fax:** (716)594-6480
**Email:** descoteauxw@roberts.edu
**Website:** http://www.rwc.edu/academic/social_w_s/index.htm
William R. Descoteaux, Director

### ★ 19030 ★ State University of New York, Albany
**School of Social Welfare**
**Graduate Program in Social Work**
135 Western Ave.
Albany, NY 12222
**Phone:** (518)442-5320      **Fax:** (518)442-5380
**Email:** kbl@csc.albany.edu
**Website:** http://www.albany.edu/ssw/index.html
Katharine Briar-Lawson, Director

**★ 19031 ★ State University of New York, Buffalo**
**School of Social Work**
**Graduate Program in Social Work**
685 Baldy Hall
PO Box 601050
Buffalo, NY 14260-1050
**Phone:** (716)645-3381     **Fax:** (716)645-3883
**Email:** shulman@acsu.buffalo.edu
**Website:** http://www.socialwork.buffalo.edu/
Lawrence Shulman, Director

**★ 19032 ★ State University of New York, Stony Brook**
**School of Social Welfare**
**Graduate Program in Social Work**
Health Sciences Center, Level 2, Rm. 093
Stony Brook, NY 11794-8231
**Phone:** (631)444-2139     **Fax:** (631)444-8908
**Email:** francesb@ssw.hsc.sunysb.edu
**Website:** http://www.uhmc.sunysb.edu/socwelf/
Frances L. Brisbane, Director

**★ 19033 ★ Syracuse University**
**School of Social Work**
**Graduate Program in Social Work**
Sims Hall
Syracuse, NY 13244-1230
**Phone:** (315)443-5550     **Fax:** (315)443-5576
**Email:** wlpoll@social.syr.edu
**Website:** http://www.social.syr.edu/
Bruce W. Lagay, Director

**★ 19034 ★ Yeshiva University**
**Wurzweiler School of Social Work**
**Graduate Program in Social Work**
Belfer Hall
2495 Amsterdam Ave.
New York, NY 10033
**Phone:** (212)960-0820     **Fax:** (212)960-0822
**Email:** srgelman@ymail.yu.edu
**Website:** http://www.yu.edu/wurzweiler
Sheldon R. Gelman, Director

### North Carolina

**★ 19035 ★ East Carolina University**
**School of Social Work and Criminal Justice Studies**
**Graduate Program in Social Work**
Ragsdale Bldg., Rm. 134
Greenville, NC 27858-4353
**Phone:** (252)328-4208     **Fax:** (252)328-4196
**Email:** griffinl@mail.ecu.edu
**Website:** http://www.ecu.edu/
W. David Harrison, Director

**★ 19036 ★ University of North Carolina, Chapel Hill**
**School of Social Work**
**Graduate Program in Social Work**
Tate-Turner-Kuralt Bldg.
301 Pittsboro St.
CB 3550
Chapel Hill, NC 27599-3550
**Phone:** (919)962-1225     **Fax:** (919)962-0890
**Email:** stromgot@email.unc.edu
**Website:** http://ssw.unc.edu
Jack Richman, Director

**★ 19037 ★ University of North Carolina, Greensboro/North Carolina A & T State University**
**Joint Master of Social Work Program**
PO Box 26170
Greensboro, NC 27402-6170
**Phone:** (336)334-4100     **Fax:** (336)334-5210
**Email:** jcrife@uncg.edu

**Website:** http://www.uncg.edu/swk/joint_msw.htm
John C. Rife, Director

### North Dakota

**★ 19038 ★ University of North Dakota**
**Department of Social Work**
**Graduate Program in Social Work**
Gillette Hall
Box 7135
Grand Forks, ND 58202-7135
**Phone:** (701)777-2669     **Fax:** (701)777-4257
**Email:** mike_jacobsen@mail.und.nodak.edu
**Website:** http://www.und.nodak.edu
Ralph Woehle, Director

### Ohio

**★ 19039 ★ Case Western Reserve University**
**Mandel School of Applied Social Sciences**
**Master in Social Work Program**
10900 Euclid Ave.
Cleveland, OH 44106-7164
**Phone:** (216)368-2270     **Fax:** (216)368-2850
**Email:** msassdean@po.cwru.edu
**Website:** http://msass.cwru.edu
Darlyne Bailey, Director

**★ 19040 ★ Ohio State University**
**College of Social Work**
**Graduate Program in Social Work**
300 Stillman Hall
1947 College Rd.
Columbus, OH 43210-1162
**Phone:** (614)292-2972     **Fax:** (614)292-6940
**Email:** tripodi.5@osu.edu
**Website:** http://www.csw.ohio-state.edu/
Tony Tripodi, Director

**★ 19041 ★ University of Akron/Cleveland State University**
**School of Social Work**
**Joint Master of Social Work Program**
Polsky Bldg., Room 411
Akron, OH 44325-8001
**Phone:** (330)972-5275     **Fax:** (330)972-5739
**Email:** vfitch@uakron.edu
Virginia Fitch, Director

**★ 19042 ★ University of Cincinnati**
**School of Social Work**
**Graduate Program in Social Work**
PO Box 210108
Cincinnati, OH 45221-0108
**Phone:** (513)556-4615     **Fax:** (513)556-2077
**Email:** philip.jackson@uc.edu
**Website:** http://www.uc.edu/socialwork/
Philip Jackson, Director

### Oklahoma

**★ 19043 ★ University of Oklahoma**
**School of Social Work**
**Graduate Program in Social Work**
1005 Jenkins Ave.
Norman, OK 73019
**Phone:** (405)325-2821     **Fax:** (405)325-7072
**Website:** http://www.ou.edu/socialwork/
Roosevelt Wright, Jr., Director

### Oregon

**★ 19044 ★ Portland State University**
**Graduate School of Social Work**
PO Box 751
Portland, OR 97207-0751
**Phone:** (503)725-4712     **Fax:** (503)725-5545
**Email:** wardj@rri.pdx.edu

**Website:** http://www.ssw.pdx.edu/
James H. Ward, Director

### Pennsylvania

**★ 19045 ★ Bryn Mawr College**
**Graduate School of Social Work and Social Research**
300 Airdale Rd.
Bryn Mawr, PA 19010-1697
**Phone:** (610)520-2600     **Fax:** (610)520-2655
**Email:** rmayden@brnymawr.edu
**Website:** http://www.brynmawr.edu/gsswsr
Ruth W. Mayden, Director

**★ 19046 ★ Marywood University**
**School of Social Work**
**Graduate Program in Social Work**
2300 Adams Ave.
Scranton, PA 18509-1598
**Phone:** (570)348-6282     **Fax:** (570)961-4742
**Email:** whitaker@ac.marywood.edu
**Website:** http://www.marywood.edu/goals.htm
William H. Whitaker, Director

**★ 19047 ★ Temple University**
**School of Social Administration**
**Graduate Program in Social Work**
Ritter Hall Annex, Rm. 555
1301 Cecil B. Moore Ave.
Philadelphia, PA 19122
**Phone:** (215)204-8623     **Fax:** (215)204-9606
**Email:** leonard@vm.temple.edu
**Website:** http://www.temple.edu/socialwork/
Curtis A. Leonard, Director

**★ 19048 ★ University of Pennsylvania**
**School of Social Work**
**Graduate Program in Social Work**
3701 Locust Walk
Philadelphia, PA 19104-6214
**Phone:** (215)898-5511     **Fax:** (215)573-2099
**Email:** iram@ssw.upenn.edu
**Website:** http://www.ssw.upenn.edu/
Roberta R. Iversen, Director

**★ 19049 ★ University of Pittsburgh**
**School of Social Work**
**Graduate Program in Social Work**
2117 Cathedral of Learning
Pittsburgh, PA 15260
**Phone:** (412)624-6304     **Fax:** (412)624-6323
**Email:** deesw@vms.cis.pitt.edu
**Website:** http://www.pitt.edu/~pittssw/
Sandra Wexler, Director

**★ 19050 ★ West Chester University**
**Department of Graduate Social Work**
Reynolds Hall
West Chester, PA 19383
**Phone:** (610)436-2664     **Fax:** (610)738-0375
**Website:** http://www.wcupa.edu
Ann A. Abbott, Chairman of the Board

**★ 19051 ★ Widener University**
**Center for Social Work Education**
**Graduate Program in Social Work**
1 University Place
Chester, PA 19013
**Phone:** (610)499-1153     **Fax:** (610)499-4617
**Email:** paula.t.silver@.widener.edu
**Website:** http://muse.widener.edu/socialwork/
Paula T. Silver, Director

## Puerto Rico

**★ 19052 ★ Universidad Interamericana de Puerto Rico, Recinto Metropolitano**
**Graduate Social Work Program**
PO Box 191293
San Juan, PR 00919-1293
**Phone:** (787)250-1912 **Fax:** (787)250-6843
Rosalie Rosa Soderal, Director

**★ 19053 ★ University of Puerto Rico, Rio Piedra Campus**
**Beatriz Lassalle Graduate School of Social Work**
PO Box 23345
San Juan, PR 00931-3345
**Phone:** (787)763-3725 **Fax:** (787)763-3725
**Website:** http://www.upr.edu/
Norma Rodriguez-Roldan, Director

## Rhode Island

**★ 19054 ★ Rhode Island College**
**School of Social Work**
**Graduate Program in Social Work**
600 Mt. Pleasant Dr.
Providence, RI 02908
**Phone:** (401)456-8042 **Fax:** (401)456-8620
**Website:** http://www.ric.edu/socwk/
George D. Metrey, Director

## South Carolina

**★ 19055 ★ University of South Carolina**
**College of Social Work**
**Graduate Program in Social Work**
Columbia, SC 29208
**Phone:** (803)777-5291 **Fax:** (803)777-3498
**Email:** frank.raymond@sc.edu
**Website:** http://www.sc.edu/cosw/
Frank B. Raymond, III, Director

## Tennessee

**★ 19056 ★ University of Tennessee**
**College of Social Work**
**Graduate Program in Social Work**
109 Henson Hall
Knoxville, TN 37996-3333
**Phone:** (865)974-3176 **Fax:** (865)974-4803
**Email:** jfiene@utk.edu
**Website:** http://www.csw.utk.edu/
Karen M. Sowers, Director

## Texas

**★ 19057 ★ Baylor University**
**School of Social Work**
**Graduate Program in Social Work**
PO Box 97320
Waco, TX 76798-7320
**Phone:** (254)710-6400 **Fax:** (254)710-6455
**Website:** http://www.baylor.edu
Diana R. Garland, Chairman of the Board

**★ 19058 ★ Our Lady of the Lake University**
**Worden School of Social Service**
**Graduate Program in Social Work**
411 SW 24th St.
San Antonio, TX 78207-4689
**Phone:** (210)434-3969 **Fax:** (210)431-4028
**Email:** zimmc@lake.ollusa.edu
**Website:** http://www.ollusa.edu/academic/worden/worden.htm
James Allen, Director

**★ 19059 ★ Southwest Texas State University**
**School of Social Work**
**Graduate Program in Social Work**
601 University Dr.
San Marcos, TX 78666-4616
**Phone:** (512)245-8833 **Fax:** (512)245-8097
**Email:** kb01@swt.edu
Dorinda N. Noble, Director

**★ 19060 ★ Stephen F. Austin State University**
**School of Social Work**
**Master of Social Work Program**
SFA Station
PO Box 6104
Nacogdoches, TX 75962-6104
**Phone:** (936)468-4020 **Fax:** (936)468-7201
**Website:** http://www.sfasu.edu/aas/socwk
Michael R. Daley, Director

**★ 19061 ★ University of Houston**
**Graduate School of Social Work**
237 Social Work Bldg.
Houston, TX 77204-4013
**Phone:** (713)743-8085 **Fax:** (713)743-3267
**Email:** lcolby@uh.edu
**Website:** http://www.sw.uh.edu/
Ira C. Colby, Director

**★ 19062 ★ University of Texas, Arlington**
**School of Social Work**
**Graduate Program in Social Work**
Box 19129
Arlington, TX 76019
**Phone:** (817)272-3181 **Fax:** (817)272-5229
**Email:** granvold@uta.edu
**Website:** http://www.uta.edu/ssw/utassw.html
Santos H. Hernandez, Director

**★ 19063 ★ University of Texas, Austin**
**School of Social Work**
**Graduate Program in Social Work**
1925 San Jacinto Blvd.
Austin, TX 78712
**Phone:** (512)471-1937 **Fax:** (512)471-7268
**Email:** bwwhite@mail.utexas.edu
**Website:** http://utexas.edu/depts/sswork/
Barbara W. White, Director

## Utah

**★ 19064 ★ Brigham Young University**
**School of Social Work**
**Master of Social Work Program**
217 Knight Mangum Bldg.
PO Box 24476
Provo, UT 84602-4476
**Phone:** (801)378-3282 **Fax:** (801)378-4049
**Email:** socialwork@byu.edu
**Website:** http://fhss.byu.edu/socwork/
Elaine Walton, Director

**★ 19065 ★ University of Utah**
**Graduate School of Social Work**
395 S 1500 E, Rm. 111
Salt Lake City, UT 84112-0260
**Phone:** (801)581-6192 **Fax:** (801)585-3219
**Email:** jmather@ocwk.utah.edu
**Website:** http://www.socwk.utah.edu
Jannah Hurn Mather, Director

## Vermont

**★ 19066 ★ University of Vermont**
**Department of Social Work**
**Graduate Program in Social Work**
288 Waterman Bldg.
Burlington, VT 05405
**Phone:** (802)656-8800 **Fax:** (802)656-8565
**Email:** dmpratt@zoo.uvm.edu
**Website:** http://www.uvm.edu/~socwork/index.html
Gale Burford, Director

## Virginia

**★ 19067 ★ Norfolk State University**
**Ethelyn R. Strong School of Social Work**
**Graduate Program in Social Work**
700 Park Ave.
Norfolk, VA 23504
**Phone:** (757)823-8668 **Fax:** (757)823-2556
**Website:** http://www.nsu.edu/schools/swork/index.htm
Marvin D. Feit, Director

**★ 19068 ★ Radford University**
**School of Social Work**
**Graduate Program in Social Work**
Box 6958
Radford, VA 24142
**Phone:** (540)831-7689 **Fax:** (540)831-7670
**Email:** mrigby@runet.edu
**Website:** http://www.runet.edu/~sowk-web/
Marilyn A. Rigby, Director

**★ 19069 ★ Virginia Commonwealth University**
**School of Social Work**
**Graduate Program in Social Work**
1001 W Franklin St.
PO Box 842027
Richmond, VA 23284-2027
**Phone:** (804)828-1030 **Fax:** (804)828-7541
**Email:** fbaskind@vcu.edu
**Website:** http://www.vcu.edu/slwweb/index.htm
Frank R. Baskind, Director

## Washington

**★ 19070 ★ Eastern Washington University**
**Inland Empire School of Social Work and Human Services**
**Graduate Program in Social Work**
526 5th St.
Cheney, WA 99004-2431
**Phone:** (509)359-6482 **Fax:** (509)359-6475
**Email:** socialwork@ewu.edu
**Website:** http://sswhs.ewu.edu/socialwork.html
Michael L. Frumkin, Director

**★ 19071 ★ University of Washington**
**School of Social Work**
**Graduate Program in Social Work**
4101 15th Ave. NE
Seattle, WA 98105-6299
**Phone:** (206)685-1662 **Fax:** (206)543-1228
**Email:** hooy@u.washington.edu
**Website:** http://depts.u.washington.edu/sswweb
Dorothy Van Soest, Director

**★ 19072 ★ Walla Walla College**
**Graduate School of Social Work**
204 S College Ave.
College Place, WA 99324-1198
**Phone:** (509)527-2590 **Fax:** (509)527-2434
**Website:** http://www.wwc.edu
Wilma Hepker, Director

## West Virginia

**★ 19073 ★ West Virginia University**
**School of Applied Social Sciences**
**Division of Social Work**
**Graduate Program in Social Work**
PO Box 6830
Morgantown, WV 26506-6830
**Phone:** (304)293-3501 **Fax:** (304)293-5936

**Email:** blocke2@wvu.edu
**Website:** http://www.wvu.edu/~socialwk/
Virginia Stadler Majewski, Director

### Wisconsin

★ 19074 ★  **University of Wisconsin, Madison**
**School of Social Work**
**Graduate Program in Social Work**
1350 University Ave.
Madison, WI 53706-1510
**Phone:** (608)263-3561        **Fax:** (608)263-3836
**Email:** socwork@macc.wisc.edu
**Website:** http://www.wisc.edu
Daniel R. Meyer, Director

★ 19075 ★  **University of Wisconsin, Milwaukee**
**School of Social Welfare**
**Graduate Program in Social Work**
PO Box 786
Milwaukee, WI 53201
**Phone:** (414)229-4400        **Fax:** (414)229-5311
**Email:** jmj2@cds.wm.edu
**Website:** http://www.uwm.edu/Dept/SSW/
James A. Blackburn, Director

### Wyoming

★ 19076 ★  **University of Wyoming**
**Division of Social Work**
**Graduate Program in Social Work**
Box 3632
Laramie, WY 82071
**Phone:** (307)766-6112        **Fax:** (307)766-6839
**Email:** debval@uwyo.edu
**Website:** http://uwacadweb.uwyo.edu/SocialWork/sowk.html
Deborah Valentine, Director

## National & International Organizations

**American Association of Spinal Cord Injury Psychologists and Social Workers (AASCIPSW)**
*See:* Entry 12344

**Association for Applied Poetry (AAP)**
*See:* Entry 12389

★ 19077 ★  **Association of Pediatric Oncology Social Workers (APOSW)**
c/o Marilyn Lees Reinish
Ronald McDonald Childrens Hospital
Loyola University Medical Center
2160 S First Ave.
Maywood, IL 60153
**Phone:** (708)216-3639        **Fax:** (708)216-5044
**Email:** mreinis@luc.edu
**Website:** http://www.aposw.org
Nancy Barbach, Pres.
**Fnded:** 1977. **Mem:** 200. **Desc:** Social workers involved with pediatric cancer patients in medical settings nationwide. Purposes are to: advance the practice, enhance knowledge, and develop policy and programs of pediatric oncology social work; foster quality and effectiveness of the social work practice of pediatric oncology; promote solidarity among social workers; provide community and professional education; formulate and record local and federal legislation related to pediatric oncology. **Pub:** Brochure. • Newsletter, quarterly.

**Cancer Care (CC)**
*See:* Entry 10142

**National Coalition of Psychiatrists Against Motorcoach Therapy (NCPAMT)**
*See:* Entry 12577

**Society for the Psychological Study of Social Issues (SPSSI)**
*See:* Entry 12654

---

## State & Regional Organizations

### <u>Social Work</u>

*Listed below are chapters of the National Association of Social Workers, 750 1st St. NE, Ste. 700, Washington, DC 20002, (202)408-8600, http://www.naswdc.org/.*

#### AE

★ 19078 ★  **National Association of Social Workers**
**International Chapter**
CMR 419 Box 1913
APO, AE 09102
**Phone:** 011-49-622-131-5915
**Email:** naswintl@aol.com
**Website:** http://www.naswintl.org

#### Alabama

★ 19079 ★  **National Association of Social Workers**
**Alabama Chapter**
Governors Park II
2921 Marti Ln., No. G
Montgomery, AL 36116
**Phone:** (334)288-2633        **Fax:** (334)288-1398
**Email:** naswal@earthlink.net

#### Alaska

★ 19080 ★  **National Association of Social Workers**
**Alaska Chapter**
4161 Patterson Circle
Anchorage, AK 99504-4680
**Phone:** (907)332-6279        **Fax:** (907)332-6270
**Email:** naswak@alaska.net
**Website:** http://www.naswak.org

#### Arizona

★ 19081 ★  **National Association of Social Workers**
**Arizona Chapter**
1050 E Southern Ave., Ste. F-5
Tempe, AZ 85282
**Phone:** (480)968-4595        **Fax:** (480)894-9726
**Email:** chapter@naswaz.com
**Website:** http://www.naswaz.com

#### Arkansas

★ 19082 ★  **National Association of Social Workers**
**Arkansas Chapter**
1123 S University 1010
Little Rock, AR 72204
**Phone:** (501)663-0658        **Free:** 800-797-6279
**Fax:** (501)663-6406
**Email:** naswar@cei.net
**Website:** http://www.naswar.org

#### California

★ 19083 ★  **National Association of Social Workers**
**California Chapter**
1016 23rd St.
Sacramento, CA 95816
**Phone:** (916)442-4565        **Free:** 800-538-2565
**Fax:** (916)442-2075
**Email:** naswca@naswca.org
**Website:** http://www.naswca.org

★ 19084 ★  **National Association of Social Workers**
**California Chapter**
**Los Angeles Office**
315 W 9th St., Ste. 321
Los Angeles, CA 90015
**Phone:** (213)452-0090        **Fax:** (213)452-0094
**Email:** membership@naswca.org
**Website:** http://www.naswca.org

#### Colorado

★ 19085 ★  **National Association of Social Workers**
**Colorado Chapter**
2345 S Federal Blvd., Ste. 200
Denver, CO 80219
**Phone:** (303)753-8890        **Free:** 800-595-NASW
**Fax:** (303)753-8891
**Email:** naswco@qwest.net
**Website:** http://www.naswco.org

#### Connecticut

★ 19086 ★  **National Association of Social Workers**
**Connecticut Chapter**
2139 Silas Deane Hwy., Ste. 205
Rocky Hill, CT 06067
**Phone:** (860)257-8066        **Fax:** (860)257-8074
**Email:** naswct@snet.net
**Website:** http://www.naswct.org

#### Delaware

★ 19087 ★  **National Association of Social Workers**
**Delaware Chapter**
3301 Green St.
Claymont, DE 19703
**Phone:** (302)792-0646        **Fax:** (302)792-0678
**Email:** naswde@dca.net
**Website:** http://www.geocities.com/HotSprings/6271/DENASW.html

#### District of Columbia

★ 19088 ★  **National Association of Social Workers**
**DC Metro Washington Chapter**
PO Box 75236
Washington, DC 20013
**Phone:** (202)371-8282        **Fax:** (202)371-6578
**Email:** office@naswmetro.org
**Website:** http://www.naswmetro.org

#### Florida

★ 19089 ★  **National Association of Social Workers**
**Florida Chapter**
345 S Magnolia Dr., Ste. 14-B
Tallahassee, FL 32301
**Phone:** (850)224-2400        **Free:** 800-352-6279
**Fax:** (850)561-6279
**Email:** naswfl@unr.net
**Website:** http://www.naswfl.org

## Georgia

**★ 19090 ★ National Association of Social Workers**
Georgia Chapter
3070 Presidential Dr., Ste. 226
Atlanta, GA 30340
Phone: (770)234-0567    Fax: (770)234-0565
Email: naswga@mindspring.com
Website: http://www.naswga.org

## Guam

**★ 19091 ★ National Association of Social Workers**
Guam Chapter
Rm. 205, HSS Bldg., UOG
PO Box 5176
UOG Station
Mangilao, GU 96923
Phone: (671)735-2877
Email: naswgu@netpci.com

## Hawaii

**★ 19092 ★ National Association of Social Workers**
Hawaii Chapter
677 Ala Moana Blvd., No. 911
Honolulu, HI 96813
Phone: (808)521-1787    Fax: (808)521-3299
Email: info@naswhi.org
Website: http://www.naswhi.org

## Idaho

**★ 19093 ★ National Association of Social Workers**
Idaho Chapter
PO Box 7393
Boise, ID 83707
Phone: (208)345-4060    Fax: (208)345-4062
Email: naswid@qwest.net
Website: http://www.naswid.20m.com

## Illinois

**★ 19094 ★ National Association of Social Workers**
Illinois Chapter
180 N Michigan Ave., Ste. 400
Chicago, IL 60601
Phone: (312)236-8308    Fax: (312)236-6627
Email: office@naswil.org
Website: http://www.naswil.org

## Indiana

**★ 19095 ★ National Association of Social Workers**
Indiana Chapter
1100 W 42nd St., Ste. 375
Indianapolis, IN 46208
Phone: (317)923-9878    Fax: (317)925-9364
Email: naswind@aol.com

## Iowa

**★ 19096 ★ National Association of Social Workers**
Iowa Chapter
4211 Grand Ave., Level 3
Des Moines, IA 50312
Phone: (515)277-1117    Fax: (515)277-2277
Email: naswiowa@aol.com
Website: http://www.angelfire.com/ia2/nasw

## Kansas

**★ 19097 ★ National Association of Social Workers**
Kansas Chapter
Jayhawk Towers
700 SW Jackson St., Ste. 801
Topeka, KS 66603-3740
Phone: (785)354-4804    Fax: (785)354-1456
Email: knasw@birch.net
Website: http://www.knasw.com

## Kentucky

**★ 19098 ★ National Association of Social Workers**
Kentucky Chapter
310 St. Clair, Ste. 104
Frankfort, KY 40601
Phone: (502)223-0245    Fax: (502)223-0525
Email: naswky@dcr.net
Website: http://www.naswky.org

## Louisiana

**★ 19099 ★ National Association of Social Workers**
Louisiana Chapter
700 N 10th St., Ste. 200
Baton Rouge, LA 70802
Phone: (225)346-1234    Free: 800-899-1984
Fax: (225)346-5035
Email: admin@naswla.org
Website: http://www.naswla.org

## Maine

**★ 19100 ★ National Association of Social Workers**
Maine Chapter
222 Water St.
Hallowell, ME 04347-1397
Phone: (207)622-7592    Fax: (207)623-4860
Email: naswmaine@aol.com
Alt. Contact: PO Box 5065, Augusta, ME 04332.

## Maryland

**★ 19101 ★ National Association of Social Workers**
Maryland Chapter
5710 Executive Dr., No. 105
Baltimore, MD 21228
Phone: (410)788-1066    Fax: (410)747-0635
Email: mdnasw@aol.com
Website: http://www.nasw-md.org

## Massachusetts

**★ 19102 ★ National Association of Social Workers**
Massachusetts Chapter
14 Beacon St., No. 409
Boston, MA 02108
Phone: (617)227-9635    Fax: (617)227-9877
Email: chapter@naswma.org
Website: http://www.naswma.org

## Michigan

**★ 19103 ★ National Association of Social Workers**
Michigan Chapter
741 N Cedar St., Ste. 100
Lansing, MI 48906
Phone: (517)487-1548    Fax: (517)487-0675
Email: office@nasw-michigan.org
Website: http://www.nasw-michigan.org

## Minnesota

**★ 19104 ★ National Association of Social Workers**
Minnesota Chapter
1885 University Ave. W, Ste. 340
Saint Paul, MN 55104
Phone: (651)293-1935    Fax: (651)293-0952
Email: email@naswmn.org
Website: http://www.naswmn.org

## Mississippi

**★ 19105 ★ National Association of Social Workers**
Mississippi Chapter
PO Box 4228
Jackson, MS 39216
Phone: (601)981-8359    Free: 800-543-7098
Fax: (601)981-6922
Email: naswms@aol.com
Website: http://members.aol.com/naswms

## Missouri

**★ 19106 ★ National Association of Social Workers**
Missouri Chapter
Parkade Ctr., Ste. 138
601 Business Loop 70 W
Columbia, MO 65203
Phone: (573)874-6140    Free: 800-333-6279
Fax: (573)874-8738
Email: chapter@nasw-mo.org
Website: http://www.nasw-mo.org

## Montana

**★ 19107 ★ National Association of Social Workers**
Montana Chapter
25 S Ewing St., Ste. 406
Helena, MT 59601
Phone: (406)449-6208    Fax: (406)449-2533
Email: naswmt@mt.net
Website: http://www.naswmt.com

## Nebraska

**★ 19108 ★ National Association of Social Workers**
Nebraska Chapter
PO Box 83732
Lincoln, NE 68501
Phone: (402)477-7344    Free: 877-816-6279
Fax: (402)476-6547
Email: naswne@assocoffice.net
Website: http://www.naswne.org

## Nevada

**★ 19109 ★ National Association of Social Workers**
Nevada Chapter
1555 E Flamingo Rd., Ste. 158
Las Vegas, NV 89119
Phone: (702)791-5872    Fax: (702)791-5873
Email: naswnv@worldnet.att.net
Website: http://www.nasw-nv.com

## New Hampshire

**★ 19110 ★ National Association of Social Workers**
New Hampshire Chapter
c/o New Hampshire Association for the Blind
25 Walker St.
Concord, NH 03301
Phone: (603)226-7135    Fax: (603)228-3836
Email: naswnh@worldpath.net

Website: http://www.naswnh.org

## New Jersey

**★ 19111 ★ National Association of Social Workers**
**New Jersey Chapter**
2 Quarterbridge Plaza
Hamilton, NJ 08619
**Phone:** (609)584-5686          **Fax:** (609)584-5681
**Email:** naswnj@aol.com
**Website:** http://www.naswnj.org

## New Mexico

**★ 19112 ★ National Association of Social Workers**
**New Mexico Chapter**
1503 University Blvd. NE
Albuquerque, NM 87102
**Phone:** (505)247-2336          **Fax:** (505)243-0446
**Email:** nasw@qwest.net
**Website:** http://www.naswnm.org
**Remarks:** Send faxes "Attn: Dolores."

## New York

**★ 19113 ★ National Association of Social Workers**
**New York City Chapter**
50 Broadway, 10th Fl.
New York, NY 10004
**Phone:** (212)668-0050          **Fax:** (212)668-0305
**Email:** schachter@naswnyc.org
**Website:** http://www.naswnyc.org/

**★ 19114 ★ National Association of Social Workers**
**New York State Chapter**
188 Washington Ave.
Albany, NY 12210
**Phone:** (518)463-4741          **Free:** 800-724-6279
**Fax:** (518)463-6446
**Email:** naswnys@aol.com
**Website:** http://www.naswnys.org

## North Carolina

**★ 19115 ★ National Association of Social Workers**
**North Carolina Chapter**
PO Box 27582
Raleigh, NC 27611-7581
**Phone:** (919)828-9650          **Free:** 800-280-6207
**Fax:** (919)828-1341
**Email:** naswnc@aol.com
**Website:** http://www.naswnc.org

## North Dakota

**★ 19116 ★ National Association of Social Workers**
**North Dakota Chapter**
PO Box 1775
Bismarck, ND 58502-1775
**Phone:** (701)223-4161          **Fax:** (701)224-9824
**Email:** naswnd@aptnd.com
**Website:** http://www.naswdakotas.com

## Ohio

**★ 19117 ★ National Association of Social Workers**
**Ohio Chapter**
118 E Main St., Ste. 3 W
Columbus, OH 43215
**Phone:** (614)461-4484          **Fax:** (614)461-9793
**Email:** ohnasw@ameritech.net
**Website:** http://www.naswoh.org

## Oklahoma

**★ 19118 ★ National Association of Social Workers**
**Oklahoma Chapter**
2801 N Lincoln Blvd.
Oklahoma City, OK 73105
**Phone:** (405)239-7017          **Fax:** (405)236-3638
**Email:** naswok@ionet.net
**Website:** http://www.ionet.net/~naswok/

## Oregon

**★ 19119 ★ National Association of Social Workers**
**Oregon Chapter**
7688 SW Capitol Hwy.
Portland, OR 97219
**Phone:** (503)452-8420          **Fax:** (503)452-8506
**Email:** nasworegon@nasworegon.org
**Website:** http://www.nasworegon.org

## Pennsylvania

**★ 19120 ★ National Association of Social Workers**
**Pennsylvania Chapter**
1337 N Front St.
Harrisburg, PA 17102
**Phone:** (717)232-4125          **Fax:** (717)232-4140
**Email:** exec@nasw-pa.org
**Website:** http://www.nasw-pa.org

## Puerto Rico

**★ 19121 ★ National Association of Social Workers**
**Puerto Rico Chapter**
PO Box 192051
San Juan, PR 00919-2051
**Phone:** (787)758-3588          **Fax:** (787)281-8433

## Rhode Island

**★ 19122 ★ National Association of Social Workers**
**Rhode Island Chapter**
260 W Exchange St., Ste. 306
Providence, RI 02903
**Phone:** (401)274-4940          **Fax:** (401)274-4941
**Email:** rinasw@aol.com

## South Carolina

**★ 19123 ★ National Association of Social Workers**
**South Carolina Chapter**
PO Box 5008
Columbia, SC 29250
**Phone:** (803)256-8406          **Fax:** (803)254-4116
**Email:** scnasw@earthlink.net
**Website:** http://www.scnasw.org

## South Dakota

**★ 19124 ★ National Association of Social Workers**
**South Dakota Chapter**
1000 N West Ave., No. 360
Spearfish, SD 57783
**Phone:** (605)339-9104          **Fax:** (605)339-9104
**Email:** naswsd@aptnd.com
**Website:** http://www.naswdakotas.com

## Tennessee

**★ 19125 ★ National Association of Social Workers**
**Tennessee Chapter**
1808 W End Ave., Ste. 805
Nashville, TN 37203
**Phone:** (615)321-5095          **Fax:** (615)327-2676
**Email:** tnnasw@aol.com
**Website:** http://www.naswtn.com

## Texas

**★ 19126 ★ National Association of Social Workers**
**Texas Chapter**
810 W 11th St.
Austin, TX 78701
**Phone:** (512)474-1454          **Free:** 800-888-6279
**Fax:** (512)474-1317
**Email:** naswtex@naswtx.org
**Website:** http://www.naswtx.org/

## Utah

**★ 19127 ★ National Association of Social Workers**
**Utah Chapter**
University of Utah GSSW No. 229
395 S 1500 E
Salt Lake City, UT 84112-0260
**Phone:** (801)583-8855          **Fax:** (801)583-6218
**Email:** utnasw@aros.net
**Website:** http://www.utnasw.org/

## Vermont

**★ 19128 ★ National Association of Social Workers**
**Vermont Chapter**
PO Box 1348
Montpelier, VT 05601
**Phone:** (802)223-1713          **Fax:** (802)223-1713
**Email:** naswvt@madriver.com
**Website:** http://www.naswvt.org

## Virgin Islands

**★ 19129 ★ National Association of Social Workers**
**Virgin Islands Chapter**
Havensight Secretarial Services
2 Buccaneer Mall
St Thomas, VI 00802
**Phone:** (340)776-3424          **Fax:** (340)777-8108

## Virginia

**★ 19130 ★ National Association of Social Workers**
**Virginia Chapter**
1506 Staples Mill Rd.
Richmond, VA 23230
**Phone:** (804)204-1339          **Fax:** (804)204-1539
**Email:** naswva@naswva.com
**Website:** http://www.naswva.com

## Washington

**★ 19131 ★ National Association of Social Workers**
**Washington Chapter**
8711 15th Ave. NW
Seattle, WA 98117
**Phone:** (206)706-7084          **Fax:** (206)706-7085
**Email:** admin@nasw-wa.org
**Website:** http://www.nasw-wa.org

### West Virginia

**★ 19132 ★ National Association of Social Workers**
**West Virginia Chapter**
1608 Virginia St. E
Charleston, WV 25311
**Phone:** (304)345-6279          **Fax:** (304)343-3295
**Email:** mail@naswwv.org
**Website:** http://www.naswwv.org/

### Wisconsin

**★ 19133 ★ National Association of Social Workers**
**Wisconsin Chapter**
16 N Carroll St., Ste. 220
Madison, WI 53703
**Phone:** (608)257-6334          **Free:** (866)462-7994
**Fax:** (608)257-8233
**Email:** naswwi@tds.net
**Website:** http://www.naswwi.org

### Wyoming

**★ 19134 ★ National Association of Social Workers**
**Wyoming Chapter**
PO Box 701
Cheyenne, WY 82003
**Phone:** (307)634-2118          **Fax:** (307)778-9518
**Email:** wynasw@worldnet.att.net

# Chapter 62
# Sports Medicine

## Foundations & Other Funding Organizations

### Other Funding Organizations

**American Orthopaedic Society for Sports Medicine (AOSSM)**
*See:* Entry 16904

**Surfer's Medical Association**
*See:* Entry 1565

## National & International Organizations

**★ 19135 ★ African Union of Sports Medicine (AUSM)**
Faculte Medecine
Boite Postale V 166
Abidjan, Cote d'Ivoire
**Phone:** 225 466704    **Fax:** 225 466727
**Email:** smacentral@aol.com
**Website:** http://www.damoon.net/sma/index.html
**Lang(s):** English, French. **Desc:** Physicians and other health care professionals with an interest in sports medicine. Promotes excellence in the practice of sports medicine; seeks to advance scholarship and expertise in the field. Facilitates exchange of information among members; sponsors research and educational programs.

**★ 19136 ★ American Academy of Podiatric Sports Medicine (AAPSM)**
PO Box 723
Rockville, MD 20848-0723
**Free:** 800-438-3355    **Fax:** (301)962-3850
**Email:** info@aapsm.org
**Website:** http://www.aapsm.org
Rita J. Yates, Exec. Dir.
**Fnded:** 1970. **Mem:** 600. **Desc:** Podiatrists, medical doctors, and athletic trainers interested in promoting professional participation and research in sports medicine. Directs 12 committees that deal with individual sports. Compiles statistics. **Pub:** *AAPSM Newsletter*, quarterly. Newsletter. Features articles on the treatment of sports injuries in the field of podiatry. Includes calendar of events and research updates.

**★ 19137 ★ American Academy of Sports Physicians (AASP)**
17445 Oak Creek Court
Encino, CA 91316
**Phone:** (818)501-4433    **Fax:** (818)501-8855
Janie Zimmer, Coord.

**Fnded:** 1979. **Mem:** 150. **Desc:** Clinical physicians engaged in the practice of sports medicine who have made contributions in research, academics, or related fields. Objectives are to educate and inform physicians whose practices comprise mainly sports medicine and to register and recognize physicians who have expertise in sports medicine. Sponsors seminars. **Pub:** Newsletter, quarterly.

**American Canine Sports Medicine Association (ACSMA)**
*See:* Entry 20555

**American Chiropractic Association - Council on Sports Injuries and Physical Fitness (ACA)**
*See:* Entry 5908

**★ 19138 ★ American College of Sports Medicine (ACSM)**
401 W Michigan St.
Indianapolis, IN 46202-3233
**Phone:** (317)637-9200    **Fax:** (317)634-7817
**Email:** mkeckhaver@acsm.org
**Website:** http://www.acsm.org
James R. Whitehead, Exec. VP
**Fnded:** 1954. **Mem:** 17,500. **Reg. Groups:** 12. **Desc:** Promotes and integrates scientific research, education, and practical applications of sports medicine and exercise science to maintain and enhance physical performance, fitness, health, and quality of life. Certifies fitness leaders, fitness instructors, exercise test technologists, exercise specialists, health/fitness program directors, and U.S. military fitness personnel. Grants continuing medical education (CME) and continuing education credits (CEC). Operates more than 50 committees. **Pub:** *ACSM Fitness Book*. Book. Gives Guidelines on Daily Fitness Programs and Training Regimens. *Price:* $13.95. • *ACSM's Guidelines for Exercise Testing and Prescription*. • *ACSM's Health/Fitness Facility Standards and Guidelines*. • *ACSM's Resource Manual for Guidelines for Exercise Testing and Prescription*. Manual. • *American College of Sports Medicine Directory of Graduate Programs in Sports Medicine and Exercise Science*, annual. Directory. Lists graduate programs in fields related to exercise science and sports medicine at North American institutions. *Price:* $15. • *American College of Sports Medicine Guidelines for the Team Physician*. • *Exercise and Sport Sciences Reviews*, annual. Monographs. *Price:* Included in membership dues; $49.95/year for nonmembers. • *Medicine and Science in Sports and Exercise*, monthly. Journal. *Price:* Included in membership dues; $45/year for nonmembers. • *Medicine and Science in Sports and Exercise Cumulative Index*. • *Sports Medicine Bulletin*, quarterly. Magazine. Covers association activities and professional topics. Includes book reviews, calendar of events, and information on membership and fellowship. *Price:* Included in membership dues. • Also publishes position statements.

**★ 19139 ★ American Medical Equestrian Association (AMEA)**
PO Box 130848
Birmingham, AL 35213-0848
**Free:** (866)441-2632    **Fax:** (866)441-2632
**Email:** amea@charter.net
**Website:** http://www.ameaonline.org
Rusty Lowe, Exec. Dir.
**Fnded:** 1990. **Mem:** 175. **Nat'l Groups:** 1. **Desc:** Physicians, health personnel, and individuals interested in equestrian safety. Seeks to decrease accidents related to horseback riding through education and awareness programs. Advocates use of headgear for riders. Offers recommendations, consultations, and leadership to equestrian organizations. Conducts studies and surveys. Compiles statistics. **Pub:** *AMEA News*, quarterly. Newsletter. Includes articles and statistics on horse-related human injuries. *Price:* Included in membership dues. • *Planning Event Coverage*. Booklet. • *When Can My Child Ride a Horse*. Brochure.

**★ 19140 ★ American Medical Society for Sports Medicine (AMSSM)**
11639 Earnshaw
Overland Park, KS 66210
**Phone:** (913)327-1415    **Fax:** (913)327-1491
**Email:** office@amssm.org
**Website:** http://www.amssm.org
**Fnded:** 1991. **Desc:** Sports medicine specialists. Provides a forum specific for primary care non-surgical sports medicine physicians.

**★ 19141 ★ American Sports Medicine Association Board of Certification (ASMA)**
660 W Duarte Rd.
Arcadia, CA 91007
**Phone:** (626)445-1978    **Fax:** (626)574-1999
**Email:** americansportsmedicine@hotmail.com
Joe S. Borland, Bd. Chm.
**Fnded:** 1978. **Mem:** 1,400. **Desc:** Verifies and qualifies the educational competency of active athletic trainers and sports medicine trainers for certification. Establishes competency standards of education required for the prevention and care of athletic injuries and sports medicine. Maintains speakers' bureau. **Pub:** *ASMA News*, quarterly. Newsletter. *Price:* Included in membership dues. • *Special Bulletin*, periodic. Bulletin. • *Why be a Sport Medicine Trainer*. Brochure.

**★ 19142 ★ Arab Federation of Sports Medicine (AFSM)**
PO Box 7559
Doha, Qatar
**Lang(s):** Arabic, English. **Desc:** Physicians specializing in sports medicine. Seeks to advance the practice of sports medicine; encourages continuing professional development of members. Facilitates exchange of information among members; conducts educational programs.

**Asian Committee for Standardization of Physical Fitness Tests (ACSPFT)**
*See:* Entry 17796


**★ 19143 ★ Asian Federation of Sports Medicine (AFSM)**
u.s. department oft. of Orthopaedics and Traumatology
Faculty of Medicine
Chinese University of Hong Kong
Hong Kong, People's Republic of China
**Phone:** 852 26096893          **Fax:** 852 26035821
**Email:** chan6150@cuhk.edu.hk
**Lang(s):** Chinese, English. **Desc:** Health care professionals specializing in sports medicine. Seeks to advance the study, teaching, and practice of sports medicine. Facilitates exchange of information among members; sponsors research and educational programs.


**★ 19144 ★ Asian-South Pacific Association for Sport Psychology (ASPASP)**
Faculty of Social Sciences
Hong Kong Baptist University
224 Waterloo Rd.
Hong Kong, People's Republic of China
**Lang(s):** Chinese, English. **Desc:** Sports psychologists. Promotes sports psychology as a means to the enhancement of athletic performance. Serves as a clearinghouse on sports psychology; provides services to athletes and athletic clubs; sponsors research and educational programs.


**★ 19145 ★ Association for the Advancement of Applied Sport Psychology**
801 Main St., Ste. 010
Louisville, CO 80027
**Phone:** (303)494-5931          **Fax:** (303)499-2599
**Email:** webmaster@aaasponline.org
**Website:** http://www.aaasponline.org
Karen Cogan, Sec. /Treas.
**Fnded:** 1986. **Mem:** 1,100. **Desc:** Promotes the development of research, theory, and intervention strategies in sport psychology. Concerned with ethical and professional issues related to the development of sport psychology and to the provision of psychological services in sport and exercise settings. Sponsors research and educational programs. **Pub:** *AAASP Newsletter*, 3/year. Newsletter. Contains professional articles, organization information, and book reviews. • *Journal of Applied Sport Psychology*, quarterly. Journal.


**★ 19146 ★ Association of Visually Impaired Chartered Physiotherapists**
c/o Guildford Physiotherapy and Sports Clinic
Matthews House
85 Epsom Rd.
Guildford GU1 3PA, United Kingdom
**Phone:** 44 1483 575876     **Fax:** 44 1483 302691
**Fnded:** 1919. **Mem:** 125. **Desc:** Visually impaired chartered physiotherapists. To supply support and encouragement and benefits to its members. **Pub:** *Physiotherapist*, monthly. Audiotapes.


**★ 19147 ★ Big Picture Alliance**
1315 Walnut St., Ste. 1616
Philadelphia, PA 19107-4716
**Phone:** (215)735-5750          **Fax:** (215)735-9291
**Email:** BPAinfo@aol.com
**Website:** http://www.bigpicturealliance.com/newsite/frame/index_2.html
Jeffrey A. Seder, Exec. Dir.
**Fnded:** 1976. **Mem:** 50. **Desc:** Supports projects on anti-violence. Conducts research; compiles statistics. Supports vocational education in media field in inner-city minority communities via a project called "The Childrens Film Festival". **AKA:** (1995) Association for

The Advancement of Social Potential. **Frmly:** (1997) Association for the Advancement of Sports Potential.


**★ 19148 ★ Bulgarian Society of Sport Medicine and Kinestherapy**
Gurguliat 1
BG-1000 Sofia, Bulgaria
**Phone:** 359 2 894145          **Fax:** 359 2 894145
**Fnded:** 1953. **Mem:** 140. **State Groups:** 1. **Lang(s):** English. **Desc:** Fosters research in sport medicine and kinestherapy. **Pub:** *Sport i Nauka.* • *Vaprosi na Fizicheskata Kultura*, quarterly. Journal. Features information on sports and nauka.


**★ 19149 ★ Canadian Academy of Sport Medicine (CASM)**
1010 Poytek St., Unit 14
Gloucester, ON, Canada K1B 5N4
**Phone:** (613)748-5851          **Fax:** (613)748-5792
**Email:** info@casm-acms.org
**Website:** http://www.casm-acms.org
**Fnded:** 1970. **Mem:** 500. **Lang(s):** English, French. **Desc:** Physicians committed to excellence in the practice of medicine as it applies to all aspects of physical activity. Seeks to be a leader in advancing the art and science of sport medicine, including health promotion and disease prevention, for the benefit of all Canadians through programs of education, research, and service. **Pub:** *Clinical Journal of Sport Medicine*, quarterly. Journal.


**★ 19150 ★ Canadian Athletic Therapists Association (CATA)**
**(Association Canadienne des Therapeutes du Sport — ACTS)**
902 11th Ave. SW, Ste. 312
Calgary, AB, Canada T2R 0E7
**Phone:** (403)509-2282          **Fax:** (403)509-2280
**Email:** cata12@telusplanet.net
**Website:** http://www.athletictherapy.org
**Fnded:** 1965. **Mem:** 1,200. **Reg. Groups:** 7. **Lang(s):** English, French. **Desc:** Athletic therapists and other individuals engaged in the practice of sports medicine. Promotes advancement of the study and practice of sports medicine and athletic therapy; seeks to enhance the professional status of members. Encourages adoption of healthy and active lifestyles. Facilitates communication among members. Develops standards of conduct and practice and bestows certification in athletic therapy. Delivers sports medical services to grass roots sports organizations throughout Canada. Conducts educational programs; maintains hall of fame. **Pub:** *Canadian Athletic Therapists Association*, quarterly. Newsletter. • Directory, periodic.


**Canadian Fitness and Lifestyle Research Institute (CFLRI)**
**(Institute Canadien de la Recherche sur la Condition Physique et le Mode de Vie — ICRCP)**
*See:* Entry 17798


**Canadian Society for Psychomotor Learning and Sport Psychology**
**(Societe Canadienne d'Apprentissage Psychomoteur et de Psychologie du Sport)**
*See:* Entry 12441


**★ 19151 ★ Canadian Sport Massage Therapists Association**
PO Box 121
Maple Creek, SK, Canada S0N 1N0
**Phone:** (306)662-4920          **Fax:** (306)662-4951
**Email:** natoffice@csmta.ca
**Website:** http://www.csmta.ca
**Fnded:** 1987. **Desc:** Works to enhance the health care of Canadian athletes through the affective application of sport massage during all phases of athletic

training, performance and competition. Promotes a professional climate for the growth of sport massage therapy in Canada.


**★ 19152 ★ Center for Sports and Osteopathic Medicine (CDM)**
c/o Dr. Richard Bachrach
317 Madison Ave.
New York, NY 10017
**Phone:** (212)685-8113          **Fax:** (212)697-4541
**Email:** info@bonesdoctor.com
**Website:** http://www.bonesdoctor.com/
Richard Bachrach, Pres.
**Fnded:** 1978. **Desc:** Educates dancers about their bodies and preventive medicine in order to help them avoid injuries. Activities are currently concentrated in New York City area. **Frmly:** (1997) CTR for Dance Medicine.


**★ 19153 ★ Chinese Association of Sports Medicine**
11 Tiyuguan Rd.
Beijing 100061, People's Republic of China
**Phone:** 852 10 7120293     **Fax:** 852 10 7146035


**★ 19154 ★ Danish Association of Sports Medicine**
**(Dansk Idraetsmedicinsk Selskab)**
Italiensvej 1
DK-2300 Copenhagen, Denmark
**Phone:** 45 32343292          **Fax:** 45 32343964
**Email:** louice@ah.hosp.dk
**Website:** www.sportsmedicin.dk


**★ 19155 ★ European Society of Knee Surgery Sports Traumatology and Arthroscopy**
7 Av. Krieg
case postale 139
CH-1211 Geneva 17, Switzerland
**Phone:** 41 22 7034808          **Fax:** 41 22 3474769
**Email:** esska200@gve.ch
**Desc:** Surgeons involved in sports traumatology, knee surgery, and arthroscopy. Fosters communication and exchange among members.


**★ 19156 ★ Fellowship of Sports Masseurs and Therapists**
c/o FSMT
PO Box 81
Hertford SG13 7WJ, United Kingdom
**Phone:** 44 1992 537778
**Email:** admin@fsmt-uk.org
**Fnded:** 1975. **Mem:** 500. **Desc:** Sports masseurs and therapists having produced evidence of skills and knowledge in dealing with sports persons in competition, industry, rehabilitation. Sets and maintains standards in sports massage and therapy; advises on courses, helps to set up specific courses for national sports governing bodies, educational establishments sports centres and local authorities. **Pub:** Newsletter, quarterly.


**★ 19157 ★ German Association of Sport Psychology**
c/o Prof. Dr. Henning Allmer
Deutsche Sprothochschule
Psychologisches Institut
Carl-Diem-Weg 6
D-50933 Cologne, Germany
**Phone:** 49 221 4982571     **Fax:** 49 221 4982817
**Email:** allmer@hrz.dshs-koeln.de
**Website:** http://www.uni-leipzig.de/~asp/english
**Fnded:** 1969. **Mem:** 250. **Desc:** Promotes and furthers development of sport psychology through research, teaching, and application. Fosters communication and exchange among members. **Pub:** *Psychologie & Sport*. Journal.

**Institute of Athletic Motivation (IAM)**
*See:* Entry 12497

**International Academy for Sports Dentistry (IASD)**
*See:* Entry 6541

**International Academy of Sports Vision (NASV)**
*See:* Entry 20979

**★ 19158 ★ International Olympic Association for Medico-Sport Research (IOAMSR)**
**(Association Olympique Internationale pour la Recherche MedicoSportive — AOIRMS)**
c/o COI
Chateau de Vidy
CH-1007 Lausanne, Switzerland
**Phone:** 41 21 6216111    **Fax:** 41 21 6216116
**Email:** nasv@mindspring.com
**Website:** http://www.iasv.net
**Lang(s):** English, French, German, Italian. **Desc:** Medical research programs sponsored by the International Olympic Committee. Seeks to advance sports medical research and practice. Conducts research programs; serves as a clearinghouse on sports medicine.

**International Society of Arthroscopy, Knee Surgery and Orthopaedic Sports Medicine (ISAKOS)**
*See:* Entry 19570

**★ 19159 ★ International Society for Ski Traumatology and Medicine of Winter Sports**
**(Societe Internationale de Traumatologie du Ski et de Medecine des Sports d'Hiver)**
c/o Dr. M.H. Binet
Centre Medical
F-74110 Avoriaz, France
**Phone:** 33 4 50740542    **Fax:** 33 4 50740758
**Email:** binet@mdem.org
**Website:** http://www.isakos.com
**Fnded:** 1956. **Lang(s):** English, French, German, Italian, Spanish. **Desc:** Encourages an international exchange of medical experiences and ideas on the treatment of injuries resulting from mountaineering and other winter sports. **Pub:** *Congress Reports*, biennial.

**★ 19160 ★ International Society of Sports Psychology (ISSP)**
c/o Gershon Tenenbaum
Department of Educational Research
Florida State University
307 Stone Bldg.
Tallahassee, FL 32306
**Phone:** (850)644-8780    **Fax:** (850)644-8776
**Email:** tenenbaum@mail.coe.fsu.edu
**Website:** http://www.issponline.org
Gershon Tenenbaum, Pres.
**Fnded:** 1965. **Mem:** 3,000. **Desc:** Professionally qualified individuals in 47 countries interested in sports psychology. Supports and promotes scientific research and professional relations between scholars in the field; participates in information and documentation services in sports psychology; advises and facilitates the establishment of other continental, regional, and national societies of sport psychology. Provides the International Olympic Committee and United States Olympic Committee with information on sport psychology services. Maintains speakers' bureau; operates children's services. **Pub:** *International Journal of Sport Psychology*, 3/year. Journal. • *ISSP Newsletter*, semiannual. Newsletter. Covers profes-

sional issues in sports psychology; includes conference reports, employment opportunities, and membership list. *Price:* Included in membership dues. • *The Sport Psychologist*, quarterly. Journal. For those who teach or provide psychological services to athletes; covers research, practice, and professionals in the field. *Price:* $24/year for members; $28/year for non-members. • Also publishes proceedings.

**★ 19161 ★ International Sports Massage Federation (ISMF)**
2156 Newport Blvd.
Costa Mesa, CA 92627
**Phone:** (949)642-0735    **Fax:** (949)642-1729
**Email:** doctorh@aimt-inc-smti.com
**Website:** http://www.aimt-inc-smti.com
M. K. Hungerford, PhD, Pres.
**Fnded:** 1989. **Mem:** 43. **Desc:** National sports massage federations. Facilitates exchange of techniques and ideas among members; emphasizes improving relations between Socialist and non-Socialist countries. Conducts international exchange programs. Plans to publish newsletter and hold annual meeting. **Pub:** *Sports Massage Journal*, quarterly. Journal. *Price:* $35/year.

**★ 19162 ★ Joint Commission on Sports Medicine and Science (JCSMS)**
401 W Michigan St.
Indianapolis, IN 46202-3233
**Phone:** (317)637-9200    **Fax:** (317)634-7817
**Email:** jwhitehead@acsm.org
James R. Whitehead, MD, Exec. Advisor
**Fnded:** 1966. **Desc:** Provides a forum and acts as a catalyst for the promotion of increased communication among the various organizations interested in the health and safety of sports participants and to help them convey to the public the necessary information on that subject. Seeks to stimulate various organizations for continuous research on pertinent questions and problems in the field of sports injury prevention and care and for the acquisition of valid statistics on the incidence and epidemiology of injuries in sports activities. Also plays a role in helping corporations contact those sports organizations so that they can be of mutual benefit to each other. **Frmly:** (1988) Joint Commission on Competitive Safeguards and the Medical Aspects of Sports.

**★ 19163 ★ Latin and Mediterranean Group for Sport Medicine (LMGSM)**
**(Groupement Latin et Mediterraneen de Medecine du Sport — GLMMS)**
23, blvd. Carabacel
F-06000 Nice, France
**Phone:** 33 4 93328991    **Fax:** 33 4 93130762
**Email:** glmms@libertymsf.fr
**Fnded:** 1956. **Mem:** 2,000. **Lang(s):** English, French. **Desc:** Physicians in 27 Mediterranean countries interested in the medical study of sports and exercise. Objectives are to further sports medicine and to conduct studies on medical problems related to amateur and professional sports and physical activity in general. Offers continuing education classes to members. Operates speakers' bureau. **Pub:** *Apunto*, periodic. • *Archivos de Medicina del Deporte*, quarterly. • *Cinesiologie*, bimonthly. • *SMM Medecine du Sport*, bimonthly.

**★ 19164 ★ Mediterranean Association of Locomotor Pathology Connected to Sport**
**(Association Mediterraneene de Pathologies de l'Appareil Locomoteur Liees au Sport)**
20 avenue Notre Dame
F-06000 Nice, France
**Phone:** 33 4 93854677
**Lang(s):** English, French. **Desc:** Physicians specializing in locomotive sports medicine. Seeks to advance the diagnosis and treatment of locomotor sports

injuries. Serves as a clearinghouse on locomotor sports medicine; sponsors research programs and continuing professional education courses.

**★ 19165 ★ National Youth Sports Safety Foundation (NYSSF)**
One Beacon St., Ste. 3333
Boston, MA 02108
**Phone:** (617)277-1171    **Fax:** (617)722-9999
**Email:** nyssf@aol.com
**Website:** http://www.nyssf.org
Michelle Klein, Exec. Dir.
**Fnded:** 1989. **Desc:** Works to promote the safety and well-being of children and adolescents participating in sports. Strives to reduce the number and severity of injuries youth sustain in sports activities. Sponsors educational programs. Maintains speakers' bureau. **Pub:** *Sidelines*, quarterly. Newsletter. *Price:* $9.5/year. • *Yearbook of Youth Sports Safety*. **Frmly:** National Youth Sports Foundation for the Prevention of Athletic Inuries.

**★ 19166 ★ North American Society for the Psychology of Sport and Physical Activity (NASPSPA)**
c/o Jill Whitall
University of Maryland
Department of Physical Therapy
1 Penn St.
Baltimore, MD 21201
**Email:** jwhitall@som.umaryland.edu
**Website:** http://www.naspspa.org
Jill Whitall, PhD, Sec. -Treas.
**Fnded:** 1966. **Mem:** 600. **Desc:** Kinesiologists, psychologists and physical educators. Promotes scientific research and relations within the behavioral sciences with an application to sport psychology, motor learning, control, and development through meetings, investigations, and other activities.

**★ 19167 ★ Society of Sports Therapists**
c/o Graham N Smith
45c Carrick St.
Glasgow G2 8PJ, United Kingdom
**Phone:** 44 141 2213660    **Fax:** 44 141 2211525
**Email:** admin@society-of-sports.therapists.org
**Website:** http://www.society-of-sports-therapists.org
**Fnded:** 1990. **Mem:** 1,500. **Desc:** Open to anyone over the age of 18 years who has successfully completed a course in sports therapy and satisfies the criteria for membership of the Society. Aims to provide a professional body for sports therapists which will educate, monitor and legislate on all matters pertaining to sports therapy.

**★ 19168 ★ United States Sports Massage Federation (USMF)**
2156 Newport Blvd.
Costa Mesa, CA 92627
**Phone:** (949)642-0735    **Fax:** (949)642-1729
**Email:** doctorh@aimt-inc-smti.com
**Website:** http://www.aimt-inc-smti.com
M. K. Hungerford, PhD, Pres.
**Fnded:** 1989. **Mem:** 17. **Desc:** Sports massage therapists. Facilitates exchange of techniques and ideas among members. Promotes more widespread use of massage therapy by U.S. professional sports teams.

**★ 19169 ★ World Sports Medicine Association of Registered Therapists (WORLD SMAR)**
206 Marine Ave.
PO Box 5642
Newport Beach, CA 92662
**Phone:** (626)574-1999    **Fax:** (626)574-1999
**Email:** americansportsmedicine@hotmail.com
**Fnded:** 1993. **Mem:** 4,000. **Desc:** Sports medicine therapist, trainer, technician, and individuals involved in sports medicine and certified by any nationally recognized athletic trainers association. Establishes

standards of competency for trainers, therapists, and sports medicine care providers that are recognized worldwide. **Pub:** *World Smart News.* • Brochure.*Price:* Free. • Bulletin, periodic. • Newsletter, quarterly. *Price:* Included in membership dues. **AKA:** World Smart.

## Research Centers

**★ 19170 ★ Adelphi University**
**Human Performance Laboratory**
Woodruff Hall
South Ave.
Garden City, NY 11530
**Phone:** (516)877-4276          **Fax:** (516)877-4274
**Email:** otto@adelphi.edu
Dr. Robert Otto, Dir.

**Activities/Fields:** Human performance as it relates to exercise.

**★ 19171 ★ Arizona State University**
**Exercise and Sport Research Institute**
Exercise Science & Physical Education Department
PO Box 870404
Tempe, AZ 85287-0404
**Phone:** (480)965-3913          **Fax:** (480)965-8108
**Email:** philip.martin@asu.edu
**Website:** http://www.asu.edu/clas/espe/
Dr. Philip E. Martin, Ch.

**Activities/Fields:** Exercise, and human movement sport, including exercise physiology, sports psychology, exercise biochemistry, biomechanics, and motor behavior of various populations (children, athletes, elderly, adults). **Frmly:** Human Performance Laboratory.

**★ 19172 ★ Ball State University**
**Human Performance Laboratory**
Muncie, IN 47306
**Phone:** (765)285-1158          **Fax:** (765)285-3238
**Email:** strappe@bsu.edu
**Website:** http://www.bsu.edu/hpl
Dr. Scott Trappe, Actg. Dir.

**Activities/Fields:** Human performance, including studies on effects of physical training on skeletal muscular metabolism, strength development, aging, research, biomechanics, youth fitness and health, nutritional studies, endocrine mechanisms (e.g. GH), fluid replacement during and following acute dehydration, muscle glycogen utilization during prolonged exertion, and swimming research.

**★ 19173 ★ Baylor University Medical**
**Center**
**Baylor-Tom Landry Sport and Wellness**
**Science Lab**
411 N Washington, Ste. 3000
Dallas, TX 75246
**Phone:** (214)820-1513          **Fax:** (214)820-1682
**Email:** dg.mcbrayer@baylordallas.edu
Darvin G. McBrayer, Coord.

**Activities/Fields:** Sports/fitness science, including body composition, basal metabolism, exercise physiology, nutrition and biochemistry for athletes and non-athletes. **Frmly:** Human Performance Center.

**★ 19174 ★ Bridgewater State College**
**Human Performance Lab**
Bridgewater, MA 02325
**Phone:** (508)531-1200          **Fax:** (508)531-1717
**Email:** rhaslam@bridgew.edu
Dr. Robert Haslam, Dir.

**Activities/Fields:** Exercise physiology, including metabolic responses to exercise, blood flow responses to exercise, prediction of athlete success, and police and fire fighter fitness.

**★ 19175 ★ Brigham Young University**
**Human Performance Research Center**
Richards Bldg.
Provo, UT 84602
**Phone:** (801)378-3980          **Fax:** (801)378-5254
**Email:** mark_ricard@byu.edu
Dr. Mark Ricard, Dir.

**Activities/Fields:** Exercise physiology, including studies of cardiovascular changes due to exercise, energy cost of various types of exercise, and body composition changes due to exercise.

**★ 19176 ★ Cincinnati Sports Medicine**
**Research and Education Foundation**
Deaconess Hospital
311 Straight St.
Cincinnati, OH 45219
**Phone:** (513)559-2818          **Fax:** (513)475-5263
**Email:** sbwestin@csmref.org
**Website:** http://www.cincinnatisportsmed.com
Frank R. Noyes, MD, Dir.

**Activities/Fields:** Orthopedic and sports medicine with emphasis on clinical problems and surgical treatment. Areas of interest include rehabilitation protocols; autograft revision knee ligament reconstruction; meniscal allografts; osteochondral autograft transfer; carticel, posterior cruciate and posterolateral reconstruction; biomechanics of the knee and shoulder; and gait analysis.

**★ 19177 ★ Colorado State University**
**Human Performance Laboratory**
Department of Health and Exercise Science
Fort Collins, CO 80523
**Phone:** (970)491-3847          **Fax:** (970)491-7677
**Email:** israel@cahs.colostate.edu
**Website:** http://www.colostate.edu
Dr. Richard Gay Israel, Exec. Dir.

**Activities/Fields:** Human performance, body composition, metabolism, nutrition and sports performance, and exercise physiology.

**★ 19178 ★ Delaware All-Sports Research**
1601 Milltown Rd., Ste. 24
Wilmington, DE 19808
**Phone:** (302)998-0178          **Fax:** (302)999-0700
Dr. J.P. Contompasis, Dir.

**Activities/Fields:** Sports medicine, including clinical and biomechanics research and etiology, treatment, and prevention of sports injuries. Biomechanics research is primarily concerned with lower extremity functions and pathomechanics.

**★ 19179 ★ Grand Valley State University**
**Human Performance Laboratory**
132 Fieldhouse
Allendale, MI 49401
**Phone:** (616)895-3228          **Fax:** (616)895-3232
**Email:** scottj@gvsu.edu
James R. Scott, Coord.

**Activities/Fields:** Human performance studies, including elite athlete performance profiles (wrestlers), functional electro-stimulation exercise with quadriplegic participants, and faculty/staff fitness and lifestyle assessments.

**★ 19180 ★ High Technology Research**
**Institute**
1510 W Montana St.
Chicago, IL 60614
**Phone:** (773)528-1000          **Fax:** (773)528-1043
**Email:** bgoldman@worldhealth.net
**Website:** http://www.worldhealth.net
Dr. Bob Goldman, Dir.

**Activities/Fields:** Effects of drugs and ergogenetics on human performance and analysis of health and fitness products and programs on the market, including fitness technology applications in the treatment and prevention of lifestyle-induced pathologies. Programs include training methods for athletes, the

development of protocols and standards for fitness technology evaluation, drug dependency, longevity, and aids to conventional physical therapy for patients with chronic back pain. Acts as a forum for professionals interested in controversial topics such as the use of hormone drugs, anti-aging medicine, dairy supplemental calicum and estrogen supplements for prevention or reversal of osteoporosis in women, fad diets, and high-impact versus nonballistic low-impact aerobics.

**★ 19181 ★ Human Performance**
**International (HPI)**
402-1228 Hamilton St.
Vancouver, BC, Canada V6B 6L2
**Phone:** (604)684-6192          **Fax:** (604)684-6194
**Email:** info@humanperformance.ca
**Website:** http://www.humanperformance.ca
Dr. Dan Q. Marisi, Dir.

**Activities/Fields:** Biomechanical, physiological, and psychological and medical factors affecting human performance during competitive racing and other athletic activities, such as the influence of body heat on cardiovascular stress.

**Indiana University-Purdue University at**
**Indianapolis**
**Human Performance and Biomechanics**
**Laboratory**
*See:* Entry 4648

**★ 19182 ★ International Center for**
**Aquatic Research**
1 Olympic Plz.
Colorado Springs, CO 80909
**Phone:** (719)578-4578          **Fax:** (719)578-4669
**Email:** jskinner@usa-swimming.org
**Website:** http://www.usa-swimming.org
Jonty Skinner, Contact

**Activities/Fields:** Human performance studies, including training methodology, exercise biochemistry, physiology of performance, muscle strength/power and conditioning, motion and computer analysis, and sports psychology. **Pub:** *Coaching Development Series.* • *IBM compatible software on Human Performance Programs.* • *Nutrition Logbook and Analysis.* • *Performance Profiles of Developing and Elite Swimmers.* • *Sports Medicine Informational Pamphlets: Volumes One and Two.* Pamphlet. • *Sports Participation and Excercise Induced Asthma.* • *Stretching and Warmup Techniques.* • *Training Agenda.* • *Training Methodology.* • *Winning Spirit Instructional Series.*

**★ 19183 ★ International Council of Motor**
**Sport Sciences**
3905 Vincennes Rd., Ste. 303
Indianapolis, IN 46268
**Phone:** (317)471-3596          **Fax:** (317)471-3508
**Email:** icmsin@aol.com
**Website:** http://motorsportsafety.org
Jon Potter, Bus. Admin.

**Activities/Fields:** Enhancement of performance and safety in automobile racing, including the physical and psychological aspects of race performance as well as the role of diet, exercise, and mental preparation in performance. **Frmly:** Motor Sport Research Council.

**★ 19184 ★ Kent State University**
**Exercise Physiology Lab**
162 Gym Annex
Sch. of Exercise, Leisure & Sport
Kent, OH 44242
**Phone:** (330)672-2857          **Fax:** (330)672-2250
**Email:** wglickma@kent.edu
Dr. Ellen Glickman, Contact

**Activities/Fields:** Exercise physiology, body composition, and physical fitness, including studies of protein metabolism and exercise, cardiovascular/respiratory responses during exercise in heat and cold, an neuromuscular integration/biomechanics, and psychosocial reactivity to behavioral stressors. **Frmly:** Applied Physiology Research Laboratory.


**Laban/Bartenieff Institute of Movement Studies, Inc.**
*See:* Entry 20195


**★ 19185 ★ Laval University**
**Division of Kinesiology**
Department of Social Science et Preventive Medicine
Faculty of Medicine
PEPS Rm. 2142
Quebec, QC, Canada G1K 7P4
**Phone:** (418)656-7831　　　　**Fax:** (418)656-3044
**Email:** louis.perusse@kin.msp.ulaval.ca
Louis Perusse, Dir.

**Activities/Fields:** Genetic and molecular basis of obesity and its co-morbidities. Genetics of performance and adaptation to exercise training. Research focuses on the quantification of heritability levels and the identification of genes and molecular markers through association and linkage analyses.


**★ 19186 ★ Melpomene Institute for Women's Health Research**
1010 University Ave.
Saint Paul, MN 55104
**Phone:** (651)642-1951　　　　**Fax:** (651)642-1871
**Email:** health@melpomene.org
**Website:** http://www.melpomene.org
Judy Mahle Lutter, Pres.

**Activities/Fields:** Physically active women and girls, including effects of exercise on menstruation, pregnancy, adolescent girls, self-esteem and physical activity, menopause, body image, osteoporosis, stress and aging, children's introduction to physical activity. **Pub:** *The Bodywise Woman.* • *Breast Cancer: A Handbook.* • *A Guide for Physically Active Women.* • *Level Playing Fields.* • *Melpomene Journal,* 3/year. • *Of Heroes Hopes.* • *Reliable Information about Physical Activity and Health.*


**★ 19187 ★ National Institute for Fitness and Sport**
250 University Blvd.
Indianapolis, IN 46202-5192
**Phone:** (317)274-3432　　　　**Fax:** (317)274-7408
**Website:** http://www.nifs.org
Jerry Taylor, Pres.

**Activities/Fields:** Exercise physiology, sports medicine, and health and fitness education. **Pub:** *NIF Source,* bimonthly. Newsletter.


**★ 19188 ★ Nicholas Institute of Sports Medicine and Athletic Trauma**
Department of Orthopedic Surgery
Lenox Hill Hospital
100 E 77th St.
New York, NY 10021
**Phone:** (212)434-2710　　　　**Fax:** (212)434-2687
**Email:** mchugh@nismat.org
**Website:** http://www.nismat.org
Dr. Malachy P. McHugh, Res. Dir.

**Activities/Fields:** Sports medicine in the areas of orthopedics and trauma, fluid and electrolyte balance, nutrition, endocrinology and physical therapy, cardiology, and biomechanics.


**Orthopedic Biomechanics Institute**
*See:* Entry 16956


**★ 19189 ★ Pennsylvania State University**
**Biomechanics Laboratory**
39 Recreation Hall
University Park, PA 16802
**Phone:** (814)865-3445　　　　**Fax:** (814)865-2440
Dr. Vladimir Zatisiorsky, Dir.

**Activities/Fields:** Human movement, including scientific study and analysis of human motion as observed in sports, industry, and activities of daily living. Analyzes gymnastics, diving, cross-country skiing, swimming, and other sports through use of high-speed video, force measuring devices, and online computer techniques. Studies of elite athletes in Olympic and world championships are conducted with support of U.S. Olympic Committee and the Medical Commission of the International Olympic Committee. Testing, evaluation, and development of sports equipment and playground surface materials are also conducted.


**★ 19190 ★ Pennsylvania State University**
**Center for Sports Medicine**
1850 E Park Ave., Ste. 112
State College, PA 16803
**Phone:** (814)865-3566　　　　**Fax:** (814)865-7803
**Email:** wsebastianell@psu.edu
Dr. Wayne Sebastianelli, Dir.

**Activities/Fields:** Physiology of human performance, sports conditioning, and the role of exercise in the prevention and rehabilitation of sports injuries. Areas of investigation include molecular biology, physiology, biomechanics, locomotion studies, nutrition, bioengineering, and epidemiology. **Pub:** *Penn State Sports Medicine Newsletter,* monthly.


**★ 19191 ★ Pennsylvania State University**
**Noll Physiological Research Center**
129 Noll Laboratory Bldg.
University Park, PA 16802
**Phone:** (814)865-3453　　　　**Fax:** (814)865-4602
**Email:** paf4@psu.edu
**Website:** http://www.noll.psu.edu/
Dr. Peter A. Farrell, Dir.

**Activities/Fields:** Metabolic adaptations to stress, biology of aging, and environmental and exercise physiology. Studies the effects of aging, physical inactivity, nutritional status, and heat, cold, and altitude stress on muscle metabolism and function, thermoregulation and cardiovascular control, reproduction, function and carbohydrate, insulin, and protein metabolism. **Frmly:** Laboratory for Human Performance Research.


**★ 19192 ★ Temple University**
**Biokinetics Research Laboratory**
Pearson Hall
Philadelphia, PA 19122
**Phone:** (215)204-8753　　　　**Fax:** (215)204-4662
Dr. Zebulon Kendricks, Dir.

**Activities/Fields:** Exercise physiology, biomechanics, and motor learning, including studies on biochemical adaptations to exercise, muscular strength and endurance, longitudinal effects of regular vigorous physical activity, environmental influences on physical work, metabolism, and perceptual motor behavior.


**★ 19193 ★ Temple University**
**Center for Sports Medicine and Science**
Health Science Center Campus
3401 N Broad St.
Philadelphia, PA 19140
**Phone:** (215)707-2111　　　　**Fax:** (215)707-2324
Dr. Joseph J. Thoder, Chm.

**Activities/Fields:** Post-operative knee surgery follow-up, post-operative arthroscopic shoulder surgery follow-up, and development of instrument for arthroscopic knee reconstruction.


**★ 19194 ★ United States Sports Academy (USSA)**
1 Academy Dr.
Daphne, AL 36526
**Phone:** (251)626-3303　　　　**Fax:** (251)625-1035
**Email:** academy@.ussa.edu
**Website:** http://www.ussa.edu
Robert C. Campbell, III, Chair

**Activities/Fields:** Sport and sport education in an effort to upgrade sports medicine, sport coaching, sport management, and fitness management, including studies of athletic injuries, body composition of adults, motor performance of youth, physical fitness of adults, ECG abnormalities and changes due to exercise, biomechanical analysis of gross motor skills and three-dimensional gait analysis, product and equipment evaluation and drug use/abuse in sports evaluation and analysis. Research is carried on with local high school athletes, members of the USSA student body, youth involved in the Academy's overseas projects, and selected off-campus program participants. **Pub:** *Sport Supplement,* quarterly. • *USSA Academy News,* quarterly.


**★ 19195 ★ University of British Columbia**
**Allan McGavin Sports Medicine Centre**
3055 Wesbrook Mall
Vancouver, BC, Canada V6T 1Z3
**Phone:** (604)822-4045　　　　**Fax:** (604)822-9058
**Website:** http://sportsmed.cstudies.ubc.ca/

**Activities/Fields:** Iron metabolism in exercise, growth hormone and exercise, biomechanics of running and use of foot orthotic devices, anaerobic threshold in runners, overuse injuries in running, and overuse injuries in aerobic fitness classes. The unit also functions as a clinical service and education center.


**★ 19196 ★ University of Calgary**
**Human Performance Laboratory**
Faculty of Kinesiology
2500 University Dr. NW
Calgary, AB, Canada T2N 1N4
**Phone:** (403)220-3436　　　　**Fax:** (403)284-3553
**Email:** nigg@ucalgary.ca
**Website:** http://www.kin.ucalgary.ca
Dr. Benno M. Nigg, Dir.

**Activities/Fields:** Mobility and longevity; biomechanics, including load on the musculoskeletal system, basic muscle mechanics, joint mechanics, lower back biomechanics, orthoses, sport shoes, and sports equipment; exercise physiology, including muscle physiology, limiting factors in performance and biochemistry of high performance; and neuromotor psychology, including studies involving ice hockey video discs and studies of eye movement in sports. **Pub:** *Annual Report.* **Frmly:** Laboratory for Human Performance Studies.


**★ 19197 ★ University of Calgary**
**Sport Medicine Centre**
2500 University Dr. NW
Calgary, AB, Canada T2N 1N4
**Phone:** (403)220-8232　　　　**Fax:** (403)282-6170
**Email:** rcjackso@ucalgary.ca
**Website:** http://www.kin.ucalgary.ca/SMC/html/index.html
Roger Jackson, Dir.

**Activities/Fields:** Human movement and sport, including anthropometry, athletic therapy, biochemistry, biomechanics, epidemiology, growth and development, nutrition, orthopedics, orthotics, physiology, physiotherapy, and sport medicine.


**★ 19198 ★ University of Delaware**
**Sports Science Laboratory**
S College Ave.
Newark, DE 19716
**Phone:** (302)831-8006　　　　**Fax:** (302)831-3693
**Email:** provost@udel.edu
Michelle Provost-Craig, PhD, Co-Dir.

**Activities/Fields:** Sports science, biomechanics, exercise physiology, bone density, and elite skaters.


**★ 19199 ★ University of Florida**
**Center for Exercise Science**
25 Florida Gym
Gainesville, FL 32611
**Phone:** (352)392-9575　　　　**Fax:** (352)392-0316
**Email:** spowers@hhp.ufl.edu
Scott Powers, PhD, Dir.

**Activities/Fields:** Fitness as it relates to athletic performance, as well as the general population, including research on biomechanics and skill acquisition; health risk factors; exercise and. the lumbar and cervical spine, sports, aging, menopause, diabetes, and athletic performance. **Pub:** *Journal of Cardiopulmonary Rehabilitation.* **Frmly:** Center for Physical and Motor Fitness.


### ★ 19200 ★ University of Illinois at Urbana-Champaign
### Athletic Training Research Lab

906 S Goodwin
Urbana, IL 61801
**Phone:** (217)333-7699          **Fax:** (217)244-7322
**Email:** g-bell@uiuc.edu
**Website:** http://www.kines.uiuc.edu/atcentral/
Prof. Gerald W. Bell, Dir.

**Activities/Fields:** Therapeutic affects of exercise on musculoskeletal injuries, medical supervision of sports programs, response of wheelchair athletes to exercise and training programs, and epidemiological aspects of sports injuries for high school participants, intramural sports participants, and dance students. **Pub:** *Journal of Athletic Training.* • *Journal of the Illinois Athletic Trainers Association.* • *Journal of Orthopedic Sports PT.* **Frmly:** Sports Injuries/Therapeutic Exercise Research Unit.


### ★ 19201 ★ University of Illinois at Urbana-Champaign
### Biomechanics Research Laboratory of Illinois

Freer Hall
Department of Kinesiology
906 S Goodwin
Urbana, IL 61801
**Phone:** (217)333-2461          **Fax:** (217)244-7322

**Activities/Fields:** Sports biomechanics (tennis, fencing, athletics, volleyball, and rope jumping), biomechanics of sports safety and injury potential, force production, occupational biomechanics (firefighting tasks), movement patterns of the elderly, and strength training.


### ★ 19202 ★ University of Manitoba
### Health, Leisure, and Human Performance Research Institute (HLHP)

307 Max Bell Centre
Winnipeg, MB, Canada R3T 2N2
**Phone:** (204)474-7087          **Fax:** (204)261-4802
**Email:** hjanzen@cc.umanitoba.ca
**Website:** http://www.umanitoba.ca/faculties/physed/research/
Dr. Henry Janzen, Actg. Dir.

**Activities/Fields:** Health and Wellness Research Group, Lifespan and Disability Research Group, Exercise and Environmental Medicine Research Group, Leisure and Tourism Research Group, Sport and Human Performance Research Group. **Frmly:** Sport and Exercise Sciences Research Institute.


### ★ 19203 ★ University of Miami
### Laboratory of Clinical and Applied Physiology

PO Box 248065
Coral Gables, FL 33124-8065
**Phone:** (305)284-3024          **Fax:** (305)284-5168
**Email:** aperry@miami.edu
**Website:** http://www.education.miami.edu
Dr. Arlette Perry, Dir.

**Activities/Fields:** Kinesiology, muscle cell and cardiovascular physiology, sports nutrition, obesity, electromyography, lipid physiology, exercise biochemistry, and health/exercise prescription. **Pub:** *American Journal of Clinical Nutrition.* • *International Journal of Sports Nutrition.* • *Journal of Applied Physiology.* • *Medicine and Science in Sports and Exercise.* **Frmly:** Human Performance Laboratory.


### ★ 19204 ★ University of Michigan
### Health Management Research Center

1027 E Huron St.
Ann Arbor, MI 48104-1688
**Phone:** (734)763-2462          **Fax:** (734)763-2206
**Email:** dwe@umich.edu
**Website:** http://www.umich.edu/~hmrc
Dr. D.W. Edington, Dir.

**Activities/Fields:** Examines the relationships between lifestyle behaviors, quality of life, organizational productivity, and health care costs. **Pub:** *Cost Benefit Analysis,* annually. **Frmly:** Fitness Research Center.


### ★ 19205 ★ University of Missouri—Columbia
### Exercise Physiology Graduate Program

217 Gwynn Hall
Department of Nutritional Sciences
Columbia, MO 65211
**Phone:** (573)882-4288          **Fax:** (573)884-6992
**Email:** thomastr@missouri.edu
**Website:** http://www.missouri.edu/~nutsci/exphy.htm
Tom R. Thomas, PhD, Dir.

**Activities/Fields:** Exercise physiology, including calorie expenditure and different modes of exercise; exercise and blood lipoproteins.


### ★ 19206 ★ University of Nevada, Las Vegas
### Exercise Physiology Laboratory

Box 3034
4505 Maryland Pky.
Las Vegas, NV 89154-3034
**Phone:** (702)895-3766          **Fax:** (702)895-4191
**Email:** golding@ccmail.nevada.edu
**Website:** http://www.lagolding.com
Dr. Lawrence A. Golding, Dir.

**Activities/Fields:** Primary function and research emphasis is the study of the biology of exercise. Studies include the physiological effect of both the immediate effect of exercise and the long range effect of physical training, the effect of the environment on physical performance (heat, humidity, cold, altitude, and pollution), the effect of aging on physical performance, and the impact of exercise on the older adult, the effects of drug use and diet supplement on physical performance, and a longitudinal study on the effect of regular exercise on coronary risk factors and aging.


### ★ 19207 ★ University of North Carolina at Chapel Hill
### National Center for Catastrophic Sports Injury Research

CB 8700
204 Fetzer Gymnasium
Chapel Hill, NC 27599-8700
**Phone:** (919)962-5171          **Fax:** (919)962-0489
**Email:** mueller@email.unc.edu
**Website:** http://www.unc.edu/depts/nccsi
Dr. Frederick O. Mueller, Dir.

**Activities/Fields:** Fatality and permanent injury in sports, especially football. **Pub:** *Annual Report.*


### ★ 19208 ★ University of Pittsburgh
### Center for Exercise and Health-Fitness Research

A149B Trees Hall
Pittsburgh, PA 15261
**Phone:** (412)648-8251          **Fax:** (412)648-7092
Dr. Robert J. Robertson, Dir.

**Activities/Fields:** Physiology of exercise and work, perception of physical exertion, cardiac rehabilitation, and ergogenic aids, including studies conducted by full-time faculty members and graduate students of the University. **Frmly:** Human Energy Research Laboratory.


### ★ 19209 ★ University of Rhode Island
### Exercise Science Laboratories

Independence Sq. 2
25 W Independence Way
Kingston, RI 02881
**Phone:** (401)874-2976          **Fax:** (401)874-5630
**Email:** manfredi@uri.edu
Thomas Manfredi, PhD, Co-Dir.

**Activities/Fields:** Physiological profiles of athletic populations, diet and weight loss, aging and exercise. **Frmly:** Human Performance Laboratory.


### ★ 19210 ★ University of Utah
### Human Performance Research Laboratory

250 South 1850 East, Rm. 235
Salt Lake City, UT 84112
**Phone:** (801)585-6172          **Fax:** (801)585-3992
Dr. Andrea T. White, Dir.

**Activities/Fields:** Effects of exercise and environment on muscular, cardiovascular, respiratory, nervous, and thermoregulatory systems of the human body. Programs are conducted on exercise and multiple sclerosis patients, women at risk for osteoporosis, exercise and functional abilities and health benefits.


### University of Vermont
### McClure Musculoskeletal Research Center
*See:* Entry 13737


### ★ 19211 ★ Vanderbilt University
### Energy Balance Laboratory

Clinical Research Center
21st Ave. S
Nashville, TN 37232-2195
**Phone:** (615)343-8497          **Fax:** (615)343-8915
**Email:** kong.chen@mcmail.vanderbilt.edu
**Website:** http://www.uvm.edu/~ortho
Dr. Kong Chen, Dir.

**Activities/Fields:** Use of indirect calorimetry to measure energy expenditure, and metabolic rate and physical activities under a variety of conditions, including exercise, dietary intake, and environmental changes. Emphasis is on the identification of determinants of energy expenditure and body weight regulation. Uses hydrostatic weighing, bioelectrical impedance, and other methods to measure body composition.

# Federal Government Agencies

★ 19212 ★ **U.S. Department of Health and Human Services**
**National Institutes of Health (NIH)**
**National Institute on Alcohol Abuse and Alcoholism (NIAAA)**
9000 Rockville Pike
Bethesda, MD 20892
**Phone:** (301)443-3885
**Website:** http://www.niaaa.nih.gov/
Enoch Gordis, MD, Director
**Desc:** The Institute conducts and supports biomedical and behavioral research, in order to provide science-based approaches to the prevention and treatment of alcohol abuse and alcoholism. It provides a national focus for the Federal effort to increase knowledge and disseminate research findings to the scientific community, health care system ,and the public.

★ 19213 ★ **U.S. Department of Health and Human Services**
**National Institutes of Health (NIH)**
**National Institute on Drug Abuse (NIDA)**
9000 Rockville Pike
Bethesda, MD 20892
**Phone:** (301)443-1124
**Website:** http://www.nida.nih.gov/
Kenneth Olden, Director
**Desc:** The Institute's mission is to lead the Nation in bringing the power of science to bear on drug abuse and addiction, through the strategic support and conduct of research across a broad range of disciplines, and the rapid and effective dissemination and use of the results of that research to significantly improve drug abuse and addiction prevention, treatment, and policy.

★ 19214 ★ **U.S. Department of Health and Human Services (SAMHSA)**
**Substance Abuse and Mental Health Services Administration (SAMHSA)**
5600 Fishers Ln.
Rockville, MD 20857
**Phone:** (301)443-4797
**Website:** http://www.samhsa.gov/
Joseph H. Autry, Acting Administrator
**Desc:** The mission of SAMHSA is to ensure that knowledge, based on science and state-of-the-art practice is effectively used for the prevention and treatment of addictive and mental disorders. Major components include: Center for Substance Abuse Prevention , Center for Substance Abuse Treatment, and the Center for Mental Health Services.

★ 19215 ★ **U.S. Department of Health and Human Services**
**Substance Abuse and Mental Health Services Administration**
**Center for Substance Abuse Prevention**
5600 Fishers Lane
Rockville, MD 20857
**Phone:** (301)443-0365
**Website:** http://www.samhsa.gov/centers/csap/csap.html
Ruth Sanchez-Way, PhD, Director
**Desc:** The Center provides a national focus for the federal effort to prevent alcohol and other drug abuse. To this end, it develops and reviews policy; administers grants; helps disseminate research findings; and supports training for substance abuse practitioners.

★ 19216 ★ **U.S. Department of Health and Human Services**
**Substance Abuse and Mental Health Services Administration**
**Center for Substance Abuse Treatment**
5600 Fishers Lane
Rockville, MD 20857
**Phone:** (301)443-8956
**Website:** http://www.samhsa.gov/centers/csat2002/csat_frame.html
H. Westley Clarke, MD, Director
**Desc:** The principal function of the Center is to provide national leadership for the federal effort to enhance approaches and provide resources to ensure provision of services and programs focusing on the treatment of substance abuse and the co-occurring physical and/or psychiatric conditions.

# Foundations & Other Funding Organizations

## Private Foundations

★ 19217 ★ **Arca Foundation**
1308 19th St., NW
Washington, DC 20036
**Phone:** (202)822-9193      **Fax:** (202)785-1446
**Email:** arca@crosslink.net
**Website:** http://www.arcafoundation.org
Donna Edwards, Executive Director
**Fnded:** 1952. **Philosophy:** "The purpose of the foundation is to support not-for-profit organizations in the United States whose work encourages a more open foreign policy, based on respect for international law, human rights and the sovereignty of all nations. The foundation also supports projects concerned with domestic social change. In 1999, the Arca Foundation continued its focus on U.S. policy toward Cuba, building on a decade of experience in supporting citizen participation in policy debates and peaceful change in the hemisphere. Our grantmaking has emphasized issues and countries where a shift in U.S. policy or public opinion can make a significant, if not decisive difference. Arca's grantmaking in 1999 continued to emphasize the urgent need for campaign finance reform supporting educational efforts at the state and national level. Other domestic grants reflected the board's concern with the dramatic deterioration of conditions for working people in this country, and the need to build strong coalitions to level the playing field for everyone." 1999 Annual Report **Priorities:** *Civic & Public Affairs:* 19%. For issues concerning U.S. domestic policy, musgrove seminars, and campaign reform. *Environment:* 36%. Funds domestic social change. *Note:* Total contributions made in 1999. **Typ. Recipients:** Health Policy/Cost Containment, Substance Abuse. **Geo. Dist:** national.

★ 19218 ★ **Atlantic Foundation**
14 Fairgrounds Rd., Ste. A
Hamilton, NJ 08619
**Phone:** (609)689-1040      **Fax:** (609)689-1059
J. Seward Johnson, Jr., Chairman
**Fnded:** 1964. **Philosophy:** The Atlantic Foundation primarily funds organizations affiliated with science, specifically oceanography and marine science. The foundation's major recipient is the Harbor Branch Oceanographic Institute. Technical educational institutes also are funded on occasion. **Priorities:** *Arts & Humanities:* About 1%. Funds a film festival. *Education:* 23%. Supports educational facilities, and fellowship programs. *Religion:* 72%. Emphasis on the Harbor Branch Oceanographic Institution. *Note:* Total contributions made in 1998. **Typ. Recipients:** Substance Abuse. **Geo. Dist:** eastern United States.

**Christ is Our Salvation Foundation (CIOS)**
*See:* Entry 11374

**Corbett Foundation**
*See:* Entry 17782

**Courtney S. Turner Charitable Trust**
*See:* Entry 147

★ 19219 ★ **Edward E. Ford Foundation**
1912 Sunderland Pl. NW
Washington, DC 20036-1608
**Phone:** (202)955-1028      **Fax:** (202)955-8097
**Email:** office@eeford.org
**Website:** http://www.eeford.org
Walter Burgin, Executive Director
**Fnded:** 1957. **Philosophy:** Although the charter is broad in its scope, the "major objective of the Foundation is to encourage and improve secondary education as provided by independent private schools in the United States." The foundation believes that the most significant impact stems from a narrow focus. The foundation's interest in education stems from Mr. Ford's notion that students who graduate from such institutions go on to become productive, motivated contributors to our society, and that schools provide a choice in education for both students and their par-

ents. Since 1957, the board has given almost $52 million to a variety of issues affecting secondary private education without favoring any one type of school or project. In recent years, more funding has gone to co-educational schools and non-boarding institutions, and matching grants have been slightly more common than outright grants. Grants have been made for scholarships, professional development for teachers, summer workshops, buildings, curriculum, and computer education for faculty. Grants always are made to individual schools. Applicants must be members of the National Association of Independent Schools (NAIS). Presently, the board has an interest in supporting projects designed to benefit faculty in NAIS schools. The foundation also is interested in computer education and related technology for faculty. The foundation initiated a students grant program in 1993 for regional and state associations of NAIS. **Priorities:** *Education:* 100%. Supports faculty enrichment, capital and building projects, scholarships, and educational programs. *Note:* Total contributions made in fiscal 1999. **Typ. Recipients:** Substance Abuse. **Geo. Dist:** nationally, including United States territories.

**F. B. Heron Foundation**
*See:* Entry 5466

**Ford Family Foundation**
*See:* Entry 246

**Frances and Benjamin Benenson Foundation**
*See:* Entry 253

**Freed Foundation**
*See:* Entry 12272

**★ 19220 ★ J. Roderick MacArthur Foundation**
9333 North Milwaukee Ave.
Niles, IL 60714
**Phone:** (847)966-0143          **Fax:** (847)581-8730
**Website:** http://www.tfff.org
Marylou Bane, Administrator
**Fnded:** 1976. **Philosophy:** The foundation supports charitable organizations that protect human rights, civil liberties, social justice, and freedom of expression. **Priorities:** *Arts & Humanities:* 65%. Supports Harper's Magazine Foundation. *Civic & Public Affairs:* 8%. Supports public policy and initiatives to abolish the death penalty. *Education:* 2%. Funds media education and a school. *Environment:* 22%. Supports Vietnam Veterans of America Foundation. *International:* Less than 1%. *Note:* Total contributions made in 1999. **Typ. Recipients:** Home-Care Services, Substance Abuse. **Geo. Dist:** nationally.

**John G. and Marie Stella Kenedy Memorial Foundation**
*See:* Entry 418

**John P. McGovern Foundation**
*See:* Entry 423

**John Randolph and Dora Haynes Foundation**
*See:* Entry 426

**★ 19221 ★ Joseph Rowntree Charitable Trust**
The Garden House
Water End
York 403 6WQ, United Kingdom
**Email:** info@haynesfoundation.org
**Website:** http://www.jrct.org.uk
**Fnded:** 1996. **Priorities:** *Civic & Public Affairs:* 30%. Foundations, public policy, anti-poverty groups, and legal assistance receive support. *Education:* 15%.

Supports higher education. *Environment:* 30%. Child protection receives funding. *Note:* Total contributions made in 1999. **Typ. Recipients:** Substance Abuse.

**Lilly Endowment**
*See:* Entry 18213

**Louise Taft Semple Foundation**
*See:* Entry 7872

**Maclellan Foundation**
*See:* Entry 18214

**Whitehall Foundation**
*See:* Entry 756

## Corporate Foundations

**ABC Foundation**
*See:* Entry 795

**AFLAC Inc.**
*See:* Entry 802

**AGL Resources Inc.**
*See:* Entry 803

**Amerus Group Co.**
*See:* Entry 831

**Anheuser-Busch Foundation/Anheuser-Busch Charitable Trust**
*See:* Entry 839

**Appleton Papers Inc.**
*See:* Entry 843

**Bank of New York Co., Inc.**
*See:* Entry 868

**Bank One, Texas-Houston Office**
*See:* Entry 869

**Bechtel Foundation**
*See:* Entry 10059

**Boise Cascade Corp.**
*See:* Entry 8547

**Briggs & Stratton Corp. Foundation**
*See:* Entry 903

**★ 19222 ★ Brown & Williamson Tobacco Corp.**
Brown & Williamson Tower 200
401 S Fourth St.
PO Box 35090
Louisville, KY 40202
**Phone:** (502)568-7451          **Fax:** (502)568-8262
**Email:** lmlang@bechtel.com
**Website:** http://www.bw.com
Gail Strange, Sr. Mgr., Corp. and Community Relations
**Typ. Recipients:** Substance Abuse. **Geo. Dist:** headquarters and operating communities.

**Commonwealth Edison Co.**
*See:* Entry 960

**CSR America Companies Foundation**
*See:* Entry 10063

**Edison Family Foundation**
*See:* Entry 17871

**Fabri-Kal Foundation**
*See:* Entry 1037

**General Mills Foundation**
*See:* Entry 1081

**Guardian Life Insurance Co. of America**
*See:* Entry 1103

**★ 19223 ★ GuideOne Foundation**
1111 Ashworth Rd.
West Des Moines, IA 50265
**Phone:** (515)225-5156          **Fax:** (515)267-5588
**Email:** karen_olvany@glic.com
**Website:** http://www.glic.com
Mark McDougal, Foundation Coordinator
**Typ. Recipients:** Substance Abuse. **Geo. Dist:** nationally.

**Halliburton Foundation, Inc.**
*See:* Entry 1109

**Hershey Foods Corp.**
*See:* Entry 11437

**Household International Inc.**
*See:* Entry 1132

**International Multifoods Charitable Foundation**
*See:* Entry 7881

**Kirkland & Ellis Foundation**
*See:* Entry 1188

**Louisiana Land & Exploration Co. Foundation**
*See:* Entry 1211

**Mallinckrodt Inc.**
*See:* Entry 11449

**MGIC Investment Corp.**
*See:* Entry 1240

**Monroe Auto Equipment Co. Foundation**
*See:* Entry 10066

**National Fuel Gas Co.**
*See:* Entry 11454

**National Life Group**
*See:* Entry 1257

**★ 19224 ★ New York Times Co. Foundation**
229 W 43rd St.
New York, NY 10036-3959
**Phone:** (212)556-1091          **Fax:** (212)556-4450
**Email:** john_ludwick@mgic.com
**Website:** http://www.nationallife.com
Jack Rosenthal, President
**Priorities:** *Arts & Humanities:* 32%. Majority supports the performing arts, particularly the Metropolitan Museum of Art and Lincoln Center and its constituent

institutions. Other interests include museums, libraries, public broadcasting, and literary arts. *Civic & Public Affairs:* 13%. Supports urban and economic development, community clubs, food distribution, youth services, foreign and domestic policy, a police foundation, civil rights, minority and women's affairs, and services for the elderly. *Education:* 40%. Particular interest in minority education, arts and journalism programs, scholarships, and precollege education. Supports colleges and universities near operating locations, particularly New York. *Note:* Total contributions made in 2000. **Typ. Recipients:** Substance Abuse. **Geo. Dist:** communities served by company affiliates; some internationally; some nationally; New York, NY, metropolitan area.

**OMC Foundation**
*See:* Entry 11458

**Oshkosh Truck Foundation**
*See:* Entry 10067

**Public Service Electric & Gas Foundation**
*See:* Entry 8553

**Salomon Smith Barney**
*See:* Entry 18224

**Scripps Howard Foundation**
*See:* Entry 8555

**Solo Cup Foundation**
*See:* Entry 1397

**Southern New England Telephone Co.**
*See:* Entry 11463

**Springs Industries, Inc.**
*See:* Entry 1402

**Star Tribune Foundation**
*See:* Entry 5475

**Sunoco Inc.**
*See:* Entry 11465

**SunTrust Banks Foundation**
*See:* Entry 1420

**SuperValu Foundation**
*See:* Entry 7885

**The Timken Co. Charitable Trust**
*See:* Entry 1438

**Toro Foundation**
*See:* Entry 10070

**Toyota U.S.A. Foundation**
*See:* Entry 1444

**UST Inc.**
*See:* Entry 1471

**Xerox Foundation**
*See:* Entry 5476

## Other Funding Organizations

**★ 19225 ★ American Academy of Addiction Psychiatry (AAAP)**
7301 Mission Rd., Ste. 252
Prairie Village, KS 66208
**Phone:** (913)262-6161 **Fax:** (913)262-4311
**Email:** info@aaap.org
**Website:** http://www.aaap.org
Jeanne G. Trumble, Exec. Dir.
**Desc:** Psychiatrists and other health care and mental health professionals treating people with addictive behaviors. Promotes accessibility to highest quality treatment for all who need it; promotes excellence in clinical practice in addiction psychiatry; educates the public to influence public policy regarding addictive illness; provides continuing education for addiction professionals; disseminates new information in the field of addiction psychiatry; and encourages research on the etiology, prevention, identification, and treatment of the addictions. **Awards:** Founders Award (annual); Medical Student Award (annual); monetary (annual); Resident Award (annual).

**International Nurses Society on Addictions (NNSA)**
*See:* Entry 14924

**★ 19226 ★ Jewish Alcoholics, Chemically Dependent Persons and Significant Others (JACS)**
850 Seventh Ave.
New York, NY 10019
**Phone:** (212)397-4197 **Fax:** (212)399-3525
**Email:** jacs@jacsweb.org
**Website:** http://www.jacsweb.org
Maxine Uttal, Dir.
**Desc:** Jewish alcoholics and addicts, family members, and concerned friends. Acts as an additional resource to promote and enhance recovery from chemical dependency. Provides research and information on chemical addiction in the Jewish community. Maintains speakers' bureau. **Awards:** Retreat Scholarships (semiannual) for recovering alcoholics, addicts, family members in financial need.

**★ 19227 ★ National Alliance of Methadone Advocates (NAMA)**
435 2nd Ave.
New York, NY 10010
**Phone:** (212)595-6262 **Fax:** (212)595-6262
**Email:** nama4u@mail-x-change.com
**Website:** http://www.methadone.org/
Joycelyn Woods, Pres.
**Desc:** Methadone maintenance patients and supporters of methadone maintenance treatment. Promotes quality methadone maintenance treatment as the most effective modality for the treatment of heroin addiction. **Awards:** National Methadone Conference (periodic) to patient or family member interested in methadone advocacy.

## National & International Organizations

**★ 19228 ★ Addiction Research and Treatment Corp. (ARTC)**
22 Chapel St.
Brooklyn, NY 11201
**Phone:** (718)260-2900 **Fax:** (718)260-8276
**Email:** rsage@artcny.org
**Website:** http://www.Artcny.org
Dr. Beny J. Primm, Pres.
**Fnded:** 1969. **Mem:** 250. **Desc:** Operates a multimodality drug treatment program with nine ambulatory treatment clinics and a Vocational Evaluation Center. Funded by the state of New York Substance Abuse Services and Medicaid reimbursements. Treatments

employed are primarily detoxification, methadone maintenance, and drug-free services. Other services include: individual counseling, group therapy, job development, vocational counseling, mental health care, and recreation. Participates in national research programs. Sponsors substance abuse and AIDS research projects. Maintains speakers' bureau. Publishes abstracts.

**★ 19229 ★ Al Anon/Alateen/Alcoholics Anonymous**
Box 1672
Yellowknife, NT, Canada X1A 2N1
**Phone:** (867)873-5096
**Lang(s):** English, French. **Desc:** Alcoholics and their families. Promotes abstinence from liquor. Assists individuals wishing to abstain from drinking using a twelve-step program facilitated by participation in support groups; provides assistance to families of alcoholics. **Pub:** Report, periodic.

**★ 19230 ★ Al-Anon - Children of Alcoholics**
Box 9
Yellowknife, NT, Canada X1A 2N1
**Phone:** (867)873-5096
**Lang(s):** English, French. **Desc:** Children of alcoholics. Seeks to improve the quality of life of members; encourages abstinence from drinking for alcoholic parents. Provides support and services to children of alcoholics.

**★ 19231 ★ Al-Anon Family Group Headquarters, World Service Office (AFG)**
1600 Corporate Landing Pkwy.
Virginia Beach, VA 23454-5617
**Phone:** (757)563-1600 **Free:** 888-4AL-ANON
**Fax:** (757)563-1655
**Email:** wso@al-anon.org
**Website:** http://www.al-anon.alateen.org
**Fnded:** 1951. **Reg. Groups:** 30000. **Desc:** Relatives and friends of individuals with an alcohol problem. Operates Alateen for members 12-20 years of age whose lives have been adversely affected by someone else's drinking problem, usually a parent's. **Pub:** *Al-Anon Family Group Headquarters–The Forum: A Meeting in My Pocket*, monthly. Magazine. Written by Al-Anon members. Includes calendar of events. *Price:* $10/year. ● *Al-Anon Speaks Out*, semiannual. For the professional community regarding alcohol abuse. *Price:* Free. ● *Alateen Talk*, bimonthly. Newsletter. Contains written and artistic contributions from Alateen members. Includes articles written by adult Alateen sponsors and coordinators. *Price:* Included in Alateen Group Registration; $2.50/year for individuals; $.15/copy. ● *Inside Al-Anon: World Service Office Highlights*, bimonthly. Newsletter. Presents news, policy, and commentary from Al-Anon volunteers, staff, and readers sharing experiences of individual and group growth. ● *Loner's Letter Box*, bimonthly. Newsletter. *Price:* available to members only. ● Also publishes leaflets, pamphlets, and books.

**★ 19232 ★ Al-Anon Family Groups - United Kingdom and Eire**
61 Great Dover St.
London SE1 4YF, United Kingdom
**Phone:** 44 207 4030888 **Fax:** 44 207 3789910
**Email:** alanonuk@aol.com
**Website:** http://www.hexnet.co.uk/alanon/
**Fnded:** 1951. **Nat'l Groups:** 900. **Lang(s):** English, Irish. **Desc:** Family and friends of problem drinkers. Offers support and hope for members, whether the alcoholic is still drinking or not. Offers Alateen programs for young people aged 12-20 who have been affected by someone else's drinking, usually that of a parent. **Pub:** *Al-Anon - A Community Resource*. Brochure. ● *Facts About Al-Anon and Alateen*. Brochure.

**★ 19233 ★ Alateen**
426 Major MacKenzie Dr. E, Unit 1A
Richmond Hill, ON, Canada L4C 1J2
**Phone:** (905)770-1060

**Lang(s):** English, French. **Desc:** Alcoholic teens. Promotes abstinence from alcohol among members. Facilitates recovery among members using a 12step program utilizing support groups. **Pub:** *SDSA News*, quarterly. Newsletter. • *You See Down's Syndrome. We See Potential.* Brochure.

**★ 19234 ★ Alateen**
1600 Corporate Landing Pkwy.
Virginia Beach, VA 23454-5617
**Phone:** (757)563-1600          **Free:** 888-425-2666
**Fax:** (757)563-1655
**Email:** wso@al-anon.org
**Website:** http://www.alateen.org
Ric Buchanan, Exec. Dir.

**Fnded:** 1957. **Nat'l Groups:** 3000. **Local Groups:** 1826. **Desc:** Individuals ages 12-19 who have been adversely affected by a relative or friend with an alcohol problem. **Pub:** *Alateen Talk*, quarterly. Newsletter.

**★ 19235 ★ Alcohol and Drug Concerns (ADC)**
112-4500 Sheppard Ave. E
Toronto, ON, Canada M1S 3R6
**Phone:** (416)293-3400          **Fax:** (416)293-1142
**Email:** info@concerns.ca
**Website:** http://www.concerns.ca

**Fnded:** 1876. **Mem:** 1,200. **Reg. Groups:** 1. **Lang(s):** English, French. **Desc:** Individuals and organizations. Seeks to eliminate the harm associated with substance abuse among youth. Serves as a clearinghouse on substance abuse and related social problems; makes available support and services to teens, their families, and schools. **Pub:** *Concerns*, quarterly. Newsletter. Contains information for those interested in helping youth learn responsible drug use.

**★ 19236 ★ Alcohol and Drug Free Traffic - International (ADFTI)**
Gammelgardsvagen 38
S-112 64 Stockholm, Sweden
**Phone:** 46 8 6726165          **Fax:** 46 8 6726167
**Email:** landsradet@sobernet.org

**Lang(s):** English, Swedish. **Desc:** Individuals and organizations. Seeks to eliminate driving while under the influence of alcohol or other substances. Lobbies for heavier penalties for individuals convicted of driving under the influence; conducts educational programs to raise public awareness of the dangers of drinking and driving.

**★ 19237 ★ Alcohol and Drug Problems Association of North America (ADPA)**
307 N Main
Saint Charles, MO 63301
**Phone:** (314)589-6702          **Fax:** (314)940-2358
**Email:** blefilm@juno.com
**Website:** http://www.adpana.com
Barbara Eisenstadt, EdD, Contact

**Fnded:** 1949. **Mem:** 1,325. **Desc:** Individuals (1100), official state or provincial alcoholism program members (75), and other alcoholism and/or drug agencies and institutions (150). Seeks to facilitate governmental and professional activities in the fields of alcoholism, alcohol-related problems, and drug abuse by exchange of information, promotion of legislation and standards which will contribute to the care and control of alcoholism, and research and cooperation. Maintains continuing education program and placement service. **Pub:** *ADPA Professional*, bimonthly. Newsletter. On public policy concerning drug and alcohol abuse. Includes book reviews; calendar of events; educational opportunities. *Price:* Included in membership dues. • *Special Reports*, periodic. **Frmly:** (1956) National States Conference on Alcoholism; (1972) North American Association of Alcoholism Programs.

**★ 19238 ★ Alcohol and Other Drugs Council of Australia (ADCA)**
PO Box 269
Woden, ACT 2606, Australia
**Phone:** 61 2 62810686          **Fax:** 61 2 62810995
**Email:** adca@adca.org.au
**Website:** http://www.adca.org.au

**Fnded:** 1967. **Mem:** 400. **Desc:** Develops and promotes national policies and advises on all issues concerning alcohol and other drugs. Conducts research. Runs media campaigns on alcohol and drug use. **Pub:** *ADCA Annual Report*, annual. • *ADCA Update*, monthly. Newsletter. • *AIM.* • *Drug Contents.*

**★ 19239 ★ Alcohol Research Information Service (ARIS)**
430 Lathrop St.
Lansing, MI 48912
**Phone:** (517)485-9900          **Fax:** (517)485-1928
**Email:** alcoholisadrugtoo@voyager.net
Robert Hammond, Exec. Dir.

**Fnded:** 1931. **Desc:** Individual and corporate contributors. Collects, correlates, and disseminates information regarding alcohol and alcoholic products, their manufacture, sale, and use for beverage, industrial, or other purposes, and their relation to the health and well-being of the people of the United States. Operates clearinghouse for information on alcohol, drugs, and compulsive and problem gambling. Compiles statistics. **Pub:** *Monday Morning Report*, bimonthly. Newsletter. Contains six pages. *Price:* $100 first class mail. • Newsletter, semimonthly. *Price:* $60/year. Also provides teaching materials for elementary and secondary school levels, and adults. **Frmly:** (1984) American Business Men's Research Foundation.

**★ 19240 ★ Alcoholics Anonymous Australia**
National Office
48 Firth St.
Arncliffe, NSW 2205, Australia
**Phone:** 61 2 95998866          **Fax:** 61 2 95998844
**Email:** national.office@aa.org.au
**Website:** http://www.alcoholicsanonymous.org.au

**Lang(s):** English. **Desc:** Individuals recovering from alcoholism in Australia. Members believe that they can free themselves from alcohol abuse by following a 12-step program that includes sharing of experiences, strength, and hope with fellow members. Refuses alliance with any sect, denomination, political organization, or institution and does not endorse or oppose any cause.

**★ 19241 ★ Alcoholics Anonymous - Brazil (Junaab-Junta de Servicos Gerais de A.A. do Brasil)**
Av. Senador Queiros 101, 2 cj 205
01026-001 Sao Paulo, SP, Brazil
**Phone:** 55 11 2293611          **Fax:** 55 11 2293611
**Email:** aa@alcoolicosanonimos.org.br
**Website:** http://www.alcoolicosanonimos.org.br

**Fnded:** 1947. **Mem:** 120,000. **Nat'l Groups:** 5300. **Reg. Groups:** 130. **State Groups:** 420. **Lang(s):** Dutch, English, Portuguese. **Desc:** Individuals recovering from alcoholism in Brazil. Members believe that they can free themselves from alcohol by following a 12-step program that includes sharing of experiences, strength, and hope with fellow members. Refuses alliance with any sect, denomination, political organization, or institution and does not endorse or oppose any cause. **Pub:** *Bob Mural*, bimonthly. Newsletter. • *Revista Vivencia*, bimonthly. Magazine. • Books. • Pamphlets.

**★ 19242 ★ Alcoholics Anonymous - England**
PO Box 1
Stonebow House
Stonebow
York YO1 7NJ, United Kingdom

**Phone:** 44 1904 644026          **Fax:** 44 1904 629091
**Website:** http://www.alcoholics-anonymous.org.uk

**Lang(s):** English. **Desc:** Individuals recovering from alcoholism in the United Kingdom and the Republic of Ireland. Members believe that they can free themselves from alcohol abuse by following a 12step program that includes sharing of experiences, strength, and hope with fellow members. Refuses alliance with any sect, denomination, political organization, or institution and does not endorse or oppose any cause. **Frmly:** Alcoholics Anonymous World Services - United Kingdom and Eire General Services Office.

**★ 19243 ★ Alcoholics Anonymous - French General Services Office**
21, rue Trousseau
F-75011 Paris, France
**Phone:** 33 1 48064368          **Fax:** 33 1 40210535
**Email:** aaf2@club_internet.fr
**Website:** http://perso.club-internet.fr/aafr/

**Fnded:** 1960. **Mem:** 11,000. **Reg. Groups:** 23. **Local Groups:** 560. **Lang(s):** French. **Desc:** Individuals recovering from alcoholism in France. Members believe that they can free themselves from alcohol abuse by following a 12-step program that includes sharing of experiences, strength, and hope with fellow members. Refuses alliance with any sect, denomination, political organization, or institution and does not endorse or oppose any cause. **Frmly:** (1997) Alcoholics Anonymous World Services - French General Services Office; (1997) Services Generaux Al-Anon.

**★ 19244 ★ Alcoholics Anonymous World Services (AA)**
Box 459
Grand Central Sta.
475 Riverside Dr., 11th Fl.
New York, NY 10163
**Phone:** (212)870-3400          **Fax:** (212)870-3003
**Website:** http://www.aa.org
Greg Muth, Gen. Service Mgr.

**Fnded:** 1935. **Desc:** Individuals recovering from alcoholism. AA maintains that members can solve their common problem and help others achieve sobriety through a twelve step program that includes sharing their experience, strength, and hope with each other. Self-supported through members' contributions, AA is not allied with any sect, denomination, political organization, or institution and does not endorse nor oppose any cause. **Pub:** *AA Comes of Age.* • *Alcoholics Anonymous.* • *As Bill Sees It.* • *Dr. Bob and the Good Oldtimers.* • *Pass it On.* • *Twelve Steps and Twelve Traditions.*

**★ 19245 ★ Alcoholics Anonymous World Services - General Service Board for French-Speaking Belgium**
rue du Boulet, 11
B-1000 Brussels, Belgium
**Phone:** 32 2 5114030          **Fax:** 32 1 1844658
**Email:** aa.bsg@skynet.be
**Website:** http://www.alcooliquesanonymes.be

**Fnded:** 1953. **Nat'l Groups:** 230. **Reg. Groups:** 8. **Lang(s):** French. **Desc:** French-speaking individuals recovering from alcoholism in Belgium. Members believe that they can free themselves from alcohol abuse by following a 12-step program that includes sharing of experiences, strength, and hope with fellow members. Refuses alliance with any sect, denomination, political organization, or institution and does not endorse or oppose any cause.

**★ 19246 ★ Alcoholics Anonymous World Services - New Zealand General Services Office**
PO Box 6458, level 2, Unit 4
The Harbour City Centre
Panana, New Zealand
**Phone:** 64 9 47924250

**Lang(s):** English. **Desc:** Individuals recovering from alcoholism in New Zealand. Members believe that they can free themselves from alcohol abuse by following a 12-step program that includes sharing of experiences, strength, and hope with fellow members. Refuses alliance with any sect, denomination, political organization, or institution and does not endorse or oppose any cause.

★ **19247** ★ **Alcoholics Anonymous World Services - Swedish General Services Office**
**(Al-Anon Familjegrupper i Sverige)**
Erstagatan 1
S-116 28 Stockholm, Sweden
**Phone:** 46 8 6431393  **Fax:** 46 8 6431393
**Email:** afg@al-anon.a.se
**Website:** http://www.al-anon.a.se

**Lang(s):** Swedish. **Desc:** Individuals recovering from alcoholism in Sweden. Members believe that they can free themselves from alcohol abuse by following a 12-step program that includes sharing of experiences, strength, and hope with fellow members. Refuses alliance with any sect, denomination, political organization, or institution and does not endorse or oppose any cause.

★ **19248** ★ **American Academy of Addiction Psychiatry (AAAP)**
7301 Mission Rd., Ste. 252
Prairie Village, KS 66208
**Phone:** (913)262-6161  **Fax:** (913)262-4311
**Email:** info@aaap.org
**Website:** http://www.aaap.org
Jeanne G. Trumble, Exec. Dir.

**Fnded:** 1985. **Mem:** 1,000. **Reg. Groups:** 9. **Desc:** Psychiatrists and other health care and mental health professionals treating people with addictive behaviors. Promotes accessibility to highest quality treatment for all who need it; promotes excellence in clinical practice in addiction psychiatry; educates the public to influence public policy regarding addictive illness; provides continuing education for addiction professionals; disseminates new information in the field of addiction psychiatry; and encourages research on the etiology, prevention, identification, and treatment of the addictions. **Pub:** *AAAP News*, quarterly. Journal. • *American Journal on Addictions*, quarterly. Journal.

**American Academy of Health Care Providers**
*See:* Entry 12333

★ **19249** ★ **American Academy of Health Care Providers (AACHP)**
875 Massachusetts Ave., Fl. 7
Cambridge, MA 02139-3015
**Phone:** (617)661-6248  **Fax:** (617)492-3183
**Email:** info@americanacademy.org
**Website:** http://www.americanacademy.org

**Fnded:** 1989. **Desc:** Health care professionals, mental health care providers, and social workers treating individuals with addictive disorders. Promotes excellence in the care of people with addictions. Develops and enforces standards of ethics and practice for addiction medicine; facilitates exchange of information among members; holds examination and confers certification to qualified addiction care providers.

**American College of Addiction Treatment Administrators (ACATA)**
*See:* Entry 9691

★ **19250** ★ **American Council on Alcohol Problems (ACAP)**
2376 Lakeside Dr.
Birmingham, AL 35244
**Phone:** (205)989-8177  **Fax:** (205)985-9015
**Email:** dliacap@aol.com

**Website:** http://americancouncilonalcoholproblems.com
Dr. D.L. Ireland, Contact

**Fnded:** 1895. **Desc:** Federation of 36 state affiliates and 22 denominational judicatories; 1000 associate members. Seeks long-range solutions to the problems posed by alcohol. Employs educational, and legislative approaches for the prevention of alcoholism and other alcohol-related problems. Coordinates the work of state affiliates who carry on their programs under provisions of the 21st Amendment, putting alcohol control largely at state level. Denominations channel their cooperative social concerns through elected directors who guide the program and activities of ACAP. **Pub:** *The American Issue*, quarterly. • Directory, annual. **Frmly:** (1948) Anti-Saloon League of America; (1950) Temperance League of America; (1964) National Temperance League.

★ **19251** ★ **American Council on Alcoholism (ACA)**
3900 N Fairfax Dr., Ste. 401
Arlington, VA 22203
**Phone:** (703)248-9005  **Free:** 800-527-5344
**Fax:** (703)248-9007
**Email:** aca2@earthlink.net
**Website:** http://www.aca-usa.org
Chuck Pena, Exec. Dir.

**Fnded:** 1953. **Mem:** 400. **Desc:** Works to educate the public about the effects of alcohol, alcoholism, alcohol abuse, and the need for prompt, effective, affordable, and available treatment. Provides a toll-free Helpline for alcoholism treatment and recovery referral and assistance. **Pub:** *Frequently Asked Questions About Alcoholism*. • *Recovery*, quarterly. Newsletter. Publicizes issues concerning alcoholism; promotes the understanding that alcoholism is a treatable disease; contains research results. *Price:* Included in membership dues. • *Teenage Drinking*. **Frmly:** Maryland Society on Alcoholism; (1974) Baltimore Area Council on Alcoholism.

★ **19252** ★ **American Council for Drug Education (ACDE)**
164 W 74th St.
New York, NY 10023
**Free:** 800-488-DRUG  **Fax:** (212)595-2553
**Email:** acde@phoenixhouse.org
**Website:** http://www.acde.org
Robert Balster, PhD, Advisor

**Fnded:** 1977. **Desc:** Doctors, mental health counselors, teachers, clergymen, policymakers, school librarians, parent groups, industry leaders, and concerned individuals. Disseminates information and research on all drugs of abuse. Makes available resource information kits that include both written and audiovisual materials. Provides prevention materials such as "How to Speak to Your Kids about Marijuana." **Pub:** *Free Catalog.* For parents, children, schools, and other professionals. • Brochures. • Handbooks. **Frmly:** (1983) American Council on Marijuana and Other Psychoactive Drugs.

★ **19253** ★ **American Osteopathic Academy of Addiction Medicine**
142 E Ontario St.
Chicago, IL 60611
**Phone:** (312)202-8163  **Fax:** (312)202-8483
**Email:** nvidmer@aoa-net.org
Nina Vidmer, Exec. Dir.

**Fnded:** 1986. **Mem:** 100. **Desc:** Physicians. Conducts research into the diagnosis, intervention, and treatment of substance abuse problems. Seeks to educate society, and to influence the passage of legislation regarding drug abuse. Provides seminars and lectures to students, physicians, medical and dental societies, civic groups, religious organizations, bar associations, and law enforcement bodies. **Pub:** *AOAAM News and Advocate*, quarterly. Newsletter. **Frmly:** (1996) American Osteopathic Academy Addictionology.

★ **19254** ★ **American Outreach Association (AOA)**
PO Box 25042
Colorado Springs, CO 80936
**Phone:** (719)592-1134  **Fax:** (719)592-1134
**Email:** aoa_cs@hotmail.com
**Website:** http://www.americanoutreach.org
Charles Prusch, Dir.

**Fnded:** 1989. **Reg. Groups:** 5. **Desc:** Collects and disseminates information on subjects such as alcoholism, drug abuse, inhalants, and smoking to the public. Organizes community awareness activities and presentations. Reviews drug policies, programs, and educational material. Assists business and industry in establishing drug-free work environments. Sponsors Project HOLD, a program that fosters a change of attitudes, values, and behaviors in the home away from drug abuse. Operates placement service; maintains speakers' bureau. **Pub:** *Health Watch*, quarterly. Newsletter. • *Mommy, What are Drugs?*. • *Mommy What are Inhalants?*. • *Mommy, What is Alcohol?*. • *Mommy, What is Smoking?*. • *Mother Earth, What is Cultural Diversity?*.

★ **19255** ★ **American Society of Addiction Medicine (ASAM)**
4601 N Park Ave., Arcade Ste. 101
Chevy Chase, MD 20815
**Phone:** (301)656-3920  **Fax:** (301)656-3815
**Email:** email@asam.org
**Website:** http://www.asam.org
Dr. James F. Callahan, Exec. VP/CEO

**Fnded:** 1954. **Mem:** 3,000. **State Groups:** 28. **Desc:** Physicians with special interest and experience in the field of alcoholism and other drug dependencies and who wish to share this experience with other professionals in order to extend their knowledge of addictive diseases; promote dissemination of that knowledge; enlighten the public regarding these problems; advance education and research in the field of addiction. Holds annual Ruth Fox Course for Physicians, annual Medical-Scientific Conference and five other conferences/courses. **Pub:** *ASAM News*, bimonthly. Newsletter. *Price:* $25. • *ASAM Patient Placement Criteria for the Treatment of Substance-Related Disorders*. • *Guidelines for Facilities Treating Chemically Dependent Patients at Risk for AIDS*. • *Journal of Addictive Diseases*, quarterly. Journal. • *Principles of Addiction Medicine*. *Price:* $155. **Frmly:** (1967) New York City Medical Society on Alcoholism; (1989) American Medical Society on Alcoholism and Other Drug Dependencies.

★ **19256** ★ **Association of Halfway House Alcoholism Programs of North America (AHHAP)**
5 Ridgeview Rd.
Box 610
Kerhonkson, NY 12446-9603
**Phone:** (845)626-2684  **Fax:** (845)626-2685
**Email:** ahhap@aol.com
**Website:** http://www.ahhap.org
John Curtiss, Pres.

**Fnded:** 1965. **Mem:** 450. **Reg. Groups:** 13. **State Groups:** 50. **Desc:** Halfway house corporations, staff, board members, and individuals closely related to the halfway house movement. Charitable organization dedicated to educating and serving halfway house programs through technical assistance, consultant services, workshops, conferences, and related services. Operates placement service. Disseminates information and materials. **Pub:** *AHHAP Membership Directory*, annual. Membership Directory. • *Communications and Services Newsletter*, quarterly. Newsletter. • *Conference Proceedings*, annual. Proceedings.

★ **19257** ★ **Association of Medical Education and Research in Substance Abuse (AMERSA)**
125 Whipple, 3rd Fl., Ste. 300
Providence, RI 02908
**Phone:** (401)349-0000  **Fax:** 877-418-8769
**Email:** isabel@amersa.org

**Website:** http://www.amersa.org
Isbell Vieira, MD, Exec. Dir.

**Fnded:** 1976. **Mem:** 300. **Desc:** Multidisciplinary organization of health care professionals dedicated to improving education in the care of individuals with substance abuse problems. **Pub:** *Substance Abuse*, quarterly. Journal. *Price:* Included in membership dues; $40/year for nonmembers. • Membership Directory, biennial.

★ 19258 ★ **Association of Recovering Motorcyclists (ARM)**
1503 Market St.
La Crosse, WI 54601
**Phone:** (608)784-8462　　　　**Fax:** (608)784-9085
**Email:** armintl86@aol.com
**Website:** http://arm-intl.com
Jerry Scudder, Pres.

**Fnded:** 1985. **Mem:** 500. **State Groups:** 44. **Desc:** Support group for motorcyclists who are recovering from alcohol or drug addiction. Helps members enjoy the hobby of motorcycling; tries to eliminate the notion of motorcycling as a negative lifestyle. Sponsors motorcycle runs, picnics, and dances. Operates speakers' bureau. **Pub:** *ARM Newsletter*, quarterly. Newsletter. *Price:* Free to inmates; Included in membership dues. • Directory, periodic.

★ 19259 ★ **Australian Drug Foundation (ADF)**
409 King St.
West Melbourne, VIC 3003, Australia
**Phone:** 61 3 92788100　　　　**Fax:** 61 3 93283008
**Email:** adf@adf.org.au
**Website:** http://www.adf.org.au

**Fnded:** 1959. **Lang(s):** English. **Desc:** Educators, journalists, librarians, health workers, and researchers. Seeks to prevent and reduce alcohol and other drug problems in the Australian community through the provision of quality information and practical assistance in a professional manner. Assists in the development of school and community programs; conducts research and training; and sponsors art and sporting events as part of outreach efforts.

★ 19260 ★ **BACCHUS and Gamma Peer Education Network**
National Headquarters
PO Box 100430
Denver, CO 80250
**Phone:** (303)871-0901　　　　**Fax:** (303)871-0907
**Email:** bacgram@aol.com
**Website:** http://www.bacchusgamma.org
Drew Hunter, Exec. Dir.

**Fnded:** 1975. **Mem:** 24,500. **Nat'l Groups:** 3. **Reg. Groups:** 13. **State Groups:** 49. **Local Groups:** 750. **Desc:** Students, advisors, faculty, and staff of colleges and universities in the U.S., Canada, and Mexico. Primary mission is to deliver alcohol abuse prevention and health education to college students and their communities. Promotes responsible decisions and healthy lifestyles and discourages irresponsible or illegal use of alcohol. Encourages year-round prevention and education programs and activities. Operates: Project GAMMA (Greeks Advocating Mature Management of Alcohol), a cooperative effort between BACCHUS and national greek-letter organizations to increase undergraduate participation in alsohol education programs; National Collegiate Alcohol Awareness Week; and Safe Spring Break. Offers the Certified Peer Educator Training Progam, a skill-based training curriculum for students. (Bacchus is the acronym for Boost Alcohol Consciousness Concerning the Health of University Students and the name of the Roman god of wine.) **Pub:** *The Bacchus Beat*, monthly. Newsletter. *Price:* Free for members. • *CPE Training Series*. • Catalog.Lists educational materials. • Newsletter, 10/year. • Pamphlets. • Videos. **Frmly:** (1993) BACCHUS of the U.S.

★ 19261 ★ **Calix Society (CS)**
2555 Hazelwood Ave.
Saint Paul, MN 55109-2030
**Phone:** (651)773-3117　　　　**Free:** 800-398-0524
Jim Billigmeier, Pres.

**Fnded:** 1947. **Mem:** 3,000. **State Groups:** 14. **Local Groups:** 22. **Desc:** Catholic alcoholics who are maintaining sobriety through their own participation in Alcoholics Anonymous. Non-Catholic alcoholics and interested individuals are welcome. Promotes total abstinence for Catholic alcoholics and encourages their spiritual development. ("Calix" means "chalice" in Latin and refers to the society's belief in "substituting the cup that sanctifies for the cup that stupefies.") **Pub:** *Calix and the Twelve Steps*. Book. *Price:* $7. • *The Chalice*, bimonthly. Newsletter. Contains contributed stories regarding spiritual and physical recovery. Includes book reviews, obituaries, research reports, and statistics. *Price:* $15/year. • *Directory of Calix Units in the U.S. and Canada*, periodic. Directory. • *The Light of Faith*. Book. *Price:* $7. • *What and Why*. Brochure.

★ 19262 ★ **Canadian Association for Children of Alcoholics (CACA) (Association Canadienne pour Enfants d'Alcooliques — ACEA)**
Hospital for Sick Children
555 University Ave.
Toronto, ON, Canada M5G 1X8
**Phone:** (416)813-1500
**Website:** http://www.sickkids.on.ca

**Lang(s):** English, French. **Desc:** Individuals providing services to alcoholics and their families; children of alcoholics. Promotes increased awareness of issues faced by children of alcoholics and other substance abusers. Encourages research; advocates for expansion of services available to children of substance abusers.

★ 19263 ★ **Canadian Centre on Substance Abuse (CCSA) (Centre Canadien de Lutte Contre l'Alcoolisme et les Toxicomanies — CCLCAT)**
75 Albert St., Ste. 300
Ottawa, ON, Canada K1P 5E7
**Phone:** (613)235-4048　　　　**Fax:** (613)235-8101
**Email:** info@ccsa.ca
**Website:** http://www.ccsa.ca

**Lang(s):** English, French. **Desc:** Individuals and organizations. Seeks to prevent substance abuse; promotes recovery among substance abusers. Seeks to raise awareness of substance abuse issues among policy makers and the public; makes available support and services to substance abusers and their families. **Pub:** *Action News*. Newsletter.

★ 19264 ★ **Canadian Women's Temperance Union (CWTU)**
Charles Prom Bldg., Ste. 203
730 Yonge St.
Toronto, ON, Canada M4T 2B7
**Phone:** (416)921-4909

**Lang(s):** English, French. **Desc:** Women opposed to alcohol abuse. Promotes abstinence from alcohol consumption. Provides support and assistance to alcohol abusers and their families; lobbies for stricter laws regulating the sale and consumption of alcohol.

★ 19265 ★ **Canadians for Safe and Sober Driving**
199 Advance Blvd., Unit 207
Brampton, ON, Canada L6T 4N2
**Phone:** (905)793-4233　　　　**Fax:** (905)793-7035
**Email:** add@attcanada.ca
**Website:** http://www.add.ca

**Fnded:** 1983. **Lang(s):** English, French. **Desc:** Seeks to promote public safety and eliminate deaths and injuries caused by impaired or drunk driving. Conducts educational programs to raise public awareness of the dangers of driving while intoxicated. **Frmly:** (2000) Against Drunk Driving.

★ 19266 ★ **Children of Alcoholics Foundation (COAF)**
164 W 74th St.
New York, NY 10023-2301
**Phone:** (212)595-5810　　　　**Fax:** (212)595-2553
**Email:** coaf@phoenixhouse.org
**Website:** http://www.coaf.org

**Fnded:** 1982. **Desc:** Seeks to educate the public and professionals about children of substance abusers and the effects of parental substance abuse, and stimulate interest in seeking solutions to their problems. Promotes research, educational and informational programs, and public discussion on alcoholism, substance abuse, and its effects on children; disseminates reports and research results; investigates the effectiveness of public policies, programs, and laws; encourages participation and assists government and community agencies in providing assistance to children of substance abusers and seeking solutions to the problems of these children. Facilitates research and educational and informational programs on other aspects of childhood, the parent-child relationship, physiological and psychological aspects of human development, child abuse and neglect, and substance abuse of other psychoactive substances. **Pub:** *Free Catalog*. Catalog.

★ 19267 ★ **Christian Addiction Rehabilitation Association (CARA)**
c/o Dr. Robert A. Emberger
Whosoever Gospel Mission and Rescue Home
101 E Chelten Ave
Philadelphia, PA 19144
**Phone:** (215)438-3094　　　　**Fax:** (215)438-4327
**Website:** http://www.iugm.org/cara.html
Dr. Robert Emberger, Contact

**Fnded:** 1967. **Mem:** 48. **Desc:** Provides support and serves as a clearinghouse of information for individuals involved in ministry to addicts. Conducts two conferences per year. **Pub:** Newsletter, monthly. *Price:* Free w/membership. **Frmly:** Christian Alcoholic Rehabilitation Association.

★ 19268 ★ **Co-Anon Family Groups**
PO Box 12722
Tucson, AZ 85732
**Free:** 800-898-9985
**Email:** info@co-anon.org
**Website:** http://www.co-anon.org/

**Fnded:** 1985. **Desc:** Spouses, relatives, and friends of people who are chemically dependent. Seeks to help individuals affected by another's cocaine addiction by applying the Twelve Steps and Twelve Traditions of Alcoholics Anonymous. Assists in the formation of Co-Anon groups. **Pub:** Brochure.

★ 19269 ★ **Cocaine Anonymous World Services (CAWS)**
3740 Overland Ave., Ste. C
Los Angeles, CA 90034
**Phone:** (310)559-5833　　　　**Free:** 800-347-8998
**Fax:** (310)559-2554
**Email:** cawso@ca.org
**Website:** http://www.ca.org
Mary Hukill, Dir. of Operations

**Fnded:** 1982. **Mem:** 15,000. **Reg. Groups:** 2000. **Desc:** Fellowship of men and women who share their experience, strength, and hope with each other that they may solve their common problem and help others to recover from addiction, remaining free from cocaine and all other mind-altering drugs. Applies the Alcoholics Anonymous World Services' 12-step approach to persons addicted to cocaine. **Pub:** *A Guide to the Twelve Steps*. Pamphlet. *Price:* $.15. • *A Higher Power*. Pamphlet. *Price:* $.15. • *And All Other Mind Altering Substances*. Pamphlet. *Price:* $.15. • *Choosing Your Sponsor*. Pamphlet. *Price:* $.15. • *Crack*. Pamphlet. *Price:* $.15. • *The First 30 Days*. Pamphlet. *Price:* $.15. • *Hope, Faith, and Courage*. Book. *Price:*

$12.95 hard cover; $9.95 soft cover. • *The Newsgram*, quarterly. Newsletter. *Price:* Free. • *Self Test for Cocaine Addiction.* Pamphlet. *Price:* $.15. • *Suggestions for Relapse Prevention and Recovery.* Pamphlet. *Price:* $.15. • *Tips on Staying Clean and Sober.* Pamphlet. *Price:* $.15. • *To the Newcomer.* Pamphlet. *Price:* $.15. • *Tools of Recovery.* Pamphlet. *Price:* $.15. • *What Is C.A.?.* Pamphlet. *Price:* $.15.

**★ 19270 ★ Community Anti-Drug Coalitions of America (CADCA)**
901 N Pitt St., Ste. 300
Alexandria, VA 22314
**Free:** 800-54-CADCA　　　**Fax:** (703)706-0565
**Email:** info@cadca.org
**Website:** http://www.cadca.org
**Fnded:** 1992. **Mem:** 5,000. **Desc:** Working to create and strengthen the capacity of new and existing coalitions to build safe, healthy and drug-free communities.

**★ 19271 ★ D.A.R.E. America**
PO Box 512090
Los Angeles, CA 90051-0090
**Website:** http://www.dare.com/
**Desc:** Seeks to provide students with a knowledge base on the effects of drug abuse that go beyond the physical ramifications and extend to emotional, social, and economic aspects of life. Aims to build decision-making and problem solving skills and strategies to help students make informed decisions and resist drug use, peer pressure, and violence. Provides students with alternatives to drug use. Sponsors National D.A.R.E. Day. **Pub:** *Keeping Kids Drug Free: The Official Parents Guide.* Book.

**★ 19272 ★ Do It Now Foundation (DINF)**
PO Box 27568
Tempe, AZ 85285
**Phone:** (480)736-0599　　　**Free:** 877-515-9411
**Fax:** (480)736-0771
**Email:** info@doitnow.org
**Website:** http://www.doitnow.org
James D. Parker, Exec. Dir.
**Fnded:** 1968. **Mem:** 40. **Desc:** Works to provide factual information to students and adults about prescription drugs, over-the-counter drugs, street drugs, alcohol, eating disorders, AIDS, and related health issues. Assists organizations engaged in alcohol and drug abuse education. Publishes educational materials; offers pamphlets, posters, books, and radio public service tapes.

**★ 19273 ★ Drug and Alcohol Testing Industry Association (DATIA)**
1600 Duke St., Ste. 220
Alexandria, VA 22314
**Free:** 800-355-1257　　　**Fax:** (703)519-1716
**Email:** datia@wpa.org
**Website:** http://www.datia.org
Dean Klassy, Chm.
**Fnded:** 1995. **Mem:** 1,000. **Desc:** Drug and alcohol service providers including collection sites, laboratories, consortiums/TPA's, MRO's and testing equipment manufacturers.

**★ 19274 ★ Drug Free Kids: America's Challenge**
PO Box 60865
Washington, DC 20039
**Phone:** (301)681-7861
**Email:** info@drugfreekids.org
**Website:** http://www.ourdrugfreekids.org
Joyce Nalepka, Pres.
**Desc:** Promote protection of children against drugs. Hold vigils and rallies.

**★ 19275 ★ DrugScope**
32-36 Loman St.
London SE1 0EE, United Kingdom

**Phone:** 44 20 79281211　　　**Fax:** 44 20 79281771
**Email:** services@drugscope.org.uk
**Website:** http://www.drugscope.org.uk
**Fnded:** 2000. **Mem:** 900. **Desc:** One of UK's leading centres of expertise on the misuse of drugs. Aims to inform policy development and reduce drug-related risk. Offers self-help information through website. **Pub:** Directories.

**★ 19276 ★ Dual Disorders Anonymous**
PO Box 681264
Schaumburg, IL 60168-1264
**Phone:** (847)490-9379
**Email:** pat63659@cs.com
**Website:** http://ourworld.cs.com/pat63659/myhome-page/business.html
Pat Kent, Pres.
**Fnded:** 1982. **Mem:** 500. **Nat'l Groups:** 20. **Reg. Groups:** 3. **State Groups:** 1. **Local Groups:** 21. **Desc:** Individuals with alcohol or drug addictions as well as mental or emotional disorders. Provides support group opportunities to emotionally or mentally disordered alcoholics and addicts; conducts volunteer programs for dually diagnosed patients. Utilizes the 12-step method of self-help. **Pub:** Booklet. • Brochures.

**★ 19277 ★ 800-COCAINE**
c/o Jack Routleoge
Phoenix House
164 W 74th St.
New York, NY 10023
**Phone:** (212)595-5810　　　**Free:** 800-262-2463
Jack Routleoge, Contact
**Desc:** Provides general information about substance abuse, treatment referrals, and in emergency situations, crisis intervention. **Pub:** Pamphlets.

**★ 19278 ★ Entertainment Industries Council (EIC)**
1760 Reston Pky., Ste. 415
Reston, VA 20190
**Phone:** (703)481-1414　　　**Fax:** (703)481-1418
**Email:** eiceast@eiconline.org
**Website:** http://eiconline.org
Brian L. Dyak, Pres.
**Fnded:** 1983. **Mem:** 130. **Desc:** Corporations and representatives of the entertainment industry including actors, agents, publicists, producers, directors, and writers. Goal is to utilize the power and influence of the entertainment industry in a national campaign to combat and deglamorize substance abuse, especially among young people. Seeks to identify and provide celebrity role models for young people. Hopes to increase youth awareness of drug abuse through television, radio, music, and motion pictures. Develops projects to aid in eliminating substance abuse problems within the entertainment industry. Conducts seminars and training sessions on drug abuse prevention; also conducts radio interview series, television specials, outreach programs, and employee assistance and fundraising programs. Collects and disseminates information on progress made by the entertainment industry in drug abuse prevention. In conjunction with IMMEDIA Foundation, coordinates network of 400 radio stations involved in public affairs projects designed to discourage substance abuse. Provides celebrity speakers' bureau on drug prevention, seat belt awareness, and intravenous drug use/AIDS. Bestows EIC Drug Prevention Award annually to a leader from entertainment industry contributing to drug awareness. **Pub:** *Profile*, monthly. • *Spotlight on Depiction*, annual. • Annual Report, quarterly.

**★ 19279 ★ Ethos Foundation (EF)**
5201 Leesburg Pike, Ste. 100
Falls Church, VA 22041
**Phone:** (703)671-5335　　　**Fax:** (703)671-5352
**Email:** ethosfndtn@aol.com
Megan L. Fraser, Admin.
**Fnded:** 1978. **Reg. Groups:** 1. **Desc:** Provides counseling, education, and rehabilitation services and crisis

intervention in the area of substance abuse. Aims to educate alcohol and drug abusers, their families, and the public on substance abuse. Conducts training programs for counselors, physicians, clergy, social workers, and employees; offers programs for hospitals, federal and local governments, and the private and public sectors. Cooperates with criminal justice departments. Conducts research. Sponsors workshops and seminars. Maintains speakers' bureau; compiles statistics. (Ethos is the Greek word for sentiment, values, and moral nature.)

**★ 19280 ★ Eurocare: Advocacy for the Prevention of Alcohol Harm in Europe**
Rue des Confederes 96-98
B-1000 Brussels, Belgium
**Phone:** 32 2 7367351　　　**Fax:** 32 2 7360572
**Email:** eurocare@village.uunet.be
**Website:** http://www.eurocare.org/
**Fnded:** 1990. **Desc:** An alliance of agencies set up to tackle problems associated with alcohol use at European level, presenting its views to the European Commission and Parliament as well as decision making bodies of national member states.

**★ 19281 ★ European Association for the Treatment of Addiction - U.K. (EATA)**
Waterbridge House
32-36 Loman St.
London SE1 0EE, United Kingdom
**Phone:** 44 20 79228753　　　**Fax:** 44 20 79284644
**Email:** secretariat@eata.org.uk
**Website:** http://www.box-1.freeserve.co.uk
**Fnded:** 1992. **Mem:** 80. **Lang(s):** English. **Desc:** Substance abuse treatment centers; health care and other professionals with an interest in the treatment of people who abuse substances. Seeks to advance the treatment of people with substance abuse problems; promotes increased understanding of the scientific, psychological, and medical aspects of substance abuse. Facilitates communication and cooperation among members; facilitates research and educational programs.

**★ 19282 ★ European Society for Biomedical Research on Alcoholism (ESBRA)**
Place Croix du Sud 1
1348 Louvain-la-Neuve, Belgium
**Phone:** 32 10474094　　　**Fax:** 32 10474384
**Email:** Dewittte@bani.ucl.ac.be
**Website:** http://www.imm.ki.se/moltox/esbra/es-bra.htm
**Fnded:** 1987. **Desc:** Fosters biomedical research on alcoholism in Europe; assists in prevention and education in matters related to alcoholism.

**★ 19283 ★ Families Anonymous (FA)**
PO Box 3475
Culver City, CA 90231-3475
**Phone:** (310)815-8010　　　**Free:** 800-736-9805
**Fax:** (310)815-9682
**Email:** famanon@familiesanonymous.org
**Website:** http://www.familiesanonymous.org
**Fnded:** 1971. **Nat'l Groups:** 300. **Desc:** Twelve-step groups of parents, relatives, and friends concerned about drug abuse, alcoholism, or related behavioral problems. Self-supported, self-help modeled after Al-Anon Family Groups and Alcoholics Anonymous programs. Assists families in overcoming over-protectiveness of substance abusers and developing a better understanding of their problems, thereby improving interfamily relationships. Aids in establishing community meetings; makes referrals to other agencies. Can provide speakers on request. **Pub:** *Today A Better Way*. Book. FA's daily thought book, written entirely by the fellowship. *Price:* $6.50/copy. • *The Twelve Step Rag: For Relatives and Friends Concerned about the Use of Drugs or Related Behavioral Problems*, bi-monthly. Newsletter. Contains articles, poetry and organizational information. *Price:* Free to FA groups; $4.50/year for individuals; $8.50/2 yrs.; $12/3 yrs. •

Catalog. • Directory, periodic. • Pamphlets. • Publishes over 80 items of literature for member inspiration and recovery. Prices vary by size and pages.

**★ 19284 ★ Families Worldwide**
5248 Pinemont Dr., Ste. C-190
Salt Lake City, UT 84123
**Phone:** (801)268-6461          **Fax:** (801)268-6471
**Email:** bstone81@ix.netcom.com
**Website:** http://www.fww.org
Brad Stone, Chm.

**Fnded:** 1972. **Desc:** Strengthens family bonds through programs which promote well-researched wellness skills and traditional family values. The program can be used in alcohol/substance abuse prevention with at-risk families and also in bolstering stronger families. Volunteers work as facilitators in presenting the program to families, school, civic and church groups, and other community organizations. Conducts workshops for family care professional. Currently developing chapters to extend outreach and a family center program which will strenghen families and provide humanitarian services. **Pub:** *Solutions for Families.* Available online for download. **Frmly:** (1997) The Cottage Program International, Inc.

**★ 19285 ★ Family Council on Drug Awareness (FCDA)**
PO Box 1716
El Cerrito, CA 94530
**Phone:** (510)215-8326          **Fax:** (510)215-8326
**Email:** director@fcda.org
**Website:** http://www.fcda.org
Chris Conrad, Dir.

**Fnded:** 1989. **Desc:** Promotes "legal reforms that recognize human rights, encourage responsible behavior, separate cannabis from hard drugs, and protect children from the unregulated and indiscriminate market of illegal drugs." Serves as an information clearinghouse on medical marijuana, illegal substances and drug law reform; distributes educational materials and supports 18 years, age of consent, for cannabis use. **Pub:** Brochures.

**★ 19286 ★ Friends of Temperance (FT) (Raittiuden Ystavat — RY)**
Annankatu 29 A 9
FIN-00100 Helsinki, Finland
**Phone:** 358 9 6944177          **Fax:** 358 9 6944407
**Email:** tom.anthoni-koivuluhta@raitis.fi
**Website:** http://www.raitis.fi

**Fnded:** 1853. **Mem:** 10,000. **Lang(s):** English, Finnish, Swedish. **Desc:** Temperance and substance abuse prevention and treatment organizations. Promotes increased involvement in temperance issues by the public and by development organizations worldwide. Conducts temperance education courses; facilitates cooperation among temperance organizations. **Pub:** *Ystavien Kesken*, QRT. Newsletter.

**Fundacion Antidrogas de El Salvador**
*See:* Entry 5683

**★ 19287 ★ Hazelden Foundation (HF)**
15245 Pleasant Valley Rd.
PO Box 11
Center City, MN 55012-0011
**Phone:** (651)213-4000          **Free:** 800-257-7800
**Fax:** (651)213-4544
**Email:** info@hazelden.org
**Website:** http://www.hazelden.org
Nick Hilger, Pres. /CEO

**Fnded:** 1949. **Desc:** Provides treatment, recovery, education, and professional services for chemical dependency and other addictive behaviors. Operates: Hazelden Foundation Center, a treatment center; Fellowship Club in New York, St. Paul and West Palm Beach, Florida, an intermediate care facility; Hazelden Center for Youth and Families for adolescents and young adults; Hazelden Renewal Center for individuals recovering from addictive behaviors and their

families; Hanley-Hazelden Center in West Palm Beach, Florida, for inpatient and outpatient treatment; Also provides: aftercare therapy; counselor training; 5-7 day, live-in family program that acquaints relatives and other associates of chemically-dependent individuals with problems of chemical dependency; continuing education programs for professionals; and communities. **Pub:** *Hazelden Voice*, semiannual. Newsletter. Provides information on health and recovery from addictive behavior. • *Publishing Catalog*, monthly. Catalog. • Books. • Pamphlets. • Makes available educational and audiovisual materials.

**★ 19288 ★ Health Connection**
55 W Oak Ridge Dr.
Hagerstown, MD 21740
**Phone:** (301)393-3267          **Free:** 800-548-8700
**Fax:** 888-294-8405
**Email:** sales@healthconnection.org
**Website:** http://www.healthconnection.org
Bob Smith, Pres.

**Fnded:** 1954. **Desc:** Promotes nationwide education for the prevention of drug addiction and alcoholism through direct mailings of materials to schools, churches, and civic organizations. Participates, through exhibits, in conferences and conventions of teachers and school personnel. **Pub:** *Catalogue*, annual. • *Listen*, monthly. Magazine. • *Teaching Guide to Winner Magazine*, 9/year. Magazine. • *Winner*, 9/year. • Books. • Films. • Pamphlets. • Reprints. • Videos. • Also publishes teaching aids, posters, and filmstrips. Distributes puppets/puppet programs. **Frmly:** (1993) Narcotics Education.

**★ 19289 ★ Impaired Physician Program (IPP)**
c/o Georgia Impaired Health Professionals Program
5448 Yorketown Dr.
Atlanta, GA 30349
**Phone:** (770)994-0185          **Free:** 800-445-4232
**Fax:** (770)994-2024
G. Douglas Talbott, MD, Founder & Dir.

**Fnded:** 1975. **Desc:** Purpose is to provide assistance to physicians, other health professionals, and their spouses with problems such as alcoholism, substance abuse, or codependence; seeks to locate and identify persons in need of help and to provide assistance. Conducts in- and outpatient treatment programs. Offers counseling; maintains advocacy program to assist physicians and other health professionals in re-entering their profession. Maintains speakers' bureau.

**★ 19290 ★ Institute for a Drug-Free Workplace**
1225 I St. NW, Ste. 1000
Washington, DC 20005-3914
**Phone:** (202)842-7400          **Fax:** (202)842-0022
**Email:** pizanias@drugfreeworkplace.org
**Website:** http://www.drugfreeworkplace.org/
Mark A. de Bernardo, Exec. Dir.

**Fnded:** 1989. **Mem:** 90. **Desc:** Businesses, organizations, and individuals united to preserve the rights of employers and employees involved in corporate drug abuse prevention programs. Seeks to influence public policy pertaining to drug-abuse prevention in the workplace. Conducts surveys. **Pub:** *Avoiding Legal Liability: The 25 Most Common Employer Mistakes in Addressing Drug Abuse.* Book. *Price:* $40. • *Does Drug Testing Work?.* Book. *Price:* $36. • *Drug and Alcohol Abuse Prevention and the ADA: An Employer's Guide.* Book. *Price:* $32. • *Drug Testing in the Workplace: Basic Issues, Answers, and Options for Employees.* Booklet. *Price:* $4.50. • *Employee Assistance Programs: An Employer's Development and Implementation Guide.* Booklet. *Price:* $4.50. • *Employee Drug Education and Awareness and Supervisor Training: An Employer's Development and Implementation Guide.* Booklet. *Price:* $4.50. • *Guide to Dangerous Drugs.* Booklet. *Price:* $2.40. • *Guide to State and Federal Drug Testing Laws*, annual. Book. *Price:* $295. • *International Guide to Workplace Substance Abuse Prevention.* Book. *Price:* $80. • *Policy*

*on Drug and Alcohol Abuse Prevention: An Employer's Development and Implementation Guide.* Booklet. *Price:* $4.50. • *What Every Employee Should Know About Alcohol Abuse: Answer to 25 Good Questions.* Booklet. *Price:* $2.30.

**★ 19291 ★ Institute for Integral Development (IID)**
PO Box 2172
Colorado Springs, CO 80901
**Phone:** (719)634-7943          **Free:** 800-544-9562
**Fax:** (719)630-7025
**Email:** iidevo@aol.com
**Website:** http://www.institutefortraining.com
Dan Barmettler, Dir.

**Fnded:** 1977. **Desc:** Provides a forum for discussion of issues pertaining to alcoholism and other addictions; seeks to train educators, medical professionals, and mental health practitioners in understanding and assisting addicted individuals. Sponsors seminars and workshops; provides educational audiotapes; offers consulting services. Maintains speakers' bureau; operates small library.

**★ 19292 ★ Inter-Association Task Force on Alcohol and Other Substance Abuse Issues (IATF)**
c/o Bacchus and Gamma Peer Education Network
PO Box 100430
Denver, CO 80250
**Phone:** (303)871-0901          **Fax:** (303)871-0907
**Email:** dhunter@du.edu
**Website:** http://www.iatf.org
Drew Hunter, Convener

**Fnded:** 1983. **Mem:** 20. **Desc:** Associations of college professionals and student leaders. Purposes are to enhance the development and implementation of alcohol and other substance abuse education activities in institutions of higher education throughout the U.S. and to encourage collaboration among professionals and student associations. Sponsors National Collegiate Alcohol Awareness Week and National Collegiate Health and Wellness Week. **Pub:** *First National Conference on Alcohol Policy Initiatives.* • *Guidelines for Marketing of Alcohol Beverage on Campus.* Pamphlet. • *National Collegiate Alcohol Awareness Week Mailing Handbook.* Handbook. **Frmly:** Inter-Association Task Force on Alcohol Issues; (2002) Inter-Association Task Force on Campus Alcohol and Other Substance Abuse Issues.

**★ 19293 ★ International Association for Education to a Life Without Drugs - Norway**
Odinsvei 13
N-4846 Arendal, Norway
**Email:** dag-magne.johannessen@tyholmen.vgs.no

**Lang(s):** Norwegian. **Desc:** National branch of the international organization. Individuals and organizations interested in preventing substance abuse among youth. Promotes international cooperation among alcohol and drug abuse education programs. Gathers and disseminates information on drug abuse and youth; facilitates contact among members and between members and organizations with similar goals worldwide. Conducts educational programs.

**★ 19294 ★ International Commission for the Prevention of Alcoholism and Drug Dependency (ICPA)**
12501 Old Columbia Pike
Silver Spring, MD 20904
**Phone:** (301)680-6719          **Fax:** (301)680-6707
**Email:** 74617.1663@compuserve.com
Dr. Peter N. Landless, Exec. Dir.

**Fnded:** 1952. **Desc:** Representatives of national public health committees and other individuals interested in the physical and social effects of alcoholism and drug dependency. Fosters the scientific study of alcohol and drugs, their effects on the physical, mental, and moral powers of the individual, and their effects on social, economic, political, and religious life.

Encourages preventive education; disseminates information on drug and alcohol abuse. Serves as a liaison with similar groups around the world. Sponsors exchange and research programs. Conducts film shows, forums, and radio and television events. **Pub:** *ICPA Dispatch*, periodic. • *ICPA Reporter*, periodic. Newsletter. Describes worldwide activities of ICPA and local communities. **Frmly:** (1982) International Commission for the Prevention of Alcoholism.

**★ 19295 ★ International Council on Alcohol, Drugs and Traffic Safety (ICADTS)**
Mississippi State, MS 39762
**Phone:** (601)325-7959    **Fax:** (601)325-7966
**Email:** bwparker@ssrc.msstate.edu
Barry M. Sweedler, Pres.

**Fnded:** 1950. **Mem:** 150. **Desc:** Working to reduce mortality and morbidity brought about by misuse of alcohol and drugs by operators of vehicles in all modes of transportation. Sponsors international and regional conferences to collect, disseminate and share essential information among professionals in the fields of law, medicine, public health, economics, law enforcement, public information and education, human factors and public policy. **Pub:** *ICADTS Reporter*, quarterly. Newsletter. • *Journal of Traffic Medicine*, quarterly. Journal.

**★ 19296 ★ International Doctors in Alcoholics Anonymous (IDAA)**
PO Box 199
Augusta, MO 63332
**Phone:** (636)482-4548    **Fax:** (636)228-4102
**Website:** http://www.idaa.org
C. Richard McKinley, MD, Exec. Dir.

**Fnded:** 1949. **Mem:** 5,100. **Desc:** Doctors who are alcoholics; doctors interested in Alcoholics Anonymous World Services. Seeks to exchange knowledge and experience in the recovery from and management of alcoholism for members and persons who fall within their sphere of influence. Supports AA-type group activities. **Pub:** *International Doctors in Alcoholics Anonymous–Newsletter*, quarterly. Newsletter. *Price:* Included in membership dues. • *Letter*, 3/year.

**★ 19297 ★ International Drug Strategy Institute**
901 Garfield
Topeka, KS 66606
**Fax:** (785)368-0713
**Email:** cfay@dfap.org
**Website:** http://www.estreet.com/orgs/dsi/
Dr. Eric Voth, Chm.

**Mem:** 40. **Desc:** Works to develop effective international policies and strategies to discourage drug use and legalization of illicit drugs. Disseminates accurate scientific information on drugs.

**★ 19298 ★ International Group for Research on Drug Abuse (GRITO)**
21, rue d'Assas
F-75270 Paris, France
**Phone:** 33 1 44395227    **Fax:** 33 1 44395228
**Email:** fiuc@club-internet.fr
**Website:** http://

**★ 19299 ★ International Lawyers in Alcoholics Anonymous (ILAA)**
c/o Ben Graham
PO Box 552212
Las Vegas, NV 89155-2212
**Phone:** (702)870-5466    **Fax:** (702)455-9597
**Email:** grahamr@co.clark.nv.us
**Website:** http://www.ilaa.org
Ben Graham, Sec.

**Fnded:** 1975. **Mem:** 1,300. **Desc:** Alcoholic lawyers who are seeking sobriety through their affiliation with Alcoholics Anonymous World Services. Seeks to: spread the message of AA to alcoholic attorneys; work to educate the judiciary and lawyers on the problem of

alcoholism; support attorneys in their recovery. **Pub:** *ILAA*, 3-4/year. Newsletter.

**★ 19300 ★ International Nurses Anonymous (INA)**
c/o Pat Green
1020 Sunset Dr.
Lawrence, KS 66044
**Phone:** (785)842-3893
**Email:** patlgreen@aol.com
**Website:** http://www.crml.uab.edu/~jah/ina.html
Pat Green, Sec. -Treas.

**Fnded:** 1988. **Mem:** 500. **Desc:** Nurses, nursing students, and former nurses who are involved in a 12-step recovery program. Provides mutual support and networking; serves as a resource for newly recovering nurses. **Pub:** *INA Newsletter*, semiannual. Newsletter. *Price:* Free to members.

**International Nurses Society on Addictions (NNSA)**
*See:* Entry 15723

**★ 19301 ★ International Society for Biomedical Research on Alcoholism (ISBRA)**
PO Box 2023332
Denver, CO 80220-8332
**Phone:** (303)355-6420    **Fax:** (303)355-1207
**Email:** isbra@usa.net
**Website:** http://www.isbra.com
Phillipe De Witte, Pres.

**Fnded:** 1980. **Mem:** 730. **Reg. Groups:** 3. **Desc:** Physicians, psychologists, biologists, and other scientists in over 20 countries who conduct research on biological factors in the etiology and treatment of alcoholism and its medical complications. Official collaborating agency of the World Health Organization. Conducts international collaborative research projects and training courses. **Pub:** *Advances in Biomedical Alcohol Research*, biennial. Book. Contains proceedings of the biennial congresses. • *Alcoholism: Clinical and Experimental Research*, bimonthly. Journal. *Price:* $55 members; $110 nonmembers.

**★ 19302 ★ Israel Society for the Prevention of Alcoholism (ISPA)**
4 Nordau St.
52464 Ramat Gan, Israel
**Phone:** 972 3 6720457    **Fax:** 972 3 6700725
**Email:** aweiss@shani.net
**Website:** http://www.ias.org.uk/ispa/
**Fnded:** 1976. **Lang(s):** English, Hebrew. **Desc:** Psychiatrists, physicians, nurses, social workers, recovering alcoholics. Works to develop and advance research, prevention and treatment of alcoholism in Israel. Participates in the "Drugs and Alcohol" committee in the Israeli parliament; offers advice to police on the enforcement of alcohol regulations. **Pub:** *Alcohol in Israel*, semiannual. Journal. Contains summaries in English. • *ISPA Bulletin*, quarterly. Bulletin.

**★ 19303 ★ Jewish Alcoholics, Chemically Dependent Persons and Significant Others (JACS)**
850 Seventh Ave.
New York, NY 10019
**Phone:** (212)397-4197    **Fax:** (212)399-3525
**Email:** jacs@jacsweb.org
**Website:** http://www.jacsweb.org
Maxine Uttal, Dir.

**Fnded:** 1980. **Mem:** 1,000. **State Groups:** 28. **Desc:** Jewish alcoholics and addicts, family members, and concerned friends. Acts as an additional resource to promote and enhance recovery from chemical dependency. Provides research and information on chemical addiction in the Jewish community. Maintains speakers' bureau. **Pub:** *JACS Journal*, annual. Journal. • *JACS Newsletter*, monthly. Newsletter. *Price:* Free.

**★ 19304 ★ Join Together (JTO)**
441 Stuart St., 7th Fl.
Boston, MA 02116
**Phone:** (617)437-1500    **Fax:** (617)437-9394
**Email:** info@jointogether.org
**Website:** http://www.jointogether.org/about/

**Fnded:** 1991. **Desc:** Committed to reduce, prevent, and treat substance abuse. Offers reports, newsletters, and community action toolkits. Sponsors the National Leadership Fellows program.

**★ 19305 ★ Kids In a Drug-Free Society (K.I.D.S.)**
c/o Ron Sconyers
6515 George Washington Memorial Hwy.
Ste. 105
Yorktown, VA 23692
**Phone:** (757)833-0833    **Fax:** (757)833-0835
**Email:** ron.sconyers@keepkidsdrugfree.com
Ron Sconyers, Pres.

**Desc:** Behavioral change program offered to corporate America as a public service or an employee benefit that helps teach parents how to talk with their 11-13 year old children about substance abuse.

**★ 19306 ★ Luz Social Services**
2797 N Introspect Dr.
Tucson, AZ 85745
**Phone:** (520)882-6216    **Fax:** (520)623-9291
**Email:** luz@luzsocialservices.org
**Website:** http://www.luzsocialservices.org
Dr. Pepe Barron, CEO

**Fnded:** 1989. **Mem:** 18. **Desc:** Assists with family issues, specifically substance abuse. Maintains a speakers' bureau. Conducts research and educational programs. **Pub:** *Adelante Juntous*, monthly. Newsletter.

**★ 19307 ★ Moderation Management (MM)**
c/o HRC
22 W 27th St.
New York, NY 10001
**Phone:** (212)871-0974    **Fax:** (212)213-6582
**Email:** mm@moderation.org
**Website:** http://www.moderation.org/
**Fnded:** NNsi. **Mem:** I,ver. **Desc:** People concerned about their drinking. Behavioral change program and national support group to aid people to reduce drinking and make positive lifestyle changes; empowers individuals to accept responsibility for their actions, whether its moderation or abstinence; promotes early self-recognition of risky drinking behavior.

**★ 19308 ★ NAADAC The Association for Addiction Professionals (NAADAC)**
901 N Washington St., Ste. 600
Alexandria, VA 22314
**Phone:** (703)741-7686    **Free:** 800-548-0497
**Fax:** (703)741-7698
**Email:** naadac@naadac.org
**Website:** http://www.naadac.org
Pat Ford Roegner, Exec. Dir.

**Fnded:** 1972. **Mem:** 14,000. **Reg. Groups:** 8. **State Groups:** 47. **Desc:** Counselors providing addiction treatment. Objective is to provide national representation for counselors as well as for their training and education. Works to gain public recognition of alcoholism as a disease. Seeks legislation establishing accreditation standards for counselors. Informs the public about chemical dependency and the availability of assistance. **Pub:** *Counseling Lesbian, Gay and Bisexual Persons with Alcohol and Drug Problems.* Papers. • *The Counselor*, bimonthly. Magazine. For counselors on alcohol and drug abuse. Includes book, pamphlet, and film list. Also contains notices of employment and educational opportunities. *Price:* Included in membership dues. • *NAADAC Ethical Standards.* • *NAADAC Newsletter*, bimonthly. Newsletter. *Price:* Included in membership. • *NAADAC Study Guide on Additional Counseling.* • Also publishes annual conference papers. **Frmly:** (2001) National

Association of Alcoholism and Drug Abuse Counselors.

**★ 19309 ★ Narcotic Educational Foundation of America (NEFA)**
28245 Ave. Crocker, Ste. 230
Santa Clarita, CA 91355-1201
**Phone:** (661)775-6968          **Fax:** (661)775-1648
**Email:** lwhite@cnoa.org
**Website:** http://www.cnoa.org/nefa.htm
Lorraine White, Exec. Sec.
**Fnded:** 1924. **Desc:** Conducts an education program revealing the dangers that result from the illicit and abusive use of narcotics and dangerous drugs, so that youth and adults will be protected from both mental and physical drug dependency and harm. **Pub:** *Alcohol-A Potent Drug.* Brochure. • *Am I Addicted or Dependent?.* • *Designer Drugs: The Analog Game.* • *The Heroin Story.* • *Huffing: Inhalants.* • *Lysergic Acid Diethylamide: Is it a Dream or Nightmare?.* • *The PCP Story.* • *Rohypnol: The Date Rape Drug.* • *Speed: Amphetamines.* • *The Story of Cocaine.* • *Tobacco: Smoke or Chew.* • *Understanding Anabolic Steroids.* • *Use of Marijuana as a 'Medicine'.* • *Valium & Other Depressants.* • *What About Marijuana?.*

**★ 19310 ★ Narcotics Anonymous (NA)**
PO Box 9999
Van Nuys, CA 91409
**Phone:** (818)773-9999          **Fax:** (818)700-0700
**Email:** fsmail@na.org
**Website:** http://www.na.org
Jeff Gershoff, Fellowship Svcs.
**Fnded:** 1953. **Mem:** 500,000. **Reg. Groups:** 105. **State Groups:** 50. **Local Groups:** 27400. **Desc:** Recovering addicts throughout the world meet to offer help to fellow addicts seeking recovery. Members meet regularly to facilitate and stabilize their recovery. Uses 12-step program adapted from Alcoholics Anonymous to aid in the recovery process. **Pub:** *It Works: How and Why.* Book. Guide to NA primary principles. • *Just For Today: Daily Meditations for Recovering Addicts.* Book. • *NA Way Magazine: The International Journal of the Fellowship of Narcotics Anonymous,* quarterly. Magazine. Recounts experiences of members during their recoveries. Includes calendar of events and annual index. *Price:* Free. • *Narcotics Anonymous.* Book. Basic textbook of NA. • *Narcotics Anonymous: It Works How and Why.* Books.

**★ 19311 ★ National Acupuncture Detoxification Association (NADA)**
PO Box 1927
Vancouver, WA 98668-1927
**Phone:** (360)254-0186          **Fax:** (360)260-8620
**Email:** webmaster@acudetox.com
**Website:** http://www.acudetox.com
Jay Renaud, MPA, Office Mgr.
**Fnded:** 1985. **Mem:** 880. **Nat'l Groups:** 1. **State Groups:** 2. **Desc:** Works to promote the use of acupuncture in the treatment of addictions. Provides training and educational materials. **Pub:** *Guidepoints: Acupuncture in Recovery,* monthly. Newsletter. *Price:* $180/year.

**★ 19312 ★ National Alliance of Methadone Advocates (NAMA)**
435 2nd Ave.
New York, NY 10010
**Phone:** (212)595-6262          **Fax:** (212)595-6262
**Email:** nama4u@mail-x-change.com
**Website:** http://www.methadone.org/
Joycelyn Woods, Pres.
**Fnded:** 1988. **Mem:** 15,000. **Nat'l Groups:** 5. **Reg. Groups:** 20. **State Groups:** 10. **Local Groups:** 27. **Desc:** Methadone maintenance patients and supporters of methadone maintenance treatment. Promotes quality methadone maintenance treatment as the most effective modality for the treatment of heroin addiction. **Pub:** *Manual Series - Starting A Methadone Advocacy Group.* • *NAMA Advocate,* quarterly. Newsletter.

*Price:* $25/year, U.S.; $40 international. • Educational Series - 2.00 each.

**★ 19313 ★ National Asian Pacific American Families Against Substance Abuse (NAPAFASA)**
340 E Second St., Ste. 409
Los Angeles, CA 90012
**Phone:** (213)625-5795          **Fax:** (213)625-5796
**Email:** jmori@aars-inc.org
**Website:** http://www.napafasa.org
Jeff Mori, Chm.
**Fnded:** 1988. **Nat'l Groups:** 200. **Desc:** Members include AAPI and human service organizations. Works to involve service providers, families, and youth to reach API communities in the promotion of health, social justice and the reduction of substance abuse and related problems. Special projects offer organizations technical assistance, training, program planning and clinical training.

**★ 19314 ★ National Association of Addiction Treatment Providers (NAATP)**
313 E Liberty St., Ste. 129
Lancaster, PA 17603-2748
**Phone:** (717)392-8480          **Fax:** (717)392-8481
**Email:** rhunsicker@naatp.org
**Website:** http://www.naatp.org
Ronald J. Hunsicker, Pres. /CEO
**Fnded:** 1978. **Mem:** 210. **State Groups:** 12. **Desc:** Corporate and private institutional alcohol and/or drug dependency treatment facilities. Promotes awareness of chemical dependency as a treatable disease; advocates high standards of health care in substance abuse treatment facilities. Encourages member education. Maintains contact with U.S. Congress and state and local governments. Serves in an advisory capacity to the Joint Commission on Accreditation of Healthcare Organizations and to the Commission on Accreditation of Rehabilitation Facilities. Compiles statistics on chemical dependency treatment and recovery. **Pub:** *NAATP Visions,* monthly. Newsletter. *Price:* Free. For members only. **Frmly:** (1987) National Association of Alcoholism Treatment Programs.

**★ 19315 ★ National Association of Alcohol and Drug Abuse Counsellors**
1 Plato Pl.
72-74 St. Dionis Rd.
London SW6 4TU, United Kingdom
**Phone:** 44 20 76109102      **Fax:** 44 20 73842636
**Email:** office@naadac.org.uk
**Website:** http://www.naadac.org.uk
**Fnded:** 1984. **Mem:** 160. **Desc:** Individual counsellors dedicated to the development of the professional specialism of alcoholism and drug abuse counselling as a means of securing the provision of quality care to those who experience primary and secondary addiction problems, their families and dependants and others significant to them. Promotes recognition of the qualified alcoholism and drug abuse counsellor as a health care professional; fosters interaction and exchange of knowledge and experience between counsellor associations; advocates on a national level for alcoholism and drug abuse counsellors on issues affecting the profession; promotes a code of ethics. **Pub:** *NAADAC News,* quarterly. Newsletter.

**★ 19316 ★ National Association on Alcohol, Drugs and Disability (NAADD)**
2165 Bunker Hill Dr.
San Mateo, CA 94402-3801
**Phone:** (650)578-8047          **Fax:** (650)286-9205
**Email:** jdem@aimnet.com
**Website:** http://www.naadd.org/
John deMiranda, Exec. Dir.
**Desc:** Promotes awareness and education about substance abuse among people with co-existing disabilities; aims to create public awareness of issues related to alcoholism, drug addition, and substance abuse faced by persons with co-existing disabilities; provides a peer approach to enhance access to

services, information, education and prevention through collaborative efforts of individuals and organizations. Sponsors the California Technology Assistance & Training Project. **Pub:** *The NAADD Report: The Newsletter on Alcohol, Drugs and Disability,* annual. Newsletter.

**★ 19317 ★ National Association of Athletes Against Drugs (NAAAD)**
2481 Pacific Ave., Ste. C
Long Beach, CA 90806-2953
**Phone:** (562)424-6542          **Fax:** (562)426-9863
**Email:** educat2100@aol.com
Elliott Smith, Chm.
**Fnded:** 1992. **Mem:** 1,293. **Reg. Groups:** 3. **Desc:** Professional athletes in motor sports. Promotes use of the fame enjoyed by racing drivers to deter youth from substance abuse. Seeks to increase participation by African-Americans in professional motor sports. Conducts educational programs; participates in charitable activities; makes available children's services; compiles statistics; maintains speakers' bureau. **Pub:** *The Informer,* periodic. Newsletter. *Price:* for members.

**★ 19318 ★ National Association for Children of Alcoholics (NACoA)**
11426 Rockville Pike, St. 100
Rockville, MD 20852
**Phone:** (301)468-0985          **Free:** 888-554-2627
**Fax:** (301)468-0987
**Email:** nacoa@nacoa.org
**Website:** http://www.nacoa.org
Sis Wenger, Exec. Dir.
**Fnded:** 1983. **Mem:** 4,000. **Desc:** Authors, educators, physicians, psychologists, therapists, and children of alcoholics. Supports and serves as a resource for individuals of all age groups who are COAs. Objectives are to increase public and professional awareness and recognition of the special needs of children of alcoholics; to provide leadership in public policy at the national, state, and local level; to act as an informational and educational resource to academic and other community systems; to create networks that facilitate the exchange of information and resources; to initiate and advance professional knowledge and understanding; to advocate for accessible programs and services. Compiles statistics; conducts educational programs. **Pub:** *Children of Alcoholics: Selected Readings, Vol. II.* Book. • *It's Elementary: Meeting the Needs of High Risk Youth in the School Setting.* Booklet. • *NACoA Network,* bimonthly. Newsletter. *Price:* $20. • *Poor Jennifer: She's Always Losing Her Hat.* Video. • Also makes available posters, videos, booklets, brochures.

**National Association of County Behavioral Health Directors (NACBHD)**
*See:* Entry 12569

**★ 19319 ★ National Association on Drug Abuse Problems (NADAP)**
355 Lexington Ave.
New York, NY 10017
**Phone:** (212)986-1170          **Fax:** (212)697-2939
**Email:** info@NADAP.com
**Website:** http://www.nadap.org
John Darin, Pres.
**Fnded:** 1971. **Desc:** Sponsored by business and labor organizations. Serves as an information clearinghouse and referral bureau for corporations and local communities interested in prevention of substance abuse and treatment of substance abusers. Provides: resources to local communities seeking to combat drug and alcohol abuse; corporate services for employers interested in creating a drug-free workplace. Community education and development services include: development of drug and alcohol awareness presentations for community organizations; identification of local substance abuse treatment resources; consultation on development of local prevention, treatment, and vocational programs. Corporate services include: provision of drug and alcohol information seminars in the

workplace and through union organizations; assistance in formulation of company drug and alcohol policies; aid in the development and implementation of employee assistance programs; training of supervisors; assistance for companies and labor unions wishing to make full use of local treatment agency networks. Makes available vocational education services including training in job hunting, job interview workshops, training programs for substance abuse treatment professionals, and individual consultations for recovering substance abusers seeking to return to the job market. Provides placement services; has conducted surveys on the employability of rehabilitated drug users and found that former addicts perform comparably with others hired for similar jobs. Operates Neighborhood Prevention Network, through which local communities develop parent support groups and youth peer leadership groups dedicated to combatting drug and alcohol abuse. NPN provides substance abuse prevention and early intervention services for children and youth and ongoing training and materials dealing with specific issues in urban substance abuse. Maintains speakers' bureau. **Pub:** *Conference Proceedings*, biennial. Proceedings. • *NADAP News/Report*, quarterly. Newsletter. Covers current issues in the field of substance abuse. *Price:* Free. • Reports.

★ 19320 ★ **National Association for Families and Addiction Research and Education**
200 S Michigan Ave, Ste. 1430
Chicago, IL 60604-2404
**Phone:** (312)541-1272          **Fax:** (312)431-8697
Judith C. Burnison, Exec. Officer
**Fnded:** 1987. **Mem:** 750. **Reg. Groups:** 3. **Desc:** Conducts educational and research programs on substance abuse during pregnancy, and the effects of substance abuse on the fetus. Sponsors training forums and charitable programs; operates cocaine baby helpline. Compiles statistics; maintains speakers' bureau. **Pub:** *Update*, quarterly. Newsletter. Contains information on model programs and research. *Price:* Included in membership dues. **Frmly:** (1996) National Association Perinatal Addiction and Research Education.

**National Association of Lesbian/Gay Addiction Professionals (NALGAP)**
*See:* Entry 18904

**National Association of State Alcohol and Drug Abuse Directors (NASADAD)**
*See:* Entry 9752

★ 19321 ★ **National Association of Substance Abuse Trainers and Educators (NASATE)**
1521 Hillary St.
New Orleans, LA 70118
**Phone:** (504)286-5234
**Email:** dcoffice@nasadad.org
**Website:** http://www.nasadad.org
Dr. Tom Lief, Chairperson
**Fnded:** 1982. **Mem:** 100. **Reg. Groups:** 2. **Desc:** Accredited colleges and universities offering 12 or more course credit hours in the field of substance abuse. Goal is to provide a network for exchange on courses, student population, degreed and nondegreed programs, and graduate study in chemical dependency training. Acts as a clearinghouse for students interested in substance abuse training programs; assists universities with the development of such programs. Provides for the exchange of information among universities concerning certificates, continuing education units, degrees, and opportunities for transfer and enrollment in undergraduate, graduate, and professional schools. Examines the educational and training needs of students and their career mobility as substance abuse practitioners. **Pub:** *Annual Directory*. Directory.

★ 19322 ★ **National Catholic Council on Alcoholism and Related Drug Problems (NCCA)**
1550 Hendrickson St.
Brooklyn, NY 11234-3514
**Phone:** (718)951-7177          **Fax:** (718)951-7233
**Email:** kieranncca@aol.com
**Website:** http://www.nccatoday.org
Msgr. K. Martin, Contact
**Fnded:** 1949. **Mem:** 300. **Desc:** Promotes adequate treatment for all clergy and religious men and women suffering from alcoholism and drug dependency through consultation and supportive services. Cooperates with treatment programs for the spiritual, physical, and mental rehabilitation of alcoholics and drug dependent persons, especially with Alcoholics Anonymous World Services. Promotes pastoral ministry to alcoholics and their families. Educates Catholics, especially priests and religious men and women in pastoral ministries, on alcohol and alcohol problems as well as the use and abuse of alcohol and drugs. Sponsors workshops; conducts alcohol and drug abuse education programs in houses of formation and seminaries. Maintains speakers' bureau. **Pub:** *Alcoholism A Source Book for the Priest-Reprint of 1960 edition in 1998*. Book. • *The Best of the Blue Book Vol II 196-1997 publised 1999*. Book. • *The Blue Book*, annual. Book. Proceedings of annual symposium. *Price:* $15 donation. • *Newsnotes*, quarterly. Newsletter. **Frmly:** National Clergy Conference on Alcoholism; (1988) National Clergy Council on Alcoholism and Related Drug Problems.

★ 19323 ★ **National Committee for the Prevention of Alcoholism and Drug Dependency (NCPADD)**
c/o Thomas R. Neslund
12501 Old Columbia Pike
Silver Spring, MD 20904-6600
**Phone:** (301)680-6719          **Fax:** (301)680-6707
**Email:** 74617.1663@compuserve.com
Dr. Peter N. Landless, Exec. Dir.
**Fnded:** 1950. **Mem:** 50. **Desc:** Health officials, physicians, educators, social workers, youth leaders, clergymen, temperance leaders, businessmen, judges, and others. To further the study of the effects of alcohol and other drugs on the physical, mental and moral powers of the individual citizen and on the social, economic, political, and religious life of the nation. Fosters nationwide educational program through films, lectures, forums, radio, and television programs. **Pub:** *ICPA Reporter*, quarterly. Bulletin. Describes worldwide activities of ICPA and local communities. **Frmly:** National Committee for the Prevention of Alcoholism.

★ 19324 ★ **National Council on Alcoholism and Drug Dependence (NCADD)**
20 Exchange Pl., Ste. 2902
New York, NY 10005-3201
**Phone:** (212)269-7797          **Free:** 800-622-2255
**Fax:** (212)269-7510
**Email:** national@ncadd.org
**Website:** http://www.ncadd.org
Stacia Murphy, Pres.
**Fnded:** 1944. **State Groups:** 11. **Local Groups:** 90. **Desc:** Works for the prevention and treatment of alcoholism and other drug dependence through programs of public education, information, and public policy advocacy. Sponsors National Alcohol Awareness Month each April. **Pub:** *NCADD Amethyst*, quarterly. Newsletter. *Price:* $50. • *NCADD Washington Report*, monthly. Newsletter. Newsletter reporting on washington issues related to alcolholism/drug dependence. *Price:* $97/year; $174/2 years; $259/3 years. • *Resource and Referral Guide*, annual. • *What Are the Signs of Alcoholism?*. • *What Can You Do About Someone Else's Drinking?*. • *Whos' Got the Power? You...or Drugs?*. Pamphlets. • Annual Report. **Frmly:** (1949) National Committee for Education on Alcoholism; (1955) National Committee on Alcoholism; (1990) National Council on Alcoholism.

★ 19325 ★ **National Families in Action (NFIA)**
Century Plaza II
2957 Clairmont Rd., Ste.150
Atlanta, GA 30329-1647
**Phone:** (404)248-9676          **Fax:** (404)248-1312
**Email:** nfia@nationalfamilies.org
**Website:** http://www.nationalfamilies.org
Sue Rusche, Exec. Dir.
**Fnded:** 1977. **Desc:** Parents and other adults concerned about preventing drug abuse. Seeks to: educate parents, children, and the community about the use of drugs; counteract social pressures that condone and promote drug use; stop drug use. Worked for passage of statewide drug paraphernalia statutes. Collects and disseminates information about the effects of drugs. Maintains Drug Information Center, which contains more than 500,000 documents, studies, books, brochures, and films and videos relating to drug abuse. Operates after-school program for parents and youth. **Pub:** *Crack Update*. Brochure. Describes the effects of this highly addictive form of cocaine. *Price:* $35/100. • *False Messengers: How Addictive Drugs Change the Brain*. • *Guide to the Legalization Movement and How You Can Stop It*. Book. *Price:* $10. • *12 Reasons Not to Legalize Drugs*. *Price:* $15/100. • *12 Tips for Helping Your Children Stay Drug-Free*. *Price:* $15/100. • *You Have the Right to Know Curriculum Series*. Books. *Price:* $10/each. • Also publishes Inhalant Update. **Frmly:** (1982) DeKalb Families in Action; (1983) Families in Action; (1984) Families in Action Drug Information Center; (1990) Families in Action National Drug Information Center.

★ 19326 ★ **National Family Partnership (NFP)**
c/o Informed Families Education Center
2490 Coral Way, Ste. 501
Miami, FL 33145
**Phone:** (305)856-4886          **Free:** 800-705-8997
**Fax:** (305)856-4815
**Email:** mosendorf@informedfamilies.org
**Website:** http://www.nfp.org
Peggy B. Sapp, Pres.
**Fnded:** 1980. **Mem:** 65. **Reg. Groups:** 32. **State Groups:** 22. **Desc:** Provides services, resources, and drug prevention programs for local parent and youth groups across the country. Sponsors Annual Red Ribbon Celebration in October; serves as a clearinghouse for state and federal legislation. **Pub:** *NFP Update*, quarterly. Newsletter. *Price:* $25/year for individuals; $100/year for groups. • Manuals. **Frmly:** National Federation of Parents for Drug-Free Youth.

★ 19327 ★ **National Hispanic Family**
1559 Sherman Way
North Hollywood, CA 91605
**Phone:** (818)503-6300          **Fax:** (818)764-8414
Soledad Alatoue, Dir.
**Fnded:** 1951. **Desc:** Works to help Hispanic families, particularly in the area of drug abuse prevention. Organizes English language and citizenship classes. **Pub:** Directory, annual.

★ 19328 ★ **National Parents' Resource Institute for Drug Education (PRIDE)**
4684 Evergreen Dr.
Newaygo, MI 49337
**Phone:** (231)652-4400          **Free:** 800-668-9277
**Fax:** (231)652-2461
**Email:** prideyouth@ncats.net
**Website:** http://www.prideyouthprograms.org
Marsha Keith Schucharfd, PhD, Founder
**Fnded:** 1977. **Desc:** Parents, youth groups, educators, law enforcement officials, community groups, and corporations. Promotes drug abuse prevention through education. Provides current research information on drug abuse and facilitates the organization of parent peer groups, parent-school teams, and community action groups to reduce adolescent drug abuse. Gathers and disseminates information on the latest medical and scientific findings on the effects of drugs on youth, current patterns of drug and alcohol use

among youth, social and cultural pressures that encourage youth to use drugs, and institutional and legal efforts being made to prevent drug abuse, reduce drug supplies, and prosecute drug traffickers. Conducts the PRIDE Community Action Plan to assist communities in establishing an effective drug abuse program and the PRIDE's Parent Training Program to assist concerned parents. Offers America's PRIDE, ClubPRIDE, and PRIDE Junior youth programs. Develops workplace drug training programs for corporations. Sponsors the annual PRIDE World Drug Conference, which seeks to bring parents, youth, and the public into contact with scientists, physicians, and policymakers dealing with adolescent drug abuse; also sponsors a series of one-day conferences for local community teams who are trained to return to their neighborhoods to organize workshops. Operates speakers' bureau; conducts educational programs and children's services; compiles statistics. Maintains library. **Pub:** *PRIDE Quarterly.* Newsletter. Discusses the legal, pharmacological, psychological, social, cultural, and physiological effects of adolescent drug use. Includes overviews. *Price:* $25/year. • Also publishes books and pamphlets. **AKA:** PRIDE (Parents' Resource Institute for Drug Education). **Frmly:** (1982) Parent Resources and Information on Drug Education.

★ **19329** ★ **National Prevention Network (NPN)**
808 17th St. NW, Ste. 410
Washington, DC 20006
**Phone:** (202)293-0090　　**Fax:** (202)293-1250
**Email:** amoghul@nasadad.org
**Website:** http://www.nasadad.org
Alan Moghul, PhD, Dir., Prevention Svcs.

**Fnded:** 1982. **Mem:** 61. **Reg. Groups:** 5. **State Groups:** 50. **Desc:** Officials of state alcohol and drug agencies. Works to enhance national, state, and local programs for drug and alcohol abuse prevention; serves as a network among state agency personnel and other prevention professionals to assist in the development of effective and innovative substance abuse prevention strategies; seeks to establish guidelines for quality service. Collects and disseminates information and statistics on prevention services, programs, trends, activities, and issues. Provides consultation on technical matters; conducts research. **Pub:** *NPN Membership List,* quarterly.

★ **19330** ★ **New Hope Foundation**
51 Throckmorton St.
Freehold, NJ 07728
**Phone:** (732)308-0113　　**Fax:** (732)308-0115
**Website:** http://www.newhopefoundation.org
Alicia Goodhue, Contact

**Desc:** Private citizens, businesses, and organizations. Strives to serve those in need of treatment of alcoholism, drug addition, and gambling. Offers both inpatient and outpatient services.

★ **19331** ★ **Nordic Council for Alcohol and Drug Research (NCADR) (Nordiska Namnden for Alkohol- och Drogforskning — NAD)**
Annegatan 29 A 23
FIN-00100 Helsinki 10, Finland
**Phone:** 358 9 6948082　　**Fax:** 358 9 6949081
**Email:** nads@kaapeli.fi
**Website:** http://www.kaapeli.fi/nad
**Fnded:** 1978. **Mem:** 5. **Lang(s):** Danish, Norwegian, Swedish. **Desc:** Researchers from Denmark, Finland, Iceland, Norway, and Sweden. Coordinates alcohol and drug research within Scandinavia; initiates new research projects. Organizes seminars. Disseminates information. **Pub:** Book.

★ **19332** ★ **Partnership for a Drug Free America (DFA)**
405 Lexington Ave., 16th Fl.
New York, NY 10174
**Phone:** (212)922-1560　　**Fax:** (212)922-1570

**Website:** http://www.drugfreeamerica.org
Richard Bonnette, Pres.

**Fnded:** 1986. **Mem:** 2,500. **Desc:** A coalition of individuals and organizations representing the advertising, production, and communications industries. Seeks to utilize the creative skills of members to change social attitudes towards illegal drugs. Believes that drug abuse is a major crisis affecting American families and work environments. Works to evoke a social revulsion to what the group views as current public acceptance and complacency toward illegal drugs. Focuses on advertising strategies that will "unsell" illegal drugs, "de-normalize" drug usage in the U.S., and reinforce positive factors of life without drugs. Creates advertising campaigns targeted toward preteens, teenagers, young adults, and "influencers" (peers, parents, health care professionals, teachers, and opinion leaders). Is currently running media anti-drug advertisements, including an advertisement depicting an egg being fried as an analogy to the effects of drugs on the human brain. Conducts research evaluation program to assess attitudinal changes of targeted groups toward illegal drugs, monitor usage trends, and evaluate the effectiveness of these advertisments. **Pub:** *Partnership for a Drug-Free America Newsletter,* quarterly. Newsletter. • Bulletin, periodic. **Frmly:** (1990) Media-Advertising Partnership for a Drug-Free America.

★ **19333** ★ **People Against Impaired Driving (PAID)**
10015 103rd Ave., Ste. 1405
Edmonton, AB, Canada T5J 0H1
**Phone:** (780)462-2426　　**Fax:** (780)462-2596
**Fnded:** 1982. **Mem:** 300. **Lang(s):** English, French. **Desc:** Volunteers opposed to impaired driving. Seeks to erradicate drunken and impaired driving; works to strengthen impaired driving statutes and improve their enforcement. Provides support and services to victims of impaired drivers and their families. Lobbies government agencies for more punitive measures against repeat impaired driving offenders. Conducts educational campaigns to raise public awareness of impaired driving and its effects; maintains speakers' bureau. **Pub:** *People Against Impaired Driving.* Brochure. • Newsletter, periodic.

★ **19334** ★ **Phoenix House of New York**
164 W 74th St.
New York, NY 10023
**Phone:** (212)595-5810　　**Fax:** (212)496-6035
**Email:** phcomm@phoenixhouse.org
**Website:** http://www.phoenixhouse.org
Mitchell S. Rosenthal, MD, Pres.

**Fnded:** 1967. **Mem:** 760. **Desc:** Provides drug abuse treatment, vocational and educational services through individual, group and family counseling, and self help rehabilitation programs. Operates 20 facilities for adolescents and adults in New York, New Jersey and California and Texas. Operates extensive range of drug-free treatment programs including: Phoenix Academy (Board of Education certified, residential high school for adolescents); Step One (Board of Education certified day-school); IMPACT (outpatient intervention for teenagers and their parents); long-term residential treatment for adults; short-term out-patient and in-patient adult drug treatment. Also operates programs geared to specific populations, such as PORTAL program for homeless mothers and their children living in shelter accommodation; prison-based and community aftercare programs for male and female criminal offenders. Phoenix House Drug Education and Prevention Unit conducts adult and adolescent drug education workshops in public and private schools, corporations and other workplaces. **Pub:** *Phoenix House News,* quarterly. Newsletter. *Price:* Free. • Brochures. • Newsletter, quarterly. • Pamphlets. • Annual Report. **Frmly:** (2000) Phoenix House Foundation.

★ **19335** ★ **Pill Addicts Anonymous (PAA)**
PO Box 13738
Reading, PA 19612-3738
**Fnded:** 1979. **Mem:** 100. **State Groups:** 2. **Local Groups:** 2. **Desc:** Individuals who wish to recover from pill and drug addiction. Provides support through group sessions. **Pub:** Pamphlets. *Price:* Free.

★ **19336** ★ **Pills Anonymous (PA)**
PO Box 772
Bronx, NY 10451
**Phone:** (212)874-0700
**Website:** http://www.pillsanonymous.com
**Fnded:** 1975. **Local Groups:** 3. **Desc:** Persons addicted to drugs including tranquilizers, stimulants, analgesics, sedatives, cocaine, and marijuana. Purpose is to apply the Alcoholics Anonymous World Services' 12-step approach to persons dependent on addictive drugs. Provides emotional support to members, many of whom became addicted after using the drugs for legitimate reasons (for example, to alleviate the chronic pain of migraine headaches or arthritis) and teaches them methods of coping with pain that do not require drugs. **Frmly:** (1984) Pills Anonymous; (1992) Drugs Anonymous.

★ **19337** ★ **Pioneer Total Abstinence Association**
27 Upper Sherrard St.
Dublin 1, Ireland
**Phone:** 353 1 8749464　　**Fax:** 353 1 8748485
**Email:** pioneer@s-j.ie
**Website:** http://www.pioneertotal.ie
**Fnded:** 1895. **Mem:** 500,000. **Desc:** Promotes sobriety, principally by prayer and consecrated abstinence from alcohol of members. Encourages members to engage in good works.

★ **19338** ★ **Project Renewal**
c/o Carrie VanDusen
200 Varick St., 9th Fl.
New York, NY 10014
**Phone:** (212)620-0340　　**Fax:** (212)243-4868
**Website:** http://www.projectrenewal.org
Carrie VanDusen, Dir. Development

**Fnded:** 1967. **Desc:** Provides care for homeless adults in New York City. Funded by the New York City Department of Mental Health, Mental Retardation and Alcoholism Services, the U.S. Department of Housing and Urban Development, the New York State Office of Mental Health, the New York City Department of Homeless Services, the New York City Human Resources Administrative Divison of AIDS Service, the New York State Office of Alcoholism and Substance Abuse Services; private individuals, and corporations and foundations. Main components of the program are: a 48 bed alcohol detoxification facility for homeless male alcoholics; a 150 person alcoholism outpatient clinic for sober homeless alcoholics; a 20 person, year-long program offering therapy and work rehabilitation for homeless alcoholics and other substance abusers; Midtown Outreach Program, which sends medical and outreach teams to homeless people on the streets and in shelters. Offers training, job placement, and permanent supported housing. **Frmly:** (1995) Manhattan Bowery Corporation.

★ **19339** ★ **Rational Recovery Systems (RRS)**
PO Box 800
Lotus, CA 95651
**Phone:** (530)621-2667　　**Free:** 800-303-CURE
**Fax:** (530)622-4296
**Email:** rr@rational.org
**Website:** http://www.rational.org
Jack Trimpey, Pres.

**Fnded:** 1986. **Desc:** Rational Recovery means self-recovery from substance addiction through planned abstinence. Leads to complete abstinence from substance abuse using Addictive Voice Recognition Technique (AVRT). **Pub:** *AVRT Live (Addictive Voice*

*Recognition Technique).* Videos. Complete 12-video VHS set. *Price:* $995. • *The Final Fix.* Audiotapes. *Price:* $39.95. • *Greater Expectations.* Video. *Price:* $89.95. • *Journal of Rational Recovery,* quarterly. Journal. Contains articles by recovered addicts of alcohol, drugs, and eating disorders and others. *Price:* $36/year. • *Rational Recovery/The New Cure for Substance Addiction. Price:* $14.95. • *The Small Book: A Revolutionary Alternative for Overcoming Alcohol and Drug Dependence. Price:* $14.95. • *Taming the Feast Beast. Price:* $14.95. • *There's Nothing Wrong With You.* Video. *Price:* $89.95.

**★ 19340 ★   Recovered Alcoholic Clergy Association (RACA)**
Emmanuel Episcopal Church
498 Prince Ave.
Athens, GA 30601
**Fax:** (706)208-3790
**Email:** petercourtney@charter.net
**Website:** http://www.geocities.com/HotSprings/8872
Peter Courtney, Pres.

**Fnded:** 1968. **Mem:** 350. **Nat'l Groups:** 2. **Local Groups:** 100. **Desc:** Clergy in the Episcopal church orders and persons attending or teaching at Episcopal seminaries who have drinking problems. Recommends alcohol addiction treatment centers for members; trains individuals involved in confronting persons with drinking problems. Seeks to provide moral support to members; provides guidance to the families and/or colleagues of problem drinkers; maintains speakers' bureau. **Pub:** *No foolin,* monthly. Newsletter. • *RACA Directory,* annual. Directory. • Pamphlets.

**★ 19341 ★   Recovery Ministries**
876 Market Way
Clarkston, GA 30021
**Phone:** (516)997-0476
Virginia M. King, Exec. Dir.

**Fnded:** 1982. **Mem:** 600. **Desc:** A network of individuals, parishes, and Episcopal church diocesan committees addressing the issue of alcohol and drug use and addiction. Seeks to involve the Episcopal church in alcohol and other drug addiction issues. Serves as a resource clearinghouse. Sponsors annual Alcohol-Drug Awareness Sunday to provide information to congregations. **Pub:** *Alcohol-Drug Awareness Sunday Information Packet,* annual. Educational material. *Price:* $6. • *The NECAD News,* quarterly. *Price:* available to members only. • Brochures. • Newsletter. **Frmly:** (1997) National Episcopal Coalition on Alcohol and Drugs.

**★ 19342 ★   Remembering ADAM**
PO Box 665
Hastings, PA 16646
**Free:** 877-767-2326
**Email:** adam51988@aol.com
**Website:** http://www.rememberingadam.com
Deborah A. Fowler, Contact

**Fnded:** 1999. **Mem:** 16. **Desc:** Volunteers. Provide speakers for events. Promote drug use awareness.

**★ 19343 ★   Research and Education on Impaired Driving (REID)**
1912-10015 103rd Ave., Ste. 1405
Edmonton, AB, Canada T5S 0H1

**Fnded:** 1982. **Mem:** 300. **Lang(s):** English, French. **Desc:** Volunteers opposed to drunk and impaired driving. Promotes increased public awareness of the dangers of impaired driving; seeks to improve enforcement of laws prohibiting drunken and impaired driving. Conducts educational pograms; sponsors research; maintains speakers' bureau.

**★ 19344 ★   Research Society on Alcoholism (RSA)**
4314 Medical Pkwy., No. 12
Austin, TX 78756-3332
**Phone:** (512)454-0022          **Fax:** (512)454-0812
**Email:** debbyrsa@bga.com

**Website:** http://www.RSOA.org
Debra Sharp, Exec. Dir.

**Fnded:** 1976. **Mem:** 1,400. **Desc:** Scientists who hold an M.D. or Ph.D. degree and others actively engaged in research on alcoholism and alcohol-related problems; doctoral students; professionals in related fields who are interested in supporting alcohol research. Purposes are to: serve as a forum for researchers working in the field; aid and further the application of research to problems related to alcoholism; disseminate scientific information; protect the rights of researchers and human research subjects; assess research priorities; enlighten the public about problems of alcoholism. Provides opportunities for communication and discussion among scientists, clinicians, and lay workers in alcoholism research, diagnosis, and treatment. Conducts lectures. **Pub:** *Alcoholism: Clinical and Experimental Research,* monthly. Journal. Includes book reviews and research reports. *Price:* $105 members; $145 members, foreign; $318 nonmembers. • *Recent Developments in Alcoholism,* annual. Monograph. *Price:* $382 Canada and Mexico; $406 nonmembers, foreign. • *RSA Directory,* periodic. Directory. *Price:* available to members only; available to members only.

**★ 19345 ★   Scottish Council on Alcohol (SCA)**
166 Buchanan St.
Glasgow G1 2NH, United Kingdom
**Phone:** 44 141 3339677          **Fax:** 44 141 3331606

**Fnded:** 1973. **Lang(s):** English. **Desc:** Seeks to reduce the level of alcohol abuse in Scotland. Conducts educational and training programs for health care professionals and therapists working with people who abuse alcohol; serves as a clearinghouse on alcohol abuse programs and services. Participates in charitable activities; compiles statistics. **Pub:** *Alcohol Update,* quarterly. Newsletter. • *Scottish Council on Alcohol Annual Report,* annual. Annual Report. • Books. • Reports.

**★ 19346 ★   Secular Organizations for Sobriety (SOS)**
4773 Hollywood Blvd.
Hollywood, CA 90027
**Phone:** (323)666-4295          **Fax:** (323)666-4271
**Email:** sos@CFIWest.org
**Website:** http://cfiwest.org/sos
James R. Christopher, Founder

**Fnded:** 1986. **Mem:** 20,000. **Desc:** Recovering alcoholics and drug addicts; families and friends of alcoholics or drug addicts. Serves as a support system free of any religious or spiritual undercurrent; believes sobriety is a process of personal responsibility. Espouses "a healthy skepticism" and encourages self-reliance and free thought. Maintains speakers' bureau. Compiles statistics. **Pub:** *Save Our Selves,* quarterly. Newsletter.

**★ 19347 ★   Society for Prevention Research (SPR)**
1300 I St., NW, Ste. 250 West
Washington, DC 20005
**Phone:** (202)216-9670          **Fax:** (202)216-9671
**Email:** cedarspr@pitt.edu
**Website:** http://www.preventionresearch.org
Ralph E. Tarter, PhD, Admin.

**Fnded:** 1992. **Mem:** 400. **Desc:** Scientists, practitioners, and adminstrators working in the field of substance abuse prevention. Works to improve prevention intervention through empirical investigation. Facilitates communication and cooperation among prevention interventionists working in fields including etiology, epidemiology, and the social sciences. Serves as a clearinghouse on prevention intervention. Sponsors multidisciplinary studies of factors influencing substance abusers, including social maladjustment, crime, and behavioral disorders. **Pub:** *Prevention Science,* quarterly. Journal.

**★ 19348 ★   Society for the Study of Addiction to Alcohol and Other Drugs (SSA)**
c/o Liz Smedley
Centre for Health Economics
University of York
Heslington
York YO10 5DD, United Kingdom
**Phone:** 44 1904 434255          **Fax:** 44 1904 432700
**Email:** eas8@york.ac.uk
**Website:** http://www.addiction-ssa.org

**Fnded:** 1884. **Mem:** 293. **Reg. Groups:** 1. **Lang(s):** English. **Desc:** Medical and allied health professionals seeking to stimulate scientific study of alcohol and drug addiction. Conducts research and educational programs. **Pub:** *Addiction,* monthly. Journal. • Monographs.

**★ 19349 ★   Triangle Club**
2030 P St. NW
Washington, DC 20035
**Phone:** (202)659-8641
**Website:** http://www.triangleclub.org

**Fnded:** 1980. **Mem:** 1,000. **Desc:** Regular groups of Alcoholics Anonymous World Services specifically composed of gays and lesbians. Purpose is to serve the gay and lesbian members of AA and to provide advice and support to other members of AA. Works for unity and service with AA for the betterment of the gay and lesbian members and AA; advocates freedom in communication as an important aid to recovery. Provides alcoholism professionals with information about gay and lesbian AA groups for use in counseling lesbian and gay alcoholics. Assists in the exchange of recorded tapes of lesbian and gay AA speakers. **Pub:** *World Directory of Gay/Lesbian Groups of Alcoholics Anonymous,* annual. Directory. • Newsletter, 4/year. • Also publishes calendar of events and pamphlet. **Frmly:** International Advisory Council for Homosexual Men and Women in Alcoholics Anonymous.

**★ 19350 ★   Women for Sobriety (WFS)**
PO Box 618
Quakertown, PA 18951
**Phone:** (215)536-8026          **Fax:** (215)538-9026
**Email:** newlife@nni.com
**Website:** http://www.womenforsobriety.org
Becky Fenner, Dir.

**Fnded:** 1975. **Mem:** 5,000. **Nat'l Groups:** 200. **Desc:** Self-help groups of women alcoholics who use a program "based on abstinence, comprised of Thirteen Acceptance Statements that, when accepted and used, will provide each woman with a new way of life through a new way of thinking. Starts with coping first but then moves on to overcoming and a whole change in the approach to each day." Recognizes differences between male and female alcoholics in the method of successful recovery. Small groups organize and meet independently. Maintains speakers' bureau. **Pub:** *Sobering Thoughts,* monthly. Newsletter. Contains calendar of events, research updates, membership articles, and news on WFS meetings. *Price:* $14.95/year. • Also publishes tapes, workbooks, booklets, and videos.

**★ 19351 ★   Women's Drug Research Project (WDR)**
c/o Beth G. Reed
University of Michigan
School of Social Work
1065 Frieze Bldg.
Ann Arbor, MI 48109-1285
**Phone:** (734)763-5958
Beth G. Reed, Coord.

**Fnded:** 1973. **Desc:** Has investigated differences in the needs and problems of men and women entering drug abuse treatment programs. Studied two outpatient methadone programs and two residential therapeutic communities, which were established to gather new information about women addicts, their needs, and possible methods for meeting those needs. Also collected data from 20 programs in five cities for studies on treatment organization and psychosocial characteristics of addicts.

★ **19352** ★ **Youth Power**
2000 Franklin St., Ste.400
Oakland, CA 94612-2908
**Free:** 800-258-2766　　　　**Fax:** (510)451-9360
**Email:** youth@youthpower.org
John Demiranda, Exec. Dir.
**Fnded:** 1985. **Mem:** 56,000. **Reg. Groups:** 50. **Desc:** Local clubs comprised of children aged 5-18. Develops, promotes, and evaluates the work of member and affiliate clubs. Conducts research-based programs in youth development and primary prevention including tobacco, alcohol, and illegal substance abuse, dropouts, and teenage pregnancy programs. Sponsors "Just Say No" Awareness Week. **Pub:** *Powerlines*, quarterly. *Price:* Free. • Annual Reports. • Also publishes fact sheets. **Frmly:** (1988) Just Say No Foundation; (1999) Just Say No International.

---

## Research Centers

★ **19353** ★ **Addiction Research and Treatment Corp.**
22 Chapel St.
Brooklyn, NY 11201
**Phone:** (718)260-2917　　　**Fax:** (718)522-3186
**Email:** lbrown@artcny.org
Dr. Lawrence S. Brown, Jr., Sr. VP
**Activities/Fields:** Alcohol and drug addiction, including studies on alcoholism among those addicted to opiates, immunological parameters of drug abuse, stress among patients and staff, and the relationship of patterns of drug abuse and sexual practices to the frequency of human immunodeficiency virus (HIV) infection (exposure to AIDS virus). Conducts clinical trials of drugs for drug abuse and the treatment of HIV disease.

★ **19354** ★ **Arkansas Health Department Alcohol and Drug Abuse Prevention Bureau**
5800 W 10th, Ste. 907
Little Rock, AR 72204
**Phone:** (501)280-4500　　　**Fax:** (501)280-4519
**Email:** rstephen@healthyarkansas.com
Ray L. Stephens, Dir.
**Activities/Fields:** Substance abuse prevention.

★ **19355** ★ **Brown University Center for Alcohol and Addiction Studies**
PO Box G - BH
Providence, RI 02912
**Phone:** (401)444-1800　　　**Fax:** (401)444-1850
**Email:** caas@brown.edu
**Website:** http://www.caas.brown.edu
Peter M. Monti, PhD, Dir.
**Activities/Fields:** Alcohol and addiction studies, including an individual's relationship to alcohol and the effectiveness of community reinforcement on treatment, the relationship between smoking and drinking among alcoholics, matching treatment focus to dysfunction, social skills treatment of cocaine abusers, cue exposure and social skills treatment for alcoholics, deterring preadolescent drug and AIDS-risky behavior, time dynamics of alcohol treatment outcome, treatment research validation and extension program, substance abuse prevention program for Native American youth, hospital intervention services, and healthcare policy. **Pub:** *Digest of Addiction Theory and Application*, monthly.

**Department of Veterans Affairs Medical Center (Portland, OR)**
**Research & Development Service**
*See:* Entry 2482

★ **19356** ★ **Friends Research Institute**
505 Baltimore Ave.
PO Box 10676
Baltimore, MD 21285
**Phone:** (410)823-5116　　　**Fax:** (410)823-5131
**Email:** fri@friendsresearch.org
**Website:** http://www.friendsresearch.org
Patrick F. Bogan, Exec. Dir.
**Activities/Fields:** Studies narcotic addiction to provide statistical documentation of its relation to crime, effectiveness of addiction treatment programs, and HIV as a result of lifestyle. Also conducts pharmaceutical and medical device research. **Pub:** *Newsletter*. **Frmly:** Friends Medical Science Research Center, Inc.

★ **19357** ★ **Johns Hopkins University Behavioral Pharmacology Research Unit**
Johns Hopkins Bayview Campus
5510 Nathan Shock Dr.
Baltimore, MD 21224-6823
**Phone:** (410)550-0035　　　**Fax:** (410)550-0030
**Email:** bigelow@jhmi.edu
George E. Bigelow, PhD, Sci. Dir.
**Activities/Fields:** Human behavioral pharmacology of substance abuse and dependence, including clinical studies on abuse liability assessment, performance effects, and applied treatment interventions for opioids (analgesics) and narcotics, sedatives, anxiolytics, alcohol, tobacco, nicotine, caffeine, and cocaine.

**Legacy Clinical Research and Technology Center**
*See:* Entry 5801

★ **19358** ★ **National Development and Research Institutes, Inc.**
71 W 23rd St., 8th Fl.
New York, NY 10010
**Phone:** (212)845-4400　　　**Fax:** (212)845-4698
**Email:** wagoner@ndri.org
**Website:** http://www.ndri.org
Dr. Fred Streit, Exec. Dir
**Activities/Fields:** Drug abuse, including evaluations of treatment and prevention programs; AIDS research as it relates to substance abuse; epidemiology of drug abuse; drugs and crime; drug abuse and the criminal justice system; street studies of drug sales, use, and prevention; evaluation and enhancement of AIDS outreach; and intervention services for high-risk adolescents. **Frmly:** Narcotic and Drug Research Inc.

★ **19359** ★ **Pittsburgh Adolescent Alcohol Research Center (PAARC)**
3811 O'Hara St.
Pittsburgh, PA 15213
**Phone:** (412)624-2636　　　**Fax:** (412)624-0850
**Email:** clarkdb@msx.upmc.edu
**Website:** http://www.pitt.edu/~paarc/paarc.html
Dr. Duncan B. Clark, Dir.
**Activities/Fields:** Adolescent alcohol abuse and dependence, including biobehavioral manifestations. **Pub:** *Newsletter*.

★ **19360** ★ **Rockefeller University Laboratory of the Biology of Addictive Diseases**
1230 York Ave.
New York, NY 10021-6399
**Phone:** (212)327-8247　　　**Fax:** (212)327-8574
**Email:** kreek@mail.rockefeller.edu
**Website:** http://www.rockefeller.edu
Dr. Mary Jeanne Kreek, Hd.
**Activities/Fields:** Biological basis of opiate, alcohol, and cocaine addiction; the biological correlates of addictive disease, including the physiological and pharmacological effects of chronic drug use; and the medical complications of drug use, especially hepatitis B and C, hepatitis delta, and human immunodeficiency viral infections. Other areas include molecular neurobiology and human molecular genetics of the addictive diseases with special attention on the role of the endogenous opioid system in these disorders, including cocaine dependency and alcoholism, as well as opiate addition; and the role of the endogenous opioids and the specific opioid receptors in the addictive diseases and in normal and abnormal physiology of the neuroendocrine and gastrointestinal systems.

★ **19361** ★ **Rutgers University Center of Alcohol Studies**
607 Allison Rd.
Piscataway, NJ 08854-8001
**Phone:** (732)445-2190　　　**Fax:** (732)445-3500
**Email:** cas2@rci.rutgers.edu
**Website:** http://www.rci.rutgers.edu/~cas2
Robert J. Pandina, PhD, Dir.
**Activities/Fields:** Causes and treatment of alcoholism and drug abuse, diverse actions of alcohol and other drugs on the body, means to prevent alcohol and other drug misuse, and the incidence and prevalence of normal and problem alcohol consumption in the U.S. and the world, including human enzyme systems important in alcohol metabolism, development of tolerance and physical dependence on alcohol, and hormonal changes. **Pub:** *Journal of Studies on Alcohol*, bimonthly. • *Monographs of the Rutgers Center of Alcohol Studies*. • *National Institute of Alcohol Abuse and Alcoholism-Rutgers University Center of Alcohol Studies (NIAAA-RUCAS) Treatment Series*.

★ **19362** ★ **Southern California Research Institute**
11914 W Washington Blvd.
Los Angeles, CA 90066
**Phone:** (310)390-8481　　　**Fax:** (310)398-6651
**Email:** mburns5573@aol.com
**Website:** http://www.scri.org
Dr. Marcelline Burns, Dir.
**Activities/Fields:** Effects of alcohol and drugs on behavior, including effects of alcohol and drugs on driving.

★ **19363** ★ **State University of New York at Buffalo Research Institute on Addictions**
1021 Main St.
Buffalo, NY 14203-1016
**Phone:** (716)887-2566　　　**Fax:** (716)887-2252
**Email:** connors@ria.org
**Website:** http://www.ria.org/
Gerard J. Connors, PhD, Dir.
**Activities/Fields:** Etiology, course, treatment, and prevention of alcoholism and substance abuse. Studies the following six aspects of substance abuse: normative patterns; biochemical, physiological, psychological, and social antecedents and consequences; biopsychosocial aspects of consumption in early and middle adulthood; family aspects; alcohol-drug interactions; and treatment and prevention strategies. **Pub:** *RIA Publications*, annually. • *RIA Report*, quarterly. **Frmly:** Research Institute on Alcoholism.

★ **19364** ★ **U.S. Department of Health and Human Services National Institute on Alcohol Abuse and Alcoholism**
Willco Bldg., Ste. 400
6000 Executive Blvd.
Bethesda, MD 20892-7003
**Phone:** (301)443-3885　　　**Fax:** (301)443-7043
**Email:** rkington@mail.nih.gov
**Website:** http://www.niaaa.nih.gov
Raynard S. Kington, MD, Actg. Dir.
**Activities/Fields:** Prevention and treatment of alcohol-related problems and alcoholism. Seeks to develop new scientific knowledge that will reduce the incidence and prevalence of alcohol abuse and alcoholism and the associated morbidity and mortality. Conducts and supports research aimed at determining the causes of alcoholism, discovering how alcohol damages the organs of the body, and developing

prevention and treatment strategies for application in the nation's health care system. Conducts policy studies with broad implications for alcohol prevention and treatment; and conducts epidemiological studies to assess the risks for and problems among various population groups.

**★ 19365 ★ U.S. Department of Health and Human Services**
**National Institute on Alcohol Abuse and Alcoholism**
**Basic Research Division**
Willco Bldg., Rm. 402
6000 Exec. Blvd.
Bethesda, MD 20892
**Phone:** (301)443-0799 **Fax:** (301)594-0673
**Email:** sz14w@nih.gov
**Website:** http://www.niaaa.nih.gov/extramural/resch-pro.htm
Samir Zakhari, Ch.

**Activities/Fields:** Multiple determinants and processes of alcoholism and other alcohol-related problems. Division administers the Institute's National Alcohol Research Centers Program as well as its research scientists development and training programs. In addition, it collaborates with other national and international agencies, universities, and scientific organizations and provides technical assistance to universities, federal agencies, state and local governments, and community and voluntary organizations. Principal Division components are: Biomedical Research Branch and Neurosciences Research Branch. Research Branch and Neurosciences Research Branch.

**★ 19366 ★ U.S. Department of Health and Human Services**
**National Institute on Alcohol Abuse and Alcoholism**
**Basic Research Division**
**Biomedical Research Branch**
Willco Bldg., St. 402
6000 Executive Blvd., MSC 7003
Bethesda, MD 20892-7003
**Phone:** (301)443-4224 **Fax:** (301)594-0673
Dr. Samir Zakhari, PhD, Dir.

**Activities/Fields:** Supports and administers NIAAA extramural research grants and training programs on the effects of alcohol abuse and alcoholism as related to the central nervous system, the fetal alcohol syndrome, and neuroendocrine and pathological conditions. Research is aimed at reduction of morbidity and mortality associated with alcoholism and alcohol abuse and includes research in the areas of etiology, pathogenesis, identification, treatment, and prevention as well as in the development of basic research tools and methodologies. **Pub:** *Alcohol and Health Monograph Series.*

**★ 19367 ★ U.S. Department of Health and Human Services**
**National Institute on Alcohol Abuse and Alcoholism**
**Basic Research Division**
**Neurosciences and Behavioral Research Branch**
6000 Executive Blvd.
Bethesda, MD 20892-7003
**Phone:** (301)443-4223 **Fax:** (301)594-0673
**Email:** ewitt@willco.niaaa.nih.gov
**Website:** http://www.niaaa.nih.gov/extramural/resch-pro.htm
Ellen Witt, PhD, Contact
**Activities/Fields:** Effect of alcohol on the brain and behavior.

**★ 19368 ★ U.S. Department of Health and Human Services**
**National Institute on Alcohol Abuse and Alcoholism**
**Biometry and Epidemiology Division**
6000 Executive Blvd., MSC 7003
Bethesda, MD 20892-7003
**Phone:** (301)443-3306 **Fax:** (301)443-8614
Mary Dufor, MD, Actg. Dir.

**Activities/Fields:** Incidence and prevalence of alcohol abuse and alcoholism (both nationally and in specific population groups); conducts national surveillance activities to collect and analyze alcohol-related program data through various information systems; and develops and maintains information systems to collect and analyze alcohol-related data. Division also collaborates with other organizations engaged in alcohol data collection activities, such as state-based information systems, in order to exchange pertinent data and to utilize existing data systems where appropriate.

**★ 19369 ★ U.S. Department of Health and Human Services**
**National Institute on Alcohol Abuse and Alcoholism**
**Division of Clinical and Prevention Research**
6000 Executive Blvd.
Willco Bldg., St. 505
Bethesda, MD 20892-7003
**Phone:** (301)443-1206 **Fax:** (301)443-8774
**Email:** rfuller@arswillco.niaaa.nih.gov
**Website:** http://www.niaaa.nih.gov/extramural/resch-pro.htm
Richard K. Fuller, MD, Dir.

**Activities/Fields:** Supports alcohol abuse and alcoholism treatment, prevention, and health services research through grants and cooperative agreements. Principal Division components are the Prevention Research Branch, the Treatment Research Branch, and the Health Services Research Program.

**★ 19370 ★ U.S. Department of Health and Human Services**
**National Institute on Alcohol Abuse and Alcoholism**
**Intramural Clinical and Biological Research Division**
NIH Bldg. 10, Rm. 3C103
9000 Rockville Pike
Bethesda, MD 20892
**Phone:** (301)496-8996 **Fax:** (301)402-0445
**Email:** gkunos@mail.nih.gov
Dr. George Kunos, Dir.

**Activities/Fields:** Multiple determinants and processes of alcoholism and other alcohol-related problems and on prevention, diagnosis, treatment, and rehabilitation. It also provides in-house research scientist training in a variety of disciplines for work in alcohol-related research and collaborates with other agencies, universities, and scientific organizations. Division comprises laboratories of Clinical Studies; Metabolism; Membrane Biochemistry and Biophysics; Molecular and Cellular Neurobiology; and Neurogenetics.

**★ 19371 ★ U.S. Department of Health and Human Services**
**National Institute on Alcohol Abuse and Alcoholism**
**Intramural Clinical and Biological Research Division**
**Clinical Studies Laboratory**
NIH Bldg. 10, Rm. 3C114
9000 Rockville Pike
Bethesda, MD 20892
**Phone:** (301)496-5353 **Fax:** (301)402-0445
Paul Andreas, Contact

**Activities/Fields:** Neuroscience, clinical pharmacology, analytical biochemistry, internal medicine, and psychiatry, all as related to alcoholism.

**★ 19372 ★ U.S. Department of Health and Human Services**
**National Institute on Alcohol Abuse and Alcoholism**
**Intramural Clinical and Biological Research Division**
**Laboratory of Molecular and Cellular Neurobiology**
Park Bldg., Rm. 158
Bethesda, MD 20892-8115
**Phone:** (301)443-1234 **Fax:** (301)480-6882
**Email:** fweight@niaaa.nih.gov
Dr. Forrest Weight, Chf.

**Activities/Fields:** Alcohol and alcoholism, physiology, and pharmacology.

**★ 19373 ★ U.S. Department of Health and Human Services**
**National Institute on Alcohol Abuse and Alcoholism**
**Prevention Research Center**
Pacific Institute for Research and Evaluation
2150 Shattuck Ave., Ste. 900
Berkeley, CA 94704
**Phone:** (510)486-1111 **Fax:** (510)644-0594
**Email:** holder@prev.org
Dr. Harold D. Holder, PhD, Dir.

**Activities/Fields:** Prevention of alcohol-related problems. Research focuses on better understanding the social and physical environment that influences individual behavior and problems relating to alcohol abuse. Objectives are to: develop innovative research and approaches that contribute to informed decisions about cost-effective prevention programs and policies at the local, state, and national levels; contribute to broader theoretical frameworks in the prevention of alcohol-related problems, especially in the area of environmental factors; summarize new and existing knowledge about prevention theories, policies, and programs and disseminate information to professional, academic, and community audiences; and provide.

**U.S. Department of Veterans Affairs**
**Veterans Health Administration**
**Office of Research and Development**
**Medical Research Service**
**(Alcoholism Research Center )**
*See:* Entry 13508

**★ 19374 ★ University of California, Los Angeles**
**Alcohol Research Center**
Neuropsychiatric Institute
760 Westwood Plz.
Los Angeles, CA 90024
**Phone:** (310)825-1891 **Fax:** (310)206-7309
Dr. Ernest P. Noble, Dir.

**Activities/Fields:** Causes of alcoholism, including genetic predisposition.

**★ 19375 ★ University of California, San Francisco**
**Ernest Gallo Clinic and Research Center**
5858 Horton St., Ste. 200
Emeryville, CA 94608
**Phone:** (510)985-3100 **Fax:** (510)985-3888
**Email:** diamond@itsa.ucsf.edu
**Website:** http://www.egcrc.org
Dr. Ivan Diamond, Dir.

**Activities/Fields:** Alcoholism, with special emphasis on molecular, cellular, physiological and genetic mechanisms of tolerance, dependence and addiction to ethanol.

**University of Colorado**
**National Center for American Indian and Alaska Native Mental Health Research**
*See:* Entry 12757

**★ 19376 ★ University of Colorado—Denver**
**Alcohol Research Center**
4200 E 9th Ave.
CB C236
Denver, CO 80262
**Phone:** (303)315-7076     **Fax:** (303)315-7097
**Email:** richard.deitrich@uchsc.edu
**Website:** http://www.uchsc.edu/ctrsinst/alcrc/index.html
Dr. Richard A. Deitrich, Sci. Dir.
**Activities/Fields:** Mechanism of the action of alcohol to determine the ways in which alcohol affects the brain during both acute and chronic periods of intake, including studies on alcohol as a stimulus, different responses elicited by alcohol, and the products of alcohol metabolism. Uses genetic manipulation in animal models to define the acute and chronic affects of alcohol in relation to heredity.

**★ 19377 ★ University of Connecticut**
**Alcohol Research Center**
MC-2103
263 Farmington Ave.
Farmington, CT 06030-1410
**Phone:** (860)679-3423     **Fax:** (860)679-1296
**Email:** hesselb@psych.uchc.edu
Victor Hesselbrock, PhD, Sci. Dir. Prod.
**Activities/Fields:** Genetic, psychiatric, biological, behavioral, and cross-cultural aspects of alcoholism, including alcoholic typologies, treatment matching, familial alcoholism, alcohol dependence syndrome, and early intervention. Activities focus on clinical trials of new psychotherapies and pharmacotherapies, biological responses to alcohol-related stimuli, diagnosis of alcohol dependence, animal studies of neurobiological correlates of alcohol consumption, ASP and family history variables as risk factors in the development of alcohol dependence, and research on treatment services for alcoholics.

**★ 19378 ★ University of Kentucky**
**Center on Drug and Alcohol Research**
643 Maxwelton Ct.
Lexington, KY 40506-0350
**Phone:** (859)257-2355     **Fax:** (859)323-1193
**Email:** cleukef@uky.edu
**Website:** http://www.uky.edu/RGS/cdar/cdar2.htm
Dr. Carl G. Leukefeld, Dir.
**Activities/Fields:** Biological, social, and psychological aspects of alcohol and drug abuse; and HIV/AIDS. Conducts household and other surveys. **Frmly:** Multidisciplinary Research Center on Drug and Alcohol Abuse.

**★ 19379 ★ University of Manitoba**
**Alcohol and Tobacco Research Unit**
Department of Community Health Sciences
MS-740B
S111-750 Bannatyne Ave.
Winnipeg, MB, Canada R3E 0W3
**Phone:** (204)789-3473     **Fax:** (204)789-3905
**Email:** rmurray@hsc.mb.ca
**Website:** http://www.umanitoba.ca/faculties/medicine/chs/department/alcoh.html
Dr. Robert P. Murray, Contact
**Activities/Fields:** Health, behavioral, social and economic correlates and consequences of the use of alcohol, tobacco and other drugs consumed for non-therapeutic purposes.

**★ 19380 ★ University of Michigan**
**Addiction Research Center**
Bldg. 2, Ste. A
Substance Abuse Div.
Department of Psychiatry
400 E Eisenhower Pky.
Ann Arbor, MI 48108-0740
**Phone:** (734)615-6060     **Fax:** (734)615-6085
**Email:** zuckerra@umich.edu
**Website:** http://www.med.umich.edu/psych/sub/index.html
Dr. Robert A. Zucker, Dir.
**Activities/Fields:** Developmental psychopathology and genetics of substance use disorders, alcohol problems among the elderly, etiology and treatment of alcoholism, treatment outcomes and other health services research with alcohol and other substance abusing patients, pharmacotherapy trials, efficacy of brief intervention techniques with alcohol abusing populations. **Frmly:** Alcohol Research Center.

**★ 19381 ★ University of North Carolina at Chapel Hill**
**Bowles Center for Alcohol Studies**
CB 7178
Thurston-Bowles Bldg.
Chapel Hill, NC 27599-7178
**Phone:** (919)966-5678     **Fax:** (919)966-5679
**Email:** ftcrews@med.unc.edu
**Website:** http://www.med.unc.edu/alcohol/
Fulton T. Crews, PhD, Dir.
**Activities/Fields:** Broad range of studies on alcohol effects on brain, liver and fetus. **Pub:** *Centerline Newsletter.* **Frmly:** Center for Alcohol Studies.

**★ 19382 ★ University of Pennsylvania**
**Substance Abuse Treatment Unit**
Bldg. 7, 116-D
VA Medical Center
28 Woodland Ave.
Philadelphia, PA 19104
**Phone:** (215)823-5188     **Fax:** (215)823-4248
James Kurtz, MD, Dir.
**Activities/Fields:** Alcohol and drug dependence, including research on psychotherapy, endocrine system, alcoholism and schizophrenia, methadone-maintained cocaine abusers, and outpatient versus inpatient detoxification.

**University of Texas—Houston Health Science Center**
**Mental Sciences Institute**
*See:* Entry 12777

**University of Toronto**
**Centre for Health Promotion**
**Ontario Tobacco Research Unit**
*See:* Entry 9082

**University of Washington**
**Alcohol and Drug Abuse Institute**
*See:* Entry 12780

**★ 19383 ★ Wright State University**
**Rehabilitation Research and Training Center on Drugs and Disability**
Sch. of Medicine
PO Box 927
Dayton, OH 45401-0927
**Phone:** (937)775-1484     **Fax:** (937)775-1495
**Email:** sardi@wright.edu
**Website:** http://www.med.wright.edu/SOM/SARDI/
Dennis Moore, EdD, Dir.
**Activities/Fields:** Substance abuse issues among individuals qualifying for vocational rehabilitation services. **Pub:** *Online newsletter,* 3/year.

# State Government Agencies

## Substance Abuse

**★ 19384 ★ Alabama Department of Mental Health and Mental Retardation**
**Substance Abuse Services Division**
100 N Union St.
PO Box 301410
Montgomery, AL 36130-1410
**Phone:** (334)242-3107
**Website:** http://www.mh.state.al.us/services/sa/samain.html
John Houston, Contact

**★ 19385 ★ Alaska Department of Health and Social Services**
**Alcoholism and Drug Abuse Division**
240 Main St., Ste. 701
PO Box 110607
Juneau, AK 99811-0607
**Phone:** (907)465-2071     **Free:** 800-478-2072
**Fax:** (907)465-2185
**Website:** http://www.hss.state.ak.us/dada/
Carl Lewis, Contact

**★ 19386 ★ Arizona Department of Health Services**
**Behavioral Health Services Division**
**Substance Abuse Office**
2122 E Highland
Phoenix, AZ 85016
**Phone:** (602)381-8999     **Fax:** (602)553-9143
**Email:** cdye@hs.state.az.us
**Website:** http://www.hs.state.az.us/bhs/bsagmh.htm

**★ 19387 ★ Arkansas Department of Health**
**Alcohol and Drug Abuse Prevention Division**
4815 W Markham
Little Rock, AR 72205
**Phone:** (501)280-4500     **Fax:** (501)280-4519
**Website:** http://health.state.ar.us/
Tommie J. Waters, Contact

**★ 19388 ★ California Health and Welfare Agency**
**Alcohol and Drug Programs Department**
1700 K St.
Sacramento, CA 95814
**Phone:** (916)445-1943
**Website:** http://www.adp.cahwnet.gov

**★ 19389 ★ Colorado Department of Human Services**
**Alcohol and Drug Abuse Division**
4055 S Lowell Blvd.
Denver, CO 80236
**Phone:** (303)866-7480     **Fax:** (303)866-7481
**Email:** randall.deyle@state.co.us
**Website:** http://www.cdhs.state.co.us/ohr/adad/index.html
Janet Wood, Director

**★ 19390 ★ Connecticut Department of Mental Health and Addiction Services**
**Addiction Services**
410 Capitol Ave., 4th Fl.
PO Box 341431
Hartford, CT 06134
**Phone:** (860)418-7000     **Free:** 800-446-7348
**Website:** http://www.dmhas.state.ct.us/

★ 19391 ★ **Delaware Department of Health and Social Services**
**Alcoholism, Drug Abuse, and Mental Health Division**
1901 N Dupont Hwy.
New Castle, DE 19720
**Phone:** (302)255-9247          **Fax:** (302)255-4427
**Email:** dhssinfo@state.de.us
**Website:** http://www.state.de.us/dhss/dadamh/dmhhome.htm
Renata J. Henry, Director

★ 19392 ★ **District of Columbia Department of Human Services**
**Public Health Commission**
**Alcohol and Drug Abuse Administration**
1300 1st St., NE
Washington, DC 20002
**Phone:** (202)727-9393          **Fax:** (202)727-0092
**Website:** http://www.dchealth.com/welcome.htm

★ 19393 ★ **Florida Department of Children and Families**
**Human Services Program Office**
**Alcohol, Drug Abuse and Mental Health Office**
1317 Winewood Blvd. Bldg. 6 Room 300
Tallahassee, FL 32399-0700
**Phone:** (850)487-2920
**Website:** http://www5.myflorida.com/cf_web/myflorida2/healthhuman/ddp/

★ 19394 ★ **Georgia Department of Human Resources**
**Mental Health, Developmental Disabilities, Addictive Diseases**
**Alcohol and Drug Abuse Services Office**
2 Peachtree St., NW
Atlanta, GA 30303
**Phone:** (404)657-2272          **Fax:** (404)657-2107
**Email:** xwiggins@dmh.dhr.state.ga.us
**Website:** http://www2.state.ga.us/departments/dhr/mhmrsa.html

★ 19395 ★ **Hawaii Department of Health**
**Behavioral Health Administration**
**Alcohol and Drug Abuse Division**
601 Kamokila Blvd.
Kapolei, HI 96707
**Phone:** (808)692-7506
**Website:** http://www.state.hi.us/health/resource/drug_abuse.html
Elaine J. Wilson, Director

★ 19396 ★ **Idaho Department of Health and Welfare**
**Family and Community Services Division**
**Substance Abuse Bureau**
450 W State St., 5th Fl.
PO Box 83720
Boise, ID 83720-0036
**Phone:** (208)334-5593          **Free:** 800-926-2588
**Fax:** (208)334-6699
**Email:** connorc@idhw.state.id.us
**Website:** http://www2.state.id.us/dhw/mentalhealth/index.htm
Pharis Stanger, Contact

★ 19397 ★ **Indiana Family and Social Services Administration**
**Addiction Services Division**
**Division of Mental Health**
402 W Washington St., Rm. W353
Indianapolis, IN 46204-2739
**Phone:** (317)232-7939          **Free:** 800-901-1133
**Fax:** (317)233-3472
**Website:** http://www.ai.org/fssa/dmh/index.html
Janet Corson, Director

★ 19398 ★ **Iowa Department of Public Health**
**Substance Abuse and Health Promotion Division**
Lucas State Office Bldg.
321 E 12th St.
Des Moines, IA 50319
**Phone:** (515)281-4417
**Email:** webmaster@idph.state.ia.us
**Website:** http://idph.state.ia.us/SA.HTM

★ 19399 ★ **Kansas Department of Social and Rehabilitation Services**
**Alcohol and Drug Abuse Services**
915 SW Harrison St.
Topeka, KS 66612
**Phone:** (785)296-3271
**Website:** http://www.srskansas.org/hcp/mhsatr/mhsatr.htm
Janet Schalansky, Contact

★ 19400 ★ **Kentucky Health Services Cabinet**
**Mental Health and Mental Retardation Department**
**Substance Abuse Division**
100 Fair Oaks Ln., 4E-D
Frankfort, KY 40621-0001
**Phone:** (502)564-2880          **Fax:** (502)564-7152
**Email:** webmaster@rdmc.org
**Website:** http://dmhmrs.chr.state.ky.us/SA/

★ 19401 ★ **Louisiana Department of Health and Hospitals**
**Louisiana Office for Addictive Disorders**
1201 Capitol Access Rd.
PO Box 2790, Bin 18
Baton Rouge, LA 70821-2790
**Phone:** (225)342-6717          **Fax:** (225)342-3875
**Email:** webmaster@dhh.state.la.us
**Website:** http://www.dhh.state.la.us/OADA/index.htm

★ 19402 ★ **Maine Office of the Governor**
**Substance Abuse Office**
159 State House Station
A.M.H.I. Complex, Marquardt Buidling
Augusta, ME 04333-0159
**Phone:** (207)287-2595          **Fax:** (207)287-4334
**Email:** kimberly.johnson@state.me.us
**Website:** http://www.state.me.us/dmhmrsa/osa/
Kimberly Johnson, Contact

★ 19403 ★ **Maryland Department of Health and Mental Hygiene**
**Alcohol and Drug Abuse Administration**
55 Wade Ave.
Catonsville, MD 21228
**Phone:** (410)402-8600          **Fax:** (410)402-8601
**Email:** adaainfo@dhmh.state.md.us
**Website:** http://maryland-adaa.org/
Peter F. Luongo, PhD, Director

★ 19404 ★ **Massachusetts Executive Office of Health and Human Services**
**Public Health Department**
**Substance Abuse Services Bureau**
250 Washington St., 3rd Fl.
Boston, MA 02108
**Phone:** (617)624-5111          **Fax:** (617)624-5185
**Email:** BSAS.questions@state.ma.us
**Website:** http://www.state.ma.us/dph/bsas/bsas.htm
Deborah Klein Walker, Director

★ 19405 ★ **Michigan Community Health Department**
**Drug Control and Substance Abuse Services Office**
Lewis Cass Bldg, 6th floor
320 S Walnut St.
Lansing, MI 48913
**Phone:** (517)373-3500          **Fax:** (517)335-2671
**Email:** yaldooc@michigan.gov
**Website:** http://www.michigan.gov/mdch/
Craig Yaldoo, Director

★ 19406 ★ **Minnesota Department of Human Services**
**Health and Continuing Care Strategies**
**Chemical Health Division**
444 Lafayette Rd. N
Saint Paul, MN 55155
**Phone:** (651)582-1832
**Email:** dhs.info@state.mn.us
**Website:** http://www.dhs.state.mn.us/contcare/default.htm

★ 19407 ★ **Missouri Department of Mental Health**
**Alcohol and Drug Abuse Division**
1706 E Elm St.
PO Box 687
Jefferson City, MO 65102
**Phone:** (573)751-4942
**Email:** dmhmail@mail.dmh.state.mo.us
**Website:** http://www.modmh.state.mo.us/ada/index.html
Michael Couty, Director

★ 19408 ★ **Montana Department of Public Health and Human Services**
**Addictive and Mental Disorders Division**
PO Box 202905
PO Box 202951
Helena, MT 59620-2905
**Phone:** (406)444-3964          **Fax:** (406)444-4435
**Email:** daanderson@state.mt.gov
**Website:** http://www.dphhs.state.mt.us/divisions/amd/amd.htm
Dan Anderson, Director

★ 19409 ★ **Nebraska Department of Health and Human Services**
**Mental Health, Substance Abuse and Addiction Services Office**
PO Box 98925
Lincoln, NE 68509-8925
**Phone:** (402)479-5166
**Email:** hhsinfo@www.hhs.state.ne.us
**Website:** http://www.hhs.state.ne.us/sua/beh_sua.htm
Ron Sorensen, Director

★ 19410 ★ **Nevada Department of Employment Training and Rehabilitation**
**Rehabilitation Division**
**Alcohol and Drug Abuse Bureau**
500 E 3rd St.
Carson City, NV 89713-0021
**Phone:** (775)687-4790
**Email:** detrvr@nvdetr.org
**Website:** http://detr.state.nv.us/rehab/reh%5Fgen.htm

★ 19411 ★ **New Hampshire Department of Health and Human Services**
**Alcohol & Drug Abuse Prevention & Recovery Division**
105 Pleasant St.
Concord, NH 03301-3857
**Phone:** (603)271-6100          **Fax:** (603)271-6116
**Website:** http://www.dhhs.state.nh.us/

**★ 19412 ★ New Jersey Department of Health**
**Addiction Services Division**
120 S Stockton St.
PO Box 362
Trenton, NJ 08625-0362
**Phone:** (609)984-0895
**Email:** tpb@doh.state.nj.us
**Website:** http://www.state.nj.us/health/as/addsrvs.htm
Theodore P. Bucon, Director

**★ 19413 ★ New Mexico Department of Health**
**Behavioral Health Services Division**
Harold Runnels Bldg.
1190 S St. Francis Dr.
PO Box 26110
Santa Fe, NM 87502-6110
**Phone:** (505)827-2601          **Free:** 800-362-2013
**Email:** pbrown@health.state.nm.us
**Website:** http://www.health.state.nm.us/

**★ 19414 ★ New York State Office of Alcohol and Substance Abuse Services**
1450 Western Ave.
Albany, NY 12203-3526
**Phone:** (518)473-3460
**Email:** info@oasas.state.ny.us
**Website:** http://www.oasas.state.ny.us/

**★ 19415 ★ North Carolina Department of Health and Human Services**
Mental Health, Developmental Disabilities and Substance Abuse Services Division
**Substance Abuse Services Section**
3007 Mail Service Ctr.
325 N Salisbury St.
Raleigh, NC 27699-3007
**Phone:** (919)733-4670          **Fax:** (919)733-9455
**Email:** jo.yarbrough@ncmail.net
**Website:** http://www.dhhs.state.nc.us/mhddsas/
Jo Yarbrough, Contact

**★ 19416 ★ North Dakota Department of Human Services**
Mental Health and Substance Abuse Services
**Alcoholism and Drug Abuse Issues**
600 S Second St., Ste 1E
Bismarck, ND 58504
**Phone:** (701)328-8920          **Free:** 800-642-6042
**Fax:** (701)328-8979
**Email:** soerhk@state.nd.us
**Website:** http://lnotes.state.nd.us/dhs/dhsweb.nsf/88f6de947ec9f2778625663c006afc52/83f8cbc7e20b76398625666d007f3b73?OpenDocument

**★ 19417 ★ Ohio Department of Alcohol and Drug Addiction Services**
280 N High St., 12th Fl.
Columbus, OH 43215-2537
**Phone:** (614)466-3445          **Fax:** (614)752-8645
**Email:** general@ada.state.oh.us
**Website:** http://www.state.oh.us/ada/odada.htm
Luceille Fleming, Director

**★ 19418 ★ Oklahoma Department of Mental Health**
**Substance Abuse Services**
1200 NE 13th St.
PO Box 53277
Oklahoma City, OK 73152-3277
**Phone:** (405)522-3908
**Email:** rbrown@odmhsas.org
**Website:** http://www.odmhsas.org/subab.htm
Terry Cline, PhD, Director

**★ 19419 ★ Oregon Department of Human Resources**
**Alcohol and Drug Abuse Programs Office**
500 Summer St. NE, E86
Salem, OR 97301-1118
**Phone:** (503)945-5763          **Fax:** (503)378-8467
**Email:** oadap.info@state.or.us
**Website:** http://www.oadap.hr.state.or.us/
Ann Brand, PhD, Director

**★ 19420 ★ Pennsylvania Department of Health**
Health Promotion, Disease and Substance Abuse Prevention
**Drug and Alcohol Programs Bureau**
Health and Welfare Bldg.
PO Box 90
Harrisburg, PA 17108
**Phone:** (717)783-8200
**Email:** webmaster@health.state.pa.us
**Website:** http://www.health.state.pa.us/PHP/SCA/default.htm

**★ 19421 ★ Rhode Island Division of Behavioral Healthcare**
**Substance Abuse Treatment and Prevention Services**
14 Harrington Rd.
Cranston, RI 02920
**Phone:** (401)462-2338          **Fax:** (401)462-6078
**Website:** http://www.mhrh.state.ri.us/Behavioral_Health.htm
Craig S. Stenning, Director

**★ 19422 ★ South Carolina Department of Alcohol and Other Drug Abuse Services**
101 Business Park Blvd.
Columbia, SC 29203-9498
**Phone:** (803)896-5555          **Fax:** (803)896-5557
**Email:** lgrant@daodas.state.sc.us
**Website:** http://www.daodas.state.sc.us./web/
Wendell Price, Director

**★ 19423 ★ South Dakota Department of Human Services**
**Alcohol and Drug Abuse Division**
Hillsview Plaza, E Hwy 34
c/o 500 E Capitol
Pierre, SD 57501
**Phone:** (605)773-3123          **Fax:** (605)773-7076
**Email:** infodada@dhs.state.sd.us
**Website:** http://www.state.sd.us/dhs/ADA/index.htm
Gilbert Sudbeck, Director

**★ 19424 ★ Tennessee Department of Health**
**Alcohol and Drug Abuse Services Bureau**
Cordell Hull Bldg.
425 5th Ave. N
Nashville, TN 37247-4401
**Phone:** (615)741-1921          **Fax:** (615)532-2419
**Website:** http://www2.state.tn.us/health/A&D/information.htm

**★ 19425 ★ Texas Commission on Alcohol and Drug Abuse**
9001 N IH 35, Ste. 105
PO Box 80529
Austin, TX 78708
**Phone:** (512)349-6600          **Free:** 800-832-9623
**Email:** contact@tcada.state.tx.us
**Website:** http://www.tcada.state.tx.us/

**★ 19426 ★ Utah Department of Human Services**
**Substance Abuse Division**
120 N 200 W, Rm. 201
PO Box 45500
Salt Lake City, UT 84103
**Phone:** (801)538-3939          **Fax:** (801)538-4696
**Website:** http://www.hsdsa.state.ut.us/

**★ 19427 ★ Vermont Agency of Human Services**
**Alcohol and Drug Abuse Programs Division**
108 Cherry St.
PO Box 70
Burlington, VT 05402-0070
**Phone:** (802)651-1550          **Fax:** (802)651-1573
**Email:** vtadap@vdh.state.vt.us
**Website:** http://www.state.vt.us/adap/
Marcia LaPlante, Director

**★ 19428 ★ Virginia Office of Health and Human Resources**
Mental Health, Retardation and Substance Abuse Services Department
**Substance Abuse Services Division**
PO Box 1797
Richmond, VA 23218
**Phone:** (804)786-3906          **Fax:** (804)371-0091
**Email:** rjohnson@dmhmrsas.state.va.us
**Website:** http://www.dmhmrsas.state.va.us/
Robert L. Johnson, Contact

**★ 19429 ★ Washington Department of Social and Health Services**
Health and Rehabilitative Services Office
**Alcohol and Substance Abuse Division**
PO Box 45130
Olympia, WA 98504-5130
**Free:** 877-301-4557
**Email:** askdshs@dshs.wa.gov
**Website:** http://www.wa.gov/dshs/hrsa/hrsa3ov.html

**★ 19430 ★ West Virginia Department of Health and Human Resources**
Community Support Bureau
Behavioral Health Services Office
**Alcoholism and Drug Abuse Division**
350 Capitol St., Rm. 350
Charleston, WV 25301-3702
**Phone:** (304)558-4224          **Fax:** (304)558-1008
**Email:** stevemason@wvdhhr.org
**Website:** http://www.wvdhhr.org/obhs/
Steve Mason, Director

**★ 19431 ★ Wisconsin Department of Health and Family Services**
Supportive Living Division
**Substance Abuse Bureau**
1 Wilson St., Rm. 434
Madison, WI 53702
**Phone:** (608)266-0040
**Email:** langkj@dhfs.state.wi.us
**Website:** http://www.dhfs.state.wi.us/substabuse/index.htm
Keith Lang, Contact

**★ 19432 ★ Wyoming Department of Health**
Behavioral Health Community Programs Division
**Substance Abuse Division**
2424 Pioneer Ave., Ste. 306
Cheyenne, WY 82002
**Free:** 800-535-4006          **Fax:** (307)777-7006
**Email:** info@state.wy.us
**Website:** http://substanceabuse.state.wy.us/
Diane Galloway, PhD, Director

## Foundations & Other Funding Organizations

### Other Funding Organizations

**★ 19433 ★ Academy of Surgical Research (ASR)**
13355 10th Ave. N, Ste. 108
Minneapolis, MN 55441-5510
**Phone:** (763)765-2300     **Fax:** (763)765-2329
**Email:** director@surgicalresearch.org
**Website:** http://www.surgicalresearch.org
Patricia Nolt, Exec. Dir.

**Desc:** Individuals, organizations, and corporations with an interest in surgical research. Seeks to advance surgical techniques and equipment through improved research. Facilitates cooperation and exchange of information among members; fosters interdisciplinary transfer of ideas to advance surgical research. **Awards:** Barry Sauer Award (annual); C. William Hall Award (annual); Markowitz Award (annual) various; Von Recum Award (annual).

**★ 19434 ★ America Society of Plastic Surgeons (ASPS)**
444 E Algonquin Rd.
Arlington Heights, IL 60005
**Phone:** (847)228-9900     **Free:** 888-4-PLASTIC
**Fax:** (847)228-9131
**Website:** http://www.plasticsurgery.org
Edward Luce, MD, Pres.

**Desc:** Plastic surgeons. Dedicated to quality patient care and to maintain professional and ethical standards through education, research, and advocacy of socioeconomic and other professional activities. **Awards:** Circle of Excellence Media Awards (annual) offered to newspapers, magazines, radio, television, news services, and news web sites.

**★ 19435 ★ American Academy of Facial Plastic and Reconstructive Surgery (AAFPRS)**
310 S Henry St.
Alexandria, VA 22314
**Phone:** (703)299-9291     **Free:** 800-332-FACE
**Fax:** (703)299-8898
**Email:** info@aafprs.org
**Website:** http://www.facemd.org
Stephen C. Duffy, Exec. VP

**Desc:** Physicians specializing in facial plastic surgery. Promotes research and study in the field. Maintains speakers' bureau. Conducts educational and charitable programs; compiles statistics. **Awards:** Ben Shuster Memorial (annual) for the most outstanding research paper by a resident or fellow in trainig on any clinical work or research in facial plastc and reconstructive surgery delivered at a national meeting (or its equivalent) between March 1 and February 28; Bernstein Award (annual) for an AAFPRS Fellow member who is conducting original research which will advance facial plastic and reconstructive surgery; Community Service (annual) for any member who has distinguished himself/herself by providing and/or making possible free medical service to the poor in his/her community; F. Mark Rafaty Memorial (annual) for any member who has made outstanding contributions to facial plastic and reconstructive surgery; Investigator Development Award (annual) for AAFPRS member who is conducting significant clinical or labo ratory research and for the training of resident surgeons in research; Ira Tresley Research Award (annual) for the best original research in facial plastic surgery by an AAFPRS member who has been board certified for at least three years; John Dickinson Teacher (annual) for a Fellow member for sharing knowledge about facial plastic surgery with the effective use of audiovisuals over a number of years; John Orlando Roe (annual) for the graduate fellow who submits the best scholarly paper written during fellowship; Resident Research Award (annual) for residents who are AAFPRS members; Sir Harold Delf Gillies (annual) for the graduate fellow who submits the best research paper written during fellowship; William Wright (annual) for a member who has made outstanding contributions to facial plastic and reconstructive surgery.

**★ 19436 ★ American Academy of Orthopaedic Surgeons (AAOS)**
6300 N River Rd.
Rosemont, IL 60018-4262
**Phone:** (847)823-7186     **Free:** 800-346-AAOS
**Fax:** (847)823-8125
**Email:** custserv@aaos.org
**Website:** http://www.aaos.org
Dr. William Tipton, Exec. VP

**Desc:** Professional society of orthopedic surgeons certified by the American Board of Orthopedic Surgery to practice orthopedic (bone and joint) surgery. Promotes physician education and skills enhancement by offering textbooks, clinical videotapes, courses and self-assessment exams. **Awards:** Humanitarian Award (annual); International Award (annual); Kappa Delta (annual); National Award (annual).

**★ 19437 ★ American Academy of Otolaryngology - Head and Neck Surgery (AAO-HNS)**
1 Prince St.
Alexandria, VA 22314-3357
**Phone:** (703)836-4444     **Fax:** (703)683-5100
**Email:** webmaster@enthet.org
**Website:** http://www.entnet.org
KJ Lee, MD, Exec. VP

**Desc:** Professional society of medical doctors specializing in otolaryngology (diseases of the ear, nose, and throat) and head and neck surgery. Represents otolaryngology in governmental and socioeconomic areas and provides high-quality medical education for otolaryngologists. Coordinates Combined Otolaryngological Spring Meetings for ten national otolaryngological societies. Operates job information exchange service and museum. **Awards:** Grant for research; Honor Award (annual); Humanitarian Efforts Award (annual); Presidential Award (annual).

**★ 19438 ★ American Association for Hand Surgery (AAHS)**
20 N Michigan Ave., Ste. 700
Chicago, IL 60602
**Phone:** (312)236-3307     **Fax:** (312)782-0553
**Email:** contact@handsurgery.org
**Website:** http://www.handsurgery.org
Laura Downes Leeper, CAE, Exec. Dir.

**Desc:** Plastic, orthopedic, general surgeons, and physical and occupational therapists having a specific interest in hand surgery; individuals in the medical profession, basic sciences, or allied services interested in the improvement of hand surgery. Purpose is to advance hand surgery. Conducts symposia; offers specialized education. **Awards:** Research Grants (annual) based on proposal submission.

**American Association of Oral and Maxillofacial Surgeons (AAOMS)**
*See:* Entry 6331

**★ 19439 ★ American College of Foot and Ankle Surgeons (ACFAS)**
515 Busse Hwy.
Park Ridge, IL 60068
**Phone:** (847)292-2237     **Free:** 800-421-2237
**Fax:** (847)292-2022
**Email:** mail@acfas.org
**Website:** http://www.acfas.org/
Thomas R. Schedler, CAE, Exec. Dir.

**Desc:** Objectives are to: promote and disseminate information on podiatric surgery among the public, podiatric surgeons, and other health professionals; encourage and publish research findings and related literature; provide intensive programs for clinical and experimental research to improve podiatric surgery and to promote our members' professional and socioeconomic activities. **Awards:** Abstract Award (annual); Journal Article Award (annual); Research Award (annual).

**★ 19440 ★ American College of Surgeons (ACS)**
633 N Saint Clair St.
Chicago, IL 60611-3211
**Phone:** (312)202-5000     **Fax:** (312)202-5001
**Email:** postmaster@facs.org
**Website:** http://www.facs.org
Thomas Russell, MD, Exec. Dir.

**Desc:** Professional association of surgeons worldwide organized primarily to improve the quality of care for surgical patients by elevating the standards of surgical education and practice. Conducts nationwide programs to improve emergency medical services and hospital cancer programs. Sponsors continuing education and self-assessment courses for surgeons in practice. **Awards:** Australia/New Zealand Traveling Fellowship (periodic); Distinguished Service Award (annual); International Guest Scholarship (periodic) surgeons from overseas; Research Scholarship (periodic).

**★ 19441 ★ American Foundation for Surgery of the Hand (AFSH)**
6300 N River Rd., Ste. 600
Rosemont, IL 60018-4256
**Phone:** (847)384-8300          **Fax:** (847)384-1435
**Email:** info@hand-surg.org
**Website:** http://www.assh.org
Mark Anderson, Exec. Dir.
**Desc:** Awards grants to medical, educational, research, and public education programs related to the field of hand and upper extremity surgery. **Awards:** Grant bestowed to medical, educational, research, and public education programs related to the field of hand and upper extremity surgery.

**★ 19442 ★ American Head and Neck Society (AHNS)**
601 N Caroline, Rm. 6254
Baltimore, MD 21287
**Phone:** (410)647-2227          **Fax:** (410)647-8944
**Email:** rwagner@pitt.edu
**Website:** http://www.headandneckcancer.org
Keith S. Heller, MD, Pres.
**Desc:** Otolaryngologists and other physicians with board certification whose primary interest is head and neck oncology. Associate membership is for other other practioners who treat head and neck cancer. Seeks to advance knowledge relevant to treatment of diseases of the head and neck, including reconstruction and rehabilitation. Promotes development of programs of training in head and neck oncology. **Awards:** Research Award (annual) competition for best head and neck cancer research; Resident Awards.

**★ 19443 ★ American Society for Bariatric Surgery (ASBS)**
7328 W University Ave., Ste. F
Gainesville, FL 32607
**Phone:** (352)331-4900          **Fax:** (352)331-4975
**Email:** info@asbs.org
**Website:** http://www.asbs.org
Georgeann Mallory, Exec. Dir.
**Desc:** Works to advance the art and science of bariatric surgery. Supports clinical and laboratory investigations; promotes guidelines for ethical patient care; conducts educational programs for physicians, paramedicals and lay people; provides a forum for the exchange of ideas. **Awards:** Resident/Trainee Award (annual) for a resident or trainee in the field of bariatric surgery.

**★ 19444 ★ American Society of Maxillofacial Surgeons (ASMS)**
4900B S 31st. St.
Arlington, VA 22206-1656
**Phone:** (703)820-7400          **Fax:** (703)931-4520
**Email:** admin@maxface.org
**Website:** http://www.maxface.org
Thomas F. Fise, Exec. Dir.
**Desc:** Professional society of doctors of medicine and doctors of dental surgery who have at least five years of recognized graduate training and experience in maxillofacial surgery. Seeks to stimulate and advance knowledge of the science and art of maxillofacial surgery and improve and elevate the standard of practice. **Awards:** Research Grant Awards (annual).

**★ 19445 ★ American Society of Plastic Surgeons and Plastic Surgery Education Foundation (ASPRS)**
444 E Algonquin Rd.
Arlington Heights, IL 60005
**Phone:** (847)228-9900          **Free:** 888-4-PLASTIC
**Fax:** (847)228-9131
**Website:** http://www.plasticsurgery.org
Edward Luce, MD, Pres.
**Desc:** Professional society of plastic surgeons. Works in \cooperation with the Plastic Surgery Educational Foundation to promote optimal care for plastic surgery patients through research, service, and education activities. Sponsors public/patient education program,

clinical symposia, and professional development workshops. Acts as a liaison between members and government and medical organizations. Conducts charitable activities; maintains speakers' bureau; compiles statistics. **Awards:** Circle of Excellence Journalism Award (annual) to newspapers, wire services, magazines, radio, or TV.

**American Society of Plastic Surgical Nurses (ASPSN)**
*See:* Entry 14919

**★ 19446 ★ American Surgical Association (ASA)**
c/o Robert P. Jones, Jr., Ed.D.
13 Elm St.
Manchester, MA 01944-1314
**Phone:** (978)526-8330          **Fax:** (978)526-7521
**Email:** asa@prri.com
Carlos A. Pellegrini, MD, Sec.
**Desc:** Surgeons organized to promote the science and art of surgery. Bestows medallion for scientific achievement. **Awards:** American Surgical Association Foundation Fellowship (annual) US citizen or permanent resident with a M.D. or equivalent medical degree who has completed an ACGME approved residency and hold a faculty appointment in an accredited medical school or similar medical institution.

**Association of Bone and Joint Surgeons (ABJS)**
*See:* Entry 16905

**★ 19447 ★ Association for Surgical Education (ASE)**
SIU School of Medicine
Department of Surgery
PO Box 19655
Springfield, IL 62794-9655
**Phone:** (217)545-3835          **Fax:** (217)524-2431
**Email:** membershipo@surgicaleducation.com
**Website:** http://www.surgicaleducation.com
Susan Kepner, Exec. Dir.
**Desc:** Surgeons and individuals involved or interested in undergraduate surgical education. Purpose is to develop and disseminate information on motivation, techniques, research, and applications for presenting curricula in undergraduate surgical education. Acts as forum for research in surgical education; serves as information clearinghouse. Compiles statistics; maintains speakers' bureau. Conducts educational programs. **Awards:** Best Paper Award (annual); Presidential Teaching Award (annual) for research in surgical education.

**★ 19448 ★ Association of Surgical Technologists (AST)**
7108-C S Alton Way
Englewood, CO 80112-2106
**Phone:** (303)694-9130          **Fax:** (303)694-9169
**Email:** kludwig@ast.org
**Website:** http://www.ast.org
William J. Teutsch, Exec. Dir.
**Desc:** Individuals who have received specific education and training to deliver surgical patient care in the operating room. Membership categories are available for both certified and student surgical technologists. Emphasis is placed on encouraging members to participate actively in a continuing education program. Aims are: to study, discuss, and exchange knowledge, experience, and ideas in the field of surgical technology; to promote a high standard of surgical technology performance in the community for quality patient care; to stimulate interest in continuing education. Local groups sponsor workshops and institutes. Conducts research. **Awards:** AST Scholarship (annual) for students enrolled in CAAHEP-accredited programs.

**Foundation for Hand Research and Education**
*See:* Entry 13525

**★ 19449 ★ International Society of Arthroscopy, Knee Surgery and Orthopaedic Sports Medicine (ISAKOS)**
145 Town and Country Dr., Ste. 106
Danville, CA 94526-3963
**Phone:** (925)314-7920          **Fax:** (925)314-7922
**Email:** isako@isakos.com
**Website:** http://www.isakos.com
Michelle Johnson, Soc. Mgr.
**Desc:** Orthopaedic surgeons specializing in problems of the knee, arthroscopy, orthopaedic sports medicine. **Awards:** Albert Trillot Award (biennial); John T. Joyce Award (biennial).

**★ 19450 ★ Interplast**
300-B Pioneer Way
Mountain View, CA 94041-1506
**Phone:** (650)962-0123          **Free:** 888-467-5278
**Fax:** (650)962-1619
**Email:** ipnews@interplast.org
**Website:** http://www.interplast.org
Susan W. Hayes, Pres. /CEO
**Desc:** Sends volunteer teams of medical professionals to developing countries to perform free reconstructive surgery on patients with birth defects, burns, and other crippling deformities. Plans include travel to foreign sites such as Mongolia, Peru, Ecuador, Vietnam, Thailand, Chile, Nepal, Honduras, Brazil, Dominican Republic, Bangladesh, Ukraine and the Phillippines to perform an estimate of 2000 free surgeries. Conducts teaching programs during trips to developing countries. **Awards:** Medical Scholar Program (annual) medical scholarship for foreign medical personnel.

**★ 19451 ★ Plastic Surgery Educational Foundation (PSEF)**
444 E Algonquin Rd.
Arlington Heights, IL 60005
**Phone:** (847)228-9900          **Free:** 888-4-PLASTIC
**Fax:** (847)228-9131
**Email:** memserv@plasticsurgery.org
**Website:** http://www.plasticsurgery.org
Dave Fellers, CAE, Exec. Dir.
**Desc:** Plastic and reconstructive surgeons. Purpose is to identify and respond to the educational needs of members and their patients. Sponsors regional and national demonstrations, lectures, educational seminars, symposia, and workshops focusing on plastic surgery techniques and procedures. Conducts annual in-service and self-assessment examinations dealing with topics such as aesthetic and breast surgery, hand and extremities, integument, maxillofacial surgery, and pediatric plastic surgery. Administers Visiting Professors Program; compiles statistics; sponsors charitable programs. **Awards:** Scholarship bestowed in basic science, clinical research, and senior categories.

**Ruth Jackson Orthopaedic Society (RJOS)**
*See:* Entry 16907

**Scoliosis Research Society (SRSO)**
*See:* Entry 16908

**★ 19452 ★ Society of Air Force Clinical Surgeons**
839 W Lincoln Ave., No. 716
Woodland, CA 95695
**Phone:** (530)661-0352          **Fax:** (530)661-0352
**Email:** rosepreuit@aol.com
**Website:** http://atech.org/SAFCS/
Rose A. Thomas, Exec. Dir.
**Desc:** Air Force Clinical Surgeons. Promotes excellence in surgery within the Air Force, serves as a forum for the presentation of scientific papers, fosters

esprit de corps, and promulgates military surgical objectives. **Awards:** Clinical Surgeons Award (annual) for the best original paper written and presented by a resident or fellow at the annual meeting; Trauma/ Critical Care Award (annual) for the best scientific and best clinical paper presented.

## ★ 19453 ★ Society for Clinical Vascular Surgery
13 Elm St.
Manchester, MA 01944-1314
**Website:** http://www.vascsurg.org/doc/Jvonliebig.html
**Desc:** Academic and community vascular surgeons. Promotes vascular surgery in the U.S. **Awards:** William J. von Liebig Foundation Award for Excellence in Vascular Surgical Research (annual) to individuals early in their training to pursue a career in research.

## ★ 19454 ★ Society of Reproductive Surgeons (SRS)
1209 Montgomery Hwy.
Birmingham, AL 35216-2809
**Phone:** (205)978-5000          **Fax:** (205)978-5005
**Email:** finch@asrm.org
**Website:** http://www.reprodsurgery.org
Cheryl Finch, Admin.
**Desc:** Reproductive surgeons. Gathers and disseminates information on reproductive surgery; conducts continuing education programs for members. Makes available referrals list. **Awards:** SRS Prize Paper (annual) based on peer review.

## ★ 19455 ★ Society for Surgery of the Alimentary Tract (SSAT)
13 Elm St.
Manchester, MA 01944
**Phone:** (978)526-8330          **Fax:** (978)526-4018
**Email:** ssat@prri.com
**Website:** http://www.ssat.com
Robert P. Jones, Jr., Exec. Dir.
**Desc:** Licensed physicians with an interest in surgical aspects of digestive diseases. Seeks to advance the study, teaching, and practice of surgery of the alimentary tract; promotes continuing professional development of members. Serves as a forum for the discussion of new alimentary surgical techniques; encourages training opportunities and funding for alimentary surgical research. **Awards:** Career Development Award (annual) to young researchers.

## Society of Surgical Oncology (SSO)
*See:* Entry 10092

## ★ 19456 ★ United Ostomy Association (UOA)
19772 MacArthur Blvd., Ste. 200
Irvine, CA 92612-2405
**Free:** 800-826-0826
**Email:** director@uoa.org
**Website:** http://www.uoa.org
Nancy Italia, Exec. Dir.
**Desc:** Individuals who have lost the normal function of their bowel or bladder necessitating colostomy, ileostomy, ileal conduit, or ureterostomy surgery, known as ostomy. Aids in rehabilitation of these persons through mutual aid, moral support, and exchange of practical information in managing the stoma and its necessary prosthetic appliances; sponsors visiting program allowing patients to ask non-medical questions of individuals who have experienced a similar condition. Works to educate the public as to the nature of ostomy, with a view to ending job and insurance discrimination. Encourages research on management of ostomy and prosthetic equipment and appliances; also encourages study of the costs for rehabilitating ostomy patients. Prepares exhibits for medical conventions. Maintains speakers' bureau; compiles statistics. **Awards:** AVET Scholarship (semiannual).

## ★ 19457 ★ Western Surgical Association (WSA)
c/o Richard C. Thirlby, MD
Virginia Mason Medical Clinic
1100 Ninth Ave., C6-GSUR
Seattle, WA 98111
**Phone:** (206)223-6636          **Free:** 800-354-9527
**Fax:** (206)625-7245
**Email:** Richard.Thirlby@vmmc.org
**Website:** http://www.vmmc.org
Dr. Richard Thirlby, MD, Sec.
**Desc:** Surgeons who have contributed to surgical education and advancement. Objectives are to cultivate, promote, and diffuse knowledge of the art and science of surgery; to sponsor and maintain the highest standards of practice; to deliver the best possible care to all people. **Awards:** J. Bradley Aust Award (annual) for best paper presented by a new member.

## World Federation of Neurosurgical Societies (WFNS)
*See:* Entry 13883

# National & International Organizations

## Academy of Ambulatory Foot and Ankle Surgery (AAFS)
*See:* Entry 17698

## Academy of Medical Surgical Nurses (AMSN)
*See:* Entry 15630

## ★ 19458 ★ Academy of Surgical Research (ASR)
13355 10th Ave. N, Ste. 108
Minneapolis, MN 55441-5510
**Phone:** (763)765-2300          **Fax:** (763)765-2329
**Email:** director@surgicalresearch.org
**Website:** http://www.surgicalresearch.org
Patricia Nolt, Exec. Dir.
**Fnded:** 1982. **Mem:** 425. **Desc:** Individuals, organizations, and corporations with an interest in surgical research. Seeks to advance surgical techniques and equipment through improved research. Facilitates cooperation and exchange of information among members; fosters interdisciplinary transfer of ideas to advance surgical research. **Pub:** *Journal of Investigative Surgery*, periodic. Journal. Discusses advances in surgical research techniques and education. *Price:* $29.95.

## Accreditation Review Committee on Education in Surgical Technology (ARC-ST)
*See:* Entry 4793

## ★ 19459 ★ America Society of Plastic Surgeons (ASPS)
444 E Algonquin Rd.
Arlington Heights, IL 60005
**Phone:** (847)228-9900          **Free:** 888-4-PLASTIC
**Fax:** (847)228-9131
**Email:** acollinsworth@ast.org
**Website:** http://www.plasticsurgery.org
Edward Luce, MD, Pres.
**Fnded:** 1931. **Mem:** 5,000. **Reg. Groups:** 29. **State Groups:** 35. **Desc:** Plastic surgeons. Dedicated to quality patient care and to maintain professional and ethical standards through education, research, and advocacy of socioeconomic and other professional activities. **Pub:** *Plastic and Reconstructive Surgery*, monthly. Journal. Includes research reports and book reviews. *Price:* $420 for non-members. **Frmly:** ASPRS

- American Society of Plastic and Reconstructive Surgery.

## ★ 19460 ★ American Academy of Cosmetic Surgery (AACS)
737 N Michigan Ave., Ste. 820
Chicago, IL 60611
**Phone:** (312)981-6760
**Website:** http://www.cosmeticsurgery.org
Jeffrey P. Knezovich, Exec. VP
**Fnded:** 1985. **Mem:** 1,400. **Desc:** Licensed cosmetic surgeons. Seeks to encourage high-quality cosmetic medical and dental care; provides continuing education for cosmetic surgeons; promotes research. Compiles statistics. Maintains hall of fame and speakers' bureau. **Pub:** *American Journal of Cosmetic Surgery*, quarterly. Journal. *Price:* $110 in U.S.; $130 outside U.S. • *Membership Roster*, annual. Membership Directory. • *Newsline*, bimonthly. Newsletter.

## ★ 19461 ★ American Academy of Facial Plastic and Reconstructive Surgery (AAFPRS)
310 S Henry St.
Alexandria, VA 22314
**Phone:** (703)299-9291          **Free:** 800-332-FACE
**Fax:** (703)299-8898
**Email:** info@aafprs.org
**Website:** http://www.facemd.org
Stephen C. Duffy, Exec. VP
**Fnded:** 1964. **Mem:** 2,600. **Desc:** Physicians specializing in facial plastic surgery. Promotes research and study in the field. Maintains speakers' bureau. Conducts educational and charitable programs; compiles statistics. **Pub:** *The Face Book: The Pros and Cons of Facial Plastic Surgery*. • *Face Facts*, quarterly. • *Facial Plastic Surgery Today*, quarterly. • *Facial Plastic Times*, monthly. Newsletter. Includes calendar of events and book reviews. *Price:* available to members only. • Brochures. • Membership Directory, annual. Includes buyers' guide. *Price:* $35/copy for members; $75/copy for nonmember physicians; $300/copy for others. • Monographs. • Videos.

## ★ 19462 ★ American Academy of Neurological and Orthopaedic Surgeons (AANOS)
2300 S Rancho Dr., Ste. 202
Las Vegas, NV 89102-4508
**Phone:** (702)388-7390          **Fax:** (702)388-7395
**Email:** aanos@lasvegas.net
**Website:** http://www.aanos.org
Dr. Kazem Fathie, MD, Chair
**Fnded:** 1977. **Mem:** 280. **Desc:** Neurological and orthopaedic surgeons, neurologists, physiatrists, and professionals in allied medical or surgical specialties. Provides and encourages information about and understanding of neurological and orthopaedic medicine and surgery, a branch of medicine that deals with diseases and injuries to the human neuromusculoskeletal system; seeks to improve patient care. Maintains American Board of Neurological and Orthopaedic Medicine and Surgery and American Board of Spinal Surgery. Sponsors charitable program. Maintains a complete collection of recordings of scientific meetings since 1977. Operates 40 colleges of experts in individual disciplines related to neurological and orthopaedic medicine and surgery. Acronym stands for Fellowship of the American Academy of Neurological and Orthopaedic Surgeons. **Pub:** *Journal of Neurological and Orthopaedic Medicine and Surgery (JONOMS)*, quarterly. Journal. *Price:* $125/year in U.S.; $135/year outside U.S.

## ★ 19463 ★ American Academy of Neurological Surgery
c/o Mayo Clinic
200 1st. St. SW
Rochester, MN 55905
**Phone:** (507)284-2511          **Fax:** (507)284-5206
Dr. David Piepgras, Sec.

Fnded: 1938. Mem: 168. Desc: Leaders in the field of neurological surgery united for neurosurgical education.

★ 19464 ★ **American Academy of Orthopaedic Surgeons (AAOS)**
6300 N River Rd.
Rosemont, IL 60018-4262
Phone: (847)823-7186    Free: 800-346-AAOS
Fax: (847)823-8125
Email: custserv@aaos.org
Website: http://www.aaos.org
Dr. William Tipton, Exec. VP

Fnded: 1933. Mem: 24,000. Reg. Groups: 6. State Groups: 30. Desc: Professional society of orthopedic surgeons certified by the American Board of Orthopedic Surgery to practice orthopedic (bone and joint) surgery. Promotes physician education and skills enhancement by offering textbooks, clinical videotapes, courses and self-assessment exams. Pub: *Journal of the American Academy of Orthopaedic Surgeons: A Comprehensive Review.* • Bulletin, bimonthly.

★ 19465 ★ **American Academy of Otolaryngology - Head and Neck Surgery (AAO-HNS)**
1 Prince St.
Alexandria, VA 22314-3357
Phone: (703)836-4444    Fax: (703)683-5100
Email: webmaster@enthet.org
Website: http://www.entnet.org
KJ Lee, MD, Exec. VP

Fnded: 1982. Mem: 10,000. Desc: Professional society of medical doctors specializing in otolaryngology (diseases of the ear, nose, and throat) and head and neck surgery. Represents otolaryngology in governmental and socioeconomic areas and provides high-quality medical education for otolaryngologists. Coordinates Combined Otolaryngological Spring Meetings for ten national otolaryngological societies. Operates job information exchange service and museum. Pub: *American Academy of Otolaryngology-Head and Neck Surgery–Bulletin,* monthly. Magazine. Includes academy news, calendar of events, employment opportunity listings, legislative news, and research updates. *Price:* Included in membership dues; $55/year for nonmembers. • *Conjoint Directory of the American Academy of Otolaryngology - Head and Neck Surgery,* semiannual. Directory. • *Otolaryngology - Head and Neck Surgery,* monthly. Journal. *Price:* Included in membership dues; $93/year for domestic nonmembers; $158/year for domestic institutions. • Monographs. • Videos.

★ 19466 ★ **American Association for Accreditation of Ambulatory Surgery Facilities (AAAASF)**
1202 Allanson Rd.
Mundelein, IL 60060
Phone: (847)949-6058    Free: 888-545-5222
Fax: (847)566-4580
Email: aaaasf@sprynet.com
Website: http://www.aaaasf.org
Ronald E. Iverson, Pres.

Fnded: 1981. Mem: 720. Desc: Board-certified surgeon-operated ambulatory surgical facilities. To maintain high standards through adherence to a voluntary program of inspection and accreditation of ambulatory surgery facilities. Pub: Newsletter, semiannual. Frmly: (1994) American Association for Accreditation of Ambulatory Plastic Surgery Facilities.

★ 19467 ★ **American Association of Ambulatory Surgery Centers (AAASC)**
PO Box 23220
San Diego, CA 92193
Phone: (858)490-8085    Free: 800-237-3768
Fax: (858)490-9016
Email: aaasc@mtgsunlimited.com
Website: http://www.aaasc.org
Michelle Freeland, Admin. Dir.

Fnded: 1978. Mem: 500. Desc: Assists physicians, corporations, healthcare administrators to provide excellence in ambulatory care; provides information to build free-standing surgery center by addressing legal, accreditation and leadership issues. Pub: *Monitor,* quarterly. Newsletter. • Membership Directory, annual. For members only on website. *Price:* Free to members. Frmly: (1986) Society for Office-Based Surgery; (1996) American Society of Outpatient Surgeons.

★ 19468 ★ **American Association for Hand Surgery (AAHS)**
20 N Michigan Ave., Ste. 700
Chicago, IL 60602
Phone: (312)236-3307    Fax: (312)782-0553
Email: contact@handsurgery.org
Website: http://www.handsurgery.org
Laura Downes Leeper, CAE, Exec. Dir.

Fnded: 1970. Mem: 1,081. Desc: Plastic, orthopedic, general surgeons, and physical and occupational therapists having a specific interest in hand surgery; individuals in the medical profession, basic sciences, or allied services interested in the improvement of hand surgery. Purpose is to advance hand surgery. Conducts symposia; offers specialized education. Pub: *Annual Program.* • *Hand Surgery Newsletter,* quarterly. Newsletter. *Price:* Included in membership dues.

★ 19469 ★ **American Association of Neurological Surgeons (AANS)**
5550 Meadowbrook Dr.
Rolling Meadows, IL 60008
Phone: (847)378-0500    Free: 888-566-2267
Fax: (847)378-0600
Email: info@aans.org
Website: http://www.neurosurgery.org/aans/
Julian T. Hoff, MD, Chmn.

Fnded: 1931. Mem: 5,011. State Groups: 50. Desc: Neurological surgeons united to promote excellence in neurological surgery and its related sciences. Provides funding to foster research in the neurosciences. Conducts specialized education. The largest publisher of neurosurgical books in the world. Pub: *American Association of Neurological Surgeons Bulletin,* quarterly. Bulletin. *Price:* Included in membership dues. • *Directory of Neurological Surgery,* annual. Directory. *Price:* $50 for members. • *Journal of Neurosurgery,* monthly. Journal. *Price:* $100/year for members; $110/year for nonmembers; $60/year for residents. • *Neurosurgical Operative Atlas.* Booklets. • *Neurosurgical Topics,* quarterly. Books. *Price:* $85 for members; $95 for nonmembers; $75 for residents. • *Neurosurgical Topics Series.* Books. • *Self-Assessment in Neurological Surgery,* triennial. Booklet. Contains multiple choice and patient management tests. *Price:* $175/copy for members; $225/copy for nonmembers; $145 for residents. Frmly: (1966) Harvey Cushing Society.

**American Association of Oral and Maxillofacial Surgeons (AAOMS)**
*See:* Entry 6430

★ 19470 ★ **American Association of Plastic Surgeons (AAPS)**
c/o R. Barrett Noone, M.D.
444 E Algonquin Rd.
Arlington Heights, IL 60005
Phone: (847)228-9900    Free: 888-475-2784
Fax: (847)228-9131
Email: executivesecretary@aaps1921.org
Website: http://www.aaps1921.org
Dr. Ronald Iverson, MD, Pres.

Fnded: 1921. Mem: 425. Desc: Professional society of plastic surgeons. Frmly: (1942) American Association of Oral and Plastic Surgeons.

**American Association of Podiatric Physicians and Surgeons (AAPPS)**
*See:* Entry 17701

★ 19471 ★ **American Association for the Surgery of Trauma (AAST)**
Department of Surgery
UCLA Medical Center
10833 LeConte Ave. CHS 72-178
Los Angeles, CA 90095
Phone: (310)794-4210    Fax: (310)794-4251
Email: hcryer@mednet.ucla.edu
Website: http://www.aast.org
H. Gill Cryer, MD, Sec.

Fnded: 1938. Mem: 844. Desc: Professional society of surgeons interested in the cultivation and improvement of the science and art of the surgery of trauma and allied sciences. Pub: *Journal of Trauma,* monthly. Journal.

★ 19472 ★ **American Association of Surgical Physician Assistants (AASPA)**
PO Box 867
Bernardsville, NJ 07924
Free: 888-882-2772    Fax: (732)805-9582
Email: TheAASPA@aol.com
Website: http://www.aaspa.com
Susan E. Lusty, Exec. Dir.

Fnded: 1973. Mem: 600. Nat'l Groups: 1. Desc: Surgical physician assistants, students in accredited physician assistant programs, and allied health professionals. Purposes are to promote academic and clinical excellence among members, to respond to the needs of surgical physician assistants, and to educate the medical community and the public about the role of surgical physician assistants in health care. Pub: *Surgical Physician Assistant,* monthly. Journal. • *The Sutureline,* quarterly. Newsletter. *Price:* Included in membership dues. Frmly: (1996) American Association of Surgeon Assistants.

★ 19473 ★ **American Association for Thoracic Surgery (AATS)**
13 Elm St.
Manchester, MA 01944
Phone: (978)526-8330    Fax: (978)526-7521
Email: aats@prri.com
Website: http://www.aats.org
William T. Maloney, Exec. Dir.

Fnded: 1917. Mem: 1,200. Desc: Specialists in surgery of the chest region, including cardiovascular surgeons. Encourages investigation and study of intrathoracic physiology, pathology, and therapy. Pub: *Journal of Thoracic and Cardiovascular Surgery,* monthly. Journal. • Membership Directory, annual.

★ 19474 ★ **American Board of Abdominal Surgery (ABAS)**
675 Main St.
Melrose, MA 02176
Phone: (617)665-6102    Fax: (617)665-4127
Email: office@abdominalsurg.org
Website: http://www.abdominalsurg.org
Louis F. Alfano, MD, Exec. Sec.

Fnded: 1957. Mem: 2,402. Desc: Specialists in abdominal surgery. Improves the quality of graduate education for abdominal surgery. Establishes minimum educational and training standards for the specialty. Determines whether candidates have received adequate preparation as cefined by the board. Provides comprehensive examinations to determine the ability and fitness of candidates. Certifies surgeons who have satisfied the requirements of the board as a protection to the public and the profession. Gives oral and written examinations in abdominal surgery. Pub: *ASAS Journal,* annual. Journal. *Price:* for members. • *Surgeon,* semiannual. *Price:* for members.

★ 19475 ★ **American Board of Colon and Rectal Surgery (ABCRS)**
20600 Eureka Rd., Ste. 600
Taylor, MI 48180
Phone: (734)282-9400    Fax: (734)282-9402
Email: admin@abcrs.org
Website: http://www.abcrs.org
Irene Babcock, Exec. Asst.

**Fnded:** 1934. **Desc:** Certification board established to investigate qualifications, administer examinations, and provide certification as diplomates for medical doctors specializing in colon and rectal surgery. **Pub:** *American Board of Colon and Rectal Surgery–Newsletter to Diplomates*, annual. Newsletter. Includes research updates. *Price:* Included in membership dues. **Frmly:** American Board of Proctology.


★ **19476** ★ **American Board of Neurological Surgery (ABNS)**
6550 Fannin St., No. 2139
Houston, TX 77030-2722
**Phone:** (713)790-6015          **Fax:** (713)794-0207
**Email:** abns@tmb.tmc.edu
**Website:** http://www.abns.org
Mary Louise, Admin.

**Fnded:** 1940. **Desc:** Certification board to investigate qualifications of, administer examinations to, and certify as diplomates medical doctors specializing in neurological surgery. Works to stimulate development of adequate training facilities and aids in evaluating residencies under consideration by the Accreditation Council on Graduate Medical Education of the American Medical Association. **Pub:** *Newsletter to Diplomates*, annual. Newsletter. *Price:* Free.


★ **19477** ★ **American Board of Oral and Maxillofacial Surgery (ABOMS)**
625 N Michigan Ave., Ste. 1820
Chicago, IL 60611
**Phone:** (312)642-0070          **Fax:** (312)642-8584
**Email:** CPena@aboms.org
**Website:** http://www.aboms.org
David E. Frost, DDS, Pres.

**Fnded:** 1946. **Mem:** 3,580. **Desc:** Certification board to establish qualifications, conduct examinations, and certify surgeons whom the board finds qualified to practice oral and maxillofacial medicine, including diagnostic, surgical, and adjunctive treatment of the diseases, injuries, and defects of the oral and maxillofacial regions. **Frmly:** (1978) American Board of Oral Surgery.


★ **19478** ★ **American Board of Orthopaedic Surgery (ABOS)**
400 Silver Cedar Ct.
Chapel Hill, NC 27514
**Phone:** (919)929-7103          **Fax:** (919)942-8988
**Website:** http://www.abos.org
Dr. G. Paul DeRosa, Exec. Dir.

**Fnded:** 1934. **Mem:** 12. **Desc:** Certification board to establish qualifications, conduct annual examinations, and certify as diplomates those whom the board finds qualified to practice orthopaedic surgery. **Pub:** *Directory of Diplomates*, annual. Directory. *Price:* $25 plus shipping and handling.


★ **19479** ★ **American Board of Plastic Surgery (ABPS)**
7 Penn Center, Ste. 400
1635 Market St.
Philadelphia, PA 19103-2204
**Phone:** (215)587-9322          **Fax:** (215)587-9622
**Email:** info@abplsurg.org
**Website:** http://www.abplsurg.org
Dr. R. Barrett Noone, Exec. Dir.

**Fnded:** 1937. **Mem:** 20. **Desc:** Certification board established to investigate the qualifications of, administer examinations to, and certify as diplomates medical doctors specializing in the entire field of plastic and reconstructive surgery. **Pub:** *Booklet of Information*, annual.


**American Board of Podiatric Surgery (ABPS)**
*See:* Entry 17704

★ **19480** ★ **American Board of Surgery (ABS)**
1617 John F. Kennedy Blvd., Ste. 860
Philadelphia, PA 19103
**Phone:** (215)568-4000          **Fax:** (215)563-5718
**Email:** info@abps.org
**Website:** http://www.absurgery.org
Dr. Wallace P. Ritchie, Jr., Exec. Dir.

**Fnded:** 1937. **Mem:** 29. **Desc:** Examining and certifying board in general surgery; also certifies in Pediatric Surgery, Vascular Surgery, Surgical Critical Care, and Hand Surgery. Membership is drawn from 23 national and regional surgical and specialty societies and organizations. Currently offers Recertification in General Surgery, Pediatric Surgery, Vascular Surgery, and Surgical Critical Care. **Pub:** *ABMS Directories of Certified Specialists*. Directory. • *Directory of Medical Specialists*. • *Service Booklets of Information*, annual.


★ **19481** ★ **American Board of Thoracic Surgery (ABTS)**
1 Rotary Center, Ste. 803
Evanston, IL 60201
**Phone:** (847)475-1520          **Fax:** (847)475-6240
**Email:** abts_evanston@msn.com
**Website:** http://www.abts.org/
William A. Gay, Jr. MD, Sec. -Treas.

**Fnded:** 1948. **Desc:** Medical certification board that certifies surgeons specializing in thoracic surgery. **Frmly:** Board of Thoracic Surgery.


**American College of Angiology (ACA)**
*See:* Entry 4957


**American College of Eye Surgeons (ACES)**
*See:* Entry 20859


★ **19482** ★ **American College of Foot and Ankle Surgeons (ACFAS)**
515 Busse Hwy.
Park Ridge, IL 60068
**Phone:** (847)292-2237          **Free:** 800-421-2237
**Fax:** (847)292-2022
**Email:** mail@acfas.org
**Website:** http://www.acfas.org/
Thomas R. Schedler, CAE, Exec. Dir.

**Fnded:** 1942. **Mem:** 5,000. **Reg. Groups:** 14. **Desc:** Objectives are to: promote and disseminate information on podiatric surgery among the public, podiatric surgeons, and other health professionals; encourage and publish research findings and related literature; provide intensive programs for clinical and experimental research to improve podiatric surgery and to promote our members' professional and socioeconomic activities. **Pub:** *American College of Foot and Ankle Surgeons–Newsletter*, bimonthly. Bulletin. *Price:* Included in membership dues. • *Complications in Foot and Ankle Surgery*, bimonthly. Journal. Includes book reviews and journal abstracts. *Price:* Included in membership dues; $73/year for nonmember individuals; $97/year for nonmember institutions. • *Membership Roster*, annual. Membership Directory. **Frmly:** (1993) American College of Foot Surgeons.


**American College of MOHS Micrographic Surgery and Cutaneous Oncology (ACMMSCO)**
*See:* Entry 10100


★ **19483** ★ **American College of Oral and Maxillofacial Surgeons (ACOMS)**
c/o Emelie C. Schnettler
1100 NW Loop 410, Ste. 420
San Antonio, TX 78213-2266
**Phone:** (210)344-5674          **Free:** 800-522-6676
**Fax:** (210)344-9754
**Email:** info@acoms.org

**Website:** http://www.acoms.org
Debbie E. Wilson, Dir.

**Fnded:** 1975. **Mem:** 2,500. **Desc:** Diplomates of the American Board of Oral and Maxillofacial Surgery who practice oral and maxillofacial surgery. To advance the integrity of the profession through continuing education, exchange of ideas, certification procedures, and cooperation with allied groups. **Pub:** *ACOMS Review*, quarterly. **Frmly:** (1975) Association of Diplomates of the American Board of Oral Surgery.


**American College of Osteopathic Surgeons (ACOS)**
*See:* Entry 16993


★ **19484** ★ **American College of Surgeons (ACS)**
633 N Saint Clair St.
Chicago, IL 60611-3211
**Phone:** (312)202-5000          **Fax:** (312)202-5001
**Email:** postmaster@facs.org
**Website:** http://www.facs.org
Thomas Russell, MD, Exec. Dir.

**Fnded:** 1913. **Mem:** 63,400. **Local Groups:** 67. **Desc:** Professional association of surgeons worldwide organized primarily to improve the quality of care for surgical patients by elevating the standards of surgical education and practice. Conducts nationwide programs to improve emergency medical services and hospital cancer programs. Sponsors continuing education and self-assessment courses for surgeons in practice. **Pub:** *ACS Publications and Services Catalog*, annual. Catalog. Lists ACS publications. *Price:* Free. • *American College of Surgeons Yearbook*, triennial. Yearbook. Lists ACS fellows. *Price:* Free. For members only. • *Bulletin of the American College of Surgeons*, monthly. Bulletin. Includes ACS and Washington news. *Price:* Included in membership dues. • *Journal of the American College of Surgeons*, monthly. Journal. Includes The Surgeon at Work Section, collective literature reviews, and book reviews. • *Resources for Optimal Care of the Injured Patient*. *Price:* $15. • *Surgical Forum*, annual. Abstracts of research papers presented during clinical congress. *Price:* $25/issue.


**American College of Veterinary Surgeons (ACVS)**
*See:* Entry 20564


**American Council of Certified Podiatric Physicians and Surgeons**
*See:* Entry 17709


★ **19485** ★ **American Foundation for Surgery of the Hand (AFSH)**
6300 N River Rd., Ste. 600
Rosemont, IL 60018-4256
**Phone:** (847)384-8300          **Fax:** (847)384-1435
**Email:** info@hand-surg.org
**Website:** http://www.assh.org
Mark Anderson, Exec. Dir.

**Fnded:** 1986. **Desc:** Awards grants to medical, educational, research, and public education programs related to the field of hand and upper extremity surgery.


**American Osteopathic College of Ophthalmology and the American Osteopathic College of Otolaryngology-Head and Neck Surgery (AOCOO-HNS)**
*See:* Entry 20872


★ **19486** ★ **American Pediatric Surgical Association (APSA)**
60 Revere Dr., Ste. 500
Northbrook, IL 60062
**Phone:** (847)480-9576          **Fax:** (847)480-9282
**Email:** eapsa@eapsa.org

**Website:** http://www.eapsa.org
Keven Cuff, Exec. Sec.

**Fnded:** 1970. **Mem:** 488. **Desc:** Pediatric surgeons who are certified by the American Board of Surgery for competence in dealing with surgical problems of infancy and childhood. Seeks to provide competent medical care for children. Serves as a forum for discussion of ethics involving child care. Presents new concepts and advances in surgical care of infants and children. **Pub:** *Annual Program Booklet*, annual. Booklet. • *APSA Membership Directory*, annual. Membership Directory. • *Business Meeting Minutes*, annual. • *Cancer Newsletter*, annual. Newsletter. • *Journal of Pediatric Surgery*, monthly. Journal. • *Newsletter*, semiannual.

### ★ 19487 ★ American Shoulder and Elbow Surgeons (ASES)

c/o American Academy of Orthopaedic Surgeons
6300 N River Rd., Ste. 727
Rosemont, IL 60018-4226
**Phone:** (847)698-1629 **Fax:** (847)823-0536
**Email:** leffevt@mqh.harvard.edu
**Website:** http://www.aaos.org/wordhtml/ases/homeases.htm
Karen Jared, Dir.

**Fnded:** 1982. **Mem:** 146. **Desc:** Orthopedic surgeons. Purpose is to promote the exchange and dissemination of information on shoulder and elbow surgery and treatment. Sponsors educational courses.

### ★ 19488 ★ American Society of Abdominal Surgeons (ASAS)

675 Main St.
Melrose, MA 02176
**Phone:** (617)665-6102 **Fax:** (617)665-4127
**Email:** office@abdominalsurg.org
**Website:** http://www.abdominalsurg.org
Louis F. Alfano, MD, Exec. Sec.

**Fnded:** 1959. **Mem:** 2,842. **Desc:** Medical doctors specializing in abdominal surgery. Sponsors extensive program of surgical education including study courses, postgraduate programs, lectures, and demonstrations. **Pub:** *American Society of Abdominal Surgeons*, annual. Journal. *Price:* available to members only. • *The Surgeon*, semiannual. Newsletter. Includes calendar of events. *Price:* available to members only. • Books.

### ★ 19489 ★ American Society for Aesthetic Plastic Surgery (ASAPS)

11081 Winners Cir.
Los Alamitos, CA 90720-2813
**Phone:** (562)799-2356 **Fax:** (562)799-1098
**Email:** asaps@surgery.org
**Website:** http://www.surgery.org
Sue Dykema, Dep. Exec. Dir.

**Fnded:** 1864. **Mem:** 1,052. **Desc:** Board-certified plastic surgeons. Provides continuing education to members in the area of aesthetic plastic surgery, through presentation of papers, study sessions, and scientific sessions. Operates grant program. Provides speakers; conducts research programs. **Pub:** *Aesthetic Society News*, quarterly. Newsletter. • *Aesthetic Surgery Journal*, semiannual. Journal. Reviews developments in the field and research results; includes society news. *Price:* Included in membership dues.

### ★ 19490 ★ American Society for Bariatric Surgery (ASBS)

7328 W University Ave., Ste. F
Gainesville, FL 32607
**Phone:** (352)331-4900 **Fax:** (352)331-4975
**Email:** info@asbs.org
**Website:** http://www.asbs.org
Georgeann Mallory, Exec. Dir.

**Fnded:** 1983. **Mem:** 1,000. **Desc:** Works to advance the art and science of bariatric surgery. Supports clinical and laboratory investigations; promotes guidelines for ethical patient care; conducts educational programs for physicians, paramedicals and lay people; provides a forum for the exchange of ideas. **Pub:** *ASBS Newsletter*, periodic. Newsletter. • *Obesity*

*Surgery*, bimonthly. Journal. International, interdisciplinary forum for communicating latest research and surgical techniques. *Price:* $350/institute; $180/personal.

### ★ 19491 ★ American Society of Colon and Rectal Surgeons (ASCRS)

85 W Algonquin Rd., Ste. 550
Arlington Heights, IL 60005
**Phone:** (847)290-9184 **Fax:** (847)290-9203
**Email:** ascrs@ascrs.org
**Website:** http://www.fascrs.org/
Robert D. Fry, Pres.

**Fnded:** 1899. **Mem:** 2,100. **Reg. Groups:** 19. **Desc:** Professional society of surgeons specializing in the diagnosis and treatment of diseases of the colon, rectum, and anus. Offers placement service; conducts research programs. **Pub:** *Diseases of the Colon and Rectum*, monthly. Journal. *Price:* $177 U.S. individual; $263 institution; $222 foreign individual; $308 foreign institution.

### ★ 19492 ★ American Society for Dermatologic Surgery (ASDS)

5550 Meadowbrook Dr., No. 102
Rolling Meadows, IL 60008
**Phone:** (847)956-0900 **Free:** 800-441-2737
**Fax:** (847)956-0999
**Email:** asds@neton-line.com
**Website:** http://www.asds-net.org
Cheryl K. Nordstedt, Exec. Dir.

**Fnded:** 1970. **Mem:** 2,400. **Desc:** Physicians specializing in dermatologic surgery. Purpose is to maintain the highest possible standards in medical education, clinical practice, and patient care. Seeks to promote high standards in allied health professions and services as they relate to dermatology. **Pub:** *Dermatologic Surgery Journal*, monthly. Journal. • *Roster*, annual.

### ★ 19493 ★ American Society of General Surgeons

2122 Grove
Glenview, IL 60025
**Phone:** (847)391-9770 **Free:** 800-998-8322
**Fax:** (847)391-9711
**Email:** asgs-info@theasgs.org
**Website:** http://www.theasgs.org
Peter A. Duhamel, MDFACS, Pres.

**Fnded:** 1993. **Mem:** 3,600. **Desc:** Board certified general surgeons who perform procedures within the scope of general surgery. **Pub:** *Surgfax*, monthly. Features timely updates on current issues.

### ★ 19494 ★ American Society of Hair Restoration Surgery (ASHRS)

c/o American Academy of Cosmetic Surgery
737 N Michigan Ave., Ste. 820
Chicago, IL 60611
**Phone:** (312)981-6760 **Fax:** (312)981-6787
**Email:** info@cosmeticsurgery.org
**Website:** http://www.cosmeticsurgery.org
Jeffrey P. Knezovich, Exec. VP

**Fnded:** 1985. **Mem:** 1,800. **Desc:** Dedicated to fostering the growth and quality of hair restoration surgery worldwide; promotes exchange of information among surgeons and allied professionals in the area of hair restoration surgery; advances the latest scientific data and techniques in clinical practice.

### ★ 19495 ★ American Society for Laser Medicine and Surgery (ASLMS)

2404 Stewart Sq.
Wausau, WI 54401
**Phone:** (715)845-9283 **Fax:** (715)848-2493
**Email:** information@aslms.org
**Website:** http://www.aslms.org
Richard O. Gregory, MD, Sec.

**Fnded:** 1980. **Mem:** 3,050. **Desc:** Physicians, physicists, and other scientists; nurses, dentists, podiatrists, veterinarians, and other paramedical personnel; technicians and commercial representatives concerned

with the medical applications of lasers. Facilitates exchange of information concerning lasers. **Pub:** *Lasers in Surgery and Medicine*, bimonthly. Journal. *Price:* Included in membership dues. • *Official ASLMS Newsletter*, periodic. Newsletter.

### ★ 19496 ★ American Society of Lipo-Suction Surgery (ASLSS)

737 N Michigan Ave., Ste. 820
Chicago, IL 60611-6659
**Phone:** (312)981-6760 **Fax:** (312)981-6787
**Email:** info@cosmeticsurgery.org
**Website:** http://www.cosmeticsurgery.org
Jeffery P. Knezozich, Exec. VP

**Fnded:** 1982. **Mem:** 400. **Desc:** Surgeons specializing in dermatology, general surgery, gynecology, otolaryngology, plastic and reconstructive surgery, and cosmetic surgery. Trains surgeons in the art and methods of lipo-suction surgery. (Lipo-suction surgery is a procedure wherein fatty tissue is removed from the body by suction. It is not meant to reduce weight but to adjust body contours. Lipo-suction surgery is not currently part of the ordinary medical school curriculum.) Conducts workshops and seminars. **Pub:** *American Journal of Cosmetic Surgery*, quarterly. Journal. *Price:* $128 U.S.; $154 Intl. • *Membership Roster*, annual. Membership Directory. • *Newsline*, bimonthly. Newsletter.

### ★ 19497 ★ American Society of Maxillofacial Surgeons (ASMS)

4900B S 31st. St.
Arlington, VA 22206-1656
**Phone:** (703)820-7400 **Fax:** (703)931-4520
**Email:** admin@maxface.org
**Website:** http://www.maxface.org
Thomas F. Fise, Exec. Dir.

**Fnded:** 1947. **Mem:** 385. **Desc:** Professional society of doctors of medicine and doctors of dental surgery who have at least five years of recognized graduate training and experience in maxillofacial surgery. Seeks to stimulate and advance knowledge of the science and art of maxillofacial surgery and improve and elevate the standard of practice. **Pub:** *Maxillofacial News*, quarterly. Newsletter.

### American Society of Ophthalmic Plastic and Reconstructive Surgery (ASOPRS)

*See:* Entry 20876

### ★ 19498 ★ American Society of Plastic Surgeons and Plastic Surgery Education Foundation (ASPRS)

444 E Algonquin Rd.
Arlington Heights, IL 60005
**Phone:** (847)228-9900 **Free:** 888-4-PLASTIC
**Fax:** (847)228-9131
**Website:** http://www.plasticsurgery.org
Edward Luce, MD, Pres.

**Fnded:** 1931. **Mem:** 5,000. **Reg. Groups:** 29. **State Groups:** 35. **Desc:** Professional society of plastic surgeons. Works in cooperation with the Plastic Surgery Educational Foundation to promote optimal care for plastic surgery patients through research, service, and education activities. Sponsors public/patient education program, clinical symposia, and professional development workshops. Acts as a liaison between members and government and medical organizations. Conducts charitable activities; maintains speakers' bureau; compiles statistics. **Pub:** *American Society of Plastic and Reconstructive Surgeons Combined Roster*, annual. Directory. Administrative, member alpha/geo, bylaws and related organization listing. *Price:* First copy free to members; $35 additional copies; $750 nonmembers. • *Journal of Plastic and Reconstructive Surgery*, monthly. Journal. Includes research reports and book reviews. *Price:* Free to members; $303 for nonmembers. • *Plastic Surgery News*, monthly. Tabloid including information on employment opportunities and current events. *Price:* Free to members; $75 for nonmembers. **Frmly:** (2000) American Society of Plastic and Reconstructive Surgeons.

**American Society of Plastic Surgical Nurses (ASPSN)**
*See:* Entry 15658

**★ 19499 ★ American Society for Reconstructive Surgery (ASRM)**
20 N Michigan Ave., Ste. 700
Chicago, IL 60602
**Phone:** (312)456-9579  **Fax:** (312)782-0553
**Email:** contact@microsurg.org
**Website:** http://www.microsurg.org
Erika Monroe Kane, Exec. Dir.

**Desc:** Healthcare professionals. Strives to facilitate information flow for reconstructive microsurgery professionals. **Pub:** Newsletters. • Membership Directory.

**★ 19500 ★ American Society for Surgery of the Hand (ASSH)**
6300 N River Rd., Ste. 600
Rosemont, IL 60018-4256
**Phone:** (847)384-8300  **Fax:** (847)384-1435
**Email:** info@assh.org
**Website:** http://www.assh.org
Mark Anderson, Exec. Dir.

**Fnded:** 1946. **Mem:** 1,800. **Desc:** Surgeons specializing in surgery of the hand. Funds research in the field of hand surgery. Sponsors educational programs. Maintains a website that offers information on common hand problems **Pub:** *Essentials of Hand Surgery.* Book. • *Global Service Information for Hand Surgery.* Manual. • *Hand Surgery Guide to the ICD-9-CM-Second Edition.* Book. • *Hand Surgery Update.* Book. • *Hand Surgery Update 2.* Booklet. • *The Journal of Hand Surgery,* bimonthly. Journal. • *Patient Education Brochures.* Brochures. Series of 16 brochures with information for patients. • *Self-assessment Examination in Hand Surgery,* annual.

**★ 19501 ★ American Society of Transplant Surgeons**
1020 N Fairfax St., No. 200
Alexandria, VA 22314-1537
**Phone:** (703)684-5990  **Free:** 888-990-2787
**Fax:** (703)684-6303
**Email:** shaked@mail.med.upenn.edu
Arthur J. Matas, MD, Sec.

**Fnded:** 1975. **Mem:** 850. **Desc:** Surgeons specializing in transplantation. Promotes and encourages education and research, especially in transplantation surgery; collaborates with public and private organizations; participates and assists in developing programs and coordinates efforts on projects that will benefit organ recipients. **Pub:** *Chimera,* quarterly. • *Transplantation,* monthly.

**★ 19502 ★ American Surgical Association (ASA)**
c/o Robert P. Jones, Jr., Ed.D.
13 Elm St.
Manchester, MA 01944-1314
**Phone:** (978)526-8330  **Fax:** (978)526-7521
**Email:** asa@prri.com
Carlos A. Pellegrini, MD, Sec.

**Fnded:** 1880. **Mem:** 949. **Desc:** Surgeons organized to promote the science and art of surgery. Bestows medallion for scientific achievement. **Pub:** *Annals of Surgery,* monthly. • *Transactions,* annual.

**★ 19503 ★ Argentine Academy of Surgery (Academia Argentina de Cirugia)**
Marcelo T. de Alvear 2415
1122 Buenos Aires, Argentina
**Phone:** 54 1 9253649
**Fnded:** 1911.

**★ 19504 ★ Arthroscopy Association of North America (AANA)**
6300 N River Rd., Ste. 104
Rosemont, IL 60018
**Phone:** (847)292-2262  **Fax:** (847)292-2268
**Email:** ed@aana.org
**Website:** http://www.aana.org
Edward A. Goss, Exec. Dir.

**Fnded:** 1982. **Mem:** 1,500. **Desc:** Orthopedic surgeons. To advance arthroscopy, a diagnostic or surgical procedure in which an arthroscope, is inserted into a joint. The surgeon can either look directly into the arthroscope or observe on a screen the view projected by the arthroscope. In this way the surgeon can diagnose a condition using only a small incision for insertion of the arthroscope. The arthroscope also allows certain surgical procedures to be performed within viewing range of the scope. Sponsors research and continuing education programs. **Pub:** *AANA Membership Directory,* annual. Membership Directory. *Price:* Included in membership dues. • *Arthroscopy: The Journal of Arthroscopic and Related Surgery,* quarterly. Journal. *Price:* $170/year for individuals; $220/year for institutions. • *Inside AANA,* quarterly. Newsletter.

**★ 19505 ★ Asian Association of Oral and Maxillo Facial Surgeons (AAOMFS)**
Maxillo-Facial Unit
Ripas Hospital
Bandar Seri Begawan, Brunei Darussalam
**Phone:** 673 2 447583

**Lang(s):** Arabic, English. **Desc:** Oral and maxillofacial surgeons. Seeks to advance the practice of oral and maxillofacial surgery. Facilitates exchange of information among members; conducts research and continuing professional development programs.

**★ 19506 ★ Asian Association of Pediatric Surgeons (AAPS)**
c/o Department of Pediatric Surgery
Juntendo University School of Medicine
2-1-1 Hongo
Bunkyo-Hu
Tokyo 113-8421, Japan
**Phone:** 81 3 38133111  **Fax:** 81 3 58022033

**Lang(s):** English, Japanese. **Desc:** Pediatric surgeons working in Asia. Seeks to advance the practice of pediatric surgery in Asia. Facilitates exchange of information among members.

**★ 19507 ★ Asian-Australasian Society of Neurological Surgeons (AASNS)**
23, Bharathidasan Rd.
Teynampet
Chennai
Madras 600 018, India
**Phone:** 91 44 4364150  **Fax:** 91 44 4335050
**Email:** kganap@hotmail.com
**Website:** http://aasns.com

**Mem:** 15,000. **Lang(s):** English. **Desc:** Neurological surgeons. Seeks to advance the practice of neurological surgery; promotes continuing professional development among members. Serves as a clearinghouse on neurological surgery; sponsors training courses. **Pub:** Newsletter, annual.

**Asian - Australasian Society of Neurological Surgeons (AASNS)**
*See:* Entry 13930

**★ 19508 ★ Asian Pacific Federation of Societies for Surgery of the Hand (APFSSH)**
c/o Australian Hand Surgery Society
PO Box 304
Lutwycher, QLD 4030, Australia
**Phone:** 61 7 38576033  **Fax:** 61 7 38576822
**Email:** austhandsurgery@bigpond.com
**Website:** http://www.apfss.org

**Lang(s):** English. **Desc:** Orthopedic surgeons specializing in surgery on the hands. Seeks to advance the practice of hand surgery; promotes continuing professional development of members. Facilitates exchange of information among members; sponsors research and training programs.

**★ 19509 ★ Asian Society for Cardiovascular Surgery (ASCS)**
c/o Department of Cardiac Surgery
University of Tokyo
Bunkyo-ku
Tokyo 113-8655, Japan
**Phone:** 81 3 58008855  **Fax:** 81 3 58008854

**Lang(s):** English, Korean. **Desc:** Cardiovascular surgeons. Seeks to advance the practice of cardiovascular surgery; promotes continuing professional development among members. Facilitates exchange of information among members; sponsors research and educational programs.

**★ 19510 ★ Asian Society for Hepato-Biliary-Pancreatic Surgery (ASHBPS)**
Department of Surgery
Chinese University of Hong Kong
Hong Kong, People's Republic of China
**Phone:** 852 26322952  **Fax:** 852 26473074
**Email:** hbp2001@cuhk.edu.hk

**Lang(s):** Chinese, English. **Desc:** Surgeons specializing in operations on the liver, biliary system, and pancreas. Seeks to advance the practice of hepatic, biliary, and pancreatic surgery; promotes continuing professional development of members. Serves as a forum for the exchange of information among members; sponsors research and educational programs.

**★ 19511 ★ Asian Society for Stereotactic Functional and Computer Assisted Neurosurgery**
Functional and Gamma Knife
Surgery Center
Nakao-machi
Takasaki 886, Japan
**Phone:** 81 272 3626201  **Fax:** 81 272 3628901
**Fnded:** 1994. **Mem:** 300. **Nat'l Groups:** 7. **Lang(s):** English, Japanese. **Desc:** Neurosurgeons. Promotes increased use of stereotactic and computer assisted neurosurgical techniques; seeks to advance surgical assistive technologies. Facilitates exchange of information among members; provides support to surgical technology research programs; sponsors continuing professional development courses. **Pub:** *Stereotactic and Functional Neurosurgery,* bimonthly. Journal.

**★ 19512 ★ Asian Surgical Association (ASA)**
Department of Surgery
University of Hong Kong Medical Centre
Queen Mary Hospital
Pokfulam Rd.
Hong Kong, People's Republic of China
**Phone:** 852 28554235  **Fax:** 852 28181186
**Email:** info@asiansurgassoc.org
**Website:** http://www.AsianSurgAssoc.org

**Fnded:** 1976. **Mem:** 1,030. **Lang(s):** Chinese, English. **Desc:** Surgeons. Seeks to advance surgical practice. Facilitates exchange of information among members; sponsors continuing professional development courses. **Pub:** *Asian Journal of Surgery,* quarterly. Journal. Includes original scientific contributions in clinical and experimental surgery, features the latest surgical advances and developments in Asia.

**★ 19513 ★ Association of Academic Chairmen of Plastic Surgery (AACPS)**
4900 B South 31st St.
Arlington, VA 22206
**Phone:** (703)820-7400  **Fax:** (703)931-4520
**Email:** aacps@mindspring.com
**Website:** http://www.aacplasticsurgery.org

**Fnded:** 1985. **Mem:** 270. **Desc:** Chairmen of plastic and reconstructive surgery education and residency programs. Seeks to advance the study and teaching of plastic and reconstructive surgery. Facilitates establishment of graduate medical education and residency programs in plastic and reconstructive surgery. Conducts educational programs.


### ★ 19514 ★ Association for Academic Surgery (AAS)

60 Revere Dr., Ste. 500
Northbrook, IL 60062
**Phone:** (847)509-1945          **Fax:** (847)480-9282
**Email:** aas@aasurg.org
**Website:** http://www.aasurg.org
Melanie Epel, Exec. Dir.

**Fnded:** 1966. **Mem:** 2,736. **Desc:** Active (700) and senior (1250) surgeons with backgrounds in all surgical specialties in academic surgical centers at chief resident level or above. Encourages young surgeons to pursue careers in academic surgery; supports them in establishing themselves as investigators and educators by providing a forum in which senior surgical residents and junior faculty members may present papers on subjects of clinical or laboratory investigations; promotes interchange of ideas between senior surgical residents, junior faculty, and established academic surgeons; facilitates communication among academic surgeons in all surgical fields. Maintains placement service. service. **Pub:** *Journal of Surgical Research*, monthly. Journal. *Price:* Included in membership dues.


### ★ 19515 ★ Association of Coloprociology of Great Britain and Ireland

c/o The Royal College of Surgeons of England
35-43 Lincoln's Inn Fields
London WC2A 3PE, United Kingdom
**Phone:** 44 20 79730307          **Fax:** 44 20 74309235
**Email:** acpgbi@asgbi.org.uk
**Website:** http://www.acpgbi.org.uk

**Fnded:** 1990. **Mem:** 1,200. **Reg. Groups:** 20. **Lang(s):** English. **Desc:** A multidisciplinary association to promote standards and training in coloproctology. **Pub:** *Colorectal Disease*, bimonthly. Journal. • *Guidelines for the Management of Colorectal Cancer.* Handbook.


**Association of Neurosurgical Physician Assistants (ANSPA)**
*See:* Entry 13946


**Association of PeriOperative Registered Nurses (AORN)**
*See:* Entry 15667


### ★ 19516 ★ Association of Physician Assistants in Cardiovascular Surgery (APACVS)

PO Box 4834
Englewood, CO 80155
**Phone:** (303)221-5651          **Free:** 877-221-5651
**Fax:** (303)771-2550
**Email:** padns@aol.com
**Website:** http://www.apacvs.org
David Gray, Pres.

**Fnded:** 1981. **Mem:** 600. **Desc:** Physician assistants who work with cardiovascular surgeons. Objective is to assist in defining the role of physician assistants in the field of cardiovascular surgery through educational forums. **Pub:** *CardioVision*, quarterly. Newsletter. • *Salary and Benefits Survey*, annual. Survey. • Membership Directory, annual.


**Association of Police Surgeons**
*See:* Entry 12232


### ★ 19517 ★ Association of Program Directors in Surgery

4900B 31st St.
Arlington, VA 22206
**Phone:** (703)820-7400          **Fax:** (703)931-4520
**Email:** veldenz@jax.ufl.edu
**Website:** http://www.apds.org
Thomas F. Fise, Contact

**Fnded:** 1978. **Mem:** 507. **Desc:** Program directors in surgery. Conducts educational programs and scientific meetings. **Pub:** *Current Surgery*, 9/year. *Price:* $40 for members.


### ★ 19518 ★ Association for Research in Vascular Surgery (ARVS) (Association de Recherche en Chirurgie Vasculaire — ARCV)

Clinique de Franciscaines
9, impasse Jean-Bouin
F-30000 Nimes, France
**Phone:** 33 66 766048          **Fax:** 33 66 269812
**Email:** jeanmariecardon@hotmail.com

**Fnded:** 1986. **Mem:** 30. **Lang(s):** French. **Desc:** Vascular and cardiac surgeons, vascular radiologists, and anesthesiologists. Conducts research in the field, particularly on the uses of endovascular devices. Members exchange information on technological advancement in the field.


### ★ 19519 ★ Association of Surgeons of Great Britain and Ireland

c/o The Royal College of Surgeons of England
35-43 Lincoln's Inn Fields
London WC2A 3PE, United Kingdom
**Phone:** 44 20 79730303          **Fax:** 44 20 74309235
**Email:** admin@asgbi.org.uk
**Website:** http://www.asgbi.org.uk

**Fnded:** 1920. **Mem:** 2,000. **Lang(s):** English. **Desc:** General surgeons. Concerned with the advancement of the science and art of surgery and the promoting of friendship amongst surgeons. The Association is the specialty association for general surgery and is recognized as such by Government as well as by the profession. **Pub:** *British Journal of Surgery*, monthly. Journal.


### ★ 19520 ★ Association of Surgeons of India

Adams Rd., Chepauk
Madras 600 005, India
**Phone:** 91 44 567095
**Fnded:** 1938.


### ★ 19521 ★ Association for Surgical Education (ASE)

SIU School of Medicine
Department of Surgery
PO Box 19655
Springfield, IL 62794-9655
**Phone:** (217)545-3835          **Fax:** (217)524-2431
**Email:** membership@surgicaleducation.com
**Website:** http://www.surgicaleducation.com
Susan Kepner, Exec. Dir.

**Fnded:** 1980. **Mem:** 700. **Desc:** Surgeons and individuals involved or interested in undergraduate surgical education. Purpose is to develop and disseminate information on motivation, techniques, research, and applications for presenting curricula in undergraduate surgical education. Acts as forum for research in surgical education; serves as information clearinghouse. Compiles statistics; maintains speakers' bureau. Conducts educational programs. **Pub:** *Focus on Surgical Education*, quarterly. Journal. *Price:* Included in membership dues.


### ★ 19522 ★ Association of Surgical Technologists (AST)

7108-C S Alton Way
Englewood, CO 80112-2106
**Phone:** (303)694-9130          **Fax:** (303)694-9169
**Email:** kludwig@ast.org
**Website:** http://www.ast.org
William J. Teutsch, Exec. Dir.

**Fnded:** 1969. **Mem:** 17,700. **Desc:** Individuals who have received specific education and training to deliver surgical patient care in the operating room. Membership categories are available for both certified and student surgical technologists. Emphasis is placed on encouraging members to participate actively in a continuing education program. Aims are: to study, discuss, and exchange knowledge, experience, and ideas in the field of surgical technology; to promote a high standard of surgical technology performance in the community for quality patient care; to stimulate interest in continuing education. Local groups sponsor workshops and institutes. Conducts research. **Pub:** *AST Core Curriculum for Surgical First Assisting.* Book. • *AST Core Curriculum for Surgical Technology.* Book. • *The Surgical Technologist*, monthly. Journal. Covers surgical procedures and equipment, aseptic techniques, medical law, and legislation. Also includes association news, and annual subject index. *Price:* Included in membership dues; $36/year for nonmembers. • *Surgical Technologist Certifying Exam Study Guide.* Book. **Frmly:** (1978) Association of Operating Room Technicians.


### ★ 19523 ★ Association of Women Surgeons (AWS)

414 Plaza Dr., Ste. 209
Westmont, IL 60559
**Phone:** (630)655-0392          **Fax:** (630)655-0391
**Email:** info@womensurgeons.org
**Website:** http://www.womensurgeons.org
Judith Keel, Exec. Dir.

**Fnded:** 1981. **Mem:** 1,300. **Desc:** Women surgeons, interns, and residents; retired women surgeons; women in medical school interested in a career in surgery; interested individuals. Promotes the professional and personal goals of women surgeons and women involved and interested in the medical profession. Encourages interaction between women surgeons internationally. Serves as a network for the exchange of ideas and information. **Pub:** *AWS Connexions*, quarterly. Newsletter. Includes notice of meetings, lists employment opportunities, profiles of outstanding women surgeons. • *Pocket Mentor.* Handbook. Features information for residents and interns. • *Resource Manual*, annual. Membership Directory. Serves as a networking device among members.


### ★ 19524 ★ Australian Society of Otolaryngology Head and Neck Surgery (ASOHNS)

level 4, 68 Alfred St., Ste. 403
Missions Pointe, NSW 2061, Australia
**Phone:** 61 2 99545856          **Fax:** 61 2 99576863
**Email:** enquiries@asohns.org.au
**Website:** http://www.asohns.org.au

**Fnded:** 1950. **Mem:** 427. **Nat'l Groups:** 1. **State Groups:** 6. **Lang(s):** English. **Desc:** Ear, nose, and throat surgeons. Represents member interests. Provides registrar training. **Pub:** *Australian Journal of Oto-Laryngology*, 3/year. Journal. • *Australian Otolaryngology*, quarterly. Newsletter.


### ★ 19525 ★ BeNeLux Association of Bariatric Surgeons (BABS)

Vromenhove 13
B-2070 Zwijdrecht, Belgium
**Phone:** 32 3 2528103          **Fax:** 32 3 2528103
**Email:** luc.lemmens@pandora.be
**Website:** http://www.babsweb.org/

**Fnded:** 1996. **Desc:** Promotes discussion on surgical treatment; brings together health care specialists of all disciplines to improve treatment; provides standards and guidelines of treatment.

**★ 19526 ★ British Association of Aesthetic Plastic Surgeons (BAAPS)**
Royal College of Surgeons of England
35-43 Lincoln's Inn Fields
London WC2A 3PN, United Kingdom
**Phone:** 44 207 4052234    **Fax:** 44 207 4301840
**Email:** info@baaps.org.uk
**Website:** http://www.baaps.org.uk
**Fnded:** 1980. **Mem:** 140. **Lang(s):** English. **Desc:** Fosters exchange of information among surgeons for the advancement of aesthetic plastic surgery. Encourages specialized training among plastic surgeons. Develops and advocates high standards of professional conduct; advises, promotes, and disseminates information on aesthetic plastic surgery. Provides educational programs for general practitioners and the press; conducts semiannual educational program for trainees and consultants. **Pub:** *Directory*, annual. Membership Directory. **Frmly:** (1979) Association of Cosmetic Plastic Surgeons of Great Britain.

**★ 19527 ★ British Association of Day Surgery**
35-43 Lincoln's Inn Fields
London WC2A 3PN, United Kingdom
**Phone:** 44 207 9730308    **Fax:** 44 207 9730314
**Email:** bads@bads.co.uk
**Website:** http://www.bads.co.uk
**Fnded:** 1990. **Mem:** 720. **Lang(s):** English. **Desc:** Nurses, managers, surgeons and anaesthetists. To encourage the expansion of day surgery and to promote education, research and high-quality treatment in this field. Organizes seminars, meetings and holds an annual conference. Advice is provided to Royal Colleges, NHS Executive, regional commissions and trusts including private health organizations. **Pub:** *Journal of One Day Surgery*, quarterly. Journal.

**★ 19528 ★ British Association of Oral and Maxillofacial Surgeons**
c/o Royal College of Surgeons
35-43 Lincoln's Inn Fields
London WC2A 3PN, United Kingdom
**Phone:** 44 20 74058074    **Fax:** 44 20 74309997
**Website:** http://www.baoms.org.uk
**Fnded:** 1962. **Mem:** 1,200. **Desc:** Aims to promote the advancement of education and research into the development of oral and maxillofacial surgery in the British Isles; to encourage, and assist postgraduate education, study and research in oral and maxillofacial surgery. Arranges regular meetings at which lectures and demonstrations will be given. **Pub:** *British Journal of Oral & Maxillofacial Surgery*, bimonthly. Journal.

**★ 19529 ★ British Association of Otorhinolaryngologists - Head and Neck Surgeons**
c/o Royal College of Surgeons
35-43 Lincoln's Inn Fields
London WC2A 3PE, United Kingdom
**Phone:** 44 20 74048373    **Fax:** 44 20 74044200
**Email:** orl@bao-hns.demon.co.uk
**Website:** http://www.orl-baohns.org
**Fnded:** 1943. **Mem:** 1,019. **Lang(s):** English. **Desc:** Consultant ENT and head and neck surgeons, consultant audiological physicians as well as medical practitioners engaged in the practice of otorhinolaryngology and head and neck surgery in grades other than that of consultant. Aims to support and encourage education, research, development, and audit in otorhinolaryngology, head and neck surgery. Promotes the highest standards or medical and surgical practice within otorhinolarynglogy, head and neck surgery, for the benefit of patients. **Pub:** *Clinical Otolaryngology*, bimonthly. • Newsletter, bimonthly.

**British Association of Paediatric Surgeons (BAPS)**
*See:* Entry 5635

**★ 19530 ★ British Association of Plastic Surgeons**
The Royal College of Surgeons
35-43 Lincoln's Inn Fields
London WC2A 3PN, United Kingdom
**Phone:** 44 20 78315161    **Fax:** 44 20 78314041
**Email:** secretariat@baps.co.uk
**Website:** http://www.baps.co.uk
**Fnded:** 1946. **Mem:** 596. **Desc:** Plastic Surgeons. Promotes and directs the development of plastic surgery and aims to foster and co-ordinate education, study and research in plastic surgery. **Pub:** *British Journal of Plastic Surgery*, 8/year. Journal.

**★ 19531 ★ British Association of Urological Surgeons**
c/o Royal College of Surgeons
35-43 Lincoln's Inn Fields
London WC2A 3PN, United Kingdom
**Phone:** 44 20 7405 1390    **Fax:** 44 207 4045048
**Email:** pneville@baus.demon.co.uk
**Website:** http://www.baus.org.uk
**Fnded:** 1945. **Mem:** 1,400. **Desc:** Urological surgeons from the UK and overseas. Medical practitioners in other specialties with an interest in urology. Aims to promote a high standard in the practice of urology. **Pub:** *Members Handbook*. Handbook.

**★ 19532 ★ British Institute of Dental and Surgical Technologists**
School of Dentristry, Rm. 888
St. Chads Queensway
Birmingham B4 6NN, United Kingdom
**Fnded:** 1935. **Mem:** 300. **Desc:** Maintains standards as a professional institute for dental and surgical technicians. **Pub:** *Journal of the British Institute of Surgical Technologists*, annual. Journal. **Frmly:** (1998) British Institute of Surgical Technologists.

**British Society of Periodontology**
*See:* Entry 6484

**★ 19533 ★ British Society for Surgery of the Hand**
The Royal College of Surgeons of England
37-42 Lincoln's Inn Fields
London WC2A 3PN, United Kingdom
**Phone:** 44 20 78315162    **Fax:** 44 20 78314041
**Email:** secretariat@bssh.ac.uk
**Website:** http://www.bssh.ac.uk
**Fnded:** 1970. **Mem:** 653. **Desc:** The membership is drawn from the two major parent specialties of orthopedic and plastic surgery; all members share an interest in the hand. To promote and direct the development of hand surgery and to foster and co-ordinate education, study and research in hand surgery including the dissemination and diffusion of knowledge of hand surgery among members of the Society and the medical profession. **Pub:** *Journal of Hand Surgery*, bimonthly. Journal.

**★ 19534 ★ Bulgarian Society of Aesthetic Surgery and Aesthetic Medicine**
ii, 20th April Str.
BG-1606 Sofia, Bulgaria
**Phone:** 359 2 9524652    **Fax:** 359 2 9515668
**Email:** uservdev@infocom.bg
**Website:** http://www.ijacbs.com
**Fnded:** 1993. **Mem:** 47. **Lang(s):** Bulgarian, English. **Desc:** Fosters research in aesthetic, comestic surgery and medicine.

**★ 19535 ★ Canadian Academy of Facial Plastic and Reconstructive Surgery (Academie Canadienne de Chirurgie Plastique et Reconstructive Faciale)**
c/o Mt. Sinai Hospital
600 University Ave., Rm. 401
Toronto, ON, Canada M5G 1X5
**Phone:** (905)569-6965    **Fax:** (905)569-6965
**Email:** info@facialcosmeticsurgery.org
**Website:** http://www.facialcosmeticsurgery.org
**Fnded:** 1981. **Mem:** 50. **Lang(s):** English, French. **Desc:** Plastic and reconstructive surgeons specializing in facial procedures. Seeks to advance the practice of facial cosmetic surgery. Facilitates exchange of information among members; conducts continuing professional education courses. **Frmly:** CAFPRS.

**★ 19536 ★ Canadian Association of General Surgeons (CAGS)**
PO Box 1011
Saint Anthony, NF, Canada A0K 4S0
**Phone:** (709)454-3333    **Fax:** (709)454-2052
**Email:** gwn.fitz@nf.sympatico.ca
**Website:** http://cags.medical.org
**Lang(s):** English, French. **Desc:** General surgeons. Promotes professional development of members; seeks to advance the practice of general surgery. Represents members' collective interests; conducts continuing professional education courses.

**★ 19537 ★ Canadian Association of Oral and Maxillofacial Surgeons (CAOMS) (Association canadienne des specialistes en chirurgie buccale et maxillo-faciale — ACSCBMF)**
No. 1, 1380 W 7th Ave.
Vancouver, BC, Canada V6H 3W5
**Phone:** (604)733-6676    **Fax:** (604)733-4416
**Website:** http://www.caoms.ca
**Lang(s):** English, French. **Desc:** PPX Promotes and represents oral and maxillofacial surgeons in Canada.

**Canadian Association of Paediatric Surgeons (CAPS) (Association Canadienne de la Chirurgie Pediatrique — ACCP)**
*See:* Entry 5639

**Canadian Association of Pediatric Surgeons (CAPS)**
*See:* Entry 5641

**★ 19538 ★ Canadian Neurosurgery Society (CNS) (Societe Canadienne de Neurochirurgie — SCN)**
c/o Canadian Congress of Neurological Sciences
PO Box 5456, Sta. A
Calgary, AB, Canada T2H 1X8
**Phone:** (403)229-9544    **Fax:** (403)229-1661
**Email:** brains@ccns.org
**Website:** http://www.ccns.org/cnsspage.htm
**Lang(s):** English, French. **Desc:** Neurosurgeons, neurologists, and other individuals with an interest in neurosurgery. Seeks to improve neurosurgical techniques; promotes professional development of members. Sponsors research and educational programs; facilitates communication and cooperation among members.

**★ 19539 ★ Canadian Society for Aesthetic (Cosmetic) Plastic Surgery (CSACPS)**
2334 Heska Rd.
Pickering, ON, Canada L1V 2P9
**Phone:** (905)831-7750    **Fax:** (905)831-7248
**Email:** information@csaps.ca

**Website:** http://www.csaps.ca
**Fnded:** 1972. **Mem:** 136. **Lang(s):** English, French. **Desc:** Educates plastic surgeons and residents, in the United States and Canada, on cosmetic surgery techniques. Conducts educational programs.

**★ 19540 ★ Canadian Society of Otolaryngology - Head and Neck Surgery**
221 Millford Cres. 554
Elora, ON, Canada N0B 1S0
**Phone:** (519)846-0630　　　**Free:** 800-655-9533
**Fax:** (519)846-9529
**Email:** cso.hns@sympatico.ca
**Website:** http://www.csohns.com
**Fnded:** 1947. **Mem:** 650. **Nat'l Groups:** 1. **Lang(s):** English, French. **Desc:** Professional society of practicing and retired otolaryngologists; otolaryngology residents join as associates. Provides for the discussion of professional issues. Arranges educational programs and competitions. **Pub:** *Canadian Journal of Otolaryngology*, bimonthly. • Brochure, annual. • Membership Directory, periodic. • Newsletter, semiannual.

**★ 19541 ★ Canadian Society of Plastic Surgeons (CSPS)**
30 St. Joseph Blvd. E, No. 917
Montreal, QC, Canada H2T 1G9
**Phone:** (514)843-5415　　　**Fax:** (514)843-7005
**Email:** csps_sccp@sympatico.ca
**Website:** http://www.plasticsurgery.ca
**Fnded:** 1947. **Mem:** 503. **Lang(s):** English, French. **Desc:** Plastic surgeons, medical educators, and students. Seeks to advance the study and practice of cosmetic surgery. Serves as a clearinghouse on plastic surgery. **Pub:** *CSPS News*, 3/year. Newsletter.

**★ 19542 ★ Canadian Thoracic Society (CTS)**
**(Societe Canadienne de Thoracologie — SCT)**
The Lung Association Nation Office
3 Raymond St., Ste. 300
Ottawa, ON, Canada K1R 1A3
**Phone:** (613)569-6411　　　**Fax:** (613)569-8860
**Email:** info@lung.ca
**Website:** http://www.lung.ca/cts
**Lang(s):** English, French. **Desc:** Physicians and other health care professionals with an interest in thoracic surgery. Seeks to advance the study and practice of thoracic medicine. Serves as a clearinghouse on thoracic medicine; conducts continuing professional education programs for members.

**Clinical Orthopaedic Society (COS)**
*See:* Entry 16925

**★ 19543 ★ Congress of Neurological Surgeons (CNS)**
10 N Martingale Rd., Ste. 190
Schaumburg, IL 60173
**Phone:** (847)240-2500　　　**Free:** 877-517-1267
**Fax:** (847)240-0804
**Email:** info@1cns.org
**Website:** http://www.neurosurgery.org
Gerald E. Rodts, Jr., Sec.
**Fnded:** 1951. **Mem:** 3,500. **Desc:** Professional society of neurological surgeons in the United States and 55 other countries who meet annually to express their views on various aspects of the principles and practice of neurological surgery; to exchange technical information and experience; to join study of the developments in scientific fields allied to neurological surgery. Promotes interest of neurological surgeons in their practice; provides placement service; honors a living leader in the field of neurological surgery annually. **Pub:** *Clinical Neurosurgery*, annual. • *Neurosurgery*, monthly. • *U.S. and Canada Directory*, annual. Directory. • *World Directory*, biennial. Directory. • Newsletter, quarterly.

**EngenderHealth**
*See:* Entry 18272

**★ 19544 ★ European Academy of Facial Plastic Surgery (EAFPS)**
c/o BAO-HNS
The Royal College of Surgeons
35-43 Lincoln's Inn Fields
London WC2A 3PE, United Kingdom
**Phone:** 44 20 78313916　　**Fax:** 44 20 74044200
**Email:** eafps@bao-hns.demon.co.uk
**Website:** http://www.orl-baohns.org
**Fnded:** 1977. **Mem:** 500. **Lang(s):** English. **Desc:** Practicing and student facial and neck surgeons. Aims to further plastic and reconstructive surgery by stimulating research in neurosurgery, ophthalmology, otorhinolaryngology, and maxillofacial surgery; encourages cooperation among members, particularly between surgeons working in different specialties. Offers program on techniques in reconstructive surgery. **Pub:** *Facial Plastic Surgery*, quarterly. Monograph. • *Membership List*, periodic. **Frmly:** Joseph Society.

**★ 19545 ★ European Association for Cranio-Maxillo-Facial Surgery (EACMFS)**
The Clock House
39 North St.
Midhurst GU29 9DS, United Kingdom
**Phone:** 44 1730 815726　　　**Fax:** 44 1730 812042
**Email:** ea.cms@virgin.net
**Fnded:** 1970. **Mem:** 800. **Nat'l Groups:** 2. **Reg. Groups:** 5. **Lang(s):** English, French, German. **Desc:** Surgeons involved in oral and cranio-maxillofacial surgery. Encourages discussion and conducts medical courses on subjects such as orthognathic and temporomandibular joint surgery and plastic and aesthetic surgery. Maintains speakers' bureau. **Pub:** *Journal of Cranio-maxillo-facial Surgery*, bimonthly. Journal.

**★ 19546 ★ European Board of Plastic, Reconstructive and Aesthetic Surgery (EBOPRAS)**
3, rue du Languedoc
F-31000 Toulouse, France
**Email:** costagliola.m@chu-toulouse.fr
**Website:** http://www.uems.be/ebopras2.htm
**Fnded:** 1991. **Desc:** Guarantees highest standards of care in the field of plastic surgery.

**European Rhinologic Society (ERS)**
*See:* Entry 6041

**★ 19547 ★ European Society for Cardiovascular Surgery (ESCVS)**
**(Societe Europeenne de Chirurgie Cardiovasculaire)**
c/o Prof. C. Muneretto
Spedali Civili, U.D.A. Cardiochirurgia
P.le Spedali Civili 1
I-25123 Brescia, Italy
**Phone:** 39 30 3996400　　　**Fax:** 39 30 3996096
**Email:** munerett@master.cci.unibs.it
**Website:**　　　　　　http://www.esvs.org/esvs/ESCVSbudapest2001.html
**Fnded:** 1952. **Mem:** 1,230. **Nat'l Groups:** 40. **Lang(s):** English. **Desc:** European Chapter of the International Society of Cardiovascular Surgery. Members are cardiac and vascular surgeons. Promotes the study of cardiovascular diseases; facilitates exchange of information and ideas concerning cardiovascular diseases. **Pub:** *Cardiovascular Surgery*, bimonthly. Journal.

**★ 19548 ★ European Society for Cataract and Refractive Surgeons (ESCRS)**
**(Club International d'Implants Oculaires)**
10 Hagan Court
Lad Lane
Dublin 2, Ireland
**Phone:** 353 1 6618904　　　**Fax:** 353 1 6785047
**Email:** escrs@agewda-comm.ie
**Website:** http://www.escrs.com
**Fnded:** 1958. **Mem:** 3,000. **Lang(s):** English. **Desc:** Strives to advance scientific knowledge in the field of intraocular lens implantation and in the art and practice of such surgery.

**European Society for Gynecological Endoscopy (ESGE)**
*See:* Entry 16674

**European Society of Knee Surgery Sports Traumatology and Arthroscopy**
*See:* Entry 19155

**★ 19549 ★ European Society of Ophthalmic Plastic and Reconstructive Surgery (ESOPRS)**
c/o Prof. Rolph Guthoff
Universitats Augenlink
Doberaner St. 140
Post Box 10 08 88
D-18055 Rostock, Germany
**Email:** esska200@gve.ch
**Fnded:** 1981. **Mem:** 225. **Nat'l Groups:** 15. **Lang(s):** English. **Desc:** Coordinates activities in the field of plastic and reconstructive surgery of the eye. Disseminates information on the latest scientific advancements. **Pub:** *Orbit*, monthly. Journal.

**European Society of Ophthalmic Plastic and Reconstructive Surgery**
*See:* Entry 20950

**★ 19550 ★ European Society of Surgery**
Nordre Ringgade 1
DK-8000 Arhus, Denmark
**Email:** rudolf.gurhoff@med.uni-rostock.de
**Website:** http://www.esoprs.com

**★ 19551 ★ European Society for Surgery of Shoulder and Elbow (ESSE)**
50-52, av Chanoine Cartellier
F-69230 Saint-Genis-Laval, France
**Fnded:** 1987.

**★ 19552 ★ European Society of Surgical Geriatrics**
25, av Charles de Gaulle
F-91150 Etampes, France

**European Society of Surgical Oncology (ESSO)**
*See:* Entry 10166

**★ 19553 ★ European Society of Thoracic Surgeons (ESTS)**
Solidtudstr. 18
Stuttgart
D-70839 Gerlingen, Germany
**Phone:** 49 7156 2032241　　**Fax:** 49 7156 2032003
**Email:** sue@ests.org.uk
**Website:** http://www.esso-surgeonline.be
**Desc:** Thoracic surgeons in Europe. Seeks to improve the study and practice of thoracic surgery.

**★ 19554 ★ European Society for Vascular Surgery (ESVS)**
University of Bath, Rm. L2.27
Clavertown Down
Bath BA2 7AY, United Kingdom
**Phone:** 44 1225 323770　　**Fax:** 44 1225 323669
**Email:** s.needham@bath.ac.uk
**Website:** http://www.esvs.org

**Fnded:** 1987. **Lang(s):** English. **Desc:** Vascular surgeons and national vascular societies. Seeks to advance vascular surgical techniques; promotes continuing professional development among vascular surgeons. Serves as a clearinghouse on vascular surgery; facilitates exchange of information among members; sponsors research and educational programs. **Pub:** *European Journal of Vascular and Endovascular Surgery,* monthly.

**★ 19555 ★ European Union of Paediatric Surgical Associations (EUPSA)**
Division of Pediatric Surgery
Academic Hospital Free University de Brussels
B-1090 Brussels, Belgium
**Phone:** 32 24776061          **Fax:** 32 24776074
**Email:** hlkdbra@az.vub.ac.be
**Fnded:** 1972. **Mem:** 24. **Lang(s):** English. **Desc:** National associations of pediatric surgeons. Promotes high standards of practice. Works to: standardize educational requirements in pediatric surgery; define the scope of pediatric surgery. Participates in the exchange of trainees among member associations.

**Faculty of Dental Surgery (FDS)**
*See:* Entry 6523

**★ 19556 ★ Federated Ambulatory Surgery Association (FASA)**
700 N Fairfax St., No. 306
Alexandria, VA 22314
**Phone:** (703)836-8808          **Fax:** (703)549-0976
**Email:** fasa@fasa.org
**Website:** http://www.fasa.org
Kathy Bryant, Exec. Dir.
**Fnded:** 1974. **Mem:** 1,200. **Desc:** Physicians, nurses, health administrators, and other individuals representing more than 800 outpatient surgery facilities. Promotes the concept of ambulatory (outpatient) surgical care. Facilitates exchange of knowledge and ideas regarding the care of ambulatory surgical patients. Represents members' interests at national level. Provides information to members, other organizations, and the public regarding government activities, legislation, statistical studies, group purchase programs, and the availability of malpractice insurance. Sponsors seminars, educational programs, and panel discussions; conducts studies and surveys in the field. **Pub:** *FASA Update,* bimonthly. Newsletter. • Membership Directory, annual. **Frmly:** Society for the Advancement of Freestanding Ambulatory Surgical Care; (1986) Freestanding Ambulatory Surgery Association.

**★ 19557 ★ French-Speaking Association of Surgical Endocrinology (FSASE) (Association Francophone de Chirurgie Enocrinienne — AFCE)**
Hopital de la Timone
Service de Chirurgie Generale et Endocrinienne
Centre Hospitalier Reg Universite de Lyon
1, rue de l'Antiquaille
F-69321 Lyon Cedex 5, France
**Phone:** 33 4 72385036          **Fax:** 33 4 72386540
**Fnded:** 1988. **Mem:** 125. **Lang(s):** English, French. **Desc:** Surgical endocrinologists. Seeks to advance the study, teaching, and practice of surgical endocrinology. Sponsors research programs and continuing professional development courses. **Pub:** *Anales de chisurgie,* 10/year. Journal.

**Gynecologic Surgery Society (GSS)**
*See:* Entry 16680

**Hong Kong Association of Dental Surgery Assistants (HKADSA)**
*See:* Entry 6531

**★ 19558 ★ Hong Kong Society of Minimal Access Surgery**
Duke of Windsor Social Service Bldg., 4/F
15 Hennessy Rd.
Hong Kong, People's Republic of China
**Email:** info@hksmas.org
**Website:** http://www.gynecologicsurgerysociety.org
**Fnded:** 1992. **Mem:** 369. **Lang(s):** Chinese, English. **Desc:** Medical practitioners, scientists and researchers, and other individuals with an interest in laparoscopy and other minimal access surgical techniques. Seeks to advance the practice of minimal access surgery. Promotes continuing professional advancement of members. Conducts public education programs and continuing professional development courses; facilitates international exchange among minimal access surgeons; sponsors research projects; makes available scholarships and other assistance to minimal access surgery students. Provides charitable medical care; assists in the development of hospitals and other health care facilities. **Pub:** *Elsa Journal,* quarterly. Journal.

**★ 19559 ★ Hong Kong Thoracic Society**
New Clinical Bldg., Rm. 302
University Department of Medicine
Queen Mary Hospital
Pokfulam
Hong Kong, People's Republic of China
**Phone:** 852 28554542          **Fax:** 852 28725828
**Email:** tamcy@ha.org.hk
**Website:** http://www.fmshk.com.hk/hkts
**Fnded:** 1987. **Mem:** 600. **Lang(s):** Chinese, English. **Desc:** Thoracic physicians, surgeons, and other medical personnel. Seeks to improve the study and practice of thoracic surgery and related disciplines. Conducts research and educational programs. **Pub:** *HKTS/ACCP Joint Newsletter,* periodic. Newsletter.

**★ 19560 ★ Indian Association of Paediatric Surgeons (IAPS)**
Department of Paediatric Surgery
B.J. Wadia Hospital for Children
Parel
Bombay 400 012, Maharashtra, India
**Phone:** 91 22 4172543          **Fax:** 91 22 4143435
**Email:** santoshjk@yahoo.com
**Fnded:** 1965. **Mem:** 600. **Desc:** Pediatric surgeons in India. Promotes continuing professional advancement of members. **Pub:** Journal, periodic.

**Indian Association of Surgical Oncology (IASO)**
*See:* Entry 10183

**★ 19561 ★ International Academy of Cosmetic Surgery (IACS)**
Via della Camilluccia 643
I-00135 Rome, Italy
**Phone:** 39 6 36304792          **Fax:** 39 6 36304165
**Email:** ravibina@hotmail.com
**Fnded:** 1970. **Mem:** 410. **Desc:** Cosmetic and reconstructive surgeons. Conducts training programs for doctors from underdeveloped countries. **Pub:** *Bulletin,* quarterly. Bulletin.

**★ 19562 ★ International Association for Ambulatory Surgery**
Ave du Duc Jean 71-73
1083 Brussels, Belgium
**Phone:** 32 2 4257076          **Fax:** 32 2 4224271
**Email:** c.delathouwer@baas.be
**Website:** http://www.iaas-med.org/
**Fnded:** 1995. **Desc:** Promotes exchange of information on and advancement of ambulatory surgery; encourages its high quality development and expansion; fosters education and research in the field and disseminates research results; establishes close relations with relevant organizations and stimulates development of national societies in the field.

**International Association of Ocular Surgeons (IAOS)**
*See:* Entry 20983

**★ 19563 ★ International Association of Oral and Maxillofacial Surgeons (IAOMS)**
9700 W Bryn Mawr, Ste. 210
Rosemont, IL 60018-5701
**Phone:** (847)678-9370          **Fax:** (847)878-9380
**Email:** lsayler@iaoms.org
**Website:** http://www.iaoms.org/
Victor Moncarz, Exec. Dir.
**Fnded:** 1965. **Mem:** 4,000. **Nat'l Groups:** 63. **Desc:** Seeks to improve the quality of healthcare worldwide through the advancement of patient care, education, and research in oral and maxillofacial surgery. **Pub:** *I.A.O.M.S.,* semiannual. Newsletter. • *International Journal of Oral and Maxillofacial Surgery,* bimonthly. Journal. • *Registry of Fellows.* • *Rules and Regulations of the IAOMS.*

**★ 19564 ★ International College of Surgeons (ICS)**
1516 N Lake Shore Dr.
Chicago, IL 60610
**Phone:** (312)642-3555          **Fax:** (312)787-1624
**Email:** max@icsglobal.org
**Website:** http://www.icsglobal.org
Max Downham, Exec. Dir.
**Fnded:** 1935. **Mem:** 10,000. **Nat'l Groups:** 70. **Reg. Groups:** 6. **Desc:** General surgeons and surgical specialists in 110 countries maintaining official relations with the World Health Organization. Promotes the universal teaching and advancement of surgery and its allied sciences. Maintains International Museum of Surgical Sciences containing specialty rooms showing the growth and perfection of many surgical specialties. Maintains library open to researchers, individuals working in the profession, and the public. Organizes postgraduate clinics around the world; conducts lecture series and periodic congresses; offers grants, scholarships, and loans for residencies, research, and advanced study in surgery. Sends surgical teaching teams to developing countries. Bestows honorary fellowship. **Pub:** *International College of Surgeons Newsletter,* quarterly. Newsletter. Covers college news and business. • *International Surgery,* quarterly. Journal. Presents papers on clinical, experimental, cultural, and historical topics pertinent to surgery and related fields. Contains book reviews. *Price:* $25/year for members; $50/year for nonmembers.

**★ 19565 ★ International Confederation for Plastic, Reconstructive and Aesthetic Surgery (IPRAS)**
4 Exec. Pk. Dr.
Albany, NY 12203
**Phone:** (518)438-1434          **Fax:** (518)489-1205
**Email:** ipras@ipras.org
Dr. James G. Hoehn, MD, Gen. Sec.
**Fnded:** 1955. **Mem:** 90. **Nat'l Groups:** 90. **Reg. Groups:** 3. **Desc:** National associations representing 13000 plastic surgeons. Promotes plastic surgery both clinically and scientifically. Encourages closer relationships between international members and direct contact between national societies. Disseminates information on developments in other countries. Seeks to widen the scope of understanding and knowledge in the field and reinforce the worldwide fraternity of plastic surgeons. **Pub:** *Globe Plast,* 3/year. Newsletter. *Price:* Free to members.

**★ 19566 ★ International Confederation for Plastic Reconstructive and Aesthetic Surgery - Asian-Pacific Section**
22 Bakhtawar Annexe
22 Narayan Dabholkar Rd.
Bombay 400 006, Maharashtra, India

**Phone:** 91 22 3675431          **Fax:** 91 22 3686368
**Email:** bmdaver@bom8.v5nl.net.in
**Website:** http://worldplasticsurgery.org
**Fnded:** 1970. **Mem:** 2,282. **Nat'l Groups:** 18.
**Lang(s):** English. **Desc:** Plastic and reconstructive
surgeons who are members of national societies of the
International Confederation for Plastic, Reconstructive
and Aesthetic Surgery. Promotes high standards of
practice and continuing education for members. **Pub:**
*Newsletter of the Asian Pacific Section*, annual. News-
letter.

★ 19567 ★ **International Federation of
  Societies for Surgery of the Hand
  (IFSSH)**
4, bd du President Edwards
F-67000 Strasbourg, France
**Phone:** 33 3 88354500          **Fax:** 33 3 88240707
**Email:** ifssh@handlibrary.org
**Website:** http://www.thehand.com/ifssh
**Fnded:** 1966. **Desc:** Exchanges knowledge, improv-
ing education and research, furthering availability of
hand surgery and cooperation among hand surgeons.

★ 19568 ★ **International Federation of
  Societies for Surgery of the Hand
  (IFSSH)**
c/o Dr. James R. Urbaniak
PO Box 2912
Duke University Medical Center
Durham, NC 27710
**Phone:** (919)684-5388          **Fax:** (919)681-7378
**Email:** urban006@mc.duke.edu
**Website:**      http://www.handlibrary.org/handsocieties/
ifssh/ifsshmain.html
James R. Urbaniak, MD, Sec. Gen.
**Fnded:** 1966. **Mem:** 5,000. **Reg. Groups:** 43. **Desc:**
Individuals involved in hand surgery. Coordinates
activities by maintaining liaison among member societies; promotes the exchange of information; attempts
to improve opportunities for study and observation on
an international level. Establishes and recommends
standards of nomenclature, classification of malformations, and disability evaluation; promotes a bibliography of world literature on surgery of the hand. Conducts scientific sessions; maintains committees to
develop standards and agreements on special areas
of hand surgery. **Pub:** Newsletter, annual.

★ 19569 ★ **International Federation of
  Surgical Colleges (IFSC)**
c/o SWA. Gunn, M.D., M.S, FRCSC, Hon. Sec.-
Gen.
CH-1279 Bogis-Bossey, Switzerland
**Phone:** 41 22 7762161          **Fax:** 41 22 7766417
**Email:** ifsc.us-muldoon@mail.med.upenn.edu
**Fnded:** 1958. **Mem:** 795. **Nat'l Groups:** 64. **Lang(s):**
English. **Desc:** National colleges, academies, and
associations of surgery in 70 countries. Works to
improve standards of surgery throughout the world.
Promotes cooperation and exchange of medical and
surgical information among surgical institutions. Encourages high standards of education, training, and
research in surgery and its allied sciences. Supports
clinical and scientific congresses in the surgical community. Fosters cooperation in developing the best
possible standards of surgical facilities and treatment,
and in providing appropriate scholarships and surgical
training in countries requesting aid. Collaborates with
the World Health Organization to strengthen rural
surgical health services in developing countries; maintains distribution facility for journals to Third World
nations. **Pub:** *IFSC News*, biennial. Newsletter. •
*World Journal of Surgery*, monthly. Journal. Additional
publications include collected papers.

**International Oculoplastic Society (IOSI)**
*See:* Entry 20992

**International Pediatric Endosurgery Group
  (IPEG)**
*See:* Entry 5697

★ 19570 ★ **International Society of
  Arthroscopy, Knee Surgery and
  Orthopaedic Sports Medicine (ISAKOS)**
145 Town and Country Dr., Ste. 106
Danville, CA 94526-3963
**Phone:** (925)314-7920          **Fax:** (925)314-7922
**Email:** isako@isakos.com
**Website:** http://www.isakos.com
Michelle Johnson, Soc. Mgr.
**Fnded:** 1978. **Mem:** 1,100. **Desc:** Orthopaedic sur-
geons specializing in problems of the knee, arthosco-
py, orthopaedic sports medicine. **Pub:** *The Journal of
Athroscopic and Related Surgery*. Journal. • Newslet-
ter, semiannual. **Frmly:** International Arthroscopy As-
sociation; (1995) International Society of the Knee.

**International Society for Cardiovascular
  Surgery (ISCVS)**
*See:* Entry 5026

**International Society for Dermatologic
  Surgery (ISDS)**
*See:* Entry 6829

★ 19571 ★ **International Society for
  Digestive Surgery**
13 Elm St.
Manchester, MA 01944
**Phone:** (978)526-8330          **Fax:** (978)526-4018
**Email:** ssat@prri.com
**Website:** http://www.isdsworld.org
E.H. Farthmann, MD, Pres.
**Fnded:** 1969. **Mem:** 1,205. **Desc:** Dedicated to presenting current information to the medical world concerning advances in gastrointestinal surgery, to permit
the free exchange of new knowledge, to allow comparison of experiences, to stimulate clinical studies, and
to seek improved diagnostic and therapeutic measures. **Pub:** *Digestive Surgery*, bimonthly. Journal.
Contains information concerned with diseases of the
alimentary tract.

★ 19572 ★ **International Society of Hair
  Restoration Surgery (ISHRS)**
930 N Meacham Rd.
Schaumburg, IL 60173
**Free:** 800-444-2737          **Fax:** (847)330-1135
**Email:** info@ishrs.org
**Website:** http://www.ishrs.org
**Fnded:** 1992. **Mem:** 700. **Desc:** Hair restoration
specialists. Endeavors to advance the art and science
of hair restoration. **Pub:** *Dermatologic Surgery*, month-
ly. Journal. • *Hair Transplant Forum International*,
bimonthly. Newsletter.

★ 19573 ★ **International Society for
  Minimal Intervention in Spinal Surgery**
c/o Prof. Hansjoerg F. Leu, Sec.
Spital Neumunster
Prsima Spine Unit
Trichtenhauserstrasse 12
CH-8125 Zollikerberg, Switzerland
**Fax:** 41 1 3912646
**Fnded:** 1989. **Mem:** 361. **Reg. Groups:** 9. **State
Groups:** 8. **Lang(s):** English. **Desc:** Promotes the
development of minimally invasive spinal surgery.

**International Society for Minimally
  Invasive Cardiac Surgery (ISMICS)**
*See:* Entry 5029

**International Society of Refractive
  Surgery (ISRS)**
*See:* Entry 21000

★ 19574 ★ **International Society of
  Surgery (ISS)
  (Societe Internationale de Chirurgie —
  SIC)**
Netzibodenstr. 34
PO Box 1527
CH-4133 Pratteln, Switzerland
**Phone:** 41 61 8159666          **Fax:** 41 61 8114775
**Email:** surgery@iss-sic.ch
**Website:** http://www.iss-sic.ch
**Fnded:** 1902. **Mem:** 3,700. **Nat'l Groups:** 105.
**Lang(s):** English. **Desc:** Surgeons from 105 countries
wishing to contribute to the progress of science by
researching and discussing surgical problems at con-
gresses and general assemblies. **Pub:** *ISS/SIC*, 2-3/
year. Newsletter. Contains membership information. •
*Membership Booklet*, biennial. Booklet. • *World Journal of Surgery*, monthly. Scientific publication on
general surgery.

★ 19575 ★ **Interplast**
300-B Pioneer Way
Mountain View, CA 94041-1506
**Phone:** (650)962-0123          **Free:** 888-467-5278
**Fax:** (650)962-1619
**Email:** ipnews@interplast.org
**Website:** http://www.interplast.org
Susan W. Hayes, Pres. /CEO
**Fnded:** 1969. **Reg. Groups:** 3. **State Groups:** 5.
**Desc:** Sends volunteer teams of medical professionals to developing countries to perform free reconstructive surgery on patients with birth defects, burns, and
other crippling deformities. Plans include travel to
foreign sites such as Mongolia, Peru, Ecuador, Vietnam, Thailand, Chile, Nepal, Honduras, Brazil, Dominican Republic, Bangladesh, Ukraine and the Phillippines to perform an estimate of 2000 free surgeries.
Conducts teaching programs during trips to developing countries. **Pub:** *Healing Hand*, quarterly. Newsletter.

★ 19576 ★ **Japan Society of Plastic and
  Reconstructive Surgery (JSPRS)**
c/o Business Center for Academy Societies of
  Japan
5-16-9, Honkomagome
Bunkyo-ku
Tokyo 113-8622, Japan
**Phone:** 81 3 58145801          **Fax:** 81 3 58145820
**Fnded:** 1958. **Mem:** 1,010. **Lang(s):** English, Japanese. **Desc:** Promotes practice of plastic and reconstructive surgery in Japan. Maintains high professional
standards. Disseminates information among members. **Pub:** *Journal of JSPRS*. Journal.

★ 19577 ★ **Korean Society of Plastic and
  Reconstructive Surgery (KSPRS)
  (Dae Han Sung Hyung Owe Gua)**
c/o Korean Medical Association Bldg. 601
302-75 Ichon-Dong Yongsan-ku
Seoul 140-30, Republic of Korea
**Phone:** 82 2 7901443          **Fax:** 82 2 7901442
**Email:** kprs@chollan.net
**Website:** http://www.plasticsurgery.or.kr
**Fnded:** 1966. **Mem:** 600. **Local Groups:** 5. **Lang(s):**
Korean. **Desc:** Aims to: increase scientific knowledge
in the field of plastic and reconstructive surgery;
promote friendship and communication between sur-
geons. Conducts continuing medical education, resi-
dent teaching program, courses, and symposia. Spon-
sors research. **Pub:** *Journal of the Korean Society of
Plastic and Reconstructive Surgery*, periodic. Journal.
• *List of Members KSPRS*, periodic. • *Newsletter
KSPRS*, quarterly.

★ 19578 ★ **Michael E. DeBakey
  International Surgical Society (MEDISS)**
c/o Kenneth L. Mattox
1 Baylor Plz.
Department of Surgery
Houston, TX 77030

**Phone:** (713)798-4557    **Fax:** (713)796-9605
**Email:** mediss@aol.com
**Website:** http://www.mediss.org
George P. Noon, Pres.

**Fnded:** 1976. **Mem:** 640. **Desc:** Physicians organized to encourage, advance, and promote scientific research relating to the treatment of general vascular, cardiac and cardiovascular defects and diseases through general vascular and cardiovascular surgery. **Frmly:** (1983) Michael E. DeBakey International Cardiovascular Society.

---

**★ 19579 ★  Middle East Neurosurgical Society**
**(Societe de Neurochirurgie du Moyen Orient)**
American Univ. Medical Center
PO Box 113-6044
Beirut, Lebanon
**Phone:** 961 1 353486    **Fax:** 961 1 373 1450231
**Fnded:** 1958. **Mem:** 545. **Lang(s):** English. **Desc:** Individuals in 12 countries. Disseminates information to the medical profession and to the public on clinical advancements and scientific research in neurosurgery and similar disciplines.

---

**★ 19580 ★  National Academy of Surgery**
**(Academie nationale de chirurgie)**
15, rue de l'Ecole de Medecine
F-75006 Paris, France
**Phone:** 33 1 43540232    **Fax:** 33 1 43293444
**Fnded:** 1731. **Desc:** Promotes research and progress in surgery.

---

**National College of Foot Surgeons (NCFS)**
See: Entry 17723

---

**★ 19581 ★  National Foundation for Facial Reconstruction (NFFR)**
317 E 34th St.
New York, NY 10016
**Phone:** (212)263-6656    **Fax:** (212)263-7534
**Email:** info@nffr.org
**Website:** http://www.nffr.org
Whitney Burnett, Exec. Dir.

**Fnded:** 1951. **Desc:** Assists individuals with a craniofacial deformity. Supports the treatment and rehabilitation efforts of the Institute of Reconstructive Plastic Surgery at New York University Medical center. Assists in patient care, research, the training and education of personnel engaged in reconstructive plastic surgery, conducts public education campaigns that promote national awareness of the problems of facial deformities and available treatment methods, and initiates and stimulates research. **Pub:** *NFFR Newsletter*, annual. Newsletter. Reports on the rehabilitation of individuals with facial disfigurement. Includes case histories and research updates. *Price:* Free. • *Out of the Shadows. . .Into a Bright New Future.* Brochure. • Proceedings. **Frmly:** (1986) Society for the Rehabilitation of the Facially Disfigured.

---

**★ 19582 ★  National Surgical Assistant Association (NSAA)**
740 B2 E Flynn Ln.
Phoenix, AZ 85014-1031
**Free:** 888-633-0479    **Fax:** (602)212-9692
**Email:** nsaa@namgmt.com
**Website:** http://www.nsaa.net
Ruth Helein, Exec. Dir.

**Fnded:** 1983. **Mem:** 650. **Desc:** Professional surgical assistants throughout the United States. Provides standard guidelines and regulations. Establishes rules for those who practice and function as surgical assistants. Examines, reviews, and certifies the training, duration, experience, skills, and knowledge of its members. **Pub:** *CSA Node*, quarterly. Newsletter. Provides articles on latest surgical techniques and trends in the operating room. • Membership Directory.

---

**Neurosurgical Society of Australasia**
See: Entry 14090

---

**★ 19583 ★  Operation Smile International - Vietnam (OSIV)**
Cityuate Bldg., Ste. 34C
Tran Hung Dao 104
Hanoi, Vietnam
**Phone:** 84 4 9420347    **Fax:** 84 4 9420051
**Email:** vietopsmile@netnam.org.vn
**Website:** http://www.operationsmile.org

**Lang(s):** English, French, Vietnamese. **Desc:** Reconstructive surgeons and other health care professionals. Seeks to increase the availability of cosmetic and reconstructive surgery among impoverished children. Performs free reconstructive surgery on needy children; conducts training programs for surgeons; distributes medical equipment and supplies to indigenous health care centers.

---

**★ 19584 ★  Outpatient Ophthalmic Surgery Society (OOSS)**
793 A. Foothill Blvd., pmb 119
San Luis Obispo, CA 93405
**Phone:** 877-220-3585    **Fax:** 877-220-2793
**Email:** info@ooss.org
**Website:** http://www.ooss.org
Karen S. Morgan, Admin. Dir.

**Fnded:** 1981. **Mem:** 700. **Desc:** Ophthalmic surgeons. Purpose is to gather and share information about outpatient eye surgery in order to promote high-quality, low-cost patient care. **Pub:** *Dollars and Disease: The True Cost of Cataracts.* • Journal, annual. • Newsletter, quarterly. • Also publishes books; produces videotapes.

---

**★ 19585 ★  Plastic Surgery Administrative Association (PSAA)**
4900 B S 31st St.
Arlington, VA 22206-1656
**Phone:** (703)931-4520
**Email:** psaa@mindspring.com
**Website:** http://www.plasticadmin.org/

**Fnded:** 1975. **Desc:** Plastic surgery administrators in all practices areas, including solo, group, academic, and surgi-center environments. Promotes the professional development of managers of plastic surgery practices; provides resources in order to achieve competency and efficiency; advocates for members on issues that affect the delivery of plastic surgery care; provides platform for networking. **Pub:** *Administrator Review*, quarterly. Educational publication that informs members of new product information, clinical and administrative updates, and organization activities. • Newsletter, quarterly. Contains educational information.

---

**★ 19586 ★  Plastic Surgery Educational Foundation (PSEF)**
444 E Algonquin Rd.
Arlington Heights, IL 60005
**Phone:** (847)228-9900    **Free:** 888-4-PLASTIC
**Fax:** (847)228-9131
**Email:** memserv@plasticsurgery.org
**Website:** http://www.plasticsurgery.org
Dave Fellers, CAE, Exec. Dir.

**Fnded:** 1948. **Mem:** 4,500. **Desc:** Plastic and reconstructive surgeons. Purpose is to identify and respond to the educational needs of members and their patients. Sponsors regional and national demonstrations, lectures, educational seminars, symposia, and workshops focusing on plastic surgery techniques and procedures. Conducts annual in-service and self-assessment examinations dealing with topics such as aesthetic and breast surgery, hand and extremities, integument, maxillofacial surgery, and pediatric plastic surgery. Administers Visiting Professors Program; compiles statistics; sponsors charitable programs. **Pub:** *Plastic and Reconstructive Surgery.* Journal. • *Plastic Surgery News.* • Booklets. **Frmly:** (1981) Education Foundation of American Society of Plastic and Reconstructive Surgeons.

---

**★ 19587 ★  Plastic Surgery Research Council (PSRC)**
45 Lyme Rd., Ste. 304
Hanover, NH 03755
**Phone:** (603)643-2325    **Fax:** (603)643-1444
**Email:** psrc@sover.net
**Website:** http://www.ps-rc.org
William A. Zamboni, MD, Chair

**Fnded:** 1955. **Mem:** 232. **Desc:** To foster fundamental research in the fields of plastic and reconstructive surgery. **Pub:** *Meeting Abstracts*, annual.

---

**Portuguese Society of Stomatology and Dental Medicine (PSSDM)**
**(Sociedade Portugesa de Estomatolgia Emedicina Dentaria — SPEMD)**
See: Entry 6583

---

**Puerto Rico Association of Pediatric Surgeons**
See: Entry 5746

---

**Royal Australasian College of Dental Surgeons**
See: Entry 6584

---

**★ 19588 ★  Royal Australasian College of Surgeons (RACS)**
Spring St.
Melbourne, VIC 3000, Australia
**Phone:** 61 3 92491200    **Fax:** 61 3 92491219
**Email:** registrar@racds.org
**Website:** http://www.racds.org
**Fnded:** 1927.

---

**★ 19589 ★  Royal College of Surgeons of Edinburgh**
Nicolson St.
Edinburgh EH8 9DW, United Kingdom
**Phone:** 44 131 5271600    **Fax:** 44 131 5576406
**Email:** information@rcsed.ac.uk
**Website:** http://www.rcsed.ac.uk
**Fnded:** 1505. **Desc:** Promotes the education, training and examination, the raising of standards in surgical practice.

---

**★ 19590 ★  Royal College of Surgeons of England (RCS Eng)**
35/43 Lincoln's Inn Fields
London WC2A 3PN, United Kingdom
**Phone:** 44 20 74053474    **Fax:** 44 20 78319438
**Email:** external@rcseng.ac.uk
**Website:** http://www.rcseng.ac.uk

**Fnded:** 1800. **Mem:** 15,000. **Lang(s):** English. **Desc:** Surgeons and dental surgeons in the United Kingdom. Aims to promote and encourage the study and practice of surgery as an art and a science. Maintains professional standards through examinations; establishes criteria for the qualification of consultant and dental surgeons in the National Health Service; advises government and other professional bodies on surgical matters; conducts research. Offers postgraduate courses in surgery and related subjects; sponsors seminars and workshops. Operates the Hunterian Museum. **Pub:** *Annals of the Royal College of Surgeons of England*, bimonthly. Report.

---

**★ 19591 ★  Scandinavian Association of Paediatric Surgeons (SCAPS)**
**(Nordisk Barnkirurgisk Forening — NBF)**
c/o Torbjorn Kufaas
Department of Pediatric Surgery
Regionsykehuset
N-7006 Trondheim, Norway
**Phone:** 47 7 3998000    **Fax:** 47 7 3997428
**Fnded:** 1964. **Mem:** 146. **Nat'l Groups:** 5. **Lang(s):** Danish, English, Norwegian, Swedish. **Desc:** Pediatric surgeons in 5 countries. Promotes the development of

pediatric surgery and cooperation among members; represents members internationally. Encourages co-operative studies.


★ **19592** ★ **Scandinavian Association of Plastic Surgeons (SAPS) (Nordisk Plastikkirurgisk Forening — NPF)**
c/o Dr. Mikael Relander
Bokbackgranden 4B
FIN-20900 Turku, Finland
**Phone:** 358 2 2581560          **Fax:** 358 2 6102984
**Email:** mihael.relander@pp-timnet.fi

**Fnded:** 1951. **Mem:** 225. **Lang(s):** Danish, Finnish, Icelandic, Norwegian, Swedish. **Desc:** Plastic surgeons in 5 countries. Promotes the advancement of plastic surgery. Keeps members informed of developments in plastic surgery. Sponsors courses. **Pub:** *List of Members*, periodic. • *Scandinavian Journal of Plastic and Reconstructive Surgery and Hand Surgery*, quarterly. Journal.


★ **19593** ★ **Scandinavian Association for Thoracic Surgery (SATS) (Nordisk Thoraxkirurgisk Forening — NTF)**
c/o Prof. Hostrup Nielsen, MD
Department of Cardio-Thoracic Surgery
Skejby University Hospital
Brendstrupgaardsvej
DK-8200 N Arhus, Denmark
**Phone:** 45 89 495410          **Fax:** 45 89 496005
**Email:** phn@sks.aaa.dk
**Website:** http://www.scandinavian-ats.org

**Fnded:** 1949. **Mem:** 250. **Lang(s):** English. **Desc:** Scandinavian thoracic and cardiovascular surgeons. Conducts graduate lectures and presentations of scientific papers. **Frmly:** Scandinavian Association for Thoracic and Cardiovascular Surgery.


**Scandinavian Neurosurgical Society (SNS) (Nordisk Neurokirurgisk Forening — NNF)**
*See:* Entry 14107


★ **19594** ★ **Scandinavian Surgical Society (SSS)**
c/o Jon Haffner, M.D., Ph.D.
Univ. of Turku
Lemminkaisenkatu 14-18 B
FIN-20520 Turku, Finland
**Phone:** 358 2 2612203          **Fax:** 358 2 2612284
**Email:** tiitmathiesen@neuro.ks.se

**Fnded:** 1893. **Mem:** 4,352. **Nat'l Groups:** 5. **Lang(s):** Danish, English, Finnish, Icelandic, Norwegian, Swedish. **Desc:** Surgeons in Denmark, Finland, Iceland, Norway, and Sweden. Seeks to: promote clinical and research work and training in the field of surgery; encourage scientific and clinical communication between surgeons in the Scandinavian countries and elsewhere. Offers courses in surgical disciplines. **Pub:** *European Journal of Surgery*, semiannual. Journal. **Frmly:** (1994) Nordic Surgical Society.


★ **19595** ★ **Scandinavian Work Group on Reconstructive Microsurgery**
Department of Plastic Surgery
Herlev Hospital
University of Copenhagen
DK-2730 Herlev, Denmark
**Phone:** 45 44535300          **Fax:** 45 44535332


★ **19596** ★ **Slovak Society of Plastic Surgery**
c/o Centre of Burns
Hospital
Lucna 57
SK-040 15 Kosice, Slovakia
**Phone:** 42 195 6842129      **Free:** 42 195 6841311
**Fax:** 42 195 6842129

**Fnded:** 1989. **Mem:** 8. **Lang(s):** English, German, Russian, Slovak. **Desc:** Plastic surgeons. Promotes professional advancement of members and continued improvement in the practice of cosmetic surgery; represents members' interests.


★ **19597** ★ **Society of Air Force Clinical Surgeons**
839 W Lincoln Ave., No. 716
Woodland, CA 95695
**Phone:** (530)661-0352          **Fax:** (530)661-0352
**Email:** rosepreuit@aol.com
**Website:** http://atech.org/SAFCS/
Rose A. Thomas, Exec. Dir.

**Fnded:** 1958. **Mem:** 640. **Desc:** Air Force Clinical Surgeons. Promotes excellence in surgery within the Air Force, serves as a forum for the presentation of scientific papers, fosters esprit de corps, and promulgates military surgical objectives.


**Society of American Gastrointestinal Endoscopic Surgeons (SAGES)**
*See:* Entry 9153


★ **19598** ★ **Society for Clinical Vascular Surgery**
13 Elm St.
Manchester, MA 01944-1314
**Email:** sagesmail@aol.com
**Website:** http://www.vascsurg.org/doc/Jvonliebig.html

**Fnded:** 1969. **Desc:** Academic and community vascular surgeons. Promotes vascular surgery in the U.S.


**Society of Eye Surgeons (SES)**
*See:* Entry 21077


★ **19599** ★ **Society of Graduate Surgeons (SGS)**
4929 Wilshire Blvd., No. 428
Los Angeles, CA 90010
**Phone:** (323)937-5514          **Fax:** (323)937-0959
**Email:** ief@iefusa.org
**Website:** http://www.iefusa.org
C. James Dowden, Exec. Dir.

**Fnded:** 1950. **Mem:** 375. **Desc:** Surgeons who have completed general surgery residencies at USC-LA County Medical Center. Conducts post-graduate educational programs for members and surgeons.


★ **19600** ★ **Society of Laparoendoscopic Surgeons (SLS)**
7330 SW 62nd Pl., Ste. 410
Miami, FL 33143-4825
**Phone:** (305)665-9959          **Free:** 800-446-2659
**Fax:** (305)667-4123
**Email:** info@sls.org
**Website:** http://www.sls.org
Paul A. Wetter, MD, Contact

**Fnded:** 1990. **Mem:** 6,700. **Desc:** Laparoscopic and endoscopic surgeons from all specialties and other health care professionals. Promotes improvement in laparoscopic and endoscopic surgical techniques; facilitates professional growth of members. Conducts educational programs. **Pub:** *Journal of the Society of Laparoendoscopic Surgeons*, quarterly. Journal. This is a multi-disciplinary journal of laparoscopy, endoscopy and minimally invasive surgery. *Price:* $195 in U.S. • *SLS Report*, semiannual. Newsletter. Membership newsletter. *Price:* $85.


**Society of Neurological Surgeons (SNS)**
*See:* Entry 14113


**Society of Neurosurgical Anesthesia and Critical Care (SNACC)**
*See:* Entry 4471


★ **19601** ★ **Society of Reproductive Surgeons (SRS)**
1209 Montgomery Hwy.
Birmingham, AL 35216-2809
**Phone:** (205)978-5000          **Fax:** (205)978-5005
**Email:** finch@asrm.org
**Website:** http://www.reprodsurgery.org
Cheryl Finch, Admin.

**Fnded:** 1984. **Mem:** 450. **Desc:** Reproductive surgeons. Gathers and disseminates information on reproductive surgery; conducts continuing education programs for members. Makes available referrals list. **Pub:** *SRS Newsletter*, semiannual. Newsletter.


★ **19602** ★ **Society for Surgery of the Alimentary Tract (SSAT)**
13 Elm St.
Manchester, MA 01944
**Phone:** (978)526-8330          **Fax:** (978)526-4018
**Email:** ssat@prri.com
**Website:** http://www.ssat.com
Robert P. Jones, Jr., Exec. Dir.

**Fnded:** 1960. **Mem:** 2,500. **Desc:** Licensed physicians with an interest in surgical aspects of digestive diseases. Seeks to advance the study, teaching, and practice of surgery of the alimentary tract; promotes continuing professional development of members. Serves as a forum for the discussion of new alimentary surgical techniques; encourages training opportunities and funding for alimentary surgical research. **Pub:** *Journal of Gastrointestinal Surgery*, bimonthly. Journal. • *Patient Care Guidelines*. Handbook.


**Society of Surgical Oncology (SSO)**
*See:* Entry 10253


★ **19603** ★ **Society of Thoracic Surgeons (STS)**
633 N St. Clair St., No. 2320
Chicago, IL 60611
**Phone:** (312)202-5800          **Fax:** (312)202-5801
**Email:** sts@sba.org
**Website:** http://www.sts.org
Donald A. Turney, Exec. Dir.

**Fnded:** 1964. **Mem:** 4,700. **Desc:** Surgeons who confine their practice to the field of thoracic-cardiovascular surgery. Objectives are: to improve the quality and practice of thoracic and cardiovascular surgery as a specialty; to strengthen and establish basic standards in training programs; to encourage clinical and basic research; to promote the professional development of those surgeons specializing in the field; to represent and sponsor those surgeons who have recently entered the field. Conducts annual postgraduate program and three-day scientific session. **Pub:** *Annals of Thoracic Surgery*, monthly.


**Society of United States Air Force Flight Surgeons**
*See:* Entry 4486


★ **19604** ★ **Society of University Otolaryngologists - Head and Neck Surgeons (SUO-HNS)**
c/o Marvin Fried
USC School of Medicine
Department of Otolaryngology
1200 N State St.
Box 795
Los Angeles, CA 90033
**Phone:** (323)226-7315          **Fax:** (323)226-2780
**Email:** Robert.Yono@brooksaf.mil
**Website:** http://www.sousaffs.org
Donna Hoffman, M.A., Exec. Dir.

**Fnded:** 1964. **Mem:** 500. **Desc:** Otolaryngologists affiliated with universities through an approved residency training program, faculty appointment, or teaching or research position. Promotes the advancement of the art and science of otolaryngology by the development and improvement of undergraduate and graduate teaching programs. Encourages basic research and clinical investigation as an integral part of university training programs. Sponsors annual course; maintains society records. **Pub:** Directory, annual. **Frmly:** (1983) Society of University Olodaryngologists.


★ 19605 ★ **Society of University Surgeons (SUS)**
c/o Administrative Office
PO Box 16549
West Haven, CT 06516
**Phone:** (203)932-0541     **Fax:** (203)937-7716
**Email:** samokar@1-2000.com
Mary E. Samokar, Admin. Dir.

**Fnded:** 1938. **Mem:** 1,280. **Desc:** Professional society of surgeons connected with university teaching. Works to advance the art and science of surgery by encouraging original investigations both in the clinic and in the laboratory and by developing methods of graduate teaching of surgery with particular reference to the resident system. **Pub:** *Surgery*, monthly. Journal.


★ 19606 ★ **Society for Vascular Surgery (SVS)**
13 Elm St.
Manchester, MA 01944
**Phone:** (978)526-8330     **Fax:** (978)526-4018
**Email:** svs@prri.com
**Website:** http://www.vascularweb.org
David M. Cloud, Exec. Dir.

**Fnded:** 1945. **Mem:** 594. **Desc:** Professional society of board-certified surgeons interested in promoting the study of and research in the circulatory system. **Pub:** *Journal of Vascular Surgery*, monthly.


**South African Association of Paediatric Surgeons (SAAPS)**
**(Suid-Afrikaanse Vereniging van Kinderchirurge — SAVK)**
*See:* Entry 5762


★ 19607 ★ **Surgical Research Society**
Academic Surgical Unit
The University of Hull
Castle Hill Hospital
Cottingham HU6 5JQ, United Kingdom
**Phone:** 44 1482 623225     **Fax:** 44 1482 623274
**Email:** h.binks@hull.ac.uk
**Website:** http://www.surgicalresearchsociety.org.uk
**Mem:** 547. **Desc:** Surgeons. To provide for the interchange of information about research related to surgery and surgical disease. **Pub:** *British Journal of Surgery*. Journal.


★ 19608 ★ **Surgical Research Society of Southern Africa (SRSSA)**
**(Chirurgiese Navorsingsvereniging van Suide Afrika — CNSA)**
PO Box 231
Medunsa 0204, Republic of South Africa
**Phone:** 27 12 5214153     **Fax:** 27 12 5124467
**Email:** jferreira@medunsa.ac.za
**Website:** http://www.wits.ac.za/surgery/srs/
**Fnded:** 1972. **Mem:** 270. **Local Groups:** 5. **Lang(s):** Afrikaans, English. **Desc:** Surgeons and surgeons in training. Promotes research, particularly among younger members, in clinical and experimental surgery. Sets surgical research standards. Provides funding to surgery departments of South African universities; offers grants and scholarships; sponsors competitions. **Pub:** *Abstracts of Society Meeting*, annual. • *South Africa Journal of Surgery*, periodic.


**Tunisian Society of Cardiology and Cardiovascular Surgery**
*See:* Entry 5077


**Union of Middle Eastern and Mediterranean Pediatric Societies (UMEMPS)**
**(Union des Societes de Pediatrie du Moyen-Orient et de la Mediterranee — USPMOM)**
*See:* Entry 5769


★ 19609 ★ **Western Surgical Association (WSA)**
c/o Richard C. Thirlby, MD
Virginia Mason Medical Clinic
1100 Ninth Ave., C6-GSUR
Seattle, WA 98111
**Phone:** (206)223-6636     **Free:** 800-354-9527
**Fax:** (206)625-7245
**Email:** Richard.Thirlby@vmmc.org
**Website:** http://www.vmmc.org
Dr. Richard Thirlby, MD, Sec.

**Fnded:** 1891. **Mem:** 700. **Desc:** Surgeons who have contributed to surgical education and advancement. Objectives are: to cultivate, promote, and diffuse knowledge of the art and science of surgery; to sponsor and maintain the highest standards of practice; to deliver the best possible care to all people. **Pub:** *Western Surgical Association Newsletter*, quarterly. Newsletter. Includes information on new members and information on upcoming meetings. *Price:* Free. • *Western Surgical Association Program*, annual. Book. Contains abstracts of papers to be presented at annual meeting, also includes transactions.


**Women's Healthcare Educational Network (WHEN)**
*See:* Entry 10260


★ 19610 ★ **World Federation of Associations of Pediatric Surgeons**
c/o Prof. J. Boix-Ochoa
Clinica Infantil 'Vall d'Hebron, Dpto. de Cirugia Pediatrica
Fac. de Medicina
University Autonoma
PO Vall d'Hebron, s/n
E-08035 Barcelona, Spain
**Email:** info@whenusa.org
**Website:** http://www.whenusa.org
**Lang(s):** English, Spanish. **Desc:** Pediatric surgeons and other medical professionals with an interest in pediatric surgery. Seeks to advance pediatric surgical procedures. Serves as a clearinghouse on pediatric surgery; conducts research and continuing professional development programs.


★ 19611 ★ **World Federation of Neurosurgical Societies (WFNS)**
c/o Dr. Edward Laws
University of Virginia Health Systems
Department of Neuro-Societies
PO Box 800212
Charlottesville, VA 22908
**Phone:** (804)924-2650     **Fax:** (804)924-5894
**Website:** http://www.wfns.org
Dr. Edward Laws, Sec.

**Fnded:** 1957. **Mem:** 64. **Reg. Groups:** 5. **Desc:** National neurosurgical societies representing approximately 17,400 neurosurgeons. Works for the advancement of neurological surgery. **Pub:** *Critical Reviews in Neurosurgery*. Journal. • *Federation News*, quarterly. Newsletter. *Price:* $75. • *Proceedings of International Congress*, quadrennial. Proceedings. • *World Directory*, periodic. Directory.


★ 19612 ★ **World Society for Stereotactic and Functional Neurosurgery (WSSFN)**
c/o New York University Medical Center
Department of Neurosurgery
500 First St.
New York, NY 10016
**Fax:** (212)263-8031


**Email:** kelly@mcns04.nyu.edu
**Website:** http://www.wssfn.org/
Patrick J. Kelly, VP

**Fnded:** 1963. **Mem:** 600. **Nat'l Groups:** 3. **Reg. Groups:** 4. **Desc:** Neurosurgeons and professors dedicated to the advancement of stereotactic studies and procedures. Original manuscripts submitted at meetings are published and used as reference books throughout the world. **Pub:** *Stereotactic and Functional Neurosurgery*, quarterly. Journal. • *Studies in Stereoencephalotomy*, quadrennial. **AKA:** World Stereotactic Society; WSSFN. **Frmly:** (1973) International Society for Research in Stereoencephalotomy.


**World Society for Stereotactic and Functional Neurosurgery (WSSFN)**
*See:* Entry 14134


# Research Centers


★ 19613 ★ **Agnes Barr Chase Surgical Research Foundation**
Parkinson Pavilion, 4th Fl.
Department of Surgery
Temple University
Broad & Ontario Sts.
Philadelphia, PA 19140
**Phone:** (215)707-5080     **Fax:** (215)707-1915
**Email:** jrudy@vm.temple.edu
**Website:** http://www.wssfn.org
Dr. Daniel T. Dempsey, Chm., Dept. of Surgery

**Activities/Fields:** Provides support for research in the Department of Surgery, with emphasis on the specialties of gastrointestinal, vascular, and cardio-thoracic surgery.


**Christine M. Kleinert Institute for Hand and Microsurgery, Inc.**
*See:* Entry 13686


★ 19614 ★ **Duke University Frank Hawkins Kenan Plastic Surgery Research Laboratories**
Medical Center
016 Research Park 4
PO Box 3906
Durham, NC 27710
**Phone:** (919)684-3929     **Fax:** (919)681-2670
**Email:** klitz@acpub.duke.edu
**Website:** http://www.duke.edu/~klitz
Prof. Bruce Klitzman, Sr. Dir.

**Activities/Fields:** Microvascular physiology, tissue engineering, plastic surgery, including wound healing monitoring tissue viability, thrombolytic therapy, preservation of organs, and biocompatibility of synthetic vascular grafts (prostheses). Also conducts studies on microcirculation, skin cancer, and aging skin. **Frmly:** Plastic Surgery Research Laboratories.


★ 19615 ★ **Edward Dana Mitchell Surgical Research Laboratory**
956 Court, E228
Department of Surgery
University of Tennessee
Memphis, TN 38163
**Phone:** (901)448-8370     **Fax:** (901)448-7306
**Activities/Fields:** Surgery, transplantation, sepsis, shock, nutrition, hepatic dysfunction, and gut immunology.


**Georgetown University Division of Comparative Medicine**
*See:* Entry 2496

**★ 19616 ★ Institute for Applied Laser Surgery**
2 Bala Plz., Ste. PL-13
Bala Cynwyd, PA 19004
**Phone:** (610)667-4080    **Fax:** (610)667-2748
Dr. Ronald A. Kirschner, Dir.

**Activities/Fields:** Surgical applications of lasers and laser-related accessory development. Activities include development of new procedures in cardiovascular, peripheral vascular, cutaneeur, plastic, urologic, gynocologic, orthopedic surgery, and endoscopic surgery. **Pub:** *Newsletter.* **Frmly:** Medical Laser Technology Center.

**★ 19617 ★ New York University**
**Institute of Reconstructive Plastic Surgery**
560 1st Ave.
New York, NY 10016
**Phone:** (212)263-5209    **Fax:** (212)263-2838
**Email:** joseph.mccarthy@med.nyu.edu
Joseph G. McCarthy, MD, Dir.

**Activities/Fields:** Etiology and treatment of craniofacial anomalies, bone physiology, including distraction, computer graphics, microvascular surgery, and wound healing, including studies of cleft lip and cleft palate, jaw deformities, ear malformations, hand injuries, and allied problems.

**Oral and Maxillofacial Surgery Foundation**
*See:* Entry 6611

**★ 19618 ★ Plastic Surgery Research Council (Hanover, NH)**
45 Lyme Rd., Ste. 304
Hanover, NH 03755
**Phone:** (603)643-2325    **Fax:** (603)643-1444
**Email:** psrc@sover.net
**Website:** http://www.ps-rc.org
Catherin B. Foss, Contact

**Activities/Fields:** Plastic surgery.

**★ 19619 ★ Plastic Surgery Research Council (Pittsburgh, PA)**
Scaife Hall, 676
University of Pittsburgh Medical Center
3550 Terrace St.
Pittsburgh, PA 15261
**Phone:** (412)648-8100    **Fax:** (412)648-1987
**Email:** manders@upmc.msx.edu
Ernest K. Manders, Contact

**Activities/Fields:** Tissue engineering.

**★ 19620 ★ St. Louis University**
**Theodore Cooper Surgical Research Institute**
Department of Surgery
1402 S Grand Blvd.
Saint Louis, MO 63104
**Phone:** (314)577-8561    **Fax:** (314)268-5180
**Email:** smithp2@slu.edu
Dr. Gregory S. Smith, Dir.

**Activities/Fields:** Gastrointestinal and hepatic physiology, bioartificial liver, myocardial revascularization, drug metabolism, pharmacokinetics, toxicokinetics, organ transplantation and preservation, cardiac assist and replacement, myocardial preservation and pulmonary function, islet cell transplantation, immunology/nutrition, shock and multiple organ failure, neuropharmacology, transplantation immunogenetics, image guided surgery, and molecular biology. **Pub:** *Research Prospectus,* annually. • *SRI Insights,* quarterly. **Frmly:** Vallee Willman Surgical Research Institute; Institute of Experimental Surgery.

**★ 19621 ★ Stanford University**
**Image Guidance Laboratories (IGL)**
Department of Neurosurgery
School of Medicine
300 Pasteur Dr., MC No. 5327 at S-008
Stanford, CA 94305-5327
**Phone:** (650)498-7958    **Fax:** (650)724-4846
**Email:** info@igl.stanford.edu
**Website:** http://neurosurgery.stanford.edu/igl/
Prof. Ramin Shahidi, Dir.

**Activities/Fields:** Surgical navigation techniques and minimally invasive surgical technology. **Pub:** *Papers.*

**U.S. Department of Defense**
**Army Medical Research and Materiel Command**
**Army Institute of Surgical Research**
*See:* Entry 13471

**★ 19622 ★ U.S. Department of Defense**
**Army Medical Research and Materiel Command**
**Walter Reed Army Institute of Research**
**Surgery Division**
503 Robert Grant Ave., Rm. 1A34
Silver Spring, MD 20910-7500
**Phone:** (301)319-9761    **Fax:** (301)319-9839
**Email:** frederick.pearce@na.amedd.army.mil
**Website:** http://wrair-www.army.mil
Frederick Pearce, PhD, Chf.

**Activities/Fields:** Military medical problems of combat injury, shock, wounding, and resuscitation (singly or in combination) in order to establish optimal prophylactic and therapeutic care of severely injured patients. Division also develops adjuncts for the diagnosis and management of blast-induced injury to the lung and/or gastrointestinal tract; and develops and provides laboratory models for biomedical assessment of medical material systems. Branch components include Physiology of Combat Trauma, and Field Biomedical Engineering. **Frmly:** (2000) Surgery Division.

**U.S. Department of Health and Human Services**
**National Cancer Institute**
**Division of Clinical Sciences**
**Surgery Branch**
*See:* Entry 10471

**U.S. Department of Health and Human Services**
**National Institute of Neurological Disorders and Stroke**
**Division of Intramural Research (Clinical Neurosciences Program)**
**Surgical Neurology Branch**
*See:* Entry 14315

**★ 19623 ★ University of Alberta**
**Surgical-Medical Research Institute**
1074 Dentistry Pharmacy Centre
Edmonton, AB, Canada T6G 2N8
**Phone:** (780)492-3386    **Fax:** (780)492-1627
**Email:** rrajotte@ualberta.ca
Dr. Ray V. Rajotte, Dir.

**Activities/Fields:** Institute is composed of multidisciplinary teams carrying out biomedical research. Principal fields of study include: islet transplantation, the immunology of diabetes, glucose regulation studies, experiments for extending the application of laparoscopic surgery and including a minimal access laboratory, and metabolic aspects of organ preservation (liver, heart, small bowel).

**★ 19624 ★ University of Illinois at Chicago**
**Surgical Oncology**
MC 820
Clinical Science Bldg., MC 820
College of Medicine
840 S Wood St.
Chicago, IL 60612
**Phone:** (312)996-6666    **Fax:** (312)996-9365
**Email:** ncornel@uic.edu
Dr. Nancy Tapas K. Cornelius Das Gupta, Prog. Coord.

**Activities/Fields:** Tumor biology, including molecular biology and molecular genetics, drug development, chemoprevention, drug resistance, genetic rearrangement, gene regulation, signal transduction, epidemiology prevention, and clinical research. Center specializes in the study of cancers of the head and neck region, breast, esophagus, stomach, small and large bowel, colon and rectum, liver and pancreas, skin, and soft body tissue.

**★ 19625 ★ University of Kentucky**
**Center for Minimally Invasive Surgery**
Chandler Medical Center
800 Rose St., C-344
Lexington, KY 40536-0293
**Phone:** (859)323-6278    **Fax:** (859)257-1428
**Email:** apark@uky.edu
**Website:** http://www-mis.uky.edu/
Adrian Park, MD, Dir.

**Activities/Fields:** Surgery using an endoscope and its benefits especially regarding recovery time and economic impact.

**★ 19626 ★ University of Manitoba**
**Health Sciences Centre**
**Surgical Research Office**
Department of Surgery
GE 611-820 Sherbrook St.
Winnipeg, MB, Canada R3A 1R9
**Phone:** (204)787-3791    **Fax:** (204)787-1342
**Email:** hunruh@hsc.mb.ca
Dr. Helmut Unruh, Res. Dir.

**Activities/Fields:** Orthopedics, oncology, gastrointestinal surgery, neurosurgery, respirology, urology, cardiology, and pediatric and general surgery.

**★ 19627 ★ University of Michigan**
**Pediatric Surgery Research Laboratories**
F3970 Mott Children's Hospital
Ann Arbor, MI 48109-0245
**Phone:** (734)764-4151    **Fax:** (734)936-9784
**Email:** acoran@umich.edu
Arnold G. Coran, MD, Dir.

**Activities/Fields:** Pediatric surgery, including physiological and biochemical changes during septic and hemorrhagic shock in puppies, physiology and metabolism of patients receiving total parenteral nutrition, physiology of endorectal pull-through operations for Hirschprung's disease in dogs, determination of trace element levels in infants receiving oral feedings or total parenteral nutritional solutions, and bacterial translocation in newborn babies.

**★ 19628 ★ University of Michigan**
**Thoracic Surgery Research Lab**
University Medical Center
Ann Arbor, MI 48109
**Phone:** (734)936-5800    **Fax:** (734)615-2656
**Email:** morrin@umich.edu
Dr. Mark Orringer, Dir.

**Activities/Fields:** Cardiovascular and pulmonary physiology and transplantations, cellular and molecular aspects of allograft rejection and tolerance, molecular genetics of human lung and esophageal cancer, regional ventricular function (using sonomicrometry measurements) in conditions of ischemia, infarction, and reperfusion, neonatal myocardial performance and protection of the neonatal heart during ischemia, and role of cytokines in cardiac and pulmonary injury.

**University of Minnesota**
**Experimental Surgical Services Laboratories**
*See:* Entry 5189

**University of Missouri—Columbia
Division of Cardiothoracic Surgery**
*See:* Entry 5190

**★ 19629 ★ University of Pennsylvania
Harrison Department of Surgical
  Research**
Margarett M. Clark Laboratories
313 Stemmler Hall
Philadelphia, PA 19104-6070
**Phone:** (215)898-8081          **Fax:** (215)573-2001
**Email:** curtisj@health.missouri.edu
**Website:** http://www.surgery.missouri.edu
Clyde F. Barker, MD, Dir.

**Activities/Fields:** Cancer, cardiovascular disease, gastrointestinal physiology, shock and surgical bacteriology, nutrition of surgical patients, and surgical specialities, including studies of stomach and duodenum, pancreas, colon, liver, blood flow, hypertension, equilibrium tissue oxygen requirements, tissue oxygen, oxygen supply in shock and shock-like states, chemotherapy, patient antitumor agents, immunology, ultraviolet light in protection against wound infection, transplantation of tissues and organs, and role of electronics in surgical research. **Pub:** *Annual report.*

**University of Vermont
General Clinical Research Center**
*See:* Entry 2738

**★ 19630 ★ University of Virginia
Surgical Therapeutic Advancement Center
  (STAC)**
MR 4 Bldg., Rm. 3122
University of Virginia Health System
PO Box 801373
Charlottesville, VA 22908-1373
**Phone:** (434)243-0315          **Fax:** (434)243-0318
**Email:** uvatac@virginia.edu
**Website:**          http://www.vtmednet.org/~g195040/
gcrcpage.htm
William D. Spotnitz, MD, Dir.

**Activities/Fields:** Development of innovations in the field of surgery to improve the clinical care of patients.
**Pub:** *Journal manuscripts.*

**★ 19631 ★ University of Washington
Center for Videoendoscopic Surgery
  (CVES)**
Department of Surgery, Box 356410
1959 NE Pacific St., Rm. BB-487
Seattle, WA 98195

**Phone:** (206)685-9076          **Fax:** (206)685-6912
**Email:** cwesterg@u.washington.edu
**Website:** http://depts.washington.edu/cves/
Prof. Carlos A. Pellegrini, MD, Dir.

**Activities/Fields:** Development of new minimally invasive surgical techniques.

**★ 19632 ★ Vanderbilt University
S.R. Light Laboratory for Surgical
  Research**
MCN, Rm. CC-2307
Nashville, TN 37232
**Phone:** (615)322-2096          **Fax:** (615)343-1355
**Email:** phil.williams@mcmail.vanderbilt.edu
**Website:** http://www.mc.vanderbilt.edu/surgery/rsrch-div.htm
Phillip E. Williams, Dir.

**Activities/Fields:** All phases of medicine involving use of experimental animals. Specific research includes studies of metabolism, particularly mechanisms of stress-related changes in glucose and amino acids; cardiothoracic study of pathophysiology of ischemic myocardium; and renovascular physiology. Also develops new surgical instrumentation and techniques.

# Chapter 65
# Therapy & Rehabilitation

## Foundations & Other Funding Organizations

### Private Foundations

**★ 19633 ★ Arthur S. DeMoss Foundation**
Phillips Point West Tower, Ste. 1600
777 South Flagler Dr.
West Palm Beach, FL 33401
**Phone:** (561)804-9011  **Fax:** (561)804-9025
Mrs. Arthur DeMoss, Contact
**Fnded:** 1955. **Philosophy:** The foundation's focus is conducting its own projects, staffed by its own people. Additionally, a few grants are awarded. Sponsored projects are Power for Living, a multi-national evangelical outreach, which promotes the free book, *Power for Living: Executive Ministries,* dedicated to "winning and discipling business and professional executives to Jesus Christ;" Life Action Ministries, which is concerned with "teaching Biblical principles regarding the building of Christian families and Christian homes;" and Rebirth of America, which promotes the free book of the same name, and is concerned with the departure of present day America from "our founding fathers' respect for God's moral law." Foundation grantmaking is restricted to Christian evangelical causes. **Priorities:** *Note:* Total contributions made in 1998. **Typ. Recipients:** Family Planning, Medical Rehabilitation, Medical Research. **Geo. Dist:** nationally and internationally.

**Clara Blackford Smith and W. Aubrey Smith Charitable Foundation**
*See:* Entry 128

**Dora Roberts Foundation**
*See:* Entry 177

**Hattie M. Strong Foundation**
*See:* Entry 329

**Irving I. Moskowitz Foundation**
*See:* Entry 379

**Lannan Foundation**
*See:* Entry 5467

**Mericos Foundation**
*See:* Entry 541

**Ordean Foundation**
*See:* Entry 570

**Paul Ogle Foundation**
*See:* Entry 4920

**Paul Stock Foundation**
*See:* Entry 578

**Perkins-Prothro Foundation**
*See:* Entry 583

**Swalm Foundation**
*See:* Entry 713

**Tozer Foundation**
*See:* Entry 730

**★ 19634 ★ Wieboldt Foundation**
53 West Jackson Boulevard, Ste. 838
Chicago, IL 60604
**Phone:** (312)786-9377  **Fax:** (312)786-9232
**Email:** *reginamc@corecomm.net*
**Website:** http://www.swalm.org
Carmen Prieto, Assistant Director
**Fnded:** 1921. **Philosophy:** Over 15 years ago, the directors adopted a creed that states the central purpose and direction of the foundation: "Our recognition of community organizing or community action as the foundation's prime concern is promoted by our conviction that a sense of powerlessness and the apathy and alienation bred of this sense are at the root of many of the ills of our time. We believe that funding those efforts that give people hope that they can exercise a degree of control over their lives and that involve them working together toward jointly defined ends is an important contribution to the resolution of social ills." The Wieboldt Foundation has three noteworthy characteristics: a grant-making program aimed at developing the capacity of local citizens in Chicago's poorest neighborhoods, a board of directors directly involved in the work of the foundation, and a propensity to fund new areas of interest. Community organizing has been a steadily increasing focus over the past 15 years. Grants have been awarded to organizations in low-income neighborhoods that foster leadership development and get neighborhood citizens involved in problem solving. The foundation recognizes that the difficulty of such efforts requires long-term commitment. A majority of grants, therefore, are renewals. The foundation also funds groups that develop policy, advocate, carry on research, and bring their technical expertise to the service of community groups. Such civic groups have been especially active in issues of equality and justice. Since 1988, the board has been deeply involved with school reform. It also focused on deepening its understanding of community organizations by greatly increasing the number of on-site visits and by holding board meetings in neighborhood settings with community leaders. The foundation also developed a Program Related Investments initiative. This initiative makes available loans, loan guarantees, and equity investments to housing, community development, and community service organizations. In 1992, the foundation in conjunction with the Woods Charitable Fund, established an annual "Community Organizing" award to recognize excellent and effective community organizing in the Chicago area. The award will be an unrestricted grant of $10,000 to $15,000.

*Priorities: Civic & Public Affairs:* About 63%. Community organizations, leadership development, and ethnic groups. *Education:* About 7%. Primary and secondary school enrichment programs. *Environment:* 7%. Neighborhood organizations. *International:* 4%. Healthcare issues. *Note:* Total contributions made in 1997. **Typ. Recipients:** Health Policy/Cost Containment, Medical Rehabilitation, Public Health. **Geo. Dist:** Chicago, IL, including metropolitan area.

### Corporate Foundations

**Ameritech Foundation**
*See:* Entry 8546

**Amsted Industries Foundation**
*See:* Entry 837

**Carrier Corp.**
*See:* Entry 918

**Excel Corp.**
*See:* Entry 1033

**NEC Foundation of America**
*See:* Entry 5583

**Torchmark Corp.**
*See:* Entry 1443

**USX Foundation, Inc.**
*See:* Entry 1472

### Other Funding Organizations

**★ 19635 ★ American Art Therapy Association (AATA)**
1202 Allanson Rd.
Mundelein, IL 60060-3808
**Phone:** (847)949-6064  **Free:** 888-290-0878
**Fax:** (847)566-4580
**Email:** info@arttherapy.org
**Website:** http://www.arttherapy.org
Shaun McNiff, Pres.
**Desc:** Art therapists, students, and individuals in related fields. Supports the progressive development of therapeutic uses of art, the advancement of research, and improvements in the standards of practice. Has established specific professional criteria for training art therapists. Facilitates the exchange of information and experience. Compiles statistics.
**Awards:** Cay Drachnik Minorities Fund (annual) bestowed to members of a minority group who are enrolled in an AATA approved program and who can demonstrate financial need; Distinguished Service Awards (annual); Gladys Agell Award for Excellence in Research (annual) bestowed to the most outstanding project, completed within the past year, by an art therapist using a statistical measure in the area of

applied art therapy; Myra Levick Scholarship Fund (annual) bestowed to students who demonstrate financial need, acceptance into an AATA approved graduate art therapy program, and an undergraduate GPA of at least 3.0; Rawley Silver Scholarship Fund (annual) bestowed to persons whose academic record or prior experience is deemed excellent and who are enrolled in an AATA approved art therapy program.

★ **19636** ★ **Association for Play Therapy**
2050 N Winery Ave., Ste. 101
Fresno, CA 93703
**Phone:** (559)252-2278          **Fax:** (559)252-2297
**Email:** info@a4pt.org
**Website:** http://www.a4pt.org
William M. Burns, Contact
**Desc:** Professionals and students involved in play therapy. Promotes interests of members. Provides books and materials at a discount to members. **Awards:** Student Research Award (annual) for graduate students who have completed research on play therapy while enrolled in an accredited program.

**Association of Rehabilitation Nurses (ARN)**
*See:* Entry 14920

★ **19637** ★ **Foundation for Physical Therapy (FPT)**
c/o American Physical Therapy Association
1111 Fairfax St.
Alexandria, VA 22314-1488
**Phone:** (703)683-6743          **Free:** 800-875-1378
**Fax:** (703)684-7343
**Email:** foundation@apta.org
**Website:** http://www.apta.org/Foundation
Christine A. Williams, Vice Pres.
**Desc:** Supports the physical therapy profession's research needs by funding scientific and clinically-relevant physical therapy research. **Awards:** Doctoral Opportunities for Clinicians and Scholars (annual) for physical therapists who have completed one full year of doctoral coursework.; Research Grants for individuals and groups of researchers to pursue scientifically based and clinically related physical therapy research.

★ **19638** ★ **National Rehabilitation Administration Association (NRAA)**
c/o National Rehabilitation Association
633 S Washington St.
Alexandria, VA 22314
**Phone:** (703)836-0850          **Fax:** (703)836-0848
**Email:** info@nationalrehab.org
**Website:** http://www.nationalrehab.org
**Desc:** Nonprofit rehabilitation instructors, state agency vocational rehabilitation instructors, and private instructors. Promotes continuing professional development of members. Conducts professional training sessions. **Awards:** Grant (periodic) Professional programs in the fields of rehabilitation administration and supervision.

★ **19639** ★ **Neuro-developmental Treatment Association (NDTA)**
1540 S Coast Hwy., Ste. 203
Laguna Beach, CA 92651
**Free:** 800-869-9295          **Fax:** (949)376-3456
**Email:** membership@ndta.org
**Website:** http://www.ndta.org
Howard Adler, Principal Dir.
**Desc:** Physical and occupational therapists, speech pathologists, special educators, physicians, parents, and others interested in neurodevelopmental treatment. (NDT is a form of therapy for individuals who suffer from central nervous system disorders resulting in abnormal movement. Treatment attempts to initiate or refine normal stages and processes in the development of movement.) Informs members of new developments in the field and with ideas that will eventually improve fundamental independence. Locates articles related to NDT. Regional groups maintain libraries.

**Awards:** Award of Excellence (annual); Certificate of Appreciation; Research Grant Award (annual).

**Vocational Evaluation and Work Adjustment Association (VEWAA)**
*See:* Entry 7896

# Medical & Allied Health Schools

## Occupational Therapy

*The following programs (baccalaureate and graduate) for the occupational therapist are accredited by the Accreditation Council for Occupational Therapy Education of the American Occupational Therapy Association. For career information, and for a listing of approved entry level programs (associate and certificate) for occupational therapy assistants, contact the American Occupational Therapy Association at 4720 Montgomery Lane, Bethesda, MD 20824, (301)652-2682, http://www.aota.org/.*

### Alabama

★ **19640** ★ **Alabama State University**
**College of Health Sciences**
**Occupational Therapy Program**
915 S Jackson St.
Montgomery, AL 36101-0271
**Phone:** (334)229-4615          **Fax:** (334)229-4964
**Email:** dtoole@asunet.alasu.edu
**Website:** http://www.alasu.edu
Donna R. Toole, EdD, Director

★ **19641** ★ **Tuskegee University**
**Department of Allied Health**
**Occupational Therapy Program**
Basil O'Connor Hall
Tuskegee University, AL 36088-1696
**Phone:** (334)727-8696          **Fax:** (334)727-8259
**Email:** grayg@tusk.edu
**Website:** http://svmc107.tusk.edu/tu/nah/occutherapy.html
Gwendolyn Gray, Director

★ **19642** ★ **University of Alabama, Birmingham**
**School of Health Related Professions**
**Occupational Therapy Program**
102 Bishop Bldg.
1530 3rd Ave. S
Birmingham, AL 35294-2030
**Phone:** (205)934-3568          **Fax:** (205)975-7787
**Email:** cpeyton@uab.edu
**Website:** http://www.uab.edu
Claudia Peyton, Director

★ **19643** ★ **University of South Alabama**
**Springhill Academic Campus**
**Occupational Therapy Program**
1504 Springhill Ave., Rm. 5108
Mobile, AL 36604
**Phone:** (334)434-3939          **Fax:** (334)434-3934
**Email:** mscaffa@jaguar1.usouthal.edu
**Website:** http://www.southal.edu
Marjorie E. Scaffa, PhD, Director

### Arizona

★ **19644** ★ **Kirksville College**
**Arizona School of Health Sciences**
**Occupational Therapy Program**
5850 E Still Cir.
Mesa, AZ 85206

**Phone:** (480)219-6000
**Email:** melvinj@az.swc.kcom.edu
**Website:** http://www.ashs.edu
Judith A. Melvin, PhD, Director

★ **19645** ★ **Midwestern University, Glendale**
**Occupational Therapy Program**
19555 N 59th Ave.
Glendale, AZ 85308
**Phone:** (623)572-3630          **Free:** 888-247-9277
**Fax:** (623)572-3635
**Email:** cmerch@arizona.midwestern.edu
**Website:** http://www.midwestern.edu
Christine Merchant, Director

### Arkansas

★ **19646** ★ **University of Central Arkansas**
**Occupational Therapy Program**
201 Donaghey Ave., HSC Ste. 300
Box 5001
Conway, AR 72035-0001
**Phone:** (501)450-3192          **Fax:** (501)450-3622
**Email:** LindaS@mail.uca.edu
**Website:** http://www.uca.edu/divisions/academic/chas/ot.html
Linda D. Shalik, PhD, Director

### California

★ **19647** ★ **California State University, Dominguez Hills**
**Occupational Therapy Program**
1000 E Victoria St., LCH B-102
Carson, CA 90747
**Phone:** (310)243-2726          **Fax:** (310)516-3317
**Email:** mnoriega@soh.csudh.edu
**Website:** http://www.csudh.edu
Marilyn Masunaka-Noriega, Director

★ **19648** ★ **Dominican University of California**
**Occupational Therapy Program**
50 Acacia Ave.
San Rafael, CA 94901-2298
**Phone:** (415)458-3731          **Fax:** (415)458-3774
**Email:** rramsey@dominican.edu
**Website:** http://www.dominican.edu
Ruth Ramsey, Director

★ **19649** ★ **Loma Linda University**
**School of Allied Health Professions**
**Occupational Therapy Program**
SAHP-Nichol Hall, Rm. A902
Loma Linda, CA 92350-0001
**Phone:** (909)558-4628          **Fax:** (909)558-0239
**Email:** liane-hewitt@sahp.llu.edu
**Website:** http://www.llu.edu
Liane Hewitt, Director

★ **19650** ★ **Samuel Merritt College**
**Occupational Therapy Program**
370 Hawthorne Ave.
Oakland, CA 94609-3108
**Phone:** (510)869-8925          **Fax:** (510)869-6282
**Email:** gmccorma@samuelmerritt.edu
**Website:** http://www.samuelmerritt.edu
Guy L. McCormack, PhD, Director

★ **19651** ★ **San Jose State University**
**College of Applied Sciences and Arts**
**Occupational Therapy Program**
1 Washington Sq.
San Jose, CA 95192-0059
**Phone:** (408)924-3070          **Fax:** (408)924-3088
**Email:** guburton@email.sjsu.edu
**Website:** http://www.sjsu.edu
Gordon V. Burton, PhD, Director

**★ 19652 ★ University of Southern California**
**Department of Occupational Science and Occupational Therapy**
**Occupational Therapy Program**
1540 Alcazar, CHP 133
Los Angeles, CA 90089-9003
**Phone:** (323)442-2850          **Fax:** (323)442-1540
**Email:** otdept@usc.edu
**Website:** http://www.usc.edu/OT
Florence A. Clark, PhD, Director

## Colorado

**★ 19653 ★ Colorado State University**
**Occupational Therapy Program**
228 Occupational Therapy Bldg.
Fort Collins, CO 80523
**Phone:** (970)491-6253          **Fax:** (970)491-6290
**Email:** hanzlik@cahs.colostate.edu
**Website:** http://www.cahs.colostate.edu/ot
Jodie Redditi-Hanzlik, PhD, Director

## Connecticut

**★ 19654 ★ Quinnipiac University**
**School of Health Sciences**
**Occupational Therapy Program**
275 Mt. Carmel Ave.
Hamden, CT 06518-0569
**Phone:** (203)582-8204          **Fax:** (203)281-8706
**Email:** hartmann@quinnipiac.edu
**Website:** http://www.quinnipiac.edu
Kimberly D. Hartmann, Director

**★ 19655 ★ University of Hartford**
**College of Education, Nursing and Health Professions**
**Occupational Therapy Program**
Dana Hall, Rm. 232
200 Bloomfield Ave.
West Hartford, CT 06117-1599
**Phone:** (860)768-4377          **Fax:** (860)768-5244
**Email:** bsmith@mail.hartford.edu
**Website:** http://uhavax.hartford.edu/~healthpro
Betsey C. Smith, Director

## District of Columbia

**★ 19656 ★ Howard University**
**Division of Allied Health Sciences**
**Occupational Therapy Program**
6th and Bryant Sts. NW
Washington, DC 20059-0001
**Phone:** (202)806-7614          **Fax:** (202)462-5248
**Email:** sjackson@fac.howard.edu
**Website:** http://www.howard.edu
Shirley Jackson, Director

## Florida

**★ 19657 ★ Barry University**
**Occupational Therapy Program**
11300 NE 2nd Ave.
Miami Shores, FL 33161-6695
**Phone:** (305)899-3213          **Fax:** (305)899-2958
**Email:** mmitchell@mail.barry.edu
**Website:** http://www.barry.edu/snhs/Msprograms/OccupationalTherapy
Douglas Mitchell, Director

**★ 19658 ★ Florida Agricultural and Mechanical (A&M) University**
**Occupational Therapy Program**
223 Ware-Rhaney Bldg.
Tallahassee, FL 32307
**Phone:** (850)561-2185          **Fax:** (850)561-2457
**Website:** http://www.famu.edu
Jacquelyn Anderson Bolden, PhD, Director

**★ 19659 ★ Florida Gulf Coast University**
**Occupational Therapy Program**
10501 FGCU Blvd. S
Fort Myers, FL 33965-6565
**Phone:** (941)590-7550          **Fax:** (941)590-7474
**Email:** lcampani@fgcu.edu
**Website:** http://www.fgcu.edu
Loredana Campanile, Director

**★ 19660 ★ Florida International University**
**Occupational Therapy Program**
University Park Campus, CH-101
Miami, FL 33199
**Phone:** (305)348-2263          **Fax:** (305)348-1240
**Email:** shaffner@fiu.edu
**Website:** http://w3.fiu.edu/ot
Pamela Shaffner, Director

**★ 19661 ★ Nova Southeastern University**
**College of Allied Health**
**Health Professions Division**
**Occupational Therapy Program**
3200 S University Dr.
Fort Lauderdale, FL 33328
**Phone:** (954)262-1110          **Fax:** (954)262-2290
**Email:** reba@hpd.acast.nova.edu
**Website:** http://www.nova.edu/cwis/centers/hpd/ot/index.html
Carol Niman Reed, EdD, Director

**★ 19662 ★ University of Florida**
**Occupational Therapy Program**
PO Box 100164, HSC
Gainesville, FL 32610-0164
**Phone:** (352)392-2617          **Fax:** (352)846-1042
**Email:** walker.hrp@mail.health.efl.edu
**Website:** http://www.hp.ufl.edu/ot
William C. Mann, PhD, Director

**★ 19663 ★ University of St. Augustine for Health Sciences**
**Institute of Occupational Therapy**
1 University Blvd.
Saint Augustine, FL 32086
**Phone:** (904)826-0084          **Free:** 800-241-1027
**Fax:** (904)827-0069
**Email:** ksclayto@usa.edu
**Website:** http://www.usa.edu
Karen S. Clayton, PhD, Director

## Georgia

**★ 19664 ★ Brenau University**
**Occupational Therapy Program**
1 Centennial Cir.
Gainesville, GA 30501
**Phone:** (770)534-6139          **Fax:** (770)534-6186
**Email:** bschell@lib.brenau.edu
**Website:** http://www.brenau.edu/OT
Barbara A. Schell, PhD, Director

**★ 19665 ★ Medical College of Georgia**
**School of Allied Health Sciences**
**Occupational Therapy Program**
EF 102
1120 15th St.
Augusta, GA 30912-0700
**Phone:** (706)721-2725          **Fax:** (706)721-9718
**Email:** kbradley@mail.mcg.edu
**Website:** http://www.mcg.edu/sah/ot/index.html
Kathy P. Bradley, EdD, Director

**★ 19666 ★ Medical College of Georgia/ Columbus State University**
**Occupational Therapy Program**
Illges Hall, Rm. 107
4225 University Ave.
Columbus, GA 31907

**Phone:** (706)568-2242          **Fax:** (706)568-2073
**Email:** jjedlick@mail.mcg.edu
**Website:** http://www.mcg.edu/sah/ot/index.html
Kathy Bradley, EdD, Director

## Idaho

**★ 19667 ★ Idaho State University**
**Occupational Therapy Program**
Campus Box 8045
Pocatello, ID 83209-8045
**Phone:** (208)282-4095
**Website:** http://www.isu.edu/departments/dpot

## Illinois

**★ 19668 ★ Chicago State University**
**College of Health Sciences**
**Occupational Therapy Program**
9501 S King Dr.
Chicago, IL 60628-1598
**Phone:** (773)995-2366          **Fax:** (773)995-2839
**Email:** bahgkks@csu.edu
**Website:** http://www.csu.edu
Kuzhilethu K. Kshepakaran, Director

**★ 19669 ★ Governors State University**
**College of Health Professions**
**Occupational Therapy Program**
University Park, IL 60466-0975
**Phone:** (708)534-7293          **Fax:** (708)534-1647
**Email:** b-cada@govst.edu
**Website:** http://www.govst.edu
Elizabeth Cada, Director

**★ 19670 ★ Midwestern University**
**College of Health Sciences**
**Occupational Therapy Program**
555 31st St.
Downers Grove, IL 60515
**Phone:** (630)515-6188          **Fax:** (630)515-7224
**Email:** tlaster@midwestern.edu
**Website:** http://www.midwestern.edu
Thomas Evans Laster, Director

**★ 19671 ★ Rush University**
**Rush-Presbyterian-St. Luke's Medical Center**
**Occupational Therapy Program**
600 S Paulina, Ste. 1009-B
Chicago, IL 60612-3833
**Phone:** (312)942-5099          **Fax:** (312)942-6989
**Email:** jbachelder@rushu.rush.edu
**Website:** http://www.rushu.rush.edu
Judy Bachelder, PhD, Director

**★ 19672 ★ University of Illinois, Chicago**
**College of Health and Human Development Sciences**
**Occupational Therapy Program**
1919 W Taylor St., M/C 811
Chicago, IL 60612
**Phone:** (312)996-6901          **Fax:** (312)413-0256
**Email:** Kielhfnr@uic.edu
**Website:** http://www.uic.edu/ahp/OT
Gary Kielhofner, DrPH, Director

## Indiana

**★ 19673 ★ Indiana University**
**School of Allied Health Sciences**
**Occupational Therapy Program**
Coleman Hall 316
1140 W Michigan St.
Indianapolis, IN 46202-5119
**Phone:** (317)274-8006          **Fax:** (317)274-2150
**Email:** chamant@iupui.edu
**Website:** http://www.iupui.edu/it/iusahs
Celestine Hamant, Director

## ★ 19674 ★ University of Indianapolis
**School of Occupational Therapy**
1400 E Hanna Ave.
Indianapolis, IN 46227-3697
**Phone:** (317)788-3432          **Fax:** (317)788-3542
**Email:** moyers@uindy.edu
**Website:** http://www.ot.uindy.edu
Penelope A. Moyers, EdD, Director

## ★ 19675 ★ University of Southern Indiana
**Occupational Therapy Program**
8600 University Blvd.
Evansville, IN 47712-3534
**Phone:** (812)465-1179          **Fax:** (812)465-7092
**Email:** otinfo@usi.edu
**Website:** http://health.usi.edu/acadprog/ot/index.htm
Aimee J. Luebben, EdD, Director

### Iowa

## ★ 19676 ★ Saint Ambrose University
**Occupational Therapy Program**
518 W Locust
Davenport, IA 52803-2898
**Phone:** (563)333-6277          **Fax:** (563)333-6410
**Email:** pwenthe@saunix.sau.edu
**Website:** http://www.sau.edu
Phyllis Wenthe, Director

### Kansas

## ★ 19677 ★ Newman University
**Occupational Therapy Program**
3100 McCormick Ave.
Wichita, KS 67213-2097
**Phone:** (316)942-4291          **Fax:** (316)942-4483
**Email:** sowersj@newmanu.edu
**Website:** http://www.newmanu.edu/ot
Jeanne Sowers, Director

## ★ 19678 ★ University of Kansas Medical Center
**School of Allied Health**
**Occupational Therapy Program**
3033 Robinson
3901 Rainbow Blvd.
Kansas City, KS 66160-7602
**Phone:** (913)588-7174          **Fax:** (913)588-4568
**Email:** wdunn@kumc.edu
**Website:** http://www.kumc.edu/SAH/OTEd/index.html
Winnie Dunn, PhD, Director

### Kentucky

## ★ 19679 ★ Eastern Kentucky University
**Occupational Therapy Program**
Dizney 103
Richmond, KY 40475-3135
**Phone:** (859)622-3300          **Fax:** (859)622-1605
**Email:** otsbenne@acs.eku.edu
**Website:** http://www.health.eku.edu
Onda Bennett, PhD, Director

## ★ 19680 ★ Spalding University
**Occupational Therapy Program**
851 S 4th St.
Louisville, KY 40203-2188
**Phone:** (502)585-7125          **Fax:** (502)588-7175
**Email:** rstrickland@spalding.edu
**Website:** http://www.spalding.edu
L. Randy Strickland, EdD, Director

### Louisiana

## ★ 19681 ★ Louisiana State University Health Sciences Center, New Orleans
**School of Allied Health Professions**
**Occupational Therapy Program**
1900 Gravier St.
New Orleans, LA 70112-2223
**Phone:** (504)568-4302          **Fax:** (504)568-4306
**Email:** taylor@lsuhsc.edu
**Website:** http://www.lsumc.edu
Eve Taylor, PhD, Director

## ★ 19682 ★ Louisiana State University Health Sciences Center, Shreveport
**School of Allied Health Professions**
**Occupational Therapy Program**
1501 Kings Hwy.
PO Box 33932
Shreveport, LA 71130-3932
**Phone:** (318)675-6827          **Fax:** (318)675-6937
**Email:** kseidn@lsumc.edu
**Website:** http://www.lsumc.edu
Kristin Seidner, Director

## ★ 19683 ★ University of Louisiana, Monroe
**College of Allied Health and Rehabilitation Professions**
**Occupational Therapy Program**
Monroe, LA 71209-0430
**Phone:** (318)342-1610          **Fax:** (318)342-5584
**Email:** aldavis@alpha.ulm.edu
**Website:** http://www.ulm.edu/ot/OT.html
Kathryn H. Davis, Director

### Maine

## ★ 19684 ★ University of New England
**College of Arts and Sciences**
**Occupational Therapy Program**
Biddeford, ME 04005-9599
**Phone:** (207)283-0171          **Fax:** (207)282-6379
**Email:** nmacrae@mailbox.une.edu
**Website:** http://www.une.edu
Nancy MacRae, Director

## ★ 19685 ★ University of Southern Maine
**Lewiston-Auburn College**
**Occupational Therapy Program**
51 Westminster St.
Lewiston, ME 04240-3534
**Phone:** (207)753-6523          **Fax:** (207)753-6555
**Email:** rblack@usm.maine.edu
**Website:** http://www.usm.maine.edu/~lac/ot
Roxie M. Black, Director

### Maryland

## ★ 19686 ★ Towson University
**Department of Occupational Therapy and Occupational Science**
**Occupational Therapy Program**
8000 York Rd.
Towson, MD 21252-0001
**Phone:** (410)704-4170
**Email:** mreitz@towson.edu
**Website:** http://www.towson.edu/OT
S. Maggie Reitz, PhD, Director

### Massachusetts

## ★ 19687 ★ American International College
**Occupational Therapy Program**
1000 State St.
Box 46
Springfield, MA 01109-3189
**Phone:** (413)205-3321
**Email:** dowroyer@acad.aic.edu
**Website:** http://www.aic.edu
Cathy A. Dow-Royer, Director

## ★ 19688 ★ Bay Path College
**Occupational Therapy Program**
588 Longmeadow St.
Longmeadow, MA 01106
**Phone:** (413)565-1331          **Fax:** (413)565-1102
**Email:** ksladyk@baypath.edu
**Website:** http://www.baypath.edu
Karen Sladyk, PhD, Director

## ★ 19689 ★ Boston University
**Sargent College of Health and Rehabilitation Sciences**
**Occupational Therapy Program**
635 Commonwealth Ave.
Boston, MA 02215
**Phone:** (617)353-2000          **Fax:** (617)353-2926
**Email:** wjcoster@bu.edu
**Website:** http://www.bu.edu/sargent/ot
Wendy Coster, PhD, Director

## ★ 19690 ★ Springfield College
**Occupational Therapy Program**
263 Alden St.
Springfield, MA 01109-3797
**Phone:** (413)748-3762          **Fax:** (413)748-3796
**Email:** kpost@spfldcol.edu
**Website:** http://www.spfldcol.edu/ot
Katherine M. Post, Director

## ★ 19691 ★ Tufts University
**Boston School of Occupational Therapy**
**Occupational Therapy Program**
26 Winthrop St.
Medford, MA 02155-7084
**Phone:** (617)627-3720          **Fax:** (617)627-3722
**Email:** sschwartz@emerald.tufts.edu
**Website:** http://www.tufts.edu
Sharan Schwartzberg, EdD, Director

## ★ 19692 ★ Worcester State College
**Occupational Therapy Program**
486 Chandler St.
Worcester, MA 01602-2597
**Phone:** (508)929-8624          **Fax:** (508)929-8178
**Email:** djoss@worcester.edu
**Website:** http://www.worc.mass.edu
Mark S. Rosenfeld, PhD, Director

### Michigan

## ★ 19693 ★ Baker College of Flint
**Occupational Therapy Program**
G-1050 W Bristol Rd.
Flint, MI 48507-5508
**Phone:** (810)766-4100          **Fax:** (810)766-4049
**Email:** hagen_d@flint.baker.edu
**Website:** http://www.baker.edu
Darrell Hagen, Director

## ★ 19694 ★ Eastern Michigan University
**Department of Associated Health Professions**
**Occupational Therapy Program**
322 Everett Marshall Hall
Ypsilanti, MI 48197-2239
**Phone:** (734)487-4094          **Fax:** (734)487-4095
**Website:** http://www.emich.edu
Betsy Francis, PhD, Director

## ★ 19695 ★ Saginaw Valley State University
**Occupational Therapy Program**
Ryder Center W, Rm. 105
7400 Bay Rd.
University Center, MI 48710-0001

**Phone:** (989)791-7356          **Fax:** (989)790-0545
**Website:** http://www.svsu.edu
Alfred G. Bracciano, EdD, Director

**★ 19696 ★ Wayne State University**
**Eugene Applebaum College of Pharmacy**
   **and Health Sciences**
**Occupational Therapy Program**
Detroit, MI 48202-3489
**Phone:** (313)577-1435          **Fax:** (313)577-5822
**Website:** http://wizard.pharm.wayne.edu/OT
Nancy J. Powell, PhD, Director

**★ 19697 ★ Western Michigan University**
**Occupational Therapy Program**
EWB Bldg.
1903 W Michigan Ave.
Kalamazoo, MI 49008-5051
**Phone:** (616)387-7260          **Fax:** (616)387-7262
**Email:** petersonc@wmich.edu
**Website:** http://www.wmich.edu
Cindee Peterson, PhD, Director

## Minnesota

**★ 19698 ★ College of Saint Catherine**
**Occupational Therapy Program**
2004 Randolph Ave.
Mail No. 4092
Saint Paul, MN 55105-1794
**Phone:** (651)690-6606          **Fax:** (651)690-8804
**Email:** jdbhaugen@stkate.edu
**Website:** http://www.stkate.edu/ot
Julie D. Bass Haugen, PhD, Director

**★ 19699 ★ College of Saint Scholastica**
**Occupational Therapy Program**
1200 Kenwood Ave.
Duluth, MN 55811
**Phone:** (218)723-6099          **Fax:** (218)723-6472
**Email:** rberkela@css.edu
**Website:** http://www.css.edu
Ron Berkeland, Director

**★ 19700 ★ University of Minnesota**
**Occupational Therapy Program**
MMC 388
420 Delaware St. SE
Minneapolis, MN 55455-0392
**Phone:** (612)626-5887          **Fax:** (612)625-7192
**Email:** otprog@tc.umn.edu
**Website:** http://www.ot.umn.edu
Judith Reisman, PhD, Director

## Mississippi

**★ 19701 ★ University of Mississippi**
   **Medical Center**
**School of Related Health Professions**
**Occupational Therapy Program**
2500 N State St.
Jackson, MS 39216-4505
**Phone:** (601)984-6350          **Fax:** (601)984-6344
**Email:** bgroat@shrp.umsmed.edu
**Website:** http://shrp.umc.edu
Bette A. Groat, Director

## Missouri

**★ 19702 ★ Maryville University**
**Occupational Therapy Program**
13550 Conway Rd.
Saint Louis, MO 63141
**Phone:** (314)529-9515          **Fax:** (314)529-9085
**Email:** lhunt@maryville.edu
**Website:**    http://www.maryville.edu/sohp/programs/
ot.htm
Linda Hunt, Director

**★ 19703 ★ Rockhurst University**
**College of Arts and Sciences**
**Occupational Therapy Program**
1100 Rockhurst Rd.
Kansas City, MO 64110-2561
**Phone:** (816)501-4635          **Fax:** (816)501-4643
**Email:** jane.rues@rockhurst.edu
**Website:** http://www.rockhurst.edu/ot
Jane P. Rues, EdD, Director

**★ 19704 ★ Saint Louis University (SLU)**
**Edward and Margaret Doisey School of**
   **Allied Health Professions**
**Occupational Therapy Program**
3437 Caroline St.
Saint Louis, MO 63104
**Phone:** (314)577-8514          **Fax:** (314)268-5414
**Email:** behrsk@slu.edu
**Website:** http://www.slu.edu/colleges/AH/OT
Shirley K. Behr, PhD, Director

**★ 19705 ★ University of Missouri,**
   **Columbia**
**School of Health Related Professions**
**Occupational Therapy Program**
407 Lewis Hall
Columbia, MO 65211
**Phone:** (573)882-3988          **Fax:** (573)884-2610
**Email:** baldwin@healthmissouri.edu
**Website:** http://www.missouri.edu
Diana J. Baldwin, Director

**★ 19706 ★ Washington University**
**School of Medicine**
**Occupational Therapy Program**
4444 Forest Park Ave.
Campus Box 8505
Saint Louis, MO 63108
**Phone:** (314)286-1600          **Fax:** (314)286-1601
**Email:** cbaum@ot-link.wustl.edu
**Website:** http://www.ot.wustl.edu
M. Carolyn Baum, PhD, Director

## Nebraska

**★ 19707 ★ College of Saint Mary**
**Occupational Therapy Program**
1901 S 72nd St.
Omaha, NE 68124-2377
**Phone:** (402)399-2400          **Free:** 800-926-5534
**Fax:** (402)399-2647
**Email:** pgromak@csm.edu
**Website:** http://www.csm.edu
Patricia A. Gromak, Director

**★ 19708 ★ Creighton University**
**School of Pharmacy and Allied Health**
**Occupational Therapy Program**
2500 California Plaza
Omaha, NE 68178-0259
**Phone:** (402)280-5957          **Free:** 800-325-2830
**Fax:** (402)280-5692
**Email:** rpadilla@creighton.edu
**Website:** http://ot.creighton.edu
Rene Padilla, Director

## New Hampshire

**★ 19709 ★ University of New Hampshire**
**School of Health and Human Services**
**Occupational Therapy Program**
Hewitt Hall
4 Library Way
Durham, NH 03824-3563
**Phone:** (603)862-2167          **Fax:** (603)862-0778
**Email:** acseidel@christa.unh.edu
**Website:** http://www.unh.edu
Alice Seidel, EdD, Director

## New Jersey

**★ 19710 ★ Kean University**
**School of Natural Applied and Health**
   **Sciences**
**Occupational Therapy Program**
Townsend T209
PO Box 411
Union, NJ 07083-9982
**Phone:** (908)527-2590          **Fax:** (908)527-3222
**Email:** ot@turbo.kean.edu
**Website:** http://www.kean.edu/~ot
Karen Stern, EdD, Director

**★ 19711 ★ Richard Stockton College of**
   **New Jersey**
**Professional Studies Division**
**Occupational Therapy Program**
Jim Leeds Rd.
PO Box 195
Pomona, NJ 08240-0195
**Phone:** (609)652-4687
**Website:** http://www.stockton.edu

**★ 19712 ★ Seton Hall University**
**Occupational Therapy Program**
McQuaid Hall
400 S Orange Ave.
South Orange, NJ 07079-2689
**Phone:** (973)761-7145
**Email:** breinees@shu.edu
**Website:**    http://gradmeded.shu.edu/graduatepro-
grams/msot.html
Estelle B. Breines, PhD, Director

## New Mexico

**★ 19713 ★ University of New Mexico**
**School of Medicine**
**Occupational Therapy Program**
Health Science and Services Bldg., Rm. 215
Albuquerque, NM 87131-5641
**Phone:** (505)272-1753          **Fax:** (505)272-8079
**Email:** tkcrowe@salud.unm.edu
**Website:** http://hsc.unm.edu/ot
Terry K. Crowe, PhD, Director

## New York

**★ 19714 ★ Columbia University**
**Occupational Therapy Program**
Neurological Institute, 8th Fl.
710 W 168th St.
New York, NY 10032
**Phone:** (212)305-3781          **Fax:** (212)305-4569
**Email:** jf6@columbia.edu
**Website:** http://columbiaOT.org
Janet Falk-Kessler, EdD, Director

**★ 19715 ★ Dominican College**
**Occupational Therapy Program**
470 Western Hwy.
Orangeburg, NY 10962-1299
**Phone:** (845)359-7800          **Fax:** (845)359-2313
**Website:** http://www.dc.edu
Sandra F. Countee, PhD, Director

**★ 19716 ★ D'Youville College**
**Occupational Therapy Program**
320 Porter Ave.
Buffalo, NY 14201-1084
**Phone:** (716)881-7600          **Fax:** (716)881-8137
**Email:** gingherm@dyc.edu
**Website:** http://www.dyc.edu
Merlene C. Gingher, EdD, Director

**★ 19717 ★ Ithaca College**
**Occupational Therapy Program**
200 Smiddy Hall
Ithaca, NY 14850
**Phone:** (607)274-1975          **Fax:** (607)274-3055
**Email:** catheyg@ithaca.edu
**Website:** http://www.ithaca.edu/hshp/ot
Catherine Y. Gordon, EdD, Director

**★ 19718 ★ Keuka College**
**Occupational Therapy Program**
Keuka Park, NY 14478-0098
**Phone:** (315)279-5255
**Email:** ptalty@mail.keuka.edu
**Website:** http://www.keuka.edu
Peter M. Talty, Director

**★ 19719 ★ Long Island University,**
**Brooklyn**
**Occupational Therapy Program**
1 University Plaza
Brooklyn, NY 11201
**Phone:** (718)488-1011
**Website:** http://www.liu.edu

**★ 19720 ★ Mercy College**
**Occupational Therapy Program**
555 Broadway
Dobbs Ferry, NY 10522-1189
**Phone:** (914)674-9331          **Fax:** (914)674-9457
**Email:** otprogram@mercy.edu
**Website:** http://grad.mercy.edu/occupationaltherapy
Joan Toglia, Director

**★ 19721 ★ New York Institute of**
**Technology**
**Occupational Therapy Program**
PO Box 8000
Old Westbury, NY 11568-8000
**Phone:** (516)686-3738          **Fax:** (516)686-3795
**Email:** hplotnick@iris.nyit.edu
**Website:** http://www.nyit.edu
Hermine Plotnick, Director

**★ 19722 ★ New York University**
**School of Education**
**Occupational Therapy Program**
35 W 4th St., 11th Fl.
New York, NY 10012-1172
**Phone:** (212)998-5825          **Fax:** (212)995-4044
**Email:** labovitz@is2.nyu.edu
**Website:** http://www.nyu.edu/education/ot
Jim Hinojosa, PhD, Director

**★ 19723 ★ Sage Colleges**
**Occupational Therapy Program**
45 Ferry St.
Troy, NY 12180-4115
**Phone:** (518)244-2217          **Free:** 800-999-3772
**Fax:** (518)244-4524
**Email:** frankm@sage.edu
**Website:** http://www.sage.edu
Martha M. Frank, Director

**★ 19724 ★ State University of New York,**
**Buffalo**
**Occupational Therapy Program**
515 Stockton Kimball Tower
3435 Main St.
Buffalo, NY 14214-3079
**Phone:** (716)829-3141          **Fax:** (716)829-3217
**Email:** nochajsk@buffalo.edu
**Website:** http://wings.buffalo.edu/academic/department/hrp/ot
Susan M. Nochajski, PhD, Director

**★ 19725 ★ State University of New York**
**Health Science Center, Brooklyn**
**(SUNY)**
**College of Health Related Professions**
**Occupational Therapy Program**
450 Clarkson Ave., Box 81
Brooklyn, NY 11203-2098
**Phone:** (718)270-7730          **Fax:** (718)270-7464
**Email:** jsabari@netmail.hscbklyn.edu
**Website:** http://www.downstate.edu/chrp.ot
Joyce Sabari, PhD, Director

**★ 19726 ★ State University of New York,**
**Stony Brook**
**School of Health Technology and**
**Management**
**Division of Rehabilitation Sciences**
**Occupational Therapy Program**
L2-031
Stony Brook, NY 11794-8201
**Phone:** (631)444-8160          **Fax:** (631)444-7621
**Email:** dcosta@epo.hsc.sunysb.edu
**Website:** http://www.sunysb.edu
Donna M. Costa, Director

**★ 19727 ★ Syracuse University**
**Utica College**
**Division of Health and Human Studies**
**Occupational Therapy Program**
1600 Burrstone Rd.
Utica, NY 13502-4892
**Phone:** (315)792-3006          **Fax:** (315)792-3248
**Email:** pcarey@utica.ucsu.edu
**Website:** http://www.utica.edu
Paula D. Carey, Director

**★ 19728 ★ Touro College, Bay Shore**
**Occupational Therapy Program**
1700 Union Blvd.
Bay Shore, NY 11706
**Phone:** (631)665-1600          **Fax:** (631)665-6084
**Email:** tonyh@touro.edu
**Website:** http://www.touro.edu/shs
Anthony Hollander, PhD, Director

**★ 19729 ★ Touro College, Manhattan**
**School of Health Sciences**
**Occupational Therapy Program**
27-33 W 23rd St.
New York, NY 10010-4202
**Phone:** (212)463-0400
**Email:** tonyh@touro.edu
**Website:** http://www.touro.edu/shs
Anthony C. Hollander, PhD, Director

**★ 19730 ★ York College of the City**
**University of New York (CUNY)**
**Occupational Therapy Program**
94-20 Guy R. Brewer Blvd.
Jamaica, NY 11451-9902
**Phone:** (718)262-2720          **Fax:** (718)262-2767
**Email:** kaplan@york.cuny.edu
**Website:** http://www.york.cuny.edu/~healthsci/index.html
Lillian Kaplan, Director

## North Carolina

**★ 19731 ★ East Carolina University**
**School of Allied Health Sciences**
**Occupational Therapy Program**
Greenville, NC 27858-4353
**Phone:** (252)328-4441          **Fax:** (252)328-4470
**Email:** dickersona@mail.ecu.edu
**Website:** http://www.ecu.edu/ot
Anne Dickerson, PhD, Director

**★ 19732 ★ Lenoir-Rhyne College**
**Occupational Therapy Program**
Box 7547
Hickory, NC 28603
**Phone:** (828)328-7300          **Fax:** (828)328-7364
**Email:** sssahler@lrc.edu
**Website:** http://www.lrc.edu/departments/ot/oth_department.html
Susan Stallings-Sahler, PhD, Director

**★ 19733 ★ University of North Carolina,**
**Chapel Hill**
**Division of Occupational Science**
**Occupational Therapy Program**
Medical School, Wing E
Campus Box 7120
Chapel Hill, NC 27599-7120
**Phone:** (919)966-2451          **Fax:** (919)966-9007
**Website:** http://www.alliedhealth.unc.edu/ocsci
Cathy Nielson, Director

**★ 19734 ★ Winston-Salem State**
**University**
**Occupational Therapy Program**
601 Martin Luther King, Jr. Dr.
Campus Box 19368
Winston-Salem, NC 27110
**Phone:** (336)750-3170          **Fax:** (336)750-3173
**Email:** baldwinlc@wssu.edu
**Website:** http://www.wssu.edu
Lynda C. Baldwin, Director

## North Dakota

**★ 19735 ★ University of Mary**
**Occupational Therapy Program**
7500 University Dr.
Bismarck, ND 58504-9652
**Phone:** (701)255-7500          **Free:** 800-408-6279
**Fax:** (701)255-7687
**Email:** ikensl@umary.edu
**Website:** http://www.umary.edu
Stacie L. Iken, Director

**★ 19736 ★ University of North Dakota**
**Occupational Therapy Program**
Box 7126, University Station
Grand Forks, ND 58202-7126
**Phone:** (701)777-2209          **Fax:** (701)777-2212
**Email:** smcintyr@mail.med.und.nodak.edu
**Website:** http://www.med.und.nodak.edu/depts/ot/home.htm
Sue McIntyre, Director

## Ohio

**★ 19737 ★ Cleveland State University**
**Occupational Therapy Program**
Health Sciences 103
1983 E 24th St.
Cleveland, OH 44115-2440
**Phone:** (216)687-3567          **Fax:** (216)687-9316
**Email:** j.bazyk@csuohio.edu
**Website:** http://www.csuohio.edu/healthsci/hs.htm
John J. Bazyk, Director

**★ 19738 ★ Medical College of Ohio,**
**Toledo**
**School of Allied Health**
**Occupational Therapy Program**
3015 Arlington Ave.
Toledo, OH 43614-5803
**Phone:** (419)383-4160          **Fax:** (419)383-5880
**Email:** jthomas@mco.edu
**Website:** http://www.mco.edu
Julie J. Thomas, PhD, Director

★ **19739** ★ **Ohio State University**
**School of Allied Medical Professions**
**Occupational Therapy Program**
1583 Perry St., 406 SAMP
Columbus, OH 43210-1234
**Phone:** (614)292-1706　　**Fax:** (614)292-0210
**Website:** http://www.amp.ohio-state.edu
H. Kay Grant, PhD, Director

★ **19740** ★ **Shawnee State University**
**Occupational Therapy Program**
940 2nd St.
Portsmouth, OH 45662-4303
**Phone:** (740)351-3209
**Email:** swheeler@shawnee.edu
**Website:** http://www.shawnee.edu
Steve D. Wheeler, Director

★ **19741** ★ **University of Findlay**
**Occupational Therapy Program**
1000 N Main St.
Findlay, OH 45840-3695
**Phone:** (419)424-5314　　**Free:** 800-472-9502
**Fax:** (419)424-6977
**Email:** owens@mail.findlay.edu
**Website:** http://www.findlay.edu
Peggy Owens, Director

★ **19742** ★ **Xavier University**
**Occupational Therapy Program**
3800 Victory Pkwy.
Cincinnati, OH 45207-7341
**Phone:** (513)745-3150　　**Fax:** (513)745-3261
**Email:** jpecin@aol.com
**Website:** http://www.xu.edu
Joanne Phillips Estes, Director

### Oklahoma

★ **19743** ★ **University of Oklahoma**
**Schusterman Health Sciences Center**
**Occupational Therapy Program**
4502 E 41st St.
Tulsa, OK 74135
**Phone:** (918)838-4660
**Website:** http://w3.uokhsc.edu/rehab

★ **19744** ★ **University of Oklahoma**
　**Health Sciences Center, Oklahoma City**
**College of Allied Health**
**Occupational Therapy Program**
801 NE 13th St.
Oklahoma City, OK 73190-1090
**Phone:** (405)271-2411　　**Fax:** (405)271-2432
**Email:** toby-hamilton@uokhsc.edu
**Website:** http://w3.uokhsc.edu/rehab
Toby B. Hamilton, Director

### Oregon

★ **19745** ★ **Pacific University**
**School of Occupational Therapy**
2043 College Way
Forest Grove, OR 97116-1797
**Phone:** (503)359-2789　　**Free:** 800-933-9308
**Fax:** (503)359-2980
**Email:** mcewenm@pacificu.edu
**Website:** http://www.ot.pacificu.edu
Molly McEwen, Director

### Pennsylvania

★ **19746** ★ **Alvernia College**
**Occupational Therapy Program**
400 St. Bernardine St.
Reading, PA 19607-1799
**Phone:** (610)796-8339　　**Fax:** (610)796-8422
**Email:** pennyne@alvernia.edu
**Website:** http://www.alvernia.edu
Neil Penny, Director

★ **19747** ★ **Chatham College**
**Occupational Therapy Program**
Woodland Rd.
Pittsburgh, PA 15233
**Phone:** (412)365-1290　　**Fax:** (412)365-1213
**Email:** henry@chatham.edu
**Website:** http://www.chatham.edu
Eileen Henry, EdD, Director

★ **19748** ★ **College Misericordia**
**Division of Health Sciences**
**Occupational Therapy Program**
301 Lake St.
Dallas, PA 18612-1098
**Phone:** (866)262-6363
**Email:** jcipiran@miseri.edu
**Website:** http://www.misericordia.edu
Joseph A. Cipriani Jr., EdD, Director

★ **19749** ★ **Duquesne University**
**John G. Rangos, Sr. School of Health**
**Sciences**
**Occupational Therapy Program**
Health Sciences Bldg., Rm. 234
Pittsburgh, PA 15282-0020
**Phone:** (412)396-5945　　**Fax:** (412)396-4343
**Email:** crist@duq.edu
**Website:** http://www.healthsciences.duq.edu/ot/oth-ome.html
Patricia Crist, PhD, Director

★ **19750** ★ **Elizabethtown College**
**Occupational Therapy Program**
1 Alpha Dr.
Elizabethtown, PA 17022-2298
**Phone:** (717)361-1174　　**Fax:** (717)361-1176
**Email:** gillardm@etown.edu
**Website:** http://www.etown.edu
Marian Gillard, PhD, Director

★ **19751** ★ **Gannon University**
**Occupational Therapy Program**
109 University Sq.
Erie, PA 16541-0001
**Phone:** (814)871-7663　　**Fax:** (814)871-5662
**Email:** dijoseph@gannon.edu
**Website:** http://www.gannon.edu
Linda M. DiJoseph, Director

★ **19752** ★ **Mount Aloysius College**
**Occupational Therapy Program**
7373 Admiral Peary Hwy.
Cresson, PA 16630
**Phone:** (814)886-6522　　**Fax:** (814)886-4906
**Email:** tclark@mtaloy.edu
**Website:** http://www.mtaloy.edu
Threese A. Clark, Director

★ **19753** ★ **Pennsylvania State University,**
　**Mont Alto**
**Occupational Therapy Program**
1 Campus Dr.
Mont Alto, PA 17237-9703
**Phone:** (717)749-6130　　**Fax:** (717)749-6166
**Email:** jvd102@psu.edu
**Website:** http://www.ma.psu.edu/ot.htm
Janet DeLany, D Ed, Director

★ **19754** ★ **Philadelphia University**
**Occupational Therapy Program**
School House Ln. and Henry Ave.
Philadelphia, PA 19144-5497
**Phone:** (215)951-2943
**Email:** admissions@philacol.edu
**Website:** http://www.philau.edu

★ **19755** ★ **Saint Francis University**
**Occupational Therapy Program**
PO Box 600
Loretto, PA 15940-0600
**Phone:** (814)472-3899
**Website:** http://www.saintfrancisuniversity.edu

★ **19756** ★ **Temple University**
**College of Allied Health Professions**
**Occupational Therapy Program**
3307 N Broad St.
Philadelphia, PA 19140
**Phone:** (215)707-4813　　**Fax:** (215)707-7656
**Email:** mkinneal@astro.temple.edu
**Website:** http://www.temple.edu/OT
Moya Kinnealey, PhD, Director

★ **19757** ★ **Thomas Jefferson University**
**College of Health Professions**
**Occupational Therapy Program**
Edison Bldg., Rm. 810
130 S 9th St.
Philadelphia, PA 19107-5233
**Phone:** (215)503-8010　　**Fax:** (215)503-3499
**Email:** janice.burke@mail.tju.edu
**Website:** http://jeffline.tju.edu/cwis/chp/index2.html
Janice P. Burke, PhD, Director

★ **19758** ★ **University of Pittsburgh**
**School of Health and Rehabilitation**
　**Sciences**
**Occupational Therapy Program**
5012 Forbes Tower
Pittsburgh, PA 15260
**Phone:** (412)383-6620
**Email:** jcr@pitt.edu
**Website:** http://www.shrs.pitt.edu/ot/index.html
Joan Rogers, PhD, Director

★ **19759** ★ **University of the Sciences in**
　**Philadelphia**
**Occupational Therapy Program**
600 S 43rd St.
Box 24
Philadelphia, PA 19104-4495
**Phone:** (215)596-8810　　**Fax:** (215)596-8690
**Email:** r.ideish@usip.edu
**Website:** http://www.usip.edu
Paula Kramer, PhD, Director

★ **19760** ★ **University of Scranton**
**Occupational Therapy Program**
Scranton, PA 18510-4501
**Phone:** (570)941-7540　　**Fax:** (570)941-4380
**Email:** kasarjl@uofs.edu
**Website:** http://www.scranton.edu
Jack Kasar, PhD, Director

### Puerto Rico

★ **19761** ★ **University of Puerto Rico**
**Occupational Therapy Program**
Medical Sciences Campus - CHRP
PO Box 365067
San Juan, PR 00936-5067
**Phone:** (787)758-2525　　**Fax:** (787)282-8174
**Website:** http://www.upr.clu.edu/englishv2/home.htm
Migdalia Morales, Director

### South Carolina

★ **19762** ★ **Medical University of South**
　**Carolina**
**College of Health Professions**
**Occupational Therapy Program**
171 Ashley Ave., Rm. 123-CHP
Charleston, SC 29425-2701
**Phone:** (843)792-2961
**Email:** trickeyb@musc.edu

**Website:** http://www.musc.edu/chp-rehab/ot/oth-ome.htm
Becki A. Trickey, PhD, Director

### South Dakota

**★ 19763 ★ University of South Dakota**
**Occupational Therapy Program**
414 E Clark St.
Vermillion, SD 57069-2390
**Phone:** (605)677-5600　　　　**Fax:** (605)677-6581
**Website:** http://www.usd.edu/usdot
Barbara Brockevelt, Director

### Tennessee

**★ 19764 ★ Belmont University**
**School of Occupational Therapy**
1900 Belmont Blvd.
Nashville, TN 37212-3757
**Phone:** (615)460-6700　　　　**Fax:** (615)460-6475
**Email:** mcphees@mail.belmont.edu
**Website:** http://www.belmont.edu/ot
Scott D. McPhee, DrPH, Director

**★ 19765 ★ Milligan College**
**Occupational Therapy Program**
PO Box 130
Milligan College, TN 37682
**Phone:** (423)975-8010　　　　**Fax:** (423)975-8019
**Email:** dwpoff@milligan.edu
**Website:** http://www.milligan.edu
Daniel W. Poff, PhD, Director

**★ 19766 ★ Tennessee State University**
**School of Allied Health Professions**
**Occupational Therapy Program**
3500 John A. Merritt Blvd.
Nashville, TN 37209-1561
**Phone:** (615)963-5891　　　　**Fax:** (615)963-5926
**Email:** snyderl@harpo.tnstate.edu
**Website:** http://duke.tnstate.edu/ot
Larry Snyder, Director

**★ 19767 ★ University of Tennessee, Chattanooga**
**Occupational Therapy Program**
1 Provident W Bldg.
Chattanooga, TN 37402
**Phone:** (423)785-2357
**Website:** http://www.utc.edu/~chhs.rehab.htm

**★ 19768 ★ University of Tennessee, Memphis**
**Health Science Center**
**Occupational Therapy Program**
822 Beale St., Rm. 350
Memphis, TN 38163
**Phone:** (901)448-8393　　　　**Fax:** (901)448-7545
**Email:** anolen@utmem.edu
**Website:** http://www.utmem.edu/occ_therapy/home.html
Ann H. Nolen, PsyD, Director

### Texas

**★ 19769 ★ Texas Tech University Health Sciences Center, Amarillo**
**School of Allied Health Professions**
**Occupational Therapy Program**
1300 Wallace Blvd.
Amarillo, TX 79106
**Phone:** (806)743-3220
**Website:** http://www.ttuhsc.edu

**★ 19770 ★ Texas Tech University Health Sciences Center, Lubbock**
**School of Allied Health**
**Occupational Therapy Program**
STOP 6220, Rm. 2C212
3601 4th St.
Lubbock, TX 79430
**Phone:** (806)743-3220　　　　**Fax:** (806)743-2515
**Email:** alhsb@ttuhsc.edu
**Website:** http://www.ttuhsc.edu
Susan C. Burwash, Director

**★ 19771 ★ Texas Tech University Health Sciences Center, Odessa**
**School of Allied Health**
**Occupational Therapy Program**
800 W 4th St.
Odessa, TX 79763
**Phone:** (906)743-3220
**Website:** http://www.ttuhsc.edu

**★ 19772 ★ Texas Woman's University, Dallas**
**Occupational Therapy Program**
Dallas, TX
**Phone:** (940)898-2801
**Email:** ot@twu.edu
**Website:** http://www.twu.edu/ot

**★ 19773 ★ Texas Woman's University, Denton**
**School of Occupational Therapy**
Box 425648, TWU Station
Denton, TX 76204-5648
**Phone:** (940)898-2801　　　　**Fax:** (940)898-2806
**Email:** ot@twu.edu
**Website:** http://www.twu.edu/ot
Janette Schkade, PhD, Director

**★ 19774 ★ Texas Woman's University, Houston**
**Occupational Therapy Program**
Houston, TX
**Phone:** (940)898-2801
**Email:** ot@twu.edu
**Website:** http://www.twu.edu/ot

**★ 19775 ★ University of Texas, El Paso**
**College of Health Professions**
**Occupational Therapy Program**
1101 N Campbell St.
El Paso, TX 79902
**Phone:** (915)747-7270
**Website:** http://www.utep.edu

**★ 19776 ★ University of Texas Health Science Center, San Antonio**
**Occupational Therapy Program**
7703 Floyd Curl Dr.
Mail Code 6245
San Antonio, TX 78229-3900
**Phone:** (210)567-8880　　　　**Fax:** (210)567-8893
**Email:** haradon@uthscsa.edu
**Website:** http://www.uthscsa.edu
Gale L. Haradon, PhD, Director

**★ 19777 ★ University of Texas Medical Branch, Galveston**
**School of Allied Health Sciences**
**Occupational Therapy Program**
301 University Blvd.
Galveston, TX 77555-1028
**Phone:** (409)772-3060　　　　**Fax:** (409)747-1615
**Email:** laprimea@utmb.edu
**Website:** http://www.sahs.utmb.edu/programs/ot
Loree Primeau, PhD, Director

**★ 19778 ★ University of Texas, Pan-American**
**Occupational Therapy Program**
1201 W University Dr.
Edinburg, TX 78539-2999
**Phone:** (956)381-2475　　　　**Fax:** (956)381-2476
**Email:** jebowen@panam.edu
**Website:** http://www.panam.edu
Judith E. Bowen, Director

### Utah

**★ 19779 ★ University of Utah**
**Occupational Therapy Program**
520 Wakara Way
Salt Lake City, UT 84108-1290
**Phone:** (801)585-9135
**Website:** http://www.health.utah.edu/octh

### Virginia

**★ 19780 ★ College of Health Sciences**
**Community Hospital of Roanoke Valley**
**Occupational Therapy Program**
920 S Jefferson St.
Roanoke, VA 24016
**Phone:** (540)985-8594　　　　**Fax:** (540)985-9773
**Website:** http://www.chs.edu
David A. Hayes, Director

**★ 19781 ★ James Madison University**
**College of Integrated Science and Technology**
**Department of Health Sciences**
**Occupational Therapy Program**
MSC 4301
Harrisonburg, VA 22807
**Phone:** (540)568-2399
**Website:** http://www.jmu.edu

**★ 19782 ★ Shenandoah University**
**Occupational Therapy Program**
333 W Cork St., 5th Fl.
Winchester, VA 22601
**Phone:** (540)665-5559　　　　**Fax:** (540)665-5564
**Email:** gstone@su.edu
**Website:** http://www.su.edu
Gretchen V.M. Stone, PhD, Director

**★ 19783 ★ Virginia Commonwealth University**
**Occupational Therapy Program**
PO Box 980008
Richmond, VA 23298-0008
**Phone:** (804)828-2219　　　　**Fax:** (804)828-0782
**Email:** sjlane@vcu.edu
**Website:** http://views.vcu.edu/sahp/occu
Shelly J. Lane, PhD, Director

### Washington

**★ 19784 ★ Eastern Washington University**
**Occupational Therapy Program**
Riverpoint Higher Education Park, Health Sciences Bldg.
310 N Riverpoint Blvd., Box R
Spokane, WA 99202-1675
**Phone:** (509)368-6560
**Website:** http://www.csmt.ewu.edu/csmt/ot/ot-dept.htm

**★ 19785 ★ University of Puget Sound**
**School of Occupational Therapy**
1500 N Warner
Tacoma, WA 98416-0510
**Phone:** (253)879-3281　　　　**Fax:** (253)879-2933
**Email:** tomlin@ups.edu
**Website:** http://www.ups.edu/ot
George Tomlin, PhD, Director

★ **19786 ★ University of Washington**
**Department of Rehabilitation Medicine**
**Occupational Therapy Program**
Box 356490
Seattle, WA 98195
**Phone:** (206)598-5410 **Fax:** (206)685-3244
**Email:** ot@u.washington.edu
**Website:** http://depts.washington.edu/rehab/education/ot.shtml
Elizabeth M. Kanny, PhD, Director

### West Virginia

★ **19787 ★ West Virginia University**
**Occupational Therapy Program**
Robert C. Byrd Health Sciences Center
PO Box 9139 - HSN
Morgantown, WV 26506-9139
**Phone:** (304)293-8828 **Fax:** (304)293-7105
**Email:** rmccombi@wvu.edu
**Website:** http://www.hsc.wvu.edu/som/ot
Randy McCombie, PhD, Director

### Wisconsin

★ **19788 ★ Concordia University,**
**Wisconsin**
**Occupational Therapy Program**
12800 N Lake Shore Dr.
Mequon, WI 53092-2402
**Phone:** (414)243-4429 **Fax:** (414)243-4506
**Email:** peggy.denton@cuw.edu
**Website:** http://www.cuw.edu/occupationaltherapy
Peggy L. Denton, PhD, Director

★ **19789 ★ Mount Mary College**
**Occupational Therapy Program**
2900 N Menomonee River Pkwy.
Milwaukee, WI 53222-4597
**Phone:** (414)256-1246 **Fax:** (414)256-1224
**Email:** olsonj@mtmary.edu
**Website:** http://www.mtmary.edu
Jane Olson, PhD, Director

★ **19790 ★ University of Wisconsin,**
**LaCrosse**
**Occupational Therapy Program**
4043 Health Science Center
1725 State St.
La Crosse, WI 54601
**Phone:** (608)785-6620 **Fax:** (608)785-6647
**Email:** marti_pm@mail.uwlax.edu
**Website:** http://perth.uwlax.edu/ot
Peggy M. Martin, Director

★ **19791 ★ University of Wisconsin,**
**Madison**
**Occupational Therapy Program**
1300 University Ave., 2110 MSC
Madison, WI 53706-1532
**Phone:** (608)262-2936
**Email:** hohlstein@education.wisc.edu
**Website:** http://www.soemadison.wisc.edu/kinesiology/ugrad/ot.htm
Rita Hohlstein, Director

★ **19792 ★ University of Wisconsin,**
**Milwaukee**
**School of Allied Health Professions**
**Occupational Therapy Program**
PO Box 413
Milwaukee, WI 53201-0413
**Phone:** (414)229-4713 **Fax:** (414)229-3930
**Email:** smithro@uwm.edu
**Website:** http://www.uwm.edu/SAHP
Roger O. Smith, PhD, Director

### Wyoming

★ **19793 ★ University of North Dakota**
**Casper College**
**Occupational Therapy Program**
125 College Dr.
Casper, WY 82601
**Phone:** (307)268-2867 **Fax:** (307)268-3099
**Email:** mwonser@acad.cc.whecn.edu
**Website:** http://www.cc.whecn.edu
Marla Wonser, Director

## Physical Therapy

*The following programs for physical therapists are accredited by the American Physical Therapy Association (APTA), 1111 N Fairfax St., Alexandria, VA 22314, (800)999-APTA, http://www.apta.org/. The APTA also accredits and maintains a listing of educational programs for physical therapy assistants.*

### Alabama

★ **19794 ★ University of Alabama,**
**Birmingham**
**School of Health Related Professions**
**Physical Therapist Program**
Bishop Bldg., Rm. 102
1530 3rd Ave. S
Birmingham, AL 35294-2030
**Phone:** (205)934-3566 **Fax:** (205)975-7787
**Email:** sshaw@uab.edu
**Website:** http://main.uab.edu/show.asp?durki=3415
Sharon Shaw, DrPH, Director

★ **19795 ★ University of South Alabama**
**Department of Physical Therapy**
**Physical Therapist Program**
1504 Springhill Ave., Rm. 1214
Mobile, AL 36604
**Phone:** (251)434-3575 **Fax:** (251)434-3822
**Website:** http://www.usouthal.edu/usa/allhealth/pt.htm
Dennis W. Fell, MD, Director

### Arizona

★ **19796 ★ Arizona School for Health**
**Sciences**
**Kirksville College of Osteopathic**
**Medicine**
**Physical Therapy Program**
5850 E Still Cir.
Mesa, AZ 85206
**Phone:** (480)219-6000 **Fax:** (480)219-6100
**Email:** sbrown@ashs.edu
**Website:** http://www.ashs.edu/discpl_pt.htm
Suzanne Robben Brown, Director

★ **19797 ★ Northern Arizona University**
**Department of Physical Therapy**
**Physical Therapist Program**
PO Box 15105
Flagstaff, AZ 86011
**Phone:** (928)523-4092 **Fax:** (928)523-9289
**Email:** carl.derosa@nau.edu
**Website:** http://www.nau.edu
Carl DeRosa, PhD, Director

### Arkansas

★ **19798 ★ Arkansas State University**
**College of Nursing and Health**
**Professions**
**Physical Therapy Program**
PO Box 910
State University, AR 72467-0910
**Phone:** (870)972-3591 **Fax:** (870)972-3652
**Email:** jguffey@astate.edu
**Website:** http://pt.astate.edu
J. Stephen Guffey, EdD, Director

★ **19799 ★ University of Central**
**Arkansas**
**Department of Physical Therapy**
**Physical Therapist Program**
201 Donaghey, PTC 300
Conway, AR 72035-0001
**Phone:** (501)450-3611 **Fax:** (501)450-5822
**Email:** venitaL@mail.uca.edu
**Website:** http://www.uca.edu/divisions/academic/pt
Venita Lovelace-Chandler, PhD, Director

### California

★ **19800 ★ Azusa Pacific University**
**Physical Therapist Program**
901 E Alosta Ave.
Azusa, CA 91702-7000
**Phone:** (626)815-5020 **Fax:** (626)815-5017
**Email:** mlaymon@apu.edu
**Website:** http://www.apu.edu/clas/grad/pt
Michael Laymon, Director

★ **19801 ★ California State University,**
**Fresno**
**Physical Therapist Program**
2345 E San Ramon Ave., MS-MH 29
Fresno, CA 93740-8031
**Phone:** (559)278-2625 **Fax:** (559)278-3635
**Email:** janetd@csufresno.edu
**Website:** http://www.csufresno.edu/physicaltherapy
Janet K. Duttarer, PhD, Director

★ **19802 ★ California State University,**
**Long Beach**
**College of Health and Human Services**
**Physical Therapist Program**
1250 Bellflower Blvd.
Long Beach, CA 90840
**Phone:** (562)985-4072 **Fax:** (562)985-4069
**Email:** rjmorris@csulb.edu
**Website:** http://www.csulb.edu
Ray J. Morris, Director

★ **19803 ★ California State University,**
**Northridge**
**Department of Health Sciences**
**Physical Therapist Program**
Northridge, CA 91330-8285
**Phone:** (818)677-4081 **Fax:** (818)677-3101
**Email:** george.wolfe@csun.edu
**Website:** http://www.csun.edu
George A. Wolfe, PhD, Director

★ **19804 ★ California State University,**
**Sacramento**
**College of Health and Human Services**
**Physical Therapist Program**
6000 J St.
Sacramento, CA 95819-6020
**Phone:** (916)278-6426 **Fax:** (916)278-5053
**Email:** mcgintys@csus.edu
**Website:** http://www.hhs.csus.edu
Susan M. McGinty, EdD, Director

★ **19805 ★ Chapman University**
**Department of Physical Therapy**
**Physical Therapist Program**
1 University Dr.
Orange, CA 92866
**Phone:** (714)744-7620 **Fax:** (714)744-7621
**Email:** gabard@chapman.edu
**Website:** http://www.chapman.edu/wilkinson/pt
Donald L. Gabard, PhD, Director

**★ 19806 ★ Loma Linda University**
**School of Allied Health Professions**
**Department of Physical Therapy**
**Physical Therapist Program**
Loma Linda, CA 92350
**Phone:** (909)824-4632          **Fax:** (909)824-4291
**Email:** lchinnock@sahp.llu.edu
**Website:** http://www.llu.edu
Larry Chinnock, EdD, Director

**★ 19807 ★ Mount Saint Mary's College**
**Department of Physical Therapy**
**Physical Therapist Program**
12001 Chalon Rd.
Los Angeles, CA 90049-1599
**Phone:** (310)954-4171          **Fax:** (310)954-4179
**Email:** cmoore@msmc.la.edu
**Website:** http://www.msmc.la.edu/Academics/Majors-
Programs/Master%20Physical%20Therapy/PT.htm
Cynthia L. Moore, Director

**★ 19808 ★ Samuel Merritt College**
**Physical Therapist Program**
370 Hawthorne Ave.
Oakland, CA 94609
**Phone:** (510)869-6241          **Fax:** (510)869-6282
**Email:** mjewell@samuelmerritt.edu
**Website:** http://www.samuelmerritt.edu
Martha J. Jewell, PhD, Director

**★ 19809 ★ University of California, San**
**Francisco/San Francisco State**
**University**
**Department of Physical Therapy and**
**Rehabilitation Science**
**Physical Therapist Program**
1320 7th Ave.
Box 0736
San Francisco, CA 94143-0736
**Phone:** (415)338-2001          **Fax:** (415)338-0907
**Email:** gppt@sfsu.edu
**Website:** http://www.ucsf.edu
Nancy Byl, PhD, Director

**★ 19810 ★ University of the Pacific**
**School of Pharmacy and Health Sciences**
**Department of Physical Therapy**
**Physical Therapist Program**
Stockton, CA 95211
**Phone:** (209)946-2886          **Fax:** (209)946-2367
**Email:** dumphred@uop.edu
**Website:** http://www.uop.edu
Darcy Umphred, PhD, Director

**★ 19811 ★ University of Southern**
**California**
**Department of Biokinesiology & Physical**
**Therapy**
**Physical Therapist Program**
1540 E Alcazar St., CHP 155
Los Angeles, CA 90089-9006
**Phone:** (323)442-2890          **Fax:** (323)442-1515
**Email:** jamesgor@usc.edu
**Website:** http://www.usc.edu
James Gordon, EdD, Director

**★ 19812 ★ Western University of Health**
**Sciences**
**Department of Physical Therapy**
**Education**
**Physical Therapist Program**
309 E 2nd St.
Pomona, CA 91766-1854
**Phone:** (909)469-5294          **Fax:** (909)469-5692
**Email:** dredmanbentley@westernu.edu
**Website:** http://www.westernu.edu/cahp.html
Donna Redman-Bentley, PhD, Director

## Colorado

**★ 19813 ★ Regis University**
**Department of Physical Therapy**
**Physical Therapist Program**
3333 Regis Blvd.
Mail Code G-4
Denver, CO 80221-1099
**Phone:** (303)458-4066          **Fax:** (303)964-5474
**Email:** btschoep@regis.edu
**Website:** http://www.regis.edu
Barbara A. Tschoepe, PhD, Director

**★ 19814 ★ University of Colorado**
**Health Science Center**
**Physical Therapist Program**
4200 E 9th Ave.
Box C244
Denver, CO 80262
**Phone:** (303)372-9144          **Fax:** (303)372-9016
**Email:** carolyn.heriza@uchsc.edu
**Website:** http://www.uchsc.edu/gs/pt
Carolyn B. Heriza, EdD, Director

## Connecticut

**★ 19815 ★ Quinnipiac University**
**School of Health Sciences**
**Physical Therapist Program**
Mt. Carmel Ave.
Hamden, CT 06518
**Phone:** (203)582-5251          **Fax:** (203)582-8706
**Email:** tantorski@quinnipiac.edu
**Website:** http://www.quinnipiac.edu
Edward P. Tantorski, Director

**★ 19816 ★ Sacred Heart University**
**Physical Therapist Program**
5151 Park Ave.
Fairfield, CT 06432-1000
**Phone:** (203)365-7656          **Fax:** (203)365-4723
**Email:** emerym@sacredheart.edu
**Website:** http://www.sacredheart.edu
Michael J. Emery, EdD, Director

**★ 19817 ★ University of Connecticut**
**School of Allied Health Professions**
**Department of Physical Therapy**
**Physical Therapist Program**
358 Mansfield Rd., U-101
Storrs, CT 06269-2101
**Phone:** (860)486-2834          **Fax:** (860)486-1588
**Email:** hasson@uconnvm.uconn.edu
**Website:** http://www.alliedhealth.uconn.edu
Scott Hasson, EdD, Director

**★ 19818 ★ University of Hartford**
**Department of Physical Therapy**
**Physical Therapist Program**
200 Bloomfield Ave.
West Hartford, CT 06117-1599
**Phone:** (860)768-5303          **Fax:** (860)768-5244
**Email:** certo@hartford.edu
**Website:** http://www.hartford.edu
Catherine M. E. Certo, ScD, Director

## Delaware

**★ 19819 ★ University of Delaware**
**Department of Physical Therapy**
**Physical Therapist Program**
303 McKinly Laboratory
Newark, DE 19716
**Phone:** (302)831-8910          **Fax:** (302)831-4234
**Email:** sbinder@udel.edu
**Website:** http://www.udel.edu/PT/index.html
Stuart A. Binder-MacLeod, PhD, Director

## District of Columbia

**★ 19820 ★ The George Washington**
**University**
**School of Medicine and Health Sciences**
**Program in Physical Therapy**
2100 M St. NW, Ste. 203
Washington, DC 20037
**Phone:** (202)496-8370          **Fax:** (202)496-6288
**Email:** hspglr@gwumc.edu
**Website:** http://www.gwumc.edu/healthsci
Gloria L. Rogers, Director

**★ 19821 ★ Howard University**
**College of Pharmacy, Nursing, and Allied**
**Health Sciences**
**Physical Therapist Program**
6th and Bryant Sts. NW
Washington, DC 20059
**Phone:** (202)806-7613          **Fax:** (202)806-2820
**Email:** ktavakol@howard.edu
**Website:** http://www.howard.edu
Kamran Tavakol, PhD, Director

## Florida

**★ 19822 ★ Florida Agricultural and**
**Mechanical (A&M) University**
**School of Allied Health Sciences**
**Physical Therapist Program**
Ware-Rhaney Bldg., Rm. 223
Tallahassee, FL 32307-3500
**Phone:** (850)599-3820          **Fax:** (850)561-2457
**Email:** dowery@lycos.com
**Website:** http://www.famu.edu
Evelyn S. Dowery, EdD, Director

**★ 19823 ★ Florida Gulf Coast University**
**Department of Physical Therapy**
10501 FGCU Blvd. S
Fort Myers, FL 33965-6565
**Phone:** (941)590-1000          **Fax:** (941)590-1010
**Email:** ekwill@fgcu.edu
**Website:** http://www.fgcu.edu/chp/pt
Ellen Kroog Williamson, Chairman of the Board

**★ 19824 ★ Florida International**
**University**
**College of Health Sciences**
**Department of Physical Therapy**
**Physical Therapist Program**
Miami, FL 33199
**Phone:** (305)348-3831          **Fax:** (305)348-1240
**Email:** elbauml@fiu.edu
**Website:** http://w3.fiu.edu/pt
Leonard Elbaum, EdD, Director

**★ 19825 ★ Nova Southeastern University**
**College of Allied Health**
**Health Profession Division**
**Physical Therapist Program**
3200 S University Dr.
Fort Lauderdale, FL 33328
**Phone:** (954)262-1662          **Fax:** (954)262-1783
**Email:** hill@nova.edu
**Website:** http://www.nova.edu/pt
Cheryl J. Hill, Director

**★ 19826 ★ University of Central Florida**
**Physical Therapist Program**
4000 Central Florida Blvd.
HPAI, Ste. 256
Orlando, FL 32816-2205
**Phone:** (407)823-3462          **Fax:** (407)823-3464
**Email:** kparry@mail.ucf.edu
**Website:** http://www.cohpa.ucf.edu/health.pro
Katherine K. Parry, PhD, Director

★ 19827 ★ **University of Florida**
**College of Health Professions**
**Department of Physical Therapy**
**Physical Therapist Program**
Box 100154 HSC
Gainesville, FL 32610-0154
**Phone:** (352)265-0085     **Fax:** (352)265-0731
**Email:** rgarrigu@hp.ufl.edu
**Website:** http://www.ufl.edu
Robert Garrigues, PhD, Director

★ 19828 ★ **University of Miami**
**School of Medicine**
**Physical Therapist Program**
5915 Ponce de Leon Blvd., 5th Fl.
Coral Gables, FL 33146
**Phone:** (305)284-4535     **Fax:** (305)284-6128
**Email:** shayes@miami.edu
**Website:** http://www.miami.edu
Sherrill H. Hayes, PhD, Director

★ 19829 ★ **University of North Florida**
**College of Health**
**Physical Therapist Program**
4567 St. John's Bluff Rd. S
Jacksonville, FL 32224
**Phone:** (904)620-2841     **Fax:** (904)620-2848
**Email:** mnonnema@unf.edu
**Website:** http://www.unf.edu
Margaret Nonnemacher, PhD, Director

★ 19830 ★ **University of Saint Augustine**
**for Health Sciences**
**Institute of Physical Therapy**
**Physical Therapist Program**
1 University Blvd.
Saint Augustine, FL 32086
**Phone:** (904)826-0084     **Fax:** (904)826-0085
**Email:** gcgornia@usa.edu
**Website:** http://www.usa.edu
Gerard C. Gorniak, PhD, Director

★ 19831 ★ **University of South Florida**
**School of Physical Therapy**
12901 Bruce B Downs Blvd., MDC 77
Tampa, FL 33612
**Phone:** (813)974-8870     **Fax:** (813)974-8915
**Email:** mclenden@hsc.usf.edu
**Website:** http://www.hsc.usf.edu/COM/physicaltherapy
Martha Clendenin, PhD, Director

## Georgia

★ 19832 ★ **Armstrong Atlantic State**
**University**
**Physical Therapist Program**
11935 Abercorn St.
Savannah, GA 31419-1997
**Phone:** (912)921-2327     **Fax:** (912)921-5838
**Email:** lakedavi@mail.armstrong.edu
**Website:** http://www.pt.armstrong.edu
David A. Lake, PhD, Director

★ 19833 ★ **Emory University**
**Division of Physical Therapy**
**Physical Therapist Program**
1441 Clifton Rd. NE, Ste. 423
Atlanta, GA 30322
**Phone:** (404)712-5660     **Fax:** (404)712-4130
**Email:** pcatlin@emory.edu
**Website:** http://www.cc.emory.edu/MED/AH/PT
Pamela A. Catlin, EdD, Director

★ 19834 ★ **Georgia State University**
**Department of Physical Therapy**
**Physical Therapist Program**
University Plaza
Atlanta, GA 30303

**Phone:** (404)651-3091     **Fax:** (404)651-1584
**Email:** mpearl@gsu.edu
**Website:** http://www.gsu.edu
Marcia Pearl, PhD, Director

★ 19835 ★ **Medical College of Georgia**
**School of Allied Health Sciences**
**Department of Physical Therapy**
**Physical Therapist Program**
Augusta, GA 30912-0800
**Phone:** (706)721-2141     **Fax:** (706)721-3209
**Email:** dkeskula@mail.mcg.edu
**Website:** http://www.mcg.edu
Douglas R. Keskula, PhD, Director

★ 19836 ★ **North Georgia College and**
**State University**
**Physical Therapist Program**
Barnes Hall, Rm. A-8
Dahlonega, GA 30597
**Phone:** (706)864-1422     **Fax:** (706)864-1493
**Email:** rlaird@ngcsu.edu
**Website:** http://www.ngc.peachnet.edu/academic/sciences/pt/pthome.htm
Robert J. Laird, PhD, Director

## Idaho

★ 19837 ★ **Idaho State University**
**Kasiska College of Health Professions**
**Department of Physical and Occupational**
**Therapy**
**Physical Therapist Program**
Box 8045
Pocatello, ID 83209
**Phone:** (208)282-4095     **Fax:** (208)282-4962
**Email:** physther@isu.edu
**Website:** http://www.isu.edu/departments/dpot
Alexander G. Urfer, PhD, Director

## Illinois

★ 19838 ★ **Bradley University**
**Department of Physical Therapy**
**Physical Therapist Program**
1501 W Bradley Ave.
Peoria, IL 61625
**Phone:** (309)677-3489     **Fax:** (309)677-4053
**Email:** jun@bumail.bradley.edu
**Website:** http://www.bradley.edu/academics/ehs/pt/pt_index.html
Mary Jo Mays, PhD, Director

★ 19839 ★ **Governors State University**
**College of Health Professions**
**Physical Therapist Program**
University Park, IL 60466
**Phone:** (708)534-7290     **Fax:** (708)534-1647
**Email:** r-carter@govst.edu
**Website:** http://www.govst.edu/mpt
Russell E. Carter, EdD, Director

★ 19840 ★ **The Herman M. Finch**
**University of Health Sciences /Chicago**
**Medical School**
**School of Related Health Sciences**
**Physical Therapist Program**
3333 Green Bay Rd.
North Chicago, IL 60064
**Phone:** (847)578-3307     **Fax:** (847)578-8816
**Email:** schuitd@finchcms.edu
**Website:** http://www.finchcms.edu
Dale Schuit, PhD, Director

★ 19841 ★ **Midwestern University**
**College of Health Sciences**
**Physical Therapist Program**
555 31st St.
Downers Grove, IL 60515

**Phone:** (630)515-6462     **Free:** 800-458-6253
**Fax:** (630)515-7224
**Email:** dcechx@midwestern.edu
**Website:** http://www.midwestern.edu/Pages/PTP.html
Donna Cech, Director

★ 19842 ★ **Northern Illinois University**
**School of Allied Health Professions**
**Physical Therapist Program**
DeKalb, IL 60115
**Phone:** (815)753-1383     **Fax:** (815)753-0720
**Email:** mblascha@niu.edu
**Website:** http://www.niu.edu
M. J. Blaschak, PhD, Director

★ 19843 ★ **Northwestern University**
**Medical School**
**Department of Physical Therapy and**
**Human Movement Sciences**
**Physical Therapist Program**
645 N Michigan Ave., Ste. 1100
Chicago, IL 60611-2814
**Phone:** (312)908-8160     **Fax:** (312)908-0741
**Email:** k-hayes@northwestern.edu
**Website:** http://www.nupt.nwu.edu
Karen W. Hayes, PhD, Director

★ 19844 ★ **University of Illinois, Chicago**
**College of Applied Health Sciences**
**Physical Therapist Program**
1919 W Taylor St., M/C 898
Chicago, IL 60612
**Phone:** (312)996-7764     **Fax:** (312)996-3807
**Email:** astorto@uic.edu
**Website:** http://www.uic.edu/ahp/pt
Suzann K. Campbell, PhD, Director

## Indiana

★ 19845 ★ **Indiana University**
**School of Allied Health Sciences**
**Physical Therapist Program**
Coleman Hall 120
1140 W Michigan St.
Indianapolis, IN 46202-5119
**Phone:** (317)278-1875     **Fax:** (317)278-1876
**Email:** wsquille@iupui.edu
**Website:** http://www.indiana.edu/
William S. Quillen, PhD, Director

★ 19846 ★ **University of Evansville**
**Department of Physical Therapy**
**Physical Therapist Program**
1800 Lincoln Ave.
Evansville, IN 47722
**Phone:** (812)479-2345     **Free:** 800-423-8633
**Fax:** (812)479-2717
**Email:** mk43@evansville.edu
**Website:** http://www.evansville.edu
Mary P. Kessler, Director

★ 19847 ★ **University of Indianapolis**
**Krannert School of Physical Therapy**
**Physical Therapist Program**
1400 E Hanna Ave.
Indianapolis, IN 46227-3697
**Phone:** (317)788-3500     **Fax:** (317)788-3542
**Email:** cgraham@uindy.edu
**Website:** http://www.uindy.edu
Cecilia Graham, PhD, Director

## Iowa

★ 19848 ★ **Clarke College**
**Department of Physical Therapy**
**Physical Therapist Program**
1550 Clarke Dr.
Dubuque, IA 52001-3198
**Phone:** (319)588-6382     **Fax:** (319)588-6789

**Email:** jbrasseu@clarke.edu
**Website:** http://www.clarke.edu
Jeannette Brasseur, PhD, Director


★ 19849 ★ **Des Moines University,**
**Osteopathic Medical Center**
**College of Health Sciences**
**Physical Therapist Program**
3200 Grand Ave.
Des Moines, IA 50312
**Phone:** (515)271-1634          **Free:** 800-240-2767
**Fax:** (515)271-1714
**Email:** Susan.Cigelman@dmu.edu
**Website:** http://www.dmu.edu/pt/index.htm
M. Susan Cigelman, EdD, Director


★ 19850 ★ **Saint Ambrose University**
**College of Human Services**
**Department of Physical Therapy**
**Physical Therapist Program**
518 W Locust
Davenport, IA 52803
**Phone:** (563)333-6403          **Fax:** (563)333-6410
**Email:** pt@sau.edu
**Website:** http://web.sau.edu/mpt
Sandra L. Cassady, PhD, Director


★ 19851 ★ **University of Iowa**
**College of Medicine**
**Physical Therapist Program**
2600 Steindler Bldg.
Iowa City, IA 52242-1008
**Phone:** (319)335-9791          **Fax:** (319)335-9707
**Email:** david-nielsen@uiowa.edu
**Website:** http://www.uiowa.edu
David H. Nielsen, PhD, Director


### Kansas

★ 19852 ★ **University of Kansas Medical**
**Center**
**Department of Physical Therapy**
**Education**
**Physical Therapist Program**
3056 Robinson Hall
3901 Rainbow Blvd.
Kansas City, KS 66160-7601
**Phone:** (913)588-6799          **Fax:** (913)588-4568
**Email:** Enwemeka@kumc.edu
**Website:** http://www.kumc.edu/SAH/pted/
Chukuka Enwemeka, PhD, Director


★ 19853 ★ **Wichita State University**
**College of Health Professions**
**Physical Therapist Program**
1845 Fairmont
Wichita, KS 67260-0043
**Phone:** (316)978-3604          **Fax:** (316)978-3025
**Email:** wilson@chp.twsu.edu
**Website:** http://chp.wichita.edu/pt
Camilla M. Wilson, PhD, Director


### Kentucky

★ 19854 ★ **Bellarmine University**
**Lansing School of Nursing and Health**
**Sciences**
**Physical Therapist Program**
Miles Hall, Rm. 105
2001 Newburg Rd.
Louisville, KY 40205
**Phone:** (502)852-7816          **Fax:** (502)852-4597
**Email:** mwiegand@bellarmine.edu
Mark Wiegand, PhD, Director


★ 19855 ★ **University of Kentucky**
**Physical Therapist Program**
213 CAHP Bldg.
121 Washington Ave.
Lexington, KY 40506-0003
**Phone:** (859)323-1100          **Fax:** (859)257-1816
**Email:** trmalo1@pop.uky.edu
**Website:** http://www.uky.edu/
Terry R. Malone, EdD, Director


### Louisiana

★ 19856 ★ **Louisiana State University**
**Health Sciences Center, New Orleans**
**School of Allied Health Professions**
**Physical Therapist Program**
1900 Gravier St.
LSU Health Sciences Center
New Orleans, LA 70112
**Phone:** (504)568-4288          **Fax:** (504)568-6552
**Website:** http://www.lsumc.edu
Elizabeth Weiss, PhD, Director


★ 19857 ★ **Louisiana State University**
**Health Sciences Center, Shreveport**
**School of Allied Health Professions**
**Physical Therapist Program**
1501 Kings Hwy.
PO Box 33932
Shreveport, LA 71130-3932
**Phone:** (318)675-6820          **Fax:** (318)675-6937
**Email:** sdunn2@lsumc.edu
**Website:** http://www.lsumc.edu
Sharon Dunn, Director


### Maine

★ 19858 ★ **Husson College**
**Physical Therapist Program**
1 College Circle
Bangor, ME 04401
**Phone:** (207)941-7101          **Fax:** (207)941-7883
**Email:** sidaway@husson.edu
**Website:** http://www.husson.edu/pt
Ben Sidaway, PhD, Director


★ 19859 ★ **University of New England**
**Department of Physical Therapy**
**Physical Therapist Program**
11 Hills Beach Rd.
Biddeford, ME 04005
**Phone:** (207)283-0171          **Fax:** (207)294-5926
**Email:** msheldon@une.edu
**Website:** http://www.une.edu
Mike Sheldon, Director


### Maryland

★ 19860 ★ **University of Maryland,**
**Baltimore**
**School of Medicine**
**Physical Therapist Program**
100 Penn St., Rm. 115
Baltimore, MD 21201
**Phone:** (410)706-7720          **Fax:** (410)706-6387
**Email:** mrodgers@umaryland.edu
**Website:** http://pt.umaryland.edu
Mary M. Rodgers, PhD, Director


★ 19861 ★ **University of Maryland,**
**Eastern Shore**
**Department of Physical Therapy**
**Physical Therapist Program**
Kiah Hall, 1st Fl.
Princess Anne, MD 21853-1299
**Phone:** (410)651-6360          **Fax:** (410)651-6259
**Email:** rlblakely@mail.umes.edu
**Website:** http://www.umes.edu/pt
Raymond L. Blakely, PhD, Director


### Massachusetts

★ 19862 ★ **American International**
**College**
**Physical Therapist Program**
1000 State St.
Springfield, MA 01109-9983
**Phone:** (413)205-3412          **Fax:** (413)788-9961
**Email:** eswanson@acad.aic.edu
**Website:** http://www.aic.edu/web/ptherapy/index.htm
Edward Swanson, Director


★ 19863 ★ **Boston University**
**Sargent College of Health and**
**Rehabilitation Sciences**
**Department of Physical Therapy**
**Physical Therapist Program**
635 Commonwealth Ave.
Boston, MA 02215
**Phone:** (617)353-2720          **Fax:** (617)353-9463
**Email:** fetters@bu.edu
**Website:** http://www.bu.edu/sargent
Linda Fetters, PhD, Director


★ 19864 ★ **MGH Institute of Health**
**Professions**
**Physical Therapist Program**
Charleston Navy Yard
36 1st Ave.
Boston, MA 02129
**Phone:** (617)724-4841          **Fax:** (617)724-4854
**Email:** Lportney@mghihp.edu
**Website:** http://www.mghihp.edu
Leslie G. Portney, PhD, Director


★ 19865 ★ **Northeastern University**
**Physical Therapist Program**
Mugar Life Science Bldg., Rm. 117-A
360 Huntington Ave.
Boston, MA 02115
**Phone:** (617)373-3160          **Fax:** (617)373-3161
**Email:** mharris@neu.edu
**Website:** http://www.northeastern.edu/
Meredith H. Harris, EdD, Director


★ 19866 ★ **Simmons College**
**Graduate School for Health Studies**
**Program in Physical Therapy**
300 The Fenway
Boston, MA 02115
**Phone:** (617)521-2635          **Fax:** (617)521-3137
**Email:** djette@simmons.edu
**Website:** http://www.simmons.edu/gshs
Diane Jette, Director


★ 19867 ★ **Springfield College**
**Department of Physical Therapy**
**Physical Therapist Program**
263 Alden St.
Springfield, MA 01109
**Phone:** (413)748-3590          **Fax:** (413)748-3371
**Email:** ltsoumas@spfldcol.edu
**Website:** http://www.spfldcol.edu/pt
Linda J. Tsoumas, Director


★ 19868 ★ **University of Massachusetts,**
**Lowell**
**Physical Therapist Program**
Weed Hall
3 Solomon Way, Ste. 5
Lowell, MA 01854-5095
**Phone:** (978)934-4517          **Fax:** (978)934-3006
**Email:** sally_healey@uml.edu
**Website:** http://www.uml.edu/
Joseph A. Dorsey, EdD, Director

## Michigan

**★ 19869 ★ Andrews University**
**Department of Physical Therapy**
**Physical Therapist Program**
Berrien Springs, MI 49104-0420
**Phone:** (616)471-6551  **Free:** 800-827-2878
**Fax:** (616)471-2866
**Email:** perryw@andrews.edu
**Website:** http://www.andrews.edu/PHTH
Wayne L. Perry, PhD, Director

**★ 19870 ★ Central Michigan University**
**Physical Therapist Program**
134 Pearce Hall
Mount Pleasant, MI 48859
**Phone:** (517)774-2347  **Fax:** (517)774-2908
**Email:** herman.l.triezenberg@cmich.edu
**Website:** http://www.cmich.edu/~physther/
Herm Triezenberg, PhD, Director

**★ 19871 ★ Grand Valley State University**
**Physical Therapist Program**
328 Henry Hall
Allendale, MI 49401
**Phone:** (616)895-3356  **Fax:** (616)895-3350
**Email:** peckj@gvsu.edu
**Website:** http://www.gvsu.edu/pt
John Peck, PhD, Director

**★ 19872 ★ Oakland University**
**School of Health Sciences**
**Physical Therapist Program**
Rochester, MI 48309-4482
**Phone:** (248)370-4041  **Fax:** (248)370-4287
**Email:** marcoux@oakland.edu
**Website:** http://www.acs.oakland.edu
Beth C. Marcoux, PhD, Director

**★ 19873 ★ University of Michigan, Flint**
**School of Health Professions and Studies**
**Physical Therapist Program**
Flint, MI 48502-1950
**Phone:** (810)762-3373  **Fax:** (810)766-6668
**Email:** pkc@umflint.edu
**Website:** http://www.flint.umich.edu/Departments/PT
Paulette Cebulski, PhD, Director

**★ 19874 ★ Wayne State University**
**Physical Therapist Program**
439 Shapero Hall
Detroit, MI 48202
**Phone:** (313)577-1432  **Fax:** (313)577-8586
**Email:** aa4944@wayne.edu
**Website:** http://www.wayne.edu
Louis R. Amundsen, PhD, Director

## Minnesota

**★ 19875 ★ College of Saint Catherine,**
**Minneapolis**
**Physical Therapist Program**
601 25th Ave. S
Minneapolis, MN 55454
**Phone:** (651)690-7822  **Fax:** (651)690-7876
**Email:** dosellheim@stkate.edu
**Website:** http://www.stkate.edu/
Debra Sellheim, PhD, Director

**★ 19876 ★ College of Saint Scholastica**
**Department of Physical Therapy**
**Graduate Physical Therapist Program**
1200 Kenwood Ave.
Duluth, MN 55811
**Phone:** (218)723-6786  **Fax:** (218)723-6472
**Email:** dwise@css.edu
**Website:** http://www.css.edu
Denise Wise, PhD, Director

**★ 19877 ★ Mayo Foundation**
**Mayo School of Sciences**
**Physical Therapist Program**
200 1st St. SW
Rochester, MN 55905
**Phone:** (507)284-2054  **Fax:** (507)284-0656
**Email:** cummings.john@mayo.edu
**Website:** http://www.mayo.edu
John P. Cummings, PhD, Director

**★ 19878 ★ University of Minnesota**
**Physical Therapist Program**
Box 388 UMHC
Minneapolis, MN 55455
**Phone:** (612)624-0427  **Fax:** (612)625-7192
**Email:** carey007@maroon.tc.umn.edu
**Website:** http://www.physther.med.umn.edu/
James R. Carey, PhD, Director

## Mississippi

**★ 19879 ★ University of Mississippi**
**Medical Center**
**School of Health Related Professions**
**Physical Therapist Program**
2500 N State St.
Jackson, MS 39216-4505
**Phone:** (601)984-6330  **Fax:** (601)815-1715
**Email:** ngreenwald@shrp.umsmed.edu
**Website:** http://shrp.umc.edu/programs/pt.html
Neva F. Greenwald, Director

## Missouri

**★ 19880 ★ Maryville University, Saint**
**Louis**
**Department of Physical Therapy**
**Physical Therapist Program**
13550 Conway Rd.
Saint Louis, MO 63141
**Phone:** (314)529-9523  **Fax:** (314)529-9495
**Email:** chuckpt@maryville.edu
**Website:** http://www.maryville.edu
Charles Gulas, Director

**★ 19881 ★ Rockhurst University**
**Physical Therapist Program**
1100 Rockhurst Rd.
Kansas City, MO 64110
**Phone:** (816)501-4059  **Fax:** (816)501-4643
**Email:** spake@vax1.rockhurst.edu
**Website:** http://www.rockhurst.edu
Ellen Spake, Director

**★ 19882 ★ Saint Louis University**
**Department of Physical Therapy**
**Physical Therapist Program**
3437 Caroline St., Rm. 1026
Saint Louis, MO 63104
**Phone:** (314)577-8505  **Fax:** (314)577-8513
**Email:** ruebling@slu.edu
**Website:** http://www.slu.edu/colleges/AH/PTH
Irma S. Ruebling, Director

**★ 19883 ★ Southwest Baptist University**
**Department of Physical Therapy**
**Physical Therapist Program**
1600 University Ave.
Bolivar, MO 65613-2496
**Phone:** (417)328-1672  **Fax:** (417)328-1658
**Email:** dhash@sbuniv.edu
**Website:** http://falcon.sbuniv.edu/pt/index.html
Dorothy Hash, DPT, Director

**★ 19884 ★ University of Missouri,**
**Columbia**
**School of Health Professions**
**Physical Therapist Program**
106 Lewis Hall
Columbia, MO 65211
**Phone:** (573)882-7103  **Fax:** (573)884-8369
**Email:** denbighb@ext.missouri.edu
**Website:** http://www.missouri.edu
Marilyn K. Sanford, PhD, Director

**★ 19885 ★ Washington University**
**Department of Physical Therapy**
**Physical Therapist Program**
4444 Forest Park Blvd., Ste. 1101
Saint Louis, MO 63108
**Phone:** (314)286-1400  **Fax:** (314)286-1410
**Email:** deusingers@msnotes.wustl.edu
**Website:** http://medicine.wustl.edu/~ptprog/
Susan S. Deusinger, PhD, Director

## Montana

**★ 19886 ★ University of Montana,**
**Missoula**
**Department of Physical Therapy**
**Physical Therapist Program**
Skaggs Bldg. 135
Missoula, MT 59812
**Phone:** (406)243-4753  **Fax:** (406)243-2795
**Email:** williams@selway.umt.edu
**Website:** http://www.umt.edu/pt
Ann K. Williams, PhD, Director

## Nebraska

**★ 19887 ★ Creighton University**
**School of Pharmacy and Allied Health**
**Professions**
**Physical Therapist Program**
2500 California Plaza
Omaha, NE 68178
**Phone:** (402)280-5675  **Fax:** (402)280-5692
**Email:** rsandstr@creighton.edu
**Website:** http://spahp.creighton.edu
Robert Sandstrom, PhD, Director

**★ 19888 ★ University of Nebraska**
**Medical Center**
**Division of Physical Therapy Education**
**Physical Therapist Program**
984420 Nebraska Medical Ctr.
Omaha, NE 68198-4420
**Phone:** (402)559-4259  **Fax:** (402)559-8626
**Email:** phageman@unmc.edu
**Website:** http://www.unmc.edu/PhysicalTherapy/pte-du.htm
Patricia A. Hageman, PhD, Director

## Nevada

**★ 19889 ★ University of Nevada, Las**
**Vegas**
**Physical Therapist Program**
4505 Maryland Pkwy.
Box 453029
Las Vegas, NV 89154-3029
**Phone:** (702)895-3003  **Fax:** (702)895-4883
**Email:** hwallmann@ccmail.nevada.edu
**Website:** http://www.unlv.edu/Colleges/Health_Sciences/Physical_Therapy/index.html
Harvey Wallmann, Chairman of the Board

## New Hampshire

**★ 19890 ★ Notre Dame College**
**Physical Therapist Program**
2321 Elm St.
Manchester, NH 03104-2299
**Phone:** (603)647-5500  **Fax:** (603)222-7520

Email: Ehaskvitz@notredame.edu
Esther Haskvitz, PhD, Director

### New Jersey

**★ 19891 ★ Richard Stockton College of New Jersey**
Physical Therapist Program
Jim Leeds Rd.
Pomona, NJ 08240
Phone: (609)652-4261     Fax: (609)652-4858
Email: bkathrins@stockton.edu
Website: http://loki.stockton.edu/index.html
Bess Kathrins, Director

**★ 19892 ★ Rutgers, the State University of New Jersey/University of Medicine and Dentistry of New Jersey**
Camden Campus
Physical Therapist Program
Primary Care Center, Ste. 228
40 E Laurel Rd.
Stratford, NJ 08084-1353
Phone: (856)566-6456     Fax: (856)566-6458
Email: mnardone@umdnj.edu
Website: http://camden-www.rutgers.edu/
Marie Koval Nardone, Director

**★ 19893 ★ University of Medicine and Dentistry of New Jersey**
School of Health Related Professions
Physical Therapist Program
65 Bergen St.
Newark, NJ 07107-3001
Phone: (973)972-5454     Fax: (973)972-3717
Email: merians@umdnj.edu
Website: http://www.umdnj.edu/~shrpweb
Alma S. Merians, PhD, Director

### New Mexico

**★ 19894 ★ University of New Mexico**
Physical Therapist Program
Health Sciences and Services Bldg., Rm. 204
Albuquerque, NM 87131-5661
Phone: (505)272-5755     Fax: (505)272-8079
Email: randrews@salud.unm.edu
Website: http://www.unm.edu/
Ronald Andrews, PhD, Director

### New York

**★ 19895 ★ City University of New York**
College of Staten Island
Physical Therapist Program
2800 Victory Blvd.
Staten Island, NY 10314
Phone: (718)982-3153     Fax: (718)982-2984
Email: rothmanj@postbox.csi.cuny.edu
Website: http://www.library.csi.cuny.edu/dept/pt/main.htm
Jeffrey Rothman, EdD, Director

**★ 19896 ★ Clarkson University**
Department of Physical Therapy
PO Box 5880
Potsdam, NY 13699-5880
Phone: (315)268-3786     Fax: (315)268-1539
Email: feitelsb@clarkson.edu
Website: http://www.clarkson.edu
Samuel B. Feitelberg, Director

**★ 19897 ★ Columbia University**
Physical Therapist Program
710 W 168th St., 8th Fl.
New York, NY 10032
Phone: (212)305-3781     Fax: (212)305-4569
Email: kh111@columbia.edu
Website: http://cpmcnet.columbia.edu/dept/pt
Kenneth J. Harwood, PhD, Director

**★ 19898 ★ Daemen College**
Physical Therapist Program
4380 Main St.
Amherst, NY 14226-3592
Phone: (716)839-8345     Fax: (716)839-8537
Email: mbrogan@daemen.edu
Website: http://www.daemen.edu/departments/pt/default.html
Michael S. Brogan, Director

**★ 19899 ★ D'Youville College**
Physical Therapist Program
1 D'Youville Sq.
320 Porter Ave.
Buffalo, NY 14201-1084
Phone: (716)881-7702     Fax: (716)881-8137
Email: riversl@dyc.edu
Website: http://www.koolnet.org
Lynn Rivers, Director

**★ 19900 ★ Hunter College**
School of Health Sciences
Physical Therapist Program
425 E 25th St.
New York, NY 10010
Phone: (212)481-4469     Fax: (212)481-8618
Email: gkrasilo@hunter.cuny.edu
Website: http://www.hunter.cuny.edu/health/pt
Gary Krasilovsky, PhD, Director

**★ 19901 ★ Ithaca College**
Department of Physical Therapy
Physical Therapist Program
332 Smiddy Hall
Ithaca, NY 14850-7183
Phone: (607)274-3342     Fax: (607)274-1137
Email: rbrown@ithaca.edu
Website: http://www.ithaca.edu/hshp/pt/pt2/icpt2/html
Renee Brown, PhD, Director

**★ 19902 ★ Long Island University, Brooklyn**
Zeckendorf Health Sciences Center
Division of Physical Therapy
1 University Plaza
Brooklyn, NY 11201-5372
Phone: (718)488-1063     Fax: (718)780-4002
Email: wsusman@liu.edu
Website: http://www.brooklyn.liunet.edu/cwis/bklyn/health/bsphythe.html
William M. Susman, PhD, Director

**★ 19903 ★ Mercy College**
Physical Therapist Program
Graduate Center
555 Broadway
Dobbs Ferry, NY 10522
Phone: (914)674-9331     Free: 800-637-2969
Fax: (914)674-9457
Email: cfendersn@mercy.edu
Website: http://www.mercynet.edu/programs/index.htmlgrad
Claudia B. Fenderson, EdD, Director

**★ 19904 ★ Nazareth College of Rochester**
Physical Therapy Department
4245 East Ave.
Rochester, NY 14618-3790
Phone: (716)389-2900     Fax: (716)389-2908
Email: jwbloss@naz.edu
Website: http://www.naz.edu/dept/physical_therapy/index.html
Jill W. Bloss, Director

**★ 19905 ★ New York Institute of Technology**
Department of Physical Therapy
Wheatley Rd.
Box 8000
Old Westbury, NY 11568-8000
Phone: (516)686-7696     Fax: (516)686-7699
Email: pdouris@nyit.edu
Website: http://iris.nyit.edu/~physther
Peter C. Douris, EdD, Director

**★ 19906 ★ New York Medical College**
Graduate School of Health Sciences
Physical Therapist Program
Learning Center, Rm. 302
Valhalla, NY 10595
Phone: (914)594-4517     Fax: (914)594-4292
Email: michael_majsak@nymc.edu
Website: http://www.nymc.edu/admit/gshs/phys_therapy.htm
Michael J. Majsak, EdD, Director

**★ 19907 ★ New York University**
Physical Therapist Program
380 2nd Ave., 4th Fl.
New York, NY 10010-4086
Phone: (212)998-9400     Fax: (212)995-4190
Email: wk1@is2.nyu.edu
Website: http://www.nyu.edu/education/pt
Wen Ling, PhD, Director

**★ 19908 ★ The Sage Colleges**
Division of Health and Rehabilitation Sciences
Physical Therapist Program
Troy, NY 12180
Phone: (518)244-2266     Fax: (518)244-4524
Email: sellem@sage.edu
Website: http://www.sage.edu/html/RSC/prrsc.html
Marjane Selleck, Director

**★ 19909 ★ State University of New York, Brooklyn (SUNY)**
Health Science Center
Physical Therapist Program
450 Clarkson Ave., Box 16
Brooklyn, NY 11203-2098
Phone: (718)270-7720     Fax: (718)270-7439
Email: jkatz@downstate.edu
Website: http://www.hscbklyn.edu/CHRP/pt.html
Joanne S. Katz, PhD, Director

**★ 19910 ★ State University of New York, Buffalo**
Department of Physical Therapy, Exercise and Nutrition Sciences
Physical Therapist Program
405 Kimball Tower
3435 Main St.
Buffalo, NY 14214-3079
Phone: (716)829-2941     Fax: (716)829-2428
Email: sbennett@buffalo.edu
Website: http://wings.buffalo.edu
Susan E. Bennett, EdD, Director

**★ 19911 ★ State University of New York, Stony Brook**
School of Health Technology and Management
Physical Therapist Program
Health Sciences Center
Stony Brook, NY 11794-8201
Phone: (631)444-3250     Fax: (631)444-7621
Email: rjohnson@epo.hsc.sunysb.edu
Website: http://www.sunysb.edu
Richard W. Johnson, Director

**★ 19912 ★ State University of New York**
**Upstate Medical Center**
**College of Health Professions**
**Physical Therapist Program**
750 E Adams St.
Syracuse, NY 13210
**Phone:** (315)464-0881  **Fax:** (315)464-6887
**Email:** grametp@upstate.edu
**Website:** http://www.ec.hscsyr.edu/CHRP/pt/physical_therapy.html
Pamela Gramet, PhD, Director


**★ 19913 ★ Syracuse University**
**Utica College**
**Health and Human Studies Division**
**Physical Therapist Program**
1600 Burrstone Rd.
Utica, NY 13502-4892
**Phone:** (315)792-3059  **Fax:** (315)792-3248
**Email:** dscalise-smith@utica.ucsu.edu
**Website:** http://www.ucsu.edu/academic/majors/ptmajor.html
Dale Scalise-Smith, PhD, Director


**★ 19914 ★ Touro College**
**School of Health Sciences**
**Physical Therapist Program**
1700 Union Blvd.
Bay Shore, NY 11706
**Phone:** (631)665-1600  **Fax:** (631)665-4986
**Email:** josephw@touro.edu
**Website:** http://www.touro.edu/HEALTH/pt.htm
Kevin Wong, Director


### North Carolina

**★ 19915 ★ Duke University Medical**
**Center**
**Physical Therapist Program**
PO Box 3965
Durham, NC 27710
**Phone:** (919)684-2445  **Fax:** (919)684-6708
**Email:** richa052@mc.duke.edu
Jan K. Richardson, PhD, Director


**★ 19916 ★ East Carolina University**
**Department of Physical Therapy**
**Physical Therapist Program**
Greenville, NC 27858-4353
**Phone:** (252)328-4450  **Fax:** (252)328-0707
**Email:** albrightb@ecu.edu
**Website:** http://www.ecu.edu/pt/
Bruce C. Albright, PhD, Director


**★ 19917 ★ Elon University**
**Department of Physical Therapy**
**Education**
**Physical Therapist Program**
Campus Box 2085
Elon, NC 27244-2010
**Phone:** (336)278-6400  **Free:** 800-334-8448
**Fax:** (336)278-6414
**Email:** rogers@elon.edu
Elizabeth Rogers, EdD, Director


**★ 19918 ★ University of North Carolina,**
**Chapel Hill**
**Division of Physical Therapy**
**Physical Therapist Program**
Medical School Wing E
CB 7135
Chapel Hill, NC 27599-7135
**Phone:** (919)966-4708  **Fax:** (919)966-3678
**Email:** dsekerak@med.unc.edu
**Website:** http://www.med.unc.edu/mahp/physical/
Darlene K. Sekerak, PhD, Director


**★ 19919 ★ Western Carolina University**
**Physical Therapist Program**
312 Moore Bldg.
Cullowhee, NC 28723-9646
**Phone:** (828)227-7070  **Fax:** (828)227-7071
**Email:** klunnen@email.wcu.edu
**Website:** http://www.wcu.edu/aps/pt/
Karen Y. Lennen, EdD, Director


**★ 19920 ★ Winston-Salem State**
**University**
**Physical Therapist Program**
601 Martin Luther King Jr. Dr.
Winston-Salem, NC 27110
**Fax:** (336)750-2192
**Email:** greengj@wssu.edu
Gloria J. Green, Director


### North Dakota

**★ 19921 ★ University of Mary**
**Division of Human Performance Sciences**
**Physical Therapist Program**
7500 University Dr.
Bismarck, ND 58504-9652
**Phone:** (701)255-7500  **Free:** 800-408-6279
**Fax:** (701)255-7687
**Email:** mparker@umary.edu
**Website:** http://www.umary.edu/pt.htm
Michael G. Parker, PhD, Director


**★ 19922 ★ University of North Dakota**
**School of Medicine and Health Sciences**
**Physical Therapist Program**
501 N Columbia Rd.
PO Box 9037
Grand Forks, ND 58202-9037
**Phone:** (701)777-2831  **Fax:** (701)777-4199
**Email:** tommohr@medicine.nodak.edu
**Website:** http://www.med.und.nodak.edu/depts/pt/home.htm
Thomas M. Mohr, PhD, Director


### Ohio

**★ 19923 ★ Andrews University, Dayton**
**Department of Physical Therapy**
**Physical Therapist Program**
2912 Springboro W, Ste. 301
Dayton, OH 45439
**Phone:** (937)298-2878  **Fax:** (937)298-9500
**Email:** daryls@andrews.edu
**Website:** http://www.andrews.edu/PHTH/
Daryl Stuart, EdD, Director


**★ 19924 ★ Cleveland State University**
**Department of Health Sciences**
**Physical Therapist Program**
Health Sciences Bldg., No. 109
2121 Euclid Ave.
Cleveland, OH 44115
**Phone:** (216)687-3567  **Fax:** (216)687-9316
**Email:** m.wagner@csuohio.edu
**Website:** http://www.csuohio.edu
Marilyn B . Wagner, PhD, Director


**★ 19925 ★ College of Mount St. Joseph**
**Physical Therapist Program**
5701 Delhi Rd.
Cincinnati, OH 45233-1672
**Phone:** (513)244-4890  **Fax:** (513)451-2547
**Email:** terri_glenn@mail.msj.edu
Terri M. Glenn, PhD, Director


**★ 19926 ★ Medical College of Ohio**
**Physical Therapist Program**
4418 Collier Bldg.
3015 Arlington Ave.
Toledo, OH 43614
**Phone:** (419)383-3518  **Fax:** (419)383-5880

**Email:** chornbeck@mco.edu
**Website:** http://www.mco.edu/
Catherine L. Hornbeck, Director


**★ 19927 ★ Ohio State University**
**Physical Therapist Program**
306 Allied Medical Professions
1583 Perry St.
Columbus, OH 43210
**Phone:** (614)292-5921  **Fax:** (614)292-0210
**Email:** nichols.3@osu.edu
**Website:** http://www.amp.ohio-state.edu/
Deborah S. Nichols, PhD, Director


**★ 19928 ★ Ohio University**
**School of Physical Therapy**
**Physical Therapist Program**
Grover Center, W290
Athens, OH 45701
**Phone:** (740)593-1225  **Fax:** (740)593-0292
**Email:** overbya@ohio.edu
**Website:** http://www.ohiou.edu/
Averell S. Overby, DrPH, Director


**★ 19929 ★ University of Cincinnati**
**College of Allied Health Sciences**
**Physical Therapy Program**
French East
PO Box 670394
Cincinnati, OH 45267-0394
**Phone:** (513)558-7477  **Fax:** (513)558-7474
**Email:** mulligea@uc.edu
**Website:** http://www.uc.edu/cahs/
Lizanne Mulligan, PhD, Director


**★ 19930 ★ University of Findlay**
**Physical Therapist Program**
1000 N Main St.
Findlay, OH 45840
**Phone:** (419)424-4863  **Fax:** (419)424-6977
**Email:** dutton@lucy.findlay.edu
**Website:** http://www.findlay.edu/academic/science/health/index.html
Lisa L. Dutton, Director


**★ 19931 ★ Walsh University**
**Division of Physical Therapy**
2020 Easton St. NW
North Canton, OH 44720-3396
**Phone:** (330)490-7286  **Fax:** (330)490-7371
**Email:** sbemis@alex.walsh.edu
Susan A. Bemis, EdD, Director


**★ 19932 ★ Youngstown State University**
**Physical Therapist Program**
B080 Cushwa Hall
Youngstown, OH 44555-2558
**Phone:** (330)742-2558  **Fax:** (330)742-1898
**Email:** mmcclell@cc.ysu.edu
**Website:** http://www.ysu.edu/colleges/hhs/hhsindex.htm
Marleen McClelland, PhD, Director


### Oklahoma

**★ 19933 ★ University of Oklahoma**
**Health Sciences Center**
**Physical Therapist Program**
PO Box 26901
Oklahoma City, OK 73190
**Phone:** (405)271-2131  **Fax:** (405)271-2432
**Website:** http://w3.ouhsc.edu/ahealth/rehab.htm
Martha J. Ferretti, Director

## Ontario

### ★ 19934 ★ University of Toronto
**Physical Therapist Program**
256 McCaul St.
Toronto, ON, Canada M5T 1W5
**Phone:** (416)978-2769
**Fax:** (416)978-4363
**Email:** m.verrier@utoronto.ca
Molly Verrier, Director

## Oregon

### ★ 19935 ★ Pacific University
**School of Physical Therapy**
**Physical Therapist Program**
2043 College Way
Forest Grove, OR 97116
**Phone:** (503)352-2846
**Fax:** (503)352-2995
**Email:** banaitid@pacificu.edu
**Website:** http://nellie.pacificu.edu/PT/index.html
Daiva A. Banaitis, PhD, Director

## Pennsylvania

### ★ 19936 ★ Arcadia University
**Department of Physical Therapy**
**Physical Therapist Program**
450 S Easton Rd.
Glenside, PA 19038-3295
**Phone:** (215)572-2950
**Fax:** (215)572-2157
**Email:** craik@arcadia.edu
Rebecca L. Craik, PhD, Director

### ★ 19937 ★ Chatham College
**Physical Therapist Program**
Woodland Rd.
Pittsburgh, PA 15232-2826
**Phone:** (412)365-1409
**Fax:** (412)365-1213
**Email:** rpatterson@chatham.edu
**Website:** http://www.chatham.edu/academic/pt/physther1.htm
Ray M. Patterson, EdD, Director

### ★ 19938 ★ College Misericordia
**Physical Therapist Program**
301 Lake St.
Dallas, PA 18612-1098
**Phone:** (570)674-6465
**Fax:** (570)674-3052
**Email:** cwilkins@miseri.edu
**Website:** http://www.miseri.edu/academic/Undergrad/healthweb/PTWeb/DeptHome.htm
Catherine Perry Wilkinson, EdD, Director

### ★ 19939 ★ Duquesne University
**School of Health Sciences**
**Physical Therapist Program**
109 Health Sciences Bldg.
Pittsburgh, PA 15282
**Phone:** (412)396-5541
**Fax:** (412)396-4399
**Email:** morgan@duq2.cc.duq.edu
**Website:** http://www.duq.edu/
Robert C. Morgan, PhD, Director

### ★ 19940 ★ Gannon University
**College of Sciences, Engineering and Health Sciences**
**Physical Therapist Program**
109 University Sq.
Erie, PA 16541-0001
**Phone:** (814)871-5639
**Fax:** (814)871-5662
**Email:** meacci001@gannon.edu
**Website:** http://www.gannon.edu/
Charles Meacci, EdD, Director

### ★ 19941 ★ MCP Hahnemann University
**Programs in Rehabilitation Sciences**
**Physical Therapist Program**
Mail Stop 502
245 N 15th St.
Philadelphia, PA 19102-1192
**Phone:** (215)762-4973
**Fax:** (215)762-3886
**Email:** jane.k.oeffner@drexel.edu
**Website:** http://www.auhs.edu/shp/depts/pt
Jane K. Oeffner, Director

### ★ 19942 ★ Neumann College
**Division of Nursing and Health Sciences**
**Physical Therapy Program**
1 Neumann Dr.
Aston, PA 19014-1298
**Phone:** (610)558-5534
**Fax:** (610)361-5290
**Email:** postr@neumann.edu
**Website:** http://www.neumann.edu
Robert E. Post, PhD, Director

### ★ 19943 ★ Saint Francis University
**Physical Therapist Program**
PO Box 600
Loretto, PA 15940-0600
**Phone:** (814)472-3123
**Fax:** (814)472-3140
**Email:** episarski@francis.edu
Edward M. Pisarski, EdD, Director

### ★ 19944 ★ Slippery Rock University of Pennsylvania
**Graduate School of Physical Therapy**
**Physical Therapist Program**
Physical Therapy Bldg.
North Rd.
Slippery Rock, PA 16057
**Phone:** (724)738-2080
**Fax:** (724)738-2113
**Email:** barbara.billek@sru.edu
**Website:** http://www.sru.edu/
Barbara Billek-Sawhney, EdD, Director

### ★ 19945 ★ Temple University
**College of Allied Health Professions**
**Physical Therapist Program**
3307 N Broad St.
Philadelphia, PA 19140
**Phone:** (215)707-4816
**Fax:** (215)707-7500
**Email:** lhack001@astro.ocis.temple.edu
**Website:** http://astro.ocis.temple.edu/
Laurita M. Hack, PhD, Director

### ★ 19946 ★ Thomas Jefferson University
**College of Health Professions**
**Physical Therapist Program**
130 S 9th St., Ste. 830 Edison
Philadelphia, PA 19107-5233
**Phone:** (215)503-8025
**Fax:** (215)503-3499
**Email:** marcus.besser@mail.tju.edu
**Website:** http://www.tju.edu
Marcus P. Besser, PhD, Director

### ★ 19947 ★ University of Pittsburgh
**School of Health and Rehabilitation Sciences**
**Physical Therapist Program**
6035 Forbes Tower
Pittsburgh, PA 15260
**Phone:** (412)647-1252
**Fax:** (412)647-1222
**Email:** delitto@pitt.edu
**Website:** http://www.pitt.edu/
Anthony Delitto, PhD, Director

### ★ 19948 ★ University of the Sciences in Philadelphia
**Physical Therapist Program**
600 S 43rd St.
Philadelphia, PA 19104
**Phone:** (215)596-8849
**Fax:** (215)895-3121
**Email:** a.iglars@usip.edu
**Website:** http://www.pcps.edu
Annette Iglarsh, PhD, Director

### ★ 19949 ★ University of Scranton
**Physical Therapist Program**
800 Linden St.
Scranton, PA 18510-4586
**Phone:** (570)941-7499
**Fax:** (570)941-7940
**Email:** kosmahle1@scranton.edu
**Website:** http://academic.uofs.edu/department/pt/default.htm
Edmund M. Kosmahl, EdD, Director

### ★ 19950 ★ Widener University
**School of Human Service Professions**
**Physical Therapist Program**
1 University Pl.
Chester, PA 19013
**Phone:** (610)499-1277
**Fax:** (610)499-1231
**Email:** robin.l.dole@widener.edu
**Website:** http://www.widener.edu/widener1.html
Robin L. Dole, EdD, Director

## Rhode Island

### ★ 19951 ★ University of Rhode Island
**Physical Therapist Program**
Independence Square II
25 W Independence Way
Kingston, RI 02881-0180
**Phone:** (401)874-5001
**Fax:** (401)874-5630
**Email:** rowinski@uri.edu
**Website:** http://www.uri.edu/hss/pt/index.html
Mark J. Rowinski, PhD, Director

## South Carolina

### ★ 19952 ★ Medical University of South Carolina
**Department of Rehabilitation Sciences**
**Physical Therapist Program**
171 Ashley Ave.
Charleston, SC 29425-2730
**Phone:** (843)792-2961
**Fax:** (843)792-0710
**Email:** morrisetted@musc.edu
**Website:** http://www.musc.edu/chp-rehab/
David Morrisette, PhD, Director

## South Dakota

### ★ 19953 ★ University of South Dakota
**Department of Physical Therapy**
**Physical Therapist Program**
414 E Clark St.
Vermillion, SD 57069
**Phone:** (605)677-5915
**Fax:** (605)677-6529
**Website:** http://www.usd.edu/med/som/somdept/pt/
Lana R. Svien, Director

## Tennessee

### ★ 19954 ★ Belmont University
**Physical Therapist Program**
1900 Belmont Blvd.
Nashville, TN 37212-3757
**Phone:** (615)460-6727
**Fax:** (615)460-6729
**Email:** greathoused@mail.belmont.edu
David G. Greathouse, PhD, Director

### ★ 19955 ★ East Tennessee State University
**Physical Therapist Program**
Box 70624
Johnson City, TN 37614-1709
**Phone:** (423)439-8793
**Fax:** (423)439-8077
**Email:** williada@etsu.edu
**Website:** http://www.etsu.edu/cpah/physther/pt/index.htm
Duane A. Williams, Director

**★ 19956 ★ University of Tennessee, Chattanooga**
**School of Rehabilitation Professions**
**Physical Therapist Program**
302 Health and Human Services Bldg.
615 McCallie Ave.
Chattanooga, TN 37403-2598
**Phone:** (423)755-4747      **Fax:** (423)785-2215
**Email:** randy-walker@utc.edu
**Website:** http://www.utc.edu/
J. Randy Walker, PhD, Director

**★ 19957 ★ University of Tennessee**
**Health Science Center**
**Physical Therapist Program**
822 Beale St., Ste. 337
Memphis, TN 38163
**Phone:** (901)448-5888      **Fax:** (901)448-7545
**Email:** bconnolly@utmem.edu
**Website:** http://www.utmen.edu/physther/intro.html
Barbara H. Connolly, EdD, Director

### Texas

**★ 19958 ★ Hardin-Simmons University**
**Physical Therapist Program**
2200 Hickory
PO Box 16065
Abilene, TX 79698-6065
**Phone:** (915)670-5860      **Free:** 888-820-0218
**Fax:** (915)670-5868
**Email:** joconnel@hsutx.edu
**Website:** http://www.hsutx.edu/grad/pt.htm
Janelle O'Connell, PhD, Director

**★ 19959 ★ Southwest Texas State**
**University**
**Health Science Center**
**Physical Therapist Program**
601 University Dr.
San Marcos, TX 78666-4616
**Phone:** (512)245-8351      **Fax:** (512)245-8736
**Email:** bs04@swt.edu
**Website:** http://www.swt.edu
Barbara Sanders, PhD, Director

**★ 19960 ★ Texas Tech University Health**
**Sciences Center, Lubbock**
**Physical Therapist Program**
3601 4th St.
Lubbock, TX 79430
**Phone:** (806)743-3220      **Fax:** (806)743-1262
**Email:** alhap@ttuhsc.edu
**Website:** http://www.ttuhsc.edu/pages/alhpt/alhpt_homepage.html
Andrew Priest, EdD, Director

**★ 19961 ★ Texas Woman's University**
**School of Physical Therapy**
**Physical Therapist Program**
PO Box 425766, TWU Station
Denton, TX 76204-5766
**Phone:** (940)898-2460      **Fax:** (940)898-2486
**Email:** crozier@twu.edu
**Website:** http://www.twu.edu/pt/
Carolyn Rozier, PhD, Director

**★ 19962 ★ U.S. Army/Baylor University**
**Academy of Health Sciences**
**MCCS-HMT Physical Therapy Branch**
**Physical Therapist Program**
3151 Scott Rd.
Fort Sam Houston, TX 78234-6138
**Phone:** (210)221-8410      **Fax:** (210)221-7585
**Email:** timothy.flynn@cen.amedd.army.mil
**Website:** http://www.cs.amedd.army.mil/baylorpt/65b.htm
Lt. Col. Timothy W. Flynn, PhD, Director

**★ 19963 ★ University of Texas, El Paso**
**Physical Therapist Program**
1101 N Campbell
El Paso, TX 79902-0581
**Phone:** (915)747-8207      **Fax:** (915)747-8211
**Email:** ryberg@miners.utep.edu
**Website:** http://www.nurse.utep.edu/pt/index.htm
J. Alan Ryberg, PhD, Director

**★ 19964 ★ University of Texas Health**
**Science Center, San Antonio**
**Physical Therapist Program**
7703 Floyd Curl Dr.
San Antonio, TX 78229-3900
**Phone:** (210)567-8862      **Fax:** (210)567-8774
**Email:** dedomenico@uthscsa.edu
**Website:** http://www.uthscsa.edu/sah_main.html
Giovanni de Domenico, PhD, Director

**★ 19965 ★ University of Texas Medical**
**Branch, Galveston**
**School of Allied Health Sciences**
**Physical Therapist Program**
301 University Blvd.
Galveston, TX 77555-1028
**Phone:** (409)772-3068      **Fax:** (409)747-1613
**Email:** mhinman@utmb.edu
**Website:** http://www.utmb.edu
Martha Hinman, EdD, Director

**★ 19966 ★ University of Texas**
**Southwestern Medical Center, Dallas**
**Southwestern Allied Health Sciences**
**School**
**Physical Therapist Program**
5323 Harry Hines Blvd.
Dallas, TX 75390-8876
**Phone:** (214)648-1551      **Fax:** (214)648-1511
**Email:** pwinch@mednet.swmed.edu
**Website:** http://www.swmed.edu/
Patricia Winchester, PhD, Director

### Utah

**★ 19967 ★ University of Utah**
**Division of Physical Therapy**
**Physical Therapist Program**
520 Wakara Way, Ste. 302
Salt Lake City, UT 84108
**Phone:** (801)581-8681      **Fax:** (801)585-5629
**Email:** scott.ward@hsc.utah.edu
**Website:** http://www.utah.edu/
R. Scott Ward, PhD, Director

### Vermont

**★ 19968 ★ University of Vermont**
**School of Allied Health Sciences**
**Physical Therapist Program**
305 Rowell Bldg.
Burlington, VT 05405-0068
**Phone:** (802)656-3252      **Fax:** (802)656-6586
**Email:** jheld@zoo.uvm.edu
**Website:** http://www.uvm.edu/
Jean M. Held, EdD, Director

### Virginia

**★ 19969 ★ Marymount University**
**Physical Therapist Program**
2807 N Glebe Rd.
Arlington, VA 22207-4299
**Phone:** (703)284-5980      **Fax:** (703)284-5981
**Email:** diana.venskus@marymount.edu
Diana Gilroy Venskus, Director

**★ 19970 ★ Old Dominion University**
**School of Community Health Professions**
**and Physical Therapy**
**Physical Therapist Program**
Health Science Bldg.
Norfolk, VA 23529-0288
**Phone:** (757)683-4519      **Fax:** (757)683-4410
**Email:** gmaihafe@odu.edu
**Website:** http://www.odu.edu
George Maihafer, PhD, Director

**★ 19971 ★ Shenandoah University**
**School of Health Professions**
**Physical Therapist Program**
333 W Cork St.
Winchester, VA 22601
**Phone:** (540)665-5520      **Free:** 800-432-2266
**Fax:** (540)665-5530
**Email:** stepper@su.edu
**Website:** http://www.su.edu/pt/
Steven H. Tepper, PhD, Director

**★ 19972 ★ Virginia Commonwealth**
**University**
**Medical College of Virginia**
**Physical Therapist Program**
Box 980224
Richmond, VA 23298-0224
**Phone:** (804)828-0234      **Fax:** (804)828-8111
**Email:** tmayhew@hsc.vcu.edu
**Website:** http://views.vcu.edu/pt/
Thomas Mayhew, PhD, Director

### Washington

**★ 19973 ★ Eastern Washington**
**University**
**Department of Physical Therapy**
310 N Riverpoint Blvd.
Box T
Spokane, WA 99202-1675
**Phone:** (509)368-6601      **Fax:** (509)368-6623
**Email:** deldin@mail.ewu.edu
**Website:** http://www.ewu.edu
Donna El-Din, PhD, Chairman of the Board

**★ 19974 ★ University of Puget Sound**
**Physical Therapist Program**
1500 N Warner
Tacoma, WA 98416
**Phone:** (253)879-3281      **Fax:** (253)879-2933
**Email:** hummel@ups.edu
**Website:** http://www.ups.edu
Kathie Hummel-Berry, PhD, Director

**★ 19975 ★ University of Washington**
**Department of Rehabilitation Medicine**
**Physical Therapist Program**
1959 NE Pacific St.
Seattle, WA 98195-6490
**Phone:** (206)598-5333      **Fax:** (206)685-3244
**Email:** mguthrie@u.washington.edu
**Website:** http://weber.u.washington.edu/~rehab
Mark R. Guthrie, PhD, Director

### West Virginia

**★ 19976 ★ West Virginia University**
**School of Medicine**
**Physical Therapist Program**
PO Box 9226
Morgantown, WV 26506-9226
**Phone:** (304)293-3610      **Fax:** (304)293-7105
**Email:** mmandich@hsc.wvu.edu
**Website:** http://www.hsc.wvu.edu/som/pther
MaryBeth Mandich, PhD, Director

**★ 19977 ★ Wheeling Jesuit University**
**Physical Therapist Program**
316 Washington Ave.
Wheeling, WV 26003
**Phone:** (304)243-2432     **Free:** (866)243-2068
**Fax:** (304)243-2042
**Email:** lezook@wju.edu
Letha Zook, EdD, Director

## Wisconsin

**★ 19978 ★ Carroll College**
**Physical Therapist Program**
100 N East Ave.
Waukesha, WI 53186
**Phone:** (262)524-1294     **Fax:** (262)524-7690
**Email:** jhopp@carroll1.cc.edu
**Website:** http://www.cc.edu/pt
Jane F. Hopp, PhD, Director

**★ 19979 ★ Concordia University,**
**Wisconsin**
**Physical Therapist Program**
12800 N Lake Shore Dr.
Mequon, WI 53092-7699
**Phone:** (262)243-4433     **Fax:** (414)243-4506
**Email:** terry.steffen@cuw.edu
**Website:** http://www.cuw.edu
Teresa M. Steffen, PhD, Director

**★ 19980 ★ Marquette University**
**Physical Therapist Program**
PO Box 1881
Milwaukee, WI 53201-1881
**Phone:** (414)288-7194     **Fax:** (414)288-5987
**Email:** lawrence.pan@marquette.edu
**Website:** http://www.marquette.edu/chs
Lawrence G. Pan, PhD, Director

**★ 19981 ★ University of Wisconsin, La**
**Crosse**
**Department of Physical Therapy**
**Physical Therapist Program**
4071 Health Science Ctr.
1725 State St.
La Crosse, WI 54601
**Phone:** (608)785-8470     **Fax:** (608)785-8460
**Email:** straker.gwyn@uwlax.edu
**Website:** http://www.uwlax.edu/SAH/PT/PhysicalTherapy.html
Gwyneth Straker, Director

**★ 19982 ★ University of Wisconsin,**
**Madison**
**Physical Therapist Program**
5175 Medical Sciences Ctr.
1300 University Ave.
Madison, WI 53706-1532
**Phone:** (608)263-7131     **Fax:** (608)263-6434
**Email:** steinkam@surgery.wisc.edu
**Website:** http://www.medsch.wisc.edu/pt
Lisa Steinkamp, Director

## Rehabilitation

*The institutions listed below offer programs in rehabilitation education. All are members of the National Council on Rehabilitation Education, c/o California State University—Fresno, Rehabilitation Counseling Program, 5005 N Maple Ave., MS 3, Fresno, CA 93740-8025, (559)278-0325, http:// www.nchrtm.okstate.edu/ncre/.*

## Alabama

**★ 19983 ★ Auburn University**
**Department of Rehabilitation and Special**
**Education**
**Rehabilitation Counseling Program**
1228 Haley Center
Auburn, AL 36849
**Phone:** (334)844-5943     **Fax:** (334)844-2080
**Email:** mcdanrs@mail.auburn.edu
**Website:** http://www.auburn.edu/academic/education/rse/
Randall McDaniel, Contact

**★ 19984 ★ Troy State University**
**Department of Human Services**
**Rehabilitation Program**
104 McCartha Hall
Troy, AL 36082
**Phone:** (334)670-3366     **Fax:** (334)670-3473
**Email:** rmillard@p-c-net.net
Richard P. Millard, RhD, Contact

**★ 19985 ★ University of Alabama**
**Rehabilitation Counseling Program**
Box 870231
Tuscaloosa, AL 35487-0231
**Phone:** (205)348-1190     **Fax:** (205)348-7584
**Email:** jsatcher@bamaed.ua.edu
**Website:** http://www.bamaed.ua.edu/Counsed.htm
Jamie Satcher, PhD, Contact

## Alberta

**★ 19986 ★ University of Calgary**
**Community Rehabilitation and Disability**
**Studies**
**Community Rehabilitation Program**
2500 University Dr. NW
Calgary, AB, Canada T2N 1N4
**Phone:** (403)220-3543     **Fax:** (403)220-6494
**Email:** marlett@ucalgary.ca
Nancy Marlett, PhD, Director

## Arizona

**★ 19987 ★ University of Arizona**
**College of Education**
**Department of Special Education,**
**Rehabilitation and School Psychology**
**Rehabilitation Counseling Program**
Rm. 412
PO Box 210069
Tucson, AZ 85721
**Phone:** (520)621-7822     **Fax:** (520)621-3821
**Email:** sales@email.arizona.edu
**Website:** http://www.ed.arizona.edu/departs/SER/serinfo.htm
Amos Sales, EdD, Contact

## Arkansas

**★ 19988 ★ Arkansas State University**
**Department of Psychology and**
**Counseling**
**Rehabilitation Counseling Program**
PO Box 1560
State University, AR 72467
**Phone:** (870)972-3064     **Fax:** (870)972-3828
**Email:** tturner@kiowa.astate.edu
**Website:** http://147.97.11.245/cep/mrc/index.html
Tyra Turner, RhD, Contact

**★ 19989 ★ Arkansas Tech University**
**Rehabilitation Science**
348 Witherspoon Hall
Russellville, AR 72801
**Phone:** (501)968-0283     **Fax:** (501)964-0544
**Email:** penny.willmering@mail.atu.edu
Penny Willmering, Director

**★ 19990 ★ University of Arkansas,**
**Fayetteville**
**Department of Rehabilitation Education**
**and Research**
**Rehabilitation Counseling Program**
346 N West Ave.
WAAX 319
Fayetteville, AR 72701
**Phone:** (501)575-3658     **Fax:** (501)575-3253
**Email:** jandrew@comp.uark.edu
**Website:** http://comp.uark.edu/~rehab/grad.html
Jason D. Andrew, PhD, Contact

## California

**★ 19991 ★ California State University,**
**Fresno**
**School of Education and Human**
**Development**
**Rehabilitation Counseling Program**
5005 N Maple Ave., MS 3
Fresno, CA 93740-8025
**Phone:** (559)278-0325     **Fax:** (559)278-0404
**Email:** charlesa@csufresno.edu
**Website:** http://caracas.soehd.csufresno.edu/
Charles Arokiasamy, RhD, Contact

**★ 19992 ★ California State University,**
**Los Angeles**
**Division of Administration and**
**Counseling**
**Rehabilitation Counseling Program**
5151 State University Dr.
King Hall C1065
Los Angeles, CA 90032
**Phone:** (323)343-4250     **Fax:** (323)343-4252
**Email:** mbrodwi@calstatela.edu
**Website:** http://www.calstatela.edu/dept/edac/index.htm
Martin Brodwin, Contact

**★ 19993 ★ California State University,**
**Sacramento**
**School of Education**
**Department of Special Education,**
**Rehabilitation and School Psychology**
**Vocational Rehabilitation and Counseling**
**Programs**
6000 J St.
Eureka Hall, Rm. 316
Sacramento, CA 95819-6079
**Phone:** (916)278-6622     **Fax:** (916)278-3498
**Email:** kochr@educserver.educ.csus.edu
**Website:** http://edweb.csus.edu/eds/default.html
Richard A. Koch, EdD, Contact

**★ 19994 ★ San Diego State University**
**Department of Administration,**
**Rehabilitation and Post-secondary**
**Education**
**Rehabilitation Counseling Program**
Interwork Institute
5850 Hardy Ave., No. 112
San Diego, CA 92182-5313
**Phone:** (619)594-6406     **Fax:** (619)594-4208
**Email:** fmcfarla@mail.sdsu.edu
**Website:** http://www.interwork.sdsu.edu/~dwright/EdLdr/
Fred McFarlane, PhD, Contact

**★ 19995 ★ San Francisco State**
**University**
**Department of Counseling**
**Rehabilitation Counseling Program**
1600 Holloway Ave.
San Francisco, CA 94132
**Phone:** (415)338-2005     **Fax:** (415)338-0594
**Email:** ali1212@sfsu.edu

**Website:** http://www.sfsu.edu/~counsel/html/program/RC.htm
Anita Leal-Idrogo, PhD, Contact

## Colorado

**★ 19996 ★ University of Northern Colorado**
**Department of Human Services**
**Rehabilitation Counseling Program**
Gunter Hall, Rm. 1250
Greeley, CO 80639
**Phone:** (970)351-2403    **Fax:** (970)351-1255
**Email:** jfried@hhs.unco.edu
**Website:** http://www.hhs.unco.edu/Rehab.htm
Juliet H. Fried, EdD, Contact

## District of Columbia

**★ 19997 ★ George Washington University**
**Rehabilitation Counseling Program**
2011 Eye St. NW
Ste. 300
Washington, DC 20052
**Phone:** (202)973-1550    **Fax:** (202)775-0053
**Email:** garcia@gwu.edu
**Website:** http://www.gwu.edu/~chaos/
Jorge Garcia, RhD, Director

## Florida

**★ 19998 ★ Florida State University**
**Department of Human Services and Studies**
**Rehabilitation Counseling**
College of Education
215 Stone Bldg.
Tallahassee, FL 32306
**Phone:** (850)644-3854    **Fax:** (850)644-4335
**Email:** debener@garnet.acns.fsu.edu
**Website:** http://www.fsu.edu/~coe/departments/hss.html
Deborah Ebener, PhD, Contact

**★ 19999 ★ University of Florida**
**Department of Rehabilitation Counseling**
**Rehabilitation Counseling Program and Rehabilitative Services**
PO Box 100175
University of Florida Health Sciences Center
Gainesville, FL 32610-0175
**Phone:** (352)265-0745    **Fax:** (352)265-0744
**Email:** horace-sawyer@ufl.edu
Horace W. Sawyer, Contact

**★ 20000 ★ University of North Florida**
**Department of Health Science**
**Rehabilitation Counseling Program**
4567 St. Johns Bluff Rd. S
Jacksonville, FL 32224-2645
**Phone:** (904)620-2840    **Fax:** (904)620-2848
**Email:** jpatters@unf.edu
**Website:** http://www.unf.edu  or  http://www.unf.edu/coh/cohrehab.htm
Jeanne Patterson, EdD, Contact

**★ 20001 ★ University of South Florida**
**College of Arts and Sciences**
**Department of Rehabilitation Counseling**
4202 E Fowler Ave., SOC 107
Tampa, FL 33620-8100
**Phone:** (813)974-2855    **Fax:** (813)974-8080
**Email:** emener@chuma1.cas.usf.edu
**Website:** http://www.cas.usf.edu/rehab_counseling/index.html
William G. Emener, PhD, Contact

## Georgia

**★ 20002 ★ Georgia State University**
**Department of Counseling and Psychological Services**
**Rehabilitation Counseling Program**
College of Education, 9th Fl.
Atlanta, GA 30303-3083
**Phone:** (404)651-2550    **Fax:** (404)651-1160
**Email:** rweed@gsu.edu
**Website:** http://www.gsu.edu/~wwwcps/
Roger O. Weed, PhD, Contact

**★ 20003 ★ Thomas University**
**Division of Human Services**
**Rehabilitation Services Program**
1501 Millpond Rd.
Thomasville, GA 31792-7499
**Phone:** (912)226-1621    **Fax:** (912)226-1653
**Email:** schandler@thomascollege.edu
Shirley K. Chandler, PhD, Director

**★ 20004 ★ University of Georgia**
**Department of Counseling and Human Development Services**
**Rehabilitation Counseling Program**
402 Aderhold Hall
Athens, GA 30602-7142
**Phone:** (706)542-1812    **Fax:** (706)542-4130
**Email:** ygetch@coe.uga.edu
**Website:** http://www.coe.uga.edu/dev/echd/rehabhp.htm
Yvette Getch, PhD, Contact

## Hawaii

**★ 20005 ★ University of Hawaii, Manoa**
**Department of Counselor Education**
**Rehabilitation Counseling Program**
1776 University Ave.
Wist Annex 2-221
Honolulu, HI 96822
**Phone:** (808)956-7904    **Fax:** (808)956-3814
**Email:** oda@hawaii.edu
**Website:** http://www.hawaii.edu/97catalog/education/counseling.html
E. Aiko Oda, PhD, Contact

## Idaho

**★ 20006 ★ University of Idaho**
**Division of Adult, Counselor, and Technology Education**
**Rehabilitation/Community Counseling Program**
College of Education, Rm. 211-C
Moscow, ID 83843-3083
**Phone:** (208)885-6556    **Fax:** (208)885-6869
**Email:** jfischer@uidaho.edu
**Website:** http://www.uidaho.edu/ed/acte/
Jerry Fischer, RhD, Contact

## Illinois

**★ 20007 ★ Illinois Institute of Technology**
**Institute of Psychology**
**Rehabilitation Counseling Program**
Life Sciences Bldg., Rm. 252
3101 S Dearborn St.
Chicago, IL 60616
**Phone:** (312)567-3515    **Fax:** (312)567-3493
**Email:** psychlam@minna.cns.iit.edu
**Website:** http://www.iit.edu/colleges/psych/
Chow Lam, PhD, Director

**★ 20008 ★ Northern Illinois University**
**Department of Communicative Disorders**
**Rehabilitation Counseling Program**
DeKalb, IL 60115-2899
**Phone:** (815)753-1484    **Fax:** (815)753-9123
**Email:** glong@niu.edu
**Website:** http://www.chhs.niu.edu/comd/
Gregory Long, PhD, Contact

**★ 20009 ★ Southern Illinois University, Carbondale**
**Rehabilitation Institute**
**Rehabilitation Counseling and Rehabilitation Services Programs**
Rehn Hall 317
Carbondale, IL 62901-4609
**Phone:** (618)536-7704    **Fax:** (618)453-8271
**Email:** dmadams@siu.edu
**Website:** http://www.siu.edu/~rehabrct/
David Adams, Director

**★ 20010 ★ University of Illinois**
**Department of Community Health**
**Rehabilitation Counseling Program**
120 Huff Hall
MC-588
Champaign, IL 61820
**Phone:** (217)333-2307    **Fax:** (217)333-2766
**Email:** alston@uiuc.edu
**Website:** http://www.als.uiuc.edu/chlth/chlth-home.html
Reginald Alston, PhD, Contact

## Iowa

**★ 20011 ★ Drake University**
**School of Education**
**Rehabilitation Counseling Program**
3206 University Ave.
Des Moines, IA 50311
**Phone:** (515)271-3061    **Fax:** (515)271-4848
**Email:** bs6991r@acad.drake.edu
**Website:** http://www.educ.drake.edu/nri/default.html
Robert Stensrud, EdD, Contact

**★ 20012 ★ University of Iowa**
**Rehabilitation Counseling Program**
N362 Lindquist Center N
Iowa City, IA 52242-1529
**Phone:** (319)335-5275    **Fax:** (319)335-5291
**Email:** vilia-tarvydas@uiowa.edu
**Website:** http://www.uiowa.edu/~counsed/
Vilia Tarvydas, PhD, Contact

## Kansas

**★ 20013 ★ Emporia State University**
**Division of Counselor Education and Rehabilitation Programs**
1200 Commercial
Campus Box 4036
Emporia, KS 66801-5807
**Phone:** (316)341-5220    **Fax:** (316)341-6200
**Email:** kuehnmar@emporia.edu
**Website:** http://www.emporia.edu/counre/index.htm
Marvin D. Kuehn, EdD, Contact

## Kentucky

**★ 20014 ★ University of Kentucky**
**Rehabilitation Counseling Program**
224 Taylor Education Bldg.
Lexington, KY 40506
**Phone:** (859)257-3834    **Fax:** (859)257-3835
**Email:** rec002@pop.uky.edu
**Website:** http://www.uky.edu/Education/EDP/cpoption.html
Ralph Crystal, PhD, Contact

## Louisiana

**★ 20015 ★  Louisiana State University
Health Sciences Center**
**School of Allied Health Professions**
**Department of Rehabilitation Counseling**
**Rehabilitation Counseling Program**
1900 Gravier St.
Rm. 8C1, Box G6-2
New Orleans, LA 70112-2262
**Phone:** (504)568-4315          **Fax:** (504)568-4324
**Email:** dstroh@lsuhsc.edu
**Website:** http://AlliedHealth.lsuhsc.edu
Douglas Strohmer, PhD, Contact

**★ 20016 ★  Southern University**
**Rehabilitation Counseling and Services**
**Department of Psychology**
**Rehabilitation Counseling Program**
Baton Rouge, LA 70813
**Phone:** (225)771-2819          **Fax:** (225)771-2293
**Email:** kundusubr@aol.com
**Website:** http://www.subr.edu/academic/science/
Madan M. Kundu, PhD, Contact

## Maine

**★ 20017 ★  University of Maine,
Farmington**
**Department of Health and Rehabilitation**
**Rehabilitation Services**
228 Main St.
Farmington, ME 04938
**Phone:** (207)778-7097          **Fax:** (207)778-7045
**Email:** kbarrett@maine.edu
Karen Barrett, RhD, Contact

**★ 20018 ★  University of Southern Maine**
**Rehabilitation Counseling Program**
400 Bailey Hall
Gorham, ME 04038
**Phone:** (207)780-5319          **Fax:** (207)780-5043
**Email:** smurphy@usm.maine.edu
**Website:** http://www.usm.maine.edu/~coe/hrd/ce.htm
Stephen Murphy, PhD, Contact

## Maryland

**★ 20019 ★  Coppin State College**
**Department of Applied Psychology and
Rehabilitation Counseling**
**Rehabilitation Counseling Program**
2500 W North Ave.
Baltimore, MD 21216-3698
**Phone:** (410)383-5791          **Fax:** (410)383-5791
**Email:** jspry@coe.coppin.umd.edu
**Website:** http://www.coppin.edu/academic/academ-
ic.html
Janet Denise Spry, PhD, Contact

**★ 20020 ★  University of Maryland**
**Counseling and Personnel Services
Department**
**Rehabilitation Counseling Program**
College of Education
Benjamin Bldg., Rm. 3214
College Park, MD 20742
**Phone:** (301)405-2858          **Fax:** (301)405-9995
**Email:** ef24@umail.umd.edu
**Website:** http://www.inform.umd.edu/EDUC/Depts/
EDCP/Rehab/index.html
Ellen Fabian, PhD, Contact

**★ 20021 ★  University of Maryland
Eastern Shore**
**Department of Rehabilitation Services**
**Rehabilitation Services and Counseling
Programs**
934-5 Backbone Rd.
Princess Anne, MD 21853-1299
**Phone:** (410)651-6262          **Fax:** (410)651-6736
**Email:** dw.edwards@mail.umes.edu
Dothel W. Edwards, Jr., Contact

## Massachusetts

**★ 20022 ★  Assumption College**
**Institute for Social and Rehabilitation
Services**
500 Salisbury St.
Worcester, MA 01609
**Phone:** (508)767-7370          **Fax:** (508)798-2872
**Email:** wtalley@assumption.edu
**Website:** http://www.assumption.edu:80/dept/SocRe-
hab/socmain.html
William B. Talley, RhD, Director

**★ 20023 ★  Boston University**
**Sargent College of Health and
Rehabilitation Sciences**
**Department of Rehabilitation Counseling**
635 Commonwealth Ave.
Boston, MA 02215
**Phone:** (617)353-2725          **Fax:** (617)353-8914
**Email:** ado@bu.edu
**Website:** http://www.bu.edu/sargent/RC
Arthur E. Dell Orto, PhD, Exec Director

**★ 20024 ★  Springfield College**
**Rehabilitation Services Department**
**Rehabilitation Counseling Program**
263 Alden St.
Springfield, MA 01109
**Phone:** (413)748-3318          **Fax:** (413)748-3787
**Email:** thomas_ruscio_jr@spfldcol.edu
**Website:**    http://www.springfieldcollege.edu/home-
page.nsf
Thomas Ruscio, Contact

**★ 20025 ★  University of Massachusetts**
**Counseling and School Psychology**
**Rehabilitation Counseling**
100 Morrissey Blvd.
Boston, MA 02125
**Phone:** (617)287-7602          **Fax:** (617)287-7664
**Email:** rick.houser@umb.edu
**Website:**   http://www.umb.edu/academic_programs/
Graduate_Programs/Counseling/Counselin g.html
Rick Houser, PhD, Contact

## Michigan

**★ 20026 ★  Michigan State University**
**Office of Rehabilitation and Disability
Studies**
**Counseling, Educational Psychology and
Special Education**
**Rehabilitation Counseling Program**
College of Education
237 Erickson Hall
East Lansing, MI 48824-1034
**Phone:** (517)355-1838          **Fax:** (517)353-6393
**Email:** leahym@pilot.msu.edu
**Website:**    http://ed-web3.educ.msu.edu/ord/de-
fault.htm
Michael Leahy, PhD, Director

**★ 20027 ★  Wayne State University**
**Rehabilitation Counseling and Community
Inclusion**
**Rehabilitation Counseling Program**
5425 Gullen Mall
311 College of Education
Detroit, MI 48202
**Phone:** (313)577-1743          **Fax:** (313)577-5235
**Email:** a_coven@wayne.edu
**Website:** http://www.coe.wayne.edu/org/TBF/tbf.html
Arnold B. Coven, EdD, Contact

**★ 20028 ★  Western Michigan University**
**Departments of Counselor Education and
Counseling Psychology and Blind
Rehabilitation**
**Rehabilitation Counseling Program**
3404 Sangren Hall
Kalamazoo, MI 49008-5111
**Phone:** (616)387-3455          **Fax:** (616)387-3567
**Email:** matt.rushlau@wmich.edu
**Website:** http://www.wmich.edu/hhs/blrh/html/rtc.htm
Matthew Rushlau, EdD, Director

## Minnesota

**★ 20029 ★  Minnesota State University,
Mankato**
**Department of Speech, Hearing and
Rehabilitation Services**
**Rehabilitation Counseling Program**
103 Armstrong Hall
Mankato, MN 56001
**Phone:** (507)389-1414          **Fax:** (507)389-2821
**Email:** gschneck@mankato.msus.edu
**Website:**      http://www.mankato.msus.edu/dept/re-
habcnslg/index.htm
Gerald Schneck, PhD, Contact

**★ 20030 ★  Saint Cloud State University**
**Department of Educational Research,
School Counseling and Rehabilitation**
**Rehabilitation Counseling Program**
720 Fourth Ave. S
Saint Cloud, MN 56301
**Phone:** (320)255-2240          **Fax:** (320)255-4082
**Email:** jhotz@stcloudstate.edu
**Website:**    http://condor.stcloudstate.edu/~bulletin/
apsy/brochure1.html
John C. Hotz, RhD, Contact

## Mississippi

**★ 20031 ★  Jackson State University**
**Rehabilitation Counseling Program**
PO Box 17501
Jackson, MS 39217
**Phone:** (601)968-2380          **Fax:** (601)974-6050
**Email:** fgiles@ccaix.jsums.edu
**Website:**    http://ccaix.jsums.edu/~www/soe/html/sp-
ed-rehab.html
Frank L. Giles, PhD, Contact

**★ 20032 ★  Mississippi State University**
**Department of Counselor Education and
Educational Psychology**
**Rehabilitation Counseling Program**
Mail Stop 9727
Mississippi State, MS 39762
**Phone:** (662)325-3426          **Fax:** (662)325-3263
**Email:** ghendren@colled.msstate.edu
**Website:** http://www.educ.msstate.edu/CEdEPy/ce-
depy.html
Glen Hendren, PhD, Contact

## Missouri

**★ 20033 ★ Maryville University, Saint Louis**
**Department of Rehabilitation Counseling**
**Rehabilitation Counseling Program**
13550 Conway Rd.
Saint Louis, MO 63141-7299
**Phone:** (314)529-9625     **Fax:** (314)529-9139
**Email:** lcarlucc@maryville.edu
Lance W. Carluccio, PhD, Director

**★ 20034 ★ University of Missouri, Columbia**
**Department of Educational and Counseling Psychology**
**Rehabilitation Counseling Program**
16 Hill Hall
Columbia, MO 65211
**Phone:** (573)882-7731     **Fax:** (573)884-5989
**Email:** robertsc@missouri.edu
**Website:** http://tiger.coe.missouri.edu/~ecp/
C. David Roberts, PhD, Director

## Montana

**★ 20035 ★ Montana State University, Billings**
**Department of Counseling and Human Services**
**Rehabilitation Counseling Program**
1500 N 30th St.
Billings, MT 59101-0298
**Phone:** (406)657-2075     **Fax:** (406)657-2807
**Email:** ed_davis@vixen.emcmt.edu
**Website:** http://www.msubillings.edu/chs/rehab.html
Alan H. Davis, PhD, Contact

## New Jersey

**★ 20036 ★ University of Medicine and Dentistry of New Jersey**
**Department of Psychiatric Rehabilitation**
**School of Health-Related Professions**
1776 Raritan Rd.
Rm. 517
Scotch Plains, NJ 07076
**Phone:** (908)889-2430     **Fax:** (908)889-2432
Kenneth J. Gill, PhD, Contact

## New York

**★ 20037 ★ Cornell University**
**Program on Employment and Disability**
**School of Industrial and Labor Relations**
106 ILR Extension Bldg.
Ithaca, NY 14853-3901
**Phone:** (607)255-7727     **Fax:** (607)255-2763
**Email:** smb23@cornell.edu
Susanne M. Bruyere, PhD, Director

**★ 20038 ★ Hofstra University**
**Department of Counseling, Research, Special Education and Rehabilitation**
**Rehabilitation Counseling Program**
124 Hofstra University
111 Mason Hall
Hempstead, NY 11549
**Phone:** (516)463-5782     **Fax:** (516)463-6415
**Email:** edajsl@hofstra.edu
**Website:** http://www.hofstra.edu/Communities/?uri=/Graduate&bounce=/Graduate
Joseph Lechowicz, PhD, Director

**★ 20039 ★ Hunter College**
**City University of New York**
**Department of Educational Foundations and Counseling Programs**
**Rehabilitation Counseling Program**
695 Park Ave.
New York, NY 10021
**Phone:** (212)772-4755     **Fax:** (212)650-3198
**Website:** http://discovery.hunter.cuny.edu/~bettye/couns.html
John O'Neill, PhD, Contact

**★ 20040 ★ New York University**
**Rehabilitation Counseling Program**
35 W Fourth St.
Room 1200
New York, NY 10012-1172
**Phone:** (212)998-5293     **Fax:** (212)995-4192
**Email:** david.peterson@nyu.edu
**Website:** http://www.nyu.edu/education/health/rehab/index.html
David B. Peterson, PhD, Director

**★ 20041 ★ State University of New York, Albany**
**Department of Counseling Psychology**
**Rehabilitation Counseling Program**
1400 Washington Ave.
(Education 220)
Albany, NY 12222
**Phone:** (518)442-5050     **Fax:** (518)442-4953
**Email:** sgrand@nycap.rr.com
**Website:** http://www.albany.edu/counseling_psych/
Sheldon Grand, PhD, Contact

**★ 20042 ★ State University of New York, Brooklyn**
**Department of Counseling and Educational Psychology**
**Rehabilitation Counseling Program**
409 Christopher Baldy Hall
Buffalo, NY 14260-1000
**Phone:** (716)645-2484     **Fax:** (716)645-6661
**Email:** tjanikow@buffalo.edu
**Website:** http://www.gse.buffalo.edu/DC/CEP/RC.html
Timothy P. Janikowski, PhD, Contact

**★ 20043 ★ Syracuse University**
**Rehabilitation Counseling Program**
259 Huntington Hall
Syracuse, NY 13244-2340
**Phone:** (315)443-9624     **Fax:** (315)443-5732
**Email:** jlbellin@sued.syr.edu
**Website:** http://soeweb.syr.edu/chs/index.htm
James Bellini, PhD, Contact

## North Carolina

**★ 20044 ★ East Carolina University**
**School of Allied Health Sciences**
**Department of Rehabilitation Studies**
**Rehabilitation Counseling Program**
Greenville, NC 27858-4353
**Phone:** (252)328-4455     **Fax:** (252)328-4470
**Email:** thomass@mail.ecu.edu
**Website:** http://www.ecu.edu/rehb/rc.htm
Stephen W. Thomas, EdD, Contact

**★ 20045 ★ University of North Carolina, Chapel Hill**
**Division of Rehabilitation Psychology and Counseling**
**Rehabilitation Psychology and Counseling Program**
224 Medical School Wing E, CB 7205
Chapel Hill, NC 27599-7205
**Phone:** (919)966-3351     **Fax:** (919)966-9125
**Email:** eburker@css.unc.edu
**Website:** http://www.alliedhealth.unc.edu/rps/
Eileen Burker, PhD, Contact

## Ohio

**★ 20046 ★ Bowling Green State University**
**Department of Special Education**
**Rehabilitation Counseling Program**
451 Education Bldg.
Bowling Green, OH 43403-0255
**Phone:** (419)372-7293     **Fax:** (419)372-8265
**Email:** jstewar@bgnet.bgsu.edu
**Website:** http://www.bgsu.edu/colleges/edhd/EIS/DIS/
Jay R. Stewart, PhD, Director

**★ 20047 ★ Kent State University**
**Educational Foundations and Special Services**
**Rehabilitation Counseling Program**
405 White Hall
Kent, OH 44242
**Phone:** (330)672-2294
**Email:** prumrill@educ.kent.edu
**Website:** http://www.educ.kent.edu/CoE/EFSS/Programs/RCE/rce.html
Phillip Rumrill, PhD, Contact

**★ 20048 ★ Ohio State University**
**Rehabilitation Services**
**Rehabilitation Counseling Program**
356 Arps Hall
1945 N High St.
Columbus, OH 43210
**Phone:** (614)292-8183     **Fax:** (614)292-4255
**Email:** klein.3@osu.edu
**Website:** http://www.coe.ohio-state.edu/paes/Default.htm
Michael Klein, PhD, Contact

**★ 20049 ★ Ohio University**
**Department of Counseling and Higher Education**
**Rehabilitation Counseling Program**
201 McCracken Hall
Athens, OH 45701-2979
**Phone:** (740)593-4440     **Fax:** (740)593-0799
**Email:** olsheski@oak.cats.ohiou.edu
**Website:** http://www.ohiou.edu/che/index.html
Jerry Olsheski, PhD, Contact

**★ 20050 ★ Wright State University**
**Rehabilitation Counseling Programs**
MO52 Creative Arts Center
3640 Colonel Glenn Hwy.
Dayton, OH 45435-0001
**Phone:** (937)775-2075     **Fax:** (937)775-2042
**Email:** stephen.fortson@wright.edu
**Website:** http://www.ed.wright.edu/departments/hs/programs.html
Stephen Fortson, PhD, Contact

## Oklahoma

**★ 20051 ★ East Central University**
**Department of Human Resources**
**Rehabilitation Counseling Program**
Box Z-2
Ada, OK 74820
**Phone:** (580)332-8000     **Fax:** (580)436-3329
**Email:** rbmgrtnr@mailclerk.ecok.edu
**Website:** http://www.ecok.edu/acaddept/humres/rehbmast.html
Richard Baumgartner, EdD, Contact

**★ 20052 ★ Langston University, Oklahoma City**
**Rehabilitation Counseling Program**
4205 N Lincoln Blvd.
Oklahoma City, OK 73105
**Phone:** (405)962-1671    **Fax:** (405)962-1621
**Email:** clmoore@lunet.edu
Corey Moore, RhD, Director

**★ 20053 ★ Oklahoma State University**
**National Clearinghouse of Rehabilitation Training Materials**
5202 N Richmond Hill Dr.
Stillwater, OK 74078-4080
**Phone:** (405)624-7650    **Free:** 800-223-5219
**Fax:** (405)624-0695
**Email:** brookdj@okstate.edu
David J. Brooks, Director

**★ 20054 ★ University of Oklahoma**
**National Center for Disability Education and Training**
106 W Constitution, Bldg. 158
Norman, OK 73072-7820
**Phone:** (405)325-4913    **Fax:** (405)325-1632
C. Owen Pollard, Director

### Oregon

**★ 20055 ★ Portland State University**
**School of Education**
**Rehabilitation Counseling Program**
PO Box 751
Portland, OR 97207
**Phone:** (503)725-4619    **Fax:** (503)725-5599
**Email:** livnehh@ed.pdx.edu
**Website:** http://www.ed.pdx.edu/spedcoun/rehab/
Hanoch Livneh, PhD, Contact

**★ 20056 ★ Western Oregon University**
**Division of Special Education**
**Rehabilitation Counselor Education Program**
Education Bldg., Rm. 220
345 N Monmouth Ave.
Monmouth, OR 97361
**Phone:** (503)838-8444    **Fax:** (503)838-8228
**Email:** kellerl@wou.edu
**Website:** http://www.wou.edu/education/sped/rc.html
Linda Keller, PhD, Contact

### Pennsylvania

**★ 20057 ★ East Stroudsburg University**
**Department of Special Education/ Rehabilitation**
**Rehabilitative Services**
200 Prospect St.
East Stroudsburg, PA 18301-2999
**Phone:** (570)422-3558    **Fax:** (570)422-3777
**Email:** dsteere@po-box.esu.edu
Daniel Steere, PhD, Contact

**★ 20058 ★ Pennsylvania State University**
**Department of Counselor Education, Counseling Psychology and Rehabilitation Services**
**Rehabilitation Counseling Program**
327 Cedar Bldg.
University Park, PA 16802-3110
**Phone:** (814)865-6643    **Fax:** (814)863-7750
**Email:** bbh2@psu.edu
**Website:** http://www.ed.psu.edu/cned/rehab/
Brandon Hunt, PhD, Contact

**★ 20059 ★ University of Scranton**
**Department of Counseling and Human Services**
**Rehabilitation Counseling Programs**
435 McGurrin Hall
Scranton, PA 18510-4523
**Phone:** (570)941-4236    **Fax:** (570)941-5882
**Email:** bruchl1@uofs.edu
**Website:** http://academic.uofs.edu/department/chs/grad.html
Lori A. Bruch, EdD, Contact

### Puerto Rico

**★ 20060 ★ University of Puerto Rico**
**Rio Piedras Campus**
**Rehabilitation Counseling Program**
PO Box 23345
San Juan, PR 00931-3345
**Phone:** (787)764-0000    **Fax:** (787)763-4199
Hilda E. Gonzalez de Perez, Contact

### South Carolina

**★ 20061 ★ South Carolina State University**
**Department of Human Services**
**Rehabilitation Counseling Program**
300 College St.
PO Box 7356
Orangeburg, SC 29117-0001
**Phone:** (803)536-8600    **Fax:** (803)533-3636
**Email:** underwood@scsu.edu
**Website:** http://www.scsu.edu/academic/S_Applie/Rehib_Co/index.htm
C. Brannon Underwood, PhD, Contact

**★ 20062 ★ University of South Carolina**
**School of Medicine**
**Rehabilitation Counseling Program**
3555 Harden St. Extension, Ste. B-20
Columbia, SC 29208
**Phone:** (803)434-4296    **Fax:** (803)434-4231
**Email:** mkress@medpark.sc.edu
**Website:** http://www.med.sc.edu/REHAB/PROGRAM/HOMEPG.htm
Manuela K. Kress-Shull, Director

### Tennessee

**★ 20063 ★ University of Memphis**
**Department of Counseling, Educational Psychology and Research**
**Rehabilitation Counseling Program**
Ball Education Bldg., Rm. 100
Memphis, TN 38152
**Phone:** (901)678-2841    **Fax:** (901)678-4778
**Email:** strauser.david@coe.memphis.edu
**Website:** http://www.people.memphis.edu/~coe_cepr/rehab.htm
David Strauser, Contact

**★ 20064 ★ University of Tennessee, Knoxville**
**Counseling, Deafness and Human Services**
**Rehabilitation Counseling Program**
133 Claxton Education Addition
Knoxville, TN 37996-3400
**Phone:** (423)974-2321    **Fax:** (423)974-8674
**Email:** askinner@utk.edu
**Website:** http://www.coe.utk.edu/units/rdhs.html
Amy Skinner, PhD, Contact

### Texas

**★ 20065 ★ Stephen F. Austin State University**
**Department of Counseling and Special Education Programs**
**Rehabilitation Counseling Program**
PO Box 13019, SFA Sta.
Nacogdoches, TX 75962
**Phone:** (409)468-2906    **Fax:** (409)468-5837
**Email:** rchoate@sfasu.edu
**Website:** http://www.education.sfasu.edu/csped/rehabcn.htm
Robert Choate, EdD, Director

**★ 20066 ★ University of North Texas**
**Department of Rehabilitation, Social Work and Addictions**
**Rehabilitation Counseling Program**
PO Box 310919
Denton, TX 76203-0919
**Phone:** (940)565-2488    **Fax:** (940)565-3960
**Email:** pleung@scs.cmm.unt.edu
**Website:** http://www.scs.unt.edu/depts/rswa/msrhab.htm
Paul Leung, PhD, Contact

**★ 20067 ★ University of Texas**
**Southwestern Medical Center at Dallas**
**Department of Rehabilitation Science**
**Rehabilitation Counseling Program**
5323 Harry Hines Blvd.
Dallas, TX 75235-9088
**Phone:** (214)648-1740    **Fax:** (214)648-1771
**Email:** dpool@mednet.swmed.edu
**Website:** http://www.swmed.edu/home_pages/publish/ahs_catalog/rehab.html
Donald A. Pool, PhD, Contact

**★ 20068 ★ University of Texas, Austin**
**Rehabilitation Counselor Education**
**Rehabilitation Counseling Program**
Special Education, D5300
Austin, TX 78712
**Phone:** (512)471-4161    **Fax:** (512)471-4061
**Email:** r.parker@mail.utexas.edu
**Website:** http://www.edb.utexas.edu/coe/depts/sped/Rehab/homepage.html
Randall M. Parker, PhD, Director

**★ 20069 ★ University of Texas, Pan American**
**College of Health Sciences and Human Services**
**Rehabilitative Services Program**
1201 W University Dr.
Edinburg, TX 78539-2999
**Phone:** (956)316-7036    **Fax:** (956)384-5237
**Email:** bjreed@panam.edu
Bruce Reed, PhD, Contact

### Utah

**★ 20070 ★ Utah State University**
**Department of Special Education and Rehabilitation**
**Rehabilitation Counseling Program**
2865 Old Main Hill
Logan, UT 84322-2865
**Phone:** (435)797-3243    **Fax:** (435)797-3572
**Email:** garthe@coe.usu.edu
**Website:** http://www.rce.usu.edu/
Garth M. Eldredge, PhD, Contact

## Virginia

★ **20071** ★ **Virginia Commonwealth University**
**Medical College of Virginia**
**Department of Rehabilitation Counseling**
1121 E Clay St.
McGuire Hall, Rm. 218
PO Box 980330
Richmond, VA 23298-0330
**Phone:** (804)828-1132 **Fax:** (804)828-1321
**Email:** bmcbull@vcu.edu
**Website:** http://views.vcu.edu/sahp/rehab/
Brian T. McMahon, PhD, Contact

## Washington

★ **20072** ★ **Western Washington University**
**Center for Continuing Education in Rehabilitation**
**Rehabilitation Counseling Program**
6912 220th St. SW, Ste. 105
Mountlake Terrace, WA 98043
**Phone:** (425)774-4446 **Free:** 888-377-0100
**Fax:** (425)774-9303
**Email:** geri.hansen@wwu.edu
Geraldine Hansen, EdD, Director

## West Virginia

★ **20073** ★ **West Virginia University**
**Department of Counseling, Rehabilitation Counseling and Counseling Psychology**
**Rehabilitation Counseling Program**
PO Box 6122
502 Allen Hall
Morgantown, WV 26506-6122
**Phone:** (304)293-3807 **Fax:** (304)293-4082
**Email:** mglenn@wvu.edu
**Website:** http://www.wvu.edu/~hre/
Margaret Glenn, EdD, Contact

## Wisconsin

★ **20074** ★ **University of Wisconsin, Madison**
**Department of Rehabilitation Psychology and Special Education**
**Rehabilitation Counseling Program**
432 N Murray St.
Madison, WI 53706-1496
**Phone:** (608)263-5860 **Fax:** (608)262-8108
**Email:** rlynch@education.wisc.edu
**Website:** http://www.soemadison.wisc.edu/rpse/
Ruth Torkelson Lynch, PhD, Contact

★ **20075** ★ **University of Wisconsin, Milwaukee**
**Department of Educational Psychology**
**Rehabilitation Counseling Program**
773 Enderis Hall
PO Box 53201
Milwaukee, WI 53201
**Phone:** (414)229-4767 **Fax:** (414)229-4939
**Website:** http://www.uwm.edu/Dept/EdPsych/msinf.html
Douglas J. Mickelson, Contact

★ **20076** ★ **University of Wisconsin, Stout**
**Department of Rehabilitation and Counseling**
**Rehabilitation Counseling Program**
214 10th Ave., Rm. 405
Menomonie, WI 54751
**Phone:** (715)232-2499 **Fax:** (715)232-2356
**Email:** stewarts@uwstout.edu
**Website:** http://www.uwstout.edu/programs/bsvr/
Shirley Stewart, Contact

# National & International Organizations

★ **20077** ★ **American Academy of Physical Medicine and Rehabilitation (AAPM&R)**
1 IBM Plz., Ste. 2500
Chicago, IL 60611-3604
**Phone:** (312)464-9700 **Fax:** (312)464-0227
**Email:** info@aapmr.org
**Website:** http://www.aapmr.org
Ronald A. Henrichs, CAE, Exec. Dir.
**Fnded:** 1938. **Mem:** 6,300. **Desc:** National medical specialty society of physical medicine and rehabilitation physicians whose patients include people with physical disabilities and chronic, disabling illnesses. Mission is to maximize quality of life, minimize the incidence and prevalence of impairments, disability, and handicaps, promote societal health, and enhance the understanding and development of psychiatry. Offers educational opportunities and advocacy support to members and provides information, referrals, and patient education materials. **Pub:** *AAPM&R Membership Directory*, annual. Membership Directory. Arranged alphabetically, geographically, and by special interest group. *Price:* Included in membership dues. • *Archives of Physical Medicine and Rehabilitation*, monthly. Journal. Provides original research and clinical reports to health professionals who work with the disabled, elderly, and handicapped. *Price:* Included in membership dues; $159/year for nonmembers; $200/year for institutions; $72/year for students. • *The Physiatrist*, 10/year. Newsletter. Provides information on organizational activities, legislative and practice issues. Includes research updates, calendar, and quarterly inserts. *Price:* Included in membership dues. • *Study Guide*. Published part of Self-Directed Medical Knowledge Program. **Frmly:** (1956) American Society of Physical Medicine and Rehabilitation.

★ **20078** ★ **American Association for Therapeutic Humor (AATH)**
4534 W Butler Dr.
Glendale, AZ 85302
**Phone:** (623)934-6068 **Fax:** (623)934-5902
**Email:** office@aath.org
**Website:** http://www.aath.org
April Becerra, Exec. Dir.
**Fnded:** 1987. **Mem:** 500. **Desc:** Health care providers, clergy, and educators; other interested individuals. Promotes the use of humor as a therapeutic technique; disseminates public information about laughter and humor; offers networking service to further understanding of therapeutic humor; conducts research programs that incorporate therapeutic uses of humor. Maintains speakers' bureau. **Pub:** *Laugh It Up*, quarterly. Newsletter. • *Laugh It Update*, bimonthly. Monograph. • Bibliographies. • Also makes available tapes.

★ **20079** ★ **American Board of Physical Medicine and Rehabilitation (ABPMR)**
Norwest Center, Ste. 674
21 1st St. SW
Rochester, MN 55902-3092
**Phone:** (507)282-1776 **Fax:** (507)282-9242
**Email:** info@abpmr.org
**Website:** http://www.abpmr.org/
Nicholas E. Walsh, MD, Chair
**Fnded:** 1947. **Mem:** 6,515. **Desc:** Certification board to establish qualifications, conduct examinations, and certify physicians who have completed the requirements in physical medicine and rehabilitation. **Pub:** Booklet, annual. *Price:* Free.

★ **20080** ★ **American Center for the Alexander Technique (ACAT)**
39 W 14th St. No. 507
New York, NY 10011
**Phone:** (212)633-2229

**Email:** acatusa@aol.com
**Website:** http://www.acatnyc.org
Jane Tomkiewicz, Exec. Dir.
**Fnded:** 1964. **Mem:** 80. **Desc:** Promotes the Alexander Technique, an educational technique that enables individuals to use their bodies with ease, grace, flexibility, and freedom from strain in any physical activity. Formed to assure further development of the technique in this country and to maintain its standards. Answers requests for information and refers interested people to certified teachers. Sponsors Teacher Certification Program consisting of 1600 hours over nine ten-week terms, the last a teaching apprenticeship, to certify students who have demonstrated, to the satisfaction of the faculty, a high standard both of teaching skills and of personal use. **Pub:** *ACAT News*, periodic. Newsletter. • *Annual Certified Member/Teacher List*.

★ **20081** ★ **American Congress of Rehabilitation Medicine (ACRM)**
6801 Lake Plz. Dr., No. B-205
Indianapolis, IN 46220-4049
**Phone:** (317)915-2250 **Fax:** (317)915-2245
**Email:** acrm@acrm.org
**Website:** http://www.acrm.org
Ric Morgan, MBA, Exec. Dir.
**Fnded:** 1923. **Mem:** 1,100. **Desc:** Physicians, nurses, physical therapists, psychologists, occupational therapists, social workers, speech/language pathologists, and other allied health specialists active in and contributing to advancement in the field of medical rehabilitation. **Pub:** *ACRM Membership Directory*, annual. Membership Directory. • *Archives of Physical Medicine and Rehabilitation*, monthly. Journal. • *Rehabilitation Outlook*, quarterly. Newsletter. **Frmly:** American Congress of Physical Medicine; American Congress of Physical Medicine and Rehabilitation.

**American Fracture Association (AFA)**
*See:* Entry 16994

★ **20082** ★ **American Horticultural Therapy Association (AHTA)**
909 York St.
Denver, CO 80206
**Phone:** (303)370-8087 **Free:** 800-634-1603
**Fax:** (303)331-5776
**Email:** ahtaadmin@earthlink.net
**Website:** http://www.ahta.org
Stephanie Shulman, Contact
**Fnded:** 1973. **Mem:** 800. **Reg. Groups:** 13. **Desc:** Professional horticultural therapists and rehabilitation specialists; horticultural therapy students; institutions and commercial organizations. Promotes and encourages the development of horticulture and related activities as a therapeutic and rehabilitative medium. Coordinates efforts of professional and educational organizations and conducts regional workshops and seminars. Provides resource information; offers papers at various conferences. Registers professional horticultural therapists. **Pub:** *AHTA Annual Membership Directory*, annual. Membership Directory. *Price:* $15 for members; $25 for nonmembers. • *Journal of Therapeutic Horticulture*, annual. Journal. Contains research and programmatic articles. *Price:* $15; $15 for members; $25 for nonmembers. • *Newsletter American Horticultural Therapy Association*, biennial. Newsletter. Includes association news, program features, horticultural therapy activities, and member profiles. *Price:* $35/year; $3/issue.

★ **20083** ★ **American Israeli Lighthouse (AIL)**
276 5th Ave, Rm. 713
New York, NY 10001-4509
**Phone:** (212)838-5322
Mrs. Leonard F. Dank, Pres.
**Fnded:** 1927. **Mem:** 1,500. **State Groups:** 8. **Local Groups:** 7. **Desc:** Works to raise funds for the maintenance of a rehabilitation center in Kiriat Haim, Israel for adult blind and physically handicapped persons. Promotes research in the development of

techniques in education, vocational training, and rehabilitation. **Pub:** *The Tower*, annual.

★ **20084** ★ **American Kinesiotherapy Association (AKTA)**
One IBM Plaza, Ste. 2500
2801 W Bancroft St.
Chicago, IL 60611-3604
**Free:** 800-296-AKTA          **Fax:** (312)464-0227
**Email:** ccbkt@aol.com
**Website:** http://www.akta.org
Michael Westmoreland, Pres.

**Fnded:** 1946. **Mem:** 450. **Reg. Groups:** 7. **State Groups:** 50. **Desc:** Professional society of kinesiotherapists, and associate and student members with interest in physical and mental rehabilitation and adapted physical education. (Kinesiology is the study of human movement; kinesiotherapists use kinesiology to design and implement therapeutic exercise to meet the rehabilitative needs of persons with disease, injury, and/or physical disorders.) Goal is to promote the profession of kinseotherapy by working toward public recognition of kinesiotherapy and to pursue and support legislative concerns of the profession. Works to maintain and advance the standard of care through educational opportunities. **Pub:** *Career in Kinesiology*. Brochure. • *Cinical Kinesiology*, quarterly. Journal. Publishes manuscripts of professional and scientific nature in disciplines relates to kinesiotherapy. *Price:* $25 individuals; $45 library or institution. • *Mobility*, quarterly. Newsletter. • Also publishes rehabilitation brochures. **Frmly:** (1968) Association for Physical and Mental Rehabilitation; (1987) American Corrective Therapy Association.

★ **20085** ★ **American Massage Therapy Association (AMTA)**
820 Davis St., Ste. 100
Evanston, IL 60201-4444
**Phone:** (847)864-0123          **Free:** 888-843-2682
**Fax:** (847)864-1178
**Email:** info@amtamassage.org
**Website:** http://www.amtamassage.org
Ronald Precht, Communications Mgr.

**Fnded:** 1943. **Mem:** 46,000. **State Groups:** 52. **Desc:** Massage therapists and massage schools. Promotes standards for the profession, has a Code of Ethics, and supports chapter efforts for state regulation of massage. Sponsors National Massage Therapy Awareness Week to promote public education on the benefits of massage; offers educational literature. Supports research on the efficacy of massage. Offers free Find A Message Therapists National locater service to help consumers and healthcare professionals find qualified, professional massage therapists. **Pub:** *Finding A Qualified Massage Therapist*. Brochure. • *Hands On*, bimonthly. Newsletter. Features association and member news. *Price:* Free for members. • *Massage Therapy*. Brochure. • *Massage Therapy Journal*, quarterly. Journal. Contains scholarly articles on massage therapy. *Price:* $25/year in U.S.; $70/year outside U.S. • *Sports Massage*. Brochure. • *Stress*. Brochure. • Product brochure of AMTA products and publications. **Frmly:** (1983) American Massage and Therapy Association.

★ **20086** ★ **American Medical Rehabilitation Providers Association (AMRPA)**
1710 N St. NW
Washington, DC 20009
**Phone:** (202)223-1920          **Free:** 888-346-4624
**Fax:** (202)223-1925
**Email:** czollar@amrpa.org
**Website:** http://www.amrpa.org
Carolyn C. Zollar, VP for Government Relations & Policy Dev

**Fnded:** 1997. **Mem:** 300. **State Groups:** 29. **Desc:** Rehabilitation facilities in the U.S. and Canada; agencies operating established medical, residential and vocational rehabilitation facilities. Promotes expansion and improvement of rehabilitation services to disabled persons as provided in rehabilitation facilities. Repre-

sents the concerns of rehabilitation providers before Congress and government agencies. Is concerned with quality operation of rehabilitation centers and facilities. Conducts research and development programs in national rehabilitation policy. Sponsors seminars and provides specialized education programs. **Pub:** *Rehabilitation Insurance Report*, monthly. Newsletter. Analyzes insurance issues relevant to rehabilitation services. *Price:* $50/year to members; $65/year to nonmembers. • *Rehabilitation Review*, weekly. Newsletter. Monitors developments in the rehabilitation industry. Includes research updates and a calendar of events. *Price:* Included in membership dues; $125/year for nonmembers. • Books. • Monographs. • Videos. **Frmly:** (1975) International Association of Rehabilitation Facilities; (1980) Association of Rehabilitation Facilities; (1994) National Association of Rehabilitation Facilities; (1998) American Rehabilitation Association.

★ **20087** ★ **American Occupational Therapy Association (AOTA)**
4720 Montgomery Ln.
PO Box 31220
Bethesda, MD 20824-1220
**Phone:** (301)652-2682          **Free:** 800-377-8555
**Fax:** (301)652-7711
**Email:** praota@aota.org
**Website:** http://www.aota.org
Joseph C. Isaacs, Exec. Dir.

**Fnded:** 1917. **Mem:** 41,000. **Desc:** Occupational therapists and occupational therapy assistants who provide services to people whose lives have been disrupted by physical injury or illness, developmental problems, the aging process, or social or psychological difficulties. Occupational therapy focuses on the active involvement of the patient in specially designed therapeutic tasks and activities to improve function, performance capacity, and the ability to cope with demands of daily living. **Pub:** *American Journal of Occupational Therapy*, bimonthly. Journal. • *OT Practice*, biweekly. • *Publications Catalog*. Catalog. • Also publishes more than 100 single titles. **Frmly:** National Society for the Promotion of Occupational Therapy.

**American Osteopathic College of Physical Medicine and Rehabilitation (AOCPMR)**
*See:* Entry 17004

★ **20088** ★ **American Physical Therapy Association (APTA)**
1111 N Fairfax St.
Alexandria, VA 22314-1488
**Phone:** (703)684-2782          **Free:** 800-999-2782
**Fax:** (703)684-7343
**Email:** benmassey@apta.org
**Website:** http://www.apta.org
Ben F. Massey, Jr., Pres.

**Fnded:** 1921. **Mem:** 72,000. **Reg. Groups:** 52. **Desc:** Professional organization of physical therapists and physical therapist assistants and students. Fosters the development and improvement of physical therapy service, education, and research; evaluates the organization and administration of curricula; directs the maintenance of standards and promotes scientific research. Acts as an accrediting body for educational programs in physical therapy and is responsible for establishing standards. Offers advisory and consultation services to schools of physical therapy and facilities offering physical therapy services; provides placement services at conference. **Pub:** *Physical Therapy*, monthly. Journal. Features peer-reviewed scientific and professional articles, continuing education course listings, abstracts of current literature, and book reviews. *Price:* Included in membership dues; $60/year for nonmembers. • *PT Bulletin Online*, weekly. Newsletter. Includes employment listings and information on upcoming seminars. *Price:* Included in membership dues. • *PT Magazine*, monthly. Journal. Features columns on risk management and reimbursement strategies. Contains advertisers' index and information on new products and literature. *Price:* Included in membership dues; $55/year for nonmem-

bers; $7/copy. • Brochures. • Monographs. • Also issues bulletins to chapters and publishes anthologies, handbooks, and educational resource guides. **Frmly:** (1921) American Women's Physical Therapeutic Association; (1948) American Physiotherapy Association.

★ **20089** ★ **American Rehabilitation Counseling Association (ARCA)**
c/o American Counseling Association
5999 Stevenson Ave.
Alexandria, VA 22304-3300
**Phone:** (703)823-9800          **Free:** 800-545-2223
**Fax:** (703)823-0252
**Website:** http://www.nchrtm.okstate.edu/arca/
Ellen Fabian, Pres.

**Fnded:** 1958. **Mem:** 2,329. **Desc:** A division of the American Counseling Association. Rehabilitation counselors and interested professionals and students. Purpose is to improve the rehabilitation counseling profession and its services to individuals with disabilities. Promotes high standards in rehabilitation counseling, practice, research, and education. Encourages the exchange of information between rehabilitation professionals and consumer groups. Serves as liaison among members and public and private rehabilitation counselors across the country. Sponsors educational and training programs. **Pub:** *ARCA News*, quarterly. Newsletter. Provides information on the procedures and problems involved in rehabilitation counseling and special education for the disabled and the aged. *Price:* Included in membership dues. • *Rehabilitation Counseling Bulletin*, quarterly. Journal. *Price:* Included in membership dues; $18/year for nonmembers.

★ **20090** ★ **American Rehabilitation Economics Association (AREA)**
127 N Westwind Dr.
El Cajon, CA 92020-2955
**Free:** 800-317-AREA          **Fax:** (619)593-9989
**Email:** areaorg@cox.net
**Website:** http://www.a-r-e-a.org
Margy Ashby, Sec.-Treas.

**Fnded:** 1989. **Mem:** 105. **Nat'l Groups:** 1. **Desc:** Forensic specialists with expertise in evaluating the medical, vocational, and economic aspects of injury. Strives to bring recognition to the combined use of vocational rehabilitation and earnings loss assessment as a distinct discipline. Also provides a peer-exchange forum for vocational, economic, and legal experts who practice in this field. **Pub:** *The Earnings Analyst*, annual. Journal. *Price:* $25.

★ **20091** ★ **American Society for the Alexander Technique (AMSAT)**
PO Box 60008
Florence, MA 01062-0008
**Phone:** (413)584-2359          **Free:** 800-473-0620
**Fax:** (413)584-3097
**Email:** alexandertech@earthlink.net
**Website:** http://www.alexandertech.org/
Cheryl Pleskow, Office Mgr.

**Fnded:** 1987. **Mem:** 600. **Desc:** Individuals who have completed a three-year training course and have been certified by AMSAT; students currently enrolled in an approved AMSAT teacher training course. Promotes and trains teachers of the Alexander Technique. (Created by Australian actor F. M. Alexander (1863-1955), the technique employs reeducation of habitual movement patterns so the body is used efficiently with the least amount of "wear and tear.") Seeks to: promote proficiency, knowledge, and skill in the field of psycho-physical reeducation; encourage education and study in the Alexander Technique; approve the establishment and continuation of teacher training courses. Promotes communication and the interchange of skills and information between the society and other organizations of teachers in the Alexander Technique; works to achieve reciprocal memberships between such organizations. Promotes and conducts research. Compiles information regarding teacher members and members of affiliated societies and disseminates this information to the public. Maintains speakers' bureau. **Pub:** *AMSAT News*, quarterly. *Price:* $30/year. • *List of Certified Training Courses*, semiannual. • *Teaching Members List*, semiannual.

**★ 20092 ★ American Society of Hand Therapists (ASHT)**
401 N Michigan Ave.
Chicago, IL 60611-4267
**Phone:** (312)321-6866　　　**Fax:** (312)673-6670
**Email:** asht@sba.com
**Website:** http://www.asht.org
Lisa Keckich, Exec. Dir.

**Fnded:** 1977. **Mem:** 2,700. **Desc:** Registered and licensed occupational and physical therapists specializing in hand therapy and committed to excellence and professionalism in hand rehabilitation. Purposes are to promote research, publish information, improve treatment techniques, and standardize hand evaluation and care. Fosters education and communication between therapists in the U.S. and abroad. Compiles statistics; conducts research and education programs and continuing education seminars. **Pub:** *ASHT Times*, quarterly. Newsletter. *Price:* Included in membership dues. • *Journal of Hand Therapy*, quarterly. Journal. *Price:* Included in membership dues.

**American Society of Neurorehabilitation**
*See:* Entry 13924

**★ 20093 ★ American Therapeutic Recreation Association (ATRA)**
1414 Prince St., Ste. 204
Alexandria, VA 22314
**Phone:** (703)683-9420　　　**Fax:** (703)683-9431
**Email:** membership@atra-tr.org
**Website:** http://www.atra-tr.org/atra.htm
Ann D. Huston, Exec. Dir.

**Fnded:** 1984. **Mem:** 3,750. **Reg. Groups:** 25. **Desc:** Therapeutic recreation professionals and students; interested others. (Therapeutic recreation is often referred to as recreational therapy and uses treatment modalities to improve the physical, mental, and emotional functions of persons with illnesses or disabling conditions.) Promotes the use of therapeutic recreation in hospitals, mental rehabilitation centers, physical rehabilitation centers, senior citizen treatment centers, and other public health facilities. Conducts discussions on certification and legislative and regulatory concerns that affect the industry. Sponsors seminars and workshops; conducts research. **Pub:** *Annual in Therapeutic Recreation*, annual. Journal. Published in conjunction with American Association for Leisure and Recreation. *Price:* Included in membership dues. • *ATRA Newsletter*, bimonthly. Newsletter. *Price:* Included in membership dues. • *Employment Update*, monthly. Features employment and internship opportunities for therapeutic recreation professionals. *Price:* Included in membership dues. • *Evaluation of Therapeutic Recreation through Quality Assurance*. • *Risk Management in Therapeutic Recreation*.

**Arab Forum for Primary Health Care and Community Based Rehabilitation**
*See:* Entry 1937

**★ 20094 ★ Asian Confederation of Physical Therapy (ACPT)**
Indonesian Therapy Association
Jalan Puskesmas 20
Otista
Jakarta, Indonesia
**Lang(s):** English, Indonesian. **Desc:** Physical therapists and health care institutions. Seeks to advance the study, teaching, and practice of physical therapy. Serves as a clearinghouse on physical therapy; sponsors research and continuing professional development programs.

**★ 20095 ★ Asian-Pacific Federation of Therpeutic Communities (APFTC)**
Mahidol Bldg.
NGO-ANCC
Rajvithi Rd.
Bangkok 10400, Thailand
**Phone:** 66 2 2455522　　　**Fax:** 66 2 2455522
**Lang(s):** English, Thai. **Desc:** Institutions offering therapeutic services. Seeks to improve the quality and availability of therpeutic services in Asia and the Pacific. Serves as a clearinghouse on therapy and therapeutic communities; sponsors research and educational programs.

**★ 20096 ★ Asociacion para la Luch contra la Paralisis Infantil (ALPI)**
Salguero 1639
1425 Buenos Aires, Argentina
**Phone:** 54 1 841034

**Fnded:** 1943. **Desc:** Devoted to rehabilitating adults and children with motor disabilities resulting from accidents or illness, furthers research in this field, especially complex cases of disability such as brain or spinal injuries.

**★ 20097 ★ Association of Academic Physiatrists (AAP)**
1106 N Charles St., Ste. 201
Baltimore, MD 21201
**Phone:** (410)637-8300　　　**Fax:** (410)637-8399
**Email:** aap@physiatry.org
**Website:** http://www.physiatry.org
Carolyn L. Braddom, EdD, Exec. Dir.

**Fnded:** 1967. **Mem:** 1,400. **Desc:** Academic physicians practicing physical medicine and rehabilitation and certified by the American Board of Physical Medicine and Rehabilitation. Objectives are: to advance teaching and research in physical medicine and rehabilitation within the area of academic medicine; to promote the dissemination of information to future physicians planning to work in this field; to become involved in the exchange of information from other areas of medicine both in basic sciences and in the clinical areas of teaching and research. **Pub:** *American Journal of Physical Medicine and Rehabilitation*, monthly. Journal. • *Residency Program Directory*, annual. Directory. • Membership Directory, annual. • Newsletter, quarterly.

**★ 20098 ★ Association of Caribbean Occupational Therapists (ACOT)**
PO Box 8677
CSO
Kingston, Jamaica
**Phone:** (876)928-1280　　　**Fax:** (876)928-1236
**Email:** leanycam@hotmail.com

**Fnded:** 1991. **Mem:** 25. **Lang(s):** English. **Desc:** Occupational therapists. Seeks to advance the practice of occupational therapy; promotes adherence to high standards of professional conduct and ethics by members. Facilitates exchange of information among members; sponsors continuing professional development courses. **Pub:** *Association of Caribbean Occupational Therapists' Scientific Conferen ce*, biannual. Newsletter.

**★ 20099 ★ Association for Dance Movement Therapy - United Kingdom (ADMTUK)**
c/o Quaker Meeting House
Wedmore Vale
Bristol BS3 5HX, United Kingdom
**Email:** query@dmtuk.demon.co.uk
**Website:** http://www.admt.org.uk
**Fnded:** 1982. **Mem:** 200. **Lang(s):** English. **Desc:** Individuals united to promote dance movement therapy. Monitors and promotes training. Offers professional services. Organizes summer schools, workshops and seminars. **Pub:** *ADMTUK Quartly - "E-Motion"*, quarterly. Newsletter. • Articles, periodic. • Pamphlets, periodic.

**★ 20100 ★ Association of Independent Physical Therapists (Bundesverband Selbstandiger PhysiotherapeutInnen)**
Konigsallee 178A
D-44799 Bochum, Germany
**Phone:** 49 234 977450　　　**Fax:** 49 234 9774545
**Email:** ifk@ifk.de
**Website:** http://www.ifk-ev.de
**Fnded:** 1981. **Mem:** 3,400. **Lang(s):** English. **Desc:** Physical therapists in Germany. Promotes the physical therapy industry. Represents the interests of freelance physical therapists. **Pub:** *KG-Intern*, bimonthly. Magazine.

**★ 20101 ★ Association for Play Therapy**
2050 N Winery Ave., Ste. 101
Fresno, CA 93703
**Phone:** (559)252-2278　　　**Fax:** (559)252-2297
**Email:** info@a4pt.org
**Website:** http://www.a4pt.org
William M. Burns, Contact

**Fnded:** 1982. **Mem:** 3,500. **Desc:** Professionals and students involved in play therapy. Promotes interests of members. Provides books and materials at a discount to members. **Pub:** *Association for Play Therapy Newsletter*, quarterly. Newsletter. *Price:* Included in membership dues. • *International Journal of Play Therapy*, semiannual. Journal. *Price:* Included in membership dues.

**★ 20102 ★ Association of Professional Music Therapists**
26 Hamlyn Rd.
Glastonbury BA6 8HT, United Kingdom
**Phone:** 44 1458 834919　　　**Fax:** 44 1458 834919
**Email:** APMToffice@aol.com
**Website:** http://www.apmt.org.uk
**Fnded:** 1976. **Mem:** 470. **Reg. Groups:** 12. **Lang(s):** French. **Desc:** Professional music therapists and music therapy students. To fulfill the needs of qualified music therapists in Great Britain. Focuses on employment and sharing of information. Works to protect music therapists already in work and to assist in the creation of new posts. Sets standards of practice and training. **Pub:** *APMT Newsletter*, quarterly. Newsletter. • *British Journal of Music Therapy*, semiannual. Journal. • *Job List*, monthly.

**★ 20103 ★ Association for the Rehabilitation of the Brain Injured (ARBI)**
3412 Spruce Dr. SW
Calgary, AB, Canada T3C 3A4
**Phone:** (403)242-7116　　　**Fax:** (403)242-7478
**Email:** arbi@cadvision.com
**Website:** http://www.arbi.ca
**Lang(s):** English, French. **Desc:** Individuals with brain injuries and their families; health care professionals working with people with brain injuries. Seeks to improve the quality of life of people with brain injuries and their families; promotes advancement in the treatment of brain injuries. Makes available support and services to people with brain injuries and their families.

**Association of Rehabilitation Nurses (ARN)**
*See:* Entry 15668

**★ 20104 ★ Association of Rehabilitation Programs in Computer Technology (ARPCT)**
503 S York St.
Denver, CO 80209-4640
**Phone:** (303)733-2111　　　**Fax:** (303)733-2225
**Email:** stevelawrence@2111usa.com
**Website:** http://www.arpct.org
Steve Lawrence, Pres.

**Fnded:** 1978. **Mem:** 40. **Desc:** Rehabilitation training programs; business and community leaders and rehabilitation trainers are associate members. Dedicated to providing data processing as a career path for handicapped persons. Purposes are to: promote communications among the programs designed to train and place handicapped persons in the data processing field; foster and provide assistance for new projects and programs; establish standards and procedures for programs to ensure the maximum benefit for the disabled persons served. Promotes the involvement of the education and research communities. Offers professional training; compiles statistics; sponsors competitions. **Pub:** *Handbook for Implementing New Projects.* • *Viewpoint*, quarterly. Newsletter. • Membership Directory, annual. **Frmly:** (1996) Association of Rehabilitation Programs in Data Processing.

★ 20105 ★ **Australian Music Therapy Association (AMTA)**
PO Box 79
Turramurra, NSW 2074, Australia
**Phone:** 61 2 94495279          **Fax:** 61 2 99883856
**Email:** info@austmta.org
**Website:** http://www.austmta.org.au
**Fnded:** 1975. **Mem:** 450. **State Groups:** 3. **Lang(s):** English. **Desc:** Registered music therapists, students, and interested others. Promotes the theory and practice of music therapy. Offers registration accreditation of training program and in-service education for other professional groups; provides printed resources; conducts research. **Pub:** *Australian Journal of Music Therapy*, annual. Journal. Contains clinical documentation and research information. • *Bulletin*, 3/year. Newsletter. • *Network*, 3/year. Newsletter. For RMTs only.

★ 20106 ★ **Back Association of Canada (BAC)**
83 Cottingham St.
Toronto, ON, Canada M4V 1B9
**Phone:** (416)967-4670
**Fnded:** 1981. **Lang(s):** English, French. **Desc:** Back pain sufferers; health care professionals interested in the treatment of back pain. Seeks to improve the quality of life of people with back pain; promotes advancement in the diagnosis and treatment of back disorders. Serves as a clearinghouse on back pain; provides services to back pain sufferers; conducts research and educational programs.

★ 20107 ★ **Biomagnetic Therapy Association (BTA)**
PO Box 394
Lyons, CO 80540
**Phone:** (303)823-0307
**Email:** info@biomagnetic.org
**Website:** http://www.biomagnetic.org
Suzy Balliett, Contact
**Fnded:** 1995. **Mem:** 150. **Desc:** Health care professionals and other individuals with an interest in biomagnetic therapy. Biomagnetic therapy is the art and science of applying and removing magnetic fields for health benefits. Seeks to advance the study and practice of biomagnetic therapy; promotes increased use of biomagnetic therapy in the treatment of a wide variety of disorders. Serves as a clearinghouse on biomagnetic and related therapies; conducts continuing professional education programs; sponsors research. **Pub:** *Biomagnetic Therapy Association Newsletter*, quarterly. **Price:** $45/year.

★ 20108 ★ **Blue Heron Support Services Association (BHSSA)**
PO Box 4238
Barrhead, AB, Canada T7N 1A2
**Phone:** (780)674-4944          **Fax:** (780)674-6294
**Email:** bhssa@telvsplanet.net
**Website:** http://www.bhssa.com
**Lang(s):** English, French. **Desc:** Rehabilitation centers. Seeks to advance rehabilitative therapies; promotes increased availability of rehabilitation services.

Represents members' interests; conducts research and educational programs.

★ 20109 ★ **British Association of Art Therapists**
c/o Mary Ward House
5 Tavistock Pl.
London WC1H 9SN, United Kingdom
**Phone:** 44 207 3833774          **Fax:** 44 207 3875513
**Fnded:** 1964. **Desc:** Art therapists. **Pub:** *Art Therapy in Education.* Brochure. • *Code of Ethics.* • *Inscape*, semiannual. Journal. • *Register of Therapists.* • Brochure. Discusses art therapy as a profession in Great Britain.

**British Association and College of Occupational Therapists**
*See:* Entry 16765

**British Association of Occupational Therapists**
*See:* Entry 16766

★ 20110 ★ **British Society for Music Therapy**
25 Rosslyn Ave.
East Barnet
Barnet EN4 8DH, United Kingdom
**Phone:** 44 208 3688879          **Fax:** 44 208 3688879
**Email:** info@bsmt.org
**Website:** http://www.bsmt.org
**Fnded:** 1958. **Mem:** 800. **Lang(s):** English. **Desc:** Open to all interested in music therapy. Promotes the use and development of music therapy in treatment, and rehabilitation of children and adults suffering from emotional, physical or mental handicap. Holds meetings and conferences. **Pub:** *British Journal of Music Therapy*, semiannual. Journal. • *BSMT Bulletin*, 3/year. • Papers. Related to conference proceedings. • Newsletter, periodic.

★ 20111 ★ **Canadian Association of Physical Medicine and Rehabilitation (CAPM&R)**
774 Echo Dr.
Ottawa, ON, Canada K1S 5N8
**Phone:** (613)730-6245          **Fax:** (613)730-1116
**Email:** capm&r@rcpsc.edu
**Website:** http://capmr.medical.org
**Fnded:** 1962. **Mem:** 285. **Lang(s):** English, French. **Desc:** Organizes scientific retreats. **Pub:** *CAPM&R Newsletter*, 3/year. Newsletter.

**Canadian Association of Psychoanalytic Child Therapists**
*See:* Entry 5642

★ 20112 ★ **Canadian Association of Rehabilitation Professionals (CARP)**
201 Consumers Rd., Ste. 302
Toronto, ON, Canada M2J 4G8
**Phone:** (416)494-4700          **Free:** 888-876-9992
**Fax:** (416)494-9139
**Email:** info@carpnational.org
**Website:** http://www.interlog.com/~capct/
**Fnded:** 1970. **Mem:** 2,600. **Reg. Groups:** 7. **Lang(s):** English, French. **Desc:** Professional association for people working in the field of rehabilitation. Promotes excellence in rehabilitation education, training, and practice. Formulates and enforces Code of Ethics. Facilitates communication to its members and stakeholders. Responsible for professional development, promotion of the Canadian Certified Rehabilitation Counselling (CCRC), Certified Vocational Evaluator (CVE), and the granting of the Registered Rehabilitation Professional (RRP) designation to qualified members. **Pub:** *Rehab Review*, quarterly. Newsletter. • *Rehabilitation Journal*, quarterly. Journal. Two international and two Canadian publication per year. **Frmly:**

(1995) Canadian Association of Rehabilitation Personnel.

**Canadian Council on Rehabilitation and Work (CCRW) (Conseil Canadien de la Readaptation et du Travail — CCRT)**
*See:* Entry 16770

★ 20113 ★ **Canadian Occupational Therapy Foundation (COTF) (Fondation Canadienne d'Ergotherapie — FCE)**
150 Eglinton Av, Ste. 207
Toronto, ON, Canada M4P 1E8
**Phone:** (416)487-5438          **Fax:** (416)487-5407
**Email:** pat@cotfcanada.org
**Website:** http://www.cotfcanada.org
**Lang(s):** English, French. **Desc:** Occupational therapists and other health care professionals. Seeks to advance the study and practice of occupational therapy. Conducts fundraising activities; provides support and assistance to occupational therapy research programs; sponsors educational courses.

★ 20114 ★ **Canadian Orthopractic Manual Therapy Association (COMTA)**
No. 207, 11520-100 Ave.
Edmonton, AB, Canada T5K 0J7
**Phone:** (780)482-7428          **Fax:** (780)488-2463
**Email:** info@orthopractic.org
**Website:** http://orthopractic.org
**Lang(s):** English. **Desc:** Professional groups that support orthopractic philosophy, including clinical specialists, basic scientists, and educators. Works to provide the public, healthcare professionals, government and funding agencies with guidelines on the provision of safe and effective manual therapy, including mobilization and manipulation.

★ 20115 ★ **Canadian Physiotherapy Association (CPA) (Association Canadienne de Physiotherapie — ACP)**
2345 Younge St., Ste. 410
Toronto, ON, Canada M4P 2E5
**Phone:** (416)932-1888          **Free:** 800-387-8679
**Fax:** (416)932-9708
**Email:** information@physiotherapy.ca
**Website:** http://www.physiotherapy.ca
**Lang(s):** English, French. **Desc:** Physiotherapists and educational institutions. Seeks to advance the study, teaching, and practice of physiotherapy. Facilitates communication and cooperation among members; sponsors research and educational programs.

★ 20116 ★ **Canadian Play Therapy Institute (CPTI)**
11E-900 Greenbank Rd., Ste. 527
Nepean, ON, Canada K2J 4P6
**Phone:** (613)634-3125          **Fax:** (613)634-0866
**Email:** information@playtherapy.org
**Website:** http://www.playtherapy.org
**Fnded:** 1990. **Mem:** 700. **Lang(s):** English. **Desc:** Play therapists, psychologists, and others with an interest in play therapy. Promotes excellence in the practice of play therapy; seeks to advance the profession of child psychology. Facilitates exchange of information among members; sponsors research and continuing professional development programs.

**Canadian Society of Respiratory Therapists (CSRT) (Societe Canadienne des Therapeutes Respiratoires — SCTR)**
*See:* Entry 18739

**★ 20117 ★ CARF, The Rehabilitation Accreditation Commission (CARF)**
4891 E Grant Rd.
Tucson, AZ 85712
**Phone:** (520)325-1044        **Fax:** (520)318-1129
**Email:** info@carf.org
**Website:** http://www.carf.org
Brian J. Boon, Pres.

**Fnded:** 1966. **Desc:** Sponsored by rehabilitation organizations. The commission is the standard setting and accrediting authority for organizations providing rehabilitation services. Encourages development and improvement of uniformly high standards of performance for all organizations serving individuals with developmental, physical, or emotional disabilities. Surveys and accredits rehabilitation organizations; conducts research and educational activities related to standards for organizations offering programs in comprehensive inpatient rehabilitation, spinal cord injury, chronic pain management, brain injury, outpatient medical rehabilitation, work hardening, infant and early childhood development, vocational evaluation, work adjustment, occupational skill training, job placement, work services, supported employment, industry-based programs, community living, psychosocial programs, respite programs, alcoholism and other drug abuse rehabilitation programs, and community mental health programs. Accreditation Program is administered by a 53-member appointed board of trustees. **Pub:** *CARF Connection*, semiannual. Covers commission activities. *Price:* Free. • *Standards Manual for Employment Community Services*, annual. Describes accreditation standards for programs providing services to the disabled; includes glossary. *Price:* $90/year. **Frmly:** (1998) Commission on Accreditation of Rehabilitation.

**★ 20118 ★ Certification Board for Music Therapists (CBMT)**
506 E Lancaster Ave., Ste. 102
Downingtown, PA 19335
**Phone:** (610)269-8900        **Free:** 800-765-CBMT
**Fax:** (610)269-9232
**Email:** info@cbmt.com
**Website:** http://www.cbmt.com
Joy S. Schneck, Exec. Dir.

**Fnded:** 1982. **Mem:** 3,330. **Desc:** Board-certified professional music therapists. Certifies and recertifies (every 5 years) professional music therapists through examination and continuing professional education. Monitors competence and professional growth of certificants. **Pub:** *BC-Status*, semiannual. Newsletter. Includes list of new members and updates on recertification process. *Price:* Free for members. • *Candidate Handbook.* Handbook. • *Recertification Manual.* Manual. • *Recertification, Self-Growth, and You.*

**★ 20119 ★ Chartered Society of Physiotherapy (CSP)**
14 Bedford Row
London WC1R 4ED, United Kingdom
**Phone:** 44 207 3066666        **Fax:** 44 207 3066611
**Website:** http://www.csp.org.uk

**Fnded:** 1894. **Mem:** 32,000. **Desc:** The professional association, educational body and trade union of the United Kingdom's 32,000 chartered psychotherapists, physical students and assistants. Aims to protect member's interests and help them to achieve the best possible patient care. **Pub:** *Frontline*, bimonthly. • *Physiotherapy Journal*, monthly. Journal.

**Committee on Accreditation for Respiratory Care (COARC)**
*See:* Entry 18741

**Council on Chiropractic Physiological Therapeutics and Rehabilitation (CCPT)**
*See:* Entry 5925

**★ 20120 ★ Council on Rehabilitation Education (CORE)**
1835 Rohlwing Rd., Ste. E
Rolling Meadows, IL 60008
**Phone:** (847)394-1785        **Fax:** (847)394-2108
**Email:** nchrtm@okstate.edu
**Website:** http://www.core-rehab.org
Donald C. Linkowski, Exec. Dir.

**Fnded:** 1972. **Mem:** 90. **Desc:** Sponsored by the American Rehabilitation Counseling Association, Council of State Administrators of Vocational Rehabilitation, American Rehabilitation Association, National Council on Rehabilitation Education, and the National Rehabilitation Counseling Association. Promotes effective delivery of rehabilitation services to people with disabilities. Surveys, critiques, and works to improve rehabilitation educational programs at the postgraduate level; bestows recognition on programs judged effective. **Pub:** *CORE News*, annual. Lists recognized rehabilitation counselor education programs.

**★ 20121 ★ Council of State Administrators of Vocational Rehabilitation (CSAVR)**
4733 Bethesda Ave., Ste. 330
Bethesda, MD 20814
**Phone:** (301)654-8414        **Fax:** (301)654-5542
Carl Suter, Exec. Dir.

**Fnded:** 1940. **Mem:** 81. **Reg. Groups:** 10. **State Groups:** 81. **Desc:** Administrators of state vocational rehabilitation agencies. Serves as an advisory body to federal agencies and the public in the development of policies affecting rehabilitation of handicapped persons; acts as a forum for discussion on the provision of quality rehabilitation services. Compiles statistics. **Pub:** *CSAVR Memorandum*, semimonthly. • *Proceedings of Conferences*, semiannual. • *State Rehabilitation Directors*, periodic. Directory. • Manuals. • Reports.

**★ 20122 ★ Danish Occupational Therapy Association**
c/o Scandinavian Journal of Occupational Therapy
Department of Social Medicine and Rehabilitation
Umea University
S-901 87 Umea, Sweden
**Phone:** 46 90 7869272        **Fax:** 46 90 7869267

**Lang(s):** Danish. **Desc:** Occupational therapists and other health care professionals engaged in occupational medicine in Denmark. Promotes scientific inquiry in the field of occupational therapy and serves as a forum for the dissemination of research results. Areas of inquiry include: physical disability; mental health and disabilities; therapeutic equipment, environments, and techniques; assessment and evaluation of disabilities; vocational and educational training.

**★ 20123 ★ Delta Society (DS)**
289 Perimeter Rd. E
Renton, WA 98055-1329
**Phone:** (425)226-7357        **Fax:** (425)235-1076
**Email:** info@deltasociety.org
**Website:** http://www.deltasociety.org
Linda M. Hines, Pres. /CEO

**Fnded:** 1977. **Mem:** 6,000. **Desc:** Doctors, nurses, veterinarians, therapists, nursing home personnel, animal trainers and breeders, pet owners, academicians, and students of gerontology, psychology, therapeutic recreation, and other health fields. Assesses the role of animal companions in society and the effect of human-animal interaction on the mental and physical well-being of people. Seeks to establish an interdisciplinary approach to studying human-animal interactions, and to increase awareness of these interactions among health and social care professionals. Provides training to for persons seeking to establish and maintain programs that involve animals in animal-assisted activities/therapy. Operates National Service Dog Center serving people with disabilities in conjunction with the American Humane Association; and Pet Partners, a national registration for volunteers and animals involved in programs. Creating Service Dog

Education System to train trainers of service dogs. Distributes information on research, programs, and legislation concerning human-animal relationships. Maintains collection of article reprints. **Pub:** *Alert*, bimonthly. Newsletter. • *InterActions*, quarterly. Magazine. • *Pet Partners Newsletter*, bimonthly. Newsletter. Includes practical information for volunteers in animal-assisted activities and therapy programs. • Journal.

**★ 20124 ★ Finnish Occupational Therapy Association**
c/o Scandinavian Journal of Occupational Therapy
Department of Social Medicine and yRehabilitation
Umea University
S-901 87 Umea, Sweden
**Phone:** 46 90 7869272        **Fax:** 46 90 7869267

**Lang(s):** Finnish. **Desc:** Occupational therapists and other health care professionals engaged in occupational medicine in Finland. Promotes scientific inquiry in the field of occupational therapy and serves as a forum for the dissemination of research results. Areas of inquiry include: physical disability; mental health and disabilities; therapeutic equipment, environments, and techniques; assessment and evaluation of disabilities; vocational and educational training.

**★ 20125 ★ Foundation for Physical Therapy (FPT)**
c/o American Physical Therapy Association
1111 Fairfax St.
Alexandria, VA 22314-1488
**Phone:** (703)683-6743        **Free:** 800-875-1378
**Fax:** (703)684-7343
**Email:** foundation@apta.org
**Website:** http://www.apta.org/Foundation
Christine A. Williams, Vice Pres.

**Fnded:** 1979. **Nat'l Groups:** 1. **Desc:** Supports the physical therapy profession's research needs by funding scientific and clinically-relevant physical therapy research.

**★ 20126 ★ German Association for Physiotherapy (Deutscher Verband fur Physiotherapie)**
Deutzer Freiheit 72-74
D-50679 Cologne, Germany
**Phone:** 49 221 9810270        **Fax:** 49 221 98102725
**Email:** info@zvk.org
**Website:** http://www.zvk.org

**Fnded:** 1949. **Mem:** 32,000. **Nat'l Groups:** 16. **Reg. Groups:** 15. **Lang(s):** English, French. **Desc:** Promotes physical therapy education. Maintains contacts with medical and scientific associations. Represents the interests of physical therapists. Contracts with national health organizations (HMO's). **Pub:** *Curriculum, 4 vols..* Journal. • *Krankengymnastik*, monthly. Brochure. Includes news from the Association. Provides summaries in English and French. • *Physiotherapy Profession.* Brochure. Special information brochures and sheets.

**★ 20127 ★ Hong Kong Society of Certified Prosthetist-Orthotists**
Hong Kong Polytechnic University
Hung Hom
Hong Kong, People's Republic of China
**Phone:** 852 27667676        **Fax:** 852 23624365
**Email:** rcaaron@polyu.edu.hk
**Website:** http://www.polyu.edu.hk/~hkscpo

**Fnded:** 1995. **Mem:** 90. **Lang(s):** Chinese, English. **Desc:** Individuals who have successfully completed an accredited program in prosthetics and orthotics and have passed the organization's examination. Promotes high standards of ethics and professional practice in the field of orthotics and prosthetics. Conducts continuing professional development and scientific education programs; makes available certification examinations.

**★ 20128 ★ The Hong Kong Society for Rehabilitation (HKSR)**
7 Sha Wan Dr.
Hong Kong, People's Republic of China
**Phone:** 852 28176277        **Fax:** 852 28551947
**Email:** hksr@rehabsociety.org.hk
**Website:** http://www.renet.org
**Fnded:** 1959. **Mem:** 120. **Lang(s):** Chinese, English. **Desc:** Works to restore victims of physical or visceral disability brought on by disease or injury to economic self-sufficiency. Promotes continued professional advancement by members. Conducts research, educational, and charitable programs. **Pub:** Pamphlet, periodic. • Report, periodic.

**★ 20129 ★ Icelandic Occupational Therapy Association**
c/o Scandinavian Journal of Occupational Therapy
Department of Social Medicine and Rehabilitation
Umea University
S-901 87 Umea, Sweden
**Phone:** 46 90 7869272        **Fax:** 46 90 7869267
**Lang(s):** Icelandic. **Desc:** Occupational therapists and other health care professionals engaged in occupational medicine in Iceland. Promotes scientific inquiry in the field of occupational therapy and serves as a forum for the dissemination of research results. Areas of inquiry include: physical disability; mental health and disabilities; therapeutic equipment, environments, and techniques; assessment and evaluation of disabilities; vocational and educational training.

**Infusion Nurses Society (INS)**
*See:* Entry 15719

**★ 20130 ★ International Art Therapy Association (IATA)**
**(Association Internationale - Art-Therape — AIAT)**
14 rue des Freres Morane, Espace 15
F-75015 Paris, France
**Phone:** 33 1 45545192        **Fax:** 33 1 45545192
**Email:** chris.hunt@ins1.org
**Website:** http://www.ins1.org
**Lang(s):** English, French. **Desc:** Art therapists. Seeks to advance the practice of art therapy. Promotes art therapy; conducts continuing professional development courses for members.

**International Association of Colon Therapy (I-ACT)**
*See:* Entry 9133

**★ 20131 ★ International Association of Human-Animal Interaction Organizations (IAHAIO)**
c/o Linda Hines
289 Perimeter Rd. E
Renton, WA 98055-1329
**Phone:** (425)226-7357        **Fax:** (425)235-1076
**Email:** info@deltasociety.org
**Website:** http://www.iahaio.org
Linda M. Hines, Sec. -Treas.
**Fnded:** 1990. **Mem:** 22. **Nat'l Groups:** 22. **Desc:** Provides a forum for exchange of ideas and information among organizations concerned with the study of the mutual welfare of people and animals. Encourages research and promotes educational and practical developments in the field of human-animal interactions. Hosts and international conference every three years. **Pub:** *Proceedings of International Conference*, triennial. Proceedings. Includes papers presented at international conference. • Also contributes to and distributes *Anthrozoos: Journal of the Delta Society*. **Frmly:** (1990) International Society for the Study of the Human-Companion Animal Bond.

**★ 20132 ★ International Association for Oxygen Therapy (IAOT)**
3801 Northampton St. NW, Ste. 2
Washington, DC 20012
**Phone:** (202)537-0771        **Free:** 877-367-2654
**Fax:** (202)443-4319
**Email:** info@oxytherapies.com
**Website:** http://www.oxytherapies.com
A. Ann Steiner, Contact
**Fnded:** 1898. **Mem:** 3,500. **Nat'l Groups:** 1. **Reg. Groups:** 12. **State Groups:** 24. **Local Groups:** 150. **Desc:** Oxidation therapists. Promotes the use of oxidation enhancing therapies to physicians and the general public. Compiles statistics. Conducts research, educational, and charitable programs. Maintains museum and speakers' bureau. **Pub:** *IAOT Newsletter (Oxidation News)*, quarterly. Newsletter. Features international journal of WNHO. *Price:* Free sample; included in membership dues.

**★ 20133 ★ International Association for Regression Research and Therapies (IARRT)**
PO Box 20151
Riverside, CA 92516
**Phone:** (909)784-1570        **Fax:** (909)784-8440
**Email:** info@iarrt.org
**Website:** http://www.aprt.org
Connie Brooks, Exec. Dir.
**Fnded:** 1980. **Mem:** 800. **State Groups:** 20. **Desc:** Psychiatrists, psychologists, counselors, and students; organizations and individuals interested in past-life regression therapy. Promotes past-life therapy as a means of helping individuals realize their capacity to change and improve their lives. Works for progressive application of the therapy and the establishment of clinical standards for training therapists. Acts as a communications network for the exchange of information and experiences. Disseminates information to the public about benefits of the therapy. Registers therapists. Promotes research in the field. **Pub:** *Journal of Regression Therapy*, annual. Journal. *Price:* $26/volume. • *Past Life Research and Therapies*, quarterly. Newsletter. Contains editorials, Open Forum, reviews, and calender of events. *Price:* $10/year. • Audiotapes. • Directory, periodic. • Videos. **Frmly:** Association for Past Life Research and Therapies; (1991) Association for Past-Life Research and Therapy; (2002) Association for Past-Life Research and Therapies.

**★ 20134 ★ International Association of Rehabilitation Professionals (IARP)**
3540 Soqel Ave., Ste. A
Santa Cruz, CA 95062-1769
**Free:** 800-240-9059
**Email:** gzimmermann@rehabpro.org
**Website:** http://www.rehabpro.org
Glenn Zimmermann, Exec. Dir.
**Mem:** 2,800. **Desc:** Members of the rehabilitation industry. Promotes effective interdisciplinary rehabilitation, disability management and return-to-work services for the disabled and disadvantaged. Provides continuing education and career enhancement programs for members. Works to influence government and industry policy.

**★ 20135 ★ International Association of Trichologists (IAT)**
185 Elizabeth St., Ste. 919
Sydney, NSW 2000, Australia
**Phone:** 61 2 92671384        **Fax:** 61 8 82968450
**Email:** dsalinger@ozemail.com.au
**Website:** http://www.trichology.edu.au
**Fnded:** 1973. **Mem:** 125. **Lang(s):** English. **Desc:** Individuals licensed to practice or perform manipulative, electrical, light, or cosmetic therapy upon the scalp. Promotes the study, research, and legitimate practice of the treatment and care of the human hair and scalp. Prescribes and administers course of study of trichology. Conducts testing; grants certification; offers placement service. Has established code of ethics. **Pub:** *Guide to Hair Loss*. Book. • *Picture Guide to Scalp & Hair Problems*. Book. • Newsletter, bi-monthly.

**★ 20136 ★ International Board for Regression Therapy (IBRT)**
9091 Beach Rd.
Canastota, NY 13032
**Email:** freedman@dreamscape.com
**Website:** http://www.ibrt.org
Russell Davis, PhD, Contact
**Desc:** Therapists, researchers, training programs. Provide documentation, training and certificates. Promote public awareness of regression therapy.

**★ 20137 ★ International Brain Injury Association**
c/o Stig Tomasen
Hjerneskadeforeningen
Brondby Mollevej 8
DK-2605 Brondby, Germany
**Phone:** 45 43 432433        **Fax:** 45 43 422430
**Email:** info@hjerneskadeforeningen.dk
**Website:** http://www.hjerneskadeforeningen.dk
**Fnded:** 1985. **Mem:** 1,500. **Reg. Groups:** 10. **State Groups:** 1. **Lang(s):** English. **Desc:** Supports those with brain injuries and their families in the rehabilitation process of resuming normal activities.

**★ 20138 ★ International Federation of Physical Medicine and Rehabilitation (IFPMR)**
c/o Werner Van Cleemputte
Medicongress
28-34 Waal poel
B-9960 Asseneole, Belgium
**Phone:** 32 9 3443959        **Fax:** 32 9 3444010
**Email:** isprm@medicongress.com
**Website:** http://www.isprm.org
**Fnded:** 1950. **Mem:** 40. **Lang(s):** English. **Desc:** National societies of physical medicine and rehabilitation composed of qualified physicians and surgeons, and approved by the Federation's Board of Governors. Promotes high standards in education and training and the importance of physical medicine and rehabilitation; encourages the exchange of information between medical and nonmedical workers in the field of rehabilitation. Collects and distributes data on rehabilitation; encourages contact between members. **Pub:** *Regulations and List of Members*, quadrennial. Directory. • *White Book on Education and Training*, periodic. Book.

**★ 20139 ★ International Federation of Societies for Hand Therapy**
c/o Corrianne van Velze
PO Box 846
Groenkloof
Pretoria 0027, Republic of South Africa
**Phone:** 27 12 3462700        **Fax:** 27 12 3462700
**Email:** vanvelze@afnca.com
**Website:** http://www.ifsht.org
**Fnded:** 1985. **Mem:** 26. **Desc:** Works to develop the field of hand therapy. Promotes continuing education, training and networking among members.

**★ 20140 ★ International Foundation for Stutterers (IFS)**
PO Box 462
Belle Mead, NJ 08502
**Phone:** (609)275-3806
**Website:** http://www.medhelp.org/amshc/amshc701.htm
Edward D. Riordan, Pres.
**Fnded:** 1980. **Mem:** 1,100. **Desc:** Individuals who stutter, their families, speech therapists, and other interested persons. Goal is to provide for the treatment and cure of stuttering through speech therapy in conjunction with selfhelp groups. Believes it is imperative for stutterers to reinforce techniques learned through speech therapy in an atmosphere outside of clinics and with the support of other stutterers. Establishes, maintains, and encourages formation of region-

al selfhelp groups for individuals undergoing therapy. Aims to make the public aware of the availability of professional treatment for stutterers. Conducts research to examine the causes and treatments of stuttering and to provide findings to the public. Sponsors seminars for speech therapists. Maintains speakers' bureau. **Pub:** *Look Who's Talking*, quarterly. Newsletter. *Price:* $18/year.

**★ 20141 ★ International French-Speaking Association of Paraplegic Therapy Groups (AFIGAP)**
**(Association Francophone Internationale des Groupes d'Animation de la Paraplegie — AFIGAP)**
Service de Reeducation Foutionelle
C.H.U. de Nantes
F-44093 Saint Jacques, France
**Phone:** 33 1 64422081          **Fax:** 33 1 64422082
**Fnded:** 1976. **Mem:** 180. **Reg. Groups:** 6. **Lang(s):** French. **Desc:** Doctors, nurses, physical therapists, occupational therapists, social workers, and others who have an interest in the treatment and rehabilitation of paraplegics. Purpose is to study and develop all means of advancing the knowledge and treatment of paraplegia. Provides for the exchange of information, publications, and research. Organizes professional training for nurses, physiotherapists, and occupational therapists. **Pub:** *Annuales de Medecine de Reeducation, Readaptation, et Medecin Physique*, periodic. • *Congress Proceedings*, annual. • *Early Treatment of Paraplegia*. Book. • Brochures, periodic.

**★ 20142 ★ International Massage Association (IMA)**
PO Drawer 421
Warrenton, VA 20188
**Phone:** (540)351-0800          **Free:** 800-933-7113
**Fax:** (540)351-0816
**Email:** massage@his.com
**Website:** http://www.imagroup.com
Will Green, Pres.
**Fnded:** 1994. **Mem:** 41,000. **Desc:** Professional massage practitioners and massage schools. Promotes unification of massage practitioners, regardless of technique or training. Provides services to members including credit card merchant accounts, industry discounts, personal business assistance and free internet advertising. Makes available professional insurance policies and health care plan to members. **Pub:** *IMA Success*. Newsletter.

**★ 20143 ★ International Phototherapy Association (IPA)**
c/o Judy Weiser
PhotoTherapy Centre
1300 Richards St., Ste. 205
Vancouver, BC, Canada V6B 3G6
**Phone:** (604)689-9709     **Fax:** (604)633-1505
**Email:** jweiser@istar.ca
**Website:** http://www.phototherapy-centre.com
**Fnded:** 1981. **Mem:** 225. **Lang(s):** English. **Desc:** Art therapists, psychologists, social workers, psychiatric nurses, other human service professionals (150), and students (75) in 9 countries. Fosters the development and use of still photographs, films, videotapes, discs, and holography in human service interventions including mental health and social welfare services. Seeks to: increase the effectiveness of phototherapy through research and practice; train and supervise students and professionals in behavioral and psychological phototherapy. Conducts training workshops. **Pub:** Booklets, annual.

**★ 20144 ★ International Union of Therapeutics**
**(Union Therapeutique Internationale)**
c/o Prof. A. Pradalier
Hopital Universitaire Louis Mourier
178, rue des Renouillers
F-92701 Colombes Cedex, France
**Phone:** 33 47 606705       **Fax:** 33 47 606072

**Email:** secretariat.medecine4@lmr.ap-hop-paris.fr
**Fnded:** 1934. **Mem:** 350. **Lang(s):** English, French. **Desc:** International organizations in 22 countries interested in the development of therapeutics. Conducts training, research, and exchange programs. **Pub:** *Abstracts or Communications' Book of the Congress*, biennial.

**Israeli Association of Creative and Expressive Therapies (ICET)**
*See:* Entry 4290

**★ 20145 ★ Latin American Vocational Rehabilitation Group (GLARP)**
**(Grupo Latinoamericano de Rehabilitacion Profesional — GLARP)**
Carerra 9 No. 93
Zona Postal 8
Bogota, Colombia
**Phone:** 57 1 2183015          **Fax:** 57 1 6184196
**Email:** glarp@cable.net.co
**Website:** http://www.yahat.org
**Fnded:** 1977. **Mem:** 110. **Nat'l Groups:** 78. **Lang(s):** English, French, Portuguese, Spanish. **Desc:** Private institutions in 18 countries offering professional rehabilitation services. Promotes vocational rehabilitation and adjunctive professions throughout Latin America; encourages the growth of member groups. Coordinates projects in the interest of members, including courses, seminars, and consulting sessions; offers scholarships. Sponsors research and educational programs. Works in conjunction with Centro de Documentation e Informacion en Rehabilitacion.

**★ 20146 ★ National Association of Multicultural Rehabilitation Concerns (NAMRC)**
c/o National Rehabilitation Association
633 S Washington St.
Alexandria, VA 22314
**Phone:** (703)836-0850          **Fax:** (703)836-0848
**Email:** info@nationalrehab.org
**Website:** http://www.nationalrehab.org/website/divs/namrc.html
**Desc:** Rehabilitation professionals, human services providers, educators, researchers, students, and other individuals with an interest in rehabilitation and people with disabilities. Promotes increased awareness of the barriers created by cultural insensitivity; seeks to ensure availability and quality of rehabilitation services to people of all cultural and ethnic backgrounds. Conducts continuing education courses and certification programs for rehabilitation professionals; supports legislation that encourages multiculturalism in American society and benefits people with disabilities. **Pub:** *Cultural Network Newsletter*, periodic. Newsletter.

**National Association of Nurse Massage Therapists (NANMT)**
*See:* Entry 15732

**★ 20147 ★ National Association of Rehabilitation Instructors (NARI)**
c/o Nancy Marie-Luce
2939 Johnson Rd. SW
Huntsville, AL 35805-5844
**Free:** 800-671-6837          **Fax:** (205)533-1464
**Email:** simpson@nebi.com
**Website:** http://members.aol.com/nanmt1/about.html
Julie Brock, Contact
**Mem:** 87. **State Groups:** 50. **Desc:** Objective is to promote rehabilitation of all persons with disabilities. Acts as a medium through which rehabilitation instructors can coordinate their efforts with other instructors, facilities, workshops, individuals, and organizations serving persons with disabilities. Conducts training workshops at the state level. **Pub:** *NARI Newsletter*, 3/year. Bulletin.

**★ 20148 ★ National Association of Rehabilitation Professionals in the Private Sector (NARPPS)**
783 Rio DelMar Blvd., Ste. 61
Aptos, CA 95003
**Phone:** (831)662-0310          **Free:** 800-240-9059
**Fax:** (831)662-8487
**Email:** gzimmermann@rehabpro.org
**Website:** http://www.rehabpro.com
Glenn Zimmermann, Exec. Dir.
**Fnded:** 1977. **Mem:** 3,300. **State Groups:** 36. **Desc:** Private rehabilitation companies, insurance companies, rehabilitation nurses, and rehabilitation professionals in the private sector. Seeks to promote the field of private rehabilitation and to provide for information exchange on rehabilitation issues and techniques. **Pub:** *NARPPS Journal*, quarterly. Journal. Includes book reviews and case studies. *Price:* Included in membership dues; $60/year for nonmembers; $35/year for libraries and schools. • *NARPPS National Directory*, annual. Directory. Contains membership listings by state; includes member name and advertisers indexes. *Price:* Included in membership dues; $50/copy for nonmembers. • *Rehabilitation Professional*, bimonthly. Newsletter.

**★ 20149 ★ National Association of Rehabilitation Providers and Agencies**
11250 Roger Bacon Dr., Ste. 8
Reston, VA 20190-5202
**Phone:** (703)437-4377          **Fax:** (703)435-4390
**Email:** nara@naranet.org
**Website:** http://www.naranet.org
Rick Guggolz, Exec. Dir.
**Fnded:** 1978. **Mem:** 100. **Desc:** Members are rehabilitation companies servicing patients (including Medicare recipients) with physical therapy, occupational therapy and speech pathology services in outpatient and long-term care settings. Associate members are rehabilitation vendors. **Pub:** *NARA News*, quarterly. Newsletter. Provides legislative news for rehabilitation companies; contains articles on Medicare, business management, etc.

**★ 20150 ★ National Association of Rehabilitation Support Staff (NARSS)**
c/o National Rehabilitation Association
633 S Washington St.
Alexandria, VA 22314
**Phone:** (703)836-0850          **Fax:** (703)836-0848
**Email:** info@nationalrehab.org
**Website:** http://www.nationalrehab.org/website/divs/narss.html
**Desc:** Office support staff in a rehabilitation setting. Promotes professional advancement of members; seeks to insure more effective rehabilitation services for people with disabilities. Conducts advocacy activities on behalf of people with disabilities; sponsors training courses for rehabiltation support staff; provides support and services to organizations representing people with disabilities. **Pub:** *NARSS Newsletter*, periodic. Newsletter.

**★ 20151 ★ National Association of Service Providers in Private Rehabilitation (NASPPR)**
c/o National Rehabilitation Association
633 S Washington St.
Alexandria, VA 22314
**Phone:** (703)836-0850          **Fax:** (703)836-0848
**Email:** info@nationalrehab.org
**Website:** http://www.nationalrehab.org/website/divs/nasppr.html
**Desc:** Rehabilitation nurses and counselors, physical therapists, job placement professionals, and other individuals with an interest in the rehabilitation and employment of people with disabilities. Seeks to improve practice and outcomes in both the medical and placement phases of the rehabilitation process. Serves as a forum for the exchange of information among rehabilitation professionals; facilitates coopera-

tion among members; sponsors educational and training programs.

★ **20152** ★ **National Board for Certification in Occupational Therapy (NBCOT)**
800 S Frederick Ave., Ste. 200
Gaithersburg, MD 20877-4150
**Phone:** (301)990-7979   **Fax:** (301)869-8492
**Email:** webmaster@nbcot.org
**Website:** http://www.nbcot.org
Maria Reed, Exec. Dir.

**Fnded:** 1986. **Desc:** Participants are occupational therapists and occupational therapy assistants. Administers certification program and maintains certification records of certificants; operates disciplinary mechanisms. **Pub:** *Report to the Profession*, 2/yr. Newsletters. • Brochures. • Reports. **Frmly:** (1996) AOTCB; (1998) American Occupational Therapy Certification Board.

**National Board for Respiratory Care (NBRC)**
*See:* Entry 18752

★ **20153** ★ **National Center for Therapeutic Riding (NCTR)**
PO Box 434
Burtonsville, MD 20866
**Phone:** (301)421-0380   **Fax:** (301)421-0384
**Email:** nctriding@aol.com
**Website:** http://www.nctrriding.org
Robyn Douglas-Watts, Exec. Dir.

**Fnded:** 1973. **Desc:** Nonprofit center that provides specialized horseback riding lessons to students with disabilities and other individuals from the Washington, DC area. Using the horse as a motivator, classes focus on teaching techniques for the physically handicapped, emotionally disturbed, learning disabled, or mentally retarded person. **Pub:** *NCTR Horsemanship Manual*. Manual. **Frmly:** (1980) Rock Creek Park Horse Centre.

★ **20154** ★ **National Council on Rehabilitation Education (NCRE)**
c/o Dr. Garth Eldredge
Utah State University
Department of Special Education and
Rehabilitation
Logan, UT 84322-2870
**Phone:** (435)797-3241   **Fax:** (435)797-3572
**Email:** garth@coe.usu.edu
**Website:**   http://www.nchrtm.okstate.edu/ncre/ncre.html
Dr. Garth Eldredge, Admin. Sec.

**Fnded:** 1961. **Mem:** 540. **Desc:** Academic institutions and organizations; professional educators, researchers, and students. Goals are to: assist in the documentation of the effect of education in improving services to persons with disability; determine the skills and training necessary for effective rehabilitation services; develop role models, standards, and uniform licensure and certification requirements for rehabilitation personnel; interact with consumers and public and private sector policy makers. Disseminates information and provides forum for discussion. Sponsors specialized education and placement service. Compiles statistics. Works closely with agencies and associations serving persons with disabilities. **Pub:** *NCRE Newsletter*, quarterly. Newsletter. • *Rehabilitation Education*, quarterly. Journal. *Price:* $90/year for institutions. • Membership Directory, annual. *Price:* $25. • Monographs. • Report, quarterly. **Frmly:** (1976) Council of Rehabilitation Counselor Educators.

★ **20155** ★ **National Council for Therapeutic Recreation Certification (NCTRC)**
7 Elmwood Dr.
New City, NY 10956
**Phone:** (845)639-1439   **Fax:** (845)639-1471

**Email:** nctrc@nctrc.org
**Website:** http://www.nctrc.org
Peg Connolly, PhD, Exec. Dir.

**Fnded:** 1981. **Mem:** 17,170. **Desc:** Objectives are to: establish standards for certification and recertification of individuals who work in the therapeutic recreation field; grant recognition to individuals who voluntarily apply and meet established standards; monitor adherence to standards by certified personnel. **Pub:** *National Council for Therapeutic Recreation Certification: Certification Standards*. Book. • *NCTRC Newsletter*, semiannual. Newsletter.

★ **20156** ★ **National Rehabilitation Administration Association (NRAA)**
c/o National Rehabilitation Association
633 S Washington St.
Alexandria, VA 22314
**Phone:** (703)836-0850   **Fax:** (703)836-0848
**Email:** info@nationalrehab.org
**Website:** http://www.nationalrehab.org

**Desc:** Nonprofit rehabilitation instructors, state agency vocational rehabilitation instructors, and private instructors. Promotes continuing professional development of members. Conducts professional training sessions. **Pub:** *Journal of Rehabilitation Administration*, periodic. Journal. • *NRAA Newsletter*, periodic. Newsletter.

★ **20157** ★ **National Rehabilitation Association (NRA)**
633 S Washington St.
Alexandria, VA 22314
**Phone:** (703)836-0850   **Fax:** (703)836-0848
**Email:** info@nationalrehab.org
**Website:**   http://www.nationalrehab.org/website/index.html

**Fnded:** 1925. **Mem:** 11,000. **Nat'l Groups:** 9. **Reg. Groups:** 7. **State Groups:** 52. **Desc:** Mission is providing opportunities through knowledge and diversity for professionals in the fields of rehabilitation of people with disabilities. **Pub:** *Contemporary Rehab Magazine*, 8/year. Magazine. Includes calendar of events, listing of employment opportunities, chapter news, human interest stories, and practice information. *Price:* Included in membership dues. • *Journal of Rehabilitation*, quarterly. Journal. Includes articles on rehabilitation research and new technology. Also includes book reviews and annual index. *Price:* Included in membership dues; $65/year for nonmembers. • *Report of the Annual Mary E. Switzer Memorial Seminar*. Monographs. *Price:* $15/monograph.

★ **20158** ★ **National Rehabilitation Counseling Association (NRCA)**
8807 Sudley Rd., Ste. 102
Manassas, VA 20110-4719
**Phone:** (703)361-2077   **Fax:** (703)361-2489
**Email:** nrcaoffice@aol.com
**Website:** http://nrca-net.org/
Dr. Betty Hedgeman, Admin.

**Fnded:** 1958. **Mem:** 2,500. **Desc:** A division of the National Rehabilitation Association. Professional and student rehabilitation counselors. Works to expand the role of counselors in the rehabilitation process and seeks to advance members' professional development. Supports legislation favoring the profession. **Pub:** *Journal of Applied Rehabilitation Counseling*, quarterly. Journal. Includes research information and literature and book reviews. *Price:* Included in membership dues; $15 for nonmembers; $30 for institutions. • *With One Voice*, quarterly. Newsletter. Membership activities newsletter; includes legislative news and listing of employment opportunities. *Price:* Included in membership dues.

★ **20159** ★ **National Rehabilitation Information Center (NARIC)**
4200 Forbes Blvd., Ste. 202
Lanham, MD 20706
**Phone:** (301)459-5900   **Free:** 800-346-2742
**Fax:** (301)459-5900

**Email:** naricinfo@heitechservices.com
**Website:** http://www.naric.com
Mark X. Odum, Dir.

**Fnded:** 1977. **Desc:** Purpose is to improve delivery of information to the rehabilitation community. Disseminates the findings of programs funded by the National Institute on Disability and Rehabilitation Research; prepares custom bibliographies; helps locate answers to reference questions; searches for relevant materials in other commercially available databases. **Pub:** *Compendium of Products by NIDRR Grantees and Contractors*, annual. Directory. *Price:* $5. • *NIDRR Program Directory*, annual. *Price:* $5. • *REHABDATA Thesaurus*. *Price:* $25.

★ **20160** ★ **National Therapeutic Recreation Society (NTRS)**
22377 Belmont Ridge Rd.
Ashburn, VA 20148-4501
**Phone:** (703)858-0784   **Free:** 800-626-6772
**Fax:** (703)858-0794
**Email:** ntrsnrpa@aol.com
**Website:** http://www.nrpa.org/branches/ntrs.htm
Rikki S. Epstein, Exec. Dir.

**Fnded:** 1966. **Mem:** 2,000. **Desc:** Professionals, educators, and students involved in the provision of therapeutic recreation services for persons with disabilities in clinical and residential facilities and in the community. Offers technical assistance services to agencies, institutions, and individuals. **Pub:** *Management of Therapeutic Recreation Services*. • *NTRS Report*, quarterly. Newsletter. *Price:* Included in membership dues. • *Parks and Recreation*, monthly. Magazine. *Price:* Included in membership dues. • *Philosophy of Therapeutic Recreation: Ideas and Issues*. • *Preparing for a Career in Therapeutic Recreation*.

★ **20161** ★ **Neuro-developmental Treatment Association (NDTA)**
1540 S Coast Hwy., Ste. 203
Laguna Beach, CA 92651
**Free:** 800-869-9295   **Fax:** (949)376-3456
**Email:** membership@ndta.org
**Website:** http://www.ndta.org
Howard Adler, Principal Dir.

**Fnded:** 1967. **Mem:** 3,800. **Reg. Groups:** 14. **Desc:** Physical and occupational therapists, speech pathologists, special educators, physicians, parents, and others interested in neurodevelopmental treatment. (NDT is a form of therapy for individuals who suffer from central nervous system disorders resulting in abnormal movement. Treatment attempts to initiate or refine normal stages and processes in the development of movement.) Informs members of new developments in the field and with ideas that will eventually improve fundamental independence. Locates articles related to NDT. Regional groups maintain libraries. **Pub:** *NDTA Network*, bimonthly. Newsletter. *Price:* for members. **Frmly:** International Bobath Alumni Association.

★ **20162** ★ **New Zealand Society for Music Therapy (NZSMT)**
47 The Crows Nest
Whitby
Porirua 6006, New Zealand
**Phone:** 64 4 2347192   **Fax:** 64 4 2347191
**Email:** lewishome@xtra.w.nz
**Website:** http://www.nzsme.org.nz/therapy.html

**Fnded:** 1974. **Mem:** 150. **Reg. Groups:** 4. **Local Groups:** 4. **Lang(s):** English. **Desc:** Music therapy professionals. Promotes the therapeutic use of music as an educational tool for the intellectually and physically disabled, rehabilitation patients, and special education students. Initiates discussions with government departments concerning professional training courses and job establishment for music therapists. Encourages hospitals and community groups to consider employment of music therapists. Offers training courses; local branches conduct workshops and provide speakers. **Pub:** *Journal*, annual. Journal. • *MusT*, periodic. Newsletter.

**★ 20163 ★ North American Hyperthermia Society**
820 Jorie Blvd.
Oak Brook, IL 60523
**Phone:** (630)571-2904      **Fax:** (630)571-7837
**Website:** http://www.thermaltherapy.org
**Fnded:** 1986. **Desc:** Promotes researchers in the field of thermal therapy; seeks to advance communication between theoreticians, experimentalists, and clinical practitioners; aims to increase understanding and use of hyperthermia; disseminates research findings. **Pub:** *International Journal of Hyperthermia*, bimonthly. Journal. Features research and clinical studies and trials on hyperthermia. *Price:* $905 for institutions; $548 for institutions.

**Nursing Touch and Massage Therapy Association International (NTMTAI)**
*See:* Entry 15764

**★ 20164 ★ Orthopaedic Section, American Physical Therapy Association**
2920 E Ave. S, Ste. 200
La Crosse, WI 54601-7202
**Phone:** (608)788-3982      **Fax:** (608)788-3965
**Email:** tfred@centurytel.net
**Website:** http://www.orthopt.org
Terri A. DeFlonan, Exec. Dir.
**Fnded:** 1974. **Mem:** 13,000. **Desc:** Orthopaedic physical therapists and physical therapist assistants who belong to the American Physical Therapy Association; physical therapy educators and students. Supports the continued growth of the physical therapy profession through education and research; promotes development of a standard certification procedure for the field. Seeks to assure the quality of physical therapy curricula at both the undergraduate and postgraduate levels. Facilitates communication among orthopedic physical therapists and other health care professionals. Gathers and disseminates information on the care of musculoskeletal disorders. Provides access to a network of orthopaedic study groups. **Pub:** *Journal of Orthopaedic and Sports Physical Therapy*, monthly. Journal. • *Orthopaedic Physical Therapy Practice*, quarterly. • *Orthopaedic Section of the American Physical Therapy Association*. Newsletter. Describes orthopaedic physical therapy and what the section is all about.

**★ 20165 ★ Outpatient Intravenous Infusion Therapy Association (OPIVITA)**
401 Broadway
Tacoma, WA 98402
**Phone:** (253)627-1850      **Fax:** (253)274-0877
**Email:** opivita1@aol.com
**Website:** http://www.opivita.com/
**Desc:** Strives to educate physicians and their team members in the provision of safe and effective outpatient parenteral infusion therapy (OPAT).

**★ 20166 ★ P.R.I.D.E. Foundation - Promote Real Independence for the Disabled and Elderly (P.R.I.D.E.)**
391 Long Hill Rd.
Box 1293
Groton, CT 06340-1293
**Phone:** (860)445-1448      **Free:** 800-332-9122
**Fax:** (860)445-1448
**Email:** dresspride@aol.com
**Website:** http://members.aol.com/sewtique/pride/home.htm
Evelyn S. Kennedy, Exec. Dir.
**Fnded:** 1978. **Desc:** Provides rehabilitation assistance for the handicapped and elderly in the areas of home management, independent dressing, and personal grooming. Designs and develops special garments that will help the handicapped feel more comfortable and dress independently; designs assistive devices for use in the kitchen, bedroom, and bathroom. Provides discussion leaders for community outreach and assistance to health agencies, social service groups, and volunteer organizations. Conducts

workshops and educational forums for rehabilitation centers, educational institutions, and community agencies. Sponsored Project Pride, an in-class training program providing physically and mentally handicapped individuals with entry-level occupational skills in the sewing field. Conducts public exhibitions and demonstrations of clothing and adaptive devices. **Pub:** *Children's Fashions and Special Needs*. Paper. • *Dressing With Pride*. Book. • *Fashion and Clothing Accessibility*. Book. • *Resources and Clothing for Special Needs*. • *Scoliosis and Fashion*. Paper.

**★ 20167 ★ People-Animals-Love (PAL)**
3201 New Mexico Ave. NW, Ste. 350
Washington, DC 20016
**Phone:** (202)895-1395      **Fax:** (202)274-1995
**Email:** palemail@aol.com
**Website:** http://www.peopleanimalslove.com
Susan L. Wellman, Exec. Dir.
**Fnded:** 1981. **Desc:** Purpose is to improve the quality of life of the elderly, the widowed, and the institutionalized by providing them with visits from pets and trained volunteers. Has initiated programs in nursing homes, prisons, hospices, and hospitals. Preliminary studies suggest that: pets may positively affect a person's blood pressure and general well-being; prisoners with pets often require less disciplinary action and medical attention; pets help lessen loneliness, hopelessness, and boredom; and that animals may be used effectively to reach at-risk children. Conducts summer P.A.L. camp to acquaint urban children with animals. Also visits inner city schools with farm animal program. Conducts P.A.L. Club, an after-school program targeting at-risk youth. **Pub:** *PAL Newsletter*, quarterly. Newsletter. • Brochure.

**★ 20168 ★ Play Therapy International (PTI)**
11E-900 Greenbank Rd., Ste. 527
Nepean, ON, Canada K2J 4P6
**Phone:** (613)634-3125      **Fax:** (613)634-0866
**Email:** pti@playtherapy.org
**Website:** http://www.playtherapy.org/
**Fnded:** 1996. **Mem:** 1,200. **Lang(s):** English, French. **Desc:** Professional child psychotherapists and play therapists, students, and other individuals with an interest in child psychology. Promotes advancement in the teaching, theory, and practice of play therapy and child psychotherapy. Conducts examinations and bestows certification to child psychotherapists and play therapists; makes available continuing professional advancement programs to members. Serves as a clearinghouse on play therapy; represents members within the psychological community and before public bodies. Sponsors research; provides children's services; maintains speakers' bureau. **Pub:** *Play News*, quarterly. Newsletter. • *World of Children*, semiannual. Journal.

**★ 20169 ★ Private Practice Section/ American Physical Therapy Association (PPS)**
1710 Rhode Island NW, 8th Fl.
Washington, DC 20036
**Phone:** (202)457-1115      **Fax:** (202)457-9191
**Email:** info@ppsapta.org
**Website:** http://www.ppsapta.org
Joanne E. Dunne, CAE, Exec. Dir.
**Fnded:** 1955. **Mem:** 3,500. **Desc:** Physical therapists who are members of the American Physical Therapy Association and who are in private practice. Purposes are: to provide physical therapists with information on establishing and managing a private practice; to promote high standards of private practice physical therapy; to represent private practitioners before governmental and professional agencies; to disseminate information relating to private practice. Monitors federal and state legislation. Holds forums and seminars. Bestows Robert G. Dicus Award to recognize individuals for achievement in and commitment to the private practice of physical therapy. **Pub:** *An Employers Guide to Obtaining Physical Therapy Services*. • *How to Start a PT Private Practice*. • *IMPACT*, monthly.

Magazine. Covers practice management, marketing, clinical developments, legislative and regulatory news, and research and professional issues. • *Private Practice Section Membership Directory*, annual. Membership Directory. Arranged alphabetically and geographically. Includes meeting schedule. *Price:* Included in membership dues; $300 for nonmembers. • *Private Practice Valuation Primer - How to Value a Practice for Sale or Purchase*. • *Twenty Questions About Private Practice*. Pamphlet. • Also makes available blood borne pathogen kit.

**★ 20170 ★ Project Magic (PM)**
Kansas Rehabilitation Hospital
1504 SW 8 St.
Topeka, KS 66606
**Phone:** (913)235-6600      **Free:** 888-221-8199
**Website:** http://www.dcopperfield.com
Julie DeJean, Dir.
**Fnded:** 1982. **Desc:** Provides information and facilitates communication between magicians, occupational therapists, and patients with physical, psychosocial, and developmental disabilities. Created by television magician David Copperfield, the project works to rehabilitate patients by teaching them magic tricks instead of, or in addition to, traditional therapy techniques. Seeks to motivate patients to develop new skills and improve their self-image by demonstrating magical tricks. Tricks such as sleight-of-hand teach physical dexterity and mental puzzles help people to improve memory, concentration, and the ability to think sequentially. Provides interested magicians and occupational therapists with information and written material on the therapeutic value of magic for disabled persons. Sponsors educational seminars and workshops for rehabilitation facilities and health professionals. **Pub:** *David Copperfield's Project Magic Booklet*, periodic.

**★ 20171 ★ Rehabilitation Engineering and Assistive Technology Society of North America (RESNA)**
1700 N Moore St., Ste. 1540
Arlington, VA 22209-1903
**Phone:** (703)524-6686      **Fax:** (703)524-6630
**Email:** info@resna.org
**Website:** http://www.resna.org/
Larry Pencak, Exec. Dir.
**Fnded:** 1980. **Mem:** 1,250. **Desc:** Rehabilitation professionals, providers, and consumers. An interdisciplinary association for the advancement of rehabilitation and assistive technologies. Objectives are to improve the quality of life for disabled persons through the application of science and technology; influence policy relating to delivery of technology to disabled persons. Is concerned with the design and development of rehabilitation devices and the modification of housing and transportation systems. **Pub:** *Assistive Technology*, semiannual. Journal. • *Assistive Technology Sourcebook*. *Price:* $30. • *Augmentative Communication: Finding a Voice*. Video. Contains information on augmentative and alternative communication systems for funding sources and case managers. *Price:* $30. • *Backs: Correction or Accommodation*. Video. Contains information about static and adjustable back supports for funding sources and case managers. *Price:* $30. • *Communication: The Key to Teamwork*. Video. Includes explanations of assistive technology by rehabilitation experts for funding sources and case managers. *Price:* $30. • *Manual Mobility: Finding the Right Wheels*. Video. Contains information about rigid, folding, and lightweight wheelchairs for funding sources and case managers. *Price:* $30. • *RESNA News*, quarterly. • *Understanding the Technology When Selecting Wheelchairs*. *Price:* $10. • Brochures. • Manuals. • Membership Directory, annual. • Monographs. • Proceedings, annual. • Reports. • Also publishes an education series. **Frmly:** (1988) RESNA: Association for the Advancement of Rehabilitation Technology.

## ★ 20172 ★ Rehabilitation International (RI)

25 E 21st St.
New York, NY 10010
**Phone:** (212)420-1500　　**Fax:** (212)505-0871
**Email:** rehabintl@rehab-international.org
**Website:** http://www.rehab-international.org/
Lex Frieden, Sr. VP

**Fnded:** 1922. **Mem:** 150. **Desc:** Organizations in 90 countries conducting programs for the rehabilitation of people with physical and mental disabilities. Disseminates information on every phase of disability prevention and rehabilitation. Assists experts in planning work or study programs outside their own countries; aids in practical development of national rehabilitation programs. **Pub:** *International Journal of Rehabilitation Research*, quarterly. Journal. • *International Rehabilitation Review*, triennial. Newsletter. Provides coverage of United Nations agencies, discusses the elimination of architectural and environmental barriers for the disabled. *Price:* $30/year. • *One-In-Ten*, quarterly. Newsletter. • *Proceedings of World Congress*, quadrennial. • *Rehabilitation*, semiannual. • Directory, annual. • Also publishes booklets and papers. **Frmly:** (1939) International Society for Crippled Children; (1960) International Society for the Welfare of Cripples; (1976) International Society for Rehabilitation of the Disabled.

## ★ 20173 ★ Rehabilitation and Resource Centre for Torture Victims (RCT) (Rehabiliterings-og Forskningscentret for Torturofre)

Borgergade 13
PO Box 90409
DK-1022 Copenhagen K, Denmark
**Phone:** 45 33 760600　　**Fax:** 45 33 760500
**Email:** irct@irct.org
**Website:** http://www.irct.org

**Fnded:** 1982. **Desc:** Medical doctors, nurses, psychologists, social workers, physiotherapists, interpreters and administrative staff. Studies and develops optimal treatment and rehabilitation programs for victims of torture. Provides, on outpatient basis, traditional medical treatment and personal and social counseling. Participates in information campaigns against torture. Sponsors seminars and symposia. Maintains documentation center. **Pub:** *Annual Report*, annual. • *Torture*, quarterly. Journal. Includes information on rehabilitation of torture victims and prevention of torture.

## ★ 20174 ★ Rehabilitation Technology Association

c/o Dave Whipp
West Virginia Rehabilitation Research and Training Center
806 Allen Hall
PO Box 6122
Morgantown, WV 26506-6122
**Phone:** (304)293-5314　　**Free:** 800-624-8284
**Fax:** (304)766-2689
**Email:** director@icdi.wvu.edu
**Website:** http://www.icdi.wvu.edu
Ranjit K. Majumder, Contact

**Fnded:** 1982. **Mem:** 1,000. **Desc:** Individuals involved in the rehabilitation field. Uses technology to enhance performance in their jobs. **Pub:** *RTA Online Newsletter*, quarterly. Newsletter. Contains articles on rehabilitation and information technologies. *Price:* Free.

## Scandinavian Association of Zone-Therapeutists (S.F.2.) (Skandinavisk Forening for Zoneterapeutes — S.F.2.)

*See:* Entry 4312

## ★ 20175 ★ Section for Long Term Care and Rehabilitation

c/o American Hospital Association
1 N Franklin St.
Chicago, IL 60606
**Phone:** (312)422-3302　　**Fax:** (312)422-4590
**Email:** ssonik@aha.org
**Website:** http://www.aha.org
Susanne Sonik, Dir.

**Fnded:** 1984. **Mem:** 2,600. **Desc:** Functions as part of the American Hospital Association. Promotes understanding of the health and continuing care needs of persons of all ages and issues pertinent to health care provider organizations. Seeks to improve continuity of care between acute, pre- and post-acute, and long-term services; supports efforts to improve health care delivery to chronically ill, elderly and disabled. research.

## ★ 20176 ★ Sister Kenny Rehabilitation Services (SKRS)

800 E 28th St.
Minneapolis, MN 55407
**Phone:** (612)863-4457　　**Fax:** (612)863-2591
Mark Dixon, Exec. Dir.

**Fnded:** 1942. **Desc:** To investigate, evaluate, promote, and support projects in rehabilitation and provide rehabilitative patient care. (Named for Elizabeth Kenny, 1886-1952, an Australian nurse who developed a method for treating poliomyelitis with thermal compresses and physical therapy.) Compiles statistics on research activities and patient care activities. Specializes in the treatment of acutely and chronically disabled patients. A large number of patients are stroke victims, spinal cord-injured, or brain-damaged. Rehabilitation services are also used by patients with arthritis, cerebral palsy, Parkinson's disease, polio residuals, or other neuromuscular disorders or musculoskeletal injuries. Offers professional education programs to instruct medical and allied health profession als in the most recent and most relevant rehabilitation practices. Teaches rehabilitation personnel nursing skills needed to fill the special requirements of chronically ill and physically disabled people. **Frmly:** (1965) Sister Kenny Foundation; (1976) American Rehabilitation Foundation; (2002) Sister Kenny Institute.

## ★ 20177 ★ Society for Companion Animal Studies (SCAS)

10B Leny Rd.
Callander FK17 8BA, United Kingdom
**Phone:** 44 1877 330996　　**Fax:** 44 1877 330996
**Website:** http://www.scas.org.uk

**Fnded:** 1979. **Mem:** 350. **Nat'l Groups:** 1. **Lang(s):** English. **Desc:** Academics, physicians, psychologists, veterinarians, and laypersons in 13 countries interested in the study of the relationship between people and companion animals. Examines the effects animals have on the emotional and physical well being of individuals. Studies and disseminates results on the benefits companion animals bring to the clients of health and social care professionals. Conducts surveys and research projects. **Pub:** *Death of an Animal Friend*. Booklet. • *Guidelines for the Introduction of Pets in Nursing Homes and Other Institutions*. • *Issues in Research in Companion Animal Studies*. Report. • *Journal of Society for Companion Animal Studies*, quarterly. Journal. • *Pet Loss and Support for Bereaved Pet Owners*. Report. • *Pets, Health and Quality of Life for Older People*. • *When a Pet Dies*. Manual. **Frmly:** (1979) Group for the Study of the Human/Companion Animal Bond.

## ★ 20178 ★ Society for Light Treatment and Biological Rhythms (SLTBR)

PO Box 591687
174 Cook St.
San Francisco, CA 94159-1687
**Phone:** (415)876-0716　　**Fax:** (415)751-2758
**Email:** sltbrinfo@aol.com
**Website:** http://www.sltbr.org
Kathleen Matikonis, Exec. Dir.

**Fnded:** 1988. **Mem:** 400. **Desc:** Fosters research, professional development, and clinical applications in the fields of light therapy and biological rhythms. **Pub:** *Light Treatment and Biological Rhythms*, quarterly. Bulletin.

## Spinal Injuries Action Association (SIAA)

*See:* Entry 14117

## ★ 20179 ★ Swedish Association of Occupational Therapists (SAOT) (Forbundet Sveriges Arbetsterapeuter — FSA)

Planiavagen 13
Box 760
S-131 24 Nacka, Sweden
**Phone:** 46 8 4662440　　**Fax:** 46 8 4662424
**Email:** fsa@akademikerhuset.se
**Website:** http://www.fsa.akademikerhuset.se

**Fnded:** 1979. **Mem:** 9,000. **Reg. Groups:** 31. **Lang(s):** English, Swedish. **Desc:** Union of occupational therapists in Sweden. Compiles statistics; conducts research and educational programs; negotiates working conditions and wages. **Pub:** *Arbetsterapeuten*, monthly. Journal. Contains information about occupational therapy and employment listings. • *Arbetsterapeuten Publicerar Sig.* • *FOU-Rapporter*, semiannual.

## ★ 20180 ★ Swedish Association of Registered Physical Therapists (Legitimerade Sjukgymnasters Riksforbund — LSR)

Vasagatan 48
Box 3196
S-103 63 Stockholm, Sweden
**Phone:** 46 8 56706100　　**Fax:** 46 8 56706199
**Email:** kansli@lsr.se
**Website:** http://www.lsr.se

**Fnded:** 1943. **Mem:** 11,000. **Lang(s):** English, Swedish. **Desc:** Union of physical therapists in Sweden. Sponsors educational programs; compiles statistics. **Pub:** *Nordisk Fysioterapi*, quarterly. Journal. • *Sjukgymnasten*, monthly. Magazine.

## ★ 20181 ★ Swedish Occupational Therapy Association

c/o Scandinavian Journal of Occupational Therapy
Planiavagen 13, Box 760
Umea University
S-131 24 Nacka, Sweden
**Phone:** 46 8 4662440　　**Fax:** 46 8 4662424
**Email:** fsa@akademikerhuset.se
**Website:** http://www.fsa.akademikerhuset.se

**Lang(s):** Swedish. **Desc:** Occupational therapists and other health care professionals engaged in occupational medicine in Sweden. Promotes scientific inquiry in the field of occupational therapy and serves as a forum for the dissemination of research results. Areas of inquiry include: physical disability; mental health and disabilities; therapeutic equipment, environments, and techniques; assessment and evaluation of disabilities; vocational and educational training.

## ★ 20182 ★ Therapeutic Communities of America (TCA)

1601 Connecticut Ave. NW, Ste. 803
Washington, DC 20009
**Phone:** (202)296-3503　　**Fax:** (202)518-5475
**Email:** tcanet@erols.org
**Website:** http://www.tcanet.org
Kevin McEneaney, Pres.

**Fnded:** 1975. **Mem:** 100. **Desc:** Selfhelp treatment and rehabilitation agencies in the U.S. and Canada involving a highly structured treatment environment. Therapeutic community (TC) programs blend primary care, counseling and social services with resocialization, milieu therapy, behavior modification, progression through a hierarchy of occupational training and responsibility with the TC, and community re-entry. May include outpatient, day treatment, aftercare services, and prevention, as well as programs for individuals involved with the juvenile and criminal justice systems. Works with, and for, clients, their families, and their employers. Interacts with health agencies, federal and state governments, law enforcement, the judiciary, community organizations, business, labor, and media. Provides leadership for national and international conferences. Maintains staff code of ethics and offers counselor certification program. *Pub: Data Bank Updates*, periodic. • *Legislative Updates*, periodic. • Monographs. • Newsletter, bimonthly. • Proceedings.


**★ 20183 ★ Therapy Dogs International (TDI)**
88 Bartley Rd.
Flanders, NJ 07836
**Phone:** (973)252-9800          **Fax:** (973)252-7171
**Email:** tdi@gti.net
**Website:** http://www.tdi-dog.org
Ursula Kempe, CEO

**Fnded:** 1976. **Mem:** 7,000. **Reg. Groups:** 32. **Desc:** Dedicated to the regulation, testing, selection, and registration of qualified dogs and handlers for the purpose of visitations to hospitals, nursing homes, and other institutions where therapy dogs are needed. **Pub:** *Therapy Dogs International*, 3/year. Newsletter. • Brochures.


**★ 20184 ★ Vocational Evaluation and Work Adjustment Association (VEWAA)**
PO Box 26273
Colorado Springs, CO 80936
**Phone:** (719)380-1412          **Fax:** (719)638-6153
**Email:** sjctcm@aol.com
**Website:** http://www.vewaa.org
Robin Cook, Pres.

**Fnded:** 1967. **Mem:** 1,600. **Reg. Groups:** 7. **Desc:** A division of the National Rehabilitation Association. Specialists in vocational evaluation and work adjustment whose goals are to improve and advance the field and to promote high ethical practices through training and research. Conducts educational programs at state, regional, and national levels. Works with other organizations to develop a certification program for vocational evaluators and work adjustment personnel. Keeps legislators informed of the needs of persons with disabilities; promotes adequate funding of state and federal programs benefiting persons with disabilities. Disseminates employment information to members. **Pub:** Bulletin, quarterly. • Newsletter, quarterly. • National Directory of Vocational Evaluation and Assessment Professionals.


**★ 20185 ★ World Confederation for Physical Therapy (WCPT) (Confederation Mondiale pour la Therapie Physique)**
46-48 Grosvenor Gardens
London SW1W 0EB, United Kingdom
**Phone:** 44 207 8819234     **Fax:** 44 207 8819239
**Email:** wcpt@dial.pipex.com
**Website:** http://www.wcpt.org

**Fnded:** 1951. **Mem:** 83. **Nat'l Groups:** 65. **Reg. Groups:** 5. **Desc:** Confederation of 83 national associations representing physical therapists around the world supported mainly by subscriptions from its member organizations. Works to improve global health by: representing physical therapy and physical therapists internationally, collaborating with international and national organisations, encouraging high standards of physical therapy research, education and practice, and supporting communications of WCPT. **Pub:** *Annual Report.* • *Key Notes: Opinion Papers on a Variety of Professional Matters*, periodic. Reports. • *WCPT News*, semiannual. Newsletter. • Books, periodic.


**★ 20186 ★ World Federation of Occupational Therapists (WFOT) (Federation Mondiale des Ergotherapeutes)**
PO Box 30
Forrestfield, WA 6058, Australia
**Phone:** 61 8 94269200          **Fax:** 61 8 94815223
**Email:** wfot@multiline.com.au
**Website:** http://www.wfot.org.au

**Fnded:** 1952. **Mem:** 50. **Lang(s):** English. **Desc:** Membership is comprised of 50 countries which have Occupational Therapy Associations with approved constitutions and educational programmes; associate members, which are countries with approved constitutions; and individual members, who are qualified occupational therapists. Objectives are to: promote the occupational therapy profession; provide for exchange of information and publications; encourage international cooperation; establish standards of education for occupational therapists; maintain professional ethics; facilitate international exchange and placement of therapists and students. Promotes research; assists developing countries in formulating education programs for occupational therapists. **Pub:** *Conference Proceedings*, quadrennial. • *WFOT Bulletin*, semiannual. Journal. • Bibliographies, periodic. Contains information on standards and requirements. • Manuals, periodic. Contains information on study courses. • Pamphlets, periodic. Contains information on standards and requirements.


**★ 20187 ★ World Rehabilitation Fund (WRF)**
386 Park Ave. S, Ste. 500
New York, NY 10016
**Phone:** (212)725-7875          **Fax:** (212)725-8402
**Email:** wrfnewyork@msn.com
**Website:** http://www.worldrehabfund.org
Heather Burns, Pres.

**Fnded:** 1955. **Mem:** 19. **Desc:** Assist governmental and voluntary agencies in establishing, improving and expanding rehabilitation care services for persons with disabilities caused by landmines and other ordinance, national disasters and other causes. Provides technical assistance, training, medical equipment and supplies. Have offices in New York, Brussels, Beirut, Kampala, Guatemala City, Manila and Madras. Also have projects in Haiti and Pakistan.


**World Sports Medicine Association of Registered Therapists (WORLD SMAR)**
*See:* Entry 19169


**★ 20188 ★ Wound, Ostomy and Continence Nurses Society: An Association of E.T. Nurses (WOCN)**
4700 W Lake Ave.
Glenview, IL 60025
**Phone:** (847)375-6730          **Free:** 888-224-9626
**Email:** membership@wocn.org
**Website:** http://www.wocn.org
Maureen O'Connor, Senior Mgr.

**Fnded:** 1969. **Mem:** 4,000. **Nat'l Groups:** 10. **Reg. Groups:** 11. **Local Groups:** 20. **Desc:** Enterostomal therapy (ET) nurses, wound, ostomy and continence care nurses in 10 countries trained in WOCN accredited schools; individuals interested in objectives of the association who hold a valid license in medicine or nursing; health-related firms. Seeks to support ET, wound, ostomy, and continence, nurses by promoting educational, clinical, and research opportunities and to guide the delivery of expert health care to individuals with wounds, ostomies, and incontinence. **Pub:** *Journal of Wound, Ostomy and Continence Nursing*, bimonthly. Journal. • *Management of Urinary Incontinence*. Slides and handout. *Price:* $50 for members; $85 for nonmembers. • *Patient Information Data System*. *Price:* $95 for members; $125 for nonmembers. • *Professional Practice Manual*. Manual. *Price:* $85 for members; $125 for nonmembers. • *Standards of Care Guidelines for Management*. Booklets. • *WOCN News*, quarterly. Newsletter. • Membership Directory, annual. *Price:* $35 for members; $50 for

nonmembers. • Fact Sheets and Position Statements N/C. **Frmly:** Wound, Ostomy and Continence Nurses Society, An Association of E.T. Nurses; (1993) International Association for Enterostomal Therapy.


# Research Centers


**★ 20189 ★ Boston University Center for Rehabilitation Effectiveness (CRE)**
Sargent College of Health & Rehabilitation Sciences
635 Commonwealth Ave., 6th Fl.
Boston, MA 02215-1605
**Phone:** (617)353-3277          **Fax:** (617)358-1355
**Email:** pandres@bu.edu
**Website:** http://www.bu.edu/cre/
Patricia Andres, Mgr.

**Activities/Fields:** Rehabilitative care and its effectiveness across the lifespan, specifically studies on human performance, motor learning and physiological processes underlying clinical improvement; investigations of psychosocial and interpersonal factors affecting rehabilitation outcome; evaluation of rehabilitation protocols on all types of facilities; etc. **Pub:** *Technical manuals.*


**★ 20190 ★ Colorado State University Colorado Injury Control Research Center (CICRC)**
Department of Environmental Health
College of Veterinary Medicine and Biomedical Sciences
Environmental Health Bldg.
Fort Collins, CO 80523-1676
**Phone:** (970)491-0670          **Fax:** (970)491-1032
**Email:** loranns@colostate.edu
**Website:** http://www.cvmbs.colostate.edu/EnHealth/CICRC
Dr. Lorann Stallones, Dir.

**Activities/Fields:** Acute care, rehabilitation, prevention, and epidemology in injury control and prevention of injuries in the Rocky Mountain Region.


**★ 20191 ★ Georgia Institute of Technology Center for Assistive Technology and Environmental Access (CATEA)**
490 10th St.
Atlanta, GA 30332-0156
**Phone:** (404)894-4960          **Free:** 800-726-9119
**Fax:** (404)894-9320
**Email:** hunter.ramseur@arch.gatech.edu
**Website:** http://www.arch.gatech.edu/crt/
Joe Koncelik, Dir.

**Activities/Fields:** Develops procedures to help persons with disabilities. Coordinates research and services related to rehabilitation technology within the University System of Georgia. **Pub:** *Newsletter*, quarterly. **Frmly:** Center for Rehabilitation Technology.


**★ 20192 ★ The Heuga Center**
27 Main St., Ste. 303
PO Box 491
Edwards, CO 81632-0491
**Phone:** (970)926-1290          **Free:** 800-367-3101
**Fax:** (970)926-1295
**Email:** bhutchinson@heuga.org
**Website:** http://www.heuga.org
Brian Hutchinson, Exec. VP

**Activities/Fields:** Improvement of the quality of life for those with multiple sclerosis (MS) and other potentially debilitating neurological disorders. Focuses on the effects of goal-oriented exercise on the fitness of those with MS.

**★ 20193 ★ The Institute for Rehabilitation and Research (TIRR)**
1333 Moursund Ave.
Houston, TX 77030
**Phone:** (713)799-5000  **Free:** 800-447-3422
**Fax:** (713)799-7095
**Website:** http://www.tirr.org
Louisa F. Adelung, Pres.

**Activities/Fields:** Clinical neurophysiologic, neuroendocrinologic, psychoecologic, and exercise tolerance studies of patients with severe spinal cord injuries; development and assessment of mechanical and electronic assistive devices for neurologically impaired individuals; research and technical developments concerned with the effects of pressure on human tissue; provision of personal assistance for persons with severe physical disabilities; and program evaluations to improve services for persons with head injury, amputation, or spinal cord injury. **Pub:** *TIRR Research Projects Guide.*

**★ 20194 ★ Kennedy Krieger Institute**
707 N Broadway
Baltimore, MD 21205
**Phone:** (410)502-9483  **Fax:** (410)502-9524
**Email:** goldstein@kennedykrieger.org
**Website:** http://www.kennedykrieger.org
Dr. Gary W. Goldstein, Pres.

**Activities/Fields:** Pediatric rehabilitation evaluation, treatment, and research, including interdisciplinary studies in genetics, biochemistry, toxicology, neurochemistry, metabolic diseases, speech and hearing, pharmacology, behavioral sciences, and special education. Major emphasis is placed on physical rehabilitation, effectiveness of drug support, behavior modification, evaluation of neurological disorders in children, and developing and testing training techniques.

**★ 20195 ★ Laban/Bartenieff Institute of Movement Studies, Inc.**
234 5th Ave., Rm. 201
New York, NY 10001
**Phone:** (212)477-4299  **Fax:** (212)477-3702
**Email:** limsinfo@erols.com
Lucy Rumack, Dir. of Certificate Prog.

**Activities/Fields:** Perception, description, and analysis of human movement for applications in dance and theater, physical therapy, psychotherapy, nonverbal communication, management consulting, anthropology, and fitness and sports training. The Institute's mission is to further the studies of the principles of movement formulated by Rudolf Laban (1879-1958), an Austro-Hungarian dancer, choreographer, and philosopher, and Irmgard Bartenieff (1900-1981), who applied her Laban training to physical therapy, dance therapy, anthropology, and dance. **Pub:** *Member's Newsletter.* • *Movement Studies Journal.*

**Louisiana Tech University**
**Center for Biomedical Engineering and Rehabilitation Science**
*See:* Entry 4531

**Massachusetts Institute of Technology**
**Eric P. and Evelyn E. Newman Laboratory for Biomechanics and Human Rehabilitation**
*See:* Entry 4533

**National Institute for Rehabilitation Engineering**
*See:* Entry 4538

**★ 20196 ★ New York University Medical Rehabilitation Research and Training Center**
400 E 34th St.
New York, NY 10016
**Phone:** (212)263-6547  **Fax:** (212)263-8815
**Email:** Mathew.Lee@mcrks.med.nyu.edu

**Website:** http://www.theoffice.net/nire
Dr. Mathew Lee, Chm.

**Activities/Fields:** Rehabilitation for Parkinson's disease, Alzheimer's disease, brain trauma and stroke victims, spinal cord injuries, and comprehensive management of neuromuscular disease. Seeks to identify and validate specific treatment modalities applied to persons disabled by these neuromuscular disorders and to develop and improve new and existing treatment modalities, and to quantify and standardize methods of evaluating disease activity and remission.

**★ 20197 ★ New York University Rusk Institute of Rehabilitation Medicine**
400 E 34th St.
New York, NY 10016
**Phone:** (212)263-5870  **Fax:** (212)263-8510
**Website:** http://www.med.nyu.edu/rusk/
Dr. Mathew Lee, Chm.

**Activities/Fields:** Management of neuromuscular disease, Parkinson's disease, Alzheimer's disease, brain trauma and stroke victims.

**★ 20198 ★ New York University Medical Center**
**Head Trauma Program**
660 1st Ave.
New York, NY 10010
**Phone:** (212)263-7156  **Fax:** (212)263-6807
**Email:** yehuda.ben-yishay@med.nyu.edu
Dr. Yehuda Ben-Yishay, Dir.

**Activities/Fields:** Young adults suffering from head injuries. Conducts systematic remedial training in attention and concentration, various aspects of perception, perceptual-motor integration (eye-hand integration), and logical reasoning and interpersonal skills. Provides individual and family counseling and prevocational explorations. **Pub:** *Working Approaches to Remediation of Cognitive Deficits in Brain Damaged Persons,* annually.

**Northwestern University**
**Prosthetics Research Laboratory**
*See:* Entry 16954

**Packard Children's Hospital at Stanford**
**Rehabilitation Technology Center**
*See:* Entry 8197

**★ 20199 ★ Rancho Rehabilitation Engineering Program**
Los Amigos Research & Education Institute, Inc.
7503 Bonita St.
Downey, CA 90242
**Phone:** (562)401-7994  **Fax:** (562)803-6117
**Email:** ve.hzo@lpch.stanford.edu
**Website:** http://www.ranchorep.org
Dr. Donald McNeal, Co-Dir.

**Activities/Fields:** Develops appropriate technology and assessment procedures in the field of rehabilitation engineering and assures their availability to individuals with physical disabilities.

**★ 20200 ★ Rehabilitation Institute of Chicago**
345 E Superior, Ste. 1406
Chicago, IL 60611
**Phone:** (312)238-3919  **Fax:** (312)238-2208
**Email:** w-rymer@northwestern.edu
**Website:** http://www.smpp.nwu.edu
Dr. William Z. Rymer, Dir. of Res.

**Activities/Fields:** Rehabilitation medicine, brain trauma, stroke, atherosclerosis, neuromuscular diseases, applied neurophysiology, deep venous thrombosis, spinal cord injury, arthritis, prosthetics/orthotics, rehabilitation nursing, allied health, and communicative disorders.

**★ 20201 ★ Rehabilitation Institute of Michigan**
261 Mack Ave.
Detroit, MI 48201
**Phone:** (313)745-9735  **Fax:** (313)966-7502
**Email:** mwayland@dmc.org
**Website:** http://www.rimrehab.org/rim/
Dr. Marilyn Wayland, Dir.

**Activities/Fields:** Physical medicine and rehabilitation medicine, including electromyography, rehabilitation engineering, neuropsychology, measures of rehabilitation outcome, and methods of evaluation and treatment of patients with closed head injuries, spinal cord injuries, cerebrovascular accidents, and other diagnoses. **Pub:** *Research report,* annually. • *Thinking Cap.*

**Research and Development Institute**
*See:* Entry 8198

**★ 20202 ★ Revici Foundation for Lipid Research**
200 W 57th St.
New York, NY 10019
**Phone:** (212)246-5122  **Fax:** (212)246-1535
**Email:** aweissberg@aol.com
Anita Weissberg, MD, Dir.

**Activities/Fields:** Develops lipid therapy for various physiopathological conditions. Conducts studies on experimental theories in oncology, particulary the use of lipid therapy in physiopathological conditions. Investigates alternatives to the traditional treatments for cancer and other degenerative diseases, including AIDS. **Frmly:** Institute of Applied Biology.

**★ 20203 ★ Roosevelt Warm Springs Institute for Rehabilitation**
PO Box 1000
Warm Springs, GA 31830-0268
**Phone:** (706)655-5616  **Fax:** (706)655-5630
**Email:** evprather@dhr.state.ga.us
**Website:** http://www.rooseveltrehab.org
Evelyn Prather, Res. Spec.

**Activities/Fields:** Clinical aspects of rehabilitation, marketing, administration, and product development. **Pub:** *Research Brief,* annually. • *The Spirit Newsletter,* quarterly.

**Stanford University**
**Stanford Cardiac Rehabilitation Program**
*See:* Entry 5140

**★ 20204 ★ Thomas Jefferson University Regional Spinal Cord Injury System of Delaware Valley**
132 S 10th St., Ste. 375 Main Bldg.
Philadelphia, PA 19107-5099
**Phone:** (215)955-6579  **Fax:** (215)955-5152
**Email:** john.ditunno@mail.tju.edu
**Website:** http://www.spinalcordcenter.org
Dr. John F. Ditunno, Jr., Proj. Dir.

**Activities/Fields:** Acute care and rehabilitation for individuals disabled by spinal cord injury, including recovery of upper and lower extremity strength and function and the development of international standards to measure improvements in walking. The center is one of five nationwide participating in a study utilizing body weight-supported ambulation therapy funded by the National Institute of Child Health and Human Development of the National Institutes of Health. The center is also involved in multi-center drug trials and other therapeutic interventions and participates in the collection and storage of training and educational materials for spinal cord injury. **Pub:** *Newsletter.* • *SCI Research Update,* annually.

**★ 20205 ★ U.S. Department of Education**
**National Institute on Disability and**
 **Rehabilitation Research**
**Southeastern Michigan Spinal Cord Injury**
 **System (SEMSCIS)**
Rehabilitation Institute of Michigan
261 Mack Blvd.
Detroit, MI 48201
**Phone:** (313)745-9770  **Fax:** (313)966-7502
**Email:** mdijkers@med.wayne.edu
**Website:** http://www.neurosurg.wayne.edu
Dr. Marcel Dijkers, Co-Project Dir.
**Activities/Fields:** Spinal cord injuries, including reha-
bilitation for patients with such injuries, reduction of
such injuries, and new treatments.

**U.S. Department of Veterans Affairs**
**Veterans Health Administration**
**Office of Research and Development**
**Rehabilitation and Development Service**
**(Center for Rehabilitative Auditory**
 **Research)**
*See:* Entry 13513

**U.S. Department of Veterans Affairs**
**Veterans Health Administration**
**Office of Research and Development**
**Rehabilitation and Development Service**
**(Center for Mobility)**
*See:* Entry 13514

**U.S. Department of Veterans Affairs**
**Veterans Health Administration**
**Office of Research and Development**
**Rehabilitation and Development Service**
**(Center for Healthy Aging with**
 **Disabilities)**
*See:* Entry 13515

**U.S. Department of Veterans Affairs**
**Veterans Health Administration**
**Office of Research and Development**
**Rehabilitation and Development Service**
**(Center for Functional Electric**
 **Stimulation)**
*See:* Entry 13516

**★ 20206 ★ University of Alabama at**
 **Birmingham**
**Model Regional Spinal Cord Injury Care**
 **System**
Spain Rehab Center, Rm. 529
619 19th St. S
Birmingham, AL 35249-7330
**Phone:** (205)934-3334  **Fax:** (205)975-4691
**Email:** jacksona@uab.edu
**Website:** http://main.uab.edu/show.asp?durki=10712
Amie Jackson, MD, Proj. Dir. & Ch.
**Activities/Fields:** Rehabilitation needs of those with
spinal cord injury (SCI), including urological studies.
System objectives include: to deliver and improve
comprehensive medical, vocational, and psychosocial
rehabilitation services for individuals with SCI; to
evaluate both the effectiveness of services and their
costs and benefits; to produce new and useful information; to demonstrate and evaluate the application of
improved methods and equipment; and to participate
in national studies of the benefits of a spinal cord injury
service system. **Pub:** *Spinal Cord Injury: Clinical
Outcomes.*

**★ 20207 ★ University of Alabama at**
 **Birmingham**
**National Spinal Cord Injury Statistical**
 **Center**
1717 6th Ave. S, Rm. 515
Birmingham, AL 35233-7330

**Phone:** (205)934-5049  **Fax:** (205)934-2709
**Email:** nscisc@uab.edu
**Website:** http://www.spinalcord.uab.edu
Vicki Farris, Contact
**Activities/Fields:** Data collection, storage, and analy-
ses of national spinal cord injury statistics, submitted
by 16 federally sponsored Spinal Cord Injury Care
Systems. **Pub:** *Reports.* • *SCI: The Facts and Figures.*
Book.

**★ 20208 ★ University of Alabama at**
 **Birmingham**
**Rehabilitation Research and Training**
 **Center on Secondary Conditions of**
 **Spinal Cord Injury**
Department of Physical Medicine & Rehabilitation
Spain Rehab Ctr.
1717 6th Ave. S, Rm. 190
Birmingham, AL 35233-7330
**Phone:** (205)934-3450  **Fax:** (205)975-4691
**Email:** richards@uab.edu
**Website:** http://main.uab.edu/show.asp?darki=8762
J. Scott Richards, PhD, Contact
**Activities/Fields:** Prevention and treatment of secon-
dary conditions of spinal cord injury (SCI), including
urologic, respiratory and pulmonary complications;
pain; psycho-social conditions; nutrition; and assess-
ment of secondary conditions. **Pub:** *Pushin' On.*

**★ 20209 ★ University of Alabama at**
 **Birmingham**
**Traumatic Brain Injury Care System**
 **(TBICS)**
619 19th St. S, SRC529
Birmingham, AL 35249-7330
**Phone:** (205)934-3454  **Free:** 800-346-2742
**Fax:** (205)975-4691
**Email:** novack@uab.edu
**Website:** http://main.uab.edu/show.asp?durki=9505
Thomas Novack, PhD, Prin. Investigator
**Activities/Fields:** Effectiveness of care, rehabilitation,
and recovery outcomes for people with traumatic brain
injuries. **Pub:** *TBI Research Update.*

**★ 20210 ★ University of California, San**
 **Diego**
**Hyperbaric Medicine Center**
USCD Medical Center
200 W Arbor Dr.
San Diego, CA 92103-8688
**Phone:** (619)543-6463
**Email:** tneuman@ucsd.edu
Dr. Tom Neuman, Dir.
**Activities/Fields:** Hyperbaric oxygen therapy, includ-
ing application in burns, infectious diseases, wound
healing, and diving medicine.

**University of Illinois at Chicago**
**Rehabilitation Research and Training**
 **Center on Aging with Developmental**
 **Disabilities (RRTCADD)**
*See:* Entry 3105

**★ 20211 ★ University of Montana**
**Research and Training Center on Rural**
 **Rehabilitation Services**
52 Corbin Hall
Missoula, MT 59812
**Phone:** (406)243-5467  **Free:** 888-268-2743
**Fax:** (406)243-2743
**Email:** ruraldoc@selway.umt.edu
**Website:** http://ruralinstitute.umt.edu/rtcrural
Tom Seekins, PhD, Dir.
**Activities/Fields:** Employment and vocational rehabil-
itation service needs of people with disabilities in rural
areas; intervention development to improve employ-
ment outcomes; rural self-employment models; rural
independent living; improvment of transportation,
health care, housing, and accessibility; rural models
for prevention of secondary disabilities; disability legis-

lation and American Indian tribes; and alternative
models of delivery of rural rehabilitation services. **Pub:**
*Newsletter,* quarterly.

**★ 20212 ★ University of Montreal**
**Rehabilitation Institute of Montreal**
6300 Darlington Ave.
Montreal, QC, Canada H3S 2J4
**Phone:** (514)340-2085  **Fax:** (514)340-2091
**Email:** treeves@ssss.gouv.qc.ca
**Website:** http://ireadapt.qc.ca
Mindy Levin, Sci. Dir.
**Activities/Fields:** Biomedical research, focusing on
rehabilitation of patients suffering from spinal cord
injury, amputation, stroke, and traumatic head injuries;
behavioral research, including studies of the physical,
psychological, and occupational obstacles that prevent brain-injured persons from being reintegrated into
society; and rehabilitation engineering for upper- and
lower-limb amputees.

**University of Wisconsin—Stout**
**Research and Training Center on**
 **Community Rehabilitation Programs to**
 **Improve Employment Outcomes**
*See:* Entry 8231

**Wake Forest University**
**J. Paul Sticht Center on Aging and**
 **Rehabilitation**
*See:* Entry 3120

**★ 20213 ★ West Virginia University**
**University Affiliated Center for**
 **Developmental Disabilities (UACDD)**
955 Hartman Run Rd.
Morgantown, WV 26505
**Phone:** (304)293-4692  **Fax:** (304)293-7294
**Email:** adey@wvu.edu
**Website:** http://www.wfubmc.edu
Ashok S. Dey, Dir.
**Activities/Fields:** Developmental disabilities, mental
retardation (all ages), nutrition, under nutrition, brain
development, speech and language development,
medical aspects of developmental disabilities, high-
risk families, and program evaluation. Graduate re-
search assistants come from various University disciplines to participate in applied research activities. **Pub:**
*Quarterly Report.*

**★ 20214 ★ Western Michigan University**
**Occupational Therapy Teaching Research**
 **Clinic**
Occupational Therapy Department
1201 Oliver St.
Kalamazoo, MI 49008
**Phone:** (616)387-7260  **Fax:** (616)387-7262
**Email:** berit.miller@wmich.edu
Berit Miller, Coord.
**Activities/Fields:** Occupational therapy and clinical
research on developmental disabilities and learning
disabilities.

# State Government Agencies

## Rehabilitation

**★ 20215 ★ Alabama Department of**
 **Rehabilitation Services**
2129 E S Blvd.
Montgomery, AL 36116
**Phone:** (334)281-8780  **Free:** 800-441-7607
**Fax:** (334)281-1973
**Email:** webinfo@rehab.state.al.us
**Website:** http://www.rehab.state.al.us/
Steve Shivers, Director

**★ 20216 ★ Alaska Department of Labor and Workforce Development**
**Vocational Rehabilitation Division**
801 W 10th St., Ste. 1A
Juneau, AK 99801-1894
**Phone:** (907)465-2814  **Free:** 800-478-2815
**Fax:** (907)465-2856
**Email:** Vikki_Parson@labor.state.ak.us
**Website:** http://www.labor.state.ak.us/dvr/home.htm
Duane French, Director

**★ 20217 ★ Arizona Department of Economic Security**
**Employment and Rehabilitation Services Division**
**Rehabilitation Services Administration**
Site Code 733A
PO Box 6123
Phoenix, AZ 85005
**Phone:** (602)542-3871  **Fax:** (602)542-6474
**Email:** azrsa@cirs.org
**Website:** http://www.de.state.az.us/links/economic/webpage/page6.html

**★ 20218 ★ Arkansas Department of Education**
**Rehabilitation Services Division**
1616 Brookwood Dr.
Little Rock, AR 72203
**Phone:** (501)296-1600  **Free:** 800-330-0632
**Fax:** (501)296-1655
**Website:** http://www.ark.org/ars/

**★ 20219 ★ California Health and Welfare Agency**
**Rehabilitation Department**
PO Box 944222
Sacramento, CA 94244-2220
**Phone:** (916)263-8681  **Fax:** (916)327-4567
**Email:** suggest@rehab.cahwnet.gov
**Website:** http://www.rehab.ca.gov/

**★ 20220 ★ Colorado Department of Human Services**
**Rehabilitation Services Division**
2211 West Evans, Bldg. B
Denver, CO 80223
**Phone:** (720)884-1234  **Fax:** (720)884-1213
**Email:** debbie.powell@state.co.us
**Website:** http://www.cdhs.state.co.us/ods/dvr/index.html
Diana Huerta, Director

**★ 20221 ★ Connecticut Department of Social Services**
**Rehabilitation Services Bureau**
25 Sigourney St.
Hartford, CT 06105-5033
**Phone:** (860)424-4848  **Free:** 800-842-1508
**Email:** brs.dss@po.state.ct.us
**Website:** http://www.dss.state.ct.us/svcs/rehab.htm

**★ 20222 ★ Delaware Department of Labor**
**Vocational Rehabilitation Division**
4425 N Market St.
P.O.Box 9969
Wilmington, DE 19801
**Phone:** (302)761-8275  **Fax:** (302)761-6611
**Email:** dlabor@state.de.us
**Website:** http://www.delawareworks.com/divisions/dvr/welcome.htm
Andrea S. Guest, Director

**★ 20223 ★ Florida Department of Labor and Employment Security**
**Vocational Rehabilitation Division**
2002 Old St. Augustine Rd., Bldg. A
Tallahassee, FL 32399-0696
**Phone:** (850)488-6210  **Free:** 800-451-4327
**Fax:** (850)921-7215
**Website:** http://www.rehabworks.org/

**★ 20224 ★ Georgia Department of Human Resources**
**Rehabilitation Services Division**
2 Peachtree St. NW, Ste. 376-S
Atlanta, GA 30303
**Phone:** (404)206-6000  **Fax:** (404)206-6011
**Email:** defennel@dhr.state.ga.us
**Website:** http://www.vocrehabga.org/

**★ 20225 ★ Idaho Board of Education**
**Vocational Education Division**
650 W State St., Rm. 324
PO Box 83720
Boise, ID 83720-0095
**Phone:** (208)334-3216  **Fax:** (208)334-2365
**Email:** bmoench@pte.state.id.us
**Website:** http://www.pte.state.id.us/
Dr. Mike Rush, Director

**★ 20226 ★ Illinois Department of Human Services**
**Rehabilitation Services Bureau**
100 S Grand Ave. East 3rd Flr.
PO Box 19429
Springfield, IL 62762
**Phone:** (217)785-0234  **Free:** 800-225-3607
**Fax:** (217)558-4270
**Email:** ors@dhs.state.il.us
**Website:** http://WWW.STATE.il.us/agency/dhs/rsnp.html
Carl Suter, Director

**★ 20227 ★ Indiana Family and Social Services Administration**
**Disability, Aging and Rehabilitative Services Division**
402 W Washington St.
PO Box 7083
Indianapolis, IN 46207-7083
**Phone:** (317)232-1147  **Free:** 800-545-7763
**Fax:** (317)233-4693
**Email:** webmaster@ai.org
**Website:** http://www.state.in.us/fssa/HTML/PROGRAMS/2b.html

**★ 20228 ★ Iowa Department of Education**
**Vocational Rehabilitation Division**
510 E 12th St.
Des Moines, IA 50319
**Phone:** (515)281-6731  **Free:** 800-532-1486
**Fax:** (515)281-4703
**Email:** dcarlson@dvrs.state.ia.us
Dwight R. Carlson, Director

**★ 20229 ★ Kansas Department of Social and Rehabilitation Services**
**Rehabilitation Services Division**
915 SW Harrison St.
Topeka, KS 66612
**Phone:** (785)296-3959  **Fax:** (785)296-2173
**Website:** http://www.srskansas.org/ISD.htm

**★ 20230 ★ Kentucky Workforce Development Cabinet**
**Vocational Rehabilitation Department**
209 St. Clair St., 2d Fl.
Frankfort, KY 40601
**Phone:** (502)564-4440  **Free:** 800-372-7172
**Fax:** (502)564-6742
**Email:** wfd.vocrehab@mail.state.ky.us

**Website:** http://kydvr.state.ky.us/

**★ 20231 ★ Louisiana Department of Social Services**
**Rehabilitation Services Division**
8225 Florida Blvd.
PO Box 94371
Baton Rouge, LA 70806
**Phone:** (225)725-4131  **Free:** 800-737-2958
**Fax:** (225)925-4484
**Email:** webmaster@dss.state.la.us
**Website:** http://www.dss.state.la.us/offlrs/index.htm
Ed Barras, Contact

**★ 20232 ★ Maine Department of Labor**
**Rehabilitation Services Office**
150 State House Station
Augusta, ME 04333-0150
**Phone:** (207)624-5950  **Fax:** (207)624-5980
**Email:** John.G.Shattuck@state.me.us
**Website:** http://janus.state.me.us/labor/brs/vr.htm

**★ 20233 ★ Maryland Department of Education**
**Vocational Rehabilitation Division**
2301 Argonne Dr.
Baltimore, MD 21218-1696
**Phone:** (410)554-9385  **Fax:** (410)554-9412
**Email:** dors@msde.state.md.us
**Website:** http://www.dors.state.md.us/voc_rehab.html

**★ 20234 ★ Massachusetts Rehabilitation Commission**
Fort Point Pl. Ste. 600
27 Wormwood St.
Boston, MA 02210-1616
**Phone:** (617)204-3600  **Free:** 800-245-6543
**Fax:** (617)727-1354
**Email:** Robert.Donahue@mrc.state.ma.us
**Website:** http://www.magnet.state.ma.us/mrc/mrc.htm

**★ 20235 ★ Michigan Jobs Commission**
**Rehabilitation Services Division**
**The Open Door Employment & Disability Network**
608 W Allegan
PO Box 30010
Lansing, MI 48909
**Phone:** (517)373-3390  **Free:** 800-605-6722
**Fax:** (517)373-0565
**Website:** http://www.mrs.mjc.state.mi.us/

**★ 20236 ★ Minnesota Economic Security Department**
**Rehabilitation Services Division**
390 N Robert St.
Saint Paul, MN 55101
**Phone:** (651)296-5616  **Free:** 800-328-9095
**Email:** Howard.Glad@state.mn.us
**Website:** http://www.mnworkforcecenter.org/burgundy/rehab.htm
Howard Glad, Contact

**★ 20237 ★ Mississippi Department of Rehabilitation Services**
1281 Hwy. 51 N
Madison, MS 39110
**Phone:** (601)853-5100  **Free:** 800-443-1000
**Fax:** (601)853-5205
**Email:** bmcmillan@mdrs.state.ms.us
**Website:** http://www.mdrs.state.ms.us/
H.S. McMillan, Director

★ 20238 ★ **Missouri Department of Elementary and Secondary Education**
**Vocational Rehabilitation Division**
3024 Dupont Cir.
Jefferson City, MO 65109-0525
**Phone:** (573)751-3251    **Free:** 877-222-8963
**Fax:** (573)751-1441
**Email:** kkendle@movr.dese.state.mo.us
**Website:** http://www.dese.state.mo.us/divvocrehab/

★ 20239 ★ **Montana Department of Public Health and Human Services**
**Vocational Rehabilitation Program**
111 N Sanders, Ste. 307
PO Box 4210
Helena, MT 59604-4210
**Phone:** (406)444-2590    **Free:** 877-296-1197
**Fax:** (406)444-3632
**Email:** jmathews@state.mt.gov
**Website:** http://www.dphhs.state.mt.us/dsd/govt_programs/vrp/index.htm

★ 20240 ★ **Nebraska Department of Education**
**Rehabilitation Services Division**
301 Centennial Mall S
PO Box 94987
Lincoln, NE 68509-4987
**Phone:** (402)471-6329    **Free:** 800-472-3382
**Fax:** (402)471-0117
**Email:** a_sumner@vocrehab.state.ne.us
**Website:** http://www.vocrehab.state.ne.us/
Frank C. Lloyd, Director

★ 20241 ★ **Nevada Department of Employment Training and Rehabilitation**
**Rehabilitation Division**
**Vocational Rehabilitation Bureau**
505 E King St., Rm. 501
Carson City, NV 89701-3704
**Phone:** (775)684-4070    **Fax:** (775)684-4161
**Email:** detrinfo@govmail.state.nv.us
**Website:** http://detr.state.nv.us/rehab/reh_vorh.htm

★ 20242 ★ **New Hampshire Department of Education**
**Vocational Rehabilitation Bureau**
78 Regional Dr., Bldg.2
Concord, NH 03301
**Phone:** (603)271-3471    **Free:** 800-299-1647
**Fax:** (603)271-7095
**Email:** jchaput@ed.state.nh.us
**Website:** http://www.ed.state.nh.us/adulted/adult.htm
Paul K. Leather, Director

★ 20243 ★ **New Jersey Department of Labor**
**Vocational Rehabilitation Services Division**
135 E State St.
PO Box 398
Trenton, NJ 08625-0398
**Phone:** (609)292-5987    **Fax:** (609)292-8347
**Email:** dvradmin@dol.state.nj.us
**Website:** http://www.state.nj.us/labor/dvrs/dvr.html
Thomas G. Jennings, Director

★ 20244 ★ **New Mexico Department of Education**
**Vocational Rehabilitation Division**
435-D St. Michaels Dr., Bldg. D
Santa Fe, NM 87505
**Phone:** (505)954-8500    **Free:** 800-224-7005
**Fax:** (505)954-8562
**Email:** afox@state.nm.us
**Website:** http://www.state.nm.us/dvr/
Amber Fox, Contact

★ 20245 ★ **New York State Department of Education**
**Developmental Disabilities Planning Council**
155 Washington Ave., 2nd Fl.
Albany, NY 12210
**Phone:** (518)486-7505    **Free:** 800-395-3372
**Fax:** (518)402-3505
**Email:** ddpc@ddpc.state.ny.us
**Website:** http://www.ddpc.state.ny.us/

★ 20246 ★ **North Carolina Department of Health and Human Services**
**Vocational Rehabilitation Services Division**
805 Ruggles Dr.
2801 Mail Service Ctr.
Raleigh, NC 27603-2038
**Phone:** (919)733-3364    **Fax:** (919)733-7968
**Email:** dvr.information@ncmail.net
**Website:** http://dvr.dhhs.state.nc.us/
Bob Philbeck, Director

★ 20247 ★ **North Dakota Department of Human Services**
**Disability Services**
600 S Second St.
Bismarck, ND 58504-5729
**Phone:** (701)328-8930    **Free:** 800-755-8529
**Fax:** (701)328-8969
**Email:** soperc@state.nd.us
**Website:** http://lnotes.state.nd.us/dhs/dhsweb.nsf/ServicePages/DisabilityServices

★ 20248 ★ **Ohio Rehabilitation Services Commission**
**Vocational Rehabilitation Bureau**
400 E Campus View Blvd., SW3C
Columbus, OH 43235-4604
**Phone:** (614)438-1250    **Free:** 800-282-4536
**Fax:** (614)438-1257
**Email:** beverly.jennings@rsc.state.oh.us
**Website:** http://www.state.oh.us/rsc/VR_Services/BVR/bvr.html
June K. Gutterman, Director

★ 20249 ★ **Oklahoma Department of Rehabilitation Services**
**Rehabilitative Services Bureau**
3535 NW 58th St., Ste 500
Oklahoma City, OK 73112
**Phone:** (405)951-3400    **Free:** 800-845-8476
**Fax:** (405)951-3259
**Website:** http://www.okrehab.org/

★ 20250 ★ **Oregon Department of Human Resources**
**Vocational Rehabilitation Division**
500 Summer St., NE
E87
Salem, OR 97301-1120
**Phone:** (503)945-5880    **Fax:** (503)947-5010
**Email:** dhr.info@state.or.us
**Website:** http://vrdweb.hr.state.or.us/

★ 20251 ★ **Pennsylvania Department of Labor and Industry**
**Vocational Rehabilitation Office**
909 Green St.
Harrisburg, PA 17102
**Phone:** (717)787-5244    **Free:** 800-442-6351
**Email:** ovr@dli.state.pa.us
**Website:** http://www.dli.state.pa.us/landi/cwp/view.asp?a=128&Q=168255

★ 20252 ★ **Puerto Rico Department of Social Services**
**Vocational Rehabilitation Administration**
PO Box 191118
San Juan, PR 00919-1118
**Phone:** (787)729-0160    **Fax:** (787)728-8070
**Email:** webmaster@govpr.org
**Website:** http://fortaleza.govpr.org/

★ 20253 ★ **Rhode Island Department of Human Services**
**Community Services**
**Vocatonal Rehabilitation Services**
40 Fountain St.
Providence, RI 02903
**Phone:** (401)421-7005    **Fax:** (401)222-3574
**Website:** http://www.ors.state.ri.us/vocpage.htm

★ 20254 ★ **South Carolina Department of Vocational Rehabilitation**
1410 Boston Ave.
PO Box 15
West Columbia, SC 29171
**Phone:** (803)896-6504    **Fax:** (803)896-6529
**Email:** info@scvrd.state.sc.us
**Website:** http://www.scvrd.net
Larry Bryant, Director

★ 20255 ★ **South Dakota Department of Human Services**
**Rehabilitation Services Division**
Hillsview Plaza, E Hwy 34
500 E Capitol
Pierre, SD 57501-5070
**Phone:** (605)773-3195    **Fax:** (605)773-5483
**Email:** eric.weiss@state.sd.us
**Website:** http://www.state.sd.us/dhs/drs/
Grady Kickul, Director

★ 20256 ★ **Tennessee Department of Human Services**
**Rehabilitation Services Division**
400 Deaderick St.
15th floor
Nashville, TN 37248-0060
**Phone:** (615)313-4714    **Fax:** (615)741-4165
**Website:** http://www.state.tn.us/humanserv/
Carl Brown, Contact

★ 20257 ★ **Texas Rehabilitation Commission**
4900 N Lamar Blvd.
Austin, TX 78751
**Phone:** (512)424-4000    **Free:** 800-628-5115
**Website:** http://www.rehab.state.tx.us/
Vernon Arrell, Director

★ 20258 ★ **Utah Rehabilitation Office**
**Rehabilitation Services Division**
250 E 500 S
Salt Lake City, UT 84111
**Phone:** (801)538-7530    **Fax:** (801)538-7522
**Website:** http://www.usor.state.ut.us/

★ 20259 ★ **Vermont Agency of Human Services**
**Social and Rehabilitation Services Department**
**Vocational Rehabilitation Division**
**Planning and Evaluation Division**
103 S Main St.
Waterbury, VT 05671-2401
**Phone:** (802)241-2131    **Fax:** (802)241-2407
**Email:** webmaster@srs.state.vt.us
**Website:** http://www.state.vt.us/srs
Don Mandelkorn, Director

**★ 20260 ★ Virgin Islands Department of Human Services**
**Disabilities and Rehabilitation Services Division**
Roy Lester Schneider Hospital
Knud Hansen Complex, Bldg. A 1303
Hospital Ground
Saint Thomas, VI 00802
**Phone:** (340)774-0930　　　**Fax:** (340)774-3466
**Email:** humanservices@usvi.org
**Website:** http://www.usvi.org/humanservices/index.html

**★ 20261 ★ Virginia Office of Health and Human Resources**
**Rehabilitative Services Department**
8004 Franklin Farms Dr.
PO Box K300
Richmond, VA 23288
**Phone:** (804)662-7000　　　**Free:** 800-552-5019
**Fax:** (804)662-9140
**Email:** drs@drs.state.va.us
**Website:** http://www.vadrs.org/

**★ 20262 ★ Washington Department of Social and Health Services**
**Health and Rehabilitative Services Office**
**Vocational Rehabilitation Division**
PO Box 45340
Olympia, WA 98504-5060
**Phone:** (360)438-8000　　　**Free:** 800-637-5627
**Fax:** (360)438-8007
**Website:** http://www1.dshs.wa.gov/dvr/index.htm

**★ 20263 ★ West Virginia State Board of Education and the Arts**
**Rehabilitation Services Division**
State Capitol Complex
PO Box 50890
Charleston, WV 25305-0890
**Phone:** (304)766-4600　　　**Free:** 800-642-8207
**Fax:** (304)766-4905
**Email:** penneyh@mail.drs.state.wv.us
**Website:** http://www.wvdrs.org/
Janice Holland, Director

**★ 20264 ★ Wisconsin Department of Workforce Development**
**Vocational Rehabilitation Division**
2917 International Ln., Ste. 300
PO Box 7852
Madison, WI 53707-7852
**Phone:** (608)243-5600　　　**Free:** 800-442-3477
**Fax:** (608)243-5680
**Email:** dwddvr@dwd.state.wi.us
**Website:** http://www.dwd.state.wi.us/dvr/

**★ 20265 ★ Wyoming Department of Employment**
**Vocational Rehabilitation Division**
1100 Herschler Bldg.
122 W 25th St.
Cheyenne, WY 82002
**Phone:** (307)777-7389　　　**Fax:** (307)777-5939
**Email:** jmcint@state.wy.us
**Website:** http://wydoe.state.wy.us/doe.asp?ID=5
Gary W. Child, Director

## State & Regional Organizations

### Physical Therapy

*The following are state chapters of the American Physical Therapy Association, 1111 N Fairfax St.,* Alexandria, VA 22314-1488, (800)999-APTA, http://www.apta.org/.

## Alabama

**★ 20266 ★ American Physical Therapy Association**
**Alabama Chapter**
323 De La Mare Ave.
Fairhope, AL 36532-2319
**Phone:** (251)990-9666　　　**Fax:** (251)990-8019
**Email:** rhonda@pradcom.com
**Website:** http://www.ptalabama.org
Rhonda Wilkinson, Contact
Karen Moore, Contact

## Alaska

**★ 20267 ★ American Physical Therapy Association**
**Alaska Chapter**
8970 Northwood Park Cir.
Eagle River, AK 99577
**Phone:** (907)566-3749
**Email:** runwithstrength@gci.net
Bethany Lawso, Contact

## Arizona

**★ 20268 ★ American Physical Therapy Association**
**Arizona Chapter**
4035 E Fanfol
Phoenix, AZ 85028
**Phone:** (602)569-9101　　　**Free:** 800-264-APTA
**Fax:** (602)996-3966
**Email:** info@azapta.org
**Website:** http://www.azapta.org
Pauline Wampler, Director

## Arkansas

**★ 20269 ★ American Physical Therapy Association**
**Arkansas Chapter**
PO Box 2068
Conway, AR 72033-2068
**Phone:** (501)269-8247　　　**Fax:** (501)327-1370
**Email:** arpta@cyberback.com
**Website:** http://www.arpta.org
Lauren Maxwell, Director

## California

**★ 20270 ★ American Physical Therapy Association**
**California Chapter**
2520 Venture Oaks Way, Ste. 150
Sacramento, CA 95833-4228
**Phone:** (916)929-2782　　　**Fax:** (916)646-5960
**Email:** pevans@ccapta.org
**Website:** http://www.ccapta.org
Patricia Evans, Contact

## Colorado

**★ 20271 ★ American Physical Therapy Association**
**Colorado Chapter**
7853 E Arapahoe Ct., Ste. 2100
Englewood, CO 80112-1361
**Phone:** (303)694-4728　　　**Free:** 800-875-2782
**Fax:** (303)694-4869
**Email:** apta@assnoffice.com
**Website:** http://www.assnoffice.com/apta
Ellen Caruso, Exec Director

## Connecticut

**★ 20272 ★ American Physical Therapy Association**
**Connecticut Chapter**
330 Main St., 3rd Fl.
Hartford, CT 06106-5408
**Phone:** (860)246-4414　　　**Fax:** (860)541-6484
**Email:** abrunetti@tcor.com
**Website:** http://www.ctpt.org
Allyson J. Brunetti, Contact

## District of Columbia

**★ 20273 ★ American Physical Therapy Association**
**District of Columbia Chapter**
6981 32nd St. NW
Washington, DC 20015
**Phone:** (202)723-2819　　　**Fax:** (202)537-1388
**Email:** tmsgloria@aol.com
Gloria Rogers, President

## Florida

**★ 20274 ★ American Physical Therapy Association**
**Florida Chapter**
1705 S Gadsden St.
Tallahassee, FL 32301
**Phone:** (850)222-1243　　　**Fax:** (850)224-5281
**Email:** ccrosby@fpta.org
**Website:** http://www.fpta.com
Craig Crosby, Director

## Georgia

**★ 20275 ★ American Physical Therapy Association**
**Georgia Chapter**
1260 Winchester Pkwy., Ste. 205
Smyrna, GA 30080
**Phone:** (770)433-2418　　　**Fax:** (770)433-2907
**Email:** ptagexec@bellsouth.net
**Website:** http://www.ptagonline.org
Kathy Brooks, Director

## Hawaii

**★ 20276 ★ American Physical Therapy Association**
**Hawaii Chapter**
1360 S Bertania St., Ste. 301
Honolulu, HI 96814-1514
**Phone:** (808)247-0105　　　**Fax:** (808)523-7809
**Email:** jgold@hillandknowlton.com
**Website:** http://www.hapta.org
Joanne Reid, PT, Contact

## Idaho

**★ 20277 ★ American Physical Therapy Association**
**Idaho Chapter**
PO Box 1273
Boise, ID 83701-1273
**Phone:** (208)342-6647　　　**Fax:** (208)342-6647
**Email:** ipta@aol.com
**Website:** http://www.ptidaho.org
Jill Cooper, Director

## Illinois

**★ 20278 ★ American Physical Therapy Association**
**Illinois Chapter**
1010 Jorie Blvd., Ste. 134
Oak Brook, IL 60523
**Phone:** (630)571-1400　　　**Free:** 800-552-4782
**Fax:** (630)571-1406
**Email:** staylor@ipta.org

**Website:** http://www.ipta.org
Stephanie Taylor, Contact

## Indiana

★ **20279** ★ American Physical Therapy
   Association
**Indiana Chapter**
PO Box 26692
Indianapolis, IN 46226-0692
**Phone:** (317)823-3681          **Fax:** (317)823-3681
**Email:** schroeder@inapta.org
**Website:** http://www.inapta.org
Teresa Schroeder, Director

## Iowa

★ **20280** ★ American Physical Therapy
   Association
**Iowa Chapter**
1228 8th St., Ste. 106
West Des Moines, IA 50265-2622
**Phone:** (515)222-9838          **Free:** 800-925-3064
**Fax:** (515)222-9839
**Email:** mail@iowaapta.org
**Website:** http://www.iowaapta.org
Michael C. Mandel, Director

## Kansas

★ **20281** ★ American Physical Therapy
   Association
**Kansas Chapter**
214 SW 6th St., Ste. 300
Topeka, KS 66603-3719
**Phone:** (785)233-5400          **Fax:** (785)290-0476
**Email:** executivedirector@kpta.kscoxmail.com
**Website:** http://www.kpta.com
Brenda Straub, Contact

## Kentucky

★ **20282** ★ American Physical Therapy
   Association
**Kentucky Chapter**
4010 Dupont Cir., Ste. 584
Louisville, KY 40207
**Phone:** (502)899-9341          **Fax:** (502)899-9342
**Email:** kpta@bluegrass.net
**Website:** http://www.KPTA.org
Maria Gray, Director

## Louisiana

★ **20283** ★ American Physical Therapy
   Association
**Louisiana Chapter**
8550 United Plaza Blvd., Ste. 1001A
Baton Rouge, LA 70809-2256
**Phone:** (225)922-4614          **Fax:** (225)922-4611
**Email:** bconnor@pncpa.com
**Website:** http://www.lpta.org
Bland O'Connor, Director

## Maine

★ **20284** ★ American Physical Therapy
   Association
**Maine Chapter**
PO Box 1783
Portland, ME 04104-1783
**Phone:** (207)799-1584          **Fax:** (207)799-1584
**Email:** jangeyer1@aol.com
**Website:** http://www.maineapta.org
Jan Geyer, Contact

## Maryland

★ **20285** ★ American Physical Therapy
   Association
**Maryland Chapter**
PO Box 1099
Laurel, MD 20725-1099
**Phone:** (301)362-4290          **Free:** 800-306-5596
**Fax:** 800-675-9438
**Email:** aptamd@erols.com
**Website:** http://www.aptamd.org
Wayne Becraft, President

## Massachusetts

★ **20286** ★ American Physical Therapy
   Association
**Massachusetts Chapter**
34 Atlantic St.
Gloucester, MA 01930-1625
**Phone:** (978)281-5393          **Fax:** (978)282-4384
**Email:** kag@shore.net
**Website:** http://aptaofma.org
Karen A. Gallagher, Director

## Michigan

★ **20287** ★ American Physical Therapy
   Association
**Michigan Chapter**
PO Box 21236
Lansing, MI 48909-1236
**Phone:** (517)347-0880          **Free:** 800-242-8131
**Fax:** (517)347-4720
**Email:** mpta@mpta.org
**Website:** http://www.mpta.com
Terry Warren, Director

## Minnesota

★ **20288** ★ American Physical Therapy
   Association
**Minnesota Chapter**
1711 W County Rd. B, Ste. 101 S
Roseville, MN 55113-4036
**Phone:** (651)635-0902          **Fax:** (651)635-0903
**Email:** mnapta@isd.net
Judy Hawley, Contact

## Mississippi

★ **20289** ★ American Physical Therapy
   Association
**Mississippi Chapter**
921 N Congress St.
Jackson, MS 39202-2554
**Phone:** (601)354-3629          **Free:** 800-247-1106
**Fax:** (601)355-1506
**Email:** insightltd@msn.com
Deirdre McGowan, PhD, Director

## Missouri

★ **20290** ★ American Physical Therapy
   Association
**Missouri Chapter**
205 E Capitol, Ste. 100
Jefferson City, MO 65101
**Phone:** (573)556-6730          **Free:** 888-222-6782
**Fax:** (573)556-6731
**Email:** mcapta@aol.com
**Website:** http://www.mopt.org
Debbie Stover, Director

## Montana

★ **20291** ★ American Physical Therapy
   Association
**Montana Chapter**
PO Box 4553
Missoula, MT 59806-4553

**Phone:** (406)251-5232          **Fax:** (406)251-5270
**Email:** mapta@montana.com
**Website:** http://www.mapta.com
Robin Childers, Director

## Nebraska

★ **20292** ★ American Physical Therapy
   Association
**Nebraska Chapter**
PO Box 540427
Omaha, NE 68154-0427
**Phone:** (402)491-3660          **Fax:** (402)431-1372
**Email:** npta@npta.org
**Website:** http://www.npta.org
Judy Kramolisch, Director

## Nevada

★ **20293** ★ American Physical Therapy
   Association
**Nevada Chapter**
8665 W Flamingo Rd., Ste. 131
PMB 105
Las Vegas, NV 89147
**Phone:** (702)571-1535          **Fax:** (702)889-1674
**Email:** npta@infi.net
**Website:** http://www.nvapta.org
Carolyn Muse Grant, Contact

## New Hampshire

★ **20294** ★ American Physical Therapy
   Association
**New Hampshire Chapter**
PO Box 978
Manchester, NH 03105-0978
**Phone:** (603)627-7970          **Fax:** (603)627-3970
**Email:** nhapta@xtdl.com
**Website:** http://www.nhapta.org
James H. Bradley, Director

## New Jersey

★ **20295** ★ American Physical Therapy
   Association
**New Jersey Chapter**
1100 US Hwy. 130, Ste. 3
Robbinsville, NJ 08691-1108
**Phone:** (609)208-0200          **Fax:** (609)208-1000
**Email:** aptanj@aptanj.org
**Website:** http://www.aptanj.org
Judy Oiler, Director

## New York

★ **20296** ★ American Physical Therapy
   Association
**New York Chapter**
5 Palisades Dr., Ste. 330
Albany, NY 12205
**Phone:** (518)459-4499          **Free:** 800-459-4489
**Fax:** (518)459-8953
**Email:** lesliew@nypta.org
**Website:** http://www.nypta.org
Leslie J. Wood, Director

## North Carolina

★ **20297** ★ American Physical Therapy
   Association
**North Carolina Chapter**
316 W Millbrook Rd., Ste. 105
Raleigh, NC 27609
**Phone:** (919)841-0268          **Free:** 800-948-2672
**Fax:** (919)841-0269
**Email:** NCPTAHQ1@aol.com
**Website:** http://www.ncpt.org
Donna Willis, Contact

## North Dakota

★ **20298** ★ **American Physical Therapy Association**
**North Dakota Chapter**
Department of Physical Therapy
University of North Dakota
Grand Forks, ND 58202-9037
**Phone:** (701)777-3873     **Fax:** (701)777-4199
**Email:** awhite@medicine.nodak.edu
Alyson White, Director

## Ohio

★ **20299** ★ **American Physical Therapy Association**
**Ohio Chapter**
2066 W Henderson Rd., Ste. 202
Columbus, OH 43220-2452
**Phone:** (614)538-9612     **Fax:** (614)538-9614
**Email:** opt@ohiopt.org
**Website:** http://www.ohiopt.org
Nancy Garland, Contact

## Oklahoma

★ **20300** ★ **American Physical Therapy Association**
**Oklahoma Chapter**
223 W Ridgewood
Shawnee, OK 74801
**Phone:** (405)275-7588     **Fax:** (405)275-7588
**Email:** JGSecret@aol.com
Joyce Gowin, CPS, Director

## Oregon

★ **20301** ★ **American Physical Therapy Association**
**Oregon Chapter**
147 SE 102nd
Portland, OR 97216
**Phone:** (503)262-9247     **Free:** 877-492-4919
**Fax:** (503)253-9172
**Email:** opta@teleport.com
**Website:** http://www.opta.org
Sandra Fisher, CAE, Director

## Pennsylvania

★ **20302** ★ **American Physical Therapy Association**
**Pennsylvania Chapter**
4701 Devonshire Rd., Ste. 106
Harrisburg, PA 17109
**Phone:** (717)541-9169     **Fax:** (717)541-9182
**Email:** PAPTASSN@aol.com
**Website:** http://www.ppta.org
Kim Annibali, Director

## Puerto Rico

★ **20303** ★ **American Physical Therapy Association**
**Puerto Rico Chapter**
Prodriquez Olmo K-26
Arecibo, PR 00612
**Phone:** (787)854-3700     **Fax:** (787)817-6037
**Email:** damarisv@coqui.net
Damaris Vazquez, PT, President

## Rhode Island

★ **20304** ★ **American Physical Therapy Association**
**Rhode Island Chapter**
PO Box 1409
Kingston, RI 02881-0492
**Phone:** (401)874-5391     **Fax:** (401)874-5630
**Email:** RIAPTA@email.com
Bruce Goodeluck, President

## South Carolina

★ **20305** ★ **American Physical Therapy Association**
**South Carolina Chapter**
3650-A Center Cir.
Fort Mill, SC 29715
**Phone:** (803)802-5454     **Fax:** (815)371-1499
**Email:** executiveofficer@scapta.org
**Website:** http://www.scapta.org
Jane Boston, Exec Director

## South Dakota

★ **20306** ★ **American Physical Therapy Association**
**South Dakota Chapter**
PO Box 88033
Sioux Falls, SD 57109-0033
**Phone:** (605)339-4839     **Fax:** (605)357-8780
**Email:** sodakpt@aol.com
**Website:** http://www.sdpta.org
Deby McCauley, Contact

## Tennessee

★ **20307** ★ **American Physical Therapy Association**
**Tennessee Chapter**
PO Box 23071
Nashville, TN 37202
**Phone:** (615)269-5312     **Fax:** (615)297-5852
**Email:** tpta1@aol.com
**Website:** http://www.tptaonline.org
Debbie Lowenthal, Contact

## Texas

★ **20308** ★ **American Physical Therapy Association**
**New Mexico Chapter**
5125 Highlands
McKinney, TX 75070
**Email:** hjhammonds@msn.com
**Website:** http://www.nmapta.org
Holly Hammonds, Director

★ **20309** ★ **American Physical Therapy Association**
**Texas Chapter**
400 W 15th St., Ste. 805
Austin, TX 78701-1647
**Phone:** (512)477-1818     **Fax:** (512)477-1434
**Email:** weitz@tpta.org
**Website:** http://www.tpta.org
Tim Weitz, Exec Director

## Utah

★ **20310** ★ **American Physical Therapy Association**
**Utah Chapter**
2101 East 3870 South
Salt Lake City, UT 84109

**Phone:** (801)278-4016     **Fax:** (801)278-2752
**Email:** uapta@softsolutions.com
Diane Buma, Director

## Vermont

★ **20311** ★ **American Physical Therapy Association**
**Vermont Chapter**
1878 Mountain Rd., Ste. 1
Stowe, VT 05672-4775
**Phone:** (802)253-2273     **Fax:** (802)253-7754
**Email:** psweat@zoo.uvm.edu
Philip L. Sweet, PT, President

## Virginia

★ **20312** ★ **American Physical Therapy Association**
**Virginia Chapter**
1111 N Fairfax St.
Alexandria, VA 22314-1488
**Free:** 800-999-2782     **Fax:** (703)706-8575
**Email:** debbiekelly@apta.org
**Website:** http://www.vpta.org
Debbie Kelly, Director

## Washington

★ **20313** ★ **American Physical Therapy Association**
**Washington Chapter**
208 NW Rogers
Olympia, WA 98502-4940
**Phone:** (360)352-7290     **Free:** 800-554-5569
**Fax:** (206)352-7298
**Email:** caryn.porter@ptwa.org
**Website:** http://www.ptwa.org
Caryn Porter, Director

## West Virginia

★ **20314** ★ **American Physical Therapy Association**
**West Virginia Chapter**
2110 Kanawha Blvd. E, Ste. 220
Charleston, WV 25311
**Phone:** (304)345-6808     **Fax:** (304)344-4139
**Email:** jrm@wvapta.org
**Website:** http://www.movementscience.com/host_wvpta/
Nancy Tonkin, Contact

## Wisconsin

★ **20315** ★ **American Physical Therapy Association**
**Wisconsin Chapter**
802 W Broadway, Ste. 208
Madison, WI 53713
**Phone:** (608)221-9191     **Fax:** (608)221-9697
**Email:** wpta@wpta.org
**Website:** http://www.wpta.org
Karen Oshman, Director

## Wyoming

★ **20316** ★ **American Physical Therapy Association**
**Wyoming Chapter**
13475 Wisconsin
Casper, WY 82609
**Phone:** (307)235-3910
**Email:** kjbpt@touchtronics.net
**Website:** http://www.wypta.org
Kathy Brunken, PT, President

# Chapter 66
# Transplantation

## Foundations & Other Funding Organizations

### Other Funding Organizations

**★ 20317 ★ American Society of Transplantation (ASTA)**
7000 Commerce Pkwy., Ste. C
Mount Laurel, NJ 08054
**Phone:** (856)439-9986          **Fax:** (856)439-9982
**Email:** ast@ahint.com
**Website:** http://www.a-s-t.org/
Lawrence Turka, MD, Pres.
**Desc:** Promotes and encourages education and research with respect to transplantation medicine and immunology; provides a forum for exchange of scientific information related to transplantation across solid organ specialties. **Awards:** AST Fujisawa Fellowship in Transplantation (annual); AST President's Award (annual); AST Sandoz Fellowship in Transplantation (biennial); Faculty Development (annual); Novartis Fellowship in Transplantation (annual); Roche New Investigator Award (annual); Upjohn Young Investigators Award.

**★ 20318 ★ International Society for Heart and Lung Transplantation (ISHLT)**
14673 Midway Rd., Ste. 200
Addison, TX 75001
**Phone:** (972)490-9495          **Fax:** (972)490-9499
**Email:** ishlt@ishlt.org
**Website:** http://www.ishlt.org
Amanda W. Rowe, Exec. Dir.
**Desc:** Medical doctors, Ph.D.s, nurses, researchers, and others interested in artificial hearts and in heart and heart-lung failure and transplantation. Provides a center for discussion, exchange of information, and activities that promote the interests of heart and lung transplantation. Seeks to heighten awareness of public and governmental agencies regarding developments in the field. Maintains the International Heart and Lung Transplantation Registry. **Awards:** Caves Award (annual) best abstract by student/resident; Ortho Biotech/ISHLT Research Fellowship Award (annual) for young researchers; Roche/ISHLT Research Fellowship Award (annual) for young researchers.

**International Transplant Nurses Society (ITNS)**
*See:* Entry 14926

**★ 20319 ★ National Foundation for Transplants**
1102 Brookfield, Ste. 200
Memphis, TN 38119
**Phone:** (901)684-1697          **Free:** 800-489-3863
**Fax:** (901)684-1128
**Email:** jhill@transplants.org
**Website:** http://www.transplants.org
Gary McMahan, Dir.
**Desc:** Works to guide and assist fundraising for transplant patients and their families. Offers grants for smaller emergency transplants and medication needs. Provides financial support and advocacy. **Awards:** Medications Grants and Emergency Grants (monthly) transplant candidates or transplant recipients with one-time (not ongoing) need for medications or other transplant-related emergencies. Must be verified by a medical professional.

**★ 20320 ★ Transplant Recipients International Organization (TRIO)**
2117 L St. NW, Ste. 353
Washington, DC 20037-1524
**Phone:** (202)293-0980          **Free:** 800-TRIO-386
**Fax:** (202)239-8727
**Email:** TRIOIntl@aol.com
**Website:** http://www.trioweb.org
Lisa Kory, Exec. Dir.
**Desc:** Transplant candidates, recipients, family members, donor families, and medical personnel. Provides support and medical information to patients and their families. Conducts educational programs. **Awards:** Scholarship (annual); Thomas Starzl Humanitarian Award (annual) for a person who has greatly influenced the field of transplantation.

## National & International Organizations

**★ 20321 ★ American Association of Tissue Banks (AATB)**
1350 Beverly Rd., Ste. 220-A
Mc Lean, VA 22101
**Phone:** (703)827-9582          **Free:** 800-635-2282
**Fax:** (703)356-2198
**Email:** aatb@aatb.org
**Website:** http://www.aatb.org
Duke Kasprisin, MD, Pres.
**Fnded:** 1976. **Mem:** 1,200. **Desc:** Goals are to encourage the development of regional tissue banks and the establishment of guidelines and standards for the retrieval, preservation, storage, and distribution of tissues for transplantation. **Pub:** *AATB Membership Directory*, annual. Membership Directory. Lists individuals and institutions. *Price:* Included in membership dues. • *AATB Newsletter*, quarterly. Newsletter. *Price:* Available to members only. • *American Association of Tissue Banks–Technical Manual*, periodic. • *Standards for Tissue Banking*, periodic.

**American Society of Transplant Surgeons**
*See:* Entry 19501

**★ 20322 ★ American Society of Transplantation (ASTA)**
7000 Commerce Pkwy., Ste. C
Mount Laurel, NJ 08054
**Phone:** (856)439-9986          **Fax:** (856)439-9982
**Email:** ast@ahint.com
**Website:** http://www.a-s-t.org/
Lawrence Turka, MD, Pres.
**Fnded:** 1982. **Mem:** 1,300. **Desc:** Promotes and encourages education and research with respect to transplantation medicine and immunology; provides a forum for exchange of scientific information related to transplantation across solid organ specialties. **Pub:** *AST Newsletter*, quarterly. Newsletter. *Price:* Included in membership dues. • *AST Primer on Transplantation.* • *AST Washington Round-Up*, monthly.

**★ 20323 ★ American Transplant Association (ATA)**
980 N Michigan Ave., Ste. 1400
Chicago, IL 60611
**Free:** 800-494-4527          **Fax:** 800-494-4527
**Email:** ata@americantransplant.org
**Website:** http://www.americantransplant.org/
John Butorac, Exec. Dir.
**Fnded:** 1995. **Mem:** 1,200. **Desc:** Provides patient-oriented education, services and support to transplant patients and their families and friends. **Pub:** *A Patient's Guide to Transplantation*. Book. *Price:* $10 nonmember. • *reOrganized!*, monthly. Newsletter. • *Transcend*, 3/year. Newsletter. For contributors and supporters.

**★ 20324 ★ Asian Society of Transplantation (AST)**
Department of General Surgery
College of Medicine
Yonsei University
CPO Box 8044
Seoul 120-752, Republic of Korea
**Lang(s):** English, Korean. **Desc:** Physicians and other health care personnel with an interest in transplantation. Promotes advancement in transplantation techniques and technologies. Serves as a clearinghouse on transplantation; conducts research and educational programs.

**★ 20325 ★ Association of Nurses Endorsing Transplantation (ANET)**
PO Box 541234
Merritt Island, FL 32954-1234
**Phone:** (321)459-3777          **Fax:** (321)459-3777
**Website:** http://www.anetonline.org
Mary Gainey, RNC, Exec. Dir.
**Fnded:** 1983. **Mem:** 75. **Desc:** Registered nurses, LVNs, LPNs, student nurses, chaplains, social workers, hospitals, health care facilities. Promotes organ and tissue donation for transplantation and research. **Pub:** *ANET Newsletter*, quarterly. Newsletter. • *Handbook*, annual. **Frmly:** (1983) Consortium of Registered Nurses for Eye Acquisition.

**★ 20326 ★ Association of Organ Procurement Organizations (AOPO)**
1364 Beverly Rd., Ste. 100
Mc Lean, VA 22101
**Phone:** (703)573-2676          **Fax:** (703)573-0578

**Email:** organdonation@aopo.org
**Website:** http://www.aopo.org
Paul M. Schwab, Exec. Dir.
**Fnded:** 1984. **Mem:** 59. **Desc:** Works to represent and serve organ procurement organizations to maximize the availability of organs and tissues and enhance the quality and effectiveness of the donation process. Establishes organizational and ethical standards for OPOs; offers accreditation; provides status reports of federal legislative activities; disseminates information on federal policies and technical advancements; conducts educational programs. **Pub:** *AOPO Update*, monthly. Newsletter. • Membership Directory.

★ **20327** ★ **British Association of Hair Transplant Surgeons**
125 Worlds End Land
Quinton
Birmingham B32 1JX, United Kingdom
**Desc:** Promotes the science of hair transplantation.

★ **20328** ★ **Center for Organ Recovery and Education (CORE)**
204 Sigma Dr.
Ridc Park
Pittsburgh, PA 15238
**Free:** 800-366-6777    **Fax:** (412)963-3563
**Email:** pkornick@core.org
**Website:** http://www.core.org
Pat Kornick, VP, Corporate Development
**Fnded:** 1977. **Desc:** Manages organ, tissue and eye donation activities. Offers families the opportunity to donate; coordinates the surgical recovery of the organs, tissue and eyes, and facilitates the computerized matching of donating organs and placement of corneas. Maintains permanent tribute to donors. Sponsors continuing education programs for health professionals in regional hospitals and associations. Also provides speakers for presentation to civic organizations and schools or corporations. **Pub:** *The COREnection*, quarterly. Newsletter. • Pamphlets. • Also publishes protocols. **Frmly:** (1984) Transplant Organ Procurement Organization; (1992) Pittsburgh Transplant Foundation.

**Children's Organ Transplant Association (COTA)**
*See:* Entry 5663

**European Dialysis and Transplant Nurses Association/European Renal Care Association (EDTNA/ERCA)**
*See:* Entry 15708

**European Federation for Immunogenetics (EFI)**
*See:* Entry 3210

★ **20329** ★ **European Heart Transplant Federation (EHTF)**
Rue St Eleuthere 52
7500 Tournai, Belgium
**Phone:** 32 6 9235179    **Fax:** 32 6 9235157
**Email:** ihbsecr@euronet.nl
**Website:** http://www.edtna-erca.org
**Fnded:** 1994. **Desc:** Encourages education and research relevant to organ transplantation.

★ **20330** ★ **European Transplant Coordinators Organization (ETCO)**
Steenveldstraat 18
B-3210 Linden, Belgium
**Phone:** 32 16 622110    **Fax:** 32 16 622981
**Email:** etco.trekels@unicall.be
**Website:** http://www.etco.org
**Lang(s):** Dutch, English, French. **Desc:** Professionals working in the field of tissue procurement and transplantation; other interested individuals. Seeks to increase the availability of human tissues and organs for

transplantation; promotes professional advancement of members. Serves as a clearinghouse on tissue procurement and transplantation; facilitates communication and cooperation among members; sponsors educational programs; compiles statistics. **Pub:** Journal, periodic.

★ **20331** ★ **Eurotransplant International Foundation (EIF)**
c/o Mrs. V. Diepeveen, Sec.
PO Box 2304
NL-2301 CH Leiden, Netherlands
**Phone:** 31 71 5795795    **Fax:** 31 71 5790057
**Email:** verena@eurotransplant.nl
**Website:** http://www.eurotransplant.nl
**Fnded:** 1966. **Lang(s):** English. **Desc:** International non-profit organ exchange organization. **Pub:** *Eurotransplant Newsletter*, monthly.

**Eye Bank Association of America (EBAA)**
*See:* Entry 20952

**Eye-Bank for Sight Restoration (EBSR)**
*See:* Entry 20953

★ **20332** ★ **International Bone Marrow Transplant Registry (IBMTR)**
8701 Watertown Plank Rd.
PO Box 26509
Milwaukee, WI 53226
**Phone:** (414)456-8325    **Fax:** (414)456-6530
**Email:** ibmtr@mcw.edu
**Website:** http://www.ibmtr.org
Mary M. Horowitz, MD, MS, Scientific Dir.
**Fnded:** 1972. **Mem:** 450. **Desc:** Voluntary organizations of basic and clinical scientists. Working to address important issues in blood and marrow transplantation. Gathers information on results of blood and marrow transplants; Information is used to guide clinical decisions and identify the most effective treatment strategies for individual patients based on a number of variables including age, disease type and stage, prior treatment, etc. **Pub:** *IBMTR/ABMTR Newsletter*, semiannual. Newsletter.

★ **20333** ★ **International Liver Transplantation Society (ILTS)**
17000 Commerce Parkway, Ste. C
Mount Laurel, NJ 08054
**Phone:** (856)439-0500    **Fax:** (856)439-0524
**Email:** ilts@ahint.com
**Website:** http://www.ilts.org
William T. Merritt, MD, Pres.
**Fnded:** 1992. **Mem:** 700. **Desc:** Individuals interested in liver transplantation. Seeks to educate members on liver transplantation. Offers post graduate courses and mini-symposia. **Pub:** *Liver Transplantation and Surgery*, bimonthly. Journal.

★ **20334** ★ **International Society for Heart and Lung Transplantation (ISHLT)**
14673 Midway Rd., Ste. 200
Addison, TX 75001
**Phone:** (972)490-9495    **Fax:** (972)490-9499
**Email:** ishlt@ishlt.org
**Website:** http://www.ishlt.org
Amanda W. Rowe, Exec. Dir.
**Fnded:** 1981. **Mem:** 2,250. **Desc:** Medical doctors, Ph.D.s, nurses, researchers, and others interested in artificial hearts and in heart and heart-lung failure and transplantation. Provides a center for discussion, exchange of information, and activities that promote the interests of heart and lung transplantation. Seeks to heighten awareness of public and governmental agencies regarding developments in the field. Maintains the International Heart and Lung Transplantation Registry. **Pub:** *The Journal of Heart and Lung Transplantation*, monthly. Journal. **Frmly:** (1991) International Society for Heart Transplantation.

★ **20335** ★ **International Transplant Coordinators Society (ITCS)**
CPTC, Univ Hospital Gasthuisberg
3000 Leuven, Belgium
**Phone:** 32 1 6344596    **Fax:** 32 1 6344590
**Email:** donoraction_lr@compuserve.com
**Website:** http://www.kuleuven.ac.be/facdep/medicine/itcs/Home.html
**Desc:** Creates a structure that could respond to transplant coordination issues at international meetings.

**International Transplant Nurses Society (ITNS)**
*See:* Entry 15725

★ **20336** ★ **Japanese Society for Artificial Organs**
Society Center C21
5-16-9 honkomagome
Bunkyo-ku
Tokyo 113, Japan
**Phone:** 81 3 58145801    **Fax:** 81 3 58145820
**Email:** itns@msn.com
**Website:** http://www.itns.org
**Fnded:** 1962. **Mem:** 4,000. **Desc:** Promotes the use of artificial organs in transplantation. **Pub:** *Journal of Artificial Organs*, semiannual. Journal.

★ **20337** ★ **LifeBanc**
20600 Chagrin Blvd., Ste. 350
Cleveland, OH 44122-5343
**Phone:** (216)752-5433    **Free:** 888-558-5433
**Fax:** (216)751-4204
**Email:** info@lifebanc.org
**Website:** http://www.lifebanc.org
Debbie May-Johnson, Exec. Dir.
**Fnded:** 1986. **Desc:** Responsible for all aspects of the organ donation program - evaluation, management, procurement and subsequent use of organs and tissue for transplantation, as well as providing bereavement services for donor families. Mission is to increase organ and tissue donation for those awaiting transplant, to provide community and professional education to people of all ages about the need for, and the benefits of, organ and tissue donation, and to respect and support those individuals and families whose generosity and compassion make it possible to improve and save the lives of others. **Pub:** Pamphlets.

★ **20338** ★ **The Living Bank International (TLB)**
PO Box 6725
Houston, TX 77265-6725
**Phone:** (713)961-9431    **Free:** 800-528-2971
**Fax:** (713)961-0979
**Email:** info@livingbank.org
**Website:** http://www.livingbank.org
Jon Echie, Pres. /CEO
**Fnded:** 1968. **Mem:** 326,000. **Desc:** Open to anyone who wishes to donate organs and/or tissues at time of death. Provides a centralized registry for people who want to donate organs/tissues at the time of death. Those interested in becoming donors can request donor registration forms on which they specify which organs and/or tissues they will donate and any limitations or special wishes. Document must be signed by two witnesses. Donors receive an organ donor card which is carried by the individual at all times and which indicates that the person is registered with The Living Bank. If death is imminent or has occurred, The Living Bank is notified and one of their staff members refers the situation to the closest organ procurement organization or other appropriate agency. The organ procurement organization makes the decision regarding what can and cannot be used for transplant. The major types of transplants that are currently being performed include cornea, skin, heart, liver, kidney, intestine, pancreas, and lung transplants. For individuals wishing to donate their whole bodies for anatomical research and study, they should contact The Living Bank for information on how to register with the

nearest medical school. Due to many of the body donor programs being full, many medical schools now require that you be pre-registered. Operates speakers bureau in communities throughout the country. **Pub:** *Bank Account*, quarterly. Newsletter. Includes news updates on advances in the fields of organ donation and transplantation. *Price:* Free. • Brochures. • Also publishes educational and informational materials. **Frmly:** (2001) The Living Bank.

**★ 20339 ★ Mexican Association for Promoting Kidney Transplant (Asociacio Mexicana Protransplante Renal — AMPRAC)**
Yacatas 387
Col. Navarte
03020 Mexico City, Mexico
**Phone:** 52 55 435946     **Fax:** 52 55 432818
**Fnded:** 1997. **Desc:** Offers support to kidney patients and their families. Promotes organ donation. Disseminates information.

**★ 20340 ★ National Foundation for Transplants**
1102 Brookfield, Ste. 200
Memphis, TN 38119
**Phone:** (901)684-1697     **Free:** 800-489-3863
**Fax:** (901)684-1128
**Email:** jhill@transplants.org
**Website:** http://www.transplants.org
Gary McMahan, Dir.

**Fnded:** 1983. **Desc:** Works to guide and assist fundraising for transplant patients and their families. Offers grants for smaller emergency transplants and medication needs. Provides financial support and advocacy. **Frmly:** (1999) Organ Transplant Fund.

**★ 20341 ★ National Marrow Donor Program (NMDP)**
3001 Broadway NE, Ste. 500
Minneapolis, MN 55413-1753
**Phone:** 888-999-6743     **Free:** 800-627-7692
**Website:** http://www.marrow.org
Jeffrey W. Chell, MD, CEO

**Fnded:** 1986. **Mem:** 450. **Desc:** Facilitates unrelated donor stem cell transplants for patients with life-threatening blood diseases who do not have matching donors in their families. Facilitates more than 100 transplants each month. Provides a single point of access for all sources of blood stem cells used in transplantation: marrow, peripheral blood, and umbilical cord blood. The Registry is able to search its own database and provides physicians with information on multiple stem cell sources for life-saving transplants. Since 1987, the NMDP has recruited a diverse Registry of approximately four million potential volunteer marrow and blood stem cell donors, provided transplants to more than 9,000 patients, developed education and recruitment initiatives to increase the diversity of the Registry, increased the number of minority patients receiving transplants each year, developed patient advocacy services, established a system of listing cord blood units within its own national Registry. Materials are available free of charge for both potential donors and patients. There is access to interpreters in over 141 languages for these materials. **Pub:** *Living Gift of Life*. Brochure. • *Marrow Messenger*, annual. • *Medical Professionals's Guide to Unrelated Marrow Transplantation*. • *The Missing Piece*, annual. Brochure. • Brochures. **Frmly:** National Bone Marrow Donor Registry.

**★ 20342 ★ North American Society for Dialysis and Transplantation (NASDT)**
c/o Dr. Wadi Suki
6550 Fannin, Ste. 1273
Houston, TX 77030
**Phone:** (713)790-3275     **Fax:** (713)790-5053
**Website:** http://www.asts.org/ethics.cfm
Dr. Wadi Suki, Sec.-Treas.

**Fnded:** 1981. **Mem:** 200. **Desc:** Professionals active in the area of teaching, manufacturing, and administra-

tion in the fields of nephrology and transplantation including nephrologists, transplant surgeons and physicians, registered nurses, dialysis nurses, and transplant coordinators. Promotes education and research and disseminates current knowledge and technology in the field of kidney dialysis and transplantation.

**★ 20343 ★ North American Transplant Coordinators Organization (NATCO)**
PO Box 15384
Shawnee Mission, KS 66285-5384
**Phone:** (913)492-3600     **Fax:** (913)599-5340
**Email:** natco-info@goamp.com
**Website:** http://www.natco1.org
Judy M. Graham, Pres.

**Fnded:** 1979. **Mem:** 1,800. **Desc:** Nurses and allied health professionals working with organ recipients and those working to obtain and distribute human organs and tissues to waiting victims of end-stage organ failure. Seeks to influence increased procurement and use of transplantable organs and tissues under the direction of individuals and institutions responsible for the employment of members. Disseminates information to members, medical personnel, technicians, and the public regarding the benefits of organ transplantation, new techniques in organ procurement, advancements in immunology and preservation, transplant surgery, and other aspects of organ transplantation. Promotes and supports training and development programs for new transplant coordinators. Sponsors seminars, workshops, and annual training course on procurement for transplant coordinators. Offers job referral information. **Pub:** *NATCO–InTouch*, bimonthly. Newsletter. Includes calendar of events, employment opportunity listings, legislative updates, and conference reports. *Price:* Included in membership dues. • *North American Transplant Coordinators Organization–Membership Directory*, annual. Directory. *Price:* Included in membership dues. • *Progress in Transplantation*, QRT. Journal. Includes clinical articles addressing transplantation issues.

**★ 20344 ★ Tissue Banks International (TBI)**
815 Park Ave.
Baltimore, MD 21201-4887
**Phone:** (410)783-0183     **Free:** 800-756-4824
**Fax:** (410)454-4457
**Email:** tbi@tbionline.org
**Website:** http://www.tbionline.org
Gerald Cole, Pres. /CEO

**Fnded:** 1962. **Mem:** 76. **Desc:** A non-profit network of medical eye and tissue banks. Provides eye tissue for sight-restoring corneal transplant surgery. Also distributes bone, skin, and other soft tissues. Assists members with operational areas. Provides grants for research into the causes and cures of blindness. Distributes information on eye, tissue, and organ donation. Conducts educational and charitable programs. **Pub:** Brochure.

**★ 20345 ★ Transplant Recipients International Organization (TRIO)**
2117 L St. NW, Ste. 353
Washington, DC 20037-1524
**Phone:** (202)293-0980     **Free:** 800-TRIO-386
**Fax:** (415)239-8727
**Email:** TRIOIntl@aol.com
**Website:** http://www.trioweb.org
Lisa Kory, Exec. Dir.

**Fnded:** 1987. **Mem:** 3,500. **Nat'l Groups:** 1. **Reg. Groups:** 6. **Desc:** Transplant candidates, recipients, family members, donor families, and medical personnel. Provides support and medical information to patients and their families. Conducts educational programs. **Pub:** *TRIO Lifelines*, bimonthly. Newsletter. Includes chapter activities and current transplantation news.

**★ 20346 ★ Transplantation Society (TS)**
Central Business Office
205 Viger Ave. W, Ste. 201
Montreal, QC, Canada H2Z 1G2
**Phone:** (514)874-1998     **Fax:** (514)874-1580
**Email:** info@transplantation-soc.org
**Website:** http://www.transplantation-soc.org/new/default4.htm

**Fnded:** 1966. **Mem:** 1,400. **Lang(s):** English. **Desc:** Physicians and scientists who have made significant contributions to the advancement of knowledge in transplantation biology and medicine. Purpose is to further information in the general area of transplantation biology and medicine, with related interests in cancer immunology and host responses to infectious microorganisms. **Pub:** *Transplantation Proceedings*, bimonthly. Proceedings.

**★ 20347 ★ United Network for Organ Sharing (UNOS)**
1100 Boulders Pky., Ste. 500
PO Box 13770
Richmond, VA 23225-8770
**Phone:** (804)327-1432     **Free:** 888-TX1-NF01
**Fax:** (804)323-7343
**Email:** editor@unos.org
**Website:** http://www.unos.org
Jeremiah G. Turcotte, MD, Pres.

**Fnded:** 1984. **Mem:** 434. **Reg. Groups:** 11. **Desc:** Transplant and organ procurement centers, tissue-typing labs, and health care professionals engaged in organ transplant operations. Administers the National Organ Procurement and Transplantation Network and the U.S. Scientific Registry for Organ Transplantation, as mandated by law under contract with the U.S. Department of Health and Human Services. Maintains national waiting list for transplant candidates. Operates the Organ Center, which matches patients in need of transplants with donated organs. Formulates and implements national policies on equitable access and organ allocation and organ procurement standards. Conducts professional education courses for transplant personnel. Maintains and publicizes national statistics on organ donation and transplantation. **Pub:** *UNOS Update*, monthly. Magazine. *Price:* Free to domestic subscribers. **AKA:** UNOS.

# Research Centers

**★ 20348 ★ Baylor University Medical Center**
**Blood and Bone Marrow Transplant Program**
3535 Worth St., Ste. 185
Dallas, TX 75246
**Phone:** (214)820-2610     **Fax:** (214)820-7346
**Website:** http://www.bhcs.com/bits/bonemarrow/bonemarrow.html
Joseph W. Fay, MD, Dir.

**Activities/Fields:** Bone marrow transplantation research in leukemia/lymphoma studies, including graft-vs-host disease, evaluation of immune recovery post transplant, evaluation of growth factors in transplantation, and applications of molecular biology/gene rearrangement in marrow transplantation, and dendritic cell transplantation.

**★ 20349 ★ Blood and Marrow Transplant Laboratory**
Children's Hospital of Orange County
455 S Main St.
Orange, CA 92868
**Phone:** (714)289-4060     **Fax:** (714)516-4277
**Email:** vslone@choc.org
Dr. Leonard Sender, Dir.

**Activities/Fields:** Bone marrow immunology experiments, including tumor purging using chemotherapy and monoclonal antibodies, molecular detection of minimal residual disease, purification of hematopoietic stem cells, and purging and cultivation of bone marrow. Also studies umbilical cord blood harvesting, storage, and expansion; and T-cell depletion for unrelated bone marrow transplantation. **Frmly:** Bone Marrow Transplant Laboratory.

**Connecticut Eye Bank and Visual Research Foundation, Inc.**
*See:* Entry 21096

**Edward Dana Mitchell Surgical Research Laboratory**
*See:* Entry 19615

★ **20350** ★ **Loyola University Chicago**
**Heart Transplant and Heart Failure Program**
2160 S 1st Ave.
Maywood, IL 60153
**Phone:** (708)216-4810 **Fax:** (708)327-2770
**Email:** mmullen@luc.edu
**Website:** http://www.cteyebank.org
Dr. G. Martin Mullen, Dir.
**Activities/Fields:** Cardiac transplantation and immunology, including allograft rejection, vascular diseases, and transplant tolerance.

★ **20351** ★ **McGill University**
**Division of Transplantation**
687 Ave. des Pins Ouest
Montreal, QC, Canada H3A 1A1
**Phone:** (514)843-1649 **Fax:** (514)843-1708
**Email:** rolf.loertscher@mcgill.ca
Rolf Loertscher, MD, Dir.
**Activities/Fields:** Performs joint clinical trials in organ transplantation, conducts autoimmunity and other immunobiology/immunogenetics studies, formulates public policy objectives regarding organ grafting, examines the ethical and legal aspects of transplantation and allocation of scarce resources, and evaluates the cost-effectiveness of transplantation programs. Develops computer expert systms for medical diagnosis and medical education. Also centralizes patient data and results of McGill Teaching Hospital programs, serves as an administrative clearinghouse for patient samples and data, and facilitates interaction among the basic science laboratories at the University's Medical School.

★ **20352** ★ **Microsurgical Transplantation Research Foundation**
Davies Medical Center, Mob Annex 140
45 Castro St.
San Francisco, CA 94114
**Phone:** (415)565-6136 **Fax:** (415)864-1654
**Email:** pps@the-buncke-clinic.com
Dr. Harry J. Buncke, Dir.
**Activities/Fields:** Physiological and technical outcomes of microvascular replantation and transplantation; reconstructive microsurgery, and hand surgery; cryopreservation of tissues; hyperbaric oxygen therapy; and tissue oximetry with ischemia/perfusion injury.

★ **20353** ★ **National Institute of Transplantation**
2200 W 3rd St., Ste. 100
Los Angeles, CA 90057-1922
**Phone:** (213)413-2779 **Fax:** (213)484-6652

**Website:** http://www.transplantation.com
Robert Mendez, MD, Dir.
**Activities/Fields:** Kidney and pancreas transplantation and new approaches to organ transplantation and avoiding organ rejection. **Pub:** *Miracle of Life Newsletter*, quarterly. • *NIT Newsletter*, biennially.

★ **20354** ★ **Oregon Health and Science University**
**Transplant and Immunogenetics Laboratory**
2611 SW 3rd, Ste. 360
Portland, OR 97201
**Phone:** (503)494-8394 **Fax:** (503)494-7695
**Email:** normand@ohsu.edu
Douglas Norman, MD, Dir.
**Activities/Fields:** Human immunobiology of organ transplantation.

★ **20355** ★ **Stanford University**
**Laboratory for Transplantation Immunology**
Falk Cardiovascular Research Bldg.
Department of Cardiothoracic Surgery
School of Medicine
300 Pasteur Dr.
Palo Alto, CA 94305-5407
**Phone:** (650)498-6391 **Fax:** (650)725-3826
**Email:** rem@stanfordl.edu
Dr. Randall E. Morris, Dir.
**Activities/Fields:** Development of compounds to reduce rejection of transplanted organs. Studies focus on small molecules, monoclonal antibodies, and naturally occurring substances.

**U.S. Department of Health and Human Services**
**National Institute of Allergy and Infectious Diseases (NIAID)**
**Division of Allergy, Immunology, and Transplantation**
**Genetics and Transplantation Branch**
*See:* Entry 3276

★ **20356** ★ **University of Calgary**
**Joint Injury and Arthritis Research Group**
436 Heritage Medical Research Bldg.
3330 Hospital Dr. NW
Calgary, AB, Canada T2N 4N1
**Phone:** (403)220-8666
**Email:** rcbray@ucalgary.ca
**Website:** http://joint.mccaig.ucalgary.ca/jiarg/
Dr. Robert Bray, Ch.
**Activities/Fields:** Biological and nonbiological transplants of joints and ligaments and electrical stimulation of injured tissues, including studies of joint reconstruction, gait analysis, sports medicine and athletic injuries, inherited connective tissue diseases, osteoarthritis and rheumatism.

★ **20357** ★ **University of California, Los Angeles**
**Marrow and Stem Cell Transplantation Program**
Center for Health Science
Los Angeles, CA 90095-1678
**Phone:** (310)206-5755 **Fax:** (310)206-5511
**Email:** mterrito@medmet.ucla.edu

**Website:** http://www.cancer.mednet.ucla.edu/hematbmt/
Mary Territo, MD, Dir.
**Activities/Fields:** Treatment of leukemia, lymphoma, myeloma, breast cancer, solid tumors, and aplastic anemia. Evaluates the use of bone marrow, cord blood, and stem cell transplantation as treatment for a number of hematologic and malignant diseases. **Frmly:** University of California, Los Angeles - Bone Marrow Transplantation Program.

★ **20358** ★ **University of California, San Diego**
**Center for Transplantation**
200 W Arbor Dr.
San Diego, CA 92103-8745
**Phone:** (619)294-6257
**Email:** kkrzeminski@ucsd.edu
**Website:** http://www.health.ucsd.edu/transplant/
Mary Cunanan, Exec. Dir.
**Activities/Fields:** Immunosuppressive and anti-infection drugs, the development of extra conporeal liver assist technologies, the biology of rejection, organ preservation, and the long-term medical problems of transplant recipients.

**University of California, San Francisco**
**Immunogenetics and Transplantation Laboratory**
*See:* Entry 3299

★ **20359** ★ **University of Louisville**
**Institute for Cellular Therapeutics**
570 S Preston St., Ste. 404
Louisville, KY 40202
**Phone:** (502)453-7823
**Email:** stilds01@gwise.edu
**Website:** http://louisville.edu
Suzanne T. Ildstad, MD, Dir.
**Activities/Fields:** Stem cell biology and bone marrow transplantation to fight disease. **Pub:** *Newsletter*, semiannually.

★ **20360** ★ **University of Pittsburgh Medical Center**
**Thomas E. Starzl Transplantation Institute**
Falk Medical Bldg., 4th Fl.
3601 5th Ave.
Pittsburgh, PA 15213
**Phone:** (412)648-3200 **Free:** 877-640-6746
**Fax:** (412)648-3085
**Email:** sticlinic@msx.upmc.edu
**Website:** http://www.sti.upmc.edu/Overview/about_sti.htm
John J. Fung, MD, CEO
**Activities/Fields:** All aspects of the transplantation of organs, including islet cell transplantation, bioartificial organ development, xenotransplantation, immunosuppression, organ preservation, immunobiology of rejection, mechanisms of tolerance and chronic rejection, autoimmunity. **Pub:** *Manuscripts.* • *Chapters.* • *Books.*

## Federal Government Agencies

**U.S. Department of Health and Human Services**
**National Institutes of Health (NIH)**
**National Institute of Diabetes, Digestive and Kidney Diseases (NIDDK)**
*See:* Entry 8657

## Foundations & Other Funding Organizations

### Corporate Foundations

**Genentech Foundation for Biomedical Sciences**
*See:* Entry 1079

### Other Funding Organizations

**★ 20361 ★ American Urogynecologic Society (AUGS)**
2025 M St. NW, Ste. 800
Washington, DC 20036
**Phone:** (202)367-1167      **Fax:** (202)367-2167
**Email:** augs@dc.sba.com
**Website:** http://www.augs.org
Steven C. Kemp, Exec. Dir.
**Desc:** Physicians and health professionals actively engaged in providing quality urogynecologic care to women. Dedicated to research and education in urogynecology and to improved care for women with lower urinary tract disorders. **Awards:** Health Science Award (annual).

**★ 20362 ★ Interstitial Cystitis Association (ICA)**
110 N Washington St., No. 340
Rockville, MD 20850-2239
**Phone:** (301)610-5300      **Free:** 800-HEL-PICA
**Fax:** (301)610-5308
**Email:** icamail@ichelp.org
**Website:** http://www.ichelp.org
**Desc:** Support network for patients suffering or suspected of suffering from interstitial cystitis, an inflammation of the bladder wall that primarily affects women; its cause and cure are unknown. Works to inform the public and especially the medical profession about the seriousness of IC. Raises funds for research into treatments and cures; maintains a medical advisory board. Is establishing a national registry to record facts about IC. **Awards:** Pilot Award for worthy research connected.

**★ 20363 ★ Society of Women in Urology**
c/o Wendy J. Weiser
1111 N Plaza Dr., Ste. 550
Schaumburg, IL 60173-4946
**Phone:** (847)517-7225      **Fax:** (847)517-7229
**Email:** swiu@wjweiser.com
Wendy Weiser, Contact
**Desc:** Women working in the field of urology. **Awards:** Elisabeth Pickett Research Award (annual) for urology based.

## National & International Organizations

**★ 20364 ★ African Association of Nephrology (AAN)**
Service de Medecine Interne et de Nephrologie
Hopital Charles Nicolle
PO Box 290 Mahrajene
1082 Tunis, Tunisia
**Lang(s):** Arabic, English, French. **Desc:** Nephrologists and other scientists and health care professionals with an interest in nephrology. Seeks to advance the study, teaching, and practice of nephrology; promotes continuing professional development of members. Facilitates communication and cooperation among members; sponsors research and educational programs; makes available health care services.

**★ 20365 ★ American Association of Clinical Urologists (AACU)**
1111 N Plaza Dr., No. 550
Schaumburg, IL 60173-6021
**Phone:** (847)517-1050      **Fax:** (847)517-7229
**Email:** aacu@wjweiser.com
**Website:** http://aacuweb.org
Wendy J. Weiser, Exec. Dir.
**Fnded:** 1970. **Mem:** 5,600. **Desc:** Clinical urologists who are members of the American Urological Association or its sections and the American Medical Association. Purposes are to stimulate interest in the science and practice of urology and to promote understanding of socioeconomic and political affairs affecting medical practice. Does not abstract statistical information or function as a referral service for people with urological/medical problems. **Pub:** *AACU Fax*, 3-4/year. Newsletter. • *AACU News*. • *Membership Roster*, annual. • Journal, bimonthly.

**★ 20366 ★ American Association of Kidney Patients (AAKP)**
3505 E Frontage Rd., Ste. 315
Tampa, FL 33607
**Phone:** (813)636-8100      **Free:** 800-749-2257
**Fax:** (813)636-8100
**Email:** info@aakp.org
**Website:** http://www.aakp.org
Kris Robinson, Exec. Dir.
**Fnded:** 1969. **Mem:** 8,000. **Local Groups:** 24. **Desc:** Persons on hemodialysis, peritoneal dialysis, and with kidney transplants; their families and friends; professionals in the renal community. Educates the patient and the public regarding kidney disease; works for improved quality of care for all patients; promotes a donor program. **Pub:** *AAKPRENALIFE*, bimonthly. Magazine. *Price:* $25. • *Americans with Disabilities Act of 1990*. Brochure. Explains the Americans with Disabilities Act. • *Blood Chemistry Levels*. Brochure. • *Dietary Counters*. Brochure. • Also publishes other informational materials including care of the kidneys, treatment options and conditions that may affect the kidneys. **Frmly:** National Association of Patients on Hemodialysis; National Association of Patients on Hemodialysis and Transplantation.

**★ 20367 ★ American Board of Urology (ABU)**
2216 Ivy Rd., Ste. 210
Charlottesville, VA 22903
**Phone:** (804)979-0059      **Fax:** (804)979-0266
**Website:** http://www.abu.org
Stuart S. Howards, MD, Exec. Sec.
**Fnded:** 1935. **Mem:** 12. **Desc:** Conducts examinations and certifies physicians in the specialty of urology (branch of medicine that is concerned with the genito-urinary tract). **Pub:** *Information for Applicants and Candidates*, annual. Includes certification details and schedule of exams.

**★ 20368 ★ American Foundation for Urologic Disease (AFUD)**
1128 N Charles St.
Baltimore, MD 21201
**Phone:** (410)468-1800      **Free:** 800-242-2383
**Fax:** (410)468-1808
**Email:** admin@afud.org
**Website:** http://www.afud.org
Thomas Bruckman, Exec. Dir.
**Fnded:** 1987. **Desc:** Medical research and education organization working to broaden the base of urological research and enhance public and health care providers awareness of urologic disease in the U.S. Conducts public educational programs on topics including childhood urological problems, prostate disease, and bladder disorders. Encourages advocacy among prostate cancer survivors. Makes available research fellowships and grants.

**★ 20369 ★ American Kidney Fund (AKF)**
6110 Executive Blvd., Ste. 1010
Rockville, MD 20852
**Phone:** (301)881-3052      **Free:** 800-638-8299
**Fax:** (301)881-0898
**Email:** helpline@akfinc.org
**Website:** http://www.akfinc.org
Karen M. Sendelback, CFRE, Exec. Dir.
**Fnded:** 1971. **Reg. Groups:** 1. **Desc:** Works to alleviate the financial burdens caused by kidney disease; improve the quality of life for kidney patients; promote kidney health care nationwide. Provides direct financial assistance to needy kidney disease

victims with costs specific to their treatment. Funds are raised through direct mail from the public. Supports dialysis center emergency funds. Programs include: American Kidney Fund Clinical Scientist in Nephrology program, which provides assistance to nephrology students pursuing scholarship in the provision of clinical care; patient and community services; public and professional education; kidney donor development; and clinical research. **Pub:** *American Kidney Fund–Annual Report*, annual. Annual Report. *Price:* Free. • *Clinical Strategies Newsletter for Health Professionals*, semiannual. Newsletter. *Price:* Free. • Brochures.

**American Nephrology Nurses' Association (ANNA)**
*See:* Entry 15650

★ **20370** ★ **American Society of Nephrology (ASN)**
2025 M St. NW, No. 800
Washington, DC 20036-2422
**Phone:** (202)367-1190          **Fax:** (202)367-2190
**Email:** asn@dc.sba.com
**Website:** http://www.asn-online.org/
Karen Campbell, Exec. Dir.
**Fnded:** 1966. **Mem:** 7,500. **Desc:** Nephrologists united for the exchange of scientific information. Seeks to contribute to the education of members and to improve the quality of patient care. Conducts educational courses. Maintains placement service. **Pub:** *Abstracts and Program*, annual. Journal. Program and abstracts for annual scientific meeting. *Price:* $35. • *ASN Highlights*, quarterly. Newsletter. • *Journal of the American Society of Nephrology*, monthly. Journal. • *Member Resource Directory*, periodic. Membership Directory.

★ **20371** ★ **American Urogynecologic Society (AUGS)**
2025 M St. NW, Ste. 800
Washington, DC 20036
**Phone:** (202)367-1167          **Fax:** (202)367-2167
**Email:** augs@dc.sba.com
**Website:** http://www.augs.org
Steven C. Kemp, Exec. Dir.
**Fnded:** 1979. **Mem:** 950. **Desc:** Physicians and health professionals actively engaged in providing quality urogynecologic care to women. Dedicated to research and education in urogynecology and to improved care for women with lower urinary tract disorders. **Pub:** *Quarterly Report*, quarterly. Newsletter. Describe Case Reports-Articles. *Price:* $30/subscription.

★ **20372** ★ **American Urological Association (AUA)**
1120 N Charles St.
Baltimore, MD 21201
**Phone:** (410)727-1100          **Fax:** (410)223-4370
**Email:** aua@auanet.org
**Website:** http://www.auanet.org
G. James Gallagher, Exec. Dir.
**Fnded:** 1902. **Mem:** 13,000. **Reg. Groups:** 8. **Desc:** Professional society of physicians specializing in urology. Provides education and formulation of health casre policy for urologists. **Pub:** *AUA News*, monthly. Magazine. • *Health Policy Brief*, monthly. Newsletter. • *Journal of Urology*, monthly. Journal. • *Membership Roster*, biennial.

★ **20373** ★ **Arab Society of Nephrology and Renal Transplantation (ASNRT)**
El Mahrajene
PO box 290
1082 Tunis, Tunisia
**Phone:** 216 1 889293          **Fax:** 216 1 889293
**Fnded:** 1988. **Lang(s):** Arabic, English. **Desc:** Nephrologists and other physicians and surgeons with an interest in renal transplantation. Seeks to advance the study and practice of nephrology and renal transplantation. Serves as a clearinghouse on nephrology and

related surgery; sponsors continuing professional development courses; conducts research. **Pub:** *Nephrology Forum*, semiannual. Journal.

★ **20374** ★ **Asian-Pacific Society of Nephrology (APSN)**
Monash Medical Centre
246 Clayton Rd.
Clayton, VIC 3168, Australia
**Lang(s):** English. **Desc:** Nephrologists. Seeks to advance the study, teaching, and practice of nephrology. Facilitates exchange of information among members; sponsors research programs and continuing professional development courses.

★ **20375** ★ **Association of German Urologists (Berufsverband der Deutschen Urologen)**
Erdinger Str. 19
D-84405 Dorfen, Germany
**Phone:** 49 8081 41313          **Fax:** 49 8081 4468
**Fnded:** 1956. **Mem:** 6,980. **State Groups:** 19. **Desc:** Urologists practicing in Germany. Promotes the advancement of the field of urology. **Pub:** *Urologeb*, bimonthly. Journal. • *Urotelegramm*, bimonthly. Newsletter.

**Board of Nephrology Examiners Nursing and Technology (BONENT)**
*See:* Entry 15673

★ **20376** ★ **British Association for Paediatric Nephrology**
c/o Dr. Lesley Rees
Renal Office
St. Ormond St. Hospital fo Children
London WC1N 3JH, United Kingdom
**Phone:** 44 207 8138346          **Fax:** 44 207 8298841
**Email:** reesl@gosh.nhs.uk
**Website:** http://www.uwcm.ac.uk/uwcm/ch/bapn
**Fnded:** 1973. **Mem:** 60. **Desc:** Paediatricians participating in the care of children with kidney diseases. Aims to promote policies concerning the care of children with renal disease, to conduct scientific meetings, to consider manpower and training issues and to conduct multicentre trials and other collaborative research.

**British Association of Urological Surgeons**
*See:* Entry 19531

★ **20377** ★ **Canadian Association of Nephrology Nurses and Technicians**
1255 Sheppard E
North York, ON, Canada M2K 1E2
**Phone:** (416)496-8633          **Fax:** (416)496-8634
**Email:** info@naturopath.assoc.ca
**Website:** http://www.cannt.ca
**Lang(s):** English, French. **Desc:** Nephrology nurses and technicians. Promotes professional development of members; seeks to advance the treatment of individuals with nephrological conditions. Serves as a clearinghouse on nephrology treatment centers; conducts continuing professional education courses.

★ **20378** ★ **Canadian Continence Foundation**
PO Box 30
Victoria Branch
Westmount, QC, Canada H3Z 2V4
**Phone:** (514)488-8379          **Fax:** (514)488-1379
**Email:** help@continence-fdn.ca
**Website:** http://www.continence-fdn.ca
**Fnded:** 1986. **Mem:** 14,000. **Lang(s):** English, French. **Desc:** People suffering from incontinence, health care professionals, and other individuals with an interest in incontinence and related health problems. Seeks to improve the quality of life of people with

incontinence. Facilitates formation of support groups; conducts research and educational programs; participates in charitable activities. **Pub:** *Informer*, 3/year. Newsletter. **Frmly:** Simon Foundation - Canada.

★ **20379** ★ **Canadian Interstitial Cystitis Society**
PO Box 51008
8697 10th Ave.
Burnaby, BC, Canada V3N 5B9
**Phone:** (250)758-3207          **Fax:** (250)758-4894
**Email:** smcnicol@pacificcoast.net
**Website:** http://ic-network.com/canada
**Fnded:** 1989. **Mem:** 700. **Lang(s):** English, French. **Desc:** Support group for patients suffering or suspected of suffering from interstitial cystitis, an inflammation of the bladder wall that primarily affects women, and whose causes and cure are unknown. Works to inform the public and the medical profession about the seriousness of IC. Raises funds for research into treatments and cures. **Pub:** *Bladdertalk*, quarterly. Newsletter. **Frmly:** British Columbia Interstitial Cystitis Association.

★ **20380** ★ **Canadian Liver Foundation (CLF)**
2235 Sheppard Ave. E, Ste. 1500
Toronto, ON, Canada M2J 5B5
**Phone:** (416)491-3353          **Free:** 800-563-5483
**Fax:** (416)491-4952
**Email:** clf@liver.ca
**Website:** http://www.liver.ca
**Fnded:** 1969. **Lang(s):** English, French. **Desc:** Health care professionals and researchers with an interest in hepatic diseases. Promotes increased understanding of the causes, prevention, and treatment of diseases of the liver; facilitates professional advancement of members. Works to lessen the incidence of hepatic disease through public education; provides support and services to people with hepatic diseases and their families. Conducts charitable programs; maintains speakers' bureau. **Pub:** Pamphlets.

★ **20381** ★ **Canadian Urological Association (CUA) (Association Canadienne d'Urologie — ACU)**
Dept of Surgery
University of Alberta 2D2.13
WMH Centre, 8440-112th St.
Edmonton, AB, Canada T6G 2B7
**Phone:** (780)407-3282          **Fax:** (780)407-2694
**Email:** cua@cua.org
**Website:** http://www.cua.org
**Lang(s):** English, French. **Desc:** Urologists, scientists, and other health care professionals with an interest in urology. Seeks to advance the study and practice of urology. Facilitates exchange of information among members; sponsors research and educational programs.

★ **20382** ★ **Certification Board for Urologic Nurses and Associates**
East Holly Ave., Box 56
Pitman, NJ 08071-0056
**Phone:** (856)256-2351          **Fax:** (856)589-7463
**Email:** cbuna@ajj.com
**Website:** http://www.suna.org
Karen Graf, Pres.
**Fnded:** 1972. **Mem:** 500. **Desc:** Conducts certification exam for urologic professionals. **Frmly:** American Board of Urologic Allied Health Professionals.

★ **20383** ★ **Chinese Association of Urine Therapy**
72 Wu Kon Lio Rd.
Wuki Industrial Park
Taipei, Taiwan
**Phone:** 886 2 22988446          **Fax:** 886 2 22996990
**Email:** webmaster@autourine.com
**Website:** http://www.auto-urine.com

**Desc:** Promotes urine therapy and medical research on urine therapy. **Pub:** *Urine Therapy Association Magazine*, quarterly. Magazine.

**★ 20384 ★ Continence Restored, Inc. (CRI)**
407 Strawberry Hill Ave.
Stamford, CT 06902
**Phone:** (203)348-0601
Anne Smith-Young, Pres.
**Fnded:** 1985. **State Groups:** 2. **Desc:** Participants are people with bladder control problems and interested individuals. Organizes support groups. Provides information on incontinence devices and treatment; offers referrals. Compiles statistics.

**European Dialysis and Transplant Nurses Association/European Renal Care Association (EDTNA/ERCA)**
*See:* Entry 15708

**European Society for Pediatric Nephrology (ESPN)**
*See:* Entry 5680

**★ 20385 ★ Hong Kong Society of Nephrology**
Department of Medicine
Prince of Wales Hospital
Hong Kong, People's Republic of China
**Fax:** 852 26 375396
**Email:** philipli@cuhk.edu.hk
**Website:** http://www.fmshk.com.hk/hksnephrol
**Fnded:** 1979. **Mem:** 606. **Lang(s):** Chinese, English. **Desc:** Doctors of medicine specializing in nephrology (152) are full members; nurses, other health care professionals, and students with an interest in nephrology (454) are associate members. Seeks to advance the study and practice of nephrology; encourages professional development of members. Promotes organ donation. Serves as a forum for discussion of nephrology and related medical and scientific topics; functions as liaison linking members with related scientific and professional bodies; holds interhospital renal meetings. Conducts research and educational programs. Sponsors competitions and charitable, recreational, and social activities. **Pub:** *Hong Kong Journal of Nephrology*, semiannual. Journal. • Newsletter, quarterly.

**Hong Kong Stoma Association**
*See:* Entry 9129

**International Pediatric Nephrology (IPNA)**
*See:* Entry 5698

**★ 20386 ★ International Society for Peritoneal Dialysis (ISPD)**
66 Martin St.
Milton, ON, Canada L9T 2R2
**Phone:** (905)875-2456 **Fax:** (905)875-2864
**Email:** jwinch@ix.netcom.com
**Website:** http://www.ispd.org
**Fnded:** 1984. **Mem:** 1,500. **Lang(s):** English. **Desc:** Physicians, nurses, and biomedical engineers involved in peritoneal dialysis, a procedure similar to artificial kidney machine dialysis but involving insertion of a tube into the abdomen to cleanse blood within the body. Seeks to advance knowledge of peritoneal dialysis through exchange and research. **Pub:** *Peritoneal Dialysis International*, bimonthly. Journal.

**★ 20387 ★ International Society of Urology (ISU)**
**(Societe Internationale d'Urologie — SIU)**
10, ave. Hippocrate
B-1200 Brussels, Belgium
**Phone:** 33 3 20576389 **Fax:** 33 3 20379893

**Email:** siusecretarita@wanadoo.fr
**Fnded:** 1907. **Mem:** 4,708. **Nat'l Groups:** 100. **Lang(s):** English. **Desc:** Surgeons and other specialists in the field of urology. Promotes research in urology; fosters communication among members. Sponsors meetings and programs in postgraduate education. **Pub:** *Membership List*, annual. Newsletter. • *Newsletter*, annual. Monograph. • Monograph, triennial.

**★ 20388 ★ Interstitial Cystitis Association (ICA)**
110 N Washington St., No. 340
Rockville, MD 20850-2239
**Phone:** (301)610-5300 **Free:** 800-HEL-PICA
**Fax:** (301)610-5308
**Email:** icamail@ichelp.org
**Website:** http://www.ichelp.org
**Fnded:** 1984. **Desc:** Support network for patients suffering or suspected of suffering from interstitial cystitis, an inflammation of the bladder wall that primarily affects women; its cause and cure are unknown. Works to inform the public and especially the medical profession about the seriousness of IC. Raises funds for research into treatments and cures; maintains a medical advisory board. Is establishing a national registry to record facts about IC. **Pub:** *ICA Update*, quarterly. Newsletter. Covers IC research and political and educational activities of the ICA. *Price:* $45/year.

**★ 20389 ★ Irish Kidney Association (IKA)**
Renal Transplant Support Centre
Beaumont Hospital
Dublin 9, Ireland
**Phone:** 353 1 6689788 **Fax:** 353 1 6683820
**Email:** info@ika.ie
**Website:** http://www.ika.ie
**Fnded:** 1978. **Mem:** 3,000. **Lang(s):** English, Irish. **Desc:** Individuals and organizations. Seeks to improve the quality of life of people with kidney disease and their families. Serves as a clearinghouse on kidney transplantation and available donors. Makes available counseling services; conducts educational and advocacy campaigns. Distributes organ donor cards.

**★ 20390 ★ National Association for Continence**
PO Box 8310
Spartanburg, SC 29305-8310
**Phone:** (864)579-7900 **Free:** 800-BLA-DDER
**Fax:** (864)579-7902
**Email:** memberservices@nafc.org
**Website:** http://www.nafc.org
Nancy Muller, Exec. Dir.
**Fnded:** 1982. **Mem:** 140,000. **Nat'l Groups:** 1. **Desc:** Works to help individuals who have bladder control problems. Acts as a clearinghouse of information and services involving incontinence and assistive devices for consumers and their families as well as medical, nursing, and social service organizations. **Pub:** *Quality Care*, quarterly. Newsletter. *Price:* $20/year. • *Resource Guide-Continence Products and Services*. **Frmly:** Help for Incontinent People.

**★ 20391 ★ National Association of Nephrology Technicians/Technologists (NANT)**
PO Box 2307
Dayton, OH 45401-2307
**Phone:** (937)586-3705 **Free:** 877-607-NANT
**Fax:** (937)586-3699
**Email:** nant@nant.melnet.com
**Website:** http://www.dialysistech.org
Francine W. Rickenbach, CAE
**Fnded:** 1983. **Mem:** 1,200. **State Groups:** 22. **Desc:** Nephrology technicians and technologists. Promotes the recognition, job security, and employment opportunities of nephrology technicians and technologists. Sets forth standards for the dialysis industry; educates dialysis practitioners; promotes research; disseminates new ideas; addresses technician and technolo-

gist practice issues. **Pub:** *A Manual on Water Treatment for Hemodialysis*. Book. Discusses each component of a hemodialysis water treatment system. *Price:* $17.50 for members; $34.50 for nonmembers. • *Core Curriculum for the Reprocessing of Dialyzers*. *Price:* $15 for members; $20 for nonmembers. • *Dialysis Technology, Second Edition*. *Price:* $40 member; $50 nonmember. • *Nant News*, bimonthly. Newsletter. • *Study Guide for Technologists, Second Edition*. *Price:* $20 member; $30 nonmember. **Frmly:** (1994) National Association of Nephrology Technologists.

**★ 20392 ★ National Kidney Foundation (NKF)**
30 E 33rd St., Ste. 1100
New York, NY 10016
**Phone:** (212)889-2210 **Free:** 800-622-9010
**Fax:** (212)779-0068
**Email:** info@kidney.org
**Website:** http://www.kidney.org
John Davis, Chief Exec. Officer
**Fnded:** 1950. **Local Groups:** 200. **Desc:** Supports research, patient services, professional and public education, organ and tissue donor program, and community service. Affiliates conduct community and patient services including: drug banks; transportation; early screening; patient seminars. Sponsors symposium for health care professionals. Maintains speakers' bureau and biographical archives; compiles statistics. **Pub:** *Advances in Renal Replacement Therapy*, quarterly. Journal. • *American Journal of Kidney Diseases*, monthly. Journal. Covers research in kidney and urinary tract diseases. Includes annual index and conference reports. *Price:* Included in membership dues. • *CNNT Newsletter*, quarterly. Newsletter. Contains employment opportunity listings and regional news. *Price:* Included in membership dues. • *CNSW Newsletter*, quarterly. Newsletter. Includes calendar of events, information on current literature, employment opportunities, and legislative and regional reports. *Price:* Included in membership dues. • *CRN News and Briefs*, quarterly. Newsletter. Contains employment opportunity listings, legislative news, and research reports. *Price:* Included in membership dues. • *Journal of Nephrology Social Work*, annual. Journal. • *Journal of Renal Nutrition*, quarterly. Journal. • *National Kidney Foundation–Clinical Nephrology Meetings Proceedings Book*. **Frmly:** (1958) National Nephrosis Foundation; (1964) National Kidney Disease Foundation.

**★ 20393 ★ National Kidney and Urologic Diseases Information Clearinghouse (NKUDIC)**
3 Information Way
Bethesda, MD 20892-3580
**Phone:** (301)654-4415 **Free:** 800-891-5390
**Fax:** (301)907-8906
**Email:** nkudic@info.niddk.nih.gov
**Website:** http://www.niddk.nih.gov
**Fnded:** 1987. **Desc:** An information and referral service of the National Institute of Diabetes and Digestive Kidney Diseases. Responds to written inquiries, develops and distributes publications about kidney and urologic diseases, and provides referrals to kidney and urologic organizations, including support groups. Maintains a database of patient and professional educational materials and performs searches. Provides bulk orders of publications to health and information professionals planning patient health education programs. Established by the National Institutes of Health. **Pub:** *Research Updates in Kidney and Urologic Health*, semiannual. Newsletter. • Booklets. • Directories. • Also publishes a variety of patient education materials including fact sheets and literature searches from the Combined Health Information Database (CHID).

**National Renal Administrators Association (NRAA)**
*See:* Entry 9759

**North American Society for Dialysis and Transplantation (NASDT)**
*See:* Entry 20342

---

**★ 20394 ★ Renal Physicians Association (RPA)**
4701 Randolph Rd., Ste. 102
Rockville, MD 20852
**Phone:** (301)468-3515 **Free:** 800-RPA-7525
**Fax:** (301)468-3511
**Email:** rpa@renalmd.org
**Website:** http://www.renalmd.org/
Dale Singer, Exec. Dir.

**Fnded:** 1973. **Mem:** 2,100. **Desc:** Physicians specializing in the treatment of renal (kidney) diseases. Promotes optimal care and high standards of treatment for patients. Serves as a national representative for physicians engaged in the study and management of patients with kidney and related disorders; specifically, expresses the concerns and needs of renal physicians to congressional and governmental agencies legislating, executing, and regulating the federal End Stage Renal Disease Program. Provides resources for the development of national policies concerning kidney disease such as ESRD legislative and network activities, federal funding for related research, and studies relative to treatment procedures and clinical practices. Conducts educational programs. Associate membership is open to practice managers who are responsible for billing and coding in nephrologists' offices. **Pub:** *RPA News*, bimonthly. Newsletter. *Price:* Included in membership dues.

**★ 20395 ★ Scandinavian Association of Urology (SAU)**
**(Nordisk Urologisk Forening — NUF)**
Rikshospitalet
Kir avd A
N-0027 Oslo A, Norway
**Email:** alxsch@online.no

**Fnded:** 1957. **Mem:** 750. **Lang(s):** Danish, English, Finnish, Icelandic, Norwegian, Swedish. **Desc:** Scandinavian physicians specializing in urology or having an interest in the field. Maintains international working groups. **Pub:** *NUF-Bulletinen*, semiannual. • *Scandinavian Journal of Urology and Nephrology*, quarterly.

**★ 20396 ★ Scientific Society of Nephrology**
Klinichen Tsentar po Nephrologia
Dame Gruev 8
BG-1303 Sofia, Bulgaria
**Email:** delijska@sbline.net

**Fnded:** 1973. **Mem:** 250. **Lang(s):** English, French, German. **Desc:** Fosters research in nephrology. **Pub:** *Jouranl of Nephrology*, monthly. Journal.

**★ 20397 ★ Simon Foundation for Continence (SFC)**
Box 835-F
Wilmette, IL 60091
**Phone:** (847)864-3913 **Free:** 800-23-SIMON
**Fax:** (847)864-9758
**Email:** simoninfo@simonfoundation.org
**Website:** http://www.simonfoundation.org
Cheryle B. Gartley, Pres.

**Fnded:** 1983. **Mem:** 140,000. **Desc:** Persons with urinary and bowel incontinence; family members, doctors, medical personnel, and others concerned with the condition. Seeks to educate the public on urinary and bowel problems, to provide information to persons with incontinence, and to remove the stigma attached to the condition. Acts as support group. Organizes "I Will Manage" selfhelp groups. Conducts research on the manufacture and usability of incontinency products, the number of people who have the problems, and the types and causes of incontinence; compiles statistics. Maintains speakers' bureau. **Pub:** *A Time for Action.* Video. • *The Choice Is Yours.* Video. • *The Informer: Helping People with Incontinence*, quarterly. Newsletter. *Price:* Included in membership dues. • *Managing Incontinence: A Guide to*

*Living with the Loss of Bladder Control.* Book. • *The Solution Starts with You.* Video. **Frmly:** Simon Foundation.

**★ 20398 ★ Sociedad Chilena de Urologia**
Esmeralda 678
Santiago, Chile
**Phone:** 56 2 6642469
**Email:** luicoz@entelchile.net
**Fnded:** 1935.

**★ 20399 ★ Society of Government Service Urologists**
7027 Weathered Post
PO Box 681965
San Antonio, TX 78268
**Phone:** (210)681-0587 **Fax:** (210)680-7725
**Email:** sgsu@txdirect.net
**Website:** http://www.txdirect.net/~sgsu
Preston Littrell, Admin.

**Fnded:** 1952. **Mem:** 731. **Desc:** Urologists. Promotes exchange of information on advancements in urological research. **Pub:** *SGSU*, quarterly. Newsletter. *Price:* Free.

**Society for Pediatric Urology (SPU)**
*See:* Entry 5760

**Society of Urologic Nurses and Associates (SUNA)**
*See:* Entry 15777

**★ 20400 ★ Society of Women in Urology**
c/o Wendy J. Weiser
1111 N Plaza Dr., Ste. 550
Schaumburg, IL 60173-4946
**Phone:** (847)517-7225 **Fax:** (847)517-7229
**Email:** swiu@wjweiser.com
**Website:** http://www.suna.org
Wendy Weiser, Contact

**Fnded:** 1991. **Mem:** 260. **Desc:** Women working in the field of urology. **Pub:** *SWIU News.* Newsletter.

## Research Centers

**★ 20401 ★ Columbia University Molecular Urology Laboratory**
College of Physicians and Surgeons
Department of Urology
630 W 168th St.
New York, NY 10032
**Phone:** (212)305-5727 **Fax:** (212)305-1564
**Email:** rb46@colombia.edu
Dr. Ralph Buttyan, Dir.

**Activities/Fields:** Molecular biology, focusing on prostate cancer, bladder disease, renal disease, erectile dysfunction, and cell death research.

**★ 20402 ★ PKD Foundation**
4901 Main St., Ste. 200
Kansas City, MO 64112-2634
**Phone:** (816)931-2600 **Free:** 800-753-2873
**Fax:** (816)931-8655
**Email:** pkdcure@pkdcure.org
**Website:** http://www.pkdcure.org
Dave Switzer, Mktg. /PR Dir.

**Activities/Fields:** Cause, treatment, and cure of polycystic kidney disease (PKD). Activities include identification of gene defect responsible for PKD, analysis of abnormal cell and cyst growth, and analysis of kidney function and progressive kidney failure. **Pub:** *The Family and ADPKD: A Guide for Children and Parents.* • *Health Tips for Living with PKD.* • *PKD Patients Manual "Your Child, Your Family and ARPKD".* • *PKR Progress Newsletter.* • *Q&A on PKD.* **Frmly:** Polycystic Kidney Research Foundation.

**U.S. Department of Health and Human Services**
**National Heart, Lung, and Blood Institute**
**Laboratory of Kidney and Electrolyte Metabolism**
*See:* Entry 8767

**U.S. Department of Health and Human Services**
**National Institute of Diabetes and Digestive and Kidney Diseases**
**Division of Extramural Activities**
*See:* Entry 8781

**★ 20403 ★ U.S. Department of Health and Human Services**
**National Institute of Diabetes and Digestive and Kidney Diseases**
**Division of Kidney, Urologic, and Hematologic Diseases**
NIH Bldg. 31, Rm. 9A-17
31 Center Dr.
MSC 2510
Bethesda, MD 20892-2510
**Phone:** (301)496-6325 **Fax:** (301)402-4874
**Email:** briggsj@hq.niddk.nih.gov
**Website:** http://www.niddk.nih.gov/fund/divisions/kuh/kuhintro.htm
Josephine P. Briggs, MD, Dir.

**Activities/Fields:** Kidney, urinary, and hematologic disorders, including epidemiologic studies and clinical trials. Offers investigator-initiated research grants and awards, program/project grants, center grants, and cooperative agreements. Also sponsors research fellowships, training grants, career development awards, and resource and research and development contracts. Scientific activities conducted through eleven major programs: Renal Physiology/Cell Biology Program, which focuses on the underlying mechanisms of kidney disease; Urology Program, which focuses on basic and clinical studies of normal and disease states of genitourinary system; Centers Program, which focuses on clinical studies in nephrology and urology; Manpower Program, which offers research training and career development awards; Chronic Renal Diseases Program, which supports basic and clinical research on chronic kidney diseases; End-Stage Renal Disease (ESRD) Program, which focuses on the mechanisms involved in ESRD; Clinical Trial Program, which focuses on clinical trials in urologicc and renal kidney diseases; Diabetic Nephropathy Program, which focuses on mechanisms of diabetic kidney disease and development of new therapies; Hematology Program, which focuses on normal and disease states of hematopoietic system; Epidemiology Program, which supports development of epidemiologic data related to major kidney, urologic, and hematologic diseases; HIV Program, which focuses on effects of HIV infection on renal, urinary, and hematopoietic function; and Small Business Innovation Research Program, which promotes commercialization of and small business involvement in federally funded research.

**★ 20404 ★ U.S. Department of Health and Human Services**
**National Institute of Diabetes and Digestive and Kidney Diseases (NIDDK)**
**Division of Kidney, Urologic, and Hematologic Diseases (DKUHD)**
**Chronic Renal Diseases Program**
6707 Democracy Blvd. Ste. 601
Bethesda, MD 20892-5458
**Phone:** (301)594-7717 **Fax:** (301)480-3510
**Email:** gladys_hirschman@nih.gov
Dr. Gladys H. Hirschman, MD, Prog. Dir.

**Activities/Fields:** Kidney diseases and develops treatments to prevent their onset and progression. Focuses on pathophysiology (including immunopathogenic mechanisms) of chronic renal diseases such as lupus nephritis, polycystic kidney disease, or interstitial nephritis, IgA nephropathy, and other glomerulopathies/glomerulonephritis; progressive renal disease; renial diseases of congenital and genetic origins i.e., polycystic kidney disease; kidney disease in children and in minority populations; role of nutrition in renal disease; kidney disease caused by diabetes mellitus, including studies on pathogenic mechanisms, genetic morphologic and functional markers; and natural history of diabetic nephropathy, hypertensive renal disease and all of the above in the pediatric population.


### ★ 20405 ★ U.S. Department of Health and Human Services
**National Institute of Diabetes and Digestive and Kidney Diseases**
**Division of Kidney, Urologic, and Hematologic Diseases**
**Renal Physiology / Cell Biology Program**
Natcher Bldg. 5458
6707 Democracy Blvd.
Bethesda, MD 20892-5458
**Phone:** (301)594-7719 **Fax:** (301)480-3510
**Activities/Fields:** Underlying mechanisms of kidney disease. Studies in this program examine the normal structure and function of the kidney, including its biochemistry, metabolism, transport, and fluid-electrolyte dynamics. Research supported is on the metabolic and physiologic transport processes that regulate solute and water excretion, as are studies on the adverse effects of drugs, nephrotoxins, and environmental toxins on the kidney. The program also has a primary interest in studies on analgesic abuse and heavy metal toxicities, as well as studies certain causes of acute renal failure such as hyppoxic injury.


### ★ 20406 ★ U.S. Department of Health and Human Services
**National Institute of Diabetes and Digestive and Kidney Diseases**
**Division of Kidney, Urologic, and Hematologic Diseases**
**Urology and Women's Urological Health Program**
Two Democracy Plaza Rm. 600
6707 Democracy Blvd. MSC 5458
Bethesda, MD 20892-5458
**Phone:** (301)594-7717 **Fax:** (301)480-3510
**Email:** nybergl@extra.niddk.nih.gov
Dr. Leroy M. Nyberg, Dir.
**Activities/Fields:** Normal and disease states of genitourinary system, including structure and function of the bladder, urethra, and prostate. Program interests include pyelonephritis, interstitial cystitis, urolithiasis, benign prostatic hyperplasia, prostatitis, impotence and sexual dysfunction, and urinary incontinence.


**U.S. Department of Health and Human Services**
**National Institutes of Health**
**National Cancer Institute**
**Division of Clinical Sciences**
**(Urologic Oncology Branch)**
*See:* Entry 10560


### ★ 20407 ★ University of Alabama at Birmingham
**Nephrology Research and Training Center**
Division of Nephrology
1900 University Blvd., Rm. 647 THT
Birmingham, AL 35294-0007
**Phone:** (205)934-3585 **Fax:** (205)934-1879
**Email:** dwarnock@nrtc.dom.uab.edu
**Website:** http://www.nrtc.uab.edu
David G. Warnock, MD, Dir.
**Activities/Fields:** Membrane transport, renal tubular transport, acid base physiology, renal hypertension, renal ultrastructure, epithelial ion transport, electron microprobe, erythropoietin, and population studies of genetic factors in hypertension.


### ★ 20408 ★ University of Alabama at Birmingham
**Urological Rehabilitation and Research Center**
The Kirklin Clinic
UAB Medical Center
2000 6th Ave. S
Birmingham, AL 35249
**Phone:** (205)934-9999 **Fax:** (205)934-2709
**Email:** klloyd@uab.edu
**Website:** http://www.health.uab.edu/show.asp?durki=10551
L. Keith Lloyd, MD, Dir.
**Activities/Fields:** Urological dysfunctions.


### ★ 20409 ★ University of Kansas
**Division of Nephrology and Hypertension**
3901 Rainbow Blvd.
Kansas City, KS 66160-7382
**Phone:** (913)588-6074 **Fax:** (913)588-3867
**Email:** ddiederi@kumc.edu
Dennis Diederich, MD, Dir.
**Activities/Fields:** Laboratory and clinical investigations into kidney physiology, polycystic kidney disease, basement membrane structure and function, kidney stones, acute renal failure, and diuretics. Research methods include tubule microperfusion, amino acid analyses, peptide synthesis, and morphometrics.


### ★ 20410 ★ University of Louisville
**Kidney Disease Program**
615 S Preston St.
Louisville, KY 40202-1718
**Phone:** (502)852-5757 **Fax:** (502)852-7643
**Email:** gra@louisville.edu
**Website:** http://kdp01.kdp-baptist.louisville.edu
George R. Aronoff, MD, Ch.
**Activities/Fields:** Kidney disease, focusing on the following areas: proteomics, cellular physiology, second messengers, biological transport, cellular immunology, transplantation, artificial membranes, dialysis, clinical pharmacology, pharmacokinetics, nephrotoxicity, drug metabolism, hypertension, and tissue typing.
**Frmly:** Bioengineering Laboratory.


### ★ 20411 ★ University of Medicine and Dentistry of New Jersey
**Urology Research Laboratory**
185 S Orange Ave., Rm. H516
Newark, NJ 07103-2714
**Phone:** (973)972-7728 **Fax:** (973)972-3892
Dr. Robert Irwin, Ch.
**Activities/Fields:** Interaction between retinoids and audiogens in the control of prostate cells and its role in prostate cancer. Effects of spinal cord injury on male reproduction and testing regimens to prevent such effects.


### ★ 20412 ★ University of Rochester
**Nephrology Research Program**
601 Elmwood Ave.
PO Box 675
Rochester, NY 14642
**Phone:** (716)275-4517 **Fax:** (716)442-9201
**Email:** david_bushinsky@urmc.rochester.edu
Dr. David Bushinsky, Dir.
**Activities/Fields:** Physiological regulation of water and salt excretion, renal potassium handling in vivo and in the isolated perfused kidney, regulation of intrarenal blood flow, fluorescence videomicroscopy studies of inner medullary blood flow, role of nucleosides as regulators of kidney function and hemodynamics, renal microvascular endothelium and epithelial cell cultures, in vivo perfusion of capillaries from the renal microcirculation, pathogenesis of acute renal failure, modulators of renal ischemic injury, and studies of tubular functioning in humans.


### ★ 20413 ★ University of Southern California
**Division of Nephrology**
1200 N State St., Rm. GNH 4250
Los Angeles, CA 90033
**Phone:** (323)226-7307 **Fax:** (323)226-5390
**Email:** campese@hsc.usc.edu
Dr. Vito Campese, Ch.
**Activities/Fields:** Hypertension, renal disease, hypertension and the progression of renal disese.


### ★ 20414 ★ Washington University in St. Louis
**Chromalloy American Kidney Center**
660 S Euclid, CB 8129
Saint Louis, MO 63110
**Phone:** (314)362-8231 **Fax:** (314)362-7232
**Email:** jdelmez@im.wustl.edu
Dr. James Delmez, Dir.
**Activities/Fields:** Lipid abnormalities in uremia, muscle protein metabolism in uremia, metabolic bone disease in uremia, parathyroid hormone, and vitamin D and aluminum metabolism.


# State & Regional Organizations

## Kidney

*The following organizations are affiliates of the National Kidney Foundation, 30 E 33rd St., Ste. 1100, New York, NY 10016, (800)622-9010, http://www.kidney.org/.*

### Alabama

### ★ 20415 ★ National Kidney Foundation of Alabama, Inc.
562 Clay St.
PO Box 342
Montgomery, AL 36101
**Phone:** (334)265-1033 **Fax:** (334)264-6296
**Email:** nkfal@bellsouth.net
**Website:** http://www.nkfalabama.org

### Arizona

### ★ 20416 ★ National Kidney Foundation of Arizona, Inc.
Arizona Kidney Foundation
4203 E Indian School Rd., Ste. 140
Phoenix, AZ 85018
**Phone:** (602)840-1644 **Fax:** (602)840-2360
**Website:** http://www.azkidney.org

### Arkansas

### ★ 20417 ★ National Kidney Foundation of Arkansas, Inc.
1 Lile Ct., Ste. 201
PO Box 453
Little Rock, AR 72203
**Phone:** (501)664-4343 **Fax:** (501)664-7145
**Email:** nkfa@aristotle.net
**Website:** http://www.kidneyar.com

### California

### ★ 20418 ★ National Kidney Foundation of Northern California, Inc.
11 Mission St., 3rd Fl.
San Francisco, CA 94105
**Phone:** (415)543-3303 **Fax:** (415)543-3331
**Website:** http://www.kidneynca.org

**★ 20419 ★ National Kidney Foundation of Southern California, Inc.**
5777 W Century Blvd., Ste. 1450
Los Angeles, CA 90045
**Phone:** (310)641-8152    **Free:** 800-747-5527
**Fax:** (310)641-5246
**Email:** jmartinez@kidneysocal.org
**Website:** http://www.kidneysocal.org

## Colorado

**★ 20420 ★ National Kidney Foundation of Colorado, Idaho, Montana, and Wyoming, Inc.**
Cherry Creek Place III
3151 S Vaughn, Ste. 505
Aurora, CO 80014
**Phone:** (720)748-9991    **Fax:** (720)748-1273
**Email:** mlhanson@kidneycimw.org
**Website:** http://www.kidneycimw.org

## Connecticut

**★ 20421 ★ National Kidney Foundation of Connecticut, Inc.**
920 Farmington Ave.
West Hartford, CT 06107
**Phone:** (860)232-6054    **Free:** 800-441-1280
**Fax:** (860)236-1367
**Email:** info@kidneyct.org
**Website:** http://www.kidneyct.org

## District of Columbia

**★ 20422 ★ National Kidney Foundation of the National Capital Area, Inc.**
5335 Wisconsin Ave. NW, Ste. 300
Washington, DC 20015
**Phone:** (202)244-7900    **Fax:** (202)244-7405
**Email:** penglert@kidneywdc.org
**Website:** http://www.kidneywdc.org

## Florida

**★ 20423 ★ National Kidney Foundation of Florida, Inc.**
Palmetto Bldg., No. 119
1040 Woodcock Rd.
Orlando, FL 32803
**Phone:** (407)894-7325    **Free:** 800-927-9659
**Fax:** (407)895-0051
**Email:** nkf@kidneyfla.org
**Website:** http://www.kidneyfla.org

## Georgia

**★ 20424 ★ National Kidney Foundation of Georgia, Inc.**
2951 Flowers Rd. S, Ste. 221
Atlanta, GA 30341
**Phone:** (770)452-1539    **Free:** 800-633-2339
**Fax:** (770)452-7564
**Email:** cstarr@nkfg.org
**Website:** http://www.kidneyga.org

## Hawaii

**★ 20425 ★ National Kidney Foundation of Hawaii, Inc.**
1314 S King St., No. 305
Honolulu, HI 96814
**Phone:** (808)593-1515    **Fax:** (808)593-8096
**Email:** stacey@kidneyhi.org
**Website:** http://www.kidneyhi.org

## Illinois

**★ 20426 ★ National Kidney Foundation of Illinois, Inc.**
215 W Illinois, Ste. 1-C
Chicago, IL 60610
**Phone:** (312)321-1500    **Fax:** (312)321-1505

**Email:** kidney@nkfi.org
**Website:** http://www.nkfi.org/

## Indiana

**★ 20427 ★ National Kidney Foundation of Indiana, Inc.**
911 E 86th St., No. 100
Indianapolis, IN 46240
**Phone:** (317)722-5640    **Free:** 800-382-9971
**Fax:** (317)722-5650
**Email:** NKFI@in.net
**Website:** http://www.kidneyindiana.org

## Iowa

**★ 20428 ★ National Kidney Foundation of Iowa, Inc.**
c/o Mercy Medical Center
Mercy Medical Center
701 10th St. SE, No. 5618
Cedar Rapids, IA 52402
**Phone:** (319)369-4474    **Free:** 800-369-3619
**Fax:** (319)369-4419
**Email:** info@kidneyia.org
**Website:** http://www.kidneyia.org

## Kansas

**★ 20429 ★ National Kidney Foundation of Kansas and Western Missouri, Inc.**
1900 W 47th Pl., Ste. 310
Westwood, KS 66205
**Phone:** (913)262-1551    **Free:** 800-444-8113
**Fax:** (913)722-4841
**Email:** info@kidneyksmo.org
**Website:** http://www.kidneyksmo.org

## Kentucky

**★ 20430 ★ National Kidney Foundation of Kentucky, Inc.**
250 E Liberty St., No. 710
Louisville, KY 40202
**Phone:** (502)585-5433    **Fax:** (502)585-1445
**Email:** nkfk@nkfk.org
**Website:** http://www.nkfk.org

## Louisiana

**★ 20431 ★ National Kidney Foundation of Louisiana, Inc.**
8200 Hampson, Ste. 425
New Orleans, LA 70118
**Phone:** (504)861-4500    **Free:** 800-462-3694
**Fax:** (504)861-1976
**Email:** kidneyla@gnofn.org
**Website:** http://www.kidneyla.org

## Maine

**★ 20432 ★ National Kidney Foundation of Maine, Inc.**
630 Congress St.
PO Box 1134
Portland, ME 04104
**Phone:** (207)772-7270    **Free:** 800-639-7220
**Fax:** (207)772-4202
**Website:** http://www.kidney.me.org

## Maryland

**★ 20433 ★ National Kidney Foundation of Maryland, Inc.**
1107 Kenilworth Dr., No. 202
Baltimore, MD 21204
**Phone:** (410)494-8545    **Free:** 800-671-5369
**Fax:** (410)494-8549
**Website:** http://www.kidneymd.org

## Massachusetts

**★ 20434 ★ National Kidney Foundation of Massachusetts, Rhode Island, New Hampshire, and Vermont, Inc.**
129 Morgan Dr.
Norwood, MA 02062
**Phone:** (781)278-0222    **Fax:** (781)278-0333
**Email:** blinden@kidneyhealth.org
**Website:** http://www.kidneyhealth.org

## Michigan

**★ 20435 ★ National Kidney Foundation of Michigan, Inc.**
1169 Oak Valley Dr.
Ann Arbor, MI 48108
**Phone:** (734)222-9800    **Free:** 800-482-1455
**Fax:** (734)222-9801
**Email:** kbergquist@nkfm.org
**Website:** http://www.nkfm.org

## Minnesota

**★ 20436 ★ National Kidney Foundation of Minnesota, Inc.**
920 S 7th St.
Minneapolis, MN 55415
**Phone:** (612)337-7300    **Fax:** (612)904-4268
**Remarks:** Also serves North and South Dakota.

## Mississippi

**★ 20437 ★ National Kidney Foundation of Mississippi, Inc.**
3000 Old Canton Rd., Ste. 100
PO Box 55802
Jackson, MS 39296
**Phone:** (601)981-3611    **Fax:** (601)981-3612
**Email:** gailgsweat@yahoo.com
**Website:** http://www.kidneyms.org

## Missouri

**★ 20438 ★ National Kidney Foundation of Eastern Missouri and Metro-East, Inc.**
1423 Hanley Industrial Dr.
Saint Louis, MO 63144
**Phone:** (314)961-2828    **Free:** 800-489-9585
**Fax:** (314)961-0888
**Email:** mherrmann@nkfstl.com
**Website:** http://www.nkfstl.com

## Nebraska

**★ 20439 ★ National Kidney Foundation of Nebraska, Inc.**
7101 Newport Ave., No. 301
Omaha, NE 68152
**Phone:** (402)572-3180    **Free:** 800-642-1255
**Fax:** (402)572-3211
**Website:** http://www.kidneyne.org

## Nevada

**★ 20440 ★ National Kidney Foundation of Nevada, Inc.**
3050 E Desert Inn Rd., No. 121
Las Vegas, NV 89121
**Phone:** (702)735-9222    **Fax:** (702)735-9224
**Email:** nkfnv@aol.com
**Website:** http://vegasonline.com/NKF/NKFHP.htm

## New Mexico

**★ 20441 ★ National Kidney Foundation of New Mexico, Inc.**
PO Box 14238
Albuquerque, NM 87191-4238
**Phone:** (505)293-5298

**Email:** connieqb@kidney-nm.org

### New York

**★ 20442 ★ National Kidney Foundation of Central New York, Inc.**
731 James St., No. 200
Syracuse, NY 13203
**Phone:** (315)476-0311     **Free:** 877-854-3639
**Fax:** (315)476-3707
**Email:** NKF@CNYKidney.org
**Website:** http://www.cnykidney.org

**★ 20443 ★ National Kidney Foundation of Greater New York, Inc.**
30 E 33rd St.
New York, NY 10016
**Phone:** (212)889-2210     **Free:** 800-622-9010
**Fax:** (212)689-9261
**Website:** http://www.nkfofgreaterny.org
**Frmly:** National Kidney Foundation of New York /New Jersey, Inc.

**★ 20444 ★ National Kidney Foundation of Northeast New York, Inc.**
23 Computer Dr. E
Albany, NY 12205
**Phone:** (518)458-9697     **Free:** 800-999-9697
**Fax:** (518)458-9690
**Email:** nkfneny@crisny.org
**Website:** http://www.nkfneny.org

**★ 20445 ★ National Kidney Foundation of Upstate New York, Inc.**
3300 Monroe Ave., Ste. 100D
Rochester, NY 14618
**Phone:** (716)264-0420     **Free:** 800-724-9421
**Fax:** (716)264-0109
**Email:** nkfnyup@rochester.rr.com
**Website:** http://www.kidneynyup.org

**★ 20446 ★ National Kidney Foundation of Western New York, Inc.**
3871 Harlem Rd., No. 11
Buffalo, NY 14215
**Phone:** (716)835-1323     **Fax:** (716)835-2281
**Email:** nkfwny@hotmail.com
**Website:** http://www.nkfofwny.org

### North Carolina

**★ 20447 ★ National Kidney Foundation of North Carolina, Inc.**
5950 Fairview Rd., No. 708
Charlotte, NC 28210
**Phone:** (704)552-1351     **Free:** 800-356-5362
**Fax:** (704)552-7870
**Email:** lskipper@nkfnc.org
**Website:** http://www.nkfnc.org

### Ohio

**★ 20448 ★ National Kidney Foundation of Ohio, Inc.**
1373 Grandview Ave., No. 200
Columbus, OH 43212
**Phone:** (614)481-4030     **Fax:** (614)481-4038
**Email:** info@nkfofohio.org
**Website:** http://www.nkfofohio.org

### Oklahoma

**★ 20449 ★ National Kidney Foundation of Oklahoma, Inc.**
3617 NW 58th St., No. 101
Oklahoma City, OK 73112
**Phone:** (405)947-6405     **Free:** 800-946-6405
**Fax:** (405)947-6463
**Website:** http://www.nkfo.org

### Oregon

**★ 20450 ★ National Kidney Foundation of Oregon and Washington, Inc.**
1006 SE Grand Ave., Ste. 100
PO Box 15149
Portland, OR 97293-9149
**Phone:** (503)963-5364     **Free:** 888-3-KIDNEY
**Fax:** (503)238-1754
**Email:** help@kidneywa.org
**Website:** http://www.kidneyorwa.org

**★ 20451 ★ National Kidney Foundation of Oregon and Washington, Inc. Medford Chapter**
33 N Central Ave., No. 406
Medford, OR 97501
**Phone:** (541)773-8930     **Fax:** (541)773-8964
**Email:** medford@kidneyorwa.org
**Website:** http://www.kidneyorwa.org

### Pennsylvania

**★ 20452 ★ National Kidney Foundation of the Delaware Valley, Inc.**
325 Chestnut St.
Philadelphia, PA 19106
**Phone:** (215)923-8611     **Fax:** (215)923-2199
**Email:** info@nkfdv.org
**Website:** http://www.nkfdv.org

**★ 20453 ★ National Kidney Foundation of Western Pennsylvania, Inc.**
555 Grant St., No. 380
Pittsburgh, PA 15219
**Phone:** (412)261-4115     **Fax:** (412)261-1405
**Email:** bonnieg@kidneywp.org
**Website:** http://www.kidneywp.org
**Remarks:** Also serves northern West Virginia.

### South Carolina

**★ 20454 ★ National Kidney Foundation of South Carolina, Inc.**
5000 Thurmond Mall, Ste. 106
Columbia, SC 29201
**Phone:** (803)799-3870     **Free:** 800-488-2277
**Fax:** (803)799-3871
**Email:** bhughes@kidney-sc.org
**Website:** http://www.kidney-sc.org

### South Dakota

**★ 20455 ★ National Kidney Foundation of South Dakota, Inc.**
400 S Sycamore, No. 104
Sioux Falls, SD 57110
**Phone:** (605)338-0518

### Tennessee

**★ 20456 ★ National Kidney Foundation of East Tennessee, Inc.**
4450 Walker Blvd., No. 2
Knoxville, TN 37917
**Phone:** (865)688-5481     **Fax:** (865)688-0196
**Email:** helen@kidneyetn.org
**Website:** http://www.kidneyetn.org

**★ 20457 ★ National Kidney Foundation of Middle Tennessee, Inc.**
2120 Crestmoor Rd.
Nashville, TN 37215
**Phone:** (615)383-3887     **Fax:** (615)383-2647
**Email:** nkfmdtn@bellsouth.net
**Website:** http://www.nkfmdtn.org

**★ 20458 ★ National Kidney Foundation of West Tennessee, Inc.**
857 Mt. Moriah Rd., Ste. 201
Memphis, TN 38117
**Phone:** (901)683-6185     **Free:** 800-273-3869
**Fax:** (901)683-6189
**Email:** nkf@bellsouth.net

### Texas

**★ 20459 ★ National Kidney Foundation of North Texas, Inc.**
3530 Forest Ln., Ste. 105
Dallas, TX 75234
**Phone:** (214)351-2393     **Free:** 877-543-6397
**Fax:** (214)351-3797
**Email:** info@nkft.org
**Website:** http://www.nkft.org

**★ 20460 ★ National Kidney Foundation of South and Central Texas, Inc.**
1919 Oakwell Farms Pkwy., Ste. 135
San Antonio, TX 78218
**Phone:** (210)829-1299     **Free:** 800-829-1299
**Fax:** (210)829-1248
**Email:** nkf@kidneytx.org
**Website:** http://www.kidneytx.org

**★ 20461 ★ National Kidney Foundation of Southeast Texas, Inc.**
2400 Augusta Dr., No. 252
Houston, TX 77057
**Phone:** (713)952-5499     **Free:** 800-961-5683
**Fax:** (713)952-5497
**Website:** http://nkfset.org

**★ 20462 ★ National Kidney Foundation of the Texas Coastal Bend, Inc.**
719 N Upper Broadway
PO Box 9172
Corpus Christi, TX 78469
**Phone:** (512)884-5892     **Fax:** (512)884-2332

**★ 20463 ★ National Kidney Foundation of West Texas, Inc.**
4601 50th St., Ste. 101
Lubbock, TX 79414
**Phone:** (806)799-7753     **Fax:** (806)799-0277
**Email:** nkfwt@nts-online.net
**Website:** http://www.nkfwt.org

### Utah

**★ 20464 ★ National Kidney Foundation of Utah, Inc.**
Edgemont Professional Plaza
3707 N Canyon Rd., 1-D
Provo, UT 84604
**Phone:** (801)226-5111     **Fax:** (801)226-8278
**Email:** NKFU@KidneyUT.org
**Website:** http://www.KidneyUT.org

### Virginia

**★ 20465 ★ National Kidney Foundation of the Virginias, Inc.**
2601 Willard Rd., Ste. 103
Richmond, VA 23294
**Phone:** (804)288-8342     **Free:** 888-543-6398
**Fax:** (804)282-7835
**Email:** randallm@kidneyva.org
**Website:** http://www.kidneyva.org

### Washington

**★ 20466 ★ National Kidney Foundation of Oregon and Washington, Inc.**
2889 152nd Ave. NE, Ste. C
Redmond, WA 98052

**Phone:** (425)883-2869          **Free:** 888-4-KIDNEY
**Fax:** (425)883-3869
**Email:** help@kidneyorwa.org
**Website:** http://www.kidneyorwa.org

★ **20467** ★ **National Kidney Foundation of Oregon and Washington, Inc.**
**Yakima Chapter**
32 N 3rd St., No. 412
Yakima, WA 98901
**Phone:** (509)452-2024          **Fax:** (509)225-6387
**Email:** yakima@kidneyorwa.org
**Website:** http://www.kidneyorwa.org

## West Virginia

★ **20468** ★ **National Kidney Foundation of Western Pennsylvania, Inc.**
**Charleston Area Chapter**
PO Box 2024
Charleston, WV 25327
**Phone:** (304)345-6998
**Remarks:** Also serves middle and southern West Virginia.

## Wisconsin

★ **20469** ★ **National Kidney Foundation of Wisconsin, Inc.**
280 Regency Ct., No. 100
Brookfield, WI 53045
**Phone:** (262)821-0705          **Free:** 800-543-6393
**Fax:** (414)821-5641
**Email:** nkfw@kidneywi.org
**Website:** http://www.kidneywi.org

## <u>Urological</u> <u>Diseases</u>

*State chapters of the American Urological Association are listed below. The national office is located at 1120 N Charles St., Baltimore, MD 21201. Additional information can be obtained by calling the national office at (410) 727-1100, or by consulting their web site at http://auanet.org/.*

## California

★ **20470** ★ **American Urological Association**
**Western Section**
1950 Old Tustin Ave.
Santa Ana, CA 92705
**Phone:** (714)550-9155          **Fax:** (714)550-9234
**Email:** urologyusa@aol.com
**Website:** http://www.urologyusa.com
Frank J. DeSantis, Exec Director

**Remarks:** The Western section comprises the states of Alaska, Arizona, California, Hawaii, Idaho, Montana, Nevada, Oregon, Utah, Washington and Wyoming; the Canadian provinces of Alberta, British Columbia and Saskatchewan; and the island possessions of the United States in the Pacific Ocean.

## Illinois

★ **20471** ★ **American Urological Association**
**North Central Section**
1111 N Plaza Dr., Ste. 550
Schaumburg, IL 60173-4950
**Phone:** (847)517-1544          **Fax:** (847)517-7229
**Email:** ncs@wjweiser.com
Wendy Weiser, Exec Director

**Remarks:** Comprises the states of Illinois, Indiana, Iowa, Michigan, Minnesota, North Dakota, Ohio, South Dakota and Wisconsin.

★ **20472** ★ **American Urological Association**
**South Central Section**
1111 N Plaza Dr., Ste. 550
Schaumburg, IL 60173-4950
**Phone:** (847)605-0850          **Fax:** (847)517-7229
**Email:** scs@wjweiser.com
Wendy Weiser, Exec Director

**Remarks:** Comprises the states of Arkansas, Colorado, Kansas, Missouri, Nebraska, New Mexico, Oklahoma and Texas, in addition to Mexico, Belize and the Republics of Costa Rica, El Salvador, Honduras and Nicaragua.

★ **20473** ★ **American Urological Association**
**Southeastern Section**
1111 N Plaza Dr., Ste. 550
Schaumburg, IL 60173-4950
**Phone:** (847)969-0248          **Fax:** (847)517-7229
**Email:** ses@wjweiser.com
**Website:** http://www.sesaua.org
Wendy Weiser, Contact

**Remarks:** Comprises the states of Alabama, Florida, Georgia, Kentucky, Louisiana, Mississippi, North Carolina, South Carolina and Tennessee, in addition to Puerto Rico, the Virgin Islands and the Republic of Panama.

## Massachusetts

★ **20474** ★ **American Urological Association**
**Mid-Atlantic Section**
13 Elm St.
Manchester, MA 01944-1314

**Phone:** (978)526-8330          **Fax:** (978)526-4018
**Email:** maaua@prri.com
**Website:** http://www.auanet.org/membership/sections/midatlantic/
Robert P. Jones, EdD, Exec Director

**Remarks:** Comprises the southern portion of the state of New Jersey and the eastern portion of the state of Pennsylvania. The states of Delaware, Maryland, Virginia and West Virginia are also included, as well as Washington, D.C.

★ **20475** ★ **American Urological Association**
**New England Section**
13 Elm St.
Manchester, MA 01944
**Phone:** (978)526-8330          **Fax:** (978)526-4018
**Email:** neaua@prri.com
Aurelie M. Alger, JD, Exec Director

**Remarks:** Comprises the states of Connecticut, Maine, Massachusetts, New Hampshire, Rhode Island and Vermont.

★ **20476** ★ **American Urological Association**
**Northeastern Section**
13 Elm St.
Manchester, MA 01944
**Phone:** (978)526-8330          **Fax:** (978)526-4018
**Email:** nsaua@prri.com
David Cloud, Exec Director

**Remarks:** Comprises the state of New York (except the southeastern portion) and the western portion of the state of Pennsylvania. The eastern portion of Canada, including the provinces of Ontario, Quebec, New Brunswick, Nova Scotia, Prince Edward Island, Newfoundland and Manitoba are also included.

## New York

★ **20477** ★ **American Urological Association**
**New York Section**
1216 Fifth Ave., Rm. 554
New York, NY 10029
**Phone:** (212)722-4300          **Fax:** (212)722-1842
**Email:** auany@aol.com
Ida Flores, Exec Director

**Remarks:** Comprises the southeastern portion of the state of New York, including Long Island, and the northern portion of the state of New Jersey.

# Chapter 68
# Veterinary Medicine

## Federal Government Agencies

**★ 20478 ★ U.S. Department of Agriculture**
**Agricultural Research Service (ARS)**
**National Agricultural Library (NAL)**
5601 Sunnyside Ave., Rm. 1-2250
Beltsville, MD 20705-5128
**Phone:** (301)504-1638 **Fax:** (301)504-1648
**Website:** http://www.usda.gov
**Desc:** The National Agricultural Library provides information services over a broad range of agricultural interests to a wide cross-section of users, from research scientists to the general public. The Library assists users through a variety of specialized information centers.

**★ 20479 ★ U.S. Department of Agriculture**
**Animal and Plant Health Inspection Service**
**Veterinary Services**
Legislative and Public Affairs
Washington, DC 20250
**Phone:** (202)720-2511
**Website:** http://www.usda.gov
**Desc:** Animal health officials are responsible for programs to protect and improve the health, quality, and marketability of U.S. animals and animal products. The programs are carried out through cooperative links with States, foreign governments, livestock producers, and other Federal agencies. Service officials exclude, control, and eradicate animal pests and diseases by carrying out eradication and control programs for certain diseases, providing diagnostic services, and gathering and disseminating information regarding animal health in the United States through land, air and ocean ports. They also certify as to the health status of animals and animal products being exported to other countries and respond to animal disease incursions or epidemics which threaten the health status of U.S. livestock and poultry. The service also administers a Federal law intended that all veterinary biological products, whether developed by conventional or new biotechnological procedures, used in the diagnosis, prevention and treatment of animal diseases are safe, pure, potent and effective. The Service regulates firms that manufacture veterinary biological products subject to the act, including licensing the manufacturing establishment and its products, inspecting production facilities and production methods, and testing products under a surveillance program.

**★ 20480 ★ U.S. Department of Health and Human Services**
**Food and Drug Administration**
**Center for Veterinary Medicine**
7519 Standish Pl.
Rockville, MD 20855
**Phone:** (301)827-3800
**Website:** http://www.fda.gov/cvm/default.html
Stephen F. Sundlof, DVM, Director
**Desc:** The Center develops and conducts programs with respect to the safety and efficacy of veterinary preparations and devices; evaluates proposed use of veterinary preparations for animal safety and efficacy; and evaluates FDA's surveillance and compliance programs relating to veterinary drugs and other veterinary medical matters.

## Foundations & Other Funding Organizations

### Private Foundations

**★ 20481 ★ Animal Assistance Foundation**
455 Sherman St., Ste. 462
Denver, CO 80203
**Phone:** (303)744-8396 **Fax:** (303)744-7065
**Email:** info@aaf-fd.org
**Website:** http://www.aaf-fd.org
David Gies, Executive Director
**Fnded:** 1975. **Philosophy:** The Animal Assistance Foundation is a nonprofit organization dedicated to domestic pet population control and to the enhancement of animal welfare through charitable, scientific, and educational means. This will be accomplished by providing leadership on animal welfare issues, assuring the continuing operation of the Harrison Memorial Animal Hospital, contributing funds and other assistance to animal welfare organizations, and supporting veterinary, scientific, and social domestic pet research. **Priorities:** *Environment:* 100%. Provides support for pet population control, research, and humane education. All grants relate in some way to helping companion animals. *Note:* Total contributions made in fiscal 2000. **Typ. Recipients:** AIDS/HIV, Substance Abuse. **Geo. Dist:** CO.

### Other Funding Organizations

**★ 20482 ★ American Association of Equine Practitioners (AAEP)**
4075 Iron Works Parkway
Lexington, KY 40511
**Phone:** (859)233-0147 **Free:** 800-443-0177
**Fax:** (859)233-1968
**Email:** dfoley@aaep.org
**Website:** http://www.aaep.org
David L. Foley, Exec. Dir.
**Desc:** Veterinarians who specialize in equine medicine and surgery. Disseminates the latest scientific information relative to the practice of equine medicine; promotes research on horses. Maintains 10 professional committees. **Awards:** AAEP/American Live Stock Insurance Co. (annual); AAEP Research Program (annual); AAEP/United States Pony Club (annual).

**★ 20483 ★ American Association of Feline Practitioners (AAFP)**
200 4th Ave. N, No. 900
Nashville, TN 37219
**Phone:** (615)257-7788 **Free:** 800-204-3514
**Fax:** (615)254-7047
**Email:** aafp@walkermgmt.com
**Website:** http://www.aafponline.org
Dr. Diane Eigner, Pres.
**Desc:** Doctors of veterinary medicine who specialize or have a general interest in the field of feline medicine and surgery. Works to promote the interests and improve the public stature of feline practice and to increase the knowledge of veterinarians in the field. Cooperates with other veterinary and cat fancier organizations. **Awards:** Grant for feline research; recognition for student achievement.

**★ 20484 ★ American Board of Veterinary Toxicology (ABVT)**
School of Veterinary Medicine
382 W St. Rd.
Kennett Square, PA 19348
**Phone:** (610)444-5800 **Fax:** (610)925-8117
**Email:** roder@amaonline.com
**Website:** http://www.abvt.org
Carl T. Olsonnga, Exec. Sec.
**Desc:** Seeks to: further education and scientific progress in veterinary toxicology; encourage research and training; establish and maintain the highest possible standards of training and experience for qualification in toxicology; recognize qualified specialists through certification. Conducts annual examination. **Awards:** Lloyd Laboratories Pfizer Student Paper Award (annual) for best paper relating to veterinary toxicology.

**★ 20485 ★ American College of Veterinary Dermatology (ACVD)**
c/o Alexis Borich, Exec. Sec.
5610 Kearny Mesa Rd., Ste. B
San Diego, CA 92111
**Phone:** (858)560-9393 **Fax:** (858)560-0206
**Website:** http://www.acvd.org
Dr. Donna W Angarano, Pres.
**Desc:** Specialists in veterinary dermatology who have satisfied examination requirements; individuals with national reputation and standing are charter diplomates. promotes veterinary dermatology enhances the competencey of professionals in the field. Seeks to develop guidelines for postdoctoral education and to establish experience prerequisites for certification in veterinary dermatology. Administers examinations and certifies veterinarians as veterinary dermatology specialists. Encourages research and other contributions in areas of pathogenesis, diagnosis, therapy, prevention, and control of diseases affecting the skin of animals. Authorizes training programs in the field.

**Awards:** ACVD Award of Excellence (annual) for excellence in research, teaching, and service in the field of veterinary dermatology.

### ★ 20486 ★ American College of Veterinary Radiology (ACVR)

c/o Dr. M. Bernstein
PO Box 87
Glencoe, IL 60022
**Phone:** (847)251-5517          **Fax:** (847)446-8618
**Email:** tgnyland@usdavis.edu
**Website:** http://www.acvr.ucdavis.edu/
Dr. M. Bernstein, Exec. Dir.

**Desc:** Diplomate members (215) are veterinarians certified by the college in veterinary radiology; associate members (6) are individuals distinguished in radiological science but who are not certified veterinary radiologists. Educational association working to advance the art and science of radiology. Certifies candidates who have demonstrated proficiency in veterinary radiology. Encourages the development of teaching personnel and training facilities in veterinary radiology. Aids in the evaluation of residencies and fellowships in veterinary radiology under consideration by the Council on Education of the American Veterinary Medical Association. Advises veterinarians who desire certification in veterinary radiology. Conducts continuing education seminars in conjunction with other veterinary organizations. **Awards:** Research Grant (annual) publishes in Journal Veterinary Radiology and Ultrasound; Resident Authored Paper (annual) for best resident-authored paper.

### ★ 20487 ★ American Veterinary Society of Animal Behavior (AVSAB)

c/o Steven Feldman
9414 Brandywine Rd.
Clinton, MD 20735
**Phone:** (301)868-1180
**Email:** avsabe@yahoo.com
**Website:** http://www.avma.org/avsab/
Steve Feldman, Sec. /Treas.

**Desc:** Veterinarians and veterinary students. Promotes inquiry and research into animal behavior. Seeks to advance ethological knowledge regarding the care and utilization of captive, domesticated, and free-living animals. Promotes and facilitates the exchange of information among those concerned with animal behavior and well-being; encourages discussion on veterinary aspects of animal behavior and the publication of materials in the field. **Awards:** Student Excellence in Applied Animal Research (annual).

### ★ 20488 ★ Association of Zoo Veterinary Technicians

White Oak Conservation Center
3823 Owens Rd.
Yulee, FL 32097
**Phone:** (386)879-7636          **Fax:** (386)879-7637
**Email:** cheryl_purnell@ncmail.net
**Website:** http://www.AZVT.org
Cheryl Purnell, Exec. Dir.

**Desc:** Zoo veterinary technicians. **Awards:** Laurie Page-Peck Scholarship (annual) for veterinary technician students with interest in zoo medicine; must write a paper for presentation at annual conference.

### ★ 20489 ★ International Veterinary Acupuncture Society (IVAS)

PO Box 271395
Fort Collins, CO 80527-1395
**Phone:** (970)266-0660          **Fax:** (970)266-0777
**Email:** office@ivas.org
**Website:** http://www.ivas.org/
Edward C. Boldt, Jr., Exec. Dir.

**Desc:** Veterinarians and veterinary students. Encourages knowledge and research of the philosophy, technique, and practice of veterinary acupuncture. Fosters high standards in the field; promotes scientific investigation. Accumulates resources for scientific research and education; collects data concerning clinical and research cases where animals have been treated with acupuncture; disseminates information to veterinary students, practitioners, other scientific groups, and the public. Offers 100 contact hour basic veterinary acupuncture course; administers certification examination. **Awards:** Research Grant (annual).

### ★ 20490 ★ Mid-Atlantic States Association of Avian Veterinarians (MASAAV)

Memorial Bldg., Ste. 291
610 N Main St.
Blacksburg, VA 24060-3311
**Phone:** (540)951-2559          **Fax:** (540)953-0230
**Email:** office@masaav.org
**Website:** http://www.masaav.org
Keath L. Marx, DVM, Exec. Dir.

**Desc:** Works to address the needs of the avian veterinarian and technicians. innovative veterinary medicine and surgery to improve the health of avian patients. Conducts educational programs; makes donations for avian research; keeps members informed regarding legislation of interest to the profession. **Awards:** E. L. Stubbs Research Grant (periodic) researchers in avian medicine and surgery; Pamela Slack Award for Excellence (annual) veterinary college junior.

### ★ 20491 ★ National Association of Federal Veterinarians (NAFV)

1101 Vermont Ave. NW, Ste. 710
Washington, DC 20005-6308
**Phone:** (202)289-6334          **Fax:** (202)842-4360
**Email:** nafv@erols.com
**Website:** http://users.erols.com/nafv/
Alice M. Thaler, Pres.

**Desc:** Professional society of veterinarians employed by the U.S. Government. Maintains speakers' bureau. **Awards:** Dr. Daniel E. Salmon Award (annual) for federally employed veterinarians with no more than 10 years service.

### ★ 20492 ★ Orthopedic Foundation for Animals (OFA)

2300 Nifong Blvd.
Columbia, MO 65201-3856
**Phone:** (573)442-0418          **Fax:** (573)875-5073
**Email:** ofa@offa.org
**Website:** http://www.offa.org
Dr. G.G. Keller, Project Dir.

**Desc:** National and local dog clubs and individual breeders. Acts as a clearinghouse for information on orthopedic diseases of animals, particularly hip dysplasia in dogs (a hereditary condition resulting in abnormal development of the hip joints). Is attempting to develop a national control program through monitoring animals and conducting selective breeding and research. Conducts educational seminars; compiles statistics; sponsors a national referral service for animal breeders. Maintains library of all breed canine pelvic radiographs. **Awards:** Grant for research.

### ★ 20493 ★ Veterinary Orthopedic Society (VOS)

PO Box 313
Newmarket, NH 03857-0313
**Phone:** (603)659-7989          **Fax:** (603)659-7989
**Email:** vosclarkmt@aol.com
**Website:** http://www.vet.ohio-state.edu/docs/vos
Mary Tuson Clark, Exec. Sec.

**Desc:** Veterinarians interested in orthopedic surgery. Promotes education and research in veterinary orthopedic surgery. Provides a forum for the exchange of ideas among veterinarians in academia, research, and practice. **Awards:** Hohn-Johnson Research Awards (annual) for research; Mark S. Blomberg Memorial Resident Research Award (annual) outstanding resident abstract submitted to the VOS scientific program.

# Medical & Allied Health Schools

## Veterinary Medicine

*Colleges of veterinary medicine listed in this section are accredited by the American Veterinary Medical Association, 1931 N Meacham Rd., Ste. 100, Schaumburg, IL 60173, (847)925-8070, http://www.avma.org/.*

### Alabama

### ★ 20494 ★ Auburn University College of Veterinary Medicine

Auburn University, AL 36849
**Phone:** (334)844-3691
**Website:** http://www.vetmed.auburn.edu

### ★ 20495 ★ Tuskegee University School of Veterinary Medicine

Tuskegee University, AL 36088
**Phone:** (334)727-8173
**Website:** http://svmc107.tusk.edu

### California

### ★ 20496 ★ University of California, Davis School of Veterinary Medicine

Davis, CA 95616-8734
**Phone:** (530)752-1360
**Website:** http://www.vetmed.ucdavis.edu

### ★ 20497 ★ Western University of Health Sciences College of Veterinary Medicine

309 E 2nd St., College Plaza
Pomona, CA 91766
**Phone:** (909)469-5628
**Website:** http://www.westernu.edu/cvm.html

### Colorado

### ★ 20498 ★ Colorado State University College of Veterinary Medicine and Biomedical Sciences

Fort Collins, CO 80523
**Phone:** (970)491-7051
**Website:** http://www.cvmbs.colostate.edu

### Florida

### ★ 20499 ★ University of Florida College of Veterinary Medicine

Gainesville, FL 32610-0125
**Phone:** (352)392-4700
**Website:** http://www.vetmed.ufl.edu

### Georgia

### ★ 20500 ★ University of Georgia College of Veterinary Medicine

Athens, GA 30602
**Phone:** (706)542-3461
**Website:** http://www.vet.uga.edu

### Illinois

### ★ 20501 ★ University of Illinois College of Veterinary Medicine

2001 S Lincoln
Urbana, IL 61801
**Phone:** (217)333-2760
**Website:** http://www.cvm.uiuc.edu

## Indiana

**★ 20502 ★ Purdue University**
**School of Veterinary Medicine**
1240 Lynn Hall
West Lafayette, IN 47907-1240
**Phone:** (765)494-7607
**Website:** http://www.vet.purdue.edu

## Iowa

**★ 20503 ★ Iowa State University**
**College of Veterinary Medicine**
Ames, IA 50011
**Phone:** (515)294-1242
**Website:** http://www.vetmed.iastate.edu

## Kansas

**★ 20504 ★ Kansas State University**
**College of Veterinary Medicine**
Manhattan, KS 66506
**Phone:** (785)532-6011
**Website:** http://www.vet.ksu.edu

## Louisiana

**★ 20505 ★ Louisiana State University**
**School of Veterinary Medicine**
Baton Rouge, LA 70803
**Phone:** (225)346-3100
**Website:** http://www.vetmed.lsu.edu

## Massachusetts

**★ 20506 ★ Tufts University**
**School of Veterinary Medicine**
200 Westboro Rd.
North Grafton, MA 01536
**Phone:** (508)839-5302
**Website:** http://www.tufts.edu/vet

## Michigan

**★ 20507 ★ Michigan State University**
**College of Veterinary Medicine**
East Lansing, MI 48824-1314
**Phone:** (517)355-6509
**Website:** http://www.cvm.msu.edu

## Minnesota

**★ 20508 ★ University of Minnesota**
**College of Veterinary Medicine**
Saint Paul, MN 55108
**Phone:** (612)624-9227
**Website:** http://www.cvm.umn.edu

## Mississippi

**★ 20509 ★ Mississippi State University**
**College of Veterinary Medicine**
Mississippi State, MS 39762
**Phone:** (662)325-3432
**Website:** http://www.cvm.msstate.edu

## Missouri

**★ 20510 ★ University of Missouri**
**College of Veterinary Medicine**
Columbia, MO 65211
**Phone:** (573)882-3877
**Website:** http://www.cvm.missouri.edu

## New York

**★ 20511 ★ Cornell University**
**College of Veterinary Medicine**
Ithaca, NY 14853-6401
**Phone:** (607)253-3700
**Website:** http://www.vet.cornell.edu

## North Carolina

**★ 20512 ★ North Carolina State University**
**College of Veterinary Medicine**
4700 Hillsborough St.
Raleigh, NC 27606
**Phone:** (919)513-6200
**Website:** http://www.cvm.ncsu.edu

## Ohio

**★ 20513 ★ Ohio State University**
**College of Veterinary Medicine**
Columbus, OH 43210
**Phone:** (614)292-1171
**Website:** http://www.vet.ohio-state.edu

## Oklahoma

**★ 20514 ★ Oklahoma State University**
**College of Veterinary Medicine**
Stillwater, OK 74078
**Phone:** (405)744-6648
**Website:** http://www.cvm.okstate.edu

## Ontario

**★ 20515 ★ University of Guelph**
**Ontario Veterinary College**
Guelph, ON, Canada N1G 2W1
**Fax:** (519)837-3230

## Oregon

**★ 20516 ★ Oregon State University**
**College of Veterinary Medicine**
Corvallis, OR 97331-4801
**Phone:** (541)737-2141
**Website:** http://www.vet.orst.edu

## Pennsylvania

**★ 20517 ★ University of Pennsylvania**
**School of Veterinary Medicine**
3800 Spruce St.
Philadelphia, PA 19104-6044
**Phone:** (215)898-5434
**Website:** http://www.vet.upenn.edu

## Prince Edward Island

**★ 20518 ★ University of Prince Edward Island**
**Atlantic Veterinary College**
Charlottetown, PE, Canada C1A 4P3
**Phone:** (902)566-0800    **Fax:** (902)566-0958

## Quebec

**★ 20519 ★ University of Montreal**
**Faculty of Veterinary Medicine**
Saint Hyancinthe, QC, Canada J2S 7C6
**Phone:** (514)345-8521    **Fax:** (514)778-8114

## Saskatchewan

**★ 20520 ★ University of Saskatchewan**
**Western College of Veterinary Medicine**
52 Campus Dr.
Saskatoon, SK, Canada S7N 5B4
**Fax:** (306)966-8747

## Tennessee

**★ 20521 ★ University of Tennessee**
**College of Veterinary Medicine**
Knoxville, TN 37901
**Phone:** (865)974-7262
**Website:** http://www.vet.utk.edu

## Texas

**★ 20522 ★ Texas A&M University**
**College of Veterinary Medicine**
College Station, TX 77843-4461
**Phone:** (409)845-5051
**Website:** http://www.cvm.tamu.edu

## Virginia

**★ 20523 ★ Virginia Tech/University of Maryland**
**Virginia-Maryland Regional College of Veterinary Medicine**
Blacksburg, VA 24061-0442
**Phone:** (540)231-4621
**Website:** http://www.vetmed.vt.edu

## Washington

**★ 20524 ★ Washington State University**
**College of Veterinary Medicine**
Pullman, WA 99164-7010
**Phone:** (509)335-9515
**Website:** http://www.vetmed.wsu.edu

## Wisconsin

**★ 20525 ★ University of Wisconsin, Madison**
**School of Veterinary Medicine**
Madison, WI 53706
**Phone:** (608)263-6716
**Website:** http://www.vetmed.wisc.edu

---

# National & International Organizations

**★ 20526 ★ Academia Nacional de Agronomia y Veterinaria**
Av Alvear 1711
1014 Buenos Aires, Argentina
**Phone:** 54 1 8124168    **Fax:** 54 1 8124168
**Fnded:** 1909.

**★ 20527 ★ Academy of Veterinary Allergy and Clinical Immunology (AVA)**
c/o Richard Rossman, Treas.
330 Waukegan Rd.
Glenview, IL 60025
**Phone:** (847)729-5200    **Fax:** (847)729-5214
**Email:** richlge@aol.com
**Website:** http://www.avaci.org
Dr. Richard Rossman, DVM, Treas.

**Fnded:** 1960. **Mem:** 300. **Desc:** Veterinarians, research M.D.s, and allergy extract firms. Promotes education and research in veterinary and comparative allergy and immunology. **Pub:** *Membership List*, periodic. • *Veterinary Allergist*, quarterly.

**★ 20528 ★ Academy of Veterinary Cardiology (AVC)**
48 Notch Rd.
Little Falls, NJ 07424
**Fax:** (973)890-5617
Andrew Beardow, Exec. VP

**Fnded:** 1967. **Mem:** 600. **Desc:** Persons with an interest in veterinary or comparative cardiology. Purpose is to disseminate literature, reviews, and materials of interest to veterinary practitioners. Maintains specialized education program. **Pub:** Membership Directory, biennial. • Newsletter, periodic. • Also publishes abstracts and bibliography.

## ★ 20529 ★ Academy of Veterinary Homeopathy (AVH)

PO Box 9280
Wilmington, DE 19809
**Free:** (866)652-1590 **Fax:** (302)653-7244
**Email:** webmaster@theavh.org
**Website:** http://www.theavh.org/
Susan H. Pitcaim, Off. Mgr.

**Fnded:** 1996. **Desc:** Works to promote education and research in veterinary homeopathy. Offers an accreditation training program for veterinarians; provides referrals to the public; sponsors continuing education conferences; supports practical and clinical research.

## ★ 20530 ★ Academy of Zoology

Church Rd. 2/95, Civil Lines
Agra 282 002, India
**Fnded:** 1954.

## ★ 20531 ★ American Academy of Veterinary and Comparative Toxicology (AAVCT)

c/o Dr. Ramesh Gupta
Murray State University in Kentucky
Breathitt Veterinary Center
715 North Dr.
PO Box 2000
Hopkinsville, KY 42240
**Phone:** (270)886-3959 **Fax:** (270)886-4295
**Email:** ramesh.gupta@murraystate.edu
Dr. Ramesh Gupta, Contact

**Fnded:** 1957. **Mem:** 178. **Desc:** Veterinarians specializing in toxicology and others interested in veterinary comparative toxicology. Sponsors and encourages scientific and technical meetings and promotes discussion and interchange of information in the following fields of veterinary comparative toxicology: teaching, research and development, diagnosis, nomenclature, public health, and other problems of common interest. Reviews manuscripts and literature pertaining to toxicology and keeps a file of such literature for use by its members. Encourages the use of uniform toxicologic nomenclature. Facilitates and implements the exchange of proven methods among veterinary comparative toxicologists. **Pub:** *Veterinary and Human Toxicology*, quarterly. Journal. Contains annual directory. **Frmly:** American College of Veterinary Toxicologists.

## ★ 20532 ★ American Academy of Veterinary Nutrition (AAVN)

1080 North Cobb Pky.
Marietta, GA 30062
**Email:** s.wynn@mindspring.com
Susan G. Wynn, DVM, Sec. -Treas.

**Fnded:** 1956. **Mem:** 475. **Desc:** Veterinarians and nutritional scientists interested in animal nutrition and health. Works to promote research and discussion in fields where health of animals may be influenced by nutrition. Sponsors programs on animal nutrition. Maintains speakers' bureau. **Pub:** Membership Directory, annual. **Frmly:** (1978) American Association of Veterinary Nutritionists.

## ★ 20533 ★ American Academy of Veterinary Pharmacology and Therapeutics (AAVPT)

c/o Dr. Vernon "Cory" Langston
Mississippi State University
College of Veterinary Medicine
PO Box 9825
Mississippi State, MS 39762
**Phone:** (662)325-1265 **Fax:** (662)325-4011
**Email:** langston@cvm.msstate.edu
**Website:** http://www.aavpt.org/
Vernon "Cory" Langston, DVM, Sec. -Treas.

**Fnded:** 1977. **Mem:** 187. **Desc:** Veterinary pharmacologists and clinicians interested in clinical therapeutics; representatives of academia, industry, and government; private practitioners. Supports and promotes education and research in comparative pharmacology, clinical veterinary pharmacology, and other aspects of pharmacology of interest to the veterinary profession; aims to enhance the exchange of educational materials and ideas among veterinary pharmacologists. Organizes committees of experts to research and make recommendations to the profession on current problems in veterinary therapeutics. Sponsors and conducts workshops and other scientific and educational meetings. **Pub:** *Journal of Veterinary Pharmacology and Therapeutics*, 8/year. Journal. • Directory, periodic. • Newsletter, quarterly.

## ★ 20534 ★ American Animal Hospital Association (AAHA)

12575 West Bayaud Ave.
Lakewood, CO 80228
**Phone:** (303)986-2800 **Free:** 800-252-2242
**Fax:** (303)986-1700
**Email:** katie.valentine@aahanet.org
**Website:** http://www.aahanet.org
John W. Albers, D.V.M., Exec. Dir.

**Fnded:** 1933. **Mem:** 17,000. **Desc:** Veterinarians engaged in small animal practice who own or staff small animal hospitals. Works for the promotion of excellence in small animal medicine and improvement of hospital facilities. Operates AAHA Foundation, which gives grants for small animal medical research. Compiles statistics. **Pub:** *American Animal Hospital Association Scientific Proceedings*, annual. Proceedings. Includes manuscripts of papers delivered at AAHA meeting. Contains authors index. *Price:* Included in membership dues; $55 for nonmembers plus shipping and handling. • *Journal of the American Animal Hospital Association*, bimonthly. Journal. Includes advertisers' index. *Price:* Included in membership dues; $107/year U.S. & Canada; $127/year Foreign Countries. • *TRENDS Magazine*, bimonthly. Magazine. Covers management trends, social issues, paraprofessional topics in veterinary medicine; includes association news, and CE calendar. *Price:* Included in membership dues; $60/year for nonmembers. • Membership Directory, annual. • Has also published atlases for ophthalmology, behavior, oncology, dermatology, cytology, and cardiology and a manual of standards.

## ★ 20535 ★ American Association of Avian Pathologists (AAAP)

382 West St. Rd.
New Bolton Center
Kennett Square, PA 19348
**Phone:** (610)444-4282 **Fax:** (610)925-8106
**Email:** aaap@vet.upenn.edu
**Website:** http://www.aaap.info/
Dr. Robert J. Eckroade, Sec. -Treas.

**Fnded:** 1957. **Mem:** 1,100. **Desc:** Membership limited to graduates of recognized veterinary colleges. Associate members are not veterinarians but are engaged in some form of avian medicine. Maintains 29 committees. **Pub:** *Avian Diseases*, quarterly. Journal. Contains case reports. *Price:* Included in membership dues; $110/year for nonmembers in U.S.; $120/year for nonmembers outside U.S. • Manuals. • Videos.

## ★ 20536 ★ American Association of Bovine Practitioners (AABP)

Box 1755
Rome, GA 30162
**Phone:** (706)232-2220 **Fax:** (706)232-2232
**Email:** aabphq@aabp.org
**Website:** http://www.aabp.org
James A Jarrett, Exec. Dir.

**Fnded:** 1965. **Mem:** 5,800. **Desc:** Veterinarians who practice bovine medicine. Aims to elevate standards in the field; cooperates with veterinary and agricultural organizations and regulatory agencies. **Pub:** *AABP Newsletter*, monthly. Newsletter. Contains meetings calendar. *Price:* Included in membership dues. • *American Association of Bovine Practitioners Directory*, annual. Directory. Includes annual supplements. *Price:* Included in membership dues; $25/copy for select others. • *American Association of Bovine Practitioners Proceedings of Annual Meeting*. *Price:* Included in membership dues; $40/copy for nonmembers. •

*Bovine Practitioner*, annual. Covers new developments in bovine practice. *Price:* Included in membership dues; $20/copy for nonmembers.

## ★ 20537 ★ American Association of Equine Practitioners (AAEP)

4075 Iron Works Parkway
Lexington, KY 40511
**Phone:** (859)233-0147 **Free:** 800-443-0177
**Fax:** (859)233-1968
**Email:** dfoley@aaep.org
**Website:** http://www.aaep.org
David L. Foley, Exec. Dir.

**Fnded:** 1954. **Mem:** 6,500. **Desc:** Veterinarians who specialize in equine medicine and surgery. Disseminates the latest scientific information relative to the practice of equine medicine; promotes research on horses. Maintains 10 professional committees. **Pub:** *AAEP Report*, monthly. Newsletter. • *Annual Convention Proceedings*, annual. Proceedings. *Price:* $37 for members; $74 for nonmembers. • Directory, annual.

## ★ 20538 ★ American Association of Feline Practitioners (AAFP)

200 4th Ave. N, No. 900
Nashville, TN 37219
**Phone:** (615)257-7788 **Free:** 800-204-3514
**Fax:** (615)254-7047
**Email:** aafp@walkermgmt.com
**Website:** http://www.aafponline.org
Dr. Diane Eigner, Pres.

**Fnded:** 1970. **Mem:** 1,400. **Desc:** Doctors of veterinary medicine who specialize or have a general interest in the field of feline medicine and surgery. Works to promote the interests and improve the public stature of feline practice and to increase the knowledge of veterinarians in the field. Cooperates with other veterinary and cat fancier organizations. **Pub:** Newsletter, semiannual.

## ★ 20539 ★ American Association of Industrial Veterinarians (AAIV)

PO Box 488
Oskaloosa, KS 66066-0488
**Phone:** (785)863-2389 **Fax:** (785)863-3141
**Email:** aaiv@rualnet.com
Peggy Miller, Admin. Coord.

**Fnded:** 1954. **Mem:** 450. **Desc:** Veterinarians, many of whom are members of the American Veterinary Medical Association and are employed in a professional capacity in industrial activities, for example, with drug and chemical firms, in livestock and poultry enterprises, or in independent research. Holds workshops. **Pub:** *AAIV Highlights*, semiannual. Newsletter. Membership activities newsletter. Includes member biographical sketches. *Price:* Included in membership dues. • Directory, annual. **Frmly:** Industrial Veterinarians Association.

## ★ 20540 ★ American Association for Laboratory Animal Science (AALAS)

9190 Crestwyn Hills Dr.
Memphis, TN 38125
**Phone:** (901)754-8620 **Fax:** (901)753-0046
**Email:** info@aalas.org
**Website:** http://www.aalas.org
Ann Tourigny Turner, PhD, Exec. Dir.

**Fnded:** 1950. **Mem:** 12,000. **Reg. Groups:** 8. **Local Groups:** 48. **Desc:** Persons and institutions professionally concerned with the production, use, care, and study of laboratory animals. Serves as clearinghouse for collection and exchange of information on all phases of laboratory animal care and management and on the care, use, and procurement of laboratory animals used in biomedical research. Conducts examinations and certification through its Animal Technician Certification Program. **Pub:** *American Association for Laboratory Animal Science–Reference Directory*, annual. Membership Directory. Arranged alphabetically by name and geographically. *Price:* Included in membership dues. • *Comparative Medicine*, bimonthly. Journal. Covers comparative and experimental medicine related to laboratory animal science. *Price:* $150 subscription rate. • *Contemporary Topics in Laboratory Animal Science*, bimonthly. Contains refereed papers covering topics in laboratory animal science; covers association activities. *Price:* Included in membership dues. • Also publishes educational materials. **Frmly:** (1967) Animal Care Panel.

**★ 20541 ★ American Association of Medical Milk Commissions (AAMMC)**
c/o Paul Fleiss, M.D.
1824 N Hillhurst Ave.
Los Angeles, CA 90027
**Phone:** (323)664-1977 **Fax:** (323)664-0870
**Email:** fleiss@hsc.usc.edu
Paul Fleiss, MD, Pres.

**Fnded:** 1907. **Mem:** 35. **Desc:** Professional society of physician members of local Medical Milk Commissions, including veterinarians, sanitarians, and bacteriologists who supervise production of certified milk (milk from dairies conforming to official standards of sanitation). **Pub:** *Methods and Standards for the Production of Certified Milk*, annual.

**★ 20542 ★ American Association of Public Health Veterinarians (AAPHV)**
c/o Dr. Joe Horman
5649 Horman Ln.
Frederick, MD 21701
**Fax:** (410)333-6333
**Email:** jthdvmmph@aol.com
**Website:** http://www.avma.org/aaphv
Dr. Joe Horman, Treas.

**Fnded:** 1953. **Mem:** 100. **Desc:** Executive veterinary public health administrators in each state. Work to guide and develop veterinary public health programs in the states and on the national level. **Pub:** *Annual National Compendium of Animal Rabies Control*, annual. **Frmly:** (1968) Association of State Public Health Veterinarians; (1979) Association of State and Territorial Public Health Veterinarians; (1984) National Association of State and Territorial Public Health Veterinarians; (2002) National Association of State Public Health Veterinarians.

**★ 20543 ★ American Association of Retired Veterinarians**
PO Box 4826
Ithaca, NY 14852
**Phone:** (607)533-4114
Dr. Walter J. Martin, Jr., Pres.

**Fnded:** 1986. **Mem:** 425. **Desc:** Individuals with a degree in veterinary medicine who are retired or considering retiring, and their spouses. Seeks to advance the science and art of veterinary medicine. Encourages friendship among those in the profession. Promotes social and professional lives of retired veterinarians. Attempts to assist future retirees in achievement of their goals in retirement life. Organizes group trips and cruises. **Pub:** *AARV Newsletter*. Newsletter. • Membership Directory, periodic.

**★ 20544 ★ American Association of Small Ruminant Practitioners (AASRP)**
1910 Lyda Ave., No. 200
Bowling Green, KY 42104
**Phone:** (270)793-0781 **Fax:** (270)782-0188
**Email:** aasrp@assrp.org
**Website:** http://www.aasrp.org
Richard W. Stobaeus, Jr., Pres.

**Fnded:** 1968. **Mem:** 1,200. **Desc:** Practicing veterinarians and veterinary students; associate members are producers, feeders, hobbyists, and others interested in sheep, goats, llamas, deer, and exotic small ruminants. Aims are to: elevate standards of practice in the field; further research programs that will assist in solving small ruminant health problems; foster communication between veterinarians, owners, and researchers in order to improve small ruminant health management programs. Sponsors specialized education programs. Conducts educational programs. Maintains speakers' bureau. **Pub:** *AASRP Newsletter*

(*Wool & Wattles*), quarterly. Newsletter. *Price:* Included in membership dues. • *Proceedings of Symposium on Health and Disease of Small Ruminants*, annual. Proceedings. *Price:* Included in membership dues. • Also publishes fact sheets and abstracts. **Frmly:** (1988) American Association of Sheep and Goat Practitioners.

**★ 20545 ★ American Association of Swine Veterinarians (AASV)**
902 1st Ave.
Perry, IA 50220-1703
**Phone:** (515)465-5255 **Fax:** (515)465-3832
**Email:** aasv@netins.net
**Website:** http://www.aasv.org
Dr. Tom Burkgren, Exec. Dir.

**Fnded:** 1969. **Mem:** 1,550. **Desc:** Veterinarians concerned with swine health and nutrition. To improve public stature and increase the knowledge of veterinarians in the field of swine practice. **Pub:** *Proceedings*, annual. *Price:* $60 plus s/h. • *Swine Health and Production*, bimonthly. Journals. *Price:* $85/year.

**★ 20546 ★ American Association of Veterinary Clinicians (AAVC)**
37 W Broad St., Ste. 480
Columbus, OH 43215-4132
**Phone:** (614)228-6599 **Fax:** (614)228-1216
**Website:** http://cvm.msu.edu/~judy/aavc1.htm

**Fnded:** 1958. **Desc:** Veterinary clinicians engaged in teaching and/or research at the professional, graduate or postgraduate level. Strives to enhance the quality of teaching, service and research, provides a forum for exploration and creative resolution of clinical issues. Hosts annual meetings, educational programs and sponsors achievement awards.

**★ 20547 ★ American Association of Veterinary Immunologists (AAVI)**
c/o Dr. Will Goff
USDA, ARS
3003 ADBF
Washington State University
Pullman, WA 99164-6630
**Phone:** (509)335-6029 **Fax:** (509)335-8328
**Email:** wgoff@vetmed.wsu.edu
**Website:** http://www.cvm.missouri.edu/aavi
Will Goff, Sec. -Treas.

**Fnded:** 1979. **Mem:** 260. **Desc:** Holders of BS or DVM degrees with an interest in veterinary immunology. Promotes development and dissemination of knowledge in the field of veterinary immunology. Conducts research and educational programs. **Pub:** *AAVI Newsletter*, periodic. Newsletter.

**★ 20548 ★ American Association of Veterinary Laboratory Diagnosticians (CVDLS:SVM)**
c/o UC Davis
PO Box 1522
Turlock, CA 95381
**Phone:** (209)634-5837 **Fax:** (209)667-4261
**Email:** abickfor@cvdls.ucdavis.edu
**Website:** http://www.aavld.org
Dr. Arthur Bickford, Sec. -Treas.

**Fnded:** 1957. **Mem:** 1,100. **Desc:** Each state has an official delegate and alternate to the association's executive board. Individual membership is open to persons active in veterinary laboratory diagnostic medicine. Disseminates information on diagnosis of animal disease; coordinates diagnostic activities of regulatory, research, and service laboratories; establishes uniform diagnostic techniques; seeks to improve existing diagnostic techniques and facilitate the development of new ones; establishes guides for personnel qualifications and facilities; acts as consultant to the U.S. Animal Health Association on uniform diagnostic criteria. **Pub:** *AAVLD Newsletter*, 3/year. Newsletter. Contains association news and information on employment opportunities. *Price:* Included in membership dues. • *Journal of Veterinary Diagnostic Investigation*,

bimonthly. Journal. *Price:* Included in membership dues.

**★ 20549 ★ American Association of Veterinary State Boards (AAVSB)**
3100 Main St., Ste. 208
Kansas City, MO 64111-1918
**Phone:** (816)931-1504 **Free:** 877-698-8482
**Fax:** (816)931-1604
**Email:** info@aavsb.org
**Website:** http://www.aavsb.org
Charlotte P. Ronan, Exec. Dir.

**Fnded:** 1957. **Mem:** 56. **Desc:** State boards of examiners in veterinary medicine. Aids state boards of veterinary medicine in the protection of the public health and welfare. Acts as a clearing house for research, collects and disseminates information about legal regulation of the veterinary profession. Works to simplify and standardize licensing and certification processes for veterinarians and veterinary technicians. Interacts with other veterinary organizations; legislative, judicial, regulatory, and executive governmental bodies; and other associations whose areas of interest may coincide. Assists member boards in fulfilling statutory, public, and ethical obligations in legal regulation and enforcement. Cooperates with the National Board Examination Committee in the design and use of entry level, relicensure and disciplinary examinations regarding the practice of veterinary medicine and regulation. Collects and disseminates information regarding disciplinary actions taken by member boards. Provides veterinary medical educational programs. **Frmly:** (1968) Association of American Board of Examiners in Veterinary Medicine; (1974) American Association State Boards, Veterinary.

**★ 20550 ★ American Association of Wildlife Veterinarians (AAWV)**
c/o Dr. Kirsten Gilardi
Wildlife Health Center
University of California
1 Shields Ave.
Davis, CA 95616
**Phone:** (530)752-4896 **Fax:** (530)752-3318
**Email:** kvgilardi@ucdavis.edu
**Website:** http://www.aawv.net
Dr. Kirsten Gilardi, Sec.

**Fnded:** 1979. **Mem:** 350. **Desc:** Veterinarians in state and federal wildlife resource agencies, universities, private practice, public health service agencies, agricultural agencies, and diagnostic laboratories; veterinary students; and interested individuals. To deal with problems confronting veterinarians who work with free-ranging wildlife. Encourages colleges of veterinary medicine to increase emphasis on management of and preventive medicine for free-ranging species; educates governmental agencies and wildlife resource interest groups; promotes utilization of veterinarians in the field of wildlife resource management and research; encourages cooperation among resource management professionals and wildlife veterinarians; promotes continuing education programs for wildlife veterinarians; emphasizes interrelationships of man, domestic animals, and wildlife with disease; encourages recognition of disease syndromes as potentially influenced by habitat succession, alteration, and pollution. **Pub:** *AAWV Newsletter*, quarterly. Newsletter. • Membership Directory, periodic.

**★ 20551 ★ American Association of Zoo Veterinarians (AAZV)**
c/o Dr. Wilbur Amand
6 N Pennell Rd.
Media, PA 19063
**Phone:** (610)892-4812 **Fax:** (610)892-4813
**Email:** aazv@aol.com
**Website:** http://www.aazv.org/aazv_001.htm
Dr. Wilbur Amand, Exec. Dir.

**Fnded:** 1947. **Mem:** 1,200. **Desc:** Veterinarians actively engaged in the practice of zoo and wildlife medicine for at least four years; veterinarians who do not qualify for active membership; persons interested in diseases of wildlife; students of veterinary medicine in any accredited veterinary school. Purposes are to: advance programs for preventive medicine, husbandry, and scientific research dealing with captive and free-ranging wild animals; provide a forum for the presentation and discussion of problems related to the field; enhance and uphold the professional ethics of veterinary medicine. **Pub:** *Conference Proceedings*, annual. Proceedings. Contains papers presented at the annual conference. *Price:* $45. • *Journal of Zoo and Wildlife Medicine*, quarterly. Journal. Contains original manuscripts, book and paper reviews and research notes/case reports. *Price:* Included in membership dues. • *Zoo Vet News*, quarterly. Newsletter. • Membership Directory, annual.

★ **20552** ★ **American Board of Veterinary Practitioners (ABVP)**
c/o Dee Ann Walker, CAE
200 4th Ave. N, Ste. 900
Nashville, TN 37219
**Phone:** (615)254-3687        **Fax:** (615)254-7047
**Email:** abvp@walkermgt.com
**Website:** http://www.abvp.com
Dee Ann Walker, CAE, Exec. Officer
**Fnded:** 1978. **Mem:** 750. **Desc:** Veterinarians. Seeks to recognize excellence in clinical, species-oriented specialty practice. Works to insure delivery of superior, comprehensive, multidisciplinary veterinary services. Confers certification; conducts educational programs. **Pub:** *ABVP News*, quarterly. Newsletter. Includes directory.

★ **20553** ★ **American Board of Veterinary Specialties (ABVS)**
c/o American Veterinary Medical Association
1931 N Meacham Rd., Ste. 100
Schaumburg, IL 60173-4360
**Phone:** (847)925-8070        **Fax:** (847)925-1329
**Email:** avmainfo@avma.org
**Website:** http://www.avma.org
Beth A. Sabin, DVM, Asst. Dir.,Educ. &Res.
**Fnded:** 1959. **Mem:** 22. **Desc:** A board of the American Veterinary Medical Association. Organization of veterinarians with advanced training in one or more specialty areas of veterinary practice, research, or study whose purpose is to recognize and supervise organizations that provide certification to qualified specialists. **Pub:** *Policies and Procedures Manual*, periodic. Manual. *Price:* First copy free; $1/additional copy. **Frmly:** Advisory Board on Veterinary Specialties.

★ **20554** ★ **American Board of Veterinary Toxicology (ABVT)**
School of Veterinary Medicine
382 W St. Rd.
Kennett Square, PA 19348
**Phone:** (610)444-5800        **Fax:** (610)925-8117
**Email:** roder@amaonline.com
**Website:** http://www.abvt.org
Carl T. Olsonnga, Exec. Sec.
**Fnded:** 1967. **Mem:** 100. **Desc:** Seeks to: further education and scientific progress in veterinary toxicology; encourage research and training; establish and maintain the highest possible standards of training and experience for qualification in toxicology; recognize qualified specialists through certification. Conducts annual examination. **Pub:** *American Board of Veterinary Toxicology–Directory of Diplomates*, annual. Directory. Lists diplomates certified as veterinary toxicologists by the board.

★ **20555** ★ **American Canine Sports Medicine Association (ACSMA)**
PO Box 82433
Baton Rouge, LA 70884
**Email:** postmaster@acsma.org
**Website:** http://www.acsma.org
Robert L. Gillette, Contact
**Fnded:** 1991. **Mem:** 200. **Desc:** Promotes interests of members. Conducts research and educational pro-

grams. **Pub:** *Newsletter of the ACSMA*, quarterly. Newsletter. *Price:* Included in membership dues.

★ **20556** ★ **American College of Laboratory Animal Medicine (ACLAM)**
c/o Dr. Melvin W. Balk
96 Chester St.
Chester, NH 03036
**Phone:** (603)887-2467        **Fax:** (603)887-0096
**Email:** mwbaclam@gsinet.net
**Website:** http://www.aclam.org
Dr. Melvin W. Balk, Exec. Dir.
**Fnded:** 1957. **Mem:** 360. **Desc:** Veterinarians specializing in laboratory animal medicine. Establishes standards of training and experience for qualification of specialists in the field, administers examinations, and certifies eligible specialists. Encourages education, training, and research in laboratory animal medicine. Sponsors symposia on infectious and metabolic diseases of laboratory animals. Conducts continuing education forums for diplomates on topics including quality assurance, biohazards, and animal production. **Pub:** *The Biology of the Laboratory Rabbit*. • *Membership Directory*, annual. Directory. • Newsletter, 4/year. **Frmly:** American Board of Laboratory Animal Medicine.

★ **20557** ★ **American College of Theriogenologists**
200 4th Ave. N, Ste. 900
Nashville, TN 37219
**Phone:** (615)244-3060        **Fax:** (615)254-7047
**Email:** act@walkermgt.com
**Website:** http://www.theriogenology.org
Tate Elder, Admin.
**Fnded:** 1970. **Mem:** 350. **Desc:** Veterinarians specializing in animal reproduction. Advances knowledge, education, and services in theriogenology. Acts as certifying agency for theriogenologists. Sponsors scientific programs. Conducts educational programs. **Pub:** *Newsletter of ACT*, bimonthly. Newsletter. *Price:* Free. • Directory, annual.

★ **20558** ★ **American College of Veterinary Anesthesiologists (ACVA)**
c/o Ron Mandsager, DVM
College of Veterinary Medicine
Oklahoma State University
Public Relations Office
308 McElroy Hall
Stillwater, OK 74078
**Phone:** (405)744-8468        **Fax:** (405)744-6265
**Website:** http://www.acva.org
Ron Mandsager, DVM, Contact
**Fnded:** 1975. **Desc:** Veterinary anesthesiologists and other individuals with an interest in the field. Promotes high standards of practice in veterinary anesthesiology; facilitates continuing professional development of members. Establishes practice guidelines and certification criteria; conducts examinations; bestows certification. Advises the American Veterinary Medical Association regarding accreditation of veterinary anesthesiology training programs.

★ **20559** ★ **American College of Veterinary Dermatology (ACVD)**
c/o Alexis Borich, Exec. Sec.
5610 Kearny Mesa Rd., Ste. B
San Diego, CA 92111
**Phone:** (858)560-9393        **Fax:** (858)560-0206
**Website:** http://www.acvd.org
Dr. Donna W Angarano, Pres.
**Fnded:** 1982. **Mem:** 133. **Desc:** Specialists in veterinary dermatology who have satisfied examination requirements; individuals with national reputation and standing are charter diplomates. promotes veterinary dermatology enhances the competencey of professionals in the field. Seeks to develop guidelines for postdoctoral education and to establish experience prerequisites for certification in veterinary dermatology. Administers examinations and certifies veterinarians as veterinary dermatology specialists. Encour-

ages research and other contributions in areas of pathogenesis, diagnosis, therapy, prevention, and control of diseases affecting the skin of animals. Authorizes training programs in the field.

★ **20560** ★ **American College of Veterinary Internal Medicine (ACVIM)**
1997 Wadsworth
Lakewood, CO 80215
**Phone:** (303)231-9933        **Free:** 800-245-9081
**Fax:** (303)231-0880
**Email:** acvim@acvim.org
**Website:** http://www.acvim.org
Dr. Guy Pidgeon, Pres.
**Fnded:** 1972. **Mem:** 1,277. **Desc:** Veterinarians certified in internal medicine and related specialties such as cardiology, neurology, and oncology. Works to advance the scope and ideals of veterinary internal medicine and to increase the competence of those practicing in the field. Issues certifying diplomas. **Pub:** *ACVIM Proceedings*, annual. Proceedings. Contains papers submitted by speakers at annual conference. *Price:* $49 in U.S.; $49 outside U.S. • *Journal of Veterinary Internal Medicine*, bimonthly. Journal.

★ **20561** ★ **American College of Veterinary Ophthalmologists (ACVO)**
c/o Dr. Mary B. Glaze
Louisiana State University
Veterinary Teaching Hospital
S Stadium Dr.
Baton Rouge, LA 70803
**Phone:** (225)346-3333        **Fax:** (225)346-3295
**Email:** info@acvo.com
**Website:** http://www.acvo.com
Dr. Mary B. Glaze, Sec. -Treas.
**Fnded:** 1969. **Mem:** 166. **Desc:** Veterinarians certified by examination in veterinary ophthalmology. Purposes are: continuing education, research, and practice in veterinary ophthalmology; establishment of standards of training and experience; recognition of individuals who have fulfilled such standards; certification of qualified veterinarians. **Pub:** *Directory of Diplomates*, quinquennial. Directory. *Price:* $10.

★ **20562** ★ **American College of Veterinary Pathologists (ACVP)**
7600 Terrace Ave., No. 203
Middleton, WI 53562-3174
**Phone:** (608)833-8725        **Fax:** (608)831-5122
**Email:** info@acvp.org
**Website:** http://www.acvp.org/
Mary Schumacher, Exec. Dir.
**Fnded:** 1948. **Mem:** 1,200. **Desc:** Professional society of specialists in veterinary pathology (origin, nature, and course of diseases in animals). Aims to further scientific progress in the specialty of veterinary pathology; to establish standards of training and experience for qualification of specialists in veterinary pathology; to further the recognition of such qualified specialists by suitable certification and other means. Recognized as the certifying agency for the specialty of veterinary pathology in the U.S. and Canada. Conducts specialized education programs and certifying exams. **Pub:** *American College of Veterinary Pathologists–Newsletter*, bimonthly. Newsletter. Covers developments in veterinary pathology; also includes association news, calendar of events, obituaries, and listing of employment opportunities. *Price:* Included in membership dues. • *Membership List*, annual. Directory. • *Veterinary Pathology: An International Journal of Natural and Experimental Disease in Animals*, bimonthly. Includes book reviews and periodic special supplements on a scientific topic. *Price:* $75/year. • Proceedings, annual.

★ **20563** ★ **American College of Veterinary Radiology (ACVR)**
c/o Dr. M. Bernstein
PO Box 87
Glencoe, IL 60022
**Phone:** (847)251-5517        **Fax:** (847)446-8618

**Email:** tgnyland@usdavis.edu
**Website:** http://www.acvr.ucdavis.edu/
Dr. M. Bernstein, Exec. Dir.

**Fnded:** 1964. **Mem:** 215. **Desc:** Diplomate members (215) are veterinarians certified by the college in veterinary radiology; associate members (6) are individuals distinguished in radiological science but who are not certified veterinary radiologists. Educational association working to advance the art and science of radiology. Certifies candidates who have demonstrated proficiency in veterinary radiology. Encourages the development of teaching personnel and training facilities in veterinary radiology. Aids in the evaluation of residencies and fellowships in veterinary radiology under consideration by the Council on Education of the American Veterinary Medical Association. Advises veterinarians who desire certification in veterinary radiology. Conducts continuing education seminars in conjunction with other veterinary organizations. **Pub:** *Veterinary Radiology and Ultrasound*, bimonthly. Journal. Covers diagnostic and therapeutic radiology, ultrasound, MR, CT, and scintigraphy. *Price:* Included in membership dues; $78/year for institutions. • Brochure. **Frmly:** (1969) American Board of Veterinary Radiology.

★ **20564** ★ **American College of Veterinary Surgeons (ACVS)**
4401 E W Hwy., No. 205
Bethesda, MD 20814-4523
**Phone:** (301)913-9550 **Fax:** (301)913-2034
**Email:** acvs@aol.com
**Website:** http://www.acvs.org
Ann Loew, Exec. Dir.

**Fnded:** 1965. **Mem:** 933. **Desc:** Acts as certification board for veterinary surgeons. **Pub:** *ACVS Newsletter*, 3/year. Newsletter. • *American College of Veterinary Surgeons–Directory of Diplomates*, biennial. Membership Directory. Includes photographic and biographical information on each member; includes alphabetical name and geographic region indexes. *Price:* Included in membership dues. • *Veterinary Surgery*, bimonthly. Journal. Presents clinical and research papers on veterinary surgery; topics include surgical techniques and management of the surgical patient. *Price:* $69/year for individuals; $100/year for institutions.

★ **20565** ★ **American Heartworm Society (AHS)**
Executive Office
PO Box 667
Batavia, IL 60510-0667
**Phone:** (630)844-9676 **Fax:** (630)892-0818
**Email:** heartwormsociety@aol.com
**Website:** http://www.heartwormsociety.org
Eve C. Larocca, Admin.

**Fnded:** 1974. **Mem:** 1,200. **Desc:** Veterinarians, physicians, parasitologists, and other scientists. Promotes scientific programs for the study of heartworm disease, caused by the filarial parasite, dilofilaria immitis. Encourages standardization of procedures for diagnosis, treatment, and prevention of heartworm disease. Keeps members abreast of current research and recent developments concerning the disease. **Pub:** *AHS Bulletin*, quarterly. Bulletin. Contains topical commentary, synopsis of clinical and scientific literature and society news. *Price:* Included in membership dues; $38/year for nonmembers. • *Recent Advances in Heartworm Disease: Symposium '98*. Proceedings.

**American Holistic Veterinary Medical Association (AHVMA)**
*See:* Entry 4216

★ **20566** ★ **American Society of Veterinary Ophthalmology (ASVO)**
1416 W Liberty Ave.
Stillwater, OK 74075
**Phone:** (405)377-4388
**Email:** membership@asvo.org
**Website:** http://www.asvo.org/
Dr, Virginia Schultz, D.V.M., Sec. -Treas.

**Fnded:** 1957. **Mem:** 250. **Desc:** Veterinarians with a special interest in ophthalmology (the science of the eye and its diseases). Sponsors research proposal competition. **Pub:** Directory, annual. • Newsletter, periodic. • Proceedings, annual.

★ **20567** ★ **American Veterinary Chiropractic Association**
PO Box 563
Port Byron, IL 61275
**Phone:** (309)658-2958 **Fax:** (309)658-2958
**Email:** amvetchiro@aol.com
**Website:** http://www.animalchiropractic.org/
Sharon L. Willoughby, DVM, Contact

**Fnded:** 1989. **Mem:** 302. **Desc:** Sponsors animal chiropractic basic certification course. Organizes other related courses.

★ **20568** ★ **American Veterinary Dental Society (AVDS)**
200 4th Ave. North, Ste. 900
Nashville, TN 37219
**Phone:** (615)251-0082 **Free:** 800-332-2837
**Fax:** (615)254-7047
**Email:** avds@walkermgt.com
Dee Ann Walker, Exec. Sec.

**Fnded:** 1976. **Mem:** 1,000. **Reg. Groups:** 1. **Desc:** Dentists, veterinarians, and others dedicated to the scientific advancement of dentistry for animals. Conducts continuing education seminars on veterinary dentistry; serves as a forum for exchange of experience and ideas. **Pub:** *Journal of Veterinary Dentistry*, quarterly. Journal. Includes association news and clinical reports. *Price:* Included in membership dues. • *Membership List*, periodic.

★ **20569** ★ **American Veterinary Medical Association (AVMA)**
1931 N Meacham Rd., Ste. 100
Schaumburg, IL 60173-4360
**Phone:** (847)925-8070 **Free:** 800-248-2862
**Fax:** (847)925-1329
**Email:** avmainfo@avma.org
**Website:** http://www.avma.org
Bruce Little, DVM, Contact

**Fnded:** 1863. **Mem:** 62,000. **State Groups:** 52. **Local Groups:** 433. **Desc:** Professional society of veterinarians. Conducts educational and research programs. Provides placement service. Sponsors American Veterinary Medical Association Foundation (also known as AVMF Foundation) and Educational Commission for Foreign Veterinary Graduates. Compiles statistics. **Pub:** *American Journal of Veterinary Research*, monthly. Journal. • *Journal of the AVMA*, semimonthly. Journal. • Directory, annual. **Frmly:** (1988) United States Veterinary Medical Association.

★ **20570** ★ **American Veterinary Society of Animal Behavior (AVSAB)**
c/o Steven Feldman
9414 Brandywine Rd.
Clinton, MD 20735
**Phone:** (301)868-1180
**Email:** avsabe@yahoo.com
**Website:** http://www.avma.org/avsab/
Steve Feldman, Sec. /Treas.

**Fnded:** 1975. **Mem:** 440. **Desc:** Veterinarians and veterinary students. Promotes inquiry and research into animal behavior. Seeks to advance ethological knowledge regarding the care and utilization of captive, domesticated, and free-living animals. Promotes and facilitates the exchange of information among those concerned with animal behavior and well-being; encourages discussion on veterinary aspects of animal behavior and the publication of materials in the field. **Pub:** *American Veterinary Society of Animal Behavior*, quarterly. Newsletter. *Price:* Included in membership dues; $30/year for nonmembers. **Frmly:** (1984) American Society of Veterinary Ethology.

★ **20571** ★ **Animal Care College**
Ascot House
High St.
Ascot SL5 7JG, United Kingdom
**Phone:** 44 1344 28269 **Fax:** 44 1344 622771
**Email:** admin@rtc-associates.freeserve.co.uk
**Website:** http://www.corsini.co.uk/animalcare/

**Fnded:** 1980. **Desc:** Open to all those who have gained certification in course recognized by the Animal Care College. To improve the quality of training in and standards of animal care. **Pub:** *Dogs Monthly*, monthly. Magazine.

★ **20572** ★ **Animal Health Distributors Association (AHDA)**
Gable Court
8 Parsons Hill
Hollesley
Woodbridge IP12 3RB, United Kingdom
**Phone:** 44 1394 410444 **Fax:** 44 1394 410455
**Email:** info@ahda.org.uk
**Website:** http://www.ahda.org.uk

**Fnded:** 1985. **Mem:** 150. **Desc:** Agricultural Merchants who are registered and qualified to distribute animal medicines to farmers and horse owners together with several wholesalers of such products. Aims to prevent the EC legislating members out of business and to ensure an appropriate number of animal medicines are classified for distribution by registered distributors and that new products are so classified. **Pub:** Newsletter, monthly.

★ **20573** ★ **Animal Health Foundation (AHF)**
3615 Bassett Rd.
Pacific, MO 63069
**Website:** http://www.animalhealthfoundation.com
Donald M. Walsh, D.V.M., Pres.

**Fnded:** 1984. **Mem:** 1,000. **Desc:** Individuals interested in finding the causes, treatments, and cure for the crippling equine disease laminitis/founder syndrome. (Laminitis is an inflammation of the laminae, the semirigid internal supporting structures of the horse's foot; founder is the crippling result of laminitis in which the coffin bone in the horse's foot puts pressure on the sole of the foot, and sometimes actually penetrates the sole.) These ailments affect horses of any age or breed, and are counted by the AHF as the second ranking disease leading to the need to euthanize horses. Supports extensive research and collects a range of related data. **Pub:** *AHF Newsletter*, periodic. Newsletter. • Brochure.

★ **20574** ★ **Animal Health Trust**
Lanwades Park
Kentford
Newmarket CB8 7UU, United Kingdom
**Phone:** 44 8700 502424 **Fax:** 44 1638 555601
**Email:** info@aht.org.uk
**Website:** http://www.aht.org.uk

**Fnded:** 1942. **Mem:** 1,000. **Reg. Groups:** 15. **Desc:** Aims to push back the frontiers of veterinary science. Develops new technology and knowledge for the better diagnosis, prevention and cure of disease. Provides a referral service for veterinary surgeons in practice. **Pub:** *AHT News*, quarterly. Newsletter. • *Annual Review*, annual. Annual Report. • *Scientific Report*, triennial. Report.

★ **20575** ★ **Animals First**
153 E 18th St., Ste. 22
New York, NY 10003
**Phone:** (212)505-1073
John Zeigler, Exec. Dir.

**Fnded:** 1972. **Nat'l Groups:** 1. **Desc:** Seeks to demonstrate to nations that their interests are best served by putting the rights of animals first. Believes that if the needs of animals are addressed as the first priority, a saner and more humane civilization would then be closer to eradicating overpopulation and environmental destruction. **Frmly:** (2000) Speak Out!.

### ★ 20576 ★ Association for Assessment and Accreditation of Laboratory Animal Care International (AAALAC)
11300 Rockville Pike, Ste. 1211
Rockville, MD 20852-3035
**Phone:** (301)231-5353　　**Free:** 800-926-0066
**Fax:** (301)231-8282
**Email:** accredit@aaalac.org
**Website:** http://www.aaalac.org
Dr. John G. Miller, DVM, Exec. Dir.

**Fnded:** 1965. **Mem:** 50. **Desc:** Promotes the humane treatment of animals in science thourgh a voluntary accrediation program. More than 600 institutions around the world have earned AAALAC International accreditation, demonstrating their commitment to responsible animal care and use. **Pub:** *AAALAC Connection*, 4/year. Newsletter. **Frmly:** American Association for Accreditation of Laboratory Animal Care.

### ★ 20577 ★ Association of Avian Medicine and Surgery (AAMS)
Yalelaan 8
NL-3584 CM Utrecht, Netherlands
**Phone:** 31 30 2539411　　**Fax:** 31 30 2518126
**Email:** n.j.schoemaker@vet.uu.nl

**Lang(s):** Dutch, English. **Desc:** Veterinarians specializing in the care of birds. Seeks to advance the study, teaching, and practice of avian medicine. Serves as a clearinghouse on veterinary and avian medicine; sponsors research programs and continuing professional development courses. **Pub:** *AAV Newsletter & Clinical Forum*, quarterly. Newsletter. • *Journal of Avian Medicine and Surgery*, quarterly. Journal. **Frmly:** (2000) Association of Avian Veterinarians - Europe.

### ★ 20578 ★ Association of British Veterinary Acupuncture
c/o Bishopton Veterinary Group
Mill Farm
Studley Rd.
Ripon HG4 2QR, United Kingdom
**Phone:** 44 1765 602396　　**Fax:** 44 1765 690505
**Email:** ldc@bishoptonvets.demon.co.uk

**Fnded:** 1987. **Mem:** 70. **Desc:** Ordinary members are veterinary surgeons. To further advancement of veterinary acupuncture in the UK. **Pub:** *Newsletter*, semiannual. Newsletter.

### ★ 20579 ★ Association for Equine Sports Medicine (AESM)
3579 E Foothill Blvd., No. 288
Pasadena, CA 91107
**Phone:** (909)869-4849　　**Fax:** (909)869-6788
**Email:** aesm@relaypoint.net
**Website:** http://www.aesm.org
Holly M. Greene, M.S., Exec. Dir.

**Fnded:** 1982. **Mem:** 400. **Desc:** Members are veterinarians, sports physiology researchers, other health professionals, or anyone who has special interest in understanding and/or application of scientific knowledge in the area of equine sports medicine and who will promote the well being of the athletic horse. **Pub:** *Equine Review*, quarterly. Newsletter. • *Proceedings of Annual Conference.*

### ★ 20580 ★ Association of Holistic Animal Practitioners (AHAP)
c/o Mary DeBono
PO Box 7906
San Diego, CA 92167-0906
**Phone:** 888-858-6862
**Email:** animalsense@msn.com
**Website:** http://www.debonosense.com
Mary DeBono, Dir.

**Fnded:** 1997. **Desc:** Works to promote practitioners of holistic animal treatments. Provides a referral service; sponsors continuing education. **Pub:** *Association of Holistic Animal Practitioners*, quarterly. Newsletter.

### ★ 20581 ★ Association of Institutions Teaching Veterinary Medicine Totally or Partially in the French Language (Association des Etablissements d'Enseignement Veterinaire Totalement ou Partiellement de Langue Francaise)
Faculte de Medicine Veterinaire
Universite de Montreal
Campus St.-Hyacinthe
CP 5000
St.-Hyacinthe, QC, Canada J2S 7C6
**Phone:** (514)343-6111　　**Fax:** (514)778-8101
**Email:** raymond.s.roy@umontreal.ca
**Website:** http://www.medvet.umontreal.ca

**Lang(s):** English, French. **Desc:** Institutions offering veterinary medical education programs in French. Promotes excellence in French-language veterinary medical education. Facilitates communication and exchange among members; conducts training programs for veterinary medical educators.

### ★ 20582 ★ Association of Reptilian and Amphibian Veterinarians (ARAV)
c/o Wilbur B. Amand
Box 605
Chester Heights, PA 19017
**Phone:** (610)892-4812　　**Fax:** (610)892-4813
**Email:** aravets@aol.com
**Website:** http://www.arav.org
Wilbur B. Amand, VMD, Exec. Dir.

**Fnded:** 1991. **Mem:** 1,250. **Desc:** Veterinarians specializing in the treatment of reptiles and amphibians. Seeks to advance the study and practice of reptilian and amphibian veterinary medicine; promotes ongoing professional development of members. Serves as a clearinghouse on reptilian and amphibian veterinary medicine; sponsors educational programs; facilitates communication and cooperation among members. **Pub:** *Journal of Herpetological Medicine and Surgery*, quarterly. Journal. • *Membership Directory*. Directory.

### ★ 20583 ★ Association of Veterinary Anaesthetists
c/o Royal Veterinary College
Hawkshead Ln.
North Mymms
Hatfield AL9 7TA, United Kingdom
**Phone:** 44 1707 666297　　**Fax:** 44 1707 660671
**Email:** kclarke@ruc.ac.uk
**Website:** http://www.aveta.org.uk

**Fnded:** 1964. **Mem:** 400. **Desc:** Veterinary surgeons; medics, anaesthetists, those with medical university qualifications and scientists, Animal technicians and veterinary nurses. Furthers teaching and research in veterinary anaesthetics. **Pub:** *Journal of Veterinary Anaesthesia and Analgesia*, quarterly. Journal. **Frmly:** Association of Veterinary Anaesthetists of Great Britian and Ireland.

### ★ 20584 ★ Association of Veterinary Teachers and Research Workers
Department of Agriculture and Rural Development for Northern
Veterinary Sciences Division
Stoney Rd.
Stormont
Belfast BT4 3SD, United Kingdom
**Phone:** 44 28 90525606　　**Fax:** 44 28 90525753
**Email:** john.mcevoy@dardni.gov.uk
**Website:** http://www.avtrw.org

**Fnded:** 1946. **Mem:** 800. **Reg. Groups:** 4. **Lang(s):** English. **Desc:** Individuals engaged primarily in veterinary teaching and research in UK and Eire. To further contact between research workers and teachers in animal research; promote and influence veterinary education; provide for and maintain the technical excellence of veterinary teaching and research. **Pub:** *AVT and RW Annual Conference*, annual. Proceedings. • Proceedings.

### ★ 20585 ★ Association for Women Veterinarians (AWV)
PO Box 2039
Starkville, MS 39760-2039
**Phone:** (662)312-0893　　**Fax:** (662)323-3280
**Email:** lapancho@ra.msstate.edu
**Website:** http://www.awv-women-veterinarians.org
Dr. Shirley Johnston, Pres.

**Fnded:** 1947. **Mem:** 400. **Desc:** Works to support veterinary medicine by providing leadership in women's issues. **Pub:** *AWV Bulletin*, quarterly. Bulletin. *Price:* Included in membership dues; $10/year for nonmembers. • *Roster of Women Veterinarians*, periodic. **Frmly:** (1981) Women's Veterinary Medical Association.

### ★ 20586 ★ Association of Zoo Veterinary Technicians
White Oak Conservation Center
3823 Owens Rd.
Yulee, FL 32097
**Phone:** (386)879-7636　　**Fax:** (386)879-7637
**Email:** cheryl_purnell@ncmail.net
**Website:** http://www.AZVT.org
Cheryl Purnell, Exec. Dir.

**Fnded:** 1981. **Mem:** 350. **Nat'l Groups:** 1. **Desc:** Zoo veterinary technicians. **Pub:** *AZVT News*, quarterly. Newsletter.

### ★ 20587 ★ Australian Veterinary Association (AVA)
Ava House
134 Hampden Rd.
Artarmon, NSW 2064, Australia
**Phone:** 61 2 94112733　　**Fax:** 61 2 94115089
**Email:** avahq@ava.com.au
**Website:** http://www.ava.com.au

**Fnded:** 1921. **Mem:** 4,500. **State Groups:** 8. **Local Groups:** 52. **Lang(s):** English. **Desc:** Graduates of Australian veterinary schools; graduates of overseas veterinary schools qualified for registration in Australia; veterinary students; associate members are non-veterinarians with close ties to the veterinary profession. Promotes the professional practice of veterinary medicine; seeks improvements in the areas of animal health, productivity, and welfare. Represents members' interests; lobbies governmental bodies on matters related to animal welfare, quarantine, and agricultural problems. Maintains 23 special interest groups offering continuing education programs. Maintains museum. **Pub:** *Australian Veterinary Journal*, monthly. Journal. • *Members Directory and Policy Compendium*, triennial. Directory. • Report, annual.

### ★ 20588 ★ British Cattle Veterinary Association
c/o BCVA Office
The Green
Frampton-on-Severn
Gloucester GL2 7EP, United Kingdom
**Phone:** 44 1452 740816　　**Fax:** 44 1452 741117
**Email:** office@cattlevet.co.uk
**Website:** http://www.bcva.org.uk

**Fnded:** 1967. **Mem:** 1,500. **Desc:** Veterinary surgeons, research workers; mostly professional veterinary surgeons in practice. Concerned with education; promotion; research into cattle topics; promotion of cattle veterinarian; political opinion on cattle matters; source of information and reference on cattle topics. **Pub:** *Cattle Practice*, quarterly. Journal. • Newsletters, quarterly.

### ★ 20589 ★ British Equine Veterinary Association
5 Finlay St.
London SW6 6HE, United Kingdom
**Phone:** 44 20 76106080　　**Fax:** 44 20 76106823
**Email:** info@beva.org.uk
**Website:** http://www.beva.org.uk

**Fnded:** 1961. **Mem:** 1,400. **Desc:** Practising equine vets, members of academia, Veterinary universities and members of pharmaceutical companies, home and overseas. Promotes the cultural, scientific and professional activities of veterinary surgeons and others interested in equine practice, welfare, teaching and research. **Pub:** *Equine Veterinary Education*, bimonthly. Journal. • *Equine Veterinary Journal*, bimonthly. Journal. • *Supplement*, periodic.

**★ 20590 ★ British Small Animal Veterinary Association (BSAVA)**
Woodrow House
1 Telford Way
Waterwells Business Pk.
Quedgeley
Gloucester GL2 4AB, United Kingdom
**Phone:** 44 1452 726700    **Fax:** 44 1452 726701
**Email:** adminoff@bsava.com
**Website:** http://www.bsava.com
**Fnded:** 1957. **Mem:** 5,100. **Local Groups:** 13. **Lang(s):** English. **Desc:** Veterinarians in 20 countries. Operates speakers' bureau; sponsors educational programs. Compiles statistics. Sponsors competitions; conducts charitable activities. **Pub:** *BSAVA Handbook*, annual. Handbook. • *BSAVA News*, monthly. Newsletter. • *Journal of Small Animal Practice*, monthly. Journal.

**★ 20591 ★ British Veterinary Association (BVA)**
7 Mansfield St.
London W1G 9NQ, United Kingdom
**Phone:** 44 207 6366541    **Fax:** 44 207 4362970
**Email:** bvahq@bva.co.uk
**Website:** http://www.bva.co.uk
**Fnded:** 1882. **Mem:** 10,000. **Nat'l Groups:** 20. **Local Groups:** 31. **Desc:** Veterinarians and veterinary students. Promotes interests of members and the animals in their care. Monitors activities of, provides advice to, and develops and maintains contact with organizations interested in animal health including government agencies, local authorities, professional societies, animal rights groups, and universities. Disseminates information to the public and the media. Conducts charitable programs. Sponsors seminars and symposia. Maintains 20 specialist divisions. **Pub:** *Annual Report*, annual. • *In Practice*, monthly. • *Journal of Small Animal Practice*. Journal. • *Veterinary Nursing*. • *Veterinary Record*, weekly. • *You and Your Vet*, quarterly. **Frmly:** (1952) National Veterinary Medical Association.

**★ 20592 ★ British Veterinary Nursing Association**
Terminus House, Level 15
Terminuc St.
Harlow CM20 1XA, United Kingdom
**Phone:** 44 1279 450567    **Fax:** 44 1279 420866
**Email:** bvna@bvna.co.uk
**Website:** http://www.bvna.org.uk
**Fnded:** 1965. **Mem:** 2,100. **Reg. Groups:** 32. **State Groups:** 1. **Desc:** Full membership qualified veterinary nurses; students; associate; supporter. To foster and promote the status of the veterinary nurse; representation on associated professional committees, and government committees. Gives advice on a career as a veterinary nurse. Membership benefits include an employment register, annual congress, reduced entry into BVNA regional and national meetings and BVNA Educational Courses. **Pub:** *Veterinary Nurse Journal, bimonthly, through membership or subscription,* bimonthly. Journal.

**★ 20593 ★ Canadian Animal Health Institute (CAHI)**
160 Research Lane, Ste. 102
Guelph, ON, Canada N1G 5B2
**Phone:** (519)763-7777    **Fax:** (519)763-7407
**Email:** cahi@cahi-icsa.ca
**Website:** http://www.cahi-icsa.ca
**Fnded:** 1968. **Mem:** 60. **Lang(s):** English, French. **Desc:** Trade association representing companies that develop and manufacture pharmaceuticals, biologi-

cals, feed additives, and animal pesticides used in veterinary medicine and livestock production. Member firms collectively manufacture approximately 90 percent of all animal health products manufactured in Canada. **Pub:** *Inforum*, bimonthly. Bulletin. Deals with current issues in the animal health industry.

**★ 20594 ★ Canadian Veterinary Medical Association (CVMA) (Association Canadienne des Medecins Veterinaires — ACMV)**
339 Booth St.
Ottawa, ON, Canada K1R 7K1
**Phone:** (613)236-1162    **Fax:** (613)236-9681
**Email:** info@canadianveterinarians.net
**Website:** http://www.cvma-acmv.org
**Fnded:** 1948. **Mem:** 4,300. **Lang(s):** English, French. **Desc:** Veterinarians in Canada. Encourages excellence in the field of veterinary medicine; seeks to increase awareness of the importance of animals; represents the interests of members. **Pub:** *Canadian Journal of Veterinary Research*, quarterly. • *Canadian Veterinary Journal*, monthly. • *CVMA Directory*, annual.

**★ 20595 ★ Chinese Association of Animal Science and Veterinary Medicine**
33 Dongdaqiao Nongfengli, Chao Yang District
Beijing 10020, People's Republic of China
**Phone:** 852 10 65066533   **Fax:** 852 10 65005670

**★ 20596 ★ Commonwealth Veterinary Association (CVA)**
c/o Centre for Animal and Plant Health
93 Mount Edward Rd.
Charlottetown, PE, Canada C1A 5T1
**Phone:** (902)368-0950    **Fax:** (902)368-0960
**Email:** stevenson@inspection.gc.ca
**Website:** http://www.freenet.edmonton.ab.ca/cva/
**Fnded:** 1967. **Mem:** 50. **Reg. Groups:** 6. **Lang(s):** English. **Desc:** National veterinary medical associations of Commonwealth countries. Promotes the veterinary profession through "encouraging the highest professional standards of education, ethics, and service." Seeks to advance animal health. Facilitates communication and cooperation among members; sponsors continuing professional education courses for veterinarians; serves as a clearinghouse on veterinary medicine. **Pub:** *CVA News*, semiannual. Journal.

**★ 20597 ★ Conference of Research Workers in Animal Diseases (CRWAD)**
c/o Dr. Robert Ellis
Colorado State University
Department of Microbiology, Rm. A102
Fort Collins, CO 80523-1677
**Phone:** (970)491-5740    **Fax:** (970)491-1815
**Email:** robert.ellis@colostate.edu
**Website:** http://www.cvmbs.colostate.edu/microbiology/crwad/crwad.htm
Dr. Robert P. Ellis, Exec. Dir.
**Fnded:** 1920. **Mem:** 550. **Desc:** Research workers in animal diseases. **Pub:** *Proceedings of the Annual Meeting–CRWAD*, annual. Journal. Contains abstracts presented at annual meeting. *Price:* $15/year.

**★ 20598 ★ Cornell Feline Health Center**
c/o Dr. James R. Richards Dir.
New York State College of Veterinary Medicine
Cornell University
Ithaca, NY 14853
**Phone:** (607)253-3414    **Fax:** (607)253-3419
**Website:** http://web.vet.cornell.edu/Public/FHC/FelineHealth.html
Dr. James R. Richards, Dir.
**Fnded:** 1975. **Mem:** 6,000. **Desc:** Professionals devoted to cats. Seeks to unravel the mysteries of feline health, nutrition, and behavior. Works to educate veterinarians and cat owners, and to aid veterinarians when new or unknown diseases occur. Provides

educational programs. **Pub:** *CatWatch*, monthly. Newsletter. Informs cat fanciers of news on cat diseases and activities at the center. • *The Cornell Book of Cats, Second Edition*. • *Feline Health Topics*.

**★ 20599 ★ Danish Veterinary History Society (Dansk Veterinaerhistorisk Samfund)**
Svalgaardsvej 20, Sjorring
DK-7700 Thisted, Denmark
**Phone:** 45 97971001    **Fax:** 45 97971701
**Fnded:** 1934. **Desc:** Supports meetings, seminars, congresses, excursions relating to the history of veterinary medicine.

**★ 20600 ★ Dog Guides Canada**
PO Box 907
Oakville, ON, Canada L6J 5E8
**Phone:** (905)842-2891    **Fax:** (905)842-3373
**Email:** info@dogguides.com
**Website:** http://www.dogguides.com
**Lang(s):** English, French. **Desc:** Breeders and trainers of hearing dogs. Promotes the use of special assistance dogs by people with disabilities. Breeds, raises, and trains hearing ear and seeing eye dogs; maintains registry of special assistance dogs for people with hearing and visual impairment.

**★ 20601 ★ European Association of Establishments for Veterinary Education (EAEVE) (Association Europeenne des Etablissements d'Enseignment Veterinaire)**
c/o Prof. T.H. Fernandes
Universidade Tecnica de Lisboa
Polo da Ajuda
Rua Prof Cid dos Santos
P-1300-477 Lisbon, Portugal
**Phone:** 351 21 3652820    **Fax:** 351 21 3652889
**Email:** eaeve@ed.ac.uk
**Desc:** Promotes veterinary education in Europe.

**★ 20602 ★ European Association of Veterinary Anatomists (EAVA)**
c/o Dr. Ignacio Salazar
Departmento de Anatomia y Embriologia
Facultad de Veterinaria
Universidad de Santiago de Compostela
E-27002 Lugo, Spain
**Phone:** 34 982 252239    **Fax:** 34 982 285939
**Email:** anigsabe@lugo.usc.es
**Website:** http://www.vetmed.uni-muenchen.de/anat1/eava/eava.html
**Fnded:** 1963. **Mem:** 270. **Lang(s):** English, French, German, Spanish. **Desc:** European and international veterinarians from 44 countries interested in morphologic research on domestic animals. **Pub:** *Vademecum of the European Association of Veterinary Anatomists*. Monographs.

**★ 20603 ★ European Association of Veterinary Diagnostic Imaging (EAVDI)**
c/o Ruth Dennis
Department of Radiology
The Animal Health Trust
Lanwades Park
Newmarket CB8 7UU, United Kingdom
**Phone:** 44 1638 555600
**Email:** ruth.dennis@aht.org.uk
**Desc:** Promotes the use of diagnostic imaging technology in veterinary medicine.

**★ 20604 ★ European College of Veterinary Diagnostic Imaging**
32 Dyrlaegevej
DK-1870 Frederiksberg, Denmark
**Phone:** 45 35282921    **Fax:** 45 35282929
**Email:** jar@kvl.dk

**Website:** http://www.vet.gla.uk/EVDI/ecvdi.htm
**Fnded:** 1993. **Desc:** Improves the quality of animal health care through specialized knowledge and skills in veterinary diagnostic imaging.

★ **20605** ★ **European Society of Feline Medicine (ESFM)**
Taeselbury High St.
Tisbury
Salisbury SP3 6LD, United Kingdom
**Phone:** 44 1747 871872    **Fax:** 44 1747 871873
**Email:** esfm@fabcats.org
**Website:** http://www.fabcats.org
**Lang(s):** English. **Desc:** Veterinarians with an interest in feline medicine. Seeks to advance the medical treatment of cats; promotes continuing professional development of members. Facilitates exchange of information among veterinarians and researchers working in the field of feline medicine; sponsors educational courses. **Pub:** *Journal of Feline Medicine and Surgery*, quarterly.

★ **20606** ★ **European Society for Laboratory Animal Veterinarians (ESLAV)**
BP 159
F-37401 Amboise, France
**Email:** pnowlan@tcd.ie
**Website:** http://www.eslav.org/
**Fnded:** 1996. **Desc:** Disseminates expert veterinary knowledge in the field of laboratory animal science.

★ **20607** ★ **European Society of Veterinary Cardiology**
c/o Michele Borgarelli
Via Cont Rosso 3
I-10121 Turin, Italy
**Desc:** Veterinarians interested animal cardiology. Works to improve methods of diagnosis, treatment, and prevention of heart disease in animals. Seeks to improve cardiology training in veterinary colleges. Promotes exchange of information and further scientific progress in veterinary cardiology. **Pub:** *Journal of Veterinary Cardiology*, periodic. Journal.

★ **20608** ★ **European Society of Veterinary Clinical Ethology (ESVCE)**
Av du Cosmonaute 3
1150 Brussels, Belgium
**Phone:** 32 2 7704008    **Fax:** 32 2 7704008
**Email:** joel.dehasse@advalvas.be
**Website:** http://www.esvce.org/
**Fnded:** 1994. **Desc:** Promotes scientific progress in veterinary and comparative clinical ethology; furthers education in veterinary clinical ethology and behavior medicine, facilitates exchange of information.

★ **20609** ★ **European Society of Veterinary Dermatology (ESVD)**
43, av Aristide-Briand
F-94110 Arcueil, France
**Phone:** 33 1 49858300    **Fax:** 33 1 49858301
**Email:** secretary@www.esvd.org
**Website:** www.esvd.org
**Fnded:** 1984. **Desc:** Fosters exchange of information with veterinary dermatologists; promotes veterinary dermatology in Europe.

★ **20610** ★ **European Society of Veterinary Orthopaedics and Traumatology (ESVOT)**
c/o Dr. Herman A.W. Hazewinkel
Faculty of Veterinary Medicine
University of Utrecht
NL-3508 TD Utrecht, Netherlands
**Desc:** Disseminates basic principles of veterinary orthopedics and traumatology through continuing education programs.

★ **20611** ★ **European Society of Veterinary Pathology (ESVP)**
c/o Dr. Manfred Reinacher
Department Vet. Pathol.
Univ. Giessen
Frankfurter Str. 96
D-35392 Giessen, Germany
**Phone:** 49 641 9938200
**Email:** manfred.reinacher@vetmed.uni-giessen.de
**Website:** http://www.bris.ac.uk/Depts/PathAndMicro/EuroVet/esvp.htm
**Fnded:** 1952. **Mem:** 500. **Lang(s):** English, French, German. **Desc:** Veterinary pathologists in 33 countries. Promotes the exchange of information and research findings. **Pub:** *European Journal of Veterinary Pathology*, 3/year. Journal.

★ **20612** ★ **European Society of Veterinary Virology**
c/o Moredun Research Institute
Pentlands Science Park, Bush Loan.
Edinburgh EH26OPZ, United Kingdom
**Phone:** 44 131 4455111    **Fax:** 44 131 4456111
**Email:** nettp@mri.sari.ac.uk
**Website:** http://www.ploufragan.afssa.fr/esvv/fee_member.html
**Fnded:** 1985. **Mem:** 250. **Desc:** Researchers and teachers in veterinary virology. Seeks to further progress in veterinary virology. Fosters communication and exchange between members. **Pub:** Newsletter, annual.

★ **20613** ★ **European Union of Veterinary Practitioners (Union europeenne des veterinaires praticiens — UEVP)**
Rosenlunds Allee 8
DK- 2720 Vanlose, Denmark
**Fnded:** 1970. **Desc:** Coordinates the work of European veterinary practitioners, relations with farmers, consumers and the European courts.

★ **20614** ★ **European Veterinary Society for Small Animal Reproduction (EVSSAR)**
Bd Colonster 20, B44
4000 Liege, Belgium
**Phone:** 32 4 3664231    **Fax:** 32 4 3664236
**Email:** j.verstegen@ulg.ac.be
**Website:** http://www.ulg.ac.be/fmv/EVSSAR/
**Desc:** Promotes research of small animal reproduction.

★ **20615** ★ **Federation of European Veterinarians in Industry and Research (FEVIR)**
Pfizer Animal Health SA.
Mercuriusstraat 20
B-1930 Zaventem, Belgium
**Fnded:** 1975. **Nat'l Groups:** 7. **Lang(s):** English, French. **Desc:** Organizations representing 4000 veterinarians working in industry and research. Represents members before the Federation of Veterinarians in Europe and provides expert opinions to European Economic Community groups. Works to improve the status of salaried veterinarians. Maintains a file on positions available for veterinarians in Europe. Conducts seminars and symposia.

★ **20616** ★ **Federation of Veterinarians of Europe (FVE)**
1 rue Defacqz
B-1000 Brussels, Belgium
**Phone:** 32 2 5337020    **Fax:** 32 2 5372828
**Email:** nancy@fve.org
**Website:** http://www.fve.org
**Fnded:** 1961. **Mem:** 42. **Lang(s):** English, French, German. **Desc:** Professional organizations of veterinarians and interested individuals in more than 30 countries. Serves as a liaison to the European Eco-

nomic Community. Works toward the unification of veterinary programmes in member countries of the EU and its observers. **Pub:** *FVE Newsletter*, monthly. Newsletter. • Manual, annual.

★ **20617** ★ **Feline Advisory Bureau (FABCFFS)**
Taeselbury,
High St.
Tisbury
Salisbury SP3 6LD, United Kingdom
**Phone:** 44 1747 871872    **Fax:** 44 1747 871873
**Email:** fab.fab@ukonline.co.uk
**Website:** http://www.fabcats.org
**Fnded:** 1958. **Mem:** 3,000. **Lang(s):** English. **Desc:** Veterinary surgeons, cat breeders, and pet owners. Promotes humane behavior toward cats and provides information on feline health and care. Raises funds for feline clinical research. Provides cat boarding information service. **Pub:** *Fab Journal*, quarterly. Journal. Information, news articles, scientific articles, letters. • *Journal of Feline Medicine and Surgery*, quarterly. Journal.

★ **20618** ★ **Finnish Veterinary Association (Finlands Veterinarforbund)**
Makelank 2C
FIN-00520 Helsinki, Finland
**Phone:** 358 9 7011388    **Fax:** 358 9 7018397
**Fnded:** 1892. **Mem:** 1,350. **Lang(s):** English, Finnish, Swedish. **Desc:** Practitioners of veterinary medicine in Finland. Seeks to develop veterinary medicine in Finland. Encourages exchange and cooperation among members; promotes and represents the professional, social, and economic welfare of members. Makes recommendations to authorities on policy matters affecting veterinary medicine; fosters international contacts. Holds Annual veterinary seminar and talks and lectures. Conducts research. Operates charitable program. **Pub:** *Suomen Elainlaakarilehti*, monthly. Journal. Also publishes report of about 400 pages from lectures of the Finnish Veterinary Congress.

★ **20619** ★ **Flying Veterinarians Association (FVA)**
101 Bingham Rd.
Columbia, MO 65203-3577
**Phone:** (573)449-4497    **Fax:** (573)449-4497
**Email:** mcclurer@missouri.edu
Robert C. McClure, D.V.M., Sec. -Treas.
**Fnded:** 1966. **Mem:** 328. **Desc:** Veterinarians holding valid private pilot certificates; individuals in the field who have an interest in flying; nonveterinarians who either teach in veterinary schools or who represent companies serving the veterinary industry. Promotes aviation safety through example and education; seeks to increase knowledge and proficiency in the operation of aircraft. Seeks to heighten awareness of and interest in aviation among young people. Emphasizes utilization of aircraft in veterinary practice. Sponsors two to four educational programs per year in conjunction with other professional veterinary medical meetings; organizes fly-ins. fly-ins. **Pub:** Directory, periodic. • Newsletter, periodic.

★ **20620** ★ **French Committee of the World Veterinary Association (FCWVA) (Comite Francais de l'Association Mondiale Veterinaire — CFAMV)**
Ecole Natl. Veterinaire d'Alfort
F-94704 Maisons-Alfort Cedex, France
**Phone:** 33 1 43967021    **Fax:** 33 1 43967022
**Email:** cfamv@vet-alfort.fr
**Fnded:** 1964. **Desc:** No further information was available for this edition.

★ **20621** ★ **Hong Kong Veterinary Association (HKVA)**
c/o Secretary
Laboratory Animal Services Centre

Chinese University
Hong Kong, People's Republic of China
**Phone:** 852 26096036  **Fax:** 852 26035723
**Email:** tonyjames@cuhk.edu.hk
**Website:** http://www.hkva.org
**Fnded:** 1982. **Mem:** 75. **Lang(s):** Cantonese, Chinese, English. **Desc:** Veterinary surgeons. Fosters advancement in the field of veterinary science. Sponsors clinical lectures. Seeks to liaise with veterinary surgeons registration board on matters affecting veterinary science in Hong Kong. **Pub:** *HKVA Newsletter*, quarterly. Contains news, reports, and abstract reprints.


**★ 20622 ★ Ibero-American Equine
Veterinary Association
(Asociacion Ibero-Americana Veterinaria
Equina)**
R Nicolau Maeder 330/62
Curitiba, Brazil
**Phone:** 55 41 3664492
**Email:** arsvet@bsi.com.br


**★ 20623 ★ Indonesia Veterinary Drug
Association (IVDA)
(Asosiasi Obat Hewan Indonesia)**
Jakarta Animal Hospital
2nd Fl., Jl. Harsono, Rm. 28
Ragunan
12550 Jakarta, Indonesia
**Phone:** 62 21 7982679  **Fax:** 62 21 7891092
**Email:** infovet@rad.net.id
**Fnded:** 1979. **Mem:** 1,344. **Lang(s):** English, Indonesian. **Desc:** Organizes veterinary industry activities in Indonesia. Maintains regulations and policies for the production of veterinary medicines. Compiles statistics. **Pub:** *Directory of Veterinary Company*, biennial. Book. • *Infovet*, monthly. Magazine. Includes information on veterinary medicine and animal husbandry. • *Veterinary Drug Index of Indonesia*. Book.


**★ 20624 ★ Institute for Laboratory
Animal Research (ILAR)**
National Research Council
2101 Constitution Ave. NW
Washington, DC 20418
**Phone:** (202)334-2590  **Fax:** (202)334-1687
**Email:** ilar@nas.edu
**Website:** http://www.national-academies.org/ilar
Joanne Zurlo, PhD, Dir.
**Fnded:** 1952. **Desc:** Organized under the auspices of the National Academy of Sciences. Acts in an advisory capacity to the federal government, upon request, and to other public and private agencies. Maintains information center and answers inquiries concerning animal models for biomedical research, location of unique animal colonies, availability of genetically defined animals from those colonies and from animal breeders, and nonanimal alternatives. Committees develop guidelines on breeding, conservation, and humane care and use of animals, including species-specific documents on cats, nonhuman primates, and rodents. Also prepares documents on guidelines and poicy issues of biotechnology and use of animals in precollege education, facilities, disease prevention, and other topics in laboratory animal science. Sources of financial support include government agencies and private organizations. Maintains advisory council and several committees comprising scientists from universities, research organizations, and medical schools. **Pub:** *Guide for the Care and Use of Laboratory Animals*. Book. • *ILAR Journal*, quarterly. • Proceedings. • Reports.Laboratory animal management documents. **Frmly:** (1997) Institute of Laboratory Animal Resources.


**★ 20625 ★ Inter-African Bureau for
Animal Resources (IBAR)**
PO Box 30786
Nairobi, Kenya
**Phone:** 254 2 338544  **Fax:** 254 2 332046

**Fnded:** 1951. **Mem:** 53. **Reg. Groups:** 5. **Lang(s):** Arabic, English, French, Portuguese. **Desc:** Countries belonging to the Organization of African Unity. Aims to control widespread animal diseases; seeks improvements in animal health and production in Africa. **Pub:** *Bulletin of Animal Health and Production in Africa*, quarterly. Bulletin. • *Information Leaflet*, weekly. • *Proceedings of ISCTRC Meeting*, biennial. **Frmly:** (1960) Inter-American Bureau for Epizootic Diseases.


**★ 20626 ★ International Association for
Aquatic Animal Medicine (IAAAM)**
c/o Donald W. Stremme, VMD
1129 Pine St.
Philadelphia, PA 19107-6035
**Phone:** (215)928-9289  **Fax:** (215)925-1510
**Email:** donstremme@aol.com
**Website:** http://iaaam.org
Donald W. Stremme, VMD, Sec. -Treas.
**Fnded:** 1969. **Mem:** 450. **Desc:** Veterinarians, Ph.D.s, and marine biologists involved in aquatic animal medicine and husbandry. Objectives are: to advance the art of aquatic animal medicine; to promote the free exchange of knowledge in the interest of improving the health care and husbandry of domestic aquatic animals and the proper management of aquatic animal resources in the wild; to provide an organization in which interested and professionally qualified individuals can work together to achieve these objectives; to provide a setting in which the development of the practice of aquatic animal medicine may be facilitated and enhanced; to promote the application of veterinary medical principles to aquatic animal disease problems. **Pub:** *IAAAM Conference Proceedings*, annual. Contains Annual Conference abstracts. • *IAAAM Directory*, annual. Directory. Included in proceedings book. • *IAAAM News*, 3/year. Newsletter. Includes association news, book reviews, calendar of events, and research updates. *Price:* Included in membership dues.


**★ 20627 ★ International Association of
Equine Dental Technicians (IAEDT)**
c/o Toots Banner
PO Box 410855
Melbourne, FL 32941
**Phone:** (321)242-9216
**Email:** rqhydedvm@anent.com
**Website:** http://www.iaeqd.org/
Toots Banner, DVM, Pres.
**Fnded:** 1987. **Mem:** 60. **Desc:** Equine dental technicians, veterinarians, and others interested in equine dental maintenance. Promotes the health and welfares of horses, and high standards and recognition in the field of equine dentistry. Acts as a forum for the exchange of information and experiences in the field. Sponsors educational programs. Offers certification program and testing. Maintains hall of fame. **Pub:** *IAEDT Newsletter*, quarterly. Newsletter. *Price:* Included in membership dues.


**★ 20628 ★ International Commission on
Protozoology (ICOP)**
010
Guangzhou 510515, People's Republic of China
**Fax:** 852 10 85148324
**Email:** tropmed@fimmu.edu.cn

**Desc:** Promotes the exchange of ideas among protozoologists throughout the world, and helps to arrange periodic International Congresses of Protozoology.


**★ 20629 ★ International Committee on
Veterinary Gross Anatomical
Nomenclature
(Committee Internationale de la
Nomeclature Macroanatomique
Veterinaire)**
Department of Veterinary Anatomy
Anatomisches Institut
Tierarfliche Hochschule
Binchofsholer Damm 15
D-30173 Hannover, Switzerland

**Lang(s):** English, French, German, Italian. **Desc:** Veterinarians. Promotes international standardization of veterinary anatomical nomenclature. Develops standard nomenclature; sponsors research; facilitates cooperation among veterinary anatomists worldwide.


**★ 20630 ★ International Embryo Transfer
Society (IETS)**
1111 N Dunlap Ave.
Savoy, IL 61874
**Phone:** (217)356-3182  **Fax:** (217)398-4119
**Email:** iets@assochq.org
**Website:** http://www.iets.org
Jennifer Gavel, Exec. Sec.
**Fnded:** 1974. **Mem:** 1,100. **Desc:** Veterinarians; researchers in reproductive physiology, animal science, genetics, endocrinology, and immunology; representatives of regulatory agencies such as government agencies and breed associations; sales representatives of drugs or equipment; students. Works to disseminate scientific and educational information; to promote more effective research; to foster and maintain high standards of education and ethics. Conducts Code Numbers to Identify Units Freezing Embryos Program, through which containers of frozen embryos are labeled with a permanent, recognized identification number. Sponsors exhibits of drugs and equipment used in embryo transfer. Conducts student competition to promote excellence in research. Maintains speakers' bureau. **Pub:** *IETS Manual*. Manuals. Covers information on minimum sanitary standards for embryo transfer procedures. *Price:* $35. • *IETS Newsletter*, quarterly. Newsletter. • *Proceedings of Annual Symposium and Conference.*


**★ 20631 ★ International Laboratory for
Research on Animal Diseases**
PO Box 30709
Nairobi, Kenya
**Phone:** 254 2 632311  **Fax:** 254 2 631499
**Lang(s):** English. **Desc:** Individuals with an interest in animal diseases. Promotes development of improved veterinary medical and animal husbandry practice to reduce the incidence of disease in livestock. Facilitates communication and cooperation among members; sponsors research and educational programs.


**★ 20632 ★ International Regional
Organization of Plant Protection and
Animal Health (OIRSA)
(Organismo Internacional Regional de
Sanidad Agropecuaria — OIRSA)**
No 14 Colonia San Francisco
San Salvador, El Salvador
**Phone:** 503 2790174  **Fax:** 503 2790189
**Website:** http://www.oirsa.org.sv
**Fnded:** 1953. **Mem:** 9. **Lang(s):** Spanish. **Desc:** Ministries of agriculture and livestock from the countries of Costa Rica, Dominican Republic, El Salvador, Guatemala, Honduras, Mexico, Belize, Nicaragua, and Panama. Objective is to prevent epidemics and exotic diseases among crops and farm animals in Central America. Informs and advises members and coordinates their activities. Special programs include: plant and animal quarantine; a regional effort to prevent Foot and Mouth Disease and a joint effort with Honduras and Guatemala to control Coffee Berry Borer; and a cooperative. Cooperative projects with the United States Department of Agriculture include identification and classification of fruit flies and the eradication of the Africanized bee. Presents national and international courses on the quarantining of cattle. **Pub:** *Animal Health*. Bulletin. • *NOTI-OIRSA*, bimonthly. Bulletin. Contains technical information.


**★ 20633 ★ International Society for
Applied Ethology (ISAE)
(Societe International d'Ethologie Applie)**
c/o Dr. Ute Knierim
International Animal Hygiene Welfare & Farm
Animal Behavior

Buenteweg 17p
D-30559 Hannover, Germany
**Phone:** 49 511 9538449     **Fax:** 49 511 9538588
**Email:** ute.knierim@tiho0hannover.de
**Website:** http://www.applied-ethology.org
**Fnded:** 1966. **Mem:** 620. **Lang(s):** English. **Desc:** Veterinarians; scientists and individuals with special knowledge of ethology, the study of animal behavior. Purpose is to advance the study of ethology as it affects animal health and welfare. Seeks to: stimulate ethological teaching and research in the veterinary and related professions; encourage discussion among members and publication of original works; further ethological knowledge on domesticated, captive, and wild animals; acts as clearinghouse for veterinarians and other interested individuals. **Pub:** *ISAE Newsletter*, semiannual. Newsletter. • *Proceedings.* **Frmly:** (1991) Society for Veterinary Ethology; (1993) Societe d'Ethologie Veterinaire.

★ 20634 ★ **International Standing Committee of the International Congress on Animal Reproduction (ICAR)**
c/o Prof. Gareth Evans
Faculty of Veterinary Science
University of Sydney
Sydney, NSW 2006, Australia
**Phone:** 61 2 93513363     **Fax:** 61 2 93513957
**Email:** garethe@vetsci.usyd.edu.au
**Fnded:** 1948. **Lang(s):** English. **Desc:** Scientists from 50 countries. Primary activity is to conduct an international congress dealing with agricultural problems such as the fundamental study and practical application of reproduction in farm animals. Congresses concentrate on physiology, pathology, and biotechnology. Other discussion topics include: techniques of artificial insemination and embryo transfer; intensification of animal reproduction; and the control and prevention of animal diseases. Fosters information exchange among scientists on an international level. **Pub:** *Congress Proceedings*, quadrennial. • *Report Booklet*, periodic. Booklet. **Frmly:** International Standing Committee of the International Congress of Phsyiology and Pathology of Animal Reproduction; International Standing Committee of International Congress on Animal Reproduction and Artificial Insemination.

★ 20635 ★ **International Veterinary Acupuncture Society (IVAS)**
PO Box 271395
Fort Collins, CO 80527-1395
**Phone:** (970)266-0660     **Fax:** (970)266-0777
**Email:** office@ivas.org
**Website:** http://www.ivas.org/
Edward C. Boldt, Jr., Exec. Dir.
**Fnded:** 1974. **Nat'l Groups:** 6. **Desc:** Veterinarians and veterinary students. Encourages knowledge and research of the philosophy, technique, and practice of veterinary acupuncture. Fosters high standards in the field; promotes scientific investigation. Accumulates resources for scientific research and education; collects data concerning clinical and research cases where animals have been treated with acupuncture; disseminates information to veterinary students, practitioners, other scientific groups, and the public. Offers 100 contact hour basic veterinary acupuncture course; administers certification examination. **AKA:** IVAS.

★ 20636 ★ **Irish Veterinary Association**
53 Lansdowne Rd.
Ballsbridge 4, Dublin, Ireland
**Fnded:** 1888. **Desc:** Promotes the veterinary profession.

**Laboratory Animal Management Association (LAMA)**
*See:* Entry 9745

★ 20637 ★ **Mid-Atlantic States Association of Avian Veterinarians (MASAAV)**
Memorial Bldg., Ste. 291
610 N Main St.
Blacksburg, VA 24060-3311
**Phone:** (540)951-2559     **Fax:** (540)953-0230
**Email:** office@masaav.org
**Website:** http://www.masaav.org
Keath L. Marx, DVM, Exec. Dir.
**Fnded:** 1979. **Mem:** 200. **Reg. Groups:** 1. **State Groups:** 9. **Desc:** Works to address the needs of the avian veterinarian and technicians. innovative veterinary medicine and surgery to improve the health of avian patients. Conducts educational programs; makes donations for avian research; keeps members informed regarding legislation of interest to the profession. **Pub:** *Conference Proceedings Book*, annual. Book. Annual conference, avian medicine and surgery. *Price:* $40; $56 overseas air. • *MASAAV Veterinary Directory for Pet Stores*, annual. Directory. • *MASAAView*, 3/year. Newsletter.

**National Association for Biomedical Research (NABR)**
*See:* Entry 4610

★ 20638 ★ **National Association of Federal Veterinarians (NAFV)**
1101 Vermont Ave. NW, Ste. 710
Washington, DC 20005-6308
**Phone:** (202)289-6334     **Fax:** (202)842-4360
**Email:** nafv@erols.com
**Website:** http://users.erols.com/nafv/
Alice M. Thaler, Pres.
**Fnded:** 1918. **Mem:** 1,600. **State Groups:** 30. **Desc:** Professional society of veterinarians employed by the U.S. Government. Maintains speakers' bureau. **Pub:** *Federal Veterinarian*, monthly. Newsletter. Includes abstracts, obituaries, federal regulatory and legislative news, and association news. *Price:* Included in membership dues; $40/year for nonmembers. • *National Association of Federal Veterinarians–Directory*, annual. Directory. *Price:* $4 for members only. **Frmly:** Bureau of Animal Industry Veterinarians; (1943) National Association of Bureau of Animal Industry Veterinarians.

★ 20639 ★ **National Association for Veterinary Acupuncture (NAVA)**
951 W Bastanchury Rd.
Fullerton, CA 92835
**Phone:** (714)871-3000     **Fax:** (714)278-9335
**Email:** drdick@e-vet.com
Richard S. Glassberg, D.V.M., Pres.
**Fnded:** 1973. **Mem:** 60. **Desc:** Veterinarians, medical doctors, acupuncturists, and interested laymen. Purpose is to educate veterinarians and laymen in the field of veterinary acupuncture and to translate material into English. Conducts seminars; maintains speakers' bureau. **Pub:** *Compendium of Human and Veterinary Acupuncture.* • *Equine Acupuncture.*

★ 20640 ★ **National Mastitis Council (NMC)**
2820 Walton Commons West, Ste. 131
Madison, WI 53718-6797
**Phone:** (608)224-0622     **Fax:** (608)224-0644
**Email:** nmc@nmconline.org
**Website:** http://www.nmconline.org
Anne Saeman, Exec. Dir.
**Fnded:** 1961. **Mem:** 2,000. **Desc:** Seeks to resolve the problem of bovine mastitis (inflammation of the udder) by developing and distributing factual information on mastitis control and encouraging mastitis research. Conducts research and education programs. Helps organize and coordinate the activities of state councils. **Pub:** *National Mastitis Council–Annual Meeting Proceedings.* Proceedings. Contains papers on topics related to the production of high quality milk and the prevention of mastitis. *Price:* Included in membership dues; $15 to nonmembers. • *Udder*

*Topics*, bimonthly. Newsletter. For people working in the dairy industry concerned with milk production. Covers topics related to the production of high quality milk. *Price:* Included in membership dues. • Also publishes books, brochures, flyers, and monographs.

★ 20641 ★ **New Zealand Veterinary Association (NZVA)**
PO Box 11-212
Manners St.
Wellington, New Zealand
**Phone:** 64 4 4710484     **Fax:** 64 4 4710494
**Email:** nzva@vets.org.nz
**Website:** http://www.vets.org.nz
**Fnded:** 1923. **Mem:** 1,500. **Reg. Groups:** 14. **Local Groups:** 15. **Lang(s):** English. **Desc:** Promotes excellence in the veterinary profession through service to its members. **Pub:** *New Zealand Veterinary Journal*, bimonthly. Journal. • *New Zealand Vetscript*, monthly.

★ 20642 ★ **Nordic Society for Veterinary Pathology**
Blowsvej 13
DK-1870 Frederiksberg, Denmark
**Phone:** 45 35283117     **Fax:** 45 35283111
**Fnded:** 1977.

★ 20643 ★ **Norwegian Veterinary Association (DNV) (Norske Veterinarforening — DNV)**
Postboks 6781
St Olavs pl
N-0130 Oslo, Norway
**Phone:** 47 22 591650     **Fax:** 47 22 690450
**Email:** dnv@vetnett.no
**Website:** http://www.vetnett.no
**Fnded:** 1888. **Mem:** 2,175. **Nat'l Groups:** 5. **Local Groups:** 15. **Lang(s):** English, Norwegian. **Desc:** Promotes the advancement of veterinary science in Norway. Sponsors educational and research programs. Compiles statistics; conducts charitable projects. **Pub:** *Norsk Veterinartidsskrift*, monthly. Journal.

★ 20644 ★ **Office International des Epizooties (OIE)**
12, rue de Prony
F-75017 Paris, France
**Phone:** 33 1 44151888     **Fax:** 33 1 42670987
**Email:** oie@oie.int
**Website:** http://www.oie.int
**Fnded:** 1924. **Mem:** 155. **Reg. Groups:** 5. **Lang(s):** English, French, Spanish. **Desc:** Veterinary services of national ministries of agriculture. Promotes and coordinates activities and research involving the epidemiology and control of contagious diseases in livestock. Collects and presents to governmental agencies data pertaining to epizootic diseases. Examines governmental agreements regarding animal health measures and assists in the supervision of their enforcement. Conducts specialized conferences and disease reporting seminars for chief veterinary officers and epidemiologists of member countries. Compiles statistics. **Pub:** *International Animal Health Code*, annual. Includes recommendations for import/export of animals, animal products, diagnostic techniques, and vaccines. • *Manual of Standards for Diagnostic Tests and Vaccines*, periodic. Manual. Outlines standards for the surveillance and control of the most imortant animal diseases. • *World Animal Health*, annual.

★ 20645 ★ **Orthopedic Foundation for Animals (OFA)**
2300 Nifong Blvd.
Columbia, MO 65201-3856
**Phone:** (573)442-0418     **Fax:** (573)875-5073
**Email:** ofa@offa.org
**Website:** http://www.offa.org
Dr. G.G. Keller, Project Dir.

**Fnded:** 1967. **Desc:** National and local dog clubs and individual breeders. Acts as a clearinghouse for information on orthopedic diseases of animals, particularly hip dysplasia in dogs (a hereditary condition resulting in abnormal development of the hip joints). Is attempting to develop a national control program through monitoring animals and conducting selective breeding and research. Conducts educational seminars; compiles statistics; sponsors a national referral service for animal breeders. Maintains library of all breed canine pelvic radiographs. **Pub:** *Proceedings of Canine Hip Dysplasia Symposium and Workshop.*

★ **20646** ★ **Phi Zeta**
c/o Dr. Robert McClure
University of Missouri
Department of Veterinary Biomedical Sciences
101 Bingham Rd.
Columbia, MO 65203-3577
**Phone:** (314)449-4497
**Email:** mcclurerc@hotmail.com
Robert McClure, Sec. -Treas.
**Fnded:** 1925. **Local Groups:** 27. **Desc:** Honor society for veterinary medicine.

★ **20647** ★ **Polish Society of Veterinary Science (PSVS) (Polskie Towarzystwo Nauk Weterynaryjnych)**
Faculty of Veterinary Medicine in Warsaw
ul. Grochowska 272
PL-03-849 Warsaw, Poland
**Phone:** 48 22 8103397    **Fax:** 48 22 8103397
**Website:** http://www.sggw.waw.pl/~ptnw/content.html
**Fnded:** 1952. **Mem:** 2,400. **Nat'l Groups:** 12. **Reg. Groups:** 17. **Lang(s):** English, Polish. **Desc:** Veterinarians in Poland. Promotes excellence in veterinary medicine. Maintains museum. **Pub:** *Medycyna Weterynaryjna*, monthly. Journal. Also publishes periodic congress and conference materials of divisions.

★ **20648** ★ **Royal College of Veterinary Surgeons**
Belgravia House
62-64 Horseferry Rd.
London SW1P 2AF, United Kingdom
**Phone:** 44 207 2222001    **Fax:** 44 207 2222004
**Email:** admin@rcvs.org.uk
**Website:** http://www.rcvs.org.uk
**Fnded:** 1844. **Mem:** 19,800. **Lang(s):** Dutch, French, German. **Desc:** Graduates possessing a veterinary degree, registerable with the RCVS who intend to practice in the UK. Statutory body governing the veterinary profession in the UK. Responsible for quality of veterinary undergraduate education at the UK veterinary schools, provision of membership examination, and discipline of members. Establishment of certificate and diploma examinations. **Pub:** *Directory of Veterinary Practices*, annual. Directory. • *Guide to Professional Conduct*, 3/year. • *RCVS Annual Report*, annual. Annual Report. • *RCVS News*, quarterly. • *RCVS Register and Directories*, annual. Directory.

★ **20649** ★ **Royal Netherlands Veterinary Association (RNVA) (Koninklijke Nederlandse Maatschappij voor Diergeneeskunde — KNMVD)**
Julianalaan 8-10
Postbus 14031
NL-3508 SB Utrecht, Netherlands
**Phone:** 31 30 2510111    **Fax:** 31 30 511787
**Email:** info@knmvd.nl
**Website:** http://www.knmvd.nl
**Fnded:** 1862. **Mem:** 4,500. **Nat'l Groups:** 10. **Reg. Groups:** 10. **Local Groups:** 27. **Lang(s):** Dutch, English, German. **Desc:** Veterinary surgeons in the Netherlands. Promotes veterinary science; protects the interests of members. Compiles statistics. **Pub:** *Annual Yearbook*, annual. Book. • *Tijdschrift voor Diergeneeskunde*, semimonthly. • *Veehouder en Dierenarts*, quarterly. • *Veterinary Quarterly*. Journal.

Includes veterinary research results and studies and case reports.

★ **20650** ★ **Singapore Veterinary Association (SVA)**
c/o Agri-Food and Veterinary Authority
5 Maxwell Rd., Ste. 03-00
Tower Block, MND Complex
Singapore 069110, Singapore
**Phone:** 65 2270670    **Fax:** 65 2276403
**Email:** sva@sva.org.sg
**Website:** http://www.sva.org.sg
**Desc:** Represents interests of veterinary surgeons and the veterinary profession in Singapore. Liaises with government agencies regarding veterinary science.

★ **20651** ★ **Society for Theriogenology (ST)**
200 4th Ave. N, No. 900
Nashville, TN 37219
**Phone:** (615)244-3060    **Fax:** (615)254-7047
**Email:** sft@walkermgt.com
**Website:** http://www.therio.org
James Alexander, Pres.
**Fnded:** 1954. **Mem:** 2,508. **Desc:** Veterinarians united to promote the practice of qualified veterinarians examining animals for breeding soundness; to facilitate these procedures by standardization of the criteria used by veterinarians; to assemble and evaluate the measurements of breeding soundness from literature and from unbiased records accumulated from all sources and distribute this information to all members. (Theriogenology is a branch of veterinary medicine that deals with reproduction, veterinary obstetrics, gynecology, and seminology.) Distributes morphology stain for use in making breeding soundness evaluations and standard forms for use in recording such evaluations. Maintains speakers' bureau. **Pub:** *Proceedings of Annual Meeting*, annual. *Price:* $50. • Newsletter, bimonthly. **Frmly:** (1975) American Veterinary Society for the Study of Breeding Soundness.

★ **20652** ★ **Standing Committee of the International Congress on Animal Reproduction (ICAR) (Comite Permanent International du Congres de Physiologie et Pathologie de la Reproduction Animale)**
Gunn Bldg., Rm. 346
Faculty of Veterinary Science
University of Sydney
Sydney, NSW 2006, Australia
**Phone:** 61 2 93513363    **Fax:** 61 2 93513957
**Email:** garethe@vetsci.su.oz.au
**Fnded:** 1948. **Lang(s):** English. **Desc:** Veterinarians and agricultural scientists with an interest in the reproduction of farm animals and wildlife. Seeks to develop new breeding and animal husbandry techniques to insure efficient propagation of livestock and conservation of wildlife. **Pub:** *ICAR Conference Proceedings*, quarterly.

★ **20653** ★ **Swedish Veterinary Association (Sveriges Veterinarforbund — SVF)**
Box 12709
S-112 94 Stockholm, Sweden
**Phone:** 46 8 54555820    **Fax:** 46 8 54555839
**Email:** office@svf.se
**Website:** http://www.svf.se
**Fnded:** 1860. **Mem:** 2,200. **Lang(s):** English, Swedish. **Desc:** Swedish veterinarians. Functions as a trade union and professional organization. Conducts continuing education courses for members. **Pub:** *Svensk Veterinartidning - SVT*, 15/year. Journal.

★ **20654** ★ **Union of Veterinarians in Bulgaria**
15A 'P. Slaveikov'Ave.
BG-1606 Sofia, Bulgaria
**Phone:** 359 2 513243    **Fax:** 359 2 542925
**Fnded:** 1893. **Mem:** 2,500. **Reg. Groups:** 36. **Local Groups:** 56. **Lang(s):** Bulgarian, English, Russian. **Desc:** Promotes and protects members' interests. **Pub:** *Veterinarna Zbirka*, monthly. Journal.

★ **20655** ★ **United States Animal Health Association (USAHA)**
PO Box K227
8100 Three Chopt Rd., Ste. 203
Richmond, VA 23288
**Phone:** (804)285-3210    **Fax:** (804)285-3367
**Email:** usaha@usaha.org
**Website:** http://www.usaha.org
Linda B. Ragland, Contact
**Fnded:** 1897. **Mem:** 1,100. **Reg. Groups:** 4. **Desc:** Veterinarians, livestock producers, and transportation and livestock companies concerned with the improvement of the health of livestock and poultry through disease control and eradication. **Pub:** *Foreign Animal Diseases Diagnosis and Control*, quarterly. Newsletter. • *Proceedings*, annual. *Price:* $30. **Frmly:** Association of State Sanitary Boards; United States Livestock Sanitary Association.

★ **20656** ★ **Veterinary Cancer Society (VCS)**
PO Box 1763
Spring Valley, CA 91979-1763
**Phone:** (619)460-2002    **Fax:** (619)741-1117
**Email:** bmcgehee@cts.com
**Website:** http://www.vetcancersociety.org
Dr. Barbara McGehee, Exec. Dir.
**Fnded:** 1974. **Mem:** 800. **Desc:** Veterinarians and others who have an interest in cancer in animals. Goals are to: achieve and maintain high standards of diagnosis, treatment, and prevention of animal cancers; advance interdisciplinary research in neoplastic diseases of animals; collect and disseminate information about animal tumors; conduct and evaluate studies, including cooperative clinical trials, of animal neoplasms. **Pub:** *VCS Newsletter*, quarterly. Newsletter. • Directory, periodic.

★ **20657** ★ **Veterinary Hospital Managers Association (VHMA)**
48 Howard St.
Albany, NY 12207
**Phone:** (518)433-8911    **Fax:** (518)463-8656
**Email:** vhma@caphill.com
**Website:** http://www.vhma.org
Christine M. Quinn, Exec. Dir.
**Fnded:** 1981. **Desc:** Individuals involved in veterinary practice management. Seeks to advance the study, teaching, and practice of veterinary practice management. Serves as a forum for the exchange of information among members; sponsors continuing professional development courses; formulates standards of ethics and practice for veterinary medical managers.

★ **20658** ★ **Veterinary Infectious Disease Organization (VIDO)**
120 Veterinary Rd.
Saskatoon, SK, Canada S7N 5E3
**Phone:** (306)966-7465    **Fax:** (306)966-7478
**Email:** vido_comm.@sask.uscsk.ca
**Website:** http://www.usask.ca/vido/
**Fnded:** 1975. **Lang(s):** English, French. **Desc:** Promotes animal health through diagnosis and prevention of production-limiting diseases. Conducts research focusing on development of new vaccines to better treat infectious diseases and the discovery and application of biotechnologies. Serves as a clearinghouse on commercial veterinary diagnosis and treatment techniques; makes available laboratory and field study services. Makes available educational and extension services. **Pub:** Brochures.

## ★ 20659 ★ Veterinary Orthopedic Society (VOS)

PO Box 313
Newmarket, NH 03857-0313
**Phone:** (603)659-7989 **Fax:** (603)659-7989
**Email:** vosclarkmt@aol.com
**Website:** http://www.vet.ohio-state.edu/docs/vos
Mary Tuson Clark, Exec. Sec.
**Fnded:** 1972. **Mem:** 600. **Desc:** Veterinarians interested in orthopedic surgery. Promotes education and research in veterinary orthopedic surgery. Provides a forum for the exchange of ideas among veterinarians in academia, research, and practice. **Pub:** *Membership List*, periodic. Journal. • *VOS Newsletter*, annual. Newsletter. *Price:* Included in membership dues.

## ★ 20660 ★ Western Veterinary Conference (WVC)

2425 E Oquendo Rd.
Las Vegas, NV 89120-2406
**Phone:** (702)739-6698 **Fax:** (702)739-6420
**Email:** info@westernveterinary.org
**Website:** http://www.wvc.org
Dr. Steven Crane, Exec. Dir.
**Fnded:** 1928. **Mem:** 4,500. **Desc:** International veterinarians attending annual conference. Provides practical continuing education for veterinarians and technicians. Topics of study at conference include small and large animal medicine and surgery, general medicine, emergency clinic operation, radiographic and clinical pathologic methods, and current research. Autotutorial programs are available. **Frmly:** (1986) Intermountain Veterinary Medical Association.

## ★ 20661 ★ World Association for the Advancement of Veterinary Parasitology (WAAVP)

PO Box 8
North Aurora, IL 60542
**Phone:** (630)844-9676 **Fax:** (630)892-0818
**Email:** isvma@aol.com
Ann R. Donoghue, DVM, Sec. -Treas.
**Fnded:** 1963. **Mem:** 560. **Desc:** Veterinarians and other scientists in 60 countries interested in veterinary parasitology. Objectives are to encourage research in veterinary parasitology, to promote the exchange of information and material between organizations and individuals, and to organize meetings for the study of parasites of veterinary importance. Maintains scientific committees. **Pub:** *Membership Directory*, annual. Membership Directory. • *Newsletter*, 3/year. Newsletter. • *Proceedings of Scientific Conferences*, biennial. • *Statutes - List of Members*, biennial. **AKA:** Association Mondiale pour l'Advancement de Parasitologie Veterinaire.

## ★ 20662 ★ World Association for Buiatrics (WAB) (Welt-Gesellschaft fur Buiatrik)

c/o Professor P. Lekeux
Faculty of Veterinary Medicine
University of Liege
Bat. B42, Sart Tilman
B-4000 Liege, Belgium
**Phone:** 32 4 3664030 **Fax:** 32 4 3662935
**Email:** pierre.lekeux@ulg.ac.be
**Website:** http://www.ulg.ac.be/fmv/wab.htm
**Fnded:** 1962. **Mem:** 10,000. **Lang(s):** English, French, German, Spanish. **Desc:** Veterinarians, practitioners, and scientists working with cattle in 48 countries. Seeks to study the diseases of cattle, including diagnosis, treatment, and prevention, and factors influencing cattle production. **Pub:** *Congress Reports*, biennial. • Newsletter, quarterly.

## ★ 20663 ★ World Association of Veterinary Anatomists (WAVA)

Department of Veterinary Anatomy & Embryology
University of Antwerp
Slachthuislaan 68
B-2060 Antwerp, Belgium
**Phone:** 32 3 2356111 **Fax:** 32 3 2724080
**Email:** weyns@ruca.ua.ac.be
**Fnded:** 1957. **Mem:** 350. **Reg. Groups:** 8. **Lang(s):** English, French, German, Spanish. **Desc:** Veterinarians and other professionals teaching and researching at veterinary institutions. Promotes the study and teaching of domestic animal anatomy. Seeks to establish a uniform nomenclature. Maintains International Committee on Veterinary Anatomical Nomenclature. **Pub:** *Anatomia, Histologia, Embryologia (Zentralblatt for Veterinarmedizin, Section C)*, quarterly. Journal. • *Nomina Anatomica Veterinaria - Nomina Histologica - Nomina Embryologica*. Book. • *WAVA-News*, annual.

## ★ 20664 ★ World Association of Veterinary Laboratory Diagnosticians (WAVLD)

PO Drawer 3040
College Station, TX 77841-3040
**Phone:** (979)845-3414 **Free:** 888-646-5623
**Fax:** (979)845-1794
**Email:** keugster@tvmdl.edu
**Website:** http://wwwtvmdl.tamu.edu
A. K. Eugster, Sec. Treas.
**Fnded:** 1977. **Mem:** 650. **Nat'l Groups:** 5. **Desc:** Individuals in 30 countries engaged in laboratory diagnosis of animal diseases. Coordinates activities of regulatory, research, and service laboratories. Maintains guidelines for personnel qualifications and facility standards. Establishes uniform laboratory methods and seeks to improve and develop existing diagnostic techniques. Disseminates information; maintains speakers' bureau. **Pub:** *Symposium Proceedings*, triennial. Proceedings.

## ★ 20665 ★ World Association of Veterinary Microbiologists, Immunologists, and Specialists in Infectious Diseases (WAVMI) (Association Mondiale des Veterinaires Microbiologistes, Immunologistes et Specialistes des Maladies Infectieuses — AMVMI)

7, ave. du General de Gaulle
F-94704 Maisons-Alfort Cedex, France
**Phone:** 33 1 43967021 **Fax:** 33 1 43967022
**Fnded:** 1968. **Lang(s):** English, French. **Desc:** Facilitates international exchange among veterinary microbiologists, immunologists, and specialists in infectious diseases. Sponsors international course in animal immunology; conducts symposia. **Pub:** *Comparative Immunology, Microbiology and Infectious Diseases*, quarterly.

## ★ 20666 ★ World Association of Veterinary Pathologists (WAVP)

Ecole Nationale Veterinaire
F-94704 Maisons-Alfort, France
**Phone:** 33 1 43967109 **Fax:** 33 1 43967112
**Email:** parodi@net-alfort.fr
**Fnded:** 1952. **Desc:** Promotes the study of pathomorphology and pathophysiology of animal diseases and their pathogenesis.

## ★ 20667 ★ World Small Animal Veterinary Association (WSAVA)

c/o Dr. Bryan Moore
76 Kohu Rd.
Titragi
Auckland, New Zealand
**Phone:** 64 9 8173444
**Website:** http://www.wsava.org
**Fnded:** 1959. **Mem:** 39. **Desc:** WSAVA is an association of Veterinary associations, representing 47,000 individuals in 35 countries involved in practice, teaching, and research related to dogs, cats, caged birds, and other small animals. Primary purpose is to advance quality and availability of veterinary medicine and surgery relating to small animals. Encourages research; conducts surveys; sponsors meetings for studying conditions and matters affecting small animals; furthers international relationships between all veterinarians dealing with small animal health and welfare. **Pub:** *Journal of Small Animal Practice*, monthly. Journal. • *Proceedings of Congress*, annual. Papers.

## ★ 20668 ★ World Veterinary Association (WVA) (Welt-Tierarztegesellschaft)

Rosenlunds Alle 8
DK-2720 Vanlose, Denmark
**Phone:** 45 38710156 **Fax:** 45 38710322
**Email:** wva@ddd.dk
**Website:** http://www.worldvet.org
**Fnded:** 1959. **Mem:** 96. **Lang(s):** English, French, German, Spanish. **Desc:** Association of national (70), international (20), and commercial (4) organizations. Purposes are to: unify and promote the veterinary profession; encourages high standards of health and welfare in all species of animals; improve veterinary science through the exchange of information and education; establish uniform nomenclature. Sends volunteers to developing countries to assist in food production, processing and distribution, to teach basic techniques in disease control and eradication and to develop national veterinary services. **Pub:** *Report on Resolutions*, periodic. • *World Veterinary Directory*, periodic. Directory. • Bulletin, semiannual. • Membership Directory, annual.

## ★ 20669 ★ World Veterinary Poultry Association (WVPA) (Asociacion Mundial Veterinaria de Avicola — AMVA)

c/o Prof. E.F. Kaleta
Justus-Liebig-Universitat Giessen
Frankfurter Str. 91
D-35392 Giessen, Germany
**Phone:** 49 641 9938430 **Fax:** 49 641 201548
**Email:** erhard.f.kaleta@vetmed.uni-giessen.de
**Website:** http://www.wvpa.net
**Fnded:** 1959. **Mem:** 1,684. **Nat'l Groups:** 31. **Lang(s):** English, French, German. **Desc:** Veterinarians and other scientists in 56 countries engaged in practice, research, or education connected with avian pathology. Objectives are to: organize meetings for studying diseases and conditions; encourage research; promote the exchange of information and material for study between individuals and organizations; establish and maintain liaisons with other groups. Organizes avian medicine sections of the World Veterinary Congresses. **Pub:** *Aerosols*, annual. Newsletter. • *Avian Pathology*, bimonthly. Journal.

## ★ 20670 ★ Zimbabwe Veterinary Association (ZVA)

PO Box CY 168
Causeway
Harare, Zimbabwe
**Phone:** 263 4 495859 **Fax:** 263 4 495859
**Email:** bvickers@esanet.zw
**Fnded:** 1920. **Mem:** 180. **Local Groups:** 1. **Lang(s):** English. **Desc:** Veterinarians practicing in Zimbabwe. Encourages contact and information exchange among members. Conducts clinical meetings and seminars. **Pub:** *The Burdizzo*, quarterly. Newsletter. • *Zimbabwe Veterinary Journal*, quarterly. Journal. **Frmly:** (1980) Rhodesian Veterinary Association.

---

# Research Centers

## ★ 20671 ★ Harvard University New England Regional Primate Research Center

1 Pine Hill Dr.
PO Box 9102
Southborough, MA 01772-9102
**Phone:** (508)624-8042 **Fax:** (508)624-8190
**Email:** ronald_desrosiers@hms.harvard.edu

**Website:** http://www.hms.harvard.edu/nerprc/
Dr. Ronald C. Desrosiers, Dir.

**Activities/Fields:** Diseases of simian primates, as they relate to clinical and comparative pathology, behavioral biology, immunology, molecular virology, microbiology, viral oncology, nutrition, and primatology.

## ★ 20672 ★ The Jackson Laboratory
**Mouse Mutant Resource**
600 Main St.
Bar Harbor, ME 04609
**Phone:** (207)288-6235 **Fax:** (207)288-6149
**Email:** mtd@jax.org
**Website:** http://www.jax.org/resources/documents/mmr/mmrhome.html
Muriel T. Davisson, PhD, Contact

**Activities/Fields:** Identifies, characterizes, and genetically maps new inherited endocrine, neurological, immunological, skeletal, and other mutations of the laboratory mouse.

## ★ 20673 ★ Johns Hopkins University
**Center for Alternatives to Animal Testing**
School of Hygiene & Public Health
111 Market Pl., Ste. 840
Baltimore, MD 21202-6709
**Phone:** (410)233-1692 **Fax:** (410)223-1603
**Email:** caat@jhsph.edu
**Website:** http://caat.jhsph.edu
Dr. Alan M. Goldberg, Dir.

**Activities/Fields:** Fosters development of scientifically acceptable in vitro and other alternatives to animal testing for use in development and safety evaluation of commercial and therapeutic products. Catalyzes validation of alternative methods. **Pub:** *Alternative Methods in Toxicology Book Series*. Book. • *Newsletter*. • *Technical Report Series*.

## ★ 20674 ★ Ohio State University
**Laboratory Animal Center**
6089 Godown Rd.
Columbus, OH 43235
**Phone:** (614)292-8541 **Fax:** (614)292-9282
**Email:** stone.4@osu.edu
Douglas Stone, DVM, Assoc. Dir.

**Activities/Fields:** Supports University biomedical research activities of all laboratory animals, quarantining of all nonhuman primates and other species depending upon the nature of the study, and long-term housing of nonhuman primates, canines, swine, and other species. Serves as a teaching resource for the College of Veterinary Medicine.

## ★ 20675 ★ Oregon Health and Science University
**Oregon Regional Primate Research Center**
505 NW 185th Ave.
Beaverton, OR 97006
**Phone:** (503)645-1141 **Fax:** (503)690-5532
**Email:** smithsu@ohsu.edu
**Website:** http://www.ohsu.edu/orprc
Dr. M. Susan Smith, PhD, Dir.

**Activities/Fields:** Nonhuman primates, particularly reproductive biology, neuroscience, and experimental pathology. Specific projects include studies on the events that control fertility in primates, causes and control of premature labor, mechanisms of steroid action, and factors affecting neural differentiation, function and plasticity. Other projects seek to understand physiological mechanisms involved in atherosclerosis and immune deficiency diseases. Provides research facilities for staff and collaborative scientists.

## ★ 20676 ★ Purdue University
**Center for Paralysis Research**
Sch. of Veterinary Medicine
1244 VCPR
West Lafayette, IN 47907-1244

**Phone:** (765)494-7600 **Fax:** (765)494-7605
**Email:** cpr@vet.purdue.edu
**Website:** http://www.vet.purdue.edu/cpr
Dr. Richard Borgens, Dir.

**Activities/Fields:** Treatments for spinal cord injury, focusing on recruitment of spared pathways in the spinal cord through the use of 4-Aminopyridine (4-AP), reconnection and regeneration of severely damaged nerve pathways through the use of oscillating electrical fields and treatment with injectable polymers that seak damaged cells, and replacement of spinal cord using enteric neuron transplantation.

## ★ 20677 ★ State University of New York Health Science Center at Brooklyn
**Primate Behavior Laboratory**
450 Clarkson Ave., Box 120
Brooklyn, NY 11203
**Phone:** (718)270-3355 **Fax:** (718)270-3355
**Email:** lrosenbl@downstate.edu
Dr. Leonard A. Rosenblum, Dir.

**Activities/Fields:** Normative and experimental studies of the development of bonnet and pigtail macaques and squirrel monkeys, including the development of mother-infant relations and infant social development, environmental factors and social development, psychosocial factors, nonhuman primate sexual behavior, primate models of psychopathology, and experimental studies of environmental enrichment, learning, and perception with computer-mediated video tasks in individual and group settings.

## Trinity University
**Genetics Laboratory for Typing Nonhuman Primates**
*See:* Entry 9436

## ★ 20678 ★ Tulane University
**Tulane Regional Primate Research Center**
18703 Three Rivers Rd.
Covington, LA 70433
**Phone:** (504)892-2040 **Fax:** (504)893-1352
**Email:** gerone@tpc.tulane.edu
**Website:** http://www2.tulane.edu/primate_center.cfm
Dr. Peter J. Gerone, Dir.

**Activities/Fields:** Use of nonhuman primates in biomedical research projects in fields of cancer, immunology, infectious diseases, primate medicine, parasitology, primatology, pathology, reproductive physiology, urology, gene therapy and veterinary science. **Frmly:** Delta Regional Primate Research Center.

## ★ 20679 ★ U.S. Department of Health and Human Services
**National Center for Research Resources**
**Comparative Medicine Program**
**Laboratory Animal Sciences Program**
9000 Rockville Pike
Bldg 12A Rm 4007, MSC5662
Bethesda, MD 20892
**Phone:** (301)496-5795 **Fax:** (301)402-0006
Dr. Judith Vaitukaitis, Dir.

**Activities/Fields:** New animal models, to improve the care and health of animals used in research, and to train veterinarians in laboratory animal medicine. Focus is on the development of improved methods for diagnosing and controlling diseases among laboratory animals; and providing support to special breeding programs to ensure an adequate supply of animals that have been shown to be good models of human diseases or that serve as important research subjects.

## ★ 20680 ★ University of California at Davis
**California Regional Primate Research Center**
1 Shields Ave.
Davis, CA 95616-8542
**Phone:** (530)752-0447 **Fax:** (530)752-2880
**Email:** crprc@ucdavis.edu

**Website:** http://www.crprc.ucdavis.edu/
Dr. Andrew G. Hendrickx, Dir.

**Activities/Fields:** Developmental and reproductive biology, behavioral and neurology, genetics, neurosciences, virology and immunology, infectious diseases, pulmonary and respiratory diseases, primate medicine, and primate pathology. Focuses on preventive medicine for humans through the use of nonhuman primates as animal models in such studies as the effects of toxic compounds, developmental toxicology, metabolic diseases, infectious agents, altered environments, and pharmacokinetics of various drugs. **Pub:** *Annual Progress Report*.

## ★ 20681 ★ University of Chicago
**Animal Resources Center**
MC 1030
5841 S Maryland Ave.
Chicago, IL 60637-1030
**Phone:** (773)702-9368 **Fax:** (773)702-9152
**Email:** gus@arc_1_bsd.uchicago.edu
Dr. August Battles, Dir.

**Activities/Fields:** Supports research on animals and animal models. **Frmly:** Office of Animal Care; A.J. Carson Animal Research Facility.

## University of Hawaii at Manoa
**Kewalo Marine Laboratory**
*See:* Entry 4751

## ★ 20682 ★ University of Illinois at Chicago
**Biologic Resource Laboratory**
MC 533
1840 W Taylor St.
Chicago, IL 60612-0533
**Phone:** (312)996-7040 **Fax:** (312)996-8065
**Email:** btb@uic.edu
**Website:** http://www.kewalo.hawaii.edu/
Dr. B. Taylor Bennett, Dir.

**Activities/Fields:** Houses animals and provides research and teaching support involving animal models for Colleges of Medicine, Dentistry, Pharmacy, and Nursing of the University.

## ★ 20683 ★ University of Kansas
**Animal Care Unit**
B054 Malott
Lawrence, KS 66045
**Phone:** (785)864-5587 **Fax:** (785)864-5305
**Email:** acu@ku.edu
**Website:** http://www.ukans.edu/~acu/acu.html
James F. Bresnahan, DVM, Dir.

**Activities/Fields:** Provides care to animals used in research, teaching, and public education at the Lawrence campus. Provides animal care, diagnostic, treatment, and necropsy services to control disease conditions and monitor health status of animal colonies. **Pub:** *Handbook for the Use of Animals in Research and Education*.

## ★ 20684 ★ University of Kansas
**Laboratory Animal Resources**
University of Kansas Medical Center
2010 W 39th St.
Kansas City, KS 66160-7185
**Phone:** (913)588-7015 **Fax:** (913)588-7277
**Email:** dpinson@kumc.edu
David M. Pinson, DVM, Dir.

**Activities/Fields:** Houses and maintains many species of animals required for various facets of biomedical research and for teaching purposes at the University. Supports a wide variety of research projects involving laboratory animals and operates a comprehensive laboratory animal program.

## University of Louisiana at Lafayette
**New Iberia Research Center**
*See:* Entry 2690

**★ 20685 ★ University of Michigan**
**Unit for Laboratory Animal Medicine**
Animal Research Facility
Ann Arbor, MI 48109-0614
**Phone:** (734)764-0277 **Fax:** (734)936-3235
**Email:** dringler@umich.edu
**Website:** http://www.ulam.umich.edu
Dr. D.H. Ringler, Dir.
**Activities/Fields:** Biomedical sciences including comparative medicine, laboratory animal medicine, animal models for biomedical research, and proper use and care of laboratory animals. Provides veterinary care for all vertebrate animals used in research and education at the University.

**★ 20686 ★ University of Missouri—**
**Columbia**
**Research Animal Diagnostic Laboratory**
1600 E Rollins
Columbia, MO 65211
**Phone:** (573)882-5983 **Free:** 800-669-0825
**Fax:** (573)884-7521
**Email:** radil@missouri.edu
**Website:** http://www.radil.missouri.edu
Dr. Lela K. Riley, Dir.
**Activities/Fields:** Human health research through the use of animals. **Pub:** *Infectious Diseases.*

**★ 20687 ★ University of Missouri—**
**Kansas City**
**Laboratory Animal Center**
1015 E 50th St.
Kansas City, MO 64110
**Phone:** (816)235-1681 **Fax:** (816)235-5275
**Email:** petersd@umkc.edu
David K. Peters, DVM, Dir.
**Activities/Fields:** Physiology, exploratory surgery, and immunology.

**★ 20688 ★ University of Montana**
**Primate Laboratory**
Department of Psychology
Missoula, MT 59812-1584
**Phone:** (406)243-2091 **Fax:** (406)243-6366
**Email:** pyadp@selway.umt.edu
**Website:** http://www.cas.umt.edu/psych
Dr. Allen D. Szalda-Petree, Dir.
**Activities/Fields:** Social and learning behaviors of developing monkeys, specifically rhesus monkeys (Macaca mulatta). Also conducts research in the use of computer video tasks to study discrimination learning, foraging behavior, and perceptual motor skills in primates. **Frmly:** Animal Behavior Laboratory.

**★ 20689 ★ University of Oklahoma**
**Animal Resources**
Health Science Center, BMSB 203
PO Box 26901
Oklahoma City, OK 73190
**Phone:** (405)271-5185 **Fax:** (405)271-2660
**Email:** gary-white@ouhsc.edu
Gary L. White, DVM, Dir.
**Activities/Fields:** Biomedical studies in general areas of physiology, pathology, microbiology, surgery, and internal medicine.

**★ 20690 ★ University of Pennsylvania**
**Referral Center for Animal Models of**
**Human Genetic Disease**
Rosenthal Bldg., Rm. 307
Veterinary School
3800 Spruce St.
Philadelphia, PA 19104-6051
**Phone:** (215)898-4852 **Fax:** (215)898-0719
**Email:** mhaskins@vet.upenn.edu
Dr. Mark Haskins, Prin. Investigator
**Activities/Fields:** Identification, characterization, evaluation, and dissemination of animal models of human genetic disease, particularly models that occur in domestic animals, with emphasis on hereditary

metabolic diseases, hereditary defects in sexual development, congenital malformations, and hereditary diseases of blood. Activities include characterization of mutant genes at the molecular level.

**★ 20691 ★ University of Pittsburgh**
**Center for Research in Reproductive**
**Physiology**
Biomedical Science Tower, S 330
Pittsburgh, PA 15261
**Phone:** (412)648-9281 **Fax:** (412)383-7159
**Email:** plant1@vms.cis.pitt.edu
Tony M. Plant, PhD, Dir.
**Activities/Fields:** Neuroendocrine control of reproduction in rhesus monkeys. **Frmly:** Center for Research in Primate Reproduction.

**★ 20692 ★ University of Puerto Rico**
**Caribbean Primate Research Center**
Medical Science Campus
PO Box 1053
Sabana Seca, PR 00952-1053
**Phone:** (787)784-0322 **Fax:** (787)795-6700
**Email:** mkessler@coqui.net
**Website:** http://cprc.rcm.upr.edu/
Dr. Matthew J. Kessler, Interim Dir.
**Activities/Fields:** General primate behavior and biology with emphasis on sociobiology and diseases of nonhuman primates. The nonhuman primate populations and associated genealogical records make possible an evaluation of genetic, ecological, and social influences on the incidence and progress of disorders of adaptation and enable research to be conducted on control of population growth, evolution of social interaction by family selection, inbreeding potential of confined populations, reproductive behavior, positional behaviors and the development of degenerative joint disease, diabetes, obesity, and macular degeneration. The Center has been active as a site for dissertation research and for long-term, follow-up studies on a collaborative basis with research investigators.

**★ 20693 ★ University of South Alabama**
**Primate Research Laboratory**
Department of Comparative Medicine, MSB 992
College of Medicine
Mobile, AL 36688-0002
**Phone:** (334)460-6293 **Fax:** (334)460-6286
**Email:** lwilliam@usouthal.edu
Bob Ricker, Lab. Supv.
**Activities/Fields:** Primates, especially as animal models of human diseases.

**★ 20694 ★ University of Texas at Austin**
**Animal Resources Center**
CMC A2500
2701 Speedway
Austin, TX 78705
**Phone:** (512)471-7534 **Fax:** (512)471-4336
**Email:** j.fineg@mail.utexas.edu
**Website:** http://www.utexas.edu/research/arc/
Jerry Fineg, DVM, Dir.
**Activities/Fields:** Provides a facility for research and housing of research animals. Also involved in diagnostic and procedural manipulation of the animals used in research and teaching elsewhere in the University. Research laboratories are provided for studies in anthropology, biochemistry, pharmaceutics, biomedical engineering, microbiology, nutrition, pharmocology, kienesiology, and zoology.

**University of Utah**
**Radiobiology Laboratory**
*See:* Entry 18095

**★ 20695 ★ University of Wisconsin—**
**Madison**
**Animal Care Unit, Gnotobiotic Section**
600 Highland Ave., CSC K4/1141
Madison, WI 53792

**Phone:** (608)262-0456 **Fax:** (608)265-6765
**Email:** southard@surgery.wisc.edu
**Website:** http://www.utah.edu/radiobiology
James H. Southard, PhD, Dir.
**Activities/Fields:** Host/parasite interactions, implicating immunology, kidney and thymus transplants, caries, bladder cancer, and toxicology; provides investigators with the technology and equipment necessary to carry out their research on animals that are either completely free of viable microorganisms or have a known microbial flora (flora-defined or gnotobiotic); improves methods used in the care of gnotobiotes, the units housing them, and equipment maintaining them; offers germfree foster mothers, rats, and mice, athymic and euthymic, to qualified researchers; performs caesarian derivations for affiliated organizations and commercial suppliers to upgrade the quality of research animals. **Pub:** *Investigator's Manual*, triennially. **Frmly:** Gnotobiotic Laboratory.

**★ 20696 ★ University of Wisconsin—**
**Madison**
**Research Animal Resources Center**
396 Enzyme Institute
1710 University Ave.
Madison, WI 53705
**Phone:** (608)262-1238 **Fax:** (608)265-2698
**Email:** parks@rarc.wisc.edu
**Website:** http://www.rarc.wisc.edu
Christine M. Parks, Dir.
**Activities/Fields:** Laboratory animal diseases. **Pub:** *Animals Newsletter.*

**★ 20697 ★ University of Wisconsin—**
**Madison**
**Wisconsin Regional Primate Research**
**Center**
1220 Capitol Ct.
Madison, WI 53715-1299
**Phone:** (608)263-3500 **Fax:** (608)263-4031
**Email:** kemnitz@primate.wisc.edu
**Website:** http://www.primate.wisc.edu
Dr. Joseph W. Kemnitz, Dir.
**Activities/Fields:** Reproduction and development, neurobiology, physiological ethology, psychobiology, aging and metabolic diseases, immunogenetics and immunology and virology. Emphasizes biomedical research and studies on captive and wild primate conservation; rhesus colonies for research in aging, AIDS, and developmental biology; and common marmosets, for research in reproduction and aging behavior. **Pub:** *Audio Visual Catalog*, biennially. • *Centerline Newsletter.* • *International Directory of Primatology*, biennially.

# State Government Agencies

## Veterinarians

**★ 20698 ★ Alabama Department of**
**Agriculture and Industries**
**State Veterinarian**
PO Box 3336
Montgomery, AL 36107
**Phone:** (334)240-7255 **Fax:** (334)223-7352
**Email:** stvet@agi.state.al.us
**Website:** http://www.agi.state.al.us/ANIMAL.htm
Dr. Tony Frazier, Contact
Dr. J. Lee Alley, Contact

**★ 20699 ★ Alaska Department of**
**Environmental Conservation**
**Environmental Health Division**
**State Veterinarian**
500 S Alaska St.
Animal Industries Program
Palmer, AK 99645
**Phone:** (907)745-3236 **Fax:** (907)745-8125

**Email:** bgore@envircon.state.ak.us
**Website:** http://www.state.ak.us/dec/deh/animal/home.htm
Bert, Gore, Contact

**★ 20700 ★ Arizona Department of Agriculture**
**Animal Services Division**
**State Veterinarian**
1688 W Adams
Phoenix, AZ 85007
**Phone:** (602)542-4293      **Fax:** (602)542-4290
**Email:** statevet@agric.state.az.us
**Website:** http://agriculture.state.az.us/ASD/state_vet.htm
Dr. R.D. Willer, DIR

**★ 20701 ★ Arkansas Livestock and Poultry Commission**
**State Veterinarian**
1 Natural Resources Dr.
PO Box 5497
Little Rock, AR 72205
**Phone:** (501)224-2836
**Website:** http://www.arlpc.org/stats.asp

**★ 20702 ★ California Department of Food and Agriculture**
**Animal Industry Division**
**Animal Health Bureau**
1220 N St., Rm. A-114
PO Box 942871
Sacramento, CA 95814
**Phone:** (916)654-0881      **Fax:** (916)653-4249
**Email:** ahbfeedback@cdfa.ca.gov
**Website:** http://www.cdfa.ca.gov/
Richard Breitmeyer, Director

**★ 20703 ★ Colorado Department of Agriculture**
**Animal Industry Division**
**State Veterinarian**
700 Kipling St., Ste. 4000
Lakewood, CO 80215-5894
**Phone:** (303)239-4158      **Fax:** (303)239-4164
**Email:** comments@ag.state.co.us
**Website:** http://www.ag.state.co.us/animals/bureau.html
Dr. John Maulsby, DVM, Contact

**★ 20704 ★ Connecticut Department of Agriculture**
**State Veterinarian**
State Office Bldg., Rm. 283
765 Asylum Ave.
Hartford, CT 06105
**Phone:** (860)713-2504      **Fax:** (860)713-2514
**Email:** ctdeptag@po.state.ct.us
**Website:** http://www.state.ct.us/doag/regsinsp/livestok.htm
Mary Jane Liss, D.V.M., Contact

**★ 20705 ★ Delaware Department of Agriculture**
**Poultry and Animal Health Section**
2320 S DuPont Hwy.
Dover, DE 19901-5515
**Phone:** (302)698-4500      **Fax:** (302)697-6287
**Email:** wes@dda.state.de.us
**Website:** http://www.state.de.us/deptagri/poultryah/index.htm

**★ 20706 ★ Florida Department of Agriculture and Consumer Services**
**Animal Industry Division**
**State Veterinarian**
Nathan Mayo Bldg., Rm. 335
407 S Calhoun St.
Tallahassee, FL 32399-0800
**Phone:** (850)410-0900      **Fax:** (850)410-0907
**Email:** coffmal@doacs.state.fl.us
**Website:** http://doacs.state.fl.us/ai/ai.html
Leroy M. Coffman, Contact

**★ 20707 ★ Georgia Department of Agriculture**
**Animal Industry Division**
**State Veterinarian**
19 Martin Luther King Jr. Dr. SW Room 106
Atlanta, GA 30334
**Phone:** (404)656-3671      **Fax:** (404)657-1357
**Email:** lbrooks@agr.state.ga.us
**Website:** http://www.agr.state.ga.us/html/animal_industry.html
Lee M. Meyers, Director

**★ 20708 ★ Idaho Department of Agriculture**
**Animal Industries Division**
**Animal Health Bureau**
2270 Old Penitentiary Rd.
PO Box 790
Boise, ID 83701
**Phone:** (208)332-8534      **Fax:** (208)334-2170
**Email:** pmamer@agri.state.id.us
**Website:** http://www.agri.state.id.us/animal/vet_services.htm
Christina Morrison, DVM, Contact

**★ 20709 ★ Illinois Department of Agriculture**
**Animal Health Bureau**
State Fairgrounds
PO Box 19281
Springfield, IL 62794-9281
**Phone:** (217)782-4944      **Free:** 800-273-4763
**Fax:** (217)524-7702
**Email:** pio@agr084r1.state.il.us
**Website:** http://www.agr.state.il.us/ahwf.html

**★ 20710 ★ Iowa Department of Agriculture**
**Regulatory Division**
**Animal Health Bureau**
Wallace Bldg.
Des Moines, IA 50319
**Phone:** (515)281-8615
**Email:** John.Schiltz@idals.state.ia.us
**Website:** http://www2.state.ia.us/agriculture/regulatory.html
Dr. John Schiltz, Contact

**★ 20711 ★ Kansas Department of Animal Health**
708 SW Jackson
Topeka, KS 66603-3714
**Phone:** (785)296-2326      **Fax:** (785)296-1765
**Website:** http://www.ink.org/public/kahd/

**★ 20712 ★ Kentucky Department of Agriculture**
**Division of Animal Health**
**State Veterinarian**
100 Fair Oaks Ln., Ste. 252
Frankfort, KY 40601
**Phone:** (502)564-3956      **Fax:** (502)564-7852
**Email:** don.notter@kyagr.com
**Website:** http://www.state.ky.us/agencies/agr/statevet.htm
Don Notter, DVM, Director

**★ 20713 ★ Louisiana Deparment of Agriculture**
**Office of Animal Health Services**
**State Veterinarian**
PO Box 1951
Baton Rouge, LA 70821-1951
**Phone:** (225)925-3980      **Fax:** (225)925-4103
**Email:** maxwel_l@ldaf.state.la.us
**Website:** http://www.ldaf.state.la.us
Maxwell A. Lea, DVM, Director

**★ 20714 ★ Maine Department of Agriculture, Food and Rural Resources**
**Veterinary Services Division**
28 State House Station Deering Bldg.
AMHI Complex
Augusta, ME 04333-0028
**Phone:** (207)287-3701
**Email:** Donald.E.Hoenig@state.me.us
**Website:** http://janus.state.me.us/agriculture/animals/homepage.htm
Donald E. Hoenig, VMD, Contact

**★ 20715 ★ Maryland Department of Agriculture**
**Food Safety Consumer Services Office**
**Animal Health Division**
50 Harry S Truman Pkwy.
Annapolis, MD 21401-7080
**Phone:** (410)841-5810      **Fax:** (410)841-4914
**Email:** olsonre@mda.state.md.us
**Website:** http://www.mda.state.md.us/geninfo/genera4.htm
Roger Olson, DVM, Director

**★ 20716 ★ Massachusetts Executive Office of Environmental Affairs**
**Food and Agriculture Department**
**Animal Health Bureau**
251 Causeway St., Ste. 500
Boston, MA 02114-2151
**Phone:** (617)626-1795
**Email:** esther.wegman@state.ma.us
**Website:** http://www.massdfa.org/animalhealth/index.htm
Fred Mach, Director

**★ 20717 ★ Michigan Department of Agriculture**
**Animal Industry Division**
**State Veterinarian**
PO Box 30017
Lansing, MI 48909
**Phone:** (517)373-1077      **Free:** 800-292-3939
**Fax:** (517)373-6015
**Email:** mda-info@michigan.gov
**Website:** http://www.michigan.gov/mda
Joan M. Arnold, Director

**★ 20718 ★ Minnesota Board of Animal Health**
90 W Plato Blvd
Saint Paul, MN 55107
**Phone:** (651)296-2942      **Fax:** (651)296-7417
**Email:** bill.hartmann@bah.state.mn.us
**Website:** http://www.bah.state.mn.us/
Bill Hartmann, DVM, Director

**★ 20719 ★ Mississippi Department of Agriculture and Commerce**
**Animal Health Board**
**State Veterinarian**
121 N Jefferson
PO Box 3889
Jackson, MS 39207
**Phone:** (601)359-1170      **Free:** 888-646-8731
**Fax:** (601)359-1177
**Email:** jimw@mdac.state.ms.us
**Website:** http://www.mbah.state.ms.us/
James A. Watson, DVM, Director

**★ 20720 ★ Missouri Department of Agriculture**
**Animal Health Division and State Veterinarian**
PO Box 630
Jefferson City, MO 65102
**Phone:** (573)751-3377 **Fax:** (573)751-6919
**Email:** taylor.woods@mail.state.mo.us
**Website:** http://www.mda.state.mo.us/i4.htm
Taylor Woods, DVM, Director

**★ 20721 ★ Montana Department of Livestock**
**Animal Health Division**
PO Box 202001
Helena, MT 59620-2001
**Phone:** (406)444-2043 **Fax:** (406)444-1929
**Email:** agertonson@state.mt.gov
**Website:** http://agr.state.mt.us/
Dr. Arnold Gertonson, Contact

**★ 20722 ★ Nebraska Department of Agriculture**
**Animal Industry**
**State Veterinarian**
301 Centennial Mall S
PO Box 94787
Lincoln, NE 68509-4787
**Phone:** (402)471-2351 **Fax:** (402)471-6893
**Email:** larrylw@agr.state.ne.us
**Website:** http://www.agr.state.ne.us/division/bai/bai.htm
Larry Williams, DVM, Director

**★ 20723 ★ Nevada Department of Business and Industry**
**Agriculture Division**
**Animal Industry Bureau**
**State Veterinarian**
350 Capitol Hill Ave.
Reno, NV 89502
**Phone:** (702)688-1180 **Fax:** (702)688-1178
**Email:** dthain@govmail.state.nv.us
**Website:** http://agri.state.nv.us/indexa.htm
David Thain, DVM, Contact

**★ 20724 ★ New Hampshire Department of Agriculture**
**Animal Industry Division**
**State Veterinarian**
PO Box 2042.
Concord, NH 03302
**Phone:** (603)271-2404 **Fax:** (603)271-1109
**Email:** cwmcginnis@agr.state.nh.us
**Website:** http://www.state.nh.us/agric/anin.html
Clifford W. McGinnis, DVM, Director

**★ 20725 ★ New Jersey Department of Agriculture**
**Animal Health Division**
John Fitch Plaza
PO Box 330
Trenton, NJ 08625-0330
**Phone:** (609)292-3965 **Fax:** (609)633-2550
**Email:** ernest.zirkle@ag.state.nj.us
**Website:** http://www.state.nj.us/agriculture/animal.htm
Ernest Zirkle, DVM, Director

**★ 20726 ★ New Mexico Livestock Board**
**State Veterinarian**
300 San Mateo NE, Ste. 1000
Albuquerque, NM 87108-1500
**Phone:** (505)841-6161 **Fax:** (505)841-6160
Steven England, DVM, Contact

**★ 20727 ★ New York Department of Agriculture and Markets**
**Animal Industry Division**
**State Veterinarian**
1 Winners Circle
Albany, NY 12235
**Phone:** (518)457-3502 **Fax:** (518)457-7773
**Email:** huntleyj@nysnet.net
**Website:** http://www.agmkt.state.ny.us/
John Huntley, DVM, Director

**★ 20728 ★ North Carolina Department of Agriculture**
**Veterinary Division**
2 W Edenton St., Rm. 472
PO Box 26026
Raleigh, NC 27611
**Phone:** (919)733-7601 **Fax:** (919)733-6431
**Email:** Joe.Web@ncmail.net
**Website:** http://www.agr.state.nc.us/vet/
David Marshall, DVM, Director

**★ 20729 ★ North Dakota Board of Animal Health**
600 E Boulevard Ave., 6th Fl.
Bismarck, ND 58505-0020
**Phone:** (701)328-2654 **Fax:** (701)328-4567
**Email:** lschuler@state.nd.us
**Website:** http://www.state.nd.us/agr/
Larry A. Schuler, D.V.M., Director

**★ 20730 ★ Ohio Department of Agriculture**
**Animal Industry Division**
**State Veterinarian**
8995 E Main St.
Bldg. 6
Reynoldsburg, OH 43068
**Phone:** (614)728-6220 **Fax:** (614)728-6310
**Email:** agri@odant.agri.state.oh.us
**Website:** http://www.state.oh.us/agr/AnimalIndustryDiv.html
Dr. R. David Glauer, Director

**★ 20731 ★ Oklahoma Department of Agriculture**
**Animal Industry Division**
**State Veterinarian**
2800 N Lincoln Blvd.
Oklahoma City, OK 73152
**Phone:** (405)522-6131 **Fax:** (405)522-0756
**Email:** bhealey@oda.state.ok.us
**Website:** http://www.oda.state.ok.us/aind.htm
Burke L. Healey, DVM, Contact

**★ 20732 ★ Oregon Department of Agriculture**
**State Veterinarian**
635 Capitol St. NE
Salem, OR 97301-2532
**Phone:** (503)986-4680
**Email:** csorrels@oda.state.or.us
**Website:** http://www.oda.state.or.us/Livestock_Health_ID/animal_health/ah_main.html
Andrew Clark, D.V.M., Director

**★ 20733 ★ Pennsylvania Department of Agriculture**
**Animal Industry Bureau**
**State Veterinarian**
2301 N Cameron St.
Harrisburg, PA 17110-9408
**Phone:** (717)783-6677
**Website:** http://www.pda.state.pa.us/

**★ 20734 ★ Rhode Island Department of Environmental Management**
**Agriculture Division**
**Animal Health Section**
235 Promenade St.
Providence, RI 02908-5767
**Phone:** (401)222-2781 **Fax:** (401)222-6047
**Website:** http://www.state.ri.us/dem/org/agric.htm

**★ 20735 ★ South Carolina State Veterinarian**
PO Box 102406
Columbia, SC 29224-2406
**Phone:** (803)788-2260 **Fax:** (803)788-8058
**Email:** jbryn@clemson.edu
Dr. Jones W. Bryan, Director

**★ 20736 ★ South Dakota Animal Industry Board**
**State Veterinarian**
411 S Fort St.
Pierre, SD 57501-4503
**Phone:** (605)773-3321 **Fax:** (605)773-5459
**Email:** Dr.Holland@state.sd.us
**Website:** http://www.state.sd.us/doa/boards.htm
Sam D. Holland, Contact

**★ 20737 ★ Tennessee Department of Agriculture**
**Animal Industries Division**
**State Veterinarian**
Ellington Agricultural Ctr.
PO Box 40627
Nashville, TN 37204
**Phone:** (615)837-5120 **Fax:** (615)837-5335
**Email:** twomack@mail.state.tn.us
**Website:** http://www.state.tn.us/agriculture/regulate/regulat2.html
Ron Wilson, D.V.M., Director

**★ 20738 ★ Texas Animal Health Commission**
2105 Kramer Ln.
PO Box 12966
Austin, TX 78711
**Phone:** (512)719-0700 **Free:** 800-550-8242
**Fax:** (512)719-0719
**Email:** comments@tahc.state.tx.us
**Website:** http://www.tahc.state.tx.us/
Linda M. Logan, D.V.M., Director

**★ 20739 ★ Utah Department of Agriculture**
**Animal Health Division, State Veterinarian**
350 N Redwood Rd.
PO Box 146500
Salt Lake City, UT 84114-6500
**Phone:** (801)538-7162 **Fax:** (801)538-7169
**Email:** agmain.erogers@email.state.ut.us
**Website:** http://www.ag.state.ut.us/divisns/animind/animalmp.htm
Dr. Earl Rogers, Director

**★ 20740 ★ Vermont Department of Agriculture**
**State Veterinarian**
116 State St.
Drawer 20
Montpelier, VT 05620-2901
**Phone:** (802)828-2421 **Fax:** (802)828-2361
**Email:** vtstatevet@aol.com
**Website:** http://www.state.vt.us/agric/animal.htm
Todd Johnson, D.V.M., Director

**★ 20741 ★ Virgin Islands Department of Economic Development and Agriculture**
**Veterinary Services Division**
Estate Lower Love, Kingshill
St Croix, VI 00850

Phone: (340)778-0997　　Fax: (340)778-3101
Email: agriculture@usvi.org
Website: http://www.usvi.org/agriculture/index.html

**★ 20742 ★ Virginia Office of Commerce and Trade**
**Agriculture and Consumer Services Department**
**Animal Health Division**
1100 Bank St., Rm. 220
PO Box 1163
Richmond, VA 23218
Phone: (804)786-2483　　Free: 800-786-2373
Fax: (804)371-2380
Email: cowhite@vdacs.state.va.us
Website: http://www.vdacs.state.va.us/animals/index.html

**★ 20743 ★ Washington Department of Agriculture**
**Food Safety and Animal Health Division**
**State Veterinarian**
PO Box 42577
Olympia, WA 98504-2577
Phone: (360)902-1878　　Fax: (360)902-2087
Email: ahealth@agr.wa.gov
Website: http://www.wa.gov/agr/FoodAnimal/AnimalHealth/default.htm
Dr. Robert W. Mead, Director

**★ 20744 ★ West Virginia Department of Agriculture**
**Animal Health Division**
1900 Kanawha Blvd. E
Charleston, WV 25305
Phone: (304)558-2214　　Fax: (304)558-2231
Email: lthomas@ag.state.wv.us
Website: http://www.state.wv.us/agriculture/Departments_Descriptions/Animal_Health_Division/animal_health_division.html
Dr. Lewis Thomas, Director

**★ 20745 ★ Wisconsin Department of Agriculture, Trade and Consumer Protection**
**Animal Health Division**
ATTN: Interstate
PO Box 8911
Madison, WI 53708-8911
Phone: (608)224-4872　　Fax: (608)224-4871
Email: datcp_web@wheel.datcp.state.wi.us
Website: http://datcp.state.wi.us/static/ah/

**★ 20746 ★ Wyoming Livestock Board**
**State Veterinarian**
2020 Carey Ave., 4th Fl.
Cheyenne, WY 82002-0051
Phone: (307)777-7515　　Fax: (307)777-6561
Email: jlogan1@state.wy.us
Website: http://wlsb.state.wy.us/
Jim Logan, D.V.M., Director

# State & Regional Organizations

## Veterinary Medicine

*The following are state groups of the American Veterinary Medical Association, 1931 N Meacham Rd., Ste. 100, Schaumburg, IL 60173, (847)925-8070, http://www.avma.org/.*

## Alabama

**★ 20747 ★ Alabama Veterinary Medical Association**
PO Box 3514
Montgomery, AL 36109-0514
Phone: (334)261-3012　　Fax: (334)261-3013
Email: franzc55@cs.com
Website: http://www.alvma.com
Charles F. Franz, DVM, Exec Director

## Alaska

**★ 20748 ★ Alaska State Veterinary Medical Association**
PO Box 112269
Anchorage, AK 99511-2269
Phone: (907)344-7913　　Fax: (907)349-1255
Dr. Paul Frederickson, Contact

## Arizona

**★ 20749 ★ Arizona Veterinary Medical Association**
5502 N 19th Ave.
Phoenix, AZ 85015-7936
Phone: (602)242-7936　　Fax: (602)249-3828
Email: ekane@azvma.org
Website: http://www.azvma.org
Emily Kane, Exec Director

## Arkansas

**★ 20750 ★ Arkansas Veterinary Medical Association**
8 Shackleford Plaza, Ste. 208
Little Rock, AR 72211
Phone: (501)221-1477　　Fax: (501)221-6691
Email: info@arkvetmed.org
Website: http://www.arkvetmed.org
Mr. Robert Blount, Exec Director

## California

**★ 20751 ★ California Veterinary Medical Association**
1400 River Park Dr., Ste. 100
Sacramento, CA 95815-4505
Phone: (916)649-0599　　Fax: (916)646-9156
Email: dschumacher@cvma.net
Website: http://www.cvma.net
Dr. Richard Schumacher, Exec Director

## Colorado

**★ 20752 ★ Colorado Veterinary Medical Association**
**Denver Area Veterinary Medical Society**
789 Sherman St., Ste. 550
Denver, CO 80203
Phone: (303)318-0447　　Fax: (303)318-0450
Email: info@colovma.com
Website: http://www.colovma.com
Ralph Johnson, Exec Director

## Connecticut

**★ 20753 ★ Connecticut Veterinary Medical Association**
731 Hebron Ave.
Glastonbury, CT 06033
Phone: (860)659-9683　　Fax: (860)657-8244
Email: connveterinary@aol.com
Website: http://www.ctvma.org
Simon Flynn, Exec Director

## Delaware

**★ 20754 ★ Delaware Veterinary Medical Association**
937 Monroe Terrace
Dover, DE 19904
Phone: (302)674-8581　　Fax: (302)674-8581
Email: appelplej@aol.com
Website: http://www.avma.org/statevma/devma
Lynn Appel, Exec Director

## District of Columbia

**★ 20755 ★ District of Columbia Veterinary Medical Association**
2501 Que St. NW, No. 320
Washington, DC 20007
Phone: (301)734-5873　　Fax: (301)734-4314
Website: http://www.avma.org/statevma/dcvma
Dr. Michele April, Contact

## Florida

**★ 20756 ★ Florida Veterinary Medical Association**
7131 Lake Ellenor Dr.
Orlando, FL 32809-5738
Phone: (407)851-3862　　Fax: (407)240-3710
Email: fvma@bellsouth.net
Website: http://www.fvma.org
Donald N. Schaefer, Exec Director

## Georgia

**★ 20757 ★ Georgia Veterinary Medical Association**
2814 Spring Rd., Ste. 217
Atlanta, GA 30339
Phone: (678)309-9800　　Fax: (678)309-3361
Email: gvma@mindspring.com
Website: http://www.gvma.net
Beth Monte, Exec Director

## Hawaii

**★ 20758 ★ Hawaii Veterinary Medical Association**
4400 Kalanianaole Hwy., Ste. 6
Honolulu, HI 96821
Phone: (808)733-8828　　Fax: (808)733-8829
Website: http://www.hawaiivetmed.org
Dr. Eric Ako, Exec VP

## Idaho

**★ 20759 ★ Idaho Veterinary Medical Association**
PO Box 6573
Boise, ID 83707
Phone: (208)375-1551　　Fax: (208)376-4430
Email: msvicki1@mindspring.com
Website: http://www.ivma.org
Vicki Smith, Exec Director

**★ 20760 ★ Utah Veterinary Medical Association**
PO Box 6573
Boise, ID 83707
Phone: (208)375-1551　　Fax: (208)375-4430
Email: msvicki1@mindspring.com
Vicki Smith, Exec Director

**★ 20761 ★ Wyoming Veterinary Medical Association**
PO Box 6573
Boise, ID 83707
Phone: (208)375-1551　　Fax: (208)376-4430
Email: msvicki1@mindspring.com
Website: http://www.wyvma.org
Vicki Smith, Exec Director

## Illinois

**★ 20762 ★ Illinois State Veterinary Medical Association**
161 S Lincolnway, Ste. 302
North Aurora, IL 60542
**Phone:** (630)892-2321          **Fax:** (630)892-0818
**Email:** isvma@aol.com
**Website:** http://www.isvma.org
Eve C. Larocca, Exec Director

## Indiana

**★ 20763 ★ Indiana Veterinary Medical Association**
309 W Washington St., Ste. 202
Indianapolis, IN 46204
**Phone:** (317)974-0888          **Fax:** (317)974-0985
**Email:** ivma@iquest.net
**Website:** http://www.invma.org
Lisa Perius, Exec Director

## Iowa

**★ 20764 ★ Iowa Veterinary Medical Association**
5921 Fleur Dr.
Des Moines, IA 50321
**Phone:** (515)285-6701          **Fax:** (515)285-7809
**Email:** ivma@netins.net
**Website:** http://www.iowavma.org
Dave Furneaux, Exec Director

## Kansas

**★ 20765 ★ Kansas Veterinary Medical Association**
816 SW Tyler, Ste. 200
Topeka, KS 66612-1635
**Phone:** (785)233-4141          **Fax:** (785)233-2534
**Email:** 74253.653@compuserve.com
**Website:** http://www.vet.ksu.edu/links/KVMA
Gary Reser, CAE, Exec VP

## Kentucky

**★ 20766 ★ Kentucky Veterinary Medical Association**
PO Box 4067
Frankfort, KY 40604-4067
**Phone:** (502)226-5862          **Fax:** (502)226-6177
**Email:** kvma@aol.com
**Website:** http://www.avma.org/statevma/kyvma
Louise Cook, Exec Director

## Louisiana

**★ 20767 ★ Louisiana Veterinary Medical Association**
8550 United Plaza Blvd., Ste. 1001
Baton Rouge, LA 70809
**Phone:** (225)928-5862          **Fax:** (225)922-4611
**Email:** lvma@pncpa.com
**Website:** http://www.lvma.org
Bland O'Connor, Exec Director

## Maine

**★ 20768 ★ Maine Veterinary Medical Association**
PO Box 8
Rumford Center, ME 04278
**Phone:** (207)364-8660          **Fax:** (207)364-7209
**Email:** hersey@megalink.net
**Website:** http://www.avma.org/statevma/mevma
Dr. Charles Hersey, Exec Director

## Maryland

**★ 20769 ★ Maryland Veterinary Medical Association**
5024 R Campbell Blvd.
Nottingham, MD 21236-5943
**Free:** 888-884-6882          **Fax:** (410)931-8111
**Email:** MDVMA@aol.com
**Website:** http://www.mdvma.org
Buzz Thomas, Exec Director

## Massachusetts

**★ 20770 ★ Massachusetts Veterinary Medical Association**
169 Lakeside Ave.
Marlborough, MA 01752-4503
**Phone:** (508)460-9333          **Fax:** (508)460-9969
**Email:** staff@massvet.org
**Website:** http://www.ultranet.com/~massvet
Susan Weinstein, Exec Director

## Michigan

**★ 20771 ★ Michigan Veterinary Medical Association**
2144 Commons Pkwy.
Okemos, MI 48864-3986
**Phone:** (517)347-4710          **Fax:** (517)347-4666
**Email:** prescott@michvma.org
**Website:** http://www.michvma.org
Dr. Peter A. Prescott, Exec Director

## Minnesota

**★ 20772 ★ Minnesota Veterinary Medical Association**
393 N Dunlap St., Ste. 400
Saint Paul, MN 55104
**Phone:** (651)645-7533          **Fax:** (651)645-7539
**Email:** info@mvma.org
**Website:** http://www.mvma.org
Sharon Vangsness, CAE, Exec Director

## Mississippi

**★ 20773 ★ Mississippi Veterinary Medical Association**
209 S Lafayette St.
Starkville, MS 39759
**Phone:** (662)324-9380          **Fax:** (662)324-9380
**Email:** msvma@futuresouth.com
Dr. Harvey F. McCrory, Contact

## Missouri

**★ 20774 ★ Missouri Veterinary Medical Association**
2500 Country Club Dr.
Jefferson City, MO 65109
**Phone:** (573)636-8612          **Fax:** (573)659-7175
**Email:** movma@mchsi.com
**Website:** http://www.movma.org
Richard Antweiler, Exec Director

## Montana

**★ 20775 ★ Montana Veterinary Medical Association**
PO Box 6322
Helena, MT 59604
**Phone:** (406)447-4259          **Fax:** (406)442-8018
**Email:** stuart@initco.net
**Website:** http://www.avma.org/statevma/mtvma
Stuart Doggett, Exec Director

## Nebraska

**★ 20776 ★ Nebraska Veterinary Medical Association**
PO Box 2118
Hastings, NE 68902-2118
**Phone:** (402)463-4704          **Fax:** (402)463-5683
**Email:** gmo@inebraska.com
**Website:** http://www.nvma.org
Don Ellerbee, Exec Director

## Nevada

**★ 20777 ★ Nevada Veterinary Medical Association**
PO Box 34420
Reno, NV 89533
**Phone:** (775)324-5344          **Fax:** (775)747-9170
**Email:** nvma@775.net
**Website:** http://www.aci.net/nvma
Michelle Wagner, Exec Director

## New Hampshire

**★ 20778 ★ New Hampshire Veterinary Medical Association**
PO Box 616
Concord, NH 03302-0616
**Phone:** (603)224-2432          **Fax:** (603)225-0556
**Email:** nhvmaip@mediaone.net
JoAnn Poole, Exec Director

## New Jersey

**★ 20779 ★ New Jersey Veterinary Medical Association**
66 Morris Ave., Ste. 2A
Springfield, NJ 07081
**Phone:** (973)379-1100          **Fax:** (973)379-6507
**Email:** rickaaamac@earthlink.com
**Website:** http://www.njvma.org
Richard Alampi, Exec Director

## New Mexico

**★ 20780 ★ New Mexico Veterinary Medical Association**
3037 San Patricia NW
Albuquerque, NM 87107
**Phone:** (505)343-1691          **Fax:** (505)294-9958
**Email:** nmvma@earthlink.net
**Website:** http://home.earthlink.net/~nmvma/
Marjorie Nelson, Contact

## New York

**★ 20781 ★ New York City Veterinary Medical Association**
331 W 57th St., S293
New York, NY 10019-3101
**Phone:** (212)246-0057          **Fax:** (212)586-3949
**Email:** VMANYC@aol.com
Effie Cooper, Contact

**★ 20782 ★ New York State Veterinary Medical Society**
9 Highland Ave.
Albany, NY 12205-5417
**Phone:** (518)437-0787          **Fax:** (518)437-0957
**Email:** INFO@NYSVMS.org
**Website:** http://www.nysvms.org
Julie Lawton, Exec Director
**Frmly:** New York State Veterinary Medical Association.

## North Carolina

**★ 20783 ★ North Carolina Veterinary Medical Association**
138 Spring Ave.
Fuquay-Varina, NC 27526

**Phone:** (919)557-9385    **Fax:** (919)557-9389
**Email:** mprasor@cs.com
**Website:** http://www.ncvma.org
Mollie Rasor, Exec Director

★ **20784** ★ **South Carolina Association of Veterinarians**
PO Box 505
Hwy 903/123
Maury, NC 28554
**Phone:** (252)747-8180    **Fax:** (252)747-4100
**Email:** vetmeeting@aol.com
Ralph Lee, Exec VP

## North Dakota

★ **20785** ★ **North Dakota Veterinary Medical Association**
921 S 9th St.
Bismarck, ND 58504
**Phone:** (701)221-7740    **Fax:** (701)258-9005
**Email:** nkopp@btigate.com
Nancy Kopp, Contact

## Ohio

★ **20786** ★ **Ohio Veterinary Medical Association**
3168 Riverside Dr.
Columbus, OH 43221
**Phone:** (614)486-7253    **Fax:** (614)486-1325
**Email:** ohiovma@ohiovma.org
**Website:** http://www.ohiovma.org
Jack Advent, CAE, Exec Director

## Oklahoma

★ **20787** ★ **Oklahoma Veterinary Medical Association**
PO Box 14521
Oklahoma City, OK 73113
**Phone:** (405)478-1002    **Fax:** (405)478-7193
**Email:** okvma@compuserve.com
**Website:** http://www.okvma.org
Dr. Charles Helwig, Exec Director

## Oregon

★ **20788** ★ **Oregon Veterinary Medical Association**
1880 Lancaster Dr. NE, Ste. 118
Salem, OR 97305
**Phone:** (503)399-0311    **Fax:** (503)363-4218
**Email:** ovma@teleport.com
Glenn M. Kolb, Exec Director

## Pennsylvania

★ **20789** ★ **Pennsylvania Veterinary Medical Association**
PO Box 8820
Harrisburg, PA 17105-8820
**Phone:** (717)588-7841    **Free:** 888-550-7862
**Fax:** (717)558-7845
**Email:** pvma@pamedsoc.org
**Website:** http://www.pavma.org
Charlene Wandzilak, Exec Director

## Puerto Rico

★ **20790** ★ **Puerto Rico Veterinary Medical Association**
352 Ave. San Claudio, Ste. 248
San Juan, PR 00926-4107
**Phone:** (787)283-2840    **Fax:** (787)761-3440
**Email:** cmvpr@prw.net
Sandra Sanchez, Contact

## Rhode Island

★ **20791** ★ **Rhode Island Veterinary Medical Association**
PO Box 3
Cumberland, RI 02864
**Phone:** 877-521-0103    **Fax:** (508)399-6908
**Email:** rivma@rivma.org
**Website:** http://www.rivma.org
Nancy Klaffky, Contact

## South Dakota

★ **20792** ★ **South Dakota Veterinary Medical Association**
South Dakota VMA
Box 2175, SDU
Brookings, SD 57007-1396
**Phone:** (605)688-6649    **Fax:** (605)688-6003
**Email:** janice_kampmann@sdstate.edu
Dr. Daryl K. Thorpe, Exec Director

## Tennessee

★ **20793** ★ **Tennessee Veterinary Medical Association**
200 4th Ave. N, Ste. 900
Nashville, TN 37219
**Phone:** (615)254-3687    **Fax:** (615)254-7047
**Email:** tvma@wmgt.org
**Website:** http://www.tvmanet.org
Dee Ann Walker, CAE, Exec Director

## Texas

★ **20794** ★ **Texas Veterinary Medical Association**
6633 Hwy 290 E, Ste. 201
Austin, TX 78723
**Phone:** (512)452-4224    **Fax:** (512)452-6633
**Email:** tvma@tvma.org
**Website:** http://www.tvma.org
Dr. Elbert Hutchins, Exec Director

## Vermont

★ **20795** ★ **Vermont Veterinary Medical Association**
2073 Spear St.
Charlotte, VT 05445
**Phone:** (802)425-3495    **Fax:** (802)425-3495
**Email:** vvma@together.net
**Website:** http://www.vtvets.org
Sue Moraska, Exec Director

## Virginia

★ **20796** ★ **Virginia Veterinary Medical Association**
4001 Springfield Rd.
Glen Allen, VA 23060
**Phone:** (804)270-9013    **Fax:** (804)270-2160
**Email:** vavma@aol.com
**Website:** http://www.vvma.org
Robin R. Schmitz, Exec Director

## Washington

★ **20797** ★ **Washington State Veterinary Medical Association**
PO Box 962
Bellevue, WA 98009-0962
**Phone:** (425)454-8381    **Fax:** (425)454-8382
**Email:** wsvma1@aol.com
**Website:** http://www.wsvma.org
Sandra J. Bertelsen, Exec VP

## West Virginia

★ **20798** ★ **West Virginia Veterinary Medical Association**
35 Turner Rd.
Elkview, WV 25071
**Phone:** (304)965-3373
**Website:** http://www.avma.org/statevma/wvvma
Gail Jones, Contact

## Wisconsin

★ **20799** ★ **Wisconsin Veterinary Medical Association**
301 N Broom St.
Madison, WI 53703
**Phone:** (608)257-3665    **Fax:** (608)257-8989
**Email:** wvma@wvma.org
**Website:** http://www.wvma.org
Leslie Grendahl, Exec Director

## Federal Government Agencies

★ 20800 ★ **U.S. Department of Health and Human Services**
**National Institutes of Health (NIH)**
**National Eye Institute (NEI)**
9000 Rockville Pike
Bethesda, MD 20892
**Phone:** (301)496-2234        **Fax:** (301)496-9970
**Website:** http://www.nei.nih.gov/
Paul A. Sieving, Director

**Desc:** The Institute conducts, fosters, and supports research on the causes, natural history, prevention, diagnosis and treatment of disorders of the eye and visual system; directs the National Eye Health Education Program; provides research grants and individual and institutional research training awards; works in cooperation and collaboration with voluntary organizations and other institutions engaged in research and training in the special health problems of the blind; and collects and disseminates information on research and findings.

**U.S. Library of Congress**
**National Library Service for the Blind and Physically Handicapped**
*See:* Entry 11998

## Foundations & Other Funding Organizations

### Private Foundations

★ 20801 ★ **Christian A. Johnson Endeavor Foundation**
1060 Park Ave.
New York, NY 10128-1033
**Phone:** (212)534-6620        **Fax:** (212)410-0568
**Website:** http://www.edlead.org
Julie Kidd, President

**Fnded:** 1952. **Philosophy:** The foundation is primarily interested in supporting educational projects and educational outreach arts programs. It concentrates its giving on private institutions of higher learning at the baccalaureate level and on educational outreach programs of visual and performing arts organizations. The foundation also funds the Educational Leadership Program, which sponsors seminars and meetings for leaders in the education world. **Priorities:** *Arts & Humanities:* 10%. Funds museums, theater, music, and opera. *Education:* 81%. Supports colleges, universities, and scholarship funds. *Environment:* 2%. Funds Boys' Harbor. *Note:* Total contributions made in fiscal 2000. **Typ. Recipients:** Eyes/Blindness, Heart, People with Disabilities. **Geo. Dist:** U.S. Eastern Region.

**Mary Stuart Rogers Foundation**
*See:* Entry 5560

**Park Foundation**
*See:* Entry 10052

**Solon E. Summerfield Foundation, Inc.**
*See:* Entry 688

**Wayne and Gladys Valley Foundation**
*See:* Entry 753

**William and Mary Greve Foundation**
*See:* Entry 10058

### Corporate Foundations

★ 20802 ★ **Alcon Foundation**
6201 S Fwy.
Fort Worth, TX 76134
**Phone:** (817)293-0450        **Fax:** (817)568-7000
**Email:** Mary.Dulle@alconlabs.com
**Website:** http://www.alconlabs.com
Mary Dulle, Director, Corporate Communications

**Fnded:** 1962. **Priorities:** *Arts & Humanities:* 12%. Major support goes to theaters, music, and symphonies in the Ft. Worth area. Also contributes to libraries and public broadcasting. *Civic & Public Affairs:* 7%. Supports a variety of community organizations. *Education:* 33%. Funding supports colleges, universities, and education associations for ophthalmic or optometric research. Also funds minority education, and secondary public and private education, Junior Achievement, and the Adopt-a-School program. *Environment:* 4%. Supports a variety of social service organizations in the Ft. Worth, TX, area with grants ranging from $250 to $1,000. Majority of contributions fund child welfare and youth organizations. Other priorities include community centers, food distribution, homes, shelters, and religious welfare. *International:* 43%. Majority of contributions support eye-related health funds and health associations. *Note:* Total contributions in 2000. **Typ. Recipients:** Cancer, Cancer, Children's Health/Hospitals, Clinics/Medical Centers, Emergency/Ambulance Services, Eyes/Blindness, Health Funds, Health Organizations, Hospitals, Medical Education, Medical Research, Mental Health, People with Disabilities, Prenatal Health Issues, Public Health, Single-Disease Health Associations. **Geo. Dist:** nationally; Fort Worth, TX.

**Central Newspapers Foundation**
*See:* Entry 10062

**D.B. Reinhart Family Foundation**
*See:* Entry 985

**Ladish Co. Foundation**
*See:* Entry 11446

**MDU Resources Foundation**
*See:* Entry 5581

**NEC Foundation of America**
*See:* Entry 5583

**Spang & Co. Charitable Trust**
*See:* Entry 5588

**Susquehanna-Pfaltzgraff Foundation**
*See:* Entry 1421

**Warren Alpert Foundation**
*See:* Entry 11470

**Wolverine World Wide Foundation**
*See:* Entry 1512

### Other Funding Organizations

★ 20803 ★ **American Action Fund for Blind Children and Adults (AAFBCA)**
1800 Johnson St.
Baltimore, MD 21230
**Phone:** (410)659-9314        **Fax:** (410)685-5653
**Email:** acc@roundley.com
**Website:** http://www.actionfund.org
Dr. Marc Maurer, Exec. Dir.

**Desc:** Works to assist blind persons in securing reading material, to educate the public about blindness, to give aid to the deaf-blind and to improve the quality of life for blind persons. Provides information and referral services on Social Security Disability Insurance, employment, civil rights, products and aids, education of blind children and public rehabilitation agencies; disseminates information on Braille and sign language; distributes publications free of charge to libraries and schools. **Awards:** Kenneth Jernigan Scholarship (annual).

★ 20804 ★ **American Council of the Blind (ACB)**
1155 15th St. NW, Ste. 1004
Washington, DC 20005
**Phone:** (202)467-5081        **Free:** 800-424-8666
**Fax:** (202)467-5085
**Email:** info@acb.org
**Website:** http://www.acb.org
Charles Crawford, Exec. Dir.

**Desc:** Blind and visually impaired persons. Serves as a national information clear Security and supplemental security income programs, radio reading services, special library services, eye research, and low vision technology. Offers group insurance plans, professional assistance in public interest, class action litigation, and public education about blindness and the abilities of visually impaired people. **Awards:** Floyd Qualls Memorial Scholarships (annual) for blind postsecondary students; scholarship.

★ **20805** ★ **American Foundation for the Blind (AFB)**
11 Penn Plz., Ste. 300
New York, NY 10001
**Phone:** (212)502-7600          **Free:** 800-232-5463
**Fax:** (212)502-7777
**Email:** afbinfo@afb.net
**Website:** http://www.afb.org
Carl R. Augusto, Pres.

**Desc:** Mission is to eliminate the inequities faced by the ten million Americans who are blind or visually impaired; Helen Keller dedicated 40 years of her life to the organization. Develops, collects, and disseminates information that benefits people who are blind or visually impaired, their families and friends, professionals in the blindess field, and the general public. Takes a leadership role in identifying issues critical to people who are blind or visually impaired; conducts research, and acts as a catalyst for change. Educates the public and policymakers as to the needs and capabilities of people who are blind or visually impaired; records and duplicates Talking Books for the Library of Congress and other audio materials for various corporations and organizations; and develops public education programs. Maintains offices in Atlanta, Chicago, Dallas and San Francisco, and a governmental relations office in Washington, DC. **Awards:** Delta Gamma Foundation Memorial Scholarship (annual) to undergraduate juniors, seniors, or graduate students who are legally blind, of good character, have exhibited academic excellence, and are studying in the field of rehabilitation and/or education of persons who are visually impaired or blind; Ferdinand Torres AFB Scholarship (annual) to a full-time post-secondary student who is legally blind and who presents evidence of economic need; Frederick A. Downes Scholarship to persons who are 22 years of age or younger, legally blind, and enrolled in a course of study leading to credentials in a profession or vocation; Gladys C. Anderson Memorial Scholarship to a woman who is legally blind, studying religious or classical music at the college level; Rudolph Dillman Memorial Scholarship (annual) to graduate and undergraduate students who are legally blind and studying in the field of rehabilitation and/or education of persons who are visually impaired or blind; Telesensory Scholarship to a full-time undergraduate student who is legally blind and does not meet criteria for other AFB scholarships.

★ **20806** ★ **American Foundation for Vision Awareness (AFVA)**
243 N Lindbergh Blvd.
Saint Louis, MO 63141
**Free:** 800-927-2382          **Fax:** (314)991-4101
**Email:** afva@aol.com
**Website:** http://www.afva.org

**Desc:** Seeks to educate people of all ages about their vision; to create awareness of quality eye and vision care; and to support vision-related scientific research. **Awards:** Grant for postgraduate study and research; recognition.

★ **20807** ★ **American Optometric Foundation (AOF)**
6110 Executive Blvd., Ste. 506
Rockville, MD 20852
**Phone:** (301)984-4734          **Free:** 800-368-6AOF
**Fax:** (301)984-4737
**Email:** christine@aapotom.org
**Website:** http://www.aaopt.org/aof/about/index.asp
Christine Armstrong, Dir.

**Desc:** Optometrists, optometric organizations, corporations, and the public. Promotes research, education, literature, and professional advancement in the visual sciences. Supports fellowships in graduate research. **Awards:** Vincent Salierno Memorial Scholarship (annual) to colleges and institutions; Vistaken Research Grants (annual) for optometric research in soft disposable contact lenses; William Ezell Fellowship (annual) for post-graduate research.

**American Society of Ophthalmic Administrators (ASOA)**
*See:* Entry 9594

★ **20808** ★ **Association of Schools and Colleges of Optometry (ASCO)**
6110 Executive Blvd., Ste. 510
Rockville, MD 20852
**Phone:** (301)231-5944          **Fax:** (301)770-1828
**Email:** mwall@opted.org
**Website:** http://www.opted.org
Martin A. Wall, CAE, Exec. Dir.

**Desc:** Committed to achieving excellence in optometric education and to helping its member schools prepare well-qualified graduates for entrance into the profession of optometry. Mission is to serve the American public through the continued advancement and promotion of all aspects of academic optometry. **Awards:** Student Endowment Program (annual) recipients are chosen by each school.

★ **20809** ★ **Blind Service Association (BSA)**
22 W Monroe, 11th Fl.
Chicago, IL 60603
**Phone:** (312)236-0808          **Fax:** (312)236-8679
**Email:** blindsrvc@aol.com
Debbie Grossman, Exec. Dir.

**Desc:** Organization that has supported the independence of blind and partially blind Chicago residents since 1924. The association maintains reading rooms for daily oral readings of textbooks and work-related material primarily to blind students, senior citizens, and business and professional people; records textbooks on cassette tapes for blind people's home, study, work and leisure needs; supplies visual aids, field trips, and other assistance to blind and visually handicapped children in Chicago, IL schools; operates senior program and a consortium of blind computer users. **Awards:** Grant for blind college students; Harry G. Hershenson Memorial Award for outstanding contribution to blind people; scholarship (annual).

★ **20810** ★ **Blinded Veterans Association (BVA)**
477 H St. NW
Washington, DC 20001
**Phone:** (202)371-8880          **Free:** 800-669-7079
**Fax:** (202)371-8258
**Email:** bva@bva.org
**Website:** http://www.bva.org
Thomas H. Miller, Exec. Dir.

**Desc:** Veterans who lost their sight as a result of military service in the armed forces of the U.S.; associate members are veterans whose loss of sight was not connected with military service. Assists blinded veterans in attaining benefits and employment and with reestablishing themselves as adjusted, active, and productive citizens in their communities. Offers placement service; supports research programs; compiles statistics. **Awards:** Kathern F. Gruber Scholarship (annual) for spouses and dependent children of blinded veterans; Major General Melvin T. Maas Achievement Award (annual) for service-connected blinded veteran.

★ **20811** ★ **Catholic Association of Persons With Visual Impairment (CAPVI)**
c/o Msgr. Paul M. Lackner
Catholic Guild for the Blind
Cardinal Dearden Center
4721 Fifth Ave.
Pittsburgh, PA 15213
**Phone:** (412)687-1409          **Fax:** (412)826-8377
Msgr. Paul Lackner, Pres.

**Desc:** To assist, support, and further the vocational, spiritual, and social integration of blind and visually impaired persons in local parishes and in the community. CAPVI focuses on: raising awareness of the ability and spiritual needs, promotes active participation in the spiritual and social life of the church and

within the community; exchanges ideas, resources and other pertinent information, assists in obtaining religious material in accessible format; and works toward establishing programs within dioceses to serve this group. activities; instructs volunteers to act as guides. Assists in obtaining audiotapes and religious materials printed in braille and large type. large type. A national CAPVI office is open in New York City. **Awards:** Koch Foundation (annual).

★ **20812** ★ **Christian Record Services (CRS)**
4444 S 52nd St.
Lincoln, NE 68516-1302
**Phone:** (402)488-0981          **Fax:** (402)488-7582
**Email:** info@christianrecord.org
**Website:** http://www.christianrecord.org
Ron Bowes, Contact

**Desc:** Assists blind, visually impaired individuals. Sponsors Bible correspondence courses. Representatives visit about 40,000 blind people annually. Conducts glaucoma screening clinics in cooperation with local physicians and organizations; provides home visitation program. Sponsors National Camps for Blind Children; maintains speakers' bureau. **Awards:** Scholarship bestowed to qualified individuals who cannot obtain finacial assistance from other sources.

★ **20813** ★ **Contact Lens Association of Ophthalmologists (CLAO)**
c/o John S. Massare
721 Papworth Ave., Ste. 206
Metairie, LA 70005
**Phone:** (504)835-3937          **Fax:** (504)833-5884
**Email:** eyes@clao.org
**Website:** http://www.clao.org
John S. Massare, PhD, Exec. Dir.

**Desc:** To advance quality medical eyecare for the public by providing comprehensive ophthalmologists and other eye care professionals with education and training in contact lenses, refractive surgery, and related eyecare science. **Awards:** Grant bestowed to residents for traveling.

★ **20814** ★ **Council of Citizens With Low Vision (CCLV)**
c/o American Council of the Blind
1155 15th St. NW, Ste. 1004
Washington, DC 20005
**Phone:** (202)467-5081          **Free:** 800-733-2258
**Email:** badkron@aol.com
**Website:** http://www.cclvi.org
Ken Stewart, Pres.

**Desc:** Partially sighted and low-vision individuals, their families, and professional workers. Provides a vehicle through which partially sighted people may voice their needs, preferences, and interests. Promotes the concept that partially sighted and low-vision individuals are not blind and that they have the right to maximize the use of residual vision through the use of any visual aid, service, or technology. Keeps abreast of all developments benefiting partially sighted persons. Promotes educational, engineering, medical, rehabilitative, scientific, and social research that facilitates the lives of individuals with residual vision. Supports the development of pre-service professional training programs for the establishment and expansion of multidisciplinary low-vision services. Strives to educate the public about the existence, capabilities, and needs of such individuals. Establishes outreach programs to insure access to available services for partially sighted persons. Maintains speakers' bureau. **Awards:** Carl Foley Scholarship (annual); Telesensory Scholarship (annual).

★ **20815** ★ **Eye Bank Association of America (EBAA)**
1015 18th St., NW, Ste. 1010
Washington, DC 20036
**Phone:** (202)775-4999          **Fax:** (202)429-6036
**Email:** patricia@restoresight.org

**Website:** http://www.restoresight.org
Patricia Aiken-O'Neill, Pres.

**Desc:** Eye banks working to restore sight through the promotion and advancement of eye banking. Makes possible over 46,000 corneal transplants annually. Establishes standards for the procurement and distribution of eyes and corneal tissue. Offers training and certification programs for eye banking personnel. Compiles statistics; maintains speakers' bureau. Conducts research and educational programs. **Awards:** Gift of Sight Award (annual); Heise Award (annual); Paton Award (annual); Scientific Award (annual).

★ 20816 ★ **Glaucoma Foundation**
116 John St., Ste. 1605
New York, NY 10038
**Phone:** (212)285-0080     **Fax:** (212)504-1933
**Email:** info@glaucoma-foundation.org
**Website:** http://www.glaucoma-foundation.org/
Scott R. Christensen, Pres. /CEO

**Desc:** Individuals who have been affected by glaucoma and interested others. Works to increase public awareness and to provide research funding. Provides information about glaucoma to the medical and lay communities. Targets and funds the following areas for research: optic nerve regeneration; molecular genetics. Sponsors scientific research. **Awards:** Award of Merit; grant.

★ 20817 ★ **Glaucoma Research Foundation**
200 Pine St., Ste. 200
San Francisco, CA 94104-2712
**Phone:** (415)986-3162     **Free:** 800-826-6693
**Fax:** (415)986-3763
**Email:** info@glaucoma.org
**Website:** http://www.glaucoma.org
Rita Loskill, Dir. of Education

**Desc:** Dedicated to protecting the sight and independence of individuals with glaucoma through research and education, with the ultimate goal of finding a cure. Funds pilot project grants. **Awards:** Catalyst (annual); Pilot Project (annual) for research.

★ 20818 ★ **John Milton Society for the Blind (JMS)**
475 Riverside Dr., Rm. 455
New York, NY 10115
**Phone:** (212)870-3335     **Fax:** (212)870-3226
**Email:** order@jmsblind.org
**Website:** http://www.jmsblind.org
Robert R. Pegg, Pres.

**Desc:** Non-denominational Christian worldwide service to persons who cannot see to read regular print. Works to make Christian religious materials available to blind and visually impaired persons worldwide. Operates referral service. Provides materials for displays and exhibits. **Awards:** JMS Scholarship (annual) blind students and individuals who work with blind persons recommended to us by two US schools for the blind; New York Scholarship (annual) blind students recommended to JMS by the New York State Commission for the Blind and Visually Handicapped.

★ 20819 ★ **National Children's Eye Care Foundation (NCECF)**
c/o American Association for Pediatric
    Ophthalmology and Strabismus
PO Box 193832
San Francisco, CA 94119-3832
**Phone:** (415)561-8505     **Fax:** (415)561-8531
**Email:** aapos@aao.org
**Website:** http://med-aapos.bu.edu
Suzanne C. Beauchamp, Admin.

**Desc:** Seeks to optimize the quality of life of infants, children, and families by fostering normal development and protection of vision through promoting programs of prevention, detection, treatment, research and education. **Awards:** Fellowship Loans (annual) to fund fellowships in pediatric opthalmology; grant (annual) for research in children's eye disorders and diseases.

★ 20820 ★ **National Federation of the Blind (NFB)**
1800 Johnson St.
Baltimore, MD 21230
**Phone:** (410)659-9314     **Fax:** (410)685-5653
**Email:** nfb@nfb.org
**Website:** http://www.nfb.org
Marc Maurer, Pres.

**Desc:** Federation of state (50 plus Washington, DC and Puerto Rico) and local (600) organizations representing 50,000 blind people. Seeks the complete equality and integration of the blind into society. Monitors all legislation affecting the blind; evaluates present programs for the blind; stimulates and assists in promoting needed services. Supports and conducts scholarly research and publication of results. Works to improve policies toward the blind in such places as the U.S. Office of Personnel Management. Sponsors National White Cane Week annually for fundraising and educational purposes. Distributes information. Maintains National Blindness Information Center. **Awards:** Hermione Grant Calhoun Scholarship (annual) for blind women students; Howard Brown Rickard Scholarship for blind students of the professions; recognition for greatest contribution to the welfare of the blind; scholarship for blind postsecondary students; scholarship given to blind students.

★ 20821 ★ **Opticians Association of America (OAA)**
7023 Little River Turnpike, No. 207
Annandale, VA 22003
**Phone:** (703)916-8856     **Free:** 800-443-8997
**Fax:** (703)916-7966
**Email:** oaa@opticians.org
**Website:** http://www.opticians.org
Earl M. Cleveland, Pres.

**Desc:** Retail dispensing opticians who fill prescriptions for glasses or contact lenses written by a vision care specialist. Works to advance the science of ophthalmic optics. Conducts research and educational programs. Maintains museum and speakers' bureau. Compiles statistics. **Awards:** Russell Fritz Memorial Scholarship (annual) for a first-year student in an opticianry program accredited by the Commission on Opticianry Accreditation.

★ 20822 ★ **Pan-American Association of Ophthalmology (PAAO)**
1301 S Bowen Rd., Ste. 365
Arlington, TX 76013
**Phone:** (817)265-2831     **Fax:** (817)275-3961
**Email:** info@paao.org
**Website:** http://www.paao.org
J. Bronwyn Bateman, MD, Pres.

**Desc:** Ophthalmologists throughout the Western Hemisphere. Seeks to improve the treatment of eye diseases and prevention of blindness in the Americas through the exchange of ideas and treatments. **Awards:** Benjamin F. Boyd Humanitarian Award (biennial) for ophthalmological service and blindness prevention activities; fellowship; Gillingham - Pan American Fellowship (annual) for education.

★ 20823 ★ **Prevent Blindness America**
500 E Remington Rd.
Schaumburg, IL 60173-5611
**Phone:** (847)843-2020     **Free:** 800-331-2020
**Fax:** (847)843-8458
**Email:** info@preventblindness.org
**Website:** http://www.preventblindness.org
Elaine Barber, COO

**Desc:** Charitable organization committed to preventing blindness and preserving sight through nationwide comprehensive programs of public and professional education, research, industrial, and community services. Services include promotion and support of local glaucoma screening programs, preschool vision testing, industrial eye safety, and collection of statistical and other data on nature and extent of causes of blindness and defective vision. Operates a toll-free information center dealing with eye health and safety topics. Through the Fight for Sight Research Division,

the organization awards student fellowships, postdoctoral awards and grants in aid for medical research. Sponsors Wise Owl Program to promote widespread use of safety eyewear for various activities and occupations. Compiles statistics. **Awards:** Grant-In-Aid (annual) for funding of research in vision and ophthalmology; Postdoctoral Fellowship (annual) for basic or clinical research in vision and ophthalmology; Student Fellowship (annual) for undergraduate, graduate, and medical students interested in eye-related basic or clinical research.

★ 20824 ★ **Research to Prevent Blindness (RPB)**
645 Madison Ave.
New York, NY 10022-1010
**Phone:** (212)752-4333     **Free:** 800-621-0026
**Fax:** (212)688-6231
**Email:** info@rpbusa.org
**Website:** http://www.rpbusa.org/hc2/index.asp
Diane S. Swift, Pres.

**Desc:** National voluntary health foundation supported by foundations, corporations, and voluntary gifts and bequests from individuals. Established to stimulate basic and applied research into the causes, prevention, and treatment of blinding eye diseases. Grants funds for equipment, eye research professorships with up to 7 year salary support, assistance in financing construction campaigns for eye research laboratory facilities, and travel expenses for international scholars for short-term collaborative research in the U.S. Through seminars and other means, encourages communication among scientists, practicing ophthalmologists, and the public. Maintains scientific advisory panel. **Awards:** Career Development Award to young physicians and scientists who wish to conduct eye research; grant (annual) for eye research to departments of ophthalmology at university medical schools; Jules and Doris Stein Professorship for outstanding basic scientists from other disciplines who conduct relavent clinical research in ophthalmology; Lew R. Wasserman Merit Award for mid-career scientists who hold primary positions within departments of ophthalmology and who are actively engaged in eye research; Physician-Scientist Award for nationally recognized and established M.D.'s engaged in clinical eye research; Senior Scientific Investigator Award for investigators who have deeply influenced the course of eye research; Special Research Scholars Award for outstanding young scientists conducting research of exceptional merit and promise.

# Medical & Allied Health Schools

## Optometry

*Schools and colleges listed below are accredited by the Council on Optometric Education of the American Optometric Association (AOA), 243 N Lindbergh Blvd., St. Louis, MO 63141, (314)991-4100, http://www.aoanet.org. For general information about the profession, contact the AOA or the Association of Schools and Colleges of Optometry, 6110 Executive Blvd., Ste. 510, Rockville, MD 20852, (301)231-5944, http://home.opted.org/.*

### Alabama

★ 20825 ★ **University of Alabama, Birmingham**
**School of Optometry**
HPB 124
1530 3rd Ave. S
Birmingham, AL 35294-0010
**Phone:** (205)934-6150
**Email:** admissions@icare.opt.uab.edu
**Website:** http://www.icare..opt.uab.edu

## California

★ **20826** ★ **Southern California College of Optometry**
2575 Yorba Linda Blvd.
Fullerton, CA 92831
**Phone:** (714)449-7444
**Email:** leswalls@scco.edu
**Website:** http://www.scco.edu/second.html

★ **20827** ★ **University of California, Berkeley**
**School of Optometry**
360 Minor Hall
Berkeley, CA 94720-2020
**Phone:** (510)642-9537
**Email:** ubcso@spectacle.berkeley.edu
**Website:** http://spectacle.berkeley.edu

## Florida

★ **20828** ★ **Nova Southeastern University Health Professions Division College of Optometry**
3200 S University Dr.
Fort Lauderdale, FL 33328
**Phone:** (954)723-1125
**Email:** astella@hpd.nov.edu
**Website:** http://www.nova.edu/cwis/centers/hpd/optometry

## Illinois

★ **20829** ★ **Illinois College of Optometry**
3241 S Michigan Ave.
Chicago, IL 60616
**Phone:** (312)225-1700
**Email:** admissions@eyecare.ico.edu
**Website:** http://www.ico.edu/ico2/flindex.html

## Indiana

★ **20830** ★ **Indiana University School of Optometry**
800 E Atwater Ave.
Bloomington, IN 47405
**Phone:** (812)855-1917
**Email:** iuopt@indiana.edu
**Website:** http://www.opt.indiana.edu

## Massachusetts

★ **20831** ★ **New England College of Optometry**
424 Beacon St.
Boston, MA 02115
**Phone:** (617)266-2030
**Email:** admissio@ne-optometry.edu
**Website:** http://www.ne-optometry.edu

## Michigan

★ **20832** ★ **Ferris State University Michigan College of Optometry**
1310 Cramer Cir.
Big Rapids, MI 49307
**Phone:** (231)591-3700
**Email:** olsonc@ferris.edu
**Website:** http://www.ferris.edu/mco

## Missouri

★ **20833** ★ **University of Missouri, Saint Louis**
**School of Optometry**
8001 Natural Bridge Rd.
Saint Louis, MO 63121
**Phone:** (314)516-6263
**Email:** sdavis@umsl.edu
**Website:** http://www.umsl.edu/~optometry.html

## New York

★ **20834** ★ **State University of New York State College of Optometry**
33 W 42nd St.
New York, NY 10036
**Phone:** (212)780-5100
**Email:** admissions@sunyopt.edu
**Website:** http://www.sunyopt.edu

## Ohio

★ **20835** ★ **Ohio State University College of Optometry**
320 W 10th Ave.
PO Box 182342
Columbus, OH 43218-2342
**Phone:** (614)292-2647
**Email:** optometry@osu.edu
**Website:** http://www.optometry.ohio-state.edu

## Oklahoma

★ **20836** ★ **Northeastern State University College of Optometry**
600 N Grand Ave.
Tahlequah, OK 74464
**Phone:** (918)456-5511
**Email:** stratton@cherokee.nsuok.edu
**Website:** http://arapaho.nsuok.edu/~optometry

## Ontario

★ **20837** ★ **University of Waterloo School of Optometry**
Waterloo, ON, Canada N2L 3G1
**Phone:** (519)888-4567
Graham Strong, OD,PhD, Director

## Oregon

★ **20838** ★ **Pacific University College of Optometry**
2043 College Way
Forest Grove, OR 97116
**Phone:** (503)359-2900          **Free:** 800-933-9308
**Fax:** (503)359-2900
**Email:** admissions@pacificu.edu
**Website:** http://www.opt.pacificu.edu/opt/index.shtml

## Pennsylvania

★ **20839** ★ **Pennsylvania College of Optometry**
8360 Old York Rd.
Elkins Park, PA 19027
**Phone:** (215)780-1301          **Free:** 800-824-6262
**Email:** admissions@pco.edu
**Website:** http://www.pco.edu

## Puerto Rico

★ **20840** ★ **Inter American University of Puerto Rico School of Optometry**
PO Box 191049
San Juan, PR 00919-1049
**Phone:** (787)765-1915
**Email:** jcolon@inter.edu
**Website:** http://www.optonet.inter.edu

## Quebec

★ **20841** ★ **University of Montreal School of Optometry**
3744 Jean-Brillant, Ste. 260-7
Montreal, QC, Canada H3T 1P1
**Phone:** (514)343-6325
Pierre Simonet, PhD, Director

## Tennessee

★ **20842** ★ **Southern College of Optometry**
1245 Madison Ave.
Memphis, TN 38104
**Phone:** (901)722-3225          **Free:** 800-238-0180
**Email:** jhauser@sco.edu
**Website:** http://www.sco.edu

## Texas

★ **20843** ★ **University of Houston College of Optometry**
4800 Calhoun Rd.
Houston, TX 77204-6052
**Phone:** (713)743-2040
**Website:** http://www.opt.uh.edu

---

# National & International Organizations

★ **20844** ★ **Accreditation Council on Optometric Education (ACOE)**
243 N Lindbergh Blvd.
Saint Louis, MO 63141
**Phone:** (314)991-4100          **Fax:** (314)991-4101
**Email:** acoe@aoa.org
**Website:** http://www.aoanet.org
Joyce L. Urbeck, Admin. Dir.
**Fnded:** 1934. **Mem:** 11. **Desc:** Accrediting body for professional optometric degree (O.D.) programs (examination, diagnosis, and treatment of the conditions or impairments of the vision system), paraoptometric educational programs, and optometric residency programs. Members are appointed by the president of the American Optometric Association. Works to ensure the quality of optometric education and announces list of accredited programs. **Frmly:** (2002) Council on Optometric Education.

★ **20845** ★ **Achromatopsia Network**
PO Box 214
Berkeley, CA 94701-0214
**Phone:** (510)540-4700          **Fax:** (510)540-4767
**Email:** publications@acromat.org
**Website:** http://www.achromat.org/
Frances Futterman, Contact
**Fnded:** 1994. **Desc:** Provides information and support for individuals and families concerned with the vision disorder achromatopsia, including both rod monochromacy and blue cone monochromacy.

★ **20846** ★ **Action for Blind People**
14-16 Verney Rd.
London SE16 3DZ, United Kingdom
**Phone:** 44 171 76354800   **Fax:** 44 171 76354900
**Email:** info@afbp.org
**Website:** http://www.afbp.org
**Fnded:** 1857. **Desc:** Provides services for visually impaired people in the UK, including employment services, hotels and holidays, accommodation and residential care, and information and welfare rights advice.

**Advocates for Communication Technology for Deaf/Blind People (ACT)**
*See:* Entry 5969

★ **20847** ★ **African Union of the Blind - Kenya (AUB)**
Airport Rd.
PO Box 72872
Embakasi
Nairobi, Kenya
**Phone:** 254 2 823989          **Fax:** 254 2 823776

**Email:** afub@form-net.com
**Website:** http://www.afub.net
**Fnded:** 1987. **Mem:** 42. **Nat'l Groups:** 44. **Reg. Groups:** 6. **State Groups:** 44. **Lang(s):** English, French. **Desc:** Works to improve the quality of life of the blind and people with visual impairments in Africa. Represents the interests of people with visual impairments before government agencies, international organizations, and the public. **Pub:** *AFUB Newsletter*, semiannual. Newsletter. Contains exchange of information between national organizations.

★ **20848** ★ **All-India Ophthalmological Society**
Kotla Rd.
New Delhi 110 002, India
**Phone:** 91 11 3318813
**Fnded:** 1937.

★ **20849** ★ **All Russia Association of the Blind (Vserossiiskoe Obschestvo Slepykn — VOS)**
Novaya ploschad' 14
103672 Moscow, Russia
**Phone:** 7 95 9253730      **Fax:** 7 95 9237600
**Email:** info@vos.org.ru
**Website:** http://www.vos.org.ru
**Fnded:** 1925. **Mem:** 274,341. **Nat'l Groups:** 147. **Reg. Groups:** 74. **Local Groups:** 932. **Lang(s):** Russian. **Desc:** People with visual impairments, health care professionals, and others with an interest in the situation of people with visual impairments. Promotes the rights of people with visual impairments; represents members' interests. **Pub:** *Dialogue*, bimonthly. Audiotape. • *Literary Reading*, monthly. Magazine. Arts digest. Provides the readers with the most recent literary publications. • *Modern Prose, Modern Poetry, In the World of Music, Culture and Health, The Knowledge, Computer Technologies*, quarterly. Magazine. Covers the life of the association and international relations. • *Our Life*, monthly. Covers the life of the association and international relations. **Frmly:** (1999) All Russian Association of the Blind.

**Alstrom Syndrome International**
*See:* Entry 9297

★ **20850** ★ **American Academy of Ophthalmology (AAO)**
PO Box 7424
San Francisco, CA 94120-7424
**Phone:** (415)561-8500      **Fax:** (415)561-8533
**Email:** federal@aao.org
**Website:** http://www.aao.org
H. Dunbar Hoskins Jr.,, MD, Exec. VP
**Fnded:** 1896. **Mem:** 26,000. **Desc:** Works to achieve accessible, appropriate and affordable eye care for the public by serving the educational and professional needs of the ophthalmologist. Provides clinical education, ophthalmic practice, federal and state advocacy, patient information, and other services to its members. Provides accurate, appropriate and timely information to the public through its media and public information programs. Current activities of the foundation include National Eye Care Project; Oral Histories Program. **Pub:** *Basic and Clinical Science Course.* • *Eye Net*, monthly. Magazine. *Price:* Free to members; $128/year US non-members. • *Member Directory*, biennial. Directory. • *Ophthalmology*, monthly. Journal. • Manuals. • Videos. • Also publishes slide script packages and study guides, special interest newsletters, modules, procedures assessments, issue briefs, brochures.

★ **20851** ★ **American Academy of Optometry (AAO)**
6110 Executive Blvd., Ste. 506
Rockville, MD 20852
**Phone:** (301)984-1441      **Fax:** (301)984-4737
**Email:** loiss@aaoptom.org
**Website:** http://www.aaopt.org
Lois Schoenbrun, Exec. Dir.
**Fnded:** 1921. **Mem:** 5,000. **Local Groups:** 20. **Desc:** Optometrists, educators, and scientists interested in optometric education, and standards of care in visual problems. Conducts continuing education for optometrists and visual scientists. Sponsors 5-day annual meeting. **Pub:** *Geographic Directory of Members*, biennial. Membership Directory. Complete geographical/alphabetical listing of academy fellows. *Price:* $15. • *Optometry and Vision Science*, monthly. Includes academy news, book reviews, and periodic index. *Price:* Included in membership dues; $55/year for nonmembers; $70/year for institutions; $30/year for students. • Newsletter, bimonthly.

★ **20852** ★ **American Academy of Optometry - British Chapter (ACABC)**
2 Doric Lodge
Doric Pl.
Woodbridge IP12 1BT, United Kingdom
**Phone:** 44 1394 380139      **Fax:** 44 7967 446413
**Email:** academy@debenlogic.co.uk
**Website:** http://www.academy.org.uk
**Fnded:** 1952. **Mem:** 110. **Lang(s):** English. **Desc:** Optometrists. Seeks to advance the study, teaching, and practice of optometry. Maintains standards of training, ethics, and practice for members; conducts continuing professional development courses for optometrists.

★ **20853** ★ **American Action Fund for Blind Children and Adults (AAFBCA)**
1800 Johnson St.
Baltimore, MD 21230
**Phone:** (410)659-9314      **Fax:** (410)685-5653
**Email:** acc@roundley.com
**Website:** http://www.actionfund.org
Dr. Marc Maurer, Exec. Dir.
**Fnded:** 1919. **Desc:** Works to assist blind persons in securing reading material, to educate the public about blindness, to give aid to the deaf-blind and to improve the quality of life for blind persons. Provides information and referral services on Social Security Disability Insurance, employment, civil rights, products and aids, education of blind children and public rehabilitation agencies; disseminates information on Braille and sign language; distributes publications free of charge to libraries and schools. **Pub:** *Great Documents Series.* Books. Features Braille copies of Great American documents. • *Twin Vision.* Books. Childrens' books containing Braille and print side by side. • Also publishes Braille calendars. **Frmly:** (1990) American Brotherhood for the Blind.

★ **20854** ★ **American Association of Certified Orthoptists (AACO)**
c/o St. Louis Children's Hospital Eye Center
2 South 89
One Children's Place
Saint Louis, MO 63110
**Phone:** (314)454-6026      **Fax:** (314)454-2368
**Email:** arnoldi@vision.wustl.edu
**Website:** http://www.orthoptics.org
Kyle Arnoldi, Pres.
**Fnded:** 1940. **Mem:** 350. **Reg. Groups:** 4. **Desc:** Orthoptists certified by the American Orthoptic Council, after completing a minimum of 24 months' special training, to treat defects in binocular function. Assists in postgraduate instruction courses; conducts programs and courses at international, national, and regional meetings; helps individual orthoptists with special or unusual problem cases; trains new orthoptists. Operates a placement listing. **Pub:** *American Association of Certified Orthoptists–Directory*, annual. Directory. *Price:* Included in membership dues. • *American Orthoptic Journal*, annual. Journal. Presents new material in the fields of amblyopia and strabismus. Includes book reviews and abstracts of current English and French literature. *Price:* $25/copy for individuals; $56/copy for institutions. • *The Prism*, quadrennial. Newsletter. **Frmly:** (1963) American Association of Orthopic Technicians.

**American Association for Pediatric Ophthalmology and Strabismus**
*See:* Entry 5607

★ **20855** ★ **American Blind Bowling Association (ABBA)**
315 N Main St.
Houston, PA 15342
**Phone:** (724)745-5986
**Email:** refos@bellatlantic.net
**Website:** http://med-aapos.bu.edu/
Judy Refosco, Sec. -Treas.
**Fnded:** 1951. **Mem:** 2,000. **Reg. Groups:** 4. **State Groups:** 125. **Local Groups:** 140. **Desc:** Legally blind men and women, 18 years of age and older, competing in organized tenpin bowling. Promotes bowling as a recreational activity for adult blind persons. Sanctions member leagues; sponsors annual mail-o-graphic. Presents awards. **Pub:** *The Blind Bowler*, 3/year.

★ **20856** ★ **American Blind Skiing Foundation (ABSF)**
227 E North Ave.
Elmhurst, IL 60126
**Phone:** (847)255-1739
**Email:** absf@bigfoot.com
**Website:** http://www.absf.org/
Sam Skobel, Founder
**Fnded:** 1972. **Mem:** 175. **Desc:** Volunteers who teach downhill and cross-country recreational and competitive skiing to the blind and visually handicapped. Holds giant slalom, downhill, and cross-country races; awards trophies. Travels with blind skiers to skiing areas in Colorado, Wisconsin, and Michigan. Sponsors international races in Canada, World Cup for Disabled in Switzerland, and Olympics for Disabled in Austria.

★ **20857** ★ **American Board of Ophthalmology (ABO)**
111 Presidential Blvd., Ste. 241
Bala Cynwyd, PA 19004-1075
**Phone:** (610)664-1175      **Fax:** (610)664-6503
**Email:** info@abop.org
**Website:** http://www.abop.org
Denis O'Day, MD, Exec. Dir.
**Fnded:** 1916. **Mem:** 17. **Desc:** Medical specialty board to determine the adequacy of training, the professional preparation, and ophthalmic knowledge of ophthalmologists who wish to be certified. Works to improve the standards of graduate medical education and the facilities for special ophthalmic training. **Pub:** *Qualifications Brochure*, annual. Brochure. **Frmly:** (1933) American Board for Ophthalmic Examinations.

★ **20858** ★ **American Board of Opticianry (ABO)**
6506 Loisdale Rd., Ste. 209
Springfield, VA 22150-1815
**Phone:** (703)719-5800      **Free:** 800-296-1379
**Fax:** (703)719-9144
**Email:** mail@abo-ncle.org
**Website:** http://www.abo.org
Michael H. Robey, Exec. Dir.
**Fnded:** 1979. **Mem:** 30,000. **Desc:** Provides uniform standards for dispensing opticians by administering the National Opticianry Competency Examination and by issuing the Certified Optician Certificate to those passing the exam. Also administers the Master in Ophthalmic Optics Examination and issues certificates to opticians at the advanced level passing the exam. Maintains records of persons certified for competency in eyeglass dispensing. Adopts and enforces continuing education requirements; assists and encourages state licensing boards in the use of the National Opticianry Competency Examination for licensure purposes.

**★ 20859 ★ American College of Eye Surgeons (ACES)**
2265 Oak Ridge Court, Ste. A
Fort Myers, FL 33901
**Phone:** (941)275-8881          **Free:** 888-335-0077
**Fax:** (941)275-9969
**Email:** quality@aces-abes.org
**Website:** http://www.aces-abes.org
Brenda S. Sheets, Exec. Dir.

**Fnded:** 1986. **Mem:** 700. **Desc:** Ophthalmic surgeons. Promotes and seeks to "sustain excellence in eye surgery while supporting self-direction and self-regulation" in the field of ophthalmic surgery. Works to ensure the quality and availability of ophthalmic health and surgical services. Conducts examinations and certifies qualified surgeons in ophthalmic surgical subspecialties; conducts continuing professional education courses for members; serves as a clearinghouse on emerging ophthalmic surgical techniques and technologies. **Pub:** *American Board of Eye Surgery Directory*, annual. Directory. *Price:* $2. • *Synergism*, periodic. Newsletter.

**American College of Veterinary Ophthalmologists (ACVO)**
*See:* Entry 20561

**★ 20860 ★ American Council of the Blind (ACB)**
1155 15th St. NW, Ste. 1004
Washington, DC 20005
**Phone:** (202)467-5081          **Free:** 800-424-8666
**Fax:** (202)467-5085
**Email:** info@acb.org
**Website:** http://www.acb.org
Charles Crawford, Exec. Dir.

**Fnded:** 1961. **Mem:** 20,000. **Nat'l Groups:** 19. **State Groups:** 51. **Desc:** Blind and visually impaired persons. Serves as a national information clear Security and supplemental security income programs, radio reading services, special library services, eye research, and low vision technology. Offers group insurance plans, professional assistance in public interest, class action litigation, and public education about blindness and the abilities of visually impaired people. **Pub:** *Braille Forum*, monthly. Newsletter. Concerned with legislative developments, new products and services, medical and technological advances, and human interest stories for the blind. *Price:* Free for individuals in U.S.; $25/yr. for organizations & international subscribers.

**★ 20861 ★ American Council of the Blind Enterprises and Services (ACBES)**
120 S 6th St., Ste. 1005
Minneapolis, MN 55402-1839
**Phone:** (612)332-3242          **Free:** 800-866-3242
**Fax:** (612)332-7850
**Email:** acbesall@ix.netcom.com
**Website:** http://www.acb.org
James R. Olsen, CFO

**Fnded:** 1978. **Mem:** 16. **Desc:** Board of directors of the American Council of the Blind. Owns and operates 11 ACB thrift stores which help finance ACB and its programs and aid the blind and visually impaired in leading productive and independent lives.

**★ 20862 ★ American Council of Blind Government Employees (ACBGE)**
c/o America Council of the Blind
1155 15th St. NW, Ste. 1004
Washington, DC 20005
**Phone:** (202)467-5081          **Free:** 800-424-8666
**Fax:** (202)467-5085
**Email:** mpomerantz@mailbox.lacity.org
**Website:** http://www.acb.org/affiliates/
Mitch Pomerantz, Pres.

**Fnded:** 1978. **Mem:** 50. **Desc:** Government employees, retirees from government employment who are blind or visually handicapped, and other interested persons. Strives to improve opportunities in govern-

ment employment for the blind and visually impaired; provides career development material; works with personnel policymakers. Members participate as speakers and panelists in workshops and other meetings. Offers technical assistance through specialized education program. **Pub:** Newsletter, periodic. Available in large print or cassette. **Frmly:** (1991) American Council of Blind Federal Employees.

**★ 20863 ★ American Council of Blind Lions (ACBL)**
c/o American Council of the Blind
1155 15th St. NW, Ste. 1004
Washington, DC 20005
**Phone:** (202)467-5081          **Free:** 800-424-8666
**Email:** jabeatty1@yahoo.com
**Website:** http://www.acb.org/affiliates/
Alan Beatty, Pres.

**Fnded:** 1970. **Mem:** 141. **Desc:** Legally blind members of Lions Clubs International. Informs the public of the needs and capabilities of blind persons; exchanges information on club activities benefiting work for the blind; encourages blind people to join Lions Clubs and other civic organizations. Supports speakers' bureau. **Pub:** Newsletter, quarterly. **Frmly:** (1985) World Council of Blind Lions; (1986) Council of Blind Lions.

**★ 20864 ★ American Foundation for the Blind (AFB)**
11 Penn Plz., Ste. 300
New York, NY 10001
**Phone:** (212)502-7600          **Free:** 800-232-5463
**Fax:** (212)502-7777
**Email:** afbinfo@afb.net
**Website:** http://www.afb.org
Carl R. Augusto, Pres.

**Fnded:** 1921. **Desc:** Mission is to eliminate the inequities faced by the ten million Americans who are blind or visually impaired; Helen Keller dedicated 40 years of her life to the organization. Develops, collects, and disseminates information that benefits people who are blind or visually impaired, their families and friends, professionals in the blindness field, and the general public. Takes a leadership role in identifying issues critical to people who are blind or visually impaired; conducts research, and acts as a catalyst for change. Educates the public and policymakers as to the needs and capabilities of people who are blind or visually impaired; records and duplicates Talking Books for the Library of Congress and other audio materials for various corporations and organizations; and develops public education programs. Maintains offices in Atlanta, Chicago, Dallas and San Francisco, and a governmental relations office in Washington, DC. **Pub:** *AFB Directory of Services for Blind and Visually Impaired Persons in the U.S. and Canada*. Directory. Lists over 3000 local, state, regional, and national services, including educational, informational, rehabilitative, low-vision, and aging services. *Price:* $100/copy. • *AFB News*, semiannual. Newsletter. Covers programs and activities of the AFB. *Price:* Free. • *Journal of Visual Impairment and Blindness*, monthly. Journal. Contains articles on research and practice in the areas of rehabilitation, psychology, education, legislation, medicine, and sensory devices. *Price:* $74/year for individuals in the U.S. and Canada; $99/year for individuals outside the U.S. and Canada; $104/year for institutions in the U.S. and Canada; $129/year for institutions outside the U.S. and Canada. • Also publishes textbooks, training manuals, and resource guides, videos, and educational materials for teachers.

**★ 20865 ★ American Foundation for Vision Awareness (AFVA)**
243 N Lindbergh Blvd.
Saint Louis, MO 63141
**Free:** 800-927-2382          **Fax:** (314)991-4101
**Email:** afva@aol.com
**Website:** http://www.afva.org
**Fnded:** 1927. **Mem:** 5,000. **Desc:** Seeks to educate people of all ages about their vision; to create aware-

ness of quality eye and vision care; and to support vision-related scientific research. **Pub:** *In Focus*, quarterly. **Frmly:** (1970) Women's Auxiliary to the American Optometric Association; (1989) Auxiliary to the American Optometric Association.

**★ 20866 ★ American-Israeli Ophthalmological Society**
130 E 67th St., Ste. 1C
New York, NY 10021-6136
**Fax:** (212)734-2682

**Fnded:** 1974. **Mem:** 450. **Nat'l Groups:** 1. **Desc:** Ophthalmologists. Seeks to facilitate communication between American and Israeli ophthalmologists. Provides training for Israeli opthalmologists in the United States. Organizes conventions.

**★ 20867 ★ American Ophthalmological Society (AOS)**
PO Box 19340
San Francisco, CA 94119-3940
**Phone:** (415)561-8578          **Fax:** (415)561-8531
**Email:** admin@aosonline.org
**Website:** http://www.aosonline.org
Charles P. Wilkinson, MD, Sec. Treas.

**Fnded:** 1864. **Mem:** 319. **Desc:** Professional honorary society of physicians specializing in the functions and treatment of the eye. **Pub:** *Transactions of the American Ophthalmological Society*, annual.

**★ 20868 ★ American Optometric Association (AOA)**
243 N Lindbergh Blvd.
Saint Louis, MO 63141
**Phone:** (314)991-4100          **Fax:** (314)991-4101
**Website:** http://www.aoanet.org/
Michael D. Jones, Exec. Dir.

**Fnded:** 1898. **Mem:** 32,000. **State Groups:** 53. **Local Groups:** 500. **Desc:** Professional association of optometrists, students of optometry, and paraoptometric assistants and technicians. Purposes are: to improve the quality, availability, and accessibility of eye and vision care; to represent the optometric profession; to help members conduct their practices; to promote the highest standards of patient care. Monitors and promotes legislation concerning the scope of optometric practice, alternate health care delivery systems, health care cost containment, Medicare, and other issues relevant to eye/vision care. Supports the International Library, Archives and Museum of Optometry which includes references on ophthalmic and related sciences with emphasis on the history and socioeconomic aspects of optometry. Operates Vision U.S.A. program, which provides free eye care to the working poor. Conducts specialized education programs; operates placement service; compiles statistics. Maintains museum. Conducts Seal of Certification and Acceptance Program. **Pub:** *American Optometric Association–News*, semimonthly. Magazine. Includes employment listings, classified ads, promotional news, and obituaries. *Price:* $80/year for nonmembers; $95 in Canada; $103 outside U.S. and Canada. • *Optometry: Journal of the American Optometric Association*, monthly. Journal. Includes research articles, book reviews, calendar of events, legislative news, new products information, and advertisers' index. *Price:* $95/year for nonmembers; $130/year in Canada; $145/year outside U.S. and Canada. **Frmly:** (1903) American Optical Association.

**★ 20869 ★ American Optometric Foundation (AOF)**
6110 Executive Blvd., Ste. 506
Rockville, MD 20852
**Phone:** (301)984-4734          **Free:** 800-368-6AOF
**Fax:** (301)984-4737
**Email:** christine@aapotom.org
**Website:** http://www.aaopt.org/aof/about/index.asp
Christine Armstrong, Dir.

**Fnded:** 1947. **Desc:** Optometrists, optometric organizations, corporations, and the public. Promotes research, education, literature, and professional advancement in the visual sciences. Supports fellowships in graduate research. **Pub:** *The Torch*, quarterly. Newsletter. Updates on foundation's activities. *Price:* Free.

★ **20870** ★ **American Optometric Student Association (AOSA)**
243 N Lindbergh
Saint Louis, MO 63141
**Phone:** (314)991-4100          **Fax:** (314)991-4101
**Website:** http://www.theaosa.org/frameset2.htm
Chad Fleming, Pres.

**Fnded:** 1972. **Mem:** 5,600. **Nat'l Groups:** 1. **Local Groups:** 19. **Desc:** Optometric students, state optometric associations, and family members of optometric students. Collects updated information on progress in the optometry field. Provides members with opportunities to work in areas of health care need such as local community health projects, school curriculum changes, and health manpower legislation. Works to improve optometric education and health care for the general population. Maintains active liaison with other optometric associations. Conducts communications program. **Pub:** *AOSA Foresight: Optometry Looking Forward*, semiannual. Reports information concerning scholarships, grants, internships, and other educational issues related to the study of optometry. *Price:* Included in membership dues. • *Communicator*, 9/year. Newsletter.

★ **20871** ★ **American Orthoptic Council (AOC)**
c/o Leslie France
3914 Nakoma Rd.
Madison, WI 53711
**Phone:** (608)233-5383          **Fax:** (608)263-4247
**Email:** orthopticsaaco@aol.com
**Website:** http://www.orthoptics.org
Kyle Arnoldi, CO, Pres.

**Fnded:** 1935. **Mem:** 20. **Desc:** Ophthalmologists and orthoptists. Directs practice of orthoptists; determines qualifications of candidates; regulates training and certification of orthoptists; supervises the practice of orthoptists after certification. **Pub:** *A Career in Orthoptics*, annual. Pamphlet. Contains list of current programs and general description of profession. • *American Orthoptic Journal*, annual. Journal. Covers ocular motility and visual physiology. Contains abstracts of ophthalmic literature. *Price:* Included in membership dues; $20/year for nonmembers; $35/year for institutions. • *Orthoptic Training Centers*, annual. Pamphlet.

★ **20872** ★ **American Osteopathic College of Ophthalmology and the American Osteopathic College of Otolaryngology-Head and Neck Surgery (AOCOO-HNS)**
405 W Grand Ave.
Dayton, OH 45405
**Phone:** (937)222-8820          **Free:** 800-455-9404
**Fax:** (937)222-8840
**Email:** info@aocoohns.org
**Website:** http://www.aocoohns.org
Debra L. Bailey, Admin. Dir.

**Fnded:** 1918. **Mem:** 670. **Desc:** Osteopathic ophthalmologists and osteopathic otolaryngologists/facial plastic surgeons. Created to improve quality of training, education and practice of osteopathic ophthalmologists and facial plastic surgeons. Provides "members only" access for a wealth of information.

**American Printing House for the Blind (APH)**
*See:* Entry 12068

★ **20873** ★ **American Society of Cataract and Refractive Surgery (ASCRS)**
4000 Legato Rd. No., 850
Fairfax, VA 22033
**Phone:** (703)591-2220          **Fax:** (703)591-0614
**Email:** ascrs@ascrs.org

**Website:** http://www.ascrs.org
I. Howard Fine, MD, Pres.

**Fnded:** 1974. **Mem:** 8,000. **Desc:** Ophthalmologists interested in anterior segment surgery and refractive corneal surgery. Offers continuing medical education to ophthalmologists on cataract and refractive surgery techniques, intraocular lens designs, and related research areas; assists allied health care professionals in ophthalmology on medical and surgical care of pseudophakic (lens implant) patients. Works to improve public education in the field of eye care. Conducts research in ocular pathology in cataract and refractive surgery. Compiles statistics. **Pub:** *Administrative Eyecare*, quarterly. *Price:* Included in membership dues; $60/year for nonmembers. • *ASCRS Roster*, biennial. Membership Directory. *Price:* Free for members. • *Journal of Cataract and Refractive Surgery*, bimonthly. Journal. *Price:* Included in membership dues; $105/year for nonmembers. • Newsletter, monthly. **Frmly:** (1986) American Intra-Ocular Implant Society.

★ **20874** ★ **American Society of Contemporary Ophthalmology (ASCO)**
820 N Orleans, Ste. 208
Chicago, IL 60610
**Phone:** (312)440-0699          **Free:** 800-621-4002
**Fax:** (312)440-0580
**Email:** iaos@aol.com
**Website:** http://www.ASCMSO.com
Randall T. Bellows, MD, Dir.

**Fnded:** 1966. **Mem:** 1,000. **Desc:** Ophthalmologists interested in promoting clinical investigative advances in ophthalmology. Offers continuing medical education courses approved by the American Council for Continuing Medical Education (ACCME) on new opthalmic developments in medical, therapeutic, diagnostic, and surgical procedures. **Pub:** *Annals of Ophthalmology*, quarterly. Journal. Includes book reviews and information on educational activities and new products. A continuing medical education publication for ophthalmologist. *Price:* $160. **Frmly:** (1970) Society for Cryo-Opthamology.

★ **20875** ★ **American Society of Ocularists (ASO)**
493 8th Ave.
San Francisco, CA 94118
**Phone:** (415)221-5765
**Email:** aso@ocularist.org
**Website:** http://www.ocularist.org

**Fnded:** 1957. **Desc:** Technicians specializing in artificial eyes. Promotes research in the field of ophthalmic prosthetics and provides education and support to their members. **Pub:** *Journal of Ophthalmic Prosthetics*, annual. Journal. Published in conjunction with the ABI Professional Publications. *Price:* $35 in North America; $45 outside North America.

**American Society of Ophthalmic Administrators (ASOA)**
*See:* Entry 9707

★ **20876** ★ **American Society of Ophthalmic Plastic and Reconstructive Surgery (ASOPRS)**
1133 W Morse Blvd., Ste. 201
Winter Park, FL 32789
**Phone:** (407)647-8839
**Email:** aso@asoa.org
**Website:** http://www.asoprs.org
Barbara Beatty, Exec.

**Fnded:** 1969. **Mem:** 400. **Desc:** Physicians specializing in ophthalmic plastic and reconstructive surgery. Seeks to "advance education, research, and the quality of clinical practice in the fields of plastic and reconstructive surgery involving the eyelids, orbits, and lacrimal system." Facilitates exchange of information among members; conducts fellowship training programs.

**American Society of Ophthalmic Registered Nurses (ASORN)**
*See:* Entry 15655

★ **20877** ★ **American Society of Pediatric Nephrology**
c/o James Whitcomb Riley Hospital for Children
Wells Research Center, 2600A
702 Barnhill Dr.
Indianapolis, IN 46202
**Phone:** (317)278-0854          **Fax:** (317)278-3599
**Email:** rmatteso@lupul.edu
**Website:** http://www.aspneph.com
Kristie Matteson, Offce Coord.

**Fnded:** 1969. **Mem:** 500. **Desc:** Committed to optimal are for children with renal disease and to disseminate advances in the clinical practice and basic science of pediatric nephrology.

**American Society of Veterinary Ophthalmology (ASVO)**
*See:* Entry 20566

**Anne Sullivan Foundation for Deafblind**
*See:* Entry 5987

★ **20878** ★ **Applied Vision Association**
c/o The College of Optometrists
42 Craven St.
London WC2N 5NG, United Kingdom
**Phone:** 44 207 8396000     **Fax:** 44 207 8396800
**Email:** ndebrunner@college-optometrists.org
**Website:** http://www.dmu.ac.uk/ava/

**Fnded:** 1975. **Mem:** 240. **Desc:** Works to advance, promote, develop and improve the study and knowledge of human vision including medical problems relating to vision. **Pub:** *Bulletin of the Applied Vision Association*, bimonthly. Newsletter.

★ **20879** ★ **Asia Pacific Academy of Ophthalmology (APAO)**
Gleneagles Hospital
Annexe Block 02-38
6A Napier Rd.
Singapore 258500, Singapore
**Phone:** 65 4666666          **Fax:** 65 7333360

**Lang(s):** Chinese, English. **Desc:** Ophthalmologists. Seeks to advance ophthalmological study, teaching, and practice. Facilitates exchange of information among members; conducts continuing professional development courses.

★ **20880** ★ **Asia-Pacific Council of Optometry (APCO)**
c/o Prof. Willard B. Bleything, Sec.Gen.
2043 College Way
Forest Grove, OR 97116
**Phone:** (503)352-2170          **Free:** 877-722-8648
**Fax:** (503)352-2929
**Email:** bleythiw@pacificu.edu
Prof. Willard B. Bleything, Sec. Gen.

**Fnded:** 1978. **Mem:** 26. **Desc:** National associations of optometrists in 20 countries. Purpose is to improve the delivery of eye care and standards of visual welfare to people in the the Asian-Pacific region. **Frmly:** International Federation of Asian and Pacific Associations of Optometrists.

★ **20881** ★ **Asia Pacific Intraocular Implant Association (APIIA)**
Annexe Block 02-38
Gleneagles Hospital
6A Napier Rd.
Singapore 258500, Singapore
**Phone:** 65 4666666          **Fax:** 65 7333360

**Lang(s):** Chinese, English. **Desc:** Ophthalmologists and ocular surgeons with an interest in intraocular implants. Seeks to advance the study, teaching, and practice of intraocular implantology. Facilitates exchange of information among members; sponsors research and continuing professional development programs.

### ★ 20882 ★ Asian Blind Union (ABU)

Mezar Manil 5-E 20/13
Nazimabad
Karachi 74600, Pakistan
**Phone:** 92 21 6612391     **Fax:** 92 21 7729935
**Lang(s):** Arabic, English. **Desc:** People with visual impairment. Seeks to improve the quality of life of people with impaired vision; promotes increased awareness of issues of concern to people with visual impairment. Represents members' social, political, and legal interests; sponsors training programs to increase the self-sufficiency of people with visual impairment.

### ★ 20883 ★ Asian Foundation for the Prevention of Blindness (AFPB)

248 Nam Cheong St.
Shamshuipo
Hong Kong, People's Republic of China
**Phone:** 852 7788332     **Fax:** 852 7880040
**Lang(s):** Chinese, English. **Desc:** Medical professionals and eye care institutions. Seeks to prevent blindness and improve the quality of life of people with impaired vision. Makes available visual health screening and other eye care services to needy individuals.

### ★ 20884 ★ Asian-Oceanic Glaucoma Society (AOGS)

Singapore National Eye Centre
11 Third Hospital Ave.
Singapore 168751, Singapore
**Phone:** 65 2277255     **Fax:** 65 2277290
**Lang(s):** Chinese, English. **Desc:** Ophthalmologists specializing in the treatment of glaucoma. Promotes early diagnosis and effective treatment of glaucoma; seeks to advance the science and practice of glaucomatology. Serves as a clearinghouse on the diagnosis and treatment of glaucoma; sponsors research and continuing professional development programs.

### ★ 20885 ★ Assistance Dogs International (ADI)

PO Box 5174
Santa Rosa, CA 95402
**Phone:** (707)571-0427
**Email:** info@adionline.org
**Website:** http://www.adionline.org
Suzi Hall, Coord.
**Fnded:** 1986. **Mem:** 50. **Desc:** ADI is a coalition of not-for-profit organizations that train and place Assistance Dogs. Purpose is to improve the areas of training, placement, and utilization of Assistance Dogs, as well as staff and volunteer education. Members of ADI meet annually to share ideas, attend seminars and conduct business regarding such things as educating the public about Assistance Dogs, and the legal rights of people with disabilities partnered with Assistance Dogs, setting standards and establishing guidelines and ethics for the training of these dogs, and improving the utilization and bonding of each team.

### ★ 20886 ★ Associated Blind

110 William St., 9th Fl.
New York, NY 10011
**Phone:** (212)766-6800     **Fax:** (212)766-6809
**Email:** MemberServices@eSightCareers.net
**Website:** http://www.tabinc.org
Ruth-Ellen Simmonds, Exec. Dir.
**Fnded:** 1938. **Reg. Groups:** 1. **Local Groups:** 1. **Desc:** Individuals with an interest in people with blindness or visual disabilities. Seeks to advance the independence and social and economic acceptance of people with visual disabilities and the blind. Identifies the needs and develops practical solutions to problems faced by people with visual disabilities; conducts career preparedness programs; provides support and

assistance to entrepreunuerial ventures operated by or employing people with visual disabilities. **Pub:** *TAB News*, weekly. • *Volunteer News*, monthly.

### ★ 20887 ★ Associated Services for the Blind (ASB)

919 Walnut St.
Philadelphia, PA 19107
**Phone:** (215)627-0600     **Fax:** (215)922-0692
**Email:** asbinfo@libertynet.org
**Website:** http://www.asb.org/
Patricia C. Johnson, Chief Exec. Officer
**Fnded:** 1984. **Desc:** Multiservice agency that provides services to blind and visually impaired people. Objective is to help blind and visually impaired people live independently. Activities include: operating a braille printing house that transcribes print materials into braille; radio reading service that reads newspapers and magazines over closed-circuit radio. Offers rehabilitation program, social services, and recorded periodicals. **Pub:** *ASB Visions*, 3/year. Newsletter. • *Annual Report*, annual. Reports on services, board, financials. • Brochure.

### Association for the Advancement of Blind and Retarded (AABR)
*See:* Entry 6868

### ★ 20888 ★ Association of African Optometric Educators (AAOE)

Morny Optical Centre
PO Box 1814
Kumasi, Ghana
**Phone:** 233 51 22511     **Fax:** 233 51 25306
**Email:** blm@aabr.org
**Website:** http://aabr.org
**Lang(s):** English. **Desc:** Optometry educators. Seeks to advance optometric scholarship and practice. Sponsors training programs for optometric personnel; makes available continuing professional development courses for members.

### ★ 20889 ★ Association of Blind and Partially Sighted Teachers and Students

BM Box 6727
London WC1N 3XX, United Kingdom
**Fnded:** 1970. **Mem:** 350. **Nat'l Groups:** 1. **Desc:** Visually impaired teachers, trainers, students, people looking for work or who have an interest in education. Provides mutual support through the exchange of ideas and experience of education and employment, promotes the needs and strengths of visually impaired teachers and students, and campaigns on relevant issues. **Pub:** *ABAPSTS Bulletin*, monthly. Bulletin. Features education employment issues.

### ★ 20890 ★ Association of Blind Piano Tuners (ABPT)

24 Fairlawn Grove
Chiswick
London W4 5EH, United Kingdom
**Phone:** 44 20 89950295     **Fax:** 44 20 87422396
**Email:** abpt@uk-piano.org
**Website:** http://www.uk-piano.org/abpt/
**Mem:** 110. **Desc:** Serves the professional and particular needs of blind and partially sighted piano tuners.

### ★ 20891 ★ Association for Education and Rehabilitation of the Blind and Visually Impaired (AERBVI)

4600 Duke St., Ste. 430
Alexandria, VA 22304-9239
**Phone:** (703)823-9690     **Fax:** (703)823-9695
**Email:** aer@aerbvi.org
**Website:** http://www.aerbvi.org
Mark Richert, Exec. Dir.
**Fnded:** 1984. **Mem:** 5,500. **State Groups:** 44. **Desc:** Provides support and assistance to professionals

"who work in all phases of education and rehabilitation of blind and visually impaired persons of all ages." **Pub:** *AER Report*, bimonthly. Newsletter. For professionals in the field of service to blind and visually impaired persons; includes legislative and membership news. *Price:* Included in membership dues. • *Association for Education and Rehabilitation of the Blind and Visually Impaired–Job Exchange*, monthly. Bulletin. Lists job openings in the field of services to blind and visually impaired children and and adults. *Price:* Free to members for first 6 months. • *Careers Video*. Videos. • *Don't Settle for Just a Job: Choose a Career*, quarterly. Brochures. • *Re:View*, quarterly. Journal.

### ★ 20892 ★ Association of European Schools and Colleges of Optometry

134, rte de Chartres
F- 91440 Bures-sur-Yvette, France
**Phone:** 33 4 69076737     **Fax:** 33 4 69287806
**Fnded:** 1979.

### ★ 20893 ★ Association for Macular Diseases (AMD)

210 E 64th St., 8th Fl.
New York, NY 10021
**Phone:** (212)605-3719     **Fax:** (212)605-3795
**Email:** association@retinalresearch.org
**Website:** http://www.macula.org/
Nikolai Stevenson, Pres.
**Fnded:** 1977. **Mem:** 8,000. **Desc:** Individuals afflicted with macular diseases, and their families. (The macula of the eye is the posterior middle portion of the retina responsible for central vision. Disorders involving the macula include inflammations, tumors, retinal growths, and degenerative problems.) Purposes are to: disseminate information on available resources such as recorded material and low vision aids; promote public awareness of macular diseases; encourage growth of research into the causes, treatment, and possible prevention of macular diseases; inform the public of the need for postmortem donation of eyes having a history of macular disease and advise on procedures for making such a donation. Provides counseling programs and group sharing for afflicted persons and their families. **Pub:** *Eyes Only*, quarterly. Newsletter. *Price:* $20. **Frmly:** Association for Mascular Degeneration.

### ★ 20894 ★ Association of Optometric Educators (AOE)

NSU College of Optometry
1001 N Grand Ave.
Tahlequah, OK 74464-7017
**Phone:** (918)456-5511     **Fax:** (918)458-2104
**Website:** http://www.nsuok.edu
Dr. George Foster, Dean
**Fnded:** 1972. **Mem:** 100. **Desc:** Teachers in schools and colleges of optometry. Works to enhance the professional and academic status and conditions of service of optometric educators and to promote communication among members. Concerned with faculty welfare, faculty-administration relations, faculty-student relations, and faculty-professional relations.

### ★ 20895 ★ Association of Optometrists

61 Southwark St.
London SE1 0HL, United Kingdom
**Phone:** 44 20 72619661     **Fax:** 44 20 72610228
**Email:** postbox@assoc-optometrists.org
**Website:** http://www.assoc-optometrists.org
**Fnded:** 1946. **Mem:** 7,000. **Desc:** Optometrists and dispensing opticians and students. Aims to support, promote and protect interests of members individually and corporately; to encourage high standards of practice; to make suitable arrangements for the defence of members in disciplinary and professional matters. Advises on commercial, legal and administrative aspects of practice. **Pub:** *Optometry Today*. Journal.

**★ 20896 ★ Association Professionelle des Opticiens et Optometristes de Belgique**
rue Capitaine Crespel 26
B-1050 Brussels, Belgium
**Phone:** 32 2 5125526 **Fax:** 32 2 5023402
**Email:** apob@apob.be
**Website:** http://www.apob.be
**Fnded:** 1923. **Desc:** Promotes the profession of optometry. Provides educational opportunities for optometrists.

**★ 20897 ★ Association of Regulatory Boards of Optometry (ARBO)**
4340 East West Hwy., Ste. 1010
Bethesda, MD 20814
**Phone:** (301)913-0641 **Fax:** (301)986-1150
**Email:** arbo@arbo.org
**Website:** http://www.arbo.org
Jonette Cahoon Vaughan, Programs Coord.
**Fnded:** 1919. **Mem:** 56. **Nat'l Groups:** 4. **State Groups:** 50. **Desc:** ARBO's members are North American regulatory boards of optometry; our mission is to represent and assist member licensing agencies in regulating the practice of optometry for the public welfare. **Pub:** *ARBO Greensheet*, 3/year. Newsletter. • *Directory of Boards of Optometry*, annual. Directory. Lists members of state boards with addresses and phone/fax. *Price:* $50/copy. **Frmly:** (1999) International Association of Boards of Examiners in Optometry.

**★ 20898 ★ Association for Research in Vision and Ophthalmology (ARVO)**
12300 Twinbrook Parkway, Ste. 250
Rockville, MD 20852-1606
**Phone:** (240)221-2900 **Fax:** (240)221-0370
**Email:** mem@arvo.org
**Website:** http://www.arvo.org
Joanne G. Angle, Exec. Dir.
**Fnded:** 1928. **Mem:** 10,800. **Desc:** Professional society of researchers in vision and ophthalmology. To encourage ophthalmic research in the field of blinding eye disease. Administers Scientific Review Fight for Sight/Prevent Blindness America research program. Operates placement service. Maintains 13 scientific sections. **Pub:** *Abstract Book*, annual. Journal. Supplement to investigative ophthalmology and visual science. *Price:* $50 for nonmembers. • *ARVO Membership Directory*, annual. Directory. *Price:* $20. • *ARVO Newsletter*, biennial. Newsletter. *Price:* Free. • *Investigative Ophthalmology and Visual Science*, 13/year. Includes announcements and information for authors. *Price:* Included in membership dues for qualified members. • Also publishes membership brochure; makes available posters. **Frmly:** (1970) Association for Research in Ophthalmology.

**★ 20899 ★ Association of Schools and Colleges of Optometry (ASCO)**
6110 Executive Blvd., Ste. 510
Rockville, MD 20852
**Phone:** (301)231-5944 **Fax:** (301)770-1828
**Email:** mwall@opted.org
**Website:** http://www.opted.org
Martin A. Wall, CAE, Exec. Dir.
**Fnded:** 1941. **Mem:** 19. **Desc:** Committed to achieving excellence in optometric education and to helping its member schools prepare well-qualified graduates for entrance into the profession of optometry. Mission is to serve the American public through the continued advancement and promotion of all aspects of academic optometry. **Pub:** *Eye on Education*, quarterly. Newsletter. Reports on association and member news. • *Faculty Data Report*, annual. Report. A survey report. • *Faculty Directory*. Directory. • *Optometric Education*, quarterly. Journal. • *Residency*. Directory.

**★ 20900 ★ Association of Technical Personnel in Ophthalmology (ATPO)**
2025 Woodlane Dr.
Saint Paul, MN 55125
**Phone:** (651)731-7239 **Fax:** (651)731-0410

**Email:** atpomembership@jcahpo.org
**Website:** http://www.atpo.org
Jennifer Anderson Warwick, Mgr.
**Fnded:** 1969. **Mem:** 1,200. **Nat'l Groups:** 1. **State Groups:** 4. **Desc:** Ophthalmic assistants, technicians, technologists, surgical and keratorefractive techs, photographers, nurses, and orthoptists. Promotes high standards and professional ethics dedicated to quality ophthalmic medical care under the direction of an ophthalmologist. Recognizes the utilization of ophthalmalic medical personnel to perform certain non-medical procedures or tests as a means of enhancing the productivity of ophthalmologists and thereby increasing the availability of ophthalmologists to provide the highest level of medical service and comprehensive vision care to their patients. **Pub:** *Viewpoints*, quarterly. Newsletter. *Price:* Free for members. **Frmly:** (1989) American Association of Certified Allied Health Personnel in Ophthalmology.

**★ 20901 ★ Association of University Professors of Ophthalmology (AUPO)**
PO Box 420369
San Francisco, CA 94142-0369
**Phone:** (415)561-8548 **Fax:** (415)561-8531
**Email:** aupo@aao.org
Steve M. Podos, MD, Exec. VP
**Fnded:** 1966. **Mem:** 246. **Desc:** Heads of departments or divisions of ophthalmology in accredited medical schools throughout the U.S. and Canada; directors of ophthalmology residency programs in institutions not connected to medical schools. Promotes medical education, research, and patient care relating to ophthalmology. Operates Ophthalmology Matching Program and faculty placement service, which aids ophthalmologists interested in being associated with university ophthalmology programs to locate such programs. **Pub:** *News & Views*, quarterly. • Membership Directory, annual.

**Association of Visually Impaired Chartered Physiotherapists**
*See:* Entry 19146

**★ 20902 ★ Bates Association for Vision Education**
PO Box 25
Shoreham-by-Sea BN43 6ZF, United Kingdom
**Phone:** 44 1273 422090 **Fax:** 44 1273 1279983
**Email:** bave@seeing.org
**Website:** http://www.seeing.org
**Fnded:** 1954. **Mem:** 35. **Lang(s):** English. **Desc:** Teachers of Bates Method vision education. To advance the knowledge and practice of vision education. **Pub:** *Seeing*, quarterly. Journal. • *Vision Education News*, quarterly. Newsletter. **Frmly:** (1989) London Association of Eyesight Training; (1999) Bates Association of Great Britain.

**★ 20903 ★ Better Vision Institute (BVI)**
1700 Diagonal Rd., Ste. 500
Alexandria, VA 22314
**Phone:** (703)548-4560 **Free:** 877-642-3253
**Fax:** (703)548-4580
**Email:** vca@visionsite.org
**Website:** http://www.visionsite.org
Richard L. Elias, Exec. VP
**Fnded:** 1929. **Mem:** 500. **Desc:** Advisory council of the Vision Council of America. Carried out in consultation with a board of eye care professionals who inform the public of the need for more adequate vision care. **Pub:** *BVI News Bureau*, periodic. Contains press releases of various eyecare and eyewear information. *Price:* Free. • *Perspective*. Article. • Pamphlets. • Also publishes charts, posters, and press releases; produces school kits and counter displays for vision care practitioners, schools, and the public.

**★ 20904 ★ Blind Children's Fund (BCF)**
4740 Okemos Rd.
Okemos, MI 48864-1459

**Phone:** (517)347-1357 **Fax:** (517)347-1459
**Email:** blindchildren@aol.com
**Website:** http://www.blindchildrensfund.org
Karla B. Storrer, Exec. Dir.
**Fnded:** 1978. **Mem:** 1,300. **Reg. Groups:** 1. **Desc:** Parents and teachers of visually handicapped children from birth to seven years old. Provides parents and professionals information, materials, and resources that help them successfully teach and nurture blind, visually impaired and multi-impaired children. **Pub:** *Get A Wiggle On*. Booklet. For parents of blind or visually impaired infants with suggestions for assisting development form birth to the walking stage. *Price:* $5. • *Get Ready. . .Get Set. . .Go!* Teaches techniques for the parent or educator of the blind child, focusing on self-help skills. *Price:* $7. • *Learning to Look.* Book. For parents of severely visually impaired children. Contains specific suggestions on how to help your child use what vision she/he has or may have. *Price:* $9. • *Move It.* Booklet. Contains suggestions for the development of a preschool blind or visually impaired child from walking to school entrance age. *Price:* $5. • *Movement Education.* A movement curriculum for preschoolers. *Price:* $13. • *Parent Packet #1.* Booklet. Includes activities to teach skills at home, toys to make, how to stimulate language, and readings on blindness for parents and children. *Price:* $7. • *Our Kids Are Great!.* Parents of visually impaired children share short stories about what their children can do because of their help, love, and attention. *Price:* $3. • *VIP Newsletter*, quarterly. Newsletter. Contains information and articles for parents of blind or visually impaired children. *Price:* $10/year; $15/year outside of US. • *Watch Me Grow.* Book. Contains month by month suggestions for assisting the development of a blind or visually impaired infant from birth to age three. *Price:* $12. **Frmly:** (1987) International Institute for Visually Impaired.

**★ 20905 ★ Blind Citizens Australia (BCA)**
87 High St.
Prahran, VIC 3181, Australia
**Phone:** 61 3 95213433 **Fax:** 61 3 95213732
**Email:** bca@bca.org.au
**Website:** http://www.bca.org.au
**Fnded:** 1975. **Mem:** 3,000. **Lang(s):** English. **Desc:** Blind and vision impaired people in Australia. Seeks to achieve equity and equality by empowering members, by promoting positive community attitudes, and by striving for high quality and accessible services. Provides advocacy, information dissemination, peer support, and consultancy and advice to governments, corporations and the community.

**★ 20906 ★ Blind Service Association (BSA)**
22 W Monroe, 11th Fl.
Chicago, IL 60603
**Phone:** (312)236-0808 **Fax:** (312)236-8679
**Email:** blindsrvc@aol.com
Debbie Grossman, Exec. Dir.
**Fnded:** 1924. **Mem:** 550. **Desc:** Organization that has supported the independence of blind and partially blind Chicago residents since 1924. The association maintains reading rooms for daily oral readings of textbooks and work-related material primarily to blind students, senior citizens, and business and professional people; records textbooks on cassette tapes for blind people's home, study, work and leisure needs; supplies visual aids, field trips, and other assistance to blind and visually handicapped children in Chicago, IL schools; operates senior program and a consortium of blind computer users.

**★ 20907 ★ Blinded Veterans Association (BVA)**
477 H St. NW
Washington, DC 20001
**Phone:** (202)371-8880 **Free:** 800-669-7079
**Fax:** (202)371-8258
**Email:** bva@bva.org
**Website:** http://www.bva.org
Thomas H. Miller, Exec. Dir.

**Fnded:** 1945. **Mem:** 9,600. **Reg. Groups:** 51. **Desc:** Veterans who lost their sight as a result of military service in the armed forces of the U.S.; associate members are veterans whose loss of sight was not connected with military service. Assists blinded veterans in attaining benefits and employment and with reestablishing themselves as adjusted, active, and productive citizens in their communities. Offers placement service; supports research programs; compiles statistics. **Pub:** *BVA Bulletin*, bimonthly. Newsletter. Reports on legislation, benefits, and Department of Veterans Affairs programs affecting blind veterans; also includes association news. *Price:* Free to blind veterans.


★ **20908** ★ **Braille Authority of North America (BANA)**
919 Walnut St.
Philadelphia, PA 19107
**Phone:** (215)627-0600          **Free:** 800-223-1839
**Fax:** (215)922-0692
**Email:** dfgodz@asb.org
**Website:** http://www.brailleauthority.org/
Eileen Curran, Chairperson

**Fnded:** 1976. **Mem:** 12. **Desc:** Braille publishers, producers, and transcribers; representatives of consumer groups; educators of the visually handicapped; professional organizations. To promote and facilitate the use, teaching, and production of braille texts and other braille items. Promulgates rules, makes interpretations, and renders opinions concerning literary and technical braille codes and related forms and formats of embossed materials for the blind. **Pub:** *Braille Textbook Code Formats and Techniques*. Book. • *English Braille, American Edition*. • *Learning the Nemeth Code*. • *Nemeth Code of Braille Mathematics and Scientific Notation*. • Directory, annual.


★ **20909** ★ **Braille Foundation of Uruguay (Fundacion Braille del Uruguay — FBU)**
Durazno 1772
Blanes 1132
11200 Montevideo, Uruguay
**Phone:** 598 2 4095943          **Fax:** 598 2 4000789
**Email:** fbu@fbraille.com.uy
**Website:** http://www.fbraille.com.uy

**Fnded:** 1978. **Lang(s):** English, Spanish. **Desc:** Braille publishers, producers, transcribers, and others with an interest in the production of reading materials for the blind. Promotes the use, teaching, and production of braille texts and other braille items. Works to insure availability of braille materials nationwide.


★ **20910** ★ **Braille Revival League (BRL)**
57 Grandview Ave.
Watertown, MA 02472
**Phone:** (617)926-9198          **Free:** 800-424-8666
**Fax:** (617)923-0004
**Email:** kimcharlson@earthlink.net
Kim Charlson, Contact

**Fnded:** 1981. **Mem:** 1,000. **State Groups:** 6. **Desc:** Blind and visually impaired persons; professionals interested in promoting the use, production, and teaching of Braille. Encourages blind people to read and write in Braille; advocates the mandatory use of Braille instruction in educational facilities for the blind; promotes use of Braille material available through libraries and printing houses. Lends support to the Braille Authority of North America. Conducts research into Braille efficiency. **Pub:** *BRL Memorandum*, quarterly. Newsletter. Volumes are in Braille, large print, and computer diskette.


★ **20911** ★ **British Association of Behavioral Optometrists**
Greygarth
Littleworth
Winchcombe
Cheltenham GL54 5BT, United Kingdom
**Phone:** 44 1242 602689     **Fax:** 44 1242 602689
**Email:** greygarth@compuserve.com
**Website:** http://www.babo.co.uk

**Fnded:** 1990. **Mem:** 93. **Reg. Groups:** 6. **Desc:** Seeks to improve understanding of Behavioral Optometry, through continuing education and training and by providing an accredited list of trained optometrists.


★ **20912** ★ **British Computer Association of the Blind (BDS)**
BM Box 950
London WC1N 3XX, United Kingdom
**Email:** info@bcab.org.uk
**Website:** http://www.bcab.org.uk

**Fnded:** 1969. **Mem:** 230. **Desc:** Provides general assistance and advice on information technology issues for blind and visually impaired persons. Organizes training courses. Engages in lobbying. **Pub:** Newsletter, quarterly.


★ **20913** ★ **British Orthoptic Society**
Tavistock House North
Tavistock Sq.
London WC1H 9HX, United Kingdom
**Phone:** 44 207 3877992     **Fax:** 44 207 3832584
**Email:** bos@orthoptics.org.uk
**Website:** http://www.orthoptics.org.uk

**Fnded:** 1937. **Mem:** 1,200. **Desc:** Orthoptists, including students and retired orthoptists. Members work in both NHS and private practice. **Pub:** *British Orthoptic Journal*, annual. Journal.


★ **20914** ★ **British Retinitis Pigmentosa Society**
PO Box 350
Buckingham MK18 1GZ, United Kingdom
**Phone:** 44 1280 821334     **Fax:** 44 1280 815900
**Email:** lynda@brps.demon.co.uk
**Website:** http://www.brps.demon.co.uk

**Fnded:** 1976. **Mem:** 3,000. **Desc:** RP sufferers and their families and interested multidisciplinary members. Aims to help RP sufferers and their families cope with living with RP and to raise money for medical research. **Pub:** Handbook, annual. • Newsletter, quarterly.


★ **20915** ★ **Bulgarian Society of Opthalmology**
c/o Eye Clinic, Fifth City Clinical Hospital
Stolebov 67 - A
1233 Sofia, Bulgaria
**Phone:** 359 2 9268195          **Fax:** 359 2 9808546
**Email:** bso_pashev@excite.com

**Fnded:** 1927. **Mem:** 600. **Local Groups:** 5. **Lang(s):** English, French, Russian. **Desc:** Ophthalmologists. Fosters research in fundamental ophtalmic studies. **Pub:** *Bulgarian Review of Opthalmology*, 3/year. Magazine.


★ **20916** ★ **Canadian Association of Optometrists (CAO)**
234 Argyle Ave.
Ottawa, ON, Canada K2P 1B9
**Phone:** (613)235-7924          **Fax:** (613)235-2025
**Email:** reception@opto.ca
**Website:** http://www.opto.ca

**Fnded:** 1948. **Mem:** 3,100. **Reg. Groups:** 10. **Lang(s):** English, French. **Desc:** Optometrists, educators, and students. Promotes professional advancement of members and improvement in the teaching and practice of optometry. Conducts research and educational programs; compiles statistics. **Pub:** *CJO*, quarterly. Journal. • *FYI*, quarterly. Newsletter. • Directory, annual.


★ **20917** ★ **Canadian Council of the Blind (CCB) (Conseil Canadien des Aveugles — CCA)**
396 Cooper St., Ste. 401
Ottawa, ON, Canada K2P 2H7
**Phone:** (613)567-0311          **Free:** 877-304-0968
**Fax:** (613)567-2728
**Email:** ccb@ccbnational.net

**Website:** http://www.ccbnational.net

**Fnded:** 1944. **Mem:** 4,000. **Local Groups:** 95. **Lang(s):** English, French. **Desc:** National consumer organization representing legally blind and vision impaired individuals in Canada. Offers support through social and recreational activities. Represents members' interests in relation to government, business and industry. **Pub:** *CCB Newsletter*, monthly. Newsletter.


★ **20918** ★ **Canadian Guide Dogs for the Blind (Chiens Guides Canadiens pour Aveugles)**
PO Box 280
4120 Rideau Valley Dr. N
Manotick, ON, Canada K4M 1A3
**Phone:** (613)692-7777          **Fax:** (613)692-0650
**Email:** cgdb@sympatico.ca
**Website:** http://www.guidedogs.ca

**Fnded:** 1984. **Lang(s):** English, French. **Desc:** Works to assist visually impaired Canadians with their mobility by providing and training them in the use of professionally trained guide dogs.


★ **20919** ★ **Canadian National Institute for the Blind (CNIB) (L'Institut National Canadien pour les Aveugles — INCA)**
1929 Bayview Ave.
Toronto, ON, Canada M4G 3E8
**Phone:** (416)480-2500          **Free:** 800-513-7813
**Fax:** (416)480-7453
**Website:** http://www.cnib.ca

**Fnded:** 1918. **Mem:** 100,000. **Nat'l Groups:** 2. **Reg. Groups:** 9. **Local Groups:** 57. **Lang(s):** English, French. **Desc:** Rehabilitation organizations serving people with visual impairment. Seeks to improve the quality of life of people with visual impairment and their families. Promotes full integration of people with visual impairment into Canadian society. Makes available support and assistance to people with visual impairment; conducts educational programs. **Pub:** *Vision Magazine*, semiannual. Magazine. Provides publications in braille, on tape, and in large print.


★ **20920** ★ **Canadian Ophthalmological Society (COS) (Societe Canadienne d'Ophthalmologie — SCO)**
1525 Carling Ave., Ste. 610
Ottawa, ON, Canada K1Z 8R9
**Phone:** (613)729-6779          **Free:** 800-267-5763
**Fax:** (613)729-7209
**Email:** cos@eyesite.ca
**Website:** http://www.eyesite.ca

**Fnded:** 1937. **Mem:** 950. **Nat'l Groups:** 1. **Lang(s):** English, French. **Desc:** Ophthalmologists and ophthalmology students. Seeks to advance the study and practice of ophthalmology. Facilitates exchange of information among members; sponsors research and educational programs. **Pub:** *Canadian Journal of Ophthalmology*, 7/year. Journal.


★ **20921** ★ **Canadian Orthoptic Council (COC) (Conseil Canadien d'Orthoptique — CCO)**
506 71st Ave. SW, Ste. 5
Calgary, AB, Canada T2V 4V4
**Phone:** (403)253-6700          **Fax:** (403)253-2102

**Lang(s):** English, French. **Desc:** Health care professionals specializing in orthoptics and occular surgery. Seeks to advance the study and practice of orthoptics. Serves as a forum for the exchange of information among members; sponsors research and educational programs.


★ **20922** ★ **Care Ministries**
PO Box 1830
Starkville, MS 39760-1830
**Phone:** (662)323-4999          **Free:** 800-336-2232

**Email:** care@careministries.org
**Website:** http://www.careministries.org/
B.J. LeJeune, Dir.

**Fnded:** 1989. **Desc:** Provides information, spiritual support, community resources to blind and visually impaired. **Pub:** *Our Daily Bread*, monthly. Devotional and the Evangelical Sunday School Teachers Edition of lessons on cassette tape. • Catalog.Cassette catalog containing a variety of Christian materials, Bible studies and publications on cassette tape.

★ **20923** ★ **Carroll Center for the Blind (CCB)**
770 Centre St.
Newton, MA 02458
**Phone:** (617)969-6200          **Free:** 800-852-3131
**Fax:** (617)969-6204
**Email:** intake@carroll.org
**Website:** http://www.carroll.org
Rev. Thomas J. Carroll, Founder

**Fnded:** 1936. **Desc:** Rehabilitation center that specializes in services for adults ages 16 and up who have become blind. Provides programs for resident and commuter clients. Offers diagnostic evaluation, personal adjustment training, low vision, and children's services. Trains professionals in work with the blind through supervision of student internships and seminars for workers in the field. Maintains information and referral service. Offers computer training in specialized access devices for blind and job training. Operates charitable program. Manages statewide materials center of books in braille and large print, books for ages Kindergarten through 12th grade. **Pub:** *Blindess: What It Is, What It Does, and How to Live With It. Price:* $15. • *Carroll Center for the Blind–Focus*, semiannual. Newsletter. Covers membership activities. Includes information for donors and new program information. *Price:* Free. • *Computer Access, Resource Manual. Price:* $20. • *Educational Software, Compiled Listing. Price:* $5. • *Facing the Wind. Price:* $25. • *Mapping. Price:* $15. • *Medical Transcription Training Manual. Price:* 125. • *Resource Manual for Teaching Blind Persons to Use Computers*, annual. *Price:* $20/year; $10 for tape. • *Selected Exercises in Sensory Training. Price:* $15. • *Sensory Training, Principles of. Price:* $15. • *Videation and Spatial Orientation, Vols. I & II. Price:* $50. **Frmly:** (1972) Catholic Guild for All the Blind; (1974) Carroll Rehabilitation Center for the Visually Impaired.

★ **20924** ★ **Catholic Association of Persons With Visual Impairment (CAPVI)**
c/o Msgr. Paul M. Lackner
Catholic Guild for the Blind
Cardinal Dearden Center
4721 Fifth Ave.
Pittsburgh, PA 15213
**Phone:** (412)687-1409          **Fax:** (412)826-8377
Msgr. Paul Lackner, Pres.

**Fnded:** 1984. **Mem:** 150. **Desc:** To assist, support, and further the vocational, spiritual, and social integration of blind and visually impaired persons in local parishes and in the community. CAPVI focuses on: raising awareness of the ability and spiritual needs, promotes active participation in the spiritual and social life of the church and within the community; exchanges ideas, resources and other pertinent information, assists in obtaining religious material in accessible format; and works toward establishing programs within dioceses to serve this group. activities; instructs volunteers to act as guides. Assists in obtaining audiotapes and religious materials printed in braille and large type. large type. A national CAPVI office is open in New York City. **Pub:** *CAPVI Newsletter*, quarterly. Newsletter. Contains information regarding visually impaired persons active in the life of the church. Printed in large type, cassettes and braile upon request. *Price:* Free.

★ **20925** ★ **Challenge Aspen at Snowmass**
PO Box M
Aspen, CO 81612-9119
**Phone:** (970)923-0578          **Fax:** (970)923-7338
**Email:** possibilities@challengeaspen.com
**Website:** http://www.challengeaspen.com
Sarah Williams, Prog. Dir.

**Fnded:** 1995. **Desc:** Persons with a physical or mental disability. Assists in appreciating outdoor recreation. Operates on the "can-do" theory for people. Provides volunteer guides to help enjoy the outdoors by skiing, skating, hiking, fishing, horseback riding, swimming, and biking. Designs and conducts training courses for activity leaders in downhill skiing. **Frmly:** (2000) Blind Outdoor Leisure Development; (2000) BOLD/Challenge Aspen.

★ **20926** ★ **China Optometric and Optical Association (COOA)**
No. 6, East Changan St.
Beijing 100740, People's Republic of China
**Phone:** 86 10 63022411          **Fax:** 86 10 63185325
**Email:** optics@public.bta.net.cn
**Website:** http://www.chinaoptics.com

**Fnded:** 1985. **Lang(s):** English. **Desc:** Manufacturers, optometrists, research institutes, and other companies and organizations within the optical industry. Represents and promotes the optical industry in China. **Pub:** *China Glasses Science and Technology*. Magazine.

★ **20927** ★ **Christian Blind Mission International (CBMI)**
450 E Park Ave.
PO Box 19000
Greenville, SC 29601
**Phone:** (864)239-0065          **Free:** 800-YES-CBMI
**Fax:** (864)239-0069
**Email:** info@cbmi-usa.org
**Website:** http://www.cbmi-usa.org/
Alan Harkey, Dir.

**Fnded:** 1908. **Mem:** 7. **Nat'l Groups:** 12. **Desc:** Interdenominational Christian organization dedicated to service of the blind, visually impaired, and physically handicapped in more than 100 countries. Supports national activities of missions, churches, and voluntary organizations in developing countries with financial aid to cover operational expenses and the provision of equipment, drugs, medicines, and instruments. Fosters prevention of visually disabling ailments such as glaucoma, trachoma, and blinding cataracts. Assists in education and rehabilitation of all disabled indiviudals through establishment of vocational training centers and a corps of community volunteers to coordinate and stimulate project participation. Contributes to international efforts in the battle against blindness; conducts research on onchocerciasis, xerophthalmia, and glaucoma. Sponsors rural education programs on personal and environmental hygiene and nutrition. **Pub:** *CBMI Report*, annual. Report. • *Human Interest Stories*, monthly. • *Light*, quarterly. Newsletter.

★ **20928** ★ **Christian Record Services (CRS)**
4444 S 52nd St.
Lincoln, NE 68516-1302
**Phone:** (402)488-0981          **Fax:** (402)488-7582
**Email:** info@christianrecord.org
**Website:** http://www.christianrecord.org
Ron Bowes, Contact

**Fnded:** 1899. **Desc:** Assists blind, visually impaired individuals. Sponsors Bible correspondence courses. Representatives visit about 40,000 blind people annually. Conducts glaucoma screening clinics in cooperation with local physicians and organizations; provides home visitation program. Sponsors National Camps for Blind Children; maintains speakers' bureau. **Pub:** *Christian Record*, quarterly. In braille; for adults. • *Christian Record Talking Magazine*, quarterly. Magazine. On cassette; for adults. • *Encounter*, bimonthly. On cassette; for late teens and adults. • *Lifeglow*, quarterly. In large print; for adults. • *The Student*, monthly. In braille and on cassette. • *Young and Alive*, quarterly. In braille and large print; for teenagers/ young adults. • Also publishes braille cards. **Frmly:** Christian Record Benevolent Association; (1989) Christian Record Braille Foundation.

★ **20929** ★ **Christian Services for the Blind**
1124 Fair Oaks
PO Box 26
South Pasadena, CA 91031
**Phone:** (626)799-3935          **Fax:** (626)403-9460
**Email:** frank@csbonline.org
**Website:** http://www.csbonline.org
Frank Tucker, Contact

**Fnded:** 1949. **Nat'l Groups:** 1. **Local Groups:** 1. **Desc:** Makes available books on cassette for blind and braille books for deaf-blind individuals. **Pub:** *Bartimaeus Review*, 3/year. Newsletter. *Price:* Free. **Frmly:** Christian Fellowship for the Blind.

★ **20930** ★ **Christoffel Blindenmission (CBM)**
Nibelungenstr. 124
D-64625 Bensheim, Germany
**Phone:** 49 6251 131131          **Fax:** 49 6251 131122
**Email:** overseas@cbm-i.org
**Website:** http://www.christoffel-blindenmission.de

**Fnded:** 1908. **Mem:** 60. **Lang(s):** English, French, German, Spanish. **Desc:** Seeks to prevent and cure blindness and improve the quality of life for blind and partially sighted people. Represents the interests of visually impaired people; works to combat discrimination. Seeks to educate and rehabilitate blind and other handicapped persons. **Pub:** *Fam.-Album*, bimonthly. Newsletter. • *Light*, bimonthly. Newsletter. • Report, periodic. **Frmly:** Christian Blind Mission International.

★ **20931** ★ **College of Opticians of Chile (COC)**
**(Colegio de Opticos de Chile — COC)**
Casilla 53542
Santiago, Chile

**Lang(s):** English, Spanish. **Desc:** Opticians and opticianry students and educators. Seeks to advance the study, teaching, and practice of opticianry; promotes continuing professional development of members. Serves as a forum for the exchange of information among members; sponsors research and educational programs.

★ **20932** ★ **College of Optometrists**
42 Craven St.
London WC2N 5NG, United Kingdom
**Phone:** 44 207 8396000          **Fax:** 44 207 8396800
**Email:** optometry@college-optometrists.org
**Website:** http://www.college-optometrists.org

**Fnded:** 1980. **Mem:** 10,560. **Desc:** Consists of Fellows and Members, both home and overseas, Associate Members who do not hold full qualifications, non-practising Fellows, Honorary and Life Fellows. Concerned with the improvement and conservation of human vision, advancement for the public benefit of the study of and research into optometry and publication of the results, promotion of the science and practice of optometry and encouragement of the highest possible standards of professional competence and conduct for the public benefit. **Pub:** *Ophthalmic and Physiological Optics*, bimonthly. **Frmly:** British College of Optometrists.

★ **20933** ★ **College of Optometrists in Vision Development (COVD)**
243 N Lindbergh Blvd., Ste. 310
Saint Louis, MO 63141
**Phone:** (314)991-4007          **Free:** 888-COVD-770
**Fax:** (314)991-1167
**Email:** info@covd.org
**Website:** http://www.covd.org
Stephen C. Miller, O.D., Exec. Dir.

**Fnded:** 1970. **Mem:** 1,600. **Reg. Groups:** 3. **State Groups:** 50. **Desc:** Optometrists involved in orthoptics and optometric vision therapy with emphasis on visual information processing in visually related learning problems. Seeks to establish a body of practitioners who are knowledgeable in functional and developmental concepts of vision, to insure that the public will receive continually improving vision care; to promote, foster, and engage in interdisciplinary cooperation; to enable members to maintain the highest standards of professional knowledge and competency; to educate and encourage optometrists to qualify for membership and fellowship in the college; to certify optometrists skilled in this specialty. Conducts national educational programs and public information programs. **Pub:** *College of Optometrists in Vision Development–Membership Directory*, annual. Directory. Listings of associate and fellow members. *Price:* Included in membership dues; $3.50/copy for nonmembers. • *Journal of Optometric Vision Development*, quarterly. *Price:* $55/year. • *Visions Newsletter*, bimonthly. Newsletter. *Price:* Included in membership dues. • Brochures. • Monographs. • Also publishes research reviews.

★ **20934** ★ **Commission on Opticianry Accreditation (COA)**
PO Box 3073
Merrifield, VA 22116-3073
**Email:** coa@erols.com
**Website:** http://www.coaccreditation.com
Amy J. Hammer, Dir. of Accreditation
**Fnded:** 1979. **Mem:** 26. **Desc:** Accrediting agency for ophthalmic dispensing and ophthalmic laboratory technology programs in postsecondary institutions. Conducts an evaluator's workshop to train on-site evaluators. **Pub:** *Accreditation Guide for Laboratory Technician Programs*. Manual. *Price:* $10. • *Accreditation Guide for Ophthalmic Dispensing Programs*. Manual. *Price:* $10. • *Essentials of an Accredited Educational Program for Ophthalmic Laboratory Technician Programs*. Handbook. • *Essentials of an Accredited Educational Program for Opticianry Programs*. Handbook. • *Evaluator's Checklist for Ophthalmic Dispensing Programs*. Manual. • *Evaluator's Checklist for Ophthalmic Laboratory Technology Programs*. Manual. • *Evaluator's Handbook for Ophthalmic Dispensing Programs*. Handbook. • *Evaluator's Handbook for Ophthalmic Laboratory Technology Programs*. Handbook. • *Self-Study Report Format for Ophthalmic Dispensing Programs*. Manual. • *Self-Study Report Format for Ophthalmic Laboratory Technology Program*. Manual.

★ **20935** ★ **Contact Lens Association of Ophthalmologists (CLAO)**
c/o John S. Massare
721 Papworth Ave., Ste. 206
Metairie, LA 70005
**Phone:** (504)835-3937          **Fax:** (504)833-5884
**Email:** eyes@clao.org
**Website:** http://www.clao.org
John S. Massare, PhD, Exec. Dir.
**Fnded:** 1963. **Mem:** 1,700. **Desc:** To advance quality medical eyecare for the public by providing comprehensive ophthalmologists and other eye care professionals with education and training in contact lenses, refractive surgery, and related eyecare science. **Pub:** *CLAO Journal*, quarterly. Journal. • *CLAOgram*, monthly. Bulletin. • *Refractive Trends*, quarterly. Magazine. • *Who's Who in CLAO*, biennial. Membership Directory. *Price:* $24.95 for nonmembers. • Report. • Also publishes Contact Lenses: The CLAO Guide to Basic Science and Clinical practice Third Edition and The CLAO Pocket Guide to Contact Lens Fitting.

★ **20936** ★ **Contact Lens Council (CLC)**
8201 Corporate Dr., Ste. 850
Landover, MD 20785
**Phone:** (301)459-2618          **Fax:** (301)459-1802
**Email:** clc@us.net
**Website:** http://www.contactlenscouncil.org
**Desc:** Working to promote the safe use of contact lenses and provide opportunities for both current and prospective contact lens consumers to learn about the variety of lens options available to meet their vision and lifestyle needs.

★ **20937** ★ **Council of Citizens With Low Vision (CCLV)**
c/o American Council of the Blind
1155 15th St. NW, Ste. 1004
Washington, DC 20005
**Phone:** (202)467-5081          **Free:** 800-733-2258
**Email:** badkron@aol.com
**Website:** http://www.cclvi.org
Ken Stewart, Pres.
**Fnded:** 1978. **Mem:** 2,000. **State Groups:** 11. **Desc:** Partially sighted and low-vision individuals, their families, and professional workers. Provides a vehicle through which partially sighted people may voice their needs, preferences, and interests. Promotes the concept that partially sighted and low-vision individuals are not blind and that they have the right to maximize the use of residual vision through the use of any visual aid, service, or technology. Keeps abreast of all developments benefiting partially sighted persons. Promotes educational, engineering, medical, rehabilitative, scientific, and social research that facilitates the lives of individuals with residual vision. Supports the development of pre-service professional training programs for the establishment and expansion of multidisciplinary low-vision services. Strives to educate the public about the existence, capabilities, and needs of such individuals. Establishes outreach programs to insure access to available services for partially sighted persons. Maintains speakers' bureau. **Pub:** *Vision Access*, quarterly. Newsletter. Reports on research and resources. Available on audiocassete and in large print. *Price:* Included in membership dues.

★ **20938** ★ **Council of Families with Visual Impairment (CFVI)**
c/o American Council of the Blind
1155 15th St. NW, Ste. 1004
Washington, DC 20005
**Phone:** (202)467-5081          **Free:** 800-424-8666
**Fax:** (202)467-5085
**Email:** info@acb.org
**Website:** http://www.acb.org/affiliates/
Roy Ward, Contact
**Fnded:** 1979. **Mem:** 400. **Desc:** Sighted parents of blind and visually impaired children; blind and visually impaired parents, professionals, and interested individuals. Offers forum for support and outreach, sharing of experiences in parent-child relationships, and educational and cultural information about child development. Monitors developments in technical and legislative arenas. **Pub:** *Reflections*, 3/year. Newsletter. Published in large print. *Price:* $6; $8 for tape. **Frmly:** (1990) American Council of the Blind Parents.

★ **20939** ★ **Danish Ophthalmological Society**
**(Dansk Oftalmologisk Selskab)**
Blegdamsvej 9
DK-2100 Copenhagen, Denmark
**Fnded:** 1901.

★ **20940** ★ **DB-Link**
345 N Monmouth Ave.
Monmouth, OR 97361
**Free:** 800-854-7013          **Fax:** (503)838-8150
**Email:** dblink@tr.wou.edu
**Website:** http://www.tr.wou.edu/dblink/
Dr. John Reiman, Dir.
**Fnded:** 1992. **Desc:** Parents, service providers, administrators, and others interested in services. Identifies, coordinated, and disseminates information related to children and youth who are deaf-blind. Collaborative effort of the Helen Keller National Center, Perkins School for the Blind, and Teaching Research of Western Oregon University. **Pub:** *Deaf-Blind Perspectives*, 3/year. Newsletter. Available in standard print, Braille, large print and ASCII. *Price:* Free to subscribers. • Also publishes 10 fact sheets related to deaf-blindness. (7 of which are also in Spanish) Available full text also on web site.

**Deaf-Blind Association**
*See:* Entry 6027

**Deafblind International (Dbl)**
*See:* Entry 6031

**Deafblind UK**
*See:* Entry 6032

★ **20941** ★ **English National Association of Visually Handicapped Bowlers**
18 Hervey St.
Lowestoft NR32 2JG, United Kingdom
**Email:** rwsilson@aol.com
**Website:** http://www.deafblinduk.org.uk
**Fnded:** 1974. **Mem:** 600. **Desc:** Males and females who are visually impaired, and sighted helpers. Promotes bowls throughout the UK and the international arena. **Pub:** Newsletter, quarterly.

★ **20942** ★ **European Association of Universities, Schools and Colleges of Optometry (AEUSCO) (Association Europeenne des Universites Ecoles et Colleges d'Optometrie — AEUSCO)**
134, rte. de Chartres
F-91440 Bures-sur-Yvette, France
**Phone:** 33 1 64861213          **Fax:** 33 1 69284999
**Email:** ico.direction@wanadoo.fr
**Fnded:** 1979. **Mem:** 38. **Lang(s):** English, French. **Desc:** Schools in 16 countries providing education for optometrists and opticians. Promotes the development of optometry in Europe; seeks the standardization of optometric instruction and qualifications on a European level. Encourages cooperation and information exchange among teaching institutions. Compiles scientific and pedagogic documentation concerning optometric education in Europe. **Pub:** Newsletter, semiannual. **Frmly:** (1999) European Association of Schools and Colleges of Optometry.

★ **20943** ★ **European Association for Vision and Eye Research (EVER)**
Postbus 74
B-3000 Leuven, Belgium
**Phone:** 32 1 6336785
**Email:** luc.missotten@uz.kuleuven.ac.be
**Website:** http://www.ever.be/
**Fnded:** 1997. **Desc:** Encourages research and disseminates knowledge concerning eye and vision.

★ **20944** ★ **European Blind Union (EBU) (Union Europeenne des Aveugles — UEA)**
c/o Mokrane Boussaid
58 avenue Bosquet
F-75007 Paris, France
**Phone:** 33 1 47053820          **Fax:** 33 1 47053821
**Email:** ebu_uea@compuserve.com
**Website:** http://www.euroblind.org
**Fnded:** 1984. **Mem:** 44. **Lang(s):** English, French, German. **Desc:** European national associations of/for the blind. Works to enhance the quality of life of blind and visually impaired persons. Fosters equality and full participation of such individuals in society; promotes the prevention of blindness and visual impairment in Europe. Serves as a forum for the exchange of information concerning blindness. Encourages provisions of social rights advocacy and specialized technical aids. **Pub:** *Europa-Cassette: EEC Informations*, 5/year. • *Proceedings*, triennial. • *Review of the European Blind Union*, quarterly.

**★ 20945 ★ European Board of Ophthalmology (EBO)**
40a, av de Verdun
F-94010 Creteil, France
**Phone:** 33 1 45175266 **Fax:** 33 1 45175222
**Email:** 1063752207@compuserve.com
**Fnded:** 1992. **Desc:** Improves the training of ophthalmologists.

**★ 20946 ★ European Centre of Ophthalmology**
99932 Rue du Meridien
B-1030 Brussels, Belgium
**Fnded:** 1990.

**★ 20947 ★ European Contact Lens Society of Ophthalmologists (ECLSO)**
2 Pl. Victor Hugo
F-38000 Grenoble, France
**Phone:** 33 4 76120210 **Fax:** 33 4 76120218
**Email:** eclso@eclso.org
**Website:** http://www.eclso.org
**Fnded:** 1970. **Mem:** 3,000. **State Groups:** 20. **Desc:** Ophthalmologists in Europe. Provides information on contact lenses.

**★ 20948 ★ European Opthalmological Society (EOS)**
Moorfields Eye Hospital
City Rd.
London EC1V 2PD, United Kingdom
**Phone:** 44 171 2533411 **Fax:** 44 171 5662048
**Fnded:** 1956. **Nat'l Groups:** 45. **Lang(s):** English. **Desc:** National associations of ophthalmologists. Seeks to advance ophthalmological research, study, teaching, and practice. Promotes continuing professional development among ophthalmologists. Facilitates exchange of information among members; conducts research and educational programs.

**★ 20949 ★ European Optical Society**
Centre Universitaire, Bat. 503
PO Box 147
F-91403 Orsay Cedex, France
**Phone:** 33 1 6935 8816 **Fax:** 33 1 6985 3565
**Email:** joelle.bourges@iota.u-psud.fr
**Website:** http://www.europeanopticalsociety.org
**Fnded:** 1991. **Mem:** 600. **Desc:** Contributes to programs in optics and related sciences, and to promote their applications at the European and international levels, by bringing together individuals and legal activities involved in these disciplines and their applications.

**European Society of Ophthalmic Plastic and Reconstructive Surgery (ESOPRS)**
*See:* Entry 19549

**★ 20950 ★ European Society of Ophthalmic Plastic and Reconstructive Surgery**
c/o Rostock University Eye Dept.
PO Box 100888
Doberaner Str. 40
D-18055 Postock, Germany
**Phone:** 49 381 4948501 **Fax:** 49 381 4948502
**Email:** rudolf.gurhoff@med.uni-rostock.de
**Website:** http://www.esoprs.org
**Fnded:** 1981. **Mem:** 250. **Lang(s):** English. **Desc:** Surgeons interested in plastic surgery around the eyes. Aims to promote teaching of ophthalmic plastic surgery and to exchange new ideas. **Pub:** *Orbit Journal*, quarterly. Journal.

**★ 20951 ★ European Society of Public Health Ophthalmology (ESPHO)**
Ecole de sante publique
United des deficiencies sensorielles
ULB, route de Lennik 808
B-1070 Brussels, Belgium
**Phone:** 32 2 5554070 **Fax:** 32 2 5554049
**Fnded:** 1996. **Mem:** 49. **Desc:** Aims to promote, in cooperation with affiliated members or institutions, studies on eye and vision related topics.

**★ 20952 ★ Eye Bank Association of America (EBAA)**
1015 18th St., NW, Ste. 1010
Washington, DC 20036
**Phone:** (202)775-4999 **Fax:** (202)429-6036
**Email:** patricia@restoresight.org
**Website:** http://www.restoresight.org
Patricia Aiken-O'Neill, Pres.
**Fnded:** 1961. **Mem:** 109. **Desc:** Eye banks working to restore sight through the promotion and advancement of eye banking. Makes possible over 46,000 corneal transplants annually. Establishes standards for the procurement and distribution of eyes and corneal tissue. Offers training and certification programs for eye banking personnel. Compiles statistics; maintains speakers' bureau. Conducts research and educational programs. **Pub:** *Eye Bank Association of America–Eye Bank Statistics Report*, annual. Annual Report. Includes statistics on eye donations and corneal transplants. • *Eye Bank Association of America–Insight*, periodic. Newsletter. Contains association and industry news. • *Eye Bank Association of America–Membership Directory*, annual. Membership Directory. Lists member eye banks; listed geographically by state. • *Guidelines and Resources for Successful Public and Professional Relations and Development.*

**★ 20953 ★ Eye-Bank for Sight Restoration (EBSR)**
120 Wall St., 3rd Fl.
New York, NY 10005-3902
**Phone:** (212)742-9000 **Fax:** (212)269-3139
**Email:** info@ebsr.org
**Website:** http://www.eyedonation.org
Patricia Dahl, Exec. Dir. /CEO
**Fnded:** 1944. **Desc:** Collects and distributes healthy corneal tissue obtained from individuals who have arranged to donate their eyes, or whose relatives have authorized such donation, at the time of death. Provides speakers to explain the eye-bank program to hospital, professional, and civic groups. **Pub:** *Eye-Bank for Sight Restoration–Eye to Eye*, 3/year. Newsletter. Includes annual report. *Price:* Free.

**★ 20954 ★ Eyecare Information Service**
PO Box
Lincolnshire
Market Rasen LN8 5TS, United Kingdom
**Phone:** 44 1673 857847 **Fax:** 44 1673 857696
**Email:** eis@btinternet.com
**Website:** http://www.eyecare-trust.org.uk
**Fnded:** 1993. **Desc:** Individual optometrists and dispensing opticians, multiples, manufacturing and importing companies, who subscribe voluntarily to fund the EIS's public relations work. Concerned with the generic promotion of eyecare services and products available from professionally qualified, registered UK optical practitioners.

**★ 20955 ★ Fidelco Guide Dog Foundation (FGDF)**
PO Box 142
Bloomfield, CT 06002
**Phone:** (860)243-5200 **Fax:** (860)243-7215
**Email:** training@fidelco.org
**Website:** http://www.fidelco.org
Laurie J. Bonneau, Public Relations Mgr.
**Fnded:** 1960. **Mem:** 25,000. **Desc:** Purpose is to breed, train, and place Fidelco German shepherd guide dogs with blind persons (the Fidelco shepherd is a special breed ideally suited for guide work because of its intelligence, strength, health, and stability). Provides "In-Community" training services to blind persons; reviews performance of the guide dog teams (dog and blind individual) to see that satisfactory level of achievement is maintained; utilizes genetic processes and clinical methods to improve and refine the breed; maintains an ongoing program for development and improvement of training methods. Fidelco puppies are raised in a volunteer family for the first 12-14 months, then trained by FGDF staff for six months before final introduction to and training in the workplace and home environment of the blind recipient with a trainer's help. Maintains speakers' bureau. **Pub:** *Fidelco Audio News*, 3/year. Newsletter. • *Fidelco News*, 4/year. Newsletter. • Annual Report, annual. **Frmly:** Fidelco Foundation; (1981) Fidelco Breeder's Foundation.

**★ 20956 ★ Fiji Optometric Association (FOA)**
GPO Box 1217
Suva, Fiji
**Phone:** 679 311955 **Fax:** 679 305408
**Email:** razak@is.com.fij
**Fnded:** 1982. **Mem:** 6. **Lang(s):** English. **Desc:** Optometrists. Promotes continuing professional development of members; seeks to advance the study and practice of optometry. Sponsors eye care programs; conducts educational courses for optometrists.

**★ 20957 ★ Finnish Federation of the Visually Impaired (Nakovammaisten Keskusliitto)**
Makelankatu 50
FIN-00510 Helsinki, Finland
**Phone:** 358 9 396041 **Fax:** 358 9 39604200
**Email:** nkl@nkl.fi
**Website:** http://www.nkl.fi
**Fnded:** 1928. **Mem:** 25. **Local Groups:** 100. **Lang(s):** English, Finnish, German, Swedish. **Desc:** Works to improve the quality of life of the blind and people with visual impairment. Promotes increased availability of services for people with visual impairment in Namibia, Zambia, Ecuador, Palestine, Estonia, and Russia. Conducts educational programs for personnel working with the blind; develops, produces, and distributes braille and talking books. **Pub:** *AIRUT*, 33/year. Magazine. **Frmly:** Fissish Central Federation of the Visually Handicapped.

**★ 20958 ★ Focus**
c/o Marilyn T. Miller
1855 W Taylor St.
Chicago, IL 60612
**Phone:** (312)996-7445 **Fax:** (312)413-7895
**Email:** marimill@uic.edu
Marilyn T. Miller, MD, Contact
**Fnded:** 1961. **Mem:** 400. **Desc:** Volunteer eye surgeons. Allows American ophthalmologists the opportunity to represent their profession and country by working overseas in an area of desperate need. Doctors pay their own transportation and expenses, and contribute two working weeks of their vacation time to treating patients in Nigeria, where eye care would otherwise not be available. Medical equipment and drugs have been donated by U.S. drug and medical supply firms to the clinics operated by Focus in these countries. Group is unrelated to association of same name. **Pub:** Newsletter, 4-6/month.

**★ 20959 ★ Foundation Fighting Blindness**
11435 Cronhill Dr.
Owings Mills, MD 21117-2220
**Phone:** (410)568-0150 **Free:** 800-683-5555
**Fax:** (410)363-2393
**Email:** mpalmer@blindness.org
**Website:** http://www.blindness.org
Mitsy Palmer, Constituent Serv. Coord.
**Fnded:** 1971. **Mem:** 65,000. **Local Groups:** 35. **Desc:** Works to fund research on causes, treatments, preventive methods and cures for Retinitis Pigmentosa, macular degeneration, Usher Syndrome, Stargardt disease, and the entire spectrum of retinal degenerative diseases. Provides information and referral services; promotes public awareness; sponsors research

programs; conducts fundraisers. **Pub:** *Fighting Blindness News*, semiannual. Newsletter. Includes articles on coping, Foundation activites and research updates. *Price:* Free. • *Macular Update*, 3/year. Newsletter. Includes informational articles and research updates on macular degeneration. *Price:* Free. • Also disseminates comprehensive information kits or retinitis pigmentosa (RP), macular degeneration and Usher Syndrome. **Frmly:** RP Foundation Fighting Blindness.

★ 20960 ★ **French Society of History of Ophthalmology**
**(Societe francophone d'histoire de l'ophtalmologie — SFHO)**
22 A, rue de l'Aqueduc
F-67500 Haguenau, France
**Email:** heitz@sdv.fr
**Website:** http://www.histoph.org
**Fnded:** 1980.

★ 20961 ★ **Glaucoma Foundation**
116 John St., Ste. 1605
New York, NY 10038
**Phone:** (212)285-0080          **Fax:** (212)504-1933
**Email:** info@glaucoma-foundation.org
**Website:** http://www.glaucoma-foundation.org/
Scott R. Christensen, Pres. /CEO
**Fnded:** 1984. **Desc:** Individuals who have been affected by glaucoma and interested others. Works to increase public awareness and to provide research funding. Provides information about glaucoma to the medical and lay communities. Targets and funds the following areas for research: optic nerve regeneration; molecular genetics. Sponsors scientific research. **Pub:** *Doctor, I Have a Question....* Booklet. Answers the basic questions about glaucoma and treatments. • *Eye to Eye*, quarterly. Newsletter. Provides up to date information on advances in research and development. • *Glaucoma: What You Need To Know.* Brochure. • *You and Your Medication.* Brochure.

★ 20962 ★ **Glaucoma Research Foundation**
200 Pine St., Ste. 200
San Francisco, CA 94104-2712
**Phone:** (415)986-3162          **Free:** 800-826-6693
**Fax:** (415)986-3763
**Email:** info@glaucoma.org
**Website:** http://www.glaucoma.org
Rita Loskill, Dir. of Education
**Fnded:** 1978. **Desc:** Dedicated to protecting the sight and independence of individuals with glaucoma through research and education, with the ultimate goal of finding a cure. Funds pilot project grants. **Pub:** *Childhood Glaucoma.* Provides information for people with glaucoma and their families. *Price:* Free. • *Gleams*, quarterly. Newsletter. Includes research updates, foundation news, and medical column. *Price:* Free. • *Living With Glaucoma.* Reference guides for people with glaucoma. • *Understanding and Living with Glaucoma. Price:* Free. **Frmly:** (1993) Foundation for Glaucoma Research.

★ 20963 ★ **Gospel Association for the Blind (GAB)**
PO Box 1162
Bunnell, FL 32110
**Phone:** (386)586-5885
George Montanus, Pres.
**Fnded:** 1947. **Desc:** Religious corporation supported by contributions "to evangelize the physically blind by presenting the Gospel of the Lord Jesus Christ." Provides counseling; summer camp. **Pub:** *Jottings*, monthly. Newsletter. Christian-oriented; includes profiles of blind people. *Price:* Free. • *"The Gospel Messenger"*, monthly. Newsletter. Carries the message of the Gospel to the blind. Contains religious stories, poems, and articles. Available on cassette. *Price:* Free to the blind.

★ 20964 ★ **Guide Dog Foundation for the Blind (GDFB)**
371 E Jericho Tpke.
Smithtown, NY 11787
**Phone:** (631)265-2121          **Free:** 800-548-4337
**Fax:** (631)361-5192
**Email:** info@guidedog.org
**Website:** http://www.guidedog.org
Wells B. Jones, CAE, CEO
**Fnded:** 1946. **Mem:** 160,000. **Desc:** Works to provide independence and mobility for qualified blind applicants free of charge. Dogs are raised in volunteer homes for the first year, then trained for an additional four to six months with qualified instructor. Conducts 25-day residential training program for blind persons and guide dogs at Smithtown, NY. **Pub:** *Guideways*, 3-5/year. Newsletter. Updates the foundation's activities. *Price:* Free. • Annual Report, annual. **AKA:** Second Sight; Guiding Eyes; Guide Dog Foundation.

★ 20965 ★ **Guide Dog Users, Inc. (GDUI)**
57 Grandview Ave.
Watertown, MA 02472
**Phone:** (617)926-9198          **Free:** 888-858-1008
**Fax:** (617)923-0004
**Email:** kimcharlson@earthlink.net
**Website:** http://www.gdui.org
Kim Charlson, Contact
**Fnded:** 1969. **Mem:** 950. **State Groups:** 17. **Desc:** Persons who are visually handicapped or blind and who use guide dogs; other interested individuals. Conducts seminars, workshops, and public relations programs. Encourages promotion of aids for mobility skills and employment of the blind; promotes self-help concept for blind persons. Operates speakers' bureau. **Pub:** *Pawtracks*, quarterly. Newsletter. Provides medical, legal, and financial information on canine maintenance on audiocassette, with specific emphasis on the needs of guide dog users. *Price:* Included in membership dues; $10/year for nonmembers. • Brochures.

★ 20966 ★ **Guide Dogs of America (GDA)**
13445 Glenoaks Blvd.
Sylmar, CA 91342
**Phone:** (818)362-5834          **Free:** 800-459-4843
**Fax:** (818)362-6870
**Email:** mail@guidedogsofamerica.org
**Website:** http://www.guidedogsofamerica.org
Jay A. Bormann, Pres. /Dir.
**Fnded:** 1948. **Desc:** GDA breeds, raises and trains guide dogs for legally blind men and women throughout the U.S. and Canada and provides instruction in the use of these "special" dogs for safe mobility. All GDA services which include guide dog, specially designed harness, individualized 28 day in-residence training, and life-time follow up is free of charge. GDA is supported by donations from individuals, companies, foundations, organizations, and service clubs. Maintains speakers' bureau. Tours available by appointment. **Pub:** *Partners*, quarterly. Newsletter. **AKA:** (2001) International Guiding Eyes. **Frmly:** (1993) International Guiding Eyes.

★ 20967 ★ **Guide Dogs for the Blind (GDB)**
PO Box 151200
San Rafael, CA 94915-1200
**Phone:** (415)499-4000          **Free:** 800-295-4050
**Fax:** (415)499-4035
**Email:** information@guidedogs.com
**Website:** http://www.guidedogs.com
Richard A. Bobb, Pres. & CEO
**Fnded:** 1942. **Desc:** Supported by individuals, firms, foundations, clubs, and bequests. Provides guide dogs and in-residence training on their use to qualified blind persons, free of charge. **Pub:** *Guide Dog News*, quarterly. Newsletter. *Price:* $12/year.

★ 20968 ★ **Guide Dogs for the Blind Association**
Hillfields
Burghfield Common
Reading RG7 3YG, United Kingdom
**Phone:** 44 118 9835555     **Fax:** 44 118 9835433
**Email:** guidedogs@gdba.org.uk
**Website:** http://www.guidedogs.org.uk
**Fnded:** 1934. **Mem:** 5,000. **Local Groups:** 450. **Lang(s):** English. **Desc:** Provides guide dogs, mobility and other rehabilitation services that meet the needs of blind and partially sighted people. **Pub:** *FORWARD*, quarterly. Magazine. Also available in Braille and on audiotape.

★ 20969 ★ **Guiding Eyes for the Blind (GEB)**
611 Granite Springs Rd.
Yorktown Heights, NY 10598
**Phone:** (914)245-4024          **Free:** 800-942-0149
**Fax:** (914)245-1609
**Email:** webmaster@guiding-eyes.org
**Website:** http://guidingeyes.org
William D. Badger, Pres. /CEO
**Fnded:** 1954. **Desc:** Breeds and provides fully trained guide dogs and instruction in their use to visually impaired and blind individuals including special needs students with additional challenges. Conducts 3-year course for instructors and 4-week training programs for blind persons in proper use and care of guide dogs at Yorktown Heights, NY. Provides in-service education for staff and seminars for orientation and mobility instructors and other rehabilitation professionals. Maintains speakers' bureau of program graduates; provides home training. **Pub:** *Guide Lines*, quarterly. Newsletter. • *Insight*, biennial. Magazine. • *Lions Connection*, quarterly.

★ 20970 ★ **Helen Keller International - Indonesia (HKII)**
PO Box 4338
12950 Jakarta Pusat, Indonesia
**Phone:** 62 21 7198147     **Fax:** 62 21 7198148
**Email:** info@hkiasiapacific.org
**Website:** http://www.hkiasiapacific.org
**Desc:** National branch of the international organization. Fosters community-based blindness prevention and rehabilitation programs and services. Provides technical assistance and materials for the design and implementation of eye care within the existing primary health care system. Conducts projects and disseminates information on: preventing nutritional blindness; reducing cataract blindness; combatting onchocerciasis ("river blindness"); and improving the quality of life of the blind. Distributes medicine for eye disease treatment. Offers educational services.

★ 20971 ★ **Helen Keller International - Morocco (HKI)**
3, rue Sekkoura
Rabat, Morocco
**Phone:** 212 7 756636
**Email:** info@hkworld.org
**Website:** http://www.hki.org
**Fnded:** 1915. **Lang(s):** Arabic, French. **Desc:** Fosters community-based blindness prevention and rehabilitation programs and services. Provides technical assistance and materials for the design and implementation of eye care within the existing primary health care system. Conducts projects and disseminates information on: preventing nutritional blindness; reducing cataract blindness; combatting onchocerciasis ("river blindness"); and improving the quality of life of the blind. Distributes medicine for eye disease treatment. Offers educational services.

★ 20972 ★ **Helen Keller International - Nepal (HKIN)**
PO Box 3752
Min Bhawan
New Baneshwor
Kathmandu, Nepal

**Phone:** 977 1 480921          **Fax:** 977 1 480234
**Email:** zaman@hkinepal.wlink.com.np
**Website:** http://www.hkiasiapacific.org
**Fnded:** 1988. **Desc:** Works to prevent blindness; provides rehabilitative services to the blind. Cooperates with nongovernment agencies to devise and implement vision care initiatives. Programs focus on preventing nutritional and other preventable forms of blindness. Makes available routine eye care services; collaborates with government and nongovernment agencies to reduce micronutrient deficiencies which lead to an increase in morbidity and mortality in women and children.

### ★ 20973 ★ Helen Keller National Center for Deaf-Blind Youths and Adults (HKNC)

111 Middle Neck Rd.
Sands Point, NY 11050
**Phone:** (516)944-8900          **Fax:** (516)944-7302
**Email:** hkncdir@aol.com
**Website:** http://helenkeller.org/national/
Joseph J. McNulty, Exec. Dir.
**Fnded:** 1969. **Reg. Groups:** 10. **Desc:** Provides diagnostic evaluations, comprehensive vocational and personal adjustment training, job preparation and placement for people who are deaf-blind from every state and territory. Field services include information and referral and advocacy and technical assistance to professionals, consumers, and families. Sponsors annual National Helen Keller Deaf-Blind Awareness Week. **Pub:** *Giving.* Newsletter. • *Guidelines for Helping Deaf-Blind Persons.* Brochure. • *HKNC Description of Services.* Booklet. • *Nat-Cent News,* periodic. Magazine. • *National Family Association for the Deaf-Blind Newsletter,* periodic. Newsletter. • *Older Adult Program.* Brochure. • Also publishes many other free materials about the annual Deaf-Blind Awareness week. **Frmly:** National Rehabilitation of Deaf-Blind Adults.

### ★ 20974 ★ Helen Keller Worldwide (HKW)

352 Park Ave. S, Ste. 1200
New York, NY 10010
**Phone:** (212)532-0544          **Free:** 877-535-5374
**Fax:** (212)532-6014
**Email:** info@hkworld.org
**Website:** http://www.hkworld.org
John M. Palmer, Pres.
**Fnded:** 1915. **Desc:** Assists governments and voluntary agencies throughout Asia, Africa, and the Americas (including the United States) to establish and integrate, into their national health and welfare systems, services to prevent or cure eye diseases and blindness and to rehabilitate and educate visually disabled persons. Focuses on programs in the prevention and treatment of blindness caused by malnutrition, trachoma, onchocerciasis and cataracts. Trains health workers at all levels in the use of specially developed materials to diagnose and treat eye problems and to refer patients to hospitals. Conducts courses for teachers of blind children and for vocational and mobility instructors of blind adults; offers training for indigenous field workers who instruct the rural blind in daily living skills and provide vocational education. Provides information on programs and services on the problem of blindness throughout the world. Compiles statistics. Provides free prescription eyeglasses to junior high school students through the Childsight Program. **Pub:** *Helen Keller Annual Report,* annual. Annual Report. *Price:* Free. • *Insight,* 4/year. Newsletter. *Price:* Free. • Also publishes fact sheets, technical reports, training materials on nutritional blindness detection and treatment, and educational materials. **Frmly:** (1925) Permanent Blind Relief War Fund; (1946) American Braille Press for War and Civilian Blind; (1977) American Foundation for Overseas Blind; (1999) Helen Keller International; (2000) Helen Keller Worldwide; (2002) Helen Keller International.

**HIKE Fund**
*See:* Entry 6048

### ★ 20975 ★ Hong Kong Society of Professional Optometrists

PO Box 98603
Tsimshatsui Post Office
Hong Kong, People's Republic of China
**Fax:** 852 27826755
**Email:** query@hkspo.org.hk
**Website:** http://www.hkspo.org.hk
**Fnded:** 1982. **Mem:** 250. **Lang(s):** Chinese, English. **Desc:** Optometrists. Seeks to insure high standards of ethics and practice in optometry; facilitates professional advancement of members. Conducts continuing professional education courses; sponsors research; makes available optometric services. Participates in charitable activities; maintains speakers' bureau; compiles statistics. **Pub:** Newsletter, quarterly.

### ★ 20976 ★ In Touch Networks (ITN)

15 W 65th St.
New York, NY 10023
**Phone:** (212)769-6270          **Fax:** (212)769-4148
**Website:** http://www.intouchnetworks.net
Pete Williamson, Gen. Mgr.
**Fnded:** 1974. **Mem:** 1000,000. **Desc:** Volunteer service that allows blind or physically impaired people to listen to readings of articles from more than 100 newspapers and magazines via closed-circuit radio. Broadcasts nationally accessible on Galaxy 4 satellite. **Pub:** *Program Guide,* annual.

### ★ 20977 ★ Independent Visually Impaired Enterprisers (IVIE)

c/o American Council of the Blind
1155 15th St. NW, Ste. 1004
Washington, DC 20005
**Phone:** (202)467-5081          **Free:** 800-424-8666
**Fax:** (202)467-5085
**Email:** citowers@attbi.com
**Website:** http://www.acb.org/resources/parents.html
Cynthia Towers, Pres.
**Fnded:** 1980. **Mem:** 50. **Desc:** Blind and visually impaired people who own or operate small businesses. Seeks to: broaden vocational opportunities in business for the blind and visually impaired; improve rehabilitational facilities for all types of business enterprises; publicize capabilities of the blind and visually impaired. Maintains speakers' bureau. **Pub:** *IVIE Motivator,* quarterly. Newsletter. *Price:* $15 for non-members.

### ★ 20978 ★ Institute of Ophthalmology

Bath St.
London EC1V 9EL, United Kingdom
**Phone:** 44 207 6086800          **Fax:** 44 207 6086954
**Email:** k.higgs@ucl.ac.uk
**Website:** http://www.ucl.ac.uk/ioo
**Fnded:** 1948. **Desc:** Teaching and research into eye diseases and other causes of blindness.

### ★ 20979 ★ International Academy of Sports Vision (NASV)

3721 Redmont Rd.
Birmingham, AL 35213
**Email:** nasv@mindspring.com
**Website:** http://www.iasv.net
Dr. A. I. Garner, Exec. Dir.
**Fnded:** 1984. **Mem:** 1,000. **Desc:** Optometrists and opthalmologists; athletic trainers; team physicians, coaches, and students; educational institutions and eyewear manufacturers. Purpose is to: provide comprehensive vision care for individuals active in sports and fitness programs; foster the promotion and advancement of research, development, and education in the field; facilitate the design, development, and fitting of both protective and corrective contact lenses and eyewear for athletes; advance and enhance the role of the sports specialist to the public through a public relations program. Acts as a forum for the discussion and exchange of information in the areas of developmental vision, vision training, and therapy. Offers referral services. **Pub:** *Journal of the International Academy of Sports Vision.* Journal. • *SportsVi-*

*sion,* quarterly. Magazine. • *Update,* quarterly. • Audiotapes. • Membership Directory, annual. • Videos. **Frmly:** (1991) National Academy of Sports Vision.

### ★ 20980 ★ International Agency for the Prevention of Blindness (IAPB)

c/o Dr. Gullapalli N. Rao, Sec.Gen.
LV Prasad Eye Institute
LV Prasad Marg
Banjara Hills
Hyderabad 500034, India
**Phone:** 91 40 3545389          **Fax:** 91 40 3548271
**Email:** iapb@lvpeye.stph.net
**Fnded:** 1975. **Lang(s):** English. **Desc:** Ophthalmic societies and societies for the prevention of blindness whose members include ophthalmologists, public health officers, nutritionists, geneticists, and other health workers. Coordinates international research into the causes of impaired vision or blindness; promotes measures calculated to eliminate such causes; disseminates knowledge worldwide on preventing blindness and on matters pertaining to care of the eyes. Cooperates with the World Health Organization, United Nations Children's Fund, and other international agencies. **Pub:** *IAPB Fifth General Assembly.* Proceedings document. • *IAPB News.* Newsletter. • *World Blindness and Its Prevention Vols. 1-4.* Proceedings. Based on proceedings of respective General Assemblies.

### ★ 20981 ★ International Association of Audio Information Services (IAAIS)

c/o WVTF Radio Reading Service
4235 Electric Rd. NW, Ste. 105
Roanoke, VA 24014
**Phone:** (540)989-8900          **Free:** 800-280-5325
**Fax:** (540)776-2727
**Email:** aiblink@ak.net
**Website:** http://www.iaais.org
Ben Martin, Pres.
**Fnded:** 1977. **Mem:** 140. **Desc:** Helps members provide access to current printed information not available to print disabled people. Volunteers broadcast daily newspapers, community news updates, grocery ads, and death notices. Advocates access to printed material as a key issue under the Americans with Disabilities Act and that the Internet needs to be accessible to people with disabilities. Compiles statistics; holds competitions; maintains speakers' bureau. **Pub:** *Directory of Radio Reading Services,* annual. Directory. *Price:* $150. • *HEARSSAY,* quarterly. Newsletter. • *IAAIS Newsletter,* quarterly. Newsletter. Audio information industry news. *Price:* Free. • *Members,* annual. Directory. **Frmly:** National Association of Radio Reading Services.

### ★ 20982 ★ International Association of Contact Lens Educators (IACLE)

PO Box 328
Randwick
Sydney, NSW 2031, Australia
**Phone:** 61 2 93857466          **Fax:** 61 2 93857467
**Email:** iacle@cclru.unsw.edu.au
**Website:** http://www.iacle.org
**Fnded:** 1979. **Mem:** 513. **Lang(s):** English. **Desc:** Optometrists, Ophthalmologists, Opticians and Contactologists from 60 countries who are involved either full-time or part-time in contact lens education. Also includes staff members of recognized teaching institutions. Works to raise the standard of contact lens education worldwide and promotes the widespread, safe use of contact lenses. Provides educational infrastructure; cooperates with any organization that advances ophthalmic education.

### ★ 20983 ★ International Association of Ocular Surgeons (IAOS)

820 N Orleans St., Ste. 208
Chicago, IL 60610
**Phone:** (312)440-0699          **Free:** 800-621-4002
**Fax:** (312)440-0580

**Email:** iaos@aol.com
Randall T. Bellows, MD, Dir.

**Fnded:** 1981. **Mem:** 900. **Desc:** A division of the American Society of Contemporary Ophthalmology. Seeks to develop a global community of ophthalmic surgeons who examine and deliberate on all aspects of ocular surgery; encourage information exchange among members; and disseminate information about contemporary diagnostic and surgical procedures. **Pub:** *Annals of Ophthalmology*, quarterly. Journal. Continuing medical education for ophthalmologists. *Price:* $120.

**★ 20984 ★ International Association of Optometric Executives (IAOE)**
1505 Price, Ste. 3
Alexandria, VA 22314
**Phone:** (703)739-9200 **Free:** 800-678-9262
**Fax:** (703)739-9497 ·
**Email:** khipp@theaoa.org
**Website:** http://www.aoanet.org
Kelly Hipp, Contact

**Mem:** 75. **Desc:** Executives of optometric associations in 10 countries. Promotes continuing education in optometric association management. **Frmly:** Society of Association Optometric Executives.

**★ 20985 ★ International Blind Sports Federation (IBSF) (Association Internationale pour le Sport des Aveugles)**
c/Jose Ortega y Gasset, 18
E-28006 Madrid, Spain
**Phone:** 34 91 4365335 **Fax:** 34 91 4365354
**Email:** ibsa@ibsa.es
**Website:** http://www.ibsa.es

**Fnded:** 1981. **Mem:** 100. **Reg. Groups:** 5. **Lang(s):** English, French, Spanish. **Desc:** National organizations, institutions, and committees involved in sports for the blind. Objectives are to: involve and inspire blind persons in regular sports activities; encourage friendship among blind athletes; promote and disseminate the ideas of competitive sport and recreational sport for the blind; uphold the Olympic ideal and act in accordance with its principles. Plans, promotes and coordinates international sports events for the blind; registers records and best performances. Sponsors competitions. **Frmly:** International Blind Sports Association.

**★ 20986 ★ International Color Vision Society**
c/o Prof. J.D. Mollon
Department of Experimental Psychology
University of Cambridge
Downing St.
Stafford CB2 3EB, United Kingdom
**Phone:** 44 1782 583060 **Fax:** 44 1782 583055
**Email:** jm123@cam.ac.uk

**Fnded:** 1971. **Mem:** 200. **Lang(s):** English. **Desc:** Ophthalmologists, optometrists, physicists, physiologists, psychologists, and zoologists. Seeks to collaborate on the study of congenital and acquired color vision deficiencies. **Pub:** *Daltoniana*, quarterly. Newsletter. • *Proceedings of the IRGCVD Symposia*, biennial. **Frmly:** (2000) International Research Group on Coloru Vision Deficiencies.

**International Council for Education of People with Visual Impairment (ICEVI)**
*See:* Entry 8004

**★ 20987 ★ International Ergophthalmological Society (Societas Ergophthalmologica Internationalis — SEI)**
c/o Goldschleger Eye Insitute
Sheba Med. Center
IL-52621 Tel-Hashaner, Israel
**Phone:** 972 3 5302957

**Email:** mrosner@post.tav.ac.il
**Website:** http://www.icevi.org

**Fnded:** 1966. **Mem:** 150. **Lang(s):** English. **Desc:** National ergophthalmological associations in 47 countries; interested individuals. Promotes scientific research in the area of industrial ophthalmology (ergophthalmology) and the establishment and development of professional contacts. Conducts periodic symposia. **Pub:** *Newsletter of the International Ergophthalmologic Society*, periodic. Newsletter.

**★ 20988 ★ International Eye Foundation (IEF)**
7801 Norfolk Ave., Ste. 200
Bethesda, MD 20814
**Phone:** (301)986-1830 **Fax:** (301)986-1876
**Email:** info@iefusa.org
**Website:** http://www.iefusa.org
Victoria M. Sheffield, Exec. Dir.

**Fnded:** 1961. **Desc:** Works to restore sight and prevent blindness in poor countries around the world. Focuses on making eye clinics financially self-sufficient. Developed eye health services. Trains ophthalmologists and para-medicals, and fights vitamin A deficiency, trachoma and river blindness. Strives to help clinics become less dependent on outside donors and government funds. **Pub:** *International Eye Foundation–Eye to Eye*, semiannual. Newsletter. Concerned with the prevention of blindness in the developing countries; includes information on foundation programs. *Price:* Free. • Annual Report, annual. • Also publishes fact sheets. Primary Eye Care Manual Eye Care in Developing Nations

**★ 20989 ★ International Federation of Ophthalmological Societies (IFOS)**
c/o Bruce E. Spivey. MD, Sec.-General
Columbia-Cornell Care, L.L.C.
900 Third Ave., Ste. 500
New York, NY 10022
**Phone:** (212)588-7301 **Fax:** (212)588-7307
**Email:** info@icoph.org
**Website:** http://www.icoph.org
Bruce E. Spivey, MD, Sec. -Gen.

**Fnded:** 1857. **Nat'l Groups:** 125. **Desc:** ICO (the executive body of IFOS) represents opthalmologic organizations throughout the world. Dedicated to international exchange in ophthalmology. Encourages the study and improvement of ophthalmologic education; formulates international standards. Advocates the prevention and treatment of preventable blindness in developing nations, particularly Africa. Supports the International Agency for the Prevention of Blindness.

**★ 20990 ★ International Friendly Circle of the Blind (IFCB)**
PO Box 222
Berkeley, CA 94704
**Phone:** (415)388-3905
Don Brown, Pres.

**Fnded:** 1987. **Desc:** Individuals who collect braille writers, braille paper, pens, pencils, and other writing materials and send this material to blind or visually impaired students in developing countries.

**★ 20991 ★ International Glaucoma Association (IGA)**
108C Warner Rd.
Camberwell Hill
London SE5 9HQ, United Kingdom
**Phone:** 44 20 77373265 **Fax:** 44 20 73465929
**Website:** http://www.iga.org.uk/home.htm

**Fnded:** 1974. **Mem:** 14,500. **Lang(s):** English. **Desc:** Glaucoma patients. Seeks to educate the public about glaucoma, its causes, detection, and treatment. Provides patients, doctors, opticians, optometrists, and others a forum for the exchange of ideas on glaucoma. Supports research; bestows grants. Conducts surveys; disseminates information. **Pub:** *Glaucoma 98 - A Guide for Patients*, annual. Booklet. • Newsletter, semiannual. • Pamphlets. Leaflets. **Frmly:** (1974) Glaucoma Association.

**★ 20992 ★ International Oculoplastic Society (IOSI)**
c/o Pierre Guibor, M.D.
55 Meadowland Parkway
Hackensack, NJ 07601
**Phone:** (201)392-3438 **Fax:** (201)392-3526
**Email:** pguibor@aol.com
Pierre Guibor, MD, Dir.

**Fnded:** 1978. **Mem:** 3,000. **Reg. Groups:** 4. **Local Groups:** 2. **Desc:** Surgeons specializing in ophthalmology, otolaryngology, dermatology, and plastic surgery. Sponsors professional education and clinically applied research in the prevention, diagnosis, and treatment of disorders of the eye, orbit, adnexa, face, and skin. Seeks to promote and establish successful forms of patient care and treatment through open discussions, seminars, and instructional courses on clinical research, surgery, and medical advances. Conducts educational and charitable programs. Maintains speakers' bureau and placement servic. Compiles statistics. **Pub:** *Oculoplastic Newsletter*, semiannual. Newsletter. *Price:* Free.

**★ 20993 ★ International Organization Against Trachoma (IOAT) (Organisation Internationale pour la Lutte Contre le Trachome)**
Hospital de Creteil
Universite de Paris-Val de Marne
40, ave. de Verdun
F-94010 Creteil, France
**Phone:** 33 1 45175225 **Fax:** 33 1 45175227
**Email:** coscasgabriel@compuserve.com
**Website:** http://www.who.int/ina-ngo/ngo/ngo098.htm

**Fnded:** 1923. **Mem:** 1,200. **Lang(s):** English, French. **Desc:** Circulates information in 20 countries on current trachoma research (trachoma is a chronic, contagious eye disease) and supplies the latest information on etiology, diagnosis, epidemiology, prevention, and treatment, thus providing a scientific basis for the fight against the disease. Promotes research on trachoma; facilitates the adoption of sanitary and other regulations aimed at implementing the fight against trachoma. Maintains close contact with the World Health Organization and other institutions engaged in the fight against trachoma. **Pub:** *Revue Internationale du Trachome*, semiannual. Journal.

**★ 20994 ★ International Orthoptic Association (IOA)**
c/o Mrs. Bronia Unwin
Moorfields Eye Hospital
Orthoptic Department
City Rd.
London EC1V 2PD, United Kingdom
**Phone:** 44 207 5662163 **Fax:** 44 207 3885066
**Website:** http://home.vicnet.net.au/~ioaorth/

**Fnded:** 1967. **Mem:** 4,000. **Lang(s):** English. **Desc:** Orthoptists in 22 countries certified to treat defects in binocular vision, faulty visual habits, and low visual acuity. Organizes and conducts an international congress of orthoptists; shares information through newsletters. **Pub:** *Abstracts of Congress*, quadrennial. Journal. • *Newsletter*, annual. Newsletter.

**★ 20995 ★ International Perimetric Society (IPS)**
c/o Michael Wall, M.D.
Department of Neurology
200 Hawkins Dr., No. 2007 RCP
Iowa City, IA 52242
**Phone:** (319)356-8758 **Fax:** (319)356-4505
**Email:** michael-wall@uiowa.edu
**Website:** http://www.perimetry.org
Michael Wall, MD, Sec.

**Fnded:** 1974. **Mem:** 200. **Desc:** Ophthalmologists, scientists, and technicians in 20 countries working in the field of perimetry (visual field testing) and related areas. Promotes the study of normal and abnormal visual function and encourages worldwide cooperation and friendship among those working in the field. **Pub:** *Perimetry Update*, biennial. Proceedings.

**★ 20996 ★ International Society for Clinical Electrophysiology of Vision**
Nagoya University School of Medicine
65 Tsurumai, Cho
Showa-ku
Nagoya 466, Japan
**Phone:** 81 52 7442276     **Fax:** 81 52 7442273
**Email:** ymiyake@med.nagoya-u.ac.jp
**Website:** http://www.iscev.org
**Fnded:** 1962. **Mem:** 700. **Nat'l Groups:** 34. **Reg. Groups:** 5. **State Groups:** 34. **Local Groups:** 34. **Lang(s):** English, Japanese. **Desc:** Ophthalmologists and other individuals with an interest in the electrophysiology of vision. Seeks to advance understanding of the mechanics of vision; promotes development of new ophthalmologic techniques and technologies. Functions as a clearinghouse on the electrophysiology of vision; facilitates cooperation and communication among workers in the field of the clinical and basic electrophysiology of vision; formulates standards of terminology, research, and practice in the field. **Pub:** *Documents of Ophthalmology*, annual. Newsletter.

**★ 20997 ★ International Society of Contact Lens Specialists**
c/o Dr. Theo F. Gumpelmayer
Landstr. 49
A-4020 Linz, Austria
**Phone:** 43 70 773660     **Fax:** 43 70 7736703
**Fnded:** 1952. **Mem:** 74. **Lang(s):** German. **Desc:** Contact lens specialists.

**★ 20998 ★ International Society of Geographical and Epidemiological Ophthalmology (ISGEO)**
St. Paul's Hospital
1081 Burrard St.
Vancouver, BC, Canada V6Z 1Y6
**Phone:** (604)631-5169     **Fax:** (604)631-5058
**Email:** pcourtright@providencehealth.bc.ca
**Website:** http://www.interchg.ubc.ca/bceio/isgeo/
**Desc:** Open to all professionals who have an interest in the scientific aspects of international ophthalmology in particular and epidemiology and geographical medicine in general. Aims to promote the science of geographic and epidemiological ophthalmology among all people and nations.

**★ 20999 ★ International Society on Metabolic Eye Disease (ISMED)**
1125 Park Ave.
New York, NY 10128
**Phone:** (212)427-1246     **Fax:** (212)360-7009
Heskel M. Haddad, MD, Sec. -Treas.
**Fnded:** 1971. **Mem:** 600. **Desc:** Ophthalmologists, pediatricians, endocrinologists, internists, and paramedical personnel in 20 countries. Promotes the study of metabolic eye problems and biochemical and genetic aspects of such problems. **Pub:** *Metabolic, Pediatric, and Systemic Ophthalmology*, quarterly. Journal. **Price:** $160/year. • Book.

**★ 21000 ★ International Society of Refractive Surgery (ISRS)**
1180 Springs Centre South Blvd., No. 116
Altamonte Springs, FL 32714-1954
**Phone:** (407)786-7446     **Fax:** (407)786-7447
**Email:** isrshq@isrs.org
**Website:** http://www.isrs.org
Julia Lewis, Exec. Dir.
**Fnded:** 1979. **Mem:** 4,000. **Desc:** Eye care professionals. Provides scientific research, knowledge, and information to all individuals who are interested in refractive surgery. The association is committed to supporting and advancing the ethical practice of refractive surgery by providing quality education, stimulating information exchange, and promoting scientific research worldwide. **Pub:** *Journal of Refractive Surgery*, 6/yr.Journal. Features original research and a review of refractive and corneal surgical procedures.

*Price:* $125 per year. **Frmly:** (1996) International Society Refractive Keratplasty.

**★ 21001 ★ Interprofessional Fostering of Ophthalmic Care for Underserved Sectors (InFOCUS)**
327 Tealwood Dr.
Houston, TX 77024
**Phone:** (713)468-3040     **Fax:** (713)468-7704
**Email:** infocus@houston.rr.com
**Website:** http://www.infocusonline.org
Barbara Kazdan, Dir.
**Fnded:** 1988. **Desc:** Works in cooperation with eye care specialists, public health care professionals, health care providers and humanitarian organizations to develop sustainable eye care practices in areas with underserved populations; encourages community self-reliance. Conducts educational and charitable programs; sponsors research on appropriate technology for primary eye care.

**★ 21002 ★ Irish Guide Dogs for the Blind (IGDB)**
Model Farm Rd.
Cork, Cork, Ireland
**Phone:** 353 21 4878200     **Fax:** 353 21 4874152
**Email:** info@guidedogs.ie
**Website:** http://www.guidedogs.ie
**Lang(s):** English, Irish. **Desc:** Dog trainers and individuals providing support and services to people with impaired vision. Seeks to improve the quality of life of people with impaired vision. Makes available trained guide dogs to people with impaired vision; conducts training programs for people wishing to use guide dogs.

**★ 21003 ★ Italian Union of the Blind (Unione Italiana Ciechi — UIC)**
via Borgognona 38
I-00187 Rome, Italy
**Phone:** 39 6 699881     **Fax:** 39 6 6786815
**Website:** http://www.uiciechi.it
**Lang(s):** English, Italian. **Desc:** Seeks to improve the quality of life of people with visual impairment in Italy. Represents the interests of people with visual impairment before government agencies and the public. Conducts health education programs. Sponsors projects in the Czech Republic.

**★ 21004 ★ Japan Optometric Association (JOA)**
2-5-5 Izumi Higashiku
Nagoya 461-0001, Japan
**Phone:** 81 52 9320610     **Fax:** 81 52 9320629
**Email:** joa@pop01.odn.ne.jp
**Fnded:** 1979. **Mem:** 1,140. **Lang(s):** English, Japanese. **Desc:** Optometrists. Seeks to advance the study, teaching, and practice of optometry; promotes continuing professional development of members. Serves as a clearinghouse on optometry; sponsors research and educational programs. **Pub:** *Journal of the Japan Optometric Association*, semiannual. Journal.

**★ 21005 ★ Jewish Braille Institute of America (JBI)**
110 E 30th St.
New York, NY 10016
**Phone:** (212)889-2525     **Free:** 800-433-1531
**Fax:** (212)689-3692
**Email:** admin@jbilibrary.org
**Website:** http://www.jbilibrary.org
Dr. Ellen Isler, Exec. VP
**Fnded:** 1931. **Desc:** Jewish Braille Institute is the only library of Jewish interest in the world serving the cultural, religious, educational and communal needs of the visually impaired and blind in over 40 countries, including the U.S., Israel and the former Soviet Union, and in six languages (English, Russian, Hebrew, Hungarian, Yiddish, Polish). JBI materials are distributed free on audio cassette, in large print and in braille.

Collection includes 9,000 titles covering fiction and non-fiction, liturgical materials, and 7 monthly magazines. JBI is an affiliated library of the United States Library of Congress and is accredited as a nongovernmental organization of the United Nations. **Pub:** *Hebrew Braille Bible*. • *Hebrew Self-Taught*. Braille primer. • *JBI Voice*, 10/year. Magazine. Cassette format for non-braille reading blind and visually impaired. Includes articles on Jewish-related topics, politics, stories, and poetry. *Price:* Free to blind and visually impaired persons. • *Jewish Reference Calendar*, annual. Large print, 18-month with secular holidays and candle lighting times. • *Passover Haggadah*. Large print edition. • Also publishes prayer books and religious texts in Hebrew.

**★ 21006 ★ Jewish Guild for the Blind (JGB)**
15 W 65th St.
New York, NY 10023
**Phone:** (212)769-6200     **Free:** 800-284-4422
**Fax:** (212)769-6266
**Email:** info@jgb.org
**Website:** http://www.jgb.org
Alan R. Morse, Pres. & CEO
**Fnded:** 1914. **Desc:** Medical and vision services for blind, visually handicapped, and multihandicapped people of all ages, races, and creeds. Provides social work, counseling, and AIDS case management; job development, placement, and training; support group services; rehabilitation, including vocational, high school equivalency training, orientation and mobility, activities of daily living, and computer training; adapted physical education; communication skills; adult day healthcare program, GuildCare, in New York City, Yonkers, Bronx, Buffalo, Niagara Falls, and Albany, New York. Operates Early Intervention Program for infants and preschoolers (up to age 5); school for multihandicapped children; state licensed psychiatric clinic for emotionally disturbed blind persons and their families; day treatment programs for multihandicapped blind adults; Low Vision Services; Comprehensive Outpatient Rehabilitation Facility (C.O.R.F.). J.G.B. Facilities Corporation, the residential health care affiliate, operates the Home for Aged Blind (a nursing home), the Newman Center for Alzheimer's Care, and Center for AIDS Care, a specialized facility for visually impaired persons with AIDS, in Yonkers, NY. Cosponsors health fairs/vision screenings for the community. **Pub:** Newsletter, quarterly. Contains guild programs and events involving professional and volunteer supporters of Guild services. *Price:* Included in membership dues. **Frmly:** (1960) New York Guild for the Jewish Blind.

**★ 21007 ★ John Milton Society for the Blind (JMS)**
475 Riverside Dr., Rm. 455
New York, NY 10115
**Phone:** (212)870-3335     **Fax:** (212)870-3226
**Email:** order@jmsblind.org
**Website:** http://www.jmsblind.org
Robert R. Pegg, Pres.
**Fnded:** 1928. **Desc:** Non-denominational Christian worldwide service to persons who cannot see to read regular print. Works to make Christian religious materials available to blind and visually impaired persons worldwide. Operates referral service. Provides materials for displays and exhibits. **Pub:** *Directory of Resources for the Blind and Visually Impaired*, biennial. Directory. Lists other organizations that provide religious and other publications for the blind and visually imparied. *Price:* Free. • *Discovery*, quarterly. Religious digest for young people 8-18, in braille. *Price:* Free to blind persons. • *John Milton Adult Lesson Quarterly*. Contains Bible studies in braille and on cassette tape. *Price:* Free to blind persons. • *John Milton Magazine*, quarterly. Magazine. Reprints of reading material offered in over 50 religiou s periodicals for the sighted. Available in large print. *Price:* Free to blind persons. • *Motto Calendar*, annual. Braille reproduction of the ink-print Motto Calendar published by a Quaker family in Pennsylvania. • *Special Bible Study*, annual. Available in braille. • *World Community Day Service*, annual.

Transcript of the November service prepared by Church Women United. Available in large print. • *World Day of Prayer Service*, annual. Transcript of the March service prepared by Church Women United. Available in large print. • Also publishes publications brochure in print and in Braille. **Frmly:** John Milton Society.

---

★ **21008** ★ **John Milton Society for the Blind in Canada**
40 St. Clair Ave. E, Ste. 202
Toronto, ON, Canada M4T 1M9
**Phone:** (416)960-3953          **Fax:** (416)960-3570
**Email:** jmscan@netcom.ca
**Website:** http://www.jmscan.org
**Fnded:** 1970. **Lang(s):** English. **Desc:** National ecumenical Organization. Provides Christian materials to blind, deafblind, and visually impaired Canadians. **Pub:** *In Touch*, quarterly. Newsletter. Braille newspaper. • *Insight*, bimonthly. Newsletter. • *Insound*, bimonthly. Audiotape.

---

★ **21009** ★ **Joint Commission on Allied Health Personnel in Ophthalmology (JCAHPO)**
2025 Woodlane Dr.
Saint Paul, MN 55125-2995
**Phone:** (651)731-2944          **Free:** 800-284-3937
**Fax:** (651)731-0410
**Email:** jcahpo@jcahpo.org
**Website:** http://www.jcahpo.org
Lynn D. Anderson, Exec. Dir.
**Fnded:** 1969. **Desc:** A certifying agency for allied health personnel. Objectives are: to encourage the establishment of medically oriented programs for training allied health personnel in ophthalmology; to develop standards of education and training in the field; to examine, certify, and recertify ophthalmic medical personnel, and encourage their continued occupational development. Conducts national certifying examinations. **Pub:** *Career of Ophthalmic Medical Assisting*. • *Certification - Why & How*. • *Criteria for Certification & Recertification - Ophthalmic Assistant, Ophthalmic Technician, Ophthalmic Medical Technologist*. • *Directory of Certified Ophthalmic Medical Personnel*, annual. Directory. Arranged alphabetically and geographically. *Price:* Free to certified ophthalmic allied health staff. • *Educational Programs for Ophthalmic Medical Personnel*. • *JCAHPO CEC Matters*, quarterly. Newspaper. *Price:* Free to ophthalmic medical personnel; $20/year. • *The President's Report*, annual. Annual Report. *Price:* Free.

---

★ **21010** ★ **Kenya Society for the Blind (KSB)**
PO Box 46656
Nairobi, Kenya
**Phone:** 254 2 503757          **Fax:** 254 2 501733
**Email:** ksblind@africaonline.co.ke
**Fnded:** 1956. **Mem:** 400. **Lang(s):** English. **Desc:** Promotes the welfare, education, training, and employment of the blind and people with visual impairment. Works to prevent and cure blindness; advises public agencies in matters concerning the blind and people with visual impairment. **Pub:** Annual Report, annual. Summarizes activities and financial report for the year.

---

★ **21011** ★ **Kerato-Refractive Society (KRS)**
PO Box 601149
Dallas, TX 75360-1149
**Phone:** (972)601-5750          **Fax:** (972)713-9722
Ronald A. Schachar, MD, Exec. Sec.
**Fnded:** 1979. **Mem:** 2,000. **Desc:** Ophthalmologists and scientists interested in the latest advances in keratorefractive and laser techniques. (Keratorefraction is a surgical procedure in which the shape of the cornea and iris is changed in order to correct nearsightedness and astigmatism. The procedure is now performed with a diamond knife; use of lasers is still in the investigational stage.) Purpose is to keep profes-

sionals and others informed of the most recent advances and developments in ophthalmologic care. Conducts research and raises funds. Sponsors training programs. **Pub:** *Keratorefraction*. Book. • *Radical Keratotomy*. Book. • *Refractive Keratoplasty*. Book. • *Refractive Modulation of the Cornea*. Book. • Newsletter, biennial.

---

**Keren-Or, Inc. (K-OI)**
*See:* Entry 5708

---

★ **21012** ★ **Latin American Association of Optometrics and Opticianry (LAAOO) (Asociacion Latinoamericana de Optometria y Optica — ALOO)**
c/o Colegio de Opticos de Chile
Casilla 53542
Santiago, Chile
**Email:** info@keren-or.org
**Website:** http://www.keren-or.org/
**Lang(s):** English, Spanish. **Desc:** Optometrists and opticians. Seeks to advance optometric and optical scholarship and practice; promotes continuing professional development of members. Serves as a forum for the exchange of information among members; sponsors research and educational programs.

---

★ **21013** ★ **Latin American Blind Union - Uruguay (LABU) (Union Latinoamericana de Ciegos — ULAC)**
c/o Fundacion Braille del Uruguay
Duranzo 1772
Blanes 1132
11200 Montevideo, Uruguay
**Phone:** 598 2 4095943          **Fax:** 598 2 4000789
**Email:** fbu@fbraille.co.uy
**Website:** http://www.fbraille.com.uy
**Fnded:** 1985. **Mem:** 155. **Lang(s):** Spanish. **Desc:** Organizations of and for the blind in Latin American countries. Works for the prevention of blindness. Promotes the welfare of the blind and seeks to put them in control of their lives through the abolition of laws that discriminate against the visually handicapped. Sponsors educational programs in coordination with the International Agency for the Prevention of Blindness and the International Council for the Education of the Visually Handicapped. **Pub:** *America Latina*, quarterly. Newsletter.

---

★ **21014** ★ **Latin American Club of Neuro Ophthalmology (Club Latinoamericano de Neuroftalmologia — CLAN)**
Las Hualtatas 5951
Santiago, Chile
**Phone:** 56 2 3704600          **Fax:** 56 2 3718934
**Email:** luco@atscmet.net
**Fnded:** 1989. **Desc:** Fosters communication among scientists concerned with neuroophthalmology.

---

★ **21015** ★ **Leader Dogs for the Blind (LDB)**
PO Box 5000
Rochester, MI 48308
**Phone:** (248)651-9011          **Free:** 888-777-5332
**Fax:** (248)651-5812
**Email:** leaderdog@leaderdog.org
**Website:** http://www.leaderdog.org
William C. Hansen, Pres.
**Fnded:** 1939. **Desc:** Trains dogs to serve as guides for blind persons and conducts a supervised course of training to coordinate blind persons and their Leader Dogs as operating units; there is no charge for the service. Conducts research to determine the most satisfactory breed of dog for Leader Dog purposes. Places puppies into volunteer homes in preparation for formal adult dog training. Facilities include a dormitory, kennel, veterinary hospital, and training center. **Pub:** *Leader Dog Overview and Tour*. Videos. *Price:* Free. •

*Leader Dog Update*, quarterly. Newsletter. Available in large print, braille, and tape. *Price:* Free. • *Orientation of Dog Guide Users to New Environments*. • Also produces taped cassettes of all written materials available to the visually impared. **Frmly:** Path-Finder Guide Dogs; (1952) Leader Dog League for the Blind.

---

★ **21016** ★ **Lighthouse International**
111 E 59th St.
New York, NY 10022
**Phone:** (212)821-9200          **Free:** 800-829-0500
**Fax:** (212)821-9713
**Email:** info@lighthouse.org
**Website:** http://www.lighthouse.org
Barbara M. Silverstone, Pres. /CEO
**Fnded:** 1906. **Desc:** Works to build confidence, independence, opportunity, quality of life and hope for people with impaired vision. Provides information and resources to individuals and professionals. Operates the Lighthouse National Center for Vision and Aging and the Lighthouse National Center for Vision and Child Development; conducts continuing education programs for eye care providers; provides educational and advocacy services; offers training and employment to individuals with impaired vision; conducts laboratory research and studies on the consequences of vision impairment in everyday life. **Pub:** *Lighthouse News*, 3/year. Newsletter. *Price:* Free. • Annual Report; "Aging & Vision News"; literature on eye conditions and other aspects of vision loss.

---

★ **21017** ★ **Lutheran Braille Evangelism Association (LBEA)**
1740 Eugene St.
White Bear Lake, MN 55110
**Phone:** (651)426-0469
**Email:** lbeassoc@aol.com
**Website:** http://www.careministries.org/lbea.html
Rev. Dennis Hawkinson, Exec. Dir.
**Fnded:** 1952. **Mem:** 2,000. **Desc:** Fosters provision of religious material to the visually impaired. Supported by contributions of members. **Pub:** *Braille Evangelism Bulletin*, quarterly. Newsletter. Contains membership activities, and services and materials available. *Price:* Free. • *Christian Magnifier: A Christian Magazine in Magnified Print & Cassette*, monthly. Magazine. Contains large-print Christian inspirational readings. *Price:* $7/year. • *Tract Messenger*, monthly. Braille publication of Christian devotional readings and LBEA news. *Price:* Free. • Also provides religious material in braille, large print and audio cassette, such as the Holy Bible.

---

★ **21018** ★ **Lutheran Braille Workers (LBW)**
13471 California St.
Yucaipa, CA 92399
**Phone:** (909)795-8977          **Fax:** (909)795-8970
**Email:** lbw@lbwinc.org
**Website:** http://www.lbwinc.org
Loyd Coppenger, Exec. Dir.
**Fnded:** 1943. **Mem:** 7,000. **Desc:** Volunteers staffing 103 work centers worldwide, through which they seek to bring the Bible to the blind and visually impaired. Teaches sighted volunteers to transcribe printed material into braille and large print. Produces and distributes free biblical and devotional material in braille and large print in 40 languages. Works to constantly upgrade the systems necessary for the production of braille materials. **Pub:** *Lutheran Braille Workers–Newsletter*, quarterly. Newsletter. Covers association activities. *Price:* Free. • *Work Center Directory*, annual. Directory. • *Work Center Memo*, monthly. Newsletter. Provides information to LBW work centers.

---

★ **21019** ★ **Macular Disease Society**
PO Box 16
Denbigh LL16 5ZA, United Kingdom
**Phone:** 44 175816999
**Email:** info@maculardisease.org
**Website:** http://www.maculardisease.org

**Fnded:** 1986. **Mem:** 10,000. **Local Groups:** 100. **Desc:** Aims to provide information, fellowship and support to those with macular disease.

★ **21020** ★ **National Academy of Opticianry (NAO)**
8401 Corporate Dr No. 605
Landover, MD 20785
**Phone:** (301)577-4828          **Free:** 800-229-4828
**Fax:** (301)577-3880
**Website:** http://www.nao.org
Jim Iciek, Jr., Exec. Dir.

**Fnded:** 1973. **Mem:** 5,000. **Desc:** Offers review courses for national certification and state licensure examinations to members. Maintains speakers' bureau and Career Progression Program. **Pub:** *Academy Newsletter*, quarterly. Newsletter. • *Exam Review for Ophthalmic Dispensing.* • *Ophthalmic Dispensing Review Book.* Book. • *Optical Math Review.* • Brochure. • Videos.

★ **21021** ★ **National Accreditation Council for Agencies Serving the Blind and Visually Handicapped (NAC)**
16920 Detroit Ave., No. 100
Lakewood, OH 44107
**Email:** mundy260@aol.com
Gerald M. Mundy, Ed.D., Exec. Dir.

**Fnded:** 1966. **Desc:** Develops standards and administers a voluntary system of accreditation for school and organizations providing direct services to blind and visually disabled people. Sponsors training seminars for members and chairpersons of on-site review teams that visit organizations applying for accreditation. **Pub:** *The Standard-Bearer*, annual. • Annual Report. • Also publishes self-study and evaluation guides, incorporating standards for management and services of agencies and schools for people who are blind and visually handicapped; publications are available in print, braille, and recorded editions.

★ **21022** ★ **National Alliance of Blind Students (NABS)**
c/o American Council of the Blind
1155 15th St. NW, Ste. 1004
Washington, DC 20005
**Phone:** (202)467-5081          **Free:** 800-424-8666
**Fax:** (202)467-5085
**Email:** jsimeone1@sattbi.com
**Website:** http://www.acb.org/affiliates/
Jonathan Simeone, Pres.

**Fnded:** 1974. **Mem:** 150. **State Groups:** 8. **Desc:** Postsecondary students in academic, vocational, trade, and professional programs as well as disabled student service personnel. Aims to educate agencies, governments, institutions, and the public dealing with blind students as to their needs and educational pursuits in accredited postsecondary educational programs. Acts to protect rights and interests of blind students. Participates in annual National Student Seminar at the national convention of the American Council of the Blind. **Pub:** *Student Advocate*, quarterly. Newsletter. *Price:* Free to members.

★ **21023** ★ **National Association of Optometrists and Opticians (NAOO)**
PO Box 459
Marblehead, OH 43440
**Phone:** (419)798-2031          **Fax:** (419)798-8548
**Email:** fdrozak@cros.net
Franklin D. Rozak, Sec./Treas.

**Fnded:** 1960. **Mem:** 13,225. **Desc:** Licensed optometrists, opticians, and corporations. Conducts public affairs programs of mutual importance to members; serves as an organizational center for special purpose programs; acts as a clearinghouse for information affecting the retail optical industry. **Frmly:** National Optical Association.

★ **21024** ★ **National Association for Parents of the Visually Impaired (NAPVI)**
PO Box 317
Watertown, MA 02471
**Phone:** (617)972-7441          **Free:** 800-562-6265
**Fax:** (617)972-7444
**Email:** napvi@perkins.pvt.k12.ma.us
**Website:** http://www.spedex.com/napvi
Susan LaVenture, Exec. Dir.

**Fnded:** 1980. **Mem:** 2,000. **Reg. Groups:** 7. **State Groups:** 16. **Desc:** Parents and families of visually impaired children; community groups and agencies; interested individuals. Goals are to provide support for members and to promote public understanding of the needs and rights of the visually impaired child. Seeks to address parental needs for: emotional support; information about care, education, and treatment for their children; aid in establishing local, state, and regional groups; quality services for blind and impaired children; communication of their expertise and expectations with other parents and federal, state, and local service agencies; assurance that their children are accepted by society. Conducts workshops for parents. Conducts research programs. **Pub:** *Awareness*, quarterly. Newsletter. *Price:* Included in membership dues. • *How to Pack 'Em In: A Guide to Planning Workshops.* • *Mainstreaming Your Visually Impaired Child: Legislative Handbook for Parents.* Handbook. • *Parents to the Rescue.* Book. • *Preschool Learning Activities for the Visually Impaired Child: A Guide for Parents.* Book. • *Take Charge!: A Resource Guide for Parents of the Visually Impaired.* • *Your Child's Information Journal.* • Audiotapes. • Brochures. • Reprints. • Videos.

★ **21025** ★ **National Association of Vision Professionals (NAVP)**
c/o Prevention of Blindness Soc.
1775 Church St. NW
Washington, DC 20036
**Phone:** (202)234-1010          **Fax:** (202)234-1020
**Email:** mail@youreyes.org
**Website:** http://members.tripod.com/charlie216/
Michele Hartlove, Exec. Sec.

**Fnded:** 1976. **Mem:** 200. **Desc:** Individuals responsible for or connected with vision conservation and eye health programs in public or private agencies and institutions. Serves as a forum for ideas and programs, cooperates with other agencies, and promotes professional standards. Certifies vision screening personnel. **Pub:** *National Association of Vision Professionals–Newsletter*, quarterly. Newsletter. *Price:* Included in membership dues. **Frmly:** (1986) National Association of Vision Program Consultants.

★ **21026** ★ **National Association for Visually Handicapped (NAVH)**
22 W 21st St.
New York, NY 10010
**Phone:** (212)889-3141          **Fax:** (212)727-2931
**Email:** staff@navh.org
**Website:** http://www.navh.org
Lorraine Marchi, CEO

**Fnded:** 1954. **Mem:** 7,530. **Reg. Groups:** 2. **Desc:** Individuals, clubs, organizations, and foundations support NAVH's work in publishing and distributing large-print informational literature for the partially seeing. Acts as information clearinghouse regarding all public and private services available to the partially seeing. Offers guidance and counseling to parents of partially seeing children and to partially seeing adults. Educates the public and the professional community about the needs of the partially seeing. **Pub:** *About Children's Eyes. Price:* Free. • *It's All Right to Be Angry.* • *Knitting Instructions.* • *Large Print Loan Library Catalog*, biennial. Catalog. Lists books in large print commercial publishers available from NAVH. • *National Association for Visually Handicapped–Bulletin: Annual Program Report*, annual. Newsletter. Reports on association activities and programs. Includes obituaries. • *NAVH Update*, quarterly. Newsletter. Provides updates on issues and devices for the visually handicapped. • *Visual Aids & Information Materials.* Catalog. Features visual aids available from NAVH. • Also publishes (in English and Russian) pamphlets, guides, booklets, and manuals on eye diseases and services for visually impaired. **Frmly:** (1972) National Aid to Visually Handicapped.

★ **21027** ★ **National Beep Baseball Association (NBBA)**
2231 W 1st Ave.
Topeka, KS 66606-1304
**Phone:** (785)234-2156
**Email:** jb4208@aol.com
**Website:** http://www.nbba.org
Jeanette Bigger, Sec.

**Fnded:** 1975. **Mem:** 500. **Local Groups:** 20. **Desc:** Blind and visually impaired athletes, sighted volunteers, and others interested in participating in beep baseball. (Beep baseball uses a ball and two bases which emit sounds. Once the batter hits the ball, he or she must get to whichever base buzzes before one of the six other players fields the ball. The pitcher and catcher are sighted volunteers.) Promotes the development of amateur beep baseball and other recreational and competitive programs for the blind and visually impaired; holds tournaments. Sponsors speakers' bureau; conducts research programs. **Pub:** *Beep Baseball In A Nutshell.* Bulletin. *Price:* Free. • *History of NBBA.* Bulletin. • Newsletter, quarterly. Includes score statistics, tournament information and rule changes. *Price:* Included in membership dues.

★ **21028** ★ **National Board of Examiners in Optometry**
4340 E West Hwy., Ste. 1010
Bethesda, MD 20814
**Phone:** (301)652-5192          **Free:** 800-969-EXAM
**Fax:** (301)907-0013
**Email:** nbeo@optometry.org
**Website:** http://www.optometry.org
Dr. Norman E. Wallis, Exec. Dir.

**Fnded:** 1951. **Desc:** Administers entry-level criterion-referenced credentialing examinations to students and graduates of accredited schools and colleges of optometry for use by individual state licensing boards. Provides other evaluation, assessment, and survey services to the profession. **Pub:** *Candidates Guide*, annual. • *Test Points*, 3/year. Newsletter. • Annual Report. • Manuals.

★ **21029** ★ **National Braille Association (NBA)**
3 Townline Cir.
Rochester, NY 14623-2513
**Phone:** (585)427-8260          **Fax:** (585)427-0263
**Email:** nbaoffice@compuserve.com
**Website:** http://nationalbraille.org
Angela Coffaro, Exec. Dir.

**Fnded:** 1945. **Mem:** 1,500. **Desc:** Provides continuing education to those who prepare braille, and provides braille materials to persons who are visually impaired. Cooperates with other organizations in developing and expanding use of advanced braille codes; offers training workshops for transcribers. NBA Braille Book Bank maintains over 2000 titles and 500 standard technical tables for immediate thermoform duplication and embossing. recreation, and daily living. Cooperates with other organizations in developing and expanding use of advanced braille codes; offers training workshops for transcribers. NBA Braille Book Bank maintains over 2000 titles and 500 standard technical tables for immediate thermoform duplication and embossing. **Pub:** *Braille Technical Table Catalog*, periodic. Catalog. Contains technical tables in the NBA collection. Covers the fields of mathematics, statistics, chemistry, physics, computer science, and business. *Price:* Free. • *National Braille Association–Bulletin*, quarterly. Newsletter. Features articles of interest to members and persons working in the field of services to the visually impaired. Contains calendar of events. *Price:* Included in membership dues; $40/year for nonmembers in U.S.; $50/year outside U.S. • *National Braille Association–General Interest Catalog*, periodic. Catalog. Topics include work, recreation, and daily living. Directory of titles available in braille from NBA collection. Available in print and braille. *Price:* Free. • *National Braille Association–Music Catalog*, periodic. Catalog. Directory of music titles available in braille from NBA collection. Available in print and braille. *Price:* Free. • *National Braille Association–Textbook Catalog*, periodic. Catalog. Directory of titles of braille books from NBA collection of college-level and technical materials. Available in print and braille. *Price:* Free. • *NBA Publications*. Manuals. Cover tape recording, tactile graphics, mathematics and science brail le, textbook format braille, computer-assisted transcription, and large type. **Frmly:** (1964) National Braille Club.

★ **21030** ★ **National Braille Press (NBP)**
88 St. Stephen St.
Boston, MA 02115
**Phone:** (617)266-6160 **Free:** 888-965-8965
**Fax:** (617)437-0456
**Email:** lissa@nbp.org
**Website:** http://www.nbp.org
William M. Raeder, Pres.

**Fnded:** 1927. **Desc:** Publishes books and magazines in braille, including booklets on computers, self-help, and children's books (also in print). Supported by private gifts and legacies. Sponsors Children's Braille Book Club, offering monthly selections of print-braille books. **Pub:** *National Braille Press Release*, semiannual. Newsletter. • *Our Special*, bimonthly. • *Syndicated Columnists Weekly*.

**National Children's Eye Care Foundation (NCECF)**
*See:* Entry 5724

★ **21031** ★ **National Church Conference of the Blind**
PO Box 163
Denver, CO 80201
**Phone:** (303)455-3430
**Email:** care@careministries.org
**Website:** http://www.careministries.org/nccb.html
B.J. LeJeune, Contact
**Desc:** Blind Christians united to address accessibility issues; encourages members in faith.

★ **21032** ★ **National Contact Lens Examiners (NCLE)**
6506 Loisdale Rd., Ste.209
Springfield, VA 22150-1815
**Website:** http://www.abo.org
Michael H. Robey, Exec. Dir.
**Fnded:** 1974. **Mem:** 7,500. **Desc:** National certifying agency promoting continued development of opticians and technicians as contact lens fitters by formulating standards and procedures for determination of entry-level competency. Assists in the continuation, development, administration, and monitoring of a national Contact Lens Registry Examination (CLRE), which verifies entry-level competency of contact lens fitters. Issues certificates. Activities include: maintaining records of those certified in contact lens fitting; encouraging state occupational licensing and credentialing agencies to use the CLRE for licensure purposes; identifying contact lens dispensing education needs as a result of findings of examination programs; disseminating information to sponsors of contact lens continuing education programs.

★ **21033** ★ **National Council for the Blind of Ireland (NCBI)**
Whitworth Rd.
Druncomdra 9, Dublin, Ireland
**Phone:** 353 1 8307033 **Fax:** 353 1 8307787
**Email:** ncbi@iol.ie
**Website:** http://www.ncbi.ie
**Lang(s):** English, Irish. **Desc:** Individuals and organizations. Seeks to improve the quality of life of people with visual impairments; promotes increased independence for people with impaired vision. Makes available

support and services; conducts educational and advocacy campaigns.

★ **21034** ★ **National Eye Care Project (NECP)**
c/o American Academy of Opthalmology
PO Box 7424
San Francisco, CA 94142-7424
**Phone:** (415)561-8520 **Free:** 800-222-3937
**Email:** gnyman-york@aao.org
Gail Nyman-York, Public Svc. Mgr.
**Fnded:** 1986. **Desc:** Ophthalmologists dedicated to ensuring eye care for the elderly, particularly those who are economically disadvantaged. Provides medical and surgical eye care to individuals 65 and over who normally would not have access or the means to consult an ophthalmologist. Disseminates information on participating physicians and eye diseases. Offers referral services. A project of the Foundation of the American Academy of Ophthalmology. Publishes a fact sheet and information packet.

★ **21035** ★ **National Eye Research Foundation (NERF)**
c/o Andrew Kim
910 Skokie Blvd., No. 207A
Northbrook, IL 60062
**Phone:** (847)564-4652 **Free:** 800-621-2258
**Fax:** (847)564-0807
**Email:** nerf@eyemac.com
**Website:** http://www.nerf.org
Andrew K. Kin, Exec. Dir.
**Fnded:** 1955. **Mem:** 300. **Desc:** Persons with graduate degrees in the eye professions; persons without graduate degrees but employed in the field of eye care; others participating in the work of the foundation for charitable or public welfare purposes. Works to sponsor research and education relating to the eye and contact lenses and to promote interprofessional relations for better eye care. Serves as public information center for questions on eye care. Supports Vision Foundation for Blind Youth. Conducts research and certification program. **Pub:** *Contacto*, quarterly. Journal. *Price:* Included in membership dues; $85/year for nonmembers. • *The Pinnacle*, monthly. Newsletter.

★ **21036** ★ **National Federation of the Blind (NFB)**
1800 Johnson St.
Baltimore, MD 21230
**Phone:** (410)659-9314 **Fax:** (410)685-5653
**Email:** nfb@nfb.org
**Website:** http://www.nfb.org
Marc Maurer, Pres.
**Fnded:** 1940. **Mem:** 50,000. **State Groups:** 50. **Local Groups:** 700. **Desc:** Federation of state (50 plus Washington, DC and Puerto Rico) and local (600) organizations representing 50,000 blind people. Seeks the complete equality and integration of the blind into society. Monitors all legislation affecting the blind; evaluates present programs for the blind; stimulates and assists in promoting needed services. Supports and conducts scholarly research and publication of results. Works to improve policies toward the blind in such places as the U.S. Office of Personnel Management. Sponsors National White Cane Week annually for fundraising and educational purposes. Distributes information. Maintains National Blindness Information Center. **Pub:** *Braille Monitor*, monthly. Reports on action by the NFB on current legislative issues, legal cases, and social concerns affecting the blind; gives news of aids and appliances. *Price:* Included in membership dues; Available to nonmembers by donation. • *Future Reflections*, quarterly. Magazine. Offers guidance in the day-to-day aspects of raising a blind child. Includes literature reviews, calendar of events, and new product list. *Price:* Included in membership dues; $15/year for nonmembers. • *Voice of the Diabetic*, quarterly. Personal stories and practical guidance from blind diabetics and medical professionals; medical news; resource column; recipe corner. *Price:* Included in membership dues. • Brochures. • Pamphlets.

★ **21037** ★ **National Industries for the Blind (NIB)**
1901 N Beauregard St., Ste. 200
Alexandria, VA 22311-1727
**Phone:** (703)998-0770 **Fax:** (703)998-8268
**Email:** info@nib.org
**Website:** http://www.nib.org
Allan J. Clelland, Chm.
**Fnded:** 1938. **Mem:** 123. **Desc:** Association of agencies employing blind persons who undertake the production of certain goods and services for the federal government under the Javits-Wagner-O'Day Act. Offers gainful employment in these industries, located in 38 states, Puerto Rico, and the District of Columbia for those blind or multidisabled blind persons who are able and willing to work. Researches and recommends new products, prices, and price revisions to the Committee for Purchase From People Who Are Blind or Severely Disabled; allocates federal work orders among these agencies. Devises quality control systems; provides management and engineering services to increase plant efficiency and broaden opportunities for blind persons; assists the industries in procurement of raw materials. Marketing Division offers marketing, subcontracting, and industrial engineering expertise; Division of Rehabilitation Services works to establish evaluation and training programs to make possible the greater employment of multidisabled blind persons; Government Business Division deals with federal government contract administration, quality control, and pricing. Compiles statistics. **Pub:** *Opportunity*, quarterly. Magazine. Covers news and feature articles on agencies for the blind; describes industries, agencies, and projects that employ blind workers. • *60 Years of Success*, annual. Annual Report. • Report.

★ **21038** ★ **National League of the Blind of Ireland (NLBI)**
21 Hillstreet
Dublin 1, Ireland
**Phone:** 353 1 8742792 **Fax:** 353 1 8787139
**Fnded:** 1898. **Mem:** 150. **Lang(s):** English. **Desc:** A self-administered organization of blind individuals in the Republic of Ireland. Conducts advocacy activities, negotiating with local authorities and utility companies for better services for blind people. Offers income support programs to provide financial assistance with optical, medical, dental, clothing, and educational expenses. Advises members on their rights regarding entitlement programs; offers free legal aid. Organizes hospital visitations and sporting and social events including debates and lectures.

★ **21039** ★ **National Optometric Association (NOA)**
3723 Main St.
PO Box F
East Chicago, IN 46312
**Phone:** (219)398-1832 **Free:** 877-394-2020
**Fax:** (219)398-1077
**Email:** marshall@indiana.edu
**Website:** http://www.natoptassoc.org
Keith Howard, Pres.
**Fnded:** 1969. **Mem:** 450. **Nat'l Groups:** 1. **Reg. Groups:** 5. **Desc:** Optometrists dedicated to increasing awareness of the status of eye/vision health in the minority community and the national community at-large; and strives to make known the impact of the eye/vision dysfunction on the effectiveness and productivity of citizens and the academic proficiency of students. Conducts national minority recruiting programs, job placement, assistance programs for graduates, practitioners, and optometric organizations, and the promotion of delivery of care. Maintains speakers' bureau. Offers specialized education program. **Pub:** *NOA Newsletter*, semiannual. Newsletter. *Price:* Free.

★ **21040** ★ **National Optometry Association (NOA)**
PO Box 35189
Chicago, IL 60707-0189
**Phone:** (708)453-0080 **Fax:** (708)453-0083

**Email:** noa@rentamark.com
**Website:** http://www.medicalassociation.net
**Fnded:** 1975. **Mem:** 68,786. **Desc:** Optometrists. Seeks to increase members' public visibility and professional influence. Provides members with further education and recommends books to help the profession. Provides benefits. **Pub:** NOA-E Journal, monthly. Journal.

★ **21041** ★ **National Pro-Life Religious Council (RPIFB)**
6 Belvedere Pl., off Mountjoy Sq.
Dublin 1, Ireland
**Phone:** 353 1 8559330      **Fax:** 353 1 8559331
**Lang(s):** English, Irish. **Desc:** Religious individuals supporting the right to life of the unborn. Seeks to "see every denomination or fellowship proclaim and obey the Biblical teaching and religious tradition that affirm the value of all human life." Articulates the "historic Judeo-Christian perspective concerning human life issues" to the public; supports efforts to discourage and prevent abortion and voluntary euthanasia; ministers to people considering abortion or voluntary euthanasia. Serves as a clearinghouse on right to life issues; facilitates communication and cooperation among right to life organizations.

★ **21042** ★ **New Zealand Association of Optometrists**
PO Box 1978
Wellington, New Zealand
**Phone:** 64 4 4732322      **Fax:** 64 4 4732328
**Email:** nzao@inca.co.nz
**Website:** http://www.nzao.co.nz
**Fnded:** 1930. **Mem:** 800. **Reg. Groups:** 8. **Desc:** Optometrists in New Zealand. Seeks to ensure high standards of ethics and practice in optometry.

★ **21043** ★ **Operation Eyesight Universal (OEU)**
4 Parkdale Cres. NW
Calgary, AB, Canada T2N 3T8
**Phone:** (403)283-6323      **Fax:** (403)270-1899
**Email:** oeuca@giftofsight.com
**Website:** http://www.giftofsight.com
**Fnded:** 1963. **Mem:** 65,000. **Reg. Groups:** 3. **Lang(s):** English. **Desc:** Individuals, firms, churches, schools, service clubs, and other organizations united to promote sight restoration and blindness prevention through programs in developing countries. Provides medical, educational, assistance to needy individuals. Assists in the establishment of: special programs to combat blindness due to malnutrition; eye care hospitals; eye care departments in health care institutions; rural mobile eye programs. Works with local blindness prevention societies. Operates training programs. **Pub:** Gift of Sight, quarterly. Newsletter.

★ **21044** ★ **Ophthalmic Photographers' Society (OPS)**
c/o Barbara McCalley
1869 W Ranch Rd.
Nixa, MO 65714-9230
**Phone:** (417)725-0181      **Free:** 800-403-1677
**Fax:** (417)724-8450
**Email:** opsmember@aol.com
**Website:** http://www.opsweb.org
Jeffery A. Sobel, CRA, Contact
**Fnded:** 1969. **Mem:** 1,200. **Reg. Groups:** 9. **Desc:** Ophthalmologists, pathologists, medical and ophthalmic photographers, nurses, ophthalmic assistants, technicians, technologists, researchers, and engineers; organizations and individuals who are actively involved with ophthalmology or ophthalmic photography. Objective is to encourage the highest quality of ophthalmic photography and to promote development of new and improved techniques and equipment. (Ophthalmic photography involves photography of the eye for documentation and diagnostic purposes.) Provides continuing education and technical information. Serves as a forum for the discussion of ophthalmic photography. Provides testing, and subsequent

certification as Certified Retinal Angiographer in performance of ophthalmic photography. **Pub:** Journal of Ophthalmic Photography, semiannual. Journal. Price: $26 US; $31 International. • OPS Directory, annual. Directory. • OPS Newsletter, bimonthly. Newsletter.

★ **21045** ★ **Opticians Association of America (OAA)**
7023 Little River Turnpike, No. 207
Annandale, VA 22003
**Phone:** (703)916-8856      **Free:** 800-443-8997
**Fax:** (703)916-7966
**Email:** oaa@opticians.org
**Website:** http://www.opticians.org
Earl M. Cleveland, Pres.
**Fnded:** 1926. **Mem:** 10,000. **State Groups:** 48. **Desc:** Retail dispensing opticians who fill prescriptions for glasses or contact lenses written by a vision care specialist. Works to advance the science of ophthalmic optics. Conducts research and educational programs. Maintains museum and speakers' bureau. Compiles statistics. **Pub:** American Optician, quarterly. Magazine. Contains calendar of events and research reports. Price: Included in membership dues. **Frmly:** (1972) Guild of Prescription Opticians of America.

★ **21046** ★ **Optometric Extension Program Foundation (OEPF)**
1921 E Carnegie, Ste. 3L
Santa Ana, CA 92705-5510
**Phone:** (949)250-8070      **Fax:** (949)250-8157
**Email:** oepl@oep.org
**Website:** http://www.healthy.net/oep
Robert A. Williams, Exec. Dir.
**Fnded:** 1928. **Mem:** 4,000. **Desc:** Registered optometrists and optometric assistants enrolled for continuing education courses. Maintains speakers' bureau. Sponsors educational programs. **Pub:** Journal of Behavioral Optometry, bimonthly. Journal. Includes professional articles, calendar of events, and current affairs. Price: $65/year. • Optometric Extension Program Foundation–Curriculum II, annual. Text of 6-8 courses covering various optometry subjects. Includes literature and research reviews and annual index. Price: $350. • Reference Directory, biennial. Directory.

★ **21047** ★ **Optometric Historical Society (OHS)**
243 N Lindbergh Blvd.
Saint Louis, MO 63141
**Phone:** (314)991-4100      **Free:** 800-365-2219
**Fax:** (314)991-4101
**Email:** mdjones-od@phd.aol.org
Dr. Michael Johns, Exec. Dir.
**Fnded:** 1969. **Desc:** Optometrists and other individuals or groups interested in optometry, optics, and related disciplines. Purposes are to encourage the collection and preservation of materials relating to the history of optometry and to assist in the care of archives of optometric interest. **Pub:** Newsletter, quarterly.

★ **21048** ★ **Optometrists Association Australia**
204 Drummond St.
Carlton, VIC 3053, Australia
**Phone:** 61 3 96636833      **Fax:** 61 3 96637478
**Email:** oaanat@optometrists.asn.au
**Website:** http://www.optometrists.asn.au
**State Groups:** 6. **Lang(s):** English. **Desc:** Optometrists. Seeks to advance the profession of optometry; promotes ongoing professional development of members. Represents members' interests before government agencies and other organizations; provides resources to assist optometric practices. Makes available to the public information and services.

★ **21049** ★ **ORBIS International**
520 8th Ave, 11th Fl.
New York, NY 10018

**Phone:** (646)674-5500      **Free:** 800-ORBIS-US
**Fax:** (646)674-5599
**Email:** executive@ny.orbis.org
**Website:** http://www.orbis.org
Kathy Spahn, Pres. and Exec. Dir.
**Fnded:** 1973. **Desc:** Dedicated to saving sight and eliminating avoidable blindness worldwide. Responds to the needs of developing nations, where eighty percent of blind people live, with hands-on training for eye care professionals, public education about blindness, and technical assistance to improve access to quality ophthalmic services. Has the world's only flying eye hospital, a DC-10 that has been converted into a state-of-the-art medical facility, and flies to developing countries to provide intensive, comprehensive eye care training. Has long-term country programs in Bangladesh, China, Ethiopia, India and Vietnam. **Pub:** ORBIS Observer, quarterly. Newsletter. Price: Free. • ORBIS Observer - Hong Kong. Newsletter. • ORBIS Observer - U.K.. Newsletter. **Frmly:** Project Orbis.

★ **21050** ★ **Organization of Icelandic Optometrists (Felag Islenskra Sjontakatradinga)**
c/o Gleraugnaverslunin EGC
Haraborg 10
PO Box 403
IS-200 Kopavogi, Iceland
**Mem:** 40.

★ **21051** ★ **Orthoptic and Binocular Vision Association (OBVA)**
48 Church St.
Tamworth B79 7DE, United Kingdom
**Phone:** 44 1827 61600
**Email:** d.b.stidwill@aston.ac.uk
**Fnded:** 1958. **Mem:** 150. **Nat'l Groups:** 1. **Lang(s):** English. **Desc:** Optometrists are full members; optometry students and other health care professionals are associate members. Promotes orthoptic and vision training among health care professionals. Conducts educational programs in orthoptics and binocular vision. **Pub:** OBVA Newsletter, quarterly. Newsletter. Contains abstracts, cases, and comment.

**Outpatient Ophthalmic Surgery Society (OOSS)**
See: Entry 19584

★ **21052** ★ **Pan-American Association of Ophthalmology (PAAO)**
1301 S Bowen Rd., Ste. 365
Arlington, TX 76013
**Phone:** (817)265-2831      **Fax:** (817)275-3961
**Email:** info@paao.org
**Website:** http://www.paao.org
J. Bronwyn Bateman, MD, Pres.
**Fnded:** 1939. **Mem:** 14,000. **Desc:** Ophthalmologists throughout the Western Hemisphere. Seeks to improve the treatment of eye diseases and prevention of blindness in the Americas through the exchange of ideas and treatments. **Pub:** Noticiero, quarterly. • Pan-American Association of Ophthalmology-The Pan American, semiannual. Newsletter. Includes obituaries and conference calendar. Price: Free.

★ **21053** ★ **Pan-American Implant Association (PAIA)**
5591 Cote des Neiges Rd., Ste. 1
Montreal, QC, Canada H3T 1Y8
**Phone:** (514)735-1133      **Fax:** (514)731-0651
**Email:** uvision@generation.net
**Mem:** 250. **Desc:** Eye surgeons from North, Central, and South America dedicated to improving their skills and disseminating information to the medical communities in their homelands.

## ★ 21054 ★ Panhellenic Association of Opticians and Optometrists
49 Menadrou St., 4th Fl.
GR-10437 Athens, Greece
**Phone:** 30 1 5232616          **Fax:** 30 1 5232664
**Fnded:** 1926. **Mem:** 700. **Desc:** Opticians and optometrists. Promotes members' interests. Conducts training courses.

## ★ 21055 ★ Parents Active for Vision Education (PAVE)
4135 54th Pl.
San Diego, CA 92105-2303
**Phone:** (619)287-0081          **Free:** 800-PAVE-988
**Fax:** (619)287-0084
**Email:** info@pavevision.org
**Website:** http://www.pave-eye.com/vision
Marjie Thompson, Pres.
**Fnded:** 1988. **Local Groups:** 1. **Desc:** Parents and teachers with children in their homes and classrooms who suffer or have suffered from the effects of undiagnosed vision problems. Works to raise public awareness of learning related vision problems. Supports the development of comprehensive learning related vision screenings, vision education, and vision hygiene programs in schools and communities. Maintains speakers' bureau **Pub:** *The Hidden Disability: Undetected Vision Problems.* Pamphlet. *Price:* $23.50 100 copies, includes shipping and handling. • *Pavestones,* semiannual. Newsletter. *Price:* Free. • *Some Heroes Are Small.* Book. *Price:* $3.50 plus shipping and handling. • *Vision Alert: 20/20 is NOT Enough.* Video. *Price:* $40.

## ★ 21056 ★ Partially Sighted Society (PSS)
9 Plato Pl.
72-74 St. Dionis Rd.
London SW6 4TU, United Kingdom
**Phone:** 44 1302 323132          **Fax:** 44 171 3170289
**Fnded:** 1973. **Mem:** 2,000. **Local Groups:** 20. **Desc:** Strives to improve social, medical, and domestic services available to the visually impaired in the United Kingdom and to increase educational and employment opportunities. Offers information and advice; provides visual aids and special printing and enlargement services. Operates 3 sight centers that offer vision assessment and training services. Arranges conferences, exhibitions, and displays. **Pub:** *Oculus,* quarterly. Newsletter. In large print. • Brochures, periodic. • Catalog, periodic.

## ★ 21057 ★ Pilot Dogs (PD)
625 W Town St.
Columbus, OH 43215
**Phone:** (614)221-6367          **Fax:** (614)221-1577
**Website:** http://www.pilotdogs.org/
J. Jay Gray, Exec. Dir.
**Fnded:** 1950. **Mem:** 20,841. **Desc:** Provides guide dogs and training for the blind. **Pub:** *Pilot Light,* quarterly.

## ★ 21058 ★ Prevent Blindness America
500 E Remington Rd.
Schaumburg, IL 60173-5611
**Phone:** (847)843-2020          **Free:** 800-331-2020
**Fax:** (847)843-8458
**Email:** info@preventblindness.org
**Website:** http://www.preventblindness.org
Elaine Barber, COO
**Fnded:** 1908. **Nat'l Groups:** 1. **Reg. Groups:** 2. **State Groups:** 20. **Desc:** Charitable organization committed to preventing blindness and preserving sight through nationwide comprehensive programs of public and professional education, research, industrial, and community services. Services include promotion and support of local glaucoma screening programs, preschool vision testing, industrial eye safety, and collection of statistical and other data on nature and extent of causes of blindness and defective vision. Operates a toll-free information center dealing with eye health and safety topics. Through the Fight for Sight Research Division, the organization awards student fellowships, postdoctoral awards and grants in aid for medical research. Sponsors Wise Owl Program to promote widespread use of safety eyewear for various activities and occupations. Compiles statistics. **Pub:** *Prevent Blindness America–Annual Report.* Covers highlights and accomplishments of the previous fiscal year. Includes financial statements. *Price:* Free. • *Prevent Blindness News,* 3/year. Newsletter on eye health and safety. *Price:* $10/year. **Frmly:** (1915) National Committee for the Prevention of Blindness; (1928) National Society for the Prevention of Blindness; (1978) National Society to Prevent Blindness.

## ★ 21059 ★ Protestant Guild for Human Services (PGHS)
411 Waverley Oaks Rd., Ste. 104
Waltham, MA 02452-8405
**Phone:** (781)893-6000          **Fax:** (781)893-1171
**Email:** admin@protestantguild.org
**Website:** http://www.protestantguild.org
Edmund T. Hagerty, Exec. Dir.
**Fnded:** 1945. **Local Groups:** 2. **Desc:** Non-sectarian organization with a volunteer board and highly-trained professional staff dedicated to serving individuals with special needs. Provides a wide spectrum of services to children, adolescents and young adults with a variety of developmental disabilities. **Pub:** *Annual Report,* annual. • *PGHS News,* semiannual. Newsletter. **Frmly:** Protestant Guild for the Blind.

## ★ 21060 ★ Recording for the Blind and Dyslexic (RFB)
20 Roszel Rd.
Princeton, NJ 08540
**Phone:** (609)452-0606          **Free:** 800-803-7201
**Fax:** (609)987-8116
**Email:** info@rfbd.org
**Website:** http://www.rfbd.org
Anne T. Macdonald, Founder
**Fnded:** 1948. **Mem:** 40,000. **Reg. Groups:** 31. **Desc:** Provides library services, computerized books, books on audiotape, and other educational materials free of charge to individuals who are unable to read standard print because of a visual, physical, or perceptual disability. Materials are produced by 4800 volunteers at 31 recording studios throughout the U.S. Titles recorded supplement, but do not duplicate, those of the Library of Congress Talking Book program. **Pub:** *Catalog of Titles,* annual. Contains listings of our audio and e-text titles. *Price:* $69.95 for set. • *Disk Catalog,* quarterly. *Price:* $16/year. • *Recorded Catalog,* quarterly. *Price:* $16/year. • *Recording for the Blind–Annual Report,* annual. Annual Report. Includes financial statements for the fiscal year as well as highlights from the previous year. *Price:* Free. • *Recording for the Blind–Catalog Supplement,* periodic. • *RFB and D Impact,* quarterly. Newsletter. For donors, agencies, and schools serving the blind and print-disabled. *Price:* Free. **Frmly:** (1951) National Committee for Recording for the Blind; (2000) Recording for the Blind.

## ★ 21061 ★ Rehabilitated Blind Youth Club of Cameroon (RBYCC) (Club de Jeunes Aveugles Rehabiltes du Cameroun — CJARC)
Boite Postale 2315
Yaounde, Cameroon
**Phone:** 237 222422          **Fax:** 237 223859
**Fnded:** 1988. **Mem:** 110. **Lang(s):** English, French. **Desc:** Blind and visually impaired youth; providers of support and services to people with visual impairment. Promotes integration of people with visual impairment into the social and economic mainstream. Conducts educational and vocational training programs. **Pub:** *Bartimee,* annual. Journal. News of the RBYCC activities.

## ★ 21062 ★ Research to Prevent Blindness (RPB)
645 Madison Ave.
New York, NY 10022-1010
**Phone:** (212)752-4333          **Free:** 800-621-0026
**Fax:** (212)688-6231
**Email:** info@rpbusa.org
**Website:** http://www.rpbusa.org/hc2/index.asp
Diane S. Swift, Pres.
**Fnded:** 1960. **Desc:** National voluntary health foundation supported by foundations, corporations, and voluntary gifts and bequests from individuals. Established to stimulate basic and applied research into the causes, prevention, and treatment of blinding eye diseases. Grants funds for equipment, eye research professorships with up to 7 year salary support, assistance in financing construction campaigns for eye research laboratory facilities, and travel expenses for international scholars for short-term collaborative research in the U.S. Through seminars and other means, encourages communication among scientists, practicing ophthalmologists, and the public. Maintains scientific advisory panel. **Pub:** *Eye Research News Briefs,* annual. Newsletter. Contain reports on latest developments in eye research. *Price:* Free. • *Eye Research Seminar Papers,* biennial. Papers. • *Research to Prevent Blindness–Annual Report.* Contains information on RPB's activities in support of scientific research into the causes, treatment, and prevention of blindness. *Price:* Free.

## ★ 21063 ★ Retinitis Pigmentosa International (RPI)
c/o Helen Harris
PO Box 900
Woodland Hills, CA 91365
**Phone:** (818)992-0500          **Free:** 800-FIGHT-RP
**Fax:** (818)992-3265
**Email:** rpint@pacbell.net
**Website:** http://www.rpinternational.org
Helen Harris, Pres.
**Fnded:** 1972. **Mem:** 30,000. **State Groups:** 4. **Local Groups:** 1. **Desc:** Seeks to raise funds to support research and provide human service programs to assist the visually impaired. Offers charitable services. Maintains research programs. Also describes motion picture and television programs for the blind. Produces annual television special "The Eyes of Christmas" with celebrity memories and a motion picture described for the blind and vision impaired. **Pub:** *Nightlighter, Sound Bites,* annual. Newsletter.

## ★ 21064 ★ Retinoblastoma Society (RS)
St. Bartholomew's Hospital
London EC1A 7BE, United Kingdom
**Phone:** 44 207 6003309          **Fax:** 44 207 6008579
**Email:** rbinfo@rbsociety.org.uk
**Website:** http://www.rbsociety.org.uk
**Fnded:** 1986. **Mem:** 1,000. **Lang(s):** English. **Desc:** Children with retinoblastoma (eye cancer) and their families; other interested individuals. Seeks to improve the quality of life of people with eye cancer; promotes advancement in the prevention, diagnosis, and treatment of retinoblastoma. Provides support for people with retinoblastoma and their families; fundraising activities to support eye cancer research. **Pub:** *ORBS,* 3/year. Newsletter.

## ★ 21065 ★ Royal Australian College of Ophthalmologists
27 Commonwealth St.
Sydney, NSW 2010, Australia
**Phone:** 61 2 92677006          **Fax:** 61 92676534
**Email:** racosec@medeserv.cem.au
**Fnded:** 1969.

## ★ 21066 ★ Royal College of Ophthalmologists
17 Cornwall Terr.
London NW1 4QW, United Kingdom
**Phone:** 44 207 9350702          **Fax:** 44 207 9359838
**Email:** margaret@rcophth.btinternet.com

**Website:** http://www.rcophth.ac.uk
**Fnded:** 1988. **Mem:** 3,027. **Desc:** Medical Practitioners (ophthalmologists). **Pub:** *EYE*, bimonthly. Journal.


## Royal Institute for Deaf and Blind Children (RIDBC)
*See:* Entry 6102


## ★ 21067 ★ Royal National Institute for the Blind England (RNIB)
105 Judd St.
London WC1H 9NE, United Kingdom
**Phone:** 44 207 3881266
**Email:** cservices@rnib.org.uk
**Website:** http://www.rnib.org.uk
**Fnded:** 1868. **Reg. Groups:** 10. **Local Groups:** 40. **Lang(s):** English. **Desc:** "Wants a world in which blind and partially sighted people enjoy the same rights, freedoms, and responsibilities and quality of life as people who are fully sighted." Mission is to challenge blindness. Challenges the disabling effects of blindness by providing services to help people determine their own lives. Challenges society's actions, attitudes, and assumptions. Works to dismantle barriers that are put into the path of the blind and partially sighted people. Works to prevent, cure, and alleviate blindness. **Pub:** *Publications Catalogue*.


## ★ 21068 ★ Scandinavian Society of Cataract and Refractive Surgery
c/o Ingrid Floren
Department of Ophthalmology
University Hospital
S-221 85 Lund, Sweden
**Phone:** 46 46 171470    **Fax:** 46 46 2115074
**Email:** ingrid.floren@oft.lu.se
**Desc:** Strives to advance scientific knowledge in the field of intraocular lens implantation and the practice of refractive surgery.


## ★ 21069 ★ Schweizerische Berufsverband fur Augenoptik und Optometrie (SBAO)
Sonnmattrain 7
CH-6043 Adligenswil, Switzerland
**Phone:** 41 41 3720682    **Fax:** 41 41 3720683
**Website:** http://www.sbao.ch
**Fnded:** 1980. **Mem:** 740. **Lang(s):** English, French, German, Italian. **Desc:** Optometrists. Seeks to improve standards of optometric study, teaching, and practice. Conducts continuing professional development courses for members.


## ★ 21070 ★ Scottish Committee of Optometrists
7 Queens Bldgs.
Queensferry Rd.
Rosyth
Fife
Saint Andrews KY11 2RA, United Kingdom
**Phone:** 44 383 419444    **Fax:** 44 383 416778
**Fnded:** 1935. **Mem:** 760. **Lang(s):** English. **Desc:** All optometrists in Scotland. Represents interests of independent optometrists in Scotland. **Pub:** *Look North*, bimonthly. Newsletter.


## ★ 21071 ★ Scottish National Federation for the Welfare of the Blind
Thomas Herd House
10/12 Ward Rd.
Dundee DD1 1LX, United Kingdom
**Phone:** 44 1307 460359    **Fax:** 44 1307 460359
**Email:** snfwb@dsvip.co.uk
**Fnded:** 1917. **Mem:** 63. **Lang(s):** English. **Desc:** Parent body for numerous charities and local authorities in Scotland concerned with the welfare of blind and partially sighted people. Provides information on social work, education, and employment services. **Pub:** Annual Report.


## ★ 21072 ★ Seeing Eye
PO Box 375
Morristown, NJ 07963-0375
**Phone:** (973)539-4425    **Fax:** (973)539-0922
**Website:** http://www.seeingeye.org
**Fnded:** 1929. **Desc:** Seeks to enhance the independence, dignity, and self-confidence of blind and visually impaired persons; provides assistance to graduates and their seeing-eyed dogs; educates the public in consideration of public policy. **Pub:** Annual Report.


## SENSE
*See:* Entry 6106


## ★ 21073 ★ Sight Savers International - East, Central and Southern Africa Region
Mai Mahiu Rd., off Langata Rd.
Nairobi West
PO Box 34690
GPO
Nairobi, Kenya
**Phone:** 254 2 505750    **Fax:** 254 2 505548
**Email:** info@sightsavers.or.ke
**Website:** http://www.sightsavers.org
**Fnded:** 1949. **Desc:** Promotes programs for the blind and visually impaired in Kenya, Uganda, Tanzania, Malawi, Zimbabwe. Fosters public awareness. Programmes in eye care, education and rehabilitation for the blind and visually impaired. **Pub:** *Horizons*, quarterly. Update on SSI activities worldwide. • *Xerophthaimia Bulletin*, periodic. Bulletin.


## ★ 21074 ★ Sight Savers International - England
Grosvenor Hall
Bolnore Rd.
Haywards Heath RH16 4BX, United Kingdom
**Phone:** 44 1444 446600    **Fax:** 44 1444 446688
**Email:** information@sightsaversint.org.uk
**Website:** http://www.sightsavers.org.uk
**Fnded:** 1950. **Mem:** 30. **Lang(s):** English. **Desc:** Works to prevent and cure blindness and also to provide education and rehabilitation for blind people in economically developing countries. Concentrates on comprehensive eye services which link the sectors together. Cooperates with indigenous government agencies and local leadership to develop and implement vision care programs. Conducts leadership development and educational programs to make projects sustainable using local resources and expertise. **Pub:** *Horizons*, 3/year. Newsletter. Donor newsletter.


## ★ 21075 ★ Sociedad Argentina de Oftalmologia
Santa Fe 1171
1059 Buenos Aires, Argentina
**Phone:** 54 1 2410392
**Fnded:** 1920.


## ★ 21076 ★ Society for Excellence in Eyecare
4400 Jenifer St., NW, Ste. 230
Washington, DC 20015
**Phone:** (202)244-7334    **Fax:** (202)362-4730
**Email:** peter@see.anasmm.com
**Website:** http://www.excellenteyesurgery.com
Peter Anas, Exec. Dir.
**Fnded:** 1989. **Mem:** 100. **Desc:** Seeks excellence in eye surgery and peri-operative care and is committed that patients with ocular problems are afforded safe, high quality and cost-effective care of the eye. Endeavors to seek education, training and advocacy, those policies, procedures and technologies that promote patient access to vision restoring treatment.


## ★ 21077 ★ Society of Eye Surgeons (SES)
7801 Norfolk Ave.
Bethesda, MD 20814

**Phone:** (301)986-1830    **Fax:** (301)986-1876
**Email:** ief@iefusa.org
**Website:** http://www.iefusa.org
Kelvin Baervldd, Public Affairs Officer
**Fnded:** 1969. **Mem:** 1,000. **Desc:** Ophthamologists promoting the science of ophthalmic surgery worldwide. Supports the blindness prevention efforts of the International Eye Foundation. Provides educational, training, and eye care services by sponsoring teaching teams and professors to visit countries worldwide; fosters social exchange among physicians and scientists in the field of ophthalmology. **Pub:** *Eye to Eye*, semiannual. Newsletter. Provides program news.


## ★ 21078 ★ Surgical Eye Expeditions International (SEE Int'l)
27 C-2 E De La Guerra St.
Santa Barbara, CA 93101
**Phone:** (805)963-3303    **Free:** 800-20T-0SEE
**Fax:** (805)965-3564
**Email:** seeintl@seeintl.org
**Website:** http://www.seeintl.org
Jorge Rodriguez, MD,MPH, Contact
**Fnded:** 1974. **Mem:** 756. **Local Groups:** 1. **Desc:** Provides free sight-restoring surgery to indigent and disadvantaged blind individuals in the United States and throughout the developing world. Recruits volunteer opthalmologists, nurses, and technicians. Maintains speakers' bureau. Conducts charitable and educational programs. Provides children's services. Compiles statistics. Organizes symposia. **Pub:** *Affiliate Action*, bimonthly. Newsletter. Provides recap of current and future programs for professional members. • *SEE Scan*, annual. Newsletter. Includes news on surgical expeditions, vision care programs, and group activities. • Annual Report.


## ★ 21079 ★ Talking Newspaper Association of the United Kingdom
10 Browning Rd.
Heathfield TN21 8DB, United Kingdom
**Phone:** 44 1435 866102    **Fax:** 44 1435 865422
**Email:** info@tnauk.org.uk
**Website:** http://www.tnauk.org.uk
**Fnded:** 1974. **Mem:** 18,000. **Local Groups:** 430. **Lang(s):** English. **Desc:** Records newspapers and magazine on audio tape, computer disk, or CD-ROM for visually impaired persons. **Pub:** *Talking Newspaper News*, quarterly. Magazine.


## ★ 21080 ★ Tanzania Society for the Blind
PO Box 2254
Dar es Salaam, United Republic of Tanzania
**Phone:** 255 51 460858    **Fax:** 255 51 460857
**Desc:** Seeks to meet the special needs of the visually-impaired in Tanzania. Offers educational, training, and rehabilitation programs.


## ★ 21081 ★ Thyroid Eye Disease (TED)
Solstice
Sea Rd.
Winchelsea Beach
Winchelsea TN36 4LH, United Kingdom
**Phone:** 44 179 222338
**Email:** tedassn@eclipse.co.uk
**Fnded:** 1989. **Mem:** 700. **Lang(s):** English. **Desc:** Endocrinologists, ophthalmologists, radiologists, and other health care professionals; people with thyroid eye disease and their families. Seeks to advance the diagnosis and treatment of thyroid eye disease. Promotes increased awareness of thyroid eye disease in the medical community. Provides information, care, and support to people with thyroid eye disease; provides financial assistance to thyroid eye disease research. Maintains medical helpline. **Pub:** Newsletter, quarterly. • Bulletin, periodic.

**★ 21082 ★ U.S. Association for Blind Athletes (USABA)**
33 N Institute St.
Colorado Springs, CO 80903
**Phone:** (719)630-0422     **Fax:** (719)630-0616
**Email:** usaba@usa.net
**Website:** http://www.usaba.org/
Dr. Charly Huebner, Exec. Dir.
**Fnded:** 1976. **Mem:** 3,000. **Reg. Groups:** 4. **State Groups:** 49. **Desc:** Visually impaired athletes; fully sighted physical educators, coaches, and special education teachers; interested volunteers. Aims to develop individual independence through athletic competition. Promotes sports for the legally blind and visually impaired, organizes regional, national, and international competitions; works with other international organizations to promote goodwill and independence through friendly competition. Sports contested include alpine skiing, goalball, gymnastics, judo, nordic skiing, powerlifting, speed skating, swimming, tandem cycling, track and field and wrestling. Has sponsored 14 National Championships and 4 North American Games for the Blind between Canada and the U.S. Competed in the Paralympics in Seoul, Korea in 1988. Sent paralympic teams to Barcelona, Spain and Albertville, France in 1992. Sponsors coaches' training seminars, panel discussions, and training groups. Offers children's services; compiles statistics. **Pub:** *Directory of Organization Representatives*, quarterly. Directory. • *USABA Agenda*, monthly. Includes information on upcoming events. • *Vision*, quarterly. Magazine. Includes results of competitions and calender of events. **Price:** Included in membership dues. • Also publishes programs and grant proposals.

**★ 21083 ★ United States Blind Golfers' Association (USBGA)**
3094 Shamrock St. N
Tallahassee, FL 32308-2735
**Phone:** (850)893-4511     **Fax:** (850)893-4511
**Email:** usbga@blindgolf.com
**Website:** http://www.blindgolf.com
Bob Andrews, Pres.
**Fnded:** 1953. **Mem:** 145. **Desc:** Blind and vision impaired golfers who compete for a national championship and U.S. Open, and various other tournaments around the country and internationally. Tournaments raise funds for various blind charities. Blind Junior Golf Program. **Pub:** *The Midnight Golfer*, semiannual. Newsletter. Includes information on blind golf; some international coverage. **Price:** Free. • Also provides learning packets and information on blind golf.

**★ 21084 ★ Vision Australia Foundation**
454 Glenferrie Rd.
Kooyong, VIC 3144, Australia
**Phone:** 61 3 98649222     **Fax:** 61 3 98649210
**Email:** info@visionaustralia.org.au
**Website:** http://www.visionaustralia.org.au
**Lang(s):** English. **Desc:** Blind and vision impaired people in Australia. Provides assistance to members so that they may go on living lives they value.

**★ 21085 ★ Vision Community Services - A Division of the Massachusetts Association for the Blind (VCS)**
23A Elm St.
Watertown, MA 02472-2821
**Phone:** (617)926-4232     **Free:** 800-852-3029
**Fax:** (617)926-1412
**Email:** fweisse@mablind.org
**Website:** http://www.mablind.org
Fran Weisse, Dir. /Info. Svcs.
**Fnded:** 1903. **State Groups:** 3. **Desc:** Serves individuals who are newly blind or partially sighted, and those with progressive eye disease, as well as individuals who are blind. Provides information and referral services, individualized advocacy, self-help support groups, buddy telephone network, special services for elders, community volunteer services, recording studio, braille program, Newsline Boston, and a store of assistive devices. **Pub:** *VCS Resource List*, biennial. Catalog. In large print. Lists print, large print, cassette,

disc, and braille brochures, pamphlets, fact sheets, and catalogs. Also available on cassette. *Price:* Free. • *VCS Resource Update*, bimonthly. Newsletter. In large print. Describes services and adaptive equipment for visually impaired individuals. Also available on cassette. *Price:* Free. **Frmly:** (2001) Vision Community Services.

**★ 21086 ★ Visually Impaired Data Processors International (VIDPI)**
c/o American Council of the Blind
1155 15th St. NW, Ste. 1004
Washington, DC 20005
**Phone:** (202)467-5081     **Free:** 800-424-8666
**Email:** rrrogers@one.net
**Website:** http://www.acb.org/vidpi/
Robert R. Rogers, Pres.
**Fnded:** 1970. **Mem:** 75. **Desc:** Visually impaired electronic data processing employees; those seeking employment; employers, instructors, manufacturers, and students in the electronic data processing field. Advocates high standards in training visually impaired students. Seeks to increase employment opportunities; encourages the exchange of work technique ideas and the development of new equipment. Works with agencies to increase the availability of braille and recorded materials. Supports a speakers' bureau. **Pub:** *Views*, quarterly.

**★ 21087 ★ Visually Impaired Veterans of America (VIVA)**
c/o American Council of the Blind
1155 15th St. NW, Ste. 1004
Washington, DC 20005
**Phone:** (202)467-5081     **Free:** 800-424-8666
**Email:** rrrogers@one.net
**Website:** http://www.acb.org/vidpi/
David Dowland, Pres.
**Fnded:** 1975. **Mem:** 117. **Desc:** Veterans of the armed forces of the U.S. who have blindness or visual impairment. Purposes are: to maintain and foster the well-being and rehabilitation of all visually impaired veterans; to preserve the legal rights of all visually impaired veterans on the local, state, and national levels; to maintain, promote, and foster the social, economic, and cultural level of these veterans and to promote opportunities to increase their knowledge of educational, professional, and rehabilitation standards and methods. Seeks to acquire, preserve, and disseminate information relative to the functions and accomplishments of visually impaired veterans. Encourages research and development of new products for the blind. Maintains speakers' bureau; offers specialized education program. **Pub:** *VIVA Membership List*, annual. Membership Directory. Includes newsletter. • *VIVA Viewpoints*, quarterly. Newsletter. For blind veterans. *Price:* Included in membership dues.

**★ 21088 ★ World Blind Union (WBU) (Union Mondiale des Aveugles — UMA)**
La Coruna, 18
E-28020 Madrid, Spain
**Phone:** 34 91 5713685     **Fax:** 34 91 5715777
**Email:** umc@once.es
**Website:** http://www.once.es/wbu
**Fnded:** 1984. **Mem:** 155. **Reg. Groups:** 7. **Lang(s):** English, French, Spanish. **Desc:** National associations of the blind and international agencies for the blind. Fosters international cooperation among organizations working for the welfare of the blind and the prevention of blindness in 155 countries. Encourages creation and development of national organizations of and for the blind; seeks to provide necessary technical and material aid to such groups. Provides guidance in fields of education, rehabilitation, vocational training, and employment. Works toward the introduction and improvement of minimum standards for the welfare of the blind worldwide. Encourages and conducts studies in the field of service to the blind and the prevention of blindness. Collects and disseminates information on the conditions of the blind in different coutries; informs members of social and legislative matters relating to blindness and its prevention. Maintains relations with

numerous United Nations agencies including the World Health Organization, the International Council on Disability, and the International Agency for the Prevention of Blindness; sponsors the International Council for the Education of the Visually Impaired. **Pub:** *General Assembly Proceedings*, periodic. • *Review of the European Blind*, semiannual. • *The World Blind*, biennial. Magazine. Also available in braille and on casette.

**★ 21089 ★ World Council of Optometry (WCO)**
c/o Anthony F Di Stefano OD
8360 Old York Rd.
Elkins Park, PA 19027
**Phone:** (215)780-1320     **Fax:** (215)780-1325
**Email:** wco@pco.edu
**Website:** http://www.worldoptometry.org/
Anthony F. Di Stefano, Exec. Dir.
**Fnded:** 1927. **Mem:** 84. **Nat'l Groups:** 54. **Reg. Groups:** 3. **Desc:** National optical and optometric organizations in 60 countries. Promotes optometry and vision care worldwide. Works to develop optometry through education, legal and legislative advice, discussion with authorities, and support of similar associations. Is concerned with protecting optometry from what the league sees as proposed restrictive legislation, and apathy toward the profession. Establishes educational standards; offers evaluation program for schools and colleges of optometry; provides consulting services. **Pub:** *International Country Contact Register*, periodic. • *Interoptics*, quarterly. Newsletter. • *Members Journals*, periodic. • *Optometric Mailing Directory*, periodic. Directory. Lists information on optometric organizations. • *Publications List*, periodic. • *Register of Schools and Colleges of Optometry*, periodic. • Brochure, periodic.

**★ 21090 ★ Xavier Society for the Blind (XSB)**
154 E 23rd St.
New York, NY 10010
**Phone:** (212)473-7800     **Fax:** (212)473-7801
Alfred Caruana, Dir.
**Fnded:** 1900. **Mem:** 10,000. **Desc:** A center for publications, primarily Catholic, for the blind and visually handicapped, supported by charitable contributions. Transcribes numerous titles, including religious textbooks. Maintains a circulating library of books and other materials in braille, large type, and on tape. Items are loaned by mail from catalogs of titles in each of 3 formats. Tapes are also circulated to the physically handicapped. **Pub:** *Catholic Review*, monthly.

## Research Centers

**★ 21091 ★ Baylor College of Medicine Cullen Eye Institute**
6565 Fannin St., NC205
Houston, TX 77030
**Phone:** (713)798-5940     **Fax:** (713)798-3026
**Email:** danj@bcm.tmc.edu
**Website:** http://www.bcm.tmc.edu/ophth/
Dr. Dan B. Jones, Chm.
**Activities/Fields:** Restoring vision and preventing blindness through a better understanding of the structure, function, and diseases of the eye. Current areas of study include retina research, retinitis pigmentosa, amblyopia, ocular infections, corneal transplantation, genetic diseases of the eye, ocular trauma, cataract, glaucoma, ocular tumors, optic neuritis, laser treatment, vision processing, ocular surface disorders.

**★ 21092 ★ Baylor College of Medicine Vision Research Center**
Cullen Eye Institute
6565 Fannin St., Ste. NC200
Houston, TX 77030

**Phone:** (713)798-5942　　　**Fax:** (713)798-3026
Dr. Dan B. Jones, Hd.
**Activities/Fields:** Diseases of the retina and choroid, the cornea, and the sensory motor visual system, including studies of the anatomy, biochemistry, physiology, and pathology of the neural retina, retinal pigment epithelium and choroid, retinal organization and information processing, the role of herpes virus in corneal disease, endogenous fungal endophthalmitis and studies of cytomegolovirus in the ocular complications of AIDS, and visual dysfunction of strabismus and amblyopia.

★ 21093 ★ **Brooklyn College of City**
　　　　　　**University of New York**
**Applied Vision Institute (AVI)**
William James Hall, Rm. 4311
Department of Psychology
2900 Bedford Ave.
Brooklyn, NY 11210-2889
**Phone:** (718)951-5033
**Email:** louiseh@brooklyn.cuny.edu
**Website:** http://depthome.brooklyn.cuny.edu/psych/
infant/avl.htm
Dr. Louise Hainline, Co-Dir.
**Activities/Fields:** Adult vision.

**Brooklyn College of City University of**
　　**New York**
**Infant Study Center**
*See:* Entry 5777

★ 21094 ★ **Columbia University**
**Edward S. Harkness Eye Institute**
Columbia-Presbyterian Medical Center
635 W 165th St., Rm. 218
New York, NY 10032-3784
**Phone:** (212)305-2725　　　**Fax:** (212)305-5962
**Email:** sc434@columbia.edu
**Website:** http://cpmcnet.columbia.edu/dept/eye
Stanley Chang, MD, Chm.
**Activities/Fields:** Ophthalmology, including excimer lasers, new pulsed infrared lasers, patholophysiology and surgical management of orbitopathy, topical and depot corticosteriods in the treatment of post-cataract cystoid macular edema, glaucoma, endothelial growth factors for wound healing in animal models, and effects of diabetes mellitus upon the retinal microvasculature.

**Columbia University**
**Eye Radiation and Environmental**
　　**Research Laboratory**
*See:* Entry 4488

★ 21095 ★ **Columbia University**
**Retina Research Laboratory**
Columbia-Presbyterian Medical Center
635 W 165th St.
New York, NY 10032-3784
**Phone:** (212)305-5688　　　**Fax:** (212)305-9087
**Email:** pg10@columbia.edu
**Website:** http://cpmcnet.columbia.edu/dept/eye/rad
Peter Gouras, MD, Dir.
**Activities/Fields:** Retinal transplantation, biochemical markers for vitamin A metabolism in cultured human retinal epithelial cells, and gene insertion technology.

★ 21096 ★ **Connecticut Eye Bank and**
　　　　　　**Visual Research Foundation, Inc.**
100 Grand St.
New Britain, CT 06052
**Phone:** (860)224-5550　　　**Free:** 800-355-5520
**Fax:** (860)224-5720
**Email:** mrineh@aol.com
**Website:** http://www.cteyebank.org
Michael J. Rinehart, Pres. /CEO
**Activities/Fields:** Production of eye material for use in corneal transplantation surgery, surgical study, and

for research on blindness. Projects include the Vision Immunology Program, a study of how the eye defends against disease.

★ 21097 ★ **Dean A. McGee Eye Institute**
608 Stanton L. Young Blvd.
Oklahoma City, OK 73104-5065
**Phone:** (405)271-6060　　　**Fax:** (405)271-4442
**Email:** david-parke@ouhsc.edu
**Website:** http://www.dmei.org
Dr. David W. Parke, II, Pres. /CEO
**Activities/Fields:** Basic and clinical investigation in visual sciences; studies also include retinal biochemistry, molecular biology, and ocular microbiology.

★ 21098 ★ **Detroit Institute of**
　　　　　　**Ophthalmology**
15415 E Jefferson Ave.
Grosse Pointe Park, MI 48230-1328
**Phone:** (313)824-4710　　　**Fax:** (313)822-4233
**Website:** http://www.eyeson.org
Dr. Philip C. Hessburg, Pres.
**Activities/Fields:** Ophthalmology, low vision rehabilitation, and studies related to the relationship between vision and the operation of motorized vehicles.

★ 21099 ★ **Doheny Eye Institute**
1450 San Pablo St.
Los Angeles, CA 90033
**Phone:** (323)442-6300　　　**Fax:** (323)442-6688
**Email:** sryan@hsc.usc.edu
**Website:** http://www.usc.edu/hsc/doheny
Stephen J. Ryan, MD, Pres.
**Activities/Fields:** Eyebank, medical clinic group, tonography, electrophysiology, laser surgery center, contact lenses and ocular research facilities for experimental pathology, tissue culture, molecular biology, specialized microscopy, and biostatistics. **Pub:** *Annual Report.* • *Postscript Alumni Newsletter*, biennially. • *Update Newsletter*, quarterly.

★ 21100 ★ **Dry Eye and Tear Research**
　　　　　　**Center**
Department of Ophthalmology
Regions Hospital
640 Jackson St.
Saint Paul, MN 55101
**Phone:** (651)221-8745　　　**Fax:** (651)292-4040
**Email:** jdnelson@mis2.sprmc.healthpartners.com
J. Daniel Nelson, MD, Dir.
**Activities/Fields:** Basic and clinical studies of dry eye and tearing disorders, focusing on ocular surface diseases, the effects of chemicals and nutrients on corneal epithelium, and the role of hormones in the development of dry eye states.

★ 21101 ★ **Duke University**
**Eye Center**
PO Box 3802
Durham, NC 27710
**Phone:** (919)684-5846　　　**Fax:** (919)681-6343
**Email:** walla023@mc.duke.edu
David Epstein, MD, Ch.
**Activities/Fields:** Eye disorders, with special focus on retinal detachment, corneal diseases, and proliferative diabetic retinopathy.

★ 21102 ★ **Emory University**
**Emory Eye Center**
Emory Clinic, Bldg. B
1365B Clifton Rd. NE
Atlanta, GA 30322
**Phone:** (404)778-4456　　　**Fax:** (404)778-5128
**Email:** ophttma@emory.edu
**Website:** http://www.emory.edu/EYE_CENTER/emory_welcome_frame.html
Thomas M. Aaberg, Sr.,MD, Dir.
**Activities/Fields:** Prevention, diagnosis and treatment of eye diseases. **Pub:** *Molecular Vision Web journal.*

★ 21103 ★ **Emory University**
**Emory Eye Center**
**Division of Ophthalmic Research**
School of Medicine
1365-B Clifton Rd. NE, Ste. 2600
Atlanta, GA 30322
**Phone:** (404)778-4140　　　**Fax:** (404)778-4143
**Email:** ophthfe@emory.edu
**Website:** http://www.emory.edu/EYE_CENTER
Dr. Henry F. Edelhauser, Dir.
**Activities/Fields:** Various biochemical, pathobiochemical, physiological, and pathophysiological aspects of fundamental causes of blindness-producing diseases, especially cataract, glaucoma, retinal detachment, diabetes, and diabetic vasculopathy. Maintains strong clinical liaison in research programming.

★ 21104 ★ **Eye-Bank for Sight**
　　　　　　**Restoration**
120 Wall St.
New York, NY 10005-3902
**Phone:** (212)742-9000　　　**Fax:** (212)269-3139
**Email:** info@ebsr.org
**Website:** http://www.eyedonation.org
Patricia Dahl, Exec. Dir.
**Activities/Fields:** Collection and distribution of eye tissue to the scientific community. **Pub:** *Eye-to-Eye Newsletter*, 3/year.

★ 21105 ★ **Eye Institute of New Jersey**
New Jersey Medical School
90 Bergen St., 6th Fl.
Newark, NJ 07103-2499
**Phone:** (973)972-2050　　　**Fax:** (973)972-7986
**Email:** heinrige@umdnj.edu
George F. Heinrich, MD, Pres.
**Activities/Fields:** Ophthalmology, including cornea, retina, uveitis, glaucoma, pediatric ophthalmolgy, and neuro-ophthalmology.

★ 21106 ★ **Florida Ophthalmic Institute**
7106 NW 11th Pl., Ste. B
Gainesville, FL 32605-3192
**Phone:** (352)331-2020　　　**Fax:** (352)331-2019
**Email:** afn22025@afn.org
**Website:** http://www.see.yourmd.com
Dr. Norman S. Levy, Dir.
**Activities/Fields:** Understanding and treatment of human ocular diseases, including glaucoma and external ocular pathology.

★ 21107 ★ **Foundation for Education and**
　　　　　　**Research in Vision**
College of Optometry
University of Houston
PO Box 9246
Houston, TX 77261
**Phone:** (713)743-2044　　　**Fax:** (713)743-2053
Marilyn Levi, Contact
**Activities/Fields:** Optometry, focusing on the study of human vision. Also provides financial assistance for relevant research projects.

★ 21108 ★ **Georgetown University**
**Center for Sight**
Medical Center
3800 Reservoir Rd. NW
Washington, DC 20007
**Phone:** (202)687-4448　　　**Fax:** (202)687-5218
Dr. Howard Cupples, Dir.
**Activities/Fields:** Effectiveness, outcomes, and utilization of eye care; epidemiology of eye care delivery; functional status and utility assessment. Research includes outcomes of cataract, glaucoma, diabetic eye disease, and barrier reduction related to eye care use. **Frmly:** Worthen Center for Eye Research.

**★ 21109 ★ Glaucoma Laser Trabeculoplasty Study**
Associated Vision Consultants
29275 Northwestern Hwy., Ste. 200
Southfield, MI 48034-5744
**Phone:** (248)353-1750  **Fax:** (248)353-7645
**Email:** mnc@avc2020.com
**Website:** http://www.avc2020.com
Marshall N. Cyrlin, MD, Dir.

**Activities/Fields:** Glaucoma pharmaceuticals, laser and surgery treatments.


**★ 21110 ★ Glaucoma Research Foundation**
200 Pine St., Ste. 200
San Francisco, CA 94104-2712
**Phone:** (415)986-3162  **Free:** 800-826-6693
**Fax:** (415)986-3763
**Email:** info@glaucoma.org
**Website:** http://www.glaucoma.org
Patrick K. Hines, Pres. /CEO

**Activities/Fields:** Glaucoma. **Pub:** *Childhood Glaucoma.* • *Gleams Newsletter*, quarterly. Newsletter. • *Understanding and Living with Glaucoma.*


**★ 21111 ★ Harvard University Berman-Gund Laboratory for the Study of Retinal Degenerations**
Massachusetts Eye & Ear Infirmary
243 Charles St.
Boston, MA 02114
**Phone:** (617)573-3600  **Fax:** (617)573-3216
Eliot L. Berson, MD, Dir.

**Activities/Fields:** Effects of nutrition and light on the retina, gene detection of different forms of retinitis pigmentosa and gene therapy for animal models of hereditary retinal degenerations, human age-related macular degeneration.


**★ 21112 ★ Harvard University Howe Laboratory of Ophthalmology**
Massachusetts Eye & Ear Infirmary
243 Charles St.
Boston, MA 02114
**Phone:** (617)573-3963  **Fax:** (617)573-4290
**Website:** http://www.howelaboratory.harvard.edu
Frederick A. Jakobiec, Actg. Dir.

**Activities/Fields:** Programs to study development, structure, function, and malfunction of the mammalian, visual system. Current investigations focus on mechanisms of retinal functioning, development, and degeneration; ocular tumors; glaucoma; corneal wound healing; and ocular inflammatory diseases.


**★ 21113 ★ Helen Keller Worldwide**
90 West St., 2nd Fl.
New York, NY 10006
**Phone:** (212)776-5266  **Free:** 877-535-5374
**Fax:** (212)791-7590
**Website:** http://www.hkworld.org
John M. Palmer, Pres.

**Activities/Fields:** Etiology, prevalence, incidence, and treatment of xerophthalmia (nutritional blindness), trachoma, cataract, onchocerciasis (river blindness), and other eye diseases in developing nations. Research and technical assistance conducted in Bangladesh, Brazil, Burkina Faso, Cambodia, Cameroon, China, Cote d'Ivoire, Ghana, Indonesia, Mali, Mexico, Morocco, Mozambique, Nepal, Niger, Nigeria, The Philippines, South Africa, Tanzania, United States, and Vietnam. **Pub:** *Annual report.* **Frmly:** American Foundation for the Overseas Blind.


**★ 21114 ★ Indiana University Bloomington Borish Center for Ophthalmic Research (BCOR)**
OPT, 2nd Fl.
Bloomington, IN 47405
**Phone:** (812)855-4093  **Fax:** (812)855-5417
**Email:** sonip@indiana.edu
**Website:** http://www.opt.indiana.edu/bcor/bcor.html
P. Sarita Soni, Co-Dir.

**Activities/Fields:** Visual disorders, ocular pathologies, and systemic disease that affect the eye and its adnexia. Recent studies include contact lens comparison trials, extended wear contact lens trial, and decreasing dryness in contact lenses, collaborative longitudinal evaluation of keratoconus, teens and contact lenses, and development of confocal microscopy.


**★ 21115 ★ Indiana University Bloomington Cornea Contact Lens Research Laboratory**
OPT, 2nd Fl.
Bloomington, IN 47405
**Phone:** (812)855-8912  **Fax:** (812)855-1683
**Email:** pence@indiana.edu
**Website:** http://www.indiana.edu/~rugs/ctrdir/cclrl.html
Dr. Neil Pence, Dir.

**Activities/Fields:** Corneal topography, physiology, and pathology; contact lenses; contact lens care products; contact lens education.


**Johns Hopkins University Biomedical Optics Laboratory**
*See:* Entry 4651


**★ 21116 ★ Johns Hopkins University Center for Hereditary Eye Diseases**
Maumenee Bldg., Rm. 517
Wilmer Ophthalmological Institute
600 N Wolfe St.
Baltimore, MD 21287-9237
**Phone:** (410)955-5214  **Fax:** (410)614-4363
**Email:** jhched@jhmi.edu
**Website:** http://www.wilmer.jhu.edu/heredmee.htm
Dr. Irene H. Maumenee, Dir.

**Activities/Fields:** Studies of molecular mechanisms underlying genetic eye diseases. Emphasis on diagnosis and management of common as well as rare genetic eye diseases, and the prevention of vision loss through early medical or surgical intervention.


**★ 21117 ★ Johns Hopkins University Dana Center for Preventive Ophthalmology**
Wilmer 122
Wilmer Eye Institute
600 N Wolfe St.
Baltimore, MD 21287
**Phone:** (410)955-2777  **Fax:** (410)955-2542
**Email:** ptracey@jhmi.edu
**Website:** http://www.wilmer.jhu.edu/dana1.htm
Harry A. Quigley, MD, Dir.

**Activities/Fields:** Aims to identify eye disorders amenable to intervention and to develop intervention strategies. Studies concentrate on cataract and glaucoma, including the role of ultraviolet light in the development of cataract, evaluation of new techniques for diagnosing glaucoma at its earlier stages, and why black Americans develop glaucoma nine times more frequently than white Americans. Other studies focus on diet and measles and other infections as causes of blindness in Asia and Africa, including the effectiveness of periodic, massive dosing with vitamin A, vitamin A fortification of commonly consumed foods, nutritional education to reduce eye disorders caused by vitamin A deficiency in children, and vitamin A in relation to childhood morbidity and mortality; infrequent washing of the face as a cause of trachoma in such water-poor nations as Mexico; and evaluation of the safety and efficacy of drugs used to combat river blindness or onchocerciasis.


**★ 21118 ★ Johns Hopkins University Retinal Degenerations Research Center**
Maumenee Research Bldg., Rm. 519
Wilmer Ophthalmological Institute
600 N Wolfe St.
Baltimore, MD 21287-9257
**Phone:** (410)955-7589  **Fax:** (410)955-0749
**Email:** radler@jhmi.edu
**Website:** http://www.wilmer.jhu.edu
Dr. Ruben Adler, Dir.

**Activities/Fields:** Biochemistry of essential constituents of the retina and its adjacent tissues and potential interactions among them as related to retinitis pigmentosa and other retinal degenerations. **Frmly:** Michael M. Wynn Center for the Study of Retinal Degenerations.


**★ 21119 ★ Johns Hopkins University Retinal Vascular Center**
Maumenee Bldg., Rm. 711
Wilmer Eye Insitute
601 N Wolfe St.
Baltimore, MD 21287-9275
**Phone:** (410)955-7411  **Fax:** (410)614-1683
**Email:** aschachat@jhmi.edu
**Website:** http://www.wilmer.jhu.edu
Dr. Andrew Schachat, Dir.

**Activities/Fields:** Focuses on halting the progression of a variety of retinal-damaging disorders, including macular degeneration, diabetic retinopathy, and eye tumors. Studies the use of lasers in treating retinal, vascular, and macular disorders and explores the underlying causes of retinal, blood vessel, pigment epithelial, and photoreceptor diseases.


**★ 21120 ★ Johns Hopkins University Wilmer Ophthalmological Institute**
600 N Wolfe St.
Baltimore, MD 21287-9278
**Phone:** (410)955-6846  **Fax:** (410)955-0675
**Email:** mgoldbrg@gwgatel.jhmi.jhu.edu
**Website:** http://www.wilmer.jhu.edu
Morton F. Goldberg, MD, Chm.

**Activities/Fields:** Ophthalmology, including studies of macular degeneration, diabetic retinopathy, cataracts and the cornea, ocular immunology, uveitis (inflammatory eye diseases), retinal-damaging disorders, retinal degenerations, glaucoma, preventive ophthalmology, strabismus (misaligned or crossed eyes), double vision, amblyopia (reduced vision in one eye), hereditary eye diseases, neuroophthalmology, oculomotor functions, correlation of changes in the structure and form of eye tissue with symptoms of illness, development of new technology and techniques to study visual function disorders, development of new optical aids for the visually handicapped, immunohistochemical analysis of the blood retina barrier, retinal gene expression, genetics of eye diseases, molecular biology of eye development, molecular biology of glaucoma, and retinal pigment epithelium (RPE).


**★ 21121 ★ Laval University Medical Research Centre Ophthalmology Research Group**
2705 Blvd. Laurier
Sainte Foy, QC, Canada G1V 4G2
**Phone:** (418)654-2105  **Fax:** (418)654-2131
**Email:** groupe.ophtalmo@crchul.ulaval.ca
Dr. Alain Rousseau, Dir.

**Activities/Fields:** Laser corneal surgery, ocular melanoma, corneal wound healing and corneal transplantation, retinal pigment epethelium, genetics in melanoma glaucoma, and liver metastases from melanoma.


**★ 21122 ★ Lighthouse International Arlene R. Gordon Research Institute**
111 E 59th St.
New York, NY 10022
**Phone:** (212)821-9200  **Free:** 800-829-0500
**Email:** research@lighthouse.org
**Website:** http://www.lighthouse.org
Amy Horowitz, Sr. VP, Res.

**Activities/Fields:** Physical, functional, and psychological consequences of vision impairment. Vision research areas include helping individuals with low vision maximize their remaining vision, understanding how best to assess visual function, and devising ways of modifying environments for the safety and comfort of people who are visually impaired. Social research areas include the effects of visual impairment on the ability of people of all ages to function, the processes of adaption to a vision loss, and the social and psychological characteristics that influence adaptive and rehabilitation outcomes. **Pub:** *Lighthouse Research Monograph and Technical Series.*

**★ 21123 ★ Louisiana State University Eye Center**
2020 Gravier St., Ste. B
New Orleans, LA 70112
**Phone:** (504)412-1200 **Fax:** (504)412-1315
**Email:** pgebha@lsuhsc.edu
**Website:** http://www.lsu-eye.lsumc.edu/
Dr. Claude F. Burgoyne, Chm.

**Activities/Fields:** Ophthalmology, including lasers in ophthalmology, ocular surgery techniques, biomaterials and drug delivery, graft rejection, neurobiology and neurochemisty, and viral infection, latency, and treatment.

**★ 21124 ★ Macula Foundation, Inc.**
Manhattan Eye, Ear & Throat Hospital, 8th Fl.
210 E 64th St.
New York, NY 10021
**Phone:** (212)605-3777 **Free:** 800-622-8524
**Fax:** (212)605-3795
**Email:** foundation@retinalresearch.org
**Website:** http://www.macula.org/foundation/foundation.html
Lawrence A. Yannuzzi, MD, Pres.

**Activities/Fields:** Macular diseases, including epidemiologic, immunologic, biochemical, and clinical therapeutic studies. **Frmly:** Retinal Research Fund.

**★ 21125 ★ MCP Hahnemann University of the Health Sciences**
**Center for the Preservation of Vision**
Division of Ophthalmology
3300 Henry Ave.
Philadelphia, PA 19129
**Free:** 888-898-4746
**Email:** visioncenter@mcphu.edu
Dr. Jay L. Federman, Dir.

**Activities/Fields:** Laser applications in the treatment of eye diseases, development of a vision sensing device capable of transmitting light impulses to the brain.

**MCP Hahnemann University of the Health Sciences**
**Computer Vision Center for Vertebrate Brain Mapping**
*See:* Entry 14235

**★ 21126 ★ Medical College of Wisconsin**
**Froedtert and Medical College Eye Institute**
925 N 87th St.
Milwaukee, WI 53226
**Phone:** (414)456-7915 **Fax:** (414)456-6563
**Email:** dheuer@mcw.edu
**Website:** http://www.mcw.edu/ophthalmology
Dr. Dale Heuer, MD, Dir.

**Activities/Fields:** Ophthalmology, including anterior segment reconstruction, cataract, color vision, corneal and external eye diseases, genetics, glaucoma, ocular oncology, ophthalmic pathology, ophthalmic reconstructive surgery, orbital diseases, neuro-ophthalmology, refractive surgery, strabismus and pediatric ophthalmology, visual rehabilitation and vitreoretinal diseases.

**★ 21127 ★ Medical University of South Carolina**
**Storm Eye Institute**
167 Ashley Ave.
Charleston, SC 29425
**Phone:** (843)792-3134 **Fax:** (843)792-1723
**Email:** crossonc@musc.edu
Dr. Craig Crosson, Dir. of Res.

**Activities/Fields:** Causes of blinding diseases and development of new treatments to prevent or ameliorate disease progression, including targeting macular degeneration, diabetic retinopathy, glaucoma, cataract and refractive surgery.

**★ 21128 ★ Mississippi State University**
**Rehabilitation Research and Training Center on Blindness and Low Vision**
PO Box 6189
Mississippi State, MS 39762-6189
**Phone:** (662)325-2001 **Free:** 800-675-7782
**Fax:** (662)325-8989
**Email:** rrtc@colled.msstate.edu
**Website:** http://www.blind.msstate.edu
Dr. J. Elton Moore, Dir.

**Activities/Fields:** Career development intervention strategies for people who are blind or severely visually impaired; employment aspects of blindness and low vision. **Pub:** *Monographs.*

**★ 21129 ★ Mount Sinai School of Medicine of City University of New York**
**Vision Research Center in Ophthalmology**
1 Gustave L. Levy Pl., Box 1183
New York, NY 10029
**Phone:** (212)241-6249 **Fax:** (212)289-5945
**Email:** oscar.candia@mssm.edu
**Website:** http://www.mssm.edu/ophth/
Dr. Oscar A. Candia, Dir.

**Activities/Fields:** Ophthalmology.

**★ 21130 ★ National Eye Research Foundation**
910 Skokie Blvd., No. 207A
Northbrook, IL 60062
**Phone:** (847)564-4652 **Free:** 800-621-2258
**Fax:** (847)564-0807
**Email:** nerf@eyemac.com
**Website:** http://www.nerf.org
Andrew Kim, Contact

**Activities/Fields:** Vision, focusing on better eye care. Also promotes education relating to the eye care and contact lenses. **Pub:** *Quarterly Research Journal.*

**★ 21131 ★ New England College of Optometry**
**Myopia Research Center**
424 Beacon St.
Boston, MA 02115
**Phone:** (617)266-2030 **Fax:** (617)369-0174
**Email:** heldd@ne-optometry.edu
**Website:** http://www.ne-optometry.edu/info/research_info.htm
Richard Held, Res. Dir.

**Activities/Fields:** Human and animal studies on the development of myopia, resolution limits of human eye, and autoimimune response in diabetes. **Pub:** *Perspectives Magazine*, 3/year.

**★ 21132 ★ Oakland University**
**Eye Research Institute**
422 Dodge Hall
Rochester, MI 48309-4480
**Phone:** (248)370-2391 **Fax:** (248)370-2006
**Email:** blanks@oakland.edu
Dr. Janet C. Blanks, Dir.

**Activities/Fields:** Biochemistry, biophysics, cell biology, physiology, pharmacology, and photobiology. Research focuses on ocular tissues and includes the following topics of interest: molecular genetics of lens

proteins, ion transport and radiation damage of the cornea, light damage of the retina, signal transduction in photoreceptors, ocular drug metabolism and detoxification, and experimental models of proliferative vitreoretinopathy, uveoretinitis, cataracts (radiation and oxidation and calcium), and diabetic complications of the eye. **Frmly:** Institute of Biological Sciences.

**★ 21133 ★ Ohio Wesleyan University**
**Eye Research Projects**
Delaware, OH 43015
**Phone:** (740)368-3801 **Fax:** (740)368-3812
**Email:** dorobbin@cc.owu.edu
David O. Robbins, PhD, Dir.

**Activities/Fields:** Visual psychophysics and electrophysiology, color vision, and effects of laser irradiation on retinal morphology and function.

**★ 21134 ★ Ophthalmic Research Institute**
6110 Executive Blvd., Ste. 506
Rockville, MD 20852
**Phone:** (301)984-4735 **Fax:** (301)984-4737
Helen Viksnins, Contact

**Activities/Fields:** Vision research, instumentation and procedure evaluation, and new treatment methods.

**★ 21135 ★ Oregon Health and Science University**
**Elks' Children's Eye Clinic**
Casey Eye Institute
3375 SW Terwilliger Blvd.
Portland, OR 97201-4197
**Phone:** (503)494-7675 **Fax:** (503)494-5347
**Email:** palmere@ohsu.edu
**Website:** http://www.ohsu.edu/~cei/casey.html
Earl A. Palmer, MD, Contact

**Activities/Fields:** Pediatric ophthalmology with particular reference to abnormalities of binocular vision. Studies in strabismus, infantile and congenital glaucoma, retinopathy in premature infants, congenital cataract, and genetic diseases. Participation in multicenter clinical trials. Programs are clinically oriented, including retrospective and prospective studies of patients. Develops instruments and techniques to advance pediatric ophthalmology.

**★ 21136 ★ Pennsylvania College of Optometry**
**Cornea and Specialty Contact Lens Service (CASCLS)**
1200 W Godfrey Ave.
Philadelphia, PA 19141
**Phone:** (215)276-6000 **Fax:** (215)276-6111
**Email:** joel@pco.edu
Joel A. Silbert, Chief

**Activities/Fields:** Progression of the corneal warpage syndrome known as keratoconus; cornea and contact lenses studies, including testing lenses and lens care products for various manufacturers. The study on keratoconus, known as the Collaborative Longitudinal Evaluation of Keratoconus, is funded by the National Eye Institute.

**★ 21137 ★ Pennsylvania College of Optometry**
**Glaucoma Research Center**
1200 W Godfrey Ave.
Philadelphia, PA 19141
**Phone:** (215)276-6000
**Email:** glaucdoc@aol.com
G. Richard Bennett, OD, Dir.

**Activities/Fields:** Determining whether patients with ocular hypertension (elevated eye pressure but without glaucoma) benefit over the longer term from medical management of their pressure. This study, known as the Ocular Hypertension Treatment Study, is funded by the National Eye Institute for eight years.

**★ 21138 ★ Pennsylvania College of Optometry**
**Hafter Family Light and Laser Institute**
Old York Rd. & Township Line Rd.
Philadelphia, PA 19141
**Phone:** (215)780-1427     **Fax:** (215)780-1325
**Email:** felix@pco.edu
Dr. Felix M. Barker, Dir.

**Activities/Fields:** Corneal and retinal light damage effects, especially from short wavelength energy sources; ocular photosensitization; laser effects; excimer laser studies, including corneal wound healing in normal and diabetic individuals; glaucoma; myopia; keratoconus.

**★ 21139 ★ Pennsylvania College of Optometry**
**Institute for the Visually Impaired (IVI)**
8360 Old York Rd.
Elkins Park, PA 19027
**Phone:** (215)780-1360     **Fax:** (215)780-1336
**Email:** nancy@pco.edu
**Website:** http://www.pco.edu
Audrey J. Smith, Exec. Dir.

**Activities/Fields:** Partial sight or low vision, including rehabilitation teaching, and low vision rehabilitation, orientation, and mobility.

**★ 21140 ★ Research to Prevent Blindness**
645 Madison Ave., 21st Fl.
New York, NY 10022-1010
**Phone:** (212)752-4333     **Free:** 800-621-0026
**Fax:** (212)688-6231
**Email:** tfurlong@rpbusa.org
**Website:** http://www.rpbusa.org/hc2/index.asp
Diane S. Swift, Contact

**Activities/Fields:** Blinding eye-diseases, focusing on causes, prevention, and treatment. **Pub:** *Eye Research Newsletter.* • *Report*, annually. • *Research reports.* • *Visual Acuity/Macular Degeneration Test Card.* Brochure.

**★ 21141 ★ Schepens Eye Research Institute**
20 Staniford St.
Boston, MA 02114-2500
**Phone:** (617)912-0100     **Fax:** (617)912-0101
**Email:** geninfo@vision.eri.harvard.edu
**Website:** http://www.eri.harvard.edu
Dr. J. Wayne Streilein, Pres.

**Activities/Fields:** Retina, vitreous, cornea, glaucoma, immunology, neuroscience, transplantation, physiological optics, biomedical physics, ocular tumors, and pharmacology with strong collaboration between clinic and laboratory studies on diseases of the retina and cornea, and on glaucoma. Develops ophthalmic instruments and devices for diagnosis and treatment of eye disease, and for low vision aids. **Pub:** *Sundial*, semiannually. **Frmly:** Retina Foundation; Eye Research Institute of Retina Foundation.

**★ 21142 ★ Smith-Kettlewell Eye Research Institute**
2318 Fillmore St.
San Francisco, CA 94115
**Phone:** (415)345-2000     **Fax:** (415)345-8455
**Email:** abs@ski.org
**Website:** http://www.ski.org
Alan B. Scott, MD, Dir.

**Activities/Fields:** Visual sciences, oculomotor functioning, and rehabilitation engineering, including long-term study of the surgical and pharmacological treatment of strabismus; development of diagnostic tests for glaucoma, retinitis pigmentosa, diabetic retinopathy, and senile macular degeneration; research on the physiological basis of eye movements; studies in motion detection, pattern perception, and stereopsis; and development and evaluation of sensory aids and devices for the deaf, blind, deaf/blind, and sensory-

impaired individuals. **Pub:** *Rehabilitation Engineering Center Annual Report.*

**★ 21143 ★ Smith-Kettlewell Rehabilitation Engineering Research Institute**
18 Fillmore St.
San Francisco, CA 94115
**Phone:** (415)345-2110     **Fax:** (415)345-8455
**Email:** rerc@ski.org
**Website:** http://www.ski.org/Rehab/
Dr. John A. Brabyn, Dir.

**Activities/Fields:** Technology for blindness, visual impairment, and multi-sensory loss. **Pub:** *Annual Report.* • *IBM diskette.* • *Smith-Kettlewell Technical File Journal (in braille)*, quarterly.

**★ 21144 ★ Texas A&M University**
**Institute of Ocular Pharmacology**
College of Medicine
College Station, TX 77843-1114
**Phone:** (979)845-2817     **Fax:** (979)845-0699
Dr. George C.Y. Chiou, Dir.

**Activities/Fields:** Ocular pharmacology (the use of drugs for treating eye disease), including glaucoma, ocular inflamation, retinal degeneration, myopia, and cataract treatment. **Pub:** *Journal of Ocular Pharmacology.* • *Opthalmic Toxicology.*

**★ 21145 ★ U.S. Department of Health and Human Services**
**National Eye Institute**
**Division of Biometry and Epidemiology**
NIH Bldg. 31, Rm. 6A52
31 Center Dr. MSC 2510
Bethesda, MD 20892-2510
**Phone:** (301)496-1331     **Fax:** (301)496-2297
**Website:** http://www.nei.nih.gov
Fredrick Ferris, MD, Dir.

**Activities/Fields:** Plan, develop, and conduct human population studies concerned with the cause, prevention, and treatment of eye disease and vision disorders, with emphasis on the major causes of blindness. This includes studies of incidence and prevalence in defined populations, prospective and retrospective studies of risk factors, natural history studies, clinical trials, genetic studies, and studies to evaluate diagnostic procedures.

**★ 21146 ★ U.S. Department of Health and Human Services**
**National Eye Institute**
**Division of Biometry and Epidemiology**
**Clinical Trials Branch**
NIH Bldg. 31, Rm. 6A52
31 Center Dr. MSC 2510
Bethesda, MD 20892
**Phone:** (301)496-6583     **Fax:** (301)496-2297
**Website:** http://www.nei.nih.gov
Frederick L. Ferris, Chf.

**Activities/Fields:** Plan, develop, and conduct human population studies concerned with the cause, prevention, and treatment of eye disease and vision disorders, with emphasis on the major causes of blindness. This includes studies of incidence and prevalence on defined populations, prospective and retrospective studies of risk factors, natural history studies, clinical trials, genetic studies, and studies to evaluate diagnostic procedures.

**★ 21147 ★ U.S. Department of Health and Human Services**
**National Eye Institute**
**Extramural Research**
NIH EPS, Ste. 350
6120 Executive Blvd., MSC 7164
Bethesda, MD 20892-7164
**Phone:** (301)496-5301     **Fax:** (301)402-0528
**Email:** rh27v@nih.gov
**Website:** http://www.nei.nih.gov/
Dr. Ralph Helmsen, Res. Rsrcs. Off.

**Activities/Fields:** Improving the prevention, diagnosis, and treatment of visual disorders. This support includes the award of grants, cooperative agreements, fellowships, and contracts for research in retinal and choroidal diseases, corneal diseases, cataract, glaucoma, strabismus, amblyopia, visual processing, and low vision.

**★ 21148 ★ U.S. Department of Health and Human Services**
**National Eye Institute**
**Extramural Research**
**Corneal Diseases Program**
2020 Vision Place
Bethesda, MD 20892
**Phone:** (301)451-2020     **Fax:** (301)402-0528
**Email:** lam@nei.nih.gov/funding/nprp.htm
**Website:** http://www.nei.nih.gov
Richard S. Fischer, PhD, Contact

**Activities/Fields:** Ophthalmic research relating to corneal diseases and focusing on diseases of the cornea and the external ocular structures, including the conjunctiva and eyelids; corneal transplantation and wound healing; and contact lenses and surgical correction of refractive problems.

**★ 21149 ★ U.S. Department of Health and Human Services**
**National Eye Institute**
**Extramural Research**
**Retinal Diseases Program**
2020 Vision Place
Bethesda, MD 20892-7164
**Phone:** (301)451-2020     **Fax:** (301)402-0528
**Email:** pad@.nei.nih.gov
**Website:** http://www.nei.nih.gov/funding/nprp.htm
Peter A. Dudley, PhD, Contact

**Activities/Fields:** Structure and function of the retina and choroid in health and disease. NEI-fostered investigations include studies of the structure and metabolism of photoreceptor cells and their relationship to the underlying pigment epithelium; the retina's response to light and the initial processing of visual information transmitted to the visual centers of the brain; inflammation of the uveal tract (the iris, choroid, and ciliary body); and of the vitreous gel that fills the center of the eye. NEI also supports studies aimed at understanding causes of blindness such as developmental and hereditary retinal disorders; diabetic retinopathy and other vascular and circulatory abnormalities; myopia; ocular tumors; macular degeneration; retinal detachment; and inflammatory disorders, including uveitis. Also conducts clinical trials of the effects of treatment on retinal diseases.

**★ 21150 ★ U.S. Department of Health and Human Services**
**National Eye Institute**
**Extramural Research**
**Strabismus, Amblyopia, Visual Processing, and Low Vision**
NIH
Executive Plaza S, Ste. 350
6120 Executive Blvd., MSC 7164
Bethesda, MD 20892-7164
**Phone:** (301)496-5301     **Fax:** (301)402-0528
**Email:** oberdorfer@nei.nih.gov
**Website:** http://www.nei.nih.gov/
Michael D. Oberdorfer, PhD, Prog. Dir.

**Activities/Fields:** Contact person for extramural support for basic and clinical research on a broad range of studies concerned with the development and function of the neural pathways from the eye to the brain, the central processing of visual information, visual perception, optical properties of the eye, oculomotor function, functioning of the pupil, and control of the ocular muscles. A large number of congenital, developmental, and degenerative abnormalities affect the visual sensorimotor system, but two disorders are of primary concern–strabismus and amblyopia. These are frequent causes of visual impairment among children which may persist for life. Additional emphasis is placed on, and support provided for, research on optic neuropathies, eye movement disorders, the development of myopia, and the contact person for all research applications regarding low vision and blindness rehabilitation.


**★ 21151 ★ U.S. Department of Health and Human Services**
**National Eye Institute**
**Intramural Research Program**
NIH Bldg. 10, Rm. 10N202
9000 Rockville Pike
Bethesda, MD 20892-1858
**Phone:** (301)496-3123          **Fax:** (301)480-1122
**Email:** drbob@nei.nih.gov
Dr. Robert B. Nussenblatt, Scientific Dir.

**Activities/Fields:** In-house research aimed at improving the prevention, diagnosis, and treatment of visual disorders. Major subject of research include retinal and choroidal diseases, corneal diseases, cataract, glaucoma, and sensory and motor disorders of vision. Program comprises a Clinical Branch and laboratories of Mechanisms of Ocular Diseases, Molecular and Developmental Biology, Ophthalmic Pathology, Retinal Cell and Molecular Biology, and Sensorimotor Research. **Pub:** *NEI's Annual Report*.


**★ 21152 ★ U.S. Department of Health and Human Services**
**National Eye Institute**
**Intramural Research Program**
**Laboratory of Immunology**
NIH Bldg. 10, Rm. 10/10 N 112
9000 Rockville Pike
Bethesda, MD 20892
**Phone:** (301)496-3123          **Fax:** (301)480-1122
**Email:** drbob@nei.nih.gov
Dr. Robert B. Nussenblatt, Sci. Dir.

**Activities/Fields:** Clinical research into the causes, preventions, diagnosis, and treatment of visual system disorders. It translates laboratory research results into clinical application, directs and administers the Institute's clinical care program, and assures functioning of the eye ward and clinic in the NIH Clinical Center. Principal Branch components are: the Cataract Section, Neuro-Ophthalmology Section, Ocular Immunology Section, Ophthalmic Genetics and Pediatric Ophthalmology Section, and Retinal and Ocular Connective Tissue Diseases Section.


**★ 21153 ★ U.S. Department of Health and Human Services**
**National Eye Institute**
**Laboratory on Mechanisms of Ocular Diseases**
NIH Bldg. 6, Rm. 237/ 6 Center Dr. MSC 2735
9000 Rockville Pike
Bethesda, MD 20892-2735
**Phone:** (301)496-6669          **Fax:** (301)496-1759
**Website:** http://www.nei.nih.gov/intramural/lmod.htm
Dr. J. Samuel Zigler, Actg. Chf.

**Activities/Fields:** Mechanisms involved in cataract formation, pharmacologic and pathophysiologic aspects of aldose reductase in diabetic complications, molecular biology of a retinal dystrophy, and cataract caused by an enzyme deficiency. Laboratory also provides training opportunities in related diabetes and cataract research.


**★ 21154 ★ U.S. Department of Health and Human Services**
**National Eye Institute**
**Laboratory of Molecular and Developmental Biology**
NIH Bldg. 6, Rm. 201
6 Center Dr., MSC-2730
Bethesda, MD 20892
**Phone:** (301)496-9467          **Fax:** (301)402-0781
**Email:** joramp@nei.nih.gov
Dr. Joram Piatigorsky, Chf.

**Activities/Fields:** Cellular and molecular biology, with emphasis on molecular and developmental genetics. The research is designed to elucidate both normal and disease processes, and particular attention is given to hereditary diseases that can be studied at the gene level. Much (but not all) of the work uses eye tissue as models for general problems concerning cellular differentiation and gene expression. In addition, normal and pathogenic visual processes are related to the structure and function of genes; and phospholipid metabolism—particularly at the cell membrane—is investigated in order to advance knowledge of cellular differentiation and differential gene expression.


**★ 21155 ★ U.S. Department of Health and Human Services**
**National Eye Institute**
**Laboratory of Retinal Cell and Molecular Biology**
NIH Bldg. 6, Rm. 310
6 Center Dr. MSC 2740
Bethesda, MD 20892-2740
**Phone:** (301)496-3448          **Fax:** (301)402-1883
**Email:** bnwigg@helix.nih.gov
**Website:** http://www.nei.nih.gov/intramural/lrcmb.htm
Dr. Barbara N. Wiggert, Ch.

**Activities/Fields:** Biochemistry, molecular biology, and neurobiology of the retina.


**★ 21156 ★ U.S. Department of Health and Human Services**
**National Institutes of Health**
**National Eye Institute (NEI)**
2020 Vision Pl.
Bethesda, MD 20892-3655
**Phone:** (301)496-5248          **Fax:** (301)496-9970
**Website:** http://www.nei.nih.gov/
Dr. Paul Sieving, Dir.

**Activities/Fields:** Improving prevention, diagnosis, and treatment of visual disorders. Specifically, the Institute: supports research and research training through grants, fellowships, and contracts to medical schools and research institutions; conducts laboratory and clinical research in its own facilities and fosters statistical and epidemiological studies of visual disorders in human populations; fosters research on rehabilitation of the visually handicapped; encourages the application of research findings to clinical practice; heightens public awareness of vision problems; and cooperates with voluntary organizations that engage in related activities. The NEI organization includes a Biometry and Epidemiology Program, Extramural and Collaborative Programs, and an Intramural Research Program. **Pub:** *Strategic Plan*, quinquenially.


**U.S. Department of Health and Human Services**
**National Institutes of Health**
**National Eye Institute**
**Intramural Research**
**(Ophthalmic Genetics and Visual Function Branch)**
*See:* Entry 9445


**★ 21157 ★ U.S. Department of Health and Human Services**
**National Institutes of Health**
**National Eye Institute**
**Intramural Research**
**(Section on Molecular Structure and Function)**
Bldg. 10
10 Center Dr.
Bethesda, MD 20892
**Phone:** (301)402-3452
**Email:** graeme@helix.nih.gov
**Website:** http://www.nei.nih.gov/intramural/molstr.htm
Graeme J. Wistow, PhD, Hd.

**Activities/Fields:** Understanding important classes of proteins associated with the eye, using molecular biology, genomics, structural biology, and molecular evolution.


**★ 21158 ★ U.S. Department of Health and Human Services**
**National Institutes of Health**
**National Eye Institute**
**Intramural Research**
**((Laboratory of Mechanisms of Ocular Diseases)**
**Pathophysiology Group)**
Bldg. 6, Rm. 316
6 Center Dr., MSC 2735
Bethesda, MD 20892-2735
**Phone:** (301)496-3161          **Fax:** (301)402-1570
**Email:** robisong@nei.nih.gov
**Website:** http://www.nei.nih.gov/intramural/patho.htm
W. Gerald Robison, Jr.,Ph, Hd.

**Activities/Fields:** Human tissues and experimental animals to elucidate underlying pathogenic mechanisms of ocular diseases, including retinopathy cataracts, and keratopathy, with emphasis on prevention of ocular complications of diabetes.


**★ 21159 ★ U.S. Department of Health and Human Services**
**National Institutes of Health**
**National Eye Institute**
**Intramural Research**
**(Laboratory of Ocular Therapeutics)**
Bldg. 6, Rm. 201
6 Center Dr., MSC 2730
Bethesda, MD 20892-2730
**Phone:** (301)496-4343          **Fax:** (301)402-0781
**Email:** kador@mge1.nei.nih.gov
**Website:** http://www.nei.nih.gov/intramural/lot.htm
Peter F. Kador, PhD, Ch.

**Activities/Fields:** Development, evaluation, and mechanism of action of new ophthalmic drugs to treat eye diseases, including aldose reductase inhibitors (ARI) and anticataract agents.


**★ 21160 ★ U.S. Department of Health and Human Services**
**National Institutes of Health (NIH)**
**National Eye Institute (NEI)**
**Intramural Research**
**((Laboratory of Mechanisms of Ocular Diseases)**
**Molecular Therapeutics)**
Bldg. 6, Rm. 226
6 Center Dr., MSC 2735
Bethesda, MD 20892-2735
**Phone:** (301)496-2144
**Email:** carperd@intra.nei.nih.gov
**Website:** http://www.nei.nih.gov/intramural/mt.htm
Deborah Carper, Hd.

**Activities/Fields:** Mechanisms responsible for cataract formation, including regulation of gene expression in oxidative stress models of cataract and in mechanisms responsible for gender-based differences in cataract development in aging populations.


**★ 21161 ★ U.S. Department of Health and Human Services**
**National Institutes of Health (NIH)**
**National Eye Institute (NEI)**
**Intramural Research**
**((Laboratory of Mechanisms of Ocular Diseases)**
**Aging and Ocular Disease)**
Bldg. 6, Rm. 226
6 Center Dr., MSC 2735
Bethesda, MD 20892-2735
**Phone:** (301)496-7471
**Email:** russelp@intra.nei.nih.gov

**Website:** http://www.nei.nih.gov/intramural/aging.htm
Paul Russell, PhD, Hd.

**Activities/Fields:** Examination of changes in the eye, particularly the anterior segment, that occur with age and how some of these alterations may cause ocular disease. Research interests include cataract formation and primary open angle glaucoma.


**★ 21162 ★ U.S. Department of Health and Human Services**
**National Institutes of Health**
**National Eye Institute**
**Intramural Research**
**((Laboratory of Mechanisms of Ocular Diseases)**
**Lens and Cataract Biology Section)**
Bldg. 6, Rm. 226
6 Center Dr., MSC 2735
Bethesda, MD 20892-2735
**Phone:** (301)496-6669          **Fax:** (301)402-1759
**Email:** szigler@helix.nih.gov
**Website:** http://www.nei.nih.gov/intramural/lens.htm
J. Samuel Zigler, Jr.,Ph, Ch.

**Activities/Fields:** Structure, function, and evolution of lens crystallins and molecular mechanisms underlying cataract formation.


**★ 21163 ★ U.S. Department of Health and Human Services**
**National Institutes of Health**
**National Eye Institute**
**Intramural Research**
**(Division of Epidemiology and Clinical Research)**
Bldg. 31, Rm. 6A52
31 Center Dr., MSC 2510
Bethesda, MD 20892-2510
**Phone:** (301)496-6583          **Fax:** (301)496-2297
**Website:** http://www.nei.nih.gov/intramural/biometry.htm
Frederick L. Ferris, III,MD, Dir.

**Activities/Fields:** Human population studies concerned with cause, prevention, and treatment of eye disease and vision disorders, with emphasis on major causes of blindness.


**★ 21164 ★ U.S. Department of Veterans Affairs**
**Rehabilitation Research and Development Service**
**Center of Excellence for Innovative Visual Rehabilitation**
Neuro-Op/9th Fl.
Massachusetts Eye & Ear Infirmary
Boston VA Medical Center
243 Charles St.
Boston, MA 02114
**Email:** jrizzo@meei.harvard.edu
**Website:** http://www.vard.org/cent/boston.htm
Dr. Joseph F. Rizzo, III, Dir.

**Activities/Fields:** Development of a retinal prosthesis to restore vision in patients with retinitis pigmentosa and with age-related macular degeneration, the leading cause of blindness among veterans and the general population.


**★ 21165 ★ University of British Columbia**
**VGH/UBC Eye Care Centre**
Department of Ophthalmology
2550 Willow St.
Vancouver, BC, Canada V5Z 3N9
**Phone:** (604)875-4199          **Fax:** (604)875-4663
**Email:** jrootman@vanhosp.bc.ca
Dr. Jack Rootman, Hd.

**Activities/Fields:** Effects of diabetes on the eye with specific emphasis on circulation, electroneurophysiology of the retina, glaucoma epidemiology, visual perception, ocular therapeutics, color vision in ocular diseases, ocular oncology, orbital disease, thyroid orbitopathy, congenital glaucoma, neurophysiology

and neuropharmacology of cortical vision, experimental pathology, central nervous system development, neural mechanisms underlying amblyopia and strabismus, computational vision, anatomical connections of the central visual system, molecular biological studies of neurotransmitters, receptors, and growth factors in the visual system.


**★ 21166 ★ University of Calgary**
**Lions Sight Centre**
Faculty of Medicine
313-4411 16th Ave NW
Calgary, AB, Canada T3B 0M3
**Phone:** (403)286-3335          **Fax:** (403)286-3316
**Email:** huangp@cadvision.com
Dr. Peter T. Huang, Dir.

**Activities/Fields:** Structure, function, molecular genetics, chemistry, and development of vertebrate photoreceptors (rods and cones) and neural retina. Also studies retinal development and regeneration; myopia and regulation of ocular growth; diabetic retinopathy; and molecular genetics of human vision disorders.


**University of Calgary**
**Vision and Aging Laboratory**
*See:* Entry 3100


**★ 21167 ★ University of California, Los Angeles**
**Jules Stein Eye Institute**
Box 957000
Department of Opthalmology
100 Stein Plz.
Los Angeles, CA 90095-7000
**Phone:** (310)825-5000          **Fax:** (310)206-7488
**Email:** mondino@jsei.ucla.edu
**Website:** http://www.medsch.ucla.edu/som/jsei
Bartly J. Mondino, MD, Dir.

**Activities/Fields:** Research and study in sciences related to vision, care of patients with eye disease, and education in ophthalmology. **Pub:** *Annual Report.* • *Clinical Update,* 3/year. Newsletter. • *EYE,* 3/year. Newsletter.


**★ 21168 ★ University of California, San Francisco**
**Francis I. Proctor Foundation for Research in Ophthalmology**
95 Kirkham St.
San Francisco, CA 94143-0944
**Phone:** (415)476-1441          **Fax:** (415)502-2521
Todd P. Margolis, MD, Contact

**Activities/Fields:** Infectious and inflammatory diseases of the eye with particular emphasis on chlamydial infections, trachoma, herpetic eye infections, dry eye conditions, and uveitis.


**★ 21169 ★ University of California, San Francisco**
**Ocular Oncology Research Unit**
Beckman Vision Center-Department of Ophthalmology
10 Koret Way, Box 730
San Francisco, CA 94143
**Phone:** (415)476-0779          **Fax:** (415)502-3230
Joan M. O'Brien, MD, Dir.

**Activities/Fields:** Molecular biology and immunology of intracolar tumors, new treatment protocols, genetic testing and therapy.


**★ 21170 ★ University of Chicago**
**Visual Sciences Center**
939 E 57th St.
Chicago, IL 60637
**Phone:** (773)702-8888          **Fax:** (773)702-8094
**Email:** jernest@midway.uchicago.edu
**Website:** http://ophthalmology.bsd.uchicago.edu
Dr. J. Terry Ernest, Chm., Ophthalmology

**Activities/Fields:** Ophthalmology, visual physiology and function of the retina, color vision, evoked occipital response, laser and xenon photocoagulation for retinal disease, and pharmacology of the retinal pigment epithelium. Also conducts electron microscopy and visual molecular biology studies. **Frmly:** Eye Research Laboratories.


**★ 21171 ★ University of Florida**
**Center for Vision Research**
JHMHC
PO Box 100284
Gainesville, FL 32610-0284
**Phone:** (352)392-3451          **Fax:** (352)392-8554
**Email:** sherwood@eye1.eye.ufl.edu
**Website:** http://www.eye.ufl.edu
Mark B. Sherwood, MD, Dir.

**Activities/Fields:** Electrophysiology of the retina and biochemistry, immunology, molecular genetics, and oncology of ocular diseases.


**★ 21172 ★ University of Illinois at Chicago**
**Lions of Illinois Eye Research Institute**
UIC Eye Center
1855 W Taylor
Chicago, IL 60612
**Phone:** (312)996-6590          **Fax:** (312)996-7770
**Email:** josepuli@uic.edu
**Website:** http://www.uic.edu/com/eye/
Prof. Jose S. Pulido, Hd.

**Activities/Fields:** Diabetic retinopathy, glaucoma, cataracts, macular degeneration, retinitis pigmentosa, corneal biochemistry, molecular biology, and retinal photoreceptors. Houses the clinical trials of the UIC Department of Ophthalmology and Visual Sciences, including the Advanced Glaucoma Intervention Study, Collaborative Ocular Melanoma Study, Herpetic Eye Disease Study, and Retinopathy of Prematurity; research studies of the Applied Physics Laboratory, Lens Biochemistry Laboratory, Ophthalmic Pathology Laboratory, Ocular Molecular Biology Laboratories, Ocular Biochemistry Laboratory, Photoreceptor Research Laboratory, Laboratory of Retinal Physiology and Neurobiology, and Retinal Cell Biology Laboratory. **Pub:** *Annual Report.* • *Eye Facts.* • *Eyewitness News.*


**★ 21173 ★ University of Illinois at Chicago**
**Low Vision Rehabilitation Laboratory**
Department of Ophthalmology
1855 W Taylor
Chicago, IL 60612
**Phone:** (312)996-7179
**Email:** janeszly@uic.edu
Janet Szlyk, Dir.

**Activities/Fields:** Physiology of normal and pathologic retinas utilizing computer analyzed digitized images.


**★ 21174 ★ University of Louisville**
**Kentucky Lions Eye Center**
301 E Muhammad Ali Blvd.
Louisville, KY 40202
**Phone:** (502)852-3716          **Fax:** (502)852-4595
**Email:** hank.kaplan@louisville.edu
**Website:** http://www.louisville.edu/medschool/ophthalmology
Dr. Henry J. Kaplan, Chm.

**Activities/Fields:** Visual sciences and eye diseases.


**★ 21175 ★ University of Miami**
**Bascom Palmer Eye Institute**
School of Medicine
Department of Ophthalmology
900 Nw 17th St.
Miami, FL 33136
**Phone:** (305)326-6000          **Fax:** (305)326-6417
**Website:** http://www.bpei.med.miami.edu
Dr. Carmen A. Puliafito, Dir.

**Activities/Fields:** Glaucoma, infectious and external corneal diseases, molecular biology and genetics, neurophysiology, ocular virology, ocular immunology, hereditary retinal diseases with special emphasis on Retinitis Pigmentosa, and ophthalmic applications of lasers and polymers. Also conducts studies to improve the techniques and technology related to patient care and the prevention of blindness.

**★ 21176 ★ University of Miami**
**Bascom Palmer Eye Institute**
**Ophthalmic Biophysics Center**
Department of Ophthalmology
PO Box 016880
Miami, FL 33101-6880
**Phone:** (305)326-6069 **Fax:** (305)326-6139
**Email:** jmparel@bpei.med.miami.edu
Prof. Jean-Marie Parel, Dir.

**Activities/Fields:** Research activities involve the development and refinement of ophthalmic devices, including testing and design of the Phaco-Ersatz, a lens substitute for intraocular lenses commonly used after cataract surgery, and the development of an implant to permit the sustained release of small amounts of medication over an extended period of time, as well as several glaucoma shunt-valves devices, a controlled iontophoresis system designed to non-invasively transfer drugs into the eye to avoid systemic side effects, and an artificial cornea. Additional research includes selection of individual lasers for ophthalmic use and testing of two high speed laser cutting systems designed to offer new precision and beam control for delicate surgeries.

**★ 21177 ★ University of Miami**
**Bascom Palmer Eye Institute**
**Retinis Pigmentosa Center**
School of Medicine
Department of Ophthalmology
PO Box 016880
Miami, FL 33101-6880
**Phone:** (305)243-6545 **Fax:** (305)243-4888
**Email:** jclarkso@med.net.med.miami.edu
**Website:** http://www.miami.edu
Dr. John G. Clarkson, Dean, Sch. of Med.

**Activities/Fields:** Treatment and prevention of retinis pigmentosa, a group of disorders that cause degeneration of the retina's light-sensing cells (photoreeptors) responsible for sending visual information to the brain. Areas of specialization include diagnostics, retinal photochemistry and physiology, and molecular and cell biology.

**★ 21178 ★ University of North Texas**
**Health Science Center at Fort Worth**
**North Texas Eye Research Institute**
**(NTERI)**
3500 Camp Bowie Blvd., ME2-202
Fort Worth, TX 76107-2699
**Phone:** (817)735-2045 **Fax:** (817)735-2610
**Email:** pcammara@hsc.unt.edu
**Website:** http://www.hsc.unt.edu/research/ntrei/eye_home.asp
Patrick R. Cammarata, PhD, Dir.

**Activities/Fields:** Eye diseases, including studies on the retina, RPE cells, trophic factors, ocular diabetes, autoimmune diseases, optic nerve regeneration, glaucoma, corneal wound healing, cell death, and aging.

**★ 21179 ★ University of Pennsylvania**
**Vision Research Center**
143 Anatomy-Chemistry Bldg.
School of Medicine
36th & Hamilton Walk
Philadelphia, PA 19104
**Phone:** (215)898-6917 **Fax:** (215)573-8093
**Email:** liebmanp@mail.med.upenn.edu
**Website:** http://vrc.med.upenn.edu/
Dr. Paul Liebman, Dir.

**Activities/Fields:** Serves as a branch of the National Eye Institute of the National Institutes of Health to fund eye research projects at the University. Studies concentrate on mechanisms of normal and defective vision, including their molecular, genetic, developmental, electrophysiological, neural, and cognitive aspects.

**★ 21180 ★ University of Rochester**
**Center for Visual Science**
274 Meliora Hall
Rochester, NY 14627
**Phone:** (716)275-2459 **Fax:** (716)271-3043
**Email:** david@cvs.rochester.edu
**Website:** http://www.cvs.rochester.edu/
Dr. David Williams, Dir.

**Activities/Fields:** Optical, physiological, perceptual, and computational aspects of visual science. Encourages research in vision in Departments of Brain and Cognitive Sciences, Optics, Neurology, Neurobiology and Anatomy, Ophthalmology, and Computer Science.

**★ 21181 ★ University of Texas—Houston**
**Health Science Center**
**Hermann Eye Center**
Department of Ophthalmology & Visual Science
6431 Fannin St., Rm. 7024
Houston, TX 77030
**Phone:** (713)704-1777 **Fax:** (713)500-0682
Richard S. Ruiz, MD, Dir.

**Activities/Fields:** Cataracts, corneal disease, glaucoma, neuroophthalmology, ophthalmic surgery, pediatric ophthalmology, strabismus, and retinal disease. Additional studies include ocular melanoma, retinitis pigmentosa, diabetes, retinal pigment epithelial transplantation, ischemic optic neuropathy decompression, and pattern electrogram in Alzheimer's disease.

**★ 21182 ★ University of Waterloo**
**Centre for Contact Lens Research**
Sch. of Optometry
Waterloo, ON, Canada N2L 3G1
**Phone:** (519)888-4742 **Fax:** (519)884-8769
**Email:** dfonn@sciborg.uwaterloo.ca
**Website:** http://www.optometry.uwaterloo.ca/~cclr/
Dr. Desmond Fonn, Dir.

**Activities/Fields:** All areas related to contact lenses in order to monitor and understand the effects of contact lenses on the eye, the development of methods for evaluating and measuring the reactions to contact lens wear, and the safety and efficacy of pre and post market release of new lens materials and related products.

**★ 21183 ★ Wayne State University**
**Kresge Eye Institute**
4717 St. Antoine
Detroit, MI 48201
**Phone:** (313)577-8900 **Fax:** (313)577-5482
**Email:** gabrams@med.wayne.edu
**Website:** http://www.med.wayne.edu/kresgeeye/
Gary W. Abrams, MD, Chm.

**Activities/Fields:** Cellular and molecular biology, electron microscopy, electrophysiology, neuro-ophthalmology, ophthalmic pathology, orthoptics, biochemistry of phototransduction in the vertebrate retina, cornea, glaucoma, vitreoretinal, and biochemistry and immunology of the eye.

**★ 21184 ★ Wills Eye Hospital**
**Research Division**
900 Walnut St.
Philadelphia, PA 19107
**Phone:** (215)928-3268 **Fax:** (215)592-4628
Larry A. Donoso, Co-Dir.

**Activities/Fields:** Vitreoretinal surgery, and vitreoretinal disease management and research. Develops new instrumentation and surgical techniques and ocular application of various laser wavelengths in the various ophthalmic subspecialties in addition to vitreoretinal diseases.

**★ 21185 ★ Yale University**
**Vision Research Center**
Boardman Bldg., Box 208061
330 Cedar St.
PO Box 208061
New Haven, CT 06520-8061
**Phone:** (203)785-2405 **Fax:** (203)785-7401
**Email:** Nigel.Daw@yale.edu
**Website:** http://www.info.med.yale.edu/ophtha/
Nigel W. Daw, Dir.

**Activities/Fields:** Vision including studies on transduction, transport, myopia, neurobiology of growth and development, glaucoma, and diabetic retinopathy.

**★ 21186 ★ York University**
**Centre for Vision Research**
103 Farquharson Bldg.
4700 Keele St.
North York, ON, Canada M3J 1P3
**Phone:** (416)736-5659 **Fax:** (416)736-5857
**Email:** manini@hpl.crestech.ca
**Website:** http://cvr.yorku.ca
John Tsotsos, Dir.

**Activities/Fields:** Human and animal vision using psychophysical, physiological and computational procedures, focusing on spatial vision as applied to work in aviation, medicine, and space research.

# State Government Agencies

## Blind

**★ 21187 ★ Alabama Department of**
**Rehabilitation Services**
2129 E South Blvd.
PO Box 11586
Montgomery, AL 36116-2455
**Phone:** (334)281-8780 **Free:** 800-441-7607
**Fax:** (334)281-1973
**Email:** webinfo@rehab.state.al.us
**Website:** http://www.rehab.state.al.us/
Steve Shivers, Director

**★ 21188 ★ Alaska Department of Labor**
**and Workforce Development**
**Vocational Rehabilitation Division**
801 W 10th St., Ste. A
Juneau, AK 99801-1894
**Phone:** (907)465-2814 **Free:** 800-478-2815
**Fax:** (907)465-2856
**Email:** anne_knight@labor.state.ak.us
**Website:** http://www.labor.state.ak.us/dvr/home.htm
Duane French, Director

**★ 21189 ★ Arkansas Department of**
**Human Services**
**Division of Services for the Blind**
522 Main St.
PO Box 3237
Little Rock, AR 72203
**Phone:** (501)682-5463 **Free:** 800-960-9270
**Fax:** (501)682-0366
**Email:** charlie.cain@mail.state.ar.us
**Website:** http://www.state.ar.us/dhs/dsb/index.html
James C. Hudson, Director

**★ 21190 ★ Blind Industries and Services**
**of Maryland**
2901 Strickland St.
Baltimore, MD 21223-2796
**Phone:** (410)233-4567 **Free:** 888-322-4567
**Fax:** (410)233-0544
**Email:** dors@msde.state.md.us
**Website:** http://www.bism.com/

**★ 21191 ★ California Health and Welfare Agency**
**Rehabilitation Department**
PO Box 944222
2000 Evergreen St.
Sacramento, CA 95815
**Phone:** (916)263-8981          **Fax:** (916)327-4567
**Email:** suggest@rehab.cahwnet.gov
**Website:** http://www.rehab.ca.gov/

**★ 21192 ★ Colorado Department of Human Services**
**Division of Vocational Rehabilitation**
2211 West Evans, Bldg. B
Denver, CO 80223
**Phone:** (720)884-1234          **Fax:** (720)884-1213
**Email:** debbie.powell@state.co.us
**Website:** http://www.cdhs.state.co.us/ods/dvr/index.html
Diana Huerta, Director

**★ 21193 ★ Connecticut Board of Education and Services for the Blind**
184 Windsor Ave.
Windsor, CT 06095
**Phone:** (860)602-4000          **Free:** 800-842-4510
**Fax:** (860)602-4020
**Email:** besb@po.state.ct.us
**Website:** http://www.besb.state.ct.us/
Donna Balaski, Director

**★ 21194 ★ Delaware Department of Health and Social Services**
**Visually Impaired Division**
Biggs Bldg.
1901 N DuPont Hwy.
New Castle, DE 19720
**Phone:** (302)255-9800          **Fax:** (302)255-4441
**Email:** dhssinfo@state.de.us
**Website:** http://www.state.de.us/dhss/dvi/dvi-home.htm
Harry B. Hill, III, Director

**★ 21195 ★ Florida Department of Labor and Employment Security**
**Division of Blind Services**
Douglas Bldg.
2551 Executive Center Circle W, Ste. 200
Tallahassee, FL 32399
**Phone:** (850)487-1260          **Free:** 800-342-1330
**Fax:** (850)487-1804
**Email:** craig_kiser@dbs.doe.state.fl.us
**Website:** http://www.state.fl.us/dbs/
Craig Kiser, Director
**Frmly:** Florida Department of Education, Blind Services Division. **Program(s):** Talking Book Program; Children and Families Program; Independent Living Adult Program; Rehabilitation Center for the Blind; Business Enterprise Program; Vocational Rehabilitation Program.

**★ 21196 ★ Hawaii Department of Human Services**
**Vocational Rehabilitation and Blind Services Division**
601 Kamokila Blvd., Rm. 515
Kapolei, HI 96707
**Phone:** (808)692-7719          **Fax:** (808)692-7727
**Website:** http://www.state.hi.us/dhs/
Neil Shim, Director

**★ 21197 ★ Idaho Commission for the Blind and Visually Impaired**
341 W Washington St.
PO Box 83720
Boise, ID 83720-0012
**Phone:** (208)334-3220          **Free:** 800-542-8688
**Fax:** (208)334-2963
**Email:** dard@icbvi.state.id.us

**Website:** http://www.icbvi.state.id.us/
Dana Ard, Contact

**★ 21198 ★ Illinois Department of Human Services**
**Aid to the Aged, Blind, or Disabled**
100 S Grand Ave. E
Springfield, IL 62762
**Phone:** (217)557-1564          **Free:** 800-252-8635
**Fax:** (217)557-2112
**Email:** nsanchez@dhs.state.il.us
**Website:** http://www.state.il.us/agency/dhs/aabdnp.html

**★ 21199 ★ Iowa Department for the Blind**
524 4th St.
Des Moines, IA 50309-2364
**Phone:** (515)281-1333          **Free:** 800-362-2587
**Fax:** (515)281-1263
**Email:** harris.allen@blind.state.ia.us
**Website:** http://www.blind.state.ia.us/
Allen Harris, Director

**★ 21200 ★ Kansas Department of Social and Rehabilitation Services**
**Rehabilitation Services Division**
915 SW Harrison St.
Topeka, KS 66612
**Phone:** (785)267-5301          **Fax:** (785)296-2173
**Website:** http://www.srskansas.org/
Dale L. Barnum, Director

**★ 21201 ★ Kentucky Department for the Blind**
**Blind Department**
209 St. Clair St.
PO Box 757
Frankfort, KY 40602-0757
**Phone:** (502)564-4754          **Free:** 877-592-5463
**Fax:** (502)564-2951
**Email:** wayne.thompson@mail.state.ky.us
**Website:** http://kyblind.state.ky.us/

**★ 21202 ★ Louisiana Department of Social Services**
**Rehabilitation Services Division**
8225 Florida Blvd.
Baton Rouge, LA 70806
**Phone:** (225)925-4131          **Free:** 800-737-2958
**Fax:** (225)925-4484
**Email:** webmaster@dss.state.la.us
**Website:** http://www.dss.state.la.us/offlrs/index.htm
James Wallace, Director

**★ 21203 ★ Maine Department of Labor**
**Rehabilitation Services Bureau**
**Blind and Visually Impaired Division**
150 State House Station
Augusta, ME 04333-0150
**Phone:** (207)624-5950          **Free:** 800-698-4440
**Fax:** (207)624-5980
**Email:** Webmaster.BRS@state.me.us
**Website:** http://www.state.me.us/rehab/

**★ 21204 ★ Massachusetts Commission for the Blind**
88 Kingston St.
Boston, MA 02111
**Phone:** (617)727-5550          **Free:** 800-392-6450
**Fax:** (617)727-5960
**Email:** david.jansen@state.ma.us
**Website:** http://www.state.ma.us/mcb/
David Govostes, Director

**★ 21205 ★ Michigan Commission for the Blind**
201 N Washington Sq.
PO Box 30652
Lansing, MI 48909
**Phone:** (517)373-6425          **Free:** 800-292-4200
**Fax:** (517)335-5140
**Website:** http://www.mfia.state.mi.us/mcb/
Patrick D. Cannon, Director

**★ 21206 ★ Minnesota Department of Economic Security**
**State Services for the Blind**
390 N Robert St. Fifth Floor
Saint Paul, MN 55101
**Phone:** (651)296-1822          **Free:** 800-652-9000
**Email:** belsey@ngwmail.des.state.mn.us
**Website:** http://www.mnworkforcecenter.org/burgundy/ssb.htm
Bonnie Elsey, Contact

**★ 21207 ★ Mississippi Department of Rehabilitation Services**
1281 Hwy. 51 N
PO Box 1698
Jackson, MS 39215-1698
**Phone:** (601)853-5100          **Free:** 800-443-1000
**Fax:** (601)853-5205
**Email:** bmcmillan@mdrs.state.ms.us
**Website:** http://www.mdrs.state.ms.us/
H.S. McMillan, Director

**★ 21208 ★ Missouri Department of Social Services**
**Family Services Division**
**Rehabilitation Services for the Blind**
3418 Knipp
PO Box 88
Jefferson City, MO 65103-0088
**Phone:** (573)751-4249          **Free:** 800-592-6004
**Fax:** (573)751-4984
**Email:** mgiboney@mail.state.mo.us
**Website:** http://www.dss.state.mo.us/dfs/rehab/rehab.htm

**★ 21209 ★ Montana Disability Services Division**
**Vocational Rehabilitation Programs**
111 N Sanders, Ste. 307
PO Box 4210
Helena, MT 59604-4210
**Phone:** (406)444-2590          **Free:** 877-296-1197
**Fax:** (406)444-3632
**Email:** jmathews@state.mt.gov
**Website:** http://www.dphhs.state.mt.us/dsd/govt_programs/vrp/index.htm

**★ 21210 ★ Nebraska Department of Health and Human Services**
**Rehabilitation Services for the Visually Impaired**
PO Box 95044
Lincoln, NE 68509-5044
**Phone:** (402)471-2306          **Fax:** (402)471-0820
**Email:** hhss_system_information@hhss.state.ne.us
**Website:** http://www.hhs.state.ne.us/vii/viiindex.htm

**★ 21211 ★ Nevada Department of Employment, Training and Rehabilitation**
**Rehabilitation Division**
**Bureau of Services to the Blind and Visually Impaired**
505 E King St., Rm. 505
Carson City, NV 89701
**Phone:** (775)684-4244
**Email:** detrbsb@nvdetr.org
**Website:** http://detr.state.nv.us/rehab/reh_bvi.htm

★ 21212 ★ **New Hampshire Bureau of Adult Education**
**Division of Adult Learning and Rehabilitation**
101 Pleasant St.
Concord, NH 03301
**Phone:** (603)271-6698     **Free:** 800-299-1647
**Fax:** (603)271-1114
**Email:** jchaput@ed.state.nh.us
**Website:** http://www.ed.state.nh.us/adulted/adult.htm
Jeanne Chaput, Contact

★ 21213 ★ **New Jersey Department of Human Services**
**Commission for the Blind and Visually Impaired**
153 Halsey St.
PO Box 47017
Newark, NJ 07102
**Phone:** (973)648-2324     **Fax:** (973)648-7364
**Website:** http://www.state.nj.us/humanservices/cbvi/index.html
Jamie Casabianca Hilton, Director

★ 21214 ★ **New Mexico Commission for the Blind**
PERA Bldg., Rm. 553
Santa Fe, NM 87501
**Phone:** (505)827-4479     **Free:** 888-513-7968
**Fax:** (505)827-4475
**Email:** greg.trapp@state.nm.us
**Website:** http://www.state.nm.us/cftb/
Greg Trapp, Director

★ 21215 ★ **New York State Department of Social Services**
**Blind and Visually Handicapped Commission**
40 N Pearl St.
155 Washington Ave.
Albany, NY 12243
**Phone:** (518)473-1675     **Fax:** (518)473-9255
**Email:** cbvh@dfa.state.ny.us
**Website:** http://www.ocfs.state.ny.us/main/cbvh/default.htm
John A. Johnson, Director

★ 21216 ★ **North Carolina Department of Health and Human Services**
**Divison of Services for the Blind**
2601 Mail Service Ctr.
309 Ashe Ave. - Fisher Bldg.
Raleigh, NC 27699-2601
**Phone:** (919)733-9822     **Fax:** (919)733-9769
**Email:** john.deluca@ncmail.net
**Website:** http://www.dhhs.state.nc.us/dsb/
John DeLuca, Director

★ 21217 ★ **North Dakota Department of Human Services**
**Disability Services Division**
600 S Second St.
Bismarck, ND 58504-5729
**Phone:** (701)328-8930     **Free:** 800-755-8529
**Fax:** (701)328-8969
**Email:** dhsds@state.nd.us
**Website:** http://lnotes.state.nd.us/dhs/dhsweb.nsf/ServicePages/DisabilityServices

★ 21218 ★ **Ohio Rehabilitation Services Commission**
**Services for the Visually Impaired Bureau**
400 E Campus View Blvd., SW3A
Columbus, OH 43235-4604
**Phone:** (614)438-1255     **Free:** 800-282-4536
**Fax:** (614)438-1257
**Email:** RSC_wac@rscnet.al.state.oh.us
**Website:** http://www.state.oh.us/rsc/VR_Services/BSVI/bsvi.html
William A. Casto, II, Director

★ 21219 ★ **Oklahoma Department of Rehabilitation Services**
**Visual Services Bureau**
3535 NW 58th St., Ste. 500
Oklahoma City, OK 73112-4815
**Phone:** (405)951-3400     **Free:** 800-845-8476
**Fax:** (405)951-3529
**Email:** drspiowm@onenet.net
**Website:** http://www.okrehab.org/

★ 21220 ★ **Oregon Commission for the Blind**
535 SE 12th Ave.
Portland, OR 97214
**Phone:** (503)731-3221     **Free:** 888-202-5463
**Fax:** (503)731-3230
**Email:** ocbmail@state.or.us
**Website:** http://www.cfb.state.or.us

★ 21221 ★ **Pennsylvania Department of Public Welfare**
**Blindness and Visual Services Bureau**
2923 N 7th St.
Harrisburg, PA 17102
**Phone:** (717)787-7500
**Website:** http://www.aging.state.pa.us/aging/cwp/view.asp?a=277&Q=176872

★ 21222 ★ **Rhode Island Department of Human Services**
**Office of Rehabilitation Services**
**Services for the Blind and Visually Impaired**
40 Fountain St.
Providence, RI 02903
**Phone:** (401)222-2300     **Free:** 800-752-8088
**Fax:** (401)222-1328
**Website:** http://www.ors.state.ri.us/sbvipage.htm

★ 21223 ★ **South Carolina Commission for the Blind**
1430 Confederate Ave.
PO Box 79
Columbia, SC 29202
**Phone:** (803)898-8800     **Free:** 800-922-2222
**Fax:** (803)898-8800
**Email:** publicinfo@sccb.state.sc.us
**Website:** http://www.sccb.state.sc.us/

★ 21224 ★ **South Dakota Department of Human Services**
**Services to the Blind and Visually Impaired Division**
Hillsview Plaza, E Hwy 34
500 E Capitol Ave.
Pierre, SD 57501-5070
**Phone:** (605)773-5990     **Fax:** (605)773-5483
**Email:** jeff.kisecker@state.sd.us
**Website:** http://www.state.sd.us/dhs/sbvi/
Gaye Mattke, Director

★ 21225 ★ **Tennessee Department of Human Services**
**Rehabilitation Services Division**
**Services for the Blind and Visually Impaired**
400 Deaderick St.
Citizens Plaza Bldg, 11th Floor
Nashville, TN 37248-6200
**Phone:** (615)313-4914     **Fax:** (615)741-4165
**Email:** lgallon@mail.state.tn.us
**Website:** http://www.state.tn.us/humanserv/vishome.html

★ 21226 ★ **Texas Commission for the Blind**
4800 N Lamar Blvd., Ste. 340
PO Box 12866
Austin, TX 78756-3178
**Phone:** (512)459-2500     **Free:** 800-252-5204
**Fax:** (512)377-0685
**Email:** judy.adams@tcb.state.tx.us
**Website:** http://www.tcb.state.tx.us/

★ 21227 ★ **Vermont Agency of Human Services**
**Aging and Disabilities Department**
**Blind and Visually Impaired Division**
Osgood Bldg.
103 S Main St.
Waterbury, VT 05671-2304
**Phone:** (802)241-2210     **Fax:** (802)241-3359
**Email:** fredj@dad.state.vt.us
**Website:** http://www.dad.state.vt.us/dbvi/
Fred Jones, Director

★ 21228 ★ **Virgin Islands Department of Human Services**
**Disabilities and Rehabilitation Services Division**
Knud Hansen Complex, Bldg. A 1303
Hospital Ground
Saint Thomas, VI 00802
**Phone:** (340)774-0930     **Fax:** (340)774-3466
**Email:** humanservices@usvi.org
**Website:** http://www.usvi.org/humanservices/index.html

★ 21229 ★ **Virginia Office of Health and Human Resources**
**Department for the Blind and Visually Impaired**
397 Azalea Ave.
Richmond, VA 23227
**Phone:** (804)371-3353     **Free:** 800-622-2155
**Fax:** (804)371-3351
**Email:** bowmanja@dbvi.state.va.us
**Website:** http://www.vdbvi.org//
Joseph A. Bowman, Director

★ 21230 ★ **Washington State Department of Services for the Blind**
402 Legion Way SE, Ste. 100
PO Box 40933
Olympia, WA 98504-0933
**Phone:** (360)586-1224     **Free:** 800-552-7103
**Fax:** (360)586-7627
**Email:** dsb_info@listserv.wa.gov
**Website:** http://www.wa.gov/dsb/

★ 21231 ★ **West Virginia State Board of Rehabilitation**
**Rehabilitation Services Division**
State Capitol Complex
PO Box 50890
Charleston, WV 25305-0890
**Phone:** (304)766-4799     **Free:** 800-642-8207
**Fax:** (304)766-4905
**Email:** penneyh@mail.drs.state.wv.us
**Website:** http://www.wvdrs.org/
Janice Holland, Director

★ 21232 ★ **Wisconsin Department of Workforce Development**
**Vocational Rehabilitation Division**
2917 International Ln., Ste. 300
PO Box 7852
Madison, WI 53707-7852
**Phone:** (608)243-5600     **Free:** 800-442-3477
**Fax:** (608)243-5680
**Email:** charlene.dwyer@dwd.state.wi.us
**Website:** http://www.dwd.state.wi.us/dvr/
Charlene Dwyer, Director

**★ 21233 ★ Wyoming Department of Employment**
**Vocational Rehabilitation Division**
1100 Herschler Bldg.
122 W 25th St.
Cheyenne, WY 82002
**Phone:** (307)777-7389          **Fax:** (307)777-5939
**Email:** jmcint@state.wy.us
**Website:** http://wydoe.state.wy.us/doe.asp?ID=5
Gary W. Child, Director


## Optometry Boards

**★ 21234 ★ Alabama State Board of Optometry**
1431 Second Ave.
PO Box 448
Bessemer, AL 35020
**Phone:** (205)481-9993          **Fax:** (205)481-9959
**Email:** fwallace@al-optometry.org
**Website:** http://www.al-optometry.org
Dr. Fred Wallace, Contact


**★ 21235 ★ Alaska Board of Examiners in Optometry**
PO Box 110806
Juneau, AK 99811-0806
**Phone:** (907)465-2580          **Fax:** (907)465-2974
**Email:** steve_snyder@dced.state.ak.us
**Website:** http://www.dced.state.ak.us/occ/popt.htm
Steve Snyder, Contact


**★ 21236 ★ Arizona State Board of Optometry**
1400 W Washington, Ste. 230
Phoenix, AZ 85007
**Phone:** (602)542-3095
**Email:** jccnfer@webmail.state.az.us
**Website:** http://www.asbo.state.az.us/


**★ 21237 ★ Arkansas Board of Examiners in Optometry**
407 N Elm
Searcy, AR 72143
**Phone:** (501)268-4351          **Fax:** (501)268-5631
**Email:** bjsmall@cei.net
**Website:** http://www.state.ar.us/opt/arkopt.html
Robert Smalling, Director


**★ 21238 ★ California Board of Optometry**
400 R St., Ste. 4090
Sacramento, CA 95814
**Phone:** (916)323-8720          **Free:** 800-547-4576
**Fax:** (916)445-8711
**Email:** boardemail@optometry.ca.gov
**Website:** http://www.optometry.ca.gov/


**★ 21239 ★ Colorado Board of Examiners in Optometry**
1560 Broadway, Rm. 1310
Denver, CO 80202
**Phone:** (303)894-7751
**Email:** optometry@dora.state.co.us
**Website:** http://www.dora.state.co.us/Optometry/
Susan Warren, Contact


**★ 21240 ★ Connecticut Board of Examiners in Optometry**
410 Capitol Ave.
PO Box 340308
MS 12APP
Hartford, CT 06134-0308
**Phone:** (860)509-7562
**Website:**          http://www.ct-clic.com/detail.asp?code=1750


**★ 21241 ★ Delaware Board of Examiners in Optometry**
Cannon Bldg., Ste. 203
861 Silver Lake Blvd.
PO Box 1401
Dover, DE 19904
**Phone:** (302)739-4512          **Fax:** (302)739-2711
**Email:** jyoumans@state.de.us
**Website:** http://professionallicensing.state.de.us/boards/optometry/index.shtml
Jane Youmans, Contact


**★ 21242 ★ District of Columbia Board of Optometry**
825 North Capitol St., NE
2nd floor
Washington, DC 20002
**Phone:** (202)442-4775          **Fax:** (202)442-9431
**Website:** http://dchealth.dc.gov/prof_license/services/boards_main_action.asp?


**★ 21243 ★ Florida Board of Optometry**
4052 Bald Cypress Way, Bin C-07
PO Box 6330
Tallahassee, FL 32314-6330
**Phone:** (850)245-4355          **Fax:** (850)922-8876
**Email:** mqa_optometry@doh.state.fl.us
**Website:** http://www9.myflorida.com/mqa/optometry/op_home.html


**★ 21244 ★ Georgia State Board of Examiners in Optometry**
237 Coliseum Dr.
Macon, GA 31217-3858
**Phone:** (478)207-1686
**Email:** rfthompson@sos.state.ga.us
**Website:** http://www.sos.state.ga.us/ebd-optometry/
Anita Martin, Director


**★ 21245 ★ Hawaii Board of Examiners in Optometry**
1010 Richards St.
DCCA-PVL
PO Box 3469
Honolulu, HI 96801
**Phone:** (808)587-3295
**Website:** http://www.state.hi.us/dcca/pvl/areas_optometry.html


**★ 21246 ★ Idaho State Optometry Board**
Owyhee Plaza, 2nd Fl.
1109 Main St., Ste. 220
Boise, ID 83702-5642
**Phone:** (208)334-3233          **Fax:** (208)334-3945
**Email:** drandall@ibol.state.id.us
**Website:** http://www2.state.id.us/ibol/opt.htm


**★ 21247 ★ Illinois Optometry Examining Committee**
320 W Washington, 3rd. Fl.
Springfield, IL 62786
**Phone:** (217)782-8556          **Fax:** (217)782-7645
**Website:** http://www.dpr.state.il.us/


**★ 21248 ★ Indiana Optometry Board**
402 Washington St., Rm. W041
Indianapolis, IN 46204
**Phone:** (317)234-2054          **Fax:** (317)233-4236
**Email:** hpb8@hpb.state.in.us
**Website:** http://www.in.gov/hpb/boards/iob/
Cindy Vaught, Director


**★ 21249 ★ Iowa Board of Optometry Examiners**
Lucas State Office Bldg., 5th Fl.
321 E 12th St.
Des Moines, IA 50319-0075
**Phone:** (515)242-6385          **Fax:** (515)281-3121
**Email:** scook@idph.state.ia.us
**Website:** http://www.iowaccess.org/idph_pl/optometry/index.html


**★ 21250 ★ Kansas Board of Optometry Examiners**
3111 W 6th St.
Lawrence, KS 66049
**Phone:** (785)296-0824
**Email:** kssbeo@terraworld.net


**★ 21251 ★ Kentucky Board of Optometric Examiners**
301 E Main St., Ste. 850
Lexington, KY 40507
**Phone:** (859)246-2744          **Fax:** (859)246-2746
**Email:** KyOptometry@mail.state.ky.us
**Website:** http://optometry.state.ky.us/


**★ 21252 ★ Louisiana State Board of Optometric Examiners**
115B N 13th St.
PO Box 555
Oakdale, LA 71463
**Phone:** (318)335-2989          **Fax:** (318)335-4090
**Email:** Webmaster@dhhmail.dhh.state.la.us
**Website:** http://www.dhh.state.la.us/boards.HTM
Dr. James Sandifer, Contact


**★ 21253 ★ Maine Board of Registration and Examination in Optometry**
113 State House Station
Augusta, ME 04333-0035
**Phone:** (207)624-8691          **Fax:** (207)624-8692
**Email:** susan.a.giampetruzzi@state.me.us
**Website:**          http://www.state.me.us/pfr/auxboards/opthome.htm


**★ 21254 ★ Maryland Board of Examiners in Optometry**
4201 Patterson Ave.
Baltimore, MD 21215-2299
**Phone:** (410)764-4710          **Fax:** (410)358-2906
**Email:** optometry@dhmh.state.md.us
**Website:** http://mdoptometryboard.org/
Patricia Bennett, Contact


**★ 21255 ★ Massachusetts Board of Registration in Optometry**
239 Causeway St., Ste. 500
Boston, MA 02114
**Phone:** (617)727-3093          **Fax:** (617)727-2669
**Email:** gladys.m.clifton@state.ma.us
**Website:**          http://www.state.ma.us/reg/boards/op/default.htm
Gladys Clifton, Contact


**★ 21256 ★ Michigan State Board of Optometry Examiners**
PO Box 30670
Lansing, MI 48909-8170
**Phone:** (517)335-0918          **Fax:** (517)373-2179
**Email:** bhserinfo@cis.state.mi.us
**Website:** http://www.cis.state.mi.us/bhser/lic/boards/bdopt.htm


**★ 21257 ★ Minnesota State Board of Optometry**
2829 University Ave. SE, Ste. 550
Minneapolis, MN 55414
**Phone:** (612)617-2173          **Free:** 800-627-3529
**Fax:** (612)617-2174
**Email:** lmi@ngwmail.des.state.mn.us
**Website:**          http://www.mnworkforcecenter.org/lmi/lic_occ/optometr.htm
Laurie Mickelson, Contact

**★ 21258 ★ Mississippi State Board of Optometry**
PO Box 12370
Jackson, MS 39236-2370
**Phone:** (601)853-4338     **Fax:** (601)853-0336
Dr. Beverly Limbaugh, Contact

**★ 21259 ★ Missouri State Board of Optometry**
3605 Missouri Blvd.
PO Box 1335
Jefferson City, MO 65102-0423
**Phone:** (573)751-0814     **Fax:** (573)751-8216
**Email:** optom@mail.state.mo.us
**Website:** http://www.ecodev.state.mo.us/pr/optom/
Sharlene Rimiller, Contact

**★ 21260 ★ Montana Board of Optometry**
301 S Park, 4th Fl.
PO Box 200513
Helena, MT 59620-0513
**Phone:** (406)841-2395     **Fax:** (406)841-2305
**Email:** compolopt@state.mt.gov
**Website:** http://www.discoveringmontana.com/dli/bsd/license/contact_us.htm
Linda Grief, Contact

**★ 21261 ★ Nebraska Board of Examiners in Optometry**
PO Box 94986
Lincoln, NE 68509-4986
**Phone:** (402)471-2118     **Fax:** (402)471-3577
**Email:** Becky.Wisell@hhss.state.ne.us
**Website:** http://www.hhs.state.ne.us/crl/crlindex.htm
Becky Wisell, Contact

**★ 21262 ★ Nevada Board of Optometry**
PO Box 1824
Carson City, NV 89702
**Phone:** (775)883-8367     **Fax:** (775)883-1938
**Email:** kennedy@govmail.state.nv.us
**Website:** http://www.state.nv.us/optometry/

**★ 21263 ★ New Hampshire Board of Registration in Optometry**
2 Industrial Park Dr., Ste. 8
Concord, NH 03301-8520
**Phone:** (603)271-2428     **Fax:** (603)271-6702
**Website:** http://webster.state.nh.us/optometry/
Penny Taylor, Director

**★ 21264 ★ New Jersey Board of Optometrists**
PO Box 45012
Newark, NJ 07101
**Phone:** (973)504-6411     **Fax:** (973)648-3536
**Email:** askconsumeraffairs@smtp.lps.state.nj.us
**Website:** http://www.state.nj.us/lps/ca/medical.htmopt9
Susan Gartland, Director

**★ 21265 ★ New Mexico Board of Examiners in Optometry**
2055 Pacheco St., Ste. 400
Santa Fe, NM 87504
**Phone:** (505)476-7121
**Email:** OptometryBd@state.nm.us
**Website:** http://www.rld.state.nm.us/b&c/optometry/index.htm
Carmen E. Payne, Contact

**★ 21266 ★ New York State Board of Optometry**
Office of the Professions
State Education Bldg., 2nd Fl.
Albany, NY 12234
**Phone:** (518)474-3817
**Email:** optombd@mail.nysed.gov
**Website:** http://www.op.nysed.gov/optom.htm
Peter Ferguson, Contact

**★ 21267 ★ North Carolina State Board of Examiners in Optometry**
109 N Graham St.
Wallace, NC 28466
**Phone:** (910)285-3160     **Fax:** (910)285-4546
**Email:** ncsbeo@duplin.net
**Website:** http://www.ncoptometry.org/
John D. Robinson, Director

**★ 21268 ★ North Dakota State Board of Optometry**
341 1st St. E
Dickinson, ND 58601
**Phone:** (701)483-9141     **Fax:** (701)483-9501
**Email:** ndsbopt@dickinson.ctctel.com
**Website:** http://home.ctctel.com/ndsbopt/

**★ 21269 ★ Ohio State Board of Optometry**
77 S High St., 16th Fl.
Columbus, OH 43215-6108
**Phone:** (614)466-5115     **Free:** 888-565-3044
**Fax:** (614)644-3937
**Email:** Optometry.Board@exchange.state.oh.us
**Website:** http://www.state.oh.us/opt
Nancy L. Ott, Contact

**★ 21270 ★ Oklahoma State Board of Examiners in Optometry**
6912 E Reno, Ste. 302
Oklahoma City, OK 73110
**Phone:** (405)733-7836     **Fax:** (405)741-3060
**Website:** http://www.state.ok.us/~optometry/
Dr. Russell Laverty, Director

**★ 21271 ★ Oregon Board of Optometry**
3218 Pringle Rd. SE, Ste.270
Salem, OR 97302-6306
**Phone:** (503)373-7721     **Fax:** (503)378-3616
**Email:** David.PLUNKETT@state.or.us
**Website:** http://www.obo.state.or.us/
David W. Plunkett, Contact

**★ 21272 ★ Pennsylvania State Board of Optometry**
PO Box 2649
Harrisburg, PA 17105-2649
**Phone:** (717)783-7155     **Fax:** (717)787-7769
**Email:** optometr@pados.dos.state.pa.us
**Website:** http://www.dos.state.pa.us/bpoa/optbd/mainpage.htm
Deb Smith, Contact

**★ 21273 ★ Puerto Rico Board of Examiners in Optometry**
Call Box 10200
Santurce, PR 00908-0200
**Phone:** (787)725-8161     **Fax:** (787)725-7903

**★ 21274 ★ Rhode Island State Board of Optometry**
3 Capitol Hill, Rm. 104
Providence, RI 02908
**Phone:** (401)222-2827     **Fax:** (401)222-1272
**Email:** RussellS@doh.state.ri.us
**Website:** http://www.health.state.ri.us/hsr/optom.htm
Russell Spaight, Contact

**★ 21275 ★ South Carolina Board of Examiners in Optometry**
Kingstree Bldg.
110 Centerview Dr
PO Box 11329
Columbia, SC 29210
**Phone:** (803)896-4679     **Fax:** (803)896-4719
**Email:** combsa@mail.llr.state.sc.us
**Website:** http://www.llr.state.sc.us/POL/Optometry/Default.htm

**★ 21276 ★ South Dakota Board of Optometry**
PO Box 370
Sturgis, SD 57785-0370
**Phone:** (605)347-2136     **Fax:** (605)347-5823
**Email:** sdoptbd_99@yahoo.com
**Website:** http://www.state.sd.us/dcr/optometry/optom-ho.htm
Dr. Daniel A. Watson, Contact

**★ 21277 ★ Tennessee State Board of Optometry**
Cordell Hull Bldg., 3rd Fl.
425 Fifth Ave. N
Nashville, TN 37247
**Phone:** (615)532-3202     **Free:** 888-310-4650
**Email:** DDenton@mail.state.tn.us
**Website:** http://170.142.76.180/bmf-bin/BMFprof-gen.pl

**★ 21278 ★ Texas Optometry Board**
333 Guadalupe St., Ste. 2-420
Austin, TX 78701
**Phone:** (512)305-8500
**Email:** lois.ewald@mail.capnet.state.tx.us
**Website:** http://www.tob.state.tx.us/
Lois Ewald, Contact

**★ 21279 ★ Utah Division of Occupational and Professional Licensing Utah Optometry Board**
160 E 300 S
PO Box 146741
Salt Lake City, UT 84114-6741
**Phone:** (801)530-6621     **Fax:** (801)530-6511
**Website:** http://www.commerce.utah.gov/opl/index.html
Lynn Bernhard, Contact

**★ 21280 ★ Vermont Board of Optometry**
26 Terrace St.
Drawer 09
Montpelier, VT 05609-1101
**Phone:** (802)828-2373     **Fax:** (802)828-2465
**Email:** patkins@sec.state.vt.us
**Website:** http://vtprofessionals.org/opr1/optometrists/
Peggy Atkins, Contact

**★ 21281 ★ Virgin Islands Board of Optometrical Examiners**
Roy Lester Schneider Hospital
48 Sugar Estate
St Thomas, VI 00802
**Phone:** (340)774-0117     **Fax:** (340)777-4001
Lydia Scott, Contact

**★ 21282 ★ Virginia Board of Optometry**
6606 W Broad St., 4th Fl.
Richmond, VA 23230-1717
**Phone:** (804)662-9910     **Free:** 800-533-1560
**Fax:** (804)662-7098
**Email:** optbd@dhp.state.va.us
**Website:** http://www.dhp.state.va.us/optometry/default.htm
Elizabeth A. Carter, Director

**★ 21283 ★ Washington State Optometry Board**
1300 SE Quince St.
PO Box 47860
Olympia, WA 98504-7860
**Phone:** (360)236-4700     **Fax:** (360)236-4818
**Website:** http://www.doh.wa.gov/hsqa/hpqad/Optometry/default.htm
Ben H. Wong, Contact

## ★ 21284 ★ West Virginia Board of Optometry
101 Michael St.
Clarksburg, WV 26301-3937
**Phone:** (304)627-2106
**Website:** http://www.state.wv.us/bep/lmi/license/LI-COCCMS.HTMoptometrist

## ★ 21285 ★ Wisconsin Optometry Examining Board
1400 E Washington Ave.
PO Box 8935
Madison, WI 53708-8935
**Phone:** (608)266-0145          **Fax:** (608)267-0644
**Email:** dorl@drl.state.wi.us
**Website:** http://www.drl.state.wi.us/Regulation/applicant_information/dod272.html

## ★ 21286 ★ Wyoming State Board of Optometric Examiners
2020 Carey Ave., Ste. 201
Cheyenne, WY 82002
**Phone:** (307)777-3507
**Website:** http://www.state.wy.us/governor/boards/bdlist.html
Nanette M. Brown, Contact

# State & Regional Organizations

## Blind

*The following are state affiliates of Prevent Blindness America, 500 E Remington Rd., Schaumburg, IL 60173, (800)331-2020, http://www.preventblindness.org/. For states that do not have affiliates listed, contact the national organization for help with inquiries.*

### Arizona

## ★ 21287 ★ Prevent Blindness America Arizona Division
240 W Osborn Rd., Ste. 232
Phoenix, AZ 85015
**Phone:** (602)636-1112
**Email:** pbaarizona1@prodigy.net

## ★ 21288 ★ Prevent Blindness America Arizona Division
240 W Osborn Rd., Ste. 232
Phoenix, AZ 85015
**Phone:** (602)636-1112
**Email:** info@pbaaz.org
**Website:** http://www.prevent-blindness.org/Phoenix/index.html

### California

## ★ 21289 ★ Prevent Blindness America Northern California Affiliate
4200 California St., Ste. 101
San Francisco, CA 94118
**Phone:** (415)387-0934          **Free:** 800-338-3041
**Email:** PBNoCa@aol.com
**Website:** http://www.prevent-blindness.org/nca/

### Connecticut

## ★ 21290 ★ Prevent Blindness America Connecticut Affiliate
984 Southford Rd.
Middletown, CT 06457
**Phone:** (860)347-2020          **Free:** 800-850-2020
**Email:** info@preventblindnessct.org
**Website:** http://www.prevent-blindness.org/ct/index.html

### Florida

## ★ 21291 ★ Prevent Blindness America Florida Affiliate
3825 Henderson Blvd., Ste. 402
Tampa, FL 33629
**Phone:** (813)874-2020
**Email:** jtobin@preventblindnessfl.org
**Website:** http://www.prevent-blindness.org/florida

### Georgia

## ★ 21292 ★ Prevent Blindness America Georgia Affiliate
455 E Paces Ferry Rd., Ste. 222
Atlanta, GA 30305
**Phone:** (404)266-0071
**Email:** pbgeorgia@aol.com
**Website:** http://www.prevent-blindness.org/georgia

### Illinois

## ★ 21293 ★ Prevent Blindness America Illinois Division
39 S LaSalle St., Ste. 1224
Chicago, IL 60603
**Phone:** (312)346-9110          **Fax:** (312)346-9126
**Email:** jstolzenbach@pba-illinois.org

### Indiana

## ★ 21294 ★ Prevent Blindness America Indiana Affiliate
603 E Washington St., 5th Fl.
Indianapolis, IN 46204
**Phone:** (317)955-9580          **Free:** 800-232-2551
**Email:** jwagner@pbeye.org
**Website:** http://www.pbeye.org

### Iowa

## ★ 21295 ★ Prevent Blindness America Iowa Affiliate
1111 9th St., Ste. 250
Des Moines, IA 50314
**Phone:** (515)244-4341
**Email:** pbiowa@netins.net
**Website:** http://www.prevent-blindness.org/iowa

### Kentucky

## ★ 21296 ★ Prevent Blindness America Kentucky Division
117 Coral Ave.
Louisville, KY 40206
**Phone:** (502)895-8899          **Free:** 800-828-1179
**Email:** lrepperson@aol.com

### Massachusetts

## ★ 21297 ★ Prevent Blindness America Massachusetts Affiliate
100 Cummings Ctr., Ste. 330C
Beverly, MA 01915
**Phone:** (978)524-9500
**Email:** preventblind@aol.com
**Website:** http://www.prevent-blindness.org/MA/

### Nebraska

## ★ 21298 ★ Prevent Blindness America Nebraska Affiliate
7101 Newport Ave., Ste. 308
Omaha, NE 68152-2172
**Phone:** (402)572-3520          **Fax:** (402)572-3522
**Email:** preventblindnessnebraska@mb3.net
**Website:** http://www.prevent-blindness.org/ne/

### New Jersey

## ★ 21299 ★ Prevent Blindness America New Jersey Affiliate
2525 Rte. 130 S, Bldg. D
Cranbury, NJ 08512
**Phone:** (609)409-0770
**Email:** pblindness@aol.com
**Website:** http://www.preventblindnessnj.org

### New York

## ★ 21300 ★ Fight For Sight, Inc.
381 Park Ave. S, Ste. 809
New York, NY 10016
**Phone:** (212)679-6060
**Email:** info@fightforsight.com
**Website:** http://www.fightforsight.com

## ★ 21301 ★ Prevent Blindness America New York Division
375 Hudson St., 12th Fl.
New York, NY 10014-3660
**Phone:** (212)463-3682
**Email:** lbrenig@preventblindness.org
**Website:** http://www.preventblindness.org

### North Carolina

## ★ 21302 ★ Prevent Blindness America North Carolina Affiliate
3801 Lake Boone Trail, Ste. 410
Raleigh, NC 27607
**Phone:** (919)571-1014
**Email:** dmanley@pbnc.org
**Website:** http://www.prevent-blindness.org/nc/

### Ohio

## ★ 21303 ★ Prevent Blindness America Ohio Affiliate
1500 W 3rd Ave., Ste. 200
Columbus, OH 43212-2874
**Phone:** (614)464-2020
**Email:** preventblindnessohio@compuserve.com
**Website:** http://www.prevent-blindness.org/Ohio/

### Oklahoma

## ★ 21304 ★ Prevent Blindness America Oklahoma Affiliate
6 NE 63rd St., Ste. 150
Oklahoma City, OK 73105
**Phone:** (405)848-7123
**Email:** shan_pbo@swbell.net
**Website:** http://www.preventblindnessok.org

### Tennessee

## ★ 21305 ★ Prevent Blindness America Tennessee Affiliate
95 White Bridge Rd., Ste. 513
Nashville, TN 37205
**Phone:** (615)352-0450
**Email:** foryereyes@aol.com
**Website:** http://www.prevent-blindness.org/TN/

### Texas

## ★ 21306 ★ Prevent Blindness America Texas Affiliate
3211 W Dallas
Houston, TX 77019
**Phone:** (713)526-2559          **Free:** 888-987-4448
**Email:** pbtxhouston@compuserve.com
**Website:** http://www.prevent-blindness.org/TX/

## Utah

**★ 21307 ★ Prevent Blindness America Utah Affiliate**
661 South 200 East
Salt Lake City, UT 84111
**Phone:** (801)524-2020    **Free:** 800-675-5665
**Email:** preventblindness@uswest.net
**Website:** www.prevent-blindness.org/Utah

## Virginia

**★ 21308 ★ Prevent Blindness America Virginia Affiliate**
9840 Midlothian Turnpike, Ste. R
Richmond, VA 23235
**Phone:** (804)330-3195
**Email:** tim@pbv.org
**Website:** http://www.pbv.org

## West Virginia

**★ 21309 ★ Prevent Blindness America West Virginia Division**
729 9th Ave., No. 149
Huntington, WV 25701-2718
**Phone:** (304)529-1966    **Fax:** (304)525-4443
**Email:** prevent.blindness@verizon.net

## Wisconsin

**★ 21310 ★ Prevent Blindness America Wisconsin Affiliate**
759 N Milwaukee St.
Milwaukee, WI 53202
**Phone:** (414)765-0505
**Email:** info@preventblindnesswisconsin.org
**Website:** www.prevent-blindness.org/wi/

## Optometry

*The state optometric organizations listed below are affiliated with the American Optometric Association, 243 N Lindbergh Blvd., St. Louis, MO 63141, (314)991-4100, http://www.aoanet.org/.*

## Alabama

**★ 21311 ★ Alabama Optometric Association, Inc.**
400 S Union St., Ste. 435
Montgomery, AL 36104
**Phone:** (334)834-1057    **Fax:** (334)834-1691
**Email:** optometry@mindspring.com
**Website:** http://www.eyesite-aloa.org

## Alaska

**★ 21312 ★ Alaska Optometric Physicians Association**
1689 C St., Ste. 222
Anchorage, AK 99501-5126
**Phone:** (907)770-3777    **Fax:** (907)272-7532
**Email:** akoa@alaska.com
**Website:** http://www.akoa.org

## Alberta

**★ 21313 ★ Alberta Association of Optometrists**
10724-113 St.
Edmonton, AB, Canada T5H 3H8
**Phone:** (780)451-6824    **Fax:** (780)452-9918
**Email:** Psloan@optometrists.ab.ca
**Website:** http://www.optometrists.ab.ca

## Arizona

**★ 21314 ★ Arizona Optometric Association**
1702 E Highland Ave., No. 213
Phoenix, AZ 85016
**Phone:** (602)279-0055    **Fax:** (602)264-6356
**Email:** Jane@azoa.org
**Website:** http://www.azoa.org

## Arkansas

**★ 21315 ★ Arkansas Optometric Association**
441 S Victory St., Ste. 202
Little Rock, AR 72201
**Phone:** (501)661-7675    **Fax:** (501)661-1039
**Email:** aropt@swbell.net

**★ 21316 ★ Southwest Council of Optometry**
PO Box 1869
Alma, AR 72921
**Phone:** (501)632-2360    **Fax:** (501)632-4283
**Email:** swco@ipa.net

## British Columbia

**★ 21317 ★ British Columbia Association of Optometrists**
No. 100-10751 Shellbridge Way
Richmond, BC, Canada V6X 2W8
**Phone:** (604)270-9909    **Fax:** (604)270-4950
**Email:** cwilliams@optometrists.bc.ca
**Website:** http://www.optometrists.bc.ca

## California

**★ 21318 ★ California Optometric Association**
2415 K St.
Sacramento, CA 95816-5001
**Phone:** (916)441-3990    **Free:** 800-877-5738
**Fax:** (916)448-1423
**Email:** ELBrutvan@coavision.org
**Website:** http://www.coavision.org

## Colorado

**★ 21319 ★ Colorado Optometric Association, Inc.**
1600 Broadway, Ste. 1320
Denver, CO 80202
**Phone:** (303)863-9778    **Fax:** (303)863-9775
**Email:** ghume@visioncare.org
**Website:** http://www.visioncare.org

## Connecticut

**★ 21320 ★ Connecticut Association of Optometrists**
342 N Main St.
West Hartford, CT 06117-2507
**Phone:** (860)586-7508    **Fax:** (860)586-7550
**Email:** pberry@cao.org
**Website:** http://www.cao.org

## Delaware

**★ 21321 ★ Delaware Optometric Association, Inc.**
PO Box 1009
Selbyville, DE 19975
**Phone:** (302)436-2020    **Fax:** (302)436-8846
**Email:** Jphilov@intercom.net

## Florida

**★ 21322 ★ Florida Optometric Association**
PO Box 13429
Tallahassee, FL 32317
**Phone:** (850)877-4697    **Fax:** (850)878-0933
**Email:** Ken@floridaeyes.org
**Website:** http://www.floridaeyes.org

## Georgia

**★ 21323 ★ Georgia Optometric Association**
1000 Corporate Ctr. Dr., No. 240
Morrow, GA 30260
**Phone:** (770)961-9866    **Fax:** (770)961-9965
**Email:** GBear79180@aol.com
**Website:** http://www.goaeyes.com

**★ 21324 ★ Southern Council of Optometrists**
4661 N Shallowford Rd.
Atlanta, GA 30338
**Phone:** (770)451-8206    **Fax:** (770)451-3156
**Email:** SJGSOCO@aol.com

## Hawaii

**★ 21325 ★ Hawaii Optometric Association**
220 S King St., No. 801
Honolulu, HI 96813-4526
**Phone:** (808)537-5678    **Fax:** (808)537-1509
**Email:** Hoaopt@earthlink.net

## Idaho

**★ 21326 ★ Idaho Optometric Association, Inc.**
25095 Homedale Rd.
Wilder, ID 83676-5811
**Phone:** (208)461-2000    **Fax:** (208)337-5613
**Email:** LEBenton@aol.com

## Illinois

**★ 21327 ★ Illinois Optometric Association**
304 W Washington St.
Springfield, IL 62701
**Phone:** (217)525-8012    **Fax:** (217)525-8018
**Email:** ioa@ioaweb.org
**Website:** http://www.ioaweb.org

## Indiana

**★ 21328 ★ Indiana Optometric Association**
201 N Illinois St., Ste. 1920
PO Box 44975
Indianapolis, IN 46244-0975
**Phone:** (317)237-3560    **Fax:** (317)237-3564
**Email:** rwuensc@attglobal.net
**Website:** http://www.ioa.org

## Iowa

**★ 21329 ★ Iowa Optometric Association**
1454 30th St., Ste. 204
West Des Moines, IA 50266-1312
**Phone:** (515)222-5679    **Fax:** (515)222-9073
**Email:** IOAAED@aol.com
**Website:** http://www.iowaoptometry.org

## Kansas

**★ 21330 ★ Kansas Optometric Association**
1266 SW Topeka Blvd.
Topeka, KS 66612

**Phone:** (785)232-0225          **Fax:** (785)232-6151
**Email:** Garykoa@cjnetworks.com

## Kentucky

### ★ 21331 ★ Kentucky Optometric Association
PO Box 572
Frankfort, KY 40602
**Phone:** (502)875-3516          **Fax:** (502)875-3782
**Email:** Darleneeakin@kyeyes.org
**Website:** http://www.kyeyes.org

## Louisiana

### ★ 21332 ★ Louisiana State Association of Optometrists
115-B N 13th St.
Oakdale, LA 71463
**Phone:** (318)335-0675          **Fax:** (318)335-0677
**Email:** LSAO@bellsouth.net

## Maine

### ★ 21333 ★ Maine Optometric Association, Inc.
61A Pleasant Pond Lake
Litchfield, ME 04350
**Phone:** (207)582-9910          **Fax:** (207)582-1652
**Email:** nanmoa@aol.com
**Website:** http://www.MaineEyeDoctors.com

## Manitoba

### ★ 21334 ★ Manitoba Association of Optometrists
200B-392 Academy Rd.
Winnipeg, MB, Canada R3N 0B8
**Phone:** (204)943-9811
**Email:** mboptom@aol.com

## Maryland

### ★ 21335 ★ Maryland Optometric Association
720 Light St.
Baltimore, MD 21230
**Phone:** (410)727-7801          **Fax:** (410)752-8295
**Email:** moa@assnhqtrs.com
**Website:** http://www.marylandeyes.org

### ★ 21336 ★ The Optometric Society of the District of Columbia
7705 Cayuga Ave.
Bethesda, MD 20817
**Phone:** (301)229-4990

## Massachusetts

### ★ 21337 ★ Massachusetts Society of Optometrists, Inc.
1071 Worcester Rd., No. 12
Framingham, MA 01701-5298
**Phone:** (508)875-7900          **Fax:** (508)875-0010
**Email:** Rich@massoptom.org
**Website:** http://www.massoptom.org

## Michigan

### ★ 21338 ★ Michigan Optometric Association
530 W Ionia St., Ste. A
Lansing, MI 48933-1062
**Phone:** (517)482-0616          **Fax:** (517)482-1611
**Email:** mioptoassn@aol.com
**Website:** http://www.mioptassn.org

## Minnesota

### ★ 21339 ★ Minnesota Optometric Association, Inc.
13355 10th Ave. N, Ste. 108
Minneapolis, MN 55441-5510
**Phone:** (763)765-2393          **Fax:** (763)765-2329
**Email:** Jim@mneyedocs.org
**Website:** http://www.mneyedocs.org

## Mississippi

### ★ 21340 ★ Mississippi Optometric Association, Inc.
5420 I-55 N, Ste. D
Jackson, MS 39211
**Phone:** (601)956-7412          **Fax:** (601)956-7468
**Email:** MSOptometr@aol.com

## Missouri

### ★ 21341 ★ American Optometric Student Association
243 N Lindbergh Blvd.
Saint Louis, MO 63141
**Phone:** (314)991-4100          **Fax:** (314)991-4101
**Email:** cmfrei@aol.com
**Website:** http://www.theaosa.org

### ★ 21342 ★ Missouri Optometric Association, Inc.
100 E High St., Ste. 301
Jefferson City, MO 65101-2960
**Phone:** (573)635-6151          **Fax:** (573)635-7989
**Email:** MOOPT@socket.net
**Website:** http://www.moeyecare.org

## Montana

### ★ 21343 ★ Armed Forces Optometric Association
411 Sweetgrass Ct.
Great Falls, MT 59405
**Phone:** (406)452-5688          **Fax:** (406)452-5740
**Email:** execdir@afos2020.org
**Website:** http://www.afos2020.org

### ★ 21344 ★ Montana Optometric Association, Inc.
36 S Last Chance Gulch, Ste. A
Helena, MT 59601
**Phone:** (406)443-1160          **Fax:** (406)443-4614
**Email:** Suew@mteyes.com
**Website:** http://www.mteyes.com

## Nebraska

### ★ 21345 ★ Nebraska Optometric Association, Inc.
PO Box 81706
Lincoln, NE 68501-1706
**Phone:** (402)474-7716          **Fax:** (402)476-6547
**Email:** noa@assocoffice.net
**Website:** http://www.noaonline.org

## Nevada

### ★ 21346 ★ Nevada Optometric Association, Inc.
9101 W Sahara Ave., No. 105, PMB 172
Las Vegas, NV 89117-5772
**Phone:** (702)220-7444          **Fax:** (702)220-7444
**Email:** NOALV@aol.com
**Website:** http://www.nevadaoptometric.com

## New Brunswick

### ★ 21347 ★ New Brunswick Association of Optometrists
364 York St., Ste. 230
Fredericton, NB, Canada E3B 3P7
**Phone:** (506)458-8759          **Fax:** (506)450-1271
**Email:** nbao@nbnet.nb.ca

## New Hampshire

### ★ 21348 ★ New Hampshire Optometric Association, Inc.
767 Islington St., Ste. B
Portsmouth, NH 03801
**Phone:** (603)436-3717          **Fax:** (603)433-8815
**Email:** optometrist@attbi.com
**Website:** http://www.nhoptometry.org

## New Jersey

### ★ 21349 ★ New Jersey Optometric Association, Inc.
20 Texas Ave.
Lawrenceville, NJ 08648
**Phone:** (609)671-0900          **Fax:** (609)671-1820
**Email:** njoa@aol.com
**Website:** http://www.eyecare.org

## New Mexico

### ★ 21350 ★ New Mexico Optometric Association, Inc.
1008 Paseo del Pueblo Sur, PMB No. 241
Taos, NM 87571
**Phone:** (505)751-7242          **Fax:** (505)751-7243
**Email:** fleece@laplaza.org
**Website:** http://www.laplaza.org

## New York

### ★ 21351 ★ New York State Optometric Association, Inc.
90 S Swan St.
Albany, NY 12210
**Phone:** (518)449-7300          **Free:** 800-231-9826
**Fax:** (518)432-5902
**Email:** NYSOA2020@aol.com
**Website:** http://www.nysoa.org

## Newfoundland

### ★ 21352 ★ Newfoundland Association of Optometrists
PO Box 2284, Stn. C
Saint John's, NF, Canada A1C 6E6
**Phone:** (709)739-8284          **Fax:** (709)739-8378
**Email:** nao@roadrunner.nf.net

## North Carolina

### ★ 21353 ★ North Carolina State Optometric Society, Inc.
Box 1206
Wilson, NC 27894-1206
**Phone:** (252)237-6197          **Fax:** (252)237-9233
**Email:** nceyecare@aol.com
**Website:** http://www.nceyes.org

## North Dakota

### ★ 21354 ★ North Dakota Optometric Association, Inc.
921 S 9th St.
Bismarck, ND 58504
**Phone:** (701)258-6766          **Fax:** (701)258-9005
**Email:** ndoa@btigate.com

## Nova Scotia

**★ 21355 ★ Nova Scotia Association of Optometrists**
PO Box 21074
Cole Harbour RPO
Dartmouth, NS, Canada B2W 6B2
**Phone:** (902)435-2845          **Fax:** (902)435-2846
**Email:** nsao@accesswave.ca

## Ohio

**★ 21356 ★ Ohio Optometric Association**
PO Box 6036
Worthington, OH 43085
**Phone:** (614)781-0708          **Fax:** (614)781-6521
**Email:** rcornett@ooa.org
**Website:** http://www.ooa.org

## Oklahoma

**★ 21357 ★ Oklahoma Association of Optometric Physicians**
4545 N Lincoln Blvd., No. 105
Oklahoma City, OK 73105
**Phone:** (405)524-1075          **Fax:** (405)524-1077
**Email:** saundra@ix.netcom.com
**Website:** http://www.oaop.com

## Ontario

**★ 21358 ★ Canadian Association of Optometrists**
234 Argyle Ave.
Ottawa, ON, Canada K2P 1B9
**Phone:** 888-263-4676          **Fax:** (613)235-2025
**Email:** gcampbell@opto.ca
**Website:** http://www.opto.ca

**★ 21359 ★ Ontario Association of Optometrists**
290 Lawrence Ave. W
Toronto, ON, Canada M5M 1B3
**Phone:** (416)256-4411          **Fax:** (416)256-9881
**Email:** master@optom.on.ca
**Website:** http://www.optom.on.ca

## Oregon

**★ 21360 ★ Oregon Optometric Physicians Association**
4404 SE King Rd.
Milwaukie, OR 97222
**Phone:** (503)654-5036          **Free:** 800-922-2045
**Fax:** (503)659-4189
**Email:** Oopa@AssoMgt.com
**Website:** http://www.oregonoptometry.org

## Pennsylvania

**★ 21361 ★ Pennsylvania Optometric Association, Inc.**
PO Box 3312
Harrisburg, PA 17105
**Phone:** (717)233-6455          **Fax:** (717)233-6833
**Email:** Charlie@poaeyes.org
**Website:** http://www.poaeyes.org

## Prince Edward Island

**★ 21362 ★ Prince Edward Island Association of Optometrists**
216 Water St.
Summerside, PE, Canada C1N 1B3
**Phone:** (902)436-8549

## Quebec

**★ 21363 ★ Quebec Optometric Association**
1265 Berri St., Ste. 740
Montreal, QC, Canada H2L 4X4
**Phone:** (514)288-6272
**Email:** aoq@login.net

## Rhode Island

**★ 21364 ★ Rhode Island Optometric Association**
2484 Warwick Ave.
PMB 117
Warwick, RI 02889
**Phone:** (401)732-1752          **Fax:** (401)732-1771
**Email:** astanelun@aol.com
**Website:** http://www.rioa.org

## Saskatchewan

**★ 21365 ★ Saskatchewan Association of Optometrists**
125-3rd Ave. S
Saskatoon, SK, Canada S7K 1L6
**Phone:** (306)652-2069
**Email:** saskop@sk.sympatico.ca

## South Carolina

**★ 21366 ★ South Carolina Optometric Association, Inc.**
2730 Devine St.
Columbia, SC 29205
**Phone:** (803)799-6721          **Fax:** (803)799-2305
**Email:** optichk1@aol.com
**Website:** http://www.sc-eyecare.org

## South Dakota

**★ 21367 ★ South Dakota Optometric Society**
PO Box 1173
Pierre, SD 57501
**Phone:** (605)224-8199          **Fax:** (605)224-6047
**Email:** Sdeyes3@home.com

## Tennessee

**★ 21368 ★ Tennessee Optometric Association, Inc.**
2727 Branford Ave.
Nashville, TN 37204
**Phone:** (615)269-9092          **Fax:** (615)269-5986
**Email:** Garylodom@aol.com
**Website:** http://www.toaonline.org

## Texas

**★ 21369 ★ Texas Optometric Association, Inc.**
1503 S I-35
Austin, TX 78741
**Phone:** (512)707-2020          **Fax:** (512)326-8504
**Email:** Spirit7651@aol.com
**Website:** http://www.texas.optometry.net

## Utah

**★ 21370 ★ Utah Optometric Association**
230 W 200 S, Ste. 2110
Salt Lake City, UT 84101-3409
**Phone:** (801)364-9103          **Fax:** (801)364-9613
**Email:** uoa@xmission.com
**Website:** http://www.utaheyedoc.org

## Vermont

**★ 21371 ★ Vermont Optometric Association**
PO Box 2027
120 Western Ave.
Brattleboro, VT 05303
**Phone:** (802)254-9012          **Fax:** (802)258-4705
**Email:** Dreye@together.net

## Virginia

**★ 21372 ★ Virginia Optometric Association**
118 N 8th St.
Richmond, VA 23219-2305
**Phone:** (804)643-0309          **Fax:** (804)643-0311
**Email:** VOAEyeDocs@aol.com
**Website:** http://www.voanet.org

## Washington

**★ 21373 ★ Washington Association of Optometric Physicians**
555-116th NE, No. 166
Bellevue, WA 98004-5205
**Phone:** (425)455-0874          **Fax:** (425)646-9646
**Email:** waop@eyes.org
**Website:** http://www.eyes.org

## West Virginia

**★ 21374 ★ The West Virginia Optometric Association, Inc.**
815 Quarrier St., Ste. 345
Charleston, WV 25301-2616
**Phone:** (304)345-4710          **Fax:** (304)346-6416
**Email:** rprice0851@aol.com
**Website:** http://www.wvoa.com

## Wisconsin

**★ 21375 ★ Wisconsin Optometric Association, Inc.**
5721 Odana Rd., Ste. 110
Madison, WI 53719
**Phone:** (608)274-4322          **Fax:** (608)274-8646
**Email:** Brownlowod@aol.com
**Website:** http://www.woa-eyes.org

## Wyoming

**★ 21376 ★ Wyoming Optometric Association**
PO Box 3050
Cheyenne, WY 82003
**Phone:** (307)632-8819          **Fax:** (307)634-0804
**Email:** mgmtassn@aol.com
**Website:** http://www.optometry.wyoming.net

# Alphabetical Name and Keyword Index

*This is an alphabetical listing of all resources included in this directory as well as former or alternate names of the resources. Index references are to entry numbers rather than page numbers. Entry numbers appear in lightface type if the reference is to a former or alternate name; otherwise, entry numbers appear in boldface type. Consult the "User's Guide" at the beginning of this directory for more detailed information about the index.*

## A

Alpha One Foundation **9296**
Alpha 1 National Association **18727**
Alpha Resource Center of Santa Barbara **7002**
Alpha School of Massage, Inc. **3600**
Alpha Tau Delta **14915**, **15632**
ALS Association 13927
    ALS of Michigan Inc. **14594**
    Arizona Chapter **14575**
    Bay Area Chapter **14576**
    Central Tennessee Chapter **14609**
    Connecticut Chapter **14581**
    Evergreen Chapter **14613**
    Florida Chapter **14582**
    Florida East Coast Regional Office **14583**
    Georgia Chapter **14586**
    Greater Los Angeles Chapter **14577**
    Greater New York Chapter **14602**
    Greater Philadelphia Chapter **14606**
    Greater Sacramento Chapter **14578**
    Greater Saint Louis Chapter **14597**
    Indiana Chapter **14587**
    Keith Worthington Chapter **14588**
        Central Missouri Branch Office **14598**
        Central/Western Kansas - Branch Office **14589**
    Kentucky CIO **14590**
    Massachusetts Chapter **14592**
    Massachusetts Chapter - Wakefield Office **14593**
    Minnesota Chapter **14596**
    National Capital Area Chapter **14591**
    Nevada Chapter **14600**
    New Mexico CIO **14601**
    North Carolina Chapter **14603**
    North Texas Chapter **14610**
    Northeast Ohio Chapter **14604**
    Northern New England CIO **14612**
    Orange County Chapter **14579**
    Rhode Island Chapter **14608**
    Rocky Mountain Chapter **14580**
    St. Louis Regional Chapter **14599**
    South Texas Chapter **14611**
    Southeast Wisconsin Chapter **14614**
    Southern Florida Chapter **14584**
    Tampa Bay Chapter **14585**
    West Michigan Chapter **14595**
    Western Ohio Chapter **14605**
    Western Pennsylvania Chapter **14607**
ALS Diagnostic Support Group **13538** -
ALS Forbes Norris Research Center 14008, **14135**
ALS and Neuromuscular Research Foundation 14008
ALS Research Center; Forbes Norris MDA- **14008**
ALS Support Group - Belgium **13539**
ALS Zelfhulpgroep Belgie 13539
ALSAC - St. Jude Children's Research Hospital **5602**
Alsam Foundation **38**
Alstrom Syndrome Families; International Society for 9297
Alstrom Syndrome International **9297**
Alternative Cancer Therapies; Foundation for 4258
Alternative Conjunction Clinic and School of Massage
  Therapy **4018**
Alternative Health Care; American Foundation for 4211
Alternative Health Care, Research and Development; American
  Foundation for **4211**
Alternative Health Insurance Services 4200
Alternative Medicine; National Center for Complementary and **3334**,
  **4298**
Alternative Therapists; American Society of **4223**
Altman Foundation **39**
Alton Ochsner Medical Foundation 2456
Alumni Association; International Bobath 20161
Alvernia College
    Department of Nursing **15452**
    Occupational Therapy Program **19746**
Alverno College • Division of Nursing **15615**

Alvin Community College • Advanced Respiratory Therapist
  Program **18679**
Alzheimer Angehorige Austria **13885**
Alzheimer Disease Center and Related Neuropsychiatric
  Disorders 14205
Alzheimer Europe **13886**
Alzheimer Keskuslitto **13887**
Alzheimer Scotland-Action on Dementia **13888**
Alzheimer Society of Canada **2915**
Alzheimer Society of Ireland **13889**
Alzheimer Society Romania **13890**
Alzheimer Treatment Research Center **3042**
Alzheimerforeningen **13891**
Alzheimerforeningen I Sverige **13892**
Alzheimer's Association **13859**, **13893**
    Aloha Chapter **14502**
    Big Sioux Chapter **14507**
    California Central Coast Chapter **14488**
    Central Illinois Chapter **14503**
    Central Indiana Chapter **14505**
    Central New York Chapter **14532**
    Central and North Florida Chapter **14497**
    Central Ohio Chapter **14541**
    Central and Western Virginia Chapter **14565**
    Cleveland Area Chapter **14542**
    Delaware Valley Chapter **14550**
    Desert Southwest Chapter **14487**
    East Central Iowa Chapter **14508**
    East Central Ohio Chapter **14543**
    Eastern North Carolina Chapter **14539**
    Eastern Tennessee Chapter **14555**
    Florida Gulf Coast Chapter **14498**
    Georgia Chapter **14501**
    Great Plains Chapter **14528**
    Greater Austin Chapter **14559**
    Greater Cincinnati Chapter **14544**
    Greater Dallas Chapter **14560**
    Greater East Ohio Area Chapter **14545**
    Greater Illinois Chapter **14504**
    Greater Iowa Chapter **14509**
    Greater Kentucky and Southern Indiana Chapter **14513**
    Greater Maryland Chapter **14517**
    Greater Michigan Chapter **14519**
    Greater New Jersey Chapter **14530**
    Greater New Orleans Chapter **14514**
    Greater Pennsylvania Chapter **14551**
    Greater Richmond Chapter **14566**
    Greater Wisconsin Chapter **14572**
    Heart of America Chapter **14511**
    Hudson Valley/Rockland/Westchester, NY Chapter **14533**
    Inland Northwest Chapter **14569**
    Long Island Chapter **14534**
    Los Angeles, Riverside, and San Bernardino Counties
      Chapter **14489**
    Maine Chapter **14516**
    Massachusetts Chapter **14518**
    Miami Valley Chapter **14546**
    Michigan Great Lakes Chapter **14520**
    Mid-Missouri Chapter **14524**
    Mid South Chapter **14556**
    Midlands Chapter **14529**
    Minnesota-Dakotas Chapter **14522**
    Mississippi Chapter **14523**
    Montana Chapter **14527**
    National Capital Area Chapter **14567**
    New Mexico Chapter **14531**
    New York City Chapter **14535**
    North Central Texas Chapter **14561**
    North/West Michigan Chapter **14521**
    Northeast/Central Louisiana Chapter **14515**
    Northeast Tennessee Chapter **14557**
    Northeastern New York Chapter **14536**
    Northern California and Northern Nevada Chapter **14490**

Index

American Association of Women Dentists **6432**
American Association of Women Emergency Physicians **8567**
American Association for Women Podiatrists **17686, 17702**
American Association of Women Radiologists 18102, **18102**
American Association for World Health **1882**
American Association of Zoo Veterinarians **20551**
American Athletic Association for the Deaf  6124
American Audiology Society 5974
American Auditory Society **5953, 5974**
American Autoimmune Related Diseases Association **3175, 13540**
American Back Society **13541**
American Behcet's Association 13542
American Behcet's Disease Association **13542**
American Birth Control League 18356
American Blind Bowling Association **20855**
American Blind Skiing Foundation **20856**
American Board of Abdominal Surgery **19474**
American Board of Allergy and Immunology  **3194**
American Board of Alternative Medicine  **4208**
American Board of Anesthesiology  **4439**
American Board of Cardiovascular Perfusion  **4956**
American Board for Certification in Orthotics and Prosthetics  **7912**
American Board of Chelation Therapy  **10098**
American Board of Chiropodical Dermatology  17712
American Board of Colon and Rectal Surgery  **19475**
American Board of Dental Public Health  **17915**
American Board of Dermatology  **6790**
American Board of Emergency Medicine  **8568**
American Board of Endodontics  **6433**
American Board of Examiners in Professional Psychology  12347
American Board of Examiners of Psychodrama, Sociometry, and
  Group Psychotherapy  **12346**
American Board of Examiners in Psychological Hypnosis  11658
American Board of Family Practice  **1883**
American Board of Forensic Anthropology  **12228**
American Board of Genetic Counseling  **9298**
American Board of Health Physics  **1884**
American Board of Industrial Hygiene  **16755**
American Board of Internal Medicine  **1885**
American Board of Laboratory Animal Medicine  20556
American Board of Managed Care Nursing  **15644**
American Board of Medical Specialties  **1886**
American Board of Medical Toxicology  17323
American Board of Neurological Surgery  **19476**
American Board of Neuroscience Nursing  **15645**
American Board of Nuclear Medicine  **18103**
American Board of Nursing Specialties  **15646**
American Board of Nutrition  **16456**
American Board of Obstetrics and Gynecology  **16640**
American Board for Occupational Health Nurses  **15647, 16752**
American Board for Ophthalmic Examinations  20857
American Board of Ophthalmology  **20857**
American Board of Opticianry  **20858**
American Board of Oral and Maxillofacial Pathology  **17126**
American Board of Oral and Maxillofacial Surgery  **19477**
American Board of Oral Pathology  17126
American Board of Oral Surgery  19477
American Board of Orthodontia  6434
American Board of Orthodontics  **6434**
American Board of Orthodontics; College of Diplomates of
  the  **6499**
American Board of Orthopaedic Surgery  **19478**
American Board of Otolaryngology  **5975**
American Board of Pain Medicine  **13905**
American Board of Pathology  **17127**
American Board of Pediatric Dentistry  **5608**
American Board of Pediatrics  **5609**
American Board of Pedodontics  5608
American Board of Peri Anesthesia Nursing Certification  **4440**
American Board of Periodontology  **6435**
American Board of Physical Medicine and Rehabilitation  **20079**
American Board of Plastic Surgery  **19479**
American Board of Podiatric Orthopedics  17703

American Board of Podiatric Orthopedics and Primary
  Medicine  **17703**
American Board of Podiatric Surgery  **17704**
American Board of Preventive Medicine  **17788**
American Board of Preventive Medicine and Public Health  17788
American Board of Proctology  19475
American Board of Professional Neuropsychology  **13906**
American Board of Professional Psychology  **12347**
American Board of Professional Psychology in Hypnosis  11658
American Board of Prosthodontics  **6436**
American Board of Psychiatry and Neurology  **12348**
American Board of Psychological Hypnosis  **11658**
American Board of Quality Assurance and Utilization Review
  Physicians  **1887**
American Board of Radiology  **18104**
American Board of Registration of EEG and EP
  Technologists  **13907**
American Board of Registration of EEG Technologists  13907
American Board of Sleep Medicine  **13908**
American Board of Surgery  **19480**
American Board of Thoracic Surgery  **19481**
American Board of Tropical Medicine  **11730**
American Board of Urologic Allied Health Professionals  20382
American Board of Urology  **20367**
American Board of Veterinary Practitioners  **20552**
American Board of Veterinary Radiology  20563
American Board of Veterinary Specialties  **20553**
American Board of Veterinary Toxicology  **20484, 20554**
American Braille Press for War and Civilian Blind  20974
American Brain Tumor Association  **13861, 13909, 14136**
American Broncho-Esophagological Associat ion  **18417, 18729**
American Bronchoscopic Society  18729
American Brotherhood for the Blind  20853
American Bureau for Medical Advancement in China  **1888**
American Burn Association  **4903, 4904**
American Burn Research Corporation  4911
American Business Clubs Spastic Paralysis Fund  8027
American Business Men's Research Foundation  19239
American Cancer Institutes; Association of  10272
American Cancer Society  10099
  Aberdeen Office  **11181**
  Abilene Office  **11193**
  Abingdon Office  **11228**
  Adams Office  **11120**
  Aiken Office  **11174**
  Alachua Unit  **10791**
  Albany Office  **10857**
  Albuquerque Regional Office  **11047**
  Alexandria Office  **10948**
  Allen Area Office  **11087**
  Amador County Office  **10671**
  Amarillo Office  **11194**
  Anchorage Branch  **10663**
  Antelope Valley-Eastern Sierra Unit  **10672**
  Appleton Office  **11248**
  Arkansas Division  **10670**
  Asheville Administrative Resource Center  **11076**
  Ashland Office  **10938**
  Athens Office  **10858**
  Atlanta Office  **10859**
  Auburn Unit  **10673**
  Augusta Office  **10860**
  Austin Office  **11195**
  Baker Office  **10792**
  Bakersfield Unit  **10674**
  Baldwin County Office  **10655**
  Barry County Office  **10972**
  Bartow Office  **10793**
  Baton Rouge Office  **10949**
  Bay Area Office  **10794**
  Bay Area Service Center  **10973**
  Beaumont Office  **11196**
  Bedford Office  **11121**

American Cancer Society  **10099**
    Greater North Unit  **10698**
    Greater Petaluma Area  **10699**
    Greater Salt Lake Office  **11219**
    Greater San Bernardino Area  **10700**
    Greater Tampa Office  **10814**
    Greater Ventura Unit  **10701**
    Green Bay Office  **11251**
    Green River Office  **11261**
    Greenville Administrative Resource Center  **11077**
    Greenville Office  **11177**
    Greenwood Office  **11178**
    Guam Unit  **10872**
    Gulf Coast Area Office  **10815**
    Gulf Office  **10816**
    Gulfport Office  **11002**
    Gwinnett Office  **10866**
    Hagerstown Office  **10960**
    Hamilton County Office  **11094**
    Hancock Office  **11095**
    Hannibal Office  **11008**
    Hanover Office  **11141**
    Hardee/Manatee/Highlands Unit  **10817**
    Harrisonburg Office  **11231**
    Hattiesburg Office  **11003**
    Heartland Division [Kansas City, MO]  **11009**
    Hernando Office  **10818**
    High Desert Unit  **10702**
    High-Five Unit  **10819**
    Hilton Head Office  **11179**
    Holmes/Emerald Coast Office  **10820**
    Honolulu Office  **10875**
    Hope Lodge Office  **11078**
    Houma Office  **10950**
    Houston Office  **11202**
    Hudson Valley Region
        Kingston Office  **11056**
        Middletown Office  **11057**
        Poughkeepsie Office  **11058**
        Suffern Office  **11059**
    Humboldt-Del Norte Counties Unit  **10703**
    Huntingdon Office  **11142**
    Huntington Office  **11245**
    Huntsville Office  **10659**
    Huron Valley Area Service Center  **10977**
    Imperial Central Unit  **10704**
    Indian River Office  **10821**
    Indian Wells Valley Unit  **10705**
    Indianapolis Office  **10902**
    Inland Mendocino Unit  **10706**
    Ionia County Office  **10978**
    Iowa City Office  **10928**
    Irvine Unit  **10707**
    Jackson Office  **10822, 11004, 11188**
    Jacksonville Beaches/Ponte Vedra Office  **10823**
    Jefferson City Office  **11010**
    Jefferson Office  **11143**
    Jersey Shore Region
        Shrewsbury Office  **11029**
        Toms River Office  **11030**
    Johnson City Office  **11189**
    Joplin Office  **11011**
    Kansas City Metro Office  **10933**
    Kauai Unit  **10876**
    Kearney Office  **11021**
    Kenner Office  **10951**
    Kennewick Office  **11240**
    Kings County Unit  **10708**
    Knoxville Office  **11190**
    La Crosse Office  **11252**
    Lafayette Office  **10952**
    Lake Charles Office  **10953**
    Lake County Regional Office  **10889**

American Cancer Society  **10099**
    Lake/Sumter Office  **10824**
    Lakeport Unit  **10709**
    Lakes Region Office  **11060**
    Lakeshore Area Service Center  **10979**
    Lancaster Office  **11144**
    Laredo Office  **11203**
    Larimer County Office  **10781**
    Lawton Office  **11113**
    Lebanon Office  **11145**
    Lee/Cape Coral Office  **10825**
    Lehigh Valley Office  **11146**
    Leon Office  **10826**
    Lexington Office  **10940**
    Liberty Office  **10827**
    Lincoln Office  **11022**
    Livingston County Office  **10980**
    Lodi Unit  **10710**
    Lompoc Valley Unit  **10711**
    Long Beach-Harbor-Southeast Unit  **10712**
    Lorain Area Office  **11096**
    Los Angeles Coastal Cities, South Bay Branch  **10713**
    Los Angeles Coastal Cities Unit  **10714**
    Los Angeles Region  **10715**
    Los Banos Unit  **10716**
    Louisville Area • Clark, Floyd Counties  **10941**
    Louisville Office  **10942**
    Lower Eastern Indiana Area Service Center  **10903, 10904**
    Lubbock Office  **11204**
    Lucas County Office  **11097**
    Lufkin Office  **11205**
    Lynchburg Office  **11232**
    Macomb Office  **10981**
    Macon Office  **10867**
    Madera County Unit  **10717**
    Madison Office  **11253**
    Magic Valley Office  **10882**
    Mahoning County Office  **11098**
    Manhattan/Bronx Regional Office  **11061, 11062**
    Manhattan Office  **10934**
    Mankato Office  **10994**
    Marco Island Office  **10828**
    Marietta Office  **10868**
    Marin County Unit  **10718**
    Marion Area Office  **11099**
    Marion Unit  **10829**
    Marshall Office  **10995**
    Martin Office  **10830**
    Martinsville Office  **11233**
    Mason City Office  **10929**
    Massachusetts Bay Regional Office  **10965**
    Maui-Molokai-Lanai Unit  **10877**
    McKean Office  **11147**
    Medford Office  **11118**
    Memphis Office  **11191**
    Mendocino Coast Area  **10719**
    Merced/Mariposa County Unit  **10720**
    Mercer Area Office  **11100**
    Mercer Office  **11148**
    Meridian Office  **11005**
    Metro Detroit Area Service Center  **10982**
    Metro East Regional Office  **10890**
    Metro New Jersey Region
        Elizabeth Office  **11031**
        Secaucus Office  **11032**
        West Orange Office  **11033**
    Metrolina Administrative Resource Center  **11079**
    Miami Beach/North Dade Office  **10831**
    Mid-Indiana Area Service Center  **10905, 10906**
        Kokomo Office  **10907**
        Lafayette Office  **10908**
        Marion Office  **10909**
    Mid-Southwestern Area Service Center  **10910**

American Cancer Society  **10099**
    Saint Johns Office  **10843**
    St. Joseph Office  **11014**
    St. Louis Office  **11015**
    Saint Lucie Office  **10844**
    St. Paul Office  **11000**
    Saint Thomas/Saint John Office  **11227**
    Salisbury Office  **10961**
    San Angelo Office  **11209**
    San Antonio Office  **11210**
    San Diego County Unit  **10742**
    San Fernando Valley Unit  **10743**
    San Francisco County Unit  **10744**
    San Gabriel Valley Unit  **10745**
    San Joaquin/Calaveras Unit  **10746**
    San Luis Obispo Unit  **10747**
    San Mateo County Unit  **10748**
    Santa Barbara Unit  **10749**
    Santa Clara County Unit  **10750**
    Santa Clarita Valley Unit  **10751**
    Santa Cruz County Unit  **10752**
    Santa Maria Valley Unit  **10753**
    Santa Rosa Unit  **10754, 10845**
    Sarasota Office  **10846**
    Savannah Office  **10869**
    Schuylkill Office  **11160**
    Seminole Unit  **10847**
    Sheboygan Office  **11256**
    Shreveport Office  **10955**
    Sierra View Unit  **10755**
    Sikeston Office  **11016**
    Silicon Valley/Central Coast Regional Office  **10756**
    Silver Spring Office  **10962**
    Simi Valley Unit  **10757**
    Sioux City Office  **10930**
    Sioux Falls Office  **11185**
    Siskiyou County Unit  **10758**
    Solano County Unit  **10759**
    Somerset Kentucky Office  **10947**
    Somerset Office  **11161**
    Sonoma Valley Area Office  **10760**
    South Central Indiana Area Service Center  **10916**
    South Central Los Angeles Unit  **10761**
    South Central Michigan Service Center  **10986**
    South Contra Costa County Unit  **10762**
    South Jersey Region
        Absecon Office  **11043**
        Cape May Court House Office  **11044**
        Cherry Hill Office  **11045**
        Vineland Office  **11046**
    South Palm Beach Office  **10848**
    South Placer Unit  **10763**
    South Sarasota Office  **10849**
    Southeast Indiana Area Service Center  **10917**
    Southeast New England Regional Division • Brockton
      Office  **10968**
    Southeast New England Regional Office  **10969**
    Southeast Philadelphia Regional Office  **11162**
    Southeastern Arizona Region  **10668**
    Southern New England Regional Office  **10787**
    Southern New York Region
        Elmira Office  **11066**
        Endicott Office  **11067**
        Sidney Office  **11068**
    Southern Regional Office  **10897**
    Southern Utah Office  **11222**
    Southwest Colorado Office  **10784**
    Southwest Kansas/Northwest Oklahoma Office  **10935**
    Southwest Michigan Area Service Center  **10987**
    Southwest New England Regional Office  **10788**
    Southwest Ohio Area Office  **11106**
    Southwest Region • Beaver Unit  **11163**
    Southwest Regional Office  **11164**

American Cancer Society  **10099**
    Southwestern Indiana Area Service Center  **10918**
    Spokane Office  **11241**
    Springfield Office  **11017**
    Stanislaus Unit  **10764**
    Stark Area Office  **11107**
    Staten Island Regional Office  **11069**
    Statesboro Office  **10870**
    Storm Lake Office  **10931**
    Suburban Hillsborough Unit  **10850**
    Suffolk Regional Office  **11070, 11071**
    Summit Area Office  **11108**
    Tacoma Office  **11242**
    Tehama County Unit  **10765**
    Temecula/Murrieta Unit  **10766**
    Texarkana Office  **11211**
    Texas City Office  **11212**
    Topeka Office  **10936**
    Treasure Valley Office  **10884**
    Trenton Office  **11018**
    Tri-Cities Unit  **10767**
    Tri-City Office  **10851**
    Tri-County Office  **10852**
    Tri-Valley Unit  **10768**
    Triad Administrative Resource Center .  **11081**
    Trumbull Area Office  **11109**
    Tulare County Unit  **10769**
    Tulsa Office  **11116**
    Tuolumne County Unit  **10770**
    Tuscaloosa Office  **10662**
    Tuscarawas Area Office  **11110**
    Tyler Office  **11213**
    Upper Napa Valley/Lake County Area Office  **10771**
    Upper Peninsula Area Office  **10988**
    Upper Valley Office  **11214**
    Venango-Forest Office  **11165**
    Victoria Office  **11215**
    Vienna Office  **11237**
    Wabash Valley Indiana Area Service Center  **10919**
    Waco Office  **11216**
    Warren Office  **11166**
    Washington Area Office  **11111**
    Washington Office  **10853**
    Waterloo Office  **10932**
    Watertown Office  **11186**
    Wausau Office  **11257**
    Waycross Office  **10871**
    Weld County Office  **10785**
    West Bay Regional Office  **10772**
    West Bend Office  **11258**
    West Central Regional Office  **10898**
    West Contra Costa County Unit  **10773**
    West Hawaii Unit  **10879**
    West Inland Valley Unit  **10774**
    West Michigan Area Service Center  **10989**
    West Palm Beach Office  **10854**
    West Polk Unit  **10855**
    West Unit  **10775**
    West Volusia Office  **10856**
    Westchester Regional Office  **11072**
    Western Illinois Regional Office  **10899**
    Western New England Region
        Pittsfield Office  **10970**
        West Springfield Office  **10971**
    Western New York Region
        Amherst Office  **11073**
        Buffalo Office  **11074**
        Jamestown Office  **11075**
    Western Yavapai and Mingus Verde Office  **10669**
    White Marsh Office  **10963**
    Wichita Falls Office  **11217**
    Wichita Office  **10937**
    Willmar Office  **11001**

Anorexia Nervosa and Associated Disorders; National Association
 of **12566**
Anorexia Nervosa Association; Bulimia **12429**
Anorexia Nervosa; Center for the Research and Treatment
 of **12682**
Anorexia Nervosa and Related Eating Disorders **12374**
Anschutz Family Foundation **46**
Anthem Foundation, Inc. **840**
Anthropology; American Board of Forensic **12228**
Anthroposophical Medicine; Physicians Association for **4308**
Anthroposophical Nurses Association of America **15659**
Anti-Tuberculosis Association Afghanistan Programme **11737**
Anti-Aging Medicine; American Academy of **2916**
Antibiotics; Alliance for the Prudent Use of **17317**
Anticancereuse; Groupe Europeen de Chimiotherapie **10163**
Antigen Immunochemistry; Laboratory of Tumor **10363**
Antigua Planned Parenthood Association **18230**
Antimicrobial Chemotherapy; British Society for **4596**
Antioxidant Research; Webb-Waring Institute for Cancer, Aging,
 and **4789**
Anti-Saloon League of America **19250**
Antisocial and Violent Behavior Branch **12725**
Antitrypsin Support Group; Alpha 1 **18727**
Anxiety and Affective Disorders Unit **12733**
Anxiety Research Society; Stress and **12659**
Aoki Diabetes Research Institute **8741**
AOL Foundation **5569**
AOL Time Warner Foundation **5569**
Aon Foundation **841**
AOTCB **20152**
Apartment Clearinghouse; National Accessible **8026**
Aphasia; Academy of **5963**
Aphasia Association; International **14025**
Aphasia Association; National **6071**
Aphasia Research Center **14149**
Apheresis; American Society for **12191**
Apheresis Group; Canadian **6008**
Apio-Therapy Society; North American **3191**
Apitherapy Society; American **3191**
APL Ltd. **842**
Aplastic Anemia of Canada **10112**
Aplastic Anemia Foundation of America **10111**
Aplastic Anemia and MDS International Foundation **10075, 10111**
Aplastic Anemia and Myeldysphasia Association of Canada **10112**
Apnea Association; American Sleep **13920**
Apollo College • Mesa Campus • Advanced Respiratory Therapist
 Program **18423**
Apollo College, Phoenix Campus • Advanced Respiratory Therapist
 Program **18424**
Apothecaries; American College of **17505**
Apothecaries of London; Society of **2397**
Appalachian State University
    Department of Family and Consumer Sciences • Dietetics-
     Didactic Program **16307**
    Family and Consumer Sciences • Dietetic Internship
     Program **16308**
Applebaum Foundation **47**
Appleton Papers Inc. **843**
Applied Kinesthetic Studies School of Massage **4136**
Applied Osteopathy; Academy of **16985**
Applied Physiology Research Laboratory **19184**
Applied Physiology Section **3081**
Applied Poetry; Association for **12389**
Applied Psychophysiology and Biofeedback; Association for **3329,
 4507**
Applied Research Ethics National Association **1935**
Applied and Services Research Division **12717**
Applied Vision Association **20878**
Appropriate Health Resources and Technologies Action Group **2151**
APS Foundation, Inc. **844**
Aquatic Animal Medicine; International Association for **20626**
Aquatic Research; International Center for **19182**
Aquatics Bodywork Association; Worldwide **4320**

Arab Academy of Pharmacy **17513**
Arab Americam Medical Association **2270**
Arab American Medical Association; National **1552, 2270**
Arab Centre for Medical Literature **1936**
Arab Disabled Confederation **7919**
Arab Federation of Organizations for the Deaf **5988**
Arab Federation of Sports Medicine **19142**
Arab Forum for Primary Health Care and Community Based
 Rehabilitation **1937**
Arab Medical Union **1938**
Arab Society of Nephrology and Renal Transplantation **20373**
Arapahoe Community College • Mortuary Science Program **6215**
Arbutus Vocational Society **12662**
The Arc
    Ocean County Chapter **7481**
    Warren County Chapter **7482**
The Arc [Alvin, TX] **7722**
The Arc of Adams/Clay Counties **7453**
The Arc of Adams County **7027, 7124, 7431, 7635**
The Arc of Alabama **6944**
The Arc of Alachua County, Inc. **7064**
The Arc of Alamance County, Inc. **7533**
The Arc of Alameda County **7003**
The Arc of Alexandria **7405**
The Arc of Allamakee County **7214**
The Arc of Allegan **7359**
Arc Allegheny **7634**
The Arc of Allen County **7586**
The Arc of Amador and Calaveras Counties **7004**
The Arc of Anchorage **6978**
The Arc of Anderson **7685**
The Arc of Anderson and Cherokee Counties **7723**
The Arc of Anderson County **7244, 7702**
The Arc of Anne Arundel County, Inc. **7325**
The Arc of Anoka, Ramsey, and Suburban Counties **7406**
The Arc of Appanoose County **7215**
The Arc of Arapahoe and Douglas Counties **7028**
The Arc of Arenac Area **7360**
The Arc of Arizona **6979**
The Arc of Arkansas **6997**
The Arc of Arro/Berrien County **7361**
The Arc of Artesia **7501**
The Arc of Ashtabula County **7587**
The Arc of Atchison County **7245**
The Arc of Athens-Limestone **6945**
The Arc of Atlantic County **7483**
The Arc of Auglaize County **7588**
The Arc of Augusta **7776**
The Arc of Aurora **7029**
The Arc of Autauga and Western Elmore Counties **6946**
The Arc of Bakersfield **7005**
The Arc of Baldwin County, Inc. **6947**
The Arc of Baltimore **7326**
The Arc of Barnes County **7578**
The Arc of Barren County **7262**
The Arc of Barron County **7819**
The Arc of Bartholomew County **7166**
The Arc of Baton Rouge **7276**
The Arc of the Bay Area **7724**
The Arc of Bay County **7362**
The Arc of Baytown **7725**
The Arc of Beaufort County Inc. **7534**
The Arc of Beauregard **7277**
The Arc of Beaver County **7636**
The Arc of Bell County **7726**
The Arc of Benton County **7615**
The Arc of Benzie County **7363**
The Arc of Bergen and Passaic Counties, Inc. **7484**
The Arc of Berks County **7637**
The Arc of the Big Country **7727**
The Arc of Biloxi **7432**
The Arc of Bismarck **7579**
The Arc of Black Hawk County **7216**

The Arc of Glenkirk  7125
The Arc of Gloucester  7490
The Arc of Gogebic County  7371
The Arc of Graham County  6983
The Arc of the Grand Traverse Area  7372
The Arc of Grant County  7692
The Arc of Gratiot County  7373
The Arc of Greater Corpus Christi  7741
The Arc of Greater Enfield  7041
The Arc of Greater Fall River  7342
The Arc of Greater Houston  7742
The Arc of Greater Lawrence  7343
The Arc of Greater Manchester  7478
The Arc of Greater New Orleans  7283
The Arc of Greater Plymouth  7344
The Arc of Greater Prince William/Insight, Inc.  7780
The Arc of Greater Providence  7676
The Arc of Greater Tarrant County  7743
The Arc of Greater Waltham  7345
The Arc of Greater Williamsburg  7781
The Arc of Green Valley  7308
The Arc of Greensboro, Inc.  7544
The Arc of Gregg County  7744
The Arc of Grosse Point/Harper Woods  7374
The Arc of Grundy County  7223
The Arc of the Gulf  7073
The Arc of the Habersham Area  7105
The Arc of Halifax  7782
The Arc of Halifax County  7545
The Arc of Hamblen County  7707
The Arc of Hamilton County  7224, 7594
The Arc of Hamilton County, Inc.  7708
The Arc of Hamilton/Merrick Counties  7461
The Arc of Hancock County  7173
The Arc of Hanover County  7783
The Arc of Hardin County  7225
The Arc of Harnett County  7546
The Arc of Harrison County  7813
The Arc of Harrisonburg/Rockingham County  7784
The Arc in Hawaii  7114
The Arc of Haywood County, Inc.  7547
The Arc of the Headwaters  7414
The Arc of Hennepin-Carver  7415
The Arc of Henry County  7226
The Arc of Hickman County  7709
The Arc of High Point  7548
The Arc of Hilo  7115
The Arc of Hopkins County  7745
The Arc of Horry County  7687
The Arc of Howard County  7746
The Arc of Howard County, Inc.  7329
The Arc of Hunt County  7747
The Arc of Hunterdon County  7491
The Arc of Iberia  7284
The Arc of Iberville  7285
The Arc of Idaho, Inc.  7120
The Arc of Illinois  7126
The Arc of Imperial Valley  7010
The Arc of Indian River  7074
The Arc of Indiana  7174
The Arc of Indiana County  7651
The Arc of Ionia County  7375
The Arc of Iosco  7376
The Arc of Iowa  7227
The Arc of Iowa County  7228
The Arc of Iredell County  7549
The Arc of Iroquois County  7127
The Arc of Irwin County  7106
The Arc of Isabella  7377
The Arc of Itawamba County  7435
The Arc of Jackson County  6960, 7075, 7229, 7550, 7618
The Arc of Jackson County, Inc.  7175
The Arc of Jackson Parish  7286

The Arc of Jacksonville  7076
The Arc of Jefferson County  6961, 7033, 7652
The Arc of Jefferson and Nearby Counties  7230
The Arc of Johnson County  7231
The Arc of Jones County  7436
The Arc of Josephine County  7619
The Arc of Juneau County  7826
The Arc of Juniata County  7653
The Arc of Kampeska  7693
The Arc of Kanawha Putnam  7814
The Arc of Kandiyohi County  7416
The Arc of Katy  7748
The Arc of Kauai  7116
The Arc of Kenosha County, Inc.  7827
The Arc of Kent County  7378
The Arc of Kentucky  7264
The Arc of Kerrville  7749
The Arc of the Keys, Inc.  7077
The Arc of King County  7805
The Arc of Kitsap and Jefferson Counties  7806
The Arc of Knox County  7595, 7710
The Arc of Kona  7117
The Arc of Lackawanna County  7654
The Arc of Lafayette  7287
The Arc of Lafourche  7288
The Arc of Lake County  7034, 7694
The Arc of Lake Cumberland  7265
The Arc of Lancaster County  7655
The Arc of Lander/Riverton  7843
The Arc of Lane County  7620
The Arc of Langlade County  7828
The Arc of Laramie County  7844
The Arc of Las Cruces  7504
The Arc of Lawrence County  6962
The Arc of Leavenworth County  7252
The Arc of Lee County  7078, 7128, 7232, 7551
The Arc of Lehigh and Northampton Counties Inc.  7656
The Arc of Lenawee  7379
The Arc of Lenoir County  7552
The Arc of Lenowisco  7785
The Arc of LeSueur County  7417
The Arc of Levy County  7079
The Arc of Licking County  7596
The Arc of Lincoln County  7553, 7711, 7829
The Arc of Lincoln-Lancaster County  7462
The Arc of Linn County  7621
The Arc of Little Missouri  7581
The Arc of Livingston  7289, 7380
The Arc of Logan County  7266
The Arc of Loudoun County  7786
The Arc of Louisiana  7290
The Arc of Lucas County  7233, 7597
The Arc of Luna County  7505
The Arc of Luzerne County  7657
The Arc of Lycoming County  7658
The Arc of Lyman-Brule  7695
The Arc of Macon  7107
The Arc of Madison County  6963
The Arc of Madison County, Inc.  7267
The Arc of Madison-Jefferson  7080
The Arc of Madison-Leon County  7750
The Arc, Magic City Enterprises Inc.  7845
The Arc of Manistee  7381
The Arc of Marinette Area  7830
The Arc of Marion County  7081, 7622, 7815
The Arc of Marshall  7751
The Arc of Marshall County  6964, 7253, 7712
The Arc of Maryland, Inc.  7330
Arc Massachusetts  7346
The Arc of Matagorda County  7752
The Arc of Maui  7118
The Arc of McLean County • MARC  7129
The Arc of McLennan County  7753

Association of Educators for Homebound and Hospitalized Children  8185
Association des Epidemiologistes de Langue Francaise  9032
Association for Equine Sports Medicine  **20579**
Association Espanola de ELA  14115
Association des Etablissements d'Enseignement Veterinaire Totalement ou Partiellement de Langue Francaise  20581
Association of European Cancer Leagues  **10120**
Association of European Coeliac Societies  **9100**
Association for European Paediatric Cardiology  **5624**
Association of European Psychiatrists  **12394**
Association of European Schools and Colleges of Optometry  **20892**
Association of the European Self-Medication Industry  **9957**
Association Europeene pour l'Etude de l'Alimentation et du Developpement de l'Enfant  5673
Association Europeene des Pharmaciens des Hopitaux  17535
Association Europeene de Pratiques Multidisciplinaires en Sante Mentale de l'Enfant, l'Adolescent et de la Familie  12465
Association Europeene des Universites Ecoles et Colleges d'Optometrie  20942
Association Europeenne des Centres Anti-Poisons et de Toxicologie Clinique  17335
Association Europeenne des Etablissements d'Enseignment Veterinaire  20601
Association Europeenne pour l'Etude de l'Alimentation et du Developpement de l'Enfant  16476
Association Europeenne de Methodes Medicales Nouvelles  2089
Association Executives; National Council of State Pharmacy  **9757**
Association des Facultes Dentaires du Canada  6466
Association des Facultes de Medecine du Canada  1958
Association of Faculties of Pharmacy of Canada  **17518**
Association of Family Practice Administrators  **1962**
Association of Family Practice Residency Directors  **9710**
Association for Fitness Professionals; IDEA: The  17805
Association Francaise des Diabetiques  8701
Association France Alzheimer  **13940**
Association Francophone de Chirurgie Enocrinienne  19557
Association Francophone Internationale des Groupes d'Animation de la Paraplegie  20141
Association of Freestanding Radiation Oncology Centers  **18124**
Association of French Language Epidemiologists  **9032**
Association of French-Language Leprologists  **11740**
Association of French-Speaking Dermatologists  **6797**
Association of French-Speaking Physicians of Canada  **1963**
Association of Gastrointestinal Motility Disorders  **9101**
Association Generale des Hygienistes et Techniciens Municipaux  17944
Association Generale des Ingenieurs, Architectes et Hygienistes Municipaux de France, Algerie, Tunisie, Belgique, Suisse et Luxembourg  17944
Association of German Dental Manufacturers  **9958**
Association of German Urologists  **20375**
Association of Gerontology (India)  **2928**
Association for Glycogen Storage Disease  **8676, 8677, 9274**
Association of Government Nursing Staff  15664
Association of Halfway House Alcoholism Programs of North America  **19256**
Association of the Handicapped Children of Romania  **7926**
Association for Health-Care Institutions  **1964**
Association of Healthcare Internal Auditors  **9711**
Association for Healthcare Philanthropy  **11483**
Association for Healthcare Resource and Materials Management  **9959**
Association of Health Facility Licensure and Certification Directors  9712
Association of Health Facility Survey Agencies  **9712**
Association of Health Insurance Advisors  **9855**
Association for Health Services Research  1840
Association of Healthcare Philanthropy  **1965**
Association for the Help of Retarded Children  **6862, 6869**
Association for Higher Education Access and Disability  **7927**
Association on Higher Education and Disability  **7928**
Association for the History of Chiropractic  **5914**

Association of Holistic Animal Practitioners  **20580**
Association of Hong Kong Nursing Staff  **15664**
Association of Hospital Directors of Medical Education  11484
Association of Hospital Health and Fitness  17808
Association for Hospital Medical Education  **11484**
Association of Hospital Superintendents of U.S. and Canada  11477
Association for Humanistic Psychology  **12395**
Association of Humanistic Psychology Practitioners  **12396**
Association of Independent Care Advisors  **1966**
Association of Independent Physical Therapists  **20100**
Association for Individual Development  **7135**
Association of Industrial Laser Users  **4796**
Association des Infirmieres et Infirmiers du Canada  15691
Association of Institutions Teaching Veterinary Medicine Totally or Partially in the French Language  **20581**
Association for International Cancer Research  **10121**
Association of International Health Researchers  **1967, 2460**
Association Internationale Aphasie  14025
Association Internationale - Art-Therape  20130
Association Internationale Francophone des Aines  **2929**
Association Internationale Francophone de Recherche Odontologique  6553
Association Internationale pour l'Etude du Foie  9135
Association Internationale de Medecine Agricole et de Sante Rurale  16778
Association Internationale de Medecine et de Biologie de l'Environnement  8914
Association Internationale de Psychiatrie de l'Enfant et de l'Adolescent et des Professions Associees  5691
Association Internationale de Psychologie du Travail de Langue Francais  12512
Association Internationale de Psychologie du Travail de Langue Francaise  **12397**
Association Internationale pour la Recherche Medicale et les Echanges Culturels  2187
Association Internationale des Registres du Cancer  12088
Association Internationale pour le Sport des Aveugles  20985
Association Internationale des Technologistes de Laboratoire Medical  12204
Association Ivoirienne de Bien-Etre Familial  **18240**
Association of Jewish Aging Services  **2930**
Association of Labor Assistants and Childbirth Educators  **3741**
Association de Langue Francaise pour l'Etude du Diabete et des Maladies Metaboliques  8702
Association of Late-Deafened Adults  **5991**
Association of Latin Languages Allergologists and Immunologists  **3199**
Association des Leprologues de Lange Francaise  11740
Association of Life Insurance Medical Directors of America  9852
Association of Local Official Health Agencies  17921
Association of Local Public Health Agencies  **17921**
Association Luxembourg Alzheimer  **13941**
Association for Macomb-Oakland Regional Center  **7401**
Association for Macular Diseases  **20893**
Association of Managed Care Dentists  **6471**
Association of Managed Care Providers  6471
Association of Managed Healthcare Organizations  9854
Association for Mascular Degeneration  20893
Association of Massage Therapists Australia  **1968**
Association of Maternal and Child Health Programs  **5625**
Association canadienne des specialistes en chirurgie buccale et maxillo-faciale  19537
Association of Medical Deans in Europe  1975
Association of Medical Doctors of Asia  **1969**
Association for Medical Education in the Eastern Mediterranean Region  **1970**
Association for Medical Education in Europe  **1971**
Association of Medical Education and Research in Substance Abuse  **19257**
Association for Medical Education in the Western Pacific Region  **1972**
Association of Medical Illustrators  **12000, 12071**

Australian and New Zealand Society of Nuclear Medicine  **2000**
Australian Nursing Federation  **15671**
Australian Orthopedic Association  **16920**
Australian Physiotherapy Association  **2001**
Australian Private Hospitals Association  **11486**
Australian Psychological Society  **12412**
Australian Quadriplegic Association  **7932**
Australian Rheumatology Association  **13567**
Australian Self-Medication Industry  **17521**
Australian Society of Anaesthetists  **4453**
Australian Society of Clinical Hypnotherapists  **11665**
Australian Society of Hypnosis  **4228**
Australian Society for Medical Research  **2002**
Australian Society of Orthodontists  **6474**
Australian Society of Otolaryngology Head and Neck
  Surgery  **19524**
Australian Society for Reproductive Biology  **18246**
Australian Society of Sex Educators, Researchers and
  Therapists  **18888**
Australian Veterinary Association  **20587**
Australian Women's Health Network  **2003**
Austrian Neuroscience Association  **13951**
Austrian Society of Acupuncture  **4229**
Austrian Society of Cardiology  **4973**
Autism and Brain Development Research Laboratory  14221
Autism-Europe  **6870**
Autism Hotline; National  12414
Autism Independent UK  **6871**
Autism; Laboratory for Research on the Neuroscience of  **14221**
Autism Network International  **12413**
Autism; NSAC, The National Society for Children and Adults
  with  12415
Autism Research Institute  **12680**
Autism Research; National Alliance for  **2268, 6865**
Autism Services Center  **12414**
Autism Society of Alabama  **12838**
Autism Society of America  **12415**
    Greater Phoenix Chapter  **12839**
    Inland Empire Chapter  **12840**
    San Diego County Chapter  **12841**
Autism Society of Canada  **6872**
Autism Society of Connecticut  **12843**
Autism Society of Delaware  **12844**
Autism Society of Greater Cincinnati  **12850**
Autism Society of Los Angeles • United Autism Alliance  **12842**
Autism Society of Michigan  **12847**
Autism Society of Middle Tennessee  **12852**
Autism Society of North Carolina, Inc.  **12849**
Autism Society of Oregon  **12851**
Autism Society of Washington  **12853**
Autism Society of Western Kentucky  **12846**
Autism Society of Wisconsin  **12854**
Autism Treatment Services of Canada  **5997**
Autistic Association - Singapore  **6873**
Autistic Children; National Society for  12415
Autoradiographic Image Processing Center  14235
Autry Foundation  **59**
Auxiliary to the American Dental Association  6406
Auxiliary to the American Optometric Association  20865
Auxiliary to the American Osteopathic Association  16965, 17011
Auxiliary to the National Medical Association  1534, 2004
Avenues, National Support Group for Arthrogryposis Multiplex
  Congenita  **4877**
Avery Dennison Foundation  **5570**
Avian Medicine and Surgery; Association of  **20577**
Avian Pathologists; American Association of  **20535**
Avian Veterinarians; Mid-Atlantic States Association of  **20490,
  20637**
Aviation Medical Association; Civil  **4483**
Aviation Pathology and Toxicology Laboratory  4497
Aviation and Space Medicine; German Society for  **4484**
Avila College • Department of Nursing  15273
Avon Products Foundation, Inc.  **857**

AVSC International  18272
Axion Research Foundation, Inc.  **14141**
Ayur-vedic Medicine, Yoga Therapy, UltraNutrition School  **4159**
Ayurveda Holistic Center  **3887**
Ayurveda Institute of Massage and Spa Services  **3387**
Ayurvedic Institute  **3861**
Azusa Pacific University
    Physical Therapist Program  **19800**
    School of Nursing  **14985**


# B

B. B. Owen Trust  **11365**
B. C. McCabe Foundation  **60**
B.F. Goodrich Foundation, Inc.  **858**
Babies Coalition; National Healthy Mothers, Healthy  **5727**
BACCHUS and Gamma Peer Education Network  **19260**
BACCHUS of the U.S.  19260
Bach International Education Program  **3742**
Back Association of Canada  **20106**
Back Society; American  **13541**
BackCare, The National Organisation for Healthy Backs  **13952**
Bacterial Diseases Network; Canadian  **9033, 11847**
Rose M. Badgeley Charitable Trust  642
Badger Meter Foundation  **859**
Bahrain Diabetic Association  **8679**
Baird & Co. Foundation; Robert W.  **1357**
Baker Cancer Centre; Tom  **10427**
Baker College of Flint
    Health Information Administrator Program  **12027**
    Occupational Therapy Program  **19693**
Baker Hughes Foundation  **860**
Baker University • School of Nursing  **15157**
Balance Disorders Association; Dizziness and  6125
Balgarsko Dermatologichno Drujestvo  6805
Ball Brothers Foundation  **61**
Ball Corp.  **861**
Ball State University
    Department of Family and Consumer Sciences • Dietetics-
      Didactic Program  **16173**
    Family and Consumer Sciences • Dietetic Internship
      Program  **16174**
    Human Performance Laboratory  **19172**
    Public Health Entomology Laboratory  **17976**
    School of Nursing  **15124**
Ballistocardiographic Research; European Society for  5007
Ballistocardiography and Cardiovascular Dynamics; European Society
  for  5007
Baltimore Area Council on Alcoholism  19251
Baltimore Gas & Electric Foundation  **862**
Baltimore Headache Institute  **14142**
Baltimore School of Massage  **3729**
Banbury Fund  **62**
Bancroft School of Massage Therapy  **3743**
Bandag, Inc.  **863**
Bandai Foundation  **11694**
Banfi Vintners Foundation  **864**
Bangladesh Dental Society  **6475**
Bangladesh Medical Association of North America  **2005**
Bangladesh Medical Studies and Research Institute  **2006**
Banja la Mtsogolo  18276
Bank of America Foundation  **865**
Bank of Hawaii Charitable Foundation  **866**
Bank of Louisville Charities  **867**
Bank of New York Co., Inc.  **868**
Bank One Foundation  **7876**
Bank One, Texas-Houston Office  **869**
BankAtlantic Foundation  **5470**
Banks International; Tissue  **1566, 20344**
Banks Program of The DRF; National Temporal Bone  6091
Banque Canadienne de Tissue du Cerveau  13968
Banque Europeenne de Sange Congele de Groupes Rares  12203
Banta Corp. Foundation  **870**

British Institute of Industrial Therapy **16767**
British Institute of Learning Disabilities **6875**
British Institute of Musculoskeletal Medicine **13570**
British Institute of Radiology **18130**
British Institute of Surgical Technologists **19532**
British League Against Rheumatism **13571**
British Lung Foundation **18737**
British Medical Acupuncture Society **4235**
British Medical Association **2014**
British Medical Ultrasound Group **18131**
British Medical Ultrasound Society **18131**
British Microcirculation Society **4977**
British Migraine Association **14047**
British Neuroscience Association **13961**
British Nutrition Foundation **16467**
British Occupational Hygiene Society **16768**
British Orthodontic Society **6481**
British Orthopaedic Association **16921**
British Orthoptic Society **20913**
British Osteopathic Association **17012**
British Paediatric Association **5750**
British Pensioners Association **2936**
British Performing Arts Medicine Trust **2015**
Brush Pharmacological Society **17332**
British Psycho-Analytical Society **12426**
British Psychodrama Association **12427**
British Psychological Society **12428**
British Reflexology Association **4236**
British Retinitis Pigmentosa Society **20914**
British Rheumatism and Arthritis Association **13547**
British Small Animal Veterinary Association **20590**
British Society for Antimicrobial Chemotherapy **4596**
British Society of Audiology **6004**
British Society for Clinical Neurophysiology **13962**
British Society of Dental Hypnosis **11668**
British Society for Dental and Maxillofacial Radiology **6482**
British Society for Dental Research **6483**
British Society of Experimental and Clinical Hypnosis **11666**
British Society of Gastroenterology **9105**
British Society of Gerontology **2909**
British Society for Haematology **10132**
British Society of Hearing Aid Audiologists **6005**
British Society of Hypnotherapists **11667**
British Society for Immunology **3202**
British Society of Medical and Dental Hypnosis **11668**
British Society for Music Therapy **20110**
British Society of Periodontology **6484**
British Society for Research on Ageing **2934**
British Society for Rheumatology **3203**
British Society for the Study of Infection **11747**
British Society for the Study of Prosthetic Dentistry **6485**
British Society for Surgery of the Hand **19533**
British Sports Association for the Disabled **7967**
British Stammering Association **6006**
British Support Group - Inter-African Committee Against Harmful
  Traditional Practices **2016**
British Tinnitus Association **6007**
British Veterinary Association **20591**
British Veterinary Nursing Association **20592**
British Wheelchair Sports Foundation **7938**
Brittle Bone Society **13572**
Britton Fund **89**
Broncho-Esophagological Associat ion; American **18417**, **18729**
Bronchoesophagological Society; International **18747**
Bronchoscopic Society; American **18729**
Bronx Aging Study **3121**
Bronx Lebanon Hospital Center • Physician Assistant
  Program **1774**
Brookdale Community College • Advanced Respiratory Therapist
  Program **18587**
Brooklyn College of City University of New York
    Applied Vision Institute **21093**
    Infant Study Center **5777**

Brooklyn College of City University of New York (continued)
    Speech and Hearing Center **6135**
Brooklyn Hospital Center/Long Island University • Physician
  Assistant Program **1775**
Brooks Advisory Centres **18252**
Broward Community College • Advanced Respiratory Therapist
  Program **18467**
Brown Foundation **90**
Brown Information Center; The Arlin J. **10114**
Brown Shoe Co. Charitable Trust **11422**
Brown University
    Center for Alcohol and Addiction Studies **19355**
    Center for Neural Sciences **14163**
    Division of Biology and Medicine • Graduate Program in
      Molecular Pharmacology and Physiology **17290**
    Institute for Brain and Neural Systems **14164**
    International Health Institute **4625**
    School of Medicine **1687**
Brown & Williamson Tobacco Corp. **19222**
Browning-Ferris Industries Inc. **905**
Broyhill Family Foundation **91**
Bruce McMillan, Jr. Foundation **10041**
Brunswick Foundation **906**
Brush Cancer Research Institute; Geraldine **10335**
Bryan LGH Medical Center/University of Kansas • School of Nurse
  Anesthesia **4389**
The Bryant Foundation **92**
Bryn Mawr College • Graduate School of Social Work and Social
  Research **19045**
BSHAA **6005**
BSSC **4975**
Buchanan Family Foundation **93**
Buck Institute **3046**
Bucknell University • Immunobiology Research Laboratory **3240**
Bucyrus-Erie Foundation **907**
Buffett Foundation **18202**
Bugher Foundation **4917**
Buhl Foundation (PA) **94**
Bulgarian Association of Surgeons and Gastroenterologists **9151**
Bulgarian Dermatological Society **6805**
Bulgarian Family Planning and Sexual Health Association **18253**
Bulgarian Gastro-Surgical Club **9151**
Bulgarian Neuromuscular Disease Association **13573**
Bulgarian Pediatric Association **5636**
Bulgarian Society of Aesthetic Surgery and Aesthetic
  Medicine **19534**
Bulgarian Society of Cardiology **4978**
Bulgarian Society of Endocrinology **8681**
Bulgarian Society for Immunology of Reproduction **3204**
Bulgarian Society of Opthalmology **20915**
Bulgarian Society of Sport Medicine and Kinestherapy **19148**
Bulimia Anorexia Nervosa Association **12429**
Bulimia Nervosa Association; Anorexia **12373**
Bullitt Foundation **17780**
Bunbury Co., Inc. **95**
Bund Freiberuflicher Hebammen Deutschlands eV **16725**
Bundesverband der Deutschen Zahnarzte **6528**
Bundesverband Praktischer Tierarzte **2274**
Bundesverband Selbstandiger PhysiotherapeutInnen **20100**
Bundesverband der Zahnarzte des Offentlichen
  Gesundheitsdienstes **6564**
BundeszahnArztekammer-BZAK **6528**
Bundle Branch Block Association; International **5021**
Burdine Johnson Foundation **18203**
Bureau of Animal Industry Veterinarians **20638**
Bureau Appui Sante Environnement **2419**
Bureau Central pour le SIDA **11719**
Bureau of Health Services • Michigan Board of Medicine **2778**
Bureau International pour l'Epilepsie **14028**
Bureau of Legal Dentistry **6600**
Bureau of Professional Education of the American Osteopathic
  Association **17013**
Burlington Industries Foundation **11423**

Center for Interdisciplinary Research on Immunologic
 Diseases  3247
Center for Medical Consumers  **2041, 2469**
Center for Medical Consumers and Health Care Information  2041
Center for Medical Ethics  12264
Center for Mental Retardation [Cleveland, OH]  **7608**
Center for Molecular Medicine and Immunology  **3242**
Center for Neurochemistry  **14169**
Center for Neurodevelopmental Studies, Inc.  **14170**
Center for Neurologic Study  **14171**
Center for Non-Invasive Diagnosis  18190
Center for Nursing Research  2771
Center for Oral Health Research  6648
Center for Organ Recovery and Education  **20328**
Center on the Organization and Financing of Care for the Severely
 Mentally Ill  9771
Center for Pain Research and Neuromagnetics  14474
Center Perzent  **8909**
Center for Pharmaceutical Economics  17388
Center for Physical and Motor Fitness  19199
Center for Population Options  18225
Center for Professional Well-Being  **12443**
Center for Progressive Atherosclerosis Management  5172
Center on Promoting Employment  8188
Center for Radiation Therapy  **10303**
Center for Recombinant Gamete Contraceptive Vaccinogens  18415
Center for Rehabilitation Science and Biomedical Engineering  4531
Center for Rehabilitation Technology  20191
Center for Rehabilitative Auditory Research  13513
Center for Reproductive and Family Health  **18258**
Center for Reproductive Health and Family Health  18258
Center for Research in Ambulatory Health Care
 Administration  9732, 9781
Center for Research on Population and Security  **18391**
Center for Research in Primate Reproduction  20691
Center for Research on Services for Severe Mental Illness  **9771**
Center for Research on Teaching and Learning  8210
Center for Research in Thrombolysis  **10304**
Center for the Research and Treatment of Anorexia
 Nervosa  **12682**
Center for Senility Studies: Alzheimer's Disease Treatment
 Research  3042
The Center for Social Gerontology  **2941**
Center for Speech Pathology  6081
Center for Sports and Osteopathic Medicine  **19152**
Center on State Systems and Employment  **8188**
Center for the Study of Aging  3114
Center for the Study of Aging of Albany  **2942**
Center for the Study of Aging, Inc.  **3048**
Center for the Study of Cerebrovascular Disease and Stroke  14427
Center for the Study of Drug Development  17565
Center for Study of Multiple Birth  **16736, 18259**
Center for Study of Multiple Gestation  18259
Center for Study of Patient Care and Community Health  2684
Center for the Study of Pharmacy and Therapeutics for the
 Elderly  17394
Center for the Study of Psychiatry  12444
Center for the Study of Psychiatry and Psychology  **12444**
Center for the Study of Rochester's Health  **17978**
Center for the Study of Sleep  14290
Center for Substance Abuse Services Research  9770
Center for Thanatology Research  **6273**
Center for Therapeutic Massage and Wellness  **3677**
Center for Traditional Medicine  **3748**
Center for TransPersonal BodyMind Studies  **3835**
Center for Ulcer Research and Education  9184
Center for Understanding Aging  2995
Center for Universal and Holistic Studies, Paramus  **3836**
Center for Universal and Holistic Studies, Worcester  **3749**
Center for VDT and Health Research  16791
Center on Vulnerable Populations  9770
Center for the Well Being of Health Professionals  **16771**
Center for Wellbeing  **3363**

Center for the Well-Being of Health Professionals  12443
Center for Youth with Disabilities; National  **8038**
Centers and Community Oncology Program  10447
Centex Corp.  **924**
Centra-Cam Vocational Training Association  **2042**
Central American Health Institute  **2043**
Central California Hemophilia Foundation  **11265**
Central California School of Body Therapy  **3408**
Central Connecticut Arc, Inc.  **7047**
Central Connecticut State University
 Department of Health and Human Service Professions  **15030**
 New Britain School of Nurse Anesthesia  **4355**
Central Florida Hypnosis Institute  **3611**
Central Institute for the Deaf  **6136**
 Center for Childhood Deafness and Adult Aural
  Rehabilitation  **6137**
 Fay and Carl Simons Center for Biology of Hearing and
  Deafness  **6138**
Central Louisiana School of Therapeutic Massage  **3721**
Central Maine Power Co.  **925**
Central Mass School of Massage and Therapy  **3750**
Central Michigan University
 Human Environmental Studies • Dietetics-Didactic Program or
  Dietetic Internship Program  **16225**
 Physical Therapist Program  **19870**
 Physician Assistant Program  **1756**
Central Missouri State University
 Department of Human Environmental Sciences • Dietetics-
  Didactic Program  **16255**
 Department of Nursing  **15274**
Central National-Gottesman Foundation  **926**
Central Nervous System; Harvey W. Peters Research Center for the
 Study of Parkinson's Disease and Disorders of the  **14201**
Central Newspapers Foundation  **10062**
Central Ohio School of Massage  **3955**
Central Oregon Arc, Inc.  **7629**
Central Pennsylvania School of Massage, Inc.  **4023**
Central Piedmont Community College • Advanced Respiratory
 Therapist Program  **18611**
Central Regional Dental Testing Service, Inc. • CRDTS  **6657**
Central Service Professionals; American Society for
 Healthcare  **4795**
Central & South West Foundation  **927**
Central Vermont Public Service Corp.  **12280**
Central Washington University • Department of Family and
 Consumer Sciences • Dietetics-Didactic Program or Dietetic
 Internship Program  **16433**
Centre for Addiction and Mental Health • Clarke Division  **12683**
Centre for African Family Studies  **18260**
Centre Canadien de Lutte Contre l'Alcoolisme et les
 Toxicomanies  19263
Centre d'Etudes de la Famille Africaine  18260
Centre for Development and Population Activities - Egypt  **18261**
Centre for Development and Population Activities - India  **18262**
Centre for Development and Population Activities - Nigeria  **18263**
Centre for Health Education, Training and Nutrition
 Awareness  **2044**
Centre for Integrated Genomics  **10305**
Centre International de Recherche sur le Cancer  10186
Centre Muraz  **2045**
Centre for Policy on Ageing  **2943**
Centre Psycho-Corporel, Inc.  **4051**
Centre de Recherches sur les Meningites et les
 Schistosomiases  14105
Centre for Women's Health  **2046**
Centro Gerontologico Latino/Latino Gerontological Center  **2944**
Centro Internazionale di Ipnosi Medica e Psicologica  11672, 11675
Centro Nacional para la Prevencion y Control del VIH/SIDA  11806
Centro Obstetrico Familiar  18348
Centro Obstetrico Familiar COF  18348
Centura Health/Penrose-St. Francis Health Services • Nutrition
 Services • Dietetic Internship Program  **16104**
Century 21 Associates Foundation  **11425**

Duluth Clinic Education and Research Foundation  **14192**
Dumont Foundation  **184**
Dun & Bradstreet Corp. Foundation, Inc.  **1008**
Duncan Research Foundation, Inc.; Garfield G.  **8749**
Dunspaugh-Dalton Foundation  **185**
Duquesne University
    Department of Health Management Systems • Health
      Information Administrator Program  **12043**
    Graduate School of Pharmaceutical Sciences • Pharmacy
      Department  **17280**
    John G. Rangos School of Health Sciences • Department of
      Perfusion Technology  **4946**
    John G. Rangos, Sr. School of Health Sciences
      Occupational Therapy Program  **19749**
      Physician Assistant Program  **1807**
    Mylan School of Pharmacy  **17475**
    School of Health Sciences • Physical Therapist
      Program  **19939**
    School of Nursing  **15460**
Duracell International  **1009**
Durango/Purgatory Adaptive Sports Association  7902
Durham Technical Community College • Advanced Respiratory
    Therapist Program  **18612**
Dutch Association of Abortion Doctors  **18270**
Dutch Association for Dermatology and Venereology  6840
Dutch Council of the Chronically Ill and Disabled  **7981**
Dutch DeafAssociation  6035
Dutch Deafship  **6035**
Dutch Parents Organization of Hearing and Speech Impaired
    Children  **6036**
Dutch Society of Cardiology  5049
Dutton Society; Damien-  11765
Dutton Society for Leprosy Aid; Damien  **11765**
Dwight David Eisenhower Army Medical Center • Department of
    Clinical Investigation  **2487**
Dying; Americans for Better Care of the  **6263**
Dynamet, Inc.  **1010**
D'Youville College
    Coordinated Program in Dietetics  **16290**
    Department of Nursing  **15340**
    Occupational Therapy Program  **19716**
    Physical Therapist Program  **19899**
    Physician Assistant Program  **1778**
Dysautonomia Foundation  **9277, 13984**
Dysfunction Syndrome (CFIDS) Activation Network; Chronic Fatigue
    Immune  **2057**
Dyslexia Association; British  **6874**
Dyslexia Association; Canadian  **6877**
Dyslexia Association; International  **6057**
Dyslexia Association; Norwegian  **8060**
Dyslexia Institute  **6880**
Dyslexia Research Institute  **8189**
Dyslexia Society; Orton  6057
Dyslexia; Tennessee Center for the Study and Treatment of  **6170**
Dyslexic Pupils; Council for the Registration of Schools
    Teaching  **6878**
Dyslexic; Recording for the Blind and  **21060**
Dyson Foundation  **186**
Dysphagia Foundation  2499
Dysplasia; International Center for Skeletal  **9401**
dysplasia Ossificans Progressiva Association; International
    Fibro  **9336**
Dysplasias; National Foundation for Ectodermal  **9349**
Dyspraxia Association of Ireland  **5671**
Dystonia Clinical Research Center  14180
Dystonia Medical Research Foundation  **13870, 13985, 14193**
Dystrophic Epidermolysis Bullosa Research Association of
    America  **6813, 6849, 9278**
Dystrophy Association of America; Reflex Sympathetic  **13881,
14104**
dystrophy Foundation; United Leuko  **14129**

# E

E.I. du Pont de Nemours & Co.  **1011**
E. J. Grassmann Trust  **11382**
E. K. and Lillian F. Bishop Foundation  **5551**
E. L. Cord Foundation  **187**
E.L. Craig Foundation  **1012**
E. L. Wiegand Foundation  **188**
E and M Charities  **189**
E. M. Lynn Foundation  **190**
E. Rhodes and Leona B. Carpenter Foundation  **191**
Ear Dog Program; Hearing  6085
Ear Foundation  **6037**
Ear Hospitals; American Association of Eye and  **11476**
Ear Institute; House  **5107, 6051**
Ear Institute, Inc.; Midwest  **6157**
Ear, Nose, and Throat Advances in Children; Society for  **6109**
Ear Research Foundation  **6142**
Ear Research Foundation; Houston  **6147**
Ear Research Group  6159
Ear Research Institute  5107, 6051
Earhart Foundation  **7867**
Earl C. Sams Foundation  **192**
Early Intervention Infant Toddler Program, Inc.  **6994**
Ears for the Deaf  8067
Earth-Spirit, Inc.  4256
East Carolina University
    Brody School of Medicine  **1656**
    Center for Health Services Research and Development  **2488**
    Department of Environmental Health Sciences, Safety, and
      Technology • School of Industry and Technology  **8896**
    Department of Physical Therapy • Physical Therapist
      Program  **19916**
    Office of Research and Evaluation  **15781**
    School of Allied Health Sciences
      Department of Rehabilitation Studies • Rehabilitation
        Counseling Program  **20044**
      Health Information Administrator Program  **12038**
      Occupational Therapy Program  **19731**
      Physician Assistant Program  **1793**
    School of Human Environmental Sciences • Department of
      Nutrition and Hospitality Management • Dietetics-Didactic
      Program or Dietetic Internship Program  **16310**
    School of Medicine • Department of Pharmacology  **17265**
    School of Nursing  **3937, 15379**
      Nurse-Midwifery Graduate Program  **16619**
    School of Social Work and Criminal Justice Studies • Graduate
      Program in Social Work  **19035**
East Central Arc  7699
East Central University
    Department of Human Resources • Rehabilitation Counseling
      Program  **20051**
    Department of Nursing  **15424**
    Health Information Administrator Program  **12041**
East Los Angeles College • Advanced Respiratory Therapist
    Program  **18438**
East Mississippi Community College • Funeral Service
    Technology  **6235**
East Stroudsburg University • Department of Special Education/
    Rehabilitation • Rehabilitative Services  **20057**
East Stroudsburg University of Pennsylvania • Department of
    Nursing  **15461**
East Tennessee State University
    College of Nursing  **15532**
    Department of Applied Human Sciences • Dietetics-Didactic
      Program  **16380**
    Environmental Health Department  **8902**
    James H. Quillen College of Medicine  **1691**
      Department of Pharmacology  **17294**
    Physical Therapist Program  **19955**
East Tennessee State University (LB) • Advanced Respiratory
    Therapist Program  **18674**
East Texas Baptist University • Department of Nursing  **15547**

# G

# H

Helpern Institute of Forensic Medicine; Milton  **2265**, **12255**
Helping Hand Rehabilitation Center  **7143**
Hematology; American Society of  **10110**
Hematology/Oncology; American Society of Pediatric  **5614**
Hematology Research Laboratory  10625
Hematopathology Section  10495
Hematopathology; Society for  **10252**
Hemochromatosis Foundation  **8706**
Hemochromatosis Research Foundation  8706
Hemochromatosis Society; Canadian  **8686**
Hemodialysis; National Association of Patients on  20366
Hemodialysis and Transplantation; National Association of Patients on  20366
Hemophilia Association of the Capital Area  **11301**
Hemophilia Association, Inc.  **11263**
Hemophilia Association of San Diego  **11266**
Hemophilia Center of Western New York, Inc.  **11285**
Hemophilia Foundation  10233
Hemophilia Foundation of Arkansas, Inc.  **11264**
Hemophilia Foundation of Greater Florida  **11270**
Hemophilia Foundation of Hawaii  **11273**
Hemophilia Foundation of Illinois  **11274**
Hemophilia Foundation of Michigan  **11279**
Hemophilia Foundation of Minnesota & the Dakotas  **11280**
Hemophilia Foundation; National  **10233**
Hemophilia Foundation of Nevada  **11282**
Hemophilia Foundation of Northern California  **11267**
Hemophilia Foundation of Southern California  **11268**
Hemophilia of Georgia, Inc.  **11272**
Hemophilia of Indiana, Inc.  **11275**
Hemophilia of North Carolina  **11287**
Hemophilia Society; Canadian  **10138**
Hemophilia Society of Colorado  **11269**
Hemophilia Society; Swedish  **10255**
Hemophilia of South Carolina  **11297**
Hemophilia; World Federation of  **10261**
Hemostasis; International Society on Thrombosis and  10203
Hemostasis and Thrombosis Research Unit  10327
Hemp; Business Alliance for Commerce in  **2017**
Henderson State University
    Department of Family and Consumer Sciences • Dietetics-Didactic Program  **16057**
    Department of Nursing  **14970**
Henry Ford Community College • Health Careers Education Center • Advanced Respiratory Therapist Program  **18552**
Henry Ford Hospital • Sleep Disorders Center  **17359**
Henry Ford Hospital/University of Detroit Mercy • Graduate Program of Nurse Anesthesiology  **4377**
Henry Ford II Fund  **337**
Henry J. Kaiser Family Foundation  **338**
Henry Luce Foundation  **339**
Henry and Lucy Moses Fund  **340**
Henry M. Jackson Foundation for the Advancement of Military Medicine  **13468**
Henry and Marilyn Taub Foundation  **341**
Henry P. and Susan C. Crowell Trust  **342**
Hepatitis C Coalition; National  **9146**
Hepatitis Foundation International  **9127**, **10081**
Hepato-Biliary Pancreatic Association; International  9138
Hepato-Biliary-Pancreatic Surgery; Asian Society for  **19510**
Hepato-Pancreato-Biliary Association; International  **9138**
Hepatology and Nutrition; European Society of Paediatric Gastroenterology,  **9122**
Heptachlor Research and Education Foundation; Hawaii  **17358**
Herb Association; International Aromatherapy and  **4273**
Herbal Association of South Africa  **4264**
Herbal Practitioners Association; Fook Sang Acupuncture and Chinese  **4257**
Herbal Therapeutics School of Botanical Medicine  **3843**
Herbalists Guild; American  **4212**
Herbalists; National Institute of Medical  **4303**
Herbert H. and Grace A. Dow Foundation  **343**

Herbert H. Lehman College; City University of New York • Department of Health Services • Dietetic Internship Program  **16285**
Herbert L. Orlowitz Institute for Cancer and Blood Diseases  10349
Herbst Foundation  **344**
Hercules Inc.  **1126**
Hereditary Disease Foundation  **9280**, **9332**
Hereditary Metabolic Diseases; Canadian Association of Centers for the Management of  **8682**
Heritable Disorders Of Connective Tissue; Coalition For  **9311**
Heritage Centers • Erie County Chapter  **7520**
Herkimer Area Resource Center  **7521**
Herman Goldman Foundation  **345**
The Herman M. Finch University of Health Sciences /Chicago Medical School • School of Related Health Sciences • Physical Therapist Program  **19840**
Herman O. West Foundation  **11436**
Herman T. and Phenie R. Pott Foundation  **346**
Hernia Research; CHERUBS - Association of Congenital Diaphragmatic  **9306**
Hernia Society; American  **1904**
HERO  12084
Herpes Resource Center - American Social Health Association  **11701**, **11777**
Herpes Viruses Association  **11778**
Herrick Foundation  **347**
HERS Foundation  16682
Hershey Foods Corp.  **11437**
Hesperian Foundation  **2152**
Hess Foundation  **348**
Heublein Foundation Inc.  1105
The Heuga Center  **20192**
Hewlett Foundation; William and Flora  **766**
Hewlett-Packard Co. Foundation  **1127**
HHT Foundation International  **5014**
Hickory Tech Corp. Foundation  **11438**
High Meadow Foundation  **1128**
High Technology Research Institute  **19180**
Highline Community College • Advanced Respiratory Therapist Program  **18712**
HIKE Fund  **5957**, **6048**
Hill Crest Foundation  **349**
Hillcrest Foundation  **350**
Hillman Foundation  **351**
Hillsborough Community College • Advanced Respiratory Therapist Program  **18472**
Hillsdale Fund  **352**
Himalayan Institute  **4029**
Hinds Community College (LB) • Advanced Respiratory Therapist Program  **18568**
Hip and Knee Surgery; Center for  **16945**
Hipple Cancer Research Center  **10342**
Hispanic Council on Aging; National  **3012**
Hispanic Dental Association  **6333**, **6529**
Hispanic Family; National  **19327**
Hispanic Medical Association; National  **2296**
Hispanic Nurses; National Association of  **14928**, **15730**
Hispanic Senior Services; Canadian  **2940**
Hispanic-Serving Health Professions Schools; National Association of  **2277**
Histiocytosis Association of America  **10082**, **10177**
Histiocytosis-X Association of America  10177
Histochemical Society  **4605**
Histochemistry and Cytochemistry; International Federation of Societies for  **1544**, **2202**
Histocompatibility and Immunogenetics; American Society for  **3197**
Histopharmacology Section  12738
Historical Society; Optometric  21047
History of Chiropractic; Association for the  **5914**
History of Dentistry; American Academy of the  **6328**, **6416**
history Forum; Psycho  **12297**, **12609**
History of Pharmacy; American Institute of the  **17412**, **17509**
History Research in Psychopathology; Society for Life  12647

Illinois Osteopathic Medical Association **17092**
Illinois Pharmacists Association **17646**
Illinois State Dental Society **6746**
Illinois State Medical Society **2846**
Illinois State Psychiatric Institute **5821**
Illinois State University
    Department of Biological Sciences **17199**
    Department of Family and Consumer Sciences
        Dietetic Internship Program **16156**
        Dietetics-Didactic Program **16157**
    Environmental Health Program • Department of Health
      Sciences **8888**
    Health Information Administrator Program **12019**
    Mennonite College of Nursing **15102**
Illinois State Veterinary Medical Association **20762**
Illinois Tool Works Foundation **1146**
Illinois Wesleyan University • School of Nursing **15103**
Illness and Disability Statistics Branch **8200**
Illness; National Foundation for Depressive **12583**
Illustrators; Association of Medical **12000, 12071**
Imagine World Health **2159**
Imaging; Council on Diagnostic **18136**
Imaging; North American Society for Cardiac **5051, 18098**
Imaging Resource; Mayo Biomedical **4534**
Imaging Society; Computerized Medical **18135**
Imaging Technology; Japanese Society of Medical **4807**
Immaculata College
    Department of Fashion, Foods and Nutrition • Dietetics-Didactic
      Program **16353**
    Nursing Department **15467**
    Nutrition Education • Dietetic Internship Program **16354**
IMMI Word and Deed Foundation **15908**
Immune Deficiency Foundation **3179, 3219**
Immune Deficiency Foundation; Norwegian **3229**
Immune Disorder Research Centre; Arthritis and **13680**
Immune Dysfunction Syndrome (CFIDS) Activation Network; Chronic
  Fatigue **2057**
Immunization Action Coalition **11783**
Immunization; National Coalition for Adult **3223**
Immunobiology and Immunochemistry Branch **3274**
Immunochemistry; Laboratory of Tumor Antigen **10363**
Immunogenetics; American Society for Histocompatibility and **3197**
Immunogenetics; European Federation for **3210**
Immunologic Toxicology Group **8970**
Immunological Research; Irvington Institute for **11859**
Immunological Societies; International Union of **3221**
Immunologists; American Association of **3193**
Immunologists; American Association of Veterinary **20547**
Immunologists; Association of Latin Languages Allergologists
  and **3199**
Immunologists, and Specialists in Infectious Diseases; World
  Association of Veterinary Microbiologists, **20665**
Immunology Allergic, and Immunologic Diseases Program, Allergy,
  Immunology, and Transplantation Program **3272**
Immunology; American Academy of Allergy, Asthma and **3174,
3188**
Immunology; American Board of Allergy and **3194**
Immunology; American College of Allergy and **3195**
Immunology; American College of Allergy, Asthma and **3195**
Immunology; Center for Molecular Medicine and **3242**
Immunology; European Society of Paediatric Allergy and
  Clinical **3213**
Immunology; Gladstone Institute of Virology and **3248**
Immunology; Hungarian Society of Allergology and Clinical **3218**
Immunology; International Association of Allergology and
  Clinical **3236**
Immunology; Joint Council of Allergy, Asthma and **3222**
Immunology; La Jolla Institute for Allergy and **3254**
Immunology of Reproduction; Bulgarian Society for **3204**
Immunology of Reproduction; International Society for **3220**
Immunology Research; Center for Allergy and **3241**
Immunology and Respiratory Medicine; National Jewish Center
  for **18753**

Immunology Section; Clinical **3081**
Immunology Section; Ocular **21152**
Immunology Society; American In-Vitro Allergy/ **3196**
Immunology Society; Clinical **3178, 3207**
Immunology; Society for Mucosal **3234**
immunomodulation; International Society for Neuro **3180, 14038**
Immunopathology Section **10487**
Immunotherapy Cancer Research Foundation; National **10234**
Impaired; Association for Education and Rehabilitation of the Blind
  and Visually **20891**
Impaired Driving; People Against **19333**
Impaired Driving; Research and Education on **19343**
Impaired Enterprisers; Independent Visually **20977**
Impaired; Idaho Commission for the Blind and Visually **21197**
Impaired; National Association for Parents of the Visually **21024**
Impaired Physician Program **19289**
Impairment; Catholic Association of Persons With Visual **20811,
20924**
Impairment; Council of Families with Visual **20938**
Implant Association; Cochlear **5955, 6019**
Implant Association; Pan-American **21053**
Implant Dentistry; American Academy of **6417**
Implant Dentures; American Academy of **6417**
Implant Prosthodontics; American Academy of **6418**
Implant Society; American Intra- Ocular **20873**
Implanted Defibrilator Association of Scotland **5017**
Implantologists; International College of Oral **6550**
Implantologists; International Congress of Oral **6550**
Implantology Center; Asia-Pacific **6460**
Implantology; Hong Kong Society of Oral **6534**
Implants and Transplants; Academy for **6401**
Impotence Anonymous **18909**
Impotence Association **18897**
Impotence Institute of America **18898**
Impotence Research; International Society for **18900**
In Touch Networks **20976**
In Vitro Diagnostics Association; British **2013, 18251**
In Vivo Physiology; Very Low Frequency Electron Paramagnetic
  Resonance Imaging for **4869**
Inclusion Uganda **12664**
Income Association; Retirement **3026**
Incontinent People; Help for **20390**
Incontinentia Pigmenti Foundation; National **2297**
Inconvenienced Sportsmen's Association; National **7977**
Incurably Ill for Animal Research **2160**
INDENT, Dutch Dental Association **9977**
Independence Arc **7317**
Independence for the Disabled and Elderly; P.F.I.D.E. Foundation -
  Promote Real **20166**
Independence Dogs **7997**
Independence; Extensions for **7985**
Independence Foundation **372**
Independent Academic Medical Centers; Alliance of **1862**
Independent Agencies • U.S. International Development Cooperation
  Agency • U.S. Agency for International Development • Bureau for
  Global Programs, Field Support and Research **11856**
Independent Association of German Dentists **6536**
Independent Citizens Research Foundation for the Study of
  Degenerative Diseases **2161**
Independent Healthcare Association **2162**
Independent Living Centre **7998**
Independent Living; National Council on **8041**
Independent Living; Research and Training Center on **8073**
Independent Midwives Association **16683**
Independent Practice; American Psychological Association Division
  of **12363**
Independent Visually Impaired Enterprisers **20977**
India; Multiple Sclerosis Society of **13625**
Indian AIDS Hotline; National **11817**
Indian and Alaska Native Mental Health Research; National Center
  for American **12575**
Indian Association of General Practitioners **2163**
Indian Association of Paediatric Surgeons **19550**

# L

## M

Montefiore Medical Center  10265
Monterey Fund  **5561**
Monterey Institute of Touch  **3482**
Monterey Peninsula College  **3483**
Montgomery Hospital • Frank J. Tornetta School of
 Anesthesia  **4409**
Montgomery Street Foundation  **550**
Montreal Cancer Institute  **10378**
Montreal Research Centre, Hotel-Dieu  2701
The MONY Life Insurance of New York  **1249**
Mood Disorders Association of Manitoba, Inc.  **12979**
Mood Disorders Association of Ontario  **13044**
Moody Foundation  **551**
Moraine Valley Community College • Advanced Respiratory
 Therapist Program  **18499**
Moral Support; Mothrs United for  9347
Morehead State University
    College of Science and Technology • Dietetics-Didactic
     Program or Dietetic Internship Program  **16190**
    Department of Nursing and Allied Health Sciences  **15173**
Morehouse College • Prevention Research Center  **17987**
Morehouse Consortium Cancer Center; Drew/ Meharry/  **10320**
Morehouse School of Medicine  **1599**
    Office of Graduate Education in the Biomedical Sciences •
     Doctoral Program in Biomedical Sciences  **17194**
Morgan Charitable Trust; J.P.  **1156**
Morgan Memorial and Cooperative Industries and Stores  7990
Morgan Stanley Dean Witter Foundation  **11452**
Morgan State University • Department of Human Ecology •
 Dietetics-Didactic Program  **16211**
Moriah Fund, Inc.  **552**
Morningside College • Department of Nursing Education  **15154**
Morningside House  2911
Moroccan Society of Cardiology  **5044**
Morphology; European Federation for Experimental  **4602**
Morris Goldseker Foundation of Maryland  **553**
Morris and Gwendolyn Cafritz Foundation  **554**
Morris Institute of Natural Therapeutics  **3847**
Morris Stulsaft Foundation  **555**
Moscow School of Massage  **3675**
Vince Moseley Center for Children with Developmental
 Disabilities  8191
Mother and Child International  16687
Mother Love, Doula Training  **3848**
MotherCare Doula Training  **3707**
MotherMassage  **3905**
Mothers Against Munchausen Syndrome by Proxy
 Allegations  **12561**
Mothers of Asthmatics  5601
Mothers, Healthy Babies Coalition; National Healthy  **5727**
Mothers Supporting Daughters with Breast Cancer  **10219**
Mothers' Voices  **11803**
Mothrs United for Moral Support  9347
Motility Disorders Society; Pediatric Digestion and  **5742**
Motility; Scandinavian Association for Gastrointestinal  **9150**
Motility Society; American  **9094**
Motivation Institute of America Association; Fitness  **17803**
Motivation; Institute of Athletic  **12497**
Motivation and Institute of Athletic Motivation; Institute for the Study
 of Athletic  12497
Motivation; Institute for the Study of Athletic  12497
Motor Neuron Disease Association; Taiwan  **13670**
Motor Neurone Disease Association  **14050**
Motor Neurone Disease Association of Australia  **14051**
Motor Neurone Disease Association of India  **14052**
Motor Neurone Disease Association; Irish  **14042**
Motor Neurone Disease Association of New Zealand  **14053**
Motor Neurone Disease Association of South Africa  **14054**
Motor Neurone Disease and Esclerosis Lateral Amiotrofica in
 Uruguay  **14055**
Motor Neurone Disease Research Institute of Australia  **14056**
Motor Sport Research Council  19183
Motor Sport Sciences; International Council of  **19183**

Motorcoach Therapy; National Coalition of Psychiatrists
 Against  **12577**
Motorcycle Association; Wheelchair  **8180**
Motorcyclists; Association of Recovering  **19258**
Motorola Foundation  **1250**
Mott Community College • Advanced Respiratory Therapist
 Program  **18557**
Mount Aloysius College
    Department of Nursing  **15477**
    Occupational Therapy Program  **19752**
Mount Carmel College of Nursing
    Baccalaureate Nursing Program  **15413**
    Dietetic Internship Program  **16328**
Mount Hood Community College
    Advanced Respiratory Therapist Program  **18645**
    Department of Funeral Service Education  **6249**
Mount Ida College • New England Institute of Funeral Service
 Education  **6232**
Mount Madonna Center  **3484**
Mount Marty College
    Department of Nutrition and Food Science • Dietetics-Didactic
     Program or Coordinated Program in Dietetics  **16375**
    Graduate Program in Nurse Anesthesiology  **4422**
    Nursing Program  **15525**
Mount Mary College
    Graduate Program in Dietetics • Dietetic Internship Program or
     Coordinated Program in Dietetics  **16443**
    Occupational Therapy Program  **19789**
Mount Mercy College • Department of Nursing  **15155**
Mount Nittany Institute of Natural Health  **4036**
Mount Royal College Centre for Complementary Haelth
 Education  **3343**
Mount Saint Mary College • Division of Nursing  **15352**
Mount St. Mary's College
    Department of Nursing  **15003**
    Department of Physical Therapy • Physical Therapist
     Program  **19807**
Mount San Antonio College • Advanced Respiratory Therapist
 Program  **18446**
Mount Sinai Hospital • Samuel Lunenfeld Research Institute  **2555**
Mount Sinai Hospital Research Institute  2555
Mount Sinai School of Medicine • Graduate Program in the
 Biomedical Sciences • Department of Pharmacology  **17254**
Mount Sinai School of Medicine of City University of New York
    Alzheimer's Disease Research Center  **14241**
    Brookdale Center for Molecular Biology  **4661**
    Computational Neurobiology and Imaging Center  **14242**
    General Clinical Research Center  **2556**
    Vision Research Center in Ophthalmology  **21129**
Mount Sinai Spinal Cord Injury Model System  **14243**
Mountain Empire Community College • Advanced Respiratory
 Therapist Program  **18707**
Mountain Medicine; International Society for  **1545, 2218**
Mountain Research Institute; Rocky  **4336**
Mountain State School of Massage  **4183**
Mountain State University
    Physician Assistant Program  **1836**
    Program in Nursing  **15608**
Mountain States Tumor Institute, Inc.  **10379**
MountainHeart School of Bodywork and Transformational
 Therapy  **3571**
Mouvement Francais pour le Planning Familial  **18337**
Movement Analysis in Adults and Children; European Society
 for  **16930**
Movement Disorder Institute; Parkinson's and  **14261**
Movement Disorder Society  **13620**
Movement for the Handicapped; Adventures in  **7903**
Movement Studies, Inc.; Laban/ Bartenieff Institute of  **20195**
Movement Studies Institute  **3485**
Mozambique Association for Family Development  **18338**
MPS; Parents for  8723
MPS Society  8723
MPS Society; National  8723

Network for Organ Sharing; United  **20347**
Networking Institute; Gazette International  **7989**, **12003**
Networking Project for Young Adults with Disabilities  **8056**
Neumann Association; Victor C.  **7163**
Neumann College
 Division of Nursing and Health Sciences • Physical Therapy
  Program  **19942**
 Program in Nursing  **15478**
Neural Network Assembly; Asian Pacific  **13933**
Neural Network Society; International  **14035**
Neuralgia Association; Trigeminal  **14125**
Neuro Immuno Therapeutic Research Foundation  **2559**
Neuro-Linguistic Programming; International Association of  2189
Neuro-Linguistic Programming; North American Association of  2189
Neuro-Ophthalmology Section  21152
Neuro-Psychopharmacologicum; Collegium Internationale  **13978**
Neuro Therapeutics; American Society for Experimental  **13923**
Neurobiology and Anesthesiology Branch  6624
Neurobiology; Arthur M. Fishberg Research Center in  **14139**
Neurobiology and Cell Biology; Canadian Association for
 Anatomy,  **2018**
Neurobiology Section; Molecular  12733
Neurobiology Unit  14231
Neurochemistry; Asian Pacific Society for  **13934**
Neurochemistry and Brain Transport Section  3083
Neurochemistry; Center for  **14169**
Neurochemistry; European Society for  **14002**
Neurodegeneration Research Group  14211
Neurodevelopmental Studies, Inc.; Center for  **14170**
Neuro-developmental Treatment Association  **19639**, **20161**
Neuroendocrinology Research Program; Pituitary and  8774
Neuroendocrinology; Society for Behavioral  **8734**
Neurofibromatosis  **9288**, **14087**
Neurofibromatosis Association of Ireland  **14088**
Neurofibromatosis; European  **13998**
Neurofibromatosis Foundation; National  **9286**, **14077**
Neuroimaging; American Society of  **18115**
Neuroimaging and Applied Neuroscience Research Branch  12746
Neuroimaging; Society for Computerized Tomography and  18115
Neuroimmunomodulation; International Society for  **3180**, **14038**
Neurologic Study; Center for  **14171**
Neurological Association; American  **13915**
Neurological Association; ASEAN  **13929**
Neurological Association; Scandinavian  **14106**
Neurological and Communicative Disorders; National Coalition for
 Research in  14073
Neurological Disorders; National Coalition for Research in  **14073**,
 **14244**
Neurological Disorders; National Committee for Research in  14073
Neurological Institute; Barrow  **14143**
Neurological Institute; Colorado  **14176**
Neurological and Orthopaedic Surgeons; American Academy
 of  **19462**
Neurological Sciences; Canadian Congress of  **13969**
Neurological Sciences; Pan-African Association of  **14099**
Neurological Surgeons; American Association of  **19469**
Neurological Surgeons; Asian - Australasian Society of  **13930**,
 **19507**
Neurological Surgeons; Congress of  **19543**
Neurological Surgeons; Society of  **14113**
Neurological Surgery; American Board of  **19476**
Neurologically Disabled of Canada; Association for the  **13943**
Neurologically Disabled; Swedish Association of  **14122**
Neurologiskt Handikappades Riksforbund  **13642**, 14122
Neurologists; Australian Association of  **13950**
Neurology; American Academy of  **13860**, **13901**
Neurology; American Board of Psychiatry and  **12348**
Neurology Research Center  14202
Neurology Society; Child  **5653**
Neuroma Association; Acoustic  **5966**
Neuroma Association of Canada; Acoustic  **13884**
Neuromodulation Society; American  **13916**
Neuromodulation Society; International  **14036**

Neuromuscular Concepts School of Massage  **4101**
Neuromuscular Disease Association; Bulgarian  **13573**
Neuromuscular Diseases Association of Romania  **13643**
Neuromuscular Disorders; Association of  **13561**
Neuromuscular Disorders Associations; European Alliance of  **13586**
Neuromuscular Disorders; International Research Council of  **14037**,
 **14210**
Neuromuscular Research Foundation; ALS and  14008
Neuromusculoskeletel Institute  14430
Neurone Disease Association of Australia; Motor  **14051**
Neurone Disease Association of India; Motor  **14052**
Neurone Disease Association; Irish Motor  **14042**
Neurone Disease Association; Motor  **14050**
Neurone Disease Association of New Zealand; Motor  **14053**
Neurone Disease Association; Scottish Motor  **14108**
Neurone Disease Association of South Africa; Motor  **14054**
Neurone Disease and Esclerosis Lateral Amiotrofica in Uruguay;
 Motor  **14055**
Neurone Disease Research Institute of Australia; Motor  **14056**
NeuroOncology; European Association for  **10161**
Neuropathologists; American Association of  **17124**
Neuropathologists; Canadian Association of  **13964**
Neuropathologists; Club of  17124
Neuropathology; International Society of  **17144**
Neuropathy Association  **13880**, **14089**
Neuropharmacology Section; Clinical  12738
Neurophysiology; American Academy of Clinical  **13900**
Neurophysiology; British Society for Clinical  **13962**
Neurophysiology; International Federation of Clinical  **14029**
Neuropsychiatric Association; American  **12357**
Neuropsychiatric Research Institute  **14247**
Neuropsychiatric Research Society  12401
Neuropsychiatrists; American College of  **16988**
Neuropsychology; American Board of Professional  **13906**
Neuropsychology; National Academy of  **14069**
Neuropsychopharmacology; American College of  **17324**
Neuroradiology; American Society of  **18116**
Neuroradiology; American Society of Pediatric  **5615**
Neuroradiology; European Society of  **14003**
Neurorehabilitation; American Society of  **13924**
Neuroresearch; Chicago Institute of Neurosurgery and  **14173**
Neuroscience and Aging; Institute of Developmental  **14207**
Neuroscience of Autism; Laboratory for Research on the  **14221**
Neuroscience and Behavioral Science Review Branch  12720
Neuroscience Departments and Programs; Association of  **13945**
Neuroscience Nurses; American Association of  **15640**
Neuroscience Nurses; British Association of  **15675**
Neuroscience Nurses; Canadian Association of  **13965**
Neuroscience Nursing; American Board of  **15645**
The Neurosciences Institute  **14248**
Neurosciences Institute; Blanchette Rockefeller  **14148**
Neurosciences; Israel Society for  **14043**
Neurosciences Research Center  14234
Neurosurgery; Asian Society for Stereotactic Functional and
 Computer Assisted  **19511**
Neurosurgery and Neuroresearch; Chicago Institute of  **14173**
Neurosurgery Society; Canadian  **19538**
Neurosurgery; World Society for Stereotactic and Functional  **19612**
Neurosurgical Anesthesia and Critical Care; Society of  **4471**
Neurosurgical Nurses  15645
Neurosurgical Physician Assistants; Association of  **13946**
Neurosurgical Societies; European Association of  **13992**
Neurosurgical Societies; World Federation of  **13883**, **19611**
Neurosurgical Society of Australasia  **14090**
Neurosurgical Society; Middle East  **19579**
Neurosurgical Society; Scandinavian  **14107**
NeuroTherapy; Association for Comprehensive  **13939**
Neurotology Society; American  **5981**, **13863**
Neurowissenschaftliche Gesellschaft e.V.  **14012**
Neva and Wesley West Foundation  **559**
Nevada Board of Dental Examiners  **6675**
Nevada Board of Optometry  **21262**
Nevada Dental Association  **6760**

## Q



## R

Specialty Nursing Organizations and the American Nurses Association; Federation of  15751

Specialty Nursing Organizations; National Federation for  **14931, 15751**

Spectrum Center School of Massage  **4177**

Speech Action; National Association for Hearing and  5985

Speech Agencies; National Association of Hearing and  5985

Speech Association for the Deaf; Volta  5971

Speech Association; National Cued  **6082**

Speech Center; Cleveland Hearing and  **6139**

Speech to the Deaf; American Association to Promote the Teaching of  5971

Speech Foundation of America  6116

Speech and Hearing Association; National Student  6089

Speech and Hearing Center  6199

Speech Impaired Children; Dutch Parents Organization of Hearing and  **6036**

Speech Language Hearing Association; American  **5985**

Speech Language Hearing Association; National Student  **6089**

Speech-Language and Hearing; National Black Association for  **6078**

Speech Pathology Australia  **6114**

Speech Research; International Center for Hearing and  **6149**

Spencer County Association for Retarded Citizens  **7209**

Spencer Foundation  **12276**

Spencer T. and Ann W. Olin Foundation  **691**

Spina Bifida Association of America  **4896**

Spina Bifida and Hydrocephalus; Association for  **4876**

Spina Bifida and Hydrocephalus; Irish Association for  **4886**

Spina Bifida; Society for Research into Hydrocephalus and  **4895**

Spinal Cord Injury Association; National  **14084**

Spinal Cord Injury Care System; Georgia Regional  **14197**

Spinal Cord Injury Foundation; National  14084

Spinal Cord Injury Model System; Mount Sinai  **14243**

Spinal Cord Injury Nurses; American Association of  **15643**

Spinal Cord Injury Psychologists and Social Workers; American Association of  **12344**

Spinal Cord Injury Research; Craig Center for  **14186**

Spinal Cord Injury System; Northern New Jersey  **14254**

Spinal Cord Research Foundation; Kent Waldrep International  13977

Spinal Cord Society  **14116**

Spinal Injuries Action Association  **14117**

Spinal Injuries Association  **14118**

Spinal Injury Association; American  **13865, 13925**

Spine Radiology; American Society of  **18118**

Spine Research Society; Cervical  13973

Spine Society; North American  **13529, 14093**

Spirit and Breath  18101

SpiriTouch Institute, Inc.  **4193**

Spiritual Emergence Network  **12658**

Spiritual Healers; National Federation of  **4302**

Spokane Community College • Advanced Respiratory Therapist Program  18714

Spondylitis Association of America  **13669**

Spondylitis Association; Ankylosing  13669

Sport and Exercise Sciences Research Institute  19202

Sport; National Association of Governor's Councils on Physical Fitness and  17809

Sport; National Institute for Fitness and  **19187**

Sport and Physical Activity; North American Society for the Psychology of  **19166**

Sport Psychology; Association for the Advancement of Applied  **19145**

Sport Sciences; International Council of Motor  **19183**

Sports Academy; United States  **19194**

Sports Alliance; National Disability  **14074**

Sports Association; Adaptive  **7902**

Sports Association; Diabetes Exercise and  **8690, 10080**

Sports Association for the Disabled; British  7967

Sports for the Deaf; International Committee of  **6056**

Sports Dentistry; Academy for  6541

Sports Dentistry; International Academy for  **6541**

Sports Federation; USA Deaf  **6124**

Sports Injuries and Physical Fitness; American Chiropractic Association - Council on  **5908**

Sports Injuries/Therapeutic Exercise Research Unit  19200

Sports; Joint Commission on Competitive Safeguards and the Medical Aspects of  19162

Sports Massage Federation; International  **19161**

Sports Massage Federation; United States  **19168**

Sports Medicine; American Academy of Podiatric  **19136**

Sports Medicine; American College of  **19138**

Sports Medicine; American Medical Society for  **19140**

Sports Medicine; American Orthopaedic Society for  **16904, 16914**

Sports Medicine; American Osteopathic Academy of  **16996**

Sports Medicine Association; American Canine  **20555**

Sports Medicine Association Board of Certification; American  **19141**

Sports Medicine; Association for Equine  **20579**

Sports Medicine Association of Registered Therapists; World  **19169**

Sports Medicine and Athletic Trauma; Nicholas Institute of  **19188**

Sports Medicine Research and Education Foundation; Cincinnati  **19176**

Sports Medicine and Science; Joint Commission on  **19162**

Sports and Osteopathic Medicine; Center for  **19152**

Sports Physicians; American Academy of  **19137**

Sports Potential; Association for the Advancement of  19147

Sports Psychology; International Society of  **19160**

Sports and Recreation Association; National Handicapped  7977

Sports Research; Delaware All-  **19178**

Sports Safety Foundation; National Youth  **19165**

Sports USA; Disabled  **7977**

Sports, USA; Wheelchair  **8181**

Sports Vision; International Academy of  **20979**

Sports Vision; National Academy of  20979

Sportsmen's Association; National Inconvenienced  7977

Spouse Foundation; Well  **12666**

Spring/Close Foundation  **692**

Spring Hill College • Division of Nursing  **14946**

Springfield Association for Retarded Citizens  **7160**

Springfield College

    Department of Physical Therapy • Physical Therapist Program  **19867**

    Occupational Therapy Program  **19690**

    Rehabilitation Services Department • Rehabilitation Counseling Program  **20024**

    School of Social Work • Graduate Program in Social Work  **18997**

Springfield College/Baystate Health System • Physician Assistant Program  **1755**

Springfield Technical Community College • Advanced Respiratory Therapist Program  **18549**

Springs Foundation, Inc.  **693**

Springs Industries, Inc.  **1402**

Sprint Foundation  **10069**

Sprint/United Telephone  **1403**

Sprue Association; Midwestern Celiac  9109

Spunk Fund Inc.  **694**

SPX Foundation  **1404**

Square D Foundation  **1405**

Stackpole-Hall Foundation  **695**

Staff Development Organization; National Nursing  **14933, 15755**

Standard Products Co. Charitable Foundation  **1406**

Standing Committee of the Hospitals of the European Union  **11511**

Standing Committee of the International Congress on Animal Reproduction  20652

Standing Liaison Committee of EU Speech and Language Therapists and Logopedists  6115

Stanford Heart Disease Prevention Program  17826

Stanford University

    AIDS Clinical Trials Unit  **11876**

    Beckman Center for Molecular and Genetic Medicine  9430

    Center for Advanced Magnetic Resonance Technology  **4830**

    Center for Biomedical Ethics  **12259**

    Center for Research in Disease Prevention  **17826**

    Center for Research on Sleep and Circadian Rhythm  **14275**

    General Clinical Research Center  **2593**

# U

University of California, San Francisco/San Francisco State
  University • Department of Physical Therapy and Rehabilitation
  Science • Physical Therapist Program  **19809**
University of California, Santa Barbara • Autism Research
  Center  **14407**
University of Central Arkansas
    Department of Nursing  **14975**
    Department of Physical Therapy • Physical Therapist
      Program  **19799**
    Family and Consumer Sciences
        Dietetic Internship Program  **16062**
        Dietetics-Didactic Program  **16063**
    Occupational Therapy Program  **19646**
University of Central Florida
    Center for Discovery of Drugs and Diagnostics  **2668**
    College of Health and Public Affairs • Health Services
      Administration Program  **9613**
    Department of Health Professions and Physical Therapy •
      Advanced Physical Therapist Program  **18482**
    Health Information Administrator Program  **12014**
    Physical Therapist Program  **19826**
    School of Nursing  **15056**
    School of Social Work • Graduate Program in Social
      Work  **18961**
University of Central Oklahoma
    College of Education • Department of Human Environmental
      Sciences • Dietetics-Didactic Program  **16343**
    Department of Funeral Service Education  **6248**
    Department of Nursing  **15435**
    Human Environmental Sciences • Dietetic Internship
      Program  **16344**
University of Charleston • Department of Nursing  **15610**
University of Charleston (LB) • Advanced Respiratory Therapist
  Program  **18718**
University of Chicago
    Animal Resources Center  **20681**
    Ben May Institute for Cancer Research  **10593**
    BioCARS: A Synchrotron Structural Biology Resource  **4747**
    Brain Research Institute  **14408**
    Cancer Research Center  **10594**
    Center for Clinical Medical Ethics  **12262**
    Clinical Nutrition Research Unit  **16522**
    Diabetes Research and Training Center  **8817**
    Division of the Biological Sciences
        Department of Neurobiology, Pharmacology, and
          Physiology  **17205**
        Pritzker School of Medicine  **1606**
    EM Core Facility for Biological Research  **4748**
    General Clinical Research Center  **2669**
    Graduate Program in Health Administration and Policy  **9621**
    Gwen Knapp Center for Lupus and Immunology
      Research  **13723**
    Inflammatory Bowel Disease Research Center  **9186**
    Institute for Mind and Biology  **2670**
    Joseph B. Kirsner Center for the Study of Digestive
      Diseases  **9187**
    Joseph P. Kennedy, Jr., Mental Retardation Research
      Center  **6905**
    Kurt Rossmann Laboratories for Radiologic Image
      Research  **18093**
    Lipoprotein Study Unit  **4749**
    Liver Study Unit  **9188**
    Perinatal Center  **16741**
    School of Social Service Administration • Graduate Program in
      Social Work  **18973**
    Visual Sciences Center  **21170**
University of Cincinnati
    Barrett Cancer Center  **10595**
    Cardio-Vascular Laboratory  **5178**
    Cardiovascular Research and Education Center  **5179**
    Center for Environmental Genetics  **8979**
    Cincinnati Rheumatic Disease Study Group  **13724**

University of Cincinnati (continued)
    College of Allied Health Sciences • Physical Therapy
      Program  **19929**
    College of Medicine  **1665**
        Department of Pharmacology and Cell Biophysics  **17276**
    College of Nursing  **15418**
        Masters Program in Nurse Anesthesia  **4404**
    College of Nursing and Health • Nurse-Midwifery Graduate
      Program  **16622**
    College of Pharmacy  **17470**
        Pharmacology and Toxicology Program  **17277**
    Department of Health Sciences • Dietetics-Didactic
      Program  **16335**
    Division of Epidemiology and Biostatistics  **9075**
    Education and Research Center  **16836**
    Headache Center  **14409**
    Institute for Health Policy and Health Services Research  **9789**
        Center for Clinical Effectiveness  **9790**
        Child Policy Research Center  **5818**
    Noyes-Giannestres Biomechanics Laboratories  **2671**
    School of Social Work • Graduate Program in Social
      Work  **19042**
    Shriners Hospitals for Children—Cincinnati  **4914**
University of Cincinnati, College of Nursing and Health  **3973**
University of Cincinnati Medical Center • Hoxworth Blood Center •
  Specialist in Blood Bank Technology Program  **12177**
University College of the Cariboo • School of Nursing  **14982**
University of Colorado
    B.F. Stolinsky Research Laboratories  **6906**
    Cancer Center  **10596**
    Center for Health Services Research  **9888**
    Center for Human Nutrition  **2672**
    Clinical Mass Spectrometry Research Resource  **4559**
    General Clinical Research Center—Adults  **2673**
    General Clinical Research Center—Pediatric  **5819**
    Health Science Center • Physical Therapist Program  **19814**
    Health Sciences Center
        Department of Pharmacology  **17182**
        School of Nursing  **15025**
            Nurse-Midwifery Graduate Program  **16598**
    Immunology Center  **3301**
    National Center for American Indian and Alaska Native Mental
      Health Research  **12757**
    Rocky Mountain Prevention Research Center  **18008**
    School of Medicine • Child Health Associate/Physician Assistant
      Program  **1725**
    School of Nursing • Nurse-Midwifery Option  **3578**
University of Colorado at Boulder
    Institute for Behavioral Genetics  **9502**
    Speech, Language, and Hearing Center  **6181**
University of Colorado, Colorado Springs • Beth El College of
  Nursing and Health Sciences  **15026**
University of Colorado—Denver
    Alcohol Research Center  **19376**
    Center for Human Investment Policy  **9791**
    Graduate School of Business Administration • Programs in
      Health Services Administration  **9607**
    Network for Healthcare Management • Executive Master of
      Business Administration in Health Administration  **9608**
    Rocky Mountain Taste and Smell Center  **14410**
    School of Medicine  **1587**
University of Colorado Health Sciences Center • School of
  Pharmacy  **17425**
University of Colorado Medical Center • School of Dentistry  **6349**
University of Connecticut
    A.J. Pappanikou Center for Developmental Disabilities  **8213**
    Alcohol Research Center  **19377**
    Center for Environmental Health  **8980**
    Center for Health Fitness  **2674**
    Center for Neurological Sciences  **14411**
    Connecticut Chemosensory Clinical Research Center  **14412**
    Dietetics-Didactic Program  **16113**

University of Minnesota (continued)
    Dental Research Institute  **6643**
    Department of Food Science and Nutrition • Dietetic Internship
      Program or Dietetics-Didactic Program  **16248**
    Division of Health Services Research and Policy  **9796**
    Experimental Surgical Services Laboratories  **5189**
    General Clinical Research Center  **2699**
    Hematology, Oncology and Transplantation Division  **10609**
    Hormel Institute  **4764**
    Institute of Human Genetics  **9509**
    Institute of Medical Biotechnology  **4765**
    KDWB Variety Family Center  **5827**
    Medical School • Department of Pharmacology  **17233**
    Midwest Center for Occupational Health and Safety  **16841**
    Minnesota Dental Research Center for Biomaterials and
      Biomechanics  **6644**
    Minnesota Molecular and Cellular Therapeutics Facility  **4766**
    Minnesota Oral Health Clinical Research Center  **6645**
    National Teen Pregnancy Prevention Research Center  **18015**
    Occupational Therapy Program  **19700**
    Physical Therapist Program  **19878**
    Program in Healthcare Administration  **9633**
    Program of Mortuary Science  **6234**
    School of Dentistry  **6368**
    School of Nursing • Nurse-Midwifery Graduate Program  **16611**
    School of Public Health  **17893**
University of Minnesota, Duluth
    Department of Social Work • Graduate Program in Social
      Work  **19007**
    School of Medicine  **1628**
University of Minnesota, Minneapolis • Medical School  **1629**
University of Minnesota, Twin Cities
    School of Nursing  **15264**
    School of Social Work • Graduate Program in Social
      Work  **19008**
University of Mississippi
    Department of Family and Consumer Sciences • Dietetics-
      Didactic Program  **16252**
    National Center for Natural Products Research  **17398**
    Pharmaceutical Marketing and Management Research
      Program  **17577**
    Research Institute of Pharmaceutical Sciences  **17578**
      Environmental Toxicology Research Program  **8989**
    School of Dentistry  **6369**
    School of Medicine  **1630**
      Graduate Programs in the Basic Medical Sciences •
        Department of Pharmacology and Toxicology  **17234**
    School of Pharmacy  **17453**
      Department of Pharmacology  **17235**
University of Mississippi Medical Center
    Health Information Administrator Program  **12030**
    School of Health Related Professions • Physical Therapist
      Program  **19879**
    School of Nursing  **15270**
    School of Related Health Professions • Occupational Therapy
      Program  **19701**
University of Missouri
    College of Veterinary Medicine  **20510**
    Mutant Mouse Regional Resource Center  **4767**
University of Missouri, Columbia
    Coordinated Program in Dietetics  **16264**
    Cosmopolitan International Diabetes Center  **8826**
    Cystic Fibrosis Research Center  **9510**
    Department of Educational and Counseling Psychology •
      Rehabilitation Counseling Program  **20034**
    Division of Cardiothoracic Surgery  **5190**
    Exercise Physiology Graduate Program  **19205**
    Health Services Management  **9635**
    John M. Dalton Cardiovascular Research Center  **4562**
    Missouri Arthritis Rehabilitation Research and Training
      Center  **13732**
    Missouri Institute of Mental Health  **12763**
    Missouri Model Spinal Cord Injury System  **14441**

University of Missouri, Columbia (continued)
    Radiation Oncology Program  **18189**
    Research Animal Diagnostic Laboratory  **20686**
    School of Health Professions • Physical Therapist
      Program  **19884**
    School of Health Related Professions • Occupational Therapy
      Program  **19705**
    School of Medicine  **1632**
      Department of Pharmacology  **17237**
    School of Nursing  **15288**
    School of Social Work • Graduate Program in Social
      Work  **19013**
    Sinclair School of Nursing  **3815**
      Nurse-Midwifery Graduate Program  **16612**
University of Missouri, Columbia (LB) • Advanced Respiratory
  Therapist Program  **18579**
University of Missouri—Kansas City
    Dental Research Program  **6646**
    Laboratory Animal Center  **20687**
    School of Dentistry  **6370**
    School of Medicine  **1633**
    School of Nursing  **15289**
    School of Pharmacy  **17455**
      Department of Pharmaceutical Science  **17238**
University of Missouri—St. Louis
    Center for Neurodynamics  **14442**
    Center for Trauma Recovery  **12764**
    College of Nursing  **15290**
    School of Optometry  **20833**
University of Mobile • School of Nursing  **14952**
University of Montana
    Primate Laboratory  **20688**
    Research and Training Center on Rural Rehabilitation
      Services  **20211**
    Rural Institute: Center for Excellence in Developmental
      Disabilities Education, Research, and Service  **8223**
    School of Pharmacy and Allied Health Sciences  **17456**
University of Montana, Missoula • Department of Physical Therapy •
  Physical Therapist Program  **19886**
University of Montevallo • Family and Consumer Sciences •
  Dietetics-Didactic Program  **16044**
University of Montreal
    Acoustics Group  **6193**
    Biomedical Modeling Research Group  **4563**
    Centre for Occupational Stress and Health  **16842**
    Clinical Research Institute of Montreal • Multidisciplinary
      Research Group on Hypertension  **5191**
    Experimental Neuropsychology Research Group  **14443**
    Faculty of Medicine  **1685**
    Faculty of Veterinary Medicine  **20519**
    Fernand Seguin Research Centre  **17399**
    Institute of Biomedical Engineering  **4564**
    Interdisciplinary Health Research Group  **18016**
    Membrane Transport Research Group  **4768**
    Montreal Heart Institute • Research Centre  **5192**
    Neurological Sciences Research Centre  **14444**
    Rehabilitation Institute of Montreal  **20212**
    Research Centre, Hospital du Sacre-Coeur  **2700**
    Research Group on the Autonomic Nervous System  **14445**
    Riviere-des-Prairies Hospital Research Centre  **12765**
    Sainte-Justine Hospital Research Centre  **16742**
    School of Optometry  **20841**
University of Montreal Health Centre • Research Centre  **2701**
University of Nebraska
    College of Medicine  **1636**
    Medical Center • College of Pharmacy  **17458**
University of Nebraska, Kearney • Department of Family and
  Consumer Sciences • Dietetics-Didactic Program  **16266**
University of Nebraska—Lincoln
    Barkley Memorial Center  **6194**
    Department of Nutritional Science and Dietetics • Dietetics-
      Didactic Program  **16267**

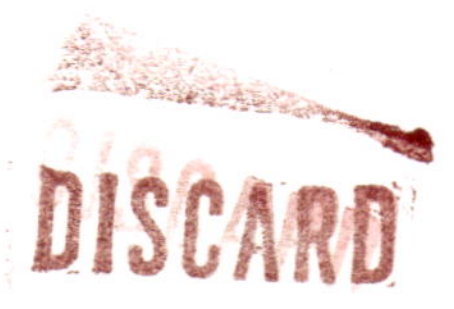